Nelson
TEXTBOOK *of*
PEDIATRICS

Nelson
TEXTBOOK *of*
PEDIATRICS

EDITION 20

Robert M. Kliegman, MD
Professor and Chair Emeritus
Department of Pediatrics
Medical College of Wisconsin
Milwaukee, Wisconsin

Bonita F. Stanton, MD
Vice-Dean of Research
Professor of Pediatrics
Wayne State University School of Medicine
Detroit, Michigan

Joseph W. St Geme III, MD
Chair, Department of Pediatrics
Professor of Pediatrics and Microbiology
Perelman School of Medicine at the University of
    Pennsylvania
Physician-in-Chief
Leonard and Madlyn Abramson Endowed Chair in
    Pediatrics
Children's Hospital of Philadelphia
Philadelphia, Pennsylvania

Nina F. Schor, MD, PhD
William H. Eilinger Professor and Chair
Department of Pediatrics
Professor
Department of Neurology
Pediatrician-in-Chief
Golisano Children's Hospital
University of Rochester Medical Center
Rochester, New York

Editor Emeritus
Richard E. Behrman, MD
Nonprofit Healthcare and Educational
Consultants to Medical Institutions
Santa Barbara, California

ELSEVIER

ELSEVIER

1600 John F. Kennedy Blvd.
Ste. 1800
Philadelphia, PA 19103-2899

NELSON TEXTBOOK OF PEDIATRICS, TWENTIETH EDITION ISBN: 978-1-4557-7566-8
International Edition ISBN: 978-0-323-35307-6

Previous editions copyrighted 2011, 2007, 2004, 2000, 1996, 1992, 1987, 1983, 1979, 1975, 1969, 1964, 1959

International Standard Book Number: 978-1-4557-7566-8

Content Strategy Director: Mary Gatsch
Executive Content Strategist: Kate Dimock
Content Development Specialist: Jennifer Shreiner
Publishing Services Manager: Patricia Tannian
Senior Project Manager: John Casey

Printed in Canada

Last digit is the print number: 9 8 7 6 5 4 3 2 1

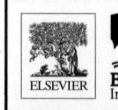

To the Child's Physician and especially to those who through their expressed confidence
in past editions of this book have provided the stimulus for this revision.
Waldo E. Nelson, 9/e, 1969

This is as true in 2015 as it was in 1969.
R.M. Kliegman, 20/e, 2015

Contributors

Mark J. Abzug, MD
Professor of Pediatrics
Division of Pediatric Infectious Diseases
University of Colorado School of Medicine
Children's Hospital Colorado
Aurora, Colorado
Nonpolio Enteroviruses

David R. Adams, MD, PhD
National Human Genome Research Institute
National Institutes of Health
Bethesda, Maryland
*Genetic Approaches to Rare and Undiagnosed
    Diseases*

Stewart L. Adelson, MD
Assistant Clinical Professor
Department of Psychiatry
Columbia University College of Physicians and
    Surgeons
Adjunct Clinical Assistant Professor
Weill Cornell Medical College of Cornell
    University
New York, New York
Gay, Lesbian, and Bisexual Adolescents

John J. Aiken, MD, FACS, FAAP
Professor of Surgery
Division of Pediatric General and Thoracic Surgery
Medical College of Wisconsin
The Children's Hospital of Wisconsin
Milwaukee, Wisconsin
Acute Appendicitis
Inguinal Hernias
Epigastric Hernia

Begum Akay, MD
Assistant Professor of Surgery
Division of Pediatric Surgery
Oakland University William Beaumont School of
    Medicine
Beaumont Health
Royal Oak, Michigan
Surgical Conditions of the Anus and Rectum

Cezmi A. Akdis, MD
Professor of Immunology
Swiss Institute of Allergy and Asthma Research
Christine Kühne Center for Allergy Research and
    Education
Davos, Switzerland;
Medical Faculty, University of Zurich
Zurich, Switzerland
Allergy and the Immunologic Basis of Atopic Disease

Evaline A. Alessandrini, MD, MSCE
Professor of Clinical Pediatrics
University of Cincinnati College of Medicine
Division of Emergency Medicine
Director, Quality Scholars Program in Health Care
    Transformation
Cincinnati Children's Hospital Medical Center
Cincinnati, Ohio
*Emergency Medical Services for Children: Outcomes
    and Risk Adjustment*

Michael A. Alexander, MD
Professor of Pediatrics and Rehabilitation Medicine
Thomas Jefferson Medical College
Philadelphia, Pennsylvania;
Emeritus Medical Staff
Alfred I. duPont Hospital for Children
Wilmington, Delaware
Evaluation of the Child for Rehabilitative Services

Omar Ali, MD
Assistant Professor
Department of Pediatrics
Medical College of Wisconsin
Division of Endocrinology
Children's Hospital of Wisconsin
Milwaukee, Wisconsin
*Hyperpituitarism, Tall Stature, and Overgrowth
    Syndromes*
Hypofunction of the Testes
Pseudoprecocity Resulting from Tumors of the Testes
Gynecomastia

Namasivayam Ambalavanan, MD
Professor of Pediatrics
Division of Neonatology
University of Alabama, Birmingham
Birmingham, Alabama
High-Risk Pregnancies
The Fetus
Nervous System Disorders
Hypoxia-Ischemic Encephalopathy
Respiratory Tract Disorders
Jaundice and Hyperbilirubinemia in the Newborn
Kernicterus
Genitourinary System
The Umbilicus
Metabolic Disturbances
The Endocrine System

Karl E. Anderson, MD, FACP
Professor
Departments of Preventive Medicine, Community
    Health, Internal Medicine, and Pharmacology
    and Toxicology
Director, Porphyria Laboratory and Center
University of Texas Medical Branch
Galveston, Texas
The Porphyrias

Peter M. Anderson, MD, PhD
Curtis Distinguished Professor
Department of Pediatrics
University of Texas MD Anderson Cancer Center
Houston, Texas
Neoplasms of the Kidney

Kelly K. Anthony, PhD, PLLC
Assistant Professor
Department of Psychiatry and Behavioral Sciences
Duke University Medical Center
Durham, North Carolina
Musculoskeletal Pain Syndromes

Alia Y. Antoon, MD
Assistant Clinical Professor
Department of Pediatrics
Harvard Medical School
Chief of Pediatrics
Shriners Hospital for Children
Boston, Massachusetts
Burn Injuries
Cold Injuries

Susan D. Apkon, MD
Associate Professor
Department of Rehabilitation Medicine
University of Washington School of Medicine
Director, Rehabilitation Medicine
Seattle Children's Hospital
Seattle, Washington
Ambulation Assistance

Stacy P. Ardoin, MD, MHS
Associate Professor of Clinical Medicine
Adult and Pediatric Rheumatology
The Ohio State University Wexner Medical Center
Nationwide Children's Hospital
Columbus, Ohio
Systemic Lupus Erythematosus
Vasculitis Syndromes

Monica I. Ardura, DO, MSCS
Assistant Professor of Pediatrics
Section of Infectious Disease and Immunology
The Ohio State University College of Medicine
Nationwide Children's Hospital
Columbus, Ohio
Hansen Disease (Mycobacterium leprae)

Michelle M. Ariss, MD
Assistant Professor
Department of Ophthalmology
University of Missouri—Kansas City School of
    Medicine
Children's Mercy Hospital
Kansas City, Missouri
Growth and Development (Eye)
Examination of the Eye
Abnormalities of Refraction and Accommodation
Disorders of Vision
Abnormalities of Pupil and Iris
Disorders of Eye Movement and Alignment
Abnormalities of the Lids
Disorders of the Lacrimal System
Disorders of the Conjunctiva
Abnormalities of the Cornea
Abnormalities of the Lens
Disorders of the Uveal Tract
Disorders of the Retina and Vitreous
Abnormalities of the Optic Nerve
Childhood Glaucoma
Orbital Abnormalities
Orbital Infections
Injuries to the Eye

Thaís Armangué, MD
Clinical Fellow and Predoctoral Researcher
ICREA-IDIBAPS Neuroimmunology Program
Hospital Clinic
Barcelona, Spain
Autoimmune Encephalitis

Carola A.S. Arndt, MD
Professor of Pediatrics
Department of Pediatrics and Adolescent Medicine
Division of Pediatric Hematology-Oncology
Mayo Clinic
Rochester, Minnesota
Soft Tissue Sarcomas
Neoplasms of Bone

Stephen S. Arnon, MD, MPH
Chief, Infant Botulism Treatment and Prevention
    Program Branch
Division of Communicable Disease Control
Center for Infectious Diseases
California Department of Public Health
Richmond, California
Botulism (Clostridium botulinum)
Tetanus (Clostridium tetani)

Stephen C. Aronoff, MD, MBA
Professor and Waldo E. Nelson Chair
Department of Pediatrics
Temple University School of Medicine
Philadelphia, Pennsylvania
Cryptococcus neoformans
Histoplasmosis (Histoplasma capsulatum)
Paracoccidioides brasiliensis
Sporotrichosis (Sporothrix schenckii)
Zygomycosis (Mucormycosis)
Nonbacterial Food Poisoning

David M. Asher, MD
Supervisory Medical Officer
Chief, Laboratory of Bacterial and Transmissible
    Spongiform Encephalopathy Agents
Center for Biologics Evaluation and Research
    (CBER)
United States Food and Drug Administration
Silver Spring, Maryland
Transmissible Spongiform Encephalopathies

Ann Ashworth, PhD, Hon FRCPCH
Professor Emeritus
Department of Population Health
Nutrition Group
London School of Hygiene and Tropical Medicine
London, United Kingdom
Nutrition, Food Security, and Health

Barbara L. Asselin, MD
Professor of Pediatrics and Oncology
Department of Pediatrics
University of Rochester School of Medicine
Golisano Children's Hospital
Rochester, New York
Epidemiology of Childhood and Adolescent Cancer

Joann L. Ater, MD
Associate Professor
Department of Pediatrics
University of Texas MD Anderson Cancer Center
Houston, Texas
Brain Tumors in Childhood
Neuroblastoma

Erika F. Augustine, MD
Assistant Professor of Neurology and Pediatrics
Division of Child Neurology
University of Rochester Medical Center
Rochester, New York
Dystonia

Marilyn C. Augustyn, MD
Professor of Pediatrics
Boston University School of Medicine
Boston Medical Center
Boston, Massachusetts
Impact of Violence on Children

Ellis D. Avner, MD
Professor
Departments of Pediatrics and Physiology
Medical College of Wisconsin
Milwaukee, Wisconsin
Introduction to Glomerular Diseases
Clinical Evaluation of the Child with Hematuria
*Isolated Glomerular Diseases with Recurrent Gross
    Hematuria*
Glomerulonephritis Associated with Infections
Membranous Nephropathy
Membranoproliferative Glomerulonephritis
*Glomerulonephritis Associated with Systemic Lupus
    Erythematosus*
Henoch-Schönlein Purpura Nephritis
Rapidly Progressive (Crescentic) Glomerulonephritis
Goodpasture Disease
Hemolytic-Uremic Syndrome
Upper Urinary Tract Causes of Hematuria
Hematologic Diseases Causing Hematuria
Anatomic Abnormalities Associated with Hematuria
Lower Urinary Tract Causes of Hematuria
Introduction to the Child with Proteinuria
Transient Proteinuria
Orthostatic (Postural) Proteinuria
Fixed Proteinuria
Nephrotic Syndrome
Tubular Function
Renal Tubular Acidosis
Nephrogenic Diabetes Insipidus
*Bartter and Gitelman Syndromes and Other
    Inherited Tubular Transport Abnormalities*
Tubulointerstitial Nephritis
Toxic Nephropathy
Cortical Necrosis
Renal Failure

Carlos A. Bacino, MD
Professor of Molecular and Human Genetics
Baylor College of Medicine
Chief, Genetics Service
Director, Pediatric Genetics Clinic
Texas Children's Hospital
Houston, Texas
Cytogenetics

Robert N. Baldassano, MD
Colman Family Chair in Pediatric Inflammatory
    Bowel Disease and Professor of Pediatrics
University of Pennsylvania Perelman School of
    Medicine
Director, Center for Pediatric Inflammatory Bowel
    Disease
The Children's Hospital of Philadelphia
Philadelphia, Pennsylvania
Inflammatory Bowel Disease
Eosinophilic Gastroenteritis

Keith D. Baldwin, MD, MSPT, MPH
Assistant Professor
Department of Orthopaedic Surgery
University of Pennsylvania Perelman School of
    Medicine
Neuromuscular Orthopaedics and Orthopaedic
    Trauma
Children's Hospital of Philadelphia
Philadelphia, Pennsylvania
Growth and Development
Evaluation of the Child
Torsional and Angular Deformities
Common Fractures

Christina Bales, MD
Assistant Professor of Pediatrics
University of Pennsylvania Perelman School of
    Medicine
Attending Physician
Division of Gastroenterology, Hepatology, and
    Nutrition
The Children's Hospital of Philadelphia
Philadelphia, Pennsylvania
Intestinal Atresia, Stenosis, and Malrotation

William F. Balistreri, MD
Medical Director Emeritus, Pediatric Liver Care
    Center
Division of Pediatric Gastroenterology, Hepatology,
    and Nutrition
Cincinnati Children's Hospital Medical Center
Cincinnati, Ohio
Morphogenesis of the Liver and Biliary System
Manifestations of Liver Disease
Cholestasis
Metabolic Diseases of the Liver
Viral Hepatitis
Liver Disease Associated with Systemic Disorders
Mitochondrial Hepatopathies

Robert S. Baltimore, MD
Professor of Pediatrics and Epidemiology
Clinical Professor of Nursing
Associate Director of Hospital Epidemiology (for
    Pediatrics)
Yale-New Haven Hospital
New Haven, Connecticut
Listeria monocytogenes
*Pseudomonas, Burkholderia, and
    Stenotrophomonas*

Manisha Balwani, MBBS, MS
Assistant Professor
Departments of Medicine and Genetics and
    Genomic Sciences
Icahn School of Medicine at Mount Sinai
New York, New York
The Porphyrias

Christine E. Barron, MD
Associate Clinical Professor
Department of Pediatrics
Brown University Alpert Medical School
Rhode Island Hospital
Providence, Rhode Island
Adolescent Rape

Karyl S. Barron, MD
Deputy Director
Division of Intramural Research
National Institute of Allergy and Infectious
    Diseases
National Institutes of Health
Bethesda, Maryland
Amyloidosis

Dorsey M. Bass, MD
Associate Professor of Pediatrics
Division of Pediatric Gastroenterology
Stanford University School of Medicine
Palo Alto, California
Rotaviruses, Caliciviruses, and Astroviruses

Mark L. Batshaw, MD
Professor and Chairman
Department of Pediatrics
Associate Dean, Academic Affairs
George Washington University
School of Medicine and Health Sciences
Executive Vice-President
Chief Academic Officer and Physician-in-Chief
Children's National Medical Center
Washington, DC
Intellectual Disability

Nerissa S. Bauer, MD, MPH
Assistant Professor
Department of General and Community Pediatrics
Section of Children's Health Services Research
Indiana University School of Medicine
Indianapolis, Indiana
*Developmental-Behavioral Screening and
Surveillance*

Michelle L. Bayer, MD
Resident Physician
Department of Dermatology
Medical College of Wisconsin
Children's Hospital of Wisconsin
Milwaukee, Wisconsin
Disorders of the Mucous Membranes

Richard E. Behrman, MD
Nonprofit Healthcare and Educational Consultants
to Medical Institutions
Santa Barbara, California
Overview of Pediatrics

Michael J. Bell, MD
Professor
Departments of Critical Care Medicine, Neurologic
Surgery, and Pediatrics
University of Pittsburgh School of Medicine
Director, Pediatric Neurocritical Care
Director, Pediatric Neurotrauma Center
University of Pittsburgh Medical Center
Pittsburgh, Pennsylvania
Neurologic Emergencies and Stabilization

John W. Belmont, MD, PhD
Professor
Departments of Molecular and Human Genetics,
Pediatrics, and Pathology and Immunology
Baylor College of Medicine
Houston, Texas
Genetics of Common Disorders

**Daniel K. Benjamin Jr., MD, PhD,
MPH**
Professor of Pediatrics
Division of Pediatric Infectious Diseases
Faculty Associate Director, Duke Clinical Research
Institute
Duke University Medical Center
Durham, North Carolina
Principles of Antifungal Therapy
Candida

**Michael J. Bennett, PhD, FRCPath,
FACB**
Professor of Pathology and Laboratory Medicine
University of Pennsylvania Perelman School of
Medicine
Director, Michael J. Palmieri Metabolic Disease
Laboratory
Children's Hospital of Philadelphia
Philadelphia, Pennsylvania
Disorders of Mitochondrial Fatty Acid β-Oxidation

Susanne M. Benseler, MD, PhD
Associate Professor, Faculty of Medicine
University of Calgary
Pediatric Rheumatologist, Section Chief
Rheumatology
Alberta Children's Hospital
Calgary, Alberta, Canada
Central Nervous System Vasculitis

Daniel Bernstein, MD
Alfred Woodley Salter and Mabel Smith Salter
Endowed Professor in Pediatrics
Stanford University School of Medicine
Director, Division of Pediatric Cardiology
Lucile Packard Children's Hospital
Palo Alto, California
Cardiac Development
The Fetal to Neonatal Circulatory Transition
History and Physical Examination
Laboratory Evaluation
*Epidemiology and Genetic Basis of Congenital Heart
Disease*
*Evaluation and Screening of the Infant or Child with
Congenital Heart Disease*
*Acyanotic Congenital Heart Disease: Left-to-Right
Shunt Lesions*
*Acyanotic Congenital Heart Disease: Obstructive
Lesions*
*Acyanotic Congenital Heart Disease: Regurgitant
Lesions*
*Cyanotic Congenital Heart Disease: Evaluation of
the Critically Ill Neonate with Cyanosis and
Respiratory Distress*
*Cyanotic Congenital Heart Lesions: Lesions
Associated with Decreased Pulmonary Blood
Flow*
*Cyanotic Congenital Heart Disease: Lesions
Associated with Increased Pulmonary Blood Flow*
*Other Congenital Heart and Vascular
Malformations*
Pulmonary Hypertension
*General Principles of Treatment of Congenital Heart
Disease*
Infective Endocarditis
Rheumatic Heart Disease
Heart Failure
Pediatric Heart and Heart-Lung Transplantation
*Diseases of the Blood Vessels (Aneurysms and
Fistulas)*

**Zulfiqar Ahmed Bhutta, MBBS, PhD,
FRCPCH, FAAP**
Professor of Paediatrics, Nutritional Sciences, and
Public Health
University of Toronto Faculty of Medicine
Robert Harding Chair in Global Child Health and
Policy
Co-Director, SickKids Centre for Global Child
Health
The Hospital for Sick Children
Toronto, Ontario, Canada;
Founding Director, Centre of Excellence in Women
and Child Health
The Aga Khan University, South Central Asia and
East Africa
Karachi, Pakistan
*Innovations in Addressing Child Health and
Survival in Low-Income Settings*
Salmonella
Acute Gastroenteritis in Children

Samra S. Blanchard, MD
Associate Professor of Pediatrics
University of Maryland School of Medicine
Baltimore, Maryland
Peptic Ulcer Disease in Children

Joshua A. Blatter, MD, MPH
Instructor in Pediatrics
Division of Pediatric Allergy, Immunology, and
Pulmonary Medicine
Associate Director, Pediatric Lung Transplantation
Center
Washington University School of Medicine in
St. Louis
St. Louis, Missouri
Congenital Disorders of the Lung

Archie Bleyer, MD, FRCP (Glasg)
Clinical Research Professor
Knight Cancer Center
Oregon Health & Science University
Chair, Institutional Review Board for St. Charles
Health System
Portland, Oregon;
Professor of Pediatrics
University of Texas MD Anderson Cancer Center
Houston, Texas
Principles of Treatment (Cancer and Benign Tumors)
The Leukemias
Congenital Disorders of the Lung

Steven R. Boas, MD, FAAP, FACSM
Director, The Cystic Fibrosis Center of Chicago
President and CEO, The Cystic Fibrosis Institute
Glenview, Illinois;
Clinical Associate Professor of Pediatrics
Northwestern University Feinberg School of
Medicine
Chicago, Illinois
Emphysema and Overinflation
α_1-Antitrypsin Deficiency and Emphysema
Other Distal Airway Diseases
Skeletal Diseases Influencing Pulmonary Function

Walter O. Bockting, PhD
Professor of Medical Psychology (in Psychiatry and
Nursing)
Research Scientist, New York State Psychiatric
Institute
Division of Gender, Sexuality, and Health
Department of Psychiatry
Columbia University College of Physicians and
Surgeons
New York, New York
Sexual Identity Development

Neal F. Boerkoel, MD, PhD
National Human Genome Research Institute
National Institutes of Health
Bethesda, Maryland
*Genetic Approaches to Rare and Undiagnosed
Diseases*

Natalija Bogdanovic, MD
Department of Psychiatry
Boston Medical Center
Boston, Massachusetts
Mood Disorders

Mark Boguniewicz, MD
Professor of Pediatrics
Division of Pediatric Allergy-Immunology
University of Colorado School of Medicine
National Jewish Health
Denver, Colorado
Ocular Allergies
Adverse Reactions to Drugs

Daniel J. Bonthius, MD, PhD
Professor of Pediatrics and Neurology
University of Iowa School of Medicine
Iowa City, Iowa
Lymphocytic Choriomeningitis Virus

Brett J. Bordini
Assistant Professor
Department of Pediatrics
Medical College of Wisconsin
Pediatric Hospitalist
Children's Hospital of Wisconsin
Milwaukee, Wisconsin
Plastic Bronchitis

Kenneth M. Boyer, MD
Woman's Board Professor and Chairman
Rush Medical College of Rush University
Chicago, Illinois
Toxoplasmosis (Toxoplasma gondii)

Amanda M. Brandow, DO, MS
Associate Professor of Pediatrics
Division of Pediatric Hematology/Oncology
Medical College of Wisconsin
Milwaukee, Wisconsin
Polycythemia
Non-Clonal Polycythemia
Anatomy and Function of the Spleen
Splenomegaly
Hyposplenism, Splenic Trauma, and Splenectomy

†David Branski, MD
Professor Emeritus
The Hebrew University–Hadassah School of
  Medicine
Jerusalem, Israel
Disorders of Malabsorption
Chronic Diarrhea

David T. Breault, MD, PhD
Assistant Professor of Pediatrics
Harvard Medical School
Division of Endocrinology
Boston Children's Hospital
Boston, Massachusetts
Diabetes Insipidus
*Other Abnormalities of Arginine Vasopressin
  Metabolism and Action*

William J. Britt, MD
Charles A. Alford Professor of Pediatric Infectious
  Diseases
Professor of Pediatrics and Microbiology and
  Neurobiology
University of Alabama Birmingham School of
  Medicine
Birmingham, Alabama
Cytomegalovirus

Angela R. Bryan, MD
Fellow in Pediatric Rheumatology
Duke University Health System
Durham, North Carolina
Juvenile Idiopathic Arthritis

Rebecca H. Buckley, MD
J. Buren Sidbury Professor of Pediatrics
Professor of Immunology
Duke University School of Medicine
Durham, North Carolina
Evaluation of Suspected Immunodeficiency
The T-, B-, and NK-Cell Systems
*T Lymphocytes, B Lymphocytes, and Natural Killer
  Cells*
Primary Defects of Antibody Production
Primary Defects of Cellular Immunity
*Primary Combined Antibody and Cellular
  Immunodeficiencies*

**Cynthia Etzler Budek, MS, APN/NP,
CPNP-AC/PC**
Pediatric Nurse Practitioner
Department of Pulmonary and Critical Care
  Medicine
Transitional Care/Pulmonary Habilitation Unit
Ann & Robert H. Lurie Children's Hospital of
  Chicago
Chicago, Illinois
Chronic Severe Respiratory Insufficiency

E. Stephen Buescher, MD
Professor of Pediatrics
Eastern Virginia Medical School
Medical Director, Infection Control
Medical Director, Clinical Microbiology
  Laboratory
Children's Hospital of the King's Daughters
Norfolk, Virginia
Diphtheria (Corynebacterium diphtheriae)

Supinda Bunyavanich, MD, MPH
Assistant Professor
Departments of Pediatrics and Genetics and
  Genomic Sciences
Jaffe Food Allergy Institute
Mindich Child Heath and Development Institute
Ichan School of Medicine at Mount Sinai
New York, New York
Diagnosis of Allergic Disease
Principles of Treatment of Allergic Disease

Carey-Ann D. Burnham, PhD
Assistant Professor of Pathology and Immunology
Assistant Professor of Pediatrics
Washington University School of Medicine in St.
  Louis
Medical Director, Clinical Microbiology
Barnes-Jewish Hospital
St. Louis, Missouri
Diagnostic Microbiology

Gale R. Burstein, MD, MPH
Clinical Professor
Department of Pediatrics
State University of New York at Buffalo
School of Medicine and Biomedical Sciences
Commissioner
Erie County Department of Health
Buffalo, New York
Adolescent Physical and Social Development
The Epidemiology of Adolescent Health Problems
Delivery of Healthcare to Adolescents
The Breast
Menstrual Problems
Contraception
Sexually Transmitted Infections

**Amaya L. Bustinduy, MD, MPH, FAAP,
FRCPCH**
Paediatric Infectious Diseases Research Group
  (PIDRG)
St. George's University of London
London, United Kingdom
Schistosomiasis (Schistosoma)
Flukes (Liver, Lung, and Intestinal)

Miguel M. Cabada, MD, MSc
Research Associate, Tropical Medicine Institute
Universidad Peruana Cayetano Heredia
Lima, Peru;
Adjunct Instructor of Medicine
Division of Infectious Diseases
University of Texas Medical Branch at Galveston
Galveston, Texas
*Echinococcosis (Echinococcus granulosus and
  Echinococcus multilocularis)*

Derya Caglar, MD
Assistant Professor
Department of Pediatrics
University of Washington School of Medicine
Attending Physician
Division of Emergency Medicine
Seattle Children's Hospital
Seattle, Washington
Drowning and Submersion Injury

Mitchell S. Cairo, MD
Professor
Departments of Pediatrics, Medicine, Pathology,
  Microbiology and Immunology and Cell
  Biology and Anatomy
New York Medical College
Chief, Division of Pediatric Hematology, Oncology,
  and Stem Cell Transplantation
Maria Fareri Children's Hospital at Westchester
  Medical Center
New York Medical College
Valhalla, New York
Lymphoma

Lauren E. Camarda, MD
Instructor in Pediatrics
Northwestern University Feinberg School of
  Medicine
Division of Pediatric Pulmonary Medicine
Ann & Robert H. Lurie Children's Hospital of
  Chicago
Chicago, Illinois
Wheezing, Bronchiolitis, and Bronchitis

Bruce M. Camitta, MD
Rebecca Jean Slye Professor of Pediatrics
Division of Pediatric Hematology/Oncology
Medical College of Wisconsin
Midwest Children's Cancer Center
Milwaukee, Wisconsin
Polycythemia
Non-Clonal Polycythemia
Anatomy and Function of the Spleen
Splenomegaly
Hyposplenism, Splenic Trauma, and Splenectomy
Anatomy and Function of the Lymphatic System
Abnormalities of Lymphatic Vessels
Lymphadenopathy

Angela J.P. Campbell, MD, MPH
Medical Officer
Epidemiology and Prevention Branch, Influenza
  Division
National Center for Immunization and Respiratory
  Diseases
Centers for Disease Control and Prevention
Atlanta, Georgia
Influenza Viruses
Parainfluenza Viruses

Waldemar A. Carlo, MD
Edwin M. Dixon Professor of Pediatrics
Director, Division of Neonatology
University of Alabama, Birmingham Hospital
Birmingham, Alabama
Overview of Mortality and Morbidity
The Newborn Infant
High-Risk Pregnancies
The Fetus
The High-Risk Infant
Clinical Manifestations of Diseases in the Newborn Period
Nervous System Disorders
Delivery Room Emergencies
Respiratory Tract Disorders
Digestive System Disorders
Blood Disorders
Genitourinary System
The Umbilicus
Metabolic Disturbances
The Endocrine System

Robert B. Carrigan, MD
Assistant Clinical Professor
Department of Orthopaedic Surgery
University of Pennsylvania Perelman School of Medicine
Pediatric Hand Surgeon
Children's Hospital of Philadelphia
Philadelphia, Pennsylvania
The Upper Limb

Mary T. Caserta, MD
Professor of Pediatrics
Division of Pediatric Infectious Diseases
University of Rochester School of Medicine and Dentistry
Rochester, New York
Roseola (Human Herpesviruses 6 and 7)
Human Herpesvirus 8

Denise Casey, MD
Medical Officer
Pediatric Oncology, Neuro-Oncology, and Rare Tumors Team
Office of Hematology and Oncology Products
Food and Drug Administration
U.S. Department of Health and Human Services
Silver Spring, Maryland
Hereditary Spherocytosis

Ellen Gould Chadwick, MD
Irene Heinz Given and John LaPorte Given Chair in Pediatrics
Professor and Associate Chair for Education
Department of Pediatrics
Northwestern University Feinberg School of Medicine
Associate Director, Section of Pediatric, Adolescent, and Maternal HIV Infection
Ann & Robert H. Lurie Children's Hospital of Chicago
Chicago, Illinois
Acquired Immunodeficiency Syndrome (Human Immunodeficiency Virus)

Lisa J. Chamberlain, MD, MPH
Assistant Professor of Pediatrics
Stanford University School of Medicine
Center for Health Policy
Center for Primary Care and Outcomes Research
Stanford, California
Chronic Illness in Childhood

Jennifer I. Chapman, MD
Assistant Professor of Pediatrics
George Washington University School of Medicine and Health Sciences
Program Director, Pediatric Emergency Medicine Fellowship
Children's National Medical Center
Washington, DC
Principles Applicable to the Developing World

Ira M. Cheifetz, MD, FCCM, FAARC
Professor of Pediatrics and Anesthesiology
Chief, Pediatric Critical Care Medicine
Duke University School of Medicine
Chief Medical Officer, Children's Services
Associate Chief Medical Officer, Duke Hospital
Duke Children's Hospital
Durham, North Carolina
Pediatric Emergencies and Resuscitation
Shock

Wassim Chemaitilly, MD
Director, Endocrinology Division
St. Jude Children's Research Hospital
Memphis, Tennessee
Physiology of Puberty
Disorders of Pubertal Development

Yuan-Tsong Chen, MD, PhD
Professor
Departments of Pediatrics and Genetics
Duke University Medical Center
Durham, North Carolina
Defects in Metabolism of Carbohydrates

Russell W. Chesney, MD
Le Bonheur Professor and Former Chair
Department of Pediatrics
University of Tennessee Health Science Center
Children's Foundation Research Institute
Memphis, Tennessee
Rickets Associated with Renal Tubular Acidosis
Bone Structure, Growth, and Hormonal Regulation
Primary Chondrodystrophy (Metaphyseal Dysplasia)
Hypophosphatasia
Hyperphosphatasia
Osteoporosis

Jennifer A. Chiriboga, PhD
Pediatric and School Psychologist
Assistant Professor
Department of Counseling, Psychology, and Special Education
Duquesne University School of Psychology
Pittsburgh, Pennsylvania
Anxiety Disorders

Yvonne E. Chiu, MD
Assistant Professor of Dermatology and Pediatrics
Medical College of Wisconsin
Milwaukee, Wisconsin
Morphology of the Skin
Evaluation of the Patient
Eczematous Disorders
Photosensitivity
Diseases of the Epidermis

Christine B. Cho, MD
Assistant Professor of Pediatrics
Division of Pediatric Allergy and Clinical Immunology
National Jewish Health
University of Colorado School of Medicine
Denver, Colorado
Ocular Allergies
Adverse Reactions to Drugs

Robert D. Christensen, MD
Professor and Presidential Endowed Chair
Divisions of Neonatology and Hematology/Oncology
Department of Pediatrics
University of Utah School of Medicine
Director of Neonatology Research
Intermountain Healthcare
Salt Lake City, Utah
Development of the Hematopoietic System

Andrew Chu, MD
Attending Physician
Division of Gastroenterology
Children's Hospital of Pittsburgh of UPMC
Pittsburgh, Pennsylvania
Superior Mesenteric Artery Syndrome (Wilkie Syndrome, Cast Syndrome, Arteriomesenteric Duodenal Compression Syndrome)
Ileus, Adhesions, Intussusception, and Closed-Loop Obstructions

Michael J. Chusid, MD
Professor of Pediatrics
Chief, Pediatric Infectious Diseases
Medical College of Wisconsin
Medical Director, Infectious Diseases
Children's Hospital of Wisconsin
Milwaukee, Wisconsin
Infection Prevention and Control
Other Anaerobic Infections

Col. Theodore J. Cieslak, MD, FAAP, FIDSA
Pediatric Infectious Diseases
San Antonio Military Medical Center
Department of Pediatrics
Fort Sam Houston, Texas
Biologic and Chemical Terrorism

Jeff A. Clark, MD
Associate Professor
Department of Pediatrics
Wayne State University School of Medicine
Pediatric ICU Fellowship Director
Children's Hospital of Michigan
Detroit, Michigan
Respiratory Distress and Failure
Respiratory Pathophysiology and Regulation

Thomas G. Cleary, MD
Professor of Pediatrics (Retired)
University of Texas Health Sciences Center
Houston, Texas
Shigella
Escherichia coli

John David Clemens, MD
Director
International Vaccine Institute
Seoul, South Korea
International Immunization Practices

Bria M. Coates, MD
Instructor in Pediatrics
Northwestern University Feinberg School of
    Medicine
Division of Pediatric Critical Care Medicine
Ann & Robert H. Lurie Children's Hospital of
    Chicago
Chicago, Illinois
Wheezing, Bronchiolitis, and Bronchitis

Thomas D. Coates, MD
Professor of Pediatrics and Pathology
University of Southern California Keck School of
    Medicine
Head, Section of Hematology
Children's Center for Cancer and Blood Diseases
Children's Hospital of Los Angeles
Los Angeles, California
Neutrophils
Disorders of Phagocyte Function

Joanna S. Cohen, MD
Adjunct Assistant Professor of Emergency
    Medicine
George Washington University School of Medicine
Division of Pediatric Emergency Medicine
Children's National Medical Center
Washington, DC
Care of Abrasions and Minor Lacerations

Mitchell B. Cohen, MD
Professor and Chair, Department of Pediatrics
University of Alabama at Birmingham
Physician-in-Chief, Children's of Alabama
Birmingham, Alabama
Clostridium difficile Infection

Michael Cohen-Wolkowiez, MD
Associate Professor of Pediatrics
Division of Pediatric Infectious Diseases
Duke University School of Medicine
Durham, North Carolina
Principles of Antifungal Therapy

Robert A. Colbert, MD, PhD
Deputy Clinical Director
National Institute of Arthritis and Musculoskeletal
    and Skin Diseases
Chief, Pediatric Translational Branch
National Institutes of Health
Bethesda, Maryland
*Ankylosing Spondylitis and Other
    Spondyloarthritides*
Reactive and Postinfectious Arthritis

F. Sessions Cole III, MD
Assistant Vice-Chancellor for Children's Health
Park J. White Professor of Pediatrics
Professor of Cell Biology and Physiology
Washington University School of Medicine in St.
    Louis
Chief Medical Officer
Vice-Chairman, Department of Pediatrics
Director of Newborn Medicine
St. Louis Children's Hospital
St. Louis, Missouri
Diffuse Lung Diseases in Childhood

John L. Colombo, MD
Professor of Pediatrics
University of Nebraska College of Medicine
Division of Pediatric Pulmonology
Nebraska Regional Cystic Fibrosis Center
University of Nebraska Medical Center
Omaha, Nebraska
Aspiration Syndromes
Chronic Recurrent Aspiration

Joseph A. Congeni, MD
Director, Sports Medicine Center
Akron Children's Hospital
Akron, Ohio;
Associate Professor of Pediatrics and Sports
    Medicine
Northeast Ohio Medical University
Rootstown, Ohio;
Clinical Associate Professor of Pediatrics and
    Sports Medicine
Ohio University College of Osteopathic Medicine
Athens, Ohio
Sports-Related Traumatic Brain Injury (Concussion)
Cervical Spinal Injuries

Christine M. Conroy, BS
Villanova University
Villanova, Pennsylvania
Arthrogryposis

Amber R. Cooper, MD, MSCI
Assistant Professor
Division of Reproductive Endocrinology and
    Infertility
Department of Obstetrics and Gynecology
Washington University School of Medicine in St.
    Louis
St. Louis, Missouri
Vulvovaginal and Müllerian Anomalies

Ronina A. Covar, MD
Associate Professor
Department of Pediatrics
National Jewish Health
University of Colorado School of Medicine
Denver, Colorado
Childhood Asthma

James E. Crowe Jr., MD
Professor of Pediatrics and Microbiology and
    Immunology
Ingram Professor of Research
Director, Vanderbilt Vaccine Center
Vanderbilt University Medical Center
Nashville, Tennessee
Respiratory Syncytial Virus
Human Metapneumovirus

Steve J. Czinn, MD
Professor and Chair
Department of Pediatrics
University of Maryland School of Medicine
Baltimore, Maryland
Peptic Ulcer Disease in Children

Josep O. Dalmau, MD, PhD
Research Professor ICREA-IDIBAPS
Department of Neurology
Hospital Clinic
Barcelona, Spain;
Adjunct Professor of Neurology
University of Pennsylvania Perelman School of
    Medicine
Philadelphia, Pennsylvania
Autoimmune Encephalitis

Toni Darville, MD
Professor of Pediatrics and Microbiology and
    Immunology
University of North Carolina at Chapel Hill School
    of Medicine
Vice-Chair for Pediatric Research
Chief, Division of Pediatric Infectious Diseases
NC Children's Hospital
Chapel Hill, North Carolina
Neisseria gonorrhoeae (Gonococcus)

Robert S. Daum, MD, CM
Professor of Pediatrics, Microbiology, and
    Molecular Medicine
University of Chicago Pritzker School of Medicine
Department of Pediatric Infectious Diseases
The University of Chicago Medicine Comer
    Children's Hospital
Chicago, Illinois
Haemophilus influenzae

Loren T. Davidson, MD
Assistant Clinical Professor
Department of Physical Medicine and
    Rehabilitation
University of California, Davis
Davis, California;
Director, Spinal Cord Injury
Shriner's Hospital for Children
Sacramento, California
Spasticity

Richard S. Davidson, MD
Clinical Professor
Department of Orthopaedic Surgery
University of Pennsylvania Perelman School of
    Medicine
Attending Orthopaedic Surgeon
Children's Hospital of Philadelphia
Philadelphia, Pennsylvania
The Foot and Toes
Leg-Length Discrepancy
Arthrogryposis

H. Dele Davies, MD, MS, MHCM
Vice-Chancellor for Academic Affairs
Dean for Graduate Studies
University of Nebraska Medical Center
Omaha, Nebraska
Chancroid (Haemophilus ducreyi)
Syphilis (Treponema pallidum)
Nonvenereal Treponemal Infections
Leptospira
Relapsing Fever (Borrelia)

Najat C. Daw, MD
Professor
Division of Pediatrics
University of Texas MD Anderson Cancer Center
Houston, Texas
Neoplasms of the Kidney

Peter S. Dayan, MD
Assistant Professor of Clinical Pediatrics
Columbia University College of Physicians and
    Surgeons
Associate Director and Fellowship Director
Division of Pediatric Emergency Medicine
Morgan Stanley Children's Hospital of New
    York–Presbyterian
New York, New York
Acute Care of the Victim of Multiple Trauma

Michael R. DeBaun, MD, MPH
Professor of Pediatrics and Medicine
J.C. Peterson Chair in Pediatric Pulmonology
Vice-Chair for Clinical Research
Pediatrics Director, Vanderbilt-Maherry Center of
    Excellence in Sickle Cell Disease
Vanderbilt University
Nashville, Tennessee
Hemoglobinopathies

David R. DeMaso, MD
George P. Gardner and Olga E. Monks Professor of
 Child Psychiatry
Professor of Pediatrics
Harvard Medical School
Psychiatrist-in-Chief and Chairman of Psychiatry
The Leon Eisenberg Chair in Psychiatry
Boston Children's Hospital
Boston, Massachusetts
Assessment and Interviewing
Psychological Treatment of Children and Adolescents
Psychopharmacology
Psychotherapy
Psychiatric Hospitalization
Somatic Symptom and Related Disorders
Rumination and Pica
Motor Disorders and Habits
Mood Disorders
Suicide and Attempted Suicide
Disruptive, Impulse-Control, and Conduct Disorders
Autism Spectrum Disorder
Childhood Psychoses

Mark R. Denison, MD
Craig-Weaver Professor of Pediatrics
Division of Pediatric Infectious Disease
Vanderbilt University Medical Center
Nashville, Tennessee
Coronaviruses

Arlene E. Dent, MD, PhD
Assistant Professor of Pediatrics
Division of Infectious Diseases
Case Western Reserve University School of
 Medicine
Cleveland, Ohio
Ascariasis (Ascaris lumbricoides)
Trichuriasis (Trichuris trichiura)
Enterobiasis (Enterobius vermicularis)
Strongyloidiasis (Strongyloides stercoralis)
Lymphatic Filariasis (Brugia malayi, Brugia timori,
 and Wuchereria bancrofti)
Other Tissue Nematodes
Toxocariasis (Visceral and Ocular Larva Migrans)
Trichinosis (Trichinella spiralis)

Robert J. Desnick, MD, PhD
Dean for Genetics and Genomic Medicine
Professor and Chair Emeritus, Genetics and
 Genomic Sciences
Professor, Departments of Pediatrics, Oncological
 Sciences, and Obstetrics, Gynecology, and
 Reproductive Science
Icahn School of Medicine at Mount Sinai
New York, New York
Lipidoses (Lysosomal Storage Disorders)
Mucolipidoses
Disorders of Glycoprotein Degradation and
 Structure
The Porphyrias

Gabrielle A. deVeber, MD, MHSc
Professor of Paediatrics
Director, Children's Stroke Program
University of Toronto Faculty of Medicine
Staff Neurologist
Senior Scientist, Child Health Evaluative Sciences
The Hospital for Sick Children
Toronto, Ontario, Canada
Pediatric Stroke

Anil Dhawan, MD
Consultant Paediatric Hepatologist
Pediatric Liver Centre
King's College London School of Medicine
King's College Hospital NSH Foundation Trust
London, United Kingdom
Liver and Biliary Disorders Causing Malabsorption

André A.S. Dick, MD, MPH, FACS
Assistant Professor of Surgery
Division of Transplantation
University of Washington School of Medicine
Division of Transplant Surgery
Seattle Children's Hospital
Seattle, Washington
Intestinal Transplantation in Children with
 Intestinal Failure

Brianne Z. Dickey, MD
Resident Physician
Department of Dermatology
Medical College of Wisconsin
Milwaukee, Wisconsin
Morphology of the Skin
Evaluation of the Patient
Eczematous Disorders
Photosensitivity
Diseases of the Epidermis

Harry C. Dietz III, MD
Victor A. McKusick Professor of Medicine and
 Genetics
Departments of Pediatrics, Medicine, and
 Molecular Biology and Genetics
Investigator, Howard Hughes Medical Institute
Director, William S. Smilow Center for Marfan
 Syndrome Research
Institute of Genetic Medicine
Johns Hopkins University School of Medicine
Baltimore, Maryland
Marfan Syndrome

Lydia J. Donoghue, MD
Director, Trauma Center
Children's Hospital of Michigan
Detroit, Michigan
Tumors of the Digestive Tract

Patricia A. Donohoue, MD
Professor of Pediatrics
Chief, Section of Endocrinology and Diabetes
Medical College of Wisconsin
Program Director, Endocrine and Diabetes
Children's Hospital of Wisconsin
Milwaukee, Wisconsin
Development and Function of the Gonads
Hypofunction of the Testes
Pseudoprecocity Resulting from Tumors of the Testes
Gynecomastia
Hypofunction of the Ovaries
Pseudoprecocity Resulting from Lesions of the Ovary
Disorders of Sex Development

Mary K. Donovan, RN, CS, PNP
Pediatric Nurse Practitioner and Care Coordinator
Shriners Hospital for Children
Shriners Burns Hospital
Boston, Massachusetts
Burn Injuries
Cold Injuries

John P. Dormans, MD
Professor and The Richard M. Armstrong Jr.
 Endowed Chair
Department of Orthopaedic Surgery
University of Pennsylvania Perelman School of
 Medicine
Chief, Division of Orthopaedic Surgery
Children's Hospital of Philadelphia
Philadelphia, Pennsylvania
Growth and Development
Evaluation of the Child
The Hip
Common Fractures

Kelly A. Dougherty, PhD
Assistant Professor of Pediatrics
University of Pennsylvania Perelman School of
 Medicine
Division of Gastroenterology, Hepatology, and
 Nutrition
Children's Hospital of Philadelphia
Philadelphia, Pennsylvania
Nutritional Requirements

Alexander Doyle, MBBS
HHMI Postdoctoral Research Fellow
Institute of Genetic Medicine
Johns Hopkins University School of Medicine
Baltimore, Maryland
Marfan Syndrome

Daniel A. Doyle, MD
Chief, Division of Endocrinology
Alfred I. duPont Hospital for Children
Nemours Children's Health System
Wilmington, Delaware
Hormones and Peptides of Calcium Homeostasis
 and Bone Metabolism
Hypoparathyroidism
Pseudohypoparathyroidism (Albright Hereditary
 Osteodystrophy)
Hyperparathyroidism

**Jefferson J. Doyle, MBBChir, MHS,
MA**
Postdoctoral Research Fellow
Institute of Genetic Medicine
Johns Hopkins University School of Medicine
Baltimore, Maryland
Marfan Syndrome

Patrick C. Drayna, MD
Assistant Professor of Pediatrics
Division of Pediatric Emergency Medicine
Medical College of Wisconsin
Children's Hospital of Wisconsin
Milwaukee, Wisconsin
Evaluation of the Sick Child in the Office and Clinic

Stephen C. Dreskin, MD, PhD
Professor of Medicine and Immunology
Division of Allergy and Clinical Immunology
Department of Medicine
University of Colorado School of Medicine
Aurora, Colorado
Urticaria (Hives) and Angioedema

Beth A. Drolet, MD
Professor of Dermatology
Medical College of Wisconsin
Children's Hospital of Wisconsin
Milwaukee, Wisconsin
Principles of Therapy (Skin)
Hyperpigmented Lesions
Diseases of Subcutaneous Tissue
Disorders of the Mucous Membranes
Cutaneous Bacterial Infections
Cutaneous Fungal Infections
Cutaneous Viral Infections
Arthropod Bites and Infestations

Yigal Dror, MD, FRCP(C)
Professor of Paediatrics
University of Toronto Faculty of Medicine
Head, Hematology Section Director, Marrow
  Failure and Myelodysplasia Program
The Hospital for Sick Children
Toronto, Ontario, Canada
The Inherited Pancytopenias

Howard Dubowitz, MD, MS, FAAP
Professor of Pediatrics
Chief, Division of Child Protection
Director, Center for Families
Department of Pediatrics
University of Maryland School of Medicine
Baltimore, Maryland
Abused and Neglected Children

J. Stephen Dumler, MD
Professor of Pathology and Microbiology and
  Immunology
University of Maryland School of Medicine
Baltimore, Maryland
Spotted Fever Group Rickettsioses
Scrub Typhus (Orientia tsutsugamushi)
Typhus Group Rickettsioses
Ehrlichioses and Anaplasmosis
Q Fever (Coxiella burnetii)

Aubrey N. Duncan, MD
Resident Physician
Department of Pediatrics
University of Rochester Medical Center
Rochester, New York
Deformational Plagiocephaly

Janet Duncan, MSN, CPNP
Department of Psychosocial Oncology and
  Palliative Care
Boston Children's Hospital
Dana-Farber Cancer Institute
Boston, Massachusetts
Pediatric Palliative Care

Paula M. Duncan, MD
Professor
Department of Pediatrics
University of Vermont College of Medicine
Burlington, Vermont
*Maximizing Children's Health: Screening,
  Anticipatory Guidance, and Counseling*

Jeffrey A. Dvergsten, MD
Assistant Professor of Pediatrics
Duke University School of Medicine
Division of Pediatric Rheumatology
Duke University Health System
Durham, North Carolina
Treatment of Rheumatic Diseases

Michael G. Earing, MD
Professor of Internal Medicine and Pediatrics
Division of Adult Cardiovascular Medicine and
  Division of Pediatric Cardiology
Medical College of Wisconsin
Director, Wisconsin Adult Congenital Heart
  Disease Program (WAtCH)
Children's Hospital of Wisconsin
Milwaukee, Wisconsin
Congenital Heart Disease in Adults

Matthew D. Eberly, MD
Assistant Professor of Pediatrics
Uniformed Services University of the Health
  Sciences
Bethesda, Maryland
Primary Amebic Meningoencephalitis

Elizabeth A. Edgerton, MD, MPH
Assistant Professor
Departments of Pediatrics and Preventive and
  Community Health
George Washington University School of Medicine
Division of Emergency Medicine
Children's National Medical Center
Washington, DC
*Interfacility Transport of the Seriously Ill or Injured
  Pediatric Patient*

Marie E. Egan, MD
Associate Professor of Pediatrics (Respiratory) and
  of Cellular and Molecular Physiology
Director, Cystic Fibrosis Center
Yale School of Medicine
New Haven, Connecticut
Cystic Fibrosis

Jack S. Elder, MD, FACS
Chief of Pediatric Urology
Massachusetts General Hospital
Boston, Massachusetts
Congenital Anomalies and Dysgenesis of the Kidneys
Urinary Tract Infections
Vesicoureteral Reflux
Obstruction of the Urinary Tract
Anomalies of the Bladder
Neuropathic Bladder
Enuresis and Voiding Dysfunction
Anomalies of the Penis and Urethra
Disorders and Anomalies of the Scrotal Contents
Trauma to the Genitourinary Tract
Urinary Lithiasis

Dianne S. Elfenbein, MD
Professor of Pediatrics
Director, Division of Adolescent Medicine
St. Louis University School of Medicine
St. Louis, Missouri
Adolescent Pregnancy

Stephen C. Eppes, MD, FAAP
Professor of Pediatrics
Jefferson Medical College of Thomas Jefferson
  University
Philadelphia, Pennsylvania;
Director, Pediatric Infectious Diseases
Christiana Care Health System
Wilmington, Delaware
Lyme Disease (Borrelia burgdorferi)

Jessica Ericson, MD
Pediatric Infectious Diseases Fellow
Duke University Medical Center
Durham, North Carolina
Candida

Alessio Fasano, MD
Visiting Professor of Pediatrics
Harvard Medical School
Chief, Division of Pediatric Gastroenterology and
  Nutrition
Associate Chief, Department of Pediatrics, Basic,
  Clinical, and Translational Research
Director, Center for Celiac Research
MassGeneral Hospital for Children
Boston, Massachusetts
Celiac Disease (Gluten-Sensitive Enteropathy)

Susan Feigelman, MD
Professor, Department of Pediatrics
University of Maryland School of Medicine
Baltimore, Maryland
Overview and Assessment of Variability
Assessment of Fetal Growth and Development
The First Year
The Second Year
The Preschool Years
Middle Childhood

Marianne E. Felice, MD
Professor
Departments of Pediatrics and Obstetrics and
  Gynecology
University of Massachusetts Medical School
Principle Investigator, National Children's Study
UMass Study Center
Worcester, Massachusetts
Adolescent Pregnancy
Adolescent Rape

Eric I. Felner, MD, MSCR
Associate Professor of Pediatrics
Division of Pediatric Endocrinology
Director, Pediatric Endocrinology Fellowship
  Program
Director, Pediatric Clerkships
Emory University School of Medicine
Atlanta, Georgia
Hormones of the Hypothalamus and Pituitary
Hypopituitarism

Edward C. Fels, MD
Pediatric and Adult Rheumatology
Rheumatology Associates, PA
Portland, Maine
Vasculitis Syndromes

Kora N. Felsch, MD
Hospitalist
Cardinal Glennon Children's Medical Center
St. Louis, Missouri
Breast Concerns

Thomas W. Ferkol Jr., MD
Alexis Hartmann Professor of Pediatrics
Director, Division of Pediatric Allergy,
  Immunology, and Pulmonary Medicine
Washington University School of Medicine in
  St. Louis
St. Louis, Missouri
*Primary Ciliary Dyskinesia (Immotile Cilia
  Syndrome, Kartagener Syndrome)*

Can H. Ficicioglu, MD, PhD
Associate Professor
Department of Pediatrics
University of Pennsylvania Perelman School of
  Medicine
Director, Newborn Metabolic Screening Program
Children's Hospital of Philadelphia
Philadelphia, Pennsylvania
Phenylalanine

Jonathan D. Finder, MD
Professor of Pediatrics
University of Pittsburgh School of Medicine
Attending Pediatric Pulmonologist
Division of Pediatric Pulmonology
Children's Hospital of Pittsburgh of UPMC
Pittsburgh, Pennsylvania
Bronchomalacia and Tracheomalacia
Congenital Disorders of the Lung

Kristin N. Fiorino, MD
Assistant Professor of Clinical Pediatrics
University of Pennsylvania Perelman School of
    Medicine
Attending Physician
Division of Gastroenterology, Hepatology, and
    Nutrition
The Children's Hospital of Philadelphia
Philadelphia, Pennsylvania
Motility Disorders and Hirschsprung Disease

Philip R. Fischer, MD
Professor of Pediatrics
Mayo Clinic
Rochester, Minnesota
Adult Tapeworm Infections
Cysticercosis
Echinococcosis (Echinococcus granulosus and
    Echinococcus multilocularis)

Veronica H. Flood, MD
Associate Professor of Pediatrics
Division of Pediatric Hematology/Oncology
Medical College of Wisconsin
Milwaukee, Wisconsin
Hereditary Clotting Factor Deficiencies (Bleeding
    Disorders)
von Willebrand Disease
Thrombocytopenia from Acquired Disorders Causing
    Decreased Production

Patricia M. Flynn, MD
Deputy Clinical Director
Arthur Ashe Chair in Pediatric AIDS Research
Director, Clinical Research, Infectious Diseases
St. Jude Children's Research Hospital
Professor of Pediatrics and Preventive Medicine
University of Tennessee College of Medicine
Memphis, Tennessee
Infection Associated with Medical Devices
Cryptosporidium, Isospora, Cyclospora, and
    Microsporidia

Joel A. Forman, MD
Associate Professor of Pediatrics and Preventive
    Medicine
Vice-Chair for Education
Department of Pediatrics
Icahn School of Medicine at Mount Sinai
New York, New York
Chemical Pollutants

Michael M. Frank, MD
Samuel L. Katz Professor of Pediatrics, Medicine,
    and Immunology
Duke University School of Medicine
Durham, North Carolina
Urticaria (Hives) and Angioedema

**Melvin H. Freedman, MD, FRCP(C),
FAAP**
Professor Emeritus of Pediatrics
University of Toronto Faculty of Medicine
Honorary Consultant, Hematology/Oncology
The Hospital for Sick Children
Toronto, Ontario, Canada
The Inherited Pancytopenias

Megan Culler Freeman, PhD
Departments of Pediatrics and Pathology,
    Microbiology, and Immunology
Vanderbilt University School of Medicine
Nashville, Tennessee
Coronaviruses

Melissa J. Frei-Jones, MD, MSCI
Assistant Professor of Pediatrics
Division of Pediatric Hematology/Oncology
University of Texas Health Sciences Center
Santa Rosa Children's Hospital
San Antonio, Texas
Hemoglobinopathies

Deborah Friedman, MD
Assistant Clinical Professor of Pediatrics
Case Western Reserve University School of
    Medicine
Cleveland, Ohio
Neonatal Lupus

Erika Friehling, MD
Assistant Professor of Pediatrics
University of Pittsburgh School of Medicine
Division of Pediatric Hematology/Oncology
Children's Hospital of Pittsburgh of UPMC
Pittsburgh, Pennsylvania
Principles of Diagnosis (Cancer and Benign
    Tumors)
Principles of Treatment (Cancer and Benign
    Tumors)
The Leukemias

Donald P. Frush, MD
Professor of Radiology
Chief, Division of Pediatric Radiology
Duke University Medical Center
Durham, North Carolina
Biologic Effects of Radiation on Children

James T. Gaensbauer, MD, MSc
Assistant Professor of Pediatrics
University of Colorado School of Medicine
Divisions of Hospital Medicine and Infectious
    Diseases
Children's Hospital Colorado
Aurora, Colorado
Staphylococcus

Sheila Gahagan, MD, MPH
Professor and Chief
Academic General Pediatrics, Child Development,
    and Community Health
Martin Stein Endowed Chair, Developmental-
    Behavioral Pediatrics
University of California, San Diego
La Jolla, California
Overweight and Obesity

William A. Gahl, MD, PhD
Clinical Director, National Human Genome
    Research Institute
Director, NIH Undiagnosed Diseases Program
National Institutes of Health
Bethesda, Maryland
Genetic Approaches to Rare and Undiagnosed
    Diseases

Sheila S. Galbraith, MD
Associate Professor of Dermatology
Medical College of Wisconsin
Children's Hospital of Wisconsin
Milwaukee, Wisconsin
Hypopigmented Lesions
Diseases of the Dermis
Acne

William B. Gallentine, DO
Assistant Professor of Pediatrics
Duke University School of Medicine
Division of Pediatric Neurology
Duke University Health System
Durham, North Carolina
Central Nervous System Vasculitis

Paula M. Gardiner, MD, MPH
Assistant Professor
Department of Family Medicine
Boston University School of Medicine
Assistant Director, Integrative Medicine
Boston Medical Center
Boston, Massachusetts
Complementary Therapies and Integrative Medicine

Luigi R. Garibaldi, MD
Professor of Pediatrics
University of Pittsburgh School of Medicine
Clinical Director
Division of Pediatric Endocrinology
Children's Hospital of UPMC
Pittsburgh, Pennsylvania
Physiology of Puberty
Disorders of Pubertal Development

Gregory M. Gauthier, MD, MS
Assistant Professor of Medicine
Division of Infectious Diseases
University of Wisconsin School of Medicine
Madison, Wisconsin
Blastomycosis (Blastomyces dermatitidis)

K. Michael Gibson, PhD
Allen I. White Distinguished Professor and Chair
Experimental and Systems Pharmacology
Washington State University College of
    Pharmacology
Spokane, Washington
Genetic Disorders of Neurotransmitters

Mark Gibson, MD
Professor (Clinical) Emeritus
Department of Obstetrics and Gynecology
Chief, Division of Reproductive Endocrinology
University of Utah School of Medicine
Salt Lake City, Utah
Polycystic Ovary Syndrome and Hirsutism

Francis Gigliotti, MD
Professor of Pediatrics and Microbiology and
    Immunology
Lindsey Distinguished Professor for Pediatric
    Research
University of Rochester School of Medicine and
    Dentistry
Division of Pediatric Infectious Diseases
University of Rochester Medical Center
Rochester, New York
Pneumocystis jiroveci (Pneumocystis carinii)

Walter S. Gilliam, MSEd, PhD
Associate Professor
Department of Psychology
Child Study Center
Director, The Edward Zigler Center in Child
    Development and Social Policy
Yale School of Medicine
New Haven, Connecticut
*Childcare: How Pediatricians Can Support Children
    and Families*

Salil Ginde, MD, MPH
Assistant Professor of Pediatrics
Division of Pediatric Cardiology
Medical College of Wisconsin
Milwaukee, Wisconsin
Congenital Heart Disease in Adults

Charles M. Ginsburg, MD
Senior Associate Dean for Academic
    Administration
Professor of Pediatrics
Marilyn R. Corrigan Distinguished Chair in
    Pediatric Research
University of Texas Southwestern Medical Center
Houston, Texas
Animal and Human Bites

**John A. Girotto, MD, MMA, FAAP,
FACS**
Associate Professor of Pediatrics, Neurosurgery,
    and Plastic and Reconstructive Surgery
Director, Cleft and Craniofacial Anomalies Center
Golisano Children's Hospital at Strong
University of Rochester Medical Center
Rochester, New York
Deformational Plagiocephaly

Lisa Giulino-Roth, MD
Assistant Professor of Pediatrics
Division of Pediatric Hematology/Oncology
Weill Cornell Medical College
New York, New York
Lymphoma

Frances Page Glascoe, PhD
Professor
Department of Pediatrics
Vanderbilt University School of Medicine
Nashville, Tennessee
*Developmental-Behavioral Screening and
    Surveillance*

Denise M. Goodman, MD, MS
Professor
Department of Pediatrics
Northwestern University Feinberg School of
    Medicine
Ann & Robert H. Lurie Children's Hospital of
    Chicago
Chicago, Illinois
Wheezing, Bronchiolitis, and Bronchitis

Alison Gopnik, PhD
Professor of Psychology and Affiliate Professor of
    Philosophy
University of California at Berkeley
Berkeley, California
Cognitive Development: Domains and Theories

Leslie B. Gordon, MD, PhD
Associate Professor of Pediatrics Research
Warren Alpert Medical School of Brown University
Providence, Rhode Island;
Department of Anesthesia
Boston Children's Hospital
Harvard Medical School
Boston, Massachusetts;
Medical Director, The Progeria Research
    Foundation
Peabody, Massachusetts
Hutchinson-Gilford Progeria Syndrome

Marc H. Gorelick, MD, MSCE
Professor of Pediatrics
Medical College of Wisconsin
Children's Hospital of Wisconsin
Milwaukee, Wisconsin
Evaluation of the Sick Child in the Office and Clinic

Jane M. Gould, MD, FAAP
Associate Professor of Pediatrics
Drexel University College of Medicine
Attending Physician, Infectious Diseases
St. Christopher's Hospital for Children
Philadelphia, Pennsylvania
Cryptococcus neoformans
Histoplasmosis (Histoplasma capsulatum)
Paracoccidioides brasiliensis
Zygomycosis (Mucormycosis)

Olivier Goulet, MD
Professor of Pediatrics
University of Paris V—René Descartes
Head, Division of Pediatric Gastroenterology-
    Hepatology and Nutrition
Hôpital Necker-Enfants Malades/AP-HP
Paris, France
Other Malabsorptive Syndromes

Deanna M. Green, MD, MHS
Assistant Professor of Pediatrics
Division of Pediatric Pulmonary and Sleep
    Medicine
Duke University School of Medicine
Durham, North Carolina
Cystic Fibrosis

Michael Green, MD, MPH
Professor of Pediatrics and Surgery
University of Pittsburgh School of Medicine
Division of Pediatric Infectious Diseases
Children's Hospital of Pittsburgh of UPMC
Pittsburgh, Pennsylvania
Infections in Immunocompromised Persons

Thomas P. Green, MD
Founders' Board Centennial Professor and Chair
Department of Pediatrics
Northwestern University Feinberg School of
    Medicine
Physician-in-Chief
Ann & Robert H. Lurie Children's Hospital of
    Chicago
Chicago, Illinois
Diagnostic Approach to Respiratory Disease
Chronic or Recurrent Respiratory Symptoms
Pulmonary Edema

Larry A. Greenbaum, MD, PhD
Marcus Professor of Pediatrics
Director, Division of Pediatric Nephrology
Emory University School of Medicine
Children's Healthcare of Atlanta
Atlanta, Georgia
Rickets and Hypervitaminosis D
Vitamin E Deficiency
Vitamin K Deficiency
Micronutrient Mineral Deficiencies
Electrolyte and Acid-Base Disorders
Maintenance and Replacement Therapy
Deficit Therapy
Fluid and Electrolyte Treatment of Specific Disorders

Anne G. Griffiths, MD
Instructor in Pediatrics
Northwestern University Feinberg School of
    Medicine
Hospitalist, Neonatal Intensive Care Unit
Ann & Robert H. Lurie Children's Hospital of
    Chicago
Chicago, Illinois
Chronic or Recurrent Respiratory Symptoms

Allison Grimes, MD
Fellow in Pediatric Hematology/Oncology
University of Texas Health Sciences Center
San Antonio, Texas
Abnormal Hemoglobins Causing Cyanosis
Hereditary Methemoglobinemia
*Hereditary Methemoglobinemia with Deficiency of
    NADH Cytochrome B5 Reductase*

Natalia M. Grindler, MD
Resident Physician
Department of Obstetrics and Gynecology
Washington University School of Medicine in St.
    Louis
St. Louis, Missouri
Vulvovaginal and Müllerian Anomalies

Kenneth L. Grizzle, PhD
Associate Professor
Child Development Center—Brookfield
Medical College of Wisconsin
Brookfield, Wisconsin
*Childhood-Onset Fluency Disorder: Dysfluency
    (Stuttering, Stammering)*

Veronique Groleau, MD
Fellow
Division of Gastroenterology, Hepatology, and
    Nutrition
Children's Hospital of Philadelphia
Philadelphia, Pennsylvania
Nutritional Requirements
Feeding Healthy Infants, Children, and Adolescents

Andrew B. Grossman, MD
Assistant Professor of Clinical Pediatrics
University of Pennsylvania Perelman School of
    Medicine
Co-Director, Center for Pediatric Inflammatory
    Bowel Disease
The Children's Hospital of Philadelphia
Philadelphia, Pennsylvania
Inflammatory Bowel Disease

David C. Grossman, MD, MPH
Senior Investigator Group Health Research Institute
Professor of Health Services
University of Washington School of Public Health
Adjunct Professor of Pediatrics
University of Washington School of Medicine
Seattle, Washington
Injury Control

Alfredo Guarino, MD
Professor
Department of Pediatrics
University of Naples Federico II
Napoli, Italy
Chronic Diarrhea

Reut Gurion, DO
Pediatric Rheumatology Fellow
Division of Rheumatology
University Hospitals Case Medical Center
Rainbow Babies & Children's Hospital
Cleveland, Ohio
Miscellaneous Conditions Associated with Arthritis

Lisa R. Hackney, MD
Assistant Professor of Pediatrics
Division of Pediatric Hematology/Oncology
Cleveland Clinic Foundation
Cleveland, Ohio
Hereditary Stomatocytosis
Glucose-6-Phosphate Dehydrogenase Deficiency and Related Deficiencies

Gabriel G. Haddad, MD
Distinguished Professor and Chair
Department of Pediatrics
University of California, San Diego
Physician-in-Chief
Chief Scientific Officer
Rady Children's Hospital
San Diego, California
Diagnostic Approach to Respiratory Disease

Joseph Haddad Jr., MD
Howard W. Smith Professor and Interim Chair
Lawrence Savetsky Professor
Department of Otolaryngology—Head and Neck Surgery
Columbia University College of Physicians and Surgeons
Director, Pediatric Otolaryngology—Head and Neck Surgery
New York-Presbyterian Morgan Stanley Children's Hospital
New York, New York
Congenital Disorders of the Nose
Acquired Disorders of the Nose
Nasal Polyps
General Considerations and Evaluation (Ear)
Hearing Loss
Congenital Malformations
External Otitis (Otitis Externa)
The Inner Ear and Diseases of the Bony Labyrinth
Traumatic Injuries of the Ear and Temporal Bone
Tumors of the Ear and Temporal Bone

Joseph F. Hagan Jr., MD
Clinical Professor
Department of Pediatrics
University of Vermont College of Medicine
Hagan, Rinehart, and Connolly Pediatricians, PLLC
Burlington, Vermont
Maximizing Children's Health: Screening, Anticipatory Guidance, and Counseling

Scott B. Halstead, MD
Professor of Pediatrics and Medical Genetics
University of British Columbia Faculty of Medicine
British Columbia's Children's Hospital
Vancouver, British Columbia, Canada
Arboviral Infections in North America
Arboviral Infections Outside North America
Dengue Fever and Dengue Hemorrhagic Fever
Yellow Fever
Ebola and Other Viral Hemorrhagic Fevers
Hantavirus Pulmonary Syndrome

Margaret R. Hammerschlag, MD
Professor of Pediatrics and Medicine
Director, Division of Pediatric Infectious Diseases
SUNY Down State Medical Center
Brooklyn, New York
Chlamydia (Chlamydophila) pneumoniae
Chlamydia trachomatis
Psittacosis (Chlamydia psittaci)

Aaron Hamvas, MD
Raymond and Hazel Speck Barry Professor of Neonatology
Head, Division of Neonatology
Ann & Robert H. Lurie Children's Hospital of Chicago
Northwestern University Feinberg School of Medicine
Chicago, Illinois
Diffuse Lung Diseases in Childhood

Abeer J. Hani, MD
Resident Physician
Division of Pediatric Neurology
Duke University Medical Center
Durham, North Carolina
Seizures in Childhood

James C. Harris, MD
Professor of Pediatrics, Psychiatry and Behavioral Sciences, Mental Health, and History of Medicine
Division of Child and Adolescent Psychiatry
Director, Developmental Neuropsychiatry
Johns Hopkins University School of Medicine
Baltimore, Maryland
Disorders of Purine and Pyrimidine Metabolism

Mary E. Hartman, MD, MPH
Assistant Professor of Pediatrics
Washington University in St. Louis
Pediatric Critical Care Medicine
St. Louis Children's Hospital
St. Louis, Missouri
Pediatric Emergencies and Resuscitation

David B. Haslam, MD
Associate Professor of Pediatrics
University of Cincinnati College of Medicine
Director, Antimicrobial Stewardship Program
Clinical Director, Division of Infectious Diseases
Cincinnati Children's Hospital Medical Center
Cincinnati, Ohio
Non–Group A or B Streptococci
Enterococcus

H. Hesham Abdel-Kader Hassan, MD
Professor of Pediatrics
Chief, Division of Pediatric Gastroenterology and Nutrition
The University of Arizona College of Medicine
Tucson, Arizona
Cholestasis

Lindsay A. Hatzenbuehler, MD, MPH
Pediatric Infectious Diseases Fellow
Baylor College of Medicine
Texas Children's Hospital
Houston, Texas
Tuberculosis (Mycobacterium tuberculosis)

Fern R. Hauck, MD, MS
Spencer P. Bass MD Twenty-First Century Professor of Family Medicine
Departments of Family Medicine and Public Health Sciences
Director, International Family Medicine Clinic
University of Virginia School of Medicine
Charlottesville, Virginia
Sudden Infant Death Syndrome

Fiona P. Havers, MD, MHS
Epidemic Intelligence Service Office
Epidemiology and Prevention Branch, Influenza Division
National Center for Immunization and Respiratory Diseases
Centers for Disease Control and Prevention
Atlanta, Georgia
Influenza Viruses

Jacqueline T. Hecht, PhD
Professor and Division Head
Leah L. Lewis Distinguished Chair
Pediatric Research Center
Vice-Chair for Research
Department of Pediatrics
UT Health Medical School of Houston
Associate Dean for Research
UT Health School of Dentistry
Houston, Texas
General Considerations (Bone and Joint Disorders)
Disorders Involving Cartilage Matrix Proteins
Disorders Involving Transmembrane Receptors
Disorders Involving Ion Transporters
Disorders Involving Transcription Factors
Disorders Involving Defective Bone Resorption
Disorders for Which Defects Are Poorly Understood or Unknown

Sabrina M. Heidemann, MD
Professor
Department of Pediatrics
Wayne State University School of Medicine
Director, Intensive Care Unit
Co-Director of Transport
Children's Hospital of Michigan
Detroit, Michigan
Respiratory Pathophysiology and Regulation

J. Owen Hendley, MD
Professor
Department of Pediatrics
University of Virginia School of Medicine
Charlottesville, Virginia
Sinusitis
Retropharyngeal Abscess, Lateral Pharyngeal (Parapharyngeal) Abscess, and Peritonsillar Cellulitis/Abscess

Frederick M. Henretig, MD
Division of Emergency Medicine
Children's Hospital of Philadelphia
Professor Emeritus of Pediatrics
Perelman School of Medicine
University of Pennsylvania
Philadelphia, Pennsylvania
Biologic and Chemical Terrorism

Gloria P. Heresi, MD
Professor of Pediatrics
Director, Division of Pediatric Infectious Diseases
University of Texas Health Sciences Center
Houston, Texas
Campylobacter
Yersinia
Aeromonas and Plesiomonas

Andrew D. Hershey, MD, PhD, FAHS
Professor of Pediatrics and Neurology
University of Cincinnati College of Medicine
Endowed Chair, Division of Neurology
Cincinnati Children's Hospital Medical Center
Cincinnati, Ohio
Headaches

Cynthia E. Herzog, MD
Professor of Pediatrics
University of Texas MD Anderson Cancer Center
Houston, Texas
Retinoblastoma
Gonadal and Germ Cell Neoplasms
Neoplasms of the Liver
Benign Vascular Tumors
Melanoma
Nasopharyngeal Carcinoma
Adenocarcinoma of the Colon and Rectum
Desmoplastic Small Round Cell Tumor

Jessica Hochberg, MD
Assistant Professor of Pediatrics
Division of Pediatric Hematology, Oncology, and
    Stem Cell Transplant
New York Medical College
Maria Fareri Children's Hospital at Westchester
    Medical Center
Valhalla, New York
Lymphoma

Holly R. Hoefgen, MD
Fellow, Department of Obstetrics and Gynecology
Washington University School of Medicine in St.
    Louis
St. Louis, Missouri
Vulvovaginitis

Lauren D. Holinger, MD, FAAP, FACS
Paul H. Holinger MD Professor and Interim Head,
    Division of Otolaryngology
Department of Pediatrics
Northwestern University Feinberg School of
    Medicine
Ann & Robert H. Lurie Children's Hospital of
    Chicago
Chicago, Illinois
*Congenital Anomalies of the Larynx, Trachea, and
    Bronchi*
Foreign Bodies in the Airway
Laryngotracheal Stenosis and Subglottic Stenosis
Neoplasms of the Larynx, Trachea, and Bronchi

Cynthia Holland-Hall, MD, MPH
Associate Clinical Professor of Clinical Pediatrics
The Ohio State University College of Medicine
Section of Adolescent Medicine
Nationwide Children's Hospital
Columbus, Ohio
Adolescent Physical and Social Development
Transitioning to Adult Care
The Breast

Jeffrey D. Hord, MD
Director, Showers Family Center for Childhood
    Cancer and Blood Disorders
Associate Chair of Pediatrics for Subspecialty
    Practices
Akron Children's Hospital
Akron, Ohio
The Acquired Pancytopenias

B. David Horn, MD
Assistant Professor
Department of Orthopaedic Surgery
University of Pennsylvania Perelman School of
    Medicine
Attending Orthopaedic Surgeon
Children's Hospital of Philadelphia
Philadelphia, Pennsylvania
The Hip

Helen M. Horstmann, MD
Associate Professor
Department of Orthopaedic Surgery
University of Pennsylvania Perelman School of
    Medicine
Attending Physician
Children's Hospital of Philadelphia
Philadelphia, Pennsylvania
Arthrogryposis

William A. Horton, MD
Professor
Department of Molecular Medical Genetics
Oregon Health & Science University
Director of Research
Shriners Hospitals for Children
Portland, Oregon
General Considerations (Bone and Joint Disorders)
Disorders Involving Cartilage Matrix Proteins
Disorders Involving Transmembrane Receptors
Disorders Involving Ion Transporters
Disorders Involving Transcription Factors
Disorders Involving Defective Bone Resorption
*Disorders for Which Defects Are Poorly Understood
    or Unknown*

**Peter J. Hotez, MD, PhD, FASTMH,
FAAP**
Founding Dean, National School of Tropical
    Medicine
Professor of Pediatrics and Molecular Virology and
    Microbiology
Baylor College of Medicine
Endowed Chair in Tropical Pediatrics
Texas Children's Hospital
Houston, Texas
Hookworms (Necator americanus *and* Ancylostoma
    spp.)

Evelyn Hsu, MD
Assistant Professor of Pediatrics
Seattle Children's Hospital
Seattle, Washington
Liver Transplantation

Stephen A. Huang, MD
Assistant Professor of Pediatrics
Harvard Medical School
Director, Thyroid Program
Division of Endocrinology
Boston Children's Hospital
Boston, Massachusetts
Thyroid Development and Physiology
Defects of Thyroxine-Binding Globulin
Hypothyroidism
Thyroiditis
Goiter
Hyperthyroidism
Carcinoma of the Thyroid

Heather G. Huddleston, MD
Assistant Professor
Department of Obstetrics, Gynecology, and
    Reproductive Sciences
University of California, San Francisco School of
    Medicine
San Francisco, California
Polycystic Ovary Syndrome and Hirsutism

Vicki Huff, PhD
Professor
Department of Molecular Genetics/Cancer
    Genetics
University of Texas MD Anderson Cancer Center
Houston, Texas
Neoplasms of the Kidney

Denise Hug, MD
Associate Professor
Department of Ophthalmology
University of Missouri—Kansas City School of
    Medicine
Children's Mercy Hospital
Kansas City, Missouri
Growth and Development (Eye)
Examination of the Eye
Abnormalities of Refraction and Accommodation
Disorders of Vision
Abnormalities of Pupil and Iris
Disorders of Eye Movement and Alignment
Abnormalities of the Lids
Disorders of the Lacrimal System
Disorders of the Conjunctiva
Abnormalities of the Cornea
Abnormalities of the Lens
Disorders of the Uveal Tract
Disorders of the Retina and Vitreous
Abnormalities of the Optic Nerve
Childhood Glaucoma
Orbital Abnormalities
Orbital Infections
Injuries to the Eye

Dennis P.M. Hughes, MD, PhD
Associate Professor of Pediatrics
University of Texas MD Anderson Cancer Center
Houston, Texas
Melanoma

Winston W. Huh, MD
Assistant Professor of Pediatrics
University of Texas MD Anderson Cancer Center
Houston, Texas
Gonadal and Germ Cell Neoplasms
Adenocarcinoma of the Colon and Rectum

Stephen R. Humphrey, MD
Resident Physician
Department of Dermatology
Medical College of Wisconsin
Children's Hospital of Wisconsin
Milwaukee, Wisconsin
Principles of Therapy (Skin)

David A. Hunstad, MD
Associate Professor of Pediatrics and Molecular
    Microbiology
Washington University School of Medicine in St.
    Louis
St. Louis, Missouri
Animal and Human Bites

Carl E. Hunt, MD
Research Professor of Pediatrics
Uniformed Services University of the Health
    Sciences
Division of Neonatology
Walter Reed National Military Medical Center
Bethesda, Maryland;
Adjunct Professor of Pediatrics
George Washington University School of Medicine
Washington, DC
Sudden Infant Death Syndrome

Anna K. Hunter, MD
Assistant Clinical Professor of Pediatrics
University of California, San Francisco
UCSF Fresno Center for Medical Education and
    Research
Fresno, California;
Pediatric Gastroenterologist
Children's Hospital Central California
Madera, California
*Pyloric Stenosis and Other Congenital Anomalies of
    the Stomach*

Stacey S. Huppert, PhD
Associate Professor of Pediatrics
University of Cincinnati College of Medicine
Division of Gastroenterology, Hepatology, and
    Nutrition
Division of Developmental Biology
Cincinnati Children's Hospital Medical Center
Cincinnati, Ohio
Morphogenesis of the Liver and Biliary System

Patricia I. Ibeziako, MD
Assistant Professor of Psychiatry
Harvard Medical School
Director, Psychiatry Consultation Service
Boston Children's Hospital
Boston, Massachusetts
Somatic Symptom and Related Disorders

Samar H. Ibrahim, MBChB
Assistant Professor of Pediatrics
Division of Pediatric Gastroenterology and
    Hepatology
Mayo Clinic
Rochester, Minnesota
Mitochondrial Hepatopathies

Richard F. Jacobs, MD, FAAP
Robert H. Fiser Jr. MD Endowed Chair in
    Pediatrics
Professor and Chair, Department of Pediatrics
University of Arkansas for Medical Sciences
Pediatrician-in-Chief
Arkansas Children's Hospital
Little Rock, Arkansas
Actinomyces
Nocardia
Tularemia (Francisella tularensis)
Brucella

Tara Jatlaoui, MD, MPH
Research Assistant Professor
Department of Obstetrics and Gynecology
The University of North Carolina at Chapel Hill
Guest Researcher, Division of Reproductive Health
Centers for Disease Control and Prevention
Atlanta, Georgia
Contraception

M. Kyle Jensen, MD
Assistant Professor of Pediatrics
University of Utah School of Medicine
Division of Pediatric Gastroenterology
Primary Children's Hospital
Salt Lake City, Utah
Viral Hepatitis

Hal B. Jenson, MD, MBA
Founding Dean
Professor, Department of Pediatric and Adolescent
    Medicine
Western Michigan University
Homer Stryker M.D. School of Medicine
Kalamazoo, Michigan
Chronic Fatigue Syndrome
Epstein-Barr Virus
Human T-Lymphotropic Viruses (1 and 2)

Chandy C. John, MD, MS
Ryan White Professor of Pediatrics
Professor of Pediatrics, Microbiology and
    Immunology
Director, Ryan White Center for Pediatric
    Infectious Diseases and Global Health
Indiana University School of Medicine
Riley Hospital for Children at Indiana University
    Health
Indianapolis, Indiana
Health Advice for Children Traveling Internationally
Giardiasis and Balantidiasis
Malaria (Plasmodium)

Collin C. John, MD, MPH, FAAP
Assistant Professor of Internal Medicine and
    Pediatrics
Medical Director, West Virginia Birth Score
    Program
West Virginia University School of Medicine
Morgantown, West Virginia
Disorders of Lipoprotein Metabolism and Transport

Michael V. Johnston, MD
Professor of Neurology, Pediatrics, and Physical
    Medicine and Rehabilitation
Johns Hopkins University School of Medicine
Kennedy Krieger Institute
Baltimore, Maryland
Congenital Anomalies of the Central Nervous System
Encephalopathies

Richard B. Johnston Jr., MD
Professor of Pediatrics
Associate Dean for Research Development
University of Colorado School of Medicine
Aurora, Colorado;
National Jewish Health
Denver, Colorado
Monocytes, Macrophages, and Dendritic Cells
The Complement System
Disorders of the Complement System

Bridgette L. Jones, MD
Associate Professor of Pediatrics
Division of Allergy, Asthma, and Immunology
University of Missouri—Kansas City School of
    Medicine
Section of Clinical Pharmacology and Medical
    Toxicology
Children's Mercy Hospitals and Clinics
Kansas City, Missouri
Principles of Drug Therapy

James F. Jones, MD
Research Medical Officer
Viral Exanthems and Herpesvirus Branch
Division of Viral and Rickettsial Diseases
National Center for Infectious Diseases
Centers for Disease Control and Prevention
Atlanta, Georgia
Chronic Fatigue Syndrome

Marsha Joselow, MSW, LICSW
Department of Psychosocial Oncology and
    Palliative Care
Boston Children's Hospital
Dana-Farber Cancer Institute
Boston, Massachusetts
Pediatric Palliative Care

Nicholas Jospe, MD
Professor of Pediatrics
Division of Pediatric Endocrinology
Golisano Children's Hospital
University of Rochester Medical Center
Rochester, New York
Diabetes Mellitus

Joel C. Joyce, MD
Pediatric Dermatology
NorthShore University HealthSystem
Skokie, Illinois;
Clinician Educator
University of Chicago Pritzker School of Medicine
Chicago, Illinois
Vesiculobullous Disorders
Nutritional Dermatoses

Anna M. Juern, MD
Division of Pediatric Dermatology
Medical College of Wisconsin
Milwaukee, Wisconsin
Hyperpigmented Lesions
Cutaneous Bacterial Infections
Cutaneous Fungal Infections
Cutaneous Viral Infections
Arthropod Bites and Infestations

Marielle A. Kabbouche, MD
Associate Professor of Pediatrics and Neurology
University of Cincinnati College of Medicine
Division of Neurology
Cincinnati Children's Hospital Medical Center
Cincinnati, Ohio
Headaches

Linda Kaljee, PhD, MAA
Associate Professor
Department of Pediatrics
Prevention Research Center
Wayne State University School of Medicine
Detroit, Michigan
Cultural Issues in Pediatric Care

Deepak Kamat, MD, PhD, FAAP
Professor and Vice-Chair of Education
Department of Pediatrics
Wayne State University School of Medicine
Designated Institutional Official
Children's Hospital of Michigan
Detroit, Michigan
Fever
Fever Without a Focus

Alvina R. Kansra, MD
Assistant Professor of Pediatrics
Medical College of Wisconsin
Division of Endocrinology
Children's Hospital of Wisconsin
Milwaukee, Wisconsin
Hypofunction of the Ovaries
Pseudoprecocity Resulting from Lesions of the Ovary

Sheldon L. Kaplan, MD
Professor and Vice-Chair for Clinical Affairs
Department of Pediatrics
Baylor College of Medicine
Head, Department of Pediatric Medicine
Chief, Section of Infectious Disease
Texas Children's Hospital
Houston, Texas
Osteomyelitis
Septic Arthritis

Aaron M. Karlin, MD
Clinical Associate Professor
Department of Physical Medicine and
    Rehabilitation
Louisiana State University School of Medicine
Section Head, Pediatric Rehabilitation
Ochsner Clinic Medical Center
Ochsner Children's Health Center
New Orleans, Louisiana
Management of Musculoskeletal Injury
Specific Sports and Associated Injuries

Daniel L. Kastner, MD, PhD
Scientific Director
National Human Genome Research Institute
Distinguished Investigator
Medical Genetics Branch
National Institutes of Health
Bethesda, Maryland
Hereditary Periodic Fever Syndromes and Other
    Systemic Autoinflammatory Diseases

Emily R. Katz, MD
Clinical Assistant Professor
Department of Psychiatry and Human Behavior
Brown University Alpert Medical School
Director, Consultation Liaison Service
Hasbro Children's Hospital
Providence, Rhode Island
Rumination and Pica

James W. Kazura, MD
Professor of Medicine in International Health
Division of Geographic Medicine
Case Western Reserve University School of
    Medicine
Cleveland, Ohio
Ascariasis (Ascaris lumbricoides)
Trichuriasis (Trichuris trichiura)
Enterobiasis (Enterobius vermicularis)
Strongyloidiasis (Strongyloides stercoralis)
Lymphatic Filariasis (Brugia malayi, Brugia timori,
    and Wuchereria bancrofti)
Other Tissue Nematodes
Toxocariasis (Visceral and Ocular Larva Migrans)
Trichinosis (Trichinella spiralis)

Virginia A. Keane, MD
Associate Professor
Department of Pediatrics
University of Maryland School of Medicine
Baltimore, Maryland
Assessment of Growth

Gregory L. Kearns, PharmD, PhD
Marion Merrell Dow / Missouri Chair of Medical
    Research
Professor of Pediatrics and Pharmacology
University of Missouri—Kansas City School of
    Medicine
Chief Scientific Officer and Chairman, Research
    Development and Clinical Investigation
Associate Chair, Department of Pediatrics
Director, Pediatric Trial Network
Children's Mercy Hospitals and Clinics
Kansas City, Missouri;
Clinical Professor of Pediatrics
University of Kansas School of Medicine
Kansas City, Kansas
Principles of Drug Therapy

Sarah E. Keesecker, MD
Postdoctoral Residency Fellow
Department of Otolaryngology—Head and Neck
    Surgery
Columbia University College of Physicians and
    Surgeons
New York, New York
Congenital Disorders of the Nose
Acquired Disorders of the Nose
Nasal Polyps
General Considerations and Evaluation (Ear)
Hearing Loss
Congenital Malformations
External Otitis (Otitis Externa)
The Inner Ear and Diseases of the Bony Labyrinth
Traumatic Injuries of the Ear and Temporal Bone
Tumors of the Ear and Temporal Bone

Desmond P. Kelly, MD
Professor of Clinical Pediatrics
Vice-Chair for Academics, Department of
    Pediatrics
University of South Carolina School of Medicine
    Greenville
Greenville, South Carolina
Neurodevelopmental Function and Dysfunction in
    the School-Age Child

Kevin J. Kelly, MD
Professor of Pediatrics
Division of Pediatric Allergy, Immunology, and
    Rheumatology
University of North Carolina School of Medicine
Vice-Chair, Clinical Operations
Pediatrician-in-Chief
North Carolina Children's Hospital
Chapel Hill, North Carolina
Immune and Inflammatory Lung Disease

Matthew S. Kelly, MD, MPH
Pediatric Global Health Fellow
Children's Hospital of Philadelphia
Philadelphia, Pennsylvania;
Princess Marina Hospital
Gaborone, Botswana, Africa
Community-Acquired Pneumonia

Judith R. Kelsen, MD
Assistant Professor of Pediatrics
University of Pennsylvania Perelman School of
    Medicine
Attending Physician
Division of Gastroenterology, Hepatology, and
    Nutrition
The Children's Hospital of Philadelphia
Philadelphia, Pennsylvania
Foreign Bodies and Bezoars

Kathi J. Kemper, MD, MPH
Director, OSU Center for Integrative Health and
    Wellness
Professor of Pediatrics, Nursing, and Health and
    Rehabilitation Sciences
Ohio State University Wexner Medical Center
Nationwide Children's Hospital
Columbus, Ohio
Complementary Therapies and Integrative Medicine

Melissa Kennedy, MD
Attending Physician
Division of Gastroenterology, Hepatology, and
    Nutrition
The Children's Hospital of Philadelphia
Philadelphia, Pennsylvania
Malrotation
Meckel Diverticulum and Other Remnants of the
    Omphalomesenteric Duct
Intussusception
Malformations
Ascites

Eitan Kerem, MD
Professor and Chair
Department of Pediatrics
Hadassah University Medical Center
Jerusalem, Israel
Effects of War on Children

**Joseph E. Kerschner, MD, FACS,
FAAP**
Professor of Pediatrics
Dean and Executive Vice-President
Medical College of Wisconsin
Milwaukee, Wisconsin
Otitis Media

Seema Khan, MD
Associate Professor of Pediatrics
George Washington University School of Medicine
    and Health Sciences
Division of Gastroenterology and Nutrition
Children's National Medical Center
Washington, DC
Embryology, Anatomy, and Function of the
    Esophagus
Congenital Anomalies: Esophageal Atresia and
    Tracheoesophageal Fistula
Obstructing and Motility Disorders of the Esophagus
Dysmotility
Hiatal Hernia
Gastroesophageal Reflux Disease
Eosinophilic Esophagitis and Non–Gastroesophageal
    Reflux Disease Esophagitis
Esophageal Perforation
Esophageal Varices
Ingestions

Jennifer S. Kim, MD
Assistant Professor of Pediatrics
Jaffe Food Allergy Institute
Icahn School of Medicine at Mount Sinai
New York, New York
Diagnosis of Allergic Disease
Principles of Treatment of Allergic Disease

Charles H. King, MD
Professor of International Health
Center for Global Health and Diseases
Case Western Reserve University School of
    Medicine
Cleveland, Ohio
Schistosomiasis (Schistosoma)
Flukes (Liver, Lung, and Intestinal)

Stephen L. Kinsman, MD
Associate Professor of Pediatrics
Division of Pediatric Neurology
Medical University of South Carolina
Charleston, South Carolina
Congenital Anomalies of the Central Nervous System

Adam Kirton, MD, MSc, FRCPC
Associate Professor of Pediatrics and Clinical
    Neurosciences
University of Calgary Faculty of Medicine
Director, Calgary Pediatric Stroke Program
Alberta Children's Hospital Research Institute
Calgary, Alberta, Canada
Pediatric Stroke

Priya S. Kishnani, MD, MBBS
C.L. and Sue Chen Professor of Pediatrics
Chief, Division of Medical Genetics
Duke University Medical Center
Durham, North Carolina
Defects in Metabolism of Carbohydrates

Robert L. Kitts, MD
Assistant Professor of Psychiatry
Harvard Medical School
Director, Child and Adolescent Psychiatry
    Fellowship
Boston Children's Hospital
Boston, Massachusetts
Rumination and Pica

Martin B. Kleiman, MD
Ryan White Professor of Pediatrics
Indiana University School of Medicine
Riley Children's Hospital
Indianapolis, Indiana
Coccidioidomycosis (Coccidioides species)

Bruce L. Klein, MD
Visiting Associate Professor of Pediatrics
Johns Hopkins University School of Medicine
Associate Director, Pediatric Emergency Medicine
Director, Pediatric Transport
Johns Hopkins Children's Center
Baltimore, Maryland
*Interfacility Transport of the Seriously Ill or Injured
    Pediatric Patient*
Acute Care of the Victim of Multiple Trauma

Bruce S. Klein, MD
Professor of Pediatrics and Medical Microbiology
University of Wisconsin School of Medicine
Madison, Wisconsin
Blastomycosis (Blastomyces dermatitidis)

Michael D. Klein, MD, FACS, FAAP
Arvin I. Philippart MD Endowed Chair of
    Pediatric Surgical Research
Professor of Surgery
Wayne State University School of Medicine
Children's Hospital of Michigan
Detroit, Michigan
Surgical Conditions of the Anus and Rectum

Robert M. Kliegman, MD
Professor and Chairman Emeritus
Department of Pediatrics
Medical College of Wisconsin
Children's Hospital of Wisconsin
Milwaukee, Wisconsin
Refeeding Syndrome
Liver Abscess
*Generalized Arterial Calcification of Infancy/
    Idiopathic Infantile Arterial Calcification*
*Arterial Calcifications Caused by Deficiency of
    CD73*
Female Genital Mutilation/Cutting
Reflex Seizures (Stimulus Precipitated Seizures)
Nodding Syndrome

William C. Koch, MD, FAAP, FIDSA
Associate Professor of Pediatrics
Medical College of Virginia / Virginia
    Commonwealth University
Richmond, Virginia
Parvoviruses

Patrick M. Kochanek, MD, MCCM
Ake N. Grenvik Professor of Critical Care
    Medicine
Vice-Chairman, Department of Critical Care
    Medicine
Professor of Anesthesiology, Pediatrics,
    Bioengineering, and Clinical and Translational
    Science
Director, Safar Center for Resuscitation Research
University of Pittsburgh School of Medicine
Pittsburgh, Pennsylvania
Neurologic Emergencies and Stabilization

Eric Kodish, MD
Professor and Chairman
Department of Bioethics
The Cleveland Clinic Foundation
Cleveland, Ohio
Ethics in Pediatric Care

Stephan A. Kohlhoff, MD
Assistant Professor of Pediatrics and Medicine
Associate Director, Pediatric Infectious Diseases
SUNY Downstate Medical Center
Brooklyn, New York
Chlamydia (Chlamydophila) pneumoniae
Psittacosis (Chlamydia psittaci)

Mark A. Kostic, MD
Associate Professor of Pediatrics and Emergency
    Medicine
Division of Pediatric Emergency Medicine
Medical College of Wisconsin
Associate Medical Director
Wisconsin Poison Center
Milwaukee, Wisconsin
Poisoning

Linda E. Krach, MD
Adjunct Professor
Department of Physical Medicine and
    Rehabilitation
University of Minnesota School of Medicine
President, Courage Kenny Rehabilitation Institute
    (part of Allina Health)
Minneapolis, Minnesota
Severe Traumatic Brain Injury

Elliot J. Krane, MD, FAAP
Professor of Pediatrics, and Anesthesiology,
    Perioperative, and Pain Medicine
Stanford University School of Medicine
Chief, Pediatric Pain Management
Stanford Children's Health
Lucile Packard Children's Hospital at Stanford
Stanford, California
Pediatric Pain Management

Peter J. Krause, MD
Senior Research Scientist
Department of Epidemiology and Microbial
    Diseases
Yale School of Public Health
Department of Medicine and Department of
    Pediatrics
Yale School of Medicine
New Haven, Connecticut
Babesiosis (Babesia)

**Richard E. Kreipe, MD, FACCP,
FSAHM, FAED**
Dr. Elizabeth R. McArnarney Professor in
    Pediatrics funded by Roger and Carolyn
    Friedlander
Division of Adolescent Medicine
University of Rochester School of Medicine
Golisano Children's Hospital
Medical Director, Western New York
    Comprehensive Care Center for Eating
    Disorders
Rochester, New York
Eating Disorders

Steven E. Krug, MD
Professor of Pediatrics
Division of Pediatric Emergency Medicine
Northwestern University Feinberg School of
    Medicine
Ann & Robert H. Lurie Children's Hospital of
    Chicago
Chicago, Illinois
Emergency Medical Services for Children

John F. Kuttesch Jr., MD, PhD
Chief, Division of Pediatric Hematology/Oncology
Department of Pediatrics
University of New Mexico School of Medicine
Albuquerque, New Mexico
Brain Tumors in Childhood

Jennifer M. Kwon, MD, MPH
Associate Profess or of Pediatrics and Neurology
University of Rochester School of Medicine
Associate Director, Clinic for Inherited Metabolic
    Diseases
Golisano Children's Hospital
Rochester, New York
Neurodegenerative Disorders of Childhood

Catherine S. Lachenauer, MD
Assistant Professor of Pediatrics
Harvard Medical School
Division of Infectious Diseases
Boston Children's Hospital
Boston, Massachusetts
Group B Streptococcus

Stephan Ladisch, MD
Professor of Pediatrics and Biochemistry/Molecular
Biology
Department of Pediatrics
George Washington University School of Medicine
Children's Research Institute
Department of Hematology and Oncology
Children's National Medical Center
Washington, DC
Histiocytosis Syndromes of Childhood

Stephen H. LaFranchi, MD
Professor of Pediatrics
Division of Pediatric Endocrinology
Oregon Health & Science University
Portland, Oregon
Thyroid Development and Physiology
Defects of Thyroxine-Binding Globulin
Hypothyroidism
Thyroiditis
Goiter
Hyperthyroidism
Carcinoma of the Thyroid

Oren J. Lakser, MD
Assistant Professor of Pediatrics
Northwestern University Feinberg School of
Medicine
Associate Clinician Specialist
Division of Pulmonary Medicine
Ann & Robert H. Lurie Children's Hospital of
Chicago
Chicago, Illinois
Bronchiectasis
Pulmonary Abscess

Marc B. Lande, MD, MPH
Professor of Pediatrics
Division of Pediatric Nephrology
University of Rochester Medical Center
School of Medicine and Dentistry
Rochester, New York
Systemic Hypertension

Philip J. Landrigan, MD, MSc, FAAP
Dean for Global Health
Ethel H. Wise Professor and Chair, Department of
Preventive Medicine
Director, Children's Environmental Health Center
Icahn School of Medicine at Mount Sinai
New York, New York
Chemical Pollutants

Gregory L. Landry, MD
Professor
Department of Pediatrics
University of Wisconsin—Madison
School of Medicine and Public Health
Madison, Wisconsin
Epidemiology and Prevention of Injuries
Heat Injuries
*Female Athletes: Menstrual Problems and the Risk
of Osteopenia*
Performance-Enhancing Aids

Wendy G. Lane, MD, MPH, FAAP
Assistant Professor
Departments of Pediatrics and Epidemiology and
Preventive Medicine
University of Maryland School of Medicine
Baltimore, Maryland
Abused and Neglected Children

Phillip S. LaRussa, MD
Professor of Pediatrics
Columbia University Medical Center
New York, New York
Varicella-Zoster Virus Infections

J. Todd R. Lawrence, MD, PhD
Assistant Professor
Department of Orthopaedic Surgery
University of Pennsylvania Perelman School of
Medicine
Attending Orthopaedic Surgeon
Children's Hospital of Philadelphia
Philadelphia, Pennsylvania
The Knee

Brendan Lee, MD, PhD
Robert and Janice McNair Endowed Chair in
Molecular and Human Genetics
Professor, Department of Molecular and Human
Genetics
Baylor College of Medicine
Houston, Texas
Integration of Genetics into Pediatric Practice
The Genetic Approach in Pediatric Medicine
The Human Genome
Patterns of Genetic Transmission
Cytogenetics
Genetics of Common Disorders

K. Jane Lee, MD, MA
Associate Professor
Department of Pediatrics
Medical College of Wisconsin
Division of Pediatric Critical Care
Children's Hospital of Wisconsin
Milwaukee, Wisconsin
Brain Death

J. Steven Leeder, PharmD, PhD
Marion Merrell Dow / Missouri Endowed Chair in
Pediatric Pharmacology
Chief, Division of Pediatric Pharmacology and
Medical Toxicology
Children's Mercy Hospitals and Clinics
Kansas City, Missouri;
Adjunct Professor
Department of Pharmacology, Toxicology, and
Therapeutics
Kansas University School of Medicine
Kansas City, Kansas
*Pediatric Pharmacogenetics, Pharmacogenomics,
and Pharmacoproteomics*

Rebecca K. Lehman, MD
Assistant Professor of Pediatrics
Division of Pediatric Neurology
Medical University of South Carolina
Charleston, South Carolina
Neurologic Evaluation
Chorea, Athetosis, Tremor

Michael J. Lentze, MD
Professor of Pediatrics
Division of Pediatric Gastroenterology
Medizinische Universität Bonn
Bonn, Germany
*Evaluation of Children with Suspected Intestinal
Malabsorption*
Enzyme Deficiencies

Norma B. Lerner, MD, MPH
Special Advisor to the Director
Division of Blood Diseases and Resources
National Heart, Lung, and Blood Institute
National Institutes of Health
Bethesda, Maryland
The Anemias
*Congenital Hypoplastic Anemia (Diamond-Blackfan
Anemia)*
Pearson Syndrome
Acquired Pure Red Blood Cell Anemia
Anemia of Chronic Disease and Renal Disease
Congenital Dyserythropoietic Anemias
Physiologic Anemia of Infancy
Megaloblastic Anemias

Steven O. Lestrud, MD
Assistant Professor of Pediatrics
Northwestern University Feinberg School of
Medicine
Medical Director, Respiratory Care
Ann & Robert H. Lurie Children's Hospital of
Chicago
Chicago, Illinois
Bronchopulmonary Dysplasia

Donald Y.M. Leung, MD, PhD
Edelstein Family Chair of Pediatric
Allergy-Immunology
National Jewish Health
Professor of Pediatrics
University of Colorado School of Medicine
Denver, Colorado
Atopic Dermatitis (Atopic Eczema)

Chris A. Liacouras, MD
Professor of Pediatrics
University of Pennsylvania Perelman School of
Medicine
Co-Director, Center for Pediatric Eosinophilic
Disorders
The Children's Hospital of Philadelphia
Philadelphia, Pennsylvania
Normal Digestive Tract Phenomena
*Major Symptoms and Signs of Digestive Tract
Disorders*
*Normal Development, Structure, and Function
(Stomach)*
*Pyloric Stenosis and Other Congenital Anomalies of
the Stomach*
Intestinal Atresia, Stenosis, and Malrotation
*Intestinal Duplications, Meckel Diverticulum, and
Other Remnants of the Omphalomesenteric Duct*
Motility Disorders and Hirschsprung Disease
*Ileus, Adhesions, Intussusception, and Closed-Loop
Obstructions*
Foreign Bodies and Bezoars
*Functional Abdominal Pain (Nonorganic Chronic
Abdominal Pain)*
Malformations
Ascites
Peritonitis

Christopher W. Liebig, MD
Pediatric Sports Medicine Fellow
Akron Children's Hospital
Akron, Ohio
Sports-Related Traumatic Brain Injury (Concussion)

Timothy P. Lindquist, MD
Pediatric Ophthalmologist
Children's Mercy Hospital
Kansas City, Missouri
Growth and Development (Eye)
Examination of the Eye
Abnormalities of Refraction and Accommodation
Disorders of Vision
Abnormalities of Pupil and Iris
Disorders of Eye Movement and Alignment
Abnormalities of the Lids
Disorders of the Lacrimal System
Disorders of the Conjunctiva
Abnormalities of the Cornea
Abnormalities of the Lens
Disorders of the Uveal Tract
Disorders of the Retina and Vitreous
Abnormalities of the Optic Nerve
Childhood Glaucoma
Orbital Abnormalities
Orbital Infections
Injuries to the Eye

Andrew H. Liu, MD
Professor
Department of Pediatrics
National Jewish Health
University of Colorado School of Medicine
Denver, Colorado
Childhood Asthma

Stanley F. Lo, PhD
Associate Professor of Pathology
Medical College of Wisconsin
Co-Director, Clinical Laboratories
Co-Director, Biochemical Genetics Laboratory
Technical Director, Chemistry and Point of Care
   Testing Laboratories
Children's Hospital of Wisconsin
Milwaukee, Wisconsin
Laboratory Testing in Infants and Children
*Reference Intervals for Laboratory Tests and
   Procedures*

Franco Locatelli, MD
Professor of Pediatrics
University of Pavia
Pavia, Italy;
Director, Department of Pediatric Hematology and
   Oncology
IRCCS Ospedale Pediatrico Bambino Gesù
Rome, Italy
*Principles and Clinical Indications of Hematopoietic
   Stem Cell Transplantation*
*Hematopoietic Stem Cell Transplantation from
   Alternative Sources and Donors*
*Graft-Versus-Host Disease, Rejection, and
   Venoocclusive Disease*
*Infectious Complications of Hematopoietic Stem Cell
   Transplantation*
*Late Effects of Hematopoietic Stem Cell
   Transplantation*

John H. Lockhart, MD
Clinical Assistant Professor
Departments of Orthopedics and Sports Medicine
Seattle Children's Hospital
Seattle, Washington
Cervical Spinal Injuries

Sarah S. Long, MD
Professor of Pediatrics
Drexel University College of Medicine
Chief, Section of Infectious Diseases
St. Christopher's Hospital for Children
Philadelphia, Pennsylvania
Pertussis (Bordetella pertussis *and* Bordetella
   parapertussis)

Anna Lena Lopez, MD, MPH
Research Associate Professor
Institute of Child Health and Human Development
University of the Philippines Manila—National
   Institutes of Health
Clinical Associate Professor, Department of
   Pediatrics
University of the Philippines College of Medicine
Manila, Philippines
Cholera

Steven V. Lossef, MD
Head, Pediatric Interventional Radiology
Division of Diagnostic Imaging and Radiology
Children's National Medical Center
Washington, DC
Pertussis (Bordetella pertussis *and* Bordetella
   parapertussis)
Pleurisy, Pleural Effusions, and Empyema
Pneumothorax
Hemothorax
Chylothorax

Jennifer A. Lowry, MD
Associate Professor of Pediatrics
University of Missouri—Kansas City School of
   Medicine
Section Chief, Medical Toxicology
Division of Clinical Pharmacology and Therapeutic
   Innovations
Medical Director, Center for Environmental Health
Children's Mercy Hospitals and Clinics
Kansas City, Missouri
Principles of Drug Therapy

Nora T. MacZura, MD
Division of Gynecologic Oncology
Department of Obstetrics and Gynecology
Springfield Clinic
Springfield, Illinois
*Neoplasms and Adolescent Screening for Human
   Papillomavirus*

Prashant V. Mahajan, MD, MPH, MBA
Professor of Pediatrics and Emergency Medicine
Carman and Ann Adams Department of Pediatrics
Wayne State University School of Medicine
Division Chief and Research Director
Director, Center for Quality and Innovation
Pediatric Emergency Medicine
Children's Hospital of Michigan
Detroit, Michigan
Heavy Metal Intoxication

Akhil Maheshwari, MD
Associate Professor of Pediatrics and
   Pharmacology
University of Illinois, Chicago
Chief, Division of Neonatology
Director, Center for Neonatal and Pediatric
   Gastrointestinal Disease
Medical Director, Neonatal Intensive Care Unit
   and Intermediate Care Nursery
Children's Hospital of University of Illinois
Chicago, Illinois
Diaphragmatic Hernia
Foramen of Morgagni Hernia
Paraesophageal Hernia
Eventration
Digestive System Disorders
Blood Disorders

Joseph A. Majzoub, MD
Thomas Morgan Rotch Professor of Pediatrics
Professor of Medicine
Harvard Medical School
Chief, Division of Endocrinology
Boston Children's Hospital
Boston, Massachusetts
Diabetes Insipidus
*Other Abnormalities of Arginine Vasopressin
   Metabolism and Action*

Asim Maqbool, MD
Assistant Professor of Pediatrics
University of Pennsylvania Perelman School of
   Medicine
Division of Gastroenterology, Hepatology, and
   Nutrition
Children's Hospital of Philadelphia
Philadelphia, Pennsylvania
Nutritional Requirements

Ashley M. Maranich, MD
Pediatric Infectious Disease
Director, Transitional Year Program
San Antonio Military Medical Center
Fort Sam Houston, Texas
Malassezia

Mona Marin, MD
Medical Epidemiologist
Epidemiology Branch, Division of Viral Diseases
National Center for Immunization and Respiratory
   Diseases
Centers for Disease Control and Prevention
Atlanta, Georgia
Varicella-Zoster Virus Infections

Joan C. Marini, MD, PhD
Chief, Bone and Extracellular Matrix Branch
National Institute for Child Health and
   Development
National Institutes of Health
Bethesda, Maryland
Osteogenesis Imperfecta

Thomas C. Markello, MD, PhD
National Human Genome Research Institute
National Institutes of Health
Bethesda, Maryland
*Genetic Approaches to Rare and Undiagnosed
   Diseases*

Morri Markowitz, MD
Professor of Pediatrics and Medicine
Albert Einstein College of Medicine
Clinical Director, Pediatric Environmental Sciences
The Children's Hospital at Montefiore
Bronx, New York
Lead Poisoning

Kevin P. Marks, MD
Clinical Assistant Professor
Department of Pediatrics
Oregon Health & Science University School of
   Medicine
General Pediatrician
PeaceHealth Medical Group
Portland, Oregon
*Developmental-Behavioral Screening and
   Surveillance*

Stacene R. Maroushek, MD, PhD, MPH
Assistant Professor of Pediatrics
Division of Pediatric Infectious Diseases and
    Immunology
University of Minnesota Medical School
Pediatric Infectious Diseases and General
    Pediatrics
Hennepin County Medical Center
Minneapolis, Minnesota
*Medical Evaluation of Immigrant (Foreign-Born)
    Children for Infectious Diseases*
Principles of Antimycobacterial Therapy

Kari L. Martin, MD
Assistant Professor of Dermatology and Child
    Health
Associate Residency Program Director Department
    of Dermatology
University of Missouri School of Medicine
Columbia, Missouri
Diseases of the Neonate
Cutaneous Defects
Ectodermal Dysplasias
Vascular Disorders
Cutaneous Nevi
Disorders of Keratinization
Disorders of the Sweat Glands
Disorders of Hair
Disorders of the Nails
Tumors of the Skin

Wilbert H. Mason Jr., MD, MPH
Professor Emeritus of Clinical Pediatrics
University of Southern California Keck School of
    Medicine
Chief, Pediatric Infectious Diseases
Children's Hospital of Los Angeles
Los Angeles, California
Measles
Rubella
Mumps

Christopher Mastropietro, MD
Assistant Professor
Department of Pediatrics
Wayne State University School of Medicine
Associate Fellowship Director
Division of Critical Care
Children's Hospital of Michigan
Detroit, Michigan
Mechanical Ventilation

Kimberlee M. Matalon, PhD
Associate Professor
Department of Health and Human Performance
University of Houston
Houston, Texas
Aspartic Acid (Canavan Disease)

Reuben K. Matalon, MD, PhD
Professor
Department of Pediatrics and Genetics
University of Texas Medical Branch
University of Texas Children's Hospital
Galveston, Texas
Aspartic Acid (Canavan Disease)

Roshni Mathew, MD
Clinical Instructor in Pediatrics
Division of Pediatric Infectious Diseases
Stanford University School of Medicine
Stanford, California
Central Nervous System Infections
Brain Abscess

Dennis J. Matthews, MD
Professor and Chair
Department of Physical Medicine and
    Rehabilitation
University of Colorado School of Medicine
Medical Director
Children's Hospital Rehabilitation Center
PPAARDI-in-Chief
Children's Hospital Colorado
Denver, Colorado
Principles of Rehabilitation Medicine

Robert L. Mazor, MD
Clinical Associate Professor
Department of Pediatrics
University of Washington School of Medicine
Division of Critical Care and Cardiac Surgery
Clinical Director, CICU
Seattle Children's Hospital and Regional Medical
    Center
Seattle, Washington
Pulmonary Edema

Megan E. McCabe, MD
Assistant Professor
Department of Pediatrics
Yale School of Medicine
New Haven, Connecticut
Loss, Separation, and Bereavement

Susanna A. McColley, MD
Professor of Pediatrics
Northwestern University Feinberg School of
    Medicine
Director, Clinical and Translational Research
Stanley Manne Children's Research Institute
Ann & Robert H. Lurie Children's Hospital of
    Chicago
Chicago, Illinois
Pulmonary Tumors
*Extrapulmonary Diseases with Pulmonary
    Manifestations*

Margaret M. McGovern, MD, PhD
Professor and Chair
Department of Pediatrics
Stony Brook University School of Medicine
Physician-in-Chief, Stony Brook Long Island
    Children's Hospital
Stony Brook, New York
Lipidoses (Lysosomal Storage Disorders)
Mucolipidoses
*Disorders of Glycoprotein Degradation and
    Structure*

Heather S. McLean, MD
Associate Professor of Pediatrics
Duke University School of Medicine
Medical Director
Pediatric Hospital Medicine
Duke Children's Hospital
Durham, North Carolina
Failure to Thrive

Rima McLeod, MD
Jules and Doris Stein Research to Prevent
    Blindness Professor of Ophthalmology
Departments of Ophthalmology and Visual
    Sciences and Pediatrics
Medical Director, Toxoplasmosis Center
University of Chicago School of Medicine
Chicago, Illinois
Toxoplasmosis (Toxoplasma gondii)

Mary A. McMahon, MD
Assistant Professor
Department of Pediatrics
University of Cincinnati College of Medicine
Director, Division of Physical Medicine and
    Rehabilitation
Director, Physical Medicine and Rehabilitation
    Residency Program
Cincinnati Children's Hospital Medical Center
Cincinnati, Ohio
*Spinal Cord Injury and Spinal Cord Autonomic
    Crisis Management*

Asuncion Mejias, MD, PhD, MSCS
Assistant Professor of Pediatrics
Section of Infectious Diseases and Immunology
The Ohio State University College of Medicine
The Research Institute at Nationwide Children's
    Hospital
Columbus, Ohio
Hansen Disease (Mycobacterium leprae)
Mycoplasma pneumoniae
*Genital Mycoplasmas (Mycoplasma hominis,
    Mycoplasma genitalium, and Ureaplasma
    urealyticum)*

Peter C. Melby, MD
Professor of Internal Medicine (Infectious
    Diseases), Microbiology and Immunology, and
    Pathology
Director, Center for Tropical Diseases
University of Texas Medical Branch at Galveston
Galveston, Texas
Leishmaniasis (Leishmania)

Alexandra N. Menchise, MD
Pediatric Gastroenterology Fellow
Cincinnati Children's Hospital Medical Center
Cincinnati, Ohio
Metabolic Diseases of the Liver

Diane F. Merritt, MD
Professor
Department of Obstetrics and Gynecology
Director, Pediatric and Adolescent Gynecology
Washington University School of Medicine in St.
    Louis
St. Louis, Missouri
History and Physical Examination (Gynecology)
Vulvovaginitis
Bleeding
Breast Concerns
*Neoplasms and Adolescent Screening for Human
    Papillomavirus*

Ethan A. Mezoff, MD
Pediatric Gastroenterology Fellow
Cincinnati Children's Hospital Medical Center
Cincinnati, Ohio
Clostridium difficile Infection

Marian G. Michaels, MD, MPH
Professor of Pediatrics and Surgery
University of Pittsburgh School of Medicine
Division of Pediatric Infectious Diseases
Children's Hospital of Pittsburgh of UPMC
Pittsburgh, Pennsylvania
Infections in Immunocompromised Persons

Mohamad A. Mikati, MD
Wilburt C. Davison Professor of Pediatrics and
    Professor of Neurobiology
Chief, Division of Pediatric Neurology
Duke University Medical Center
Durham, North Carolina
Seizures in Childhood
Conditions That Mimic Seizures

Henry Milgrom, MD
Professor of Pediatrics
National Jewish Health
University of Colorado School of Medicine
Denver, Colorado
Allergic Rhinitis

E. Kathryn Miller, MD, MPH
Assistant Professor
Departments of Pediatrics and Allergy and
    Immunology
Vanderbilt University School of Medicine
Nashville, Tennessee
The Common Cold
Rhinoviruses

Jonathan W. Mink, MD, PhD
Frederick A. Horner MD Endowed Professor in
    Pediatric Neurology
Professor of Neurology, Neurobiology and
    Anatomy, Brain and Cognitive Sciences, and
    Pediatrics
Chief, Division of Child Neurology
Vice-Chair, Department of Neurology
University of Rochester Medical Center
Rochester, New York
Movement Disorders

R. Justin Mistovich, MD
Clinical Fellow
Division of Pediatric Orthopaedic Surgery
University of Pennsylvania Perelman School of
    Medicine
Children's Hospital of Philadelphia
Philadelphia, Pennsylvania
The Spine

Grant A. Mitchell, MD
Professor of Pediatrics
Division of Medical Genetics
University of Montreal Faculty of Medicine
Service de Genetique Medicale
Hospital Ste-Justine
Montreal, Quebec, Canada
Tyrosine

Esi Morgan-DeWitt, MD, MSCE
Associate Professor of Pediatrics
University of Cincinnati College of Medicine
Division of Rheumatology
James M. Anderson Center for Health Systems
    Excellence
Cincinnati Children's Hospital Medical Center
Cincinnati, Ohio
Treatment of Rheumatic Diseases
Sarcoidosis

Anna-Barbara Moscicki, MD
Professor of Pediatrics
University of California, San Francisco
Senior Director, Pediatric Glaser Clinic
San Francisco, California
Human Papillomaviruses

Lovern R. Moseley, PhD
Department of Psychiatry
Boston Medical Center
Boston, Massachusetts
Mood Disorders
Disruptive, Impulse-Control, and Conduct Disorders

Beth Moughan, MD
Professor of Clinical Pediatrics
Assistant Dean, Affiliate Faculty Development
Associate Chair, Clinical Affairs
Section Chief, Ambulatory Pediatrics
Temple University School of Medicine
Philadelphia, Pennsylvania
Sporotrichosis (Sporothrix schenckii)

James R. Murphy, PhD
Professor of Pediatrics
Director, Pediatric Infectious Disease Research
University of Texas Health Science Center
Houston, Texas
Campylobacter
Yersinia

Kevin P. Murphy, MD
Medical Director Pediatric Rehabilitation
Sanford Health Systems
Bismarck, North Dakota;
Medical Director, Gillette Children's Specialty
    Healthcare
Duluth Clinic
Duluth, Minnesota
Management of Musculoskeletal Injury
Specific Sports and Associated Injuries

Timothy F. Murphy, MD
Distinguished Professor
Director, UB Clinical and Translational Research
    Center
University at Buffalo, State University of New York
School of Medicine and Biomedical Sciences
Buffalo, New York
Moraxella catarrhalis

Thomas S. Murray, MD, PhD
Associate Professor of Medical Sciences
Quinnipiac University Frank H Netter MD School
    of Medicine
Hamden, Connecticut
Listeria monocytogenes
Pseudomonas, Burkholderia, and
    Stenotrophomonas

René P. Myers, MD
Chief Resident
Department of Plastic Surgery
University of Rochester Medical Center
Rochester, New York
Deformational Plagiocephaly

Mindo J. Natale, PsyD
Assistant Professor of Psychology
University of South Carolina School of Medicine
Senior Staff Psychologist
GHS Children's Hospital
Greenville, South Carolina
Neurodevelopmental Function and Dysfunction in
    the School-Age Child

William A. Neal, MD
Professor of Pediatrics
Division of Pediatric Cardiology
West Virginia University School of Medicine
Morgantown, West Virginia
Disorders of Lipoprotein Metabolism and Transport

Maureen R. Nelson, MD
Pediatric Subspecialty Services
Dell's Children's Medical Center of Central Texas
Austin, Texas
Birth Brachial Plexus Palsy

Jayne M. Ness, MD, PhD
Associate Professor of Pediatrics
Division of Pediatric Neurology
University of Alabama, Birmingham
Birmingham, Alabama
Demyelinating Disorders of the Central Nervous
    System

Kathleen A. Neville, MD, MS
Associate Professor of Pediatrics
University of Missouri—Kansas City School of
    Medicine
Director, Experimental Therapeutics in Pediatric
    Cancer
Department of Pediatric Hematology/Oncology
Children's Mercy Hospitals and Clinics
Kansas City, Missouri
Pediatric Pharmacogenetics, Pharmacogenomics,
    and Pharmacoproteomics

Mary A. Nevin, MD
Associate Professor of Pediatrics
Northwestern University Feinberg School of
    Medicine
Department of Pulmonary and Critical Care
    Medicine
Ann & Robert H. Lurie Children's Hospital of
    Chicago
Chicago, Illinois
Pulmonary Hemosiderosis
Pulmonary Embolism, Infarction, and Hemorrhage

Jane W. Newburger, MD
Commonwealth Professor of Pediatrics
Harvard Medical School
Associate Cardiologist-in-Chief, Research and
    Education
Director, Cardiac Neurodevelopmental Program
Director, Kawasaki Program
Children's Hospital Boston
Boston, Massachusetts
Kawasaki Disease

Peter E. Newburger, MD
Ali and John Pierce Professor of Pediatric
    Hematology/Oncology
Vice-Chair for Research
Department of Pediatrics
University of Massachusetts Medical School
Worcester, Massachusetts
Leukopenia
Leukocytosis

Linda S. Nield, MD
Professor of Pediatrics
Director, Pediatrics Residency Program
West Virginia University School of Medicine
Morgantown, West Virginia
Fever
Fever Without a Focus

Susan Niermeyer, MD, MPH, FAAP
Professor of Pediatrics
Section of Neonatology
University of Colorado School of Medicine
Aurora, Colorado
Altitude-Associated Illness in Children (Acute
    Mountain Sickness)

Zehava L. Noah, MD
Associate Professor of Pediatrics
Northwestern University Feinberg School of
Medicine
Division of Pediatric Critical Care Medicine
Ann & Robert H. Lurie Children's Hospital of
Chicago
Chicago, Illinois
Chronic Severe Respiratory Insufficiency

Lawrence M. Nogee, MD
Professor of Pediatrics
Department of Pediatrics
Division of Neonatology and Perinatology
Johns Hopkins University School of Medicine
Baltimore, Maryland
Diffuse Lung Diseases in Childhood

Robert L. Norris, MD, FACEP, FAAEM
Professor of Surgery
Chief, Division of Emergency Medicine
Stanford University Medical Center
Stanford, California
Envenomations

Anna Nowak-Węgrzyn, MD
Associate Professor of Pediatrics
Jaffe Food Allergy Institute
Icahn School of Medicine at Mount Sinai
New York, New York
Serum Sickness
Food Allergy and Adverse Reactions to Foods

Stephen K. Obaro, MD, PhD, FRCPCH
Professor of Pediatrics
Division of Infectious Diseases
University of Nebraska Medical Center
Omaha, Nebraska
Nonvenereal Treponemal Infections
Relapsing Fever (Borrelia)

Makram M. Obeid, MD
Clinical Fellow in Neurology
Boston Children's Hospital
Boston, Massachusetts
Conditions That Mimic Seizures

Hope L. O'Brien, MD
Assistant Professor of Pediatrics and Neurology
University of Cincinnati College of Medicine
Director, Young Adult Headache Program
Division of Neurology
Cincinnati Children's Hospital Medical Center
Cincinnati, Ohio
Headaches

Theresa J. Ochoa, MD
Associate Professor of Epidemiology and Pediatrics
The University of Texas Health Science Center at
Houston
Houston, Texas;
Universidad Peruana Cayetano Heredia
Lima, Peru
Shigella
Escherichia coli

Robin K. Ohls, MD
Professor of Pediatrics
University of New Mexico School of Medicine
Albuquerque, New Mexico
Development of the Hematopoietic System

Jean-Marie Okwo-Bele, MD, MPH
Director
Immunization, Vaccines, and Biologicals
Department
World Health Organization
Geneva, Switzerland
International Immunization Practices

Keith T. Oldham, MD
Professor and Chief
Division of Pediatric Surgery
Medical College of Wisconsin
Children's Hospital of Wisconsin
Milwaukee, Wisconsin
Acute Appendicitis
Inguinal Hernias
Epigastric Hernia

Joyce L. Oleszek, MD
Associate Professor
Department of Physical Medicine and
Rehabilitation
University of Colorado School of Medicine
Attending Physician
Children's Hospital Colorado
Denver, Colorado
Spasticity

Scott E. Olitsky, MD
Professor of Ophthalmology
University of Kansas School of Medicine
University of Missouri—Kansas City School of
Medicine
Section Chief, Ophthalmology
Children's Mercy Hospitals and Clinics
Kansas City, Missouri
Growth and Development (Eye)
Examination of the Eye
Abnormalities of Refraction and Accommodation
Disorders of Vision
Abnormalities of Pupil and Iris
Disorders of Eye Movement and Alignment
Abnormalities of the Lids
Disorders of the Lacrimal System
Disorders of the Conjunctiva
Abnormalities of the Cornea
Abnormalities of the Lens
Disorders of the Uveal Tract
Disorders of the Retina and Vitreous
Abnormalities of the Optic Nerve
Childhood Glaucoma
Orbital Abnormalities
Orbital Infections
Injuries to the Eye

John M. Olsson, MD, CPE
Professor of Pediatrics
Division Chief, General Pediatrics
Brody School of Medicine
East Carolina University
Greenville, North Carolina
The Newborn

Amanda K. Ombrello, MD
Staff Clinician
National Human Genome Research Institute
National Institutes of Health
Bethesda, Maryland
*Hereditary Periodic Fever Syndromes and Other
Systemic Autoinflammatory Diseases*
Amyloidosis

Susan R. Orenstein, MD
Professor Emerita
University of Pittsburgh School of Medicine
Division of Pediatric Gastroenterology
Children's Hospital of Pittsburgh of UPMC
Pittsburgh, Pennsylvania
*Embryology, Anatomy, and Function of the
Esophagus*
*Congenital Anomalies: Esophageal Atresia and
Tracheoesophageal Fistula*
Obstructing and Motility Disorders of the Esophagus
Dysmotility
Hiatal Hernia
Gastroesophageal Reflux Disease
*Eosinophilic Esophagitis and Non–Gastroesophageal
Reflux Disease Esophagitis*
Esophageal Perforation
Esophageal Varices
Ingestions

Walter A. Orenstein, MD, DSc (Hon)
Professor of Medicine and Pediatrics
Associate Director, Emory Vaccine Center
Emory University
Atlanta, Georgia
Immunization Practices

Marisa Osorio, DO
Acting Assistant Professor
Department of Rehabilitation Medicine
University of Washington School of Medicine
Seattle Children's Hospital
Seattle, Washington
Ambulation Assistance

Patrick O'Toole, MD
Clinical Fellow
Division of Pediatric Orthopaedic Surgery
University of Pennsylvania Perelman School of
Medicine
Children's Hospital of Philadelphia
Philadelphia, Pennsylvania
The Neck

Judith A. Owens, MD, MPH
Associate Professor
Harvard Medical School
Director of Sleep Medicine
Boston Children's Hospital
Boston, Massachusetts
Sleep Medicine

Seza Özen, MD
Professor of Paediatrics
Division of Paediatric Rheumatology
Hacettepe University
Ankara, Turkey
Behçet Disease

Charles H. Packman, MD
Professor of Medicine
University of North Carolina School of Medicine
Levine Cancer Institute, Hematologic Oncology
and Blood Disorders
Charlotte, North Carolina
*Hemolytic Anemias Resulting from Extracellular
Factors—Immune Hemolytic Anemias*

Priya Pais, MBBS, MS
Assistant Professor of Pediatrics
Division of Nephrology
Medical College of Wisconsin
Wauwatosa, Wisconsin
Lower Urinary Tract Causes of Hematuria
Introduction to the Child with Proteinuria
Fixed Proteinuria
Nephrotic Syndrome
Cortical Necrosis

Tonya M. Palermo, PhD
Professor
Department of Anesthesiology
University of Washington School of Medicine
Seattle Children's Hospital Research Institute
Seattle, Washington
Pediatric Pain Management

Cynthia G. Pan, MD
Professor of Pediatrics
Section Head, Pediatric Nephrology
Medical College of Wisconsin
Medical Director, Pediatric Dialysis and Transplant
 Services
Children's Hospital of Wisconsin
Milwaukee, Wisconsin
Introduction to Glomerular Diseases
Clinical Evaluation of the Child with Hematuria
*Isolated Glomerular Diseases with Recurrent Gross
 Hematuria*
Glomerulonephritis Associated with Infections
*Glomerulonephritis Associated with Systemic Lupus
 Erythematosus*

Diane E. Pappas, MD, JD
Professor
Department of Pediatrics
University of Virginia School of Medicine
Charlottesville, Virginia
Sinusitis
*Retropharyngeal Abscess, Lateral Pharyngeal
 (Parapharyngeal) Abscess, and Peritonsillar
 Cellulitis/Abscess*

Elizabeth P. Parks, MD, MSCE
Assistant Professor of Pediatrics
Division of Gastroenterology, Hepatology, and
 Nutrition
University of Pennsylvania Perelman School of
 Medicine
Children's Hospital of Philadelphia
Philadelphia, Pennsylvania
Nutritional Requirements
Feeding Healthy Infants, Children, and Adolescents

John S. Parks, MD, PhD
Professor of Pediatrics
Division of Pediatric Endocrinology
Emory University School of Medicine
Atlanta, Georgia
Hormones of the Hypothalamus and Pituitary
Hypopituitarism

Maria Jevitz Patterson, MD, PhD
Professor Emeritus of Microbiology and Molecular
 Genetics
Michigan State University College of Human
 Medicine
East Lansing, Michigan
Syphilis (Treponema pallidum)

Timothy R. Peters, MD
Associate Professor of Pediatrics
Section of Pediatric Infectious Diseases
Wake Forest University School of Medicine
Winston-Salem, North Carolina
Streptococcus pneumoniae (Pneumococcus)

Larry K. Pickering, MD
Senior Advisor to the Director
National Center for Immunization and Respiratory
 Diseases
Executive Secretary
Advisory Committee for Immunization Practices
Centers for Disease Control and Prevention
Adjunct Professor of Pediatrics
Emory University School of Medicine
Atlanta, Georgia
Immunization Practices

Misha L. Pless, MD
Associate Professor of Neurology
Harvard Medical School
Chief, Division of Neuro-ophthalmology
Chief, Division of General Neurology
Director, Neurology Urgent Access Center
Massachusetts General Hospital
Boston, Massachusetts
*Idiopathic Intracranial Hypertension/Pseudotumor
 Cerebri*

Laura S. Plummer, MD
Assistant Professor
Department of Ophthalmology
University of Missouri—Kansas City School of
 Medicine
Children's Mercy Hospital
Kansas City, Missouri
Growth and Development (Eye)
Examination of the Eye
Abnormalities of Refraction and Accommodation
Disorders of Vision
Abnormalities of Pupil and Iris
Disorders of Eye Movement and Alignment
Abnormalities of the Lids
Disorders of the Lacrimal System
Disorders of the Conjunctiva
Abnormalities of the Cornea
Abnormalities of the Lens
Disorders of the Uveal Tract
Disorders of the Retina and Vitreous
Abnormalities of the Optic Nerve
Childhood Glaucoma
Orbital Abnormalities
Orbital Infections
Injuries to the Eye

**Andrew J. Pollard, MBBS, BSc,
FRCP(UK), FRCPCH, PhD**
Professor of Paediatric Infection and Immunity
Department of Paediatrics
Director of the Oxford Vaccine Group
University of Oxford
Honorary Consultant Paediatrician
Children's Hospital
Oxford, United Kingdom
Neisseria meningitidis (Meningococcus)

Craig C. Porter, MD
Professor and Vice-Chair for Faculty
Department of Pediatrics
Division of Nephrology
Medical College of Wisconsin
Milwaukee, Wisconsin
Upper Urinary Tract Causes of Hematuria
Hematologic Diseases Causing Hematuria
Anatomic Abnormalities Associated with Hematuria
Transient Proteinuria
Orthostatic (Postural) Proteinuria
Tubulointerstitial Nephritis
Toxic Nephropathy

Diego Preciado, MD, PhD
Joseph E. Robert Jr. Professor of Otolaryngology
Children's National Medical Center
Associate Professor of Pediatrics and Surgery
George Washington University School of Medicine
Washington, DC
Otitis Media

David T. Price, MD
Clinical Professor
Department of Pediatrics
East Carolina University
Greenville, North Carolina
Failure to Thrive

Charles G. Prober, MD
Professor of Pediatrics, Microbiology, and
 Immunology
Senior Associate Dean, Medical Education
Stanford University School of Medicine
Stanford, California
Central Nervous System Infections
Brain Abscess

David W. Pruitt, MD
Assistant Professor
Department of Pediatrics
University of Cincinnati College of Medicine
Medical Director, Inpatient Pediatric Rehabilitation
 Unit
Director, Pediatric Rehabilitation Medicine
 Fellowship
Cincinnati Children's Hospital Medical Center
Cincinnati, Ohio
*Spinal Cord Injury and Spinal Cord Autonomic
 Crisis Management*

Linda Quan, MD
Professor
Department of Pediatrics
University of Washington School of Medicine
Attending Physician
Division of Emergency Medicine
Seattle Children's Hospital
Seattle, Washington
Drowning and Submersion Injury

Elisabeth H. Quint, MD
Professor of Obstetrics and Gynecology
Director, Fellowship in Pediatric and Adolescent
 Gynecology
Van Voightlander Women's Hospital
University of Michigan Medical School
Ann Arbor, Michigan
Gynecologic Care for Girls with Special Needs

C. Egla Rabinovich, MD, MPH
Associate Professor of Pediatrics
Duke University School of Medicine
Co-Chief, Division of Pediatric Rheumatology
Duke University Health System
Durham, North Carolina
Evaluation of Suspected Rheumatic Disease
Treatment of Rheumatic Diseases
Juvenile Idiopathic Arthritis
Scleroderma and Raynaud Phenomenon
Sjögren Syndrome
Miscellaneous Conditions Associated with Arthritis

Leslie J. Raffini, MD
Associate Professor of Pediatrics
University of Pennsylvania Perelman School of
Medicine
Division of Hematology
Children's Hospital of Philadelphia
Philadelphia, Pennsylvania
Hemostasis
Hereditary Predisposition to Thrombosis
Thrombotic Disorders in Children
Disseminated Intravascular Coagulation

Octavio Ramilo, MD
Henry G. Cramblett Chair in Medicine
Professor of Pediatrics
The Ohio State University College of Medicine
Chief, Section of Infectious Diseases and
Immunology
Nationwide Children's Hospital
Columbus, Ohio
Mycoplasma pneumoniae

Denia Ramirez-Montealegre, MD
Assistant Professor of Neurology
University of Virginia School of Medicine
Division of Pediatric Neurology
UVA Children's Hospital
Charlottesville, Virginia
Ataxias

Asma Rashid, MD, MPH
Department of Psychiatry
Boston Medical Center
Boston, Massachusetts
Disruptive, Impulse-Control, and Conduct Disorders

Giuseppe J. Raviola, MD
Assistant Professor of Psychiatry and Global
Health and Social Medicine
Harvard Medical School
Director, Psychiatry Quality Program
Boston Children's Hospital
Boston, Massachusetts
Autism Spectrum Disorder
Childhood Psychoses

Gerald V. Raymond, MD
Professor of Neurology
University of Minnesota School of Medicine
Chief of Pediatric Neurology
University of Minnesota Medical Center, Fairview
Minneapolis, Minnesota
Disorders of Very Long Chain Fatty Acids

Ann M. Reed, MD
Professor of Pediatrics
Chair, Department of Pediatrics
Physician-in-Chief, Duke Children's
Duke University
Durham, North Carolina
Juvenile Dermatomyositis

Harold L. Rekate, MD, FACS, FAAP
Professor of Neurosurgery
Hofstra Northshore School of Medicine
Director, The Chiari Institute
Harvey Cushing Neurosciences Institute
Great Neck, New York
Spinal Cord Disorders

Megan E. Reller, MD, PhD, MPH
Assistant Professor of Pathology, Medicine, and
International Health
Johns Hopkins University School of Medicine
Baltimore, Maryland
Spotted Fever Group Rickettsioses
Scrub Typhus (Orientia tsutsugamushi)
Typhus Group Rickettsioses
Ehrlichioses and Anaplasmosis
Q Fever (Coxiella burnetii)

Jorges D. Reyes, MD
Assistant Professor of Surgery
Division of Transplantation
University of Washington School of Medicine
Chief, Division of Transplant Surgery
Seattle Children's Hospital
Seattle, Washington
*Intestinal Transplantation in Children with
Intestinal Failure*
Liver Transplantation

Geoffrey A. Rezvani, MD
Assistant Professor
Department of Pediatrics
Drexel University College of Medicine
Section of Endocrinology, Diabetes, and
Metabolism
St. Christopher's Hospital for Children
Philadelphia, Pennsylvania;
Novo Nordisk, Inc.
Princeton, New Jersey
An Approach to Inborn Errors of Metabolism

Iraj Rezvani, MD
Professor of Pediatrics (Emeritus)
Temple University School of Medicine
Adjunct Professor
Department of Pediatrics
Drexel University College of Medicine
Section of Endocrinology, Diabetes, and
Metabolism
St. Christopher's Hospital for Children
Philadelphia, Pennsylvania
An Approach to Inborn Errors of Metabolism
Defects in Metabolism of Amino Acids

A. Kim Ritchey, MD
Professor of Pediatrics
Vice-Chair for Clinical Affairs
Department of Pediatrics
University of Pittsburgh School of Medicine
Division of Hematology/Oncology
Children's Hospital of Pittsburgh of UPMC
Pittsburgh, Pennsylvania
Principles of Diagnosis (Cancer)
Principles of Treatment
The Leukemias

Frederick P. Rivara, MD, MPH
Seattle Children's Guild Endowed Chair in
Pediatrics
Professor and Vice-Chair, Department of Pediatrics
University of Washington School of Medicine
Seattle, Washington
Injury Control

Elizabeth V. Robilotti, MD, MPH
Associate Director, Infection Control
Memorial Hospital Division of Infectious Diseases
Memorial Sloan Kettering Cancer Center
New York, New York
Legionella

Angela Byun Robinson, MD, MPH
Assistant Professor
Department of Pediatrics
Case Western Reserve University School of
Medicine
Program Director, Pediatric Rheumatology
University Hospitals Case Medical Center
Cleveland, Ohio
Juvenile Dermatomyositis
Miscellaneous Conditions Associated with Arthritis

Genie E. Roosevelt, MD, MPH
Associate Professor of Pediatrics
Department of Emergency Medicine
University of Colorado School of Medicine
Denver Health Medical Center
Denver, Colorado
*Acute Inflammatory Upper Airway Obstruction
(Croup, Epiglottitis, Laryngitis, and Bacterial
Tracheitis)*

David R. Rosenberg, MD
Professor and Chair, Department of Psychiatry
Miriam L. Hamburger Endowed Chair of Child
Psychiatry
Psychiatrist-in-Chief
Wayne State University and the Detroit Medical
Center
Detroit, Michigan
Anxiety Disorders

David S. Rosenblatt, MD
Holder, Dodd Q. Chu and Family Chair in Medical
Genetics
Professor, Departments of Human Genetics,
Medicine, Pediatrics, and Biology
Faculties of Medicine and Science
McGill University
Montreal, Quebec, Canada
Methionine
*Valine, Leucine, Isoleucine, and Related Organic
Acidemias*

Cindy Ganis Roskind, MD
Assistant Clinical Professor
Division of Pediatric Emergency Medicine
Columbia University College of Physicians and
Surgeons
New York, New York
Acute Care of the Victim of Multiple Trauma

A. Catharine Ross, PhD
Professor and Dorothy Foehr Huck Chair
Department of Nutritional Sciences
The Pennsylvania State University
University Park, Pennsylvania
Vitamin A Deficiencies and Excess

Mary M. Rotar, RN, BSN, CIC
Infection Prevention and Control Coordinator
Children's Hospital of Wisconsin
Milwaukee, Wisconsin
Infection Prevention and Control

Ranna A. Rozenfeld, MD
Associate Professor of Pediatrics and Medical
  Education
Northwestern University Feinberg School of
  Medicine
Division of Pediatric Critical Care Medicine
Ann & Robert H. Lurie Children's Hospital of
  Chicago
Chicago, Illinois
Atelectasis

Colleen A. Ryan, MD
Instructor in Psychiatry
Harvard Medical School
Medical Director, Psychiatry Inpatient Service
Boston Children's Hospital
Boston, Massachusetts
Motor Disorders and Habits

**H.P.S. Sachdev, MD, FIAP, FAMS,
FRCPCH**
Senior Consultant
Departments of Pediatrics and Clinical
  Epidemiology
Sitaram Bhartia Institute of Science and Research
New Delhi, India
Vitamin B Complex Deficiencies and Excess
Vitamin C (Ascorbic Acid)

**Ramesh C. Sachdeva, MD, PhD, FAAP,
FCCM**
Professor of Pediatrics (Critical Care)
Medical College of Wisconsin
Milwaukee, Wisconsin;
Associate Executive Director
Medical Director, Quality Initiatives
Director, Department of Subspecialty Pediatrics
American Academy of Pediatrics
Elk Grove Village, Illinois
Quality and Safety in Healthcare for Children

**Manish Sadarangani, BM BCh, DPhil,
MRCPCH**
Clinical Lecturer and Honorary Specialist Registrar
Paediatric Infectious Diseases and Immunology
Children's Hospital
Oxford, United Kingdom
Neisseria meningitidis (Meningococcus)

Rebecca E. Sadun, MD, PhD
Adult and Pediatric Rheumatology Fellow
Departments of Medicine and Pediatrics
Duke University School of Medicine
Durham, North Carolina
Systemic Lupus Erythematosus

Mustafa Sahin, MD, PhD
Associate Professor of Neurology
Harvard Medical School
F.M. Kirby Neurobiology Center
Boston Children's Hospital
Boston, Massachusetts
Neurocutaneous Syndromes

Robert A. Salata, MD
Professor and Executive Vice-Chair, Department of
  Medicine
Case Western Reserve University School of
  Medicine
Chief, Division of Infectious Diseases and HIV
  Medicine
University Hospitals Case Medical Center
Cleveland, Ohio
Amebiasis
Trichomoniasis (Trichomonas vaginalis)
African Trypanosomiasis (Sleeping Sickness;
  Trypanosoma brucei complex)
American Trypanosomiasis (Chagas Disease;
  Trypanosoma cruzi)

Denise A. Salerno, MD, FAAP
Professor of Clinical Pediatrics
Temple University School of Medicine
Philadelphia, Pennsylvania
Nonbacterial Food Poisoning

Edsel Maurice T. Salvana, MD
Clinical Associate Professor of Medicine
University of the Philippines College of Medicine
Director, Institute of Molecular Biology and
  Biotechnology
National Institutes of Health
Manila, The Philippines;
Adjunct Professor of Global Health
University of Pittsburgh School of Medicine
Pittsburgh, Pennsylvania
Amebiasis
Trichomoniasis (Trichomonas vaginalis)
African Trypanosomiasis (Sleeping Sickness;
  Trypanosoma brucei complex)
American Trypanosomiasis (Chagas Disease;
  Trypanosoma cruzi)

Hugh A. Sampson, MD
Kurt Hirschhorn Professor of Pediatrics
Jaffe Food Allergy Institute
Icahn School of Medicine at Mount Sinai
New York, New York
Anaphylaxis
Food Allergy and Adverse Reactions to Foods

Thomas J. Sandora, MD, MPH
Assistant Professor of Pediatrics
Harvard Medical School
Medical Director, Infection Prevention and Control
Division of Infectious Diseases
Boston Children's Hospital
Boston, Massachusetts
Community-Acquired Pneumonia

Tracy L. Sandritter, PharmD
Pharmacy Resident
Transplant Pharmacy
Children's Mercy Hospitals and Clinics
Kansas City, Missouri
Principles of Drug Therapy

Wudbhav N. Sankar, MD
Assistant Professor
Department of Orthopaedic Surgery
University of Pennsylvania Perelman School of
  Medicine
Attending Orthopaedic Surgeon
Children's Hospital of Philadelphia
Philadelphia, Pennsylvania
The Hip

Eric J. Sarkissian, MD
Ben Fox Clinical Fellow
Department of Orthopaedics
Children's Hospital of Philadelphia
Philadelphia, Pennsylvania
The Knee

Ajit A. Sarnaik, MD
Assistant Professor
Department of Pediatrics
Wayne State University School of Medicine
Associate Director, Pediatric Residency Program
Children's Hospital of Michigan
Detroit, Michigan
Respiratory Distress and Failure

Ashok P. Sarnaik, MD
Professor and Interim Chair
Department of Pediatrics
Wayne State University School of Medicine
Pediatrician in Chief
Children's Hospital of Michigan
Detroit, Michigan
Respiratory Distress and Failure
Respiratory Pathophysiology and Regulation

Harvey B. Sarnat, MD, MS, FRCPC
Professor of Pediatrics, Pathology
  (Neuropathology), and Clinical Neurosciences
Division of Pediatric Neurology
University of Calgary Faculty of Medicine
Alberta Children's Hospital
Calgary, Alberta, Canada
Evaluation and Investigation (Neuromuscular
  Disorders)
Developmental Disorders of Muscle
Muscular Dystrophies
Endocrine and Toxic Myopathies
Metabolic Myopathies
Disorders of Neuromuscular Transmission and of
  Motor Neurons
Hereditary Motor-Sensory Neuropathies
Toxic Neuropathies
Autonomic Neuropathies
Guillain-Barré Syndrome
Bell Palsy

**Minnie M. Sarwal, MD, PhD, FRCP,
DCH**
Professor, Transplant Nephrology and Pediatrics
California Pacific Medical Center
Director, The BIOMARC Institute for Personalized
  Medicine, Sutter Health Care
Director, The Sarwal Lab, CPMC-Research
  Institute
San Francisco, California;
Consulting Professor
Stanford University
Palo Alto, California
Renal Transplantation

Laura E. Schanberg, MD
Professor of Pediatrics
Duke University School of Medicine
Co-Chief, Division of Pediatric Rheumatology
Duke University Medical Center
Durham, North Carolina
Systemic Lupus Erythematosus
Musculoskeletal Pain Syndromes

Mark R. Schleiss, MD
Professor of Pediatrics
American Legion and Auxiliary Heart Foundation
    Research Chair
Director, Division of Pediatric Infectious Diseases
    and Immunology
University of Minnesota School of Medicine
Minneapolis, Minnesota
Principles of Antibacterial Therapy
Principles of Antiviral Therapy
Principles of Antiparasitic Therapy

Nina F. Schor, MD, PhD
William H. Eilinger Professor and Chair
Department of Pediatrics
Professor, Department of Neurology
Pediatrician-in-Chief
Golisano Children's Hospital
University of Rochester Medical Center
Rochester, New York
Neurologic Evaluation

Bill J. Schroeder, DO
Pediatric Emergency Medicine
Advocate Christ Medical Center
Oak Lawn, Illinois
Envenomations

James W. Schroeder Jr., MD, FACS, FAAP
Associate Professor
Department of Otolaryngology—Head and Neck
    Surgery
Northwestern University Feinberg School of
    Medicine
Ann & Robert H. Lurie Children's Hospital of
    Chicago
Chicago, Illinois
Congenital Anomalies of the Larynx, Trachea, and Bronchi
Foreign Bodies in the Airway
Laryngotracheal Stenosis and Subglottic Stenosis
Neoplasms of the Larynx, Trachea, and Bronchi

Mark A. Schuster, MD, PhD
William Berenberg Professor of Pediatrics
Harvard Medical School
Chief of General Pediatrics and Vice-Chair for
    Health Policy
Department of Medicine
Children's Hospital Boston
Boston, Massachusetts
Gay, Lesbian, and Bisexual Adolescents

Gordon E. Schutze, MD
Executive Vice-Chairman
Professor of Pediatrics
Martin I. Lorin MD Chair in Medical Education
Vice-President of International Medical Programs
Baylor International Pediatric AIDS Initiative
Baylor College of Medicine
Texas Children's Hospital
Houston, Texas
Actinomyces
Nocardia
Tularemia (Francisella tularensis)
Brucella

Daryl A. Scott, MD, PhD
Associate Professor
Department of Molecular and Human Genetics
Baylor College of Medicine
Houston, Texas
The Genetic Approach in Pediatric Medicine
The Human Genome
Patterns of Genetic Transmission

J. Paul Scott, MD
Professor of Pediatrics
Division of Pediatric Hematology/Oncology
Medical College of Wisconsin
Blood Center of Southeastern Wisconsin
Milwaukee, Wisconsin
Hemostasis
*Hereditary Clotting Factor Deficiencies (Bleeding
    Disorders)*
von Willebrand Disease
Hereditary Predisposition to Thrombosis
Thrombotic Disorders in Children
Postneonatal Vitamin K Deficiency
Liver Disease
Acquired Inhibitors of Coagulation
Disseminated Intravascular Coagulation
Platelet and Blood Vessel Disorders

Patrick C. Seed, MD, PhD
Associate Professor of Pediatrics
Division of Pediatric Infectious Diseases
Assistant Professor of Molecular Genetics and
    Microbiology
Duke University Medical Center
Durham, North Carolina
The Microbiome and Pediatric Health

George B. Segel, MD
Professor of Medicine
Professor Emeritus of Pediatrics
University of Rochester Medical Center
Rochester, New York
Definitions and Classification of Hemolytic Anemias
Hereditary Spherocytosis
Hereditary Elliptocytosis
Hereditary Stomatocytosis
*Paroxysmal Nocturnal Hemoglobinuria and
    Acanthocytosis*
Enzymatic Defects
*Hemolytic Anemias Resulting from Extracellular
    Factors—Immune Hemolytic Anemias*
*Hemolytic Anemias Secondary to Other
    Extracellular Factors*

Ernest G. Seidman, MDCM, FRCPC, FACG
Professor of Medicine and Pediatrics
Bruce Kaufman Endowed Chair in IBD
McGill University Faculty of Medicine
Director, McGill Centre of IBD
McGill University Health Center
Montreal, Quebec, Canada
Immunodeficiency Disorders
Immunoproliferative Small Intestinal Disease
Malabsorption in Eosinophilic Gastroenteritis
Malabsorption in Inflammatory Bowel Disease

Janet R. Serwint, MD
Professor
Department of Pediatrics
Johns Hopkins University School of Medicine
Baltimore, Maryland
Loss, Separation, and Bereavement

Dheeraj Shah, MD, FIAP, MAMS
Professor
Department of Pediatrics
University College of Medical Sciences
Guru Teg Bahadur Hospital
New Delhi, India
Vitamin B Complex Deficiencies and Excess
Vitamin C (Ascorbic Acid)

Ala Shaikhkhalil, MD
Fellow
Division of Gastroenterology, Hepatology, and
    Nutrition
Children's Hospital of Philadelphia
Philadelphia, Pennsylvania
Nutritional Requirements
Feeding Healthy Infants, Children, and Adolescents

Raanan Shamir, MD
Professor of Pediatrics
Sackler Faculty of Medicine
Tel-Aviv University
Tel-Aviv, Israel;
Chairman, Institute of Gastroenterology, Nutrition,
    and Liver Diseases
Schneider Children's Medical Center of Israel
Petach Tikvah, Israel
*Intestinal Infections and Infestations Associated with
    Malabsorption*
Chronic Malnutrition

Andi L. Shane, MD, MPH, MSc
Associate Professor of Pediatrics
Division of Pediatric Infectious Diseases
Emory University School of Medicine
Atlanta, Georgia
Infections of the Neonatal Infant

Bruce K. Shapiro, MD
Professor of Pediatrics
The Arnold J. Capute MD, MPH Chair in
    Neurodevelopmental Disabilities
The Johns Hopkins University School of Medicine
Vice-President, Training
Kennedy Krieger Institute
Baltimore, Maryland
Intellectual Disability

Amanda N. Shaw, MD
Pediatric Endocrinology Fellow
University of Texas Health Sciences Center
Houston, Texas
Campylobacter
Aeromonas and Plesiomonas

Bennett A. Shaywitz, MD
Charles and Helen Schwab Professor in Dyslexia
    and Learning Development
Co-Director, Center for Dyslexia and Creativity
Chief, Child Neurology
Yale University School of Medicine
New Haven, Connecticut
Dyslexia

Sally E. Shaywitz, MD
Audrey G. Ratner Professor in Learning
    Development
Co-Director, Center for Dyslexia and Creativity
Department of Pediatrics
Yale University School of Medicine
New Haven, Connecticut
Dyslexia

Philip M. Sherman, MD, FRCP(C), FAAP
Professor of Paediatrics, Microbiology, and
    Dentistry
University of Toronto Faculty of Medicine
Division of Gastroenterology, Hepatology, and
    Nutrition
Senior Scientist, Cell Biology Research Program
The Hospital for Sick Children
Toronto, Ontario, Canada
Other Malabsorptive Syndromes

Benjamin L. Shneider, MD
Professor of Pediatrics
University of Pittsburgh School of Medicine
Director, Pediatric Hepatology
Children's Hospital of Pittsburgh of UPMC
Pittsburgh, Pennsylvania
Autoimmune Hepatitis

Stanford T. Shulman, MD
Virginia H. Rogers Professor of Pediatric Infectious
    Diseases
Northwestern University Feinberg School of
    Medicine
Chief, Division of Infectious Diseases
Ann & Robert H. Lurie Children's Hospital of
    Chicago
Chicago, Illinois
Group A Streptococcus

Scott H. Sicherer, MD
Elliot and Roslyn Jaffe Professor of Pediatrics,
    Allergy, and Immunology
Jaffe Food Allergy Institute
Icahn School of Medicine at Mount Sinai
New York, New York
Allergy and the Immunologic Basis of Atopic Disease
Diagnosis of Allergic Disease
Principles of Treatment of Allergic Disease
Allergic Rhinitis
Childhood Asthma
Atopic Dermatitis (Atopic Eczema)
Insect Allergy
Ocular Allergies
Urticaria (Hives) and Angioedema
Anaphylaxis
Serum Sickness
Food Allergy and Adverse Reactions to Foods
Adverse Reactions to Drugs

Richard Sills, MD
Professor of Pediatrics
Director, Pediatric Hematology/Oncology
Upstate Medical University
Syracuse, New York
Iron-Deficiency Anemia
Other Microcytic Anemias

Mark D. Simms, MD, MPH
Professor of Pediatrics
Medical College of Wisconsin
Medical Director
Child Development Center
Children's Hospital of Wisconsin
Milwaukee, Wisconsin
*Language Development and Communication
    Disorders*
Adoption

Eric A.F. Simões, MBBS, DCH, MD
Professor of Pediatrics
University of Colorado School of Medicine
Professor of Epidemiology
Center for Global Health
Colorado School of Public Health
Division of Infectious Diseases
The Children's Hospital
Aurora, Colorado
Polioviruses

Kari A. Simonsen, MD
Assistant Professor of Pediatrics
Division of Infectious Diseases
University of Nebraska Medical Center
Omaha, Nebraska
Leptospira

Anne Slavotinek, MBBS, PhD
Professor of Clinical Pediatrics
University of California, San Francisco
San Francisco, California
Dysmorphology

Thomas L. Slovis, MD
Professor Emeritus of Radiology and Pediatrics
Wayne State University School of Medicine
Department of Pediatric Imaging
Children's Hospital of Michigan
Detroit, Michigan
Biologic Effects of Radiation on Children

P. Brian Smith, MD, MHS, MPH
Associate Professor of Pediatrics
Division of Neonatology
Duke University School of Medicine
Durham, North Carolina
Candida

Mary Beth F. Son, MD
Instructor in Pediatrics
Department of Pediatrics
Harvard Medical School
Staff Physician, Division of Immunology
Boston Children's Hospital
Boston, Massachusetts
Kawasaki Disease

Laura Stout Sosinsky, PhD
Senior Research Scientist
Early Childhood Development
Child Trends, Inc.
Bethesda, Maryland
*Childcare: How Pediatricians Can Support Children
    and Families*

Joseph D. Spahn, MD
Professor
Department of Pediatrics
National Jewish Health
University of Colorado School of Medicine
Denver, Colorado
Childhood Asthma

Rivkie Spalter
Director
Mequon Jewish Preschool
Mequon, Wisconsin
*The Reggio Emilia Educational Approach and Child
    Development and Learning*

Mark A. Sperling, MD
Professor and Chair Emeritus
Department of Pediatrics
University of Pittsburgh School of Medicine
Division of Endocrinology, Metabolism, and
    Diabetes Mellitus
Children's Hospital of Pittsburgh
Pittsburgh, Pennsylvania
Hypoglycemia

Robert L. Spicer, MD
Professor of Pediatrics
University of Nebraska Medical Center College of
    Medicine
Clinical Professor of Pediatrics
Creighton University School of Medicine
Clinical Service Chief, Cardiology
Children's Hospital and Medical Center
Omaha, Nebraska
Diseases of the Myocardium
Diseases of the Pericardium
Tumors of the Heart

David A. Spiegel, MD
Associate Professor
Department of Orthopaedic Surgery
University of Pennsylvania Perelman School of
    Medicine
Attending Orthopaedic Surgeon
Children's Hospital of Philadelphia
Philadelphia, Pennsylvania
Hypermobile Pes Planus (Flexible Flatfeet)
Toe Deformities
Shoes
The Spine
The Neck

Helen Spoudeas, MD
Honorary Senior Lecturer in Paediatric
    Endocrinology
University College London
Consultant in Neuro-Endocrine Late Effects of
    Childhood Cancer
University College London Hospital
Great Ormond Street Hospital
London, United Kingdom
Diarrhea from Neuroendocrine Tumors

Jürgen W. Spranger, MD
Professor Emeritus of Pediatrics
University of Mainz School of Medicine
Children's Hospital
Mainz, Germany
Mucopolysaccharidoses

James E. Squires, MD
Pediatric Gastroenterology Fellow
Cincinnati Children's Hospital Medical Center
Cincinnati, Ohio
Manifestations of Liver Disease

**Rajasree Sreedharan, MBBS, DCH,
MRCPCH**
Assistant Professor of Clinical Pediatrics
University of Pennsylvania Perelman School of
    Medicine
Division of Gastroenterology and Nutrition
The Children's Hospital of Philadelphia
Philadelphia, Pennsylvania
Tubular Function
Renal Tubular Acidosis
Nephrogenic Diabetes Insipidus
*Bartter and Gitelman Syndromes and Other
    Inherited Tubular Transport Abnormalities*
Renal Failure

**Raman Sreedharan, MD, DCH,
MRCPCH**
Clinical Assistant Professor of Pediatrics
University of Pennsylvania Perelman School of
    Medicine
EHR Medical Director, Specialty Care
The Children's Hospital of Philadelphia
Philadelphia, Pennsylvania
*Major Symptoms and Signs of Digestive Tract
    Disorders*
*Functional Abdominal Pain (Nonorganic Chronic
    Abdominal Pain)*

Nivedita Srinivas, MD
Clinical Instructor in Pediatrics
Division of Pediatric Infectious Diseases
Stanford University School of Medicine
Stanford, California
Central Nervous System Infections

Margaret M. Stager, MD, FAAP
Associate Professor
Department of Pediatrics
Case Western Reserve University School of
  Medicine
Director, Division of Adolescent Medicine
MetroHealth Medical Center
Cleveland, Ohio
Violent Behavior
Substance Abuse

Erin D. Stahl, MD
Assistant Professor
Department of Ophthalmology
University of Missouri—Kansas City School of
  Medicine
Children's Mercy Hospital
Kansas City, Missouri
Growth and Development (Eye)
Examination of the Eye
Abnormalities of Refraction and Accommodation
Disorders of Vision
Abnormalities of Pupil and Iris
Disorders of Eye Movement and Alignment
Abnormalities of the Lids
Disorders of the Lacrimal System
Disorders of the Conjunctiva
Abnormalities of the Cornea
Abnormalities of the Lens
Disorders of the Uveal Tract
Disorders of the Retina and Vitreous
Abnormalities of the Optic Nerve
Childhood Glaucoma
Orbital Abnormalities
Orbital Infections
Injuries to the Eye

Amy P. Stallings, MD
Assistant Professor of Pediatrics
Division of Pediatric Allergy and Immunology
Duke University School of Medicine
Durham, North Carolina
Urticaria (Hives) and Angioedema

Virginia A. Stallings, MD
Professor of Pediatrics
Division of Gastroenterology, Hepatology, and
  Nutrition
University of Pennsylvania Perelman School of
  Medicine
Director, Nutrition Center
Children's Hospital of Philadelphia
Philadelphia, Pennsylvania
Nutritional Requirements
Feeding Healthy Infants, Children, and Adolescents

Kathryn C. Stambough, MD
Resident Physician
Department of Obstetrics and Gynecology
Washington University School of Medicine in St.
  Louis
St. Louis, Missouri
History and Physical Examination (Gynecology)

Lawrence R. Stanberry, MD, PhD
Reuben S. Carpentier Professor and Chairman
Department of Pediatrics
Columbia University College of Physicians and
  Surgeons
New York, New York
Herpes Simplex Virus

Charles A. Stanley, MD
Professor of Pediatrics
University of Pennsylvania Perelman School of
  Medicine
Division of Endocrinology
Children's Hospital of Philadelphia
Philadelphia, Pennsylvania
Disorders of Mitochondrial Fatty Acid ß-Oxidation

Bonita F. Stanton, MD
Vice-Dean of Research
Professor of Pediatrics
Wayne State University School of Medicine
Detroit, Michigan
Overview of Pediatrics
Cultural Issues in Pediatric Care
Childhood Psychoses
Catatonia in Children and Adolescents

Jeffrey R. Starke, MD
Professor of Pediatrics
Division of Infectious Diseases
Baylor College of Medicine
Infection Control Officer
Texas Children's Hospital
Houston, Texas
Tuberculosis (Mycobacterium tuberculosis)

Barbara W. Stechenberg, MD
Professor of Pediatrics
Tufts University School of Medicine
Boston, Massachusetts;
Pediatric Infectious Diseases
Baystate Children's Hospital
Springfield, Massachusetts
Bartonella

William J. Steinbach, MD
Associate Professor of Pediatrics and Molecular
  Genetics and Microbiology
Duke University Medical Center
Durham, North Carolina
Principles of Antifungal Therapy
Aspergillus

Janet Stewart, MD
Associate Professor Emerita
Department of Pediatrics
University of Colorado School of Medicine
Spina Bifida Clinic
Children's Hospital Colorado
Denver, Colorado
Meningomyelocele (Spina Bifida)

Barbara J. Stoll, MD
George W. Brumley Jr. Professor and Chair
Department of Pediatrics
Emory University School of Medicine
Director, The Pediatric Center of Emory and
  Children's Healthcare of Atlanta
Atlanta, Georgia
Infections of the Neonatal Infant

Gregory A. Storch, MD
Professor of Pediatrics
Washington University in St. Louis School of
  Medicine
St. Louis, Missouri
Diagnostic Microbiology
Polyomaviruses

Ronald G. Strauss, MD
Professor Emeritus
Departments of Pediatrics and Pathology
University of Iowa Carver College of Medicine
Iowa City, Iowa
Red Blood Cell Transfusions and Erythropoietin
  Therapy
Platelet Transfusions
Neutrophil (Granulocyte) Transfusions
Plasma Transfusions
Risks of Blood Transfusions

Gina S. Sucato, MD, MPH
Associate Professor of Pediatrics
University of Pittsburgh School of Medicine
Fellowship Director, Division of Adolescent
  Medicine
Children's Hospital of Pittsburgh of UPMC
Pittsburgh, Pennsylvania
Menstrual Problems

Frederick J. Suchy, MD
Professor of Pediatrics
Associate Dean for Child Health Research
University of Colorado
Denver, Colorado;
Chief Research Officer and Director
Children's Hospital Colorado Research Institute
Aurora, Colorado
Autoimmune Hepatitis
Drug- and Toxin-Induced Liver Injury
Fulminant Hepatic Failure
Cystic Diseases of the Biliary Tract and Liver
Diseases of the Gallbladder
Portal Hypertension and Varices

Britta M. Svoren, MD
Assistant Professor of Pediatrics
Division of Pediatric Endocrinology
University of Rochester Medical Center
Rochester, New York
Diabetes Mellitus

Stephen J. Swanson, MD
Associate Professor of Pediatrics
Divisions of Global Pediatrics and Pediatric
  Infectious Diseases
University of Minnesota Medical School
Minneapolis, Minnesota
Health Advice for Children Traveling Internationally

Moira Szilagyi, MD, PhD
Professor of Pediatrics
University of Rochester School of Medicine
Rochester, New York
Foster and Kinship Care

Libo Tan, PhD
Postdoctoral Fellow
Department of Nutritional Sciences
The Pennsylvania State University
University Park, Pennsylvania
Vitamin A Deficiencies and Excess

Robert R. Tanz, MD
Professor of Pediatrics
Division of Academic General Pediatrics and
  Primary Care
Northwestern University Feinberg School of
  Medicine
Ann & Robert H. Lurie Children's Hospital of
  Chicago
Chicago, Illinois
Acute Pharyngitis

Nidale Tarek, MD
Assistant Professor of Pediatrics
University of Texas MD Anderson Cancer Center
Houston, Texas
Retinoblastoma
Neoplasms of the Liver

Cynthia J. Tifft, MD, PhD
National Human Genome Research Institute
National Institutes of Health
Bethesda, Maryland
Genetic Approaches to Rare and Undiagnosed
Diseases

Norman Tinanoff, DDS, MS
Professor
Department of Orthodontics and Pediatric
Dentistry
Chief, Division of Pediatric Dentistry
University of Maryland School of Dentistry
Baltimore, Maryland
Development and Developmental Anomalies of the
Teeth
Disorders of the Oral Cavity Associated with Other
Conditions
Malocclusion
Cleft Lip and Palate
Syndromes with Oral Manifestations
Dental Caries
Periodontal Diseases
Dental Trauma
Common Lesions of the Oral Soft Tissues
Diseases of the Salivary Glands and Jaws
Diagnostic Radiology in Dental Assessment

James K. Todd, MD
Professor of Pediatrics and Microbiology
University of Colorado School of Medicine
Professor of Epidemiology
University of Colorado School of Public Health
Director, Epidemiology and Clinical Microbiology
Children's Hospital Colorado
Aurora, Colorado
Staphylococcus

Lucy S. Tompkins, MD, PhD
Lucy Becker Professor of Medicine
Division of Infectious Diseases/Geographic
Medicine
Stanford University School of Medicine
Stanford, California
Legionella

Richard L. Tower II, MD, MS
Assistant Professor of Pediatrics
Division of Pediatric Hematology, Oncology, and
Transplant
Medical College of Wisconsin
Milwaukee, Wisconsin
Anatomy and Function of the Lymphatic System
Abnormalities of Lymphatic Vessels
Lymphadenopathy

Michael L. Trieu, MD
Instructor in Psychiatry
Harvard Medical School
Assistant in Psychiatry
Boston Children's Hospital
Boston, Massachusetts
Motor Disorders and Habits
Autism Spectrum Disorder
Childhood Psychoses
Schizophrenia Spectrum and Other Psychotic
Disorders
Acute Phobic Hallucinations of Childhood

Riccardo Troncone, MD
Professor and Director
Department of Pediatrics
University of Naples Federico II
Napoli, Italy
Celiac Disease (Gluten-Sensitive Enteropathy)

David G. Tubergen, MD
Medical Director for Host Program
MD Anderson Physicians Network
Houston, Texas
The Leukemias

Margaret A. Turk, MD
Professor
Departments of Physical Medicine and
Rehabilitation and Pediatrics
State University of New York
SUNY Upstate Medical University
Syracuse, New York
Health and Wellness for Children with Disabilities

David A. Turner, MD
Associate Professor
Department of Pediatrics
Duke University School of Medicine
Director, Pediatric Critical Care Fellowship
Program
Medical Director, Pediatric Intensive Care Unit
Duke University Medical Center
Durham, North Carolina
Shock

Christina Ullrich, MD, MPH
Assistant Professor in Pediatrics
Department of Psychosocial Oncology and
Palliative Care
Department of Pediatric Hematology/Oncology
Harvard Medical School
Boston Children's Hospital
Dana-Farber Cancer Institute
Boston, Massachusetts
Pediatric Palliative Care

David K. Urion, MD
Charles F. Barlow Chair
Department of Neurology
Harvard University
Boston Children's Hospital
Boston, Massachusetts
Attention-Deficit/Hyperactivity Disorder

Douglas Vanderbilt, MD
Associate Professor of Clinical Pediatrics
Associate Professor of Occupational Science/
Occupational Therapy
University of Southern California Keck School of
Medicine
Director, MCHB Developmental-Behavioral
Pediatrics Training Program
Children's Hospital Los Angeles
Director, California Leadership Education in
Neurodevelopmental Disabilities Program
University Center for Excellence in Developmental
Disabilities
Los Angeles, California
Bullying, Cyberbullying, and School Violence

Jon A. Vanderhoof, MD
Professor Emeritus of Pediatrics
University of Nebraska Medical Center
Omaha, Nebraska;
Lecturer in Pediatrics, Harvard Medical School
Staff Gastroenterologist, Children's Hospital Boston
Boston, Massachusetts;
Vice-President for Global Medical Affairs
Mead Johnson Nutritionals
Evansville, Indiana
Short Bowel Syndrome

George F. Van Hare, MD
Louis Larrick Ward Professor of Pediatrics
Director, Division of Pediatric Cardiology
Washington University in St. Louis
St. Louis Children's Hospital
St. Louis, Missouri
Syncope
Disturbances of Rate and Rhythm of the Heart

Jakko van Ingen, MD, PhD
Clinical Microbiology Resident
Radboud University Medical Centre
Nijmegen, The Netherlands
Nontuberculous Mycobacteria

Heather A. Van Mater, MD, MS
Assistant Professor of Pediatrics
Duke University School of Medicine
Division of Pediatric Rheumatology
Duke University Health System
Durham, North Carolina
Scleroderma and Raynaud Phenomenon
Central Nervous System Vasculitis

Dick van Soolingen, PhD
Professor of Translational Tuberculosis Research
Radboud University Medical Centre
Nijmegen, The Netherlands;
Head, Mycobacteria Reference Laboratory
National Institute for Public Health and the
Environment (RIVM)
Bilthoven, The Netherlands
Nontuberculous Mycobacteria

Christine VanTubbergen, BA
Former Coordinator, National Collaborative
Congenital Toxoplasmosis Study
The University of Chicago School of Medicine
Chicago, Illinois;
Current ORISE Fellow
Centers for Disease Control and Prevention
Atlanta, Georgia
Toxoplasmosis (Toxoplasma gondii)

Scott K. Van Why, MD
Professor of Pediatrics
Medical College of Wisconsin
Wauwatosa, Wisconsin
Membranous Nephropathy
Membranoproliferative Glomerulonephritis
Henoch-Schönlein Purpura Nephritis
Rapidly Progressive (Crescentic) Glomerulonephritis
Goodpasture Disease
Hemolytic-Uremic Syndrome

Andrea Velardi, MD
Professor of Hematology
Division of Hematology and Clinical Immunology
University of Perugia
Ospedale Santa Maria della Misericordia
Perugia, Italy
Principles and Clinical Indications of Hematopoietic
*   Stem Cell Transplantation*
Hematopoietic Stem Cell Transplantation from
*   Alternative Sources and Donors*
Graft-Versus-Host Disease, Rejection, and
*   Venoocclusive Disease*
Infectious Complications of Hematopoietic Stem Cell
*   Transplantation*
Late Effects of Hematopoietic Stem Cell
*   Transplantation*

Elliott P. Vichinsky, MD
Professor of Pediatrics
University of California, San Francisco
San Francisco, California;
Medical Director
Hematology/Oncology Programs
Children's Hospital of Oakland
Oakland, California
Hemoglobinopathies

Brian P. Vickery, MD
Assistant Professor of Pediatrics
University of North Carolina at Chapel Hill School
   of Medicine
Chapel Hill, North Carolina
Eosinophils

Bernadette E. Vitola, MD, MPH
Assistant Professor of Pediatrics
Medical College of Wisconsin
Children's Hospital of Wisconsin
Milwaukee, Wisconsin
Liver Disease Associated with Systemic Disorders

Judith A. Voynow, MD
Professor of Pediatrics
Virginia Commonwealth University
Edwin L. Kendig Jr. Chair, Division of Pediatric
   Pulmonology
Children's Hospital of Richmond at VCU
Richmond, Virginia
Cystic Fibrosis

Linda A. Waggoner-Fountain, MD
Associate Professor of Pediatrics
Division of Infectious Diseases
University of Virginia Health System
Charlottesville, Virginia
Childcare and Communicable Diseases

Steven G. Waguespack, MD, FAAP,
FACE
Professor and Deputy Department Chair
Department of Endocrine Neoplasia and
   Hormonal Disorders
University of Texas MD Anderson Cancer Center
Houston, Texas
Thyroid Tumors
Adrenal Tumors

David M. Walker, MD
Division of Pediatric Emergency Medicine
Yale University School of Medicine
New Haven, Connecticut
Principles Applicable to the Developing World

Kelly J. Walkovich, MD
Assistant Professor of Pediatrics and
   Communicable Diseases
Division of Pediatric Hematology/Oncology
University of Michigan Medical School
Ann Arbor, Michigan
Leukopenia
Leukocytosis

Rebecca Wallihan, MD
Assistant Professor of Pediatrics
Section of Infectious Diseases and Immunology
The Ohio State University College of Medicine
Nationwide Children's Hospital
Columbus, Ohio
Genital Mycoplasmas (Mycoplasma hominis,
   Mycoplasma genitalium, *and* Ureaplasma
   urealyticum)

Heather J. Walter, MD, MPH
Professor of Psychiatry and Pediatrics
Vice-Chair, Department of Psychiatry
Boston University School of Medicine
Chief, Child and Adolescent Psychiatry
Boston Medical Center
Senior Lecturer on Psychiatry
Harvard Medical School
Senior Associate in Psychiatry
Boston Children's Hospital
Boston, Massachusetts
Assessment and Interviewing
Psychological Treatment of Children and Adolescents
Motor Disorders and Habits
Psychopharmacology
Psychotherapy
Psychiatric Hospitalization
Mood Disorders
Suicide and Attempted Suicide
Disruptive, Impulse-Control, and Conduct Disorders
Autism Spectrum Disorder
Childhood Psychoses

Julie Wang, MD
Associate Professor of Pediatrics
Jaffe Food Allergy Institute
Icahn School of Medicine at Mount Sinai
New York, New York
Insect Allergy
Anaphylaxis

Stephanie M. Ware, MD, PhD,
FACMG
Associate Professor
Department of Pediatrics
University of Cincinnati College of Medicine
Co-Director, Cardiovascular Genetics
Associate Medical Director and Director of
   Research and Development
The Heart Institute Diagnostic Laboratory
Cincinnati Children's Hospital Medical Center
Cincinnati, Ohio
Diseases of the Myocardium
Diseases of the Pericardium
Tumors of the Heart

Debra E. Weese-Mayer, MD
Professor of Pediatrics
Northwestern University Feinberg School of
   Medicine
Division of Pediatric Neurology
Ann & Robert H. Lurie Children's Hospital of
   Chicago
Chicago, Illinois
Congenital Central Hypoventilation Syndrome

Jason B. Weinberg, MD
Assistant Professor of Pediatrics and Microbiology
   and Immunology
Division of Pediatric Infectious Diseases
University of Michigan Medical School
Ann Arbor, Michigan
Adenoviruses

Kathryn L. Weise, MD, MA
Program Director, Cleveland Fellowship in
   Advanced Bioethics
Department of Bioethics
The Cleveland Clinic Foundation
Cleveland, Ohio
Ethics in Pediatric Care

Pamela F. Weiss, MD, MSCE
Assistant Professor of Pediatrics
University of Pennsylvania Perelman School of
   Medicine
Division of Rheumatology
Children's Hospital of Philadelphia
Philadelphia, Pennsylvania
Ankylosing Spondylitis and Other
*   Spondyloarthritides*
Reactive and Postinfectious Arthritis

Martin E. Weisse, MD
Chief, Department of Pediatrics
Tripler Army Medical Center
Honolulu, Hawaii;
Professor of Pediatrics
Uniformed Services University of the Health
   Sciences
Bethesda, Maryland
Malassezia
Primary Amebic Meningoencephalitis

Lawrence Wells, MD
Associate Professor
Department of Orthopaedic Surgery
University of Pennsylvania Perelman School of
   Medicine
Attending Orthopaedic Surgeon
Children's Hospital of Philadelphia
Philadelphia, Pennsylvania
Growth and Development
Evaluation of the Child
Torsional and Angular Deformities
The Hip
Common Fractures

Jessica W. Wen, MD
Assistant Professor of Pediatrics
University of Pennsylvania Perelman School of
   Medicine
Attending Physician
The Children's Hospital of Philadelphia
Philadelphia, Pennsylvania
Chylous Ascites
Peritonitis

Danielle Wendel, MD
Fellow
Division of Gastroenterology, Hepatology, and
   Nutrition
Children's Hospital of Philadelphia
Philadelphia, Pennsylvania
Feeding Healthy Infants, Children, and Adolescents

Steven L. Werlin, MD
Professor of Pediatrics (Gastroenterology)
The Medical College of Wisconsin
Milwaukee, Wisconsin
Embryology, Anatomy, and Physiology (Pancreas)
Pancreatic Function Tests
Disorders of the Exocrine Pancreas
Treatment of Pancreatic Insufficiency
Pancreatitis
Pseudocyst of the Pancreas
Pancreatic Tumors

Michael R. Wessels, MD
John F. Enders Professor of Pediatrics
Professor of Medicine (Microbiology and
    Immunobiology)
Harvard Medical School
Chief, Division of Infectious Diseases
Boston Children's Hospital
Boston, Massachusetts
Group B Streptococcus

Ralph F. Wetmore, MD
Professor
Department of Otorhinolaryngology—Head and
    Neck Surgery
University of Pennsylvania Perelman School of
    Medicine
E. Mortimer Newlin Professor and Chief
Division of Pediatric Otolaryngology
Children's Hospital of Pennsylvania
Philadelphia, Pennsylvania
Tonsils and Adenoids

Randall C. Wetzel, MD
Chairman, Department of Anesthesiology Critical
    Care Medicine
The Anne O'M elveney Wilson Professor of
    Critical Care Medicine
Children's Hospital of Los Angeles
Professor of Pediatrics and Anesthesiology
University of Southern California Keck School of
    Medicine
Director, The Laura P. and Leland K. Whittier
    Virtual PICU
Los Angeles, California
Anesthesia, Perioperative Care, and Sedation

Isaiah D. Wexler, MD, PhD
Associate Professor
Department of Pediatrics
Hadassah University Medical Center
Jerusalem, Israel
Effects of War on Children

Elizabeth A. Wharff, PhD, LICSW
Assistant Professor of Psychiatry
Harvard Medical School
Director, Emergency Psychiatry Service
Boston Children's Hospital
Boston, Massachusetts
Suicide and Attempted Suicide

A. Clinton White Jr., MD
Paul R. Stalnaker MD Distinguished Professor of
    Medicine
Director, Infectious Disease Division
University of Texas Medical Branch
Galveston, Texas
Adult Tapeworm Infections
Cysticercosis
Echinococcosis (Echinococcus granulosus and
    Echinococcus multilocularis)

Perrin C. White, MD
Professor of Pediatrics
Audre Newman Rapoport Distinguished Chair in
    Pediatric Endocrinology
University of Texas Southwestern Medical Center
Dallas, Texas
Physiology of the Adrenal Gland
Adrenocortical Insufficiency
Congenital Adrenal Hyperplasia and Related
    Disorders
Cushing Syndrome
Primary Aldosteronism
Adrenocortical Tumors
Pheochromocytoma
Adrenal Masses

John V. Williams, MD
Assistant Professor of Pediatrics and of Pathology,
    Microbiology, and Immunology
Division of Pediatric Infectious Disease
Vanderbilt University School of Medicine
Nashville, Tennessee
Adenoviruses
Rhinoviruses
The Common Cold

Rodney E. Willoughby Jr., MD
Professor of Pediatrics
Medical College of Wisconsin
Pediatric Infectious Diseases
Children's Hospital of Wisconsin
Milwaukee, Wisconsin
Rabies

Michael Wilschanski, MBBS
Professor of Pediatrics
The Hebrew University–Hadassah School of
    Medicine
Director, Pediatric Gastroenterology Unit
Hadassah University Hospitals
Jerusalem, Israel
Embryology, Anatomy, and Physiology (Pancreas)
Pancreatic Function Tests
Disorders of the Exocrine Pancreas
Treatment of Pancreatic Insufficiency
Pancreatitis
Pseudocyst of the Pancreas
Pancreatic Tumors

Pamela Wilson, MD
Associate Professor
Department of Physical Medicine and
    Rehabilitation
University of Colorado School of Medicine
Children's Hospital Colorado
Denver, Colorado
Meningomyelocele (Spina Bifida)

Samantha L. Wilson, PhD
Associate Professor
Department of Pediatrics
Medical College of Wisconsin
Children's Hospital of Wisconsin
Child Development Center, International Adoption
    Clinic
Milwaukee, Wisconsin
Adoption

Jennifer J. Winell, MD
Attending Orthopaedic Surgeon
Department of Orthopaedic Surgery
Children's Hospital of Philadelphia
Philadelphia, Pennsylvania
The Foot and Toes

Glenna B. Winnie, MD
Director, Pediatric and Adolescent Sleep Center
Fairfax Neonatal Associates, PC
Fairfax, Virginia
Emphysema and Overinflation
α_1-*Antitrypsin Deficiency and Emphysema*
Pleurisy, Pleural Effusions, and Empyema
Pneumothorax
Pneumomediastinum
Hydrothorax
Hemothorax
Chylothorax

Harland S. Winter, MD
Associate Professor of Pediatrics
Harvard Medical School
Director, Pediatric Inflammatory Bowel Disease
    Center
MassGeneral Hospital for Children
Boston, Massachusetts
Chronic Diarrhea

Paul H. Wise, MD, MPH
Richard E. Behrman Professor of Child Health and
    Society
Professor of Pediatrics
Stanford University School of Medicine
Director, Center for Policy, Outcomes, and
    Prevention
Senior Fellow, Freeman-Spogli Institute for
    International Studies
Stanford, California
Chronic Illness in Childhood

Joshua Wolf, MBBS, FRACP
Assistant Member
Department of Infectious Diseases
St. Jude's Children's Research Hospital
Memphis, Tennessee
Infection Associated with Medical Devices

Joanne Wolfe, MD, MPH
Associate Professor of Pediatrics
Harvard Medical School
Chief, Division of Pediatric Palliative Care
Dana-Farber Cancer Institute
Director, Pediatric Palliative Care
Boston Children's Hospital
Boston, Massachusetts
Pediatric Palliative Care

James B. Wood, MD
Clinical Fellow
Pediatric Infectious Diseases
Vanderbilt University Medical Center
Nashville, Tennessee
Streptococcus pneumoniae (Pneumococcus)

Laura L. Worth, MD, PhD
Associate Professor of Pediatrics
University of Texas MD Anderson Cancer Center
Center Medical Director
The Children's Cancer Hospital
Houston, Texas
Molecular and Cellular Biology of Cancer

Joseph L. Wright, MD, MPH
Professor and Chair
Department of Pediatrics
Professor of Emergency Medicine
Howard University College of Medicine
Washington, DC
Emergency Medical Services for Children

Terry W. Wright, PhD
Associate Professor of Pediatrics
Division of Pediatric Infectious Diseases
University of Rochester School of Medicine and
    Dentistry
Rochester, New York
Pneumocystis jiroveci (Pneumocystis carinii)

Eveline Y. Wu, MD
Assistant Professor
Department of Pediatrics
Division of Allergy, Immunology, and
    Rheumatology
University of North Carolina at Chapel Hill
Chapel Hill, North Carolina
Juvenile Idiopathic Arthritis
Sarcoidosis

Pablo Yagupsky, MD
Professor of Pediatrics and Clinical Microbiology
Goldman School of Medicine
Ben-Gurion University of the Negev
Beer-Sheva, Israel
Kingella kingae

Michael Yaron, MD
Professor
Department of Emergency Medicine
University of Colorado School of Medicine
Aurora, Colorado
*Altitude-Associated Illness in Children (Acute
    Mountain Sickness)*

Ram Yogev, MD
Susan B. DePree Founders' Board Professor of
    Pediatrics
Northwestern University Feinberg School of
    Medicine
Director, Pediatric, Adolescent, and Maternal HIV
    Infection
Ann & Robert H. Lurie Children's Hospital of
    Chicago
Chicago, Illinois
*Acquired Immunodeficiency Syndrome (Human
    Immunodeficiency Virus)*

JiaDe Yu, MD
Resident Physician
Department of Dermatology
Medical College of Wisconsin
Children's Hospital of Wisconsin
Milwaukee, Wisconsin
Diseases of Subcutaneous Tissue

Marc Yudkoff, MD
William T. Grant Professor in Pediatrics
University of Pennsylvania Perelman School of
    Medicine
Institute for Translational Medicine and
    Therapeutics
Division of Developmental and Behavioral
    Pediatrics
Children's Hospital of Philadelphia
Philadelphia, Pennsylvania
*Urea Cycle and Hyperammonemia (Arginine,
    Citrulline, Ornithine)*

Peter E. Zage, MD, PhD
Assistant Professor of Pediatrics
Section of Pediatric Hematology/Oncology
Baylor College of Medicine
Houston, Texas
Neuroblastoma

Ramia Zakhour, MD
Pediatric Infectious Diseases Fellow
University of Texas Health Sciences Center
Houston, Texas
Yersinia

Lonnie K. Zeltzer, MD
Distinguished Professor
Departments of Anesthesiology, Psychiatry, and
    Biobehavioral Sciences
David Geffen School of Medicine at UCLA
Director, Children's Pain and Comfort Care
    Program
Mattel Children's Hospital UCLA
Los Angeles, California
Pediatric Pain Management

Klaus-Peter Zimmer, MD
Abt. Allgemeine Pädiatrie und Neonatologie
Zentrum für Kinderheilkunde und Jugendmedizin
Universitätsklinikum Gießen und Marburg GmbH
Gießen, Germany
Rare Inborn Defects Causing Malabsorption

Naama Zoran, PhD
Developmental Psychologist
International Educational Systems Consultant
Mequon, Wisconsin
*The Reggio Emilia Educational Approach and Child
    Development and Learning*

Barry S. Zuckerman, MD
Professor of Pediatrics and Chair Emeritus
Boston University School of Medicine
Boston Medical Center
Boston, Massachusetts
Impact of Violence on Children

Preface

Whoever saves one life it is considered as if they saved an entire world.
— Babylonian Talmud

The 20th edition of *Nelson Textbook of Pediatrics* continues in its tradition of being an essential resource for pediatricians as they diagnose and treat the infants, children, and adolescents of the 21st century. The 20th edition has been thoroughly revised, updated, and edited to keep up with the growing data accumulated from basic, clinical, and population-based research. The promise that translational medicine will improve the lives of all children is greater than ever. Knowledge of human development, behavior, and diseases from the molecular to sociologic levels is increasing at fantastic rates, leading to greater understanding of health and illness in children and substantial improvements in health quality for those who have access to health care. These exciting scientific advances also provide hope to effectively address prevention and treatment of new and emerging diseases threatening children and their families.

The field of pediatrics encompasses advocacy for all children throughout the world and must address societal inequalities of important resources required for normal development, as well as protection from natural and manmade disasters. Unfortunately, many children throughout the world have not benefited from the significant advances in the prevention and treatment of health-related problems, primarily because of a lack of political will and misplaced priorities. For our increasing knowledge to benefit all children and youth, medical advances and good clinical practice must always be coupled with effective advocacy.

This new edition of *Nelson Textbook of Pediatrics* attempts to provide the essential information that practitioners, house staff, medical students, and other care providers involved in pediatric health care throughout the world need to understand to effectively address the enormous range of biologic, psychologic, and social problems that our children and youth may face. Our goal is to be comprehensive yet concise and reader friendly, embracing both the new advances in clinical science and the time-honored art of pediatric practice.

The 20th edition is reorganized and revised from the previous edition. There are many additions of new diseases and new chapters, as well as substantial expansion or significant modification of others. In addition many more tables, photographs, imaging studies, and illustrative figures, as well as up-to-date references, have been added. Although, to an ill child and his or her family and physician, even the rarest disorder is of central importance, all health problems cannot possibly be covered with the same degree of detail in one general textbook of pediatrics. Thus, leading articles and subspecialty texts are referenced and should be consulted when more information is desired.

The outstanding value of the 20th edition of the textbook is due to its expert and authoritative contributors. We are all indebted to these dedicated authors for their hard work, knowledge, thoughtfulness, and good judgment. Our sincere appreciation also goes to Kate Dimock and Jennifer Shreiner at Elsevier and to Carolyn Redman at the Pediatric Department of the Medical College of Wisconsin. In addition, we thank Barbara Ruggeri for her excellent library science skills and for keeping us up to date with the literature. We have all worked hard to produce an edition that will be helpful to those who provide care for children and youth and to those desiring to know more about children's health worldwide.

In this edition we have had informal assistance from many faculty and house staff of the departments of pediatrics at the Medical College of Wisconsin, Wayne State University School of Medicine, University of Pennsylvania School of Medicine, and University of Rochester School of Medicine. The help of these individuals and of the many practicing pediatricians from around the world who have taken the time to offer thoughtful feedback and suggestions is always greatly appreciated and helpful.

Last and certainly not least, we especially wish to thank our families for their patience and understanding, without which this textbook would not have been possible.

Robert M. Kliegman, MD
Bonita F. Stanton, MD
Joseph W. St Geme III, MD
Nina F. Schor, MD, PhD

Contents

PART XIII

Adolescent Medicine

VOLUME 2

PART XVIII

The Digestive System

†Deceased.

| Contents

PART **XIX**

Respiratory System

PART **XXI**

Diseases of the Blood

PART XXIV

Urologic Disorders in Infants and Children

PART XXV

Gynecologic Problems of Childhood

PART XXVI

The Endocrine System

PART XXVIII

Neuromuscular Disorders

PART XXIX

Disorders of the Eye

PART **XXX**

The Ear

PART **XXXI**

The Skin

PART XXXII

Bone and Joint Disorders

PART XXXIII

Rehabilitation Medicine

PART XXXIV

Environmental Health Hazards

Nelson
TEXTBOOK *of*
PEDIATRICS

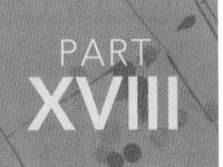
Section 1

Clinical Manifestations of Gastrointestinal Disease

Chapter 305

Normal Digestive Tract Phenomena

Chris A. Liacouras

Gastrointestinal function varies with maturity; what is a physiologic event in a newborn or infant might be a pathologic symptom at an older age. A fetus can swallow amniotic fluid as early as 12 wk of gestation, but nutritive sucking in neonates first develops at about 34 wk of gestation. The coordinated oral and pharyngeal movements necessary for swallowing solids develop within the 1st few mo of life. Before this time, the tongue thrust is upward and outward to express milk from the nipple, instead of a backward motion, which propels solids toward the esophageal inlet. By 1 mo of age, infants appear to show preferences for sweet and salty foods. Infants' interest in solids increases at approximately 4 mo of age. The recommendation to begin solids at 6 mo of age is based on nutritional and cultural concepts rather than maturation of the swallowing process (see Chapter 45). Infants swallow air during feeding, and burping is encouraged to prevent gaseous distention of the stomach.

A number of normal anatomic variations may be noted in the mouth. A **short lingual frenulum** ("tongue-tie") may be worrisome to parents but only rarely interferes with eating or speech, generally requiring no treatment. **Surface furrowing** of the tongue (a geographic or scrotal tongue) is usually a normal finding. A **bifid uvula** may be normal or associated with a submucous cleft of the soft palate.

Regurgitation, the result of gastroesophageal reflux, occurs commonly in the 1st yr of life. Effortless regurgitation can dribble out of an infant's mouth but also may be forceful. In an otherwise healthy infant with regurgitation, volumes of emesis are commonly approximately 15-30 mL but occasionally are larger. Most often, the infant remains happy, although possibly hungry, after an episode of regurgitation. Episodes can occur from one to several times per day. Regurgitation gradually resolves in 80% of infants by 6 mo of age and in 90% by 12 mo. If complications develop or regurgitation persists, gastroesophageal reflux is considered pathologic rather than merely developmental and deserves further evaluation and treatment. Complications of gastroesophageal reflux include failure to thrive, pulmonary disease (apnea or aspiration pneumonitis), and esophagitis with its sequelae (see Chapters 323 and 324).

Infants and young children may be erratic eaters; this may be a worry to parents. A toddler might eat insatiably or refuse to consume food during a meal. Toddlers and young children also tend to eat only a limited variety of foods. Parents should be encouraged to view nutritional intake over several days and not be overly concerned about individual meals. Infancy and adolescence are periods of rapid growth; high nutrient requirements for growth may be associated with vora-

cious appetites. The reduced appetite of toddlers and preschool children is often a worry to parents who are used to the relatively greater dietary intake during infancy. Demonstration of age-appropriate growth on a growth curve is reassuring.

The number, color, and consistency of stools can vary greatly in the same infant and between infants of similar age without apparent explanation. The earliest stools after birth consist of meconium, a dark, viscous material that is normally passed within the 1st 48 hr of life. With the onset of feeding, meconium is replaced by green-brown transition stools, often containing curds, and, after 4-5 days, by yellow-brown milk stools. **Stool frequency** is extremely variable in normal infants and can vary from none to 7 per day. Breastfed infants can have frequent small, loose stools early (transition stools), and then after 2-3 wk can have very infrequent soft stools. Some nursing infants might not pass any stool for 1-2 wk and then have a normal soft bowel movement. The color of stool has little significance except for the presence of blood or absence of bilirubin products (white-gray rather than yellow-brown). The presence of vegetable matter, such as peas or corn, in the stool of an older infant or toddler ingesting solids is normal and suggests poor chewing and not malabsorption. A pattern of intermittent loose stools, known as **toddler's diarrhea,** occurs commonly between 1 and 3 yr of age. These otherwise healthy growing children often drink excessive carbohydrate-containing beverages. The stools typically occur during the day and not overnight. The volume of fluid intake is often excessive; limiting sugar and unabsorbable carbohydrate-containing beverages and increasing fat in the diet often leads to resolution of the pattern of loose stools.

A protuberant abdomen is often noted in infants and toddlers, especially after large feedings. This can result from the combination of weak abdominal musculature, relatively large abdominal organs, and lordotic stance. In the 1st yr of life, it is common to palpate the liver 1-2 cm below the right costal margin. The normal liver is soft in consistency and percusses to normal size for age. A Riedel lobe is a thin projection of the right lobe of the liver that may be palpated low in the right lateral abdomen. A soft spleen tip might also be palpable as a normal finding. In thin young children, the vertebral column is easily palpable, and an overlying structure may be mistaken for a mass. Pulsation of the aorta can be appreciated. Normal stool can often be palpated in the left lower quadrant in the descending or sigmoid colon.

Blood loss from the gastrointestinal tract is never normal, but swallowed blood may be misinterpreted as gastrointestinal bleeding. Maternal blood may be ingested at the time of birth or later by a nursing infant if there is bleeding near the mother's nipple. Nasal or oropharyngeal bleeding is occasionally mistaken for gastrointestinal bleeding (see Chapter 103.4). Red dyes in foods or drinks can turn the stool red but do not produce a positive test result for occult blood.

Jaundice is common in neonates, especially among premature infants, and usually results from the inability of an immature liver to conjugate bilirubin, leading to an elevated indirect component (see Chapter 102.4). Persistent elevation of indirect bilirubin levels in nursing infants may be a result of breast milk jaundice, which is usually a benign entity in full-term infants. An elevated direct bilirubin is not normal and suggests liver disease, although in infants it may be a result of extrahepatic infection (urinary tract infection). The direct bilirubin fraction should account for no more than 15-20% of the total serum bilirubin. Elevations in direct bilirubin levels can follow indirect hyperbilirubinemia as the liver converts excessive indirect to direct bilirubin and the rate-limiting step in bilirubin excretion shifts from the glucuronidation of bilirubin to excretion of direct bilirubin into the bile canaliculus. Indirect hyperbilirubinemia, which occurs commonly in normal newborns, tends to tint the sclerae and skin golden yellow, whereas direct hyperbilirubinemia produces a greenish yellow hue.

Chapter 306

Major Symptoms and Signs of Digestive Tract Disorders

Raman Sreedharan and Chris A. Liacouras

Disorders of organs outside the gastrointestinal (GI) tract can produce symptoms and signs that mimic digestive tract disorders and should be considered in the differential diagnosis (Table 306-1). In children with normal growth and development, treatment may be initiated without a formal evaluation based on a presumptive diagnosis after taking a history and performing a physical examination. Poor weight gain or weight loss is often associated with a significant pathologic process and usually necessitates a more formal evaluation.

DYSPHAGIA

Difficulty in swallowing is termed *dysphagia*. Painful swallowing is termed **odynophagia**. **Globus** is the sensation of something stuck in the throat without a clear etiology. Swallowing is a complex process that starts in the mouth with mastication and lubrication of food that is formed into a bolus. The bolus is pushed into the pharynx by the tongue. The pharyngeal phase of swallowing is rapid and involves protective mechanisms to prevent food from entering the airway. The epiglottis is lowered over the larynx while the soft palate is elevated against the nasopharyngeal wall; respiration is temporarily arrested while the upper esophageal sphincter opens to allow the bolus to enter the esophagus. In the esophagus, peristaltic coordinated muscular contractions push the food bolus toward the stomach. The lower esophageal sphincter relaxes shortly after the upper esophageal sphincter, so liquids that rapidly clear the esophagus enter the stomach without resistance.

Dysphagia is classified as oropharyngeal dysphagia and esophageal dysphagia. **Oropharyngeal dysphagia** occurs when the transfer of the food bolus from the mouth to the esophagus is impaired (also termed *transfer dysphagia*). The striated muscles of the mouth, pharynx, and upper esophageal sphincter are affected in oropharyngeal dysphagia. Neurologic and muscular disorders can give rise to oropharyngeal dysphagia (Table 306-2). The most serious complication of oropharyngeal dysphagia is life-threatening aspiration.

A complex sequence of neuromuscular events is involved in the transfer of foods to the upper esophagus. Abnormalities of the muscles involved in the ingestion process and their innervation, strength, or coordination are associated with transfer dysphagia in infants and children. In such cases, an oropharyngeal problem is usually part of a more generalized neurologic or muscular problem (botulism, diphtheria, neuromuscular disease). Painful oral lesions, such as acute viral stomatitis or trauma, occasionally interfere with ingestion. If the nasal air passage is seriously obstructed, the need for respiration causes severe distress when suckling. Although severe structural, dental, and salivary abnormalities would be expected to create difficulties, ingestion proceeds relatively well in most affected children if they are hungry.

Esophageal dysphagia occurs when there is difficulty in transporting the food bolus down the esophagus. Esophageal dysphagia can result from neuromuscular disorders or mechanical obstruction (Table 306-3). Primary motility disorders causing impaired peristaltic function and dysphagia are rare in children. Achalasia is an esophageal motility disorder with associated inability of relaxation of the lower esophageal sphincter, and it rarely occurs in children. Motility of the distal esophagus is disordered after surgical repair of

Table 306-1	Some Nondigestive Tract Causes of Gastrointestinal Symptoms in Children

ANOREXIA
Systemic disease: inflammatory, neoplastic
Cardiorespiratory compromise
Iatrogenic: drug therapy, unpalatable therapeutic diets
Depression
Anorexia nervosa

VOMITING
Inborn errors of metabolism
Medications: erythromycin, chemotherapy, nonsteroidal anti-inflammatory drugs
Increased intracranial pressure
Brain tumor
Infection of the urinary tract
Labyrinthitis
Adrenal insufficiency
Pregnancy
Psychogenic
Abdominal migraine
Toxins
Renal disease

DIARRHEA
Infection: otitis media, urinary
Uremia
Medications: antibiotics, cisapride
Tumors: neuroblastoma
Pericarditis
Adrenal insufficiency

CONSTIPATION
Hypothyroidism
Spina bifida
Developmental delay
Dehydration: diabetes insipidus, renal tubular lesions
Medications: narcotics
Lead poisoning
Infant botulism

ABDOMINAL PAIN
Pyelonephritis, hydronephrosis, renal colic
Pneumonia (lower lobe)
Pelvic inflammatory disease
Porphyria
Angioedema
Endocarditis
Abdominal migraine
Familial Mediterranean fever
Sexual or physical abuse
Systemic lupus erythematosus
School phobia
Sickle cell crisis
Vertebral disk inflammation
Psoas abscess
Pelvic osteomyelitis or myositis
Medications

ABDOMINAL DISTENTION OR MASS
Ascites: nephrotic syndrome, neoplasm, heart failure
Discrete mass: Wilms tumor, hydronephrosis, neuroblastoma, mesenteric cyst, hepatoblastoma, lymphoma
Pregnancy

JAUNDICE
Hemolytic disease
Urinary tract infection
Sepsis
Hypothyroidism
Panhypopituitarism

tracheoesophageal fistula or achalasia. Abnormal motility can accompany collagen vascular disorders. Mechanical obstruction can be intrinsic or extrinsic. Intrinsic structural defects cause a fixed impediment to the passage of food bolus because of a narrowing within the esophagus, as in a stricture, web, or tumor. Extrinsic obstruction is

Table 306-2	Causes of Oropharyngeal Dysphagia

NEUROMUSCULAR DISORDERS
Cerebral palsy
Brain tumors
Cerebrovascular accidents
Polio and postpolio syndromes
Multiple sclerosis
Myositis
Dermatomyositis
Myasthenia gravis
Muscular dystrophies
Acquired or inherited dystonia syndrome
Dysautonomia

METABOLIC AND AUTOIMMUNE DISORDERS
Hyperthyroidism
Systemic lupus erythematosus
Sarcoidosis
Amyloidosis

INFECTIOUS DISEASE
Meningitis
Botulism
Diphtheria
Lyme disease
Neurosyphilis
Viral infection: polio, Coxsackievirus, herpes, cytomegalovirus

STRUCTURAL LESIONS
Inflammatory: abscess, pharyngitis
Congenital web
Cricopharyngeal bar
Dental problems
Bullous skin lesions
Plummer-Vinson syndrome
Zenker diverticulum
Extrinsic compression: osteophytes, lymph nodes, thyroid swelling

OTHER
Corrosive injury
Side effects of medications
After surgery
After radiation therapy

Adapted from Gasiorowska A, Faas R: Current approach to dysphagia, Gastroenterol Hepatol 5(4):269–279, 2009.

Table 306-3	Causes of Esophageal Dysphagia

NEUROMUSCULAR DISORDERS
GERD
Achalasia cardia
Diffuse esophageal spasm
Scleroderma

MECHANICAL
Intrinsic Lesions
Foreign bodies including pills
Esophagitis: GERD, eosinophilic esophagitis
Stricture: corrosive injury, pill induced, peptic
Esophageal webs
Esophageal rings
Esophageal diverticula
Neoplasm
Extrinsic Lesions
Vascular compression
Mediastinal lesion
Cervical osteochondritis
Vertebral abnormalities

GERD, gastroesophageal reflux disease.
Adapted from Gasiorowska A, Faas R: Current approach to dysphagia, Gastroenterol Hepatol 5(4):269–279, 2009.

caused by compression from vascular rings, mediastinal lesions, or vertebral abnormalities. Structural defects typically cause more problems in swallowing solids than liquids. In infants, esophageal web, tracheobronchial remnant, or vascular ring can cause dysphagia. An esophageal stricture secondary to esophagitis (chronic gastroesophageal reflux, eosinophilic esophagitis, chronic infections) occasionally has dysphagia as the first manifestation. An esophageal foreign body or a stricture secondary to a caustic ingestion also causes dysphagia. A Schatzki ring, a thin ring of mucosal tissue near the lower esophageal sphincter, is another mechanical cause of recurrent dysphagia, and again is rare in children.

When dysphagia is associated with a delay in passage through the esophagus, the patient may be able to point to the level of the chest where the delay occurs, but esophageal symptoms are usually referred to the suprasternal notch. When a patient points to the suprasternal notch, the impaction can be found anywhere in the esophagus.

REGURGITATION

Regurgitation is the effortless movement of stomach contents into the esophagus and mouth. It is not associated with distress, and infants with regurgitation are often hungry immediately after an episode. The lower esophageal sphincter prevents reflux of gastric contents into the esophagus. Regurgitation is a result of gastroesophageal reflux through an incompetent or, in infants, immature lower esophageal sphincter. This is often a developmental process, and regurgitation or "spitting" resolves with maturity. Regurgitation should be differentiated from

vomiting, which denotes an active reflex process with an extensive differential diagnosis (Table 306-4).

ANOREXIA

Anorexia means prolonged lack of appetite. Hunger and satiety centers are located in the hypothalamus; it seems likely that afferent nerves from the GI tract to these brain centers are important determinants of the anorexia that characterizes many diseases of the stomach and intestine (see Chapter 47). Satiety is stimulated by distention of the stomach or upper small bowel, the signal being transmitted by sensory afferents, which are especially dense in the upper gut. Chemoreceptors in the intestine, influenced by the assimilation of nutrients, also affect afferent flow to the appetite centers. Impulses reach the hypothalamus from higher centers, possibly influenced by pain or the emotional disturbance of an intestinal disease. Other regulatory factors include hormones, ghrelin, leptin, and plasma glucose, which, in turn, reflect intestinal function (see Chapter 47).

VOMITING

Vomiting is a highly coordinated reflex process that may be preceded by increased salivation and begins with involuntary retching. Violent descent of the diaphragm and constriction of the abdominal muscles with relaxation of the gastric cardia actively force gastric contents back up the esophagus. This process is coordinated in the medullary vomiting center, which is influenced directly by afferent innervation and indirectly by the chemoreceptor trigger zone and higher central nervous system (CNS) centers. Many acute or chronic processes can cause vomiting (see Tables 306-1 and 306-4).

Vomiting caused by obstruction of the GI tract is probably mediated by intestinal visceral afferent nerves stimulating the vomiting center (Table 306-5). If obstruction occurs below the second part of the duodenum, vomitus is usually bile stained. Emesis can also become bile stained with repeated vomiting in the absence of obstruction when duodenal contents are refluxed into the stomach. Nonobstructive lesions of the digestive tract can also cause vomiting; this includes diseases of the upper bowel, pancreas, liver, or biliary tree. CNS or metabolic derangements can lead to severe, persistent emesis.

Cyclic vomiting is a syndrome with numerous episodes of vomiting interspersed with well intervals. The North American Society for Pediatric Gastroenterology, Hepatology and Nutrition consensus statement on the diagnosis and management of cyclic vomiting criteria are listed in Table 306-6. Rome III criteria for functional GI disorders have 2 criteria for cyclic vomiting in children, and both these criteria have to

Table 306-4	Differential Diagnosis of Emesis During Childhood	
INFANT	**CHILD**	**ADOLESCENT**
COMMON		
Gastroenteritis	Gastroenteritis	Gastroenteritis
Gastroesophageal reflux	Systemic infection	GERD
Overfeeding	Gastritis	Systemic infection
Anatomic obstruction*	Toxic ingestion	Toxic ingestion
Systemic infection†	Pertussis syndrome	Gastritis
Pertussis syndrome	Medication	Sinusitis
Otitis media	Reflux (GERD)	Inflammatory bowel disease
	Sinusitis	Appendicitis
	Otitis media	Migraine
	Anatomic obstruction*	Pregnancy
	Eosinophilic esophagitis	Medications
		Ipecac abuse, bulimia
		Concussion
RARE		
Adrenogenital syndrome	Reye syndrome	Reye syndrome
Inborn errors of metabolism	Hepatitis	Hepatitis
Brain tumor (increased intracranial pressure)	Peptic ulcer	Peptic ulcer
Subdural hemorrhage	Pancreatitis	Pancreatitis
Food poisoning	Brain tumor	Brain tumor
Rumination	Increased intracranial pressure	Increased intracranial pressure
Renal tubular acidosis	Middle ear disease	Concussion
Ureteropelvic junction obstruction	Chemotherapy	Middle ear disease
Pseudoobstruction	Achalasia	Chemotherapy
	Cyclic vomiting (migraine)	Cyclic vomiting (migraine)
	Esophageal stricture	Biliary colic
	Duodenal hematoma	Renal colic
	Inborn error of metabolism	Diabetic ketoacidosis
	Pseudoobstruction	Pseudoobstruction
		Intestinal tumor
		Achalasia

*Includes malrotation, pyloric stenosis, intussusception, Hirschsprung disease.
†Meningitis, sepsis.
GERD, gastroesophageal reflux disease, inguinal hernia.

Table 306-5	Causes of Gastrointestinal Obstruction	
ESOPHAGUS	Ileal atresia	
Congenital	Meconium ileus	
Esophageal atresia	Meckel diverticulum with volvulus or intussusception	
Vascular rings	Inguinal hernia	
Schatzki ring	Internal hernia	
Tracheobronchial remnant	Intestinal duplication	
Acquired	Pseudoobstruction	
Esophageal stricture	*Acquired*	
Foreign body	Postsurgical adhesions	
Achalasia	Crohn disease	
Chagas disease	Intussusception	
Collagen vascular disease	Distal ileal obstruction syndrome (cystic fibrosis)	
	Duodenal hematoma	
STOMACH	Superior mesenteric artery syndrome	
Congenital		
Antral webs	**COLON**	
Pyloric stenosis	*Congenital*	
Acquired	Meconium plug	
Bezoar, foreign body	Hirschsprung disease	
Pyloric stricture (ulcer)	Colonic atresia, stenosis	
Chronic granulomatous disease of childhood	Imperforate anus	
Eosinophilic gastroenteritis	Rectal stenosis	
Crohn disease	Pseudoobstruction	
Epidermolysis bullosa	Volvulus	
	Colonic duplication	
SMALL INTESTINE	*Acquired*	
Congenital	Ulcerative colitis (toxic megacolon)	
Duodenal atresia	Chagas disease	
Annular pancreas	Crohn disease	
Malrotation/volvulus	Fibrosing colonopathy (cystic fibrosis)	
Malrotation/Ladd bands		

be present for a diagnosis of cyclic vomiting: 2 or more periods of intense nausea and unremitting vomiting or retching lasting hours to days and return to usual state of health lasting weeks to months.

The onset of cyclic vomiting is usually between 2 and 5 yr of age but has been observed in infants and adults. The frequency of vomiting episodes is variable (average of 12 episodes per yr) with each episode typically lasting 2-3 days and 4 or more emesis episodes per hour. The episodes usually occur in the early hours of the morning or upon wakening. Patients can have a prodrome of nausea, pallor, intolerance of noise or light, lethargy, and headache. Epigastric pain, abdominal pain, diarrhea, and fever are seen in many patients, making the diagnosis difficult. Precipitants include infection, physical stress, and psychologic stress.

Several theories have been proposed as causative factors, including a migraine-related mechanism, mitochondrial disorders, and autonomic dysfunction. More than 80% of affected children have a 1st-degree relative with migraines; many patients develop migraines later in life. Many children show evidence for sympathetic autonomic dysfunction of sudomotor systems. The differential diagnosis includes GI anomalies (malrotation, duplication cysts, choledochal cysts, recurrent intussusceptions), CNS disorders (neoplasm, epilepsy, vestibular pathology), nephrolithiasis, cholelithiasis, hydronephrosis, metabolic-endocrine disorders (urea cycle, fatty acid metabolism, Addison disease, porphyria, hereditary angioedema, familial Mediterranean fever), chronic appendicitis, and inflammatory bowel disease. Laboratory evaluation is based on a careful history and physical examination and may include, if indicated, endoscopy, contrast GI radiography, brain MRI, and metabolic studies (lactate, organic acids, ammonia). Treatment includes hydration and antiemetics (e.g., ondansetron). Prevention may be possible with lifestyle changes and prophylactic medications (cyproheptadine, propranolol, amitriptyline, phenobarbital) based on the patient's age.

Potential complications of emesis are noted in Table 306-7. Broad management strategies for vomiting in general and specific causes of emesis are noted in Tables 306-8 and 306-9.

DIARRHEA

Diarrhea is best defined as excessive loss of fluid and electrolyte in the stool. Acute diarrhea is defined as sudden onset of excessively loose stools of >10 mL/kg/day in infants and >200 g/24 hr in older children, which lasts <14 days. When the episode lasts longer than 14 days, it is called *chronic* or *persistent diarrhea*.

Normally, a young infant has approximately 5 mL/kg/day of stool output; the volume increases to 200 g/24 hr in an adult. The greatest volume of intestinal water is absorbed in the small bowel; the colon concentrates intestinal contents against a high osmotic gradient. The small intestine of an adult can absorb 10-11 L/day of a combination of ingested and secreted fluid, whereas the colon absorbs approximately 0.5 L. Disorders that interfere with absorption in the small bowel tend to produce voluminous diarrhea, whereas disorders compromising colonic absorption produce lower-volume diarrhea. **Dysentery** (small-volume, frequent bloody stools with mucus, tenesmus, and urgency) is the predominant symptom of colitis.

The basis of all diarrheas is disturbed intestinal solute transport and water absorption. Water movement across intestinal membranes is passive and is determined by both active and passive fluxes of solutes, particularly sodium, chloride, and glucose. The pathogenesis of most episodes of diarrhea can be explained by secretory, osmotic, or motility abnormalities or a combination of these (Table 306-10).

Secretory diarrhea occurs when the intestinal epithelial cell solute transport system is in an active state of secretion. It is often caused by a secretagogue, such as cholera toxin, binding to a receptor on the

---

Table 306-6	Criteria for Cyclical Vomiting Syndrome

All of the criteria must be met for the consensus definition of cyclic vomiting syndrome:
- At least 5 attacks in any interval, or a minimum of 3 episodes during a 6-mo period
- Recurrent episodes of intense vomiting and nausea lasting 1 hr to 10 days and occurring at least 1 wk apart
- Stereotypical pattern and symptoms in the individual patient
- Vomiting during episodes occurs ≥4 times/hr for ≥1 hr
- Return to baseline health between episodes
- Not attributed to another disorder

Li, B UK, Lefevre F, Chelimsky GG, et al: North American Society for Pediatric Gastroenterology, Hepatology, and Nutrition consensus statement on the diagnosis and management of cyclic vomiting syndrome, J Pediatr Gastroenterol Nutr 47:379–393, 2008.

Table 306-7	Complications of Vomiting	
COMPLICATION	**PATHOPHYSIOLOGY**	**HISTORY, PHYSICAL EXAMINATION, AND LABORATORY STUDIES**
Metabolic	Fluid loss in emesis HCl loss in emesis Na, K loss in emesis Alkalosis → • Na into cells	Dehydration Alkalosis; hypochloremia Hyponatremia; hypokalemia
Nutritional	Emesis of calories and nutrients Anorexia for calories and nutrients	Malnutrition; "failure to thrive"
Mallory-Weiss tear	Retching → tear at lesser curve of gastroesophageal junction	Forceful emesis → hematemesis
Esophagitis	Chronic vomiting → esophageal acid exposure	Heartburn; Hemoccult + stool
Aspiration	Aspiration of vomitus, especially in context of obtundation	Pneumonia; neurologic dysfunction
Shock	Severe fluid loss in emesis or in accompanying diarrhea	Dehydration (accompanying diarrhea can explain acidosis?)
	Severe blood loss in hematemesis	Blood volume depletion
Pneumomediastinum, pneumothorax	Increased intrathoracic pressure	Chest x-ray
Petechiae, retinal hemorrhages	Increased intrathoracic pressure	Normal platelet count

From Kliegman RM, Greenbaum LA, Lye PS, editors: Practical strategies in pediatric diagnosis and therapy, ed 2, Philadelphia, 2004, Elsevier, p 318.

Table 306-8	Pharmacologic Therapies for Vomiting Episodes	
THERAPEUTIC DRUG CLASS	**DRUG**	**DOSAGE**
REFLUX		
Dopamine antagonist	Metoclopramide (Reglan)	0.1-0.2 mg/kg PO or IV qid
GASTROPARESIS		
Dopamine antagonist	Metoclopramide (Reglan)	0.1-0.2 mg/kg PO or IV qid
Motilin agonist	Erythromycin	3-5 mg/kg PO or IV tid-qid
INTESTINAL PSEUDOOBSTRUCTION		
Stimulation of intestinal migratory myoelectric complexes	Octreotide (Sandostatin)	1 µg/kg SC bid-tid
CHEMOTHERAPY		
Dopamine antagonist	Metoclopramide	0.5-1.0 mg/kg IV qid, with antihistamine prophylaxis of extrapyramidal side effects
Serotoninergic 5-HT$_3$ antagonist	Ondansetron (Zofran)	0.15-0.3 mg/kg IV or PO tid
Phenothiazines (extrapyramidal, hematologic side effects)	Prochlorperazine (Compazine)	≈0.3 mg/kg PO bid-tid
	Chlorpromazine (Thorazine)	>6 mo of age: 0.5 mg/kg PO or IV tid-qid
Steroids	Dexamethasone (Decadron)	0.1 mg/kg PO tid
Cannabinoids	Tetrahydrocannabinol (Nabilone)	0.05-0.1 mg/kg PO bid-tid
POSTOPERATIVE		
	Ondansetron, phenothiazines	See under chemotherapy
MOTION SICKNESS, VESTIBULAR DISORDERS		
Antihistamine	Dimenhydrinate (Dramamine)	1 mg/kg PO tid-qid
Anticholinergic	Scopolamine (Transderm Scop)	Adults: 1 patch/3 days
ADRENAL CRISIS		
Steroids	Cortisol	2 mg/kg IV bolus followed by 0.2-0.4 mg/kg/hr IV (±1 mg/kg IM)
CYCLIC VOMITING SYNDROME		
Supportive		
Analgesic	Meperidine (Demerol)	1-2 mg/kg IV or IM q 4-6 hr
Anxiolytic, sedative	Lorazepam (Ativan)	0.05-0.1 mg/kg IV q 6 hr
Antihistamine, sedative	Diphenhydramine (Benadryl)	1.25 mg/kg IV q 6 hr
Abortive		
Serotoninergic 5-HT$_3$ antagonist	Ondansetron	See above
	Granisetron (Kytril)	10 µg/kg IV q 4-6 hr
Nonsteroidal antiinflammatory agent (GI ulceration side effect)	Ketorolac (Toradol)	0.5-1.0 mg/kg IV q 6-8 hr
Serotoninergic 5-HT$_{1D}$ agonist	Sumatriptan (Imitrex)	>40 kg: 20 mg intranasally or 25 mg PO, 1 time only
PROPHYLACTIC*		
Antimigraine, β-adrenergic blocker	Propranolol (Inderal)	0.5-2.0 mg/kg PO bid
Antimigraine, antihistamine	Cyproheptadine (Periactin)	0.25-0.5 mg/kg/day PO ÷ bid-tid
Antimigraine, tricyclic antidepressant	Amitriptyline (Elavil)	0.33-0.5 mg/kg PO tid, and titrate to maximum of 3.0 mg/kg/day as needed
		Obtain baseline ECG at start of therapy, and consider monitoring drug levels
Antimigraine antiepileptic	Phenobarbital (Luminal)	2-3 mg/kg qhs
	Erythromycin (see above)	
Low-estrogen oral contraceptives	Consider for catamenial CVS episodes	

*If >1 CVS bout/mo or symptoms are extremely disabling; taken daily.
  CVS, cyclic vomiting syndrome; ECG, electrocardiogram; GI, gastrointestinal.
  From Kliegman RM, Greenbaum LA, Lye PS, editors: Practical strategies in pediatric diagnosis and therapy, ed 2, Philadelphia, 2004, Elsevier, p 317.

surface epithelium of the bowel and thereby stimulating intracellular accumulation of cyclic adenosine monophosphate or cyclic guanosine monophosphate. Some intraluminal fatty acids and bile salts cause the colonic mucosa to secrete through this mechanism. Diarrhea not associated with an exogenous secretagogue can also have a secretory component (congenital microvillus inclusion disease). Secretory diarrhea is usually of large volume and persists even with fasting. The stool osmolality is predominantly indicated by the electrolytes and the ion gap is 100 mOsm/kg or less. The ion gap is calculated by subtracting the concentration of electrolytes from total osmolality:

$$\text{Ion gap} = \text{Stool osmolality} - [(\text{Stool Na} + \text{stool K}) \times 2]$$

Osmotic diarrhea occurs after ingestion of a poorly absorbed solute. The solute may be one that is normally not well absorbed (magnesium, phosphate, lactulose, or sorbitol) or one that is not well absorbed because of a disorder of the small bowel (lactose with lactase deficiency or glucose with rotavirus diarrhea). Malabsorbed carbohydrate is fermented in the colon, and short-chain fatty acids are produced. Although short-chain fatty acids can be absorbed in the colon and used as an energy source, the net effect is increase in the osmotic solute load. This form of diarrhea is usually of lesser volume than a secretory diarrhea and stops with fasting. The osmolality of the stool will not be explained by the electrolyte content, because another osmotic component is present and so the anion gap is >100 mOsm.

Table 306-9	Supportive and Nonpharmacologic Therapies for Vomiting Episodes
DISEASE	**THERAPY**
All	Treat cause • Obstruction: operate • Allergy: change diet (±steroids) • Metabolic error: Rx defect • Acid peptic disease: H2RAs, PPIs, etc.
COMPLICATIONS	
Dehydration	IV fluids, electrolytes
Hematemesis	Transfuse, correct coagulopathy
Esophagitis	H₂RAs, PPIs
Malnutrition	NG or NJ drip feeding useful for many chronic conditions
Meconium ileus	Gastrografin enema
DIOS	Gastrografin enema; balanced colonic lavage solution (e.g., GoLYTELY)
Intussusception	Barium enema; air reduction enema
Hematemesis	Endoscopic: injection sclerotherapy or banding of esophageal varices; injection therapy, fibrin sealant application, or heater probe electrocautery for selected upper GI tract lesions
Sigmoid volvulus	Colonoscopic decompression
Reflux	Positioning; dietary measures (infants: rice cereal, 1 tbs/oz of formula)
Psychogenic components	Psychotherapy; tricyclic antidepressants; anxiolytics (e.g., diazepam: 0.1 mg/kg PO tid-qid)

DIOS, distal intestinal obstruction syndrome; GI, gastrointestinal; H₂RA, H₂-receptor antagonist; NG, nasogastric; NJ, nasojejunal; PPIs, proton pump inhibitors; tbs, tablespoon.
From Kliegman RM, Greenbaum LA, Lye PS, editors: Practical strategies in pediatric diagnosis and therapy, ed 2, Philadelphia, 2004, Elsevier, p 319.

Table 306-10	Mechanisms of Diarrhea

PRIMARY MECHANISM	DEFECT	STOOL EXAMINATION	EXAMPLES	COMMENT
Secretory	Decreased absorption, increased secretion, electrolyte transport	Watery, normal osmolality with ion gap < 100 mOsm/kg	Cholera, toxigenic *Escherichia coli*; carcinoid, VIP, neuroblastoma, congenital chloride diarrhea, *Clostridium difficile*, cryptosporidiosis (AIDS)	Persists during fasting; bile salt malabsorption can also increase intestinal water secretion; no stool leukocytes
Osmotic	Maldigestion, transport defects ingestion of unabsorbable substances	Watery, acidic, and reducing substances; increased osmolality with ion gap > 100 mOsm/kg	Lactase deficiency, glucose-galactose malabsorption, lactulose, laxative abuse	Stops with fasting; increased breath hydrogen with carbohydrate malabsorption; no stool leukocytes
Increased motility	Decreased transit time	Loose to normal-appearing stool, stimulated by gastrocolic reflex	Irritable bowel syndrome, thyrotoxicosis, postvagotomy dumping syndrome	Infection can also contribute to increased motility
Decreased motility	Defect in neuromuscular unit(s) stasis (bacterial overgrowth)	Loose to normal-appearing stool	Pseudoobstruction, blind loop	Possible bacterial overgrowth
Decreased surface area (osmotic, motility)	Decreased functional capacity	Watery	Short bowel syndrome, celiac disease, rotavirus enteritis	Might require elemental diet plus parenteral alimentation
Mucosal invasion	Inflammation, decreased colonic reabsorption, increased motility	Blood and increased WBCs in stool	*Salmonella*, *Shigella* infection; amebiasis; *Yersinia*, *Campylobacter* infection	Dysentery evident in blood, mucus, and WBCs

VIP, vasoactive intestinal peptide; WBC, white blood cell.
From Kliegman RM, Greenbaum LA, Lye PS, editors: Practical strategies in pediatric diagnosis and therapy, ed 2, Philadelphia, 2004, Elsevier, p 274.

Motility disorders can be associated with rapid or delayed transit and are not generally associated with large-volume diarrhea. Slow motility can be associated with bacterial overgrowth leading to diarrhea. The differential diagnosis of common causes of acute and chronic diarrhea is noted in Table 306-11.

CONSTIPATION

Any definition of constipation is relative and depends on stool consistency, stool frequency, and difficulty in passing the stool. A normal child might have a soft stool only every 2nd or 3rd day without

difficulty; this is not constipation. A hard stool passed with difficulty every 3rd day should be treated as constipation. Constipation can arise from defects either in filling or emptying the rectum (Table 306-12).

A nursing infant might have very infrequent stools of normal consistency; this is usually a normal pattern. True constipation in the neonatal period is most likely secondary to Hirschsprung disease, intestinal pseudoobstruction, or hypothyroidism.

Defective rectal filling occurs when colonic peristalsis is ineffective (in cases of hypothyroidism or opiate use and when bowel obstruction is caused either by a structural anomaly or by Hirschsprung disease).

Table 306-11	Differential Diagnosis of Diarrhea

INFANT	CHILD	ADOLESCENT
ACUTE		
Common		
Gastroenteritis (viral > bacterial > protozoal)	Gastroenteritis (viral > bacterial > protozoal)	Gastroenteritis (viral > bacterial > protozoal)
Systemic infection	Food poisoning	Food poisoning
Antibiotic associated	Systemic infection	Antibiotic associated
Overfeeding	Antibiotic associated	
Rare		
Primary disaccharidase deficiency	Toxic ingestion	Hyperthyroidism
Hirschsprung toxic colitis	Hemolytic uremic syndrome	Appendicitis
Adrenogenital syndrome	Intussusception	
Neonatal opiate withdrawal		
CHRONIC		
Common		
Postinfectious secondary lactase deficiency	Postinfectious secondary lactase deficiency	Irritable bowel syndrome
Cow's milk or soy protein intolerance (allergy)	Irritable bowel syndrome	Inflammatory bowel disease
Chronic nonspecific diarrhea of infancy	Celiac disease	Lactose intolerance
Excessive fruit juice (sorbitol) ingestion	Cystic fibrosis	Giardiasis
Celiac disease	Lactose intolerance	Laxative abuse (anorexia nervosa)
Cystic fibrosis	Excessive fruit juice (sorbitol) ingestion	Constipation with encopresis
AIDS enteropathy	Giardiasis	
	Inflammatory bowel disease	
	AIDS enteropathy	
Rare		
Primary immune defects	Primary and acquired immune defects	Secretory tumor
Autoimmune enteropathy	Secretory tumors	Primary bowel tumor
IPEX and IPEX-like syndromes	Pseudoobstruction	Parasitic infections and venereal diseases
Glucose-galactose malabsorption	Sucrase-isomaltase deficiency	Appendiceal abscess
Microvillus inclusion disease (microvillus atrophy)	Eosinophilic gastroenteritis	Addison disease
Congenital transport defects (chloride, sodium)	Secretory tumors	
Primary bile acid malabsorption		
Factitious syndrome by proxy		
Hirschsprung disease		
Shwachman syndrome		
Secretory tumors		
Acrodermatitis enteropathica		
Lymphangiectasia		
Abetalipoproteinemia		
Eosinophilic gastroenteritis		
Short bowel syndrome		

From Kliegman RM, Greenbaum LA, Lye PS, editors: Practical strategies in pediatric diagnosis and therapy, ed 2, Philadelphia, 2004, Elsevier, p 272.

The resultant colonic stasis leads to excessive drying of stool and a failure to initiate reflexes from the rectum that normally trigger evacuation. Emptying the rectum by spontaneous evacuation depends on a defecation reflex initiated by pressure receptors in the rectal muscle. Stool retention, therefore, can also result from lesions involving these rectal muscles, the sacral spinal cord afferent and efferent fibers, or the muscles of the abdomen and pelvic floor. Disorders of anal sphincter relaxation can also contribute to fecal retention.

Constipation tends to be self-perpetuating, whatever its cause. Hard, large stools in the rectum become difficult and even painful to evacuate; thus, more retention occurs and a vicious circle ensues. Distention of the rectum and colon lessens the sensitivity of the defecation reflex and the effectiveness of peristalsis. Fecal impaction is common and leads to other problems. Eventually, watery content from the proximal colon might percolate around hard retained stool and pass per rectum unperceived by the child. This involuntary **encopresis** may be mistaken for diarrhea. Constipation itself does not have deleterious systemic organic effects, but urinary tract stasis can accompany severe long-standing cases and constipation can generate anxiety, having a marked emotional impact on the patient and family.

ABDOMINAL PAIN

There is considerable variation among children in their perception and tolerance for abdominal pain. This is one reason the evaluation of chronic abdominal pain is difficult. A child with **functional abdomi-** **nal pain** (no identifiable organic cause) may be as uncomfortable as one with an organic cause. It is very important to distinguish between organic and nonorganic (functional) abdominal pain because the approach for the management is based on this. Normal growth and physical examination (including a rectal examination) and the absence of anemia or hematochezia are reassuring in a child who is suspected of having functional pain.

A specific cause may be difficult to find, but the nature and location of a pain-provoking lesion can usually be determined from the clinical description. Two types of nerve fibers transmit painful stimuli in the abdomen. In skin and muscle, A fibers mediate sharp localized pain; C fibers from viscera, peritoneum, and muscle transmit poorly localized, dull pain. These afferent fibers have cell bodies in the dorsal root ganglia, and some axons cross the midline and ascend to the medulla, midbrain, and thalamus. Pain is perceived in the cortex of the postcentral gyrus, which can receive impulses arising from both sides of the body. In the gut, the usual stimulus provoking pain is tension or stretching. Inflammatory lesions can lower the pain threshold, but the mechanisms producing pain of inflammation are not clear. Tissue metabolites released near nerve endings probably account for the pain caused by ischemia. Perception of these painful stimuli can be modulated by input from both cerebral and peripheral sources. Psychologic factors are particularly important. Tables 306-13 and 306-14 list features of abdominal pain. Pain that suggests a potentially serious organic etiology is associated with age younger than 5 yr; fever; weight loss;

Table 306-12	Causes of Constipation

NONORGANIC (FUNCTIONAL)—RETENTIVE

ANATOMIC
Anal stenosis, atresia with fistula
Imperforate anus
Anteriorly displaced anus
Intestinal stricture (postnecrotizing enterocolitis)
Anal stricture

ABNORMAL MUSCULATURE
Prune-belly syndrome
Gastroschisis
Down syndrome
Muscular dystrophy

INTESTINAL NERVE OR MUSCLE ABNORMALITIES
Hirschsprung disease
Pseudoobstruction (visceral myopathy or neuropathy)
Intestinal neuronal dysplasia
Spinal cord defects
Tethered cord
Spinal cord trauma
Spina bifida

DRUGS
Anticholinergics
Narcotics
Methylphenidate
Phenytoin
Antidepressants
Chemotherapeutic agents (vincristine)
Pancreatic enzymes (fibrosing colonopathy)
Lead
Vitamin D intoxication

METABOLIC DISORDERS
Hypokalemia
Hypercalcemia
Hypothyroidism
Diabetes mellitus, diabetes insipidus

INTESTINAL DISORDERS
Celiac disease
Cow's milk protein intolerance
Cystic fibrosis (meconium ileus equivalent)
Inflammatory bowel disease (stricture)
Tumor
Connective tissue disorders
Systemic lupus erythematosus
Scleroderma

PSYCHIATRIC DIAGNOSIS
Anorexia nervosa

bile or blood-stained emesis; jaundice; hepatosplenomegaly; back or flank pain or pain in a location other than the umbilicus; awakening from sleep in pain; referred pain to shoulder, groin or back; elevated erythrocyte sedimentation rate, white blood cell count, or C-reactive protein; anemia; edema; hematochezia, or a strong family history of inflammatory bowel disease or celiac disease.

Visceral pain tends to be dull and aching and is experienced in the dermatome from which the affected organ receives innervations. So, most often, the pain and tenderness is not felt over the site of the disease process. Painful stimuli originating in the liver, pancreas, biliary tree, stomach, or upper bowel are felt in the epigastrium; pain from the distal small bowel, cecum, appendix, or proximal colon is felt at the umbilicus; and pain from the distal large bowel, urinary tract, or pelvic organs is usually suprapubic. The pain from the cecum, ascending colon, and descending colon sometimes is felt at the site of the lesion because of the short mesocecum and corresponding mesocolon. The pain caused by appendicitis is initially felt in the periumbilical region, and pain from the transverse colon is usually felt in the supra pubic region. The shifting (localization) of pain is a pointer toward diagnosis; for example, periumbilical pain of a few hours localizing to the right lower quadrant suggests appendicitis. Radiation of pain can be helpful in diagnosis; for example, in biliary colic the radiation of pain is toward the inferior angle of the right scapula, pancreatic pain radiated to the back, and the renal colic pain is radiated to the inguinal region on the same side.

Somatic pain is intense and is usually well localized. When the inflamed viscus comes in contact with the somatic organ like the parietal peritoneum or the abdominal wall, pain is localized to that site. Peritonitis gives rise to generalized abdominal pain with rigidity, involuntary guarding, rebound tenderness, and cutaneous hyperesthesia on physical examination.

Referred pain from extraintestinal locations, from shared central projections with the sensory pathway from the abdominal wall, can give rise to abdominal pain, as in pneumonia when the parietal pleural pain is referred to the abdomen.

GASTROINTESTINAL HEMORRHAGE

Bleeding can occur anywhere along the GI tract, and identification of the site may be challenging (Table 306-15). Bleeding that originates in the esophagus, stomach, or duodenum can cause **hematemesis.** When exposed to gastric or intestinal juices, blood quickly darkens to resemble coffee grounds; massive bleeding is likely to be red. Red or maroon blood in stools, **hematochezia,** signifies either a distal bleeding site or massive hemorrhage above the distal ileum. Moderate to mild bleeding from sites above the distal ileum tends to cause blackened stools of tarry consistency **(melena);** major hemorrhages in the duodenum or above can also cause melena.

Erosive damage to the mucosa of the GI tract is the most common cause of bleeding, although variceal bleeding secondary to portal hypertension occurs often enough to require consideration. Prolapse gastropathy producing subepithelial hemorrhage and Mallory-Weiss lesions secondary to mucosal tears associated with emesis are causes of upper intestinal bleeds. Vascular malformations are a rare cause in children; they are difficult to identify. Upper intestinal bleeding is evaluated with esophagogastroduodenoscopy. Evaluation of the small intestine is facilitated by capsule endoscopy. The capsule-sized imaging device is swallowed in older children or placed endoscopically in younger children. Lower GI bleeding is investigated with a colonoscopy. In brisk intestinal bleeding of unknown location, a tagged red blood cell scan is helpful in locating the site of the bleeding. Occult blood in stool is usually detected by using commercially available fecal occult blood testing cards, which are based on a chemical reaction between the chemical guaiac and oxidizing action of a substrate (hemoglobin), giving a blue color. The guaiac test is very sensitive, but random testing can miss chronic blood loss, which can lead to iron-deficiency anemia. GI hemorrhage can produce hypotension and tachycardia but rarely causes GI symptoms; brisk duodenal or gastric bleeding can lead to nausea, vomiting, or diarrhea. The breakdown products of intraluminal blood might tip patients into hepatic coma if liver function is already compromised and can lead to elevation of serum bilirubin.

ABDOMINAL DISTENTION AND ABDOMINAL MASSES

Enlargement of the abdomen can result from diminished tone of the wall musculature or from increased content: fluid, gas, or solid. Ascites, the accumulation of fluid in the peritoneal cavity, distends the abdomen both in the flanks and anteriorly when it is large in volume. This fluid shifts with movement of the patient and conducts a percussion wave. Ascitic fluid is usually a transudate with a low protein concentration resulting from reduced plasma colloid osmotic pressure of hypoalbuminemia and/or from raised portal venous pressure. In cases of portal hypertension, the fluid leak probably occurs from lymphatics on the liver surface and from visceral peritoneal capillaries, but ascites does not usually develop until the serum albumin level falls. Sodium excretion in the urine decreases greatly as the ascitic fluid accumulates and, thus, additional dietary sodium goes directly to the peritoneal space, taking with it more water. When ascitic fluid contains a high protein

Table 306-13	Chronic Abdominal Pain in Children

DISORDER	CHARACTERISTICS	KEY EVALUATIONS
NONORGANIC		
Functional abdominal pain	Nonspecific pain, often periumbilical	Hx and PE; tests as indicated
Irritable bowel syndrome	Intermittent cramps, diarrhea, and constipation	Hx and PE
Nonulcer dyspepsia	Peptic ulcer–like symptoms without abnormalities on evaluation of the upper GI tract	Hx; esophagogastroduodenoscopy
GASTROINTESTINAL TRACT		
Chronic constipation	Hx of stool retention, evidence of constipation on examination	Hx and PE; plain x-ray of abdomen
Lactose intolerance	Symptoms may be associated with lactose ingestion; bloating, gas, cramps, and diarrhea	Trial of lactose-free diet; lactose breath hydrogen test
Parasite infection (especially *Giardia*)	Bloating, gas, cramps, and diarrhea	Stool evaluation for O&P; specific immunoassays for *Giardia*
Excess fructose or sorbitol ingestion	Nonspecific abdominal pain, bloating, gas, and diarrhea	Large intake of apples, fruit juice, or candy or chewing gum sweetened with sorbitol
Crohn disease	See Chapter 336	
Peptic ulcer	Burning or gnawing epigastric pain; worse on awakening or before meals; relieved with antacids	Esophagogastroduodenoscopy, upper GI contrast x-rays, or MRI enteroscopy
Esophagitis	Epigastric pain with substernal burning	Esophagogastroduodenoscopy
Meckel diverticulum	Periumbilical or lower abdominal pain; may have blood in stool (usually painless)	Meckel scan or enteroclysis
Recurrent intussusception	Paroxysmal severe cramping abdominal pain; blood may be present in stool with episode	Identify intussusception during episode or lead point in intestine between episodes with contrast studies of GI tract
Internal, inguinal, or abdominal wall hernia	Dull abdomen or abdominal wall pain	PE, CT of abdominal wall
Chronic appendicitis or appendiceal mucocele	Recurrent RLQ pain; often incorrectly diagnosed, may be rare cause of abdominal pain	Barium enema, CT
GALLBLADDER AND PANCREAS		
Cholelithiasis	RUQ pain, might worsen with meals	Ultrasound of gallbladder
Choledochal cyst	RUQ pain, mass ± elevated bilirubin	Ultrasound or CT of RUQ
Recurrent pancreatitis	Persistent boring pain, might radiate to back, vomiting	Serum amylase and lipase ± serum trypsinogen; ultrasound, CT, or MRI-ERCP of pancreas
GENITOURINARY TRACT		
Urinary tract infection	Dull suprapubic pain, flank pain	Urinalysis and urine culture; renal scan
Hydronephrosis	Unilateral abdominal or flank pain	Ultrasound of kidneys
Urolithiasis	Progressive, severe pain; flank to inguinal region to testicle	Urinalysis, ultrasound, IVP, CT
Other genitourinary disorders	Suprapubic or lower abdominal pain; genitourinary symptoms	Ultrasound of kidneys and pelvis; gynecologic evaluation
MISCELLANEOUS CAUSES		
Abdominal migraine	See text; nausea, family Hx migraine	Hx
Abdominal epilepsy	Might have seizure prodrome	EEG (can require > 1 study, including sleep-deprived EEG)
Gilbert syndrome	Mild abdominal pain (causal or coincidental?); slightly elevated unconjugated bilirubin	Serum bilirubin
Familial Mediterranean fever	Paroxysmal episodes of fever, severe abdominal pain, and tenderness with other evidence of polyserositis	Hx and PE during an episode, DNA diagnosis
Sickle cell crisis	Anemia	Hematologic evaluation
Lead poisoning	Vague abdominal pain ± constipation	Serum lead level
Henoch-Schönlein purpura	Recurrent, severe crampy abdominal pain, occult blood in stool, characteristic rash, arthritis	Hx, PE, urinalysis
Angioneurotic edema	Swelling of face or airway, crampy pain	Hx, PE, upper GI contrast x-rays, serum C1 esterase inhibitor
Acute intermittent porphyria	Severe pain precipitated by drugs, fasting, or infections	Spot urine for porphyrins

EEG, electroencephalogram; GI, gastrointestinal; Hx, history; IVP, intravenous pyelography; O&P, ova and parasites; PE, physical exam; RLQ, right lower quadrant; RUQ, right upper quadrant.

Table 306-14	Distinguishing Features of Acute Gastrointestinal Tract Pain in Children				
DISEASE	ONSET	LOCATION	REFERRAL	QUALITY	COMMENTS
Pancreatitis	Acute	Epigastric, left upper quadrant	Back	Constant, sharp, boring	Nausea, emesis, tenderness
Intestinal obstruction	Acute or gradual	Periumbilical-lower abdomen	Back	Alternating cramping (colic) and painless periods	Distention, obstipation, emesis, increased bowel sounds
Appendicitis	Acute	Periumbilical, then localized to lower right quadrant; generalized with peritonitis	Back or pelvis if retrocecal	Sharp, steady	Anorexia, nausea, emesis, local tenderness, fever with peritonitis
Intussusception	Acute	Periumbilical-lower abdomen	None	Cramping, with painless periods	Hematochezia, knees in pulled-up position
Urolithiasis	Acute, sudden	Back (unilateral)	Groin	Sharp, intermittent, cramping	Hematuria
Urinary tract infection	Acute	Back	Bladder	Dull to sharp	Fever, costovertebral angle tenderness, dysuria, urinary frequency

Table 306-15	Differential Diagnosis of Gastrointestinal Bleeding in Childhood	
INFANT	CHILD	ADOLESCENT
COMMON		
Bacterial enteritis	Bacterial enteritis	Bacterial enteritis
Milk protein allergy intolerance	Anal fissure	Inflammatory bowel disease
Intussusception	Colonic polyps	Peptic ulcer/gastritis
Swallowed maternal blood	Intussusception	Prolapse (traumatic) gastropathy secondary to emesis
Anal fissure	Peptic ulcer/gastritis	Mallory-Weiss syndrome
Lymphonodular hyperplasia	Swallowed epistaxis	Colonic polyps
	Prolapse (traumatic) gastropathy secondary to emesis	Anal fissure
	Mallory-Weiss syndrome	
RARE		
Volvulus	Esophageal varices	Hemorrhoids
Necrotizing enterocolitis	Esophagitis	Esophageal varices
Meckel diverticulum	Meckel diverticulum	Esophagitis
Stress ulcer, gastritis	Lymphonodular hyperplasia	Pill ulcer
Coagulation disorder (hemorrhagic disease of newborn)	Henoch-Schönlein purpura	Telangiectasia-angiodysplasia
Esophagitis	Foreign body	Graft-vs-host disease
	Hemangioma, arteriovenous malformation	Duplication cyst
	Sexual abuse	
	Hemolytic-uremic syndrome	
	Inflammatory bowel disease	
	Coagulopathy	
	Duplication cyst	

concentration, it is usually an exudate caused by an inflammatory or neoplastic lesion.

When fluid distends the gut, either obstruction or imbalance between absorption and secretion should be suspected. The factors causing fluid accumulation in the bowel lumen often cause gas to accumulate, too. The result may be audible gurgling noises. The source of gas is usually swallowed air, but endogenous flora can increase considerably in malabsorptive states and produce excessive gas when substrate reaches the lower intestine. Gas in the peritoneal cavity (pneumoperitoneum) is usually caused by a perforated viscus and can cause abdominal distention depending on the amount of gas leak. A tympanitic percussion note, even over solid organs such as the liver, indicates a large collection of gas in the peritoneum.

An abdominal organ can enlarge diffusely or be affected by a discrete mass. In the digestive tract, such discrete masses can occur in the lumen, wall, omentum, or mesentery. In a constipated child, mobile, nontender fecal masses are often found. Congenital anomalies, cysts, or inflammatory processes can affect the wall of the gut. Gut wall neoplasms are extremely rare in children. The pathologic enlargement of liver, spleen, bladder, and kidneys can give rise to abdominal distention.

JAUNDICE
See Chapters 102.3 and 356.

Bibliography is available at Expert Consult.

Section **2**

The Oral Cavity

Chapter **307**

Development and Developmental Anomalies of the Teeth

Norman Tinanoff

INITIATION

The primary teeth form in dental crypts that arise from a band of epithelial cells incorporated into each developing jaw. By 12 wk of fetal life, each of these epithelial bands (**dental laminae**) has 5 areas of rapid growth on each side of the maxilla and the mandible, seen as rounded, bud-like enlargements. Organization of adjacent mesenchyme takes place in each area of epithelial growth, and the 2 elements together are the beginning of a tooth.

After the formation of these crypts for the 20 primary teeth, another generation of tooth buds forms lingually (toward the tongue); these will develop into the succeeding permanent incisors, canines, and premolars that eventually replace the primary teeth. This process takes place from approximately 5 mo of gestation for the central incisors to approximately 10 mo of age for the 2nd premolars. The permanent 1st, 2nd, and 3rd molars, on the other hand, arise from extension of the dental laminae distal to the 2nd primary molars; buds for these teeth develop at approximately 4 mo of gestation, 1 yr of age, and 4-5 yr of age, respectively.

HISTODIFFERENTIATION–MORPHODIFFERENTIATION

As the epithelial bud proliferates, the deeper surface invaginates and a mass of mesenchyme becomes partially enclosed. The epithelial cells differentiate into the ameloblasts that lay down an organic matrix that forms enamel; the mesenchyme forms the dentin and dental pulp.

CALCIFICATION

After the organic matrix has been laid down, the deposition of the inorganic mineral crystals takes place from several sites of calcification that later coalesce. The characteristics of the inorganic portions of a tooth can be altered by disturbances in formation of the matrix, decreased availability of minerals, or the incorporation of foreign materials. Such disturbances can affect the color, texture, or thickness of the tooth surface. Calcification of primary teeth begins at 3-4 mo in utero and concludes postnatally at approximately 12 mo with mineralization of the 2nd primary molars (Table 307-1).

ERUPTION

At the time of tooth bud formation, each tooth begins a continuous movement toward the oral cavity. Table 307-1 lists the times of eruption of the primary and permanent teeth.

ANOMALIES ASSOCIATED WITH TOOTH DEVELOPMENT

Both failures and excesses of tooth initiation are observed. Developmentally missing teeth can result from environmental insult, a genetic defect involving only teeth, or the manifestation of a syndrome. **Anodontia,** or absence of teeth, occurs when no tooth buds form (ectodermal dysplasia, or familial missing teeth) or when there is a disturbance

Table 307-1	Calcification, Crown Completion, and Eruption		
TOOTH	**FIRST EVIDENCE OF CALCIFICATION**	**CROWN COMPLETED**	**ERUPTION**
PRIMARY DENTITION			
Maxillary			
Central incisor	3-4 mo in utero	4 mo	7.5 mo
Lateral incisor	4.5 mo in utero	5 mo	8 mo
Canine	5.5 mo in utero	9 mo	16-20 mo
First molar	5 mo in utero	6 mo	12-16 mo
Second molar	6 mo in utero	10-12 mo	20-30 mo
Mandibular			
Central incisor	4.5 mo in utero	4 mo	6.5 mo
Lateral incisor	4.5 mo in utero	4¼ mo	7 mo
Canine	5 mo in utero	9 mo	16-20 mo
First molar	5 mo in utero	6 mo	12-16 mo
Second molar	6 mo in utero	10-12 mo	20-30 mo
PERMANENT DENTITION			
Maxillary			
Central incisor	3-4 mo	4-5 yr	7-8 yr
Lateral incisor	10 mo	4-5 yr	8-9 yr
Canine	4-5 mo	6-7 yr	11-12 yr
First premolar	1.5-1¾ yr	5-6 yr	10-11 yr
Second premolar	2-2¼ yr	6-7 yr	10-12 yr
First molar	At birth	2.5-3 yr	6-7 yr
Second molar	2.5-3 yr	7-8 yr	12-13 yr
Third molar	7-9 yr	12-16 yr	17-21 yr
Mandibular			
Central incisor	3-4 mo	4-5 yr	6-7 yr
Lateral incisor	3-4 mo	4-5 yr	7-8 yr
Canine	4-5 mo	6-7 yr	9-10 yr
First premolar	1¾-2 yr	5-6 yr	10-12 yr
Second premolar	2¼-2.5 yr	6-7 yr	11-12 yr
First molar	At birth	2.5-3 yr	6-7 yr
Second molar	2.5-3 yr	7-8 yr	11-13 yr
Third molar	8-10 yr	12-16 yr	17-21 yr

Modified from Logan WHG, Kronfeld R: Development of the human jaws and surrounding structures from birth to age 15 years, J Am Dent Assoc 20:379, 1993.

of a normal site of initiation (the area of a palatal cleft). The teeth that are most commonly absent are the 3rd molars, the maxillary lateral incisors, and the mandibular 2nd premolars.

If the dental lamina produces more than the normal number of buds, **supernumerary teeth** occur, most often in the area between the maxillary central incisors. Because they tend to disrupt the position and eruption of the adjacent normal teeth, their identification by radiographic examination is important. Supernumerary teeth also occur with cleidocranial dysplasia (see Chapter 311) and in the area of cleft palates.

Twinning, in which 2 teeth are joined together, is most often observed in the mandibular incisors of the primary dentition. It can result from gemination, fusion, or concrescence. **Gemination** is the result of the division of 1 tooth germ to form a bifid crown on a single root with a common pulp canal; an extra tooth appears to be present in the dental arch. **Fusion** is the joining of incompletely developed teeth that, owing to pressure, trauma, or crowding, continue to develop as 1 tooth. Fused teeth are sometimes joined along their entire length; in other cases, a single wide crown is supported on 2 roots. **Concrescence** is the attachment of the roots of closely approximated adjacent teeth by an excessive deposit of cementum. This type of twinning, unlike the others, is found most often in the maxillary molar region.

Disturbances during differentiation can result in alterations in dental morphology, such as **macrodontia** (large teeth) or **microdontia** (small teeth). The maxillary lateral incisors can assume a slender, tapering shape (**peg-shaped laterals**).

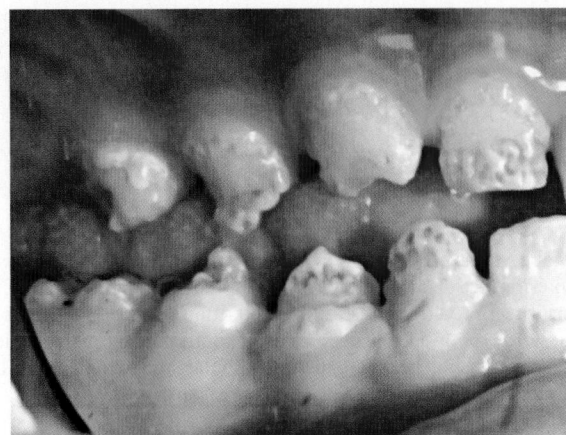

Figure 307-1 Amelogenesis imperfecta, hypoplastic type. The enamel defect results in areas of missing or thin enamel as well as grooves and pits.

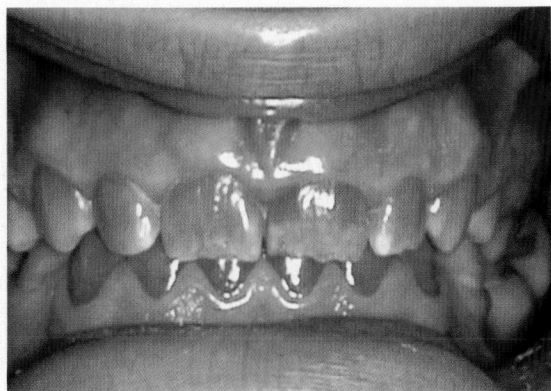

Figure 307-2 Dentinogenesis imperfecta. The bluish, opalescent sheen on several of these teeth results from genetically defective dentin. This condition may be associated with osteogenesis imperfecta. *(From Nazif MM, Martin BS, McKibben DH, et al: Oral disorders. In Zitelli BJ, Davis HW, editors: Atlas of pediatric physical diagnosis, ed 4, Philadelphia, 2002, Mosby, p. 703.)*

Amelogenesis imperfecta represents a group of hereditary conditions that manifest in enamel defects of the primary and permanent teeth without evidence of systemic disorders (Fig. 307-1). The teeth are covered by only a thin layer of abnormally formed enamel through which the yellow underlying dentin is seen. The primary teeth are generally affected more than the permanent teeth. Susceptibility to caries is low, but the enamel is subject to destruction from abrasion. Complete coverage of the crown may be indicated for dentin protection, to reduce tooth sensitivity, and for improved appearance.

Dentinogenesis imperfecta, or hereditary opalescent dentin, is a condition analogous to amelogenesis imperfecta in which the odontoblasts fail to differentiate normally, resulting in poorly calcified dentin (Fig. 307-2). This autosomal dominant disorder can also occur in patients with **osteogenesis imperfecta.** The enamel-dentin junction is altered, causing enamel to break away. The exposed dentin is then susceptible to abrasion, in some cases worn to the gingiva. The teeth are opaque and pearly, and the pulp chambers are generally obliterated by calcification. Both primary and permanent teeth are usually involved. If there is excessive wear of the teeth, selected complete coverage of the teeth may be indicated to prevent further tooth loss and improve appearance.

Localized disturbances of calcification that correlate with periods of illness, malnutrition, premature birth, or birth trauma are common. **Hypocalcification** appears as opaque white patches or horizontal lines on the tooth; **hypoplasia** is more severe and manifests as pitting or areas devoid of enamel. Systemic conditions, such as renal failure and cystic fibrosis, are associated with enamel defects. Local trauma to the primary incisors can also affect calcification of permanent incisors.

Fluorosis (mottled enamel) can result from systemic fluoride consumption > 0.05 mg/kg/day during enamel formation. This high fluoride consumption can be caused by residing in an area of high fluoride content of the drinking water (>2.0 ppm), swallowing excessive fluoridated toothpaste, or inappropriate fluoride prescriptions. Excessive fluoride during enamel formation affects ameloblastic function, resulting in inconspicuous white, lacy patches on the enamel to severe brownish discoloration and hypoplasia. The latter changes are usually seen with fluoride concentrations in the drinking water > 5.0 ppm.

Discolored teeth can result from incorporation of foreign substances into developing enamel. Neonatal hyperbilirubinemia can produce blue to black discoloration of the primary teeth. Porphyria produces a red-brown discoloration. Tetracyclines are extensively incorporated into bones and teeth and, if administered during the period of formation of enamel, can result in brown-yellow discoloration and hypoplasia of the enamel. Such teeth fluoresce under ultraviolet light. The period at risk extends from approximately 4 mo of gestation to 7 yr of life. Repeated or prolonged therapy with tetracycline carries the highest risk.

Delayed eruption of the 20 primary teeth can be familial or indicate systemic or nutritional disturbances such as hypopituitarism, hypothyroidism, cleidocranial dysplasia, trisomy 21, and multiple syndromes. Failure of eruption of single or small groups of teeth can arise from local causes such as malpositioned teeth, supernumerary teeth, cysts, or retained primary teeth. Premature loss of primary teeth is most commonly caused by premature eruption of the permanent teeth. If the entire dentition is advanced for age and sex, precocious puberty or hyperthyroidism should be considered.

Natal teeth are observed in approximately 1 in 2,000 newborn infants usually in the position of the mandibular central incisors. Natal teeth are present at birth, whereas **neonatal teeth** erupt in the 1st mo of life. Attachment of natal and neonatal teeth is generally limited to the gingival margin, with little root formation or bony support. They may be a supernumerary or a prematurely erupted primary tooth. A radiograph can easily differentiate between the two conditions. Natal teeth are associated with cleft palate, Pierre Robin syndrome, Ellis-van Creveld syndrome, Hallermann-Streiff syndrome, pachyonychia congenita, and other anomalies. A family history of natal teeth or premature eruption is present in 15-20% of affected children.

Natal or neonatal teeth occasionally result in pain and refusal to feed and can produce maternal discomfort because of abrasion or biting of the nipple during nursing. If the tooth is mobile there is a danger of detachment, with aspiration of the tooth. Because the tongue lies between the alveolar processes during birth, it can become lacerated **(Riga-Fede disease).** Decisions regarding extraction of prematurely erupted primary teeth must be made on an individual basis.

Exfoliation failure occurs when a primary tooth is not shed before the eruption of its permanent successor. Most often the primary tooth exfoliates eventually, but in some cases, the primary tooth needs to be extracted. This occurs most commonly in the mandibular incisor region.

Bibliography is available at Expert Consult.

Chapter 308
Disorders of the Oral Cavity Associated with Other Conditions
Norman Tinanoff

Disorders of the teeth and surrounding structures can occur in isolation or in combination with other systemic conditions (Table 308-1). Most commonly, medical conditions that occur during tooth development can affect tooth formation or appearance. Damage to teeth during their development is permanent.

Table 308-1	Dental Problems Associated with Selected Medical Conditions
MEDICAL CONDITION	**COMMON ASSOCIATED DENTAL OR ORAL FINDINGS**
Cleft lip and palate	Missing teeth, extra (supernumerary) teeth, shifting of arch segments, feeding difficulties, speech problems
Kidney failure	Mottled enamel (permanent teeth), facial dysmorphology
Cystic fibrosis	Stained teeth with extensive medication, mottled enamel
Immunosuppression	Oral candidiasis with potential for systemic candidiasis, cyclosporine-induced gingival hyperplasia
Low birthweight	Palatal groove, narrow arch with prolonged oral intubation; enamel defects of primary teeth
Heart defects with susceptibility to bacterial endocarditis	Bacteremia from dental procedures or trauma
Neutrophil chemotactic deficiency	Juvenile periodontitis (loss of supporting bone around teeth)
Juvenile diabetes (uncontrolled)	Juvenile periodontitis
Neuromotor dysfunction	Oral trauma from falling; malocclusion (open bite); gingivitis from lack of hygiene
Prolonged illness (generalized) during tooth formation	Enamel hypoplasia of crown portions forming during illness
Seizures	Gingival enlargement if phenytoin is used
Maternal infections	Syphilis: abnormally shaped teeth
Vitamin D–dependent rickets	Enamel hypoplasia

Chapter 309
Malocclusion
Norman Tinanoff

The oral cavity is essentially a masticatory instrument. The purpose of the anterior teeth is to bite off portions of large amounts of food. The posterior teeth reduce foodstuff to a soft, moist bolus. The cheeks and tongue force the food onto the areas of tooth contact. Establishing a proper relationship between the mandibular and maxillary teeth is important for physiologic and cosmetic reasons.

VARIATIONS IN GROWTH PATTERNS
Growth patterns are classified into 3 main types of occlusion, determined when the jaws are closed and the teeth are held together (Fig. 309-1). According to the Angle Classification of Malocclusion, in **class I occlusion** (normal), the cusps of the posterior mandibular teeth interdigitate ahead of and inside of the corresponding cusps of the opposing maxillary teeth. This relationship provides a normal facial profile.

In **class II malocclusion,** "buck teeth," the cusps of the posterior mandibular teeth are behind and inside the corresponding cusps of the maxillary teeth. This common occlusal disharmony is found in ~45% of the population. The facial profile can give the appearance of a "receding chin" (retrognathia) (mandibular deficiency) or protruding front teeth. The resultant increased space between upper and lower anterior teeth encourage finger sucking and tongue-thrust habits. Additionally, children with pronounced class II malocclusions are at greater risks of damage to the incisors as a consequence of trauma. Treatment includes orthodontic retraction of the maxilla or stimulation of the mandible.

In **class III malocclusion,** "underbite," the cusps of the posterior mandibular teeth interdigitate a tooth or more ahead of their opposing maxillary counterparts. The anterior teeth appear in cross bite with the mandibular incisors protruding beyond the maxillary incisors. The facial profile gives the appearance of a "protruding chin" (**prognathia**) with or without an appearance of maxillary deficiency. If necessary, treatment includes mandibular excess reduction osteotomy or orthodontic maxillary facial protrusion.

CROSSBITE
Normally, the mandibular teeth are in a position just inside the maxillary teeth, so that the outside mandibular cusps or incisal edges meet the central portion of the opposing maxillary teeth. A reversal of this relation is referred to as a crossbite. Crossbites can be anterior, involving the incisors; can be posterior, involving the molars; or can involve single or multiple teeth.

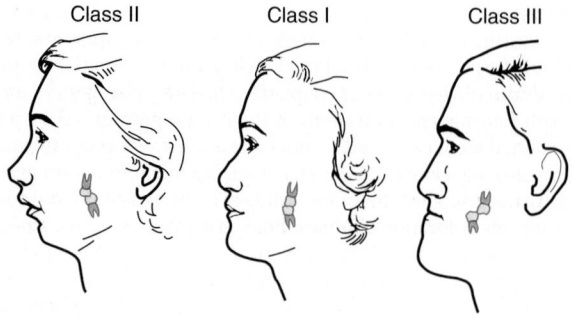

Figure 309-1 Angle classification of occlusion. The typical correspondence between the facial-jaw profile and molar relationship is shown.

OPEN AND CLOSED BITES

If the posterior mandibular and maxillary teeth make contact with each other, but the anterior teeth are still apart, the condition is called an *open bite*. Open bites can result from skeletal growth pattern or digit sucking. If digit sucking is terminated before skeletal and dental growth is complete, the open bite might resolve naturally. If mandibular anterior teeth occlude inside the maxillary anterior teeth in an overclosed position, the condition is referred to as a *closed* or *deep bite*.

Treatment of open and closed bites consists of orthodontic correction, generally performed in the preteen or teenage years. Some cases require orthognathic surgery to position the jaws optimally in a vertical direction.

DENTAL CROWDING

Overlap of incisors can result when the jaws are too small or the teeth are too large for adequate alignment of the teeth. Growth of the jaws is mostly in the posterior aspects of the mandible and maxilla, and therefore inadequate space for the teeth at 7 or 8 yr of age will not resolve with growth of the jaws. Spacing in the primary dentition is normal and favorable for adequate alignment of successor teeth.

DIGIT SUCKING

Various and conflicting etiologic theories and recommendations for correction have been proposed for digit sucking in children. Prolonged digit sucking can cause flaring of the maxillary incisor teeth, an open bite, and a posterior crossbite. The prevalence of digit sucking decreases steadily from the age of 2 yr to ≈10% by the age of 5 yr. The earlier the habit is discontinued after the eruption of the permanent maxillary incisors (age 7-8 yr), the greater the likelihood that there will be lessening effects on the dentition.

A variety of treatments have been suggested, from behavioral modification to insertion of an appliance with extensions that serves as a reminder when the child attempts to insert the digit. The greatest likelihood of success occurs in cases in which the child desires to stop. Stopping of the habit will not rectify a malocclusion caused by a prior deviant growth pattern.

Chapter **310**
Cleft Lip and Palate
Norman Tinanoff

Clefts of the lip and palate are distinct entities closely related embryologically, functionally, and genetically. It is thought that cleft of the lip appears because of hypoplasia of the mesenchymal layer, resulting in a failure of the medial nasal and maxillary processes to join. Cleft of the palate appears to represent failure of the palatal shelves to approximate or fuse.

INCIDENCE AND EPIDEMIOLOGY

The incidence of cleft lip with or without cleft palate is approximately 1 in 750 white births; the incidence of cleft palate alone is approximately 1 in 2,500 white births. Clefts of the lip are more common in males. Possible causes include maternal drug exposure, a syndrome-malformation complex, or genetic factors. Although clefts of lips and palates appear to occur sporadically, the presence of susceptible genes appears important. There are approximately 400 syndromes associated with cleft lip and palates. There are families in which a cleft lip or palate, or both, is inherited in a dominant fashion (**van der Woude syndrome**), and careful examination of parents is important to distinguish this type from others, because the recurrence risk is 50%. Ethnic factors

also affect the incidence of cleft lip and palate; the incidence is highest among Asians (~1 in 500) and Native Americans (~1 in 300), and lowest among blacks (~1 in 2,500). Cleft lip may be associated with other cranial facial anomalies, whereas cleft palate may be associated with central nervous system anomalies.

CLINICAL MANIFESTATIONS

Cleft lip can vary from a small notch in the vermilion border to a complete separation involving skin, muscle, mucosa, tooth, and bone. Clefts of the lip may be unilateral (more often on the left side) or bilateral and can involve the alveolar ridge (Fig. 310-1).

Isolated cleft palate occurs in the midline and might involve only the uvula or can extend into or through the soft and hard palates to the incisive foramen. When associated with cleft lip, the defect can involve the midline of the soft palate and extend into the hard palate on one or both sides, exposing one or both of the nasal cavities as a unilateral or bilateral cleft palate. The palate can also have a submucosal cleft indicated by a bifid uvula, partial separation of muscle with intact mucosa, or a palpable notch at the posterior of the palate.

TREATMENT

A complete program of habilitation for the child with a cleft lip or palate can require years of special treatment by a team consisting of a pediatrician, plastic surgeon, otolaryngologist, oral and maxillofacial surgeon, pediatric dentist, prosthodontist, orthodontist, speech therapist, geneticist, medical social worker, psychologist, and public health nurse.

The immediate problem in an infant born with a cleft lip or palate is feeding. Although some advocate the construction of a plastic obturator to assist in feedings, most believe that with the use of soft artificial nipples with large openings, a squeezable bottle, and proper instruction, feeding of infants with clefts can be achieved.

Surgical closure of a cleft lip is usually performed by 3 mo of age, when the infant has shown satisfactory weight gain and is free of any oral, respiratory, or systemic infection. Modification of the Millard rotation–advancement technique is the most commonly used technique; a staggered suture line minimizes notching of the lip from retraction of scar tissue. The initial repair may be revised at 4 or 5 yr of age. Corrective surgery on the nose may be delayed until adolescence. Nasal surgery can also be performed at the time of the lip repair. Cosmetic results depend on the extent of the original deformity, healing potential of the individual patient, absence of infection, and the skill of the surgeon.

Because clefts of the palate vary considerably in size, shape, and degree of deformity, the timing of surgical correction should be individualized. Criteria such as width of the cleft, adequacy of the existing palatal segments, morphology of the surrounding areas (width of the oropharynx), and neuromuscular function of the soft palate and pharyngeal walls affect the decision. The goals of surgery are the union of the cleft segments, intelligible and pleasant speech, reduction of nasal regurgitation, and avoidance of injury to the growing maxilla.

In an otherwise healthy child, closure of the palate is usually done before 1 yr of age to enhance normal speech development. When surgical correction is delayed beyond the 3rd yr, a contoured speech bulb can be attached to the posterior of a maxillary denture so that contraction of the pharyngeal and velopharyngeal muscles can bring tissues into contact with the bulb to accomplish occlusion of the nasopharynx and help the child develop intelligible speech.

A cleft palate usually crosses the alveolar ridge and interferes with the formation of teeth in the maxillary anterior region. Teeth in the cleft area may be displaced, malformed, or missing. Missing teeth or teeth that are nonfunctional are replaced by prosthetic devices.

POSTOPERATIVE MANAGEMENT

During the immediate postoperative period, special nursing care is essential. Gentle aspiration of the nasopharynx minimizes the chances of the common complications of atelectasis or pneumonia. The primary considerations in postoperative care are maintenance of a clean suture line and avoidance of tension on the sutures. The infant is fed with a

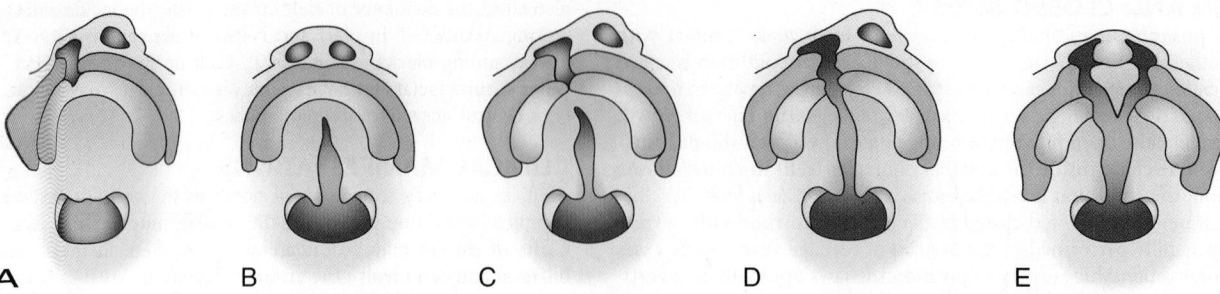

Figure 310-1 Nonsyndromic orofacial clefts. **A,** Cleft lip and alveolus. **B,** Cleft palate. **C,** Incomplete unilateral cleft lip and palate. **D,** Complete unilateral cleft lip and palate. **E,** Complete bilateral cleft lip and palate. *(From Shaw WC:* Orthodontics and occlusal management, *Oxford, England, 1993, Butterworth-Heinemann.)*

Mead Johnson bottle and the arms are restrained with elbow cuffs. A fluid or semifluid diet is maintained for 3 wk. The patient's hands, toys, and other foreign bodies must be kept away from the surgical site.

SEQUELAE

Recurrent otitis media and subsequent hearing loss are frequent with cleft palate. Displacement of the maxillary arches and malposition of the teeth usually require orthodontic correction. Misarticulations and velopharyngeal dysfunction are often associated with cleft lip and palate and may be present or persist because of physiologic dysfunction, anatomic insufficiency, malocclusion, or inadequate surgical closure of the palate. Such speech is characterized by the emission of air from the nose and by a hypernasal quality with certain sounds or by compensatory misarticulations (glottal stops). Before and sometimes after palatal surgery, the speech defect is caused by inadequacies in function of the palatal and pharyngeal muscles. The muscles of the soft palate and the lateral and posterior walls of the nasopharynx constitute a valve that separates the nasopharynx from the oropharynx during swallowing and in the production of certain sounds. If the valve does not function adequately, it is difficult to build up enough pressure in the mouth to make such explosive sounds as p, b, d, t, h, y, or the sibilants s, sh, and ch, and such words as "cats," "boats," and "sisters" are not intelligible. After operation or the insertion of a speech appliance, speech therapy is necessary.

VELOPHARYNGEAL DYSFUNCTION

The speech disturbance characteristic of the child with a cleft palate can also be produced by other osseous or neuromuscular abnormalities where there is an inability to form an effective seal between oropharynx and nasopharynx during swallowing or phonation. In a child who has the potential for abnormal speech, adenoidectomy can precipitate overt hypernasality. If the neuromuscular function is adequate, compensation in palatopharyngeal movement might take place and the speech defect might improve, although speech therapy is necessary. In other cases, slow involution of the adenoids can allow gradual compensation in palatal and pharyngeal muscular function. This might explain why a speech defect does not become apparent in some children who have a submucous cleft palate or similar anomaly predisposing to palatopharyngeal incompetence.

Clinical Manifestations

Although clinical signs vary, the symptoms of velopharyngeal dysfunction are similar to those of a cleft palate. There may be hypernasal speech (especially noted in the articulation of pressure consonants such as p, b, d, t, h, v, f, and s); conspicuous constricting movement of the nares during speech; inability to whistle, gargle, blow out a candle, or inflate a balloon; loss of liquid through the nose when drinking with the head down; otitis media; and hearing loss. Oral inspection might reveal a cleft palate or a relatively short palate with a large oropharynx; absent, grossly asymmetric, or minimal muscular activity of the soft palate and pharynx during phonation or gagging; or a submucous cleft.

Velopharyngeal dysfunction may also be demonstrated radiographically. The head should be carefully positioned to obtain a true lateral view; one film is obtained with the patient at rest and another during continuous phonation of the vowel u as in "boom." The soft palate contacts the posterior pharyngeal wall in normal function, whereas in velopharyngeal dysfunction such contact is absent.

In selected cases of velopharyngeal dysfunction, the palate may be retropositioned or pharyngoplasty may be performed using a flap of tissue from the posterior pharyngeal wall. Dental speech appliances have also been used successfully. The type of surgery used is best tailored to the findings on nasoendoscopy.

Bibliography is available at Expert Consult.

Chapter **311**
Syndromes with Oral Manifestations
Norman Tinanoff

Many syndromes have distinct or accompanying facial, oral, and dental manifestations (see Apert syndrome, Chapter 591.12; Crouzon disease, Chapter 591.12; Down syndrome, Chapter 81.2).

Osteogenesis imperfecta is often accompanied by effects on the teeth, termed dentinogenesis **imperfecta** (see Chapter 307, Fig. 307-2). Depending on the severity of presentation, treatment of the dentition varies from routine preventive and restorative monitoring to covering affected posterior teeth with stainless steel crowns, to prevent further tooth loss and improve appearance. Dentinogenesis imperfecta can also occur in isolation without the bony effects.

Another syndrome, **cleidocranial dysplasia,** has orofacial features such as frontal bossing, hypoplastic maxilla and supernumerary teeth. The primary teeth can be over retained and the permanent teeth remain unerupted. Supernumerary teeth are common, especially in the premolar area. Extensive dental rehabilitation may be needed to correct severe tooth crowding, unerupted and supernumerary teeth.

Ectodermal dysplasias (see Chapter 649) are a heterogeneous group of conditions in which oral manifestations range from little or no involvement (the dentition is completely normal) to cases in which the teeth can be totally or partially absent or malformed. Because alveolar bone does not develop in the absence of teeth, the alveolar processes can be either totally or partially absent, and the resultant overclosure of the mandible causes the lips to protrude. Facial development is otherwise not disturbed. Teeth, when present, can range from normal to small and conical. If aplasia of the buccal and labial salivary glands

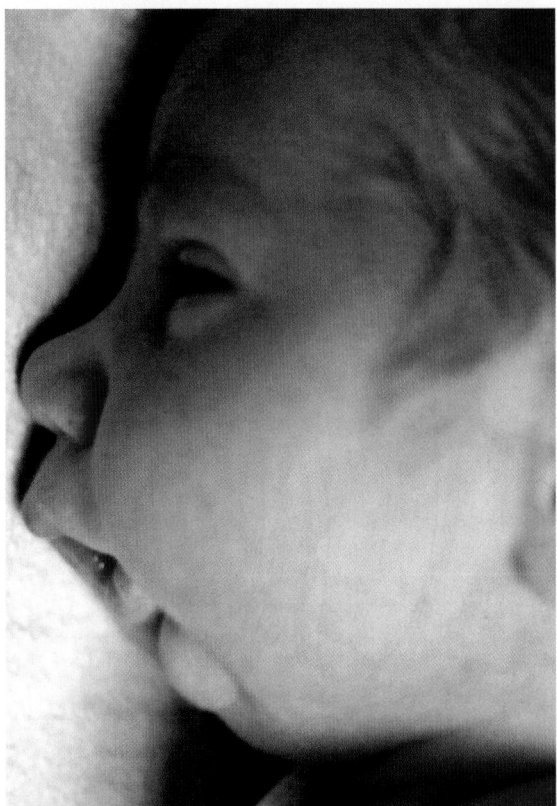

Figure 311-1 Pierre Robin syndrome. *(From Clark DA:* Atlas of neonatology, *ed 7, Philadelphia, 2000, WB Saunders, p. 144.)*

is present, dryness and irritation of the oral mucosa can occur. People with ectodermal dysplasia might need partial or full dentures, even at a very young age. The vertical height between the jaws is thus restored, improving the position of the lips and facial contours as well as restoring masticatory function.

Pierre Robin syndrome consists of micrognathia usually accompanied by a high arched or cleft palate (Fig. 311-1). The tongue is usually of normal size, but the floor of the mouth is foreshortened. The air passages can become obstructed, particularly on inspiration, usually requiring treatment to prevent suffocation. The infant should be maintained in a prone or partially prone position so that the tongue falls forward to relieve respiratory obstruction. Some patients require tracheostomy. Mandibular distraction procedures in the neonate can improve mandibular size, enhance respiration, and facilitate oral feedings.

Sufficient spontaneous mandibular growth can take place within a few months to relieve the potential airway obstruction. Often the growth of the mandible achieves a normal profile in 4-6 yr. Of children with Pierre Robin syndrome, 30-50% have **Stickler syndrome**, an autosomal dominant condition that includes other findings such as prominent joints, arthritis, hypotonia, hypermobile joints, mitral valve prolapse, hearing loss, and ocular problems (myopia, glaucoma, cataracts, retinal detachment). Mutations are noted in the genes that produce types II, IX, and XI collagen in many, but not all, patients with Stickler syndrome. Other syndromes are associated with Pierre Robin syndrome including 22Q11.2 deletion syndrome (Velocardio facial syndrome).

Mandibulofacial dysostosis (Treacher Collins syndrome or Franceschetti syndrome) is an autosomal dominant syndrome that primarily affects the face. The facial appearance varies but is characterized by downward sloping palpebral fissures, colobomas of the lower eyelids, sunken cheekbones, blind fistulas opening between the angles of the mouth and the ears, deformed pinnae, atypical hair growth extending toward the cheeks, receding chin, and large mouth. Facial clefts,

abnormalities of the ears, and deafness are common. The mandible is usually hypoplastic; the ramus may be deficient, and the coronoid and condylar processes are flat or even aplastic. The palatal vault may be either high or cleft. Dental malocclusions are common. The teeth may be missing, hypoplastic, or displaced or be in an open bite position. Initially, the primary concern is breathing and feeding problems. Surgery to restore normal structure of the face can be performed, which may include repair of cleft palate, zygomatic and orbit reconstruction, reconstruction of the lower eyelid, external ear reconstruction, and orthognathic surgery.

Hemifacial microsomia presentation can be quite variable but is usually characterized by unilateral hypoplasia of the mandible and can be associated with partial paralysis of the facial nerve, underdeveloped ear, and blind fistulas between the angles of the mouth and the ears. Severe facial asymmetry and malocclusion can develop because of the absence or hypoplasia of the mandibular condyle on the affected side. Congenital condylar deformity tends to increase with age. Early craniofacial surgery may be indicated to minimize the deformity. This disorder can be associated with ocular and vertebral anomalies (oculo-auriculo-vertebral spectrum, including Goldenhar syndrome); therefore, radiographs of the vertebrae and ribs should be considered to determine the extent of skeletal involvement.

Bibliography is available at Expert Consult.

Chapter **312**
Dental Caries
Norman Tinanoff

ETIOLOGY
The development of dental caries depends on interrelationships among the tooth surface, dietary carbohydrates, and specific oral bacteria. Organic acids produced by bacterial fermentation of dietary carbohydrates reduce the pH of dental plaque adjacent to the tooth to a point where demineralization occurs. The initial demineralization appears as an opaque **white spot lesion** on the enamel, and with progressive loss of tooth mineral, cavitation of the tooth occurs (Fig. 312-1).

The group of microorganisms, mutans streptococci, is associated with the development of dental caries. These bacteria have the ability to adhere to enamel, produce abundant acid, and survive at low pH. Once the enamel surface cavitates, other oral bacteria (lactobacilli) can colonize the tooth, produce acid, and foster further tooth demineralization. Demineralization from bacterial acid production is determined by the frequency of carbohydrate consumption and by the type of carbohydrate. Sucrose is the most cariogenic sugar because one of its by-products during bacterial metabolism is glucan, a polymer that enables bacteria to adhere more readily to tooth structures. Dietary behaviors, such as consuming sweetened beverages in a nursing bottle or frequently consuming sticky candies, increase the cariogenic potential of foods because of the long retention of sugar in the mouth.

EPIDEMIOLOGY
The incidence of dental caries has decreased in developed countries in the past 30 yr but has not decreased and remains highly prevalent among low-income children and children from developing countries. More than half of the children in the United States have dental caries, with most of those having caries primarily in the pits and fissures of the occlusal (biting) surfaces of the molar teeth.

CLINICAL MANIFESTATIONS
Dental caries of the primary dentition usually begins in the pits and fissures. Small lesions may be difficult to diagnose by visual inspection,

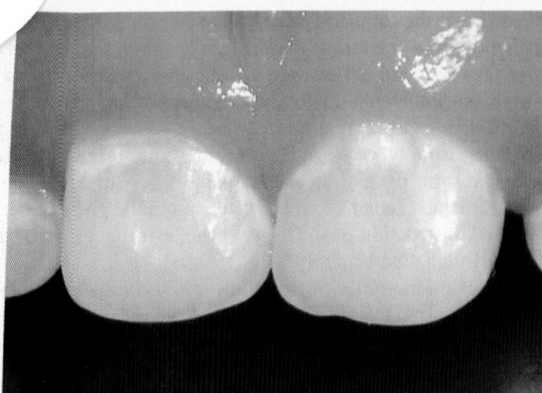

Figure 312-1 Initial carious lesions (white spot lesions) around the necks of the maxillary central incisors.

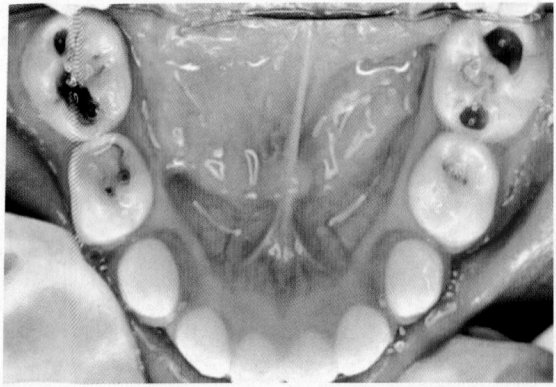

Figure 312-2 Rampant caries in a 3 yr old child. Note darkened and cavitated lesions on the fissure surfaces of mandibular molars.

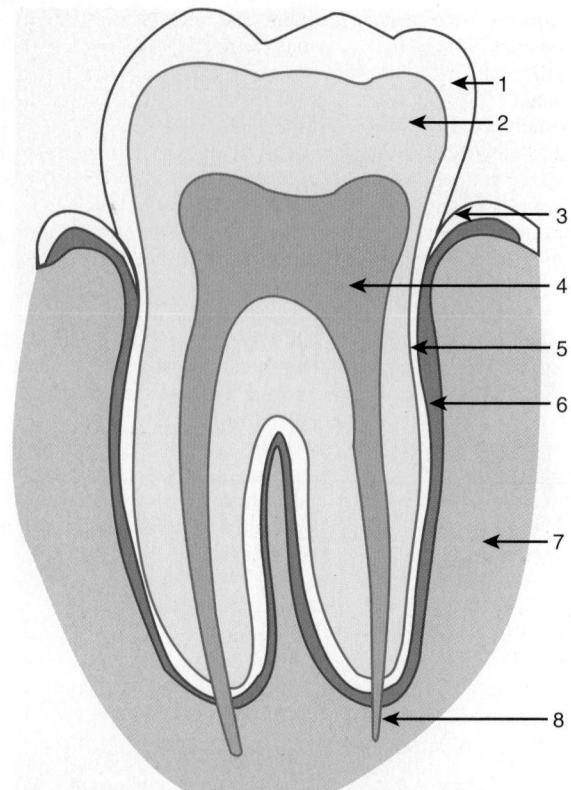

Figure 312-3 Basic dental anatomy: **1**, enamel; **2**, dentin; **3**, gingival margin; **4**, pulp; **5**, cementum; **6**, periodontal ligament; **7**, alveolar bone; **8**, neurovascular bundle.

but larger lesions are evident as darkened or cavitated lesions on the tooth surfaces (Fig. 312-2). Rampant dental caries in infants and toddlers, referred to as **early childhood caries**, is the result of early colonization of the child with cariogenic bacteria and the frequent ingestion of sugar, either in the bottle or in solid foods. The carious process in this situation is initiated earlier and consequently can affect the maxillary incisors first and then progress to the molars as they erupt.

The prevalence of early childhood caries is 30-50% in children from low socioeconomic backgrounds and as high as 70% in some Native American groups. Besides high frequency of sugar consumption and colonization with cariogenic bacteria, other enabling factors include low socioeconomic status of the family, other family member with carious teeth, recent immigrant status of the child, and the visual presence of dental plaque on the child's teeth. Children who develop caries at a young age are known to be at high risk for developing further caries as they get older. Therefore, the appropriate prevention of early childhood caries can result in the elimination of major dental problems in toddlers and less decay in later childhood.

COMPLICATIONS

Left untreated, dental caries usually destroy most of the tooth and invade the dental pulp (Fig. 312-3), leading to an inflammation of the pulp (**pulpitis**) and significant pain. Pulpitis can progress to pulp necrosis, with bacterial invasion of the alveolar bone causing a dental abscess (Fig. 312-4). Infection of a primary tooth can disrupt normal development of the successor permanent tooth. In some cases, this process leads to sepsis and infection of the facial space.

TREATMENT

The age at which dental caries occurs is important in dental management. Children younger than 3 yr of age lack the developmental ability

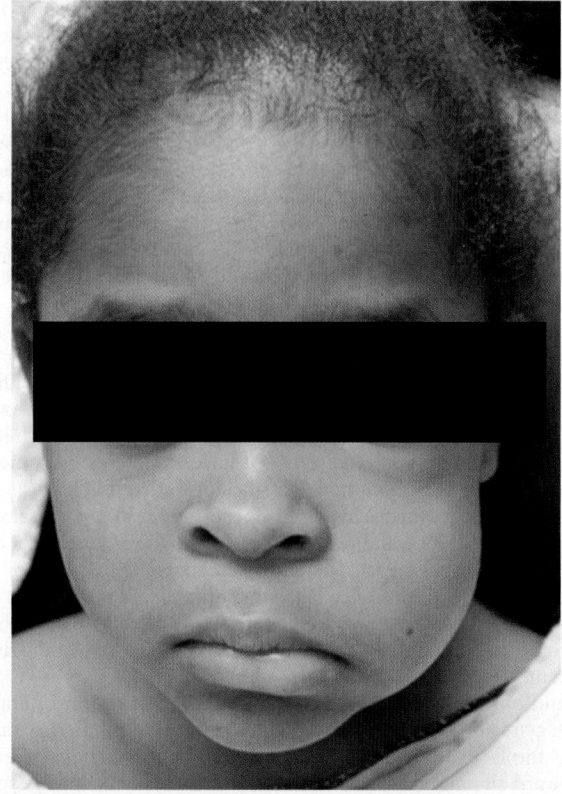

Figure 312-4 Facial swelling from an abscessed primary molar. Resolution of the inflammation can be achieved by a course of antibiotics, followed by either extraction or root canal of the offending tooth.

to cooperate with dental treatment and often require sedation, or general anesthesia to repair carious teeth. After age 4 yr, children can generally cope with dental restorative care with the use of local anesthesia.

Dental treatment, using silver amalgam, plastic composite, or stainless steel crowns, can restore most teeth affected with dental caries. If caries involves the dental pulp, a partial removal of the pulp (pulpotomy) or complete removal of the pulp (pulpectomy) may be required. If a tooth requires extraction, a space maintainer may be indicated to prevent migration of teeth, which subsequently leads to malposition of permanent successor teeth.

Clinical management of the pain and infection associated with untreated dental caries varies with the extent of involvement and the medical status of the patient. Dental infection localized to the dento-alveolar unit can be managed by local measures (extraction, pulpectomy). Oral antibiotics are indicated for dental infections associated with fever, cellulitis, and facial swelling, or if it is difficult to anesthetize the tooth in the presence of inflammation. Penicillin is the antibiotic of choice, except in patients with a history of allergy to this agent. Clindamycin and erythromycin are suitable alternatives. Oral analgesics, such as ibuprofen, are usually adequate for the pain control.

PREVENTION

Because they are seeing infants and toddlers on a periodicity schedule, physicians have an important role in screening children younger than 3 yr of age for dental caries; providing preventive instructions; applying preventive measures, such as fluoride varnish; and referring the child to a dentist if problems exist.

Fluoride

The most effective preventive measure against dental caries is communal water supplies with optimal fluoride content. Water fluoridation at the level of 0.7-1.2 mg fluoride per liter (ppm F) was introduced in the United States in the 1940s. Because fluoride from water supplies is now one of several sources of fluoride, the Department of Health and Human Services proposes to not have a fluoride range, but instead to limit the recommendation to the lower limit of 0.7 ppm F. The rationale is to balance the benefits of preventing dental caries with reducing the chance of fluorosis. Children who reside in areas with fluoride-deficient water supplies and are at risk for caries benefit from dietary fluoride supplements (Table 312-1). If the patient uses a private water supply, it is necessary to get the water tested for fluoride levels before prescribing fluoride supplements. To avoid potential overdoses, no fluoride prescription should be written for more than a total of 120 mg of fluoride. However, because of confusion regarding fluoride supplements among practitioners and parents, association of supplements with fluorosis, and lack of parent compliance with the daily administration, supplements may no longer be the first-line approach for preventing caries in preschool-aged children.

Topical fluoride on a daily basis can be achieved by using fluoridated toothpaste. Supervised use of less than a "pea-sized" amount of toothpaste (approximately 0.25 g) on the toothbrush in children younger than 6 yr of age reduces the risk of fluorosis. Children younger than 4 yr of age should brush with less than a "smear or grain-sized" amount of fluoridated toothpaste. Professional topical fluoride applications performed semiannually reportedly reduce caries by approximately

30%. Fluoride varnish is ideal for professional applications in preschool children because of ease of use, even with non–dental health providers, and its safety because of single-dose dispensers. Products that are available now come in containers of 0.25, 0.4, or 0.6 mL of varnish, corresponding to 5.6, 9.0, and 13.6 mg fluoride, respectively. Fluoride varnish should be administered twice a year for preschool children at moderate caries risk and 4 times a year for children at high caries risk.

Oral Hygiene

Daily brushing, especially with fluoridated toothpaste, helps prevent dental caries. Most children younger than 8 yr of age do not have the coordination required for adequate tooth brushing. Accordingly, parents should assume responsibility for the child's oral hygiene, with the degree of parental involvement appropriate to the child's changing abilities.

Diet

Frequent consumption of sweetened fruit drinks is not generally recognized by parents for its high cariogenic potential. Consuming sweetened beverages in a nursing bottle or sippy cup should be discouraged, and special efforts made to instruct parents that their child should only consume sweetened beverages at meal times and not exceed 6 oz per day.

Dental Sealant

Plastic dental sealants have been shown to be effective in preventing caries on the pit and fissure of the primary and permanent molars. Sealants are most effective when placed soon after teeth erupt and used in children with deep grooves and fissures in the molar teeth.

Bibliography is available at Expert Consult.

Chapter 313
Periodontal Diseases
Norman Tinanoff

The periodontium includes the gingiva, alveolar bone, cementum, and periodontal ligament (see Fig. 312-3).

GINGIVITIS

Poor oral hygiene results in the accumulation of dental plaque at the tooth–gingival interface that activates an inflammatory response, expressed as localized or generalized reddening and swelling of the gingiva. More than half of American school children experience gingivitis. In severe cases, the gingiva spontaneously bleeds and there is oral malodor. Treatment is proper oral hygiene (careful tooth brushing and flossing); complete resolution can be expected. Fluctuations in hormonal levels during the onset of puberty can increase inflammatory response to plaque. Gingivitis in healthy children is unlikely to progress to periodontitis (inflammation of the periodontal ligament resulting in loss of alveolar bone).

AGGRESSIVE PERIODONTITIS IN CHILDREN (PREPUBERTAL PERIODONTITIS)

Periodontitis in children before puberty is a rare disease that often begins between the time of eruption of the primary teeth and the age of 4 or 5 yr. The disease occurs in localized and generalized forms. There is rapid bone loss, often leading to premature loss of primary teeth. It is often associated with systemic problems, including

Table 312-1	Supplemental Fluoride Dosage Schedule		
	FLUORIDE IN HOME WATER		
AGE	**<0.3 (ppm)**	**0.3-0.6 (ppm)**	**>0.6 (ppm)**
6 mo-3 yr	0.25*	0	0
3-6 yr	0.50	0.25	0
6-16 yr	1.00	0.50	0

*Milligrams of fluoride per day.

penia, leukocyte adhesion or migration defects, hypophospha-
Papillon-Lefèvre syndrome, leukemia, and histiocytosis X. In
many cases, however, there is no apparent underlying medical problem.
Nonetheless, diagnostic work-ups are necessary to rule out underlying
systemic disease.

Treatment includes aggressive professional teeth cleaning, strategic
extraction of affected teeth, and antibiotic therapy. There are few
reports of long-term successful treatment to reverse bone loss surrounding primary teeth.

AGGRESSIVE PERIODONTITIS IN ADOLESCENTS (LOCALIZED JUVENILE PERIODONTITIS)

Aggressive periodontitis in adolescents is characterized by rapid alveolar bone loss, especially around the permanent incisors and 1st molars.
Overall prevalence in the United States is <1%, but the prevalence
among African-Americans is reportedly 2.5%. This form of periodontitis is associated with a strain of Aggregatibacter (Actinobacillus)
bacteria. In addition, the neutrophils of patients with aggressive periodontitis can have chemotactic or phagocytic defects. If left untreated,
affected teeth lose their attachment and can exfoliate. Treatment varies
with the degree of involvement. Patients whose disease is diagnosed at
onset are usually managed by surgical or nonsurgical debridement in
conjunction with antibiotic therapy. Prognosis depends on the degree
of initial involvement and compliance with therapy.

TEETHING

Teething can lead to intermittent localized discomfort in the area of
erupting primary teeth, irritability, low-grade fevers, and excessive
salivation; many children have no apparent difficulties. Treatment of
symptoms includes oral analgesics and ice rings for the child to "gum."
Similar manifestations can also arise when the 1st permanent molars
erupt at about age 6 yr.

CYCLOSPORINE- OR PHENYTOIN-INDUCED GINGIVAL OVERGROWTH

The use of cyclosporine to suppress organ rejection or phenytoin for
anticonvulsant therapy, and in some cases calcium channel blockers,
is associated with generalized enlargement of the gingiva. Phenytoin
and its metabolites have a direct stimulatory action on gingival fibroblasts, resulting in accelerated synthesis of collagen. Phenytoin induces
less gingival hyperplasia in patients who maintain meticulous oral
hygiene.

Gingival hyperplasia occurs in 10-30% of patients treated with phenytoin. Severe manifestations can include gross enlargement of the
gingiva, sometimes covering the teeth; edema and erythema of the
gingiva; secondary infection, resulting in abscess formation; migration
of teeth; and inhibition of exfoliation of primary teeth and subsequent
impaction of permanent teeth. Treatment should be directed toward
prevention and, if possible, discontinuation of cyclosporine or phenytoin. Patients undergoing long-term treatment with these drugs
should receive frequent dental examinations and oral hygiene care.
Severe forms of gingival overgrowth are treated by gingivectomy, but
the lesion recurs if drug use is continued.

ACUTE PERICORONITIS

Acute inflammation of the flap of gingiva that partially covers the
crown of an incompletely erupted tooth is common in mandibular
permanent molars. Accumulation of debris and bacteria between the
gingival flap and tooth precipitates the inflammatory response. A
variant of this condition is a gingival abscess caused by entrapment of
bacteria because of orthodontic bands or crowns. Trismus and severe
pain may be associated with the inflammation. Untreated cases can
result in facial space infections and facial cellulitis.

Treatment includes local debridement and irrigation, warm saline
rinses, and antibiotic therapy. When the acute phase has subsided,
resection of the gingival flap prevents recurrence. Early recognition of
the partial impaction of mandibular 3rd molars and their subsequent
extraction prevents these areas from developing pericoronitis.

NECROTIZING PERIODONTAL DISEASE (ACUTE NECROTIZING ULCERATIVE GINGIVITIS)

Necrotizing periodontal disease, in the past sometimes referred to as
"trench mouth," is a distinct periodontal disease associated with oral
spirochetes and fusobacteria. It is not clear, however, whether bacteria
initiate the disease or are secondary. It rarely develops in healthy children in developed countries, with a prevalence in the United States of
<1%, but is seen more often in children and adolescents from develop-
ing areas of Africa, Asia, and South America. In certain African countries, where affected children usually have protein malnutrition, the
lesion can extend into adjacent tissues, causing necrosis of facial structures (cancrum oris, or noma).

Clinical manifestations of necrotizing periodontal disease include
necrosis and ulceration of gingiva between the teeth, an adherent
grayish pseudomembrane over the affected gingiva, oral malodor, cervical lymphadenopathy, malaise, and fever. The condition may be mistaken for acute herpetic gingivostomatitis. Dark-field microscopy of
debris obtained from necrotizing lesions demonstrates dense spiro-
chete populations.

Treatment of necrotizing periodontal disease is divided into an acute
management with local debridement, oxygenating agents (direct application of 10% carbamide peroxide in anhydrous glycerol qid), and
analgesics. Dramatic resolution usually occurs within 48 hr. If a patient
is febrile, antibiotics (penicillin or metronidazole) may be an important
adjunctive therapy. A second phase of treatment may be necessary if
the acute phase of the disease has caused irreversible morphologic
damage to the periodontium. The disease is not contagious.

Bibliography is available at Expert Consult.

Chapter 314
Dental Trauma
Norman Tinanoff

Traumatic oral injuries may be categorized into 3 groups: injuries to
teeth, injuries to soft tissue (contusions, abrasions, lacerations, punctures, avulsions, and burns), and injuries to jaw (mandibular and/or
maxillary fractures).

INJURIES TO TEETH

Approximately 10% of children between 18 mo and 18 yr of age sustain
significant tooth trauma. There appear to be 3 age periods of greatest
predilection: toddlers (1-3 yr), usually from falls or child abuse; school-
age children (7-10 yr), usually from bicycle and playground accidents;
and adolescents (16-18 yr), often the result of fights, athletic injuries,
and automobile accidents. Injuries to teeth are more common among
children with protruding front teeth. Children with craniofacial abnormalities or neuromuscular deficits are also at increased risk for dental
injury. Injuries to teeth can involve the hard dental tissues, the dental
pulp (nerve), and injuries to the periodontal structure (surrounding
bone and attachment apparatus) (Fig. 314-1 and Table 314-1).

Fractures of teeth may be uncomplicated (confined to the hard
dental tissues) or complicated (involving the pulp). Exposure of the
pulp results in its bacterial contamination, which can lead to infection
and pulp necrosis. Such pulp exposure complicates therapy and can
lower the likelihood of a favorable outcome.

The teeth most often affected are the maxillary incisors. Uncomplicated crown fractures are treated by covering exposed dentin and by
placing an aesthetic restoration. Complicated crown fractures involving the tooth pulp usually require **endodontic therapy** (root canal).
Crown-root fractures and root fractures usually require extensive

dental therapy. Such injuries in the primary dentition can interfere with normal development of the permanent dentition, and therefore significant injuries of the primary incisor teeth are usually managed by extraction.

Traumatic oral injuries should be referred to a dentist as soon as possible. Even when the teeth appear intact, a dentist should promptly evaluate the patient. Baseline data (radiographs, mobility patterns, responses to specific stimuli) enable the dentist to assess the likelihood of future complications.

INJURIES TO PERIODONTAL STRUCTURES

Trauma to teeth with associated injury to periodontal structures that hold the teeth usually manifests as mobile or displaced teeth. Such injuries are more common in the primary than in the permanent dentition. Categories of trauma to the periodontium include concussion, subluxation, intrusive luxation, extrusive luxation, and avulsion.

Concussion

Injuries that produce minor damage to the periodontal ligament are termed *concussions*. Teeth sustaining such injuries are not mobile or

displaced but react markedly to percussion (gentle hitting of the tooth with an instrument). This type of injury usually requires no therapy and resolves without complication. Primary incisors that sustain concussion can change color, indicating pulpal degeneration, and should be evaluated by a dentist.

Subluxation

Subluxated teeth exhibit mild to moderate horizontal mobility and/or vertical mobility. Hemorrhage is usually evident around the neck of the tooth at the gingival margin. There is no displacement of the tooth. Many subluxated teeth need to be immobilized by splints to ensure adequate repair of the periodontal ligament. Some of these teeth develop pulp necrosis.

Intrusion

Intruded teeth are pushed up into their socket, sometimes to the point where they are not clinically visible. Intruded primary incisors can give the false appearance of being avulsed (knocked out). To rule out avulsion, a dental radiograph is indicated (Figs. 314-2 and 314-3).

Extrusion

Extrusion injury is characterized by displacement of the tooth from its socket. The tooth is usually displaced to the lingual (tongue) side, with fracture of the wall of the alveolar socket. These teeth need immediate treatment; the longer the delay, the more likely the tooth will be fixed in its displaced position. Therapy is directed at reduction (repositioning the tooth) and fixation (splinting). The pulp of such teeth often becomes necrotic and requires endodontic therapy. Extrusive luxation in the primary dentition is usually managed by extraction because

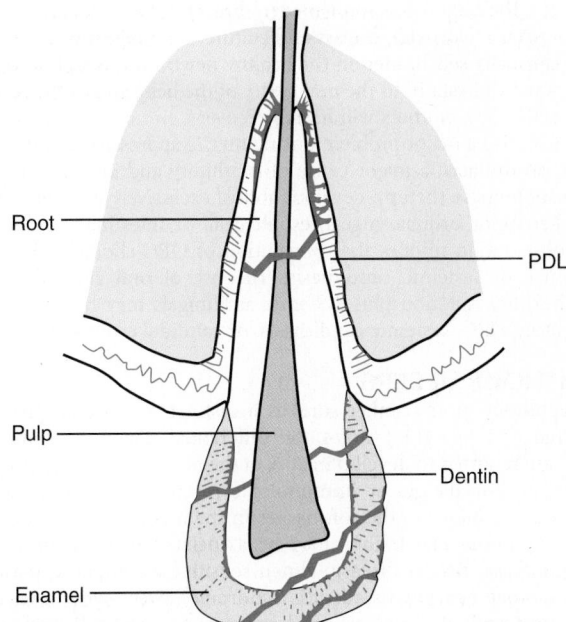

Figure 314-1 Tooth fractures can involve enamel, dentin, or pulp and can occur in the crown or root of a tooth. *PDL,* periodontal ligament. *(From Pinkham JR: Pediatric dentistry: infancy through adolescence, Philadelphia, 1988, WB Saunders, p. 172.)*

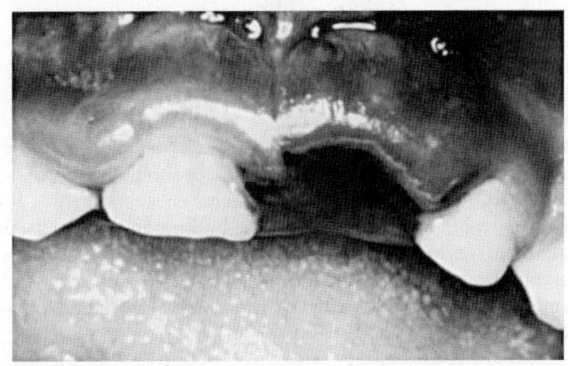

Figure 314-2 Intruded primary incisor that appears avulsed (knocked out).

Table 314-1	Injuries to Crowns of Teeth	
TYPE OF TRAUMA	**DESCRIPTION**	**TREATMENT AND REFERRAL**
Enamel infraction (crazing)	Incomplete fracture of enamel without loss of tooth structure	Initially might not require therapy but should be assessed periodically by dentist
Enamel fractures	Fracture of only the tooth enamel	Tooth may be smoothed or treated to replace fragment
Enamel and dentin fracture	Fracture of enamel and dentinal layer of the tooth. Tooth may be sensitive to cold or air. Pulp may become necrotic, leading to periapical abscess	Refer as soon as possible. Area should be treated to preserve the integrity of the underlying pulp
Enamel, dentin fracture involving the pulp	Bacterial contamination can lead to pulpal necrosis and periapical abscess. The tooth might have the appearance of bleeding or might display a small red spot	Refer immediately. The dental therapy of choice depends on the extent of injury, the condition of the pulp, the development of the tooth, time elapsed from injury, and any other injuries to the supporting structures. Therapy is directed toward minimizing contamination in an effort to improve the prognosis

From Josell SD, Abrams RG: *Managing common dental problems and emergencies,* Pediatr Clin North Am *38:1325–1342, 1991.*

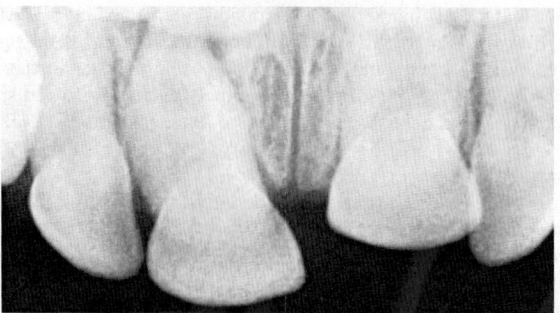

Figure 314-3 Occlusal radiograph documents intrusion of "missing tooth" presented in Figure 314-2.

complications of reduction and fixation can result in problems with development of permanent teeth.

Avulsion

If avulsed permanent teeth are replanted as soon as possible after injury, there is a good chance that normal reattachment will follow and the tooth will have a good prognosis. However, if the tooth is in a dry environment for longer than 1 hr, the ligament that holds the tooth in place has little chance for survival and failure (root resorption, ankylosis) is common. Parents confronted with this emergency situation can be instructed to do the following:

◆ Find the tooth.
◆ Briefly rinse the tooth. (Do not scrub the tooth. Do not touch the root. After plugging the sink drain, hold the tooth by the crown and rinse it under running tap water.)
◆ Insert the tooth into the socket. (Gently place it back into its normal position. Do not be concerned if the tooth extrudes slightly. If the parent or child is too apprehensive for replantation of the tooth, the tooth should be placed in cold cow's milk or other cold isotonic solution.)
◆ Go directly to the dentist. (In transit, the child should hold the tooth in its socket with a finger. The parent should buckle a seatbelt around the child and drive safely.)

After the tooth is replanted, it must be immobilized to facilitate reattachment; endodontic therapy is always required. The initial signs of complications associated with replantation can appear as early as 1 wk after trauma or as late as several years later. Close dental follow-up is indicated for at least 1 yr.

PREVENTION

To minimize the likelihood of dental injuries:

◆ Every child or adolescent who engages in contact sports should wear a mouth guard, which may be constructed by a dentist or purchased at any athletic goods store.
◆ Helmets with face guards should be worn by children or adolescents with neuromuscular problems or seizure disorders to protect the head and face during falls.
◆ Helmets should also be used during biking, skiing, skating, and skateboarding.
◆ All children or adolescents with protruding incisors should be evaluated by a pediatric dentist or orthodontist.

ADDITIONAL CONSIDERATIONS

Children who experience dental trauma might also have sustained head or neck trauma, and therefore neurologic assessment is warranted. Tetanus prophylaxis should be considered with any injury that disrupts the integrity of the oral tissues. The possibility of child abuse should always be considered.

Bibliography is available at Expert Consult.

Chapter **315**

Common Lesions of the Oral Soft Tissues

Norman Tinanoff

OROPHARYNGEAL CANDIDIASIS

Oropharyngeal infection with *Candida albicans* (thrush, moniliasis) (see Chapter 234.1) is common in neonates from contact with the organism in the birth canal or breast. The lesions of oropharyngeal candidiasis (OPC) appear as white plaques covering all or part of the oropharyngeal mucosa. These plaques are removable from the underlying surface, which is characteristically inflamed and has pinpoint hemorrhages. The diagnosis is confirmed by direct microscopic examination on potassium hydroxide smears and culture of scrapings from lesions. OPC is usually self-limited in the healthy newborn infant, but topical application of nystatin to the oral cavity of the baby and to the nipples of breastfeeding mothers will hasten recovery.

OPC is also a major problem during myelosuppressive therapy. **Systemic candidiasis**, a major cause of morbidity and mortality during myelosuppressive therapy, develops almost exclusively in patients who have had prior oropharyngeal, esophageal, or intestinal candidiasis. This observation implies that prevention of OPC should reduce the incidence of systemic candidiasis. The use of oral rinses of 0.2% chlorhexidine solution plus systemic antifungals may be effective in preventing OPC, systemic candidiasis, or candidal esophagitis.

APHTHOUS ULCERS

The aphthous ulcer (canker sore) is a distinct oral lesion, prone to recurrence; Table 315-1 notes the differential diagnosis. Aphthous ulcers are reported to develop in 20% of the population. Their etiology is unclear, but allergic or immunologic reactions, emotional stress, genetics, and injury to the soft tissues in the mouth have been implicated. Aphthous-like lesions may be associated with inflammatory bowel disease, Behçet disease, gluten-sensitive enteropathy, periodic fever-aphthae-pharyngitis-adenitis syndrome, Sweet syndrome, HIV infection (especially if ulcers are large and slow to heal), and cyclic neutropenia. Clinically, these ulcers are characterized by well-circumscribed, ulcerative lesions with a white necrotic base surrounded by a red halo. The lesions last 10-14 days and heal without scarring. Nonprescription palliative therapies, such as benzocaine and topical lidocaine, are effective, as are topical steroids. Tetracycline has benefit with severe outbreaks, but caution is necessary in pregnant women and young children to prevent tetracycline tooth staining during a child's tooth development.

HERPETIC GINGIVOSTOMATITIS

After an initial incubation period of approximately 1 wk, the initial infection with herpes simplex virus manifests as fever and malaise, usually in a child younger than 5 yr (see Chapter 252). The oral cavity can show various expressions, including the gingiva becoming erythematous, mucosal hemorrhages, and clusters of small vesicles erupting throughout the mouth. There is often involvement of the mucocutaneous margin and perioral skin (Fig. 315-1). The oral symptoms generally are accompanied by fever, lymphadenopathy, and difficulty eating and drinking. The symptoms usually regress within 2 wk without scarring. Fluids should be encouraged because the child may become dehydrated. Analgesics and anesthetic rinses can make the child more comfortable. Oral acyclovir if taken within the 1st 3 days of symptoms may be beneficial in shortening the duration of symptoms. Caution should be exercised to prevent autoinoculation or transmission of infection to the eyes.

RECURRENT HERPES LABIALIS

Approximately 90% of the population develops antibodies to herpes simplex virus. In periods of quiescence, the virus is thought to remain latent in sensory neurons. Unlike primary herpetic gingivostomatitis, which manifests as multiple painful vesicles on the lips, tongue, palate, gingiva, and mucosa, recurrent herpes is generally limited to the lips. Other than the annoyance of causing pain and an unattractive appearance, there are generally no systemic symptoms. Reactivation of the virus is thought to be the result of exposure to ultraviolet light, tissue trauma, stress, or fevers. There is little advantage of antiviral therapy over palliative therapies in an otherwise healthy patient affected by recurrent herpes.

BOHN NODULES

Bohn nodules are small developmental anomalies located along the buccal and lingual aspects of the mandibular and maxillary ridges and in the hard palate of the neonate. These lesions arise from remnants of mucous gland tissue. Treatment is not necessary, because the nodules disappear within a few weeks.

DENTAL LAMINA CYSTS

Dental lamina cysts are small cystic lesions located along the crest of the mandibular and maxillary ridges of the neonate. These lesions arise from epithelial remnants of the dental lamina. Treatment is not necessary; they disappear within a few weeks.

FORDYCE GRANULES

Almost 80% of adults have multiple yellow-white granules in clusters or plaque-like areas on the oral mucosa, most commonly on the buccal mucosa or lips. They are aberrant sebaceous glands. The glands are present at birth, but they can hypertrophy and first appear as discrete yellowish papules during the preadolescent period in approximately 50% of children. No treatment is necessary.

PARULIS

The parulis (gum boil) is a soft reddish papule located adjacent to the root of a chronically abscessed tooth. It occurs at the end-point of a draining dental sinus tract. Treatment consists of diagnosing which tooth is abscessed and extracting it or performing root canal on the offending tooth.

CHEILITIS

This dryness of the lips followed by scaling and cracking and accompanied by a characteristic burning sensation is common in children. Cheilitis may be caused by sensitivity to contact substances, lip licking, vitamin deficiency, weakened immune system, or fungal or bacterial infections. Cheilitis often occurs in association with fever. Treatment may include antifungal or antibacterial agents and frequent application of petroleum jelly.

ANKYLOGLOSSIA

Ankyloglossia or "tongue-tie" is characterized by an abnormally short lingual frenum that can hinder the tongue movement but rarely interferes with feeding or speech. The frenum might spontaneously lengthen as the child gets older. If the extent of the ankyloglossia is severe, speech may be affected and surgical correction may be indicated.

GEOGRAPHIC TONGUE

Geographic tongue (migratory glossitis) is a benign and asymptomatic lesion and is characterized by 1 or more smooth, bright red patches, often showing a yellow, gray, or white membranous margin on the dorsum of an otherwise normally roughened tongue. The condition has no known cause, and no treatment is indicated (see Chapter 664).

FISSURED TONGUE

The fissured tongue (scrotal tongue) is a malformation manifested clinically by numerous small furrows or grooves on the dorsal surface (see Chapter 664). If the tongue is painful, brushing the tongue or irrigating with water can reduce the bacteria in the fissures.

Table 315-1	Differential Diagnosis of Oral Ulceration
CONDITION	**COMMENT**
COMMON	
Aphthous (canker sore)	Painful, circumscribed lesions; recurrences
Traumatic	Accidents, chronic cheek biter, or after dental local anesthesia
Hand, foot, mouth disease	Painful; lesions on tongue, anterior oral cavity, hands, and feet
Herpangina	Painful; lesions confined to soft palate and oropharynx
Herpetic gingivostomatitis	Vesicles on mucocutaneous borders; painful, febrile
Recurrent herpes labialis	Vesicles on lips; painful
Chemical burns	Alkali, acid, aspirin; painful
Heat burns	Hot food, electrical
UNCOMMON	
Neutrophil defects	Agranulocytosis, leukemia, cyclic neutropenia; painful
Systemic lupus erythematosus	Recurrent, may be painless
Behçet syndrome	Resembles aphthous lesions; associated with genital ulcers, uveitis
Necrotizing ulcerative gingivostomatitis	Vincent stomatitis; painful
Syphilis	Chancre or gumma; painless
Oral Crohn disease	Aphthous-like; painful
Histoplasmosis	Lingual
Pemphigus	May be isolated to the oral cavity
Stevens-Johnson syndrome	May be isolated or appear initially in the oral cavity

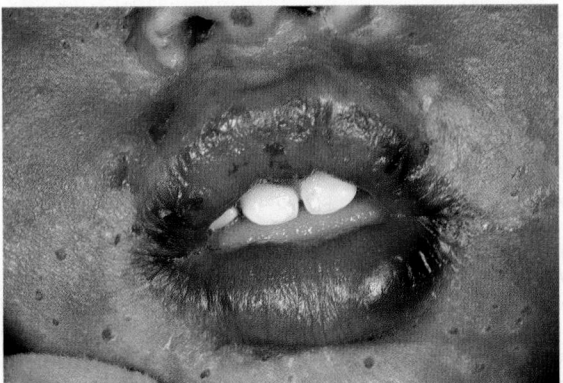

Figure 315-1 Herpetic gingivostomatitis. Lip erosions with multiple perioral herpetic lesions involving the mucotaneous borders. *(From Paller AS, Mancini AJ, editors: Hurwitz clinical pediatric dermatology, ed 3, Philadelphia, 2006, WB Saunders, p. 398.)*

Chapter **316**
Diseases of the Salivary Glands and Jaws
Norman Tinanoff

With the exception of mumps (see Chapter 248), disease of the salivary glands is rare in children. Bilateral enlargement of the submaxillary glands can occur in AIDS, cystic fibrosis, Epstein-Barr virus infection, and malnutrition, and, transiently, during acute asthmatic attacks. Chronic vomiting can be accompanied by enlargement of the parotid glands. Benign salivary gland hypertrophy has been associated with endocrinopathies: thyroid disease, diabetes, and Cushing syndrome. Infiltrative disease or tumors are uncommon; red flags include facial nerve palsy, rapid growth, fixed skin, paresthesias, ulceration, or a history of radiation to the head or neck region.

PAROTITIS
Acute parotitis is often caused by blockage, with further inflammation due to bacterial infection. The blockage may be due to a salivary stone or mucous plug. Stones can be removed by physical manipulation, surgery, or lithotripsy. **Recurrent parotitis** is an idiopathic swelling of the parotid gland that can occur in otherwise healthy children. The swelling is usually unilateral, but both glands can be involved simultaneously or alternately. There is little pain; the swelling is limited to the gland and usually lasts 2-3 wk. Treatment may include local heat, massaging the gland, and antibiotics. **Suppurative parotitis** is usually caused by *Staphylococcus aureus*. It is usually unilateral and may be accompanied by fever. The gland becomes swollen, tender, and painful. Suppurative parotitis responds to antibacterial therapy based on culture obtained from the Stensen duct or by surgical drainage. Viral causes of parotitis include mumps (often in epidemics), EBV, human herpes virus 6, enteroviruses, and HIV.

RANULA
A ranula is a cyst associated with a major salivary gland in the sublingual area. It is a large, soft, mucus-containing swelling in the floor of the mouth. It occurs at any age, including infancy. The cyst should be excised, and the severed duct should be exteriorized.

MUCOCELE
Mucocele is a salivary gland lesion caused by a blockage of a salivary gland duct. It is most common on the lower lip and has the appearance of a fluid-filled vesicle or a fluctuant nodule with the overlying mucosa normal in color. Treatment is surgical excision, with removal of the involved accessory salivary gland.

CONGENITAL LIP PITS
Congenital lip pits are caused by fistulous tracts that lead to embedded mucous glands in the lower lip. They leak saliva, especially with salivary stimulation. Lip pits can be isolated anomalies, or they can be found in patients with cleft lip or palate. Treatment is surgical excision of the glandular tissue.

ERUPTION CYST
Eruption cyst is a smooth, painless swelling over the erupting tooth. If bleeding occurs in the cyst space, it may appear blue or blue-black. In most cases, no treatment is indicated and the cyst resolves with the full eruption of the tooth.

XEROSTOMIA
Also known as dry mouth, xerostomia may be associated with fever, dehydration, anticholinergic drugs, chronic graft-versus-host disease, Mikulicz disease (leukemia infiltrates), Sjögren syndrome, or tumoricidal doses of radiation when the salivary glands are within the field. Long-term xerostomia is a high-risk factor for dental caries.

SALIVARY GLAND TUMORS
See Chapter 500.

HISTIOCYTIC DISORDERS
See Chapter 507.

TUMORS OF THE JAW
Ossifying fibroma is a common benign tumor of the jaw. It is often asymptomatic, being discovered on routine radiographic examinations. Treatment is resection because of the possibility of recurrence. **Central giant cell granuloma** is another common lesion thought to be reactive rather than neoplastic. Although usually asymptomatic, it can be expansile, with or without resorption of the roots of teeth and perforation of the cortical plate. Treatment is complete curettage or surgical excision. **Dentigerous cysts** are common lesions associated with the crown of an impacted or unerupted tooth. Although usually asymptomatic, they can become large and destructive. Treatment is surgical removal.

The malignant primary tumors of the jaw in children include Burkitt lymphoma, osteogenic sarcoma, lymphosarcoma, ameloblastoma, and, more rarely, fibrosarcoma.

Bibliography is available at Expert Consult.

Chapter **317**
Diagnostic Radiology in Dental Assessment
Norman Tinanoff

The **panoramic radiograph** provides a single tomographic image of the upper and lower jaw, including all the teeth and supporting structures. The x-ray tube rotates about the patient's head with reciprocal movement of the film or image receptor during the exposure. The panoramic image shows the teeth, mandibular bodies, rami, and condyles; maxillary sinuses; and a majority of the facial buttresses. Such images are used to show abnormalities of tooth number, development and eruption pattern, cystic and neoplastic lesions, bone infections, and fracture, as well as dental caries and periodontal disease (Fig. 317-1).

Cephalometric radiographs are posteroanterior and lateral skull films that are taken using a **cephalostat** (head positioner) and employ techniques that clearly demonstrate the facial skeleton and soft facial tissues. Similar protocols for positioning children are used throughout the world. From these images, cranial and facial points and planes can be determined and compared with standards derived from thousands of images. A child's facial growth can be assessed serially when cephalometric radiographs are taken sequentially. Relationships among the maxilla, mandible, cranial base, and facial skeleton can be determined in a quantitative manner. Additionally, the alignment of the teeth and the relation of the teeth to the supporting bone can be serially measured.

Intraoral dental radiographs are highly detailed, direct-exposure films that demonstrate sections of the child's teeth and supporting bone structures. The film or image receptor is placed lingual to the teeth,

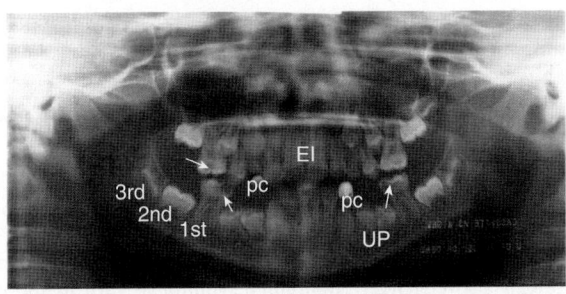

Figure 317-1 A panoramic radiograph of a 10 yr old child showing extensive dental caries of the 1st permanent molars (arrows), as well as normal structures: erupted 1st permanent molar, unerupted 2nd molar, and unerupted 3rd molar; erupted incisors (EI), unerupted premolars (UP), and erupted primary canines (pc).

and the x-ray beam is directed through the teeth and supporting structures. The resulting images are used to detect dental caries, loss of alveolar bone (periodontal disease), abscesses at the roots of the teeth, and trauma to the teeth and alveolar bone and to demonstrate the developmental status of permanent teeth within the bone.

Section 3
The Esophagus

Chapter 318
Embryology, Anatomy, and Function of the Esophagus
Seema Khan and Susan R. Orenstein

The esophagus is a hollow muscular tube, separated from the pharynx above and the stomach below by 2 tonically closed sphincters. Its primary function is to convey ingested material from the mouth to the stomach. Largely lacking digestive glands and enzymes, and exposed only briefly to nutrients, it has no active role in digestion.

EMBRYOLOGY
The esophagus develops from the postpharyngeal foregut and can be distinguished from the stomach in the 4 wk old embryo. At the same time, the trachea begins to bud just anterior to the developing esophagus; the resulting laryngotracheal groove extends and becomes the lung. Disturbance of this stage can result in congenital anomalies such as **tracheoesophageal fistula.** The length of the esophagus is 8-10 cm at birth and doubles in the 1st 2-3 yr of life, reaching approximately 25 cm in the adult. The abdominal portion of the esophagus is as large as the stomach in an 8 wk old fetus but gradually shortens to a few millimeters at birth, attaining a final length of approximately 3 cm by a few years of age. This intraabdominal location of both the distal esophagus and the **lower esophageal sphincter** (LES) is an important antireflux mechanism, because increases in intraabdominal pressure are also transmitted to the sphincter, augmenting its defense. Swallowing can be seen in utero as early as 16-20 wk of gestation, helping to

circulate the amniotic fluid; **polyhydramnios** is a hallmark of lack of normal swallowing or of esophageal or upper gastrointestinal tract obstruction. Sucking and swallowing are not fully coordinated before 34 wk of gestation, a contributing factor for feeding difficulties in premature infants.

ANATOMY
The luminal aspect of the esophagus is covered by thick, protective, nonkeratinized stratified squamous epithelium, which abruptly changes to simple columnar epithelium at the stomach's upper margin at the **gastroesophageal junction (GEJ).** This squamous epithelium is relatively resistant to damage by gastric secretions (in contrast to the ciliated columnar epithelium of the respiratory tract), but chronic irritation by gastric contents can result in morphometric changes (thickening of the basal cell layer and lengthening of papillary ingrowth into the epithelium) and subsequent metaplasia of the cells lining the lower esophagus from squamous to columnar. Deeper layers of the esophageal wall are composed successively of lamina propria, muscularis mucosae, submucosa, and the 2 layers of muscularis propria (circular surrounded by longitudinal). The 2 delimiting sphincters of the esophagus, the **upper esophageal sphincter (UES)** at the cricopharyngeus muscle and the **LES** at the **GEJ,** constrict the esophageal lumen at its proximal and distal boundaries. The muscularis propria of the upper third of the esophagus is predominantly striated, and that of the lower two-thirds is smooth muscle. Clinical conditions involving striated muscle (cricopharyngeal dysfunction, cerebral palsy) affect the upper esophagus, whereas those involving smooth muscle (achalasia, reflux esophagitis) affect the lower esophagus. The muscular LES and the mucosal "Z-line" of the GEJ may be discrepant up to several centimeters.

FUNCTION
The esophagus can be divided into 3 areas: the UES, the esophageal body, and the LES. At rest, the tonic LES pressure is normally approximately 20 mm Hg; values <10 mm Hg are usually considered abnormal, although it seems that competence against retrograde flow of gastric material is maintained if the LES pressure is >5 mm Hg. The LES pressure rises during intragastric pressure amplifications, whether caused by gastric contractions, abdominal wall muscle contractions ("straining"), or external pressure applied to the abdominal wall. It also rises in response to cholinergic stimuli, gastrin, gastric alkalization, and certain drugs (bethanechol, metoclopramide, cisapride). The UES pressure is more variable and often higher than that of the LES; it decreases almost to zero during deep sleep and it increases markedly during stress and straining. The UES and LES relax briefly to allow material to pass through during swallowing, belching, reflux, and vomiting. They can contract in response to subthreshold levels of reflux (esophagoglottal closure reflex).

Swallowing is initiated by elevation of the tongue, propelling the bolus into the pharynx. The larynx elevates and moves anteriorly, pulling open the relaxing UES, while the opposed aryepiglottic folds close. The epiglottis drops back to cover the larynx and direct the bolus over the larynx and into the UES. The soft palate occludes the nasopharynx. The primary peristalsis thus initiated is a contraction originating in the oropharynx that clears the esophagus aborally (Fig. 318-1). The LES, tonically contracted as a barrier against gastroesophageal reflux (GER), relaxes as swallowing is initiated, at nearly the same time as the UES relaxation. The LES relaxation persists considerably longer, until the peristaltic wave traverses it and closes it. The normal esophageal peristaltic speed is approximately 3 cm/sec; the wave takes 4 sec or longer to traverse the 12 cm esophagus of a young infant and considerably longer in a larger child. Facial stimulation by a puff of air can induce swallowing and esophageal peristalsis in healthy young infants, a reflex termed the **Santmyer swallow.**

In addition to relaxing to move swallowed material past the GEJ into the stomach, the LES normally relaxes to vent swallowed air or to allow retrograde expulsion of material from the stomach. Perhaps as an extension of these functions, the normal LES also permits physiologic reflux episodes, brief events that occur approximately 5 times in the

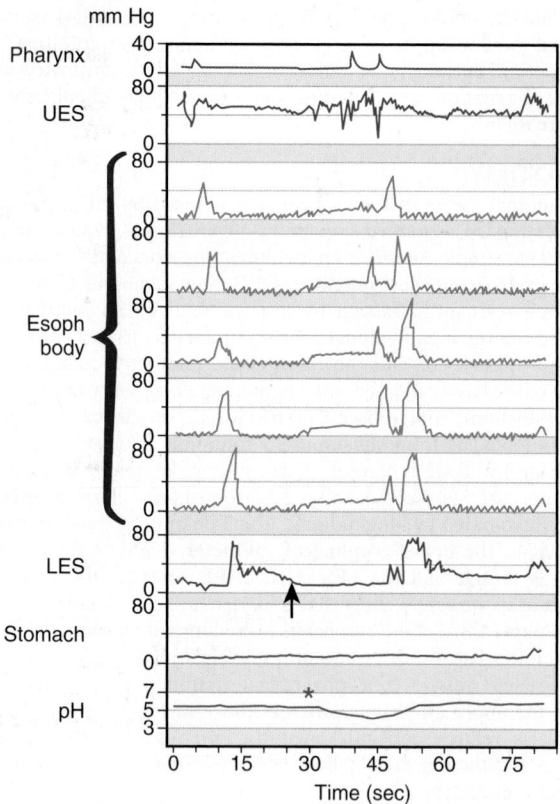

Figure 318-1 A continuous tracing of esophageal motility showing 2 swallows, as indicated by the pharyngeal contraction associated with relaxation of the upper esophageal sphincter (UES) and followed by peristalsis in the body of the esophagus. The lower esophageal sphincter (LES) also displays a transient relaxation *(arrow)* unassociated with a swallow. There is an episode of gastroesophageal reflux (*) recorded by a pH probe at the time of the transient LES relaxation. *(Courtesy of John Dent, FRACP, PhD, and Geoffrey Davidson, MD.)*

first postprandial hour, particularly in the awake state, but are otherwise uncommon. **Transient LES relaxation,** not associated with swallowing, is the major mechanism underlying **pathologic reflux** (see Fig. 318-1).

The close linkage of the anatomy of the upper digestive and respiratory tracts has mandated intricate functional protections of the respiratory tract during retrograde movement of gastric contents as well as during swallowing. The protective functions include the LES tone, the bolstering of the LES by the surrounding diaphragmatic crura, and the "backup protection" of the UES tone. Secondary peristalsis, akin to primary peristalsis but without an oral component, originates in the upper esophagus, triggered mainly by GER, and thereby also clears refluxed gastric contents from the esophagus. Another protective reflex is the "pharyngeal swallow" (initiated above the esophagus, but without lingual participation). Multiple levels of protection against aspiration include the rhythmic coordination of swallowing and breathing and a series of protective reflexes with esophagopharyngeal afferents and efferents that close the UES or larynx. These reflexes include the esophago-UES contractile reflex, the pharyngo-UES contractile reflex, the esophagoglottal closure reflex, and 2 pharyngoglottal adduction reflexes. The last 2 reflexes have chemoreceptors on the laryngeal surface of the epiglottis and mechanoreceptors on the aryepiglottic folds as their sites of stimulus. It is likely that interactions between the esophagus and the respiratory tract, which cause extraesophageal manifestations of gastroesophageal reflux disease (GERD), will be explained by subtle abnormalities in these protective reflexes.

Bibliography is available at Expert Consult.

318.1 Common Clinical Manifestations and Diagnostic Aids

Seema Khan and Susan R. Orenstein

COMMON CLINICAL MANIFESTATIONS

Manifestations of esophageal disorders include pain, obstruction or difficulty swallowing, abnormal retrograde movement of gastric contents (reflux, regurgitation, or vomiting), or bleeding; esophageal disease can also engender respiratory symptoms. Pain in the chest unrelated to swallowing (**heartburn**) can be a sign of esophagitis, but similar pain might also represent cardiac, pulmonary, or musculoskeletal disease or visceral hyperalgesia. Pain during swallowing (**odynophagia**) localizes the disease more discretely to the pharynx and esophagus and often represents inflammatory mucosal disease. Complete esophageal obstruction can be produced acutely by esophageal foreign bodies, including food impactions; can be congenital, as in esophageal atresia; or can evolve over time as a peptic stricture occludes the esophagus. Difficulty swallowing (**dysphagia**) can be produced by incompletely occlusive esophageal obstruction (by extrinsic compression, intrinsic narrowing, or foreign bodies) but can also result from dysmotility of the esophagus (whether primary/idiopathic or secondary to systemic disease). Inflammatory lesions of the esophagus without obstruction or dysmotility are a third cause of dysphagia; eosinophilic esophagitis, most often afflicting older boys, is relatively common.

The most common esophageal disorder in children is **GERD,** which is from retrograde return of gastric contents into the esophagus. **Esophagitis** can be caused by GERD, by eosinophilic disease, by infection, or by caustic substances. Esophageal **bleeding** can result from severe esophagitis that produces erosions or ulcerations and can manifest as anemia or Hemoccult-positive stools. More acute or severe bleeding can be from ruptured **esophageal varices.** The resulting hematemesis must be differentiated from more distal bleeding (gastric ulcer) and from more proximal bleeding (a nosebleed or hemoptysis). Respiratory symptoms of esophageal disease can result from luminal contents incorrectly being directed into the respiratory tract or to reflexive respiratory responses to esophageal stimuli.

DIAGNOSTIC AIDS

The esophagus can be evaluated by radiography, endoscopy, histology, scintigraphy, manometry, pH-metry (linked as indicated with other polysomnography), and multichannel intraluminal impedance. Contrast (usually barium) radiographic study of the esophagus usually incorporates fluoroscopic imaging over time so that motility and anatomy can be assessed. Although most often requested to evaluate for GERD, it is neither sensitive nor specific for this purpose; it can detect complications of GERD (stricture or hiatal hernia) or conditions mimicking GERD (pyloric stenosis or malrotation with intermittent volvulus).

Barium fluoroscopy is optimal for evaluating for structural anomalies, such as duplications, strictures, or external esophageal compression by an aberrant blood vessel, or for causes of dysmotility, such as achalasia. Modifications of the routine barium fluoroscopic study are used in special situations. When an "H-type" tracheoesophageal fistula is suspected, the test is most sensitive if the radiologist, with the patient prone, distends the esophagus with barium via a nasogastric tube. The videofluoroscopic evaluation of swallowing performed with varying consistencies of barium ("modified barium swallow," oropharyngeal videoesophagram, or "cookie swallow") optimally evaluates children with dysphagia by demonstrating incoordination of the pharyngeal and esophageal phases of swallowing and any associated aspiration.

In some centers, fiberoptic endoscopic evaluation of swallowing uses nasopharyngeal endoscopy to visualize the pharynx and larynx during swallowing of dye-enhanced foods when dysphagia, laryngeal penetration, or aspiration are suspected. This is often combined with sensory testing of the laryngeal adductor reflex in response to a calibrated puff of air through the endoscope to the arytenoids, generating the composite fiberoptic endoscopic evaluation of swallowing sensory testing that examines the mechanisms of any aspiration that is present. Endoscopy allows direct visualization of esophageal mucosa and helps therapeutically in the removal of foreign bodies and treatment of esophageal varices. Endoscopy also allows biopsy samples to be taken, thus improving the diagnosis of "endoscopy-negative" GERD, differentiating GERD from eosinophilic esophagitis, and identifying viral or fungal causes of esophagitis.

Radionuclide scintigraphy scans are helpful in evaluating the efficiency of peristalsis and demonstrating reflux episodes. They can be specific, although not very sensitive, for aspiration and can quantify gastric emptying, thus hinting at a cause for GERD. The related radionuclide salivagram can demonstrate aspiration of even minute amounts of saliva.

Esophageal manometry evaluates for dysmotility from the pharynx to the stomach; by synchronized quantitative pressure measurements along the esophagus, it detects and characterizes dysfunctions sometimes missed radiographically. Manometry is often challenging in young infants, and sphincters are optimally evaluated with special Dent sleeves, rather than the simple ports available for the esophageal body.

Extended pH monitoring of the distal esophagus is a sensitive test for acidic GER episodes that can quantify duration and degree of acidity, but not volume, of the reflux episodes. It is linked with polysomnography (a "pneumogram") when GER is suspected to cause apnea or similar symptoms.

Multichannel intraluminal impedance is a method for pH-independent detection of bolus movements in the esophagus; with a pH probe incorporated, it can distinguish between acid and nonacid liquid and gaseous reflux, the proximal extent of reflux, and several aspects of esophageal function, such as direction of bolus flow, duration of bolus presence, and bolus clearance.

Chapter 319
Congenital Anomalies

319.1 Esophageal Atresia and Tracheoesophageal Fistula

Seema Khan and Susan R. Orenstein

Esophageal atresia (EA) is the most common congenital anomaly of the esophagus, with a prevalence of 1.7 per 10,000 live births. Of these, >90% have an associated tracheoesophageal fistula (TEF). In the most common form of EA, the upper esophagus ends in a blind pouch and the TEF is connected to the distal esophagus (type C). Figure 319-1 shows the types of EA and TEF and their relative frequencies. The exact cause is still unknown; associated features include advanced maternal age, European ethnicity, obesity, low socioeconomic status, and tobacco

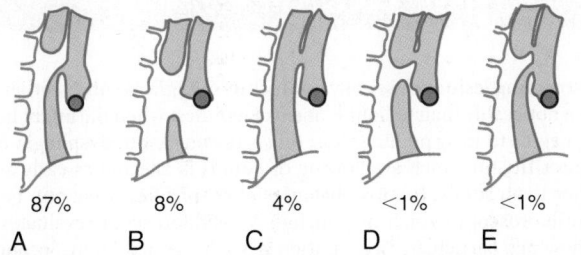

| 87% | 8% | 4% | <1% | <1% |
| A | B | C | D | E |

Figure 319-1 Diagrams of the 5 most commonly encountered forms of esophageal atresia and tracheoesophageal fistula, shown in order of frequency.

smoking. This defect has survival rates of >90%, owing largely to improved neonatal intensive care, earlier recognition, and appropriate intervention. Infants weighing < 1,500 g at birth and those with severe cardiac anomalies have the highest risk for mortality. Fifty percent of infants are nonsyndromic without other anomalies, and the rest have associated anomalies, most often associated with the VATER or VACTERL (vertebral, anorectal, [cardiac], tracheal, esophageal, renal, radial, [limb]) syndrome. Cardiac and vertebral anomalies are seen in 32% and 24%, respectively. These syndromes generally are associated with normal intelligence. Despite low concordance among twins and the low incidence of familial cases, genetic factors have a role in the pathogenesis of TEF in some patients as suggested by discrete mutations in syndromic cases: Feingold syndrome *(N-MYC)*, CHARGE syndrome *(c*oloboma of the eye, *c*entral nervous system anomalies; *h*eart defects; *a*tresia of the choanae; *r*etardation of growth and/or development; *g*enital and/or urinary defects [hypogonadism]; *e*ar anomalies and/or deafness) *(CHD7)*, and anophthalmia-esophageal-genital syndrome *(SOX2)*.

PRESENTATION

The neonate with EA typically has frothing and bubbling at the mouth and nose after birth as well as episodes of coughing, cyanosis, and respiratory distress. Feeding exacerbates these symptoms, causes regurgitation, and can precipitate aspiration. Aspiration of gastric contents via a distal fistula causes more damaging pneumonitis than aspiration of pharyngeal secretions from the blind upper pouch. The infant with an isolated TEF in the absence of EA ("H-type" fistula) might come to medical attention later in life with chronic respiratory problems, including refractory bronchospasm and recurrent pneumonias.

DIAGNOSIS

In the setting of early-onset respiratory distress, the inability to pass a nasogastric or orogastric tube in the newborn suggests EA. Perinatal radiographic findings of absence of the infant stomach bubble and maternal polyhydramnios might alert the physician to EA. Plain radiography in the evaluation of respiratory distress might reveal a coiled feeding tube in the esophageal pouch and/or an air-distended stomach, indicating the presence of a coexisting TEF (Fig. 319-2). Conversely, pure EA can manifest as an airless scaphoid abdomen. In isolated TEF (H type), an esophagogram with contrast medium injected under pressure can demonstrate the defect (Fig. 319-3). Alternatively, the orifice may be detected at bronchoscopy or when methylene blue dye injected into the endotracheal tube during endoscopy is observed in the esophagus during forced inspiration.

MANAGEMENT

Initially, maintaining a patent airway, pre-operative proximal pouch decompression to prevent aspiration of secretions and use of antibiotics to prevent consequent pneumonia are paramount. Prone positioning minimizes movement of gastric secretions into a distal fistula, and esophageal suctioning minimizes aspiration from a blind pouch. Endotracheal intubation with mechanical ventilation is to be avoided if possible because it can worsen distention of abdominal viscera. Surgical ligation of the TEF and primary end-to-end anastomosis of the esophagus via right-sided thoracotomy constitute the current standard surgical approach. In the premature or otherwise complicated infant, a primary closure may be delayed by temporizing with fistula ligation and gastrostomy tube placement. If the gap between the atretic ends of the esophagus is >3-4 cm, primary repair cannot be done; options include using gastric, jejunal, or colonic segments interposed as a neoesophagus. Careful search must be undertaken for the common associated cardiac and other anomalies. Thoracoscopic surgical repair is now considered feasible and associated with favorable long-term outcomes.

OUTCOME

The majority of children with EA and TEF grow up to lead normal lives, but complications are often challenging, particularly during the 1st 5 yr of life. Complications of surgery include anastomotic leak, refistulization, and anastomotic stricture. Gastroesophageal reflux

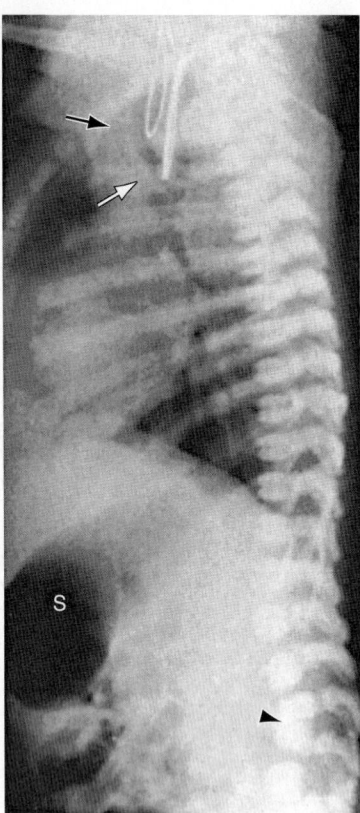

Figure 319-2 Tracheoesophageal fistula. Lateral radiograph demonstrating a nasogastric tube coiled *(arrows)* in the proximal segment of an atretic esophagus. The distal fistula is suggested by gaseous dilation of the stomach *(S)* and small intestine. The *arrowhead* depicts vertebral fusion, whereas a heart murmur and cardiomegaly suggest the presence of a ventricular septal defect. This patient demonstrated elements of the VATER (vertebral, anorectal, tracheal, esophageal, renal, radial) anomalad. *(From Balfe D, Ling D, Siegel M: The esophagus. In Putman CE, Ravin CE, editors: Textbook of diagnostic imaging, Philadelphia, 1988, WB Saunders.)*

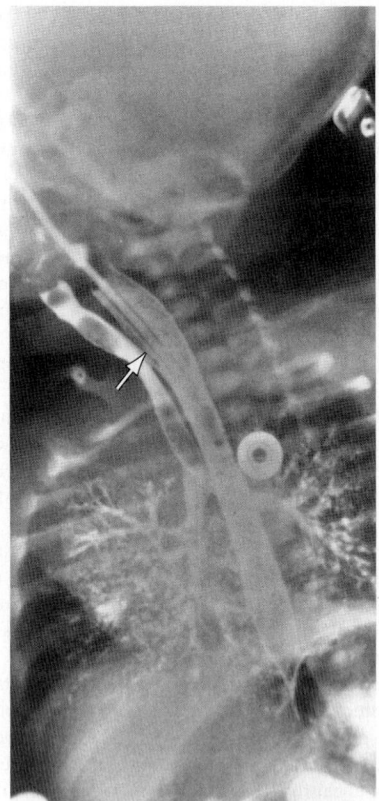

Figure 319-3 H-type fistula *(arrow)* demonstrated in an infant after barium swallow on frontal-oblique chest x-ray. The tracheal aspect of the fistula is characteristically superior to the esophageal aspect. Barium is seen to outline the tracheobronchial tree. *(From Wyllie R, Hyams JS, editors: Pediatric gastrointestinal and liver disease, ed 3, Philadelphia, 2006, Saunders Elsevier, p. 299.)*

material is often seen in the esophagus and trachea. Treatment is surgical repair, which can be complex if the defects are long.

Bibliography is available at Expert Consult.

disease, resulting from intrinsic abnormalities of esophageal function, often combined with delayed gastric emptying, contributes to management challenges in many cases. Gastroesophageal reflux disease contributes significantly to the respiratory disease (**reactive airway disease**) that often complicates EA and TEF and also worsens the frequent anastomotic strictures after repair of EA.

Many patients have an associated tracheomalacia that improves as the child grows.

Bibliography is available at Expert Consult.

319.2 Laryngotracheoesophageal Clefts
Seema Khan and Susan R. Orenstein

Laryngotracheoesophageal clefts are uncommon anomalies that result when the septum between the esophagus and trachea fails to develop fully, leading to a common channel defect between the pharyngoesophagus and laryngotracheal lumen, thus making the laryngeal closure incompetent during swallowing or reflux. Other developmental anomalies, such as EA and TEF, are seen in 20% of patients with clefts. The severity of presenting symptoms depends on the type of cleft; they are commonly classified as 4 types (I-IV) according to the inferior extent of the cleft. Early in life, the infant presents with stridor, choking, cyanosis, aspiration of feedings, and recurrent chest infections. The diagnosis is difficult and usually requires direct endoscopic visualization of the larynx and esophagus. When contrast radiography is used,

Chapter 320
Obstructing and Motility Disorders of the Esophagus
Seema Khan and Susan R. Orenstein

Obstructing lesions classically produce **dysphagia** to **solids** earlier and more noticeably than to liquids and can manifest when the infant liquid diet begins to incorporate solids; this is in contrast to **dysphagia** from **dysmotility,** in which swallowing of liquids is affected as early as, or earlier than, solids. In most instances of dysphagia, evaluation begins with fluoroscopy, which may include videofluoroscopic evaluation of swallowing, particularly if aspiration is a primary symptom. Secondary studies are often endoscopic if intrinsic obstruction is suspected or manometric if dysmotility is suspected; other imaging studies may be used in particular cases. Congenital lesions can require surgery, whereas webs and peptic strictures might respond adequately to endoscopic (or bougie) dilation. Peptic strictures, once dilated, should prompt consideration of fundoplication for ongoing prophylaxis.

EXTRINSIC

Esophageal duplication cysts are the most commonly encountered foregut duplications. These cysts are lined by intestinal epithelium, have a well-developed smooth muscle wall, and are attached to the normal gastrointestinal tract. Most of these affect the distal half of the esophagus on the right side. The most common presentation is respiratory distress caused by compression of the adjacent airways. Dysphagia is a common symptom in older children. Upper gastrointestinal bleeding can occur as a result of acid-secreting gastric mucosa in the duplication wall. **Neuroenteric cysts** might contain glial elements and are associated with **vertebral anomalies.** Diagnosis is made using modalities, such as barium swallow, chest CT, and MRI, or endosonography. Treatment is surgical; laparoscopic approach to excision is also possible.

Enlarged mediastinal or subcarinal **lymph nodes,** caused by infection (tuberculosis, histoplasmosis) or neoplasm (lymphoma), are the most common external masses that compress the esophagus and produce obstructive symptoms. **Vascular anomalies** can also compress the esophagus; *dysphagia lusoria* is a term denoting the dysphagia produced by a developmental vascular anomaly, which is often an aberrant right subclavian artery or right-sided or double aortic arch (see Chapter 432.1).

INTRINSIC

Intrinsic narrowing of the esophageal lumen can be congenital or acquired. The etiology is suggested by the location, the character of the lesion, and the clinical situation. The lower esophagus is the most common location for peptic strictures, which are generally somewhat ragged and several cm long. Thin membranous rings, including the Schatzki ring at the squamocolumnar junction, can also occlude this area. In the midesophagus, congenital narrowing may be associated with the esophageal atresia–tracheoesophageal fistula complex, in which some of the lesions might incorporate cartilage and might be impossible to dilate safely; alternatively, reflux esophagitis can induce a ragged and extensive narrowing that appears more proximal than the usual peptic stricture, often because of an associated hiatal hernia. Congenital webs or rings can narrow the upper esophagus. The upper esophagus can also be narrowed by an inflammatory stricture occurring after a caustic ingestion or due to epidermolysis bullosa. Cricopharyngeal achalasia can appear radiographically as a cricopharyngeal "bar" posteriorly in the upper esophagus. **Eosinophilic esophagitis** is one of the most common causes for esophageal obstructive symptoms. Although the pathogenesis of obstructive eosinophilic esophagitis is not yet completely explained and seems to vary among individual patients, endoscopy or radiology demonstrates stricture formation in some children with eosinophilic esophagitis, and in others a noncompliant esophagus is evident, with thickened wall layers demonstrable by ultrasonography.

Bibliography is available at Expert Consult.

Chapter **321**
Dysmotility

Seema Khan and Susan R. Orenstein

UPPER ESOPHAGEAL AND UPPER ESOPHAGEAL SPHINCTER DYSMOTILITY (STRIATED MUSCLE)

Cricopharyngeal **achalasia** signifies a failure of complete relaxation of the upper esophageal sphincter (UES), whereas cricopharyngeal **inco-**

ordination implies full relaxation of the UES but incoordination of the relaxation with the pharyngeal contraction. These entities are usually detected on videofluoroscopic evaluation of swallowing (sometimes accompanied by visible cricopharyngeal prominence, termed a *bar*), but often the most precise definition of the dysfunction is obtained with manometry. A self-limited form of cricopharyngeal incoordination occurs in infancy and remits spontaneously in the 1st yr of life if nutrition is maintained despite the dysphagia. In children, treatment options for non–self-limited cricopharyngeal achalasia consist of dilation, botox injection, and transcervical myotomy. It is important to evaluate such children thoroughly, including cranial MRI to detect **Arnold-Chiari malformations,** which can manifest in this way but are best treated by cranial decompression, rather than esophageal surgery. Cricopharyngeal spasm may be severe enough to produce posterior pharyngeal (Zenker) **diverticulum** above the obstructive sphincter; this entity occurs rarely in children.

Systemic causes of swallowing dysfunction that can affect the oropharynx, UES, and upper esophagus include cerebral palsy, Arnold-Chiari malformations, syringomyelia, bulbar palsy or cranial nerve defects (Möbius syndrome, transient infantile paralysis of the superior laryngeal nerve), transient pharyngeal muscle dysfunction, spinal muscular atrophy (including Werdnig-Hoffmann disease), muscular dystrophy, multiple sclerosis, infections (botulism, tetanus, poliomyelitis, diphtheria), inflammatory and autoimmune diseases (dermatomyositis, myasthenia gravis, polyneuritis, scleroderma), and familial dysautonomia. All of these can produce dysphagia. Medications (nitrazepam, benzodiazepines) and tracheostomy can adversely affect the function of the UES and thereby produce dysphagia.

LOWER ESOPHAGEAL AND LOWER ESOPHAGEAL SPHINCTER DYSFUNCTION (SMOOTH MUSCLE)

Causes of dysphagia resulting from more distal primary esophageal dysmotility include achalasia, diffuse esophageal spasm, nutcracker esophagus, and hypertensive lower esophageal sphincter (LES); all but achalasia are rare in children. Secondary causes include Hirschsprung disease, pseudoobstruction, inflammatory myopathies, scleroderma, and diabetes.

Achalasia is a primary esophageal motor disorder of unknown etiology characterized by loss of LES relaxation and loss of esophageal peristalsis, both contributing to a functional obstruction of the distal esophagus. Degenerative, autoimmune (antibodies to Auerbach plexus), and infectious (Chagas disease caused by *Trypanosoma cruzi*) factors are possible causes. In rare cases, achalasia is familial or part of the achalasia, alacrima, and adrenal insufficiency, known as triple A syndrome or **Allgrove syndrome**. *Pseudoachalasia* refers to achalasia caused by various forms of cancer via obstruction of the gastroesophageal junction, infiltration of the submucosa and muscularis of the LES, or as part of the paraneoplastic syndrome with formation of anti-Hu antibodies. Pathologically, in achalasia, inflammation surrounds ganglion cells, which are decreased in number. There is selective loss of postganglionic inhibitory neurons that normally lead to sphincter relaxation, leaving postganglionic cholinergic neurons unopposed. This imbalance produces high basal LES pressures and insufficient LES relaxation. The loss of esophageal peristalsis can be a secondary phenomenon.

Achalasia manifests with regurgitation and dysphagia for solids and liquids and may be accompanied by undernutrition or chronic cough; retained esophageal food can produce esophagitis. *The presentations of chronic regurgitation/vomiting with weight loss, and chronic cough have led to misdiagnoses of anorexia nervosa and asthma, respectively.* The mean age in children is 8.8 yr, with a mean duration of symptoms before diagnosis of 23 mo; it is uncommon before school age. Chest radiograph shows an air–fluid level in a dilated esophagus. **Barium fluoroscopy** reveals a smooth tapering of the lower esophagus leading to the closed LES, resembling a bird's beak (Fig. 321-1). Loss of primary peristalsis in the distal esophagus with retained food and poor emptying are often present. **Manometry** is the most sensitive diagnostic test; it reveals the defining features of aperistalsis in the distal esophageal body and incomplete or absent LES relaxation, often accompanied by high pressure LES and low-amplitude esophageal body contractions.

The goals of achalasia therapy are relief of symptoms, improvement of esophageal emptying, and prevention of megaesophagus. The 2 most effective treatment options are pneumatic dilation and laparoscopic or surgical (Heller) myotomy. Pneumatic dilation is the initial treatment of choice, and does not preclude a future myotomy. Surgeons often supplement a myotomy with an antireflux procedure to prevent the gastroesophageal reflux disease that otherwise often ensues when the sphincter is rendered less competent. Laparoscopic myotomy is a particularly effective procedure in adolescent and young adult males. Peroral endoscopic myotomy may be a feasible, safe, and an effective alternative to the laparoscopic method. Calcium channel blockers (nifedipine) and phosphodiesterase inhibitors offer temporary relief of dysphagia. Endoscopic injection of the LES with **botulinum toxin** counterbalances the selective loss of inhibitory neurotransmitters by inhibiting the release of acetylcholine from nerve terminals and may be an effective therapy. Botulinum toxin is effective in 50-65% of patients and is expensive; half the patients might require a repeat injection within 1 yr. Most eventually require dilation or surgery.

Diffuse esophageal spasm causes chest pain and dysphagia and affects adolescents and adults. It is diagnosed **manometrically** and can be treated with nitrates or calcium-channel-blocking agents.

Gastroesophageal reflux disease constitutes the most common cause of nonspecific abnormalities of esophageal motor function, probably through the effect of the esophageal inflammation on the musculature.

Bibliography is available at Expert Consult.

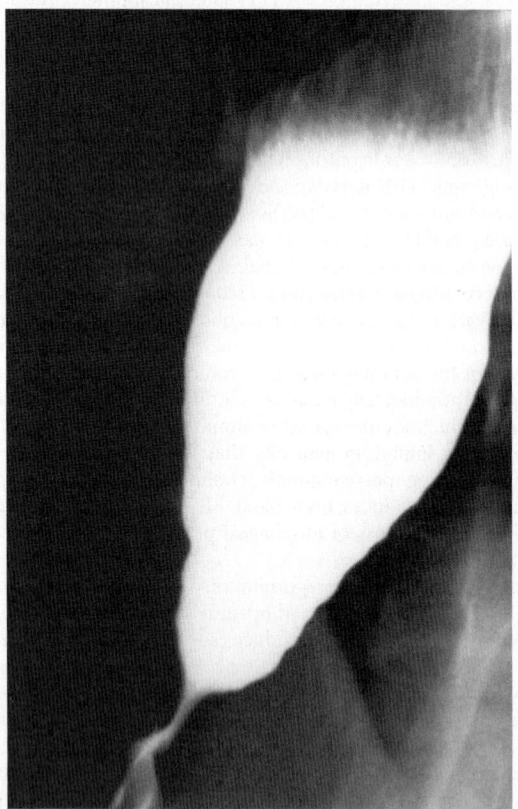

Figure 321-1 Barium esophagogram of a patient with achalasia demonstrating dilated esophagus and narrowing at the lower esophageal sphincter. Note retained secretions layered on top of barium in the esophagus.

Chapter 322
Hiatal Hernia
Seema Khan and Susan R. Orenstein

Herniation of the stomach through the esophageal hiatus can occur as a common sliding hernia (type 1), in which the gastroesophageal junction slides into the thorax, or it can be paraesophageal (type 2), in which a portion of the stomach (usually the fundus) is insinuated next to the esophagus inside the gastroesophageal junction in the hiatus (Figs. 322-1 and 322-2). A combination of sliding and paraesophageal types (type 3) is present in some patients. Sliding hernias are often associated with gastroesophageal reflux, especially in developmentally delayed children. The relationship to hiatal hernias in adults is unclear. Diagnosis is usually made by an upper gastrointestinal series and upper endoscopy. Medical treatment is not directed at the hernia but at the gastroesophageal reflux, unless failure of medical therapy prompts correction of the hernia at the time of fundoplication.

A paraesophageal hernia can be an isolated congenital anomaly or associated with gastric volvulus, or it may be encountered after fundoplication for gastroesophageal reflux, especially if the edges of a dilated esophageal diaphragmatic hiatus have not been approximated. Fullness after eating and upper abdominal pain are the usual symptoms. Infarction of the herniated stomach is rare.

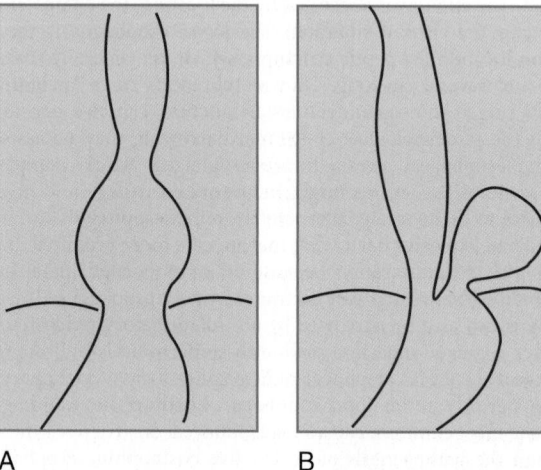

A   B

Figure 322-1 Types of esophageal hiatal hernia. **A,** Sliding hiatal hernia, the most common type. **B,** Paraesophageal hiatal hernia.

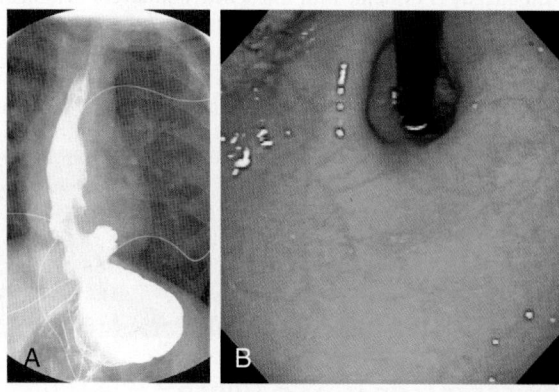

Figure 322-2 A, An upper gastrointestinal series shows a large hiatal hernia that extends above the diaphragm and impedes the exit of contrast from the esophagus into the stomach. Contrast is also noted to reflux to the upper esophagus. **B,** A retroflexed view of the hernia from the stomach during an upper endoscopy.

Gastroesophageal Reflux Disease

Seema Khan and Susan R. Orenstein

Gastroesophageal reflux disease (GERD) is the most common esophageal disorder in children of all ages. Gastroesophageal reflux (GER) signifies the retrograde movement of gastric contents across the lower esophageal sphincter (LES) into the esophagus, which occurs physiologically every day in all infants, older children, and adults. Physiologic GER is exemplified by the effortless regurgitation of normal infants. The phenomenon becomes **pathologic GERD** in infants and children who manifest or report bothersome symptoms because of frequent or persistent GER, producing esophagitis-related symptoms, or extraesophageal presentations, such as respiratory symptoms or nutritional effects.

PATHOPHYSIOLOGY

Factors determining the esophageal manifestations of reflux include the duration of esophageal exposure (a product of the frequency and duration of reflux episodes), the causticity of the refluxate, and the susceptibility of the esophagus to damage. The LES, defined as a high-pressure zone by manometry, is supported by the crura of the diaphragm at the gastroesophageal junction, together with valve-like functions of the esophagogastric junction anatomy, form the antireflux barrier. In the context of even the normal intraabdominal pressure augmentations that occur during daily life, the frequency of reflux episodes is increased by insufficient LES tone, by abnormal frequency of LES relaxations, and by hiatal herniation that prevents the LES pressure from being proportionately augmented by the crura during abdominal straining. Normal intraabdominal pressure augmentations may be further exacerbated by straining or respiratory efforts. The duration of reflux episodes is increased by lack of swallowing (e.g., during sleep) and by defective esophageal peristalsis. Vicious cycles ensue because chronic esophagitis produces esophageal peristaltic dysfunction (low-amplitude waves, propagation disturbances), decreased LES tone, and inflammatory esophageal shortening that induces hiatal herniation, all worsening reflux.

Transient LES relaxation (TLESR) is the primary mechanism allowing reflux to occur, and is defined as simultaneous relaxation of both LES and the surrounding crura. TLESRs occur independent of swallowing, reduce LES pressure to 0-2 mm Hg (above gastric), and last 10-60 sec; they appear by 26 wk of gestation. A vagovagal reflex, composed of afferent mechanoreceptors in the proximal stomach, a brainstem pattern generator, and efferents in the LES, regulates TLESRs. Gastric distention (postprandially, or from abnormal gastric emptying or air swallowing) is the main stimulus for TLESRs. Whether GERD is caused by a higher frequency of TLESRs or by a greater incidence of reflux during TLESRs is debated; each is likely in different persons. Straining during a TLESR makes reflux more likely, as do positions that place the gastroesophageal junction below the air–fluid interface in the stomach. Other factors influencing gastric pressure–volume dynamics, such as increased movement, straining, obesity, large-volume or hyperosmolar meals, gastroparesis, a large sliding hiatal hernia, and increased respiratory effort (coughing, wheezing) can have the same effect.

EPIDEMIOLOGY AND NATURAL HISTORY

Infant reflux becomes evident in the 1st few mo of life, peaks at 4 mo, and resolves in up to 88% by 12 mo and in nearly all by 24 mo. Symptoms in **older children** tend to be chronic, waxing and waning, but completely resolving in no more than half, which resembles adult patterns (Table 323-1). The histologic findings of esophagitis persist in infants who have naturally resolving symptoms of reflux. GERD likely has genetic predispositions: family clustering of GERD symptoms, endoscopic esophagitis, hiatal hernia, Barrett esophagus, and adenocarcinoma have been identified. As a continuously variable and common disorder, complex inheritance involving multiple genes and environmental factors is likely. Genetic linkage is indicated by the strong evidence of GERD in studies with monozygotic twins. A pediatric autosomal dominant form with otolaryngologic and respiratory manifestations has been located to chromosome 13q14, and the locus is termed GERD1.

CLINICAL MANIFESTATIONS

Most of the common clinical manifestations of esophageal disease can signify the presence of GERD and are generally thought to be mediated by the pathogenesis involving acid GER (Table 323-2). Although less noxious for the esophageal mucosa, nonacid reflux events are recognized to play an important role in extraesophageal disease manifestations. **Infantile reflux** manifests more often with regurgitation (especially postprandially), signs of esophagitis (irritability, arching, choking, gagging, feeding aversion), and resulting failure to thrive; symptoms resolve spontaneously in the majority of infants by 12-24 mo. **Older children** can have regurgitation during the preschool years; this complaint diminishes somewhat as children age, and complaints of abdominal and chest pain supervene in later childhood and adolescence. Occasional children present with food refusal or neck contortions (arching, turning of head) designated **Sandifer syndrome.** The respiratory presentations are also age dependent: GERD in infants can manifest as obstructive apnea or as stridor or lower airway disease in which reflux complicates primary airway disease such as laryngomalacia or bronchopulmonary dysplasia. Otitis media, sinusitis, lymphoid hyperplasia, hoarseness, vocal cord nodules, and laryngeal edema have all been associated with GERD. Airway manifestations in older children are more commonly related to asthma or to otolaryngologic disease such as laryngitis or sinusitis. Despite the high prevalence of GERD symptoms in asthmatic children, data showing direction of causality are conflicting.

DIAGNOSIS

For most of the typical GERD presentations, particularly in older children, a thorough history and physical examination suffice initially to reach the diagnosis. This initial evaluation aims to identify the pertinent positives in support of GERD and its complications and the negatives that make other diagnoses unlikely. The history may be facilitated and standardized by questionnaires (e.g., the Infant Gastroesophageal Reflux Questionnaire, the I-GERQ, and its derivative, the I-GERQ-R), which also permit quantitative scores to be evaluated for their diagnostic discrimination and for evaluative assessment of improvement or worsening of symptoms. The clinician should be alerted to the possibility of other important diagnoses in the presence of any alarm or warning signs: bilious emesis, frequent projectile emesis, gastrointestinal bleeding, lethargy, organomegaly, abdominal distention, micro- or macrocephaly, hepatosplenomegaly, failure to thrive, diarrhea, fever, bulging fontanelle, and seizures. The important differential diagnoses to consider in the evaluation of an infant or a child with chronic vomiting are milk and other food allergies, eosinophilic esophagitis, pyloric stenosis, intestinal obstruction (especially malrotation with intermittent volvulus), nonesophageal inflammatory diseases, infections, inborn errors of metabolism, hydronephrosis, increased intracranial pressure, rumination, and bulimia. Focused diagnostic testing, depending on the presentation and the differential diagnosis, can then supplement the initial examination.

Most of the esophageal tests are of some use in particular patients with suspected GERD. **Contrast (usually barium) radiographic** study of the esophagus and upper gastrointestinal tract is performed in children with vomiting and dysphagia to evaluate for achalasia, esophageal strictures and stenosis, hiatal hernia, and gastric outlet or intestinal obstruction (Fig. 323-1). It has poor sensitivity and specificity in the diagnosis of GERD as a result of its limited duration and the inability

Table 323-1	Symptoms According to Age		
MANIFESTATIONS	**INFANTS**	**CHILDREN**	**ADOLESCENTS AND ADULTS**
Impaired quality of life	+++	+++	+++
Regurgitation	++++	+	+
Excessive crying/irritability	+++	+	−
Vomiting	++	++	+
Food refusal/feeding disturbances/anorexia	++	+	+
Persisting hiccups	++	+	+
Failure to thrive	++	+	−
Abnormal posturing/Sandifer syndrome	++	+	−
Esophagitis	+	++	+++
Persistent cough/aspiration pneumonia	+	++	+
Wheezing/laryngitis/ear problems	+	++	+
Laryngomalacia/stridor/croup	+	++	−
Sleeping disturbances	+	+	+
Anemia/melena/hematemesis	+	+	+
Apnea/ALTE/desaturation	+	−	−
Bradycardia	+	?	?
Heartburn/pyrosis	?	++	+++
Epigastric pain	?	+	++
Chest pain	?	+	++
Dysphagia	?	+	++
Dental erosions/water brush	?	+	+
Hoarseness/globus pharyngeus	?	+	+
Chronic asthma/sinusitis	−	++	+
Laryngostenosis/vocal nodule problems	−	+	+
Stenosis	−	(+)	+
Barrett/esophageal adenocarcinoma	−	(+)	+

+++, Very common; ++ common; + possible; (+) rare; − absent; ? unknown; ALTE, apparent life-threatening event.
From Wyllie R, Hyams JS, Kay M, editors: Pediatric gastrointestinal and liver disease, *ed 4, Philadelphia, 2011, WB Saunders, Table 22-3, p. 235.*

to differentiate physiologic GER from GERD. Furthermore, contrast radiography neither accurately assesses mucosal inflammation nor correlates with severity of GERD.

Extended **esophageal pH monitoring** of the distal esophagus, no longer considered the sine qua non of a GERD diagnosis, provides a quantitative and sensitive documentation of acidic reflux episodes, the most important type of reflux episodes for pathologic reflux. The distal esophageal pH probe is placed at a level corresponding to 87% of the nares-LES distance, based on regression equations using the patient's height, on fluoroscopic visualization, or on manometric identification of the LES. Normal values of distal esophageal acid exposure (pH < 4) are generally established as <5-8% of the total monitored time, but these quantitative normals are insufficient to establish or disprove a diagnosis of pathologic GERD. The most important indications for esophageal pH monitoring are for assessing efficacy of acid suppression during treatment, evaluating apneic episodes in conjunction with a pneumogram and perhaps impedance, and evaluating atypical GERD presentations such as chronic cough, stridor, and asthma. Dual pH probes, adding a proximal esophageal probe to the standard distal one, are used in the diagnosis of extraesophageal GERD, identifying upper esophageal acid exposure times of 1% of the total time as threshold values for abnormality.

Endoscopy allows diagnosis of erosive esophagitis (Fig. 323-2) and complications such as strictures or Barrett esophagus; esophageal biopsies can diagnose histologic reflux esophagitis in the absence of erosions while simultaneously eliminating allergic and infectious causes. Endoscopy is also used therapeutically to dilate reflux-induced strictures. Radionucleotide scintigraphy using technetium can demonstrate aspiration and delayed gastric emptying when these are suspected.

The multichannel **intraluminal impedance** is a cumbersome test, but with potential applications both for diagnosing GERD and for understanding esophageal function in terms of bolus flow, volume clearance, and (in conjunction with manometry) motor patterns associated with GERD. Owing to the multiple sensors and a distal pH sensor, it is possible to document acidic reflux (pH < 4), weakly acidic reflux (pH 4-7), and weakly alkaline reflux (pH > 7) with multichannel intraluminal impedance. It is an important tool in those with respiratory symptoms, particularly for the determination of nonacid reflux, but must be cautiously applied in routine clinical evaluation because of limited evidence-based parameters for GERD diagnosis and symptom association.

Laryngotracheobronchoscopy evaluates for visible airway signs that are associated with extraesophageal GERD, such as posterior laryngeal inflammation and vocal cord nodules; it can permit diagnosis of silent aspiration (during swallowing or during reflux) by bronchoalveolar lavage with subsequent quantification of lipid-laden macrophages in airway secretions. Detection of pepsin in tracheal fluid is a marker of reflux-associated aspiration of gastric contents. Esophageal manometry permits evaluation for dysmotility, particularly in preparation for antireflux surgery.

Empirical antireflux therapy, using a time-limited trial of high-dose proton pump inhibitor (PPI), is a cost-effective strategy for diagnosis in adults; although not formally evaluated in older children, it has also been applied to this age group. Failure to respond to such empirical treatment, or a requirement for the treatment for prolonged periods, mandates formal diagnostic evaluation.

MANAGEMENT

Conservative therapy and lifestyle modifications that form the foundation of GERD therapy can be effectively implemented through education and reassurance for parents. Dietary measures for infants include normalization of any abnormal feeding techniques, volumes, and frequencies. Thickening of feeds or use of commercially prethickened formulas increases the percentage of infants with no regurgitation, decreases the frequency of daily regurgitation and emesis, and increases

the infant's weight gain. However, caution should be exercised when managing preterm infants because of the possible association between xanthan gum-based thickened feeds and necrotizing enterocolitis. The evidence does not clearly favor 1 type of thickener over another; the addition of a Tbsp of rice cereal per oz of formula results in a greater caloric density (30 kcal/oz) and reduced crying time, although it might not modify the number of nonregurgitant reflux episodes. A short trial of a hypoallergenic diet in infants may be used to exclude milk or soy protein allergy before pharmacotherapy. A combination of modified feeding volumes, hydrolyzed infant formulas, proper positioning, and avoidance of smoke exposure satisfactorily improve GERD symptoms in 24-59% infants with GERD. Older children should be counseled to

Table 323-2	Symptoms and Signs That May Be Associated with Gastroesophageal Reflux

Symptoms
  Recurrent regurgitation with or without vomiting
  Weight loss or poor weight gain
  Irritability in infants
  Ruminative behavior
  Heartburn or chest pain
  Hematemesis
  Dysphagia, odynophagia
  Wheezing
  Stridor
  Cough
  Hoarseness

Signs
  Esophagitis
  Esophageal stricture
  Barrett esophagus
  Laryngeal/pharyngeal inflammation
  Recurrent pneumonia
  Anemia
  Dental erosion
  Feeding refusal
  Dystonic neck posturing (Sandifer syndrome)
  Apnea spells
  Apparent life-threatening events

From Wyllie R, Hyams JS, Kay M, editors: Pediatric gastrointestinal and liver disease, ed 4, Philadelphia, 2011, WB Saunders, Table 22-1, p. 235.

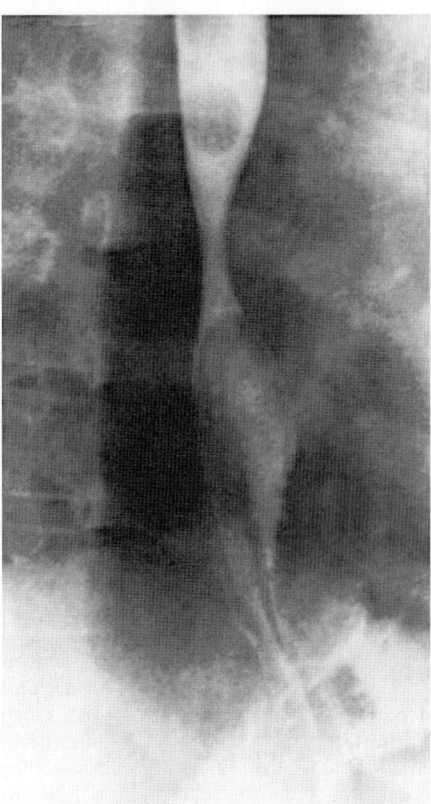

Figure 323-1 Barium esophagogram demonstrating free gastroesophageal reflux. Note stricture caused by peptic esophagitis. Longitudinal gastric folds above the diaphragm indicate the unusual presence of an associated hiatal hernia.

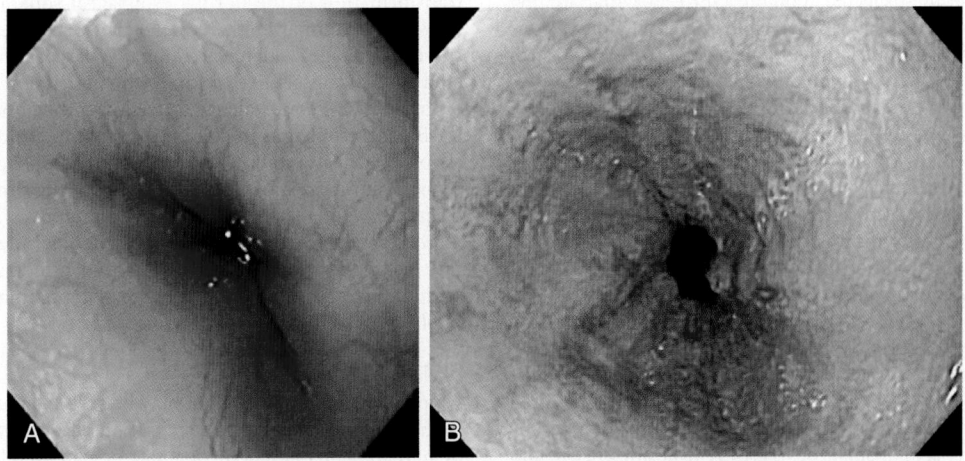

Figure 323-2 Endoscopic image of a normal esophagus **(A)** and erosive peptic esophagitis **(B)**.

avoid acidic or reflux-inducing foods (tomatoes, chocolate, mint) and beverages (juices, carbonated and caffeinated drinks, alcohol). Weight reduction for obese patients and elimination of smoke exposure are other crucial measures at all ages.

Positioning measures are particularly important for infants, who cannot control their positions independently. Seated position worsens infant reflux and should be avoided in infants with GERD. Esophageal pH monitoring demonstrates more reflux episodes in infants in supine and side positions compared with the prone position, but evidence that the supine position reduces the risk of sudden infant death syndrome has led the American Academy of Pediatrics and the North American Society of Pediatric Gastroenterology and Nutrition to recommend supine positioning during sleep. When the infant is awake and observed, prone position and upright carried position can be used to minimize reflux. Lying in the flat supine position and semi-seated positions (e.g., car seats, infant carriers) in the postprandial period are considered provocative positions for GER and therefore should be avoided. The efficacy of positioning for older children is unclear, but some evidence suggests a benefit to left side position and head elevation during sleep. The head should be elevated by elevating the head of the bed, rather than using excess pillows, to avoid abdominal flexion and compression that might worsen reflux.

Pharmacotherapy is directed at ameliorating the acidity of the gastric contents or at promoting their aboral movement, and should be considered for those symptomatic infants and children who are either highly suspected or proven to have GERD. **Antacids** are the most commonly used antireflux therapy and are readily available over the counter. They provide rapid but transient relief of symptoms by acid neutralization. The long-term regular use of antacids cannot be recommended because of side effects of diarrhea (magnesium antacids) and constipation (aluminum antacids) and rare reports of more serious side effects of chronic use.

Histamine-2 receptor antagonists (H2RAs: cimetidine, famotidine, nizatidine, and ranitidine) are widely used antisecretory agents that act by selective inhibition of histamine receptors on gastric parietal cells. There is a definite benefit of H2RAs in treatment of mild-to-moderate reflux esophagitis. H2RAs have been recommended as first-line therapy because of their excellent overall safety profile, but they are superseded by PPIs in this role, as increased experience with pediatric use and safety, FDA approval, and pediatric formulations and dosing are available.

PPIs (omeprazole, lansoprazole, pantoprazole, rabeprazole, and esomeprazole) provide the most potent antireflux effect by blocking the hydrogen–potassium adenosine triphosphatase channels of the final common pathway in gastric acid secretion. PPIs are superior to H2RAs in the treatment of severe and erosive esophagitis. Pharmacodynamic studies indicate that children require higher doses of PPIs than adults on a per-weight basis. The use of PPIs to treat infants and children deemed to have GERD on the basis of symptoms is now the standard of care. An important systematic review of the efficacy and safety of PPI therapy in pediatric GERD reveals no clear benefit for PPI over placebo use in suspected infantile GERD (crying, arching behavior). Limited pediatric data are available to draw definitive conclusions about potential complications implicated with PPI use, such as respiratory infections, *Clostridium difficile* infection, bone fractures (noted in adults), and hypomagnesemia.

Prokinetic agents available in the United States include metoclopramide (dopamine-2 and 5-HT$_3$ antagonist), bethanechol (cholinergic agonist), and erythromycin (motilin receptor agonist). Most of these increase LES pressure; some improve gastric emptying or esophageal clearance. None affects the frequency of TLESRs. The available controlled trials have not demonstrated much efficacy for GERD. In 2009, the FDA announced a black box warning for metoclopramide, linking its chronic use (longer than 3 mo) with tardive dyskinesia, the rarely reversible movement disorder. Baclofen is a centrally acting γ-aminobutyric acid agonist that decreases reflux by decreasing TLESRs in healthy adults and in a small number of neurologically impaired children with GERD. New agents of great interest include peripherally acting γ-aminobutyric acid agonists devoid of central side effects, and metabotropic glutamate receptor 5 antagonists that are reported to

reduce TLESRs but are as yet inadequately studied for this indication in children.

Surgery, usually **fundoplication,** is effective therapy for intractable GERD in children, particularly those with refractory esophagitis or strictures and those at risk for significant morbidity from chronic pulmonary disease. It may be combined with a gastrostomy for feeding or venting. The availability of potent acid-suppressing medication mandates more-rigorous analysis of the relative risks (or costs) and benefits of this relatively irreversible therapy in comparison to long-term pharmacotherapy. Some of the risks of fundoplication include a wrap that is "too tight" (producing dysphagia or gas-bloat) or "too loose" (and thus incompetent). Surgeons may choose to perform a "tight" (360 degrees, Nissen) or variations of a "loose" (<360 degrees, Thal, Toupet, Boix-Ochoa) wrap, or to add a gastric drainage procedure (pyloroplasty) to improve gastric emptying, based on their experience and the patient's disease. Preoperative accuracy of diagnosis of GERD and the skill of the surgeon are 2 of the most important predictors of successful outcome. Long-term studies suggest that fundoplications often become incompetent in children, as in adults, with reflux recurrence rates of up to 14% for Nissen and up to 20% for loose wraps; this fact currently combines with the potency of PPI therapy that is now available to shift practice toward long-term pharmacotherapy in many cases. Fundoplication procedures may be performed as open operations, by laparoscopy, or by endoluminal (gastroplication) techniques. Pediatric experience is limited with endoscopic application of radiofrequency therapy (Stretta procedure) to a 2-3 cm area of the LES and cardia to create a high-pressure zone to reduce reflux.

Bibliography is available at Expert Consult.

323.1 Complications of Gastroesophageal Reflux Disease

Seema Khan and Susan R. Orenstein

ESOPHAGEAL: ESOPHAGITIS AND SEQUELAE—STRICTURE, BARRETT ESOPHAGUS, ADENOCARCINOMA

Esophagitis can manifest as irritability, arching, and feeding aversion in infants; chest or epigastric pain in older children; and, rarely, as hematemesis, anemia, or Sandifer syndrome at any age. Erosive esophagitis is found in approximately 12% of children with GERD symptoms and is more common in boys, older children, neurologically abnormal children, children with severe chronic respiratory disease, and in those with hiatal hernia. Prolonged and severe esophagitis leads to formation of strictures, generally located in the distal esophagus, producing dysphagia, and requiring repeated esophageal dilations and often fundoplication. Long-standing esophagitis predisposes to metaplastic transformation of the normal esophageal squamous epithelium into intestinal columnar epithelium, termed **Barrett esophagus,** a precursor of esophageal adenocarcinoma. A large multicenter prospective study of 840 consecutive children who underwent elective endoscopies reported a 25.7% prevalence for reflux esophagitis, and a mere 0.12% for Barrett esophagus in children without neurologic disorders or tracheoesophageal anomalies. Both Barrett esophagus and adenocarcinoma occur more in white males and in those with increased duration, frequency, and severity of reflux symptoms. This transformation increases with age to plateau in the 5th decade; adenocarcinoma is thus rare in childhood. Barrett esophagus, uncommon in children, warrants periodic surveillance biopsies, aggressive pharmacotherapy, and fundoplication for progressive lesions.

NUTRITIONAL

Esophagitis and regurgitation may be severe enough to induce failure to thrive because of caloric deficits. Enteral (nasogastric or nasojejunal, or percutaneous gastric or jejunal) or parenteral feedings are sometimes required to treat such deficits.

EXTRAESOPHAGEAL: RESPIRATORY ("ATYPICAL") PRESENTATIONS

GERD should be included in the differential diagnosis of children with unexplained or refractory otolaryngologic and respiratory complaints. GERD can produce respiratory symptoms by direct contact of the refluxed gastric contents with the respiratory tract (aspiration, laryngeal penetration, or microaspiration) or by reflexive interactions between the esophagus and respiratory tract (inducing laryngeal closure or bronchospasm). Often, GERD and a primary respiratory disorder, such as asthma, interact and a vicious cycle between them worsens both diseases. Many children with these extraesophageal presentations do not have typical GERD symptoms, making the diagnosis difficult. These atypical GERD presentations require a thoughtful approach to the differential diagnosis that considers a multitude of primary otolaryngologic (infections, allergies, postnasal drip, voice overuse) and pulmonary (asthma, cystic fibrosis) disorders. Therapy for the GERD must be more intense (usually incorporating a PPI) and prolonged (usually at least 3-6 mo). Subspecialist assistance from the perspective of the airway disease (otolaryngology, pulmonology) and the reflux disease (gastroenterology) is often warranted for specialized diagnostic testing and for optimizing intensive management.

APNEA AND STRIDOR

These upper airway presentations have been linked with GERD in case reports and epidemiologic studies; temporal relationships between them and reflux episodes have been demonstrated in some patients by esophageal pH–multichannel intraluminal impedance studies, and a beneficial response to therapy for GERD provides further support in a number of case series. An evaluation of 1,400 infants with apnea attributed the apnea to GERD in 50%, but other studies have failed to find an association. Apnea and apparent life-threatening event caused by reflux is generally obstructive, owing to laryngospasm that may be conceived of as an abnormally intense protective reflex. At the time of such apnea, infants have often been provocatively positioned (supine or flexed seated), have been recently fed, and have shown signs of obstructive apnea, with unproductive respiratory efforts. *The evidence suggests that for the large majority of infants presenting with apnea and an apparent life-threatening event, GERD is not causal.* Stridor triggered by reflux generally occurs in infants anatomically predisposed toward stridor (laryngomalacia, micrognathia). Spasmodic croup, an episodic frightening upper airway obstruction, can be an analogous condition in older children. Esophageal pH probe studies might fail to demonstrate linkage of these manifestations with reflux owing to the buffering of gastric contents by infant formula and the episodic nature of the conditions. Pneumograms can fail to identify apnea if they are not designed to identify obstructive apnea by measuring nasal airflow.

Reflux laryngitis and other otolaryngologic manifestations (also known as laryngopharyngeal reflux) can be attributed to GERD. **Hoarseness,** voice fatigue, throat clearing, chronic cough, pharyngitis, sinusitis, otitis media, and a sensation of globus have been cited. Laryngopharyngeal signs of GERD include edema and hyperemia (of the posterior surface), contact ulcers, granulomas, polyps, subglottic stenosis, and interarytenoid edema. The paucity of well-controlled evaluations of the association contributes to the skepticism with which these associations may be considered. Other risk factors irritating the upper respiratory passages can predispose some patients with GERD to present predominantly with these complaints.

Many studies have reported a strong association between asthma and reflux as determined by history, pH–multichannel intraluminal impedance, endoscopy, and esophageal histology. **GERD symptoms are present in an average of 23% (19-80%) of children with asthma** as observed in a systematic review of 19 studies examining the prevalence of GERD in asthmatics. The review also reported abnormal pH results in 63%, and esophagitis in 35% of asthmatic children. However, this association does not clarify the direction of causality in individual cases and thus does not indicate which patients with asthma are likely to benefit from anti-GERD therapy. Children with asthma who are particularly likely to have GERD as a provocative factor are those with symptoms of reflux disease, those with refractory or steroid-dependent

asthma, and those with nocturnal worsening of asthma. Endoscopic evaluation that discloses esophageal sequelae of GERD provides an impetus to embark on the aggressive (high dose and many months' duration) therapy of GERD.

Dental erosions constitute the most common oral lesion of GERD, the lesions being distinguished by their location on the lingual surface of the teeth. The severity seems to correlate with the presence of reflux symptoms and the presence of an acidic milieu as the result of reflux in the proximal esophagus and oral cavity. The other common factors that can produce similar dental erosions are juice consumption and bulimia.

Bibliography is available at Expert Consult.

Chapter **324**
Eosinophilic Esophagitis and Non–Gastroesophageal Reflux Disease Esophagitis

Seema Khan and Susan R. Orenstein

EOSINOPHILIC ESOPHAGITIS

Eosinophilic esophagitis (EoE) is a chronic esophageal disorder characterized by infiltration of the esophageal epithelium by eosinophils, typically in a density exceeding 15 per high-power field. While infants and toddlers present commonly with vomiting, feeding problems, and poor weight gain, older children and adolescents usually experience solid food dysphagia with occasional food impactions or strictures and may complain of chest or epigastric pain. Most patients are male. The mean age at diagnosis is 7 yr (range: 1-17 yr), and the duration of symptoms is 3 yr. Many patients have other atopic diseases (or a positive family history) and associated food allergies; laboratory abnormalities can include peripheral eosinophilia and elevated immunoglobulin E (IgE) levels. The pathogenesis involves mainly T-helper type 2 cytokine-mediated pathways leading to production of a potent eosinophil chemoattractant, eotaxin-3, by esophageal epithelium. Endoscopically, the esophagus presents a granular, furrowed, ringed, or exudative appearance (Fig. 324-1); esophageal histology reveals eosinophilia, with cutpoints for diagnosis variably chosen at 15-20/high-power field. Up to 30% children with EoE have grossly normal esophageal mucosa. EoE is differentiated from gastroesophageal reflux disease by its general lack of erosive esophagitis, its greater eosinophil density, and its normal esophageal pH-multichannel intraluminal impedance results. A favorable response to proton pump inhibitor therapy should no longer be considered diagnostic of gastroesophageal reflux disease, as a subgroup of EoE patients with normal esophageal pH-multichannel intraluminal impedance also demonstrate histologic response, and constitute a proton pump inhibitor–responsive EoE group. This response may be because of an antieosinophil effect of the proton pump inhibitor class that is mediated by inhibition of eotaxin-3 secretion. Gastroesophageal reflux disease may be an important coexisting diagnosis. Evaluation of EoE should include a thorough search for food and environmental allergies via skin prick (IgE mediated) and patch (non–IgE mediated) tests.

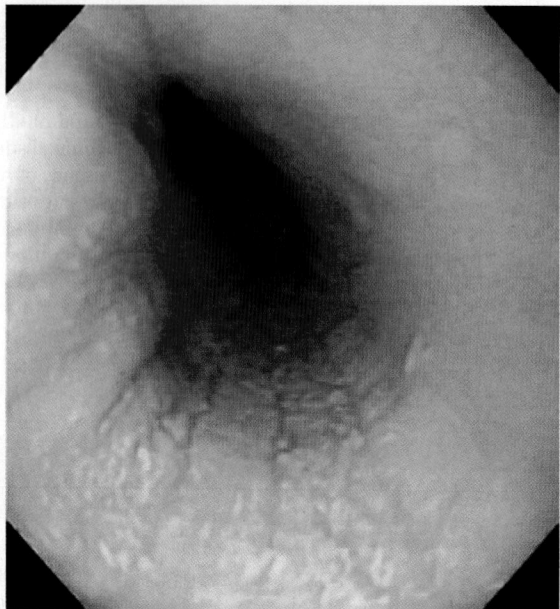

Figure 324-1 Endoscopic image of eosinophilic esophagitis with characteristic mucosal appearance of furrowing and white specks.

Treatment involves dietary restrictions that take one of 3 forms: elimination diets guided by circumstantial evidence and food allergy test results; "6 food elimination diet" removing the major food allergens (milk, soy, wheat, egg, peanuts and tree nuts, seafood); and elemental diet composed exclusively of an amino acid–based formula. Successful clinical and histologic remission is observed in 70-98% patients. Topical and systemic corticosteroids have been used successfully for nonresponders and for nonallergic ("primary") EoE, with symptomatic and histologic remission rates reaching 90%. Therapies under investigation include anti–interleukin-5 antibody (mepolizumab, reslizumab). Little is yet known about its natural history, but it seems that EoE is a chronic remitting and relapsing disorder with a potential for complications such as stricture formation.

INFECTIVE ESOPHAGITIS
Uncommon, and most often affecting immunocompromised children, infective esophagitis is caused by fungal agents, such as *Candida* and *Torulopsis glabrata*; viral agents, such as herpes simplex, cytomegalovirus, HIV, and varicella zoster; and, rarely, bacterial infections, including diphtheria and tuberculosis. The typical presenting signs and symptoms are odynophagia, dysphagia, and retrosternal pain; there may also be fever, nausea, and vomiting. Candida is the leading cause of infective esophagitis in immunocompetent and immunocompromised children, and presents with concurrent oropharyngeal infection in the majority of immunocompromised patients. Esophageal viral infections can also manifest in immunocompetent hosts as an acute febrile illness. Infectious esophagitis, like other forms of esophageal inflammation, occasionally progresses to esophageal stricture. Diagnosis of infectious esophagitis is made by endoscopy, usually notable for white plaques in candida, multiple superficial ulcers in herpes simplex virus, and single deep ulcer in cytomegalovirus, and histopathologic examination; adding polymerase chain reaction, tissue-viral culture, and immunocytochemistry enhances the diagnostic sensitivity and precision. Treatment is with appropriate antimicrobial agents, analgesics, and antacids.

"PILL" ESOPHAGITIS
This acute injury is produced by contact with a damaging agent. Medications implicated in "pill" esophagitis include tetracycline, potassium chloride, ferrous sulfate, nonsteroidal antiinflammatory medications, and alendronate. Most often the offending tablet is ingested at bedtime with inadequate water. This practice often produces acute discomfort followed by progressive retrosternal pain, odynophagia, and dysphagia. Endoscopy shows a focal lesion often localized to one of the anatomic narrowed regions of the esophagus or to an unsuspected pathologic narrowing. Treatment is supportive; lacking much evidence, antacids, topical anesthetics, and bland or liquid diets are often used.

Bibliography is available at Expert Consult.

Chapter **325**
Esophageal Perforation
Seema Khan and Susan R. Orenstein

The majority of esophageal perforations in children are from blunt trauma (automobile injury, gunshot wounds, child abuse) or are iatrogenic. Cardiac massage, the Heimlich maneuver, nasogastric tube placement, traumatic laryngoscopy or endotracheal intubation, excessively vigorous postpartum suctioning of the airway during neonatal resuscitation, difficult upper endoscopy, sclerotherapy of esophageal varices, esophageal compression by a cuffed endotracheal tube, and dilation for therapy of achalasia and strictures have all been implicated. Esophageal rupture has followed forceful vomiting in patients with anorexia and has followed esophageal injury due to caustic ingestion, foreign body ingestion, food impactions, pill esophagitis, or eosinophilic esophagitis. Drinking cold, carbonated beverages rapidly is also known to cause esophageal perforation.

Spontaneous esophageal rupture (**Boerhaave syndrome**) is less common and is associated with sudden increases in intraesophageal pressure wrought by situations such as vomiting, coughing, or straining at stool. Children and adults with eosinophilic esophagitis have also been described with Boerhaave syndrome in the setting of forceful emesis in the aftermath of esophageal food impaction. In older children, as in adults, the tear occurs on the distal left lateral esophageal wall, because the smooth muscle layer here is weakest; in neonates (neonatal Boerhaave syndrome), spontaneous rupture is on the right.

Symptoms of esophageal perforation include pain, neck tenderness, dysphagia, subcutaneous crepitus, fever, and tachycardia; several patients with cervical perforations have displayed cold water polydipsia in an attempt to soothe pain in the throat. Perforations in the proximal thoracic esophagus tend to create signs (pneumothorax, effusions) in the left chest, whereas the signs of distal tears are more often on the right. Cervical spine and chest radiographs are often diagnostic, showing mediastinal widening or paracervical free air. If these x-rays are normal, an esophagogram using water-soluble contrast media should be performed, but esophagograms miss >30% of cervical perforations. Therefore, a negative water-soluble contrast esophagogram should be followed by a barium study; the greater density of barium can better demonstrate a small defect, though with a higher risk of inflammatory mediastinitis. Endoscopy may also be useful but carries a 30% false-negative rate. CT of the chest can assist in difficult cases.

Treatment must be individualized. Small tears in contained perforations with minimal mediastinal contamination in hemodynamically stable patients can be treated conservatively with broad-spectrum antibiotics, nothing given orally, gastric drainage, and parenteral nutrition. Chest exploration and direct surgical repair is infrequently indicated these days. Mortality rates range between 20% and 28%, with poor prognosis correlated with delayed diagnosis and interventions.

Bibliography is available at Expert Consult.

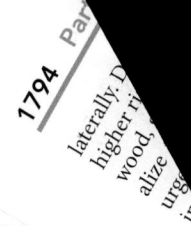

laterally. D...
higher ri...
wood,...
alize...
urg...
in...

Chapter **326**
Esophageal Varices
Seema Khan and Susan R. Orenstein

Esophageal varices form in adults with portal hypertension with hepatic venous pressure gradient above 10 mm Hg and pose a risk for bleeding at above 12 mm Hg (see Chapter 367). Spontaneous decompression of this hypertension through portosystemic collateral circulation via the coronary vein, in conjunction with the left gastric veins, gives rise to esophageal varices. Most esophageal varices are "uphill varices"; less commonly, those that arise in the absence of portal hypertension and with superior vena cava obstruction are "downhill varices." Their treatment is directed at the underlying cause of the superior vena cava abnormality. Hemorrhage from esophageal varices is the major cause of morbidity and mortality from portal hypertension. Presentation is with significant hematemesis and melena; whereas most patients have liver disease, some children with entities such as extrahepatic portal venous thrombosis might have been previously asymptomatic. Any child with hematemesis and splenomegaly should be presumed to have esophageal variceal bleeding until proved otherwise.

Upper endoscopy is the preferred diagnostic test for esophageal varices, as it provides definitive diagnosis and delineation of details that aid in predicting the risk for bleeding, as well as enabling therapy for acute bleeding episodes via either sclerotherapy or band ligation. A report comprising a large series of children with biliary atresia and portal hypertension described endoscopic findings of large varices, red marks, and the presence of gastric varices as predictive of bleeding. Non-invasive methods of evaluating varices include barium contrast studies, ultrasound, computerized tomography, magnetic resonance, and elastography, but they are not recommended for routine diagnostic evaluation because of suboptimal accuracy compared to endoscopy.

Primary prophylaxis with the goal of preventing an initial hemorrhage can decrease the incidence of esophageal bleeding; the various modalities used are nonselective β blockade (e.g., propranolol or nadolol), sclerotherapy, ligation, and portosystemic shunt surgery. Treated patients can bleed from congestive gastropathy, and no improvement in survival rate may be seen. Endoscopic variceal ligation in adults reduces the risk of first-time variceal bleeding when compared with untreated controls as well as patients treated with β blockade; a decrease in mortality is only noted in comparison to the control group (see Chapter 367). The management of acute variceal bleeding must include attention to hemodynamic stability through blood transfusion, vasoactive drugs (e.g., octreotide), short-term antibiotic use, and endoscopy to perform ligation or sclerotherapy, as needed. Transjugular intrahepatic portosystemic shunt should be considered for variceal bleeding refractory to medical and endoscopic therapy. Secondary prophylaxis to reduce recurrence of bleeding uses nonselective β blockade and obliteration of varices through serial treatment via ligation or sclerotherapy. The only randomized controlled pediatric study has shown superiority of ligation over sclerotherapy in reducing the risk for rebleeding and complications.

Bibliography is available at Expert Consult.

Chapter **327**
Ingestions

327.1 Foreign Bodies in the Eso...
Seema Khan and Susan R. Orenstein

The majority (80%) of foreign-body ingestions occur in children, mo... of whom are between 6 mo and 3 yr of age. Older children and adolescents with developmental delays and those with psychiatric disorders are also at increased risk. The presentation of a foreign body lodged in the esophagus constitutes an emergency and is associated with significant morbidity and mortality because of the potential for perforation and sepsis. Coins and small toy items are the most commonly ingested foreign bodies. Food impactions are less common in children than in adults, and usually occur in children in association with eosinophilic esophagitis, repair of esophageal atresia, and Nissen fundoplication. Most esophageal foreign bodies lodge at the level of the cricopharyngeus (upper esophageal sphincter), the aortic arch, or just superior to the diaphragm at the gastroesophageal junction (lower esophageal sphincter).

At least 30% of children with esophageal foreign bodies may be totally asymptomatic, so any history of foreign body ingestion should be taken seriously and investigated. An initial bout of choking, gagging, and coughing may be followed by excessive salivation, dysphagia, food refusal, emesis, or pain in the neck, throat, or sternal notch regions. Respiratory symptoms such as stridor, wheezing, cyanosis, or dyspnea may be encountered if the esophageal foreign body impinges on the larynx or membranous posterior tracheal wall. Cervical swelling, erythema, or subcutaneous crepitations suggest perforation of the oropharynx or proximal esophagus.

Evaluation of the child with a history of foreign body ingestion starts with plain anteroposterior radiographs of the neck, chest, and abdomen, along with lateral views of the neck and chest. The flat surface of a coin in the esophagus is seen on the anteroposterior view and the edge on the lateral view (Fig. 327-1). The reverse is true for coins lodged in the trachea; here, the edge is seen anteroposteriorly and the flat side is seen

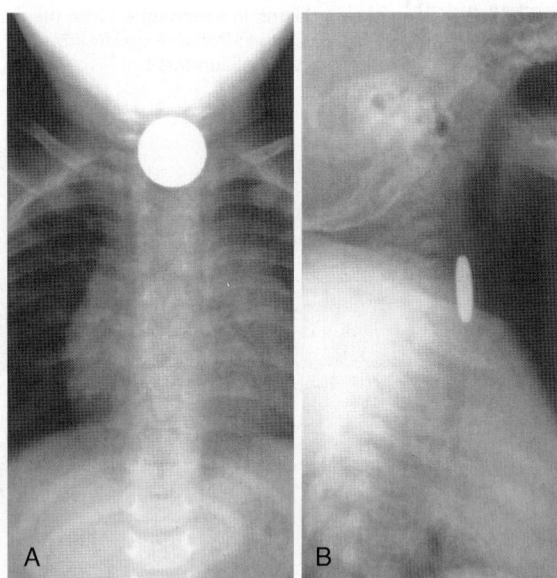

A   B

Figure 327-1 Radiographs of a coin in the esophagus. When foreign bodies lodge in the esophagus, the flat surface of the object is seen in the anteroposterior view **(A)** and the edge is seen in the lateral view **(B).** The reverse is true for objects in the trachea. (*Courtesy of Beverley Newman, MD.*)

...isk batteries can look like coins (Fig. 327-2) and have a much ...sk of burns and necrosis (Fig. 327-3). Materials such as plastic, ...glass, aluminum, and bones may be radiolucent; failure to visu-...the object with plain films in a symptomatic patient warrants ...nt endoscopy. CT scan with 3-dimensional reconstruction may ...crease the sensitivity of imaging a foreign body. Although barium ...ontrast studies may be helpful in the occasional asymptomatic patient with negative plain films, their use is to be discouraged because of the potential of aspiration as well as making subsequent visualization and object removal more difficult.

In managing the child with an esophageal foreign body, it is important to assess risk for airway compromise and to obtain a chest CT scan and surgical consultation in cases of suspected airway perforation. Treatment of esophageal foreign bodies usually merits endoscopic visualization of the object and underlying mucosa and removal of the object using an appropriately designed foreign-body-retrieving accessory instrument through the endoscope, and with an endotracheal tube protecting the airway. Sharp objects in the esophagus, disk button batteries, or foreign bodies associated with respiratory symptoms mandate urgent removal. Button (disk) batteries, in particular, must be expediently removed because they can induce mucosal injury in as little as 1 hr of contact time and involve all esophageal layers within 4 hr (see Fig. 327-3). Asymptomatic blunt objects and coins lodged in the esophagus can be observed for up to 24 hr in anticipation of passage into the stomach. If there are no problems in handling secretions, meat impactions can be observed for up to 12 hr. In patients without prior esophageal surgeries, glucagon (0.05 mg/kg IV) can sometimes be useful in facilitating passage of distal esophageal food boluses by decreasing the lower esophageal sphincter pressure. The use of meat tenderizers or gas-forming agents can lead to perforation and are not recommended. An alternative technique for removing esophageal coins impacted for <24 hr, performed most safely by experienced radiology personnel, consists of passage of a Foley catheter beyond the coin at fluoroscopy, inflating the balloon, and then pulling the catheter and coin back simultaneously with the patient in a prone oblique position. Concerns about the lack of direct mucosal visualization and, when tracheal intubation is not used, the lack of airway protection prompt caution in the use of this technique. Bougienage of esophageal coins toward the stomach in selected uncomplicated pediatric cases has been suggested to be an effective, safe, and economical modality where endoscopy might not be routinely available.

Bibliography is available at Expert Consult.

327.2 Caustic Ingestions
Seema Khan and Susan R. Orenstein

Ingestion of caustic substances is a world-wide public health problem accounting for a significant burden on healthcare resources. According to an inpatient database of U.S. pediatric hospital discharges in 2009, the estimated number of caustic ingestions was 807 (95% CI, 731-882) cases, amounting to $22,900,000 in total hospital charges. The medical sequelae of caustic ingestions are esophagitis, necrosis, perforation, and stricture formation (see Chapter 63). Most cases (70%) are accidental ingestions of liquid alkali substances that produce severe, deep liquefaction necrosis; drain decloggers are most common, and because they are tasteless, more is ingested (Table 327-1). **Acidic agents** (20% of cases) are bitter, so less may be consumed; they produce coagulation necrosis and a somewhat protective thick eschar. They can produce severe gastritis, and volatile acids can result in respiratory symptoms. Children younger than 5 yr of age account for half of the cases of caustic ingestions, and boys are far more often involved than girls.

Caustic ingestions produce signs and symptoms such as vomiting, drooling, refusal to drink, oral burns, dysphagia, dyspnea, abdominal pain, hematemesis, and stridor. Twenty percent of patients develop esophageal strictures. Absence of oropharyngeal lesions does not exclude the possibility of significant esophagogastric injury, which can

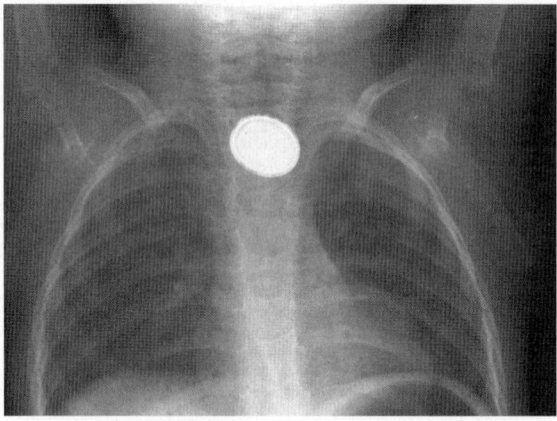

Figure 327-2 Disk battery impacted in esophagus. Note the double rim. *(From Wyllie R, Hyams JS, editors: Pediatric gastrointestinal and liver disease, ed 3, Philadelphia, 2006, Saunders.)*

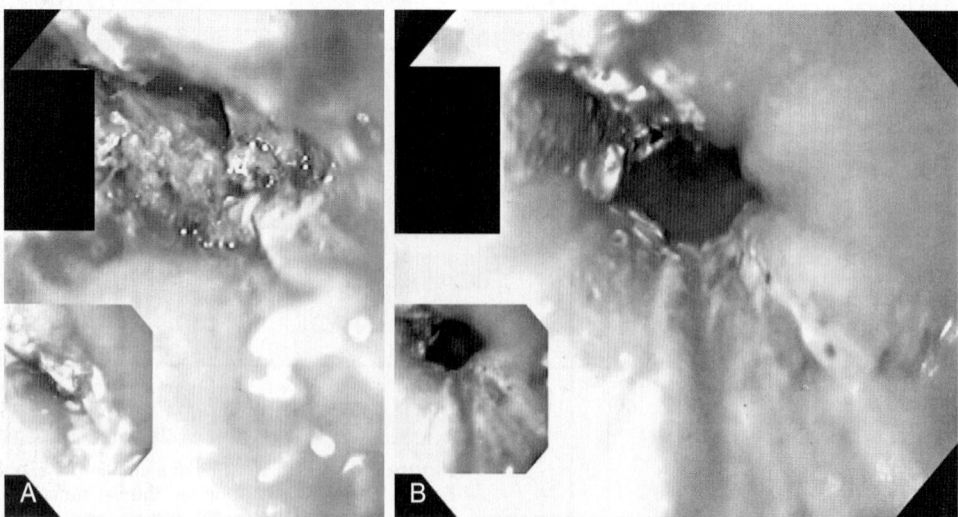

Figure 327-3 A, Disk battery in esophagus with necrotic debris at burn sites. **B,** Typical bilateral esophageal burn after removal of disk battery. *(From Wyllie R, Hyams JS, editors: Pediatric gastrointestinal and liver disease, ed 3, Philadelphia, 2006, Saunders.)*

Table 327-1	Ingestible Caustic Materials Around the House	
CATEGORY	**MOST DAMAGING AGENTS**	**OTHER AGENTS**
Alkaline drain cleaners, milking machine pipe cleaners	Sodium or potassium hydroxide	Ammonia Sodium hypochlorite Aluminum particles
Acidic drain openers	Hydrochloric acid Sulfuric acid	
Toilet cleaners	Hydrochloric acid Sulfuric acid Phosphoric acid Other acids	Ammonium chloride Sodium hypochlorite
Oven and grill cleaners	Sodium hydroxide Perborate (borax)	
Denture cleaners	Persulfate (sulfur) Hypochlorite (bleach)	
Dishwasher detergent • Liquid • Powdered • Packaged	Sodium hydroxide Sodium hypochlorite Sodium carbonate	
Bleach	Sodium hypochlorite	Ammonia salt
Swimming pool chemicals	Acids, alkalis, chlorine	
Battery acid (liquid)	Sulfuric acid	
Disk batteries	Electric current	Zinc or other metal salts
Rust remover	Hydrofluoric, phosphoric, oxalic, and other acids	
Household delimers	Phosphoric acid Hydroxyacetic acid Hydrochloric acid	
Barbeque cleaners	Sodium and potassium hydroxide	
Glyphosate surfactant (RoundUp) acid	Glyphosate herbicide	Surfactants
Hair relaxer	Sodium hydroxide	
Weed killer	Dichlorophenoxyacetate, ammonium phosphate, propionic acid	

Source: National Library of Medicine: Health and safety information on household products (website). http://householdproducts.nlm.nih.gov/
From Wylie R, Hyams JS, Kay M, editors: Pediatric gastrointestinal and liver disease, ed 4, Philadelphia, 2011, WB Saunders, Table 19-1, p. 198.

Table 327-2	Classification of Caustic Injury	
GRADE	**VISIBLE APPEARANCE**	**CLINICAL SIGNIFICANCE**
Grade 0	History of ingestion, but no visible damage or symptoms	Able to take fluids immediately
Grade 1	Edema, loss of normal vascular pattern, hyperemia, no transmucosal injury	Temporary dysphagia, able to swallow within 0-2 days, no long-term sequelae
Grade 2a	Transmucosal injury with friability, hemorrhage, blistering, exudate, scattered superficial ulceration	Scarring, no circumferential damage (no stenosis), no long-term sequelae
Grade 2b	Grade 2a plus discrete ulceration and/or circumferential ulceration	Small risk of perforation, scarring that may result in later stenosis
Grade 3a	Scattered deep ulceration with necrosis of the tissue	Risk of perforation, high risk of later stenosis
Grade 3b	Extensive necrotic tissue	High risk of perforation and death, high risk of stenosis

From Wylie R, Hyams JS, Kay M, editors: Pediatric gastrointestinal and liver disease, ed 4, Philadelphia, 2011, WB Saunders, Table 19-2, p. 199.

lead to perforation or stricture. The absence of symptoms is usually associated with no or minimal lesions; hematemesis, respiratory distress, or presence of at least 3 symptoms predicts severe lesions. An upper endoscopy is recommended as the most efficient means of rapid identification of tissue damage and must be undertaken in all symptomatic children.

Dilution by water or milk is recommended as acute treatment, but neutralization, induced emesis, and gastric lavage are contraindicated. Treatment depends on the severity and extent of damage (Table 327-2).

Stricture risk is increased by circumferential ulcerations, white plaques, and sloughing of the mucosa. Strictures can require treatment with dilation, and in some severe cases, surgical resection and colon or small bowel interposition are needed. Silicone stents (self-expanding) placed endoscopically after a dilation procedure can be an alternative and conservative approach to the management of strictures. Rare late cases of superimposed esophageal carcinoma are reported. The role of corticosteroids is controversial; they are not recommended in 1st-degree burns, but they can reduce the risk of strictures in more-advanced caustic esophagitis. Some centers also use antibiotics in the initial treatment of caustic esophagitis on the premise that reducing superinfection in the necrotic tissue bed will, in turn, lower the risk of stricture formation. However, multiple studies examining the role of antibiotics in caustic esophagitis have not reported a clinically significant benefit even in those with grade 2 or greater severity of esophagitis.

Bibliography is available at Expert Consult.

Section 4
Stomach and Intestines

Chapter **328**
Normal Development, Structure, and Function
Chris A. Liacouras

DEVELOPMENT

The primitive gut is recognizable by the 4th wk of gestation and is composed of the foregut, midgut, and hindgut. The **foregut** gives rise to the upper gastrointestinal tract, which includes the esophagus, stomach, and duodenum to the level of the insertion of the common bile duct. The **midgut** gives rise to the rest of the small bowel and the large bowel to the level of the midtransverse colon. The **hindgut** forms the remainder of the colon and upper anal canal. The rapid growth of the midgut causes it to protrude out of the abdominal cavity through the umbilical ring during fetal development. The midgut subsequently returns to the peritoneal cavity and rotates counterclockwise until the cecum lies in the right lower quadrant. The process is normally complete by the 8th wk of gestation.

The liver derives from the hepatic diverticulum that evolves into parenchymal cells, bile ducts, vascular structures, and hematopoietic and Kupffer cells. The extrahepatic bile ducts and gallbladder develop first as solid cords that canalize by the 3rd mo of gestation. The dorsal and ventral pancreatic buds grow from the foregut by the 4th wk of gestation. The 2 buds fuse by the 6th wk. Exocrine secretory capacity is present by the 5th mo.

Cis-regulatory genomic sequences govern gene expression during development. Modules of *cis* sequences are linked and allow a cascade of gene regulation that controls functional development. Extrinsic factors have the capacity to influence gene expression. In the gut, several growth factors, including growth factor-β, insulin-like growth factor, and growth factors found in human colostrum (human growth factor and epidermal growth factor), influence gene expression.

Propulsion of food down the gastrointestinal tract relies on the coordinated action of muscles in the bowel wall. The contractions are regulated by the enteric nervous system under the influence of a variety of peptides and hormones. The enteric nervous system is derived from neural crest cells that migrate in a cranial to caudal fashion. Migration of the neural crest tissue is complete by the 24th wk of gestation. Interruption of the migration results in **Hirschsprung disease**. Newborn bowel motor patterns are different from adults. Normal fasting upper gastrointestinal motility is characterized by a triphasic pattern known as the migrating motor complex. Migrating motor complexes occur less often in neonates and they have more nonmigrating phasic activity.

This leads to ineffective propulsion, particularly in premature infants. Motility in the fed state consists of a series of ring contractions that spread caudad over variable distances.

DIGESTION AND ABSORPTION

The wall of the stomach, small bowel, and colon consists of 4 layers: the mucosa, submucosa, muscularis, and serosa. Eighty-five percent of the gastric mucosa is lined by oxyntic glands containing cells that secrete hydrochloric acid, pepsinogen, and intrinsic factor, and mucous and endocrine cells that secrete peptides having paracrine and endocrine effects. Pepsinogen is a precursor of the proteolytic enzyme pepsin, and intrinsic factor is required for the absorption of vitamin B_{12}. Pyloric glands are located in the antrum and contain gastrin-secreting cells. Acid production and gastrin levels are inversely related to each other except in pathologic secretory states. Acid secretion is low at birth but increases dramatically by 24 hr. Acid and pepsin secretion peak in the 1st 10 days and decrease from 10-30 days after birth. Intrinsic factor secretion rises slowly in the 1st 2 wk of life.

The small bowel is approximately 270 cm long at birth in a term neonate and grows to an adult length of 450-550 cm by 4 yr of age. The mucosa of the small intestine is composed of villi, which are finger-like projections of the mucosa into the bowel lumen that significantly expand the absorptive surface area. The mucosal surface is further expanded by a brush border containing digestive enzymes and transport mechanisms for monosaccharides, amino acids, dipeptides and tripeptides, and fats. The cells of the villi originate in adjacent crypts and become functional as they migrate from the crypt up the villus. The small bowel mucosa is completely renewed in 4-5 days, providing a mechanism for rapid repair after injury, but in young infants or malnourished children, the process may be delayed. Crypt cells also secrete fluid and electrolytes. The villi are present by 8 wk of gestation in the duodenum and by 11 wk in the ileum.

Disaccharidase activities are measurable at 12 wk, but lactase activity does not reach maximal levels until 36 wk. Even premature infants usually tolerate lactose-containing formulas because of carbohydrate salvage by colonic bacteria. In children of African and Asian ethnicity, lactase levels may begin to fall at 4 yr of age, leading to intolerance to mammalian milk. Mechanisms to digest and absorb protein, including pancreatic enzymes and mucosal mechanisms to transport amino acids, dipeptides, and tripeptides, are in place by the 20th wk of gestation.

Carbohydrates, protein, and fat are normally absorbed by the upper half of the small intestine; the distal segments represent a vast reserve of absorptive capacity. Most of the sodium, potassium, chloride, and water are absorbed in the small bowel. Bile salts and vitamin B_{12} are selectively absorbed in the distal ileum, and iron is absorbed in the duodenum and proximal jejunum. Intraluminal digestion depends on the exocrine pancreas. Secretin and cholecystokinin stimulate synthesis and secretion of bicarbonate and digestive enzymes, which are released by the upper intestinal mucosa in response to various intraluminal stimuli, among them components of the diet.

Carbohydrate digestion is normally an efficient process that is completed in the distal duodenum. Starches are broken down to glucose, oligosaccharides, and disaccharides by pancreatic amylase. Residual glucose polymers are broken down at the mucosal level by glucoamylase. Lactose is broken down at the brush border by lactase, forming glucose and galactose; sucrose is broken down by sucrase-isomaltase to fructose and glucose. Galactose and glucose are primarily transported into the cell by a sodium- and energy-dependent process, whereas fructose is transported by facilitated diffusion.

Proteins are hydrolyzed by pancreatic enzymes, including trypsin, chymotrypsin, elastase, and carboxypeptidases, into individual amino acids and oligopeptides. The pancreatic enzymes are secreted as proenzymes, which are activated by release of the mucosal enzyme enterokinase. Oligopeptides are further broken down at the brush border by peptidases into dipeptides, tripeptides, and amino acids. Protein can enter the cell by separate noncompetitive carriers that can transport individual amino acids or dipeptides and tripeptides similar to those in the renal tubule. The human gut is capable of absorbing antigenic intact proteins in the 1st few wk of life because of "leaky" junctions between enterocytes. Entry of potential protein antigens through the mucosal barrier might have a role in later food- and microbe-induced symptoms.

Fat absorption occurs in 2 phases. Dietary triglycerides are broken down into monoglycerides and free fatty acids by pancreatic lipase and colipase. The free fatty acids are subsequently emulsified by bile acids, forming micelles with phospholipids and other fat-soluble substances, and are transported to the cell membrane, where they are absorbed. The fats are re-esterified in the enterocyte, forming chylomicrons that are transported through the intestinal lymphatics to the thoracic duct. Medium-chain fats are absorbed more efficiently and can directly enter the cell. They are subsequently transported to the liver via the portal system. Fat absorption can be affected at any stage of the digestion and absorption process. Decreased pancreatic enzymes occur in cystic fibrosis, cholestatic liver disease leads to poor bile salt production and micelle formation, celiac disease affects mucosal surface area, abnormal chylomicron formation occurs in abetalipoproteinemia, and intestinal lymphangiectasia affects transport of the chylomicrons.

Fat absorption is less efficient in the neonate compared with adults. Premature infants can lose up to 20% of their fat calories compared with up to 6% in the adult. Decreased synthesis of bile acids and pancreatic lipase and decreased efficiency of ileal absorption are contributing factors. Fat digestion in the neonate is facilitated by lingual and gastric lipases. Bile salt–stimulated lipase in human milk augments the action of pancreatic lipase. Infants with malabsorption of fat are usually fed with formulas that have a greater percentage of medium-chain triglycerides, which are absorbed independently of bile salts.

The colon is a 75-100 cm sacculated tube formed by 3 strips of longitudinal muscle called *taenia coli* that traverse its length and fold the mucosa into haustra. Haustra and taenia appear by the 12th wk of gestation. The most common motor activity in the colon is nonpropulsive rhythmic segmentation that acts to mix the chyme and expose the contents to the colonic mucosa. Mass movement within the colon typically occurs after a meal. The colon extracts additional water and electrolytes from the luminal contents to render the stools partially or completely solid. The colon also acts to scavenge by-products of bacterial degradation of carbohydrates. Stool is stored in the rectum until distention triggers a defecation reflex that, when assisted by voluntary relaxation of the external sphincter, permits evacuation.

Chapter **329**
Pyloric Stenosis and Other Congenital Anomalies of the Stomach

329.1 Hypertrophic Pyloric Stenosis
Anna K. Hunter and Chris A. Liacouras

Hypertrophic pyloric stenosis occurs in 1-3 per 1,000 infants in the United States. It is more common in whites of northern European ancestry, less common in blacks, and rare in Asians. Males (especially firstborns) are affected approximately 4-6 times as often as females. The offspring of a mother and, to a lesser extent, the father who had pyloric stenosis are at higher risk for pyloric stenosis. Pyloric stenosis develops in approximately 20% of the male and 10% of the female descendants of a mother who had pyloric stenosis. The incidence of pyloric stenosis is increased in infants with B and O blood groups. Pyloric stenosis is occasionally associated with other congenital defects, including tracheoesophageal fistula and hypoplasia or agenesis of the inferior labial frenulum.

ETIOLOGY
The cause of pyloric stenosis is unknown, but many factors have been implicated. Pyloric stenosis is usually not present at birth and is more concordant in monozygotic than dizygotic twins. It is unusual in stillbirths and probably develops after birth. Pyloric stenosis has been associated with eosinophilic gastroenteritis, Apert syndrome, Zellweger syndrome, trisomy 18, Smith-Lemli-Opitz syndrome, and Cornelia de Lange syndrome. An association has been found with the use of erythromycin in neonates with highest risk if the medication is given within the 1st 2 wk of life. There have also been reports of higher incidence of pyloric stenosis among mostly female infants of mothers treated with macrolide antibiotics during pregnancy and breastfeeding. Abnormal muscle innervation, elevated serum levels of prostaglandins, and infant hypergastrinemia has been implicated. Reduced levels of neuronal nitric oxide synthase have been found with altered expression of the neuronal nitric oxide synthase exon 1c regulatory region, which influences the expression of the neuronal nitric oxide synthase gene. Reduced nitric oxide might contribute to the pathogenesis of pyloric stenosis.

CLINICAL MANIFESTATIONS
Nonbilious vomiting is the initial symptom of pyloric stenosis. The vomiting may or may not be projectile initially but is usually progressive, occurring immediately after a feeding. Emesis might follow each feeding, or it may be intermittent. The vomiting usually starts after 3 wk of age, but symptoms can develop as early as the 1st wk of life and as late as the 5th mo. Approximately 20% have intermittent emesis from birth that then progresses to the classic picture. After vomiting, the infant is hungry and wants to feed again. As vomiting continues, a progressive loss of fluid, hydrogen ion, and chloride leads to hypochloremic metabolic alkalosis. Greater awareness of pyloric stenosis has led to earlier identification of patients with fewer instances of chronic malnutrition and severe dehydration and at times a subclinical self-resolving hypertrophy.

Hyperbilirubinemia is the most common clinical association of pyloric stenosis, also known as *icteropyloric syndrome*. Unconjugated hyperbilirubinemia is more common than conjugated and usually resolves with surgical correction. It may be associated with a decreased level of glucuronyl transferase as seen in approximately 5% of affected infants; mutations in the bilirubin uridine diphosphate glucuronosyltransferase gene (*UGT1A1*) have also been implicated. If conjugated hyperbilirubinemia is a part of the presentation, other etiologies need to be investigated. Other coexistent clinical diagnoses have been described, including eosinophilic gastroenteritis, hiatal hernia, peptic ulcer, congenital nephrotic syndrome, congenital heart disease, and congenital hypothyroidism.

The diagnosis has traditionally been established by palpating the pyloric mass. The mass is firm, movable, approximately 2 cm in length, olive shaped, hard, best palpated from the left side, and located above and to the right of the umbilicus in the midepigastrium beneath the liver's edge. The olive is easiest palpated after an episode of vomiting. After feeding, there may be a visible gastric peristaltic wave that progresses across the abdomen (Fig. 329-1).

Two imaging studies are commonly used to establish the diagnosis. Ultrasound examination confirms the diagnosis in the majority of cases. Criteria for diagnosis include pyloric thickness 3-4 mm, an overall pyloric length 15-19 mm, and pyloric diameter of 10-14 mm (Fig. 329-2). Ultrasonography has a sensitivity of approximately 95%. When contrast studies are performed, they demonstrate an elongated pyloric channel (string sign), a bulge of the pyloric muscle into the antrum (shoulder sign), and parallel streaks of barium seen in the narrowed channel, producing a "double tract sign" (Fig. 329-3).

DIFFERENTIAL DIAGNOSIS

Gastric waves are occasionally visible in small, emaciated infants who do not have pyloric stenosis. Infrequently, gastroesophageal reflux, with or without a hiatal hernia, may be confused with pyloric stenosis. Gastroesophageal reflux disease can be differentiated from pyloric stenosis by radiographic studies. Adrenal insufficiency from the adrenogenital syndrome can simulate pyloric stenosis, but the absence of a metabolic acidosis and elevated serum potassium and urinary sodium concentrations of adrenal insufficiency aid in differentiation (see Chapter 576). Inborn errors of metabolism can produce recurrent emesis with alkalosis (urea cycle) or acidosis (organic acidemia) and lethargy, coma, or seizures. Vomiting with diarrhea suggests gastroenteritis, but patients with pyloric stenosis occasionally have diarrhea. Rarely, a pyloric membrane or pyloric duplication results in projectile vomiting, visible peristalsis, and, in the case of a duplication, a palpable mass. Duodenal stenosis proximal to the ampulla of Vater results in the clinical features of pyloric stenosis but can be differentiated by the presence of a pyloric mass on physical examination or ultrasonography.

TREATMENT

The preoperative treatment is directed toward correcting the fluid, acid–base, and electrolyte losses. Correction of the alkalosis is essential to prevent postoperative apnea, which may be associated with anesthesia. Most infants can be successfully rehydrated within 24 hr. Vomiting usually stops when the stomach is empty, and only an occasional infant requires nasogastric suction.

The **surgical procedure of choice** is pyloromyotomy. The traditional Ramstedt procedure is performed through a short transverse skin incision. The underlying pyloric mass is cut longitudinally to the layer of the submucosa, and the incision is closed. Laparoscopic technique is equally successful and in one study resulted in a shorter time to full feedings and discharge from the hospital as well as greater parental satisfaction. The success of laparoscopy depends on the skill of the

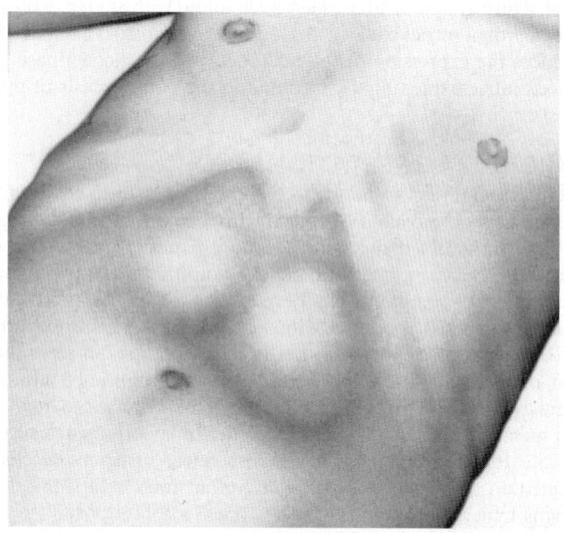

Figure 329-1 Gastric peristaltic wave in an infant with pyloric stenosis.

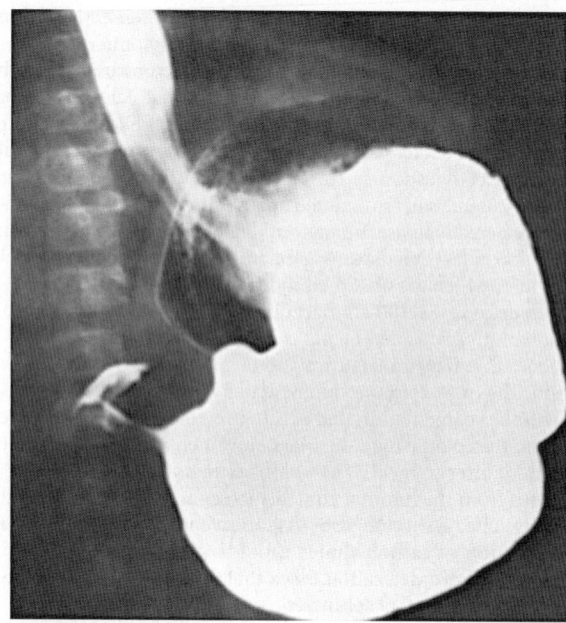

Figure 329-3 Barium in the stomach of an infant with projectile vomiting. The attenuated pyloric canal is typical of congenital hypertrophic pyloric stenosis.

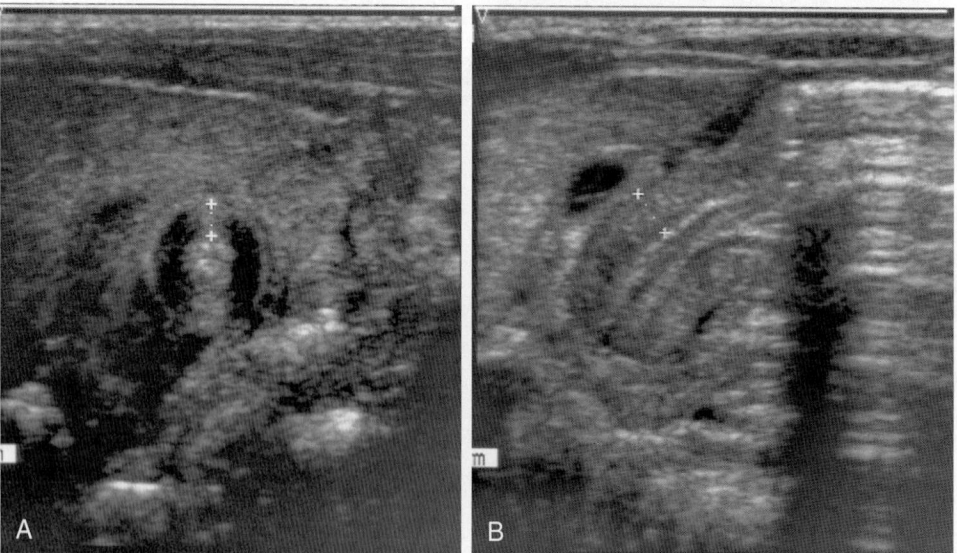

Figure 329-2 A, Transverse sonogram demonstrating a pyloric muscle wall thickness of >4 mm (distance between *crosses*). **B,** Horizontal image demonstrating a pyloric channel length >14 mm (wall thickness outlined between *crosses*) in an infant with pyloric stenosis.

surgeon. Postoperative vomiting occurs in half the infants and is thought to be secondary to edema of the pylorus at the incision site. In most infants, however, feedings can be initiated within 12-24 hr after surgery and advanced to maintenance oral feedings within 36-48 hr after surgery. Persistent vomiting suggests an incomplete pyloromyotomy, gastritis, gastroesophageal reflux disease, or another cause of the obstruction. The surgical treatment of pyloric stenosis is curative, with an operative mortality of 0-0.5%. Endoscopic balloon dilation has been successful in infants with persistent vomiting secondary to incomplete pyloromyotomy.

Conservative management with nasoduodenal feedings is advisable in patients who are not good surgical candidates. Oral and intravenous atropine sulfate (pyloric muscle relaxant) has also been described when surgical treatment is not available with 80% success rate described in some studies. In conservative protocols atropine is administered intravenously at a dose of 0.01 mg/kg 6 times a day 5 min before feeding. During atropine infusion, the heart rate needs to be continuously monitored by electrocardiography. Oral feeding is started at a volume of 10 mL formula, 6 times a day. The volume is increased day by day until patients tolerate 150 mL/kg/day unless vomiting occurs more than twice a day. When patients are able to tolerate the full volume of formula without vomiting more than twice a day, 0.02 mg/kg atropine is administered orally 6 times a day before feeding. As the conservative management takes longer and oral feedings may not be tolerated at first, worsening of the nutrition status may occur and total parenteral nutrition may be required. It was also postulated that surgical management is more time and cost effective.

Bibliography is available at Expert Consult.

329.2 Congenital Gastric Outlet Obstruction
Anna K. Hunter and Chris A. Liacouras

Gastric outlet obstruction resulting from pyloric atresia and antral webs is uncommon and accounts for <1% of all the atresias and diaphragms of the alimentary tract. The cause of the defects is unknown. Pyloric atresia has been associated with **epidermolysis bullosa** and usually presents in early infancy. The gender distribution is equal.

CLINICAL MANIFESTATIONS
Infants with pyloric atresia present with nonbilious vomiting, feeding difficulties, and abdominal distention during the 1st day of life. **Polyhydramnios** occurs in the majority of cases, and low birth weight is common. The gastric aspirate at birth is large (>20 mL fluid) and should be removed to prevent aspiration. Rupture of the stomach may occur as early as the 1st 12 hr of life. Infants with antral web may present with less dramatic symptoms, depending on the degree of obstruction. Older children with antral webs present with nausea, vomiting, abdominal pain, and weight loss.

DIAGNOSIS
The diagnosis of congenital gastric outlet obstruction is suggested by the finding of a large, dilated stomach on abdominal plain radiographs or in utero ultrasonography. Upper gastrointestinal (GI) contrast series is usually diagnostic and demonstrates a pyloric dimple. When contrast studies are performed, care must be taken to avoid possible aspiration. An antral web may appear as a thin septum near the pyloric channel. In older children, endoscopy has been helpful in identifying antral webs.

TREATMENT
The treatment of all causes of gastric outlet obstruction in neonates starts with the correction of dehydration and hypochloremic alkalosis. Persistent vomiting should be relieved with nasogastric decompression. Surgical or endoscopic repair should be undertaken when a patient is stable.

329.3 Gastric Duplication
Anna K. Hunter and Chris A. Liacouras

Gastric duplications are uncommon cystic or tubular structures that usually occur within the wall of the stomach. They account for 2-7% of all GI duplications. They are most commonly located on the greater curvature. Most are <12 cm in diameter and do not usually communicate with the stomach lumen; however, they do have common blood supply. Associated anomalies occur in as many as 35% of patients. Several hypotheses for the etiology of the duplication cysts have been developed including the splitting notochord theory, diverticulation, canalization defects, and caudal twinning.

The most common clinical manifestations are associated with partial or complete gastric outlet obstruction. In 33% of patients, the cyst may be palpable. Communicating duplications can cause gastric ulceration and be associated with hematemesis or melena.

Radiographic studies usually show a paragastric mass displacing stomach. Ultrasound can show the inner hyperechoic mucosal and outer hypoechoic muscle layers that are typical of GI duplications. Surgical excision is the treatment for symptomatic gastric duplications.

Bibliography is available at Expert Consult.

329.4 Gastric Volvulus
Anna K. Hunter and Chris A. Liacouras

The stomach is tethered longitudinally by the gastrohepatic, gastrosplenic, and gastrocolic ligaments. In the transverse axis, it is tethered by the gastrophrenic ligament and the retroperitoneal attachment of the duodenum. A volvulus occurs when one of these attachments is absent or elongated, allowing the stomach to rotate around itself. In some children, other associated defects are present, including intestinal malrotation, diaphragmatic defects, hiatal hernia, or adjacent organ abnormalities such as asplenia. Volvulus can occur along the longitudinal axis, producing organoaxial volvulus, or along the transverse axis, producing mesenteroaxial volvulus. Combined volvulus occurs if the stomach rotates around both organoaxial and mesenteroaxial axes.

The clinical presentation of gastric volvulus is nonspecific and suggests high intestinal obstruction. Gastric volvulus in infancy is usually associated with nonbilious vomiting and epigastric distention. It has also been associated with episodes of dyspnea and apnea in this age group. Acute volvulus can advance rapidly to strangulation and perforation. Chronic gastric volvulus is more common in older children; the children present with a history of emesis, abdominal pain and distention, early satiety, and failure to thrive.

The diagnosis is suggested in plain abdominal radiographs by the presence of a dilated stomach. Erect abdominal films demonstrate a double fluid level with a characteristic "beak" near the lower esophageal junction in mesenteroaxial volvulus. The stomach tends to lie in a vertical plane. In organoaxial volvulus, a single air–fluid level is seen without the characteristic beak with stomach lying in a horizontal plane. Upper GI series has also been used to aid the diagnosis.

Treatment of acute gastric volvulus is emergent surgery once a patient is stabilized. Laparoscopic gastropexy is the most common surgical approach. In selected cases of chronic volvulus in older patients, endoscopic correction has been successful.

Bibliography is available at Expert Consult.

329.5 Hypertrophic Gastropathy
Anna K. Hunter and Chris A. Liacouras

Hypertrophic gastropathy in children is uncommon and, in contrast to that in adults (Ménétrier disease), is usually a transient, benign, and self-limited condition.

PATHOGENESIS

The condition is most often secondary to cytomegalovirus (CMV) infection, but other agents, including herpes simplex virus, *Giardia*, and *Helicobacter pylori*, are also implicated. The pathophysiologic mechanisms underlying the clinical picture are not completely understood but might involve widening of gap junctions between gastric epithelial cells with resultant fluid and protein losses. There is an association with increased expression of transforming growth factor-α in gastric mucosal tissue shown in CMV induced gastropathy. *H. pylori* infection can cause the elevation of serum glucagon-like peptide-2 levels, a mucosal growth-inducing gut hormone.

CLINICAL MANIFESTATIONS

Clinical manifestations include vomiting, anorexia, upper abdominal pain, diarrhea, edema (hypoproteinemic protein- losing enteropathy), ascites, and, rarely, hematemesis if ulceration occurs.

DIAGNOSIS AND DIFFERENTIAL DIAGNOSIS

The mean age at diagnosis is 5 yr (range: 2 days-17 yr); the illness usually lasts 2-14 wk, with complete resolution being the rule. Endoscopy with biopsy and tissue CMV polymerase chain reaction is diagnostic. Endoscopy shows characteristic enlarged gastric folds. The upper GI series might show thickened gastric folds. The differential diagnosis includes eosinophilic gastroenteritis, gastric lymphoma or carcinoma, Crohn disease, and inflammatory pseudotumor.

TREATMENT

Therapy is supportive and should include adequate hydration, antisecretory agents (H₂ receptor blockade, acid suppression with proton pump inhibitors), and albumin replacement if the hypoalbuminemia is symptomatic. When *H. pylori* are detected, appropriate treatment is recommended. Ganciclovir in CMV-positive gastropathy is indicated only in severe cases. There are no official guidelines as far as the length of treatment. In practice, IV therapy is initiated for the 1st 24-48 hr. Treatment in continued with oral valganciclovir for a total of 3 wk. Complete recovery is the rule. Hypertrophic gastropathy should be considered in a previously healthy child with new onset edema and no other causes of protein losses. This is not a chronic condition in children. Disease tends to have much more severe course in adult patients.

Bibliography is available at Expert Consult.

Chapter 330

Intestinal Atresia, Stenosis, and Malrotation

Christina Bales and Chris A. Liacouras

Approximately 1 in 1,500 children is born with intestinal obstruction. Obstruction may be partial or complete, and it may be characterized as simple or strangulating. Luminal contents fails to progress in an aboral direction in simple obstruction, whereas blood flow to the intestine is also impaired in strangulating obstruction. If strangulating obstruction is not promptly relieved, it can lead to bowel infarction and perforation.

Intestinal obstruction can be further classified as either intrinsic or extrinsic based on underlying etiology. Intrinsic causes include inherent abnormalities of intestinal innervation, mucus production, or tubular anatomy. Among these, congenital disruption of the tubular structure is most common and can manifest as obliteration (atresia) or narrowing (stenosis) of the intestinal lumen. More than 90% of intestinal stenosis and atresia occurs in the duodenum, jejunum, and ileum. Rare cases occur in the colon, and these may be associated with more proximal atresias.

Extrinsic causes of congenital intestinal obstruction involve compression of the bowel by vessels (e.g., preduodenal portal vein), organs (e.g., annular pancreas), and cysts (e.g., duplication, mesenteric). Abnormalities in intestinal rotation during fetal development also represent a unique extrinsic cause of congenital intestinal obstruction. Malrotation is associated with inadequate mesenteric attachment of the intestine to the posterior abdominal wall, which leaves the bowel vulnerable to autoobstruction as a result of intestinal twisting or volvulus. Malrotation is commonly accompanied by congenital adhesions that can compress and obstruct the duodenum as they extend from the cecum to the right upper quadrant.

Obstruction is typically associated with bowel distention, which is caused by an accumulation of ingested food, gas, and intestinal secretions proximal to the point of obstruction. As the bowel dilates, absorption of intestinal fluid is decreased and secretion of fluid and electrolytes is increased. This shift results in isotonic intravascular depletion, which is usually associated with hypokalemia. Bowel distention also results in a decrease in blood flow to the obstructed bowel. As blood flow is shifted away from the intestinal mucosa, there is loss of mucosal integrity. Bacteria proliferate in the stagnant bowel, with a predominance of coliforms and anaerobes. This rapid proliferation of bacteria, coupled with the loss of mucosal integrity, allows bacterial to translocate across the bowel wall and potentially lead to endotoxemia, bacteremia, and sepsis.

The clinical presentation of intestinal obstruction varies with the cause, level of obstruction, and time between the obstructing event and the patient's evaluation. Classic symptoms of obstruction in the neonate include vomiting, abdominal distention, and obstipation. Obstruction high in the intestinal tract results in large-volume, frequent, bilious emesis with little or no abdominal distention. Pain is intermittent and is usually relieved by vomiting. Obstruction in the distal small bowel leads to moderate or marked abdominal distention with emesis that is progressively feculent. Both proximal and distal obstructions are eventually associated with obstipation. However, meconium stools can be passed initially if the obstruction is in the upper part of the intestinal tract or if the obstruction developed late in intrauterine life.

The diagnosis of congenital bowel obstruction relies on a combination of history, physical examination, and radiologic findings. In certain cases, the diagnosis is suggested in the prenatal period. Routine prenatal ultrasound can detect polyhydramnios, which often accompanies high intestinal obstruction. The presence of polyhydramnios should prompt aspiration of the infant's stomach immediately after birth. Aspiration of more than 15-20 mL of fluid, particularly if it is bile stained, is highly indicative of proximal intestinal obstruction.

In the postnatal period, a plain radiograph is the initial diagnostic study and can provide valuable information about potential associated complications. With completely obstructing lesions, plain radiographs reveal bowel distention proximal to the point of obstruction. Upright or crosstable lateral views typically demonstrate a series of air–fluid levels in the distended loops. Caution must be exercised in using plain films to determine the location of intestinal obstruction. Because colonic haustra are not fully developed in the neonate, small and large bowel obstructions may be difficult to distinguish with plain films. In these cases, contrast studies of the bowel or computed tomography images may be indicated. Oral or nasogastric contrast medium may be used to identify obstructing lesions in the proximal bowel, and contrast enemas may be used to diagnose more-distal entities. Indeed, enemas may also play a therapeutic role in relieving distal obstruction caused by meconium ileus or meconium plug syndrome.

Initial treatment of infants and children with bowel obstruction must be directed at fluid resuscitation and stabilizing the patient. Nasogastric decompression usually relieves pain and vomiting. After appropriate cultures, broad-spectrum antibiotics are usually started in ill-appearing neonates with bowel obstruction and those with suspected strangulating infarction. Patients with strangulation must have immediate surgical relief before the bowel infarcts, resulting in gangrene and intestinal perforation. Extensive intestinal necrosis results in short bowel syndrome (see Chapter 330.7). Nonoperative conservative management is usually limited to children with suspected adhesions or inflammatory strictures that might resolve with nasogastric decompression or anti-inflammatory medications. If clinical signs of improvement are not evident within 12-24 hr, then operative intervention is usually indicated.

Bibliography is available at Expert Consult.

330.1 Duodenal Obstruction

Christina Bales and Chris A. Liacouras

Congenital duodenal obstruction occurs in 2.5-10 per 100,000 live births. In most cases, it is caused by atresia, an intrinsic defect of bowel formation. It can also result from extrinsic compression by abnormal neighboring structures (e.g., annular pancreas, preduodenal portal vein), duplication cysts, or congenital bands associated with malrotation. Although intrinsic and extrinsic causes of duodenal obstruction occur independently, they can also coexist. Thus, a high index of suspicion for more than one underlying etiology may be critical to avoiding unnecessary reoperations in these infants.

Duodenal atresia complicates 1 per 10,000 live births and accounts for 25-40% of all intestinal atresias. In contrast to more-distal atresias, which likely arise from prenatal vascular accidents, duodenal atresia results from failed recanalization of the intestinal lumen during gestation. Throughout the 4th and 5th wk of normal fetal development, the duodenal mucosa exhibits rapid proliferation of epithelial cells. Persistence of these cells, which should degenerate after the 7th wk of gestation, leads to occlusion of the lumen (atresia) in approximately two-thirds of cases and narrowing (stenosis) in the remaining one-third. Duodenal atresia can take several forms, including a thin membrane that occludes the lumen, a short fibrous cord that connects 2 blind duodenal pouches, or a gap that spans 2 nonconnecting ends of the duodenum. The membranous form is most common, and it almost invariably occurs near the ampulla of Vater. In rare cases, the membrane is distensible and is referred to as a *windsock web*. This unusual form of duodenal atresia causes obstruction several centimeters distal to the origin of the membrane.

Approximately 50% of infants with duodenal atresia are premature. Concomitant congenital anomalies are common and include congenital heart disease (30%), malrotation (20-30%), annular pancreas (30%), renal anomalies (5-15%), esophageal atresia with or without tracheoesophageal fistula (5-10%), skeletal malformations (5%), and anorectal anomalies (5%). Of these anomalies, only complex congenital heart disease is associated with increased mortality. Annular pancreas is associated with increased late complications, including gastroesophageal reflux disease, peptic ulcer disease, pancreatitis, gastric outlet and recurrent duodenal obstruction, and gastric cancer. Thus, long-term follow-up of these patients into adulthood is warranted. Nearly half of patients with duodenal atresia have chromosome abnormalities; trisomy 21 is identified in up to one-third of patients.

CLINICAL MANIFESTATIONS AND DIAGNOSIS

The hallmark of duodenal obstruction is bilious vomiting without abdominal distention, which is usually noted on the 1st day of life. Peristaltic waves may be visualized early in the disease process. A history of polyhydramnios is present in half the pregnancies and is caused by inadequate absorption of amniotic fluid in the distal intestine. This fluid may be bile stained because of intrauterine vomiting. Jaundice is present in one-third of the infants.

The diagnosis is suggested by the presence of a "double-bubble" sign on a plain abdominal radiograph (Fig. 330-1). The appearance is caused by a distended and gas-filled stomach and proximal duodenum, which are invariably connected. Contrast studies are occasionally needed to exclude malrotation and volvulus because intestinal

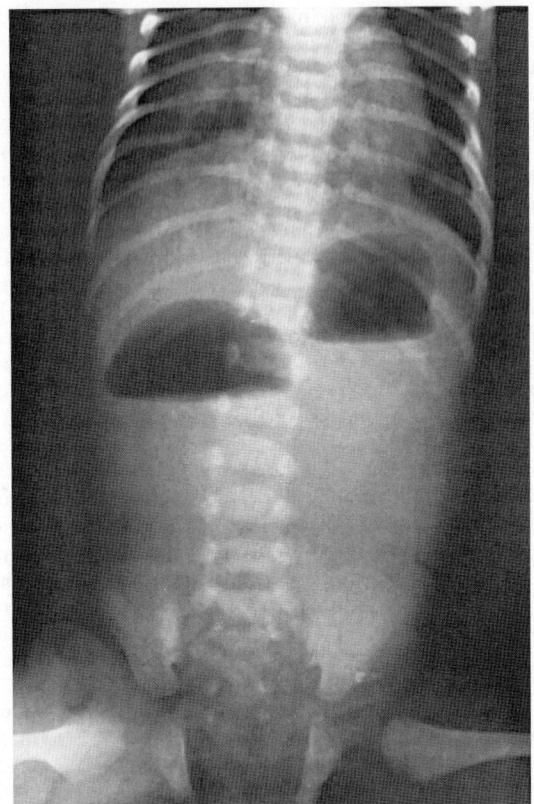

Figure 330-1 Abdominal radiograph of a newborn infant held upright. Note the "double-bubble" gas shadow above and the absence of gas in the distal bowel in this case of congenital duodenal atresia.

infarction can occur within 6-12 hr if the volvulus is not relieved. Contrast studies are generally not necessary and may be associated with aspiration. Prenatal diagnosis of duodenal atresia is readily made by fetal ultrasonography, which reveals a sonographic double-bubble. Prenatal identification of duodenal atresia is associated with decreased morbidity and fewer hospitalization days.

TREATMENT

The initial treatment of infants with duodenal atresia includes nasogastric or orogastric decompression and intravenous fluid replacement. Echocardiography, renal ultrasound, and radiology of the chest and spine should be performed to evaluate for associated anomalies. Definitive correction of the atresia is usually postponed until life-threatening anomalies are evaluated and treated.

The typical surgical repair for duodenal atresia is duodenoduodenostomy. This procedure is also preferred in cases of concomitant or isolated annular pancreas. In these instances, the duodenoduodenostomy is performed without dividing the pancreas. The dilated proximal bowel might have to be tapered to improve peristalsis. Postoperatively, a gastrostomy tube can be placed to drain the stomach and protect the airway. Intravenous nutritional support or a transanastomotic jejunal tube is needed until an infant starts to feed orally. Long-term prognosis is excellent, approaching 90% survival in most series.

Bibliography is available at Expert Consult.

330.2 Jejunal and Ileal Atresia and Obstruction

Christina Bales and Chris A. Liacouras

The primary etiologies of congenital small bowel obstruction involve intrinsic abnormalities in anatomic development (jejunoileal stenosis and atresia), mucus secretion (meconium ileus), and bowel wall innervation (long-segment Hirschsprung disease).

Jejunoileal atresias are generally attributed to intrauterine vascular accidents, which result in segmental infarction and resorption of the fetal intestine. Underlying events that potentiate vascular compromise include intestinal volvulus, intussusception, meconium ileus, and strangulating herniation through an abdominal wall defect associated with gastroschisis or omphalocele. Maternal behaviors that promote vasoconstriction, such as cigarette smoking and cocaine use, might also have a role. Only a few cases of familial inheritance have been reported. In these families, multiple intestinal atresias have occurred in an autosomal recessive pattern. Jejunoileal atresias have been linked with multiple births, low birthweight, and prematurity. Unlike atresia in the duodenum, they are not commonly associated with extraintestinal anomalies.

Five types of jejunal and ileal atresias are encountered (Fig. 330-2). In type I, a mucosal web occludes the lumen but continuity is maintained between the proximal and distal bowel. Type II involves a small-diameter solid cord that connects the proximal and distal bowel. Type III is divided into 2 subtypes. Type IIIa occurs when both ends of the bowel end in blind loops, accompanied by a small mesenteric defect. Type IIIb is similar, but it is associated with an extensive mesenteric defect and a loss of the normal blood supply to the distal bowel. The distal ileum coils around the ileocolic artery, from which it derives its entire blood supply, producing an "apple-peel" appearance. This anomaly is associated with prematurity, an unusually short distal ileum, and significant foreshortening of the bowel. Type IV involves multiple atresias. Types II and IIIa are the most common, each accounting for 30-35% of cases. Type I occurs in approximately 20% of patients. Types IIIb and IV account for the remaining 10-20% of cases, with IIIb being the least-common configuration.

Meconium ileus occurs primarily in newborn infants with cystic fibrosis, an exocrine gland defect of chloride transport that results in abnormally viscous secretions. Approximately 80-90% of infants with meconium ileus have cystic fibrosis, but only 10-15% of infants with cystic fibrosis present with meconium ileus. In simple cases, the distal 20-30 cm of ileum is collapsed and filled with pellets of pale stool. The proximal bowel is dilated and filled with thick meconium that resembles sticky syrup or glue. Peristalsis fails to propel this viscid material forward, and it becomes impacted in the ileum. In complicated cases, a volvulus of the dilated proximal bowel can occur, resulting in intestinal ischemia, atresia, and/or perforation. Perforation in utero results in meconium peritonitis, which can lead to potentially obstructing adhesions and calcifications.

Both intestinal atresia and meconium ileus must be distinguished from **long-segment Hirschsprung disease**. This condition involves congenital absence of ganglion cells in the myenteric and submucosal plexuses of the bowel wall. In a small subset (5%) of patients, the aganglionic segment includes the terminal ileum in addition to the entire length of the colon. Infants with long-segment Hirschsprung disease present with a dilated small intestine that is ganglionated but has hypertrophied walls, a funnel-shaped transitional hypoganglionic zone, and a collapsed distal aganglionic bowel.

CLINICAL MANIFESTATION AND DIAGNOSIS

Distal intestinal obstruction is less likely than proximal obstruction to be detected in utero. Polyhydramnios is identified in 20-35% of jejunoileal atresias, and it may be the first sign of intestinal obstruction. Abdominal distention is rarely present at birth, but it develops rapidly after initiation of feeds in the 1st 12-24 hr. Distention is often accompanied by vomiting, which is often bilious. Up to 80% of infants fail to pass meconium in the 1st 24 hr of life. Jaundice, associated with unconjugated hyperbilirubinemia, is reported in 20-30% of patients.

In patients with obstruction caused by jejunoileal atresia or long-segment Hirschsprung disease, plain radiographs typically demonstrate multiple air-fluid levels proximal to the obstruction in the upright or lateral decubitus positions (Fig. 330-3). These levels may be absent in patients with meconium ileus because the viscosity of the secretions in the proximal bowel prevents layering. Instead, a typical hazy or ground-glass appearance may be appreciated in the right lower quadrant. This haziness is caused by small bubbles of gas that become trapped in inspissated meconium in the terminal ileal region. If there is meconium peritonitis, patchy calcification may also be noted, particularly in the flanks. Plain films can reveal evidence of pneumoperitoneum due to intestinal perforation. Air may be seen in the subphrenic regions on the upright view and over the liver in the left lateral decubitus position.

Because plain radiographs do not reliably distinguish between small and large bowel in neonates, contrast studies are often required to localize the obstruction. Water-soluble enemas (Gastrografin, Hypaque) are particularly useful in differentiating atresia from meconium ileus and Hirschsprung disease. A small "microcolon" suggests disuse and the presence of obstruction proximal to the ileocecal valve. Abdominal ultrasound may be an important adjunctive study, which

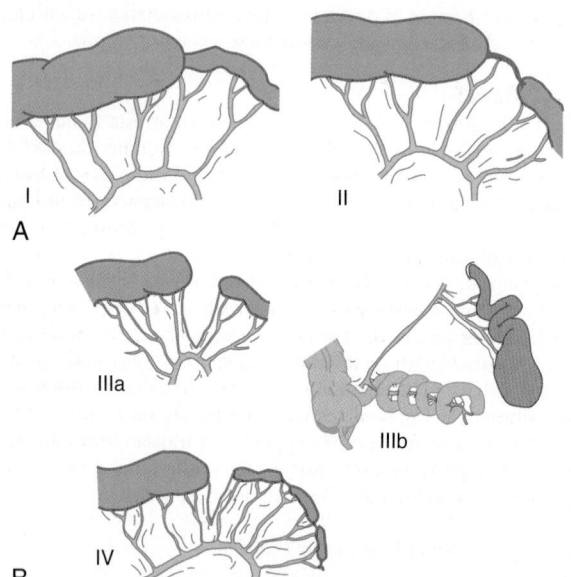

A

B

Figure 330-2 A and B, Classification of intestinal atresia. Type I: Mucosal obstruction caused by an intraluminal membrane with intact bowel wall and mesentery. Type II: Blind ends are separated by a fibrous cord. Type IIIa: Blind ends are separated by a V-shaped mesenteric defect. Type IIIb: "Apple-peel" appearance. Type IV: Multiple atresias. *(From Grosfeld J: Jejunoileal atresia and stenosis. In Welch KJ, Randolph JG, Ravitch MM, editors: Pediatric surgery, ed 4, Chicago, 1986, Year Book Medical Publishers.)*

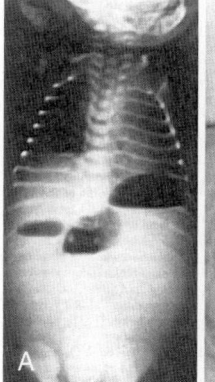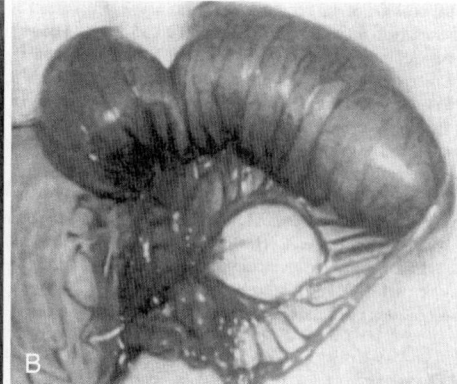

Figure 330-3 A, Abdominal radiograph in a neonate with bilious vomiting shows a few loops of dilated intestine with air–fluid levels. **B,** At laparotomy, a type I (mucosal) jejunal atresia was observed. *(From O'Neill JA Jr, Grosfeld JL, Fonkalsrud EW, et al, editors: Principles of pediatric surgery, ed 2, St. Louis, 2003, Mosby, p. 493.)*

can distinguish meconium ileus from ileal atresia and also identify concomitant intestinal malrotation.

TREATMENT

Patients with small bowel obstruction should be stable and in adequate fluid and electrolyte balance before operation or radiographic attempts at disimpaction unless volvulus is suspected. Documented infections should be treated with appropriate antibiotics. Prophylactic antibiotics are usually given before surgery.

Ileal or jejunal atresia requires resection of the dilated proximal portion of the bowel followed by end-to-end anastomosis. If a simple mucosal diaphragm is present, jejunoplasty or ileoplasty with partial excision of the web is an acceptable alternative to resection. In uncomplicated meconium ileus, Gastrografin enemas diagnose the obstruction and wash out the inspissated material. Gastrografin is hypertonic, and care must be taken to avoid dehydration, shock, and bowel perforation. The enema may have to be repeated after 8-12 hr. Resection after reduction is not needed if there have been no ischemic complications.

Approximately 50% of patients with simple meconium ileus do not adequately respond to water-soluble enemas and need laparotomy. Operative management is indicated when the obstruction cannot be relieved by repeated attempts at nonoperative management and for infants with complicated meconium ileus. The extent of surgical intervention depends on the degree of pathology. In simple meconium ileus, the plug can be relieved by manipulation or direct enteral irrigation with *N*-acetylcysteine following an enterotomy. In complicated cases, bowel resection, peritoneal lavage, abdominal drainage, and stoma formation may be necessary. Total parenteral nutrition is generally required.

Bibliography is available at Expert Consult.

330.3 Malrotation
Melissa Kennedy and Chris A. Liacouras

Malrotation is incomplete rotation of the intestine during fetal development and involves the intestinal nonrotation or incomplete rotation around the superior mesenteric artery. The gut starts as a straight tube from stomach to rectum. Intestinal rotation and attachment begins in the 5th wk of gestation when the midbowel (distal duodenum to midtransverse colon) begins to elongate and progressively protrudes into the umbilical cord until it lies totally outside the confines of the abdominal cavity. As the developing bowel rotates in and out of the abdominal cavity, the superior mesenteric artery, which supplies blood to this section of gut, acts as an axis. The duodenum, on reentering the abdominal cavity, moves to the region of the ligament of Treitz, and the colon that follows is directed to the left upper quadrant. The cecum subsequently rotates counterclockwise within the abdominal cavity and comes to lie in the right lower quadrant. The duodenum becomes fixed to the posterior abdominal wall before the colon is completely rotated. After rotation, the right and left colon and the mesenteric root become fixed to the posterior abdomen. These attachments provide a broad base of support to the mesentery and the superior mesenteric artery, thus preventing twisting of the mesenteric root and kinking of the vascular supply. Abdominal rotation and attachment are completed by the 12th wk of gestation.

Nonrotation occurs when the bowel fails to rotate after it returns to the abdominal cavity. The 1st and 2nd portions of the duodenum are in their normal position, but the remainder of the duodenum, jejunum, and ileum occupy the right side of the abdomen and the colon is located on the left. The most common type of malrotation involves failure of the cecum to move into the right lower quadrant (Fig. 330-4). The usual location of the cecum is in the subhepatic area. Failure of the cecum to rotate properly is associated with failure to form the normal broad-based adherence to the posterior abdominal wall. The mesentery, including the superior mesenteric artery, is tethered by a

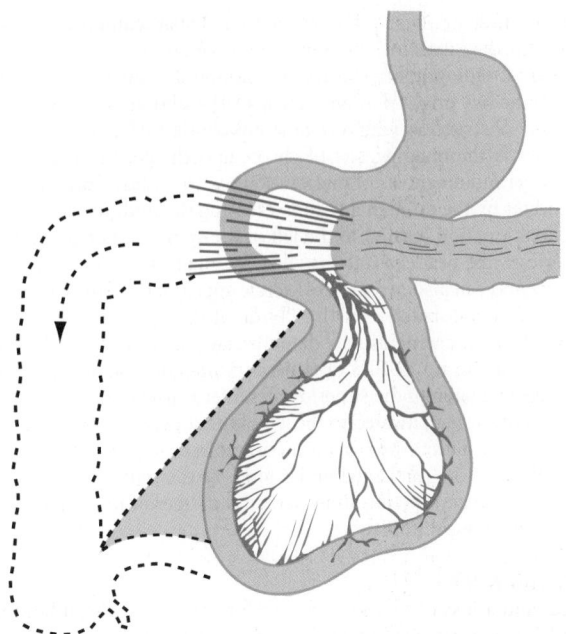

Figure 330-4 The mechanism of intestinal obstruction with incomplete rotation of the midgut (malrotation). The *dotted lines* show the course the cecum should have taken. Failure to rotate has left obstructing bands across the duodenum and a narrow pedicle for the midgut loop, making it susceptible to volvulus. *(From Nixon HH, O'Donnell B: The essentials of pediatric surgery, Philadelphia, 1961, JB Lippincott.)*

narrow stalk, which can twist around itself and produce a midgut volvulus. Bands of tissue (**Ladd bands**) can extend from the cecum to the right upper quadrant, crossing, and possibly obstructing, the duodenum.

Malrotation and nonrotation are often associated with other anomalies of the abdominal wall such as diaphragmatic hernia, gastroschisis, and omphalocele. Malrotation is also associated with the heterotaxy syndrome, which is a complex of congenital anomalies including congenital heart malformations, malrotation, biliary atresia, and either asplenia or polysplenia (see Chapter 431.11).

CLINICAL MANIFESTATIONS

The reported incidence of malrotation is approximately 1 in 500 infant population. The majority, about 75-85% of patients, present in the 1st yr of life, and more than 50% present within the 1st mo of life, with symptoms of acute or chronic obstruction. Vomiting is the most common symptom in this age group. Infants often present in the 1st wk of life with **bilious emesis** and acute bowel obstruction. Older infants present with episodes of recurrent abdominal pain that can mimic colic and suggest intermittent volvulus. Malrotation in older children can manifest with recurrent episodes of vomiting and/or abdominal pain. Patients occasionally present with **malabsorption** or **protein-losing enteropathy** associated with bacterial overgrowth. Symptoms are caused by intermittent volvulus or duodenal compression by Ladd bands or other adhesive bands affecting the small and large bowel. Approximately 25-50% of adolescents with malrotation are asymptomatic. Adolescents who become symptomatic present with acute intestinal obstruction or history of recurrent episodes of abdominal pain or postprandial bloating and occasional vomiting. Patients of any age with a rotational anomaly can develop acute bowel-threatening volvulus without preexisting symptoms.

An acute presentation of small bowel obstruction in a patient without previous bowel surgery can be the result of **volvulus** associated with malrotation. This is a life-threatening complication of malrotation, which resembles an acute abdomen or sepsis and is the main reason that symptoms suggesting malrotation should always be investigated. Volvulus occurs when the small bowel twists around the superior mesenteric artery leading to vascular compromise of the bowel. The diagnosis may be suggested by ultrasound but is confirmed by contrast radiographic studies. The abdominal plain film is usually nonspecific but might demonstrate a gasless abdomen or evidence of duodenal obstruction with a double-bubble sign. Upper gastrointestinal series is the imaging test of choice and the gold standard in the evaluation and diagnosis of malrotation and volvulus. Normal rotation is indicates by the duodenal C-loop crossing the midline and a duodenojejunal junction located to the left of the spine. Upper gastrointestinal series is the best exam to visualize the malposition of the ligament of Treitz and can also reveal a corkscrew appearance of the small bowel or a duodenal obstruction with a "bird's beak" appearance of the duodenum. Barium enema usually demonstrates malposition of the cecum but is normal in up to 20% of patients. Ultrasonography can demonstrate the inversion of the superior mesenteric artery and vein. A superior mesenteric vein located to the left of the superior mesenteric artery suggests malrotation. Malrotation with volvulus is suggested by duodenal obstruction, thickened bowel loops to the right of the spine, the superior mesenteric vein coiling around the superior mesenteric artery, and free peritoneal fluid.

TREATMENT

Surgical intervention is recommended for any patient with a significant rotational abnormality, regardless of age. If a volvulus is present, surgery is done immediately as an acute emergency, the volvulus is reduced, and the duodenum and upper jejunum are freed of any bands and remain in the right abdominal cavity. The colon is freed of adhesions and placed in the right abdomen with the cecum in the left lower quadrant, usually accompanied by incidental appendectomy. The Ladd procedure may be done laparoscopically for malrotation without volvulus and if gut ischemia is not present, but it is generally done as an open procedure if volvulus is present. The purpose of surgical intervention is to minimize the risk of subsequent volvulus rather than to return the bowel to a normal anatomic configuration. Extensive intestinal ischemia from volvulus can result in short bowel syndrome (see Chapter 330.7).

Bibliography is available at Expert Consult.

Chapter 331
Intestinal Duplications, Meckel Diverticulum, and Other Remnants of the Omphalomesenteric Duct

331.1 Intestinal Duplication
Chris A. Liacouras

Duplications of the intestinal tract are rare anomalies that consist of well-formed tubular or spherical structures firmly attached to the intestine with a common blood supply. The lining of the duplications resembles that of the gastrointestinal (GI) tract. Duplications are located on the mesenteric border and can communicate with the intestinal lumen. Duplications can be classified into 3 categories: localized duplications, duplications associated with spinal cord defects and vertebral malformations, and duplications of the colon. Occasionally (10-15% of cases), multiple duplications are found.

Localized duplications can occur in any area of the GI tract but are most common in the ileum and jejunum. They are usually cystic or tubular structures within the wall of the bowel. The cause is unknown, but their development has been attributed to defects in recanalization of the intestinal lumen after the solid stage of embryologic development. Duplication of the intestine occurring in association with **vertebral and spinal cord anomalies** (hemivertebra, anterior spina bifida, band connection between lesion and cervical or thoracic spine) is thought to arise from splitting of the notochord in the developing embryo. **Duplication of the colon** is usually associated with anomalies of the urinary tract and genitals. Duplication of the entire colon, rectum, anus, and terminal ileum can occur. The defects are thought to be secondary to caudal twinning, with duplication of the hindgut, genital, and lower urinary tracts.

CLINICAL MANIFESTATIONS

Symptoms depend on the size, location, and mucosal lining. Duplications can cause bowel obstruction by compressing the adjacent intestinal lumen, or they can act as the lead point of an intussusception or a site for a volvulus. If they are lined by acid-secreting mucosa, they can cause ulceration, perforation, and hemorrhage of or into the adjacent bowel. Patients can present with abdominal pain, vomiting, palpable mass, or acute GI hemorrhage. Intestinal duplications in the thorax (**neuroenteric cysts**) can manifest as respiratory distress. Duplications of the lower bowel can cause constipation or diarrhea or be associated with recurrent prolapse of the rectum.

The diagnosis is suspected on the basis of the history and physical examination. Radiologic studies such as barium studies, ultrasonography, CT, and MRI are helpful but usually nonspecific, demonstrating cystic structures or mass effects. Radioisotope technetium scanning can localize ectopic gastric mucosa. The treatment of duplications is surgical resection and management of associated defects.

331.2 Meckel Diverticulum and Other Remnants of the Omphalomesenteric Duct
Melissa Kennedy and Chris A. Liacouras

Meckel diverticulum is the most common congenital anomaly of the GI tract and is caused by the incomplete obliteration of the omphalomesenteric duct during the 7th wk of gestation. The omphalomesenteric duct connects the yolk sac to the gut in a developing embryo and provides nutrition until the placenta is established. Between the 5th and 7th wk of gestation, the duct attenuates and separates from the intestine. Just before this involution, the epithelium of the yolk sac develops a lining similar to that of the stomach. Partial or complete failure of involution of the omphalomesenteric duct results in various residual structures. Meckel diverticulum is the most common of these structures and is the most common congenital GI anomaly, occurring in 2-3% of all infants. A typical Meckel diverticulum is a 3-6 cm outpouching of the ileum along the antimesenteric border 50-75 cm (approximately 2 feet) from the ileocecal valve (Fig. 331-1). The distance from the ileocecal valve depends on the age of the patient. Meckel diverticulum has been conveniently referred to by the "rule of 2s," which explains the classic presentation of this congenital anomaly. Meckel diverticulum are found in approximately 2% of the general population, are usually located 2 feet proximal to the ileocecal valve and are approximately 2 inches in length, can contain 2 types of ectopic tissue (pancreatic or gastric), generally present before the age

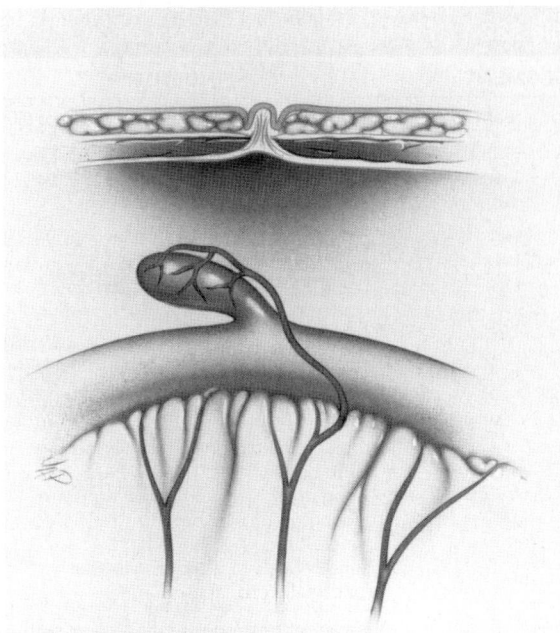

Figure 331-1 Typical Meckel diverticulum located on the antimesenteric border.

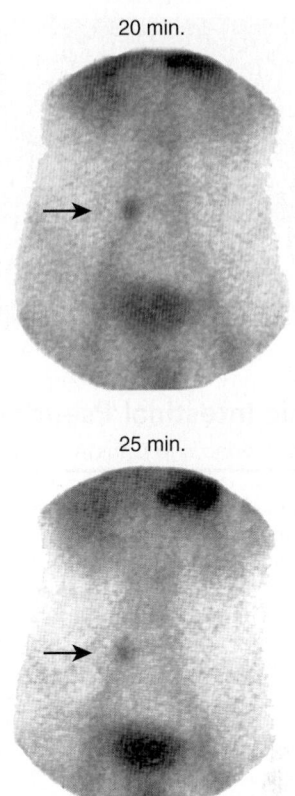

20 min.

25 min.

Figure 331-2 Meckel scan demonstrating accumulation of technetium in the stomach superior bladder (inferior) and in the acid-secreting mucosa of a Meckel diverticulum.

of 2 yr, and are found twice as commonly in females. Although intraabdominal in location, a rare presentation of a Meckel diverticulum is entrapment in an inguinal, umbilical, or femoral hernia (Littre hernia). Other omphalomesenteric duct remnants occur infrequently, including a persistently patent duct, a solid cord, or a cord with a central cyst or a diverticulum associated with a persistent cord between the diverticulum and the umbilicus.

CLINICAL MANIFESTATIONS
Symptoms of a Meckel diverticulum usually arise in the 1st or 2nd yr of life (average: 2.5 yr), but initial symptoms can occur in the 1st decade. The majority of symptomatic Meckel diverticula are lined by an ectopic mucosa, including an acid-secreting mucosa that causes intermittent painless rectal bleeding by ulceration of the adjacent normal ileal mucosa. This ectopic mucosa is most commonly of gastric origin, but it can also be pancreatic, jejunal, or a combination of these tissues. Unlike the upper duodenal mucosa, the acid is not neutralized by pancreatic bicarbonate.

The stool is typically described as brick colored or currant jelly colored. Bleeding can cause significant anemia but is usually self-limited because of contraction of the splanchnic vessels, as patients become hypovolemic. Bleeding from a Meckel diverticulum can also be less dramatic, with melanotic stools.

Less often, a Meckel diverticulum is associated with partial or complete bowel obstruction. The most common mechanism of obstruction occurs when the diverticulum acts as the lead point of an intussusception. The mean age of onset of obstruction is younger than that for patients presenting with bleeding. Obstruction can also result from intraperitoneal bands connecting residual omphalomesenteric duct remnants to the ileum and umbilicus. These bands cause obstruction by internal herniation or volvulus of the small bowel around the band. A Meckel diverticulum occasionally becomes inflamed (**diverticulitis**) and manifests similarly to acute appendicitis. These children are older, with a mean of 8 yr of age. Diverticulitis can lead to perforation and peritonitis.

DIAGNOSIS
The diagnosis of omphalomesenteric duct remnants depends on the clinical presentation. If an infant or child presents with significant

painless rectal bleeding, the presence of a Meckel diverticulum should be suspected because Meckel diverticulum accounts for 50% of all lower GI bleeds in children younger than 2 yr of age.

Confirmation of a Meckel diverticulum can be difficult. Plain abdominal radiographs are of no value, and routine barium studies rarely fill the diverticulum. The most sensitive study is a Meckel radionuclide scan, which is performed after intravenous infusion of technetium-99m pertechnetate. The mucus-secreting cells of the ectopic gastric mucosa take up pertechnetate, permitting visualization of the Meckel diverticulum (Fig. 331-2). The uptake can be enhanced with various agents, including cimetidine, ranitidine, glucagon, and pentagastrin. The sensitivity of the enhanced scan is approximately 85%, with a specificity of approximately 95%. A false-negative scan may be seen in anemic patients; although false-positive results are uncommon, they have been reported with intussusception, appendicitis, duplication cysts, arteriovenous malformations, and tumors. Other methods of detection include radiolabeled tagged red blood cell scan (the patient must be actively bleeding), abdominal ultrasound, superior mesenteric angiography, abdominal CT scan, or exploratory laparoscopy. In patients who present with intestinal obstruction or a picture of appendicitis with omphalomesenteric duct remnants, the diagnosis is rarely made before surgery.

The treatment of a symptomatic Meckel diverticulum is surgical excision. A diverticulectomy can be performed safely as either a laparoscopic or open procedure, although most continue to be performed as open procedures. There is significant debate regarding the proper management of an asymptomatic Meckel's diverticulum and whether excision vs observation is appropriate. However, the risk of serious complications does seem to exceed the operative risk in children younger than 8 yr old.

Bibliography is available at Expert Consult.

Chapter 332

Motility Disorders and Hirschsprung Disease

332.1 Chronic Intestinal Pseudoobstruction

Kristin N. Fiorino and Chris A. Liacouras

Chronic intestinal pseudoobstruction comprises a group of disorders characterized as a motility disorder with a primary defect of impaired peristalsis; symptoms are consistent with intestinal obstruction in the absence of mechanical obstruction. The natural history of pseudoobstruction is that of a primary progressive disorder, although there are occasional cases of secondary pseudoobstruction caused by conditions that can transiently or permanently alter bowel motility. The most common cause of acute pseudoobstruction is Ogilvie syndrome (acute pseudoobstruction of the colon). Pseudoobstruction represents a wide spectrum of pathologic disorders from abnormal myoelectric activity to abnormalities of the nerves (intestinal neuropathy) or musculature (intestinal myopathy) of the gut. The organs involved can include the entire gastrointestinal tract or be limited to certain components, although almost always include the small bowel. The distinctive pathologic abnormalities are considered together because of their clinical similarities.

Most congenital forms of pseudoobstruction occur sporadically, although autosomal dominant, autosomal recessive, X-linked, and familial patterns of inheritance have been identified. Patients with autosomal dominant forms of pseudoobstruction have variable expressions of the disease. Acquired pseudoobstruction can follow episodes of acute gastroenteritis, presumably resulting in injury to the myenteric plexus.

In congenital pseudoobstruction, abnormalities of the muscle or nerves can be demonstrated in the majority of cases. In myopathies, the smooth muscle is involved, in which the outer longitudinal muscle layer is replaced by fibrous material. The enteric nervous system is usually altered in neuropathies and may involve disorganized ganglia, hypoganglionosis, or hyperganglionosis. Abnormalities in the interstitial cells of Cajal, the intestinal pacemaker, are classified as mesenchymopathies. In others, mitochondrial defects have been identified. Genetic defects have been identified in the transcription factor *SOX10* and the DNA polymerase gamma gene (*POLG*) in mitochondriopathies.

CLINICAL MANIFESTATIONS

More than half the children with congenital pseudoobstruction experience symptoms in the 1st few mo of life. Two-thirds of the infants presenting in the 1st few days of life are born prematurely, and approximately 40% have malrotation of the intestine. In 75% of all affected children, symptoms occur in the 1st yr of life, while the remainder are usually symptomatic within the next several years. The most common symptoms are abdominal distention and vomiting, which are present in 75% of affected infants. Constipation, growth failure, and abdominal pain occur in approximately 60% of patients, and diarrhea in 30-40%. The symptoms wax and wane in the majority of the patients; poor nutrition, psychologic stress, and intercurrent illness tend to exacerbate symptoms. Urinary tract and bladder involvement occurs in 80% of children with myopathic pseudoobstruction and in 20% of those with neuropathic disease. Symptoms can manifest as recurrent urinary tract infection, megacystis, or obstructive symptoms.

Table 332-1	Findings in Pseudoobstruction
GI SEGMENT	**FINDINGS***
Esophageal motility	Abnormalities in approximately half of CIPO, although in some series up to 85% demonstrate abnormalities Decreased LES pressure Failure of LES relaxation Esophageal body: low-amplitude waves, poor propagation, tertiary waves, retrograde peristalsis, occasionally aperistalsis
Gastric emptying	May be delayed
EGG	Tachygastria or bradygastria may be seen
ADM	Postprandial antral hypomotility is seen and correlates with delayed gastric emptying Myopathic subtype: low-amplitude contractions, <10-20 mm Hg Neuropathic subtype: contractions are uncoordinated, disorganized Absence of fed response Fasting MMC is absent, or MMC is abnormally propagated
Colonic	Absence of gastrocolic reflex because there is no increased motility in response to a meal
ARM	Normal rectoanal inhibitory reflex

*Findings can vary according to the segment(s) of the GI tract that are involved.
ADM, Antroduodenal manometry; ARM, anorectal manometry; CIPO, chronic intestinal pseudoobstruction; EGG, electrogastrography; GI, gastrointestinal; LES, lower esophageal sphincter; MMC, migrating motor complex.
From Steffen R: Gastrointestinal motility. In Wyllie R, Hyams JS, Kay M, editors: Pediatric gastrointestinal and liver disease, ed 3, Philadelphia, 2006, WB Saunders, p. 66.

DIAGNOSIS

The diagnosis of pseudoobstruction is based on the presence of compatible symptoms in the absence of mechanical obstruction. Plain abdominal radiographs demonstrate air–fluid levels in the intestine. Neonates with evidence of obstruction at birth may have a microcolon. Contrast studies demonstrate slow passage of barium; water-soluble agents should be considered. Esophageal motility is abnormal in about half the patients. Antroduodenal (small intestinal) motility and gastric emptying studies have abnormal results if the upper gut is involved (Table 332-1). Manometric evidence of a normal migrating motor complex and postprandial activity should redirect the diagnostic evaluation. Anorectal motility is normal and differentiates pseudoobstruction from Hirschsprung disease. Full-thickness intestinal biopsy might show involvement of the muscle layers or abnormalities of the intrinsic intestinal nervous system.

The differential diagnosis is broad and includes such etiologies as Hirschsprung disease, mitochondrial neurogastrointestinal encephalomyopathy, other causes of mechanical obstruction, psychogenic constipation, neurogenic bladder, and superior mesenteric artery syndrome. Secondary causes of ileus or pseudoobstruction, such as hypothyroidism, opiates, scleroderma, Chagas disease, hypokalemia, diabetic neuropathy, amyloidosis, porphyria, angioneurotic edema, mitochondrial disorders, and radiation, must be excluded.

TREATMENT

Nutritional support is the mainstay of treatment for pseudoobstruction. Thirty percent to 50% of patients require partial or complete parenteral nutrition. Some patients can be treated with intermittent enteral supplementation, whereas others can maintain themselves on selective oral diets. Prokinetic drugs are generally used although studies have not shown definitive evidence of their efficacy. Isolated gastroparesis can follow episodes of viral gastroenteritis and spontaneously resolves, usually in 6-24 mo. Erythromycin, a motilin receptor agonist, and cisapride, a serotonin 5-HT₄ receptor agonist, can enhance gastric emptying and proximal small bowel motility and may be useful in this select group of patients. Metoclopramide, a prokinetic and antinausea agent, is effective in gastroparesis, although side effects, such as tardive dyskinesia, limit its use. Domperidone, an antidopaminergic agent, is a prokinetic agent available though the government in special circumstances. Pain management is difficult and requires a multidisciplinary approach.

Symptomatic small bowel bacterial overgrowth is usually treated with rotated non-absorbable oral antibiotics and/or probiotics. Bacterial overgrowth can be associated with steatorrhea and malabsorption. Octreotide, a long-acting somatostatin analog, has been used in low doses to treat small bowel bacterial overgrowth. Patients with acid peptic symptoms are generally treated with acid suppression. Many benefit from a gastrostomy and some benefit from decompressive enterostomies. Colectomy with ileorectal anastomosis is beneficial if the large bowel is the primary site of the motility abnormality. Bowel transplantation may benefit selected patients.

Bibliography is available at Expert Consult.

332.2 Mitochondrial Neurogastrointestinal Encephalomyopathy

Kristin N. Fiorino and Chris A. Liacouras

Mitochondrial neurogastrointestinal encephalomyopathy (MNGIE) is a multisystem autosomal recessive disease that initially presents with severe gastrointestinal disturbances; the neurologic manifestations usually occur later in the illness and may initially be subtle or asymptomatic.

MNGIE is caused by a mutation in the nuclear DNA *TYMP* gene encoding thymidine phosphorylase that results in abnormalities in intergenomic communication with resulting instability of mitochondrial DNA. There are at least 50 individual mutations with a poor genotype–phenotype correlation and varying manifestations within each family. Consanguinity is present in 30% of families.

MNGIE affects both males and females and is usually diagnosed in the 2nd and 3rd decade (average age: 18 yr; range: 5 mo-35 yr). Onset is usually around age 12 yr, but there is often a 5-10 yr delay in the diagnosis.

MNGIE initially presents with gastrointestinal symptoms. Severe intestinal dysmotility and gastroparesis is associated with early satiety, postprandial emesis, episodic pseudoobstruction, diarrhea, constipation and abdominal pain and cramping, which leads to significant cachexia. Because of the age of onset, emesis, early satiety, and cachexia patients are often misdiagnosed with an eating disorder.

Most often following the onset of gastrointestinal manifestations, ptosis, progressive external ophthalmoplegia, hearing loss and peripheral neuropathy may develop. The neuropathy is either demyelinating or a mixed axonal demyelinating type and manifests as weakness, decreased or absent deep tendon reflexes, and paresthesias. Leukoencephalopathy is initially asymptomatic and noted on MRI as patchy lesions predominantly in the cortex but also in the basal ganglia and brainstem. Eventually the central nervous system lesions become diffuse and confluent. A small number of patients develop cognitive impairment or dementia.

The diagnosis is suggested by the constellation of gastrointestinal and neurologic symptoms, lactic acidosis, ragged red fibers, and cytochrome C oxidase deficient fibers seen in most patients on muscle biopsy.

Treatment is focused on providing sufficient nutritional support and avoidance of infectious complications and of nutritional deficiencies. Stem cell transplantation has been successful in a small number of patients.

Overall the prognosis is poor with few surviving into the 4th or 5th decade.

Bibliography is available at Expert Consult.

332.3 Encopresis and Functional Constipation

Kristin N. Fiorino and Chris A. Liacouras

Constipation is defined as a delay or difficulty in defecation present for 2 wk or longer and significant enough to cause distress to the patient. Another approach to the definition is the Rome Criteria, outlined in Table 332-2. Functional constipation, also known as idiopathic constipation or fecal withholding, can usually be differentiated from constipation secondary to organic causes on the basis of a history and physical examination. Unlike anorectal malformations and Hirschsprung disease, functional constipation typically starts after the neonatal period. Usually, there is an intentional or subconscious withholding of stool. An acute episode usually precedes the chronic course. The acute episode may be a dietary change from human milk to cow's milk, secondary to the change in the protein and carbohydrate ratio or an allergy to cow's milk. The stool becomes firm, smaller, and difficult to pass, resulting in anal irritation and often an anal fissure. In toddlers, coercive or inappropriately early toilet training is a factor that can initiate a pattern of stool retention. In older children, retentive constipation can develop after entering a situation that makes stooling inconvenient such as school. Because the passage of bowel movements is painful, voluntary withholding of feces to avoid the painful stimulus develops.

CLINICAL MANIFESTATIONS
When children have the urge to defecate, typical behaviors include contracting the gluteal muscles by stiffening the legs while lying down, holding onto furniture while standing, or squatting quietly in corners, waiting for the call to stool to pass. The urge to defecate passes as the rectum accommodates to its contents. A vicious cycle of retention develops, as increasingly larger volumes of stool need to be expelled. Caregivers may misinterpret these activities as straining, but it is withholding behavior. There is often a history of blood in the stool noted with the passage of a large bowel movement. Findings suggestive of

Table 332-2	Chronic Constipation: Rome III Criteria

INFANTS AND TODDLERS
Must include 1 mo of **at least 2** of the following in infants up to 4 yr of age:
- ≤2 Defecations per week
- ≥1 Episode of incontinence after the acquisition of toilet training skills
- History of excessive stool retention
- History of painful or hard bowel movements
- Presence of a large fecal mass in the rectum
- History of a large-diameter stool that might obstruct the toilet
  Accompanying symptoms may include irritability, decreased appetite, and/or early satiety. The accompanying symptoms disappear immediately following passage of a large stool.

CHILDREN WITH A DEVELOPMENTAL AGE OF 4-18 YR
Must include **2 or more** of the following in a child with a developmental age of at least 4 yr with insufficient criteria for diagnosis of irritable bowel syndrome*:
- ≤2 Defecations per week
- ≥1 Episode of fecal incontinence per week
- History of retentive posturing or excessive volitional stool retention
- History of painful or hard bowel movements
- Presence of a large fecal mass in the rectum
- History of a large-diameter stool that might obstruct the toilet

*Criteria fulfilled at least once per week for at least 2 mo before diagnosis.
From Hyman P, Milla P. Benninga M, et al: Childhood functional gastrointestinal disorders: neonate/toddler, Gastroenterology 130:1519–1526, 2006; and Rasquin A, DiLorenzo C, Forbes D, et al: Childhood functional gastrointestinal disorders: child/adolescent, Gastroenterology 130:1527–1537, 2006.

underlying pathology include failure to thrive, weight loss, abdominal pain, vomiting, or persistent anal fissure or fistula.

In functional constipation, daytime encopresis is common. Encopresis is defined as voluntary or involuntary passage of feces into inappropriate places at least once a month for 3 consecutive months once a chronologic or developmental age of 4 yr has been reached. Encopresis is not diagnosed when the behavior is exclusively the result of the direct effects of a substance (e.g., laxatives) or a general medical condition (except through a mechanism involving constipation). Subtypes include retentive encopresis (with constipation and overflow incontinence) representing 65-95% of cases, and nonretentive encopresis (without constipation and overflow incontinence). **Nonretentive fecal incontinence** is defined as no evidence of fecal retention (impaction), ≥1 episodes per week in the previous 2 mo in a child at a developmental age >4 yr, defecation in places inappropriate to the social context and no evidence of anatomic, inflammatory, metabolic, endocrine, or neoplastic process that could explain the symptoms. Encopresis can persist from infancy onward (primary) or can appear after successful toilet training (secondary).

DIAGNOSIS

The physical examination often demonstrates a large volume of stool palpated in the suprapubic area; rectal examination demonstrates a dilated rectal vault filled with guaiac-negative stool. Children with encopresis often present with reports of underwear soiling, and many parents initially presume that diarrhea, rather than constipation, is the cause. In **retentive encopresis**, associated complaints of difficulty with defecation, abdominal or rectal pain, impaired appetite with poor growth, and urinary (day and/or night) incontinence are common. Children often have large bowel movements that obstruct the toilet. There may also be retentive posturing or recurrent urinary tract infections. **Nonretentive encopresis** is more likely to occur as a solitary symptom and have associated primary underlying psychological etiology. Children with encopresis can present with poor school performance and attendance that is triggered by the scorn and derision from schoolmates because of the child's offensive odor.

The presence of a hair tuft over the spine or spinal dimple, or failure to elicit a cremasteric reflex or anal wink suggests spinal pathology. A tethered cord is suggested by decreased or absent lower leg reflexes. Spinal cord lesions can occur with overlying skin anomalies. Urinary tract symptoms include recurrent urinary tract infection and enuresis. Children with no evidence of abnormalities on physical examination rarely require radiologic evaluation.

In refractory patients (intractable constipation), specialized testing should be considered to rule out conditions such as hypothyroidism, hypocalcemia, lead toxicity, celiac disease, and allergy testing. Colonic transit studies using radio-opaque markers or scintigraphy techniques may be useful. Selected children can benefit from MRI of the spine to identify an intraspinal process, motility studies to identify underlying myopathic or neuropathic bowel abnormalities, or a contrast enema to identify structural abnormalities. In patients with severe functional constipation, water-soluble contrast enema reveals the presence of a megarectosigmoid (Fig. 332-1). Anorectal motility studies can demonstrate a pattern of paradoxical contraction of the external anal sphincter during defecation, which can be treated by behavior modification and biofeedback. Colonic motility can guide therapy in refractory cases, demonstrating segmental problems that might require surgical intervention.

Complications of retentive encopresis include day and night urinary incontinence, urinary retention, urinary tract infection, megacystis, and rarely toxic megacolon.

TREATMENT

Therapy for functional constipation and encopresis includes patient education, relief of impaction, and softening of the stool. Caregivers must understand that soiling associated with overflow incontinence is

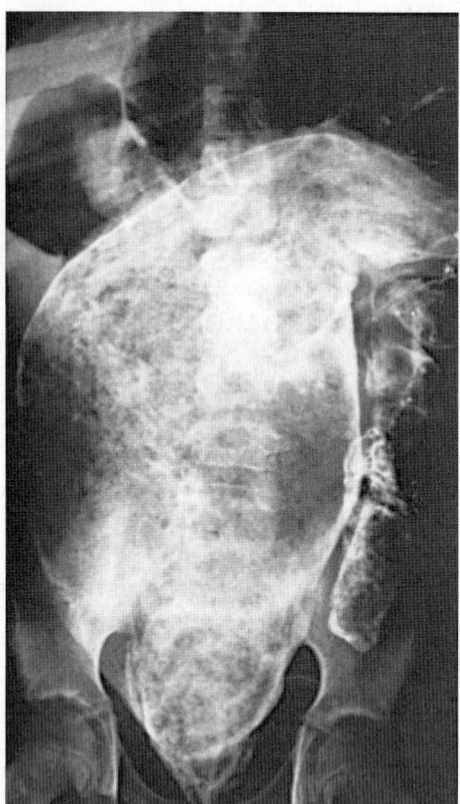

Figure 332-1 Barium enema in a 14 yr old boy with severe constipation. The enormous dilation of the rectum and distal colon is typical of acquired functional megacolon.

associated with loss of normal sensation and not a willful act. There needs to be a focus on adherence with regular postprandial toilet sitting and adoption of a balanced diet. In addition, caregivers should be instructed not to respond to soiling with retaliatory or punitive measures, because children are likely to become angry, ashamed, and resistant to intervention. From the outset, parents should be actively encouraged to reward the child for adherence to a healthy bowel regimen and to avoid power struggles.

If an impaction is present on the initial physical examination, an enema is usually required to clear the impaction while stool softeners are started as maintenance medications. Typical regimens include the use of polyethylene glycol preparations, lactulose, or mineral oil (Tables 332-3 and 332-4). Prolonged use of stimulants such as senna or bisacodyl should be avoided.

Compliance can wane, and failure of this standard treatment approach sometimes requires more intensive intervention. In cases where behavioral or psychiatric problems are evident, involvement of a psychologist or behavioral management (e.g., behavior programs and/or biofeedback). Maintenance therapy is generally continued until a regular bowel pattern has been established and the association of pain with the passage of stool is abolished.

For children with chronic diarrhea and/or irritable bowel syndrome where stress and anxiety play a major role, stress reduction and learning effective coping strategies can play an important role in responding to the encopresis. Relaxation training, stress inoculation, assertiveness training, and/or general stress management procedures can be helpful. Children with spinal problems can be successfully managed with low volumes of fluid through a cecostomy or sigmoid tube.

Bibliography is available at Expert Consult.

Table 332-3	Suggested Medications and Dosages for Disimpaction	
MEDICATION	**AGE**	**DOSAGE**
RAPID RECTAL DISIMPACTION		
Glycerin suppositories	Infants and toddlers	
Phosphate enema	<1 yr	60 mL
	>1 yr	6 mL/kg bodyweight, up to 135 mL twice
Milk of molasses enema	Older children	(1:1 milk:molasses) 200-600 mL
SLOW ORAL DISIMPACTION IN OLDER CHILDREN		
Over 2-3 Days		
Polyethylene glycol with electrolytes		25 mL/kg bodyweight/hr, up to 1000 mL/hr until clear fluid comes from the anus
Over 5-7 Days		
Polyethylene without electrolytes		1.5 g/kg bodyweight/day for 3 days
Milk of magnesia		2 mL/kg bodyweight twice/day for 7 days
Mineral oil		3 mL/kg bodyweight twice/day for 7 days
Lactulose or sorbitol		2 mL/kg bodyweight twice/day for 7 days

From Loening-Baucke V: Functional constipation with encopresis. In Wyllie R, Hyams JS, Kay M, editors: Pediatric gastrointestinal and liver disease, ed 3, Philadelphia, 2006, WB Saunders, p 183.

Table 332-4	Suggested Medications and Dosages for Maintenance Therapy of Constipation	
MEDICATION	**AGE**	**DOSE**
FOR LONG-TERM TREATMENT (YEARS)		
Milk of magnesia	>1 mo	1-3 mL/kg bodyweight/day, divided into 1-2 doses
Mineral oil	>12 mo	1-3 mL/kg bodyweight/day, divided into 1-2 doses
Lactulose or sorbitol	>1 mo	1-3 mL/kg bodyweight/day, divided into 1-2 doses
Polyethylene glycol 3350 (MiraLAX)	>1 mo	0.7 g/kg bodyweight/day, divided into 1-2 doses
FOR SHORT-TERM TREATMENT (MONTHS)		
Senna (Senokot) syrup, tablets	1-5 yr	5 mL (1 tablet) with breakfast, max 15 mL daily
	5-15 yr	2 tablets with breakfast, maximum 3 tablets daily
Glycerin enemas	>10 yr	20-30 mL/day (½ glycerin and ½ normal saline)
Bisacodyl suppositories	>10 yr	10 mg daily

From Loening-Baucke V: Functional constipation with encopresis. In Wyllie R, Hyams JS, Kay M, editors: Pediatric gastrointestinal and liver disease, ed 3, Philadelphia, 2006, WB Saunders, p. 185.

332.4 Congenital Aganglionic Megacolon (Hirschsprung Disease)
Kristin N. Fiorino and Chris A. Liacouras

Hirschsprung disease, or congenital aganglionic megacolon, is a developmental disorder (neurocristopathy) of the enteric nervous system, characterized by the absence of ganglion cells in the submucosal and myenteric plexus. It is the most common cause of lower intestinal obstruction in neonates, with an overall incidence of 1 in 5,000 live births. The male:female ratio for Hirschsprung disease is 4:1 for short-segment disease, and approximately 2:1 with total colonic aganglionosis. Prematurity is uncommon.

There is an increased familial incidence in long-segment disease. Hirschsprung disease may be associated with other congenital defects, including trisomy 21, Joubert syndrome, Goldberg-Shprintzen syndrome, Smith-Lemli-Opitz syndrome, Shah-Waardenburg syndrome, cartilage-hair hypoplasia, multiple endocrine neoplasm 2 syndrome, neurofibromatosis, neuroblastoma, congenital hypoventilation (Ondine's curse), and urogenital or cardiovascular abnormalities. Hirschsprung disease has been seen in association with microcephaly, mental retardation, abnormal facies, autism, cleft palate, hydrocephalus, and micrognathia.

PATHOLOGY
Hirschsprung disease is the result of an absence of ganglion cells in the bowel wall, extending proximally and continuously from the anus for a variable distance. The absence of neural innervation is a consequence of an arrest of neuroblast migration from the proximal to distal bowel. Without the myenteric and submucosal plexus, there is inadequate relaxation of the bowel wall and bowel wall hypertonicity, which can lead to intestinal obstruction.

Hirschsprung disease is usually sporadic, although dominant and recessive patterns of inheritance have been demonstrated in family groups. Genetic defects have been identified in multiple genes that encode proteins of the RET signaling pathway *(RET, GDNF,* and *NTN)* and involved in the endothelin (EDN) type B receptor pathway *(EDNRB, EDN3,* and *EVE-1).* Syndromic forms of Hirschsprung disease have been associated with the *L1CAM, SOX10,* and *ZFHX1B* (formerly *SIP1)* genes.

The aganglionic segment is limited to the rectosigmoid in 80% of patients. Approximately 10-15% of patients have long-segment disease, defined as disease proximal to the sigmoid colon. Total bowel aganglionosis is rare and accounts for approximately 5% of cases. Observed histologically is an absence of Meissner's and Auerbach's plexuses and hypertrophied nerve bundles with high concentrations of acetylcholinesterase between the muscular layers and in the submucosa.

CLINICAL MANIFESTATIONS
Hirschsprung disease is usually diagnosed in the neonatal period secondary to a distended abdomen, failure to pass meconium, and/or bilious emesis or aspirates with feeding intolerance. In 99% of healthy full-term infants, meconium is passed within 48 hr of birth. Hirschsprung disease should be suspected in any full-term infant (the disease is unusual in preterm infants) with delayed passage of stool. Some neonates pass meconium normally but subsequently present with a history of chronic constipation. Failure to thrive with hypoproteinemia from protein-losing enteropathy is a less common presentation because Hirschsprung disease is usually recognized early in the course of the illness. Breastfed infants might not suffer disease as severe as formula-fed infants.

Failure to pass stool leads to dilation of the proximal bowel and abdominal distention. As the bowel dilates, intraluminal pressure

Table 332-5	Distinguishing Features of Hirschsprung Disease and Functional Constipation	
VARIABLE	**FUNCTIONAL**	**HIRSCHSPRUNG DISEASE**
HISTORY		
Onset of constipation	After 2 yr of age	At birth
Encopresis	Common	Very rare
Failure to thrive	Uncommon	Possible
Enterocolitis	None	Possible
Forced bowel training	Usual	None
EXAMINATION		
Abdominal distention	Uncommon	Common
Poor weight gain	Rare	Common
Rectum	Filled with stool	Empty
Rectal examination	Stool in rectum	Explosive passage of stool
Malnutrition	None	Possible
INVESTIGATIONS		
Anorectal manometry	Relaxation of internal anal sphincter	Failure of internal anal sphincter relaxation
Rectal biopsy	Normal	No ganglion cells, increased acetylcholinesterase staining
Barium enema	Massive amounts of stool, no transition zone	Transition zone, delayed evacuation (>24 hr)

From Imseis E, Gariepy C: Hirschsprung disease. In Walker WA, Goulet OJ, Kleinman RE et al, editors: Pediatric gastrointestinal disease, ed 4, Hamilton, Ontario, 2004, BC Decker, p. 1035.

increases, resulting in decreased blood flow and deterioration of the mucosal barrier. Stasis allows proliferation of bacteria, which can lead to enterocolitis (*Clostridium difficile, Staphylococcus aureus,* anaerobes, coliforms) with associated diarrhea, abdominal tenderness, sepsis and signs of bowel obstruction. Early recognition of Hirschsprung disease before the onset of enterocolitis is essential in reducing morbidity and mortality.

Hirschsprung disease in older patients must be distinguished from other causes of abdominal distention and chronic constipation (Table 332-5 and Fig. 332-2). The history often reveals constipation starting in infancy that has responded poorly to medical management. Fecal incontinence, fecal urgency, and stool-withholding behaviors are usually not present. The abdomen is tympanitic and distended, with a large fecal mass palpable in the left lower abdomen. Rectal examination demonstrates a normally placed anus that easily allows entry of the finger but feels snug. The rectum is usually empty of feces, and when the finger is removed, there may be an explosive discharge of foul-smelling feces and gas. The stools, when passed, can consist of small pellets, be ribbon-like, or have a fluid consistency, unlike the large stools seen in patients with functional constipation. Intermittent attacks of intestinal obstruction from retained feces may be associated with pain and fever. Urinary retention with enlarged balder or hydronephrosis can occur secondary to urinary compression.

In neonates, Hirschsprung disease must be differentiated from meconium plug syndrome, meconium ileus, and intestinal atresia. In older patients, the **Currarino triad** must be considered, which includes anorectal malformations (ectopic anus, anal stenosis, imperforate anus), sacral bone anomalies (hypoplasia, poor segmentation), and presacral anomaly (anterior meningoceles, teratoma, cyst).

DIAGNOSIS

Rectal suction biopsy is the gold standard for diagnosing Hirschsprung disease. The biopsy material should contain an adequate amount of submucosa to evaluate for the presence of ganglion cells. To avoid obtaining biopsies in the normal area of hypoganglionosis, which ranges from 3-17 mm in length, the suction rectal biopsy should be obtained no closer than 2 cm above the dentate line. The biopsy specimen should be stained for acetylcholinesterase to facilitate interpretation. Patients with aganglionosis demonstrate a large number of hypertrophied nerve bundles that stain positively for acetylcholinesterase with an absence of ganglion cells. Calretinin staining may provide a diagnosis of Hirschsprung disease when acetylcholinesterase staining may not be sufficient.

Anorectal manometry evaluates the internal anal sphincter while a balloon is distended in the rectum. In healthy individuals, rectal

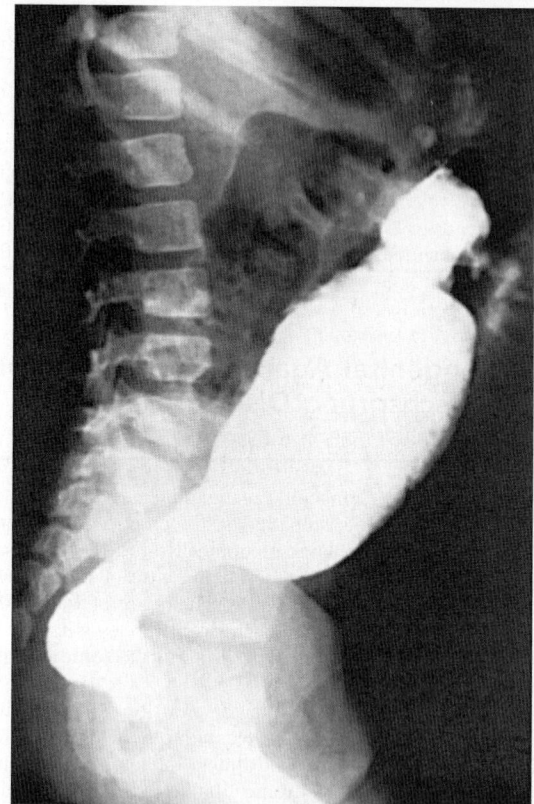

Figure 332-2 Lateral view of a barium enema in a 3 yr old girl with Hirschsprung disease. The aganglionic distal segment is narrow, with distended normal ganglionic bowel above it.

distention initiates relaxation of the internal anal sphincter in response to rectal distention. In patients with Hirschsprung disease, the internal anal sphincter fails to relax in response to rectal distention. Although the sensitivity and specificity can vary widely, in experienced hands, the test can be quite sensitive. The test, however, can be technically difficult to perform in young infants. A normal response in the course of manometric evaluation precludes a diagnosis of Hirschsprung disease; an equivocal or paradoxical response requires a repeat motility or rectal biopsy.

An unprepared contrast enema is most likely to aid in the diagnosis in children older than 1 mo of age because the proximal ganglionic segment might not be significantly dilated in the 1st few wk of life. Classic findings are based on the presence of an abrupt narrow transition zone between the normal dilated proximal colon and a smaller-caliber obstructed distal aganglionic segment. In the absence of this finding, it is imperative to compare the diameter of the rectum to that of the sigmoid colon, because a rectal diameter that is the same as or smaller than the sigmoid colon suggests Hirschsprung disease. Radiologic evaluation should be performed without preparation to prevent transient dilation of the aganglionic segment. As many as 10% of newborns with Hirschsprung disease have a normal contrast study. Twenty-four-hour delayed films are helpful in showing retained contrast (see Fig. 332-2). If significant barium is still present in the colon, it increases the suspicion of Hirschsprung disease even if a transition zone is not identified. Barium enema examination is useful in determining the extent of aganglionosis before surgery and in evaluating other diseases that manifest as lower bowel obstruction in a neonate. Full-thickness rectal biopsies can be performed at the time of surgery to confirm the diagnosis and level of involvement.

TREATMENT

Once the diagnosis is established, the definitive treatment is operative intervention. Previously, a temporary ostomy was placed and definitive surgery was delayed until the child was older. Currently, many infants undergo a primary pull-through procedure except if there is associated enterocolitis or other complications, when a decompressing ostomy is usually required.

There are 3 basic surgical options. The first successful surgical procedure, described by Swenson, was to excise the aganglionic segment and anastomose the normal proximal bowel to the rectum 1-2 cm above the dentate line. The operation is technically difficult and led to the development of 2 other procedures. Duhamel described a procedure to create a neorectum, bringing down normally innervated bowel behind the aganglionic rectum. The neorectum created in this procedure has an anterior aganglionic segment with normal sensation and a posterior ganglionic segment with normal propulsion. The endorectal pull-through procedure described by Soave involves stripping the mucosa from the aganglionic rectum and bringing normally innervated colon through the residual muscular cuff, thus bypassing the abnormal bowel from within. Advances in techniques have led to successful laparoscopic single-stage endorectal pull-through procedures, which are the treatment of choice.

In ultrashort-segment Hirschsprung disease, also known as anal achalasia, the aganglionic segment is limited to the internal sphincter. The clinical symptoms are similar to those of children with functional constipation. Ganglion cells are present on rectal suction biopsy, but the anorectal manometry is abnormal, with failure of relaxation of the internal anal sphincter in response to rectal distention. Current treatment, although controversial, includes anal botulism injection to relax the anal sphincter and anorectal myectomy if indicated.

Long-segment Hirschsprung disease involving the entire colon and, at times, part of the small bowel presents a difficult problem. Anorectal manometry and rectal suction biopsy demonstrate findings of Hirschsprung disease, but radiologic studies are difficult to interpret because a colonic transition zone cannot be identified. The extent of aganglionosis can be determined accurately by biopsy at the time of laparotomy. When the entire colon is aganglionic, often together with a length of terminal ileum, ileal-anal anastomosis is the treatment of choice, preserving part of the aganglionic colon to facilitate water absorption, which helps the stools to become firm.

The prognosis of surgically treated Hirschsprung disease is generally satisfactory; the great majority of patients achieve fecal continence. Long-term postoperative problems include constipation, recurrent enterocolitis, stricture, prolapse, perianal abscesses, and fecal soiling. Some children require myectomy or a redo pull-through procedure.

Bibliography is available at Expert Consult.

332.5 Intestinal Neuronal Dysplasia
Kristin N. Fiorino and Chris A. Liacouras

Intestinal neuronal dysplasia (IND) describes different quantitative (hypo- or hyperganglionosis) and qualitative (immature or heterotropic ganglion cells) abnormalities of the myenteric and/or submucosal plexus. The typical histology is that of hyperganglionosis and giant ganglia. Type A occurs very rarely and is characterized by congenital aplasia or hypoplasia of the sympathetic innervation. Patients present early in the neonatal period with episodes of intestinal obstruction, diarrhea, and bloody stools. Type B, which accounts for more than 95% of cases, is characterized by malformation of the parasympathetic submucous and myenteric plexus with giant ganglia and thickened nerve fibers, increased acetylcholinesterase staining, and isolated ganglion cells in the lamina propria. IND type B mimics Hirschsprung disease, and patients present with chronic constipation.

Clinical manifestations include abdominal distention, constipation, and enterocolitis. Various lengths of bowel may be affected from segmental to the entire intestinal tract. IND has been observed in an isolated form and proximal to an aganglionic segment. Other intra- and extraintestinal manifestations are present in patients with IND. It has been reported in all age groups, most commonly in infancy, but is also seen in adults who have had constipation not dating back to childhood.

Associated diseases and conditions include Hirschsprung disease, prematurity, small left colon syndrome, and meconium plug syndrome. Studies have identified a deficiency in substance P in patients with IND. No mutations in the coding regions of the *RET*, *GDNF*, *EDNRB*, or *EDN3* genes have been identified.

Management includes that for functional constipation and, if unsuccessful, surgery is indicated.

Bibliography is available at Expert Consult.

332.6 Superior Mesenteric Artery Syndrome (Wilkie Syndrome, Cast Syndrome, Arteriomesenteric Duodenal Compression Syndrome)
Andrew Chu and Chris A. Liacouras

Superior mesenteric artery syndrome results from compression of the 3rd duodenal segment by the artery against the aorta. Malnutrition or catabolic states may cause mesenteric fat depletion, which collapses the duodenum within a narrowed aortomesenteric angle. Other etiologies include extraabdominal compression (e.g., body cast) and mesenteric tension, as can occur from ileoanal pouch anastomosis.

Symptoms include intermittent epigastric pain, anorexia, nausea, and vomiting. Risk factors include thin body habitus, prolonged bed rest, abdominal surgery, and exaggerated lumbar lordosis. Onset can be within weeks of a trigger, but some patients have chronic symptoms that evade diagnosis. A classic example is an underweight adolescent who begins vomiting 1-2 wk following scoliosis surgery. Recognition may be delayed in the context of an eating disorder.

The diagnosis is established radiologically by demonstrating a duodenal cutoff just right of midline along with proximal duodenal dilation, with or without gastric dilation. Although the upper gastrointestinal series remains a mainstay, modalities including CT, MR angiography, or ultrasound may be more appropriate if there is concern for other etiologies like malignancy. Upper endoscopy should be considered to rule out intraluminal pathology.

Treatment focuses on obstructive relief, nutritional rehabilitation, and correction of associated fluid and electrolyte abnormalities. Lateral or prone positioning can shift the duodenum away from obstructing structures and allow resumption of oral intake. In such cases, prokinetic agents (e.g., erythromycin) may be helpful. If repositioning is unsuccessful, patients require nasojejunal enteral nutrition past the obstruction or parenteral nutrition if this is not tolerated. Patients with refractory courses may require surgery to bypass the obstruction.

Bibliography is available at Expert Consult.

Chapter 333
Ileus, Adhesions, Intussusception, and Closed-Loop Obstructions

333.1 Ileus
Andrew Chu and Chris A. Liacouras

Ileus is the failure of intestinal peristalsis caused by loss of coordinated gut motility without evidence of mechanical obstruction. In children, it is most often associated with abdominal surgery or infection (gastroenteritis, pneumonia, peritonitis). Ileus also accompanies metabolic abnormalities (e.g., uremia, hypokalemia, hypercalcemia, hypermagnesemia, acidosis) or administration of certain drugs, such as opiates, vincristine, and antimotility agents such as loperamide when used during gastroenteritis.

Ileus manifests with nausea, vomiting, feeding intolerance, abdominal distention with associated pain, and delayed passage of stool and bowel gas. Bowel sounds are minimal or absent, in contrast to early mechanical obstruction, when they are hyperactive. Abdominal radiographs demonstrate multiple air–fluid levels throughout the abdomen. Serial radiographs usually do not show progressive distention as they do in mechanical obstruction. Contrast radiographs, if performed, demonstrate slow movement of barium through a patent lumen. Ileus after abdominal surgery generally resolves in within 72 hr.

Treatment involves correcting the underlying abnormality, supportive care of comorbidities, and mitigation of iatrogenic contributions. Electrolyte abnormalities should be identified and corrected, and narcotic agents, when used, should be weaned as tolerated. Nasogastric decompression can relieve recurrent vomiting or abdominal distention associated with pain; resultant fluid losses should be corrected with isotonic crystalloid solution. Prokinetic agents such as erythromycin are not routinely recommended. Selective peripheral opioid antagonists such as methylnaltrexone hold promise in decreasing postoperative ileus, but pediatric data are lacking.

Bibliography is available at Expert Consult.

333.2 Adhesions
Andrew Chu and Chris A. Liacouras

Adhesions are fibrous tissue bands that result from peritoneal injury. They can constrict hollow organs and are a major cause of postoperative small bowel obstruction. Most remain asymptomatic, but problems can arise anytime after the 2nd postoperative week to years after surgery, regardless of surgical extent. In one study, the 5-year readmission risk because of adhesions varied by operative region (2.1% for colon to 9.2% for ileum) and procedure (0.3% for appendectomy to 25% for ileostomy formation/closure). The overall risk was 5.3% excluding appendectomy and 1.1% when appendectomy was included.

The diagnosis is suspected in patients with abdominal pain, constipation, emesis, and a history of intraperitoneal surgery. Nausea and vomiting quickly follow onset of pain. Initially, bowel sounds are hyperactive, and the abdomen is flat. Subsequently, bowel sounds disappear, and bowel dilation can cause abdominal distention. Fever and leukocytosis suggest bowel necrosis and peritonitis. Plain radiographs demonstrate obstructive features, and a CT scan or contrast studies may be needed to define the etiology.

Management includes nasogastric decompression, intravenous fluid resuscitation, and broad-spectrum antibiotics in preparation for surgery. Nonoperative intervention is contraindicated unless a patient is stable with obvious clinical improvement. In children with repeated obstruction, fibrin-glued plication of adjacent small bowel loops can reduce the risk of recurrent problems. Long-term complications include female infertility, failure to thrive, and chronic abdominal and/or pelvic pain.

Bibliography is available at Expert Consult.

333.3 Intussusception
Melissa Kennedy and Chris A. Liacouras

Intussusception occurs when a portion of the alimentary tract is telescoped into an adjacent segment. It is the most common cause of intestinal obstruction between 5 mo and 3 yr of age and the most common abdominal emergency in children younger than 2 yr. Sixty percent of patients are younger than 1 yr of age, and 80% of the cases occur before age 24 mo; it is rare in neonates. The incidence varies from 1 to 4 per 1,000 live births. The male : female ratio is 3 : 1. Many small bowel–small bowel and a few small bowel–colonic intussusceptions reduce spontaneously; if left untreated, ileal–colonic intussusception may lead to intestinal infarction, perforation, peritonitis, and death.

ETIOLOGY AND EPIDEMIOLOGY
Approximately 90% of cases of intussusception in children are idiopathic. The seasonal incidence has peaks in fall and winter. Correlation with prior or concurrent respiratory adenovirus (type C) infection has been noted, and the condition can complicate otitis media, gastroenteritis, Henoch-Schönlein purpura, or other upper respiratory tract infections. The risk of intussusception was increased in infants 1 yr of age or younger after receiving a tetravalent rhesus-human reassortant rotavirus vaccine within 2 wk of immunization. The Advisory Committee on Immunization Practices no longer recommends this vaccine, and it is no longer available. Although rotavirus produces an enterotoxin, there is no association between wild-type human rotavirus and intussusception. The currently approved rotavirus vaccines are associated with a slightly increased risk of intussusception.

It is postulated that gastrointestinal infection or the introduction of new food proteins results in swollen Peyer patches in the terminal ileum. Lymphoid nodular hyperplasia is another related risk factor. Prominent mounds of lymph tissue lead to mucosal prolapse of the ileum into the colon, thus causing an intussusception. In 2-8% of patients, **recognizable lead points** for the intussusception are found, such as a Meckel diverticulum, intestinal polyp, neurofibroma, intestinal duplication cysts, inverted appendix stump, leiomyomas, hamartomas, ectopic pancreatic tissue, anastomotic suture line, enterostomy tube, posttransplant lymphoproliferative disease, hemangioma, or malignant conditions such as lymphoma, or Kaposi sarcoma. Lead points are more common in children older than 2 yr of age; the older the child, the higher the risk of a lead point. In adults, lead points are present in 90%. Intussusception can complicate mucosal hemorrhage, as in Henoch-Schönlein purpura, idiopathic thrombocytopenic purpura, or hemophilia. Cystic fibrosis, celiac disease, and Crohn disease are other risk factors. Postoperative intussusception is ileoileal and usually occurs within several days of an abdominal operation. Intrauterine intussusception may be associated with the development of intestinal atresia. Intussusception in premature infants is rare.

Ileal–ileal intussusception may be more common than previously believed, is often idiopathic or associated with Henoch-Schönlein purpura, and usually resolves spontaneously.

PATHOLOGY

Intussusceptions are most often ileocolic, less commonly cecocolic, and occasionally ileal. Very rarely, the appendix forms the apex of an intussusception. The upper portion of bowel, the **intussusceptum,** invaginates into the lower, the **intussuscipiens,** pulling its mesentery along with it into the enveloping loop. Constriction of the mesentery obstructs venous return; engorgement of the intussusceptum follows, with edema, and bleeding from the mucosa leads to a bloody stool, sometimes containing mucus. The apex of the intussusception can extend into the transverse, descending, or sigmoid colon, even to and through the anus in neglected cases. This presentation must be distinguished from rectal prolapse. Most intussusceptions do not strangulate the bowel within the 1st 24 hr but can eventuate in intestinal gangrene and shock.

CLINICAL MANIFESTATIONS

In typical cases, there is sudden onset, in a previously well child, of severe paroxysmal colicky pain that recurs at frequent intervals and is accompanied by straining efforts with legs and knees flexed and loud cries. The infant may initially be comfortable and play normally between the paroxysms of pain; but if the intussusception is not reduced, the infant becomes progressively weaker and lethargic. At times, the **lethargy** is disproportionate to the abdominal signs. Eventually, a shock-like state, with fever and peritonitis, can develop. The pulse becomes weak and thready, the respirations become shallow and grunting, and the pain may be manifested only by moaning sounds. Vomiting occurs in most cases and is usually more frequent in the early phase. In the later phase, the vomitus becomes bile stained. Stools of normal appearance may be evacuated in the 1st few hr of symptoms. After this time, fecal excretions are small or more often do not occur, and little or no flatus is passed. Blood is generally passed in the 1st 12 hr, but at times not for 1-2 days, and infrequently not at all; 60% of infants pass a stool containing red blood and mucus, the currant jelly stool. Some patients have only irritability and alternating or progressive lethargy. The classic triad of pain, a palpable sausage-shaped abdominal mass, and bloody or currant jelly stool is seen in <30% of patients with intussusception. The combination of paroxysmal pain, vomiting and a palpable abdominal mass has a positive predictive value of >90%; the presence of rectal bleeding increases this to approximately 100%.

Palpation of the abdomen usually reveals a slightly tender sausage-shaped mass, sometimes ill defined, which might increase in size and firmness during a paroxysm of pain and is most often in the right upper abdomen, with its long axis cephalocaudal. If it is felt in the epigastrium, the long axis is transverse. Approximately 30% of patients do not have a palpable mass. The presence of bloody mucus on rectal examination supports the diagnosis of intussusception. Abdominal distention and tenderness develop as intestinal obstruction becomes more acute. On rare occasions, the advancing intestine prolapses through the anus. *This prolapse can be distinguished from prolapse of the rectum by the separation between the protruding intestine and the rectal wall, which does not exist in prolapse of the rectum.*

Ileoileal intussusception in children younger than 2 yr can have a less-typical clinical picture, the symptoms and signs being chiefly those of small intestinal obstruction; these often resolve without treatment. **Recurrent intussusception** is noted in 5-8% and is more common after hydrostatic than surgical reduction. Chronic intussusception, in which the symptoms exist in milder form at recurrent intervals, is more likely to occur with or after acute enteritis and can arise in older children as well as in infants.

DIAGNOSIS

When the clinical history and physical findings suggest intussusception, an ultrasound is typically performed. A plain abdominal radiograph might show a density in the area of the intussusception. Screening

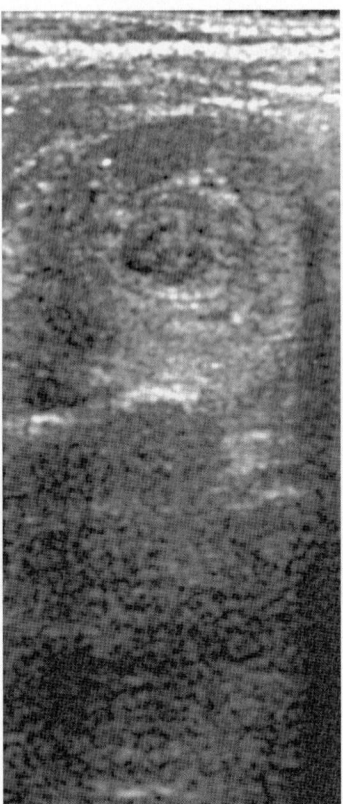

Figure 333-1 Transverse image of an ileocolic intussusception. Note the loops within the loops of bowel.

ultrasounds for suspected intussusception increases the yield of diagnostic or therapeutic enemas and reduces unnecessary radiation exposure in children with negative ultrasound examinations. The diagnostic findings of intussusception on ultrasound include a tubular mass in longitudinal views and a doughnut or target appearance in transverse images (Fig. 333-1). Ultrasound has a sensitivity of approximately 98-100% and a specificity of approximately 98% in diagnosing intussusception. Air, hydrostatic (saline), and, less often, water-soluble contrast enemas have replaced barium examinations. Contrast enemas demonstrate a filling defect or cupping in the head of the contrast media where its advance is obstructed by the intussusceptum (Fig. 333-2). A central linear column of contrast media may be visible in the compressed lumen of the intussusceptum, and a thin rim of contrast may be seen trapped around the invaginating intestine in the folds of mucosa within the intussuscipiens (coiled-spring sign), especially after evacuation. Retrogression of the intussusceptum under pressure and visualized on x-ray or ultrasound documents successful reduction. Air reduction is associated with fewer complications and lower radiation exposure than traditional contrast hydrostatic techniques.

DIFFERENTIAL DIAGNOSIS

It may be particularly difficult to diagnose intussusception in a child who already has gastroenteritis; a change in the pattern of illness, in the character of pain, or in the nature of vomiting or the onset of rectal bleeding should alert the physician. The bloody stools and abdominal cramps that accompany enterocolitis can usually be differentiated from intussusception because in enterocolitis the pain is less severe and less regular, there is diarrhea, and the infant is recognizably ill between pains. Bleeding from a Meckel diverticulum is usually painless. Joint symptoms, purpura, or hematuria usually but not invariably accompany the intestinal hemorrhage of Henoch-Schönlein purpura. Because intussusception can be a complication of this disorder, ultrasonography may be needed to distinguish the conditions.

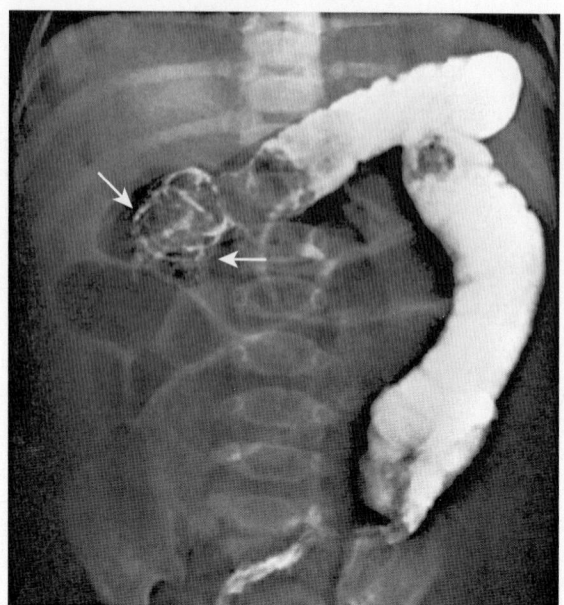

Figure 333-2 Intussusception in an infant. The obstruction is evident in the proximal transverse colon. Contrast material between the intussusceptum and the intussuscipiens is responsible for the coiled-spring appearance.

It is important in patients with cystic fibrosis to distinguish intussusception from distal intestinal obstruction syndrome. Distal intestinal obstruction syndrome requires antegrade treatment, which would be harmful if there was an intussusception.

TREATMENT

Reduction of an acute intussusception is an emergency procedure and should be performed immediately after diagnosis in preparation for possible surgery. In patients with prolonged intussusception and signs of shock, peritoneal irritation, intestinal perforation, or pneumatosis intestinalis, hydrostatic reduction should not be attempted.

The success rate of radiologic hydrostatic reduction under fluoroscopic or ultrasonic guidance is approximately 80-95% in patients with ileocolic intussusception. Spontaneous reduction of intussusception occurs in approximately 4-10% of patients. Bowel perforations occur in 0.5-2.5% of attempted barium and hydrostatic (saline) reductions. The perforation rate with air reduction is 0.1-0.2%. Surgical reduction is indicated in the presence of refractory shock, suspected bowel necrosis or perforation, peritonitis, and multiple recurrences (suspected lead point).

An **ileoileal intussusception** is best demonstrated by abdominal ultrasonography. Reduction by instillation of contrast agents, saline, or air might not be possible. Such intussusceptions can develop insidiously after bowel surgery and require reoperation if they do not spontaneously reduce. Ileoileal disease is common with Henoch-Schönlein purpura and other unidentifiable disorders and usually resolves without the need for any specific treatment. If manual operative reduction is impossible or the bowel is not viable, resection of the intussusception is necessary, with end-to-end anastomosis.

PROGNOSIS

Untreated intussusception in infants is usually fatal; the chances of recovery are directly related to the duration of intussusception before reduction. Most infants recover if the intussusception is reduced in the 1st 24 hr, but the mortality rate rises rapidly after this time, especially after the 2nd day. Spontaneous reduction during preparation for operation is not uncommon.

The **recurrence rate** after reduction of intussusceptions is approximately 10%, and after surgical reduction it is 2-5%; none has recurred after surgical resection. Most recurrences occur within 72 hr of reduction. Corticosteroids may reduce the frequency of recurrent intussusception. Repeated reducible episodes caused by lymphonodular hyperplasia may respond to treatment of identifiable food allergies if present. A single recurrence of intussusception can usually be reduced radiologically. In patients with multiple ileal–colonic recurrences, a lead point should be suspected and laparoscopic surgery considered. It is unlikely that an intussusception caused by a lesion such as lymphosarcoma, polyp, or Meckel diverticulum will be successfully reduced by radiologic intervention. With adequate surgical management, laparoscopic reduction carries a very low mortality.

Bibliography is available at Expert Consult.

333.4 Closed-Loop Obstructions
Andrew Chu and Chris A. Liacouras

Closed-loop obstructions (i.e., **internal hernia**) result from bowel loops that enter windows created by mesenteric defects or adhesions and become trapped. Vascular engorgement of the strangulated bowel results in intestinal ischemia and necrosis unless promptly relieved. Prior abdominal surgery is an important risk factor. Symptoms include abdominal pain, distention, and bilious emesis. Symptoms can be intermittent if the herniated bowel slides in and out of the defect. Peritoneal signs suggest ischemic bowel. Plain radiographs demonstrate signs of small bowel obstruction or free air if the bowel has perforated. CT scan can identify and delineate internal hernias. Supportive management includes intravenous fluids, antibiotics, and nasogastric decompression. Prompt surgical relief of the obstruction is indicated to prevent bowel necrosis.

Bibliography is available at Expert Consult.

Chapter 334
Foreign Bodies and Bezoars

334.1 Foreign Bodies in the Stomach and Intestine
Judith R. Kelsen and Chris A. Liacouras

Once in the stomach, 95% of all ingested objects pass without difficulty through the remainder of the gastrointestinal tract. Perforation after ingestion of a foreign body is estimated to be <1% of all objects ingested. Perforation tends to occur in areas of physiologic sphincters (pylorus, ileocecal valve), acute angulation (duodenal sweep), congenital gut malformations (webs, diaphragms, diverticula), or areas of previous bowel surgery.

Most patients who ingest foreign bodies are between the ages of 6 mo and 6 yr. Coins are the most commonly ingested foreign body in children, and meat or food impactions are the most common accidental foreign body in adolescents and adults. Patients with nonfood foreign bodies often describe a history of ingestion. Young children might have a witness to ingestion. Immediate concerns are what is the foreign body, location of the foreign body, what is the size of the foreign body, and the time that the ingestion occurred. Approximately 90% of foreign bodies are opaque. Radiologic examination is routinely performed to determine the type, number, and location of the suspected objects. Contrast radiographs may be necessary to demonstrate some objects, such as plastic parts or toys.

Conservative management is indicated for most foreign bodies that have passed through the esophagus and entered the stomach. Most objects pass though the intestine in 4-6 days, although some take as long as 3-4 wk. While waiting for the object to pass, parents are instructed to continue a regular diet and to observe the stools for the appearance of the ingested object. Cathartics should be avoided. Exceptionally long or sharp objects are usually monitored radiologically. Parents or patients should be instructed to report abdominal pain, vomiting, persistent fever, and hematemesis or melena immediately to their physicians. Failure of the object to progress within 3-4 wk seldom implies an impeding perforation but may be associated with a congenital malformation or acquired bowel abnormality.

Certain objects pose more risk than others. In cases of sharp foreign bodies, such as straight pins, weekly assessments are required. Surgical removal is necessary if the patient develops symptoms or signs of obstruction or perforation or if the foreign body fails to progress for several weeks. Small magnets used to secure earrings or parts of toys are associated with bowel perforation. Whereas a single magnet in the stomach may not require intervention in a asymptomatic child, a magnet in the esophagus requires immediate removal. When the multiple magnets disperse after ingestion, they may be attracted to each other across bowel wall, leading to pressure necrosis and perforation (Fig. 334-1). Inexpensive toy medallions containing lead can lead to **lead toxicity.** Newer coins can also decompose when subjected to prolonged acid exposure. Unless multiple coins are ingested; however, the metals released are unlikely to pose a clinical risk.

Ingestion of batteries rarely leads to problems, but symptoms can arise from leakage of alkali or heavy metal (mercury) from battery degradation in the gastrointestinal tract. Batteries can also generate electrical current and thereby cause low-voltage electrical burns to the intestine. If patients experience symptoms such as vomiting or abdominal pain, if a large-diameter battery (>20 mm in diameter) remains in the stomach for longer than 48 hr, or if a lithium battery is ingested, the battery should be removed. Batteries larger than 15 mm that do not pass the pylorus within 48 hr are less likely to pass spontaneously and generally require removal. In children younger than 6 yr of age, batteries larger than 15 mm are not likely to pass spontaneously and should be removed endoscopically. If the patient develops peritoneal signs, surgical removal is required. Batteries beyond the duodenum pass per rectum in 85% within 72 hr. The battery should be identified by size and imprint code or by evaluation of a duplicate measurement of the battery compartment. The National Button Battery Ingestion Hotline (202-625-3333) can be called for help in identification. The Poison Control Center (800-222-1222) can be called as well for ingestion of batteries and caustic materials. Lithium batteries result in more severe injury than a button alkali battery, with damage occurring in

minutes. Button batteries in a symptomatic child should be removed, or if there are multiple batteries, they should be removed.

In older children and adults, oval objects larger than 5 cm in diameter or 2 cm in thickness tend to lodge in the stomach and should be endoscopically retrieved. Thin long objects >6 cm in length fail to negotiate the pylorus or duodenal sweep and should also be removed. In infants and toddlers, objects >3 cm in length or >20 mm in diameter do not usually pass through the pylorus and should be removed. An open safety pin presents a major problem and requires urgent endoscopic removal if within reach. Razor blades can be managed with a rigid endoscope by pulling the blade into instrument. The endoscopist can alternatively use a rubber hood on the head of the endoscope to protect the esophagus. Other sharp objects (needles, bones, pins) usually pass the stomach but complications may be as high as 35%; if possible they should be removed by endoscope if in the stomach or proximal duodenum. If sharp objects are not able to be removed but no progress is observed in location during 3 days, surgical removal is indicated. Drugs (aggregated iron pills, cocaine) may have to be surgically removed; initial management can include oral polyethylene glycol lavage. Drug body packing (heroin, cocaine) is usually seen on kidneys-ureters-bladder or CT imaging and often pass without incident. Endoscopic procedures may rupture the material causing severe toxicity. Surgery is indicated if toxicity develops or if the packages fail to progress or if there are signs of obstruction.

Ingestion of magnets poses a danger to children. The number of magnets is thought to be critical. If a single magnet is ingested, there is the least likelihood of complications. If 2 or more magnets are ingested, the magnetic poles are attracted to each other and create the risk of obstruction, fistula development, and perforation. Endoscopic retrieval is emergent after films are taken when multiple magnets are ingested. Abdominal pain or peritoneal signs require urgent surgical intervention. If all magnets are located in the stomach, immediate endoscopic removal is indicated. If the ingestion occurred greater than 12 hr prior to evaluation, General Surgery should be consulted. If the magnets are beyond the stomach and the patient is symptomatic, General Surgery should be consulted. If the patient is asymptomatic, endoscopic or colonoscopic removal may be considered along with a surgical evaluation.

Lead-based foreign bodies can cause symptoms from lead intoxication. Early endoscopic removal is indicated of an object suspected to contain lead. A lead level should be obtained.

Water-absorbing polymer balls (beads) can expand to approximately 400 times its starting size and if ingested may produce intestinal obstruction. Initially of a small diameter, they pass the pylorus only to rapidly enlarge in the small intestine. Surgical removal is indicated.

Children occasionally place objects in their rectum. Small blunt objects usually pass spontaneously, but large or sharp objects typically need to be retrieved. Adequate sedation is essential to relax the anal sphincter before attempted endoscopic or speculum removal. If the object is proximal to the rectum, observation for 12-24 hr usually allows the object to descend into the rectum.

Bibliography is available at Expert Consult.

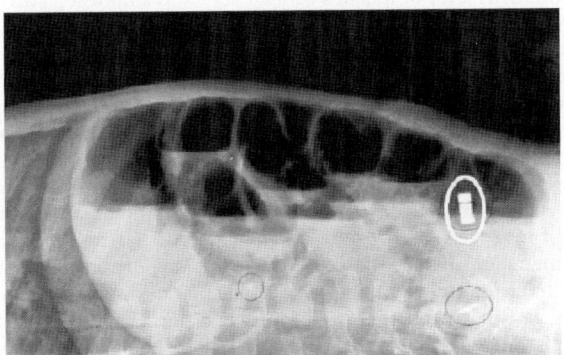

Figure 334-1 Abdominal radiograph of a boy aged 3 yr, noting 3 attached magnets that resulted in volvulus (i.e., twisting of the bowel) and multiple bowel perforations. *(Courtesy of the U.S. Consumer Product Safety Commission. From Centers for Disease Control and Prevention: Gastrointestinal injuries from magnet ingestion in children—United States, 2003–2006, MMWR Morb Mortal Wkly Rep 55:1296–1300, 2006.)*

334.2 Bezoars
Judith R. Kelsen and Chris A. Liacouras

A bezoar is an accumulation of exogenous matter in the stomach or intestine. They are predominantly composed of food or fiber. Most bezoars have been found in females with underlying personality problems or in neurologically impaired persons. Patients who have undergone abdominal surgery are at higher risk for the development of bezoars. The peak age at onset of symptoms is the 2nd decade of life.

Bezoars are classified on the basis of their composition. **Trichobezoars** are composed of the patient's own hair. It is most frequently it is a complication of the psychiatric disorders trichotillomania and the most severe form is known as Rapunzel syndrome. **Phytobezoars** are composed of a combination of plant and animal material, and gastric phytobezoars are the most common in patients with poor motility. **Lactobezoars** were previously found most often in premature infants and can be attributed to the high casein or calcium content of some premature formulas. Swallowed chewing gum can occasionally lead to a bezoar.

Trichobezoars can become large and form casts of the stomach; they can enter into the proximal duodenum. They manifest as symptoms of gastric outlet or partial intestinal obstruction including vomiting, anorexia, and weight loss. Patients might complain of abdominal pain, distention, and severe halitosis. Physical examination can demonstrate patchy baldness and a firm mass in the left upper quadrant. Patients occasionally have iron-deficiency anemia, hypoproteinemia, or steatorrhea caused by an associated chronic gastritis. Phytobezoars manifest in a similar manner. Detached segments of the bezoar or trichobezoar can migrate to the small intestine as a "satellite masses" and result in small bowel obstruction.

An abdominal plain film can suggest the presence of a bezoar, which can be confirmed on ultrasound or CT examination. On CT a bezoar appears a nonhomogeneous, nonenhancing mass within the lumen of the stomach or intestine. Oral contrast circumscribes the mass.

Bezoars in the stomach can usually be removed endoscopically. If endoscopy is unsuccessful, surgical intervention may be needed. Lactobezoars usually resolve when feedings are withheld for 24-48 hr. Coca-Cola has been used as a dissolution therapy for gastric phytobezoar and has been shown to be effective when used with endoscopy.

Sunflower seed bezoars are reported to cause rectal pain and constipation as a result of the seed shells being associated with fecal impaction. Endoscopic removal is indicated, as these bezoars are refractory to enema or lavage management.

Bibliography is available at Expert Consult.

Chapter 335
Peptic Ulcer Disease in Children
Samra S. Blanchard and Steven J. Czinn

Peptic ulcer disease, the end result of inflammation caused by an imbalance between cytoprotective and cytotoxic factors in the stomach and duodenum, manifests with varying degrees of gastritis or frank ulceration. The pathogenesis of peptic ulcer disease is multifactorial, but the final common pathway for the development of ulcers is the action of acid and pepsin-laden contents of the stomach on the gastric and duodenal mucosa and the inability of mucosal defense mechanisms to allay those effects. Abnormalities in the gastric and duodenal mucosa can be visualized on endoscopy, with or without histologic changes. Deep mucosal lesions that disrupt the muscularis mucosa of the gastric or duodenal wall define **peptic ulcers.** Gastric ulcers are generally located on the lesser curvature of the stomach, and 90% of duodenal ulcers are found in the duodenal bulb. Despite the lack of large population-based pediatric studies, rates of peptic ulcer disease in childhood appear to be low. Large pediatric centers anecdotally report an incidence of 5-7 children with gastric or duodenal ulcers per 2,500 hospital admissions each year.

Ulcers in children can be classified as **primary** peptic ulcers, which are chronic and more often duodenal, or **secondary,** which are usually more acute in onset and are more often gastric (Table 335-1). Primary ulcers are most often associated with *Helicobacter pylori* infection; idiopathic primary peptic ulcers account for up to 20% of duodenal

Table 335-1	Etiologic Classification of Peptic Ulcers

Positive for *Helicobacter pylori* infection
Drug (NSAID)-induced
H. pylori and NSAID-positive
H. pylori and NSAID-negative*
Acid hypersecretory state (Zollinger-Ellison syndrome)
Anastomosis ulcer after subtotal gastric resection
Tumors (cancer, lymphoma)
Rare specific causes
Crohn disease of the stomach or duodenum
Eosinophilic gastroduodenitis
Systemic mastocytosis
Radiation damage
Viral infections (cytomegalovirus or herpes simplex infection, particularly in immunocompromised patients)
Colonization of stomach with *Helicobacter heilmannii*
Severe systemic disease
Cameron ulcer (gastric ulcer where a hiatal hernia passes through the diaphragmatic hiatus)
True idiopathic ulcer

*Requires search for other specific causes.
NSAID, nonsteroidal anti-inflammatory drug.
From Vakil N, Megraud F: Eradication therapy for Helicobacter pylori, Gastroenterology 133:985–1001, 2007.

ulcers in children. Secondary peptic ulcers can result from stress caused by sepsis, shock, or an intracranial lesion (Cushing ulcer), or in response to a severe burn injury (Curling ulcer). Secondary ulcers are often the result of using aspirin or nonsteroidal antiinflammatory drugs (NSAIDs); hypersecretory states like Zollinger-Ellison syndrome (see Chapter 335.1), short bowel syndrome, and systemic mastocytosis are rare causes of peptic ulceration.

PATHOGENESIS
Acid Secretion
By 3-4 yr of age, gastric acid secretion approximates adult values. Acid initially secreted by the oxyntic cells of the stomach has a pH of approximately 0.8, whereas the pH of the stomach contents is 1-2. Excessive acid secretion is associated with a large parietal cell mass, hypersecretion by antral G cells, and increased vagal tone, resulting in increased or sustained acid secretion in response to meals and increased secretion during the night. The secretagogues that promote gastric acid production include acetylcholine released by the vagus nerve, histamine secreted by enterochromaffin cells, and gastrin released by the G cells of the antrum. Mediators that decrease gastric acid secretion and enhance protective mucin production include prostaglandins.

Mucosal Defense
A continuous layer of mucous gel that serves as a diffusion barrier to hydrogen ions and other chemicals covers the gastrointestinal (GI) mucosa. Mucus production and secretion are stimulated by prostaglandin E_2. Underlying the mucous coat, the epithelium forms a second-line barrier, the characteristics of which are determined by the biology of the epithelial cells and their tight junctions. Another important function of epithelial cells is to secrete chemokines when threatened by microbial attack. Secretion of bicarbonate into the mucous coat, which is regulated by prostaglandins, is important for neutralization of hydrogen ions. If mucosal injury occurs, active proliferation and migration of mucosal cells occurs rapidly, driven by epithelial growth factor, transforming growth factor-α, insulin-like growth factor, gastrin, and bombesin, and covers the area of epithelial damage.

CLINICAL MANIFESTATIONS
The presenting symptoms of peptic ulcer disease vary with the age of the patient. Hematemesis or melena is reported in up to half of the patients with peptic ulcer disease. School-age children and adolescents more commonly present with epigastric pain and nausea, presentations generally seen in adults. Dyspepsia, epigastric abdominal pain or fullness, is seen in older children. Infants and younger children usually

present with feeding difficulty, vomiting, crying episodes, hematemesis, or melena. In the neonatal period, gastric perforation can be the initial presentation.

The classic symptom of peptic ulceration, epigastric pain alleviated by the ingestion of food, is present only in a minority of children. Many pediatric patients present with poorly localized abdominal pain, which may be periumbilical. The vast majority of patients with periumbilical or epigastric pain or discomfort do not have a peptic ulcer, but rather a functional GI disorder, such as irritable bowel syndrome or nonulcer (functional) dyspepsia. Patients with peptic ulceration rarely present with acute abdominal pain from perforation or symptoms and signs of pancreatitis from a posterior penetrating ulcer. Occasionally, bright red blood per rectum may be seen if the rate of bleeding is brisk and the intestinal transit time is short. Vomiting can be a sign of gastric outlet obstruction.

The pain is often described as dull or aching, rather than sharp or burning, as in adults. It can last from minutes to hours; patients have frequent exacerbations and remissions lasting from weeks to months. Nocturnal pain waking the child is common in older children. A history of typical ulcer pain with prompt relief after taking antacids is found in <33% of children. Rarely, in patients with acute or chronic blood loss, penetration of the ulcer into the abdominal cavity or adjacent organs produces shock, anemia, peritonitis, or pancreatitis. If inflammation and edema are extensive, acute or chronic gastric outlet obstruction can occur.

DIAGNOSIS

Esophagogastroduodenoscopy is the method of choice to establish the diagnosis of peptic ulcer disease. It can be safely performed in all ages by experienced pediatric gastroenterologists. Endoscopy allows the direct visualization of esophagus, stomach, and duodenum, identifying the specific lesions. Biopsy specimens must be obtained from the esophagus, stomach, and duodenum for histologic assessment as well as to screen for the presence of H. pylori infection. Endoscopy also provides the opportunity for hemostatic therapy including injection and the use of a heater probe or electrocoagulation if necessary. Fecal enzyme immunoassay tests for H. pylori are available and have varying utility in children.

PRIMARY ULCERS
Helicobacter pylori Gastritis

H. pylori is among the most common bacterial infections in humans. H. pylori is a Gram-negative, S-shaped rod that produces urease, catalase, and oxidase, which might play a role in the pathogenesis of peptic ulcer disease. The mechanism of acquisition and transmission of H. pylori is unclear, although the most likely mode of transmission is fecal–oral or oral–oral. Viable H. pylori organisms can be cultured from the stool or vomitus of infected patients. Risk factors such as low socioeconomic status in childhood or affected family members also influence the prevalence. All children infected with H. pylori develop histologic chronic active gastritis but are often asymptomatic. In children, H. pylori infection can manifest with abdominal pain or vomiting and, less often, refractory iron deficiency anemia or growth retardation. H. pylori can be associated, though rarely, with chronic autoimmune thrombocytopenia. Chronic colonization with H. pylori can predispose children to a significantly increased risk of developing a duodenal ulcer, gastric cancer such as adenocarcinoma, or mucosa-associated lymphoid tissue lymphomas. The relative risk of gastric carcinoma is 2.3-8.7 times greater in infected adults as compared to uninfected subjects. H. pylori is classified by the World Health Organization as a group I carcinogen.

Anemia, idiopathic thrombocytopenic purpura, short stature, and sudden infant death syndrome (SIDS) have also been reported as extragastric manifestations of H. pylori infection. In one published study, H. pylori infection has been correlated with cases of SIDS, but there is no evidence to suggest that H. pylori plays a role in the pathogenesis of SIDS.

The **diagnosis** of H. pylori infection is made histologically by demonstrating the organism in the biopsy specimens (Fig. 335-1). Although

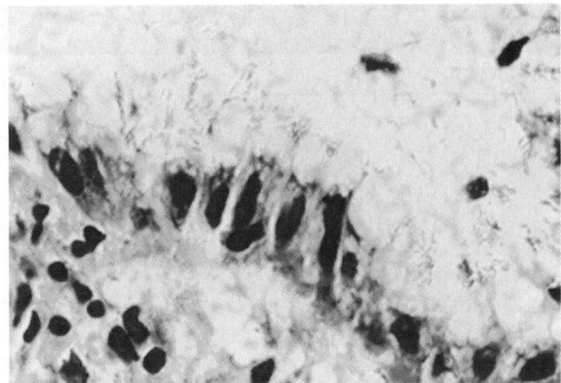

Figure 335-1 Appearance of *Helicobacter pylori* on the gastric mucosal surface with Giemsa stain (high-power view). *(From Campbell DI, Thomas JE:* Helicobacter pylori *infection in paediatric practice,* Arch Dis Child Educ Pract Ed *90:ep25–ep30, 2005.)*

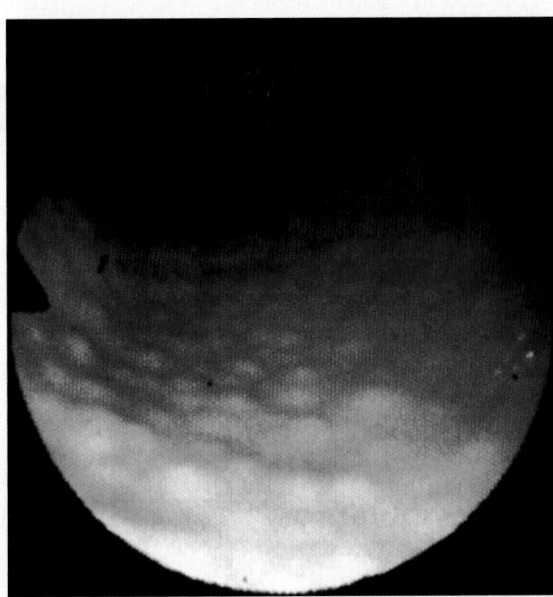

Figure 335-2 Endoscopic view of lymphoid modular hyperplasia of the gastric antrum. *(From Campbell DI, Thomas JE:* Helicobacter pylori *infection in paediatric practice,* Arch Dis Child Educ Pract Ed *90:ep25–ep30, 2005.)*

serologic assays using validated immunoglobulin G antibody detection may be helpful for screening children for the presence of H. pylori, they do not help predict active infection or assess the success of antimicrobial eradication therapy. ^{13}C-urea breath tests and stool antigen tests are also noninvasive methods of detecting H. pylori infection. Nonetheless, for children with suspected H. pylori infection, an initial upper endoscopy is recommended to evaluate and confirm H. pylori disease. The range of endoscopic findings in children with H. pylori infection varies from being grossly normal to the presence of nonspecific gastritis with prominent rugal folds, nodularity (Fig. 335-2), or ulcers. Because the antral mucosa appears to be endoscopically normal in a significant number of children with primary H. pylori gastritis, gastric biopsies should always be obtained from the body and antrum of the stomach regardless of the endoscopic appearance. If H. pylori is identified, even in a child with no symptoms, eradication therapy should be offered (Tables 335-2 and 335-3).

Idiopathic Ulcers

H. pylori–negative duodenal ulcers in children who have no history of taking NSAIDs represent 15-20% of pediatric duodenal ulcers. These patients do not have nodularity in the gastric antrum or histologic

Table 335-2 | Recommended Eradication Therapies for *Helicobacter pylori*—Associated Disease in Children

MEDICATIONS	DOSE	DURATION OF TREATMENT
Amoxicillin	50 mg/kg/day in 2 divided doses	14 days
Clarithromycin	15 mg/kg/day in 2 divided doses	14 days
Proton pump inhibitor	1 mg/kg/day in 2 divided doses	1 mo
or		
Amoxicillin	50 mg/kg/day in 2 divided doses	14 days
Metronidazole	20 mg/kg/day in 2 divided doses	14 days
Proton pump inhibitor	1 mg/kg/day in 2 divided doses	1 mo
or		
Clarithromycin	15 mg/kg/day in 2 divided doses	14 days
Metronidazole	20 mg/kg/day in 2 divided doses	14 days
Proton pump inhibitor	1 mg/kg/day in 2 divided doses	1 mo

Adapted from Gold BD, Colletti RB, Abbott M, et al: Medical position statement: The North American Society for Pediatric Gastroenterology and Nutrition. Helicobacter pylori infection in children: recommendations for diagnosis and treatment, J Pediatr Gastroenterol Nutr 31:490–497, 2000.

Table 335-3 | Antisecretory Therapy with Pediatric Dosages

MEDICATION	PEDIATRIC DOSE	HOW SUPPLIED
H₂ RECEPTOR ANTAGONISTS		
Cimetidine	20-40 mg/kg/day Divided 2-4 × a day	Syrup: 300 mg/mL Tablets: 200, 300, 400, 800 mg
Ranitidine	4-10 mg/kg/day Divided 2 or 3 × a day	Syrup: 75 mg/5 mL Tablets: 75, 150, 300 mg
Famotidine	1-2 mg/kg/day Divided twice a day	Syrup: 40 mg/5 mL Tablets: 20, 40 mg
Nizatidine	5-10 mg/kg/day divided twice a day Older than 12 yr: 150 mg twice a day	Solution: 15 mg/ml Capsule 150, 300 Tablet: 75 mg
PROTON PUMP INHIBITORS		
Omeprazole	1.0-3.3 mg/kg/day weigh <20 kg: 10 mg/day weigh >20 kg: 20 mg/day Approved for use in those older than 2 yr	Capsules: 10, 20, 40 mg
Lansoprazole	0.8-4 mg/kg/day weigh <30 kg: 15 mg/day weigh >30 kg: 30 mg/day Approved for use in those older than 1 yr	Capsules: 15, 30 mg Powder packet: 15, 30 mg SoluTab: 15, 30 mg
Rabeprazole	1-11 yr(weigh <15 kg): 5 mg/day 1-11 yr (weigh >15 kg): 10 mg/day >12 yr: 20 mg tablet	Delayed release capsule: 5, 10 mg Delayed release tablet: 20 mg
Pantoprazole	1-5 yr:0.3-1.2 mg/kg/day (limited data) >5 yr of age: weigh >15 kg to <40 kg: 20 mg/day weigh >40 kg: 40 mg/day	Tablet: 20, 40 mg Powder pack: 40 mg
CYTOPROTECTIVE AGENTS		
Sucralfate	40-80 mg/kg/day	Suspension: 1,000 mg/5 mL Tablet: 1,000 mg

evidence of gastritis. In idiopathic ulcers, acid suppression alone is the preferred effective treatment. Either proton pump inhibitors (PPIs) or H₂ receptor antagonists may be used. Idiopathic ulcers have a high recurrence rate after discontinuing antisecretory therapy. These children should be followed closely, and if symptoms recur, antisecretory therapy should be restarted. In such cases, if the child is older than 1 yr, PPIs are preferred for maintenance therapy, because they have been shown to be superior to H₂ receptor antagonists in preventing recurrent ulcers.

SECONDARY ULCERS
Aspirin and Other Nonsteroidal Antiinflammatory Drugs
NSAIDs produce mucosal injury by direct local irritation and by inhibiting cyclooxygenase and prostaglandin formation. Prostaglandins enhance mucosal resistance to injury; therefore, a decrease in

prostaglandin production increases the risk of mucosal injury. The severe erosive gastropathy produced by NSAIDs can ultimately result in bleeding ulcers or gastric perforations. The location of these ulcers is more common in the stomach than in the duodenum, and usually in the antrum.

"STRESS" ULCERATION
Stress ulceration usually occurs within 24 hr of onset of a critical illness in which physiologic stress is present. In many cases, the patients bleed from gastric erosions, rather than ulcers. Approximately 25% of the critically ill children in a pediatric intensive care unit have macroscopic evidence of gastric bleeding. Preterm and term infants in the neonatal intensive care unit can also develop gastric mucosal lesions and can present with upper GI bleeding or perforated ulcers. Although prophylactic measures to prevent stress ulcers in children are not standardized, drugs that inhibit gastric acid production are often used in the

pediatric intensive care unit to reduce the rate of gastric erosions or ulcers.

TREATMENT

The management of acute hemorrhage includes serial monitoring of pulse, blood pressure, and hematocrit to insure hemodynamic stability and avoid significant hypovolemia and anemia. Normal saline can be used to resuscitate a patient who has poor intravascular volume status. This can be followed by packed red blood cell transfusions for significant symptomatic anemia. The patient's blood should be typed and cross matched, and a large-bore catheter should be placed for fluid or blood replacement. A nasogastric tube should be placed to determine if the bleeding has stopped. Significant anemia can occur after fluid resuscitation as a consequence of equilibration or continued blood loss (which can also cause shock). In adults, a conservative threshold for transfusion (<7 g/dL vs 9 g hemoglobin) resulted in improved survival and fewer episodes of rebleeding. Fortunately, most acute peptic ulcer bleeding stops spontaneously.

Patients with suspected peptic ulcer hemorrhage should receive high-dose intravenous PPI therapy, which lowers the risk of rebleeding. Some centers also use octreotide, which lowers splanchnic blood flow and gastric acid production.

Once the patient is hemodynamically stable, endoscopy may be indicated to identify the source of bleeding and treat a potential bleeding site. Methods used for vessel hemostasis include pressure, laser, thermal or electric coagulation; clips; bands; and injections (epinephrine, saline).

Ulcer therapy has 2 goals: ulcer healing and elimination of the primary cause. Other important considerations are relief of symptoms and prevention of complications. The **first-line drugs** for the treatment of gastritis and peptic ulcer disease in children are PPIs and H$_2$ receptor antagonists (see Table 335-3). PPIs are more potent in ulcer healing. Cytoprotective agents can also be used as adjunct therapy if mucosal lesions are present. Antibiotics in combination with a PPI must be used for the treatment of *H. pylori*-associated ulcers (see Table 335-2).

H$_2$-receptor antagonists (cimetidine, ranitidine, famotidine, nizatidine) competitively inhibit the binding of histamine at the H$_2$ subtype receptor of the gastric parietal cell. PPIs block the gastric parietal cell H$^+$/K$^+$–adenosine triphosphatase pump in a dose-dependent fashion, reducing basal and stimulated gastric acid secretion. Currently, 7 PPIs are available in the United States: omeprazole, lansoprazole, pantoprazole, esomeprazole, rabeprazole, dexlansoprazole, and omeprazole/sodium bicarbonate. Apart from the last 2, they are all approved in children and adolescents. They are well tolerated with only minor adverse effects, such as diarrhea (1-4%), headache (1-3%), and nausea (1%). When one considers therapeutic efficacy, the evidence suggests that all PPIs have comparable efficacy in treatment of peptic ulcer disease using standard doses and are superior to H$_2$-receptor antagonists. PPIs have their greatest effect when given before a meal. Pantoprazole and esomeprazole are the only PPI available in United States. Intravenous PPI should be used in acute upper GI bleeding. In adults, intravenous PPI in acute upper GI bleeding setting decreases the bleeding and need of intervention during endoscopy.

Treatment of *Helicobacter pylori*–Related Peptic Ulcer Disease

In pediatrics, antibiotics and bismuth salts have been used in combination with PPIs to treat *H. pylori* infection (see Table 335-2). Eradication rates in children range from 68-92% when the dual or triple therapy is used for 4-6 wk. The ulcer healing rate ranges from 91-100%. Triple therapy yields a higher cure rate than dual therapy. The optimal regimen for the eradication of *H. pylori* infection in children has yet to be established, but the use of a PPI in combination with clarithromycin and amoxicillin or metronidazole for 2 wk is a well-tolerated and recommended triple therapy (see Table 335-2). Although children younger than 5 yr of age can become reinfected, the most common reason for treatment failure is poor compliance or antibiotic resistance. *H. pylori* has become more resistant to clarithromycin or metronida-

zole as a consequence of the extensive use of these antibiotics for other infections. In the case of resistant *H. pylori* infection, sequential treatment or rescue therapy with different antibiotics is acceptable options. The sequential treatment regimen is a 10-day treatment consisting of a PPI and amoxicillin (both twice daily) administered for the 1st 5 days followed by triple therapy consisting of a PPI, clarithromycin, and metronidazole for the remaining 5 days. Levofloxacin, rifabutin, or furazolidone can be used with amoxicillin and bismuth as a rescue therapy depending on the age of the patient. Fidaxomicin has equivalent efficacy to vancomycin in adults. Knowledge of the community's *H. pylori* resistance pattern to clarithromycin or metronidazole might help chose the initial or rescue therapy.

Surgical Therapy

Since the discovery of *H. pylori* and the availability of modern medical management, peptic ulcer disease requiring surgical treatment has become extremely rare. The indications for surgery remain uncontrolled bleeding, perforation, and obstruction. Since the introduction of H$_2$-receptor antagonists, the recognition and treatment of *H. pylori*, and the use of PPIs, the incidence of surgery for bleeding and perforation has decreased dramatically.

Bibliography is available at Expert Consult.

335.1 Zollinger-Ellison Syndrome
Samra S. Blanchard and Steven J. Czinn

Zollinger-Ellison syndrome is a rare syndrome characterized by refractory, severe peptic ulcer disease caused by gastric hypersecretion due to the autonomous secretion of gastrin by a neuroendocrine tumor, a gastrinoma. Clinical presentations are similar to those of peptic ulcer disease with the addition of diarrhea. The diagnosis is suspected by the presence of recurrent, multiple, or atypically located ulcers. More than 98% of patients have elevated fasting gastrin levels. Zollinger-Ellison syndrome is common in patients with **multiple endocrine neoplasia 1** and rare with **neurofibromatosis** and **tuberous sclerosis**. Prompt and effective management of increased gastric acid secretion is essential in the management. PPIs are the drug of choice due to their long duration of action and potency. H$_2$-receptor antagonists are also effective, but higher doses are required than those used in peptic ulcer disease.

Bibliography is available at Expert Consult.

Chapter **336**
Inflammatory Bowel Disease
Andrew B. Grossman and Robert N. Baldassano

The term *inflammatory bowel disease* (IBD) is used to represent 2 distinctive disorders of idiopathic chronic intestinal inflammation: Crohn disease and ulcerative colitis. Their respective etiologies are poorly understood, and both disorders are characterized by unpredictable exacerbations and remissions. The most common time of onset of IBD is during the preadolescent/adolescent era and young adulthood. A bimodal distribution has been shown with an early onset at 10-20 yr of age and a second, smaller peak at 50-80 yr of age. Approximately 25% of patients present before 20 yr of age. IBD may begin as early as the 1st yr of life, and an increased incidence among young children has been observed since the turn of the century. Children with early-onset IBD are more likely to have colonic involvement. In developed countries, these disorders are the major causes of chronic intestinal inflammation in children beyond the 1st few yr of life. A third, less-common category, indeterminate colitis, represents approximately 10% of pediatric patients.

IBD may be classified according to age at onset: pediatric onset (<17 yr), early onset (<10 yr), very early onset (<6 yr), infant/toddler onset (0-2 yr), and neonatal onset IBD. Children with very early onset (representing ~1% of patients) and those <1 yr of age (0.2%), have a high incidence of monogenetic causes of IBD (see Table 336-5) rather than idiopathic and probably polygenetic-environmental causes of IBD.

Genetic and environmental influences are involved in the pathogenesis of IBD. The prevalence of Crohn disease in the United States is much lower for Hispanics and Asians than for whites and blacks. The risk of IBD in family members of an affected person has been reported in the range of 7-30%; a child whose parents both have IBD has a >35% chance of acquiring the disorder. Relatives of a patient with ulcerative colitis have a greater risk of acquiring ulcerative colitis than Crohn disease, whereas relatives of a patient with Crohn disease have a greater risk of acquiring this disorder; the 2 diseases can occur in the same family. The risk of occurrence of IBD among relatives of patients with Crohn disease is somewhat greater than for patients with ulcerative colitis.

The importance of genetic factors in the development of IBD is noted by a higher chance that both twins will be affected if they are monozygotic rather than dizygotic. The concordance rate in twins is higher in Crohn disease (36%) than in ulcerative colitis (16%). Genetic disorders that have been associated with IBD include Turner syndrome, the Hermansky-Pudlak syndrome, glycogen storage disease type Ib, and various immunodeficiency disorders. In 2001, the first IBD gene, NOD2, was identified through association mapping. A few months later, the IBD 5 risk haplotype was identified. These early successes were followed by a long period without notable risk factor discovery. Since 2006, the year of the first published genome wide array study on IBD, there has been an exponential growth in the set of validated genetic risk factors for IBD.

A perinuclear antineutrophil cytoplasmic antibody is found in approximately 70% of patients with ulcerative colitis compared with <20% of those with Crohn disease and is believed to represent a marker of genetically controlled immunoregulatory disturbance. Approximately 55% of those with Crohn disease are positive for anti–Saccharomyces cerevisiae antibody. Since the importance of these were first described, multiple other serologic and immune markers of Crohn disease and ulcerative colitis have been recognized.

IBD is caused by dysregulated or inappropriate immune response to environmental factors in a genetically susceptible host. An abnormality in intestinal mucosal immunoregulation may be of primary importance in the pathogenesis of IBD, involving activation of cytokines, triggering a cascade of reactions that results in bowel inflammation. These cytokines are recognized as known or potential targets for IBD therapies.

Multiple environmental factors are recognized to be involved in the pathogenesis of IBD, none more critical than the gut microbiota. The increasing incidence of IBD over time is likely in part attributable to alterations in the microbiome. Evidence includes association between IBD and residence in or immigration to industrialized nations, with a "Western" diet, increased use of antibiotics at a younger age, high rates of vaccination, and less exposure to microbes at a young age. While gut microbes likely play an important role in the pathogenesis of IBD, the exact mechanism needs to be elucidated further. Some environmental factors are disease specific; for example, cigarette smoking is a risk factor for Crohn disease but paradoxically protects against ulcerative colitis.

It is usually possible to distinguish between ulcerative colitis and Crohn disease by the clinical presentation and radiologic, endoscopic, and histopathologic findings (Table 336-1). It is not possible to make a definitive diagnosis in approximately 10% of patients with chronic colitis; this disorder is called *indeterminate colitis*. Occasionally, a child

Table 336-1	Comparison of Crohn Disease and Ulcerative Colitis	
FEATURE	**CROHN DISEASE**	**ULCERATIVE COLITIS**
Rectal bleeding	Sometimes	Common
Diarrhea, mucus, pus	Variable	Common
Abdominal pain	Common	Variable
Abdominal mass	Common	Not present
Growth failure	Common	Variable
Perianal disease	Common	Rare
Rectal involvement	Occasional	Universal
Pyoderma gangrenosum	Rare	Present
Erythema nodosum	Common	Less common
Mouth ulceration	Common	Rare
Thrombosis	Less common	Present
Colonic disease	50-75%	100%
Ileal disease	Common	None except backwash ileitis
Stomach–esophageal disease	More common	Chronic gastritis can be seen
Strictures	Common	Rare
Fissures	Common	Rare
Fistulas	Common	Rare
Toxic megacolon	None	Present
Sclerosing cholangitis	Less common	Present
Risk for cancer	Increased	Greatly increased
Discontinuous (skip) lesions	Common	Not present
Transmural involvement	Common	Unusual
Crypt abscesses	Less common	Common
Granulomas	Common	None
Linear ulcerations	Uncommon	Common
Perinuclear antineutrophil cytoplasmic antibody–positive	<20%	70%

initially believed to have ulcerative colitis on the basis of clinical findings is subsequently found to have Crohn colitis. This is particularly true for the youngest patients, because Crohn disease in this patient population can more often manifest as exclusively colonic inflammation, mimicking ulcerative colitis. The medical treatments of Crohn disease and ulcerative colitis overlap.

Extraintestinal manifestations occur slightly more commonly with Crohn disease than with ulcerative colitis (Table 336-2). Growth retardation is seen in 15-40% of children with Crohn disease at diagnosis. Decrease in height velocity occurs in nearly 90% of patients with Crohn disease diagnosed in childhood or adolescence. Of the extraintestinal manifestations that occur with IBD, joint, skin, eye, mouth, and hepatobiliary involvement tend to be associated with colitis, whether ulcerative or Crohn. The presence of some manifestations, such as peripheral arthritis, erythema nodosum, and anemia, correlates with activity of the bowel disease. Activity of pyoderma gangrenosum correlates less well with activity of the bowel disease, whereas sclerosing cholangitis, ankylosing spondylitis, and sacroiliitis do not correlate with intestinal disease. Arthritis occurs in 3 patterns: migratory peripheral arthritis involving primarily large joints, ankylosing

Table 336-2	Extraintestinal Complications of Inflammatory Bowel Disease

MUSCULOSKELETAL
Peripheral arthritis
Granulomatous monoarthritis
Granulomatous synovitis
Rheumatoid arthritis
Sacroiliitis
Ankylosing spondylitis
Digital clubbing and hypertrophic osteoarthropathy
Periosteitis
Osteoporosis, osteomalacia
Rhabdomyolysis
Pelvic osteomyelitis
Recurrent multifocal osteomyelitis
Relapsing polychondritis

SKIN AND MUCOUS MEMBRANES
Oral lesions
Cheilitis
Aphthous stomatitis, glossitis
Granulomatous oral Crohn disease
Inflammatory hyperplasia fissures and cobblestone mucosa
Peristomatitis vegetans

DERMATOLOGIC
Erythema nodosum
Pyoderma gangrenosum
Sweet syndrome
Metastatic Crohn disease
Psoriasis
Epidermolysis bullosa acquisita
Perianal skin tags
Polyarteritis nodosa

OCULAR
Conjunctivitis
Uveitis, iritis
Episcleritis
Scleritis
Retrobulbar neuritis
Chorioretinitis with retinal detachment
Crohn keratopathy
Posterior segment abnormalities
Retinal vascular disease

BRONCHOPULMONARY
Chronic bronchitis with bronchiectasis
Chronic bronchitis with neutrophilic infiltrates
Fibrosing alveolitis
Pulmonary vasculitis
Small airway disease and bronchiolitis obliterans
Eosinophilic lung disease
Granulomatous lung disease
Tracheal obstruction

CARDIAC
Pleuropericarditis
Cardiomyopathy
Endocarditis
Myocarditis

MALNUTRITION
Decreased intake of food
• Inflammatory bowel disease
• Dietary restriction
Malabsorption
• Inflammatory bowel disease
• Bowel resection
• Bile salt depletion
• Bacterial overgrowth

Intestinal losses
• Electrolytes
• Minerals
• Nutrients
Increased caloric needs
• Inflammation
• Fever

HEMATOLOGIC
Anemia: iron deficiency (blood loss)
Vitamin B_{12} (ileal disease or resection, bacterial overgrowth, folate deficiency)
Anemia of chronic inflammation
Anaphylactoid purpura (Crohn disease)
Hyposplenism
Autoimmune hemolytic anemia
Coagulation abnormalities
Increased activation of coagulation factors
Activated fibrinolysis
Anticardiolipin antibody
Increased risk of arterial and venous thrombosis with cerebrovascular stroke, myocardial infarction, peripheral arterial, and venous occlusions

RENAL AND GENITOURINARY
Metabolic
• Urinary crystal formation (nephrolithiasis, uric acid, oxylate)
Hypokalemic nephropathy
Inflammation
• Retroperitoneal abscess
• Fibrosis with ureteral obstruction
• Fistula formation
Glomerulitis
Membrane nephritis
Renal amyloidosis, nephrotic syndrome

PANCREATITIS
Secondary to medications (sulfasalazine, 6-mercaptopurine, azathioprine, parenteral nutrition)
Ampullary Crohn disease
Granulomatous pancreatitis
Decreased pancreatic exocrine function
Sclerosing cholangitis with pancreatitis

HEPATOBILIARY
Primary sclerosing cholangitis
Small duct primary sclerosing cholangitis (pericholangitis)
Carcinoma of the bile ducts
Fatty infiltration of the liver
Cholelithiasis
Autoimmune hepatitis

ENDOCRINE AND METABOLIC
Growth failure, delayed sexual maturation
Thyroiditis
Osteoporosis, osteomalacia

NEUROLOGIC
Peripheral neuropathy
Meningitis
Vestibular dysfunction
Pseudotumor cerebri
Cerebral vasculitis
Migraine

Modified from Kugathasan S: Diarrhea. In Kliegman RM, Greenbaum LA, Lye PS, editors: Practical strategies in pediatric diagnosis and therapy, ed 2, Philadelphia, 2004, WB Saunders, p. 285.

spondylitis, and sacroiliitis. The peripheral arthritis of IBD tends to be nondestructive. Ankylosing spondylitis begins in the 3rd decade and occurs most commonly in patients with ulcerative colitis who have the human leukocyte antigen B27 phenotype. Symptoms include low back pain and morning stiffness; back, hips, shoulders, and sacroiliac joints are typically affected. Isolated sacroiliitis is usually asymptomatic but is common when a careful search is performed. Among the skin manifestations, erythema nodosum is most common. Patients with erythema nodosum or pyoderma gangrenosum have a high likelihood of having arthritis as well. Glomerulonephritis, uveitis, and a hypercoagulable state are other rare manifestations that occur in childhood. Cerebral thromboembolic disease has been described in children with IBD.

336.1 Chronic Ulcerative Colitis

Andrew B. Grossman and Robert N. Baldassano

Ulcerative colitis, an idiopathic chronic inflammatory disorder, is localized to the colon and spares the upper gastrointestinal (GI) tract. Disease usually begins in the rectum and extends proximally for a variable distance. When it is localized to the rectum, the disease is ulcerative proctitis, whereas disease involving the entire colon is pancolitis. Approximately 50-80% of pediatric patients have extensive colitis, and adults more commonly have distal disease. Ulcerative proctitis is less likely to be associated with systemic manifestations, although it may be less responsive to treatment than more-diffuse disease. Approximately 30% of children who present with ulcerative proctitis experience proximal spread of the disease. Ulcerative colitis has rarely been noted to present in infancy. Dietary protein intolerance can easily be misdiagnosed as ulcerative colitis in this age group. Dietary protein intolerance (cow's milk protein) is a transient disorder; symptoms are directly associated with the intake of the offending antigen.

The incidence of ulcerative colitis has remained relatively constant, in contrast to an increase in Crohn disease, but varies with country of origin. The age-specific incidence rates of pediatric ulcerative colitis in North America is 2 per 100,000 population. The prevalence of ulcerative colitis in northern European countries and the United States varies from 100-200 per 100,000 population. Men are slightly more likely to acquire ulcerative colitis than are women; the reverse is true for Crohn disease.

CLINICAL MANIFESTATIONS

Blood, mucus, and pus in the stool as well as diarrhea are the typical presentation of ulcerative colitis. Constipation may be observed in those with proctitis. Symptoms such as tenesmus, urgency, cramping abdominal pain (especially with bowel movements), and nocturnal bowel movements are common. The mode of onset ranges from insidious with gradual progression of symptoms to acute and fulminant (Table 336-3, Fig. 336-1). Fever, severe anemia, hypoalbuminemia, leukocytosis, and more than 5 bloody stools per day for 5 days define **fulminant colitis**. Chronicity is an important part of the diagnosis; it is difficult to know if a patient has a subacute, transient infectious

colitis or ulcerative colitis when a child has had 1-2 wk of symptoms. Symptoms beyond this duration often prove to be secondary to IBD. Anorexia, weight loss, and growth failure may be present, although these complications are more typical of Crohn disease.

Extraintestinal manifestations that tend to occur more commonly with ulcerative colitis than with Crohn disease include pyoderma gangrenosum, sclerosing cholangitis, chronic active hepatitis, and ankylosing spondylitis. Iron deficiency can result from chronic blood loss as well as decreased intake. Folate deficiency is unusual but may be accentuated in children treated with sulfasalazine, which interferes with folate absorption. Chronic inflammation and the elaboration of a variety of inflammatory cytokines can interfere with erythropoiesis and result in the anemia of chronic disease. Secondary amenorrhea is common during periods of active disease.

The clinical course of ulcerative colitis is marked by remission and relapse, often without apparent explanation. After treatment of initial symptoms, approximately 5% of children with ulcerative colitis have a prolonged remission (longer than 3 yr). Approximately 25% of children presenting with severe ulcerative colitis require colectomy within 5 yr of diagnosis, compared with only 5% of those presenting with mild disease. It is important to consider the possibility of enteric infection with recurrent symptoms; these infections can mimic a flare-up or actually provoke a recurrence. The use of nonsteroidal antiinflammatory drugs is considered by some to predispose to exacerbation.

It is generally believed that the risk of colon cancer begins to increase after 8-10 yr of disease and can then increase by 0.5-1% per year. The risk is delayed by approximately 10 yr in patients with colitis limited to the descending colon. Proctitis alone is associated with virtually no increase in risk over the general population. Because colon cancer is usually preceded by changes of mucosal dysplasia, it is recommended that patients who have had ulcerative colitis for longer than 10 yr be screened with colonoscopy and biopsies every 1-2 yr. Although this is the current standard of practice, it is not clear if morbidity and mortality are changed by this approach. Two competing concerns about this

Table 336-3	Montreal Classification of Extent and Severity of Ulcerative Colitis

- E1 (proctitis): inflammation limited to the rectum
- E2 (left-sided; distal): inflammation limited to the splenic flexure
- E3 (pancolitis): inflammation extends to the proximal splenic flexure
- S0 (remission): no symptoms
- S1 (mild): 4 or less stools per day (with or without blood), absence of systemic symptoms, normal inflammatory markers
- S2 (moderate): 4 stools per day, minimum signs of systemic symptoms
- S3 (severe): 6 or more bloody stools per day, pulse rate of ≥90 beats per min, temperature ≥37.5°C (99.5°F), hemoglobin concentration <105 g/L, erythrocyte sedimentation rate ≥30 mm/hr

E, extent; S, severity.
From Ordàs I, Eckmann L, Talamini M, et al: Ulcerative colitis, Lancet 380:1606–1616, 2012 (Panel 2, p. 1610).

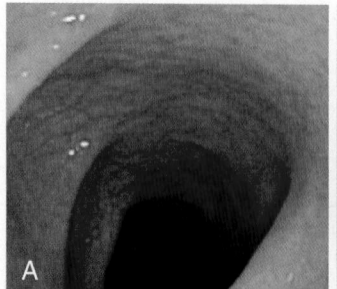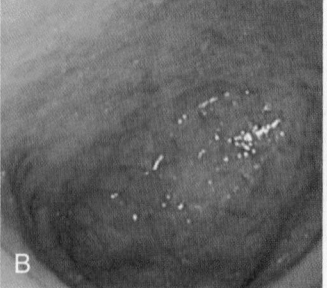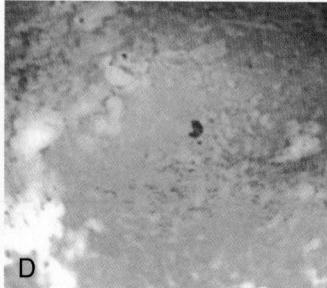

Figure 336-1 Mayo endoscopic score for ulcerative colitis. **A,** Score 0 = normal; endoscopic remission. **B,** Score 1 = mild; erythema, decreased vascular pattern, mild friability. **C,** Score 2 = moderate; marked erythema, absent vascular pattern, friability, erosions. **D,** Score 3 = severe; spontaneous bleeding, ulceration. *(Images courtesy of Elena Ricart. From Ordàs I, Eckmann L, Talamini M, et al: Ulcerative colitis, Lancet 380:1606–1616, 2012, Fig. 2, p. 1610.)*

| Table 336-4 | Infectious Agents Mimicking Inflammatory Bowel Disease |

AGENT	MANIFESTATIONS	DIAGNOSIS	COMMENTS
BACTERIAL			
Campylobacter jejuni	Acute diarrhea, fever, fecal blood, and leukocytes	Culture	Common in adolescents, may relapse
Yersinia enterocolitica	Acute → chronic diarrhea, right lower quadrant pain, mesenteric adenitis–pseudoappendicitis, fecal blood, and leukocytes	Culture	Common in adolescents as fever of unknown origin, weight loss, abdominal pain
	Extraintestinal manifestations, mimics Crohn disease		
Clostridium difficile	Postantibiotic onset, watery → bloody diarrhea, pseudomembrane on sigmoidoscopy	Cytotoxin assay	May be nosocomial Toxic megacolon possible
Escherichia coli O157:H7	Colitis, fecal blood, abdominal pain	Culture and typing	Hemolytic uremic syndrome
Salmonella	Watery → bloody diarrhea, foodborne, fecal leukocytes, fever, pain, cramps	Culture	Usually acute
Shigella	Watery → bloody diarrhea, fecal leukocytes, fever, pain, cramps	Culture	Dysentery symptoms
Edwardsiella tarda	Bloody diarrhea, cramps	Culture	Ulceration on endoscopy
Aeromonas hydrophila	Cramps, diarrhea, fecal blood	Culture	May be chronic Contaminated drinking water
Plesiomonas shigelloides	Diarrhea, cramps	Culture	Shellfish source
Tuberculosis	Rarely bovine, now *Mycobacterium tuberculosis*	Culture, purified protein derivative, biopsy	Can mimic Crohn disease
	Ileocecal area, fistula formation		
PARASITES			
Entamoeba histolytica	Acute bloody diarrhea and liver abscess, colic	Trophozoite in stool, colonic mucosal flask ulceration, serologic tests	Travel to endemic area
Giardia lamblia	Foul-smelling, watery diarrhea, cramps, flatulence, weight loss; no colonic involvement	"Owl"-like trophozoite and cysts in stool; rarely duodenal intubation	May be chronic
AIDS-ASSOCIATED ENTEROPATHY			
Cryptosporidium	Chronic diarrhea, weight loss	Stool microscopy	Mucosal findings not like inflammatory bowel disease
Isospora belli	As in *Cryptosporidium*		Tropical location
Cytomegalovirus	Colonic ulceration, pain, bloody diarrhea	Culture, biopsy	More common when on immunosuppressive medications

plan of management remain unresolved. The original studies may have overestimated the risk of colon cancer and, therefore, the need for surveillance has been overemphasized; and screening for dysplasia might not be adequate for preventing colon cancer in ulcerative colitis if some cancers are not preceded by dysplasia.

DIFFERENTIAL DIAGNOSIS

The major conditions to exclude are infectious colitis, allergic colitis, and Crohn colitis. Every child with a new diagnosis of ulcerative colitis should have stool cultured for enteric pathogens, stool evaluation for *Clostridium difficile*, ova and parasites, and perhaps serologic studies for amebae (Table 336-4). Cytomegalovirus infection can mimic ulcerative colitis or be associated with an exacerbation of existing disease, usually in immunocompromised patients. The most difficult distinction is from Crohn disease because the colitis of Crohn disease can initially appear identical to that of ulcerative colitis, particularly in younger children. The gross appearance of the colitis or development of small bowel disease eventually leads to the correct diagnosis; this can occur years after the initial presentation.

At the onset, the colitis of hemolytic uremic syndrome may be identical to that of early ulcerative colitis. Ultimately, signs of microangiopathic hemolysis (the presence of schistocytes on blood smear), thrombocytopenia, and subsequent renal failure should confirm the diagnosis of hemolytic-uremic syndrome. Although Henoch-Schönlein purpura can manifest as abdominal pain and bloody stools, it is not usually associated with colitis. Behçet disease can be distinguished by its typical features (see Chapter 161). Other considerations are radiation proctitis, viral colitis in immunocompromised patients, and ischemic colitis (Table 336-5). In infancy, dietary protein intolerance can be confused with ulcerative colitis, although the former is a transient problem that resolves on removal of the offending protein, and ulcerative colitis is extremely rare in this age group. Hirschsprung disease can produce an enterocolitis before or within months after surgical correction; this is unlikely to be confused with ulcerative colitis.

DIAGNOSIS

The diagnosis of ulcerative colitis or ulcerative proctitis requires a typical presentation in the absence of an identifiable specific cause (see Tables 336-4 and 336-5) and typical endoscopic and histologic findings (see Tables 336-1 and 336-2). One should be hesitant to make a diagnosis of ulcerative colitis in a child who has experienced symptoms for <2-3 wk until infection has been excluded. When the diagnosis is suspected in a child with subacute symptoms, the physician should make a firm diagnosis only when there is evidence of chronicity on colonic biopsy. Laboratory studies can demonstrate evidence of anemia (either iron deficiency or the anemia of chronic disease) or hypoalbuminemia. Although the sedimentation rate and C-reactive protein are often elevated, they may be normal even with fulminant colitis. An elevated white blood cell count is usually seen only with more-severe colitis. Fecal calprotectin levels are usually elevated and are increasingly recognized to be a more sensitive and specific marker of GI inflammation than typical laboratory parameters. Barium enema is suggestive but not diagnostic of acute (Fig. 336-2) or chronic burned-out disease (Fig. 336-3).

The diagnosis of ulcerative colitis must be confirmed by endoscopic and histologic examination of the colon (see Fig. 336-1). Classically, disease starts in the rectum with a gross appearance characterized by erythema, edema, loss of vascular pattern, granularity, and friability. There may be a "cutoff" demarcating the margin between inflammation and normal colon, or the entire colon may be involved. There may

Table 336-5	Chronic Inflammatory-Like Intestinal Disorders Including Monogenetic Diseases

INFECTION (see Table 336-4)
AIDS-Associated
Toxin
Immune–Inflammatory
Severe combined immunodeficiency diseases
Agammaglobulinemia
Chronic granulomatous disease
Wiskott-Aldrich syndrome
Common variable immunodeficiency diseases
Acquired immunodeficiency states
Dietary protein enterocolitis
Autoimmune polyendocrine syndrome type 1
Behçet disease
Lymphoid nodular hyperplasia
Eosinophilic gastroenteritis
Omenn syndrome
Graft-versus-host disease
IPEX (immune dysfunction, polyendocrinopathy, enteropathy, X-linked) syndromes
Interleukin-10 signaling defects
Autoimmune enteropathy*
Microscopic colitis
Hyperimmunoglobulin M syndrome
Hyperimmunoglobulin E syndromes
Mevalonate kinase deficiency
Familial Mediterranean fever
Phospholipase $C\gamma_2$ defects
Familial hemophagocytic lymphohistiocytosis type 5
X-linked lymphoproliferative syndromes types 1, 2
Congenital neutropenias
Leukocyte adhesion deficiency 1

VASCULAR–ISCHEMIC DISORDERS
Systemic vasculitis (systemic lupus erythematosus, dermatomyositis)
Henoch-Schönlein purpura
Hemolytic uremic syndrome
Granulomatosis with angiitis

OTHER
Glycogen storage disease type 1b
Dystrophic epidermolysis bullosa
X-linked ectodermal dysplasia and immunodeficiency
Dyskeratosis congenita
ADAM-17 deficiency
Prestenotic colitis
Diversion colitis
Radiation colitis
Neonatal necrotizing enterocolitis
Typhlitis
Sarcoidosis
Hirschsprung colitis
Intestinal lymphoma
Laxative abuse
Endometriosis
Hermansky-Pudlak syndrome
Trichohepatoenteric syndrome
PTEN hamartoma syndrome

*May be the same as IPEX.

be some variability in the intensity of inflammation even in those areas involved. Flexible sigmoidoscopy can confirm the diagnosis; colonoscopy can evaluate the extent of disease and rule out Crohn colitis. A colonoscopy should not be performed when fulminant colitis is suspected because of the risk of provoking *toxic megacolon* or causing a perforation during the procedure. The degree of colitis can be evaluated by the gross appearance of the mucosa. One does not generally see discrete ulcers, which would be more suggestive of Crohn colitis. The endoscopic findings of ulcerative colitis result from microulcers, which give the appearance of a diffuse abnormality. With very severe chronic colitis, pseudopolyps may be seen. Biopsy of involved bowel demonstrates evidence of acute and chronic mucosal inflammation.

Typical histologic findings are cryptitis, crypt abscesses, separation of crypts by inflammatory cells, foci of acute inflammatory cells, edema, mucus depletion, and branching of crypts. The last finding is not seen in infectious colitis. Granulomas, fissures, or full-thickness involvement of the bowel wall (usually on surgical rather than endoscopic biopsy) suggests Crohn disease.

Perianal disease, with the exception of mild local irritation or anal fissures associated with diarrhea, should make the clinician think of Crohn disease. Plain radiographs of the abdomen might demonstrate loss of haustral markings in an air-filled colon or marked dilation with toxic megacolon. With severe colitis, the colon may become dilated; a diameter of >6 cm, determined radiographically, in an adult suggests toxic megacolon. If it is necessary to examine the colon radiologically in a child with severe colitis (to evaluate the extent of involvement or to try to rule out Crohn disease), it is sometimes helpful to perform an upper GI contrast series with small bowel follow-through and then look at delayed films of the colon. A barium enema is contraindicated in the setting of a potential toxic megacolon.

TREATMENT
Medical

A medical cure for ulcerative colitis is not available; treatment is aimed at controlling symptoms and reducing the risk of recurrence, with a secondary goal of minimizing steroid exposure. The intensity of treatment varies with the severity of the symptoms.

The first drug class to be used with mild or mild-to-moderate colitis is an aminosalicylate. Sulfasalazine is composed of a sulfur moiety linked to the active ingredient 5-aminosalicylate (5-ASA). This linkage prevents the premature absorption of the medication in the upper GI tract, allowing it to reach the colon, where the 2 components are separated by bacterial cleavage. The dose of sulfasalazine is 50-75 mg/kg/24 hr (divided into 2-4 doses). Generally, the dose is not more than 2-4 g/24 hr. Hypersensitivity to the sulfa component is the major side effect of sulfasalazine and occurs in 10-20% of patients. Because of poor tolerance, sulfasalazine is used less commonly than other, better tolerated 5-ASA preparations (mesalamine, 50-100 mg/kg/day; balsalazide 110-175 mg/kg/day). Sulfasalazine and the 5-ASA preparations effectively treat active ulcerative colitis and prevent recurrence. It is recommended that the medication be continued even when the disorder is in remission. These medications might also decrease the lifetime risk of colon cancer.

Approximately 5% of patients have an allergic reaction to 5-ASA, manifesting as rash, fever, and bloody diarrhea, which can be difficult to distinguish from symptoms of a flare of ulcerative colitis. 5-ASA can also be given in enema or suppository form and is especially useful for proctitis. Hydrocortisone enemas are used to treat proctitis as well, but they are probably not as effective. A combination of oral and rectal 5-ASA as well as monotherapy with rectal preparation has been shown to be more effective than just oral 5-ASA for distal colitis. Extended release budesonide may also induce remission in patients with mild to moderate ulcerative colitis.

Probiotics are effective in adults for maintenance of remission for ulcerative colitis, although they do not induce remission during an active flare. The most promising role for probiotics has been to prevent pouchitis, a common complication following colectomy and ileal–pouch anal anastomosis surgery.

Children with moderate to severe pancolitis or colitis that is unresponsive to 5-ASA therapy should be treated with corticosteroids, most commonly, prednisone. The usual starting dose of prednisone is 1-2 mg/kg/24 hr (40-60 mg maximum dose). This medication can be given once daily. With severe colitis, the dose can be divided twice daily and can be given intravenously. Steroids are considered an effective medication for acute flares, but they are not appropriate maintenance medications because of loss of effect and side effects, including growth retardation, adrenal suppression, cataracts, osteopenia, aseptic necrosis of the head of the femur, glucose intolerance, risk of infection, mood disturbance, and cosmetic effects.

For a hospitalized patient with persistence of symptoms despite intravenous steroid treatment for 3-5 days, escalation of therapy or

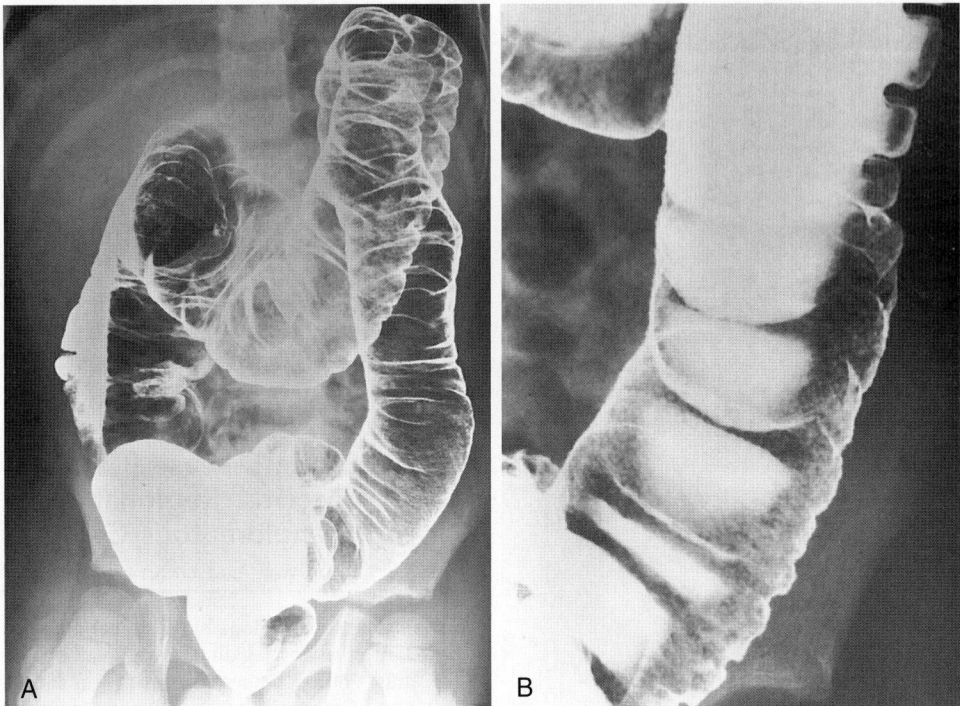

Figure 336-2 Ulcerative colitis. Double-contrast barium enema in a 5 yr old boy who had had intermittent intestinal and extraintestinal symptoms since the age of 3 yr. **A,** Small ulcerations are distributed uniformly about the colonic circumference and continuously from the rectum to the proximal transverse colon. This pattern of involvement is typical of ulcerative colitis. **B,** In this coned view of the sigmoid in the same patient, small ulcerations are represented by fine spiculation of the colonic contour in tangent and by fine stippling of the colon surface en face. *(From The child with diarrhea. In Hoffman AD, Hilton SW, Edwards DK, editors: Practical pediatric radiology, ed 2, Philadelphia, 1994, WB Saunders, p. 260.)*

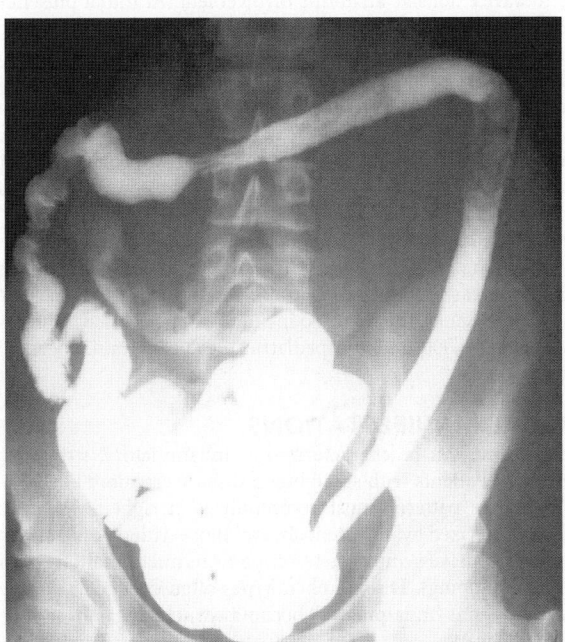

Figure 336-3 Ulcerative colitis: late changes. This single-contrast barium enema shows the late changes of ulcerative colitis in a 15 yr old girl. The colon is featureless, reduced in caliber, and shortened. Dilation of the terminal ileum (backwash ileitis) is present. *(From The child with diarrhea. In Hoffman AD, Hilton SW, Edwards DK, editors: Practical pediatric radiology, ed 2, Philadelphia, 1994, WB Saunders, p 262.)*

surgical options should be considered. The validated pediatric ulcerative colitis activity index can be utilized to help determine current disease severity based on clinical factors, and help determine who is more likely to respond to steroids and those who will likely require escalation of therapy (Table 336-6).

With medical management, most children are in remission within 3 mo; however, 5-10% continue to have symptoms unresponsive to treatment beyond 6 mo. Many children with disease requiring frequent corticosteroid therapy are started on immunomodulators such as azathioprine (2.0-2.5 mg/kg/day) or 6-mercaptopurine (1-1.5 mg/kg/day). Uncontrolled data suggest a corticosteroid-sparing effect in many treated patients. This is not an appropriate choice in a steroid nonresponsive patient with acute severe colitis because of longer onset of action. Lymphoproliferative disorders are associated with thiopurine use. Cyclosporine, which is associated with improvement in some children with severe or fulminant colitis, is rarely used owing to its high side-effect profile, its inability to change the natural history of disease, and the increasing use of infliximab, a chimeric monoclonal antibody to tumor necrosis factor (TNF)-α, which is also effective in cases of fulminant colitis. Infliximab is effective for induction and maintenance therapy in adults with moderate to severe disease. TNF blocking agents are associated with an increased risk of infection (particularly tuberculosis) and malignancies (lymphoma, leukemia). Adalimumab is also approved for treatment of moderate to severe ulcerative colitis in adults. Vedolizumab, a humanized monoclonal antibody that inhibits adhesion and migration of leukocytes into the gastrointestinal tract, is approved for the treatment of ulcerative colitis in adults. Tofacitinib, an oral Janus kinase inhibitor, is undergoing trials in adults with active moderate to severe ulcerative colitis.

Surgical

Colectomy is performed for intractable disease, complications of therapy, and fulminant disease that is unresponsive to medical management. No clear benefit of the use of total parenteral nutrition or a

Table 336-6	Pediatric Ulcerative Colitis Activity Index	
ITEM		**POINTS**
(1) *Abdominal pain*		
	No pain	0
	Pain can be ignored	5
	Pain cannot be ignored	10
(2) *Rectal bleeding*		
	None	0
	Small amount only, in <50% of stools	10
	Small amount with most stools	20
	Large amount (>50% of the stool content)	30
(3) *Stool consistency of most stools*		
	Formed	0
	Partially formed	5
	Completely unformed	10
(4) *Number of stools per 24 h*		
	0-2	0
	3-5	5
	6-8	10
	>8	15
(5) *Nocturnal stools (any episode causing wakening)*		
	No	0
	Yes	10
(6) *Activity level*		
	No limitation of activity	0
	Occasional limitation of activity	5
	Severe restricted activity	10
Sum of Index (0-85)		

continuous enteral elemental diet in the treatment of severe ulcerative colitis has been noted. Nevertheless, parenteral nutrition is used if oral intake is insufficient so that the patient will be nutritionally ready for surgery if medical management fails. With any medical treatment for ulcerative colitis, the clinician should always weigh the risk of the medication or therapy against the fact that colitis can be successfully treated surgically.

Surgical treatment for intractable or fulminant colitis is total colectomy. The optimal approach is to combine colectomy with an endorectal pull-through, where a segment of distal rectum is retained and the mucosa is stripped from this region. The distal ileum is pulled down and sutured at the internal anus with a J pouch created from ileum immediately above the rectal cuff. This procedure allows the child to maintain continence. Commonly, a temporary ileostomy is created to protect the delicate anastomosis between the sleeve of the pouch and the rectum. The ileostomy is usually closed within several months, restoring bowel continuity. At that time, stool frequency is often increased but may be improved with loperamide. The major complication of this operation is *pouchitis*, which is a chronic inflammatory reaction in the pouch, leading to bloody diarrhea, abdominal pain, and, occasionally, low-grade fever. The cause of this complication is unknown, although it is more common when the ileal pouch has been constructed for ulcerative colitis than for other indications (e.g., familial polyposis coli). Pouchitis is seen in 30-40% of patients who had ulcerative colitis. It commonly responds to treatment with oral metronidazole or ciprofloxacin. Probiotics have also been shown to decrease the rate of pouchitis as well as the recurrence of pouchitis following antibiotic therapy.

Support
Psychosocial support is an important part of therapy for this disorder. This may include adequate discussion of the disease manifestations and management between patient and physician, psychologic counseling for the child when necessary, and family support from a social worker or family counselor. Patient support groups have proved helpful for some families. Children with ulcerative colitis should be encouraged to participate fully in age-appropriate activities; however, activity may need to be reduced during periods of disease exacerbation.

PROGNOSIS
The course of ulcerative colitis is marked by remissions and exacerbations. Most children with this disorder respond initially to medical management. Many children with mild manifestations continue to respond well to medical management and may stay in remission on a prophylactic 5-ASA preparation for long periods. An occasional child with mild onset, however, experiences intractable symptoms at a later time. Beyond the 1st decade of disease, the risk of development of colon cancer begins to increase rapidly. The risk of colon cancer may be diminished with surveillance colonoscopies beginning after 8-10 yr of disease. Detection of significant dysplasia on biopsy would prompt colectomy.

Bibliography is available at Expert Consult.

336.2 Crohn Disease (Regional Enteritis, Regional Ileitis, Granulomatous Colitis)
Andrew B. Grossman and Robert N. Baldassano

Crohn disease, an idiopathic, chronic inflammatory disorder of the bowel, involves any region of the alimentary tract from the mouth to the anus. Although there are many similarities between ulcerative colitis and Crohn disease, there are also major differences in the clinical course and distribution of the disease in the GI tract (see Table 336-1). The inflammatory process tends to be eccentric and segmental, often with skip areas (normal regions of bowel between inflamed areas). Although inflammation in ulcerative colitis is limited to the mucosa (except in toxic megacolon), GI involvement in Crohn disease is often transmural.

Compared to adult-onset disease, pediatric Crohn disease is more likely to have extensive anatomic involvement. At initial presentation, more than 50% of patients have disease that involves ileum and colon (ileocolitis), 20% have exclusively colonic disease, and upper GI involvement (esophagus, stomach, duodenum) is seen in up to 30% of children. Isolated small bowel disease is much less common in the pediatric population compared to adults. Isolated colonic disease is common in children younger than 8 yr of age and may be indistinguishable from ulcerative colitis. Anatomic location of disease tends to extend over time in children.

Crohn disease tends to have a bimodal age distribution, with the first peak beginning in the teenage years. The incidence of Crohn disease has been increasing, whereas that of ulcerative colitis has been stable. In the United States, the reported incidence of pediatric Crohn disease is 4.56 per 100,000 and the pediatric prevalence is 43 per 100,000 children.

CLINICAL MANIFESTATIONS
Crohn disease can be characterized as inflammatory, stricturing, or penetrating. Patients with small bowel disease are more likely to have an obstructive pattern (most commonly with right lower quadrant pain) characterized by fibrostenosis, and those with colonic disease are more likely to have symptoms resulting from inflammation (diarrhea, bleeding, cramping). Disease phenotypes often change as duration of disease lengthens (inflammatory becomes structuring and/or penetrating) (Fig. 336-4).

Systemic signs and symptoms are more common in Crohn disease than in ulcerative colitis. Fever, malaise, and easy fatigability are common. Growth failure with delayed bone maturation and delayed sexual development can precede other symptoms by 1 or 2 yr and is at least twice as likely to occur with Crohn disease as with ulcerative colitis. Children can present with growth failure as the only manifestation of Crohn disease. Decreased height velocity occurs in about 88% of prepubertal patients diagnosed with Crohn disease, and this often precedes GI symptoms. Causes of growth failure include inadequate caloric intake, suboptimal absorption or excessive loss of nutrients, the

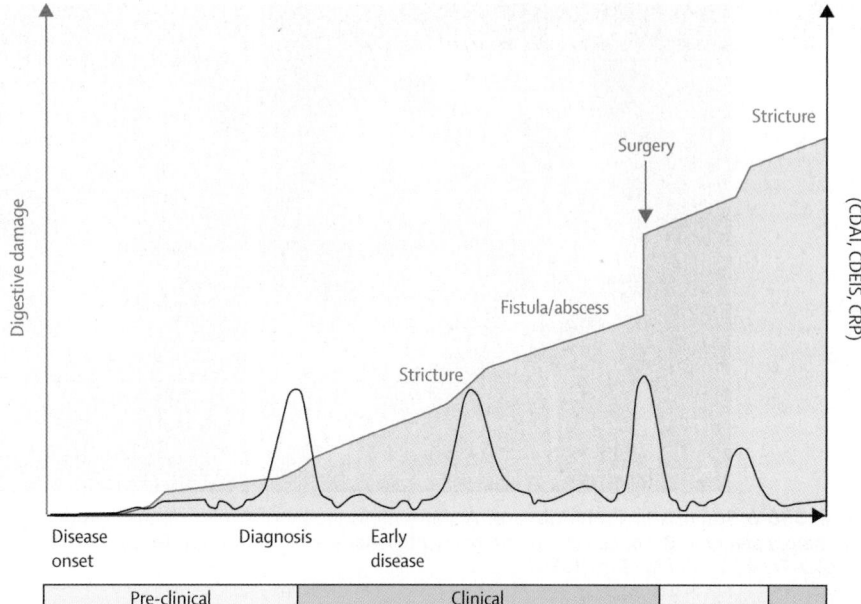

Figure 336-4 The Lémann Score. Exemplary visualization of the Lémann score, a new technique to score and study intestinal damage in Crohn disease. *CDAI,* Crohn disease activity index; *CDEIS,* Crohn disease of endoscopic severity; *CRP,* C-reactive protein. *(From Baumgart DC, Sandborn WJ: Crohn's disease. Lancet 380:1590–1602, 2012, Fig. 5, p. 1596.)*

effects of chronic inflammation on bone metabolism and appetite, and the use of corticosteroids during treatment. Primary or secondary amenorrhea and pubertal delay are common. In contrast to ulcerative colitis, perianal disease is common (tag, fistula, deep fissure, abscess). Gastric or duodenal involvement may be associated with recurrent vomiting and epigastric pain. Partial small bowel obstruction, usually secondary to narrowing of the bowel lumen from inflammation or stricture, can cause symptoms of cramping abdominal pain (especially with meals), borborygmus, and intermittent abdominal distention (Figs. 336-5 and 336-6). Stricture should be suspected if the child notes relief of symptoms in association with a sudden sensation of gurgling of intestinal contents through a localized region of the abdomen.

Penetrating disease is demonstrated by fistula formation. Enteroenteric or enterocolonic fistulas (between segments of bowel) are often asymptomatic but can contribute to malabsorption if they have high output or result in bacterial overgrowth (Fig. 336-7). Enterovesical fistulas (between bowel and urinary bladder) originate from ileum or sigmoid colon and appear as signs of urinary infection, pneumaturia, or fecaluria. Enterovaginal fistulas originate from the rectum, cause feculent vaginal drainage, and are difficult to manage. Enterocutaneous fistulas (between bowel and abdominal skin) often are caused by prior surgical anastomoses with leakage. Intraabdominal abscess may be associated with fever and pain but might have relatively few symptoms. Hepatic or splenic abscess can occur with or without a local fistula. Anorectal abscesses often originate immediately above the anus at the crypts of Morgagni. The patterns of perianal fistulas are complex because of the different tissue planes. Perianal abscess is usually painful, but perianal fistulas tend to produce fewer symptoms than anticipated. Purulent drainage is commonly associated with perianal fistulas. **Psoas abscess** secondary to intestinal fistula can present as hip pain, decreased hip extension (psoas sign), and fever.

Extraintestinal manifestations occur more commonly with Crohn disease than with ulcerative colitis; those that are especially associated with Crohn disease include oral aphthous ulcers, peripheral arthritis, erythema nodosum, digital clubbing, episcleritis, renal stones (uric acid, oxalate), and gallstones. Any of the extraintestinal disorders described in the section on IBD can occur with Crohn disease (see Table 336-2). The peripheral arthritis is nondeforming. The occurrence of extraintestinal manifestations usually correlates with the presence of colitis.

Extensive involvement of small bowel, especially in association with surgical resection, can lead to short bowel syndrome, which is rare in children. Complications of terminal ileal dysfunction or resection

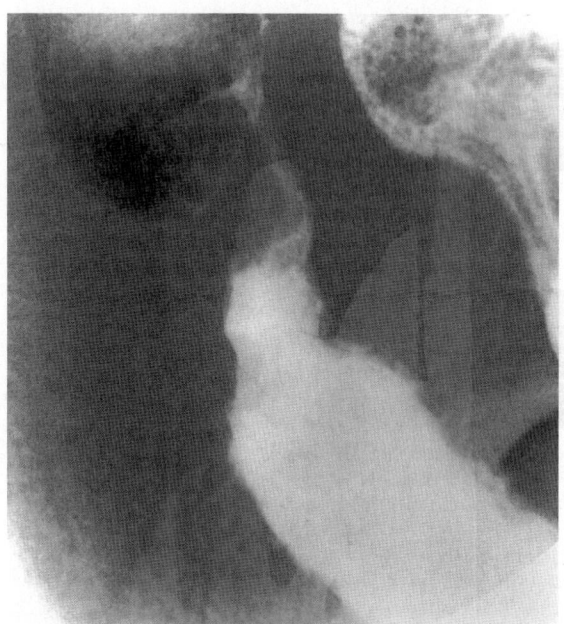

Figure 336-5 Stenotic Crohn disease. Severe stenosis of the terminal ileum is present in this 16 yr old boy. Inflammatory effacement of the mucosal folds and small ulcerations characterize the proximal nonstenotic segment. *(From The child with diarrhea. In Hoffman AD, Hilton SW, Edwards DK, editors:* Practical pediatric radiology, *ed 2, Philadelphia, 1994, WB Saunders, p. 267.)*

include bile acid malabsorption with secondary diarrhea and vitamin B_{12} malabsorption, with possible resultant deficiency. Chronic steatorrhea can lead to oxaluria with secondary renal stones. Increasing calcium intake can actually decrease the risk renal stones secondary to ileal inflammation. The risk of cholelithiasis is also increased secondary to bile acid depletion.

A disorder with this diversity of manifestations can have a major impact on an affected child's lifestyle. Fortunately, the majority of children with Crohn disease are able to continue with their normal activities, having to limit activity only during periods of increased symptoms.

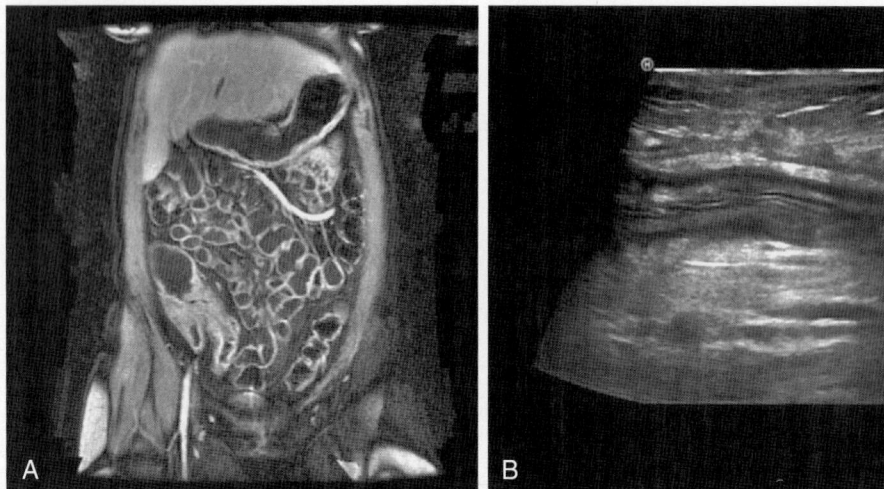

Figure 336-6 Stenosis in Crohn disease. **A,** MR enterography of Crohn disease restricted to the terminal ileum (Montreal category L1) with inflammatory stenosis. **B,** Ultrasound image of an intestinal stenosis in Crohn disease. *(From Baumgart DC, Sandborn WJ: Crohn's disease.* Lancet *380:1590–1602, 2012, Fig. 4, p. 1596.)*

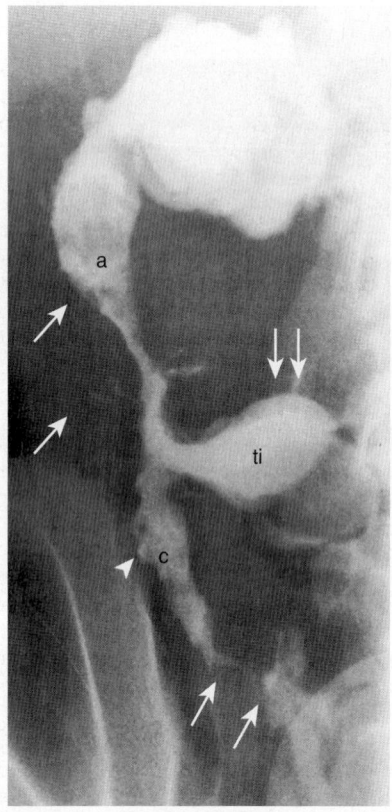

Figure 336-7 Crohn disease: sinuses and fistula. Severe ileocolitis has resulted in an ileocecal fistula *(single arrows, lower)* and sinus formation in the ascending colon (a) *(arrows on platform)*. c, Cecum *(arrowhead); ti,* terminal ileum *(paired arrows). (From The child with diarrhea. In Hoffman AD, Hilton SW, Edwards DK, editors: Practical pediatric radiology, ed 2, Philadelphia, 1994, WB Saunders, p 268.)*

DIFFERENTIAL DIAGNOSIS

The most common diagnoses to be distinguished from Crohn disease are the infectious enteropathies (in the case of Crohn disease: acute terminal ileitis, infectious colitis, enteric parasites, and periappendiceal abscess) (see Tables 336-4, 336-5, and 336-7). *Yersinia* can cause many of the radiologic and endoscopic findings in the distal small bowel that are seen in Crohn disease. The symptoms of bacterial dysentery are

more likely to be mistaken for ulcerative colitis than for Crohn disease. Celiac disease and *Giardia* infection have been noted to produce a Crohn-like presentation including diarrhea, weight loss, and protein-losing enteropathy. GI tuberculosis is rare but can mimic Crohn disease. Foreign-body perforation of the bowel (toothpick) can mimic a localized region with Crohn disease. Small bowel lymphoma can mimic Crohn disease but tends to be associated with nodular filling defects of the bowel without ulceration or narrowing of the lumen. Bowel lymphoma is much less common in children than is Crohn disease. Recurrent functional abdominal pain can mimic the pain of small bowel Crohn disease. *Lymphoid nodular hyperplasia* of the terminal ileum (a normal finding) may be mistaken for Crohn ileitis. Right lower quadrant pain or mass with fever can be the result of periappendiceal abscess. This entity is occasionally associated with diarrhea as well.

Growth failure may be the only manifestation of Crohn disease; other disorders such as growth hormone deficiency, gluten-sensitive enteropathy (celiac disease), Turner syndrome, or anorexia nervosa must be considered. If arthritis precedes the bowel manifestations, an initial diagnosis of juvenile idiopathic arthritis may be made. Refractory anemia may be the presenting feature and may be mistaken for a primary hematologic disorder. Chronic granulomatous disease of childhood can cause inflammatory changes in the bowel as well as perianal disease. Antral narrowing in this disorder may be mistaken for a stricture secondary to Crohn disease. Other immunodeficiencies or autoinflammatory conditions and monogenetic disorders may present with GI symptoms suggestive of IBD, particularly in very early or infant/toddler onset of disease (see Table 336-5).

DIAGNOSIS

Crohn disease can manifest as a variety of symptom combinations. At the onset, symptoms may be subtle (growth retardation, abdominal pain alone); this explains why the diagnosis might not be made until 1 or 2 yr after the start of symptoms. The diagnosis of Crohn disease depends on finding typical clinical features of the disorder (history, physical examination, laboratory studies, and endoscopic or radiologic findings), ruling out specific entities that mimic Crohn disease, and demonstrating chronicity. The history can include any combination of abdominal pain (especially right lower quadrant), diarrhea, vomiting, anorexia, weight loss, growth retardation, and extraintestinal manifestations. Only 25% initially have the triad of diarrhea, weight loss, and abdominal pain. Most do not have diarrhea, and only 25% have GI bleeding.

Children with Crohn disease often appear chronically ill. They commonly have weight loss and growth failure, and they are often

Table 336-7	Differential Diagnosis of Presenting Symptoms of Crohn Disease
PRIMARY PRESENTING SYMPTOM	**DIAGNOSTIC CONSIDERATIONS**
Right lower quadrant abdominal pain, with or without mass	Appendicitis, infection (e.g., *Campylobacter, Yersinia* spp.), lymphoma, intussusception, mesenteric adenitis, Meckel diverticulum, ovarian cyst
Chronic periumbilical or epigastric abdominal pain	Irritable bowel syndrome, constipation, lactose intolerance, peptic disease
Rectal bleeding, no diarrhea	Fissure, polyp, Meckel diverticulum, rectal ulcer syndrome
Bloody diarrhea	Infection, hemolytic-uremic syndrome, Henoch-Schönlein purpura, ischemic bowel, radiation colitis
Watery diarrhea	Irritable bowel syndrome, lactose intolerance, giardiasis, *Cryptosporidium* infection, sorbitol, laxatives
Perirectal disease	Fissure, hemorrhoid (rare), streptococcal infection, condyloma (rare)
Growth delay	Endocrinopathy
Anorexia, weight loss	Anorexia nervosa
Arthritis	Collagen vascular disease, infection
Liver abnormalities	Chronic hepatitis

From Kugathasan S: Diarrhea. In Kliegman RM, Greenbaum LA, Lye PS, editors: Practical strategies in pediatric diagnosis and therapy, ed 2, Philadelphia, 2004, WB Saunders, p. 287.

malnourished. The earliest sign of growth failure is decreased height velocity, which can be present in up to 88% of prepubertal patients with Crohn disease and typically precedes symptoms. Children with Crohn disease often appear pale, with decreased energy level and poor appetite; the latter finding sometimes results from an association between meals and abdominal pain or diarrhea. There may be abdominal tenderness that is either diffuse or localized to the right lower quadrant. A tender mass or fullness may be palpable in the right lower quadrant. Perianal disease, when present, may be characteristic. Large anal skin tags (1-3 cm diameter) or perianal fistulas with purulent drainage suggest Crohn disease. Digital clubbing, findings of arthritis, and skin manifestations may be present.

A complete blood cell count commonly demonstrates anemia, often with a component of iron deficiency, as well as thrombocytosis. Although the erythrocyte sedimentation rate and C-reactive protein are often elevated, they may be unremarkable. The serum albumin level may be low, indicating small bowel inflammation or protein-losing enteropathy. Fecal calprotectin and lactoferrin are increasingly being utilized as more sensitive and specific markers of bowel inflammation as compared to serologic parameters, and these are often elevated. Multiple serologic, immune, and genetic markers can also be abnormal, although the best utilization of these remains to be determined.

The small and large bowel and the upper GI tract should be examined by both endoscopic and radiologic studies in the child with suspected Crohn disease. Esophagogastroduodenoscopy and ileocolonoscopy should be performed to properly assess the upper GI tract, terminal ileum, and entire colon. Findings on colonoscopy can include patchy, nonspecific inflammatory changes (erythema, friability, loss of vascular pattern), aphthous ulcers, linear ulcers, nodularity, and strictures. Findings on biopsy may be only nonspecific chronic inflammatory changes. Noncaseating granulomas, similar to those of sarcoidosis, are the most characteristic histologic findings, although often they are not present. Transmural inflammation is also characteristic but can be identified only in surgical specimens.

Radiologic studies are necessary to assess the entire small bowel and investigate for evidence of structuring or penetrating disease. A variety of findings may be apparent on radiologic studies. Plain films of the abdomen may be normal or might demonstrate findings of partial small bowel obstruction or thumbprinting of the colon wall. An upper GI contrast study with small bowel follow-through might show aphthous ulceration and thickened, nodular folds as well as narrowing or stricturing of the lumen. Linear ulcers can give a cobblestone appearance to the mucosal surface. Bowel loops are often separated as a result of thickening of bowel wall and mesentery. Other manifestations on radiographic studies that suggest more-severe Crohn disease are

fistulas between bowel (enteroenteric or enterocolonic), sinus tracts, and strictures (see Figs. 336-5, 336-6, and 336-7).

An upper GI contrast examination with small bowel follow-through has typically been the study of choice for imaging of the small bowel, but CT and MR enterography and small bowel ultrasound are increasingly being used. MR and ultrasound have the advantage of not exposing the patient to ionizing radiation. CT and MR enterography can also assess for extraluminal findings such as abscesses and phlegmons. MR of the pelvis is also useful for delineating the extent of perianal involvement.

Video capsule endoscopy is another modality that allows for evaluation of the small bowel. This study can uncover mucosal inflammation or ulceration that might not have been detected by traditional imaging.

TREATMENT
Crohn disease cannot be cured by medical or surgical therapy. The aim of treatment is to relieve symptoms and prevent complications of chronic inflammation (anemia, growth failure), prevent relapse, minimize corticosteroid exposure, and, if possible, effect mucosal healing.

Medical
The specific therapeutic modalities used depend on geographic localization of disease, severity of inflammation, age of the patient, and the presence of complications (abscess). Traditionally, a "step-up" treatment paradigm has been utilized in the treatment of pediatric Crohn disease, whereby early disease is treated with steroids and less immunosuppressive medications. Escalation of therapy would occur if disease severity increased, the patient was refractory to current medications, or for steroid dependence. More recently, a "top-down" approach has been espoused, particularly in adults after multiple studies demonstrated superior efficacy. With this approach, patients with moderate to severe Crohn disease are treated initially with stronger, disease modifying agents, with the goal of achieving mucosal healing, or deep remission, early in the disease course. This is thought to increase the likelihood of long-term remission while decreasing corticosteroid exposure. The role for this approach in pediatrics is still being determined, but top down treatment is being increasingly utilized.

5-Aminosalicylates
For mild terminal ileal disease or mild Crohn disease of the colon, an initial trial of mesalamine (50-100 mg/kg/day, maximum 3-4 g) may be attempted. Specific pharmaceutical preparations have been formulated to release the active 5-ASA compound throughout the small bowel, in the ileum and colon, or exclusively in the colon. Rectal preparations are used for distal colonic inflammation.

Antibiotics/Probiotics

Antibiotics such as metronidazole (10-20 mg/kg/day) are used for infectious complications, are first-line therapy for perianal disease (although perianal disease usually recurs when antibiotic is discontinued), and they may be effective for treatment of mild to moderate Crohn disease. To date, probiotics have not been shown to be effective in induction or maintenance of remission for pediatric Crohn disease.

Corticosteroids

Corticosteroids are utilized for acute exacerbations of pediatric Crohn disease because they effectively suppress acute inflammation, rapidly relieving symptoms (prednisone, 1-2 mg/kg/day, maximum 40-60 mg). The goal is to taper dosing as soon as the disease becomes quiescent. Clinicians vary in their tapering schedules, and the disease can flare during this process. There is no role for continuing corticosteroids as maintenance therapy because, in addition to their side effects, tolerance develops and steroids do not change disease course or promote healing of mucosa. A special controlled ileal-release formulation of budesonide, a corticosteroid with local antiinflammatory activity on the bowel mucosa and high hepatic first-pass metabolism, is also used for mild to moderate ileal or ileocecal disease (adult dose: 9 mg daily). Ileal-release budesonide appears to be more effective than mesalamine in the treatment of active ileocolonic disease but is less effective than prednisone. Although less effective than traditional corticosteroids, budesonide does cause less steroid-related side effects.

Immunomodulators

Approximately 70% of patients require escalation of medical therapy within in the 1st yr of pediatric Crohn disease diagnosis. Immunomodulators such as azathioprine (2.0-2.5 mg/kg/day) or 6-mercaptopurine (1.0-1.5 mg/kg/day) may be effective in some children who have a poor response to prednisone or who are steroid dependent. Because a beneficial effect of these drugs can be delayed for 3-4 mo after starting therapy, they are not helpful acutely. The early use of these agents can decrease cumulative prednisone dosages over the 1st 1-2 yr of therapy. Genetic variations in an enzyme system responsible for metabolism of these agents (thiopurine S-methyltransferase) can affect response rates and potential toxicity. Lymphoproliferative disorders have developed from thiopurine use in patients with IBD. Other common toxicities include hepatitis, pancreatitis, increased risk of skin cancer, increased risk of infection, and slightly increased risk of lymphoma.

Methotrexate is another immunomodulator that is effective in the treatment of active Crohn disease and has been shown to improve height velocity in the 1st yr of administration. The advantages of this medication include once-weekly dosing by either subcutaneous or oral route (10-15 mg/m², adult dose 25 mg weekly) and a more-rapid onset of action (6-8 wk) than azathioprine or 6-mercaptopurine. Folic acid is usually administered concomitantly to decrease medication side effects. Administration of ondansetron prior to methotrexate has been shown to diminish the risk of the most common side effect of nausea. The most common toxicity is hepatitis. The immunomodulators are effective for the treatment of perianal fistulas.

Biologic Therapy

Therapy with antibodies directed against mediators of inflammation is used for patients with Crohn disease. Infliximab, a chimeric monoclonal antibody to TNF-α, is effective for the induction and maintenance of remission and mucosal healing in chronically active moderate to severe Crohn disease, healing of perianal fistulas, steroid sparing, and preventing postoperative recurrence. Pediatric data additionally support improved growth with the administration of this medication. The onset of action of infliximab is quite rapid and it is initially given as 3 infusions over a 6 wk period (0, 2, and 6 wk), followed by maintenance dosing beginning every 8 wk. The durability of response to infliximab is variable and dose escalation (higher dose and/or decreased interval) is often necessary. Measurement of serum trough infliximab level prior to an infusion can help guide dosing decisions. Side effects include infusion reactions, increased incidence of infections (especially reactivation of latent tuberculosis), increased risk of lymphoma, and the development of autoantibodies. The development of antibodies to infliximab is associated with an increased incidence of infusion reactions and decreased durability of response. Regularly scheduled dosing of infliximab, as opposed to episodic dosing on an as-needed basis, is associated with decreased levels of antibodies to infliximab. A purified protein derivative test for tuberculosis should be done before starting infliximab.

Adalimumab, a subcutaneously administered, fully humanized monoclonal antibody against TNF-α, is effective for the treatment of chronically active moderate to severe Crohn disease in adults and children. After a loading dose, this is typically administered once every 2 wk, although dose escalation is sometimes required with this medication. Vedolizumab, a humanized monoclonal antibody that inhibits adhesion and migration of leukocytes into the gastrointestinal tract, was recently approved for the treatment of Crohn disease in adults. Antibodies against interleukins 12 and 23 antiselective adhesion molecules (ustekinumab), chemokine antagonists, and antagonist to Janus kinase 3 are currently being tested.

Enteral Nutritional Therapy

Exclusive enteral nutritional therapy, whereby all of a patient's calories are delivered via formula, is an effective primary as well as adjunctive treatment. The enteral nutritional approach is as rapid in onset of response and as effective as the other treatments. Pediatric studies have suggested similar efficacy to prednisone for improvement in clinical symptoms, but enteral nutritional therapy is superior to steroids for actual healing of mucosa. Because affected patients have poor appetite and these formulas are relatively unpalatable, they are often administered via a nasogastric or gastrostomy infusion, usually overnight. The advantages are that it is relatively free of side effects, avoids the problems associated with corticosteroid therapy, and simultaneously addresses the nutritional rehabilitation. Children can participate in normal daytime activities. A major disadvantage of this approach is that patients are not able to eat a regular diet because they are receiving all of their calories from formula. A novel approach where 80-90% of caloric needs are provided by formula, allowing children to have some food intake, has been successful. For children with growth failure, this approach may be ideal, however.

High-calorie oral supplements, although effective, are often not tolerated because of early satiety or exacerbation of symptoms (abdominal pain, vomiting, or diarrhea). Nonetheless, they should be offered to children whose weight gain is suboptimal even if they are not candidates for exclusive enteral nutritional therapy. The continuous administration of nocturnal nasogastric feedings for chronic malnutrition and growth failure has been effective with a much lower risk of complications than parenteral hyperalimentation.

Surgery

Surgical therapy should be reserved for very specific indications. Recurrence rate after bowel resection is high (>50% by 5 yr); the risk of requiring additional surgery increases with each operation. Potential complications of surgery include development of fistula or stricture, anastomotic leak, postoperative partial small bowel obstruction secondary to adhesions, and short bowel syndrome. Surgery is the treatment of choice for localized disease of small bowel or colon that is unresponsive to medical treatment, bowel perforation, fibrosed stricture with symptomatic partial small bowel obstruction, and intractable bleeding. Intraabdominal or liver abscess sometimes is successfully treated by ultrasonographic or CT-guided catheter drainage and concomitant intravenous antibiotic treatment. Open surgical drainage is necessary if this approach is not successful. Growth retardation was once considered an indication for resection; without other indications, trial of medical and/or nutritional therapy is currently preferred.

Perianal abscess often requires drainage unless it drains spontaneously. In general, perianal fistulas should be managed by a combined medical and surgical approach. Often, the surgeon places a seton through the fistula to keep the tract open and actively draining while medical therapy is administered, to help prevent the formation of a perianal abscess. A severely symptomatic perianal fistula can require fistulotomy, but this procedure should be considered only if the location allows the sphincter to remain undamaged.

The surgical approach for Crohn disease is to remove as limited a length of bowel as possible. There is no evidence that removing bowel up to margins that are free of histologic disease has a better outcome than removing only grossly involved areas. The latter approach reduces the risk of short bowel syndrome. Laparoscopic approach is increasingly being used, with decreased postoperative recovery time. One approach to symptomatic small bowel stricture has been to perform a strictureplasty rather than resection. The surgeon makes a longitudinal incision across the stricture but then closes the incision with sutures in a transverse fashion. This is ideal for short strictures without active disease. The reoperation rate is no higher with this approach than with resection, whereas bowel length is preserved. Postoperative medical therapy with agents such as mesalamine, metronidazole, azathioprine, and, more recently, infliximab, is often given to decrease the likelihood of postoperative recurrence.

Severe perianal disease can be incapacitating and difficult to treat if unresponsive to medical management. Diversion of fecal stream can allow the area to be less active, but on reconnection of the colon, disease activity usually recurs.

Support

Psychosocial issues for the child with Crohn disease include a sense of being different, concerns about body image, difficulty in not participating fully in age-appropriate activities, and family conflict brought on by the added stress of this disease. Social support is an important component of the management of Crohn disease. Parents are often interested in learning about other children with similar problems, but children may be hesitant to participate. Social support and individual psychologic counseling are important in the adjustment to a difficult problem at an age that by itself often has difficult adjustment issues. Patients who are socially "connected" fare better. Ongoing education about the disease is an important aspect of management because children generally fare better if they understand and anticipate problems. The Crohn and Colitis Foundation of America has local chapters throughout the United States and supports several regional 1-wk camps for children with Crohn disease.

PROGNOSIS

Crohn disease is a chronic disorder that is associated with high morbidity but low mortality. Symptoms tend to recur despite treatment and often without apparent explanation. Weight loss and growth failure can usually be improved with treatment and attention to nutritional needs. Up to 15% of patients with early growth retardation secondary to Crohn disease have a permanent decrease in linear growth. Osteopenia is particularly common in those with chronic poor nutrition and frequent exposure to high doses of corticosteroids. Some of the extraintestinal manifestations can, in themselves, be major causes of morbidity, including sclerosing cholangitis, chronic active hepatitis, pyoderma gangrenosum, and ankylosing spondylitis.

The region of bowel involved and complications of the inflammatory process tend to increase with time and include bowel strictures, fistulas, perianal disease, and intra-abdominal or retroperitoneal abscess. A majority of patients with Crohn disease eventually require surgery for one of its many complications; the rate of reoperation is high. Surgery is unlikely to be curative and should be avoided except for the specific indications noted previously. An earlier, most aggressive medical treatment approach, with the goal of exacting mucosal healing may improve long-term prognosis, and this is an active area of investigation. The risk of colon cancer in patients with long-standing Crohn colitis approaches that associated with ulcerative colitis, and screening colonoscopy after 10 yr of colonic disease is indicated.

Despite these complications, most children with Crohn disease lead active, full lives with intermittent flare-up in symptoms.

Bibliography is available at Expert Consult.

Chapter 337
Eosinophilic Gastroenteritis
Andrew B. Grossman and Robert N. Baldassano

Eosinophilic gastroenteritis consists of a group of rare and poorly understood disorders that have in common gastric and small intestine infiltration with eosinophils and peripheral eosinophilia. The esophagus and large intestine may also be involved. Tissue eosinophilic infiltration can be seen in mucosa, muscularis, or serosa. The mucosal form is most common and is diagnosed by identifying large numbers of eosinophils in biopsy specimens of gastric antrum or small bowel. This condition clinically overlaps the dietary protein hypersensitivity disorders of the small bowel and colon. The differential diagnosis also includes celiac disease, chronic granulomatous disease, connective tissue disorders and vasculitides, multiple infections (particularly parasites), hypereosinophilic syndrome, early inflammatory bowel disease, and rarely malignancy. Many patients have allergies to multiple foods, seasonal allergies, atopy, eczema, and asthma. Serum immunoglobulin E is commonly elevated. Peripheral eosinophilia is present in approximately 5-70% of patients with this disorder. Other laboratory abnormalities can include hypoalbuminemia, iron deficiency anemia, and elevated liver enzymes.

The presentation of eosinophilic gastroenteritis is nonspecific. Clinical symptoms often correlate with which layers of the gastrointestinal tract are affected. Mucosal involvement can produce nausea, vomiting, diarrhea, abdominal pain, gastrointestinal bleeding, protein-losing enteropathy, or malabsorption. Involvement of the muscularis can produce obstruction (especially of the pylorus) or intussusception, whereas serosal activity produces abdominal distention and eosinophilic ascites. Presentation in infants can be similar to pyloric stenosis. Laboratory testing often reveals peripheral eosinophilia, elevated serum immunoglobulin E levels, hypoalbuminemia, and anemia.

The disease usually runs a chronic, debilitating course with sporadic severe exacerbations. Although almost always effective for the treatment of isolated eosinophilic esophagitis, elemental diets are not always successful for the treatment of eosinophilic gastroenteritis. Orally administered cromolyn sodium and montelukast are sometimes successful. A majority of patients require treatment with systemic corticosteroids, which are often effective.

Bibliography is available at Expert Consult.

Chapter 338
Disorders of Malabsorption
David Branski

All disorders of malabsorption are associated with diminished intestinal absorption of one or more dietary nutrients. Malabsorption can result from a defect in the nutrient **digestion** in the intestinal lumen or from defective mucosal **absorption.** Malabsorption disorders can be categorized into generalized mucosal abnormalities usually

Table 338-1	Malabsorption Disorders and Chronic Diarrhea Associated with Generalized Mucosal Defect

Mucosal disorders
  Gluten-sensitive enteropathy (celiac disease)
  Cow's milk and other protein-sensitive enteropathies
  Eosinophilic enteropathy
Protein-losing enteropathy
  Lymphangiectasia (congenital and acquired)
  Disorders causing bowel mucosal inflammation, Crohn disease
Congenital bowel mucosal defects
  Microvillous inclusion disease
  Tufting enteropathy
  Carbohydrate-deficient glycoprotein syndrome
  Enterocyte heparan sulfate deficiency
  Enteric anendocrinosis (NEUROG 3 mutation)
  Tricho-hepatic-enteric syndrome
Immunodeficiency disorders
  Congenital immunodeficiency disorders
    Selective immunoglobulin A deficiency (can be associated with celiac disease)
    Severe combined immunodeficiency
    Agammaglobulinemia
    X-linked hypogammaglobulinemia
    Wiskott-Aldrich syndrome
    Common variable immunodeficiency disease
    Chronic granulomatous disease
  Acquired immune deficiency
    HIV infection
    Immunosuppressive therapy and post–bone marrow transplantation
Autoimmune enteropathy
  IPEX (immune dysregulation, polyendocrinopathy, enteropathy, X-linked inheritance)
  IPEX-like syndromes
  Autoimmune polyglandular syndrome type 1
Miscellaneous
  Immunoproliferative small intestinal disease
  Short bowel syndrome
  Blind loop syndrome
  Radiation enteritis
  Protein–calorie malnutrition
  Crohn disease
  Pseudoobstruction

Table 338-2	Classification of Malabsorption Disorders and Chronic Diarrhea Based on the Predominant Nutrient Malabsorbed

CARBOHYDRATE MALABSORPTION
Lactose malabsorption
Congenital lactase deficiency
Hypolactasia (adult type)
Secondary lactase deficiency
Congenital sucrase-isomaltase deficiency
Glucose galactose malabsorption

FAT MALABSORPTION
Abetalipoproteinemia
Lymphangiectasia
Homozygous hypobetalipoproteinemia
Chylomicron retention disease (Anderson disease)
Cystic fibrosis
Shwachman-Diamond syndrome
Johanson-Blizzard syndrome
Pearson syndrome
Secondary exocrine pancreatic insufficiency
Isolated enzyme deficiency
Enterokinase deficiency
Trypsinogen deficiency
Lipase/colipase deficiency
Chronic pancreatitis
Protein–calorie malnutrition
Decreased pancreozymin/cholecystokinin secretion
Disrupted enterohepatic circulation of bile salts
Cholestatic liver disease
Bile acid synthetic defects
Bile acid malabsorption (terminal ileal disease)

PROTEIN/AMINO ACID MALABSORPTION
Lysinuric protein intolerance (defect in dibasic amino acid transport)
Hartnup disease (defect in free neutral amino acids)
Blue diaper syndrome (isolated tryptophan malabsorption)
Oasthouse urine disease (defect in methionine absorption)
Lowe syndrome (lysine and arginine malabsorption)
Enterokinase deficiency

MINERAL AND VITAMIN MALABSORPTION
Congenital chloride diarrhea
Congenital sodium absorption defect
Acrodermatitis enteropathica (zinc malabsorption)
Menkes disease (copper malabsorption)
Vitamin D–dependent rickets
Folate malabsorption
Congenital
Secondary to mucosal damage (celiac disease)
Vitamin B_{12} malabsorption
Autoimmune pernicious anemia
Decreased gastric acid (H_2 blockers or proton pump inhibitors)
Terminal ileal disease (e.g., Crohn disease) or resection
Inborn errors of vitamin B_{12} transport and metabolism
Primary hypomagnesemia

DRUG INDUCED
Sulfasalazine: folic acid malabsorption
Cholestyramine: calcium and fat malabsorption
Anticonvulsant drugs such as phenytoin (causing vitamin D deficiency and folic acid and calcium malabsorption)
Gastric acid suppression: vitamin B_{12}
Methotrexate: mucosal injury

resulting in malabsorption of multiple nutrients (Table 338-1) or malabsorption of specific nutrients (carbohydrate, fat, protein, vitamins, minerals, and trace elements) (Table 338-2). Almost all the malabsorption disorders are accompanied by chronic diarrhea which further worsens the malabsorption. (see Chapter 341).

CLINICAL APPROACH

The clinical features depend on the extent and type of the malabsorbed nutrient. The common presenting features, especially in toddlers with malabsorption, are diarrhea, abdominal distention, and failure to gain weight, with a fall in growth chart percentiles. Physical findings include abdominal distention, muscle wasting, and the disappearance of the subcutaneous fat, with subsequent loose skinfolds (Fig. 338-1). The nutritional consequences of malabsorption are more dramatic in toddlers because the limited energy reserves and higher proportion of calorie intake being used for weight gain and linear growth. In older children, malnutrition can result in growth retardation, as is commonly seen in children with late diagnosis of celiac disease. If malabsorption is left untreated, linear growth slows, and with prolonged malnutrition, death can follow (see Chapter 46). This extreme outcome is usually restricted to children living in the developing world, where resources to provide enteral and parenteral nutrition support may be limited. Specific findings on examination can guide toward a specific disorder; edema is usually associated with protein-losing enteropathy, digital clubbing with cystic fibrosis and celiac disease, perianal excoria-

tion and gaseous abdominal distention with carbohydrate malabsorption, perianal and circumoral rash with acrodermatitis enteropathica, abnormal hair with Menkes syndrome, and the typical facial features diagnostic of the Johanson-Blizzard syndrome.

Many children with malabsorption disorders have very good appetites as they try to compensate for the fecal protein and energy losses. In exocrine pancreatic insufficiency, fecal losses of up to 40% of ingested protein and energy do not lead to malnutrition, as long as they are compensated by an increased appetite. In conditions associated

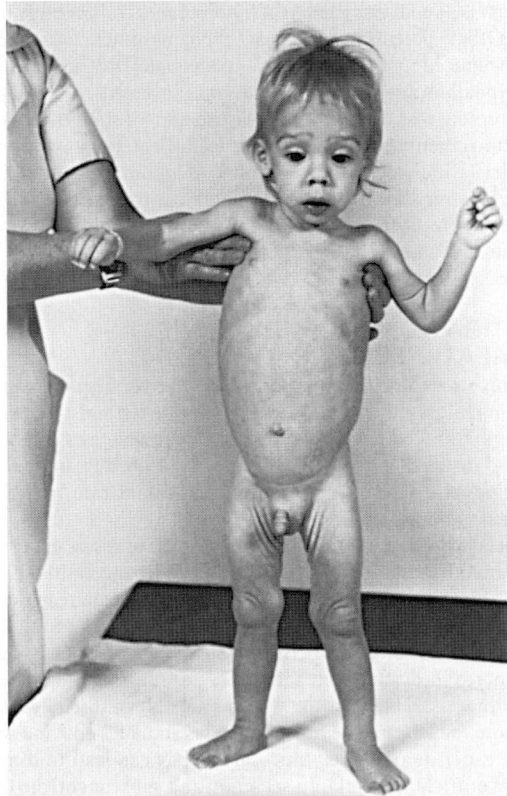

Figure 338-1 An 18 mo old boy with active celiac disease. Note the loose skinfolds, marked proximal muscle wasting and distended abdomen. The child looks ill.

Table 338-3	Diarrheal Diseases Appearing in the Neonatal Period
CONDITION	**CLINICAL FEATURES**
Microvillus inclusion disease	Secretory watery diarrhea
Tufting enteropathy	Secretory watery diarrhea
Congenital glucose-galactose malabsorption	Acidic diarrhea
Congenital lactase deficiency	Acidic diarrhea
Congenital chloride diarrhea	Hydramnion, secretory watery diarrhea Metabolic alkalosis
Congenital defective jejunal Na^+-H^+ exchange	Hydramnion, secretory watery diarrhea
Congenital bile acid malabsorption	Steatorrhea
Congenital enterokinase deficiency	Failure to thrive, edema
Congenital trypsinogen deficiency	Failure to thrive, edema
Congenital lipase and/or colipase deficiency	Failure to thrive, oily stool
Enteric anendocrinosis (NEUROG 3 mutation)	Hyperchloremic acidosis, failure to thrive
Immunodeficiency and autoinflammatory diseases (see Table 336-5)	Failure to thrive, opportunistic infections, eczema

Adapted from Schmitz J: Maldigestion and malabsorption. In Walker WA, Durie PR, Hamilton JR, et al, editors: Pediatric gastrointestinal disease, ed 3, Hamilton, Ontario, 2000, BC Decker, p. 55.

with villous atrophy or inflammation (celiac disease, postinfectious enteropathy), fecal protein and energy losses are usually modest, but associated anorexia and reduced food intake results in malnutrition.

The nutritional assessment is an important part of clinical evaluation in children with malabsorptive disorders (see Chapter 44). Long-term calcium and vitamin D malabsorption can lead to reduced bone mineral density and metabolic bone disease, with increased risk of bone fractures. Vitamin K malabsorption, irrespective of the underlying mechanism (fat malabsorption, mucosal atrophy), can result in coagulopathy. Severe protein-losing enteropathy is often associated with malabsorption syndromes (celiac disease, intestinal lymphangiectasia) and causes hypoalbuminemia and edema. Other nutrient deficiencies include iron malabsorption causing microcytic anemia and low reticulocyte count, low serum folate levels in conditions associated with mucosal atrophy, especially in the proximal part of the small intestinal tract and low serum vitamin A and vitamin E concentrations in fat malabsorption.

Clinical history alone might not be sufficient to make a specific diagnosis, but it can direct the pediatrician toward a more structured and rational investigative approach. Diarrhea is the main clinical expression of malabsorption. Onset of diarrhea in early infancy suggests a congenital defect (Tables 338-3 and 336-5). In secretory diarrhea caused by disorders such as congenital chloride diarrhea and microvillus inclusion disease, the stool is watery and voluminous and can be mistaken for urine. Onset of symptoms after introduction of a particular food into a child's diet can provide diagnostic clues, such as with sucrose in sucrase-isomaltase deficiency. The nature of the diarrhea may be helpful: explosive watery diarrhea suggests carbohydrate malabsorption; loose, bulky stools are associated with celiac disease; and pasty and yellowish offensive stools suggest an exocrine pancreatic insufficiency. Stool color is usually not helpful; green stool with undigested "peas and carrots" can suggest rapid intestinal transit in toddler's diarrhea, which is a self-limiting condition unassociated with failure to thrive.

338.1 Evaluation of Children with Suspected Intestinal Malabsorption

Michael J. Lentze and David Branski

The investigation is guided by the history and physical examination. In a child presenting with chronic or recurrent diarrhea, the initial work-up should include stool cultures and antibody tests for parasites, stool microscopy for ova and parasites such as *Giardia,* and stool occult blood and leukocytes to exclude inflammatory disorders. Stool pH and reducing substances for carbohydrate malabsorption, and quantitative stool fat examination and α_1-antitrypsin to demonstrate fat and protein malabsorption, respectively, should also be determined. Fecal stool elastase-1 can determine exocrine pancreatic insufficiency.

A complete blood count including peripheral smear for microcytic anemia, lymphopenia (lymphangiectasia), neutropenia (Shwachman syndrome), and acanthocytosis (abetalipoproteinemia) is useful. If celiac disease is suspected, serum immunoglobulin (Ig) A and tissue transglutaminase (TG2) antibody levels should be determined. Depending on the initial test results, more-specific investigations can be planned.

INVESTIGATIONS FOR CARBOHYDRATE MALABSORPTION

Measurement of carbohydrate in the stool, using a Clinitest reagent that identifies reducing substances, is a simple screening test. An acidic stool with >2+ reducing substance suggests carbohydrate malabsorption. Sucrose or starch in the stool is not recognized as a reducing sugar until after hydrolysis with hydrochloric acid, which converts them to reducing sugars.

Breath hydrogen test is used to identify the specific carbohydrate that is malabsorbed. After an overnight fast, the suspected sugar (lactose, sucrose, fructose, or glucose) is administered as an oral solution (carbohydrate load 1-2 g/kg, maximum 50 g). In malabsorption, the sugar is not digested or absorbed in the small bowel, passes on to the colon, and is metabolized by the normal bacteria flora. One of the products of this process is hydrogen gas, which is absorbed through the colon mucosa and excreted in the breath. Increased hydrogen concentration in the breath samples suggests carbohydrate malabsorption. A rise in breath hydrogen of 20 ppm above the baseline is considered a positive test. The child should not be on antibiotics at the time of the test, because colonic flora is essential for fermenting the sugar.

Small bowel mucosal biopsies can measure mucosal disaccharidase (lactase, sucrase, maltase, palatinase) concentrations directly. In primary enzyme deficiencies the mucosal enzyme levels are low and small bowel mucosal morphology is normal. Partial or total villous atrophy due to disorders such as celiac disease, or following rotavirus gastroenteritis can result in secondary disaccharidase deficiency and transient lactose intolerance. The disaccharidase levels revert to normal after mucosal healing.

INVESTIGATIONS FOR FAT MALABSORPTION

The presence of fat globules in the stool suggests fat malabsorption. The ability to assimilate fat varies with age; a premature infant can absorb only 65-75% of dietary fat, a full-term infant absorbs almost 90%, and an older child absorbs more than 95% of fat while on a regular diet. Quantitative determination of fat malabsorption requires a 3-day stool collection for evaluation of fat excretion and determination of the coefficient of fat absorption:

Coefficient of fat absorption%
$$= (fat\ intake - fecal\ fat\ losses / fat\ intake) \times 100$$

where fat intake and fat losses are in grams. Because fecal fat balance studies are cumbersome, expensive, and unpleasant to perform, simpler tests are often preferred. Among these stool tests, the acid steatocrit test is the most reliable. When bile acid deficiency is suspected of being the cause of fat malabsorption, the evaluation of bile acid levels in duodenal fluid aspirate may be useful.

Fat malabsorption and exocrine pancreatic insufficiency are usually associated with deficiencies of fat-soluble vitamins A, D, E, and K. Serum concentrations of vitamins A, D, and E can be measured. A prolonged prothrombin time is an indirect test to assess vitamin K deficiency.

INVESTIGATIONS FOR PROTEIN-LOSING ENTEROPATHY

Dietary and endogenous proteins secreted into the bowel are almost completely absorbed; <1 g of protein from these sources passes into the colon. The majority of the stool nitrogen is derived from gut bacterial proteins. Excessive bowel protein loss usually manifests as **hypoalbuminemia**. Because the most common cause of hypoalbuminemia in children is a renal disorder, urinary protein excretion must be determined. Other potential causes of hypoalbuminemia include liver disease (reduced production) and inadequate protein intake. Very rarely hypoalbuminemia can result from an extensive skin disorder causing protein loss via the skin. Measurement of stool α_1-**antitrypsin** is a useful screening test for protein-losing enteropathy. This serum protein has a molecular weight similar to albumin's; however, unlike albumin it is resistant to digestion in the gastrointestinal (GI) tract. Excessive α_1-antitrypsin excretion in the stool should prompt further investigations to identify the specific cause of gut or stomach (Menetrier disease) protein loss.

INVESTIGATIONS FOR EXOCRINE PANCREATIC FUNCTION (Fig. 338-2)

Cystic fibrosis is the most common cause of exocrine pancreatic insufficiency in children; therefore, a sweat chloride test must be performed before embarking on invasive tests to investigate possible exocrine pancreatic insufficiency. Many cases of cystic fibrosis are detected by neonatal genetic screening programs; occasional rare mutations are undetected.

Fecal elastase-1 estimation is a sensitive test to assess exocrine pancreatic function in chronic cystic fibrosis and pancreatitis. Elastase-1 is a stable endoprotease unaffected by exogenous pancreatic enzymes. One disadvantage of the fecal elastase-1 test is the lack of full differentiation between primary exocrine pancreatic insufficiency and exocrine pancreatic dysfunction secondary to intestinal villous atrophy. The proximal small bowel is the site for pancreozymin/cholecystokinin production; the latter is the hormone that stimulates enzyme secretion from the exocrine pancreas. Mucosal atrophy can lead to diminished pancreozymin/cholecystokinin secretion and subsequently to exocrine pancreatic insufficiency. Fecal elastase-1 can also give a false-positive result during acute episodes of diarrhea.

Serum trypsinogen concentration can also be used as a screening test for exocrine pancreatic insufficiency. In cystic fibrosis, the levels are greatly elevated early in life, and then they gradually fall, so that by 5-7 yr of age, most patients with cystic fibrosis with pancreatic insufficiency have subnormal levels. Patients with cystic fibrosis and adequate exocrine pancreatic function tend to have normal or elevated levels. In such patients, observing the trend in serial serum trypsinogen estimation may be useful in monitoring exocrine pancreatic function. In Shwachman syndrome, another condition associated with exocrine pancreatic insufficiency, the serum trypsinogen level is low.

Other tests for pancreatic insufficiency (nitroblue tetrazolium–paraaminobenzoic acid test and pancreolauryl test) measure urine or breath concentrations of substances released and absorbed across the mucosal surface following pancreatic digestion. These tests lack specificity and are rarely used in clinical practice.

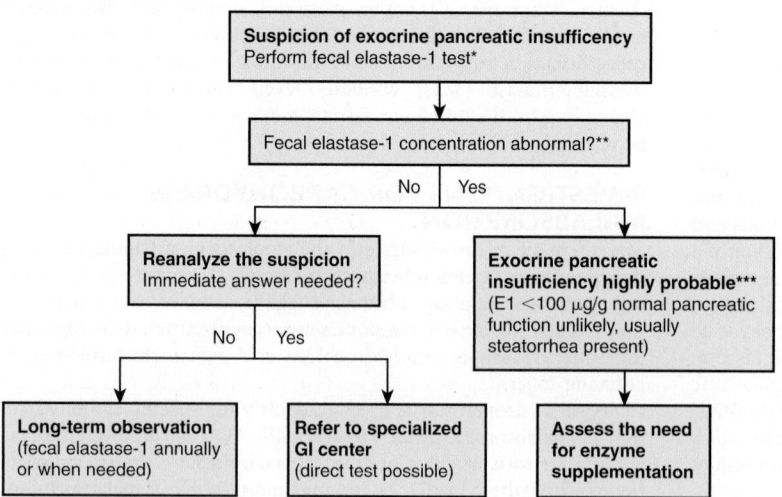

Figure 338-2 Algorithm for assessment of exocrine pancreatic function. *If not available, use other test. Perform appropriate imaging studies of the pancreas. **In case of borderline values, consider repeating the test with 3 independent samples. ***Consider differential diagnosis (especially consider mucosal villous atrophy and dilution effect of watery stool). GI, gastrointestinal. (*Adapted from Walkowiak J, Nousia-Arvanitakis S, Henker J, et al: Indirect pancreatic function tests in children. J Pediatr Gastroenterol Nutr 40:107-114, 2005.*)

The gold standard test for exocrine pancreatic function is direct analysis of **duodenal aspirate** for volume, bicarbonate, trypsin, and lipase upon secretin, and pancreozymin/cholecystokinin stimulation. This involves duodenal intubation (see Chapter 348).

INVESTIGATIONS FOR INTESTINAL MUCOSAL DISORDERS

Establishing a specific diagnosis for malabsorption often requires histologic examination of small bowel mucosal biopsies. These are obtained during endoscopy, which allows multiple biopsies to be performed, because mucosal involvement can be patchy, especially in celiac disease. Periodic acid–Schiff (PAS) staining of mucosal biopsies and electron microscopy are necessary in congenital diarrhea to assess congenital microvillus atrophy. Bowel mucosal lesions can also be segmental in cases of intestinal lymphangiectasia. In these situations, radiographic small bowel series or repeated ultrasonographies can identify a region of thickened bowel responsible for protein loss. During endoscopy, mucosal biopsies can be obtained to measure mucosal disaccharidase activities. Duodenal aspirates can be performed to measure pancreatic enzyme concentration as well as quantitative bacterial cultures. Aspirates to demonstrate other infections and infestations such as *Giardia* may be useful.

IMAGING PROCEDURES

Plain radiographs and barium contrast studies might suggest a site and cause of intestinal motility disorders. Although flocculations of barium and dilated bowel with thickened mucosal folds have been attributed to diffuse malabsorptive lesions such as celiac disease, these abnormalities are nonspecific. Diffuse fluid-filled bowel loops during sonography also suggest malabsorption.

338.2 Celiac Disease (Gluten-Sensitive Enteropathy)

David Branski, Riccardo Troncone, and Alessio Fasano

ETIOLOGY AND EPIDEMIOLOGY

Celiac disease is an immune-mediated systemic disorder elicited by gluten and related prolamines in genetically susceptible individuals and characterized by the presence of a variable combination of gluten-dependent clinical manifestations, celiac disease–specific antibodies, HLA-DQ2 or DQ8 haplotypes, and enteropathy. Celiac disease–specific antibodies comprise autoantibodies against **TG2,** including **endomysial antibodies (EMA),** and antibodies against **deamidated forms of gliadin peptides**.

Celiac disease is triggered by the ingestion of wheat gluten and related prolamines from rye and barley. In most studies oats proved to be safe; however, a few celiac disease patients have oats prolamine–reactive mucosal T cells that can cause mucosal inflammation.

Celiac disease is a common disorder (1% prevalence of biopsy-proven disease). It is thought to be rare in Central Africa and East Asia. Environmental factors might affect the risk of developing celiac disease or the timing of its presentation. Neither the delayed introduction of gluten, or breastfeeding, or the introduction of small quantities of gluten prevents celiac disease in high-risk patients. Infectious agents have been hypothesized to play a role because frequent rotavirus infections are associated with an increased risk. It is plausible that the contact with gliadin at a time when there is ongoing intestinal inflammation, altered intestinal permeability, and enhanced antigen presentation can increase the risk of developing celiac disease, at least in a subset of persons (Fig. 338-3).

GENETICS AND PATHOGENESIS

A genetic predisposition is suggested by the family aggregation and the concordance in monozygotic twins, which approaches 100%. The strongest association is with human leukocyte antigen (HLA)-DQ2.5 (1 or 2 copies encoded by DQA1 *05 [for the chain] and DQB1*02

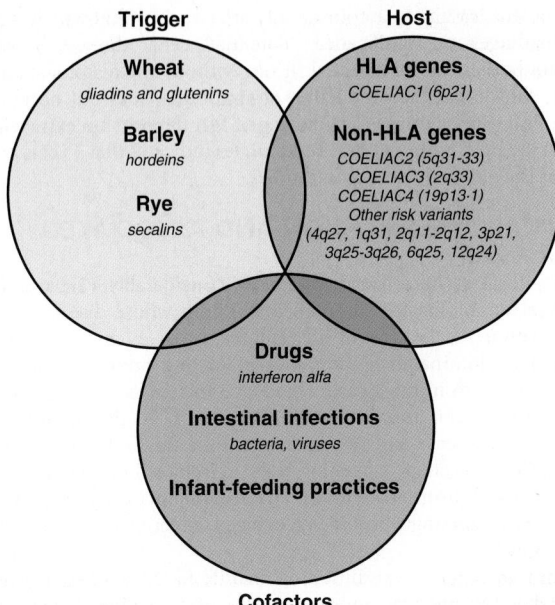

Figure 338-3 Causative factors in celiac disease. HLA, human leukocyte antigen. (*From Di Sabatino A, Corassa GR: Celiac disease. Lancet* 373:1480–1490, 2009.)

genes [for the chain]). Such a DQ molecule has been found to be present in more than 90% of celiac patients. The highly homologous DQ2.2 molecule confers a much lesser risk, while the data available on DQ2-negative celiac disease patients indicate that they almost invariably are HLA-DQ8–positive (DQA1*0301/DQB1*0302). A gene dosage effect has been suggested, and a molecular hypothesis for such a phenomenon has been proposed, based on the impact of the number and quality of the HLA-DQ2 molecules on gluten peptide presentation to T cells. Other non-HLA genes confer susceptibility to celiac disease. Genome-wide association studies have shown risk variants in genes controlling T-cell activation and recruitment, some being shared with type 1 diabetes and other autoimmune diseases. Interestingly, very few polymorphisms associated with celiac disease are in coding regions, as they often are in binding sites for transcription factors, then affecting gene expression.

Celiac disease is a T-cell–mediated chronic inflammatory disorder with an autoimmune component. Altered processing by intraluminal enzymes, changes in intestinal permeability and activation of innate immunity mechanisms precede the activation of the adaptive immune response. Immunodominant epitopes from gliadin are highly resistant to intraluminal and mucosal digestion; incomplete degradation favor the immunostimulatory and toxic effects of these sequences. Some gliadin peptides (p31-43) are able to activate innate immunity, in particular they induce interleukin (IL)-15. The latter, but also type 1 interferons, may alter the tolerogenic phenotype of dendritic cells, resulting in lamina propria T-cell activation by other peptides presented in the context of HLA-DQ2 or HLA-DQ8 molecules. Gliadin-specific T-cell responses are enhanced by the action of TG2; the enzyme converts particular glutamine residues into glutamic acid, which results in higher affinity of these gliadin peptides for HLA-DQ2 or HLA-DQ8. The pattern of cytokines produced following gliadin activation is clearly dominated by interferon-γ (T-helper type 1 skewed); IL-21 is also upregulated. Downstream T-cell activation, a complex remodeling of the mucosa takes place, involving increased levels of metalloproteinases and growth factors, which leads to the classical flat mucosa. A severe impairment of intraepitheleal lymphocytes (IELs) homeostasis is present in celiac disease. IL-15 is implicated in the expression of natural killer receptors CD94 and NKG2D, as well as in epithelial expression of stress molecules, thus enhancing cytotoxicity, cell apoptosis, and villous atrophy. The most evident expression of autoimmunity is the presence of serum antibodies to TG2. However, the mechanisms leading to autoimmunity are largely unknown, as well as their pathogenetic significance. "Potential" celiac disease, in which TG2 antibodies can be detected in situ without any histologic abnormality, shows that the production of antibodies does not necessarily lead to intestinal damage. The finding of IgA deposits on extracellular TG2 in the liver, lymph nodes, and muscles indicates that TG2 is accessible to the gut-derived autoantibodies.

CLINICAL PRESENTATION AND ASSOCIATED DISORDERS

Clinical features of celiac disease vary considerably (Table 338-4). Intestinal symptoms are common in children whose disease is diagnosed within the 1st 2 yr of life; failure to thrive, chronic diarrhea, vomiting, abdominal distention, muscle wasting, anorexia, and irritability are present in most cases (see Fig. 338-1). Occasionally there is constipation, rectal prolapse, or intussusception. As the age at presentation of the disease shifts to later in childhood, and with the more liberal use of serologic screening tests, extraintestinal manifestations and associated disorders, without any accompanying digestive symptoms, have increasingly become recognized, affecting almost all organs (Table 338-5).

The most common extraintestinal manifestation of celiac disease is iron-deficiency anemia, unresponsive to iron therapy. Osteoporosis may be present; in contrast to the situation in adults, it can be reversed by a gluten-free diet, with restoration of normal peak bone densitometric values. Other extraintestinal manifestations include short stature, arthritis and arthralgia, epilepsy with bilateral occipital calcifications, peripheral neuropathies, cardiomyopathy, isolated hypertransaminasemia, dental enamel hypoplasia, aphthous stomatitis, and alopecia. The mechanisms responsible for the severity and the variety of clinical presentations remain obscure. Nutritional deficiencies or abnormal immune responses have been advocated.

Silent celiac disease is being increasingly recognized, mainly in asymptomatic 1st-degree relatives of celiac disease patients investigated during screening studies. However, small bowel biopsy in these people reveals severe mucosal damage consistent with celiac disease. Potential celiac disease is defined when patients have positive celiac disease–specific antibodies, but without documented small bowel damage. It is important to follow these patients because they can develop established celiac disease in the future (Table 338-6).

Some diseases, many with an autoimmune pathogenesis, are found with a higher-than-normal incidence in celiac disease patients. Among these are type 1 diabetes, autoimmune thyroid disease, Addison disease, Sjögren syndrome, autoimmune cholangitis, autoimmune hepatitis, primary biliary cirrhosis. Such associations have been interpreted as a consequence of the sharing of identical HLA haplotypes.

Table 338-4	Some Clinical Manifestations of Celiac Disease in Children and Adolescents

SYSTEM	MANIFESTATION	(POSSIBLE) CAUSE
Gastrointestinal	Diarrhea Distended abdomen Vomiting Anorexia Weight loss Failure to thrive Rectal prolapse Aphthous stomatitis Intussusception	Atrophy of the small bowel mucosa Malabsorption
Hematologic	Anemia	Iron malabsorption
Skeletal	Rickets Osteoporosis Enamel hypoplasia of the teeth	Calcium/vitamin D malabsorption
Muscular	Atrophy	Malnutrition
Neurologic	Peripheral neuropathy Epilepsy Irritability Cerebral calcifications Cerebellar ataxia	Thiamine/vitamin B_{12} deficiency
Endocrinologic	Short stature Pubertas tarda Secondary hyperparathyroidism	Malnutrition Calcium/vitamin D malabsorption
Dermatologic	Dermatitis herpetiformis Alopecia areata Erythema nodosum	Autoimmunity
Respiratory	Idiopathic pulmonary hemosiderosis	

Adapted from Mearin ML: Celiac disease among children and adolescents, Curr Probl Pediatr Adolesc Health Care 37:81–112, 2007.

Table 338-5	Risk Groups for Celiac Disease Case-Finding

First-degree relatives
Dermatitis herpetiformis
Unexplained iron-deficiency anemia
Autoimmune thyroiditis
Type 1 diabetes
Unexplained infertility
Recurrent abortion
Dental enamel hypoplasia
Cryptic hypertransaminasemia
Autoimmune liver disease
Short stature
Delayed puberty
Down, Williams, and Turner syndromes
Irritable bowel syndrome
Unexplained osteoporosis
Sjögren syndrome
Epilepsy (poorly controlled) with occipital calcifications
Selective immunoglobulin A deficiency
Autoimmune endocrinopathies
Addison disease
Aphthous stomatitis
Ataxia
Alopecia
Polyneuropathy
Irritable bowel syndrome

Modified from Di Sabatino A, Corazza GR: Coeliac disease, Lancet 373:1480–1490, 2009.

Table 338-6	Clinical Spectrum of Celiac Disease

SYMPTOMATIC
Frank malabsorption symptoms: chronic diarrhea, failure to thrive, weight loss
Extraintestinal manifestations: anemia, fatigue, hypertransaminasemia, neurologic disorders, short stature, dental enamel defects, arthralgia, aphthous stomatitis

SILENT
No apparent symptoms in spite of histologic evidence of villous atrophy
In most cases identified by serologic screening in at-risk groups (see Table 330-1)

LATENT
Subjects who have a normal histology, but at some other time, before or after, have shown a gluten-dependent enteropathy

POTENTIAL
Subjects with positive celiac disease serology but without evidence of altered jejunal histology
It might or might not be symptomatic

Table 338-7	Other Causes of Flat Mucosa

Autoimmune enteropathy
Tropical sprue
Giardiasis
HIV enteropathy
Bacterial overgrowth
Crohn disease
Eosinophilic gastroenteritis
Cow's milk enteropathy
Soy protein enteropathy
Primary immunodeficiency
Graft-versus-host disease
Chemotherapy and radiation
Protein energy malnutrition
Tuberculosis
Lymphoma
Nongluten food intolerances

Modified from Di Sabatino A, Corazza GR: Coeliac disease, Lancet 373:1480–1490, 2009.

The relation between celiac disease and other autoimmune diseases is poorly defined; once those diseases are established, they are not influenced by a gluten-free diet. Other associated conditions include selective IgA deficiency and Down, Turner, and Williams syndromes.

Patients with celiac disease show increased long-term mortality, the risk rising with delayed diagnosis and/or poor dietary compliance. Non-Hodgkin lymphoma is the main cause of death. Adult patients can develop complications such a refractory celiac disease, ulcerative jejunoileitis, or enteropathy-associated T-cell lymphoma.

DIAGNOSIS

The diagnosis of celiac disease is based on a combination of symptoms, antibodies, HLA, and duodenal histology (Table 338-7). The initial approach to symptomatic patients is to test for anti-TG2 IgA antibodies and in addition for total IgA in serum to exclude IgA deficiency. As an alternative for total IgA in serum direct testing for IgG anti–deamidated forms of gliadin peptides antibodies can be performed. If IgA anti-TG2 antibodies are negative and serum total IgA is normal for age (or IgG anti–deamidated forms of gliadin peptides antibodies are negative), celiac disease is unlikely to be the cause of the symptoms. If anti-TG2 antibody testing is positive the patients should be referred to a pediatric gastroenterologist for further diagnostic workup, which depends on the serum antibody levels. Patients with positive anti-TG2 antibody levels <10 × upper limits of normal should undergo upper endoscopy with multiple biopsies. In patients with positive anti-TG2 antibody levels at or >10 × upper limits of normal, blood should be drawn for HLA and EMA testing. If the patient is positive for EMA antibodies and positive for DQ2 or DQ8 HLA testing, the diagnosis of celiac disease is confirmed, a gluten-free diet is started, and the patient is followed for improvement of symptoms and decline of antibodies. In the rare case of negative results for HLA and/or anti-EMA in a child with TG2 antibody titers ≥10 × upper limits of normal, the different possibilities for false-positive and false-negative test results need to be considered. In these circumstances, the diagnostic workup should be extended, including repeated testing and duodenal biopsies. In totally asymptomatic persons belonging to high-risk groups, celiac disease should always be diagnosed using duodenal biopsies. When biopsies are indicated at least 4 fragments should be obtained from the descending part of the duodenum and at least 1 from the duodenal bulb. The diagnosis is confirmed by an antibody decline and preferably a clinical response to a gluten-free diet. Gluten challenge and repetitive biopsies will only be necessary in selected cases in which diagnostic uncertainty remains.

TREATMENT

The only treatment for celiac disease is lifelong strict adherence to a gluten-free diet (Fig. 338-4). This requires a wheat-, barley-, and rye-free diet. Despite evidence that oats are safe for most patients with

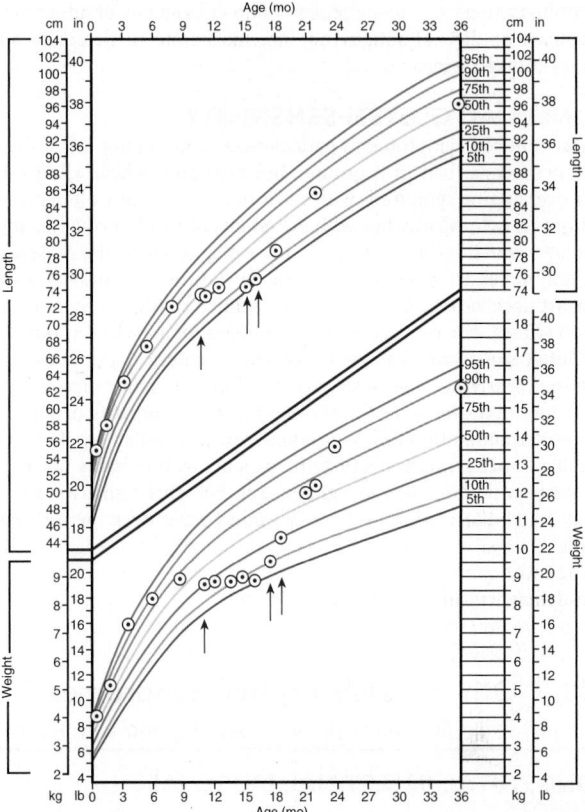

Figure 338-4 Gluten-sensitive enteropathy. Growth curve demonstrates initial normal growth from 0-9 mo, followed by onset of poor appetite with intermittent vomiting and diarrhea after initiation of gluten-containing diet (*single arrow*). After biopsy conformed diagnosis and treatment with gluten-free diet (*double arrow*), growth improves.

celiac disease, there is concern regarding the possibility of contamination of oats with gluten during harvesting, milling, and shipping. Nevertheless, it seems wise to add oats to the gluten-free diet only when the latter is well established, so that possible adverse reactions can be readily identified. There is a consensus that all celiac disease patients should be treated with a gluten-free diet regardless of the presence of symptoms. However, whereas it is relatively easy to assess the health improvement after treatment of celiac disease in patients with clinical symptoms of the disease, it proves difficult in persons with asymptomatic celiac disease. The nutritional risks, particularly osteopenia, are those mainly feared for subjects who have silent celiac disease and continue on a gluten-containing diet. Little is known about the health risks in untreated patients with minor enteropathy, which may be clinically silent. There are no guidelines concerning the need for a gluten-free diet in subjects with "potential" celiac disease (patients with positive celiac disease–associated serology but without enteropathy).

The Codex Alimentarius Guidelines define gluten-free as <20 ppm, but, although analytical methods for gluten detection have already reached a satisfactory degree of sensitivity, more information is needed on the daily gluten amount that may be tolerated by celiac disease patients. The data available so far seem to suggest that the threshold should be set to <50 mg/day, although individual variability makes it difficult to set a universal threshold.

It is important that an experienced dietician with specific expertise in celiac disease counseling educates the family and the child about dietary restriction. Compliance with a gluten-free diet can be difficult, especially in adolescents. It is recommended that children with celiac disease be monitored with periodic visits for assessment of symptoms, growth, physical examination, and adherence to the gluten-free diet. Periodic measurements of TG2 antibody levels to document reduction in antibody titers can be helpful as indirect evidence of adherence to a gluten-free diet, although they are inaccurate in detecting slight dietary transgressions.

NONCELIAC GLUTEN SENSITIVITY

Wheat-induced symptoms in patients who do not have celiac disease have been described in 2 groups. **IgE-mediated wheat allergy** may have overlapping symptoms with celiac disease but more often presents without an enteropathy but with symptoms of atopy (urticaria, angioedema, eczema, asthma, rhinitis) and is diagnosed by the presence of IgE antibodies to wheat (serum specific IgE or skin prick tests). In contrast to celiac disease and nonceliac gluten sensitivity, symptoms in IgE-mediated disease occur soon after ingestion of wheat products.

Gluten sensitivity has been defined as enteric (abdominal pain, bloating, diarrhea) and systemic (headache, fatigue, muscle aches, rash) after ingesting wheat in the absence of enteropathy or HLA risk factors and autoantibodies. Symptoms are often similar to patients with irritable bowel syndrome and some patients with irritable bowel syndrome respond positively to a gluten-free diet. This is an area of uncertainty in pediatrics because most studies have been performed in adults.

Bibliography is available at Expert Consult.

338.3 Other Malabsorptive Syndromes

Philip M. Sherman, David Branski, and Olivier Goulet

CONGENITAL INTESTINAL MUCOSAL DEFECTS
Microvillus Inclusion Disease (Congenital Microvillus Atrophy)

Microvillus inclusion disease (MVID) is an autosomal recessive disorder, which manifests *at birth* with **profuse watery secretory diarrhea**. It is the most severe cause of congenital diarrhea involving the development of intestinal mucosa. Light microscopy of the small bowel mucosa demonstrates diffuse thinning of the mucosa, with hypoplastic villus atrophy and no inflammatory infiltrate. Diagnosis may be easily performed with light microscopy using PAS and CD10 staining, which shows a very thin or absent brush border, together with positive PAS and CD10 intracellular inclusions. Electron microscopy shows enterocytes with absent or sparse microvilli. The apical cytoplasm of the enterocytes contains electron-dense secretory granules; the hallmark is presence of microvilli within involutions of the apical membrane. Polyhydramnios is not a classic presentation of MVID but is increasingly observed according to the progresses in prenatal follow up. Neonates usually present very early onset of severe watery diarrhea (up to 200-330 mL/kg/day) causing dehydration and failure to thrive. Despite parenteral nutrition, diarrhea continues and initial fluid management is difficult. The disease is fatal without long-term parenteral nutrition support. Most children die in infancy or early childhood. To date, no causal treatment exists for MVID. Trials with antiinflammatory drugs, including steroids and antisecretory medications (such as Sandostatin or loperamide), did not significantly change stool volumes over a prolonged period; colostrum and epidermal growth factor have failed as well, but octreotide has shown a partial improvement in 1 patient, supposedly via its ability to reduce intestinal fluids (see Chapter 339). Intestinal transplantation is the only definitive treatment for this rare disease. Many cases in the same family, frequently in a highly consanguineous union, gave the impression of an autosomic recessive transmission. Mutations of the *MYO5B* gene coding for a nonconventional motor protein, Myosin Vb, are associated with MVID in a cohort of patients suffering from early-onset MVID. Most early-onset MVID patients display a mutation in *MYO5B*, but there is a great allelic heterogeneity. These mutations result in a loss of function at the proteic level, with abnormal cell polarity, that would involve *MYO5B* protein in regulating intracellular protein trafficking as well as in the cytoskeleton organization.

It is likely that in very rare cases a milder phenotype may allow slow weaning from parenteral nutrition, allowing the patient to reach young adulthood and enjoy partial oral feeding.

Tufting Enteropathy (Congenital Tufting Enteropathy)

Tufting enteropathy (intestinal epithelial dysplasia) manifests in the 1st few wk of life with **persistent watery diarrhea** and accounts for a small fraction of infants with intractable diarrhea of infancy. The distinctive feature on small intestinal mucosal biopsy is focal epithelial "tufts" (teardrop-shaped groups of closely packed enterocytes with apical rounding of the plasma membrane) involving 80-90% of the epithelial surface. However, the typical pathology does not appear immediately after birth, and in other known enteropathies, tufts are seen on ≤15% of the epithelial surface. One difficulty comes from the mononuclear T cell's infiltration of the lamina propria, which can guide wrongly to a disimmune enteropathy, especially when initially lacking tufts. The increased intestinal permeability caused by cell adhesion defect could be responsible for the inflammatory reaction. Colonic epithelium shows abnormalities that are more difficult to identify. Electron microscopy does not help in establishing the diagnosis.

The pathogenesis of this severe digestive disease is from a disorder of cell–cell and cell–matrix interactions, because there is an abnormal distribution of $\alpha_2\beta_1$-integrin along the crypt–villus axis, increased expression of desmoglein, and ultrastructural changes of desmosomes. Tufting enteropathy is often associated with *punctiform keratitis* and *conjunctival dysplasia* resembling typical pictures of tufts. The genetic basis of tufting enteropathy supports this speculation, because mutations in the *EPCAM* gene, encoding an epithelial cell adhesion molecule protein, have been described. The phenotype associated with mutations of *EPCAM* is usually an isolated congenital diarrhea without associated extradigestive symptoms, except in some patients with late-onset arthritis. A founder effect at the *EPCAM* locus in congenital tufting enteropathy (CTE) has been shown in the Arabic Gulf population.

In the **syndromic form** of CTE, diarrhea is associated with one or more of these same anomalies: superficial punctate keratitis, choanal, esophageal or intestinal atresia, anal imperforation, hair dysplasia, skin hyperlaxity, bone abnormalities, hexadactylia, and facial dysmorphism. Anomalies appear isolated for most, except for superficial punctate keratitis and choanal atresia that are consistently found in the population of patients with mutated *SPINT2* for conjunctival inflammation (100%) and in 50% of cases for choanal atresia; moreover, these anomalies are never found in the population of patients with *EPCAM* mutations.

No **treatment** has been effective, so management requires permanent parenteral nutrition with possible intestinal transplantation (see Chapter 339).

Enteric Anendocrinosis

Mutations of the *NEUROG3* gene produce generalized mucosal malabsorption, vomiting, diarrhea, failure to thrive, dehydration, and a hyperchloremic metabolic acidosis. Oral alimentation with anything other than water produces diarrhea. Villus-crypt architecture in small bowel biopsies is normal, but staining for neuroendocrine cells (e.g., employing antichromogranin antibodies) demonstrates a complete absence of this secretory cell lineage with preservation of goblet cells and Paneth cells. **Treatment** is with total parenteral nutrition and small bowel transplantation.

PROPROTEIN CONVERTASE 1/3 DEFICIENCY

Chronic watery, *neonatal onset diarrhea* is described in infants with hyperinsulinism, hypoglycemia, hypogonadism, and hypoadrenalism. Small bowel biopsy reveals a nonspecific enteropathy. A clue to the autosomal recessive condition is subsequent onset of marked obesity with hyperphagia in the toddler years in both affected probands and symptomatic siblings. Elevated serum levels of proinsulin are highly supportive of this underdiagnosed disorder, which is caused by loss-of-function mutations in the *PCSK1* gene.

CARBOHYDRATE-DEFICIENT GLYCOPROTEIN SYNDROME AND ENTEROCYTE HEPARAN SULFATE DEFICIENCY

Congenital disorders of glycosylation (also carbohydrate-deficient glycoprotein [CDG]) are genetic disorders of assembly of *N*-glycans in the cytosol and endoplasmic reticulum, resulting in a variety of manifestations (see Chapter 87.6). The subtypes of CDG I are all associated with **protein-losing enteropathy.** Diagnosis can be established by isoelectric focusing of serum transferrin, enzyme analysis, and DNA analysis. Oral mannose can provide effective therapy in CDG Ib, so early identification of children presenting with hypoglycemia, hypothyroidism, and/or thyroid binding globulin deficiency is beneficial.

Congenital enterocyte heparan deficiency is a rare cause of intractable diarrhea with protein-losing enteropathy, which may be an unusual presentation of the CDG syndrome type 1 (also known as Jaeken syndrome) (see Chapter 87.6). Heparan sulfate is a glycosaminoglycan with multiple roles in the intestine, including restriction of charged macromolecules, such as albumin, in the vascular lumen.

SYNDROMIC DIARRHEA

Syndromic diarrhea (SD), also known as phenotypic diarrhea or **trichohepatoenteric** syndrome is a congenital enteropathy manifesting with *early onset* of severe diarrhea requiring parenteral nutrition. The estimated prevalence is approximately 1 per 300,000-400,000 live births in Western Europe. Patients are born small for gestational age and present with diarrhea starting in the 1st 6 mo of life (<1 mo of age in most cases). They have an abnormal phenotype, including facial dysmorphism with prominent forehead, broad nose, and hypertelorism and a distinct abnormality of hair, **trichorrhexis nodosa.** Hairs are woolly, easily removed, and poorly pigmented. Abnormal cutaneous spots including café-au-lait on the lower limbs may be observed. Liver disease affects about half of the patients with extensive fibrosis or cirrhosis. Cardiac abnormalities and colitis have been reported sporadically, as well as 1 case involving polyhydramnios, placental abnormalities, and congenital hemochromatosis. The patients have defective antibody responses despite normal serum immunoglobulin levels and defective antigen-specific skin tests despite positive proliferative responses in vitro. Microscopic analysis shows twisted hair (pili torti), aniso- and poilkilotrichosis, and trichorrhexis nodosa. Histopathologic analysis shows nonspecific villus atrophy with or without mononuclear cell infiltration of the lamina propria, and without specific histologic abnormalities involving the epithelium. The common association of the disorder with parental consanguinity and/or affected siblings indicates a genetic origin with autosomal recessive transmission. Mutations in the *TTC37* gene are the basis of the syndrome. *TTC37* encodes a protein known as Thespin, which is in many tissues (vascular endothelium, lymph, pituitary stalk, lung and intestine), but is not expressed in the liver. In patients with SD, with no mutation in *TTC37*, there are mutations in the *SKIV2L* gene. This gene encodes a protein of the Ski multiprotein complex that is involved in the control of RNA by the exosome, including the regulation of normal messenger RNA and the degradation of nonfunctional messenger RNA.

Prognosis of this type of intractable diarrhea of infancy is poor, with most patients having died between the ages of 2 and 5 yr, some of them with early-onset liver disease.

AUTOIMMUNE ENTEROPATHY

Symptoms of autoimmune enteropathy usually occur *after the 1st 6 mo of life,* presenting with chronic diarrhea, protein-losing enteropathy, malabsorption, and failure to thrive. The diagnosis is based on the endoscopic and histologic evaluation of the inflammation mainly of the small bowel but also of the colon. Histologic findings in the small bowel include partial or complete villous atrophy, crypt hyperplasia, and an increase in chronic inflammatory cells in the lamina propria. In contrast to gluten-sensitive enteropathy (celiac disease), there is no increased number in intraepithelial lymphocytes. Immunologic analyses indicate the presence of autoantibodies and, most importantly, of *anti-enterocyte antibodies,* as well as *anti-autoimmune*

enteropathy-75 kDa. Specific serum antienterocyte antibodies can be identified in 50% or more of patients by indirect immunofluorescent staining of normal small bowel mucosa and kidney. In some patients *anti-goblet cell antibodies* also can be demonstrated.

Extraintestinal autoimmune disorders are usual and include arthritis, membranous glomerulonephritis, insulin-dependent diabetes, thrombocytopenia, autoimmune hepatitis, hypothyroidism, and hemolytic anemia. It is essential to exclude an underlying primary immune deficiency, particularly in boys with other autoimmune features (e.g., diabetes mellitus), because a proportion has underlying *i*mmune dysregulation, *p*olyendocrinopathy, *e*nteropathy, *X*-linked (IPEX) syndrome (see Chapter 126.5). Different phenotypes of IPEX syndrome patients, as well as IPEX-like forms of autoimmune enteropathy that are *FOXP3*-independent are described involving girls as well with or without extraintestinal autoimmune disorders. Contrary to classical IPEX, the cause of IPEX-like or type 2 autoimmune enteropathy is only partially elucidated on a molecular basis. However, in patients who do not show genetic defects in FOXP3 or CD25, abnormal functions of CD4+CD25 high-regulatory T cells should be documented. Autoimmune enteropathy is reported in cases of Schimke immunoosseous dysplasia.

Treatment options are rather limited and based on T-cell–suppressive immunomodulation. Upon initial stabilization using steroid pulse therapy and calcineurin-dependent immunosuppressive drugs, such as tacrolimus, most often patients are maintained on rapamycin with azathioprine, methotrexate or rituximab in few patients. A theoretic alternative treatment option could be in form of hematopoietic stem cell transplantation; this treatment option is preferable in patients with a molecular defect, such as previously shown for patients with classical IPEX syndrome.

BILE ACID MALABSORPTION

In primary bile acid malabsorption, mutation of the ileal sodium–bile acid cotransporter gene, *SLC10A2,* results in *congenital diarrhea,* steatorrhea, interruption of enterohepatic circulation of bile acids, and reduced plasma cholesterol levels. Bile acids are normally synthesized from cholesterol in the liver and secreted into the small intestine, where they facilitate absorption of fat, fat-soluble vitamins, and cholesterol. Bile acids are reabsorbed in the distal ileum, return to the liver via the portal venous circulation, and resecrete into bile. Normally, the enterohepatic circulation of bile acids is an extremely efficient process; only 10% of the intestinal bile acids escape reabsorption and are eliminated in feces. Bile acid secretion is largely autoregulated, but there is only a limited capacity to increase bile acid secretion. Reduction in the bile acid pool from bile acid malabsorption causes steatorrhea, which requires restriction of dietary fat. Unabsorbed bile acids stimulate chloride excretion in the colon, resulting in diarrhea, which responds to cholestyramine, an anion-binding resin. Secondary bile acid malabsorption can result from ileal disease, such as in Crohn disease, and following an ileal resection.

Chronic neonatal-onset diarrhea has also been described in autosomal recessive **cerebrotendinous xanthomatosis,** which is caused by an inborn error of bile acid synthesis resulting from 27-hydroxylase deficiency. These children also present with juvenile-onset cataracts and developmental delay. Neonatal cholestasis has also been described as a presenting feature. Tendon xanthomas develop in the second and third decades of life. The diagnosis is important to establish, because treatment is effective when employing oral chenodeoxycholic acid.

INTESTINAL LYMPHANGIECTASIA

Obstruction of the lymphatic drainage of the intestine can be caused by either congenital defects in lymphatic duct formation or by secondary causes (Table 338-8). The **congenital** form is often associated with lymphatic abnormalities elsewhere in the body, as occur with Turner, Noonan, and Klippel-Trenaunay-Weber syndromes. Causes of **secondary** lymphangiectasia include constrictive pericarditis, heart failure, retroperitoneal fibrosis, abdominal tuberculosis, and retroperitoneal malignancies. Lymph rich in proteins, lipids, and lymphocytes leak

Table 338-8	Causes of Protein-Losing Enteropathy

Mucosal inflammation
Infection
Cytomegalovirus
Bacterial overgrowth
Invasive bacterial infection
Clostridium difficile
Helicobacter pylori
Giardiasis
Measles
Strongyloides stercoralis
Gastric inflammation
Menetrier disease
Eosinophilic gastroenteropathy
Intestinal inflammation
Celiac disease
Crohn disease
Eosinophilic gastroenteropathy
Tropical sprue
Radiation enteritis
Primary intestinal lymphangiectasia
Secondary intestinal lymphangiectasia
Constrictive pericarditis
Congestive heart failure
Post-Fontan procedure
Malrotation
Lymphoma
Noonan syndrome
Sarcoidosis
Radiation therapy
Arsenic poisoning
Colonic inflammation
Inflammatory bowel diseases
Necrotizing enterocolitis
Congenital disorders of glycosylation
Enterocyte heparin sulfate deficiency

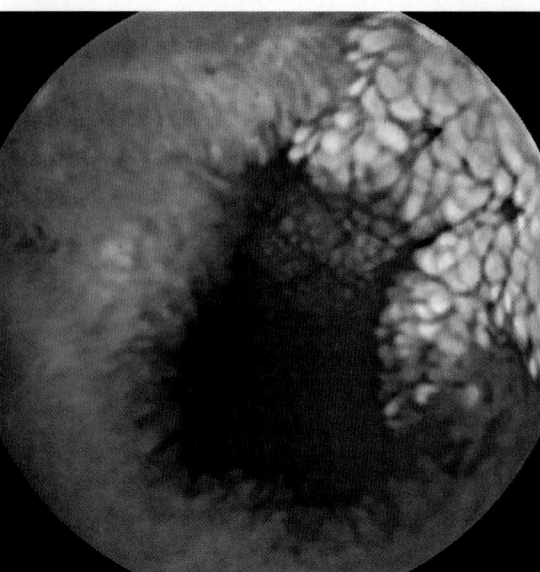

Figure 338-5 Swollen villi detected by videocapsule endoscopy in the proximal ileum. *(From Gortani G, Maschio M, Ventura A: A child with edema, lower limb deformity, and recurrent diarrhea. J Pediatr 161:1177, 2012, Fig. 1.)*

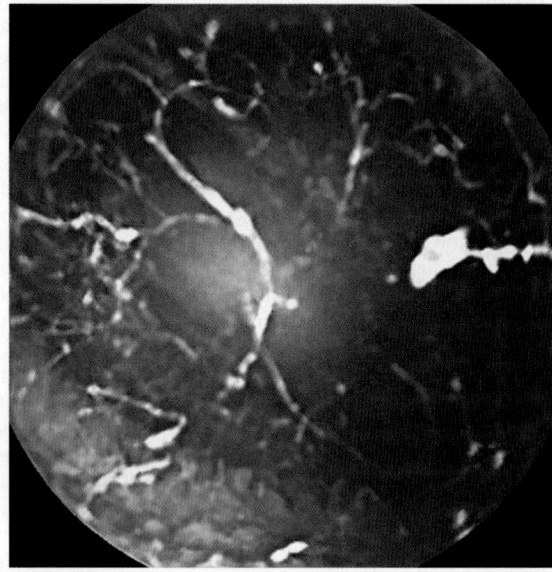

Figure 338-6 Protein-rich lymphatic fluid aggregates detected by videocapsule endoscopy in the intestinal lumen. *(From Gortani G, Maschio M, Ventura A: A child with edema, lower limb deformity, and recurrent diarrhea. J Pediatr 161:1177, 2012, Fig. 2.)*

into the bowel lumen, resulting in protein-losing enteropathy, steatorrhea, and lymphocyte depletion. Hypoalbuminemia, hypogammaglobulinemia, edema, lymphopenia, malabsorption of fat and fat-soluble vitamins, and chylous ascites often occur. Intestinal lymphangiectasia can also manifest with ascites, peripheral edema and a low serum albumin.

The diagnosis is suggested by the typical findings in association with an elevated fecal α_1-antitrypsin clearance. Radiologic findings of uniform, symmetric thickening of mucosal folds throughout the small intestine are characteristic but nonspecific. Small bowel mucosal biopsy can show dilated lacteals with distortion of villi and no inflammatory infiltrate. A patchy distribution and deeper mucosal involvement on occasion causes false-negative results on small bowel histology. Video capsule endoscopy may reveal similar lesions (Figs. 338-5 and 338-6). **Treatment** of lymphangiectasia includes restricting the amount of long-chain fat ingested and administering a formula containing protein and medium-chain triglycerides (MCTs). Supplementing a low-fat diet with MCT oil in cooking is used in the management of older children with lymphangiectasia. Rarely, parenteral nutrition is required. If only a portion of the intestine is involved, surgical resection may be considered.

ABETALIPOPROTEINEMIA

Abetalipoproteinemia is a rare autosomal recessive disorder of lipoprotein metabolism (Bassen-Kornzweig syndrome) (see Chapter 86). It is associated with severe fat malabsorption from birth. Children fail to thrive during the 1st yr of life, with stools that are pale, foul smelling, and bulky. The abdomen is distended and deep tendon reflexes are absent as a result of peripheral neuropathy, which is secondary to vitamin E (fat-soluble vitamin) deficiency. Intellectual development tends to be slow. After 10 yr of age, intestinal symptoms are less severe, ataxia develops, and there is a loss of position and vibration sensation

with the onset of intention tremors unless vitamin E levels are maintained in the normal range. These latter symptoms reflect involvement of the posterior columns, cerebellum, and basal ganglia. In adolescence, atypical retinitis pigmentosa develops without adequate supplemental of vitamin E; for instance, using a tocopheryl polyethylene glycol succinate (TPGS) formulation of the vitamin.

Diagnosis rests on the presence of acanthocytes in the peripheral blood smear and extremely low plasma levels of cholesterol (<50 mg/dL); triglycerides are also very low (<20 mg/dL). Chylomicrons and very-low-density lipoproteins are not detectable, and the low-density lipoprotein fraction is virtually absent from the circulation. Marked triglyceride accumulation in villus enterocytes occurs in the duodenal mucosa. Steatorrhea occurs in younger patients, but other processes of nutrient assimilation are intact. Rickets may be an unusual initial manifestation of abetalipoproteinemia and hypobetalipoproteinemia. Rickets is caused by steatorrhea-induced calcium losses and vitamin D deficiency. Patients have mutations of the microsomal triglyceride transfer protein gene, resulting in absence of microsomal triglyceride transfer protein function in the small bowel. This protein is required for normal assembly and secretion of very low density lipoproteins and chylomicrons.

Specific **treatment** is not available. Large supplements of the fat-soluble vitamins A, D, E, and K should be given. Vitamin E (100-200 mg/kg/24 hr) appears to arrest neurologic and retinal degeneration. Limiting long-chain fat intake can alleviate intestinal symptoms; MCTs can be used to supplement fat intake.

HOMOZYGOUS HYPOBETALIPOPROTEINEMIA

Homozygous hypobetalipoproteinemia (see Chapter 86) is transmitted as an autosomal dominant trait. The homozygous form is indistinguishable from abetalipoproteinemia. The parents of these patients, as heterozygotes, have reduced plasma low-density lipoprotein and apoprotein-β concentrations, whereas the parents of patients with abetalipoproteinemia have normal levels. On transmission electron microscopy of small bowel biopsies, the size of lipid vacuoles in enterocytes differentiates between abetalipoproteinemia and hypobetalipoproteinemia: many small vacuoles are present in hypobetalipoproteinemia, and larger vacuoles are seen in abetalipoproteinemia.

CHYLOMICRON RETENTION DISEASE (ANDERSON DISEASE)

In chylomicron retention disease, a rare recessive disorder, there is a defect in chylomicron exocytosis from enterocytes. Sar1-guanosine triphosphate promotes the formation of endoplasmic reticulum to Golgi transport carriers, and *Sar1b* is defective in Anderson disease. These patients have severe intestinal symptoms with steatorrhea, chronic diarrhea, and failure to thrive. Acanthocytosis is rare and neurologic manifestations are less severe than those observed in abetalipoproteinemia. Plasma cholesterol levels are moderately reduced (<75 mg/dL) and fasting triglycerides are normal, but the fat-soluble vitamins, particularly A and E, are very low. Treatment is early aggressive therapy with fat-soluble vitamins and modification of dietary fat intake, as in the treatment of abetalipoproteinemia.

WOLMAN DISEASE

Wolman disease is a rare, lethal lipid storage disease that leads to lipid accumulation in multiple organs, including the small intestine. In addition to vomiting, severe diarrhea, and hepatosplenomegaly, patients have steatorrhea as a result of lymphatic obstruction. Deficiency of lysosomal acid lipase is the underlying cause of disease (see Chapter 80). Successful long-term bone marrow engraftment results in normalization of peripheral blood leukocyte lysosomal enzyme acid lipase activity, with subsequent resolution of diarrhea and the restoration of developmental milestones.

DGAT1 MUTATION

Two siblings in one family with severe protracted diarrhea starting at 3 days of age had loss-of-function homozygous splice mutations in the diacylglycerol acyltransferase (*DGAT1*) gene that catalyzes the final step in the synthesis of triglycerides.

Bibliography is available at Expert Consult.

338.4 Intestinal Infections and Infestations Associated with Malabsorption

Raanan Shamir and David Branski

Malabsorption is a rare consequence of primary intestinal infection and infestation in immunocompetent children. Malabsorption is mainly seen after infection with *Campylobacter, Shigella, Salmonella, Giardia*, cryptosporidium, coccidioidosis, and rotavirus. These infectious causes of malabsorption are more common in immunocompromised children.

POSTINFECTIOUS DIARRHEA

In infants and very young toddlers chronic diarrhea can appear following infectious enteritis, regardless of the nature of the pathogen. The pathogenesis of the diarrhea is not always clear and may be related to secondary lactase deficiency, food protein allergy, antibiotic-associated colitis (including pseudomembranous colitis caused by *Clostridium difficile* toxin), or a combination of these.

Treatment is supportive and may include a lactose-free diet in the presence of secondary lactase deficiency; infants might require a semielemental diet. The beneficial effect of specific probiotic products should await well-controlled clinical trials.

BACTERIAL OVERGROWTH

Bacteria are normally present in large numbers in the colon (10^{11}-10^{13} colony-forming units [CFU]/g of feces) and have a symbiotic relationship with the host, providing nutrients and protecting the host from pathogenic organisms. Bacteria are usually present only in a small number in the stomach and small bowel and excessive numbers of bacteria in the stomach or small bowel are harmful. Gastric acid pH prevents the ingested organisms from colonizing the small bowel. Small bowel motility and the migrating motor complex cleanse the small bowel between meals and at night; the ileocecal valve prevents colonic bacteria from refluxing into the ileum. Mucosal defenses such as mucin and immunoglobulins prevent bacterial overgrowth in the small bowel. Bacterial overgrowth can result from clinical conditions that alter the gastric pH or small bowel motility, including disorders such as partial bowel obstruction, diverticula, intestinal failure, intestinal duplications, diabetes mellitus, idiopathic intestinal pseudoobstruction syndrome, and scleroderma. Prematurity, immunodeficiency, and malnutrition are other factors associated with bacterial overgrowth of the small bowel.

Diagnosis of bacterial overgrowth can be made by culturing small bowel aspirate (>10^5 CFU/mL) or by lactulose hydrogen breath test. Lactulose is a synthetic disaccharide, which is not digested by mucosal brush border enzymes but can be fermented by bacteria. High baseline hydrogen and a quick rise in hydrogen in expired breath samples support the diagnosis of bacterial overgrowth, but false-positive tests are common.

Bacterial overgrowth leads to inefficient intraluminal processing of dietary fat and to steatorrhea due to bacterial deconjugation of bile salts, vitamin B_{12} malabsorption, and microvillus brush border damage with malabsorption. Bacterial consumption of vitamin B_{12} and enhanced synthesis of folate result in decreased vitamin B_{12} and increased folate serum levels. Overproduction of D-lactate (the isomer of L-lactate) can cause stupor, neurologic dysfunction, and shock from D-lactic acidosis. Lactic acidosis should be suspected in children at risk of bacterial overgrowth, who show signs of neurologic deterioration and a high anion gap metabolic acidosis not explained by measurable acids such as L-lactate. Measurement of D-lactate is required because standard lactate assay only measures the L-isomer.

Treatment of bacterial overgrowth focuses on correction of underlying causes such as partial obstruction. The oral administration of antibiotics is the mainstay of therapy. Initial treatment with 2-4 wk of metronidazole can provide relief for many months. Cycling of antibiotics including azithromycin, trimethoprim-sulfamethoxazole, ciprofloxacin, and metronidazole may be required. Other alternatives are oral nonabsorbable antibiotics such as aminoglycosides, nitazoxanide, or rifaximin. Occasionally, antifungal therapy is required to control fungal overgrowth of the bowel.

TROPICAL SPRUE

Natives and expatriates of certain tropical regions can present with a diffuse lesion of the small intestinal mucosa—tropical sprue, even long after emigration. The endemic regions include South India, the Philippines, and some islands in the Caribbean. It is uncommon in Africa, Jamaica, and Southeast Asia. The etiology of this disorder is unclear;

because it follows outbreaks of acute diarrheal disease and improves with antibiotic therapy, an infectious etiology is suspected. The incidence is decreasing worldwide, possibly due to common use of antibiotics for gastroenteritis in developing countries. Yet, in 2011, tropical sprue was still the leading cause of malabsorption in a referral center in south India. Clinical symptoms include fever and malaise followed by watery diarrhea. After about a week the acute features subside, and anorexia, intermittent diarrhea, and chronic malabsorption result in severe malnutrition characterized by glossitis, stomatitis, cheilosis, night blindness, hyperpigmentation, and edema reflecting the various nutrient deficiencies. Muscle wasting is often marked, and the abdomen is often distended. Megaloblastic anemia results from folate and vitamin B_{12} deficiencies.

Diagnosis is made by small bowel biopsy, which shows villous flattening, crypt hyperplasia, and a chronic inflammatory cell infiltrate of the lamina propria with adjacent lipid accumulation in the surface epithelium.

Treatment requires nutritional supplementation, including supplementation of folate and vitamin B_{12}. To prevent recurrence, 6 mo of therapy with oral folic acid (5 mg) and tetracycline or sulfonamides is recommended. Relapses occur in 10-20% of patients who continue to reside in an endemic tropical region; additional courses of antibiotics may be necessary.

WHIPPLE DISEASE

Whipple disease is a chronic systemic infectious disorder. It is a rare disease, especially in childhood. The disease is caused by an infectious agent, *Tropheryma whipplei,* which can be cultured from a lymph node in the involved tissue.

The most common symptoms in Whipple disease are diarrhea, abdominal pain, weight loss, and joint pains. Malabsorption, lymphadenopathy, skin hyperpigmentation, and neurologic changes are also common. Neurologic manifestations and malabsorption are also common.

Involvement of other organs such as eyes, heart, and kidneys has been reported.

Diagnosis requires a high index of suspicion and is made upon demonstration of PAS-positive macrophage inclusions in the biopsy material, usually a duodenal biopsy. Positive identification using polymerase chain reaction for *T. whipplei confirms the diagnosis. It should not be done on stool specimens, because false-positive results were reported in healthy individuals.*

Treatment requires antibiotics such as cotrimoxazole for 1-2 yr. A 2-wk course of intravenous ceftriaxone or meropenem, followed by cotrimoxazole for 1 yr, is recommended.

Bibliography is available at Expert Consult.

338.5 Immunodeficiency Disorders
Ernest G. Seidman and David Branski

Malabsorption can occur with **congenital immunodeficiency** disorders, and chronic diarrhea with failure to thrive is often the mode of presentation. Defects of humoral and or cellular immunity may be involved, including selective IgA deficiency, agammaglobulinemia, common variable immunodeficiency disease (CVID), severe combined immunodeficiency, Wiskott-Aldrich syndrome, or chronic granulomatous disease. Although most patients with selective IgA deficiency are asymptomatic, malabsorption caused by giardiasis or nonspecific enteropathy with bacterial overgrowth can occur. Malabsorption syndrome or chronic noninfectious diarrhea has been reported in 60% of children with CVID, most often in the subgroup with low memory B cell counts. Malabsorption has also been reported in approximately 10% of patients with late-onset CVID, often secondary to giardiasis. Celiac disease is more common in patients with IgA deficiency and CVID. Paradoxically, it is more difficult to exclude the diagnosis of celiac disease because of the lack of reliability of IgA- and IgG-based

serologic tests. Malabsorption as a result of chronic rotavirus, giardiasis, bacterial overgrowth, and protein-losing enteropathy are well-recognized complications of X-linked agammaglobulinemia. Malabsorption associated with immunodeficiency is exacerbated by villus atrophy and secondary disaccharidase deficiency. In chronic granulomatous disease, phagocytic function is impaired and granulomas develop throughout the GI tract, mimicking Crohn disease. In addition to failure to thrive, it is important to consider that malabsorption associated with immunodeficiency is often complicated by micronutrient deficiencies, including vitamins A, E, and B_{12}, and calcium, zinc, and iron.

Overall, immunodeficiencies such as hypogammaglobulinemia in the pediatric age group are more often secondary to other conditions such as cancer and chemotherapy, chronic infections, malabsorption, nephrotic syndrome, or cardiac disease. Malnutrition, diarrhea, and failure to thrive are common in untreated children with **HIV infection.** The risk of GI infection is related to the depression of the CD4 count. Opportunistic infections include *Cryptosporidium parvum,* cytomegalovirus, *Mycobacterium avium-intracellulare, Isospora belli, Enterocytozoon bieneusi, Candida albicans,* astrovirus, calicivirus, adenovirus, and the usual bacterial enteropathogens. In these patients, *Cryptosporidium* can cause a chronic secretory diarrhea.

Cancer chemotherapy can damage the bowel mucosa, leading to secondary malabsorption of disaccharides such as lactose. After bone marrow transplantation, mucosal damage from **graft-versus-host disease** can cause diarrhea and malabsorption. Small bowel biopsies show nonspecific villus atrophy, mixed inflammatory cell infiltrates, and increased apoptosis. Cancer chemotherapy and bone marrow transplantation are associated with pancreatic damage leading to exocrine pancreatic insufficiency.

Bibliography is available at Expert Consult.

338.6 Immunoproliferative Small Intestinal Disease
Ernest G. Seidman and David Branski

Malignant lymphomas of the small intestine are categorized into 3 subtypes: Burkitt lymphoma, non-Hodgkin lymphomas, and Mediterranean lymphoma. Burkitt lymphoma, the most common form in children, characteristically involves the terminal ileum with extensive abdominal involvement. The relatively uncommon "Western" type of non-Hodgkin lymphomas (usually large B-cell type), can involve various parts of the small intestine. **Mediterranean lymphoma** predominantly involves the proximal small intestine. The World Health Organization recommended the term *immunoproliferative small intestinal disease* (IPSID) for the syndrome associated with Mediterranean lymphoma, because in its early stages it does not appear to be a truly malignant lymphoma. Many of the patients with "secretory" IPSID syndrome have variable levels of abnormal immunoglobulin in serum or other body fluids, identified as truncated α heavy chain. The World Health Organization classification lists IPSID with heavy chain diseases as a special variant of extranodal marginal zone B-cell small intestinal **mucosa-associated lymphoid tissue lymphoma.**

IPSID occurs most often in the proximal small intestine in older children and young adults in the Mediterranean basin, Middle East, Asia, and Africa. Poverty and frequent episodes of gastroenteritis during infancy are antecedent risk factors. The initial clinical presentation is intermittent diarrhea and abdominal pain. Later, chronic diarrhea with malabsorption (60-80%), protein-losing enteropathy, weight loss, digital clubbing, and growth failure ensue. Intestinal obstruction, abdominal masses, and ascites are common in advanced stages.

In contrast to primary nonimmunoproliferative small intestinal lymphomas, in which the pathology in the intestine is usually focal, involving specific segments of the intestine and leaving the segments between the involved areas free of disease, the pathology in IPSID is diffuse, with a mucosal cellular infiltrate involving large segments of the intestine and sometimes the entire length of the intestine, thus producing malabsorption. Molecular and immunohistochemical studies demonstrated an association with *Campylobacter jejuni* infection. The differential diagnosis includes chronic enteric infections (parasites, tropical sprue), celiac disease, and other lymphomas. Radiologic findings include multiple filling defects, ulcerations, strictures, and enlarged mesenteric lymph nodes on CT scan.

The diagnosis is usually established by endoscopic biopsies and/or laparotomy. Upper endoscopy shows thickening, erythema, and nodularity of the mucosal folds in the duodenum and proximal jejunum. As the disease progresses, tumors usually appear in the proximal small intestine and rarely in the stomach. The diagnosis requires multiple duodenal and jejunal mucosal biopsies showing dense mucosal infiltrates, consisting of centrocyte-like and plasma cells. Progression to higher-grade large-cell lymphoplasmacytic and immunoblastic lymphoma is characterized by increased plasmocytic atypia with formation of aggregates and later sheets of dystrophic plasma cells and immunoblasts invading the submucosa and muscularis propria. A serum marker of IgA, a heavy-chain paraprotein, is present in most cases.

Treatment of early-stage IPSID with antibiotics results in complete remission in 30-70% of cases. However, the majority of untreated IPSID cases progress to lymphoplasmacytic and immunoblastic lymphoma invading the intestinal wall and mesenteric lymph nodes and can metastasize to distant organs, requiring chemotherapy.

Bibliography is available at Expert Consult.

338.7 Short Bowel Syndrome
Jon A. Vanderhoof and David Branski

Short bowel syndrome results from congenital malformations or resection of the small bowel. Table 338-9 lists the causes of short bowel syndrome. Loss of >50% of the small bowel, with or without a portion of the large intestine, can result in symptoms of generalized malabsorption disorder or in specific nutrient deficiencies, depending on the region of the bowel resected. At birth, the length of small bowel is 200-250 cm; by adulthood, it grows to 300-800 cm. Bowel resection in an infant has a better prognosis than in an adult because of the potential for intestinal growth. An infant with as little as 15 cm of bowel with an ileocecal valve, or 20 cm without, has the potential to survive and be eventually weaned from total parenteral nutrition.

In addition to the length of the bowel, the anatomic location of the resection is also important. The jejunum has more circular folds and longer villi. The proximal 100-200 cm of jejunum is the main site for carbohydrate, protein, iron, and water-soluble vitamin absorption, whereas fat absorption occurs over a longer length of the small bowel. Depending on the region of the bowel resected, specific nutrient malabsorption can result. Vitamin B_{12} and bile salts are only absorbed in the distal ileum (Fig. 338-7). Jejunal resections are generally tolerated better than ileal resections because the ileum can adapt to absorb nutrients and fluids. Net sodium and water absorption is relatively much higher in the ileum. Ileal resection has a profound effect on fluid and electrolyte absorption due to malabsorption of sodium and water by the remaining ileum; ileal malabsorption of bile salts stimulates increased colonic secretion of fluid and electrolytes.

Table 338-9	Causes of Short Bowel Syndrome

CONGENITAL
Congenital short bowel syndrome
Multiple atresias
Gastroschisis

BOWEL RESECTION
Necrotizing enterocolitis
Volvulus with or without malrotation
Long segment Hirschsprung disease
Meconium peritonitis
Crohn disease
Trauma

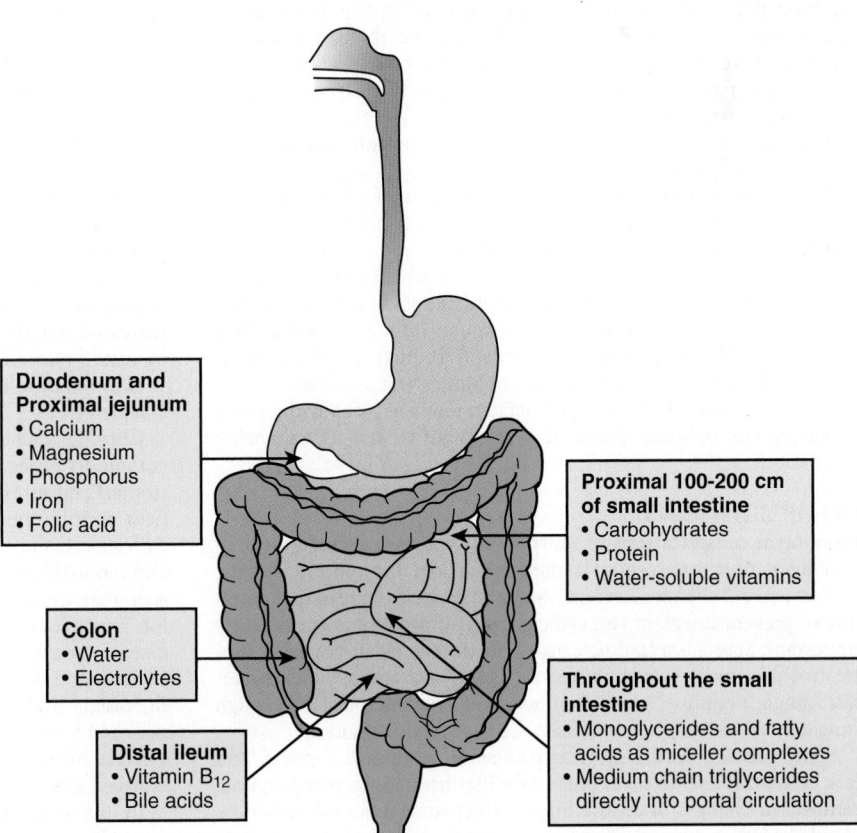

Figure 338-7 Absorption of nutrients in the small bowel varies with the region.

TREATMENT

After bowel resection, treatment of short bowel syndrome is initially focused on repletion of the massive fluid and electrolyte losses while the bowel initially accommodates to absorb these losses. Nutritional support is often provided via parenteral nutrition. A central venous catheter should be inserted to provide parenteral fluid and nutrition support. The ostomy or stool output should be measured and fluid and electrolyte losses adequately replaced. Measurement of urinary Na^+ to assess body Na^+ stores is useful to prevent Na^+ depletion. Maintaining urinary Na^+ higher than K^+ ensures that Na^+ intake is adequate. Use of oral glucose electrolyte solutions improves intestinal sodium absorption, particularly in patients without a colon.

After the initial few weeks following resection, fluid and electrolyte losses stabilize, and the focus of therapy shifts to bowel rehabilitation with the gradual reintroduction of enteral feeds. Continuous small-volume trophic enteral feeding should be initiated with a an extensively hydrolyzed protein and MCT-enriched formula or mother's milk to stimulate gut hormones and promote mucosal growth. Enteral feeding also increases pancreatobiliary flow and reduces parenteral nutrition–induced hepatotoxicity. As soon as possible, the infant should be given a small amount of water and then formula or mother's milk by mouth to maintain an interest in oral feeding and minimize or avoid the development of **oral aversion.** As intestinal adaptation occurs, enteral feeding increases and parenteral supplementation decreases. The bowel mucosa proliferates and bowel lengthens with growth.

Approximately 50% of patients with short bowel syndrome achieve enteral autonomy within 5 yr of bowel resection. Many have initial successes but then require intermittent periods of parenteral nutrition. Enteral autonomy often requires years to achieve.

Patients may require repeat surgeries for obstruction or bowel lengthening procedures (longitudinal lengthening, serial transverse enteroplasties, or both).

After achieving the maximal increase in bowel absorptive capacity, management of specific micronutrient and vitamin deficiencies and treatment of transient problems such as postinfectious mucosal malabsorption are required. GI infections such as rotavirus or small bowel bacterial overgrowth can cause setbacks in the progression to full enteral feeding in patients with marginal absorptive function. A marked increase in stool output or evidence of carbohydrate malabsorption (stool pH <5.5 and positive test for reducing substances) contraindicate further increases in enteral feeds. Slow advancement of continuous enteral feeding rates continues until all nutrients are provided enterally. Then the feeds can be altered to include increased oral or bolus feeding volumes.

In patients with large stool output, the addition of soluble fiber and antidiarrheal agents such as loperamide and anticholinergics can be beneficial, although these drugs can increase the risk of bacterial overgrowth. Cholestyramine can be beneficial for patients with distal ileal resection, but its potential depletion of the bile acid pool can increase steatorrhea. Bacterial overgrowth is common in infants with a short bowel and can delay progression of enteral feedings. Empirical treatment with metronidazole or other antibiotics (nitazoxanide, rifaximine) is often useful. Diets high in fat and lower in carbohydrate may be helpful in reducing bacterial overgrowth as well as enhancing adaptation.

COMPLICATIONS

Long-term complications of short bowel syndrome include those of parenteral nutrition: central catheter infection, thrombosis, hepatic cholestasis and cirrhosis, and gallstones. Appropriate care of the central line to prevent infection and catheter-related thrombosis is extremely important. Sepsis is a leading cause of death, can occur any time after treatment is initiated (months to years later), and is most often bacterial (single organism more common than polymicrobial), although fungal infection may be noted in 20-25% of septic episodes.

Some patients need long-term parenteral nutritional support, and lack of central line access is potentially life-threatening; inappropriate removal or changes of central lines in the neonatal period should be avoided. Other complications of terminal ileal resection include

vitamin B_{12} deficiency, which might not appear until 1-2 yr after parenteral nutrition is withdrawn. Long-term monitoring for deficiencies of vitamin B_{12}, folate, iron, fat-soluble vitamins, and trace minerals such as zinc and copper is important. **Renal stones** can occur as a result of hyperoxaluria secondary to steatorrhea (calcium binds to the excess fat and not to oxalate, so more oxalate is reabsorbed and excreted in the urine). Venous thrombosis and vitamin deficiency have been associated with hyperhomocystinemia in short bowel syndrome. Bloody diarrhea secondary to patchy, mild colitis can develop during the progression of enteral feedings. The pathogenesis of this "feeding colitis" is unknown, but it is usually benign and can improve with a hypoallergenic diet or treatment with mesalamine.

In patients who are unable to achieve full enteral feeding after several years of nutritional rehabilitation, surgical bowel lengthening procedures may be considered. In some children with complications of parenteral nutrition, especially impending liver failure, small intestinal and liver transplantation may be considered (see Chapter 331).

Bibliography is available at Expert Consult.

338.8 Chronic Malnutrition

Raanan Shamir and David Branski

Primary malnutrition (i.e., undernutrition) is very common in developing countries and is directly related to increased disease burden and mortality (see Chapter 46). In developed countries, chronic malnutrition occurs mainly as a result of decreased food intake, malabsorption syndromes, and increased nutritional needs in children with chronic diseases. Malnutrition is diagnosed in 11-50% of hospitalized children and recent reports from Europe suggest a prevalence of close to 20% in chronically ill children. Child neglect and improper preparation of formula can result in severe malnutrition. Malnutrition can be identified by evaluating dietary intake, by medical history (anorexia, vomiting, dysphagia, mood and behavioral changes, abdominal pain, diarrhea), by anthropometric measurements (e.g., reduced weight per age and weight per height, body mass index <5th percentile), and by clinical signs of nutrient deficiencies (atrophic tongue in iron-deficiency anemia or alopecia in zinc deficiency). Screening tools for malnutrition are used in adults to provide a simple and fast way of diagnosing those patients in need. Few such screening tools for the pediatric population were developed and are being studied.

Malnourished children suffer from impaired immunity, poor wound healing, muscle weakness, and diminished psychologic drive. Malnutrition has short-term consequences (increased disability, morbidity, and mortality) and long-term consequences (final adult size, lower IQ, economic productivity). Undernutrition in hospitalized children is related to increased infectious complications, delayed recovery, increased length of stay and costs, increased readmission rate, and increased mortality.

Nutritional rehabilitation in malnourished children is discussed in Chapter 46.

Chronic malnutrition complicated by diarrheal dehydration is a commonly observed phenomenon. Infectious diarrhea is common in tropical and subtropical countries, in the setting of poor hygiene practices, in immunocompromised hosts (e.g., HIV, congenital immunodeficiency), and when impairment of the immune response is due to chronic malnutrition itself. In children with chronic disorders, diarrhea may be related to the underlying disease that should be sought for. Examples include noncompliance with a gluten-free diet in celiac disease, noncompliance with pancreatic enzyme treatment in cystic fibrosis, and disease relapse in inflammatory bowel disease (IBD). In the case of IBD, relapse should be diagnosed only after infectious diarrhea and *C. difficile* infection have been ruled out. Malnutrition per se can lead to exocrine pancreatic insufficiency, which, in turn, aggravates malabsorption and diarrhea.

In infants and children with severe malnutrition, many of the signs normally used to assess the state of hydration or shock are unreliable.

Severe malnutrition might be accompanied by sepsis; thus, children with septic shock might not have diarrhea, thirst, or sunken eyes but may be hypothermic, hypoglycemic, or febrile. The electrocardiogram often shows tachycardia, low amplitude, and flat or inverted T waves. Cardiac reserve seems lowered, and heart failure is a common complication.

Despite clinical signs of dehydration, urinary osmolality may be low in the chronically malnourished child. Renal acidifying ability is also limited in patients with malnutrition.

Management of the diarrhea in chronically malnourished children is based on 3 principles: oral rehydration to correct dehydration, rapid resumption of feeds with avoidance of periods of nothing by mouth, and treating the etiology of the diarrhea.

When treating the dehydration, it must be remembered that in dehydrated and malnourished infants there appears to be overexpansion of the extracellular space accompanied by extracellular and presumably intracellular hypoosmolality. Thus, reduced or hypotonic osmolarity oral rehydration solutions are indicated in this setting. When oral rehydration is not possible, the route of choice is nasogastric, and intravenous therapy should be avoided if possible.

Initial intravenous therapy in profound dehydration is designed to improve the circulation and expand extracellular volume. For patients with edema, the quality of fluid and the rate of administration might need to be readjusted from recommended levels to avoid over hydration and pulmonary edema. Blood should be given if the patient is in shock and is severely anemic. Potassium salts can be given early if urine output is good. Clinical and electrocardiogram improvement may be more rapid with magnesium therapy.

Children with chronic malnutrition are at risk for the refeeding syndrome. Therefore, initial calorie provision should not exceed the previous daily intake and is usually begun at 50-75% of estimated resting energy expenditure, with rapid increase to caloric goals once there are no severe abnormalities in sodium, potassium, phosphorus, calcium, or magnesium. Correction of malnutrition and catch-up growth are not part of the primary treatment of these children, but a nutrition rehabilitation plan is necessary.

Bibliography is available at Expert Consult.

338.9 Enzyme Deficiencies
Michael J. Lentze and David Branski

CARBOHYDRATE MALABSORPTION

Symptoms of carbohydrate malabsorption include loose watery diarrhea, flatulence, abdominal distention, and pain. Some children are asymptomatic unless the malabsorbed carbohydrate is consumed in large amounts. Disaccharidases are present on the brush border membrane of the small bowel. Disaccharidase deficiency can be caused by a genetic defect or secondarily by damage to the small bowel epithelium, as occurs with infection or inflammatory disorders.

Unabsorbed carbohydrates enter the large bowel and are fermented by intestinal bacteria, producing organic acids and gases such as methane and hydrogen. The gases can cause discomfort and the unabsorbed carbohydrate and the organic acids cause osmotic diarrhea characterized by an acidic pH and presence of either reducing or nonreducing sugars in the stool. Hydrogen gas can be detected in the breath as a sign of fermentation of unabsorbed carbohydrates (H_2-breath test).

LACTASE DEFICIENCY

Congenital lactase deficiency is rare and is associated with symptoms occurring on exposure to lactose in milk. Fewer than 50 cases have been reported worldwide. In patients with congenital lactase deficiency, 5 distinct mutations in the coding region of the *LCT* gene were found. In most patients (84%), homozygosity for a nonsense mutation, 4170T-A (Y1390X; OMIM 223000), designated Fin (major), was found.

Primary adult type-hypolactasia is caused by a physiologic decline in lactase actively that occurs following weaning in most mammals. The brush-border lactase is expressed at low levels during fetal life; activity increases in late fetal life and peaks from term to 3 yr, after which levels gradually decrease with age. This decline in lactase levels varies between ethnic groups. Lactase deficiency occurs in approximately 15% of white adults, 40% of Asian adults, and 85% of black adults in the United States. Lactase is encoded by a single gene (*LCT*) of approximately 50 kb located on chromosome 2q21. C/T (−13910) polymorphisms of the *MCM6* gene were found to be related to adult-type hypolactasia in most European populations. In 3 African populations—Tanzanians, Kenyans, and Sudanese—3 single-nucleotide polymorphisms, G/C (−14010), T/G (−13915), and C/G (−13907), were identified with lactase persistence and have derived alleles that significantly enhance transcription from the lactase gene promoter in vitro.

Secondary lactose intolerance follows small bowel mucosal damage (celiac disease, rotavirus infection) and is usually transient, improving with mucosal healing.

Lactase deficiency can be diagnosed by H_2-breath test or by measurement of lactase activity in mucosal tissue retrieved by small bowel biopsy. Diagnostic testing is not mandatory, and often simple dietary changes that reduce or eliminate lactose from the diet relieve symptoms.

Treatment of lactase deficiency consists of a milk-free diet. A lactose-free formula (based on either soy or cow's milk) can be used in infants. In older children, low-lactose milk can be consumed. Addition of lactase to dairy products usually abbreviates the symptoms.

Live-culture yogurt contains bacteria that produce lactase enzymes and is therefore tolerated in most patients with lactase deficiency. Hard cheeses have a small amount of lactose and are generally well tolerated.

FRUCTOSE MALABSORPTION

Children consuming a large quantity of juice rich in fructose, corn syrup, or natural fructose in fruit juices can present with diarrhea, abdominal distention, and slow weight gain. Restricting the amount of juice in the diet resolves the symptoms and helps avoid unnecessary investigations. Fructose H_2 breath test can be helpful in the diagnosis of fructose malabsorption. The reason for fructose malabsorption is the reduced abundance of GLUT-5 transporter on the surface of the intestinal brush-border membrane, which occurs in approximately 5% of the population.

SUCRASE–ISOMALTASE DEFICIENCY

Sucrase–isomaltase deficiency is a rare autosomal recessive disorder with a complete absence of sucrase and reduced maltase digestive activity. The sucrase–isomaltase complex is composed of 1,927 amino acids encoded by a 3,364 bp messenger RNA. The gene locus on chromosome 3 has 30 exons spanning 106.6 kb. The majority of sucrase–isomaltase mutations result in a lack of enzyme protein synthesis (null mutation). Posttranslational processing defects are also identified.

Approximately 2% of Europeans and Americans are mutant heterozygote. Sucrase deficiency is especially common in indigenous Greenlanders (estimated 5%) in whom it is often accompanied by lactase deficiency.

Symptoms of sucrase-isomaltase deficiency usually begin when the infant is exposed to sucrose or a glucose polymer diet. This can occur with ingestion of non–lactose-based infant formula or on the introduction of pureed food, especially fruits and sweets. Diarrhea, abdominal pain, and poor growth are observed. Occasional patients present with symptoms in late childhood or even adult life, but careful history often indicates that symptoms appeared earlier. Diagnosis of sucrase-isomaltase malabsorption requires acid hydrolysis of stool for reducing substances because sucrase is a nonreducing sugar. Alternatively, diagnosis can be achieved with hydrogen breath test or direct enzyme assay of small bowel biopsy.

The mainstay of **treatment** is lifelong dietary restriction of sucrose-containing foods. Enzyme replacement with a purified yeast enzyme, sacrosidase (Sucraid), is a highly effective adjunct to dietary restriction.

GLUCOSE–GALACTOSE MALABSORPTION

More than 30 different mutations of the sodium/glucose cotransporter gene (*SGLT1*) are identified. These mutations cause a rare autosomal recessive disorder of intestinal glucose and galactose/Na$^+$ cotransport system that leads to osmotic diarrhea. Because most dietary sugars are polysaccharides or disaccharides with glucose or galactose moieties, diarrhea follows the ingestion of glucose, breast milk, or conventional lactose-containing formulas. Dehydration and acidosis can be severe, resulting in death.

The stools are acidic and contain sugar. Patients with the defect have normal absorption of fructose, and their small bowel function and structure are normal in all other aspects. Intermittent or permanent glycosuria after fasting or after a glucose load is a common finding because of the transport defect also being present in the kidney. The presence of reducing substances in watery stools and slight glycosuria despite low blood sugar levels is highly suggestive of glucose–galactose malabsorption. Malabsorption of glucose and galactose is easily identified using the breath hydrogen test. It is safe to perform the first test with a dose of 0.5 g/kg of glucose; if necessary, a second test can be performed using 2 g/kg. Breath H$_2$ will rise more than 20 ppm. The small intestinal biopsy is useful to document a normal villous architecture and normal disaccharidase activities. The identification of mutations of *SGLT1* makes it possible to perform prenatal screening in families at risk for the disease.

Treatment consists of rigorous restriction of glucose and galactose. Fructose, the only carbohydrate that can be given safely, should be added to a carbohydrate-free formula at a concentration of 6-8%. Diarrhea immediately ceases when infants are given such a formula. Although the defect is permanent, later in life, limited amounts of glucose, such as starches or sucrose may be tolerated.

EXOCRINE PANCREATIC INSUFFICIENCY

Chapter 349 discusses disorders of exocrine pancreatic insufficiency. Cystic fibrosis is the most common congenital disorder associated with exocrine pancreatic insufficiency. Although rare, the next most common cause of pancreatic insufficiency in children is Shwachman-Diamond syndrome. Other rare disorders causing exocrine pancreatic insufficiency are Johanson-Blizzard syndrome (severe steatorrhea, aplasia of alae nasi, deafness, hypothyroidism, scalp defects), Pearson bone marrow syndrome (sideroblastic anemia, variable degree of neutropenia, thrombocytopenia), and isolated pancreatic enzyme deficiency (lipase, colipase and lipase–colipase, trypsinogen, amylase). Deficiency of enterokinase—a key enzyme that is produced in the proximal small bowel and is responsible for the activation of trypsinogen to trypsin—manifests clinically as exocrine pancreatic insufficiency.

Autoimmune polyendocrinopathy syndrome type 1, a rare autosomal recessive disorder, is caused by mutation in the autoimmune regulator gene (*AIRE*). Chronic mucocutaneous candidiasis is associated with failure of parathyroid gland, adrenal cortex, pancreatic β cells, gonads, gastric parietal cells, and thyroid gland. Pancreatic insufficiency and steatorrhea are associated with this condition.

ENTEROKINASE (ENTEROPEPTIDASE) DEFICIENCY

Enterokinase (enteropeptidase) is a brush-border enzyme of the small intestine. It is responsible for the activation of trypsinogen into trypsin. Deficiency of this enzyme results in severe diarrhea, malabsorption, failure to thrive, and hypoproteinemic edema after birth.

Enterokinase deficiency is caused by mutation in the serine protease-7 gene (*PRSS7*) on chromosome 21q21. The diagnosis can be established by measuring the enzyme level in intestinal tissue. Treatment of this rare autosomal recessive disorder consists of replacement with pancreatic enzymes and administration of a protein hydrolyzed formula with added MCT oil in infancy.

TRYPSINOGEN DEFICIENCY

Trypsinogen deficiency is a rare syndrome with symptomatology similar to that of enterokinase deficiency. Enterokinase catalyzes the conversion of trypsinogen to trypsin, which, in turn, activates the various pancreatic proenzymes such as chymotrypsin, procarboxypeptidase, and proelastase for their active forms. Deficiency of trypsinogen results in severe diarrhea, malabsorption, failure to thrive, and hypoproteinemic edema soon after birth.

The trypsinogen gene is encoded on chromosome 7q35. Treatment is the same as for enterokinase deficiency, with pancreatic enzymes and protein hydrolysate formula with added MCT oil in infancy.

338.10 Liver and Biliary Disorders Causing Malabsorption

Anil Dhawan and David Branski

Absorption of fats and fat-soluble vitamins depends to a great extent on adequate bile flow providing bile acids to the small intestine. Most of the liver and biliary disorders lead to impairment of the bile flow, contributing to malabsorption of long-chain fatty acids and vitamins such as A, D, E, and K. Liver disorders that are associated with significant malabsorption and failure to thrive are: (1) progressive familial intrahepatic cholestasis (types 1, 2, and 3) and bile acid synthesis defects. Progressive familial intrahepatic cholestasis type 1 is also associated with chronic diarrhea caused by bile transport defect in the gut. It is not uncommon for these children to have symptomatic fat-soluble vitamin deficiencies like pathologic fractures and peripheral neuropathy. (2) Children with storage disorders such as Wolman disease also manifest with severe failure to thrive and multiple vitamin deficiencies. (3) Children with biliary disorders such as biliary atresia after a Kasai portoenterostomy, cystic fibrosis, neonatal sclerosing cholangitis, Alagille syndrome, and sclerosing cholangitis constitute another major group of disorders where malabsorption could be a significant problem. In addition, severe portal hypertension can lead to portal hypertensive enteropathy, resulting in poor absorption of the nutrients. Decompensated liver disease leads to anorexia and increased energy expenditures, further widening the gap between calorie intake and net absorption, leading to severe malnutrition. Adequate management of nutrition is essential to improve the outcome with or without liver transplantation. This is usually achieved by using MCT-rich milk formula, supplemental vitamins, and continuous or bolus enteral feed where oral intake is poor.

Vitamin D deficiency is commonly observed on biochemical tests, and children rarely present with pathologic fractures. Simultaneous administration of vitamin D with the water-soluble vitamin E preparation (TPGS 1,000 succinate) enhances absorption of vitamin D. In young infants, oral vitamin D$_3$ is given at a dose of 1,000 IU/kg/24 hr. After 1 mo, if the serum 25-hydroxyvitamin D level is low, the same dose of oral vitamin D is mixed with TPGS. 25-Hydroxyvitamin D is then monitored every 3 mo, with adjustment of doses as necessary.

Vitamin E deficiency in patients with chronic cholestasis is not usually symptomatic, but it can manifest as a progressive neurologic syndrome, which includes peripheral neuropathy (manifesting as loss of deep tendon reflexes and ophthalmoplegia), cerebellar ataxia, and posterior column dysfunction. Early in the course, findings are partially reversible with treatment; late features might not be reversible. It may be difficult to identify vitamin E deficiency because the elevated blood lipid levels in cholestatic liver disease can falsely elevate the serum vitamin E level. Therefore, it is important to measure the ratio of serum vitamin E to total serum lipids; the normal level for patients younger than 12 yr of age is >0.6, and for patients older than 12 yr it is >0.8. The neurologic disease can be prevented with the use of an oral water-soluble vitamin E preparation (TPGS, Liqui-E) at a dose of 25-50 IU/day in neonates and 1 IU/kg/day in children.

Vitamin K deficiency can occur as a result of cholestasis and poor fat absorption. In children with liver disease it is very important to differentiate between the coagulopathy related to vitamin K malabsorption and one secondary to the synthetic failure of the liver. A single dose of vitamin K administered intravenously does not correct the prolonged prothrombin time in liver failure, but the deficiency state responds within a few hours. Easy bruising may be the first sign. In neonatal cholestasis, coagulopathy as a result of vitamin K deficiency can manifest with intracranial bleeds with devastating consequences, and prothrombin time should be routinely measured to monitor for deficiency in children with cholestasis. All children with cholestasis should receive vitamin K supplements.

Vitamin A deficiency is rare and is associated with night blindness, xerophthalmia, and increased mortality if patients contract measles. Serum vitamin A levels should be monitored and adequate supplementation considered.

338.11 Rare Inborn Defects Causing Malabsorption

Klaus-Peter Zimmer and David Branski

Some congenital (primary) malabsorption disorders originate from a defect of integral membrane proteins, which fulfill a transport function as receptor or channel across the apical or basolateral membrane of enterocytes for nutritional components. Histologic examination of the small and large bowel is typically normal. Most of these disorders are inherited in an autosomal recessive pattern. Most are rare, and patients present with a broad phenotypic heterogeneity as a result of modifier genes and nutritional and other secondary factors.

DISORDERS OF CARBOHYDRATE ABSORPTION

Patients with **Fanconi-Bickel syndrome** present with tubular nephropathy; rickets; hepatomegaly; glycogen accumulation in liver, kidney, and small bowel; failure to thrive; and fasting hypoglycemia. The disorder is caused by homozygous mutations of GLUT2, the facilitative glucose (and galactose) transporter at the basolateral membrane of enterocytes hepatocytes, renal tubules, pancreatic islet cells, and cerebral neurons. Because severe osmotic diarrhea is not a feature of Fanconi-Bickel syndrome, a GLUT2-independent basolateral transport for glucose is suggested. GLUT2 seems to modulate insulin secretion, renal reabsorption, and glucose uptake from the apical membrane of enterocytes in response to the (postprandial) sugar environment. Diagnostic signs are elevated galactose levels in the blood (found in the neonatal screening program), neonatal bilateral cataracts, marked glycosuria, generalized aminoaciduria, and excessive renal losses of phosphate and calcium. Liver and kidneys are enlarged. Therapy includes substitution of electrolyte losses and vitamin D and supplying uncooked cornstarch to prevent hypoglycemia. Patients who present in the neonatal period need frequent small meals and galactose-free milk.

DISORDERS OF AMINO ACID AND PEPTIDE ABSORPTION

Owing to their ontogenic origins, enterocytes and renal tubules express amino acid transporter in common. Their highest intestinal transporter activity is found in the jejunum. The transporters causing Hartnup disease, cystinuria, iminoglycinuria, and dicarboxylic aminoaciduria are located in the apical membrane, and those causing lysinuric protein intolerance (LPI) and blue diaper syndrome are anchored in the basolateral membrane of the intestinal epithelium.

Dibasic amino acids, including cystine, ornithine, lysine, and arginine are taken up by the Na-independent SLC3A1/SLC7A9, which is defective in **cystinuria**. The overall prevalence of the disease is 1 in 7,000 newborns. This disorder is not associated with any GI or nutritional consequences because of compensation by alternative transporter. However, hypersecretion of cystine in the urine leads to recurrent cystine stones, which account for up to 1% of all urinary tract stones. Ample hydration, urine alkalinization, and cystine-binding thiol drugs can increase the solubility of cystine. Cystinuria type I is inherited as an autosomal recessive trait, and the transmission of type II is autosomal dominant with incomplete penetrance. Cystinuria type I has been described in association with 2p21 deletion syndrome and hypotonia–cystinuria syndrome.

Hartnup disease is characterized by malabsorption of neutral amino acids, including the essential amino acid tryptophan, with aminoaciduria, photosensitive pellagra-like rash, headaches, cerebellar ataxia, delayed intellectual development, and diarrhea. The clinical spectrum ranges from asymptomatic patients to severely affected patients with progressive neurodegeneration leading to death by adolescence. SLC6A19, which is the major luminal sodium-dependent neutral amino acid transporter of small intestine and renal tubules, has been identified as the defective protein. Its association with collectrin and angiotensin-converting enzyme II is likely to be involved in the phenotypic heterogeneity of Hartnup disorder. Tryptophan is a precursor of nicotinamide adenine dinucleotide phosphate biosynthesis; therefore the disorder can be treated by nicotinamide in addition to a diet of 4 g protein/kg. The use of lipid-soluble esters of amino acids and tryptophan ethylester has also been reported.

In the **blue diaper syndrome (indicanuria, Drummond syndrome)** tryptophan is specifically malabsorbed and the defect is expressed only in the intestine and not in the kidney, in contrast to Hartnup disease. Intestinal bacteria convert the unabsorbed tryptophan to indican, which is responsible for the bluish discoloration of the urine after its hydrolysis and oxidation. Symptoms can include digestive disturbances such as vomiting, constipation, poor appetite, failure to thrive, hypercalcemia, nephrocalcinosis, fever, irritability, and ocular abnormalities. The molecular genetic defect of this disorder has not yet been characterized.

The underlying defect of **iminoglycinuria** is the malabsorption of proline, hydroxyproline, and glycine as a consequence of the proton amino acid transporter SLC36A2 defect, with a possible participation of modifier genes, one of which (SLC6A20) is present in the intestinal epithelium. This disorder is usually benign, but sporadic cases with encephalopathy, mental retardation, deafness, blindness, kidney stones, hypertension, and gyrate atrophy have been described.

The excitatory amino acid carrier SLC1A1 is affected in **dicarboxylic aminoaciduria**. This carrier is present in the small intestine, kidney, and brain, and transports the anionic acids L-glutamate, L- and D-aspartate, and L-cysteine. There are single case reports indicating that this disorder could be associated with hyperprolinemia and neurologic symptoms such as **POLIP** (polyneuropathy, ophthalmoplegia, leukoencephalopathy, intestinal pseudoobstruction syndrome).

A histidine-specific transport system has also been proposed. A few patients have been reported with an intestinal and renal defect of this carrier. It has not been confirmed that patients with **histidinuria**, who have low plasma histidine levels, in contrast to histidinemia, develop neurologic symptoms (e.g., hearing loss, myoclonic seizures).

A methionine-preferring transporter in the small intestine was suggested to be affected in **Smith-Strang disease (oasthouse urine disease)**, which is characterized by purple, red-brown-colored urine with a cabbage-like odor, containing 2-hydroxybutyric acid, valine, and leucine. The potential symptoms of **methionine malabsorption** include neurologic signs, white hair, and diarrhea. Large amounts of methionine and branched-chain amino acids are present in the feces but not in the urine. A low-methionine diet is recommended to alleviate the symptoms.

Among the diseases (see the earlier discussion of cystinuria) with a membrane transport defect of cationic amino acids (lysine, arginine, ornithine), **LPI** is the second most common, with a prevalence in Finland of 1 in 60,000. The y$^+$LAT-1 (SLC7A7) carrier at the basolateral membrane of the intestinal and renal epithelium is affected, with failure to deliver cytosolic dibasic cationic amino acids into the paracellular space in exchange for Na$^+$ and neutral amino. This defect is not compensated by the SLC3A1/SLC7A9 transporter (at the apical membrane), the latter being affected in cystinuria. The symptoms of

LPI, which appear after weaning, include diarrhea, failure to thrive, hepatosplenomegaly, nephritis, respiratory insufficiency, alveolar proteinosis, pulmonary fibrosis, and osteoporosis. Abnormalities of bone marrow have also been described in a subgroup of LPI patients. The disorder is characterized by low plasma concentrations of dibasic amino acids (in contrast to high levels of citrulline, glutamine, and alanine) and massive excretion of lysine (as well as orotic acid, ornithine, and arginine in moderate excess) in the urine. Hyperammonemia and coma usually develop after episodic attacks of vomiting, after fasting, or following administration of large amounts of protein (or alanine load), possibly because of a deficiency of intramitochondrial ornithine. Some patients show moderate retardation. Cutaneous manifestations can include alopecia, perianal dermatitis, and sparse hair. Some patients avoid protein-containing food. Treatment includes orally administered citrulline (200 mg/kg/day), which is well absorbed from the intestine; dietary protein restriction (<1.5 g/kg/day); and carnitine supplementation. One patient with **isolated lysinuria** has been reported with growth failure, seizures, and mental retardation.

DISORDERS OF FAT TRANSPORT

Chapter 86 describes abetalipoproteinemia, hypobetalipoproteinemia, and chylomicron retention disease. The long-chain fatty acid (FATP4) and cholesterol transporters, the latter being called Niemann-Pick C1-like protein (NPC1L1), have been characterized at the intestinal brush-border in knockout mice models showing a hyperproliferative hyperkeratosis and an impaired fatty acid and cholesterol uptake. NPC1L1 is inhibited by ezetimibe, which is used to restrict the absorption of dietary cholesterol.

Tangier disease is characterized by the absence of high-density lipoprotein cholesterol, which is caused by mutations in the adenosine triphosphate–binding cassette transporter A1 (ABCA1) gene. The failure of intracellular phospholipids and cholesterol efflux to lipid-poor apolipoprotein acceptors such as high-density lipoprotein predisposes to premature coronary heart disease and accumulation of cholesterol in liver, spleen, lymph nodes (tonsils), and small intestine.

Features of Tangier disease include orange tonsils, hepatosplenomegaly, relapsing neuropathy, orange-brown spots on the colon and ileum, diarrhea in association with decreased plasma cholesterol levels (apolipoprotein A-I and A-II), and normal or elevated triglyceride levels. Specific therapy for Tangier disease has not yet been established.

In **sitosterolemia,** defective efflux of sterol leads to increased absorption of dietary sterols; normally, <5% are retained by the GI tract. Patients carry mutations of the ABCG5 (sterolin-1) and ABCG8 (sterolin-2) transporters. The disorder is associated with tendon xanthomas, increased atherosclerosis, and hemolysis. Plasma levels of phytosterols (mainly sitosterol) are typically >10 mg/dL.

Congenital diarrhea in newborns with hyperlipidemia may indicate impaired fat (bile) absorption and mutations of the microsomal enzyme acyl-coenzyme A:diacylglycerol acyltransferase 1 (DGAT1), which catalyzes the final step in triglyceride synthesis.

DISORDERS OF VITAMIN ABSORPTION

Transporters and receptors of the intestinal epithelium have been described for water-soluble but not fat-soluble vitamins, the latter being absorbed primarily by enterocytes, by passive diffusion after emulsification of fats by bile salts. Transfer proteins (retinol-binding protein, RBP4, and α-tocopherol transfer protein, TTP1) have been involved in deficiency states of vitamins E (spinocerebellar ataxia) and A (ophthalmologic signs), respectively.

Vitamin B_{12} (cobalamin) is used exclusively by microorganisms and is acquired mostly from meat and milk. Its absorption starts with the removal of cobalamin from dietary protein by gastric acidity and its binding to haptocorrin. In the duodenum, pancreatic proteases hydrolyze the cobalamin-haptocorrin complex, allowing the binding of cobalamin to intrinsic factor (IF), which originates from parietal cells. The receptor of the cobalamin-IF complex is located at the apical membrane of the ileal enterocytes and represents a heterodimer consisting of cubilin and amnionless, with endocytic uptake of this ligand into endosomes, where it binds to megalin and forms a cobalamin–transcobalamin-2 complex (after cleavage of IF) for further transcytosis. As a cofactor for methionine synthase, cobalamin converts homocysteine to methionine. Cobalamin deficiency can be caused by inadequate intake of the vitamin (e.g., breastfeeding by mothers on a vegetarian diet), primary or secondary achlorhydria including autoimmune gastritis, exocrine pancreatic insufficiency, bacterial overgrowth (see Chapter 338.4), ileal disease (Crohn disease, see Chapter 336), ileal (or gastric) resection, infections (fish tapeworm), and Whipple disease (see Chapter 341).

Clinical signs of congenital **cobalamin malabsorption**, which usually appear from a few mo to 14 yr of age, are pancytopenia including megaloblastic anemia, fatigue, failure to thrive, and neurologic symptoms, including developmental delay. Recurrent infections and bruising may be present. Laboratory evaluation indicates low serum cobalamin, hyperhomocysteinemia, methylmalonic acidemia, and mild proteinuria. The Schilling test is useful to differentiate between lack of IF and malabsorption of cobalamin. Three rare autosomal recessive disorders of congenital cobalamin deficiency affect absorption and transport of cobalamin (in addition to 7 other inherited defects of cobalamin metabolism). These include mutations of the gastric IF (GIF) gene with absence of IF (but normal acid secretion and lack of autoantibodies against IF or parietal cells), mutations of the amnionless (AMN) and cubilin (CUBN) genes (**Imerslund-Grasbeck syndrome**), and mutations in the transcobalamin 2 cDNA. These disorders require long-term parenteral cobalamin treatment: intramuscular injections of hydroxycobalamin 1 mg daily for 10 days and then once a month. High-dose substitution with oral cyanocobalamin (1 mg biweekly) does not seem to be sufficient for all patients with congenital cobalamin deficiency.

Folate is an essential vitamin required to synthesize methionine from homocysteine. It is found mainly in green leafy vegetables, legumes, and oranges. It is converted to 5- methyltetrahydrofolate after its uptake by enterocytes. Secondary folate deficiency is caused by insufficient folate intake, villous atrophy (e.g., celiac disease, IBD), treatment with phenytoin, and trimethoprim, among others (see Chapter 448.1). Several inherited disorders of folate metabolism and transport have been described.

Hereditary **folate malabsorption** is characterized by a defect of the proton-coupled folate transporter (formerly reported to be HCP1, a heme carrier) of the brush-border, leading to impaired absorption of folate in the upper small intestine as well as impaired transport of folate into the central nervous system. Mutations of the reduced folate carrier (RFC1, SLC19A1) have not been found in this entity. Sulfasalazine and methotrexate are potent inhibitors of proton-coupled folate transporter. Symptoms of congenital folate malabsorption are diarrhea, failure to thrive, megaloblastic anemia (in the 1st few mo of life), glossitis, infections (Pneumocystis jiroveci) with hypoimmunoglobulinemia, and neurologic abnormalities (seizures, mental retardation, and basal ganglia calcifications). Macrocytosis, with or without neutropenia, multilobulated polymorphonuclear cells, increased lactate dehydrogenase and bilirubin, increased saturation of transferrin, and decreased cholesterol can be found. Low levels of folate are present in serum and cerebrospinal fluid. Plasma homocysteine concentrations as well as urine excretion of formiminoglutamic acid and orotic acid are elevated. Long-lasting deficiency is best documented using red cell folate. Therapy involves large doses of oral (up to 100 mg/day) or systemic (intrathecal) folate.

The molecular basis of intestinal transport of other water-soluble vitamins such as **vitamin C** (Na$^+$-dependent vitamin C transporters 1 and 2), **pyridoxine/vitamin B_6**, and **biotin/vitamin B_5** (Na$^+$-dependent multivitamin transporter) have been described; however congenital defects of these transporter systems have not yet been found in humans. A **thiamine/vitamin B_1**-responsive megaloblastic anemia syndrome, which is associated with early-onset type 1 diabetes mellitus and sensorineural deafness, is caused by mutations of the thiamine transporter protein, THTR-1 (SLC19A2), present in the brush-border.

DISORDERS OF ELECTROLYTE AND MINERAL ABSORPTION

Congenital chloride diarrhea belongs to the more common causes of severe congenital diarrhea, with prevalence in Finland of 1:20,000. It is caused by a defect of the *SLC26A3* gene, which encodes a Na^+-independent Cl^-/HCO_3^- exchanger within the apical membrane of ileal and colonic epithelium. Founder mutations have been described in Finnish, Polish, and Arab patients: V317del, I675-676ins, and G187X, respectively. The Cl^-/HCO_3^- exchanger absorbs chloride originating from gastric acid and the cystic fibrosis transmembrane conductance regulator and secretes bicarbonate into the lumen, neutralizing the acidity of gastric secretion.

Prenatal clinical signs of this disorder are a dilated small bowel that can mislead to a diagnosis of intestinal obstruction. Newborns with congenital chloride diarrhea present with severe life-threatening secretory diarrhea during the 1st few wk of life. Laboratory findings are metabolic alkalosis, hypochloremia, hypokalemia, and hyponatremia (with high plasma renin and aldosterone activities). Fecal chloride concentrations are >90 mmol/L and exceed the sum of fecal sodium and potassium. Early diagnosis and aggressive lifelong enteral substitution of KCl in combination with NaCl (chloride doses of 6-8 mmol/kg/day for infants and 3-4 mmol/kg/day for older patients) prevent mortality and long-term complications (such as urinary infections, hyperuricemia with renal calcifications, renal insufficiency, and hypertension) and allow normal growth and development. Orally administered proton pump inhibitors, cholestyramine, and butyrate can reduce the severity of diarrhea. The diarrheal symptoms usually tend to regress with age. However, febrile diseases are likely to exacerbate symptoms as a consequence of severe dehydration and electrolyte imbalances. (See Chapter 52 for fluid and electrolyte management.)

The classic form of **congenital sodium diarrhea** manifests with polyhydramnios, massive secretory diarrhea, severe metabolic acidosis, alkaline stools (fecal pH >7.5) and hyponatremia as a result of fecal losses of Na^+ (fecal Na^+ >70 mmol/L). Urinary secretion of sodium is low to normal. There is partial villous atrophy. The molecular genetic defect could not be located in the Na^+-H^+ exchangers, which were thought to be impaired because they seem to be mainly responsible for Na^+ absorption in the small intestine. In addition, a syndromic form of congenital sodium diarrhea with choanal or anal atresia, hypertelorism, and corneal erosions has been related to mutations of *SPINT2*, encoding a serine–protease inhibitor, whose pathophysiologic action on intestinal Na^+ absorption is unclear. Some patients can be weaned from parenteral nutrition later in childhood but depend on oral sodium citrate supplementation.

The congenital form of **acrodermatitis enteropathica** manifests with severe deficiency of body zinc soon after birth in bottle-fed children or after weaning from breastfeeding. Clinical signs of this disorder are anorexia, diarrhea, failure to thrive, humoral and cell-mediated immunodeficiency (poor wound healing, recurrent infections), male hypogonadism, skin lesions (vesicobullous dermatitis on the extremities and perirectal, perigenital, and perioral regions, and alopecia), and neurologic abnormalities (tremor, apathy, depression, irritability, nystagmus, photophobia, night blindness, and hypogeusia). The genetic defect of acrodermatitis enteropathica is caused by a mutation in the Zrt-Irt-lik protein 4 (ZIP4, SLC39A4), normally expressed on the apical membrane, which enables the uptake of zinc into the cytosol of enterocytes. The zinc-dependent alkaline phosphatase and plasma zinc levels are low. Paneth cells in the crypt of the small intestinal mucosa show inclusion bodies. Acrodermatitis enteropathica requires long-term treatment with elemental zinc 1 mg/kg/day. Maternal zinc deficiency impairs embryonic, fetal, and postnatal development. Chapter 51 describes the acquired forms of zinc deficiency.

Menkes disease and **occipital horn syndrome** are both caused by mutations in the gene encoding Cu^{2+} transporting adenosine triphosphatase (ATPase), α-polypeptide (ATP7A), also called Menkes or MNK protein. ATP7A is mainly expressed by enterocytes, placental cells, and the central nervous system, and is localized in the *trans*-Golgi network for copper transfer to enzymes in the secretory pathway or to endosomes to facilitate copper efflux. Copper values in liver and brain

are low in contrast to an increase in mucosal cells, including enterocytes and fibroblasts. Plasma copper and ceruloplasmin levels decline postnatally. Clinical features of Menkes disease are progressive cerebral degeneration (convulsions), feeding difficulties, failure to thrive, hypothermia, apnea, infections (urinary tract), peculiar facies, hair abnormalities (kinky hair), hypopigmentation, bone changes, and cutis laxa. Patients with the classic form of Menkes disease usually die before the age of 3 yr. A therapeutic trial with copper-histidinase should start before the age of 6 wk. In contrast to Menkes disease, occipital horn syndrome usually manifests during adolescence with borderline intelligence, craniofacial abnormalities, skeletal dysplasia (short clavicles, pectus excavatum, genu valgum), connective tissue abnormalities, chronic diarrhea, orthostatic hypotension, obstructive uropathy, and osteoporosis. It should be differentiated from Ehlers-Danlos syndrome type V.

Active **calcium** absorption is mediated by the transient receptor potential channel 6 (TRPV6) at the brush border membrane, calbindin, and the CaATPase, or the Na^+-Ca^{++} exchanger for calcium efflux at the basolateral membrane within the proximal small bowel. A congenital defect of these transporters has not yet been described.

Intestinal absorption of dietary magnesium, which occurs via the transient receptor potential channel TRPM6 at the apical membrane, is impaired in familial **hypomagnesemia with secondary hypocalcemia**, which manifests with neonatal seizures and tetany.

Intestinal iron absorption consists of several complex regulated processes starting with the uptake of heme-containing iron by heme carrier protein 1 (HCP1) and Fe^{2+} (after luminal reduction of oxidized Fe^{3+}) by the divalent metal transporter 1 (DMT1) at the apical membrane, followed by the efflux of Fe^{2+} by ferroportin 1 (also called iron-regulated transporter) at the basolateral membrane of duodenal enterocytes. Mutations of the ferroportin 1 gene have been found in the autosomal dominant form of **hemochromatosis type 4**. Mutations of HFE (Cys282 Tyr, His63Asn, Ser65Cys) of classic hemochromatosis reduce the endocytic uptake of diferric transferrin by the transferrin receptor-1 at the basolateral membrane of the intestinal epithelium. Hepcidin antimicrobial peptide encodes hepcidin, a hepatic peptide hormone, which inhibits the efflux of iron through ferroportin and can be induced by IL-6. It is the defective gene of juvenile hemochromatosis (type 2, subtype B).

Bibliography is available at Expert Consult.

338.12 Malabsorption in Eosinophilic Gastroenteritis

Ernest G. Seidman and David Branski

Eosinophilic digestive diseases are a group of rare and heterogeneous conditions characterized by patchy or diffuse eosinophilic infiltration of GI tissue. The diagnosis of eosinophilic gastroenteritis is based on GI symptoms, GI eosinophilic infiltrates, and the absence of other causes such as parasitic infection (most commonly *Enterobius vermicularis* in children) or a specific allergic response. Peripheral eosinophilia and elevated serum IgE levels are variably present are not diagnostic criteria. The majority (50-70%) of patients have a history of other allergic disorders, and others might have associated connective tissue diseases. Approximately 10% of patients with this disorder have an immediate family member affected, suggesting that eosinophilic GI disorders stem from a genetic predisposition, common environmental factors, or, most likely, a combination. Hypersensitivity to specific food allergens has been postulated as an etiologic factor. Symptoms depend on the severity and location of eosinophilic inflammation. Any region or layer (mucosa, submucosa, and serosa) of the gut may be involved, alone or in combination.

Diagnosis requires pan-endoscopy with biopsies. Eosinophilic infiltrates dominate the histologic findings, and signs of other inflammatory diseases are absent; in particular, the crypt architecture remains normal, no parasites are identified, and no eggs or larvae are found.

Table 338-10	Common Micronutrient Deficiencies in Inflammatory Bowel Disease			
MICRONUTRIENT	**CROHN DISEASE AND/OR ULCERATIVE COLITIS**	**MALABSORPTION**	**INTESTINAL LOSSES**	**INADEQUATE INTAKE**
Iron	CD and UC	+ (CD)	+++	++
Vitamins A, D, E, K	CD > UC	++ (CD)		+++
Vitamin B$_{12}$	CD	+++		+
Vitamin B$_1$, B$_2$, B$_6$	CD > UC			++
Vitamin C, glutathione (antioxidants)	CD and UC		++	++
Folate	CD and UC	++		+
Calcium, magnesium, selenium, zinc	CD and UC	++	+++	+
Polyunsaturated fatty acids	CD	++		++

CD, Crohn disease; UC, ulcerative colitis.

An increase in mast cells and IgE-containing plasma cells may be observed. Mucosal biopsies will only establish the diagnosis in cases with mucosal involvement. Small bowel capsule endoscopy is often very useful in that it characteristically reveals denuded mucosal erythema with marked focal villous atrophy in areas out of reach of standard endoscopes. The most common sites of involvement are the stomach and small intestine.

Symptoms may include abdominal pain (90%), vomiting (60%), nausea (50%), and abdominal distention (50%). Diarrhea with weight loss because of malabsorption can occur if small bowel involvement with villous blunting is extensive. Other than peripheral eosinophilia, hypoalbuminemia as a result of protein-losing enteropathy and iron-deficiency anemia are the more common laboratory findings.

Nutritional exclusion (or elemental) diets and corticosteroids are the mainstay of treatment. Approximately 50% of cases are complex, characterized by unpredictable relapses and a chronic course. Less-well-documented treatments, such as mast cell stabilizers and leukotriene antagonists (montelukast), have been used in small, uncontrolled trials. Clinical trials using biological modalities such as monoclonal anti-IgE (omalizumab) and anti-IL-5 (SCH55700/reslizumab and mepolizumab) are anticipated for severe cases.

Bibliography is available at Expert Consult.

338.13 Malabsorption in Inflammatory Bowel Disease
Ernest G. Seidman and David Branski

Crohn disease and ulcerative colitis represent the 2 forms of chronic, immune-mediated IBD that commonly affect pediatric patients (see Chapter 336). Because the small bowel is involved in the majority of pediatric Crohn disease patients, malabsorption of nutrients is far more of a problem than in ulcerative colitis. At the time of diagnosis, significant weight loss is observed in up to 85% of pediatric patients with Crohn disease and in approximately 65% with ulcerative colitis, due to inadequate intake of energy and micronutrients as well as diarrhea and malabsorption. Consequently, growth failure as a consequence of chronic undernutrition is far more common in Crohn disease than in ulcerative colitis, affecting up to 40% of cases.

In addition to malabsorption, energy intake is lower in patients with Crohn disease compared to healthy controls, in part due to lesser appetite. Excessive levels of proinflammatory cytokines are implicated in causing the anorexia as well as in mediating impaired growth. The symptoms, including abdominal pain, nausea, vomiting, and diarrhea, can cause affected children to have a lower desire to eat, which can lead to reduced food intake. This can, in turn, negatively affect nutritional status during a child's critical period of growth and development.

Patients with IBD are also at risk of developing nutritional deficiencies because of restrictive diets imposed by caregivers or by the patients themselves.

In children with active disease, inadequate intakes of energy and of a number of micronutrients have been observed. Reduced energy intake during active disease can contribute to poor weight gain and impaired growth. Patients with IBD, particularly Crohn disease, often have multiple nutritional deficiencies and may be in negative nitrogen balance because of decreased intake and malabsorption of macro- and micronutrients. Quantifying nutrient intake, determining micronutrient deficiencies, and ascertaining requirements for nutritional supplementation are essential components of successful management in pediatric IBD.

Optimizing nutritional status and growth are key priorities in the management of IBD in children and adolescents. Energy intake should meet the added costs of catch-up growth and are usually in the range of 40-70 kcal/kg ideal body weight per day. Protein requirements are higher in Crohn disease (1-1.5 g/kg/day). Bone mineral density deficit is common, even in pediatric patients who have not been exposed to systemic corticosteroid therapy. Osteoporosis or osteopenia is best assessed by bone densitometry, and levels of vitamin 25-hydroxyvitamin D should be monitored. Table 338-10 shows other micronutrient deficiencies that result from inadequate intake, malabsorption, and gut losses.

Bile acid malabsorption is common in ileal Crohn disease, especially after small bowel resection. This leads to diarrhea and also places patients at increased risk for urolithiasis and cholelithiasis. The prevalence of recurrent calcium-oxalate urolithiasis is up to 5-fold higher in Crohn disease. Increased urinary oxalate and decreased citrate excretion, resulting from bowel resection with mainly preserved colon, were identified as crucial risk factors for stone formation. The hyperoxaluria predominantly results from increased colonic permeability to oxalate due to disturbed bile acid metabolism.

Enteral nutrition support is favored over parenteral for all but Crohn disease patients with extreme short gut. To induce remission, exclusive nutritional therapy given orally was reported to be as effective as when continuously administered by enteral feeding tube. However, weight gain was significantly greater for the latter group. Patients requiring hospitalization for a severe relapse should receive nutrition support if they are already malnourished or their intake is likely to be severely curtailed for ≥1 wk. Preoperative nutrition support is essential to the prevention of morbidity and mortality. However, clinicians must be aware of the risk of the refeeding syndrome in patients with severe malnutrition. In ulcerative colitis, nutrition support is adjunctive therapy; there is no evidence that bowel rest or total parenteral nutrition parenteral nutrition influences the outcome of severe ulcerative colitis.

Bibliography is available at Expert Consult.

Chapter **339**

Intestinal Transplantation in Children with Intestinal Failure

Jorge D. Reyes and André A.S. Dick

The introduction of tacrolimus and the development of the abdominal multiorgan procurement techniques allowed the tailoring of various types of intestine grafts that can contain other intraabdominal organs, such as the liver, pancreas, and stomach; this has been critical to the application of this type of organ transplant. The understanding that the liver protects the intestine against rejection demonstrates the interaction between recipient and donor immunocytes (host-versus-graft and graft-versus-host) which under the cover of immunosuppression allows varying degrees of graft acceptance and eventual minimization of drug therapy. Over the past several years the number of patients placed on the list for and those undergoing intestinal transplantation has decreased, which may be a result of (1) improvements in the care of patients with intestinal failure under a multidisciplinary intestinal care team management, (2) the introduction of new lipid management strategies for the treatment of cholestatic liver disease, and (3) corrective surgery enhancing absorptive surface and motility.

INDICATIONS FOR INTESTINAL TRANSPLANT

Intestinal failure describes a patient who has lost the ability to maintain nutritional support and adequate fluid requirements, needed to sustain growth, with their own intestine and is permanently dependent on total parenteral nutrition (TPN). The majority of these patients have short bowels as a result of a congenital deficiency or acquired condition (see Chapter 338.7). In others, the cause of intestinal failure is a functional disorder of motility or absorption (Table 339-1). Rarely do patients receive intestinal transplants for benign neoplasms. The complications of intestinal failure include loss of venous access, life-threatening infections, and TPN-induced cholestatic liver disease.

Table 339-1	Causes of Intestinal Failure in Children Requiring Transplantation

SHORT BOWEL
- Congenital disorders
- Volvulus
- Gastroschisis
- Necrotizing enterocolitis
- Intestinal atresia
- Trauma

INTESTINAL DYSMOTILITY
- Intestinal pseudoobstruction
- Intestinal aganglionosis (Hirschsprung disease)

ENTEROCYTE DYSFUNCTION
- Microvillus inclusion disease
- Tufting enteropathy
- Autoimmune disorders
- Crohn disease

TUMORS
- Familial polyposis
- Inflammatory pseudotumor

Paucity of Venous Access

Administration of TPN requires the insertion of a centrally placed venous catheter, there being only 6 readily accessible sites (bilateral internal jugulars, subclavians, iliac veins). The loss of venous access generally occurs in the setting of recurrent catheter sepsis and thrombosis; clinical convention suggests that loss of 50% of these venous access sites places the patient at risk of not being able to be treated with TPN.

Life-Threatening Infections

Life-threatening infections are usually catheter-related; the absence of significant lengths of intestine may be associated with abnormal motility of the residual bowel (producing both delayed or rapid emptying), with varying degrees of bacterial overgrowth and possible bacterial or fungal translocation as a consequence of loss of intestinal barrier function and/or loss of gut immunity. This situation can produce cholestatic liver disease, multisystem organ failure, and metastatic infectious foci in lungs, kidneys, liver, and the brain.

Liver Disease

The development of cholestatic liver disease is the most serious complication of intestinal failure and may be a consequence of the toxic drug effects of TPN on hepatocytes, a disruption of bile flow and bile acid metabolism, and the frequent occurrence of bacterial translocation and sepsis with endotoxin release into the portal circulation. This complication varies in frequency depending on the patient's age and the etiology of the intestinal failure; it is most common in neonates with extreme short gut. The effects on the liver include fatty transformation, steatohepatitis and necrosis, fibrosis, and then cholestasis. The development of clinical jaundice (total bilirubin >3 mg/dL) and thrombocytopenia are significant risk factors for poor outcome, because these changes portend the development of portal hypertensive gastroenteropathy, hypersplenism, coagulopathy, and uncontrollable bleeding.

TRANSPLANTATION OPERATION
Donor Selection

Intestinal grafts are usually procured from hemodynamically stable, ABO-identical brain-dead donors who have minimal clinical or laboratory evidence suggesting intraabdominal ischemia; size matching varies according to age of the recipients; present surgical techniques allow for significant reductions of the graft in order to achieve abdominal closure. Human leukocyte antigen has been random, and cross-matching has not been a determinant of graft acceptance. Exclusion criteria include a history of malignancy and intraabdominal evidence of infection; systemic viral or bacterial infections are not excluded. Donor preparation has been limited to the administration of systemic and enteral antibiotics. Prophylaxis for graft-versus-host disease with graft pretreatment using irradiation or a monoclonal antilymphocyte antibody has varied over time. Grafts have been preserved with the University of Wisconsin solution, as is the case with other types of abdominal organs.

Types of Intestinal Grafts

Intestinal allografts are used in various forms, either alone (as an **isolated intestine graft**) or as a composite graft, which can include the liver, duodenum, and pancreas (**liver–intestine graft**); when this composite graft includes the stomach, and the recipient operation requires the removal of all of the patient's gastrointestinal tract (as with intestinal pseudoobstruction) and liver, then this replacement graft is known as a **multivisceral graft**.

The procurement of these various types of grafts focuses on the preservation of the arterial vessels of celiac and/or superior mesenteric arteries, as well as appropriate venous outflow, which would include the superior mesenteric vein or the hepatic veins in the composite grafts. The larger composite grafts inherently retain the celiac and superior mesenteric arteries; this includes multivisceral grafts, liver plus small bowel grafts, and "modified multivisceral grafts" in which the liver is excluded but the entire gastrointestinal tract is replaced, including the stomach. The isolated intestine graft retains the superior mesenteric artery and vein; this graft can be accomplished with preservation of the vessels going to the pancreas, when that organ has been allocated to another recipient. The graft that is to be used in a particular recipient is dissected out in situ and then removed after cardiac arrest of the donor, with core cooling of the organs, using an infusion of preservation solution (Fig. 339-1).

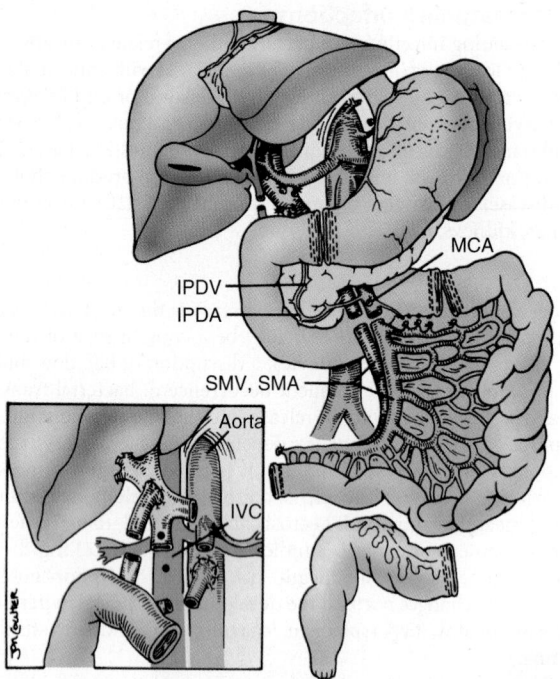

Figure 339-1 The various abdominal organs can be dissected in situ, providing isolated or composite grafts to fit the individual patient's needs. Separation of intestine and pancreas is feasible, with preservation of the inferior pancreaticoduodenal artery (*IPDA*) and vein (*IPDV*). The use of vascular grafts from the donor allow connections to the superior mesenteric pedicle (artery [*SMA*] and vein [*SMV*]) to aorta and inferior vena cava (*IVC*) or portal vein (*inset*). (*Reproduced with permission from Abu-Elmagd K, Fung J, Bueno J, et al: Logistics and technique for procurement of intestinal, pancreatic and hepatic grafts from the same donor,* Ann Surg *232:680–697, 2000.*)

Various modifications in these grafts have included the preservation of visceral ganglia at the base of the arteries, the inclusion of donor duodenum and pancreas for the liver and intestine graft, the inclusion of colon, the reduction of the liver graft (into left or right side) and variable reduction of the intestine graft, and the development of living donor intestine grafts.

The Recipient Operation
Because many children have had multiple previous abdominal operations, intestinal transplantation can be a formidable technical challenge; most children require replacement of the liver because of TPN-induced disease and often present with advanced liver failure. Transplantation of an isolated intestinal allograft involves exposure of the lower abdomen, infrarenal aorta, and inferior vena cava. Placement of vascular homografts using donor iliac artery and vein to these vessels allows arterialization and venous drainage of the intestinal graft. In patients who have retained their intestine and then undergo an enterectomy at the time of transplantation, use of the native superior mesenteric vessels is feasible.

Transplantation of a larger composite graft requires the removal and replacement of the native liver in the liver with intestine transplant, and complete abdominal exenteration in the multivisceral transplant. In a similar fashion, the infrarenal aorta is exposed for placement of an arterial conduit graft (donor thoracic aorta) for arterialization of the graft. The venous drainage is achieved to the retained hepatic veins, which are fashioned to a single conduit for anastomosis to the allograft liver.

The intestinal anastomosis to native proximal and distal bowel are performed, leaving an enterostomy of distal allograft ileum; this will be used for routine posttransplantation surveillance endoscopy and biopsy. This ostomy is closed 3-6 mo after transplantation (Fig. 339-2).

POSTOPERATIVE MANAGEMENT
Immunosuppression
Successful immunosuppression for intestinal transplantation is initiated with tacrolimus and corticosteroids. This required high levels of tacrolimus (in the nephrotoxic range), and although initial success rates were high they were followed by rejection rates of >80%, infection, and late drug toxicities, resulting in a gradual loss of grafts and patients. The next generation of protocols incorporated the addition of other agents, such as azathioprine, cyclophosphamide, induction with an interleukin-2 antibody antagonist, mycophenolate mofetil, and rapamycin. This modification resulted in a decreased incidence in the severity of initial rejection; the ability to decrease immunosuppression

Small Bowel Transplantation Surgery

Isolated Intestine   Combined with Liver   Multivisceral

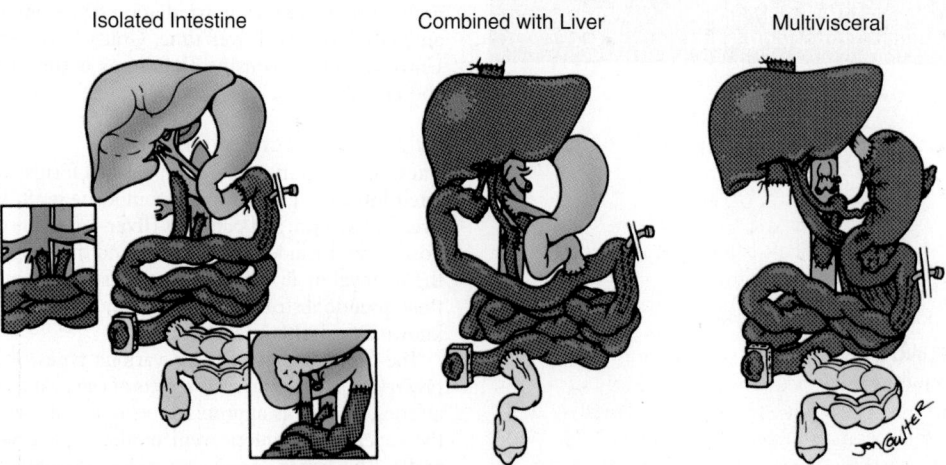

Figure 339-2 The 3 basic intestinal transplant procedures (the graft is *shaded*). With the isolated intestine, the venous outflow may be to the recipient portal vein (*main figure*), inferior vena cava (*inset left*), or superior mesenteric vein (*inset right*). With the composite grafts, which include the liver, the arterialization is from the aorta with venous drainage out from the liver graft to the recipient inferior vena cava.

later did not allow for stabilization of long-term survival. The introduction of *recipient* pretreatment using antilymphocyte antibodies and the elimination of recipient therapy with steroids have resulted in improved transplant survival as a result of a significant decrease in the incidence of rejection and infection, permitting the gradual decrease of immunosuppressive drug therapy within 3 mo, and a decline in drug toxicity events. The most common initial maintenance regimen used is tacrolimus and prednisone dual therapy. By 1 yr the majority of patients are on tacrolimus monotherapy.

Allograft Assessment

There are no simple laboratory tools that allow assessment of the intestinal allograft. The gold standard for diagnosis of intestinal allograft rejection has been serial endoscopic surveillance and biopsies through the allograft ileostomy. Clinical signs and symptoms of rejection or infection of the allograft can overlap and mimic each other, producing either rapid diarrhea or complete ileus with pseudoobstruction syndromes, or gastrointestinal bleeding. Any changes in clinical status should warrant thorough evaluation for rejection with endoscopic biopsies and an evaluation for opportunistic infection, malabsorption, and other enteral infections.

The diagnosis of acute rejection is based on seeing destruction of crypt epithelial cells from apoptosis, in association with a mixed lymphocytic infiltrate. These histologic findings may or may not correlate with endoscopic evidence of injury, which varies from diffuse erythema and friability to ulcers and, in cases of severe rejection, exfoliation of the intestinal mucosa. Chronic rejection of the allograft can be diagnosed only through full thickness sampling of the intestine, which shows the typical vasculopathy that can result in progressive ischemia of the allograft.

Rejection and Graft-Versus-Host Disease

Acute rejection rates for the intestinal allograft are significantly higher than with any other organ, in the range of 80-90%, and severe rejection requiring the use of antilymphocyte antibody preparations may be as high as 30%. Triple-drug regimens and the use of interleukin-2 antibody inhibitors have resulted in significant decreases in rejection rates; nonetheless, the amount of immunosuppression was incompatible with improvements in long-term patient and graft survival. Rejection rates of 40% are achievable with the use of antilymphocyte globulin. These protocols induce varying degrees of "proper tolerance," which can eventually allow for minimization of immunosuppression, thus reducing the risk of drug toxicity and infection. Vascular rejection has been an uncommon occurrence, and chronic rejection has been seen in approximately 15% of cases. Graft-versus-host disease is infrequent but potentially life-threatening. The mortality rate exceeds 80% and most recipients die from infectious complications from bone marrow failure. The incidence seen in intestinal transplantation is 5-6%. Although no standard treatment is available, early diagnosis, prevention of infection, and initiation of treatment as soon as possible may improve outcomes.

Infections

Infectious complications are the most significant cause of morbidity and mortality after intestinal transplantation. The most common infections (bacterial, fungal, polymicrobial) occur as a result of the continuing need for venous catheter placement for as long as 1 yr posttransplantation. Infections as a consequence of immunosuppressive drug management are from cytomegalovirus (CMV) infection (22% incidence), Epstein-Barr virus (EBV)–induced infections (21% incidence), and adenovirus enteritis (40% incidence). Despite improvements in monitoring and preventative measures, CMV remains the most common viral infection post–intestinal transplantation. CMV may be acquired from blood transfusions, reactivation of endogenous viruses, or the donated allograft. The highest risk recipients for CMV infection are those who are immunologically naïve and receive an allograft from a donor who is seropositive. The 2 mainstay CMV prevention strategies commonly employed are universal prophylaxis and preemptive therapy. Current consensus guidelines

recommend prophylaxis treatment for high-risk patients (donor+/recipient−). The preferred drugs for CMV prophylaxis are ganciclovir and oral valganciclovir.

Patients at the highest risk for EBV infection are similarly those who are seronegative at the time of transplantation and those requiring a high-burden immunosuppressive therapy to maintain their graft. EBV disease varies from asymptomatic viremia to posttransplant lymphoproliferative disorder (PTLD). The incidence of EBV-related PTLD is highest in patients receiving intestinal allografts compared to liver, heart, or kidney. Children have a higher incidence of PTLD compared to adults, and are most likely to have EBV+PTLD. Early diagnosis and prevention of PTLD is essential and the mainstay of therapy is to reduce immunosuppression, although some patients have required chemotherapy. The use of anti–B-cell monoclonal antibodies, such as the anti-CD20 antibody rituximab, in PTLD has been successful as noted in anecdotal reports. Successful management of these viral infections is achieved through early detection and preemptive therapy, for both CMV and EBV, before the development of a serious life-threatening infection. This approach has improved outcomes for CMV, eliminating the mortality in the pediatric patient population (see Chapters 178, 254, and 255).

Outcomes

Intestinal transplantation is the standard of care for children with intestinal failure who have significant complications of TPN and can no longer tolerate such therapy. Data from the Organ Procurement and Transplantation Network (OPTN)/Scientific Registry of Transplant Recipients (SRTR) Annual Report 2011, and center-specific data reports have documented significant improvements with short- and long-term survivals for transplantations occurring principally in the last 10 yr; intestinal transplantation (liver-intestine and isolated intestinal transplants) graft failure rates for deceased donor transplants in 2010-2011 were 26% at 1 yr, 46% at 3 yr for transplants in 2008-2009, and 48% at 5 yr for transplants in 2006-2007 (Fig. 339-3). It is hoped that with the minimization strategies currently used the long-term survival will plateau as occurs with other organ transplants; rehabilitation and quality-of-life studies have shown that more than 80% of survivors reach total independence from TPN and have meaningful

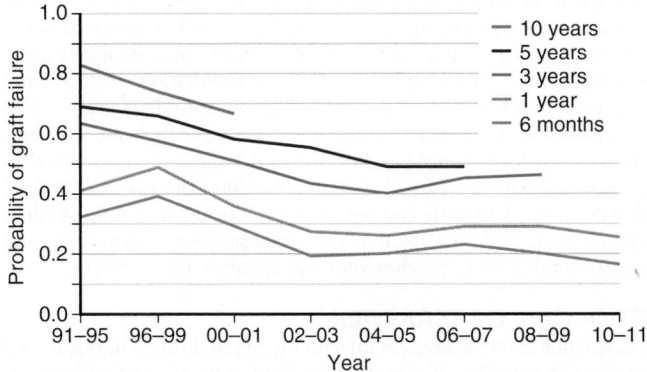

**Graft Failure Among Intestinal Transplant Recipients:
Deceased Donor**

Figure 339-3 OPTN/SRTR Annual Report demonstrating that intestine graft survival has improved significantly with the application of better immunosuppressive strategies, infection surveillance and management, and perioperative care. Cox proportional hazards models reporting probability, adjusting for age, sex, and race. *(From Organ Procurement and Transplantation Network (OPTN) and Scientific Registry of Transplant Recipients (SRTR): OPTN/SRTR 2011 Annual Data Report. Department of Health and Human Services, Health Resources and Services Administration, Healthcare Systems Bureau, Division of Transplantation; 2012. Available at http://srtr.transplant.hrsa.gov/annual_reports/2011/default.aspx)*

life activities. Consequently, there has been a shift in efforts to improve long-term outcomes and quality of life.

Bibliography is available at Expert Consult.

Chapter 340
Acute Gastroenteritis in Children
Zulfiqar Ahmed Bhutta

The term *gastroenteritis* denotes infections of the gastrointestinal tract caused by bacterial, viral, or parasitic pathogens (Tables 340-1 to 340-3). Many of these infections are foodborne illnesses. The most common manifestations are diarrhea and vomiting, which can also be associated with systemic features such as abdominal pain and fever. The term **gastroenteritis** captures the bulk of infectious cases of diarrhea. The term **diarrheal disorders** is more commonly used to denote infectious diarrhea in public health settings, although several noninfectious causes of gastrointestinal illness with vomiting and/or diarrhea are well recognized (Table 340-4).

EPIDEMIOLOGY OF CHILDHOOD DIARRHEA
Diarrheal disorders in childhood account for a large proportion (9%) of childhood deaths, with an estimated 0.71 million deaths per year globally, making it the second most common cause of child deaths worldwide. Almost 1.731 billion episodes of diarrhea occurred in 2010 in children younger than 5 yr of age in developing countries, with more than 80% of the episodes occurring in Africa and South Asia (50.5% and 32.5%, respectively) and 36 million of the total episodes progress to severe episodes. Global mortality may be declining rapidly, but the overall incidence of diarrhea has only declined from 3.4 to approximately 2.9 episodes per child-year in the past 2 decades, and it is estimated to account for 23 million childhood disability-adjusted life years.

The decline in diarrheal mortality, despite the lack of significant changes in incidence, is the result of preventive rotavirus vaccination and improved case management of diarrhea, as well as improved nutrition of infants and children. These interventions have included widespread home- and hospital-based oral rehydration therapy and improved nutritional management of children with diarrhea.

In addition to the risk of mortality, persistently high rates of diarrhea, especially prolonged and persistent diarrhea among young children may be associated with long-term adverse outcomes. Diarrheal illnesses, especially early and repeated episodes among young children can be associated with malnutrition, micronutrient deficiencies, and significant deficits in psychomotor and cognitive development.

ETIOLOGY OF DIARRHEA
Gastroenteritis is the result of infection acquired through the fecal–oral route or by ingestion of contaminated food or water. Gastroenteritis is associated with poverty, poor environmental hygiene, and development indices. Enteropathogens that are infectious in a small inoculum (*Shigella*, enterohemorrhagic *Escherichia coli*, *Campylobacter jejuni*, noroviruses, rotavirus, *Giardia lamblia*, *Cryptosporidium parvum*, *Entamoeba histolytica*) can be transmitted by person-to-person contact, whereas others, such as cholera, are generally a consequence of contamination of food or water supply (see Tables 340-1 to 340-3).

In the United States, rotavirus and the noroviruses (small round viruses such as Norwalk-like virus and caliciviruses) are the most common viral agents, followed by sapoviruses, enteric adenoviruses, and astroviruses (see Table 340-2). Foodborne outbreaks in the United States are mostly caused by norovirus, accounting for 58% of all episodes, and by bacterial causes, which are most commonly *Salmonella*, *Clostridium perfringens*, *Campylobacter*, and *Staphylococcus aureus*, followed much less often by *E. coli*, *Clostridium botulinum*, *Shigella*, *Cryptosporidium*, *Yersinia*, *Listeria*, *Vibrio*, and *Cyclospora* species, in that order. Food sources include poultry, leafy vegetables, beef, fruits and nuts, vine-stalk vegetables, and many other foods.

Direct person-to-person contact outbreaks of gastroenteritis are usually caused by norovirus and *Shigella* species. Unknown agents are seen in 30-40%; other pathogens include *Salmonella*, rotavirus, *Giardia*, *Cryptosporidium*, *Clostridium difficile*, and *C. jejuni*.

The exact etiologic fractions of diarrhea among children in developing countries are a subject of much research, and our knowledge of the various pathogens that cause moderate to severe childhood diarrhea has grown considerably (Fig. 340-1; Table 340-5). There are indications that rates of hospitalization and deaths caused by *Shigella* infections, especially *Shigella dysenteriae* type 1, the most severe form of shigellosis, may be declining; however, it accounts for nearly 28,000 deaths annually. Enteropathogenic *E. coli* is responsible for 79,000 and enterotoxigenic *E. coli* (ETEC) may be responsible for 42,000 deaths annually among children younger than 5 yr. Rotavirus infections (the most common identifiable viral cause of gastroenteritis in all children) account for 197,000 deaths annually or 28% of all deaths caused by diarrhea among children younger than 5 yr of age.

PATHOGENESIS OF INFECTIOUS DIARRHEA
Pathogenesis and severity of bacterial disease depend on whether organisms have preformed toxins *(S. aureus, Bacillus cereus)*, produce secretory (cholera, *E. coli*, *Salmonella*, *Shigella*) or cytotoxic (*Shigella*, *S. aureus*, *Vibrio parahaemolyticus*, *C. difficile*, *E. coli*, *C. jejuni*) toxins, or are invasive, and on whether they replicate in food. Enteropathogens can lead to either an inflammatory or noninflammatory response in the intestinal mucosa (Table 340-6).

Enteropathogens elicit **noninflammatory diarrhea** through **enterotoxin** production by some bacteria, destruction of villus (surface) cells by viruses, adherence by parasites, and adherence and/or translocation by bacteria. **Inflammatory diarrhea** is usually caused by bacteria that directly invade the intestine or produce cytotoxins with consequent fluid, protein, and cells (erythrocytes, leukocytes) that enter the intestinal lumen. Some enteropathogens possess more than 1 virulence property. Some viruses, such as rotavirus, target the microvillus tips of the enterocytes and can enter the cells by direct invasion or calcium-dependent endocytosis. This can result in villus shortening and loss of enterocyte absorptive surface through cell shortening and loss of microvilli (Fig. 340-2).

Most bacterial pathogens elaborate enterotoxins; the rotavirus protein NSP4 acts as a viral enterotoxin. Bacterial enterotoxins can selectively activate enterocyte intracellular signal transduction and can also affect cytoskeletal rearrangements with subsequent alterations in the water and electrolyte fluxes across enterocytes. In toxigenic diarrhea, enterotoxin produced by *Vibrio cholerae*, increased mucosal levels of cyclic adenosine monophosphate, inhibit electroneutral NaCl absorption but have no effect on glucose-stimulated Na^+ absorption. In inflammatory diarrhea (e.g., *Shigella* spp. or *Salmonella* spp.) there is extensive histologic damage, resulting in altered cell morphology and reduced glucose-stimulated Na^+ and electroneutral NaCl absorption. The role of 1 or more cytokines in this inflammatory response is critical. In secretory cells from crypts, Cl secretion is minimal in normal subjects and is activated by cyclic adenosine monophosphate in toxigenic and inflammatory diarrhea (Fig. 340-3).

ETEC colonizes and adheres to enterocytes of the small bowel via its surface fimbriae (pili) and induces hypersecretion of fluids and electrolytes into the small intestine through 1 of 2 toxins: the heat-labile enterotoxin or the heat-stable enterotoxin. Heat-labile enterotoxin is structurally similar to the *V. cholerae* toxin, and activates adenylate cyclase, resulting in an increase in intracellular cyclic guanosine monophosphate (Fig. 340-4). In contrast, *Shigella* spp. cause

Text continued on p. 1864

Table 340-1	Foodborne Bacterial Illnesses					
ETIOLOGY	INCUBATION PERIOD	SIGNS AND SYMPTOMS	DURATION OF ILLNESS	ASSOCIATED FOODS	LABORATORY TESTING	TREATMENT
Bacillus anthracis	2 days to weeks	Nausea, vomiting, malaise, bloody diarrhea, acute abdominal pain	Weeks	Insufficiently cooked contaminated meat	Blood	Penicillin is first choice for naturally acquired GI anthrax but use beta lactams with high index of suspicion for resistance Ciprofloxacin is second option
Bacillus cereus (preformed enterotoxin)	1-6 hr	Sudden onset of severe nausea and vomiting Diarrhea may be present	24 hr	Improperly refrigerated cooked or fried rice, meats	Normally a clinical diagnosis Clinical laboratories do not routinely identify this organism If indicated, send stool and food specimens to reference laboratory for culture and toxin identification	Supportive care
Bacillus cereus (diarrheal toxin)	10-16 hr	Abdominal cramps, watery diarrhea, nausea	24-48 hr	Meats, stews, gravies, vanilla sauce	Testing not necessary, self-limiting Consider testing food and stool for toxin in outbreaks	Supportive care
Brucella abortus, Brucella melitensis, and Brucella suis	7-21 days	Fever, chills, sweating, weakness, headache, muscle and joint pain, diarrhea, bloody stools during acute phase	Weeks	Raw milk, goat cheese made from unpasteurized milk, contaminated meats	Blood culture and positive serology	Acute: Rifampin and doxycycline daily for ≥6 wk Infections with complications require combination therapy with rifampin, tetracycline, and an aminoglycoside
Campylobacter jejuni	2-5 days	Diarrhea, cramps, fever, and vomiting; diarrhea may be bloody	2-10 days	Raw and undercooked poultry, unpasteurized milk, contaminated water	Routine stool culture; Campylobacter requires special media and incubation at 42°C (107.6°F) to grow	Supportive care For severe cases, antibiotics, such as azithromycin and quinolones, may be indicated early in the diarrheal disease Guillain-Barré syndrome can be a sequela
Clostridium botulinum: children and adults (preformed toxin)	12-72 hr	Vomiting, diarrhea, blurred vision, diplopia, dysphagia, descending muscle weakness	Variable (days to months) Can be complicated by respiratory failure and death	Home-canned foods with a low acid content, improperly canned commercial foods, home-canned or fermented fish, herb-infused oils, baked potatoes in aluminium foil, cheese sauce, bottled garlic, foods held warm for extended periods (e.g., in a warm oven)	Stool, serum, and food can be tested for toxin Stool and food can also be cultured for the organism These tests can be performed at some state health department laboratories and CDC	Supportive care Botulism antitoxin is helpful if given early in the course of the illness. Antitoxin for children and adults is available through CDC Contact the state health department. The 24-hr number for CDC is (800) 232-4636 (800-CDC-INFO)
Clostridium botulinum: infants	3-30 days	In infants <12 mo, lethargy, weakness, poor feeding, constipation, hypotonia, poor head control, poor gag and sucking reflex	Variable	Honey, home-canned vegetables and fruits, corn syrup	Stool, serum, and food can be tested for toxin Stool and food can also be cultured for the organism These tests can be performed at some state health department laboratories and CDC	Supportive care Botulinum antitoxin for infants can be obtained from the Infant Botulism Prevention Program, Health and Human Services, California (510-540-2646)

Continued

Table 340-1	Foodborne Bacterial Illnesses—cont'd					
ETIOLOGY	**INCUBATION PERIOD**	**SIGNS AND SYMPTOMS**	**DURATION OF ILLNESS**	**ASSOCIATED FOODS**	**LABORATORY TESTING**	**TREATMENT**
Clostridium perfringens toxin	8-16 hr	Watery diarrhea, nausea, abdominal cramps; fever is rare	24-48 hr	Meats, poultry, gravy, dried or precooked foods, time- and/or temperature-abused food	Stools can be tested for enterotoxin and cultured for organism Because *Clostridium perfringens* can normally be found in stool, quantitative cultures must be done: A count of at least 106 C. *perfringens* spores per gram of stool within 48 hr of when illness began is required to diagnose infection	Supportive care Antibiotics not indicated
Enterohemorrhagic *Escherichia coli* (EHEC) including *E. coli* O157:H7 and other Shiga toxin–producing *E. coli* (STEC)	1-8 days	Severe diarrhea that is often bloody, abdominal pain and vomiting Usually, little or no fever is present More common in children <4 yr old	5-10 days	Undercooked beef especially hamburger, unpasteurized milk and juice, raw fruits and vegetables (e.g., sprouts), salami (rarely), contaminated water	Stool culture; *E. coli* O157:H7 requires special media to grow. If *E. coli* O157:H7 is suspected, specific testing must be requested. Shiga toxin testing may be done using commercial kits; positive isolates should be forwarded to public health laboratories for confirmation and serotyping	Supportive care, monitor renal function, hemoglobin, and platelets closely. *E. coli* O157:H7 infection is also associated with hemolytic uremic syndrome (HUS), which can cause lifelong complications Studies indicate that antibiotics might promote the development of HUS. Antidiarrheal agents like Imodium may also increase the risk of developing HUS
Enterotoxigenic *E. coli* (ETEC)	1-3 days	Watery diarrhea, abdominal cramps, some vomiting	3 to >7 days	Water or food contaminated with human feces	Stool culture ETEC requires special laboratory techniques for identification that may not be widely available; consequently, physicians may make the diagnosis based on a patient's history and symptoms If ETEC is suspected, must alert microbiology laboratory that is testing the specimen	Supportive care Antibiotics are rarely needed except in severe cases Recommended antibiotics include quinolones although these are rarely required unless there is severe infection and should be administered early. Antimotility medications should be avoided by persons with high fevers or bloody diarrhea, and should be discontinued if diarrhea symptoms persist more than 48 hr. Bismuth subsalicylate compounds (e.g., Pepto-Bismol) can help reduce the number of bowel movements

Etiologic Agent	Incubation Period	Signs and Symptoms	Duration of Illness	Associated Foods	Laboratory Testing	Treatment
Listeria monocytogenes	9-48 hr for GI symptoms, 2-6 wk for invasive disease	Fever, muscle aches, and nausea or diarrhea; Pregnant women might have mild flu-like illness, and infection can lead to premature delivery or stillbirth; Elderly or immunocompromised patients can have bacteremia or meningitis	Variable	Fresh soft cheeses, unpasteurized milk, inadequately pasteurized milk, ready-to-eat deli meats, hot dogs	Blood or cerebrospinal fluid cultures. Selective enrichment media improve rates of isolation from contaminated specimens; Asymptomatic fecal carriage occurs; therefore, stool culture usually not helpful; Antibody to listeriolysin O may be helpful to identify outbreak retrospectively	Supportive care and antibiotics; intravenous ampicillin, penicillin G, or TMP-SMX is recommended for invasive disease
	At birth and infancy	Infants infected from mother at risk for sepsis or meningitis				Higher dosages of ampicillin recommended for neonatal sepsis or meningitis
Salmonella spp.	1-3 days	Diarrhea, fever, abdominal cramps, vomiting; *S. typhi* and *S. paratyphi* produce typhoid with insidious onset characterized by fever, headache, constipation, malaise, chills, and myalgia; diarrhea is uncommon, and vomiting is not usually severe	4-7 days	Contaminated eggs, poultry, unpasteurized milk or juice, cheese, contaminated raw fruits and vegetables (alfalfa sprouts, melons); *S. typhi* epidemics are often related to fecal contamination of water supplies or street-vended foods	Routine stool cultures	Supportive care; Other than for *S. typhi* and *S. paratyphi*, antibiotics are not indicated unless there is extraintestinal spread, or the risk of extraintestinal spread of the infection; Consider ampicillin, third-generation cephalosporins, or quinolones if indicated; A vaccine exists for *S. typhi* but is not completely effective. Washing hands and avoiding suspicious foods is equally useful at preventing disease as vaccination
Shigella spp.	24-48 hr	Abdominal cramps, fever, diarrhea; Stools might contain blood and mucus	4-7 days	Food or water contaminated with human fecal material; Usually person-to-person spread, fecal-oral transmission; Ready-to-eat foods touched by infected food workers, e.g., raw vegetables, salads, sandwiches	Routine stool cultures	Supportive care. Antibiotics are recommended for severe disease, bloody diarrhea, or compromised immune systems. Resistance to traditional first-line drugs like ampicillin and TMP-SMX is common. When susceptibility is unknown or when an ampicillin- or TMP-SMX–resistant strain is isolated, choices for therapy include fluoroquinolones, ceftriaxone, and azithromycin. Antidiarrheal agents such as Imodium or Lomotil can worsen the illness and should be avoided
Staphylococcus aureus (preformed enterotoxin)	1-6 hr	Sudden onset of severe nausea and vomiting; Abdominal cramps; Diarrhea and fever may be present	24-48 hr	Unrefrigerated or improperly refrigerated meats, potato and egg salads, cream pastries	Normally a clinical diagnosis; Stool, vomitus, and food can be tested for toxin and cultured if indicated	Supportive care

Continued

Table 340-1	Foodborne Bacterial Illnesses—cont'd					
ETIOLOGY	INCUBATION PERIOD	SIGNS AND SYMPTOMS	DURATION OF ILLNESS	ASSOCIATED FOODS	LABORATORY TESTING	TREATMENT
Vibrio cholerae (toxin)	24-72 hr	Profuse watery diarrhea and vomiting, which can lead to severe dehydration and death within hours	3-7 days Causes life-threatening dehydration	Contaminated water, fish, shellfish, street-vended food typically from Latin America or Asia	Stool culture *V. cholerae* requires special media to grow: Cary-Blair media is ideal for transport, and the selective thiosulfate–citrate–bile salts agar (TCBS) is ideal for isolation and identification.; if *V. cholerae* is suspected, must request specific testing. Commercially available rapid test kits (e.g., Crystal VC dipstick) are useful in epidemic settings but do not test susceptibility or subtype so should not be used for routine diagnosis	Supportive care with aggressive oral and intravenous rehydration Doxycycline is recommended as first-line treatment for adults, whereas azithromycin is recommended as first-line treatment for children and pregnant women. Ciprofloxacin and doxycycline recommended as second-line drugs for children
Vibrio parahaemolyticus	2-48 hr	Watery diarrhea, abdominal cramps, nausea, vomiting	2-5 days	Undercooked or raw seafood, such as fish, shellfish	Stool cultures. *V. parahaemolyticus* requires special media (TCBS agar) to grow; must request specific testing	Supportive care There is no evidence that antibiotic treatment decreases the severity or the length of the illness. Antibiotics are recommended in severe or prolonged cases: tetracycline or ciprofloxacin can be used
Vibrio vulnificus	1-7 days	Vomiting, diarrhea, abdominal pain, bacteremia, and wound infections More common and potentially fatal in the immunocompromised or in patients with chronic liver disease (presenting with septic shock and hemorrhagic bullous skin lesions)	2-8 days	Undercooked or raw shellfish, especially oysters, other contaminated seafood, and open wounds exposed to seawater	Stool, wound, or blood cultures *V. vulnificus* requires special media (TCBS agar) to grow; if *V. vulnificus* is suspected, must request specific testing	Supportive care and antibiotics: doxycycline, and a third-generation cephalosporin such as ceftazidime is recommended
Yersinia enterocolitica and *Yersinia pseudotuberculosis*	24-48 hr	Appendicitis-like symptoms (diarrhea and vomiting, fever, abdominal pain) occur primarily in older children and young adults Might have a scarlatiniform rash or erythema nodosum with *Y. pseudotuberculosis*	1-3 wk, usually self-limiting	Undercooked pork, unpasteurized milk, tofu, contaminated water Infection has occurred in infants whose caregivers handled chitterlings	Stool, vomitus, or blood culture, throat, lymph nodes, joint fluid, urine, and bile *Yersinia* requires special media to grow; must request specific testing Serology is available in research and reference laboratories	Supportive care If septicemia or other invasive disease occurs, antibiotic therapy with aminoglycosides, doxycycline, TMP-SMX, or fluoroquinolones may be useful

CDC, Centers for Disease Control and Prevention; GI, gastrointestinal; TMP-SMX, trimethoprim-sulfamethoxazole.
From Centers for Disease Control and Prevention: Diagnosis and management of foodborne illnesses, MMWR 53(RR-4):1-33, 2004.

Table 340-2 | Foodborne Viral Illnesses

ETIOLOGY	INCUBATION PERIOD	SIGNS AND SYMPTOMS	DURATION OF ILLNESS	ASSOCIATED FOODS	LABORATORY TESTING	TREATMENT
Hepatitis A	28 days average (15-50 days)	Diarrhea, dark urine, jaundice, and flu-like symptoms, i.e., fever, headache, nausea, and abdominal pain	Variable, 2 wk-3 mo	Shellfish harvested from contaminated waters, raw produce, contaminated drinking water, uncooked foods, and cooked foods that are not reheated after contact with infected food handler	Increase in ALT, bilirubin Positive IgM and anti–hepatitis A antibodies	Supportive care Prevention with immunization (vaccine available for persons 1 year and older)
Caliciviruses (including noroviruses and sapoviruses)	12-48 hr	Nausea, vomiting, abdominal cramping, diarrhea, fever, myalgia, and some headache Diarrhea is more prevalent in adults and vomiting is more prevalent in children Prolonged asymptomatic excretion possible	12-60 hr	Shellfish, fecally contaminated foods, ready-to-eat foods touched by infected food workers (salads, sandwiches, ice, cookies, fruit)	Routine RT-PCR. RT-PCR assays are the preferred laboratory method for detecting norovirus. Conventional RT-PCR followed by sequence analysis of the RT-PCR products is used for norovirus genotyping. Rapid commercial assays, such as enzyme immunoassays (EIAs), have poor sensitivity and are not recommended for establishing diagnosis Clinical diagnosis, negative bacterial cultures Stool is negative for WBCs	Supportive care such as rehydration. Avoid giving antimotility agents to children younger than 3 yr old. However, these agents may be helpful in older children and adults, particularly when used along with rehydration treatment Good hygiene
Rotavirus (groups A-C)	1-3 days	Vomiting, watery diarrhea, low-grade fever Temporary lactose intolerance can occur Infants and children, elderly, and immunocompromised are especially vulnerable	4-8 days	Fecally contaminated foods Ready-to-eat foods touched by infected food workers (salads, fruits)	Diagnosis may be made by rapid antigen detection of rotavirus in stool specimens.	Supportive care Severe diarrhea can require fluid and electrolyte replacement
Other viral agents (astroviruses, adenoviruses, parvoviruses)	10-70 hr	Nausea, vomiting, diarrhea, malaise, abdominal pain, headache, fever	2-9 days	Fecally contaminated foods Ready-to-eat foods touched by infected food workers Some shellfish	Identification of the virus in early acute stool samples Serology Commercial ELISA kits are available for adenoviruses and astroviruses	Supportive care, usually mild, self-limiting Good hygiene

ALT, alanine aminotransferase; ELISA, enzyme-linked immunosorbent assay; IgM, immunoglobulin M; RT-PCR, reverse transcriptase polymerase chain reaction; WBCs, white blood cells.
From Centers for Disease Control and Prevention: Diagnosis and management of foodborne illnesses. MMWR 53(RR-4):1-33, 2004.

Table 340-3	Foodborne Parasitic Illnesses					
ETIOLOGY	**INCUBATION PERIOD**	**SIGNS AND SYMPTOMS**	**DURATION OF ILLNESS**	**ASSOCIATED FOODS**	**LABORATORY TESTING**	**TREATMENT**
Angiostrongylus cantonensis	1 wk–≥1 mo	Severe headaches, nausea, vomiting, neck stiffness, paresthesias, hyperesthesias, seizures, and other neurologic abnormalities	Several weeks to several months	Raw or undercooked intermediate hosts (e.g., snails or slugs), infected paratenic (transport) hosts (e.g., crabs, freshwater shrimp), fresh produce contaminated with intermediate or transport hosts	No readily available blood tests. History is major guide to diagnosis. Examination of CSF for elevated pressure, protein, leukocytes, and eosinophils; serologic testing using ELISA to detect antibodies to *Angiostrongylus cantonensis*	Supportive care. There is no specific treatment. Repeat lumbar punctures and use of corticosteroid therapy may be used for more severely ill patients
Cryptosporidium	2-10 days	Diarrhea (usually watery), stomach cramps, upset stomach, slight fever	May be remitting and relapsing over weeks to months	Any uncooked food or food contaminated by an ill food handler after cooking; drinking water	Request specific examination of the stool for *Cryptosporidium*. Most often, stool specimens are examined microscopically using different techniques (e.g., acid-fast staining, direct fluorescent antibody [DFA], and/or enzyme immunoassays for detection of *Cryptosporidium* sp. antigens) May need to examine water or food	Supportive care, self-limited If severe, nitazoxanide can be prescribed for all patients 1 yr of age or older
Cyclospora cayetanensis	1-14 days, usually at ≥1 wk	Diarrhea (usually watery), loss of appetite, substantial loss of weight, stomach cramps, nausea, vomiting, fatigue	May be remitting and relapsing over weeks to months	Various types of fresh produce (imported berries, lettuce)	Request specific examination of the stool for *Cyclospora* May need to examine water or food	TMP-SMX for 7 days
Entamoeba histolytica	2-3 days–1-4 wk	Diarrhea (often bloody), frequent bowel movements, lower abdominal pain	May be protracted (several weeks to several months)	Any uncooked food or food contaminated by an ill food handler after cooking; drinking water	Examination of fresh stool for cysts and parasites; may need at least 3 samples Serology for long-term infections	For asymptomatic infections, paromomycin and iodoquinol are the drugs of choice. For symptomatic intestinal disease or extraintestinal infections (e.g., hepatic abscess), the drugs of choice are metronidazole and tinidazole, immediately followed by treatment with paromomycin or iodoquinol

Organism	Incubation period	Signs/Symptoms	Source	Diagnosis	Treatment
Giardia lamblia	1-2 wk	Diarrhea, stomach cramps, gas, weight loss	Any uncooked food or food contaminated by an ill food handler after cooking; drinking water	Examination of stool for ova and parasites; may need at least 3 samples	Metronidazole, tinidazole, or nitazoxanide. Alternatives to these medications include paromomycin, quinacrine, and furazolidone
Toxoplasma gondii	5-23 days	Generally asymptomatic, 20% develop cervical lymphadenopathy and/or a flu-like illness. In immunocompromised patients: CNS disease, myocarditis, or pneumonitis is often seen	Accidental ingestion of contaminated substances (e.g., soil contaminated with cat feces on fruits and vegetables); raw or partially cooked meat (especially pork, lamb, and venison)	The diagnosis of toxoplasmosis is typically made by serologic testing. however, IgM antibodies can persist for 6-18 mo and thus do not necessarily indicate recent infection. PCR of bodily fluids. Diagnosis can also be made by isolation of parasites from blood or other body fluids; observation of parasites in patient specimens via microscopy or histology. Detection of organisms is rare	Asymptomatic healthy, but infected, persons do not require treatment. Spiramycin or pyrimethamine plus sulfadiazine may be used for pregnant women. Pyrimethamine plus sulfadiazine may be used for immunocompromised persons, in specific cases. Pyrimethamine plus sulfadiazine (with or without steroids) may be given for ocular disease when indicated. Folinic acid is given with pyrimethamine plus sulfadiazine to counteract bone marrow suppression
Toxoplasma gondii (congenital infection)	In infants at birth	Treatment of the mother can reduce severity and/or incidence of congenital infection. Most infected infants have few symptoms at birth; later, they generally develop signs of congenital toxoplasmosis (mental retardation, severely impaired eyesight, cerebral palsy, seizures), unless the infection is treated	Passed from mother (who acquired acute infection during pregnancy) to child	Isolation of T. gondii from placenta, umbilical cord, or infant blood; PCR of white blood cells, CSF, or amniotic fluid, or IgM and IgA serology, performed by a reference laboratory	
Trichinella spiralis	1-2 days for initial symptoms; others begin 2-8 wk after infection	Acute: nausea, diarrhea, vomiting, fatigue, fever, abdominal discomfort followed by muscle soreness, weakness, and occasional cardiac and neurologic complications	Raw or undercooked contaminated meat, usually pork or wild game meat (e.g., bear or moose)	Positive serology or demonstration of larvae via muscle biopsy; increase in eosinophils	Supportive care plus mebendazole or albendazole. In addition to antiparasitic medication, treatment with steroids is sometimes required in more severe cases

CNS, central nervous system; CSF, cerebrospinal fluid; ELISA, enzyme-linked immunosorbent assay; IgA, immunoglobulin A; IgM, immunoglobulin M; PCR, polymerase chain reaction; TMP-SMX, trimethoprim-sulfamethoxazole.
From Centers for Disease Control and Prevention: Diagnosis and management of foodborne illnesses. MMWR 53(RR-4):1-33, 2004.

Table 340-4 | Foodborne Noninfectious Illnesses

ETIOLOGY	INCUBATION PERIOD	SIGNS AND SYMPTOMS	DURATION OF ILLNESS	ASSOCIATED FOODS	LABORATORY TESTING	TREATMENT
Antimony	5 min–8 hr usually <1 hr	Vomiting, metallic taste	Usually self-limited	Metallic container	Identification of metal in beverage or food	Supportive care
Arsenic	Few hours	Vomiting, colic, diarrhea	Several days	Contaminated food	Urine Can cause eosinophilia	Gastric lavage, BAL (dimercaprol)
Cadmium	5 min–8 hr usually <1 hr	Nausea, vomiting, myalgia, increase in salivation, stomach pain	Usually self-limited	Seafood, oysters, clams, lobster, grains, peanuts	Identification of metal in food	Supportive care
Ciguatera fish poisoning (ciguatera toxin)	2-6 hr	GI: abdominal pain, nausea, vomiting, diarrhea	Days to weeks to months	A variety of large reef fish: grouper, red snapper, amberjack, and barracuda (most common)	Radioassay for toxin in fish or a consistent history	Supportive care, IV mannitol Children more vulnerable
	3 hr	Neurologic: paresthesias, reversal of hot or cold, pain, weakness				
	2-5 days	Cardiovascular: bradycardia, hypotension, increase in T-wave abnormalities				
Copper	5 min–8 hr usually <1 hr	Nausea, vomiting, blue or green vomitus	Usually self-limited	Metallic container	Identification of metal in beverage or food	Supportive care
Mercury	1 wk or longer	Numbness, weakness of legs, spastic paralysis, impaired vision, blindness, coma Pregnant women and the developing fetus are especially vulnerable	May be protracted	Fish exposed to organic mercury, grains treated with mercury fungicides	Analysis of blood, hair	Supportive care
Mushroom toxins, short-acting (muscimol, muscarine, psilocybin, Coprinus atramentaria, ibotenic acid)	<2 hr	Vomiting, diarrhea, confusion, visual disturbance, salivation, diaphoresis, hallucinations, disulfiram-like reaction, confusion, visual disturbance	Self-limited	Wild mushrooms (cooking might not destroy these toxins)	Typical syndrome and mushroom identified or demonstration of the toxin	Supportive care
Mushroom toxins, long-acting (amanitin)	4-8 hr diarrhea; 24-48 hr liver failure	Diarrhea, abdominal cramps, leading to hepatic and renal failure	Often fatal	Mushrooms	Typical syndrome and mushroom identified and/or demonstration of the toxin	Supportive care, life-threatening, may need life support
Nitrite poisoning	1-2 hr	Nausea, vomiting, cyanosis, headache, dizziness, weakness, loss of consciousness, chocolate-brown blood	Usually self-limited	Cured meats, any contaminated foods, spinach exposed to excessive nitrification	Analysis of the food, blood	Supportive care, methylene blue

Agent	Incubation period	Symptoms	Duration	Associated foods	Laboratory testing	Treatment
Pesticides (organophosphates or carbamates)	Few minutes to few hours	Nausea, vomiting, abdominal cramps, diarrhea, headache, nervousness, blurred vision, twitching, convulsions, salivation, meiosis	Usually self-limited	Any contaminated food	Analysis of the food, blood	Atropine; 2-PAM (pralidoxime) is used when atropine is not able to control symptoms; rarely necessary in carbamate poisoning
Puffer fish (tetrodotoxin)	<30 min	Paresthesias, vomiting, diarrhea, abdominal pain, ascending paralysis, respiratory failure	Death usually in 4-6 hr	Puffer fish	Detection of tetrodotoxin in fish	Life-threatening, may need respiratory support
Scombroid (histamine)	1 min-3 hr	Flushing, rash, burning sensation of skin, mouth and throat, dizziness, urticaria, paresthesias	3-6 hr	Fish: bluefin, tuna, skipjack, mackerel, marlin, escolar, and mahi mahi	Demonstration of histamine in food or clinical diagnosis	Supportive care, antihistamines
Shellfish toxins (diarrheic, neurotoxic, amnesic)	Diarrheic shellfish poisoning: 30 min-2 hr Neurotoxic shellfish poisoning: few minutes to hours Amnesic shellfish poisoning: 24-48 hr	Nausea, vomiting, diarrhea, and abdominal pain accompanied by chills, headache, and fever Tingling and numbness of lips, tongue, and throat, muscular aches, dizziness, reversal of the sensations of hot and cold, diarrhea, and vomiting Vomiting, diarrhea, abdominal pain and neurologic problems such as confusion, memory loss, disorientation, seizure, coma	hr to 2-3 days	A variety of shellfish, primarily mussels, oysters, scallops, and shellfish from the Florida coast and the Gulf of Mexico	Detection of the toxin in shellfish; high-pressure liquid chromatography	Supportive care, generally self-limiting Elderly are especially sensitive to amnesic shellfish poisoning
Shellfish toxins (paralytic shellfish poisoning)	30 min-3 hr	Diarrhea, nausea, vomiting leading to paresthesias of mouth and lips, weakness, dysphasia, dysphonia, respiratory paralysis	Days	Scallops, mussels, clams, cockles	Detection of toxin in food or water where fish are located; high-pressure liquid chromatography	Life-threatening, may need respiratory support
Sodium fluoride	Few minutes to 2 hr	Salty or soapy taste, numbness of mouth, vomiting, diarrhea, dilated pupils, spasms, pallor, shock, collapse	Usually self-limited	Dry foods (e.g., dry milk, flour, baking powder, cake mixes) contaminated with NaF-containing insecticides and rodenticides	Testing of vomitus or gastric washings Analysis of the food	Supportive care
Thallium	Few hours	Nausea, vomiting, diarrhea, painful paresthesias, motor polyneuropathy, hair loss	Several days	Contaminated food	Urine, hair	Supportive care
Tin	5 min-8 hr usually <1 hr	Nausea, vomiting, diarrhea	Usually self-limited	Metallic container	Analysis of the food	Supportive care
Vomitoxin	Few minutes to 3 hr	Nausea, headache, abdominal pain, vomiting	Usually self-limited	Grains such as wheat, corn, barley	Analysis of the food	Supportive care
Zinc	Few hours	Stomach cramps, nausea, vomiting, diarrhea, myalgias	Usually self-limited	Metallic container	Analysis of the food, blood and feces, saliva or urine	Supportive care

BAL, bronchoalveolar lavage; GI, gastrointestinal.
From Centers for Disease Control and Prevention: Diagnosis and management of foodborne illnesses, MMWR 53(RR-4):1-33, 2004.

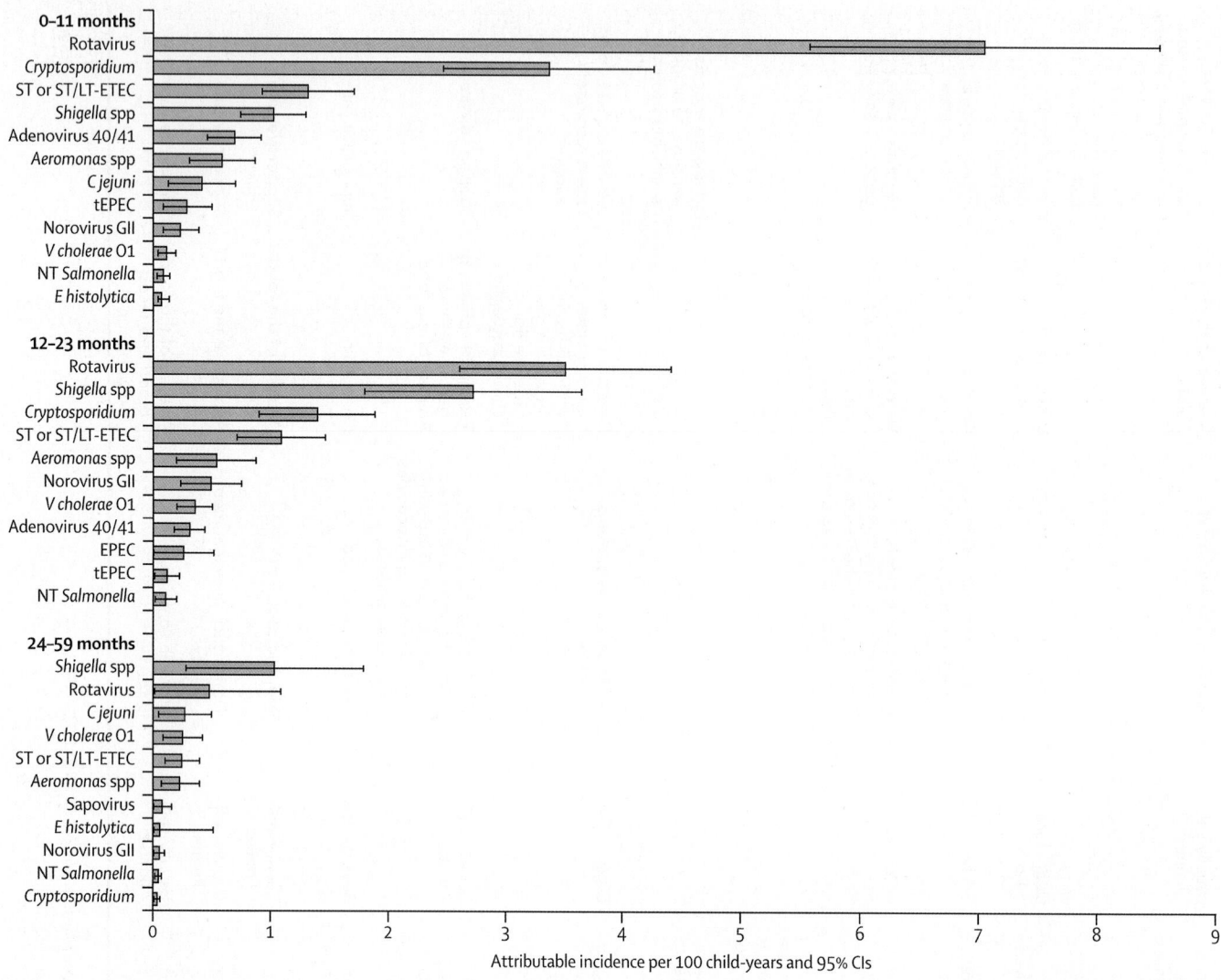

Figure 340-1 Attributable incidence of pathogen-specific moderate-to-severe diarrhea per 100 child-yr by age stratum, all sites combined. The bars show the incidence rates and the error bars show the 95% confidence intervals. *(From Kotloff KL, Nataro JP, Blackwelder WC, et al. Burden and aetiology of diarrhoeal disease in infants and young children in developing countries [the Global Enteric Multicenter Study, GEMS]: a prospective, case-control study. Lancet 382(9888):209–222, 2013, Fig. 4.)*

gastroenteritis via a superficial invasion of colonic mucosa, which they invade through M cells located over Peyer patches. After phago-cytosis, a series of events occurs, including apoptosis of macrophages, multiplication and spread of bacteria into adjacent cells, release of inflammatory mediators (interleukin-1 and -8), transmigration of neu-trophils into the lumen of the colon, neutrophil necrosis and degranu-lation, further breach of the epithelial barrier, and mucosal destruction (Fig. 340-5).

RISK FACTORS FOR GASTROENTERITIS
In developed countries, episodes of infectious diarrhea can occur through seasonal exposure to organisms such as rotavirus, or exposure to pathogens in settings of close contact (e.g., daycare centers). Major risks include environmental contamination and increased exposure to enteropathogens. Additional risks include young age, immunodefi-ciency, measles, malnutrition, and lack of exclusive or predominant breastfeeding. Malnutrition increases the risk of diarrhea and associ-ated mortality, and moderate to severe stunting increases the odds of diarrhea-associated mortality. The fraction of such infectious diarrhea deaths that are attributable to nutritional deficiencies varies with the prevalence of deficiencies; the highest attributable fractions are in sub-Saharan Africa, south Asia, and Andean Latin America. The risks are particularly higher with micronutrient malnutrition; in children with

vitamin A deficiency, and accounts for 157,000 deaths from diarrhea, measles, and malaria. **Zinc deficiency** is estimated to cause 116,000 deaths from diarrhea and pneumonia. Table 340-7 summarizes some of the key risk factors associated with childhood diarrhea globally.

The majority of cases of diarrhea resolve within the 1st wk of the illness. A smaller proportion of diarrheal illnesses fail to resolve and persist for longer than 2 wk. **Persistent diarrhea** is defined as episodes that began acutely but last for 14 or more days. Such episodes account for 3-19% of all diarrheal episodes in children younger than 5 yr of age and up to 50% of all diarrhea-related deaths; persistent diarrhea has a case fatality rate of 60%. Many children (especially infants and tod-dlers) in developing countries have frequent episodes of acute diarrhea. Although few individual episodes persist beyond 14 days, frequent episodes of acute diarrhea, as well as prolonged diarrhea (lasting between 7-13 days of age), can result in nutritional compromise and can predispose these children to develop persistent diarrhea, protein-calorie malnutrition, and secondary infections.

CLINICAL MANIFESTATION OF DIARRHEA
Most of the clinical manifestations and clinical syndromes of diarrhea are related to the infecting pathogen and the dose or inoculum (see Tables 340-1 to 340-3). Additional manifestations depend on the devel-opment of complications (e.g., dehydration and electrolyte imbalance)

Table 340-5 | Weighted Annual Incidence (Per 100 Child-Years) of Moderate-to-Severe Diarrhea Attributable to a Specific Pathogen, with 95% Confidence Interval, By Age Stratum and Country

AGE GROUP	PATHOGEN	GAMBIA	MALI	MOZAMBIQUE	KENYA	INDIA	BANGLADESH	PAKISTAN
<12 mo	**VIRUSES**							
	Rotavirus	3.2 (1.7-4.6)	8.4 (3.5-13.3)	3.5 (1.5-5.4)	10.1 (5.4-14.8)	25.4 (14.7-36.2)	2.1 (1.0-3.2)	5.5 (2.6-8.5)
	Norovirus GII	1.2 (0.4-2.0)	–	–	–	–	–	–
	Adenovirus 40/41	0.3 (0.1-0.6)	0.7 (0.1-1.3)	0.3 (0.0-0.5)	–	3.7 (1.6-5.9)	0.5 (0.2-0.8)	0.5 (0.1-0.8)
	BACTERIA							
	ST-ETEC (ST-only or LT/ST)	0.7 (0.1-1.2)	1.4 (0.3-2.5)	–	3.6 (1.4-5.8)	2.8 (0.9-4.8)	0.2 (0.0-0.4)	1.7 (0.6-2.8)
	Shigella	0.5 (0.2-0.9)	–	–	2.3 (0.8-3.8)	1.9 (0.4-3.3)	1.7 (0.8-2.6)	1.9 (0.8-2.9)
	Aeromonas	–	–	–	–	–	1.2 (0.3-2.2)	2.8 (1.0-4.5)
	Campylobacter jejuni	–	–	–	–	–	1.1 (0.1-2.2)	1.7(0.0-3.3)
	Typical EPEC	–	–	–	2.7 (0.6-4.7)		–	–
	Nontyphoidal Salmonella	–	–	–	–		0.5 (0.2-0.9)	
	Vibrio cholerae O1	–	–	–	–	–	–	0.8 (0.2-1.3)
	PROTOZOA							
	Cryptosporidium	1.6 (0.7-2.4)	5.4 (2.1-8.8)	1.8 (0.7-3.0)	4.6 (2.0-7.2)	11.1 (5.4-16.9)	0.7 (0.2-1.2)	1.4 (0.1-2.6)
	Entamoeba histolytica	–	–	–	–	–	0.5 (0.0-0.9)	–
12-23 mo	**VIRUSES**							
	Rotavirus	3.3 (1.3-5.2)	4.1 (1.0-7.1)	–	3.0 (1.6-4.3)	12.4 (7.1-17.7)	3.0 (1.1-4.9)	1.6 (0.6-2.7)
	Norovirus GII	1.7 (0.5-2.8)	–	–	–	2.3 (0.4-4.2)		–
	Adenovirus 40/41	0.4 (0.0-0.8)	–	–	–	2.2 (0.9-3.4)		0.4 (0.0-0.7)
	BACTERIA							
	ST-ETEC (ST-only or LT/ST)	1.5 (0.3-2.8)	0.8 (0.0-1.7)	0.7 (0.2-1.2)	1.5 (0.6-2.5)	2.8 (1.1-4.6)		0.9 (0.2-1.7)
	EAEC	–	–	–	–	–	1.6 (0.0-3.2)	–
	Shigella	2.5 (0.9-4.1)	0.8 (0.0-1.6)	0.5 (0.1-0.9)	1.0 (0.3-1.8)	3.5 (1.7-5.4)	8.5 (3.3-13.7)	2.1 (0.7-3.4)
	Aeromonas	–	–	–	–	–	1.9 (0.2-3.7)	1.6 (0.2-2.9)
	Campylobacter jejuni	–	–	–	–	–	–	–
	Typical EPEC	–	–	–	0.8 (0.0-1.5)	–	–	–
	Nontyphoidal Salmonella	–	–	–	0.7 (0.1-1.4)	–	–	–
	Vibrio cholerae O1	–	–	–	–	1.6 (0.6-2.7)	0.2 (0.0-0.5)	1.3 (0.4-2.1)
	PROTOZOA							
	Cryptosporidium	1.5 (0.4-2.5)	1.6 (0.0-3.3)	–	2.0 (0.9-3.0)	4.1 (1.2-6.9)	–	1.4 (0.4-2.4)
	Entamoeba histolytica	–	–	–	–	–	–	–
24–59 mo	**VIRUSES**							
	Rotavirus	0.4 (0.1-0.6)	0.4 (0.0-3.2)	–	0.3 (0.1-0.4)	3.5 (0.0-7.1)	–	–
	Norovirus GII	0.3 (0.0-0.5)	–	–	–	–	–	–
	Sapovirus	–	–	–	–	0.8 (0.0-1.8)	–	–
	Adenovirus 40/41	–	–	–	–		–	–
	BACTERIA							
	ST-ETEC (ST-only or LT/ST)	0.3 (0.0-0.5)		–	0.4 (0.1-0.6)	1.5 (0.0-3.1)	–	0.1 (0.0-0.3)
	EAEC	–	–	–	–	–	–	–
	Shigella	0.4 (0.1-0.7)	0.3 (0.0-2.9)	0.4 (0.0-0.9)	0.7 (0.4-1.1)	2.9 (0.0-5.9)	3.1 (0.0-6.3)	0.2 (0.0-0.4)
	Aeromonas	–	–	–	–	–	0.8 (0.0-1.8)	0.5 (0.2-0.9)
	Campylobacter jejuni	–	–	–	–	2.4 (0.0-5.0)	–	0.4 (0.0-0.7)
	Typical EPEC	–	–	–	–	–	–	–
	Nontyphoidal Salmonella	–	–	–	0.3 (0.1-0.5)	–	–	–
	Vibrio cholerae O1	–	–	0.2 (0.0-0.5)	–	1.8 (0.0-3.8)	0.1 (0.0-0.3)	–
	PROTOZOA							
	Cryptosporidium	–	–	–	0.2 (0.0-0.4)	–	–	–
	Entamoeba histolytica	–	0.3 (0.0-2.7)	–	–	–	–	–

EAEC, enteroadherent *Escherichia coli*; EPEC, enteropathogenic *Escherichia coli*; ETEC, enterotoxigenic *Escherichia coli*; LT, heat-labile; ST, heat stable.

Table 340-6	Comparison of 3 Types of Enteric Infection		

| | TYPE OF INFECTION | | |
PARAMETER	I	II	III
Mechanism	Noninflammatory (enterotoxin or adherence/superficial invasion)	Inflammatory (invasion, cytotoxin)	Penetrating
Location	Proximal small bowel	Colon	Distal small bowel
Illness	Watery diarrhea	Dysentery	Enteric fever
Stool examination	No fecal leukocytes Mild or no ↑ lactoferrin	Fecal polymorphonuclear leukocytes ↑↑ Lactoferrin	Fecal mononuclear leukocytes
Examples	*Vibrio cholerae* *Escherichia coli* (ETEC, LT, ST) *Clostridium perfringens* *Bacillus cereus* *Staphylococcus aureus* Also[†]: *Giardia lamblia* *Rotavirus* *Norwalk-like viruses* *Cryptosporidium parvum* *E. coli* (EPEC, EAEC) *Microsporidia* *Cyclospora cayetanensis*	*Shigella* *E. coli* (EIEC, EHEC) *Salmonella enteritidis* *Vibrio parahaemolyticus* *Clostridium difficile* *Campylobacter jejuni* *Entamoeba histolytica**	*Salmonella typhi* *Yersinia enterocolitica* ?*Campylobacter fetus*

*Although amebic dysentery involves tissue inflammation, the leukocytes are characteristically pyknotic or absent, having been destroyed by the virulent amebae.
[†]Although not typically enterotoxic, these pathogens alter bowel physiology via adherence, superficial cell entry, cytokine induction, or toxins that inhibit cell function.
EAEC, enteroaggregative *E. coli*; EHEC, enterohemorrhagic *E. coli*; EIEC, enteroinvasive *E. coli*; EPEC, enteropathogenic *E. coli*; ETEC, enterotoxigenic *E. coli*; LT, heat-labile; ST, heat-stable.
From Mandell GL, Bennett JE, Dolin R, editors: *Principles and practices of infectious diseases*, ed 7, Philadelphia, 2010, Churchill Livingstone.

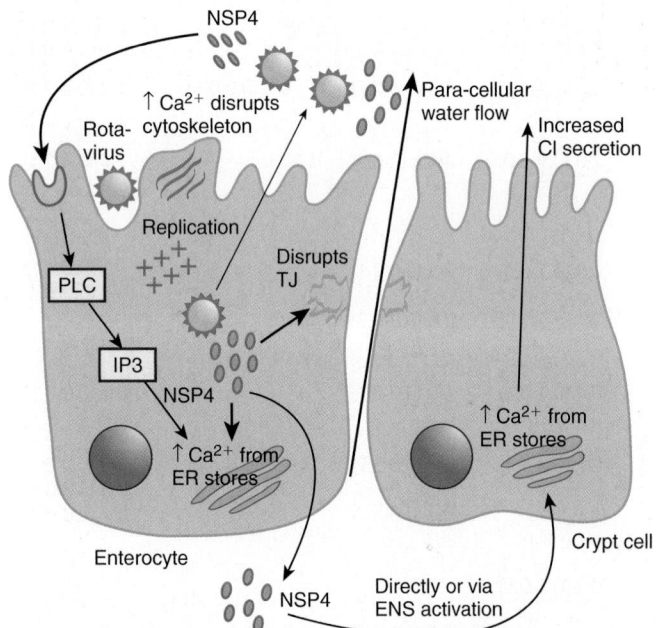

Figure 340-2 Pathogenesis of rotavirus infection and diarrhea. *ENS*, enteric nervous system; *ER*, endoplasmic reticulum; *PLC*, phospholipase C; *TJ*, tight junction. (*Adapted from Ramig RF: Pathogenesis of intestinal and systemic rotavirus infection, J Virol 78:10213–10220, 2004.*)

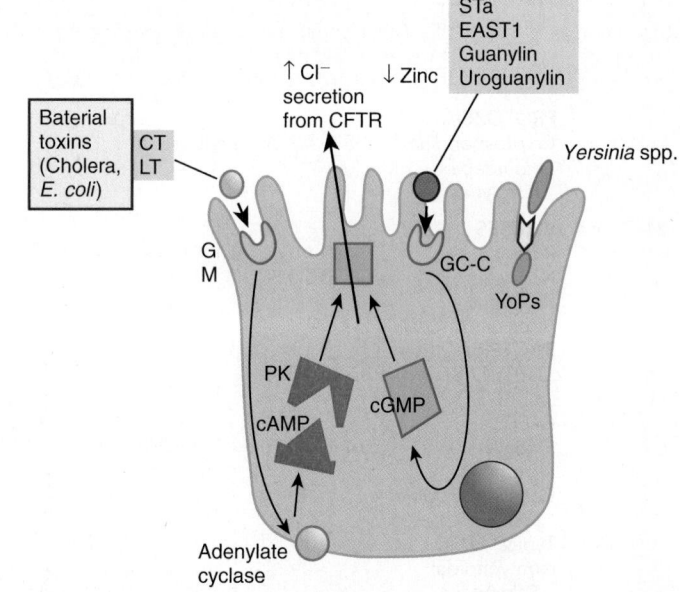

Figure 340-3 Mechanism of cholera toxin. (*Adapted from Thapar M, Sanderson IR: Diarrhoea in children: an interface between developing and developed countries, Lancet 363:641–653, 2004; and Montes M, DuPont HL: Enteritis, enterocolitis and infectious diarrhea syndromes. In Cohen J, Powderly WG, Opal SM, et al, editors: Infectious diseases, ed 2, London, 2004, Mosby, pp. 31–52.*)

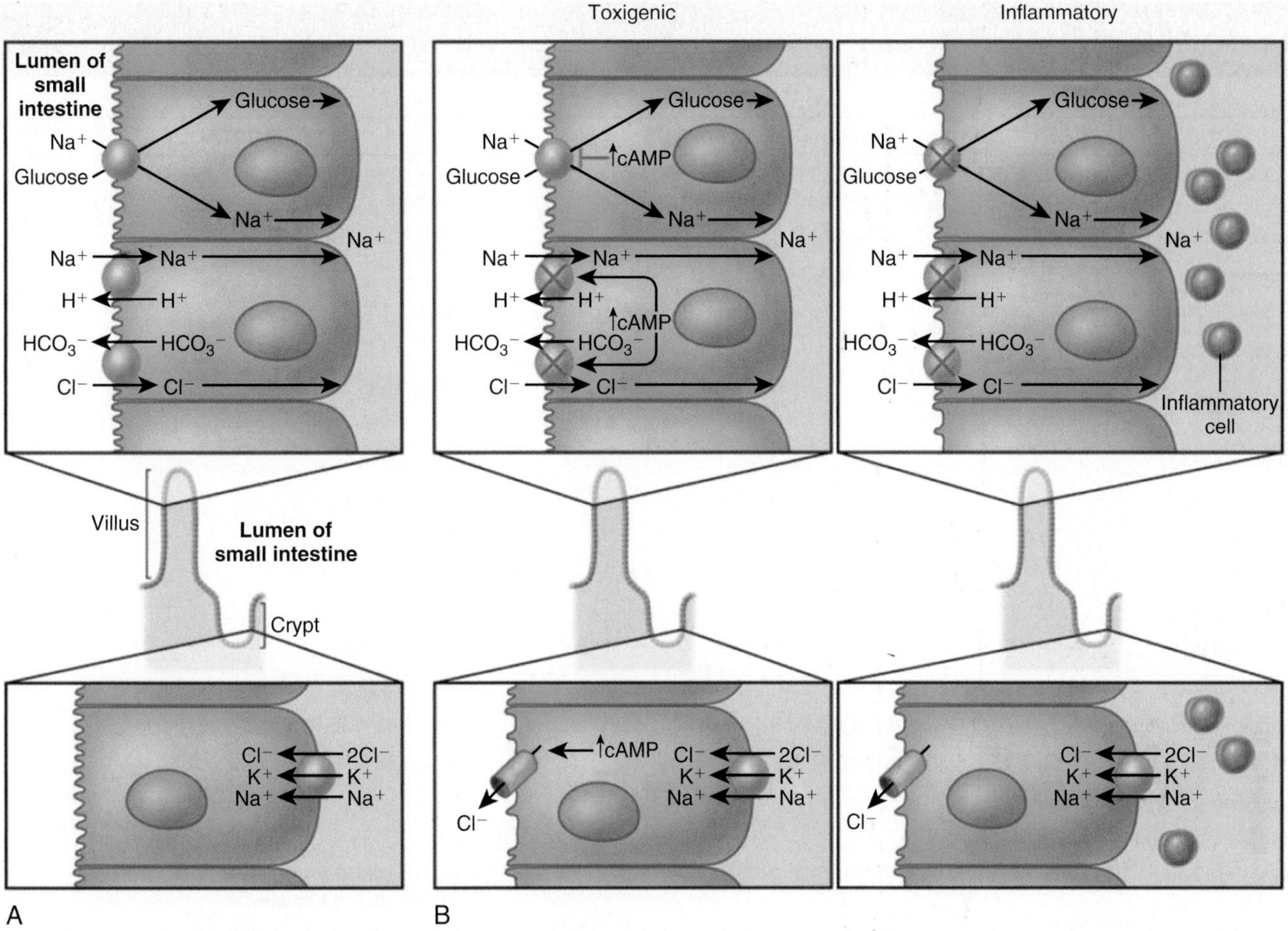

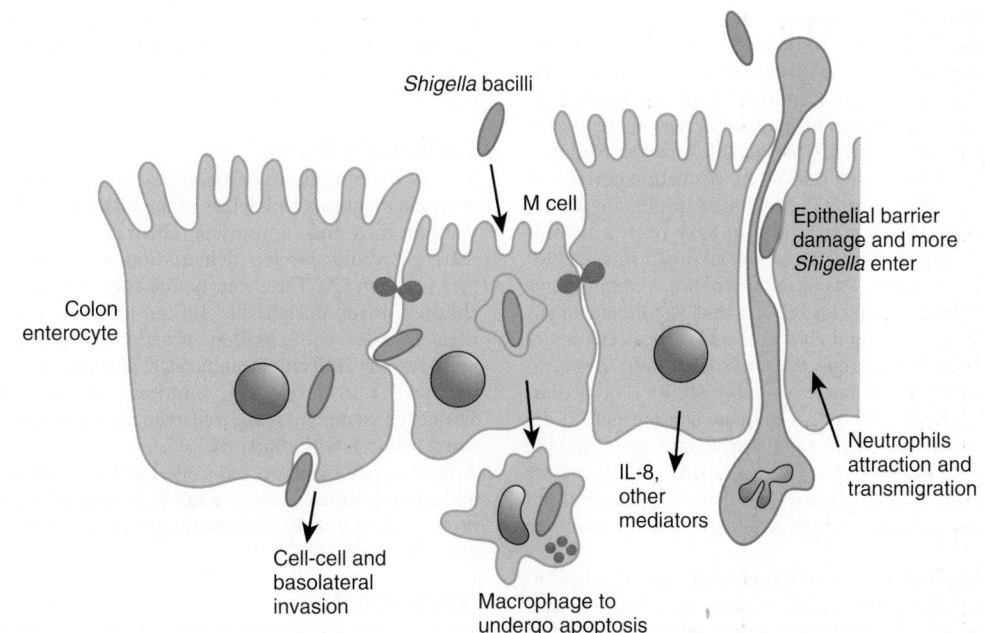

Figure 340-4 Movement of Na⁺ and Cl⁻ in the small intestine. **A,** Movement in normal subjects. Na+ is absorbed by 2 different mechanisms in absorptive cells from villi: glucose-stimulated absorption and electroneutral absorption (which represents the coupling of Na⁺/H⁺ and Cl⁻/HCO₃⁻ exchanges). **B,** Movement during diarrhea caused by a toxin and inflammation. (*From Petri WA, Miller M, Binder HJ, et al: Enteric infections, diarrhea and their impact on function and development,* J Clin Invest *118:1277–1290, 2008.*)

Figure 340-5 Pathogenesis of *Shigella* infection and diarrhea. *IL-8,* Interleukin-8. (*Adapted from Opal SM, Keusch GT: Host responses to infection. In Cohen J, Powderly WG, Opal SM, et al, editors: Infectious diseases, ed 2, London, 2004, Mosby, pp. 31–52.*)

Table 340-7	Proven Risk Factors with Direct Biologic Links to Diarrhea: Relative Risks (RR) or Odds Ratios (OR) and 95% Confidence Intervals

	DIARRHEA	
	MORBIDITY	**MORTALITY**
Lack of exclusive breastfeeding (0-5 mo)	RR = 2.65 (1.72-4.07) compared to not breastfed infants	RR = 10.52 (2.79-39.6) compared to not breastfed infants
No breastfeeding (6-23 mo)	RR = 1.32 (1.06-1.63)	RR = 2.18 (1.14-4.16)
Underweight	(<−2 WAZ) RR = 1.23 (1.12-1.35)	
−2 to <−1 WAZ		OR = 2.1 (1.6
−3 to <−2 WAZ		OR = 3.4 (2.7
<−3 WAZ		OR = 9.5 (5.5
Stunted		
−2 to <−1 HAZ		OR = 1.2 (0.9
−3 to <−2 HAZ		OR = 1.6 (1.1
<−3 HAZ		OR = 4.6 (2.7
Wasted		
−2 to <−1 WHZ		OR = 1.2 (0.7
−3 to <−2 WHZ		OR = 2.9 (1.8
<−3 WHZ		OR = 6.3 (2.7
Vitamin A deficiency	Inconsistent evidence	RR = 1.47 (1.25-175)
Zinc deficiency	RR = 0.87 (0.81-0.94)	RR = 0.82 (0.64-1.05)
Crowding (>8 persons/kitchen)		
Indoor air pollution		
Unwashed hands	RR = 0.58 (0.49–0.69)	Risk relationship suggested but studies of poor methodologic quality
Poor water quality	RR = 0.73 (0.53-1.01) Inconsistent evidence from blinded studies	Relationship suggested but few studies of sufficient quality
Inappropriate excreta disposal	Limited evidence suggests risk relationship	

HAZ, height-for-age Z-score; WAZ, weight-for-age Z score; WHZ, weight-for-height Z-score.
Adapted from Walker CL, Rudan I, Liu L, et al: Global burden of childhood pneumonia and diarrhoea. Lancet 381:1405–1416, 2013.

and the nature of the infecting pathogen (Table 340-8). Usually the ingestion of preformed toxins (e.g., those of *S. aureus*) is associated with the rapid onset of nausea and vomiting within 6 hr, with possible fever, abdominal cramps, and diarrhea within 8-72 hr. Watery diarrhea and abdominal cramps after an 8-16 hr incubation period are associated with enterotoxin-producing *C. perfringens* and *B. cereus*. Abdominal cramps and watery diarrhea after a 16-48 hr incubation period can be associated with noroviruses, several enterotoxin-producing bacteria, *Cryptosporidium,* and *Cyclospora,* and also have been a notable feature of influenza virus H1N1 infections. Several organisms, including *Salmonella, Shigella, C. jejuni, Yersinia enterocolitica,* enteroinvasive or hemorrhagic (Shigatoxin-producing) *E. coli,* and *V. parahaemolyticus,* produce diarrhea that can contain blood as well as fecal leukocytes in association with abdominal cramps, tenesmus, and fever; these features suggest **bacterial dysentery** and fever (Table 340-8). Bloody diarrhea and abdominal cramps after a 72-120 hr incubation period are associated with infections from *Shigella* and also Shigatoxin-producing *E. coli,* such as *E. coli* O157:H7. Organisms associated with dysentery or hemorrhagic diarrhea can also cause watery diarrhea alone without fever or that precedes a more complicated course that results in dysentery.

Although many of the manifestations of acute gastroenteritis in children are nonspecific, some clinical features can help identify major categories of diarrhea and allow rapid triage for antibiotic or specific dietary therapy (see Tables 340-1 to 340-4). There is considerable overlap in the symptomatology. The positive predictive values for the features of dysentery are very poor; the negative predictability for bacterial pathogens is much better in the absence of signs of dysentery. If warranted and if facilities and resources permit, the etiology can be verified by appropriate laboratory testing.

COMPLICATIONS

Most of the complications associated with gastroenteritis are related to delays in diagnosis and delays in the institution of appropriate therapy. Without early and appropriate rehydration, many children with acute diarrhea would develop dehydration with associated complications (see Chapter 57). These can be life-threatening in infants and young children. Inappropriate therapy can lead to prolongation of the diarrheal episodes, with consequent malnutrition and complications such as secondary infections and micronutrient deficiencies (iron, zinc, vitamin A). In developing countries and HIV-infected populations, associated bacteremias are well-recognized complications in malnourished children with diarrhea.

Specific pathogens are associated with extraintestinal manifestations and complications. These are not pathognomonic of the infection, nor do they always occur in close temporal association with the diarrheal episode (Table 340-9).

DIAGNOSIS

The diagnosis of gastroenteritis is based on clinical recognition, an evaluation of its severity by rapid assessment and by confirmation by appropriate laboratory investigations, if indicated.

Table 340-8	Differential Diagnosis of Acute Dysentery and Inflammatory Enterocolitis

SPECIFIC INFECTIOUS PROCESSES
Bacillary dysentery (Shigella dysenteriae, Shigella flexneri, Shigella sonnei, Shigella boydii; invasive Escherichia coli)
Campylobacteriosis (Campylobacter jejuni)
Amebic dysentery (Entamoeba histolytica)
Ciliary dysentery (Balantidium coli)
Bilharzial dysentery (Schistosoma japonicum, Schistosoma mansoni)
Other parasitic infections (Trichinella spiralis)
Vibriosis (Vibrio parahaemolyticus)
Salmonellosis (Salmonella typhimurium)
Typhoid fever (Salmonella typhi)
Enteric fever (Salmonella choleraesuis, Salmonella paratyphi)
Yersiniosis (Yersinia enterocolitica)
Spirillar dysentery (Spirillum spp.)

PROCTITIS
Gonococcal (Neisseria gonorrhoeae)
Herpetic (herpes simplex virus)
Chlamydial (Chlamydia trachomatis)
Syphilitic (Treponema pallidum)

OTHER SYNDROMES
Necrotizing enterocolitis of the newborn
Enteritis necroticans
Pseudomembranous enterocolitis (Clostridium difficile)
Typhlitis

CHRONIC INFLAMMATORY PROCESSES
Enteropathogenic and enteroaggregative E. coli
Gastrointestinal tuberculosis
Gastrointestinal mycosis
Parasitic enteritis

SYNDROMES WITHOUT KNOWN INFECTIOUS CAUSE
Idiopathic ulcerative colitis
Crohn disease
Radiation enteritis
Ischemic colitis
Allergic enteritis

From Mandell GL, Bennett JE, Dolin R, editors: Principles and practices of infectious diseases, ed 7, Philadelphia, 2010, Churchill Livingstone.

Clinical Evaluation of Diarrhea

The most common manifestations of gastrointestinal tract infection in children are diarrhea, abdominal cramps, and vomiting. Systemic manifestations are varied and associated with a variety of causes. The evaluation of a child with acute diarrhea includes:

◆ Assessing the degree of dehydration and acidosis and provide rapid resuscitation and rehydration with oral or intravenous fluids as required (Tables 340-10 and 340-11).
◆ Obtaining appropriate contact, travel, or exposure history. This includes information on exposure to contacts with similar symptoms, intake of contaminated foods or water, child-care center attendance, recent travel of patient or contact with a person who traveled to a diarrhea-endemic area, and use of antimicrobial agents.
◆ Clinically determining the etiology of diarrhea for institution of prompt antibiotic therapy, if indicated.

Although nausea and vomiting are nonspecific symptoms, they indicate infection in the upper intestine. Fever suggests an inflammatory process but also occurs as a result of dehydration or coinfection (e.g., urinary tract infection, otitis media). Fever is common in patients with inflammatory diarrhea. Severe abdominal pain and tenesmus indicate involvement of the large intestine and rectum. Features such as nausea and vomiting and absent or low-grade fever with mild to moderate periumbilical pain and watery diarrhea indicate small intestine involvement and also reduce the likelihood of a serious bacterial infection.

This clinical approach to the diagnosis and management of diarrhea in young children is a critical component of the **Integrated Management of Childhood Illnesses** package that is being implemented in developing countries that have a high burden of diarrhea mortality (Figs. 340-6 and 340-7).

Stool Examination

Microscopic examination of the stool and cultures can yield important information on the etiology of diarrhea. Stool specimens could be examined for mucus, blood, and leukocytes. Fecal leukocytes indicate bacterial invasion of colonic mucosa, although some patients with shigellosis have minimal leukocytes at an early stage of infection, as do patients infected with Shigatoxin-producing E. coli and E. histolytica. Recent advances in rapid molecular methods of diagnosis for bacterial and parasitic infections have made the role of traditional microscopy less important; however, this is still a useful test in developing countries. XTAG GPP is an FDA-approved gastrointestinal pathogen panel using multiplexed nucleic acid technology that detects Campylobacter, C. difficile, toxin A/B, E. coli 0157, enterotoxigenic E. coli, Salmonella, Shigella, Shiga-like toxin E. coli, norovirus, rotavirus A, Giardia, and Cryptosporidium. Stool cultures should be obtained as early in the course of disease as possible from children with **bloody diarrhea** in whom stool microscopy indicates **fecal leukocytes,** in **outbreaks** with suspected **hemolytic-uremic syndrome,** and in **immunosuppressed** children with diarrhea. Stool specimens for culture need to be transported and plated quickly; if the latter is not quickly available, specimens might need to be transported in special transport media. The yield and diagnosis of bacterial diarrhea is improved by using molecular diagnostic procedures such as real-time polymerase chain reaction. In most previously healthy children with uncomplicated watery diarrhea, no laboratory evaluation is needed except for epidemiologic purposes.

TREATMENT

The broad principles of management of acute gastroenteritis in children include oral rehydration therapy, enteral feeding and diet selection, zinc supplementation, and additional therapies such as probiotics.

Oral Rehydration Therapy

Children, especially infants, are more susceptible than adults to dehydration because of the greater basal fluid and electrolyte requirements per kg and because they are dependent on others to meet these demands. **Dehydration** must be evaluated rapidly and corrected in 4-6 hr according to the degree of dehydration and estimated daily requirements. A small minority of children, especially those in shock or unable to tolerate oral fluids, require initial intravenous rehydration, but oral rehydration is the preferred mode of rehydration and replacement of ongoing losses (see Tables 340-8 and 340-9). Risks associated with severe dehydration that might necessitate intravenous resuscitation include: age <6 mo; prematurity; chronic illness; fever >38°C (100.4°F) if younger than 3 mo or >39°C (102.2°F) if 3-36 mo of age; bloody diarrhea; persistent emesis; poor urine output; sunken eyes; and a depressed level of consciousness. The low-osmolality World Health Organization (WHO) oral rehydration solution (ORS) containing 75 mEq of sodium, 64 mEq of chloride, 20 mEq of potassium, and 75 mmol of glucose per liter, with total osmolarity of 245 mOsm/L, is now the global standard of care and more effective than home fluids, including decarbonated soda beverages, fruit juices, and tea. These are not suitable for rehydration or maintenance therapy because they have inappropriately high osmolalities and low sodium concentrations. Figure 340-7 and Tables 340-10 and 340-11 outline a clinical evaluation plan and management strategy for children with moderate to severe diarrhea. Oral rehydration should be given to infants and children slowly, especially if they have emesis. It can be given initially by a dropper, teaspoon, or syringe, beginning with as little as 5 mL at a time. The volume is increased as tolerated. Replacement for emesis or stool losses is noted in Table 340-11. Oral rehydration can also be given by a nasogastric tube if needed; this is not the usual route.

Limitations to oral rehydration therapy include shock, an ileus, intussusception, carbohydrate intolerance (rare), severe emesis, and

Table 340-9	Extraintestinal Manifestations of Enteric Infections

MANIFESTATION	ASSOCIATED ENTERIC PATHOGEN(S)	ONSET AND PROGNOSIS
Focal infections from systemic spread of bacterial pathogens, including vulvovaginitis, urinary tract infection, endocarditis, osteomyelitis, meningitis, pneumonia, hepatitis, peritonitis, chorioamnionitis, soft-tissue infection, and septic thrombophlebitis	All major pathogens can cause such direct extraintestinal infections, including *Salmonella, Shigella, Yersinia, Campylobacter, Clostridium difficile*	Onset usually during the acute infection but can occur subsequently Prognosis depends on infection site
Reactive arthritis	*Salmonella, Shigella, Yersinia, Campylobacter, Cryptosporidium, C. difficile*	Typically occurs 1-3 wk after infection Relapses after reinfection can develop in 15-50% of people, but most children recover fully within 2-6 mo after the first symptoms appear
Guillain-Barré syndrome	*Campylobacter*	Usually occurs a few weeks after the original infection Prognosis is good although 15-20% may have sequelae
Glomerulonephritis	*Shigella, Campylobacter, Yersinia*	Can be of sudden onset in acute, referring to a sudden attack of inflammation, or chronic, which comes on gradually In most cases, the kidneys heal with time
Immunoglobulin A (IgA) nephropathy	*Campylobacter*	Characterized by recurrent episodes of blood in the urine, this condition results from deposits of the protein IgA in the glomeruli. IgA nephropathy can progress for years with no noticeable symptoms Men seem more likely to develop this disorder than women
Erythema nodosum	*Yersinia, Campylobacter, Salmonella*	Although painful, is usually benign and more commonly seen in adolescents Resolves with 4-6 wk
Hemolytic uremic syndrome	*Shigella dysenteriae* 1, *Escherichia coli* O157:H7, others	Sudden onset, short-term renal failure In severe cases, renal failure requires several sessions of dialysis to take over the kidney function, but most children recover without permanent damage to their health
Hemolytic anemia	*Campylobacter, Yersinia*	Relatively rare complication and can have a chronic course

From Centers for Disease Control and Prevention: Managing acute gastroenteritis among children, MMWR Recomm Rep 53:1–33, 2004.

Table 340-10	Symptoms Associated with Dehydration

SYMPTOM	MINIMAL OR NO DEHYDRATION (<3% LOSS OF BODY WEIGHT)	MILD TO MODERATE DEHYDRATION (3-9% LOSS OF BODY WEIGHT)	SEVERE DEHYDRATION (>9% LOSS OF BODY WEIGHT)
Mental status	Well; alert	Normal, fatigued or restless, irritable	Apathetic, lethargic, unconscious
Thirst	Drinks normally; might refuse liquids	Thirsty; eager to drink	Drinks poorly; unable to drink
Heart rate	Normal	Normal to increased	Tachycardia, with bradycardia in most severe cases
Quality of pulses	Normal	Normal to decreased	Weak, thready, or impalpable
Breathing	Normal	Normal; fast	Deep
Eyes	Normal	Slightly sunken	Deeply sunken
Tears	Present	Decreased	Absent
Mouth and tongue	Moist	Dry	Parched
Skinfold	Instant recoil	Recoil in <2 sec	Recoil in >2 sec
Capillary refill	Normal	Prolonged	Prolonged; minimal
Extremities	Warm	Cool	Cold; mottled; cyanotic
Urine output	Normal to decreased	Decreased	Minimal

Adapted from Duggan C, Santosham M, Glass RI: The management of acute diarrhea in children: oral rehydration, maintenance, and nutritional therapy, MMWR Recomm Rep 41(RR-16):1–20, 1992; and World Health Organization: The treatment of diarrhoea: a manual for physicians and other senior health workers, Geneva, 1995, World Health Organization; Centers for Disease Control and Prevention: Diagnosis and management of foodborne illnesses, MMWR 53(RR-4):1-33, 2004.

high stool output (>10 mL/kg/hr). Ondansetron (oral mucosal absorption preparation) reduces the incidence of emesis, thus permitting more effective oral rehydration and is well established in emergency management of acute gastroenteritis in developed countries.

Enteral Feeding and Diet Selection

Continued enteral feeding in diarrhea aids in recovery from the episode, and a continued age-appropriate diet after rehydration is the norm. Although intestinal brush-border surface and luminal enzymes

can be affected in children with prolonged diarrhea, there is evidence that satisfactory carbohydrate, protein, and fat absorption can take place on a variety of diets. Once rehydration is complete, food should be reintroduced while oral rehydration is continued to replace ongoing losses from emesis or stools and for maintenance. Breastfeeding or nondiluted regular formula should be resumed as soon as possible. Foods with complex carbohydrates (rice, wheat, potatoes, bread, and cereals), lean meats, yogurt, fruits, and vegetables are also tolerated. Fatty foods or foods high in simple sugars (juices, carbonated sodas)

Table 340-11	Summary of Treatment Based on Degree of Dehydration		
DEGREE OF DEHYDRATION	**REHYDRATION THERAPY**	**REPLACEMENT OF LOSSES**	**NUTRITION**
Minimal or no dehydration	Not applicable	<10 kg body weight: 60-120 mL ORS for each diarrheal stool or vomiting episode >10 kg body weight: 120-240 mL ORS for each diarrheal stool or vomiting episode	Continue breastfeeding or resume age-appropriate normal diet after initial hydration, including adequate caloric intake for maintenance*
Mild to moderate dehydration	ORS, 50-100 mL/kg body weight over 3-4 hr	Same	Same
Severe dehydration	Lactated Ringer solution or normal saline in 20 mL/kg body weight IV until perfusion and mental status improve; then administer 100 mL/kg body weight ORS over 4 hr or 5% dextrose normal saline IV at twice maintenance fluid rates	Same; if unable to drink, administer through nasogastric tube or administer 5% dextrose in normal saline with 20 mEq/L potassium chloride IV	Same

*Overly restricted diets should be avoided during acute diarrheal episodes. Breastfed infants should continue to nurse ad libitum even during acute rehydration. Infants too weak to eat can be given milk or formula through a nasogastric tube. Lactose-containing formulas are usually well tolerated. If lactose malabsorption appears clinically substantial, lactose-free formulas can be used. Complex carbohydrates, fresh fruits, lean meats, yogurt, and vegetables are all recommended. Carbonated drinks or commercial juices with a high concentration of simple carbohydrates should be avoided.
ORS, oral rehydration solution.
From Centers for Disease Control and Prevention: Diagnosis and management of foodborne illnesses, MMWR 53(RR-4):1-33, 2004.

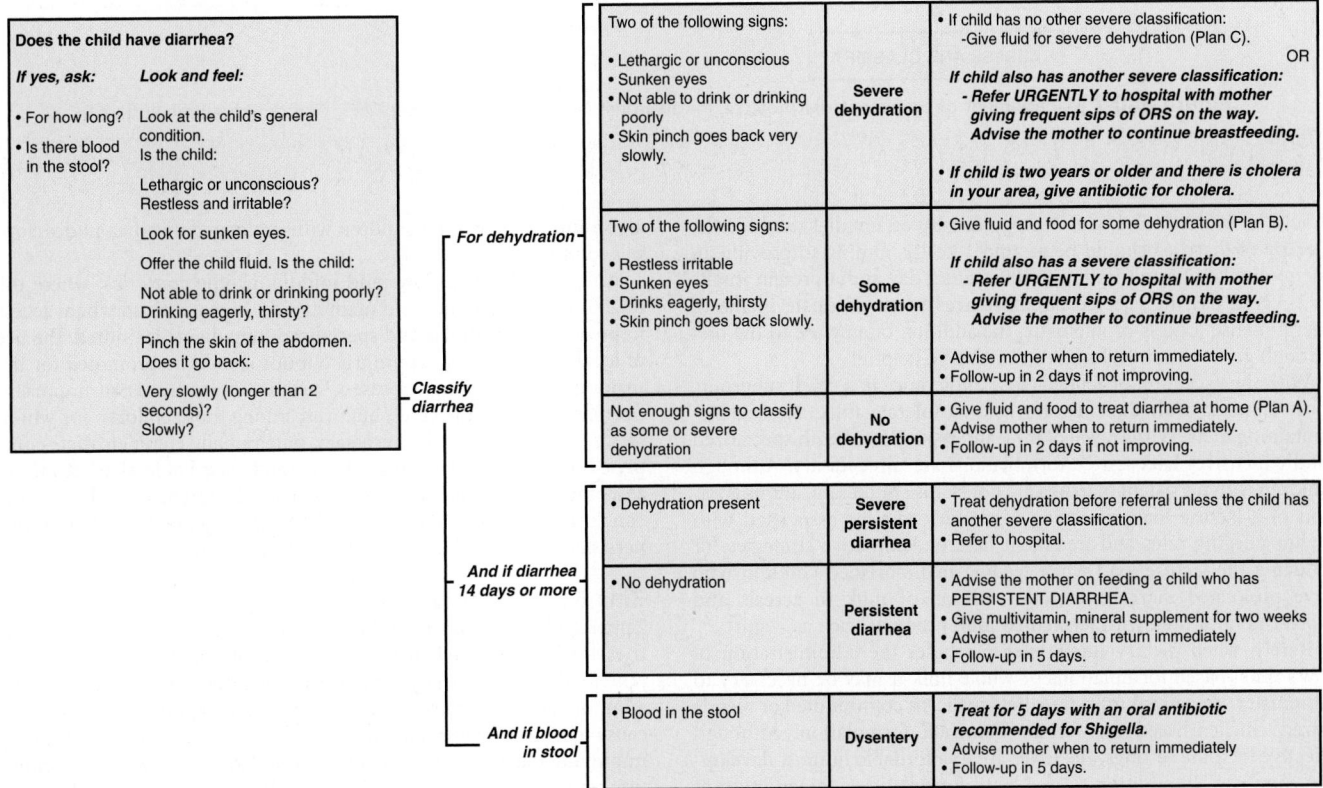

Figure 340-6 Integrated Management of Childhood Illnesses (IMCI) protocol for the recognition and management of diarrhea in developing countries. *ORS,* Oral rehydration solution.

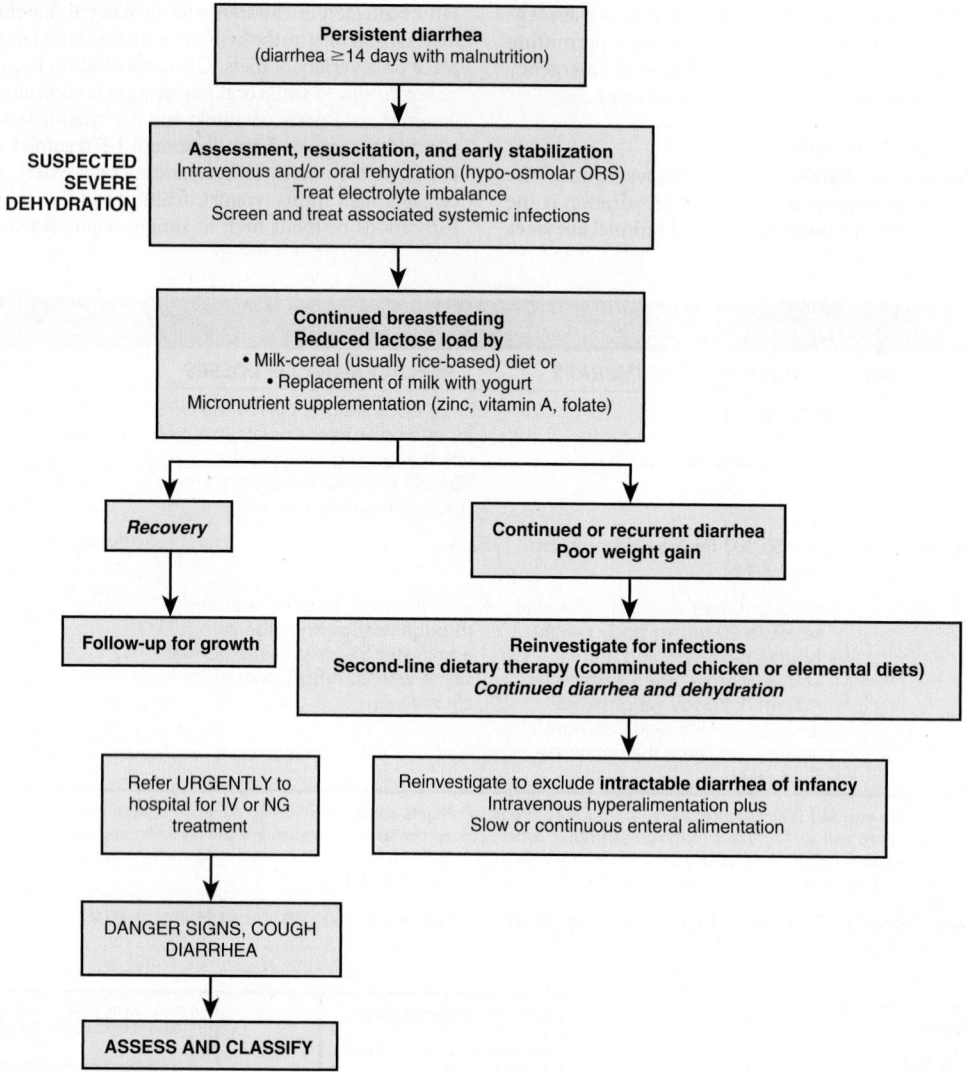

Figure 340-7 Management of persistent diarrhea. *IV*, Intravenous; *NG*, nasogastric tube; *ORS*, oral rehydration solution.

should be avoided. The usual energy density of any diet used for the therapy of diarrhea should be around 1 kcal/g, aiming to provide an energy intake of a minimum of 100 kcal/kg/day and a protein intake of 2-3 g/kg/day. In selected circumstances when adequate intake of energy-dense food is problematic, the addition of amylase to the diet through germination techniques can also be helpful.

With the exception of acute lactose intolerance in a small subgroup, most children with diarrhea are able to tolerate milk and lactose-containing diets. Withdrawal of milk and replacement with specialized (and expensive) lactose-free formulations are unnecessary. Although children with persistent diarrhea are not lactose intolerant, administration of a lactose load exceeding 5 g/kg/day may be associated with higher purging rates and treatment failure. Alternative strategies for reducing the lactose load while feeding malnourished children who have prolonged diarrhea include addition of milk to cereals and replacement of milk with fermented milk products such as yogurt.

Rarely, when dietary intolerance precludes the administration of cow's milk–based formulations or whole milk it may be necessary to administer specialized milk-free diets such as a comminuted or blenderized chicken-based diet or an elemental formulation. Although effective in some settings, the latter are unaffordable in most developing countries. In addition to rice-lentil formulations, the addition of green banana or pectin to the diet has also been shown to be effective in the treatment of persistent diarrhea. Figure 340-7 gives an

algorithm for managing children with prolonged diarrhea in developing countries.

Among children in low- and middle-income countries, where the dual burden of diarrhea and malnutrition is greatest and where access to proprietary formulas and specialized ingredients is limited, the use of locally available age-appropriate foods should be promoted for the majority of acute diarrhea cases. Lactose intolerance is an important complication in some cases, but even among those children for whom lactose avoidance may be necessary, nutritionally complete diets comprised of locally available ingredients can be used at least as effectively as commercial preparations or specialized ingredients. These same conclusions may also apply to the dietary management of children with persistent diarrhea, but the evidence remains limited.

Zinc Supplementation

Zinc supplementation in children with diarrhea in developing countries leads to reduced duration and severity of diarrhea and could potentially prevent a large proportion of cases from recurring. Zinc administration for diarrhea management can significantly reduce all-cause mortality by 46% and hospital admission by 23%. In addition to improving diarrhea recovery rates, administration of zinc in community settings leads to increased use of ORS and reduction in the inappropriate use of antimicrobials. All children older than 6 mo of age with acute diarrhea in at-risk areas should receive oral zinc (20 mg/

day) in some form for 10-14 days during and continued after diarrhea. The role of zinc in well nourished, zinc replete populations in developed countries is less certain.

Additional Therapies

The use of probiotic nonpathogenic bacteria for prevention and therapy of diarrhea has been successful in some settings although the evidence is inconclusive to recommend their use in all settings. In addition to restoring beneficial intestinal flora, probiotics can enhance host protective immunity such as downregulation of proinflammatory cytokines and upregulation of anti inflammatory cytokines. A variety of organisms (*Lactobacillus, Bifidobacterium*) have a good safety record; therapy has not been standardized and the most effective (and safe) organism has not been identified. *Saccharomyces boulardii* is effective in antibiotic-associated and in *C. difficile* diarrhea, and there is some evidence that it might prevent diarrhea in daycare centers. *Lactobacillus rhamnosus GG* is associated with reduced diarrheal duration and severity, which reduction is more evident in cases of childhood rotavirus diarrhea.

Antimotility agents (loperamide) are contraindicated in children with dysentery and probably have no role in the management of acute watery diarrhea in otherwise healthy children. Similarly, **antiemetic** agents, such as the phenothiazines, are of little value and are associated with potentially serious side effects (lethargy, dystonia, malignant hyperpyrexia). Nonetheless, ondansetron is an effective and less-toxic antiemetic agent and as indicated previously, is a useful adjunct to the treatment of vomiting in ambulatory settings with reduced risk of intravenous fluid requirements and hospitalization. Because persistent vomiting can limit oral rehydration therapy, a single sublingual dose of an oral dissolvable tablet of ondansetron (4 mg 4-11 yr and 8 mg for children older than 11 yr [generally 0.2 mg/kg]) may be given. However, most children do not require specific antiemetic therapy; careful oral rehydration therapy is usually sufficient.

Racecadotril, an enkephalins inhibitor, has inconsistently been shown to reduce stool output in patients with diarrhea. Experience with this drug in children is limited, and for the average child with acute diarrhea it may be unnecessary.

Antibiotic Therapy

Timely antibiotic therapy in select cases of diarrhea related to bacterial infections can reduce the duration and severity of illness and prevent complications (Table 340-12). Although these agents are important to use in specific cases, their widespread and indiscriminate use leads to the development of antimicrobial resistance. **Nitazoxanide**, an antiinfective agent, is effective in the treatment of a wide variety of pathogens, including *C. parvum, G. lamblia, E. histolytica, Blastocystis hominis, C. difficile*, and rotavirus.

PREVENTION

In many developed countries, diarrhea caused by pathogens such as *C. botulinum, E. coli* O157:H7, *Salmonella, Shigella, V. cholerae, Cryptosporidium*, and *Cyclospora* is a notifiable disease and, thus, contact tracing and source identification is important in preventing outbreaks.

Many developing countries struggle with huge disease burdens of diarrhea where a wider approach to diarrhea prevention may be required. Preventive strategies may be of relevance to both developed and developing countries.

Promotion of Exclusive Breastfeeding

Exclusive breastfeeding (administration of no other fluids or foods for the 1st 6 mo of life) is not common, especially in many developed countries. Exclusive breastfeeding protects very young infants from diarrheal disease through the promotion of passive immunity and through reduction in the intake of potentially contaminated food and water. Breast milk contains all the nutrients needed in early infancy, and when continued during diarrhea, it also diminishes the adverse impact on nutritional status. Exclusive breastfeeding for the 1st 6 mo of life is widely regarded as one of the most effective

interventions to reduce the risk of premature childhood mortality and the potential to prevent 12% of all deaths of children younger than 5 yr of age.

Improved Complementary Feeding Practices

There is a strong inverse association between appropriate, safe complementary feeding and mortality in children age 6-11 mo; malnutrition is an independent risk for the frequency and severity of diarrheal illness. Complementary foods should be introduced at 6 mo of age, and breastfeeding should continue for up to 2 yr. Complementary foods in developing countries are generally poor in quality and often are heavily contaminated, thus predisposing to diarrhea. Contamination of complementary foods can be potentially reduced through caregivers' education and improving home food storage. Improved vitamin A status has been shown to reduce the frequency of severe diarrhea. Vitamin A supplementation reduces all-cause childhood mortality by 25% (95% confidence interval [CI], 12-36%) and diarrhea-specific mortality by 30% (95% CI, 14-42%).

Rotavirus Immunization

Most infants acquire rotavirus diarrhea early in life; an effective rotavirus vaccine would have a major effect on reducing diarrhea mortality in developing countries. In 1998, a quadrivalent Rhesus rotavirus-derived vaccine was licensed in the United States but subsequently withdrawn because of an increased risk of intussusception. Subsequent development and testing of newer rotavirus vaccines have led to their introduction in most developed countries and approval by the WHO in 2009 for widespread use in developing countries. It is now clear that the introduction of these vaccines is associated with a significant reduction in severe diarrhea and associated mortality.

The institution of large-scale rotavirus vaccination programs has led to major reduction in the burden of disease and associated mortality. In an evaluation of large-scale rotavirus vaccine introduction, coverage rate of 74% was achieved in infants younger than 12 mo of age, with 41% reduction (95% CI, 36-47%) in diarrhea-related mortality. In an evaluation of the vaccine in Africa, overall protective efficacy against rotavirus gastroenteritis ranged from 49-61%, with 30% protective efficacy against all-cause severe gastroenteritis in infancy. Vaccine (live virus) associated rotavirus infection has been reported in children with severe combined immunodeficiency disease, but the vaccine has been shown to be safe in HIV-infected populations.

Other vaccines that could potentially reduce the burden of severe diarrhea and mortality in young children are vaccines against cholera, *Shigella*, and ETEC. Preventive use of cholera vaccines in endemic countries can reduce the risk of developing cholera by 52% (95% CI, 36-65%).

Improved Water and Sanitary Facilities and Promotion of Personal and Domestic Hygiene

Much of the reduction in diarrhea prevalence in the developed world is the result of improvement in standards of hygiene, sanitation, and water supply. Strikingly, an estimated 88% of all diarrheal deaths worldwide can be attributed to unsafe water, inadequate sanitation, and poor hygiene. Improving water quality can reduce the risk of diarrhea by 17%, whereas hand washing with soap and safe excreta disposal reduce the risk of diarrhea by 48% and 36%, respectively. Behavioral change strategies through promotion of handwashing indicate that handwashing promotion and access to soap reduces the burden of diarrhea in developing countries.

Improved Case Management of Diarrhea

Improved management of diarrhea through prompt identification and appropriate therapy significantly reduces diarrhea duration, its nutritional penalty, and risk of death in childhood. Improved management of acute diarrhea is a key factor in reducing the burden of prolonged episodes and persistent diarrhea. The WHO/UNICEF recommendations to use low-osmolality ORS and zinc supplementation for the management of diarrhea, coupled with selective and appropriate use of antibiotics, have the potential to reduce the number of diarrheal

Table 340-12	Antibiotic Therapy for Infectious Diarrhea

ORGANISM	DRUG OF CHOICE	DOSAGE AND DURATION OF TREATMENT
Shigella (severe dysentery and EIEC dysentery)	Ciprofloxacin, ampicillin, ceftriaxone, azithromycin, or TMP-SMX Most strains are resistant to several antibiotics	Ceftriaxone 50-100 mg/kg/day IV or IM, qd or bid × 7 days Ciprofloxacin 20-30 mg/kg/day PO bid × 7-10 days Ampicillin PO, IV 50-100 mg/kg/day qid × 7 days
EPEC, ETEC, EIEC	TMP-SMX or ciprofloxacin	TMP 10 mg/kg/day and SMX 50 mg/kg/day bid × 5 days Ciprofloxacin PO 20-30 mg/kg/day qid for 5-10 days
Salmonella	No antibiotics for uncomplicated gastroenteritis in normal hosts caused by nontyphoidal species **Treatment** indicated in infants younger than 3 mo, and patients with malignancy, chronic GI disease, severe colitis hemoglobinopathies, or HIV infection, and other immunocompromised patients Most strains are resistant to multiple antibiotics	See treatment of *Shigella*
Aeromonas/Plesiomonas	TMP-SMX Ciprofloxacin	TMP 10 mg/kg/day and SMX 50 mg/kg/day bid for 5 days Ciprofloxacin PO 20-30 mg/kg/day divided bid × 7-10 days
Yersinia spp.	Antibiotics are not usually required for diarrhea Deferoxamine therapy should be withheld for severe infections or associated bacteremia Treat sepsis as for immunocompromised hosts, using combination therapy with parenteral doxycycline, aminoglycoside, TMP-SMX, or fluoroquinolone	
Campylobacter jejuni	Erythromycin or azithromycin	Erythromycin PO 50 mg/kg/day divided tid × 5 days Azithromycin PO 5-10 mg/kg/day qid × 5 days
Clostridium difficile	Metronidazole (first line) Discontinue initiating antibiotic Vancomycin (second line)	PO 30 mg/kg/day divided qid × 5 days; max 2 g PO 40 mg/kg/day qid × 7 days, max 125 mg
Entamoeba histolytica	Metronidazole followed by iodoquinol or paromomycin	Metronidazole PO 30-40 mg/kg/day tid × 7-10 days Iodoquinol PO 30-40 mg/kg/day tid × 20 days Paromomycin PO 25-35 mg/kg/day tid × 7 days
Giardia lamblia	Furazolidone or metronidazole or albendazole or quinacrine	Furazolidone PO 25 mg/kg/day qid × 5-7 days Metronidazole PO 30-40 mg/kg/day tid × 7 days Albendazole PO 200 mg bid × 10 days
Cryptosporidium spp.	Nitazoxanide PO treatment may not be needed in normal hosts In immunocompromised, PO immunoglobulin + aggressively treat HIV, etc.	Children 1-3 yr: 100 mg bid × 3 days Children 4-11 yr: 200 mg bid
Isospora spp.	TMP-SMX	PO TMP 5 mg/kg/day and SMX 25 mg/kg/day, bid × 7-10 days
Cyclospora spp.	TMP/SMX	PO TMP 5 mg/kg/day and SMX 25 mg/kg/day bid × 7 days
Blastocystis hominis	Metronidazole or iodoquinol	Metronidazole PO 30-40 mg/kg/day tid × 7-10 days Iodoquinol PO 40 mg/kg/day tid × 20 days

EIEC, Enteroinvasive *Escherichia coli*; EPEC, enteropathogenic *E. coli*; ETEC, enterotoxigenic *E. coli*; GI, gastrointestinal; max, maximum; SMX, sulfamethoxazole; TMP, trimethoprim.

deaths among children through Community Case Management and Integrated Management of Childhood Illnesses.

Community-based interventions to diagnose and treat childhood diarrhea through community health workers leads to a significant rise in care seeking behaviors for diarrhea and are associated with significantly increased use of ORS and zinc at household level as well as reduction in the unnecessary use of antibiotics for diarrhea by 75%.

Bibliography is available at Expert Consult.

340.1 Traveler's Diarrhea
Zulfiqar Ahmed Bhutta

Traveler's diarrhea is a common complication of visitors to developing countries and is caused by a variety of pathogens, in part depending on the season and the region visited (see Table 340-12). Traveler's diarrhea has a high attack rate among travelers from higher-income countries visiting, during the summer, countries in a warmer climate that have a high prevalence of indigenous infectious diarrhea. Traveler's diarrhea can manifest with watery diarrhea or as dysentery. Without treatment, 90% will have resolved within a week and 98% within a month of onset. Some individuals develop more severe diarrhea and become dehydrated or unwell and may experience systemic complications that warrant further attention. Most cases of traveler's diarrhea resolve spontaneously and a simple stool culture may be the only investigation required. For those individuals with ongoing symptoms, further tests should be requested depending on the history and clinical presentation.

TREATMENT

Traveler's diarrhea is often self-limiting but requires particular attention to avoid dehydration. For infants and children, rehydration, as discussed in Chapter 340, is appropriate, followed by a standard diet. Adolescents and adults should increase their intake of electrolyte-rich fluids. Kaolin-pectin, anticholinergic agents, *Lactobacillus,* and bismuth salicylate have not been effective therapies. Loperamide, an antimotility and antisecretory agent, reduces the number of stools in older children with watery diarrhea and improves outcomes when used in combination with antibiotics in traveler's diarrhea. However, loperamide should be used with great caution or not at all in febrile or toxic patients with dysentery and in those with bloody diarrhea.

Antibiotics, with or without loperamide, can also reduce the number of unformed stools. Short-duration (3 days) therapy with fluoroquinolones, trimethoprim-sulfamethoxazole, azithromycin, or rifaximin is effective; the choice of antibiotic depends on the age of the patient, the potential organism, and the organism's local resistance patterns. However, antibiotics often have a negative risk-benefit ratio when weighing potential side effects vs treatment need for a short-lasting and self-limiting disease such as traveler's diarrhea. Azithromycin has several advantages over other antibiotics. It is taken only once (1,000 mg), the rate of antimicrobial resistance is low, and it has a good safety profile. Furthermore, in contrast to rifaximin, it can be used in severe cases of diarrhea with fever or bloody stools and can even be administered in children. Optionally, azithromycin can be combined with antimotility medications such as loperamide. Travelers should be reminded that diarrhea can be a symptom of other severe diseases, such as malaria. Therefore, if diarrhea persists or additional symptoms such as fever occur, travelers should seek medical advice. For up-to-date information on local pathogens and resistant patterns, see www.cdc.gov/travel.

PREVENTION

Travelers should drink bottled or canned beverages or boiled water. They should avoid ice, salads, and fruit they did not peel themselves. Food should be eaten hot, if possible. Raw or poorly cooked seafood is a risk, as is eating in a restaurant rather than a private home. Swimming pools and other recreational water sites can also be contaminated.

Chemoprophylaxis is not routinely recommended for previously healthy children or adults. Nonetheless, travelers should bring azithromycin (younger than 16 yr of age) or ciprofloxacin (older than 16 yr of age) and begin antimicrobial therapy if diarrhea develops.

Bibliography is available at Expert Consult.

Chapter **341**
Chronic Diarrhea
Alfredo Guarino, David Branski, and Harland S. Winter

DEFINITION AND EPIDEMIOLOGY

Chronic diarrhea is defined as stool volume of more than 10 g/kg/day in toddlers/infants and greater than 200 g/day in older children that lasts for 14 days or more. In practice, this usually means having loose or watery stools more than 3 times a day. *Awakening at night to pass stool is often a sign of an organic cause of diarrhea.* The epidemiology has 2 distinct patterns. In developing countries, chronic diarrhea is, in many cases, the result of an intestinal infection that persists longer than expected. This syndrome is often defined as *protracted diarrhea,* but there is no clear distinction between protracted and chronic diarrhea. In countries with higher socioeconomic conditions, chronic diarrhea is less frequent and the etiology often varies with age. The outcome of diarrhea depends on the cause and ranges from benign, self-limited

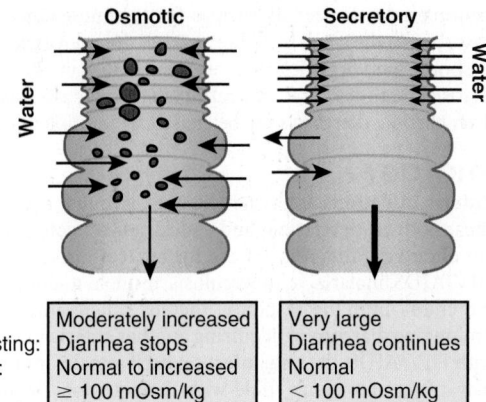

	Osmotic	Secretory
Stool volume:	Moderately increased	Very large
Response to fasting:	Diarrhea stops	Diarrhea continues
Stool osmolality:	Normal to increased	Normal
Ion gap:	≥ 100 mOsm/kg	< 100 mOsm/kg

Figure 341-1 Pathways of osmotic and secretory diarrhea. Osmotic diarrhea is caused by functional or structural damage of intestinal epithelium. Nonabsorbed osmotically active solutes drive water into the lumen. Stool osmolality and ion gap are generally increased. Diarrhea stops in children when not eating. In secretory diarrhea, ions are actively pumped into the intestine by the action of exogenous and endogenous secretagogues. Usually there is no intestinal damage. Osmolality and ion gap are within normal levels. Large volumes of stools are lost independent of food ingestion.

conditions, such as toddler's diarrhea, to severe congenital diseases, such as microvillus inclusion disease, that may lead to progressive intestinal failure.

PATHOPHYSIOLOGY

The mechanisms of diarrhea are generally divided into secretory and osmotic, but often diarrhea is a combination of both mechanisms. In addition, inflammation and motility disorders may contribute to diarrhea. Secretory diarrhea is usually associated with large volumes of watery stools and persists when oral feeding is withdrawn. Osmotic diarrhea is dependent on oral feeding, and stool volumes are usually not as massive as in secretory diarrhea (Fig. 341-1).

Secretory diarrhea is characterized by active electrolyte and water fluxes toward the intestinal lumen, resulting from either the inhibition of neutral NaCl absorption in villous enterocytes or an increase in electrogenic chloride secretion in secretory crypt cells as a result of the opening of the cystic fibrosis transmembrane regulator (CFTR) chloride channel or both. The result is more secretion from the crypts than absorption in the villous that persists during fasting. The other components of the enterocyte ion secretory machinery are (1) the Na-K 2Cl cotransporter for the electroneutral chloride entrance into the enterocyte; (2) the Na-K pump, which decreases the intracellular Na^+ concentration, determining the driving gradient for further Na^+ influx; and (3) the K^+ selective channel, that enables K^+, once it has entered the cell together with Na^+, to return to the extracellular fluid.

Electrogenic secretion is induced by an increase of intracellular concentration of cyclic adenosine monophosphate, cyclic guanosine monophosphate, or calcium in response to microbial enterotoxins, or to endogenous endocrine or nonendocrine moieties, including inflammatory cytokines. Another mechanism of secretory diarrhea is the inhibition of the electroneutral NaCl-coupled pathway that involves the Na^+/H^+ and the Cl^-/HCO_3^- exchangers. Defects in the genes of the Na^+/H^+ and the Cl^-/HCO_3^- exchangers are responsible for congenital Na^+ and Cl^- diarrhea, respectively.

Osmotic diarrhea is caused by nonabsorbed nutrients in the intestinal lumen as a result of 1 or more of the following mechanisms: (1) intestinal damage (e.g., enteric infection); (2) reduced absorptive surface area (e.g., active celiac disease); (3) defective digestive enzyme or nutrient carrier (e.g., lactase deficiency); (4) decreased intestinal transit time (e.g., functional diarrhea); and (5) nutrient overload, exceeding the digestive capacity (e.g., overfeeding, sorbitol in fruit juice). Whatever the mechanism, the osmotic force generated by nonabsorbed solutes drives water into the intestinal lumen. A very common example of osmotic diarrhea is lactose intolerance. Lactose, if not absorbed in the small intestine, reaches the colon, where it is fermented to short-chain organic acids, releasing hydrogen that is detected in the lactose breath test, and generating an osmotic overload. In many children chronic diarrhea may be caused by multiple mechanisms.

ETIOLOGY

Enteric infections are by far the most frequent cause of chronic diarrhea, both in developing and industrialized countries but, outcomes are often very different. In the former, comorbid conditions, such as HIV/AIDS, malaria, or tuberculosis, result in malnutrition that impairs the child's immune response, thereby potentiating the likelihood of prolonging diarrhea or acquiring another enteric infection. In children with HIV/AIDS, the viral infection itself impairs immune function and may trigger a vicious circle with malnutrition. Sequential infections with the same or different pathogens may also be responsible for chronic diarrhea.

In developing countries, enteroadherent *Escherichia coli* and *Giardia lamblia* have been implicated in chronic diarrhea, whereas, in developed countries, chronic infectious diarrhea usually runs a more benign course and the etiology is often viral, with a major role of rotavirus and norovirus (Table 341-1). Opportunistic microorganisms induce diarrhea exclusively, more severely or for more prolonged periods, in specific populations, such as immunocompromised children. Specific agents cause chronic diarrhea or exacerbate diarrhea in many chronic diseases. *Clostridium difficile* or cytomegalovirus act as opportunistic agents in oncologic patients as well as in patients with inflammatory bowel diseases. *Cryptosporidium* may induce severe and protracted diarrhea in AIDS patients.

In small intestinal bacterial overgrowth, diarrhea may be the result of either a direct interaction between the microorganism and the enterocyte or the consequence of deconjugation and dehydroxylation of bile salts, and hydroxylation of fatty acids due to an increased proliferation of bacteria in the proximal intestine. Postenteritis diarrhea syndrome is a clinicopathologic condition in which small intestinal mucosal damage persists after acute gastroenteritis. Sensitization to food antigens, secondary disaccharidase deficiency, persistent infections, reinfection with an enteric pathogen, or side effects of medication may be responsible for causing postenteritis diarrhea syndrome, thought to be related to perturbations of the intestinal microbiome. Functional diarrhea which may be related to the pathogenesis of irritable bowel syndrome may be caused by complications of an acute gastroenteritis. Noninfectious chronic diarrhea is the manifestation of a broad number of heterogeneous conditions that vary with the age of the patient (Table 341-2; see also Table 336-5).

Table 341-1	A Comparative List of Prevalent Agents and Conditions in Children with Persistent Infectious Diarrhea in Industrialized and Developing Countries

AGENT/DISEASE	
INDUSTRIALIZED COUNTRIES	**DEVELOPING COUNTRIES**
Clostridium difficile	Enteroaggregative *E. coli*
Enteroaggregative *Escherichia coli*	Atypical *E. coli*
	Shigella
	Heat stable/heat labile enterotoxin-producing *E. coli*
Astrovirus	Rotavirus*
Norovirus	*Cryptosporidium*
Rotavirus*	*Giardia lamblia*
Small intestinal bacterial overgrowth (SIBO)	Tropical sprue
Postenteritis diarrhea syndrome	

*More frequent in industrialized than in developing countries as agent of chronic diarrhea.

A reduction of intestinal absorptive surface is responsible for diarrhea in celiac disease, a genetically determined permanent gluten intolerance that affects as many as 1 in 100 individuals, depending on geographic origin. In the genetically susceptible host, gliadin, the major protein of gluten, reacts with the immune system to cause villous atrophy. The reduction of functional absorptive surface area is reversible upon restriction of gluten from the diet. Celiac disease presents with more severe intestinal symptoms in younger children. **Allergy to cow's milk protein** and other food proteins also may present during infancy with chronic diarrhea. Eosinophilic gastroenteritis is characterized by eosinophilic infiltration of the intestinal wall and is strongly associated with atopy. However, whereas diarrhea in food allergy responds to withdrawal of the responsible food, this does not always occur in eosinophilic gastroenteritis, in which immune suppression may be needed.

Lactose intolerance or carbohydrate malabsorption may be caused by a brush-border enzyme defect in lactase, sucrase-isomaltase, or to a defect in the sodium/glucose cotransporter protein (SGLT1) that is transcribed from the *SLC5A1* gene causing congenital glucose-galactose malabsorption. The result of these genetic mutations is chronic diarrhea. More commonly, lactose intolerance is secondary to lactase deficiency caused by intestinal mucosal damage. Depending on ethnicity, a progressive, age-related, loss of lactase activity may begin around age 7 yr and affects approximately 80% of the nonwhite population, and acquired hypolactasia may be responsible for chronic diarrhea in older children receiving cow's milk (adult-type lactase deficiency).

In older children and adolescents, **inflammatory bowel diseases, including Crohn disease, ulcerative colitis, and inflammatory bowel disease–undetermined,** cause chronic diarrhea that is often associated with abdominal pain, elevated inflammatory markers, and increased concentrations of fecal calprotectin or lactoferrin (see Chapter 336). The age of onset of inflammatory bowel disease is broad, with rare cases described in the 1st few mo of life, but the peak incidence in childhood occurring in adolescence. The severity of the symptoms is highly variable with a pattern characterised by long periods of well-being followed by exacerbations. Growth retardation and delays in sexual maturation may precede the onset of gastrointestinal symptoms by up to 18 mo.

Chronic diarrhea may be the manifestation of maldigestion caused by exocrine **pancreatic disorders**. In most patients with cystic fibrosis, exocrine pancreatic insufficiency results in steatorrhea and protein malabsorption. In Shwachman-Diamond syndrome, exocrine pancreatic hypoplasia may be associated with neutropenia, bone changes, and intestinal protein-losing enteropathy. Specific isolated pancreatic enzyme defects, such as lipase deficiency, result in fat and/or protein malabsorption. Familial pancreatitis, associated with a mutation in the trypsinogen gene, may be associated with exocrine pancreatic insufficiency and chronic diarrhea. Mutations in CFTR, CTRC, PRSS1, SPINK 1, and SPINK 5 are all associated with hereditary pancreatitis.

Liver disorders may lead to a reduction in the bile salts pool resulting in fat malabsorption. Bile acid loss may be associated with diseases affecting the terminal ileum, such as Crohn disease, or following ileal resection. In primary bile acid malabsorption, neonates and young infants present with chronic diarrhea and fat malabsorption caused by mutations of ileal bile transporter.

The most benign etiology of chronic diarrhea is nonspecific diarrhea that encompasses functional diarrhea (or toddler's diarrhea) in children younger than 4 yr of age and irritable bowel syndrome in those 5 yr of age and older. The diseases fall under the umbrella of functional disorders, in that in older children abdominal pain is often associated with diarrhea alternating with constipation and growth and weight gain are normal.

Diarrhea may be the result from an **excessive intake of fluid and carbohydrate**. If the child's fluid intake were >150 mL/kg/24 hr, fluid intake should be reduced not to exceed 90 mL/kg/24 hr. The child is often irritable in the 1st days of the fluid restriction; however, persistence results in a decrease in the stool frequency and volume. If the dietary history suggests that the child is ingesting significant amounts of fruit juice, especially apple juice, then the consumption of juice

Table 341-2	Main Etiologies of Noninfectious Chronic Diarrhea in Children Older and Younger Than 2 Yr of Age	
ETIOLOGY	**YOUNGER THAN 2 YR**	**OLDER THAN 2 YR**
Abnormal digestive processes	Shwachman-Diamond syndrome, isolated pancreatic enzyme deficiency, chronic pancreatitis, Johanson-Blizzard syndrome, Pearson syndrome. Trypsinogen and enterokinase deficiency: chronic cholestasis; use of bile acids sequestrants; primary bile acid malabsorption	Cystic fibrosis, terminal ileum resection
Nutrient malabsorption	Congenital sucrase-isomaltase deficiency; congenital lactase deficiency; glucose-galactose malabsorption; fructose malabsorption; congenital short bowel	Hypoalactasia; acquired short bowel
Immune/inflammatory	Food allergy; autoimmune enteropathy; primary and secondary immunodeficiencies; IPEX syndrome	Celiac disease; eosinophilic gastroenteritis, inflammatory bowel diseases
Structural defects	Microvillus inclusion disease, tufting enteropathy, phenotypic diarrhea, heparan-sulphate deficiency, $\alpha_2\beta_1$ and $\alpha_6\beta_4$ integrin deficiency, lymphangiectasia, enteric anendocrinosis (neurogenin-3 mutation)	Rare
Defects of electrolyte and metabolite transport	Congenital chloride diarrhea, congenital sodium diarrhea, acrodermatitis enteropathica, selective folate deficiency, abetalipoproteinemia, activating guanylate cyclase mutation	Late onset chloride diarrhea
Motility disorders	Hirschsprung disease, chronic intestinal pseudoobstruction (neurogenic and myopathic)	Thyrotoxicosis
Neoplastic diseases	Neuroendocrine hormone-secreting tumors: Apudomas such as VIPoma, Zollinger- Ellison, and mastocytosis	Neuroendocrine hormone-secreting tumors: Apudomas such as VIPoma, Zollinger-Ellison, and mastocytosis
Diarrhea associated with exogenous substances	Excessive intake of carbonated fluid, foods or drinks containing sorbitol, mannitol, or xylitol; excessive intake of antacids or laxatives containing lactulose or $Mg(OH)_2$; excessive intake of methylxanthines-containing drinks (cola, tea, coffee)	Excessive intake of carbonated fluid, foods or drinks containing sorbitol, mannitol, or xylitol; excessive intake of antacids or laxatives containing lactulose or $Mg(OH)_2$; excessive intake of methylxanthines-containing drinks (cola, tea, coffee)
Chronic nonspecific diarrhea	Functional diarrhea*	Irritable bowel syndrome†

*Until 4 yr of age, according to Rome III criteria.
†Older than 5 yr of age according to Rome III criteria.
IPEX, immunodysregulation polyendocrinopathy enteropathy X-linked syndrome; VIPoma, vasoactive intestinal polypeptide tumor.

should be decreased. Sorbitol, which is a nonabsorbable sugar, is found in apple, pear, and prune juices, and often causes diarrhea in toddlers. Moreover, apple and pear juices contain higher amounts of fructose than glucose, a feature postulated to cause diarrhea in toddlers. In older children, irritable bowel syndrome is often associated with abdominal pain and may be related to anxiety, depression, and other psychologic disturbances.

The most severe etiology of chronic diarrhea includes a number of heterogeneous congenital conditions leading to syndromes related to **intractable diarrhea.** This is often the result of a permanent defect in the structure or function of the enterocyte, leading to progressive, potentially irreversible intestinal failure. The main etiologies of intractable diarrhea include structural enterocyte defects, disorders of intestinal motility, immune-based disorders, short gut syndrome, and disorders without demonstrable abnormalities.

Structural enterocyte defects are caused by specific molecular defects responsible for early onset, severe diarrhea. In microvillus inclusion disease, microvilli are sequestered in vacuoles as a consequence of autophagocytosis because of a defect in protein trafficking disrupting enterocyte polarity (Fig. 341-2). Intestinal epithelial dysplasia (or tufting enteropathy) is caused by focal crowding of enterocytes that produce epithelial abnormalities resembling tufts (tears). Abnormal deposition of laminin and heparan sulfate proteoglycan on the basement membrane has been detected in intestinal epithelia. An abnormal intestinal distribution of $\alpha_2\beta_1$ and $\alpha_6\beta_4$ integrins is implicated in tufting enteropathy. These ubiquitous proteins are involved in cell–cell and cell–matrix interactions, and play a crucial role in cell development and differentiation.

Electrolyte transport defects are a subgroup of structural enterocyte defects that include congenital chloride diarrhea, in which a mutation in the solute carrier family 26 member 3 gene (*SLC26A3*) leads to severe intestinal Cl^- malabsorption from a defect in or absence of the Cl^-/HCO_3^- exchanger. The consequent defect in bicarbonate secretion leads to metabolic alkalosis and acidification of the intestinal content, with further inhibition of Na^+/H^+ exchanger-dependent Na^+ absorption. Patients with congenital sodium diarrhea show similar clinical features, because of a defective Na^+/H^+ exchanger in the small and large intestine, leading to massive Na^+ fecal loss and severe acidosis. Familial diarrhea syndrome caused by a mutation guanylate cyclase-C is characterized by abdominal pain, dysmotility, and inflammation coupled with mild secretory diarrhea.

Disorders of intestinal motility include abnormal development and function of the enteric nervous system, such as in Hirschsprung disease and chronic idiopathic intestinal pseudoobstruction (which encompass both the neurogenic and the myogenic forms). Other motility disorders may be secondary to extraintestinal disorders, such as in hyperthyroidism and scleroderma. Motility disorders are associated with either constipation or diarrhea or both, with the former usually dominating the clinical picture.

Autoimmune processes may target the intestinal epithelium, alone or in association with extraintestinal symptoms. Autoimmune enteropathy is associated with the production of antienterocyte and antigoblet cell antibodies, primarily immunoglobulin A, but also immunoglobulin G, directed against components of the enterocyte brush-border or cytoplasm and by a cell-mediated autoimmune response with mucosal T-cell activation. An X-linked

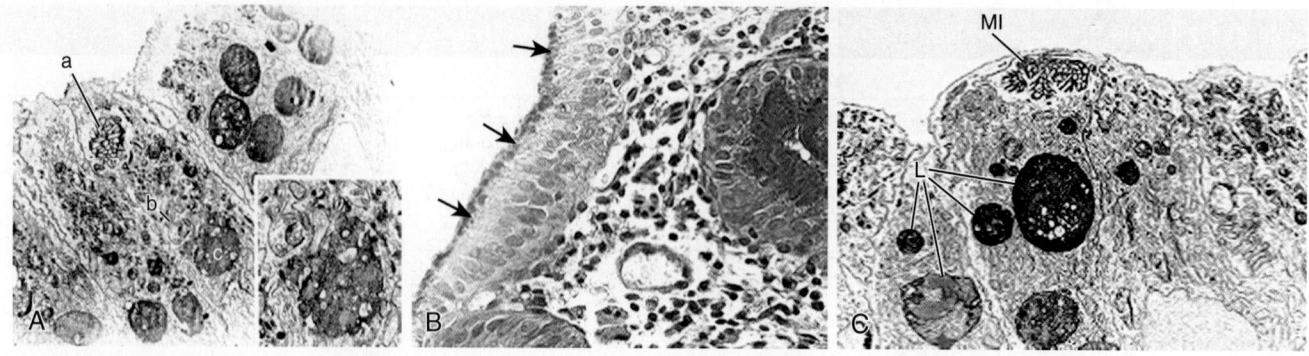

Figure 341-2 Microvillus inclusion disease. **A,** From top to bottom: microvillus inclusion *(a)*, a granule with few microvilli *(b)*, and a lysosome *(c)* detected in the same enterocyte. *Inset:* Higher magnification of *b* and *c* ×11,000, inset ×21,500. **B,** Microvillus inclusion disease. Periodic acid-Schiff (PAS) staining highlights abundant PAS-positive material *(arrows)* in the apical part of the enterocyte cytoplasm. **C,** Microvillus inclusion disease. The villous enterocyte lack brush-border microvilli, whereas their apical cytoplasm contains a microvillus inclusion *(MI)* and numerous lysosomes *(L)* ×5,500. (**A** *from Morroni M, Cangiotti AM, Guarino A, et al. Unusual ultrastructural features in microvillous inclusion disease: a report of two cases. Virchows Arch 448:805–810, 2006.*)

immune-dysregulation, polyendocrinopathy, and enteropathy (IPEX syndrome) is associated with variable gene mutations and phenotypes of chronic diarrhea. Other immunoregulatory defects, found in patients with agammaglobulinemia, isolated immunoglobulin A deficiency, and combined immunodeficiency disorders, may result in persistent infectious diarrhea.

Phenotypic diarrhea, also defined as syndromic diarrhea or trichohepatoenteric syndrome, is a rare disease presenting with facial dysmorphism, woolly hair, severe diarrhea, and malabsorption (Fig. 341-3). Half of the patients have liver disease.

Short bowel syndrome is the single most frequent etiology of chronic diarrhea and intestinal failure (see Chapter 338.7). Many intestinal abnormalities such as stenosis, segmental atresia, and malrotation may require surgical resection, but the most frequent primary cause of short bowel is necrotizing enterocolitis. In these conditions, the residual intestine may be insufficient to carry on its digestive–absorptive functions. Rarely, a child may be born with a congenitally short small bowel resulting in delayed growth. In rare cases of severe chronic diarrhea, the gastrointestinal symptoms may be the initial manifestation of mitochondrial disease, carbohydrate deficient glycoproteins, or a primary immune deficiency. **Multiple food protein hypersensitivity** also is included in the list of causes of protracted diarrhea syndrome. The disease is believed to be the result of a reaction against specific proteins contained in foods. Diarrhea often resolves with fasting or when an amino-acid–based formula is started. Although most children with food intolerance in infancy are eventually able to resume a regular diet, some require restrictions throughout their lives. When the cause of the diarrhea remains undetermined and the clinical course is inconsistent with organic disorders, factitious disorder by proxy should be considered.

GENETIC AND MOLECULAR BASIS OF THE PROTRACTED DIARRHEA SYNDROME

The genetic and molecular basis of many causes of protracted diarrhea have been identified recently and a new classification of congenital diarrheal disorders (CDDs) has been proposed (Table 341-3). CDDs are a group of rare, but severe enteropathies, with a similar clinical presentation despite a different outcome. However, diarrhea is the result of structural and functional abnormalities resulting in either secretory or osmotic diarrhea. Often diarrhea presents at birth or shortly thereafter, but in milder forms diarrhea may go unrecognized for years. CDDs are rare diseases, however in most specific disorders the specific genetic defect and transmission are known. Hereditary fructose intolerance is associated with mutations in the *ASDOB* gene that encodes for the aldolase B enzyme that is found primarily in the liver and is involved in the metabolism of fructose. Individuals with hereditary fructose intolerance may have nausea, abdominal pain/bloating, vomiting, diarrhea, and hypoglycemia. Continued ingestion

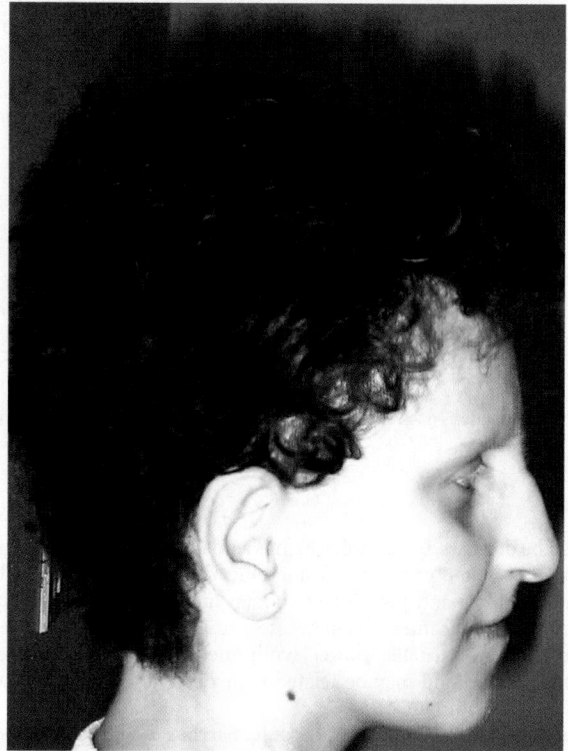

Figure 341-3 Phenotypic diarrhea. The child shows facial dysmorphism, hypertelorism, and woolly hair; etiology is unknown, but the presence of affected siblings suggests an autosomal recessive transmission.

of fructose results in hepatomegaly and eventually cirrhosis. The incidence of hereditary fructose intolerance is estimated to be 1 in 20,000-30,000. In contrast, fructose malabsorption is common in Western countries with estimates as high as 40% of the population. These individuals cannot absorb fructose and often develop bloating, abdominal pain, diarrhea, and flatulence. They do not have liver disease.

The incidence of other genetic disorders associated with CDD ranges from 1 in 2,500 for cystic fibrosis, 1 in 5,000 for sucrose-isomaltase deficiency, 1 in 60,000 for congenital lactase deficiency, to 1 in 400,000 to trichohepatoenteric syndrome. For most CDDs, such as polyendocrinopathy, X-linked (IPEX) syndrome, or autoimmune polyglandular syndrome type 1, the clinical application of exome

Table 341-3 | Classification of Congenital Diarrheal Disorders Based on Their Molecular Defect and Their Inheritance

DEFECTS OF DIGESTION, ABSORPTION, AND TRANSPORT OF NUTRIENTS AND ELECTROLYTES

DISEASE	GENE Name	Location	TRANSMISSION AND INCIDENCE	MECHANISM
Genes Encoding Brush-Border Enzymes				
Congenital lactase deficiency (LD)	LCT	2q21.3	AR, 1 in 60,000 in Finland; lower in other ethnic groups	Osmotic
Congenital sucrase-isomaltase deficiency (SID)	SI	3q26.1	AR, 1 in 5,000; higher incidence in Greenland, Alaska, and Canada	Osmotic
Congenital maltase-glucoamylase deficiency (MGD)	Not defined	—	Few cases described	Osmotic
Genes Encoding Membrane Carriers				
Glucose-galactose malabsorption (GGM)	SLC5A1	22q13.1	AR, few hundred cases described	Osmotic
Fructose malabsorption (FM)	Not defined	—	Up to 40%	Osmotic
Fanconi-Bickel syndrome (FBS)	SLC2A2	3q26.2	AR, rare, higher frequency in consanguineous	Osmotic
Acrodermatitis enteropathica (ADE)	SLC39A4	8q24.3	AR, 1 in 500,000	Osmotic
Congenital chloride diarrhea (CCD, DIAR 1)	SLC26A3	7q31.1	AR, sporadic; frequent in some ethnicities	Osmotic
Lysinuric protein intolerance (LPI)	SLC7A7	14q11.2	AR, about 1 in 60,000 in Finland and Japan; rare in other ethnic groups	Osmotic
Primary bile acid malabsorption (PBAM)	SLC10A2	13q33.1	AR	Secretory
Cystic fibrosis (CF)	CFTR	7q31.2	AR, 1 in 2,500	Osmotic
Genes Encoding Pancreatic Enzymes				
Enterokinase deficiency (EKD)	PRSS7	21q21	AR	Osmotic
Hereditary pancreatitis (HP)	PRSS1	7q34	AR, cases with compound mutations in different genes; SPINK1 mutations may also cause tropical pancreatitis	Osmotic
	SPINK1	5q32		
Congenital absence of pancreatic lipase (APL)	PNLIP	10q25.3	—	Osmotic
Genes Encoding Proteins of Lipoprotein Metabolism				
Abetalipoproteinemia (ALP)	MTTP	4q27	AR, about 100 cases described; higher frequency among Ashkenazi Jews	Osmotic
Hypobetalipoproteinemia (HLP)	Apo B	2p24.1	Autosomal codominant	Osmotic
Chylomicron retention disease (CRD)	SAR1B	5q31.1	AR, about 40 cases described	Osmotic
Genes Encoding Other Types of Proteins				
Congenital sodium diarrhea (CSD, DIAR 3)	SPINT2 (only syndromic CSD)	19q13.2	AR	Osmotic
Shwachman-Diamond syndrome (SDS)	SBDS	7q11	AR	Osmotic
Activating GUCY2C mutation	Guanylate cyclase-C	Unknown	AD	Secretory
Genes Encoding for Other Enzymes				
Defect in triglyceride synthesis	DGAT1	Splice variant (chromosome 8, 145541756 A G) in the splice donor site 32 of exon 8, altering the invariant GT to GC	AR	Protein-losing enteropathy

DISEASE	OMIM NUMBER	TRANSMISSION AND INCIDENCE	MECHANISM
DEFECTS OF ENTEROCYTE DIFFERENTIATION AND POLARIZATION			
Microvillous inclusion disease (MVID, DIAR 2)	251850	AR; rare; higher frequency among Navajo	Secretory
Congenital tufting enteropathy (CTE, DIAR 5)	613217	AR; 1 in 50,000-100,000; higher among Arabians	Secretory
Trichohepatoenteric syndrome (THE)	222470	AR; 1 in 400,000	Secretory
DEFECTS OF ENTEROENDOCRINE CELL DIFFERENTIATION			
Congenital malabsorptive diarrhea (CMD, DIAR 4)	610370	AR; few cases described	Osmotic
Proprotein convertase 1/3 deficiency (PCD)	600955	AR	Osmotic
DEFECTS OF MODULATION OF INTESTINAL IMMUNE RESPONSE			
Autoimmune polyglandular syndrome type 1 (APS1)	240300	AR; AD (1 family)	Secretory
Immune dysfunction, polyendocrinopathy, X-linked (IPEX)	601410	X-linked (autosomal cases described), very rare	Secretory
IPEX-like syndrome	—	Not X-linked	Secretory

AD, autosomal dominant; AR, autosomal recessive.

Table 341-4	Degree of Malnutrition as Estimated by Visceral Protein Concentrations in Children with Chronic Diarrhea				
VISCERAL PROTEIN	**HALF-LIFE**	**NORMAL VALUES**	**MILD MALNUTRITION**	**MODERATE MALNUTRITION**	**SEVERE MALNUTRITION**
Albumin	20 days	30-45 g/L	3.0-2.9 g/L	2.8-2.5 g/L	<2.5 g/L
Prealbumin	2 days	0.2-04 g/L	0.2-0.18 g/L	0.17-0.1 g/L	<0.1 g/L
Retinol binding protein	12 hr	2.6-7.6 g/L	2.5-2.0 g/L	1.9 -1.5 g/L	<1 g/L
Transferrin	8 days	218-411 µg/dL	200-150 µg/dL	149-100 µg/dL	<100 µg/dL
Serum iron	11-19 hr	16-124 µg/dL	15-13 µg/dL	12-10 µg/dL	<10 µg/dL

Consider also the concentrations of the following micronutrients: calcium, zinc, magnesium, iodine, vitamin A, vitamin C, vitamin B_1.

sequencing is likely to increase identification of more patients with these rare causes of chronic diarrhea.

Selected CDDs are more frequent in ethnic groups where consanguineous marriages are common, or in some geographic areas because of founder effects. For example, congenital lactase deficiency is more common in Finland; lysinuric protein intolerance has a higher incidence either in Finland and in Japan because of founder effect, and a specific mutation is typically found in each of the 2 ethnic groups. A defect in the *DGAT1* gene was identified using whole-exome sequencing in an Ashkenazi Jewish family and associated with the early onset of vomiting and nonbloody diarrhea with protein-losing enteropathy.

Most cases of protracted diarrhea syndrome are not easily treated. The natural history of protracted diarrhea is related to the primary intestinal disease and the specific defect in nutrient absorption. Treatment is more favorable for motility disorders and autoimmune enteropathy than for structural enterocyte defects. Children with motility disorders may have persistent symptoms, but they are rarely fatal; whereas children with structural enterocyte defects have a more severe course, poorer prognosis, and are more likely to be candidates for intestinal transplantation (see Chapter 339). Some late-onset CDDs may be relatively mild and are recognized only later in life.

EVALUATION OF PATIENTS
Because of the spectrum of etiologies, the medical approach should be based on diagnostic algorithms that begin with assessment for infectious causes, and then consider the age of the child, growth, and clinical and epidemiologic factors. Early onset may suggest a congenital or severe condition. In later infancy and up to 2 yr of age, infections and allergies are more common; inflammatory diseases are more frequent in older children and adolescents. Celiac disease and chronic nonspecific diarrhea should always be considered independently of age because of their relatively high frequency at all ages.

Specific clues in the family and personal history may provide useful indications, suggesting a congenital, allergic or inflammatory etiology. A history of polyhydramnios is consistent with congenital chloride-sodium diarrhea, or cystic fibrosis. An acute onset of diarrhea that runs a protracted course suggests post-enteritis diarrhea or small intestinal overgrowth or the onset of chronic nonspecific diarrhea (toddler's diarrhea). In children, with chronic nonspecific diarrhea there is often a history of an acute gastroenteritis. The association of diarrhea with specific foods may indicate a nutrient basis, such as intolerance to selected nutrients (fructose). Anthropometric evaluation is essential to understand if diarrhea has affected weight gain and growth. The amount of weight loss over time provides an estimate of the severity of diarrhea. Normal weight and growth strongly support functional diarrhea that may respond to simple dietary management.

Initial clinical examination should include the evaluation of general and nutritional status. Dehydration, marasmus, or kwashiorkor require prompt supportive interventions to stabilize the patient. Nutritional evaluation should start with the evaluation of the weight and height curves, and of the weight-for-height index to determine the impact of diarrhea on growth. Weight is generally impaired before height, but with time, linear growth also becomes affected, and both parameters may be equally abnormal in the long-term. Assessment of nutritional status includes a dietary history and biochemical and nutritional investigations. Caloric intake should be quantitatively determined and the relationship between weight modifications and energy intake should be carefully considered.

Biochemical markers may assist in grading malnutrition (Table 341-4) as the half-life of serum proteins may distinguish between short- and long-term malnutrition. Assessment of body composition may be performed by measuring mid-arm circumference and triceps skinfold thickness or, more accurately, by bioelectrical impedance analysis or dual-emission x-ray absorptiometry scans. Evaluation of micronutrient concentrations should always be considered. Zinc, magnesium, vitamin A, and folate deficiency are associated with chronic diarrhea and should be provided if needed.

Diagnosis of functional diarrhea is based on clinical assessment using established age-related criteria. It should be noted that a child with functional diarrhea may be inappropriately "treated" with a diluted hypocaloric diet in an effort to reduce the diarrhea, resulting in impaired growth.

The search for an etiology may be based on the relevant causes of diarrhea for the age of the child. Continued diarrhea with fasting or fecal electrolyte concentrations discriminate between secretory and osmotic diarrhea. Associated symptoms and selected investigations provide important diagnostic clues. Signs of general inflammation such as fever, mucoid or bloody stools, and abdominal pain may suggest inflammatory bowel disease. The presence of eczema or asthma is associated with an allergic disorder, whereas specific extraintestinal manifestations (arthritis, diabetes, thrombocytopenia, etc.) may suggest an autoimmune disease. Specific skin lesions may be suggestive of acrodermatitis enteropathica that might respond to zinc replacement. Typical facial abnormalities and woolly hair are associated with phenotypic diarrhea (see Fig. 341-3).

INVESTIGATIONS
Microbiologic investigation should include a thorough list of intestinal bacterial, viral, and protozoan pathogens. Proximal intestinal bacterial overgrowth may be determined using the hydrogen breath test, after an oral glucose or lactulose load, but either substrate may give false results.

Initial investigations of a child with chronic diarrhea should always include an assessment of intestinal inflammation using fecal calprotectin or lactoferrin, and serology for celiac disease (see Chapter 338.2). The role of a mucosal biopsy is determined by the noninvasive diagnostic evaluation in consultation with a pediatric gastroenterologist.

Noninvasive assessment of digestive-absorptive function and of intestinal inflammation plays a key role in the diagnostic work-up (Table 341-5). Abnormalities in the digestive–absorptive function tests suggest small bowel involvement, whereas intestinal inflammation, as demonstrated by increased fecal calprotectin or lactoferrin, supports colitis. Histology is important in establishing mucosal involvement, noting changes in the epithelial cells, or in identifying specific

Table 341-5	Noninvasive Tests for Intestinal Digestive–Absorptive Function and Inflammation	
TEST	**NORMAL VALUES**	**IMPLICATION**
α_1-Antitripsin concentration	<0.9 mg/g	Increased intestinal permeability/protein loss
Steatocrit	<2.5% (older than 2 yr) fold increase over age-related values (younger than 2 yr)	Fat malabsorption
Fecal-reducing substances	Absent	Carbohydrate malabsorption
Elastase concentration	>200 µg/g	Pancreatic function
Chymotrypsin concentration	>7.5 units/g >375 units/24 hr	Pancreatic function
Fecal occult blood	Absent	Blood loss in the stools/inflammation
Fecal calprotectin concentration	<100 µg/g (in children to 4 yr of age) <50 µg/g (older than 4 yr)	Intestinal inflammation
Fecal leukocytes	<5/microscopic field	Colonic inflammation
Nitric oxide in rectal dialysate	<5 µM of NO_2^-/NO_3^-	Rectal inflammation
Dual sugar (cellobiose/mannitol) absorption test	Urine excretion ratio: 0.010 ± 0.018	Increased intestinal permeability
Xylose oral load	25 mg/dL	Reduced intestinal surface

intracellular inclusion bodies caused by pathogens, such as cytomegalovirus, or the presence of parasites. Electron microscopy is essential to detect subcellular structural abnormalities such as microvillous inclusion disease. Immunohistochemistry allows the study of mucosal immunity as well as of other cell types (smooth muscle cells and enteric neuronal cells).

Imaging has a major role in the diagnostic approach. Abdominal ultrasound may help in detecting liver and pancreatic abnormalities or an increase in distal ileal wall thickness that suggests inflammatory bowel disease. A preliminary plain abdominal x-ray is useful for detection of abdominal distention, suggestive of intestinal obstruction, or increased retention of colonic feces. Intramural or portal gas may be seen in necrotizing enterocolitis or intussusception. Structural abnormalities such as diverticula, malrotation, stenosis, blind loop, inflammatory bowel disease, as well as motility disorders, may be investigated through a barium meal and a small bowel follow-through. Capsule endoscopy allows the exploration of the entire intestinal tract searching for structural changes, inflammation or bleeding and the new SmartPill measures pressure, pH, and temperature as it moves through the gastrointestinal tract, assessing motility.

Specific investigations should be carried out for specific diagnostic indications. Prick and patch test may support a diagnosis of food allergy. However, elimination diet with withdrawal of the suspected harmful food from the diet and subsequent challenge is the most reliable strategy by which to establish a diagnosis. Bile malabsorption may be explored by the retention of the bile acid analog ^{75}Se-homocholic acid-taurine (^{75}SeHCAT) in the enterohepatic circulation. A scintigraphic examination, with radio-labeled octreotide is indicated in suspected APUD cell neoplastic proliferation. In other diseases, specific imaging techniques such as computed tomography, or nuclear magnetic resonance endoscopic retrograde cholangiopancreatography and magnetic resonance cholangiopancreatography may have important diagnostic value.

Once infectious agents have been excluded and nutritional assessment performed, a stepwise approach to the child with chronic diarrhea may be applied. The main causes of chronic diarrhea should be investigated, based on the features of the diarrhea and the specific nutrient(s) that is (are) affected. The use of whole-exome sequencing is of benefit in children suspected of having mendelian-related causes of chronic diarrhea. A step-by-step diagnostic approach is important to minimize the unnecessary use of invasive procedures as well as the cost, while optimizing the yield of the diagnostic work-up (Table 341-6).

TREATMENT

Chronic diarrhea associated with impaired nutritional status should always be considered a serious disease, and therapy should be started promptly. Treatment includes general supportive measures, nutritional rehabilitation, elimination diet, and medications. The latter include therapies for specific etiologies as well as interventions aimed at counteracting fluid secretion and/or promoting restoration of disrupted intestinal epithelium. Because death in most instances is caused by dehydration, replacement of fluid and electrolyte losses is the most important early intervention.

Nutritional rehabilitation is often essential and is based on clinical and biochemical assessment. Potentially harmful nutrients must be identified and avoided. In moderate to severe malnutrition, caloric intake may be progressively increased to 50% or more above the recommended dietary allowances. The intestinal absorptive capacity should be monitored by digestive function tests. In children with steatorrhea, medium-chain triglycerides may be the main source of lipids. A lactose-free diet should be started in all children with chronic diarrhea and is recommended by the World Health Organization. Lactose is generally replaced by maltodextrin or a combination of complex carbohydrates. A sucrose-free formula is indicated in sucrase-isomaltase deficiency. Semielemental or elemental diets have the dual purpose of overcoming food intolerance, which may be the primary cause of chronic diarrhea, particularly in infancy and early childhood, and facilitating nutrient absorption. The sequence of elimination should begin from less to more restricted diets, that is, cow's milk protein hydrolysate to amino-acid–based formulas, depending on the child's situation. In severely compromised infants, it may be prudent to start with amino-acid–based feeding.

When oral nutrition is not feasible or fails, enteral or parenteral nutrition should be considered. Enteral nutrition may be performed via nasogastric or gastrostomy tube and is indicated in a child who is not able to be fed orally, either because of inability to tolerate nutrient requirements or because of extreme weakness. Continuous enteral nutrition is effective in children with a compromised absorptive capacity, such as short bowel syndrome where the remaining mucosal surface is intact. In extreme wasting, enteral nutrition may not be tolerated and parenteral nutrition is required.

Micronutrient and vitamin supplementation are part of nutritional rehabilitation, especially in malnourished children in developing countries. Zinc supplementation is important in both prevention and therapy of chronic diarrhea, since it promotes ion absorption, restores

Table 341-6	Stepwise Diagnostic Approach to Children with Diarrhea

STEP 1	STEP 2
Intestinal Microbiology	*Evaluation of Intestinal Morphology:*
Stool cultures	Endoscopy and standard jejunal/colonic histology*
Microscopy for parasites	Morphometry
Viruses	PAS staining
H_2 breath test	Electron microscopy
Screening Test for Celiac Disease:	Imaging (upper or lower bowel series, capsule endoscopy)
Serology according to age and level of IgA (including AGA IgA/IgG, EMA IgA/IgG, tTG IgA/IgG)	**STEP 3**
Noninvasive Tests for:	*Special Investigations:*
Intestinal function (including double sugar test, xylosemia, iron absorption test)	Intestinal immunohistochemistry
Pancreatic function (amylase, lipase, fecal elastase)	Antienterocyte antibodies
Intestinal inflammation (fecal calprotectin, rectal nitric oxide)	Serum chromogranin and catecholamines
Tests for Food Allergy:	Autoantibodies
Prick/patch tests for foods	[75]SeHCAT measurement
Abdominal Ultrasounds (Scan of Last Ileal Loop)	Brush-border enzymatic activities
	Motility and electrophysiologic studies

*The decision to perform an upper or a lower endoscopy may be supported by noninvasive tests.

AGA, antigliadin antibody; EMA, endomysial antibody; Ig, immunoglobulin; PAS, periodic acid–Schiff; [75]SeHCAT, ^{75}Se-homocholic acid-taurine; tTG, tissue transglutaminase.

Table 341-7	Treatment of Infectious Persistent Diarrhea

	FACTOR	INDICATIONS	DOSAGE	DURATION
Antibiotics	Trimethoprim-sulfamethoxazole	*Salmonella* spp., *Shigella*	10-50 mg/kg/day in 2 divided doses–daily os	7 days
	Azithromycin	*Shigella*	1° day: 12 mg/kg/day once–daily os 2°-5° days: 6 mg/kg/day once–daily os	5 days
	Ciprofloxacin		20-30 mg/kg/day in 2 divided doses–os or iv	7 days
	Ceftriaxone		50-100 mg/kg/day once–im or iv	7 days
	Erythromycin	*Campylobacter*	50 mg/kg/day in 2-3 divided doses–os	7 days
	Metronidazole	*Giardia, Entamoeba*	20-30 mg/kg/day in 2-3 divided doses–os	7 days Small intestinal bacterial overgrowth
Antiparasitic	Nitazoxanide Albendazole	*Amebiasis, Giardiasis, Cryptosporidiosis* and helminth infections	100 mg every 12 hr for children ages 12-47 mo 200 mg every 12 hr for children ages 4-11 yr 500 mg every 12 hr for children older than 11 yr 400 mg once	3 days
Probiotics	*Lactobacillus* GG		$1\text{-}2 \times 10^{11}$–$1 \times 10^{11}$ CFU/day–os	For a minimum period of 7 days or until diarrhea stopped
	Saccharomyces boulardii		1×10^{10} germs live (500 mg)/day–os	For a minimum period of 7 days or till diarrhea stopped
Human serum immunoglobulin		Severe *Rotavirus* diarrhea	300 mg/kg single oral administration	
Antisecretory	Racecadotril	Secretory diarrhea	1.5 mg/kg every 8 hr–os	For a minimum period of 7 days or till diarrhea stopped
Adsorbents	Diosmectite		3-6 g every 12-24 hr–os	5 days

im, Intramuscular; iv, intravenouis; os, by mouth.

epithelial proliferation, and stimulates immune response. Nutritional rehabilitation has a general beneficial effect on the patient's general condition, intestinal function, and immune response.

Functional diarrhea in children may benefit from a diet based on the "4 F" principles (reduce fructose and fluids, increase fat and fiber). Probiotics have been used with some success as adjunctive therapy based on the evidence that changes in intestinal microflora might be beneficial in several other intestinal diseases.

Pharmacologic therapy includes antiinfective drugs, immune suppression, and drugs that may inhibit fluid loss and promote cell growth. If a bacterial agent is detected, specific antibiotics should be prescribed. Empiric antibiotic therapy may be used in children with either small bowel bacterial overgrowth or with suspected infectious diarrhea. Table 341-7 summarizes the treatment of postinfectious persistent

diarrhea. Immune suppression should be considered in selected conditions such as autoimmune enteropathy.

Treatment may be also directed at modifying specific pathophysiologic processes. Secretion of ions may be reduced by proabsorptive agents, such as the enkephalinase inhibitor racecadotril. In diarrhea caused by neuroendocrine tumors, microvillus inclusion disease and enterotoxin-induced severe diarrhea, a trial of somatostatin analog octreotide may be considered. Zinc promotes both enterocyte growth and ion absorption and may be effective when intestinal atrophy and ion secretion are associated. However, when therapeutic attempts have failed, the only option to avoid intestinal failure may be parenteral nutrition or eventually intestinal transplantation.

Bibliography is available at Expert Consult.

341.1 Diarrhea from Neuroendocrine Tumors

Helen Spoudeas and David Branski

Rare tumors of the neuroendocrine cells of the gastroenteropancreatic axis and adrenal and extraadrenal sites derive from the APUD system. They are characterized by an excessive production of 1 or several peptides, which, when released into the circulation, exert their endocrine effects and can be measured by radioimmunologic methods (in the plasma or as their urinary metabolites) and hence act as tumor markers. In clinically functioning tumors, the hypersecretion causes a recognizable syndrome that can include watery diarrhea. Though rare, neuroendocrine tumor (NET) should be considered a potential cause in patients with a particularly severe or chronic course (resulting in electrolyte and fluid depletion), associated flushing, palpitations, or bronchospasm, or a positive family history of multiple endocrine neoplasia 1 or 2 syndromes (Table 341-8).

Depending on the tumor type, the peptide marker(s) in the plasma and/or the 24-hr urinary metabolite(s) measured (on 2 occasions), form the basis of the biochemical diagnosis, the prognosis (tumor load) and treatment monitoring. Baseline tests should include plasma chromogranin A and urinary 5-hydroxyindoloacetic acid, other specific biochemistry being guided by the suspected syndrome (see Table 341-8). Carcinoid tumors are gastroenteropancreatic NETs, typically of the midgut (rather than fore- or hindgut), which may cause flushing and bronchospasm in addition to diarrhea and which, because of their portal drainage, are the most prone to late presentation and malignancy. Localization of any NET is best achieved with a multimodality approach at a center of excellence. Thus whole-body CT, MRI, and somatostatin receptor scintigraphy may be required (because nearly all NETs express membrane receptors for small peptides, e.g., somatostatin), with gallium-68 positron emission tomography/CT recommended for detecting an unknown primary. Long-acting somatostatin analogs might also have a role in palliation.

Tumor resection is the treatment of choice but is potentially hazardous and can precipitate life-threatening adrenergic crises; it should only be undertaken by an endocrine surgeon with experience under carefully controlled medical and anesthetic conditions and in conjunction with an endocrinologist. Tumor histochemistry will confirm the NET type and classification of NETs should be based on the World Health Organization 2010 Union for International Cancer Control TNM criteria (7th edition). This diagnosis in a child should prompt a genetic referral to exclude a tumor predisposition syndrome in which the child is the index case and tumor registration. Management and follow-up is multidisciplinary and should be undertaken in an age-appropriate setting with access to adult specialists with expertise in these rare conditions.

Table 341-8	Diarrhea Caused by Neuroendocrine Tumors			
TUMOR AND CELL TYPE	**SITE**	**MARKERS**	**SIGNS OF HORMONE HYPERSECRETION**	**THERAPY**
Carcinoid	Intestinal argentaffin cells, typically midgut, also foregut and hindgut, ectopic bronchial tree	**Serotonin (5-HT)**, urine **5-HIAA**[†] (diagnostic) Also produce substance P, neuropeptide K, somatostatin, VIP Chromogranin A	Secretory diarrhea, crampy abdominal pain, flushing, wheezing, (and cardiac valve damage if foregut site)	Resection Somatostatin analog, (palliative) Genetic MEN-1
Gastrinoma, Zollinger-Ellison syndrome	Pancreas, small bowel, liver and spleen	**Gastrin**	Multiple peptic ulcers, secretory diarrhea	H₂-blockers, PPI, tumor resection, (gastrectomy) Genetic MEN-1
Mastocytoma	Cutaneous, intestine, liver, spleen	**Histamine, VIP**	Pruritus, flushing, apnea If VIP, diarrhea	H₁- and H₂-blockers, cromolyn, steroids, resection if solitary
Medullary carcinoma	Thyroid C-cells	**Calcitonin**, VIP, prostaglandins	Secretory diarrhea	Radical thyroidectomy ± lymphadenectomy (genetic MEN-2A/B, familial MTC)
Ganglioneuroma, pheochromocytoma, ganglioneuroblastoma, neuroblastoma	Chromaffin cells; abdominal > other sites; extraadrenal or adrenal	**Metanephrines** and **catecholamines**, VIP VMA, HMA in neuroblastoma	Hypertension, tachycardia, paroxysmal palpitations, sweating, anxiety, watery diarrhea*	Perioperative α-adrenergic (BP) and β-adrenergic blockade with volume support tumor resection Genetic MEN-2 (*RET* gene), VHL, NF-1, SDH
Somatostatinoma	Pancreas	**Somatostatin**	Secretory diarrhea, steatorrhea, cholelithiasis, diabetes	Resection Genetic MEN-1
VIPoma	Pancreas	**VIP, prostaglandins**	Secretory diarrhea, achlorhydria, hypokalemia	Somatostatin analogs, resection Genetic MEN-1

*Diarrhea has been reported only in adult patients with pheochromocytoma.
†Bold indicates major markers.
BP, blood pressure; H₁, histamine receptor type 1; H₂, histamine receptor type 2; HMA, homovanillic acid; MEN-1, multiple endocrine neoplasia type 1; MTC, medullary thyroid carcinoma; NF-1, neurofibromatosis type 1; PPI, proton pump inhibitor; SDH, succinate dehydrogenase; VHL, von Hippel-Lindau disease; VIP, vasoactive intestinal polypeptide; VMA, vanillylmandelic acid.
Adapted from Spoudeas HA, editor: Paediatric endocrine tumours. A multidisciplinary consensus statement of best practice from a working group convened under the auspices of the British Society of Paediatric Endocrinology and Diabetes (BSPED) and the United Kingdom Children's Cancer Study Group (UKCCSG), Crawley, West Sussex, 2005, Novo Nordisk.

Chapter 342

Functional Abdominal Pain (Nonorganic Chronic Abdominal Pain)

Raman Sreedharan and Chris A. Liacouras

Recurrent abdominal pain in children was defined as at least 3 episodes of pain over at least 3 mo that interfered with function. In many situations the term *recurrent abdominal pain* was used synonymously with *functional abdominal pain*. Other terms, such as *chronic abdominal pain, nonorganic abdominal pain,* and *psychogenic abdominal pain,* that were also used for describing abdominal pain in children, led to clinical confusion. The American Academy of Pediatrics Subcommittee on Chronic Abdominal Pain and the North American Society for Pediatric Gastroenterology Hepatology and Nutrition Committee on Abdominal Pain suggested that the term recurrent abdominal pain no longer be used. Table 342-1 outlines the recommended clinical

definitions for long-lasting intermittent or constant abdominal pain by the same committees.

Chronic abdominal pain can be organic or nonorganic, depending on whether a specific etiology is identified. Nonorganic abdominal pain or functional abdominal pain refers to pain without evidence of anatomic, inflammatory, metabolic, or neoplastic abnormalities. **Functional gastrointestinal disorders (FGIDs)** are a group of gastrointestinal (GI) disorders that include variable combinations of chronic or recurrent GI symptoms not explained by structural or biochemical abnormalities. The Rome Committee updates and modifies the information on FGIDs for clinical and research purposes. The Rome III process had 2 pediatric subcommittees based on age range: Neonate/Toddler (0-4 yr) and Child/Adolescent (4-18 yr). The Child/Adolescent committee categorized abdominal pain–related FGIDs under Category H2 (Table 342-2). Table 342-3 defines the Rome III criteria for the diagnosis of Childhood Functional Abdominal Pain (category H2d) and the Childhood Functional Abdominal Pain Syndrome (category H2d1).

The exact incidence and prevalence of chronic abdominal pain is not known. There are reports of chronic abdominal pain affecting 9-15% of children. There are also reports that 13% of middle school and 17% of high school children have weekly complaints of abdominal pain.

Table 342-1	Recommended Clinical Definitions of Long-Standing Intermittent or Constant Abdominal Pain in Children
DISORDER	**DEFINITION**
Chronic abdominal pain	Long-lasting intermittent or constant abdominal pain that is functional or organic (disease based)
Functional abdominal pain	Abdominal pain without demonstrable evidence of pathologic condition, such as anatomic metabolic, infectious, inflammatory or neoplastic disorder. Functional abdominal pain can manifest with symptoms typical of functional dyspepsia, irritable bowel syndrome, abdominal migraine or functional abdominal pain syndrome
Functional dyspepsia	Functional abdominal pain or discomfort in the upper abdomen
Irritable bowel syndrome	Functional abdominal pain associated with alteration in bowel movements
Abdominal migraine	Functional abdominal pain with features of migraine (paroxysmal abdominal pain associated with anorexia, nausea, vomiting or pallor as well as maternal history of migraine headaches)
Functional abdominal pain syndrome	Functional abdominal pain without the characteristics of dyspepsia, irritable bowel syndrome, or abdominal migraine

Adapted from Di Lorenzo C, Colletti RB, Lehmann HP, et al; American Academy of Pediatrics Subcommittee on Chronic Abdominal Pain; NASPGHAN Committee on Abdominal Pain: Chronic abdominal pain in children: a clinical report of the American Academy of Pediatrics and the North American Society for Pediatric Gastroenterology, Hepatology and Nutrition, J Pediatr Gastroenterol Nutr 40(3):245–248, 2005.

Table 342-2	Childhood Functional GI Disorders: Child/Adolescent (Category H)
H1.	Vomiting and aerophagia
H1a.	Adolescent rumination syndrome
H1b.	Cyclic vomiting syndrome
H1c.	Aerophagia
H2.	Abdominal pain—related functional gastrointestinal disorders
H2a.	Functional dyspepsia
H2b.	Irritable bowel syndrome
H2c.	Abdominal migraine
H2d.	Childhood functional abdominal pain
H2d1.	Childhood functional abdominal pain syndrome
H3.	Constipation and incontinence
H3a.	Functional constipation
H3b.	Nonretentive fecal incontinence

Adapted from Rome Foundation: Rome III disorders and criteria. www.romecriteria.org/criteria/.

Table 342-3	Rome III Criteria for Childhood Functional Abdominal Pain H2d and Childhood Functional Abdominal Pain Syndrome H2d1

H2d. CHILDHOOD FUNCTIONAL ABDOMINAL PAIN
Diagnostic criteria* must include **all** of the following:
• Episodic or continuous abdominal pain
• Insufficient criteria for other functional gastrointestinal disorders
• No evidence of an inflammatory, anatomic, metabolic, or neoplastic process that explains the subject's symptoms

H2d1. CHILDHOOD FUNCTIONAL ABDOMINAL PAIN SYNDROME
Diagnostic criteria* must satisfy criteria for childhood functional abdominal pain and have at least 25% of the time **one or more** of the following:
• Some loss of daily function
• Additional somatic symptoms such as headache, limb pain, or difficulty sleeping

*Criteria fulfilled at least once per week for ≥2 mo prior to diagnosis.
Adapted from Rome Foundation: Rome III disorders and criteria. http://www.romecriteria.org/criteria/.

PATHOPHYSIOLOGY

The symptoms of FGIDs may be the result of dysfunctions of the intestinal sensory and motor systems. The pathophysiology of functional abdominal pain is complex and not fully understood. Visceral hypersensitivity and motility disturbances are thought to be involved in functional abdominal pain. The traditional concept that motility disorders alone have an important role in functional pain has not been confirmed. It is believed that visceral hypersensitivity leading to abnormal bowel sensitivity to stimuli (physiologic, psychologic, noxious) might have a more dominant role in functional abdominal pain. Visceral hypersensitivity could be the result of abnormal interpretation of normal signals by the brain or aberrant signals sent to the brain or a combination. Intestinal pain receptors respond to mechanical and/or chemical stimuli. The visceral receptors can respond to both mechanical and chemical stimuli, but the mucosal receptors are primarily stimulated by chemical stimuli.

The viscera are innervated by dual set of nerves (vagal and splanchnic spinal nerves or pelvic and splanchnic spinal nerves). The spinal afferents carry impulses to the spinal cord. The dorsal horn of the spinal cord regulates conduction of impulses from peripheral nociceptive receptors to the spinal cord and brain, and the pain experience is further influenced by cognitive and emotional centers. Chronic peripheral nervous system pain can produce increased neural activity in higher central nervous system centers, leading to perpetuation of pain. Psychosocial stress can affect pain intensity and quality through these mechanisms. The child's response to pain can be influenced by stress, personality type, and the reinforcement of illness behavior within the family. The autonomic and enteric nervous systems can overlie the initiation, perception, and perpetuation of pain.

A normal functioning enteric nervous system (ENS) is important for coordination of intestinal motility, secretion, and blood flow. Abnormalities of the ENS may be an underlying factor for functional abdominal pain. Inflammation of the intestine and its role in the pathogenesis of functional abdominal pain could be a result of the effects of the inflammatory mediators and cytokines (released by the various inflammatory cells) on the ENS. The dysregulation in the brain–gut interactions can also lead to functional abdominal pain. The role of certain triggers for pain, such as lactose, sorbitol, fructose, bile acids, or fatty acids, could be a result of the altered sensitivity or motor function, because some patients have relief when eliminating these from their diet. Altered intestinal permeability enabling passage of food antigens into the mucosa leading to prolonged stimulation of the intestinal mucosal immune system and the ENS is also a possible cause for functional abdominal pain.

EVALUATION AND DIAGNOSIS

While evaluating a patient with chronic abdominal pain, distinguishing organic pain and functional pain can be challenging. A wide range of potential organic causes of chronic abdominal pain (see Table 306-13) must be considered before establishing a diagnosis of functional pain (nonorganic). Frequently cited causes of chronic abdominal pain include constipation, esophagitis, gastritis, inflammatory bowel disease, and possibly giardiasis. There is little evidence that the frequency, severity, or location of the pain helps to distinguish between organic and nonorganic pain. It is controversial whether nighttime awakening because of pain is concerning for organic disorders or if it can also be seen with functional pain syndromes.

Children with chronic abdominal pain might have associated headaches, anorexia, nausea, vomiting, excessive gas, diarrhea or constipation, and joint pain, but this does not help distinguish between functional and organic disorder. Negative lifestyle events and high life stress levels also do not help to distinguish organic and nonorganic pain, despite several reports of higher levels of life stress in children with chronic abdominal pain. Daily stressors may increase the likelihood for pain episodes, but there is no evidence that psychologic issues distinguishes between organic and nonorganic abdominal pain. Nonetheless, it is important to investigate and manage the psychologic factors because there is evidence suggesting that children with chronic

abdominal pain have more anxiety and depression symptoms. Whether this causes pain or is the result of pain is not known.

Children with functional pain do not have higher levels of conduct disorder or oppositional behavior compared to the controls but they can be more prone to emotional symptoms or psychiatric disorders later in life. Parents of patients with functional abdominal pain have more symptoms of somatization, anxiety, and depression. Both the family and the affected child (when the child gets to adult age) have a higher incidence of **irritable bowel syndrome (IBS)**.

A thorough history and physical examination will identify the alarm symptoms and signs (Tables 342-4 and 342-5). The presence of alarm symptoms and signs warrants further investigation. The absence of alarm symptoms and signs, a normal physical examination, and a normal stool Hemoccult test is sufficient for an initial diagnosis of functional abdominal pain. The laboratory, radiologic, or endoscopic approach to children with chronic abdominal pain should be individualized, depending on the findings suggested by a detailed history and physical examination.

Laboratory studies may be unnecessary if the history and physical examination lead to a diagnosis of functional abdominal pain. Nonetheless, medical tests can reassure the patient and family, and at times the physician, if there is significant functional disability and poor quality of life. A complete blood cell count, sedimentation rate, C-reactive protein, basic chemistry panel, celiac panel, stool culture, stool test for ova and parasites, and urinalysis are reasonable screening studies. *The risk of celiac disease may be 4 times higher in these patients compared with the general population.* Elevated stool calprotectin levels usually suggest an inflammatory etiology.

If indicated, an ultrasound examination of the abdomen can give information about kidneys, gallbladder, and pancreas; with lower

Table 342-4	Alarm Symptoms Usually Needing Further Investigations

Pain that wakes up the child from sleep
Persistent right upper or right lower quadrant pain
Significant vomiting (bilious vomiting, protracted vomiting, cyclical vomiting, or worrisome pattern to the physician)
Unexplained fever
Genitourinary tract symptoms
Dysphagia
Chronic severe diarrhea or nocturnal diarrhea
Gastrointestinal blood loss
Involuntary weight loss
Deceleration of linear growth
Delayed puberty
Family history of inflammatory bowel disease, celiac disease, and peptic ulcer disease

Table 342-5	Alarm Signs Usually Needing Further Investigations

Localized tenderness in the right *upper* quadrant
Localized tenderness in the right *lower* quadrant
Localized fullness or mass
Hepatomegaly
Splenomegaly
Jaundice
Costovertebral angle tenderness
Arthritis
Spinal tenderness
Perianal disease
Abnormal or unexplained physical findings
Hematochezia
Anemia

abdominal pain, a pelvic ultrasonogram may be indicated. An upper GI x-ray series is indicated if one suspects a disorder of the stomach or small intestine.

Helicobacter pylori infection does not seem to be associated with chronic abdominal pain, but in patients with symptoms suggesting gastritis or ulcer, an *H. pylori* test (fecal *H. pylori* antigen) may be performed. Breath hydrogen testing is done for ruling out lactose or sucrose malabsorption. Lactose intolerance is so common that the finding may be coincidental, and the clinician must be cautious in attributing chronic abdominal pain to this condition.

Esophagogastroduodenoscopy is indicated with symptoms that suggest persistent upper GI pathology. In the absence of this suspicion, esophagogastroduodenoscopy is unlikely to identify an abnormality and is usually not necessary.

TREATMENT

Making a positive diagnosis of functional abdominal pain is important and can be done by the primary care pediatrician in most 4-18 yr old children with chronic abdominal pain if there are no alarm symptoms or signs, a normal physical examination, and a negative stool occult blood test. In practice, on many occasions children do not get a conclusive diagnosis of functional abdominal pain. This can lead to unwarranted referrals and increased anxiety to the patient and the family. Even if a diagnostic evaluation is initiated during the initial office visit, a discussion about functional abdominal pain as the most likely diagnosis during that visit will help the patient and family to understand the diagnosis better. Close following and counseling by one consistent healthcare provider is essential.

The most important component of the treatment is reassurance and education of the child and family. The child and family need to be reassured that no evidence of a serious underlying disorder is present. The family and the child with functional pain might worry about the inability to identify an organic cause and may be resistant to a diagnosis of nonorganic disease. Explanation in simple language that although the pain is real, there is no underlying serious disorder usually alleviates the anxiety in the patient and family. Children of families that do not accept a functional cause of the symptoms are more likely to have persistent somatic complaints and school absences. The parents should be instructed to avoid reinforcing the symptoms with secondary gain. If children have missed school or have been removed from routine activities because of the pain, it is important that they return to regular activities.

Treatment goals should be set for return to function and minimizing pain. Complete disappearance of pain would be an unreasonable goal to set. Cognitive-behavioral therapy is helpful in the short term for managing pain and functional disability (Table 342-6). Biofeedback, guided imagery, and relaxation techniques have been useful in some children with functional pain. Even though studies do not show consistent benefits from medications, time-limited use of medications is usually part of the multidisciplinary approach. The commonly used

medications include acid suppressants for dyspepsia symptoms, antispasmodics, and low-dose amitriptyline. For chronic abdominal pain with IBS symptoms, antidiarrheals and nonstimulating laxatives are used. Peppermint oil for 2 wk improves IBS symptoms in children. There is no evidence that a lactose-restricted diet or fiber supplements decrease the frequency of attacks in chronic abdominal pain in children. Proton pump inhibitors or visceral muscle relaxants (anticholinergics) are used empirically but are often unhelpful in the absence of specific indication.

Irritable Bowel Syndrome

IBS is characterized as a chronic FGID associated with abdominal pain or discomfort and altered bowel function without evidence of an inflammatory, anatomic, metabolic, or neoplastic process. Table 342-7 presents the Rome III diagnostic criteria for diagnosing IBS in children and adolescents.

Abdominal pain is episodic, cramping, or aching, usually in the lower abdomen, and often relieved by defecation. There may be abdominal discomfort, bloating, and flatulence. Diarrhea and constipation alone or in an alternating pattern must be present. The diarrhea is often watery and frequent and is associated with pain, the passage of mucus per rectum, and a feeling of incomplete emptying. The constipation is associated with a decreased stooling frequency and the passage of hard stools. Symptoms may be traced back to childhood or following an episode of presumed bacterial or viral gastroenteritis. It is important to rule out organic causes of abdominal pain and altered bowel patterns, especially celiac disease, even in the absence of the classic features of this disease.

Many dietary modifications have been suggested for relief of symptoms but not proven. Restriction of dietary fermentable oligosaccharides, disaccharides, monosaccharaides, and polyols in some studies have shown symptom relief.

Table 342-7	Rome III Criteria for Child/Adolescent Irritable Bowel Syndrome H2b

Diagnostic criteria* must include **all** of the following:
1. Abdominal discomfort† or pain associated with 2 or more of the following at least 25% of the time:
   a. Improvement with defecation
   b. Onset associated with a change in frequency of stool
   c. Onset associated with a change in form (appearance) of stool
2. No evidence of an inflammatory, anatomic, metabolic, or neoplastic process that explains the subject's symptoms

*Criteria fulfilled at least once per week for at least 6 mo prior to diagnosis.
†"Discomfort" means an uncomfortable sensation not described as pain.
Adapted from Rome Foundation: Rome III disorders and criteria.
http://www.romecriteria.org/criteria/

Table 342-6	Effectiveness of Treatments for Abdominal Pain in Children	
THERAPY	**DEFINITION OF DISORDER**	**EFFECTIVENESS**
Cognitive behavioral (family) therapy	Recurrent abdominal pain	Beneficial
Famotidine	Recurrent abdominal pain and dyspeptic symptoms	Inconclusive
Added dietary fiber	Recurrent abdominal pain	Unlikely to be beneficial
Lactose-free diet	Recurrent abdominal pain	Unlikely to be beneficial
Peppermint oil	Irritable bowel syndrome	Likely to be beneficial
Amitriptyline	Functional gastrointestinal disorders, irritable bowel syndrome	Inconsistent results
Lactobacillus GG	Irritable bowel syndrome using Rome III criteria	Unlikely to be beneficial

The effectiveness of analgesics, antispasmodics, sedatives, and antidepressants is currently unknown.
From Berger MY, Gieteling MJ, Benninga MA: Chronic abdominal pain in children, BMJ 334:997–1002, 2007.

Probiotics are reported to be helpful in diarrhea predominant IBS, but larger trials are necessary to prove probiotics are beneficial. Management focuses on the dominant symptoms. Pain has been managed with cognitive-behavioral therapy, pain clinic referrals, peppermint, antispasmodic agents, and tricyclic antidepressant agents (amitriptyline). Diarrhea has been managed with loperamide, oral nonabsorbable antibiotics, and 5-HT$_3$ antagonists (alosetron). Constipation is managed with fiber (psyllium), increased fluid intake, lactulose, 5-HT$_4$ agonists (tegaserod), and selective C2 chloride channel–activating agents. In all medication trials, there is often a high response to placebo.

Bibliography is available at Expert Consult.

Chapter **343**
Acute Appendicitis
John J. Aiken and Keith T. Oldham

Acute appendicitis remains the most common acute surgical condition in children and a major cause of childhood morbidity. While prompt appendectomy remains the mainstay of treatment, management has changed substantially in the past several decades with improved antibiotic regimens, advances in imaging techniques, percutaneous drainage procedures by interventional radiologists, initial nonoperative management in select cases, and the use of laparoscopy. Approximately 100,000 children are treated in children's hospitals for appendicitis each year. The incidence of appendicitis increases with age, from a rate of 1-2 per 10,000 children from birth to 4 yr of age, to a rate of 19-28 per 10,000 children younger than age 14 yr annually. Children have a lifetime risk of ≈7% and appendicitis is diagnosed in 1-8% of children presenting to the emergency department for evaluation of abdominal pain. The misdiagnosis of appendicitis is second only to meningitis as a cause of medical malpractice suits in pediatric emergency care. Mortality is low (<1%), but morbidity remains high, mostly in association with complicated (perforated) appendicitis. Advances in surgical (laparoscopy) and imaging technology have significantly escalated treatment-related costs without demonstrable improvement in patient outcomes. In addition, there are marked variations in practice patterns and resource utilization in the evaluation and management of appendicitis. Children have a higher perforation rate than adults and up to 40% of children present with complicated disease.

PATHOLOGY
The clinical entity of acute appendiceal inflammation followed by perforation, abscess formation, and peritonitis is most likely a disease of multiple etiologies, the final common pathway of which involves invasion of the appendiceal wall by bacteria. One pathway to acute appendicitis begins with luminal obstruction; inspissated fecal material, lymphoid hyperplasia, ingested foreign body, parasites, and tumors have been implicated. Obstruction of the appendiceal lumen initiates a progressive cascade including increasing intraluminal pressures from bacterial proliferation and continued secretion of mucus, elevated intraluminal pressure, lymphatic and venous congestion and edema, impaired arterial perfusion, ischemia of the wall of the appendix, bacterial invasion of the appendiceal wall, and necrosis. This progression correlates with the clinical disease progression from simple appendicitis to gangrenous appendicitis and, thereafter, appendiceal perforation. Submucosal lymphoid follicles, which can obstruct the appendiceal lumen, are few at birth but multiply steadily during childhood, reaching a peak in number during the teen years, when acute appendicitis is most common, and declining after age 30 yr. Because of this prominence of lymphoid tissue, some have hypothesized that the appendix may have an immune function similar to that of the thymus or bursa of Fabricius. Fecaliths and appendicitis are more common in developed countries with refined, low-fiber diets than in developing countries with a high-fiber diet; no causal relationship has been established between lack of dietary fiber and appendicitis.

The finding that <50% of specimens from cases of acute appendicitis demonstrate luminal obstruction on radiographic, gross, or pathologic examination has prompted investigations of alternative etiologies. Enteric infection likely plays a role in many cases in association with mucosal ulceration and invasion of the appendiceal wall by bacteria. Bacteria such as *Yersinia*, *Salmonella*, and *Shigella* spp., and viruses such as infectious mononucleosis, mumps, coxsackievirus B, and adenovirus, are implicated. In addition, case reports demonstrate the occurrence of appendicitis from ingested foreign bodies, in association with carcinoid tumors of the appendix or *Ascaris* and following blunt abdominal trauma. Children with cystic fibrosis have an increased incidence of appendicitis; the cause is believed to be the abnormal thickened mucus. Appendicitis in neonates is rare and warrants diagnostic evaluation for cystic fibrosis and Hirschsprung disease.

A primary focus in the management of acute appendicitis is avoidance of sepsis and the infectious complications leading to increased morbidity, mostly seen in association with perforation. Bacteria can be cultured from the serosal surface of the appendix before microscopic or gross perforation and bacterial invasion of the mesenteric veins can result in portal vein or superior mesenteric vein sepsis (pylephlebitis), thrombosis, and liver abscess. Subsequent to perforation, the microbiologic fecal contamination may be localized to the right lower quadrant (RLQ) or pelvis by the omentum and adjacent loops of bowel, resulting in a localized abscess or inflammatory mass (phlegmon), or, alternatively, the fecal contamination can spread throughout the peritoneal cavity, causing diffuse peritonitis. Young children typically have a poorly developed omentum and are often unable to control the local infection. Perforation and abscess formation with appendicitis can lead to fistula formation in adjacent organs, scrotal cellulitis and abscess through a patent processus vaginalis (congenital indirect inguinal hernia), or small bowel obstruction.

CLINICAL FEATURES
Appendicitis is most common in older children, with peak incidence between the ages of 12 and 18 yr; it is rare in children younger than 5 yr of age (<5% of cases) and extremely rare (<1% of cases) in children younger than 3 yr of age. It affects boys slightly more often than girls and whites more often than blacks in the United States. There is a seasonal peak incidence in autumn and spring. There appears to be a familial predisposition in some cases, particularly in children in whom appendicitis develops before age 6 yr. Perforation in appendicitis is more common in children compared to adults, particularly in young children; with perforation rates as high as 82% for children younger than 5 yr and approaching 100% in infants. There is an increased incidence of perforated appendicitis in children of minority race and children with Medicaid health insurance.

Appendicitis in children has an immensely broad spectrum of clinical presentation. The signs and symptoms can be classic or often atypical and quite variable depending on the timing of presentation, the patient's age, the location of the appendix, and individual variability in the evolution of the disease process. Children early in the disease process can appear well and demonstrate minimal symptoms, subtle findings on physical examination, and normal laboratory studies; those with perforation and advanced peritonitis often demonstrate severe illness with bowel obstruction, renal failure, and septic shock.

While the classic presentation of acute appendicitis is well described, this represents <50% of cases; therefore, the majority of cases of appendicitis have an "atypical" presentation. The illness typically begins insidiously with a brief (several hours) period of generalized malaise and anorexia; the child does not appear ill and the family is not likely to seek consultation assuming the child has "stomach flu" or a viral syndrome. Unfortunately, if the diagnosis is appendicitis, the illness escalates rapidly with progressive abdominal pain followed by vomiting, and appendiceal perforation is likely to occur within 48 hr of the onset of illness. The opportunity for diagnosis before perforation in acute appendicitis in children is generally brief (~36-48 hr).

Abdominal pain is consistently the primary and often the first symptom; beginning shortly (hours) after the onset of illness. As with other visceral organs, there are no somatic pain fibers within the appendix; therefore, early appendiceal inflammation results in pain which is vague, poorly localized, unrelated to activity or position, often colicky, and periumbilical in location as a result of visceral inflammation from a distended appendix. Progression of the inflammatory process in the next 12-24 hr leads to involvement of the adjacent parietal peritoneal surfaces, resulting in somatic pain localized to the RLQ. It is important to note the position of the appendix can vary greatly. In 50% of the population it is located in a retrocecal position; likely resulting in a delayed presentation. In others it is located over the pelvic brim, occasionally descending low down in the pelvis. *The position of the appendix is a critical factor affecting interpretation of presenting signs and symptoms and accurate diagnosis.* The pain becomes steady and more severe and is exacerbated by movement. The child often describes marked discomfort with the "bumpy" car ride to the hospital, moves cautiously, and has difficulty getting onto the examining room stretcher. Nausea and vomiting occur in more than half the patients, and usually *follow* the onset of abdominal pain by several hours. Anorexia is a classic and consistent finding in acute appendicitis, but occasionally, affected patients are hungry. Diarrhea and urinary symptoms are also common, particularly in cases of perforated appendicitis when there is likely inflammation near the rectum and possible abscess in the pelvis. As it progresses, appendicitis is often associated with adynamic ileus; leading to the complaint of constipation and possible misdiagnosis. Because enteric infections can cause appendicitis, diarrhea may be the initial manifestation and gastroenteritis may be the assumed diagnosis. In contrast to gastroenteritis, the abdominal pain in appendicitis is constant (not cramping or relieved by defecation), the emesis may become bile stained and persistent, and the clinical course worsens steadily rather than demonstrating a waxing and waning pattern. Fever is common and typically low-grade unless perforation has occurred. Most patients demonstrate at least mild tachycardia.

The temporal progression of symptoms from vague, mild pain, malaise, and anorexia to severe localized pain, fever, and vomiting typically occurs rapidly, in 24-48 hr in the majority of cases. If the diagnosis is delayed beyond 36-48 hr, the perforation rate exceeds 65%. A period after perforation of lessened abdominal pain and acute symptoms has been described, presumably with the elimination of pressure within the appendix. If the omentum or adjacent intestine is able to wall off the infectious process, the evolution of illness is less predictable and delay in presentation is likely. If perforation leads to diffuse peritonitis, the child generally has escalating diffuse abdominal pain and rapid development of toxicity evidenced by dehydration and signs of sepsis including hypotension, oliguria, acidosis, and high-grade fever. When several days have elapsed in the progression of appendicitis, patients often develop signs and symptoms of developing small bowel obstruction. If the appendix is retrocecal, appendicitis predictably evolves more slowly and patients are likely to relate 4-5 days of illness preceding evaluation. The pain is typically more lateral and posterior and can mimic the symptoms associated with septic arthritis of the hip or a psoas muscle abscess. Occasionally patients will complain of urinary symptoms, presumably related to inflammation adjacent to the ureter and/or bladder. Painful voiding may not be from dysuria but pressure transmitted to an inflamed peritoneum.

PHYSICAL EXAMINATION

Although the hallmark of diagnosing acute appendicitis remains a careful and thorough history and physical examination, all clinicians know the arcane nature of acute appendicitis, the consistent or typical clinical features are not present in all patients, and the diagnosis can be a humbling experience even for the most experienced clinicians. A primary focus of the initial assessment is attention to the temporal

evolution of the illness in relation to specific presenting signs and symptoms. In many children, appendicitis can be confidently diagnosed based on history and physical examination alone, and the children can thus be spared the treatment delay, expense, and possible radiation exposure associated with imaging studies.

Physical examination begins with inspection of the child's demeanor as well as the appearance of the abdomen. Because appendicitis most often has an insidious onset, children rarely present <12 hr from the onset of illness, and the children who do present early are likely to have minimal findings. Children with early appendicitis (18-36 hr) typically appear mildly ill and move tentatively, hunched forward and, often, with a slight limp favoring the right side. Supine, they often lie quietly on their right side with their knees pulled up to relax the abdominal muscles, and when asked to lie flat or sit up, they move cautiously and might use a hand to protect the RLQ.

Early in appendicitis, the abdomen is typically flat; abdominal distention suggests more advanced disease characteristic of perforation or developing small bowel obstruction. Auscultation can reveal normal or hyperactive bowel sounds in early appendicitis, which are replaced by hypoactive bowel sounds as the disease progresses to perforation. *The judicious use of morphine analgesia to relieve abdominal pain does not change diagnostic accuracy or interfere with surgical decision making, and patients should receive adequate pain control.*

Localized abdominal tenderness is the single most reliable finding in the diagnosis of acute appendicitis. McBurney described the classic point of localized tenderness in acute appendicitis, which is the junction of the lateral and middle thirds of the line joining the right anterior–superior iliac spine and the umbilicus, but the tenderness can also localize to any of the aberrant locations of the appendix. Localized tenderness is a later and less-consistent finding when the appendix is retrocecal in position (>50% of cases). In cases of an appendix localized entirely in the pelvis, the tenderness on abdominal examination may be minimal and best appreciated on rectal examination.

A gentle touch on the child's arm at the beginning of the examination with the reassurance that the abdominal examination will be similarly gentle can help to establish trust and increase the chance for a reliable and reproducible examination. The examination is best initiated in the left lower abdomen, so that the immediate part of the exam is not uncomfortable, and conducted in a counterclockwise direction moving gently to the left upper abdomen, right upper abdomen, and, lastly, the right lower abdomen. This should alleviate anxiety, allow relaxation of the abdominal musculature, and enhance trust. The examiner makes several "circles" of the abdomen with sequentially more pressure. A soft, compressible, nontender abdominal wall is reassuring. In appendicitis, any abdominal wall movement, including coughing (Dunphy sign), may elicit pain. A consistent finding in acute appendicitis is guarding; rigidity of the overlying rectus muscle. This rigidity may be voluntary, to protect the area of tenderness from the examiner's hand, or involuntary, secondary to peritonitis causing spasm of the overlying muscle.

Examination findings must be interpreted relative to the temporal evolution of the illness. Abdominal tenderness may be vague or even absent early in the course of appendicitis and is often diffuse after rupture. Rebound tenderness and referred tenderness (Rovsing sign) are also consistent findings in acute appendicitis but not always present. Rebound tenderness is elicited by deep palpation of the abdomen followed by the sudden release of the examining hand. This is often very painful to the child and has demonstrated poor correlation with peritonitis, so it should be avoided. Gentle finger percussion is a better test for peritoneal irritation. Similarly, digital rectal examination is uncomfortable and unlikely to contribute to the evaluation of appendicitis in most cases of appendicitis in children. Psoas and obturator internus signs are pain with passive stretch of these muscles. The psoas sign is elicited with active right thigh flexion or passive extension of the hip and typically positive in cases of a retrocecal appendix. The obturator sign is demonstrated by adductor pain after internal rotation of the flexed thigh and typically positive in cases of a pelvic appendix. Physical examination may demonstrate a mass in the RLQ representing an inflammatory phlegmon around the appendix or a localized abscess (fluid collection).

DIAGNOSTIC STUDIES
Laboratory Findings

A variety of laboratory tests have been used in the evaluation of children with suspected appendicitis. Individually, none are very sensitive or specific for appendicitis, but collectively they can affect the clinician's level of suspicion and decision-making to proceed with pediatric surgery consultation, discharge, or imaging studies. Findings should be interpreted with attention to the temporal evolution of the illness.

A complete blood count with differential and urinalysis are commonly obtained. The leukocyte count in early appendicitis may be normal and typically is only mildly elevated with a left shift (11,000-16,000/mm^3) as the illness progresses in the initial 24-48 hr. Whereas a normal white blood cell (WBC) count never completely eliminates appendicitis, a count <8,000/mm^3 in a patient with a history of illness longer than 48 hr should be viewed as highly suspicious for an alternative diagnosis. The leukocyte count may be markedly elevated (>20,000/mm^3) in perforated appendicitis and rarely in nonperforated cases; a markedly elevated WBC count, other than in cases of advanced, perforated appendicitis, should raise suspicion of an alternative diagnosis.

Urinalysis often demonstrates a few white or red blood cells, as a result of the proximity of the inflamed appendix to the ureter or bladder, but it should be free of bacteria. The urine is often concentrated and contains ketones from diminished oral intake and vomiting. Gross hematuria is uncommon and suggests primary renal pathology such as Henoch-Schönlein purpura.

Electrolytes and liver chemistries are generally normal unless there has been a delay in diagnosis, leading to severe dehydration and/or sepsis. Amylase and liver enzymes are only helpful to exclude alternative diagnoses such as pancreatitis and cholecystitis and are not obtained if appendicitis is the strongly suspected diagnosis. Electrolytes are most helpful to assess level of illness and direct fluid resuscitation, but rarely aid accurate diagnosis.

C-reactive protein increases in proportion to the degree of appendiceal inflammation but is nonspecific and not widely used. Serum amyloid A protein is consistently elevated in patients with acute appendicitis with a sensitivity and specificity of 86% and 83%, respectively.

The Pediatric Appendicitis Score combines history, physical, and laboratory data to assist in the diagnosis (Table 343-1). Scores ≤2 suggest a very low likelihood of appendicitis, whereas scores ≥8 are highly associated with appendicitis. Scores between 3 and 7 warrant further evaluation or diagnostic studies. Nonetheless, no scoring system is perfectly sensitive or specific and none have demonstrated reliability above history and physical examination by an experienced clinician.

Radiologic Studies

Following a thorough initial evaluation; history, physical examination, and review of vital signs and laboratory studies, if the diagnosis is uncertain, advanced radiographic studies can improve diagnostic accuracy.

Plain Radiographs

Plain abdominal radiographs may be helpful in select cases of abdominal pain/suspected appendicitis. Plain abdominal x-rays can demonstrate several findings in acute appendicitis including sentinel loops of bowel and localized ileus, scoliosis from psoas muscle spasm, a colonic air–fluid level above the right iliac fossa (colon "cutoff" sign), a RLQ soft-tissue mass, or a calcified appendicolith (5-10% of cases), but they are normal in 50% of patients, have a low sensitivity, and are not generally recommended (Fig. 343-1). Plain films are most helpful in evaluating complicated cases in which small bowel obstruction or free air is suspected.

Ultrasound

Ultrasound is usually utilized for diagnostic accuracy in the evaluation of acute appendicitis and has demonstrated >90% sensitivity and specificity in pediatric centers experienced with the technique. Graded abdominal compression is used to displace the cecum and ascending colon and identify the appendix, which has a typical target appearance (Fig. 343-2). The ultrasound criteria for appendicitis include wall thickness ≥6 mm, luminal distention, lack of compressibility, a complex mass in the RLQ, or an appendicolith. The visualized appendix usually

Table 343-1	Pediatric Appendicitis Scores
FEATURE	**SCORE**
Fever >38°C (100.4°F)	1
Anorexia	1
Nausea/vomiting	1
Cough/percussion/hopping tenderness	2
Right lower quadrant tenderness	2
Migration of pain	1
Leukocytosis >10,000 (10^9/L)	1
Polymorphonuclear-neutrophilia >7,500 (10^9/L)	1
Total	10

From Acheson J, Banerjee J: Management of suspected appendicitis in children, Arch Dis Child Educ Pract Ed 95:9–13, 2010.

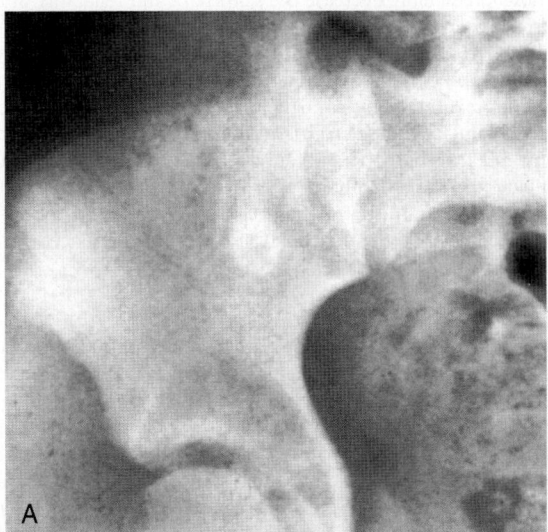
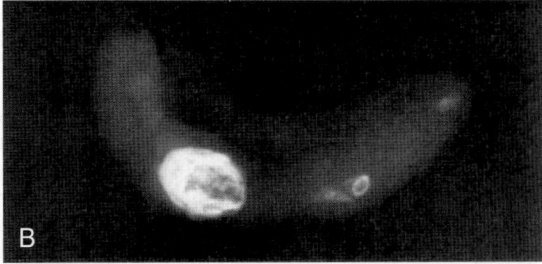

Figure 343-1 Calcified appendicoliths are seen in a coned-down anteroposterior view of the right lower quadrant **(A)** and in the resected appendix of a 10 yr old girl with acute appendicitis **(B)**. *(From Kuhn JP, Slovis TL, Haller JO:* Caffrey's pediatric diagnostic imaging, *vol 2, ed 10, Philadelphia, 2004, Mosby, p. 1682.)*

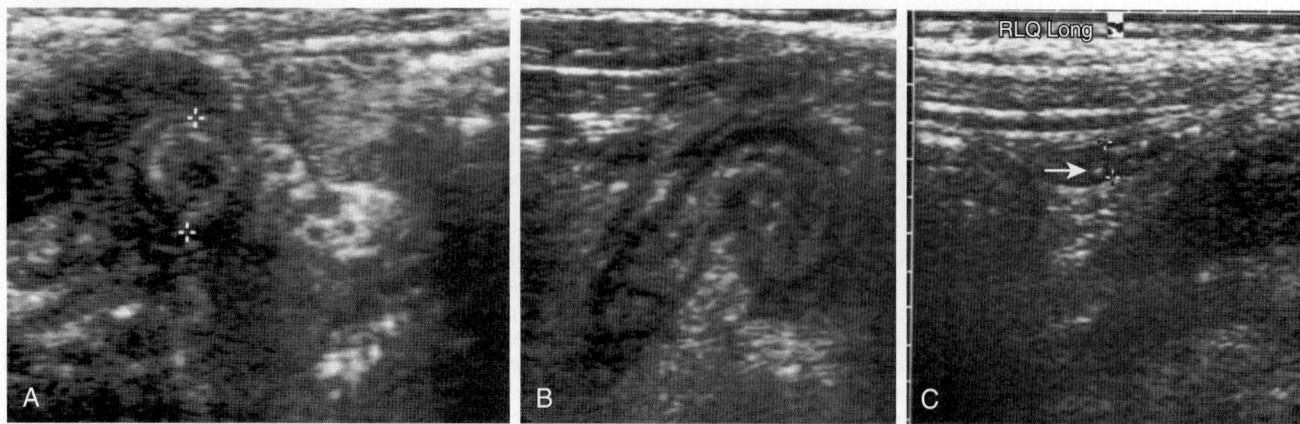

Figure 343-2 Ultrasound examination of patients with appendicitis. **A,** Transverse ultrasound scan of the appendix demonstrates the characteristic "target sign." In this case, the innermost portion is sonolucent, compatible with fluid or pus. **B,** Longitudinal view of another patient demonstrates the alternating hyperechoic and hypoechoic layers with an outermost hypoechoic layer, suggesting periappendiceal fluid. **C,** Longitudinal ultrasound scan of the right lower quadrant demonstrates a dilated, noncompressible appendix. The bright echo within the appendix represents an appendicolith with acoustic shadowing *(arrow)*. *(From Kuhn JP, Slovis TL, Haller JO: Caffrey's pediatric diagnostic imaging, vol 2, ed 10, Philadelphia, 2004, Mosby, p. 1684.)*

coincides with the site of localized pain and tenderness. Findings that suggest advanced appendicitis on ultrasound include asymmetric wall thickening, abscess formation, associated free intraperitoneal fluid, surrounding tissue edema, and decreased local tenderness to compression. *The main limitation of ultrasound is an inability to visualize the appendix, which is reported in up to 20% of cases.* **A normal appendix must be visualized to exclude appendicitis by ultrasound.** Certain conditions predictably decrease the sensitivity and reliability of ultrasound for appendicitis, including obesity, bowel distention, and pain, which interferes with the exam. Major advantages of ultrasound include its easy availability, rapid method, low cost, and freedom from need for patient preparation and ionizing radiation. Ultrasound can be particularly helpful in adolescent girls, a group with a high negative appendectomy rate (normal appendix found at surgery), because of its ability to evaluate for ovarian pathology without ionizing radiation. A diagnostic or normal ultrasound exam eliminates the need for CT and should be considered the first exam in a center experienced with the technique.

CT Scan

CT scan had been the gold standard imaging study for evaluating children with suspected appendicitis, but carries the significant negative effects of radiation exposure and increased costs. It should be used only in carefully selected patients and always observing the reduced radiation dosage recommendations for children. CT examination can be performed in many ways, including standard CT scan, helical CT scan, with or without oral and intravenous contrast, examination of both the abdomen and pelvis or pelvis alone, focused appendiceal CT scan, and focused appendiceal CT scan with rectal contrast. All of these techniques have demonstrated >95% sensitivity and specificity for acute appendicitis. Findings on CT scan consistent with appendicitis include a distended (dilated >7 mm) thick-walled appendix, inflammatory streaking of surrounding mesenteric fat, and a pericecal phlegmon or abscess (Figs. 343-3 and 343-4). In addition, appendicoliths are more readily demonstrated on CT scan (40-50%) than on plain radiographs (5-15%). CT scan may be most useful in advanced appendicitis to identify and guide percutaneous drainage of fluid collections and identification of an inflammatory mass, which might prompt a plan for initial nonoperative management. The use of CT scan to "rule out" acute appendicitis and avoid the need (and expenditures) of in-hospital admission is suspect as in early appendicitis CT findings are predictably subtle and in more advanced cases CT scan should be unnecessary as an accurate diagnosis should be able to be made on careful history and physical examination.

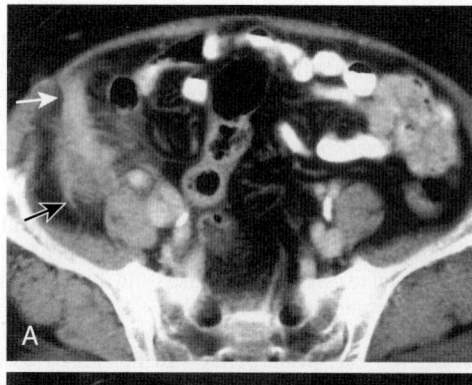

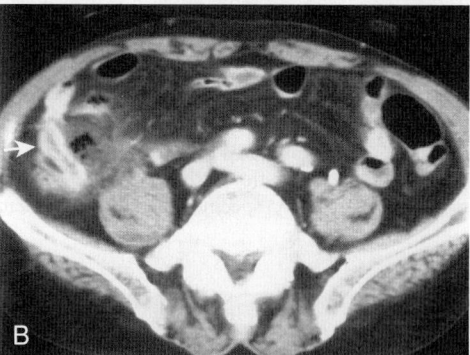

Figure 343-3 A, Phlegmon *(open arrow)* is noted around the enlarged appendix *(solid arrow)* in perforated appendicitis. **B,** Extraluminal air is shown adjacent to the wall-enhanced appendix *(arrow)* in perforated appendicitis. *(From Yeung KW, Chang MS, Hsiao CP: Evaluation of perforated and nonperforated appendicitis with CT, Clin Imaging. 28(6):422–427, 2004.)*

Disadvantages of CT scan include; greater cost; radiation exposure; possible need for intravenous, oral, or rectal contrast; and possible need for sedation. Children have an increased sensitivity to radiation and a longer life ahead to potentially develop a radiation-induced malignancy. A single CT scan has been reported to confirm a 1 in 1,000 lifetime mortality risk, and the risk has been reported as high as 1 in 550 in children younger than age 5 yr. Oral contrast is problematic if

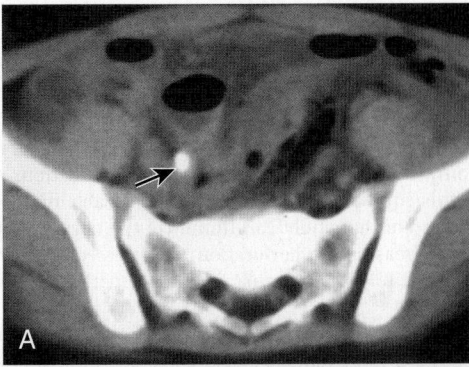

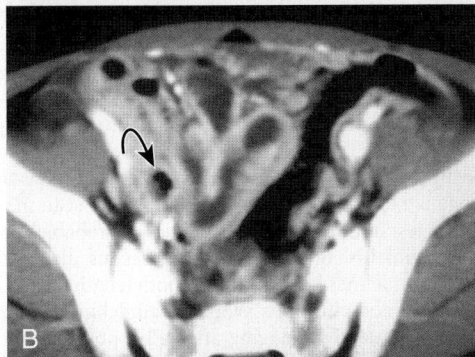

Figure 343-4 A, Precontrast-enhanced CT reveals an appendicolith *(arrow)* in perforated appendicitis. **B,** Postcontrast-enhanced CT (1 cm below the level in **A**) reveals intraluminal air in the appendix *(curved arrow)* associated with ileal wall enhancement in perforated appendicitis. *(From Yeung KW, Chang MS, Hsiao CP: Evaluation of perforated and nonperforated appendicitis with CT, Clin Imaging 28(6):422–427, 2004.)*

appendicitis is confirmed, because of the risk for aspiration at induction of anesthesia. Because the finding of fat stranding in surrounding tissues is a key component of CT evaluation for appendicitis, CT is less reliable in thin children with minimal body fat. For this reason, rectal contrast can increase diagnostic accuracy in this group. CT imaging is also helpful in demonstrating nonappendiceal causes of abdominal pain.

Following initial evaluation, if the diagnosis of acute appendicitis is suspected but uncertain, it is advisable to obtain pediatric surgical consultation before proceeding with a CT scan. An alternative approach to diminish the use of CT scans is the emerging use of observational units for a period up to 23 hr to follow clinical disease progression. Acute appendicitis is most often a rapidly progressive illness and signs and symptoms including fever, tachycardia, nausea and/or vomiting, and focal tenderness, which become more prominent despite intravenous fluids will often lower negative appendectomy rates and enable an accurate diagnosis without the need for advanced imaging.

MRI/White Blood Cell Scan

MRI is at least equivalent to CT in diagnostic accuracy for appendicitis and does not involve ionizing radiation. The use of MRI in the evaluation of appendicitis is limited because it is less available, more costly, often requires sedation, and does not offer equivalent access for drainage of fluid collections. MRI may prove most useful in adolescent girls when advanced imaging is needed. Radionuclide-labeled WBC scans have also been used in some centers in evaluating atypical cases of possible appendicitis in children and demonstrated a high sensitivity (97%) but only modest specificity (80%).

DIFFERENTIAL DIAGNOSIS

The list of illnesses that can mimic acute appendicitis is extensive because many gastrointestinal, gynecologic, and inflammatory disor-ders can manifest with similar illness history, signs, and symptoms. Differential diagnosis, even limited to common conditions, includes gastroenteritis, mesenteric adenitis, Meckel diverticulitis, inflammatory bowel disease, diabetes mellitus, sickle cell disease, streptococcal pharyngitis, lower lobe pneumonia, cholecystitis, pancreatitis, urinary tract infection, infectious enteritis, and, in girls, ovarian torsion, ectopic pregnancy, ruptured ovarian cysts, and pelvic inflammatory disease (including tuboovarian abscess). Intestinal tract lymphoma, tumors of the appendix (carcinoid in children), and ovarian tumors are rare but can also masquerade as acute appendicitis. In patients with pyelonephritis, the fever and WBC count are likely much higher, symptoms of dysuria will be present, and the tenderness is located more in the flank or costovertebral angle. Rarely, appendicitis may recur in the stump of a previous appendectomy. *Children younger than 3 yr of age and adolescent girls have historically proven to be at particularly high risk for an incorrect diagnosis.*

Most important is differentiation of the patients with gastroenteritis, which is the most common misdiagnosis in the child with appendicitis. The time course of illness (hours, days, weeks) leading to presentation is a critical component of the history. The classic patient with acute appendicitis describes abdominal pain as the preeminent symptom. In general, symptoms of systemic illness such as headache, chills, and myalgias indicate that a patient does not have appendicitis. Acute appendicitis most often begins insidiously as generalized malaise or anorexia, but there is early (within hours) onset of abdominal pain and the illness typically escalates rapidly in the initial 24-48 hr. Most patients with acute appendicitis have 1-3 episodes of vomiting in the initial 24-48 hr of illness; multiple episodes of vomiting are unusual in early appendicitis. In contrast, when gastroenteritis is the diagnosis, diarrhea and vomiting are more likely to be predominant symptoms early in the illness, and abdominal pains may seem associated with the frequent episodes of diarrhea and vomiting. In patients with an acute presentation (<72 hr of illness), vomiting preceding pain, large-volume diarrhea, large amounts of nonbilious vomiting, and high fever suggest gastroenteritis. In addition, patients with appendicitis typically have normal or hypoactive bowel sounds, whereas gastroenteritis typically produces persistently hyperactive bowel sounds. From the onset of illness, the child with appendicitis typically has a steadily deteriorating clinical course, whereas the child with gastroenteritis may have an undulating course, at times feeling better and other times feeling worse.

In the classic child with acute appendicitis who presents within 48 hr of the onset of illness, the WBC count can be low, normal, or elevated but is only rarely elevated >20,000/mm³. WBC counts in this range should prompt consideration of alternative diagnoses.

A child who presents with a history of illness of longer than 3-4 days is often more challenging. If the diagnosis is appendicitis, perforation has likely occurred and the child's presentation should evidence signs and symptoms of localized abscess/phlegmon in the RLQ or diffuse peritonitis. At this point in the illness, the WBC count should be elevated (>12,000/mm³) with a left shift; a WBC count <7,000/mm³ with a lymphocytosis is distinctly unusual in advanced appendicitis and more typical of gastroenteritis. A slightly slower progression of illness is also typical when the appendix is in a retrocecal position and symptoms and anterior abdominal wall tenderness typically are slower to evolve.

An abnormal hemogram combined with purpuric skin lesions, arthritis, and nephritis suggests a diagnosis of Henoch-Schönlein purpura or hemolytic-uremic syndrome. Torsion of an undescended testis and epididymitis are common but should be discovered on physical examination. Meckel diverticulitis is an infrequent condition, but the clinical presentation closely mimics appendicitis and the diagnosis is usually made at surgery. Primary spontaneous peritonitis is classically seen in prepubertal girls is often mistaken for appendicitis.

It should be recognized that "missed" appendicitis is the most common cause of small bowel obstruction in children without history of prior abdominal surgery. Atypical presentations of appendicitis are expected in association with other conditions such as pregnancy, Crohn disease, steroid treatment, and immunosuppressive therapy.

Appendicitis in association with Crohn disease often has a protracted presentation with an atypical pattern of recurring but localized abdominal pain.

The diagnosis of appendicitis in adolescent girls is especially challenging, and some series report negative appendectomy rates as high as 30-40%. Ovarian cysts are often acutely painful as a result of rupture, rapid enlargement, or hemorrhage. Rupture of an ovarian follicle associated with ovulation often causes mid-cycle lateralizing pain (mittelschmerz), but there is no progression of symptoms and systemic illness is absent. Ovarian tumors and torsion can also mimic acute appendicitis, although ovarian torsion is typically characterized by the acute onset of severe pain and is associated with more dramatic nausea and vomiting than is normally seen in early appendicitis. In pelvic inflammatory disease, the pain is typically suprapubic, bilateral, and of longer duration. The need for accurate urgent diagnosis in girls is influenced by concern that perforated appendicitis can predispose the patient to future ectopic pregnancy or tubal infertility, although data have not consistently demonstrated increased incidence of infertility after perforated appendicitis. For these reasons, adjunct diagnostic studies (ultrasound, CT, or diagnostic laparoscopy) should be used more liberally in this group of patients to keep negative appendectomy rates low.

DIAGNOSTIC APPROACH

A diagnosis of acute appendicitis is made in only 50-70% of children at the time of initial assessment; negative appendectomy rates remain high (10-20%) and perforation rates (30-40%) have not changed in the past few decades.

Traditionally, early surgery in equivocal cases was the standard; aimed to minimize perforation rates and complications. Negative laparotomy rates of 10-20% were common and were deemed acceptable to keep perforation rates low. Many authors have criticized these high negative laparotomy rates, citing the risks and expense of unnecessary surgery and anesthesia. In a national database, overall rupture rates for appendicitis varied from 20-76%, with a median of 36%. The median overall negative laparotomy rate (normal appendix at surgery) was 2.6%, significantly lower than traditionally reported rates of 10-20%. The lack of consensus in management approach is reflected by the fact that the use of diagnostic imaging in cases of suspected appendicitis varied from 18-89%.

Some clinicians remain steadfast to the primacy of a careful history and physical examination and rarely order advanced imaging studies. The initial assessment, along with the history and physical examination, may include a complete blood count with differential, urinalysis, and plain films (chest and abdominal series). If the initial assessment leads to a high level of suspicion for appendicitis, pediatric surgical consultation should be the next step, with the likelihood of prompt appendectomy without further studies. If the initial evaluation suggests a nonsurgical diagnosis and a low concern for appendicitis, the child may be discharged with family education regarding the natural history and progression of acute appendicitis and advice to return for repeat evaluation if the child is not improving on liquids and a bland diet in the next 24 hr. This approach has demonstrated high sensitivity and specificity (>90%) at certain institutions, but collective data from many centers have not been able to reproduce this degree of accuracy.

Previous reports recommending CT scans in all equivocal cases to minimize perforation rates and morbidity are not supported in the current climate to reduce the use of CT scan and ionizing radiation. It seems likely that if imaging studies are obtained in all patients with equivocal presentations and a brief duration of illness (<24 hr), the false-negative rate of the imaging studies will increase. Maximum benefit and effectiveness of advanced imaging is obtained when it is used selectively in children for whom the diagnosis is equivocal after careful history and physical examination by an experienced clinician and who are not too early in the temporal evolution of the illness.

In equivocal cases, some centers proceed with a plan of active observation. Many reports substantiate improved diagnostic accuracy by observation and serial examination over a period of 12-24 hr, simplifying the eventual decision to proceed with appendectomy, discharge the patient, or proceed with advanced imaging studies, and report no correlation between surgical morbidity and timing of surgery. The use of observation units, where the child may be observed with intravenous fluids, serial vital signs, and planned repeat physical examination in 6-12 hr. is a strategy gaining increased popularity. At the end of a period of observation, the clinician should decide to discharge the patient based on improved clinical status, proceed to appendectomy, or proceed to further imaging evaluation. Advanced imaging in this equivocal group will be more reliable further into the disease process and hopefully can minimize the negative laparotomy rate without increasing the perforation rate (missed or delayed diagnosis). Less than 2% of children's appendices perforate while under observation.

A thoughtful approach in equivocal cases of appendicitis is to begin with ultrasound if it is available and the hospital has experience with ultrasound for possible appendicitis. In 1 study, ultrasound decreased the need for CT scan in 22% of patients. If ultrasound imaging is inconclusive, the next diagnostic step could be pediatric surgical consultation, a brief period of observation followed by clinical reevaluation and CT scan if the diagnosis remains equivocal. The period of observation (12-24 hr) can occur at home provided the patient is physiologically well; a hospital-based observational unit has the advantage of being able to provide intravenous fluids. CT scan may be used as the first-line test in obese patients, in cases of probable advanced or perforated appendicitis, or when there is gaseous distention of the bowel. Practice guidelines have decreased both length of stay and costs without increasing complications. One such guideline employing clinical judgment and selective imaging attained a positive and negative predictive value for appendicitis of 94% and 99%, respectively.

TREATMENT

Once the diagnosis of appendicitis is confirmed or highly suspected, the standard treatment for acute appendicitis is most often prompt appendectomy. Some reports suggest initial nonoperative management (antibiotics and drainage of fluid collections) as an alternative option in late presentations, depending on the patient's general condition and the state of the appendix. In adults with simple appendicitis, broad-spectrum antibiotics alone have resulted in resolution of symptoms. Nonetheless, there is a 20% chance of recurrence within 1 year of conservative therapy, and of those 20% will present with perforation or a gangrenous appendix. One small nonrandomized trial of nonoperative therapy for uncomplicated appendicitis in children reported a success rate of ~90%. To be considered uncomplicated, patients had pain ≤48 hours, ultrasonographic or CT documentation of a nonruptured appendix, as well as an appendiceal diameter ≤1.1 cm without phlegmon, abscess, or fecalith. Management included a minimum of 24 hr of intravenous antibiotics (piperacillin-tazobactam or ciprofloxacin with metronidazole) followed by amoxicillin-clavulanate or ciprofloxacin with metronidazole to complete a 10-day total antibiotic course.

Emergency (middle of the night) surgery is rarely indicated, and most patients require preoperative supportive measures to stabilize vital signs and to ensure the safety of the procedure, anesthesia, and improve outcomes. In addition, often, unexpected pathology (appendiceal tumors, intestinal lymphoma, congenital renal anomalies, inflammatory bowel disease) is discovered at operation, and intraoperative consultation and frozen section may be needed. There is no correlation between timing of surgery and perforation rates or postoperative morbidity when the operation proceeds within 24-48 hr of diagnosis. In addition, appendectomy can be a challenging operation, with potential for major complications including injury to adjacent intestine, the iliac vessels, or the right ureter. The operation should proceed semielectively within 12-24 hr of diagnosis. Children with appendicitis are typically at least mildly dehydrated and require preoperative fluid resuscitation to correct hypovolemia and electrolyte abnormalities before anesthesia. Fever, if present, should be treated. Pain management begins even before a definitive diagnosis is made, and consultation of a pain service, if available, is appropriate once a decision is made to proceed to surgery. In the majority of cases, preoperative management can be accomplished during the period of diagnostic evaluation and prompt appendectomy can be performed.

In patients in whom perforated appendicitis is identified at the time of diagnosis, the operation is even less urgent and proper preoperative management is more critical. When the illness is protracted owing to a delay in diagnosis or presentation, patients can demonstrate significant physiologic derangements including severe dehydration, hypotension, acidosis, and renal failure. These patients require a longer period of stabilization with fluid resuscitation and antibiotics, including, in occasional cases, admission to an intensive care unit before proceeding with more definitive management. Based on the patient's status, findings on CT scan, and availability of experienced radiologists, the initial plan may be percutaneous drainage of fluid collections by interventional radiology and continued fluid resuscitation and antibiotics. An inflammatory mass (phlegmon) without an identifiable fluid component might initially respond to nonoperative management with fluids and antibiotics. Placement of 1 or more drainage catheters under imaging (CT or ultrasound) guidance has been successful in more than 80% of patients. Most pediatric surgeons recommend delayed appendectomy (during the same hospitalization) or interval appendectomy (4-6 wk after the initial presentation), to prevent recurrent appendicitis (≈20%); this is an area of some controversy.

If diffuse peritonitis exists, most surgeons proceed promptly with appendectomy after a brief period of intravenous fluids and broad spectrum antibiotics. Others continue nonoperative management provided the patient demonstrates clinical improvement by physiologic criteria including hemodynamic stability, urine output, control of fever, and declining leukocyte count. If the patient demonstrates clinical recovery by resolution of fever, sepsis, and return of bowel function, generally a 2 wk course of oral antibiotics is completed and a decision is made regarding interval appendectomy in 6-8 wk. A child who fails to improve within 24-72 hr needs an urgent appendectomy to control sepsis. Emergency appendectomy should only be performed in the occasional circumstance when physiologic resuscitation requires urgent control of advanced peritoneal sepsis not amenable to interventional drainage or this is not available.

Antibiotics

Antibiotics substantially lower the incidence of postoperative wound infections and intraperitoneal abscesses in perforated appendicitis, but their role is less well defined in simple appendicitis. The antibiotic regimen should be directed against the typical bacterial flora found in the appendix, including anaerobic organisms (*Bacteroides, Clostridia,* and *Peptostreptococcus* spp.) and Gram-negative aerobic bacteria (*Escherichia coli, Pseudomonas aeruginosa, Enterobacter,* and *Klebsiella* spp.). Gram-positive organisms are less commonly found in the colon, and the need to provide antibiotic coverage for them (primarily enterococcus) is controversial. Many antibiotic combinations have demonstrated equivalent efficacy in controlled trials in terms of wound infection rate, resolution of fever, length of stay, and incidence of complications.

For simple nonperforated appendicitis, one preoperative dose of a single broad-spectrum agent (cefoxitin) or equivalent is sufficient. The practice in perforated or gangrenous appendicitis, most surgeons prefer combination regimens such as Zosyn (piperacillin/tazobactam), ticarcillin/clavulanate, or ceftriaxone/metronidazole. The traditional "triple" antibiotic regimen (ampicillin, gentamicin, and clindamycin or metronidazole) is still effective, but adds cost and has the concern for ototoxicity. Antibiotic coverage is continued postoperatively for 3-5 days. Oral antibiotics are equally as effective as intravenous, and therefore the patient can be switched to an oral regimen and discharged once bowel function returns. This transition to oral antibiotics has significantly affected length of stay and cost in the management of perforated appendicitis.

Interval Appendectomy

Ruptured appendicitis complicated by a walled-off inflammatory mass or abscess can be treated without immediate appendectomy. This strategy is intended to avoid a predictable higher surgical complication rate and is often useful in children, in whom the overall incidence of perforation approaches 50%. In this group of patients, debate exists over the need for interval appendectomy if the child recovers well without "up front" appendectomy. The risk of developing recurrent appendicitis if the appendix is not removed is unknown, and published reports vary between 10% and 80% (most are closer to 10%). Most cases of recurrent appendicitis develop within 2 yr of the initial illness. Some authors believe interval appendectomy is unnecessary because of the low risk for recurrent appendicitis. Others support interval appendectomy to avoid recurrent appendicitis and to confirm the original diagnosis, citing an incidence of unexpected pathology in 30% of interval appendectomy specimens. The vast majority of pediatric surgeons perform interval appendectomy routinely (4-6 wk interval) after initial nonoperative management of perforated appendicitis.

Surgical Technique

Diagnostic laparoscopy and laparoscopic appendectomy (minimally invasive technique) for both simple and perforated appendicitis are the preferred approaches in most pediatric centers; the open surgery is still performed in selected cases. Laparoscopic appendectomy has significant advantages in administrative factors (cost, resource utilization, length of stay), and slight improvement in clinical outcome measures (wound infection rate, intraabdominal abscess, analgesic requirements, return to full activity), but have failed to establish an evidence-based preference between laparoscopic and open appendectomy in children. In nonperforated appendicitis, laparoscopic appendectomy appears to have lower narcotic analgesic requirements, decreased wound morbidity, and improved cosmesis, but operative times seem slightly higher and costs are almost doubled compared to the open procedure. Length of hospitalization is similar for both approaches.

The role of laparoscopy in perforated appendicitis is less-well defined. There are no convincing data to recommend one approach in all patients. Most pediatric surgeons use both approaches selectively. The laparoscopic approach is used most often for obese patients, when alternative diagnoses are suspected, and in adolescent girls to better evaluate for ovarian pathology and pelvic inflammatory disease while avoiding the ionizing radiation associated with CT imaging. Injection of local anesthetic (bupivacaine) into the wound reduces postoperative pain.

Complications

Morbidity rates for appendicitis vary widely in large series from 10-45%. The principal determinant of complications is the severity of the appendicitis. In nonperforated appendicitis, an overall complication rate of 3-7% is expected. With perforation, the complication rate rises to 15-30%. The most common complications are wound infections (3-10%) and intraabdominal abscesses; both are more common after perforation. Perforation and abscess formation can also lead to fistula formation in adjacent organs. Perforation rates are consistently >80% in children younger than 5 yr of age. Delay in return to full activity and function is also predictable in perforated appendicitis. Patients with advanced appendicitis can progress to sepsis and multisystem organ failure, but generally these patients respond promptly to antibiotics, fluids, and other supportive measures preoperatively. Other potential complications include postoperative ileus, diffuse peritonitis, portal vein pylephlebitis (rare), and adhesive small bowel obstruction. Readmission rates are significantly higher in perforated appendicitis (≈20%) and this has become an important marker in recent quality metrics. Mortality with appendicitis is rare (<0.5%) and seen mostly in neonates and immunocompromised patients.

INCIDENTAL APPENDICOLITHS

The question of the "incidental" appendicolith is an intriguing one for pediatric practitioners. These are patients who **do not** have appendicitis but are found to have an appendicolith with imaging. In adults, incidental appendicoliths identified by CT scans vary in incidence from <1% to as high as 10%. An appendicolith is defined as a calcification within the appendiceal lumen. They have a characteristic dense and laminated appearance when compared to other lower abdominal calcifications, including phleboliths (venous calcifications) and, in girls, ovarian calcifications, most commonly seen in ovarian tumors. They can be appreciated on plain film, ultrasound, and CT scan; CT scan is the most reliable. Occasionally an appendicolith is noted during laparoscopy while visualizing a noninflamed appendix.

When an appendicolith is noted in the evaluation of a child with abdominal pain and suspected appendicitis, the finding of the appendicolith confirms the diagnosis; surgical consultation and prompt appendectomy is indicated. Appendicoliths may be noted in the evaluation of patients who have no signs of appendicitis; such as imaging obtained after trauma or for nonspecific abdominal complaints. The concern in this setting is that the appendicolith may increase the eventual development of acute appendicitis. In addition, there is the concern that appendicitis that develops in association with an appendicolith may have a rapidly escalating course and early perforation. Some physicians believe that an appendicolith may be associated with recurrent RLQ/iliac fossa pain.

Incidental appendicoliths may be transient and in most short-term follow-up studies have a low risk of subsequent acute appendicitis. The risk of subsequent appendicitis may be higher in those presenting with abdominal pain or those younger than 19 yr of age. The lifetime risk for the development of appendicitis in patients with an incidental appendicolith is approximately 5%.

Radiographically detected incidental appendicoliths are usually managed with observation, planned follow up, and patient education for signs of an acute appendicitis, while those detected during laparoscopy to rule out acute appendicitis (when the appendix is normal in appearance) may or may not undergo appendectomy. After discussing the risks and benefits with the family, and persistence of the appendicolith, some conclude that an elective appendectomy may be indicated.

Bibliography is available at Expert Consult.

Chapter 344
Surgical Conditions of the Anus and Rectum

344.1 Anorectal Malformations
Begum Akay and Michael D. Klein

In understanding the spectrum of anorectal anomalies, it is necessary to consider the importance of the sphincter complex, a mass of muscle fibers surrounding the anorectum (Fig. 344-1). This complex is the combination of the puborectalis, levator ani, external and internal sphincters, and the superficial external sphincter muscles, all meeting at the rectum. Anorectal malformations are defined by the relationship of the rectum to this complex and include varying degrees of stenosis to complete atresia. The incidence is 1 per 3,000 live births. Significant long-term concerns focus on bowel control and urinary and sexual functions.

EMBRYOLOGY

The hindgut forms early as the part of the primitive gut tube that extends into the tail fold in the 2nd wk of gestation. At about day 13, it develops a ventral diverticulum, the allantois or primitive bladder. The junction of allantois and hindgut become the cloaca, into which the genital, urinary, and intestinal tubes empty. This is covered by a cloacal membrane. The urorectal septum descends to divide this common channel by forming lateral ridges, which grow in and fuse by

the middle of the 7th wk. Opening of the posterior portion of the membrane (the anal membrane) occurs in the 8th wk. Failures in any part of these processes can lead to the clinical spectrum of anogenital anomalies.

Imperforate anus can be divided into low lesions, where the rectum has descended through the sphincter complex, and high lesions, where it has not. Most patients with imperforate anus have a fistula. There is a spectrum of malformation in boys and girls. In boys, low lesions usually manifest with meconium staining somewhere on the perineum along the median raphe (Fig. 344-2A). Low lesions in girls also manifest as a spectrum from an anus that is only slightly anterior on the perineal body to a fourchette fistula that opens on the moist mucosa of the introitus distal to the hymen (Fig. 344-3A). A high imperforate anus in a boy has no apparent cutaneous opening or fistula, but it usually has a fistula to the urinary tract, either the urethra or the bladder (Fig. 344-2B). Although there is occasionally a rectovaginal fistula, in girls, high lesions are usually cloacal anomalies in which the rectum, vagina, and urethra all empty into a common channel or cloacal stem of varying length (Fig. 344-3B). The interesting category of boys with imperforate anus and no fistula occurs mainly in children with trisomy 21.

ASSOCIATED ANOMALIES

There are many anomalies associated with anorectal malformations (Table 344-1). The most common are anomalies of the kidneys and urinary tract in conjunction with abnormalities of the sacrum. This complex is often referred to as the **caudal regression syndrome.** Boys with a rectovesical fistula and patients with a persistent cloaca have a 90% risk of urologic defects. Other common associated anomalies are cardiac anomalies and esophageal atresia with or without tracheoesophageal fistula. These can cluster in any combination in a patient. When combined, they are often accompanied by abnormalities of the radial aspect of the upper extremity and are termed the VATERR

Table 344-1	Associated Malformations

GENITOURINARY
Vesicoureteric reflux
Renal agenesis
Renal dysplasia
Ureteral duplication
Cryptorchidism
Hypospadias
Bicornuate uterus
Vaginal septums

VERTEBRAL
Spinal dysraphism
Tethered chord
Presacral masses
Meningocele
Lipoma
Dermoid
Teratoma

CARDIOVASCULAR
Tetralogy of Fallot
Ventricular septal defect
Transposition of the great vessels
Hypoplastic left-heart syndrome

GASTROINTESTINAL
Tracheoesophageal fistula
Duodenal atresia
Malrotation
Hirschsprung disease

CENTRAL NERVOUS SYSTEM
Spina bifida
Tethered cord

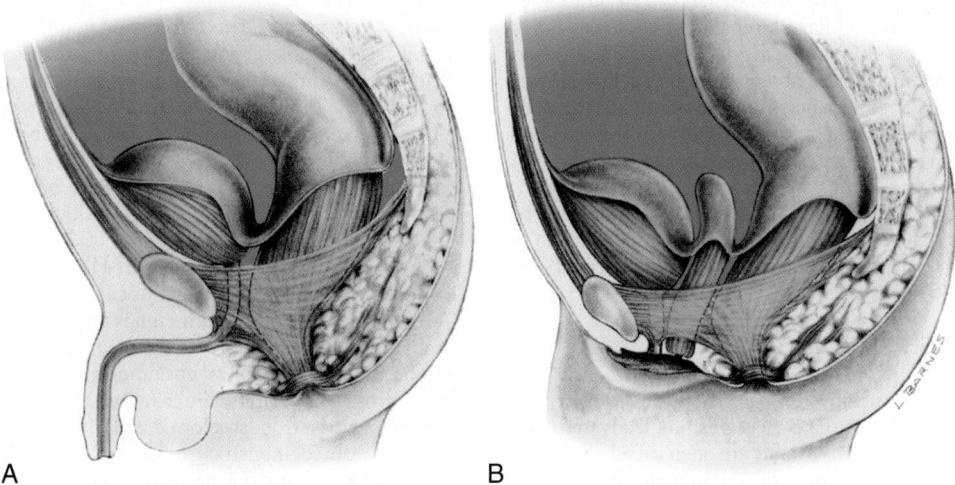

Figure 344-1 Normal anorectal anatomy in relation to pelvic structures. **A,** Male. **B,** Female. *(From Peña A: Atlas of surgical management of anorectal malformations, New York, 1989, Springer-Verlag, p. 3.)*

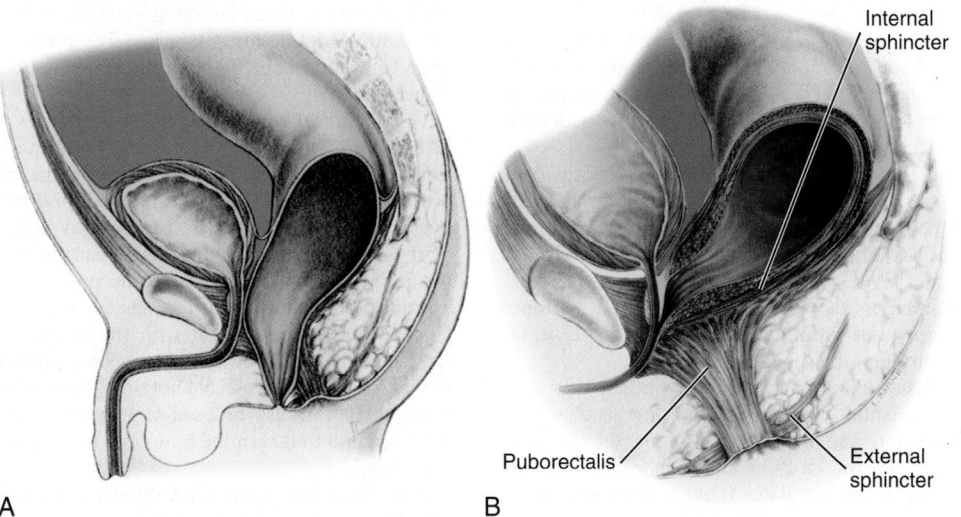

Figure 344-2 Imperforate anus in males. **A,** Low lesions. **B,** High lesions. *(From Peña A: Atlas of surgical management of anorectal malformations, New York, 1989, Springer-Verlag, pp. 7, 26.)*

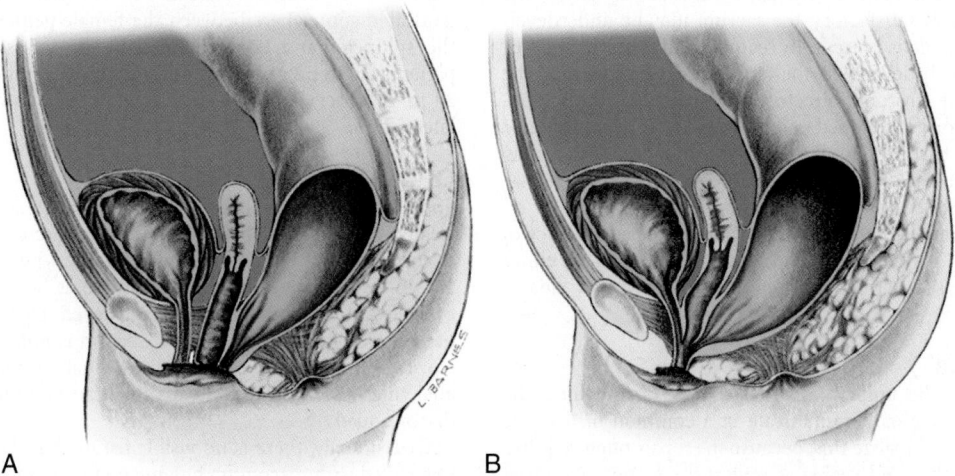

Figure 344-3 Imperforate anus in females. **A,** Vestibular fistula. **B,** Cloaca. *(From Peña A: Atlas of surgical management of anorectal malformations, New York, 1989, Springer-Verlag, pp. 50, 60.)*

(*v*ertebral, *a*nal, *t*racheal, *e*sophageal, *r*adial, *r*enal) or VACTERL (*v*ertebral, *a*nal, *c*ardiac, *t*racheal, *e*sophageal, *r*enal, *l*imb) anomalad.

A good correlation exists between the degree of sacral development and future function. Patients with an absent sacrum usually have permanent fecal and urinary incontinence. Spinal abnormalities and different degrees of dysraphism are often associated with these defects. Tethered cord occurs in approximately 25% of patients with anorectal malformations. Untethering of the cord can lead to improved urinary and rectal continence in some patients, although it seldom reverses established neurologic defects. The diagnosis of spinal defects can be established in the 1st 3 mo of life by spinal ultrasound. In older patients, MRI is needed.

MANIFESTATIONS AND DIAGNOSIS
Low Lesions
Examination of a newborn includes the inspection of the perineum. The absence of an anal orifice in the correct position leads to further evaluation. Mild forms of imperforate anus are often called *anal stenosis* or *anterior ectopic anus*. These are probably imperforate anus with a perineal fistula. The normal position of the anus on the perineum is approximately halfway (0.5 ratio) between the coccyx and the scrotum or introitus. Although symptoms, primarily constipation, have been attributed to anterior ectopic anus (ratio: <0.34 in girls, <0.46 in boys), many patients have no symptoms.

If no anus or fistula is visible, there may be a low lesion or "covered anus." In these cases, there are well-formed buttocks and often a thickened raphe or "bucket handle." After 24 hr, meconium bulging may be seen, creating a blue or black appearance. In these cases, an immediate perineal procedure can often be performed, followed by a dilation program.

In a boy, the perineal (cutaneous) fistula can track anteriorly along the median raphe across the scrotum and even down the penile shaft. This is usually a thin track, with a normal rectum often just a few millimeters from the skin. Extraintestinal anomalies are seen in <10% of these patients.

In a girl, a low lesion enters the vestibule or fourchette (the moist mucosa outside the hymen but within the introitus). In this case, the rectum has descended through the sphincter complex.

Children with a low lesion can usually be treated initially with perineal manipulation and dilation. Visualizing these low fistulas is so important in the evaluation and treatment that one should avoid passing a nasogastric tube for the 1st 24 hr to allow the abdomen and bowel to distend, pushing meconium down into the distal rectum.

High Lesions
In a boy with a high imperforate anus, the perineum appears flat. There may be air or meconium passed via the penis (urethra) when the fistula is high, entering the bulbar or prostatic urethra, or even the bladder. In **rectobulbar urethral fistulas** (the most common in boys), the sphincter mechanism is satisfactory, the sacrum may be underdeveloped, and an anal dimple is present. In **rectoprostatic urethral fistulas,** the sacrum is poorly developed, the scrotum may be bifid, and the anal dimple is near the scrotum. In **rectovesicular fistulas,** the sphincter mechanism is poorly developed and the sacrum is hypoplastic or absent. In boys with trisomy 21, all the features of a high lesion may be present, but there is no fistula, the sacrum and sphincter mechanisms are usually well developed, and the prognosis is good.

In girls with high imperforate anus, there may be the appearance of a rectovaginal fistula. A true rectovaginal fistula is rare. Most are either the fourchette fistulas described earlier or are forms of a cloacal anomaly.

Persistent Cloaca
In persistent cloaca, the embryologic stage persists in which the rectum, urethra, and vagina communicate in a common orifice, the cloaca. It is important to realize this, because the repair often requires repositioning the urethra and vagina as well as the rectum. Children of both sexes with a high lesion require a colostomy before repair.

Rectal Atresia
Rectal atresia is a rare defect occurring in only 1% of anorectal anomalies. It has the same characteristics in both sexes. The unique feature of this defect is that affected patients have a normal anal canal and a normal anus. The defect is often discovered while rectal temperature is being taken. An obstruction is present approximately 2 cm above the skin level. These patients need a protective colostomy. The functional prognosis is excellent because they have a normal sphincteric mechanism (and normal sensation), which resides in the anal canal.

APPROACH TO THE PATIENT
Evaluation includes identifying associated anomalies (see Table 344-1). Careful inspection of the perineum is important to determine the presence or absence of a fistula. If the fistula can be seen there, it is a low lesion. The invertogram or upside-down x-ray is of little value, but a prone crosstable lateral plain x-ray at 24 hr of life (to allow time for bowel distention from swallowed air) with a radiopaque marker on the perineum can demonstrate a low lesion by showing the renal gas bubble <1 cm from the perineal skin. A plain x-ray of the entire sacrum, including both iliac wings, is important to identify sacral anomalies and the adequacy of the sacrum. An abdominal-pelvic ultrasound and voiding cystourethrogram must be performed. The clinician should also pass a nasogastric tube to identify esophageal atresia and should obtain an echocardiogram. In boys with a high lesion, the voiding cystourethrogram often identifies the rectourinary fistula. In girls with a high lesion, more invasive evaluation, including vaginogram and endoscopy, is often necessary for careful detailing of the cloacal anomaly.

Good clinical evaluation and a urinalysis provide enough data in 80-90% of **male** patients to determine the need for a colostomy. Voluntary sphincteric muscles surround the most distal part of the bowel in cases of perineal and rectourethral fistulas, and the intraluminal bowel pressure must be sufficiently high to overcome the tone of those muscles before meconium can be seen in the urine or on the perineum. The presence of meconium in the urine and a flat bottom are considered indications for the creation of a colostomy. Clinical findings consistent with the diagnosis of a perineal fistula represent an indication for an anoplasty without a protective colostomy. Ultrasound is valuable not only for the evaluation of the urinary tract, but it can also be used to investigate spinal anomalies in the newborn and to determine how close to the perineum the rectum has descended.

More than 90% of the time, the diagnosis in **females** can be established on perineal inspection. The presence of a single perineal orifice is a cloaca. A palpable pelvic mass (hydrocolpos) reinforces this diagnosis. A vestibular fistula is diagnosed by careful separation of the labia, exposing the vestibule. The rectal orifice is located immediately in front of the hymen within the female genitalia and in the vestibule. A perineal fistula is easy to diagnose. The rectal orifice is located somewhere between the female genitalia and the center of the sphincter and is surrounded by skin. Less than 10% of these patients fail to pass meconium through the genitalia or perineum after 24 hr of observation. Those patients can require a prone crosstable lateral film.

OPERATIVE REPAIR
Sometimes a perineal fistula, if it opens in good position, can be treated by simple dilation. Hegar dilators are employed, starting with a No. 5 or 6 and letting the baby go home when the mother can use a No. 8. Twice-daily dilatations are done at home, increasing the size every few weeks until a No. 14 is achieved. By 1 yr of age, the stool is usually well formed and further dilation is not necessary. By the time No. 14 is reached, the examiner can usually insert a little finger. If the anal ring is soft and pliable, dilation can be reduced in frequency or discontinued.

Occasionally, there is no visible fistula, but the rectum can be seen to be filled with meconium bulging on the perineum, or a covered anus is otherwise suspected. If confirmed by plain x-ray or ultrasound of the perineum that the rectum is <1 cm from the skin, the clinician can do a minor perineal procedure to perforate the skin and then proceed with dilation or do a simple perineal anoplasty.

When the fistula orifice is very close to the introitus or scrotum, it is often appropriate to move it back surgically. This also requires postoperative dilation to prevent stricture formation. This procedure can be done any time from the newborn period to 1 yr. It is preferable to wait until dilatations have been done for several wk and the child is bigger. The anorectum is a little easier to dissect at this time. The posterior sagittal approach of Peña is used, making an incision around the fistula and then in the midline to the site of the posterior wall of the new location. The dissection is continued in the midline, using a muscle stimulator to be sure there is adequate muscle on both sides. The fistula must be dissected cephalad for several centimeters to allow posterior positioning without tension. If appropriate, some of the distal fistula is resected before the anastomosis to the perineal skin.

In children with a high lesion, a double-barrel colostomy is performed. This effectively separates the fecal stream from the urinary tract. It also allows the performance of an augmented pressure colostogram before repair to identify the exact position of the distal rectum and the fistula. The definitive repair or posterior sagittal anorectoplasty (PSARP) is performed at about 1 yr of age. A midline incision is made, often splitting the coccyx and even the sacrum. Using a muscle stimulator, the surgeon stays strictly in the midline and divides the sphincter complex and identifies the rectum. The rectum is then opened in the midline and the fistula is identified from within the rectum. This allows a division of the fistula without injury to the urinary tract. The rectum is then dissected proximally until enough length is gained to suture it to an appropriate perineal position. The muscles of the sphincter complex are then sutured around (and especially behind) the rectum.

Other operative approaches (such as an anterior approach) are used, but the most popular procedure is by laparoscopy. This operation allows division of the fistula under direct visualization and identification of the sphincter complex by transillumination of perineum. Other imaging techniques in the management of anorectal malformations include 3D endorectal ultrasound, intraoperative MRI and colonoscopy-assisted PSARPs, which may help perform a technically "better" operation. None of these other procedures or innovations has demonstrated improved outcomes.

A similar procedure can be done for female high anomalies with variations to deal with separating the vagina and rectum from within the cloacal stem. When the stem is longer than 3 cm, this is an especially difficult and complex procedure.

Usually, the colostomy can be closed 6 wks or more after the PSARP. Two weeks after any anal procedure, twice-daily dilatations are performed by the family. By doing frequent dilatations, each one is not so painful and there is less tissue trauma, inflammation, and scarring.

OUTCOME

The ability to achieve rectal continence depends on both motor and sensory elements. There must be adequate muscle in the sphincter complex and proper positioning of the rectum within the complex. There must also be intact innervation of the complex and of sensory elements as well as the presence of these sensory elements in the anorectum. Patients with low lesions are more likely to achieve true continence. They are also, however, more prone to constipation, which leads to overflow incontinence. It is very important that all these patients are followed closely, and that the constipation and anal dilation are well managed until toilet training is successful. Tables 344-2 and 344-3 outline the results of continence and constipation in relation to the malformation encountered.

Children with high lesions, especially boys with rectoprostatic urethral fistulas and girls with cloacal anomalies, have a poorer chance of being continent, but they can usually achieve a socially acceptable defecation (without a colostomy) pattern with a bowel management program. Often, the bowel management program consists of a daily

Table 344-2	Results of Surgical Treatment of Anorectal Malformations: Total Continence*	
TYPE		**PERCENTAGE**
LOW		
Perineal fistula		90
Rectal atresia/stenosis		75
Vestibular fistula		71
HIGH		
Imperforate with no fistula		60
Bulbar urethral fistula		50
Short cloaca		50
Prostatic fistula		31
Long cloaca		29
Bladder neck fistula		12

*Voluntary bowel movements, no soiling.
  Modified from Levitt MA, Peña A: Outcomes from the correction of anorectal malformations, Curr Opin Pediatr 17:394–401, 2005.

Table 344-3	Constipation and Type of Anogenital Malformation
TYPE	**PERCENTAGE**
Vestibular fistula	61
Bulbar urethral fistula	64
Rectal atresia/stenosis	50
Imperforate with no fistula	55
Perineal fistula	57
Long cloaca	35
Prostatic fistula	45
Short cloaca	40
Bladder neck fistula	16

Modified from Levitt MA, Peña A: Outcomes from the correction of anorectal malformations, Curr Opin Pediatr 17:394–401, 2005.

enema to keep the colon empty and the patient clean until the next enema. If this is successful, an *antegrade continence enema* (ACE) procedure, sometimes called the Malone or MACE procedure, can improve the patient's quality of life. These procedures provide access to the right colon either by bringing the appendix out the umbilicus in a nonrefluxing fashion or by putting a plastic button in the right lower quadrant to access the cecum. The patient can then sit on the toilet and administer the enema through the ACE, thus flushing out the entire colon. Antegrade regimens can produce successful 24 hr cleanliness rates of up to 95%. Of special interest is the clinical finding that most patients improve their control with growth. Patients who wore diapers or pull-ups to primary school are often in regular underwear by high school. Some groups have taken advantage of this evidence of psychologic influences to initiate behavior modification early with good results.

344.2 Anal Fissure

Begum Akay and Michael D. Klein

Anal fissure is a laceration of the anal mucocutaneous junction. It is an acquired lesion of unknown etiology. While likely secondary to the forceful passage of a hard stool, it is mainly seen in infants younger than 1 yr of age when the stool is frequently quite soft. Fissures may be the consequence and not the cause of constipation.

CLINICAL MANIFESTATIONS

A history of constipation is often described, with a recent painful bowel movement corresponding to the fissure formation after passing of hard stool. The patient then voluntarily retains stool to avoid another painful bowel movement, exacerbating the constipation, resulting in harder stools. Complaints of pain on defecation and bright red blood on the surface of the stool are often elicited.

The diagnosis is established by inspection of the perineal area. The infant's hips are held in acute flexion, the buttocks are separated to expand the folds of the perianal skin, and the fissure becomes evident as a minor laceration. Often a small skin appendage is noted peripheral to the lesion. This "skin tag" actually represents epithelialized granulomatous tissue, formed in response to chronic inflammation. Findings on rectal examination can include hard stool in the ampulla and rectal spasm.

TREATMENT

The parents must be counseled as to the origin of the laceration and the mechanism of the cycle of constipation. The goal is to ensure that the patient has soft stools to avoid overstretching the anus. The healing process can take several weeks or even several months. A single episode of impaction with passing of hard stool can exacerbate the problem. Treatment requires that the primary cause of the constipation be identified. The use of dietary and behavioral modification and a stool softener is indicated. Parents should titrate the dose of the stool softener based on the patient's response to treatment. Stool softening is best done by increasing water intake or using an oral polyethylene glycolate such as MiraLAX or GlycoLax. Surgical intervention, including stretching of the anus, "internal" anal sphincterotomy, or excision of the fissure, is not indicated or supported by scientific evidence.

Chronic anal fissures in older patients are associated with constipation, prior rectal surgery, Crohn disease, and chronic diarrhea. They are managed initially like fissures in infants, with stool softeners with the addition of sitz baths. Topical 0.2% glyceryl trinitrate reduces anal spasm and heals fissures, but it is often associated with headaches. Calcium channel blockers, such as 2% diltiazem ointment and 0.5% nifedipine cream, are more effective and cause fewer headaches than glyceryl trinitrate. Injection of botulinum toxin from 1.25-25 units is also effective and probably replicates chemically the action of internal sphincterotomy which is the most effective treatment in adults, although seldom used in children.

344.3 Perianal Abscess and Fistula

Begum Akay and Michael D. Klein

Perianal abscess, like all skin and soft-tissue infections, have become much more common since the year 2000 (a 4-fold increase in patients admitted to our hospital, and a 3-fold increase in patients presenting to the emergency room). These usually manifest in infancy and are of unknown etiology. Fistula appears to secondary to abscess rather than a cause. Links to congenitally abnormal crypts of Morgagni have been proposed, suggesting that deeper crypts (3-10 mm rather than the normal 1-2 mm) lead to trapped debris and cryptitis (Fig. 344-4).

Conditions associated with the risk of an anal fistula include Crohn disease, tuberculosis, pilonidal disease, hidradenitis, HIV, trauma, foreign bodies, dermal cysts, sacrococcygeal teratoma, actinomycosis, lymphogranuloma venereum and radiotherapy.

The most common organisms isolated from perianal abscesses are mixed aerobic (*Escherichia coli, Klebsiella pneumoniae, Staphylococcus aureus*) and anaerobic (*Bacteroides* spp., *Clostridium, Veillonella*) flora. Ten percent to 15% yield pure growth of *E. coli, S. aureus*, or *Bacteroides fragilis*. There is a strong male predominance in those affected who are younger than 2 yr of age. This imbalance corrects in older patients, where the etiology shifts to associated conditions such as inflammatory bowel disease, leukemia, or immunocompromised states.

CLINICAL MANIFESTATIONS

In younger patients, symptoms are usually mild and can consist of low-grade fever, mild rectal pain, and an area of perianal cellulitis. Often these spontaneously drain and resolve without treatment. In older patients with underlying predisposing conditions, the clinical course may be more serious. A compromised immune system can mask fever and allow rapid progression to toxicity and sepsis. Abscesses in these patients may be deeper in the ischiorectal fossa or even supralevator in contrast to those in younger patients, which are usually adjacent to the involved crypt.

Progression to fistula in patients with perianal abscesses occurs in up to 85% of cases and usually manifests with drainage from the perineal skin or multiple recurrences. Similar to abscess formation, fistulas have a strong male predominance. Histologic evaluation of fistula tracts typically reveals an epithelial lining of stratified squamous cells associated with chronic inflammation. It might also reveal an alternative etiology such as the granulomas of Crohn disease or even evidence of tuberculosis.

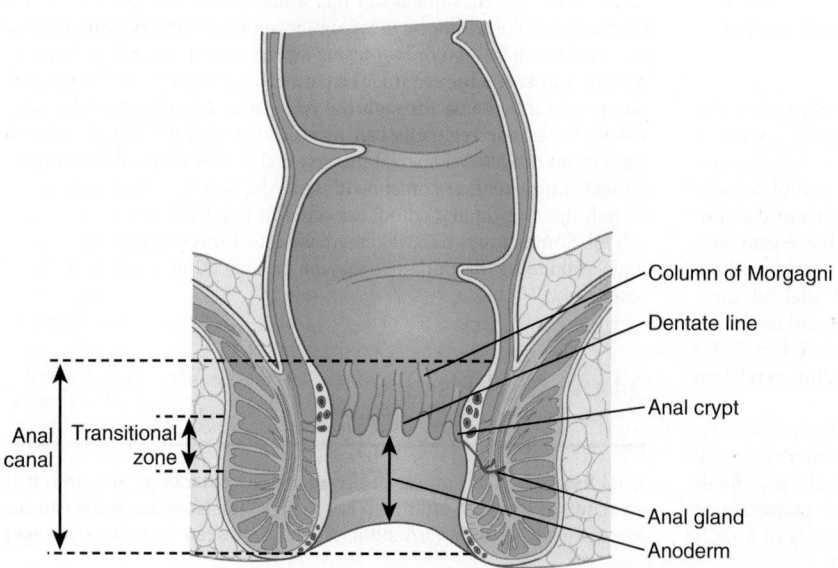

Anal canal | Transitional zone

Column of Morgagni
Dentate line
Anal crypt
Anal gland
Anoderm

Figure 344-4 Anatomy of the anal canal. *(Adapted from Brunicardi FC, Anderson DK, Billar TR, et al: Schwartz's principles of surgery, ed 8, New York, 2004, McGraw-Hill.)*

TREATMENT

Treatment is rarely indicated in infants with no predisposing disease because the condition is often self-limited. Even in cases of fistulization, conservative management (observation) is advocated because the fistula often disappears spontaneously. Antibiotics are not useful in these patients. When dictated by patient discomfort, abscesses may be drained under local anesthesia. Fistulas requiring surgical intervention may be treated by fistulotomy (unroofing or opening), fistulectomy (excision of the tract leaving it open to heal secondarily), or placement of a seton (heavy suture threaded through the fistula, brought out the anus and tied tightly to itself). In patients with inflammatory bowel disease topical tacrolimus has been effective.

Older children with predisposing diseases might also do well with minimal intervention. If there is little discomfort and no fever or other sign of systemic illness, local hygiene and antibiotics may be best. The danger of surgical intervention in an immunocompromised patient is the creation of an even larger, nonhealing wound. There certainly are such patients with serious systemic symptoms who require more aggressive intervention along with treatment of the predisposing condition. Broad-spectrum antibiotic coverage must be administered and wide excision and drainage are mandatory in cases involving sepsis and expanding cellulitis.

Fistulas in older patients are mainly associated with Crohn disease, a history of pull-through surgery for the treatment of Hirschsprung disease, or, in rare cases, tuberculosis. Those fistulas are often resistant to therapy and require treatment of the predisposing condition.

Complications of treatment include recurrence and, rarely, incontinence.

344.4 Hemorrhoids
Begum Akay and Michael D. Klein

Hemorrhoidal disease does occur in children and adolescents, often related to a diet deficient in fiber and poor hydration. In younger children, the presence of hemorrhoids should also raise the suspicion of portal hypertension. A third of patients with hemorrhoids require treatment.

CLINICAL MANIFESTATIONS

Presentation depends on the location of the hemorrhoids. External hemorrhoids occur below the dentate line (see Figs. 344-4 and 344-5)

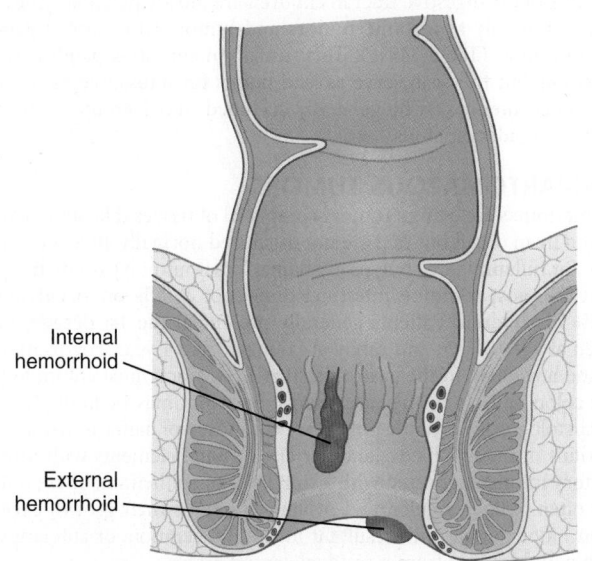

Figure 344-5 Formation of hemorrhoids.

and are associated with extreme pain and itching, often due to acute thrombosis. Internal hemorrhoids are located above the dentate line and manifest primarily with bleeding, prolapse, and occasional incarceration.

TREATMENT

In most cases, conservative management with dietary modification, decreased straining, and avoidance of prolonged time spent sitting on the toilet results in resolution of the condition. Discomfort may be treated with topical analgesics or anti-inflammatories such as Anusol (pramoxine) and Anusol-HC (hydrocortisone) and sitz baths. The natural course of thrombosed hemorrhoid involves increasing pain, which peaks at 48-72 hr, with gradual remission as the thrombus organizes and involutes over the next 1-2 wk. In cases where the patient with external hemorrhoids presents with excruciating pain soon after the onset of symptoms, thrombectomy may be indicated. This is best accomplished with local infiltration of bupivacaine 0.25% with epinephrine 1 : 200,000, followed by incision of the vein or skin tag and extraction of the clot. This provides immediate relief; recurrence is rare and further follow-up is unnecessary.

Internal hemorrhoids can become painful when prolapse leads to incarceration and necrosis. Pain usually resolves with reduction of hemorrhoidal tissue. Surgical treatment is reserved for patients failing conservative management. Techniques described in adults include excision, rubber banding, stapling, and excision using the LigaSure device. Given the infrequency of hemorrhoidal disease in children, and the need for general anesthesia to treat it, we have been quite satisfied with simple excision ligating the vein proximal and using the Bovie for hemostasis.

Complications are rare (<5%) and include recurrence, bleeding, infection, nonhealing wounds, and fistula formation.

344.5 Rectal Mucosal Prolapse
Begum Akay and Michael D. Klein

Rectal mucosal prolapse is the exteriorization of the rectal mucosa through the anus. In the unusual occurrence when all of the layers of the rectal wall are included, it is called **procidentia or rectocele.** Most cases of rectal tissue protruding through the anus are prolapse and not polyps, hemorrhoids, intussusception, or other tissue.

Most cases of prolapse are idiopathic. The onset is often between 1 and 5 yr of age. It usually occurs when the child begins standing and then resolves by approximately 3-5 yr of age when the sacrum has taken its more adult shape and the anal lumen is oriented posteriorly. Thus, the entire weight of the abdominal viscera is not pushing down on the rectum as it is earlier in development.

Other predisposing factors include intestinal parasites (particularly in endemic areas), malnutrition, diarrhea, ulcerative colitis, pertussis, Ehlers-Danlos syndrome, meningocele (more often associated with procidentia owing to the lack of perineal muscle support), cystic fibrosis, and chronic constipation. Patients treated surgically for imperforate anus can also have varying degrees of rectal mucosal prolapse. This is particularly common in patients with poor sphincteric development.

CLINICAL MANIFESTATIONS

Rectal mucosal prolapse usually occurs during defecation, especially during toilet training. Reduction of the prolapse may be spontaneous or accomplished manually by the patient or parent. In severe cases, the prolapsed mucosa becomes congested and edematous, making it more difficult to reduce. Rectal prolapse is usually painless or produces mild discomfort. If the rectum remains prolapsed after defecation, it can be traumatized by friction with undergarments, with resultant bleeding, wetness, and potentially, ulceration. The appearance of the prolapse varies from bright red to dark red and resembles a beehive. It can be as long as 10-12 cm. See Chapter 345 for a distinction from a prolapsed polyp.

TREATMENT

Initial evaluation should include tests to rule out any predisposing conditions, especially cystic fibrosis and sacral root lesions. Reduction of protrusion is aided by pressure with warm compresses. An easy method of reduction is to cover the finger with a piece of toilet paper, introduce it into the lumen of the mass, and gently push it into the patient's rectum. The finger is then immediately withdrawn. The toilet paper adheres to the mucous membrane, permitting release of the finger. The paper, when softened, is later expelled.

Conservative treatment consists of careful manual reduction of the prolapse after defecation, attempts to avoid excessive pushing during bowel movements (with patient's feet off the floor), use of laxatives and stool softeners to prevent constipation, avoidance of inflammatory conditions of the rectum, and treatment of intestinal parasitosis when present. If all this fails, surgical treatment may be indicated. Existing surgical options are associated with some morbidity, and therefore medical treatment should always be attempted first.

Sclerosing injections have been associated with complications such as neurogenic bladder. We have found linear cauterization effective and with few complications other than recurrence. In the operating room, the prolapse is recreated by traction on the mucosa. Linear burns are made through nearly the full thickness of the mucosa using electrocautery. One can usually make 8 linear burns on the outside and 4 on the inside of the prolapsed mucosa. In the immediate postoperative period, prolapse can still occur, but in the next several weeks, the burned areas contract and keep the mucosa within the anal canal. The Delorme mucosal sleeve resection addresses mucosal prolapse via a transanal approach by incising, prolapsing, and amputating the redundant mucosa. The resulting mucosal defect is then approximated with absorbable suture.

For patients with procidentia or full-thickness prolapse or intussusception of the rectosigmoid (usually from myelodysplasia or other sacral root lesions) other, more invasive options exist. Those most commonly in use by pediatric surgeons today include the following: A modification of the Thiersch procedure involves placing a subcutaneous suture to narrow the anal opening. Complications include obstruction, fecal impaction, and fistula formation. Laparoscopic rectopexy is effective and can be performed as an outpatient. The Altemeier perineal rectosigmoidectomy is a transanal, full-thickness resection of redundant bowel with a primary anastomosis to the anus.

344.6 Pilonidal Sinus and Abscess

Begum Akay and Michael D. Klein

The etiology of pilonidal disease remains unknown; 3 hypotheses explaining its origin have been proposed. The first states that trauma, such as can occur with prolonged sitting, impacts hair into the subcutaneous tissue, which serves as a nidus for infection. The second suggests that in some patients, hair follicles exist in the subcutaneous tissues, perhaps the result of some embryologic abnormality, and that they serve as a focal point for infection, especially with secretion of hair oils. The third speculates that motion of the buttocks disturbs a particularly deep midline crease and works bacteria and hair beneath the skin. This theory arises from the apparent improved short-term and long-term results of operations that close the wound off the midline, obliterating the deep natal cleft.

Pilonidal disease usually manifests in adolescents or young adults with significant hair over the midline sacral and coccygeal areas. It can occur as an acute abscess with a tender, warm, flocculent, erythematous swelling or as draining sinus tracts. This disease does not resolve with nonoperative treatment. An acute abscess should be drained and packed open with appropriate anesthesia. Oral broad-spectrum antibiotics covering the usual isolates (*S. aureus* and *Bacteroides* species) are prescribed, and the patient's family withdraws the packing over the course of a week. When the packing has been totally removed, the area can be kept clean by a bath or shower. The wound usually heals completely in 6 wk. Once the wound is healed, most pediatric surgeons feel that elective excision should be scheduled to avoid recurrence. There are some reports, however, this is only necessary if the disease recurs. Usually, patients who present with sinus tracts are managed with a single elective excision.

Most surgeons carefully identify the extent of each sinus tract and excise all skin and subcutaneous tissue involved to the fascia covering the sacrum and coccyx. Some close the wound in the midline; others leave it open and packed for healing by secondary intention. This method has been modified by the application of a vacuum-assisted (VAC sponge) dressing, This is a system that applies continuous suction to a porous dressing. It is usually changed every 3 days and can be done at home with the assistance of a nurse. Some marsupialize the wound by suturing the skin edges down to the exposed fascia covering the sacrum and coccyx. There appears to be improved success with excision and closure in such a way that the suture line is not in the midline. Currently there appears to be enthusiasm for less radical methods that Bascon has introduced, treating simple sinus tracts with small local procedures and limiting excision to only diseased tissues, while still keeping the incision off the midline. Recurrence or wound-healing problems are relatively common, occurring in 9-27% of cases. The variety of treatments and procedures currently being described indicates that all of them are associated with significant complications and delays in return to normal activity. Still, it is rare for problems to persist beyond 1-2 yr. Recalcitrant cases are treated by a large, full-thickness gluteal flap or skin grafting.

A simple dimple located in the midline intergluteal cleft, at the level of the coccyx, is seen relatively commonly in normal infants. No evidence indicates that this little sinus provokes any problems for the patient. An open dermal sinus is an asymptomatic, benign condition that does not require operative intervention.

Bibliography is available at Expert Consult.

Chapter **345**
Tumors of the Digestive Tract
Lydia J. Donoghue

Tumors of the digestive tract in children are mostly polypoid. They are also commonly syndromic tumors and tumors with known genetic identification (Table 345-1). They usually manifest as painless rectal bleeding, but they can serve as lead points for intussusception. Most intestinal tumors can be generally classified into 2 groups: hamartomatous or adenomatous.

HAMARTOMATOUS TUMORS

Hamartomas are benign tumors composed of tissues that are normally found in an organ but that are not organized normally. Juvenile, retention, or inflammatory polyps are hamartomatous polyps, which represent the most common intestinal tumors of childhood, occurring in 1-2% of children. Patients generally present in the 1st decade, most often at ages 2-5 yr, and rarely at younger than 1 year. Polyps may be found anywhere in the gastrointestinal (GI) tract, most commonly in the colon or rectum; they are often solitary but may be multiple.

Histologically, juvenile polyps are composed of hamartomatous collections of mucus-filled glandular and stromal elements with inflammatory infiltrate, covered with a thin layer of epithelium. These polyps are often bulky, vascular, and prone to bleed as their growth exceeds their blood supply with resultant mucosal ulceration, or autoamputation with bleeding from a residual central artery.

Table 345-1	General Features of the Inherited Colorectal Cancer Syndromes					
SYNDROME	**POLYP DISTRIBUTION**	**AGE OF ONSET**	**RISK OF COLON CANCER**	**GENETIC LESION**	**CLINICAL MANIFESTATIONS**	**ASSOCIATED LESIONS**
HAMARTOMATOUS POLYPS						
Juvenile polyposis	Large and small intestine, gastric polyps	1st decade	~10-50%	*PTEN, SMAD4, BMPR1A* Autosomal dominant	Possible rectal bleeding, abdominal pain, intussusception	Congenital abnormalities in 20% of the nonfamilial type, clubbing, AV malformations
Peutz-Jeghers syndrome	Small and large intestine	1st decade	Increased	*LKB1/STK11* Autosomal dominant	Possible rectal bleeding, abdominal pain, intussusception	Orocutaneous melanin pigment spots
Cowden syndrome	Colon	2nd decade	Not increased	*PTEN* gene	Macrocephaly, breast/thyroid/endometrial cancers, developmental delay	
Bannayan-Riley-Ruvalcaba syndrome	Colon	2nd decade	Not increased	*PTEN* gene	Macrocephaly, speckled penis, thyroid/breast cancers, hemangiomas, lipomas	
ADENOMATOUS POLYPS						
Familial adenomatous polyposis (FAP)	Large intestine, often >100	16 yr (range: 8-34 yr)	100%	5q (*APC* gene), autosomal dominant	Rectal bleeding, abdominal pain, bowel obstruction	Desmoids, CHRPE, upper GI polyps, osteoma, hepatoblastoma, thyroid cancer
Attenuated familial adenomatous polyposis (AFAP)	Colon (fewer in number)	>18 yr	Increased	*APC* gene	Same as FAP	Fewer associated lesions
MYH-associated polyposis	Colon	>20yr	High risk	*MYH* autosomal recessive	Same as FAP	May be confused with sporadic FAP or AFAP; few extraintestinal findings
Gardner syndrome	Large and small intestine	16 yr (range: 8-34 yr)	100%	5q (*APC* gene)	Rectal bleeding, abdominal pain, bowel obstruction	Desmoid tumors, multiple osteomas, fibromas, epidermoid cysts
Hereditary nonpolyposis colon cancer, (Lynch syndrome)	Large intestine	40 yr	30%	DNA mismatch repair genes (*MMR*) Autosomal dominant	Rectal bleeding, abdominal pain, bowel obstruction	Other tumors (e.g., ovary, ureter, pancreas, stomach)

AV, Arteriovenous; CHRPE, congenital hypertrophy of the retinal pigment epithelium; GI, gastrointestinal.

Patients often present with painless rectal bleeding after defecation. Bleeding is generally scant and intermittent; rarely iron deficiency anemia is the chief presenting symptom. Extensive bleeding can occur but is generally self-limited, requiring supportive care until the bleeding stops spontaneously after autoamputation. Occasionally endoscopic polypectomy is required for control of bleeding. Abdominal pain or cramps are uncommon unless associated with intussusception. Patients can present with prolapse, with a dark, edematous, pedunculated mass protruding from the rectum. Mucus discharge and pruritus are associated with prolapse.

Patients presenting with rectal bleeding require thorough work-up; differential diagnosis includes anal fissure, other intestinal polyposis syndromes, Meckel diverticulum, inflammatory bowel disease, intestinal infections, Henoch-Schönlein purpura, or coagulopathy.

Diagnosis and therapy are best accomplished via endoscopy. Polyps may be visualized via air-contrast barium enema, but this provides no therapeutic advantage and is uncomfortable and usually performed without sedation or anesthesia. Colonoscopy affords opportunity for biopsy, polypectomy by snare cautery, and visualization of synchronous lesions; up to 50% of children have 1 or more additional polyps,

and approximately 20% may have more than 5 polyps. Retrieved polyps should be sent for histologic evaluation for definitive diagnosis.

Juvenile Polyposis Syndrome
Patients with juvenile polyposis syndrome (JPS) present with multiple juvenile polyps, ≥5 but typically 50-200. Polyps may be isolated to the colon or distributed throughout the GI tract. There is often a family history (20-50%) with an autosomal dominant pattern of variable penetrance. Alterations in transforming growth factor-β pathways have been identified in some JPS patients and families; mutations in *SMAD4* or *BMPR1A* are found in 50-60% of patients with JPS. Genetic testing is available for both of these mutations. Clinical diagnosis of JPS is established by presence of 1 of the following: 3-10 polyps on colonoscopy; polyps outside the colon; or any number of polyps in a patient with a family history of JPS.

Histologically, these polyps are identical to solitary juvenile polyps; however, the GI malignancy risk is greatly increased (10-50%). Most malignancy is colorectal, although gastric, upper GI, and pancreatic tumors have been described. The risk of malignancy is greater in patients with >3 polyps and a positive family history. These patients should therefore undergo routine esophagogastroduodenoscopy, colonoscopy, and upper GI contrast studies. Serial polypectomy or polyp biopsy should be undertaken if possible. If dysplasia or malignant degeneration is found, a total colectomy is indicated.

Juvenile polyposis of infancy is characterized by early polyp formation (younger than 2 yr of age) and may be associated with protein-losing enteropathy, hypoproteinemia, anemia, failure to thrive, and intussusception. Early endoscopic or surgical intervention may be needed.

Peutz-Jeghers Syndrome

Peutz-Jeghers syndrome (PJS) is a rare autosomal dominant disorder (incidence: ~1:120,000 total population) characterized by mucocutaneous pigmentation and extensive GI hamartomatous polyposis. Macular pigmented lesions may be dark brown to dark blue and are found primarily around the lips and oral mucosa, although these lesions may also be found on the hands, feet, or perineum. Lesions can fade by puberty or adulthood.

Polyps are primarily found in the small intestine (in order of prevalence: jejunum, ileum, duodenum) but may also be colonic or gastric. Histologically, polyps are defined by normal epithelium surrounding bundles of smooth muscle arranged in a branching or frondlike pattern. Symptoms arising from GI polyps in PJS are similar to those of other polyposis syndromes, namely bleeding and abdominal cramping from obstruction or recurrent intussusception. Patients can require repeated laparotomies and intestinal resections.

The diagnosis of PJS is made clinically in patients with histologically proven hamartomatous polyps if 2 of 3 conditions are met: positive family history with an autosomal dominant inheritance pattern, mucocutaneous hyperpigmentation, and small bowel polyposis. Genetic testing can reveal mutations in *LKB1/STK11*; (19p13.3), a serine-threonine kinase that acts as a tumor-suppressor gene. Up to 94% of patients with clinical characteristics of PJS have a mutation at this locus. Only 50% of patients with PJS have an affected family member, suggesting a high rate of spontaneous mutations.

Patients with PJS have increased risk of GI and extraintestinal malignancies. Lifetime cancer risk has been reported from 47-93%. Colorectal, breast, and reproductive tumors are most common. GI surveillance should begin in childhood (by age 8 yr or when symptoms occur) with upper and lower endoscopy. The small bowel may be evaluated radiographically, with enteroscopy, or with wireless capsule endoscopy. Polyps larger than 1.5 cm should be removed. Screening for breast, gynecologic, and testicular cancers should be routine after age 18 yr.

PTEN Hamartoma Tumor Syndromes

Mutations in the tumor-suppressor gene protein tyrosine phosphatase and tensin homolog (*PTEN*) are associated with several rare autosomal dominant syndromes, including Cowden syndrome and Bannayan-Riley-Ruvalcaba syndrome. These patients present with multiple hamartomas in skin (99%), brain, breast, thyroid, endometrium, and GI tract (60%). Patients are at increased risk for breast and thyroid malignancies; the risk of GI cancer does not appear to be elevated.

ADENOMATOUS TUMORS
Adenomatous Polyposis Coli-Associated Polyposis Syndromes

Familial adenomatous polyposis (FAP) is the most common genetic polyposis syndrome (incidence 1:5,000 to 1:17,000 persons) and is characterized by numerous adenomatous polyps throughout the colon, as well as extraintestinal manifestations. FAP and related syndromes (attenuated FAP; Gardner and Turcot syndromes) are linked to mutations in the adenomatous polyposis coli *(APC)* gene, a tumor suppressor mapped to 5q21. *APC* regulates degradation of β-catenin, a protein with roles in regulation of the cytoskeleton, tissue architecture organization, cell migration and adherence, and numerous other functions. Intracellular accumulation of β-catenin may be responsible for colonic epithelial cell proliferation and adenoma formation. More than 400

APC mutations have been described, and up to 30% of patients present with no family history (spontaneous mutations).

Polyps generally develop late in the 1st decade of life or in adolescence (mean age of presentation is 16 yr). At the time of diagnosis, 5 or more adenomatous polyps are present in the colon and rectum. By young adulthood the number typically increases to hundreds or even thousands. Adenomatous polyps (or adenomas) are precancerous lesions within the surface epithelium of the intestine, displaying various degrees of dysplasia. Without intervention, the risk of developing colon cancer is 100% by the 5th decade of life (average age of cancer diagnosis is 40 yr). Other GI adenomas can develop, particularly in the stomach and duodenum (50-90%). The risk of periampullary or duodenal carcinoma is significantly elevated (4-12% lifetime risk). Young patients with FAP are also at increased risk for developing hepatoblastoma (1.6% before age 5 yr).

Extraintestinal manifestations of FAP may be present from birth or develop in early childhood. Lesions include congenital hypertrophy of retinal pigment epithelium, desmoid tumors, epidermoid cysts, osteomas, fibromas, and lipomas. Many of these benign soft-tissue tumors appear before intestinal polyps develop. Expression of extraintestinal findings can depend on location of mutation on the *APC* gene.

Other syndromes associated with *APC* mutations include Gardner syndrome, classically characterized by multiple colorectal polyps, desmoid tumors, and soft-tissue tumors including fibromas, osteomas (typically mandibular), epidermoid cysts, and lipomas. Once thought to be a distinct clinical entity, Gardner syndrome shares many characteristics with FAP. Up to 20% of FAP patients present with the classic extraintestinal manifestations once associated with Gardner syndrome. Some (but not all) cases of Turcot syndrome are also related to *APC*. These patients present with colorectal polyposis and primary brain tumors (medulloblastoma). Attenuated FAP is characterized by a significantly increased risk of colorectal cancer but fewer polyps than classic FAP (average: 30 polyps). The average age of cancer diagnosis in this form of FAP is 50-55 yr. Upper GI tumors and extraintestinal manifestations may be present but are less common.

The clinical presentation of FAP is variable. Polyps are generally asymptomatic initially (and might remain so). If symptoms develop, they can include rectal bleeding (possibly with secondary anemia), cramping, and diarrhea. The presence of symptoms at presentation does not correlate with malignant changes. Diagnosis should be suspected from family history, and ensuing sigmoidoscopy or colonoscopy is confirmatory. Histologic examination of biopsied polyps reveals adenomatous architecture (as opposed to inflammatory or hamartomatous polyps found in other polyposis syndromes) with varying degrees of dysplasia. Genetic testing for *APC* mutations is clinically available, and index patients should be tested. If a mutation is identified, affected family members should be screened and appropriate genetic counseling should be provided. If the index patient does not demonstrate a defined mutation, family members may undergo genetic testing, which might identify novel *APC* mutations. Children with identified *APC* mutations must undergo careful surveillance, with sigmoidoscopy every 1-2 yr. Once polyps are identified, colonoscopy should be performed annually. Patients should also have upper endoscopy after development of colonic polyps to monitor for gastric and especially duodenal lesions.

Treatment of FAP requires prophylactic proctocolectomy to prevent cancer. Ileoanal pull-through procedures restore bowel continuity, with acceptable functional outcomes. Resection should be done once polyposis has become extensive (>20-30) or by the mid-teens. Nonsteroidal antiinflammatory agents, such as sulindac, and cyclooxygenase-2 inhibitors, such as celecoxib, might inhibit polyp progression. No guidelines have been established, however, and their efficacy in preventing malignant transformation of existing polyps is unknown.

Carcinoma

Primary carcinomas of the small bowel or colon are extremely rare in children. Development of adenocarcinoma in adolescence or early adulthood may be associated with a genetic predisposition or syndrome such as FAP, hereditary nonpolyposis colon carcinoma, PJS, or inflammatory bowel disorders such as Crohn disease or ulcerative colitis.

Colorectal carcinoma, though rare (reported incidence of 1 case per 1,000,000 persons younger than 19 yr of age), is the most common primary GI carcinoma in children. Many cases are spontaneous (i.e., not associated with a genetic predisposition or syndrome). Histologically, tumors tend to be poorly differentiated and pathologically aggressive. Patients may be asymptomatic, or they present with nonspecific signs and symptoms such as abdominal pain, constipation, and vomiting. Delay in diagnosis is common. Many patients present with advanced-stage disease, with microscopic or gross metastases at the time of diagnosis. Surgical resection is the primary treatment modality, although with delayed presentation and advanced-stage disease, complete resection may not be possible. Chemotherapy and radiation have a limited role in patients with metastatic disease.

OTHER GASTROINTESTINAL TUMORS

Lymphoma

Lymphoma is the most common GI malignancy in the pediatric population. Approximately 30% of children with non-Hodgkin lymphoma present with abdominal tumors. Immunocompromised patients have an increased incidence of lymphoma. Predisposing conditions include HIV/AIDS, agammaglobulinemia, long-standing celiac disease, and bone marrow or solid-organ transplantation. Lymphoma can occur anywhere in the GI tract, but it most commonly occurs in distal small bowel and ileocecal region. Presenting symptoms include crampy abdominal pain, vomiting, obstruction, bleeding, or palpable mass. Lymphoma should be considered in patients older than 3 yr of age who present with intussusception.

Nodular Lymphoid Hyperplasia

Lymphoid follicles in the lamina propria and submucosa of the gut normally aggregate in Peyer patches, most prominently in the distal ileum. These follicles can become hyperplastic, forming nodules that protrude into the lumen of the bowel. Some suggested etiologies are infectious (classically *Giardia*), allergic, or immunologic. Nodular lymphoid hyperplasia has been described in infants with enterocolitis secondary to dietary protein sensitivity. This phenomenon has also been described in patients with inflammatory bowel disease and Castleman disease. Patients may be asymptomatic or may present with abdominal pain, rectal bleeding, diarrhea, or intussusception. Nodular lymphoid hyperplasia usually resolves spontaneously and rarely requires therapy; in cases with severe pain or bleeding, corticosteroids may be effective.

Carcinoid Tumor

Carcinoids are neuroendocrine tumors of enterochromaffin cells, which can occur throughout the GI tract, but in children they are typically found in the appendix. This is often an incidental diagnosis at the time of appendectomy. Complete resection of small tumors (<1 cm) with clear surgical margins is curative. Appendiceal tumors >2 cm mandate further bowel resection. Carcinoid tumors outside the appendix (small intestine, rectum, stomach) are more likely to metastasize. Metastatic carcinoid tumor within the liver can give rise to the carcinoid syndrome. Serotonin, 5-hydroxytryptophan, or histamine are elaborated by the tumor, and elevated serum levels cause cramps, diarrhea, vasomotor disturbances (flushing), bronchoconstriction, and right-heart failure. The diagnosis is confirmed by elevated urinary 5-hydroxyindoleacetic acid. Symptomatic relief of carcinoid symptoms may be achieved with administration of somatostatin analogs (octreotide).

Leiomyoma

Leiomyomas are rare benign tumors that can arise anywhere in the GI tract, although most often in the stomach, jejunum, or distal ileum. Age of presentation is variable, from the newborn period through adolescence. Patients may be asymptomatic or can present with an abdominal mass, obstruction, intussusception, volvulus, or pain and bleeding from central necrosis of the tumor. Surgical resection is the treatment of choice. Pathologically, these tumors may be difficult to distinguish from malignant leiomyosarcomas. Smooth muscle tumors occur with increased incidence in children with HIV or those requiring immunosuppression after transplantation.

Gastrointestinal Stromal Cell Tumors

Gastrointestinal stromal cell tumors (GISTs) are intestinal mesenchymal tumors that probably arise from interstitial cells of Cajal or their precursors. Historically, these may have been diagnosed as tumors of smooth muscle or neural cell origin. The World Health Organization recognized GIST in 1990 as a distinct neoplasm. Typically GISTs arise in adults, after the 3rd decade of life. Cases have also been reported in the pediatric population, generally in adolescents. In the pediatric population tumors are most commonly found in the stomach, though they can occur anywhere in the GI tract or even the mesentery or omentum. Patients may be asymptomatic or can present with an abdominal mass, lower GI bleeding, or obstruction. Treatment consists of surgical en bloc resection of local disease. Recurrence rates are high and early postoperative surveillance is recommended. GISTs occurring in adults are typically associated with mutation in the *KIT* oncogene. This mutation is less commonly found in pediatric GISTs (~15%). Adjuvant therapy for *KIT*⁺ lesions is imatinib or sunitinib, tyrosine kinase inhibitors that are available as oral therapy. Patients with persistent disease or metastases might benefit from treatment.

Vascular Tumors

Vascular malformations and hemangiomas are rare in children. The usual presentation is painless rectal bleeding, which may be chronic or acute, with massive or even fatal hemorrhage. There are usually no associated symptoms, although intussusception has been described. Half of patients have associated cutaneous hemangiomas or telangiectasias. These lesions may be associated with blue rubber bleb nevus syndrome or hereditary hemorrhagic telangiectasia. About half of these lesions are in the colon and can be identified on colonoscopy. During acute bleeding episodes, bleeding can be localized via nuclear medicine bleeding scans, mesenteric angiography, or endoscopy. Colonic bleeding may be controlled by endoscopic means. Surgical intervention is required only occasionally for isolated lesions.

Bibliography is available at Expert Consult.

Chapter 346
Inguinal Hernias
John J. Aiken and Keith T. Oldham

Inguinal hernias are one of the most common conditions seen in pediatric practice and the most common surgical procedure performed in pediatric surgical practice. The frequency of this condition in concert with its potential morbidity of ischemic injury to the intestine, testis, or ovary makes proper diagnosis and management an important part of daily practice for pediatric practitioners and pediatric surgeons. The overwhelming majority of inguinal hernias in infants and children are congenital **indirect** hernias (99%) as a consequence of a patent processus vaginalis (PV); a developmental structure important in testicular descent. The incidence of inguinal hernia in children is up to 10 times higher in boys than in girls. Two other types of inguinal hernia are **direct** (acquired) hernia (0.5-1.0%) and **femoral** hernia (<0.5%). Approximately 50% of inguinal hernias manifest clinically in the 1st yr of life, most in the 1st 6 mo. Premature infants have an incidence of inguinal hernia approaching 30%. The risk of incarceration and possible strangulation of an inguinal hernia is also greatest in the 1st yr of life (30-40%) and mandates prompt identification and operative repair to minimize morbidity and complications.

EMBRYOLOGY AND PATHOGENESIS

Indirect inguinal hernias in infants and children are congenital and result from an arrest of embryologic development; failure of obliteration of the PV rather than a weakness in the inguinal musculature. The pertinent developmental anatomy of indirect inguinal hernia relates to development of the gonads and descent of the testis through the internal ring and into the scrotum late in gestation. The testes descend from the urogenital ridge in the retroperitoneum to the area of the internal ring by about 28 wk of gestation. The final descent of the testes into the scrotum occurs late in gestation between weeks 28 and 36. The testis is preceded in descent to the scrotum by the gubernaculum and the PV. The PV, an outpouring of peritoneum in the lower abdomen, is present in the developing fetus at 12 wk gestation that develops lateral to the deep inferior epigastric vessels and descends anteriorly along the spermatic cord within the cremasteric fascia through the internal inguinal ring. The testis accompanies the PV as it exits the abdomen and descends into the scrotum. The gubernaculum testis forms from the mesonephros (developing kidney), attaches to the lower pole of the testis, and directs the testis through the internal ring, inguinal canal and into the scrotum. The testis passes through the inguinal canal in a few days but takes about 4 wk to migrate from the external ring to the scrotum. The cord-like structures of the gubernaculum occasionally pass to ectopic locations (perineum or femoral region), resulting in ectopic testes.

In the last few weeks of gestation or shortly after birth, the layers of the PV normally fuse together and obliterate the patency from the peritoneal cavity through the inguinal canal to the testis. The PV also obliterates just above the testes, and the portion of the PV that envelops the testis becomes the tunica vaginalis. In girls, the PV obliterates earlier, at approximately 7 mo of gestation, and may explain why girls demonstrate a much lower incidence of inguinal hernia. *Failure of the PV to close permits fluid or abdominal viscera to escape the peritoneal cavity into the extraabdominal inguinal canal and accounts for a variety of inguinal–scrotal abnormalities seen in infancy and childhood.* The ovaries descend into the pelvis from the urogenital ridge but do not exit from the abdominal cavity. The cranial portion of the gubernaculum in girls differentiates into the ovarian ligament, and the inferior aspect of the gubernaculum becomes the round ligament, which passes through the internal ring and attaches to the labia majora. The PV in girls extends into the labia majora through the inguinal canal and is also known as the canal of Nuck. Involution of the left-sided PV precedes that of the right; which is consistent with the increased incidence of indirect inguinal hernias on the right side (60%).

Androgenic hormones, adequate end-organ receptors, and mechanical factors such as increased intra-abdominal pressure influence complete descent of the testis through the inguinal canal. The testes and spermatic cord structures (spermatic vessels and vas deferens) are located in the retroperitoneum but are affected by increases in intraabdominal pressure as a consequence of their intimate attachment to the descending PV. The genitofemoral nerve also has an important role: It innervates the cremaster muscle, which develops within the gubernaculum, and experimental division or injury to both nerves in the fetus prevents testicular descent. Failure of regression of smooth muscle (present to provide the force for testicular descent) might have a role in the development of indirect inguinal hernias. Several studies have investigated genes involved in the control of testicular descent for their role in closure of the patent PV, for example, hepatocyte growth factor and calcitonin gene-related peptide. Unlike in adult hernias, there does not appear to be any change in collagen synthesis associated with inguinal hernias in children (Fig. 346-1).

A **direct inguinal hernia** originates medial to the deep inferior epigastric vessels and is external to the cremasteric fascia; the hernia sac directly through the posterior wall of the inguinal canal. A **femoral hernia** originates medial to the femoral vein and descends inferior to the inguinal ligament along the femoral canal.

GENETICS

There is some genetic risk incurred for siblings of patients with inguinal hernias; the sisters of affected girls are at the highest risk, with a relative risk of 17.8. In general, the risk of brothers of a sibling is approximately 4-5, as is the risk of a sister of an affected brother. Both a multifactorial threshold model and autosomal dominance with incomplete penetrance and sex influence have been suggested as an explanation for this pattern of inheritance.

PATHOLOGY

Failure of closure of the PV leads to a number of common inguinal–scrotal conditions in infants and children including; inguinal hernia, scrotal hydrocele (communicating and noncommunicating), and hydrocele of the spermatic cord. Closure of the PV is often incomplete at birth and continues postnatally; the rate of patency is inversely proportional to the age of the child. It has been estimated that the patency rate of the PV is as high as 80% at birth and decreases to ≈40% during the 1st yr of life, and that ≈20% of boys have a persistent patency of the PV at 2 yr of age. Patency of the PV after birth is an opening from the abdominal cavity to the inguinal region and therefore a potential hernia, but not all patients will develop a clinical hernia. An inguinal hernia occurs clinically when intraabdominal contents escape

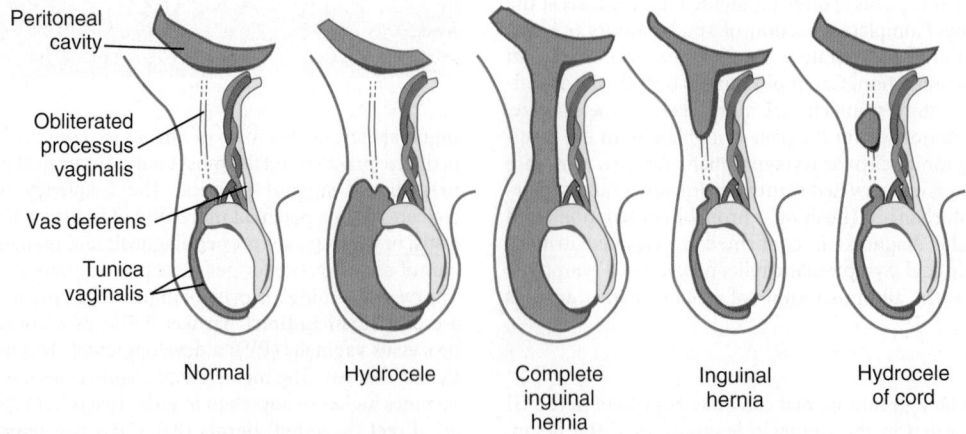

Figure 346-1 Hernia and hydroceles. *(Modified from Scherer LR III, Grosfeld JL: Inguinal and umbilical anomalies, Pediatr Clin North Am 40:1121–1131, 1993.)*

Table 346-1	Predisposing Factors for Hernias

Prematurity
Urogenital
- Cryptorchidism
- Exstrophy of the bladder or cloaca
- Ambiguous genitalia
- Hypospadias/epispadius
Increased peritoneal fluid
- Ascites
- Ventriculoperitoneal shunt
- Peritoneal dialysis catheter
Increased intraabdominal pressure
- Repair of abdominal wall defects
- Severe ascites (chylous)
- Meconium peritonitis
Chronic respiratory disease
- Cystic fibrosis
Connective tissue disorders
- Ehlers-Danlos syndrome
- Hunter-Hurler syndrome
- Marfan syndrome
- Mucopolysaccharidosis

the abdominal cavity and enter the inguinal region through the patency. Based on their location in the inguinal canal (lateral to the inferior epigastric vessels), these are **indirect** inguinal hernias but are rarely associated with a muscular weakness or defect, as is typical of an adult hernia. Depending on the extent of patency of the PV, the hernia may be confined to the inguinal region or pass down into the scrotum. Complete failure of obliteration of the PV, mostly seen in infants, predisposes to a complete inguinal hernia characterized by a protrusion of abdominal contents into the inguinal canal and possibly extending into the scrotum. Obliteration of the PV distally (around the testis) with patency proximally results in the classic indirect inguinal hernia with the protrusion in the inguinal canal.

A **hydrocele** is when only fluid enters the patent PV; the swelling may exist only in the scrotum (scrotal hydrocele), only along the spermatic cord in the inguinal region (hydrocele of the spermatic cord), or extend from the scrotum through the inguinal canal and even into the abdomen (abdominal–scrotal hydrocele). A hydrocele is termed a *communicating hydrocele* if it demonstrates fluctuation in size, often increasing in size after activity and, at other times, being smaller when the fluid decompresses into the peritoneal cavity. Occasionally, hydroceles develop in older children following trauma, inflammation, or tumors affecting the testis. Although reasons for failure of closure of the PV are unknown, it is more common in cases of testicular nondescent (cryptorchidism) and prematurity. In addition, persistent patency of the PV is twice as common on the right side, presumably related to later descent of the right testis and interference with obliteration of the PV from the developing inferior vena cava and external iliac vein. Table 346-1 lists the risk factors identified as contributing to the development of clinical inguinal hernia and that relate to conditions that predispose to failure of obliteration of the PV. Incidence of inguinal hernia in patients with cystic fibrosis is approximately 15%, believed to be related to an altered embryogenesis of the wolffian duct structures, which leads to an absent vas deferens in males with this condition. There is also an increased incidence of inguinal hernia in patients with **testicular feminization syndrome** and other disorders of sexual development. The rate of recurrence after repair of an inguinal hernia in patients with a connective tissue disorder approaches 50%, and often the diagnosis of connective tissue disorders in children results from investigation after development of a recurrent inguinal hernia.

INCIDENCE

The incidence of congenital indirect inguinal hernia in full-term newborn infants is estimated at 3.5-5.0%. The incidence of hernia in preterm and low birthweight infants is considerably higher, ranging from 9-11%, and approaches 30% in very-low birthweight infants (<1,000 g) and preterm infants (<28 wk of gestation). Inguinal hernia is much more common in boys than girls, with a male : female ratio of approximately 8 : 1. Approximately 60% of inguinal hernias occur on the right side, 30% are on the left side, and 10% are bilateral. The incidence of bilateral hernias is higher in girls and appears to be 20-40%. An increased incidence of congenital inguinal hernia has been documented in twins and in family members of patients with inguinal hernia. There is a history of another inguinal hernia in the family in 11.5% of patients.

CLINICAL PRESENTATION

An inguinal hernia typically appears as a bulge or mass in the inguinal region. In boys, the mass potentially extends through the inguinal area into the scrotum; in girls the mass typically occurs in the upper portion of the labia majora. The bulge or mass is most visible at times of irritability or increased intraabdominal pressure (crying, straining, coughing). It may be present at birth or might not appear until weeks, months, or years later. The bulge is most often first noted by the parents or on routine examination by the primary care physician. The classic history from the parents is of intermittent groin, labial, or scrotal swelling that spontaneously reduces but that is gradually enlarging or is more persistent and is becoming more difficult to reduce. The **hallmark signs** of an inguinal hernia on physical examination are a smooth, firm mass that emerges through the external inguinal ring lateral to the pubic tubercle and enlarges with increased intraabdominal pressure. When the child relaxes, the hernia typically reduces spontaneously or can be reduced by gentle pressure, first posteriorly to free it from the external ring and then upward toward the peritoneal cavity. In boys, the hernia sac contains intestines; female infants often have an ovary and fallopian tube in the hernia sac.

Methods used to demonstrate the hernia on examination vary depending on the age of the child. A quiet infant can be made to strain the abdominal muscles by stretching the infant out supine on the bed with legs extended and arms held straight above the head. Most infants struggle to get free, thus increasing the intraabdominal pressure and pushing out the hernia. Older patients can be asked to perform the Valsalva maneuver by blowing up a balloon or coughing. The older child should be examined while standing and examination after voiding also can be helpful. With increased intraabdominal pressure, the protruding mass is obvious on inspection of the inguinal region or can be palpated by an examining finger invaginating the scrotum to palpate at the external ring. Another test is the **"silk glove sign,"** which describes the feeling of the layers of the hernia sac as they slide over the spermatic cord structures with rolling of the spermatic cord beneath the index finger at the pubic tubercle. A femoral hernia appears as a protrusion on the medial aspect of the thigh, below the inguinal region and does not enter the scrotum or labia. In the absence of a bulge, the finding of increased thickness of the inguinal canal structures on palpation also suggests the diagnosis of an inguinal hernia. It is important on examination to note the position of the testes because retractile testes are common in infants and young boys and can mimic an inguinal hernia with a bulge in the region of the external ring. Because in the female patient approximately 20-25% of inguinal hernias are sliding hernias (the contents of the hernia sac are adherent within the sac and therefore not reducible), a fallopian tube or ovary can be palpated in the inguinal canal as a firm, slightly mobile, non-tender mass in the labia or inguinal canal.

As the majority of young child hernias reduce spontaneously, the physical examination in the office can be equivocal. Infants and children with a strong history suggestive of inguinal hernia and an equivocal clinical examination may be offered ultrasound or referral to a pediatric surgeon. In recent years, diagnostic laparoscopy has been increasingly used to evaluate for suspected inguinal hernia; particularly in infants where the risk of incarceration and potential injury to the intestines or testis is high. In an older child with low risk of incarceration, the parents can be educated and asked to observe for the bulge and take a digital image at home.

EVALUATION OF ACUTE INGUINAL–SCROTAL SWELLING

Commonly in pediatric practice, an inguinal–scrotal mass appears suddenly in an infant or child and is associated with discomfort. The **differential diagnosis** includes incarcerated inguinal hernia, acute hydrocele, torsion of an undescended testis, and suppurative inguinal lymphadenitis. Differentiating between the incarcerated inguinal hernia and the acute hydrocele is probably the most difficult. The infant or child with an incarcerated inguinal hernia is likely to have associated findings suggesting intestinal obstruction, such as colicky abdominal pain, abdominal distention, vomiting, and cessation of stool, and might appear ill. The infant with an acute hydrocele might have discomfort but is consolable and tolerates feedings without signs or symptoms suggesting intestinal obstruction. When the diagnosis is incarcerated inguinal hernia, plain radiographs typically demonstrate distended intestines with multiple air–fluid levels.

On examination of the child with the acute hydrocele, the clinician may note that the mass is somewhat mobile. In addition, in the area between the suspected hydrocele mass and the internal ring, the cord structures can appear only slightly thickened. With the incarcerated hernia, there is a lack of mobility of the groin mass and marked swelling or mass extending from the scrotal mass through the inguinal area and up to and including the internal ring. An experienced clinician can selectively use a bimanual examination to help differentiate groin abnormalities. The examiner palpates the internal ring per rectum, with the other hand placing gentle pressure on the inguinal region over the internal ring. In cases of an indirect inguinal hernia, an intraabdominal organ can be palpated extending through the internal ring.

Another method used in evaluation is **transillumination.** It must be noted that transillumination can be misleading because the thin wall of the infant's intestine can approximate that of the hydrocele wall and both might transilluminate. This is also the reason aspiration to determine the contents of a groin mass is discouraged. **Ultrasonography** can help distinguish between a hernia, a hydrocele, and lymphadenopathy. An expeditious diagnosis is important to avoid the potential complications of an incarcerated hernia, which can develop rapidly. Diagnostic laparoscopy has emerged as an effective and reliable tool in this setting by pediatric surgeons but requires general anesthesia.

The occurrence of suppurative adenopathy in the inguinal region can be confused with an incarcerated inguinal hernia. Examination of the watershed area of the inguinal lymph node might reveal a superficial infected or crusted lesion. In addition, the swelling associated with inguinal lymphadenopathy is typically located more inferior and lateral than the mass of an inguinal hernia, and there may be other associated enlarged nodes in the area. Torsion of an undescended testis can manifest as a painful erythematous mass in the groin. The absence of a gonad in the scrotum in the ipsilateral side should clinch this diagnosis.

Incarcerated Hernia

Incarceration is a common consequence of untreated inguinal hernia in infants and presents as a nonreducible mass in the inguinal canal, scrotum, or labia. Contained structures can include small bowel, appendix, omentum, colon, or, rarely, Meckel diverticulum. In girls, the ovary, fallopian tube, or both are commonly incarcerated. Rarely, the uterus in infants can also be pulled into the hernia sac. A **strangulated hernia** is one that is tightly constricted in its passage through the inguinal canal and, as a result, the hernia contents have become ischemic or gangrenous.

Although incarceration may be tolerated in adults for years, most nonreducible inguinal hernias in children, unless treated, rapidly progress to strangulation with potential infarction of the hernia contents or intestinal obstruction. Initially, pressure on the herniated viscera leads to impaired lymphatic and venous drainage. This leads, in turn, to

swelling of the herniated viscera, which further increases the compression in the inguinal canal, ultimately resulting in total occlusion of the arterial supply to the trapped viscera. Progressive ischemic changes take place, culminating in gangrene and/or perforation of the herniated viscera. The testis is at risk of ischemia because of compression of the testicular blood vessels by the strangulated hernia. In girls, herniation of the ovary places it at risk of strangulation and torsion. The incidence of incarceration of an inguinal hernia is between 12% and 17% throughout childhood; two-thirds of incarcerated hernias occur in the 1st yr of life. The greatest risk is in infants younger than 6 mo of age, with reported incidences of incarceration between 25% and 30%. The incidence of incarceration is slightly less in premature infants, although the reasons are unclear.

The symptoms of an incarcerated hernia are irritability, feeding intolerance, and abdominal distention in the infant; pain in the older child. Within a few hours, the infant becomes inconsolable; lack of flatus or stool signals complete intestinal obstruction. A somewhat tense, nonfluctuant mass is present in the inguinal region and can extend down into the scrotum or labia. The mass is well defined, firm, and does not reduce. With the onset of ischemic changes, the pain intensifies, and the vomiting becomes bilious or feculent. Blood may be noted in the stools. The mass is typically tender, and there is often edema and erythema of the overlying skin. The testes may be normal, demonstrate a reactive hydrocele, or may be swollen and hard on the affected side because of venous congestion resulting from compression of the spermatic veins and lymphatic channels at the inguinal ring by the tightly strangulated hernia mass. Abdominal radiographs demonstrate features of partial or complete intestinal obstruction, and gas within the incarcerated bowel segments may be seen below the inguinal ligament or within the scrotum.

Ambiguous Genitalia

Infants with disorders of sexual development commonly present with inguinal hernias, often containing a gonad, and require special consideration. In female infants with inguinal hernias, particularly if the presentation is bilateral inguinal masses, **testicular feminization syndrome** should be suspected (>50% of patients with testicular feminization have an inguinal hernia) (see Chapter 588). Conversely, the true incidence of testicular feminization in all female infants with inguinal hernias is difficult to determine but is approximately 1%. In phenotypic females, if the diagnosis of testicular feminization is suspected preoperatively, the child should be screened with a buccal smear for Barr bodies and appropriate genetic evaluation before proceeding with the hernia repair. The diagnosis of testicular feminization is occasionally made at the time of operation by identifying an abnormal gonad (testis) within the hernia sac or absence of the uterus on laparoscopy or rectal exam. In the normal female infant, the uterus is easily palpated as a distinct midline structure beneath the symphysis pubis on rectal examination. Preoperative diagnosis of testicular feminization syndrome or other disorders of sexual development such as mixed gonadal dysgenesis and selected pseudohermaphrodites enables the family to receive genetic counseling, and gonadectomy can be accomplished at the time of the hernia repair.

MANAGEMENT

The presence of an inguinal hernia in the pediatric age group constitutes the indication for operative repair. An inguinal hernia does not resolve spontaneously, and early repair eliminates the risk of incarceration and the associated potential complications, particularly in the 1st 6-12 mo of life. The timing of operative repair depends on several factors, including age, general condition of the patient, and comorbid conditions. In infants (younger than 1 yr old) with an inguinal hernia, repair should proceed promptly (within 2-3 wk) because as many as 70% of incarcerated inguinal hernias requiring emergency operation occur in infants younger than 11 mo. In addition, the incidence of complications associated with *elective* hernia repair (intestinal injury, testicular atrophy, recurrent hernia, wound infection) are low (≈1%), but rise to as high as 18-20% when repair is performed at the time of incarceration. The incidence of testicular atrophy after incarceration in infants younger than 3 mo of age has been reported as high as 30%. Therefore, an approach emphasizing prompt elective repair in infants is warranted. In children older than 1 yr, the risk of incarceration is less and the repair can be scheduled with less urgency. For the routine reducible hernia, the operation should be carried out electively shortly after diagnosis. Elective inguinal hernia repair can be safely performed in an outpatient setting with an expectation for full recovery within 48 hr. The operation should be performed at a facility with the ability to admit the patient to an inpatient unit as needed. Certain conditions can dictate postponement of repair, such as marked prematurity, intercurrent pneumonia (especially respiratory syncytial virus), other infections, or severe congenital heart disease. In cases of prematurity (1,800-2,000 g), repair is typically performed before discharge from the neonatal ICU.

The operation is most often performed under general anesthesia, but it can be performed under spinal anesthesia in selected high-risk infants in whom avoidance of intubation is preferable (because of, e.g., chronic lung disease or bronchopulmonary dysplasia). A regional caudal block or local inguinal nerve block using local anesthetic is useful to diminish perioperative pain and increase patient comfort. These techniques, along with the use of rapid-acting general anesthetics, allow the majority of infants to be discharged home within hours of operation. Prophylactic antibiotics are not routinely used except for associated conditions, such as congenital heart disease or the presence of a ventriculoperitoneal shunt. Preterm infants mandate special consideration because of their higher risk for apnea and bradycardia following general anesthesia (see Chapter 61). Infants younger than 44 wk postconceptional age and full-term infants younger than 3 mo of age and with comorbid conditions should be observed overnight with appropriate apnea and cardiorespiratory monitors.

An incarcerated, irreducible hernia without evidence of strangulation in a clinically stable patient should initially be managed nonoperatively. Unless there is clear peritonitis or bowel compromise, incarcerated hernias can usually be reduced manually using a technique called *taxis*. Manual reduction is performed first with traction caudad and posteriorly to free the mass from the external inguinal ring, and then upward to reduce the contents back into the peritoneal cavity. The attempt should not be continued if the infant is crying and resisting the pressure on the hernia. The use of cautious sedation or analgesia with experienced monitoring before attempting reduction can be helpful; this reduces intraabdominal pressure and relieves the pressure on the neck of the hernia sac at the inguinal ring. Care must be taken to avoid respiratory depression, especially common in the premature infant. Other techniques advocated to assist in the nonoperative reduction of an incarcerated inguinal hernia include elevation of the lower torso and legs. Ice packs should be avoided in infants because of the risk of hypothermia but may be used for brief periods in the older child. If reduction is successful but difficult, the patient should be observed (several hours) to ensure that feedings are tolerated and there is no concern that necrotic intestine was reduced; fortunately, this is an uncommon occurrence. Because of the high risk for early recurrent incarceration, surgical repair is performed 24-48 hr later, by which time there is less edema, handling of the sac is easier, and the risk of complications is reduced.

A common presentation in female patients is an irreducible ovary in the inguinal hernia in an otherwise asymptomatic patient. The inguinal mass is soft and nontender to gentle exam, and there is no swelling or edema; thus, there are no findings suggesting strangulation. This represents a **"sliding"** hernia with the fallopian tube and ovary fused to the wall of the hernia sac. Overzealous attempts to reduce the hernia are unwarranted and potentially harmful to the tube and ovary. The risk that incarceration of the ovary in this setting will lead to strangulation is not known. Most pediatric surgeons recommend elective repair of the hernia within 24-48 hr. For any patient who presents with a prolonged history of incarceration, signs of peritoneal irritation, or small bowel obstruction, surgery and operative reduction and repair of the hernia should be urgently performed.

Operative Management

When the hernia cannot be reduced or signs of strangulation are present, immediate operation is indicated to prevent further damage to the contents of the hernia sac or testis. If there are signs of intestinal obstruction or strangulation, urgent, initial management includes nasogastric intubation, intravenous fluids, and administration of broad-spectrum antibiotics. When fluid and electrolyte imbalance has been corrected and the child's condition is satisfactory, exploration is undertaken. The operation consists of opening of the inguinal canal, reduction of the contents of the hernia sac, separation of the hernia sac from the spermatic cord vessels and vas deferens in the inguinal canal, and high ligation of the hernia sac at the internal ring. Resection of nonviable structures within the hernia sac or of an infarcted testis may be indicated based on the experience and judgment of the surgeon. Although often the testis might appear ischemic, most testes recover after the incarceration is relieved and should not be removed.

The elective operative repair of a congenital indirect inguinal hernia is straightforward and consists of high ligation of the hernia sac (PV) at the level of the internal ring, thus preventing protrusion of abdominal contents into the inguinal canal. In boys, this requires careful separation of the sac from the spermatic cord structures and avoidance of injury to these vital structures. An associated hydrocele, present approximately 20% of the time, is released anteriorly to avoid injury to the spermatic cord structures located posteriorly. In girls, surgical repair is simpler because the hernia sac and round ligament can be ligated without concern for injury to the ovary and its blood supply, which generally remain within the abdomen. If the ovary and fallopian tube are within the sac and not reducible, the sac is ligated distal to these structures and the internal ring is closed after reducing the sac and its contents to the abdominal cavity.

Laparoscopic Inguinal Hernia Repair

Although the classic open inguinal hernia repair is most commonly performed, laparoscopic repair is increasingly used by pediatric surgeons experienced in the technique. Like the open technique, the laparoscopic technique is fundamentally a **high ligation** of the indirect inguinal hernia sac. In the open surgical technique, a small inguinal skin crease incision is employed, the inguinal canal is opened and careful identification and separation of the hernia sac from the vas deferens and the testicular blood supply is performed, followed by high ligation of the sac at the level of the internal ring (entrance point to the peritoneal cavity). In female infants, opening of the sac to visualize the ovary and fallopian tube may help avoid injury to these structures during suture ligation of the sac and also rule out testicular feminization syndrome. In laparoscopic inguinal hernia repair, the hernia sac, anterior to the vas deferens and the testicular blood vessels, is suture-ligated at the internal ring without inguinal exploration or handling of the spermatic cord structures. Proponents of the laparoscopic approach cite ease of examining the contralateral internal ring, decreased manipulation of the vas deferens and spermatic vessels, decreased operative time, and an ability to identify unsuspected direct or femoral hernias. In a prospective, randomized study, the laparoscopic approach was associated with decreased pain, parental perception of faster recovery, and parental perception of better wound cosmesis; however, complication and recurrence rates have been slightly higher for the laparoscopic approach and the approach has yet to gain wide acceptance. Laparoscopic procedures in infants should always be performed expeditiously and with low insufflations pressure to avoid the risk of cardiorespiratory compromise. Postoperative pain in both techniques is managed with oral acetaminophen for 24-48 hr; older children may require a brief period of postoperative narcotics.

Contralateral Inguinal Exploration

Controversy exists regarding when to proceed with contralateral groin exploration in infants and children with a unilateral indirect inguinal hernia. The only purpose of contralateral exploration is to avoid the occurrence of a hernia on that side at a later date. The advantages of contralateral exploration include avoidance of parental anxiety and possibly a second anesthesia, the cost of additional surgery, and the risk of contralateral incarceration. The disadvantages of exploration include potential injury to the spermatic cord vessels, vas deferens, and testis; increased operative and anesthesia time; and the fact that, in many infants, it is an unnecessary procedure. The relevant issues in the debate revolve around the frequency of occurrence of contralateral hernias after one-sided hernia repair and the relation of this to age, gender, and side of the clinically apparent hernia. Most large series noted a chance of developing a contralateral hernia following inguinal hernia repair as 30-40% in children younger than 2 yr of age; leading most pediatric surgeons to recommend routine contralateral exploration in this age group. Unfortunately, infants and young children have delicate spermatic cord structures and when boys were studied 8-20 yr after inguinal hernia repair, 5.8% of them had decreased testicular size on the side of the repair and 1% had testicular atrophy. In girls, because of the higher incidence of bilateral inguinal hernias and elimination of concern for injury to the spermatic cord or testis, routine contralateral exploration is recommended up to age 5 or 6 yr. Laparoscopy enables assessment of the contralateral side without risk of injury to the spermatic cord structures or testis. This procedure can be performed through an umbilical incision or by passing a 30-degree or 70-degree oblique scope through the open hernia sac just before ligation of the hernia sac on the involved side. If patency of the contralateral side is demonstrated, the surgeon can proceed with bilateral hernia repair, and if the contralateral side is properly obliterated, exploration and potential complications are avoided. The downside of this approach include the risks associated with laparoscopy, and that laparoscopy cannot differentiate between a patent PV and a true hernia (Figs. 346-2 and 346-3). Infants and children with risk factors for development of an inguinal hernia or with medical conditions that increase the risk of general anesthesia should be approached with a low threshold for routine contralateral exploration.

DIRECT INGUINAL HERNIA

Direct inguinal hernias are rare in children; approximately 0.5-1%. Direct hernias appear as groin masses that extend toward the femoral vessels with exertion or straining. The etiology is from a muscular defect or weakness in the floor of the inguinal canal *medial* to the epigastric vessels. Thus, direct inguinal hernias in children are generally considered an acquired defect. In one-third of cases, the patient has a history of a prior indirect hernia repair on the side of the direct hernia, which suggests a possible injury to the floor muscles of the inguinal canal at the time of the first herniorrhaphy. Patients with **connective tissue disorders** such as Ehlers-Danlos syndrome or Marfan syndrome and mucopolysaccharidosis such as Hunter-Hurler syndrome are at increased risk for the development of direct inguinal hernias either independently or after indirect inguinal hernia repair.

Operative repair of a direct inguinal hernia involves strengthening of the floor of the inguinal canal, and many standard techniques have been described, similar to repair techniques used in adults. The repair can be performed through a single limited incision and, therefore, laparoscopic repair does not offer significant advantage. Recurrence after repair, in contrast to that in adults, is extraordinarily rare. Because typically the area of muscular weakness is small and pediatric tissues have greater elasticity, primary repair is usually possible. Prosthetic material for direct hernia repair or other approaches, such as preperitoneal repair, are rarely required in the pediatric age group. The older child with a direct inguinal hernia and a connective tissue disorder may be the exception, and a laparoscopic approach and prosthetic material in such a case can be useful for repair.

FEMORAL HERNIA

Femoral hernias are also rare in children (<1% of groin hernias in children). They are more common in girls than boys, with a ratio of 2:1. They are extremely rare in infancy and occur typically in older children. Femoral hernias represent a protrusion through the femoral canal. The bulge of a femoral hernia is located below the inguinal ligament and typically projects toward the medial aspect of the proximal thigh. Femoral hernias are more often missed clinically than direct hernias on physical examination or at the time of indirect hernia repair. Repair of a femoral hernia involves closure of the defect at the femoral canal, generally suturing the inguinal ligament to the pectineal ligament/fascia.

COMPLICATIONS

Complications after elective inguinal hernia repair are uncommon (≈1.5%) but significantly higher in association with incarceration (≈10%). The major risk of elective inguinal hernia repair in infants and children relates to the need for general anesthesia. Surgical complications can be related to technical factors (recurrence, iatrogenic cryptorchidism, inadvertent injury to the vas deferens or spermatic vessels), or to the underlying process, such as bowel ischemia, gonadal infarction, and testicular atrophy following incarceration.

Wound Infection

Wound infection occurs in <1% of elective inguinal hernia repairs in infants and children, but the incidence increases to 5-7% in association with incarceration and emergent repair. The patient typically develops fever and irritability 3-5 days after the surgery, and the wound demonstrates warmth, erythema, and fluctuance. Management consists of opening and draining the wound, a short course of antibiotics, and a

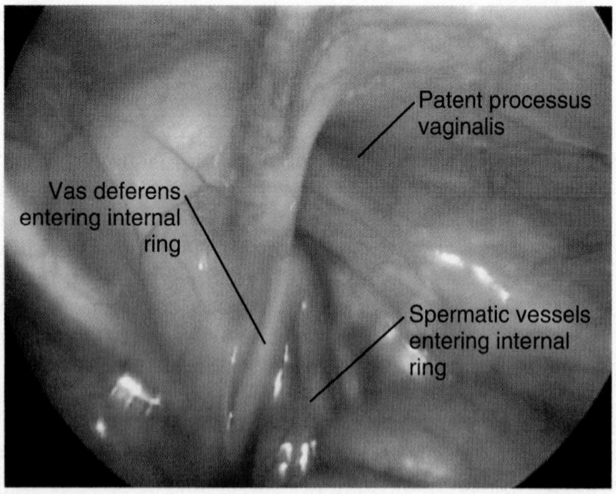

Figure 346-2 Image on laparoscopy of patent processus vaginalis on right side.

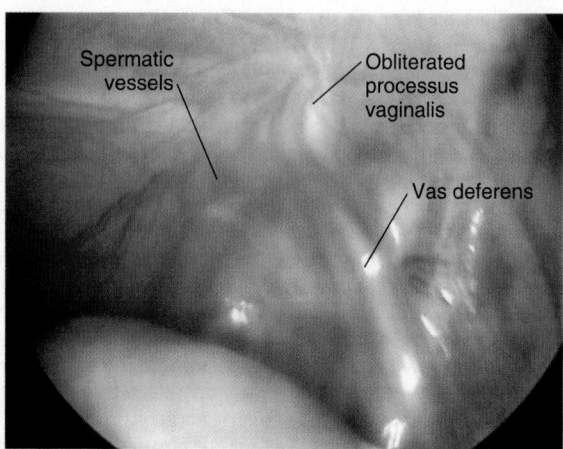

Figure 346-3 Image on diagnostic laparoscopy of obliterated processus vaginalis on left side.

daily wound dressing. Most common organisms are Gram-positive (*Staphylococcus* and *Streptococcus* spp.), and consideration should be given to coverage of methicillin-resistant *Staphylococcus aureus*. The wound generally heals in 1-2 wk with low morbidity and a good cosmetic result.

Recurrent Hernia

The recurrence rate of inguinal hernias after elective inguinal hernia repairs is generally reported as 0.5-1.0%, with rates as high as 2% for premature infants. The rate of recurrence after emergency repair of an incarcerated hernia is much higher; reported as 3-6% in most large series. The true incidence of recurrence is most certainly even higher, given the problem of accurate long-term follow-up. In the group of patients who develop recurrent inguinal hernia, the recurrence occurs in 50% within 1 yr of the initial repair and in 75% by 2 yr. Recurrence of an indirect hernia is most likely the result of a technical problem in the original procedure, such as failure to identify the sac properly, failure to perform high ligation of the sac at the level of the internal ring, or a tear in the sac that leaves a strip of peritoneum along the cord structures. Recurrence as a direct hernia can result from injury to the inguinal floor (transversalis fascia) during the original procedure or failure to identify a direct hernia during the original exploration. Patients with connective tissue disorders (collagen deficiency) or conditions that cause increased intraabdominal pressure (ventriculoperitoneal shunts, ascites, peritoneal catheter for dialysis) are at increased risk for recurrence.

Iatrogenic Cryptorchidism

Iatrogenic cryptorchidism describes malposition of the testis after inguinal hernia repair. This complication is usually related to disruption of the testicular attachment in the scrotum at the time of hernia repair or failure to recognize an undescended testis during the original procedure, allowing the testes to retract, typically to the region of the external ring. At the completion of inguinal hernia repair, the testis should be placed in a dependent intrascrotal position. If the testis will not remain in this position, proper fixation in the scrotum should be performed at the time of the hernia repair.

Incarceration

Incarceration of an inguinal hernia can result in injury to the intestines, the fallopian tube and ovary, or the ipsilateral testis. The incidence of incarceration of a congenital indirect inguinal hernia is reported as 6-18% throughout childhood and as high as 30% for infants younger than 3 mo of age. Intestinal injury requiring bowel resection is uncommon, occurring in only 1-2% of incarcerated hernias. In cases of incarceration in which the hernia is reduced nonoperatively, the likelihood of intestinal injury is low; however, these patients should be observed closely for 6-12 hr following reduction of the hernia persistent for signs and symptoms of intestinal obstruction, such as fever, vomiting, abdominal distention, or bloody stools.

The reported incidence of testicular infarction and subsequent testicular atrophy with incarceration is 4-12%, with higher rates among the irreducible cases requiring emergency operative reduction and repair. The testicular insult can be caused by compression of the gonadal vessels by the incarcerated hernia mass or as a result of damage incurred during operative repair. Young infants are at highest risk, with testicular infarction rates reported as high as 30% in infants younger than 2-3 mo of age. These problems underscore the need for prompt reduction of incarcerated hernias and early repair once the diagnosis is known to avoid repeat episodes of incarceration.

Injury to the Vas Deferens and Male Fertility

Similar to the gonadal vessels, the vas deferens can be injured as a consequence of compression from an incarcerated hernia or during operative repair. This injury is almost certainly underreported because it is unlikely to be recognized until adulthood and, even then, possibly only if the injury is bilateral. Although the vulnerability of the vas deferens has been documented in many studies, no good data exist as to the actual incidence of this problem. One review reported an incidence of injury to the vas deferens of 1.6% based on pathology demonstrating segments of the vas deferens in the hernia sac specimen; this may be overstated, because others have shown that small glandular inclusions found in the hernia sac can represent müllerian duct remnants and are of no clinical importance. The relationship between male fertility and previous inguinal hernia repair is also unknown. There appears to be an association between infertile males with testicular atrophy and abnormal sperm count and a previous hernia repair. A relationship has also been reported between infertile males with spermatic autoagglutinating antibodies and previous inguinal hernia repair. The proposed etiology is that operative injury to the vas deferens during inguinal hernia repair might result in obstruction of the vas with diversion of spermatozoa to the testicular lymphatics, and this breach of the blood–testis barrier produces an antigenic challenge, resulting in formation of spermatic autoagglutinating antibodies.

Bibliography is available at Expert Consult.

Section 5

Exocrine Pancreas

Chapter 347
Embryology, Anatomy, and Physiology

Steven L. Werlin and Michael Wilschanski

The human pancreas develops from the ventral and dorsal domains of the primitive duodenal endoderm beginning at about the 5th wk of gestation (Fig. 347-1). The larger dorsal anlage, which develops into the tail, body, and part of the head of the pancreas, grows directly from the duodenum. The smaller ventral anlage develops as 1 or 2 buds from the primitive liver and eventually forms the major portion of the head of the pancreas. At about the 17th wk of gestation, the dorsal and ventral anlagen fuse as the buds develop and the gut rotates. The ventral duct forms the proximal portion of the major pancreatic duct of Wirsung, which opens into the ampulla of Vater. The dorsal duct forms the distal portion of the duct of Wirsung and the accessory duct of Santorini, which empties independently in approximately 5% of people. Variations in fusion might account for pancreatic developmental anomalies. Pancreatic agenesis has been associated with a base pair deletion in the ipf1 *HOX* gene, *PDX1*, and possibly in the *PTF1A* and *FS123TER* genes. Other genes involved in pancreatic organogenesis include the *IHH*, *SHH* or sonic hedgehog gene, *SMAD2*, and transforming growth factor-1β genes

The pancreas lies transversely in the upper abdomen between the duodenum and the spleen in the retroperitoneum (Fig. 347-2). The head, which rests on the vena cava and renal vein, is adherent to the C loop of the duodenum and surrounds the distal common bile duct. The tail of the pancreas reaches to the left splenic hilum and passes above the left kidney. The lesser sac separates the tail of the pancreas from the stomach.

By the 13th wk of gestation, exocrine and endocrine cells can be identified. Primitive acini containing immature zymogen granules are found by the 16th wk. Mature zymogen granules containing amylase,

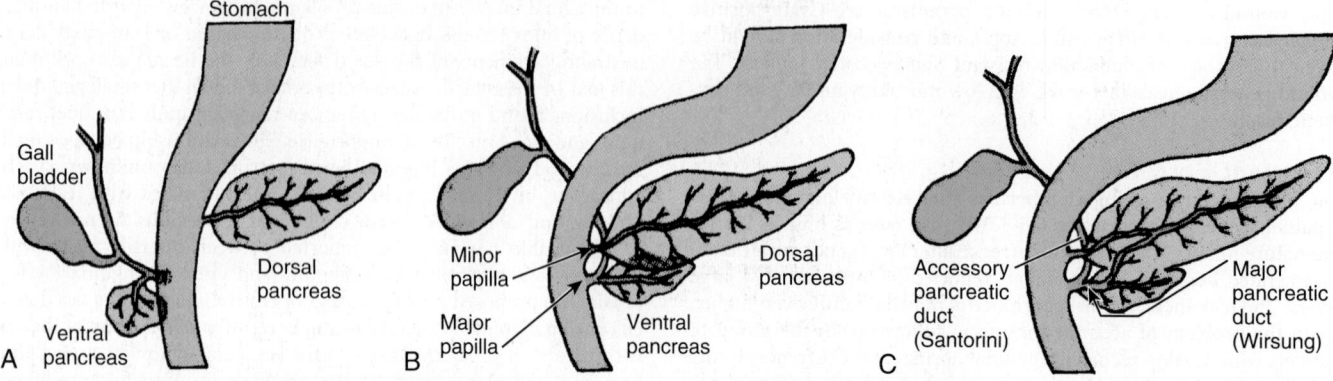

Figure 347-1 Development of the exocrine pancreas. **A,** Gestational age 6 wk. **B,** Gestational age 7-8 wk. The ventral pancreas has rotated but has not yet fused with the dorsal pancreas. **C,** The ventral and dorsal pancreatic ductal systems have fused. *(From Werlin SL: The exocrine pancreas. In Kelly VC, editor:* Practice of pediatrics, *vol 3, Hagerstown, MD, 1980, Harper and Row, Fig. 16-1.)*

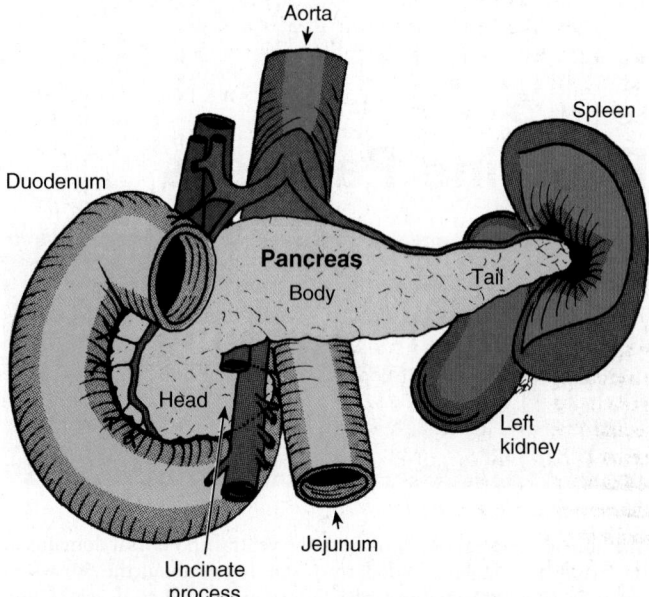

Figure 347-2 Anterior view of the pancreas: relationship to neighboring structures. *(From Werlin SL: The exocrine pancreas. In Kelly VC, editor:* Practice of pediatrics, *vol 3, Hagerstown, MD, 1980, Harper and Row, Fig. 16-2.)*

trypsinogen, chymotrypsinogen, and lipase are present at the 20th wk. Centroacinar and duct cells, which are responsible for water, electrolyte, and bicarbonate secretion, are also found by the 20th wk. The final 3-dimensional structure of the pancreas consists of a complex series of branching ducts surrounded by grape-like clusters of epithelial cells. Cells containing glucagon are present at the 8th wk. Islets of Langerhans appear between the 12th and 16th wk.

Bibliography is available at Expert Consult.

347.1 Anatomic Abnormalities
Steven L. Werlin and Michael Wilschanski

Complete or partial **pancreatic agenesis** is a rare condition. Complete agenesis is associated with severe neonatal diabetes and usually death at an early age (see Chapter 589). Partial or dorsal pancreatic agenesis is often asymptomatic but may be associated with diabetes, congenital

heart disease, polysplenia, and recurrent pancreatitis. Pancreatic agenesis is also associated with malabsorption.

An **annular pancreas** results from incomplete rotation of the left (ventral) pancreatic anlage, which may be a result of recessive mutations in the *IHH* or *SHH* genes. Patients usually present in infancy with symptoms of complete or partial bowel obstruction or in the 4th or 5th decade. There is often a history of maternal polyhydramnios. Other congenital anomalies, such as Down syndrome, tracheoesophageal fistula, intestinal atresia, imperforate anus, malrotation and cardiorenal abnormalities, and pancreatitis, may be associated with annular pancreas. Some children present with chronic vomiting, pancreatitis, or biliary colic. The treatment of choice is duodenojejunostomy. Division of the pancreatic ring is not attempted, because a duodenal diaphragm or duodenal stenosis often accompanies annular pancreas.

Ectopic pancreatic rests in the stomach or small intestine occur in approximately 3% of the population. Most cases (70%) are found in the upper intestinal tract. Recognized on barium contrast studies by their typical umbilicated appearance, they are rarely of clinical importance. On endoscopy, they are irregular, yellow nodules 2-4 mm in diameter. A pancreatic rest may rarely be the lead point of an intussusception, produce hemorrhage, or cause bowel obstruction.

Pancreas divisum, which occurs in 5-15% of the population, is the most common pancreatic developmental anomaly. As the result of failure of the dorsal and ventral pancreatic anlagen to fuse, the tail, body, and part of the head of the pancreas drain through the small accessory duct of Santorini rather than the main duct of Wirsung. Some investigators believe that this anomaly may be associated with recurrent pancreatitis when there is relative obstruction of the outflow of the ventral pancreas. Diagnosis is made by endoscopic retrograde cholangiopancreatography or by magnetic resonance cholangiopancreatography. It was recently shown that pancreatitis in patients with pancreas divisum is associated with mutations in the *CFTR* gene. Sphincterotomy is no longer recommended in these patients unless other anomalies are present.

Choledochal cysts are dilations of the biliary tract and usually cause biliary tract symptoms, such as jaundice, pain, and fever. On occasion, the presentation may be pancreatitis. The diagnosis is usually made with ultrasonography, CT or biliary scanning, or magnetic resonance cholangiopancreatography. Similarly, a choledochocele, an intraduodenal choledochal cyst may manifest with pancreatitis. The diagnosis can be difficult and require magnetic resonance cholangiopancreatography, endoscopic retrograde cholangiopancreatography, or endoscopic ultrasound.

A number of rare conditions, such as Ivemark and Johanson-Blizzard syndromes include pancreatic dysgenesis or dysfunction among their features. Many of these syndromes include renal and hepatic dysgenesis along with the pancreatic anomalies.

Bibliography is available at Expert Consult.

347.2 Physiology
Steven L. Werlin and Michael Wilschanski

The acinus is the functional unit of the exocrine pancreas. Acinar cells are arrayed in a semicircle around a lumen. Ducts that drain the acini are lined by centroacinar and ductular cells. This arrangement allows the secretions of the various cell types to mix.

The acinar cell synthesizes, stores, and secretes more than 20 enzymes, which are stored in zymogen granules, some in inactive forms. The relative concentration of the various enzymes in pancreatic juice is affected and perhaps controlled by the diet, probably by regulating the synthesis of specific messenger RNA. The main enzymes involved in digestion include *amylase*, which splits starch into maltose, isomaltose, maltotriose; dextrins; and *trypsin* and *chymotrypsin*, endopeptidases secreted by the pancreas as inactive proenzymes. Trypsinogen is activated in the gut lumen by enterokinase, a brush-border enzyme. Trypsin can then activate trypsinogen, chymotrypsinogen, and procarboxypeptidase into their respective active forms. Pancreatic lipase requires *colipase*, a coenzyme also found in pancreatic fluid, for activity. Lipase liberates fatty acids from the 1 and 3 positions of triglycerides, leaving a monoglyceride.

The stimuli for exocrine pancreatic secretion are neural and hormonal. Acetylcholine mediates the cephalic phase; cholecystokinin (CCK) mediates the intestinal phase. CCK is released from the duodenal mucosa by luminal amino acids and fatty acids. Feedback regulation of pancreatic secretion is mediated by pancreatic proteases in the duodenum. Secretion of CCK is inhibited by the digestion of a trypsin-sensitive, CCK-releasing peptide released in the lumen of the small intestine or by a monitor peptide released in pancreatic fluid.

Centroacinar and duct cells secrete water and bicarbonate. Bicarbonate secretion is under feedback control and is regulated by duodenal intraluminal pH. The stimulus for bicarbonate production is secretin in concert with CCK. Secretin cells are abundant in the duodenum.

Although normal pancreatic function is required for digestion, maldigestion occurs only after considerable reduction in pancreatic function; lipase and colipase secretion must be decreased by 90-98% before fat maldigestion occurs.

Although amylase and lipase are present in the pancreas early in gestation, secretion of both amylase and lipase is low in the infant. Adult levels of these enzymes are not reached in the duodenum until late in the 1st yr of life. Digestion of the starch found in many infant formulas depends in part on the low levels of salivary amylase that reach the duodenum. This explains the diarrhea that may be seen in infants who are fed formulas high in glucose polymers or starch. Neonatal secretion of trypsinogen and chymotrypsinogen is at approximately 70% of the level found in the 1 yr old infant. The low levels of amylase and lipase in duodenal contents of infants may be partially compensated by salivary amylase and lingual lipase. This explains the relative starch and fat intolerance of premature infants.

Bibliography is available at Expert Consult.

Chapter **348**
Pancreatic Function Tests
Steven L. Werlin and Michael Wilschanski

INDIRECT TESTING
Pancreatic function can be measured by direct and indirect methods. An indirect test, the measurement of *fecal elastase*, which has become the standard screening test for pancreatic insufficiency, has a sensitivity and specificity > 90%. A fecal elastase > 100 μg/g of stool has a 99% predictive value in ruling out pancreatic insufficiency based on an abnormal 72 hr fecal fat. Falsely abnormal results can occur in many enteropathies, such as celiac disease, and when the stool is very loose. The activity of other pancreatic enzymes in stool is now rarely measured.

DIRECT TESTING
Classically, a triple-lumen tube was used to isolate the pancreatic secretions in the duodenum. Measurement of bicarbonate concentration and enzyme activity (*trypsin, chymotrypsin, lipase,* and *amylase*) is performed on the aspirated secretions. Because this test is cumbersome and time consuming it is infrequently used except in the research setting. Although the most commonly used direct test is collection of pancreatic juice at endoscopy after stimulation with secretin and/or cholecystokinin there is controversy over this approach.

A 72 hr stool collection for quantitative analysis of fat content is the gold standard for the diagnosis of malabsorption. The collection is usually performed at home, and the parent is asked to keep a careful dietary record, from which fat intake is calculated. A preweighed, sealable plastic container is used, which the parent keeps in the freezer. Freezing helps to preserve the specimen and reduce odor. Infants are dressed in disposable diapers with the plastic side facing the skin so that the complete sample can be transferred to the container. Normal fat absorption is >93% of intake. The presence of fat malabsorption does not differentiate between pancreatic dysfunction and enteropathies, such as celiac disease. Qualitative examination of the stool for microscopic fat globules can give false-positive and false-negative results.

Pancreatic function can also be measured by a breath test using ^{13}C-triolein as the substrate. This test has not gained widespread acceptance because it is relatively insensitive in detecting mild cases of pancreatic insufficiency, and detection of $^{13}CO_2$ requires a mass spectrophotometer that is not generally available.

Bibliography is available at Expert Consult.

Chapter **349**
Disorders of the Exocrine Pancreas
Steven L. Werlin and Michael Wilschanski

DISORDERS ASSOCIATED WITH PANCREATIC INSUFFICIENCY
Other than cystic fibrosis, conditions that cause pancreatic insufficiency are very rare in children. They include Shwachman-Diamond syndrome, Johanson-Blizzard syndrome, isolated enzyme deficiencies, enterokinase deficiency (see Chapter 338), chronic pancreatitis, and protein-calorie malnutrition (see Chapters 46 and 338).

CYSTIC FIBROSIS
(See Chapter 403.)

Cystic fibrosis (CF) is the most common lethal genetic disease in white children. By the end of the 1st yr of life, 85-90% of children with CF have pancreatic insufficiency, which, if untreated, will lead to malnutrition. Treatment of the associated pancreatic insufficiency leads to improvement in absorption, better growth, and more normal stools.

Pancreatic function can be monitored in children with CF with serial measurements of fecal elastase. Ten percent to 15% of CF patients are pancreatic sufficient and their presentation tends to be later in life, including recurrent pancreatitis, male infertility, and chronic bronchiectasis. CF is part of the newborn screen in every state in the United States and in most countries in the Western world.

SHWACHMAN-DIAMOND SYNDROME
(See Chapter 131.)

Shwachman-Diamond syndrome (SDS) is an autosomal recessive syndrome (1 per 20,000 births) caused by a mutation of the Shwachman-Bodian-Diamond *(SBDS)* gene on chromosome 7, which causes ribosomal dysfunction in 90-95% of patients. Signs and symptoms of SDS include pancreatic insufficiency; neutropenia, which may be cyclic, neutrophil chemotaxis defects, metaphyseal dysostosis, failure to thrive, and short stature. Some patients with SDS have liver or kidney involvement, dental disease, or learning difficulty. SDS is a common cause of congenital neutropenia.

Patients typically present in infancy with poor growth and steatorrhea. These children can be readily differentiated from those with CF by their normal sweat chloride levels, lack of mutations in the CF gene, characteristic metaphyseal lesions, and fatty pancreas characterized by a hypodense appearance on CT and MRI scans.

Despite adequate pancreatic replacement therapy and correction of malabsorption, poor growth commonly continues. Pancreatic insufficiency is often transient, and steatorrhea frequently spontaneously improves with age. Recurrent pyogenic infections (otitis media, pneumonia, osteomyelitis, dermatitis, sepsis) are frequent and are a common cause of death. **Thrombocytopenia is found in 70% of patients and anemia in 50%.** Development of a *myelodysplastic syndrome* can occur, with transformation to *acute myeloid leukemia* in 24%. The pancreatic acini are replaced by fat with little fibrosis. Islet cells and ducts are normal. Bone marrow transplant is the treatment of choice in patients who develop acute myeloid leukemia.

PEARSON SYNDROME
Pearson syndrome is caused by a mitochondrial DNA mutation affecting oxidative phosphorylation that manifests in infants with severe **macrocytic anemia** and **variable thrombocytopenia.** The bone marrow demonstrates vacuoles in erythroid and myeloid precursors as well as ringed sideroblasts. In addition to its role in severe bone marrow failure, pancreatic insufficiency contributes to growth failure. Mitochondrial DNA mutations are transmitted through maternal inheritance to both sexes or are sporadic.

JOHANSON-BLIZZARD SYNDROME
The features of the Johanson-Blizzard syndrome include exocrine pancreatic deficiency, aplasia or hypoplasia of the alae nasi, congenital deafness, hypothyroidism, developmental delay, short stature, ectodermal scalp defects, absence of permanent teeth, urogenital malformations, and imperforate anus. This syndrome is caused by a mutation in the *UBR1* gene found on chromosome 15. The UBR1 protein acts as a ubiquitin ligase

ISOLATED ENZYME DEFICIENCIES
Isolated deficiencies of trypsinogen, enterokinase, lipase, and colipase have been reported. Although enterokinase is a brush-border enzyme, deficiency causes pancreatic insufficiency because enterokinase is required to activate trypsinogen to trypsin in the duodenum. Deficiencies of trypsinogen or enterokinase manifest with failure to thrive, hypoproteinemia, and edema. Isolated amylase deficiency is typically developmental and resolves by age 2-3 yr.

OTHER SYNDROMES ASSOCIATED WITH PANCREATIC INSUFFICIENCY
Pancreatic agenesis, congenital pancreatic hypoplasia, and congenital rubella are rare causes of pancreatic insufficiency. Pancreatic insufficiency has also been reported in duodenal atresia and stenosis and

may also be seen in an infant with familial or nonfamilial hyperinsulinemic hypoglycemia, who requires 95-100% pancreatectomy to control hypoglycemia. Pancreatic insufficiency, which may be found in children with celiac disease and undernutrition, recovers with nutritional rehabilitation.

Bibliography is available at Expert Consult.

Chapter 350
Treatment of Pancreatic Insufficiency
Steven L. Werlin and Michael Wilschanski

The most important therapy of pancreatic insufficiency is pancreatic enzyme replacement therapy (PERT). The enzymes are enterically coated to protect the enzymes from degradation by gastric acid and from autodigestion in the small intestine. It is common for patients to change from one product to another using a 1:1 lipase ratio and then titrating for maximum efficacy.

The North American Cystic Fibrosis Foundation has published dosing guidelines based on age and fat ingestion (Table 350-1). Because these products contain excess protease compared with lipase, the dosage is estimated from the lipase requirement. The final dosage of PERT for children is often established by trial and error. An adequate dose is one that is followed by resumption of normal growth and the return of the stools to normal fat content, which, when desired, can be verified by a 72-hr fecal fat collection and normalization of stool consistency color. Because there is no elastase in enzyme preparations, fecal elastase can not be used to monitor appropriateness of PERT dosage. Enzyme replacement should be divided and given at the beginning of and during the meal. Enzymes should not be chewed, crushed, or dissolved in food, which would allow gastric acid to penetrate the enteric coating and destroy the enzymes. Enzymes must also be given with snacks, which contain fat. Increasing enzyme supplements beyond the recommended dose does not improve absorption, might retard growth, and can cause **fibrosing colonopathy** (see below).

A major issue has been the ingestion of enzymes by infants. The importance of correct enzyme ingestion in infants and children is obvious but there may be difficulty in feeding the infant microspheres, however small they may be. Enterically coated microspheres can be

Table 350-1	Pancreatic Enzyme Replacement Therapy
Infants (up to 12 mo)	2000-4000 units lipase/120 mL breast milk or formula
12 mo-4 yr	1000 units lipase/kg/meal initially, then titrate per response
Children older than 4 yr and adults	500 units lipase/kg/meal initially, up to maximum of 2500 units lipase/kg/meal or 10,000 units lipase/kg/day or 4,000 units lipase/g fat ingested per day
PLUS: one half the standard meal dose to be given with snacks	

Data from Borowitz D, Baker RD, Stallings V: Consensus report in nutrition for pediatric patients with cystic fibrosis. J Pediatr Gastroenterol Nutr 35:246-259, 2002.

mixed with apple sauce for oral use or crushed for use in tube feeding. Patients treated with this approach achieve growth and weight gain, proving their efficacy

Treatment of exocrine pancreatic insufficiency by oral enzyme replacement usually corrects protein malabsorption, but steatorrhea is difficult to completely correct. Factors contributing to fat malabsorption include inadequate dosage, incorrect timing of doses in relation to food consumption or gastric emptying, lipase inactivation by gastric acid, and the observation that *chymotrypsin* in the enzyme preparation digests and thus inactivates *lipase*.

When adequate fat absorption is not achieved, gastric acid neutralization with an H_2-receptor antagonist or, more commonly, a proton pump inhibitor, decreases enzyme inactivation by gastric acid and thus improves delivery of lipase into the intestine. Enteric coating also protects lipase from acid inactivation.

Untoward effects secondary to PERT include allergic reactions, increased uric acid levels, and kidney stones. **Fibrosing colonopathy**, consisting of colonic fibrosis and strictures, can occur 7-12 mo after overdose of PERT.

Fat-soluble vitamin supplements are required by pancreatic insufficiency patients because of the ongoing mild to moderate fat malabsorption that occurs despite PERT.

Bibliography is available at Expert Consult.

Chapter **351**
Pancreatitis

351.1 Acute Pancreatitis
Steven L. Werlin and Michael Wilschanski

Acute pancreatitis, the most common pancreatic disorder in children, is increasing in incidence and at least 30-50 cases are now seen in major pediatric centers per year. In children, blunt abdominal injuries, multisystem disease such as the hemolytic uremic syndrome and inflammatory bowel disease, biliary stones or microlithiasis (sludging), and drug toxicity are the most common etiologies. Although many drugs and toxins can induce acute pancreatitis in susceptible persons, in children, valproic acid, L-asparaginase, 6-mercaptopurine, and azathioprine are the most common causes of drug-induced pancreatitis. Other cases follow organ transplantation or are caused by infections, metabolic disorders, or mutations in susceptibility genes (see Chapter 351.2). Fewer than 5% of cases are idiopathic (Table 351-1).

After an initial insult, such as ductal disruption or obstruction, there is premature activation of trypsinogen to trypsin within the acinar cell. Trypsin then activates other pancreatic proenzymes, leading to autodigestion, further enzyme activation, and release of active proteases. Lysosomal hydrolases colocalize with pancreatic proenzymes within the acinar cell. Pancreastasis (similar in concept to cholestasis) with continued synthesis of enzymes occurs. Lecithin is activated by phospholipase A_2 into the toxic lysolecithin. Prophospholipase is unstable and can be activated by minute quantities of trypsin. After the insult, cytokines and other proinflammatory mediators are released.

The healthy pancreas is protected from autodigestion by pancreatic proteases that are synthesized as inactive proenzymes; digestive enzymes that are segregated into secretory granules at pH 6.2 by low calcium concentration, which minimizes trypsin activity; the presence of protease inhibitors both in the cytoplasm and zymogen granules; and enzymes that are secreted directly into the ducts.

Histopathologically, interstitial edema appears early. Later, as the episode of pancreatitis progresses, localized and confluent necrosis, blood vessel disruption leading to hemorrhage, and an inflammatory response in the peritoneum can develop.

Criteria for the diagnosis of pancreatitis in children are defined as 2 of 3 of the following: abdominal pain; serum amylase and/or lipase activity at least 3 times greater than the upper limit of normal; and imaging findings characteristic of, or compatible with, acute pancreatitis.

CLINICAL MANIFESTATIONS
Mild Acute Pancreatitis
The patient with acute pancreatitis has severe abdominal pain, persistent vomiting, and possibly fever. The pain is epigastric or in either upper quadrant, steady, often resulting in the child's assuming an antalgic position with hips and knees flexed, sitting upright, or lying on the side. The child is very uncomfortable and irritable and appears acutely ill. The abdomen may be distended and tender and a mass may be palpable. The pain can increase in intensity for 24-48 hr, during which time vomiting may increase and the patient can require hospitalization for dehydration and might need fluid and electrolyte therapy. The prognosis for complete recovery in the acute uncomplicated case is excellent.

Severe Acute Pancreatitis
Severe acute pancreatitis is rare in children. In this life-threatening condition, the patient is acutely ill with severe nausea, vomiting, and abdominal pain. Shock, high fever, jaundice, ascites, hypocalcemia, and pleural effusions can occur. A bluish discoloration may be seen around the umbilicus (Cullen sign) or in the flanks (Grey Turner sign). The pancreas is necrotic and can be transformed into an inflammatory hemorrhagic mass. The mortality rate, which is approximately 20%, is related to the systemic inflammatory response syndrome with multiple organ dysfunction, shock, renal failure, acute respiratory distress syndrome, disseminated intravascular coagulation, massive gastrointestinal bleeding, and systemic or intraabdominal infection. The percentage of necrosis seen on CT scan and failure of pancreatic tissue to enhance on CT scan (suggesting necrosis) predicts the severity of the disease.

DIAGNOSIS
Acute pancreatitis is usually diagnosed by measurement of serum lipase and amylase activities. Serum lipase is now considered the test of choice for acute pancreatitis as it is more specific than amylase for acute inflammatory pancreatic disease and should be determined when pancreatitis is suspected. The serum lipase rises by 4-8 hr, peaks at 24-48 hr, and remains elevated 8-14 days longer than serum amylase. Serum lipase can be elevated in nonpancreatic diseases. The serum amylase level is typically elevated for up to 4 days. A variety of other conditions can also cause hyperamylasemia without pancreatitis (Table 351-2). Elevation of salivary amylase can mislead the clinician to diagnose pancreatitis in a child with abdominal pain. The laboratory can separate amylase isoenzymes into pancreatic and salivary fractions. Initially, serum amylase levels are normal in 10-15% of patients.

Other laboratory abnormalities that may be present in acute pancreatitis include hemoconcentration, coagulopathy, leukocytosis, hyperglycemia, glucosuria, hypocalcemia, elevated γ-glutamyl transpeptidase, and hyperbilirubinemia.

X-ray of the chest and abdomen might demonstrate nonspecific findings. The chest x-ray might demonstrate atelectasis, basilar infiltrates, elevation of the hemidiaphragm, left- (rarely right-) sided pleural effusions, pericardial effusion, and pulmonary edema. Abdominal x-rays might demonstrate a sentinel loop, dilation of the transverse colon (cutoff sign), ileus, pancreatic calcification (if recurrent), blurring of the left psoas margin, a pseudocyst, diffuse abdominal haziness (ascites), and peripancreatic extraluminal gas bubbles.

Table 351-1	Etiology of Acute and Recurrent Pancreatitis in Children

DRUGS AND TOXINS
Acetaminophen overdose
Alcohol
L-Asparaginase
Azathioprine
Carbamazepine
Cimetidine
Corticosteroids
Enalapril
Erythromycin
Estrogen
Furosemide
Glucagon-like peptide-1 agents
Isoniazid
Lisinopril
6-Mercaptopurine
Methyldopa
Metronidazole
Octreotide
Organophosphate poisoning
Pentamidine
Retrovirals: DDC (dideoxycytidine), DDI (dideoxyinosine), tenofovir
Sulfonamides: mesalamine, 5-aminosalicylates, sulfasalazine, trimethoprim-sulfamethoxazole
Sulindac
Tetracycline
Thiazides
Valproic acid
Venom (spider, scorpion, Gila monster lizard)
Vincristine
Volatile hydrocarbons

GENETIC
Cationic trypsinogen gene (PRSS1)
Chymotrypsin C gene (CTRC)
Cystic fibrosis gene (CFTR)
Trypsin inhibitor gene (SPINK1)

INFECTIOUS
Ascariasis
Coxsackie B virus
Epstein-Barr virus
Hepatitides A, B
Influenzae A, B
Leptospirosis
Malaria
Measles
Mumps
Mycoplasma
Rubella
Rubeola
Reye syndrome: varicella, influenza B
Septic shock

OBSTRUCTIVE
Ampullary disease
Ascariasis
Biliary tract malformations
Choledochal cyst
Choledochocele
Cholelithiasis, microlithiasis, and choledocholithiasis (stones or sludge)
Duplication cyst
Endoscopic retrograde cholangiopancreatography (ERCP) complication
Pancreas divisum
Pancreatic ductal abnormalities
Postoperative
Sphincter of Oddi dysfunction
Tumor

SYSTEMIC DISEASE
Autoimmune pancreatitis (IgG$_4$-related systemic disease)
Brain tumor
Collagen vascular diseases
Crohn disease
Diabetes mellitus (ketoacidosis)
Head trauma
Hemochromatosis
Hemolytic uremic syndrome
Hyperlipidemia: types I, IV, V
Hyperparathyroidism/hypercalcemia
Kawasaki disease
Malnutrition
Organic academia
Peptic ulcer
Periarteritis nodosa
Renal failure
Systemic lupus erythematosus
Transplantation: bone marrow, heart, liver, kidney, pancreas
Vasculitis

TRAUMATIC
Blunt injury
Burns
Child abuse
Hypothermia
Surgical trauma
Total-body cast

CT scanning has a major role in the diagnosis and follow-up of children with pancreatitis. Findings can include pancreatic enlargement, a hypoechoic, sonolucent edematous pancreas, pancreatic masses, fluid collections, and abscesses (Fig. 351-1); 20% or more of children with acute pancreatitis initially have normal imaging studies. In adults, CT findings are the basis of a widely accepted prognostic system. Ultrasonography is more sensitive than CT scanning for the diagnosis of biliary stones. Magnetic resonance cholangiopancreatography and endoscopic retrograde cholangiopancreatography are essential in the investigation of recurrent pancreatitis, nonresolving pancreatitis, and disease associated with gallbladder pathology. Endoscopic ultrasonography also helps visualize the pancreaticobiliary system.

TREATMENT

The aims of medical management are to relieve pain and restore metabolic homeostasis. Analgesia should be given in adequate doses. Fluid, electrolyte, and mineral balance should be restored and maintained. Nasogastric suction is useful in patients who are vomiting. While vomiting, the patient should be maintained with nothing by mouth. Recovery is usually complete within 4-5 days. Refeeding can commence when vomiting has resolved. Early refeeding by nasogastric tube or on demand decreases the complication rate and length of stay.

In severe pancreatitis, antibiotics are used to treat infected necrosis but prophylactic antibiotics are not recommended. Gastric acid is suppressed. Endoscopic therapy can be of benefit when pancreatitis is caused by anatomic abnormalities, such as strictures or stones. Enteral alimentation by mouth, nasogastric tube, or nasojejunal tube (in severe cases or for those intolerant of oral or nasogastric feedings), within 2-3 days of onset, reduces the length of hospitalization, complication rate and survival in adult patients with severe acute pancreatitis. In children, surgical therapy of nontraumatic, acute pancreatitis

is rarely required but may include drainage of necrotic material or abscesses.

PROGNOSIS
Children with uncomplicated acute pancreatitis do well and recover within 4-5 days. When pancreatitis is associated with trauma or systemic disease, the prognosis is typically related to the associated medical conditions.

Bibliography is available at Expert Consult.

Table 351-2	Differential Diagnosis of Hyperamylasemia

PANCREATIC PATHOLOGY
Acute or chronic pancreatitis
Complications of pancreatitis (pseudocyst, ascites, abscess)
Factitious pancreatitis

SALIVARY GLAND PATHOLOGY
Parotitis (mumps, *Staphylococcus aureus*, cytomegalovirus, HIV, Epstein-Barr virus)
Sialadenitis (calculus, radiation)
Eating disorders (anorexia nervosa, bulimia)

INTRAABDOMINAL PATHOLOGY
Biliary tract disease (cholelithiasis)
Peptic ulcer perforation
Peritonitis
Intestinal obstruction
Appendicitis

SYSTEMIC DISEASES
Metabolic acidosis (diabetes mellitus, shock)
Renal insufficiency, transplantation
Burns
Pregnancy
Drugs (morphine)
Head injury
Cardiopulmonary bypass

351.2 Chronic Pancreatitis
Steven L. Werlin and Michael Wilschanski

Chronic pancreatitis in children is often caused by genetic mutations or by congenital anomalies of the pancreatic or biliary ductal system. Mutations in the *PRSS1* gene (cationic trypsinogen) located on the long arm of chromosome 7, in *SPINK 1* gene (pancreatic trypsin inhibitor) located on chromosome 5, in the cystic fibrosis gene (*CFTR*), and in the chymotrypsin C gene (*CTRC*) may all lead to chronic pancreatitis (see Table 351-1).

Cationic trypsinogen has a trypsin-sensitive cleavage site. Loss of this cleavage site in the abnormal protein permits uncontrolled activation of trypsinogen to trypsin, which leads to autodigestion of the pancreas. Mutations in *PRSS1* act in an autosomal dominant fashion with incomplete penetrance and variable expressivity. Symptoms often begin in the 1st decade but are usually mild at the onset. Although spontaneous recovery from each attack occurs in 4-7 days, episodes become progressively severe. Clinically, hereditary pancreatitis may be diagnosed by the presence of the disease in successive generations of

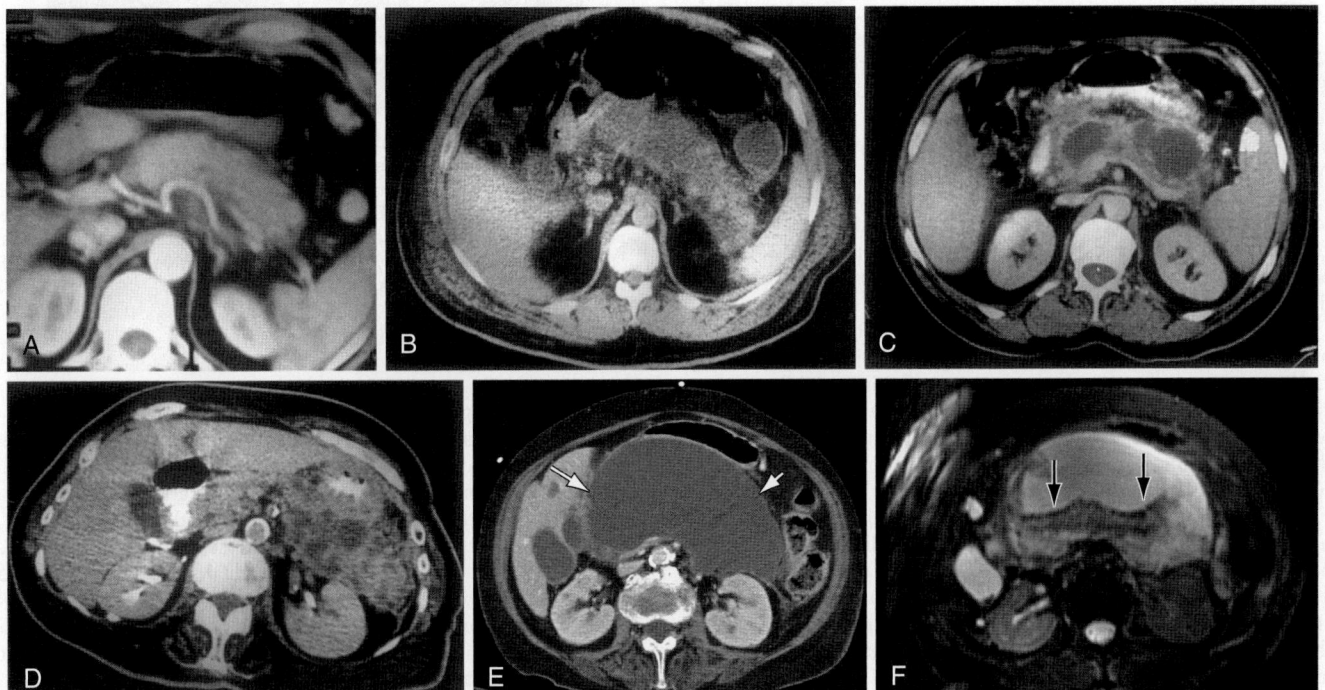

Figure 351-1 CT and MRI appearance of pancreatitis. **A,** Mild acute pancreatitis. Arterial phase spiral CT. Diffuse enlargement of pancreas without fluid accumulation. **B,** Severe acute pancreatitis. Lack of enhancement of the pancreatic parenchyma due to the necrosis of the entire pancreatic gland. **C,** Pancreatic pseudocyst. A round fluid collection with thin capsule is seen within the lesser sac. **D,** Acute severe pancreatitis and peripancreatic abscess formation. Peripancreatic abscess formation is observed within the peripancreatic and the left anterior pararenal space. **E,** Pancreatic necrosis. A well-defined fluid attenuation collection in the pancreatic bed *(white arrows)* seen on contrast-enhanced CT imaging. **F,** The same collection is more complex appearing on the corresponding T2-weighted MR image. The internal debris and necrotic tissue are better appreciated because of the superior soft-tissue contrast of MRI *(black arrows)*. (**A-D** from Elmas N: The role of diagnostic radiology in pancreatitis, Eur J Radiol 38[2]:120–132, 2001, Figs. 1, 3b, 4a, and 5. **E-F** from Soakar A, Rabinowitz CB, Sahani DV: Cross-sectional imaging in acute pancreatitis, Radiol Clin North Am 45[3]:447–460, 2007, Fig. 14.)

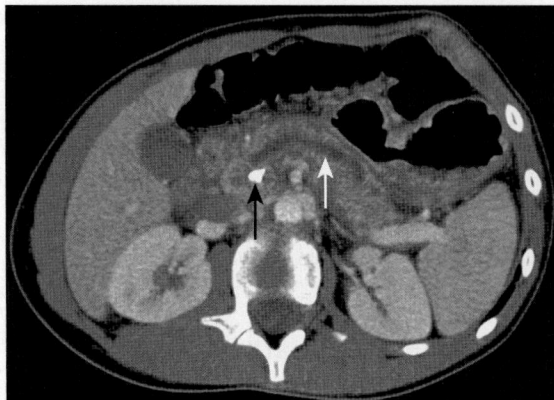

Figure 351-2 Chronic pancreatitis. Computed tomogram showing calcification in the head of the pancreas (black arrow) and dilated pancreatic duct (white arrow) in a 12 yr old patient. (Courtesy of Dr. Janet Reid. From Wyllie R, Hyams JS, editors: Pediatric gastrointestinal and liver disease, ed 3, Philadelphia, 2006, WB Saunders.)

a family. An evaluation during symptom-free intervals may be unrewarding until calcifications, pseudocysts, or pancreatic exocrine and endocrine insufficiency develops (Fig. 351-2). Chronic pancreatitis is a risk factor for future development of pancreatic cancer. Multiple mutations of the *PRSS1* gene associated with hereditary pancreatitis have been described.

Trypsin inhibitor acts as a fail-safe mechanism to prevent uncontrolled autoactivation of trypsin. Mutations in the *SPINK1* gene have been associated with recurrent or chronic pancreatitis. In *SPINK1* mutations, this fail-safe mechanism is lost; this gene may be a modifier gene and not the direct etiologic factor.

Mutations of the cystic fibrosis gene (*CFTR*), associated with pancreatic sufficiency or which do not typically produce pulmonary disease, can cause chronic pancreatitis, possibly from ductal obstruction. Patients with genotypes associated with mild phenotypic effects have a greater risk of developing pancreatitis than patients with genotypes associated with moderate-severe phenotypes.

Mutations in the chymotrypsin C (*CTRC*) gene, which cause a gain of function, may also cause recurrent pancreatitis. Indications for genetic testing include recurrent episodes of acute pancreatitis, chronic pancreatitis, a family history of pancreatitis, or unexplained pancreatitis in children.

Other conditions associated with chronic, relapsing pancreatitis are hyperlipidemia (types I, IV, and V), hyperparathyroidism, and ascariasis. Previously, most cases of recurrent pancreatitis in childhood were considered idiopathic; with the discovery of gene families associated with recurrent pancreatitis, this has changed. Congenital anomalies of the ductal systems, such as pancreas divisum are more common than previously recognized.

Autoimmune pancreatitis typically manifests with jaundice, abdominal pain, and weight loss. The pancreas is typically enlarged and the pancreas is hypodense on CT. The pathogenesis is unknown. Type 1 is a systemic disease and is associated with high serum immunoglobulin (Ig) G₄. In type 2 IgG₄, levels are normal and the disease is limited to the pancreas. Both types respond to steroids. There have been only a few case reports of this condition in children.

Juvenile tropical pancreatitis is the most common form of chronic pancreatitis in developing equatorial countries. The highest prevalence is in the Indian state of Kerala. Tropical pancreatitis occurs during late childhood or early adulthood, manifesting with abdominal pain and irreversible pancreatic insufficiency followed by diabetes mellitus within 10 yr. The pancreatic ducts are obstructed with inspissated secretions, which later calcify. This condition is associated with mutations in the *SPINK* gene in 50% of cases.

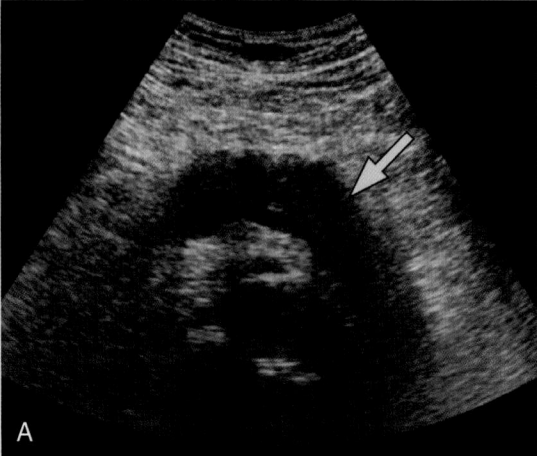

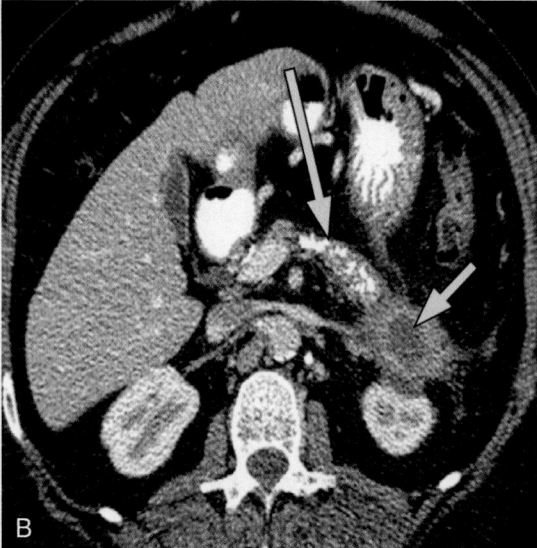

Figure 351-3 Examples of ultrasound and multidetector images in patients with chronic pancreatitis. **A,** Transabdominal ultrasound scan showing a uniformly swollen, hypoechoic pancreas (arrow), typical of autoimmune pancreatitis. **B,** Multidetector CT showing pancreatic calculi in an atrophic pancreas (long arrow) and a pseudocyst at the tail of the pancreas (short arrow). (From Braganza JM, Lee SH, McCloy RF, McMahon MJ: Chronic pancreatitis. Lancet 377:1184–1197, 2011, Fig. 5, p 1191.)

A thorough diagnostic evaluation of every child with more than 1 episode of pancreatitis is indicated. Serum lipid, calcium, and phosphorus levels are determined. Stools are evaluated for ascaris, and a sweat test is performed. Plain abdominal films are evaluated for the presence of pancreatic calcifications. Abdominal ultrasound or CT scanning is performed to detect the presence of a pseudocyst (Figs. 351-3 and 351-4). The biliary tract is evaluated for the presence of stones. After genetic counseling, evaluation of *PRSS1, SPINK1, CFTR,* and *CRTC* genotypes can be measured.

Magnetic resonance cholangiopancreatography and endoscopic retrograde cholangiopancreatography are techniques that can be used to define the anatomy of the gland and are mandatory if surgery is considered. Magnetic resonance cholangiopancreatography is the test of choice when endotherapy is not being considered and should be performed as part of the evaluation of any child with idiopathic, nonresolving, or recurrent pancreatitis and in patients with a pseudocyst before drainage. In these cases a previously undiagnosed anatomic defect that may be amenable to endoscopic or surgical therapy may be detected. Endoscopic treatments include sphincterotomy, stone

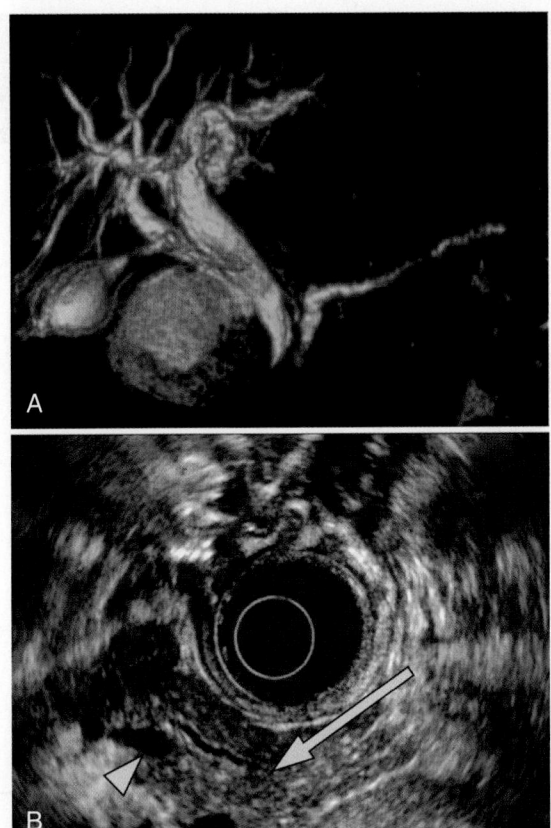

Figure 351-4 Examples of 3-dimensional magnetic resonance cholangiopancreatogram and endoscopic ultrasound in patients with chronic pancreatitis. **A,** Three-dimensional magnetic resonance cholangiopancreatogram shows a minimally dilated biliary tree and moderately dilated irregular main pancreatic duct. **B,** Endoscopic ultrasound scan shows a minimally dilated pancreatic duct in the head of pancreas *(arrow)* consistent with mild chronic pancreatitis: the distal common bile duct appears normal *(arrowhead)*. *(From Braganza JM, Lee SH, McCloy RF, McMahon MJ: Chronic pancreatitis. Lancet 377:1184–1197, 2011, Fig. 6, p. 1191.)*

extraction, drainage on pseudocysts, and insertion of pancreatic or biliary endoprosthetic stents. These treatments allow successful nonsurgical management of conditions previously requiring surgical intervention. In patients with intractable pain total pancreatectomy and islet cell transfusion is performed in specialized centers.

Bibliography is available at Expert Consult.

Chapter 352
Pseudocyst of the Pancreas
Steven L. Werlin and Michael Wilschanski

Pancreatic pseudocyst formation is an uncommon sequela to acute or chronic pancreatitis. Pseudocysts are sacs delineated by a fibrous wall in the lesser peritoneal sac. They can enlarge or extend in almost any direction, thus producing a wide variety of symptoms (see Fig. 351-1*C*).

A pancreatic pseudocyst is suggested when an episode of pancreatitis fails to resolve or when a mass develops after an episode of pancreatitis. Clinical features usually include pain, nausea, and vomiting, but many patients are asymptomatic. The most common signs are a palpable mass in 50% of patients and jaundice in 10%. Other findings include ascites and pleural effusions (usually left-sided).

Pancreatic pseudocysts can be detected by transabdominal ultrasonography, CT scanning, magnetic resonance cholangiopancreatography, endoscopic retrograde cholangiopancreatography, and endoscopic ultrasound. Because of its ease, availability, and reliability, ultrasonography is the first choice. Sequential ultrasonography studies have demonstrated that most small pseudocysts (<6 cm) resolve spontaneously. It is recommended that the patient with acute pancreatitis undergo an ultrasonographic evaluation 2-4 wk after resolution of the acute episode for an evaluation of possible pseudocyst formation.

Percutaneous and endoscopic drainage of pseudocysts have replaced open surgical drainage, except for complicated or recurrent pseudocysts. Whereas a pseudocyst must be allowed to mature for 4-6 wk before surgical drainage is attempted, percutaneous or endoscopic drainage can be attempted earlier. In some cases, endoscopic creation of a cystgastrostomy is performed. When a surgical treatment is planned an magnetic resonance cholangiopancreatography or endoscopic retrograde cholangiopancreatography is performed to define anatomic abnormalities and aid the surgeon in planning his approach. Endoscopic ultrasound is helpful when an endoscopic approach is chosen.

Bibliography is available at Expert Consult.

Chapter 353
Pancreatic Tumors
Steven L. Werlin and Michael Wilschanski

Pancreatic tumors can be of either endocrine or nonendocrine origin. Tumors of endocrine origin include insulinomas and gastrinomas. These and other functioning tumors occur in the autosomal dominantly inherited multiple endocrine neoplasia type 1 (MEN-1). Hypoglycemia accompanied by higher-than-expected insulin levels or refractory gastric ulcers (Zollinger-Ellison syndrome) indicate the possibility of a pancreatic tumor (see Chapter 345). Most gastrinomas arise outside of the pancreas. The treatment of choice is surgical removal. If the primary tumor cannot be found, or if it has metastasized, cure might not be possible. Treatment with a high dose of a proton pump inhibitor to inhibit gastric acid secretion is then indicated.

The watery diarrhea–hypokalemia–acidosis syndrome is usually produced by the secretion of vasoactive intestinal peptide by a non–α-cell tumor (VIPoma) (see Table 341-7). Vasoactive intestinal peptide levels are often, but not always, increased in the serum. Treatment is surgical removal of the tumor. When this is not possible, symptoms may be controlled by the use of octreotide acetate (cyclic somatostatin, Sandostatin), a synthetic analog of somatostatin. Pancreatic tumors secreting a variety of hormones, including glucagon, somatostatin, and pancreatic polypeptide have also been described. The treatment is surgical resection when possible.

Pancreatoblastomas, pancreatic adenocarcinomas, cystadenomas, and rhabdomyosarcomas are rarely encountered. Pancreatoblastoma, a malignant embryonal tumor that secretes α-fetoprotein and can contain both endocrine and exocrine elements, is the most common pancreatic neoplasm in young children. Presurgical chemotherapy should be considered for lesions not primarily resectable. Resection can be curative; adjuvant chemotherapy has been used but its effectiveness is not established.

Carcinoma of the exocrine pancreas is a major problem in adults, accounting for 2% of diagnoses and 5% of deaths from cancer. It is very rare in childhood. No definite causes are known. Several genetic syndromes including mutations in the *PRSS1* and *MEN-1* genes lead to an increased incidence of pancreatic cancer in adult life. The Frantz tumor is a papillary cystic tumor usually found in girls and young women. Typical presenting symptoms are abdominal pain, mass, or jaundice. The treatment of choice is total surgical removal.

Insulinomas and persistent hyperinsulinemic hypoglycemia of infancy produce symptomatic hypoglycemia caused by mutations in a variety of genes, most commonly *GUUD1* and *KATP*. Massive subtotal or total pancreatectomy is the treatment of choice when medical treatment fails (see Chapter 86). These children might then develop pancreatic insufficiency and diabetes as a complication of surgery.

Pancreatic lesions in von Hippel-Lindau disease are usually benign and cystic. Cystadenomas, familial adenocarcinomas, and islet cell tumors are less common. Metastases have been reported, but adjuvant therapy after surgical excision cannot yet be recommended. The diagnosis is suggested by CT scanning.

Prognosis is good for completely resected endocrine tumors but very poor for carcinomas, even with extensive surgery. Children who survive partial or complete pancreatectomy may have decreased pancreatic exocrine and endocrine reserve.

Bibliography is available at Expert Consult.

Table 354-1	Selected Growth Factors, Receptors, Protein Kinases, and Transcription Factors Required for Normal Liver Development in Animal Models

INDUCTION OF HEPATOCYTE FATE THROUGH CARDIAC MESODERM
Fibroblast growth factors (FGFs) 1, 2, 8
FGF receptors 1, 4

INDUCTION OF HEPATOCYTE FATE THROUGH SEPTUM TRANSVERSUM
Bone morphogenetic proteins 2, 4, 7

STIMULATION OF HEPATOBLAST GROWTH AND PROLIFERATION
Hepatocyte growth factor (HGF)
HGF receptor c-met
"Pioneer" transcription factors Foxa1, Foxa2, and Gata4, Gata6
Transcription factors Xbp1, Foxm1b, Hlx, Hex, Prox1
Wnt signalling pathway, β-catenin

SPECIFICATION OF HEPATOCYTE LINEAGE
HGF
Transforming growth factor-β and its downstream effectors Smad 2, Smad 3
Hepatocyte nuclear factors (HNFs) 1α, 4α, 6

SPECIFICATION OF CHOLANGIOCYTE LINEAGE
Jagged 1 (Notch ligand) and Notch receptors 1, 2
HNF6, HNF1β
Wnt signalling pathway, β-catenin
Vacuolar sorting protein Vps33b

Section 6
The Liver and Biliary System

Chapter **354**

Morphogenesis of the Liver and Biliary System

Stacey S. Huppert and William F. Balistreri

During the early embryonic process of gastrulation, the 3 embryonic germ layers (endoderm, mesoderm, ectoderm) are formed. The liver and biliary system arises from cells of the ventral foregut endoderm; their development can be divided into 3 distinct processes (Fig. 354-1). First, through unknown mechanisms, the ventral foregut endoderm acquires *competence* to receive signals arising from the cardiac mesoderm. These mesodermal signals, in the form of various fibroblast growth factors and bone morphogenetic proteins, lead to *specification* of cells that have the potential to form the liver and activate liver-specific genes. During this period of hepatic fate decision, "pioneer" transcription factors, including *Foxa* and *Gata4*, bind to specific binding sites in compacted chromatin, open the local chromatin structure, and mark genes as competent. But these will only be expressed if they are correctly induced by additional transcription factors. Newly specified cells then delaminate from the ventral foregut endoderm and migrate in a cranial ventral direction into the septum

transversum in the 4th wk of human gestation to initiate liver *morphogenesis.*

The growth and development of the newly budded liver require interactions with endothelial cells. Certain proteins are important for liver development in animal models (Table 354-1). In addition to these proteins, microRNAs, which consist of small noncoding, single-stranded RNAs, have a functional role in the regulation of gene expression and hepatobiliary development in zebrafish and mouse models.

Within the ventral mesentery, proliferation of migrating cells form anastomosing hepatic cords, with the network of primitive liver cells, sinusoids, and septal mesenchyme establishing the basic architectural pattern of liver lobule (Fig. 354-2). The solid *cranial* portion of the hepatic diverticulum (pars hepatis) eventually forms the hepatic parenchyma and the intrahepatic bile ducts. The hepatic lobules are identifiable in the 6th wk of human gestation. The bile canalicular structures, including microvilli and junctional complexes, are specialized loci of the liver cell membrane; these appear very early in gestation, and large canaliculi bounded by several hepatocytes are seen by 6-7 wk.

Hepatocytes and bile duct cells (cholangiocytes) originate from hepatoblasts as common precursors. Notch signaling, which is impaired in Alagille syndrome, promotes hepatoblast differentiation into biliary epithelium, whereas hepatocyte growth factor antagonizes differentiation. The development of the intrahepatic bile ducts is determined by the development and branching pattern of the portal vein. Around the 8th wk of gestation, starting at the hilum of the liver, primitive hepatoblasts adjacent to the mesenchyme around the portal vein branches form a cylindrical sleeve, termed the *ductal plate.* From 12 wk of gestation onward, a "remodeling" of the ductal plate occurs, with some segments of the ductal plate undergoing tubular dilation and excess ductal plate cells gradually disappearing. The ramification of the biliary tree continues throughout human fetal life and at the time of birth the most peripheral branches of the portal veins are still surrounded by ductal plates; these require 4 more weeks to develop into definitive portal ducts. Lack of remodeling of the ductal plate results in persistence of primitive ductal plate configurations, an abnormality called *ductal plate malformation.* This histopathologic lesion has been

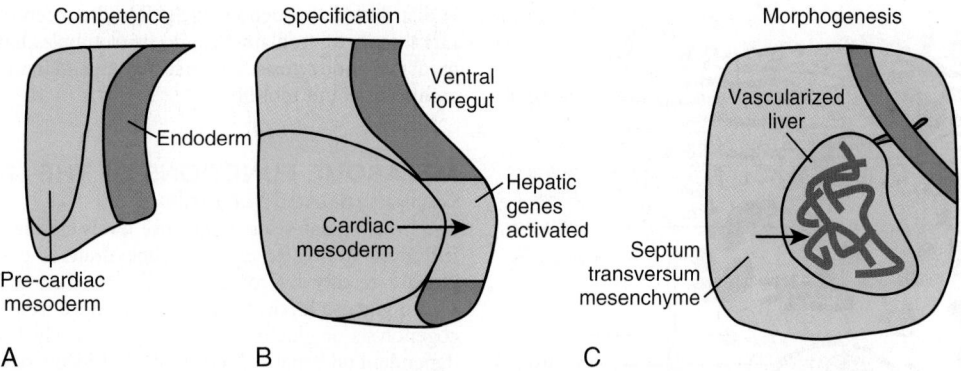

Figure 354-1 Processes involved in early liver development. **A,** The ventral foregut endoderm acquires *competence* to receive signals arising from the cardiac mesoderm. **B,** Specific cells of the ventral foregut endoderm undergo *specification* and activation of liver-specific genes under the influence of mesodermal signals. **C,** Liver *morphogenesis* is initiated as the newly specified cells migrate into the septum transversum under the influence of signaling molecules and extracellular matrix released by septum transversum mesenchymal cells and of primitive endothelial cells. *(Reprinted from Zaret KS: Liver specification and early morphogenesis, Mech Dev 92:83–88, 2000; copyright 2000, with permission from Elsevier Science.)*

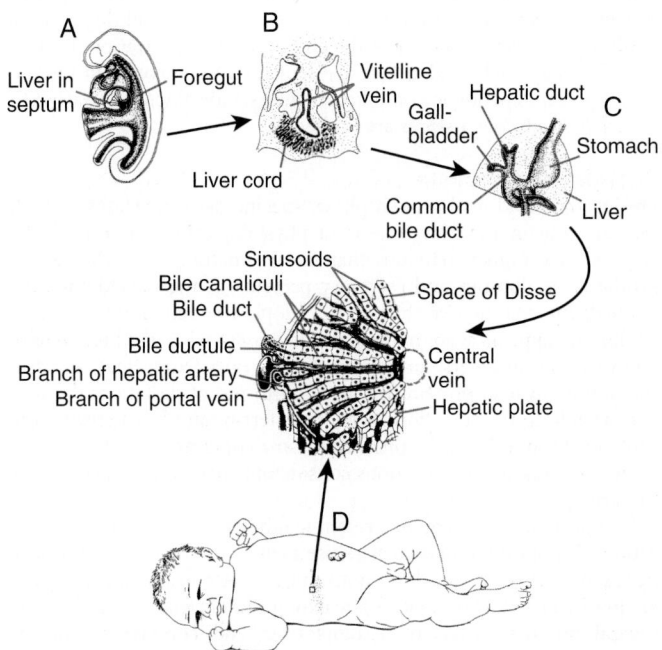

Figure 354-2 Hepatic morphogenesis. **A,** Ventral outgrowth of hepatic diverticulum from foregut endoderm in the 3.5 wk embryo. **B,** Between the 2 vitelline veins, the enlarging hepatic diverticulum buds off epithelial (liver) cords that become the liver parenchyma, around which the endothelium of capillaries (sinusoids) align (4 wk embryo). **C,** Hemisection of embryo at 7.5 wk. **D,** Three-dimensional representation of the hepatic lobule as present in the newborn. *(Reprinted from Andres JM, Mathis RK, Walker WA: Liver disease in infants. Part I: developmental hepatology and mechanisms of liver dysfunction, J Pediatr 90:686–697, 1977.)*

observed in liver biopsies of a variety of liver conditions, including congenital hepatic fibrosis, Caroli disease, and biliary atresia.

The *caudal* part (pars cystica) of the hepatic diverticulum becomes the gallbladder, cystic duct, and common bile duct. The distal portions of the right and left hepatic ducts develop from the extrahepatic ducts, whereas the proximal portions develop from the first intrahepatic ductal plates. The extrahepatic bile ducts and the developing intrahepatic biliary tree maintain luminal continuity and patency from the beginning of organogenesis (see Fig. 354-2C).

Fetal hepatic blood flow is derived from the hepatic artery and from the portal and umbilical veins, which form the portal sinus. The portal venous inflow is directed mainly to the right lobe of the liver and umbilical flow primarily to the left. The ductus venosus shunts blood from the portal and umbilical veins to the hepatic vein, bypassing the sinusoidal network. After birth, the ductus venosus becomes obliterated when oral feedings are initiated. The fetal oxygen saturation is lower in portal than in umbilical venous blood; accordingly, the right hepatic lobe has lower oxygenation and greater hematopoietic activity than the left hepatic lobe.

The transport and metabolic activities of the liver are facilitated by the structural arrangement of liver cell cords, which are formed by rows of hepatocytes, separated by sinusoids that converge toward the tributaries of the hepatic vein (the central vein) located in the center of the lobule (see Fig. 354-2D). This establishes the pathways and patterns of flow for substances to and from the liver. In addition to arterial input from the systemic circulation, the liver also receives venous input from the gastrointestinal tract via the portal system. The products of the hepatobiliary system are released by 2 different paths: through the hepatic vein and through the biliary system back into the intestine. Plasma proteins and other plasma components are secreted by the liver. Absorbed and circulating nutrients arrive through the portal vein or the hepatic artery and pass through the sinusoids and past the hepatocytes to the systemic circulation at the central vein. Biliary components are transported via the series of enlarging channels from the bile canaliculi through the bile ductule to the common bile duct.

Bile secretion is first noted at the 12th wk of human gestation. The major components of bile vary with stage of development. Near term, cholesterol and phospholipid content is relatively low. Low concentrations of bile acids, the absence of bacterially derived (secondary) bile acids, and the presence of unusual bile acids reflect low rates of bile flow and immature bile acid synthetic pathways.

The liver reaches a peak relative size of approximately 10% of the fetal weight at the 9th wk. Early in development, the liver is a primary site of hematopoiesis. In the 7th wk, hematopoietic cells outnumber functioning hepatocytes in the hepatic anlage. These early hepatocytes are smaller than at maturity (~20 μm vs 30-35 μm) and contain less glycogen. Near term, the hepatocyte mass expands to dominate the organ, as cell size and glycogen content increase. Hematopoiesis is virtually absent by the 2nd postnatal month in full-term infants. As the density of hepatocytes increases with gestational age, the relative volume of the sinusoidal network decreases. The liver constitutes 5% of body weight at birth but only 2% in an adult.

Several metabolic processes are immature in a healthy newborn infant, owing in part to the fetal patterns of activity of various enzymatic processes. Many fetal hepatic functions are carried out by the maternal liver, which provides nutrients and serves as a route of elimination of metabolic end products and toxins. Fetal liver metabolism is devoted primarily to the production of proteins required for growth.

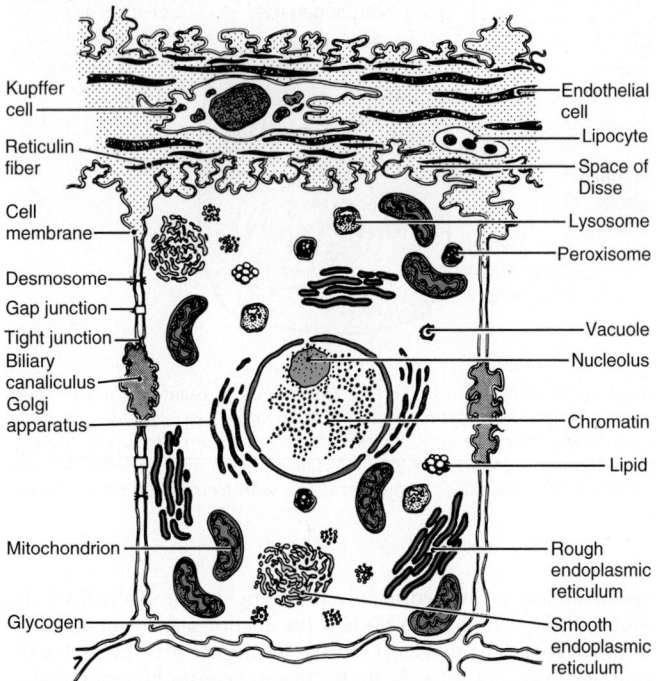

Figure 354-3 Schematic view of the ultrastructure and organelles of hepatocytes. *(Reprinted from Sherlock S: Hepatic cell structure. In Sherlock S, editor: Diseases of the liver and biliary system, ed 6, Oxford, 1981, Blackwell Scientific, p. 10, with permission from Blackwell Scientific.)*

Toward term, primary functions become production and storage of essential nutrients, excretion of bile, and establishment of processes of elimination. Extrauterine adaptation requires de novo enzyme synthesis. Modulation of these processes depends on substrate and hormonal input via the placenta and on dietary and hormonal input in the postnatal period.

HEPATIC ULTRASTRUCTURE

Hepatocytes exhibit various ultrastructural features that reflect their biologic functions (Fig. 354-3). Hepatocytes, like other epithelial cells, are polarized, meaning that their structure and function are directionally oriented. One result of this polarity is that various regions of the hepatocyte plasma membrane exhibit specialized functions. Bidirectional transport occurs at the *sinusoidal* surface, where materials reaching the liver via the portal system enter and compounds secreted by the liver leave the hepatocyte. *Canalicular* membranes of adjacent hepatocytes form bile canaliculi, which are bounded by tight junctions, preventing transfer of secreted compounds back into the sinusoid. Within hepatocytes, metabolic and synthetic activities are contained within a number of different cell organelles. The oxidation and metabolism of heterogeneous classes of substrates, fatty acid oxidation, key processes in gluconeogenesis, and the storage and release of energy occur in the abundant mitochondria.

The endoplasmic reticulum, a continuous network of rough- and smooth-surfaced tubules and cisternae, is the site of various processes, including protein and triglyceride synthesis and drug metabolism. Low fetal activity of endoplasmic reticulum–bound enzymes accounts for a relative inefficiency of xenobiotic (drug) metabolism. The Golgi apparatus is active in protein packaging and possibly in bile secretion. Hepatocyte peroxisomes are single-membrane-limited cytoplasmic organelles that contain enzymes such as oxidases and catalase and those that have a role in lipid and bile acid metabolism. Lysosomes contain numerous hydrolases that have a role in intracellular digestion. The hepatocyte cytoskeleton, composed of actin and other filaments, is distributed throughout the cell and concentrated near the plasma membrane. Microfilaments and microtubules have a role in receptor-mediated endocytosis, in bile secretion, and in maintaining hepatocyte architecture and motility.

METABOLIC FUNCTIONS OF THE LIVER
Carbohydrate Metabolism

The liver regulates serum glucose levels closely via several processes, including storage of excess carbohydrate as glycogen, a polymer of glucose readily hydrolyzed to glucose during fasting. To maintain serum glucose levels, hepatocytes produce free glucose by either glycogenolysis or gluconeogenesis. Immediately after birth, an infant is dependent on hepatic glycogenolysis. Gluconeogenic activity is present at a low level in the fetal liver and increases rapidly after birth. Fetal glycogen synthesis begins at about the 9th wk of gestation, with glycogen stores most rapidly accumulated near term, when the liver contains 2-3 times the amount of glycogen of adult liver. Most of this stored glycogen is used in the immediate postnatal period. Reaccumulation is initiated at about the 2nd wk of postnatal life, and glycogen stores reach adult levels at approximately the 3rd wk in healthy full-term infants. In preterm infants, serum glucose levels fluctuate in part because efficient regulation of the synthesis, storage, and degradation of glycogen develops only near the end of full-term gestation. Dietary carbohydrates such as galactose are converted to glucose, but there is a substantial dependence on gluconeogenesis for glucose in early life, especially if glycogen stores are limited.

Protein Metabolism

During the rapid fetal growth phase, specific decarboxylases that are rate limiting in the biosynthesis of physiologically important polyamines have higher activities than in the mature liver. The rate of synthesis of albumin and secretory proteins in the developing liver parallels the quantitative changes in endoplasmic reticulum. Synthesis of albumin appears at approximately the 7th-8th wk in the human fetus and increases in inverse proportion to that of α-fetoprotein, which is the dominant fetal protein. By the 3rd-4th mo of gestation, the fetal liver is able to produce fibrinogen, transferrin, and low-density lipoproteins. From this period on, fetal plasma contains each of the major protein classes at concentrations considerably below those achieved at maturity.

The *postnatal* patterns of protein synthesis vary with the class of protein. Lipoproteins of each class rise abruptly in the 1st wk after birth to reach levels that vary little until puberty. Albumin concentrations are low in a neonate (~2.5 g/dL), reaching adult levels (~3.5 g/dL) after several months. Levels of ceruloplasmin and complement factors increase slowly to adult values in the 1st yr. In contrast, transferrin levels at birth are similar to those of an adult, decline for 3-5 mo, and rise thereafter to achieve their final concentrations. Low levels of activity of specific proteins have implications for the nutrition of an infant. A low level of cystathionine γ-lyase (cystathionase) activity impairs the *trans*-sulfuration pathway by which dietary methionine is converted to cysteine. Consequently, the latter must be supplied in the diet. Similar dietary requirements might exist for other sulfur-containing amino acids, such as taurine.

Lipid Metabolism

Fatty acid oxidation provides a major source of energy in early life, complementing glycogenolysis and gluconeogenesis. Newborn infants are relatively intolerant of prolonged fasting, owing in part to a restricted capacity for hepatic ketogenesis. Rapid maturation of the ability of the liver to oxidize fatty acid occurs in the 1st few days of life. Milk provides the major source of calories in early life; this high-fat, low-carbohydrate diet mandates active gluconeogenesis to maintain blood glucose levels. When the glucose supply is limited, ketone body production from endogenous fatty acids can provide energy for hepatic gluconeogenesis and an alternative fuel for brain metabolism. When carbohydrates are in excess, the liver produces triglycerides. Metabolic processes involving lipids and lipoproteins are predominantly hepatic; liver immaturity or disease affects lipid concentrations and lipoproteins.

Biotransformation

Newborn infants have a decreased capacity to metabolize and detoxify certain drugs, owing to underdevelopment of the hepatic microsomal component that is the site of the specific oxidative, reductive, hydrolytic, and conjugation reactions required for these biotransformations. The major components of the monooxygenase system, such as cytochrome P450, cytochrome-*c* reductase, and the reduced form of nicotinamide-adenine dinucleotide phosphate, are present in low concentrations in fetal microsomal preparations. In full-term infants, hepatic uridine diphosphate glucuronosyltransferase and enzymes involved in the oxidation of polycyclic aromatic hydrocarbons are expressed at very low levels.

Age-related differences in pharmacokinetics vary from compound to compound. The half-life of acetaminophen in a newborn is similar to that of an adult, whereas theophylline has a half-life of approximately 100 hr in a premature infant, as compared to 5-6 hr in an adult. These differences in metabolism, as well as factors such as binding to plasma proteins and renal clearance, determine appropriate drug dosage to maximize effectiveness and to avoid toxicity. Dramatic examples of the susceptibility of newborn infants to drug toxicity are the responses to chloramphenicol (the "gray baby" syndrome) or to benzoyl alcohol and its metabolic products, which involve ineffective glucuronide and glycine conjugation, respectively. The low concentrations of antioxidants (vitamin E, superoxide dismutase, glutathione peroxidase) in the fetal and early newborn liver lead to increased susceptibility to deleterious effects of oxygen toxicity and oxidant injury through lipid peroxidation.

Conjugation reactions, which convert drugs or metabolites into water-soluble forms that can be eliminated in bile, are also catalyzed by hepatic microsomal enzymes. Newborn infants have decreased activity of hepatic uridine diphosphate glucuronosyltransferase, which converts unconjugated bilirubin to the readily excreted glucuronide conjugate and is the rate-limiting enzyme in the excretion of bilirubin. There is rapid postnatal development of transferase activity irrespective of gestational age, which suggests that birth-related, rather than age-related, factors are of primary importance in the postnatal development of activity of this enzyme. Microsomal activity can be stimulated by administration of phenobarbital, rifampin, or other inducers of cytochrome P450. Alternatively, drugs such as cimetidine can inhibit microsomal P450 activity.

Hepatic Excretory Function

Hepatic excretory function and bile flow are closely related to hepatic *bile acid* excretion and enterohepatic recirculation. Bile acids, the major products of cholesterol degradation, are incorporated into mixed micelles with cholesterol and phospholipid. These micelles act as an efficient vehicle for solubilization and intestinal absorption of lipophilic compounds, such as dietary fats and fat-soluble vitamins. Secretion of bile acids by the liver cells is the major determinant of bile flow in the mature animal. Accordingly, maturity of bile acid metabolic processes affects overall hepatic excretory function, including biliary excretion of endogenous and exogenous compounds.

In humans, the 2 primary bile acids, cholic acid and chenodeoxycholic acid, are synthesized in the liver. Before excretion, they are conjugated with glycine and taurine. In response to a meal, contraction of the gallbladder delivers bile acids to the intestine to assist in fat digestion and absorption. After mediating fat digestion, the bile acids themselves are reabsorbed from the terminal ileum through specific active transport processes. They return to the liver via portal blood, are taken up by liver cells, and are reexcreted in bile. In an adult, this enterohepatic circulation involves 90-95% of the circulating bile acid pool. Bile acids that escape ileal reabsorption reach the colon, where the bacterial flora, through dehydroxylation and deconjugation, produce the secondary bile acids, deoxycholate and lithocholate. In an

Table 354-2	Causes of Impaired Bile Acid Metabolism and Enterohepatic Circulation

DEFECTIVE BILE ACID SYNTHESIS OR TRANSPORT
Inborn errors of bile acid synthesis (reductase deficiency, isomerase deficiency)
Progressive familial intrahepatic cholestasis (PFIC1, PFIC2, PFIC3)
Intrahepatic cholestasis (neonatal hepatitis)
Acquired defects in bile acid synthesis secondary to severe liver disease

ABNORMALITIES OF BILE ACID DELIVERY TO THE BOWEL
Celiac disease (sluggish gallbladder contraction)
Extrahepatic bile duct obstruction (e.g., biliary atresia, gallstones)

LOSS OF ENTEROHEPATIC CIRCULATION OF BILE ACIDS
External bile fistula
Cystic fibrosis
Small bowel bacterial overgrowth syndrome (with bile acid precipitation, increased jejunal absorption, and "short-circuiting")
Drug-induced entrapment of bile acids in intestinal lumen (e.g., cholestyramine)

BILE ACID MALABSORPTION
Primary bile acid malabsorption (absent or inefficient ileal active transport)
Secondary bile acid malabsorption
Ileal disease or resection
Cystic fibrosis

DEFECTIVE UPTAKE OR ALTERED INTRACELLULAR METABOLISM
Parenchymal disease (acute hepatitis, cirrhosis)
Regurgitation from cells
Portosystemic shunting
Cholestasis

adult, the composition of bile reflects the excretion of the primary and also the secondary bile acids, which are reabsorbed from the distal intestinal tract.

Intraluminal concentrations of bile acids are low in newborn infants and increase rapidly after birth. The expansion of the bile acid pool is critical because bile acids are required to stimulate bile flow and absorb lipids, a major component of the diet of a newborn. Nuclear receptors, such as farnesoid X receptor, control intrahepatic bile acid homeostasis through several mechanisms, including regulation of expression of the genes encoding 2 key proteins, cholesterol 7α-hydroxylase (CYP7A1) and bile salt export pump (BSEP). These proteins are critical for bile acid synthesis and canalicular secretion, respectively. Neonatal expression of these nuclear receptors varies depending on the studied animal model and is largely unknown for humans.

Because of inefficient ileal reabsorption of bile acids and the low rate of hepatic clearance of bile acids from portal blood, serum concentrations of bile acids are commonly elevated in healthy newborns, often to levels that would suggest liver disease in older persons. Transient phases of "physiologic cholestasis" and "physiologic steatorrhea" can often be observed in low birthweight infants and in full-term infants following perinatal stress, such as hypoxia or infection, but are otherwise uncommon in healthy full-term newborns.

Many of the processes related to immaturity of the newborn in liver morphogenesis and function as discussed earlier are implied in the increased susceptibility of infants to liver disease associated with parenteral nutrition. The reduced bile salt pool, hepatic glutathione depletion, and deficient sulfation contribute to production of toxic lithocholic bile acids and cholestasis, whereas deficiencies of essential amino acids, including taurine and cysteine, and excessive lipid infusion can lead to hepatic steatosis in these infants. Beyond the neonatal period, disturbances in bile acid metabolism may be responsible for diverse effects on hepatobiliary and intestinal function (Table 354-2).

Bibliography is available at Expert Consult.

Chapter 355
Manifestations of Liver Disease

James E. Squires and William F. Balistreri

PATHOLOGIC MANIFESTATIONS

Alterations in hepatic structure and function can be acute or chronic, with varying patterns of reaction of the liver to cell injury. Hepatocyte injury can be caused by viral infection, drugs or toxins, hypoxia, immunologic disorders, or inborn errors of metabolism. The injury results in inflammatory cell infiltration or cell death (necrosis), which may be followed by a healing process of scar formation (fibrosis) and, potentially, nodule formation (regeneration). Cirrhosis is the end result of any progressive liver disease.

Cholestasis is an alternative or concomitant response to injury caused by extrahepatic or intrahepatic obstruction to bile flow. Substances that are normally excreted in bile, such as conjugated bilirubin, cholesterol, bile acids, and trace elements, accumulate in serum. Bile pigment accumulation in liver parenchyma can be seen in liver biopsy specimens. In extrahepatic obstruction, bile pigment may be visible in the intralobular bile ducts or throughout the parenchyma as bile lakes or infarcts. In intrahepatic cholestasis, an injury to hepatocytes or an alteration in hepatic physiology leads to a reduction in the rate of secretion of solute and water. Likely causes include alterations in enzymatic or canalicular transporter activity, permeability of the bile canalicular apparatus, organelles responsible for bile secretion, or ultrastructure of the cytoskeleton of the hepatocyte. The end result can be clinically indistinguishable from obstructive cholestasis.

Cirrhosis, defined histologically by the presence of bands of fibrous tissue that link central and portal areas and form parenchymal nodules, is a potential end stage of any acute or chronic liver disease. Cirrhosis can be macronodular, with nodules of various sizes (up to 5 cm) separated by broad septa, or micronodular, with nodules of uniform size (<1 cm) separated by fine septa; mixed forms occur. The progressive scarring of cirrhosis results in altered hepatic blood flow, with further impairment of liver cell function. Increased intrahepatic resistance to portal blood flow leads to portal hypertension.

The liver can be secondarily involved in neoplastic (metastatic) and nonneoplastic (storage diseases, fat infiltration) processes, as well as a number of systemic conditions and infectious processes. The liver can be affected by chronic passive congestion (congestive heart failure) or acute hypoxia, with hepatocellular damage.

CLINICAL MANIFESTATIONS
Hepatomegaly

Enlargement of the liver can be caused by several mechanisms (Table 355-1). Normal liver size estimations are based on age-related clinical indices, such as the degree of extension of the liver edge below the costal margin, the span of dullness to percussion, or the length of the vertical axis of the liver, as estimated from imaging techniques. In children, the normal liver edge can be felt up to 2 cm below the right costal margin. In a newborn infant, extension of the liver edge more than 3.5 cm below the costal margin in the right midclavicular line suggests hepatic enlargement. Measurement of liver span is carried out by percussing the upper margin of dullness and by palpating the lower edge in the right midclavicular line. This may be more reliable than an extension of the liver edge alone. The 2 measurements may correlate poorly.

The liver span increases linearly with body weight and age in both sexes, ranging from approximately 4.5-5.0 cm at 1 wk of age to approximately 7-8 cm in boys and 6.0-6.5 cm in girls by 12 yr of age. The lower edge of the right lobe of the liver extends downward (Riedel lobe) and can normally be palpated as a broad mass in some people. An

Table 355-1	Mechanisms of Hepatomegaly

INCREASE IN THE NUMBER OR SIZE OF THE CELLS INTRINSIC TO THE LIVER

Storage
Fat: malnutrition, obesity, diabetes mellitus, metabolic liver disease (diseases of fatty acid oxidation and Reye syndrome–like illnesses), lipid infusion (total parenteral nutrition), cystic fibrosis, medication related, pregnancy
Specific lipid storage diseases: Gaucher, Niemann-Pick, Wolman disease
Glycogen: glycogen storage diseases (multiple enzyme defects); total parenteral nutrition; infant of diabetic mother, Beckwith syndrome
Miscellaneous: α_1-antitrypsin deficiency, Wilson disease, hypervitaminosis A, neonatal iron storage disease

Inflammation
Hepatocyte enlargement (hepatitis)
• Viral: acute and chronic
• Bacterial: sepsis, abscess, cholangitis
• Toxic: drugs
• Autoimmune
Kupffer cell enlargement
• Sarcoidosis
• Systemic lupus erythematosus
• Macrophage activating syndrome

INFILTRATION OF CELLS

Primary Liver Tumors: Benign
Hepatocellular
• Focal nodular hyperplasia
• Nodular regenerative hyperplasia
• Hepatocellular adenoma
Mesodermal
• Infantile hemangioendothelioma
• Mesenchymal hamartoma
Cystic masses
• Choledochal cyst
• Hepatic cyst
• Hematoma
• Parasitic cyst
• Pyogenic or amebic abscess

Primary Liver Tumors: Malignant
Hepatocellular
• Hepatoblastoma
• Hepatocellular carcinoma
Mesodermal
• Angiosarcoma
• Undifferentiated embryonal sarcoma
Secondary or metastatic processes
• Lymphoma
• Leukemia
• Histiocytosis
• Neuroblastoma
• Wilms tumor

INCREASED SIZE OF VASCULAR SPACE
Intrahepatic obstruction to hepatic vein outflow
• Venoocclusive disease
• Hepatic vein thrombosis (Budd-Chiari syndrome)
• Hepatic vein web
Suprahepatic
• Congestive heart failure
• Pericardial disease
• Tamponade
Post-Fontan procedure
Constrictive pericarditis
Hematopoietic: sickle cell anemia, thalassemia

INCREASED SIZE OF BILIARY SPACE
Congenital hepatic fibrosis
Caroli disease
Extrahepatic obstruction

IDIOPATHIC
Various
• Riedel lobe
• Normal variant
• Downward displacement of diaphragm

enlarged left lobe of the liver is palpable in the epigastrium of some patients with cirrhosis. Downward displacement of the liver by the diaphragm (hyperinflation) or thoracic organs can create an erroneous impression of hepatomegaly.

Examination of the liver should note the consistency, contour, tenderness, and presence of any masses or bruits, as well as assessment of spleen size. Documentation of the presence of ascites and any stigmata of chronic liver disease is important.

Ultrasound is useful in assessment of liver size and consistency, as well as gallbladder size. Gallbladder length normally varies from 1.5-5.5 cm (average: 3 cm) in infants to 4-8 cm in adolescents; width ranges from 0.5-2.5 cm for all ages. Gallbladder distention may be seen in infants with sepsis. The gallbladder is often absent in infants with biliary atresia.

Jaundice (Icterus)

Yellow discoloration of the sclera, skin, and mucous membranes is a sign of hyperbilirubinemia (see Chapter 102.3). Clinically apparent jaundice in children and adults occurs when the serum concentration of bilirubin reaches 2-3 mg/dL (34-51 μmol/L); the neonate might not appear icteric until the bilirubin level is >5 mg/dL (>85 μmol/L). Jaundice may be the earliest and only sign of hepatic dysfunction. Liver disease must be suspected in the infant who appears only mildly jaundiced but has dark urine or acholic (light-colored) stools. Immediate evaluation to establish the cause is required.

Measurement of the total serum bilirubin concentration allows quantitation of jaundice. Bilirubin occurs in plasma in 4 forms: *unconjugated* bilirubin tightly bound to albumin; *free* or *unbound bilirubin* (the form responsible for kernicterus, because it can cross cell membranes); *conjugated bilirubin* (the only fraction to appear in urine); and *δ fraction* (bilirubin covalently bound to albumin), which appears in serum when hepatic excretion of conjugated bilirubin is impaired in patients with hepatobiliary disease. The δ fraction permits conjugated bilirubin to persist in the circulation and delays resolution of jaundice. Although the terms *direct* and *indirect* bilirubin are used equivalently with *conjugated* and *unconjugated* bilirubin, this is not quantitatively correct, because the direct fraction includes both conjugated bilirubin and δ bilirubin.

Investigation of jaundice in an infant or older child must include determination of the accumulation of both unconjugated and conjugated bilirubin. Unconjugated hyperbilirubinemia might indicate increased production, hemolysis, reduced hepatic removal, or altered metabolism of bilirubin (Table 355-2). Conjugated hyperbilirubinemia reflects decreased excretion by damaged hepatic parenchymal cells or disease of the biliary tract, which may be a result of obstruction, sepsis, toxins, inflammation, and genetic or metabolic disease (Table 355-3).

Pruritus

Intense generalized itching can occur in patients with chronic liver disease often in association with cholestasis (conjugated hyperbilirubinemia). Symptoms can be generalized or localized (commonly to palms and soles), are usually worse at night, are exacerbated with stress and heat, and are relieved by cool temperatures. Pruritus is unrelated to the degree of hyperbilirubinemia; deeply jaundiced patients can be asymptomatic. Although retained components of bile are likely important, the cause is probably multifactorial, as evidenced by the symptomatic relief of pruritus after administration of various therapeutic agents including bile acid-binding agents (cholestyramine), choleretic agents (ursodeoxycholic acid), opiate antagonists, antihistamines, and antibiotics. Plasmapheresis, molecular adsorbent recirculating system therapy, and surgical diversion of bile (partial external biliary diversion) have been used in attempts to provide relief for medically refractory pruritus.

Spider Angiomas

Vascular spiders (telangiectasias), characterized by central pulsating arterioles from which small, wiry venules radiate, may be seen in patients with chronic liver disease; these are usually most prominent

| **Table 355-2** | Differential Diagnosis of Unconjugated Hyperbilirubinemia |

INCREASED PRODUCTION OF UNCONJUGATED BILIRUBIN FROM HEME
Hemolytic Disease (Hereditary or Acquired)
Isoimmune hemolysis (neonatal; acute or delayed transfusion reaction; autoimmune)
• Rh incompatibility
• ABO incompatibility
• Other blood group incompatibilities
Congenital spherocytosis
Hereditary elliptocytosis
Infantile pyknocytosis
Erythrocyte enzyme defects
Hemoglobinopathy
• Sickle cell anemia
• Thalassemia
• Others
Sepsis
Microangiopathy
• Hemolytic-uremic syndrome
• Hemangioma
• Mechanical trauma (heart valve)
Ineffective erythropoiesis
Drugs
Infection
Enclosed hematoma
Polycythemia
• Diabetic mother
• Fetal transfusion (recipient)
• Delayed cord clamping

DECREASED DELIVERY OF UNCONJUGATED BILIRUBIN (IN PLASMA) TO HEPATOCYTE
Right-sided congestive heart failure
Portacaval shunt

DECREASED BILIRUBIN UPTAKE ACROSS HEPATOCYTE MEMBRANE
Presumed enzyme transporter deficiency
Competitive inhibition
• Breast milk jaundice
• Lucey-Driscoll syndrome
• Drug inhibition (radiocontrast material)
Miscellaneous
• Hypothyroidism
• Hypoxia
• Acidosis

DECREASED STORAGE OF UNCONJUGATED BILIRUBIN IN CYTOSOL (DECREASED Y AND Z PROTEINS)
Competitive inhibition
Fever

DECREASED BIOTRANSFORMATION (CONJUGATION)
Neonatal jaundice (physiologic)
Inhibition (drugs)
Hereditary (Crigler-Najjar)
• Type I (complete enzyme deficiency)
• Type II (partial deficiency)
Gilbert disease
Hepatocellular dysfunction

ENTEROHEPATIC RECIRCULATION
Breast milk jaundice
Intestinal obstruction
• Ileal atresia
• Hirschsprung disease
• Cystic fibrosis
• Pyloric stenosis
Antibiotic administration

Table 355-3	Differential Diagnosis of Neonatal and Infantile Cholestasis

INFECTIOUS

Generalized bacterial sepsis

Viral hepatitis
- Hepatitides A, B, C, D, E
- Cytomegalovirus
- Rubella virus
- Herpesviruses: herpes simplex, human herpesvirus 6 and 7
- Varicella virus
- Coxsackievirus
- Echovirus
- Reovirus type 3
- Parvovirus B19
- HIV
- Adenovirus

Others
- Toxoplasmosis
- Syphilis
- Tuberculosis
- Listeriosis
- Urinary tract infection

TOXIC

Sepsis

Parenteral nutrition related

Drug, dietary supplement, herbal related

METABOLIC

Disorders of amino acid metabolism
- Tyrosinemia

Disorders of lipid metabolism
- Wolman disease
- Niemann-Pick disease (type C)
- Gaucher disease

Cholesterol ester storage disease

Disorders of carbohydrate metabolism
- Galactosemia
- Fructosemia
- Glycogenosis IV

Disorders of bile acid biosynthesis

Other metabolic defects
- α_1-Antitrypsin deficiency
- Cystic fibrosis
- Hypopituitarism
- Hypothyroidism
- Zellweger (cerebrohepatorenal) syndrome

- Wilson disease
- Neonatal iron storage disease
- Indian childhood cirrhosis/infantile copper overload
- Congenital disorders of glycosylation
- Mitochondrial hepatopathies
- Citrin deficiency

GENETIC OR CHROMOSOMAL

Trisomies 17, 18, 21

INTRAHEPATIC CHOLESTASIS SYNDROMES

"Idiopathic" neonatal hepatitis

Alagille syndrome

Intrahepatic cholestasis (progressive familial intrahepatic cholestasis [PFIC])
- FIC-1 deficiency
- BSEP (bile salt export pump) deficiency
- MDR3 deficiency

Familial benign recurrent cholestasis associated with lymphedema (Aagenaes syndrome)

ARC (arthrogryposis, renal dysfunction, and cholestasis) syndrome

Caroli disease (cystic dilation of intrahepatic ducts)

EXTRAHEPATIC DISEASES

Biliary atresia

Sclerosing cholangitis

Bile duct stricture/stenosis

Choledochal–pancreaticoductal junction anomaly

Spontaneous perforation of the bile duct

Choledochal cyst

Mass (neoplasia, stone)

Bile/mucous plug ("inspissated bile")

MISCELLANEOUS

Shock and hypoperfusion

Associated with enteritis

Associated with intestinal obstruction

Neonatal lupus erythematosus

Myeloproliferative disease (trisomy 21)

Hemophagocytic lymphohistiocytosis (HLH)

COACH syndrome (coloboma, oligophrenia, ataxia, cerebellar vermis hypoplasia, hepatic fibrosis)

Cholangiocyte cilia defects

in the superior vena cava distribution area (on the face and chest). Their size varies between 1 and 10 mm and they exhibit central clearing with pressure. They presumably reflect altered estrogen metabolism in the presence of hepatic dysfunction.

Palmar Erythema

Blotchy erythema, most noticeable over the thenar and hypothenar eminences and on the tips of the fingers, is also noted in patients with chronic liver disease. Abnormal serum estradiol levels and regional alterations in peripheral circulation have been identified as possible causes.

Xanthomas

The marked elevation of serum cholesterol levels (to >500 mg/dL) associated with some forms of chronic cholestasis can cause the deposition of lipid in the dermis and subcutaneous tissue. Brown nodules can develop, first over the extensor surfaces of the extremities; rarely, xanthelasma of the eyelids develops.

Portal Hypertension

Portal hypertension occurs when there is increased portal resistance and/or increased portal flow. The portal system drains the splanchnic area (abdominal portion of the gastrointestinal tract, pancreas, and spleen) into the hepatic sinusoids. Normal portal pressure is between 3 and 6 mm Hg. Portal hypertension is defined as a portal pressure greater than 10 mm Hg. Clinically significant portal hypertension exists when pressure exceeds a threshold of 12 mm Hg or greater. Portal hypertension is the main complication of cirrhosis, directly responsible for 2 of its most common and potentially lethal complications: ascites and variceal hemorrhage.

Ascites

Ascites is a consequence of increased hydrostatic and osmotic pressures within the hepatic and mesenteric capillaries resulting in transfer of fluid from the blood vessels to the lymphatics that overcomes the drainage capacity of the lymphatic system. Ascites can also be associated with nephrotic syndrome and other urinary tract abnormalities, metabolic diseases (such as lysosomal storage diseases), congenital or acquired heart disease, and hydrops fetalis. Factors favoring the intraabdominal accumulation of fluid include decreased plasma colloid osmotic pressure, increased capillary hydrostatic pressure, increased ascitic colloid osmotic fluid pressure, and decreased ascitic fluid hydrostatic pressure. Abnormal renal sodium retention must be considered.

Gastrointestinal Bleeding

Chronic liver disease may manifest as gastrointestinal hemorrhage. Bleeding may result from portal hypertensive gastropathy, gastric antral vascular ectasia, or varix rupture. Variceal hemorrhage is classically from an esophageal origin but may be caused by gastric, duodenal, peristomal, or rectal varices. Variceal hemorrhage results from increased pressure within the varix, which leads to changes in the diameter of the varix and increased wall tension. When the variceal wall strength is exceeded, physical rupture of the varix results. Given the high blood flow and pressure in the portosystemic collateral system, coupled with the lack of a natural mechanism to tamponade variceal bleeding, the rate of hemorrhage can be striking.

Encephalopathy

Hepatic encephalopathy can involve any neurologic function, and it can be prominent or present in subtle forms such as deterioration of school performance, sleep disturbances, depression, or emotional outbursts. It can be recurrent and precipitated by intercurrent illness, drugs, bleeding, or electrolyte and acid-base disturbances. The appearance of hepatic encephalopathy depends on the presence of portosystemic shunting, alterations in the blood–brain barrier, and the interactions of toxic metabolites with the central nervous system. Postulated causes include altered ammonia metabolism, synergistic neurotoxins, decreased cerebral oxygen metabolism and blood flow, or false neurotransmitters with plasma amino acid imbalance.

Endocrine Abnormalities

Endocrine abnormalities are more common in adults with hepatic disease than in children. They reflect alterations in hepatic synthetic, storage, and metabolic functions, including those concerned with hormonal metabolism in the liver. Proteins that bind hormones in plasma are synthesized in the liver, and steroid hormones are conjugated in the liver and excreted in the urine; failure of such functions can have clinical consequences. Endocrine abnormalities can also result from malnutrition or specific deficiencies.

Renal Dysfunction

Systemic disease or toxins can affect the liver and kidneys simultaneously, or parenchymal liver disease can produce secondary impairment of renal function. In hepatobiliary disorders, there may be renal alterations in sodium and water economy, impaired renal concentrating ability, and alterations in potassium metabolism. Ascites in patients with cirrhosis may be related to inappropriate retention of sodium by the kidneys and expansion of plasma volume, or it may be related to sodium retention mediated by diminished effective plasma volume. **Hepatorenal syndrome** is defined as functional renal failure in patients with end-stage liver disease. The pathophysiology of hepatorenal syndrome is related to splanchnic vasodilation, mesenteric angiogenesis, and decreased effective blood volume with resulting decreased renal perfusion. The hallmark is intense renal vasoconstriction (mediated by hemodynamic, humoral, or neurogenic mechanisms) with coexistent systemic vasodilation. The diagnosis is supported by the findings of oliguria (<1 mL/kg/day), a characteristic pattern of urine electrolyte abnormalities (urine sodium < 10 mEq/L, fractional excretion of sodium of <1%, urine:plasma creatinine ratio <10, and normal urinary sediment), absence of hypovolemia, and exclusion of other kidney pathology. The best treatment of hepatorenal syndrome is timely liver transplantation, because complete renal recovery can be expected.

Pulmonary Involvement

Hepatopulmonary syndrome is characterized by the typical triad of hypoxemia, intrapulmonary vascular dilations, and liver disease. There is intrapulmonic right-to-left shunting of blood resulting from enlarged pulmonary vessels that prevents red blood cells traveling through the center of the vessel adequate exposure to oxygen-rich alveoli. Shunting of vasodilatory mediators from the mesentery away from the liver is thought to contribute. It should be suspected and investigated in the child with chronic liver disease with history of shortness of breath or

exercise intolerance and clinical examination findings of cyanosis (particularly of the lips and fingers), digital clubbing, and oxygen saturations <96%, particularly in the upright position. Treatment is timely liver transplantation; resolution of pulmonary involvement usually follows.

Portopulmonary hypertension is a condition characterized by an increase in the resistance to pulmonary arterial blood flow in the setting of portal hypertension. It is defined by a pulmonary arterial pressure >25 mm Hg at rest and above 30 mm Hg with exercise, elevated pulmonary vascular resistance with pulmonary arterial occlusion pressure, or a left-ventricular end-diastolic pressure of <15 mm Hg. Although the pathophysiology is unclear, symptoms suggesting a diagnosis include exertional dyspnea, fatigue, syncope, palpitations, and chest pain.

Recurrent Cholangitis

Ascending infection of the biliary system is often seen in pediatric cholestatic disorders, most commonly because of Gram-negative enteric organisms, such as *Escherichia coli*, *Klebsiella*, *Pseudomonas*, and *Enterococcus*. Liver transplantation is the definitive treatment for recurrent cholangitis, especially when medical therapy is not effective.

Miscellaneous Manifestations of Liver Dysfunction

Nonspecific signs of acute and chronic liver disease include anorexia, which often affects patients with anicteric hepatitis and with cirrhosis associated with chronic cholestasis; abdominal pain or distention resulting from ascites, spontaneous peritonitis, or visceromegaly; malnutrition and growth failure; and bleeding, which may be a result of altered synthesis of coagulation factors (biliary obstruction with vitamin K deficiency or excessive hepatic damage) or to portal hypertension with hypersplenism. In the presence of hypersplenism, there can be decreased synthesis of specific clotting factors, production of qualitatively abnormal proteins, or alterations in platelet number and function. Altered drug metabolism can prolong the biologic half-life of commonly administered medications.

Bibliography is available at Expert Consult.

355.1 Evaluation of Patients with Possible Liver Dysfunction

James E. Squires and William F. Balistreri

Adequate evaluation of an infant, child, or adolescent with suspected liver disease involves an appropriate and accurate history, a carefully performed physical examination, and skillful interpretation of signs and symptoms. Further evaluation is aided by judicious selection of diagnostic tests, followed by the use of imaging modalities or a liver biopsy. Most of the so-called liver function tests do not measure specific hepatic functions: a rise in serum aminotransferase levels reflects liver cell injury, an increase in immunoglobulin levels reflects an immunologic response to injury, or an elevation in serum bilirubin levels can reflect any of several disturbances of bilirubin metabolism (see Tables 355-2 and 355-3). Any single biochemical assay provides limited information, which must be placed in the context of the entire clinical picture. The most cost-efficient approach is to become familiar with the rationale, implications, and limitations of a selected group of tests so that specific questions can be answered. Young infants with cholestatic jaundice should be evaluated promptly to identify patients needing surgical intervention.

For a patient with suspected liver disease, evaluation addresses the following issues in sequence: Is liver disease present? If so, what is its nature? What is its severity? Is specific treatment available? How can we monitor the response to treatment? What is the prognosis?

BIOCHEMICAL TESTS

Laboratory tests commonly used to screen for or to confirm a suspicion of liver disease include measurements of serum aminotransferase, bilirubin (total and fractionated), and alkaline phosphatase (AP) levels, as well as determinations of prothrombin time (PT) or international normalized ratio (INR) and albumin level. These tests are complementary, provide an estimation of synthetic and excretory functions, and might suggest the nature of the disturbance (inflammation or cholestasis).

The severity of the liver disease may be reflected in clinical signs or biochemical alterations. Clinical signs include encephalopathy, variceal hemorrhage, worsening jaundice, apparent shrinkage of liver mass owing to massive necrosis, or onset of ascites. Biochemical alterations include hypoglycemia, acidosis, hyperammonemia, electrolyte imbalance, continued hyperbilirubinemia, marked hypoalbuminemia, or a prolonged PT or INR that is unresponsive to parenteral administration of vitamin K.

Acute liver cell injury (parenchymal disease) caused by viral hepatitis, drug- or toxin-induced liver disease, shock, hypoxemia, or metabolic disease is best reflected by a marked increase in serum aminotransferase levels. Cholestasis (obstructive disease) involves regurgitation of bile components into serum; the serum levels of total and conjugated bilirubin and serum bile acids are elevated. Elevations in serum AP, 5′ nucleotidase, and γ-glutamyl transpeptidase levels are also sensitive indicators of obstruction or inflammation of the biliary tract. Fractionation of the total serum bilirubin level into conjugated and unconjugated bilirubin fractions helps to distinguish between elevations caused by processes such as hemolysis and those caused by hepatic dysfunction. A predominant elevation in the conjugated bilirubin level provides a relatively sensitive index of hepatocellular disease or hepatic excretory dysfunction.

Alanine aminotransferase (ALT, serum glutamate pyruvate transaminase) is liver specific, whereas aspartate aminotransferase (AST, serum glutamic-oxaloacetic transaminase) is derived from other organs in addition to the liver. The most marked rises of AST and ALT levels can occur with acute hepatocellular injury; a several thousand-fold elevation can result from acute viral hepatitis, toxic injury, hypoxia, or hypoperfusion. After blunt abdominal trauma, parallel elevations in aminotransferase levels can provide an early clue to hepatic injury. A differential rise or fall in AST and ALT levels sometimes provides useful information. In acute hepatitis, the rise in ALT may be greater than the rise in AST. In alcohol-induced liver injury, fulminant echovirus infection, and various metabolic diseases, more predominant rises in the AST level are reported. In chronic liver disease or in intrahepatic and extrahepatic biliary obstruction, AST and ALT elevations may be less marked. Elevated serum aminotransferase levels are seen in patients with nonalcoholic fatty liver disease and nonalcoholic steatohepatitis (NASH), the notable characteristic is histology similar to alcoholic-induced liver injury in the absence of alcohol abuse.

Hepatic synthetic function is reflected in serum albumin and protein levels and in the PT or INR. Examination of serum globulin concentration and of the relative amounts of the globulin fractions may be helpful. Patients with autoimmune hepatitis often have high γ-globulin levels and increased titers of anti–smooth muscle, antinuclear, and anti–liver-kidney-microsome antibodies. Antimitochondrial antibodies may also be found in patients with autoimmune hepatitis. A resurgence in α-fetoprotein levels can suggest hepatoma, hepatoblastoma, or hereditary tyrosinemia. Hypoalbuminemia caused by depressed synthesis can complicate severe liver disease and serve as a prognostic factor. Deficiencies of factor V and of the vitamin K–dependent factors (II, VII, IX, and X) can occur in patients with severe liver disease or fulminant hepatic failure. If the PT or INR is prolonged as a result of intestinal malabsorption of vitamin K (resulting from cholestasis) or decreased nutritional intake of vitamin K, parenteral administration of vitamin K should correct the coagulopathy, leading to normalization within 12-24 hr. Unresponsiveness to vitamin K suggests severe hepatic disease. Persistently low levels of factor VII are evidence of a poor prognosis in fulminant liver disease.

Interpretation of results of biochemical tests of hepatic structure and function must be made in the context of age-related changes. The activity of AP varies considerably with age. Normal growing children have significant elevations of serum AP activity originating from influx into serum of the isoenzyme that originates in bone, particularly in rapidly growing adolescents. An isolated increase in AP does not indicate hepatic or biliary disease if other liver tests are normal. Other enzymes such as 5′ nucleotidase and γ-glutamyl transpeptidase are increased in cholestatic conditions and may be more specific for hepatobiliary disease. 5′ nucleotidase is not found in bone. γ-Glutamyl transpeptidase exhibits high enzyme activity in early life that declines rapidly with age. Cholesterol concentrations increase throughout life. Cholesterol levels may be markedly elevated in patients with intra- or extrahepatic cholestasis and decreased in severe acute liver disease such as hepatitis.

Interpretation of serum ammonia values must be carried out with caution because of variability in their physiologic determinants and the inherent difficulty in laboratory measurement.

LIVER BIOPSY

Liver biopsy combined with clinical data can suggest a cause for hepatocellular injury or cholestatic disease in most cases. Specimens of liver tissue can be used to determine a precise histologic diagnosis in patients with neonatal cholestasis, chronic hepatitis, nonalcoholic fatty liver disease or nonalcoholic steatohepatitis, metabolic liver disease, intrahepatic cholestasis, congenital hepatic fibrosis, or undefined portal hypertension. The sample may be subjected to enzyme analysis to detect inborn errors of metabolism and to analysis of stored material such as iron, copper, or specific metabolites. Liver biopsies can monitor responses to therapy or detect complications of treatment with potentially hepatotoxic agents, such as aspirin, antiinfectives (minocycline, ketoconazole, isoniazid), antimetabolites, antineoplastics, or anticonvulsant agents.

In infants and children, needle biopsy of the liver is easily accomplished percutaneously. The amount of tissue obtained, even in small infants, is usually sufficient for histologic interpretation and for biochemical analyses, if the latter are deemed necessary. Percutaneous liver biopsy can be performed safely in infants as young as 1 wk of age. Contraindications to the percutaneous approach include prolonged PT or INR; thrombocytopenia; suspicion of a vascular, cystic, or infectious lesion in the path of the needle; and severe ascites. If administration of fresh-frozen plasma or of platelet transfusions fails to correct a prolonged PT, INR, or thrombocytopenia, a tissue specimen can be obtained via alternative techniques. Considerations include either the open laparotomy (wedge) approach by a general surgeon or the transjugular approach under ultrasound and fluoroscopic guidance by an experienced pediatric interventional radiologist in an appropriately equipped fluoroscopy suite. The risk of development of a complication such as hemorrhage, hematoma, creation of an arteriovenous fistula, pneumothorax, or bile peritonitis is small.

HEPATIC IMAGING PROCEDURES

Various techniques help define the size, shape, and architecture of the liver and the anatomy of the intrahepatic and extrahepatic biliary trees. Although imaging might not provide a precise histologic and biochemical diagnosis, specific questions can be answered, such as whether hepatomegaly is related to accumulation of fat or glycogen or is caused by a tumor or cyst. These studies can direct further evaluation such as percutaneous biopsy and make possible prompt referral of patients with biliary obstruction to a surgeon. Choice of imaging procedure should be part of a carefully formulated diagnostic approach, with avoidance of redundant demonstrations by several techniques.

A *plain x-ray study* can suggest hepatomegaly, but a carefully performed physical examination gives a more reliable assessment of liver size. The liver might appear less dense than normal in patients with fatty infiltration or denser with deposition of heavy metals such as iron. A hepatic or biliary tract mass can displace an air-filled loop of bowel. Calcifications may be evident in the liver (parasitic or neoplastic disease), in the vasculature (portal vein thrombosis), or in the

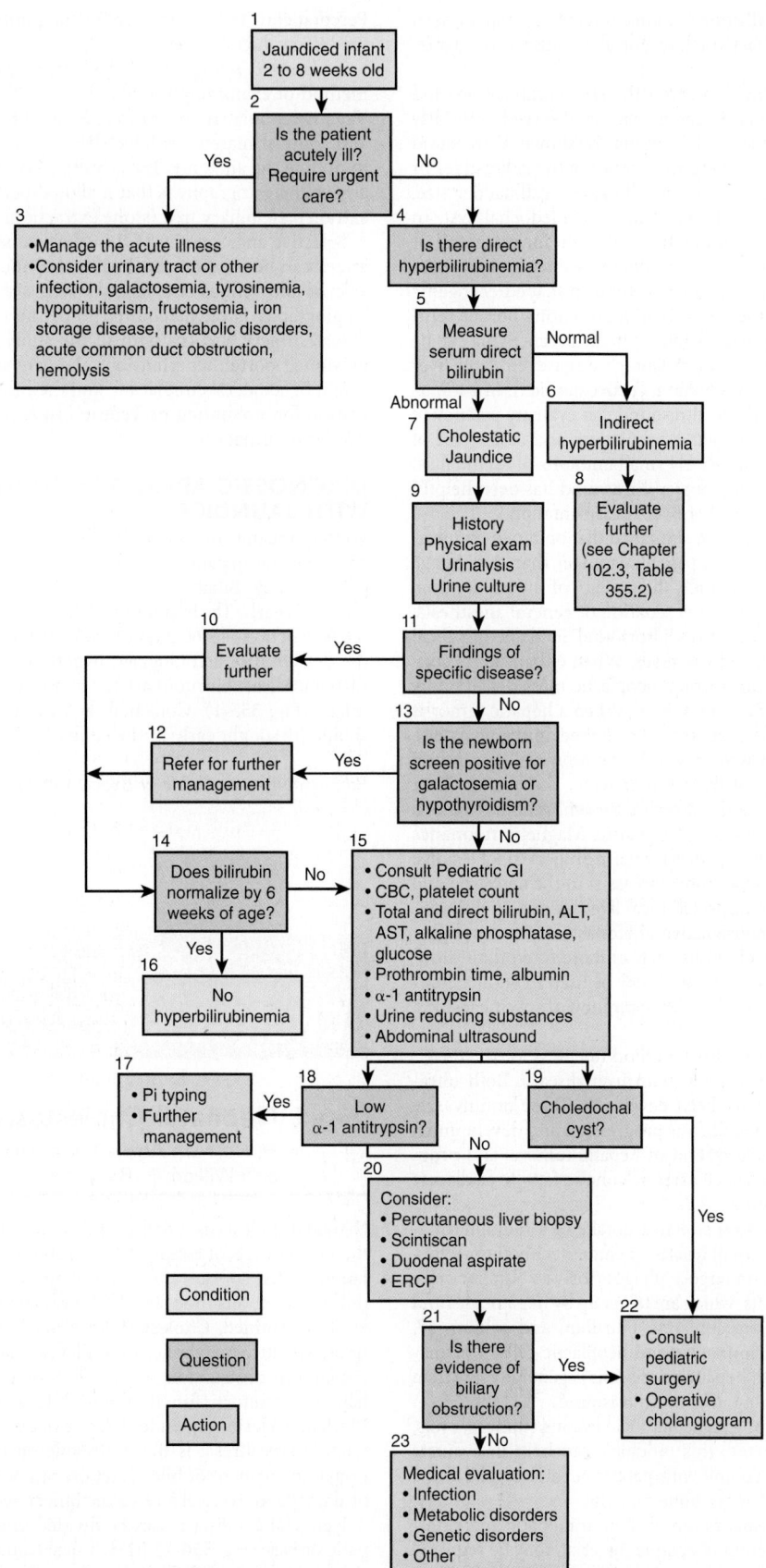

Figure 355-1 Cholestasis clinical practice guideline. Algorithm for a 2-8 wk old. ALT, alanine aminotransferase; AST, aspartate aminotransferase; ERCP, endoscopic retrograde cholangiopancreatography. *(From Moyer V, Freese DK, Whitington PF, et al; North American Society for Pediatric Gastroenterology, Hepatology and Nutrition: Guideline for the evaluation of cholestatic jaundice in infants: recommendations of the North American Society for Pediatric Gastroenterology, Hepatology and Nutrition, J Pediatr Gastroenterol Nutr 39:115–128, 2004.)*

gallbladder or biliary tree (gallstones). Collections of gas may be seen within the liver (abscess), biliary tract, or portal circulation (necrotizing enterocolitis).

Ultrasound provides information about the size, composition, and blood flow of the liver. Increased echogenicity is observed with fatty infiltration; mass lesions as small as 1-2 cm may be shown. Ultrasound has replaced cholangiography in detecting stones in the gallbladder or biliary tree. Even in neonates, ultrasound can assess gallbladder size, detect dilation of the biliary tract, and define a choledochal cyst. In infants with biliary atresia, ultrasound findings might include small or absent gallbladder; nonvisualization of the common duct; and presence of the triangular cord sign, a triangular or tubular-shaped echogenic density in the bifurcation of the portal vein, representing fibrous remnants at the porta hepatis. Hyperechogenic hepatic parenchyma can be seen with metabolic disease (glycogen storage disease) or fatty liver (obesity, malnutrition, hyperalimentation, corticosteroids). In patients with portal hypertension, Doppler ultrasound can evaluate patency of the portal vein, demonstrate collateral circulation, and assess size of spleen and amount of ascites. Relatively small amounts of ascitic fluid can also be detected. The use of Doppler ultrasound has been helpful in determining vascular patency after liver transplantation.

CT scanning provides information similar to that obtained by ultrasound but is less suitable for use in patients younger than 2 yr of age because of the small size of structures, the paucity of intraabdominal fat for contrast, and the need for heavy sedation or general anesthesia. CT scan may be more accurate than ultrasound in detecting focal lesions such as tumors, cysts, and abscesses. When enhanced by contrast medium, CT scanning can reveal a neoplastic mass density only slightly different from that of a normal liver. When a hepatic tumor is suspected, CT scanning is the best method to define anatomic extent, solid or cystic nature, and vascularity. CT scanning can also reveal subtle differences in density of liver parenchyma, the average liver attenuation coefficient being reduced with fatty infiltration. MRI is a useful alternative that limits radiation exposure. Magnetic resonance cholangiography can be of value in differentiating biliary tract lesions. MRI with Eovist (gadoxetate disodium) can assist in the detection and characterization of known or suspected focal liver lesions. In differentiating obstructive from nonobstructive cholestasis, CT scanning or MRI identifies the precise level of obstruction more often than ultrasound. Either CT scanning or ultrasound may be used to guide percutaneously placed fine needles for biopsies, aspiration of specific lesions, or cholangiography.

Elastography is a novel noninvasive method to assess for the development of hepatic fibrosis in patients with liver disease. Both ultrasound and MR methods of have been developed. These noninvasive techniques allow for monitoring fibrosis progression and development of cirrhosis, improved characterization of hepatic tumors, and prognostic stratification of diseases such as nonalcoholic fatty liver disease and nonalcoholic steatohepatitis.

Radionuclide scanning relies on selective uptake of a radiopharmaceutical agent. Commonly used agents include technetium-99m–labeled sulfur colloid, which undergoes phagocytosis by Kupffer cells; ^{99m}Tc-iminodiacetic acid agents, which are taken up by hepatocytes and excreted into bile in a fashion similar to bilirubin; and gallium-67, which is concentrated in inflammatory and neoplastic cells. The anatomic resolution possible with hepatic scintiscans is generally less than that obtained with CT scanning, MRI, or ultrasound.

The ^{99m}Tc-sulfur colloid scan can detect focal lesions (tumors, cysts, abscesses) >2-3 cm in diameter. This modality can help to evaluate patients with possible cirrhosis and with patchy hepatic uptake and a shift of colloid uptake from liver to bone marrow.

Cholangiography, direct visualization of the intrahepatic and extrahepatic biliary tree after injection of opaque material, may be required in some patients to evaluate the cause, location, or extent of biliary obstruction. Percutaneous transhepatic cholangiography with a fine needle is the technique of choice in infants and young children. The likelihood of opacifying the biliary tract is excellent in patients in whom CT scanning, MRI, or ultrasound demonstrates dilated ducts.

Percutaneous transhepatic cholangiography has been used to outline the biliary ductal system.

Endoscopic retrograde cholangiopancreatography is an alternative method of examining the bile ducts in older children. The papilla of Vater is cannulated under direct vision through a fiberoptic endoscope, and contrast material is injected into the biliary and pancreatic ducts to outline the anatomy. The advantage of endoscopic retrograde cholangiopancreatography is that it allows therapeutic interventions of the extrahepatic biliary tree (stone extraction, stent placement, etc.).

Selective angiography of the celiac, superior mesenteric, or hepatic artery can be used to visualize the hepatic or portal circulation. Both arterial and venous circulatory systems of the liver can be examined. Angiography is often required to define the blood supply of tumors before surgery and is useful in the study of patients with known or presumed portal hypertension. The patency of the portal system, the extent of collateral circulation, and the caliber of vessels under consideration for a shunting procedure can be evaluated. MRI can provide similar information.

DIAGNOSTIC APPROACH TO INFANTS WITH JAUNDICE

Well-appearing infants can have cholestatic jaundice. Biliary atresia and neonatal hepatitis are the most common causes of cholestasis in early infancy. Biliary atresia portends a poor prognosis unless it is identified early. The best outcome for this disorder is with early surgical reconstruction (45-60 days of age). History, physical examination, and the detection of a conjugated hyperbilirubinemia via examination of total and direct bilirubin are the first steps in evaluating the jaundiced infant (Fig. 355-1). Consultation with a pediatric gastroenterologist should be sought early in the course of the evaluation.

Bibliography is available at Expert Consult.

Chapter 356
Cholestasis

356.1 Neonatal Cholestasis
H. Hesham Abdel-Kader Hassan and William F. Balistreri

Neonatal cholestasis is defined biochemically as prolonged elevation of the serum levels of conjugated bilirubin beyond the 1st 14 days of life. Jaundice that appears after 2 wk of age, continues to progress, or does not resolve at this time should be evaluated and a conjugated bilirubin level determined. Cholestasis in a newborn can be caused by infectious, genetic, metabolic, or undefined abnormalities giving rise to *mechanical* obstruction of bile flow or to *functional* impairment of hepatic excretory function and bile secretion (see Table 355-3). Mechanical lesions include stricture or obstruction of the common bile duct; biliary atresia is the prototypic obstructive abnormality. Functional impairment of bile secretion can result from congenital defects or damage to liver cells or to the biliary secretory apparatus.

Neonatal cholestasis can be divided into extrahepatic and intrahepatic disease (Fig. 356-1). The clinical features of any form of cholestasis are similar. In an affected neonate, the diagnosis of certain entities, such as galactosemia, sepsis, or hypothyroidism, is relatively simple and a part of most neonatal screening programs. In most cases, the cause of cholestasis is more obscure. Differentiation among biliary atresia and idiopathic neonatal hepatitis is particularly difficult.

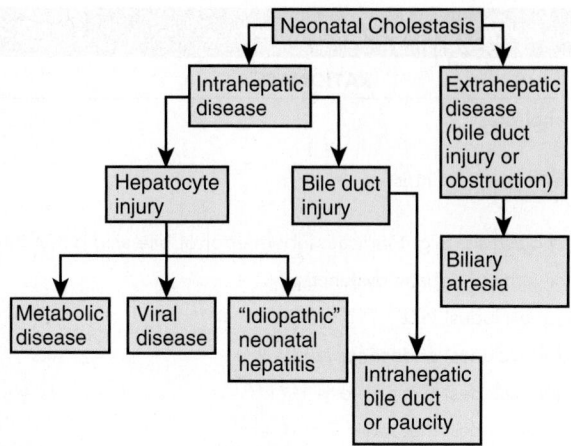

Figure 356-1 Neonatal cholestasis. Conceptual approach to the group of diseases presenting as cholestasis in the neonate. There are areas of overlap: patients with biliary atresia might have some degree of intrahepatic injury. Patients with "idiopathic" neonatal hepatitis might, in the future, be determined to have a primary metabolic or viral disease.

MECHANISMS

Metabolic liver disease caused by inborn errors of bile acid metabolism or transport is associated with accumulation of atypical toxic primitive bile acids and failure to produce normal choleretic and trophic bile acids. The clinical and histologic manifestations are nonspecific and are similar to those in other forms of neonatal hepatobiliary injury. Autoimmune mechanisms may also be responsible for some of the enigmatic forms of neonatal liver injury.

Some of the histologic manifestations of hepatic injury in early life are not seen in older patients. Giant cell transformation of hepatocytes occurs commonly in infants with cholestasis and can occur in any form of neonatal liver injury. It is more common and more severe in intra-hepatic forms of cholestasis. The clinical and histologic findings that exist in patients with neonatal hepatitis and in those with biliary atresia are quite disparate; the basic process is an undefined initiating insult causing inflammation of the liver cells or of the cells within the biliary tract. If bile duct epithelium is the predominant site of disease, chol-angitis can result and lead to progressive sclerosis and narrowing of the biliary tree, the ultimate state being complete obliteration (biliary atresia). Injury to liver cells can present the clinical and histologic picture of "neonatal hepatitis." This concept does not account for the precise mechanism, but it offers an explanation for well-documented cases of unexpected postnatal evolution of these disease processes; infants initially regarded as having neonatal hepatitis, with a patent biliary system shown on cholangiography, can later develop biliary atresia.

Functional abnormalities in the generation of bile flow can also have a role in neonatal cholestasis. Bile flow is directly dependent on effec-tive hepatic bile acid excretion by the hepatocytes. During the phase of relatively inefficient liver cell transport and metabolism of bile acids in early life, minor degrees of hepatic injury can further decrease bile flow and lead to production of atypical and potentially toxic bile acids. Selective impairment of a single step in the series of events involved in hepatic excretion produces the full expression of a cholestatic syn-drome. Specific defects in bile acid synthesis are found in infants with various forms of intrahepatic cholestasis (Table 356-1). Severe forms of familial cholestasis are associated with neonatal hemochromatosis and an aberration in the contractile proteins that compose the cyto-skeleton of the hepatocyte. **Neonatal hemochromatosis** can also be an alloimmune-mediated gestational (maternal antibodies against fetal hepatocytes) disease responsive to maternal intravenous immunoglob-ulin. Sepsis is known to cause cholestasis, presumably mediated by an endotoxin produced by *Escherichia coli*.

Table 356-1 | Proposed Subtypes of Intrahepatic Cholestasis

A. Disorders of membrane transport and secretion
  1. Disorders of canalicular secretion
    a. Bile acid transport: BSEP deficiency
      i. Persistent, progressive (PFIC type 2)
      ii. Recurrent, benign (BRIC type 2)
    b. Phospholipid transport: MDR3 deficiency (PFIC type 3)
    c. Ion transport: cystic fibrosis (*CFTR*)
  2. Complex or multiorgan disorders
    a. FIC1 deficiency
      i. Persistent, progressive (PFIC type 1, Byler disease)
      ii. Recurrent, benign (BRIC type 1)
    b. Neonatal sclerosing cholangitis (*CLDN1*)
    c. Arthrogryposis-renal dysfunction-cholestasis syndrome (*VPS33B*)
B. Disorders of bile acid biosynthesis and conjugation
  1. 3-oxoΔ-4-steroid 5β-reductase deficiency
  2. 3β-hydroxy-5-C$_{27}$-steroid dehydrogenase/isomerase deficiency
  3. Oxysterol 7α-hydroxylase deficiency
  4. Bile acid-coenzyme A (CoA) ligase deficiency
  5. BAAT deficiency (familial hypercholanemia)
C. Disorders of embryogenesis
  1. Alagille syndrome (Jagged1 defect, syndromic bile duct paucity)
  2. Ductal plate malformation (ARPKD, ADPLD, Caroli disease)
D. Unclassified (idiopathic "neonatal hepatitis"): mechanism unknown

Note: FIC1 deficiency, BSEP deficiency, and some of the disorders of bile acid biosynthesis are characterized clinically by low levels of serum GGT despite the presence of cholestasis. In all other disorders listed, the serum GGT level is elevated.
  ADPLD, autosomal dominant polycystic liver disease (cysts in liver only); ARPKD, autosomal recessive polycystic kidney disease (cysts in liver and kidney); BAAT, bile acid transporter; BRIC, benign recurrent intrahepatic cholestasis; BSEP, bile salt export pump; CFTR, cystic fibrosis transmembrane regulator; GGT, γ-glutamyl transpeptidase; PFIC, progressive familial intrahepatic cholestasis.
  From Balistreri WF, Bezerra JA, Jansen P, et al: Intrahepatic cholestasis: summary of an American Association for the Study of Liver Diseases single-topic conference, Hepatology 42:222–235, 2005.

EVALUATION

The evaluation of the infant with jaundice should follow a logical, cost-effective sequence in a multistep process (Table 356-2). Although cho-lestasis in the neonate may be the initial manifestation of numerous and potentially serious disorders, the clinical manifestations are usually similar and provide very few clues about etiology. Affected infants have icterus, dark urine, light or acholic stools, and hepatomegaly, all result-ing from decreased bile flow as a result of either hepatocyte injury or bile duct obstruction. Hepatic synthetic dysfunction can lead to hypo-prothrombinemia and bleeding. Administration of vitamin K should be included in the initial treatment of cholestatic infants to prevent hemorrhage.

In contrast to unconjugated hyperbilirubinemia, which can be phys-iologic, cholestasis (conjugated bilirubin elevation of any degree) in the neonate is **always pathologic** and prompt differentiation is imperative. Thus the initial step is to identify the infant who has cholestasis. The next step is to recognize conditions that cause cholestasis and for which specific therapy is available to prevent further damage and avoid long-term complications such as sepsis, an endocrinopathy (hypothyroid-ism, panhypopituitarism), nutritional hepatotoxicity caused by a specific metabolic illness (galactosemia), or other metabolic diseases (tyrosinemia).

Hepatobiliary disease can be the initial manifestation of homozy-gous α$_1$-antitrypsin deficiency or of cystic fibrosis. Neonatal liver disease can also be associated with congenital syphilis and specific viral infections, notably echovirus and herpesviruses including

Table 356-2	Value of Specific Tests in the Evaluation of Patients with Suspected Neonatal Cholestasis
TEST	**RATIONALE**
Serum bilirubin fractionation (i.e., assessment of the serum level of conjugated bilirubin)	Indicates cholestasis
Assessment of stool color (does the baby have pigmented or acholic stools?)	Indicates bile flow into intestine
Urine and serum bile acids measurement	Confirms cholestasis; might indicate inborn error of bile acid biosynthesis
Hepatic synthetic function (albumin, coagulation profile)	Indicates severity of hepatic dysfunction
α_1-Antitrypsin phenotype	Suggests (or excludes) PiZZ
Thyroxine and TSH	Suggests (or excludes) endocrinopathy
Sweat chloride and mutation analysis	Suggests (or excludes) cystic fibrosis
Urine and serum amino acids and urine reducing substances	Suggests (or excludes) metabolic liver disease
Ultrasonography	Suggests (or excludes) choledochal cyst; might detect the triangular cord sign, suggesting biliary atresia
Hepatobiliary scintigraphy	Documents bile duct patency or obstruction
Liver biopsy	Distinguishes biliary atresia; suggests alternative diagnosis

PiZZ, protease inhibitor ZZ phenotype; TSH, thyroid-stimulating hormone.

cytomegalovirus. These account for a small percentage of cases of neonatal hepatitis syndrome The hepatitis viruses (A, B, C) rarely cause neonatal cholestasis.

The final and critical step in evaluating neonates with cholestasis is to differentiate extrahepatic biliary atresia from neonatal hepatitis.

INTRAHEPATIC CHOLESTASIS
Neonatal Hepatitis
The term *neonatal hepatitis* implies intrahepatic cholestasis (see Fig. 356-1), which has various forms (see Tables 356-1 and 356-3).

Idiopathic neonatal hepatitis, which can occur in either a sporadic or a familial form, is a disease of unknown cause. Patients with the sporadic form presumably have a specific yet undefined metabolic or viral disease. Familial forms, on the other hand, presumably reflect a genetic or metabolic aberration; in the past, patients with α_1-antitrypsin deficiency were included in this category.

Aagenaes syndrome is a form of idiopathic familial intrahepatic cholestasis associated with lymphedema of the lower extremities. The relationship between liver disease and lymphedema is not understood and may be attributable to decreased hepatic lymph flow or hepatic lymphatic hypoplasia. Affected patients usually present with episodic cholestasis with elevation of serum aminotransferases, alkaline phosphatase, and bile acids. Between episodes, the patients are usually asymptomatic and biochemical indices improve. Compared to other types of hereditary neonatal cholestasis, patients with Aagenaes syndrome have a relatively good prognosis because more than 50% can expect a normal life span. The locus for Aagenaes syndrome is mapped to a 6.6 cM interval on chromosome 15q.

Zellweger (cerebrohepatorenal) syndrome is a rare autosomal recessive genetic disorder marked by progressive degeneration of the liver and kidneys (see Chapter 80.2). The incidence is estimated to be 1 in 100,000 births; the disease is usually fatal in 6-12 mo. Affected infants have severe, generalized hypotonia and markedly impaired neurologic function with psychomotor retardation. Patients have an abnormal head shape and unusual facies, hepatomegaly, renal cortical cysts, stippled calcifications of the patellas and greater trochanter, and ocular abnormalities. Hepatic cells on ultrastructural examination show an absence of peroxisomes. MRI performed in the 3rd trimester can allow analysis of cerebral gyration and myelination, facilitating the prenatal diagnosis of Zellweger syndrome.

Neonatal iron storage disease (neonatal hemochromatosis) is a rapidly progressive disease characterized by increased iron deposition in the liver, heart, and endocrine organs without increased iron stores in the reticuloendothelial system. Patients have multiorgan failure and shortened survival. Familial cases are reported, and repeated affected neonates in the same family are common. This is an alloimmune disorder with maternal antibodies directed against the fetal liver. Laboratory findings include hypoglycemia, hyperbilirubinemia, hypoalbuminemia, elevated ferritin and profound hypoprothrombinemia. Serum aminotransferase levels may be high initially but normalize with the progression of the disease. The diagnosis is usually confirmed by buccal mucosal biopsy or MRI demonstrating extrahepatic siderosis. The prognosis is poor; however, liver transplantation can be curative. Despite initially encouraging reports, the use of a combination of antioxidants and prostaglandin infusion with chelation might not uniformly improve outcome in patients with neonatal iron storage disease. Although recovery from neonatal iron storage disease either spontaneously or with medical therapy is unusual, the potential for histologic recovery with regression of fibrosis has been reported. The differential diagnosis includes familial hemophagocytic lymphohistiocytosis, mitochondrial respiratory chain disorders, galactosemia, tyrosinemia, viral hepatitis (HSV, CMV), congenital syphilis, and idiopathic neonatal hepatitis.

Neonatal hemochromatosis seems to be a gestational alloimmune disease, and reoccurrence of severe neonatal hemochromatosis in at-risk pregnancies may be reduced by maternal treatment with weekly (beginning gestational age 18 wk) high-dose intravenous immunoglobulin (1 g/kg) during gestation. After birth, affected neonates are treated with exchange transfusions and intravenous immunoglobulin (1 g/kg), which improves survival and reduces the need for liver transplantation.

Disorders of Transport, Secretion, Conjugation, and Biosynthesis of Bile Acids
Progressive familial intrahepatic cholestasis type 1 (PFIC 1) or FIC1 disease (formerly known as **Byler disease**) is a severe form of intrahepatic cholestasis. The disease was initially described in the Amish kindred of Jacob Byler. Affected patients present with steatorrhea, pruritus, vitamin D–deficient rickets, gradually developing cirrhosis, and **low** γ-glutamyl transpeptidase (GGT) levels. The absence of bile duct paucity and extrahepatic features differentiate this disorder from Alagille syndrome.

PFIC 1 (FIC-1 deficiency) has been mapped to chromosome 18q12 and results from defect in the gene for F1C1 (*ATP8B1*; see Tables 356-3 and 356-4). F1C1 is a P-type adenosine triphosphatase that functions as aminophospholipid flippase, facilitating the transfer of phosphatidyl

Table 356-3	Molecular Defects Causing Liver Disease		
GENE	**PROTEIN**	**FUNCTION, SUBSTRATE**	**DISORDER**
ATP8b1	FIC1	P-type ATPase; aminophospholipid translocase that flips phosphatidylserine and phosphatidylethanolamine from the outer to the inner layer of the canalicular membrane	PFIC 1 (Byler disease), BRIC 1, GFC
ABCB11	BSEP	Canalicular protein with ATP-binding cassette (ABC family of proteins); works as a pump transporting bile acids through the canalicular domain	PFIC 2, BRIC 2
ABCB4	MDR3	Canalicular protein with ATP-binding cassette (ABC family of proteins); works as a phospholipid flippase in canalicular membrane	PFIC 3, ICP, cholelithiasis
AKR1D1	5β-reductase	3-oxoΔ-4-steroid 5β-reductase gene; regulates bile acid synthesis	BAS: neonatal cholestasis with giant cell hepatitis
HSD3B7	C27-3β-HSD	3β-hydroxy-5-C$_{27}$-steroid oxidoreductase (C27-3β-HSD) gene; regulates bile acid synthesis	BAS: chronic intrahepatic cholestasis
CYP7BI	CYP7BI	Oxysterol 7α-hydroxylase; regulates the acidic pathway of bile acid synthesis	BAS: neonatal cholestasis with giant cell hepatitis
JAG1	JAG1	Transmembrane, cell-surface proteins that interact with Notch receptors to regulate cell fate during embryogenesis	Alagille syndrome
TJP2	Tight junction protein	Belongs to the family of membrane-associated guanylate kinase homologs that are involved in the organization of epithelial and endothelial intercellular junction; regulates paracellular permeability	FHC
BAAT	BAAT	Enzyme that transfers the bile acid moiety from the acyl coenzyme A thioester to either glycine or taurine	FHC
EPHX1	Epoxide hydrolase	Microsomal epoxide hydrolase regulates the activation and detoxification of exogenous chemicals	FHC
ABCC2	MRP2	Canalicular protein with ATP-binding cassette (ABC family of proteins); regulates canalicular transport of GSH conjugates and arsenic	Dubin-Johnson syndrome
ATP7B	ATP7B	P-type ATPase; function as copper export pump	Wilson disease
CLDN1	Claudin 1	Tight junction protein	NSC
CIRH1A	Cirhin	Cell signaling?	NAICC
CFTR	CFTR	Chloride channel with ATP-binding cassette (ABC family of proteins); regulates chloride transport	Cystic fibrosis
PKHD1	Fibrocystin	Protein involved in ciliary function and tubulogenesis	ARPKD
PRKCSH	Hepatocystin	Assembles with glucosidase II α subunit in endoplasmic reticulum	ADPLD
VPS33B	Vascular Protein sorting 33	Regulates fusion of proteins to cellular membrane	ARC

ADPLD, autosomal dominant polycystic liver disease; ARC, arthrogryposis–renal dysfunction–cholestasis syndrome*; ARPKD, autosomal recessive polycystic kidney disease; ATP, adenosine triphosphate; ATPase, adenosine triphosphatase; BAAT, bile acid transporter; BAS, bile acid synthetic defect; BRIC, benign recurrent intrahepatic cholestasis; BSEP, bile salt export pump; CFTR, cystic fibrosis transmembrane conductance regulator; FHC, familial hypercholanemia; GFC, Greenland familial cholestasis; GSH, glutathione; ICP, intrahepatic cholestasis of pregnancy; NAICC, North American Indian childhood cirrhosis; NSC, neonatal sclerosing cholangitis with ichthyosis, leukocyte vacuoles, and alopecia; PFIC, progressive familial intrahepatic cholestasis*. (*Low γ-glutamyl transpeptidase [PFIC types 1 and 2, BRIC types 1 and 2, ARC].)

From Balistreri WF, Bezerra JA, Jansen P, et al: Intrahepatic cholestasis: summary of an American Association for the Study of Liver Diseases single-topic conference, Hepatology 42:222–235, 2005.

serine and phosphatidyl ethanolamine from the outer to inner hemileaflet of the cellular membrane. F1C1 might also play a role in intestinal bile acid absorption, as suggested by the high level of expression in the intestine. Defective F1C1 might also result in another form of intrahepatic cholestasis: **benign recurrent intrahepatic cholestasis (BRIC) type I.** The disease is characterized by recurrent bouts of cholestasis, jaundice, and severe pruritus lasting from 2 wk to 6 mo; it can last up to 5 yr. The episodes vary from few episodes per year to 1 episode per decade and can profoundly affect the quality of life. Nonsense, frame shift, and deletional mutations cause PFIC type 1; missense and split-type mutations result in BRIC type I. Typically, patients with BRIC type I have normal cholesterol and GGT levels.

PFIC type 2 *(BSEP deficiency)* is mapped to chromosome 2q24 and is similar to PFIC 1 but is present in non-Amish families (Middle Eastern and European). The disease results from defects in the canalicular adenosine triphosphate–dependent bile acid transporter BSEP

(ABCB11). The progressive liver disease results from accumulation of bile acids secondary to reduction in canalicular bile acid secretion. Mutation in *ABC11* is also described in another disorder, BRIC type 2, characterized by recurrent bouts of cholestasis.

In contrast to PFIC 1 and PFIC 2, patients with **PFIC type 3** *(MDR3 disease)* have **high** levels of GGT. The disease results from defects in a canalicular phospholipids flippase, MDR3 *(ABCB4),* which results in deficient translocation of phosphatidylcholine across the canalicular membrane. Mothers who are heterozygous for this gene can develop intrahepatic cholestasis during pregnancy.

Familial hypercholanemia is characterized by elevated serum bile acid concentration, pruritus, failure to thrive, and coagulopathy. Familial hypercholanemia is a complex genetic trait associated with mutation of bile acid coenzyme A (CoA), amino acid N-acyltransferase (encoded by *BAAT*), as well as mutations in tight junction protein 2 (encoded by *TJP 2,* also known as *ZO-2*). Mutation of BAAT, which

Table 356-4	Progressive Familial Intrahepatic Cholestasis		
	PFIC 1	**PFIC 2**	**PFIC 3**
Transmission	Autosomal recessive	Autosomal recessive	Autosomal recessive
Chromosome	18q21-22	2q24	7q21
Gene	*ATP8B1/F1C1*	*ABCB11/BSEP*	*ABCB4/MDR3*
Protein	FIC1	BSEP	MDR3
Location	Hepatocyte, colon, intestine, pancreas; on apical membranes	Hepatocyte canalicular membrane	Hepatocyte canalicular membrane
Function	ATP-dependent aminophospholipid flippase; unknown effects on intracellular signaling	ATP-dependent bile acid transport	ATP-dependent phosphatidylcholine translocation
Phenotype	Progressive cholestasis, diarrhea, steatorrhea, growth failure, severe pruritus	Rapidly progressive cholestatic giant cell hepatitis, growth failure, pruritus	Later-onset cholestasis, portal hypertension, minimal pruritus, intraductal and gallbladder lithiasis
Histology	Initial bland cholestatic; coarse, granular canalicular bile on EM	Neonatal giant cell hepatitis, amorphous canalicular bile on EM	Proliferation of bile ductules, periportal fibrosis, eventually biliary cirrhosis
Biochemical features	Normal serum GGT; high serum, low biliary bile acid concentrations	Normal serum GGT; high serum, low biliary bile acid concentrations	Elevated serum GGT; low to absent biliary PC; absent serum LPX; normal biliary bile acid concentrations
Treatment	Biliary diversion, ileal exclusion, liver transplantation, but post-OLT diarrhea, steatorrhea, fatty liver	Biliary diversion, liver transplantation	UDCA if residual PC secretion; liver transplantation

ATP, adenosine triphosphate; BSEP, bile salt export pump; EM, electron microscopy; GGT, γ-glutamyl transpeptidase; LPX, lipoprotein X; OLT, orthotopic liver transplantation; PC, phosphatidylcholine; PFIC, progressive familial intrahepatic cholestasis; UDCA, ursodeoxycholic acid.
From Suchy FJ, Sokol RJ, Balistreri WF, editors: Liver disease in children, ed 3, New York, 2007, Cambridge University Press.

is a bile acid–conjugating enzyme, abrogates the enzyme activity. Patients who are homozygous for this mutation have only unconjugated bile acids in their bile. Mutation of both BAAT and TJP 2 can disrupt bile acid transport and circulation. Patients with familial hypercholanemia usually respond to the administration of ursodeoxycholic acid.

Defective bile acid biosynthesis is postulated to be an initiating or perpetuating factor in neonatal cholestatic disorders; the hypothesis is that inborn errors in bile acid biosynthesis lead to absence of normal trophic or choleretic primary bile acids and accumulation of atypical (hepatotoxic) metabolites. Inborn errors of bile acid biosynthesis cause acute and chronic liver disease; early recognition allows institution of targeted bile acid replacement, which reverses the hepatic injury. Several specific defects have been described:

◆ **Deficiency of Δ^4-3-oxosteroid-5β reductase,** the 4th step in the pathway of cholesterol degradation to the primary bile acids, manifests with significant cholestasis and liver failure developing shortly after birth, with coagulopathy and metabolic liver injury resembling tyrosinemia. Hepatic histology is characterized by lobular disarray with giant cells, pseudoacinar transformation, and canalicular bile stasis. Mass spectrometry is required to document increased urinary bile acid excretion and the predominance of oxo-hydroxy and oxo-dihydroxy cholenoic acids. **Treatment** with cholic acid and ursodeoxycholic acid is associated with normalization of biochemical, histologic, and clinical features.

◆ **Deficiency of 3β-hydroxy-Δ^5-C₂₇-steroid oxidoreductase (3β-HSD),** the 2nd step in bile acid biosynthesis, causes progressive familial intrahepatic cholestasis. Affected patients usually have jaundice with increased aminotransferase levels and hepatomegaly; GGT levels and serum cholylglycine levels are **normal.** The histology is variable, ranging from giant cell hepatitis to chronic hepatitis. The diagnosis, suggested by mass spectrometry detection of C^{24} bile acids in urine, which retain the 3β-hydroxy-Δ^5 structure, can be confirmed by determination of 3β-HSD activity in cultured fibroblasts using 7α-hydroxy-Δ^5 cholesterol as a substrate. Primary bile acid therapy, administered

orally to down regulate cholesterol 7α-hydroxylase activity, to limit the production of 3β-hydroxy-Δ^5 bile acids, and to facilitate hepatic clearance, has been effective in reversing hepatic injury.

BILE ACID–COENZYME A LIGASE DEFICIENCY
Conjugation with the amino acids glycine and taurine is the final step in bile acid synthesis. Two enzymes catalyze the amidation of bile acids. In the first reaction, a CoA thioester is formed by the rate-limiting bile acid–CoA ligase. The other reaction involves the coupling of glycine or taurine and is catalyzed by a cytosolic bile acid–CoA:amino acid N-acyltransferase. Several patients with bile acid–CoA ligase deficiency have been reported. The patients present with conjugated hyperbilirubinemia, growth failure, or fat-soluble vitamin deficiency, and are identified with mutation of the bile acid–CoA ligase gene. Administration of conjugates of the primary bile acid, glycocholic acid may be beneficial and can correct the fat-soluble vitamin malabsorption and improve growth.

DISORDERS OF EMBRYOGENESIS
Alagille syndrome (arteriohepatic dysplasia) is the most common syndrome with intrahepatic bile duct paucity. Bile duct "paucity" (often erroneously called *intrahepatic biliary atresia*) designates an absence or marked reduction in the number of interlobular bile ducts in the portal triads, with normal-size branches of portal vein and hepatic arteriole. Biopsy in early life often reveals an inflammatory process involving the bile ducts; subsequent biopsy specimens then show subsidence of the inflammation, with residual reduction in the number and diameter of bile ducts, analogous to the "disappearing bile duct syndrome" noted in adults with immune-mediated disorders. Serial assessment of hepatic histology often suggests progressive destruction of bile ducts.

Clinical manifestations of Alagille syndrome are expressed in various degrees and can be nonspecific; they include unusual facial characteristics (broad forehead; deep-set, widely spaced eyes; long, straight nose; and an underdeveloped mandible). There may also be

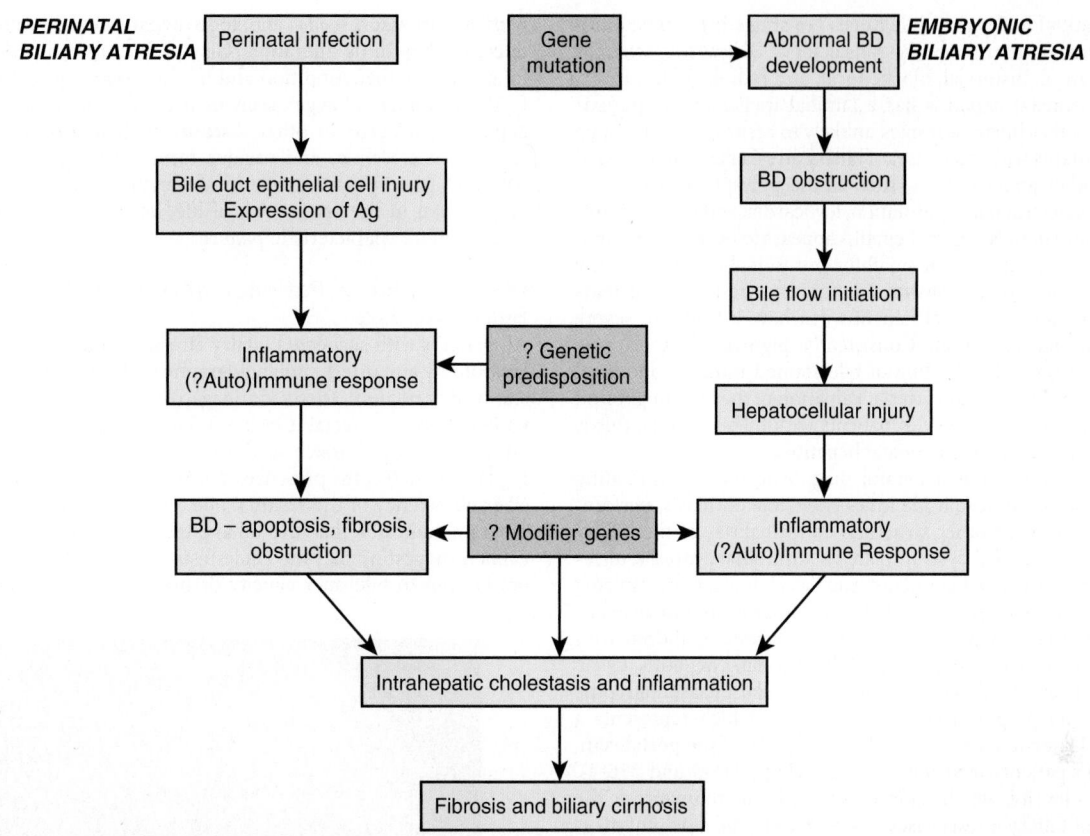

Figure 356-2 Proposed pathways for pathogenesis of 2 forms of biliary atresia (BA). *Perinatal* BA can develop when a perinatal insult, such as a cholangiotropic viral infection, triggers bile duct (BD) epithelial cell injury and exposure of self-antigens or neoantigens that elicit a subsequent immune response. The resulting inflammation induces apoptosis and necrosis of extrahepatic BD epithelium, resulting in fibro-obliteration of the lumen and obstruction of the BD. Intrahepatic bile ducts can also be targets in the ongoing TH1 immune (autoimmune?) attack and the cholestatic injury, resulting in progressive portal fibrosis and culminating in biliary cirrhosis. *Embryonic* BA may be the result of mutations in genes controlling normal bile duct formation or differentiation, which secondarily induces an inflammatory/immune response within the common bile duct and liver after the initiation of bile flow at approximately 11-13 wk of gestation. Secondary hepatocyte and intrahepatic bile duct injury ensue either as a result of cholestatic injury or as targets for the immune (autoimmune?) response that develops. The end result is intrahepatic cholestasis and portal tract fibrosis, culminating in biliary cirrhosis. Other major factors may be the role played by genetic predisposition to autoimmunity and modifier genes that determine the extent and type of cellular and immune response and the generation of fibrosis. *(From Mack CL, Sokol RJ: Unraveling the pathogenesis and etiology of biliary atresia,* Pediatr Res 57:87R–94R, 2005.)

ocular abnormalities (posterior embryotoxon, microcornea, optic disk drusen, shallow anterior chamber), cardiovascular abnormalities (usually peripheral pulmonic stenosis, sometimes tetralogy of Fallot, pulmonary atresia, ventricular septal defect, atrial septal defect, aortic coarctation), vertebral defects (butterfly vertebrae, fused vertebrae, spina bifida occulta, rib anomalies), and tubulointerstitial nephropathy. Other findings such as short stature, pancreatic insufficiency, and defective spermatogenesis can reflect or produce nutritional deficiency. The prognosis for prolonged survival is good, but patients are likely to have pruritus, xanthomas with markedly elevated serum cholesterol levels, and neurologic complications of vitamin E deficiency if untreated. Mutations in human Jagged1 gene *(JAG1)*, which encodes a ligand for the notch receptor, are linked to Alagille syndrome.

BILIARY ATRESIA

The term *biliary atresia* is imprecise because the anatomy of abnormal bile ducts in affected patients varies markedly. A more appropriate terminology would reflect the pathophysiology, namely noncystic obliterative cholangiopathy. The term *obliterative cholangiopathy* may be divided into 2 major types: cystic and noncystic. The cystic disorder will incorporate the different types of choledochal cysts, while the noncystic form will encompass the 2 types of biliary atresia (fetal and perinatal) in addition to neonatal sclerosing cholangitis.

Patients can have distal segmental bile duct obliteration with patent extrahepatic ducts up to the porta hepatis. This is a surgically correctable lesion, but it is uncommon. The most common form of biliary atresia, accounting for approximately 85% of the cases, is obliteration of the entire extrahepatic biliary tree at or above the porta hepatis. This presents a much more difficult problem in surgical management. Most patients with biliary atresia (85-90%) are normal at birth and have a postnatal progressive obliteration of bile ducts; the embryonic or fetal-onset form manifests at birth and is associated with other congenital anomalies (situs inversus, polysplenia, intestinal malrotation, complex congenital heart disease) within the polysplenia spectrum (biliary atresia splenic malformation) (Fig. 356-2; see Chapter 431.11). The postnatal onset may be an immune- or infection-mediated process.

Biliary atresia has been detected in 1 in 10,000-15,000 live births. Biliary atresia is more common in East Asian countries; patients may be born term or preterm. Screening for biliary atresia in infants after birth is not universal, but in high-risk locations, stool color cards that help detect acholic stools have been used with some success. In addition, any infant with new onset or persistent jaundice beyond 8 wk of life should be screened with a total and direct reacting bilirubin level to detect cholestasis.

Differentiation of Idiopathic Neonatal Hepatitis from Biliary Atresia

It may be difficult to clearly differentiate infants with biliary atresia, who require surgical correction, from those with intrahepatic disease (neonatal hepatitis) and patent bile ducts. No single biochemical test or imaging procedure is entirely satisfactory. Diagnostic schemas incorporate clinical, historical, biochemical, and radiologic features.

Idiopathic neonatal hepatitis has a familial incidence of approximately 20%, whereas biliary atresia is unlikely to recur within the same family. A few infants with fetal onset of biliary atresia have an increased incidence of other abnormalities, such as the polysplenia syndrome with abdominal heterotaxia, malrotation, levocardia, and intraabdominal vascular anomalies. Neonatal hepatitis appears to be more common in infants who are premature or small for gestational age. Persistently acholic stools suggest biliary obstruction (biliary atresia), but patients with severe idiopathic neonatal hepatitis can have a transient severe impairment of bile excretion. Consistently pigmented stools rule against biliary atresia. The finding of bile-stained fluid on duodenal intubation also excludes biliary atresia. Palpation of the liver might find an abnormal size or consistency in patients with biliary atresia; this is less common with idiopathic neonatal hepatitis.

Abdominal ultrasound is a helpful diagnostic tool in evaluating neonatal cholestasis because it identifies choledocholithiasis, perforation of the bile duct, or other structural abnormalities of the biliary tree such as a choledochal cyst. In patients with biliary atresia, ultrasound can detect associated anomalies such as abdominal polysplenia and vascular malformations. The gallbladder either is not visualized or is a microgallbladder in patients with biliary atresia. Children with intrahepatic cholestasis caused by idiopathic neonatal hepatitis, cystic fibrosis, or total parenteral nutrition can have similar ultrasonographic findings. Ultrasonographic triangular cord sign, which represents a cone-shaped fibrotic mass cranial to the bifurcation of the portal vein, may be seen in patients with biliary atresia (Figs. 356-3 and 356-4). The echogenic density, which represents the fibrous remnants at the porta hepatis of biliary atresia cases at surgery, may be a helpful diagnostic tool in evaluating patients with neonatal cholestasis.

Hepatobiliary scintigraphy with technetium-labeled iminodiacetic acid derivatives is a sensitive but not specific test for biliary atresia. It fails to identify other structural abnormalities of the biliary tree or vascular anomalies. The lack of the specificity of the test and the need to wait for 5 days makes this procedure less practical and of limited usefulness in the evaluation of children with suspected biliary atresia.

Percutaneous liver biopsy is the most valuable procedure in the evaluation of neonatal hepatobiliary diseases and provides the most reliable discriminatory evidence. Biliary atresia is characterized by bile ductular proliferation, the presence of bile plugs, and portal or perilobular edema and fibrosis, with the basic hepatic lobular architecture intact. In neonatal hepatitis, there is severe, diffuse hepatocellular disease, with distortion of lobular architecture, marked infiltration

with inflammatory cells, and focal hepatocellular necrosis; the bile ductules show little alteration. Giant cell transformation is found in infants with either condition and has no diagnostic specificity.

The histologic changes seen in patients with idiopathic neonatal hepatitis can occur in other diseases, including α_1-antitrypsin deficiency, galactosemia, and various forms of intrahepatic cholestasis. Although paucity of intrahepatic bile ductules may be detected on liver biopsy even in the 1st few wk of life, later biopsies in such patients reveal a more characteristic pattern.

Management of Patients with Suspected Biliary Atresia

All patients with suspected biliary atresia should undergo exploratory laparotomy and direct cholangiography to determine the presence and site of obstruction. Direct drainage can be accomplished in the few patients with a correctable lesion. When no correctable lesion is found, an examination of frozen sections obtained from the transected porta hepatis can detect the presence of biliary epithelium and determine the size and patency of the residual bile ducts. In some cases, the cholangiogram indicates that the biliary tree is patent but of diminished caliber, suggesting that the cholestasis is not due to biliary tract obliteration but to bile duct paucity or markedly diminished flow in the

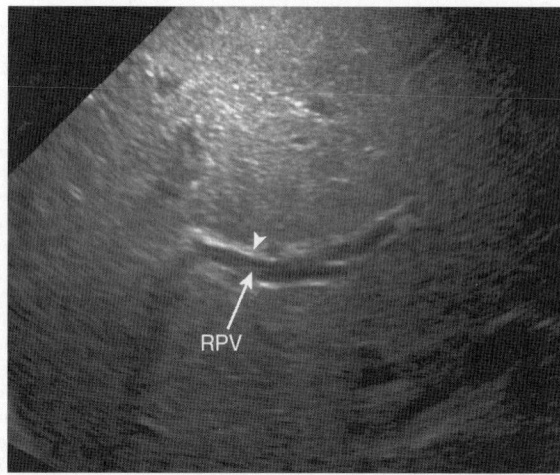

Figure 356-4 Biliary atresia in an 8 wk old male with elevated direct bilirubin. Transverse sonogram shows the triangular cord sign seen as a linear cord of echogenicity (arrowhead) along the right portal vein (RPV). (From Lowe LH: Imaging hepatobiliary disease in children, Semin Roentgenol 43:39–49, 2008, Fig. 1B.)

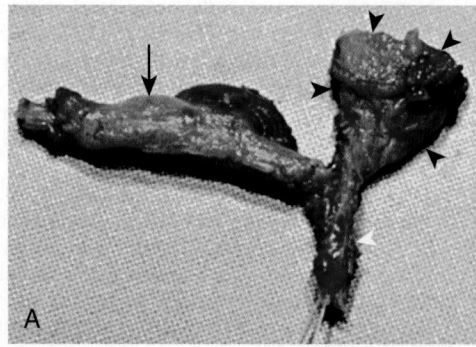 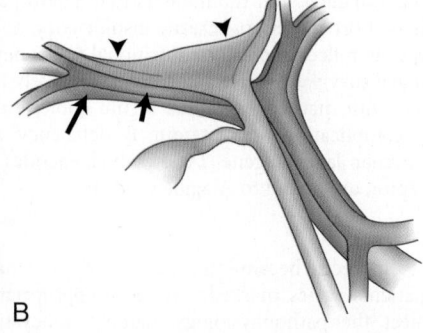

Figure 356-3 Surgical findings of biliary atresia. **A,** Photograph of surgical specimen of obliterated extrahepatic bile ducts shows the fibrous ductal remnant (black arrowheads) in the porta hepatis, atretic gallbladder (arrow), and fibrous common bile duct (white arrowhead). The fibrous ductal remnant is a triangular cone-shaped mass. **B,** Schematic represents the anatomic relationship between the fibrous ductal remnant and blood vessels around the porta hepatis. The triangular, cone-shaped, fibrous ductal remnant (black arrowheads, green) is positioned anterior and slightly superior to the portal vein (long arrow, blue) and the hepatic artery (short arrow, red). (**A** from Park WH, Choi SO, Lee HJ, et al: A new diagnostic approach to biliary atresia with emphasis on the ultrasonographic triangular cord sign: comparison of ultrasonography, hepatobiliary scintigraphy, and liver needle biopsy in the evaluation of infantile cholestasis, J Pediatr Surg 32:1555–1559, 1997.)

presence of intrahepatic disease. In these cases, transection of or further dissection into the porta hepatis should be avoided.

For patients in whom no correctable lesion is found, the **hepatoportoenterostomy (Kasai) procedure** should be performed. The rationale for this operation is that minute bile duct remnants, representing residual channels, may be present in the fibrous tissue of the porta hepatis; such channels may be in direct continuity with the intrahepatic ductule system. In such cases, transection of the porta hepatis with anastomosis of bowel to the proximal surface of the transection might allow bile drainage. If flow is not rapidly established in the 1st mo of life, progressive obliteration and cirrhosis ensue. If microscopic channels of patency > 150 μm in diameter are found, postoperative establishment of bile flow is likely. The success rate for establishing good bile flow after the Kasai operation is much higher (90%) if performed before 8 wk of life. Therefore, early referral and prompt evaluation of infants with suspected biliary atresia is important.

Some patients with biliary atresia, even of the "noncorrectable" type, derive long-term benefits from interventions such as the Kasai procedure. In most, a degree of hepatic dysfunction persists. Patients with biliary atresia usually have persistent inflammation of the intrahepatic biliary tree, which suggests that biliary atresia reflects a dynamic process involving the entire hepatobiliary system. This might account for the ultimate development of complications such as portal hypertension. The short-term benefit of hepatoportoenterostomy is decompression and drainage sufficient to forestall the onset of cirrhosis and sustain growth until a successful liver transplantation can be done.

MANAGEMENT OF CHRONIC CHOLESTASIS
With any form of neonatal cholestasis, whether the primary disease is idiopathic neonatal hepatitis, intrahepatic cholestasis, or biliary atresia, affected patients are at increased risk for progression and complications of chronic cholestasis. These reflect various degrees of residual hepatic functional capacity and are due directly or indirectly to diminished bile flow. Any substance normally excreted into bile is retained in the liver, with subsequent accumulation in tissue and in serum. Involved substances include bile acids, bilirubin, cholesterol, and trace elements. Decreased delivery of bile acids to the proximal intestine leads to inadequate digestion and absorption of dietary long-chain triglycerides and fat-soluble vitamins. Impairment of hepatic metabolic function can alter hormonal balance and utilization of nutrients. Progressive liver damage can lead to biliary cirrhosis, portal hypertension, and liver failure.

Treatment of such patients is empirical, and is guided by careful monitoring (Table 356-5). No therapy is known to be effective in halting the progression of cholestasis or in preventing further hepatocellular damage and cirrhosis.

Growth failure is a major concern and is related in part to malabsorption and malnutrition resulting from ineffective digestion and absorption of dietary fat. Use of a medium-chain triglyceride-containing formula can improve caloric balance.

With chronic cholestasis and prolonged survival, children with hepatobiliary disease can experience deficiencies of the fat-soluble vitamins (A, D, E, K). Inadequate absorption of fat and fat-soluble vitamins may be exacerbated by administration of the bile acid binder cholestyramine. Metabolic bone disease is common.

Serum vitamin A concentration can usually be maintained at normal levels in patients who have chronic cholestasis and who receive oral supplementation of vitamin A esters. It is essential to monitor the vitamin A status in such patients.

A **degenerative neuromuscular syndrome** was found in patients with chronic cholestasis, caused by fat soluble vitamin malabsorption and vitamin E deficiency; affected children experience progressive areflexia, cerebellar ataxia, ophthalmoplegia, and decreased vibratory sensation. Specific morphologic lesions were found in the central nervous system, peripheral nerves, and muscles. These lesions are preventable and are not commonly seen today; they were potentially reversible in children younger than 3-4 yr of age. Affected children have low serum vitamin E concentrations, increased hydrogen peroxide hemolysis, and low ratios of serum vitamin E to total serum lipids (<0.6 mg/g for children younger than 12 yr and <0.8 mg/g for older patients). Vitamin E deficiency may be prevented by oral administration of large doses (up to 1,000 IU/day); patients unable to absorb sufficient quantities may require administration of D-α-tocopheryl polyethylene glycol 1,000 succinate orally. Serum levels may be monitored as a guide to efficacy.

Pruritus is a particularly troublesome complication of chronic cholestasis, often with the appearance of xanthomas. Both features seem to be related to the accumulation of cholesterol and bile acids in serum and in tissues. Elimination of these retained compounds is difficult when bile ducts are obstructed, but if there is any degree of bile duct patency, administration of ursodeoxycholic acid can increase bile flow or interrupt the enterohepatic circulation of bile acids and thus decrease the xanthomas and ameliorate the pruritus (see Table 356-5). Ursodeoxycholic acid therapy can also lower serum cholesterol levels. The recommended initial dose is 15 mg/kg/24 hr.

Table 356-5	Suggested Medical Management of Persistent Cholestasis
CLINICAL IMPAIRMENT	**MANAGEMENT**
Malnutrition resulting from malabsorption of dietary long-chain triglycerides	Replace with dietary formula or supplements containing medium-chain triglycerides
Fat-soluble vitamin malabsorption:	
Vitamin A deficiency (night blindness, thick skin)	Replace with 10,000-15,000 IU/day as Aquasol A
Vitamin E deficiency (neuromuscular degeneration)	Replace with 50-400 IU/day as oral α-tocopherol or TPGS
Vitamin D deficiency (metabolic bone disease)	Replace with 5,000-8,000 IU/day of D₂ or 3-5 μg/kg/day of 25-hydroxycholecalciferol
Vitamin K deficiency (hypoprothrombinemia)	Replace with 2.5-5.0 mg every other day as water-soluble derivative of menadione
Micronutrient deficiency	Calcium, phosphate, or zinc supplementation
Deficiency of water-soluble vitamins	Supplement with twice the recommended daily allowance
Retention of biliary constituents such as cholesterol (itch or xanthomas)	Administer choleretic bile acids (ursodeoxycholic acid, 15-30 mg/kg/day)
Progressive liver disease; portal hypertension (variceal bleeding, ascites, hypersplenism)	Interim management (control bleeding; salt restriction; spironolactone)
End-stage liver disease (liver failure)	Transplantation

TPGS, D-tocopherol polyethylene glycol 1,000 succinate.

Partial external biliary diversion is efficacious in managing pruritus refractory to medical therapy and provides a favorable outcome in a select group of patients with chronic cholestasis who have not yet developed cirrhosis. The surgical technique involves resecting a segment of intestine to be used as a biliary conduit. One end of the conduit is attached to the gallbladder and the other end is brought out to the skin, forming a stoma. The main drawback of the procedure is the need to use an ostomy bag.

Progressive fibrosis and cirrhosis lead to the development of portal hypertension and consequently to ascites and variceal hemorrhage. The presence of ascites is a risk factor for the development of spontaneous bacterial peritonitis. The 1st step in the management of patients with ascites is to rule out spontaneous bacterial peritonitis and restrict sodium intake to 0.5 g (~1-2 mEq/kg/24 hr). There is no need for fluid restriction in patients with adequate renal output. Should this be ineffective, diuretics may be helpful. The diuretic of choice is spironolactone (3-5 mg/kg/24 hr in 4 doses). If spironolactone alone does not control ascites, the addition of another diuretic such as thiazide or furosemide may be beneficial. Patients with ascites but without peripheral edema are at risk for reduced plasma volume and decreased urine output during diuretic therapy. Tense ascites alters renal blood flow and systemic hemodynamics. Paracentesis and intravenous albumin infusion can improve hemodynamics, renal perfusion, and symptoms. Follow-up includes dietary counseling and monitoring of serum and urinary electrolyte concentrations.

In patients with portal hypertension, variceal hemorrhage and the development of hypersplenism are common. It is important to ascertain the cause of bleeding because episodes of gastrointestinal hemorrhage in patients who have chronic liver disease may be from gastritis or peptic ulcer disease. Because the management of these various complications differs, differentiation, perhaps via endoscopy, is necessary before treatment is initiated. If the patient is volume depleted, blood transfusion should be carefully administered, avoiding overtransfusion, which can precipitate further bleeding. Balloon tamponade is not recommended in children because it can be associated with significant complications. Sclerotherapy or endoscopic variceal ligation may be useful palliative measures in the management of bleeding varices and may be superior to surgical alternatives.

For patients with advanced liver disease, hepatic transplantation has a success rate >85%. If the operation is technically feasible, it will prolong life and might correct the metabolic error in diseases such as α1-antitrypsin deficiency, tyrosinemia, and Wilson disease. Success depends on adequate intraoperative, preoperative, and postoperative care, and on cautious use of immunosuppressive agents. Scarcity of donors of small livers severely limits the application of liver transplantation for infants and children. The use of reduced-size transplants and living donors increases the ability to treat small children successfully.

PROGNOSIS

For patients with idiopathic neonatal hepatitis, the variable prognosis might reflect the heterogeneity of the disease. In sporadic cases, 60-70% recover with no evidence of hepatic structural or functional impairment. Approximately 5-10% have persistent fibrosis or inflammation, and a smaller percentage have more severe liver disease, such as cirrhosis. Infants usually die early in the course of the illness, owing to hemorrhage or sepsis. Of infants with idiopathic neonatal hepatitis of the familial variety, only 20-30% recover; 10-15% acquire chronic liver disease with cirrhosis. Liver transplantation may be required.

Bibliography is available at Expert Consult.

356.2 Cholestasis in the Older Child

H. Hesham Abdel-Kader Hassan and William F. Balistreri

Cholestasis with onset after the neonatal period is most often caused by acute viral hepatitis or exposure to hepatotoxic drugs. However, many of the conditions causing neonatal cholestasis can also cause chronic cholestasis in older patients. Consequently, older children and adolescents with conjugated hyperbilirubinemia should be evaluated for acute and chronic viral hepatitis, α1-antitrypsin deficiency, Wilson disease, liver disease associated with inflammatory bowel disease, autoimmune hepatitis, drug-induced liver injury, and the syndromes of intrahepatic cholestasis. Other causes include obstruction caused by cholelithiasis, abdominal tumors, enlarged lymph nodes, or hepatic inflammation resulting from drug ingestion. Management of cholestasis in the older child is similar to that proposed for neonatal cholestasis (see Table 356-5).

Chapter 357
Metabolic Diseases of the Liver

Alexandra N. Menchise and William F. Balistreri

Metabolic liver diseases in children, although individually rare, altogether represent a significant cause of morbidity and mortality. The liver has a central role in synthetic, degradative, and regulatory pathways involving carbohydrate, protein, lipid, trace element, and vitamin metabolism. Inborn errors of metabolism result in metabolic abnormalities, specific enzyme deficiencies or defects, and disorders of protein transport that can have primary or secondary effects on the liver (Table 357-1). Liver disease can arise when absence of an enzyme produces a block in a metabolic pathway, when unmetabolized substrate accumulates proximal to a block, when deficiency of an essential substance produced distal to an aberrant chemical reaction develops, or when synthesis of an abnormal metabolite occurs. The spectrum of pathologic changes includes **hepatocyte injury,** with subsequent failure of other metabolic functions, often eventuating in cirrhosis, liver tumors, or both; **storage** of lipid, glycogen, or other products manifested as hepatomegaly, often with complications specific to deranged metabolism (hypoglycemia with glycogen storage disease); and absence of structural change despite profound **metabolic effects,** as with urea cycle defects. Clinical manifestations of metabolic diseases of the liver mimic infections, intoxications, and hematologic and immunologic diseases (Table 357-2). Many metabolic diseases are detected in expanded newborn metabolic screening programs (see Chapter 84). Clues are provided by family history of a similar illness or by the observation that the onset of symptoms is closely associated with a change in dietary habits; in patients with hereditary fructose intolerance, symptoms follow ingestion of fructose (sucrose). Clinical and laboratory evidence often guides the evaluation. Liver biopsy offers morphologic study and permits enzyme assays, as well as quantitative and qualitative assays of various other constituents (e.g., hepatic copper content in Wilson disease). Genetic/molecular diagnostic approaches are also available. Such studies require cooperation of experienced laboratories and careful attention to collection and handling of specimens. Treatment depends on the specific type of defect and although relatively uncommon, altogether metabolic diseases of the liver account for up to 10% of the indications for liver transplantation in children, a number that may be underestimated given the acute nature of some of these conditions, precluding complete diagnostic investigation prior to transplantation.

Table 357-1	Inborn Errors of Metabolism That Affect the Liver

DISORDERS OF CARBOHYDRATE METABOLISM
Disorders of galactose metabolism
  Galactosemia (galactose-1-phosphate uridyltransferase deficiency)
Disorders of fructose metabolism
  Hereditary fructose intolerance (aldolase deficiency)
  Fructose-1,6 diphosphatase deficiency
Glycogen storage diseases
  Type I
  Von Gierke Ia (glucose-6-phosphatase deficiency)
  Type Ib (glucose-6-phosphatase transport defect)
  Type III Cori/Forbes (glycogen debrancher deficiency)
  Type IV Andersen (glycogen branching enzyme deficiency)
  Type VI Hers (liver phosphorylase deficiency)
Congenital disorders of glycosylation (multiple subtypes)

DISORDERS OF AMINO ACID AND PROTEIN METABOLISM
Disorders of tyrosine metabolism
  Hereditary tyrosinemia type I (fumarylacetoacetate deficiency)
  Tyrosinemia, type II (tyrosine aminotransferase deficiency)
Inherited urea cycle enzyme defects
  CPS deficiency (carbamoyl phosphate synthetase I deficiency)
  OTC deficiency (ornithine transcarbamoylase deficiency)
  Citrullinemia type I (argininosuccinate synthetase deficiency)
  Argininosuccinic aciduria (argininosuccinate deficiency)Argininemia (arginase deficiency)
  N-AGS deficiency (N-acetylglutamate synthetase deficiency)
Maple serum urine disease (multiple possible defects*)

DISORDERS OF LIPID METABOLISM
Wolman disease (lysosomal acid lipase deficiency)
Cholesteryl ester storage disease (lysosomal acid lipase deficiency)
Homozygous familial hypercholesterolemia (low-density lipoprotein receptor deficiency)
Gaucher disease type I (β-glucocerebrosidase deficiency)
Niemann-Pick type C (NPC 1 and 2 mutations)

DISORDERS OF BILE ACID METABOLISM
Defects in bile acid synthesis
Zellweger syndrome—cerebrohepatorenal (multiple mutations in peroxisome biogenesis genes)

DISORDERS OF METAL METABOLISM
Wilson disease (ATP7B mutations)
Hepatic copper overload
Indian childhood cirrhosis (ICC)
Neonatal iron storage disease

DISORDERS OF BILIRUBIN METABOLISM
Crigler-Najjar (bilirubin-uridine diphosphoglucuronate glucuronosyltransferase mutations)
  Type I
  Type II
Gilbert disease (bilirubin-uridine diphosphoglucuronate glucuronosyltransferase polymorphism)
Dubin-Johnson syndrome (multiple drug-resistant protein 2 mutation)
Rotor syndrome

MISCELLANEOUS
α₁-Antitrypsin deficiency
Citrullinemia type II (citrin deficiency)
Cystic fibrosis (cystic fibrosis transmembrane conductance regulator mutations)
Erythropoietic protoporphyria (ferrochelatase deficiency)
Polycystic kidney disease

*Maple syrup urine disease can be caused by mutations in branched-chain α-keto dehydrogenase, keto acid decarboxylase, lipoamide dehydrogenase, or dihydrolipoamide dehydrogenase.

Table 357-2	Clinical Manifestations That Suggest the Possibility of Metabolic Disease

Recurrent vomiting, failure to thrive, short stature
Dysmorphic features
Jaundice, hepatomegaly (±splenomegaly), fulminant hepatic failure, edema/anasarca
Hypoglycemia, organic acidemia, lactic acidemia, hyperammonemia, bleeding (coagulopathy)
Developmental delay/psychomotor retardation, hypotonia, progressive neuromuscular deterioration, seizures, myopathy, neuropathy
Cardiac dysfunction/failure
Unusual odors
Rickets
Cataracts

357.1 Inherited Deficient Conjugation of Bilirubin (Familial Nonhemolytic Unconjugated Hyperbilirubinemia)
Alexandra N. Menchise and William F. Balistreri

Bilirubin is the metabolic end product of heme. Before excretion into bile, it is first glucuronidated by the enzyme bilirubin-uridine diphosphoglucuronate glucuronosyltransferase (UDPGT). UDPGT activity is deficient or altered in 3 genetically and functionally distinct disorders (Crigler-Najjar [CN] syndromes type I and II and Gilbert syndrome), producing congenital nonobstructive, nonhemolytic, **unconjugated** hyperbilirubinemia. UGT1A1 is the primary UDPGT isoform needed for bilirubin glucuronidation, and complete absence of UGT1A1 activity causes CN type I. CN type II is caused by decreased UGT1A1 activity.

Gilbert syndrome is caused by a common polymorphism, a TA insertion in the promoter region of UGT1A1 that leads to decreased binding of the TATA binding protein and decreases normal gene activity but only to approximately 30%. Snapback primer genotyping can distinguish all UGT1A1 promoter genotypes. Unlike the CN syndromes, Gilbert syndrome usually occurs after puberty; it is not associated with chronic liver disease and no treatment is required. However, it is more common, affecting up to 5-10% of the white population with total serum bilirubin concentrations that fluctuate from 1-6 mg/dL. Because UGT1A1 is involved in glucuronidation of multiple substrates other than bilirubin (e.g., pharmaceutical drugs, endogenous hormones, environmental toxins, and aromatic hydrocarbons) and glucuronidation leads to inactivation of these substrates, mutations in the UGT1A1 gene are implicated in cancer risk and the predisposition to drug toxicity specifically in cancer chemotherapy and episodes of jaundice when exposed to the agents.

CRIGLER-NAJJAR SYNDROME TYPE I (GLUCURONYL TRANSFERASE DEFICIENCY)
CN type I is rare and inherited as an autosomal recessive trait and is usually secondary to mutations that cause a premature stop codon or frameshift mutation and thereby abolish UGT1A1 activity. As many as 59 mutations have been identified to date. Parents of affected children have partial defects in conjugation as determined by hepatic specific enzyme assay or by measurement of glucuronide formation; their serum unconjugated bilirubin concentrations are normal.

Clinical Manifestations
Severe unconjugated hyperbilirubinemia develops in homozygous affected infants in the 1st 3 days of life, and without treatment, serum unconjugated bilirubin concentrations of 25-35 mg/dL are reached in the 1st mo. Kernicterus, an almost universal complication of this disorder, is usually first noted in the early neonatal period; some treated infants have survived childhood without clinical sequelae. Stools are

pale yellow. Persistence of unconjugated hyperbilirubinemia at levels >20 mg/dL after the 1st wk of life in the absence of hemolysis should suggest the syndrome.

Diagnosis

The diagnosis of CN type I is based on the early age of onset and the extreme level of bilirubin elevation in the absence of hemolysis. In the bile, bilirubin concentration is <10 mg/dL compared with normal concentrations of 50-100 mg/dL; there is no bilirubin glucuronide. Definitive diagnosis is established by measuring hepatic glucuronyl transferase activity in a liver specimen obtained by a closed biopsy; open biopsy should be avoided because surgery and anesthesia can precipitate kernicterus. DNA diagnosis is also available and may be preferable. Identification of the heterozygous state in parents also strongly suggests the diagnosis. The differential diagnosis of unconjugated hyperbilirubinemia is discussed in Chapter 102.3.

Treatment

The serum unconjugated bilirubin concentration should be kept to <20 mg/dL for at least the 1st 2-4 wk of life; in low birthweight infants, the levels should be kept lower. This usually requires repeated exchange transfusions and phototherapy in the immediate neonatal period. Oral calcium phosphate supplementation renders phototherapy more effective as it forms complexes with bilirubin in the gut. Phenobarbital therapy, through CYP450 enzyme induction, should be considered to determine responsiveness and differentiation between types I and II. In patients with CN type I there is no response to phenobarbital treatment.

The risk of kernicterus persists into adult life, although the serum bilirubin levels required to produce brain injury beyond the neonatal period are considerably higher (usually >35 mg/dL). Therefore, phototherapy is generally continued through the early years of life. In older infants and children, phototherapy is used mainly during sleep so as not to interfere with normal activities. Despite the administration of increasing intensities of light for longer periods, the serum bilirubin response to phototherapy decreases with age. Additional adjuvant therapy using agents that bind photobilirubin products such as cholestyramine or agar can also be used to interfere with the enterohepatic recirculation of bilirubin.

Prompt treatment of intercurrent infections, febrile episodes, and other types of illness might help prevent the later development of kernicterus, which can occur at bilirubin levels of 45-55 mg/dL. All patients with CN type I have eventually experienced severe kernicterus by young adulthood.

Orthotopic liver transplantation cures the disease and has been successful in a small number of patients; isolated hepatocyte transplantation has been reported as bridge therapy to liver transplantation, with most, but not all patients eventually requiring orthotopic transplantation. Other therapeutic modalities have included plasmapheresis and limitation of bilirubin production. The latter option, inhibiting bilirubin generation, is possible via inhibition of heme oxygenase using metalloporphyrin therapy.

CRIGLER-NAJJAR SYNDROME TYPE II (PARTIAL GLUCURONYL TRANSFERASE DEFICIENCY)

Like CN type I, CN type II is an autosomal recessive disease; it is caused by homozygous missense mutations in UGT1A1, resulting in reduced (partial) enzymatic activity. More than 45 mutations have been identified to date. Type II disease can be distinguished from type I by the marked decline in serum bilirubin level that occurs in type II disease after treatment with phenobarbital secondary to an inducible phenobarbital response element on the UGT1A1 promoter.

Clinical Manifestations

When this disorder appears in the neonatal period, unconjugated hyperbilirubinemia usually occurs in the 1st 3 days of life; serum bilirubin concentrations can be in a range compatible with physiologic jaundice or can be at pathologic levels. The concentrations characteristically remain elevated into and after the 3rd wk of life, persisting in a range of 1.5-22 mg/dL; concentrations in the lower part of this range can create uncertainty about whether chronic hyperbilirubinemia is present. Development of kernicterus is unusual. Stool color is normal, and the infants are without clinical signs or symptoms of disease. There is no evidence of hemolysis. Liver enzymes and synthetic function tests are typically normal.

Diagnosis

Concentration of bilirubin in bile is nearly normal in patients with CN type II. Jaundiced infants and young children with type II syndrome respond readily to 5 mg/kg/24 hr of oral phenobarbital, with a decrease in serum bilirubin concentration to 2-3 mg/dL in 7-10 days.

Treatment

Long-term reduction in serum bilirubin levels can be achieved with continued administration of phenobarbital at 5 mg/kg/24 hr. The cosmetic and psychosocial benefit should be weighed against the risks of an effective dose of the drug because there is a small long-term risk of kernicterus even in the absence of hemolytic disease. Orlistat, an irreversible inhibitor of intestinal lipase, increases fecal fat excretion and decreases plasma unconjugated bilirubin concentrations (~10%) in patients with CN types I and II.

INHERITED CONJUGATED HYPERBILIRUBINEMIA

Conjugated hyperbilirubinemia can be caused by a small number of rare autosomal recessive conditions characterized by mild jaundice. The transfer of bilirubin and other organic anions from the liver cell to bile is defective. Chronic mild conjugated hyperbilirubinemia is usually detected during adolescence or early adulthood but can occur as early as the second year of life. The results of routine liver function tests are normal. Jaundice can be exacerbated by infection, pregnancy, oral contraceptives, alcohol consumption, and surgery. There is usually no morbidity and life expectancy is normal, but these disorders can initially present difficult problems in the differential diagnosis of more serious diseases.

DUBIN-JOHNSON SYNDROME

Dubin-Johnson syndrome is an autosomal recessive inherited defect with variable penetrance in hepatocyte secretion of bilirubin glucuronide. The defect in hepatic excretory function is not limited to conjugated bilirubin excretion but also involves several organic anions normally excreted from the liver cell into bile. Absent function of multiple drug-resistant protein 2 (MRP2), an adenosine triphosphate–dependent canalicular transporter, is the responsible defect. More than 10 different mutations, including compound heterozygous mutation in the CMOAT gene, have been identified and either affect localization of MRP2 with resultant increased degradation or impair MRP2 transport activity in the canalicular membrane. Bile acid excretion and serum bile acid levels are normal. Total urinary coproporphyrin excretion is normal in quantity but coproporphyrin I excretion increases to approximately 80% with a concomitant decrease in coproporphyrin III excretion. Normally, coproporphyrin III is >75% of the total. Cholangiography fails to visualize the biliary tract and x-ray of the gallbladder is also abnormal. Liver histology demonstrates normal architecture, but hepatocytes contain black pigment similar to melanin. Liver function is normal and prognosis is excellent. The most commonly reported symptoms are abdominal pain and fatigue, jaundice, dark urine, and slight enlargement of the liver. Jaundice fluctuates in intensity and is aggravated by intercurrent disease.

Rotor Syndrome

Patients with Rotor syndrome have an additional deficiency in organic anion uptake. Biallelic inactivating mutations in the linked genes *SLCO1B1* and *SLCO1B3* result in functional deficiencies of both protein products (OATP1B1 and OATP1B, respectively) and are reported to cause Rotor syndrome. Importantly, these mutations may confer significant drug toxicity risk. Unlike Dubin-Johnson syndrome, total urinary coproporphyrin excretion is elevated, with a relative increase in the amount of the coproporphyrin I isomer. The gallbladder is normal by roentgenography, and liver cells contain no black pigment. In Dubin-Johnson and Rotor syndromes, sulfobromophthalein excretion is often abnormal.

Bibliography is available at Expert Consult.

357.2 Wilson Disease
Alexandra N. Menchise and William F. Balistreri

Wilson disease (hepatolenticular degeneration) is an autosomal recessive disorder that can be associated with degenerative changes in the brain, liver disease, and Kayser-Fleischer rings in the cornea (Fig. 357-1). The incidence is 1 in 55,000 births in the United States and 1 in 30,000 to 1 in 50,000 births worldwide. It is progressive and potentially fatal if untreated; specific effective treatment is available. Rapid diagnostic investigation of the possibility of Wilson disease in a patient presenting with any form of liver disease, particularly if older than 5 yr of age, not only facilitates early institution of management of Wilson disease and related genetic counseling but also allows appropriate treatment of non-Wilsonian liver disease once copper toxicosis is ruled out.

PATHOGENESIS
The abnormal gene for Wilson disease is localized to the long arm of chromosome 13 (13q14.3). The Wilson disease gene encodes a copper transporting P-type adenosine triphosphatase (ATPase), ATP7B, which is mainly but not exclusively expressed in hepatocytes and is critical for biliary copper excretion and for copper incorporation into ceruloplasmin. Absence or malfunction of ATP7B results in decreased biliary copper excretion and diffuse accumulation of copper in the cytosol of hepatocytes. With time, liver cells become overloaded and copper is redistributed to other tissues, including the brain and kidneys, causing toxicity, primarily as a potent inhibitor of enzymatic processes. Ionic copper inhibits pyruvate oxidase in brain and ATPase in membranes, leading to decreased adenosine triphosphate-phosphocreatine and potassium content of tissue.

More than 500 mutations in the gene have been identified from which 380 have a confirmed role in the pathogenesis of the disease, making diagnosis by DNA mutational analysis a difficult task unless a proband mutation is known. Most patients are compound heterozy-gotes. Mutations that completely knock out gene function are associated with an onset of disease symptoms as early as 2-3 yr of age, when Wilson disease might not typically be considered in the differential diagnosis. Milder mutations can be associated with neurologic symptoms or liver disease as late as 80 yr of age.

CLINICAL MANIFESTATIONS
Forms of Wilsonian hepatic disease include asymptomatic hepatomegaly (with or without splenomegaly), subacute or chronic hepatitis, and acute hepatic failure (with or without hemolytic anemia). Cryptogenic cirrhosis, portal hypertension, ascites, edema, variceal bleeding, or other effects of hepatic dysfunction (delayed puberty, amenorrhea, coagulation defects) can be manifestations of Wilson disease.

Disease presentations are variable, with a tendency to familial patterns. The younger the patient, the more likely hepatic involvement will be the predominant manifestation. Girls are 3 times more likely than boys to present with acute hepatic failure. Clinically evident liver disease may precede neurologic manifestations by as much as 10 yr. After 20 yr of age, neurologic symptoms predominate.

Neurologic disorders can develop insidiously or precipitously, with intention tremor, dysarthria, rigid dystonia, Parkinsonism, choreiform movements, lack of motor coordination, deterioration in school performance, or behavioral changes. Kayser-Fleischer rings are absent in young patients with hepatic Wilson disease up to 50% of the time but are present in 95% of patients with neurologic symptoms and somewhat over half of those without neurologic symptoms. **Psychiatric manifestations** include depression, personality changes, anxiety, or psychosis.

Coombs-negative **hemolytic anemia** may be an initial manifestation, possibly related to the release of large amounts of copper from damaged hepatocytes; this form of Wilson disease is usually fatal without transplantation. During hemolytic episodes, urinary copper excretion and serum copper levels (not ceruloplasmin bound) are markedly elevated. Manifestations of renal Fanconi syndrome and progressive renal failure with alterations in tubular transport of amino acids, glucose, and uric acid may be present. Unusual manifestations include arthritis, pancreatitis, nephrolithiasis, infertility or recurrent miscarriages, cardiomyopathy, and endocrinopathies (hypoparathyroidism).

PATHOLOGY
All grades of hepatic injury occur in patients with Wilson disease with steatosis, hepatocellular ballooning and degeneration, glycogen granules, minimal inflammation, and enlarged Kupffer cells being most common. The earliest histologic feature is often mild steatosis and this may be misdiagnosed as nonalcoholic fatty liver disease or nonalcoholic steatohepatitis. Additionally, the lesion may be indistinguishable from that of autoimmune hepatitis. With progressive parenchymal damage, fibrosis and cirrhosis develop. Ultrastructural changes primarily involve the mitochondria and include increased density of the matrix material, inclusions of lipid and granular material, and increased intracristal space with dilation of the tips of the cristae.

DIAGNOSIS
Wilson disease should be considered in children and teenagers with unexplained acute or chronic liver disease, neurologic symptoms of unknown cause, acute hemolysis, psychiatric illnesses, behavioral changes, Fanconi syndrome, or unexplained bone (osteoporosis, fractures) or muscle disease (myopathy, arthralgia). The clinical suspicion is confirmed by study of indices of copper metabolism.

Most patients with Wilson disease have decreased ceruloplasmin levels (<20 mg/dL). The failure of copper to be incorporated into ceruloplasmin leads to a plasma protein with a shorter half-life and, therefore, a reduced steady-state concentration of ceruloplasmin in the circulation. Caution should be used in interpreting serum ceruloplasmin levels, because they may be elevated in acute inflammation and in states of elevated estrogen such as pregnancy, estrogen supplementation, or oral contraceptive use and may be low in autoimmune hepatitis, celiac disease, familial aceruloplasminemia or in heterozygous carriers of ATP7B mutations who do not show copper overload disease.

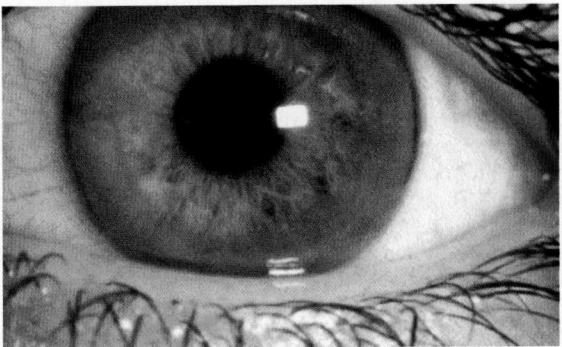

Figure 357-1 Kayser-Fleischer (K-F) ring. There is a brown discoloration at the outer margin of the cornea because of the deposition of copper in Descemet's membrane. Here it is clearly seen against the light green iris. Slit-lamp examination is required for secure detection. *(From Ala A, Walker AP, Ashkan K, et al: Wilson's disease, Lancet 369:397–408, 2007.)*

The serum "free" copper level may be elevated in early Wilson disease (>1.6 μmol/L), and urinary copper excretion (usually <40 μg/day) is increased to >100 μg/day and often up to 1,000 μg or more per day (typical findings in Wilson disease: urine copper excretion >1.6 μmol/24 hr, >0.64 μmol/24 hr in children). In equivocal cases, the response of urinary copper output to chelation may be of diagnostic help. During the 24 hr urine collection patients are given two 500 mg oral doses of D-penicillamine 12 hr apart; affected patients excrete >1,600 μg/24 hr.

Demonstration of Kayser-Fleischer rings, which might not be present in younger children, requires a slit-lamp examination by an ophthalmologist. After adequate treatment, Kayser-Fleischer rings resolve.

Liver biopsy is of value for determining the extent and severity of liver disease and for measuring the hepatic copper content (normally <10 μg/g dry weight) but is only required if clinical signs and noninvasive tests do not allow a final diagnosis or if another liver disorder is suspected. Hepatic copper accumulation is the hallmark of Wilson disease and measurement of hepatic parenchymal copper concentration is the method of choice for diagnosis. In Wilson disease, hepatic copper content usually exceeds 250 μg/g dry weight (>4 μmol/g dry weight is the best biochemical evidence for Wilson disease but lowering the threshold to 1.2 μmol/g dry weight improves sensitivity without significantly effecting specificity). In healthy heterozygotes, levels may be intermediate. In later stages of Wilson disease hepatic copper content can be unreliable because cirrhosis leads to variable hepatic copper distribution and sampling error.

Family members of patients with proven cases require screening for presymptomatic Wilson disease. Such screening should include determination of the serum ceruloplasmin level and urinary copper excretion. If these results are abnormal or equivocal, liver biopsy should be carried out to determine morphology and hepatic copper content. Genetic screening by either linkage analysis or direct DNA mutation analysis is possible, especially if the mutation for the proband case is known or the patient is from an area where a specific mutation is known (in central and eastern Europe, the *H1069Q* mutation is present in 50-80% of patients).

TREATMENT

A major attempt should be made to restrict dietary copper intake to <1 mg/day. Foods such as liver, shellfish, nuts, and chocolate should be avoided. If the copper content of the drinking water exceeds 0.1 mg/L, it may be necessary to demineralize the water. Once the diagnosis has been made, treatment needs to be lifelong.

The initial treatment in symptomatic patients is the administration of copper-chelating agents, which leads to rapid excretion of excess deposited copper. Chelation therapy is managed with oral administration of D-penicillamine (β,β-dimethylcysteine) in a dose of 1 g/day in 2 doses before meals for adults and 20 mg/kg/day for pediatric patients or triethylene tetramine dihydrochloride (Trien, TETA, trientine) at a dose of 0.5-2.0 g/day for adults and 20 mg/kg/day for children. In response to chelation, urinary copper excretion markedly increases, and with continued administration, urinary copper levels can become normal, with marked improvement in hepatic and neurologic function and the disappearance of Kayser-Fleischer rings.

Approximately 10-50% of patients initially treated with penicillamine for neurologic symptoms have a worsening of their condition. Toxic effects of penicillamine occur in 10-20% and consist of hypersensitivity reactions (i.e., Goodpasture syndrome, systemic lupus erythematosus, polymyositis), interaction with collagen and elastin, deficiency of other elements such as zinc, and aplastic anemia and nephrosis. Because penicillamine is an antimetabolite of vitamin B₆, additional amounts of this vitamin are necessary. For these reasons, triethylene tetramine dihydrochloride is a preferred alternative, and is considered first-line therapy for some patients. Trientine has few known side effects. Ammonium tetrathiomolybdate is another alternative chelating agent under investigation for patients with neurologic disease; initial results suggest that significantly fewer patients experience neurologic deterioration with this drug compared to penicillamine. The initial dose is 120 mg/day (20 mg between meals tid and 20 mg with meals tid). Side effects include anemia, leukopenia, thrombocytopenia, and mild elevations of transaminases. Because of its extensive decoppering effect, ammonium tetrathiomolybdate also has antiangiogenic effects.

Zinc has also been used as adjuvant therapy, maintenance therapy, or primary therapy in presymptomatic patients, owing to its unique ability to impair the gastrointestinal absorption of copper. Zinc acetate is given in adults at a dose of 25-50 mg of elemental zinc 3 times a day, and 25 mg 3 times a day in children older than 5 yr of age. Side effects are mostly limited to gastric irritation but also include reduced leukocyte chemotaxis and elevations in serum lipase and/or amylase. Current guidelines recommend that all symptomatic patients with Wilson disease receive a chelating agent (penicillamine or trientine). Zinc may have a role as a first-line therapy in patients with neurologic disease but exclusive monotherapy with zinc in symptomatic liver disease is controversial and not recommended.

Antioxidants (vitamin E and curcumin) and pharmacologic chaperones (4-phenylbutyrate and curcumin) may have a role as adjunctive treatment but more research is needed.

PROGNOSIS

Untreated patients with Wilson disease can die of hepatic, neurologic, renal, or hematologic complications. Medical therapy is rarely effective in those presenting with acute liver failure. The prognosis for patients receiving prompt and continuous penicillamine is variable and depends on the time of initiation of and the individual response to chelation. Liver transplantation should be considered for patients with fulminant liver disease, decompensated cirrhosis, or progressive neurologic disease; the last indication remains controversial. Liver transplantation is curative, with a survival rate of approximately 85-90%. In asymptomatic siblings of affected patients, early institution of chelation or zinc therapy can prevent expression of the disease.

Bibliography is available at Expert Consult.

357.3 Indian Childhood Cirrhosis

Alexandra N. Menchise and William F. Balistreri

Indian childhood cirrhosis (ICC) is a chronic liver disease of young children unique to the Indian subcontinent. ICC manifests with jaundice, pruritus, lethargy, and hepatosplenomegaly. Untreated ICC has a mortality of 40-50% within 4 wks. Histologically, it is characterized by hepatocyte necrosis, Mallory bodies, intralobular fibrosis, and inflammation.

The etiology has remained elusive; it was once believed that excess copper ingestion in the setting of a genetic susceptibility to copper toxicosis was the most likely cause. Epidemiologic data demonstrates that the copper toxicity theory is unlikely. The increased hepatic copper content, usually >700 μg/g dry weight, seen in ICC is only seen in the late stages of disease and is accompanied by even higher levels of zinc, a non-hepatotoxic metal. The copper-contaminated utensils used to feed babies and implicated in excess copper ingestion are found in only 10-15% of all cases. The current hypothesis implicates the postnatal use of local hepatotoxic therapeutic remedies, although the exact causative agent is unknown.

Over the last few decades, as the awareness of the disease has increased, the incidence of ICC has decreased and has even been virtually eliminated in some areas of India although established and nontypical cases are probably being missed because of lack of histologic confirmation and unawareness of the protean manifestations and natural history of this disease. Variants of this syndrome have been named according to the population where it has been described, such as Tyrolean childhood cirrhosis or North American ICC. It has also been reported in the Middle East, West Africa, and North and Central America.

Bibliography is available at Expert Consult.

357.4 Neonatal Iron Storage Disease

Alexandra N. Menchise and William F. Balistreri

Neonatal iron storage disease (NISD), also known as **neonatal hemochromatosis**, is a rare form of fulminant liver disease that manifests in the 1st few days of life. It is unrelated to the familial forms of hereditary hemochromatosis that occur later in life. NISD has a high rate of recurrence in families, with approximately 80% probability that subsequent infants will be affected. NISD is postulated to be a gestational alloimmune disease and has also been classified as **congenital alloimmune hepatitis**. Alloimmunity develops in the pregnant mother of the affected infant when she is exposed to an unknown fetal hepatocyte cell surface antigen that she does not recognize as *self*. Maternal immunoglobulin G to this fetal antigen then crosses the placenta and induces hepatic injury via immune system activation. The defining feature of gestational alloimmune liver disease is complement-mediated hepatocyte injury, the evidence for which comes from detection of the C5b-9 complex by immunohistochemistry. Additional evidence of a gestational insult is given by the fact that affected infants may be born prematurely or with intrauterine growth restriction. Several infants with NISD also have renal dysgenesis.

Excess non–transferrin-bound iron in gestational alloimmune liver disease may result from fetal liver injury that causes reduced synthesis of key iron regulatory and transport proteins. The pattern of extrahepatic siderosis appears to be determined by the normal capacity of various tissues to import non–transferrin-bound iron and not export cellular iron. It is now thought that fecal liver injury is the primary event leading to the development of the neonatal hemochromatosis phenotype providing further evidence that this is not a primary iron overload disease.

NISD is a rapidly fatal, progressive illness characterized by hepatomegaly, hypoglycemia, hypoprothrombinemia, hypoalbuminemia, hyperferritinemia, and hyperbilirubinemia. The coagulopathy is refractory to therapy with vitamin K. Liver pathology demonstrates severe liver injury with acute and chronic inflammation, fibrosis, and cirrhosis. The diagnosis can be confirmed in the neonate with severe liver injury and extrahepatic siderosis (biopsy material of buccal mucosal glands is laden with iron) or MRI determination of iron storage in organs such as the pancreas.

The prognosis for affected infants is generally poor, but some patients with NISD have been successfully treated with iron-chelating agents (deferoxamine) combined with aggressive antioxidant therapy. Combining this therapy with double volume exchange transfusion followed by administration of intravenous immunoglobulin (IVIG) has also been shown to remove the injury-causing maternal immunoglobulin G. Liver transplantation should also be an early consideration. Recurrences of NISD may be modified with IVIG administered to the mother once a wk from the 18th wk of gestation until delivery. The largest experience reports 48 women with previous infants with NISD who successfully delivered 52 babies after IVIG treatment. The majority of infants had biochemical evidence of liver disease with elevated serum α-fetoprotein and ferritin. All infants survived with medical therapy or no therapy.

Bibliography is available at Expert Consult.

357.5 Miscellaneous Metabolic Diseases of the Liver

Alexandra N. Menchise and William F. Balistreri

α₁-ANTITRYPSIN DEFICIENCY

A small percentage of patients homozygous for deficiency of the major serum protease inhibitor α₁-antitrypsin manifest neonatal cholestasis or later-onset childhood cirrhosis. α₁-Antitrypsin deficiency is caused by mutation in the SERPINA1 gene and it is an autosomal recessive disorder. α₁-Antitrypsin, a protease inhibitor synthesized by the liver, protects lung alveolar tissues from destruction by neutrophil elastase (see Chapter 393). α₁-Antitrypsin is present in more than 20 different codominant alleles, only a few of which are associated with defective protease inhibitors. The most common allele of the protease inhibitor (Pi) system is M, and the normal phenotype is PiMM. The Z allele predisposes to clinical deficiency; patients with liver disease are usually PiZZ homozygotes and have serum α₁-antitrypsin levels <2 mg/mL (~10-20% of normal). The incidence of the PiZZ genotype in the white population is estimated at 1 in 2,000-4,000 live births. Compound heterozygotes PiZ-, PiSZ, PiZI are not a cause of liver disease alone but can act as modifier genes, increasing the risk of progression in other liver disease such as nonalcoholic fatty liver disease and hepatitis C. The null phenotype because of stop codons in the coding exon of the α₁-antitrypsin gene or complete deletion of α₁-antitrypsin coding exons leads to the complete absence of any protein and causes only lung disease.

Newly formed α₁-antitrypsin peptide normally enters the endoplasmic reticulum, where it undergoes enzymatic modification and folding before transport to the plasma membrane, where it is excreted as a 55 kDa glycoprotein. In affected patients with PiZZ, the rate at which the α₁-antitrypsin peptide folds is decreased, and this delay allows the formation of polymers that are retained in the endoplasmic reticulum. How the polymers cause liver damage is not completely elucidated, but research indicates that accumulation of abnormally folded protein leads to activation of stress and proinflammatory pathways in the endoplasmic reticulum and hepatocyte programmed cell death. In liver biopsies from patients, polymerized α₁-antitrypsin peptides can be seen by electron microscopy and histochemically as periodic acid–Schiff-positive diastase-resistant globules primarily in periportal hepatocytes, but also in Kupffer cells and biliary epithelial cells. The pattern of neonatal liver injury can be highly variable, and liver biopsies might demonstrate hepatocellular necrosis, inflammatory cell infiltration, bile duct proliferation, periportal fibrosis, or cirrhosis.

In affected patients, the course of liver disease is also highly variable. Prospective studies in Sweden have shown that only 10% of patients develop clinically significant liver disease by their 4th decade. Genetic traits or environmental factors must influence the development of disease in α₁-antitrypsin–deficient patients. Infants with liver disease are indistinguishable from other infants with "idiopathic" neonatal hepatitis, of whom they constitute approximately 5-10%. Jaundice, acholic stools, and hepatomegaly are present in the 1st wk of life, but the jaundice usually clears in the 2nd-4th mo. Complete resolution, persistent liver disease, or the development of cirrhosis can follow. Older children can present with asymptomatic hepatomegaly or manifestations of chronic liver disease or cirrhosis, with evidence of portal hypertension. Emphysema is not typically observed in children but an increased risk for developing asthma is reported. Cigarette smoking promotes development of lung disease so children should be counseled on avoidance or smoking cessation as part of their anticipatory guidance. Long-term patients are at risk for hepatocellular carcinoma.

Therapy is supportive; liver transplantation has been curative.

CITRIN DEFICIENCY

Neonatal intrahepatic cholestasis caused by citrin deficiency presents in the 1st few mo of life with manifestations that initially may be indistinguishable from other causes of neonatal cholestasis, especially biliary atresia. Patients may have jaundice, hepatomegaly, liver dysfunction with coagulopathy, fatty liver infiltration, hyperammonemia with or without hypoglycemia. Presymptomatic patients may be identified from the newborn metabolic screen with hypergalactosemia, hypermethionemia, and hyperphenylalanemia, not all patients are identified by newborn screening.

Neonatal intrahepatic cholestasis caused by citrin deficiency is caused by a mutation in the *SLC25A13* gene, which encodes citrin, a mitochondrial carrier protein (calcium binding aspartate-glutamate carrier) and is involved in the urea cycle, gluconeogenesis and glycolysis. The mutation is most common among East Asian populations

Affected infants have hypergalactosemia, elevated bile acids, vitamin K–dependent coagulopathy, and elevated levels of citrulline and methionine. Treatment includes that for neonatal cholestasis and in many patients but more severely affected patients may develop progressive hepatic failure requiring liver transplantation in the 1st yr of life.

Bibliography is available at Expert Consult.

Chapter 358
Viral Hepatitis
M. Kyle Jensen and William F. Balistreri

Viral hepatitis continues to be a major health problem in both developing and developed countries. This disorder is caused by at least 5 pathogenic hepatotropic viruses recognized to date: hepatitides A (HAV), B (HBV), C (HCV), D (HDV), and E (HEV) viruses (Table 358-1). Many other viruses (and diseases) can cause hepatitis, usually as 1 component of a multisystem disease. These include herpes simplex virus, cytomegalovirus, Epstein-Barr virus, varicella-zoster virus, HIV, rubella, adenoviruses, enteroviruses, parvovirus B19, and arboviruses (Table 358-2).

The hepatotropic viruses are a heterogeneous group of infectious agents that cause similar acute clinical illness. In most pediatric patients, the acute phase causes no or mild clinical disease. Morbidity is related to rare cases of **acute liver failure** (ALF) in susceptible patients, and to the chronic disease state and attendant complications that 3 of these viruses (hepatitides B, C, and D) can cause.

ISSUES COMMON TO ALL FORMS OF VIRAL HEPATITIS
Differential Diagnosis
Often what brings the patient with hepatitis to medical attention is clinical icterus, with yellow skin and/or mucous membranes. The liver is usually enlarged and tender to palpation and percussion. Splenomegaly and lymphadenopathy may be present. Extrahepatic symptoms (rashes, arthritis) are more readily seen in HBV and HCV infections. Clinical signs of altered sensorium or hyperreflexia should be carefully sought, because they mark the onset of encephalopathy and ALF.

The differential diagnosis varies with age of presentation.

In the **newborn period,** infection is a common cause of conjugated hyperbilirubinemia; the infectious cause is either a bacterial agent (e.g., *Escherichia coli, Listeria,* syphilis) or a nonhepatotropic virus (e.g., herpes simplex virus, enteroviruses, cytomegalovirus). Metabolic (α_1-antitrypsin deficiency, cystic fibrosis, tyrosinemia), and anatomic

causes (biliary atresia, choledochal cysts) and inherited forms of intrahepatic cholestasis should always be excluded.

In later **childhood,** extrahepatic obstruction (gallstones, primary sclerosing cholangitis, pancreatic pathology), inflammatory conditions (autoimmune hepatitis, juvenile rheumatoid arthritis, Kawasaki disease), immune dysregulation (hemophagocytic lymphohistiocytosis), infiltrative disorders (malignancies), toxins and medications, metabolic disorders (Wilson disease, cystic fibrosis), and infection (Epstein-Barr virus, varicella, malaria, leptospirosis, syphilis) should be ruled out.

Pathogenesis
The acute response of the liver to hepatotropic viruses involves a direct cytopathic and an immune-mediated injury. The entire liver is involved. Necrosis is usually most marked in the centrilobular areas. An acute mixed inflammatory infiltrate predominates in the portal areas but also affects the lobules. The lobular architecture remains intact, although balloon degeneration and necrosis of single or groups of parenchymal cells commonly occurs. Fatty change is rare except with HCV infection. Bile duct proliferation but not bile duct damage is common. Diffuse Kupffer cell hyperplasia is noticeable in the sinusoids. Neonates often respond to hepatic injury by forming **giant cells.**

In **fulminant hepatitis,** parenchymal collapse occurs on the just-described background.

With recovery, the liver morphology returns to normal within 3 mo of the acute infection. If chronic hepatitis develops, the inflammatory infiltrate settles in the periportal areas and often leads to progressive scarring. Both of these hallmarks of chronic hepatitis are seen in cases of HBV and HCV.

Common Biochemical Profiles in the Acute Infectious Phase
Acute liver injury caused by the hepatotropic viruses manifests in 3 main functional liver biochemical profiles. These serve as an important guide to supportive care and monitoring in the acute phase of the infection for all viruses.

As a reflection of *cytopathic injury* to the hepatocytes, there is a rise in serum levels of alanine aminotransferase (ALT) and aspartate aminotransferase (AST). The magnitude of enzyme elevation does not correlate with the extent of hepatocellular necrosis and has little prognostic value. There is usually slow improvement over several weeks, but AST and ALT levels lag behind the serum bilirubin level, which tends to normalize first. Rapidly falling aminotransferase levels can predict a poor outcome, particularly if their decline occurs in conjunction with a rising bilirubin level and a prolonged prothrombin time; this combination of findings usually indicates that massive hepatic injury has occurred.

Cholestasis, defined by elevated serum conjugated bilirubin levels, results from abnormal bile flow at the canalicular and cellular level as a result of hepatocyte damage and inflammatory mediators. Elevation of serum alkaline phosphatase, 5′-nucleotidase, γ-glutamyl transpeptidase, and urobilinogen mark cholestasis. Improvement tends to parallel the acute hepatitis phase. Absence of cholestatic markers

Table 358-1	Features of the Hepatotropic Viruses				
VIROLOGY	**HAV RNA**	**HBV DNA**	**HCV RNA**	**HDV RNA**	**HEV RNA**
Incubation (days)	15-19	60-180	14-160	21-42	21-63
Transmission					
• Parenteral	Rare	Yes	Yes	Yes	No
• Fecal–oral	Yes	No	No	No	Yes
• Sexual	No	Yes	Yes	Yes	No
• Perinatal	No	Yes	Rare	Yes	No
Chronic infection	No	Yes	Yes	Yes	No
Fulminant disease	Rare	Yes	Rare	Yes	Yes

<table>
<tr><td colspan="2">Table 358-2   Causes and Differential Diagnosis of Hepatitis in Children</td></tr>
</table>

INFECTIOUS
Hepatotropic viruses
- HAV
- HBV
- HCV
- HDV
- HEV
- Hepatitis non–A-E viruses

Systemic infection that can include hepatitis
- Adenovirus
- Arbovirus
- Coxsackievirus
- Cytomegalovirus
- Enterovirus
- Epstein-Barr virus
- "Exotic" viruses (e.g., yellow fever)
- Herpes simplex virus
- Human immunodeficiency virus
- Paramyxovirus
- Rubella
- Varicella zoster

Other

NONVIRAL LIVER INFECTIONS
Abscess
Amebiasis
Bacterial sepsis
Brucellosis
Fitz-Hugh-Curtis syndrome
Histoplasmosis
Leptospirosis
Tuberculosis
Other

AUTOIMMUNE
Autoimmune hepatitis
Sclerosing cholangitis
Other (e.g., systemic lupus erythematosus, juvenile rheumatoid arthritis)

METABOLIC
α_1-Antitrypsin deficiency
Tyrosinemia
Wilson disease
Other

TOXIC
Iatrogenic or drug induced (e.g., acetaminophen)
Environmental (e.g., pesticides)

ANATOMIC
Choledochal cyst
Biliary atresia
Other

HEMODYNAMIC
Shock
Congestive heart failure
Budd-Chiari syndrome
Other

NONALCOHOLIC FATTY LIVER DISEASE
Idiopathic
Reye syndrome
Other

From Wyllie R, Hyams JS, editors: Pediatric gastrointestinal and liver disease, ed 3, Philadelphia, 2006, WB Saunders.

does not rule out progression to chronicity in HCV or HBV infections.

Altered synthetic function is the most important marker of liver injury. Monitoring of synthetic function should be the main focus in clinical follow-up to define the severity of the disease. In the acute phase, the degree of liver synthetic dysfunction guides treatment and helps to establish intervention criteria. Abnormal liver synthetic function is a marker of liver failure and is an indication for prompt referral to a transplant center. Serial assessment is necessary because liver dysfunction does not progress linearly. Synthetic dysfunction is reflected by a combination of abnormal protein synthesis (prolonged prothrombin time, high international normalized ratio, low serum albumin levels), metabolic disturbances (hypoglycemia, lactic acidosis, hyperammonemia), poor clearance of medications dependent on liver function, and altered sensorium with increased deep tendon reflexes (hepatic encephalopathy).

HEPATITIS A
HAV infection is the most prevalent hepatotropic virus. This virus is also responsible for most forms of acute and benign hepatitis; although fulminant hepatic failure can occur, it is rare (<1% of cases in the United States) and occurs more often in adults than in children.

Etiology
HAV is an RNA virus, a member of the picornavirus family. It is heat stable and has limited host range—namely, the human and other primates.

Epidemiology
HAV infection occurs throughout the world but is most prevalent in developing countries. In the United States, 30-40% of the adult population has evidence of previous HAV infection. Hepatitis A is thought to account for approximately 50% of all clinically apparent acute viral hepatitis in the United States. As a result of aggressive implementation of a childhood vaccination strategy, the prevalence of symptomatic HAV cases in the United States has declined significantly. However, outbreaks in daycare centers (where the spread from young, nonicteric, infected children can occur easily) as well as multiple foodborne and waterborne outbreaks have justified the implementation of a universal vaccination program.

HAV is highly contagious. Transmission is almost always by person-to-person contact through the fecal–oral route. Perinatal transmission occurs rarely. No other form of transmission is recognized. HAV infection during pregnancy or at the time of delivery does not appear to result in increased complications of pregnancy or clinical disease in the newborn. In the United States, increased risk of infection is found in contacts with infected persons, childcare centers, and household contacts. Infection is also associated with contact with contaminated food or water and after travel to endemic areas. Common source foodborne and waterborne outbreaks have occurred, including several caused by contaminated shellfish, frozen berries, and raw vegetables; no known source is found in about half of the cases. The mean incubation period for HAV is approximately 3 wk. Fecal excretion of the virus starts late in the incubation period, reaches its peak just before the onset of symptoms, and resolves by 2 wk after the onset of jaundice in older subjects. The duration of viral excretion is prolonged in infants. The patient is, therefore, contagious before clinical symptoms are apparent and remains so until viral shedding ceases.

Clinical Manifestations
HAV is responsible for acute hepatitis only. Often, this is an anicteric illness, with clinical symptoms indistinguishable from other forms of viral gastroenteritis, particularly in young children.

The illness is much more likely to be symptomatic in older adolescents or adults, in patients with underlying liver disorders, and in those who are immunocompromised. It is characteristically an acute febrile illness with an abrupt onset of anorexia, nausea, malaise, vomiting, and jaundice. The typical duration of illness is 7-14 days (Fig. 358-1).

Other organ systems can be affected during acute HAV infection. Regional lymph nodes and the spleen may be enlarged. The bone marrow may be moderately hypoplastic, and aplastic anemia has been reported. Tissue in the small intestine might show changes in villous structure, and ulceration of the gastrointestinal tract can occur, especially in fatal cases. Acute pancreatitis and myocarditis have been reported, though rarely, and nephritis, arthritis, vasculitis, and cryo-globulinemia can result from circulating immune complexes.

Diagnosis

Acute HAV infection is diagnosed by detecting antibodies to HAV, specifically, anti-HAV (immunoglobulin [Ig] M) by radioimmunoassay or, rarely, by identifying viral particles in stool. A viral polymerase chain reaction (PCR) assay is available for research use (Table 358-3). Anti-HAV is detectable when the symptoms are clinically apparent, and it remains positive for 4-6 mo after the acute infection. A neutralizing anti-HAV (IgG) is usually detected within 8 wk of symptom onset and is measured as part of a total anti-HAV in the serum. Anti-HAV (IgG) confers long-term protection. Rises in serum levels of ALT, AST, bilirubin, alkaline phosphatase, 5′-nucleotidase, and γ-glutamyl trans-peptidase are almost universally found and do not help to differentiate the cause of hepatitis.

Complications

Although most patients achieve full recovery, 2 distinct complications can occur. *ALF* from HAV infection is a rare but not infrequent complication of HAV. Those at risk for this complication are adolescents and adults, but also immunocompromised patients or those with

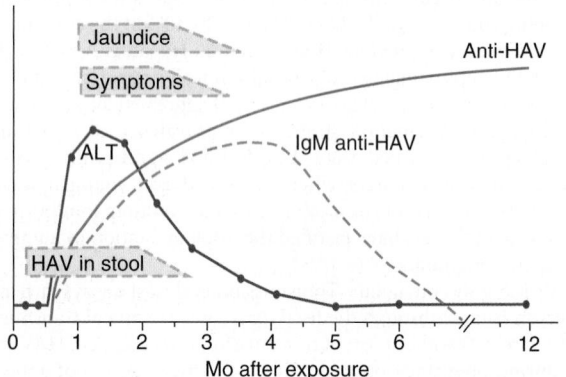

Figure 358-1 The serologic course of acute hepatitis A. *ALT*, alanine aminotransferase; *HAV*, hepatitis A virus. (*From Goldman L, Ausiello D: Cecil textbook of medicine, ed 22, Philadelphia, 2004, WB Saunders, p 913.*)

underlying liver disorders. The height of HAV viremia may be linked to the severity of hepatitis. Whereas in the United States, HAV represents < 0.5% of pediatric-age ALF, it is responsible for up to 3% mortality in the adult population with ALF. In endemic areas of the world, HAV constitutes up to 40% of all cases of pediatric ALF. HAV can also progress to a *prolonged cholestatic syndrome* that waxes and wanes over several months. Pruritus and fat malabsorption are problematic and require symptomatic support with antipruritic medications and fat-soluble vitamins. This syndrome occurs in the absence of any liver synthetic dysfunction and resolves without sequelae.

Treatment

There is no specific treatment for hepatitis A. Supportive treatment consists of intravenous hydration as needed and antipruritic agents and fat-soluble vitamins for the prolonged cholestatic form of disease. Serial monitoring for signs of ALF and, if ALF is diagnosed, a prompt referral to a transplantation center can be lifesaving.

Prevention

Patients infected with HAV are contagious for 2 wk before and approximately 7 days after the onset of jaundice and should be excluded from school, childcare, or work during this period. Careful hand-washing is necessary, particularly after changing diapers and before preparing or serving food. In hospital settings, contact and standard precautions are recommended for 1 wk after onset of symptoms.

Immunoglobulin

Indications for intramuscular administration of Ig (0.02 mL/kg) include preexposure and postexposure prophylaxis (Table 358-4).

Ig is recommended for preexposure prophylaxis for susceptible travelers to countries where HAV is endemic, and it provides effective protection for up to 3 mo. *HAV vaccine given any time before travel is preferred for preexposure prophylaxis in healthy persons, but Ig ensures an appropriate prophylaxis in children younger than 12 mo old, patients allergic to a vaccine component, or those who elect not to receive the vaccine.* If travel is planned in <2 wk, older patients, immunocompromised hosts, and those with chronic liver disease or other medical conditions should receive both Ig and the HAV vaccine.

Ig prophylaxis in postexposure situations should be used as soon as possible (not effective more than 2 wk after exposure). It is exclusively used for children younger than 12 mo old, immunocompromised hosts, those with chronic liver disease or in whom vaccine is contraindicated. Ig is preferred in patients older than 40 yr of age, with HAV

Table 358-3	Diagnostic Blood Tests: Serology and Viral PCR				
HAV	**HBV**	**HCV**	**HDV**	**HEV**
ACUTE/ACTIVE INFECTION				
Anti-HAV IgM(+)	Anti-HBc IgM(+)	Anti-HCV(+)	Anti-HDV IgM(+)	Anti-HEV IgM(+)
Blood PCR positive*	HBsAg(+)	HCV RNA(+) (PCR)	Blood PCR positive	Blood PCR positive
	Anti-HBs(–)		HBsAg(+)	
	HBV DNA(+) (PCR)		Anti-HBs(–)	
PAST INFECTION (RECOVERED)				
Anti-HAV IgG(+)	Anti-HBs(+)	Anti-HCV(–)	Anti-HDV IgG(+)	Anti-HEV IgG(+)
	Anti-HBc IgG(+)	Blood PCR(–)	Blood PCR (–)	Blood PCR(–)
CHRONIC INFECTION				
N/A	Anti-HBc IgG(+)	Anti-HCV(+)	Anti-HDV IgG(+)	N/A
	HBsAg(+)	Blood PCR (+)	Blood PCR (–)	
	Anti-HBs(–)		HBsAg(+)	
	PCR (+)or (–)		Anti-HBs(–)	
VACCINE RESPONSE				
Anti-HAV IgG(+)	Anti-HBs(+)	N/A	N/A	N/A
	Anti-HBc(–)			

*Research tool.
    HAV, hepatitis A virus; HBs, hepatitis B surface; HBsAg, hepatitis B surface antigen; Ig, immunoglobulin; PCR, polymerase chain reaction.

Table 358-4	Hepatitis A Virus Prophylaxis		
PREEXPOSURE PROPHYLAXIS (TRAVELERS TO ENDEMIC REGIONS)			
AGE	**EXPECTED EXPOSURE DURATION**		**DOSE**
<1 year of age	<3 months		Ig 0.02 mL/kg
	3-5 months		Ig 0.06 mL/kg
	Long term (>5months)		Ig 0.06 mL/kg at departure and every 5 mo thereafter
≥1 year of age	Healthy host		HAV vaccine
	Immunocompromised host, or one with chronic liver disease or chronic health problems		HAV vaccine and Ig 0.02 mL/kg
POSTEXPOSURE PROPHYLAXIS*			
EXPOSURE	**RECOMMENDATIONS**		
≤2 wk since exposure	<1 year-old: Ig 0.02 mL/kg		
	Immunocompromised host, or host with chronic liver disease or chronic health problems: Ig 0.02 mL/kg and HAV vaccine		
	>1 year and healthy host: HAV vaccine, Ig remains optional		
	Sporadic non–household or close contact exposure: prophylaxis not indicated*		
>2 wk since exposure	None		

*Decision for prophylaxis in nonhousehold contacts should be tailored to individual exposure and risk. Ig, Immunoglubulin.

vaccine preferred in healthy persons 12 mo-40 yr old. *An alternative approach is to immunize previously unvaccinated patients who are 12 mo old or older with the age-appropriate vaccine dosage as soon as possible.* Ig is not routinely recommended for sporadic nonhousehold exposure (e.g., protection of hospital personnel or schoolmates). The vaccine has several advantages over Ig, including long-term protection, availability and ease of administration, with cost similar to, or less than, that of Ig.

Vaccine

The availability of 2 inactivated, highly immunogenic, and safe HAV vaccines has had a major impact on the prevention of HAV infection. Both vaccines are approved for children older than 12 mo. They are administered intramuscularly in a 2-dose schedule, with the 2nd dose given 6-12 mo after the 1st dose. Seroconversion rates in children exceed 90% after an initial dose and approach 100% after the 2nd dose; protective antibody titer persists for longer than 10 yr in the vast majority of patients. The immune response in immunocompromised persons, older patients, and those with chronic illnesses may be suboptimal; in those patients, combining the vaccine with Ig for pre- and postexposure prophylaxis is indicated. HAV vaccine may be administered simultaneously with other vaccines. A combination HAV and HBV vaccine is approved in adults older than age 18 yr. For healthy persons at least 12 mo old, vaccine is preferable to Ig for preexposure and postexposure prophylaxis (see Table 358-3).

In the United States and some other countries, universal vaccination is now recommended for all children older than 12 mo. Nevertheless, studies show <50% of U.S. adolescents have received 1 dose of the vaccine, and <30% have received the complete vaccine series. The vaccine is effective in curbing outbreaks of HAV because of rapid seroconversion and the long incubation period of the disease.

Prognosis

The prognosis for the patient with HAV is excellent, with no long-term sequelae. The only feared complication is ALF. HAV infection remains a major cause of morbidity; it has a high socioeconomic impact during epidemics and in endemic areas.

HEPATITIS B
Etiology

HBV is a member of the Hepadnaviridae family. HBV has a circular, partially double-stranded DNA genome composed of approximately 3,200 nucleotides. Four genes have been identified: the S (surface),

C (core), X, and P (polymer) genes. The surface of the virus includes particles designated *hepatitis B surface antigen (HBsAg),* which is a 22 nm diameter spherical particle and a 22 nm wide tubular particle with a variable length of up to 200 nm. The inner portion of the virion contains hepatitis B core antigen (HBcAg), the nucleocapsid that encodes the viral DNA, and a nonstructural antigen called hepatitis B e antigen (HBeAg), a nonparticulate soluble antigen derived from HBcAg by proteolytic self-cleavage. HBeAg serves as a marker of active viral replication and usually correlates with HBV DNA levels. Replication of HBV occurs predominantly in the liver but also occurs in the lymphocytes, spleen, kidney, and pancreas.

Epidemiology

HBV has been detected worldwide, with an estimated 400 million persons chronically infected. The areas of highest prevalence of HBV infection are sub-Saharan Africa, China, parts of the Middle East, the Amazon basin, and the Pacific Islands. In the United States, the native population in Alaska had the highest prevalence rate before the implementation of universal vaccination programs. An estimated 1.25 million persons in the United States are chronic HBV carriers, with approximately 300,000 new cases of HBV occurring each year, the highest incidence being among adults 20-39 yr of age. One in 4 chronic HBV carriers will develop serious sequelae in their lifetime. The number of new cases in children reported each year is thought to be low but is difficult to estimate because many infections in children are asymptomatic. In the United States, since 1982 when the first vaccine for HBV was introduced, the overall incidence of HBV infection has been reduced by more than half. Since the implementation of universal vaccination programs in Taiwan and the United States, substantial progress has been made toward eliminating HBV infection in children in these countries. In fact, in Alaska, where HBV neared epidemic proportions, universal newborn vaccination with mass screening and immunization of susceptible Alaska Natives virtually eliminated symptomatic HBV and secondary hepatocellular carcinoma.

HBV is present in high concentrations in blood, serum, and serous exudates and in moderate concentrations in saliva, vaginal fluid, and semen. Efficient transmission occurs through blood exposure and sexual contact. Risk factors for HBV infection in children and adolescents include acquisition by intravenous drugs or blood products, contaminated needles used for acupuncture or tattoos, sexual contact, institutional care, and intimate contact with carriers. No risk factors are identified in approximately 40% of cases. HBV is not thought to be transmitted via indirect exposure, such as sharing toys.

In children, the most important risk factor for acquisition of HBV remains perinatal exposure to an HBsAg-positive mother. The risk of transmission is greatest if the mother is also HBeAg-positive; up to 90% of these infants become chronically infected if untreated. Intrauterine infection occurs in 2.5% of these infants. In most cases, serologic markers of infection and antigenemia appear 1-3 mo after birth, suggesting that transmission occurred at the time of delivery. Virus contained in amniotic fluid or in maternal feces or blood may be the source. Immunoprophylaxis with hepatitis B immunoglobulin (HBIG) and the HBV immunization, given within 12 hr of delivery is very effective in preventing infection and protects > 95% of neonates born to HBsAg-positve mothers. Of the 22,000 infants born each year to HBsAg-positive mothers in the United States, >98% receive immunoprophylaxis and are thus protected. Infants who fail to receive the complete vaccination series (e.g., homeless children, international adoptees, and children born outside the United States), however, have the highest incidence of developing chronic HBV. These and all infants born to HBsAg-positive mothers should have follow-up HBsAg and anti-HBs tested to determine appropriate follow-up.

HBsAg is inconsistently recovered in human milk of infected mothers. Breastfeeding of nonimmunized infants by infected mothers does not confer a greater risk of hepatitis than does formula feeding.

The risk of developing **chronic HBV** infection, defined as being positive for HBsAg for longer than 6 mo, is inversely related to age of acquisition. In the United States, although <10% of infections occurs in children, these infections account for 20-30% of all chronic cases. This risk of chronic infection is 90% in children younger than 1 yr; the risk is 30% for those 1-5 yr and 2% for adults. Chronic infection is associated with the development of chronic liver disease and hepatocellular carcinoma. The carcinoma risk is independent of the presence of cirrhosis and was the most prevalent cancer-related death in young adults in Asia where HBV was endemic.

HBV has 8 genotypes (A-H). A is pandemic, B and C are prevalent in Asia, D is seen in Southern Europe, E in Africa, F in the United States, G in the United States and France, and H in Central America. Genetic variants have become resistant to antiviral agents. After infection, the incubation period ranges from 45-160 days, with a mean of approximately 120 days.

Pathogenesis

The acute response of the liver to HBV is the same as for all hepatotropic viruses. Persistence of histologic changes in patients with hepatitis B indicates development of chronic liver disease. HBV, unlike the other hepatotropic viruses, is a predominantly noncytopathogenic virus that causes injury mostly by immune-mediated processes. The severity of hepatocyte injury reflects the degree of the immune response, with the most complete immune response being associated with the greatest likelihood of viral clearance but also the most severe injury to hepatocytes. The 1st step in the process of **acute hepatitis** is infection of hepatocytes by HBV, resulting in expression of viral antigens on the cell surface. The most important of these viral antigens may be the nucleocapsid antigens HBcAg and HBeAg. These antigens, in combination with class I major histocompatibility proteins, make the cell a target for cytotoxic T-cell lysis.

The mechanism for development of **chronic hepatitis** is less well understood. To permit hepatocytes to continue to be infected, the core protein or major histocompatibility class I protein might not be recognized, the cytotoxic lymphocytes might not be activated, or some other, yet unknown mechanism might interfere with destruction of hepatocytes. This **tolerance** phenomenon predominates in the perinatally acquired cases, resulting in a high incidence of persistent infection in children with no or little inflammation in the liver, normal liver enzymes, and markedly elevated HBV viral load. Although end-stage liver disease rarely develops in those patients, the inherent hepatocellular carcinoma risk is very high, possibly related, in part, to uncontrolled viral replication cycles.

ALF has been seen in infants of chronic carrier mothers who have anti-HBe or are infected with a precore-mutant strain. This fact led to the postulate that HBeAg exposure in utero in infants of chronic carriers likely induces tolerance to the virus once infection occurs postnatally. In the absence of this tolerance, the liver is massively attacked by T cells and the patient presents with ALF.

Immune-mediated mechanisms are also involved in the **extrahepatic conditions** that can be associated with HBV infections. **Circulating immune complexes** containing HBsAg can result in polyarteritis nodosa, membranous or membranoproliferative glomerulonephritis, polymyalgia rheumatica, leukocytoclastic vasculitis, and Guillain-Barré syndrome.

Clinical Manifestations

Many acute cases of HBV infection in children are asymptomatic, as evidenced by the high carriage rate of serum markers in persons who have no history of acute hepatitis. The usual acute symptomatic episode is similar to that of HAV and HCV infections but may be more severe and is more likely to include involvement of skin and joints (Fig. 358-2). The first biochemical evidence of HBV infection is elevation of serum ALT levels, which begin to rise just before development of fatigue, anorexia, and malaise, which occurs approximately 6-7 wk after exposure. The illness is preceded in a few children by a serum sickness–like prodrome marked by arthralgia or skin lesions, including urticarial, purpuric, macular, or maculopapular rashes. Papular acrodermatitis, the Gianotti-Crosti syndrome, can also occur. Other extrahepatic conditions associated with HBV infections in children include polyarteritis nodosa, glomerulonephritis, and aplastic anemia. Jaundice is present in approximately 25% of acutely infected patients and usually begins approximately 8 wk after exposure and lasts approximately 4 wk.

In the usual course of resolving HBV infection, symptoms are present for 6-8 wk. The percentage of children in whom clinical evidence of hepatitis develops is higher for HBV than for HAV, and the rate of ALF is also greater. Most patients do recover, but the "chronic carrier state" complicates up to 10% of cases acquired in adulthood. The rate of development of chronic infection depends largely on the mode and age of acquisition and occurs in up to 90% of perinatal cases. Chronic hepatitis, cirrhosis, and hepatocellular carcinoma are only seen with chronic infection. Chronic HBV infection has 3 identified phases: immune tolerant, immune active, and inactive. Most children fall in the immune-tolerant phase, against which no effective therapy has been developed. Most treatments target the immune active phase of the disease, characterized by active inflammation, elevated ALT/AST levels, and progressive fibrosis. Spontaneous HBeAg seroconversion, defined as the development of anti-HBe and becoming HBeAg-negative, occurs in the immune-tolerant phase, albeit at low rates of 4-5% per year. It is more common in childhood-acquired HBV rather than in vertically transmitted infections. Seroconversion can occur over many years, during which time significant damage to

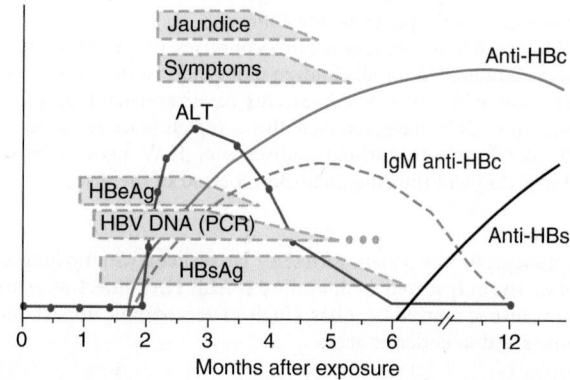

Figure 358-2 The serologic course of acute hepatitis B. *HBc,* hepatitis B core; *HBeAg,* hepatitis B e antigen; *HBs,* hepatitis B surface; *HBsAg,* hepatitis B surface antigen; *HBV,* hepatitis B virus; *PCR,* polymerase chain reaction. *(From Goldman L, Ausiello D: Cecil textbook of medicine, ed 22, Philadelphia, 2004, WB Saunders, p 914.)*

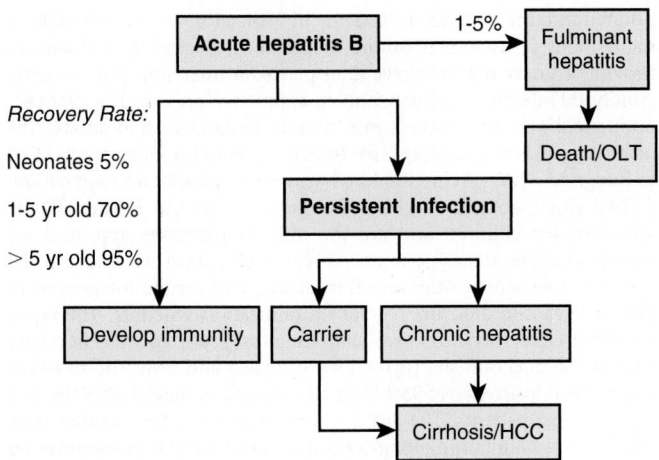

Figure 358-3 Natural history of hepatitis B virus infection. *HCC,* hepatocellular carcinoma; *OLT,* orthotopic liver transplant.

the liver may take place. There are no large studies that help accurately assess the lifetime risks and morbidities of children with chronic HBV infection, making the timing of still less-than-ideal treatments ever so hard to decide. Reactivation of chronic infection has been reported in immunosuppressed children (treated with chemotherapy, biologic immunomodulators such as infliximab, T-cell depleting agents), leading to an increased risk of ALF or to rapidly progressing fibrotic liver disease.

Diagnosis

The serologic profile of HBV infection is more complex than for HAV infection and differs depending on whether the disease is acute or chronic (Fig. 358-3). Several antigens and antibodies are used to confirm the diagnosis of acute HBV infection (see Table 358-3). Routine screening for HBV infection requires assay of multiple serologic markers (HBsAg, anti-HBc, anti-HBs). HBsAg is the first serologic marker of infection to appear and is found in almost all infected persons; its rise closely coincides with the onset of symptoms. Persistence of HBsAg beyond 6 mo defines the chronic infection state. During recovery from acute infection, because HBsAg levels fall before symptoms wane, IgM antibody to HBcAg (anti-HBc IgM) might be the only marker of acute infection. Anti-HBc IgM rises early after the infection and remains positive for many months before being replaced by anti-HBc IgG, which then persists for years. Anti-HBc is therefore a valuable serologic marker of acute HBV infection. Anti-HBs marks serologic recovery and protection. Only anti-HBs is present in persons immunized with hepatitis B vaccine, whereas both anti-HBs and anti-HBc are detected in persons with resolved infection. HBeAg is present in active acute or chronic infection and is a marker of infectivity. The development of anti-HBe, termed seroconversion, marks improvement and is a goal of therapy in chronically infected patients. HBV DNA can be detected in the serum of acutely infected patients and chronic carriers. High DNA titers are seen in patients with HBeAg, and they typically fall once anti-HBe develops.

Complications

Acute liver failure with coagulopathy, encephalopathy, and cerebral edema occurs more commonly with HBV than the other hepatotropic viruses. The risk of ALF is further increased when there is coinfection or superinfection with HDV and in an immunosuppressed host. Mortality from ALF is >30%, and liver transplantation is the only effective intervention. Supportive care aimed at sustaining patients and early referral to a liver transplantation center can be lifesaving. As mentioned, HBV infection can also result in **chronic hepatitis,** which can lead to cirrhosis, end-stage liver disease complications, and primary **hepatocellular carcinoma. Membranous glomerulonephritis** with

deposition of complement and HBeAg in glomerular capillaries is a rare complication of HBV infection.

Treatment

Treatment of *acute* HBV infection is largely supportive. Close monitoring for liver failure and extrahepatic morbidities is key.

Treatment of *chronic* HBV infection is in evolution; no one drug currently achieves consistent, complete eradication of the virus. The natural history of HBV chronic infection in children is complex, and there is a lack of reliable long-term outcome data on which to base treatment recommendations. Treatment of chronic HBV infection in children should be individualized and done under the care of a pediatric gastroenterologist experienced in treating liver disease.

The goal of treatment is to reduce viral replication defined by having undetectable HBV DNA in the serum and development of anti-HBe, termed seroconversion. The development of anti-HBe transforms the disease into an inactive form, thereby decreasing infectivity, active liver injury and inflammation, fibrosis progression, and the risk of hepatocellular carcinoma.

Currently, treatment is only indicated for patients in the immune-active form of the disease, as evidenced by elevated ALT and/or AST, who have fibrosis on liver biopsy, putting the child at higher risk for cirrhosis during childhood.

Treatment Strategies

Interferon-α2b (IFN-α2b) has immunomodulatory and antiviral effects. It has been used in children, with long-term viral response rates similar to the 25% rate reported in adults. Interferon (IFN) use is limited by its subcutaneous administration, treatment duration of 24 wk, and possible side effects (flu-like symptoms, marrow suppression, depression, retinal changes, autoimmune disorders). IFN is further contraindicated in decompensated cirrhosis. One advantage of IFN, compared to other treatments, is that viral resistance does not develop with its use.

Lamivudine is an oral synthetic nucleoside analog that inhibits the viral enzyme reverse transcriptase. In children older than age 2 yr, its use for 52 wk resulted in HBeAg clearance in 34% of patients with an ALT > 2 times normal; 88% remained in remission at 1 yr. It has a good safety profile. Lamivudine has to be used for ≥6 mo after viral clearance, and the emergence of a mutant viral strain (YMDD) poses a barrier to its long-term use. Combination therapy in children using IFN and lamivudine did not seem to improve the rates of response in most series.

Adefovir (a purine analog that inhibits viral replication) is approved for use in children older than 12 yr of age, in whom a prospective 1-year study showed 23% seroconversion. No viral resistance was noted in that study but has been reported in adults.

Entecavir (a nucleoside analog that inhibits replication) is currently approved for use in children older than age 16 yr. Prospective data has shown a 21% seroconversion rate in adults with minimal resistance developing. Patients in whom resistance to lamivudine developed, have an increased risk of resistance developing to entecavir.

Tenofovir (a nucleotide analog that inhibits viral replication) is also approved for use in children older than age 16 yr. Data have shown efficacy in children older than age 12 yr. Prospective data have shown a 21% seroconversion rate with a very low rate of resistance developing. Patients with lamivudine-resistant mutations do not appear to have an increased rate of resistance. Concern exists over long-term use and bone mineral density.

Peginterferon-α₂ has the same mechanism of action as IFN, but is given once weekly. This formulation has not been approved in the United States but is recommended for the treatment of chronic HBV in other countries. Patients most likely to respond to currently available drugs have low serum HBV DNA titers, are HBeAg-positive, have active hepatic inflammation (ALT greater than twice the upper limit of normal for at least 6 mo), and recently acquired disease.

Immune tolerant patients—those with normal ALT and AST, who are HBeAg-positive with elevated viral load—are currently not considered for treatment, although the emergence of new treatment paradigms are promising for this large, yet hard-to-treat, subgroup of patients.

Prevention

The most effective prevention strategies have resulted from the screening of pregnant mothers and the use of HBIG and hepatitis B vaccine in infants as noted earlier. In HBsAg-positive and HBeAg-positive mothers, a 10% risk of chronic HBV infection exists compared to 1% in HBeAg-negative mothers. This knowledge offers screening strategies that may affect both mother and infant through the use of antiviral medications during the 3rd trimester. Recent guidelines suggest that mothers with a HBV DNA viral load >200,000 IU/mL receive an antiviral such as telbivudine, lamivudine, or tenofovir during the 3rd trimester, especially if they had a previous child who developed chronic HBV after receiving HBIG and the hepatitis B vaccine.

Household, sexual, and needle-sharing contacts should be identified and vaccinated if they are susceptible to HBV infection. Patients should be advised about the perinatal and intimate contact risk of transmission of HBV. HBV is not spread by breastfeeding, kissing, hugging, or sharing water or utensils. Children with HBV should not be excluded from school, play, childcare, or work, unless they are prone to biting. A support group might help children to cope better with their disease. Families should not feel obligated to disclose the diagnosis as this information may lead to prejudice or mistreatment of the patient or the patient's family. All patients positive for HBsAg should be reported to the state or local health department, and chronicity is diagnosed if they remain positive past 6 mo.

Hepatitis B Immunoglobulin

HBIG is indicated only for specific postexposure circumstances and provides only temporary protection (3-6 mo; Table 358-5). It plays a pivotal role in preventing perinatal transmission when administered within 12 hr of birth.

Universal Vaccination

In 2005, the Centers for Disease Control and Prevention Advisory Committee on Immunization Practices revised its recommendations regarding HBV vaccination. These recommendations have been incorporated into the American Academy of Pediatrics Vaccine schedule. A main focus is **universal infant vaccination,** beginning at birth, to provide a safety net for preventing perinatal infection, prevent early childhood infection, facilitate implementation of universal vaccine recommendations, and prevent infection in adolescents and adults. The ultimate goal is to eliminate HBV transmission in the United States and to integrate HBV vaccination in a harmonized childhood vaccination.

Two single-antigen vaccines (Recombivax HB and Engerix-B) are approved for children and are the only preparations approved for infants younger than age 6 mo. Three combination vaccines can be used for subsequent immunization dosing and enable integration of the HBV vaccine into the regular immunization schedule. The safety profile of HBV vaccine is excellent. The most reported side effects are pain at the injection site (up to 29% of cases) and fever (up to 6% of cases). Seropositivity is >95% with all vaccines, achieved after the 2nd dose in most patients. The 3rd dose serves as a booster and may have an effect on maintaining long-term immunity. In immunosuppressed patients and infants whose birthweight is <2,000 g, a 4th dose is recommended, as is checking for seroconversion. Despite declines in the anti-HBs titer in time, most healthy vaccinated persons remain protected against HBV infection.

Current HBV vaccination recommendations are as follows (see Table 358-5):

◆ Infants born to HBsAg-negative mothers:
  ◆ For all medically stable infants weighing >2,000 g at birth and born to HBsAg-*negative* mothers, the 1st dose of HBV vaccine should be administered before hospital discharge. Single-dose antigen HBV vaccine should be used for the birth dose. Subsequent doses to complete the series are given at 1-4 mo and at 6-18 mo of age. Routine postvaccination testing of immunized infants born to HBsAg-*negative* women or with anti-HBs is not recommended.
  ◆ In rare circumstances (on a case-by-case basis), the 1st dose may be delayed (up to 2 mo) until after hospital discharge. When a decision to delay is made, however, a physician's order to withhold the birth dose, along with a copy of the original laboratory report indicating that the mother was HBsAg-*negative*, should be placed on the medical record.

Table 358-5	Indications and Dosing Schedule for Hepatitis B Vaccine and Hepatitis B Immunoglobulin		
	VACCINE DOSE		
	RECOMBIVAX HB (µg)	**ENGERIX-B (µg)**	**SCHEDULE**
UNIVERSAL PROPHYLAXIS			
Infants of HBsAg(−) women	5	10	Birth, 1-2, 6-18 mo
Children and adolescents (11-19 yr old)	5	10	0, 1, and 6 mo
POSTEXPOSURE PROPHYLAXIS IN SUSCEPTIBLE INDIVIDUALS			
Contact with HBsAg(+) Source			
Infants of HBsAg(+) women	5	10	Birth* (+HBIG[†]), 1 and 6 mo
Intimate or Identifiable Blood Exposure			
0-19 yr old	5	10	Exposure (+HBIG[†]), 1 and 6 mo
>19 yr old	10	20	Exposure (+HBIG[†]), 1 and 6 mo
Household			
0-19 yr old	5	10	Exposure, 1 and 6 mo
>19 yr old	10	20	Exposure, 1 and 6 mo
Casual	None	None	None
Immunocompromised[‡]	40	40	Exposure (+HBIG[†]), 1 and 6 mo
Contact with Unknown HBsAg Status; Intimate or Identifiable Blood Exposure			
>19 yr old	10	20	Exposure, 1 and 6 mo
Immunocompromised[‡]	40	40	Exposure (+HBIG[†]), 1 and 6 mo

*Both HBIG and vaccine should be administered within 12 hr of the infant's birth and within 24 hr of identifiable blood exposure. HBIG can be given up to 14 days after sexual exposure.
[†]HBIG dose: 0.5 µL for newborns of HBsAg-positive mothers, and 0.0 6 µL/kg for all others when recommended.
[‡]Seroconversion status of immunocompromised patients should be checked 1-2 mo after the last dose of vaccine, and yearly thereafter. Booster doses of vaccine should be administered if the anti-HBs titer is <10 mIU/mL. Nonresponsive patients should be considered at high risk for HBV acquisition and counseled about preventive measures.
HBs, hepatitis B surface; HBsAg, hepatitis B surface antigen; HBV, hepatitis B virus.

- Preterm infants weighing <2,000 g at birth and born to HBsAg-*negative* mothers should have their initial dose delayed until 1 mo of age or before hospital discharge.
- To increase coverage of children and adolescents not previously vaccinated, many states have made immunization a requirement for entry into junior high school (middle school).
- Infants born to HBsAg-positive or HBsAg-unknown mothers:
  - To prevent perinatal transmission through improved maternal screening and immunoprophylaxis, infants born to HBsAg-positive women should receive vaccine at birth, 1-2 mo, and 6 mo of age (see Table 358-4). The 1st dose should be accompanied by administration of 0.5 mL of HBIG as soon after delivery as possible (within 12 hr) because the effectiveness decreases rapidly with increased time after birth.
  - If mother's HBsAg status is unknown, the vaccine should be administered within 12 hr of birth regardless of birthweight. For infants weighing <2,000 g, HBIG and the HBV vaccine should be administered within 12 hr of birth. The mother's HBsAg status should be administered as soon as possible and, if she is HBsAg-positive, HBIG should be given for infants weighing ≥2,000 g (no later than age 1 wk).

Postvaccination testing for HBsAg and anti-HBs should be done at 9-18 mo. If the result is positive for anti-HBs, the child is immune to HBV. If the result is positive for HBsAg only, the parent should be counseled and the child evaluated by a pediatric gastroenterologist. If the result is negative for both HBsAg and anti-HBs, a second complete hepatitis B vaccine series should be administered, followed by testing for anti-HBs to determine if subsequent doses are needed.

Administration of 4 doses of vaccine is permissible when combination vaccines are used after the birth dose; this does not increase vaccine response.

Postexposure Prophylaxis
Recommendations for postexposure prophylaxis for prevention of hepatitis B infection depend on the conditions under which the person is exposed to HBV (see Table 358-5). Vaccination should never be postponed if written records of the exposed person's immunization history are not available, but every effort should still be made to obtain those records.

Special Populations
Patients with cirrhosis may not respond as well to the HBV vaccine and repeating anti-HBs titers should be performed. Adult studies suggest higher dosage or shorter interval between dosages may increase the immunization effectiveness. Recent evidence has shown patients with inflammatory bowel disease frequently have not been immunized, or did not develop complete immunity to HBV, as demonstrated by inadequate anti-HBs levels. These patients may be at risk for fulminant HBV when immunosuppression is started as part of their treatment regimen, specifically with biologic agents such as infliximab.

Prognosis
In general, the outcome after acute HBV infection is favorable, despite a risk of ALF. The risk of developing chronic infection brings the risks of liver cirrhosis and hepatocellular carcinoma to the forefront. Perinatal transmission leading to chronicity is responsible for the high incidence of hepatocellular carcinoma in young adults in endemic areas. Importantly, HBV infection and its complications are effectively controlled and prevented with vaccination and multiple clinical trials are ongoing in an effort to improve and guide treatment regimens.

HEPATITIS C
Etiology
HCV is a single-stranded RNA virus, classified as a separate genus within the Flaviviridae family, with marked genetic heterogeneity. It has 6 major genotypes and numerous subtypes and quasi-species, which permit the virus to escape host immune surveillance. Genotype variation might partially explain the differences in clinical course and

response to treatment. Genotype 1b is the most common genotype in the United States and is the least responsive to the currently available medications.

Epidemiology
In the United States, HCV infection is the most common cause of chronic liver disease in adults and causes 8,000-10,000 deaths per year. Approximately 4 million people in the United States and 170 million people worldwide are estimated to be infected with HCV. Approximately 85% of infected adults remain chronically infected. In children, seroprevalence of HCV is 0.2% in those younger than age 11 yr and 0.4% in children age 11 yr or older. However, even more children may be infected as only a small percentage of HCV-infected children are identified, and an even smaller number subsequently receive treatment. Appropriate identification, and screening, for infected individuals should be implemented.

Risk factors for HCV transmission in the United States included blood transfusion before 1992 as the most common route of infection, but, with current screening practices, the risk of HCV transmission is approximately 0.001% per unit transfused. Illegal drug use with exposure to blood or blood products from HCV-infected persons accounts for more than half of adult cases in the United States. Sexual transmission, especially through multiple sexual partners, is the second most common cause of infection. Other risk factors include occupational exposure, but approximately 10% of new infections have no known transmission source. In children, perinatal transmission is the most prevalent mode of transmission (see Table 358-1). Perinatal transmission occurs in up to 5% of infants born to viremic mothers. HIV coinfection and high viremia titers (HCV RNA-positive) in the mother can increase the transmission rate to 20%. The incubation period is 7-9 wk (range: 2-24 wk).

Pathogenesis
The pattern of acute hepatic injury is indistinguishable from that of other hepatotropic viruses. In chronic cases, lymphoid aggregates or follicles in portal tracts are found, either alone or as part of a general inflammatory infiltrate of the portal areas. Steatosis is also often seen in these liver specimens. HCV appears to cause injury primarily by cytopathic mechanisms, but immune-mediated injury can also occur. The cytopathic component appears to be mild, because the acute illness is typically the least severe of all hepatotropic virus infections.

Clinical Manifestations
Acute HCV infection tends to be mild and insidious in onset (Fig. 358-4; see also Table 358-1). ALF rarely occurs. HCV is the most likely

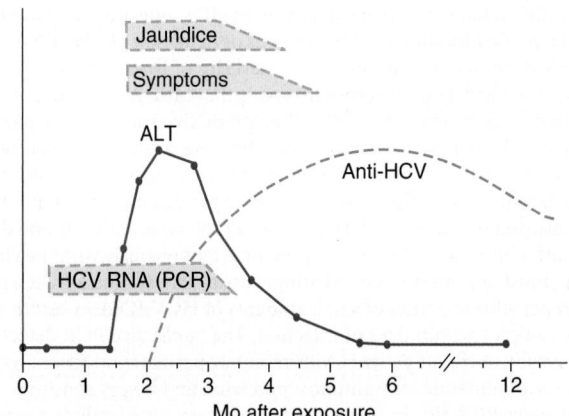

Figure 358-4 The serologic course of acute hepatitis C. *ALT*, alanine aminotransferase; *HCV*, hepatitis C virus; *PCR*, polymerase chain reaction. (*From Goldman L, Ausiello D: Cecil textbook of medicine, ed 22, Philadelphia, 2004, WB Saunders, p. 915.*)

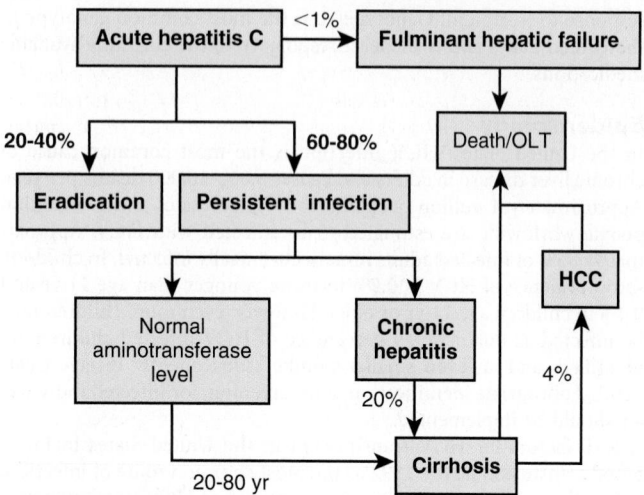

Figure 358-5 Natural history of hepatitis C virus infection. *HCC, hepatocellular carcinoma; OLT, orthotopic liver transplant. (From Hochman JA, Balistreri WF: Chronic viral hepatitis: always be current! Pediatr Rev 24:399–410, 2003.)*

hepatotropic virus to cause chronic infection (Fig. 358-5). Of affected adults, <15% clear the virus; the rest develop chronic hepatitis. In pediatric studies, 6-19% of children achieved spontaneous sustained clearance of the virus during a 6 yr follow-up.

Chronic HCV infection is also clinically silent until a complication develops. Serum aminotransferase levels fluctuate and are sometimes normal, but histologic inflammation is universal. Progression of liver fibrosis is slow over several years, unless comorbid factors are present, which can accelerate fibrosis progression. Approximately 25% of infected patients ultimately progress to cirrhosis, liver failure, and, occasionally, primary hepatocellular carcinoma (HCC) within 20-30 yr of the acute infection. Although progression is rare within the pediatric age range, cirrhosis and HCC from HCV have been reported in children. The long-term morbidities constitute the rationale for diagnosis and treatment in children with HCV.

Chronic HCV infection can be associated with **small vessel vasculitis** and is a common cause of essential mixed cryoglobulinemia. Other extrahepatic manifestations, predominantly seen in adults, include cutaneous vasculitis, peripheral neuropathy, cerebritis, membranoproliferative glomerulonephritis, and nephrotic syndrome. Antibodies to smooth muscle, antinuclear antibodies, and low thyroid hormone levels may also be present.

Diagnosis
Clinically available assays for detection of HCV infection are based on detection of antibodies to HCV antigens or detection of viral RNA (**see** Table 358-3); neither can predict the severity of liver disease.

The most widely used **serologic test** is the third-generation enzyme immunoassay to detect anti-HCV. The predictive value of this assay is greatest in high-risk populations, but the false-positive rate can be as high as 50-60% in low-risk populations. False-negative results also occur because antibodies remain negative for as long as 1-3 mo after clinical onset of illness. Anti-HCV is not a protective antibody and does not confer immunity; it is usually present simultaneously with the virus.

The most commonly used **virologic assay** for HCV is a PCR assay, which permits detection of small amounts of **HCV RNA** in serum and tissue samples within days of infection. The *qualitative* PCR detection is especially useful in patients with recent or perinatal infection, hypogammaglobulinemia, or immunosuppression and is very sensitive. The *quantitative* PCR aids in identifying patients who are likely to respond to therapy and in monitoring response to therapy.

Screening for HCV should include all patients with the following risk factors: history of illegal drug use (even if only once), receiving clotting factors made before 1987 (when inactivation procedures were

introduced) or blood products before 1992, hemodialysis, idiopathic liver disease, and children born to HCV-infected women (qualitative PCR in infancy and anti-HCV after 12-18 mo of age). In children, it is also important to consider whether the mother has any of the risk factors noted above that would increase her possibility of developing HCV. Routine screening of all *pregnant women* is not recommended. The Centers for Disease Control, did however, recommend in 2012 that all individuals born between 1945 and 1965 be screened.

Determining HCV **genotype** is also important, particularly when therapy is considered, because the response to the current therapeutic agents varies greatly. Genotype 1 is poorly responsive; genotypes 2 and 3 are more reliably responsive to therapy (as discussed later).

Aminotransferase levels typically fluctuate during HCV infection and do not correlate with the degree of liver fibrosis.

A liver biopsy is the only means to assess the presence and extent of hepatic fibrosis, outside of overt signs of chronic liver disease. A liver biopsy is indicated only before starting any treatment and to rule out other causes of overt liver disease.

Complications
The risk of ALF caused by HCV is low, but the risk of **chronic hepatitis** is the highest of all the hepatotropic viruses. In adults, risk factors for progression to hepatic fibrosis include older age, obesity, male sex, and even moderate alcohol ingestion (two 1 oz drinks per day). Progression to cirrhosis or HCC is a major cause of morbidity and the most common indication for liver transplantation in adults in the United States.

Treatment
In adults, *peginterferon* (subcutaneous, weekly) combined with ribavirin (oral, daily) was standard therapy until 2012 for genotype 1. Currently recommended first-line adult therapy for genotype 1 includes these 2 medications with the use of sofosbuvir, an oral, direct-acting antiviral agent, for only 12 wk or an oral regimen of sofosbuvir, simeprevir, and possibly ribavirin. Ongoing studies suggest that future treatments will be even more effective, with fewer side effects.

Traditionally, patients most likely to respond had mild hepatitis, shorter duration of infection, low viral titers and either genotype 2 or 3 virus. Patients with genotype 1 virus responded poorly. Response to peginterferon alfa/ribavirin may be predicted by single-nucleotide polymorphisms near the interleukin 28B gene, but with these newer treatment regimens excellent response rates are being reported with shorter duration, IFN-free regimens. The goal of treatment is to achieve a sustained viral response (SVR), as defined by the absence of viremia 6 mo after stopping the medications; SVR is associated with improved histology and decreased risk of morbidities.

The natural history of HCV infection in children is still being defined. It is believed that children have a higher rate of spontaneous clearance than adults (up to 45% by age 19 yr). A multicenter study followed 359 children infected with HCV over 10 yr. Only 7.5% had cleared the virus, and 1.8% progressed to decompensated cirrhosis. Treatment in adults with **acute** HCV in a pilot study showed an 88% SVR in genotype 1 subjects (treated with IFN and ribavirin for 24 wk). Such data, if confirmed, could actually raise the question whether children, with shorter duration of infection and fewer comorbid conditions than their adult counterparts, could be "ideal" candidates for treatment. Given the adverse effects of currently available therapy, this strategy is not recommended outside of clinical trials.

Peginterferon (Schering), IFN-α2b, and ribavirin are approved by the FDA for use in children older than 3 yr of age with HCV hepatitis. Studies of IFN monotherapy in children demonstrated a higher SVR than in adults, with better compliance and fewer side effects. An SVR up to 49% for genotype 1 was achieved in multiple studies. Factors associated with a higher likelihood of response are age younger than 12 yr, genotypes 2 and 3, and, in patients with genotype 1b, an RNA titer of <2 million copies/mL of blood, and viral response (PCR at weeks 4 and 12 of treatment). Side effects of medications lead to discontinuation of treatment in a high proportion of patients; these include influenza-like symptoms, anemia, and neutropenia. Long-term effects of these medicines also need to be evaluated as significant differences were noted in children's weight, height, body mass index, and body composition. Most of these delays improved following cessation of treatment, but height z-scores continued to lag behind.

Treatment should be considered for all children infected with genotypes 2 and 3, because they have an 80-90% response rate to therapy with peginterferon and ribavirin. If the child has genotype 1b virus, the treatment choice remains more controversial. Pediatric guidelines recommend treatment to eradicate HCV infection, prevent progression of liver disease and development of HCC, and to remove the stigma associated with HCV. Treatment should be considered for patients with evidence of advanced fibrosis or injury on liver biopsy. The currently approved treatment consists of 48 wk of peginterferon and ribavirin (therapy should be stopped if still detectable on viral PCR at 24 wk of therapy). Treatment of children with normal biochemical profile and mild histologic inflammation should be reserved to a clinical study context.

Newer Treatments
Peginterferon and direct-acting antivirals, including telaprevir and boceprevir (viral protease inhibitors), demonstrated a much improved SVR rate in adults. Telaprevir and boceprevir were the first direct-acting antiviral agents approved to combat hepatitis C. Newer medications, including sofosbuvir and simeprevir, have already replaced telaprevir and boceprevir as the treatment of choice for hepatitis C genotype 1. Studies are pending in pediatrics. Combination therapy schemes and staggered therapy is also being explored in adults. Interleukin 28B, a host marker of immune responsiveness, has also been evaluated to predict host response to treatment with standard peginterferon and ribavirin, but will become even less important as IFN free regimens become standard practice. Varying IFN-free regimens are now available for all HCV genotypes allowing even greater likelihood of achieving viral eradication, with completely oral medication regimens, and without the use of IFN and its attendant side effects. With the rapid development of new medications and regimens, frequent review of up-to-date resources, such as www.hcvguidelines.org, will be vital to provide optimal care.

Prevention
No vaccine is yet available to prevent HCV, although ongoing research suggests this will be possible in the future. Current Ig preparations are not beneficial, likely because Ig preparations produced in the United States do not contain antibodies to HCV because blood and plasma donors are screened for anti-HCV and excluded from the donor pool. Broad neutralizing antibodies to HCV were found to be protective and might pave the road for vaccine development.

Once HCV infection is identified, patients should be screened yearly with a liver ultrasound and serum α-fetoprotein for HCC, as well as for any clinical evidence of liver disease. Vaccinating the affected patient against HAV and HBV will prevent superinfection with these viruses and the increased risk of developing severe liver failure.

Prognosis
Viral titers should be checked yearly to document spontaneous remission. Most patients develop chronic hepatitis. Progressive liver damage is higher in those with additional comorbid factors such as alcohol consumption, viral genotypic variations, obesity, and underlying genetic predispositions. Referral to a pediatric gastroenterologist is strongly advised to take advantage of up-to-date monitoring regimens and to optimize their enrollment in treatment protocols when available.

HEPATITIS D
Etiology
HDV, the smallest known animal virus, is considered defective because it cannot produce infection without concurrent HBV infection. The 36 nm diameter virus is incapable of making its own coat protein; its outer coat is composed of excess HBsAg from HBV. The inner core of the virus is single-stranded circular RNA that expresses the HDV antigen.

Epidemiology
HDV can cause an infection at the same time as the initial HBV infection (coinfection), or HDV can infect a person who is already infected with HBV (superinfection). Transmission usually occurs by intrafamilial or intimate contact in areas of high prevalence, which are primarily developing countries (see Table 358-1). In areas of low prevalence, such as the United States, the parenteral route is far more common. HDV infections are uncommon in children in the United States but must be considered when ALF occurs. The incubation period for HDV superinfection is approximately 2-8 wk; with coinfection, the incubation period is similar to that of HBV infection.

Pathogenesis
Liver pathology in HDV hepatitis has no distinguishing features except that damage is usually quite severe. In contrast to HBV, HDV causes injury directly by cytopathic mechanisms. The most severe cases of HBV infection appear to result from coinfection of HBV and HDV.

Clinical Manifestations
The symptoms of hepatitis D infection are similar to, but usually more severe than those of the other hepatotropic viruses. The clinical outcome for HDV infection depends on the mechanism of infection. In coinfection, acute hepatitis, which is much more severe than for HBV alone, is common, but the risk of developing chronic hepatitis is low. In superinfection, acute illness is rare and chronic hepatitis is common. The risk of ALF is highest in superinfection. Hepatitis D should be considered in any child who experiences ALF.

Diagnosis
HDV has not been isolated and no circulating antigen has been identified. The diagnosis is made by detecting IgM antibody to HDV; the antibodies to HDV develop approximately 2-4 wk after coinfection and approximately 10 wk after a superinfection. A test for anti-HDV antibody is commercially available. PCR assays for viral RNA are available as research tools (see Table 358-2).

Complications
HDV must be considered in all cases of ALF. Coinfection with HBV can also result in a more severe chronic disease.

Treatment
The treatment is based on supportive measures once an infection is identified. There are no specific HDV-targeted treatments to date. The treatment is mostly based on controlling and treating HBV infection, without which HDV cannot induce hepatitis. Small research studies suggest that IFN is the preferred treatment regimen, but ongoing studies still seek the ideal management strategy and the regimen should be personalized for each patient.

Prevention
There is no vaccine for hepatitis D. Because HDV replication cannot occur without hepatitis B coinfection, immunization against HBV also prevents HDV infection. Hepatitis B vaccines and HBIG are used for the same indications as for hepatitis B alone.

HEPATITIS E
Etiology
HEV has been cloned using molecular techniques. This RNA virus has a nonenveloped sphere shape with spikes and is similar in structure to the caliciviruses.

Epidemiology
Hepatitis E is the epidemic form of what was formerly called non-A, non-B hepatitis. Transmission is fecal–oral (often waterborne) and is associated with shedding of 27-34 nm particles in the stool (see Table 358-1). The highest prevalence of HEV infection has been reported in the Indian subcontinent, the Middle East, Southeast Asia, and Mexico, especially in areas with poor sanitation. The prevalence, however, appears to be increasing in the United States and other developed

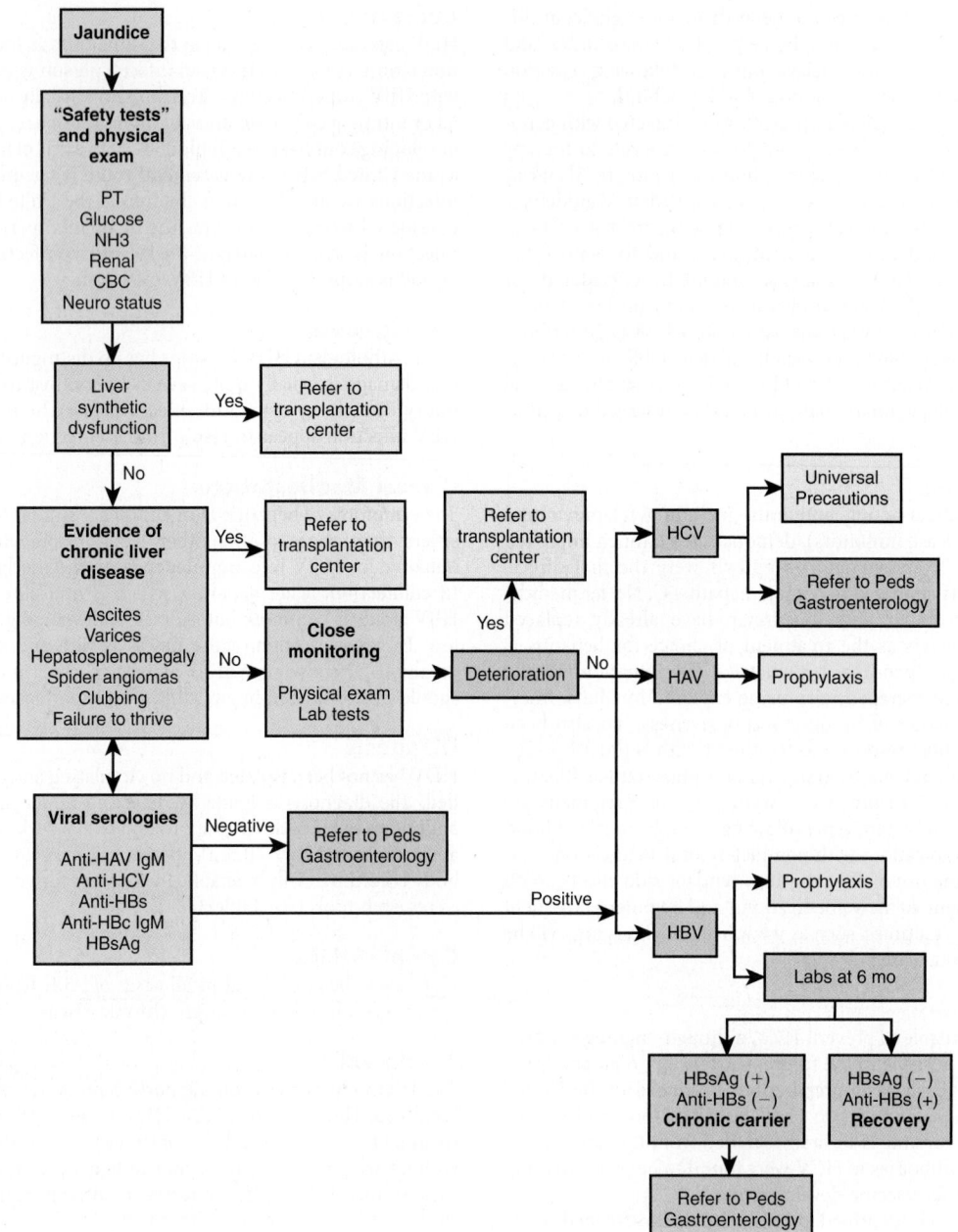

Figure 358-6 Clinical approach to viral hepatitis. *CBC*, complete blood count with differential; *HAV*, hepatitis A virus; *HBs*, hepatitis B surface; *HBsAg*, hepatitis B surface antigen; *HBV*, hepatitis B virus; *HCV*, hepatitis C virus; *IgM*, immunoglobulin M; *NH₃*, ammonia; *PT*, prothrombin time.

countries and has been postulated to be the most common cause of acute hepatitis and jaundice in the world. The mean incubation period is approximately 40 days (range: 15-60 days).

Pathogenesis
HEV appears to act as a cytopathic virus. The pathologic findings are similar to those of the other hepatitis viruses.

Clinical Manifestations
The clinical illness associated with HEV infection is similar to that of HAV but is often more severe. As with HAV, chronic illness does not occur. In addition to often causing a more severe episode than HAV, HEV tends to affect older patients, with a peak age between 15 and 34 yr. HEV is a major pathogen in pregnant women, in whom it causes ALF with a high fatality incidence. HEV could also lead to decompensation of pre-existing chronic liver disease.

Complications
HEV is associated with a high risk of death in pregnant women. No other complications are recognized in association with this virus.

Diagnosis
Recombinant DNA technology has resulted in development of antibodies to HEV particles, and IgM and IgG assays are available to distinguish between acute and resolved infections (see Table 358-3). IgM antibody to viral antigen becomes positive after approximately 1 wk of illness. Viral RNA can be detected in stool and serum by PCR.

Prevention
A recombinant hepatitis E vaccine is highly effective in adults. No evidence suggests that Ig is effective in preventing HEV infections. Ig pooled from patients in endemic areas might prove to be effective.

APPROACH TO ACUTE OR CHRONIC HEPATITIS

Although new treatment modalities for chronic viral hepatitis are continuously being developed and treatment outcomes have improved, the major medical breakthrough in regard to the pediatric population is prevention, with the availability of effective and safe vaccines for the HAV and HBV infections. The availability of more sensitive and reliable diagnostic tools may lead to improved care for affected patients. The primary care physician is at the forefront of the care and control of patients exposed to these viruses. Aggressive perinatal, childhood, and adolescent immunization strategies have already had a major impact in endemic HAV and HBV areas.

Identifying deterioration of the patient with acute hepatitis and the development of ALF is a major contribution of the primary pediatrician (Fig. 358-6). If ALF is identified, the clinician should immediately refer the patient to a transplantation center; this can be lifesaving.

Once chronic infection is identified, close follow-up and referral to a pediatric gastroenterologist is recommended to enroll the patient in appropriate treatment trials. Treatment of chronic HBV and HCV in children should preferably be delivered within, or using data from pediatric controlled trials as indications, timing, regimen, and outcomes remain to be defined and cannot simply be extrapolated from adult data. All patients with chronic viral hepatitis should avoid, as much as possible, further insult to the liver: HAV vaccine is recommended; patients must avoid alcohol consumption and obesity, and they should exercise care when taking new medications, including nonprescription drugs and herbal medications.

International adoption and ease of travel continue to change the epidemiology of hepatitis viruses. In the United States, chronic HBV and HCV have a high prevalence among international adoptee patients; vigilance is required to establish early diagnosis in order to offer appropriate treatment as well as prophylactic measures to limit viral spread.

Chronic hepatitis can be a stigmatizing disease for children and their families. The pediatrician should offer, with proactive advocacy, appropriate support for them as well as needed education for their social circle. Scientific data and information about support groups are available for families on the websites for the American Liver Foundation (www.liverfoundation.org) and the North American Society for Pediatric Gastroenterology, Hepatology and Nutrition (www.naspghan.org), as well as through pediatric gastroenterology centers.

Bibliography is available at Expert Consult.

Chapter **359**
Liver Abscess
Robert M. Kliegman

Pyogenic liver abscesses are rare in children, with an incidence of 10/100,000 hospitalizations. Pyogenic hepatic abscesses can be caused by bacteria entering the liver via the portal circulation in cases of omphalitis, portal vein pylephlebitis, intraabdominal infection, or abscess secondary to appendicitis or inflammatory bowel disease; a primary bacteremia (sepsis, endocarditis); ascending cholangitis associated with biliary tract obstruction caused by gallstones or sclerosing cholangitis, after a Kasai procedure, or secondary to choledochal cysts; contiguous infection (subphrenic abscess) or penetrating trauma; and cryptogenic biliary tract infections. Very rarely, liver abscesses occur after percutaneous liver biopsy. Hepatic abscesses can also occur in neonates in association with sepsis, umbilical vein associated infection, or cannulation; 50% are seen in children younger than 6 yr old. In adults with pyogenic liver abscesses, liver transplantation is a significant risk factor; it is not known if pediatric liver transplant patients are

also at increased risk. Children with chronic granulomatous disease, Job syndrome, or cancer are also at increased risk for a hepatic abscess.

In children with pyogenic liver abscesses, the most common pathogenic organisms include *Staphylococcus aureus, Streptococcus* spp.; *Escherichia coli, Klebsiella pneumoniae, Salmonella,* and anaerobic organisms; *Entamoeba histolytica* or *Toxocara canis*–associated liver abscesses have also been reported in developing countries or in highly endemic areas.

Amebic disease is rare in the United States and is associated with immigrants from or travel to highly endemic areas. Recovery of *E. histolytica* from the stool is pathogenic and highly suggestive of an amebic abscess, but this must be distinguished from *Entamoeba dispar,* which looks similar but is nonpathogenic; antiamebic antibodies help identify *E. histolytica.* Multiple microabscesses are most commonly secondary to bacteremia, candidemia, or cat scratch disease. Polymicrobial involvement is seen in approximately 50%; cryptogenic abscesses are often monomicrobial with *S. aureus* as the lead single agent in children without underlying liver or intestinal tract disease.

Signs and symptoms are nonspecific and can include fever, chills, night sweats, malaise, fatigue, nausea, abdominal pain with right upper quadrant tenderness, and hepatomegaly; jaundice is uncommon. Diagnosis can be challenging and is often delayed; a high index of suspicion is necessary in children with risk factors. Serum aminotransferase and more often the alkaline phosphatase levels are elevated. The erythrocyte sedimentation rate is high, and leukocytosis is common. The results of blood cultures are positive in 50% of patients. Chest x-rays might show elevation of the right hemidiaphragm with decreased mobility or a right pleural effusion. Ultrasound or CT can confirm diagnosis (Figs. 359-1 to 359-3). Solitary liver abscesses (70% of cases) in the right lobe of the liver (75% of cases) are more common than multiple abscesses or solitary left lobe abscesses. Enzyme-linked immunosorbent assay testing for *E. histolytica* Gal/GalNAc (galactose/*N*-acetyl-D-galactosamine) lectin in serum is usually positive with amebiasis.

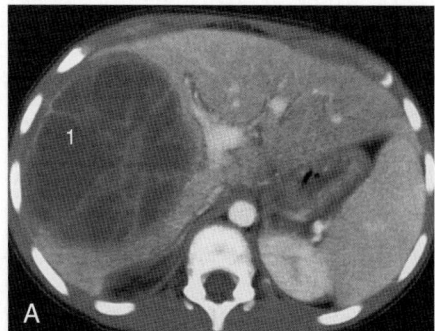

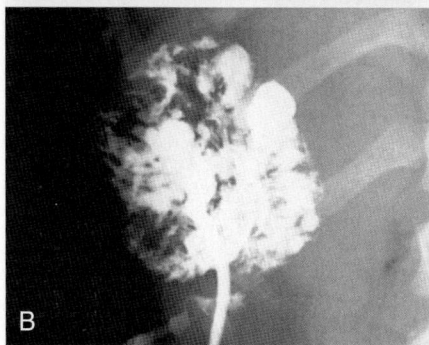

Figure 359-1 Liver abscess. **A,** Contrast-enhanced CT scan demonstrates a multiloculated septated mass of decreased attenuation in the right lobe of the liver. There is increased attenuation of the septa. There is also faintly visible edema between the abscess and the enhanced normal liver. **B,** Injection of contrast material after percutaneous drainage of this documented streptococcal abscess demonstrates the multilocular nature of the lesion and its irregularly marginated wall. *(From Kuhn JP, Slovis TL, Haller JO: Caffrey's pediatric diagnostic imaging, vol 2, ed 10, Philadelphia, 2004, Mosby, p. 1470.)*

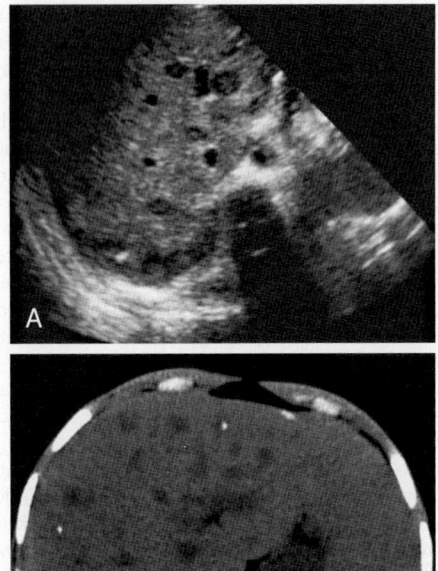

Figure 359-2 Hepatic candidiasis. Transverse sonogram **(A)** and CT scan **(B)** of the upper abdomen demonstrate "bull's-eye" lesions in the right lobe of the liver in an immunocompromised patient. The calcifications seen on the CT scan are presumed to represent sequelae of prior infection. Liver biopsy demonstrated candidiasis. *(From Kuhn JP, Slovis TL, Haller JO: Caffrey's pediatric diagnostic imaging, vol 2, ed 10, Philadelphia, 2004, Mosby, p. 1472.)*

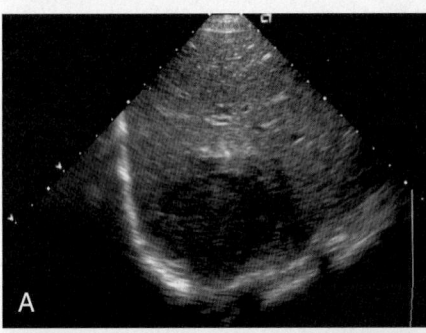

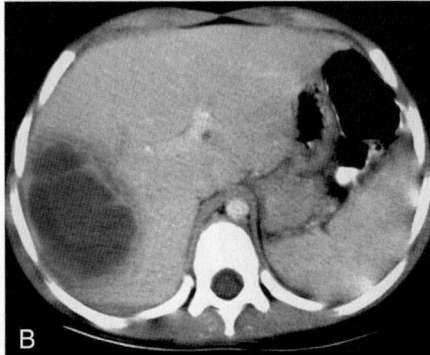

Figure 359-3 Amebic abscess. **A,** Sonogram demonstrates a hypoechogenic mass in the right lobe of the liver with a more hypoechoic surrounding rim. **B,** CT scan demonstrates a low-attenuation mass in the right lobe of the liver with a prominent halo. *(From Kuhn JP, Slovis TL, Haller JO: Caffrey's pediatric diagnostic imaging, vol 2, ed 10, Philadelphia, 2004, Mosby, p. 1473.)*

Treatment requires percutaneous ultrasound- or CT-guided needle aspiration and less often open surgical drainage, particularly if multiple or large abscesses are present. Some place a drain and leave it in until the abscess wall collapses, others just do single or repeated aspirations. Aerobic and anaerobic cultures should be obtained. Some treat empirically without aspiration or drainage. If amebic disease is present, most do not attempt aspiration.

Antibiotic therapy should initially be broad spectrum but then narrowed, based on the culture results of the abscess fluid. Empirical initial antibiotic regimens include ampicillin/sulbactam, ticarcillin/clavulanic acid, or piperacillin/tazobactam. Others recommend a combination of a third-generation cephalosporin plus metronidazole. Amebic abscesses are treated with metronidazole or tinidazole plus paromomycin (oral nonabsorbable to treat the associated intestinal amebic infection). Antibiotic therapy for pyogenic abscess is intravenous for 2-3 wk followed by oral therapy to complete a 4-6 wk course. Mortality has decreased significantly since the 1980s with early diagnosis and initiation of appropriate therapy.

Bibliography is available at Expert Consult.

Chapter 360
Liver Disease Associated with Systemic Disorders

Bernadette E. Vitola and William F. Balistreri

Liver disease is found in a wide variety of systemic illnesses, both as a result of the primary pathologic process and as a secondary complication of the disease or associated therapy.

INFLAMMATORY BOWEL DISEASE
Ulcerative colitis and Crohn disease are associated with hepatobiliary disease that includes autoimmune and inflammatory processes related to inflammatory bowel disease (IBD) (sclerosing cholangitis, autoimmune hepatitis), drug toxicity (thiopurines, methotrexate, 5-ASA, biologics), malnutrition and disordered physiology (fatty liver, cholelithiasis), bacterial translocation and systemic infections (hepatic abscess, portal vein thrombosis), hypercoagulability (infarction, Budd-Chiari), and long-term complications of these liver diseases, such as ascending cholangitis, cirrhosis, portal hypertension, and biliary carcinoma. Hepatobiliary manifestations may continue to progress even when intestinal symptoms are well-controlled and are unrelated to either the severity or duration of intestinal disease.

Sclerosing cholangitis is the most common hepatobiliary disease associated with IBD, occurring in 2-8% of adult patients with ulcerative colitis and less often in Crohn disease. Conversely, 70-90% of patients with sclerosing cholangitis have ulcerative colitis. In pediatric patients with IBD, the diagnosis typically occurs in the 2nd decade of life with a median age of 14 yr. Sclerosing cholangitis is characterized by progressive inflammation and fibrosis of segments of the intra- and extrahepatic bile ducts and can progress to complete obliteration. Genetic susceptibility, with associations with the cystic fibrosis transmembrane conductance regulator (CFTR) and several human leukocyte antigens, has been demonstrated. Many patients are asymptomatic and the disease is initially diagnosed by routine liver function testing that reveals elevated serum alkaline phosphatase (AP), 5'-nucleotidase, or γ-glutamyl transpeptidase activities. Antinuclear or anti–smooth muscle antibodies might also be present in the serum. Ten percent to 15% of adult patients present with symptoms including anorexia, weight loss, pruritus, fatigue, right upper quadrant pain, and jaundice; intermittent acute cholangitis accompanied by fever, jaundice, and right upper quadrant pain can also occur. Portal hypertension can develop with progressive disease. These symptoms are less common in children, in whom hepatobiliary disease is often recognized by routine screening of liver function tests. In children with sclerosing cholangitis, approximately 11% present initially with hepatic manifestations and the associated asymptomatic IBD is discovered only on subsequent endoscopy.

Magnetic resonance cholangiography is an established first-line diagnostic test for sclerosing cholangitis. Characteristic findings include beading and irregularity of the intrahepatic and extrahepatic bile ducts. Liver biopsy typically reveals periductal fibrosis and inflammation, fibroobliterative cholangitis, and portal fibrosis, but it is not required for the diagnosis in patients with radiologic evidence of sclerosing cholangitis.

Sclerosing cholangitis is strongly associated with hepatobiliary malignancies (cholangiocarcinoma, hepatocellular carcinoma, gallbladder carcinoma) with a reported incidence varying between 9% and 14%. In one large series, patients with IBD and sclerosing cholangitis had a 10-fold increased risk of colorectal carcinoma and a 14-fold increased risk of pancreatic cancer compared to the general population. Tumor serology (CA 19-9) and cross-sectional liver imaging may be a useful screening strategy to identify patients with sclerosing cholangitis at increased risk for cholangiocarcinoma.

There is no definitive medical treatment for sclerosing cholangitis; liver transplantation is the only long-term option for progressive cirrhosis, and autoimmune disease can recur in the allograft in 20-25% of patients. Short-term therapy aims at improving biliary drainage and attempting to slow the obliterative process. Ursodeoxycholic acid, at a dose of 15-30 mg/kg/24 hr, improves bile flow and laboratory parameters but has not been shown to improve clinical outcome. Dominant extrahepatic biliary strictures may be dilated or endoscopically stented. Immunosuppressive therapy with corticosteroids and/or azathioprine improves biochemical parameters but has been disappointing in halting long-term histologic progression. Symptomatic therapy should be initiated for pruritus (rifampin, ursodeoxycholic acid, diphenhydramine), malnutrition (enteral supplementation), and ascending cholangitis (antibiotics) as indicated. Total colectomy may not be beneficial in preventing or managing hepatobiliary complications in patients with ulcerative colitis.

IBD-associated **autoimmune hepatitis** (AIH) can closely resemble IBD-associated sclerosing cholangitis, a condition often referred to as **overlap syndrome** or autoimmune sclerosing cholangitis (ASC). These patients typically exhibit hyperglobulinemia (marked increase in serum immunoglobulin G levels). In some children, the disease is initially diagnosed as AIH and later is found to be sclerosing cholangitis after cholangiography; in other cases, AIH manifests years after diagnosis of IBD-associated sclerosing cholangitis. Liver biopsy in patients with ASC shows interface hepatitis, in addition to the bile duct injury associated with sclerosing cholangitis. Immunosuppressive medication (corticosteroids and/or azathioprine) is the mainstay of therapy for ASC; long-term response does not appear to be as favorable as in AIH alone. Long-term survival in children with ASC appears to be similar to those with sclerosing cholangitis, with an overall median (50%) survival free of liver transplantation of 12.7 yr.

Fatty liver disease might also be more prevalent in adult patients with IBD, ranging from 25-40% in 1 large series and often correlates with severity of IBD. Gallstones are more prevalent in those with Crohn disease (11%) than in those with ulcerative colitis (7.5%) and in normal subjects (5%). The true prevalence of these IBD-associated liver diseases in pediatric patients is unknown, however.

BACTERIAL SEPSIS
Sepsis can mimic liver disease and should be excluded in any critically ill patient who develops cholestasis in the absence of markedly elevated serum aminotransferase or AP levels, even when other signs of infection are not evident. Gram-negative organisms are most often isolated from blood cultures, in particular *Escherichia coli*, *Klebsiella pneumoniae*, and *Pseudomonas aeruginosa*. Lipopolysaccharides and other bacterial endotoxins are thought to interfere with bile secretion by directly altering the structure or function of bile canalicular membrane transport proteins. The serum bilirubin level, predominantly the conjugated fraction, is elevated. Serum AP and aminotransferase activities may also be elevated. Liver biopsy shows intrahepatic cholestasis with little or no hepatocyte necrosis. Kupffer cell hyperplasia and an increase in inflammatory cells are also common. Similar findings can occur with urosepsis.

CELIAC DISEASE
Celiac disease (see Chapter 338.2) may present with laboratory abnormalities, including aminotransferase elevation and prolonged prothrombin time, as well as histologic changes, such as mild periportal and lobular inflammation. These abnormalities typically all improve on a gluten-free diet. Gastrointestinal symptoms may not be present. Other autoimmune liver diseases (AIH, primary sclerosing cholangitis) are also associated with celiac disease although they do not respond as well to a gluten-free diet.

CARDIAC DISEASE
Hepatic injury can occur as a complication of severe acute or chronic congestive heart failure (see Chapter 442), cyanotic congenital heart disease (see Chapters 430 and 431), and acute ischemic shock. In all conditions, passive congestion and reduced cardiac output can contribute to liver damage. Elevated central venous pressure is transmitted to the hepatic veins, smaller venules, and, ultimately, the surrounding hepatocytes, resulting in hepatocellular atrophy in the centrilobular zone of the liver. Owing to decreased cardiac output, there is decreased hepatic arterial blood flow, and centrilobular hypoxia results. Hepatic necrosis leads to lactic acidosis, elevated aminotransferase levels, cholestasis, prolonged partial thromboplastin time, cirrhosis, and possibly hypoglycemia as a result of impaired hepatocellular metabolism. Jaundice, tender hepatomegaly, and, in some cases, ascites and splenomegaly can occur. However, aminotransferases are often minimally elevated with slowly progressive fibrosis since there is minimal inflammation or cell death.

After acute hypovolemic shock, serum aminotransferase levels can rise dramatically but rapidly return to normal when perfusion and cardiac function improve. Hepatic necrosis or acute liver failure can occur in infants with hypoplastic left heart syndrome and coarctation of the aorta. High systemic venous pressures after Fontan procedures can also lead to hepatic dysfunction, marked by prolonged prothrombin time and cardiac cirrhosis. The aim of therapy in all causes of cardiac-associated liver disease is to improve cardiac output, reduce systemic venous pressures, and monitor for other signs of hypoperfusion. Even mild liver disease can have an impact on mortality after cardiac surgery, with poorer outcomes with progressively worse liver disease. In adults with cirrhosis undergoing cardiac surgery, overall mortality was 17% but varied significantly from 5% with mild disease to 70% with advanced liver disease.

CHOLESTASIS ASSOCIATED WITH TOTAL PARENTERAL NUTRITION
Total parenteral nutrition (TPN) can cause a variety of liver diseases, including hepatic steatosis, gallbladder and bile duct damage, and cholestasis. Cholestasis is the most severe complication and can lead to progressive fibrosis and cirrhosis. It is the major factor limiting effective long-term use of TPN in children and adults. Risk factors for TPN-associated cholestasis include prolonged duration of TPN, prematurity, low birthweight, sepsis, necrotizing enterocolitis, and short bowel syndrome.

The pathogenesis of TPN-associated cholestasis is multifactorial. Sepsis; excess caloric intake; high amounts of protein, fat, or carbohydrate; specific amino acid toxicities; nutrient deficiencies; and toxicities related to components such as manganese, aluminum, and copper can all contribute to hepatic injury. Recent data implicate both the type and volume of lipid administered. Prolonged enteral fasting compromises mucosal integrity and increases bacterial mucosal translocation. Fasting also decreases release of cholecystokinin, which promotes bile flow. This leads to biliary stasis, cholestasis, and formation of biliary sludge and gallstones, which exacerbates hepatic dysfunction. Sepsis, particularly that caused by Gram-negative bacteria, and associated endotoxins, can also exacerbate liver damage.

Early histologic findings include macrovesicular steatosis, canalicular cholestasis, and periportal inflammation. These changes can regress after cessation of short-term TPN. Prolonged duration of TPN is marked by bile duct proliferation or ductopenia, portal fibrosis, and expansion of portal triads and it can progress to cirrhosis and end-stage liver disease.

Clinical onset is typically marked by gradual onset of cholestasis, developing after more than 2 wk of TPN. In low birthweight infants, the onset of jaundice can overlap the phase of physiologic (unconjugated) hyperbilirubinemia. Any icteric infant who has received TPN for more than 1 wk should have bilirubin fractionated. With prolonged duration, hepatic enlargement or splenomegaly can develop. Serum bile acid concentrations can increase. Rises in serum aminotransferase activities may be a late finding. An elevation in serum AP activity may be caused by rickets, a common complication of TPN in low birthweight infants.

In addition to cholestasis, biliary complications of intravenous nutrition include cholelithiasis and the development of biliary sludge, associated with thick, inspissated gallbladder contents. These may be asymptomatic. Hepatic steatosis or elevated serum aminotransferase levels can also occur in the absence of cholestasis, particularly in older children. This is generally mild and resolves after TPN is discontinued. Serum bilirubin and bile acid levels remain within the normal range. Other causes of liver disease should also be considered, especially if evidence of hepatic dysfunction persists despite weaning from TPN and initiating enteral feeds. If serum AP or aminotransferase levels remain elevated, liver biopsy may be necessary for accurate diagnosis.

Treatment of TPN-associated cholestasis is focused on avoiding progressive liver injury by limiting duration whenever possible. Enteral feeding should be initiated as soon as tolerated and prolonged fasting should be avoided. Even small volumes of nutrients given by intermittent oral feedings or by continuous nasogastric drip promote bile flow, enterohepatic recirculation of bile acids, and intestinal motility, and they enhance mucosal barrier function, reducing the risk of bacterial translocation. Improved TPN solutions that meet the specific needs of neonates can prevent deficiencies and toxicities. The risk of further hepatic injury should always be considered when weighing the option of continuing TPN indefinitely, and all efforts should be made to try to advance enteral feeds whenever possible. There has been concern that the soy-based emulsions provided with TPN may be a significant contributing factor to TPN-associated cholestasis as a result of proinflammatory omega-6 fatty acids. Several strategies have been employed to minimize exposure to these fatty acids by limiting total lipid and/or introducing alternate sources of lipid including fish oil and olive oil to provide more omega-3 fatty acids. The long-term effects of these strategies on essential fatty acid deficiency or growth are unclear although there is some evidence that TPN-associated cholestasis may improve.

Ursodeoxycholic acid therapy may be beneficial in improving jaundice and hepatosplenomegaly. Other therapies, such as administration of antibiotics to reduce intraluminal bacterial overgrowth or oral administration of taurine or cholecystokinin, remain experimental.

CYSTIC FIBROSIS

Cystic fibrosis (CF) (see Chapter 403) is caused by mutations in the *CFTR* gene, which impair chloride transport across the apical membranes of epithelial cells in numerous organs (including cholangiocytes). The majority of patients with CF have some evidence of hepatobiliary disease; however, less than one-third of these patients develop clinically significant liver disease. Hepatobiliary complications account for approximately 2.5% of overall mortality in patients with CF. The onset of liver disease occurs at a median age of 10 yr, and >90% occurs by 20 yr.

Focal biliary cirrhosis is the pathognomonic liver lesion in CF and is postulated to result, in part, from impaired secretory function of the bile duct epithelium. Blockage of biliary ductules secondary to viscid secretions results in periductal inflammation, bile duct proliferation, and increased fibrosis within focal portal tracts. Gradual progression to multilobular cirrhosis can occur and result in portal hypertension and end-stage liver disease in 1-8% of patients. Liver disease tends to occur mainly in males with pancreatic insufficiency and requires 2 CFTR mutations without residual function. One candidate gene modifier for clinical phenotypes of CF-related liver disease that shows a strong association is SERPINA1. However, additional study of mutational analysis is necessary before we are able to predict which patients with CF will develop liver disease. Clinical risk factors that may be associated with liver disease include older age, pancreatic insufficiency, male gender, and possibly a history of meconium ileus.

Treatment with oral ursodeoxycholic acid (10-15 mg/kg/day) may be beneficial in improving liver function, presumably by improving bile flow; further research is necessary to determine whether a true long-term benefit exists. Because it is difficult to predict which patients will develop liver disease, prophylactic therapy is not possible. Progression of liver disease is generally slow. Patients who develop end-stage liver disease might require liver transplantation for survival.

BONE MARROW TRANSPLANTATION

Liver disease is common in patients who have received hematopoietic stem cell transplantation (SCT), whether the cells are harvested from bone marrow or peripheral blood (see Chapters 135-139). The pathogenesis is varied and includes infections (viral, bacterial, or fungal); toxicity from parenteral nutrition, chemotherapy, or radiation; venoocclusive disease (VOD); graft-versus-host disease (GVHD); or hemosiderosis secondary to iron overload from frequent blood transfusions. GVHD, drug toxicity, and sepsis are the most common causes of liver dysfunction after allogeneic SCT.

Diagnosis is often challenging because of the coexistence of multiple risk factors. Clinical course, symptoms and signs, and biochemical liver function and viral serologic tests must be considered in making the correct diagnosis. Percutaneous liver biopsy may be necessary; histology can show extensive bile duct injury in GVHD, viral inclusions in cytomegalovirus disease, or the characteristic endothelial lesion in VOD. It is important to diagnose the cause accurately, because treatment for GVHD differs markedly from that of other conditions (i.e., initiating immunosuppression for GVHD) and can worsen hepatitis secondary to infections.

GVHD of the liver can be acute or chronic but often occurs with the presence of GVHD in other target organs such as the skin and gut (see Chapter 137). Hepatic GVHD is caused by immunologic reaction to bile duct epithelium, leading to a nonsuppurative cholangitis. Histologic features of GVHD include loss of intralobular bile ducts, endothelial injury of hepatic and portal venules, and hepatocellular necrosis.

Onset typically occurs at the time of donor engraftment (days 14-21 after SCT). In acute hepatic GVHD, serum aminotransferase levels can rise markedly in the absence of elevated bilirubin, AP, and γ-glutamyl transpeptidase levels, mimicking viral hepatitis. Acute hepatic GVHD can manifest both early (days 14-21) and late (after day 70) after allogeneic SCT. In chronic hepatic GVHD, serum aminotransferase levels are not as markedly elevated and cholestasis is more prominent, with marked rises in serum conjugated bilirubin, γ-glutamyl transpeptidase, and AP levels. Other signs and symptoms can include hepatic tenderness, dark urine, acholic stools, itching, and anorexia.

VOD of the liver usually develops in the 1st 3 wk after SCT. The incidence ranges from 5-39% in pediatric patients, with reported mortality rates varying from 0-47%. Risk factors include trauma, high-dose conditioning regimens, coagulopathies, sickle cell anemia, leukemia, polycythemia vera, thalassemia major, hepatic abscesses, irradiation, GVHD, iron overload, preexisting liver disease, and younger age. VOD is caused by fibrous obliteration of the terminal hepatic venules and small lobular veins, with resultant damage to the surrounding hepatocytes and sinusoids. It is not associated with thrombus formation, in contrast with Budd-Chiari syndrome, which involves occlusion of the larger hepatic veins or inferior vena cava by a web, mass, or thrombus.

Pathologic changes in patients with VOD are best demonstrated using special (trichrome) stains to highlight the central veins. The lesions may be patchy. Later in the course, hepatic venules may be completely obliterated.

Symptoms typically include jaundice, painful hepatomegaly, rapid weight gain, and ascites. VOD resolves in the majority of patients but can also lead to multisystem organ failure, hepatic encephalopathy, and fulminant hepatic failure. Less-severe forms may be characterized by jaundice and ascites with a slow resolution; in very mild cases, histologic changes may be the sole manifestation. The diagnosis rests on the exclusion of other diseases, such as GVHD, congestive cardiomyopathy, constrictive pericarditis, and Budd-Chiari syndrome.

Treatment for VOD with defibrotide has been successful in multicenter phase II trials in both adult and pediatric patients; defibrotide, an agent with antithrombotic and thrombolytic properties, is administered at doses of 20-40 mg/kg/day. Complete response rates vary between 36% and 76% and survival of longer than 100 days post-SCT ranges from 32-79%, with better outcomes in pediatric patients. Little toxicity has been noted; however, pediatric patients are at a higher risk of bleeding with treatment compared to adults. Oral ursodeoxycholic acid can decrease the incidence of severe liver disease in patients undergoing SCT and reduces the incidence of VOD and transplant-related mortality in adults. Supportive management includes maintaining intravenous hydration and renal perfusion.

HEMOGLOBINOPATHIES

Patients with sickle cell anemia (see Chapter 462.1) or thalassemia (see Chapter 462.10) can have hepatic dysfunction caused by acute or chronic viral hepatitis, hemosiderosis from frequent transfusion therapy, hepatic crises related to severe intrahepatic cholestasis, sequestration, or ischemic necrosis. Cholelithiasis and hemosiderosis are both common and treatable. Higher volume of transfusions is associated with both higher hepatic iron content and fibrosis. Chelation therapy for iron overload is usually safe and effective.

Hepatic sickle cell crisis or "sickle hepatopathy" occurs in approximately 10% of patients with sickle cell disease. It manifests with intense right upper quadrant pain and tenderness, fever, leukocytosis, and jaundice. Bilirubin levels may be markedly elevated; serum AP levels may be only moderately elevated. It can be difficult to distinguish sickle hepatopathy from viral hepatitis, acute cholecystitis or choledocholithiasis; therefore, these conditions should be excluded. Generally, hepatic sickle cell crisis is self-limited and symptoms resolve within 1-3 wk. **Sickle cell intrahepatic cholestasis** manifests as hepatomegaly, abdominal pain, hyperbilirubinemia, and coagulopathy, and can progress to acute liver failure, leaving transplantation as the only therapeutic option. Transplantation carries a high risk for graft loss from vascular complications.

On occasion, children with sickle cell disease experience a benign elevation of bilirubin levels >20 mg/dL but unaccompanied by severe pain or fever. There is no change in hematocrit or reticulocyte count nor any association with a hemolytic crisis.

HISTIOCYTIC DISORDERS

Langerhans cell histiocytosis (see Chapter 507.1) is the most common of the histiocytoses and typically affects the bone and skin. However, it can cause infiltration of high-risk organs such as the liver resulting in periportal inflammation and sclerosing cholangitis. Liver involvement often results in worse outcomes. Hemophagocytic lymphohistiocytosis (see Chapter 507.2) is a multiorgan, severe, and potentially fatal inflammatory process associated with activation of macrophages that mimics sepsis. The hepatic manifestation of hemophagocytic lymphohistiocytosis is usually acute liver failure with portal inflammatory infiltrates noted on liver biopsy.

Bibliography is available at Expert Consult.

360.1 Nonalcoholic Fatty Liver Disease

Bernadette E. Vitola and William F. Balistreri

Nonalcoholic fatty liver disease (NAFLD) is part of the spectrum of liver disease strongly associated with obesity and is the most common chronic liver disease in children. NAFLD can range from fatty liver alone to a triad of fatty infiltration, inflammation, and fibrosis, termed **nonalcoholic steatohepatitis (NASH),** which resembles alcoholic liver disease but occurs with little or no exposure to ethanol. Unlike adults, NASH in children has 2 distinct histologic types. **Type 1 NASH** resembles adult histologic findings with steatosis and balloon degeneration of hepatocytes and/or periportal fibrosis. **Type 2 NASH** includes steatosis and portal inflammation. Many patients are asymptomatic. Liver histology from autopsy data suggests that 10% of children and 38% of obese children ages 2-19 yr have NAFLD. The risk is lower in African-American children. Elevated serum aminotransferase levels are not sensitive or specific markers for NAFLD. A normal serum alanine aminotransferase level is present in 21-23% of pediatric patients with NAFLD. No biomarkers are currently a reliable alternative to biopsy. Although ultrasonography detects NAFLD, no current imaging modalities distinguish between steatosis and NASH. A liver biopsy may be required for a delimiting diagnosis. The estimated prevalence in adults is thought to be as high as 15-20% for NAFLD overall and 2-4% for NASH. Risk factors in pediatric cohorts include obesity, male gender, white or Hispanic ethnicity, hypertriglyceridemia, and insulin resistance. Hepatic steatosis alone may be benign, but up to a quarter of patients with NASH can develop progressive fibrosis with resultant cirrhosis. The long-term prognosis of NASH that has developed in childhood is unknown. Children diagnosed with NAFLD should be screened for comorbid conditions associated with the metabolic syndrome, including diabetes, hypertension, dyslipidemia, and obstructive sleep apnea. Obese children and overweight children with other risk factors who are older than 3 yr of age should be screened for NAFLD by checking aminotransferase levels and liver ultrasound, even though neither is highly sensitive or specific.

Although there is no definitive treatment for NAFLD, gradual weight loss is effective in normalizing serum alanine aminotransferase and improving NAFLD. Low glycemic index foods, avoiding fructose, and substituting polyunsaturated fatty acids for saturated fats may help. Vitamins E and C provide no additional benefit to the efficacy of lifestyle intervention (diet and exercise) in improving steatosis or biochemical abnormalities in pediatric NAFLD. However, vitamin E does improve balloon degeneration in pediatric NASH. Metformin has produced mixed results in the treatment of NAFLD. Thiazolidinediones (pioglitazone, rosiglitazone) improve liver histology in adults with NASH but have not been well studied in children. Ursodeoxycholic acid has not been efficacious. In view of the potential role of the gut microbiome in contributing to the pathogenesis of NAFLD, the role of probiotics as an adjunct to lifestyle changes is under investigation. A preliminary study using ω-3 docosahexanoic acid in children showed improved insulin sensitivity, alanine aminotransferase, triglycerides, body mass index, and histology in children with NAFLD. Cysteamine bitartrate (slow release), a potential precursor of glutathione, an antioxidant, may reduce liver enzyme levels, as well as serum leptin and adiponectin levels, and is also a potential candidate for the treatment of NAFLD.

Bibliography is available at Expert Consult.

Chapter 361
Mitochondrial Hepatopathies
Samar H. Ibrahim and William F. Balistreri

Hepatocytes contain a high density of mitochondria, because the liver, with its biosynthetic and detoxifying functions, is highly dependent on adenosine triphosphate. Defects in mitochondrial function can lead to impaired oxidative phosphorylation, increased generation of reactive oxygen species, impairment of other metabolic pathways, and activation of mechanisms of cellular death. Mitochondrial disorders can be divided into primary, in which the mitochondrial defect is the primary cause of the disorder, and secondary, in which mitochondrial function is affected by exogenous injury or a genetic mutation that affects non-mitochondrial proteins (see Chapter 87.4). Primary mitochondrial disorders can be caused by mutations affecting mitochondrial DNA (mtDNA) or by nuclear genes that encode mitochondrial proteins or cofactors (Tables 361-1 and 361-2). Secondary mitochondrial disorders include diseases with an uncertain etiology such as Reye syndrome; disorders caused by endogenous or exogenous toxins, drugs, or metals; and other conditions in which mitochondrial oxidative injury may be involved in the pathogenesis of liver injury.

EPIDEMIOLOGY
Mitochondrial respiratory chain disorders of all types affect 1 in 20,000 children younger than 16 yr of age; liver involvement has been reported in 10-20% of patients with respiratory chain defect.

More than 200 pathogenic point mutations, deletions, insertions, and rearrangements that involve mtDNA and nuclear DNA that encodes mitochondrial proteins are identified. Mitochondrial genetics are unique because mitochondria are able to replicate, transcribe, and translate their mitochondrial-derived DNA independently. A typical hepatocyte contains approximately 1000 copies of mtDNA. Oxidative phosphorylation (the process of adenosine triphosphate production) occurs in the respiratory chain located in the inner mitochondrial membrane and is divided into 5 multienzyme complexes: reduced nicotinamide adenine dinucleotide coenzyme Q reductase (complex I), succinate–coenzyme Q reductase (complex II), reduced coenzyme Q–cytochrome-*c* reductase (complex III), cytochrome-*c* oxidase (complex IV), and adenosine triphosphate synthase (complex V). The respiratory chain peptide components are encoded by both nuclear and mtDNA genes, hence mutations in either genome can result in disorders of oxidative phosphorylation. Thirteen essential polypeptides are synthesized from the small 16.5-kilobase circular double-stranded mtDNA. Mitochondrial DNA also encodes the 24 transfer RNAs required for intramitochondrial protein synthesis, whereas nuclear genes encode more than 70 respiratory chain subunits and an array of enzymes and cofactors required to maintain mtDNA, including DNA polymerase-γ (POLG), thymidine kinase 2, and deoxyguanosine kinase.

Expression of mitochondrial disorders is complex and epidemiologic studies are hampered by technical difficulties collecting and processing tissue specimens needed to make accurate diagnoses, the variability in clinical presentation, and the fact that most disorders display maternal inheritance with variable penetrance (see Chapter 80). mtDNA mutates 10 times more often than nuclear DNA secondary to a lack of introns, protective histones, and an effective repair system in mitochondria. Mitochondrial genetics also display a threshold effect in that the type and severity of mutation required for clinical expression varies among people and organ systems, this is explained by the concept of heteroplasmy, in which cells and tissues harbor both normal and mutant mtDNA in various amounts because of random partitioning during cell division.

CLINICAL MANIFESTATIONS
Defects in oxidative phosphorylation can affect any tissue to a variable degree, with the most energy-dependent organs being the most vulnerable. One should consider the diagnosis of a mitochondrial disorder in a patient of any age who presents with progressive, multisystem involvement that cannot be explained by a specific diagnosis. Gastrointestinal complaints include vomiting, diarrhea, constipation, failure to thrive, and abdominal pain; certain mitochondrial disorders have characteristic gastrointestinal presentations. Pearson marrow-pancreas syndrome manifests with sideroblastic anemia and exocrine pancreatic insufficiency, whereas mitochondrial neurogastrointestinal encephalomyopathy manifests with chronic intestinal pseudoobstruction and cachexia. Hepatic presentations range from chronic cholestasis, hepatomegaly, cirrhosis, steatosis to fulminant hepatic failure and death.

PRIMARY MITOCHONDRIAL HEPATOPATHIES
Neonatal Liver Failure
A common presentation of respiratory chain defects is severe liver failure manifested as jaundice, hypoglycemia, coagulopathy, renal dysfunction, and hyperammonemia, with onset within the 1st few wk to mo of life. The key biochemical features include a markedly elevated plasma lactate concentration, an elevated molar ratio of plasma lactate to pyruvate (>25 mol/mol), and a raised ratio of β-hydroxybutyrate to acetoacetate (2.0 mol/mol). Symptoms are nonspecific and include lethargy and vomiting. Most patients additionally have neurologic involvement manifested as a weak suck, recurrent apnea, or myoclonic epilepsy. Liver biopsy shows predominantly microvesicular steatosis, cholestasis, bile duct proliferation, glycogen depletion, and iron overload. With standard therapy, the prognosis is very poor, and most patients die from liver failure or infection in the 1st few mo of life. **Cytochrome-*c* oxidase** (complex IV) is the most common deficiency in these infants, although complexes I and III and mtDNA depletion syndromes also are implicated (see Table 361-1).

Table 361-1	Classification of Primary Mitochondrial Hepatopathies

Respiratory chain (electron transport) defects (oxidative phosphorylation)
Neonatal liver failure
Complex I deficiency
Complex IV deficiency (*SCO1* mutations)
Complex III deficiency (*BCS1L* mutations)
Coenzyme Q deficiency
Multiple complex deficiencies (transfer and elongation factor mutations)
mtDNA depletion syndrome (*DUGOK, MPV17, POLG, SUCLG1, C10orf2/Twinkle* mutations)
Later-onset liver dysfunction or failure
Alpers-Huttenlocher disease (*POLG* mutations)
Pearson marrow-pancreas syndrome (mtDNA deletion)
Mitochondrial neurogastrointestinal encephalopathy (*TYMP* mutations)
Navajo neurohepatopathy (*MPV17* mutations)
Fatty acid oxidation defects
Long-chain 3-hydroxyacyl-coenzyme A dehydrogenase
Carnitine palmitoyltransferases I and II deficiencies
Carnitine–acylcarnitine translocase deficiency
Urea cycle enzyme deficiencies
Electron transfer flavoprotein and electron transfer flavoprotein dehydrogenase deficiencies
Phosphoenolpyruvate carboxykinase (mitochondrial) deficiency; nonketotic hyperglycemia
Citrin deficiency; neonatal intrahepatic cholestasis caused by citrin deficiency (*SLC25A13* mutations)

From Lee WS, Sokol RJ: Mitochondrial hepatopathies: advances in genetics, therapeutic approaches and outcomes. J Pediatr 163:942–948, 2013 (Table 1, p. 943).

Table 361-2	Genotypic Classification of Primary Mitochondrial Hepatopathies and Organ Involvement			
GENE	**RESPIRATORY CHAIN COMPLEX**	**HEPATIC HISTOLOGY**	**OTHER ORGANS INVOLVED**	**CLINICAL FEATURES**
Deletion	Multiple (Pearson)	Steatosis, fibrosis	Kidney, heart, CNS, muscle	Sideroblastic anemia, variable thrombocytopenia and neutropenia, persistent diarrhea
MPV17	I, III, IV	Steatosis	CNS, muscle, gastrointestinal tract	Adult-onset multisystemic involvement: myopathy, ophthalmoplegia, severe constipation, parkinsonism
DGUOK	I, III, IV	Steatosis, fibrosis	Kidneys, CNS, muscle	Nystagmus, hypotonia, renal Fanconi syndrome, acidosis
MPV17	I, III, IV	Steatosis, fibrosis	CNS, PNS	Hypotonia
SUCLG1	I, III, IV	Steatosis	Kidneys, CNS, muscle	Myopathy, sensorineural hearing loss, respiratory failure
POLG1	I, III, IV	Steatosis, fibrosis	CNS, muscle	Liver failure preceded by neurologic symptoms, intractable seizures, ataxia, psychomotor regression
C10orf2/Twinkle	I, III, IV	Steatosis	CNS, muscle	Infantile-onset spinocerebellar ataxia, loss of skills
BCS1L	III (GRACILE)		CNS ±, muscle ±, kidneys	Fanconi-type renal tubulopathy
SCO1	IV	Steatosis, fibrosis	Muscle	
TRMU	I, III, IV	Steatosis, fibrosis		Infantile liver failure with subsequent recovery
EFG1	I, III, IV	Steatosis	CNS	Severe, rapidly progressive encephalopathy
EFTu	I, III, IV	Unknown	CNS	Severe lactic acidosis, rapidly fatal encephalopathy

CNS, central nervous system; GRACILE, growth restriction, aminoaciduria, cholestasis, iron overload, lactic acidosis, and early death; PNS, peripheral nervous system.
From Lee WS, Sokol RJ: Mitochondrial hepatopathies: advances in genetics, therapeutic approaches and outcomes. J Pediatr 163:942–948, 2013 (Table 2, p. 944).

Alpers Syndrome (Alpers-Huttenlocher Syndrome or Alpers Hepatopathic Poliodystrophy)

Diagnostic criteria include refractory, mixed-type seizures that include a focal component; psychomotor regression that is episodic and triggered by intercurrent infections; and hepatopathy with or without acute liver failure. Alpers syndrome manifests from infancy up to 8 yr of age with seizures, hypotonia, feeding difficulties, psychomotor regression, and ataxia. Patients develop hepatomegaly and jaundice and have a slower progression to liver failure than those with cytochrome-c oxidase deficiency. Elevated blood or cerebrospinal fluid lactate and pyruvate levels are supportive for the diagnosis, in addition to characteristic electroencephalogram findings (high-amplitude slow activity with polyspikes), asymmetric abnormal visual evoked responses, and low-density areas or atrophy in the occipital or temporal lobes on computed tomography scanning of the brain. In some patients, complex I deficiency has been found in liver or muscle mitochondria. The disease is inherited in an autosomal recessive fashion; mutations in the catalytic subunit of the nuclear gene mtDNA *POLG* have been identified in multiple families with Alpers syndrome, leading to the advent of molecular diagnosis for Alpers syndrome. *Patients with POLG mutations are susceptible to valproate-induced liver dysfunction.*

Mitochondrial DNA Depletion Syndrome

Mitochondrial DNA depletion syndrome (MDS) is characterized by a tissue-specific reduction in mtDNA copy number, leading to deficiencies in complexes I, III, and IV. MDS manifests with phenotypic heterogeneity, multisystem and localized disease forms include myopathic, hepatocerebral, and liver-restricted presentations. Infants with the hepatocerebral form present in the neonatal period. The first symptoms are metabolic and rapidly progress to hepatic failure with hypoglycemia and vomiting. This stage is followed by neurologic involvement affecting the central and peripheral systems. Laboratory studies are characterized by lactic acidosis, hypoglycemia and markedly elevated α-fetoprotein in plasma. In some patients iron overload has been found with elevated transferrin saturation, high ferritin levels, and iron accumulation in hepatocytes and Kupffer cells. Death usually occurs by 1 yr of age. Spontaneous recovery has been reported in a patient

with liver-restricted disease. Inheritance is autosomal recessive and mutations in the nuclear gene deoxyguanosine kinase gene *(DGUOK)* have been identified in many patients with hepatocerebral MDS. **Thymidine kinase 2** has been implicated in the myopathic form; no known genetic defect has been identified in liver-restricted MDS. Multiple other nuclear genes including *POLG, MPV17,* **Twinkle helicase gene,** and *SUCLG1,* have been implicated in hepatocerebral MDS. Liver biopsies of patients with MDS show microvesicular steatosis, cholestasis, focal cytoplasmic biliary necrosis, and cytosiderosis in hepatocytes and sinusoidal cells. Ultrastructural changes are characteristic with oncocytic transformation of mitochondria, which is characterized by mitochondria with sparse cristae, granular matrix, and dense or vesicular inclusions. If the native DNA-encoded complex II is normal and the activities of the other complexes are decreased, one should investigate mtDNA copy numbers for a MDS. **Diagnosis** is established by demonstration of a low ratio of mtDNA (<10%) to nuclear DNA in affected tissues and/or genetic testing. Importantly, the sequence of the mitochondrial genome is normal.

Navajo Neurohepatopathy

Navajo neurohepatopathy (NNH) is an autosomal recessive sensorimotor neuropathy with progressive liver disease found only in Navajo Indians of the southwestern United States. The incidence is 1 in 1,600 live births. Diagnostic criteria include sensory neuropathy; motor neuropathy; corneal anesthesia; liver disease; metabolic or infectious complications including failure to thrive, short stature, delayed puberty, or systemic infection; and evidence of central nervous system demyelination on radiographic imaging and peripheral nerves biopsies. *MPV17* gene mutation **is implicated** in the pathogenesis of NNH. Interestingly, this is the same gene implicated in MDS (see earlier), demonstrating that NNH may be a specific type of MDS found only in Navajo Indians. NNH is divided into 3 phenotypic variations based on age of presentation and clinical findings.

First, **classic NNH** appears in infancy with severe progressive neurologic deterioration manifesting clinically as weakness, hypotonia, loss of sensation with accompanying acral mutilation, corneal ulcerations, and poor growth. Liver disease, present in the majority of patients, is secondary and variable and includes asymptomatic elevations of liver function tests, Reye syndrome–like episodes, hepatocellular carcinoma, or cirrhosis. γ-Glutamyl transpeptidase levels tend to be higher than in other forms of NNH. Liver biopsy might show chronic portal tract inflammation and cirrhosis, but it shows less cholestasis, hepatocyte ballooning, and giant cell transformation than other forms of NNH.

Infantile NNH manifests between the ages of 1 and 6 mo with jaundice and failure to thrive, and progresses to liver failure and death by 2 yr of age. Patients have hepatomegaly with moderate elevations in aspartate aminotransferase, alanine aminotransferase, and γ-glutamyl transpeptidase. Liver biopsy demonstrates pseudoacinar formation, multinucleate giant cells, portal and lobular inflammation, canalicular cholestasis, and microvesicular steatosis. Progressive neurologic symptoms are not usually noticed at presentation but do develop later.

Childhood NNH manifests from age 1-5 yr with the acute onset of fulminant hepatic failure that leads to death within months. Most patients also have evidence of neuropathy at presentation. Liver biopsies are similar to those in infantile NNH, except significant hepatocyte ballooning and necrosis, bile duct proliferation, and cirrhosis are also seen.

There is no effective treatment for any of the forms of NNH, and neurologic symptoms often preclude liver transplantation. The identical *MPV17* mutation is seen in patients with both the infantile and classic form of NNH highlighting the clinical heterogeneity of NNH.

Pearson Syndrome

Pearson marrow-pancreas syndrome has a neonatal-onset with severe macrocytic anemia, variable neutropenia and thrombocytopenia, and ringed sideroblasts in the bone marrow. Diarrhea and fat malabsorption develop in early childhood secondary to extensive pancreatic fibrosis, acinar atrophy and partial villous atrophy of the small intestine. The liver involvement includes hepatomegaly, steatosis, and cirrhosis. Liver failure and death have been reported before the age of 4 yr. Other features of the syndrome include renal tubular disease, photosensitivity, diabetes mellitus, hydrops fetalis, and the late development of visual impairment, tremor, ataxia, proximal muscle weakness, external ophthalmoplegia, and a pigmentary retinopathy. Methylglutaconic aciduria is a useful diagnostic marker. Large deletions of mtDNA are reported in most patients resulting in complexes I and III deficiency. mtDNA deletions can be detected in patients' cultured fibroblasts as well as in peripheral blood lymphocytes.

Villous Atrophy Syndrome

Children with this disease present with severe anorexia, vomiting, chronic diarrhea, and villous atrophy in the 1st yr of life. Hepatic involvement includes mild elevation of aminotransferase levels, hepatomegaly, and steatosis. Lactic acidosis is worsened with high-dextrose intravenous infusions or enteral nutrition. Diarrhea improved by 5 yr of age in association with the normalization of intestinal biopsies. Subsequently, patients develop retinitis pigmentosa, cerebellar ataxia, sensorineural deafness, and proximal muscle weakness, with eventual death late in the 1st decade of life. The disease is attributed to a mtDNA rearrangement defect. A complex III deficiency was found in the muscle of affected patients.

GRACILE Syndrome

The acronym GRACILE sums the most important clinical features, namely fetal growth restriction (birth weight about −4 SD), aminoaciduria (caused by Fanconi-type tubulopathy), cholestasis (with steatosis and cirrhosis), iron overload, severe lactic acidosis, and early death. The syndrome is associated with mutations of the complex III assembly factor BCS1L. The liver histology shows microvesicular steatosis and cholestasis with abundant iron accumulation in hepatocytes and Kupffer cells. The liver iron content slightly decreases with age, concomitantly with increasing fibrosis and cirrhosis. Abnormal transaminases and coagulation are noted, but the cause of death seems to be related to energy depletion than to liver failure. About half of the cases die within the 1st 2 wk; the oldest infant lived to 4 mo of age.

Mutations in Nuclear Translation and Elongation Factor Genes

Mutations in nuclear translation factor genes (*TRMU*) of the respiratory chain enzyme complexes have been identified as the etiology for acute liver failure manifesting at ages 1 day to 6 mo. The respiratory chain deficit was similar to MDS, where the activity of the native DNA encoded complex II was normal, whereas complexes I, III, and IV were decreased. The elongation factor EFG1 (gene *GFM1*) mutation was associated with fetal growth restriction, lactic acidosis, liver dysfunction that progresses into liver failure and death. The mutation in the elongation factor EFTu manifests as severe lactacidosis and lethal encephalopathy with mild hepatic involvement.

SECONDARY MITOCHONDRIAL HEPATOPATHIES

Secondary mitochondrial hepatopathies are caused by a hepatotoxic metal, drug, toxin, or endogenous metabolite. In the past, the most common secondary mitochondrial hepatopathy was **Reye syndrome,** the prevalence of which peaked in the 1970s and had a mortality rate of >40%. Even though mortality has not changed, the prevalence has decreased from >500 cases in 1980 to approximately 35 cases per year since. As to the decline of Reye syndrome, recent literature data reveal that this is related to more accurate modern diagnosis of infectious, metabolic, or toxic disease, reducing the percentage of idiopathic or true cases of Reye syndrome. Reye syndrome is precipitated in a genetically susceptible person by the interaction of a viral infection (influenza, varicella) and salicylate and or antiemetic use. Clinically, it is characterized by a preceding viral illness that appears to be resolving and the acute onset of vomiting and encephalopathy (Table 361-3). Neurologic symptoms can rapidly progress to seizures, coma, and death. Liver dysfunction is invariably present when vomiting develops, with coagulopathy and elevated serum levels of aspartate aminotransferase, alanine aminotransferase, and ammonia. Importantly, patients remain anicteric and serum bilirubin levels are normal. Liver biopsies show microvesicular steatosis without evidence of liver inflammation or necrosis. Death is usually secondary to increased intracranial pressures and herniation. Patients who survive have full recovery of liver function but should be carefully screened for fatty-acid oxidation and fatty-acid transport defects (Table 361-4).

Acquired abnormalities of mitochondrial function can be caused by several drugs and toxins, including valproic acid, cyanide, amiodarone, chloramphenicol, iron, antimycin A, the emetic toxin of *Bacillus cereus*, and nucleoside analogs. Valproic acid is a branched fatty acid that can be metabolized into the mitochondrial toxin 4-envalproic acid. Children with underlying respiratory chain defects appear more sensitive to the toxic effects of this drug and valproic acid is reported to precipitate liver failure in patients with **Alpers syndrome** and **cytochrome-*c* oxidase deficiency.** Nucleoside analogs directly inhibit mitochondrial respiratory chain complexes. The reverse transcriptase inhibitors zidovudine, didanosine, stavudine, and zalcitabine used to treat HIV-infected patients inhibit DNA polymerase-γ of mitochondria and can block elongation of mtDNA, leading to mtDNA

Table 361-3	Clinical Staging of Reye Syndrome and Reye-Like Diseases

Symptoms at the time of admission:
I. Usually quiet, **lethargic** and sleepy, vomiting, laboratory evidence of liver dysfunction
II. Deep lethargy, **confusion,** delirium, combativeness, hyperventilation, hyperreflexia
III. Obtunded, **light coma** ± seizures, **decorticate** rigidity, intact pupillary light reaction
IV. Seizures, deepening coma, **decerebrate rigidity,** loss of oculocephalic reflexes, fixed pupils
V. Coma, loss of deep tendon reflexes, respiratory arrest, fixed dilated pupils, **flaccidity/decerebration** (intermittent); isoelectric electroencephalogram

Metabolic disease
- Organic aciduria
- Disorders of oxidative phosphorylation
- Urea cycle defects (carbamoyl phosphate synthetase, ornithine transcarbamylase)
- Defects in fatty acid oxidation metabolism
- Acyl–coenzyme A dehydrogenase deficiencies
- Systemic carnitine deficiency
- Hepatic carnitine palmitoyltransferase deficiency
- 3-OH, 3-methylglutaryl-coenzyme A lyase deficiency
- Fructosemia

Central nervous system infections or intoxications (meningitis), encephalitis, toxic encephalopathy
Hemorrhagic shock with encephalopathy
Drug or toxin ingestion (salicylate, valproate)

Table 362-1	Disorders Producing Chronic Hepatitis

Chronic viral hepatitis
- Hepatitis B
- Hepatitis C
- Hepatitis D

Autoimmune hepatitis
- Anti-actin antibody positive
- Anti–liver-kidney microsomal antibody positive
- Anti-soluble liver antigen antibody-positive
- Others (includes antibodies to liver-specific lipoproteins or asialoglycoprotein)
- Overlap syndrome with sclerosing cholangitis and autoantibodies
- Systemic lupus erythematosus
- Celiac disease

Drug-induced hepatitis

Metabolic disorders associated with chronic liver disease
- Wilson disease
- Nonalcoholic steatohepatitis
- α_1-Antitrypsin deficiency
- Tyrosinemia
- Niemann-Pick disease type 2
- Glycogen storage disease type iv
- Cystic fibrosis
- Galactosemia
- Bile acid biosynthetic abnormalities

depletion. Other conditions that can lead to mitochondrial oxidative stress include cholestasis, nonalcoholic steatohepatitis, α_1-antitrypsin deficiency, and Wilson disease.

TREATMENT OF MITOCHONDRIAL HEPATOPATHIES

There is no effective therapy for most patients with mitochondrial hepatopathies; neurologic involvement often precludes orthotropic liver transplantation. Several drug mixtures that include antioxidants, vitamins, cofactors, and electron acceptors have been proposed, but no randomized, controlled trials have been completed to evaluate these drug combinations. Current treatment strategies are supportive and include the infusion of sodium bicarbonate for acute metabolic acidosis, low carbohydrate diet may decrease the lactic acidosis, transfusions for anemia and thrombocytopenia, and exogenous pancreatic enzymes for pancreatic insufficiency.

Bibliography is available at Expert Consult.

Chapter **362**
Autoimmune Hepatitis
Benjamin L. Shneider and Frederick J. Suchy

Autoimmune hepatitis is a chronic hepatic inflammatory process manifested by elevated serum aminotransaminase concentrations, liver-associated serum autoantibodies, and/or hypergammaglobulinemia. The target of the inflammatory process can include hepatocytes and to a lesser extent bile duct epithelium. Chronicity is determined either by duration of liver disease (typically >3-6 mo) or by evidence of chronic hepatic decompensation (hypoalbuminemia, thrombocytopenia) or physical stigmata of chronic liver disease (clubbing, spider telangiectasia, splenomegaly, ascites). The severity is variable; the affected child might have only biochemical evidence of liver dysfunction, might have stigmata of chronic liver disease, or can present in hepatic failure.

Chronic hepatitis can also be caused by persistent viral infection (see Chapter 358), drugs (see Chapter 363), metabolic diseases (see Chapter 361), or unknown and autoimmune disorders (Table 362-1).

Approximately 5% or less of chronic cases in the United States are associated with hepatitis B infection; unusually severe disease may be caused by superimposed infection with hepatitis D (a defective RNA virus that is dependent on replicating hepatitis B virus). More than 90% of hepatitis B infections in the 1st yr of life become chronic, compared with 5-10% among older children and adults. Chronic hepatitis develops in >50% of acute hepatitis C virus infections. Patients receiving blood products or who have had massive transfusions are at increased risk. Hepatitis A does not lead to chronic liver disease. Hepatitis E can become chronic in immunosuppressed patients. **Drugs** commonly used in children that can cause chronic liver injury include isoniazid, methyldopa, pemoline, nitrofurantoin, dantrolene, minocycline, pemoline, and the sulfonamides. **Metabolic diseases** can lead to chronic hepatitis, including α_1-antitrypsin deficiency, inborn errors of bile acid biosynthesis, and Wilson disease. **Nonalcoholic steatohepatitis,** usually associated with obesity and insulin resistance, is another common cause of chronic hepatitis. It can progress to cirrhosis, but responds to weight reduction. In many cases, the cause of chronic hepatitis is unknown; in some, an autoimmune mechanism is suggested by the finding of serum antinuclear and anti–smooth muscle antibodies and by multisystem involvement (arthropathy, thyroiditis, rashes, Coombs-positive hemolytic anemia).

Autoimmune hepatitis is a clinical constellation that suggests an immune-mediated process; it is responsive to immunosuppressive therapy (Table 362-2). Autoimmune hepatitis typically refers to a primarily hepatocyte-specific process, whereas autoimmune cholangiopathy and sclerosing cholangitis are predominated by intra- and extrahepatic bile duct injury. Overlap of the process involving both hepatocyte and bile duct directed injury may be more common in children. De novo hepatitis can be seen in a subset of liver transplant recipients whose initial disease was not autoimmune.

ETIOLOGY

In **autoimmune hepatitis** a dense portal mononuclear cell infiltrate invades the surrounding parenchyma and comprises T and B lymphocytes, macrophages, and plasma cells. The immunopathogenic mechanisms underlying autoimmune hepatitis are unsettled. Triggering factors can include molecular mimicry, infections, drugs, and the environment (toxins) in a genetically susceptible host. Several human leukocyte antigen class II molecules, particularly DR3, DR4, and DR7 isoforms, confer susceptibility to autoimmune hepatitis. Self-antigenic

Table 362-2	Classification of Autoimmune Hepatitis	
VARIABLE	**TYPE 1 AUTOIMMUNE HEPATITIS**	**TYPE 2 AUTOIMMUNE HEPATITIS**
Characteristic autoantibodies	Antinuclear antibody* Smooth-muscle antibody* Antiactin antibody† Autoantibodies against soluble liver antigen and liver-pancreas antigen‡ Atypical perinuclear antineutrophil cytoplasmic antibody	Antibody against liver-kidney microsome type 1* Antibody against liver cytosol type 1* Antibody against liver-kidney microsomal type 3
Geographic variation	Worldwide	Worldwide; rare in North America
Age at presentation	Any age	Predominantly childhood and young adulthood
Gender of patients	Female in ~75% of cases	Female in ~95% of cases
Association with other autoimmune diseases	Common	Common§
Clinical severity	Broad range, variable	Generally severe
Histopathologic features at presentation	Broad range, mild disease to cirrhosis	Generally advanced
Treatment failure	Infrequent	Frequent
Relapse after drug withdrawal	Variable	Common
Need for long-term maintenance	Variable	~100%

*The conventional method of detection is immunofluorescence.
†Tests for this antibody are rarely available in commercial laboratories.
‡This antibody is detected by enzyme-linked immunosorbent assay.
§Autoimmune polyendocrinopathy-candidiasis-ectodermal dystrophy is seen only in patients with type 2 disease.
From Krawitt EL: Autoimmune hepatitis, N Engl J Med 354:54–66, 2006.

peptides are processed by populations of antigen presenting cells and presented to CD4 and CD8 effector T-cells. CD4+ T lymphocytes recognizing a self-antigenic liver peptide orchestrate liver injury. Cell-mediated injury by cytokines released by CD8+ cytotoxic T cells and/or antibody-mediated cytotoxicity can be operative. There is also evidence that regulatory T-cells from autoimmune hepatitis patients are impaired in their ability to control the proliferation of CD4 and CD8 effector cells. Cytochrome P450 2D6 is the main autoantigen in type 2 autoimmune hepatitis.

Antibody-coated hepatocytes may be lysed by complement or Fc-bearing natural killer lymphocytes. Heterozygous mutations in the **autoimmune regulator gene (AIRE),** which encodes a transcription factor controlling the negative selection of autoreactive thymocytes, can be found in some children with autoimmune hepatitis types 1 and 2. *AIRE* mutations also cause **autoimmune polyendocrinopathy-candidiasis-ectodermal dystrophy** (also called autoimmune polyendocrinopathy syndrome) in which autoimmune hepatitis occurs in approximately 20% of patients.

PATHOLOGY

The histologic features common to untreated cases include inflammatory infiltrates, consisting of lymphocytes and plasma cells that expand portal areas and often penetrate the lobule (interface hepatitis); moderate to severe piecemeal necrosis of hepatocytes extending outward from the limiting plate; variable necrosis, fibrosis, and zones of parenchymal collapse spanning neighboring portal triads or between a portal triad and central vein (bridging necrosis); and variable degrees of bile duct epithelial injury. Distortion of hepatic architecture can be severe; cirrhosis may be present in children at the time of diagnosis. Histologic features in acute liver failure may be obscured by massive necrosis and multilobular collapse. Other histologic features may suggest an alternative diagnosis: characteristic periodic acid–Schiff-positive, diastase-resistant granules are seen in α_1-antitrypsin deficiency, and macrovesicular and microvesicular steatosis is found in Nonalcoholic steatohepatitis and often in Wilson disease. Bile duct injury can suggest an autoimmune cholangiopathy. Ultrastructural analysis might suggest distinct types of storage disorders.

CLINICAL MANIFESTATIONS

The clinical features and course of autoimmune hepatitis are extremely variable. Signs and symptoms at the time of presentation comprise a wide spectrum of disease including a substantial number of asymptomatic patients and some who have an acute, even fulminant, onset. In 25-30% of patients with autoimmune hepatitis, particularly children, the illness mimics acute viral hepatitis. In most, the onset is insidious. Patients can be asymptomatic or have fatigue, malaise, behavioral changes, anorexia, and amenorrhea, sometimes for many months before jaundice or stigmata of chronic liver disease are recognized. Extrahepatic manifestations can include arthritis, vasculitis, nephritis, thyroiditis, Coombs-positive anemia, and rash. Some patients' initial clinical features reflect cirrhosis (ascites, bleeding esophageal varices, or hepatic encephalopathy).

There may be mild to moderate jaundice in severe cases. Spider telangiectasias and palmar erythema may be present. The liver may be tender and slightly enlarged but might not be felt in patients with cirrhosis. The spleen is commonly enlarged. Edema and ascites may be present in advanced cases. Evidence of involvement of other organ systems may be found.

LABORATORY FINDINGS

The findings are related to the severity of presentation. In many asymptomatic cases, serum aminotransferase ranges between 100 and 300 IU/L, whereas levels in excess of 1,000 IU/L can be seen in symptomatic young patients. Serum bilirubin concentrations may be normal in mild cases but are commonly 2-10 mg/dL in more severe cases. Serum alkaline phosphatase and γ-glutamyl transpeptidase activities are normal to slightly increased but may be more significantly elevated in autoimmune cholangiopathy or in the setting of overlap with sclerosing cholangitis. Serum γ-globulin levels can show marked polyclonal elevations. Hypoalbuminemia is common. The prothrombin time is prolonged, most often as a result of vitamin K deficiency but also as a reflection of impaired hepatocellular function. A normochromic normocytic anemia, leukopenia, and thrombocytopenia are present and become more severe with the development of portal hypertension and hypersplenism.

Most patients with autoimmune hepatitis have hypergammaglobulinemia. Serum immunoglobulin G levels usually exceed 16 g/L. Characteristic patterns of serum **autoantibodies** define distinct subgroups of autoimmune hepatitis (see Table 362-2). The most common pattern (type 1) is associated with the formation of non–organ-specific antibodies, such as antiactin (smooth muscle) and antinuclear antibodies. Approximately 50% of these patients are 10-20 yr of age. High titers of a liver-kidney microsomal antibody are detected in another form (type 2) that usually affects children 2-14 yr of age. A subgroup of primarily young women might demonstrate autoantibodies against a soluble liver antigen but not against nuclear or microsomal proteins. Antineutrophil cytoplasmic antibodies may be seen more commonly in autoimmune cholangiopathy. Autoantibodies are rare in healthy children so that titers as low as 1:40 may be significant, although nonspecific elevation in autoantibodies can be observed in a variety of liver diseases. Up to 20% of patients with apparent autoimmune hepatitis might not have autoantibodies at presentation. Antibodies to a cytochrome P450 component of liver-kidney microsomal can be found in adult patients with chronic hepatitis C infection. Homologies in antigenic peptide epitopes between the hepatitis C virus and cytochrome P450 might explain this. Other, less-common autoantibodies include rheumatoid factor, antiparietal cell antibodies, and antithyroid antibodies. A Coombs-positive hemolytic anemia may be present.

DIAGNOSIS

Autoimmune hepatitis is a clinical diagnosis based on certain diagnostic criteria; no single test will make this diagnosis. Diagnostic criteria with scoring systems have been developed for adults and modified slightly for children, although these scoring systems were developed as research and not diagnostic tools. Important positive features include female gender, primary elevation in transaminases and not alkaline phosphatase, elevated γ-globulin levels, the presence of autoantibodies (most commonly antinuclear, smooth muscle, or liver-kidney microsome), and characteristic histologic findings (Fig. 362-1). Important negative features include the absence of viral markers (hepatitides B, C, D) of infection, absence of a history of drug or blood product exposure, and negligible alcohol consumption.

Common conditions that might lead to chronic hepatitis should be excluded (see Table 362-1). The differential diagnosis includes $α_1$-antitrypsin deficiency (see Chapter 357) and Wilson disease (see Chapter 357.2). The former disorder must be excluded by performing $α_1$-antitrypsin phenotyping and the latter by measuring serum ceruloplasmin and 24 hr urinary copper excretion and/or hepatic copper levels. Chronic hepatitis may occur in patients with inflammatory bowel disease, but liver dysfunction in such patients is more commonly caused by pericholangitis or sclerosing cholangitis. Celiac disease (see

Chapter 338.2) is associated with liver disease that is akin to autoimmune hepatitis, and appropriate serologic testing should be performed, including assays for antitissue transglutaminase antibodies or antiendomysial antibodies. An ultrasonogram should be done to identify a choledochal cyst or other structural disorders of the biliary system. MR cholangiography may be very useful for screening for evidence of sclerosing cholangitis. An overlap syndrome with features of primary sclerosing cholangitis and autoimmune hepatitis is being increasingly recognized with wider application of MR cholangiography. Dilated or obliterated veins on ultrasonography suggest the possibility of the Budd-Chiari syndrome.

TREATMENT

Prednisone, with or without azathioprine or 6-mercaptopurine, improves the clinical, biochemical, and histologic features in most patients with autoimmune hepatitis and prolongs survival in most patients with severe disease. The goal is to suppress or eliminate hepatic inflammation with minimal side effects. Prednisone at an initial dose of 1-2 mg/kg/24 hr is continued until aminotransferase values return to less than twice the upper limit of normal. The dose should then be lowered in 5 mg decrements over 2-4 mo until a maintenance dose of 0.1-0.3 mg/kg/24 hr is achieved. In patients who respond poorly, who experience severe side effects, or who cannot be maintained on low-dose steroids, azathioprine (1.5-2.0 mg/kg/24 hr, up to 100 mg/24 hr) can be added, with frequent monitoring for bone marrow suppression. Measurement of thiopurine methyltransferase activity should be done prior to beginning treatment with the thiopurine drugs azathioprine and 6-mercaptopurine. Patients with low activity (10% prevalence) or absent activity (prevalence 0.3%) are at risk for developing severe drug-induced myelotoxicity from accumulation of the unmetabolized drug. Measurement of the drug metabolites, 6-thioguanine nucleotide and 6-methylmercaptopurine, is useful in determining why a patient is not responding to a standard dose of a thiopurine drug and may help in avoiding myelosuppression and hepatotoxicity. Single-agent therapy with alternate-day corticosteroids should be used with great caution, although addition of azathioprine to alternate-day steroids can be an effective approach that minimizes corticosteroid-related toxicity. In patients with a mild and relatively asymptomatic presentation, some favor a lower starting dose of prednisone (10-20 mg) coupled with the simultaneous early administration of either 6-mercaptopurine (1.0-1.5 mg/kg/24 hr) or azathioprine (1.5-2.0 mg/kg/24 hr). Patients with primary sclerosing cholangitis/autoimmune hepatitis overlap syndrome respond similarly to immunosuppressive therapy. Precise diagnostic criteria for autoimmune disease in the setting of sclerosing cholangitis do not exist. Autoimmune markers and immunoglobulin levels are often elevated in children with sclerosing cholangitis and do not necessarily indicate a diagnosis of coincident autoimmune hepatitis. The choleretic agent, ursodeoxycholic acid, is often used in biliary tract disease, but trials in adults with primary sclerosing cholangitis have not shown efficacy, and patients have experienced toxicity at higher doses. There is a potential role for budesonide combined with azathioprine in treatment of noncirrhotic patients. Budesonide is a corticosteroid with high first-pass clearance by the liver and fewer systemic side effects including suppression of hypothalamic–pituitary axis. Cyclosporine, tacrolimus, mycophenolate mofetil, and sirolimus have been used in the management of cases refractory to standard therapy. Use of these agents should be reserved for practitioners with extensive experience in their administration, because the agents have a more restricted therapeutic to toxic ratio.

Histologic progress does not necessarily need to be assessed by sequential liver biopsies, although biochemical remission does not ensure histologic resolution. Follow-up liver biopsy is an important consideration in patients for whom consideration is given to discontinuing corticosteroid therapy. In patients with disappearance of symptoms and biochemical abnormalities and resolution of the necroinflammatory process on biopsy, an attempt at gradual discontinuation of medication is justified. There is a high rate of relapse after discontinuation of therapy. Relapse can require reinstitution of induction dosing of immunosuppression to control disease relapse.

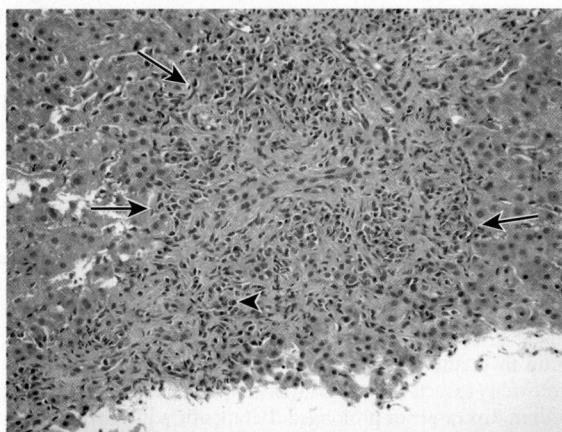

Figure 362-1 Autoimmune hepatitis. Liver biopsy showing fibrous expansion of the portal tracts with moderate portal lymphocytic infiltrates rich in plasma cells *(arrowhead)*. There is extensive interface hepatitis *(arrows)*. Original magnification ×20. *(Courtesy of Margret Magid, Mount Sinai School of Medicine.)*

PROGNOSIS

The initial response to therapy in autoimmune hepatitis is generally prompt, with a >75% rate of remission. Transaminases and bilirubin fall to near-normal levels, often in the 1st 1-3 mo. When present, abnormalities in serum albumin and prothrombin time respond over a longer period (3-9 mo). In patients meeting the criteria for tapering and then withdrawal of treatment (25-40% of children), 50% are weaned from all medication; in the other 50%, relapse occurs after a variable period. Relapse usually responds to retreatment. Many children will not meet the criteria for an attempt at discontinuation of immunosuppression and should be maintained on the smallest dose of prednisone that minimizes biochemical activity of the disease. A careful balance of the risks of continued immunosuppression and ongoing hepatitis must be continually evaluated. This requires continual screening for complications of medical therapy (monitoring of linear growth velocity, ophthalmologic examination, bone density measurement, blood pressure monitoring). Intermittent flares of hepatitis can occur and can necessitate recycling of prednisone therapy.

Some children have a relatively steroid-resistant form of hepatitis. More extensive evaluations of the etiology of their hepatitis should be undertaken, directed particularly at reassessing for the presence of either sclerosing cholangitis or Wilson disease. Nonadherence to medical therapy is one of the most common causes of "resistance" to medical therapy. Progression to cirrhosis can occur in autoimmune hepatitis despite a good response to drug therapy and prolongation of life. Corticosteroid therapy in fulminant autoimmune disease may be useful, although it should be administered with caution, given the predisposition of these patients to systemic bacterial and fungal infections.

Liver transplantation has been successful in patients with end-stage or fulminant liver disease associated with autoimmune hepatitis (see Chapter 368). Disease recurs after transplantation in approximately 30% of patients and is associated with increased concentrations of serum autoantibodies and interface hepatitis on liver biopsy.

Bibliography is available at Expert Consult.

Chapter **363**

Drug- and Toxin-Induced Liver Injury

Frederick J. Suchy

The liver is the main site of drug metabolism and is particularly susceptible to structural and functional injury after ingestion, parenteral administration, or inhalation of chemical agents, drugs, plant derivatives (home remedies), or environmental toxins. The possibility of drug use or toxin exposure at home or in the parents' workplace should be explored for every child with liver dysfunction. The clinical spectrum of illness can vary from asymptomatic biochemical abnormalities of liver function to fulminant failure. Liver injury may be the only clinical feature of an adverse drug reaction or may be accompanied by systemic manifestations and damage to other organs. In hospitalized patients, clinical and laboratory findings may be confused with the underlying illness. In a recent series after acetaminophen, antimicrobial (50%) and central nervous system agents (40%) were the most commonly implicated drug classes causing liver injury in children.

There is growing concern about environmental hepatotoxins that are insidious in their effects. Many environmental toxins including the plasticizers, biphenyl A and the phthalates, are ligands for nuclear receptors that transcriptionally activate the promoters of many genes involved in xenobiotic and lipid metabolism and may contribute to obesity and nonalcoholic fatty liver disease. Nonalcoholic fatty liver disease now affects 5-10% of all children in the United States and has the potential to evolve to cirrhosis and liver failure.

Hepatic metabolism of drugs and toxins is mediated by a sequence of enzymatic reactions that in large part transform hydrophobic, less-soluble molecules into more nontoxic, hydrophilic compounds that can be readily excreted in urine or bile (see Chapter 59). Relative liver size, liver blood flow, and extent of protein binding also influence drug metabolism. Phase 1 of the process involves enzymatic activation of the substrate to reactive intermediates containing a carboxyl, phenol, epoxide, or hydroxyl group. Mixed-function monooxygenase, cytochrome-c reductase, various hydrolases, and the cytochrome P450 (CYP) system are involved in this process. Nonspecific induction of these enzymatic pathways, which can occur during intercurrent viral infection, with starvation, and with administration of certain drugs such as anticonvulsants, can alter drug metabolism and increase the potential for hepatotoxicity. A single agent can be metabolized by >1 biochemical reaction. The reactive intermediates that are potentially damaging to the cell are enzymatically conjugated in phase 2 reactions with glucuronic acid, sulfate, acetate, glycine, or glutathione. Some drugs may be directly metabolized by these conjugating reactions without first undergoing phase 1 activation. Phase 3 is the energy-dependent excretion of drug metabolites and their conjugates by an array of membrane transporters in the liver and kidney such as the multidrug resistant protein 1.

Pathways for biotransformation are expressed early in the fetus and infant, but many phase 1 and phase 2 enzymes are immature, particularly in the 1st yr of life. CYP3A4 is the primary hepatic CYP expressed postnatally and metabolizes more than 75 commonly used therapeutic drugs and several environmental pollutants and procarcinogens. Hepatic CYP3A4 activity is poorly expressed in the fetus but increases after birth to reach 30% of adult values by 1 mo and 50% of adult values between 6 and 12 mo of age. CYP3A4 can be induced by a number of drugs, including phenytoin, phenobarbital, and rifampin. Enhanced production of toxic metabolites can overwhelm the capacity of phase 2 reactions. Conversely, numerous inhibitors of CYP3A4 from several different drug classes, such as erythromycin and cimetidine, can lead to toxic accumulations of CYP3A4 substrates. By contrast, although CYP2D6 is also developmentally regulated (maturation by 10 yr of age), its activity depends more on genetic polymorphisms than on sensitivity to inducers and inhibitors because more than 70 allelic variants of CYP2D6 significantly influence the metabolism of many drugs. Uridine diphosphateglucuronosyltransferase 1A6, a phase 2 enzyme that glucuronidates acetaminophen, is also absent in the human fetus, increases slightly in the neonate, but does not reach adult levels until sometime after 10 yr of age. Mechanisms for the uptake and excretion of organic ions can also be deficient early in life. Impaired drug metabolism via phase 1 and phase 2 reactions present in the 1st few mo of life is followed by a period of enhanced metabolism of many drugs in children through 10 yr of age compared with adults.

Genetic polymorphisms in genes encoding enzymes and transporters mediating phases 1, 2, and 3 reactions can also be associated with impaired drug metabolism and an increased risk of hepatotoxicity. Some cases of idiosyncratic hepatotoxicity can occur as a result of aberrations (polymorphisms) in phase 1 drug metabolism, producing intermediates of unusual hepatotoxic potential combined with developmental, acquired, or relative inefficiency of phase 2 conjugating reactions. Children may be more or less susceptible than adults to hepatotoxic reactions; liver injury after the use of the anesthetic halothane is rare in children, and acetaminophen toxicity is less common in infants than in adolescents, whereas most cases of fatal hepatotoxicity associated with sodium valproate use have been reported in children. Excessive or prolonged therapeutic administration of acetaminophen combined with reductions in caloric or protein intake can produce hepatotoxicity in children. In this setting, acetaminophen metabolism may be impaired by reduced synthesis of sulfated and glucuronated metabolites and reduced stores of glutathione. Immaturity of hepatic drug metabolic pathways can prevent degradation of a toxic agent; under other circumstances, the same immaturity might limit the formation of toxic metabolites. Severe sodium valproate hepatotoxicity is often associated with an underlying inherited mitochondrial disorder.

Chemical hepatotoxicity can be predictable or idiosyncratic. Predictable hepatotoxicity implies a high incidence of hepatic injury in exposed persons, with dose dependence. It is understandable that only a few drugs in clinical use fall into this category. These agents might damage the hepatocyte directly through alteration of membrane lipids (peroxidation) or through denaturation of proteins; such agents include carbon tetrachloride and trichloroethylene. Indirect injury can occur through interference with metabolic pathways essential for cell integrity or through distortion of cellular constituents by covalent binding of a reactive metabolite; examples include the liver injury produced by acetaminophen or by antimetabolites such as methotrexate or 6-mercaptopurine.

Idiosyncratic hepatotoxicity is uncommon and unpredictable but accounts for the majority of adverse reactions. In contrast to previous dogma that idiosyncratic reactions are independent of dose, there is new information that higher doses of drugs metabolized in the liver have a greater risk for hepatotoxicity.

Idiosyncratic drug reactions in certain patients can reflect aberrant pathways for drug metabolism, possibly related to genetic polymorphisms, with production of toxic intermediates (isoniazid and sodium valproate can cause liver damage through this mechanism). Duration of drug use before liver injury varies (weeks to ≥1 yr) and the response to reexposure may be delayed.

An idiosyncratic reaction can also be immunologically mediated as a result of prior sensitization (hypersensitivity); extrahepatic manifestations of hypersensitivity can include fever, rash, arthralgia, and eosinophilia. Duration of exposure before reaction is generally 1-4 wk, with prompt recurrence of injury on re-exposure. Studies indicate that arene oxides, generated through oxidative (CYP) metabolism of aromatic anticonvulsants (phenytoin, phenobarbital, carbamazepine), can initiate the pathogenesis of some hypersensitivity reactions. Arene oxides, formed in vivo, can bind to cellular macromolecules, thus perturbing cell function and possibly initiating immunologic mechanisms of liver injury.

Although the generation of chemically reactive metabolites has received great attention in the pathogenesis of hepatotoxicity, increasing evidence now exists for the multifactorial nature of the process, in particular the role played by the host immune system. Activation of liver nonparenchymal Kupffer cells and infiltration by neutrophils perpetuate toxic injury by many drugs by release of reactive oxygen and nitrogen species as well as cytokines. Stellate cells can also be activated, potentially leading to hepatic fibrosis and cirrhosis.

The pathologic spectrum of drug-induced liver disease is extremely wide, is rarely specific, and can mimic other liver diseases (Table 363-1). Predictable hepatotoxins, such as acetaminophen, produce centrilobular necrosis of hepatocytes. Steatosis is an important feature of tetracycline (microvesicular) and ethanol (macrovesicular) toxicities. A cholestatic hepatitis can be observed, with injury caused by erythromycin estolate and chlorpromazine. Cholestasis without inflammation may be a toxic effect of estrogens and anabolic steroids. Use of oral contraceptives and androgens has also been associated with benign and malignant liver tumors. Some idiosyncratic drug reactions can produce mixed patterns of injury, with diffuse cholestasis and cell necrosis. Chronic hepatitis has been associated with the use of methyldopa and nitrofurantoin.

Some herbal supplements are associated with hepatic injury or even liver failure (Table 363-2) related to their intrinsic toxicity or because of contamination with fungal toxins, pesticides, or heavy metals. The mechanism of liver injury due to these agents is unknown in the majority of cases.

Clinical manifestations can be mild and nonspecific, such as fever and malaise. Fever, rash, and arthralgia may be prominent in cases of hypersensitivity. In ill hospitalized patients, the signs and symptoms of hepatic drug toxicity may be difficult to separate from the underlying illness. The differential diagnosis should include acute and chronic viral

Table 363-1	Patterns of Hepatic Drug Injury
DISEASE	**DRUG**
Centrilobular necrosis	Acetaminophen Halothane
Microvesicular steatosis	Valproic acid
Acute hepatitis	Isoniazid
General hypersensitivity	Sulfonamides Phenytoin
Fibrosis	Methotrexate
Cholestasis	Chlorpromazine Erythromycin Estrogens
Sinusoidal obstruction syndrome (venoocclusive disease)	Irradiation plus busulfan Cyclophosphamide
Portal and hepatic vein thrombosis	Estrogens Androgens
Biliary sludge	Ceftriaxone
Hepatic adenoma or hepatocellular carcinoma	Oral contraceptives Anabolic steroids

Table 363-2	Potentially Hepatotoxic Herbal or Dietary Supplements

Celandine
Chaparral (creosote bush, greasewood, *Larrea tridentata*)
Chinese herbs
Comfrey leaves (pyrrolizidine alkaloids)
Germander extracts (*Teucrium chamaedrys*)
Kava (*Kava kava*, awa, kew)
LipoKinetix (phenylpropanolamine, sodium usinate, diiodothyronine, yohimbine, caffeine)
Ma huang (*Ephedra*)
Mushroom (*Amanita phalloides*, *Galerina*)
Senecio
Valerian with skullcap

hepatitis, biliary tract disease, septicemia, ischemic and hypoxic liver injury, malignant infiltration, and inherited metabolic liver disease.

The laboratory features of drug- or toxin-related liver disease are extremely variable. Hepatocyte damage can lead to elevations of serum aminotransferase activities and serum bilirubin levels and to impaired synthetic function as evidenced by decreased serum coagulation factors and albumin. Hyperammonemia can occur with liver failure or with selective inhibition of the urea cycle (sodium valproate). Toxicologic screening of blood and urine specimens can aid in the detecting drug or toxin exposure. Percutaneous liver biopsy may be necessary to distinguish drug injury from complications of an underlying disorder or from intercurrent infection.

Slight elevation of serum aminotransferase activities (generally <2-3 times normal) can occur during therapy with drugs, particularly anticonvulsants, capable of inducing microsomal pathways for drug metabolism. Liver biopsy reveals proliferation of smooth endoplasmic reticulum but no significant liver injury. Liver test abnormalities often resolve with continued drug therapy.

TREATMENT

Treatment of drug- or toxin-related liver injury is mainly supportive. Contact with the offending agent should be avoided. Corticosteroids might have a role in immune-mediated disease. *N*-Acetylcysteine therapy, by stimulating glutathione synthesis, is effective in preventing or attenuating hepatotoxicity when administered within 16 hr after an acute overdose of acetaminophen and appears to improve survival in patients with severe liver injury even up to 36 hr after ingestion (see Chapter 63). Intravenous L-carnitine may be of value in treating valproic acid–induced hepatotoxicity. Orthotopic liver transplantation may be required for treatment of drug- or toxin-induced hepatic failure.

PROGNOSIS

The prognosis of drug- or toxin-induced liver injury depends on its type and severity. Injury is usually completely reversible when the hepatotoxic factor is withdrawn. The mortality of submassive hepatic necrosis with fulminant liver failure can, however, exceed 50%. Hyperbilirubinemia, coagulopathy, and elevated serum creatinine are associated with an increased risk of death or need for liver transplantation. With continued use of certain drugs, such as methotrexate, effects of hepatoxicity can proceed insidiously to cirrhosis, even with normal or near normal liver tests. Neoplasia can follow long-term androgen therapy. Rechallenge with a drug suspected of having caused previous liver injury is rarely justified and can result in fatal hepatic necrosis.

PREVENTION

The prevention of drug-induced liver injury remains a challenge. Monitoring of liver biochemical tests may be useful in some cases, but it can prove difficult to sustain for agents used for many years. Such testing may be particularly important in patients with pre-existing liver disease. For drugs with particular hepatotoxic potential, even if episodes are infrequent in children, such as with the use of isoniazid, patients should be advised to immediately stop the medication with onset of nausea, vomiting, abdominal pain, and fatigue until liver damage is excluded. Obvious symptoms of liver disease such as jaundice and dark urine can lag behind severe hepatocellular injury. Monitoring for toxic metabolites and genotyping can be effective in preventing severe toxicity with the use of azathioprine. Advances in pharmacogenomics, such as the use of gene chips to detect variants in some of the CYP enzymes, hold promise of a personalized approach to prevent hepatotoxicity.

Bibliography is available at Expert Consult.

Chapter 364
Fulminant Hepatic Failure
Frederick J. Suchy

Fulminant hepatic failure (acute liver failure) is a clinical syndrome resulting from massive necrosis of hepatocytes or from severe functional impairment of hepatocytes. Synthetic, excretory, and detoxifying functions of the liver are all severely impaired. In adults, hepatic encephalopathy has been an essential diagnostic feature. This narrow definition may be problematic because early hepatic encephalopathy can be difficult to detect in infants and children. The currently accepted definition in children includes biochemical evidence of acute liver injury (usually <8 wk duration); no evidence of chronic liver disease; and hepatic-based coagulopathy defined as a prothrombin time (PT) >15 sec or international normalized ratio (INR) >1.5 not corrected by vitamin K in the presence of clinical hepatic encephalopathy, or a PT >20 sec or INR >2 regardless of the presence of clinical hepatic encephalopathy. Liver failure in the perinatal period can be associated with prenatal liver injury and even cirrhosis. Examples include neonatal iron storage (hemochromatosis) disease, tyrosinemia, and some cases of congenital viral infection. Liver disease may be noticed at birth or after several days of apparent well-being. Fulminant Wilson disease also occurs in older children who were previously asymptomatic but, by definition, have preexisting liver disease. In some cases of liver failure, particularly in the idiopathic form of acute hepatic failure, the onset of encephalopathy occurs later, from 8-28 wk after the onset of jaundice.

ETIOLOGY

Fulminant hepatic failure can be a complication of viral hepatitis (A, B, D, E). An unusually high risk of fulminant hepatic failure occurs in young people who have combined infections with the hepatitis B virus (HBV) and hepatitis D. Mutations in the precore and/or promoter region of HBV DNA are associated with fulminant and severe hepatitis. HBV is also responsible for some cases of fulminant liver failure in the absence of serologic markers of HBV infection but with HBV DNA found in the liver. Hepatitides C and E viruses are uncommon causes of fulminant hepatic failure in the United States. Patients with chronic hepatitis C are at risk if they have superinfection with hepatitis A virus. Epstein-Barr virus, herpes simplex virus, adenovirus, enteroviruses, cytomegalovirus, parvovirus B19, human herpesvirus-6, and varicella-zoster infections can also produce fulminant hepatitis in children.

Fulminant hepatic failure can also be caused by autoimmune hepatitis in approximately 5% of cases. Patients have a positive autoimmune marker (e.g., antinuclear antibody, anti–smooth muscle antibody, liver-kidney microsomal antibody, or soluble liver antigen) and possibly an elevated serum immunoglobulin G level. Liver histology, if a biopsy can be safely done, might support the diagnosis.

Acute liver failure is a common feature of hemophagocytic lymphohistiocytosis caused by several gene defects, infections by mostly viruses of the herpes group, and a variety of other conditions including organ transplantation and malignancies. Impaired function of natural killer cells and cytotoxic T-lymphocyte cells with uncontrolled hemophagocytosis and cytokine overproduction is characteristic for genetic and acquired forms of hemophagocytic lymphohistiocytosis. Biochemical markers include elevated ferritin and triglycerides and low fibrinogen.

An idiopathic form of fulminant hepatic failure accounts for 40-50% of cases in children. The disease occurs sporadically and usually without the risk factors for common causes of viral hepatitis. It is likely that the etiology of these cases is heterogeneous, including unidentified or variant viruses, excessive immune activation, and undiagnosed metabolic disorders.

Various hepatotoxic drugs and chemicals can also cause fulminant hepatic failure. Predictable liver injury can occur after exposure to carbon tetrachloride or *Amanita phalloides* mushroom or after acetaminophen overdose. Acetaminophen is the most common etiology of acute hepatic failure in children and adolescents in the United States and England. In addition to the acute intentional ingestion of a massive dose, a therapeutic misadventure leading to severe liver injury can also occur in ill children given doses of acetaminophen exceeding weight-based recommendations for many days. Such patients can have reduced stores of glutathione after a prolonged illness and a period of poor nutrition. Idiosyncratic damage can follow the use of drugs such as halothane, isoniazid, or sodium valproate. Herbal supplements are additional causes of hepatic failure (see Table 363-2).

Ischemia and hypoxia resulting from hepatic vascular occlusion, severe heart failure, cyanotic congenital heart disease, or circulatory shock can produce liver failure. Metabolic disorders associated with hepatic failure include Wilson disease, acute fatty liver of pregnancy, galactosemia, hereditary tyrosinemia, hereditary fructose intolerance, neonatal iron storage disease, defects in β-oxidation of fatty acids, and deficiencies of mitochondrial electron transport particularly mitochondrial DNA depletion disorders.

PATHOLOGY

Liver biopsy usually reveals patchy or confluent massive necrosis of hepatocytes. Multilobular or bridging necrosis can be associated with collapse of the reticulin framework of the liver. There may be little or no regeneration of hepatocytes. A zonal pattern of necrosis may be observed with certain insults. (Centrilobular damage is associated with acetaminophen hepatotoxicity or with circulatory shock.) Evidence of severe hepatocyte dysfunction rather than cell necrosis is occasionally the predominant histologic finding (microvesicular fatty infiltrate of hepatocytes is observed in Reye syndrome, β-oxidation defects, and tetracycline toxicity).

PATHOGENESIS

The mechanisms that lead to fulminant hepatic failure are poorly understood. It is unknown why only approximately 1-2% of patients with viral hepatitis experience liver failure. Massive destruction of hepatocytes might represent both a direct cytotoxic effect of the virus and an immune response to the viral antigens. One-third to one-half of patients with HBV-induced liver failure become negative for serum hepatitis B surface antigen within a few days of presentation and often have no detectable HBV antigen or HBV DNA in serum. These findings suggest a hyperimmune response to the virus that underlies the massive liver necrosis. Formation of hepatotoxic metabolites that bind covalently to macromolecular cell constituents is involved in the liver injury produced by drugs such as acetaminophen and isoniazid; fulminant hepatic failure can follow depletion of intracellular substrates involved in detoxification, particularly glutathione. Whatever the initial cause of hepatocyte injury, various factors can contribute to the pathogenesis of liver failure, including impaired hepatocyte regeneration, altered parenchymal perfusion, endotoxemia, and decreased hepatic reticuloendothelial function.

The pathogenesis of hepatic encephalopathy can relate to increased serum levels of ammonia, false neurotransmitters, amines, increased γ-aminobutyric acid receptor activity, or increased circulating levels of endogenous benzodiazepine-like compounds. Decreased hepatic clearance of these substances can produce marked central nervous system dysfunction.

CLINICAL MANIFESTATIONS

Fulminant hepatic failure can be the presenting feature of liver disease or it can complicate previously known liver disease (acute-on-chronic liver failure). A history of developmental delay and/or neuromuscular dysfunction can indicate an underlying mitochondrial or β-oxidation defect. A child with fulminant hepatic failure has usually been previously healthy and most often has no risk factors for liver disease such as exposure to toxins or blood products. Progressive jaundice, fetor hepaticus, fever, anorexia, vomiting, and abdominal pain are common. A rapid decrease in liver size without clinical improvement is an ominous sign. A hemorrhagic diathesis and ascites can develop.

Patients should be closely observed for hepatic encephalopathy, which is initially characterized by minor disturbances of consciousness or motor function. Irritability, poor feeding, and a change in sleep rhythm may be the only findings in infants; asterixis may be demonstrable in older children. Patients are often somnolent, confused, or combative on arousal and can eventually become responsive only to painful stimuli. Patients can rapidly progress to deeper stages of coma in which extensor responses and decerebrate and decorticate posturing appear. Respirations are usually increased early, but respiratory failure can occur in stage IV coma (Table 364-1).

LABORATORY FINDINGS

Serum direct and indirect bilirubin levels and serum aminotransferase activities may be markedly elevated. Serum aminotransferase activities do not correlate well with the severity of the illness and can actually decrease as a patient deteriorates. The blood ammonia concentration is usually increased, but hepatic coma can occur in patients with a normal blood ammonia level. PT and the INR are prolonged and often do not improve after parenteral administration of vitamin K. Hypoglycemia can occur, particularly in infants. Hypokalemia, hyponatremia, metabolic acidosis, or respiratory alkalosis can develop.

TREATMENT

Specific therapies for identifiable causes of acute liver failure include *N*-acetylcysteine (acetaminophen), acyclovir (herpes simplex virus), penicillin (*Amanita* mushrooms), nucleos(t)ide analogs such as entecavir or lamivudine (HBV), and prednisone (autoimmune hepatitis). Management of other types of fulminant hepatic failure is supportive. No therapy is known to reverse hepatocyte injury or to promote hepatic regeneration.

An infant or child with acute hepatic failure should be cared for in an institution able to perform a liver transplantation if necessary and managed in an intensive care unit with continuous monitoring of vital functions. Endotracheal intubation may be required to prevent aspiration, to reduce cerebral edema by hyperventilation, and to facilitate pulmonary toilet. Mechanical ventilation and supplemental oxygen are often necessary in advanced coma. Sedatives should be avoided unless needed in the intubated patient because these agents can aggravate or precipitate encephalopathy. Opiates may be better tolerated than benzodiazepines. Prophylactic use of proton pump inhibitors should be considered because of the high risk of gastrointestinal bleeding.

Hypovolemia should be avoided and treated with cautious infusions of isotonic fluids and blood products. Renal dysfunction can result from dehydration, acute tubular necrosis, or functional renal failure (hepatorenal syndrome). Electrolyte and glucose solutions should be administered intravenously to maintain urine output, to correct or prevent hypoglycemia, and to maintain normal serum potassium concentrations. Hyponatremia is common and should be avoided, but it is usually dilutional and not a result of sodium depletion. Parenteral supplementation with calcium, phosphorus, and magnesium may be required. Hypophosphatemia, probably a reflection of liver regeneration, and early phosphorus administration are associated with a better prognosis in acute liver failure, whereas hyperphosphatemia predicts a failure of spontaneous recovery.

Coagulopathy should be treated with parenteral administration of vitamin K and can require infusion of fresh-frozen plasma, cryoprecipitate, and platelets to treat clinically significant bleeding; disseminated intravascular coagulation can also occur. Plasmapheresis can permit temporary correction of the bleeding diathesis without resulting in volume overload. Recombinant factor VIIa has been used for transient correction of coagulopathy refractory to fresh frozen plasma infusions and can facilitate the performance of invasive procedures

Table 364-1	Stages of Hepatic Encephalopathy			
	STAGES			
	I	**II**	**III**	**IV**
Symptoms	Periods of lethargy, euphoria; reversal of day–night sleeping; may be alert	Drowsiness, inappropriate behavior, agitation, wide mood swings, disorientation	Stupor but arousable, confused, incoherent speech	Coma IVa responds to noxious stimuli IVb no response
Signs	Trouble drawing figures, performing mental tasks	Asterixis, fetor hepaticus, incontinence	Asterixis, hyperreflexia, extensor reflexes, rigidity	Areflexia, no asterixis, flaccidity
Electroencephalogram	Normal	Generalized slowing, q waves	Markedly abnormal, triphasic waves	Markedly abnormal bilateral slowing, d waves, electric-cortical silence

such as placement of a central line or an intracranial pressure monitor. Continuous hemofiltration is useful for managing fluid overload and acute renal failure.

Patients should be monitored closely for infection, including sepsis, pneumonia, peritonitis, and urinary tract infections. At least 50% of patients experience serious infection. Gram-positive organisms (*Staphylococcus aureus, Staphylococcus epidermidis*) are the most common pathogens, but Gram-negative and fungal infections are also observed.

Gastrointestinal hemorrhage, infection, constipation, sedatives, electrolyte imbalance, and hypovolemia can precipitate encephalopathy and should be identified and corrected. Protein intake should be initially restricted or eliminated, depending on the degree of encephalopathy. The gut should be purged with several enemas. Lactulose should be given every 2-4 hr orally or by nasogastric tube in doses (10-50 mL) sufficient to cause diarrhea. The dose is then adjusted to produce several acidic, loose bowel movements daily. Lactulose syrup diluted with 1-3 volumes of water can also be given as a retention enema every 6 hr. Lactulose, a nonabsorbable disaccharide, is metabolized to organic acids by colonic bacteria; it probably lowers blood ammonia levels through decreasing microbial ammonia production and through trapping of ammonia in acidic intestinal contents. Oral or rectal administration of a nonabsorbable antibiotic such as rifaximin or neomycin can reduce enteric bacteria responsible for ammonia production. Oral antibiotics may be more effective than lactulose in lowering serum ammonia levels. In a recent clinical trial, *N*-acetylcysteine was not effective in improving the outcome of patients with acute liver failure not associated with acetaminophen.

Cerebral edema is an extremely serious complication of hepatic encephalopathy that responds poorly to measures such as corticosteroid administration and osmotic diuresis. Monitoring intracranial pressure can be useful in preventing severe cerebral edema, in maintaining cerebral perfusion pressure, and in establishing the suitability of a patient for liver transplantation. Controlled trials have shown a worsened outcome of fulminant hepatic failure in patients treated with corticosteroids.

Temporary liver support continues to be evaluated as a bridge for the patient with liver failure to liver transplantation or regeneration. Nonbiologic systems, essentially a form of liver dialysis with an albumin-containing dialysate, and biologic liver support devices that involve perfusion of the patient's blood through a cartridge containing liver cell lines or porcine hepatocytes can remove some toxins, improve serum biochemical abnormalities, and, in some cases, improve neurologic function, but there has been little evidence of improved survival, and few children have been treated.

Orthotopic liver transplantation can be lifesaving in patients who reach advanced stages (III, IV) of hepatic coma. Reduced-size allografts and living donor transplantation have been important advances in the treatment of infants with hepatic failure. Partial auxiliary orthotopic or heterotopic liver transplantation is successful in a small number of children, and in some cases it has allowed regeneration of the native liver and eventual withdrawal of immunosuppression. Orthotopic liver transplantation should not be done in patients with liver failure and neuromuscular dysfunction secondary to a mitochondrial disorder because progressive neurologic deterioration is likely to continue after transplantation.

PROGNOSIS

Children with acute hepatic failure fare better than adults. Improved survival can be attributed to careful intensive care and if necessary liver transplantation. In the largest prospective study from the Pediatric Acute Liver Failure Study Group, 709 children were assessed at 21 days: 50.3% of patients survived with supportive care alone, 36.2% survived after liver transplantation, and 13.4% died. A scoring system based on peak values of total serum bilirubin, PT, and plasma ammonia concentration predicted transplant-free survival. Prognosis varies considerably with the cause of liver failure and stage of hepatic encephalopathy. Survival rates with supportive care may be as high as 90% in acetaminophen overdose and with fulminant hepatitis A. By contrast, spontaneous recovery can be expected in only approximately 40% of

patients with liver failure caused by the idiopathic form of acute liver failure or an acute onset of Wilson disease. In patients who progress to stage IV coma (see Table 364-1), the prognosis is extremely poor. Brainstem herniation is the most common cause of death. Major complications such as sepsis, severe hemorrhage, or renal failure increase the mortality. The prognosis is particularly poor in patients with liver necrosis and multiorgan failure.

Age <1 yr, stage 4 encephalopathy, an INR >4, and the need for dialysis before transplantation are associated with increased mortality. Pretransplantation serum bilirubin concentration or the height of hepatic enzymes is not predictive of posttransplantation survival. A plasma ammonia concentration >200 µmol/L is associated with a 5-fold increased risk of death.

Children with acute hepatic failure are more likely to die while on the waiting list compared to children with other diagnoses. Owing to the severity of their illness, the 6 mo post–liver transplantation survival of approximately 75% in most studies is significantly lower than the 90% achieved in children with chronic liver disease. Patients who recover from fulminant hepatic failure with only supportive care do not usually develop cirrhosis or chronic liver disease. Aplastic anemia occurs in approximately 10% of children with the idiopathic form of fulminant hepatic failure and is often fatal.

Bibliography is available at Expert Consult.

Chapter 365
Cystic Diseases of the Biliary Tract and Liver
Frederick J. Suchy

Cystic lesions of liver may be initially recognized during infancy and childhood (Table 365-1). Hepatic fibrosis can also occur as part of an associated developmental defect (Table 365-2). Cystic renal disease is usually associated and often determines the clinical presentation and prognosis. Virtually all proteins encoded by genes mutated in combined cystic diseases of the liver and kidney are at least partially localized to primary cilia in renal tubular cells and cholangiocytes.

CHOLEDOCHAL CYSTS

Choledochal cysts are congenital dilatations of the common bile duct that can cause progressive biliary obstruction and biliary cirrhosis. Cylindrical (fusiform) and spherical (saccular) cysts of the extrahepatic ducts are the most common types. Segmental or diffuse dilation can be observed. A diverticulum of the common bile duct or dilation of the intraduodenal portion of the common duct (*choledochocele*) is a variant. Cystic dilation of the intrahepatic bile ducts may be associated with a choledochal cyst or Caroli disease.

The pathogenesis of choledochal cysts remains uncertain. Some reports suggest that junction of the common bile duct and the pancreatic duct before their entry into the sphincter of Oddi might allow reflux of pancreatic enzymes into the common bile duct, causing inflammation, localized weakness, and dilation of the duct. It also has been proposed that a distal congenital stenotic segment of the biliary tree leads to increased intraluminal pressure and proximal biliary dilation. Other possibilities are that choledochal cysts represent malformations of the common duct or that they occur as part of the spectrum of an infectious disease that includes neonatal hepatitis and biliary

Table 365-1	Renal Disorders Associated with Fibropolycystic Liver Diseases
FIBROPOLYCYSTIC LIVER DISEASE	**ASSOCIATED RENAL DISORDER**
Congenital hepatic fibrosis (CHF)	Autosomal-recessive polycystic kidney disease* Autosomal-dominant polycystic kidney disease Cystic renal dysplasia Nephronophthisis None
Caroli syndrome (CS)	Autosomal-recessive polycystic kidney disease* Autosomal-dominant polycystic kidney disease None
Caroli disease	Autosomal-recessive polycystic kidney disease
von Meyenburg complexes (isolated)	?
von Meyenburg complexes with CHF or CS	Autosomal-recessive polycystic kidney disease
von Meyenburg complexes with polycystic liver disease	Autosomal-dominant polycystic kidney disease
Polycystic liver disease	Autosomal-dominant polycystic kidney disease* ? None

*Most common associated disorders.
From Suchy FJ, Sokol RJ, Balistreri WF, editors: Liver disease in children, ed 3, New York, 2007, Cambridge University Press, p. 27.

Table 365-2	Syndromes Associated with Congenital Hepatic Fibrosis
SYNDROME	**FEATURES**
Jeune syndrome	Asphyxiating thoracic dystrophy, with cystic renal tubular dysplasia and congenital hepatic fibrosis (15q13)
Joubert syndrome	Oculo-encephalo-hepato-renal (AH11, HPHP1)
COACH syndrome	Cerebellar vermis hypoplasia, oligophrenia, congenital ataxia, ocular coloboma, and hepatic fibrosis (MKS3, CC2D2A, RPGRIP1L)
Meckel syndrome type 1	Cystic renal dysplasia abnormal bile duct development with fibrosis, posterior encephalocele, and polydactyly (13q13, 17a21, 8q24)
Carbohydrate-deficient glycoprotein syndrome type 1b	Phosphomannose isomerase 1 deficiency (PMI)
Ivemark syndrome type 2	Autosomal-recessive renal-hepatic-pancreatic dysplasia
Miscellaneous syndromes	Intestinal lymphangiectasia, enterocolitis cystic Short rib (Beemer-Langer) syndrome Osteochondrodysplasia

From Suchy FJ, Sokol RJ, Balistreri WF, editors: Liver disease in children, ed 3, New York, 2007, Cambridge University Press, p. 931.

atresia. Consistent with this theory, reovirus RNA has been detected in liver and biliary tissues of some infants with choledochal cysts.

Approximately 75% of cases appear during childhood. The infant typically presents with cholestatic jaundice; severe liver dysfunction including ascites and coagulopathy can rapidly evolve if biliary obstruction is not relieved. An abdominal mass is rarely palpable. In an older child, the **classic triad** of abdominal pain, jaundice, and mass occurs in <33% of patients. Features of acute cholangitis (fever, right upper quadrant tenderness, jaundice, leukocytosis) may be present. The diagnosis is made by ultrasonography; choledochal cysts have been identified prenatally using this technique. Magnetic resonance cholangiography is useful in the preoperative assessment of choledochal cyst anatomy.

The **treatment of choice** is primary excision of the cyst and a Roux-en-Y choledochojejunostomy. Simple drainage into the small bowel is less satisfactory owing to a risk of development of carcinoma in the residual cystic tissue. The postoperative course can be complicated by recurrent cholangitis or stricture at the anastomotic site.

Autosomal Recessive Polycystic Kidney Disease
Autosomal recessive polycystic kidney disease (ARPKD) manifests predominantly in childhood (see Chapter 521.2). Bilateral enlargement of the kidneys is caused by a generalized dilation of the collecting tubules. The disorder is invariably associated with congenital hepatic fibrosis and various degrees of biliary ductal ectasia that are discussed in detail later.

The polycystic kidney and hepatic disease 1 (PKHD1) gene, mutated in ARPKD, encodes a protein that is called fibrocystin/polyductin, which is localized to cilia on the apical domain of renal collecting cells and cholangiocytes. The primary defect in ARPKD may be ciliary dysfunction related to the abnormality in this protein. Fibrocystin/polyductin appears to have a role in the regulation of cellular adhesion, repulsion, and proliferation and/or the regulation and maintenance of renal collecting tubules and bile ducts, but its exact role in normal and cystic epithelia remains unknown. Kidney and liver disease are independent and variability in severity and not explainable by type of PKHD1 mutation. Phenotypic variability among affected siblings suggests importance of modifier genes as well as possibly environmental influences.

In ARPKD, the cysts arise as ectatic expansions of the collecting tubules and bile ducts that remain in continuity with their structures of origin. ARPKD normally presents in early life, often shortly after birth, and is generally more severe than autosomal dominant polycystic kidney disease (ADPKD). Fetal ultrasound may visualize large echogenic kidneys, also described as "bright," with low or absent amniotic fluid (oligohydramnios). However, in many instances the features of ARPKD are not visualized on sonogram until the 3rd trimester or after birth.

Patients with ARPKD can die in the perinatal period owing to renal failure or lung dysgenesis. The kidneys in these patients are usually markedly enlarged and dysfunctional. Respiratory failure can result from compression of the chest by grossly enlarged kidneys, from fluid retention, or from concomitant pulmonary hypoplasia (see Chapter 515.2). The clinical pathologic findings within a family tend to breed true, although there has been some variability in the severity of the disease and the time for presentation within the same family. In patients surviving infancy because of a milder renal phenotype, liver disease may be a prominent part of the disorder. The liver disease in ARPKD is related to congenital malformation of the liver with varying degrees of periportal fibrosis, bile ductular hyperplasia, ectasia, and dysgenesis. Initial symptoms are liver related in approximately 26% of patients. This can manifest clinically as variable, cystic dilation of the intrahepatic biliary tree with congenital hepatic fibrosis. Congenital hepatic fibrosis and Caroli disease likely result from an abnormality in remodeling of the embryonic ductal plate of the liver. *Ductal plate malformation* refers to the persistence of excess embryonic bile duct structures in the portal tracts.

Variable abnormalities of bile ducts (irregular dilation, proliferation, cysts) and portal fibrosis can also be associated with Meckel syndrome, trisomy 17-18, tuberous sclerosis, and asphyxiating thoracic dystrophy (see Table 365-2).

Cystic Dilation of the Intrahepatic Bile Ducts (Caroli Disease)

Congenital saccular dilation can affect several segments of the intrahepatic bile ducts; the dilated ducts are lined by cuboidal epithelium and are in continuity with the main duct system, which is usually normal. Choledochal cysts have also been associated with Caroli disease. Bile duct dilation leads to stagnation of bile and formation of biliary sludge and intraductal lithiasis.

There is a marked predisposition to ascending cholangitis which may be exacerbated by calculus formation within the abnormal bile ducts.

Affected patients usually experience symptoms of acute cholangitis as children or young adults. Fever, abdominal pain, mild jaundice, and pruritus occur, and a slightly enlarged, tender liver is palpable. Elevated alkaline phosphatase activity, direct-reacting bilirubin levels, and leukocytosis may be observed during episodes of acute infection. In patients with Caroli disease, clinical features may be the result of a combination of recurring bouts of cholangitis, reflecting the intrahepatic ductal abnormalities and portal hypertensive bleeding resulting from hepatic fibrosis. Ultrasonography shows the dilated intrahepatic ducts, but definitive diagnosis and extent of disease must be determined by percutaneous transhepatic, endoscopic, or magnetic resonance cholangiography.

Cholangitis and sepsis are treated with appropriate antibiotics. Calculi can require surgery. Partial hepatectomy may be curative in rare cases in which cystic disease is confined to a single lobe. The prognosis is otherwise guarded, largely owing to difficulties in controlling cholangitis and biliary lithiasis and to a significant risk for developing cholangiocarcinoma. ARPKD patients with recurrent cholangitis or complications of portal hypertension may require combined liver-kidney transplant.

Congenital Hepatic Fibrosis

Congenital hepatic fibrosis is usually associated with ARPKD and is characterized pathologically by diffuse periportal and perilobular fibrosis in broad bands that contain distorted bile duct–like structures and that often compresses or incorporate central or sublobular veins (see Table 365-2). Irregularly shaped islands of liver parenchyma contain normal-appearing hepatocytes. Caroli disease and choledochal cysts are associated. Most patients have renal disease, mostly autosomal recessive polycystic renal disease and rarely nephronophthisis. Congenital hepatic fibrosis also occurs as part of the **COACH syndrome** (cerebellar vermis hypoplasia, oligophrenia, congenital ataxia, coloboma, and hepatic fibrosis). Congenital hepatic fibrosis has been described in children with a congenital disorder of glycosylation caused by mutations in the gene encoding phosphomannose isomerase (see Chapter 87.6).

Several different forms of congenital hepatic fibrosis have been defined clinically: portal hypertensive (most common) cholangitic, mixed, and latent. The disorder usually has its onset in childhood, with hepatosplenomegaly or with bleeding secondary to portal hypertension. In a recent study, splenomegaly, as a marker for portal hypertension, developed early in life and was present in 60% of children younger than 5 yr of age.

Cholangitis can occur in patients, as these patients have abnormal biliary tracts even without Caroli disease. Hepatocellular function is usually well preserved. Serum aminotransferase activities and bilirubin levels are usually normal in the absence of cholangitis and choledocholithiasis; serum alkaline phosphatase activity may be slightly elevated. The serum albumin level and prothrombin time are normal. Liver biopsy is rarely required for diagnosis, particularly in patients with obvious real disease.

Treatment of this disorder should focus on control of bleeding from esophageal varices and aggressive antibiotic treatment of cholangitis. Infrequent mild bleeding episodes may be managed by endoscopic sclerotherapy or band ligation of the varices. After more-severe hemorrhage, portacaval anastomosis can relieve portal hypertension. The prognosis may be greatly improved by a shunting procedure, but survival in some patients may be limited by renal failure.

AUTOSOMAL DOMINANT POLYCYSTIC KIDNEY DISEASE

ADPKD (see Chapter 521.3), a common inherited disease, affects 1 in 1,000 live births. It is characterized by progressive renal cyst development and cyst enlargement and an array of extrarenal manifestations. There is a high degree of intrafamilial and interfamilial variability in the clinical expression of the disease.

ADPKD is caused by mutation in 1 of 2 genes, *PKD1* or *PKD2*, which account for 85-90% and 10-15% of cases, respectively. The proteins encoded by these genes, polycystin-1 and polycystin-2, are expressed in renal tubule cells and in cholangiocytes. Polycystin-1 functions as a mechanosensor in cilia, detecting the movement of fluid through tubules and transmitting the signal through polycystin-2, which acts as a calcium channel.

Dilated, noncommunicating cysts are most commonly observed. Other hepatic lesions are rarely associated with ADPKD, including the ductal plate malformation, congenital hepatic fibrosis, and biliary microhamartomas (the von Meyenburg complexes). Approximately 50% of patients with renal failure have demonstrable hepatic cysts that are derived from, but not in continuity with, the biliary tract. The hepatic cysts increase with age. A recent imaging study showed that prevalence of hepatic cysts was 58% in patients 15-24 yr old. Hepatic cystogenesis appears to be influenced by estrogens. Although the frequency of cysts is similar in boys and girls, the development of large hepatic cysts is mainly a complication in girls. Hepatic cysts are often asymptomatic but can cause pain and are occasionally complicated by hemorrhage, infection, jaundice from bile duct compression, portal hypertension with variceal bleeding, or hepatic venous outflow obstruction from mechanical compression of hepatic veins, resulting in tender hepatomegaly and exudative ascites. Cholangiocarcinoma can occur. Subarachnoid hemorrhage can result from the associated cerebral arterial aneurysms.

Selected patients with severe symptomatic polycystic liver disease and favorable anatomy benefit from liver resection or fenestration. Combined liver-kidney transplantation may be required.

There is considerable evidence for a role of cyclic adenosine monophosphate in epithelial proliferation and fluid secretion in experimental renal and hepatic cystic disease. Several clinical trials in adults have shown that somatostatin analogs can blunt hepatic cyst expansion by blocking secretin-induced cyclic adenosine monophosphate generation and fluid secretion by cholangiocytes.

AUTOSOMAL DOMINANT POLYCYSTIC LIVER DISEASE

Autosomal dominant polycystic liver disease is a distinct clinical and genetic identity in which multiple cysts develop and are unassociated with cystic kidney disease. Liver cysts arise from but are not in continuity with the biliary tract. Girls are more commonly affected than boys, and the cysts often enlarge during pregnancy. Cysts are rarely identified in children. Cyst complications are related to effects of local compression, infection, hemorrhage, or rupture. Genes associated with autosomal dominant polycystic liver disease are *PRKCSH* and *SEC63*, which encode hepatocystin and Sec63, respectively. Hepatocystin is a protein kinase C substrate adK-H that is involved in the proper folding and maturation of glycoproteins. It has been localized to the endoplasmic reticulum. *SEC63* encodes a protein SEC63P, which is a component of the protein translocation machinery in the endoplasmic reticulum.

A solitary liver cyst (nonparasitic) rarely occurs in childhood. Abdominal distention and pain may be present, and a poorly defined right upper quadrant mass may be palpable. These benign lesions are best left undisturbed unless they compress adjacent structures or a complication occurs, such as hemorrhage into the cyst.

Bibliography is available at Expert Consult.

Chapter **366**
Diseases of the Gallbladder

Frederick J. Suchy

ANOMALIES

The gallbladder is congenitally absent in approximately 0.1% of the population. Hypoplasia or absence of the gallbladder can be associated with extrahepatic biliary atresia or cystic fibrosis. Duplication of the gallbladder occurs rarely. Gallbladder ectopia may occur with a transverse, intrahepatic, left-sided, or retroplaced location. Multiseptate gallbladder, characterized by the presence of multiple septa dividing the gallbladder lumen, is another rare congenital anomaly of the gallbladder.

ACUTE HYDROPS

Table 366-1 lists the conditions associated with hydrops of the gallbladder.

Acute noncalculous, noninflammatory distention of the gallbladder can occur in infants and children. It is defined by the absence of calculi, bacterial infection, or congenital anomalies of the biliary system. The disorder may complicate acute infections and Kawasaki disease, but the cause is often not identified. Hydrops of the gallbladder may also develop in patients receiving long-term parenteral nutrition, presumably as a result of gallbladder stasis during the period of enteral fasting. Hydrops is distinguished from acalculous cholecystitis by the absence of a significant inflammatory process and a generally benign prognosis.

Affected patients usually have right upper quadrant pain with a palpable mass. Fever, vomiting, and jaundice may be present and are usually associated with a systemic illness such as streptococcal infection. Ultrasonography shows a markedly distended, echo-free gallbladder, without dilation of the biliary tree. Acute hydrops is usually treated conservatively with a focus on supportive care and managing the intercurrent illness; cholecystostomy and drainage are rarely needed. Spontaneous resolution and return of normal gallbladder function usually occur over a period of several wk. If a laparotomy is required, a large, edematous gallbladder is found to contain white, yellow, or green bile. Obstruction of the cystic duct by mesenteric adenopathy is occasionally observed. Cholecystectomy is required if the gallbladder is gangrenous. Pathologic examination of the gallbladder wall shows edema and mild inflammation. Cultures of bile are usually sterile.

Table 366-1	Conditions Associated with Hydrops of the Gallbladder

Kawasaki disease
Streptococcal pharyngitis
Staphylococcal infection
Leptospirosis
Ascariasis
Threadworm
Sickle cell crisis
Typhoid fever
Thalassemia
Total parenteral nutrition
Prolonged fasting
Viral hepatitis
Sepsis
Henoch-Schönlein purpura
Mesenteric adenitis
Necrotizing enterocolitis

CHOLECYSTITIS AND CHOLELITHIASIS

Acute acalculous cholecystitis is uncommon in children and is usually caused by infection. Pathogens include streptococci (groups A and B), Gram-negative organisms, particularly *Salmonella* and *Leptospira interrogans*. Parasitic infestation with *Ascaris* or *Giardia lamblia* may be found. Calculous cholecystitis may rarely follow abdominal trauma or burn injury or is associated with a systemic vasculitis, such as periarteritis nodosa.

Clinical features include right upper quadrant or epigastric pain, nausea, vomiting, fever, and jaundice. Right upper quadrant guarding and tenderness are present. Ultrasonography discloses an enlarged, thick-walled gallbladder, without calculi. Serum alkaline phosphatase activity and direct-reacting bilirubin levels are elevated. Leukocytosis is usual.

Patients may recover with treatment of systemic and biliary infection. Because the gallbladder can become gangrenous, daily ultrasonography is useful in monitoring gallbladder distention and wall thickness. Cholecystectomy is required in patients who fail to improve with conservative management. Cholecystostomy drainage is an alternative approach in a critically ill patient.

Cholelithiasis is relatively rare in otherwise healthy children, occurring more commonly in patients with various predisposing disorders (Table 366-2). In an ultrasonographic survey of 1570 children (ages 6-19 yr) the overall prevalence of gallstone disease was 0.13% (0.27% in female subjects). In children, >70% of gallstones are the pigment type, 15-20% are cholesterol stones, and the remainder are composed of a mixture of cholesterol, organic matrix, and calcium bilirubinate. Black pigment gallstones, composed mostly of calcium bilirubinate and glycoprotein matrix, are a frequent complication of chronic hemolytic anemias. Brown pigment stones form mostly in infants as a result of biliary tract infection. Unconjugated bilirubin is the predominant component, formed by the high β-glucuronidase activity of infected bile. Cholesterol gallstones are composed purely of cholesterol or contain >50% cholesterol along with a mucin glycoprotein matrix and calcium bilirubinate. Calcium carbonate stones have also been described in children.

Patients with hemolytic disease (including sickle cell anemia, the thalassemias, and red blood cell enzymopathies) and Wilson disease are at increased risk for black pigment cholelithiasis. In sickle cell disease, pigment gallstones can develop before age 4 yr and have been reported in 17-33% of patients 2-18 yr of age. Genetic variation in the promoter of uridine diphosphate-glucuronosyltransferase 1A1 (the [TA]7/[TA]7 and [TA]7/[TA]8 genotypes) underlies **Gilbert syndrome**, a relatively common, chronic form of unconjugated hyperbilirubinemia, and is a risk factor for pigment gallstone formation in sickle cell disease.

Table 366-2	Conditions Associated with Cholelithiasis

Biliary dyskinesia
Chronic hemolytic disease (sickle cell anemia, spherocytosis, thalassemia, Gilbert disease)
Ileal resection or disease
Cystic fibrosis
Cirrhosis
Cholestasis
Crohn disease
Obesity
Insulin resistance
Prolonged parenteral nutrition
Prematurity with complicated medical or surgical course
Prolonged fasting or rapid weight reduction
Treatment of childhood cancer
Abdominal surgery
Pregnancy
Sepsis
Genetic (*ABCB4*, *ABCG5/G8*) progressive familial intrahepatic cholestasis
Cephalosporins

Cirrhosis and chronic cholestasis also increase the risk for pigment gallstones. Sick premature infants may also have gallstones; their treatment is often complicated by such factors as bowel resection, necrotizing enterocolitis, prolonged parenteral nutrition without enteral feeding, cholestasis, frequent blood transfusions, and use of diuretics. Cholelithiasis in premature infants is often asymptomatic and may resolve spontaneously. Brown pigment stones are found in infants with obstructive jaundice and infected intra- and extrahepatic bile ducts. These stones are usually radiolucent, owing to a lower content of calcium phosphate and carbonate and a higher amount of cholesterol than in black pigment stones. MDR3 deficiency caused by *ABCB4* mutations) is a cholestatic syndrome related to impaired biliary phospholipid excretion. It is associated with symptomatic and recurring cholelithiasis. Patients may show intrahepatic lithiasis, sludge, or microlithiasis along the biliary tree.

Obesity has assumed an increasingly important role as a risk factor for cholesterol cholelithiasis in children, particularly in adolescent girls. Cholesterol gallstones are also found in children with disturbances of the enterohepatic circulation of bile acids, including patients with ileal disease and bile acid malabsorption, such as those with ileal resection, ileal Crohn disease, and cystic fibrosis. Pigment stones can also occur in these patients.

Cholesterol gallstone formation seems to result from an excess of cholesterol in relation to the cholesterol-carrying capacity of micelles in bile. Supersaturation of bile with cholesterol, leading to crystal and stone formation, could result from decreased bile acid or from an increased cholesterol concentration in bile. Other initiating factors that may be important in stone formation include gallbladder stasis or the presence in bile of abnormal mucoproteins or bile pigments that may serve as a nidus for cholesterol crystallization.

Prolonged use of high-dose ceftriaxone, a third-generation cephalosporin, has been associated with the formation of calcium-ceftriaxone salt precipitates *(biliary pseudolithiasis)* in the gallbladder. Biliary sludge or cholelithiasis can be detected in >40% of children who are treated with ceftriaxone for at least 10 days. In rare cases, children become jaundiced and develop abdominal pain; precipitates usually resolve spontaneously within several months after discontinuation of the drug.

Acute or chronic cholecystitis is often associated with gallstones. The acute form may be precipitated by impaction of a stone in the cystic duct. Proliferation of bacteria within the obstructed gallbladder lumen can contribute to the process and lead to biliary sepsis. Chronic calculous cholecystitis is more common. It can develop insidiously or follow several attacks of acute cholecystitis. The gallbladder epithelium commonly becomes ulcerated and scarred.

More than 50% of patients with gallstones have symptoms, and 18% present with a complication as the first indication of cholelithiasis, such as pancreatitis, choledocholithiasis or acute calculous cholecystitis. The most important clinical feature of cholelithiasis is recurrent abdominal pain, which is often colicky and localized to the right upper quadrant. An older child may have intolerance for fatty foods. Acute cholecystitis is characterized by fever, pain in the right upper quadrant, and often a palpable mass. Jaundice occurs more commonly in children than adults. Pain may radiate to an area just below the right scapula. A plain x-ray of the abdomen may reveal opaque calculi, but radiolucent (cholesterol) stones are not visualized. Accordingly, ultrasonography is the method of choice for gallstone detection. Hepatobiliary scintography is a valuable adjunct in that failure to visualize the gallbladder provides evidence of cholecystitis.

Cholecystectomy is curative. Laparoscopic cholecystectomy is routinely performed in symptomatic infants and children with cholelithiasis. Common bile duct stones are unusual in children, occurring in 2-6% of cases with cholelithiasis, often in association with obstructive jaundice and pancreatitis. Operative cholangiography should be done at the time of surgery, however, to detect unsuspected common duct calculi. Endoscopic retrograde cholangiography with extraction of common duct stones is an option before laparoscopic cholecystectomy in older children and adolescents.

Asymptomatic patients with cholelithiasis pose a more difficult management problem. Studies in adults indicate a lag time of more than a decade between initial formation of a gallstone and development of symptoms. Spontaneous resolution of cholelithiasis has been reported in infants and children. If surgery is deferred for any patient, however, parents should be counseled about signs and symptoms consistent with cholecystitis or obstruction of the common bile duct by a gallstone. In patients with chronic hemolysis or ileal disease, cholecystectomy can be carried out at the same time as another surgical procedure. Because laparoscopic surgery can safely be performed in children with sickle cell disease, elective cholecystectomy is being done more frequently at the time of gallstone diagnosis, before symptoms or complications develop. In cases associated with liver disease, severe obesity, or cystic fibrosis, the surgical risk of cholecystectomy may be substantial so that the risks and benefits of the operation need to be carefully considered.

BILIARY DYSKINESIA

Biliary dyskinesia is a motility disorder of the biliary tract that may cause acalculous biliary colic in children, often in association with nausea and fatty food intolerance. There are usually no gallstones on imaging. Sphincter of Oddi dysfunction may be a variant that can present with chronic abdominal pain and recurrent pancreatitis. The diagnosis is based on a cholecystokinin–diisopropyl iminodiacetic acid scan demonstrating a gallbladder ejection fraction of less than 35%. Reproduction of pain on cholecystokinin administration may also be seen, as well as the absence of gallbladder filling on an otherwise normal ultrasound examination. In several recent reports, laparoscopic cholecystectomy was effective in providing both short-term and long-term improvement of symptoms in most children with biliary dyskinesia.

Bibliography is available at Expert Consult.

Chapter 367
Portal Hypertension and Varices
Frederick J. Suchy

Portal hypertension, defined as an elevation of portal pressure >10-12 mm Hg, is a major cause of morbidity and mortality in children with liver disease. The normal portal venous pressure is approximately 7 mm Hg. The clinical features of the various forms of portal hypertension may be similar, but the associated complications, management, and prognosis can vary significantly and depend on whether the process is complicated by hepatic insufficiency.

ETIOLOGY

Portal hypertension can result from obstruction to portal blood flow anywhere along the course of the portal venous system. Table 367-1 outlines the various disorders associated with portal hypertension. Portal hypertension can occur as a result of prehepatic, intrahepatic, or posthepatic obstruction to the flow of portal blood.

Extrahepatic portal vein obstruction is an important cause of portal hypertension in childhood. The obstruction can occur at any level of the portal vein. Umbilical infection (**omphalitis**) with or without a history of catheterization of the umbilical vein may be causal in neonates. The infection can potentially spread from the umbilical vein to the left branch of the portal vein and eventually to the main portal venous channel. Intraabdominal infections, including acute

EXTRAHEPATIC PORTAL HYPERTENSION
Portal vein agenesis, atresia, stenosis
Portal vein thrombosis or cavernous transformation
Splenic vein thrombosis
Increased portal flow
Arteriovenous fistula

INTRAHEPATIC PORTAL HYPERTENSION
Hepatocellular disease
Acute and chronic viral hepatitis
Cirrhosis
Congenital hepatic fibrosis
Wilson disease
α_1-Antitrypsin deficiency
Glycogen storage disease type IV
Hepatotoxicity
Methotrexate
Parenteral nutrition
Biliary tract disease
Extrahepatic biliary atresia
Cystic fibrosis
Choledochal cyst
Sclerosing cholangitis
Intrahepatic bile duct paucity
Idiopathic portal hypertension
Postsinusoidal obstruction
Budd-Chiari syndrome
Venoocclusive disease

appendicitis and primary peritonitis, can be causal in older children. Portal vein thrombosis is also associated with neonatal dehydration and systemic infection. In older children, inflammatory bowel disease can be associated with a hypercoagulable state and portal venous obstruction. Thrombosis of the portal vein has also occurred in association with biliary tract infections and primary sclerosing cholangitis. **Portal vein thrombosis** is associated with hypercoagulable states, such as deficiencies of factor V Leiden, protein C, or protein S. The portal vein can be replaced by a fibrous remnant or contain an organized thrombus. Rare developmental anomalies producing extrahepatic portal hypertension include agenesis, atresia, or stenosis of the portal vein. Obstruction by a web or diaphragm can also occur. At least half of reported cases have no defined cause.

Uncommonly, presinusoidal hypertension can be caused by increased flow through the portal system as a result of a congenital or acquired arteriovenous fistula.

The intrahepatic causes of portal hypertension are numerous. Obstruction to flow can occur on the basis of a presinusoidal process, including acute and chronic hepatitis, congenital hepatic fibrosis, and schistosomiasis. Portal infiltration with malignant cells or granulomas can also contribute. An idiopathic form of portal hypertension characterized by splenomegaly, hypersplenism, and portal hypertension without occlusion of portal or splenic veins and with no obvious disease in the liver has been described. In some patients, noncirrhotic portal fibrosis has been observed.

Cirrhosis is the predominant cause of portal hypertension and is related to obstruction of blood flow through the portal vein. The numerous causes of cirrhosis include recognized disorders such as biliary atresia, autoimmune hepatitis, chronic viral hepatitis, and metabolic liver disease such as α_1-antitrypsin deficiency, Wilson disease, glycogen storage disease type IV, hereditary fructose intolerance, and cystic fibrosis.

Postsinusoidal causes of portal hypertension are also observed in childhood. The **Budd-Chiari syndrome** occurs with obstruction to hepatic veins anywhere between the efferent hepatic veins and the entry of the inferior vena cava into the right atrium. In most cases, no specific cause can be found, but thrombosis can occur from inherited and acquired hypercoagulable states (antithrombin III deficiency,

protein C or S deficiency, factor V Leiden or prothrombin mutations, paroxysmal nocturnal hemoglobinemia, pregnancy, oral contraceptives) and can complicate hepatic or metastatic neoplasms, collagen vascular disease, infection, and trauma. Additional causes of the Budd-Chiari syndrome include Behçet syndrome, inflammatory bowel disease, aspergillosis, dacarbazine therapy, and inferior vena cava webs.

Sinusoidal obstruction syndrome (venoocclusive disease) is the most common cause of hepatic vein obstruction in children. In this disorder, occlusion of the centrilobular venules or sublobular hepatic veins occurs. The disorder occurs after total body irradiation with or without cytotoxic drug therapy that is commonly used before bone marrow transplantation. The disease has also occurred after ingestion of herbal remedies containing the pyrrolizidine alkaloids, which are sometimes taken as medicinal teas.

PATHOPHYSIOLOGY

The primary hemodynamic abnormality in portal hypertension is increased resistance to portal blood flow. This is the case whether the resistance to portal flow has an intrahepatic cause such as cirrhosis or is due to portal vein obstruction. Portosystemic shunting should decompress the portal system and thus significantly lower portal pressures. Despite the development of significant collaterals deviating portal blood into systemic veins, portal hypertension is maintained by an overall increase in portal venous flow and thus maintenance of portal hypertension. A hyperdynamic circulation is achieved by tachycardia, an increase in cardiac output, and decreased systemic vascular resistance. Splanchnic dilation also occurs. Overall, the increase in portal flow likely contributes to an increase in variceal transmural pressure. The increase in portal blood flow is related to the contribution of hepatic and collateral flow; the actual portal blood flow reaching the liver is reduced. It is also likely that hepatocellular dysfunction and portosystemic shunting lead to the generation of various humoral factors that cause vasodilation and an increase in plasma volume.

Many complications of the portal hypertension can be accounted for by the development of a remarkable collateral circulation. Collateral vessels can form prominently in areas in which absorptive epithelium joins stratified epithelium, particularly in the esophagus or anorectal region. The superficial submucosal collaterals, especially those in the esophagus and stomach and, to a lesser extent, those in the duodenum, colon, or rectum, are prone to rupture and bleeding under increased pressure. In portal hypertension, the vascularity of the stomach is also abnormal and demonstrates prominent submucosal arteriovenous communications between the muscularis mucosa and dilated precapillaries and veins. The resulting lesion, a vascular ectasia, has been called **congestive gastropathy** and contributes to a significant risk of bleeding from the stomach.

CLINICAL MANIFESTATIONS

Bleeding from esophageal varices is the most common presentation. Less commonly, patients bleed from varices around a stoma or from anorectal varices. In patients with underlying hepatic disease, physical examination might show jaundice and stigmata of cirrhosis such as palmar erythema and vascular telangiectasias. Growth retardation can occur in patients with cirrhosis and, to a lesser extent, in children with isolated extrahepatic portal vein obstruction. Ascites may be present in patients with intrahepatic causes of portal hypertension and can transiently occur with portal vein obstruction. Dilated cutaneous collateral vessels carrying blood from the portal to systemic circulation may be apparent in the periumbilical region. In the absence of clinical or biochemical features of liver disease and with a liver of normal size, portal vein obstruction is most likely. Well-compensated cirrhosis cannot be completely ruled out under these conditions. Cholestasis and liver dysfunction with elevated serum bilirubin and aminotransferases occur uncommonly in portal vein obstruction as a result of external compression of bile ducts by cavernous transformation of the portal vein. This complication is called **portal hypertensive biliopathy**.

An enlarged, hard liver with minimal disturbance of hepatic function suggests the possibility of congenital hepatic fibrosis.

Hemorrhage, particularly in children with portal vein obstruction, can be precipitated by minor febrile, intercurrent illness. The mechanism is often unclear; aspirin or other nonsteroidal antiinflammatory drugs may be a contributing factor by damaging the integrity of a congested gastric mucosa or interfering with platelet function. Coughing during a respiratory illness can also increase intravariceal pressure. The bleeding may become apparent with hematemesis or with melena. Gastrointestinal hemorrhage can also originate from portal hypertensive gastropathy or from gastric, duodenal, peristomal, or rectal varices.

Splenomegaly, sometimes with hypersplenism, is the next most common presenting feature in portal vein obstruction and may be discovered first on routine physical examination. Because more than half of patients in many series with portal vein obstruction do not experience bleeding until after age 6 yr, the diagnosis should be suggested in a child without hepatocellular disease who had a complicated neonatal course and in whom asymptomatic splenomegaly later developed. Long-term follow-up of patients with portal vein obstruction has revealed a variety of complications including variceal hemorrhage, hypersplenism, biliary obstruction, growth and development retardation, and neuropsychiatric dysfunction.

Children with portal hypertension, regardless of the underlying cause, may have recurrent bouts of life-threatening hemorrhage. In patients with portal vein obstruction and normal hepatic function, the bleeding usually stops spontaneously. In patients with intrahepatic disease, the combination of portal hypertension and poor liver synthetic ability (coagulopathy) can make bleeding much more difficult to control. Moreover, esophageal hemorrhage and cirrhosis can have injurious effects on the liver, further impairing hepatic function and sometimes precipitating jaundice, ascites, and encephalopathy. Blood in the intestinal lumen can promote bacterial translocation, leading to peritonitis. Another serious complication is the hepatopulmonary syndrome, which develops in ≥10% of patients with portal hypertension. It is defined as an arterial oxygenation defect induced by intrapulmonary microvascular dilation, resulting from release of a number of endogenous vasoactive molecules, including endothelin-1 and nitric oxide into the venous circulation.

DIAGNOSIS

In patients with established chronic liver disease or in those in whom portal vein obstruction is suspected, an experienced ultrasonographer should be able to demonstrate the patency of the portal vein, and Doppler flow ultrasonography can demonstrate the direction of flow within the portal system. The pattern of flow correlates with the severity of cirrhosis and encephalopathy. Reversal of portal vein blood flow (hepatofugal flow) is more likely to be associated with variceal bleeding. Ultrasonography is also effective in detecting the presence of esophageal varices. Another important feature of extrahepatic portal vein obstruction is cavernous transformation of the portal vein, in which an extensive complex of small collateral vessels form in the paracholedochal and epicholedochal venous system to bypass the obstruction. Other imaging techniques also contribute to further definition of the portal vein anatomy but are required less often; contrast-enhanced CT and magnetic resonance angiography provide information similar to ultrasonography. Selective arteriography of the celiac axis, superior mesenteric artery, and splenic vein may be useful in precise mapping of the extrahepatic vascular anatomy. This is not required to establish a diagnosis but can prove valuable in planning surgical decompression of portal hypertension. The platelet count, spleen length measured by ultrasonography, and serum albumin are the best noninvasive predictors of portal hypertension in children.

In a patient with hypoxia (**hepatopulmonary syndrome**), intrapulmonary microvascular dilation is demonstrated with contrast-enhanced echocardiography that shows delayed appearance in the left heart of microbubbles from a saline bolus injected into a peripheral vein.

Endoscopy is the most reliable method for detecting esophageal varices and for identifying the source of gastrointestinal bleeding.

Although bleeding from esophageal or gastric varices is most common in children with portal hypertension, up to one third of patients, particularly those with cirrhosis, have bleeding from some other source such as portal hypertensive gastropathy or gastric or duodenal ulcerations. There is a strong correlation between variceal size as assessed endoscopically and the probability of hemorrhage. Red spots apparent over varices at the time of endoscopy are a strong predictor of imminent hemorrhage.

TREATMENT

The therapy of portal hypertension can be divided into emergency treatment of potentially life-threatening hemorrhage and prophylaxis directed at prevention of initial or subsequent bleeding. It must be emphasized that the use of many therapies is based on experience in adults with portal hypertension. There is a lack of rigorous studies on the ability of endoscopy screening, endoscopic treatment of varices, and use of nonselective β-blockers to alter the outcome of portal hypertension in children.

Treatment of patients with variceal hemorrhage must focus on fluid resuscitation, initially in the form of crystalloid infusion, followed by the replacement of red blood cells. Correction of coagulopathy by administration of vitamin K and/or infusion of platelets or fresh-frozen plasma may be required. A nasogastric tube should be placed to document the presence of blood within the stomach and to monitor for ongoing bleeding. An H_2-receptor blocker or proton pump inhibitor should be given intravenously to reduce the risk of bleeding from gastric erosions. In most patients, particularly those with extrahepatic portal hypertension and with normal hepatic synthetic function, bleeding usually stops spontaneously. Care should be taken in fluid resuscitation of children after bleeding to avoid producing an excessively high venous pressure and increasing risk for further bleeding.

Pharmacologic therapy to decrease portal pressure may be considered in patients with continued bleeding. Vasopressin or one of its analogs is commonly used and is thought to act by increasing splanchnic vascular tone and thus decreasing portal blood flow. Vasopressin is administered initially with a bolus of 0.33 units/kg over 20 min, followed by a continued infusion of the same dose on an hourly basis or a continuous infusion of 0.2 units/1.73 m²/min. The drug has a half-life of approximately 30 min. Its use may be limited by the side effects of vasoconstriction, which can impair cardiac function and perfusion to the heart, bowel, and kidneys and can also, as a result, exacerbate fluid retention. Nitroglycerin, usually given as a portion of a skin patch, has also been used to decrease portal pressure and, when used in conjunction with vasopressin, can ameliorate some of its untoward effects. The somatostatin analog octreotide is more commonly used, and it decreases splanchnic blood flow with fewer side effects. It may be administered by continuous intravenous infusion of 1.0-5.0 μg/kg/hr. However, the use of octreotide in adults with variceal hemorrhage has not been associated with a reduction in rates of rebleeding or mortality. Its use and efficacy in children have not been rigorously evaluated.

After an episode of variceal hemorrhage or in patients in whom bleeding cannot be controlled, endoscopic sclerosis or elastic band ligation of esophageal varices are important options. In endoscopic sclerosis, sclerosants are injected either intravariceally or paravariceally until bleeding has stopped. Although bleeding can be controlled acutely in most cases, further sessions of sclerotherapy are required to achieve temporary obliteration of the varices. Treatments may be associated with further bleeding, bacteremia, esophageal ulceration, and stricture formation. Most centers do not perform endoscopic sclerotherapy of varices prophylactically but use the procedure as a bridge to the time of liver transplantation or a surgical shunting procedure. Endoscopic elastic band ligation of varices has been shown in adult and pediatric studies to be more effective and associated with fewer complications than is sclerotherapy.

In patients who continue to bleed despite pharmacologic and endoscopic methods to control hemorrhage, a Sengstaken-Blakemore tube may be placed to stop hemorrhage by mechanically compressing esophageal and gastric varices. The device is rarely used now, but it may be the only option to control life-threatening hemorrhage. It carries a significant rate of complications and a high rate of bleeding when the device is removed, and it poses a particularly high risk for pulmonary aspiration. The tube is not well tolerated in children without significant sedation.

Various surgical procedures have been devised to divert portal blood flow and to decrease portal pressure. A portacaval shunt diverts nearly all of the portal blood flow into the subhepatic inferior right vena cava. Although portal pressure is significantly reduced, because of the significant diversion of blood from the liver, patients with parenchymal liver disease have a marked risk for hepatic encephalopathy. Even mild hepatic encephalopathy can impair cognitive function, including school performance. More selective shunting procedures, such as mesocaval or distal splenorenal shunt, can effectively decompress the portal system while allowing a greater amount of portal blood flow to the liver. The small size of the vessels makes these operations technically challenging in infants and small children, and there is a significant risk of failure as a result of shunt thrombosis. A shunt may be good option in a child with relatively well-preserved liver function, as sometimes occurs in patients with biliary atresia, congenital hepatic fibrosis, or cystic fibrosis. Portal vein thrombosis has been managed with the Rex shunt (superior mesenteric vein to left portal vein bypass), which restores physiologic portal blood flow and inflow of hepatotrophic factors. Growth and cognitive function improve after this procedure.

A transjugular intrahepatic portosystemic shunt, in which a stent is placed by an interventional radiologist between the right hepatic vein and the right or left branch of the portal vein, can aid in the management of portal hypertension in children, especially in those needing temporary relief before liver transplantation. The transjugular intrahepatic portosystemic shunt procedure can precipitate hepatic encephalopathy and is prone to thrombosis.

Orthotopic liver transplantation represents a much better therapy for portal hypertension resulting from intrahepatic disease and cirrhosis. A prior portosystemic shunting operation does not preclude a successful liver transplantation but makes the operation technically more difficult.

Long-term treatment with nonspecific β-blockers, such as propranolol, has been used extensively in adults with portal hypertension. These agents might act by lowering cardiac output and portal perfusion. Evidence in adult patients shows that β-blockers can reduce the incidence of variceal hemorrhage and improve long-term survival. A therapeutic effect is thought to result when the pulse rate is reduced by ≥25%. There is limited published experience with the use of this therapy in children.

PROGNOSIS
Portal hypertension secondary to intrahepatic disease has a poor prognosis. Portal hypertension is usually progressive in these patients and is often associated with deteriorating liver function. Efforts should be directed toward prompt treatment of acute bleeding and prevention of recurrent hemorrhage with available methods. Patients with progressive liver disease and significant esophageal varices ultimately require orthotopic liver transplantation. Liver transplantation is the only effective therapy for hepatopulmonary syndrome and should also be considered for patients with portal hypertension secondary to hepatic vein obstruction or resulting from severe venoocclusive disease.

In patients with portal vein obstruction, episodes of bleeding can become less frequent and severe with age as a collateral circulation develops, >50% experience bleeding during adolescence. Neurocognitive defects diagnosed by careful psychologic testing indicate portosystemic encephalopathy caused by naturally occurring portosystemic shunts. Progressive liver disease can occur later as a consequence of bile duct compression from dilated collateral venous channels (portal biliopathy). These complications can be treated or prevented by the Rex shunt.

Bibliography is available at Expert Consult.

Chapter 368
Liver Transplantation
Jorge D. Reyes and Evelyn Hsu

Refinements in the management of hepatic failure, organ procurement and implantation techniques, organ preservation, perioperative care, and the development of effective immunosuppressive management (cyclosporine in 1978 and tacrolimus in 1989) survival rates for liver transplantation is now >90%. Complications inherent in the toxicity/infection profile of immunosuppressive drug therapy have occurred and enhancements in our understanding of the relationship between recipient and host immune systems have resulted in the development of tailored immunotherapy. In addition, the search for "tolerance" enhancing protocols, which could lead to transplantation without the need for long-term immunosuppression. The creation of a national system for matching these donor organs with waiting recipients (the Organ Procurement and Transplantation Network and the United Network for Organ Sharing [UNOS]) provides equitable sharing of this scarce organ resource to the neediest patients with the adoption of the Pediatric End-Stage Liver Disease and Medical End-Stage Liver Disease (for adolescents) scoring systems.

INDICATIONS
The diseases for which liver transplantation is indicated can be categorized into the following groups:
- Obstructive biliary tract disease: biliary atresia, sclerosing cholangitis, traumatic or postsurgical injury
- Metabolic disorders: α_1-antitrypsin deficiency, tyrosinemia type I, glycogen storage disease type IV, Wilson disease, neonatal hemochromatosis, Crigler-Najjar type I, familial hypercholesterolemia, primary oxalosis, organic academia, urea cycle defects
- Acute hepatitis: fulminant hepatic failure, viral, toxin, or drug induced
- Chronic hepatitis with cirrhosis: hepatitis B or C, autoimmune
- Intrahepatic cholestasis: idiopathic neonatal hepatitis, Alagille syndrome, progressive familial intrahepatic cholestasis
- Miscellaneous: cryptogenic cirrhosis, congenital hepatic fibrosis, Caroli disease, cystic fibrosis, polycystic kidney and liver disease, cirrhosis induced by total parenteral nutrition
- Primary liver tumors: benign tumors (hamartomas, hemangioendothelioma), unresectable hepatoblastoma, and hepatocellular carcinoma
- Emerging indications: graft-versus-host-disease (a complication of bone marrow transplantation), hemophilia, and portosystemic shunts

Biliary atresia is the most common indication for liver transplantation in children, followed by metabolic and inborn disorders, autoimmune and familial cholestatic disorders, and acute hepatic necrosis.

Biliary atresia may present with 2 clinical patterns: an acquired form for which there may be nonrandom clustering of potential etiologies (80% of cases), and a syndromic/embryonic form that includes other anomalies, such as polysplenia or asplenia, preduodenal portal vein, intestinal malrotation, situs anomalies, and absence of the retrohepatic vena cava. Hepatoportoenterostomy may benefit survival if performed within the 1st 30 days of life, however, some patients with successful drainage later develop cirrhosis with portal hypertension (variceal bleeding and ascites). Children with biliary atresia (or any other obstructive biliary disorder) who do not achieve successful drainage require liver transplantation within the 1st yr of life.

Inborn errors of metabolism result from a single enzyme deficiency that results in alteration of synthesis, breakdown, transport, or function of carbohydrate, fat, or protein. They can be grouped into those diseases which cause structural damage and cirrhosis, and potentially end-stage liver disease, as well as liver cancer (i.e., α_1-antitrypsin deficiency, Wilson disease, cystic fibrosis, progressive familial intrahepatic cholestasis), and those inborn errors that manifest principally by their hepatic enzyme deficiency with no hepatocellular injury; complications occur in "satellite" systems such as the brain (hyperammonemic conditions), the kidney (hyperoxaluria type 1), or heart (familial hypercholesterolemia). Some metabolic disorders place patients at risk for decompensation throughout their entire lives, and others (e.g., Crigler-Najjar) manifest principally after adolescence. Liver transplantation replaces the enzyme deficiency; the value and risk benefit of doing so in the absence of cirrhosis has prompted the pursuit of gene therapy and hepatocyte transplantation as possible alternatives, but their therapeutic benefit is yet to be determined.

Although many patients with **fulminant hepatic failure** will survive without transplant, it accounts for approximately 13% of pediatric liver transplantation and has required the most intense concentration of multimodal management/support, and organ graft options yet devised. It is a diagnosis without clear etiology in more than 50% of cases, and posttransplantation survival varies but is generally poor because of multifactorial issues related to comorbidities and listing/transplantation graft option availability.

Primary hepatic malignancies in children are rare (<2% of all pediatric malignancies), and account for a little less than 10% of transplants. Hepatoblastoma accounts for the majority of cases (75% of primary liver tumors in childhood) and is usually of an advanced stage, yet adjuvant chemotherapy and total hepatectomy with transplantation provide cure and long-term survival for the majority of patients thus treated. Survival of >85% has been reported by the International Society of Pediatric Oncology and several American centers.

Some diseases do not produce life-threatening complications, yet their impact on growth, development, and quality of life can be so devastating that liver transplantation is a valid therapy and cure. The distribution of liver grafts does follow guidelines based on severity of liver disease as reflected in the Pediatric End-Stage Liver Disease scoring system developed by UNOS, which takes into calculation the measurable values of bilirubin, creatinine, and international normalization ratio.

Contraindications to liver transplantation include uncontrolled infection of extrahepatic origin, uncontrolled extrahepatic malignancies, and severely disabling and uncorrectable disease in other organ systems, principally the heart and lungs. Although combined liver and heart or lung transplantation has been performed in adults and children, such cases require special consideration and centers dedicated to the complexities of posttransplantation management. Also, disabling neurologic disease can preclude liver transplantation if the outcome will not allow the child to develop some measure of independence and quality of life.

TECHNICAL INNOVATIONS

There are no limitations on age or weight for liver transplantation, a consequence to improved posttransplantation outcomes as a result of improvements in perioperative management (recipient selection, care, and timing of transplantation as well as intra- and posttransplantation care), and to the development and successful transplantation of segmental liver grafts.

To enhance the availability of liver grafts to children and optimize the timing of transplantation, the use of reduced-size or segmental grafts (a right or left lobe of liver, or the left lateral segment of the left lobe) were developed; this advancement allows the selection of a liver from a larger donor for implantation into a child, thus correcting the size mismatch. Because liver reduction inherently removes a potential graft for an adult recipient, techniques were developed for the use of segments from living donors (using usually the left lateral segment for small pediatric recipients), and then split-liver grafts from deceased

donors where the left lateral segment is transplanted into a child and the leftover segment of right lobe and medial segment of left lobe (essentially a right trisegment graft) are transplanted into an adult. Reduction of a liver graft is performed ex vivo; split-liver grafts can be accomplished either ex vivo or in situ (in the hemodynamically stable brain-dead donor). Donors suitable for aforementioned graft variants should ideally be young (younger than 45 yr of age), healthy, and nonobese; however, variations are guided by the severity of illness and urgency for transplantation of the recipient.

The implantation of a liver (either whole organ or segment) involves removal of the native liver and encompasses 4 anastomoses: the suprahepatic vena cava, the portal vein, the hepatic artery, and the bile duct. Modifications of the procedure generally involve retaining (or not) of the retrohepatic vena cava, the performance (or not) of a temporary portocaval shunt to decompress the splanchnic venous system during the anhepatic phase, and the use of vascular homografts of donor iliac vein or artery to replace the native inflow (guided by the presence of recipient anomalies or thrombosis of native vessels). The donor bile duct may be connected to a loop of recipient intestine (Roux-en-Y limb) or the native bile duct.

UNOS reported outcomes analyzing graft types and outcomes have shown improved graft survival in children younger than 3 yr of age for live donor grafts when compared to deceased donor whole, split, and reduced grafts. After the 1st yr, however, patient and allograft survivals were similar regardless of whether the graft was a whole liver, deceased donor segment, or living donor.

IMMUNOSUPPRESSION

The goal of effective clinical immunosuppression after solid-organ transplantation is to inhibit antigen-induced T-lymphocyte activation and cytokine production, interrupt allo–major histocompatibility complex recognition, or block effector responses. To prevent overly weakening the host response to infection, these effects should be accomplished while preserving immunocompetence. A major emphasis is the prevention of acute and chronic rejection and the ability to reverse refractory acute rejection. These efforts have been, for the most part, successful; the current challenge is long-term survival and quality of life, inherently involving strategies to minimize the long-term toxicity of immunosuppressive drug therapy, which can include renal failure, cardiovascular complications, and infections. Studies have led to a better understanding of lymphocyte subsets and function, the discovery that rejection could be reversed with steroids or antilymphocyte globulin, and then the realization that long-lasting donor-specific unresponsiveness could be achieved with less drug therapy, while preserving immunocompetence.

Immediately peri- or posttransplantation therapy may involve antilymphocyte antibody induction with depleting antibodies (monoclonal or polyclonal) such as antithymocyte globulin antibody, or the use of a chimeric mouse–human antibody that blocks the interleukin-2 receptor of the T cell, thus preventing activation and replication of antigen-selected T cells. Corticosteroids act through the suppression of antibody production and cytokine synthesis (interleukin-2, and interferon-γ), decreasing proliferation of T cells (helper, suppressor, and cytotoxic), B cells, and neutrophils. Maintenance immunosuppression is achieved through the use of calcineurin phosphatase inhibitor activity using drugs such as cyclosporine or tacrolimus; these drugs interfere with the production and release of interleukin-2 which plays a critical role in the cytotoxic T-cell response, thus inhibiting T-cell–mediated acute cellular rejection. Tacrolimus has shown to be a more powerful drug, however, the ability to progress or initiate maintenance immunosuppression in the absence of corticosteroids is of particular benefit in the children. Other drugs, such as azathioprine or mycophenolate mofetil, which inhibit the synthesis of purine nucleosides and thus the proliferation of T and B lymphocytes and antibody formation, may be added to enhance the antirejection profile, allow for decrease in the calcineurin dosage, or manage chronic rejection. Rapamycin, a macrolide which binds its' molecular target of mammalian target of rapamycin receptor, decreases interleukin-2 production, and thus T- and B-cell activation and proliferation.

COMPLICATIONS

Posttransplantation complications can be related to the pretransplantation condition of the recipient and the donor match and type, immunologic responses to the graft and the need for enhanced immunosuppressive drug therapy, and toxicity effects of these drugs or infections from over-immunosuppression. They can occur at varying specific frequencies over a fairly well-defined time course (early, late, remote).

The most predictable complications involve those inherent to the transplantation operation and include primary nonfunction of the graft (rare in pediatric recipients given the selection criteria of potential donors); hepatic artery thrombosis is the most frequent and early vascular complication, occurring in 5-10% of recipients and can have devastating consequences on the graft (acute necrosis and gangrene, and biliary leaks/stricture/bilomas), which may require urgent retransplantation; portal vein or hepatic vein strictures/occlusions are rare and generally occur later posttransplantation. Biliary strictures are the most frequent surgical complication (10-30%) after liver transplantation and should be included in the differential diagnosis of any posttransplantation liver allograft dysfunction. Management of these complication varies and may include interventional radiologic procedures, reoperation, or retransplantation.

Rejection usually occurs after the 1st 2 wk after transplantation, with the highest incidence (30-60%) within the 1st 90 days. Diagnosis is suspected based on abnormal liver function studies, and rarely are there systemic signs such as fever, abdominal pain, new-onset ascites or hydrothorax; the diagnosis requires biopsy confirmation; treatment algorithms include high doses of corticosteroids and antilymphocyte antibodies. Chronic rejection is less frequent (5-10%) and is characterized by progressive damage and loss of bile ductules with consequent cholestasis; treatment involves long-term enhancement of maintenance immunosuppression with corticosteroids and other agents.

The need to treat rejection can place the patient at a higher risk of drug toxicity or infection. The most common transplantation-related infections are cytomegalovirus and Epstein-Barr virus infections, for which there are well-developed algorithms of prophylaxis. Epstein-Barr virus-induced **posttransplant lymphoproliferative disease** represents a unique complication of over-immunosuppression and infection occurring in approximately 10% of patients, and that has been managed by withdrawal of immunosuppression and antiviral therapy; some patients require chemotherapy.

OUTCOMES

The clinical, surgical, and immunosuppressive drug therapy advances since the 1990s have dramatically improved survival of liver transplantation in children. The SPLIT registry data (1092 patients in North America transplanted since 1995) demonstrate 1-yr patient and graft survival of 86.3% and 80.2%, respectively. UNOS data reveal a 1 yr patient and graft survival for biliary atresia of 95% and 87% respectively. Longer-term survival is inherently dependent on adequacy of long term immunosuppression management, adherence to care protocols, and prevention of infection/toxicities/chronic rejection.

With longer survival times, the issues of growth, quality of life, and patient loss with a functioning graft have come to the forefront. The goals have been reset to seek the induction protocols and strategies that can foster minimization of drug therapy and even a drug-free state, the induction of tolerance.

Bibliography is available at Expert Consult.

Section 7
Peritoneum

Chapter 369
Malformations
Melissa Kennedy and Chris A. Liacouras

Congenital peritoneal bands represent anatomically unabsorbed portions of omentum and mesentery and most commonly occur in the regions of the duodenum, duodenojejunal flexure, ileocecal junction, and ascending colon. Although usually benign, they may be responsible for intestinal obstruction or midgut volvulus and resulting intestinal necrosis. Intraabdominal herniations infrequently occur through ring-like formations produced by anomalous peritoneal bands. Numerous other anomalies can occur in the course of the development of the peritoneum but are rarely of clinical importance. Absence of the omentum or its duplication occurs rarely. Omental cysts arise in obstructed lymphatic channels within the omentum. They may be congenital or can result from trauma and are usually asymptomatic. Abdominal pain or partial small bowel obstruction can result from compression or torsion of the small bowel from traction on the omentum.

Bibliography is available at Expert Consult.

Chapter 370
Ascites
Melissa Kennedy and Chris A. Liacouras

Ascites is the pathologic accumulation of fluid within the peritoneal cavity. Multiple causes of ascites have been described (Table 370-1). In children, hepatic and renal disease are the most common causes, but ascites can also be caused by cardiac disease, trauma, infection, or neoplasia.

The clinical hallmark of ascites is abdominal distention. Early satiety and dyspnea can occur with a moderate amount of ascites. Considerable intraperitoneal fluid can accumulate before ascites is detectable by the classic physical signs: bulging flanks, dullness to percussion, shifting dullness, a fluid wave, and the "puddle sign" (percussion of a supine person's abdomen over the umbilicus becomes dull as the patient is moved to a prone position and ascitic fluid puddles in dependent regions). Umbilical herniation can be associated with tense ascites. Ultrasound examination is useful for detecting small amounts of ascites.

Abdominal paracentesis can provide symptomatic relief and may be diagnostic of the cause of the ascites. Determining the serum-ascites albumin gradient can help to determine the cause of ascites. A gradient greater than 1.1 g/dL (high-gradient ascites) is consistent with ascites caused by portal hypertension, whereas a gradient <1.1 g/dL (low-gradient ascites) indicates ascites of nonportal-hypertensive etiology.

The course, prognosis, and treatment of ascites depend entirely on the cause. For most patients, treatment consists of dietary sodium restriction and diuretic therapy with spironolactone, with the addition of furosemide in more severe cases. Supplemental albumin can also aid in ascitic fluid mobilization. Refractory cases may require large volume paracentesis or transjugular intrahepatic portosystemic shunting.

Table 370-1	Causes of Ascites

HEPATIC
Cirrhosis
Congenital hepatic fibrosis
Portal vein obstruction
Fulminant hepatic failure
Budd-Chiari syndrome
Lysosomal storage disease

RENAL
Nephrotic syndrome
Obstructive uropathy
Perforation of urinary tract
Peritoneal dialysis

CARDIAC
Heart failure
Constrictive pericarditis
Inferior vena cava web

INFECTIOUS
Abscess
Tuberculosis
Chlamydia
Schistosomiasis

GASTROINTESTINAL
Infarcted bowel
Perforation
Protein-losing enteropathy

NEOPLASTIC
Lymphoma
Neuroblastoma

GYNECOLOGIC
Ovarian tumors
Ovarian torsion, rupture

PANCREATIC
Pancreatitis
Ruptured pancreatic duct

MISCELLANEOUS
Systemic lupus erythematosus
Autoinflammatory recurrent fever syndromes
Ventriculoperitoneal shunt
Eosinophilic ascites
Chylous ascites
Hypothyroidism

Patients with any type of ascites are at increased risk for spontaneous bacterial peritonitis.

Bibliography is available at Expert Consult.

370.1 Chylous Ascites
Jessica W. Wen and Chris A. Liacouras

Chylous ascites refers to peritoneal fluid that contains lymphatic drainage with a characteristic milky appearance that is rich in triglycerides. Chylous ascites can result from congenital anomaly, injury, or obstruction of the intra-abdominal portion of the thoracic duct. Although uncommon, it can occur at any age. In the pediatric population, the most common cause is lymphatic malformation. Other causes include surgical injury to the lymphatics, trauma, cirrhosis, peritoneal bands, generalized lymphangiomatosis, chronic inflammatory processes of the bowel, and mycobacterial infection. Malignancy is a fairly common cause in the adult population but uncommon in pediatrics. Congenital anomalies of the lymphatic system can be associated with Turner, Noonan, yellow nail, and Klippel-Trenaunay-Weber syndromes.

The most common presentation is painless abdominal distention, and it may be accompanied by poor weight gain and loose stools. Peripheral edema is common. Massive chylous ascites can result in scrotal edema, inguinal and umbilical herniation, and respiratory difficulties.

Diagnosis of chylous ascites depends on the demonstration of milky ascitic fluid obtained via paracentesis after a fat-containing feeding. Ascites fluid analysis reveals high protein content, elevated triglycerides, and lymphocytosis. If the patient has had nothing by mouth, the fluid may appear serous. Hypoalbuminemia, hypogammaglobulinemia, and lymphopenia are common in these patients.

Treatment includes a high-protein, low-fat diet supplemented with medium-chain triglycerides that are absorbed directly into the portal circulation and decrease lymph production. Parenteral alimentation may be necessary if nutrition remains impaired on oral feedings this may also significantly decrease lymph flow and facilitate sealing at the point of lymph leakage. Octreotide, a somatostatin analog, has been used by subcutaneous route in chylous ascites. The mechanism is not clearly understood; however, it decreases intestinal blood flow leading to decreased portal pressure and it also inhibits lymphatic secretion through somatostatin receptors in the intestinal wall. Paracentesis should be repeated only if abdominal distention causes respiratory distress. Laparotomy may be indicated to search for the site of the leakage if a trial of dietary management has been unsuccessful and a lymphangiogram demonstrates site of leakage.

Bibliography is available at Expert Consult.

Chapter 371
Peritonitis
Jessica W. Wen and Chris A. Liacouras

Inflammation of the peritoneal lining of the abdominal cavity can result from infectious, autoimmune, neoplastic, and chemical processes. Infectious peritonitis is usually defined as primary (spontaneous) or secondary. In primary peritonitis, the source of infection originates outside the abdomen and seeds the peritoneal cavity via hematogenous, lymphatic, or transmural spread. Secondary peritonitis arises from the abdominal cavity itself through extension from or rupture of an intraabdominal viscus or an abscess within an organ. Tertiary peritonitis refers to recurrent diffuse or localized disease and is associated with poorer outcomes than secondary peritonitis.

Clinically, patients have abdominal pain, abdominal tenderness, and rigidity on exam. Peritonitis can result from rupture of a hollow viscus, such as the appendix or a Meckel diverticulum; disruption of the peritoneum from trauma or peritoneal dialysis catheter; chemical peritonitis from other bodily fluid, including bile and urine; and infection. Meconium peritonitis is described in Chapters 102.1 and 330. Peritonitis is considered a surgical emergency and requires exploration and lavage of the abdomen except in spontaneous bacterial peritonitis.

Bibliography is available at Expert Consult.

371.1 Acute Primary Peritonitis
Jessica W. Wen and Chris A. Liacouras

ETIOLOGY AND EPIDEMIOLOGY
Primary peritonitis usually refers to bacterial infection of the peritoneal cavity without a demonstrable intraabdominal source. Most cases occur in children with ascites resulting from cirrhosis and nephrotic syndrome. Infection can result from translocation of gut bacteria as

well as immune dysfunction. Rarely, primary peritonitis occurs in previously healthy children. Pneumococci (most common), group A streptococci, enterococci, staphylococci, and Gram-negative enteric bacteria, especially *Escherichia coli* and *Klebsiella pneumoniae,* are most commonly found. *Mycobacterium tuberculosis, Neisseria meningitidis,* and *Mycobacterium bovis* are rare causes.

CLINICAL MANIFESTATIONS
Onset may be insidious or rapid and is characterized by fever, abdominal pain and a toxic appearance. Vomiting and diarrhea may be present. Hypotension and tachycardia are common along with shallow, rapid respirations because of discomfort associated with breathing. Abdominal palpation might demonstrate rebound tenderness and rigidity. Bowel sounds are hypoactive or absent. However, signs and symptoms may be subtle at times and increase vigilance is needed in cirrhotic patients who have ascites and present with unexplained leukocytosis, azotemia, or metabolic acidosis.

DIAGNOSIS AND TREATMENT
Peripheral leukocytosis with a marked predominance of polymorphonuclear cells is common, although the white blood cell (WBC) count can be affected by preexisting hypersplenism in patients with cirrhosis. Patients with nephrotic syndrome generally have proteinuria, and low serum albumin in these patients is associated with increased risk of peritonitis. X-ray examination of the abdomen reveals dilation of the large and small intestines, with increased separation of loops secondary to bowel wall thickening. Distinguishing primary peritonitis from appendicitis may be impossible in patients without a history of nephrotic syndrome or cirrhosis; accordingly, the diagnosis of primary peritonitis is made by CT scan, laparoscopy, or laparotomy. In a child with known renal or hepatic disease and ascites, the presence of peritoneal signs should prompt diagnostic paracentesis. Infected fluid usually reveals a WBC count of ≥250 cells/mm³, with >50% polymorphonuclear cells.

Primary peritonitis is usually monomicrobial. The presence of mixed bacterial flora on ascitic fluid examination or free air on abdominal roentgenogram in children with presumed peritonitis mandates laparotomy to localize a perforation as a likely intraabdominal source of the infection. Inoculation of ascitic fluid obtained at paracentesis directly into blood culture bottles increases the yield of positive cultures. Parenteral antibiotic therapy with broad spectrum coverage, such as cefotaxime, should be started promptly, with subsequent changes dependent on sensitivity testing (vancomycin for resistant pneumococci). Therapy should be continued for 10-14 days.

Culture-negative neutrocytic ascites is a variant of primary peritonitis with a ascetic fluid WBC count of >500 cells/mm³, a negative culture, no intraabdominal source of infection, and no prior treatment with antibiotics. It should be treated in a similar manner as primary peritonitis.

Bibliography is available at Expert Consult.

371.2 Acute Secondary Peritonitis
Jessica W. Wen and Chris A. Liacouras

Acute secondary peritonitis most often results from entry of enteric bacteria into the peritoneal cavity through a necrotic defect in the wall of the intestines or other viscus as a result of obstruction or infarction or after rupture of an intraabdominal visceral abscess. It most commonly follows perforation of the appendix. Other causes include incarcerated hernias, rupture of a Meckel diverticulum, midgut volvulus, intussusception, hemolytic uremic syndrome, peptic ulceration, inflammatory bowel disease, necrotizing cholecystitis, necrotizing enterocolitis, typhlitis, and traumatic perforation.

Peritonitis in the neonatal period most often occurs as a complication of necrotizing enterocolitis but may be associated with meconium ileus or spontaneous (or indomethacin-induced) rupture of the

stomach or intestines. In postpubertal girls, bacteria from the genital tract (*Neisseria gonorrhoeae, Chlamydia trachomatis*) can gain access to the peritoneal cavity via the fallopian tubes, causing secondary peritonitis. The presence of a foreign body, such as a ventriculoperitoneal catheter or peritoneal dialysis catheter, can predispose to peritonitis, with skin microorganisms, such as *Staphylococcus epidermidis, Staphylococcus aureus,* and *Candida albicans,* contaminating the shunt. Secondary peritonitis results from direct toxic effects of bacteria as well as local and systemic release of inflammatory mediators in response to organisms and their products (lipopolysaccharide endotoxin). The development of sepsis depends on various host and disease factors, as well as promptness of antimicrobial and surgical intervention.

CLINICAL MANIFESTATIONS
Similar to primary peritonitis, characteristic symptoms include fever, diffuse abdominal pain, nausea, and vomiting. Physical findings of peritoneal inflammation include rebound tenderness, abdominal wall rigidity, a paucity of body motion (lying still), and decreased or absent bowel sounds from paralytic ileus. Massive exudation of fluid into the peritoneal cavity, along with the systemic release of vasodilative substances, can lead to the rapid development of shock. A toxic appearance, irritability, and restlessness are common. Basilar atelectasis as well as intrapulmonary shunting can develop, with progression to acute respiratory distress syndrome.

Laboratory studies reveal a peripheral WBC count >12,000 cells/mm³, with a marked predominance of polymorphonuclear forms. X-rays of the abdomen can reveal free air in the peritoneal cavity, evidence of ileus or obstruction, peritoneal fluid, and obliteration of the psoas shadow. Other peritoneal fluid findings suggestive of secondary peritonitis include elevated total protein (>1 g/dL), low glucose (<50 mg/dL).

TREATMENT
Aggressive fluid resuscitation and support of cardiovascular function should begin immediately. Stabilization of the patient before surgical intervention is mandatory. Antibiotic therapy must provide coverage for organisms that predominate at the site of presumed origin of the infection. In contrast to primary peritonitis, secondary peritonitis is typically polymicrobial. For perforation of the lower gastrointestinal tract, a regimen of ampicillin, gentamicin, and clindamycin or metronidazole will adequately address infection by *E. coli, Klebsiella,* and *Bacteroides* spp. and enterococci. Alternative therapy could include ticarcillin-clavulanic acid and an aminoglycoside or piperacillin/tazobactam. Surgery to repair a perforated viscus should proceed after the patient is stabilized and antibiotic therapy is initiated. Intraoperative peritoneal fluid cultures will indicate whether a change in the antibiotic regimen is warranted. Empirical treatment for peritoneal dialysis catheter–related peritonitis may include intraperitoneal cefepime or cefazolin plus ceftazidime. Serious infection from peritoneal dialysis catheters can generally be prevented with good catheter hygiene and prompt removal and replacement with signs of progressive infection.

Bibliography is available at Expert Consult.

371.3 Acute Secondary Localized Peritonitis (Peritoneal Abscess)
Jessica W. Wen and Chris A. Liacouras

ETIOLOGY
Intraabdominal abscesses occur less commonly in children and infants than in adults, but can develop in visceral intraabdominal organs (hepatic, splenic, renal, pancreatic, tuboovarian abscesses) or in the interintestinal, periappendiceal, subdiaphragmatic, subhepatic, pelvic, or retroperitoneal spaces. Most commonly, periappendiceal and pelvic abscesses arise from a perforation of the appendix. Transmural

inflammation with fistula formation can result in intraabdominal abscess formation in children with inflammatory bowel disease.

CLINICAL MANIFESTATIONS

Prolonged fever, anorexia, vomiting, and lassitude suggest the development of an intraabdominal abscess. The peripheral WBC count is elevated, as is the erythrocyte sedimentation rate. With an appendiceal abscess, there is localized tenderness and a palpable mass in the right lower quadrant. A pelvic abscess is suggested by abdominal distention, rectal tenesmus with or without the passage of small-volume mucous stools, and bladder irritability. Rectal examination might reveal a tender mass anteriorly. Subphrenic gas collection, basal atelectasis, elevated hemidiaphragm, and pleural effusion may be present with a subdiaphragmatic abscess. Psoas abscess can develop from extension of infection from a retroperitoneal appendicitis, Crohn disease, perirenal or intrarenal abscess. Abdominal findings may be minimal, and presentation can include a limp, hip pain, and fever. Ultrasound examination, CT scanning, and MRI may be used to localize intraabdominal abscesses; MRI gives the best resolution of disease involvement.

TREATMENT

An abscess should be drained and appropriate antibiotic therapy provided. Drainage can be performed under radiologic control (ultrasonogram or CT guidance) and an indwelling drainage catheter left in place or surgically depending on location of abscess. Initial broad-spectrum antibiotic coverage such as a combination of ampicillin, gentamicin, and clindamycin or ciprofloxacin and metronidazole should be started and can be modified depending on the results of sensitivity testing. The treatment of appendiceal rupture complicated by abscess formation may be problematic because intestinal phlegmon formation can make surgical resection more difficult. Intensive antibiotic therapy for 4-6 wk followed by an interval appendectomy is often the treatment course followed.

Bibliography is available at Expert Consult.

Chapter **372**
Epigastric Hernia
John J. Aiken and Keith T. Oldham

Epigastric hernias are ventral hernias in the midline of the abdominal wall between the xiphoid and the umbilicus. Epigastric hernias result from defects in the decussating fibers of the linea alba and are more likely congenital than acquired. Because most epigastric hernias are small and asymptomatic, the true incidence is unknown, but the reported incidence in childhood varies from <1% to as high as 5%. Epigastric hernias may be single or multiple and are 2-3 times more common in males than females. The defect typically contains only preperitoneal fat without a peritoneal sac or abdominal viscera. Epigastric (incisional) hernias can occur in a previous incision site or be associated with ventricular-peritoneal shunts.

CLINICAL PRESENTATION

Epigastric hernias typically appear in young children as a visible or palpable mass in the midline, between the umbilicus and the xiphoid, noted by the parents or primary care practitioner. The mass is almost always small (<1 cm) and asymptomatic. The mass is typically present at all times but most apparent at times of irritability or straining. Occasionally, the mass is intermittent and the child relates pain localized to the site of the hernia. Physical examination demonstrates a firm mass, directly in the midline, anywhere between the umbilicus and the xiphoid. Epigastric hernias typically contain only preperitoneal fat and are not reducible because of the small size of the fascial defect. Rarely, a fascial defect is noted without a palpable mass. The mass may be intermittent if the fat reduces with relaxation of the abdominal muscles. Herniation of intestines or abdominal viscera in an epigastric hernia would be exceptionally rare. The mass may be tender to examination, but strangulation of the hernia contents is uncommon. Physical examination is almost always diagnostic and imaging studies are unnecessary.

The natural history of epigastric hernias is for gradual enlargement over time as intermittently more preperitoneal fat is extruded through the defect at times of straining or increased intraabdominal pressure. Left untreated, the defect can enlarge and allow herniation of intraabdominal viscera within a peritoneal sac. Epigastric hernias do not resolve spontaneously, and therefore operative repair is the recommended treatment.

The site should be carefully marked preoperatively because the mass and defect can be difficult to localize after induction of anesthesia. A limited transverse incision is made over the mass and dissection is performed to delineate the edges of the fascial defect. If herniated fat is present, it is dissected free of the subcutaneous tissues and can be reduced or ligated and excised. The defect is closed using absorbable suture. The skin is closed with an absorbable subcuticular suture. Postoperative complications are rare and the recurrence rate is low.

Bibliography is available at Expert Consult.

372.1 Incisional Hernia
John J. Aiken and Keith T. Oldham

Hernia formation at the site of a previous laparotomy is uncommon in childhood. Factors associated with an increased risk of incisional hernia include increased intraabdominal pressure, wound infection, and midline incision. Transverse abdominal incisions are favored because of their increased strength and blood supply, which reduce the likelihood of wound infection and incisional hernia. Although most incisional hernias require repair, operation should be deferred until the child is in optimal medical condition. Some incisional hernias resolve, especially those occurring in infants. Some recommend elastic bandaging to discourage enlargement of the hernia and to promote spontaneous healing. Newborns with abdominal wall defects represent the largest group of children with incisional hernias. Initial management should be conservative, with repair deferred until about 1 yr of age. Incarceration is very uncommon but is an indication for prompt repair.

Bibliography is available at Expert Consult.

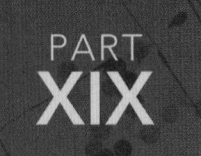
Development and Function

Chapter **373**

Respiratory Pathophysiology and Regulation

Ashok P. Sarnaik, Sabrina M. Heidemann, and Jeff A. Clark

The respiratory system serves to supply sufficient oxygen to meet metabolic demands and remove carbon dioxide. Abnormalities in any of the multiple processes (including ventilation, perfusion, and diffusion) that are involved in tissue oxygenation and carbon dioxide removal can lead to respiratory failure. The pathophysiologic manifestations of respiratory disease processes are profoundly influenced by age- and growth-dependent changes in the physiology and anatomy of the respiratory control mechanisms, airway dynamics, and lung parenchymal characteristics. Smaller airways, a more compliant chest wall, and poor hypoxic drive render a younger infant more vulnerable compared to an older child with similar severity of disease.

Respiratory distress may be diagnosed from signs such as cyanosis, nasal flaring, grunting, tachypnea, wheezing, chest wall retractions, and stridor. Respiratory failure can be present without respiratory distress; a patient with abnormalities of central nervous system (CNS) or neuromuscular disease or exhaustion might not be able to mount sufficient effort to appear in respiratory distress. A child who appears in respiratory distress might not have a respiratory illness; a patient with primary metabolic acidosis (diabetic ketoacidosis) or CNS excitatory states (encephalitis) can present in severe respiratory distress without respiratory disease.

Bibliography is available at Expert Consult.

373.1 Lung Volumes and Capacities in Health and Disease

Ashok P. Sarnaik, Jeff A. Clark, and Sabrina M. Heidemann

Traditionally, lung volumes are measured with a spirogram (Fig. 373-1). **Tidal volume (V_T)** is the amount of air moved in and out of the lungs during each breath; at rest, V_T is normally 6-7 mL/kg body weight. **Inspiratory capacity** is the amount of air inspired by maximum inspiratory effort after tidal expiration. **Expiratory reserve volume** is the amount of air exhaled by maximum expiratory effort after tidal expiration. The volume of gas remaining in the lungs after maximum expiration is **residual volume. Vital capacity** is defined as the amount of air moved in and out of the lungs with maximum inspiration and expiration. Vital capacity, inspiratory capacity, and expiratory reserve volume are decreased in lung pathology but are also effort dependent. **Total lung capacity** is the volume of gas occupying the lungs after maximum inhalation.

Flow volume relationship offers a valuable means at the bedside or in an office setting to detect abnormal pulmonary mechanics and response to therapy with relatively inexpensive and easy-to-use devices. After maximum inhalation, the patient forcefully exhales through a mouthpiece into the device until residual volume is reached followed by maximum inhalation (Fig. 373-2). Flow is plotted against volume. **Maximum forced expiratory flow (FEF$_{max}$)** is generated in the early part of exhalation, and it is a commonly used indicator of airway obstruction in asthma and other obstructive lesions. Provided maximum pressure is generated consistently during exhalation, a decrease in flow is a reflection of increased airway resistance. The total volume exhaled during this maneuver is **forced vital capacity (FVC)**. **Volume exhaled in 1 sec** is referred to as **FEV$_1$**. FEV$_1$/FVC is expressed as a percentage

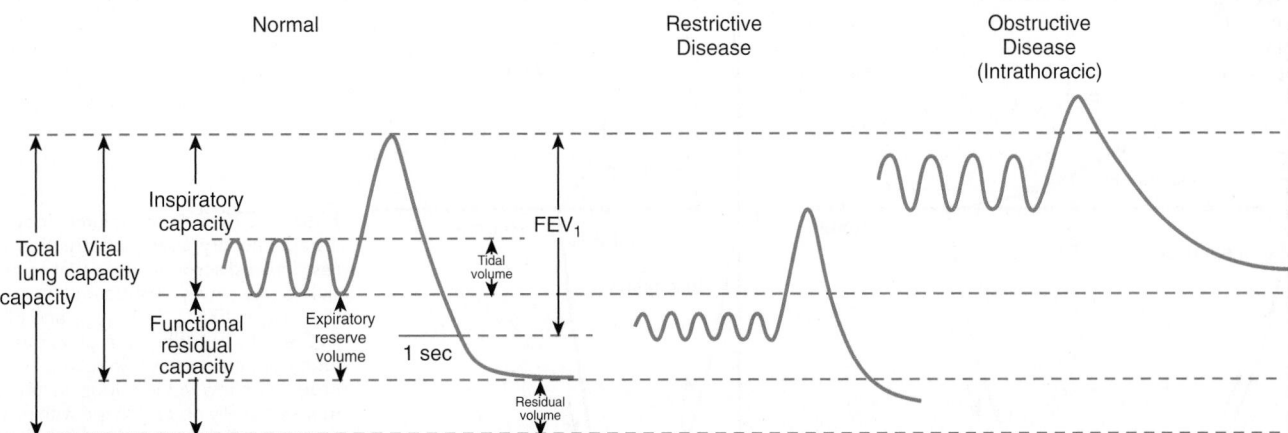

Figure 373-1 Spirogram showing lung volumes and capacities. FEV$_1$ is the maximum volume exhaled in 1 sec after maximum inspiration. Restrictive diseases are usually associated with decreased lung volumes and capacities. Intrathoracic airway obstruction is associated with air trapping and abnormally high functional residual capacity and residual volume. FEV$_1$ and vital capacity are decreased in both restrictive and obstructive diseases. The ratio of FEV$_1$ to vital capacity is normal in restrictive disease but decreased in obstructive disease. FEV, forced expiratory volume.

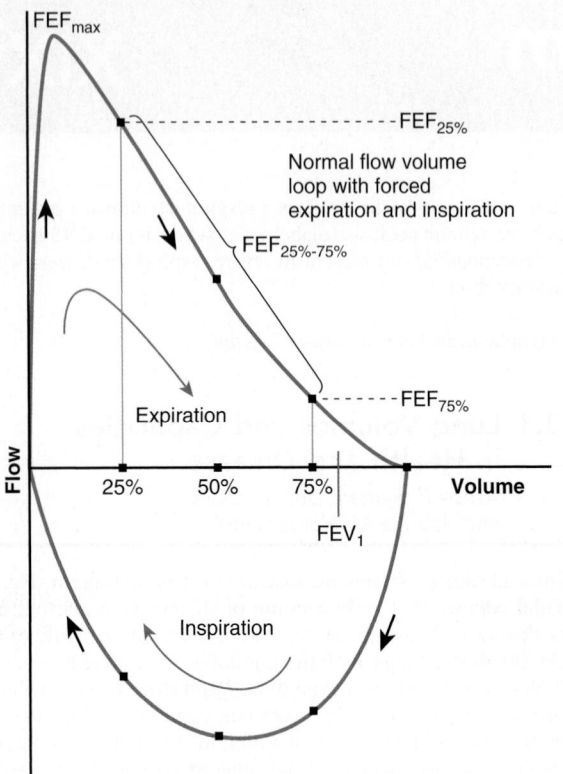

Figure 373-2 Flow volume loop in a normal person performed after maximal inspiration followed by forced complete expiration and forced complete inhalation. FEF_{max} represents maximum flow during expiration. This is attained soon after initiation of the expiration. Fall in expiratory flow is gradual until it reaches zero after exhalation is complete. $FEF_{25\%-75\%}$ represents mean flow from 25% ($FEF_{25\%}$) to 75% ($FEF_{75\%}$) of exhaled forced expiratory volume (FEV), also termed *forced vital capacity* (FVC). FEV_1 is amount of volume after 1 sec of forced exhalation. Normally FEV_1 is around 80% of FVC.

of FVC. $FEF_{25\%-75\%}$ is the mean flow between 25% and 75% of FVC and is considered relatively effort independent. Individual values and shapes of flow-volume curves show characteristic changes in obstructive and restrictive respiratory disorders (Fig. 373-3). In intrapulmonary airway obstruction such as asthma or cystic fibrosis, there is a reduction of FEF_{max}, $FEF_{25\%-75\%}$, FVC, and FEV_1/FVC. Also, there is a characteristic concavity in the middle part of the expiratory curve. In restrictive lung disease such as interstitial pneumonia (see Chapter 399.5) and kyphoscoliosis (see Chapter 417.5), FVC is decreased with relative preservation of airflow and FEV_1/FVC. The flow volume curve assumes a vertically oblong shape compared to normal. Changes in shape of the flow volume loop and individual values depend on the type of disease and the extent of severity. Serial determinations provide valuable information regarding disease evolution and response to therapy.

Functional residual capacity (FRC) is the amount of air left in the lungs after tidal expiration. FRC has important pathophysiologic implications. Alveolar gas composition changes during inspiration and expiration. **Alveolar Po_2 (PAo_2)** increases and **alveolar Pco_2 ($PAco_2$)** decreases during inspiration as fresh atmospheric gas enters the lungs. During exhalation, PAo_2 decreases and $PAco_2$ increases as pulmonary capillary blood continues to remove oxygen from and add CO_2 into the alveoli (Fig. 373-4). FRC acts as a buffer, minimizing the changes in PAo_2 and $PAco_2$ during inspiration and expiration. FRC represents the environment available for pulmonary capillary blood for gas exchange at all times.

A decrease in FRC is often encountered in alveolar interstitial diseases and thoracic deformities. The major pathophysiologic consequence of decreased FRC is **hypoxemia**. Reduced FRC results in a sharp decline in PAo_2 during exhalation because a limited volume is available for gas exchange. Po_2 of pulmonary capillary blood therefore falls excessively during exhalation, leading to a decline in **arterial** Po_2 (PAo_2). Any increase in PAo_2 (and therefore Pao_2) during inspiration cannot compensate for the decreased Pao_2 during expiration. The explanation for this lies in the shape of O_2-hemoglobin (Hb) dissociation curve, which is sigmoid shaped (Fig. 373-5). Because most of the oxygen in blood is combined with Hb, it is the percentage of **oxyhemoglobin (So_2)** that gets averaged rather than the Po_2. Although an

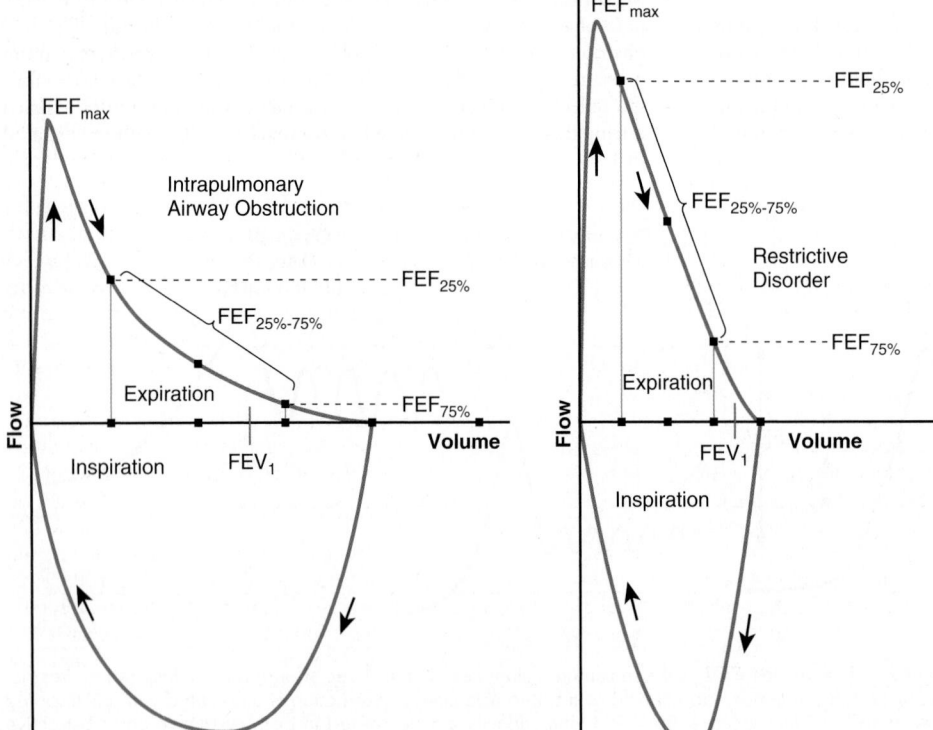

Figure 373-3 Flow volume loops in **intrapulmonary airway obstruction and restrictive disorders.** Note that in intrapulmonary airway obstruction, there is a decrease in FEF_{max}, $FEF_{25\%-75\%}$, and FEV_1/FVC%. The middle part of expiratory loop appears concave. In restrictive disorder, the flow volume loop assumes a more vertically oblong shape with reduction in FVC but not the FEV_1/FVC%. Expiratory and inspiratory flow rates are relatively unaffected. FEF, forced expiratory flow; FEV, forced expiratory volume; FVC, forced vital capacity.

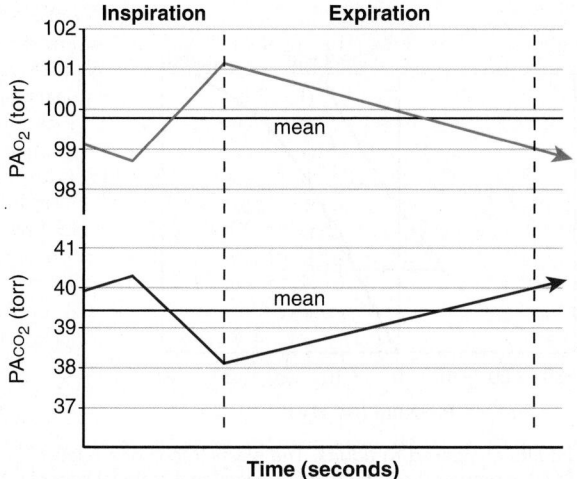

Figure 373-4 Alveolar Po_2 rises and Pco_2 falls during inspiration as fresh atmospheric gas is brought into the lungs. During expiration, the opposite changes occur as pulmonary capillary blood continues to remove O_2 and add CO_2 from the alveoli without atmospheric enrichment. Note that during the early part of inspiration, alveolar Po_2 continues to fall and Pco_2 continues to rise because of inspiration of the dead space that is occupied by the previously exhaled gas. *(Modified from Comroe JH: Physiology of respiration, ed 2, Chicago, 1974, Year Book Medical Publishers, p 12.)*

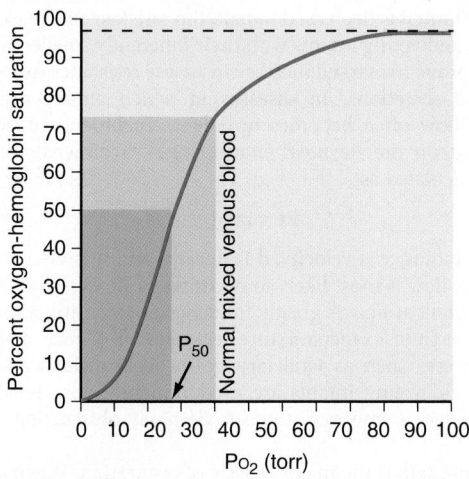

Figure 373-5 Oxygen-hemoglobin dissociation curve. P_{50} of adult blood is around 27 torr. Under basal conditions, mixed venous blood has Po_2 of 40 torr and oxygen-hemoglobin saturation of 75%. In arterial blood, these values are 100 torr and 97.5%, respectively. Note that there is a steep decline in oxygen-hemoglobin saturation at PaO_2 <50 torr, but relatively little increase in saturation is gained at PO_2 >70 torr.

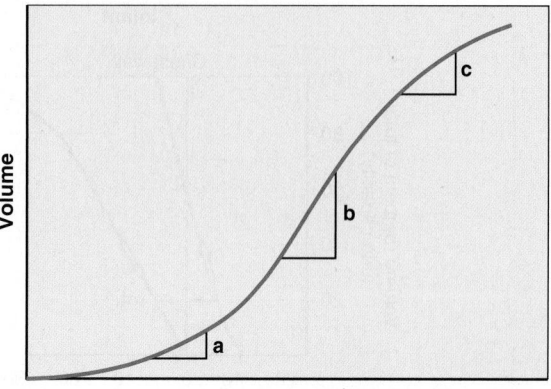

Figure 373-6 Lung compliance is significantly influenced by the functional residual capacity (FRC). The same change in pressure is associated with less change in volume when FRC is abnormally decreased *(a)* or abnormally increased *(c)* compared to the normal state *(b)*.

FRC. Abnormalities of FRC result in increased work of breathing with spontaneous respiration and increased barotrauma in mechanical ventilation.

Bibliography is available at Expert Consult.

373.2 Chest Wall

Ashok P. Sarnaik, Sabrina M. Heidemann, and Jeff A. Clark

The chest wall and diaphragm of an infant are mechanically disadvantaged compared to that of an adult when required to increase thoracic (and therefore the lung) volume. The infant's ribs are oriented much more horizontally and the diaphragm is flatter and less domed. Consequently, the infant is unable to duplicate the efficiency of upward and outward movement of obliquely oriented ribs and downward displacement of the domed diaphragm in an adult to expand the thoracic capacity. Additionally, the infant's rib cage is softer and thus more compliant compared to an adult's rib cage. Although a soft, highly compliant chest wall is beneficial to a baby in its passage through the birth canal and allows future lung growth, it places the young infant in a vulnerable situation under certain pathologic conditions. Chest wall compliance is a major determinant of FRC. Because the chest wall and the lungs recoil in opposite directions at rest, FRC is reached at the point where the outward elastic recoil of the thoracic cage counterbalances the inward lung recoil. This balance is attained at a lower lung volume in a young infant because of the extremely high thoracic compliance compared to older children (Fig. 373-7). The measured FRC in infants is higher than expected because respiratory muscles of infants maintain the thoracic cage in an inspiratory position at all times. Additionally, some amount of air trapping during expiration occurs in young infants.

The increased chest wall compliance is a distinct disadvantage to the young infant under several pathologic conditions. A decrease in muscle tone, as occurs in *rapid eye movement (REM)* sleep or with CNS depression, allows greater chest wall retraction because of less opposition to the lung recoil; the FRC decreases in such states. The respiratory muscles of infants are poorly equipped to sustain large workloads. They are more easily fatigued than those of older children, limiting their ability to maintain adequate ventilation in lung disease. In diseases of poor lung compliance (atelectasis, pulmonary edema), excessive lung recoil results in greater retraction of the soft chest wall and more loss of FRC than occurs in older children and adults with stiffer chest walls. Increased negative intrathoracic pressure required to overcome airway resistance in upper airway obstruction also produces greater chest wall

increase in arterial Po_2 cannot increase O_2-Hb saturation >100%, there is a steep desaturation of Hb below a Po_2 of 50 torr; thus, decreased So_2 during exhalation as a result of low FRC leads to overall arterial desaturation and hypoxemia. The adverse pathophysiologic consequences of decreased FRC are ameliorated by application of **positive end-expiratory pressure (PEEP)** and increasing the inspiratory time during mechanical ventilation.

The lung pressure–volume relationship is markedly influenced by FRC (Fig. 373-6). Pulmonary compliance is decreased at abnormally low or high FRC.

FRC is abnormally increased in intrathoracic airway obstruction, which results in incomplete exhalation, and abnormally decreased in alveolar-interstitial diseases. At excessively low or high FRC, tidal respiration requires higher inflation pressures compared to normal

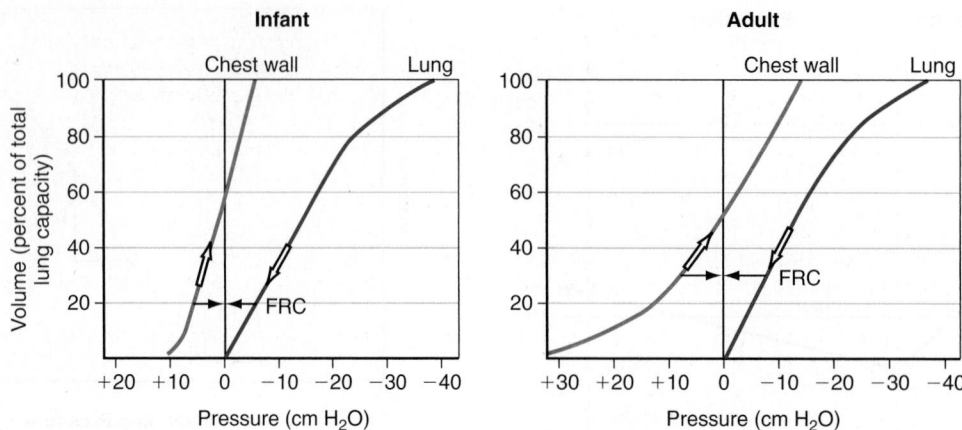

Figure 373-7 Schematic of interaction between chest wall and lung recoil in infants compared to adults. The elastic recoil of a relatively more compliant chest wall is balanced by the lung recoil at a lower volume (FRC) in infants compared to adults. FRC, functional residual capacity.

recoil and reduced FRC in young infants. Application of PEEP is beneficial in such states for stabilizing the chest wall and restoring FRC.

Young infants do not tolerate sustained respiratory loads as well as older children and adults. Respiratory muscle ontogeny is characterized by changes in the composition of muscle fiber types in the diaphragm and intercostals throughout infancy. Type I fibers are slow-twitch and high-oxidative in nature, whereas type II fibers are fast-twitch and low-oxidative. Type I fibers have low contractility but are fatigue resistant. Type II fibers have high contractility but are more prone to fatigue. The proportion of type I fibers in the diaphragm and intercostals of premature infants is only around 10%. This increases to around 25% in full-term newborns and around 50% in children older than age 2 yr. Respiratory muscles of premature babies and young infants are therefore more susceptible to fatigue, resulting in earlier decompensation.

Abnormalities of the chest wall are encountered in certain pathologic conditions. Chest wall instability can result from trauma (fractured ribs, thoracotomy) and neuromuscular diseases that lead to intercostal and diaphragmatic muscle weakness. The increased chest wall compliance makes such children more vulnerable to respiratory decompensation when faced with similar pulmonary pathology compared to older children and adults with stiffer chest walls. Children with rigid, noncompliant chest wall (asphyxiating thoracic dystrophy of Jeune [see Chapters 417.3 and 700], achondroplasia [see Chapter 417.4]) have markedly diminished lung volumes and capacities.

Bibliography is available at Expert Consult.

373.3 Pulmonary Mechanics and Work of Breathing in Health and Disease

Ashok P. Sarnaik, Sabrina M. Heidemann, and Jeff A. Clark

The movement of air in and out of the lungs requires a sufficient pressure gradient between alveoli and atmosphere during inspiration and expiration. Part of the pressure gradient is required to overcome the lung and chest wall elastance; another part is needed to overcome airway resistance. **Elastance** refers to the property of a substance to oppose deformation or stretching. It is calculated as a change in pressure (ΔP) divided by change in volume (ΔV). Elastic recoil is a property of a substance that enables it to return to its original state after it is no longer subjected to pressure. **Compliance** ($\Delta V \div \Delta P$) is the reciprocal of elastance. In the context of the pulmonary parenchyma, airways, and the chest wall, the compliance refers to their distensibility. **Resistance** is calculated as the amount of pressure required to generate flow of gas

across the airways. Resistance to laminar flow is governed by *Poiseuille's law* stated as:

$$R = 8l\eta \div \Pi r^4$$

where R is resistance, l is length, η is viscosity, and r is the radius. The practical implication of pressure-flow relationship is that airway resistance is inversely proportional to its radius raised to the 4th power. If the airway lumen is decreased in half, the resistance increases 16-fold. Newborns and young infants with their inherently smaller airways are especially prone to marked increase in airway resistance from inflamed tissues and secretions. In diseases in which airway resistance is increased, flow often becomes turbulent. **Turbulence** depends to a great extent on the *Reynolds number* (Re), a dimensionless entity, which is calculated as:

$$Re = 2rvd \div \eta$$

where r is radius, v is velocity, d is density, and η is viscosity. Turbulence in gas flow is most likely to occur when Re exceeds 2000. Resistance to turbulent flow is greatly influenced by density. A low-density gas such as helium-oxygen mixture decreases turbulence in obstructive airway diseases such as viral laryngotracheobronchitis and asthma. Neonates and young infants are predominantly nose breathers and therefore even a minimal amount of nasal obstruction is poorly tolerated.

The diaphragm is the major muscle of respiration. When additional **work of breathing (WOB)** is required, intercostal and other accessory muscles of respirations also contribute to the increased work. The V_T and respiratory rate are adjusted, both in health and disease, to maintain the required minute volume with the least amount of energy expenditure. The total WOB (necessary to create pressure gradients to move air) is divided into 2 parts. The first part is to overcome the lung and chest wall elastance and is referred to as **elastic work (W_{elast})**. The second part is to overcome airway and tissue resistance, and is referred to as **resistive work (W_{resist})**. W_{elast} is directly proportional to V_T, whereas W_{resist} is determined by the rate of airflow and, therefore, respiratory rate. The total WOB is lowest at a rate of 35-40/min for neonates and 14-16/min for older children and adults. W_{elast} is disproportionately increased in diseases with decreased compliance and W_{resist} is increased in airway obstruction. Consequently, respirations are shallow (low V_T) and rapid in diseases of low compliance and deep and relatively slow (low flow rate) in diseases of increased resistance.

Compared to older children, young infants have disproportionately greater W_{elast} because the negative intrapleural pressure during inspiration causes the retractile (more compliant) chest wall to collapse and pose an impediment to air entry. Young infants increase their respiratory rate with any mechanical abnormality. Other examples of compliant chest wall being a disadvantage include flail chest resulting from rib fractures, thoracotomy, and neuromuscular weakness. One of the salutary effects of continuous positive airway pressure in such situations is the stabilization of the chest wall. Under normal conditions, the energy cost of WOB contributes to only approximately 2% of total caloric expenditure. In children with chronic lung disease or congestive heart failure the WOB can contribute to as much as 40% of total energy expenditure during physical activity, thus increasing their caloric needs.

Time constant, measured in seconds, is a product of compliance and resistance. It is a reflection of the amount of time required for proximal airway pressure (and therefore volume) to equilibrate with alveolar pressure. It takes 3 time constants for 95%, and 5 time constants for 99% of pressure equilibration to occur. Because intrathoracic airways expand during inspiration and narrow during expiration, expiratory time constant is longer than inspiratory time constant. Diseases characterized by decreased compliance (pneumonia, pulmonary edema, atelectasis) are associated with a shorter time constant and therefore require less time for alveolar inflation and deflation. Diseases associated with increased resistance (asthma, bronchiolitis, aspiration syndromes) have prolonged time constant and therefore require more time for alveolar inflation and deflation. Pathologic alterations in time constants have practical significance during mechanical ventilation. Patients with shorter time constants are best ventilated with relatively smaller tidal volumes and faster rates to minimize peak inflation pressure. In patients with increased airway resistance, a fast respiratory rate (and, therefore, less time) does not allow enough pressure equilibration to occur between the proximal airway and the alveoli. Inadequate inspiratory time results in lower V_T, whereas insufficient exhalation time results in inadvertent PEEP, often referred to as auto-PEEP or intrinsic PEEP. Such patients are best ventilated with relatively slower rates and larger tidal volumes.

Bibliography is available at Expert Consult.

373.4 Airway Dynamics in Health and Disease

Ashok P. Sarnaik, Sabrina M. Heidemann, and Jeff A. Clark

Because the trachea and airways of an infant are much more compliant than those of older children and adults, changes in intrapleural pressure result in much greater changes in airway diameter. The airway can be divided into 3 anatomic parts: the **extrathoracic airway** extends from the nose to the thoracic inlet, the **intrathoracic–extrapulmonary airway** extends from the thoracic inlet to the main stem bronchi, and the **intrapulmonary airway** is within the lung parenchyma. During normal respirations, intrathoracic airways expand in inspiration as intrapleural pressure becomes more negative and narrow in expiration as they return to their baseline at FRC. The changes in diameter are of little significance in normal respiration. In diseases characterized by airway obstruction, much greater changes in intrapleural pressure are required to generate adequate airflow, resulting in greater changes in airway lumen. The changes in the size of airway during respiration are accentuated in young infants with their softer, more compliant airways.

In extrathoracic airway obstruction (choanal atresia [see Chapter 376], retropharyngeal abscess, laryngotracheobronchitis [see Chapter 385]), the high negative intrapleural pressure during inspiration is transmitted up to the site of obstruction, after which there is a rapid dissipation of pressure. Therefore, the extrathoracic airway below the site of obstruction has markedly increased negative pressure inside, resulting in its collapse, which makes the obstruction worse (Fig. 373-8A). This produces inspiratory difficulty, prolongation of inspiration, and inspiratory stridor. Also, the increased negative intrapleural pressure results in chest wall retractions. During expiration, the increased positive intrapleural pressure is again transmitted up the airways to the site of obstruction, leading to a distention of the extrathoracic airway and amelioration of obstruction (Fig. 373-8B).

Because of the increased positive intrapleural pressure during exhalation, the chest wall tends to bulge out, which produces the **classic paradoxical respiration,** in which the chest retracts during inspiration and bulges out during expiration. The younger the child, the softer is the chest wall and the more marked is the paradoxical respiration of extrathoracic airway obstruction. A pattern of seesaw respiration may also be evident in newborns and young infants as the compliant chest wall is sucked in and the abdomen bulges out during inspiration, with the converse happening during expiration.

In obstruction of intrathoracic–extrapulmonary airway (vascular ring [see Chapter 386.8], mediastinal tumors) and intrapulmonary airway (asthma, bronchiolitis), the increased negative intrapleural pressure results in a distention of intrathoracic airways during inspiration, thus providing some relief from obstruction (Fig. 373-9A).

During expiration, the increased positive intrathoracic pressure is transmitted up to the site of obstruction, after which it dissipates rapidly. The intrathoracic airway above the site of obstruction is

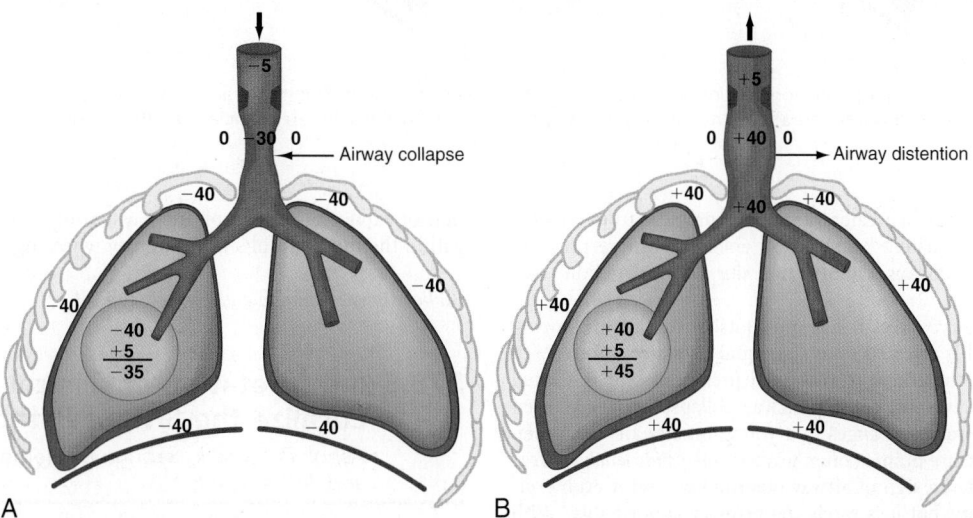

Figure 373-8 A, In extrathoracic airway obstruction, the increased negative pressure during inspiration is transmitted up to the site of obstruction. This results in collapse of the extrathoracic airway below the site of obstruction, making the obstruction worse during inspiration. Note that the pressures are compared to the atmospheric pressure, which is traditionally represented as 0 cm. Terminal airway pressure is calculated as intrapleural pressure plus lung recoil pressure. Lung recoil pressure is arbitrarily chosen as 5 cm for the sake of simplicity. **B,** During expiration, the positive pressure below the site of obstruction results in distention of extrathoracic airway and amelioration of symptoms.

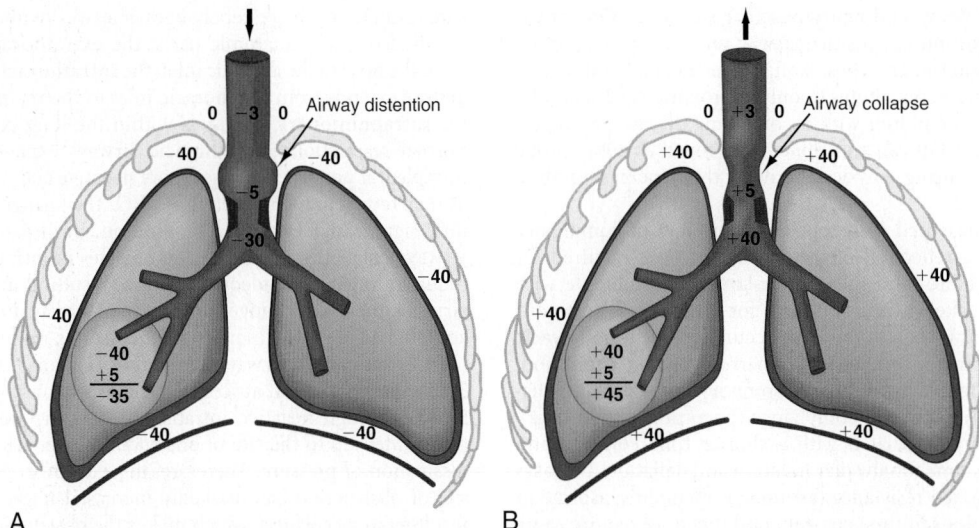

Figure 373-9 A, In intrathoracic–extrapulmonary airway obstruction, the increased negative pressure during inspiration is transmitted up to the site of obstruction. This results in the distention of the intrathoracic airway above the lesion because it is surrounded by an even greater negative intrapleural pressure. **B,** During expiration, the increased positive airway pressure rapidly dissipates above the obstruction. Consequently, there is a collapse of the intrathoracic airway above the obstruction as it is subjected to markedly increased positive intrapleural pressure, making the obstruction worse during expiration.

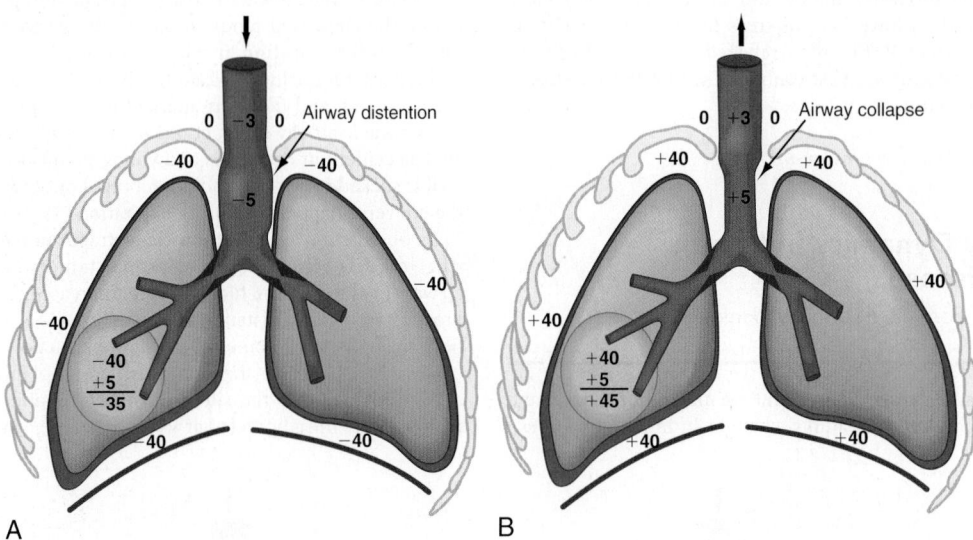

Figure 373-10 A and **B,** In intrapulmonary airway obstruction, even a wider segment of intrathoracic airway is subjected to pressure changes compared to those observed in intrathoracic-extrapulmonary airway obstruction. Such lesions are associated with marked increase in airway obstruction during expiration.

therefore subjected to much greater intrapleural pressure from outside, which cannot be adequately balanced by enough positive pressure inside, resulting in collapse above the site of obstruction (see Fig. 373-9*B*).

The site at which pressures inside and outside the airway during exhalation are equal is referred to as the **equal pressure point**. With intrathoracic airway obstruction, the equal pressure point is shifted distally toward the alveolus, causing airway collapse above. Marked inspiratory and expiratory changes in a young infant's airway lumen above the equal pressure point is often termed *collapsible trachea*. **Tracheal collapse** is often a sign of airway obstruction, and it even contributes to its severity, but it is rarely the primary abnormality. With intrapulmonary airway obstruction, an even wider portion of intrathoracic airway is subjected to pressure swings during inspiration and expiration (Fig. 373-10).

Both intrathoracic–extrapulmonary and intrapulmonary airway obstruction result in increasing difficulty during expiration, prolonga-

tion of expiration, and expiratory wheezing. Any airway obstruction within the thorax results in expiratory wheezing.

Bibliography is available at Expert Consult.

373.5 Interpretation of Clinical Signs to Localize the Site of Pathology

Ashok P. Sarnaik, Sabrina M. Heidemann, and Jeff A. Clark

The first step in establishing the diagnosis of respiratory disease is appropriate interpretation of clinical findings. Respiratory distress can occur without respiratory disease, and severe respiratory failure can be present without significant respiratory distress. Diseases characterized by CNS excitation, such as encephalitis, and neuroexcitatory drugs are associated with central neurogenic hyperventilation. Similarly, diseases that produce metabolic acidosis, such as diabetic ketoacidosis, salicylism, and shock, result in hyperventilation as a compensatory response. Patients in either group could be considered clinically to have respiratory distress; they are distinguished from patients with respiratory disease by their increased V_T as well as the respiratory rate. Their blood gas values reflect a low $PaCO_2$ and a normal PaO_2. Patients with neuromuscular diseases, such as Guillain-Barré syndrome or myasthenia gravis, and those with an abnormal respiratory drive can develop severe respiratory failure but are not able to mount sufficient effort to appear in respiratory distress. In these patients, respirations are ineffective or can even appear normal in the presence of respiratory acidosis and hypoxemia.

The rate and depth of respiration and the presence of retractions, stridor, wheezing, and grunting are valuable signs in localizing the site of respiratory pathology (Table 373-1 and Fig. 373-11). Rapid and shallow respirations (**tachypnea**) are characteristic of parenchymal pathology, in which the elastic WOB is increased disproportionately to the resistive WOB. Chest wall, intercostal, and suprasternal **retractions** are most striking, with increased negative intrathoracic pressure during inspiration. This occurs in extrathoracic airway obstruction as well as diseases of decreased compliance. Inspiratory **stridor** is a hallmark of extrathoracic airway obstruction. Expiratory **wheezing** is characteristic of intrathoracic airway obstruction, either extrapulmonary or intrapulmonary. **Grunting** is produced by expiration against a partially closed glottis and is an attempt to maintain positive airway pressure during expiration for as long as possible. Such prolongation of positive pressure is most beneficial in alveolar diseases that produce widespread loss of FRC, such as in pulmonary edema, hyaline membrane disease, and pneumonia. Grunting is also effective in small airway obstruction (bronchiolitis) to maintain a higher positive pressure in the airway during expiration, decreasing the airway collapse.

Bibliography is available at Expert Consult.

373.6 Ventilation-Perfusion Relationship in Health and Disease

Ashok P. Sarnaik, Sabrina M. Heidemann, and Jeff A. Clark

Gravitational force pulls the lung away from the nondependent part of the parietal pleura. Therefore, alveoli and airways in the nondependent

Table 373-1	Interpreting the Clinical Signs of Respiratory Disease			
SIGN	**EXTRATHORACIC AIRWAY OBSTRUCTION**	**INTRATHORACIC– EXTRAPULMONARY AIRWAY OBSTRUCTION**	**INTRAPULMONARY AIRWAY OBSTRUCTION**	**PARENCHYMAL PATHOLOGY**
Tachypnea	+	+	++	++++
Retractions	++++	++	++	+++
Stridor	++++	++	−	−
Wheezing	±	+++	++++	±
Grunting	±	±	++	++++

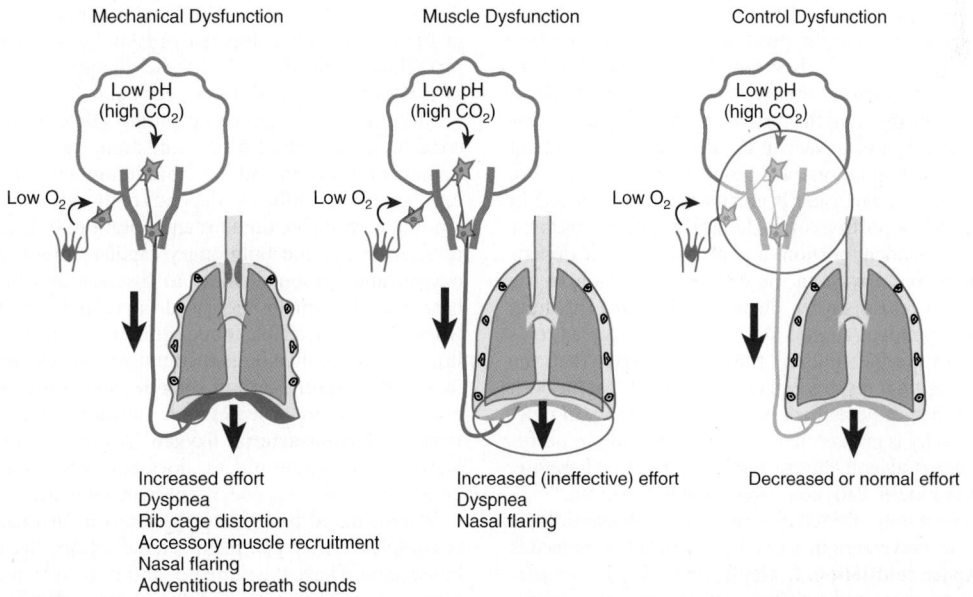

Figure 373-11 **Presentation profiles of respiratory failure in childhood.** When a mechanical dysfunction is present (by far, the most common circumstance), arterial hypoxemia and hypercapnia (and hence, pH) are sensed by peripheral (carotid bodies) and central (medullary) chemoreceptors. After being integrated with other sensory information from the lungs and chest wall, chemoreceptor activation triggers an increase in the neural output to the respiratory muscles *(vertical arrows)*, which results in the physical signs that characterize respiratory distress. When the problem resides with the respiratory muscles (or their innervation), the same increase in neural output occurs *(arrow)*, but the respiratory muscles cannot increase their effort as demanded; therefore, the physical signs of distress are more subtle. Finally, when the control of breathing is itself affected by disease, the neural response to hypoxemia and hypercapnia is absent or blunted and the gas exchange abnormalities are not accompanied by respiratory distress.

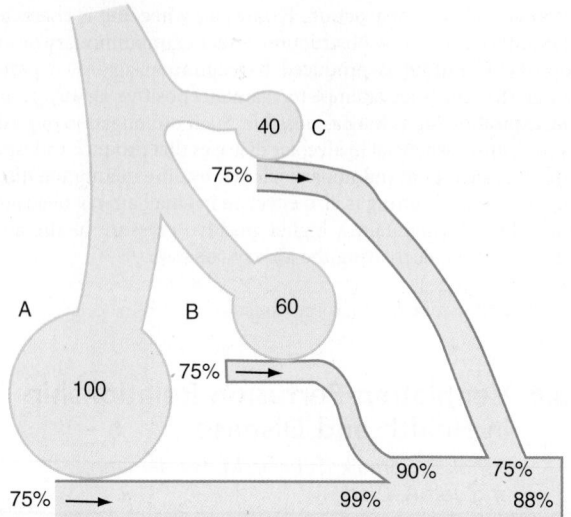

Figure 373-12 Diagram demonstrating the effects of decreased ventilation–perfusion ratios on arterial oxygenation in the lungs. Three alveolar–capillary units are illustrated. Unit A has normal ventilation and an alveolar P_{O_2} of 100 mm Hg (shown by the number in the middle of the space). The blood that circulates through this unit raises its oxygen saturation from 75% (the saturation of mixed venous blood) to 99%. Unit B has a lower ventilation–perfusion ratio and a lower alveolar P_{O_2} of 60 mm Hg. The blood that circulates through this unit reaches a saturation of only 90%. Finally, unit C is not ventilated at all. Its alveolar P_{O_2} is equivalent to that of the venous blood, which travels through the unit unaltered. The oxygen saturation of the arterial blood reflects the weighted contributions of these 3 units. If it is assumed that each unit has the same blood flow, the arterial blood would have a saturation of only 88%. Ventilation–perfusion mismatch is the most common mechanism of arterial hypoxemia in lung disease. Supplemental oxygen increases the arterial P_{O_2} by raising the alveolar P_{O_2} in lung units that, like B, have a ventilation–perfusion ratio >0.

parts (the upper lobes in upright position) of the lung are subjected to greater negative intrapleural pressure during tidal respiration and are kept relatively more inflated compared to the dependent alveoli and airways (the lower lobes in upright position). The nondependent alveoli are less compliant because they are already more inflated. During tidal inspiration, ventilation therefore occurs preferentially in the dependent portions of the lung that are more amenable to expansion. Although perfusion is also greater in the dependent portions of the lung because of greater pulmonary arterial hydrostatic pressure from gravity, the increase in perfusion is greater than the increase in ventilation in the dependent portions of the lung. Thus, the ratios favor ventilation in the nondependent portions and perfusion in the dependent portions. Because the airways in the dependent portion of the lung are narrower, they close earlier during expiration. The lung volume at which the dependent airways start to close is referred to as the **closing capacity**. In normal children, the FRC is greater than the closing capacity. During tidal respiration, airways remain patent both in the dependent and the nondependent portions of the lung. In newborns, the closing capacity is greater than the FRC, resulting in perfusion of poorly ventilated alveoli during tidal respiration; therefore, normal neonates have a lower P_{aO_2} compared to older children.

The relationship is adversely affected in a variety of pathophysiologic states (Fig. 373-12). Air movement in areas that are poorly perfused is referred to as **dead space ventilation.** Examples of dead space ventilation include pulmonary thromboembolism and hypovolemia. Perfusion of poorly ventilated alveoli is referred to as **intrapulmonary right-to-left shunting** or **venous admixture**. Examples include pneumonia, asthma, and hyaline membrane disease. In intrapulmonary airway obstruction, the closing capacity is abnormally increased and can exceed the FRC. In such situations, perfusion of poorly ventilated alveoli during tidal respiration results in venous admixture.

Bibliography is available at Expert Consult.

373.7 Gas Exchange in Health and Disease

Ashok P. Sarnaik, Sabrina M. Heidemann, and Jeff A. Clark

The main function of the respiratory system is to remove carbon dioxide from and add oxygen to the systemic venous blood brought to the lung. The composition of the inspired gas, ventilation, perfusion, diffusion, and tissue metabolism have a significant influence on the arterial blood gases.

The total pressure of the atmosphere at sea level is 760 torr. With increasing altitude, the atmospheric pressure decreases. The total atmospheric pressure is equal to the sum of partial pressures exerted by each of its component gases. Alveolar air is 100% humidified and, therefore, for alveolar gas calculations, the inspired gas is also presumed to be 100% humidified. At a temperature of 37°C (98.6°F) and 100% humidity, water vapor exerts pressure of 47 torr, regardless of altitude. In a natural setting, the atmosphere consists of 20.93% oxygen. **Partial pressure of oxygen in inspired gas (P_{IO_2})** at sea level is therefore $(760 - 47) \times 20.93\% = 149$ torr. When breathing 40% oxygen at sea level, P_{IO_2} is $(760 - 47) \times 40\% = 285$ torr. At higher altitudes, breathing different concentrations of oxygen, P_{IO_2} is less than at sea level, depending on the prevalent atmospheric pressures. In Denver (altitude of 5,000 feet and barometric pressure of 632 torr), P_{IO_2} in room air is $(632 - 47) \times 20.93\% = 122$ torr, and in 40% oxygen, it is $(632 - 47) \times 40\% = 234$ torr.

Minute volume is a product of V_T and respiratory rate. Part of the V_T occupies the conducting airways (anatomic dead space), which does not contribute to gas exchange in the alveoli. **Alveolar ventilation** is the volume of atmospheric air entering the alveoli and is calculated as $(V_T - \text{dead space}) \times$ respiratory rate. Alveolar ventilation is inversely proportional to arterial P_{CO_2} (P_{aCO_2}). When alveolar ventilation is halved, P_{aCO_2} is doubled. Conversely, doubling of alveolar ventilation decreases P_{aCO_2} by 50%. **Alveolar P_{O_2} (P_{aO_2})** is calculated by the **alveolar air equation** as follows:

$$P_{AO_2} = P_{IO_2} - (P_{ACO_2} \div R)$$

where R is the respiratory quotient. For practical purposes, P_{ACO_2} is substituted by **arterial P_{CO_2}** (P_{aCO_2}) and R is assumed to be 0.8. According to the alveolar air equation, for a given P_{IO_2}, a rise in P_{aCO_2} of 10 torr results in a decrease in P_{AO_2} by $10 \div 0.8$ or 10×1.25 or 12.5 torr. Thus, proportionately inverse changes in P_{AO_2} occur to the extent of $1.25\times$ the changes in P_{ACO_2} (or P_{aCO_2}).

After the alveolar gas composition is determined by the inspired gas conditions and process of ventilation, gas exchange occurs by the process of diffusion and equilibration of alveolar gas with pulmonary capillary blood. Diffusion depends on the alveolar capillary barrier and amount of available time for equilibration. In health, the equilibration of alveolar gas and pulmonary capillary blood is complete for both oxygen and carbon dioxide. In diseases in which alveolar capillary barrier is abnormally increased (alveolar interstitial diseases) and/or when the time available for equilibration is decreased (increased blood flow velocity), diffusion is incomplete. Because of its greater solubility in liquid medium, carbon dioxide is 20 times more diffusible than oxygen. Therefore, diseases with diffusion defects are characterized by marked **alveolar-arterial oxygen (A-aO_2)** gradients and hypoxemia. Significant elevation of CO_2 does not occur as a result of a diffusion defect unless there is coexistent hypoventilation.

Venous blood brought to the lungs is "arterialized" after diffusion is complete. After complete arterialization, the pulmonary capillary blood should have the same P_{O_2} and P_{CO_2} as in the alveoli. The arterial blood gas composition is different from that in the alveoli, even in normal conditions because there is a certain amount of dead space ventilation as well as venous admixture in a normal lung. Dead space ventilation results in a higher P_{aCO_2} than P_{ACO_2}, whereas venous admixture or right-to-left shunting results in a lower P_{aO_2} compared to the alveolar gas composition (see Fig. 373-12). P_{aO_2} is a reflection of the amount of oxygen dissolved in blood, which is a relatively minor component of total blood oxygen content. For every 100 torr P_{O_2}, there is 0.3 mL of dissolved O_2 in 100 mL of blood. The total blood oxygen content is composed of the dissolved oxygen and the oxygen bound to hemoglobin. Each gram of hemoglobin carries 1.34 mL of O_2 when 100% saturated with oxygen. Thus, 15 g of hemoglobin carries 20.1 mL of oxygen. **Arterial oxygen content (Cao_2)**, expressed as mL O_2/dL blood, can be calculated as $(Pao_2 \times 0.003) + (Hb \times 1.34 \times So_2)$, where Hb is grams of Hb per deciliter of blood and So_2 is percentage of oxyhemoglobin saturation. The relationship of Po_2 and the amount of oxygen carried by the hemoglobin is the basis of the O_2-Hb dissociation curve (see Fig. 373-5). The Po_2 at which hemoglobin is 50% saturated is referred to as P_{50}. At a normal pH, hemoglobin is 94% saturated at Po_2 of 70, and little further gain in saturation is accomplished at a higher Po_2. At Po_2 <50, there is a steep decline in saturation and therefore the oxygen content.

Oxygen delivery to the tissues is a product of oxygen content and cardiac output. When hemoglobin is near 100% saturated, the blood contains approximately 20 mL oxygen per 100 mL or 200 mL/L. In a healthy adult, the cardiac output is approximately 5 L/min, oxygen delivery 1,000 mL/min, and oxygen consumption 250 mL/min. Mixed venous blood returning to the heart has a Po_2 of 40 torr and is 75% saturated with oxygen. Blood oxygen content, cardiac output, and oxygen consumption are important determinants of mixed venous oxygen saturation. Given a steady-state blood oxygen content and oxygen consumption, the mixed venous saturation is an important indicator of cardiac output. A declining mixed venous saturation in such a state indicates decreasing cardiac output.

Bibliography is available at Expert Consult.

373.8 Interpretation of Blood Gases

Ashok P. Sarnaik, Sabrina M. Heidemann, and Jeff A. Clark

Clinical observations and interpretation of blood gas values are critical in localizing the site of the lesion and estimating its severity (Table 373-2). In airway obstruction above the carina (subglottic stenosis, vascular ring), blood gases reflect overall alveolar hypoventilation. This is manifested by an elevated $PAco_2$ and a proportionate decrease in Pao_2 as determined by the alveolar air equation. A rise in $Paco_2$ of 20 torr decreases Pao_2 by 20×1.25 or 25 torr. In the absence of significant parenchymal disease and intrapulmonary shunting, such lesions respond very well to supplemental oxygen in reversing hypoxemia. Similar blood gas values, demonstrating alveolar hypoventilation and response to supplemental oxygen, are observed in patients with a depressed respiratory center and ineffective neuromuscular function, resulting in respiratory insufficiency. Such patients can be easily distinguished from those with airway obstruction by their poor respiratory effort.

In intrapulmonary airway obstruction (asthma, bronchiolitis), blood gases reflect ventilation-perfusion imbalance and venous admixture. In these diseases, the obstruction is not uniform throughout the lungs, resulting in areas that are hyperventilated and others that are

hypoventilated. Pulmonary capillary blood coming from hyperventilated areas has a higher Po_2 and lower Pco_2, whereas that coming from hypoventilated regions has a lower Po_2 and higher Pco_2. A lower blood Pco_2 can compensate for the higher Pco_2 because the Hb-CO_2 dissociation curve is relatively linear. In mild disease, the hyperventilated areas predominate, resulting in hypocarbia. An elevated Pao_2 in hyperventilated areas cannot compensate for the decreased Pao_2 in hypoventilated areas because of the shape of the O_2-Hb dissociation curve. This results in venous admixture, arterial desaturation, and decreased Pao_2 (see Fig. 373-12). With increasing disease severity, more areas become hypoventilated, resulting in normalization of $Paco_2$ with a further decrease in Pao_2. A normal or slightly elevated $Paco_2$ in asthma should be viewed with concern as a potential indicator of impending respiratory failure. In severe intrapulmonary airway obstruction, hypoventilated areas predominate, leading to hypercarbia, respiratory acidosis, and hypoxemia. The degree to which supplemental oxygenation raises Pao_2 depends on the severity of the illness and the degree of venous admixture.

In alveolar and interstitial diseases, blood gas values reflect both intrapulmonary right-to-left shunting and a diffusion barrier. Hypoxemia is a hallmark of such conditions occurring early in the disease process. $Paco_2$ is either normal or decreased. An increase in $Paco_2$ is observed only later in the course, as muscle fatigue and exhaustion result in hypoventilation. Response to supplemental oxygen is relatively poor with shunting and diffusion disorders compared to other lesions.

Most clinical entities present with mixed lesions. A child with a vascular ring might also have an area of atelectasis; the arterial blood gas reflects both processes. The blood gas values reflect the more dominant lesion.

Bibliography is available at Expert Consult.

373.9 Pulmonary Vasculature in Health and Disease

Ashok P. Sarnaik, Sabrina M. Heidemann, and Jeff A. Clark

The tunica media of the pulmonary arteries of the fetus become more muscular in the last trimester of pregnancy (see Chapter 101.1). Up to 90% of the systemic venous return is shunted away from the pulmonary arterial circulation to the systemic arterial circulation through the foramen ovale and the ductus arteriosus. After birth, with functional closure of the foramen ovale and the ductus arteriosus, and dilation of the pulmonary arterial circulation with consequent decrease in **pulmonary vascular resistance** (**PVR**), all of the right ventricular output passes through the lung. The PVR is approximately 50% of the systemic arterial resistance 3 days after birth. In the next several wk after birth as pulmonary arterial musculature in the tunica media involutes, there is a further decline in PVR and therefore in pulmonary artery pressure. Two to 3 mo after birth, the PVR and the pulmonary artery pressure

LESION	EFFECT	TYPICAL ABG
Central (above the carina) airway obstruction, or Depressed respiratory center, or Ineffective neuromuscular function	Uniform alveolar hypoventilation	Early increase in Pco_2 Proportionate decrease in Po_2 depending on alveolar air equation Response to supplemental oxygen: Excellent
Intrapulmonary airway obstruction	Venous admixture $\dot{V}/\dot{Q}$ mismatch	Mild: ↓ Pco_2, ↓ Po_2 Moderate: "normal" Pco_2, ↓↓ Po_2 Severe: ↑↑ Pco_2, ↓↓↓ Po_2 Response to supplemental oxygen: good
Alveolar–interstitial pathology	Diffusion defect R → L shunt	Early decrease in Po_2 depending on severity Normal or low Pco_2, ↑ Pco_2 if fatigue develops Response to supplemental oxygen: fair to poor

Table 373-2 | Interpretation of Arterial Blood Gas Values

ABG, arterial blood gas; $\dot{V}/\dot{Q}$, ventilation–perfusion.

are approximately 15% of the systemic values, a relationship that exists through childhood and adolescence. Pulmonary vasculature constricts in response to hypoxemia, acidosis, and hypercarbia and dilates with increased alveolar and arterial Po_2, alkalosis, and hypocarbia. Younger infants, with their relatively muscular pulmonary arteries, are especially susceptible to pulmonary vasoconstrictive stimuli.

Failure of the pulmonary arterial circulation to dilate after birth results in **persistent pulmonary hypertension of the newborn** (see Chapter 101.7). Because of the persistently high PVR, the systemic venous blood returning to the right side of the heart continues to be shunted across the foramen ovale and the ductus arteriosus to the systemic arterial circulation, leading to a vicious cycle of hypoxemia, acidosis, and further pulmonary vasoconstriction.

The relatively high PVR opposes excessive left-to-right shunting in full-term neonates with ventricular septal defect and patent ductus arteriosus (see Chapter 426). Such infants do not usually manifest heart failure until 2-3 mo after birth, when PVR has sufficiently declined. Premature infants who have lesions capable of left-to-right shunting are susceptible to developing heart failure earlier in life because of less musculature in pulmonary artery tunica media and, therefore, a lower PVR. The gradual physiologic decline in PVR over the 1st 2-3 mo of life also explains how infants with anomalous left coronary artery arising from the pulmonary artery are asymptomatic at birth but present with signs of coronary insufficiency when PVR has fallen sufficiently to critically decrease coronary perfusion. Persistent and long-term left-to-right shunting carries the risk of developing secondary pulmonary vascular disease characterized by the postnatal development of medial muscular hypertrophy followed by intimal proliferation and increased PVR. Early changes in pulmonary vasculature are reversible with correction of the congenital heart defect responsible for left-to-right shunting. Advanced pulmonary vascular disease is characterized by irreversible intimal and medial changes. When PVR is increased to suprasystemic levels, right-to-left shunting occurs and is characterized by a cyanotic state (Eisenmenger syndrome), making the heart defect inoperable in the absence of an accompanying lung transplantation (see Chapter 433.2).

Pulmonary hypertension can develop without a well-defined etiology (primary pulmonary hypertension) or as a consequence of an underlying disease (secondary pulmonary hypertension) (see Chapter 433). Adverse effects of pulmonary hypertension are related to an increased right ventricular afterload, decreased cardiac output, and heart failure characterized by increased systemic venous pressure, hepatomegaly, and edema. In an acute situation, right ventricular failure and decreased cardiac output can worsen oxygen delivery and hypoxemia. Right ventricular failure secondary to pulmonary pathology is referred to as **cor pulmonale.** Secondary pulmonary hypertension is a common occurrence in end-stage chronic obstructive pulmonary disease such as cystic fibrosis (see Chapter 403) and bronchopulmonary dysplasia (see Chapter 416). Pulmonary arterial involvement is sometimes encountered in collagen vascular diseases such as scleroderma (see Chapter 160) and dermatomyositis (see Chapter 159). Functional or structural upper airway obstruction can also produce right ventricular failure. Children with marked obesity are also susceptible to chronic alveolar hypoventilation and right heart failure, termed **Pickwickian syndrome.** Treatment of the underlying cause is the first priority in patients with secondary pulmonary hypertension (see Chapter 433). Pulmonary hypertension is diagnosed by cardiac catheterization in order to rule out other pulmonary vascular diseases and to test for pulmonary reactivity. A diagnosis of pulmonary hypertension is a mean pulmonary artery pressure of ≥25 mm Hg at rest with a normal pulmonary capillary wedge pressure of ≤15 mm Hg and increased PVR index of ≥3 Wood units/m². Even though the etiologies are different, most of the drugs used to treat this condition in children are adapted from adult studies. Calcium channel blockers, prostanoids (epoprostenol, treprostinil, and iloprost), endothelin receptor antagonists (bosentan, ambrisentan) and phosphodiesterase 5-inhibitors (sildenafil, tadalafil) are some of the agents used for treatment.

Bibliography is available at Expert Consult.

373.10 Immune Response of the Lung to Injury
Ashok P. Sarnaik, Sabrina M. Heidemann, and Jeff A. Clark

Local and systemic diseases can potentially induce an inflammatory response in the lung. Local diseases of the lung capable of inducing the inflammatory response include infectious processes, aspiration, asphyxia, pulmonary contusion, and inhalation of chemical irritants; systemic diseases include sepsis, shock, trauma, and cardiopulmonary bypass. This inflammatory response is mediated through the release of cytokines and other mediators. In the lung, alveolar macrophages are the chief architects of the early cytokine response, producing **tumor necrosis factor-α** and **interleukin-1β.** These cytokines are involved in initiating the inflammatory cascade, resulting in the production of other cytokines, prostaglandins, reactive oxygen species, and upregulating cell adhesion molecules, which, in turn, leads to white cell migration into the lung tissue. The pathophysiologic consequences of the inflammatory response include injury to pulmonary capillary endothelium and the alveolar epithelial cells. Various cytokines and eicosanoids produce pulmonary vasoconstriction, resulting in pulmonary hypertension and increased right ventricular afterload. Injury to the capillary endothelium results in increased permeability and exudation of protein-rich fluid into the pulmonary interstitium and alveoli. Cellular debris and fibrin form the characteristic eosinophilic hyaline membranes along the walls of the alveolar duct. There is sloughing of type 1 pneumocytes. Interstitial and alveolar edema results in decreased FRC, diffusion barrier, intrapulmonary right-to-left shunting across poorly ventilating alveoli, and increase in the A-aO_2 gradient. Clinically, A-aO_2 gradient >200 is characterized as *acute lung injury* and a gradient >300 is termed **acute respiratory distress syndrome (ARDS)** (see Chapter 71). The inflammatory response to lung injury changes from the fetus to the adult. The fetus and neonate are more likely to have less of an inflammatory cytokine response as demonstrated by a decrease in tumor necrosis factor-α production when mononuclear cells are stimulated when compared to the adult.

The pediatrician must consider the potential adverse effects of therapeutic interventions such as oxygen, endotracheal intubation, and mechanical ventilation as part of the pathophysiologic consequences of ARDS. High concentrations of inspired oxygen have a risk of pulmonary capillary and epithelial cell injury; the concentration of oxygen below which it can be considered safe has not been established. In addition to the potential for nosocomial pneumonia, mechanical ventilation carries the risk of ventilator-induced lung injury from physical stress applied to terminal airways, alveolar epithelium, and pulmonary capillaries. Excessive V_T can itself result in mechanical disruption capable of perpetuating the inflammatory response. If alveoli are allowed to deflate excessively during exhalation, they are subjected to greater stress injury from alveolar recruitment and derecruitment. The mechanical ventilation strategy aimed at minimizing ventilator-induced lung injury in ARDS includes alveolar recruitment and maintenance of adequate FRC throughout the respiratory cycle with an optimum PEEP, and ventilation with relatively low (6-8 mL/kg) V_T.

373.11 Regulation of Respiration
Ashok P. Sarnaik, Sabrina M. Heidemann, and Jeff A. Clark

The main function of respiration is to maintain normal blood gas homeostasis to match the metabolic needs of the body with the least amount of energy expenditure. Respiratory rate and V_T are regulated by a complex interaction of **controllers, sensors,** and **effectors.** The central respiratory controller consists of a group of neurons in the CNS that receives and integrates the afferent information from sensors and sends motor impulses to effectors to initiate and maintain respiration. Sensors are a variety of receptors located throughout the body. They gather chemical and physical information that is sent to the controller either to stimulate or to inhibit its activity. Effectors are the various muscles of respiration that, under the influence of controllers, coordinate respiration and move air in and out of the lung at a given V$_T$ and rate. The respiratory regulatory mechanism itself undergoes a significant maturation process from the neonatal period throughout infancy and early childhood. **Sleep states** have the potential for profound influences on the control of respiration.

CENTRAL RESPIRATORY CONTROLLER

Although the respiratory cycle is often viewed as having an active phase (inspiration) and a passive phase (expiration), rhythmic breathing is a complex process controlled by interaction of numerous distinct groups of neurons. Neuronal control of respiration occurs in 3 phases—inspiration (I), early expiration (E1), and late expiration (E2)—and each may be dysfunctional in disease states. The respiratory controller mechanism comprises 2 functionally and anatomically distinct groups of neurons located in the CNS: 1 for **voluntary** and the other for **automatic control**. These areas of respiratory control can function independently but are also capable of interacting with each other.

Voluntary control of respiration resides in the cerebral motor cortex and limbic forebrain structure. Information is received from sensory neurons such as pain, touch, temperature, smell, vision, and emotions, and impulses are sent directly to the respiratory muscles through corticobulbar and corticospinal tracts. Voluntary control of respiration is important for protection from aspiration and inhalation of noxious gases. A certain level of consciousness is necessary to exercise voluntary control of respiration. Patients with CNS injury and toxic or metabolic encephalopathies may lose voluntary control of respirations to varying degrees, depending on the extent of CNS dysfunction.

Automatic control of respiration resides in the brainstem. Central pattern generators (CPGs) are neuronal circuits that generate rhythmic motor output, do not require conscious input, and are responsible for numerous coordinated motor functions such as breathing, swallowing, chewing, walking, and vomiting. The primary CPGs responsible for control of breathing are located in the pons and medulla and include the Bötzinger complex (BotC), pre-Bötzinger complex (pre-BotC), rostral ventral respiratory group and the caudal ventral respiratory group in the medulla, and the Kolliker-Fuse and lateral parabrachial areas in the pons. In addition, an area located adjacent to the facial nerve nucleus, the parafacial respiratory group, is an important modulator of respiration and dysfunction here likely plays a key role in congenital central hypoventilation syndrome (CCHS). Pre-BotC and rostral ventral respiratory group are thought to be the primary sites for inspiratory rhythm generation and BotC and caudal ventral respiratory group are thought to be the primary sites of expiratory rhythm generation under normal circumstances. However, each area is under significant influence from other areas including the nucleus tractus solitus, which is the area responsible for receiving visceral sensor afferents (see below). The genetic mutation responsible for Prader-Willi syndrome is similar to a genetic knockout in mice known to be associated with abnormal development of the pre-BotC and is likely responsible for the abnormal O$_2$ and CO$_2$ responsiveness associated with this disease.

CPG areas can also be modulated by neurotransmitters, which can stimulate, inhibit, or modify their activity; they possess receptors for substance P (neurokinin), acetylcholine (nicotinic), glutamate, and opioid μ receptors among others. The embryologic development of these areas is regulated by several genes such as Hox paralogs and Hox-regulating genes *kreisler/mafB* and *Krox20*. A group of neurons located in the lower pons is collectively termed the **apneustic center,** which stimulates pre-BotC, resulting in prolonged inspiratory gasps (apneuses) interrupted by transient expiratory efforts. Another group of neurons in the upper pons, called the *pneumotaxic center,* is involved in inhibiting the activity of pre-BotC. The role of apneustic and pneumotaxic centers is to fine-tune the rhythmic respiratory activity generated by pre-BotC neurons.

Abnormalities of respirations are commonly encountered in CNS dysfunction and have given clues to the role each of these areas plays in the regulation of respiration. Global CNS depression can manifest as slow and shallow respirations with resultant hypoventilation and respiratory acidosis. Bihemispheric and diencephalic pathology can lead to **Cheyne-Stokes respirations,** characterized by periods of apnea interspersed with hyperventilation. Injuries within the rostral brainstem or tegmentum can lead to central neurogenic hyperventilation and respiratory alkalosis. Mid to caudal pontine lesion can result in an apneustic breathing pattern characterized by a prolonged inspiratory pause. Medullary lesions result in ataxic, irregular breathing or apnea.

SENSORS

The primary responsibility of the respiratory system is to maintain a steady and adequate supply of oxygen to the blood and help maintain adequate pH by eliminating CO$_2$. Even short periods of hypoxemia or acidosis are poorly tolerated, and as such, the body has evolved multiple mechanisms to identify hypoxemia and acidosis/increased CO$_2$. Various receptors throughout the body are responsible for sensing and sending afferent information that modulates the activity of the central respiratory controller. These receptors are sensory nerve endings that respond to changes in their environment. They are termed either **chemoreceptors** or **mechanoreceptors,** depending on the type of stimulus that is sensed. Chemoreceptors are classified as central or peripheral, depending on their location.

Central chemoreceptors are so termed because of their location within the CNS. Chemoreceptors sense a change in the chemical composition of body fluid to which they are exposed. Central chemoreceptors reside over a wide area that includes the posterior hypothalamus, cerebellum, locus ceruleus, raphe, and multiple nuclei within the brainstem. Central chemoreceptors bathe in the extracellular fluid of the brain and respond to the changes in the H$^+$ concentration. Information sensing an increase in H$^+$ concentration stimulates ventilatory response of the controller, whereas a decrease inhibits it. The brain's extracellular fluid, represented by the cerebrospinal fluid (CSF), is separated from the blood by the blood-brain barrier, which is relatively impermeable to H$^+$ and HCO$_3^-$ ions but is readily permeable to CO$_2$. A rise in Paco$_2$ is quickly reflected in a similar rise in the CSF. The consequent fall in CSF pH is sensed by the central chemoreceptors, causing stimulation of the controller and increase in ventilation. Changes in Paco$_2$ result in stimulation or inhibition of ventilation by changes in CSF pH. CSF pH in normal conditions is approximately 7.32. Compared to blood, CSF has much less CO$_2$ buffering capacity because of a much lower protein concentration. Consequently, the change in CSF pH is more pronounced than that in the blood for the same change in Paco$_2$. With a persistent elevation in Paco$_2$, the CSF pH eventually tends to normalize as HCO$_3^-$ equilibrates across the blood-brain barrier. Consequently, patients with chronic obstructive pulmonary disease have a relatively normal CSF pH, and they do not show the ventilatory response that is observed with an acute rise in Paco$_2$. Although O$_2$ chemosensing has traditionally been described as a function of peripheral chemosensors, multiple brainstem areas, including those with CPG function, are oxygen responsive in the range typical to peripheral chemosensor cells.

Peripheral chemoreceptors are located in carotid bodies just above the bifurcation of the common carotid and external carotid arteries, and in the aortic bodies above and below the aortic arch; the carotid bodies are the most important in humans. The most important variable in determining the activity of the carotid bodies is changes in Pao$_2$ and much of their afferent output result from changes in membrane potential due to oxygen sensitive potassium channels. Although the carotid bodies have a relatively high metabolic rate, they receive a very high flow for their rather small size. In the setting of normal oxygen delivery, the dissolved oxygen reflected by Pao$_2$ is sufficient for their metabolism. Stimulation of carotid bodies resulting in increased ventilation occurs when their oxygen supply is decreased below their metabolic requirements. This occurs when there is decreased Pao$_2$, decreased blood flow (low cardiac output), and impaired oxygen use (cyanide poisoning). Anemia and dyshemoglobinemias do not stimulate carotid body activation unless Pao$_2$ and the cardiac output are compromised. The relationship of Pao$_2$ and the stimulation of carotid bodies is nonlinear (Fig. 373-13).

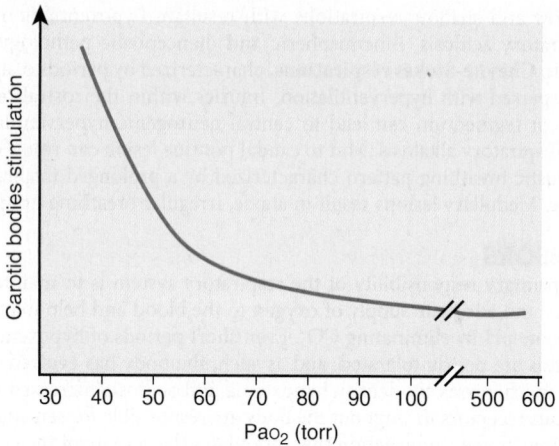

Figure 373-13 Significant stimulation of carotid bodies occurs with PaO₂ level <100 torr. A subjective feeling of dyspnea does not occur, however, until PaO₂ is <50 torr, at which point stimulation of the carotid bodies increases exponentially.

Carotid bodies are activated at a PaO₂ of <500 torr and are responsible for roughly a third of the respiratory drive during normal breathing. Their contribution to respiratory drive increases with decreasing age and may be the major determinant to respiratory drive in premature infants. Periodic breathing and other unstable respiratory patterns seen in newborns may be a result of an increased reliance of peripheral oxygen sensing in maintaining respiratory drive. As PaO₂ decreases, carotid body afferent output increases. A relatively small increase in ventilation occurs until the PaO₂ reaches 100 torr. Where the PaO₂ is <100 torr, the carotid body stimulation increases significantly. The carotid body receptor response rate is fast enough to alter their discharge rate during the respiratory cycle as a result of small cyclic changes in PaO₂ during inspiration and expiration. At PaO₂ levels <50 torr, carotid body stimulation increases exponentially. The most important effect of carotid body stimulation is an increase in respiratory rate and V_T. Additional effects include vasoconstriction, bradycardia, systemic hypertension, release of antidiuretic hormone, and stimulation of the adrenal medulla and adrenal cortex. The bradycardic effect of carotid body stimulation is overshadowed by the pulmonary reflex, which is induced by lung inflation and results in tachycardia. Patients in whom lung inflation is prevented are more likely to develop bradycardia after hypoxic stimulation of carotid bodies. Examples of such situations are fetal hypoxia, CNS depression, neuromuscular blockade, myopathy, neuropathy, and controlled ventilation. The peripheral chemoreceptors are responsible for almost all of the increase in ventilation that occurs in response to hypoxemia.

Peripheral chemoreceptors are also stimulated by an increase in PaCO₂; this response requires a relatively large change in PaCO₂ and results in a smaller rise in minute ventilation compared to the effect of CO₂ on central chemoreceptors. The peripheral chemoreceptors respond much more quickly (within 1 sec), however, whereas the central chemoreceptors can take minutes to respond. Thus peripheral chemoreceptors are important in the immediate rise in ventilation in response to a large and abrupt increase in PaCO₂. Decreased pH also stimulates the peripheral chemoreceptors. The effect of pH is regardless of whether the acidosis is a result of respiratory or metabolic causes. Decreased PaO₂, increased PaCO₂, and decreased pH act synergistically on carotid bodies. The combined effect is greater than the sum of their individual actions.

In contrast to the central chemoreceptors, the peripheral chemoreceptors are not easily depressed, such as by anesthesia or opiates. They also do not adapt easily to a persistent stimulus such as hypoxia, as do the central chemoreceptors to hypercarbia. The central chemoreceptors in hypoxic patients are relatively unresponsive to CO₂ at a time when respirations are predominantly stimulated by effects of hypoxia on peripheral chemoreceptors.

LUNG RECEPTORS

Stretch receptors are located within the airway smooth muscle. They are stimulated by lung inflation, and the impulse is conducted via the vagus nerve. The main effect of these receptors is to decrease the respiratory rate due to an inhibition of inspiratory muscle activity and an increase in exhalation time. This reflex is termed **Hering-Breuer inflation reflex**. Hering-Breuer deflation reflex stimulates inspiratory muscle activity in response to deflation of the lung. These reflexes are not operative during normal breathing in adults but may be important in newborns. Stretch receptors play an important role in minimizing the energy required for the WOB in respiratory disease. In diseases in which airway resistance is increased (asthma), more energy is needed to overcome airway resistance. Slow and deep breathing is most economical in such a situation because of relatively lower flow rate, and greater alveolar inflation is possible without stretching of the airway smooth muscle earlier during inspiration. In diseases of compliance (pulmonary edema), rapid and shallow breathing is most economical to keep the elastic work at minimum. Because of the stiffer alveoli in such situations, the transpulmonary pressure is transmitted to the airway smooth muscle earlier during inspiration, stimulating the stretch receptors and turning off inspiration.

Irritant receptors are present in between the epithelial cells in the airway mucous membrane. They are stimulated by particulate matter, noxious gases, and chemical fumes in the inspired gas, and also by cold air. The vagus nerve is responsible for conducting the impulse. Stimulation of irritant receptors results in bronchoconstriction and hyperpnea.

J receptors derive their name because of their juxtacapillary location. They lie in the alveolar walls close to the pulmonary capillaries. Pulmonary capillary engorgement and interstitial and alveolar wall edema provide stimuli for activation of the J receptors, resulting in shallow and rapid respirations and dyspnea. This is seen in left heart failure, ARDS, and interstitial diseases.

Muscle receptors important for regulation of respirations are those in the diaphragm and the intercostals. Stretch of the muscle sensed by the muscle spindle is used to control the strength of contraction. Excessive distortion of the diaphragm and the intercostals inhibits inspiratory activity when large negative intrathoracic pressure is required to move air, such as in airway obstruction. The soft chest walls of newborns and young infants are more susceptible to distortion; such children might respond to upper airway obstruction by premature cessation of inspiration and apnea rather than by the prolongation of inspiration required to move sufficient air past the obstruction.

Arterial baroreceptors located in aortic arch and carotid sinuses can influence respiration depending on arterial blood pressure. A decrease in blood pressure results in hyperventilation and an increased blood pressure causes hypoventilation.

Pain and temperature receptors also influence respirations, and they are especially pronounced in the neonates and young infants. A painful stimulus causes breath holding followed by hyperventilation. Increased skin temperature causes hyperventilation, and hypothermia results in hypoventilation. In the context of cold stimulus, the facial area is most important in causing apnea.

EFFECTORS

The most important effectors of respiration are the diaphragm, intercostals, and abdominal muscles. They receive impulses from the controller and effect ventilation. Accessory effectors such as sternocleidomastoids and paraspinal muscles may be called on to make additional contribution to the respiratory efforts in times of need. The effectors can be seriously impaired in malnutrition, spinal injury, and neuromuscular disease.

SLEEP STATES

Respiratory regulation is considerably affected by sleep. Sleep, in general, decreases central chemosensitivity to CO₂. PaCO₂ is increased by a few torr compared to that in the wakeful state. Two broad categories of sleep states exist: *non–rapid eye movement* (NREM) and **REM** sleep (see Chapter 19). NREM sleep is characterized by high-voltage, slow waves on electroencephalogram and is associated with fragmented mental activity. Muscle tone and movements are relatively unaffected. NREM sleep is likened to a "relatively inactive brain in a movable body." REM sleep is so termed because of the presence of episodic bursts of REMs.

The most clinically significant aspect of REM sleep is marked suppression of postural muscle tone and lack of spontaneous movements. REM sleep is likened to "a highly activated brain in a paralyzed body." Descending axons from the dorsal pontine tegmentum region are responsible for the REM sleep–specific characteristic atonia and paralysis. The predominant sleep pattern in premature babies is REM sleep. A full-term newborn has 50% REM sleep. Most of the sleep maturation occurs in the 1st 6 mo of life. Older children and adults spend approximately 20% of their sleep in the REM state. Sleep-related respiratory abnormalities are encountered predominantly in REM sleep.

Depression of muscle tone during REM sleep has 2 major effects. The relaxed and therefore increasingly compliant chest wall retracts inward much more during inspiration than a less-compliant chest wall would, resulting in an impediment to air inflow and a paradoxical (seesaw) pattern of breathing in which the abdomen and the chest wall move asynchronously. The second effect is that of relaxation of the genioglossus, palatal, and other upper airway muscles, causing airway obstruction. REM sleep–related respiratory abnormalities are commonly encountered in premature infants and in children with coexistent anatomic upper airway obstruction, obesity, and neuromuscular dysfunction.

REGULATION OF RESPIRATION IN SPECIAL SITUATIONS
Fetus, Newborns, and Young Infants
At various stages of development, the response to chemoreceptor and mechanoreceptor stimulation and the efficiency of effectors are markedly different. Unlike adults, who show an immediate and sustained response to hypoxemia characterized by hyperventilation, the newborn exhibits a biphasic response. After an initial brief period (1-2 min) of hyperventilation, the neonate and young infant develop hypoventilation and apnea when hypoxemia is sustained. This explains why such infants are much more prone to develop respiratory arrest in hypoxic states than are older children and adults. Lower gestational age of the infant is associated with a more pronounced and earlier apneic response to hypoxemia. Fetal respiratory activity, for example, is switched off when faced with oxygen deprivation. Maturation of carotid chemoreceptors may be an explanation for the differences in hypoxic response at various stages of development. Sensitivity of CO_2 sensors also undergoes maturation. Compared to adults and older children, neonates and young infants have decreased CO_2 responsiveness, as measured by an increase in minute alveolar ventilation for a given increase in $Paco_2$. Theophylline and caffeine increase the central chemoreceptor ventilatory response to CO_2 and decrease the number of apneic spells in premature babies.

The neonatal respiratory muscles are poorly equipped to sustain large workloads; they are more easily fatigued than in older children, and this significantly limits their ability to maintain adequate ventilation in lung disease. Also, the excessive inward retraction of the relatively soft infantile chest wall stimulates the intercostal muscles' stretch receptors, sending inhibitory impulses to the respiratory center. Young infants are therefore at greater risk of developing apnea when respiratory muscles are subjected to large elastic loads, such as in upper airway obstruction.

Many neurotransmitters involved in regulation of respiration also undergo developmental maturational changes. Serotoninergic neurons located in the raphe nuclei possess chemosensitive properties and respond to a decrease in pH. An increase in population of these neurons is associated with increasing chemosensitivity in the developing animal. Abnormalities of the arcuate nucleus, the human equivalent of the rat and cat medullary raphe, have been demonstrated at autopsy on infants dying of sudden infant death syndrome (SIDS; Chapter 375). Cohort studies of Japanese, African-American, and white victims of SIDS have implicated a homozygous gene that encodes for the long allele of the serotonin transporter promoter. SIDS victims are more likely to express the long allele of the serotonin transporter promoter and miss the short allele compared to controls. The delay in development of serotoninergic neurons or overexpression of the long allele for serotonin transporter promoter might explain the abnormal respiratory response to adverse conditions, which results in SIDS. Central chemoreception is also severely impaired in congenital central hypoventilation syndrome (**CCHS**), also known as Ondine's curse, which results in sleep-associated respiratory arrests. Mutations of *PHOX2B* gene located on chromosome 4 cause CCHS.

Chronic Hypoxia and Hypercarbia
The respiratory control mechanism is altered when exposed to chronic conditions. In patients with chronic pulmonary insufficiency with elevated $Paco_2$, the CSF pH has been normalized and the central chemoreceptors become unresponsive to CO_2. Renal compensation results in bicarbonate retention and relative normalization of blood pH. Arterial hypoxemia remains the chief stimulus for ventilation, which is predominantly dependent on peripheral chemoreceptor stimulation by a low Pao_2. Administration of a high amount of oxygen in such patients carries a risk of sudden removal of the hypoxic stimulus, cessation of breathing, exacerbation of hypercarbia and CO_2 narcosis, and coma. Patients with chronic obstructive pulmonary disease and neuromuscular disease are especially susceptible to this complication. Children with bronchopulmonary dysplasia or with muscular dystrophy who have had a high $Paco_2$, with or without supplemental oxygen, can develop serious hypoventilation and respiratory acidosis when their Pao_2 is increased more than their baseline with administration of a higher amount of oxygen.

Chronically hypoxic patients, such as those living at high altitude and those with cyanotic heart disease and interstitial lung disease, have a blunted chemoreceptor function and poor response to further hypoxemia. It is of interest to the clinician that children with poorly controlled asthma also show a blunted hypoxic response and can appear to be breathing relatively comfortably in spite of dangerously low Pao_2. Such children and their caretakers are at risk of failing to appreciate the severity of their disease, which can result in delay in instituting appropriate therapy.

Bibliography is available at Expert Consult.

Chapter **374**
Diagnostic Approach to Respiratory Disease
Gabriel G. Haddad and Thomas P. Green

A careful history and physical examination are essential to the accurate diagnosis of a child presenting with respiratory signs and/or symptoms. Sometimes, but not always, additional diagnostic tests and modalities are required.

HISTORY
The history begins with a narrative provided by the parent/caretaker with input from the patient. The history should include questions about respiratory symptoms (dyspnea, cough, pain, wheezing, snoring, apnea, cyanosis), chronicity, timing during day or night, and associations with activities including exercise or food intake. The respiratory system interacts with a number of other systems, and questions related

to cardiac, gastrointestinal, central nervous, hematologic, and immune systems may be relevant. Questions related to gastrointestinal reflux, congenital abnormalities (airway anomalies, ciliary dyskinesia), or immune status may be important in a patient with repeated pneumonia. The family history is essential and should include inquiries about siblings and other close relatives with similar symptoms or any chronic disease with respiratory components.

PHYSICAL EXAMINATION

Respiratory dysfunction usually produces detectable alterations in the pattern of breathing. Values for normal respiratory rates are presented in Table 67-1 (in Chapter 67) and depend on many factors, most importantly, age. Repeated respiratory rate measurements are necessary because respiratory rates, especially in the young, are exquisitely sensitive to extraneous stimuli. Sleeping respiratory rates are more reproducible in infants than those obtained during feeding or activity. These rates vary among infants but average 40-50 breaths/min in the 1st few wk of life and usually <60 breaths/min in the 1st few days of life.

Respiratory control abnormalities can cause the child to breathe at a low rate or periodically. Mechanical abnormalities produce compensatory changes that are generally directed at altering minute ventilation to maintain alveolar ventilation. Decreases in lung compliance require increases in muscular force and breathing rate, leading to variable increases in chest wall retractions and nasal flaring. The respiratory excursions of children with restrictive disease are shallow. An expiratory grunt is common as the child attempts to raise the *functional residual capacity* (FRC) by closing the glottis at the end of expiration. Children with obstructive disease might take slower, deeper breaths (see Chapter 373). When the obstruction is **extrathoracic** (from the nose to the mid-trachea), inspiration is more prolonged than expiration, and an inspiratory stridor can usually be heard (see Fig. 373-8 in Chapter 373). When the obstruction is **intrathoracic,** expiration is more prolonged than inspiration, and the patient often has to make use of accessory expiratory muscles. Intrathoracic obstruction results in air trapping and, therefore, a larger residual volume and, perhaps, greater FRC (see Fig. 373-10 in Chapter 373).

Lung percussion has limited value in small infants because it cannot discriminate between noises originating from tissues that are close to each other. In adolescents and adults, percussion is usually dull in restrictive lung disease, with a pleural effusion, pneumonia, and atelectasis, but it is tympanitic in obstructive disease (asthma, pneumothorax).

Auscultation confirms the presence of inspiratory or expiratory prolongation and provides information about the symmetry and quality of air movement. In addition, it often detects abnormal or adventitious sounds such as **stridor** (a predominant inspiratory monophonic noise), **crackles** (or **rales**) (high-pitched, interrupted sounds found during inspiration and more rarely during early expiration, which denote opening of previously closed air spaces), or **wheezes** (musical, continuous sounds usually caused by the development of turbulent flow in narrow airways) (Table 374-1). **Digital clubbing** is a sign of chronic hypoxia and chronic lung disease (Fig. 374-1) but may be a result of nonpulmonary etiologies (Table 374-2).

Table 374-1	Lung Sound Nomenclature
TYPE	**SOUND**
DISCONTINUOUS	
Fine (high pitch, low amplitude, short duration)	Fine crackles/rales
Coarse (low pitch, high amplitude, long duration)	Coarse crackles
CONTINUOUS	
High pitch	Wheezes
Low pitch	Rhonchi

From Cugell DW: Lung sound nomenclature, Am Rev Respir Dis 136:1016, 1987, with permission.

BLOOD GAS ANALYSIS

See also Chapters 373.7 and 373.8.

An arterial blood gas analysis is probably the single most useful rapid test of pulmonary function. Although this analysis does not specify the cause of the condition or the specific nature of the disease process, it can give an overall assessment of the functional state of the respiratory system and clues about the pathogenesis of the disease. Because the detection of cyanosis is influenced by skin color, perfusion, and blood hemoglobin concentration, the clinical detection by inspection is an unreliable sign of hypoxemia. Arterial hypertension, tachycardia, and diaphoresis are late, and not exclusive, signs of hypoventilation.

Blood gas exchange is evaluated most accurately by the direct measurement of arterial pressure of oxygen (Po_2), pressure of carbon dioxide (Pco_2), and pH. The blood specimen is best collected anaerobically in a heparinized syringe containing only enough heparin solution to displace the air from the syringe. The syringe should be sealed, placed in ice, and analyzed immediately. Although these measurements have no substitute in many conditions, they require arterial puncture and have been replaced to a great extent by noninvasive monitoring, such as capillary samples and/or oxygen saturation.

The age and clinical condition of the patient need to be taken into account when interpreting blood gas tensions. With the exception of neonates, values of arterial Po_2 <85 mm Hg are usually abnormal for a child breathing room air at sea level. Calculation of the alveolar–arterial oxygen gradient is useful in the analysis of arterial oxygenation, particularly when the patient is not breathing room air or in the presence of hypercarbia. Values of arterial Pco_2 >45 mm Hg usually indicate hypoventilation or a severe ventilation–perfusion mismatch, unless they reflect respiratory compensation for metabolic alkalosis (see Chapter 55).

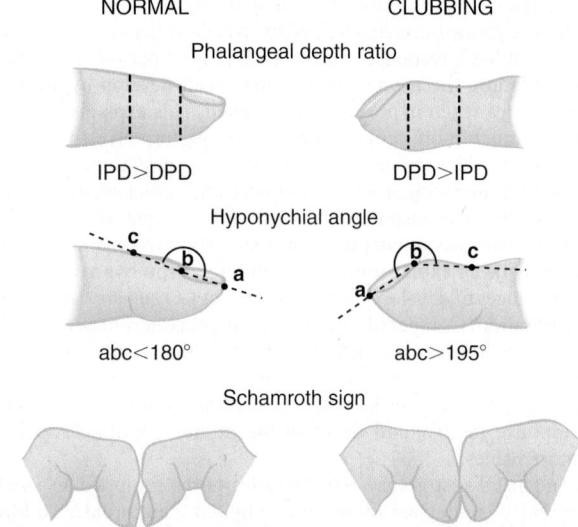

NORMAL   CLUBBING

Phalangeal depth ratio

IPD>DPD   DPD>IPD

Hyponychial angle

abc<180°   abc>195°

Schamroth sign

Figure 374-1 Finger clubbing can be measured in different ways. The ratio of the distal phalangeal diameter (DPD) over the interphalangeal diameter (IPD), or the phalangeal depth ratio, is <1 in normal subjects but increases to >1 with finger clubbing. The DPD/IPD can be measured with calipers or, more accurately, with finger casts. The hyponychial angle can be measured from lateral projections of the finger contour on a magnifying screen and is usually <180 degrees in normal subjects but >195 degrees in patients with finger clubbing. For bedside clinical assessment, the Schamroth sign is useful. The dorsal surfaces of the terminal phalanges of similar fingers are placed together. With clubbing, the normal diamond-shaped aperture or "window" at the bases of the nail beds disappears, and a prominent distal angle forms between the ends of the nails. In normal subjects, this angle is minimal or nonexistent. *(From Pasterkamp H: The history and physical examination. In Wilmott RW, Boat TF, Bush A, et al, editors: Kendig and Chernick's disorders of the respiratory tract in children, ed 8, Philadelphia, 2012, Elsevier.)*

Table 374-2	Nonpulmonary Diseases Associated with Clubbing

CARDIAC
Cyanotic congenital heart disease
Subacute bacterial endocarditis
Chronic congestive heart failure

HEMATOLOGIC
Thalassemia
Congenital methemoglobinemia (rare)

GASTROINTESTINAL
Crohn disease
Ulcerative colitis
Celiac disease
Chronic dysentery, sprue
Polyposis coli
Severe gastrointestinal hemorrhage
Small bowel lymphoma
Liver cirrhosis (including α_1-antitrypsin deficiency)

OTHER
Thyroid deficiency (thyroid acropachy)
Chronic pyelonephritis (rare)
Toxic (e.g., arsenic, mercury, beryllium)
Lymphomatoid granulomatosis
Fabry disease
Raynaud disease, scleroderma
Familial

UNILATERAL CLUBBING
Vascular disorders (e.g., subclavian arterial aneurysm, brachial arteriovenous fistula)
Subluxation of shoulder
Median nerve injury
Local trauma

From Pasterkamp H: The history and physical examination. In Wilmott RW, Boat TF, Bush A, et al, editors: Kendig and Chernick's disorders of the respiratory tract in children, ed 8, Philadelphia, 2012, Elsevier.

TRANSILLUMINATION OF THE CHEST

In infants up to at least 6 mo of age, a pneumothorax (see Chapter 101.12) can often be diagnosed by transilluminating the chest wall using a fiberoptic light probe. Free air in the pleural space often results in an unusually large halo of light in the skin surrounding the probe. Comparison with the contralateral chest is often very helpful in interpreting findings. This test is unreliable in older patients and in those with subcutaneous emphysema or atelectasis.

RADIOGRAPHIC TECHNIQUES
Chest X-Rays

A posteroanterior and a lateral view (upright and in full inspiration) should be obtained except in situations in which the child is medically unstable. Portable films, although useful in the latter situation, can give a somewhat distorted image. Expiratory films can be misinterpreted, although a comparison of expiratory and inspiratory films may be useful in evaluating a child with suspected foreign body (localized failure of the lung to empty reflects bronchial obstruction: Chapter 387). If pleural fluid is suspected (see Chapter 410), decubitus films are indicated. Films taken in a recumbent position are difficult to interpret if there is fluid within the pleural space or a cavity.

Upper Airway Film

A lateral view of the neck can yield invaluable information about upper airway obstruction (see Chapter 385) and particularly about the condition of the retropharyngeal, supraglottic, and subglottic spaces (which should also be viewed in an anteroposterior projection). Knowing the phase of respiration during which the film was taken is often essential for accurate interpretation. Magnified airway films are often helpful in delineating the upper airways. Patients with suggested obstruction should not be unattended in the radiology department.

Sinus and Nasal Films

The general utility of roentgenographic examination of the sinuses is uncertain because of the large number of films with positive findings (low sensitivity and specificity). Imaging studies are not necessary to confirm the diagnosis of sinusitis in children younger than age 6 yr. CT scans are indicated if surgery is required, in cases of complications caused by sinus infection, in immunodeficient patients, and for recurrent infections that are not responsive to medical management.

Chest Computed Tomography and Magnetic Resonance Imaging

Chest CT and MRI can potentially provide images of higher quality and sensitivity than is possible with other imaging modalities. For example, chest CT identifies early abnormalities in young children with cystic fibrosis before pathologic changes are detectable by either plain chest radiographs or pulmonary function testing. Several caveats, however, must be noted. Conventional chest CT involves considerably higher radiation doses than plain films (see Chapter 718). The time required to perform chest CT examinations and the complications of respiratory and body motion mandates the use of sedation for this procedure in many infants and young children. However, improvements in imaging hardware and software have drastically reduced required radiation doses as well as imaging time, obviating the need for sedation in many patients. Chest CT is particularly useful in evaluating very small lesions (e.g., early metastases, mediastinal and pleural lesions, solid or cystic parenchymal lesions, pulmonary embolism, and bronchiectasis). The use of intravenous contrast material during CT imaging enhances vascular structures, distinguishing vessels from other soft-tissue densities. MRI does not involve ionizing radiation, but long imaging times are still involved, and sedation will be necessary to limit spontaneous movement. The utility of MRI of the chest is largely limited to the analysis of mediastinal, hilar, and vascular anatomy. Parenchymal structures and lesions are not well evaluated by MRI.

Fluoroscopy

Fluoroscopy is especially useful for evaluating stridor and abnormal movement of the diaphragm or mediastinum. Many procedures, such as needle aspiration or biopsy of a peripheral lesion, are also best accomplished with the aid of fluoroscopy, CT, or ultrasonography. Videotape recording, which does not increase radiation exposure, can allow detailed study through replay capability during a brief exposure to fluoroscopy.

Barium Swallow

A barium swallow study, performed with fluoroscopy and spot films, is indicated in the evaluation of patients with recurrent pneumonia, persistent cough of undetermined cause, stridor, or persistent wheezing. The technique can be modified by using barium of different textures and thicknesses, ranging from thin liquid to solids, to evaluate swallowing mechanics, the presence of vascular rings (see Chapter 386), and tracheoesophageal fistulas (see Chapter 319), especially when aspiration is suspected. A contrast esophagram has been used in evaluating newborns with suggested esophageal atresia, but this procedure entails a high risk of pulmonary aspiration and is not usually recommended. Barium swallows are useful in evaluating suggested gastroesophageal reflux (see Chapter 323), but because of the high incidence of asymptomatic reflux in infants, the applicability of the findings to the clinical problem may be complicated.

Pulmonary Arteriography and Aortograms

Pulmonary arteriography has been used to allow detailed evaluation of the pulmonary vasculature; has been helpful in assessing pulmonary blood flow and in diagnosing congenital anomalies, such as lobar agenesis, unilateral hyperlucent lung, vascular rings, and arteriovenous malformations; and it is sometimes useful in evaluating solid or cystic lesions. Thoracic aortograms demonstrate the aortic arch, its major vessels, and the systemic (bronchial) pulmonary circulation. They are useful in evaluating vascular rings and suspected pulmonary sequestration. Although most hemoptysis is from the bronchial arteries, bronchial arteriography is seldom helpful in diagnosing or treating intrapulmonary bleeding in children. Real-time and Doppler echocardiography and thoracic CT with contrast are noninvasive methods that often reveal similar information and should be considered before arteriography is performed.

Radionuclide Lung Scans

The usual scan uses intravenous injection of material (macroaggregated human serum albumin labeled with ^{99m}Tc) that will be trapped in the pulmonary capillary bed. The distribution of radioactivity, proportional to pulmonary capillary blood flow, is useful in evaluating pulmonary embolism and congenital cardiovascular and pulmonary defects. Acute changes in the distribution of pulmonary perfusion can reflect alterations of pulmonary ventilation.

The distribution of pulmonary ventilation can also be determined by scanning after the patient inhales a radioactive gas such as xenon-133. After the intravenous injection of xenon-133 dissolved in saline, pulmonary perfusion and ventilation can be evaluated by continuous recording of the rate of appearance and disappearance of the xenon over the lung. Appearance of xenon early after injection is a measure of perfusion, and the rate of washout during breathing is a measure of ventilation in the pediatric population. The most important indication for this test is to demonstrate defects in the pulmonary arterial distribution that can occur with congenital malformations or pulmonary embolism. **Spiral reconstruction CT** with contrast medium enhancement is very helpful in evaluating pulmonary thrombi and emboli. Abnormalities in regional ventilation are also easily demonstrable in congenital lobar emphysema, cystic fibrosis, and asthma.

PULMONARY FUNCTION TESTING

See also Chapters 373.7 and 373.9.

The measurement of respiratory function in infants and young children can be difficult because of the lack of cooperation. Attempts have been made to overcome this limitation by creating standard tests that do not require the patient's active participation. Respiratory function tests still provide only a partial insight into the mechanisms of respiratory disease at early ages.

Whether restrictive or obstructive, most forms of respiratory disease cause alterations in lung volume and its subdivisions. Restrictive diseases typically decrease **total lung capacity (TLC)**. TLC includes residual volume, which is not accessible to direct determinations. It must therefore be measured indirectly by gas dilution methods or, preferably, by **plethysmography.** Restrictive disease also decreases **vital capacity (VC).** Obstructive diseases produce gas trapping and thus increase residual volume and FRC, particularly when these measurements are considered with respect to TLC.

Airway obstruction is most commonly evaluated from determinations of gas flow in the course of a forced expiratory maneuver. The **peak expiratory flow** is reduced in advanced obstructive disease. The wide availability of simple devices that perform this measurement at the bedside makes it useful for assessing children who have airway obstruction. Evaluation of peak flows requires a voluntary effort, and peak flows may not be altered when the obstruction is moderate or mild. Other gas flow measurements require that the child inhale to TLC and then exhale as far and as fast as possible for several seconds. Cooperation and good muscle strength are therefore necessary for the measurements to be reproducible. The **forced expiratory volume in 1 sec** (FEV_1) correlates well with the severity of obstructive diseases. The **maximal midexpiratory flow rate,** the average flow during the middle 50% of the forced VC, is a more reliable indicator of mild airway obstruction. Its sensitivity to changes in residual volume and VC, however, limits its use in children with more severe disease. The construction of flow-volume relationships during the forced VC maneuvers overcomes some of these limitations by expressing the expiratory flows as a function of lung volume.

A **spirometer** is used to measure VC and its subdivisions and expiratory (or inspiratory) flow rates (see Fig. 365-1 in Chapter 365). A simple manometer can measure the maximal inspiratory and expiratory force a subject generates, normally at least 30 cm H_2O, which is useful in evaluating the neuromuscular component of ventilation. Expected normal values for VC, FRC, TLC, and residual volume are obtained from prediction equations based on body height.

Flow rates measured by spirometry usually include the FEV_1 and the **maximal midexpiratory flow rate.** More information results from a maximal expiratory flow-volume curve, in which expiratory flow rate is plotted against expired lung volume (expressed in terms of either VC or TLC). Flow rates at lung volumes less than approximately 75% VC are relatively independent of effort. Expiratory flow rates at low lung volumes (<50% VC) are influenced much more by small airways than are flow rates at high lung volumes (FEV_1). The flow rate at 25% VC is a useful index of small airway function. Low flow rates at high lung volumes associated with normal flow at low lung volumes suggest upper airway obstruction.

Airway resistance (R_{AW}) is measured in a plethysmograph, or, alternatively, the reciprocal of R_{AW}, **airway conductance,** may be used. Because R_{AW} measurements vary with the lung volume at which they are taken, it is convenient to use **specific airway resistance,** SR_{AW} ($SR_{AW} = R_{AW}/$lung volume), which is nearly constant in subjects older than age 6 yr (normally <7 sec/cm H_2O).

The **diffusing capacity for carbon monoxide** is related to oxygen diffusion and is measured by rebreathing from a container having a known initial concentration of carbon monoxide or by using a single-breath technique. Decreases in diffusing capacity for carbon monoxide reflect decreases in effective alveolar capillary surface area or decreases in diffusibility of the gas across the alveolar-capillary membrane. Primary diffusion abnormalities are unusual in children; therefore, this test is most commonly employed in children with rheumatologic or autoimmune diseases and in children exposed to toxic drugs to the lungs (e.g., oncology patients) or chest wall radiation. Regional gas exchange can be conveniently estimated with the perfusion-ventilation xenon scan. Determining arterial blood gas levels also discloses the effectiveness of alveolar gas exchange.

Pulmonary function testing, although rarely resulting in a diagnosis, is helpful in defining the type of process (obstruction, restriction) and the degree of functional impairment, in following the course and treatment of disease, and in estimating the prognosis. It is also useful in preoperative evaluation and in confirmation of functional impairment in patients having subjective complaints but a normal physical examination. In most patients with obstructive disease, a repeat test after administering a bronchodilator is warranted.

Most tests require some cooperation and understanding by the patient, and interpretation is greatly facilitated if the test conditions and the patient's behavior during the test are known. Infants and young children who cannot or will not cooperate with test procedures can be studied in a limited number of ways, which often require sedation. Flow rates and pressures during tidal breathing, with or without transient interruption of the flow, may be useful to assess some aspects of R_{AW} or obstruction and to measure compliance of the lungs and thorax. Expiratory flow rates can be studied in sedated infants with passive compression of the chest and abdomen with a rapidly inflatable jacket. Gas dilution or plethysmographic methods can also be used in sedated infants to measure FRC and R_{AW}.

MICROBIOLOGY: EXAMINATION OF LUNG SECRETIONS

The specific diagnosis of infection in the lower respiratory tract depends on the proper handling of an adequate specimen obtained in an appropriate fashion. Nasopharyngeal or throat cultures are often used but might not correlate with cultures obtained by more-direct techniques from the lower airways. Sputum specimens are preferred and are often obtained from patients who do not expectorate by deep throat swab immediately after coughing or by saline nebulization. Specimens can also be obtained directly from the tracheobronchial tree by nasotracheal aspiration (usually heavily contaminated), by transtracheal aspiration through the cricothyroid membrane (useful in adults and adolescents but hazardous in children), and in infants and children by a sterile catheter inserted into the trachea either during direct laryngoscopy or through a freshly inserted endotracheal tube. A specimen can also be obtained at bronchoscopy. A percutaneous lung tap or an open biopsy is the only way to obtain a specimen absolutely free of oral flora.

A specimen obtained by direct expectoration is usually assumed to be of tracheobronchial origin, but often, especially in children, it is not from this source. The presence of alveolar macrophages (large mononuclear cells) is the hallmark of tracheobronchial secretions. Nasopharyngeal and tracheobronchial secretions can contain ciliated epithelial cells, which are more commonly found in sputum. Nasopharyngeal and oral secretions often contain large numbers of squamous epithelial cells. Sputum can contain both ciliated and squamous epithelial cells.

During sleep, mucociliary transport continually brings tracheobronchial secretions to the pharynx, where they are swallowed. An early-morning fasting gastric aspirate often contains material from the tracheobronchial tract that is suitable for culture for acid-fast bacilli.

The absence of polymorphonuclear leukocytes in a Wright-stained smear of sputum or **bronchoalveolar lavage** (BAL) fluid containing adequate numbers of macrophages may be significant evidence against a bacterial infectious process in the lower respiratory tract, assuming that the patient has normal neutrophil counts and function. Eosinophils suggest allergic disease. Iron stains can reveal hemosiderin granules within macrophages, suggesting pulmonary hemosiderosis. Specimens should also be examined by Gram stain. Bacteria within or near macrophages and neutrophils can be significant. Viral pneumonia may be accompanied by intranuclear or cytoplasmic inclusion bodies visible on Wright-stained smears, and fungal forms may be identifiable on Gram or silver stains.

With advances in the area of genomics and the speed with which it is possible to identify microbes, microbiologic analysis has been expanded. For example, specific bacteria in the lungs of children with cystic fibrosis (see Chapter 403) are linked to morbidity and mortality. There is a correlation between patient age and morbidity and mortality (as expected) but that there are important microbes that are correlated either negatively or positively with early or late pathogenic processes. *Haemophilus influenzae* (see Chapter 194) is negatively correlated and *Pseudomonas aeruginosa* and *Stenotrophomonas maltophilia* (see Chapter 205) have a strong positive correlation with patient age in cystic fibrosis. The microbiota diversity is much broader in those who are healthier individuals or those that are younger patients with cystic fibrosis than the older and sicker population.

In addition, the microbiomes (see Chapter 171) in the respiratory tract of smokers and nonsmokers differ substantially. In all patients, most of the bacteria found in the lungs are also present in the oral cavity, as expected, although some bacteria, such as *Haemophilus* and enterobacteria are much more represented in the lungs than in the mouth. Principal differences between smokers and nonsmokers are found in the microbiome in the mouth, for example, bacteria like *Neisseria*.

EXERCISE TESTING

Exercise testing (see Chapter 423.5) is a more-direct approach for detecting diffusion impairment as well as other forms of respiratory disease. Exercise is a strong provocateur of bronchospasm in susceptible patients, so exercise testing can be useful in the diagnosis of patients with asthma that is only apparent with activity. Measurements of heart and respiratory rate, minute ventilation, oxygen consumption, carbon dioxide production, and arterial blood gases during incremental exercise loads often provide invaluable information about the functional nature of the disease. Often a simple assessment of the patient's exercise tolerance in conjunction with other, more static forms of respiratory function testing can allow a distinction between respiratory and nonrespiratory disease in children.

SLEEP STUDIES
See Chapter 19.

AIRWAY VISUALIZATION AND LUNG SPECIMEN–BASED DIAGNOSTIC TESTS
Laryngoscopy
The evaluation of stridor, problems with vocalization, and other upper airway abnormalities usually requires direct inspection. Although indirect (mirror) laryngoscopy may be reasonable in older children and adults, it is rarely feasible in infants and small children. Direct laryngoscopy may be performed with either a rigid or a flexible instrument. The safe use of the rigid scope for examining the upper airway requires topical anesthesia and either sedation or general anesthesia, whereas the flexible laryngoscope can often be used in the office setting with or without sedation. Further advantages to the flexible scope include the ability to assess the airway without the distortion that may be introduced by the use of the rigid scope and the ability to assess airway dynamics more accurately. Because there is a relatively high incidence of concomitant lesions in the upper and lower airways, it is often prudent to examine the airways above and below the glottis, even when the primary indication is in the upper airway (stridor).

Bronchoscopy and Bronchoalveolar Lavage
Bronchoscopy is the inspection of the airways. BAL is a method used to obtain a representative specimen of fluid and secretions from the lower respiratory tract, which is useful for the cytologic and microbiologic diagnosis of lung diseases, especially in those who are unable to expectorate sputum. BAL is performed after the general inspection of the airways and before tissue sampling with a brush or biopsy forceps. BAL is accomplished by gently wedging the scope into a lobar, segmental, or subsegmental bronchus and sequentially instilling and withdrawing sterile nonbacteriostatic saline in a volume sufficient to ensure that some of the aspirated fluid contains material that originated from the alveolar space. Nonbronchoscopic BAL can be performed, although with less accuracy and, therefore, less-reliable results, in intubated patients by instilling and withdrawing saline through a catheter passed though the artificial airway and blindly wedged into a distal airway. In either case, the presence of alveolar macrophages documents that an alveolar sample has been obtained. Because the methods used to perform BAL involve passage of the equipment through the upper airway, there is a risk of contamination of the specimen by upper airway secretions. Careful cytologic examination and quantitative microbiologic cultures are important for correct interpretation of the data. BAL can often obviate the need for more-invasive procedures such as open lung biopsy, especially in immunocompromised patients.

Indications for diagnostic bronchoscopy and BAL include recurrent or persistent pneumonia or atelectasis, unexplained or localized and persistent wheeze, the suspected presence of a foreign body, hemoptysis, suspected congenital anomalies, mass lesions, interstitial disease, and pneumonia in the immunocompromised host. Indications for therapeutic bronchoscopy and BAL include bronchial obstruction by mass lesions, foreign bodies or mucus plugs, and general bronchial toilet and bronchopulmonary lavage. The patient undergoing bronchoscopy ventilates around the flexible scope, whereas with the rigid scope, ventilation is accomplished through the scope. Rigid bronchoscopy is preferentially indicated for extracting foreign bodies, for removing tissue masses, and in patients with massive hemoptysis. In other cases, the flexible scope offers the advantages that it can be passed through endotracheal or tracheostomy tubes, can be introduced into bronchi that come off the airway at acute angles, and can be safely and effectively inserted with topical anesthesia and conscious sedation.

Regardless of the instrument used, the procedure performed, or its indications, the most common complications are related to sedation. The relatively more common complications related to the bronchoscopy itself include transient hypoxemia, laryngospasm, bronchospasm, and cardiac arrhythmias. Iatrogenic infection, bleeding, pneumothorax, and pneumomediastinum are rare but reported complications of bronchoscopy or BAL. Bronchoscopy in the setting of possible pulmonary abscess or hemoptysis must be undertaken with advance preparations for definitive airway control, mindful of the possibility that pus or blood might flood the airway. Subglottic edema is a more common complication of rigid bronchoscopy than of flexible procedures, in which the scopes are smaller and less likely to traumatize the mucosa. Postbronchoscopy croup is treated with oxygen, mist, vasoconstrictor aerosols, and corticosteroids as necessary.

Thoracoscopy

The pleural cavity can be examined through a thoracoscope, which is similar to a rigid bronchoscope. The thoracoscope is inserted through an intercostal space and the lung is partially deflated, thus allowing the operator to view the surface of the lung, the pleural surface of the mediastinum and diaphragm, and the parietal pleura. Multiple thoracoscopic instruments can be inserted, allowing endoscopic biopsy of the lung or pleura, resection of blebs, abrasion of the pleura, and ligation of vascular rings.

Thoracentesis

For diagnostic or therapeutic purposes, fluid can be removed from the pleural space by needle. Generally, as much fluid as possible should be withdrawn, and an upright chest roentgenogram should be obtained after the procedure. Complications of thoracentesis include infection, pneumothorax, and bleeding. Thoracentesis on the right may be complicated by puncture or laceration of the capsule of the liver and, on the left, by puncture or laceration of the capsule of the spleen. Specimens obtained should always be cultured, examined microscopically for evidence of bacterial infection, and evaluated for total protein and total differential cell counts. Lactic acid dehydrogenase, glucose, cholesterol, triglyceride (chylous), and amylase determinations may also be useful. If malignancy is suspected, cytologic examination is imperative.

Transudates result from mechanical factors influencing the rate of formation or reabsorption of pleural fluid and generally require no further diagnostic evaluation. Exudates result from inflammation or other disease of the pleural surface and underlying lung and require a more complete diagnostic evaluation. In general, transudates have a total protein of <3 g/dL or a ratio of pleural protein to serum protein <0.5, a total leukocyte count of fewer than 2,000/mm^3 with a predominance of mononuclear cells, and low lactate dehydrogenase levels. Exudates have high protein levels and a predominance of polymorphonuclear cells (although malignant or tuberculous effusions can have a higher percentage of mononuclear cells). Complicated exudates often require continuous chest tube drainage and have a pH <7.2. Tuberculous effusions can have low glucose and high cholesterol content.

Lung Tap

Using a technique similar to that used for thoracentesis, a percutaneous lung tap is the most direct method of obtaining bacteriologic specimens from the pulmonary parenchyma and is the only technique other than open lung biopsy not associated with at least some risk of contamination by oral flora. After local anesthesia, a needle attached to a syringe containing nonbacteriostatic sterile saline is inserted using aseptic technique through the inferior aspect of an intercostal space in the area of interest. The needle is rapidly advanced into the lung; the saline is injected and reaspirated, and the needle is withdrawn. These actions are performed as quickly as possible. This procedure usually yields a few drops of fluid from the lung, which should be cultured and examined microscopically.

Major indications for a lung tap are infiltrates of undetermined cause, especially those unresponsive to therapy in immunosuppressed patients who are susceptible to unusual organisms. Complications are the same as for thoracentesis, but the incidence of pneumothorax is higher and somewhat dependent on the nature of the underlying disease process. In patients with poor pulmonary compliance, such as children with *Pneumocystis* pneumonia, the rate can approach 30%, with 5% requiring chest tubes. Bronchopulmonary lavage has replaced lung taps for most purposes.

Lung Biopsy

Lung biopsy may be the only way to establish a diagnosis, especially in protracted, noninfectious disease. In infants and small children, thoracoscopic or open surgical biopsies are the procedures of choice, and

in expert hands, there is low morbidity. Biopsy through the 3.5 mm diameter pediatric bronchoscopes limits the sample size and diagnostic abilities. As well as ensuring that an adequate specimen is obtained, the surgeon can inspect the lung surface and choose the site of biopsy. In older children, transbronchial biopsies can be performed using flexible forceps through a bronchoscope, an endotracheal tube, a rigid bronchoscope, or an endotracheal tube, usually with fluoroscopic guidance. This technique is most appropriately used when the disease is diffuse, as in the case of *Pneumocystis* pneumonia, or after rejection of a transplanted lung. The diagnostic limitations related to the small size of the biopsy specimens can be mitigated by the ability to obtain several samples. The risk of pneumothorax related to bronchoscopy is increased when transbronchial biopsies are part of the procedure; however, the ability to obtain biopsy specimens in a procedure performed with topical anesthesia and conscious sedation offers advantages to the select population for whom this procedure offers a reasonable diagnostic yield.

Sweat Testing

See Chapter 403.

Bibliography is available at Expert Consult.

Chapter 375
Sudden Infant Death Syndrome
Carl E. Hunt and Fern R. Hauck

Sudden infant death syndrome (SIDS) is defined as the sudden, unexpected death of an infant that is unexplained by a thorough postmortem examination, which includes a complete autopsy, investigation of the scene of death, and review of the medical history. An autopsy is essential to identify possible natural explanations for sudden unexpected death such as congenital anomalies or infection and to diagnose traumatic child abuse (Tables 375-1, 375-2, and 375-3; see Chapter 40). The autopsy typically cannot distinguish between SIDS and intentional suffocation, but the scene investigation and medical history may be of help if inconsistencies are evident. **Sudden unexpected infant death (SUID)** is a term that encompasses all sudden unexpected infant deaths. Unexplained SUID is equivalent to SIDS.

EPIDEMIOLOGY

SIDS is the third leading cause of infant mortality in the United States, accounting for approximately 8% of all infant deaths. It is the most common cause of postneonatal infant mortality, accounting for 40-50% of all deaths between 1 mo and 1 yr of age. The annual rate of SIDS in the United States was stable at 1.3-1.4 per 1,000 live births (approximately 7,000 infants/year) before 1992, when it was recommended that infants sleep nonprone as a way to reduce risk for SIDS. Since then, particularly after initiation of the national Back to Sleep campaign in 1994, the rate of SIDS progressively declined and then leveled off in 2001 at 0.55 per 1,000 live births (2,234 infants). The rates have remained stagnant since that time; in 2009 it was 0.54 per 1,000 live births (2,231 infants). The decline in the number of SIDS deaths in the United States and other countries has been attributed to increasing use of the supine position for sleep. In 1992, 82% of sampled infants in the United States were placed prone for sleep. Several other countries have decreased prone sleeping prevalence to ≤2%, but in the United States in 2009, 11% of infants were still being placed prone for sleep and 13% were being placed in the side position. Among black infants, these rates were even higher: 22% prone and 22% side in 2009.

Table 375-1	Differential Diagnosis of Sudden Unexpected Infant Death		
CAUSE OF DEATH	**PRIMARY DIAGNOSTIC CRITERIA**	**CONFOUNDING FACTOR(S)**	**FREQUENCY DISTRIBUTION (%)**
EXPLAINED AT AUTOPSY			
Natural			18-20*
Infections	History, autopsy, and cultures	If minimal findings: SIDS	35-46[†]
Congenital anomaly	History and autopsy	If minimal findings: SIDS	14-24[†]
Unintentional injury	History, scene investigation, autopsy	Traumatic child abuse	15*
Traumatic child abuse	Autopsy and scene investigation	Unintentional injury	13-24*
Other natural causes	History and autopsy	If minimal findings: SIDS, or intentional suffocation	12-17*
UNEXPLAINED AT AUTOPSY			
SIDS	History, scene investigation, absence of explainable cause at autopsy	Intentional suffocation	80-82%
Intentional suffocation (filicide)	Perpetrator confession, absence of explainable cause at autopsy	SIDS	Unknown, but <5% of all SUID
Accidental suffocation or strangulation in bed (ASSB)	History and scene investigation, ideally including doll re-enactment	Assigned to ICD-10 code (SIDS) for U.S. vital statistics database Unexplained Undetermined	Varies with individual medical examiners and coroners

*As a percentage of all sudden unexpected infant deaths explained at autopsy.
[†]As a percentage of all natural causes of sudden unexpected infant deaths explained at autopsy.
ICD-10, International Classification of Diseases, Version 10; SIDS, sudden infant death syndrome; SUDI, sudden unexpected death in infancy.
Adapted from Hunt CE: Sudden infant death syndrome and other causes of infant mortality: diagnosis, mechanisms and risk for recurrence in siblings, Am J Respir Crit Care Med 164:346–357, 2001.

Table 375-2	Conditions That Can Cause Apparent Life-Threatening Events or Sudden Unexpected Infant Death

CENTRAL NERVOUS SYSTEM
Arteriovenous malformation
Subdural hematoma
Seizures
Congenital central hypoventilation
Neuromuscular disorders (Werdnig-Hoffmann disease)
Chiari crisis
Leigh syndrome

CARDIAC
Subendocardial fibroelastosis
Aortic stenosis
Anomalous coronary artery
Myocarditis
Cardiomyopathy
Arrhythmias (prolonged Q-T syndrome, Wolff-Parkinson-White syndrome, congenital heart block)

PULMONARY
Pulmonary hypertension
Vocal cord paralysis
Aspiration
Laryngotracheal disease

GASTROINTESTINAL
Diarrhea and/or dehydration
Gastroesophageal reflux
Volvulus

ENDOCRINE–METABOLIC
Congenital adrenal hyperplasia
Malignant hyperpyrexia
Long- or medium-chain acyl coenzyme A deficiency
Hyperammonemias (urea cycle enzyme deficiencies)
Glutaric aciduria
Carnitine deficiency (systemic or secondary)
Glycogen storage disease type I
Maple syrup urine disease
Congenital lactic acidosis
Biotinidase deficiency

INFECTION
Sepsis
Meningitis
Encephalitis
Brain abscess
Pyelonephritis
Bronchiolitis (respiratory syncytial virus)
Infant botulism
Pertussis

TRAUMA
Child abuse
Accidental or intentional suffocation
Physical trauma
Factitious syndrome (formerly Munchausen syndrome) by proxy

POISONING (INTENTIONAL OR UNINTENTIONAL)
Boric acid
Carbon monoxide
Salicylates
Barbiturates
Ipecac
Cocaine
Insulin
Others

From Kliegman RM, Greenbaum LA, Lye PS: Practical strategies in pediatric diagnosis and therapy, ed 2, Philadelphia, 2004, Elsevier Saunders, p. 98.

Table 375-3	Differential Diagnosis of Recurrent Sudden Infant Death in a Sibship

IDIOPATHIC
Recurrent sudden infant death syndrome

CENTRAL NERVOUS SYSTEM
Congenital central hypoventilation
Neuromuscular disorders
Leigh syndrome

CARDIAC
Endocardial fibroelastosis
Wolff-Parkinson-White syndrome
Prolonged Q-T syndrome or other cardiac channelopathy
Congenital heart block

PULMONARY
Pulmonary hypertension

ENDOCRINE–METABOLIC
See Table 375-2

INFECTION
Disorders of immune host defense

CHILD ABUSE
Filicide or infanticide
Factitious syndrome (formerly Munchausen syndrome) by proxy

From Kliegman RM, Greenbaum LA, Lye PS: Practical strategies in pediatric diagnosis and therapy, ed 2, Philadelphia, 2004, Elsevier Saunders, p 101.

Table 375-4	Identified Genes for Which the Distribution of Polymorphisms Differs in Sudden Infant Death Syndrome Infants Compared to Control Infants

CARDIAC CHANNELOPATHIES (11)
Potassium ion channel genes (*KCNE2, KCNH2, KCNQ1, KCNJ8*)
Sodium ion channel gene (*SCN5A*) (long QT syndrome 3, Brugada syndrome)
GPD1-L-encoded connexin43 (Brugada syndrome)
SCN3B (Brugada syndrome)
CAV3 (long QT syndrome 9)
SCN4B (long QT syndrome 10)
SNTA-1 (long QT syndrome 11)
RyR2 (catecholaminergic polymorphic ventricular tachycardia)

SEROTONIN (5-HT) (3)
5-HT transporter protein (*5-HTT*)
Intron 2 of *SLC6A4* (variable number tandem repeat [VNTR] polymorphism)
5-HT fifth Ewing variant (FEV) gene

GENES PERTINENT TO DEVELOPMENT OF AUTONOMIC NERVOUS SYSTEM (9)
Paired-like homeobox 2a (*PHOX2A*)
PHOX2B
Rearranged during transfection factor (*RET*)
Endothelin converting enzyme-1 (*ECE1*)
T-cell leukemia homeobox (*TLX3*)
Engrailed-1 (*EN1*)
Tyrosine hydroxylase (*THO1*)
Monamine oxidase A (*MAOA*)
Sodium/proton exchanger 3 (*NHE3*) (medullary respiratory control)

INFECTION AND INFLAMMATION (8)
Complement C4A
Complement C4B
Interleukin-1RN (gene encoding IL-1 receptor antagonist [ra]; proinflammatory)
Interleukin-6 (IL-6; proinflammatory)
Interleukin-8 (IL-8; proinflammatory; associated with prone sleeping position)
Interleukin-10 (IL-10)
Vascular endothelial growth factor (VEGF) (proinflammatory)
Tumor necrosis factor (TNF)-α (proinflammatory)

OTHER (3)
Mitochondrial DNA (mtDNA) polymorphisms (energy production)
Flavin-monooxygenase 3 (*FMO3*) (enzyme metabolizes nicotine; risk factor with smoking mothers)
Aquaporin-4 (T allele and CT/TT genotype associated with maternal smoking and with increased brain/body weight ratio in SIDS infants)

Adapted from Hunt CE, Hauck FR: Sudden infant death syndrome: gene-environment interactions. In Brugada R, Brugada J, Brugada P, editors: Clinical care in inherited cardiac syndromes, Guildford, UK, 2009, Springer-Verlag London.

There is increasing evidence that infant deaths previously classified as SIDS are now being classified by medical examiners and coroners as from other causes, notably **accidental suffocation and strangulation in bed**. Between 1994 and 2004, there has been a quadrupling in the rates of accidental suffocation and strangulation in bed, from 2.8-12.5 deaths per 100,000 live births. These sudden and unexpected infant deaths are primarily associated with an unsafe sleeping environment such as prone position or in bed with parents. Based on these trends and the commonality of many of the sleep environment risk factors that are associated with both SIDS and other sleep-related SUID, risk reduction measures will be later described that are applicable to all sleep-related SUID.

PATHOLOGY

There are no autopsy findings pathognomonic for SIDS and no findings required for the diagnosis. There are some common findings. Petechial hemorrhages are found in 68-95% of cases and are more extensive than in explained causes of infant mortality. Pulmonary edema is often present and may be substantial. The reasons for these findings are unknown.

SIDS infants have several identifiable changes in the lungs and other organs and in brainstem structure and function. Nearly 65% of SIDS infants have structural evidence of preexisting, chronic, low-grade asphyxia, and other studies have identified biochemical markers of asphyxia. SIDS victims have higher levels of vascular endothelial growth factor (VEGF) in the cerebrospinal fluid. These increases may be related to VEGF polymorphisms (see "Genetic Risk Factors" below and Table 375-4) or might indicate recent hypoxemic events, because VEGF is upregulated by hypoxia. Brainstem findings include a persistent increase of dendritic spines and delayed maturation of synapses in the medullary respiratory centers, and decreased tyrosine hydroxylase immunoreactivity and catecholaminergic neurons. Cardiac muscle muscarinic receptor overexpression has also been reported in SIDS infants compared to infants who died from noncardiac causes. The regulatory mechanism may be related to increased acetylcholine esterase enzyme activity. The retrotrapezoid nucleus is one of the primary sites of central chemoreception and respiratory drive, and structural and/or PHOX2B-expression abnormalities have been reported in significantly more SIDS and other SUID cases than controls.

The ventral medulla has been a particular focus for studies in SIDS infants. It is an integrative area for vital autonomic functions including breathing, arousal, and chemosensory function. Quantitative 3-dimensional anatomic studies indicate that some SIDS infants have hypoplasia of the arcuate nucleus and up to 60% have histopathologic evidence of less-extensive bilateral or unilateral hypoplasia. Consistent with the apparent overlap between putative mechanisms for SIDS and for unexpected late fetal deaths, approximately 30% of late unexpected and unexplained stillbirths also have hypoplasia of the arcuate nucleus.

Neurotransmitter studies of the arcuate nucleus have also identified receptor abnormalities in some SIDS infants that involve several receptor types relevant to state-dependent autonomic control overall and to ventilatory and arousal responsiveness in particular. These deficits include significant decreases in binding to kainate, muscarinic cholinergic, and serotonin (5-HT) receptors. Studies of the ventral medulla have identified morphologic and biochemical deficits in 5-HT neurons and decreased γ-aminobutyric acid receptor A receptor binding in the medullary serotonergic system. Immunohistochemical analyses reveal an increased number of 5-HT neurons and an increase in the fraction of 5-HT neurons showing an immature morphology, suggesting a failure or delay in the maturation of these neurons. High neuronal levels of interleukin-1β are present in the arcuate and dorsal vagal nuclei in SIDS victims compared to controls, perhaps contributing to molecular interactions affecting cardiorespiratory and arousal responses.

The neuropathologic data provide compelling evidence for altered 5-HT homeostasis, creating an underlying vulnerability contributing to SIDS. 5-HT is an important neurotransmitter and the 5-HT neurons in the medulla project extensively to neurons in the brainstem and spinal cord that influence respiratory drive and arousal, cardiovascular control including blood pressure, circadian regulation and non–rapid eye movement (REM) sleep, thermoregulation, and upper airway reflexes. Medullary 5-HT neurons may be respiratory chemosensors and may be involved with respiratory responses to intermittent hypoxia and respiratory rhythm generation. Decreases in 5-HT_{1A} and 5-HT_{2A} receptor immunoreactivity have been observed in the dorsal nucleus of the vagus, solitary nucleus, and ventrolateral medulla. There are extensive serotoninergic brainstem abnormalities in SIDS infants, including increased 5-HT neuronal count, a lower density of 5-HT_{1A} receptor-binding sites in regions of the medulla involved in homeostatic function, and a lower ratio of 5-HT transporter (5-HTT) binding density to 5-HT neuronal count in the medulla. Male SIDS infants have lower receptor-binding density than female SIDS infants. These findings suggest that the synthesis and availability of 5-HT is decreased within 5-HT pathways and hence impairs neuronal firing. Medullary tissue levels of 5-HT and its primary biosynthetic enzyme (tryptophan hydroxylase) were observed to be lower in SIDS cases compared to age-matched controls, indicating reduced 5-HT synthesis and hence a deficiency in 5-HT.

ENVIRONMENTAL RISK FACTORS

Declines of 50% or more in rates of SIDS in the United States and around the world have occurred following national education campaigns directed at reducing risk factors associated with SIDS. The reductions in risk appear to be related primarily to decreases in placing infants prone for sleep and increases in placing them supine. A number of other risk factors also have significant associations with SIDS (Table 375-5). Although many are nonmodifiable and most of the modifiable factors have not changed appreciably, self-reported maternal smoking prevalence during pregnancy has decreased by 25% in the past decade in the United States.

Nonmodifiable Environmental Risk Factors

Lower socioeconomic status has consistently been associated with higher risk, although SIDS affects infants from all social strata. In the United States, African-American, Native American, and Alaskan Native infants are 2-3 times more likely than white infants to die of SIDS, whereas Asian, Pacific Islander, and Hispanic infants have the lowest incidence. Some of this disparity may be related to the higher concentration of poverty and other adverse environmental factors found within some, but not all, of the communities with higher incidence.

Infants are at greatest risk of SIDS at 2-4 mo of age, with most deaths having occurred by 6 mo. This characteristic age has decreased in some countries as the SIDS incidence has declined, with deaths occurring at earlier ages and with a flattening of the peak age incidence. Similarly, the commonly observed winter seasonal predominance of SIDS has declined or disappeared in some countries as prone prevalence has decreased, supporting prior findings of an interaction between sleep position and factors more common in colder months (overheating as a consequence of elevated interior temperatures or bundling with blankets and heavy clothing, or infection). Male infants are 30-50% more likely to be affected than female infants.

Table 375-5	Environmental Factors Associated with Increased Risk for Sudden Infant Death Syndrome

MATERNAL AND ANTENATAL RISK FACTORS
Elevated 2nd trimester serum α-fetoprotein
Smoking
Alcohol use
Drug use (cocaine, heroin)
Nutritional deficiency
Inadequate prenatal care
Low socioeconomic status
Younger age
Lower education
Single marital status
Shorter interpregnancy interval
Intrauterine hypoxia
Fetal growth restriction

INFANT RISK FACTORS
Age (peak 2-4 mo, but may be decreasing)
Male gender
Race and ethnicity (African-American and Native American, other minorities)
Growth failure
No breast-feeding
No pacifier (dummy)
Prematurity
Prone and side sleep position
Recent febrile illness (mild infections)
Inadequate immunizations
Smoking exposure (prenatal and postnatal)
Soft sleeping surface, soft bedding
Bed sharing with parent(s) or other children
Thermal stress, overheating
Colder season, no central heating

Modifiable Environmental Risk Factors
Pregnancy-Related Factors

An increased SIDS risk is associated with numerous obstetric factors, suggesting that the in utero environment of future SIDS infants is suboptimal. SIDS infants are more commonly of higher birth order, independent of maternal age, and of gestations after shorter interpregnancy intervals. Mothers of SIDS infants generally receive less prenatal care and initiate care later in pregnancy. Additionally, low birthweight, preterm birth, and slower intrauterine and postnatal growth rates are risk factors.

Cigarette Smoking

There is a major association between intrauterine exposure to cigarette smoking and risk for SIDS. The incidence of SIDS is approximately 3 times greater among infants of mothers who smoke in studies conducted before SIDS risk-reduction campaigns and 5 times higher in studies after implementation of risk-reduction campaigns. The risk of death is progressively greater as daily cigarette use increases. The effects of smoking by the father and other household members are more difficult to interpret because they are highly correlated with maternal smoking. There appears to be a small independent effect of paternal smoking, but data on other household members have been inconsistent.

It is very difficult to assess the independent effect of infant exposure to **environmental tobacco smoke** because parental smoking behaviors during and after pregnancy are also highly correlated. An increased risk of SIDS is also found for infants exposed only to postnatal maternal environmental tobacco smoke. There is a dose–response for the number of household smokers, number of people smoking in the same room as the infant, and the number of cigarettes smoked. These data suggest that keeping the infant free of environmental tobacco smoke can further reduce an infant's risk of SIDS.

Drug and Alcohol Use

Most studies link maternal prenatal drug use, especially opiates, with an increased risk of SIDS, ranging from a 2-15–fold increased risk. Most but not all studies have not found an association between maternal alcohol use prenatally or postnatally and SIDS. In one study of Northern Plains Indians, periconceptional alcohol use and binge drinking in the 1st trimester were associated with a 6-fold and an 8-fold increased risk of SIDS, respectively. A Danish cohort study found that mothers admitted to the hospital for an alcohol- or drug-related disorder at any time before or after the birth of their infants had a 3-times higher risk of their infant dying from SIDS, and a Dutch study reported that maternal alcohol consumption in the 24 hr before the infant died carried a 2-8–fold increased risk of SIDS. Siblings of infants with fetal alcohol syndrome have a 10-fold increased risk of SIDS compared to controls.

Infant Sleep Environment

Sleeping prone has consistently been shown to increase the risk of SIDS. As rates of prone positioning have decreased in the general population, the odds ratios for SIDS in infants still sleeping prone have increased. **The highest risk of SIDS occurs in infants who are usually placed nonprone, but placed prone for last sleep ("unaccustomed prone") or found prone ("secondary prone").** The "unaccustomed prone" position may be more likely to occur in daycare or other settings outside the home and highlights the need for all infant caretakers to be educated about appropriate sleep positioning.

Side-sleeping is also a significant risk factor. The initial SIDS risk-reduction campaign recommendations considered side sleeping to be nearly equivalent to the supine position in reducing the risk of SIDS. Subsequent studies documented that side-sleeping infants were twice as likely to die of SIDS as infants sleeping supine. This increased risk might relate to the relative instability of the position, with some infants placed on the side rolling to the prone position. With the overall decrease in rates of placing infants prone for sleep, a higher proportion of SIDS is now attributed to being placed on the side for sleeping than for being placed prone. Nevertheless, the majority of SIDS occurrences are associated with being found prone. The **current recommendations** call for **supine position for sleeping for all infants except those few with specific medical conditions** for which recommending a different position may be justified, in particular infants with apparent anatomical or functional upper airway compromise.

Many parents and healthcare providers were initially concerned that supine sleeping would be associated with an increase in adverse consequences, such as difficulty sleeping, vomiting, or aspiration. Evidence suggests that the risk of regurgitation and choking is highest for prone-sleeping infants. Some newborn nursery staff still tend to favor side positioning, which models inappropriate infant care practice to parents. Infants sleeping on their backs do not have more episodes of cyanosis or apnea, and reports of apparent life-threatening events actually decreased in Scandinavia after increased use of the supine position. Among infants in the United States who maintained the same sleep position at 1, 3, and 6 mo of age, no clinical symptoms or reasons for outpatient visits (including fever, cough, wheezing, trouble breathing or sleeping, vomiting, diarrhea, or respiratory illness) were more common in infants sleeping supine or on their sides compared with infants sleeping prone. Three symptoms were actually less common in infants sleeping supine or on their sides: fever at 1 mo, stuffy nose at 6 mo, and trouble sleeping at 6 mo. Outpatient visits for ear infection were less common at 3 and 6 mo for infants sleeping supine and also less common at 3 mo for infants sleeping on their side. These results provide reassurance for parents and healthcare providers and should contribute to universal acceptance of supine as the safest and optimal sleep position for infants.

Soft sleep surfaces or bedding, such as comforters, pillows, sheepskins, polystyrene bean pillows, and older or softer mattresses are associated with increased risk of SIDS. **Head and face covering by loose bedding,** particularly heavy comforters, is also associated with increased risk. **Overheating** has been associated with increased risk for SIDS based on indicators such as higher room temperature, a febrile history, sweating, and excessive clothing or bedding. Some studies have identified an interaction between overheating and prone sleeping, with overheating increasing the risk of SIDS only when infants are sleeping prone. Higher external environmental temperatures have not been associated with increased SIDS incidence in the United States.

Several studies have implicated **bed sharing** as a risk factor for SIDS. Bed sharing is particularly hazardous when other children are in the same bed, when the parent is sleeping with an infant on a couch or other soft or confining sleeping surface, and when the mother smokes. Infants younger than 4 mo of age are at increased risk even when mothers are nonsmokers. A meta-analysis of 19 studies found that the low-risk infants (i.e., those who were breastfed and never exposed to cigarette smoke in utero or after birth) still had a 5-fold increased risk of SIDS until the age of 3 mo if bed sharing. Risk is also increased with longer duration of bed sharing during the night, whereas returning the infant to the infant's own crib has not been associated with increased risk. Room sharing without bed sharing is associated with lower SIDS rates, and is therefore recommended.

Infant Feeding Care Practices and Exposures

It is currently believed that there is a **protective effect of breastfeeding on SIDS,** after taking into account confounding factors. A meta-analysis found that there was a 45% reduction in SIDS after adjusting for confounding variables and that this protective effect increased for exclusive breastfeeding compared with partial breastfeeding.

Pacifier (dummy) use is associated with a lower risk of SIDS in the majority of studies when used for last sleep. Although it is not known if this is a direct effect of the pacifier itself or from associated infant or parental behavior, there is increasing evidence that pacifier use even with dislodgment can increase the arousability of infants during sleep. Concerns have been expressed about recommending pacifiers as a means of reducing the risk of SIDS for fear of adverse consequences, particularly interference with breastfeeding. Well-designed studies have found no association between pacifiers and breastfeeding duration.

Upper respiratory tract infections have generally not been found to be an independent risk factor for SIDS, but these and other minor infections may still have a role in the causal pathway of SIDS when other risk factors are present. Risk for SIDS has been found to be increased after illness among prone sleepers, those who were heavily wrapped, and those whose heads were covered during sleep.

No adverse association between immunizations and SIDS has been found. Indeed, SIDS infants are less likely to be immunized than control infants and, in immunized infants, no temporal relationship between vaccine administration and death has been identified. In a meta-analysis of case-control studies that adjusted for potentially confounding factors, the risk of SIDS for infants immunized with diphtheria, tetanus, and pertussis was half that for nonimmunized infants.

SIDS rates remain higher among Native Americans, Alaskan Natives, and African-Americans. This may be due, in part, to group differences in adopting supine sleeping or other risk-reduction practices. Greater efforts are needed to address this persistent disparity and to ensure that SIDS risk-reduction education reaches all parents and all other care providers, including other family members and personnel at daycare centers.

GENETIC RISK FACTORS

As summarized in Table 375-4, there are numerous genetic differences identified in SIDS infants compared to healthy infants and to infants dying from other causes. Polymorphisms occurring at higher incidence in SIDS compared to controls include at least 11 cardiac ion channelopathy genes that are proarrhythmic, 3 5-HT genes, 8 autonomic nervous system development genes, and 8 genes related to infection that are proinflammatory.

Multiple studies confirm the importance of a final common pathway that involves cardiac sodium or potassium channel dysfunction caused by direct or indirect disturbance resulting in **either long QT syndrome (LQTS)** or other arrhythmia associated with current dysfunction. LQTS is a known cause of sudden unexpected death in adults and

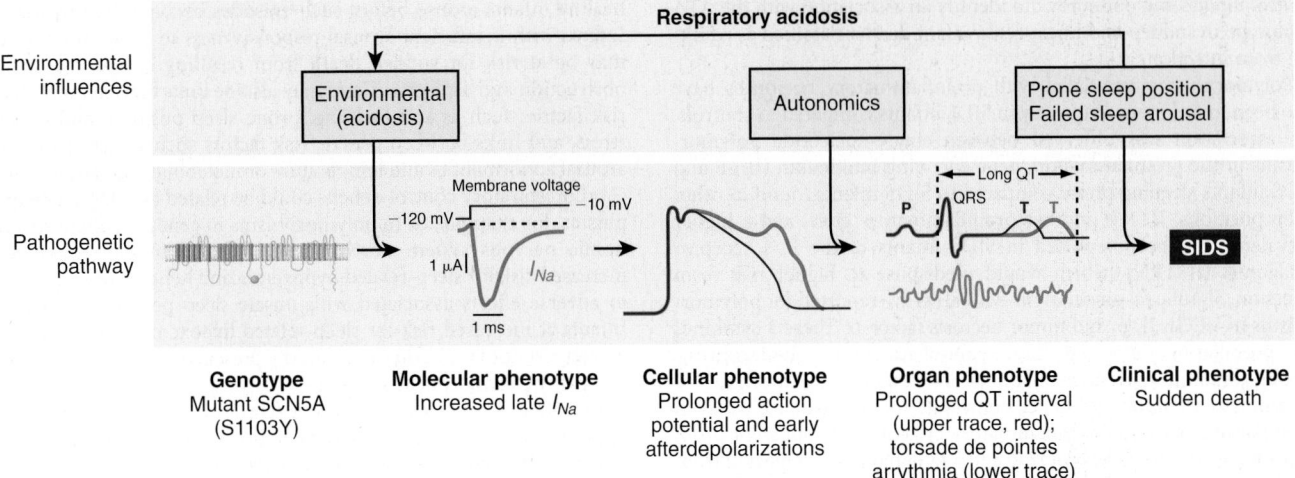

Respiratory acidosis

Environmental influences

Pathogenetic pathway

Genotype	Molecular phenotype	Cellular phenotype	Organ phenotype	Clinical phenotype
Mutant SCN5A (S1103Y)	Increased late I_{Na}	Prolonged action potential and early afterdepolarizations	Prolonged QT interval (upper trace, red); torsade de pointes arrythmia (lower trace)	Sudden death

Figure 375-1 An arrhythmogenic pathogenetic pathway for sudden infant death syndrome (SIDS) from patient genotype to clinical phenotype, with environmental influences noted. The genetic abnormality—in this instance, a polymorphism in the cardiac Na+ channel SCN5A—causes a molecular phenotype of increased late Na+ current (I_{Na}) under the influence of environmental factors such as acidosis. Interacting with other ion currents that may themselves be altered by genetic and environmental factors, the late Na+ current causes a cellular phenotype of prolonged action potential duration as well as early afterdepolarizations. Prolonged action potential in the cells of the ventricular myocardium and further interaction with environmental factors such as autonomic innervation, which, in turn, may be affected by genetic factors, produce a tissue-organ phenotype of a prolonged Q-T interval on the electrocardiogram (ECG) and torsades de pointes arrhythmia in the whole heart. If this is sustained or degenerates to ventricular fibrillation, the clinical phenotype of SIDS results. Environmental and multiple genetic factors can interact at many different levels to produce the characteristic phenotypes at the molecular, cellular, tissue, organ, and clinical levels. *(From Makielski JC: SIDS: genetic and environmental influences may cause arrhythmia in this silent killer, J Clin Invest 116:297–299, 2006.)*

children, as the result of a prolonged cardiac action potential by either increasing depolarization or decreasing repolarization current (Fig. 375-1). The first evidence supporting a causal role for LQTS in SIDS was a large Italian study in which a corrected QT interval >440 milliseconds on an electrocardiogram performed on days 3-4 of life was associated with a 41.3 odds ratio for SIDS. Several case reports have subsequently provided proof of concept that cardiac channelopathy polymorphisms are associated with SIDS. LQTS is associated with polymorphisms related mainly to gain-of-function mutations in the **sodium channel gene** *(SCN5A)* that encode critical channel pore-forming α subunits or essential channel-interacting proteins. LQTS also is associated with mainly loss-of-function polymorphisms in potassium channel genes. **Short QTS (SQTS)** is more recently recognized as another cause of life-threatening arrhythmia or sudden death, often during rest or sleep. Gain-of-function mutations in genes including *KCNH2* and *KCNQ1* have been causally linked to SQTS, and some of these deaths have occurred in infants, suggesting that SQTS may also be causally linked to SIDS.

Both LQTS and SQTS are proarrhythmic and associated with cardiac arrest and sudden death. The other cardiac ion-related channelopathy polymorphisms are also proarrhythmic, including Brugada syndrome *(BrS1, BrS2)*, and catecholaminergic paroxysmal ventricular tachycardia *(CPVT1)*. Collectively, these mutations in cardiac ion channels provide a lethal arrhythmogenic substrate in some infants at risk for SIDS (see Fig. 375-1) and may account for 10% or more of SIDS cases.

Impaired central respiratory regulation is an important biologic abnormality in SIDS and genetic polymorphisms have been identified in SIDS infants that affect both serotonergic and adrenergic neurons. Monamine oxidase A metabolizes both of these neurotransmitters and a recent study has observed a high association between SIDS and low expressing alleles in males, perhaps contributing to the higher incidence of SIDS in males. Many genes are involved in the control of 5-HT synthesis, storage, membrane uptake, and metabolism. Polymorphisms have been identified in the promoter region of the 5-HT transporter (5-HTT) protein gene that occur in greater frequency in SIDS than control infants. The long "L" allele increased effectiveness of the promoter and reduced extracellular 5-HT concentrations at nerve endings compared to the short "S" allele. White, African-American,

and Japanese SIDS infants were more likely than ethnicity-matched controls to have the "L" (long) allele, and there was also a negative association between SIDS and the S/S genotype. The L/L genotype was associated with increased 5-HT transporters on neuroimaging and postmortem binding studies. However, in a large San Diego dataset of SIDS infants, no relationship was found between SIDS and the L allele or the LL genotype.

An association has also been observed between SIDS and a 5-HTT intron 2 polymorphism, which differentially regulate *5-HTT* expression. There were positive associations between SIDS and the intron 2 genotype distributions in African-American infants compared to African-American controls. The human *FEV* gene is specifically expressed in central 5-HT neurons in the brain, with a predicted role in specification and maintenance of the serotoninergic neuronal phenotype. An insertion mutation has been identified in intron 2 of the *FEV* gene, and the distribution of this mutation differs significantly in SIDS compared to control infants.

Molecular genetic studies in SIDS victims have also identified mutations pertinent to early embryologic development of the autonomic nervous system (Table 375-4). Eleven protein-changing mutations have been identified in 14 of 92 SIDS cases among the *PHOX2a, RET, ECE1, TLX3,* and *EN1* genes. Only 1 of these mutations *(TLX3)* was found in 2 of 92 controls. African-American infants accounted for 10 of 11 mutations in SIDS infants and in both affected controls with protein-changing mutations. Eight polymorphisms in the *PHOX2B* gene occurred significantly more frequently in SIDS compared to control infants. One study has reported an association between SIDS and a distinct tyrosine hydroxylase gene *(THO1)* allele, which regulates gene expression and catecholamine production.

Genetic differences in SIDS infants compared to control infants have been reported for 2 complement *C4* genes. Some SIDS infants have loss-of-function polymorphisms in the gene promoter region for IL-10, another anti-inflammatory cytokine. Among SIDS infants compared to living controls, sudden infant death was strongly associated with the IL-10 polymorphism. These IL-10 polymorphisms were associated with decreased IL-10 levels and hence could contribute to SIDS by delaying initiation of protective antibody production or reducing capacity to inhibit inflammatory cytokine production. Other studies have not found differences in IL-10 genes in SIDS compared to control infants, but one study did identify an association with the ATA haplotype in sudden and unexpected infant deaths classified as resulting from infection.

Polymorphisms associated with proinflammatory responses have also been found more frequently in SIDS infants compared to controls. An association was observed between single-nucleotide polymorphisms in the proinflammatory gene encoding interleukin (IL)-8 and SIDS infants sleeping prone compared to SIDS infants found in other sleep positions. IL-1 is another proinflammatory gene, and a higher prevalence has been reported in SIDS infants of the IL-1 receptor antagonist (IL-1RN), which would predispose to higher risk from infection. Significant associations with SIDS are reported for polymorphisms in VEGF, IL-6, and tumor necrosis factor-α. These 3 cytokines are proinflammatory, and these gain-of-function polymorphisms would result in increased inflammatory response to infectious or inflammatory stimuli and hence contribute to an imbalance between proinflammatory and antiinflammatory cytokines. As apparent proof of principle, elevated levels of IL-6 and VEGF have been reported from cerebrospinal fluid in SIDS infants. There were no group differences in the IL6-174G/C polymorphism in a Norwegian SIDS study, but the aggregate evidence nevertheless suggests an activated immune system in SIDS and thus implicates genes involved in the immune system. Almost all SIDS infants in 1 study had positive histories for prone sleeping and fever prior to death and positive HLA-DR expression in laryngeal mucosa, and high HLA-DR expression was associated with high levels of IL-6 in cerebrospinal fluid.

Numerous reports have implicated polymorphisms in genes regulating energy production in SIDS infants, but the importance of these findings requires further study (Table 375-4). Of interest, cardiac arrhythmias, including prolonged QT intervals, have been observed in families with mitochondrial disease. However, the mitochondrial DNA polymorphism T3394C that is associated with cardiac arrhythmia has not been observed to occur with greater frequency in SIDS compared to control infants.

GENE-AND-ENVIRONMENT INTERACTIONS

Interactions between genetic and environmental risk factors determine the actual risk for SIDS in individual infants (Fig. 375-2). There appears to be an interaction between prone sleep position and impaired ventilatory and arousal responsiveness. Facedown or nearly facedown sleeping does occasionally occur in prone-sleeping infants, but normal

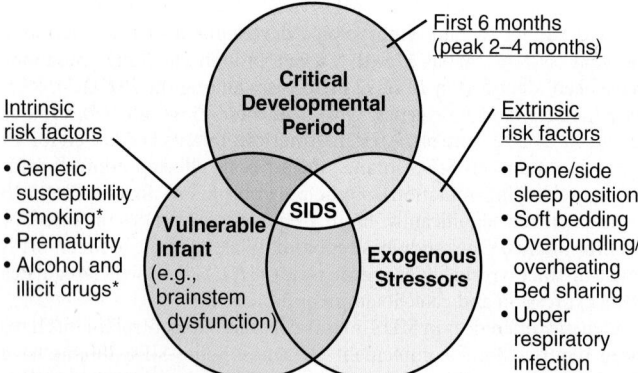

Figure 375-2 Schematic of the triple-risk model for sudden infant death syndrome (SIDS) showing the critical interactions between intrinsic risk factors (including genetic risk factors) resulting in a vulnerable infant, a critical developmental period or age, and exogenous stressors or extrinsic risk factors. *(Adapted from Filiano JJ, Kinney HC: A perspective on the neuropathologic findings in victims of the sudden infant death syndrome: the triple risk model, Biol Neonate 65:194–197, 1994.)*

healthy infants arouse before such episodes become life-threatening. Infants with insufficient arousal responsiveness to asphyxia, however, may be at risk for sudden death from resulting episodes of airway obstruction and asphyxia. There may also be links between modifiable risk factors such as soft bedding, prone sleep position, and thermal stress, and links between genetic risk factors such as ventilatory and arousal abnormalities and temperature or metabolic regulation deficits. Cardiorespiratory control deficits could be related to 5-HTT polymorphisms, for example, or to polymorphisms in genes pertinent to autonomic nervous system development. Affected infants could be at increased risk for sleep-related hypoxemia and hence more susceptible to adverse effects associated with unsafe sleep position or bedding. Infants at increased risk for sleep-related hypoxemia could also be at greater risk for fatal arrhythmias in the presence of a cardiac ion channelopathy polymorphism.

In >50% of SIDS victims, recent febrile illnesses, often related to upper respiratory infection, have been documented (see Table 375-5). Otherwise benign infections might increase risk for SIDS if interacting with genetically determined impaired immune responses, including those resulting from partial deletions in the complement C4 gene or to interleukin polymorphisms (see Table 375-4). Deficient inflammatory responsiveness can also occur as a result of mast cell degranulation, which has been reported in SIDS infants; this is consistent with an anaphylactic reaction to a bacterial toxin, and some family members of SIDS infants also have mast cell hyperreleasability and degranulation, suggesting that increased susceptibility to an anaphylactic reaction is another genetic factor influencing fatal outcomes to otherwise minor infections in infants. Interactions between upper respiratory infections or other minor illnesses and other factors such as prone sleeping might also play a role in the pathogenesis of SIDS.

The increased risk for SIDS associated with fetal and postnatal exposure to cigarette smoke may be related at least in part to genetic or epigenetic factors, including those affecting brainstem autonomic control. Human infant studies document decreased ventilatory and arousal responsiveness to hypoxia following fetal nicotine exposure, and impaired autoresuscitation after apnea has been associated with postnatal nicotine exposure. Decreased brainstem immunoreactivity to selected protein kinase C and neuronal nitric oxide synthase isoforms occurs in rats exposed to cigarette smoke prenatally, another potential cause of impaired hypoxic responsiveness. Smoking exposure also increases susceptibility to viral and bacterial infections and increases bacterial binding after passive coating of mucosal surfaces with smoke components, implicating interactions between smoking, cardiorespiratory control, and immune status. Flavin-monooxygenase 3 (FMO3) is one of the enzymes that metabolizes nicotine, and a polymorphism has recently been identified that occurs more frequently in SIDS infants compared to controls and more frequently in infants whose mothers reported heavy smoking (Table 375-4). This polymorphism thus provides a potential genetic risk factor for SIDS in infants exposed to cigarette smoke.

In infants with a cardiac ion channelopathy, risk for a fatal arrhythmia during sleep may be substantially enhanced by predisposing perturbations that increase electrical instability. These perturbations could include REM sleep with bursts of vagal and sympathetic activation, minor respiratory infections, or any other cause of sleep-related hypoxemia or hypercarbia, especially those resulting in acidosis. The prone sleeping position is associated with increased sympathetic activity.

INFANT GROUPS AT INCREASED RISK FOR SUDDEN INFANT DEATH SYNDROME
Unexplained Apparent Life-Threatening Events
Infants with an unexplained **apparent life-threatening event (ALTE)** are at increased risk for SIDS. An ALTE is defined as an episode that frightens an observer and manifests with some combination of central, obstructive, or mixed apnea; cyanotic, pallid, plethora, erythematous, color change; hypotonia (rarely hypertonia); and choking or gasping. A history of an unexplained ALTE has been reported in 5-9% of SIDS victims, and the risk of SIDS appears to be higher with 2 or more

unexplained events, but no definitive incidence rates are available. Compared with healthy control infants, the risk for SIDS may be as much as 3-5 times greater in infants having experienced an ALTE. Although most studies of ALTE have not specified gestational age, 30% of ALTE infants in the Collaborative Home Infant Monitoring Evaluation were ≤37 wk gestation at birth.

Subsequent Siblings of a Sudden Infant Death Syndrome Victim

The next-born siblings of first-born infants dying of any noninfectious natural cause are at significantly increased risk for infant death from the same cause, including SIDS. The relative risk is 9.1 for the same cause of recurrent death vs 1.6 for a different cause of death. The relative risk for recurrent SIDS (range: 5.4-5.8) is similar to the relative risk for non-SIDS causes of recurrent death (range: 4.6-12.5). The risk for recurrent infant mortality from the same cause as in the index sibling thus appears to be increased to a similar degree in subsequent siblings for both explained causes and for SIDS. This increased risk for recurrent SIDS in families is consistent with genetic risk factors interacting with environmental risk factors (see Tables 375-4 and 375-5 and Fig. 375-2).

Prematurity

Despite reductions in SIDS and SUID among infants born preterm by more than 50% since initiation of the back-to-sleep campaign in the United States 20 yr ago, the risk for death remains significantly higher than for infants born full term. This increased risk is likely related in part to immaturity of brainstem ventilatory control. Also, although the environmental risk factors for SIDS and SUID are qualitatively similar to those in full-term infants, including nonsupine sleeping position and other unsafe sleep practices, infants born preterm do have more sociodemographic risk factors overall than infants born at term. Among all gestational age groups, the postnatal age of death from SIDS and other SUID progressively decreases as gestational age at birth increases, and the postmenstrual age at death progressively increases as gestational age at birth increases. Compared with infants born at 37-42 wk, the odds ratio for SIDS is greatest for infants born at 24-28 wk gestation (2.57, 95% confidence interval 2.08, 3.17). The odds ratio progressively decreases as gestational age at birth increases, but even at 33-36 wk gestational age at birth remains significantly increased compared to infants born at term.

Physiologic Studies

Physiologic studies have been performed in healthy infants in early infancy, a few of whom later died of SIDS. Physiologic studies have also been performed on infant groups at increased risk for SIDS, especially those with ALTE and subsequent siblings of SIDS. In the aggregate, these studies have indicated brainstem abnormalities in neuroregulation of cardiorespiratory control or other autonomic functions and are consistent with the autopsy findings and genetic studies in SIDS victims (see "Pathology" and "Genetic Risk Factors" above). In addition to chemoreceptor sensitivity, these observed physiologic abnormalities also include respiratory patterns, control of heart and respiratory rate or variability, and asphyxic arousal responsiveness. A deficit in arousal responsiveness may be a necessary prerequisite for SIDS to occur but may be insufficient to cause SIDS in the absence of other genetic or environmental risk factors. **Autoresuscitation (gasping)** is a critical component of the asphyxic arousal response, and a failure of autoresuscitation in SIDS infants may be the final and most devastating physiologic failure. Most normal full-term infants younger than 9 postnatal wk of age in 1 study aroused in response to mild hypoxia, but only 10-15% aroused if older than 9 wk of age. These data thus suggest that ability to arouse to mild to moderate hypoxic stimuli may be at a nadir at the age range of greatest risk for SIDS.

The ability to shorten the QT interval as heart rate increases appears to be impaired in some SIDS victims, suggesting that such infants may be predisposed to ventricular arrhythmia. This is consistent with the observations of cardiac ion channel gene polymorphisms in other SIDS victims (see Table 375-4), but there are no antemortem QT interval

data in the SIDS infants having postmortem channelopathy polymorphisms. Infants studied physiologically and dying of SIDS a few weeks later had higher heart rates in all sleep–wake states, diminished heart rate variability during wakefulness, and significantly lower heart rate variability at the respiratory frequency across all sleep–wake cycles. Also, these SIDS infants had longer QT intervals than control infants in both REM and non-REM sleep, especially in the late hours of the night when most SIDS likely occurs. In only 1 of these SIDS infants, however, did the QT interval exceed 440 milliseconds.

Part of the decreased heart rate variability and increased heart rate observed in infants who later died of SIDS may have been related to decreased vagal tone, perhaps at least in part related to vagal neuropathy or to brainstem damage in areas responsible for parasympathetic cardiac control. In a comparison of heart rate power spectra before and after obstructive apneas in clinically asymptomatic infants, infants later dying of SIDS did not have the decreases in low-frequency to high-frequency power ratios observed in infants who survived. Some future SIDS victims thus have different autonomic responsiveness to obstructive apnea, perhaps indicating impaired autonomic nervous system control associated with higher vulnerability to external or endogenous stress factors and hence to reduced electrical stability of the heart.

Home cardiorespiratory monitors with memory capability have recorded the terminal events in some SIDS victims. These recordings did not include pulse oximetry and could not identify obstructed breaths due to reliance on transthoracic impedance for breath detection. In most instances, there has been sudden and rapid progression of severe bradycardia that was either unassociated with central apnea or appeared to occur too soon to be explained by the central apnea. These observations are consistent with an abnormality in autonomic control of heart rate variability, or with obstructed breaths resulting in bradycardia or hypoxemia and associated with impaired autoresuscitation or arousal.

CLINICAL STRATEGIES
Home Monitoring

SIDS cannot be prevented in individual infants because it is not possible to identify prospective SIDS infants, and no effective intervention has been established even if SIDS infants could be prospectively identified. Studies of cardiorespiratory pattern or other autonomic abnormalities do not have sufficient sensitivity and specificity to be clinically useful as screening tests. Home electronic surveillance using existing technology does not reduce the risk of SIDS. Although a prolonged QT interval in an infant may be treated if diagnosed, neither the role of routine postnatal electrocardiographic screening, the cost-effectiveness of diagnosis and treatment, nor the safety of treatment in infants has been established (see Chapter 429). Parental electrocardiographic screening is not helpful because spontaneous mutations are common.

Reducing the Risk of Sudden Infant Death Syndrome

Reducing risk behaviors and increasing protective behaviors among infant caregivers to achieve further reductions and eventual elimination of SIDS is a critical goal. Recent plateaus in placing infants supine for sleep in the United States at approximately 75% for all races and only 56% for African-Americans are cause for concern and require renewed educational efforts. The American Academy of Pediatrics guidelines to reduce the risk of SIDS were updated in 2011 and expanded to include reducing the risk of all sudden and unexpected sleep-related infant deaths. The guidelines are appropriate for most infants, but physicians and other healthcare providers might, on occasion, need to consider alternative approaches. The major components of the American Academy of Pediatrics guidelines are:

◆ Full-term and premature infants should be placed for sleep in the supine position. There are no adverse health outcomes from supine sleeping. Side sleeping is not recommended.

◆ It is recommended that infants sleep in the same room as their parents but in their own crib or bassinette that conforms to the safety standards of the Consumer Product Safety Commission. Placing the crib or bassinette near the mother's bed facilitates nursing and contact.

- Infants should be put to sleep on a firm mattress. Waterbeds, sofas, soft mattresses, or other soft surfaces should not be used. In addition, car seats, strollers, swings and other sitting devices should not be used for sleeping. Sleeping in an upright position can lead to gastroesophageal reflux or upper airway obstruction from head flexion.

- Soft materials in the infant's sleep environment—over, under, or near the infant—should be avoided. These include pillows, comforters, quilts, sheepskins, bumper pads, and stuffed toys. Because loose bedding may be hazardous, blankets, if used, should be tucked in around the crib mattress. Sleeping clothing, such as a sleep sack, can be used in place of blankets.

- Avoid overheating and overbundling. The infant should be lightly clothed for sleep and the thermostat set at a comfortable temperature.

- Infants should be immunized in accordance with recommendations of the American Academy of Pediatrics and the Centers for Disease Control and Prevention. There is no evidence that immunizations increase risk for SIDS. Indeed, recent evidence suggests that immunizations may have a protective effect against SIDS.

- Healthcare professionals, staff in newborn nurseries and neonatal intensive care units, and child care providers should adopt the SIDS reduction recommendations beginning at birth.

- Infants should have some time in the prone position (tummy time) while awake and observed. Alternating the placement of the infant's head as well as his or her orientation in the crib can also minimize the risk of head flattening from supine sleeping (positional plagiocephaly).

- Devices advertised to maintain sleep position, "protect" a bed-sharing infant, or reduce the risk of rebreathing are not recommended.

- Home cardiorespiratory and/or O_2 saturation monitoring may be of value for selected infants who have extreme instability, but there is no evidence that monitoring decreases the incidence of SIDS and it is therefore not recommended for this purpose.

- Breastfeeding is recommended. If possible, mothers should exclusively breastfeed or feed with expressed human milk until the infant is 6 mo of age.

- If a breastfeeding mother brings the infant into the adult bed for nursing, the infant should be returned to a separate sleep surface when the mother is ready for sleep.

- Consider offering a pacifier at bedtime and naptime. The pacifier should be used when placing the infant down for sleep and need not be reinserted once it falls out. For breastfed infants, delay introduction of the pacifier until breastfeeding is well established.

- Mothers should not smoke, drink alcohol, or use illicit drugs during pregnancy or after birth, and infants should not be exposed to secondhand smoke.

- The national Back to Sleep campaign should be expanded to emphasize the multiple characteristics of a safe sleeping environment and to focus on the groups with continuing higher rates of SIDS. Educational strategies must be tailored to each racial or ethnic group to ensure acceptance within that cultural context. Secondary care providers need to be targeted to receive these educational messages, including daycare providers, grandparents, foster parents, and babysitters.

- Research and surveillance should be continued on the risk factors, causes and pathophysiological mechanisms of SIDS and other sleep-related SUID, with the ultimate goal of preventing these deaths entirely. Federal and private funding agencies need to remain committed to this research.

Bibliography is available at Expert Consult.

Disorders of the Respiratory Tract

Chapter **376**
Congenital Disorders of the Nose

Joseph Haddad Jr. and Sarah Keesecker

NORMAL NEWBORN NOSE

In contrast to children and adults who preferentially breathe through their nose unless nasal obstruction interferes, most newborn infants are obligate nasal breathers and significant nasal obstruction presenting at birth, such as choanal atresia, may be a life-threatening situation for the infant unless an alternative to the nasal airway is established. Nasal congestion with obstruction is common in the 1st yr of life and can affect the quality of breathing during sleep; it may be associated with a narrow nasal airway, viral or bacterial infection, enlarged adenoids, or maternal estrogenic stimuli similar to rhinitis of pregnancy. The internal nasal airway doubles in size in the 1st 6 mo of life, leading to resolution of symptoms in many infants. Supportive care with a bulb syringe and saline nose drops, topical nasal decongestants, and antibiotics, when indicated, improve symptoms in affected infants.

PHYSIOLOGY

The nose is responsible for the initial warming and humidification of inspired air and olfaction. In the anterior nasal cavity, turbulent airflow and coarse hairs enhance the deposition of large particulate matter; the remaining nasal airways filter out particles as small as 6 μm in diameter. In the turbinate region, the airflow becomes laminar and the airstream is narrowed and directed superiorly, enhancing particle deposition, warming, and humidification. Nasal passages contribute as much as 50% of the total resistance of normal breathing. Nasal flaring, a sign of respiratory distress, reduces the resistance to inspiratory airflow through the nose and can improve ventilation (see Chapter 373).

Although the nasal mucosa is more vascular (especially in the turbinate region) than in the lower airways, the surface epithelium is similar, with ciliated cells, goblet cells, submucosal glands, and a covering blanket of mucus. The nasal secretions contain lysozyme and secretory immunoglobulin (Ig) A, both of which have antimicrobial activity, and IgG, IgE, albumin, histamine, bacteria, lactoferrin, and cellular debris, as well as mucous glycoproteins, which provide viscoelastic properties. Aided by the ciliated cells, mucus flows toward the nasopharynx, where the airstream widens, the epithelium becomes squamous, and secretions are wiped away by swallowing. Replacement of the mucous layers occurs about every 10-20 min. Estimates of daily mucus production vary from 0.1-0.3 mg/kg/24 hr, with most of the mucus being produced by the submucosal glands.

CONGENITAL DISORDERS

Congenital *structural nasal malformations* are uncommon compared with acquired abnormalities. The nasal bones can be congenitally absent so that the bridge of the nose fails to develop, resulting in *nasal hypoplasia*. Congenital absence of the nose *(arhinia)*, complete or partial duplication, or a single centrally placed nostril can occur in isolation but is usually part of a malformation syndrome. Rarely,

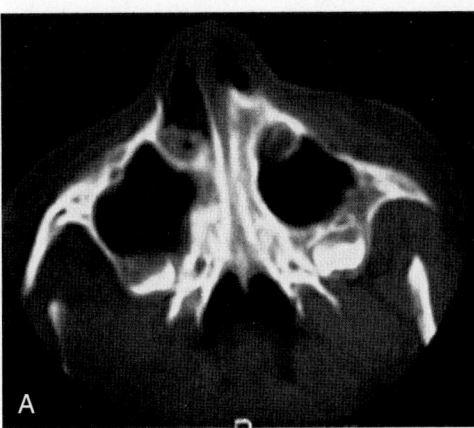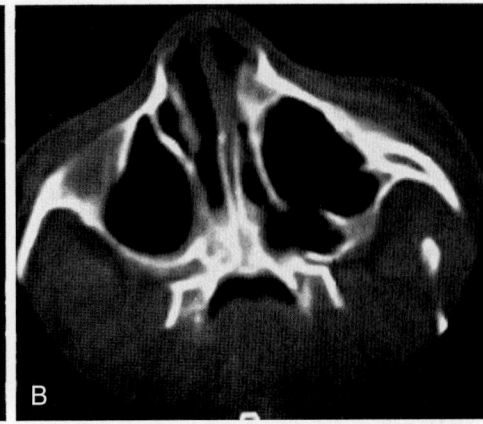

Figure 376-1 CT scan showing **(A)** hypoplastic nasal cavities and **(B)** bony and mucosal choanal atresia. *(From Altuntas A, Yilmaz MD, Kahveci OK, et al: Coexistence of choanal atresia and Tessier's facial cleft number 2, Int J Pediatr Otorhinolaryngol 68:1081–1085, 2004.)*

supernumerary teeth are found in the nose, or teeth grow into it from the maxilla.

Nasal bones can be sufficiently malformed to produce severe narrowing of the nasal passages. Often, such narrowing is associated with a high and narrow hard palate. Children with these defects can have significant obstruction to airflow during infections of the upper airways and are more susceptible to the development of chronic or recurrent hypoventilation (see Chapter 19). Rarely, the alae nasi are sufficiently thin and poorly supported to result in inspiratory obstruction, or there may be congenital nasolacrimal duct obstruction with cystic extension into the nasopharynx, causing respiratory distress.

CHOANAL ATRESIA

This is the most common congenital anomaly of the nose and has a frequency of approximately 1 in 7,000 live births. It consists of a unilateral or bilateral bony (90%) or membranous (10%) septum between the nose and the pharynx; most cases are a combination of bony and membranous atresia. The pathogenesis is unknown but theories include persistence of the buccopharyngeal membranes or failure of the oronasal membrane to rupture. The unilateral defect is more common and the female : male ratio is approximately 2 : 1. Approximately 50-70% of affected infants have other congenital anomalies (CHARGE syndrome, Treacher-Collins, Kallmann syndrome, VATER [vertebral defects, imperforate anus, tracheoesophageal fistula, and renal defects] association, Pfeiffer syndrome), with the anomalies occurring more often in bilateral cases. The **CHARGE syndrome** (*c*oloboma, *h*eart disease, *a*tresia choanae, *r*etarded growth and development or central nervous system anomalies or both, *g*enital anomalies or hypogonadism or both, and *e*ar anomalies or deafness or both) is one of the more common anomalies associated with choanal atresia— approximately 10-20% of patients with choanal atresia have it. Most patients with CHARGE syndrome have mutations in the *CHD7* gene, which is involved in chromatin organization.

Clinical Manifestations

Newborn infants have a variable ability to breathe through their mouths, so nasal obstruction does not produce the same symptoms in every infant. When the obstruction is unilateral, the infant may be asymptomatic for a prolonged period, often until the first respiratory infection, when unilateral nasal discharge or persistent nasal obstruction can suggest the diagnosis. Infants with bilateral choanal atresia who have difficulty with mouth breathing make vigorous attempts to inspire, often suck in their lips, and develop cyanosis. Distressed children then cry (which relieves the cyanosis) and become calmer, with normal skin color, only to repeat the cycle after closing their mouths. Those who are able to breathe through their mouths at once experience difficulty when sucking and swallowing, becoming cyanotic when they attempt to feed.

Diagnosis

Diagnosis is established by the inability to pass a firm catheter through each nostril 3-4 cm into the nasopharynx. The atretic plate may be seen directly with fiberoptic rhinoscopy. The anatomy is best evaluated by using high-resolution CT (Fig. 376-1).

Treatment

Initial treatment consists of prompt placement of an oral airway, maintaining the mouth in an open position, or intubation. A standard oral airway (such as that used in anesthesia) can be used, or a feeding nipple can be fashioned with large holes at the tip to facilitate air passage. Once an oral airway is established, the infant can be fed by gavage until breathing and eating without the assisted airway is possible. In bilateral cases, intubation or, less often, tracheotomy may be indicated. If the child is free of other serious medical problems, operative intervention is considered in the neonate; transnasal repair is the treatment of choice, with the introduction of small magnifying endoscopes and smaller surgical instruments and drills. Stents are usually left in place for weeks after the repair to prevent closure or stenosis. Tracheotomy should be considered in cases of bilateral atresia in which the child has other potentially life-threatening problems and in whom early surgical repair of the choanal atresia may not be appropriate or feasible. Operative correction of unilateral obstruction may be deferred for several years. In both unilateral and bilateral cases, restenosis necessitating dilation or reoperation, or both, is common. Mitomycin C has been used to help prevent the development of granulation tissue and stenosis.

CONGENITAL DEFECTS OF THE NASAL SEPTUM

Perforation of the septum is most commonly acquired after birth secondary to infection, such as syphilis or tuberculosis, or trauma; rarely, it is developmental. Continuous positive airway pressure cannulas are a cause of iatrogenic perforation. Trauma from delivery is the most common cause of septal deviation noted at birth. When recognized early, it can be corrected with immediate realignment using blunt probes, cotton applicators, and topical anesthesia. Formal surgical correction, when required, is usually postponed to avoid disturbance of midface growth.

Mild septal deviations are common and usually asymptomatic; abnormal formation of the septum is uncommon unless other malformations are present, such as cleft lip or palate.

PYRIFORM APERTURE STENOSIS

Infants with this bony abnormality of the anterior nasal aperture present at birth or shortly thereafter with severe nasal obstruction leading to noisy breathing and respiratory distress that worsen with feeding and improve with crying. It can occur in isolation or in association with other malformations including holoprosencephaly,

Nasal Pyriform Stenosis

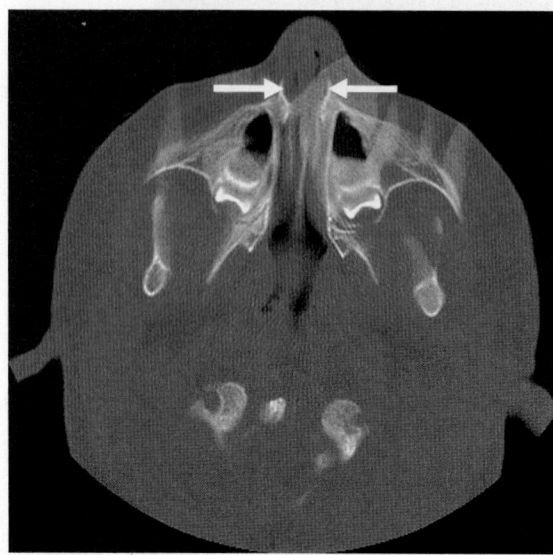

Figure 376-2 CT scan of a child who has congenital nasal pyriform aperture stenosis. Note the inward bowing of the nasal processes of the maxillary bone with the pyriform aperture measuring 7 mm *(arrows)*. *(From Tate JR, Sykes J. Congenital nasal pyriform aperture stenosis. Otolaryngol Clin North Am 42(3):521–525, 2009, Fig. 2.)*

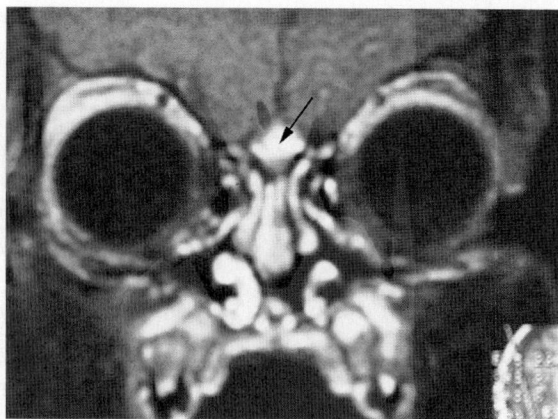

Figure 376-3 Coronal CT scan of nasal dermoid with intracranial extension (arrow). *(From Manning SC, Bloom DC, Perkins JA, et al: Diagnostic and surgical challenges in the pediatric skull base. Otolaryngol Clin North Am 38:773-794, 2005. Fig. 2.)*

hypopituitarism, and cardiac and urogenital malformations. Diagnosis is made by CT of the nose (Fig. 376-2). Medical management (nasal decongestants, humidification, nasopharyngeal airway insertion, management of reflux) can be used but surgical repair by means of an anterior, sublabial approach may be needed if the child cannot feed or breathe without difficulty. A drill is used to enlarge the stenotic anterior bone apertures.

CONGENITAL MIDLINE NASAL MASSES
Dermoids, gliomas, and *encephaloceles* (in descending order of frequency) occur intranasally or extranasally and can have intracranial connections or extend intracranially with communication to the subarachnoid space. The theory for the embryologic development of congenital midline nasal masses is faulty retraction of the dural diverticulum. Dermoids and epidermoids are the most common type of congenital midline nasal mass and have been reported to represent up to 61% of lesions. Nasal dermoids often have a dimple or pit on the nasal dorsum, sometimes with hair being present, and can predispose to intracranial infections if an intracranial fistula or sinus is present. Recurrent infection of the dermoid itself is more common. Gliomas or heterotopic brain tissue are firm, whereas encephaloceles are soft and enlarge with crying or the Valsalva maneuver. Diagnosis is based on physical examination findings and results from imaging studies. CT provides the best bony detail, but MRI is helpful also because of its superior ability to define intracranial extension (Fig. 376-3). Surgical excision of these masses is generally required, with the extent and surgical approach based on the type and size of the mass.

Other nasal masses include *hemangiomas, congenital nasolacrimal duct obstruction* (which can occur as an intranasal mass), nasal polyps, and tumors such as rhabdomyosarcoma (see Chapter 500). Nasal polyps are rarely present at birth, but the other masses often present at birth or in early infancy (see Chapter 378).

Poor development of the paranasal sinuses and a narrow nasal airway are associated with recurrent or chronic upper airway infection in Down syndrome (see Chapter 81).

DIAGNOSIS AND TREATMENT
In children with congenital nasal disorders, supportive care of the airway is given until the diagnosis is established. Diagnosis is made through a combination of flexible scoping and imaging studies,

primarily CT scan. In the case of surgically correctable congenital problems such as choanal atresia, surgery is performed once the child is deemed healthy and free of life-threatening problems such as congenital heart disease.

Bibliography is available at Expert Consult.

Chapter 377
Acquired Disorders of the Nose
Joseph Haddad Jr. and Sarah Keesecker

Tumors, septal perforations, and other acquired abnormalities of the nose and paranasal sinuses can manifest with epistaxis. Midface trauma with a nasal or facial fracture may be accompanied by epistaxis. Trauma to the nose can cause a *septal hematoma;* if treatment is delayed, this can lead to necrosis of septal cartilage and a resultant *saddle-nose deformity.* Other abnormalities that can cause a change in the shape of the nose and paranasal bones, with obstruction but few other symptoms, include *fibroosseous lesions* (ossifying fibroma, fibrous dysplasia, cementifying fibroma) and *mucoceles of the paranasal sinuses.* These conditions may be suspected on physical examination and confirmed by CT scan and biopsy. Although these are considered benign lesions, they can all greatly change the anatomy of surrounding bony structures and often require surgical intervention for management.

377.1 Foreign Body
Joseph Haddad Jr. and Sarah Keesecker

ETIOLOGY
Foreign bodies (food, beads, crayons, small toys, erasers, paper wads, buttons, batteries, beans, stones, pieces of sponge, and other small objects) are often placed in the nose by small children and developmentally delayed children and constitute ≤1% of pediatric emergency department visits. Nasal foreign bodies can go unrecognized for long periods of time because they initially produce few symptoms and

are difficult to visualize. First symptoms include unilateral obstruction, sneezing, relatively mild discomfort, and, rarely, pain. Presenting clinical symptoms include history of insertion of foreign bodies (86%), mucopurulent nasal discharge (24%), foul nasal odor (9%), epistaxis (6%), nasal obstruction (3%), and mouth breathing (2%). Irritation results in mucosal swelling because some foreign bodies are hygroscopic and increase in size as water is absorbed; signs of local obstruction and discomfort can increase with time. The patient might also present with a generalized body odor known as *bromhidrosis*.

DIAGNOSIS

Unilateral nasal discharge and obstruction should suggest the presence of a foreign body, which can often be seen on examination with a nasal speculum or wide otoscope placed in the nose. Purulent secretions may have to be cleared so that the foreign object can actually be seen; a headlight, suction, and topical decongestants are often needed. The object is usually situated anteriorly, but unskilled attempts at removal can force the object deeper into the nose. A long-standing foreign body can become embedded in granulation tissue or mucosa and appear as a nasal mass. A lateral skull radiograph assists in diagnosis if the foreign body is metallic or radiopaque.

TREATMENT

A quick examination of the nose is made to determine if a foreign body is present, and whether it needs to be removed emergently. Planning is then made for office or operating room extrication of the foreign body. Prompt removal minimizes the danger of aspiration and local tissue necrosis. This can usually be performed with topical anesthesia, using either forceps or nasal suction. Alternatively, a Katz catheter (made specifically for the removal of foreign bodies from the nose and ear) can be inserted above and distal to the object, inflated, and drawn back with gentle traction.

The "mother kiss" approach has been successful in acute situations where a person occludes the unaffected nostril and then, with a complete seal over the child's mouth attempts to dislodge the foreign body by blowing into the mouth. A similar approach uses an Ambu bag over the mouth with the unaffected nostril occluded. If there is marked swelling, bleeding, or tissue overgrowth, general anesthesia may be needed to remove the object. Infection usually clears promptly after the removal of the object and, generally, no further therapy is necessary. Magnets can be used to extract metal foreign bodies, 2% lidocaine can be used to kill live insects before removal, and irrigation should be avoided with vegetable matter or sponges because of the risk of foreign-body swelling.

COMPLICATIONS

Serious complications include posterior dislodgement and aspiration, trauma caused by the object itself or removal attempts, infection, and choanal stenosis. Infection is common and gives rise to a purulent, malodorous, or bloody discharge. Local tissue damage from long-standing foreign body, or alkaline injury from a disk battery, can lead to local tissue loss and cartilage destruction. A synechia or scar band can then form, causing nasal obstruction. Loss of septal mucosa and cartilage can cause a septal perforation. Disk batteries are especially dangerous when placed in the nose; they leach base, which causes pain and local tissue destruction in a matter of hours. Magnets also carry a risk of septal perforation and necrosis.

Tetanus is a rare complication of long-standing nasal foreign bodies in nonimmunized children (see Chapter 211). Toxic shock syndrome is also rare and most commonly occurs from nasal surgical packing (see Chapter 181.2); oral antibiotics should be administered when nasal surgical packing is placed.

PREVENTION

Tempting objects, such as round, shiny beads, should only be used under adult supervision. Disk batteries should be stored away from the reach of small children.

Bibliography is available at Expert Consult.

377.2 Epistaxis
Joseph Haddad Jr. and Sarah Keesecker

Although rare in infancy, nosebleeds are common in children older than 2 yr of age. Their incidence decreases after puberty. Diagnosis and treatment depend on the location and cause of the bleeding.

ANATOMY

The most common site of bleeding is the Kiesselbach plexus, an area in the anterior septum where vessels from both the internal carotid (anterior and posterior ethmoid arteries) and external carotid (sphenopalatine and terminal branches of the internal maxillary arteries) converge. The thin mucosa in this area, as well as the anterior location, make it prone to exposure to dry air and trauma.

ETIOLOGY

Epistaxis can be classified into primary or secondary based on cause and this has implications for diagnosis and management. Common causes of nosebleeds from the anterior septum include digital trauma, foreign bodies, dry air, and inflammation, including upper respiratory tract infections, sinusitis, and allergic rhinitis (Table 377-1). There is often a family history of childhood epistaxis. Nasal steroid sprays are commonly used in children, and their chronic use may be associated with nasal mucosal bleeding. Young infants with significant gastroesophageal reflux into the nose rarely present with epistaxis secondary to mucosal inflammation. Susceptibility is increased during respiratory infections and in the winter when dry air irritates the nasal mucosa, resulting in formation of fissures and crusting. Severe bleeding may be encountered with congenital vascular abnormalities, such as *hereditary hemorrhagic telangiectasia* (see Chapter 432.3), varicosities, hemangiomas, and, in children with thrombocytopenia, deficiency of clotting factors, particularly von Willebrand disease (see Chapter 477), hypertension, renal failure, or venous congestion. Recurrent epistaxis despite cauterization is associated with mild coagulation disorders. The family history may be positive for abnormal bleeding (epistaxis or other sites); specific testing for von Willebrand disease is indicated because the prothrombin time or partial thromboplastin time may be normal despite having a bleeding disorder. Nasal polyps or other intranasal growths may be associated with epistaxis. Recurrent, and often severe, nosebleeds may be the initial presenting symptom in **juvenile nasal angiofibroma,** which occurs in adolescent boys.

Table 377-1	Possible Causes of Epistaxis

Epistaxis digitorum (nose picking)
Rhinitis (allergic or viral)
Chronic sinusitis
Foreign bodies
Intranasal neoplasm or polyps
Irritants (e.g., cigarette smoke)
Septal deviation
Septal perforation
Trauma including child abuse
Vascular malformation or telangiectasia (hereditary hemorrhage telangiectasia)
Hemophilia
von Willebrand disease
Platelet dysfunction
Thrombocytopenia
Hypertension
Leukemia
Liver disease (e.g., cirrhosis)
Medications (e.g., aspirin, anticoagulants, nonsteroidal antiinflammatory drugs, topical corticosteroids)
Cocaine abuse

From Kucik CJ, Clenney T: Management of epistaxis, Am Fam Physician 71(2):305–311, 2005.

CLINICAL MANIFESTATIONS

Epistaxis usually occurs without warning, with blood flowing slowly but freely from 1 nostril or occasionally from both. In children with nasal lesions, bleeding might follow physical exercise. When bleeding occurs at night, the blood may be swallowed and become apparent only when the child vomits or passes blood in the stools. Posterior epistaxis can manifest as anterior nasal bleeding or, if bleeding is copious, the patient might vomit blood as the initial symptom.

TREATMENT

Most nosebleeds stop spontaneously in a few minutes. The nares should be compressed and the child kept as quiet as possible, in an upright position with the head tilted forward to avoid blood trickling back into the throat. Cold compresses applied to the nose can also help. If these measures do not stop the bleeding, local application of a solution of oxymetazoline (Afrin or Neo-Synephrine) (0.25-1%) may be useful. If bleeding persists, an anterior nasal pack may need to be inserted; if bleeding originates in the posterior nasal cavity, combined anterior and posterior packing is necessary. After bleeding is under control, and if a bleeding site is identified, its obliteration by cautery with silver nitrate may prevent further difficulties. Because the septal cartilage derives its nutrition from the overlying mucoperichondrium, only 1 side of the septum should be cauterized at a time to reduce the chance of a septal perforation. During the winter, or in a dry environment, a room humidifier, saline drops, and petrolatum (Vaseline) applied to the septum can help to prevent epistaxis. Antiseptic cream (e.g., mupirocin) significantly increases the proportion of children who have complete resolution of bleeding at 8 wk compared to no treatment. Ointments prevent infection, increase moisture, decrease bleeding, and are commonly used in clinical practice. However, the combination of silver nitrate cautery and antiseptic nasal cream is superior to antiseptic cream alone. Patients with severe epistaxis despite conservative medical measures should be considered for surgical ligation techniques or embolization. In patients with severe or repeated epistaxis, blood transfusions may be necessary. Otolaryngologic evaluation is indicated for these children and for those with bilateral bleeding or with hemorrhage that does not arise from the Kiesselbach plexus. Secondary epistaxis should be managed by identification of the cause, application of appropriate nasal therapy, and correct systemic medical management. Hematologic evaluation (for coagulopathy and anemia), along with nasal endoscopy and diagnostic imaging, may be needed to make a definitive diagnosis in cases of severe recurrent epistaxis. Replacement of deficient clotting factors may be required for patients who have an underlying hematologic disorder (see Chapter 476). Profuse unilateral epistaxis associated with a nasal mass in an adolescent boy near puberty might signal a **juvenile nasopharyngeal angiofibroma.** This unusual tumor has also been reported in a 2 yr old and in 30-40 yr olds, but the incidence peaks in adolescent and preadolescent boys. CT with contrast medium enhancement and MRI are part of the initial evaluation; arteriography, embolization, and extensive surgery may be needed.

Surgical intervention may also be needed for bleeding from the internal maxillary artery or other vessels that can cause bleeding in the posterior nasal cavity.

PREVENTION

The discouragement of nose picking, and attention to proper humidification of the bedroom during dry winter months helps to prevent many nosebleeds. Prompt attention to nasal infections and allergies is beneficial to nasal hygiene. Prompt cessation of nasal steroid sprays prevents ongoing bleeding.

Bibliography is available at Expert Consult.

Chapter **378**
Nasal Polyps
Joseph Haddad Jr. and Sarah Keesecker

ETIOLOGY

Nasal polyps are benign pedunculated tumors formed from edematous, usually chronically inflamed nasal mucosa. They commonly arise from the ethmoidal sinus and occur in the middle meatus. Occasionally, they appear within the maxillary antrum and can extend to the nasopharynx (antrochoanal polyp).

It is estimated that between 0.2% and 1% of the population will develop nasal polyps at some time; the incidence of nasal polyps increases with age. Antrochoanal polyps represent only 4-6% of all nasal polyps in the general population but account for approximately one-third of polyps in the pediatric population. Large or multiple polyps can completely obstruct the nasal passage. The polyps originating from the ethmoidal sinus are usually smaller and multiple, as compared with the large and usually single antrochoanal polyp.

Cystic fibrosis (CF; see Chapter 403) is the most common childhood cause of nasal polyposis and up to 50% of CF patients experience obstructing nasal polyposis, which is rare in non-CF children. Therefore, CF should be suspected in any child younger than 12 yr old with nasal polyps, even in the absence of typical respiratory and digestive symptoms. Cystic fibrosis patients with homozygosity for F508del and other severe mutations appear to have an elevated risk of nasal polyps. Nasal polyposis is also associated with chronic sinusitis (see Chapter 380) and allergic rhinitis. In the *Samter triad,* nasal polyps are associated with aspirin sensitivity and asthma; this condition is rare.

CLINICAL MANIFESTATIONS

Obstruction of nasal passages is prominent, with associated hyponasal speech and mouth breathing. Profuse unilateral mucoid or mucopurulent rhinorrhea may also be present. An examination of the nasal passages shows glistening, gray, grape-like masses squeezed between the nasal turbinates and the septum.

DIAGNOSIS AND DIFFERENTIAL DIAGNOSIS

Examination of the external nose and rhinoscopy is performed. Ethmoidal polyps can be readily distinguished from the well-vascularized turbinate tissue, which is pink or red; antrochoanal polyps may have a more fleshy appearance (Fig. 378-1). Antrochoanal polyps may prolapse into the nasopharynx; flexible nasopharyngoscopy can assist in

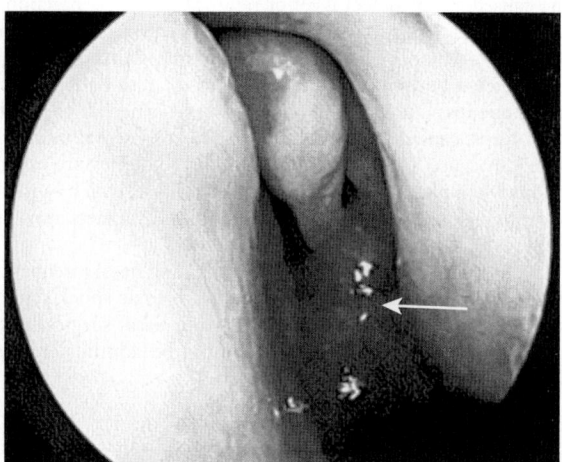

Figure 378-1 Antrochoanal polyp viewed endoscopically *(arrow).* *(From Basak S, Karaman CZ, Akdilli A, et al: Surgical approaches to antrochoanal polyps in children, Int J Pediatr Otorhinolaryngol 46:197–205, 1998.)*

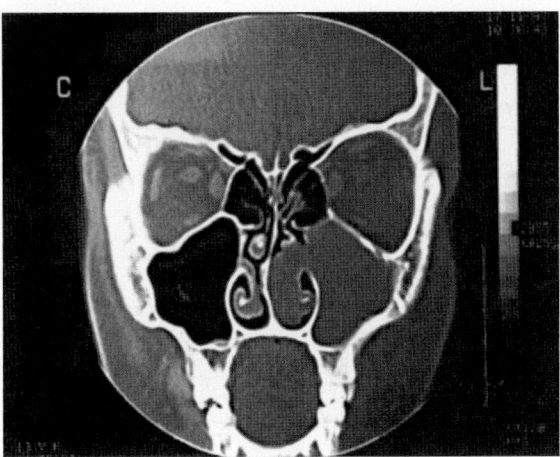

Figure 378-2 A typical CT image of an isolated antrochoanal polyp on the left side. *(From Basak S, Karaman CZ, Akdilli A, et al: Surgical approaches to antrochoanal polyps in children, Int J Pediatr Otorhinolaryngol 46:197–205, 1998.)*

making this diagnosis. Prolonged presence of ethmoidal polyps in a child can widen the bridge of the nose and erode adjacent osseous structures. Tumors of the nose cause more local destruction and distortion of the anatomy. CT scan of the midface is key to diagnosis and planning for surgical treatment (Fig. 378-2).

TREATMENT

Local or systemic decongestants are not usually effective in shrinking the polyps, although they may provide symptomatic relief from the associated mucosal edema. Intranasal steroid sprays, and sometimes systemic steroids, can provide some shrinkage of nasal polyps with symptomatic relief and have proved useful in children with CF and adults with nasal polyps. Topical nasal steroid therapy, fluticasone, mometasone, and budesonide appears to result in nasal symptom improvement. Doxycycline (200 mg on the 1st day followed by 100 mg daily) has a significant effect on the size of nasal polyps, nasal symptoms, and mucosal and systemic markers of inflammation. Polyps should be removed surgically if complete obstruction, uncontrolled rhinorrhea, or deformity of the nose appears. If the underlying pathogenic mechanism cannot be eliminated (such as CF), the polyps may soon return. Functional endoscopic sinus surgery provides more complete polyp removal and treatment of other associated nasal disease; in some cases, this has reduced the need for frequent surgeries. Nasal steroid sprays should also be started preventively, once postsurgical healing occurs.

Antrochoanal polyps do not respond to medical measures and must be removed surgically. Because these types of polyps are not associated with any underlying disease process, the recurrence rate is much less than for other types of polyps.

Bibliography is available at Expert Consult.

Chapter **379**
The Common Cold
E. Kathryn Miller and John V. Williams

The common cold is an acute viral infection of the upper respiratory tract in which the symptoms of rhinorrhea and nasal obstruction are prominent. Systemic symptoms and signs such as headache, myalgia, and fever are absent or mild. The common cold is frequently referred to as *infectious rhinitis* but may also include self-limited involvement of the sinus mucosa and is more correctly termed *rhinosinusitis*.

ETIOLOGY

The most common pathogens associated with the common cold are the more than 200 types of human rhinoviruses (see Chapter 263), but the syndrome can be caused by many different virus families (Table 379-1). Rhinoviruses are associated with more than 50% of colds in adults and children. In young children, other viral etiologies of the common cold include respiratory syncytial virus (RSV; see Chapter 260), human metapneumovirus (see Chapter 261), parainfluenza viruses (see Chapter 259), and adenoviruses (see Chapter 262). Common cold symptoms may also be caused by influenza viruses, nonpolio enteroviruses, and human coronaviruses. Many viruses that cause rhinitis are also associated with other symptoms and signs such as cough, wheezing, and fever.

EPIDEMIOLOGY

Colds occur year-round, but the incidence is greatest from the early fall until the late spring, reflecting the seasonal prevalence of the viral pathogens associated with cold symptoms. In the northern hemisphere, the highest incidence of rhinovirus infection occurs in the early fall (August-October) and in the late spring (April-May). The seasonal incidence for parainfluenza viruses usually peaks in the late fall and late spring and is highest between December and April for RSVs, influenza viruses, human metapneumoviruses, and coronaviruses. Adenoviruses are detected at a low prevalence throughout the cold season, and enteroviruses may also be detected during summer months or throughout the year.

Young children have an average of 6-8 colds per year, but 10-15% of children have at least 12 infections per year. The incidence of illness decreases with age, with 2-3 illnesses per year by adulthood. The incidence of infection is primarily a function of exposure to the virus. Children in out-of-home daycare centers during the 1st yr of life have 50% more colds than children cared for only at home. The difference in the incidence of illness between these groups of children decreases as the length of time spent in daycare increases, although the incidence of illness remains higher in the daycare group through at least the 1st 3 yr of life. When they begin primary school, children who attended daycare have less frequent colds than those who did not. Mannose-binding lectin deficiency with impaired innate immunity may be associated with an increased incidence of colds in children.

PATHOGENESIS

Viruses that cause the common cold are spread by 3 mechanisms: direct hand contact (self-inoculation of one's own nasal mucosa or conjunctivae after touching a contaminated person or object), inhalation of small-particle aerosols that are airborne from coughing, or deposition of large-particle aerosols that are expelled during a sneeze and land on nasal or conjunctival mucosa. Although the different common cold pathogens could be spread by any of these mechanisms, some routes of transmission appear to be more efficient than others for particular viruses. Studies of rhinoviruses and RSV indicate that direct contact is an efficient mechanism of transmission of these viruses, although transmission by large-particle aerosols can also occur. By contrast, influenza viruses and coronaviruses appear to be most efficiently spread by small-particle aerosols.

The respiratory viruses have evolved different mechanisms to avoid host defenses. Infections with rhinoviruses and adenoviruses result in the development of serotype-specific protective immunity. Repeated infections with these pathogens occur because there are a large number of distinct serotypes of each virus. Influenza viruses have the ability to change the antigens presented on the surface of the virus and thus behave as though there were multiple viral serotypes. The interaction of coronaviruses (see Chapter 264) with host immunity is not well defined, but it appears that multiple distinct strains of coronaviruses are capable of inducing at least short-term protective immunity. There are 4 types of parainfluenza viruses and 2 antigenic subgroups of RSV. In addition to antigenic diversity, many of these viruses are able to

Table 379-1	Pathogens Associated with the Common Cold		
ASSOCIATION	**PATHOGEN**	**RELATIVE FREQUENCY***	**OTHER COMMON SYMPTOMS AND SIGNS**
Agents primarily associated with the common cold	Human rhinoviruses Coronaviruses	Frequent Occasional	Wheezing/bronchiolitis
Agents primarily associated with other clinical syndromes that also cause common cold symptoms	Respiratory syncytial viruses Human metapneumovirus Influenza viruses Parainfluenza viruses Adenoviruses	Occasional Occasional Uncommon Uncommon Uncommon	Bronchiolitis in children <2 yr of age Pneumonia and bronchiolitis Influenza, pneumonia, croup Croup, bronchiolitis Pharyngoconjunctival fever (palpebral conjunctivitis, watery eye discharge, pharyngeal erythema)
	Enteroviruses Coxsackievirus A Other nonpolio enteroviruses	Uncommon	Herpangina (fever and ulcerated papules on posterior oropharynx Aseptic meningitis

*Relative frequency of colds caused by the agent.

reinfect the upper airway because mucosal immunoglobulin A induced by previous infection is short-lived, and the brief incubation period of these viruses allows the establishment of infection before immune memory responses. Although reinfection is not completely prevented by the adaptive host response to these viruses, the severity of illness is moderated by preexisting immunity.

Viral infection of the nasal epithelium can be associated with destruction of the epithelial lining, as with influenza viruses and adenoviruses, or there can be no apparent histologic damage, as with rhinoviruses and RSV. Regardless of the histopathologic findings, infection of the nasal epithelium is associated with an acute inflammatory response characterized by release of a variety of inflammatory cytokines and infiltration of the mucosa by inflammatory cells. This acute inflammatory response appears to be partially or largely responsible for many of the symptoms associated with the common cold. Viral shedding of most respiratory viruses peaks 3-5 days after inoculation, often coinciding with symptom onset; low levels of viral shedding may persist for up to 2 wk in the otherwise healthy host. Inflammation can obstruct the sinus ostia or eustachian tube, predisposing to bacterial sinusitis or otitis media.

The host immune system is responsible for most cold symptoms, rather than direct damage to the respiratory tract. Infected cells release cytokines, such as interleukin-8, that attract polymorphonuclear cells into the nasal submucosa and epithelium. Rhinoviruses also increase vascular permeability in the nasal submucosa, releasing albumin and bradykinin, which may contribute to symptoms.

CLINICAL MANIFESTATIONS

Symptoms of the common cold vary by age and virus. In infants, fever and nasal discharge may predominate. Fever is uncommon in older children and adults. The onset of common cold symptoms typically occurs 1-3 days after viral infection. The first symptom noted is often sore or scratchy throat, followed closely by nasal obstruction and rhinorrhea. The sore throat usually resolves quickly and, by the 2nd and 3rd day of illness, nasal symptoms predominate. Cough is associated with two-thirds of colds in children and usually begins after the onset of nasal symptoms. Cough may persist for an additional 1-2 wk after resolution of other symptoms. Influenza viruses, RSVs, human metapneumoviruses, and adenoviruses are more likely than rhinoviruses or coronaviruses to be associated with fever and other constitutional symptoms. Other symptoms of a cold may include headache, hoarseness, irritability, difficulty sleeping, or decreased appetite. Vomiting and diarrhea are uncommon. The usual cold persists for approximately 1 wk, although 10% last for 2 wk.

The physical findings of the common cold are limited to the upper respiratory tract. Increased nasal secretion is usually obvious; a change in the color or consistency of the secretions is common during the course of the illness and does not indicate sinusitis or bacterial superinfection but may indicate accumulation of polymorphonuclear cells. Examination of the nasal cavity might reveal swollen, erythematous

Table 379-2	Conditions That Can Mimic the Common Cold
CONDITION	**DIFFERENTIATING FEATURES**
Allergic rhinitis	Prominent itching and sneezing, nasal eosinophils
Vasomotor rhinitis	May be triggered by irritants, weather changes, spicy foods, etc.
Rhinitis medicamentosa	History of nasal decongestant use
Foreign body	Unilateral, foul-smelling secretions Bloody nasal secretions
Sinusitis	Presence of fever, headache or facial pain, or periorbital edema or persistence of rhinorrhea or cough for longer than 14 days
Streptococcosis	Mucopurulent nasal discharge that excoriates the nares
Pertussis	Onset of persistent or severe paroxysmal cough
Congenital syphilis	Persistent rhinorrhea with onset in the 1st 3 mo of life

nasal turbinates, although this finding is nonspecific and of limited diagnostic value. Abnormal middle ear pressure is common during the course of a cold. Anterior cervical lymphadenopathy or conjunctival injection may also be noted on exam.

DIAGNOSIS

The most important task of the physician caring for a patient with a cold is to exclude other conditions that are potentially more serious or treatable. The differential diagnosis of the common cold includes noninfectious disorders as well as other upper respiratory tract infections (Table 379-2).

LABORATORY FINDINGS

Routine laboratory studies are not helpful for the diagnosis and management of the common cold. A nasal smear for eosinophils may be useful if allergic rhinitis is suspected (see Chapter 143). A predominance of polymorphonuclear cells in the nasal secretions is characteristic of uncomplicated colds and does not indicate bacterial superinfection. Self-limited radiographic abnormalities of the paranasal sinuses are common during an uncomplicated cold; imaging is not indicated for most children with simple rhinitis.

The viral pathogens associated with the common cold can be detected by polymerase chain reaction, culture, antigen detection, or serologic methods. These studies are generally not indicated in patients with colds because a specific etiologic diagnosis is useful only when treatment with an antiviral agent is contemplated, such as for influenza viruses. Bacterial cultures or antigen detection are useful only when group A streptococcus (see Chapter 183) or *Bordetella pertussis* (see Chapter 197) is suspected. The isolation of other bacterial pathogens from nasopharyngeal specimens is not an indication of bacterial nasal infection and is not a specific predictor of the etiologic agent in sinusitis.

TREATMENT

The management of the common cold consists primarily of supportive care and anticipatory guidance as recommended by American Academy of Pediatrics and United Kingdom National Institute for Health and Clinical Excellence guidelines.

Antiviral Treatment

Specific antiviral therapy is not available for rhinovirus infections. Ribavirin, which is approved for treatment of severe RSV infections, has no role in the treatment of the common cold. The neuraminidase inhibitors oseltamivir and zanamivir have a modest effect on the duration of symptoms associated with influenza viral infections in children. Oseltamivir also reduces the frequency of influenza-associated otitis media. The difficulty of distinguishing influenza from other common cold pathogens and the necessity that therapy be started early in the illness (within 48 hr of onset of symptoms) to be beneficial are practical limitations to the use of these agents for mild upper respiratory tract infections. Antibacterial therapy is of no benefit in the treatment of the common cold and should be avoided to minimize possible adverse effects and the development of antibiotic resistance.

Supportive Care and Symptomatic Treatment

Supportive interventions are frequently recommended by providers. Maintaining adequate oral hydration may help to thin secretions and soothe respiratory mucosa. The common home remedy of ingesting warm fluids may soothe mucosa, increase nasal mucous flow, or loosen respiratory secretions. Topical nasal saline may temporarily remove secretions, and saline nasal irrigation may reduce symptoms. Cool, humidified air has not been well studied but may loosen nasal secretions; however, cool-mist humidifiers and vaporizers must be cleaned after each use. The World Health Organization suggests that neither steam nor cool-mist therapy be used in treatment of a cold.

The use of oral **nonprescription** therapies (often containing antihistamines, antitussives, and decongestants) for cold symptoms in children is controversial. Although some of these medications are effective in adults, no study demonstrates a significant effect in children, and there may be serious side effects. Young children cannot participate in the assessment of symptom severity, so studies of these treatments in children have generally been based on observations by parents or other observers, a method that is likely to be insensitive for detection of treatment effects. As a result of the lack of direct evidence for effectiveness and the potential for unwanted side effects, the American Academy of Pediatrics recommends that nonprescription cough and cold products **not** be used for infants and children younger than 6 yr of age. A decision whether to use these medications in older children must consider the likelihood of clinical benefit compared with the potential adverse effects of these drugs. The prominent or most bothersome symptoms of colds vary in the course of the illness. If symptomatic treatments are used, it is reasonable to target therapy to specific bothersome symptoms and care should be taken to ensure that caregivers understand the intended effect and can determine the proper dosage of the medications.

Zinc, given as oral lozenges to previously healthy patients, reduces the duration but not the severity of symptoms of a common cold if begun within 24 hr of symptoms. The function of the rhinovirus 3C protease, an essential enzyme for rhinovirus replication, is inhibited by zinc, but there has been no evidence of an antiviral effect of zinc in vivo. The effect of zinc on symptoms has been inconsistent, with some studies reporting dramatic treatment effects (in adults), whereas other studies find no benefit. Side effects are common and include decreased taste, bad taste, and nausea.

Fever

Fever is not usually associated with an uncomplicated common cold, and antipyretic treatment is generally not indicated.

Nasal Obstruction

Either topical or oral adrenergic agents may be used as nasal decongestants in older children and adults. Effective topical adrenergic agents such as xylometazoline, oxymetazoline, or phenylephrine are available as either intranasal drops or nasal sprays. Reduced-strength formulations of these medications are available for use in younger children, although they are not recommended for use in children younger than 6 yr old. Systemic absorption of the imidazolines (oxymetazoline, xylometazoline) has very rarely been associated with bradycardia, hypotension, and coma. Prolonged use of the topical adrenergic agents should be avoided to prevent the development of **rhinitis medicamentosa,** an apparent rebound effect that causes the sensation of nasal obstruction when the drug is discontinued. The oral adrenergic agents are less effective than the topical preparations and are occasionally associated with systemic effects such as central nervous system stimulation, hypertension, and palpitations. Aromatic vapors (such as menthol) for external rub may improve perception of nasal patency, but do not affect spirometry.

Saline nose drops (wash, irrigation) can improve nasal symptoms and may be used in all age groups.

Rhinorrhea

The first-generation antihistamines may reduce rhinorrhea by 25-30%. The effect of the antihistamines on rhinorrhea appears to be related to the anticholinergic rather than the antihistaminic properties of these drugs, and therefore the second-generation or "nonsedating" antihistamines have no effect on common cold symptoms. The major adverse effects associated with the use of the antihistamines are sedation or paradoxical hyperactivity. Overdose may be associated with respiratory depression or hallucinations. Rhinorrhea may also be treated with ipratropium bromide, a topical anticholinergic agent. This drug produces an effect comparable to the antihistamines but is not associated with sedation. The most common side effects of ipratropium are nasal irritation and bleeding.

Sore Throat

The sore throat associated with colds is generally not severe, but treatment with mild analgesics is occasionally indicated, particularly if there is associated myalgia or headache. The use of acetaminophen during rhinovirus infection is associated with suppression of neutralizing antibody responses, but this observation has no apparent clinical significance. Aspirin should not be given to children with respiratory infections because of the risk of Reye syndrome in children with influenza (see Chapter 361). **Nonsteroidal antiinflammatory drugs** are somewhat effective in relieving discomfort caused by a cold, but there is no clear evidence of their effect on respiratory symptoms. The balance of harm and benefits must be considered when using nonsteroidal antiinflammatory drugs for colds.

Cough

Cough suppression is generally not necessary in patients with colds. Cough in some patients appears to be from upper respiratory tract irritation associated with postnasal drip. Cough in these patients is most prominent during the time of greatest nasal symptoms, and treatment with a first-generation antihistamine may be helpful. Cough lozenges or hard candy may be temporarily effective and are unlikely to be harmful in children for whom they do not pose risk of aspiration (older than age 6 yr). **Honey** (5-10 mL in children ≥1 year old) has a modest effect on relieving nocturnal cough and is unlikely to be harmful in children older than 1 yr of age. Honey should be avoided in children younger than 1 yr of age because of the risk for botulism (see Chapter 210).

In some patients, cough may be a result of **virus-induced reactive airways disease**. These patients can have cough that persists for days to weeks after the acute illness and might benefit from bronchodilator or other therapy. Codeine or dextromethorphan hydrobromide has no effect on cough from colds and has potential enhanced toxicity. Expectorants such as guaifenesin are not effective antitussive agents. The combination of camphor, menthol, and eucalyptus oils may relieve nocturnal cough, but studies of their effectiveness are limited.

Ineffective Treatments

Vitamin C, guaifenesin, and inhalation of warm, humidified air are no more effective than placebo for the treatment of cold symptoms.

Echinacea is a popular herbal treatment for the common cold. Although echinacea extracts have biologic effects, echinacea is not effective as a common cold treatment. The lack of standardization of commercial products containing echinacea also presents a formidable obstacle to the rational evaluation or use of this therapy.

There is no evidence that the common cold or persistent acute purulent rhinitis of less than 10 days in duration benefits from antibiotics. In fact, there is evidence that antibiotics cause significant adverse effects when given for acute purulent rhinitis.

COMPLICATIONS

The most common complication of a cold is **acute otitis media (AOM;** see Chapter 640), which may be indicated by new-onset fever and earache after the 1st few days of cold symptoms. AOM is reported in 5-30% of children who have a cold, with the higher incidence occurring in young infants and in children cared for in a group daycare setting. Symptomatic treatment has no effect on the development of AOM, but treatment with oseltamivir might reduce the incidence of AOM in patients with influenza.

Sinusitis is another complication of the common cold (see Chapter 380). Self-limited sinus inflammation is a part of the pathophysiology of the common cold, but 0.5-2% of viral upper respiratory tract infections in adults, and 5-13% in children, are complicated by acute bacterial sinusitis. The differentiation of common cold symptoms from bacterial sinusitis may be difficult. The diagnosis of bacterial sinusitis should be considered if rhinorrhea or daytime cough persists without improvement for at least 10-14 days, if symptoms worsen over time, or if signs of more severe sinus involvement such as fever, facial pain, or facial swelling develop. There is no evidence that symptomatic treatment of the common cold alters the frequency of development of bacterial sinusitis. Bacterial pneumonia is an uncommon complication of the common cold.

Exacerbation of **asthma** is a relatively uncommon but potentially serious complication of colds. The majority of asthma exacerbations in children are associated with the common cold. There is no evidence that treatment of common cold symptoms prevents this complication; however, studies are underway in patients with underlying asthma to determine effectiveness of preventive or acute treatment at the onset of upper respiratory tract infection symptoms.

Although not a complication, another important consequence of the common cold is the inappropriate use of antibiotics for these illnesses and the associated contribution to the problem of increasing antibiotic resistance of pathogenic respiratory bacteria, as well as adverse effects from antibiotics.

PREVENTION

Chemoprophylaxis or immunoprophylaxis is generally not available for the common cold. Immunization or chemoprophylaxis against influenza can prevent colds caused by this pathogen; influenza is responsible for only a small proportion of all colds. Palivizumab is recommended to prevent RSV lower respiratory infection in high-risk infants but does not prevent upper respiratory infections from this virus. Vitamin C, garlic, or echinacea do not prevent the common cold. Vitamin C prophylaxis may shorten the duration of cold symptoms. Vitamin D deficiency is associated with increased risk of viral respiratory tract infection in some studies, nonetheless, vitamin D prophylaxis does not reduce incidence or severity of the common cold in

adults; studies in children are lacking. Zinc sulfate taken for a minimum of 5 mo may reduce the rate of cold development. However, because of duration of use and adverse effects of bad taste and nausea, this is not a recommended prevention modality in children.

Hand-to-hand transmission of rhinoviruses followed by self-inoculation may be prevented by frequent hand washing and avoiding touching one's mouth, nose, and eyes. Some studies report the use of alcohol-based hand sanitizers and virucidal hand treatments were associated with decreased transmission. In the experimental setting, virucidal disinfectants or virucidal-impregnated tissues also reduce transmission of cold viruses; under natural conditions none of these interventions prevents common colds.

Bibliography is available at Expert Consult.

Chapter **380**
Sinusitis
Diane E. Pappas and J. Owen Hendley

Sinusitis is a common illness of childhood and adolescence. There are 2 types of acute sinusitis: viral and bacterial, with significant acute and chronic morbidity as well as the potential for serious complications. The common cold produces a viral, self-limited rhinosinusitis (see Chapter 379). Approximately 0.5-2% of viral upper respiratory tract infections in children and adolescents are complicated by acute symptomatic bacterial sinusitis. Some children with underlying predisposing conditions have chronic sinus disease that does not appear to be infectious. The means for appropriate diagnosis and optimal treatment of sinusitis remain controversial.

Typically the **ethmoidal** and **maxillary** sinuses are present at birth, but only the ethmoidal sinuses are pneumatized. The maxillary sinuses are not pneumatized until 4 yr of age. The **sphenoidal** sinuses are present by 5 yr of age, whereas the **frontal sinuses** begin development at age 7-8 yr and are not completely developed until adolescence. The ostia draining the sinuses are narrow (1-3 mm) and drain into the ostiomeatal complex in the middle meatus. The **paranasal sinuses** are normally sterile, maintained by the mucociliary clearance system.

ETIOLOGY

The bacterial pathogens causing acute bacterial sinusitis in children and adolescents include *Streptococcus pneumoniae* (~30%; see Chapter 182), nontypeable *Haemophilus influenzae* (~20%; see Chapter 194), and *Moraxella catarrhalis* (~20%; see Chapter 196). Approximately 50% of *H. influenzae* and 100% of *M. catarrhalis* are β-lactamase positive. Approximately 25% of *S. pneumoniae* may be penicillin resistant. *Staphylococcus aureus*, other streptococci, and anaerobes are uncommon causes of acute bacterial sinusitis in children. Although *S. aureus* (see Chapter 181.1) is an uncommon pathogen for acute sinusitis in children, the increasing prevalence of methicillin-resistant *S. aureus* is a significant concern. *H. influenzae*, α- and β-hemolytic streptococci, *M. catarrhalis*, *S. pneumoniae*, and coagulase-negative staphylococci are commonly recovered from children with **chronic sinus disease.**

EPIDEMIOLOGY

Acute bacterial sinusitis can occur at any age. Predisposing conditions include viral upper respiratory tract infections (associated with out-of-home daycare or a school-age sibling), allergic rhinitis, and cigarette smoke exposure. Children with immune deficiencies particularly of antibody production (immunoglobulin IgG, IgG subclasses, IgA; see Chapter 124), cystic fibrosis (see Chapter 403), ciliary dysfunction (see Chapter 404), abnormalities of phagocyte function, gastroesophageal reflux, anatomic defects (cleft palate), nasal polyps, cocaine abuse, and nasal foreign bodies (including nasogastric tubes) can develop chronic or recurrent sinus disease. Immunosuppression for bone marrow transplantation or malignancy with profound neutropenia and lymphopenia predisposes to severe fungal (aspergillus, mucor) sinusitis, often with intracranial extension. Patients with nasotracheal intubation or nasogastric tubes may have obstruction of the sinus ostia and develop sinusitis with the multiple-drug resistant organisms of the intensive care unit.

Acute sinusitis is defined by duration of <30 days; subacute by duration of 1-3 mo; and chronic by duration of longer than 3 mo.

PATHOGENESIS

Acute bacterial sinusitis typically follows a viral upper respiratory tract infection. Initially, the viral infection produces a viral rhinosinusitis; MRI evaluation of the paranasal sinuses demonstrates abnormalities (mucosal thickening, edema, inflammation) of the paranasal sinuses in 68% of healthy children in the normal course of the common cold. Nose blowing has been demonstrated to generate sufficient force to propel nasal secretions into the sinus cavities. Bacteria from the nasopharynx that enter the sinuses are normally cleared readily, but during viral rhinosinusitis, inflammation and edema can block sinus drainage and impair mucociliary clearance of bacteria. The growth conditions are favorable, and high titers of bacteria are produced.

CLINICAL MANIFESTATIONS

Children and adolescents with sinusitis can present with nonspecific complaints, including nasal congestion, purulent nasal discharge (unilateral or bilateral), fever, and cough. Less-common symptoms include bad breath (halitosis), a decreased sense of smell (hyposmia), and periorbital edema. Complaints of headache and facial pain are rare in children. Additional symptoms include maxillary tooth discomfort and pain or pressure exacerbated by bending forward. Physical examination might reveal erythema and swelling of the nasal mucosa with purulent nasal discharge. Sinus tenderness may be detectable in adolescents and adults. Transillumination reveals an opaque sinus that transmits light poorly.

Differentiating bacterial sinusitis from a cold may be difficult, but certain patterns suggestive of sinusitis have been identified. These include **persistence** of nasal congestion, rhinorrhea (of any quality) and daytime cough ≥10 days without improvement; **severe symptoms** of temperature ≥39°C (102°F) with purulent nasal discharge for 3 days or longer; and **worsening symptoms** either by recurrence of symptoms after an initial improvement or new symptoms of fever, nasal discharge and daytime cough.

DIAGNOSIS

The clinical diagnosis of acute bacterial sinusitis is based on history. Persistent symptoms of upper respiratory tract infection, including nasal discharge and cough, for longer than 10 days without improvement, or severe respiratory symptoms, including temperature of at least 39°C (102°F) and purulent nasal discharge for 3-4 consecutive days, suggest a complicating acute bacterial sinusitis. Bacteria are recovered from maxillary sinus aspirates in 70% of children with such persistent or severe symptoms studied. Children with chronic sinusitis have a history of persistent respiratory symptoms, including cough, nasal discharge, or nasal congestion, lasting longer than 90 days.

Sinus aspirate culture is the only accurate method of diagnosis but is not practical for routine use for immunocompetent patients. It may be a necessary procedure for immunosuppressed patients with suspected fungal sinusitis. In adults, *rigid nasal endoscopy* is a less-invasive method for obtaining culture material from the sinus but detects a great excess of positive cultures compared to aspirates. Findings on radiographic studies (sinus plain films, CT scans) including opacification, mucosal thickening, or presence of an air–fluid level are not diagnostic (Fig. 380-1) and are not recommended in otherwise healthy children. Such findings can confirm the presence of sinus inflammation but cannot be used to differentiate among viral, bacterial, or allergic causes of inflammation.

Given the nonspecific clinical picture, differential diagnostic considerations include viral upper respiratory tract infection, allergic rhinitis, nonallergic rhinitis, and nasal foreign body. Viral upper respiratory tract infections are characterized by clear and usually nonpurulent nasal discharge, cough, and initial fever; symptoms do not usually persist beyond 10-14 days, although a few children (10%) have persistent symptoms even at 14 days. Allergic rhinitis can be seasonal; evaluation of nasal secretions should reveal significant eosinophilia.

TREATMENT

It is unclear whether antimicrobial treatment of clinically diagnosed acute bacterial sinusitis offers any substantial benefit. A randomized, placebo-controlled trial comparing 14-day treatment of children with clinically diagnosed sinusitis with amoxicillin, amoxicillin-clavulanate, or placebo found that antimicrobial therapy did not affect resolution of symptoms, duration of symptoms, or days missed from school. A similar study in adults demonstrated improved symptoms at day 7 but not day 10 of treatment. Guidelines from the American Academy of Pediatrics recommend antimicrobial treatment for acute bacterial sinusitis with severe onset or a worsening course to promote resolution of symptoms and prevent suppurative complications, although 50-60% of children with acute bacterial sinusitis recover without antimicrobial therapy.

Initial therapy with amoxicillin (45 mg/kg/day divided bid) is adequate for the majority of children with uncomplicated mild to moderate severity acute bacterial sinusitis. Alternative treatments for the penicillin-allergic patient include cefdinir, cefuroxime axetil, cefpodoxime, or cefixime. In older children, levofloxacin is an alternative antibiotic. Azithromycin and trimethoprim-sulfamethoxazole are no longer indicated because of a high prevalence of antibiotic resistance. For children with risk factors (antibiotic treatment in the preceding 1-3 mo, daycare attendance, or age younger than 2 yr) for the presence of resistant bacterial species, and for children who fail to respond to initial therapy with amoxicillin within 72 hr, or with severe sinusitis, treatment with high-dose amoxicillin-clavulanate (80-90 mg/kg/day of amoxicillin) should be initiated. Ceftriaxone (50 mg/kg, IV or IM) may be given to children who are vomiting or who are at risk for poor compliance; it should be followed by a course of oral antibiotics. Failure to respond to these regimens necessitates referral to an otolaryngologist for further evaluation because maxillary sinus aspiration for culture and susceptibility testing may be necessary. The appropriate duration of therapy for sinusitis has yet to be determined; individualization of therapy is a reasonable approach, with treatment recommended for a minimum of 10 days or 7 days after resolution of symptoms (see Fig. 380-1).

Frontal sinusitis can rapidly progress to serious intracranial complications and necessitates initiation of parenteral ceftriaxone until substantial clinical improvement is achieved (Figs. 380-2 and 380-3). Treatment is then completed with oral antibiotic therapy.

The use of decongestants, antihistamines, mucolytics, and intranasal corticosteroids has not been adequately studied in children and is not recommended for the treatment of acute uncomplicated bacterial sinusitis. Likewise, saline nasal washes or nasal sprays can help to liquefy secretions and act as a mild vasoconstrictor, but the effects have not been systematically evaluated in children.

COMPLICATIONS

Because of the close proximity of the paranasal sinuses to the brain and eyes, serious orbital and/or intracranial complications can result from acute bacterial sinusitis and progress rapidly. Orbital complications, including *periorbital cellulitis* and *orbital cellulitis* (see Chapter 634) are most often secondary to acute bacterial ethmoiditis. Infection can spread directly through the lamina papyracea, the thin bone that forms the lateral wall of the ethmoidal sinus. Periorbital cellulitis produces erythema and swelling of the tissues surrounding the globe, whereas orbital cellulitis involves the intraorbital structures and produces proptosis, chemosis, decreased visual acuity, double vision and impaired extraocular movements, and eye pain (Fig. 380-4). Evaluation should include CT scan of the orbits and sinuses with ophthalmology and otolaryngology consultations. Treatment with intravenous antibiotics

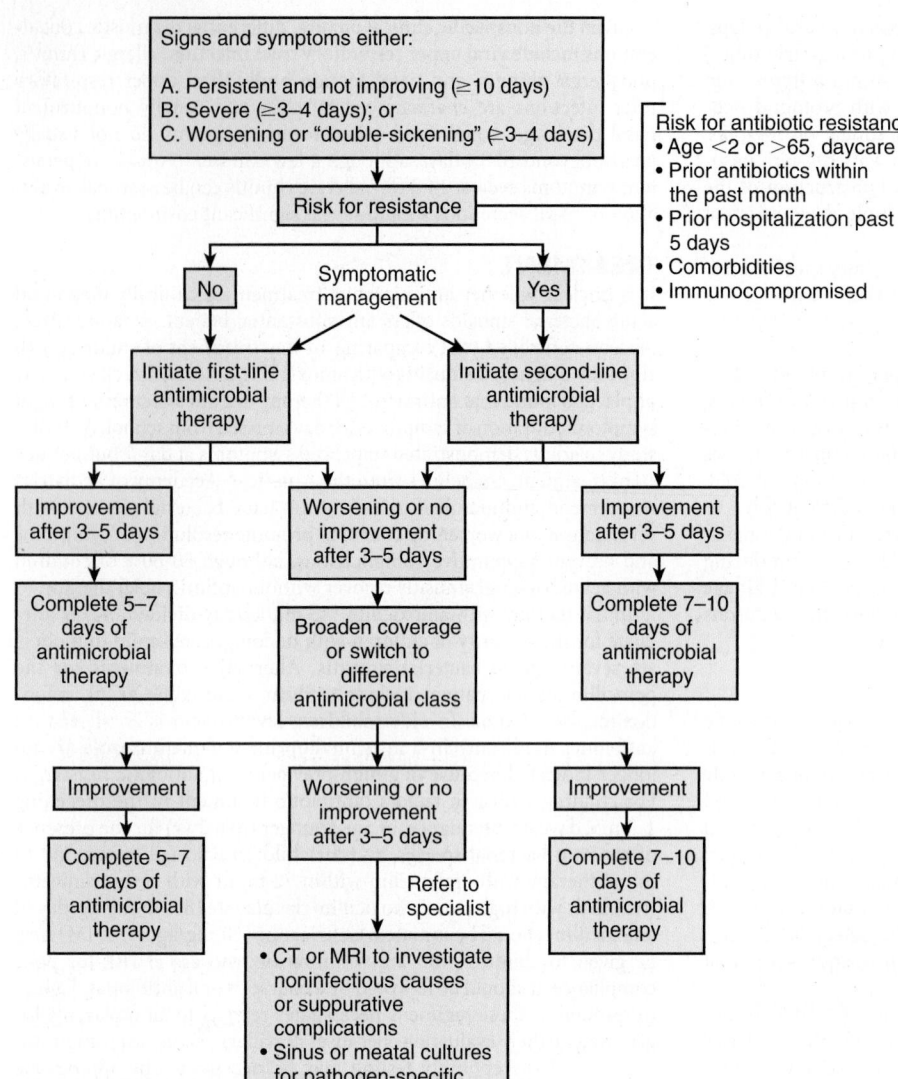

Figure 380-1 Algorithm for the management of acute bacterial rhinosinusitis. *(From Chow AW, Benninger MS, Brook I, et al: Infectious Diseases Society of America. IDSA clinical practice guideline for acute bacterial rhinosinusitis in children and adults.* Clin Infect Dis *54(8):e72–e112, 2012, Fig. 1.)*

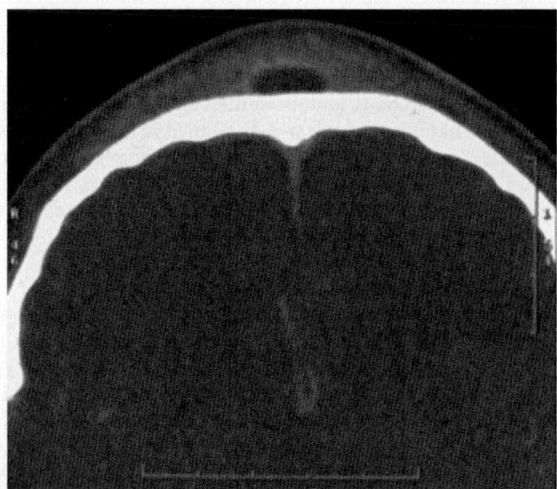

Figure 380-2 Axial plane contrast-enhanced CT scan of an 11 yr old boy with a frontal subperiosteal abscess secondary to acute frontal sinusitis. The CT scan demonstrates a ring-enhancing midline fluid density over the frontal bone. *(From Parikh SR, Brown SM: Image-guided frontal sinus surgery in children,* Operative Tech Otolaryngol Head Neck Surg *15:37–41, 2004.)*

should be initiated. Orbital cellulitis can require surgical drainage of the ethmoidal sinuses.

Intracranial complications can include epidural abscess, meningitis, cavernous sinus thrombosis, subdural empyema, and brain abscess (see Chapter 604). Children with altered mental status, nuchal rigidity, severe headache, focal neurologic findings, or signs of increased intracranial pressure (headache, vomiting) require immediate CT scan of the brain, orbits, and sinuses to evaluate for the presence of intracranial complications of acute bacterial sinusitis. Black children and males are at increased risk, but there is no evidence of increased risk due to socioeconomic status. Treatment with broad-spectrum intravenous antibiotics (usually cefotaxime or ceftriaxone combined with vancomycin) should be initiated immediately, pending culture and susceptibility results. In 50% the abscess is a polymicrobial infection. Abscesses can require surgical drainage. Other complications include osteomyelitis of the frontal bone (**Pott puffy tumor**), which is characterized by edema and swelling of the forehead (see Fig. 380-3), and **mucoceles,** which are chronic inflammatory lesions commonly located in the frontal sinuses that can expand, causing displacement of the eye with resultant diplopia. Surgical drainage is usually required.

PREVENTION

Prevention is best accomplished by frequent handwashing and avoiding persons with colds. Because acute bacterial sinusitis can complicate influenza infection, prevention of influenza infection by yearly influenza vaccine will prevent some cases of complicating sinusitis. Immunization or chemoprophylaxis against influenza with oseltamivir or zanamivir may be useful for prevention of colds caused by this pathogen and the associated complications; influenza is responsible for only a small proportion of all colds.

Bibliography is available at Expert Consult.

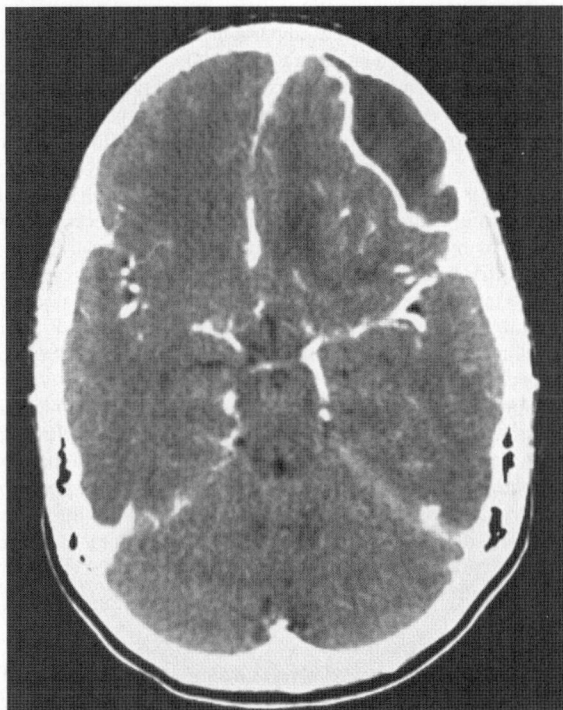

Figure 380-3 Axial plane contrast-enhanced CT scan of an 11 yr old obtunded girl with a subfrontal lobe abscess secondary to frontal sinusitis. The CT scan demonstrates an eliptiform ring-enhancing fluid-filled cavity adjacent to the frontal lobe with contralateral shift of the midline. *(From Parikh SR, Brown SM: Image-guided frontal sinus surgery in children, Operative Tech Otolaryngol Head Neck Surg 15:37–41, 2004.)*

Chapter 381
Acute Pharyngitis
Robert R. Tanz

Pharyngitis refers to inflammation of the pharynx, including erythema, edema, exudates, or an enanthem (ulcers, vesicles). Pharyngeal inflammation can be related to environmental exposures, such as tobacco smoke, air pollutants, and allergens; from contact with caustic substances, hot food, and liquids; and from infectious agents. The pharynx and mouth can be involved in various inflammatory conditions such as the periodic fever, aphthous stomatitis, pharyngitis, adenitis (PFAPA) syndrome, Kawasaki disease, inflammatory bowel disease, Stevens-Johnson syndrome, and systemic lupus erythematous. Noninfectious etiologies are typically evident from history and physical exam, but it can be more challenging to distinguish from among the numerous infectious causes of acute pharyngitis.

Acute infections of the upper respiratory tract account for a substantial number of visits to pediatricians and many feature sore throat as a symptom or evidence of pharyngitis on physical examination. The usual clinical task is to distinguish important, potentially serious, and treatable causes of acute pharyngitis from those that are self-limited and require no specific treatment or follow-up. Specifically, identifying patients who have **group A streptococcus** (GAS; *Streptococcus pyogenes;* see Chapter 183) pharyngitis and treating them with antibiotics forms the core of the management paradigm.

INFECTIOUS ETIOLOGIES
See Table 381-1.

Viruses
In North America and most industrialized countries GAS is the most important bacterial cause of acute pharyngitis, but viruses predominate as acute infectious causes of pharyngitis. Viral upper respiratory tract infections are typically spread by contact with oral or respiratory secretions and occur most commonly in fall, winter, and spring, that is, the "respiratory season." Important viruses that cause pharyngitis include influenza (see Chapter 258), parainfluenza (see Chapter 259), adenoviruses (see Chapter 262), coronaviruses (see Chapter 264), enteroviruses (see Chapter 250), rhinoviruses (see Chapter 263), respiratory

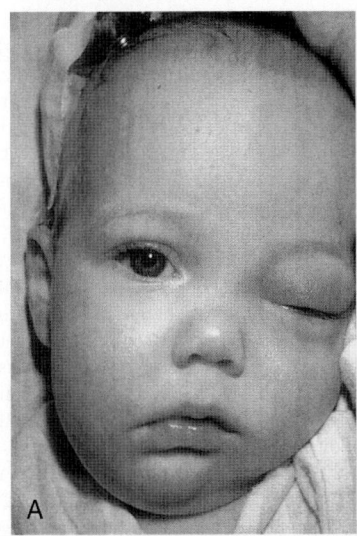
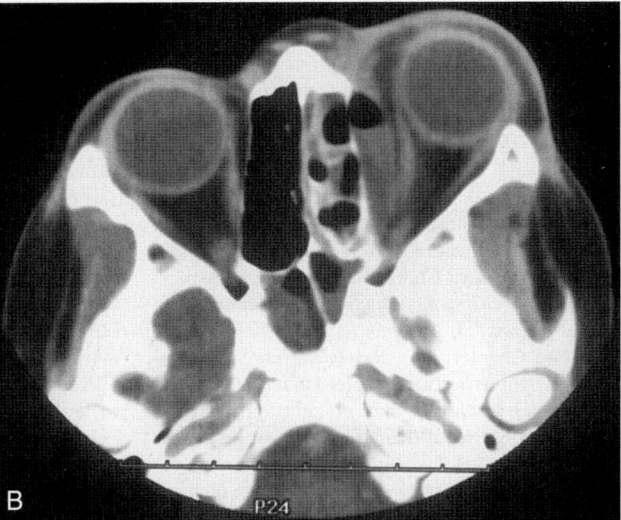

Figure 380-4 Orbital complications of acute sinusitis. **A,** An 11 mo old infant with a swollen left eye and limited ocular movement. **B,** Axial CT shows opacification of sinuses and an inflammatory mass with an air–fluid level displacing the medial rectus laterally. *(From Cooper, ML, Slovis T. The sinuses. In Slovis T, editor: Caffey's pediatric diagnostic imaging, ed 11, Philadelphia, 2008, Mosby, Fig. 43-7, p. 573.)*

Table 381-1	Infectious Agents That Cause Pharyngitis
VIRUSES	**BACTERIA**
Adenovirus	Streptococcus pyogenes
Coronavirus	(Group A streptococcus)
Cytomegalovirus	Arcanobacterium haemolyticum
Epstein-Barr virus	Fusobacterium necrophorum
Enteroviruses	Corynebacterium diphtheriae
Herpes simplex virus	Neisseria gonorrhoeae
Human immunodeficiency virus	Group C streptococci
Human metapneumovirus	Group G streptococci
Influenza viruses	Francisella tularensis
Measles virus	Chlamydophila pneumoniae
Parainfluenza viruses	Chlamydia trachomatis
Respiratory syncytial virus	Mycoplasma pneumoniae
Rhinoviruses	

syncytial virus (see Chapter 260), cytomegalovirus (see Chapter 255), Epstein-Barr virus (see Chapter 254), herpes simplex virus (see Chapter 252), and human metapneumovirus (see Chapter 261). Most viral pharyngitis, except mononucleosis, is mild. Common nonspecific symptoms such as rhinorrhea and cough develop gradually before they become prominent. However, specific findings are sometimes helpful in identifying the infectious viral agent.

Gingivostomatitis and ulcerating vesicles throughout the anterior pharynx and on the lips are seen in primary oral herpes simplex virus infection. High fever and difficulty taking oral fluids are common. This infection can last for 14 days.

Discrete **papulovesicular** lesions or **ulcerations** in the posterior oropharynx, severe throat pain, and fever are characteristic of herpangina, caused by various enteroviruses. In hand-foot-mouth disease there are vesicles or ulcers throughout the oropharynx, vesicles on the palms and soles, and sometimes on the trunk and extremities; Coxsackie A16 is the most common agent, but Enterovirus 71 and Coxsackie A6 can also cause this syndrome. Enteroviral infections are most common in the summer.

Various adenoviruses cause pharyngitis. When there is concurrent **conjunctivitis** the syndrome is called *pharyngoconjunctival fever*. The pharyngitis tends to resolve within 7 days but conjunctivitis may persist for up to 14 days. Pharyngoconjunctival fever can be epidemic or sporadic; outbreaks have been associated with exposure in swimming pools.

Intense, diffuse pharyngeal erythema and Koplik spots, the pathognomonic enanthem, occur in advance of the characteristic rash of measles. Splenomegaly or hepatomegaly may be the clue to Epstein-Barr virus infectious mononucleosis in an adolescent with exudative tonsillitis. Primary infection with HIV can manifest as the acute retroviral syndrome, with non-exudative pharyngitis, fever, maculopapular rash, arthralgia, myalgia, adenopathy, and often a maculopapular rash.

Bacteria Other Than Group A Streptococcus
In addition to GAS, bacteria that cause pharyngitis include group C and group G streptococcus (see Chapter 185), *Arcanobacterium haemolyticum*, *Francisella tularensis* (see Chapter 206), *Neisseria gonorrhoeae* (see Chapter 192), *Mycoplasma pneumoniae* (see Chapter 223), *Chlamydophila* (formerly *Chlamydia*) *pneumoniae* (see Chapter 225), *Chlamydia trachomatis* (see Chapter 226), *Fusobacterium necrophorum*, and *Corynebacterium diphtheriae* (see Chapter 187). *Haemophilus influenzae* and *Streptococcus pneumoniae* may be cultured from the throats of children with pharyngitis, but their role in causing pharyngitis has not been established.

Group C and Group G streptococcus and *A. haemolyticum* pharyngitis have been diagnosed most commonly in adolescents and adults. They resemble group A β-hemolytic streptococcus (GABHS) pharyngitis and a scarlet fever–like rash may be present with *A. haemolyticum* infections.

F. necrophorum has been suggested to be a fairly common cause of pharyngitis in older adolescents and adults (15-30 yr old). Prevalence in studies has varied from 10-48% of patients with non-GABHS pharyngitis, but large surveillance studies have not been performed. *F. necrophorum* pharyngitis is associated with development of **Lemierre syndrome**, internal jugular vein septic thrombophlebitis. Approximately 80% of cases of Lemierre syndrome are caused by this bacterium. Patients present initially with fever, sore throat, exudative pharyngitis, and/or peritonsillar abscess. The symptoms may persist, neck pain and swelling develop, and the patient appears toxic. Septic shock may ensue along with metastatic complications from septic emboli that can involve the lungs, bones and joints, central nervous system, abdominal organs, and soft tissues. The case fatality rate is 4-9%.

Gonococcal pharyngeal infections are usually asymptomatic but can cause acute pharyngitis with fever and cervical lymphadenitis. Young children with proven gonococcal disease should be evaluated for sexual abuse.

Diphtheria is extremely rare in most developed countries thanks to extensive immunization with diphtheria toxoid. However, it remains endemic in many areas of the world, including the former Soviet bloc countries, Africa, Asia, the Middle East, and Latin America. It can be considered in patients with recent travel to or from these areas and in unimmunized patients. Key physical findings are bull neck (extreme neck swelling) and a gray pharyngeal pseudomembrane that can cause respiratory obstruction.

Ingestion of water, milk, or undercooked meat contaminated by *F. tularensis* can lead to oropharyngeal tularemia. Severe throat pain, tonsillitis, cervical adenitis, oral ulcerations, and a pseudomembrane (as in diphtheria) may be present. *M. pneumoniae* and *C. pneumoniae* cause pharyngitis, but other upper and lower respiratory infections are more important and more readily recognized. Development of a severe or persistent cough subsequent to pharyngitis may be the clue to infection with one of these organisms.

Group A Streptococcus
Streptococcal pharyngitis is relatively uncommon before 2-3 yr of age, is quite common among children 5-15 yr old, and declines in frequency in late adolescence and adulthood. Illness occurs throughout the year but is most prevalent in winter and spring. It is readily spread among siblings and schoolmates. GAS causes 15-30% of pharyngitis in school-age children.

Colonization of the pharynx by GAS can result in either asymptomatic carriage or acute infection. After an incubation period of 2-5 days, pharyngeal infection with GAS classically presents as rapid onset of significant sore throat and fever. The pharynx is red, the tonsils are enlarged and often covered with a white, grayish, or yellow exudate that may be blood-tinged. There may be petechiae or "doughnut" lesions on the soft palate and posterior pharynx and the uvula may be red and swollen. The surface of the tongue can resemble a strawberry when the papillae are inflamed and prominent ("strawberry tongue"). Initially, the tongue is often side coated white, and with the swollen papillae it is called a "white strawberry tongue." When the white coating is gone after a few days, the tongue is often quite red, and is called a "red strawberry tongue." Enlarged and tender anterior cervical lymph nodes are frequently present. Headache, abdominal pain, and vomiting are frequently associated with the infection, but in the absence of clinical pharyngitis, gastrointestinal signs and symptoms should not be attributed to GAS. Ear pain is a frequent complaint but the tympanic membranes are usually normal. Diarrhea, cough, coryza, ulcerations, croup/laryngitis/hoarseness, and conjunctivitis are not associated with GAS pharyngitis and increase the likelihood of a viral etiology.

Patients infected with GAS that produce streptococcal pyrogenic exotoxin A, B, or C may demonstrate the fine red, papular ("sandpaper") rash of scarlet fever. It begins on the face and then becomes generalized. The cheeks are red and the area around the mouth is more pale, giving the appearance of circumoral pallor. The rash blanches with pressure and it may be more intense in skin creases, especially in the antecubital fossae, axillae, and inguinal creases (Pastia's lines or Pastia's sign). Pastia's lines are sometimes petechial or slightly hemorrhagic.

Capillary fragility can cause petechiae distal to a tourniquet or constriction from clothing, a positive tourniquet test or Rumpel-Leeds phenomenon. Erythema fades in a few days and when the rash resolves it typically peels like a mild sunburn. Sometimes there is sheet-like desquamation around the free margins of the finger nails. Streptococcal pyrogenic exotoxin A, encoded by the gene *spe A*, is the exotoxin most commonly associated with scarlet fever.

The M protein is an important GAS virulence factor that facilitates resistance to phagocytosis. The M protein is encoded by the *emm* gene and determines the M type (or *emm* type). Molecular methods have identified more than 200 *emm* genes (*emm* types). The M protein is immunogenic; an individual can experience multiple episodes of GAS pharyngitis in a lifetime because natural immunity is M type-specific. Numerous GAS M types can circulate in a community simultaneously and they enter and leave communities unpredictably and for unknown reasons.

DIAGNOSIS

The clinical presentations of streptococcal and viral pharyngitis often overlap. In particular, the pharyngitis of mononucleosis can be difficult to distinguish from GAS pharyngitis. Physicians relying solely on clinical judgment often overestimate the likelihood of a streptococcal etiology. Various clinical scoring systems have been described to assist in identifying patients who are likely to have GAS pharyngitis. Criteria developed for adults and modified for children by McIsaac give 1 point for each of the following criteria: history of temperature >38°C (100.4°F); absence of cough; tender anterior cervical adenopathy; tonsillar swelling or exudates; and age 3-14 yr. It subtracts a point for age ≥45 yr. At best, a McIsaac score ≥4 is associated with a positive laboratory test for GAS in less than 70% of children with pharyngitis (Table 381-2), so it, too, overestimates the likelihood of GAS. Consequently, laboratory testing is essential for accurate diagnosis. Clinical findings and/or scoring systems can best be used to assist the clinician in identifying patients in need of testing. Streptococcal antibody tests are not useful in assessing patients with acute pharyngitis.

Throat culture and **rapid antigen-detection tests** (RADTs) are the diagnostic tests for GAS available in routine clinical care. Throat culture remains the "gold standard" for diagnosing streptococcal pharyngitis. There are both false-negative cultures as a consequence of sampling errors or prior antibiotic treatment and false-positive cultures as a consequence of misidentification of other bacteria as GAS. Some laboratories prefer nucleic acid testing that is specific for GAS and no longer use culture to confirm the diagnosis. A child who is chronically colonized with GAS (streptococcal carrier) can have a positive culture if it is obtained when the child is evaluated for pharyngitis that is actually caused by a viral infection.

Streptococcal RADTs detect the group A carbohydrate of GAS. They are used by the vast majority of office-based pediatricians. All RADTs have very high specificity, generally ≥95%, so when a RADT is positive it is assumed to be accurate and throat culture is unnecessary. Because RADTs are generally less sensitive than culture, confirming a negative

rapid test with a throat culture is recommended. RADTs and throat culture exhibit spectrum bias: They are more sensitive when the pretest probability of GAS is high (signs and symptoms are typical of GAS infection) and less sensitive when the pretest probability is low. Avoidance of testing when patients have signs and symptoms more suggestive of a viral infection is recommended.

Testing for bacteria other than GAS is performed infrequently, and should be reserved for patients with persistent symptoms and symptoms suggestive of a specific non-GAS bacterial pharyngitis, for example, when there is concern for gonococcal infection or sexual abuse. Special culture media and a prolonged incubation are required to detect *A. haemolyticum*. Viral cultures are often unavailable and are generally too expensive and slow to be clinically useful. Polymerase chain reaction is more rapid and multiplex polymerase chain reaction testing for respiratory pathogens can identify a variety of viral and bacterial agents within a few hours. This may be useful in determining the isolation needs of hospitalized patients, assisting in patient prognosis, and epidemiology, but in the absence of specific treatment for most viral infections such testing is usually not necessary. A complete blood cell count showing many atypical lymphocytes and a positive mononucleosis slide agglutination test can help to confirm a clinical diagnosis of Epstein-Barr virus infectious mononucleosis.

TREATMENT

Specific therapy is unavailable for most viral pharyngitis. However, nonspecific, symptomatic therapy can be an important part of the overall treatment plan. An oral antipyretic/analgesic agent (acetaminophen or ibuprofen) can relieve fever and sore throat pain. Anesthetic sprays and lozenges (often containing benzocaine, phenol, or menthol) can provide local relief in children who are developmentally appropriate to use them. Systemic corticosteroids are sometimes used in children who have evidence of upper airway compromise due to mononucleosis. Although corticosteroids are used fairly commonly in adults with pharyngitis, large scale studies capable of providing safety and efficacy data are lacking in children. *Corticosteroids cannot be recommended for treatment of most pediatric pharyngitis.*

Antibiotic therapy of bacterial pharyngitis depends on the organism identified. On the basis of in vitro susceptibility data, oral penicillin is often suggested for patients with group C streptococcal isolates and oral erythromycin is recommended for patients with *A. haemolyticum*, but the clinical benefit of such treatment is uncertain.

Most untreated episodes of GAS pharyngitis resolve uneventfully within 5 days, but early antibiotic therapy hastens clinical recovery by 12-24 hr. The primary benefit and intent of antibiotic treatment is the prevention of acute rheumatic fever (ARF); it is highly effective when started within 9 days of onset of illness. Antibiotic therapy does not prevent acute poststreptococcal glomerulonephritis (APSGN). Antibiotic therapy should not be delayed for children with symptomatic pharyngitis and a positive GAS RADT or throat culture. Presumptive antibiotic treatment can be started when there is a clinical diagnosis of scarlet fever, a symptomatic child has a household contact with

Table 381-2	Positive Predictive Value of McIsaac Score in Children in Clinical Studies*			
SCORE	McISAAC, 2004 (N = 454)	EDMONSON, 2005 (N = 1184)	TANZ, 2009 (N = 1848)	FINE, 2012 (N = 64,789)
0	—	—	7%	17%
1	—	0.5%	19%	23%
2	20.5%	8.9%	20%	34%
3	27.5%	42.4%	29%	50%
≥4	67.8%	48.2%	49%	68%
GAS prevalence	34%	38%	30%	37%

*One point is given for each of the following criteria: history of temperature >38°C (100.4°F); absence of cough; tender anterior cervical adenopathy; tonsillar swelling or exudates; and age 3-14 yr. Note that the Centor score lacks only the age criterion. Positive predictive value refers to the proportion of patients with documented GAS by rapid antigen-detection test and/or throat culture.

Table 381-3	Recommended Treatment for Acute Streptococcal Pharyngitis

MOST PATIENTS

	WEIGHT <27 kg	WEIGHT ≥27 kg	ROUTE	DURATION
Amoxicillin	50 mg/kg once daily (maximum 1000 mg)		Oral	10 days
Penicillin V	250 mg bid	500 mg bid	Oral	10 days
Benzathine penicillin G	600,000 units	1.2 million units	IM	Once
Benzathine penicillin G + procaine penicillin G	900,000 units + 300,000 units	900,000 units + 300,000 units	IM	Once

PENICILLIN-ALLERGIC PATIENTS

	ORAL DOSE	FREQUENCY	DURATION
Cephalosporins*	Varies with agent chosen		10 days
Erythromycin			
Ethylsuccinate	40 mg/kg/day up to 1000 mg/day	bid	10 days
Estolate	20-40 mg/kg/day up to 1000 mg/day	bid	10 days
Clarithromycin	15 mg/kg/day up to 500 mg/day	bid	10 days
Azithromycin†	12 mg/kg day 1; 6 mg/kg days 2-5	qd	5 days
Clindamycin	20 mg/kg/day up to 1.8 g/day	tid	10 days

*First-generation cephalosporins are preferred; dosage and frequency vary among agents. Do not use in patients with history of immediate (anaphylactic) hypersensitivity to penicillin or other β-lactam antibiotics.
†Maximum dose is 500 mg the 1st day, 250 mg subsequent days.

documented streptococcal pharyngitis, or a history of ARF in the patient or a family member, but a diagnostic test should be performed to confirm the presence of GAS.

A variety of antimicrobial agents are effective for GAS pharyngitis (Table 381-3). Group A streptococci are universally susceptible to penicillin and all other β-lactam antibiotics. Penicillin is inexpensive, has a narrow spectrum of activity, and few adverse effects. Amoxicillin is preferred for children because of taste, availability as chewable tablets and liquid, and convenience of once-daily dosing. The duration of oral penicillin and amoxicillin therapy is 10 days. A single intramuscular dose of benzathine penicillin or a benzathine-procaine penicillin G combination is effective and ensures compliance. Follow-up testing for GAS is unnecessary after completion of therapy and is not recommended unless symptoms recur.

Patients allergic to penicillin can be treated with a 10-day course of a narrow-spectrum (first-generation) cephalosporin (cephalexin or cefadroxil) if the previous reaction to penicillin was not an immediate, type I hypersensitivity reaction. Most often, penicillin-allergic patients are treated for 10 days with erythromycin, clarithromycin, or clindamycin, or for 5 days with azithromycin.

The increased use of macrolides and related antibiotics for a variety of infections, especially the azalide, azithromycin, is associated with increased rates of resistance to these drugs among GAS in many countries. Approximately 5% of GAS in the United States and more than 10% in Canada are macrolide-resistant (macrolide resistance includes azalide resistance), but there is considerable local variation in both countries. Some macrolide-resistant GAS isolates are also resistant to clindamycin. Although not a major hindrance for treatment of pharyngitis, clindamycin resistance may be important in management of invasive GAS infections. Use of these antibiotics should be restricted to patients who cannot safely receive a β–lactam drug for GAS pharyngitis. Tetracyclines, fluoroquinolones, or sulfonamides should *not* be used to treat GAS pharyngitis.

CHRONIC GROUP A STREPTOCOCCUS CARRIERS

Patients who continue to harbor GAS in the pharynx despite appropriate antibiotic therapy are streptococcal carriers. They have little or no evidence of an immune response to the organism. The pathogenesis of chronic carriage is not known. Carriage generally poses little risk to patients and their contacts, but it can confound testing in subsequent

episodes of sore throat. Patients with repeated test-positive pharyngitis create anxiety among their families and physicians. It is usually unnecessary to attempt to eliminate chronic carriage. Instead, evaluation and treatment of pharyngitis should be undertaken without regard for chronic carriage, treating test-positive patients in routine fashion and avoiding antibiotics in patients who have negative tests. Expert opinion suggests that eradication might be attempted in select circumstances: a community outbreak of ARF or APSGN; personal or family history of ARF; an outbreak of GAS pharyngitis in a closed or semiclosed community, nursing home or healthcare facility; repeated episodes of symptomatic GAS pharyngitis in a family with "ping pong" spread among family members despite adequate therapy; when tonsillectomy is being considered because of chronic carriage or recurrent streptococcal pharyngitis; and extreme, unmanageable anxiety related to GAS carriage ("streptophobia") among family members. Clindamycin given by mouth for 10 days is effective therapy (20 mg/kg/day divided in 3 doses; adult dose 150-450 mg tid). Amoxicillin-clavulanate (40 mg amoxicillin/kg/day up to 2000 mg amoxicillin/day divided tid for 10 days) and 4 days of oral rifampin plus either intramuscular benzathine penicillin given once or oral penicillin given for 10 days have also been used.

RECURRENT PHARYNGITIS

True recurrent GAS pharyngitis can occur for several reasons: reinfection with the same M type if type-specific antibody has not developed; poor compliance with oral antibiotic therapy; macrolide resistance if a macrolide was used for treatment; and infection with a new M type. Unfortunately, determining the GAS M type in an acute infection is not available to the clinician. Treatment with intramuscular benzathine penicillin eliminates nonadherence to therapy. Apparent recurrences can represent pharyngitis of another cause in the presence of streptococcal carriage. Chronic GAS carriage is particularly likely if the illnesses are mild and otherwise atypical for GAS pharyngitis. *Undocumented histories of recurrent pharyngitis are an inadequate basis for recommending tonsillectomy.*

Tonsillectomy may lower the incidence of pharyngitis for 1-2 yr among children with frequent episodes of documented pharyngitis (≥7 episodes in the previous year or ≥5 in each of the preceding 2 yr, or ≥3 in each of the previous 3 yr). However, the frequency of pharyngitis (GAS and non-GAS) generally declines over time. By 2 yr posttonsillectomy the incidence of pharyngitis in severely affected children is similar among those who have tonsillectomy and those who do not. Few children are so severely affected and the limited clinical benefit of tonsillectomy for most must be balanced against the risks of anesthesia and surgery.

Recurrent GAS pharyngitis is rarely, if ever, a sign of an immune disorder. However, recurrent pharyngitis can be part of a recurrent fever or autoinflammatory syndrome such as PFAPA syndrome. Prolonged pharyngitis (>1 wk) can occur in infectious mononucleosis and Lemierre syndrome, but it also suggests the possibility of another disorder such as neutropenia, a recurrent fever syndrome, or an autoimmune disease such as systemic lupus or inflammatory bowel disease. In such instances, pharyngitis would be one of a number of clinical findings that together should suggest the underlying diagnosis.

COMPLICATIONS AND PROGNOSIS

Viral respiratory tract infections can predispose to bacterial middle ear infections and bacterial sinusitis. The complications of GAS pharyngitis include local suppurative complications, such as parapharyngeal abscess, and subsequent nonsuppurative illnesses, such as ARF, APSGN, poststreptococcal reactive arthritis, and possibly PANDAS (pediatric autoimmune neuropsychiatric disorders associated with *S. pyogenes*) or CANS (childhood acute neuropsychiatric symptoms).

PREVENTION

A variety of GAS vaccines are being developed. A recombinant multivalent M-type vaccine uses the terminal portions of various M proteins to take advantage of their immunogenicity. Other vaccines are based on more conserved GAS epitopes in order to avoid the necessity of matching the vaccine with the M types prevalent in a community or target population. None of the investigational GAS vaccines are near licensing for use. Antimicrobial prophylaxis with daily oral penicillin prevents recurrent GAS infections but is recommended only to prevent recurrences of ARF.

Bibliography is available at Expert Consult.

Chapter **382**

Retropharyngeal Abscess, Lateral Pharyngeal (Parapharyngeal) Abscess, and Peritonsillar Cellulitis/Abscess

Diane E. Pappas and J. Owen Hendley

The *retropharyngeal* and the *lateral pharyngeal lymph nodes* that drain the mucosal surfaces of the upper airway and digestive tracts are located in the neck within the *retropharyngeal space* (located between the pharynx and the cervical vertebrae and extending down into the superior mediastinum) and the *lateral pharyngeal space* (bounded by the pharynx medially, the carotid sheath posteriorly, and the muscles of the styloid process laterally). The lymph nodes in these deep neck spaces communicate with each other, allowing bacteria from either cellulitis or node abscess to spread to other nodes. Infection of the nodes usually occurs as a result of extension from a localized infection

of the oropharynx. A **retropharyngeal abscess** can also result from penetrating trauma to the oropharynx, dental infection, and vertebral osteomyelitis. Once infected, the nodes may progress through 3 stages: *cellulitis, phlegmon,* and *abscess.* Infection in the retropharyngeal and lateral pharyngeal spaces can result in airway compromise or posterior mediastinitis, making timely diagnosis important.

RETROPHARYNGEAL AND LATERAL PHARYNGEAL ABSCESS

Retropharyngeal abscess occurs most commonly in children younger than 3-4 yr of age; as the retropharyngeal nodes involute after 5 yr of age, infection in older children and adults is much less common.

Boys are affected more often than girls and approximately two-thirds of patients have a history of recent ear, nose, or throat infection.

Clinical manifestations of retropharyngeal abscess are nonspecific and include fever, irritability, decreased oral intake, and drooling. Neck stiffness, torticollis, and refusal to move the neck may also be present. The verbal child might complain of sore throat and neck pain. Other signs can include muffled voice, stridor, respiratory distress, or even obstructive sleep apnea. Physical examination can reveal bulging of the posterior pharyngeal wall, although this is present in <50% of infants with retropharyngeal abscess. Cervical lymphadenopathy may also be present. Lateral pharyngeal abscess commonly presents as fever, dysphagia, and a prominent bulge of the lateral pharyngeal wall, sometimes with medial displacement of the tonsil.

The differential diagnosis includes acute epiglottitis and foreign body aspiration. In the young child with limited neck mobility, meningitis must also be considered. Other possibilities include lymphoma, hematoma, and vertebral osteomyelitis.

Incision and drainage and culture of an abscessed node provides the definitive diagnosis, but CT can be useful in identifying the presence of a retropharyngeal, lateral pharyngeal, or parapharyngeal abscess (Figs. 382-1 and 382-2). With CT scans, deep neck infections can be accurately identified and localized, but CT accurately identifies abscess formation in only 63% of patients. Soft-tissue neck films taken during inspiration with the neck extended might show increased width or an air–fluid level in the retropharyngeal space. CT with contrast medium enhancement can reveal central lucency, ring enhancement, or scalloping of the walls of a lymph node. Scalloping of the abscess wall is thought to be a late finding and predicts abscess formation.

Retropharyngeal and lateral pharyngeal infections are most often polymicrobial; the usual pathogens include group A streptococcus (see Chapter 183), oropharyngeal anaerobic bacteria (see Chapter 213), and *Staphylococcus aureus* (see Chapter 181.1). In children younger than age 2 yr, there has been an increase in the incidence of retropharyngeal abscess, particularly with *S. aureus,* including methicillin-resistant strains. Mediastinitis may be identified on CT in some of these patients. Other pathogens can include *Haemophilus influenzae, Klebsiella,* and *Mycobacterium avium-intracellulare.*

Treatment options include intravenous antibiotics with or without surgical drainage. A third-generation cephalosporin combined with ampicillin-sulbactam or clindamycin to provide anaerobic coverage is effective. The increasing prevalence of methicillin-resistant *S. aureus* can influence empiric antibiotic therapy. Studies show that >50% of children with retropharyngeal or lateral pharyngeal abscess as identified by CT can be successfully treated without surgical drainage. Drainage is necessary in the patient with respiratory distress or failure to improve with intravenous antibiotic treatment. The optimal duration of treatment is unknown, but therapy for several days with intravenous antibiotics until the patient has begun to improve followed by a course of oral antibiotic is typically used.

Complications of retropharyngeal or lateral pharyngeal abscess include significant upper airway obstruction, rupture leading to aspiration pneumonia, and extension to the mediastinum. Thrombophlebitis of the internal jugular vein and erosion of the carotid artery sheath can also occur.

An uncommon but characteristic infection of the parapharyngeal space is **Lemierre disease,** in which infection from the oropharynx extends to cause septic thrombophlebitis of the internal jugular vein

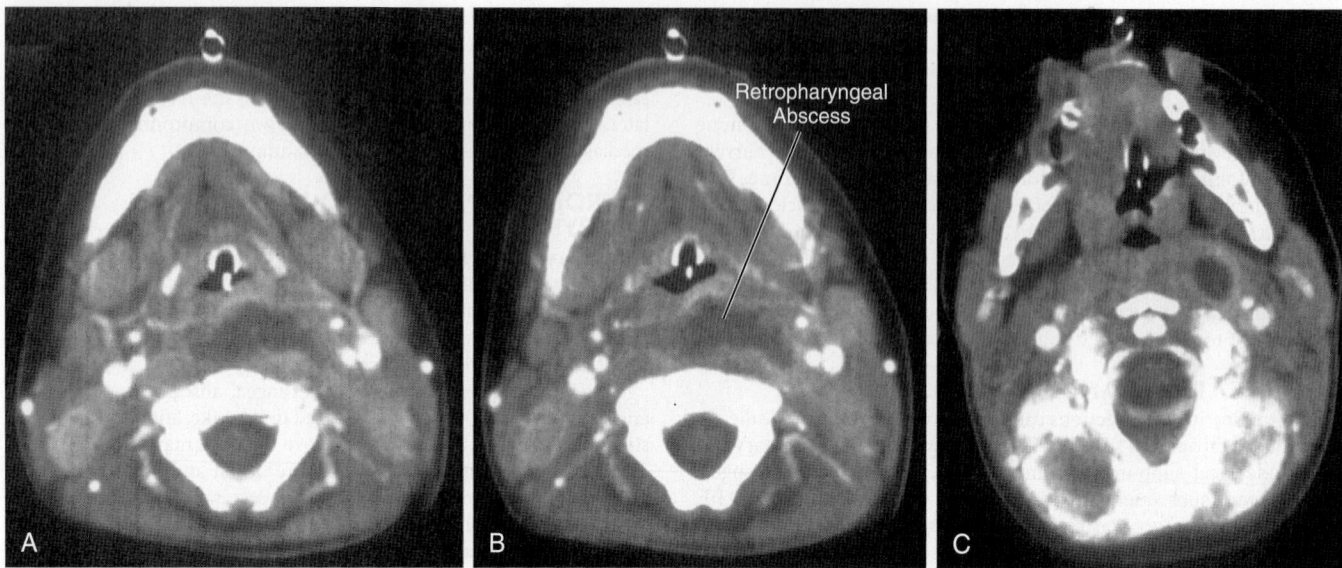

Figure 382-1 CT of retropharyngeal abscess. **A,** CT image at level of epiglottis. **B,** Sequential CT slice exhibiting ring-enhancing lesion. **C,** Further sequential CT slice demonstrating inferior extent of lesion. *(From Philpott CM, Selvadurai D, Banerjee AR: Paediatric retropharyngeal abscess,* J Laryngol Otol *118:925, 2004.)*

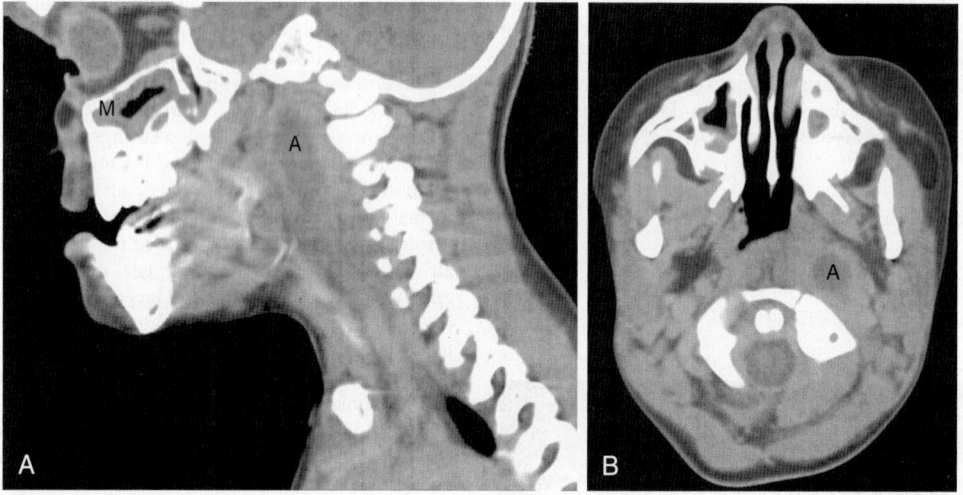

Figure 382-2 CT of parapharyngeal abscess in a 3 yr old child. **A,** Sagittal section demonstrating parapharyngeal abscess *(A)* and mucosal swelling *(M)* in the maxillary sinus. **B,** Coronal section of parapharyngeal abscess *(A).*

and embolic abscesses in the lungs (Fig. 382-3). The causative pathogen is *Fusobacterium necrophorum,* an anaerobic bacterial constituent of the oropharyngeal flora. The typical presentation is that of a previously healthy adolescent or young adult with a history of recent pharyngitis who becomes acutely ill with fever, hypoxia, tachypnea, and respiratory distress. Chest radiography demonstrates multiple cavitary nodules, often bilateral and often accompanied by pleural effusion. Blood culture may be positive. Treatment involves prolonged intravenous antibiotic therapy with penicillin or cefoxitin; surgical drainage of extrapulmonary metastatic abscesses may be necessary (see Chapters 381 and 383).

PERITONSILLAR CELLULITIS AND/OR ABSCESS

Peritonsillar cellulitis and/or abscess, which is relatively common compared to the deep neck infections, is caused by bacterial invasion through the capsule of the tonsil, leading to cellulitis and/or abscess formation in the surrounding tissues. The typical patient with a peritonsillar abscess is an adolescent with a recent history of acute pharyngotonsillitis. Clinical manifestations include sore throat, fever, trismus, and dysphagia. Physical examination reveals an asymmetric tonsillar bulge with displacement of the uvula. An asymmetric tonsillar bulge is diagnostic, but it may be poorly visualized because of trismus. CT is helpful for revealing the abscess. Group A streptococci and mixed oropharyngeal anaerobes are the most common pathogens, with more than 4 bacterial isolates per abscess typically recovered by needle aspiration.

Treatment includes surgical drainage and antibiotic therapy effective against group A streptococci and anaerobes. Surgical drainage may be accomplished through needle aspiration, incision and drainage, or tonsillectomy. Needle aspiration can involve aspiration of the superior, middle, and inferior aspects of the tonsil to locate the abscess. Intraoral ultrasound can be used to diagnose and guide needle aspiration of a peritonsillar abscess. General anesthesia may be required for the uncooperative patient. Approximately 95% of peritonsillar abscesses resolve after needle aspiration and antibiotic therapy. A small percentage of these patients require a repeat needle aspiration. The 5% with infections that fail to resolve after needle aspiration require incision and drainage. Tonsillectomy should be considered if there is failure to improve within 24 hr of antibiotic therapy and needle aspiration,

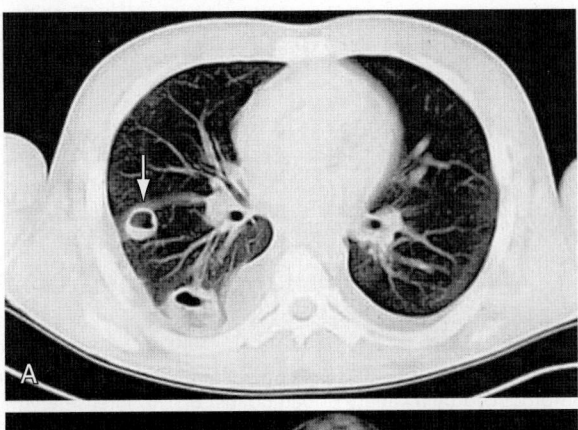

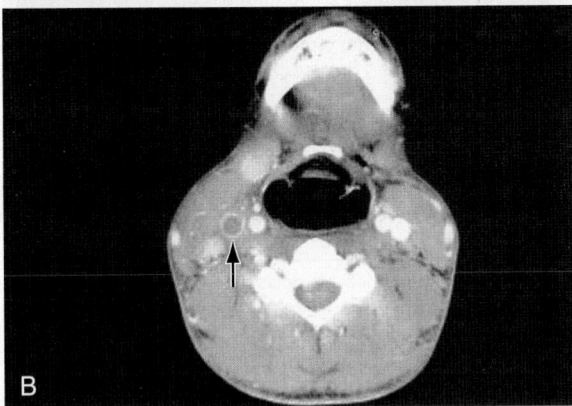

Figure 382-3 CT of Lemierre disease. **A,** CT demonstrating nodular appearance of pulmonary infiltrates *(arrow)*. **B,** CT of neck demonstrating thrombosis of right internal jugular vein *(arrow)*. *(From Plymyer MR, Zoccola DC, Tallarita G: An 18 year old man presenting with sepsis following a recent pharyngeal infection, Arch Pathol Lab Med 128:813, 2004. Reprinted with permission from Archives of Pathology & Laboratory Medicine. Copyright 2004. College of American Pathologists.)*

history of recurrent peritonsillar abscess or recurrent tonsillitis, or complications from peritonsillar abscess. The feared, albeit rare, complication is rupture of the abscess, with resultant aspiration pneumonitis. There is a 10% recurrence risk for peritonsillar abscess.

Bibliography is available at Expert Consult.

Chapter 383
Tonsils and Adenoids
Ralph F. Wetmore

ANATOMY
The *Waldeyer ring* (the lymphoid tissue surrounding the opening of the oral and nasal cavities into the pharynx) comprises the palatine tonsils, the pharyngeal tonsil or adenoid, lymphoid tissue surrounding the eustachian tube orifice in the lateral walls of the nasopharynx, the lingual tonsil at the base of the tongue, and scattered lymphoid tissue throughout the remainder of the pharynx, particularly behind the posterior pharyngeal pillars and along the posterior pharyngeal wall. The *palatine tonsil* consists of lymphoid tissue located between the

palatoglossal fold (anterior tonsillar pillar) and the palatopharyngeal fold (posterior tonsillar pillar) forms. This lymphoid tissue is separated from the surrounding pharyngeal musculature by a thick fibrous capsule. The *adenoid* is a single aggregation of lymphoid tissue that occupies the space between the nasal septum and the posterior pharyngeal wall. A thin fibrous capsule separates it from the underlying structures; the adenoid does not contain the complex crypts that are found in the palatine tonsils but rather more simple crypts. Lymphoid tissue at the base of the tongue forms the *lingual tonsil* that also contains simple tonsillar crypts.

NORMAL FUNCTION
Located at the opening of the pharynx to the external environment, the tonsils and adenoid are well situated to provide primary defense against foreign matter. The immunologic role of the tonsils and adenoids is to induce secretory immunity and to regulate the production of the secretory immunoglobulins. Deep crevices within tonsillar tissue form tonsillar crypts that are lined with squamous epithelium and host a concentration of lymphocytes at their bases. The lymphoid tissue of the Waldeyer ring is most immunologically active between 4 and 10 yr of age, with a decrease after puberty. Adenotonsillar hypertrophy is greatest between ages 3 and 6 yr; in most children tonsils begin to involute after age 8 yr. No major immunologic deficiency has been demonstrated after removal of either or both of the tonsils and adenoid.

PATHOLOGY
Acute Infection
Most episodes of acute pharyngotonsillitis are caused by viruses (see Chapter 381). Group A β-hemolytic streptococcus (GABHS) is the most common cause of bacterial infection in the pharynx (see Chapter 183).

Chronic Infection
The tonsils and adenoids can be chronically infected by multiple microbes, which can include a high incidence of β-lactamase–producing organisms. Both aerobic species, such as streptococci and *Haemophilus influenzae,* and anaerobic species, such as *Peptostreptococcus, Prevotella,* and *Fusobacterium,* contribute. The tonsillar crypts can accumulate desquamated epithelial cells, lymphocytes, bacteria, and other debris, causing cryptic tonsillitis. With time, these cryptic plugs can calcify into tonsillar concretions or tonsillolith. Biofilms appear to play a role in chronic inflammation of the tonsils.

Airway Obstruction
Both the tonsils and adenoids are a major cause of upper airway obstruction in children. Airway obstruction in children is typically manifested in sleep-disordered breathing, including obstructive sleep apnea, obstructive sleep hypopnea, and upper airway resistance syndrome (see Chapter 19). Sleep-disordered breathing secondary to adenotonsillar breathing is a cause of growth failure (see Chapter 41).

Tonsillar Neoplasm
Rapid enlargement of one tonsil is highly suggestive of a tonsillar malignancy, typically lymphoma in children.

CLINICAL MANIFESTATIONS
Acute Infection
Symptoms of GABHS infection include odynophagia, dry throat, malaise, fever and chills, dysphagia, referred otalgia, headache, muscular aches, and enlarged cervical nodes. Signs include dry tongue, erythematous enlarged tonsils, tonsillar or pharyngeal exudate, palatine petechiae, and enlargement and tenderness of the jugulodigastric lymph nodes (Fig. 383-1; see Chapters 183 and 381).

Chronic Infection
Children with chronic or cryptic tonsillitis often present with halitosis, chronic sore throats, foreign-body sensation, or a history of expelling foul-tasting and foul-smelling cheesy lumps. Examination reveals

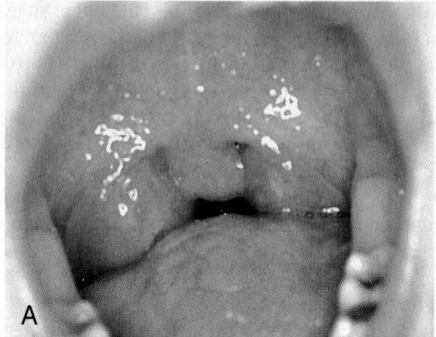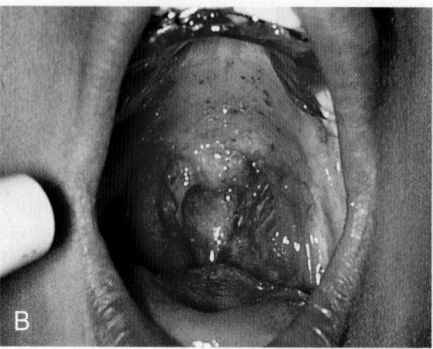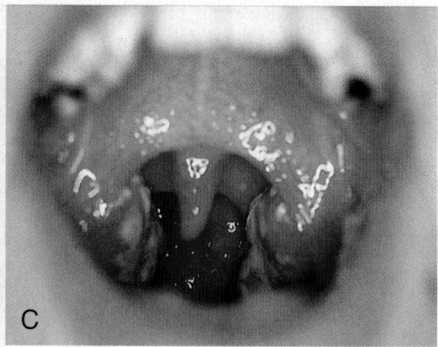

Figure 383-1 Pharyngotonsillitis. This common syndrome has a number of causative pathogens and a wide spectrum of severity. **A,** The diffuse tonsillar and pharyngeal erythema seen here is a nonspecific finding that can be produced by a variety of pathogens. **B,** This intense erythema, seen in association with acute tonsillar enlargement and palatal petechiae, is highly suggestive of group A β-streptococcal infection, though other pathogens can produce these findings. **C,** This picture of exudative tonsillitis is most commonly seen with either group A streptococcal or Epstein-Barr virus infection. (*B courtesy of Michael Sherlock, MD, Lutherville, MD. From Yellon RF, McBride TP, Davis HW: Otolaryngology. In Zitelli BJ, Davis HW, editors: Atlas of pediatric physical diagnosis, ed 4, Philadelphia, 2002, Mosby, p. 852.*)

tonsils of a range of sizes which often they contain copious debris within the crypts. The offending organism is not usually GABHS.

Airway Obstruction

The diagnosis of airway obstruction (see Chapter 19) can frequently be made by history and physical examination. Daytime symptoms of airway obstruction, secondary to adenotonsillar hypertrophy, include chronic mouth breathing, nasal obstruction, hyponasal speech, hyposmia, decreased appetite, poor school performance, and, rarely, symptoms of right-sided heart failure. Nighttime symptoms consist of loud snoring, choking, gasping, frank apnea, restless sleep, abnormal sleep positions, somnambulism, night terrors, diaphoresis, enuresis, and sleep talking. Large tonsils are typically seen on examination, although the absolute size might not indicate the degree of obstruction. The size of the adenoid tissue can be demonstrated on a lateral neck radiograph or with flexible endoscopy. Other signs that can contribute to airway obstruction include the presence of a craniofacial syndrome or hypotonia.

Tonsillar Neoplasm

The rapid unilateral enlargement of a tonsil, especially if accompanied by systemic signs of night sweats, fever, weight loss, and lymphadenopathy, is highly suggestive of a tonsillar malignancy. The diagnosis of a tonsillar malignancy should also be entertained if the tonsil appears grossly abnormal. Among 54,901 patients undergoing tonsillectomy, 54 malignancies were identified (0.087% prevalence); all but 6 malignancies had been suspected based on suspicious anatomic features preoperatively.

TREATMENT
Medical Management

The treatment of acute pharyngotonsillitis is discussed in Chapter 381 and antibiotic treatment of GABHS in Chapter 183. Because copathogens such as staphylococci or anaerobes can produce β-lactamase that can inactivate penicillin, the use of cephalosporins or clindamycin may be more efficacious in the treatment of chronic throat infections. Tonsillolith or debris may be expressed manually with either a cotton-tipped applicator or a water jet. Chronically infected tonsillar crypts can be cauterized using silver nitrate.

Tonsillectomy

Tonsillectomy alone is most commonly performed for recurrent or chronic pharyngotonsillitis. Tonsillectomy has been shown to be effective in reducing the number of infections and the symptoms of chronic tonsillitis such as halitosis, persistent or recurrent sore throats, and recurrent cervical adenitis. In resistant cases of cryptic tonsillitis, tonsillectomy may be curative. Rarely in children, tonsillectomy is indicated for biopsy of a unilaterally enlarged tonsil to exclude a neoplasm

Table 383-1	Paradise Criteria for Tonsillectomy
CRITERION	**DEFINITION**
Minimum frequency of sore throat episodes	At least 7 episodes in the previous year, at least 5 episodes in each of the previous 2 yr, or at least 3 episodes in each of the previous 3 yr
Clinical features	Sore throat plus at least 1 of the following features qualifies as a counting episode: Temperature of greater than 38.3°C (100.9°F) Cervical adenopathy (tender lymph nodes or lymph node size >2 cm) Tonsillar exudate Culture positive for group A β-hemolytic streptococcus
Treatment	Antibiotics administered in the conventional dosage for proved or suspected streptococcal episodes
Documentation	Each episode of throat infection and its qualifying features substantiated by contemporaneous notation in a medical record. If the episodes are not fully documented, subsequent observance by the physician of 2 episodes of throat infection with patterns of frequency and clinical features consistent with the initial history*

*Allows for tonsillectomy in patients who meet all but the documentation criterion. A 12 mo observation period is usually recommended before consideration of tonsillectomy.

Adapted from Baugh RF, Archer SM, Mitchell RB, et al: American Academy of Otolaryngology–Head and Neck Surgery Foundation. Clinical practice guideline: tonsillectomy in children. Otolaryngol Head Neck Surg 144(1 Suppl):S8, 2011, Table 5.

or to treat recurrent hemorrhage from superficial tonsillar blood vessels. Tonsillectomy has not been shown to offer clinical benefit over conservative treatment in children with mild symptoms.

There are large variations in surgical rates among children across countries: 144 in 10,000 in Italy; 115 in 10,000 in the Netherlands; 65 in 10,000 in England; and 50 in 10,000 in the United States. Rates are generally higher in boys. With the issuance of practice guidelines, these variations may decrease. The American Academy of Otolaryngology (AAO)–Head and Neck Surgery *Taskforce on Clinical Practice Guidelines: Tonsillectomy in Children* issued evidence-based guidelines in 2011 (Table 383-1). Table 383-2 illustrates the differences and

Table 383-2	Comparison of American, Italian, and Scottish Guidelines for Tonsillectomy in Children and Adolescents		
PARAMETER	**AAO-HNS GUIDELINES**	**ITALIAN GUIDELINES**	**SCOTTISH GUIDELINES**
Audience	Multidisciplinary	Multidisciplinary	Multidisciplinary
Target population	Children and adolescents 1-18 yr of age	Children and adults	Children 4-16 yr of age and adults
Scope	Treatment of children who are candidates for tonsillectomy	Appropriateness and safety of tonsillectomy	Management of sore throat and indications for tonsillectomy
Methods	Based on a priori protocol, systematic literature review, American Academy of Pediatrics scale of evidence quality	Systematic literature review, Italian National Program Guidelines scale of evidence quality	Based on a priori protocol, systematic literature review, Scottish Intercollegiate Guidelines Network scale of evidence quality
Recommendations			
Recurrent infection	Tonsillectomy is an option for children with recurrent throat infection that meets the Paradise criteria (see Table 383-1) for frequency, severity, treatment, and documentation of illness	Tonsillectomy is indicated in patients with at least 1 yr of recurrent tonsillitis (5 or more episodes per year) that is disabling and impairs normal activities, but only after an additional 6 mo of watchful waiting to assess the pattern of symptoms using a clinical diary	Tonsillectomy should be considered for recurrent, disabling sore throat caused by acute tonsillitis when the episodes are well documented, are adequately treated, and meet the Paradise criteria (see Table 383-1) for frequency of illness
Pain control	Recommendation to advocate for pain relief (e.g., provide information, prescribe) and educate caregivers about the importance of managing and reassessing pain	Recommendation for acetaminophen before and after surgery	Recommendation for adequate dose of acetaminophen for pain relief in children
Antibiotic use	Recommendation against perioperative antibiotics	Recommendation for short-term perioperative antibiotics*	NA
Steroid use	Recommendation for a single intraoperative dose of dexamethasone	Recommendation for a single intraoperative dose of dexamethasone	Recommendation for a single intraoperative dose of dexamethasone
Sleep-disordered breathing	Recommendation to counsel caregivers about tonsillectomy as a means to improve health in children with sleep-disordered breathing and comorbid conditions	Recommendation for diagnostic testing in children with suspected sleep respiratory disorders	NA
Polysomnography	Recommendation to counsel caregivers about tonsillectomy as a means to improve health in children with abnormal polysomnography	Recommendation for polysomnography when pulse oximetry results are not conclusive in agreement with Brouillette criteria	NA
Surgical technique	NA	Recommendation for "cold" technique	NA
Hemorrhage	Recommendation that the surgeon document primary and secondary hemorrhage after tonsillectomy at least annually	NA	NA
Adjunctive therapy	NA	NA	Recommendation against *Echinacea purpurea* for treatment of sore throat Recommendation for acupuncture in patients at risk of postoperative nausea and vomiting who cannot take antiemetic drugs

*Statement made prior to most recent Cochrane review.
  AAO-HNS, American Academy of Otolaryngology–Head and Neck Surgery; NA, not applicable.
  Adapted with permission from Baugh RF, Archer SM, Mitchell RB, et al: American Academy of Otolaryngology–Head and Neck Surgery Foundation. Clinical practice guideline: tonsillectomy in children. Otolaryngol Head Neck Surg 144(1 Suppl):S23, 2011, Table 9.

similarities between these guidelines with those of the other major professional groups across the globe.

Adenoidectomy

Adenoidectomy alone may be indicated for the treatment of chronic nasal infection (chronic adenoiditis), chronic sinus infections that have failed medical management, and recurrent bouts of acute otitis media, including those in children with tympanostomy tubes who suffer from recurrent otorrhea. Adenoidectomy may be helpful in children with chronic or recurrent otitis media with effusion. Adenoidectomy alone may be curative in the management of patients with nasal obstruction, chronic mouth breathing, and loud snoring suggesting sleep-disordered breathing. Adenoidectomy may also be indicated for children in whom upper airway obstruction is suspected of causing craniofacial or occlusive developmental abnormalities.

Tonsillectomy and Adenoidectomy

The criteria for both tonsillectomy and adenoidectomy for recurrent infection are the same as those for tonsillectomy alone. The other major indication for performing both procedures together is upper airway obstruction secondary to adenotonsillar hypertrophy that results in sleep-disordered breathing, failure to thrive, craniofacial or occlusive developmental abnormalities, speech abnormalities, or, rarely, cor pulmonale. A high proportion of children with failure to thrive in the context of adenotonsillar hypertrophy resulting in sleep disorder experiences significant growth acceleration after adenotonsillectomy.

COMPLICATIONS
Poststreptococcal Glomerulonephritis and Acute Rheumatic Fever

The 2 major complications of untreated GABHS infection are poststreptococcal glomerulonephritis and acute rheumatic fever (see Chapters 511.1 and 183).

Peritonsillar Infection

Peritonsillar infection can occur as either cellulitis or a frank abscess in the region superior and lateral to the tonsillar capsule (see Chapter 381). These infections usually occur in children with a history of recurrent tonsillar infection and are polymicrobial, including both aerobes and anaerobes. Unilateral throat pain, referred otalgia, drooling, and trismus are presenting symptoms. The affected tonsil is displaced down and medial by swelling of the anterior tonsillar pillar and palate. The diagnosis of an abscess can be confirmed by CT or by needle aspiration, the contents of which should be sent for culture.

Retropharyngeal Space Infection

Infections in the retropharyngeal space develop in the lymph nodes that drain the oropharynx, nose, and nasopharynx (see Chapter 382).

Parapharyngeal Space Infection

Tonsillar infection can extend into the parapharyngeal space, causing symptoms of fever, neck pain and stiffness, and signs of swelling of the lateral pharyngeal wall and neck on the affected side. The diagnosis is confirmed by contrast medium–enhanced CT, and treatment includes intravenous antibiotics and external incision and drainage if an abscess is demonstrated on CT (see Chapter 382). Septic thrombophlebitis of the jugular vein, **Lemierre syndrome,** manifests with fever, toxicity, neck pain and stiffness, and respiratory distress as a result of multiple septic pulmonary emboli and is a complication of a parapharyngeal space or odontogenic infection from *Fusobacterium necrophorum.* Concurrent Epstein-Barr virus mononucleosis (see Chapter 254) can be a predisposing event before the sudden onset of fever, chills, and respiratory distress in an adolescent patient. Treatment includes high-dose intravenous antibiotics (ampicillin-sulbactam, clindamycin, penicillin, or ciprofloxacin) and heparinization.

Recurrent or Chronic Pharyngotonsillitis

See Chapter 381.

CHRONIC AIRWAY OBSTRUCTION

Although rare, children with chronic airway obstruction from enlarged tonsils and adenoids can present with cor pulmonale.

The effects of chronic airway obstruction and mouth breathing on facial growth remain a subject of controversy. Studies of chronic mouth breathing, both in humans and animals, have shown changes in facial development, including prolongation of the total anterior facial height and a tendency toward a retrognathic mandible, the so-called adenoid facies. Adenotonsillectomy can reverse some of these abnormalities. Other studies have disputed these findings.

Tonsillectomy and Adenoidectomy

The risks and potential benefits of surgery must be considered (Table 383-3). Bleeding can occur in the immediate postoperative period or

Table 383-3	Risks and Potential Benefits of Tonsillectomy or Adenoidectomy or Both

RISKS
Cost*
Risk of anesthetic accidents
  Malignant hyperthermia
  Cardiac arrhythmia
  Vocal cord trauma
  Aspiration with resulting bronchopulmonary obstruction or infection
Risk of miscellaneous surgical or postoperative complications
  Hemorrhage
  Airway obstruction from edema of tongue, palate, or nasopharynx, or retropharyngeal hematoma
  Central apnea
  Prolonged muscular paralysis
  Dehydration
  Palatopharyngeal insufficiency
  Otitis media
  Nasopharyngeal stenosis
  Refractory torticollis
  Facial edema
  Emotional upset
Unknown risks

POTENTIAL BENEFITS
Reduction in frequency of ear, nose, throat illness, and thus in
  Discomfort
  Inconvenience
  School absence
  Parental anxiety
  Work missed by parents
  Costs of physician visits and drugs
Reduction in nasal obstruction with improved
  Respiratory function
  Comfort
  Sleep
  Craniofacial growth and development
  Appearance
Reduction in hearing impairment
Improved growth and overall well-being
Reduction in long-term parental anxiety

*Cost for tonsillectomy alone and adenoidectomy alone are somewhat lower.
Modified from Bluestone CD, editor: Pediatric otolaryngology, ed 4, Philadelphia, 2003, WB Saunders, p. 1213.

be delayed (consider von Willebrand disease) after separation of the eschar. The Clinical Guidelines for Tonsillectomy include a recommendation for a single intravenous dose of intraoperative dexamethasone (0.5 mg/kg), which decreases postoperative nausea and vomiting and reduces swelling. There is no evidence that use of dexamethasone in postoperative tonsillectomy patients results in an increased risk of postoperative bleeding. Routine use of antibiotics in the postoperative period is ineffective and thus the American Academy of Otolaryngology Clinical Practice Guidelines advise against its use, although this recommendation is not consistent among the major professional organizations who have issued guidelines (see Table 383-2). Codeine is associated with excessive sedation and fatalities and is not recommended.

Swelling of the tongue and soft palate can lead to acute airway obstruction in the 1st few hr after surgery. Children with underlying hypotonia or craniofacial anomalies are at greater risk for suffering this complication. Dehydration from odynophagia is not uncommon in the 1st postoperative week. Rare complications include velopharyngeal insufficiency, nasopharyngeal or oropharyngeal stenosis, and psychologic problems.

Bibliography is available at Expert Consult.

Chapter 384
Chronic or Recurrent Respiratory Symptoms

Anne G. Griffiths and Thomas P. Green

Respiratory tract symptoms, including cough, wheeze, and stridor, occur frequently or persist for long periods in a substantial number of children; other children have persistent or recurring lung infiltrates with or without symptoms. Determining the cause of these chronic findings can be difficult because symptoms can be caused by a close succession of unrelated acute respiratory tract infections or by a single pathophysiologic process. Specific and easily performed diagnostic tests do not exist for many acute and chronic respiratory conditions. Pressure from the affected child's family for a quick remedy because of concern over symptoms related to breathing may complicate diagnostic and therapeutic efforts.

A systematic approach to the diagnosis and treatment of these children consists of assessing whether the symptoms are the manifestation of a minor problem or a life-threatening process; determining the most likely underlying pathogenic mechanism; selecting the simplest effective therapy for the underlying process, which often is only symptomatic therapy; and carefully evaluating the effect of therapy. Failure of this approach to identify the process responsible or to effect improvement signals the need for more extensive and perhaps invasive diagnostic efforts, including bronchoscopy.

JUDGING THE SERIOUSNESS OF CHRONIC RESPIRATORY COMPLAINTS

Clinical manifestations suggesting that a respiratory tract illness may be life-threatening or associated with the potential for chronic disability are listed in Table 384-1. If none of these findings is detected, the chronic respiratory process is more likely to be benign. Active, well-nourished, and appropriately growing infants who present with intermittent noisy breathing but no other physical or laboratory abnormalities require only symptomatic treatment and parental reassurance. Benign-appearing but persistent symptoms are occasionally the harbinger of a serious lower respiratory tract problem. By contrast, occasionally children (e.g., infection-related asthma) have

Table 384-1	Indicators of Serious Chronic Lower Respiratory Tract Disease in Children

Persistent fever
Ongoing limitation of activity
Failure to grow
Failure to gain weight appropriately
Clubbing of the digits
Persistent tachypnea and labored ventilation
Shortness of breath and exercise intolerance
Chronic purulent sputum
Persistent hyperinflation
Substantial and sustained hypoxemia
Refractory infiltrates on chest x-ray
Persistent pulmonary function abnormalities
Family history of heritable lung disease
Cyanosis and hypercarbia

recurrent life-threatening episodes but few or no symptoms in the intervals. Repeated examinations over an extended period, both when the child appears healthy and when the child is symptomatic, may be helpful in sorting out the severity and chronicity of lung disease.

RECURRENT OR PERSISTENT COUGH

Cough is a reflex response of the lower respiratory tract to stimulation of irritant or cough receptors in the airways' mucosa. The most common cause in children is airway reactivity (asthma). Because cough receptors also reside in the pharynx, paranasal sinuses, stomach, and external auditory canal, the source of a persistent cough may need to be sought beyond the lungs. Specific lower respiratory stimuli include excessive secretions, aspirated foreign material, inhaled dust particles or noxious gases, cold or dry air, and an inflammatory response to infectious agents or allergic processes. Table 384-2 lists some of the conditions responsible for chronic cough.

Table 384-3 presents characteristics of cough that can aid in distinguishing a cough's origin. Additional useful information can include a history of atopic conditions (asthma, eczema, urticaria, allergic rhinitis), a seasonal or environmental variation in frequency or intensity of cough, and a strong family history of atopic conditions, all suggesting an allergic cause; symptoms of malabsorption or family history indicating cystic fibrosis; symptoms related to feeding, suggesting aspiration or gastroesophageal reflux; a choking episode, suggesting foreign-body aspiration; headache or facial edema associated with sinusitis; and a smoking history in older children and adolescents or the presence of a smoker in the house (Table 384-4).

The physical examination can provide much information pertaining to the cause of chronic cough. Posterior pharyngeal drainage combined with a nighttime cough suggests chronic upper airway disease such as sinusitis. An overinflated chest suggests chronic airway obstruction, as

Table 384-2	Differential Diagnosis of Recurrent and Persistent Cough in Children

RECURRENT COUGH
Reactive airway disease (asthma)
Drainage from upper airways
Aspiration
Frequently recurring respiratory tract infections in immunocompetent or immunodeficient patients
Symptomatic Chiari malformation
Idiopathic pulmonary hemosiderosis
Hypersensitivity (allergic) pneumonitis

PERSISTENT COUGH
Hypersensitivity of cough receptors after infection
Reactive airway disease (asthma)
Chronic sinusitis
Chronic rhinitis (allergic or nonallergic)
Bronchitis or tracheitis caused by infection or smoke exposure
Bronchiectasis, including cystic fibrosis, primary ciliary dyskinesia, immunodeficiency
Habit cough
Foreign-body aspiration
Recurrent aspiration owing to pharyngeal incompetence, tracheolaryngoesophageal cleft, or tracheoesophageal fistula
Gastroesophageal reflux, with or without aspiration
Pertussis
Extrinsic compression of the tracheobronchial tract (vascular ring, neoplasm, lymph node, lung cyst)
Tracheomalacia, bronchomalacia
Endobronchial or endotracheal tumors
Endobronchial tuberculosis
Hypersensitivity pneumonitis
Fungal infections
Inhaled irritants, including tobacco smoke
Irritation of external auditory canal
Angiotensin-converting enzyme inhibitors

Table 384-3	Characteristics of Cough and Other Clinical Features and Possible Causes

SYMPTOMS AND SIGNS	POSSIBLE UNDERLYING ETIOLOGY*
Auscultatory findings (wheeze, crepitations/crackles, differential breath sounds)	Asthma, bronchitis, congenital lung disease, foreign body aspiration, airway abnormality
Cough characteristics (e.g., cough with choking, cough quality, cough starting from birth)	See text; congenital lung abnormalities
Cardiac abnormalities (including murmurs)	Any cardiac illness
Chest pain	Asthma, functional, pleuritis
Chest wall deformity	Any chronic lung disease
Daily moist or productive cough	Chronic bronchitis, suppurative lung disease
Digital clubbing	Suppurative lung disease, arteriovenous shunt
Dyspnea (exertional or at rest)	Compromised lung function of any chronic lung or cardiac disease
Failure to thrive	Compromised lung function, immunodeficiency, cystic fibrosis
Feeding difficulties (including choking and vomiting)	Compromised lung function, aspiration
Hemoptysis	Bronchitis, foreign body aspiration, suctioning trauma
Immune deficiency	Atypical and typical recurrent respiratory infections
Medications or drugs	Angiotensin-converting enzyme inhibitors, puffers, illicit drug use
Neurodevelopmental abnormality	Aspiration
Recurrent pneumonia	Immunodeficiency, congenital lung problem, airway abnormality
Symptoms of upper respiratory tract infection	Can coexist or be a trigger for an underlying problem

*This is not an exhaustive list; only the more common respiratory diseases are mentioned.
From Chang AB, Landau LI, Van Asperen PP, et al: Cough in children: definitions and clinical evaluation. Thoracic Society of Australia and New Zealand, Med J Aust 184(8):399–403, 2006.

Table 384-4	Clinical Clues About Cough

CHARACTERISTIC	THINK OF
Staccato, paroxysmal	Pertussis, cystic fibrosis, foreign body, *Chlamydia* spp., *Mycoplasma* spp.
Followed by "whoop"	Pertussis
All day, never during sleep	Habit cough
Barking, brassy	Croup, habit cough, tracheomalacia, tracheitis, epiglottitis
Hoarseness	Laryngeal involvement (croup, recurrent laryngeal nerve involvement)
Abrupt onset	Foreign body, pulmonary embolism
Follows exercise	Reactive airway disease
Accompanies eating, drinking	Aspiration, gastroesophageal reflux, tracheoesophageal fistula
Throat clearing	Postnasal drip, vocal tic
Productive (sputum)	Infection, cystic fibrosis, bronchiectasis
Night cough	Sinusitis, reactive airway disease, gastroesophageal reflux
Seasonal	Allergic rhinitis, reactive airway disease
Immunosuppressed patient	Bacterial pneumonia, *Pneumocystis jiroveci, Mycobacterium tuberculosis, Mycobacterium avium-intracellulare,* cytomegalovirus
Dyspnea	Hypoxia, hypercarbia
Animal exposure	*Chlamydia psittaci* (birds), *Yersinia pestis* (rodents), *Francisella tularensis* (rabbits), Q fever (sheep, cattle), hantavirus (rodents), histoplasmosis (pigeons)
Geographic	Histoplasmosis (Mississippi, Missouri, Ohio River Valley), coccidioidomycosis (Southwest), blastomycosis (North and Midwest)
Workdays with clearing on days off	Occupational exposure

From Kliegman RM, Greenbaum LA, Lyle PS: Practical strategies in pediatric diagnosis and therapy, ed 2, Philadelphia, 2004, WB Saunders, p. 19.

in asthma or cystic fibrosis. An expiratory wheeze, with or without diminished intensity of breath sounds, strongly suggests asthma or asthmatic bronchitis but may also be consistent with a diagnosis of cystic fibrosis, bronchomalacia, vascular ring, aspiration of foreign material, or pulmonary hemosiderosis. Careful auscultation during forced expiration may reveal expiratory wheezes that are otherwise undetectable and that are the only indication of underlying reactive airways. Coarse crackles suggest bronchiectasis, including cystic fibrosis, but can also occur with an acute or subacute exacerbation of asthma. Clubbing of the digits is seen in most patients with bronchiectasis but in only a few other respiratory conditions with chronic cough (see Table 384-2). Tracheal deviation suggests foreign body aspiration or a mediastinal mass.

Allowing sufficient examination time to detect a spontaneous cough is important. If a spontaneous cough does not occur, asking the child to take a maximal breath and forcefully exhale repeatedly usually induces a cough reflex. Most children can cough on request by 4-5 yr of age. Children who cough as often as several times a minute with regularity are likely to have a habit (tic) cough (see Chapter 24). If the cough is loose, every effort should be made to obtain sputum; many older children can comply. It is sometimes possible to pick up small bits of sputum with a throat swab quickly inserted into the lower pharynx while the child coughs with the tongue protruding. Clear mucoid sputum is most often associated with an allergic reaction or asthmatic bronchitis. Cloudy (purulent) sputum suggests a respiratory tract infection but can also reflect increased cellularity (eosinophilia) from an asthmatic process. Very purulent sputum is characteristic of bronchiectasis (see Chapter 401). Malodorous expectorations suggest anaerobic infection of the lungs. In cystic fibrosis (see Chapter 403), the sputum, even when purulent, is rarely foul smelling.

Laboratory tests can help in the evaluation of a chronic cough. Only sputum specimens containing alveolar macrophages should be interpreted as reflecting lower respiratory tract processes. Sputum eosinophilia suggests asthma, asthmatic bronchitis, or hypersensitivity reactions of the lung (see Chapter 391), but a polymorphonuclear cell response suggests infection; if sputum is unavailable, the presence of eosinophilia in nasal secretions also suggests atopic disease. If most of the cells in sputum are macrophages, postinfectious hypersensitivity of cough receptors should be suspected. Sputum macrophages can be stained for hemosiderin content, which is diagnostic of pulmonary hemosiderosis (see Chapter 400), or for lipid content, which in large amounts suggests, but is not specific for, repeated aspiration. Rarely, children may expectorate partial casts of the airway which can be characterized in investigating causes of plastic bronchitis. Children whose coughs persist for more than 6 wk should be tested for cystic fibrosis regardless of their race or ethnicity (see Chapter 403). Sputum culture is helpful in evaluation of cystic fibrosis, but less so for other conditions because throat flora can contaminate the sample.

Hematologic assessment can reveal a microcytic anemia that is the result of pulmonary hemosiderosis (see Chapter 406) or hemoptysis, or eosinophilia that accompanies asthma and other hypersensitivity reactions of the lung. Infiltrates on the chest radiograph suggest cystic fibrosis, bronchiectasis, foreign body, hypersensitivity pneumonitis, or tuberculosis. When asthma-equivalent cough is suggested, a trial of bronchodilator therapy may be diagnostic. If the cough does not respond to initial therapeutic efforts, more-specific diagnostic procedures may be warranted, including an immunologic or allergic evaluation, chest and paranasal sinus imaging, esophagograms, tests for gastroesophageal reflux (see Chapter 323), and special microbiologic studies including rapid viral testing. Evaluation of ciliary morphology, nasal endoscopy, laryngoscopy and bronchoscopy may also be indicated.

Habit cough ("psychogenic cough" or "cough tic") must be considered in any child with a cough that has lasted for weeks or months, that has been refractory to treatment, and that disappears with sleep or with distraction. Typically, the cough is abrupt and loud and has a harsh, honking, or "barking" quality. A disassociation between the intensity of the cough and the child's affect is typically striking. This cough may be absent if the physician listens outside the examination room, but it will reliably appear immediately on direct attention to the child and the symptom. It typically begins with an upper respiratory infection but then lingers. The child misses many days of school because the cough disrupts the classroom. This disorder accounts for many unnecessary medical procedures and courses of medication. It is treatable with assurance that a pathologic lung condition is absent and that the child should resume full activity, including school. This assurance, together with speech therapy techniques that allow the child to reduce musculoskeletal tension in the neck and chest and that increase the child's awareness of the initial sensations that trigger cough, has been very successful. Self-hypnosis is another successful therapy, often effective with 1 session. The designation "habit cough" is preferable to "psychogenic cough" because it carries no stigma and because most of these children do not have significant emotional problems. When the cough disappears, it does not reemerge as another symptom. Nonetheless, other symptoms such as irritable bowel syndrome may be present in the patient or family.

FREQUENTLY RECURRING OR PERSISTENT STRIDOR

Stridor, a harsh, medium-pitched, inspiratory sound associated with obstruction of the laryngeal area or the extrathoracic trachea, is often accompanied by a croupy cough and hoarse voice. Stridor is most commonly observed in children with croup (see Chapter 385); foreign bodies and trauma can also cause acute stridor. A few children, however, acquire recurrent stridor or have persistent stridor from the 1st days or weeks of life (Table 384-5). Most congenital anomalies of large airways that produce stridor become symptomatic soon after

Table 384-5	Causes of Recurrent or Persistent Stridor in Children

RECURRENT
Allergic (spasmodic) croup
Respiratory infections in a child with otherwise asymptomatic anatomic narrowing of the large airways
Laryngomalacia

PERSISTENT
Laryngeal obstruction
• Laryngomalacia
• Papillomas, other tumors
• Cysts and laryngoceles
• Laryngeal webs
• Bilateral abductor paralysis of the cords
• Foreign body
Tracheobronchial disease
• Tracheomalacia
• Subglottic tracheal webs
• Endobronchial, endotracheal tumors
• Subglottic tracheal stenosis, congenital or acquired
Extrinsic masses
• Mediastinal masses
• Vascular ring
• Lobar emphysema
• Bronchogenic cysts
• Thyroid enlargement
• Esophageal foreign body
Tracheoesophageal fistula

OTHER
Gastroesophageal reflux
Macroglossia, Pierre Robin syndrome
Cri-du-chat syndrome
Paradoxical vocal cord dysfunction
Hypocalcemia
Vocal cord paralysis
Chiari crisis
Severe neonatal episodic laryngospasm caused by *SCN4A* mutation

birth. Increase of stridor when a child is supine suggests laryngomalacia or tracheomalacia. It is important to note that when evaluating for a specific anatomic cause of abnormal breath sounds, it is not uncommon to identify additional congenital anomalies of the airway. An accompanying history of hoarseness or aphonia suggests involvement of the vocal cords. Associated dysphagia may also suggest a vascular ring. In a child with intermittent stridor that accompanies physical activity and is not responsive to asthma therapies, paradoxical vocal cord dysfunction may be of consideration. Paradoxical vocal cord dysfunction may be highly supported by history and confirmed by laryngoscopy during an exercise challenge test if symptoms are successfully elicited. Speech therapy and behavior modification may be therapeutic.

Physical examination for recurrent or persistent stridor is usually unrewarding, although changes in its severity and intensity due to changes of body position should be assessed. Anteroposterior and lateral radiographs, contrast esophagography, fluoroscopy, CT, and MRI are potentially useful diagnostic tools. In most cases, direct observation by laryngoscopy is necessary for definitive diagnosis. Undistorted views of the larynx are best obtained with fiberoptic laryngoscopy.

RECURRENT OR PERSISTENT WHEEZE
See also Chapter 391.

Parents often complain that their child "wheezes," when, in fact, they are reporting respiratory sounds that are audible without a stethoscope, produce palpable resonance throughout the chest, and occur most prominently in inspiration. Some of these children have stridor, although many have audible sounds when the supraglottic airway is incompletely cleared of feedings or secretions.

True **wheezing** is a relatively common and particularly troublesome manifestation of obstructive *lower* respiratory tract disease in children. The site of obstruction may be anywhere from the intrathoracic trachea to the small bronchi or large bronchioles, but the sound is generated by turbulence in larger airways that collapse with forced expiration (see Chapter 373). Children younger than 2-3 yr are especially prone to wheezing, because bronchospasm, mucosal edema, and accumulation of excessive secretions have a relatively greater obstructive effect on their smaller airways. In addition, the compliant airways in young children collapse more readily with active expiration. Isolated episodes of acute wheezing, such as can occur with bronchiolitis, are not uncommon, but wheezing that recurs or persists for more than 4 wk suggests other diagnoses (see Table 391-1 in Chapter 391). Most recurrent or persistent wheezing in children is the result of airway reactivity. Nonspecific environmental factors such as cigarette smoke may be important contributors.

Frequently recurring or persistent wheezing starting at or soon after birth suggests a variety of other diagnoses, including congenital structural abnormalities involving the lower respiratory tract or tracheobronchomalacia (see Chapter 386.11). Wheezing that attends cystic fibrosis is most common in the 1st yr of life. Sudden onset of severe wheezing in a previously healthy child should suggest foreign-body aspiration.

Either wheezing or coughing when associated with tachypnea and hypoxemia may be suggestive of **interstitial lung disease** (see Chapter 399.5). However, many patients with interstitial lung disease demonstrate no symptoms other than rapid breathing on initial physical examination. Although chest roentgenograms may be normal in interstitial lung disease, diffuse abnormalities on chest X-ray may support further evaluation in patients suspected to have interstitial lung disease with characteristic findings described on high-resolution CT scan and lung biopsy.

Repeated examination may be required to verify a history of wheezing in a child with episodic symptoms and should be directed toward assessing air movement, ventilatory adequacy, and evidence of chronic lung disease, such as fixed overinflation of the chest, growth failure, and digital clubbing. Patients should be assessed for oropharyngeal dysphagia in cases of suspected recurrent aspiration. Clubbing suggests chronic lung infection and is rarely prominent in uncomplicated asthma. Tracheal deviation from foreign body aspiration should be sought. It is essential to rule out wheezing secondary to congestive heart failure. Allergic rhinitis, urticaria, eczema, or evidence of ichthyosis vulgaris suggests asthma or asthmatic bronchitis. The nose should be examined for polyps, which can exist with allergic conditions or cystic fibrosis.

Sputum eosinophilia and elevated serum immunoglobulin E levels suggest allergic reactions. A forced expiratory volume in 1 sec increase of 15% in response to bronchodilators confirms reactive airways. Specific microbiologic studies, special imaging studies of the airways and cardiovascular structures, diagnostic studies for cystic fibrosis, and bronchoscopy (see Chapter 366) should be considered if the response is unsatisfactory.

RECURRENT AND PERSISTENT LUNG INFILTRATES

Radiographic lung infiltrates resulting from acute pneumonia usually resolve within 1-3 wk, but a substantial number of children, particularly infants, fail to completely clear infiltrates within a 4 wk period. These children may be febrile or afebrile and may display a wide range of respiratory symptoms and signs. Persistent or recurring infiltrates present a diagnostic challenge (Table 384-6).

Symptoms associated with chronic lung infiltrates in the 1st several weeks of life (but not related to neonatal respiratory distress syndrome) suggest infection acquired in utero or during descent through the birth canal. Early appearance of chronic infiltrates can also be associated with cystic fibrosis or congenital anomalies that result in aspiration or

Table 384-6	Diseases Associated with Recurrent, Persistent, or Migrating Lung Infiltrates Beyond the Neonatal Period

Aspiration
  Pharyngeal incompetence (e.g., cleft palate)
  Laryngotracheoesophageal cleft
  Tracheoesophageal fistula
  Gastroesophageal reflux
  Lipid aspiration
  Neurologic dysphagia
  Developmental dysphagia
Congenital anomalies
  Lung cysts (cystic adenomatoid malformation)
  Pulmonary sequestration
  Bronchial stenosis or aberrant bronchus
  Vascular ring
  Congenital heart disease with large left-to-right shunt
  Pulmonary lymphangiectasia
Genetic conditions
  α_1-Antitrypsin deficiency
  Cystic fibrosis
  Primary ciliary dyskinesia (Kartagener syndrome)
  Sickle cell disease (acute chest syndrome)
Immunodeficiency, phagocytic deficiency
  Humoral, cellular, combined immunodeficiency states
  Chronic granulomatous disease and related phagocytic defects
  Complement deficiency states
Immunologic and autoimmune diseases
  Asthma
  Allergic bronchopulmonary aspergillosis
  Hypersensitivity pneumonitis
  Pulmonary hemosiderosis
  Collagen-vascular diseases
Infection, congenital
  Cytomegalovirus
  Rubella
  Syphilis
Infection, acquired
  Cytomegalovirus
  Tuberculosis
  HIV
  Other viruses
  Chlamydia
  Mycoplasma, Ureaplasma
  Pertussis
  Fungal organisms
  Pneumocystis jiroveci
  Visceral larva migrans
  Inadequately treated bacterial infection
Interstitial pneumonitis and fibrosis
  Usual interstitial pneumonitis
  Lymphoid (AIDS)
  Genetic disorders of surfactant synthesis, secretion
  Desquamative
  Acute (Hamman-Rich)
  Alveolar proteinosis
  Drug-induced, radiation-induced inflammation and fibrosis
Neoplasms and neoplastic-like conditions
  Primary or metastatic pulmonary tumors
  Leukemia
  Histiocytosis
  Eosinophilic pneumonias
Other etiologies
  Bronchiectasis
    Congenital
    Postinfectious
  Sarcoidosis

airway obstruction. A history of recurrent infiltrates, wheezing, and cough may reflect asthma, even in the 1st yr of life.

A controversial association has been posed regarding recurrent lung infiltrates in pulmonary hemosiderosis related to cow's milk hypersensitivity or unknown causes appearing in the 1st yr of life. Children with a history of bronchopulmonary dysplasia often have episodes of respiratory distress attended by wheezing and new lung infiltrates. Recurrent pneumonia in a child with frequent otitis media, nasopharyngitis, adenitis, or dermatologic manifestations suggests an immunodeficiency state, complement deficiency, or phagocytic defect (see Chapters 124-127). Primary ciliary dyskinesia is also of consideration in patients with frequent otitis media and suppurative sinopulmonary disease, with or without accompanying heterotaxy or infertility. Pulmonary sequestration may be suspected in patients with recurrent findings on radiograph that occur in the same location, both during illness and when well (see Chapter 395.4). Traction bronchiectasis may also be suggested on radiography with persistent findings in a given region of the film following history of respiratory infection. Particular attention must be directed to the possibility that the infiltrates represent lymphocytic interstitial pneumonitis or opportunistic infection associated with HIV infection (see Chapter 276). A history of paroxysmal coughing in an infant suggests pertussis syndrome or cystic fibrosis. Persistent infiltrates, especially with loss of volume, in a toddler should suggest foreign-body aspiration.

Overinflation and infiltrates suggest cystic fibrosis or chronic asthma. A "silent chest" with infiltrates should arouse suspicion of alveolar proteinosis (see Chapter 405), *Pneumocystis jiroveci* infection (see Chapter 244), genetic disorders of surfactant synthesis and secretion causing interstitial pneumonitis, or tumors. Growth should be carefully assessed to determine whether the lung process has had systemic effects, indicating substantial severity and chronicity as in cystic fibrosis or alveolar proteinosis. Cataracts, retinopathy, or microcephaly suggest in utero infection. Chronic rhinorrhea can be associated with atopic disease, cow's milk intolerance, cystic fibrosis, or congenital syphilis. The absence of tonsils and cervical lymph nodes suggests an immunodeficiency state.

Diagnostic studies should be performed selectively, based on information obtained from history and physical examination and on a thorough understanding of the conditions listed in Table 384-6. Cytologic evaluation of sputum, if available, may be helpful. Chest CT often provides more precise anatomic detail concerning the infiltrate or further characterize a region of anatomic abnormality. Bronchoscopy is indicated for detecting foreign bodies, congenital or acquired anomalies of the tracheobronchial tract, and obstruction by endobronchial or extrinsic masses (see Chapter 394). Bronchoscopy provides access to secretions that can be studied cytologically and microbiologically. Alveolar lavage fluid is diagnostic for alveolar proteinosis and persistent pulmonary hemosiderosis and can suggest aspiration syndromes. If all appropriate studies have been completed and the condition remains undiagnosed, lung biopsy might yield a definitive diagnosis, such as in interstitial lung disease or in fungal disease.

Optimal medical or surgical treatment of chronic lung infiltrates often depends on a specific diagnosis, but chronic conditions may be self-limiting (severe and prolonged viral infections in infants); in these cases, symptomatic therapy can maintain adequate lung function until spontaneous improvement occurs. Helpful measures include inhalation and physical therapy for excessive secretions, antibiotics for bacterial infections, supplementary oxygen for hypoxemia, and maintenance of adequate nutrition. Because the lung of a young child has remarkable recuperative potential, normal lung function may ultimately be achieved with treatment despite the severity of pulmonary insult occurring in infancy or early childhood.

Bibliography is available at Expert Consult.

Chapter **385**
Acute Inflammatory Upper Airway Obstruction (Croup, Epiglottitis, Laryngitis, and Bacterial Tracheitis)
Genie E. Roosevelt

Airway resistance is inversely proportional to the 4th power of the radius (see Chapter 373). Because the lumen of an infant's or child's airway is narrow, minor reductions in cross-sectional area as a result of mucosal edema or other inflammatory processes cause an exponential increase in airway resistance and a significant increase in the work of breathing. The larynx is composed of 4 major cartilages (**epiglottic, arytenoid, thyroid,** and **cricoid cartilages**, ordered from superior to inferior) and the soft tissues that surround them. The cricoid cartilage encircles the airway just below the vocal cords and defines the narrowest portion of the upper airway in children younger than 10 yr of age.

Inflammation involving the vocal cords and structures inferior to the cords is called **laryngitis, laryngotracheitis,** or **laryngotracheobronchitis,** and inflammation of the structures superior to the cords (i.e., arytenoids, aryepiglottic folds ["false cords"], epiglottis) is called **supraglottitis.** The term **croup** refers to a heterogeneous group of mainly acute and infectious processes that are characterized by a bark-like or brassy cough and may be associated with hoarseness, inspiratory stridor, and respiratory distress. **Stridor** is a harsh, high-pitched respiratory sound, which is usually inspiratory but can be biphasic and is produced by turbulent airflow; it is not a diagnosis but a sign of upper airway obstruction (see Chapter 374). Croup typically affects the larynx, trachea, and bronchi. When the involvement of the larynx is sufficient to produce symptoms, they dominate the clinical picture over the tracheal and bronchial signs. A distinction has been made between spasmodic or recurrent croup and laryngotracheobronchitis. Some clinicians believe that spasmodic croup might have an allergic component and improves rapidly without treatment, whereas laryngotracheobronchitis is always associated with a viral infection of the respiratory tract. Others believe that the signs and symptoms are similar enough to consider them within the spectrum of a single disease, in part because studies have documented viral etiologies in both acute and recurrent croup.

385.1 Infectious Upper Airway Obstruction
Genie E. Roosevelt

ETIOLOGY AND EPIDEMIOLOGY
With the exceptions of diphtheria (see Chapter 187), bacterial tracheitis, and epiglottitis, most acute infections of the upper airway are caused by viruses. The parainfluenza viruses (types 1, 2, and 3; see Chapter 259) account for approximately 75% of cases; other viruses

associated with croup include influenza A and B, adenovirus, respiratory syncytial virus, and measles. Influenza A is associated with severe laryngotracheobronchitis. *Mycoplasma pneumoniae* has rarely been isolated from children with croup and causes mild disease (see Chapter 223). Most patients with croup are between the ages of 3 mo and 5 yr, with the peak in the 2nd yr of life. The incidence of croup is higher in boys. It occurs most commonly in the late fall and winter but can occur throughout the year. Recurrences are frequent from 3-6 yr of age and decrease with growth of the airway. Approximately 15% of patients have a strong family history of croup.

In the past, *Haemophilus influenzae* type b was the most commonly identified etiology of acute epiglottitis. Since the widespread use of the *H. influenzae* type b vaccine, invasive disease caused by *H. influenzae* type b in pediatric patients has been reduced by 99% (see Chapter 194). Therefore, other agents, such as *Streptococcus pyogenes*, *Streptococcus pneumoniae*, nontypeable *H. influenzae*, and *Staphylococcus aureus*, represent a larger portion of pediatric cases of epiglottitis in vaccinated children. In the prevaccine era, the typical patient with epiglottitis caused by *H. influenzae* type b was 2-4 yr of age, although cases were seen in the 1st yr of life and in patients as old as 7 yr of age. Currently, the most common presentation of epiglottitis is an adult with a sore throat, although cases still do occur in underimmunized children; vaccine failures have been reported.

CLINICAL MANIFESTATIONS
Croup (Laryngotracheobronchitis)

Viruses typically cause croup, the most common form of acute upper respiratory obstruction. The term **laryngotracheobronchitis** refers to viral infection of the glottic and subglottic regions. Some clinicians use the term **laryngotracheitis** for the most common and most typical form of croup and reserve the term **laryngotracheobronchitis** for the more severe form that is considered an extension of laryngotracheitis associated with bacterial superinfection that occurs 5-7 days into the clinical course.

Most patients have an upper respiratory tract infection with some combination of rhinorrhea, pharyngitis, mild cough, and low-grade fever for 1-3 days before the signs and symptoms of upper airway obstruction become apparent. The child then develops the characteristic "barking" cough, hoarseness, and inspiratory stridor. The low-grade fever can persist, although temperatures may occasionally reach 39-40°C (102.2-104°F); some children are afebrile. Symptoms are characteristically worse at night and often recur with decreasing intensity for several days and resolve completely within a week. Agitation and crying greatly aggravate the symptoms and signs. The child may prefer to sit up in bed or be held upright. Older children usually are not seriously ill. Other family members might have mild respiratory illnesses with laryngitis. Most young patients with croup progress only as far as stridor and slight dyspnea before they start to recover.

Physical examination can reveal a hoarse voice, coryza, normal to moderately inflamed pharynx, and a slightly increased respiratory rate. Patients vary substantially in their degrees of respiratory distress. Rarely, the upper airway obstruction progresses and is accompanied by an increasing respiratory rate; nasal flaring; suprasternal, infrasternal, and intercostal retractions; and continuous stridor. Croup is a disease of the upper airway, and alveolar gas exchange is usually normal. Hypoxia and low oxygen saturation are seen only when complete airway obstruction is imminent. **The child who is hypoxic, cyanotic, pale, or obtunded needs immediate airway management.** Occasionally, the pattern of severe laryngotracheobronchitis is difficult to differentiate from epiglottitis, despite the usually more acute onset and rapid course of the latter.

Croup is a clinical diagnosis and does not require a radiograph of the neck. Radiographs of the neck can show the typical subglottic narrowing, or steeple sign, of croup on the posteroanterior view (Fig. 385-1). However, the steeple sign may be absent in patients with croup, may be present in patients without croup as a normal variant, and may rarely be present in patients with epiglottitis. The radiographs do not correlate well with disease severity. Radiographs should be considered only after airway stabilization in children who have an atypical presen-

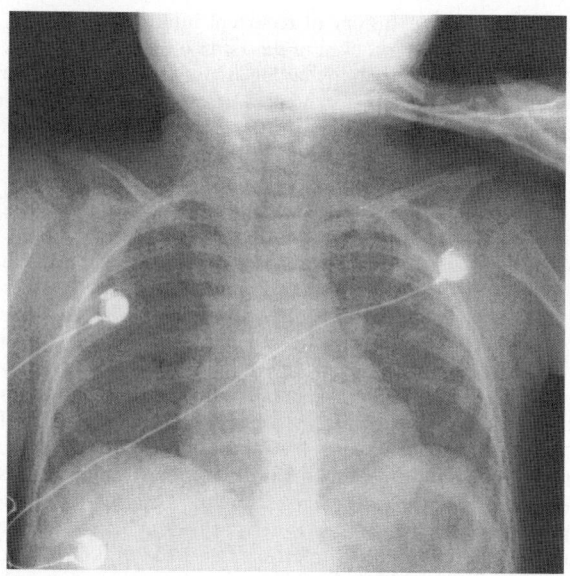

Figure 385-1 Radiograph of an airway of a patient with croup, showing typical subglottic narrowing (steeple sign).

tation or clinical course. Radiographs may be helpful in distinguishing between severe laryngotracheobronchitis and epiglottitis, but airway management should always take priority.

Acute Epiglottitis (Supraglottitis)

This now rare, but still dramatic and potentially lethal condition is characterized by an acute rapidly progressive and potentially fulminating course of high fever, sore throat, dyspnea, and rapidly progressing respiratory obstruction. The degree of respiratory distress at presentation is variable. The initial lack of respiratory distress can deceive the unwary clinician; respiratory distress can also be the first manifestation. Often, the otherwise healthy child suddenly develops a sore throat and fever. Within a matter of hours, the patient appears toxic, swallowing is difficult, and breathing is labored. Drooling is usually present and the neck is hyperextended in an attempt to maintain the airway. The child may assume the tripod position, sitting upright and leaning forward with the chin up and mouth open while bracing on the arms. A brief period of air hunger with restlessness may be followed by rapidly increasing cyanosis and coma. Stridor is a late finding and suggests near-complete airway obstruction. Complete obstruction of the airway and death can ensue unless adequate treatment is provided. The barking cough typical of croup is rare. Usually, no other family members are ill with acute respiratory symptoms.

The diagnosis requires visualization under controlled circumstances of a large, cherry red, swollen epiglottis by laryngoscopy. Occasionally, the other supraglottic structures, especially the aryepiglottic folds, are more involved than the epiglottis itself. In a patient in whom the diagnosis is certain or probable based on clinical grounds, laryngoscopy should be performed expeditiously in a controlled environment such as an operating room or intensive care unit. Anxiety-provoking interventions such as phlebotomy, intravenous line placement, placing the child supine, or direct inspection of the oral cavity should be avoided until the airway is secure. If epiglottitis is thought to be possible but not certain in a patient with acute upper airway obstruction, the patient may undergo lateral radiographs of the upper airway first. Classic radiographs of a child who has epiglottitis show the thumb sign (Fig. 385-2). Proper positioning of the patient for the lateral neck radiograph is crucial in order to avoid some of the pitfalls associated with interpretation of the film. Adequate hyperextension of the head and neck is necessary. In addition, the epiglottis can appear to be round if the lateral neck is taken at an oblique angle. If the concern for epiglottitis still exists after the radiographs, direct visualization should be performed. A physician skilled in airway management and use of

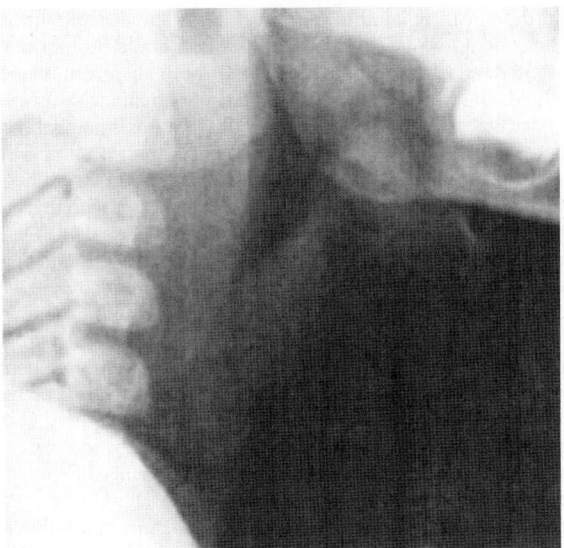

Figure 385-2 Lateral roentgenogram of the upper airway reveals the swollen epiglottis (thumb sign).

intubation equipment should accompany patients with suspected epiglottitis at all times. An older cooperative child might voluntarily open the mouth wide enough for a direct view of the inflamed epiglottis.

Establishing an airway by endotracheal or nasotracheal intubation or, less often, by tracheostomy is indicated in patients with epiglottitis, regardless of the degree of apparent respiratory distress, because as many as 6% of children with epiglottitis without an artificial airway die, compared with <1% of those with an artificial airway. No clinical features have been recognized that predict mortality. Pulmonary edema can be associated with acute airway obstruction. The duration of intubation depends on the clinical course of the patient and the duration of epiglottic swelling, as determined by frequent examination using direct laryngoscopy or flexible fiberoptic laryngoscopy. In general, children with acute epiglottitis are intubated for 2-3 days, because the response to antibiotics is usually rapid. Most patients have concomitant bacteremia; occasionally, other infections are present, such as pneumonia, cervical adenopathy, or otitis media. Meningitis, arthritis, and other invasive infections with *H. influenzae* type b are rarely found in conjunction with epiglottitis.

Acute Infectious Laryngitis
Laryngitis is a common illness. Viruses cause most cases; diphtheria is an exception but is extremely rare in industrialized countries (see Chapter 187). The onset is usually characterized by an upper respiratory tract infection during which sore throat, cough, and hoarseness appear. The illness is generally mild; respiratory distress is unusual except in the young infant. Hoarseness and loss of voice may be out of proportion to systemic signs and symptoms. The physical examination is usually not remarkable except for evidence of pharyngeal inflammation. Inflammatory edema of the vocal cords and subglottic tissue may be demonstrated laryngoscopically. The principal site of obstruction is usually the subglottic area.

Spasmodic Croup
Spasmodic croup occurs most often in children 1-3 yr of age and is clinically similar to acute laryngotracheobronchitis, except that the history of a viral prodrome and fever in the patient and family are often absent. The cause is viral in some cases, but allergic and psychologic factors may be important in others.

Occurring most commonly in the evening or nighttime, spasmodic croup begins with a sudden onset that may be preceded by mild to moderate coryza and hoarseness. The child awakens with a characteristic barking, metallic cough, noisy inspiration, and respiratory distress and appears anxious and frightened. The patient is usually afebrile. The severity of the symptoms generally diminishes within several hr, and the following day, the patient often appears well except for slight hoarseness and cough. Similar, but usually less severe, attacks without extreme respiratory distress can occur for another night or two. Such episodes often recur several times. Spasmodic croup might represent more of an allergic reaction to viral antigens than direct infection, although the pathogenesis is unknown.

DIFFERENTIAL DIAGNOSIS
These 4 syndromes must be differentiated from one another and from a variety of other entities that can present as upper airway obstruction. **Bacterial tracheitis** is the most important differential diagnostic consideration and has a high risk of airway obstruction. Diphtheritic croup is extremely rare in North America, although a major epidemic of diphtheria occurred in countries of the former Soviet Union beginning in 1990 from the lack of routine immunization. Early symptoms of diphtheria include malaise, sore throat, anorexia, and low-grade fever. Within 2-3 days, pharyngeal examination reveals the typical gray-white membrane, which can vary in size from covering a small patch on the tonsils to covering most of the soft palate. The membrane is adherent to the tissue, and forcible attempts to remove it cause bleeding. The course is usually insidious, but respiratory obstruction can occur suddenly. Measles croup almost always coincides with the full manifestations of systemic disease and the course may be fulminant (see Chapter 246).

Sudden onset of respiratory obstruction can be caused by aspiration of a **foreign body** (see Chapter 387). The child is usually 6 mo-3 yr of age. Choking and coughing occur suddenly, usually without prodromal signs of infection, although children with a viral infection can also aspirate a foreign body. A **retropharyngeal** or **peritonsillar abscess** can mimic respiratory obstruction (see Chapter 382). CT scans of the upper airway are helpful in evaluating the possibility of a retropharyngeal abscess. A peritonsillar abscess is a clinical diagnosis. Other possible causes of upper airway obstruction include extrinsic compression of the airway (laryngeal web, vascular ring) and intraluminal obstruction from masses (laryngeal papilloma, subglottic hemangioma); these tend to have chronic or recurrent symptoms.

Upper airway obstruction is occasionally associated with **angioedema** of the subglottic areas as part of anaphylaxis and generalized allergic reactions, edema after endotracheal intubation for general anesthesia or respiratory failure, hypocalcemic tetany, infectious mononucleosis, trauma, and tumors or malformations of the larynx. A croupy cough may be an early sign of asthma. Vocal cord dysfunction can also occur. Epiglottitis, with the characteristic manifestations of drooling or dysphagia and stridor, can also result from the accidental ingestion of very hot liquid.

COMPLICATIONS
Complications occur in approximately 15% of patients with viral croup. The most common is extension of the infectious process to involve other regions of the respiratory tract, such as the middle ear, the terminal bronchioles, or the pulmonary parenchyma. Bacterial tracheitis may be a complication of viral croup rather than a distinct disease. If associated with *S. aureus* or *S. pyogenes,* toxic shock syndrome can develop. Bacterial tracheitis may have a 2-phased illness, with the 2nd phase after a croup-like illness associated with high fever, toxicity, and airway obstruction. Alternatively, the onset of tracheitis occurs without a 2nd phase and appears as a continuation of the initial croup-like illness but with higher fever and worsening respiratory distress rather than the usual recovery after 2-3 days of viral croup. Pneumonia, cervical lymphadenitis, otitis media, or, rarely, meningitis or septic arthritis can occur in the course of epiglottitis. Pneumomediastinum and pneumothorax are the most common complications of tracheotomy.

TREATMENT
The mainstay of treatment for children with **croup** is airway management and treatment of hypoxia. Treatment of the respiratory distress

should take priority over any testing. Most children with either acute spasmodic croup or infectious croup can be managed safely at home. Despite the observation that cold night air is beneficial, a Cochrane review has found no evidence supporting the use of cool mist in the emergency department for the treatment of croup.

Nebulized racemic epinephrine is an accepted treatment for moderate or severe croup. The mechanism of action is believed to be constriction of the precapillary arterioles through the β-adrenergic receptors, causing fluid resorption from the interstitial space and a decrease in the laryngeal mucosal edema. Traditionally, racemic epinephrine, a 1:1 mixture of the D- and L-isomers of epinephrine, has been administered. A dose of 0.25-0.5 mL of 2.25% racemic epinephrine in 3 mL of normal saline can be used as often as every 20 min. Racemic epinephrine was initially chosen over the more active and more readily available L-epinephrine to minimize anticipated cardiovascular side effects such as tachycardia and hypertension. There is evidence that L-epinephrine (5 mL of 1:1,000 solution) is equally effective as racemic epinephrine and does not carry the risk of additional adverse effects.

The indications for the administration of nebulized epinephrine include moderate to severe **stridor at rest,** the possible need for intubation, respiratory distress, and hypoxia. The duration of activity of racemic epinephrine is <2 hr. Consequently, observation is mandated. The symptoms of croup might reappear, but racemic epinephrine does not cause rebound worsening of the obstruction. Patients can be safely discharged home after a 2-3 hr period of observation provided they have no stridor at rest; have normal air entry, normal pulse oximetry, and normal level of consciousness; and have received steroids. Nebulized epinephrine should still be used cautiously in patients with tachycardia, heart conditions such as tetralogy of Fallot, or ventricular outlet obstruction because of possible side effects.

The effectiveness of **oral corticosteroids** in viral croup is well established. Corticosteroids decrease the edema in the laryngeal mucosa through their antiinflammatory action. Oral steroids are beneficial, even in mild croup, as measured by reduced hospitalization, shorter duration of hospitalization, and reduced need for subsequent interventions such as epinephrine administration. Most studies that demonstrated the efficacy of oral dexamethasone used a *single dose of 0.6 mg/ kg,* a dose as low as 0.15 mg/kg may be just as effective. Intramuscular dexamethasone and nebulized budesonide have an equivalent clinical effect; oral dosing of dexamethasone is as effective as intramuscular administration. A single dose of oral prednisolone is less effective. There are no controlled studies examining the effectiveness of multiple doses of corticosteroids. The only adverse effect in the treatment of croup with corticosteroids is the development of *Candida albicans* laryngotracheitis in a patient who received dexamethasone, 1 mg/ kg/24 hr, for 8 days. Corticosteroids should not be administered to children with varicella or tuberculosis (unless the patient is receiving appropriate antituberculosis therapy) because they worsen the clinical course.

Antibiotics are not indicated in croup. Nonprescription cough and cold medications should not be used in children younger than 4 yr of age. A helium-oxygen mixture (heliox) may be considered in the treatment of children with severe croup for whom intubation is being considered although the evidence is inconclusive. Children with croup should be hospitalized for any of the following: progressive stridor, severe stridor at rest, respiratory distress, hypoxia, cyanosis, depressed mental status, poor oral intake, or the need for reliable observation.

Epiglottitis is a medical emergency and warrants immediate treatment with an **artificial airway** placed under controlled conditions, either in an operating room or intensive care unit. All patients should receive oxygen en route unless the mask causes excessive agitation. Racemic epinephrine and corticosteroids are ineffective. Cultures of blood, epiglottic surface, and, in selected cases, cerebrospinal fluid should be collected after the airway is stabilized. *Cefotaxime, ceftriaxone,* or *meropenem* should be given parenterally, pending culture and susceptibility reports, because 10-40% of *H. influenzae* type b cases are resistant to ampicillin. After insertion of the artificial airway, the patient should improve immediately, and respiratory distress and cyanosis

should disappear. Epiglottitis resolves after a few days of antibiotics, and the patient may be extubated; antibiotics should be continued for at least 10 days. Chemoprophylaxis is not routinely recommended for household, childcare, or nursery contacts of patients with invasive *H. influenzae* type b infections, but careful observation is mandatory, with prompt medical evaluation when exposed children develop a febrile illness. **Indications for rifampin prophylaxis** (20 mg/kg orally once a day for 4 days; maximum dose: 600 mg) for all household members include a child younger than 4 yr of age and incompletely immunized, younger than 12 mo of age and has not completed the primary vaccination series, or immunocompromised.

Acute laryngeal swelling on an allergic basis responds to epinephrine (1:1,000 dilution in dosage of 0.01 mL/kg to a maximum of 0.5 mL/dose) administered intramuscularly or racemic epinephrine (dose of 0.5 mL of 2.25% racemic epinephrine in 3 mL of normal saline) (see Chapter 149). Corticosteroids are often required (1-2 mg/ kg/24 hr of prednisone for 3-5 days). After recovery, the patient and parents should be discharged with a preloaded syringe of epinephrine to be used in emergencies. Reactive mucosal swelling, severe stridor, and respiratory distress unresponsive to mist therapy may follow endotracheal intubation for general anesthesia in children. Racemic epinephrine and corticosteroids are helpful.

Endotracheal/Nasotracheal Intubation and Tracheotomy

With the introduction of routine intubation or, less often, tracheotomy for epiglottitis, the mortality rate for epiglottis has dropped to almost zero. These procedures should always be performed in an operating room or intensive care unit if time permits; prior intubation and general anesthesia greatly facilitate performing a tracheotomy without complications. The use of an endotracheal or nasotracheal tube that is 0.5-1.0 mm smaller than estimated by age or height is recommended to facilitate intubation and reduce long-term sequelae. The choice of procedure should be based on the local expertise and experience with the procedure and postoperative care.

Intubation or tracheotomy is required for most patients with bacterial tracheitis and all young patients with epiglottitis. It is rarely required for patients with laryngotracheobronchitis, spasmodic croup, or laryngitis. Severe forms of laryngotracheobronchitis that require intubation in a high proportion of patients have been reported during severe measles and influenza A virus epidemics. Assessing the need for these procedures requires experience and judgment because they should not be delayed until cyanosis and extreme restlessness have developed (see Chapter 71). As with epiglottitis, an endotracheal or nasotracheal tube that is 0.5-1.0 mm smaller than estimated by age or height is recommended.

The endotracheal tube or tracheostomy must remain in place until edema and spasm have subsided and the patient is able to handle secretions satisfactorily. It should be removed as soon as possible, usually within a few days. Adequate resolution of epiglottic inflammation that has been accurately confirmed by fiberoptic laryngoscopy, permitting much more rapid extubation, often occurs within 24 hr. Racemic epinephrine and dexamethasone (0.5 mg/kg/dose 6-12 hr prior to extubation then every 6 hr for 6 doses with a maximum dose of 10 mg) may be useful in the treatment of upper airway edema seen postintubation.

PROGNOSIS

In general, the length of hospitalization and the mortality rate for cases of acute infectious upper airway obstruction increase as the infection extends to involve a greater portion of the respiratory tract, except in epiglottitis, in which the localized infection itself can prove to be fatal. Most deaths from croup are caused by a laryngeal obstruction or by the complications of tracheotomy. Rarely, fatal out-of-hospital arrests caused by viral laryngotracheobronchitis have been reported, particularly in infants and in patients whose course has been complicated by bacterial tracheitis. Untreated epiglottitis has a mortality rate of 6% in some series, but if the diagnosis is made and appropriate treatment is initiated before the patient is moribund, the prognosis is excellent. The outcome of acute laryngotracheobronchitis, laryngitis, and spasmodic croup is also excellent.

Bibliography is available at Expert Consult.

385.2 Bacterial Tracheitis

Genie E. Roosevelt

Bacterial tracheitis is an acute bacterial infection of the upper airway that is potentially life threatening. *S. aureus* (see Chapter 181) is the most commonly isolated pathogen with isolated reports of methicillin-resistant *S. aureus*. *S. pneumoniae*, *S. pyogenes*, *Moraxella catarrhalis*, nontypeable *H. influenzae*, and anaerobic organisms have also been implicated. The mean age is between 5 and 7 yr. There is a slight male predominance. Bacterial tracheitis often follows a viral respiratory infection (especially laryngotracheitis), so it may be considered a bacterial complication of a viral disease, rather than a primary bacterial illness. This life-threatening entity is more common than epiglottitis in vaccinated populations.

CLINICAL MANIFESTATIONS

Typically, the child has a brassy cough, apparently as part of a viral laryngotracheobronchitis. High fever and "toxicity" with respiratory distress can occur immediately or after a few days of apparent improvement. The patient can lie flat, does not drool, and does not have the dysphagia associated with epiglottitis. The usual treatment for croup (racemic epinephrine) is ineffective. Intubation or tracheostomy may be necessary, but only 50-60% of patients require intubation for management; younger patients are more likely to need intubation. The major pathologic feature appears to be mucosal swelling at the level of the cricoid cartilage, complicated by copious, thick, purulent secretions, sometimes causing pseudomembranes. Suctioning these secretions, although occasionally affording temporary relief, usually does not sufficiently obviate the need for an artificial airway.

DIAGNOSIS

The diagnosis is based on evidence of bacterial upper airway disease, which includes high fever, purulent airway secretions, and an absence of the classic findings of epiglottitis. X-rays are not needed but can show the classic findings (Fig. 385-3); purulent material is noted below the cords during endotracheal intubation (Fig. 385-4).

TREATMENT

Appropriate antimicrobial therapy, which usually includes antistaphylococcal agents, should be instituted in any patient whose course suggests bacterial tracheitis. Current empiric therapy recommendations for bacterial tracheitis include vancomycin or clindamycin and a third-generation cephalosporin (e.g., cefotaxime or ceftriaxone). When bacterial tracheitis is diagnosed by direct laryngoscopy or is strongly

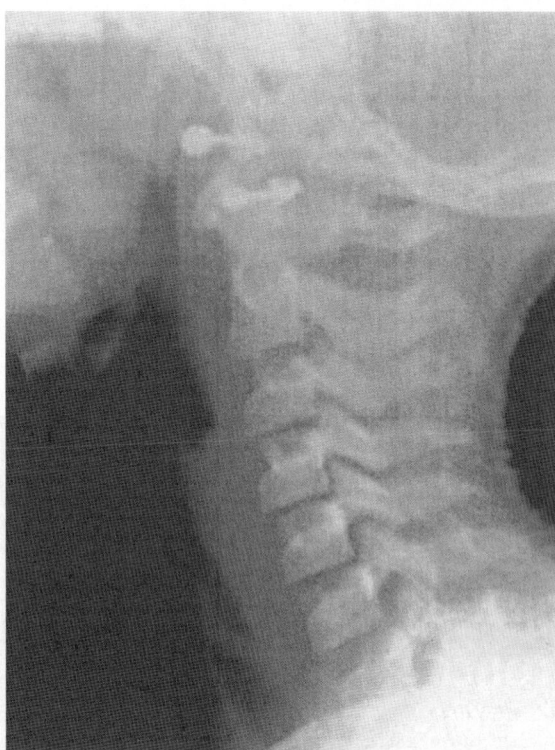

Figure 385-3 Lateral radiograph of the neck of a patient with bacterial tracheitis, showing pseudomembrane detachment in the trachea. *(From Stroud RH, Friedman NR: An update on inflammatory disorders of the pediatric airway: epiglottitis, croup, and tracheitis, Am J Otolaryngol 22:268–275, 2001. Photo courtesy of the Department of Radiology, University of Texas Medical Branch at Galveston.)*

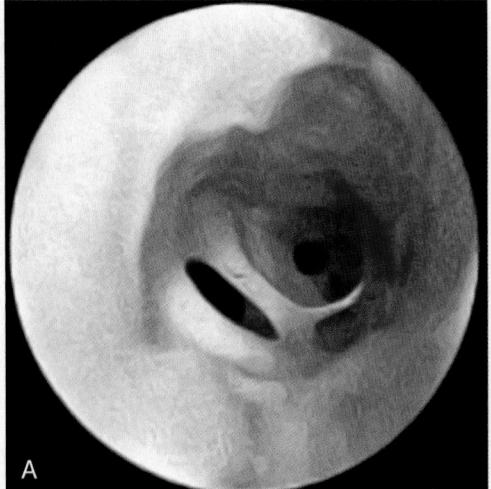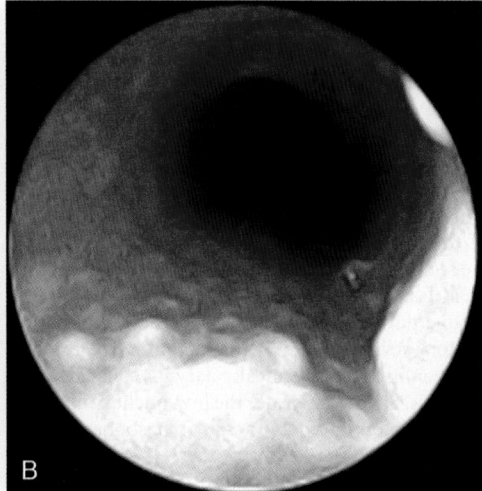

Figure 385-4 Thick tracheal membranes seen on rigid bronchoscopy. The supraglottis was normal. **A,** Thick adherent membranous secretions. **B,** The distal tracheobronchial tree is unremarkable. In contrast to croup, tenacious secretions are seen throughout the trachea, and in contrast to bronchitis, the bronchi are not affected. *(From Salamone FN, Bobbitt DB, Myer CM, et al: Bacterial tracheitis reexamined: is there a less severe manifestation? Otolaryngol Head Neck Surg 131:871–876, 2004. © 2004 American Academy of Otolaryngology–Head and Neck Surgery Foundation, Inc.)*

suspected on clinical grounds, an artificial airway should be strongly considered. Supplemental oxygen is usually necessary.

COMPLICATIONS

Chest radiographs often show patchy infiltrates and may show focal densities. Subglottic narrowing and a rough and ragged tracheal air column can often be demonstrated radiographically. If airway management is not optimal, cardiorespiratory arrest can occur. Toxic shock syndrome has been associated with staphylococcal and group A streptococcal tracheitis (see Chapter 181.2).

PROGNOSIS

The prognosis for most patients is excellent. Patients usually become afebrile within 2-3 days of the institution of appropriate antimicrobial therapy, but prolonged hospitalization may be necessary. In recent years, there appears to be a trend toward a less-morbid condition. With a decrease in mucosal edema and purulent secretions, extubation can be accomplished safely, and the patient should be observed carefully while antibiotics and oxygen therapy are continued.

Bibliography is available at Expert Consult.

Chapter **386**
Congenital Anomalies of the Larynx, Trachea, and Bronchi

James W. Schroeder Jr. and Lauren D. Holinger

The larynx functions as a breathing passage, a valve to protect the lungs, and the primary organ of communication; symptoms of laryngeal anomalies are those of airway obstruction, difficulty feeding, and abnormalities of phonation (see Chapter 373). Obstructive congenital lesions of the upper airway produce turbulent airflow according to the laws of fluid dynamics. This rapid, turbulent airflow across a narrowed segment of respiratory tract produces distinctive sounds that are diagnostically useful to the clinician. The timing of noisy breathing in relation to the sleep–wake cycle is important. Obstruction of the pharyngeal airway (by enlarged tonsils, adenoids, tongue, or syndromes with midface hypoplasia) typically produces worse obstruction during sleep than during waking. Obstruction that is worse when awake is typically laryngeal, tracheal, or bronchial, and is exacerbated by exertion. The location of the obstruction dictates the respiratory phase, tone and nature of the sound and these qualities direct the differential diagnosis. Intrathoracic lesions typically cause expiratory wheezing and stridor, often masquerading as asthma. The expiratory wheezing contrasts to the inspiratory stridor caused by the extrathoracic lesions of congenital laryngeal anomalies, specifically laryngomalacia and bilateral vocal cord paralysis. Stridor describes the low-pitched inspiratory snoring sound typically produced by nasal or nasopharyngeal obstruction.

With airway obstruction, the severity of the obstructing lesion, the work of breathing, determines the necessity for diagnostic procedures and surgical intervention. Obstructive symptoms vary from mild to severe stridor with episodes of apnea, cyanosis, suprasternal (tracheal tugging) and subcostal retractions, dyspnea, and tachypnea. Congenital anomalies of the trachea and bronchi can create serious respiratory

difficulties from the 1st few min of life. Chronic obstruction can cause failure to thrive.

Bibliography is available at Expert Consult.

386.1 Laryngomalacia
James W. Schroeder Jr. and Lauren D. Holinger

CLINICAL MANIFESTATIONS

Laryngomalacia is the most common congenital laryngeal anomaly and the most common cause of stridor in infants and children. Sixty percent of congenital laryngeal anomalies in children with stridor are due to laryngomalacia. Stridor is inspiratory, low-pitched, and exacerbated by any exertion: crying, agitation, or feeding. The stridor is caused, in part, by decreased laryngeal tone leading to supraglottic collapse during inspiration. Symptoms usually appear within the 1st 2 wk of life and increase in severity for up to 6 mo, although gradual improvement can begin at any time. Gastroesophageal reflux disease and neurologic disease influence the severity of the disease and thereby the clinical course.

DIAGNOSIS

The diagnosis is made primarily based on symptoms. The diagnosis is confirmed by outpatient flexible laryngoscopy (Fig. 386-1). When the work of breathing is moderate to severe, airway films and chest radiographs are indicated. Laryngomalacia can contribute to feeding difficulties and dysphagia in some children because of decreased laryngeal sensation and poor suck swallow breath coordination. When the inspiratory stridor sounds wet or is associated with a cough or when there is a history of repeat upper respiratory illness or pneumonia, dysphagia should be considered. When dysphagia is suspected, a contrast swallow study and/or a fiberoptic endoscopic evaluation of swallowing esophagram may be considered. Because 15-60% of infants with laryngomalacia have synchronous airway anomalies, complete bronchoscopy is undertaken for patients with moderate to severe obstruction.

TREATMENT

Expectant observation is suitable for most infants because most symptoms resolve spontaneously as the child and airway grow.

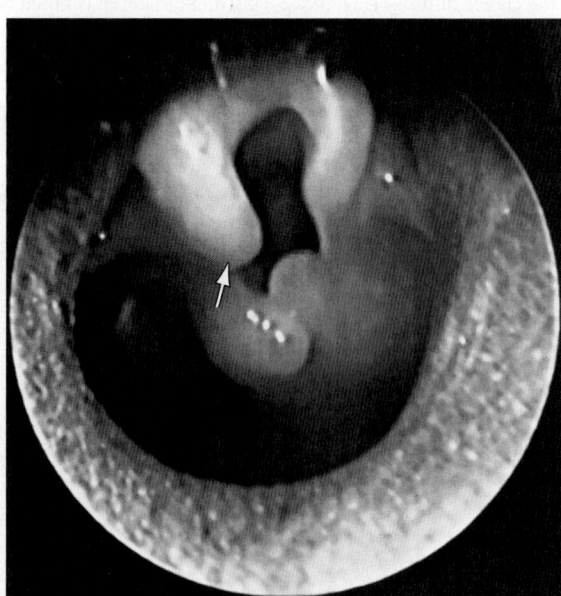

Figure 386-1 Endoscopic example of laryngomalacia. On inspiration, the epiglottic folds collapse into the airway. The lateral tips of the epiglottis are also collapsing inward *(arrow)*. *(From Slovis TL, editor: Caffey's pediatric diagnostic imaging, ed 11, Philadelphia, 2008, Mosby.)*

Laryngopharyngeal reflux is managed aggressively. In 15-20% of patients symptoms are severe enough to cause progressive respiratory distress, cyanosis, or failure to thrive. In these patients surgical intervention via supraglattoplasty is considered. Supraglattoplasty is 90% successful in relieving upper airway obstruction caused by laryngomalacia.

Bibliography is available at Expert Consult.

386.2 Congenital Subglottic Stenosis
James W. Schroeder Jr. and Lauren D. Holinger

CLINICAL MANIFESTATIONS
Congenital subglottic stenosis is the second most common cause of stridor. The subglottis is the narrowest part of the upper airway in a child. Subglottic stenosis is a narrowing of the subglottic larynx, which is the space extending from the undersurface of the true vocal cords to the inferior margin of the cricoid cartilage. It typically causes respiratory distress and biphasic or primarily inspiratory stridor. It may be congenital or acquired. Symptoms often occur with a respiratory tract infection as the edema and thickened secretions of a common cold narrow an already compromised airway leading to recurrent or persistent croup like symptoms.

Biphasic or primarily inspiratory stridor is the typical presenting symptom for congenital subglottic stenosis. Recurrent or persistent croup usually occurs in these children at 6 mo of age or younger. The edema and thickened secretions of the common cold further narrow an already marginal airway that leads to croup-like symptoms. The stenosis can be caused by an abnormally shaped cricoid cartilage; by a tracheal ring that becomes trapped underneath the cricoid cartilage; or by soft tissue thickening caused by ductal cysts, submucosal gland hyperplasia or fibrosis.

DIAGNOSIS
The diagnosis made by airway radiographs is confirmed by direct laryngoscopy. During diagnostic laryngoscopy the subglottic larynx is visualized directly and sized objectively using endotracheal tubes (Fig. 386-2). The percentage of stenosis is determined by comparing the size of the patients' larynx to a standard of laryngeal dimensions based on age. Stenosis >50% is usually symptomatic and often requires treatment. As with all cases of upper airway obstruction, tracheostomy is avoided when possible. Dilation and endoscopic laser surgery are rarely effective because most congenital stenoses are cartilaginous. Anterior laryngotracheal decompression (cricoid split) or laryngotracheal reconstruction with cartilage grafting is usually effective in avoiding tracheostomy. The differential diagnosis includes other anatomic anomalies as well as a hemangioma or papillomatosis.

Bibliography is available at Expert Consult.

386.3 Vocal Cord Paralysis
James W. Schroeder Jr. and Lauren D. Holinger

CLINICAL MANIFESTATIONS
Vocal cord paralysis is the third most common congenital laryngeal anomaly that produces stridor in infants and children. Congenital central nervous system lesions such as myelomeningocele, Chiari malformation, and hydrocephalus may be associated with bilateral paralysis.

Unilateral vocal cord paralysis is most often iatrogenic as a result of surgical treatment for gastrointestinal (tracheoesophageal fistula) and cardiovascular (patent ductus arteriosis repair) anomalies. Bilateral vocal cord paralysis produces airway obstruction manifested by high-pitched inspiratory stridor: a phonatory sound or inspiratory cry. Unilateral paralysis causes aspiration, coughing, and choking; the cry is weak and breathy, but stridor and other symptoms of airway obstruction are less common.

DIAGNOSIS
The diagnosis of vocal cord paralysis is made by awake flexible laryngoscopy. A thorough investigation for the underlying primary cause is indicated. Because of the association with other congenital lesions, evaluation includes neurology and cardiology consultations as well as diagnostic endoscopy of the larynx, trachea, and bronchi.

TREATMENT
Treatment is based on the severity of the symptoms. Vocal cord paralysis in infants usually resolves spontaneously within 6-12 mo. If it does not resolve within 2-3 yr, it is unlikely to do so. Bilateral paralysis can require temporary tracheotomy. Procedures that widen the posterior glottis to relieve the obstruction include laryngotracheal reconstruction using an endoscopically placed posterior glottis cartilage graft, or arytenoidectomy, or arytenoid lateralization. These procedures are successful in reducing the obstruction. However, they may result in aspiration that may become severe. For unilateral vocal cord paralysis with aspiration, injection laterally to the paralyzed vocal cord moves it medially to reduce aspiration and related complications.

386.4 Congenital Laryngeal Webs and Atresia
James W. Schroeder Jr. and Lauren D. Holinger

Most congenital laryngeal webs are glottic with subglottic extension and associated subglottic stenosis. Chromosomal and cardiovascular anomalies as well as chromosome 22 q 11 deletion are common in patients with congenital laryngeal web. Airway obstruction is not always present and may be related to the subglottic stenosis. Thick webs may be suspected in lateral radiographs of the airway. Diagnosis is made by direct laryngoscopy (Fig. 386-3). Treatment might require only incision or dilation. Webs with associated subglottic stenosis are likely to require cartilage augmentation of the cricoid cartilage (laryngotracheal reconstruction). Laryngeal atresia occurs as a complete glottic web and commonly is associated with tracheal agenesis and tracheoesophageal fistula.

Bibliography is available at Expert Consult.

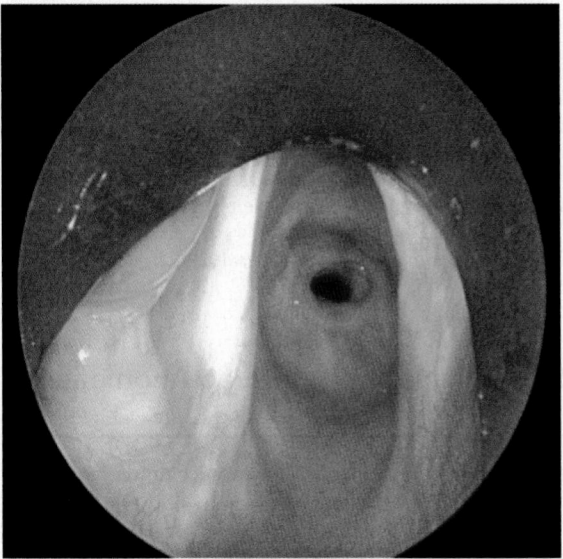

Figure 386-2 Subglottic stenosis. *(Courtesy of Rn Cantab, Wikipedia Commons.)*

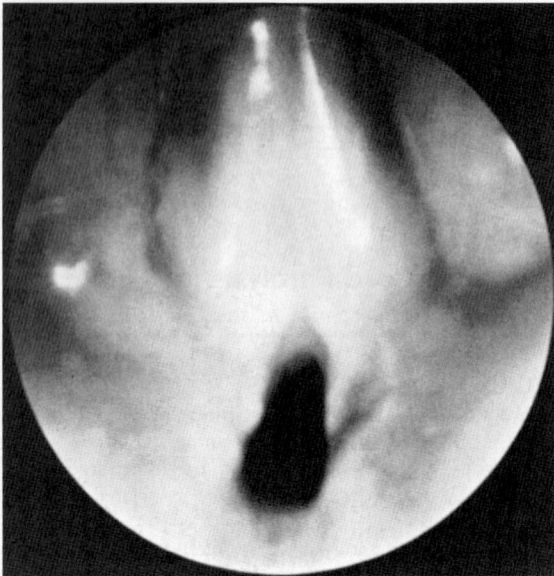

Figure 386-3 Anterior glottic web. Most of the membranous true vocal cords are involved. *(From Milczuk HA, Smith JD, Evans EC: Congenital laryngeal webs: surgical management and clinical embryology, Int J Pediatr Otorhinolaryngol 52(1):1–9, 2000.)*

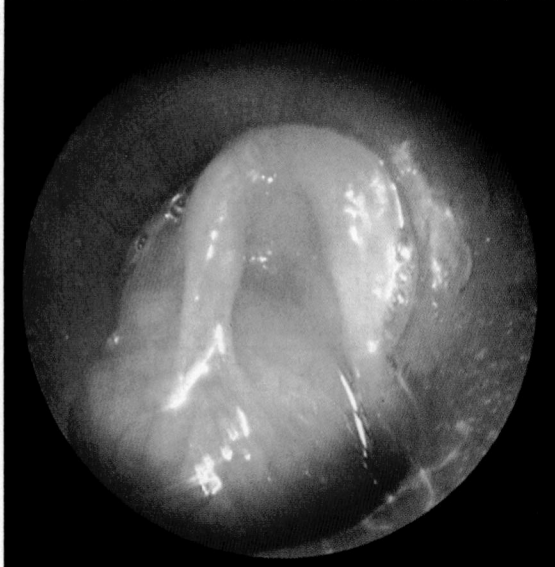

Figure 386-4 Endoscopic photograph of a saccular cyst. *(From Ahmad SM, Soliman AMS: Congenital anomalies of the larynx, Otolaryngol Clin North Am 40:177–191, 2007, Fig. 3.)*

386.5 Congenital Subglottic Hemangioma
James W. Schroeder Jr. and Lauren D. Holinger

Symptoms of airway obstruction typically occur within the 1st 2 mo. of life. Stridor is biphasic but usually more prominent during inspiration. A barking cough, hoarseness, and symptoms of recurrent or persistent croup are typical. Only 1% of children who have cutaneous hemangiomas will have a subglottic hemangioma. However, 50% of those with a subglottic hemangioma will have a cutaneous hemangioma. A facial hemangioma is not always present, but when it is evident, it is in the beard distribution. Chest and neck radiographs can show the characteristic asymmetric narrowing of the subglottic larynx. Treatment is discussed in Chapter 390.3.

Bibliography is available at Expert Consult.

386.6 Laryngoceles and Saccular Cysts
James W. Schroeder Jr. and Lauren D. Holinger

A laryngocele is an abnormal air-filled dilation of the laryngeal saccule that arises vertically between the false vocal cord, the base of the epiglottic and the inner surface of the thyroid cartilage. It communicates with the laryngeal lumen and, when intermittently filled with air, causes hoarseness and dyspnea. A saccular cyst (congenital cyst of the larynx) is distinguished from the laryngocele in that its lumen is isolated from the interior of the larynx and it contains mucus, not air in infants and children, laryngoceles cause hoarseness and dyspnea that may increase with crying. Saccular cysts may cause respiratory distress and stridor. A saccular cyst may be visible on radiography, but the diagnosis is made by laryngoscopy (Fig. 386-4). Needle aspiration of the cyst confirms the diagnosis but rarely provides a cure. Approaches include endoscopic CO_2 laser excision, endoscopic extended ventriculotomy (marsupialization or unroofing), or, traditionally, external excision.

Bibliography is available at Expert Consult.

386.7 Posterior Laryngeal Cleft and Laryngotracheoesophageal Cleft
James W. Schroeder Jr. and Lauren D. Holinger

The posterior laryngeal cleft is characterized by aspiration and is the result of a deficiency in the midline of the posterior larynx. Posterior laryngeal clefts are categorized into 4 types. Type 1 clefts are mild and the interarytenoid notch only extends down to the level of the true vocal cords; 60% of these will cause no symptoms and will not require surgical repair. In severe cases, the cleft (type 4) extends inferiorly into the cervical or thoracic trachea so there is no separation between the trachea and esophagus, creating a laryngotracheoesophageal cleft. Laryngeal clefts can occur in families and are likely to be associated with tracheal agenesis, tracheoesophageal fistula, and multiple congenital anomalies, as with G syndrome, Opitz-Frias syndrome, and Pallister-Hall syndrome.

Initial symptoms are those of aspiration and recurrent respiratory infections. Esophagogram is undertaken with extreme caution. Confirmation of the diagnosis is made by direct laryngoscopy and bronchoscopy. Treatment is based on the cleft type and the symptoms. Stabilization of the airway is the first priority. Gastroesophageal reflux must be controlled and a careful assessment for other congenital anomalies is undertaken before repair. Several endoscopic and open cervical and transthoracic surgical repairs have been described.

Bibliography is available at Expert Consult.

386.8 Vascular and Cardiac Anomalies
James W. Schroeder Jr. and Lauren D. Holinger

The aberrant innominate artery is the most common cause of secondary tracheomalacia (see Chapter 432). It may be asymptomatic and discovered incidentally or it may cause severe symptoms. Expiratory wheezing and cough occur and, rarely, reflex apnea or "dying spells." Surgical intervention is rarely necessary. Infants are treated expectantly because the problem is self-limited.

The term *vascular ring* is used to describe vascular anomalies that result from abnormal development of the aortic arch complex. The double aortic arch is the most common complete vascular ring, encircling both the trachea and esophagus, compressing both. With few exceptions, these patients are symptomatic by 3 mo of age. Respiratory symptoms predominate, but dysphagia may be present. The diagnosis is established by barium esophagram that shows a posterior indentation of the esophagus by the vascular ring (see Fig. 432-2 in Chapter 432). CT scan with contrast or MRI with angiography provides the surgeon the information needed.

Other vascular anomalies include the pulmonary artery sling, which also requires surgical correction. The most common open (incomplete) vascular ring is the aberrant right subclavian artery. Although common, it is usually asymptomatic and of academic interest only.

Congenital cardiac defects are likely to compress the left main bronchus or lower trachea. Any condition that produces significant pulmonary hypertension increases the size of the pulmonary arteries, which in turn cause compression of the left main bronchus. Surgical correction of the underlying pathology to relieve pulmonary hypertension relieves the airway compression.

Bibliography is available at Expert Consult.

386.9 Tracheal Stenoses, Webs, and Atresia
James W. Schroeder Jr. and Lauren D. Holinger

Long-segment congenital tracheal stenosis with complete tracheal rings typically occurs within the 1st yr of life, usually after a crisis has been precipitated by an acute respiratory illness. The diagnosis may be suggested by plain radiographs. CT with contrast delineates associated intrathoracic anomalies such as the pulmonary artery sling, which occurs in one third of patients; one fourth have associated cardiac anomalies. Bronchoscopy is the best method to define the degree and extent of the stenosis and the associated abnormal bronchial branching pattern. Treatment of clinically significant stenosis involves tracheal resection of short segment stenosis, slide tracheoplasty for long segment stenosis. Congenital soft-tissue stenoses and thin webs are rare. Dilation may be all that is required.

Bibliography is available at Expert Consult.

386.10 Foregut Cysts
James W. Schroeder Jr. and Lauren D. Holinger

The bronchogenic cyst, intramural esophageal cyst (esophageal duplication), and enteric cyst can all produce symptoms of respiratory obstruction and dysphagia. The diagnosis is suspected when chest radiographs or CT scan delineate the mass, and, in the case of enteric cyst, the associated vertebral anomaly. The treatment of all foregut cysts is surgical excision.

Bibliography is available at Expert Consult.

386.11 Tracheomalacia and Bronchomalacia

See Chapter 389.

Chapter 387
Foreign Bodies in the Airway
James W. Schroeder Jr. and Lauren D. Holinger

EPIDEMIOLOGY AND ETIOLOGY

Choking is a leading cause of morbidity and mortality among children, especially those younger than age 4 yr, largely because of the developmental vulnerabilities of a young child's airway and the underdeveloped ability to swallow food. Infants and toddlers use their mouths to explore their surroundings. Most victims of foreign-body aspiration are older infants and toddlers (Fig. 387-1). Children, younger than 3 yr of age, account for 73% of cases. Preambulatory toddlers can aspirate objects given to them by older siblings. The most common objects that children choke on are food, coins, balloons, and toys. One-third of aspirated objects are nuts, particularly peanuts. Fragments of raw carrot, apple, dried beans, popcorn, and sunflower or watermelon seeds are also aspirated, as are small toys or toy parts. Hard candy and chewing gum are also commonly involved objects. Adolescents may aspirate objects put in their mouth such as pins, jewelry, or blowgun darts. From 1972-1992, 449 deaths from aspirated nonfood foreign bodies among children were reported by the United States Consumer Product Safety Commission. An infant is developmentally able to suck and swallow and also is equipped with involuntary reflexes (gag, cough, and glottis closure) that help to protect against aspiration during swallowing. Dentition develops at approximately 6 mo with eruption of the incisors. Molars do not erupt until approximately 1.5 yr of age; however, mature mastication takes longer to develop. Despite a strong gag reflex, a young child's airway is more vulnerable to obstruction than an adult's airway in several ways. The smaller diameter is more likely to experience significant blockage by small foreign bodies. Mucous and secretions may form a seal around the foreign body, making it more difficult to dislodge by forced air. In addition, the force of air generated by a cough in an infant or young child is less effective in dislodging an airway obstruction. The American Academy of Pediatrics recommends that children younger than 5 yr old should avoid hard candy, chewing gum and that raw fruits and vegetables be cut into small pieces.

The most serious complication of foreign-body aspiration is complete obstruction of the airway. Globular or round food objects such

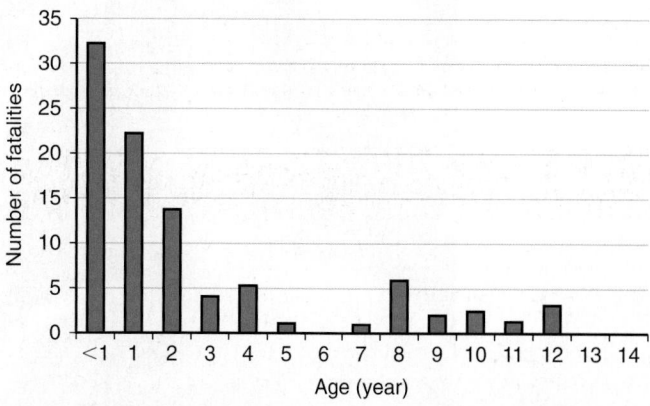

Figure 387-1 Number of fatalities vs victim age, all fatality types. *(From Milkovich SM, Altkorn R, Chen X, et al: Development of the small parts cylinder: lessons learned, Laryngoscope 118[11]:2082–2086, 2008.)*

as hot dogs, grapes, nuts, and candies are the most frequent offenders. Hot dogs are rarely seen as airway foreign bodies because toddlers who choke on hot dogs asphyxiate at the scene unless treated immediately. Complete airway obstruction is recognized in the conscious child as sudden respiratory distress followed by inability to speak or cough.

CLINICAL MANIFESTATIONS

Three stages of symptoms may result from aspiration of an object into the airway:

1. **Initial event:** Violent paroxysms of coughing, choking, gagging, and possibly airway obstruction occur immediately when the foreign body is aspirated.
2. **Asymptomatic interval:** The foreign body becomes lodged, reflexes fatigue, and the immediate irritating symptoms subside. This stage is most treacherous and accounts for a large percentage of delayed diagnoses and overlooked foreign bodies. It is during this 2nd stage, when the child is first seen, that the possibility of a foreign-body aspiration is minimized, the physician being reassured by the absence of symptoms that no foreign body is present.
3. **Complications:** Obstruction, erosion, or infection develops to direct attention again to the presence of a foreign body. In this 3rd stage, complications include fever, cough, hemoptysis, pneumonia, and atelectasis.

DIAGNOSIS

A positive history must never be ignored. A negative history may be misleading. Choking or coughing episodes accompanied by new onset wheezing are highly suggestive of an airway foreign body. Because nuts are the most common bronchial foreign body, the physician specifically questions the toddler's parents about nuts. If there is any history of eating nuts, bronchoscopy is carried out promptly.

Most airway foreign bodies lodge in a bronchus (right bronchus ~58% of cases); the location is the larynx or trachea in approximately 10% of cases. Occasionally, fragments of a foreign body may produce bilateral involvement or shifting infiltrates if it moves from lobe to lobe. An esophageal foreign body can compress the trachea and be mistaken for an airway foreign body. The patient is asymptomatic and the radiograph is normal in 15-30% of cases. Opaque foreign bodies occur in only 10-25% of cases. CT can help define radiolucent foreign bodies such as fish bones. If there is a high index of suspicion, bronchoscopy should be performed despite negative imaging studies. History is the most important factor in determining the need for bronchoscopy.

TREATMENT

The treatment of choice for airway foreign bodies is prompt endoscopic removal with rigid instruments. Bronchoscopy is deferred only until preoperative studies have been obtained and the patient has been prepared by adequate hydration and emptying of the stomach. Airway foreign bodies are usually removed the same day the diagnosis is first considered.

387.1 Laryngeal Foreign Bodies
James W. Schroeder Jr. and Lauren D. Holinger

Complete obstruction asphyxiates the child unless it is promptly relieved with the Heimlich maneuver (see Chapter 67 and Figs. 67-6 and 67-7). Objects that are partially obstructive are usually flat and thin. They lodge between the vocal cords in the sagittal plane, causing symptoms of croup, hoarseness, cough, stridor, and dyspnea.

387.2 Tracheal Foreign Bodies
James W. Schroeder Jr. and Lauren D. Holinger

Choking and aspiration occurs in 90% of patients with tracheal foreign bodies, stridor in 60%, and wheezing in 50%. Posteroanterior and lateral soft tissue neck radiographs (airway films) are abnormal in 92% of children, whereas chest radiographs are abnormal in only 58%.

387.3 Bronchial Foreign Bodies
James W. Schroeder Jr. and Lauren D. Holinger

Posteroanterior and lateral chest radiographs are standard in the assessment of infants and children suspected of having aspirated a foreign object. The abdomen is included. A good expiratory posteroanterior chest film is most helpful. During expiration the bronchial foreign body obstructs the exit of air from the obstructed lung, producing obstructive emphysema, air trapping, with persistent inflation of the obstructed lung and shift of the mediastinum toward the opposite side (Fig. 387-2). Air trapping is an immediate complication, in contrast to atelectasis, which is a late finding. Lateral decubitus chest films

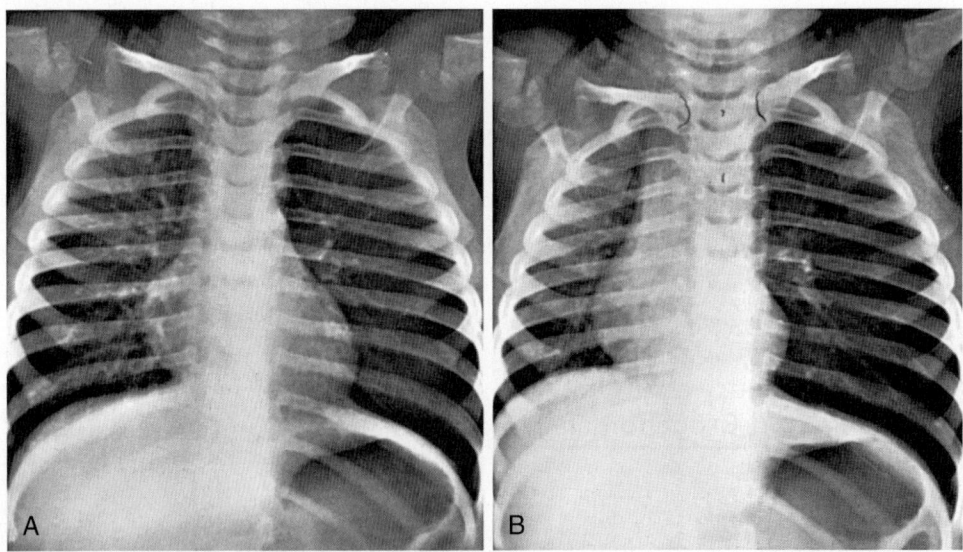

Figure 387-2 A, Normal inspiratory chest radiograph in a toddler with a peanut fragment in the left main bronchus. **B,** Expiratory radiograph of the same child showing the classic obstructive emphysema (air trapping) on the involved (left) side. Air leaves the normal right side allowing the lung to deflate. The medium shifts toward the unobstructed side.

or fluoroscopy can provide the same information but are unnecessary. History and physical examination, not radiographs, determine the indication for bronchoscopy.

Bibliography is available at Expert Consult.

Chapter **388**
Laryngotracheal Stenosis and Subglottic Stenosis

James W. Schroeder Jr.
and Lauren D. Holinger

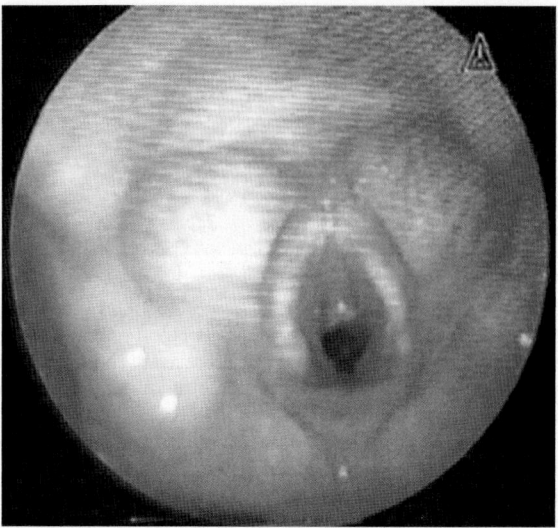

Figure 388-1 Laryngoscopy in 6 mo old infant 4 hr after extubation showing granulation in subglottic region. *(From Smith MM, Kuhl G, Carvalho PR, Marostica PJ: Flexible fiber-optic laryngoscopy in the first hours after extubation for the evaluation of laryngeal lesions due to intubation in the pediatric intensive care unit. Int J Pediatr Otorhino-laryngol 71(9):1423–1428, 2007, Fig. 4.)*

Laryngotracheal stenosis is the second most common cause of stridor in neonates and is the most common cause of airway obstruction requiring tracheostomy in infants. The glottis (vocal cords) and the upper trachea are also compromised in most laryngeal stenoses, particularly those that develop following endotracheal intubation. Subglottic stenosis is a narrowing of the subglottic larynx, which is the space extending from the undersurface of the true vocal cords to the inferior margin of the cricoid cartilage. Subglottic stenosis is considered to be congenital when there is no other apparent cause such as a history of laryngeal trauma; approximately 90% of cases manifest in the 1st yr of life.

388.1 Congenital Subglottic Stenosis

See Chapter 386.2.

388.2 Acquired Laryngotracheal Stenosis

James W. Schroeder Jr. and Lauren D. Holinger

Ninety percent of acquired stenoses are associated with endotracheal intubation, although with improved ventilatory support, the incidence of this complication is decreasing. Studies published after 1983 reported an incidence of neonatal subglottic stenosis of <4%, and those after 1990 reported an incidence of <0.63%. When the pressure of the endotracheal tube against the mucosa is greater than the capillary pressure, ischemia occurs, followed by necrosis and ulceration. Secondary infection and perichondritis develop with exposure of cartilage. Granulation tissue forms around the ulcerations (Fig. 388-1). These changes and edema throughout the larynx usually resolve spontaneously after extubation. Chronic edema and fibrous stenosis develop in only a small percentage of cases. A number of factors predispose to the development of laryngeal stenosis. Laryngopharyngeal reflux of acid and pepsin from the stomach exacerbates endotracheal tube trauma. More damage is caused in areas left unprotected, owing to loss of mucosa. Congenital subglottic stenosis narrows the larynx which makes the patient more likely to develop

acquired subglottic stenosis because significant injury is more likely to occur with use of an endotracheal tube of age-appropriate size. Other risk factors for the development of acquired subglottic stenosis include sepsis and infection, dehydration, malnutrition, chronic inflammatory disorders, and immunosuppression. An oversized endotracheal tube is the most common factor contributing to laryngeal injury. A tube that allows a small air leak at the end of the inspiratory cycle minimizes potential trauma. Other extrinsic factors—traumatic intubation, multiple reintubations, movement of the endotracheal tube, and duration of intubation—can contribute to varying degrees in individual patients.

CLINICAL MANIFESTATIONS
Symptoms of acquired and congenital stenosis are similar. Spasmodic croup, the sudden onset of severe croup in the early morning hours, is usually caused by laryngopharyngeal reflux with transient laryngospasm and subsequent laryngeal edema. These frightening episodes resolve rapidly, often before the family and child reach the emergency department.

DIAGNOSIS
The diagnosis can be made by posteroanterior and lateral airway radiographs and is confirmed by direct laryngoscopy and bronchoscopy. High-resolution CT imaging is of limited value. This is similar to the work-up associated with congenital subglottic stenosis.

TREATMENT
The severity, location, and type (cartilaginous or soft tissue) of the stenosis determine the treatment. Mild cases can be managed without operative intervention because the airway will improve as the child grows. Moderate soft-tissue stenosis is treated by endoscopy using gentle dilations or CO_2 laser. Severe laryngotracheal stenosis is likely to require laryngotracheal expansion surgery or resection of the narrowed portion of the laryngeal and tracheal airway (partial cricotracheal resection). Every effort is made to avoid tracheotomy using endoscopic techniques or open surgical procedures.

Bibliography is available at Expert Consult.

Chapter 389
Bronchomalacia and Tracheomalacia

Jonathan D. Finder

Tracheomalacia and bronchomalacia refer to chondromalacia of a central airway, leading to insufficient cartilage to maintain airway patency throughout the respiratory cycle. These are common causes of persistent wheezing in infancy. Tracheomalacia and bronchomalacia can be either primary or secondary (Table 389-1). Primary tracheomalacia and bronchomalacia are often seen in premature infants, although most affected patients are born at term. Secondary tracheomalacia and bronchomalacia refers to the situation in which the central airway is compressed by adjacent structure (e.g., vascular ring; see Chapter 432) or deficient in cartilage because of tracheoesophageal fistula (see Chapter 319). Laryngomalacia can accompany primary bronchomalacia or tracheomalacia. Involvement of the entire central airway (laryngotracheobronchomalacia) is also seen.

CLINICAL MANIFESTATIONS

Primary tracheomalacia and bronchomalacia are principally disorders of infants, with a male:female ratio of 2:1. The dominant finding, low-pitched monophonic wheezing heard predominantly during expiration, is most prominent over the central airways. Parents often describe persistent respiratory congestion even in the absence of a viral respiratory infection. When the lesion involves only 1 main bronchus

Table 389-1	Classification of Tracheomalacia

PRIMARY TRACHEOMALACIA
Congenital absence of tracheal-supporting cartilages

SECONDARY TRACHEOMALACIA
Esophageal atresia, tracheoesophageal fistula
Vascular rings (double aortic arch)
Tracheal compression from an aberrant innominate artery
Tracheal compression from mediastinal masses
Abnormally soft tracheal cartilages associated with connective
   tissue disorders
Prolonged mechanical ventilation, chronic lung disease

From McNamara VM, Crabbe DC: Tracheomalacia, Paediatr Respir Rev 5:147–154, 2004.

(more commonly the left), the wheezing is louder on that side, and there may be unilateral palpable fremitus. In cases of tracheomalacia, the wheeze is loudest over the trachea. Hyperinflation and/or subcostal retractions do not occur unless the patient also has concurrent asthma, viral bronchiolitis, or other causes of peripheral airways obstruction. In the absence of asthma, patients with tracheomalacia and bronchomalacia are not helped by administration of a bronchodilator. Acquired tracheomalacia and bronchomalacia are seen in association with vascular compression (vascular rings, slings, and innominate artery compression). Tracheomalacia is the rule following correction of tracheoesophageal fistula. Other causes of acquired tracheomalacia, which may persist after surgical correction, are cardiomegaly. Bronchomalacia is common following lung transplantation, assumed to be secondary to the loss of bronchial artery supply leading to hypoxia of the cartilage. The importance of the physical exam cannot be understated; 1 study found that pediatric pulmonologists made a correct assessment of malacia based on symptoms, history, and lung function prior to bronchoscopy in 74% of cases.

DIAGNOSIS

Definitive diagnoses of tracheomalacia and bronchomalacia are established by flexible or rigid bronchoscopy (Fig. 389-1). The lesion is difficult to detect on plain radiographs. While fluoroscopy can demonstrate dynamic collapse and avoid the need for invasive diagnostic techniques, it is poorly sensitive. Pulmonary function testing can show a pattern of decreased peak flow and flattening of the flow-volume loop. Other important diagnostic modalities include MRI and CT scanning. MRI with angiography is especially useful when there is a possibility of vascular ring and should be performed when a right aortic arch is seen on plain film radiography.

TREATMENT

Postural drainage can help with clearance of secretions. β-Adrenergic agents should be avoided in the absence of asthma, because they can exacerbate loss of airway patency due to decreased airway tone. Nebulized ipratropium bromide may be useful. Endobronchial stents have been used in severely affected patients but have a high incidence of complications, ranging from airway obstruction due to granulation tissue to erosion into adjacent vascular structures. Continuous positive airway pressure via tracheostomy may be indicated for severe cases. Surgical approach (aortopexy and bronchopexy) is rarely required and only for patients who have life-threatening apnea, cyanosis, and bradycardia ("cyanotic spells") from airway obstruction, and/or who demonstrated vascular compression.

PROGNOSIS

Primary bronchomalacia and tracheomalacia have excellent prognoses, because airflow improves as the child and the airways grow. Patients with primary airway malacia usually take longer to recover from common respiratory infections. Wheezing at rest usually resolves

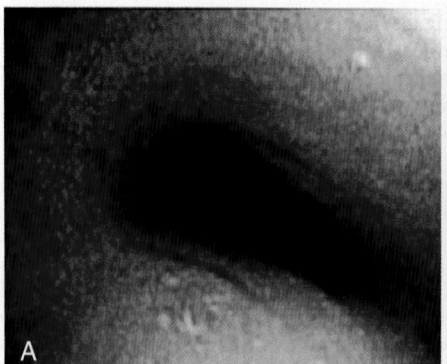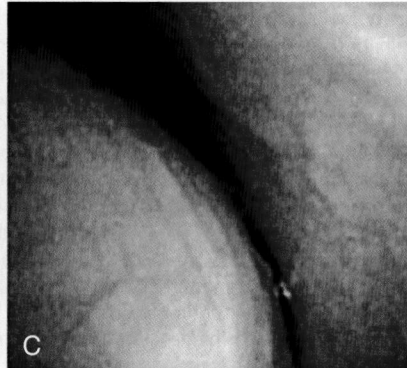

Figure 389-1 Images of tracheomalacia taken 10 mm from site. **A,** Saber-shaped or triangular appearance. **B,** Circumferential appearance. **C,** Crescent (lunate) appearance. *(From Masters IB, Zimmerman PV, Pandeya N, et al: Quantified tracheobronchomalacia disorders and their clinical profiles in children, Chest 133:461–467, 2008.)*

by age 3 yr. Prolonged bacterial bronchitis has been reported as a complication of bronchomalacia. Prognosis in secondary and acquired forms varies with cause. Patients with concurrent asthma need considerable supportive treatment and careful monitoring of respiratory status.

Bibliography is available at Expert Consult.

Chapter **390**
Neoplasms of the Larynx, Trachea, and Bronchi

390.1 Vocal Nodules
James W. Schroeder Jr. and Lauren D. Holinger

Vocal nodules, which are not true neoplasms, are the most common cause of chronic hoarseness in children. Chronic vocal abuse or misuse produces nodules at the junction of the anterior and middle thirds of the phonating edge of the vocal cords. These symmetric, bilateral swellings interfere with voice production and cause children to strain the voice. Vocal nodules can occur in infants.

When vocal abuse is the main factor, the voice is worse in the evenings. Voice therapy may be effective in the cooperative child, but for most toddlers and young children, behavioral therapy is necessary. Nodules usually resolve by early teenage years as the child matures and vocal abuse is moderated. Surgical excision is rarely indicated but may be necessary if the child is unable to communicate adequately, becomes aphonic, or requires tension and straining to make any utterance whatsoever.

When laryngopharyngeal reflux is the main factor, hoarseness is worse in the morning; laryngopharyngeal reflux commonly exacerbates vocal abuse, adding to swelling of the vocal cords. An antireflux regimen is indicated (see Chapter 323.1).

390.2 Recurrent Respiratory Papillomatosis
James W. Schroeder Jr. and Lauren D. Holinger

Papillomas are the most common respiratory tract neoplasms in children, occurring in 4.3 in 100,000. They are simply warts—benign tumors—caused by the human papillomavirus (HPV) (see Chapter 266); the same pathology is found in condylomata acuminata (vaginal warts). HPV types 6 and 11 are most commonly associated with laryngeal disease. Although it is a benign disease that usually involves the larynx, recurrent respiratory papillomatosis (RRP) has a predictable clinical course, tends to recur and spread throughout the aerodigestive tract and can undergo malignant conversion. Fifty percent of recurrent RRP cases occur in children younger than age 5 yr, but the diagnosis may be made at any age; 67% of children with RRP are born to mothers who had condylomata during pregnancy or parturition. The mode of HPV transmission is still not clear. The risk for transmission is approximately 1 in 500 vaginal births in mothers with active condylomata. Neonates have been reported to have RRP, suggesting intrauterine transmission of HPV.

CLINICAL MANIFESTATIONS
These benign squamous lesions can produce chronic hoarseness in the infant. Most occur in the larynx, specifically on the vocal cords, but in 31% these lesions occur in other areas of the respiratory tract: nose,

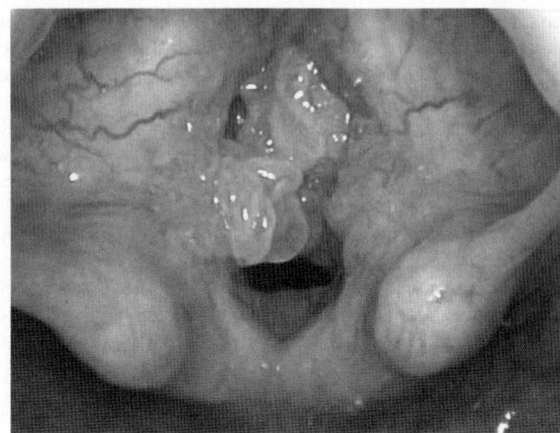
Figure 390-1 Laryngoscopic view of respiratory papillomas causing near complete obstruction at glottic level. *(From Derkay CS, Wiatrak B: Recurrent respiratory papillomatosis: a review, Laryngoscope 118: 1236–1245, 2008.)*

pharynx (especially the uvula and posterior soft palate), trachea, bronchi, and lungs. As growth of the lesions on the vocal cords progresses, hoarseness increases and communication becomes difficult. Respiratory distress develops. Surgical excision is a quality of life issue that warrants removal to improve the voice. Intervention becomes a medical necessity when airway obstruction progresses (Fig. 390-1). Symptoms often occur first during sleep with symptoms typical of obstructive sleep apnea. Progressive respiratory distress during sleep, exertion, daily activities, and finally at rest indicates the need for surgical intervention.

TREATMENT
The treatment of RRP is endoscopic surgical removal. Most surgeons in North America prefer the microdébrider. Laryngopharyngeal reflux can require treatment when reflux laryngitis is a factor. Although surgical management remains the mainstay therapy, some form of adjunct therapy may be needed in up to 20% of cases. The most widely accepted indications for adjunct therapy are a need for more than 4 surgical procedures per year, rapid regrowth of papillomata with airway compromise, or distal multisite spread of disease. Adjunct therapies include antiviral modalities (interferon, ribavirin, acyclovir, cidofovir), photodynamic therapy, dietary supplement (indole-3-carbinol), nonsteroidal antiinflammatory drug (Celebrex), retinoids, and mumps vaccination.

Bibliography is available at Expert Consult.

390.3 Congenital Subglottic Hemangioma
James W. Schroeder Jr. and Lauren D. Holinger

CLINICAL MANIFESTATIONS
Typically, congenital subglottic hemangiomas are symptomatic within the 1st 2 mo of life, almost all occurring before 6 mo of age. Stridor is biphasic but usually more prominent during inspiration. The infant may be hoarse, have a barking cough, and present with croup. Fifty percent of congenital subglottic hemangiomas are associated with facial lesions. Radiographs classically delineate an asymmetric subglottic narrowing. The diagnosis is made by direct laryngoscopy.

TREATMENT
The treatment of hemangiomas often requires input from a multispecialty vascular anomalies team. Medical management includes systemic steroids. Prednisone 2-4 mg/kg/day is given orally for 4-6 wk, less if the lesions stabilize sooner. The dosage is then tapered. If there is no response, the drug is discontinued. Propranolol 2-3 mg/kg/day is

emerging as a first-line treatment for hemangiomas with the potential to impair function (airway) or cause disfigurement if there are no cardiac or neurovascular contraindications. Although the exact mechanism of action of propranolol is unknown, it has been shown to stop progression and induce involution of hemangiomas in multiple studies. Because side effects include hypotension, bradycardia, bronchospasm, and hypoglycemia, children treated with propranolol need to be monitored closely.

Although tracheostomy establishes a safe airway, every effort should be made to find an alternative. Corticosteroids can also be injected directly into the lesion. Endoscopic excision with the CO_2 laser is effective. Combining several modalities increases the possibility of avoiding tracheotomy. External surgical excision is suitable for some lesions.

Bibliography is available at Expert Consult.

390.4 Vascular Anomalies
James W. Schroeder Jr. and Lauren D. Holinger

Vascular malformations are not true neoplastic lesions. They have a normal rate of endothelial turnover and various channel abnormalities. They are categorized by their predominant type (capillary, venous, arterial, lymphatic, or a combination thereof). Slow-flow malformations have capillary, lymphatic, or venous components. In the past, these were incorrectly called capillary hemangiomas, cystic hygromas or lymphangiomas, and cavernous hemangiomas, respectively.

Lymphatic malformations (cystic hygromas) rarely occur in the larynx. When they do, they are invariably an extension of disease from elsewhere in the head and neck. Airway obstruction can necessitate tracheostomy. The lesion can be debulked with the CO_2 laser.

Bibliography is available at Expert Consult.

390.5 Other Laryngeal Neoplasms
James W. Schroeder Jr. and Lauren D. Holinger

Neurofibromatosis (see Chapter 596.1) rarely involves the larynx. When children are affected, limited local resection is undertaken to maintain an airway and optimize the voice. Complete surgical extirpation is virtually impossible without debilitating resection of vital laryngeal structures. Most surgeons select the option of less-aggressive symptomatic surgery because of the poorly circumscribed and infiltrative nature of these fibromas. **Rhabdomyosarcoma** (see Chapter 500) and other malignant tumors of the larynx are rare. Symptoms of hoarseness and progressive airway obstruction prompt initial evaluation by flexible laryngoscopy in the office.

390.6 Tracheal Neoplasms
James W. Schroeder Jr. and Lauren D. Holinger

Tracheal tumors include malignant and benign neoplasms. The 2 most common benign tumors are inflammatory pseudotumor and hamartoma. The **inflammatory pseudotumor** is probably a reaction to a previous bronchial infection or traumatic insult. Growth is slow and the tumor may be locally invasive. Hamartomas are tumors of primary tissue elements that are abnormal in proportion and arrangement.

Tracheal neoplasms manifest with stridor, wheezing, cough, or pneumonia and are rarely diagnosed until 75% of the lumen has been obstructed (Fig. 390-2). Symptoms mimic asthma and are often misdiagnosed as such. Chest radiographs or airway films can identify the obstruction. Pulmonary function studies demonstrate an abnormal flow-volume loop. A mild response to bronchodilator therapy may be misleading. Rational treatment is based upon the histopathology.

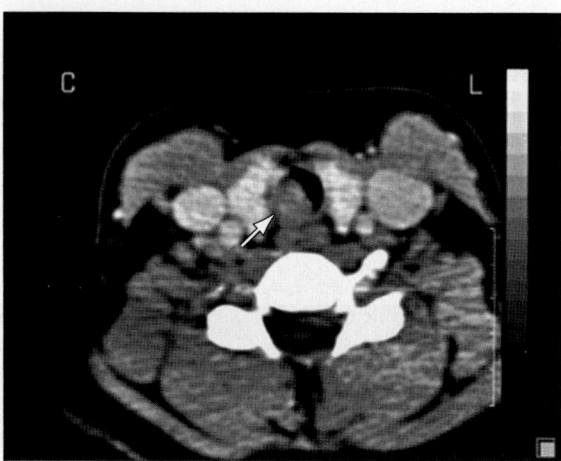

Figure 390-2 A CT scan of the trachea with a circumscribed intraluminal tracheal mass *(arrow)* in the tracheal wall. *(From Venizelos I, Papathomas T, Anagnostou E, et al: Pediatric inflammatory myofibroblastic tumor of the trachea: a case report and review of the literature, Pediatr Pulmonol 43:831–835, 2008.)*

390.7 Bronchial Tumors
James W. Schroeder Jr. and Lauren D. Holinger

Bronchial tumors are rare. Two-thirds are malignant. Bronchial "adenomas" are the most common, representing 30% of all lung tumors. Bronchogenic carcinoma is the second most common and occurs in approximately 20% of cases. Bronchial carcinoid also occurs. The diagnosis is confirmed at bronchoscopy and biopsy; treatment depends on the histopathology.

Chapter 391
Wheezing, Bronchiolitis, and Bronchitis

391.1 Wheezing in Infants: Bronchiolitis
Bria M. Coates, Lauren E. Camarda, and Denise M. Goodman

DEFINITIONS AND GENERAL PATHOPHYSIOLOGY

Wheezing, the production of a musical and continuous sound that originates from oscillations in narrowed airways, is heard mostly on expiration as a result of critical airway obstruction. **Monophonic** wheezing refers to a single-pitch sound that is produced in the larger airways during expiration, as in distal tracheomalacia or bronchomalacia. Wheezing is **polyphonic** when there is widespread narrowing of the airways, causing various pitches as air moves through different levels of obstruction to flow, as seen in asthma. When obstruction occurs in the extrathoracic airways during inspiration, the noise is referred to as **stridor.**

Infants are more likely to wheeze than older children and adults as a result of a differing set of lung mechanics. The obstruction to flow is affected by the airway caliber and compliance of the infant lung. Resistance to airflow through a tube is inversely related to the radius of the tube to the 4th power. In children younger than 5 yr old, small-caliber peripheral airways can contribute up to 50% of the total airway resistance. Marginal additional narrowing can cause further flow limitation and a subsequent wheeze.

With the very compliant newborn chest wall, the inward pressure produced in expiration subjects the intrathoracic airways to collapse. Differences in tracheal cartilage composition and airway smooth muscle tone increase the collapsibility of the infant airways in comparison to older children. These mechanisms combine to make the infant more susceptible to airway obstruction, increased resistance, and subsequent wheezing. Many of these conditions are outgrown in the 1st yr of life.

Immunologic and molecular influences can contribute to the infant's propensity to wheeze. In comparison to older children and adults, infants tend to have higher levels of lymphocytes and neutrophils, rather than mast cells and eosinophils, in bronchoalveolar lavage fluid. The childhood wheezing phenotype has been linked to many early exposures including fetal nutrition, maternal smoking, prenatal and birth maternal complications, prenatal and neonatal exposure to antibiotics, exposure to high levels of environmental allergens, and high infant adiposity. Infections during infancy have been cited as risk factors for later wheezing, including respiratory syncytial virus (RSV; see Chapter 260), rhinovirus (see Chapter 263), cytomegalovirus (see Chapter 255), human metapneumovirus (see Chapter 261), bocavirus, adenovirus, and *Chlamydia pneumoniae*.

A variety of inflammatory mediators have also been implicated in the wheezing infant such as histamine, cytokines, leukotrienes, and interleukins. Taken together, these fetal and/or early postnatal exposures may cause a "programming" of the lung that ultimately affects structure and function.

ETIOLOGY

Although wheezing in infants most frequently results from inflammation (generally bronchiolitis), there are many causes of wheezing (Table 391-1).

Acute Bronchiolitis and Inflammation of the Airway

Infection can cause obstruction to flow by internal narrowing of the airways.

Acute bronchiolitis is predominantly a viral disease. RSV is responsible for more than 50% of cases. Other agents include parainfluenza, adenovirus, rhinovirus, and *Mycoplasma*. Emerging pathogens include human metapneumovirus and human bocavirus, which may be a primary cause of viral respiratory infection or occur as a coinfection with RSV. Although bacterial pneumonia is sometimes confused clinically with bronchiolitis, there is no evidence of a bacterial cause for bronchiolitis and bronchiolitis is rarely followed by bacterial superinfection. Concurrent infection with viral bronchiolitis and pertussis has been described.

Approximately 100,000-126,000 children younger than 1 yr old are hospitalized annually in the United States because of RSV infection. The increasing rates of bronchiolitis that were seen from 1980-1996 (thought to reflect increased attendance of infants in daycare centers, changes in criteria for hospital admission, and/or improved survival of premature infants and others at risk for severe RSV-associated disease), have not continued. In fact, rates have stayed stable in subsequent years despite introduction and routine use of RSV immunoprophylaxis in high-risk populations.

Bronchiolitis is more common in boys, in those who have not been breastfed, and in those who live in crowded conditions. Risk is higher for infants with young mothers or mothers who smoked during pregnancy. Older family members are a common source of infection; they might only experience minor upper respiratory symptoms (colds). The clinical manifestations of lower respiratory tract illness seen in young infants may be minimal in older patients, in whom bronchiolar edema is better tolerated.

Not all infected infants develop lower respiratory tract illness. Host anatomic and immunologic factors play a significant role in the severity of the clinical syndrome, as does the nature of the viral pathogen.

Table 391-1	Differential Diagnosis of Wheezing in Infancy

INFECTION
Viral
Respiratory syncytial virus
Human metapneumovirus
Parainfluenza
Adenovirus
Influenza
Rhinovirus
Bocavirus
Coronavirus
Enterovirus
Other
Chlamydia trachomatis
Tuberculosis
Histoplasmosis
Papillomatosis

ASTHMA
Transient wheezer (resolved by 6 yr of age)
• Initial risk factor is primarily diminished lung size
Persistent wheezers (persists beyond 6 yr of age)
• Initial risk factors include parental asthma history, atopic dermatitis, allergen sensitization, peripheral eosinophilia (>4%) and wheezing unrelated to colds in the 1st yr of life
• At increased risk of developing clinical asthma
Late-onset wheezer (symptoms begin after age 3 yr and persist)

ANATOMIC ABNORMALITIES
Central Airway Abnormalities
Malacia of the larynx, trachea, and/or bronchi
Laryngeal or tracheal web
Tracheoesophageal fistula (specifically H-type fistula)
Laryngeal cleft (resulting in aspiration)
Extrinsic Airway Anomalies Resulting in Airway Compression
Vascular ring or sling
Mediastinal lymphadenopathy from infection or tumor
Mediastinal mass or tumor
Esophageal foreign body
Intrinsic Airway Anomalies
Airway hemangioma, other tumor
Cystic adenomatoid malformation
Bronchial or lung cyst
Congenital lobar emphysema
Aberrant tracheal bronchus
Sequestration
Congenital heart disease with left-to-right shunt (increased pulmonary edema)
Foreign body
Immunodeficiency States
Immunoglobulin A deficiency
B-cell deficiencies
AIDS
Bronchiectasis

MUCOCILIARY CLEARANCE DISORDERS
Cystic fibrosis
Primary ciliary dyskinesia
Bronchiectasis

ASPIRATION SYNDROMES
Gastroesophageal reflux disease
Pharyngeal/swallow dysfunction

OTHER
Bronchopulmonary dysplasia
Interstitial lung disease, including bronchiolitis obliterans
Heart failure
Anaphylaxis
Inhalation injury—burns

Infants with preexistent smaller airways and diminished lung function have a more severe course. In addition, RSV infection incites a complex immune response. Eosinophils degranulate and release eosinophil cationic protein, which is cytotoxic to airway epithelium. Innate immunity plays a significant role and can depend on polymorphisms in toll-like receptors, interferons, interleukins, and nuclear factor κB. Chemokines and cytokines, such as tumor necrosis factor α, may be differentially expressed, depending on the inciting virus. Coinfection with more than 1 virus can also alter the clinical manifestations and/or severity of presentation.

Acute bronchiolitis is characterized by bronchiolar obstruction with edema, mucus, and cellular debris. Even minor bronchiolar wall thickening significantly affects airflow because resistance is inversely proportional to the 4th power of the radius of the bronchiolar passage. Resistance in the small air passages is increased during both inspiration and exhalation, but because the radius of an airway is smaller during expiration, the resultant respiratory obstruction leads to early air trapping and overinflation. If obstruction becomes complete, trapped distal air will be resorbed and the child will develop atelectasis.

Hypoxemia is a consequence of ventilation–perfusion mismatch early in the course. With severe obstructive disease and tiring of respiratory effort, hypercapnia can develop.

Chronic infectious causes of wheezing should be considered in infants who seem to fall out of the range of a normal clinical course. Cystic fibrosis is one such entity; suspicion increases in a patient with persistent respiratory symptoms, digital clubbing, malabsorption, failure to thrive, electrolyte abnormalities, or a resistance to bronchodilator treatment (see Chapter 403).

Allergy and asthma are important causes of wheezing and probably generate the most questions by the parents of a wheezing infant. Asthma is characterized by airway inflammation, bronchial hyperreactivity, and reversibility of obstruction (see Chapter 144). Three identified patterns of infant wheezing are the transient early wheezer, the persistent wheezer, and the late-onset wheezer. These patterns are seen in 19.9%, 13.7%, and 15% of the general population, respectively, with the remaining 50% of the population never wheezing prior to age 6 yr. Transient early wheezers wheeze at least once with a lower respiratory infection before the age of 3 yr, but never wheeze again. The persistent wheezer has wheezing episodes before age 3 yr and is still wheezing at 6 yr of age. The late-onset wheezer does not wheeze before age 3 yr but is wheezing by 6 yr. Of all the infants who wheezed before 3 yr old, almost 60% stopped wheezing by age 6 yr.

Multiple studies have tried to predict which early wheezers will go on to have asthma in later life. Risk factors for persistent wheezing include parental history of asthma and allergies, maternal smoking, persistent rhinitis (apart from acute upper respiratory tract infections), allergen sensitization, eczema at younger than 1 yr of age, peripheral eosinophilia (>4%), and frequent episodes of wheezing during infancy.

Other Causes

Congenital malformations of the respiratory tract cause wheezing in early infancy. These findings can be diffuse or focal and can be from an external compression or an intrinsic abnormality. *External vascular compression* includes a vascular ring, in which the trachea and esophagus are surrounded completely by vascular structures, or a vascular sling, in which the trachea and esophagus are not completely encircled (see Chapter 432). *Cardiovascular causes* of wheezing include dilated chambers of the heart including massive cardiomegaly, left atrial enlargement, and dilated pulmonary arteries. Pulmonary edema caused by heart failure can also cause wheezing by lymphatic and bronchial vessel engorgement that leads to obstruction and edema of the bronchioles and further obstruction (see Chapter 442).

Foreign-body aspiration (see Chapter 397) can cause acute or chronic wheezing. It is estimated that 78% of those who die from foreign-body aspiration are between 2 mo and 4 yr old. Even in young infants, a foreign body can be ingested if given to the infant by another person, such as an older sibling. Infants who have atypical histories or misleading clinical and radiologic findings can receive a misdiagnosis of asthma or another obstructive disorder as inflammation and granu-

lation develop around the foreign body. An esophageal foreign body can transmit pressure to the membranous trachea, causing compromise of the airway lumen.

Gastroesophageal reflux (see Chapter 323.1) can cause wheezing with or without direct aspiration into the tracheobronchial tree. Without aspiration, the reflux is thought to trigger a vagal or neural reflex, causing increased airway resistance and airway reactivity. Aspiration from gastroesophageal reflux or from the direct aspiration from oral liquids can also cause wheezing.

Trauma and tumors are much rarer causes of wheezing in infants. Trauma of any type to the tracheobronchial tree can cause an obstruction to airflow. Accidental or nonaccidental aspirations, burns, or scalds of the tracheobronchial tree can cause inflammation of the airways and subsequent wheezing. Any space-occupying lesion, either in the lung itself or extrinsic to the lung, can cause tracheobronchial compression and obstruction to airflow.

CLINICAL MANIFESTATIONS
History and Physical Examination

The initial history of a wheezing infant should describe the recent event including onset, duration, and associated factors (Table 391-2). *Birth history* includes weeks of gestation, neonatal intensive care unit admission, history of intubation or oxygen requirement, maternal complications including infection with herpes simplex virus or HIV, and prenatal smoke exposure. Past medical history includes any comorbid conditions including syndromes or associations. *Family history* of cystic fibrosis, immunodeficiencies, asthma in a 1st-degree relative, or any other recurrent respiratory conditions in children should be obtained. *Social history* should include an environmental history including any smokers at home, inside or out, daycare exposure, number of siblings, occupation of inhabitants of the home, pets, tuberculosis exposure, and concerns regarding home environment (e.g., dust mites, construction dust, heating and cooling techniques, mold, cockroaches). The patient's growth chart should be reviewed for signs of failure to thrive.

On **physical examination,** evaluation of the patient's vital signs with special attention to the respiratory rate and the pulse oximetry reading for oxygen saturation is an important initial step. The **exam** is often dominated by wheezing. Auscultation might reveal fine crackles or overt wheezes, with prolongation of the expiratory phase of breathing.

Table 391-2	Pertinent Medical History in the Wheezing Infant

Did the onset of symptoms begin at birth or thereafter?
Is the infant a noisy breather and when is it most prominent?
Is the noisy breathing present on inspiration, expiration, or both?
Is there a history of cough apart from wheezing?
Was there an earlier lower respiratory tract infection?
Is there a history of recurrent upper or lower respiratory tract infections?
Have there been any emergency department visits, hospitalizations, or intensive care unit admissions for respiratory distress?
Is there a history of eczema?
Does the infant cough after crying or cough at night?
How is the infant growing and developing?
Is there associated failure to thrive?
Is there a history of electrolyte abnormalities?
Are there signs of intestinal malabsorption including frequent, greasy, or oily stools?
Is there a maternal history of genital herpes simplex virus infection?
What was the gestational age at delivery?
Was the patient intubated as a neonate?
Does the infant bottle-feed in the bed or the crib, especially in a propped position?
Are there any feeding difficulties including choking, gagging, arching, or vomiting with feeds?
Is there any new food exposure?
Is there a toddler in the home or lapse in supervision in which foreign-body aspiration could have occurred?
Change in caregivers or chance of nonaccidental trauma?

Wheezing produces an expiratory whistling sound that can be polyphonic or monophonic. Expiratory time may be prolonged. Biphasic wheezing can occur if there is a central, large airway obstruction. The degree of tachypnea does not always correlate with the degree of hypoxemia or hypercarbia, so pulse oximetry and noninvasive determination of carbon dioxide is essential. Work of breathing may be markedly increased, with nasal flaring and retractions. *Complete obstruction to airflow can eliminate the turbulence that causes wheezing; thus the lack of audible wheezing is not reassuring if the infant shows other signs of respiratory distress.* Barely audible breath sounds suggest very severe disease with nearly complete bronchiolar obstruction.

Aeration should be noted and a trial of a bronchodilator may be warranted to evaluate for any change in wheezing after treatment. Listening to breath sounds over the neck helps differentiate upper airway from lower airway sounds. The absence or presence of stridor should be noted and appreciated on inspiration. Signs of respiratory distress include tachypnea, increased respiratory effort, nasal flaring, tracheal tugging, subcostal and intercostal retractions, and excessive use of accessory muscles. In the upper airway, signs of atopy, including boggy turbinates and posterior oropharynx cobblestoning, can be evaluated in older infants. It is also useful to evaluate the skin of the patient for eczema and any significant hemangiomas; midline lesions may be associated with an intrathoracic lesion. Digital clubbing should be noted (see Chapter 374). Hyperinflation of the lungs can permit palpation of the liver and spleen.

Acute bronchiolitis is usually preceded by exposure to an older contact with a minor respiratory syndrome within the previous week. The infant first develops a mild upper respiratory tract infection with sneezing and clear rhinorrhea. This may be accompanied by diminished appetite and fever of 38.5-39°C (101-102°F), although the temperature can range from subnormal to markedly elevated. Gradually, respiratory distress ensues, with paroxysmal wheezy cough, dyspnea, and irritability. The infant is often tachypneic, which can interfere with feeding. The child does not usually have other systemic complaints, such as diarrhea or vomiting. Apnea may be more prominent than wheezing early in the course of the disease, particularly with very young infants (<2 mo old) or former premature infants.

Diagnostic Evaluation
Initial evaluation depends on likely etiology; a baseline chest radiograph, including posteroanterior and lateral films, is warranted in many cases and for any infant in acute respiratory distress, **but not routinely indicated in children with uncomplicated bronchiolitis.** Infiltrates are most often found in wheezing infants who have a pulse oximetry reading <93%, grunting, decreased breath sounds, prolonged inspiratory to expiratory ratio, and crackles. Pulse oximetry is indicated as hypoxia is common in bronchiolitis and may signify diffuse involvement, air trapping, ventilation–perfusion mismatching, and atelectasis. The chest radiograph may also be useful for evaluating hyperinflation (common in bronchiolitis and viral pneumonia), atelectasis signs of chronic disease such as bronchiectasis, or a space-occupying lesion causing airway compression. A trial of bronchodilator may be diagnostic as well as therapeutic because these medications can reverse conditions such as asthma but will not affect a fixed obstruction. Bronchodilators potentially can worsen a case of wheezing caused by tracheal or bronchial malacia. A sweat test to evaluate for cystic fibrosis and evaluation of baseline immune status are reasonable in infants with recurrent wheezing, failure to thrive, or complicated courses. Further evaluation such as upper gastrointestinal contrast x-rays, chest CT, bronchoscopy, bronchoalveolar lavage, ciliary biopsy, infant pulmonary function testing, video swallow study, and pH probe can be considered 2nd-tier diagnostic procedures in complicated patients.

The diagnosis of **acute bronchiolitis** is clinical, particularly in a previously healthy infant presenting with a 1st-time wheezing episode during a community outbreak. Chest radiography can reveal hyperinflated lungs with patchy atelectasis but is not indicated in all patients with bronchiolitis. The white blood cell and differential counts are usually normal. Viral testing (polymerase chain reaction, rapid immu-

nofluorescence, or viral culture) is helpful if the diagnosis is uncertain or for epidemiologic purposes but is not indicated in uncomplicated bronchiolitis. Because concurrent bacterial infection (sepsis, pneumonia, meningitis) is highly unlikely, confirmation of viral bronchiolitis may obviate the need for a sepsis evaluation in the febrile infant older than 28 days and assist with respiratory precautions and isolation if the patient requires hospitalization.

Treatment
Treatment of an infant with wheezing depends on the underlying etiology. Response to bronchodilators is unpredictable, regardless of cause, but suggests a component of bronchial hyperreactivity. It is appropriate to administer albuterol aerosol and objectively observe the response. For children younger than 3 yr of age, it is acceptable to continue to administer inhaled medications through a metered-dose inhaler with mask and spacer if a therapeutic benefit is demonstrated. Therapy should be continued in all patients with asthma exacerbations from a viral illness.

The use of ipratropium bromide in this population is controversial, but it appears to be somewhat effective as an adjunct therapy. It is also useful in infants with significant tracheal and bronchial malacia who may be made worse by β_2-agonists such as albuterol because of the subsequent decrease in smooth muscle tone.

A trial of inhaled steroids may be warranted in a patient who has responded to multiple courses of oral steroids and who has moderate to severe wheezing or a significant history of atopy including food allergy or eczema. Inhaled corticosteroids are appropriate for maintenance therapy in patients with known reactive airways but are controversial when used for episodic or acute illnesses. Intermittent, high-dose inhaled corticosteroids are not recommended for intermittent wheezing. Early use of inhaled corticosteroids has not been shown to prevent the progression of childhood wheezing or affect the natural history of asthma in children.

Oral steroids are generally reserved for atopic wheezing infants thought to have asthma that is refractory to other medications. Their use in 1st-time wheezing infants or in infants who do not warrant hospitalization is controversial.

Infants with **acute bronchiolitis** who are experiencing respiratory distress (hypoxia, inability to take oral feedings, apnea, extreme tachypnea) should be hospitalized; risk factors for severe disease include age <12 wk, preterm birth, or underlying comorbidity such as cardiovascular, pulmonary, neurologic, or immunologic disease. The mainstay of treatment is supportive. Hypoxemic children should receive cool humidified oxygen. Sedatives are to be avoided because they can depress respiratory drive. The infant is sometimes more comfortable if sitting with head and chest elevated at a 30-degree angle with neck extended. There is a small risk of aspiration of oral feedings in infants with bronchiolitis, owing to tachypnea and the increased work of breathing. If there is any risk for further respiratory decompensation potentially necessitating tracheal intubation, the infant should not be fed orally but be maintained with parenteral fluids. Frequent suctioning of nasal and oral secretions often provides relief of distress or cyanosis. Suctioning of secretions is an essential part of the treatment of bronchiolitis. Oxygen is definitely indicated in all infants with hypoxia. High-flow nasal cannula therapy can reduce the need for intubation in patients with impending respiratory failure.

A number of agents have been proposed as adjunctive therapies for bronchiolitis. Bronchodilators may produce short-term improvement in clinical features. This must be placed in context of potential adverse effects and the lack of any evidence indicating improvement in overall course of the disease. Systematic reviews and meta-analyses of randomized controlled trials have failed to show a benefit from bronchodilators in uncomplicated bronchiolitis. Corticosteroids, whether parenteral, oral, or inhaled, have been used for bronchiolitis despite conflicting and often negative studies. Corticosteroids are not recommended in previously healthy infants with RSV. Ribavirin, an antiviral agent administered by aerosol, has been used for infants with RSV who have congenital heart disease or chronic lung disease. There is no convincing evidence of a positive impact on clinically important outcomes such as mortality and duration of hospitalization. Antibiotics have no value unless there is coexisting bacterial infection. Likewise, there is no support for RSV immunoglobulin administration during acute episodes of RSV bronchiolitis in previously healthy children. Combined therapy with nebulized epinephrine and dexamethasone has been used with some success, but additional studies are needed to confirm its efficacy and investigate the long-term adverse effects in infants before this combination can be recommended. Nebulized hypertonic saline has been reported to have some benefit, and may shorten hospital length of stay. One study suggested that on demand therapy with inhaled epinephrine or saline was more effective than scheduled fixed dosing. Heliox delivered by tight fitting mask or by continuous positive airway pressure has been of some benefit in moderately to severely affected patients with bronchiolitis.

Certain (10%) low risk patients with bronchiolitis and an oxygen requirement may be discharged from the emergency department to receive **home oxygen therapy**. Criteria for home oxygen therapy includes: typical clinical features (no apnea, wheezing ± crackles); 2 mo-2 yr of age (>44 wk gestational age); first episode of wheezing; illness during RSV season; secretions managed by parents with bulb suctioning; smoke free home; reliable family with good access to healthcare; altitude ≤6,000 feet; absence of toxic appearance or proven bacterial disease; apparent life-threatening event; cardiac, pulmonary, immunodeficiency, or neuromuscular disorders; baseline oxygen requirement prior to current illness; mild illness as evident by feeding well and alert and active; minimal retractions; respiratory rate <50 breaths/min; oxygenation >90% on ≤0.5 L/min of oxygen. All patients must have follow-up within 24 hr of discharge from the emergency room by their primary care provider or by the emergency room staff. Chest physiotherapy does not improve disease course in hospitalized infants with bronchiolitis who are not mechanically ventilated.

PROGNOSIS

Infants with **acute bronchiolitis** are at highest risk for further respiratory compromise in the 1st 48-72 hr after onset of cough and dyspnea; the child may be desperately ill with air hunger, apnea, and respiratory acidosis. The case fatality rate is <1%, with death attributable to apnea, respiratory arrest, or severe dehydration. After this critical period, symptoms can persist. The median duration of symptoms in ambulatory patients is approximately 14 days; 10% may be symptomatic at 3 wk. There is a higher incidence of wheezing and asthma in children with a history of bronchiolitis unexplained by family history or other atopic syndromes. It is unclear whether bronchiolitis incites an immune response that manifests as asthma later or whether those infants have an inherent predilection for asthma that is merely unmasked by their episode of viral bronchiolitis.

PREVENTION

Reduction in the severity and incidence of **acute bronchiolitis** because of RSV is possible through the administration of pooled hyperimmune RSV intravenous immunoglobulin and palivizumab, an intramuscular monoclonal antibody to the RSV F protein, before and during RSV season. Palivizumab should be considered for infants younger than 2 yr of age with chronic lung disease, a history of prematurity, and some forms of congenital heart disease (see Chapter 260). Meticulous hand hygiene is the best measure to prevent nosocomial transmission.

Bibliography is available at Expert Consult.

391.2 Bronchitis

Lauren E. Camarda and Denise M. Goodman

Nonspecific bronchial inflammation is termed **bronchitis** and occurs in multiple childhood conditions. **Acute bronchitis** is a syndrome, usually viral in origin, with cough as a prominent feature.

Acute tracheobronchitis is a term used when the trachea is prominently involved. Nasopharyngitis may also be present, and a variety of viral and bacterial agents, such as those causing influenza, pertussis, and diphtheria, may be responsible. Isolation of common bacteria such as *Staphylococcus aureus* and *Streptococcus pneumoniae* from the sputum might not imply a bacterial cause that requires antibiotic therapy.

ACUTE BRONCHITIS
Clinical Manifestations

Acute bronchitis often follows a viral upper respiratory tract infection. It is more common in the winter when respiratory viral syndromes predominate. The tracheobronchial epithelium is invaded by the infectious agent, leading to activation of inflammatory cells and release of cytokines. Constitutional symptoms including fever and malaise follow. The tracheobronchial epithelium can become significantly damaged or hypersensitized, leading to a protracted cough lasting 1-3 wk.

The child first presents with nonspecific upper respiratory infectious symptoms, such as rhinitis. Three to 4 days later, a frequent, dry, hacking cough develops, which may or may not be productive. After several days, the sputum can become purulent, indicating leukocyte migration but not necessarily bacterial infection. Many children swallow their sputum which can produce emesis. Chest pain may be a prominent complaint in older children and is exacerbated by coughing. The mucus gradually thins, usually within 5-10 days, and then the cough gradually abates. The entire episode usually lasts about 2 wk and seldom longer than 3 wk.

Findings on physical examination vary with the age of the patient and stage of the disease. Early findings are absent or include low-grade fever and upper respiratory signs such as nasopharyngitis, conjunctivitis, and rhinitis. Auscultation of the chest may be unremarkable at this early phase. As the syndrome progresses and cough worsens, breath sounds become coarse, with coarse and fine crackles and scattered high-pitched wheezing. Chest radiographs are normal or can have increased bronchial markings.

The principal objective of the clinician is to exclude pneumonia, which is more likely caused by bacterial agents requiring antibiotic therapy. Absence of abnormality of vital signs (tachycardia, tachypnea, fever) and a normal physical examination of the chest reduce the likelihood of pneumonia.

Differential Diagnosis

Persistent or recurrent symptoms should lead the clinician to consider entities other than acute bronchitis. Many entities manifest with cough as a prominent symptom (Table 391-3).

Treatment

There is no specific therapy for acute bronchitis. The disease is self-limited, and antibiotics, although often prescribed, do not hasten improvement. Frequent shifts in position can facilitate pulmonary drainage in infants. Older children are sometimes more comfortable with humidity, but this does not shorten the disease course. Cough suppressants can relieve symptoms but can also increase the risk of suppuration and inspissated secretions and, therefore, should be used judiciously. Antihistamines dry secretions and are not helpful; expectorants are likewise not indicated. Nonprescription cough and cold medicines should not be used in children younger than 2 yr of age and their use is cautioned in children age 2-11 yr.

CHRONIC BRONCHITIS

Chronic bronchitis is well recognized in adults, formally defined as 3 mo or longer of productive cough each year for 2 or more yr. The disease can develop insidiously, with episodes of acute obstruction alternating with quiescent periods. A number of predisposing conditions can lead to progression of airflow obstruction or chronic obstructive pulmonary disease, with smoking as the major factor (up to 80% of patients have a smoking history). Other conditions include air pollution, occupational exposures, and repeated infections. In children, cystic fibrosis, bronchopulmonary dysplasia, and bronchiectasis must be ruled out.

The applicability of this definition to children is unclear. The existence of chronic bronchitis as a distinct entity in children is

Table 391-3	Disorders with Cough as a Prominent Finding
CATEGORY	**DIAGNOSES**
Inflammatory	Asthma
Chronic pulmonary processes	Bronchopulmonary dysplasia Postinfectious bronchiectasis Cystic fibrosis Tracheomalacia or bronchomalacia Ciliary abnormalities Other chronic lung diseases
Other chronic disease or congenital disorders	Laryngeal cleft Swallowing disorders Gastroesophageal reflux Airway compression (such as a vascular ring or hemangioma) Congenital heart disease
Infectious or immune disorders	Immunodeficiency Eosinophilic lung disease Tuberculosis Allergy Sinusitis Tonsillitis or adenoiditis *Chlamydia, Ureaplasma* (infants) *Bordetella pertussis* *Mycoplasma pneumoniae*
Acquired	Foreign-body aspiration, tracheal or esophageal

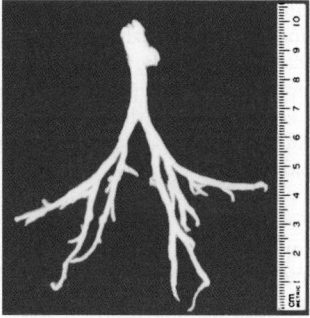

Figure 391-1 Tracheobronchial casts following bronchoscopic extraction. Casts show branched architecture corresponding to the bronchial tree. *(From Hasan RA, Black C, Reddy R: Plastic bronchitis in children. Fetal Pediatr Pathol 31;87–93, 2012, Fig. 5, p. 91.)*

controversial. Like adults, children with chronic inflammatory diseases or those with toxic exposures can develop damaged pulmonary epithelium. Thus, chronic or recurring cough in children should lead the clinician to search for underlying pulmonary or systemic disorders (see Table 391-3). One proposed entity that shares characteristics with asthma and other forms of suppurative lung disease is persistent or protracted bacterial bronchitis. Protracted bacterial bronchitis is defined as a chronic (>3 wk) wet cough, characterized by bacterial counts of 10^4 colony-forming units/mL or greater from bronchoalveolar lavage and resolution of cough within 2 wk of treatment with antimicrobial therapy.

CIGARETTE SMOKING AND AIR POLLUTION
Exposure to environmental irritants, such as tobacco smoke and air pollution, can incite or aggravate cough. There is a well-established association between tobacco exposure and pulmonary disease, including bronchitis and wheezing. This can occur through cigarette smoking or by exposure to passive smoke. Marijuana smoke and inhalants are other irritants sometimes overlooked when eliciting a history.

A number of pollutants compromise lung development and likely precipitate lung disease, including particulate matter, ozone, acid vapor, and nitrogen dioxide. Proximity to motor vehicle traffic is an important source of these pollutants. Because these substances coexist in the atmosphere, the relative contribution of any 1 to pulmonary symptoms is difficult to discern.

Bibliography is available at Expert Consult.

391.3 Plastic Bronchitis
Brett J. Bordini

Plastic bronchitis is a rare condition characterized by recurrent episodes of airway obstruction secondary to the formation of large proteinaceous branching casts that take on the shape of and obstruct the tracheobronchial tree. It is not a single disease entity, but rather represents an altered state of respiratory epithelial function and is most frequently encountered in the setting of underlying pulmonary or congenital cardiac disease, although there have been reports of plastic bronchitis complicating lymphangitic disorders, pulmonary infections, and the acute chest syndrome of sickle cell disease. In comparison to the smaller bronchial and bronchiolar casts seen with mucus plugging, the lesions of plastic bronchitis are more extensive, with casts that can outline large segments of the airway to the level of the terminal bronchioles (Fig. 391-1). These casts may be spontaneously expectorated or may require bronchoscopic removal for relief of potentially fatal airway obstruction. Cast composition varies, though typically consists of either a fibrin-predominant or mucin-predominant laminated matrix with or without inflammatory cell infiltration. Plastic bronchitis may be classified according to an associated disease, the cast histology, or a combination.

EPIDEMIOLOGY
Plastic bronchitis is rare, and its true prevalence in the pediatric population is not known but is estimated to be 6.8 cases per 100,000 patients. Prevalence does vary in relation to the underlying associated disease state, with rates as high as 14% estimated in patients who have undergone staged palliation of complex cyanotic congenital heart disease, and much lower rates seen complicating asthma and atopic disease. A slight male predominance exists for cast formation in the setting of structural heart disease, whereas cast formation in the setting of asthma and atopic disease demonstrates a female predominance.

PATHOGENESIS
The mechanism of cast formation is unclear, although it is believed to vary based on the underlying disease association and cast type. One classification system differentiates type 1 inflammatory casts, composed of primarily of fibrin with neutrophilic and more often eosinophilic infiltration, and type 2 casts, composed primarily of mucin with little to no cellular infiltration. Type 1 casts may be associated with inflammatory and infectious disorders of the lung, while type 2 casts may be associated with structural heart disease. However, these distinctions are not absolute; patients with structural heart disease can have mucin-predominant casts and patients with asthma or atopic disease can have fibrin-predominant casts, with both mucin casts and fibrin casts demonstrating various degrees of cellular infiltration.

Cast formation in the setting of structural heart disease may result from alterations in pulmonary blood flow or from alterations in lymphatic drainage, either congenital or secondary to the protein-losing enteropathy associated with Fontan physiology. Mucin-predominant casts are believed to arise secondary to mucus gland hypersecretion as well as decreased mucociliary clearance.

CLINICAL MANIFESTATIONS
Patients with plastic bronchitis may present with cough, dyspnea, wheeze, or pleuritic chest pain. Depending on the degree of airway obstruction, patients may be hypoxemic or in severe respiratory distress. The expectoration of large, branched casts that are often tan in

color and rubbery in consistency is pathognomonic for plastic bronchitis. Lung examination may reveal diminished breath sounds or wheezing in the affected area. Rarely, auscultation may reveal a sound similar to a flag flapping in the wind (*bruit de drapeau*), believed to be related to the free end of a cast striking the bronchial wall during inspiration or expiration. Further examination may provide clues to underlying comorbidities.

DIAGNOSIS

The expectoration or endoscopic discovery of large tracheobronchial casts is pathognomonic for plastic bronchitis. History should be directed at assessing for conditions known to be have an associated risk of tracheobronchial cast formation, such as uncorrected or surgically palliated complex congenital heart disease; a history of atopic disease or asthma; lymphangitic disorders such as Noonan syndrome, Turner syndrome, lymphangiectasia, and yellow nail syndrome; sickle cell disease; and infectious exposures, particularly exposure to tuberculosis or atypical mycobacteria. Other predisposing conditions include cystic fibrosis, allergic bronchopulmonary aspergillosis, bronchiectasis, toxic inhalants, and granulomatous lung diseases.

Physical examination may provide indications of an underlying diagnosis. Digital clubbing of the fingers or toes may suggest long-standing hypoxemia associated with cardiac or pulmonary disease. Cardiac examination may provide information suggesting the presence of unrecognized structural heart disease.

Chest radiography may demonstrate collapse of the involved areas of the lung, or areas of bronchiectasis distal to sites of long-standing obstruction.

There should be a high index of suspicion for plastic bronchitis in patients with known comorbidities who present with sudden respiratory decompensation. In the absence of cast expectoration, direct visualization of casts via bronchoscopy is required for diagnosis and is potentially therapeutic in relieving airway obstruction. Cast histology should be defined so as to allow for specific therapies directed at preventing recurrence. In particular, the predominant component of the cast's laminated matrix—either fibrin or mucin—should be defined, and signs of inflammation or infiltration, such as the presence of neutrophils, eosinophils, or Charcot-Leyden crystals, should be documented.

TREATMENT

Treatment is directed at correcting the underlying condition associated with the development of plastic bronchitis, at relieving acute airway obstruction secondary to the presence of casts, and at preventing the development of further casts. Rigid or flexible bronchoscopy is typically required for cast removal. If the predominant content of the cast is known, therapy with either mucolytics or fibrinolytics may be considered as an adjunct to direct removal, and aerosolized fibrinolytics such as tissue plasminogen activator or mucolytics such as N-acetylcysteine or deoxyribonuclease may be used for prevention of recurrence. Bronchodilators should be used appropriately in the setting of reactive airway disease, and inhaled or systemic corticosteroids, low-dose azithromycin, and leukotriene inhibitors may be used to minimize airway inflammation. MRI lymphangiography may identify abnormal lymphatic vessels that may benefit from lymphatic embolization procedures.

COMPLICATIONS AND PROGNOSIS

Prognosis is related primarily to the underlying condition associated with the development of plastic bronchitis. Patients whose plastic bronchitis is related to surgically palliated complex congenital heart disease are at high risk for plastic bronchitis-related mortality. Mortality can be high if casts obstruct significant portions of the airway, regardless of underlying etiology. Mortality estimates vary from 6-50% in the setting of asthma or atopic disease, and from 28-60% in the setting of complex congenital heart disease, with central airway obstruction leading to death in the majority of patients.

Bibliography is available at Expert Consult.

Chapter **392**
Emphysema and Overinflation
Steven R. Boas and Glenna B. Winnie

Pulmonary emphysema consists of distention of air spaces with irreversible disruption of the alveolar septa. It can involve part or all of a lung. **Overinflation** is distention with or without alveolar rupture and is often reversible. **Compensatory overinflation** can be acute or chronic and occurs in normally functioning pulmonary tissue when, for any reason, a sizable portion of the lung is removed or becomes partially or completely airless, which can occur with pneumonia, atelectasis, empyema, and pneumothorax. **Obstructive overinflation** results from partial obstruction of a bronchus or bronchiole, when it becomes more difficult for air to leave the alveoli than to enter. Air gradually accumulates distal to the obstruction, the so-called bypass, ball-valve, or check-valve type of obstruction.

LOCALIZED OBSTRUCTIVE OVERINFLATION

When a ball-valve type of obstruction partially occludes the main stem bronchus, the entire lung becomes overinflated; individual lobes are affected when the obstruction is in lobar bronchi. Segments or subsegments are affected when their individual bronchi are blocked. When most or all of a lobe is involved, the percussion note is hyperresonant over the area, and the breath sounds are decreased in intensity. The distended lung can extend across the mediastinum into the opposite hemithorax. Under fluoroscopic scrutiny during exhalation, the overinflated area does not decrease, and the heart and the mediastinum shift to the opposite side because the unobstructed lung empties normally.

Unilateral Hyperlucent Lung

The differential diagnosis for of this resultant **unilateral hyperlucent lung** is quite broad and can involve the lung parenchyma, airways, pulmonary vasculature, chest wall (see Chapter 417), and mediastinum. Localized obstructions that can be responsible for overinflation include airway foreign bodies and the inflammatory reaction to them (see Chapter 387), abnormally thick mucus (cystic fibrosis, Chapter 403), endobronchial tuberculosis or tuberculosis of the tracheobronchial lymph nodes (see Chapter 215), and endobronchial or mediastinal tumors.

Patients with unilateral hyperlucent lung can present with **clinical manifestations** of pneumonia, but in some patients the condition is discovered only when a chest radiograph is obtained for an unrelated reason. A few patients have hemoptysis. Physical findings can include hyperresonance and a small lung with the mediastinum shifted toward the more abnormal lung.

Swyer-James or Macleod Syndrome

The condition is thought to result from an insult to the lower respiratory tract following most commonly adenovirus (see Chapter 262), or respiratory syncytial virus (see Chapter 260), *Mycoplasma pneumoniae* (see Chapter 223), or measles (see Chapter 246). Clinically, children with this condition often have chronic cough, recurrent pneumonia, and wheezing, although some are asymptomatic. Some patients show a classic mediastinal shift away from the lesion with exhalation. CT scanning or bronchography can often demonstrate bronchiectasis. Ventilation–perfusion scans can be helpful in the diagnosis. In some patients, previous chest radiographs have been normal or have shown only an acute pneumonia, suggesting that a hyperlucent lung is an acquired lesion. No specific treatment is known; it may become less symptomatic with time. Indications as to which children would benefit from surgery remain controversial.

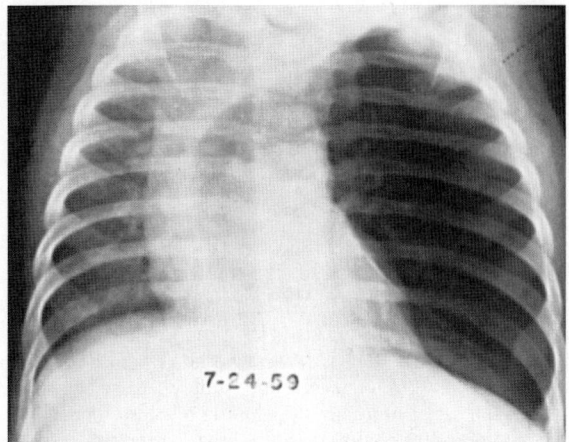

Figure 392-1 Congenital left upper lobe emphysema. Note the extension of the emphysematous lobe into the left lower lobe and its displacement of the mediastinum toward the right.

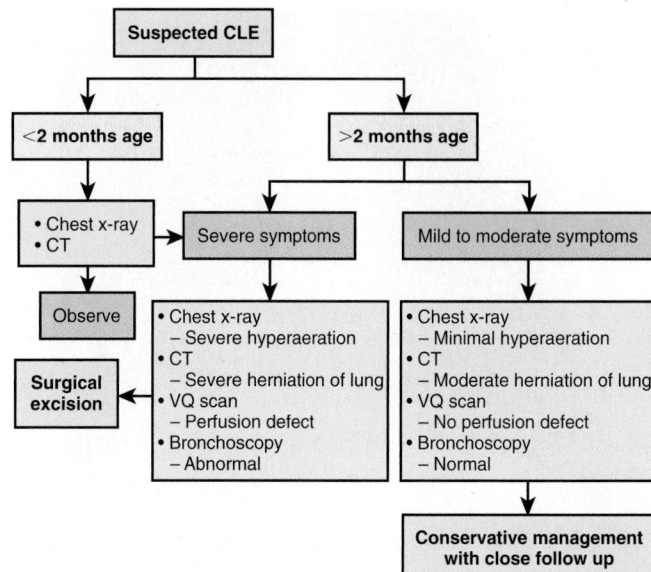

Figure 392-2 Algorithm for evaluation and treatment of congenital lobar emphysema (CLE). *(Adapted from Karnak I, Senocak ME, Ciftci AO, et al: Congenital lobar emphysema: diagnostic and therapeutic considerations, J Pediatr Surg 34:1347–1351, 1999, Fig. 4.)*

Congenital Lobar Emphysema

Congenital lobar emphysema (CLE) can result in severe respiratory distress in early infancy and can be caused by localized obstruction. Familial occurrence has been reported. In 50% of cases, a cause of CLE can be identified. Congenital deficiency of the bronchial cartilage, external compression by aberrant vessels, bronchial stenosis, redundant bronchial mucosal flaps, and kinking of the bronchus caused by herniation into the mediastinum have been described as leading to bronchial obstruction and subsequent CLE and commonly affects the left upper lobe.

Clinical manifestations usually become apparent in the neonatal period but are delayed for as long as 5-6 mo in 5% of patients. Many cases are diagnosed by antenatal ultrasonography. Babies with prenatally diagnosed cases are not always symptomatic at birth. In some patients, CLE remains undiagnosed until school age or beyond. Clinical signs range from mild tachypnea and wheeze to severe dyspnea with cyanosis. CLE can affect 1 or more lobes; it affects the upper and middle lobes, and the left upper lobe is the most common site. The affected lobe is essentially nonfunctional because of the overdistention, and atelectasis of the ipsilateral normal lung can ensue. With further distention, the mediastinum is shifted to the contralateral side, with impaired function seen as well (Fig. 392-1). A radiolucent lobe and a mediastinal shift are often revealed by radiographic examination. A CT scan can demonstrate the aberrant anatomy of the lesion, and MRI or MR angiography can demonstrate any vascular lesions, which might be causing extraluminal compression. Nuclear imaging studies are useful to demonstrate perfusion defects in the affected lobe. Figure 392-2 outlines evaluation of an infant presenting with suspected CLE. The differential diagnosis includes pneumonia with or without an effusion, pneumothorax, and cystic adenomatoid malformation.

Treatment by immediate surgery and excision of the lobe may be lifesaving when cyanosis and severe respiratory distress are present, but some patients respond to medical treatment. Selective intubation of the unaffected lung may be of value. Some children with apparent CLE have reversible overinflation, without the classic alveolar septal rupture implied in the term *emphysema*. Bronchoscopy can reveal an endobronchial lesion.

Pulmonary Vascular Abnormalities

Unilateral hyperlucency may result from **unilateral pulmonary agenesis** (see Chapter 395) that typically presents in the neonatal period. Volume loss of the affected lung results in a mediastinal shift with hyperinflation of the contralateral lung. An **anomalous origin of the left pulmonary artery** (see Chapter 432), also known as a pulmonary artery sling, can impinge the right mainstem bronchus with resultant right-sided hyperinflation or atelectasis producing hyperlucency on either the ipsilateral or contralateral side. **Pulmonary venolobar syndrome** (see Chapter 426), also known as scimitar syndrome, can also result in a hyperlucent contralateral lung dependent on the extent of hypoplasia of the right lung.

GENERALIZED OBSTRUCTIVE OVERINFLATION

Acute generalized overinflation of the lung results from widespread involvement of the bronchioles and is usually reversible. It occurs more commonly in infants than in children and may be secondary to a number of clinical conditions, including asthma, cystic fibrosis, acute bronchiolitis, interstitial pneumonitis, atypical forms of acute laryngotracheobronchitis, aspiration of zinc stearate powder, chronic passive congestion secondary to a congenital cardiac lesion, and miliary tuberculosis.

Pathology

In chronic overinflation, many of the alveoli are ruptured and communicate with one another, producing distended saccules. Air can also enter the interstitial tissue (i.e., interstitial emphysema), resulting in pneumomediastinum and pneumothorax (see Chapters 412 and 411).

Clinical Manifestations

Generalized obstructive overinflation is characterized by dyspnea, with difficulty in exhaling. The lungs become increasingly overdistended, and the chest remains expanded during exhalation. An increased respiratory rate and decreased respiratory excursion result from the overdistention of the alveoli and their inability to be emptied normally through the narrowed bronchioles. Air hunger is responsible for forced respiratory movements. Overaction of the accessory muscles of respiration results in retractions at the suprasternal notch, the supraclavicular spaces, the lower margin of the thorax, and the intercostal spaces. Unlike the flattened chest during inspiration and exhalation in cases of laryngeal obstruction, minimal reduction in the size of the overdistended chest during exhalation is observed. The percussion note is hyperresonant. On auscultation, the inspiratory phase is usually less prominent than the expiratory phase, which is prolonged and roughened. Fine or medium crackles may be heard. Cyanosis is more common in the severe cases.

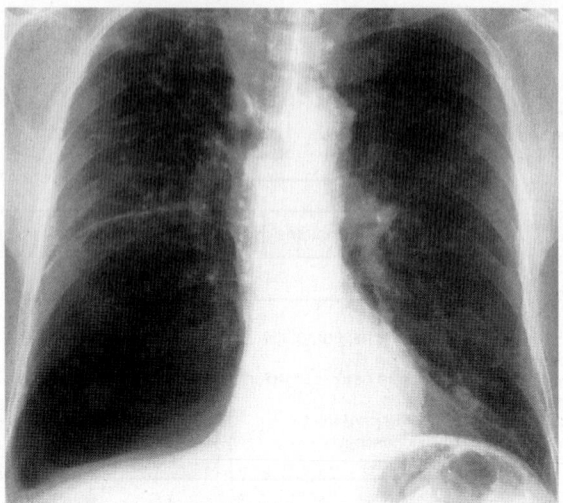

Figure 392-3 Increased transradiancy in the right lower zone. A large emphysematous bulla occupies the lower half of the right lung, and the apical changes are in keeping with previous tuberculosis. *(From Padley SPG, Hansell DM: Imaging techniques. In Albert RK, Spiro SG, Jett JR, editors:* Clinical respiratory medicine, *ed 3, Philadelphia, 2008, Mosby, Fig. 1-48.)*

Diagnosis

Radiographic and fluoroscopic examinations of the chest assist in establishing the diagnosis. Both leaves of the diaphragm are low and flattened, the ribs are farther apart than usual, and the lung fields are less dense. The movement of the diaphragm during exhalation is decreased, and the excursion of the low, flattened diaphragm in severe cases is barely discernible. The anteroposterior diameter of the chest is increased, and the sternum may be bowed outward.

Bullous Emphysema

Bullous emphysematous blebs or cysts (pneumatoceles) result from overdistention and rupture of alveoli during birth or shortly thereafter, or they may be sequelae of pneumonia and other infections. They have been observed in tuberculosis lesions during specific antibacterial therapy. These emphysematous areas presumably result from rupture of distended alveoli, forming a single or multiloculated cavity. The cysts can become large and might contain some fluid; an air–fluid level may be demonstrated on the radiograph (Fig. 392-3). The cysts should be differentiated from pulmonary abscesses. In most cases, the cysts disappear spontaneously within a few months, although they can persist for a year or more. Aspiration or surgery is not indicated except in cases of severe respiratory and cardiac compromise.

Subcutaneous Emphysema

Subcutaneous emphysema results from any process that allows free air to enter into the subcutaneous tissue (Fig. 392-4). The most common causes include pneumomediastinum or pneumothorax. Additionally, it can be a complication of fracture of the orbit, which permits free air to escape from the nasal sinuses. In the neck and thorax, subcutaneous emphysema can follow tracheotomy, deep ulceration in the pharyngeal region, esophageal wounds, or any perforating lesion of the larynx or trachea. It is occasionally a complication of thoracentesis, asthma, or abdominal surgery. Rarely, air is formed in the subcutaneous tissues by gas-producing bacteria.

Tenderness over the site of emphysema and a crepitant quality on palpation of the skin are classic manifestations. Subcutaneous emphy-

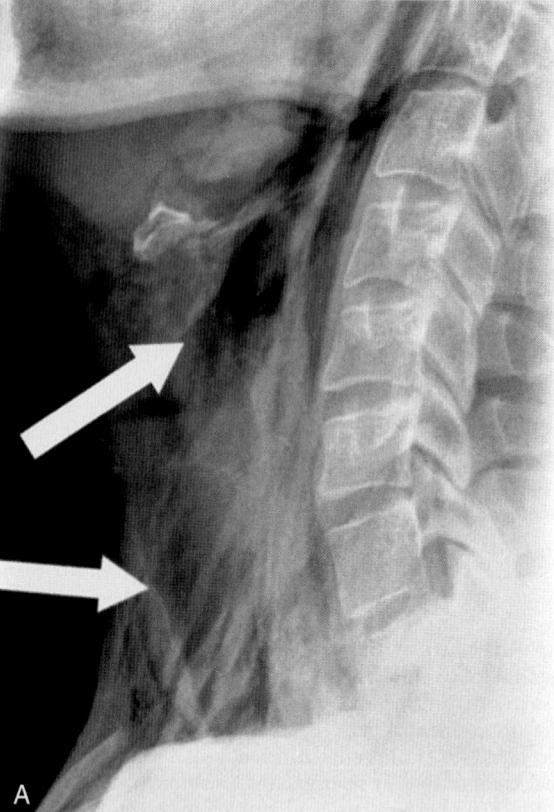

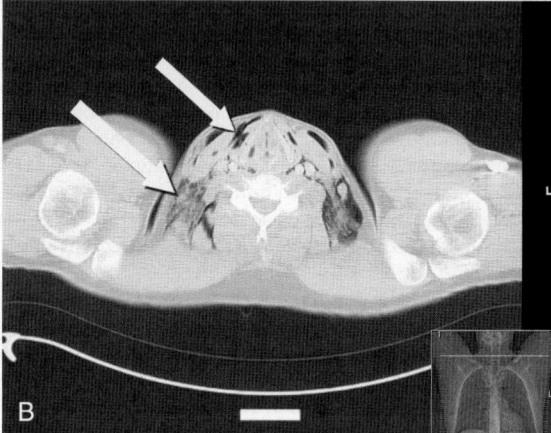

Figure 392-4 A, Lateral X-ray of neck showing subcutaneous emphysema. **B,** Axial section CT neck/thorax showing subcutaneous emphysema and pneumomediastinum. *(From Zakaria R, Khwaja H. Subcutaneous emphysema in a case of infective sinusitis: a case report.* J Med Case Rep 4:235, 2010, Figs, 1 and 2.)

sema is usually a self-limited process and requires no specific treatment. Minimization of activities that can increase airway pressure (cough, performance of high-pressure pulmonary function testing maneuvers) is recommended. Resolution occurs by resorption of subcutaneous air after elimination of its source. Rarely, dangerous compression of the trachea by air in the surrounding soft tissue requires surgical intervention.

Bibliography is available at Expert Consult.

α₁-Antitrypsin Deficiency and Emphysema

Glenna B. Winnie and Steven R. Boas

Although it rarely causes lung disease in children, homozygous deficiency of α₁-antitrypsin (α₁-AT) is an important cause of early-onset severe panacinar pulmonary emphysema in adults in the 3rd and 4th decades of life and an important cause of liver disease in children (see Chapter 357.5). It is associated with panniculitis and vasculitis in adults.

PATHOGENESIS

The type and concentration of α₁-AT are inherited as a series of codominant alleles on chromosomal segment 14q31-32.3. (See Chapter 357.5 for a discussion of genotypes and liver disease.) The autosomal recessive deficiency affects 1 in 1,600-2,500 people, or approximately 575,000 (estimated number of deficiency allele combinations) people in the United States, but is underdiagnosed. The highest risk for α₁-AT deficiency is found in whites, followed by Hispanics and Blacks, with the lowest prevalence among Mexican Americans, and little to no risk for Asians. Worldwide there are an estimated 116,000,000 carriers and 1,100,000 subjects with severe α₁-AT deficiency. The normal α₁-AT PiM protein is secreted by the liver into the circulation at a rate of approximately 34 mg/kg/day; it is also produced by lung epithelial cells and monocytes. Mutant protein is not produced (null) or is misfolded (PiZ and others); it can polymerize in the endoplasmic reticulum or be degraded, with subsequent low serum levels. Early adult-onset emphysema associated with α₁-AT deficiency occurs most commonly with PiZZ (mutation in *SERPINA1* gene), although Pi (null) (null) and, to a lesser extent, other mutant Pi types such as SZ have been associated with emphysema.

α₁-AT and other serum antiproteases help inactivate proteolytic enzymes released from dead bacteria or leukocytes in the lung. Deficiency of these antiproteases leads to an accumulation of proteolytic enzymes in the lung, resulting in destruction of pulmonary tissue with subsequent development of emphysema. Furthermore, polymerized mutant protein in the lungs may be proinflammatory. The concentration of proteases (elastase) in the patients' leukocytes may also be an important factor in determining the severity of clinical pulmonary disease with a given level of α₁-AT.

CLINICAL MANIFESTATIONS

Most patients who have the PiZZ defect have little or no detectable pulmonary disease during childhood. A few have early onset of chronic pulmonary symptoms, including dyspnea, wheezing, and cough, and panacinar emphysema has been documented by lung biopsy; it is probable that these findings occur secondarily to infection, causing inflammation with consequent early disease. Smoking greatly increases the risk of emphysema in patients with mutant Pi types. Although newborn screening to identify children with PiZZ phenotype does not affect parental smoking habits, it does decrease smoking rates among affected adolescents.

Physical examination in childhood is usually normal. It very rarely reveals growth failure, an increased anteroposterior diameter of the chest with a hyperresonant percussion note, crackles if there is active infection, and clubbing. Severe emphysema can depress the diaphragm, making the liver and spleen more easily palpable.

LABORATORY FINDINGS

Serum immunoassay measures low levels of α₁-AT; normal serum levels are 150-350 mg/dL. Serum electrophoresis reveals the pheno-type, and genotype is determined by polymerase chain reaction. In the rare patient with lung disease in adolescence, chest radiograph reveals overinflation with depressed diaphragms. Chest CT can show more hyperexpansion in the lower lung zones, with occasional bronchiectasis; CT densitometry can be a sensitive method to follow changes in lung disease. Lung function testing is usually normal in children, but it can show airflow obstruction and increased lung volumes, particularly in adolescents who smoke.

TREATMENT

Therapy for α₁-AT deficiency is intravenous replacement with enzyme derived from pooled human plasma. A level of 80 mg/dL is protective for emphysema. This target level for augmentation therapy is usually achieved with doses of 60 mg/kg IV weekly and results in the appearance of the transfused antiprotease in pulmonary lavage fluid. The Food and Drug Administration has approved the use of purified blood-derived human enzyme for ZZ and null-null patients. Replacement therapy appears most beneficial for those with moderately severe obstructive lung disease (forced expiratory volume in 1 sec is 30-65% of predicted) or those with mild lung disease experiencing a rapid decline in lung function. Augmentation therapy is not indicated for persons with the PiMZ type who have pulmonary disease, because their disease is not from enzyme deficiency. Recombinant sources of α₁-AT are under development, but current products are rapidly cleared from the circulation when given intravenously; they may be useful for inhalation therapy. Inhalation of the plasma-derived product is under evaluation. Lung transplantation has been performed for end-stage disease.

SUPPORTIVE THERAPY

Standard supportive therapy for chronic lung disease includes aggressive treatment of pulmonary infection, routine use of pneumococcal and influenza vaccines, bronchodilators, and advice about the serious risks of smoking. Such treatment is also indicated for asymptomatic family members found to have PiZZ or null-null phenotypes, but not those with PiMZ type. The clinical significance of the PiSZ type is unclear, but nonspecific treatment is reasonable. All persons with low levels of serum antiprotease should be warned that the development of emphysema is partially mediated by environmental factors and that cigarette smoking is particularly deleterious. Although identification of affected persons could help prevent development of obstructive lung disease, population screening programs are currently suspended; however, there is increased emphasis on targeted screening programs.

Bibliography is available at Expert Consult.

Other Distal Airway Diseases

394.1 Bronchiolitis Obliterans

Steven R. Boas

EPIDEMIOLOGY

Bronchiolitis obliterans (BO), a chronic obstructive lung disease of the bronchioles and smaller airways, results from an insult to the lower respiratory tract leading to fibrosis of the small airways. In the nontransplant patient, BO most commonly occurs in the pediatric population after respiratory infections, particularly adenovirus (see Chapter 262), but also *Mycoplasma pneumoniae* (see Chapter 223), measles (see Chapter 246), *Legionella pneumophila* (see Chapter 208), influenza (see Chapter 258), and pertussis (see Chapter 197); other causes

Table 394-1	Etiology of Bronchiolitis Obliterans

POSTINFECTION
Adenovirus types 3, 7, and 21
Influenza
Parainfluenza
Measles
Respiratory syncytial virus
Varicella
Mycoplasma pneumoniae

POSTTRANSPLANTATION
Chronic rejection of lung or heart/lung transplantation
Graft-versus-host disease associated with bone marrow
  transplantation

CONNECTIVE TISSUE DISEASE
Juvenile idiopathic arthritis
Sjögren syndrome
Systemic lupus erythematosus

TOXIC FUME INHALATION
NO_2
NH_3
Diacetyl flavorings (microwave popcorn)

CHRONIC HYPERSENSITIVITY PNEUMONITIS
Avian antigens
Mold

ASPIRATION
Stomach contents: gastroesophageal reflux
Foreign bodies

DRUGS
Penicillamine
Cocaine

STEVENS-JOHNSON SYNDROME
Idiopathic
Drug induced
Infection related

From Moonnumakal SP, Fan LL: Bronchiolitis obliterans in children, Curr Opin Pediatr 20:272–278, 2008.

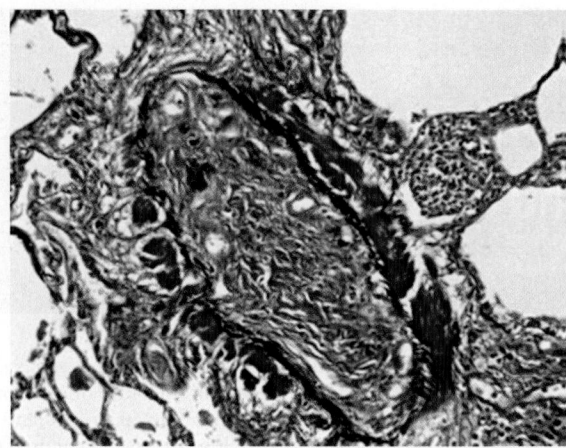

Figure 394-1 Complete obliteration of airway lumen with fibromyxoid tissue in lung transplant recipient with bronchiolitis obliterans. *(From Kurland G, Michelson P: Bronchiolitis obliterans in children, Pediatr Pulmonol 39:193–208, 2005.)*

include inflammatory diseases (juvenile idiopathic arthritis, systemic lupus erythematosus [see Chapter 158], scleroderma [see Chapter 160], Stevens-Johnson syndrome [see Chapter 152]), and inhalation of toxic fumes or particulate exposure (NO_2, incinerator fly ash, NH_3, diacetyl flavorings from microwave popcorn, papaverine, fiberglass) (Table 394-1).

Bronchiolitis obliterans syndrome (BOS), a clinical entity that relates to graft deterioration after transplantation as a result of progressive airway, is recognized as a long-term complication of lung and bone marrow transplantation; more than one-third of survivors of lung transplantation can develop this disorder. BOS occurs in all age groups, and the prevalence in 1 pediatric autopsy series was 2 per 1,000. The incidence of new cases appears to be decreasing. BOS appears to be more common among older children and adolescents than infants and toddlers. There is some evidence that postinfection obliterans may be more common in the southern hemisphere and among persons of Asian descent.

PATHOGENESIS

After the initial insult, inflammation affecting terminal bronchioles, respiratory bronchioles, and alveolar ducts can result in the obliteration of the airway lumen (Fig. 394-1). Epithelial damage resulting in abnormal repair is characteristic of BO. Complete or partial obstruction of the airway lumen can result in air trapping or atelectasis. **Bronchiolitis obliterans organizing pneumonia (BOOP)** is a fibrosing lung disease that includes the histologic features of BO with extension of the inflammatory process from distal alveolar ducts into alveoli and proliferation of fibroblasts. BOS appears histologically similar to BO.

The etiology of BOS is unclear, however, and may be unrelated to the mechanisms responsible for BO in nontransplant patients.

CLINICAL MANIFESTATIONS AND DIAGNOSIS

Cough, fever, cyanosis, dyspnea, chest pain, and respiratory distress followed by initial improvement may be the initial signs of BO. In this phase, BO is easily confused with pneumonia, bronchitis, or bronchiolitis. Progression of the disease can ensue, with increasing dyspnea, chronic cough, sputum production, and wheezing. Physical examination findings are usually nonspecific and can include wheezing, hypoxemia, and crackles. Chest radiographs may be relatively normal compared with the extent of physical findings but can demonstrate hyperlucency and patchy infiltrates. Occasionally, a Swyer-James syndrome (unilateral hyperlucent lung; see Chapter 392) develops. Pulmonary function tests demonstrate variable findings but typically show signs of airway obstruction with a variable degree of bronchodilator response. Exercise testing shows reduced exercise capacity and impaired oxygen consumption. Ventilation–perfusion scans reveal a typical moth-eaten appearance of multiple matched defects in ventilation and perfusion. High-resolution chest CT often demonstrates patchy areas or a mosaic pattern of hyperlucency, air trapping, and bronchiectasis (Fig. 394-2). (Table 394-2 provides an overview of CT findings of BO and related disorders.) Physical and radiologic signs can wax and wane over weeks or months. Open lung biopsy or transbronchial biopsy remains the best means of establishing the diagnosis of BO or BOOP.

TREATMENT

No definitive therapy exists for BO. Administration of corticosteroids may be beneficial. Immunomodulatory agents, such as sirolimus, tacrolimus, aerosolized cyclosporine, hydroxychloroquine, and macrolide antibiotics, have been used in post–lung transplantation recipients with BO with variable success. Supportive measures with oxygen, antibiotics for secondary infections, and bronchodilators are adjunct therapies. The role of gastroesophageal reflux and its association with BO has been raised, with treatment suggested whenever the diagnosis is made. Azithromycin may be effective in patients with BOS. For BOOP, use of oral corticosteroids for up to 1 yr has been advocated as first-line therapy for symptomatic and progressive disease. Patients with asymptomatic or nonprogressive BOOP can be observed.

PROGNOSIS

Some patients with BO experience rapid deterioration in their condition and die within weeks of the initial symptoms; most nontransplant patients survive with chronic disability. BOS has a higher mortality

Table 394-2	High-Resolution CT Patterns in Child with Interstitial Lung Disease					
	STUDIES (N)	GROUND-GLASS OPACITY	THICK SEPTA	NODULES	MOSAIC PATTERN	HONEYCOMBING
Bronchiolitis obliterans	4	—	—	—	X	—
Nonspecific interstitial pneumonitis	6	X	—	—	—	X
Desquamative interstitial pneumonitis	4	X	—	—	—	X
Follicular bronchitis or neuroendocrine cell hyperplasia of infancy	4	X	—	—	X	—
Lymphocytic interstitial pneumonitis	4	—	—	X	—	—
Lymphangiomatosis	2	—	X	—	—	—
Lymphangiectasia	2	—	X	—	—	—
Pulmonary alveolar proteinosis	2	X	X	—	—	—

From Long FR, Interstitial lung disease. In Slovis TL, editor: Caffey's pediatric diagnostic imaging, ed 11, Philadelphia, 2008, Mosby, Table 74-1; original data from Lynch DA, Hay T, Newell JD Jr, et al: Pediatric diffuse lung disease: diagnosis and classification using high-resolution CT. AJR Am J Roentgenol 173:713–718, 1999, and Copley SJ, Coren M, Nicholson AG, et al: Diagnostic accuracy of thin-section CT and chest radiography of pediatric interstitial lung disease. AJR Am J Roentgenol 174:549–554, 2000.

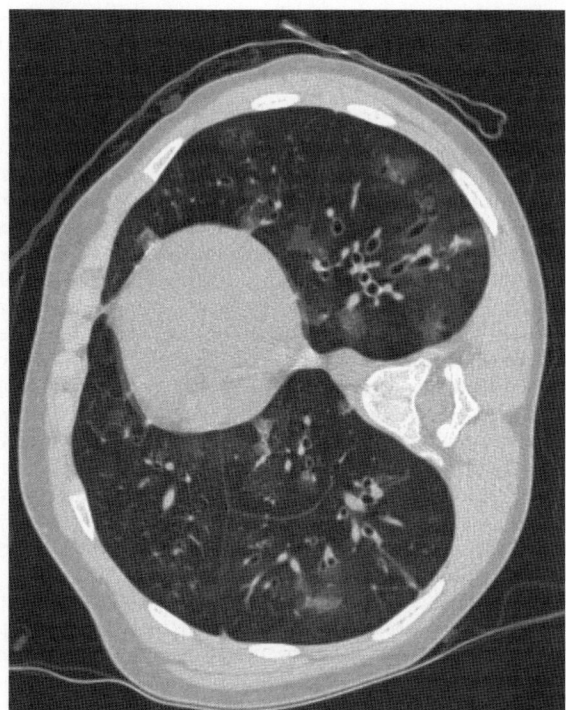

Figure 394-2 High-resolution CT scan of the chest of a child with bronchiolitis obliterans demonstrating mosaic perfusion and vascular attenuation. Air-trapping is demonstrated by lack of increase in attention or decrease in lung volume in dependent lung. *(Image courtesy of Alan Brody, MD, Cincinnati Children's Hospital Medical Center, Ohio.)*

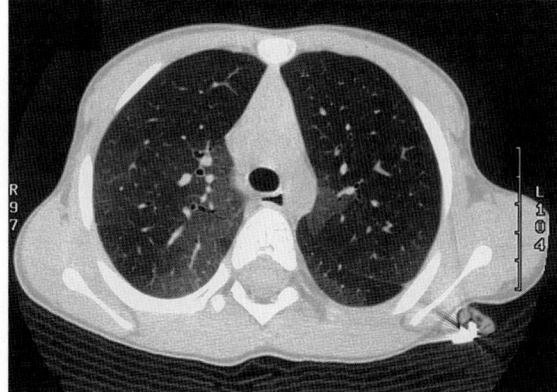

Figure 394-3 Follicular bronchiolitis in a 3 yr old girl with mosaic attenuation and cylindrical bronchiectasis. CT findings suggested BO, but a biopsy documented the presence of follicular bronchiolitis. *(From Long FR, Druhan SM, Kuhn JP. Diseases of the bronchi and pulmonary aeration. In Slovis TL, editor: Caffey's pediatric diagnostic imaging, ed 11, Philadelphia, 2008, Mosby, Fig. 73-71.)*

rate. Unlike in BO, total recovery is seen in 60-80% of patients with BOOP, although this depends on the underlying systemic disease. BOOP can relapse, especially if treatment duration is <1 yr; BOOP is amenable to repeat courses of oral corticosteroids. Unlike the more common idiopathic BOOP, progressive BOOP characterized by acute respiratory distress syndrome is rare but is aggressive in its clinical course, leading to death.

Bibliography is available at Expert Consult.

394.2 Follicular Bronchitis
Steven R. Boas

Follicular bronchitis is a lymphoproliferative lung disorder characterized by the presence of lymphoid follicles alongside the airways (bronchi or bronchioles) and infiltration of the walls of bronchi and bronchioles. Although the cause is unknown, an infectious etiology (viral, *L. pneumophila*; see Chapter 208) has been proposed. This disorder has been reported following lung transplant and in an HIV-positive child. It can occur in adults and children; in children, onset of symptoms generally occurs by 6 wk of age and peaks between 6 and 18 mo. Cough, moderate respiratory distress, fever, and fine crackles are common clinical findings. Fine crackles generally persist over time, and recurrence of symptoms is common. Chest radiographs may be relatively benign initially (air trapping, peribronchial thickening) but evolve into the typical interstitial pattern. Chest CT can show a fine reticular pattern as well as bronchiectasis and centrilobular branching but can also appear normal (see Table 394-2). Definitive diagnosis is made by open-lung biopsy (Fig. 394-3). Some patients with follicular bronchitis respond to therapy with corticosteroids. Prognosis is variable, with some patients having significant progression of pulmonary disease and others developing only mild obstructive airway disease. In children it is generally associated with immunodeficiency; the differential diagnosis includes the pulmonary complications of HIV infection (see Chapter 276).

Bibliography is available at Expert Consult.

394.3 Pulmonary Alveolar Microlithiasis
Steven R. Boas

Pulmonary alveolar microlithiasis (PAM) is a rare disease characterized by the formation of lamellar concretions of calcium phosphate or "microliths" within the alveoli, creating a classic pattern on the radiograph (Fig. 394-4).

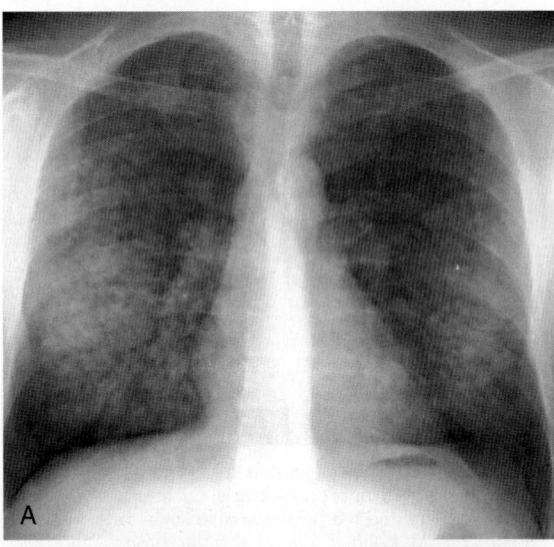

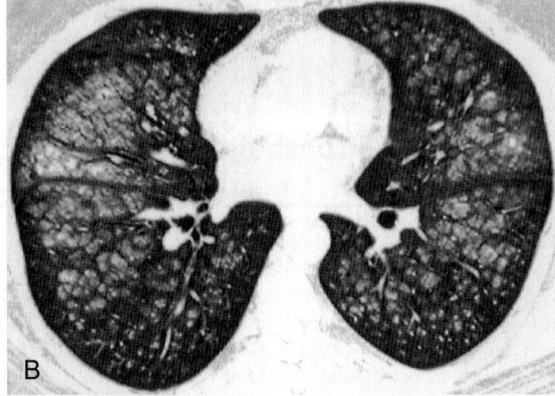

Figure 394-4 Radiographic features of pulmonary alveolar microlithiasis. **A,** Posteroanterior chest radiograph showing the classic "sandstorm" appearance of pulmonary alveolar microlithiasis, including diffuse, patchy, bilateral sharp micronodular disease. **B,** High-resolution CT scan of the chest showing micronodular densities. *(From Brandenburg VM, Schubert H. Images in clinical medicine. Pulmonary alveolar microlithiasis. N Engl J Med 348:1555, 2003.)*

EPIDEMIOLOGY AND ETIOLOGY
Although the mean age at time of diagnosis is in the mid 30s, the onset of the disease can occur in childhood. PAM is inherited in an autosomal recessive pattern. In 2006, a mutation in the gene that encodes for the type IIb sodium-phosphate cotransporter protein (SCL34A2) was discovered in people with PAM. This gene is expressed in high levels in the lungs predominantly in type 2 epithelial cells. While the precise role of this protein is unknown, it is speculated that it helps remove phosphate from the alveolar space as well as a phosphate regular in other organs.

In some families, progression of disease is rapid. An equal male and female incidence is noted. Although PAM is found throughout the world, there is a high incidence in Turkey and a lesser incidence in Italy, Japan, and India.

CLINICAL MANIFESTATIONS
When symptomatic, patients with PAM usually complain of dyspnea on exertion and nonproductive cough. Physical examination of the lungs can reveal fine inspiratory crackles and diminished breath sounds. Clubbing occurs, although this is usually a more advanced sign. Discordance between the clinical and radiographic manifestations is common. Many children are often asymptomatic on initial presentation and present with symptoms during adulthood. Complications of pneumothorax, pleural adhesions and calcifications, pleural fibrosis, apical bullae, and extrapulmonary sites of microliths have been reported (kidneys, prostate, sympathetic chain, and testes).

DIAGNOSIS
Chest radiography typically reveals bilateral infiltrates with a fine micronodular appearance or **sandstorm** appearance with greater density in the lower and middle lung fields (see Fig. 394-4). CT of the chest shows diffuse micronodular calcified densities, with thickening of the microliths along the septa and around distal bronchioles, especially in the inferior and posterior regions (see Table 394-2). Diffuse uptake of technetium-99 methylene diphosphonate by nuclear scan has been reported. Open lung and transbronchial lung biopsy reveal 0.1-0.3 mm laminated calcific concretions within the alveoli. Although the alveoli are often normal initially, progression to pulmonary fibrosis with advancing disease usually ensues. Sputum expectoration might reveal small microliths, although this finding is not diagnostic for PAM and is not typically seen in children. Detection of calcium deposits in bronchoalveolar lavage fluid on bronchoscopy supports the diagnosis. Pulmonary function testing reveals restrictive lung disease with impaired diffusing capacity as the disease progresses, whereas exercise testing demonstrates arterial oxygen desaturation. Detection of a mutation in the *SCL34A2* gene confirms the diagnosis. The differential diagnosis includes sarcoidosis, miliary tuberculosis, hemosiderosis, healed disseminated histoplasmosis, pulmonary calcinosis, and metastatic pulmonary calcifications.

TREATMENT
No specific treatment is effective, although some clinicians have used glucocorticosteroids, etidronate disodium, and bronchopulmonary lavage with limited success. Lung transplantation has been performed for this condition, although it is unknown whether the disease recurs after transplantation.

PROGNOSIS
Progressive cardiopulmonary disease can ensue, leading to cor pulmonale, superimposed infections, and subsequent death in mid-adulthood. Because of the familial nature of this disease, counseling and chest radiographs of family members are indicated.

Bibliography is available at Expert Consult.

Chapter **395**
Congenital Disorders of the Lung

395.1 Pulmonary Agenesis and Aplasia
Joshua A. Blatter and Jonathan D. Finder

ETIOLOGY AND PATHOLOGY
Pulmonary agenesis differs from hypoplasia in that agenesis entails the complete absence of a lung. Agenesis differs from aplasia by the absence of a bronchial stump or carina that is seen in aplasia. Bilateral pulmonary agenesis is incompatible with life, manifesting as severe respiratory distress and failure. Pulmonary agenesis is thought to be an autosomal recessive trait, with an estimated incidence of 1 in 10,000-15,000 births.

CLINICAL MANIFESTATIONS AND PROGNOSIS
Unilateral agenesis or hypoplasia can have few symptoms and nonspecific findings, resulting in only 33% of the cases being diagnosed while the patient is living. Symptoms tend to associated with central airway complications of compression, stenosis, and/or tracheobronchomalacia. In patients in whom the right lung is absent, the aorta can compress the trachea and lead to symptoms of central airway compression. Right lung agenesis has a higher morbidity and mortality than left lung agenesis. Pulmonary agenesis is often seen in association with other congenital anomalies such as the **VACTERL sequence** (*v*ertebral anomalies, *a*nal atresia, *c*ongenital heart disease, *t*racheoesophageal fistula, *r*enal anomalies, and *l*imb anomalies), ipsilateral facial and skeletal malformations, and central nervous system and cardiac malformations. Compensatory growth of the remaining lung allows improved gas exchange, but the mediastinal shift can lead to scoliosis and airway compression. Scoliosis can result from unequal thoracic growth.

DIAGNOSIS AND TREATMENT
Chest radiographic findings of unilateral lung or lobar collapse with a shift of mediastinal structures toward the affected side can prompt referral for suspected foreign-body aspiration, mucous plug occlusion, or other bronchial mass lesions. The diagnosis requires a high index of suspicion to avoid the unnecessary risks of bronchoscopy, including potential perforation of the rudimentary bronchus. CT of the chest is diagnostic, although the diagnosis may be suggested by chronic changes in the contralateral aspect of the chest wall and lung expansion on chest radiographs. Because pulmonary agenesis can be associated with a wide variety of congenital lesions, whole-body MRI can be useful to determine whether other systems (e.g., cardiac, gastrointestinal) are affected. Conservative treatment is usually recommended, although surgery has offered benefit in selected cases.

Bibliography is available at Expert Consult.

395.2 Pulmonary Hypoplasia
Joshua A. Blatter and Jonathan D. Finder

ETIOLOGY AND PATHOLOGY
Pulmonary hypoplasia involves a decrease in both the number of alveoli and the number of airway generations. The hypoplasia may be bilateral in the setting of bilateral lung constraint, as in oligohydramnios or thoracic dystrophy. Pulmonary hypoplasia is usually secondary to other intrauterine disorders that produce an impairment of normal lung development (see Chapter 101). Conditions such as deformities of the thoracic spine and rib cage (thoracic dystrophy), pleural effusions with fetal hydrops, congenital pulmonary airway malformation, and congenital diaphragmatic hernia physically constrain the developing lung. Any condition that produces oligohydramnios (fetal renal insufficiency or prolonged premature rupture of membranes) can also lead to diminished lung growth. In these conditions, airway and arterial branching are inhibited, thereby limiting the capillary surface area. Large unilateral lesions, such as congenital diaphragmatic hernia or pulmonary airway malformation, can displace the mediastinum and thereby produce a contralateral hypoplasia, although usually not as severe as that seen on the ipsilateral side.

CLINICAL MANIFESTATIONS
Pulmonary hypoplasia is usually recognized in the newborn period, owing to either the respiratory insufficiency or the presentation of persistent pulmonary hypertension (see Chapter 101.7). Later presentation (tachypnea) with stress or respiratory viral infection can be seen in infants with mild pulmonary hypoplasia.

DIAGNOSIS AND TREATMENT
A variety of imaging techniques, including MRI and ultrasound, with estimation of oligohydramnios, can be helpful to identify hypoplasia, but not to predict pulmonary function. Mechanical ventilation and oxygen may be required to support gas exchange. Specific therapy to control associated pulmonary hypertension, such as inhaled nitric oxide, may be useful. In cases of severe hypoplasia, the limited capacity of the lung for gas exchange may be inadequate to sustain life. Extracorporeal membrane oxygenation can provide gas exchange for a critical period of time and permit survival. Rib-expanding devices (vertically expansible prosthetic titanium ribs) can improve the survival of patients with thoracic dystrophies (see Chapter 700).

Bibliography is available at Expert Consult.

395.3 Congenital Cystic Malformation
Joshua A. Blatter and Jonathan D. Finder

PATHOLOGY
Congenital pulmonary airway malformation (CPAM), formerly known as cystic adenomatoid malformation, consists of hamartomatous or dysplastic lung tissue mixed with more normal lung, generally confined to 1 lobe. This congenital pulmonary disorder occurs in approximately 1-4 in 100,000 births. Prenatal ultrasonographic findings are classified as **macrocystic** (single or multiple cysts >5 mm) or **microcystic** (echogenic cysts <5 mm). Five histologic patterns have been described. **Type 0** (acinar dysplasia) is least common (<3%) and consists of microcystic disease throughout the lungs. The prognosis is poorest for this type, and infants die at birth. **Type 1** (60%) is macrocystic and consists of a single or several large (>2 cm in diameter) cysts lined with ciliated pseudostratified epithelium; the lesion is localized involving only a part of 1 lobe. One-third of cases have mucus-secreting cells. Presentation is in utero or in the newborn period. Cartilage is rarely seen in the wall of the cyst. This type has a good prognosis for survival. **Type 2** (20%) is microcystic and consists of multiple small cysts with histology similar to that of the type 1 lesion. Type 2 is associated with other serious congenital anomalies (renal, cardiac, diaphragmatic hernia) and carries a poor prognosis. **Type 3** (<10%) is seen mostly in males; the lesion is a mixture of microcysts and solid tissue with bronchiole-like structures lined with cuboidal ciliated epithelium and separated by areas of nonciliated cuboidal epithelium. The prognosis for this type, like type 0, is poor. **Type 4** (10%) is commonly macrocystic and lacks mucus cells. It is associated with malignancy

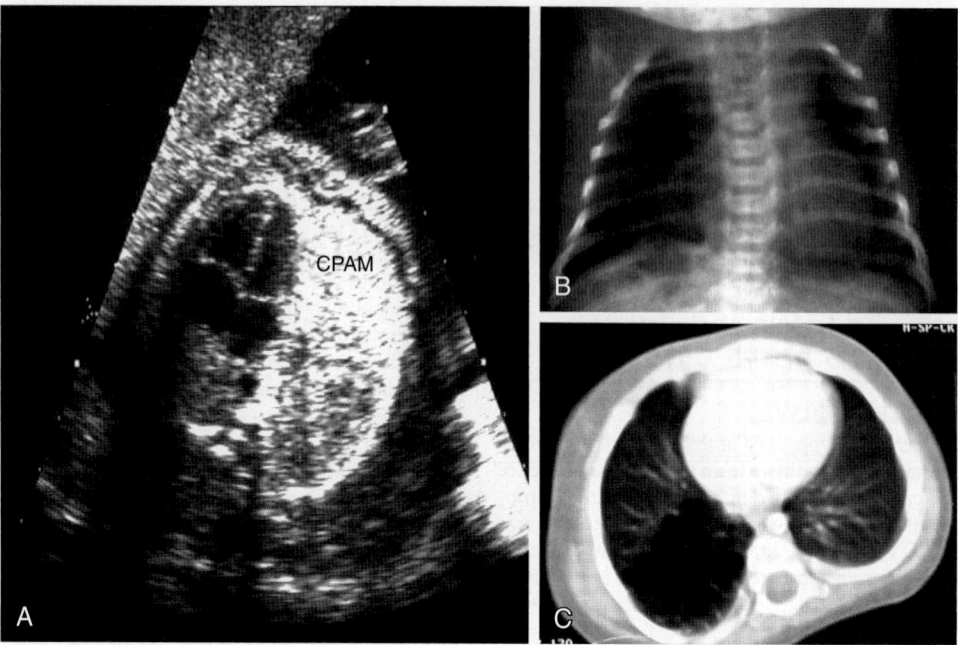

Figure 395-1 Imaging of congenital pulmonary airway malformation of the lung (CPAM) on the same patient with prenatal ultrasound scan **(A)**, chest radiograph **(B)**, and CT scan **(C)**. Note that the lesion is not visible on the chest radiograph. *(From Lakhoo K: Management of congenital cystic adenomatous malformations of the lung, Arch Dis Child Fetal Neonatal Ed 94:F73–F76, 2009.)*

(pleuropulmonary blastoma) and can present either in childhood or in asymptomatic adults.

ETIOLOGY

The lesion probably results from an embryologic injury before the 35th day of gestation, with maldevelopment of terminal bronchiolar structures. Histologic examination reveals little normal lung and many glandular elements. Cysts are very common; cartilage is rare. The presence of cartilage might indicate a somewhat later embryologic insult, perhaps extending into the 10th-24th wk. Although growth factor interactions and signaling mechanisms have been implicated in altered lung-branching morphogenesis, the exact roles in the maldevelopment seen here remain obscure.

DIAGNOSIS

Cystic airway malformations can be diagnosed in utero by ultrasonography (Fig. 395-1). Fetal cystic lung abnormalities can include CPAM (40%), pulmonary sequestration (14%) (see Chapter 395.4), or both (26%); the median age at diagnosis is usually 21 wk gestation. In 1 series, only 7% had severe signs of fetal distress including hydrops, pleural effusion, polyhydramnios, ascites, or severe facial edema; 96% of the fetuses were born alive, 2 of whom died in the neonatal period. Lesions causing fetal hydrops have a poor prognosis. Large lesions, by compressing adjacent lung, can produce pulmonary hypoplasia in non-affected lobes (see Chapter 395.2). Even lesions that appear large in early gestation can regress considerably or decrease in relative size and be associated with good pulmonary function in childhood. CT allows accurate diagnosis and sizing of the lesion and is indicated even in asymptomatic neonates.

CLINICAL MANIFESTATIONS

Patients can present in the newborn period or early infancy with respiratory distress, recurrent respiratory infection, and pneumothorax. The lesion may be confused with a diaphragmatic hernia (see Chapter 101.8). Patients with smaller lesions are usually asymptomatic until mid-childhood, when episodes of recurrent or persistent pulmonary infection or chest pain occur. Breath sounds may be diminished, with mediastinal shift away from the lesion on physical examination. Chest radiographs reveal a cystic mass, sometimes with mediastinal shift

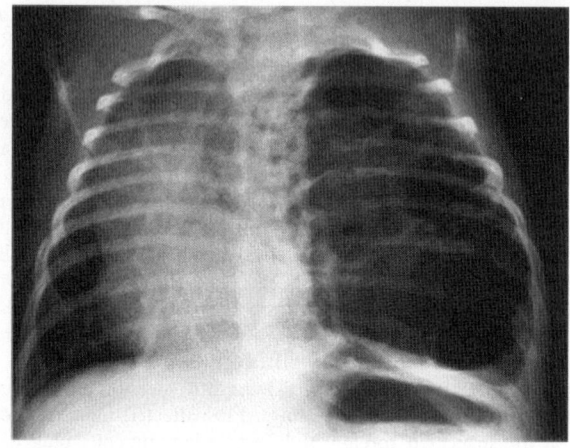

Figure 395-2 Neonatal chest x-ray showing large multicystic mass in the left hemithorax with mediastinal shift as a result of congenital pulmonary airway malformation (CPAM). *(From Williams HJ, Johnson KJ: Imaging of congenital cystic lung lesions, Paediatr Respir Rev 3:120–127, 2002.)*

(Fig. 395-2). Occasionally, an air–fluid level suggests a lung abscess (see Chapter 402).

TREATMENT

Antenatal intervention in severely affected infants is controversial but can include excision of the affected lobe for microcystic lesions, aspiration of macrocystic lesions, and, rarely, open fetal surgery. In the postnatal period, surgery is indicated for symptomatic patients. Although surgery may be delayed for asymptomatic infants because postnatal resolution has been reported, true resolution appears to be very rare in that abnormalities usually remain detectable on CT or MRI. Sarcomatous and carcinomatous degeneration have been described in patients with CPAM, so surgical resection by 1 year of age is recommended to limit malignant potential. The mortality rate is <10%. Another indication for surgery is to rule out **pleuropulmonary**

blastoma, a malignancy that can appear radiographically similar to type I CPAM.

Bibliography is available at Expert Consult.

395.4 Pulmonary Sequestration
Joshua A. Blatter and Jonathan D. Finder

Pulmonary sequestration is a congenital anomaly of lung development that can be intrapulmonary or extrapulmonary, according to the location within the visceral pleura. The majority of sequestrations are intrapulmonary.

PATHOPHYSIOLOGY
The lung tissue in a sequestration does not connect to a bronchus and receives its arterial supply from the systemic arteries (commonly off the aorta) and returns its venous blood to the right side of the heart through the inferior vena cava (**extralobar**) or pulmonary veins (**intralobar**). The sequestration functions as a space-occupying lesion within the chest; it does not participate in gas exchange and does not lead to a left-to-right shunt or alveolar dead space. Communication with the airway can occur as the result of rupture of infected material into an adjacent airway. Collateral ventilation within intrapulmonary lesions via pores of Kohn can occur. Pulmonary sequestrations can arise through the same pathoembryologic mechanism as a remnant of a diverticular outgrowth of the esophagus. Some propose that intrapulmonary sequestration is an acquired lesion primarily caused by infection and inflammation; inflammation leads to cystic changes and hypertrophy of a feeding systemic artery. This is consistent with the rarity of this lesion in autopsy series of newborns. Gastric or pancreatic tissue may be found within the sequestration. Cysts also may be present. Other associated congenital anomalies, including CPAM (see Chapter 395.3), diaphragmatic hernia (see Chapter 101.8), and esophageal cysts, are not uncommon. Some believe that intrapulmonary sequestration is often a manifestation of CPAM and have questioned the existence of intrapulmonary sequestration as a separate entity.

CLINICAL MANIFESTATIONS AND DIAGNOSIS
Physical findings in patients with sequestration include an area of dullness to percussion and decreased breath sounds over the lesion. During infection, crackles may also be present. A continuous or purely systolic murmur may be heard over the back. If findings on routine chest radiographs are consistent with the diagnosis, further delineation is indicated before surgical intervention (Fig. 395-3). CT with contrast can demonstrate both the extent of the lesion and its vascular supply. MR angiography is also useful. Ultrasonography can help rule out a diaphragmatic hernia and demonstrate the systemic artery. Surgical removal is recommended. Identifying the blood supply before surgery avoids inadvertently severing its systemic artery. Coil embolization (transumbilical in neonates; arterial in older patients) has been successful in treating patients with sequestration.

Intrapulmonary sequestration is generally found in a lower lobe and does not have its own pleura. Patients usually present with infection. In older patients, hemoptysis is common. A chest radiograph during a period when there is no active infection reveals a mass lesion; an air–fluid level may be present. During infection, the margins of the lesion may be blurred. There is no difference in the incidence of this lesion in each lung.

Extrapulmonary sequestration is much more common in boys, and almost always involves the left lung. This lesion is enveloped by a pleural covering and is associated with diaphragmatic hernia and other abnormalities such as colonic duplication, vertebral abnormalities, and pulmonary hypoplasia. Many of these patients are asymptomatic when the mass is discovered by routine chest radiography. Other patients present with respiratory symptoms or heart failure. Subdiaphragmatic extrapulmonary sequestration can manifest as an abdominal mass on prenatal ultrasonography. The advent of prenatal ultrasonography has also enabled evidence that fetal pulmonary sequestrations can spontaneously regress.

TREATMENT
Treatment of intrapulmonary sequestration is surgical removal of the lesion, a procedure that usually requires excision of the entire involved lobe. Segmental resection occasionally suffices. Surgical resection of the involved area is recommended for extrapulmonary sequestration. Coil embolization of the feeding artery has also been successful.

Bibliography is available at Expert Consult.

395.5 Bronchogenic Cysts
Joshua A. Blatter and Jonathan D. Finder

ETIOLOGY AND PATHOLOGY
Bronchogenic cysts arise from abnormal budding of the tracheal diverticulum of the foregut before the 16th wk of gestation and are originally lined with ciliated epithelium. They are more commonly found on the right and near a midline structure (trachea, esophagus, carina), but peripheral lower lobe and perihilar intrapulmonary cysts are not

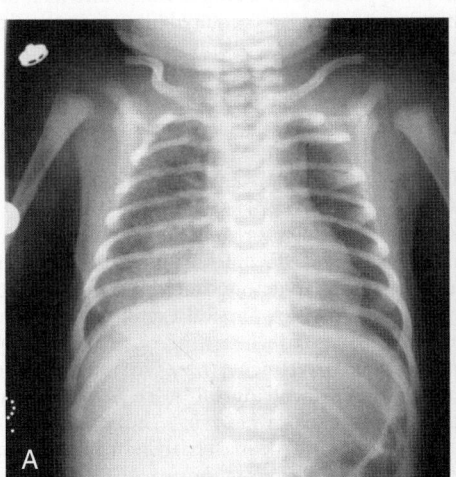
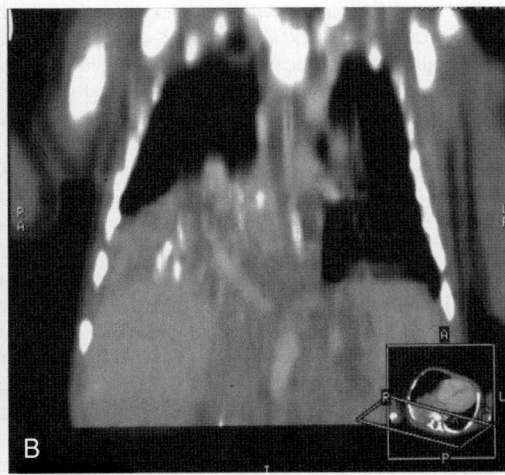

Figure 395-3 A, Plain chest x-ray showing changes in the region of the right lower/middle lobe of the lung. **B,** CT showing parenchymal changes in the right lower lobe of the lung in keeping with a sequestration. *(From Corbett HJ, Humphrey GME: Pulmonary sequestration, Paediatr Respir Rev 5:59–68, 2004.)*

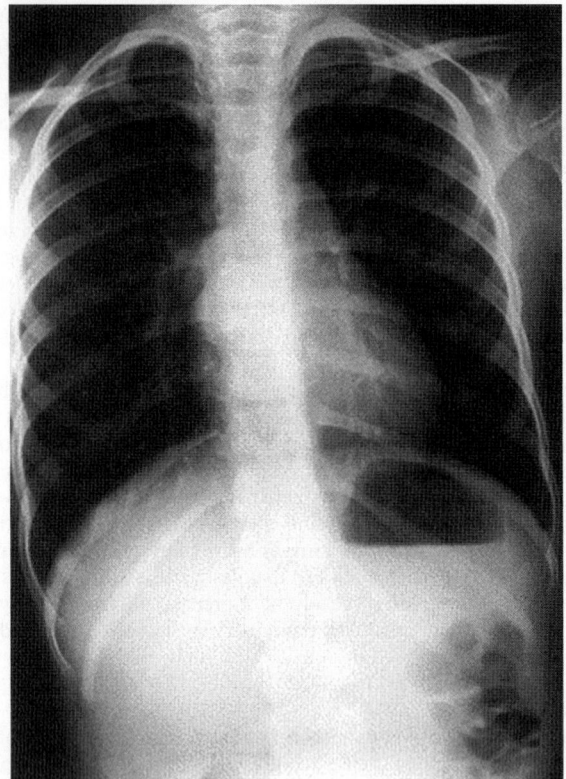

Figure 395-4 Chest x-ray showing an ovoid, well-defined, soft-tissue density causing splaying of the carina due to bronchogenic cyst. *(From Williams HJ, Johnson KJ: Imaging of congenital cystic lung lesions, Paediatr Respir Rev 3:120–127, 2002.)*

infrequent. Diagnosis may be precipitated by enlargement of the cyst, which causes symptoms by pressure on an adjacent airway. When the diagnosis is delayed until an infection occurs, the ciliated epithelium may be lost, and accurate pathologic diagnosis is then impossible. Cysts are rarely demonstrable at birth. Later, some cysts become symptomatic by becoming infected or by enlarging and compromising the function of an adjacent airway.

CLINICAL MANIFESTATIONS AND TREATMENT

Fever, chest pain, and productive cough are the most common presenting symptoms. Dysphagia may be present; some bronchogenic cysts are asymptomatic. A chest radiograph reveals the cyst, which can contain an air–fluid level (Fig. 395-4). CT scan or MRI is obtained in most cases to better demonstrate anatomy and extent of lesion before surgical resection. Treatment of symptomatic cysts is surgical excision after appropriate antibiotic management. Asymptomatic cysts are generally excised in view of the high rate of infection.

Bibliography is available at Expert Consult.

395.6 Congenital Pulmonary Lymphangiectasia
Joshua A. Blatter and Jonathan D. Finder

ETIOLOGY AND PATHOLOGY

Congenital pulmonary lymphangiectasia is characterized by greatly dilated lymphatic ducts throughout the lung. It can occur in 3 pathologic circumstances: **pulmonary venous obstruction** that produces an elevated transvascular pressure and engorges the pulmonary lymphatics; **generalized lymphangiectasia**, as a generalized disease of several organ systems, including lungs and the intestines (can be associated with Noonan syndrome); and **primary lymphangiectasia** limited to the lung as a manifestation of an abnormality in lymphatic development.

CLINICAL MANIFESTATIONS AND TREATMENT

Children with pulmonary venous obstruction or severe pulmonary lymphangiectasia present with dyspnea and cyanosis in the newborn period. Hydrops fetalis may be diagnosed antenatally. Chest radiographs reveal diffuse, dense, reticular densities with prominence of Kerley B lines. Pleural effusions are common; thoracentesis will reveal chylothorax in this setting. If the lung is not completely involved, the spared areas appear hyperlucent. Respiration is compromised because of impaired diffusion and decreased pulmonary compliance. The diagnosis can be suggested by CT scan and/or cardiac catheterization; definitive diagnosis requires lung biopsy (either thoracoscopic or open).

Treatment is supportive and includes administration of oxygen, mechanical ventilation, nutritional support (including gastrostomy placement and use of feedings containing medium-chain triglycerides), and careful fluid management with diuretics. Primary pulmonary lymphangiectasia can produce severe pulmonary dysfunction that can require long-term mechanical ventilation; long-term survival and resolution of respiratory insufficiency is possible even in severe cases. Occasionally, the pulmonary venous obstruction is secondary to left-sided cardiac lesions; relief of the latter can produce improvement in pulmonary dysfunction. Generalized lymphangiectasia produces milder pulmonary dysfunction, and survival to mid-childhood and beyond is not unusual.

Bibliography is available at Expert Consult.

395.7 Lung Hernia
Joshua A. Blatter and Jonathan D. Finder

ETIOLOGY AND PATHOLOGY

A lung hernia is a protrusion of the lung beyond its normal thoracic boundaries. Approximately 20% are congenital, with the remainder being noted after chest trauma or thoracic surgery or in patients with pulmonary diseases such as cystic fibrosis (see Chapter 403) or asthma (see Chapter 144), which cause frequent cough and generate high intrathoracic pressure. A congenital weakness of the suprapleural membrane (Sibson fascia) or musculature of the neck can play a role in the appearance of a lung hernia. More than half of congenital lung hernias and almost all acquired hernias are **cervical.** Congenital cervical hernias usually occur anteriorly through a gap between the scalenus anterior and sternocleidomastoid muscles. Cervical herniation is usually prevented by the trapezius muscle (posteriorly, at the thoracic inlet) and by the 3 scalene muscles (laterally).

CLINICAL MANIFESTATIONS AND TREATMENT

The presenting sign of a cervical hernia (Sibson hernia) is usually a neck mass noticed while straining or coughing. Some lesions are asymptomatic and detected only when a chest film is taken for another reason. Findings on physical examination are normal except during Valsalva maneuver, when a soft bulge may be noticed in the neck. In most cases, no treatment is necessary, although these hernias can cause problems during attempts to place a central venous catheter through the jugular or subclavian veins. They can resolve spontaneously.

Paravertebral or parasternal hernias are usually associated with rib anomalies. Intercostal hernias usually occur parasternally, where the external intercostal muscle is absent. Posteriorly, despite the seemingly inadequate internal intercostal muscle, the paraspinal muscles usually prevent herniation. Straining, coughing, or playing a musical instrument can have a role in causing intercostal hernias, but in most cases, there is probably a preexisting defect in the thoracic wall.

Surgical treatment for lung hernia is occasionally justified for cosmetic reasons. In patients with severe chronic pulmonary disease and chronic cough and for whom cough suppression is contraindicated, permanent correction might not be achieved.

Bibliography is available at Expert Consult.

395.8 Other Congenital Malformations of the Lung

Joshua A. Blatter and Jonathan D. Finder

CONGENITAL LOBAR EMPHYSEMA AND PULMONARY CYSTS
See Chapter 392.

PULMONARY ARTERIOVENOUS MALFORMATION
See Chapters 432 and 444.

BRONCHOBILIARY FISTULA
A bronchobiliary fistula consists of a fistulous connection between the right middle lobe bronchus and the left hepatic ductal system. Although diagnosis can be delayed until adulthood, this rare anomaly typically manifests with life-threatening bronchopulmonary infections in early infancy. Girls are more commonly affected. *Definitive diagnosis* requires endoscopy or exploratory surgery. *Treatment* includes surgical excision of the entire intrathoracic portion of the fistula. If the hepatic portion of the fistula does not communicate with the biliary system or duodenum, the involved segment might also have to be resected. Bronchobiliary communications also occur as acquired lesions resulting from hepatic disease complicated by infection.

Bibliography is available at Expert Consult.

Table 396-1	Etiology of Pulmonary Edema

INCREASED PULMONARY CAPILLARY PRESSURE
Cardiogenic, such as left ventricular failure
Noncardiogenic, as in pulmonary venoocclusive disease, pulmonary venous fibrosis, mediastinal tumors

INCREASED CAPILLARY PERMEABILITY
Bacterial and viral pneumonia
Acute respiratory distress syndrome
Inhaled toxic agents
Circulating toxins
Vasoactive substances such as histamine, leukotrienes, thromboxanes
Diffuse capillary leak syndrome, as in sepsis
Immunologic reactions, such as transfusion reactions
Smoke inhalation
Aspiration pneumonia/pneumonitis
Drowning and near drowning
Radiation pneumonia
Uremia

LYMPHATIC INSUFFICIENCY
Congenital and acquired

DECREASED ONCOTIC PRESSURE
Hypoalbuminemia, as in renal and hepatic diseases, protein-losing states, and malnutrition

INCREASED NEGATIVE INTERSTITIAL PRESSURE
Upper airway obstructive lesions, such as croup and epiglottitis
Reexpansion pulmonary edema

MIXED OR UNKNOWN CAUSES
Neurogenic pulmonary edema
High-altitude pulmonary edema
Eclampsia
Pancreatitis
Pulmonary embolism
Heroin (narcotic) pulmonary edema

Modified from Robin E, Carroll C, Zelis R: Pulmonary edema, N Engl J Med 288:239, 292, 1973; and Desphande J, Wetzel R, Rogers M: In Rogers M, editor: Textbook of pediatric intensive care, ed 3, Baltimore, 1996, Williams & Wilkins, pp. 432–442.

Chapter **396**
Pulmonary Edema
Robert L. Mazor and Thomas P. Green

A sequela of several different pathologic processes, pulmonary edema is an excessive accumulation of fluid in the interstitium and air spaces of the lung resulting in oxygen desaturation, decreased lung compliance, and respiratory distress. The condition is common in the acutely ill child.

PATHOPHYSIOLOGY
Although pulmonary edema is traditionally separated into two categories according to cause (*cardiogenic* and *noncardiogenic*), the end result of both processes is a net fluid accumulation within the interstitial and alveolar spaces. Noncardiogenic pulmonary edema, in its most severe state, is also known as **acute respiratory distress syndrome** (see Chapters 71 and 373).

The hydrostatic pressure and colloid osmotic (oncotic) pressure on either side of a pulmonary vascular wall, along with vascular permeability, are the forces and physical factors that determine fluid movement through the vessel wall. Baseline conditions lead to a net filtration of fluid from the intravascular space into the interstitium. This "extra" interstitial fluid is usually rapidly reabsorbed by pulmonary lymphat-

ics. Conditions that lead to altered vascular permeability, increased pulmonary vascular pressure, and decreased intravascular oncotic pressure increase the net flow of fluid out of the vessel (Table 396-1). Once the capacity of the lymphatics for fluid removal is exceeded, water accumulates in the lung.

To understand the sequence of lung water accumulation, it is helpful to consider its distribution among 4 distinct compartments, as follows:
- *Vascular compartment:* This compartment consists of all blood vessels that participate in fluid exchange with the interstitium. The vascular compartment is separated from the interstitium by capillary endothelial cells. Several endogenous inflammatory mediators, as well as exogenous toxins, are implicated in the pathogenesis of pulmonary capillary endothelial damage, leading to the "leakiness" seen in several systemic processes.
- *Interstitial compartment:* The importance of this space lies in its interposition between the alveolar and vascular compartments. As fluid leaves the vascular compartment, it collects in the interstitium before overflowing into the air spaces of the alveolar compartment.
- *Alveolar compartment:* This compartment is lined with type 1 and type 2 epithelial cells. These epithelial cells have a role in active fluid transport from the alveolar space, and they act as a barrier to exclude fluid from the alveolar space. The potential fluid volume of the alveolar compartment is many times greater than that of the interstitial space, perhaps providing another reason that alveolar edema clears more slowly than interstitial edema.

◆ *Pulmonary lymphatic compartment:* There is an extensive network of pulmonary lymphatics. Excess fluid present in the alveolar and interstitial compartments is drained via the lymphatic system. When the capacity for drainage of the lymphatics is surpassed, fluid accumulation occurs.

ETIOLOGY

The specific clinical findings vary according to the underlying mechanism (see Table 396-1).

Transudation of fluid as a result of increased pulmonary vascular pressure *(capillary hydrostatic pressure)* occurs in several cardiac processes. A significant left-to-right shunting lesion, such as a septal defect, leads to a pressure and volume load on the pulmonary vasculature. The resultant pulmonary edema is one of the hallmarks of congestive heart failure. Left ventricular failure, mitral valve disease, and pulmonary venous obstructive lesions cause increased "backpressure" in the pulmonary vasculature. This results in an increase in pulmonary capillary pressure.

Increased capillary permeability is usually secondary to endothelial damage. Such damage can occur secondary to direct injury to the alveolar epithelium or indirectly through systemic processes that deliver circulating inflammatory mediators or toxins to the lung. Inflammatory mediators (tumor necrosis factor, leukotrienes, thromboxanes) and vasoactive agents (nitric oxide, histamine) formed during pulmonary and systemic processes potentiate the altered capillary permeability that occurs in many disease processes, with sepsis being a common cause.

Fluid homeostasis in the lung largely depends on drainage via the lymphatics. Experimentally, pulmonary edema occurs with obstruction of the lymphatic system. Increased lymph flow and dilation of lymphatic vessels occur in chronic edematous states.

A decrease in intravascular oncotic pressure leads to pulmonary edema by altering the forces promoting fluid reentry into the vascular space. This occurs in dilutional disorders, such as fluid overload with hypotonic solutions, and in protein-losing states, such as nephrotic syndrome and malnutrition.

The excessive negative interstitial pressure seen in upper airway diseases, such as croup and laryngospasm, may promote pulmonary edema. Aside from the physical forces present in these diseases, other mechanisms may also be involved. Theories implicate an increase in CO_2 tension, decreased O_2 tension, and extreme increases in cardiac afterload, leading to transient cardiac insufficiency.

The mechanism causing neurogenic pulmonary edema is not clear. A massive sympathetic discharge secondary to a cerebral injury may produce increased pulmonary and systemic vasoconstriction, resulting in a shift of blood to the pulmonary vasculature, an increase in capillary pressure, and edema formation. Inflammatory mechanisms may also play a role by increasing capillary permeability.

The mechanism responsible for high-altitude pulmonary edema is unclear, but it may also be related to sympathetic outflow, increased pulmonary vascular pressures, and hypoxia-induced increases in capillary permeability (see Chapter 73).

Active ion transport followed by passive, osmotic water movement is important in clearing the alveolar space of fluid. There are some experimental data that β agonists and growth factors increase alveolar fluid removal. Interindividual genetic differences in the rates of these transport processes may be important in determining which individuals are susceptible to altitude-related pulmonary edema. Although the existence of these mechanisms suggests that therapeutic interventions may be developed to promote resolution of pulmonary edema, no such therapies currently exist.

CLINICAL MANIFESTATIONS

The clinical features depend on the mechanism of edema formation. In general, interstitial edema and alveolar edema prevent the inflation of alveoli, leading to atelectasis and decreased surfactant production. This results in diminished pulmonary compliance and tidal volume. The patient must increase respiratory effort and/or the respiratory rate so as to maintain minute ventilation. The earliest clinical signs of

Table 396-2	Radiographic Features That May Help Differentiate Cardiogenic from Noncardiogenic Pulmonary Edema	
RADIOGRAPHIC FEATURE	**CARDIOGENIC EDEMA**	**NONCARDIOGENIC EDEMA**
Heart size	Normal or greater than normal	Usually normal
Width of the vascular pedicle*	Normal or greater than normal	Usually normal or less than normal
Vascular distribution	Balanced or inverted	Normal or balanced
Distribution of edema	Even or central	Patchy or peripheral
Pleural effusions	Present	Not usually present
Peribronchial cuffing	Present	Not usually present
Septal lines	Present	Not usually present
Air bronchograms	Not usually present	Usually present

*The width of the vascular pedicle in adults is determined by dropping a perpendicular line from the point at which the left subclavian artery exits the aortic arch and measuring across to the point at which the superior vena cava crosses the right mainstem bronchus. A vascular pedicle width >70 mm on a portable digital anteroposterior radiograph of the chest obtained when the patient is supine is optimal for differentiating high from normal-to-low intravascular volume.
From Ware LB, Matthay MA: Acute pulmonary edema, N Engl J Med 353:2788–2796, 2005.

pulmonary edema include increased work of breathing, tachypnea, and dyspnea. As fluid accumulates in the alveolar space, auscultation reveals fine crackles and wheezing, especially in dependent lung fields. In cardiogenic pulmonary edema, a gallop may be present as well as peripheral edema and jugular venous distention.

Chest radiographs can provide useful ancillary data, although findings of initial radiographs may be normal. Early radiographic signs that represent accumulation of interstitial edema include peribronchial and perivascular cuffing. Diffuse streakiness reflects interlobular edema and distended pulmonary lymphatics. Diffuse, patchy densities, the so-called butterfly pattern, represent bilateral interstitial or alveolar infiltrates and are a late sign. Cardiomegaly is often seen with cardiogenic causes of pulmonary edema. Heart size is usually normal in noncardiogenic pulmonary edema (Table 396-2). Chest tomography demonstrates edema accumulation in the dependent areas of the lung. As a result, changing the patient's position can alter regional differences in lung compliance and alveolar ventilation.

Measurement of **brain natriuretic peptide**, often elevated in heart disease, can help differentiate cardiac from pulmonary causes of pulmonary edema. A brain natriuretic peptide level >500 pg/mL suggests heart disease; a level <100 pg/mL suggests lung disease.

TREATMENT

The treatment of a patient with noncardiogenic pulmonary edema is largely supportive, with the primary goal to ensure adequate ventilation and oxygenation. Additional therapy is directed toward the underlying cause. Patients should receive supplemental oxygen to increase alveolar oxygen tension and pulmonary vasodilation. Patients with pulmonary edema of cardiogenic causes should be managed with diuretics, inotropic agents and systemic vasodilators to reduce left ventricular afterload (see Chapter 442). Diuretics are also valuable in the treatment of pulmonary edema associated with total body fluid overload (sepsis, renal insufficiency). Morphine is often helpful as a vasodilator and a mild sedative.

Positive airway pressure improves gas exchange in patients with pulmonary edema. In tracheally intubated patients, positive end-expiratory pressure can be used to optimize pulmonary mechanics. Noninvasive forms of ventilation, such as mask or nasal prong continuous positive airway pressure, are also effective. The mechanism by which positive airway pressure improves pulmonary edema is not entirely clear but is not associated with decreasing lung water. Rather, continuous positive airway pressure prevents complete closure of alveoli at the low lung volumes present at the end of expiration. It may also recruit already collapsed alveolar units. This leads to increased functional residual capacity and improved pulmonary compliance, improved surfactant function, and decreased pulmonary vascular resistance. The net effect is to decrease the work of breathing, improve oxygenation, and decrease cardiac afterload.

When mechanical ventilation becomes necessary, especially in non-cardiogenic pulmonary edema, care must be taken to minimize the risk of development of complications from barotrauma, including pneumothorax, pneumomediastinum, and primary alveolar damage (see Chapter 71.1). Lung protective strategies include setting low tidal volumes, relatively high positive end-expiratory pressure, and allowing for permissive hypercapnia.

High-altitude pulmonary edema should be managed with altitude descent and supplemental oxygen. Portable continuous positive airway pressure or a portable hyperbaric chamber is also helpful. Nifedipine (10 mg initially, and then 20-30 mg by slow release every 12-24 hr) in adults is also helpful. If there is a history of high-altitude pulmonary edema, nifedipine and β-adrenergic agonists (inhaled) may prevent recurrence (see Chapter 73).

Bibliography is available at Expert Consult.

Chapter **397**
Aspiration Syndromes
John L. Colombo

Aspiration of material that is foreign to the lower airway produces a varied clinical spectrum ranging from an asymptomatic condition to acute life-threatening events, such as occur with massive aspiration of gastric contents or hydrocarbon products. Other chapters discuss mechanical obstruction of large- or intermediate-size airways as occurs with foreign bodies (see Chapter 387) and infectious complications of aspiration and recurrent microaspiration (see Chapter 398), such as may occur with gastroesophageal reflux (see Chapter 323.1) or dysphagia (see Chapter 306). Occult aspiration of nasopharyngeal secretions into the lower respiratory tract is a normal event in healthy people, usually without apparent clinical significance.

GASTRIC CONTENTS
Aspiration of substantial amounts of gastric contents typically occurs in the context of vomiting. It is an infrequent complication of general anesthesia, gastroenteritis, or altered level of consciousness. Among 63,180 pediatric patients undergoing general anesthesia, 24 cases of aspiration occurred, but symptoms developed in only 9. Pathophysiologic consequences can vary, depending primarily on the pH and volume of the aspirate and the amount of particulate material. Increased clinical severity is noted with volumes greater than approximately 0.8 mL/kg and/or pH <2.5. Hypoxemia, hemorrhagic pneumonitis, atelectasis, intravascular fluid shifts, and pulmonary edema all occur rapidly after massive aspiration. These occur earlier, become more severe, and last longer with acid aspiration. Most clinical changes are present within minutes to 1-2 hr after the aspiration event. In the next 24-48 hr, there is a marked increase in lung parenchymal neutrophil infiltrations, mucosal sloughing, and alveolar consolidation that often correlates with increasing infiltrates on chest radiographs. These changes tend to occur significantly later and are more prolonged after aspiration of particulate material. Although infection usually does not have a role in initial lung injury after aspiration of gastric contents, aspiration may impair pulmonary defenses, predisposing the patient to secondary bacterial pneumonia. In the patient who has shown clinical improvement but then demonstrates clinical worsening, especially with fever and leukocytosis, secondary bacterial pneumonia should be suspected.

Treatment
If large-volume or highly toxic substance aspiration occurs in a patient who already has an artificial airway in place, it is important to perform immediate suctioning of the airway. If immediate suctioning cannot be performed, later suctioning or bronchoscopy is usually of limited therapeutic value except when there is suspicion of significant particulate aspiration. Attempts at acid neutralization are not warranted because acid is rapidly neutralized by the respiratory epithelium. Patients in whom large-volume or toxic aspiration is suspected should be observed, should undergo oxygenation measurement by oximetry or blood gas analysis, and should undergo a chest radiograph, even if they are asymptomatic. If the chest radiograph findings and oxygen saturation are normal, and the patient remains asymptomatic, home observation, after a period of observation in the hospital or office, is adequate. No treatment is indicated at that time, but the caregivers should be instructed to bring the child back in for medical attention should respiratory symptoms or fever develop. For patients who present with abnormal findings or in whom such findings develop during observation, oxygen therapy is given to correct hypoxemia. Endotracheal intubation and mechanical ventilation are often necessary for more severe cases. Bronchodilators may be tried, although they are usually of limited benefit. Animal studies indicate that treatment with corticosteroids does not provide benefit, unless given nearly simultaneously with the aspiration event; use of these agents may increase the risk of secondary infection. Prophylactic antibiotics are not indicated, although in the patient with limited reserve, early antibiotic coverage may be appropriate. If used, antibiotics that cover for anaerobic microbes should be considered. If the aspiration event occurs in a hospitalized or chronically ill patient, coverage of *Pseudomonas*, *Staphylococcus aureus*, and enteric Gram-negative organisms should also be considered. If empiric antibiotics are given, they should be discontinued when cultures and course warrant. A mortality rate of ≤5% is seen if 3 or fewer lobes are involved. Unless complications develop, such as infection or barotrauma, most patients recover in 2-3 wk. Prolonged lung damage may persist, including scarring, bronchiolitis obliterans, and bronchiectasis.

Prevention
Prevention of aspiration should always be the goal when airway manipulation is necessary for intubation or other invasive procedures. Feeding with enteral tubes passed beyond the pylorus, elevating the head of the bed 30-45 degrees in mechanically ventilated patients, and oral decontamination reduce the incidence of aspiration complications in the intensive care unit. Minimizing use of sedation, monitoring for gastric residuals, and gastric acid suppression may all help prevent aspiration. However, the latter is not without some controversy. Any patient with altered consciousness, especially one who is receiving tube feedings, should be considered at high risk for aspiration. Preoperative restriction of oral fluids to otherwise normal children for 6 hr does not appear to provide benefit compared to restriction for only 2 hr in terms of risk for aspiration.

HYDROCARBON ASPIRATION
Aspiration and resulting pneumonitis are typically the most dangerous consequences of acute hydrocarbon ingestion (see Chapter 63). Although significant pneumonitis occurs in <2% of all hydrocarbon ingestions, an estimated 20 deaths occur annually from hydrocarbon aspiration in both children and adults. Some of these deaths represent suicides. Hydrocarbons with lower surface tensions (gasoline,

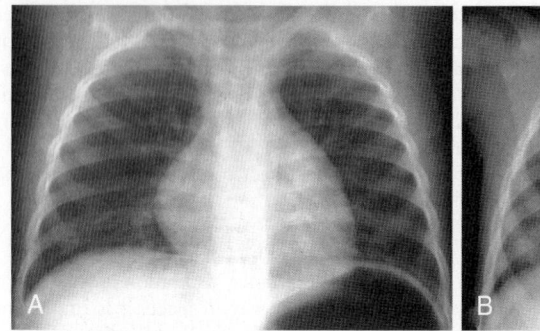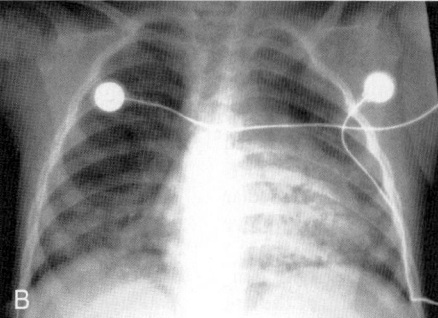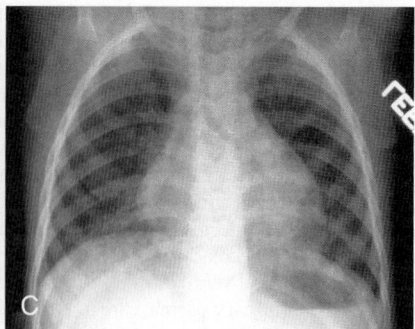

Figure 397-1 Chest radiographs of a 17 mo old who ingested furniture polish. **A,** Three hours after ingestion, the lungs are clear. **B,** At 24 hr, there are bibasilar coalescing nodular opacities. **C,** Three days later there is much clearing. *(From Slovis TL, editor:* Caffey's pediatric diagnostic imaging, *ed 11, Philadelphia, 2008, Mosby, p. 1287.)*

turpentine, naphthalene) have more potential for aspiration toxicity than heavier mineral or fuel oils. Ingestion of >30 mL (approximate volume of an adult swallow) of hydrocarbon is associated with an increased risk of severe pneumonitis. Clinical findings including chest retractions, grunting, cough, and fever may occur as soon as 30 min after aspiration or may be delayed for several hours. Lung radiographic changes usually occur within 2-8 hr, peaking in 48-72 hr (Fig. 397-1). Pneumatoceles and pleural effusions may occur. Patients presenting with cough, shortness of breath, or hypoxemia are at high risk for pneumonitis. Persistent pulmonary function abnormalities can be present many years after hydrocarbon aspiration. Other organ systems, especially the liver, central nervous system, and heart, may suffer serious injury. Cardiac dysrhythmias may occur and may be exacerbated by hypoxia and acid–base or electrolyte disturbances.

Treatment

Gastric emptying is contraindicated in nearly all situations because the risk of aspiration is greater than any systemic toxicity. Treatment is generally supportive, consisting of oxygen, fluids, and ventilatory support, and rarely extracorporeal membrane oxygenation, as necessary. Exogenous surfactant administration has been described as helpful in case reports. The child who has no symptoms and normal chest radiograph findings should be observed for 6-8 hr to ensure safe discharge. Certain hydrocarbons have more inherent systemic toxicity. The pneumonic **CHAMP** refers collectively to the following hydrocarbons: *c*amphor, *h*alogenated carbons, *a*romatic hydrocarbons, and those associated with *m*etals and *p*esticides. Patients who ingest these compounds in volumes >30 mL, such as might occur with intentional overdose, may benefit from gastric emptying. This is still a high-risk procedure that can result in further aspiration. If a cuffed endotracheal tube can be placed without inducing vomiting, this procedure should be considered, especially in the presence of altered mental status. Treatment of each case should be considered individually, with guidance from a poison control center.

Other substances that are particularly toxic and cause significant lung injury when aspirated or inhaled include baby powder, chlorine, shellac, beryllium, and mercury vapors. Repeated exposure to low concentrations of these agents can lead to chronic lung disease, such as interstitial pneumonitis and granuloma formation. Corticosteroids may help reduce fibrosis development and improve pulmonary function, although the evidence for this benefit is limited.

Bibliography is available at Expert Consult.

Chapter **398**
Chronic Recurrent Aspiration
John L. Colombo

ETIOLOGY

Repeated aspiration of even small quantities of gastric, nasal, or oral contents can lead to recurrent bronchitis or bronchiolitis; recurrent pneumonia; atelectasis; wheezing; cough; apnea; and/or laryngospasm. Pathologic outcomes include granulomatous inflammation, interstitial inflammation, fibrosis, lipoid pneumonia, and bronchiolitis obliterans. Most cases clinically manifest as airway inflammation, and are rarely associated with significant morbidity. Table 398-1 lists underlying disorders that are frequently associated with recurrent aspiration. Oropharyngeal incoordination is reportedly the most common underlying problem associated with recurrent pneumonias in hospitalized children. In 2 reports, from 26-48% of such children were found to have dysphagia with aspiration as the underlying problem. Lipoid pneumonia may occur after the use of home/folk remedies involving oral or nasal administration of animal or vegetable oils to treat various childhood illnesses. Lipoid pneumonia has been reported as a complication of these practices in the Middle East, Asia, India, Brazil, and Mexico. The initial underlying disease, language barriers, and a belief that these are not "medications" may delay the diagnosis (see Chapter 4).

Gastroesophageal reflux disease (GERD; see Chapter 323) is also a common underlying finding that may predispose to recurrent respiratory disease, but it is less frequently associated with recurrent pneumonia than is dysphagia (see Chapter 323). GERD is associated with microaspiration and bronchiolitis obliterans in lung transplant recipients. Aspiration has also been observed in infants with respiratory symptoms but no other apparent abnormalities. Recurrent microaspiration has been reported in otherwise apparently normal newborns, especially premature infants. Aspiration is also a risk in patients suffering from acute respiratory illness from other causes, especially respiratory syncytial virus infection (see Chapter 260). Modified barium swallow and videofluoroscopy reveal silent aspiration in these patients. This finding emphasizes the need for a high degree of clinical suspicion for ongoing aspiration in a child with an acute respiratory illness, being fed enterally, who deteriorates unexpectedly.

DIAGNOSIS

Some underlying predisposing factors (see Table 398-1) are frequently clinically apparent but may require specific further evaluation. Initial

Table 398-1	Conditions Predisposing to Aspiration Lung Injury in Children

ANATOMICAL AND MECHANICAL
Tracheoesophageal fistula
Laryngeal cleft
Vascular ring
Cleft palate
Micrognathia
Macroglossia
Cysts, tumors
Achalasia
Esophageal foreign body
Tracheostomy
Endotracheal tube
Nasal or oral feeding tube
Collagen vascular disease (scleroderma, dermatomyositises)
Gastroesophageal reflux disease
Obesity

NEUROMUSCULAR
Altered consciousness
Immaturity of swallowing/Prematurity
Dysautonomia
Increased intracranial pressure
Hydrocephalus
Vocal cord paralysis
Cerebral palsy
Muscular dystrophy
Hypotonia
Myasthenia gravis
Guillain-Barré syndrome
Spinal muscular atrophy
Ataxia-telangiectasia
Cerebral vascular accident

MISCELLANEOUS
Poor oral hygiene
Gingivitis
Prolonged hospitalization
Gastric outlet or intestinal obstruction
Poor feeding techniques (bottle propping, overfeeding, inappropriate foods for toddlers)
Bronchopulmonary dysplasia
Viral infection/bronchiolitis

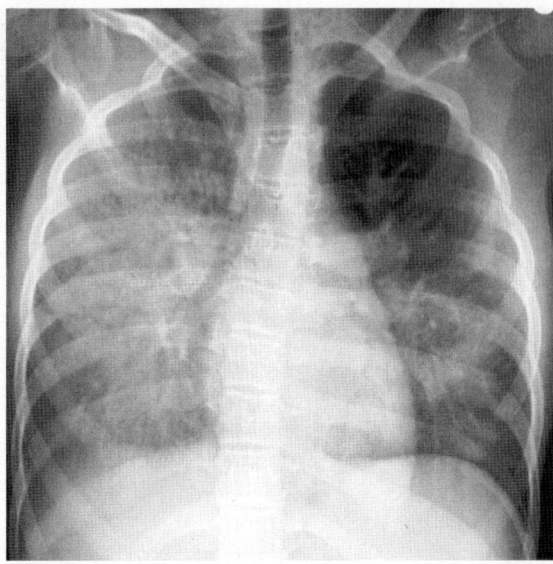

Figure 398-1 Chest radiograph of a developmentally delayed 15 yr old with chronic aspiration of oral formula. Note posterior (dependent areas) distribution with sparing of heart borders.

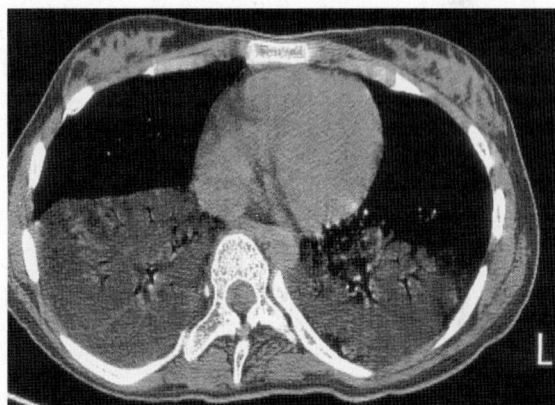

Figure 398-2 Chest CT scan of same patient as in Figure 398-1. Note lung consolidation in dependent regions is of similar density to subcutaneous fat.

assessment begins with a detailed history and physical examination. The caregiver should be asked about spitting, vomiting, arching, or epigastric discomfort in an older child; the timing of symptoms in relation to feedings; positional changes; and nocturnal symptoms, such as coughing and wheezing. It is important to remember that coughing or gagging may be minimal or absent in a child with a depressed cough or gag reflex. Observation of a feeding is an essential part of the exam when a diagnosis of recurrent aspiration is being considered. Particular attention should be given to nasopharyngeal reflux, difficulty with sucking or swallowing, and associated coughing and choking. Voice changes (wet voice) and noisy (wet) breathing should be noted. The oral cavity should be inspected for gross abnormalities and stimulated to assess the gag reflex. Drooling or excessive accumulation of secretions in the mouth suggests dysphagia. Lung auscultation may reveal transient crackles or wheezes after feeding, particularly in the dependent lung segments.

The diagnosis of recurrent microaspiration is challenging because of the lack of highly specific and sensitive tests (Table 398-2). A plain chest radiograph is the usual initial study for a child in whom recurrent aspiration is suspected. The classic findings of segmental or lobar infiltrates localized to dependent areas may be found (Fig. 398-1), but there are a wide variety of radiographic findings. These findings include diffuse infiltrates, lobar infiltrates, bronchial wall thickening, hyperinflation, and even no detectable abnormalities. CT scans, though generally not indicated to establish a diagnosis of aspiration, may show infiltrates with decreased attenuation suggestive of lipoid pneumonia (Fig. 398-2). A carefully performed barium esophagram is useful in looking for anatomic abnormalities such as vascular ring, stricture, hiatal hernia, and tracheoesophageal fistula. It also yields qualitative information about esophageal motility and, when extended, of gastric emptying. However, primarily because of the very short viewing time, the esophagram is quite insensitive and nonspecific for aspiration or GERD. A modified barium swallow study with videofluoroscopy (videofluoroscopic swallowing study) is generally considered the gold standard for evaluating the swallowing mechanism. This study is preferably done with the assistance of a pediatric feeding specialist and a caregiver in the attempt to simulate the usual feeding technique of the child. The child is seated in normal eating position, and various consistencies of barium or barium-impregnated foods are offered. This study is more sensitive for demonstrating aspiration than bedside assessment or a traditional barium swallow study. The sensitivity of the modified barium swallow study is such that it occasionally detects aspiration in patients without apparent respiratory abnormalities.

Table 398-2	Summary of Diagnostic Tests of Aspiration	
EVALUATION	**BENEFITS**	**LIMITATIONS**
Chest radiograph	Inexpensive and widely available Assesses accumulation of injury over time	Insensitive to early subtle changes of lung injury
High-resolution CT	Sensitive in detecting lung injury, such as bronchiectasis, tree-in-bud opacities, and bronchial thickening Less radiation than conventional CT Assesses accumulation of injury over time	More radiation exposure than plain radiograph Expensive
Video swallow study	Evaluates all phases of swallowing Evaluates multiple consistencies Feeding recommendations made at time of study	Information limited if child consumes only small quantities Difficult to perform in child who has not been feeding by mouth Radiation exposure proportional to study duration Cannot be performed at bedside Limited evaluation of anatomy Evaluates 1 moment in time Expensive
FEES/with sensory testing	Ability to thoroughly evaluate functional anatomy Evaluates multiple consistencies Can assess risk of aspiration in non-orally feeding child; airway protective reflexes can be assessed Feeding recommendations made at time of study Visual feedback for caregivers Can be performed at bedside No radiation exposure	Blind to esophageal phase and actual swallow Invasive and may not represent physiological swallowing conditions Evaluates 1 moment in time Not widely available Expensive
BAL	Evaluates anatomy of entire upper and lower airways Samples the end-organ of damage Sample available for multiple cytological and microbiologic tests Widely available	Uncertainty regarding interpretation of lipid-laden macrophage index Index cumbersome to calculate Requires sedation or anesthesia Invasive Expensive
Esophageal pH monitoring	Current gold standard for diagnosis of Acid gastroesophageal reflux Established normative data in children	Blind to majority of reflux (nonacid) events Difficult to establish causal relationship between gastroesophageal reflux and aspiration Somewhat invasive Evaluates short time interval
Esophageal impedance monitoring	Likely gold standard for diagnosis of GERD with supraesophageal manifestations Able to detect acid and nonacid reflux events Detects proximal reflux events Able to evaluate for GERD without stopping medications	Lack of normative data for children Somewhat invasive Expensive and cumbersome to interpret Not widely available Evaluates short time interval
Gastroesophageal scintigraphy	Performed under physiologic conditions Low radiation exposure	Poor sensitivity May not differentiate between aspiration from dysphagia or GERD
Radionuclide salivagram	Child does not have to be challenged with food bolus Low radiation exposure	Unknown sensitivity Unknown relationship to disease outcomes Evaluates 1 moment in time
Dye studies	Can be constructed as screening test or confirmatory test Can evaluate aspiration of secretions or feeds Repeating over time allows for broader evaluation	Uncertainty in interpretation owing to variability of technique Can only be performed in children with tracheostomies
Other biomarkers (pepsin, bile acids) milk protein	Theoretical high specificity and sensitivity	Limited availability and standardization Variable results to date

BAL, bronchoalveolar lavage; FEES, fiberoptic-endoscopic evaluation of swallowing; GERD, gastroesophageal reflux disease.
Modified from Boesch RP, Daines C, Willging JP, et al: Advances in the diagnosis and management of chronic pulmonary aspiration in children, Eur Respir J 28:847–861, 2006; and Tutor JD, Gosa MM: Dysphagia and aspiration in children, Pediatr Pulmonol 47(4):321–337, 2012.

A gastroesophageal "milk" scintiscan offers theoretical advantages over a barium swallow in being more physiologic and giving a longer window of viewing than the barium esophagram for detecting aspiration and GERD. However, this study has been found to have a low sensitivity and provides relatively little anatomic detail. Another radionuclide scan termed the "salivagram" may also be useful to assess aspiration of esophageal contents. When this scan is performed by experienced personnel, its sensitivity appears to be comparable to that of the modified barium swallow study. The use of fiberoptic endoscopic evaluation of swallowing has been found useful in adult and some pediatric patients, to observe swallowing directly without radiation exposure. The child's reaction to placement of the endoscope may alter the assessment of function, depending on level of comfort and cooperation.

Tracheobronchial aspirates can be examined for numerous entities to evaluate for aspiration. For patients with artificial airways, the use of an oral dye and visual examination of tracheal secretions is useful. This test should not be done on a chronic basis, such as in tube feedings, because of possible dye toxicity. In using this test acutely, the best method is to place a few drops of dye on the patient's tongue and perform subsequent suctioning of the airway over the next several minutes. Quantitation of lipid-laden alveolar macrophages from bronchial aspirates has been shown to be a sensitive test for aspiration in children, but false-positive tests occur, especially with endobronchial obstruction, use of intravenous lipids, sepsis, and pulmonary bleeding. Bronchial washings may also be examined for various food substances, including lactose, glucose, food fibers, and milk antigens, as well as pepsin. Specificity and sensitivity of these tests have not been well studied.

TREATMENT

If chronic aspiration is associated with another underlying medical condition, treatment should be directed toward that problem. The level of morbidity from respiratory problems should determine the level of intervention. Often milder dysphagia can be treated with alteration of feeding position, limiting texture of foods to those best tolerated on modified barium esophagram (usually thicker foods), or limiting quantity per feeding. Currently evidence is lacking regarding the advisability of restricting oral intake of water by children whose aspiration is largely of thin fluids. Nasogastric tube feedings can be utilized temporarily during periods of transient vocal cord dysfunction or other dysphagia. Postpyloric feedings may also be helpful, especially if gastroesophageal reflux is present, although this does not eliminate reflux. There are several surgical procedures that may be considered. Tracheostomy (see Chapter 385.1), although sometimes predisposing to aspiration, may provide overall benefit from improved bronchial hygiene and the ability to suction aspirated material. Use of a one-way (Passy-Muir) valve on a tracheostomy tube has been shown to improve swallowing. Fundoplication with gastrostomy or jejunostomy feeding tube will reduce the probability of gastroesophageal reflux-induced aspiration, but recurrent pneumonias often persist because of dysphagia and presumed aspiration of upper airway secretions. Medical treatment with anticholinergics, such as glycopyrrolate or scopolamine, may significantly reduce morbidity from salivary aspiration but often has side effects. Aggressive surgical intervention with salivary gland excision, ductal ligation, laryngotracheal separation, or esophagogastric disconnection can be considered in severe, unresponsive cases. Although usually reserved for the most severe cases, surgical therapy may significantly improve quality of life and ease of care for some patients.

Bibliography is available at Expert Consult.

Chapter **399**
Immune and Inflammatory Lung Disease

399.1 Hypersensitivity Pneumonia
Kevin J. Kelly

Hypersensitivity pneumonia (HP), aptly called *extrinsic allergic alveolitis* because the inciting agent is almost uniformly inhaled from the environment, is a complex immunologic-mediated syndrome of the pulmonary alveoli and interstitium. There are numerous specific disease names based on the origin of the offending antigen that is inhaled to describe HP. Prompt recognition of the signs and symptoms allows for complete reversal of the disease without long-term adverse consequences if the source of the exposure is recognized and abated. Failure to recognize the disease early may lead to chronic irreversible lung changes with persistent symptoms in the patient.

ETIOLOGY

The most common sources of offending agents that cause HP include agricultural aerosols, inhaled protein antigens from animals, antigens from microorganisms of bacteria, fungi, or protozoan origin, as well as chemicals of low and high molecular weight (Table 399-1). Although a large number of inciting agents are associated with *occupational diseases* in which children do not regularly work, there are many similar antigen sources in a nonoccupational environment and teenage work exposures that may occur causing the same disease. In addition to HP, the same antigens may lead to allergic asthma or chronic bronchitis as seen with animal proteins, contaminated metal working fluids, and other inhaled antigens.

Primary sources of HP in children have been the result of exposure to **pet birds** (or feathers in bedding) such as parakeets, canaries, cockatiels, or cockatoos or homes contaminated with pigeon antigens from home breeders or contamination. Humidifiers and hot tubs are notorious for contamination with **thermophilic organisms** as well as *Mycobacterium avium* complex. Mold from prior flooding or damp condensation represents an increasing problem experienced by clinicians since the building of homes with inadequate ventilation and insufficient air turnover. Allergic diseases such as asthma, chronic rhinitis, and HP may be seen from the same sources. Other family members may have symptoms of asthma or rhinitis while another may have HP.

CLASSIFICATION AND PATHOGENESIS

HP has been traditionally classified as acute, subacute, or chronic. This classification arose prior to more refined diagnostic modalities such as **high-resolution computerized tomography (HRCT)** scanning of the lungs and more refined immunologic diagnostic tests on **bronchoalveolar lavage (BAL)**. Distinguishing chronic disease from subacute disease is difficult without clear differentiating criteria, but a diagnosis of HP at any stage results in the clinician recommending very specific interventions for improvement. HP is characterized as (1) acute nonprogressive and intermittent, (2) acute progressive and intermittent, (3) chronic nonprogressive, and (4) chronic progressive (Table 399-2).

The sensitivity of the complete criteria is lower than desired as not all patients will have abnormal radiography or the findings of positive precipitins to the offending antigen. The specificity of the criteria may also be problematic. Screening for pigeon breeder's lung disease among a cohort of pigeon breeders will demonstrate that 30% or more of the pigeon breeders have immunoglobulin (Ig) G precipitins to pigeon dropping antigens while only a small number will have disease. Genetic and epigenetic factors yet to be identified are likely involved in determining who develops disease.

A diagnosis of HP is certain when the known exposure with immune response to the offending antigen is identified; the medical history and physical finding are abnormal on examination; BAL and lung biopsy are abnormal. Some clinicians have foregone the lung biopsy when a cluster of cases occurs and 1 patient biopsy is abnormal already.

The immune mechanisms involved include morphologic changes seen with immune complex-mediated disease, especially in the acute phase, accompanied complement activation followed by delayed-type hypersensitivity response. The acute phase of the disease shows alveolitis with a mixed cellular infiltration with lymphocytes, macrophage, plasma cells, and neutrophils. Continued exposure results in the formation of loose, noncaseating granuloma located near the respiratory or terminal bronchioles. It is critical when a biopsy is being performed (transbronchial or surgical) that the pathologist knows that HP is being considered as there are other **interstitial lung diseases** that produce

| Table 399-1 | Antigen Sources Associated with Specific Causes of Hypersensitivity Pneumonitis |

HYPERSENSITIVITY PNEUMONITIS	ANTIGEN SOURCE	HYPERSENSITIVITY PNEUMONITIS	ANTIGEN SOURCE
Bagassosis (mold on pressed sugar cane)	*Thermoactinomyces sacchari* *Thermoactinomyces vulgaris*	Miller's lung (dust-contaminated grain)	*Sitophilus granarius* (i.e., wheat weevil)
Bat lung (bat droppings)	Bat serum protein	Moldy hay, grain, silage (farmer's lung)	Thermophilic actinomycetes Fungi (e.g., *Aspergillus umbrosus*)
Bible printer's lung	Moldy typesetting water		
Bird fancier's lung (parakeets, budgerigars, pigeons)	Droppings, feathers, serum proteins	Mollusk shell hypersensitivity pneumonitis	Sea-snail shell
Byssinosis ("brown lung") (unclear if a true cause of hypersensitivity pneumonitis; asthma is common)	Cotton mill dust (carding and spinning areas of cotton, flax, and soft-hemp)	Mushroom worker's lung	Mushroom spores Thermophilic actinomycetes
		Paprika slicer's lung (moldy paprika pods)	*Mucor stolonifer*
Canary fancier's lung	Serum proteins	Pauli's reagent alveolitis	Sodium diazobenzene sulfate
Cheese washer's lung (moldy cheese)	*Penicillium casei* *Aspergillus clavatus*	Pearl oyster shell pneumonitis	Oyster shells
Chemical hypersensitivity pneumonitis	Diphenylmethane diisocyanate (MDI) Toluene diisocyanate (TDI)	Pituitary snuff taker's disease	Dried, powdered cattle or pig pituitary proteins)
		Potato riddler's lung (moldy hay around potatoes)	Thermophilic actinomycetes *T. vulgaris* *Faenia rectivirgula* *Aspergillus* spp.
Coffee worker's lung	Coffee-bean dust		
Composter's lung	*T. vulgaris* *Aspergillus* species		
Contaminated basement (sewage) pneumonitis	*Cephalosporium*	Poultry worker's lung (feather plucker's disease)	Serum proteins (chicken products)
Coptic lung (mummy handler's lung)	Cloth wrappings of mummies	Pyrethrum (pesticide)	Pyrethrum
		Sauna taker's lung	*Aureobasidium* spp., other sources
Detergent worker's lung (washing powder lung)	*Bacillus subtilis* enzymes	Sequoiosis (moldy wood dust)	*Graphium* *Pullularia* *Trichoderma* spp. *Aureobasidium pullulans*
Dry rot lung	*Merulius lacrymans*		
Duck fever	Feathers, serum proteins		
Epoxy resin lung	Phthalic anhydride (heated epoxy resin)	Suberosis (moldy cork dust)	*Thermoactinomyces viridis* *Penicillium glabrum* *Aspergillus conidia*
Esparto dust (mold in plaster dust)	*Aspergillus fumigatus* Thermophilic actinomycetes		
Fish meal worker's lung	Fish meal	Summer-type pneumonitis	*Trichosporon cutaneum*
Furrier's lung (sewing furs; animal fur dust)	Animal pelts	Tea grower's lung	Tea plants
		Thatched-roof lung (huts in New Guinea)	*Saccharomonospora viridis* (dead grasses and leaves)
Grain measurer's lung	Cereal grain (*Sporobolomyces*) Grain dust (mixture of dust, silica, fungi, insects, and mites)	Tobacco grower's lung	*Aspergillus* spp. *Scopulariopsis brevicaulis*
		Turkey handling disease	Serum proteins (turkey products)
Hot-tub lung (mists; mold on ceiling and around tub)	*Cladosporium* spp. *Mycobacterium avium* complex	Unventilated shower	*Epicoccum nigrum*
Humidifier fever	*Thermoactinomyces* (*T. vulgaris, T. sacchari, T. candidus*) *Klebsiella oxytoca* *Naegleria gruberi* *Acanthamoeba polyphaga* *Acanthamoeba castellani*	Upholstery fabric (nylon filament, cotton/polyester, and latex adhesive)	Aflatoxin-producing fungus, *Fusarium* spp.
		Velvet worker's lung	Unknown (? nylon velvet fiber, tannic acid, potato starch)
		Vineyard sprayer's lung	Copper sulfate (bordeaux mixture)
Laboratory worker's lung (rats, gerbils)	Urine, serum, pelts, proteins	Wine maker's lung (mold on grapes)	*Botrytis cinerea*
Lifeguard lung	Aerosolized endotoxin from pool-water sprays and fountains	Wood dust pneumonitis (oak, cedar, and mahogany dust, pine and spruce pulp)	*Alternaria* spp. *Bacillus subtilis*
Lycoperdonosis (*Lycoperdon* puffballs)	Puffball spores		
Machine operator's lung	*Pseudomonas fluorescens* Aerosolized metal working fluid	Wood pulp worker's disease (oak and maple trees)	*Penicillium* spp.
Malt worker's disease (moldy barley)	*Aspergillus fumigatus, Aspergillus clavatus*	Wood trimmer's disease (contaminated wood trimmings)	*Rhizopus* spp., *Mucor* spp.
Maple bark disease (moldy maple bark)	*Cryptostroma corticale*		

Table 399-2	Criteria Used in the Diagnosis of Hypersensitivity Pneumonitis

1. Identified exposure to offending antigen(s) by:
   - Medical history of exposure to suspected antigen in the patient's living environment
   - Investigations of the environment confirm the presence of an inciting antigen
   - Identification of specific immune responses (immunoglobulin G serum precipitin antibodies against the identified antigen) are suggestive of the potential etiology but are insufficient in isolation to confirm a diagnosis
2. Clinical, radiographic, or physiologic findings compatible with hypersensitivity pneumonitis
   - Respiratory and often constitutional signs and symptoms
     - Crackles on auscultation of the chest
     - Weight loss
     - Cough
     - Breathlessness
     - Episodic fever
     - Wheezing
     - Fatigue
   NOTE: These findings are especially suggestive of hypersensitivity pneumonitis when they appear or worsen several hours after antigen exposure.
   - A reticular, nodular, or ground glass opacities on chest radiograph or high-resolution CT
   - Abnormalities in the following pulmonary function tests
     - Spirometry (restrictive, obstructive, or mixed patterns)
     - Lung volumes (low or high)
     - Reduced diffusion capacity by carbon monoxide
     - Altered gas exchange either at rest or with exercise (reduced partial pressure of arterial oxygen by blood gas or pulse oximeter testing)
3. Bronchoalveolar lavage with lymphocytosis:
   - Usually with low CD4:CD8 ratio (i.e., CD8 is higher than normal)
   - Lymphocyte stimulation by offending antigen results in proliferation and cytokine production
4. Abnormal response to inhalation challenge testing to the offending antigen:
   - Reexposure to the environment
   - Inhalation challenge to the suspected antigen (rarely done any longer because of the risk of exacerbation of the disease)
5. Histopathology showing compatible changes with hypersensitivity pneumonitis by 1 of these findings:
   - Poorly formed, noncaseating granulomas (most often found closer to the respiratory epithelium where deposition of the offending antigen occurs)
   - Mononuclear cell infiltrate in the pulmonary interstitium

Table 399-3	Clinical History Clues Leading to a Diagnosis of Hypersensitivity Pneumonitis

Recurrent pneumonia
Pneumonia after repeat exposures (week, season, situation)
Cough, fever, and chest symptoms after making a job change or home change
Cough, fever, wheezing after return to school or only at school
Pet exposure (especially birds that shed dust such as pigeons, canaries, cockatiels, cockatoos)
Bird contaminant exposure (e.g., pigeon infestation)
Farm exposure to birds and hay
History of water damage despite typical cleaning
Use of hot tub, sauna, swimming pool
Other family members or workers with similar recurrent symptoms
Improvement after temporary environment change (e.g., vacation)

LABORATORY

Most of the abnormal laboratory findings in hypersensitivity pneumonitis are not specific and represent evidence of activated inflammatory markers or lung injury. Nonspecific elevation of immune globulins or the erythrocyte sedimentation rate and C-reactive protein may also be found. Circulating immune complexes may be detected. Lactate dehydrogenase may be elevated in the presence of lung inflammation and normalizes with response to therapy.

Serum IgG precipitins to the offending agent are frequently positive given some caveats. Commercial antigen sources from animals and birds may contain insufficient antigen for precipitation. Some laboratories performing these tests on an infrequent basis often have false-negative tests presumed to be a result of commercial antigens lacking the proper epitopes for precipitation. It is critical that laboratories familiar with the performance of these tests be utilized. Those laboratories often recognize the value of processing antigens for precipitation from the environmental source directly as the test substrate with patient serum. Skin testing for IgE-mediated disease is not warranted unless there is evidence of mixed lung pathology such as asthma and interstitial lung opacities.

BAL is one of the most sensitive tests and very helpful to the clinician in supporting the diagnosis of HP. Lymphocytosis frequently exceeding 50% of the recovered cells is seen on the BAL and should alert the clinician to the possibility of HP. Sarcoid, idiopathic pulmonary fibrosis, cryptogenic organizing pneumonia, berylliosis, granite workers lung disease, amiodarone pneumonia, lymphoma, and Langerhans cell histiocytosis may demonstrate lymphocytosis on BAL. All BAL specimens should have flow cytometry measurements of T-cell markers (CD3, CD4, and CD8 at a minimum). The predominant phenotype of the lymphocytosis is CD3+/CD8+/CD56+/CD57+/CD10−. In the normal circulation, lymphocytes with CD4 markers predominate at a ratio of approximately 2:1 compared to CD8 lymphocytes. In the lung compartment with HP, this ratio becomes approximately equal to or less than 1 (CD4:CD8 ≤1) with either an increase in CD8 lymphocytes or a decline in CD4 lymphocytes. This ratio assists the clinician in making a diagnosis of HP. This is in sharp contrast to other lymphocytic granulomatous disease, like sarcoidosis, where the CD4:CD8 is ≥2, or pulmonary fibrosis associated with connective tissue disease. Cryptogenic organizing pneumonia, a rare disease in children, also may present with BAL, where the CD4:CD8 is ≤1, and may be confused initially with HP.

Lung Biopsy

Lung biopsy is necessary to confirm a diagnosis of HP when the presence of critical elements, like antigen exposure, typical medical history, characteristic physical exam, and CD8+ cells in the BAL, are not present. Open lung biopsy is often the route of choice in young children because of the difficulty in safely obtaining satisfactory amounts of tissue by transbronchial biopsy. Lack of positive serum precipitins to offending antigen and exposure history are common reasons for obtaining lung biopsies. It is crucial to inform the

similar granulomas with subtle location differences depending on their origin.

CLINICAL MANIFESTATIONS

Heavy exposure to an offending antigen may lead to **acute HP**. This is the most common form of exposure but is still frequently not recognized. Symptoms are confused with bacterial or viral disease leading to treatment with antibiotics. Four to 6 hr after exposure the abrupt onset of cough, chest tightness, dyspnea, fever, chills, and fatigue are common (Table 399-3) Rarely, findings of wheezing are present on the initial examination. Rather, tachypnea with fine crackles may be heard by auscultation in the lung bases. However, auscultation may be normal at this stage. When **recurrent subacute disease** is present, the symptoms become progressive with weight loss, loss of appetite, and productive cough. When HP becomes **chronic** and progressive, the patient's fingers become clubbed accompanied by persistent symptoms noted above denoting a deteriorating status. If the disease progresses to interstitial fibrosis, the symptoms tend to not respond to therapy and denote a state where mortality risk is increased. Histology is hard to distinguish from **idiopathic pulmonary fibrosis** at this stage.

pathologist about the suspicion of HP so that the findings can be interpreted appropriately.

Poorly formed, noncaseating granulomas are seen near the respiratory and terminal bronchioles on histology with multinucleated giant cells. This is in sharp contrast to the granuloma of sarcoidosis that are well formed. Lymphocytes and plasma cells infiltrate the alveolar walls predominantly in a bronchocentric pattern. Fibrosis in the peribronchiole region supports a diagnosis of HP. Foamy cytoplasm accompanying large histiocytes in the alveoli and interstitium may be characteristically found.

Radiology

Chest radiograph almost always precedes the use of HRCT of the chest in children because of the need for sedation and concerns regarding risk of irradiation dose from HRCT. The plain radiograph will often demonstrate a ground-glass appearance, interstitial prominence, with a predominant location in the upper and middle lung fields. It is common for a chest radiograph to be considered normal by a radiologist early in the disease progression. Late in the disease, interstitial fibrosis may become prominent in the presence of increasing dyspnea, hypoxemia on room air, and even clubbing of the fingers. Mediastinum widening from lymphadenopathy is not usually present; when present, the lymph nodes are prominent along the airway near the carina, suggesting that the antigen source is inhaled and being responded to by the immune system.

Classical findings of mid zone and upper zone opacities with ground-glass appearance and nodularity on HRCT in the presence of typical clinical exam HP findings (lung crackles, cough, dyspnea) and lymphocytosis on BAL are almost sufficient to make a diagnosis (Fig. 399-1). These finding must prompt the clinician to identify the exposure in order to secure the diagnosis and eliminate the offending antigen. Without therapy, the progressive inflammatory response leads to air trapping, honeycombing, emphysema, and mild fibrosis in the chronic state. It is in this latter stage that idiopathic pulmonary fibrosis and nonspecific interstitial fibrosis are hard to differentiate. Whether true idiopathic pulmonary fibrosis exists in children where fibroblast foci are found on biopsy with usual interstitial fibrosis has been questioned.

Antigen Challenge By Inhalation

Inhalation challenge can be performed by 2 methods: (1) reexposure of the patient to the environment where the suspected antigen is present and (2) direct inhalation challenge at the hospital to material collected from the suspected source of the antigen. As the second method has resulted in severe exacerbation of disease in some individuals, its use is discouraged (see Chapter 399.2).

Two abnormal responses may be seen. Most commonly, where there is HP without asthma, symptoms occur 6-12 hr after direct challenge in the hospital or reexposure at source of the antigen. The challenges replicate some or all of the symptoms observed in the presenting syndrome with fever, dyspnea, fatigue, and crackles on lung auscultation. Blood drawn prior to challenge and then repeated during these symptoms often demonstrate an increased neutrophil count compared to baseline. Pulmonary function tests demonstrate a fall in **forced vital capacity** and often a concurrent fall in the **forced expiratory volume at 1 sec (FEV$_1$)** with a stable or increasing ratio of FEV$_1$:forced vital capacity percentage. Hypoxemia may accompany this decline in pulmonary function as well as a fall in the **diffusion capacity of carbon monoxide (DLCO)**. To see the complete effect, exercise during this period may show a considerable fall in oxygenation despite normal arterial blood gas oxygen tension and normal pulse oximetry at rest. This finding denotes the onset of worsening restrictive lung disease. Some patients may also demonstrate an early and late reduction in the FEV$_1$ as is seen in allergen challenge with asthma. In this dual reaction, the forced vital capacity also declines and is often accompanied by fever and leukocytosis.

TREATMENT

The control of environmental exposure to the offending antigen is a key to curing HP and remains the ideal method of treatment and

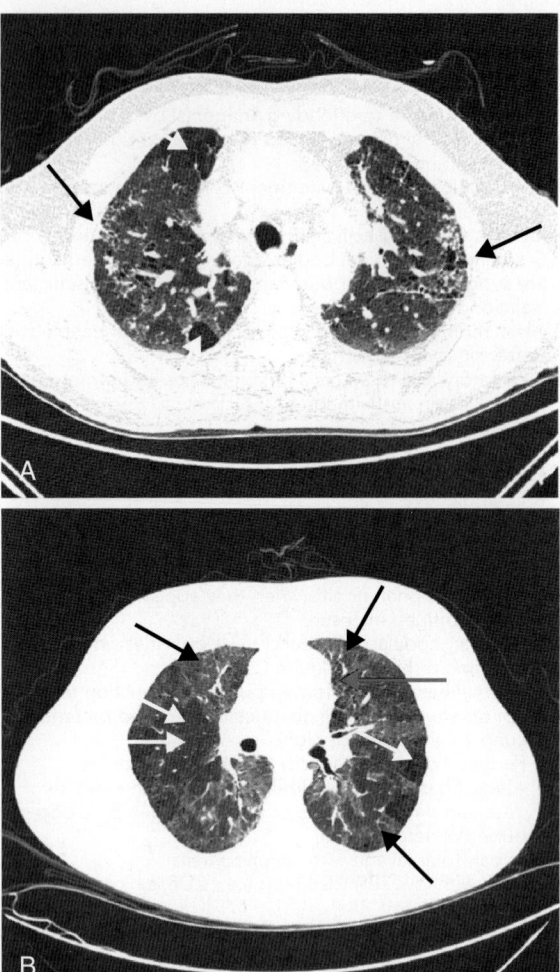

Figure 399-1 Radiologic findings in subacute (**A**) and chronic (**B**) hypersensitivity pneumonitis. **A,** Interstitial fibrosis (*black arrows*) and emphysematous changes (*white arrows*) in chronic HP with superimposed subacute HP. **B,** Ground-glass opacities (*black arrows*), mosaic perfusion (*white arrows*), and fibrosis (*red arrow*) in chronic HP caused by pigeon exposure. (*From Douglass JA, Sandrini A, Holgate ST, O'Hehir RE. Allergic bronchopulmonary aspergillosis and hypersensitivity pneumonitis. In Adkinson AF, editor: Middleton's allergy principles and practice, Philadelphia, 2014, Elsevier, Fig. 61-5.*)

prevention of recurrence. Counseling about the risk to children of exposure to birds and feathered bedding, or other environmental antigens, biologic aerosols, or agriculture dusts that are known to induce HP are important. Certainly, the source of the antigen and type of antigen appears to affect response to treatment and long-term prognosis. Older individuals who contract farmer's lung are likely to recover with minimal permanent residual effect, whereas individuals with bird fancier's lungs from antigens produced by pigeons have a worse prognosis, especially if fibrosis is detected on lung biopsy. The pediatrician should advise—in the strongest terms—removal of the antigen source from the affected child's environment. This may be an extraordinary challenge given various children's living circumstances and lack of independent control of the environment they live in.

In addition, pediatricians should be familiar with recommendations about the maintenance of heating, ventilation, and air conditioning systems, as well as of humidifiers and vaporizers. Daily drainage, cleansing of residue, and routine cleaning with hydrogen peroxide or bleach help rid humidifiers and vaporizers of harmful pathogens that cause HP.

Glucocorticosteroids at a dose of 0.5-1 mg/kg/day of prednisone or equivalent will reduce the immune inflammatory response in the lungs. Comparative trials in adults demonstrate that the use of 4 wks of therapy is as effective as 12 wks of therapy. Removal of antigen alone is sufficient to normalize lung function in most patients, but symptoms and pulmonary functions return to normal faster with the use of glucocorticoids. Because of the rapid reversal of symptoms, successful abatement of the environment is sometimes compromised when the family sees improvement prior to the antigen source removal.

Bibliography is available at Expert Consult.

399.2 Occupational and Environmental Lung Disease

Kevin J. Kelly

Occupational and environmental lung diseases constitute a larger part of primary care pediatrics, pediatric emergency medicine, and other pediatric subspecialties than most pediatric practitioners expect or realize. Although occupational and environmental lung diseases includes **occupational asthma**, **reactive airways dysfunction syndrome (RADS)**, HP, hard metal inhalation lung disease, berylliosis, and air pollution, this chapter focuses on occupational asthma and RADS. Berylliosis has a propensity to form granulomas (see Chapter 399.3). Although some diseases will be seen with regularity, the important role that a part-time workplace, school, daycare, neighbors' housing, multiple family housing, and indoor and outdoor environments may have in the causation of signs and symptoms in the patient is not always considered by the clinician.

The vast array of exposures shown to cause disease of the lungs is daunting, such as the inhalation of baking flour or household cleaning fluids causing asthma, microwave popcorn exposure to diacetyl resulting in bronchiolitis obliterans, and exposure to thermophilic organisms or mold resulting in hypersensitivity pneumonitis. The acute eosinophilic pneumonias associated with new onset of smoking and chemical inhalation of 1,1,1-trichloroethane (Scotchgard) require a high index of suspicion and unique lines of questioning. The same antigen encountered in a work, school, home, or outdoor environment may result in different disease presentation because of host factors, dose exposure, and genetic susceptibility. One of the most prominent examples is an investigation of workers who inhaled metal working fluid resulting in the development of asthma, HP, chronic bronchitis, or no symptoms at all from similar exposures. Immunologic evaluation in some exposures has shown similar immune responses in different individuals, but a wide range of disease provocation. When **high molecular weight** proteins cause asthma, symptoms of rhinoconjunctivitis frequently precede the onset of pulmonary symptoms. The medical history in occupational and environmental lung diseases has used an expanded construct with a simple acronym, WHACOS (Table 399-4).

Table 399-4	A Construct (WHACOS) That Has Been Used in Medical Interviewing of Patients, Coworkers, and Family Members When Environmental or Occupational Lung Disease Is Being Considered
W	*What* do you do?
H	*How* do you do what you do?
A	Are symptoms *Acute* or are they *Chronic*?
C	Do any *Coworkers*, family, classmates, or friends have the same symptoms?
O	Do you have any hobbies, travel, or animal/pet exposures *Outside* of school or work?
S	Are you *Satisfied* with work or school?

It is important to remember that in patients with occupational- or environmental-induced disease, the onset of symptoms has a lag time between exposure and symptoms. In occupational asthma, there may be an immediate response within 1-2 hr of exposure, demonstrated as a decline in pulmonary function, specifically the FEV_1. Usually, lung function returns to normal spontaneously unless persistent exposure occurs. Some patients demonstrate no immediate reduction in lung function, but rather experience a delayed response of 4-6 hr after the exposure. Treating physicians can take advantage of this physiology in occupational and environmental asthma by use of spirometry before and after work or school or peak flow measurements hourly during exposure and after leaving the exposure. Because workers and children in school have prolonged periods of exposure followed by a number of days without exposure, the use of pulmonary function plus bronchial hyperresponsiveness testing is helpful. Pulmonary function tests prior to starting work on a Monday of a typical work week may be normal. By Friday of a typical work or school week, the baseline pulmonary functions may have fallen and bronchial responsiveness may have become more sensitive to a lower concentration of histamine, methacholine, or mannitol. By Monday, the tests may have returned to normal or near normal with no change other than reduced exposure.

In the case of HP, a lag of 4-8 hr between the time of exposure and onset of fever, cough, and dyspnea is common. Unfortunately, the return home from hospitalization for culture-negative pneumonia to a source of antigen causing HP often results in complete reoccurrence of symptoms. Clinicians must have a high index of suspicion for HP with reoccurrence of pulmonary infiltrates shortly after reexposure (see Chapter 399.1).

CLASSIFICATION AND PATHOGENESIS

Occupational and environmental lung diseases include numerous syndromes of human lung disease such as occupational asthma, **RADS**, **reactive upper airway disease syndrome**, hypersensitivity pneumonitis (see Chapter 399.1), air pollution–induced disease, hard metal inhalation lung disease, berylliosis, occupation-induced lung cancer (e.g., mesothelioma from asbestosis), and chronic obstructive pulmonary disease without smoking. Most of these diseases are not problematic for children but adolescents may be exposed through part-time work or by single exposures as seen in RADS.

Occupational and Environmental Asthma

The general principles of diagnosis, clinical signs and symptoms, treatment, and causes of asthma are discussed in Chapter 144. High molecular weight causes of occupational and environmental asthma can be characterized as allergens, which are normally proteins and enzymes, inhaled from multiple sources (Table 399-5). These include various animals, shellfish, fish, enzymes (e.g., *Bacillus subtilis* in laundry detergent), and flour or cereals. Occupational and environmental asthma is also caused by a number of low molecular weight chemicals (Table 399-6). These chemicals are sufficient to induce an immune response but it is often not by an IgE-mediated mechanism. These chemicals appear to act as haptens that bind to human proteins, causing an immune response in the human host.

The pathogenesis of asthma in patients exposed to high molecular weight antigens follows the experience of nonoccupational asthma in patients where atopy, gender, genetics, concentration of antigen, duration of exposure, and other individual factors all contribute to the development of disease. Most individuals require a concentration and duration of exposure sufficient to cause IgE antibody sensitization to the offending allergen with development of bronchial hyperresponsiveness and airway inflammatory disease. If the allergen exposure is sufficient, these proteins can drive the immune response to a T-lymphocyte type 2 phenotype, even in patients without prior atopic disposition, as occurred in the case of latex allergy where many nonatopic individuals and patients exposed to allergen in their personal healthcare developed occupational allergy to multiple proteins from natural rubber latex. Atopic individuals are at the highest risk of developing latex allergy. A longitudinal study demonstrated that powdered latex gloves with high allergen content were the reason for the epidemic of latex allergy and

Table 399-5	High Molecular Weight Antigens Known to Induce Occupational or Environmental Asthma

OCCUPATION OR ENVIRONMENT	SOURCE	OCCUPATION OR ENVIRONMENT	SOURCE
ANIMAL-DERIVED ANTIGENS		**ACARIANS**	
Agricultural worker	Cow dander	Apple grower	Fruit tree red spider mite (*Panonychus ulmi*)
Bakery	Lactalbumin		
Butcher	Cow bone dust, pig, goat dander	Citrus farmer	Citrus red mite (*Panonychus citri*)
Cook	Raw beef	Farmer	Barn mite, two-spotted spider mite (*Tetranychus urticae*), grain mite
Dairy industry	Lactoserum, lactalbumin		
Egg producer	Egg protein	Flour handler	Mites and parasites
Farmer	Deer dander, mink urine	Grain-store worker	Grain mite
Frog catcher	Frog	Horticulturist	*Amblyseius cucumeris*
Hairdresser	Sericin	Poultry worker	Fowl mite
Ivory worker	Ivory dust	Vine grower	McDaniel spider mite (*Tetranychus mcdanieli*)
Laboratory technician	Bovine serum albumin, laboratory animal, monkey dander		
		MOLDS	
Nacre buttons	Nacre dust	Agriculture	*Plasmopara viticola*
Pharmacist	Endocrine glands	Baker	*Alternaria, Aspergillus* (unspecified)
Pork producer	Pig gut (vapor from soaking water)	Beet sugar worker	*Aspergillus* (unspecified)
Poultry worker	Chicken	Coal miner	*Rhizopus nigricans*
Tanner	Casein (cow's milk)	Coffee maker	*Chrysonilia sitophila*
Various	Bat guano	Laborer	Sooty molds (*Ascomycetes, deuteromycetes*)
Veterinarian	Goat dander		
Zookeeper	Birds	Logging worker	*Chrysonilia sitophila*
		Plywood factory worker	*Neurospora*
CRUSTACEANS, SEAFOOD, FISH		Sausage processing	*Penicillium nalgiovense*
Canning factory	Octopus	Sawmill worker	*Trichoderma koningii*
Diet product	Shark cartilage	Stucco worker	*Mucor* spp. (contaminating esparto fibers)
Fish food factory	Gammarus shrimp		
Fish processor	Clam, shrimp, crab, prawn, salmon, trout, lobster, turbot, various fishes	Technician	*Dictyostelium discoideum* (mold), *Aspergillus niger*
Fisherman	Red soft coral, cuttlefish	**MUSHROOMS**	
Jewelry polisher	Cuttlefish bone	Agriculture	*Agaricus bisporus* (white mushroom)
Laboratory grinder	Marine sponge	Baker	Baker's yeast (*Saccharomyces cerevisiae*), *Boletus edulis*
Oyster farm	Hoya (oyster farm prawn or sea-squirt)		
Restaurant seafood handler	Scallop and shrimp	Greenhouse worker	Sweet pea (*Lathyrus odoratus*)
Scallop plant processor	King scallop and queen scallop	Hotel manager	*Boletus edulis*
Technician	Shrimp meal (*Artemia salina*)	Mushroom producer	*Pleurotus cornucopiae*
		Mushroom soup processor	Mushroom unspecified
ARTHROPODS		Office worker	*Boletus edulis*
Agronomist	*Bruchus lentis*	Seller	*Pleurotus ostreatus* (spores of white spongy rot)
Bottling	Ground bug		
Chicken breeder	Herring worm (*Anisakis simplex*)	**ALGAE**	
Engineer at electric power plant	Caddis flies (*Phryganeidae*)	Pharmacist	Chlorella
		Thalassotherapist	Algae (species unspecified)
Entomologist	Lesser mealworm (*Alphitobius diaperinus* Panzer), moth, butterfly	**FLOURS**	
Farmer	Grain pests (*Eurygaster* and *Pyrale*)	Animal fodder	Marigold flour (*Tagetes erecta*)
Fish bait handler	Insect larvae (*Galleria mellonella*), mealworm larvae (*Tenebrio molitor*), green bottle fly larvae (*Lucila caesar*), daphnia, fish-feed Echinodorus larva (*Echinodorus plasmosus*), Chiromids midge (*Chironomus thummi thummi*)	Baker	Wheat, rye, soya, and buckwheat flour; Konjac flour; white pea flour (*Lathyrus sativus*)
		Food processing	White Lupin flour (*Lupinus albus*)
		POLLENS	
Fish processing	Herring worm (*Anisakis simplex*)	Florist	Cyclamen, rose
Flight crew	Screw worm fly (*Cochliomyia hominivorax*)	Gardener	Canary island date palm (*Phoenix canariensis*), Bell of Ireland (*Moluccella laevis*), Bell pepper, chrysanthemum, eggplant (*Solanum melongena*), *Brassica oleracea* (cauliflower and broccoli)
Honey processors	Honeybee		
Laboratory worker	Cricket, fruit fly, grasshopper (*Locusta migratoria*), locust		
Mechanic in a rye plant	Confused flour beetle (*Tribolium confusum*)	Laboratory worker	Sunflower (*Helianthus* spp.), thale cress (*Arabidopsis thaliana*)
Museum curator	Beetles (Coleoptera)	Olive farmers	White mustard (*Sinapis alba*)
Seed house	Mexican bean weevil (*Zabrotes subfasciatus*)	Processing worker	*Helianthus annuus*
Sericulture	Silkworm, larva of silkworm		
Sewage plant worker	Sewer fly (*Psychoda alternata*)		
Technician	Arthropods (*Chrysoperla carnea, Leptinotarsa decemlineata, Ostrinia nubilalis,* and *Ephestia kuehniella*), sheep blowfly (*Lucilia cuprina*)		
Wool worker	*Dermestidae* spp.		

Table 399-5	High Molecular Weight Antigens Known to Induce Occupational or Environmental Asthma—cont'd

OCCUPATION OR ENVIRONMENT	SOURCE	OCCUPATION OR ENVIRONMENT	SOURCE
PLANTS		Laborer	Citrus food handling (*dl*-limonene, *l*-citronellol, and dichlorophen)
Brewery chemist	Hops	Oil industry	Castor bean, olive oilcake
Brush-makers	Tampico fiber in agave leaves	Pharmaceutical	Rose hip, passion flower (*Passiflora alata*), cascara sagrada (*Rhamnus purshiana*)
Butcher	Aromatic herb		
Chemist	Linseed oilcake, *Voacanga africana* seed dust		
Cosmetics	Dusts from seeds of Sacha Inchi (*Plukenetia volubilis*), chamomile (unspecified)	Powder	Lycopodium powder
		Sewer	Kapok
		Sheller	Almond shell dust
Decorator	Cacoon seed (Entage gigas)	Stucco handler	Esparto (*Stipa tenacissima* and *Lygeum spartum*)
Floral worker	Decorative flower, safflower (*Carthamus tinctorius*) and yarrow (*Achillea millefolium*), spathe flower, statice (*Limonium tataricum*), baby's breath (*Gypsophila paniculata*), ivy (*Hedera helix*), flower (various), sea lavender (*Limonium sinuatum*)	Tobacco manufacturer	Tobacco leaf
		PLANT-DERIVED NATURAL PRODUCTS	
		Baker	Gluten, soybean lecithin
		Candy maker	Pectin
		Glove manufacturer	Latex
		Health professional	Latex
		Rose extraction	Rose oil
Food industry	Aniseed, fenugreek, peach, garlic dust, asparagus, coffee bean, sesame seed, grain dust, carrot (*Daucus carota L.*), green bean (*Phaseolus multiflorus*), lima bean (*Phaseolus lunatus*), onion, potato, swiss chard (*Beta vulgaris L.*), courgette, carob bean, spinach powder, cauliflower, cabbage, chicory, fennel seed, onion seeds (*Allium cepa*, red onion), rice, saffron (*Crocus sativus*), spices, grain dust	**BIOLOGIC ENZYMES**	
		Baker	Fungal amylase, fungal amyloglucosidase and hemicellulase
		Cheese producer	Various enzymes in rennet production (proteases, pepsine, chymosins)
		Detergent industry	Esterase, *Bacillus subtilis*
		Factory worker	*Bacillus subtilis*
		Fruit processor	Pectinase and glucanase
		Hospital personnel	Empynase (pronase B)
		Laboratory worker	Xylanase, phytase from *Aspergillus niger*
Gardener	Copperleaf (*Acalypha wilkesiana*), grass juice, weeping fig (*Ficus benjamina*), umbrella tree (*Schefflera* spp.), amaryllis (*Hippeastrum* spp.), Madagascar jasmine sap (*Stephanotis floribunda*), vetch (*Vicia sativa*)	Pharmaceutical	Bromelin, flaviastase, lactase, pancreatin, papain, pepsin, serratia peptidase, and lysozyme chloride; egg lysozyme, trypsin
		Plastic	Trypsin
Hairdresser	Henna (unspecified)	**VEGETABLE GUMS**	
Herbal tea processor	Herbal tea, sarsaparilla root, sanyak (*Dioscorea batatas*), Korean ginseng (*Panax ginseng*), tea plant dust (*Camellia sinensis*), chamomile (unspecified)	Carpet manufacturing	Guar
		Dental hygienist	*Gutta-percha*
		Gum importer	Tragacanth
		Hairdresser	Karaya
Herbalist	Liquorice roots (*Glycyrrhiza* spp.), wonji (*Polygala tenuifolia*), herb material	Printer	Acacia
Horticulture	Freesia (Freesia hybrida), paprika (*Capsicum annuum*), Brazil ginseng (*Pfaffia paniculata*)		

Table 399-6	Low Molecular Weight Chemicals Known to Induce Occupational or Environmental Asthma

CHEMICALS	OCCUPATION OR ENVIRONMENT SOURCE	CHEMICALS	OCCUPATION OR ENVIRONMENT SOURCE
Diisocyanates		Metals	Metal work
• Diphenylmethane	Polyurethane	• Chromic acid	• Plating
• Hexamethylene	Roofing materials	• Potassium dichromate	• Welding
• Naphthalene	Insulations	• Nickel sulfate	
• Toluene	Paint	• Vanadium	
		• Platinum salts	
Anhydrides	Manufacturers or users		
• Trimellitic	• Paint	Drugs	Exposure to drugs in environment
• Phthalic	• Plastics	• β-Lactams	• Pharmaceutical workers
	• Epoxy resins	• Opioids	• Farmers
		• Other	• Healthcare workers
Dyes	Personal or business use of dyes	Chemicals	Exposure in the healthcare field
• Anthraquinone	• Hair dye	• Formaldehyde	• Laboratory work
• Carmine	• Fur dye	• Glutaraldehyde	• Healthcare professionals
• Henna	• Fabric dye	• Ethylene oxide	
• Persulfate			
Glue or resin	Plastic	Wood dust	Workers/hobbyists
• Methacrylate	• Manufacturers	• Western red cedar (plicatic acid)	• Sawmill
• Acrylates	• Healthcare professionals	• Exotic woods	• Carpentry
• Epoxy	• Orthopedic specialists	• Maple	• Woodworking
		• Oak	

occupational asthma. Occupational asthma induced from multiple causes persists in individuals affected approximately 50% of the time despite primary removal of the sensitizing allergen.

Reactive Airways Disease Syndrome and Irritant-Induced Asthma

RADS presents with the development of acute respiratory symptoms within minutes or hours following a single inhalation of a *high concentration* of irritant gas, aerosol, or smoke. Table 399-7 lists the criteria for diagnosis of RADS. Asthma-like symptoms and airway hyperresponsiveness then ensue, which often persist for prolonged periods. Unlike typical asthma, RADS is often not reversible by use of a bronchodilator. This is probably a consequence of the direct injury to the epithelium and subsequent submucosal fibrosis. Chlorine gas, acetic acid, dimethylaminoethanol, chlorofluorocarbons, epichlorohydrin, and diisocyanates have been studied by experimental design of comparative groups or epidemiology studies.

Irritant induced asthma is a closely related form of asthma resulting from nonimmunologic provocation of bronchial hyperresponsiveness with airflow obstruction induced by irritant chemicals in *low concentration* after single or multiple exposures. If the resultant pulmonary symptoms occur after multiple exposures at a plant, it is termed *nonimmunologic-induced asthma*.

Predisposing factors for the development of RADS are not well characterized. Atopy and cigarette smoking may increase the risk of developing RADS when exposure through inhalation of irritant chemicals occurs. In addition to host factors, the type of chemical appears to be important. Higher concentrations of chemicals, the type of chemical (vapor or wet aerosols), and bleaching agents are the most offending agents to cause RADS. Dry particle aerosols are less likely to cause RADS. Analysis of the World Trade Center firefighters indicates that the presence of bronchial hyperresponsiveness prior to a chemical exposure does not increase the risk for an individual to develop RADS.

Pathogenesis of RADS follows a typical pattern. Initial histology demonstrates rapid denudation of the mucosa accompanied by submucosal fibrinous, hemorrhagic exudate. Subepithelial edema occurs subsequently with some regeneration of the epithelial layer, proliferation of basal and parabasal cells, and eventually areas of fibrosis. The desquamation, subepithelial fibrosis, thickening of the basement membrane, and regeneration of basal cells are all more prominent in RADS than in occupational asthma. This may explain the limited response to bronchodilator therapy in this syndrome compared to asthma.

The clinical manifestations of RADS and irritant-induced asthma are different from each other mostly in the onset of symptoms. Patients with RADS typically can pinpoint the exact time of onset of symptoms as well as the exact number of hours postexposure. The symptoms are so severe that nearly 80% of subjects in one study presented to an emergency department for care. The lower airway symptoms of cough,

Table 399-7	Criteria for the Diagnosis of Reactive Airways Disease Syndrome

Absence of previous documented respiratory symptom
Onset of symptoms most often occur after a single specific exposure
Exposure is most often to a high concentration of gas, smoke, fume, or vapor with irritant qualities
Symptoms occur within 24 hr of exposure and persist for 3 mo or longer
Symptoms mimic asthma with cough, wheezing, shortness of breath, and/or dyspnea
Pulmonary function tests may demonstrate airflow obstruction but not always
Bronchial hyperresponsiveness is documented by methacholine challenge
Alternative pulmonary diseases are not able to be found

dyspnea, chest tightness, and wheezing are prominent features in RADS, with cough being most prevalent. Because of the toxic nature of the inhaled chemical, it is predictable that an upper airway syndrome of throat and nose burning will often accompany the lower airway symptoms. This part of the complex has been referred to as **respiratory upper airway dysfunction syndrome.**

Individuals with irritant-induced asthma present with a more insidious onset of symptoms. Because of the recurrent nature of the low concentration of chemical, patients may not be able to identify the underlying trigger initially. Similar to allergic rhinitis, patients may describe nasal congestion, rhinorrhea, sneezing, postnasal drip, ocular irritation, and conjunctival injection. Pulmonary symptoms include those typically seen with asthma exacerbations.

Initial evaluation of the patient with RADS or irritant-induced asthma usually includes the medical history, physical examination, and pulse oximetry. Because of the acute nature of RADS, a chest radiograph is obtained in order to rule out other acute causes of dyspnea including pneumonia or pulmonary edema. Ideally, if the patient is not in significant distress, complete pulmonary functions with spirometry, lung volumes, and diffusion capacity are very helpful in the initial evaluation. The lack of abnormality on initial chest radiograph reassures the clinician that HRCT is not indicated.

TREATMENT

Treatment of RADS and irritant-induced asthma focuses on prevention of exposure. Because the exposure in RADS is often associated with a single known exposure, this task is readily accomplished. The low, persistent exposures are more challenging to identify and remove. Implementing treatment guidelines for asthma from all causes is recommended when intervention is required beyond antigen removal.

Bibliography is available at Expert Consult.

399.3 Granulomatous Lung Disease
Kevin J. Kelly

GRANULOMATOSIS WITH POLYANGIITIS

Granulomatosis with polyangiitis (GPA) is a disease that involves both the lower and upper respiratory tracts with granulomatous inflammation of small vessels; formerly it was known as *Wegener granulomatosis* (see Chapter 167). The pulmonary disease is frequently associated with glomerulonephritis. The simultaneous presence of pulmonary and renal disease should immediately raise the suspicion that either GPA or Goodpasture disease (see Chapter 399.5) may be causing the disease.

Etiology and Epidemiology

The prevalence of GPA disease appears to be increasing by up to 4-fold in the last 2 decades, but without male or female predominance. Diagnostic tests, such as antineutrophil antibodies, may explain some of this increased prevalence.

Pathogenesis

Clinically, the development of both upper and lower airway disease with granulomas in GPA implies that exposure to antigen in the airway of endogenous or exogenous source is involved with aberrant cell-mediated immune response. Cytokine expression by peripheral blood CD4+ lymphocytes and cells collected by BAL indicate there is a predominantly T-lymphocyte type 1 response with overexpression of interferon-γ (IFN-γ) and tumor necrosis factor (TNF). In vitro studies demonstrate a skewed T-lymphocyte type 17 response by blood CD4+ T cells in GPA, suggesting there is an immune regulatory defect that leads to excessive production of T-lymphocyte type 1/T-lymphocyte type 17 cytokines (interleukin [IL]-17, TNF, and IFN-γ) presumed to be from the environment or autoantigens. Such an inflammatory response may be sufficient to induce and sustain granuloma formation.

Detection of *autoantibodies reactive against proteins in the cytoplasmic granules of neutrophils and monocytes (antineutrophil cytoplasmic antibodies [ANCAs])* are found in 90% of the patients with GPA. The first major type of ANCA is directed against cytoplasmic proteinase-3 and is frequently named c-ANCA. The second major type of ANCA recognizes the enzyme myeloperoxidase. It is found in a small number (<10%) of patients with GPA. Antimyeloperoxidase antibodies fluoresce in a perinuclear pattern and are often referred to as perinuclear ANCA. In contrast, some patients develop the clinical phenotype of GPA in the absence of detectable ANCA.

Clinical Manifestations

Children with GPA present with respiratory complaints accompanied by fever, loss of energy, and vague joint complaints. Some may present with severe nasal disease manifested as ulceration, septal perforation, pain, sinusitis, and or epistaxis. The septal perforation may lead to deformation of the nasal bridge from erosion of the underlying cartilage but is more common in adults. Pulmonary disease occurs in the majority of patients as noted above. Symptoms range from cough, hemoptysis, dyspnea, and chest discomfort to asymptomatic infiltrates on chest radiography. Occasionally, patients with GPA will present with hemoptysis or recurrent fleeting infiltrates from **pulmonary hemorrhage**. The pathology is confusing because granulomatous disease may be difficult to demonstrate and can be confused with microscopic polyangiitis. This is found most frequently in Goodpasture disease, microscopic polyangiitis, and Henoch-Schönlein purpura. Distinguishing GPA from other pulmonary renal syndromes is easiest when there are classical symptoms of upper airway disease (nasal/sinus), lower airway disease with necrosis, granulomas on biopsy of the lung with vasculitis, and renal disease consistent with glomerulonephritis.

As many as 20% of patients with GPA will present with subglottic or endobronchial stenosis from scarring and inflammatory changes. Although it may be the presenting symptom, it often occurs in conjunction with other disease manifestations. Dyspnea and voice changes are common complaints from the patients.

Skin, ocular, and joint symptoms are common in GPA and have been found to accompany the lung and renal disease in most series 50% or more of the time. Biopsy of the skin may show nonspecific leukocytoclastic vasculitis, venulitis, or capillaritis.

Laboratory and Pathology

c-ANCA or anti–proteinase-3 antibodies are found in 90% of patients with GPA. However, they are also found in other types of vasculitis and are not sufficient in themselves to make a diagnosis without a tissue biopsy (see Chapter 167). Because of the necrotizing nature of the vasculitis, lung tissue is required for definitive diagnosis of pulmonary disease. Biopsy of the upper airway may demonstrate evidence of granulomatous disease but it is uncommon to find evidence of vasculitis; lung biopsy is warranted. Usual pathology demonstrates multiple parenchymal nodules that may be located in either the bronchial, vascular, or interstitial tissues (Fig. 399-2). The granulomatous inflammation often is found areas of necrosis and/or vasculitis.

Renal biopsy rarely is able to demonstrate granulomas or vasculitis. Rather, kidney tissues may show focal, segmental, or necrotizing glomerulonephritis without deposits of immune complexes. When the tissues fail to demonstrate classical findings, a variety of diseases (e.g., tuberculosis, sarcoid, microscopic polyangiitis, malignancy, and other autoimmune disorders) must be considered in the evaluation.

Radiology

Chest radiography in GPA will show multiple infiltrates, nodules, cavitary lesions, or interstitial lung disease. Fleeting infiltrates may be seen when recurrent hemorrhage is a part of the clinical manifestation. HRCT often demonstrates more extensive lung disease and the cavitation associated with the necrotizing nature of the disease (Fig. 399-3).

Treatment

Rapidly progressive, debilitating disease may occur when failure to diagnose GPA leads to inadequate treatment. One series of patients

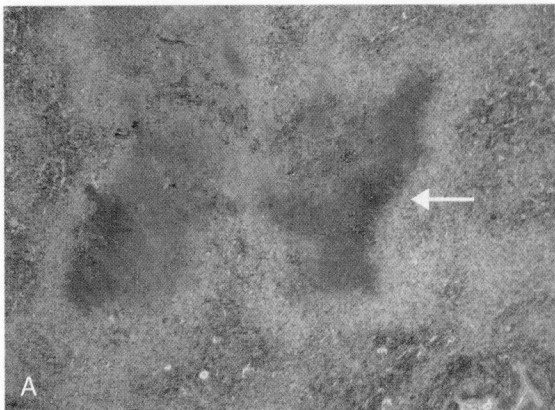
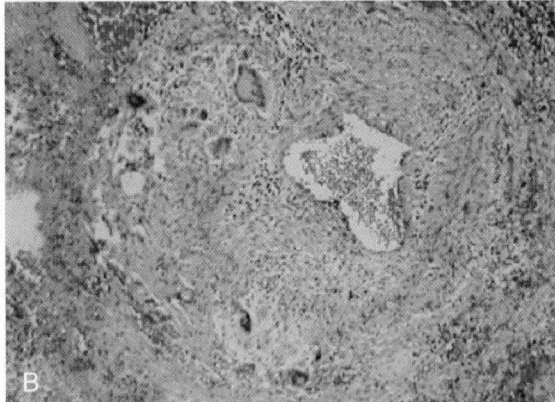

Figure 399-2 A, Low-power view of granulomatous inflammation and geographic necrosis (*arrow*) in a lung biopsy from a patient with GPA. **B,** Granulomatous vasculitis involving a small pulmonary artery in the lung of a patient with GPA. The vessel wall is markedly thickened with an inflammatory infiltrate that includes multinucleated giant cells. (*From Sneller MC, Fontana JR, Shelhamer JH. Immunologic nonasthmatic diseases of the lung. In Adkinson AF, editor:* Middleton's allergy principles and practice, *Philadelphia, 2014, Elsevier, Fig. 61-1B and C.*)

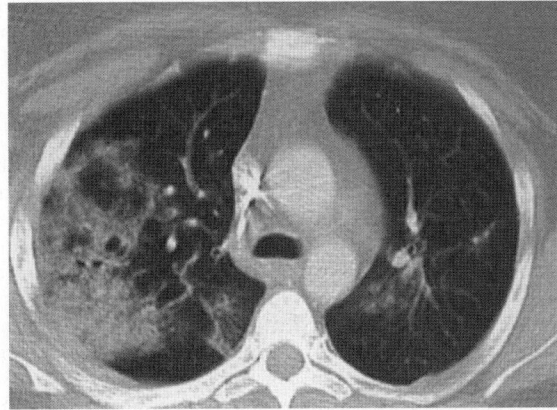

Figure 399-3 Chest CT scan of a patient with granulomatosis with polyangiitis shows typical nodular lung infiltrate with cavitation. (*From Sneller MC, Fontana JR, Shelhamer JH. Immunologic nonasthmatic diseases of the lung. In Adkinson AF, editor:* Middleton's allergy principles and practice, *Philadelphia, 2014, Elsevier, Fig. 61-1A.*)

showed death occured in 90% of patients within 2 yr of diagnosis. Glucocorticoid therapy alone resulted in relapses and inadequate control of disease in many subjects. Standard initial induction of therapy includes prednisone at 1 mg/kg/day in combination with oral cyclophosphamide at 2 mg/kg/day or intravenous dosing at 15 mg/kg monthly. This regimen is effective at induction of remission of disease process. The advantage of oral daily dosing is a reduction in relapse of disease once induction has occurred. After induction of remission (usually in 3 mo), prednisone can be tapered to an every-other-day regimen and eventually discontinued in 6-8 mo. After induction of remission, cyclophosphamide should be discontinued because of drug toxicity, serious risk of infections, risk of infertility, or cancer. In those patients with recurring relapse, cyclophosphamide has had limited use.

Once remission was achieved and cyclophosphamide discontinued; both methotrexate and azathioprine demonstrated efficacy with lowered side effects during maintenance of remission therapy for approximately 1 yr.

Adjuvant therapy with plasma exchange may be considered when life-threatening GPA disease presents. This is advocated on the premise that ANCAs are inducing disease and will be removed from the circulation with this intervention; its use has been favorably evaluated in GPA-induced renal disease. Plasmapheresis and exchange is advocated as adjuvant treatment for severe manifestations of GPA and related ANCA-associated disease based on the theoretical benefit of removing potentially pathogenic ANCA. Adjuvant plasma exchange has been studied mainly in patients with severe renal vasculitis, but there are also reports of success in severe pulmonary hemorrhage. The results of a meta-analysis of patients with renal vasculitis in 9 trials, suggest that adjuvant plasma exchange may be associated with improved renal outcome.

The removal of B-cells that produce ANCAs may be effective by reducing the production of pathogenic antibodies. Rituximab, an anti-CD20 chimeric antibody, regimens used in conjunction with glucocorticoids or glucocorticoids with a short course of cyclophosphamide are equally efficacious in inducing remission when compared to more prolonged therapy with steroid plus cyclophosphamide.

Recurrent disease remains a major problem. ANCA levels have not been shown to correlate with activity of disease or severity. Patients with isolated disease of the sinuses and nose may not warrant such toxic therapy. Therapy with topical corticosteroid and antibiotics for infection appear to be warranted. If unsuccessful, steroid with methotrexate appears to be an effective therapy.

The development of subglottic stenosis requires specific treatment. Use of cyclophosphamide with oral corticosteroid may have an incomplete or no response in the airway. Local injection of a prolonged acting corticosteroid locally appears to be indicated to reduce the inflammation and prevent further scarring. If this complication is found at presentation, simultaneous airway intervention with induction of corticosteroid and cyclophosphamide is warranted and encouraged.

SARCOIDOSIS

Sarcoidosis is an idiopathic inflammatory disease involving multiple organ systems, with characteristic histology of noncaseating granulomas (see Chapter 165). It has been postulated that sarcoidosis represents an immune response to a yet-to-be-identified agent from the environment that is likely inhaled in a susceptible host. It remains a diagnosis of exclusion from other diseases with granuloma formation on histology, such as immune deficiency of chronic granulomatous disease, granulomatous lymphocytic interstitial lung disease associated with common variable immune deficiency, HP associated with some drugs and inhalation agents, granuloma with polyangiitis, typical and atypical *Mycobacterium*, *Pneumocystis jiroveci*, and malignancy.

Epidemiology and Pathogenesis

African-American females are disproportionately affected more than any other group. Because an asymptomatic sarcoid-like distribution of noncaseating granulomas may be frequently found at autopsy, the contribution of the granulomas to the disease is not always clear. Some countries do mass chest radiograph screening for multiple diseases. In that setting, up to 50% of diagnosed sarcoidosis is asymptomatic. The severity of the disease appears to be worse in African-Americans who tend to have acute illness, whereas white subjects are more likely to be asymptomatic with a more chronic disease. There

have been clusters of disease in families and genetic testing suggests that MHC linkage on the short arm of chromosome 6 is most likely to be observed.

Sarcoidosis is rarely found in children younger than the age of 8 yr; those of African descent are most affected. The disease presentation is similar to adults with multisystem disease being the most common. Skin rash, iridocyclitis, and arthritis are seen most often without pulmonary symptoms. In northern Europe, erythema nodosum with the ocular involvement of iridocyclitis is seen most frequently. Despite the lack of symptoms, chest radiography may be abnormal in approximately 90% of children. The pulmonary disease appears to be less progressive compared to adults and patients recover spontaneously without corticosteroids. Rarely, pulmonary disease may progress to fibrosis. Ocular disease is more likely to be progressive and warrant intervention as the inflammatory response may lead to blindness from complications of iritis.

Unrecognized infection or inhalation of an immune response–inducing antigen continues to be at the forefront of consideration as a cause of the disease. Clusters of sarcoidosis in small populations, variable prevalence by geography and race, transfer of disease by organ transplant, and the reproducible granuloma formation only in patients with sarcoidosis in the skin when homogenized lymph node tissue from patients with sarcoid are injected intradermally (Kveim-Siltzbach test) have supported this hypothesis.

Clinical Manifestations

Patients with lung disease are more likely to be asymptomatic as the presentation often may be an abnormal chest radiograph. When symptomatic, patients demonstrate shortness of breath, cough, and dyspnea. Children are more likely to manifest the disease as iridocyclitis, skin rash, and arthritis. African-American children appear to have more frequent lymph node involvement, nonspecific elevations of gamma globulin, erythema nodosum, and hypercalcemia. Physical exam may reveal only an elevated respiratory rate without crackles or rales by auscultation. Pleural involvement has been seen but is uncommon. When present, a lymphocytic predominant exudate may be observed with laboratory evaluation of the pleural fluid. Unusual but reported findings include cases of pneumothorax, hemothorax, and chylothorax. One specific syndrome, **Lofgren syndrome**, with hilar lymphadenopathy, erythema nodosum, and migratory polyarthralgias, is almost exclusively seen in women. This syndrome has a strong association with HLA-DQB1*0201 and polymorphisms in the C-C chemokine receptor 2 (CCR2); these genetic markers are a predictor of a good outcome.

Although almost 90% of patients with sarcoidosis demonstrate parenchymal or mediastinal disease on chest radiography, there are many who have minimal to no symptoms. Approximately 40% of adults with stage 1 disease have endobronchial involvement found at bronchoscopy. The higher the staging level of disease, the higher the percentage of people with airway involvement.

Diagnostic Laboratory Testing

The most common but nonspecific findings are hypergammaglobulinemia, hypercalciuria, hypercalcemia, elevated alkaline phosphatase when liver disease is present, and, occasionally, anemia of chronic disease. Serum angiotensin-converting enzyme may be elevated in 75% of patients with untreated sarcoid. False-positive tests occur from other diseases so that it is not considered a diagnostic test but rather a test that strongly supports the diagnosis.

Pulmonary function tests are able to be performed accurately in most children older than the age of 4 yr. There are no specific diagnostic findings of spirometry, lung volumes, or diffusion capacity in sarcoidosis. Exercise coupled with pulmonary function tests may demonstrate a decline in diffusion capacity when alveolitis is present in hypersensitivity pneumonitis and could add diagnostic help to the clinician when attempting to differentiate sarcoidosis from HP prior to biopsy.

BAL is of great help when differentiating HP from sarcoid. BAL in sarcoid shows a marked predominance of CD4 cells. A lymphocyte

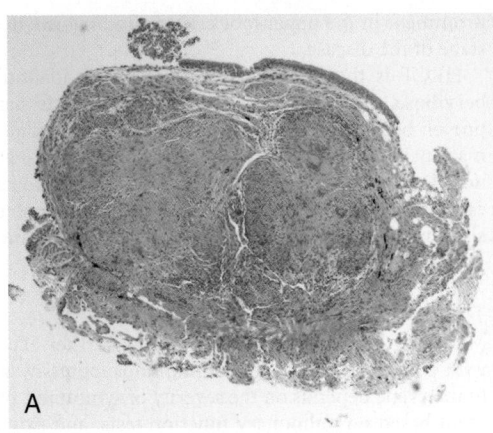 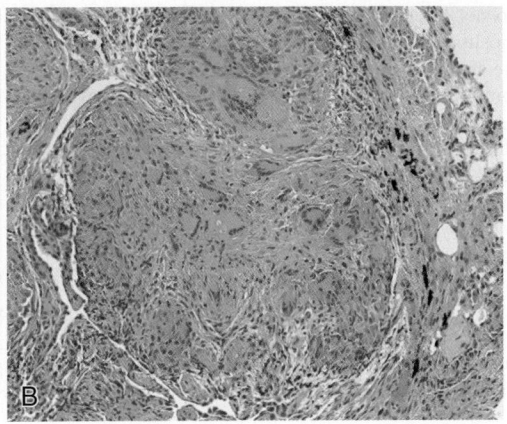

Figure 399-4 Transbronchial biopsy specimen showing a sarcoid granuloma. **A,** The granulomas are located below the bronchiolar epithelial layer that appears at the top of the frame. **B,** A higher-power view of the same biopsy specimen. The epithelioid granuloma is tightly packed and contains multiple multinucleated giant cells. There is no caseous necrosis. Special stains for acid-fast bacilli and fungi were negative. *(From Sneller MC, Fontana JR, Shelhamer JH. Immunologic nonasthmatic diseases of the lung. In Adkinson AF, editor: Middleton's allergy principles and practice, Philadelphia, 2014, Elsevier, Fig. 61-6.)*

percentage >16% on BAL, a CD4:CD8 ratio >4, and noncaseating granulomas on bronchial biopsy in the presence of abnormal angiotensin-converting enzyme levels are nearly completely diagnostic for sarcoid. In addition, T cells are activated on BAL. BAL in HP shows a significant change in the balance of CD4 to CD8 cells with the 2 cell types being nearly equal compared to the normal mild predominance of CD4 cells in the circulation. A ratio of CD4:CD8 of <1 predicts 100% of patients with BAL lymphocytosis to *not* have sarcoidosis. Neutrophil counts >2% and/or eosinophil counts >1% exclude the diagnosis of sarcoidosis.

The analysis of D-dimers in BAL fluid from subjects with sarcoidosis demonstrates an elevation in 80% of patients compared to no detectable D-dimers in unaffected control.

Histopathology

The characteristic feature of sarcoidosis is the noncaseating granuloma formation in the lung (Fig. 399-4). These granulomas are found in the bronchial walls, alveolar septa, and vascular walls of pulmonary arteries and veins. The formation of noncaseating granulomas is likely preceded by alveolitis involving the interstitium more than the alveolar spaces. There is accumulation of inflammatory cells, including monocytes, macrophages, and lymphocytes that accompany the granulomas. Multinucleated giant cells are frequently found among the epithelioid cells within the granuloma follicle. These may show cytoplasmic inclusions (e.g., asteroid bodies and Schaumann bodies) as well as some birefringent crystalline particles made of calcium oxalate and other calcium salts. These are most often identified in the upper lobes of the lungs which may lead to confusion with diseases such as hypersensitivity pneumonitis, eosinophilic granuloma, collagen vascular disease, pneumoconiosis, berylliosis, and infectious disease such as tuberculosis or histoplasmosis.

Radiology

Pulmonary imaging in sarcoid has included plain chest radiography, HRCT, **positron emission tomography** using fluorine-18-fluorodeoxyglucose, and radiotracer using gallium-67. The staging of sarcoid is performed using plain radiography and is outlined as follows:

◆ Stage I—Bilateral hilar lymphadenopathy accompanied by right paratracheal lymphadenopathy
◆ Stage II—Bilateral hilar lymphadenopathy accompanied by reticular opacities are present. If symptomatic, patients have cough and dyspnea. Occasional fever and fatigue accompany the respiratory symptoms.
◆ Stage III—Reticular opacities are found predominantly in the upper lobes with regression of hilar lymphadenopathy.

◆ Stage IV—Reticular opacities start to coalesce and lead to volume loss in the lung fields, traction bronchiectasis from conglomeration of the inflamed tissues. Extensive calcium deposits may be seen at this stage.

HRCT may be helpful in further staging of the disease, as well as in revealing abnormalities not appreciated on chest radiography. Findings in patients with sarcoidosis by HRCT include hilar lymphadenopathy, paratracheal nodules, middle to upper lung parenchymal ground-glass appearance, bronchial wall thickening, bronchiectasis, cystic changes, and fibrosis. The ground-glass appearance suggests that alveolitis, as seen in hypersensitivity pneumonitis, may be present. Biopsy has usually shown granuloma formation as the predominant histologic finding.

Treatment

Because pulmonary sarcoidosis spontaneously resolves without therapy in almost 75% of patients, clear guidelines for treatment focused on minimizing side effects of therapy is required. Glucocorticosteroids (GCSs) have long been the mainstay of therapy in sarcoid and are often used because of extra pulmonary disease. When pulmonary disease is progressive, GCS therapy is aimed at prevention of fibrosis, honeycombing, and irreversible lung disease. Assuring that disseminated infections, heart failure, thromboembolism, or pulmonary hypertension are not present is important. In addition to HRCT of the chest, performance of pulmonary function tests, electrocardiogram and echocardiogram should be considered prior to starting GCS therapy.

GCS therapy is often not started when stage I or II is present without symptoms. This scrutiny of the benefit of therapy was highlighted when prospective evaluation of GCS therapy for pulmonary disease found that nearly 50% of patients receiving GCSs had active or relapsing disease 2 yr later. In contrast, 90% of patients who did not receive GCSs had spontaneous remission of disease with the other 10% needing intervention 2 yr later. Absolute indications include progressive stage III disease with symptoms of shortness of breath, cough, or other chest symptoms such as pain. Progressive restriction shown on pulmonary function testing is an indication for therapy. Specific pulmonary function changes where lung capacity declines total 10% or greater, forced vital capacity declines 15% or more, or diffusion capacity degradation is seen of 20% or more are all indications for GCS intervention.

Dosage with oral prednisone at 0.3-0.5 mg/kg is a reasonable starting point depending on the severity of symptoms. Stability is usually achieved within 6-8 wks, after which slow progressive tapering of GCS may occur every 4-8 wks. Many favor the use of alternate-day steroids to reduce the side effects of GCSs, but little data exist to show efficacy.

Patients who do not tolerate GCSs or develop progressive disease, alternative immunosuppressive agents may add benefit to the regimen. Progressive disease also is a reminder for the clinician to reassess the diagnosis of sarcoid and review the chance that beryllium may have been the underlying reason for the progressive disease.

Inhaled GCSs have been evaluated in patients with stage I disease with variable results. Evaluation of therapy with pulmonary function testing and symptoms are the best methods to judge responsiveness to this therapy. Persistent symptoms after 4-8 wks of therapy suggest that systemic GCSs may be indicated.

BERYLLIOSIS

Chronic beryllium disease or berylliosis is an example of environmental exposure and unique granulomatous response in the lungs. Beryllium is an alkaline metal that is used in a number of industrial settings.

A diagnosis of berylliosis requires 3 criteria: (1) history of beryllium exposure; (2) positive response to lymphocyte proliferation tests to beryllium in lymphocytes obtained by BAL or blood test; and (3) noncaseating granulomas on lung biopsy. Exposure to beryllium may occur in industries such as automotive, ceramic, aerospace, metal extraction, electronics, computer, jewelry making, and dental alloys. Teenagers working summer jobs in machine work, ceramics, or wire production may be exposed. Sensitization is associated with dose and duration of exposure and has been seen to be as high as 20% in certain industries. Secretaries working in buildings where manufacturing with beryllium is active have developed berylliosis.

Pathogenesis

Genetic susceptibility coupled with immunologic response to beryllium are the 2 key contributors to the development of disease. A T-lymphocyte cell–mediated delayed hypersensitivity response to beryllium appears to be the mechanism involved with granuloma formation in the lung. The lymphocyte proliferation by T cells to beryllium is specific and does not occur to other metals. Similar to sarcoidosis, CD4+ T cells predominate on bronchoalveolar response. Beryllium appears to be inhaled and then couple with proteins in the lung or can be ingested by antigen-presenting cells. The cytokines elicited and granuloma formation suggests that sensitization is primarily a T-lymphocyte type 1 response with elevated interferon-γ and IL-2 production.

Clinical Manifestations

The clinical manifestations of berylliosis are not specific. Dry cough, fever, fatigue, weight loss, and shortness of breath all may be present. Although symptoms may occur within 3 mo, new disease has been detected up to 3 decades after exposure. Physical examination is somewhat different than the HPs and sarcoid with bibasilar crackles found on auscultation. The other mentioned diseases are more prominent in the upper lobes. Small nodule on exposed skin may also be present.

Laboratory Testing

Suspicion of berylliosis should prompt the clinician to have blood lymphocyte proliferation studies to beryllium performed as well as complete pulmonary functions. These tests need to be sent to a special center where multiple tests are run with comparison to proper positive and negative controls. When positive, the test has very high specificity for defining the presence of berylliosis at approximately 96%. However, sensitivity of the test hovers at <70%, suggesting that approximately 3 of every 10 patients who have disease may have a negative test.

Similar to other pulmonary granulomatous diseases, increased production of calcitriol is commonly found. The source of this active form of vitamin D is from activated pulmonary macrophages, which may result in hypercalciuria and hypercalcemia.

Radiography

Chest radiographs should be obtained on all patients suspected of having berylliosis. The chest radiograph may be normal, show hilar lymphadenopathy, pulmonary nodules, ground glass, or alveolar opacities. The parenchymal abnormalities may be diffuse or may be more prominent in the upper lobes. These findings are dependent upon the stage of the disease.

HRCT is the most sensitive test in the identification of chronic berylliosis. Almost 25% of the HRCT exams in patients with biopsy proven berylliosis are found to be normal. Similar to other granulomatous and HPs of the lungs, HRCT findings include parenchymal nodules of varying size, thick septal lines, ground-glass opacities, cystic cavitation, and lymphadenopathy in the hilum or mediastinum. Pleural abnormalities are less common, but thickening may be observed in proximity to parenchymal nodules.

Treatment

Managing berylliosis involves avoiding further exposure and therapy with glucocorticoids or other immunosuppressive agents. A decision to intervene depends on the severity of symptoms, physiologic impairment based on pulmonary function tests, and extent of radiographic changes. Treatment is usually started when the patient has dyspnea or cough, >10% decline in lung volumes or gas exchange, or abnormal pulmonary function tests at baseline.

Small case series have demonstrated efficacy of steroids judged by improvement of clinical symptoms, radiographic clearing of disease, and improvement in pulmonary functions, including diffusion capacity. Some patients despite improved symptoms have recurrence which may progress to fibrosis and persistent lung disease.

The differentiation between berylliosis and sarcoidosis appears to be important for long-term outcomes. It appears that the longer the delay in prescribing GCSs to patients with berylliosis may lead to a state where the lung disease is unresponsive to therapy. In contrast, use of steroids may lead to a higher rate of recurrent disease. What makes the 2 responses different is not known.

Dosing of steroids is similar to sarcoid with a starting dose of 0.5 mg/kg/day of prednisone for a duration of 6-12 wks. Once a response is established, conversion to every-other-day corticosteroid use at the same dose followed by tapering should be attempted until the lowest dose is achieved that controls the disease. Patients may require persistent therapy for the rest of their life. Genetic susceptibility to the disease may predict relapse of disease. Mutations in the HLA-DPB1 gene (homozygous for glutamate substitution at the β69 position) appear to predict specific patients who are susceptible to relapse of symptoms.

When patients fail to respond or experience recurrent relapse, methotrexate in low dose has conferred a favorable response in some patients as has been seen with sarcoidosis. Azathioprine may also be considered since sarcoidosis has responded favorably, however there are no published trials using this immunosuppressive agent. A small number of cases have also shown promise with TNF-α inhibitors both in sarcoid and beryllium-induced disease.

GRANULOMATOUS LUNG DISEASE IN PRIMARY IMMUNE DEFICIENCY

Primary immune deficiency (PID) often presents with recurrent or persistent pulmonary symptoms of recurrent infections, pneumonia, bronchiectasis, and interstitial lung disease with or without fibrosis. Immune dysregulation occurs in many of the PID with development of granulomatous lung disease and autoimmune disease. Most effort is focused on discovery of infectious pathogens in the PID causing pulmonary disturbance, but the dysregulation may be the primary problem causing symptoms and disease progression. This requires counterintuitive therapies with suppression of the immune system concurrently with immune deficiency therapy. The 2 most prominent PIDs associated with granulomatous lung disease are **chronic granulomatous disease (CGD)** (see Chapter 130) and **common variable immune deficiency (CVID)** (see Chapter 126).

The prototype organism causing granuloma formation in the lung is *Mycobacterium tuberculosis*. Nontuberculous mycobacterial infections also can cause granulomas in the presence of specific PID. These have been seen in impaired IL-12/IL-23/ IFN-γ signaling, or the presence of autoantibodies to IFN-γ. Patients with defective regulation of nuclear factor-kappa B (nuclear factor-kappa B essential modifier defects) have also been described as well with nontuberculous mycobacteria. The clinician must be certain that this low-virulence organism is not causing disease before therapy for immune dysregulation is considered.

Pathogenesis
CGD is a PID involving multiple defects in the phagocyte nicotinamide adenine dinucleotide phosphate oxidase system, which impairs the respiratory burst capacity to generate reactive species of oxygen (see Chapter 130).

Up to 25% of patients with CVID develop lung disease (see Chapter 126). These pulmonary changes include organizing pneumonia, ILD, mucosa-associated lymphoid tissue lymphoma, and noncaseating granulomas in **granulomatous and lymphocytic interstitial lung disease (GLILD)**. Elevated levels of TNF from TNF polymorphisms have been implicated as a possible mechanism. GLILD is becoming recognized more frequently in CVID. It is defined by the presence of granulomatous and a lymphocytic proliferative pattern in the lung. Granulomas may be found in other organs including bone marrow, spleen, gastrointestinal tract, skin, and liver.

The etiology of GLILD is unknown. In a case cohort study, a majority of subjects with pathology diagnostic of GLILD were found to have human herpesvirus 8 infection of the lung. These may represent a subgroup of patients with GLILD which may point to a mechanism underlying the development of pulmonary granulomas.

GLILD is sometimes misdiagnosed as sarcoidosis initially because both involve pulmonary granuloma, often accompanied by hilar and/or mediastinal lymphadenopathy. Sarcoidosis has several features that distinguish it from GLILD, such as normal or elevated serum immunoglobulin levels and frequent spontaneous remissions.

Clinical Manifestations of Granulomatous Lung Disease in Primary Immune Deficiency
Chronic respiratory disease as a result of recurrent infections is common in CGD. This is accompanied by clubbing in some patients and the other organ manifestations in the skin, liver, and genitourinary and gastrointestinal tracts. Granulomas are especially problematic in the gastrointestinal and genitourinary tracts. The inhalation of fungal spores and hyphae has led to an acute pneumonia in CGD with rapid progression to respiratory failure with hypoxemia, dyspnea, and fever. This entity, characterized as *mulch pneumonia,* appears to be best treated with antifungal medications and corticosteroids.

Radiography
Hilar and/or mediastinal lymphadenopathy occur with granulomatous lung involvement. These may manifest as parenchymal nodules and/or ground glass abnormalities and can be seen commonly in CVID and CGD. Differentiating infectious causes of pulmonary infiltration in PID is often difficult on chest radiography; HRCT is often mandatory in the initial evaluation of the patients with CVID.

Laboratory and Pulmonary Function Testing
Definitive diagnosis is made by lung biopsy. Transbronchial biopsy in children is often insufficient and lung biopsy by video-assisted thoracoscopy or open biopsy is preferred. Unless the patient's underlying immune deficiency is unknown, other laboratory testing except for infectious organisms does not contribute significantly to the diagnosis. When the child is old enough, complete pulmonary functions with spirometry, flow volume loop, lung volumes, and diffusion capacity should be obtained at baseline and then followed serially for response to therapy or progression of disease.

Therapy
The presence of GLILD in CVID can be associated with significant morbidity and possibly death. Without therapy, progressive pulmonary fibrosis and respiratory failure may occur in GLILD. The parenchymal disease may not always be controlled or relieved by glucocorticoid treatment. Other treatments include TNF antagonists, cyclosporine, or a combination therapy with rituximab and azathioprine. Response to therapy is monitored clinically and by interval HRCT of the chest, and

pulmonary function testing, including spirometry, lung volumes, and diffusing capacity.

Bibliography is available at Expert Consult.

399.4 Eosinophilic Lung Disease
Kevin J. Kelly

The eosinophilic lung diseases are a group of heterogeneous pulmonary disorders with a predominant diffuse infiltration of eosinophils in the alveolar spaces or interstitial pulmonary spaces. Lung architecture is well preserved throughout the inflammatory response, often with complete reversal of the inflammation without long-term sequelae in the majority of cases. The peripheral white blood count often (but not always) reveals elevated eosinophils. Prompt recognition of the nature of these diseases allows for lifesaving interventions in the idiopathic **acute eosinophilic pneumonia syndrome (AEP)** or resolution of persistent symptoms in the patients with chronic disease.

ETIOLOGY
Eosinophilic lung diseases are often classified under 2 subheadings: idiopathic disease and known causation (Table 399-8). They are frequently further subdivided as acute and chronic or infectious and noninfectious. The division of acute or chronic is arbitrary based on the length of symptoms present (acute = <1 mo and chronic = >1 mo) but is relevant to the clinician in determining the etiology of the symptoms in the differential diagnosis. **Löffler eosinophilic pneumonia,** induced by *Ascaris lumbricoides* and other ascarids, produces transient symptoms that self-resolve and is classified as neither acute nor chronic. Löffler syndrome has been more correctly termed pulmonary infiltrates with eosinophilia syndrome and is the most common eosinophilic infiltrative disease in children.

PATHOLOGY AND PATHOGENESIS
Eosinophilic lung disease, regardless of the stage of disease or etiology, shows mixed cellular infiltration of the alveoli and interstitial spaces with a predominance of eosinophils when transbronchial biopsy or open lung biopsy is performed. This may be accompanied by a fibrinous exudate with intact lung architecture. Other findings include eosinophilic microabscesses, a nonnecrotizing nongranulomatous vasculitis, and occasional multinucleated giant cells again without granuloma formation. BAL is the diagnostic procedure of choice, especially in the acute situation with the acute eosinophilic pneumonias; the differential cell count on the BAL is ≥25% eosinophils and is often more than 40%. This highly sensitive test and high specificity test has allowed clinicians to forego lung biopsy.

Eosinophils are filled with numerous toxic granules. Evidence of eosinophil degranulation may be found by electron microscopy, biopsy, urine excretion, and BAL fluid. Most commonly, eosinophil-derived neurotoxin, leukotriene E_4, other granule proteins, such as major basic protein, Charcot Leyden crystals, or proinflammatory cytokines, are identified and support the evidence that eosinophils are not only present but contributing to the disease process.

CLINICAL MANIFESTATIONS
Specific eosinophilic lung diseases present with a variable clinical picture; however, there are some common findings across many of the eosinophilic diseases. Dyspnea is the most common and prevalent symptom in patients with acute or chronic eosinophilic pneumonia and is accompanied by cough in the majority of patients (90%). Rhinitis and sinusitis symptoms are of lower prevalence with wide variability in children with eosinophilic pulmonary disease. Only the A specific disorder, **acute eosinophilic pneumonia,** consistently presents with respiratory failure and the requirement for mechanical ventilation at high levels of positive end expiratory pressure and high concentrations of oxygen. Although malignancy (e.g., eosinophilic leukemia) and organizing pneumonia may present with need for mechanical

Table 399-8	Key Elements in the Medical History and Physical Exam to Raise Clinical Suspicion for Diagnostic Testing to Confirm Eosinophilic Lung Disease

Medical history and examination
- Drug exposure (especially antibiotics, NSAIDs, antiepileptics, antileukotriene modifiers in EGPA)
- Environmental inhalation exposures to dust or inhaled chemicals
- New onset of smoking cigarettes
- Travel or immigration status from areas endemic with various parasites or coccidiomycosis
- Asthma (may be severe or poorly controlled with ABPA, CSS, or is relatively new in onset with IAEP)
- ABPA concurrent in 7-10% of patients with cystic fibrosis
- Extrapulmonary symptoms suggestive of vasculitis, neuropathy, heart failure, or neoplasm)
- Rash (creeping eruption in visceral larval migrans disease or ulceration in EGPA)

Diagnostic imaging and testing
- Radiography helpful in AEP, CEP, and ABPA
- Radiography not diagnostic in EGPA or drug-induced eosinophilic disease of the lung
- Simple chest radiography findings
  - Nonlobar infiltrate
  - Classic description as mirror image of pulmonary edema with peripheral infiltrates
  - Bilateral pleural effusion in AEP
  - Central bronchiectasis in ABPA
- High-resolution computerized tomography of the chest
  - Middle and upper lobe nonlobar infiltrates with areas of ground-glass appearance
  - Mucous plugging in ABPA
  - Central bronchiectasis in ABPA (confused with cystic fibrosis)
- Blood eosinophil count
  - Elevated in many eosinophilic lung diseases
  - Magnitude of eosinophil blood count does not distinguish different pulmonary diseases
  - Usually not elevated in AEP (eosinophilic disease compartmentalized to lungs)
  - May occasionally not be elevated in CEP or after use of corticosteroids
- Total serum IgE elevated in ABPA but not always in patients with cystic fibrosis with ABPA
- Serology for helminthic infections or parasites may be diagnostic but are usually not available acutely
- P-ANCA (MPO ANCA) is positive in 40-70% of EGPA (CSS)
- BAL eosinophil percentage
  - ≥25% eosinophils diagnostic in AEP
  - ≥40% eosinophils diagnostic in CEP or tropical pulmonary eosinophilia
  - Eosinophil percentages below these criteria may require lung biopsy
  - <25% eosinophils seen in connective tissue disease, sarcoid, drug-induced disease, histiocytosis X of pulmonary Langerhans cells, and interstitial pulmonary fibrosis
- Lung biopsy
  - Open lung biopsy or video-assisted thorascopic surgery when BAL nondiagnostic
  - Transbronchial biopsy is usually insufficient with peripheral infiltrative disease
  - Histology with alveolar and interstitial infiltrates of eosinophils, non-necrotizing non-granulomatous vasculitis, multinucleated giant cells without granuloma
  - EGPA shows eosinophil rich small to medium vessel, necrotizing, granulomatous vasculitis

ABPA, allergic bronchopulmonary aspergillosis; AEP, acute eosinophilic pneumonia; BAL, bronchoalveolar lavage; CEP, chronic eosinophilic pneumonia; CSS, Churg-Strauss syndrome; EGPA, eosinophilic granulomatosis with polyangiitis; IAEP, idiopathic acute eosinophilic pneumonia; MPO ANCA, myeloperoxidase antineutrophil cytoplasmic antibody; NSAID, nonsteroidal antiinflammatory drug; P-ANCA, perinuclear antineutrophil cytoplasmic antibody.

ventilation, they are less common. A history of asthma is common in the chronic eosinophilic pneumonias and in allergic bronchopulmonary aspergillosis (ABPA) and often precedes the diagnosis of these 2 conditions.

Other symptoms of fever, myalgia, fatigue, weight loss, poor appetite, and night sweats may accompany the acute or chronic eosinophilic pneumonias. When abnormalities of the liver are detected, or if arthralgia, skin changes, pericardial effusion, or peripheral neuropathy accompany the disease presentation, a diagnosis of eosinophilic GPA (formerly known as the Churg-Strauss syndrome) or the hypereosinophilic syndrome should be aggressively investigated.

Chest Imaging

The chest radiograph is one of the most helpful tests in evaluating the child with dyspnea. The characteristic feature of fluffy alveolar infiltrates in the peripheral lung field is classic (Fig. 399-5). The images may be easily recognizable by astute clinicians who have identified the etiology of the disease without eosinophil counts or BAL.

HRCT is the best advanced imaging modality for eosinophilic lung disease. Spontaneous migration of lung opacities is commonly seen in the chronic pneumonias. Most often HRCT shows simultaneous evidence of bilateral alveolar infiltrates with both confluent consolidations and ground glass appearance. The most prominent areas of abnormality are visualized in the upper lobes and subpleural regions. Specific diseases have unique findings, such as proximal bronchiectasis in ABPA and pleural effusion in acute eosinophilic pneumonia. HRCT is most sensitive in identifying the correct etiology of disease when chest radiographic findings are nonspecific.

LÖFFLER SYNDROME

The transient pulmonary infiltrates with eosinophilia syndrome that is most often seen in children (formerly known as Löffler syndrome) is characterized by migrating pulmonary infiltrates with peripheral blood eosinophilia caused by the helminthic infections. A. lumbricoides or roundworm is the most common parasite causing this disease in the United States. When a fertilized egg is ingested from contaminated food, it becomes a larval worm that can penetrate the duodenum of the small intestine and migrate in the circulation to the liver, heart, and lungs. In the pulmonary venous circulation, the larvae can break through the interstitial space to the alveoli. The juvenile larva may subsequently migrate to the trachea where they are coughed up and swallowed. The cycle may then recur with subsequent absorption of eggs that are produced in the intestinal track. Other nematodes cannot mature in the intestinal tract so their disease is limited to a single passage into the lungs.

Visceral larva migrans from multiple nematodes may cause this disease. The most common cause of these includes the dog roundworm, Toxocara canis, while Toxocara cati, Strongyloides stercoralis, Baylisascaris procyonis, and Lagochilascaris minor can all produce visceral larva migrans. Outside the United States, the common lung fluke, Paragonimus westermani, may cause a similar pulmonary disease in older children and adolescents. Western Africa, Central and South America, and the Far East are regions that paragonimiasis may be found, especially in those who eat raw crabs or crawfish. Many other parasites may have a transient pulmonary syndrome, but their diseases are most commonly manifested in other organs.

The pulmonary syndrome is classic with cough, dyspnea, migratory peripheral pulmonary infiltrates, and blood eosinophilia that is self-limited. Young children most often have a history of pica and eating dirt that is contaminated with the eggs. Because the larva can migrate to other organs as well as multiply in the intestinal and biliary tract, symptoms of abdominal pain, vomiting, rarely obstruction, cholecystitis, and pancreatitis may be found. Diagnosis is frequently made by examination of the stool where the eggs may be detected microscopically. Treatment is aimed at the intestinal disease and not the pulmonary disease per se. It is possible that antihelminthic treatment of other organ disease during the pulmonary phase of the disease will increase the inflammatory response in the lung and may require corticosteroid therapy.

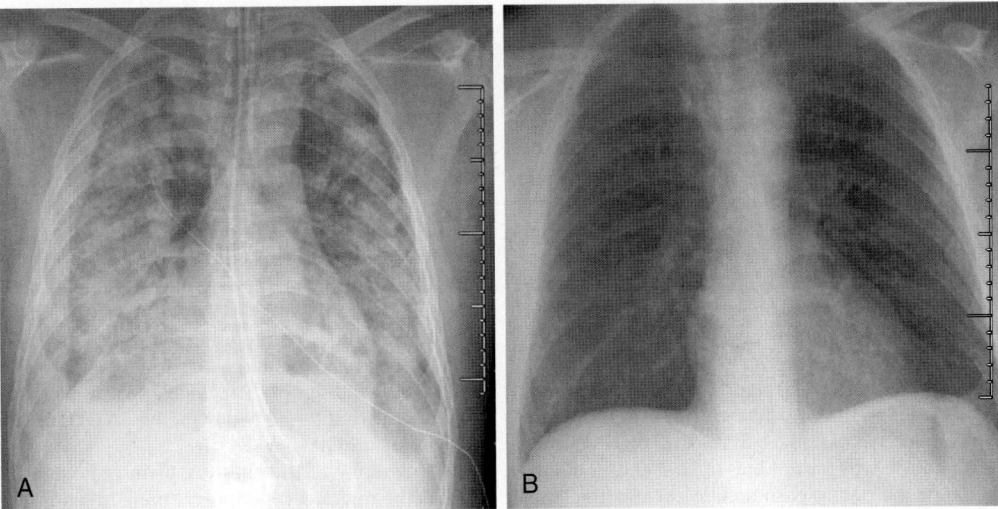

Figure 399-5 Acute eosinophilic pneumonia demonstrating the mirror image **(A)** pulmonary edema with a right pleural effusion on admission and **(B)** complete clearing upon discharge from the hospital after corticosteroid usage.

ACUTE EOSINOPHILIC PNEUMONIA

A unique and dramatic presentation of the eosinophilic pneumonias is AEP. AEP mimics infectious pneumonia or acute respiratory distress syndrome with its rapid onset and marked hypoxemia. In pediatrics, this disease most frequently occurs in the teenage population. Overall, young adults most commonly contract this idiopathic disease. Essentially all patients present within 7 days of symptom onset with dyspnea, fever, and cough, and more than 50% have chest pain. Myalgia and abdominal pain also frequently accompany this disease. Rarely, patients have presented up to 4-5 wks after onset of symptoms. Physical exam demonstrates tachypnea, tachycardia, and crackles in the lung fields on physical exam. Many patients rapidly deteriorate and require mechanical ventilation.

There is an absence of circulating eosinophilia, which contrasts the dramatic number of eosinophils seen in the BAL representing at least 25% of the inflammatory cells (often 40-55%) (Fig. 399-6). This feature helps distinguish it from the chronic pulmonary disease of eosinophilic origin.

Although this disease has been labeled as idiopathic, there have been identifiable exposures (e.g., 1,1,1-trichloroethane or Scotchgard). Numerous reports link onset of smoking tobacco, change in smoking frequency, reinitiation of smoking in young male adolescents or adults, and even massive secondary smoke exposure as critical associations with onset of AEP. World Trade Center dust is associated with development of AEP. A single smoke challenge study is associated with recurrence. Some medications are also linked to the onset of AEP. The most complete and current resource for medications linked to pulmonary disease is "The Drug-Induced Respiratory Disease Website" (http://www.pneumotox.com). When AEP is identified in a patient, the pediatrician's role in educating the patient and family about the link to smoking exposure and risk of AEP upon reexposure is warranted.

In addition to smoke exposure, AEP has been reported after smoking cocaine within hours to days after exposure. Whether this is a unique eosinophilic response to cocaine that represents one manifestation of "crack lung" or is a separate disease is unknown. "Crack lung" refers to diffuse alveolitis with pulmonary hemorrhage from an unknown mechanism that occurs within 48 hr of cocaine smoke inhalation.

Lung function has not been measured frequently in the disease because the patients have proceeded rapidly to the ICU and need for mechanical ventilation. When measured, a restrictive pattern of lung disease and reduced diffusion capacity is the usual finding arterial blood gases will show a significant increase in the alveolar–arterial gradient (see Chapter 373).

The criteria for diagnosis include the acute onset of disease, bilateral pulmonary infiltrates, reduced oxygen saturation or PaO_2 ≤60 mm Hg,

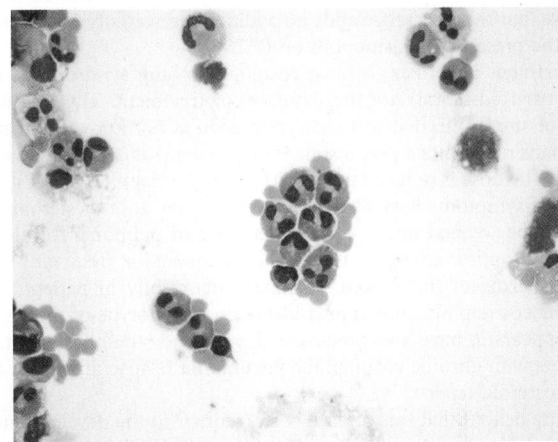

Figure 399-6 Light microscopy of eosinophils in bronchoalveolar lavage fluid.

BAL of ≥25%, and absence of a determined cause of eosinophilia. The recent onset of tobacco exposure, dust, or chemical inhalation is supporting factors in confirming a diagnosis.

Treatment has uniformly been the use of a corticosteroid (e.g., methylprednisolone 1-2 mg/kg/day) either intravenously or orally for 2-4 wks. A minimum or maximum treatment time has not been determined, but relapses or persistent symptoms are uncommon. Rare fatalities have been reported. Complete recovery has been seen in days with resolution of pleural effusions within the 4 wk treatment time. Most important, relapse has been rare, which sharply contrasts the idiopathic chronic eosinophilic pneumonias. Follow-up testing of pulmonary functions are usually normal which supports the contention that lung parenchyma heals without evidence of compromise or fibrosis.

CHRONIC EOSINOPHILIC PNEUMONIA

Chronic eosinophilic pneumonia is another idiopathic pulmonary condition without a known exposure to toxin, dust, or chemical inhalation. Eosinophils infiltrate the lung parenchyma resulting in dyspnea, cough, fever, and weight loss. It is primarily a problem for adults, with a female predominance (2:1 female:male ratio) usually in patients who are nonsmokers. Chest examination reveals tachypnea, crackles, and occasional wheezing as preceding asthma is a common finding. The classic finding on chest x-ray of the "radiographic negative of pulmonary edema" is found in these patients: central clear lung fields but fluffy, patchy peripheral infiltrates of the lung parenchyma.

When compared to AEP, the onset of disease is indolent and subtle but the accompanying fever and weight loss may lead the clinician to a concern for an underlying malignancy prior to chest radiograph and laboratory investigation. Peripheral blood eosinophilia is commonly as high as 5000/mm^3 or greater, accompanied by BAL eosinophilia >40% on the differential count. The peripheral eosinophilia sharply contrasts the lack of eosinophils seen in the blood in AEP. HRCT scan contrasts the AEP with pleural effusion as a rare finding, as well as rare cavitation.

In contrast to AEP, pulmonary function testing shows a mixed obstructive and restrictive pattern as a result of asthma occurring concurrently with pneumonia.

Inflammatory markers associated with migration and activation of eosinophils are predictably found in BAL and the urine. These include the T-lymphocyte type 2 cytokines of IL-4, IL-5, IL-6, IL-10, IL-13, and IL-18. However, T-lymphocyte type 1 cytokines of IL-2 and IL-12 are also present with many of the potent eosinophilic chemoattractants such as CCL5 (RANTES [regulated upon activation, normal T cell expressed and secreted]) and CCL11 (eotaxin-1). Toxic granule proteins of major basic protein, eosinophil-derived neurotoxin, and eosinophil cationic protein are frequently present. Unfortunately, these important molecules help confirm the eosinophilic nature of the disease, but their presence adds no additional sensitivity or specificity over the presence of eosinophils on BAL.

Treatment is similar to most eosinophilic lung syndromes where corticosteroids (oral) are the mainstay of treatment. The minimum dose of steroid needed to induce remission is not known, but most clinicians recommend prednisone (or equivalent) at 0.5 mg/kg/day for 2 wks. The dose is reduced to half (0.025 mg/kg/day) for an additional 2 wks if symptoms have abated. The remaining dose of steroid may need to be weaned over 6 mo. Symptoms and pulmonary infiltrates rapidly disappear after initiation of this treatment but frequently recur with tapering of the steroid. Asthma concurrently in patients with chronic eosinophilic pneumonia identifies a phenotype of the disease that appears to have lower relapse risk yet up to 50% of all identified patients with chronic eosinophilic pneumonia relapse during or after corticosteroid taper.

Many believe that this disease is a precursor to the development of **eosinophilic granulomatosis with polyangiitis (EGPA)** or the Churg-Strauss syndrome. The utility of inhaled corticosteroids in chronic eosinophilic pneumonia is unknown but is warranted for the persistent asthma phenotype of disease. A subset of patients develop permanent lower airway obstruction without reversibility, which requires patients with this disease to have close follow-up and monitoring of pulmonary function tests routinely.

EOSINOPHILIC GRANULOMATOSIS WITH POLYANGIITIS (THE CHURG-STRAUSS SYNDROME)

The EGPA syndrome is a systemic disease involving multiple organs but most prominently the lung. Patients present with difficult to control asthma, allergic rhinitis, and peripheral eosinophilia (>10% or >1,500 cells/µL) in the blood. Evidence of vasculitis on clinical grounds must be present in at least 2 organs. The polyangiitis appears later in the disease process with asthma being the precursor symptom in more than 90% of the cases reported. EGPA affects multiple organs including the skin, heart, gastrointestinal tract, kidneys, and central nervous system. Rhinitis is present in 75% of the patients but is not specific. Symptom complexes of fever, weight loss, fatigue, arthralgia, and myalgia may be seen in approximately two-thirds of patients. Cardiac and renal involvement is insidious in onset and should be screened for. It is the multiple organ involvement that results in the morbidity and mortality of this disease. The typical progression of the disease is in 3 phases: rhinitis and asthma first, tissue eosinophilia second, and, finally, systemic vasculitis.

The pathogenesis of EGPA is still unknown but several factors are suspected to contribute to the development of the disease. The possible link between leukotriene-receptor antagonists (zafirlukast, montelukast, or pranlukast) is controversial but still considered possible. It is suspected that use of this class of adjunctive medications in severe asthma allows for the reduction in use of corticosteroid leading to the full blown (unmasking) manifestation of EGPA. Isolated use of leukotriene-receptor antagonists may induce disease, lead to remission with cessation of leukotriene-receptor antagonists, and cause recurrence of EGPA upon reintroduction of this class of medications. Many refrain from use of leukotriene-receptor antagonists when the EGPA syndrome has been diagnosed.

Clinical and laboratory finding are able to pinpoint the diagnosis with high specificity (99.7%) and sensitivity (85%) when 4 of 6 criteria are met (asthma, eosinophilia >10%, mononeuropathy or polyneuropathy, nonfixed pulmonary infiltrates, paranasal sinus abnormalities, and biopsy findings of extravascular eosinophil infiltrates). In contrast to GPA, the rhinitis is not destructive and nasal septal perforation does not occur in EGPA.

Radiography of the chest by plain radiography or HRCT demonstrates the migratory, peripheral predominant opacities with ground-glass appearance to full consolidation. Bronchiectasis and bronchial wall thickening are reported. Pleural effusion should raise suspicion for the presence of heart failure from cardiomyopathy.

Laboratory findings include striking eosinophilia with values generally between 5,000 and 20,000/mm^3 at the time of diagnosis. These counts often parallel the vasculitis activity that is found. The BAL shows striking eosinophilia with differential counts of >60%. Other organ system levels reflect activity of eosinophils and are not specific for the EGPA diagnosis.

ANCAs are present in the EGPA syndrome. The **perinuclear-ANCA targeting myeloperoxidase** are specifically found in EGPA in approximately 40% of the patients; the absence of myeloperoxidase-ANCA does not exclude the diagnosis. Those patients with eosinophilic pneumonia, fever, and cardiac involvement are less likely to have myeloperoxidase-ANCA detected. Those with peripheral neuropathy, renal glomerular disease, and skin purpura usually have detectable myeloperoxidase-ANCAs.

Pulmonary function tests while on bronchodilators and inhaled corticosteroids for asthma show an obstructive pattern. The pulmonary obstruction is responsive to oral corticosteroid use but often has mild persistence of obstruction.

Treatment of EGPA with systemic oral corticosteroid remains the mainstay of therapy at a starting dose of 1 mg/kg/day for 4 wks. This therapy is often required for up to 12 mo or longer with a steady taper in dosage over that time. EGPA resistant to corticosteroid has responded to cyclophosphamide, IFN-α, cyclosporine, intravenous immunoglobulin, and plasmapheresis. The use of anti–IL-5 (mepolizumab) has been encouraging and may be used as a steroid-sparing agent in the future.

ALLERGIC BRONCHOPULMONARY ASPERGILLOSIS

ABPA is a complex mixed immunologic hypersensitivity reaction in the lungs and bronchi in response to exposure and colonization of *Aspergillus* species (usually *Aspergillus fumigatus*; see Chapter 237.1). This disease almost exclusively occurs in patients with preexisting asthma and up to 15% of patients with cystic fibrosis (see Chapter 402). The quantity of *Aspergillus* exposure does not correlate to the severity of disease.

The clinical pattern of disease (Table 399-9) is remarkably similar with a clinical presentation of difficult-to-treat asthma, periods of acute obstructive lung disease with bronchial mucous plugs, elevated total IgE antibody, elevated specific IgE and IgG anti-*Aspergillus* antibodies, skin prick test reactions to *Aspergillus* species, precipitating antibody to *Aspergillus* species, as well as proximal bronchiectasis. Other clinical manifestations include dyspnea, cough, shortness of breath, production of brown mucous plugs frequently characterized as "rubber" plugs, and peripheral eosinophilia, as well as pulmonary eosinophilia with infiltration of the parenchyma. The use of systemic corticosteroid may lower the total IgE antibody levels such that

Table 399-9	The Classification of the Eosinophilic Lung Diseases
IDIOPATHIC	**KNOWN ETIOLOGY**
Acute eosinophilic pneumonia	Drug-induced eosinophilic pneumonia
Chronic eosinophilic pneumonia	Infectious causes
Eosinophilic granulomatosis with polyangiitis	• Ascariasis (Löffler syndrome)*
Hypereosinophilic syndromes	• *Toxocara* (*canis* or *cati*)
• Myeloproliferative variant	• Filarial (tropical filarial eosinophilic pneumonia)
• Lymphocytic variant	• *Strongyloides stercoralis* Allergic bronchopulmonary aspergillosis Toxic
	• L-Tryptophan (eosinophilia myalgia syndrome)
	• Toxic oil syndrome Illicit drug use (cocaine, heroin, cannabis)

*Note: Löffler eosinophilic pneumonia has transient symptoms and is often classified as neither an acute or chronic eosinophilic pneumonia.

Table 399-10	Criteria for the Diagnosis of Allergic Bronchopulmonary Aspergillosis

Allergic bronchopulmonary aspergillosis–central bronchiectasis
• Medical history of asthma*
• Immediate skin prick test reaction to *Aspergillus* antigens*
• Precipitating (IgG) serum antibodies to *Aspergillus fumigatus**
• Total IgE concentration >417 IU/mL (>1000 ng/mL)*
• Central bronchiectasis on chest CT*
• Peripheral blood eosinophilia >500/mm³
• Lung infiltrates on chest x-ray or chest HRCT
• Elevated specific serum IgE and IgG to *A. fumigatus*

Allergic bronchopulmonary aspergillosis seropositive†
• Medical history of asthma†
• Immediate skin prick test reaction to *A. fumigatus* antigens†
• Precipitating (IgG) serum antibodies to *A. fumigatus*†
• Total IgE concentration >417 IU/mL (>1000 ng/mL)†

Staging of allergic bronchopulmonary aspergillosis

Stage 1	Acute	Upper and middle lob infiltration	High IgE
Stage 2	Remission	No infiltrate off steroids >6 mo	Normal to high IgE
Stage 3	Exacerbation	Upper and middle lobe in filtrations	High IgE
Stage 4	CSD asthma	Minimal infiltrate	Normal to high IgE
Stage 5	End stage	Fibrosis and/or bullae	Normal

*The criteria required for diagnosis of ABPA with central bronchiectasis.
†The first 4 criteria are required for a diagnosis of seropositive ABPA.
CSD, corticosteroid dependent.

a diagnosis may be in question when the first tests are performed at that time.

ABPA should be considered in patients with cystic fibrosis when clinical deterioration occurs without evidence of an identifiable cause. Symptoms heralding such deterioration include increasing cough, wheezing, loss of exercise tolerance, worsening exercise-induced asthma, reduction of pulmonary function, or increased sputum production without another discernible reason. Clinical findings of elevated total IgE antibody, anti-*Aspergillus* IgE, precipitating antibodies to *A. fumigatus*, and/or new abnormalities on chest radiography that fail to clear with antibiotics should alert the clinician to the possibility of ABPA.

When evaluating a child with asthma symptoms, the clinician must distinguish asthma from ABPA. If the diagnosis is suspected, skin prick test for evidence of IgE-specific antibody directed against *A. fumigatus* is essential. Intradermal skin testing when the skin prick test is negative, although not routinely performed because of poor specificity, may be performed. The absence of a positive skin prick test and intradermal test to *A. fumigatus* virtually excludes the diagnosis of ABPA. The prevalence of ABPA in patients with an existing diagnosis of asthma and an abnormal immediate skin prick test response to *A. fumigatus* has been evaluated. Between 2% and 32% of patients with asthma with concurrent skin prick test–positive reactions to *Aspergillus* have evidence of ABPA.

It is uncommon for the patient with cystic fibrosis to develop ABPA before the age of 6 yr. When the total IgE antibody in patients with cystic fibrosis exceed 500 IU/mL (1,200 ng/mL), a strong clinical suspicion of ABPA is necessary.

ABPA pathology has characteristic findings of mucoid bronchi impaction, eosinophilic pneumonia, and bronchocentric granulomas in addition to the typical histologic features of asthma. Septated hyphae are often found in the mucus-filled bronchial tree. However, the fungi do not invade the mucosa in this unique disease. *Aspergillus* may be cultured from sputum in more than 60% of ABPA patients. Interestingly, hyphae may not always be seen on microscopy.

Staging of the disease (Table 399-10) represents distinct phases of the disease but do not necessarily progress in sequence from stage 1 to stage 5. Staging of ABPA is important for treatment considerations. In many hypersensitivity diseases where IgE antibody contributes to the pathogenesis (e.g., asthma), total IgE is often used for screening for an atopic state, but is not a test that helps the clinician with serial measures. In sharp contrast, the measurement of IgE during acute exacerbations, remission, and recurrent ABPA disease is helpful in identifying the activity of disease and may herald the recurrence. During stage 1 disease, the level of IgE antibody is often very high. During stage 2 remission, a fall in the levels may be as much as 35% or more. Recurrence of activity may result in a marked rise of total IgE with a doubling of the baseline level seen during remission. During the use of glucocorticoid therapy, monthly or bimonthly levels of IgE are followed serially to assist the clinician in tapering therapy. Because exacerbations of ABPA are asymptomatic to the patient in approximately 25% of the recurrences, serial IgE accompanied by chest radiography are helpful to the clinician to guide therapy.

Radiography
Plain chest X-ray shows evidence of infiltrates especially in the upper lobes and the classic findings of bronchiectasis (Fig. 399-7). The use of HRCT demonstrates central bronchiectasis in the central regions of the lung (Fig. 399-8). HRCT may add value in the patient with a positive skin prick test and normal chest radiograph in detecting characteristic abnormalities of ABPA.

Treatment
The mainstay of therapy for ABPA has been systemic glucocorticoids with adjunct therapy with antifungal medications and anti-IgE therapy with omalizumab. Exacerbations in stages 1 and 3 are treated for 14 days with 0.5-1 mg/kg of glucocorticoid followed by every-other-day usage and tapering over 3 mo or as long as 6 mo. Stage 2 remission phase and stage 5 where fibrosis has occurred do not require glucocorticoid therapy. Stage 4 denotes a state where glucocorticoid weaning has not been successful and continued long-term therapy is required.

Antifungal therapy with a 16 wk course of itraconazole improves the response rate during exacerbations that allowed reduction of glucocorticoid dosage by 50% accompanied by a reduction of total serum IgE of 25% or more. The proposed mechanisms of action have been to either reduce the antigen load driving the immune response or possibly raising the serum levels of corticosteroid by slowing the metabolism

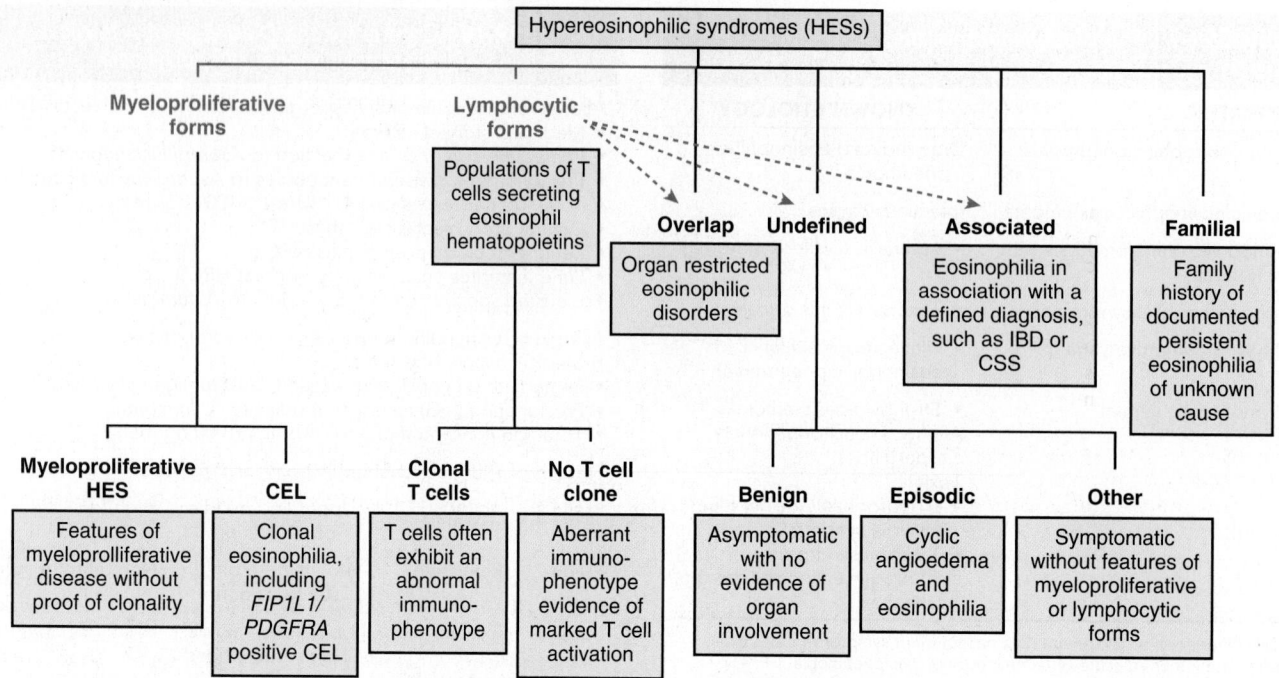

Figure 399-7 A revised classification of hypereosinophilic syndrome (HES). Changes from the previous classification are indicated in red. *Dashed arrows* identify HES forms for which at least some patients have T-cell–driven disease. Classification of myeloproliferative forms has been simplified, and patients with HES and eosinophil hematopoietin-producing T cells in the absence of a T-cell clone are included in the lymphocytic forms of HES. CSS, Churg-Strauss syndrome; IBD, inflammatory bowel disease. *(From Simon H, Rothenberg ME, Bochner BS, et al. Refining the definition of hypereosinophilic syndrome. J Allergy Clin Immunol 126:45–49, 2010, Fig. 1.)*

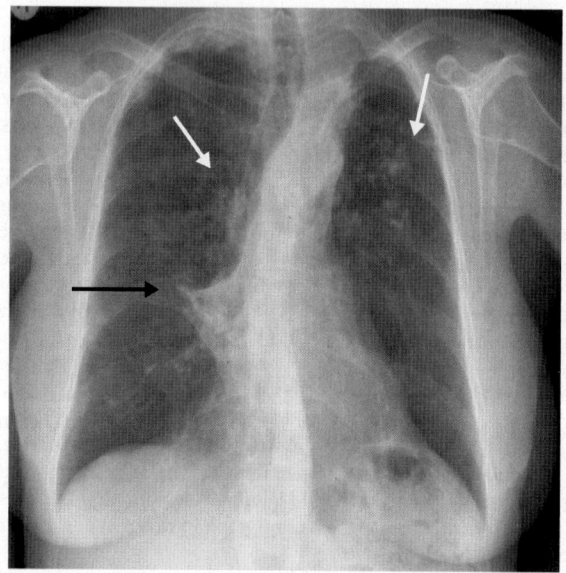

Figure 399-8 Transitory opacities *(white arrows)* and lobar collapse *(black arrow)* in patient with allergic bronchopulmonary aspergillosis. *(From Douglass JA, Sandrini A, Holgate ST, O'Hehir RE: Allergic bronchopulmonary aspergillosis and hypersensitivity pneumonitis. In Adkinson AF, editor: Middleton's allergy principles and practice, Philadelphia, 2014, Elsevier, Fig. 61-2.)*

of the steroid. This latter mechanism would be true for prednisone, which is methylated in the liver, but not for methylprednisolone, which does not require methylation.

The adult dosage recommendation for itraconazole is 200 mg 3 times per day for 3 days followed by 200 mg twice daily for the remainder of the 16 wks. Children should receive 5 mg/kg/day in a single dose. If the proper calculated dose exceeds 200 mg, then the total dose

should be divided equally and given twice daily. Serum levels of itraconazole are necessary to ensure proper absorption of the drug is occurring from the capsule form. The liquid form is more readily absorbed and has achieved levels substantially higher. The use of proton pump inhibitors and histamine 2 antagonists may reduce absorption from blockade of acid production. Voriconazole has been used as a substitute antifungal medication. Proper dosing has been established for invasive *Aspergillus* disease, but not for ABPA. Typical dosage regimen in children of 7 mg/kg/day may cause hepatotoxicity and liver function must be monitored.

Omalizumab, an anti-IgE humanized monoclonal antibody, has been used in case series of patients with cystic fibrosis and ABPA as well as a small cohort of adults without cystic fibrosis but with ABPA. Both case series demonstrated significant reductions in asthma exacerbations, ABPA exacerbations, and glucocorticoid usage. The dose prescribed has been 300-375 mg every 2 wk by subcutaneous injection.

HYPEREOSINOPHILIC SYNDROME
See Chapter 129.

The hypereosinophilic syndrome (HES) is a descriptive name of a group of disorders that are characterized by the persistent overproduction of eosinophils accompanied by eosinophil infiltration in multiple organs with end-organ damage from mediator release. The term HES should only be used when there is eosinophilia with end-organ damage from the eosinophils and not from another cause. The discovery of underlying genetic, biochemical, or neoplastic reasons for HES has led to the classification of primary, secondary, and idiopathic HES (Table 399-11). Specific syndromes such as EGPA (Churg-Strauss) have eosinophilia but the contribution of eosinophils to the organ damage is incompletely understood.

Some variants of HES have genetic mutations in tyrosine kinase receptor platelet-derived growth factor receptor-α (*PDGFRA*); males are almost exclusively affected. Otherwise, HES appears to be distributed equally among females and males.

Hypereosinophilia is defined as an absolute eosinophil number in the blood that exceeds 1.5×10^9 eosinophils on 2 separate occasions separated by at least 1 mo. Tissues are abnormal when more than 20% of nucleated cells in the bone marrow are of eosinophil origin; a pathologist determines the presence of eosinophilia; or the presence of extensive eosinophilic granule proteins are determined on biopsy to be deposited in large quantities. These disorders can be subclassified into primary (neoplastic), secondary (reactive), and idiopathic (Fig. 399-9).

Clinical manifestations of the HES include organ involvement of the heart (5%), gastrointestinal (14%), skin (37%), and pulmonary (25%-63%). The HES is complicated by thrombosis and/or neurologic disease in many patients, although the exact prevalence of this problem is incompletely categorized. Peripheral neuropathy, encephalopathy, transverse sinus thrombosis, or cerebral emboli are the most common neurologic complications. The exact mechanism of the manifestations is unclear especially in major artery thrombosis such as the femoral artery.

The most frequent pulmonary symptoms include cough and dyspnea. Many patients have obstructive lung disease with clinical wheezing. Evidence of pulmonary fibrosis and pulmonary emboli are seen with regularity. Because biopsy shows eosinophilic infiltrates similar to other pulmonary eosinophilic diseases of the lung, it is the constellation of other organ involvement or thromboembolic phenomena and other organs that must lead the clinician to a high index of suspicion for the HES.

Table 399-11	Hypereosinophilic Syndrome Variants
Myeloproliferative	Nonclonal Clonal–F1P1L1/PDGFRA-positive chronic eosinophilic leukemia
Lymphocytic	Nonclonal T cells Clonal T-cell expansion with T-cell activation
Overlap	Organ restricted
Familial	Family history of eosinophilia without known cause
Associated	Eosinophilia in chronic disease like inflammatory bowel disease or EGPA (Churg-Strauss syndrome)
Undefined	Asymptomatic Cyclic angioedema with eosinophilia (Gleich syndrome) Symptomatic without myeloproliferation or lymphocytic form

EGPA, eosinophilic granulomatosis with polyangiitis; PDGFRA, platelet-derived growth factor receptor-α.

Laboratory evaluation should include evaluation of liver enzymes, kidney function tests, creatine kinase, and troponin. The extent of cardiac involvement should be evaluated by electrocardiogram and echocardiogram. Some unique biomarkers may be tested when evaluating the myeloproliferative and T-lymphocyte HES diagnoses. Vitamin B_{12} and serum tryptase may be elevated, especially the latter, when the myeloproliferative disease is accompanied by mastocytosis. These 2 biomarkers are most frequently elevated when the mutation is present or fusion in the FIP1L1/PDGFRA sites.

Because of the extensive pulmonary disease that is seen in the HES, pulmonary function tests should be performed at diagnosis when possible to include spirometry and lung volumes. Dead space ventilation may be significantly elevated in the patients with pulmonary emboli. Pulse oximeter may be very helpful in the evaluation as well.

Chest radiography and CT are very helpful in the evaluation. Spiral chest CT should also be performed when pulmonary emboli are being considered. In one series of patients, nearly half of the patients with HES had evidence of pulmonary abnormalities including ground-glass appearing infiltrates, pulmonary emboli, mediastinal lymphadenopathy, and/or pleural effusion.

Treatment of HES depends on the type of variant (myeloproliferative, lymphocytic forms, undefined, associated with systemic diseases such as EGPA or familial). Rarely, some patients present with marked eosinophilia where the total count exceeds 100,000 cells/µL and vascular insufficiency symptoms. Prednisone at 15 mg/kg is indicated to acutely reduce the eosinophil count, after diagnostic tests are performed, when safe. If the patient is unstable, the glucocorticoid should be administered to prevent progression of symptoms. Other acute therapies aimed at reduction of eosinophil counts include vincristine, imatinib mesylate, or even leukophoresis.

When eosinophil counts are not as dramatically elevated, therapy begins with glucocorticoids at 1 mg/kg for patients who do not have the FIP1L1/PDGFRA mutation. Patients with this mutation are resistant to glucocorticoids and initial treatment should begin with imatinib, a tyrosine kinase inhibitor. Because this genetic test is often not readily available, surrogate markers for the presence of this mutation are vitamin B_{12} levels >2000 pg/mL or serum tryptase >11.5 ng/mL. It denotes the presence of resistant disease that should initially be treated with imatinib. The goal of therapy is to reduce and maintain eosinophil counts below 1.5×10^9 at the lowest dose of prednisone possible to reduce or avoid corticosteroid side effects. If corticosteroid doses can't be lowered below 10 mg/day, then imatinib can be added as combination therapy in order to spare the dose of steroid. Caution must be used in the presence of cardiac disease as introduction of imatinib has precipitated left ventricular failure.

Additional or alternative adjunct therapies that have shown promise include hydroxyurea, interferon α, anti–IL-5 monoclonal antibody therapy; and a monoclonal antibody directed against CD52. Failure of

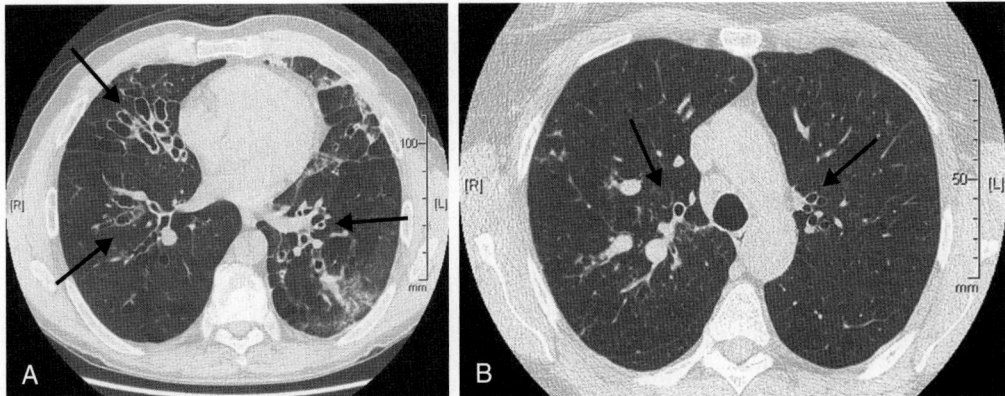

Figure 399-9 **A,** Central bronchiectasis in patient with ABPA (*arrows*). **B,** Central bronchiectasis in the upper lobes (*arrows*). (*From Douglass JA, Sandrini A, Holgate ST, O'Hehir RE: Allergic bronchopulmonary aspergillosis and hypersensitivity pneumonitis.* In Adkinson AF, editor: Middleton's allergy principles and practice, *Philadelphia, 2014, Elsevier, Fig. 61-3.*)

the above modalities may signal a need for hematopoietic stem cell transplantation. This therapy has been successful in some patients.

Bibliography is available at Expert Consult.

399.5 Interstitial Lung Disease
Kevin J. Kelly

ILD in children is caused by a large group of uncommon, heterogeneous, familial, or sporadic diseases that involve the pulmonary parenchyma and cause significant impairment of gas exchange. The ILDs in pediatrics are uncommonly caused by infectious processes and specific immunologic processes when compared to adults. The one exception to this is Goodpasture disease with classic antibasement membrane antibodies. Despite wide variations in cause, these disorders are classified together because of the similar clinical, physiologic, radiographic, and pathologic processes involving disruption of alveolar interstitium and airways. A survey of all German pediatric hospitals found a rate of occurrence of pediatric ILD of 1.3 children/million population. The pathophysiology is believed to be more complex than that of adult disease because pulmonary injury occurs during the process of lung growth and differentiation. In ILD, the initial injury causes damage to the alveolar epithelium and capillary endothelium. Abnormal healing of injured tissue may be more prominent than inflammation in the initial steps of the development of chronic ILD. Some familial cases, especially in the surfactant dysfunction disorders, involve a specific genetic mutation.

CLASSIFICATION AND PATHOLOGY
Classification of ILD in children is not standardized. It is helpful for the clinician to separate diseases into ILD on the basis of age, disorders of known and unknown etiology, and diseases related to systemic disorders (Table 399-12). A diffuse developmental disorder of the lung is likely the result of a primary aberration in lung and/or pulmonary vascular development. Growth abnormalities reflecting deficient development of alveoli are largely secondary to impaired prenatal or postnatal alveolarization from restriction of fetal thoracic space, limitation of pulmonary blood supply, or chronic lung disease of prematurity (e.g., bronchopulmonary dysplasia) (see Chapter 101). Abnormal alveolar growth may also be associated with a variety of chromosomal abnormalities such as trisomy 21. In **neuroendocrine cell hyperplasia of infancy**/persistent tachypnea of infancy, a distinct entity limited to infants and young children, the pathologic findings include hyperplasia of neuroendocrine cells within the bronchioles while the pulmonary histologic background is nearly normal. **Pulmonary interstitial glycogenosis** is characterized by diffuse accumulation of mesenchymal cells in the alveolar interstitium with accumulation of monoparticulate glycogen in the interstitial cell cytoplasm that is confirmed by ultrastructural examination.

Disorders associated with **surfactant metabolism dysfunction** explain many of formerly idiopathic pediatric ILDs. The more-severe surfactant dysfunctions, such as surfactant protein-B mutations, usually manifest as respiratory failure in neonate. **Congenital pulmonary alveolar proteinosis** is more typical of *ABCA3* mutations, and **chronic pneumonitis of infancy** is predominant histologic pattern seen in surfactant protein-C mutations. Age-related but overlapping surfactant disorders in addition to pulmonary alveolar proteinosis and chronic pneumonitis of infancy also include **desquamative interstitial pneumonia** in infants; older children and adolescents more often manifest **nonspecific interstitial pneumonia** or **usual interstitial pneumonia**. *ABCA3* mutations may produce pulmonary alveolar proteinosis, desquamative interstitial pneumonia, or nonspecific interstitial pneumonia; surfactant protein-C deficiency may also produce chronic pneumonitis of infancy in older children.

Diffuse ILD can occur without a known immunodeficiency or systemic disorder, but it can also be seen as a pulmonary manifestation of other systemic disease processes, such as collagen vascular disorders and sarcoidosis.

Table 399-12 | The Pediatric Interstitial Lung Diseases

AGE-RELATED ILDS IN INFANCY AND EARLY CHILDHOOD
Diffuse developmental disorders
• Acinar dysplasia
• Congenital alveolar dysplasia
• Alveolar capillary dysplasia with misalignment of pulmonary veins (some due to *FOXF1* mutation)
Growth abnormalities reflecting deficient alveolarization
• Pulmonary hypoplasia
• Chronic neonatal lung disease
• Chromosomal disorders
• Congenital heart disease
Neuroendocrine cell hyperplasia of infancy
Pulmonary interstitial glycogenosis (infantile cellular interstitial pneumonia)
Surfactant dysfunction disorders (pulmonary alveolar proteinosis)
• Surfactant protein–B mutation
• Surfactant protein–C mutation
• *ABCA3* mutation
• Granulocyte-macrophage colony-stimulating factor receptor (*CSF2RA*) mutation

ILD DISORDERS WITH KNOWN ASSOCIATIONS
Infectious/postinfectious processes
• Adenovirus viruses
• Influenza viruses
• *Chlamydia pneumoniae*
• *Mycoplasma pneumoniae*
Environmental agents
• Hypersensitivity pneumonitis
• Toxic inhalation
Aspiration syndromes

PULMONARY DISEASES ASSOCIATED WITH PRIMARY AND SECONDARY IMMUNE DEFICIENCY
Opportunistic infections
Granulomatous lymphocytic ILD associated with common variable immunodeficiency syndrome
Lymphoid intestinal pneumonia (HIV infection)
Therapeutic interventions: chemotherapy, radiation, transplantation, and rejection

Idiopathic ILDs
Usual interstitial pneumonitis
Desquamative interstitial pneumonitis
Lymphocytic interstitial pneumonitis and related disorders
Nonspecific interstitial pneumonitis (cellular/fibrotic)
Eosinophilic pneumonia
Bronchiolitis obliterans syndrome
Pulmonary hemosiderosis and acute idiopathic pulmonary hemorrhage of infancy
Pulmonary alveolar proteinosis
Pulmonary vascular disorders
Pulmonary lymphatic disorders
Pulmonary microlithiasis
Persistent tachypnea of infancy
Brain-thyroid-lung syndrome

SYSTEMIC DISORDERS WITH PULMONARY MANIFESTATIONS
Goodpasture disease
Gaucher disease and other storage diseases
Malignant infiltrates
Hemophagocytic lymphohistiocytosis
Langerhans cell histiocytosis
Sarcoidosis
Systemic sclerosis
Polymyositis/dermatomyositis
Systemic lupus erythematosus
Rheumatoid arthritis
Lymphangioleiomyomatosis
Pulmonary hemangiomatosis
Neurocutaneous syndromes
Hermansky-Pudlak syndrome

Modified from Deutsch GH, Young LR, Deterding RR, et al; ChILD Research Co-operative: Diffuse lung disease in young children: application of a novel classification scheme, Am J Respir Crit Care Med 176:1120–1128, 2007.

Persistent pulmonary symptoms can occur after **respiratory infections** caused by adenoviruses, influenza viruses, *Chlamydia pneumoniae*, and *Mycoplasma pneumoniae*. **Aspiration** is a frequent cause of chronic lung disease in childhood. Children with developmental delay or neuromuscular weakness are at an increased risk for aspiration of food, saliva, or foreign matter secondary to swallowing dysfunction and/or gastroesophageal reflux. An undiagnosed tracheoesophageal fistula can also result in pulmonary complications related to aspiration of gastric contents and interstitial pneumonia.

Children experiencing an exaggerated immunologic response to organic dust, molds, or bird antigens may demonstrate hypersensitivity pneumonitis. Children with malignancies may have ILD related to the primary malignancy or an opportunistic infection or secondary to chemotherapy or radiation treatment.

CLINICAL MANIFESTATIONS

A detailed history is needed to assess the severity of symptoms and the possibility of an underlying systemic disease in a patient with suspected ILD. Identification of precipitating factors, such as exposure to molds or birds and a severe lower respiratory infection, is important in establishing the diagnosis and instituting avoidance measures. A positive family history, especially in an affected infant, is suggestive of a genetic or familial disease, such as a surfactant dysfunction. Tachypnea, dyspnea, cough, and failure to thrive are commonly present. The majority of patients develop hypoxia and hypercarbia, usually a late and ominous complication. Symptoms are usually insidious and occur in a continuous, not episodic, pattern. Tachypnea, crackles on auscultation, and retractions are noted on physical examination in the majority of children with ILD, but chest physical examination findings can be normal. Wheezing and fever are uncommon findings in pediatric ILD. Cyanosis accompanied by a prominent P2 heart sound is indicative of severe disease with the development of secondary pulmonary hypertension. Anemia or hemoptysis suggests a pulmonary vascular disease or pulmonary hemosiderosis. Rashes or joint complaints are consistent with an underlying connective tissue disease.

DIAGNOSIS
Radiography

Chest radiographic abnormalities can be classified as interstitial, reticular, nodular, reticulonodular, or honeycombed. The chest radiographic appearance may also be normal despite significant clinical impairment and may correlate poorly with the extent of disease. HRCT of the chest better defines the extent and distribution of disease and can provide specific information for selection of a biopsy site. Volume-controlled full-inspiratory and end-expiratory protocols used during HRCT can provide more information, possibly showing air trapping, ground-glass patterns, mosaic patterns of attenuation, hyperinflation, bronchiectasis, cysts, and/or nodular opacities. Serial HRCT scans have been beneficial in monitoring disease progression and severity.

Pulmonary Function Tests

Pulmonary function tests are important in defining the degree of pulmonary dysfunction and in following the response to treatment. In ILD, pulmonary function abnormalities demonstrate a restrictive ventilatory deficit with decreased lung volumes and reduced lung compliance. The functional residual capacity is often reduced but is usually less affected than vital capacity and total lung capacity. The residual volume is usually maintained; therefore, ratios of functional residual capacity : total lung capacity and residual volume : total lung capacity are increased. Diffusion capacity of the lung is often reduced. Exercise testing may detect pulmonary dysfunction, even in the early stage of ILD with a decline in oxygen saturation.

Bronchoalveolar Lavage

BAL may provide helpful information regarding secondary infection, bleeding, and aspiration and allows cytology and molecular analyses. Evaluation of cell counts, differential, and lymphocyte markers may be helpful in determining the presence of hypersensitivity pneumonitis or sarcoid. Although BAL does not usually determine the exact diagnosis,

it can be diagnostic for disorders such as pulmonary alveolar proteinosis. Lung biopsy for histopathology by conventional thoracotomy or video-assisted thoracoscopy is usually the final step and is often necessary for a diagnosis. Biopsy may have a lower diagnostic yield in young children because of heterogeneous lung changes and often nonspecific histologic findings. Genetic testing for surfactant dysfunction mutational analysis is available. Evaluation for possible systemic disease may also be necessary.

TREATMENT

Supportive care of patients with ILD is essential and includes supplemental oxygen for hypoxia and adequate nutrition for growth failure. Antimicrobial treatment may be necessary for secondary infections. Some children may receive symptomatic relief from the use of bronchodilators. Antiinflammatory treatment with corticosteroids remains the initial treatment of choice. Controlled trials in children are lacking, however, and the clinical responses reported in case studies are variable. The usual dose of prednisone is 1-2 mg/kg/24 hr for 6-8 wks with tapering of dosage dictated by clinical response. Alternative, but not adequately evaluated, agents include hydroxychloroquine, azathioprine, cyclophosphamide, cyclosporine, methotrexate, intravenous immunoglobulin, granulocyte-macrophage colony-stimulating factor, and pulsed high-dose steroids. Investigational approaches involve specific agents directed against the action of cytokines, growth factors, or oxidants. Lung transplantation for progressive or end-stage ILD is successful in some infants and children. Appropriate treatment for underlying systemic disease is indicated. Preventive measures include avoidance of all inhalation irritants, such as tobacco smoke and, when appropriate, molds and bird antigens. Supervised pulmonary rehabilitation programs may be helpful.

Genetic Counseling

A high incidence of ILD in some families suggests a genetic predisposition to either development of the disease or severity of the disorder. Genetic counseling may be beneficial if a positive familial history is obtained.

PROGNOSIS

The overall mortality of ILD is very variable and depends on specific diagnosis. Some children recover spontaneously without treatment, but other children steadily progress to death. Pulmonary hypertension, failure to thrive, and severe fibrosis are considered poor prognostic indicators.

GOODPASTURE DISEASE

Goodpasture disease is the prototypical immunologic mediated interstitial lung disease (see Chapter 517). Because of the concurrent presentation of renal and pulmonary disease, the differential diagnosis focuses on distinguishing Goodpasture disease from GPA, microscopic polyangiitis, Henoch-Schönlein purpura, and idiopathic pulmonary hemorrhage syndromes.

Pathophysiology
Immunology Factors

The development of anti–glomerular basement membrane (anti-GBM) antibodies directly correlates with the development of pulmonary and renal disease. Removal of such antibodies by plasmapheresis results in improvement of the disease process in some patients but not in all. The anti-GBM antibodies are IgG_1 and IgG_4 complement-binding subclasses of IgG which activate complement. Complement fragments signal the recruitment of neutrophils and macrophage in both the lung and kidney basement membranes resulting in damage and capillaritis.

Genetic Factors

Genetics appears to contribute strongly to the development of this disease with the presence of major histocompatibility complex class II alleles DR15, DR4, DRB1*1501, DRB1*04, and DRB1*03 predisposing to disease.

Environmental Factors

Exposure to smoke appears to be a strong factor in the development Goodpasture disease. Whether smoking alters the ultrastructure of the basement membrane or exogenous particles or noxious substances in smoke alter the type IV collagen is unknown. Smokers are more likely to develop pulmonary hemorrhage than non-smokers who have Goodpasture disease. Other injuries to the alveoli from infection, hydrocarbon inhalation, or cocaine inhalation have been reported as associated events prior to development of Goodpasture disease.

Clinical Manifestations

The majority of patients present with many days or weeks of cough, dyspnea, fatigue, and sometimes hemoptysis. Young children tend to swallow small amounts of blood from hemoptysis and may present with vomiting blood. Occasionally, the hemoptysis is large and resultant anemia is a consequence of large quantities of blood loss. Renal compromise is found with abnormal renal function tests. Younger patients tend to present with both the pulmonary and renal syndrome concurrently. Adults are less likely to develop pulmonary disease.

Laboratory

Serologic detection of anti-GBM antibodies are positive in more than 90% of patients with Goodpasture disease. A complete blood count will show anemia that is normocytic and normochromic as seen in chronic inflammatory disease. Urinalysis may reveal hematuria and proteinuria and blood tests demonstrate renal compromise with elevated blood urea nitrogen and creatinine.

Studies for pANCA (antimyeloperoxidase ANCA) should also be performed and are positive in approximately 25-30% of patients concurrently with anti-GBM antibodies. Clinical disease may be more difficult to treat and the presence of these antibodies may herald a more severe form of disease.

Chest Radiography

Chest radiography in Goodpasture disease will often show widely scattered patches of pulmonary infiltrates. If these infiltrates are in the periphery of the lung, they may be difficult to distinguish from the eosinophilic lung diseases. Interstitial patterns of thickening may be found as well. HRCT is usually not performed in this disease as the constellation of pulmonary hemorrhage, renal compromise, and positive serologic tests with anti-GBM antibodies detected often preclude the need for this test.

Pulmonary Function Testing

Pulmonary spirometry often reveals a restrictive defect with reduction in forced vital capacity and forced expiratory volume at 1-second. **DLCO** is a valuable test when pulmonary hemorrhage is a strong consideration. The intent of this test is to measure the ability of the lung to transfer inhaled gas to the red blood cell in the pulmonary capillary bed. This takes advantage of the hemoglobin's high affinity to bind carbon monoxide. It was once thought that reduction of DLCO was a measure of reduced surface area of the alveoli. Current data suggests that it directly correlates with the volume of blood in the pulmonary capillary bed. In pulmonary hemorrhage syndromes, blood in the alveoli plus the blood in the capillary bed increase the DLCO significantly and should alert the clinician to the possibility of pulmonary hemorrhage.

Bronchoscopy and Bronchoalveolar Lavage

Pulmonary abnormalities can often be best assessed by a bronchoscopy with BAL. The visual presence of blood on inspection as well as BAL will be obvious. Infections must be ruled out in many cases, and this technique adds significant value. BAL cell count will show hemosiderin-laden macrophage that have engulfed and broken down the red blood cells, leaving iron in these cells.

Lung Biopsy

Lung biopsy in patients with active disease reveals capillaritis from neutrophils, hemosiderin-laden macrophages, type II pneumocyte hyperplasia, and interstitial thickening at the level of the alveolus. Staining for IgG and complement is found by immunofluorescence in along the basement membrane in a linear pattern. This antibody deposition pattern led to the investigation of endogenous antigens in the basement membrane.

Treatment

More than half of patients with Goodpasture disease who forego treatment die within 2 yr from either respiratory failure, renal failure, or both. After a diagnosis is made, therapy with corticosteroids (e.g., prednisone, 1 mg/kg/day) coupled with oral cyclophosphamide (2.5 mg/kg/day) is begun. The addition of daily plasmapheresis for 2 wks may accelerate improvement. Cyclophosphamide may be discontinued after 2-3 mo. Steroids are often weaned over a 6-9 mo period. Survival is affected by the need for ongoing dialysis. Patients who do not require persistent dialysis have a survival rate at 1 yr of 80% or more.

Bibliography is available at Expert Consult.

Chapter 400
Community-Acquired Pneumonia

Matthew S. Kelly and Thomas J. Sandora

EPIDEMIOLOGY

Pneumonia, defined as inflammation of the lung parenchyma, is the leading cause of death globally among children younger than age 5 yr, accounting for an estimated 1.2 million (18% total) deaths annually (Fig. 400-1). The incidence of pneumonia is more than 10-fold higher (0.29 episodes vs 0.03 episodes), and the number of childhood-related deaths from pneumonia ≈2,000 fold higher, in developing than in developed countries (Table 400-1). Fifteen countries account for more than three-fourths of all pediatric deaths from pneumonia.

In the United States from 1939-1996, pneumonia mortality in children declined by 97%; in 1970, pneumonia accounted for 9% of all deaths of children younger than age 5 yr compared to 2% in 2007. It is probable that this decline results from the introduction of antibiotics, vaccines, and the expansion of medical insurance coverage for children. *Haemophilus influenzae* type b (see Chapter 194) was an important cause of bacterial pneumonia in young children but became uncommon with the routine use of effective vaccines, while measles vaccine greatly reduced the incidence of measles-related pneumonia deaths in developing countries. Improved access to healthcare in rural areas of developing countries and the introduction of pneumococcal conjugate vaccines (see Chapter 182) were also important contributors to the further reductions in pneumonia-related deaths achieved over the past decade.

ETIOLOGY

Although most cases of pneumonia are caused by microorganisms, noninfectious causes include aspiration (of food or gastric acid, foreign bodies, hydrocarbons, and lipoid substances), hypersensitivity reactions, and drug- or radiation-induced pneumonitis. The cause of pneumonia in an individual patient is often difficult to determine because direct culture of lung tissue is invasive and rarely performed. Cultures performed on specimens in children obtained from the upper respiratory tract or sputum typically do not accurately reflect the cause of lower respiratory tract infection. With the use of molecular diagnostic testing, a bacterial or viral cause of pneumonia can be identified in

40-80% of children with community-acquired pneumonia. *Streptococcus pneumoniae* (pneumococcus) is the most common bacterial pathogen in children 3 wk to 4 yr of age, whereas *Mycoplasma pneumoniae* and *Chlamydophila pneumoniae* are the most frequent bacterial pathogens in children age 5 yr and older. In addition to pneumococcus, other bacterial causes of pneumonia in previously healthy children in the United States include group A streptococcus (*Streptococcus pyogenes*) and *Staphylococcus aureus* (see Chapter 181.1 and Table 400-2). *S. aureus* pneumonia often complicates an illness caused by influenza viruses.

S. pneumoniae, *H. influenzae*, and *S. aureus* are the major causes of hospitalization and death from bacterial pneumonia among children in developing countries, although in children with HIV infection, *Mycobacterium tuberculosis* (see Chapter 215), atypical mycobacteria,

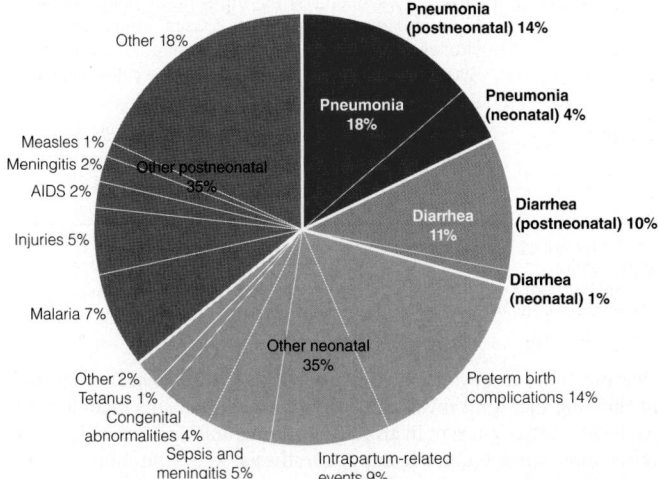

Figure 400-1 Pneumonia is the leading killer of children worldwide, as shown by this illustration of global distribution of cause-specific mortality among children younger than age 5 yr in 2010. Pneumonia causes 18% of all under-5 deaths. Values may not sum to 100% because of rounding. *(From Black RE, Allen LH, Bhutta ZA, et al: Maternal and child undernutrition: global and regional exposures and health consequences. Lancet 371:243–260, 2008; and Liu L, Johnson HL, Cousens S, et al. Global, regional, and national causes of child mortality: an updated systematic analysis for 2010 with time trends since 2000. Lancet 379:2151–2161, 2012, Fig. 2.)*

Salmonella (see Chapter 198), *Escherichia coli* (see Chapter 200), and *Pneumocystis jiroveci* (see Chapter 244) must be considered. The incidence of pneumonia caused by *H. influenzae* or *S. pneumoniae* has been significantly reduced in areas where routine immunization has been implemented.

Viral pathogens are a prominent cause of lower respiratory tract infections in infants and children older than 1 mo but younger than 5 yr of age. Viruses can be detected in 40-80% of children with pneumonia using molecular diagnostic methods. Of the respiratory viruses, respiratory syncytial virus (RSV) (see Chapter 260) and rhinoviruses are the most commonly identified pathogens, especially in children younger than 2 yr of age. However, the role of rhinoviruses in severe lower respiratory tract infection remains poorly defined as these viruses are frequently detected in infections with 2 or more pathogens and among asymptomatic children. Other common viruses causing pneumonia include influenza virus (see Chapter 258), parainfluenza viruses, adenoviruses, enteroviruses, and human metapneumovirus. Infection with more than 1 respiratory virus occurs in up to 20% of cases. The age of the patient may help identify possible pathogens (Table 400-3).

Lower respiratory tract viral infections are much more common in the fall and winter in both the northern and southern hemispheres in relation to the seasonal epidemics of respiratory viral infection that occur each year. The typical pattern of these epidemics usually begins in the fall, when parainfluenza infections appear and most often manifest as croup. Later in winter, RSV, human metapneumovirus, and influenza viruses cause widespread infection, including upper respiratory tract infections, bronchiolitis, and pneumonia. RSV is particularly severe among infants and young children, whereas influenza virus causes disease and excess hospitalization for acute respiratory illness in all age groups. Knowledge of the prevailing viral epidemic may lead to a presumptive initial diagnosis.

Immunization status is relevant because children fully immunized against *H. influenzae* type b and *S. pneumoniae* are less likely to be infected with these pathogens. Children who are immunosuppressed or who have an underlying illness may be at risk for specific pathogens, such as *Pseudomonas* spp. in patients with cystic fibrosis (see Chapter 403).

PATHOGENESIS

The lower respiratory tract is normally kept sterile by physiologic defense mechanisms, including mucociliary clearance, the properties of normal secretions such as secretory immunoglobulin (Ig) A, and

Table 400-1	Incidence of Pneumonia Cases and Pneumonia Deaths Among Children Younger Than Age 5 Yr, by UNICEF Region, 2004*			
UNICEF REGIONS	**NUMBER OF CHILDREN YOUNGER THAN 5 YR OF AGE (IN THOUSANDS)**	**NUMBER OF CHILDHOOD PNEUMONIA DEATHS (IN THOUSANDS)**	**INCIDENCE OF PNEUMONIA CASES (EPISODES PER CHILD PER YEAR)**	**TOTAL NUMBER OF PNEUMONIA EPISODES (IN THOUSANDS)**
South Asia	169,300	702	0.36	61,300
Sub-Saharan Africa	117,300	1,022	0.30	35,200
Middle East and North Africa	43,400	82	0.26	11,300
East Asia and Pacific	146,400	158	0.24	34,500
Latin America and Caribbean	56,500	50	0.22	12,200
Central and Eastern Europe and the Commonwealth of Independent States	26,400	29	0.09	2,400
Developing countries	533,000	2,039	0.29	154,500
Industrialized countries	54,200	1	0.03	1,600
World	613,600	2,044	0.26	158,500

*Regional estimates in Columns 2, 3, and 5 do not add up to the world total because of rounding.
From Wardlaw T, Salama P, White Johansson E: Pneumonia: the leading killer of children, Lancet 368:1048–1050, 2006.

Table 400-2	Causes of Infectious Pneumonia

BACTERIAL
Common

Streptococcus pneumoniae	Consolidation, empyema
Group B streptococci	Neonates
Group A streptococci	Empyema
*Mycoplasma pneumoniae**	Adolescents; summer-fall epidemics
*Chlamydophila pneumoniae**	Adolescents
Chlamydia trachomatis	Infants
Mixed anaerobes	Aspiration pneumonia
Gram-negative enterics	Nosocomial pneumonia

Uncommon

Haemophilus influenzae type b	Unimmunized
Staphylococcus aureus	Pneumatoceles, empyema; infants
Moraxella catarrhalis	
Neisseria meningitidis	
Francisella tularensis	Animal, tick, fly contact; bioterrorism
Nocardia species	Immunosuppressed persons
*Chlamydophila psittaci**	Bird contact (especially parakeets)
Yersinia pestis	Plague; rat contact; bioterrorism
Legionella species*	Exposure to contaminated water; nosocomial
*Coxiella burnetii**	Q fever; animal (goat, sheep, cattle) exposure

VIRAL
Common

Respiratory syncytial virus	Bronchiolitis
Parainfluenza types 1-3	Croup
Influenzas A, B	High fever; winter months
Adenovirus	Can be severe; often occurs between January and April
Human metapneumovirus	Similar to respiratory syncytial virus

Uncommon

Rhinovirus	Rhinorrhea
Enterovirus	Neonates
Herpes simplex	Neonates
Cytomegalovirus	Infants, immunosuppressed persons
Measles	Rash, coryza, conjunctivitis
Varicella	Adolescents or unimmunized
Hantavirus	Southwestern United States, rodents
Coronavirus (severe acute respiratory syndrome, Middle East respiratory syndrome [MERS])	Asia, Arabian peninsula

FUNGAL

Histoplasma capsulatum	Ohio/Mississippi River valley; bird, bat contact
Blastomyces dermatitidis	Ohio/Mississippi River valley
Coccidioides immitis	Southwest United States
Cryptococcus neoformans	Bird contact
Aspergillus species	Immunosuppressed persons; nodular lung infection
Mucormycosis	Immunosuppressed persons
Pneumocystis jiroveci	Immunosuppressed, steroids

RICKETTSIAL

Rickettsia rickettsiae	Tick bite

MYCOBACTERIAL

Mycobacterium tuberculosis	Travel to endemic region; exposure to high-risk persons
Mycobacterium avium complex	Immunosuppressed persons

PARASITIC

Various parasites (e.g., *Ascaris*, *Strongyloides* species)	Eosinophilic pneumonia

*Atypical pneumonia syndrome; may have extrapulmonary manifestations, low-grade fever, patchy diffuse infiltrates, poor response to β-lactam antibiotics, and negative sputum Gram stain.

From Kliegman RM, Greenbaum LA, Lye PS: Practical strategies in pediatric diagnosis & therapy, ed 2, Philadelphia, 2004, Elsevier, p. 29.

Table 400-3	Etiologic Agents Grouped by Age of the Patient

AGE GROUP	FREQUENT PATHOGENS (IN ORDER OF FREQUENCY)
Neonates (<3 wk)	Group B streptococcus, *Escherichia coli*, other Gram-negative bacilli, *Streptococcus pneumoniae*, *Haemophilus influenzae* (type b,* nontypeable)
3 wk-3 mo	Respiratory syncytial virus, other respiratory viruses (rhinoviruses, parainfluenza viruses, influenza viruses, adenovirus), *S. pneumoniae*, *H. influenzae* (type b,* nontypeable); if patient is afebrile, consider *Chlamydia trachomatis*
4 mo-4 yr	Respiratory syncytial virus, other respiratory viruses (rhinoviruses, parainfluenza viruses, influenza viruses, adenovirus), *S. pneumoniae*, *H. influenzae* (type b,* nontypeable), *Mycoplasma pneumoniae*, group A streptococcus
≥5 yr	*M. pneumoniae*, *S. pneumoniae*, *Chlamydophila pneumoniae*, *H. influenzae* (type b,* nontypeable), influenza viruses, adenovirus, other respiratory viruses, *Legionella pneumophila*

H. influenzae type b is uncommon with routine *H. influenzae* type b immunization.

Adapted from Kliegman RM, Marcdante KJ, Jenson HJ, et al: Nelson essentials of pediatrics, ed 5, Philadelphia, 2006, Elsevier, p. 504.

clearing of the airway by coughing. Immunologic defense mechanisms of the lung that limit invasion by pathogenic organisms include macrophages that are present in alveoli and bronchioles, secretory IgA, and other immunoglobulins. Trauma, anesthesia, and aspiration increase the risk of pulmonary infection.

Viral pneumonia usually results from spread of infection along the airways, accompanied by direct injury of the respiratory epithelium, which results in airway obstruction from swelling, abnormal secretions, and cellular debris. The small caliber of airways in young infants makes such patients particularly susceptible to severe infection. Atelectasis, interstitial edema, and ventilation–perfusion mismatch causing significant hypoxemia often accompany airway obstruction. Viral infection of the respiratory tract can also predispose to secondary bacterial infection by disturbing normal host defense mechanisms, altering secretions, and modifying the bacterial flora.

Bacterial pneumonia most often occurs when respiratory tract organisms colonize the trachea and subsequently gain access to the lungs, but pneumonia may also result from direct seeding of lung tissue after bacteremia. When bacterial infection is established in the lung parenchyma, the pathologic process varies according to the invading organism. *M. pneumoniae* (see Chapter 223) attaches to the respiratory epithelium, inhibits ciliary action, and leads to cellular destruction and an inflammatory response in the submucosa. As the infection progresses, sloughed cellular debris, inflammatory cells, and mucus cause airway obstruction, with spread of infection occurring along the bronchial tree, as it does in viral pneumonia.

S. pneumoniae produces local edema that aids in the proliferation of organisms and their spread into adjacent portions of lung, often resulting in the characteristic focal lobar involvement.

Group A streptococcus infection of the lower respiratory tract results in more diffuse infection with interstitial pneumonia. The pathology includes necrosis of tracheobronchial mucosa; formation of large amounts of exudate, edema, and local hemorrhage, with extension into the interalveolar septa; and involvement of lymphatic vessels and the increased likelihood of pleural involvement.

S. aureus pneumonia manifests in confluent bronchopneumonia, which is often unilateral and characterized by the presence of extensive areas of hemorrhagic necrosis and irregular areas of cavitation of the lung parenchyma, resulting in pneumatoceles, empyema, or, at times, bronchopulmonary fistulas.

Table 400-4	Differential Diagnosis of Recurrent Pneumonia

HEREDITARY DISORDERS
Cystic fibrosis
Sickle cell disease

DISORDERS OF IMMUNITY
HIV/AIDS
Bruton agammaglobulinemia
Selective immunoglobulin G subclass deficiencies
Common variable immunodeficiency syndrome
Severe combined immunodeficiency syndrome
Chronic granulomatous disease
Hyperimmunoglobulin E syndromes
Leukocyte adhesion defect

DISORDERS OF CILIA
Immotile cilia syndrome
Kartagener syndrome

ANATOMIC DISORDERS
Pulmonary sequestration
Lobar emphysema
Gastroesophageal reflux
Foreign body
Tracheoesophageal fistula (H type)
Bronchiectasis
Aspiration (oropharyngeal incoordination)
Aberrant bronchus

From Kliegman RM, Marcdante KJ, Jenson HJ, et al: Nelson essentials of pediatrics, ed 5, Philadelphia, 2006, Elsevier, p. 507.

Recurrent pneumonia is defined **as 2 or more** episodes in a single year **or 3 or more** episodes ever, with radiographic clearing between occurrences. An underlying disorder should be considered if a child experiences recurrent pneumonia (Table 400-4).

CLINICAL MANIFESTATIONS

Pneumonia is frequently preceded by several days of symptoms of an upper respiratory tract infection, typically rhinitis and cough. In viral pneumonia, fever is usually present but temperatures are generally lower than in bacterial pneumonia. Tachypnea is the most consistent clinical manifestation of pneumonia. Increased work of breathing accompanied by intercostal, subcostal, and suprasternal retractions, nasal flaring, and use of accessory muscles is common. Severe infection may be accompanied by cyanosis and lethargy, especially in infants. Auscultation of the chest may reveal crackles and wheezing, but it is often difficult to localize the source of these adventitious sounds in very young children with hyperresonant chests. It is often not possible to distinguish viral pneumonia clinically from disease caused by *Mycoplasma* and other bacterial pathogens.

Bacterial pneumonia in adults and older children typically begins suddenly with high fever, cough, and chest pain. Other symptoms that may be seen include drowsiness with intermittent periods of restlessness; rapid respirations; anxiety; and, occasionally, delirium. In many children, splinting on the affected side to minimize pleuritic pain and improve ventilation is noted; such children may lie on one side with the knees drawn up to the chest.

Physical findings depend on the stage of pneumonia. Early in the course of illness, diminished breath sounds, scattered crackles, and rhonchi are commonly heard over the affected lung field. With the development of increasing consolidation or complications of pneumonia such as pleural effusion or empyema, dullness on percussion is noted and breath sounds may be diminished. A lag in respiratory excursion often occurs on the affected side. Abdominal distention may be prominent because of gastric dilation from swallowed air or ileus. *Abdominal pain is common in lower-lobe pneumonia.* The liver may seem enlarged because of downward displacement of the diaphragm secondary to hyperinflation of the lungs or superimposed congestive heart failure.

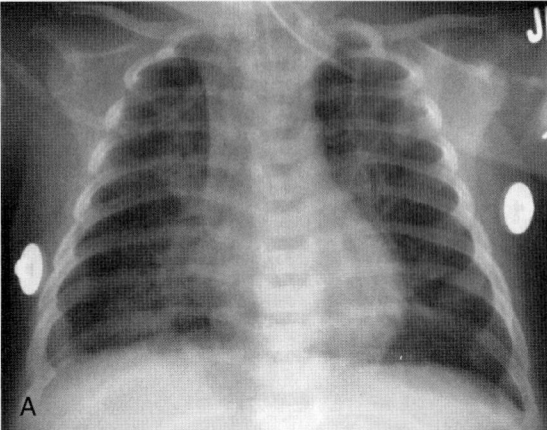
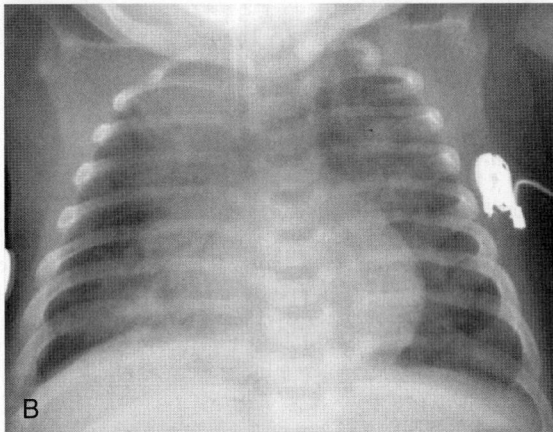

Figure 400-2 A, Radiographic findings characteristic of respiratory syncytial virus pneumonia in a 6 mo old infant with rapid respirations and fever. Anteroposterior radiograph of the chest shows hyperexpansion of the lungs with bilateral fine air space disease and streaks of density, indicating the presence of both pneumonia and atelectasis. An endotracheal tube is in place. **B,** One day later, the anteroposterior radiograph of the chest shows increased bilateral pneumonia.

Symptoms described in adults with pneumococcal pneumonia may be noted in older children but are rarely observed in infants and young children, in whom the clinical pattern is considerably more variable. In infants, there may be a prodrome of upper respiratory tract infection and diminished appetite, leading to the abrupt onset of fever, restlessness, apprehension, and respiratory distress. These infants appear ill, with respiratory distress manifested as grunting; nasal flaring; retractions of the supraclavicular, intercostal, and subcostal areas; tachypnea; tachycardia; air hunger; and often cyanosis. Results of physical examination may be misleading, particularly in young infants, with meager findings disproportionate to the degree of tachypnea. Some infants with bacterial pneumonia may have associated gastrointestinal disturbances characterized by vomiting, anorexia, diarrhea, and abdominal distention secondary to a paralytic ileus. Rapid progression of symptoms is characteristic in the most severe cases of bacterial pneumonia.

DIAGNOSIS

An infiltrate on chest radiograph (posteroanterior **and** lateral views) supports the diagnosis of pneumonia; the film may also indicate a complication such as a pleural effusion or empyema. Viral pneumonia is usually characterized by hyperinflation with bilateral interstitial infiltrates and peribronchial cuffing (Fig. 400-2). Confluent lobar consolidation is typically seen with pneumococcal pneumonia (Fig. 400-3). The radiographic appearance alone is not diagnostic, and other clinical features must be considered. Repeat chest radiographs are not required for proof of cure for patients with uncomplicated pneumonia. Some

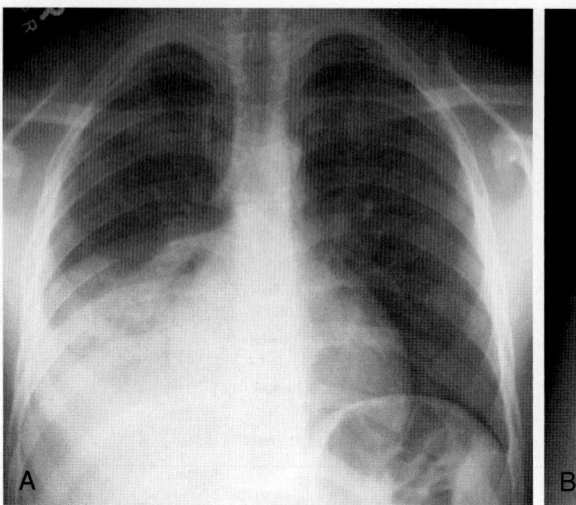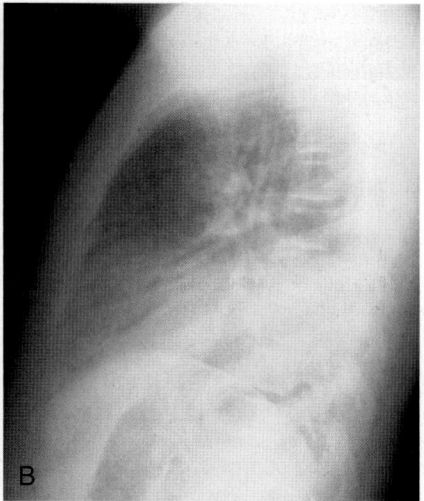

Figure 400-3 Radiographic findings characteristic of pneumococcal pneumonia in a 14 yr old boy with cough and fever. Posteroanterior (A) and lateral (B) chest radiographs reveal consolidation in the right lower lobe, strongly suggesting bacterial pneumonia.

experts suggest that a chest radiograph may not be necessary for older children with suspected pneumonia (cough, fever, localized crackles, or decreased breath sounds) who are well enough to be managed as outpatients.

Point-of-care use of portable or handheld ultrasonography is highly sensitive and specific in diagnosing pneumonia in children by determining lung consolidations and air bronchograms or effusions.

The peripheral white blood cell (WBC) count can be useful in differentiating viral from bacterial pneumonia. In viral pneumonia, the WBC count can be normal or elevated but is usually not higher than 20,000/mm^3, with a lymphocyte predominance. Bacterial pneumonia is often associated with an elevated WBC count, in the range of 15,000-40,000/mm^3, and a predominance of granulocytes. A large pleural effusion, lobar consolidation, and a high fever at the onset of the illness are also suggestive of a bacterial etiology. **Atypical pneumonia** caused by *C. pneumoniae* or *M. pneumoniae* is difficult to distinguish from pneumococcal pneumonia on the basis of radiographic and laboratory findings, and although pneumococcal pneumonia is associated with a higher WBC count, erythrocyte sedimentation rate, procalcitonin, and C-reactive protein level, there is considerable overlap, particularly with adenoviruses and enteroviruses.

The definitive diagnosis of a viral infection rests on the isolation of a virus or detection of the viral genome or antigen in respiratory tract secretions. Reliable DNA or RNA tests for the rapid detection of many respiratory pathogens, such as mycoplasma, pertussis, and viruses, including RSV, parainfluenza, influenza, and adenoviruses, are available and accurate. Serologic techniques can also be used to diagnose a recent respiratory viral infection but generally require testing of acute and convalescent serum samples for a rise in antibodies to a specific viral agent. This diagnostic technique is laborious, slow, and not generally clinically useful because the infection usually resolves by the time it is confirmed serologically. Serologic testing may be valuable as an epidemiologic tool to define the incidence and prevalence of the various respiratory viral pathogens. Patient peripheral cell gene expression patterns determined by microarray reverse transcription polymerase chain reaction is an emerging technology that may help differentiate viral from bacterial causes of pneumonia.

The definitive diagnosis of a bacterial infection requires isolation of an organism from the blood, pleural fluid, or lung. Culture of sputum is of little value in the diagnosis of pneumonia in young children, while percutaneous lung aspiration is invasive and not routinely performed. Blood culture results are positive in only 10% of children with pneumococcal pneumonia and are not recommended for nontoxic appearing children treated as an outpatient. Blood cultures are recommended for those who fail to improve or have clinical deterioration, in those

Table 400-5	Factors Suggesting Need for Hospitalization of Children with Pneumonia

Age <6 mo
Sickle cell anemia with acute chest syndrome
Multiple lobe involvement
Immunocompromised state
Toxic appearance
Moderate to severe respiratory distress
Requirement for supplemental oxygen
Complicated pneumonia*
Dehydration
Vomiting or inability to tolerate oral fluids or medications
No response to appropriate oral antibiotic therapy
Social factors (e.g., inability of caregivers to administer medications at home or follow-up appropriately)

*Pleural effusion, empyema, abscess, bronchopleural fistula, necrotizing pneumonia, acute respiratory distress syndrome, extrapulmonary infection (meningitis, arthritis, pericarditis, osteomyelitis, endocarditis), hemolytic uremic syndrome, sepsis.

Adapted from Baltimore RS: Pneumonia. In Jenson HB, Baltimore RS, editors: Pediatric infectious diseases: principles and practice, Philadelphia, 2002, WB Saunders, p. 801.

with complicated pneumonia (Table 400-5) and those requiring hospitalization. Cold agglutinins at titers >1:64 are found in the blood in ≈50% of patients with *M. pneumoniae* infections. Cold agglutinin findings are nonspecific because other pathogens such as influenza viruses may also cause increases. Acute infection caused by *M. pneumoniae* can be diagnosed on the basis of a positive polymerase chain reaction test result or seroconversion in an IgG assay. Serologic evidence, such as the antistreptolysin O titer, may be useful in the diagnosis of group A streptococcal pneumonia.

TREATMENT

Treatment of suspected bacterial pneumonia is based on the presumptive cause and the age and clinical appearance of the child. For mildly ill children who do not require hospitalization, amoxicillin is recommended. With the emergence of penicillin-resistant pneumococci, high doses of amoxicillin (80-90 mg/kg/24 hr) should be prescribed unless local data indicate a low prevalence of resistance. Therapeutic alternatives include cefuroxime axetil and amoxicillin/clavulanate. For school-age children and in children in whom infection with *M. pneumoniae* or *C. pneumoniae* is suggested, a macrolide antibiotic such as azithromycin is an appropriate choice. In adolescents, a respiratory fluoroquinolone (levofloxacin, moxifloxacin) may be considered as an alternative. Despite substantial gains over the past decade, in developing countries only ≈60% of children with symptoms of pneumonia (≈50% in sub-Saharan Africa) are taken to an appropriate caregiver, and less than one-third receive antibiotics. The World Health Organization and other international groups have developed systems to train mothers and local healthcare providers in the recognition and treatment of pneumonia.

The empiric treatment of suspected bacterial pneumonia in a hospitalized child requires an approach based on the clinical manifestations at the time of presentation. In areas without substantial high-level penicillin resistance among *S. pneumoniae*, children who are fully immunized against *H. influenzae* type b and *S. pneumoniae* and are not severely ill should receive ampicillin or penicillin G. For children who do not meet these criteria, ceftriaxone or cefotaxime should be used. If clinical features suggest staphylococcal pneumonia (pneumatoceles, empyema), initial antimicrobial therapy should also include vancomycin or clindamycin.

If viral pneumonia is suspected, it is reasonable to withhold antibiotic therapy, especially for those patients who are mildly ill, have clinical evidence suggesting viral infection, and are in no respiratory distress. However, up to 30% of patients with known viral infection, particularly influenza viruses, may have coexisting bacterial pathogens. Therefore, if the decision is made to withhold antibiotic therapy on the basis of presumptive diagnosis of a viral infection, deterioration in clinical status should signal the possibility of superimposed bacterial infection, and antibiotic therapy should be initiated.

Table 400-5 notes the indications for admission to a hospital. The optimal duration of antibiotic treatment for pneumonia has not been well-established in controlled studies. However, antibiotics should generally be continued until the patient has been afebrile for 72 hr, and the total duration should not be less than 10 days (or 5 days if azithromycin is used). Shorter courses (5-7 days) may also be effective, particularly for children managed on an outpatient basis, but further study is needed. Available data do not support prolonged courses of treatment for uncomplicated pneumonia. In developing countries, oral zinc (10 mg/day for <12 mo, 20 mg/day for ≥12 mo) reduces mortality among children with clinically defined severe pneumonia.

PROGNOSIS

Typically, patients with uncomplicated community-acquired bacterial pneumonia show response to therapy, with improvement in clinical symptoms (fever, cough, tachypnea, chest pain), within 48-96 hr of initiation of antibiotics. Radiographic evidence of improvement lags substantially behind clinical improvement. A number of possibilities must be considered when a patient does not improve with appropriate antibiotic therapy: (1) complications, such as empyema (see Table 400-5); (2) bacterial resistance; (3) nonbacterial etiologies such as viruses or fungi and aspiration of foreign bodies or food; (4) bronchial obstruction from endobronchial lesions, foreign body, or mucous plugs; (5) preexisting diseases such as immunodeficiencies, ciliary dyskinesia, cystic fibrosis, pulmonary sequestration, or congenital pulmonary airway malformation, formerly called cystic adenomatoid malformation; and (6) other noninfectious causes (including bronchiolitis obliterans, hypersensitivity pneumonitis, eosinophilic pneumonia, aspiration, and granulomatosis with polyangiitis, formerly called Wegener granulomatosis). A repeat chest radiograph is the first step in determining the reason for delay in response to treatment. Bronchoalveolar lavage may be indicated in children with respiratory failure; high-resolution CT scans may better identify complications or an anatomic reason for a poor response to therapy.

Mortality from community-acquired pneumonia in developed nations is rare, and most children with pneumonia do not experience long-term pulmonary sequelae. Some data suggest that up to 45% of children have symptoms of asthma 5 yr after hospitalization for pneumonia; this finding may reflect either undiagnosed asthma at the time of presentation or a propensity for development of asthma after pneumonia.

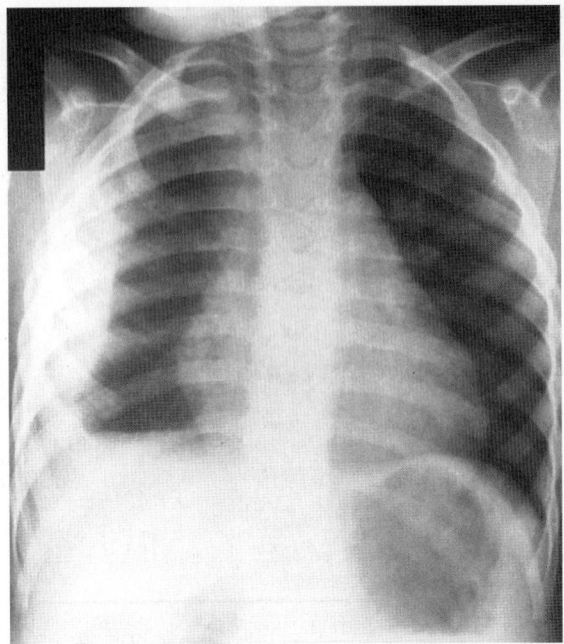

Figure 400-4 Pneumococcal empyema on the chest radiography of a 3 yr old child who has had upper respiratory symptoms and fever for 3 days. A pleural fluid collection can be seen on the right side. The patient had a positive pleural tap and blood culture result for pneumococci. The child recovered completely within 3 wk. *(From Kuhn JP, Slovis TL, Haller JO (eds): Caffrey's pediatric diagnostic imaging, ed 10, Philadelphia, 2004, Mosby, p. 1002.)*

COMPLICATIONS

Complications of pneumonia (see Table 400-5) are usually the result of direct spread of bacterial infection within the thoracic cavity (pleural effusion, empyema, and pericarditis) or bacteremia and hematologic spread (Fig. 400-4). Meningitis, suppurative arthritis, and osteomyelitis are rare complications of hematologic spread of pneumococcal or *H. influenzae* type b infection.

S. aureus, S. pneumoniae, and *S. pyogenes* are the most common causes of parapneumonic effusions and empyema (Table 400-6). Nonetheless many effusions that complicate bacterial pneumonia are sterile. Universal 16S ribosomal RNA gene polymerase chain reaction identifies the bacterial genome and can determine the bacterial etiology of the effusion if the culture is negative. The treatment of empyema is based on the stage (exudative, fibrinopurulent, organizing). Imaging studies including ultrasonography and CT are helpful in determining the stage of empyema. The mainstays of therapy include antibiotic therapy and drainage with tube thoracostomy. Additional effective approaches include the use of intrapleural fibrinolytic therapy (urokinase, streptokinase, tissue plasminogen activator) and selected video-assisted thoracoscopy to debride or lyse adhesions and drain loculated areas of pus. Early diagnosis and intervention, particularly with fibrinolysis or less often video-assisted thoracoscopy, may obviate the need for thoracotomy and open debridement. Fibrinolysis is more cost-effective than video-assisted thoracoscopy.

PREVENTION

Some evidence exists to suggest that vaccination has reduced the incidence of pneumonia hospitalizations. The annual rate of all-cause pneumonia hospitalization among children younger than 2 yr of age in the United States during the period 1997-1999 was 12.5 per 1,000 children. In February 2000, the 7-valent pneumococcal conjugate vaccine (PCV7) was licensed and recommended. In 2006, the pneumonia hospitalization rate in this age group was 8.1 per 1,000 children, a 35% decrease from the prevaccine rate. Although these data do not establish that PCV7 directly reduced pneumonia hospitalization rates,

Table 400-6	Differentiation of Pleural Fluid	
	TRANSUDATE	**EMPYEMA**
Appearance	Clear	Cloudy or purulent
Cell count (per mm³)	<1,000	Often >50,000 (cell count has limited predictive value)
Cell type	Lymphocytes, monocytes	Polymorphonuclear leukocytes (neutrophils)
Lactate dehydrogenase	<200 U/L	More than two-thirds upper limit of normal for serum lactate dehydrogenase (LDH)
Pleural fluid:serum LDH ratio	<0.6	>0.6
Protein >3 g	Unusual	Common
Pleural fluid:serum protein ratio	<0.5	>0.5
Glucose*	Normal	Low (<40 mg/dL)
pH*	Normal (7.40-7.60)	<7.10
Gram stain	Negative	Occasionally positive (less than one-third of cases)
Cholesterol		>55 mg/dL
Pleural cholesterol:serum cholesterol ratio	<0.3	>0.3

*Low glucose or pH may be seen in malignant effusion, tuberculosis, esophageal rupture, pancreatitis (positive pleural amylase), and rheumatologic diseases (e.g., systemic lupus erythematosus).
From Kliegman RM, Greenbaum LA, Lye PS: Practical strategies in pediatric diagnosis & therapy, ed 2, Philadelphia, 2004, Elsevier, p. 30.

they do suggest that vaccination has resulted in a sustained benefit in preventing hospitalization for young children with pneumonia.

In 2010, the 13-valent pneumococcal conjugate vaccine (PCV13) was licensed in the United States; it may prevent even more cases of pneumococcal disease not covered by the PCV7 vaccine.

The expansion of influenza vaccine recommendations to include all children >6 mo of age in 2010 might be expected to affect pneumonia hospitalization rates in a similar fashion, and ongoing surveillance is warranted.

Bibliography is available at Expert Consult.

Chapter 401
Bronchiectasis
Oren J. Lakser

Bronchiectasis is characterized by irreversible abnormal dilation and anatomic distortion of the bronchial tree and represents a common end stage of a many nonspecific and unrelated antecedent events. Its incidence has been decreasing overall in industrialized countries, but it persists as a problem in lower and middle income countries and among some ethnic groups in industrialized nations. Females are afflicted more frequently than males.

PATHOPHYSIOLOGY AND PATHOGENESIS

In industrialized nations, cystic fibrosis (see Chapter 403) is the most common cause of clinically significant bronchiectasis. Other conditions associated with bronchiectasis include primary ciliary dyskinesia (see Chapter 404), foreign-body aspiration (see Chapter 387), aspiration of gastric contents, immune deficiency syndromes (especially humoral immunity), and infection, especially pertussis, measles, and tuberculosis (Table 401-1). Bronchiectasis can also be congenital, as in

Table 401-1	Conditions That Predispose to Bronchiectasis in Children

PROXIMAL AIRWAY NARROWING
Airway wall compression (i.e., vascular ring, adenopathy impinging on airways)
Airway intraluminal obstruction (e.g., inhaled foreign body, granulation tissue)
Airway stenosis and malacia

AIRWAY INJURY
Bronchiolitis obliterans (e.g., postviral, after lung transplantation)
Recurrent pneumonitis or pneumonia (e.g., pneumococcal pneumonia, aspiration pneumonia)

ALTERED PULMONARY HOST DEFENSES
Cystic fibrosis
Ciliary dyskinesia
Impaired cough (e.g., neuromuscular weakness conditions)

ALTERED IMMUNE STATES
Primary abnormalities (e.g., hypogammaglobulinemia)
Secondary abnormalities (e.g., HIV infection, immunosuppressive agents)

OTHER
Allergic bronchopulmonary aspergillosis
Plastic bronchitis

From Redding GJ: Bronchiectasis in children, Pediatr Clin North Am 56:157–171, 2009, Box 1, p. 158.

Williams-Campbell syndrome, in which there is an absence of annular bronchial cartilage, and **Marnier-Kuhn syndrome** (congenital tracheobronchomegaly), in which there is a connective tissue disorder. Other disease entities associated with bronchiectasis are **right middle lobe syndrome** (chronic extrinsic compression of right middle lobe bronchus by hilar lymph nodes) and **yellow nail syndrome** (pleural effusion, lymphedema, discolored nails).

Three basic mechanisms are involved in the pathogenesis of bronchiectasis. Obstruction can occur because of tumor, foreign body, impacted mucus because of poor mucociliary clearance, external compression, bronchial webs, and atresia. Infections caused by *Bordetella pertussis*, measles, rubella, togavirus, respiratory syncytial virus, adenovirus, and *Mycobacterium tuberculosis* induce chronic inflammation, progressive bronchial wall damage, and dilation. Chronic inflammation similarly contributes to the mechanism by which obstruction leads to bronchiectasis. Activation of toll-like receptors results in the activation of nuclear factor κβ and the release of proinflammatory cytokines interleukin (IL)-1β, IL-8, and tumor necrosis factor-α. IL-8 is a chemoattractant for neutrophils, which are the main inflammatory cell involved in the pathogenesis of bronchiectasis. Once activated neutrophils produce neutrophil elastase and matrix metalloproteinases, MMP-8 and MMP-9. IL-6, IL-8, and tumor necrosis factor-α are elevated in the airways of patients with bronchiectasis. The mechanism by which bronchiectasis occurs in congenital forms is likely related to abnormal cartilage formation. The common thread in the pathogenesis of bronchiectasis consists of difficulty clearing secretions and recurrent infections with a "vicious cycle" of infection and inflammation resulting in airway injury and remodeling.

Bronchiectasis can manifest in any combination of three pathologic forms, best defined by high-resolution CT (HRCT) scan. In cylindrical bronchiectasis, the bronchial outlines are regular, but there is diffuse dilation of the bronchial unit. The bronchial lumen ends abruptly because of mucous plugging. In varicose bronchiectasis, the degree of dilation is greater, and local constrictions cause an irregularity of outline resembling that of varicose veins. There may also be small sacculations. In saccular (cystic) bronchiectasis, bronchial dilation progresses and results in ballooning of bronchi that end in fluid- or mucus-filled sacs. This is the most severe form of bronchiectasis. Bronchiectasis lies within a disease spectrum of chronic pediatric suppurative lung disease. The following definitions have been proposed: **prebronchiectasis** (chronic or recurrent endobronchial infection with nonspecific HRCT changes; may be reversible); **HRCT bronchiectasis** (clinical symptoms with HRCT evidence of bronchial dilation; may persist, progress, or improve and resolve); **established bronchiectasis**

(like the previous but with no resolution within 2 yr). Early diagnosis and aggressive therapy are important to prevent the development of established bronchiectasis.

CLINICAL MANIFESTATIONS

The most common complaints in patients with bronchiectasis are cough and production of copious purulent sputum. Younger children may swallow the sputum. Hemoptysis is seen with some frequency. Fever can occur with infectious exacerbations. Anorexia and poor weight gain may occur as time passes. Physical examination typically reveals crackles localized to the affected area, but wheezing as well as digital clubbing may also occur. In severe cases, dyspnea and hypoxemia can occur. Pulmonary function studies may demonstrate an obstructive, restrictive, or mixed pattern. Typically, impaired diffusion capacity is a late finding.

DIAGNOSIS

Conditions that can be associated with bronchiectasis should be ruled out by appropriate investigations (e.g., sweat test, immunologic workup). Chest radiographs of patients with bronchiectasis tend to be nonspecific. Typical findings can include increase in size and loss of definition of bronchovascular markings, crowding of bronchi, and loss of lung volume. In more severe forms, cystic spaces, occasionally with air–fluid levels and honeycombing, may occur. Compensatory overinflation of unaffected lung may be seen. Thin-section HRCT scanning is the gold standard, because it has excellent sensitivity and specificity. CT provides further information on disease location, presence of mediastinal lesions, and the extent of segmental involvement. The addition of radiolabeled aerosol inhalation to CT scanning can provide even more information. The CT findings in patients with bronchiectasis typically include cylindrical ("tram lines," "signet ring appearance"), varicose (bronchi with "beaded contour"), cystic (cysts in "strings and clusters"), or mixed forms (Fig. 401-1). The lower lobes are most commonly affected.

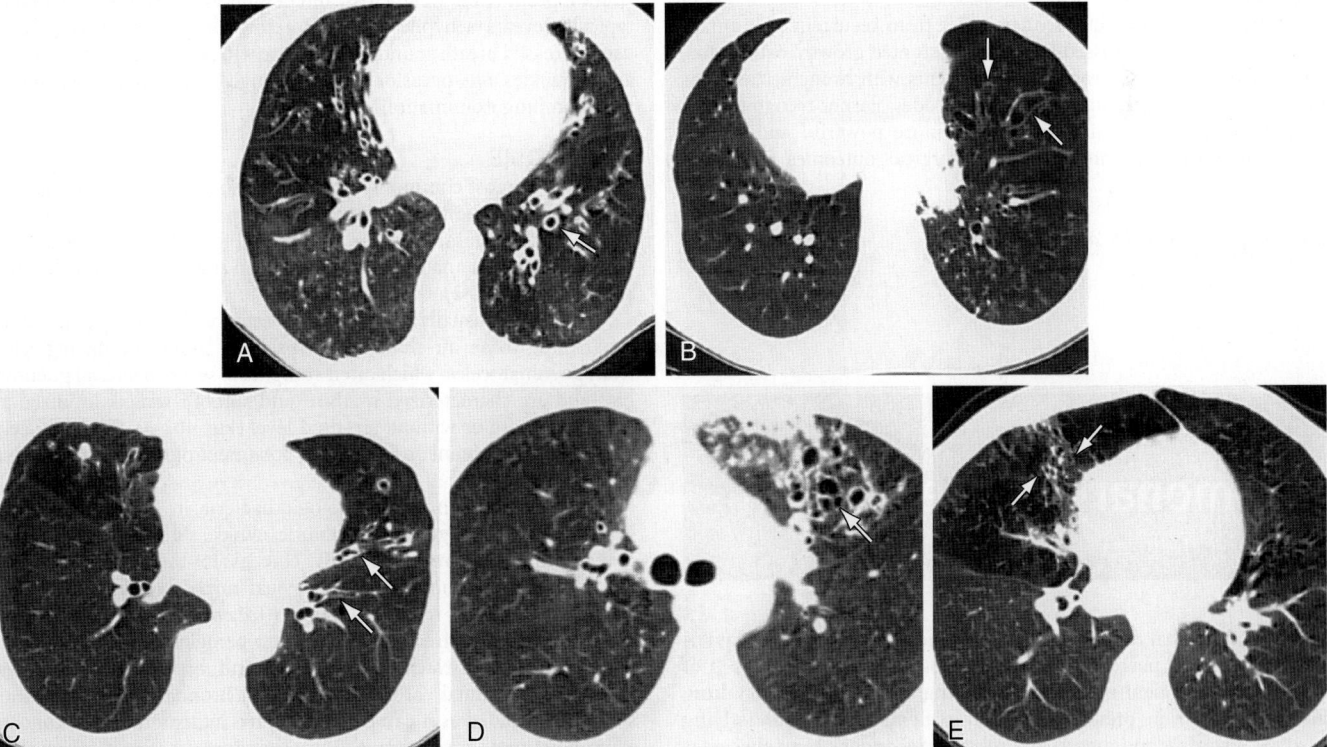

Figure 401-1 High-resolution CT scans of lungs with bronchiectasis. **A,** Dilated and thickened airways *(arrow)*. **B,** Airways do not taper *(arrows)* toward the periphery in a patient with Kartagener syndrome. **C,** Varicose changes (dilated and beaded airways *[arrows]*). **D,** Clustered cysts or saccules *(arrow)* as well as a peripheral infiltrate. **E,** Middle lobe bronchiectasis *(arrows)* in a patient with *Mycobacterium avium* complex infection. *(From Barker AF: Bronchiectasis, N Engl J Med 346:1383, 2002.)*

TREATMENT

The initial therapy for patients with bronchiectasis is medical and aims at decreasing airway obstruction and controlling infection. Chest physiotherapy (postural drainage), antibiotics, and bronchodilators are essential. Two to 4 wk of parenteral antibiotics is often necessary to manage acute exacerbations adequately. Exacerbations can be defined as the presence of 1 major criteria (wet cough enduring longer than 72 hr, increased cough frequency over 72 hr) *plus* 1 laboratory criteria (C-reactive protein >3 mg/L, serum IL-6 >2 ng/L, serum amyloid A >5 mg/L, elevated neutrophil percentage), 2 major criteria, or 1 major criteria *plus* 2 minor criteria (change in sputum color, breathlessness, chest pain, crackles/crepitations, wheeze). Antibiotic choice is dictated by the identification and sensitivity of organisms found on deep throat, sputum (induced or spontaneous), or bronchoalveolar lavage fluid cultures. The most common organisms found in children with bronchiectasis include *Streptococcus pneumoniae*, *Haemophilus influenzae* non-type b, *Moraxella catarrhalis*, and *Mycoplasma pneumoniae*. Amoxicillin/clavulanic acid (22.5 mg/kg/dose twice daily) has been particularly successful at treating most pulmonary exacerbations. Long-term prophylactic oral (macrolide) or nebulized antibiotics (e.g., tobramycin, colistin, aztreonam) may be beneficial. Airway hydration (inhaled hypertonic saline or mannitol) also improves quality of life in adults with bronchiectasis. Any underlying disorder (immunodeficiency, aspiration) that may be contributing must be addressed. When localized bronchiectasis becomes more severe or resistant to medical management, segmental or lobar resection may be warranted. Lung transplantation can also be performed in patients with bronchiectasis. A review of randomized trials among adult patients with bronchiectasis did not find strong evidence to support the routine use of inhaled corticosteroids, although some studies demonstrate improved quality of life and reduced exacerbations in patients with bronchiectasis treated with inhaled corticosteroids. Although preventative strategies, including immunization against typical respiratory pathogens (influenza, pneumococci), are generally recommended, no studies have been conducted to date to address the efficacy of these recommendations.

PROGNOSIS

Children with bronchiectasis often suffer from recurrent pulmonary illnesses, resulting in missed school days, stunted growth, osteopenia, and osteoporosis. The prognosis for patients with bronchiectasis has improved considerably in the past few decades. Earlier recognition or prevention of predisposing conditions, more powerful and broad-spectrum antibiotics, and improved surgical outcomes are likely reasons.

Bibliography is available at Expert Consult.

Chapter 402
Pulmonary Abscess
Oren J. Lakser

Lung infection that destroys the lung parenchyma, resulting in cavitations and central necrosis, can result in localized areas composed of thick-walled purulent material, called **lung abscesses**. **Primary lung abscesses** occur in previously healthy patients with no underlying medical disorders and are usually solitary. **Secondary lung abscesses** occur in patients with underlying or predisposing conditions and may be multiple. Lung abscesses are much less common in children (estimated at 0.7 per 100,000 admissions per year) than in adults.

PATHOLOGY AND PATHOGENESIS

A number of conditions predispose children to the development of pulmonary abscesses, including aspiration, pneumonia, cystic fibrosis (see Chapter 403), gastroesophageal reflux (see Chapter 323), tracheoesophageal fistula (see Chapter 319), immunodeficiencies, postoperative complications of tonsillectomy and adenoidectomy, seizures, a variety of neurologic diseases, and other conditions associated with impaired mucociliary defense. In children, aspiration of infected materials or a foreign body is the predominant source of the organisms causing abscesses. Initially, pneumonitis impairs drainage of fluid or the aspirated material. Inflammatory vascular obstruction occurs, leading to tissue necrosis, liquefaction, and abscess formation. Abscess can also occur as a result of pneumonia and hematogenous seeding from another site.

If the aspiration event occurred while the child was recumbent, the right and left upper lobes and apical segment of the right lower lobes are the dependent areas most likely to be affected. In a child who was upright, the posterior segments of the upper lobes were dependent and therefore are most likely to be affected. Primary abscesses are found most often on the right side, whereas secondary lung abscesses, particularly in immunocompromised patients, have a predilection for the left side.

Both anaerobic and aerobic organisms can cause lung abscesses. Common anaerobic bacteria that can cause a pulmonary abscess include *Bacteroides* spp., *Fusobacterium* spp., and *Peptostreptococcus* spp. Abscesses can be caused by aerobic organisms such as *Streptococcus* spp., *Staphylococcus aureus*, *Escherichia coli*, *Klebsiella pneumoniae*, *Pseudomonas aeruginosa*, and very rarely *Mycoplasma pneumoniae*. Aerobic and anaerobic cultures should be part of the work-up for all patients with lung abscess. Occasionally, concomitant viral–bacterial infection can be detected. Fungi can also cause lung abscesses, particularly in immunocompromised patients.

CLINICAL MANIFESTATIONS

The most common symptoms of pulmonary abscess in the pediatric population are cough, fever, tachypnea, dyspnea, chest pain, vomiting, sputum production, weight loss, and hemoptysis. Physical examination typically reveals tachypnea, dyspnea, retractions with accessory muscle use, decreased breath sounds, and dullness to percussion in the affected area. Crackles and, occasionally, a prolonged expiratory phase may be heard on lung examination.

DIAGNOSIS

Diagnosis is most commonly made on the basis of chest radiography. Classically, the chest radiograph shows a parenchymal inflammation with a cavity containing an air–fluid level (Fig. 402-1). A chest CT scan can provide better anatomic definition of an abscess, including location and size (Fig. 402-2).

An abscess is usually a thick-walled lesion with a low-density center progressing to an air–fluid level. Abscesses should be distinguished from pneumatoceles, which often complicate severe bacterial pneumonias and are characterized by thin- and smooth-walled, localized air collections with or without air–fluid level (Fig. 402-3). Pneumatoceles often resolve spontaneously with the treatment of the specific cause of the pneumonia.

The determination of the etiologic bacteria in a lung abscess can be very helpful in guiding antibiotic choice. Although Gram stain of sputum can provide an early clue as to the class of bacteria involved, sputum cultures typically yield mixed bacteria, and therefore are not always reliable. Attempts to avoid contamination from oral flora include direct lung puncture, percutaneous (aided by CT guidance) or transtracheal aspiration, and bronchoalveolar lavage specimens obtained bronchoscopically. Bronchoscopic aspiration should be avoided as it can be complicated by massive intrabronchial aspiration, and great care should therefore be taken during the procedure. To avoid invasive procedures in previously normal hosts, empiric therapy can be initiated in the absence of culturable material.

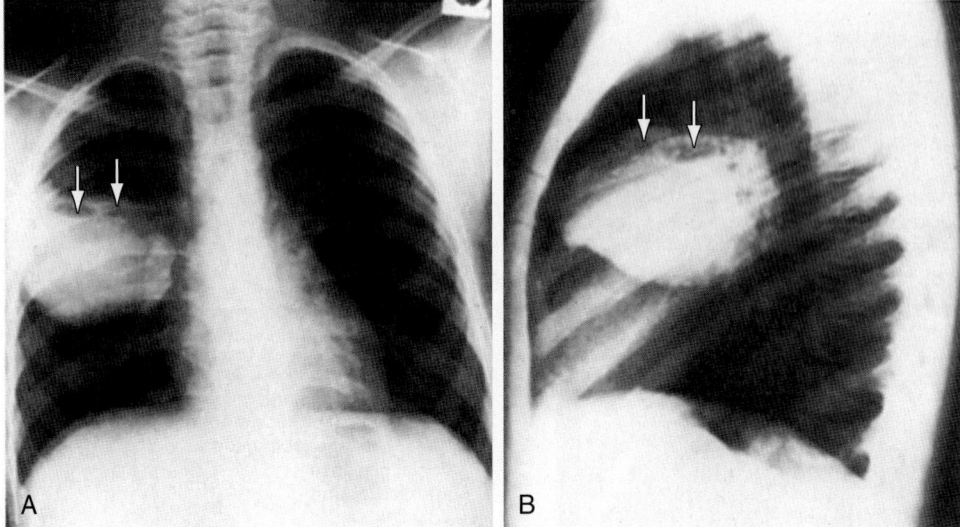

Figure 402-1 A and **B,** Multiloculated lung abscess *(arrows). (From Brook I: Lung abscess and pulmonary infections due to anaerobic bacteria. In Chernick V, Boat TF, Wilmott RW, et al, editors: Kendig's disorders of the respiratory tract in children, ed 7, Philadelphia, 2006, WB Saunders, p. 482.)*

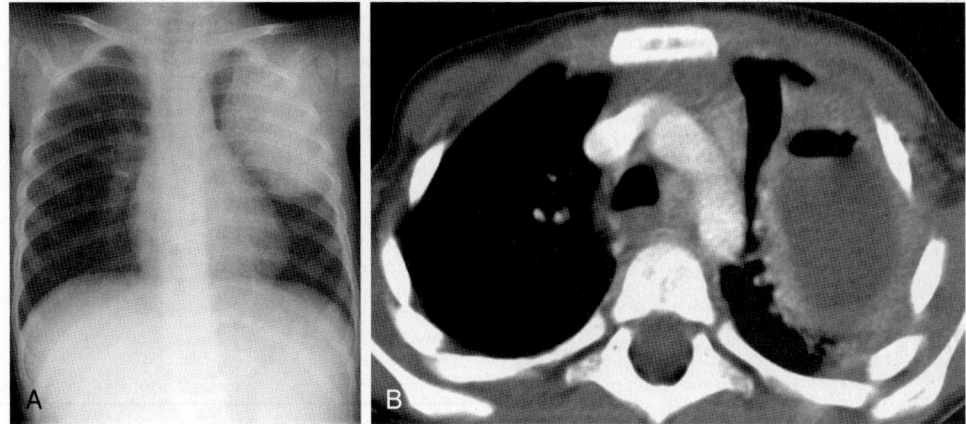

Figure 402-2 Pulmonary abscess in a 2 yr old boy with persistent cough. **A,** Chest radiograph shows large oval mass in the left upper lobe. **B,** CT scan demonstrates an abscess with a thick enhancing wall that contains both air and fluid. *(From Slovis TL, editor: Caffey's pediatric diagnostic imaging, ed 11, Philadelphia, 2008, Mosby, Fig. 78-3, p. 1297.)*

TREATMENT

Conservative management is recommended for pulmonary abscess. Most experts advocate a 2-3 wk course of parenteral antibiotics for uncomplicated cases, followed by a course of oral antibiotics to complete a total of 4-6 wk. Antibiotic choice should be guided by results of Gram stain and culture but initially should include agents with aerobic and anaerobic coverage. Treatment regimens should include a penicillinase-resistant agent active against *S. aureus* and anaerobic coverage, typically with clindamycin or ticarcillin/clavulanic acid. If Gram-negative bacteria are suspected or isolated, an aminoglycoside should be added. Early CT-guided percutaneous aspiration or drainage has been advocated as it can hasten the recovery and shorten the course of parenteral antibiotic therapy needed.

For severely ill patients or those whose status fails to improve after 7-10 days of appropriate antimicrobial therapy, surgical intervention should be considered. Minimally invasive percutaneous aspiration techniques, often with CT guidance, are the initial and, often, only intervention required. Thorascopic drainage has also been successfully utilized with minimal complications. In rare complicated cases, thoracotomy with surgical drainage or lobectomy and/or decortication may be necessary.

PROGNOSIS

Overall, prognosis for children with primary pulmonary abscesses is excellent. The presence of aerobic organisms may be a negative prognostic indicator, particularly in those with secondary lung abscesses. Most children become asymptomatic within 7-10 days, although the fever can persist for as long as 3 wk. Radiologic abnormalities usually resolve in 1-3 mo but can persist for years.

Bibliography is available at Expert Consult.

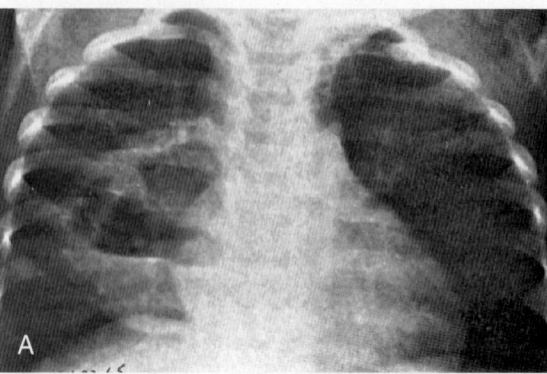

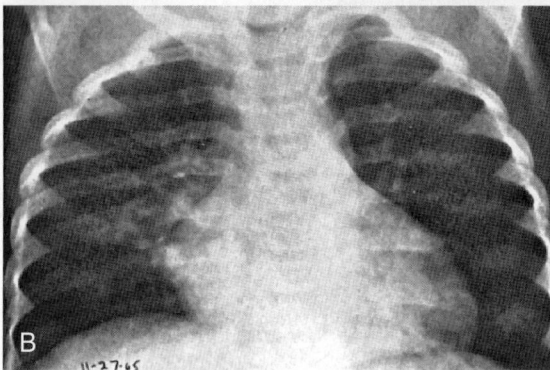

Figure 402-3 Appearance over a period of 5 days of a large multi-loculated pneumonocele in a segment of alveolar consolidation. **A,** There is a large cavity with 2 air–fluid levels in a segment of alveolar pneumonia in the right upper lobe. **B,** Five days later, the cavity and most of the pneumonic consolidation have disappeared. *(From Silverman FN, Kuhn JP: Essentials of Caffey's pediatric x-ray diagnosis, Chicago, 1990, Year Book, p. 303.)*

Chapter 403
Cystic Fibrosis

Marie E. Egan, Deanna M. Green, and Judith A. Voynow

Cystic fibrosis (CF) is an inherited multisystem disorder of children and adults; it is the most common life-limiting recessive genetic trait among whites. Dysfunction of the *cystic fibrosis transmembrane conductance regulator protein* (CFTR), the primary defect, leads to a wide and variable array of presenting manifestations and complications.

CF is responsible for most cases of exocrine pancreatic insufficiency in early life and is the major cause of severe chronic lung disease in children. It is also responsible for many cases of hyponatremic salt depletion, nasal polyposis, pansinusitis, rectal prolapse, pancreatitis, cholelithiasis, and nonautoimmune insulin-dependent hyperglycemia. Because CF may manifest as failure to thrive and, occasionally, as cirrhosis or other forms of hepatic dysfunction, this disorder enters into the differential diagnosis of many pediatric conditions (Table 403-1).

GENETICS
CF occurs most frequently in white populations of northern Europe, North America, and Australia/New Zealand. The prevalence in these populations varies but approximates 1 in 3,500 live births (1 in 9,200 individuals of Hispanic descent and 1 in 15,000 African-Americans). Although less frequent in African, Hispanic, Middle Eastern, South Asian, and eastern Asian populations, the disorder does exist in these populations as well (Fig. 403-1).

Table 403-1	Complications of Cystic Fibrosis

RESPIRATORY
Bronchiectasis, bronchitis, bronchiolitis, pneumonia
Atelectasis
Hemoptysis
Pneumothorax
Nasal polyps
Sinusitis
Reactive airway disease
Cor pulmonale
Respiratory failure
Mucoid impaction of the bronchi
Allergic bronchopulmonary aspergillosis

GASTROINTESTINAL
Meconium ileus, meconium plug (neonate)
Meconium peritonitis (neonate)
Distal intestinal obstruction syndrome (non-neonatal obstruction)
Rectal prolapse
Intussusception
Volvulus
Fibrosing colonopathy (strictures)
Appendicitis
Intestinal atresia
Pancreatitis
Biliary cirrhosis (portal hypertension: esophageal varices, hypersplenism)
Neonatal obstructive jaundice
Hepatic steatosis
Gastroesophageal reflux
Cholelithiasis
Inguinal hernia
Growth failure (malabsorption)
Vitamin deficiency states (vitamins A, K, E, D)
Insulin deficiency, symptomatic hyperglycemia, diabetes
Malignancy (rare)

OTHER
Infertility
Delayed puberty
Edema-hypoproteinemia
Dehydration–heat exhaustion
Hypertrophic osteoarthropathy-arthritis
Clubbing
Amyloidosis
Diabetes mellitus
Aquagenic palmoplantar keratoderma (skin wrinkling)

Adapted from Silverman FN, Kuhn JP: Essentials of Caffey's pediatric x-ray diagnosis, Chicago, 1990, Year Book, p. 649.

CF is inherited as an autosomal recessive trait. The CF gene codes for the CFTR protein, which is 1,480 amino acids. CFTR is expressed largely in epithelial cells of airways, the gastrointestinal tract (including the pancreas and biliary system), the sweat glands, and the genitourinary system. CFTR is a member of the adenosine triphosphate–binding cassette superfamily of proteins. It functions as a chloride channel and has other regulatory functions that are perturbed variably by the different mutations. More than 1,900 *CFTR* polymorphisms grouped into 5 main classes of mutations that affect protein function are associated with the CF syndrome (Table 403-2). The most prevalent mutation of *CFTR* is the deletion of a single phenylalanine residue at amino acid 508 (F508del). This mutation is responsible for the high incidence of CF in northern European populations and is considerably less frequent in other populations, such as those of southern Europe and Israel. Approximately 50% of individuals with CF who are of northern European ancestry are homozygous for F508del, and more than 80% carry at least 1 F508del gene. Remaining patients have an extensive array of mutations, none of which has a prevalence of more than several percentage points, except in certain populations; for example, the W1282X mutation occurs in 60% of Ashkenazi Jews with CF. The relationship between CFTR genotype and clinical phenotype is

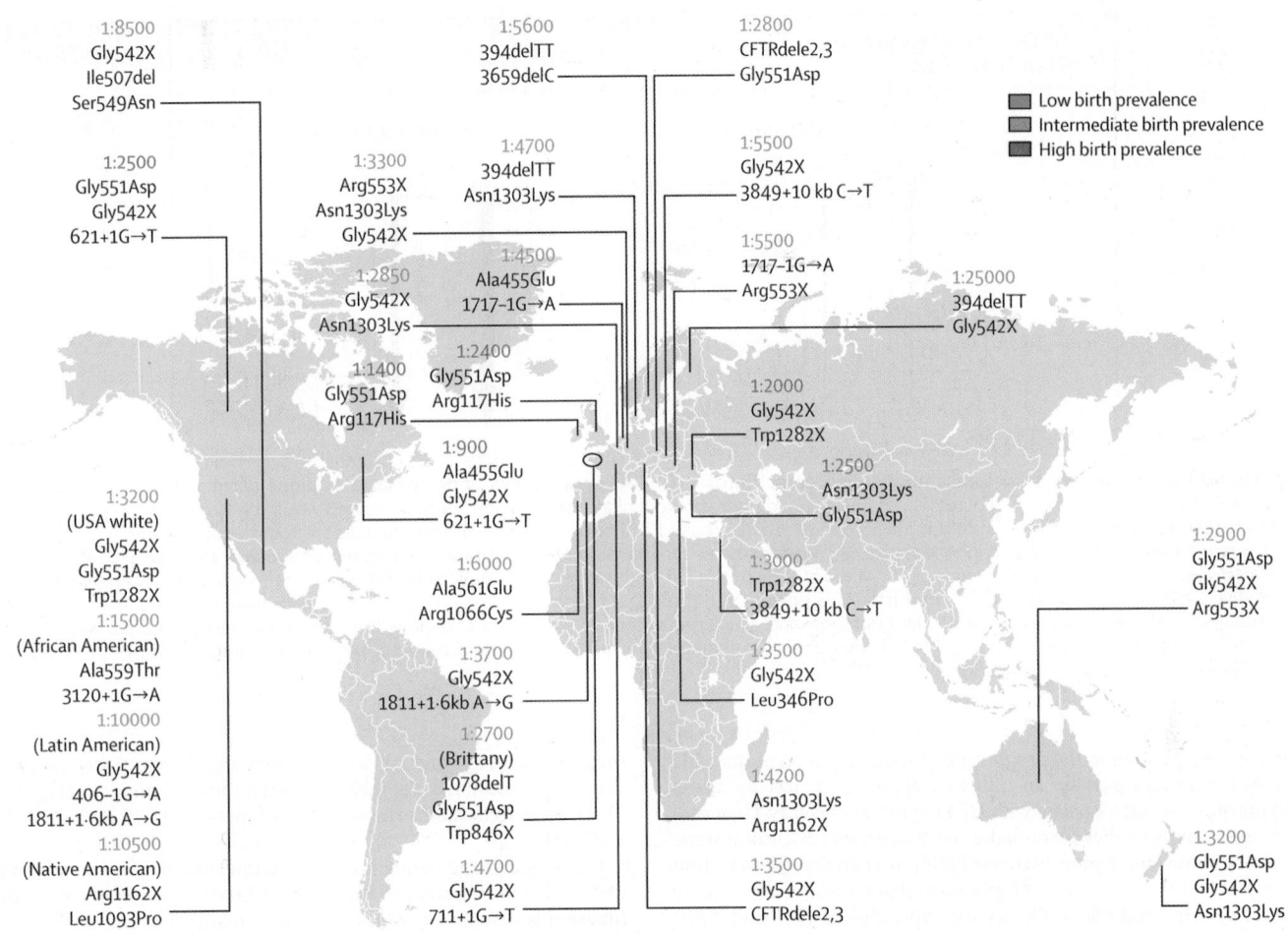

Figure 403-1 Approximate cystic fibrosis birth prevalence and common mutations for selected countries. Birth prevalence is reported as number of live births per case of cystic fibrosis. Common/important mutations in each region are listed below the prevalence figures. The birth prevalence can vary greatly among ethnic groups in a country. *(From O'Sullivan BP, Freedman SD: Cystic fibrosis, Lancet 373:1891–1902, 2009.)*

Table 403-2	One Proposed Classification of Cystic Fibrosis Transmembrane Conductance Regulator (CFTR) Mutations		
CLASS	**EFFECT ON CFTR**	**FUNCTIONAL CFTR PRESENT?**	**SAMPLE MUTATIONS**
I	Lack of protein production	No	Stop codons (designation in X; e.g., Trp1282X, Gly542X); splicing defects with no protein production (e.g., 711+1G→T, 1717-1G→A)
II	Defect in protein trafficking with ubiquitination and degradation in endoplasmic reticulum/Golgi body	No/substantially reduced	Phe508del, Asn1303Lys, Gly85Gly, leu1065Pro, Asp507, Ser549Arg
III	Defective regulation; CFTR not activated by adenosine triphosphate or cyclic adenosine monophosphate	No (nonfunction CFTR present in apical membrane)	Gly551Asp, Ser492Phe, Val520Phe, Arg553Gly, Arg560Thr, Arg560Ser
IV	Reduced chloride transport through CFTR at the apical membrane	Yes	Ala455Glu, Arg117Cys, Asp1152His, Leu227Arg, Arg334Trp, Arg117His*
V	Splicing defect with reduced production of CFTR	Yes	3849+10kbC→T, 1811+16kbA→G, IVS8-5T, 2789+5G→A

*Function of Arg117His depends on the length of the polythymidine track on the same chromosome in intron 8 (IVS8): 5T, 7T, or 9T. There is more normal CFTR function with a longer polythymidine track.

From O'Sullivan BP, Freedman SD: Cystic fibrosis, Lancet 373:1891–1902, 2009.

highly complex and is not predictable for individual patients. Mutations categorized as "severe" are associated almost uniformly with pancreatic insufficiency but only in general with more rapid progression of lung disease. *A few mutations, such as 3849 + 10kbC→T, are found in patients with normal sweat chloride concentrations.* Some individuals with polymorphisms of both *CFTR* genes have few or no CF

manifestations until adolescence or adulthood, when they present with pancreatitis, sinusitis, diffuse bronchiectasis, or male infertility. Whereas *CFTR* mutations are a sine qua non for CF, 2 mutations of *CFTR* can cause disorders that do not meet diagnostic criteria for CF and, occasionally, do not cause discernible clinical problems. Non-CFTR modifier gene polymorphisms appear to be responsible for

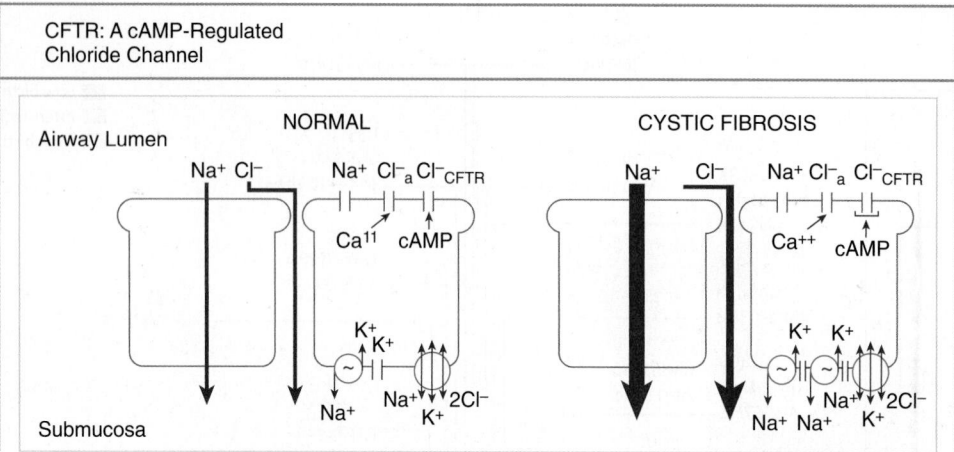

Figure 403-2 The net ion flow across normal and cystic fibrosis (CF) airway epithelia under basal conditions *(large arrows)*. Because water follows salt movement, the predicted net flux of water would be from the airway lumen to the submucosa and would be greater across CF epithelia. The increased Na^+ absorption by CF cells is associated with an increased amiloride-sensitive Na^+ conductance across the apical (luminal) membrane and increased Na^+,K^+-adenosine triphosphatase (ATPase) sites at the basolateral membrane. The cyclic adenosine monophosphate (cAMP)–mediated apical membrane conductance of Cl^- associated with the CF transmembrane regulator (CFTR) does not function in CF epithelia, but an alternative, calcium (Ca^{++})–activated Cl^- conductance is present in normal and CF cells. It is postulated that CF cells have a limited ability to secrete Cl^- and absorb $Na+$ in excessive amounts, limiting the water available to hydrate secretions and allow them to be cleared from the airways lumen. Cl^-a, Ca^{++}–activated Cl^- conductance: Cl^-CTFR, the CFTR Cl^- channel. *(From Knowles MR: Contemporary perspectives on the pathogenesis of cystic fibrosis, New Insights Cystic Fibrosis 1:1, 1993.)*

much of the variation in the progression of lung disease. Genomewide association studies provide an unbiased approach to test for novel polymorphisms that associate with CF lung disease severity. Genomewide association studies identified a polymorphism on chromosome 11 in the intergenic region between EHF (an epithelial transcription factor) and APIP (an inhibitor of apoptosis) that is associated with lung disease severity, and may influence the expression of *EHF* and *APIP*, as well as other genes in the region, including *PDHX, CD44*, and *ELF5*. A region on chromosome 20 was also found to relate to lung disease severity. This region encompasses several genes (*MC3R, CASS4, AURKA*) that may play a role in lung host-defense involving neutrophil function, apoptosis, and phagocytosis. Genomewide association studies analysis also identified genetic regions that predispose to risk for liver disease, CF-related diabetes, and meconium ileus.

Through the use of probes for 40 of the most common mutations, the genotype of 80-90% of Americans with CF can be ascertained. Genotyping using a discreet panel of mutation probes is quick and less costly than more comprehensive sequencing and is commercially available. In special cases, sequencing the entire *CFTR* gene is necessary to establish the genotype. This procedure is also available commercially and can identify polymorphisms and unique mutations of unknown clinical importance.

The high frequency of *CFTR* mutations has been ascribed to resistance to the morbidity and mortality associated with infectious dysenteries through the ages. In support of this hypothesis, cultured CF intestinal epithelial cells homozygous for the F508del mutation are unresponsive to the secretory effects of cholera toxin. CFTR heterozygous mice experience less mortality when treated with cholera toxin than their unaffected wild type littermates.

PATHOGENESIS

A number of long-standing observations of CF are of fundamental pathophysiologic importance; they include failure to clear mucous secretions, a paucity of water in mucous secretions, an elevated salt content of sweat and other serous secretions, and chronic infection limited to the respiratory tract. Additionally, there is a greater negative potential difference across the respiratory epithelia of patients with CF than across the respiratory epithelia of control subjects. Aberrant electrical properties are also demonstrated for CF sweat gland duct and rectal epithelia. The membranes of CF epithelial cells are unable to secrete chloride ions in response to cyclic adenosine monophosphate–

mediated signals, and at least in the respiratory tract, excessive amounts of sodium are absorbed through these membranes (Fig. 403-2). These defects can be traced to a dysfunction of CFTR (Figs. 403-3 and 403-4).

Cyclic adenosine monophosphate–stimulated protein kinase A regulation of chloride conductance is the primary function of CFTR; this function is absent in epithelial cells with many different mutations of the *CFTR* gene. *CFTR* mutations fall into 5 classes in another classification system, albeit with some overlap (see Fig. 403-4). Individuals with classes I, II, and III mutations, on average, have shorter survival than those with "mild" genotypes (class IV or V). The clinical importance of these functional categories is limited because they do not uniformly correlate with specific clinical features or their severity. Rather, clinical features correlate with the residual CFTR activity.

Many hypotheses have been postulated to explain how CFTR dysfunction results in the clinical phenotype. It is likely that no one hypothesis explains the full spectrum of disease. Most believe that the epithelial pathophysiology in airways involves an inability to secrete salt and secondarily to secrete water in the presence of excessive reabsorption of salt and water. The proposed outcome is insufficient water on the airway surface to hydrate secretions. Desiccated secretions become more viscous and elastic (rubbery) and are harder to clear by mucociliary and other mechanisms. In addition it has been suggested that CFTR dysfunction results in an altered microenvironment with low HCO_3^- and a more acidic pH, thus altering mucus rheology and aggravating poor mucociliary clearance. The result is that these secretions are retained and obstruct airways, starting with those of the smallest caliber, the bronchioles. Airflow obstruction at the level of small airways is the earliest observable physiologic abnormality of the respiratory system.

It is plausible that similar pathophysiologic events take place in the pancreatic and biliary ducts (and in the vas deferens), leading to desiccation of proteinaceous secretions and obstruction. Because the function of sweat gland duct cells is to absorb rather than secrete chloride, salt is not retrieved from the isotonic primary sweat as it is transported to the skin surface; chloride and sodium levels are consequently elevated.

Chronic infection in CF is limited to the airways. A likely explanation for infection is a sequence of events starting with failure to clear inhaled bacteria promptly and then proceeding to persistent colonization and an inflammatory response in airway walls. In addition, it has

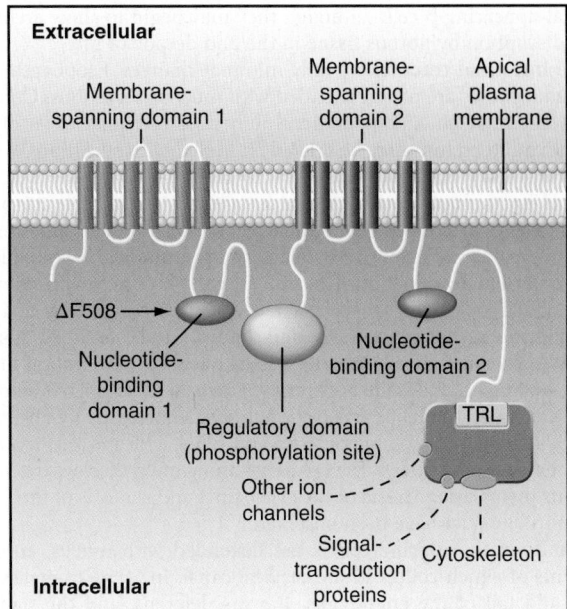

Figure 403-3 Hypothesized structure of cystic fibrosis transmembrane regulator (CFTR). The protein contains 1,480 amino acids and a number of discrete globular and transmembrane domains. Activation of CFTR relies on phosphorylation, particularly through protein kinase A but probably involving other kinases as well. Channel activity is governed by the 2 nucleotide-binding domains, which regulate channel gating. The carboxyl terminal (consisting of threonine, arginine, and leucine [TRL]) of CFTR is anchored through a PDZ-type binding interaction with the cytoskeleton and is kept in close approximation *(dashed lines)* to a number of important proteins. These associated proteins influence CFTR functions, including conductance, regulation of other channels, signal transduction, and localization at the apical plasma membrane. Each membrane-spanning domain contains 6 membrane-spanning α helixes, portions of which form a chloride-conductance pore. The regulatory domain is a site of protein kinase A phosphorylation. The common F508del mutation occurs on the surface of nucleotide-binding domain 1. *(From Rowe SM, Miller S, Sorscher EJ: Cystic fibrosis, N Engl J Med 352:1992–2001, 2005.)*

been proposed that abnormal CFTR creates a proinflammatory state or amplifies the inflammatory response to initial infections (viral or bacterial). Some investigators have identified primary differences in CF-affected immune cells and have suggested that these alterations contribute to this proinflammatory state. It appears that inflammatory events occur first in small airways, perhaps because clearance of altered secretions and microorganisms from these regions is more difficult. Chronic bronchiolitis and bronchitis are the initial lung manifestations (see Chapter 391), but after months to years, structural changes in airway walls produce bronchiolectasis and bronchiectasis. The agents of airway injury include neutrophil products, such as oxidative radicals and proteases, and immune reaction products. With advanced lung disease, infection may extend to peribronchial lung parenchyma.

A finding that is not readily explained by CFTR dysfunction is the high prevalence in patients with CF of airway colonization with *Staphylococcus aureus* (see Chapter 181.1), *Pseudomonas aeruginosa* (see Chapter 205.1), and *Burkholderia cepacia* complex (see Chapter 205.2), organisms that rarely infect the lungs of other individuals. It has been postulated that the CF airway epithelial cells or surface liquids may provide a favorable environment for harboring these organisms. CF airway epithelium may be compromised in its innate defenses against these organisms, through either acquired or genetic alterations. Antimicrobial activity is diminished in CF secretions; this diminution may be related to hyperacidic surface liquids or other effects on innate immunity. Another puzzle is the propensity for *P. aeruginosa* to undergo mucoid transformation in the CF airways. The complex polysaccharide produced by these organisms generates a biofilm that

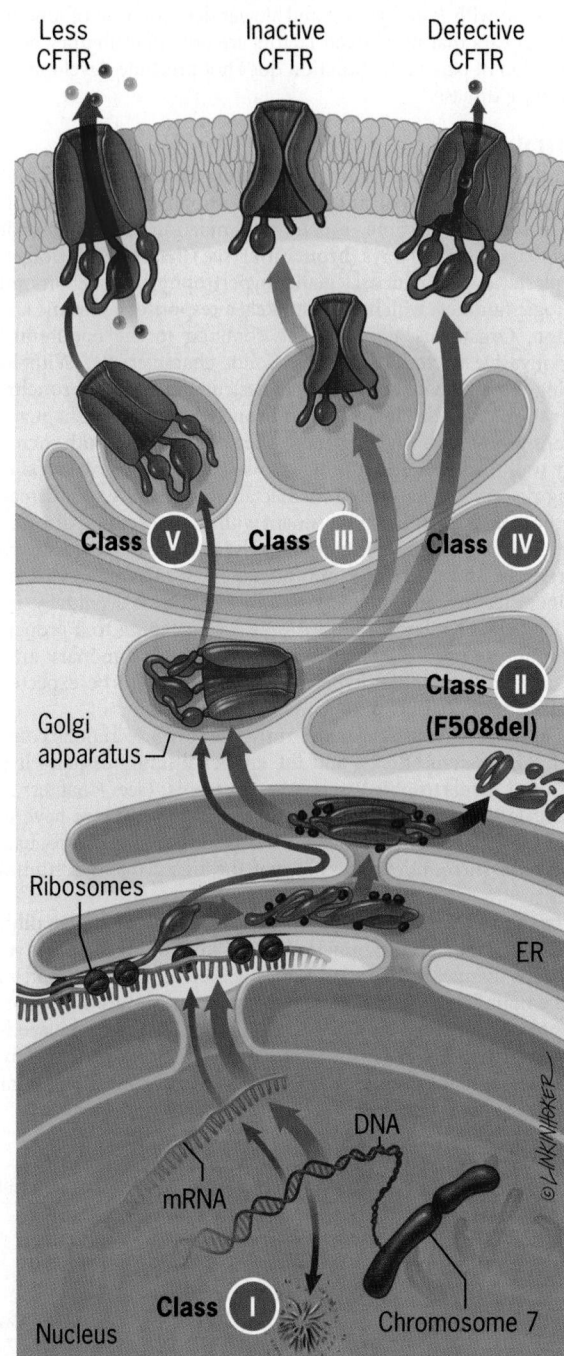

Figure 403-4 Classes of *CFTR* (cystic fibrosis transmembrane regulator) mutations. Classes of defects in the *CFTR* gene include the absence of synthesis (class I); defective protein maturation and premature degradation (class II); disordered regulation, such as diminished adenosine triphosphate (ATP) binding and hydrolysis (class III); defective chloride conductance or channel gating (class IV); and a reduced number of CFTR transcripts due to a promoter or splicing abnormality (class V) *(Copyright Michael Linkinhoker, Link Studio.)*

provides a hypoxic environment and thereby protects *Pseudomonas* against antimicrobial agents.

Nutritional deficits, including fatty acid deficiency, have been implicated as predisposing factors for respiratory tract infection. More specifically, concentrations of lipoxins—molecules that suppress neutrophilic inflammation—are suppressed in CF airways. Supporting this idea is the observation that the 10-15% of individuals with CF who retain substantial exocrine pancreatic function have delayed onset of colonization with *P. aeruginosa* and slower deterioration of lung function. It appears that nutritional factors are only contributory because preservation of pancreatic function does not preclude development of typical lung disease.

PATHOLOGY

The earliest pathologic lesion in the lung is that of **bronchiolitis** (mucous plugging and an inflammatory response in the walls of the small airways); with time, mucus accumulation and inflammation extend to the larger airways (**bronchitis**) (see Chapter 391). Goblet cell hyperplasia and submucosal gland hypertrophy become prominent pathologic findings, which is most likely a response to chronic airway infection. Organisms appear to be confined to the endobronchial space; invasive bacterial infection is not characteristic. With long-standing disease, evidence of airway destruction such as **bronchiolar obliteration, bronchiolectasis,** and **bronchiectasis** (see Chapter 401) becomes prominent. Imaging modalities demonstrate both increased airway wall thickness and luminal cross-sectional area relatively early in lung disease evaluation. Bronchiectatic cysts and emphysematous bullae or subpleural blebs are frequent with advanced lung disease, the upper lobes being most commonly involved. These enlarged air spaces may rupture and cause pneumothorax. Interstitial disease is not a prominent feature, although areas of fibrosis appear eventually. Bronchial arteries are enlarged and tortuous, contributing to a propensity for **hemoptysis** in bronchiectatic airways. Small pulmonary arteries eventually display medial hypertrophy, which would be expected in secondary pulmonary hypertension.

The **paranasal sinuses** are uniformly filled with secretions containing inflammatory products, and the epithelial lining displays hyperplastic and hypertrophied secretory elements (see Chapter 380). Polypoid lesions within the sinuses and erosion of bone have been reported. The nasal mucosa may form large or multiple polyps, usually from a base surrounding the ostia of the maxillary and ethmoidal sinuses.

The **pancreas** is usually small, occasionally cystic, and often difficult to find at postmortem examination. The extent of involvement varies at birth. In infants, the acini and ducts are often distended and filled with eosinophilic material. In 85-90% of patients, the lesion progresses to complete or almost complete disruption of acini and replacement with fibrous tissue and fat. Infrequently, foci of calcification may be seen on radiographs of the abdomen. The islets of Langerhans contain normal-appearing β cells, although they may begin to show architectural disruption by fibrous tissue in the 2nd decade of life.

The **intestinal tract** shows only minimal changes. Esophageal and duodenal glands are often distended with mucous secretions. Concretions may form in the appendiceal lumen or cecum. Crypts of the appendix and rectum may be dilated and filled with secretions.

Focal biliary cirrhosis secondary to blockage of intrahepatic bile ducts is uncommon in early life, although it is responsible for occasional cases of prolonged neonatal jaundice. This lesion becomes much more prevalent and extensive with age and is found in 70% of patients at postmortem examination. This process can proceed to symptomatic multilobular biliary cirrhosis that has a distinctive pattern of large irregular parenchymal nodules and interspersed bands of fibrous tissue. Approximately 30-70% of patients have fatty infiltration of the liver, in some cases despite apparently adequate nutrition. At autopsy, hepatic congestion secondary to cor pulmonale is frequently observed. The gallbladder may be hypoplastic and filled with mucoid material and often contains stones. The epithelial lining often displays extensive mucous metaplasia. Atresia of the cystic duct and stenosis of the distal common bile duct have been observed.

Glands of the **uterine cervix** are distended with mucus, copious amounts of which collect in the cervical canal. In >95% of males, the body and tail of the epididymis, the vas deferens, and the seminal vesicles are obliterated or atretic, resulting in male infertility.

CLINICAL MANIFESTATIONS

Mutational heterogeneity and environmental factors appear responsible for highly variable involvement of the lungs, pancreas, and other organs. A list of presenting manifestations is lengthy, although pulmonary and gastrointestinal presentations predominate (Fig. 403-5). With inclusion of CF newborn screening panels, an increasing proportion of children are diagnosed before symptoms appear.

Respiratory Tract

Cough is the most constant symptom of pulmonary involvement. At first, the cough may be dry and hacking, but eventually it becomes loose and productive. In older patients, the cough is most prominent upon arising in the morning or after activity. Expectorated mucus is usually purulent. Some patients remain asymptomatic for long periods or seem to have prolonged but intermittent acute respiratory infections. Others acquire a chronic cough in the 1st few wk of life, or they

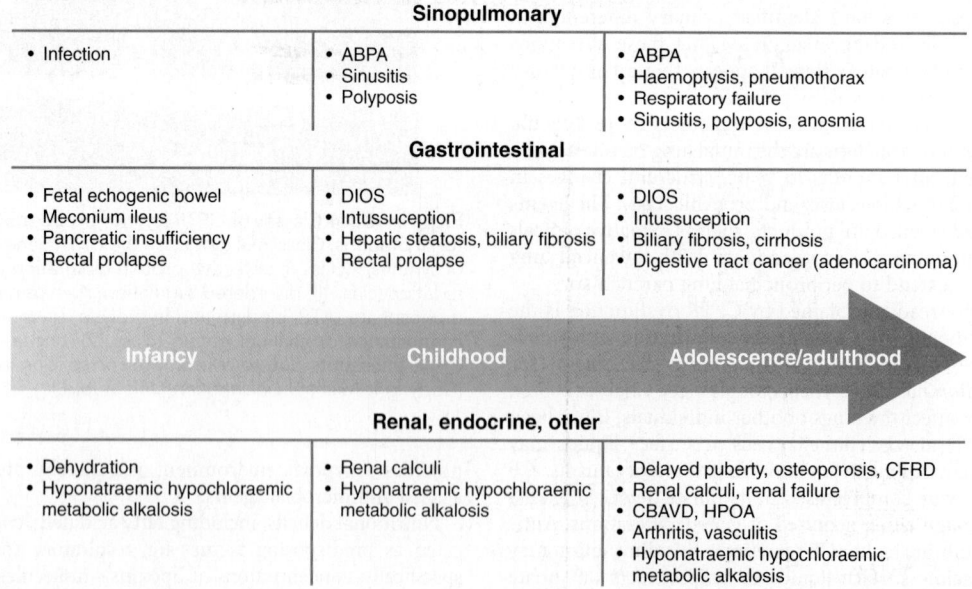

Figure 403-5 Approximate age of onset of clinical manifestations of cystic fibrosis. *ABPA,* allergic bronchopulmonary aspergillosis; *CBAVD,* congenital bilateral absence of the vas deferens; *CFRD,* cystic fibrosis-related diabetes mellitus; *DIOS,* distal intestinal obstruction syndrome; *HPOA,* hypertrophic pulmonary osteoarthritis. *(From O'Sullivan BP, Freedman SD: Cystic fibrosis,* Lancet *373:1891–1902, 2009.)*

have pneumonia repeatedly. Extensive bronchiolitis accompanied by wheezing is a frequent symptom during the 1st few yr of life. As lung disease slowly progresses, exercise intolerance, shortness of breath, and failure to gain weight or grow are noted. Exacerbations of lung symptoms, presumably owing to more active airways infection, often require repeated hospitalizations for effective treatment. Cor pulmonale, respiratory failure, and death eventually supervene unless lung transplantation is accomplished. Colonization with *B. cepacia* and other multidrug-resistant organisms may be associated with particularly rapid pulmonary deterioration and death.

The rate of progression of lung disease is the chief determinant of morbidity and mortality. The course of lung disease is largely independent of genotype. Male gender and exocrine pancreatic sufficiency are also associated with a slower rate of pulmonary function decline.

Early **physical findings** include increased anteroposterior diameter of the chest, generalized hyperresonance, scattered or localized coarse crackles, and digital clubbing. Expiratory wheezes may be heard, especially in young children. Cyanosis is a late sign. Common pulmonary complications include atelectasis, hemoptysis, pneumothorax, and cor pulmonale; these usually appear beyond the 1st decade of life.

Even though the paranasal sinuses are virtually always opacified radiographically, acute sinusitis is infrequent. Nasal obstruction and rhinorrhea are common, caused by inflamed, swollen mucous membranes or, in some cases, nasal polyposis. **Nasal polyps** are most troublesome between 5 and 20 yr of age.

Intestinal Tract

In 10-15% of newborn infants with CF, the ileum is completely obstructed by meconium (**meconium ileus**). The frequency is greater (≈30%) among siblings born subsequent to a child with meconium ileus and is particularly striking in monozygotic twins, reflecting a genetic contribution from 1 or more modifying genes. Abdominal distention, emesis, and failure to pass meconium appear in the 1st 24-48 hr of life (see Chapters 102.1 and 330.2). Abdominal radiographs (Fig. 403-6) show dilated loops of bowel with air–fluid levels and, frequently, a collection of granular, "ground-glass" material in the lower central abdomen. Rarely, **meconium peritonitis** results from intrauterine rupture of the bowel wall and can be detected radiographically as the presence of peritoneal or scrotal calcifications. **Meconium plug syndrome** occurs with increased frequency in infants with CF but is

less specific than meconium ileus. Ileal obstruction with fecal material *(distal intestinal obstruction syndrome)* occurs in older patients, causing cramping abdominal pain and abdominal distention.

More than 85% of affected children show evidence of protein and fat malabsorption from exocrine pancreatic insufficiency. Symptoms include frequent, bulky, greasy stools and failure to gain weight even when food intake appears to be large. Characteristically, stools contain readily visible droplets of fat. A protuberant abdomen, decreased muscle mass, poor growth, and delayed maturation are typical physical signs. Excessive flatus may be a problem. A number of mutations are associated with preservation of some exocrine pancreatic function, including R117H and 3849 + 10kbC→T. Virtually all individuals homozygous for F508del have pancreatic insufficiency.

Less-common gastrointestinal manifestations include intussusception, fecal impaction of the cecum with an asymptomatic right lower quadrant mass, and epigastric pain owing to duodenal inflammation. Acid or bile reflux with esophagitis symptoms is common in older children and adults. Subacute appendicitis and periappendiceal abscess have been encountered. Historically a relatively common event, rectal prolapse occurs much less frequently as the result of earlier diagnosis and initiation of pancreatic enzyme replacement therapy. Occasionally, hypoproteinemia with anasarca appears in malnourished infants, especially if children are fed soy-based preparations. Neurologic dysfunction (dementia, peripheral neuropathy) and hemolytic anemia may occur because of **vitamin E deficiency.** Deficiency of other fat-soluble vitamins is occasionally symptomatic. **Hypoprothrombinemia** caused by vitamin K deficiency may result in a bleeding diathesis. Clinical manifestations of other fat-soluble vitamin deficiencies, such as decreased bone density and night blindness, have been noted. Rickets is rare.

Biliary Tract

Evidence for liver dysfunction is most often detected in the 1st 15 yr of life and can be found in up to 30% of individuals. Biliary cirrhosis becomes symptomatic in only 5-7% of patients. Manifestations can include icterus, ascites, hematemesis from esophageal varices, and evidence of hypersplenism. A neonatal hepatitis-like picture and massive hepatomegaly owing to steatosis have been reported. Biliary colic secondary to cholelithiasis may occur in the 2nd decade or later. Liver disease occurs independent of genotype but is associated with meconium ileus and pancreatic insufficiency.

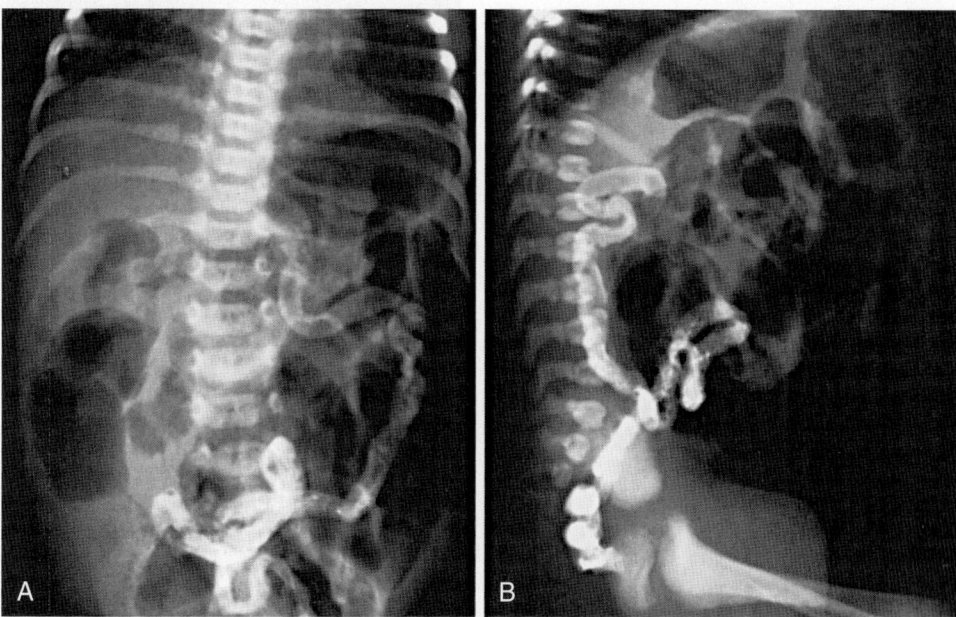

Figure 403-6 A and **B,** Contrast enema study in a newborn infant with abdominal distention and failure to pass meconium. Notice the small diameter of the sigmoid and ascending colon and dilated, air-filled loops of small intestine. Several air–fluid levels in the small bowel are visible on the upright lateral view.

Cystic Fibrosis–Related Diabetes and Pancreatitis

In addition to exocrine pancreatic insufficiency, evidence for hyperglycemia and glucosuria, including polyuria and weight loss, may appear, especially in the 2nd decade of life. Ketoacidosis usually does not occur, but eye, kidney, and other vascular complications have been noted in patients living ≥10 yr after the onset of hyperglycemia. Recurrent, acute pancreatitis occurs occasionally in individuals who have residual exocrine pancreatic function and may be the sole manifestation of 2 *CFTR* mutations.

Genitourinary Tract

Sexual development is often delayed but only by an average of 2 yr. More than 95% of males are azoospermic because of failure of development of wolffian duct structures, but sexual function is generally unimpaired. The incidence of inguinal hernia, hydrocele, and undescended testis is higher than expected. Adolescent females may experience secondary amenorrhea, especially with exacerbations of pulmonary disease. The female fertility rate is diminished. Pregnancy is generally tolerated well by women with good pulmonary function but may accelerate pulmonary progression in those with moderate or advanced lung problems. Urinary incontinence associated with cough occurs in 18-47% of female children and adolescents.

Sweat Glands

Excessive loss of salt in the sweat predisposes young children to salt depletion episodes, especially during episodes of gastroenteritis and during warm weather. These children present with **hypochloremic alkalosis.** Hyponatremia is a risk particularly in warm climates. Frequently, parents notice salt "frosting" of the skin or a salty taste when they kiss the child. A few genotypes are associated with normal sweat chloride values.

DIAGNOSIS AND ASSESSMENT

The diagnosis of CF has been based on a positive quantitative sweat test (Cl⁻ ≥60 mEq/L) in conjunction with 1 or more of the following features: typical chronic obstructive pulmonary disease, documented exocrine pancreatic insufficiency, and a positive family history. With newborn screening, diagnosis is often made prior to obvious clinical manifestations such as failure to thrive and chronic cough. Diagnostic criteria have been recommended to include additional testing procedures (Table 403-3).

Sweat Testing

The sweat test, which involves using pilocarpine iontophoresis to collect sweat and performing chemical analysis of its chloride content, is the standard approach to diagnosis of CF. The procedure requires care and accuracy. An electric current is used to carry pilocarpine into the skin of the forearm and locally stimulate the sweat glands. If an

adequate amount of sweat is collected, the specimens are analyzed for chloride concentration. Testing may be difficult in the 1st 2 wk of life because of low sweat rates but is recommended any time after the 1st 48 hr of life. Positive results should be confirmed; for a negative result, the test should be repeated if suspicion of the diagnosis remains.

More than 60 mEq/L of chloride in sweat is diagnostic of CF when 1 or more other criteria are present. Threshold levels of 30-40 mEq/L for infants have been suggested. Borderline (or intermediate) values of 40-60 mEq/L have been reported in patients of all ages who have CF with atypical involvement and require further testing. Chloride concentrations in sweat are somewhat lower in individuals who retain exocrine pancreatic function but usually remain within the diagnostic range. Table 403-4 lists the conditions associated with false-negative and false-positive sweat test results.

DNA Testing

Several commercial laboratories test for 30-96 of the most common *CFTR* mutations. This testing identifies ≥90% of individuals who carry 2 CF mutations. Some children with typical CF manifestations are found to have 1 or no detectable mutations by this methodology. Some laboratories perform comprehensive mutation analysis screening for all of the >1,900 identified mutations.

Other Diagnostic Tests

The finding of increased potential differences across nasal epithelium (nasal potential difference) that is the increased voltage response to topical amiloride application, followed by the absence of a voltage response to a β-adrenergic agonist, has been used to confirm the diagnosis of CF in patients with equivocal or frankly normal sweat chloride values.

Pancreatic Function

Exocrine pancreatic dysfunction is clinically apparent in many patients. Documentation is desirable if there are questions about the functional status of the pancreas. The diagnosis of pancreatic malabsorption can be made by the quantification of elastase-1 activity in a fresh stool sample by an enzyme-linked immunosorbent assay specific for human elastase. To determine the degree of fat malabsorption, a 72 hr stool

Table 403-3	Diagnostic Criteria for Cystic Fibrosis (CF)

Presence of typical clinical features (respiratory, gastrointestinal, or genitourinary)
or
A history of CF in a sibling
or
A positive newborn screening test
plus
Laboratory evidence for CFTR (CF transmembrane regulator) dysfunction:
  Two elevated sweat chloride concentrations obtained on separate days
  or
  Identification of two CF mutations
  or
  An abnormal nasal potential difference measurement

Table 403-4	Conditions Associated with False-Positive and False-Negative Sweat Test Results

WITH FALSE-POSITIVE RESULTS
Eczema (atopic dermatitis)
Ectodermal dysplasia
Malnutrition/failure to thrive/deprivation
Anorexia nervosa
Congenital adrenal hyperplasia
Adrenal insufficiency
Glucose-6-phosphatase deficiency
Mauriac syndrome
Fucosidosis
Familial hypoparathyroidism
Hypothyroidism
Nephrogenic diabetes insipidus
Pseudohypoaldosteronism
Klinefelter syndrome
Familial cholestasis syndrome
Autonomic dysfunction
Prostaglandin E infusions
Munchausen syndrome by proxy

WITH FALSE-NEGATIVE RESULTS
Dilution
Malnutrition
Edema
Insufficient sweat quantity
Hyponatremia
Cystic fibrosis transmembrane conductance regulator mutations with preserved sweat duct function

collection is performed for total fat quantitation with a simultaneous diet history to determine a coefficient of fat absorption. Normal fat absorption is greater than 93% of fat ingestion. Endocrine pancreatic dysfunction may be more prevalent than previously recognized. Cystic fibrosis–related diabetes affects approximately 19% of adolescents and 40-50% of adults. Many authorities advocate yearly monitoring with a modified 2 hr oral glucose tolerance test after 10 yr of age. This approach is more sensitive than spot checks of blood and urine glucose levels and glycosylated hemoglobin levels.

Radiology

Pulmonary radiologic findings suggest the diagnosis but are not specific. Hyperinflation of lungs occurs early and may be overlooked in the absence of infiltrates or streaky densities. Bronchial thickening and plugging and ring shadows suggesting bronchiectasis usually appear first in the upper lobes. Nodular densities, patchy atelectasis, and confluent infiltrate follow. Hilar lymph nodes may be prominent. With advanced disease, impressive hyperinflation with markedly depressed diaphragms, anterior bowing of the sternum, and a narrow cardiac shadow are noted. Cyst formation, extensive bronchiectasis, dilated pulmonary artery segments, and segmental or lobar atelectasis is often apparent with advanced disease. Figure 403-7 shows typical progres-

sion of lung disease. Most CF centers obtain chest radiographs (posteroanterior [PA] and lateral) at least annually. Standardized scoring of roentgenographic changes has been used to follow progression of lung disease. CT of the chest can detect and localize thickening of bronchial airway walls, mucous plugging, focal hyperinflation, and early bronchiectasis (Fig. 403-8); it is generally not used for routine evaluation of chest disease. Many children with normal lung function have bronchiectasis on CT, indicating that this imaging modality is sensitive to early lung changes.

Radiographs of paranasal sinuses reveal panopacification and, often, failure of frontal sinus development. CT provides better resolution of sinus changes if this information is required clinically. Fetal ultrasonography may suggest ileal obstruction with meconium early in the 2nd trimester, but this finding is not predictive of meconium ileus at birth.

Pulmonary Function

Standard pulmonary function studies are not obtained until patients are 4-6 yr of age, by which time many patients show the typical pattern of obstructive pulmonary involvement (see Chapter 384). Decrease in the midmaximal flow rate is an early functional change, reflecting small airway obstruction. This lesion also affects the distribution of

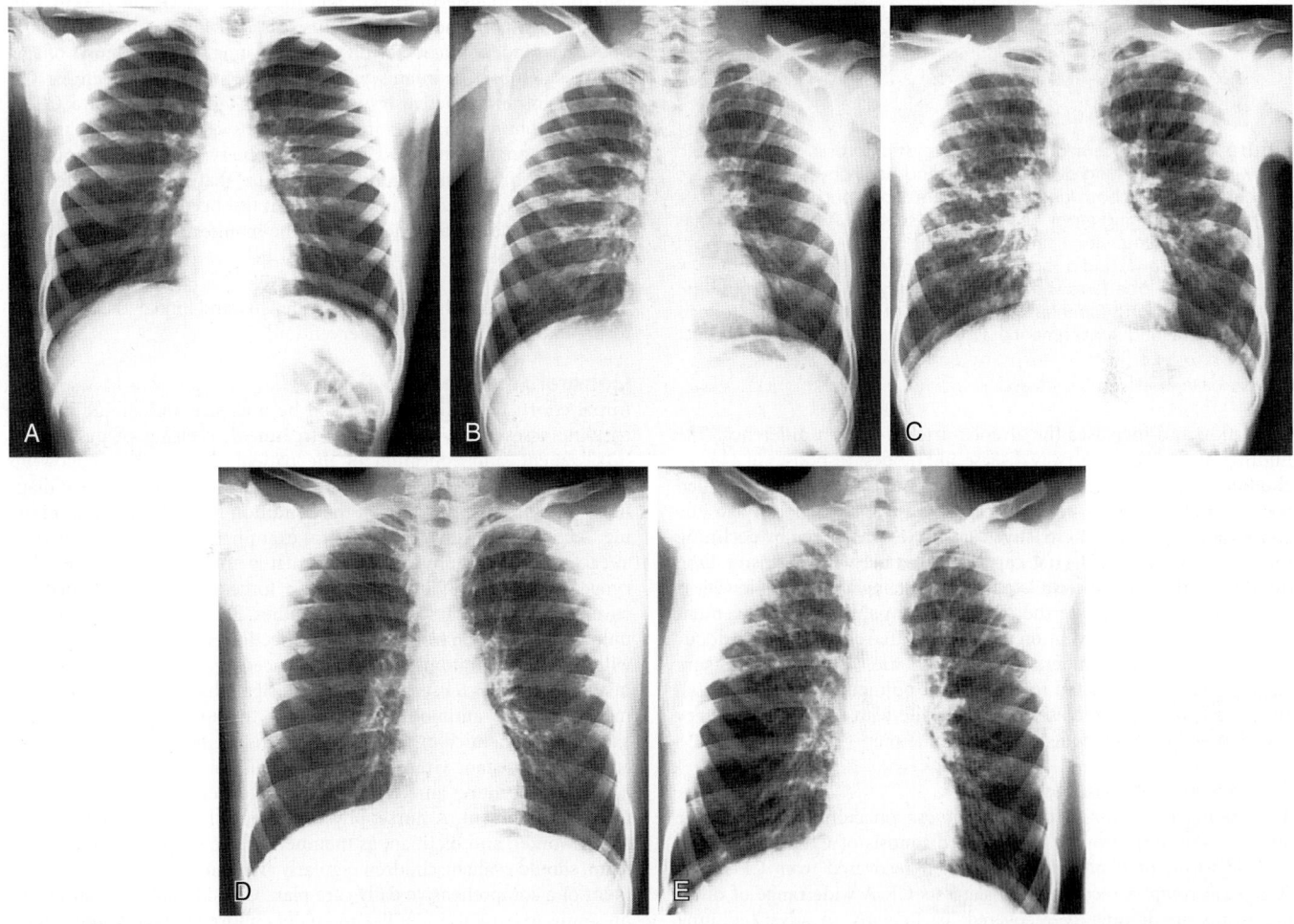

Figure 403-7 Serial radiographs in a boy show the changing appearance of cystic fibrosis over 6 yr. **A,** At 9 yr, frontal radiograph shows minimal peribronchial thickening and hyperaerated lungs indistinguishable from asthma. **B,** Nineteen months later, the radiographic picture has worsened considerably. Extensive peribronchial thickening is now noted. Mucoid impaction of the bronchus is seen in the left upper lobe and hilar shadows have become abnormally prominent. **C,** Ten months later, further deterioration is obvious. Widespread typical changes of CF are noted throughout both lungs. **D,** Follow-up studies show considerable improvement, which suggested that some of the changes evident on **C** were from superimposed infection. **E,** One year later, note the progressive changes of CF—most severe in the upper lobes bilaterally. *(From Long FR, Druhan SM, Kuhn JP. Diseases of the bronchi and pulmonary aeration. In Slovis TL, editor,* Caffey's pediatric diagnostic imaging, *ed 11, Philadelphia, 2008, Mosby, Fig. 73-54.)*

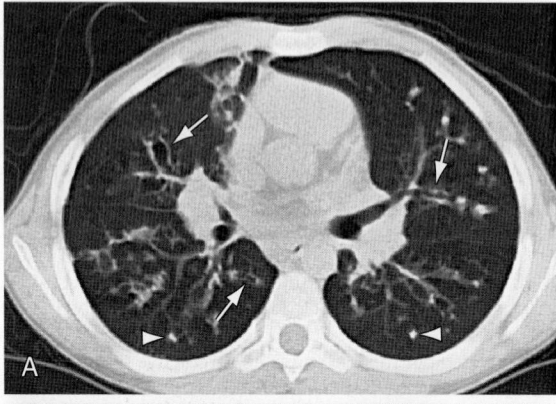

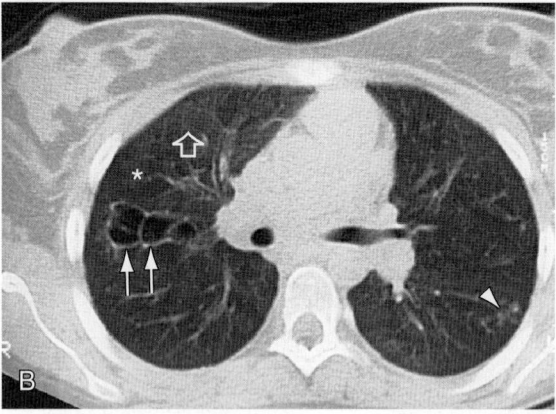

Figure 403-8 CT scans of the chest in cystic fibrosis. **A,** A 12 yr old boy with moderate lung disease. Airway and parenchymal changes are present throughout both lungs. Multiple areas of bronchiectasis *(arrows)* and mucous plugging *(arrowheads)* can be seen. **B,** A 19 yr old girl has mostly normal lung with 1 area of saccular bronchiectasis in the right upper lobe *(arrows)* and a focal area of peripheral mucous plugging in the right lower lobe *(arrowhead).* Lung density is heterogeneous with areas of normal lung *(open arrow)* and areas of low attenuation reflecting segmental and subsegmental air trapping *(asterisk).*

ventilation and increases the alveolar-arterial oxygen difference. The findings of obstructive airway disease and modest responses to a bronchodilator are consistent with the diagnosis of CF at all ages. Residual volume and functional residual capacity are increased early in the course of lung disease. Restrictive changes, characterized by declining total lung capacity and vital capacity, correlate with extensive lung injury and fibrosis and are a late finding. Testing at each clinic visit is recommended to evaluate the course of the pulmonary involvement and allow for early intervention when substantial decrements are documented. Increasing numbers of CF centers are equipped to measure airflow patterns of sedated infants (infant pulmonary function tests). Some patients reach adolescent or adult life with normal pulmonary function and without evidence of overinflation.

Microbiologic Studies
The finding of *S. aureus* or *P. aeruginosa* on culture of the lower airways (sputum) strongly suggests a diagnosis of CF. In particular, mucoid forms of *P. aeruginosa* are often recovered from CF lungs. *B. cepacia complex* recovery also suggests CF. A wide range of other organisms are frequently recovered, particularly in advanced lung disease; they include a variety of Gram-negative rods including *Stenotrophomonas maltophilia*, and *Achromobacter xylosoxidans*, fungi, and nontuberculous mycobacterial species. Failure of respiratory symptom flares to respond to usual antibiotics triggers testing for *Mycoplasma* and viruses. Fiberoptic bronchoscopy is used to gather lower respiratory tract secretions of infants and young children who do not expectorate.

Heterozygote Detection and Prenatal Diagnosis
Mutation analysis should be fully informative for testing of potential carriers or a fetus, provided that mutations within the family have been previously identified. Testing a spouse of a carrier with a standard panel of probes is ≈90% sensitive, and full CFTR sequence analysis is commercially available if further testing is warranted. Prenatal testing should be offered to all couples planning to have children in addition to individuals with a family history of CF and partners of CF women. The American College of Medical Genetics and the American College of Obstetricians and Gynecologists recommend that CF carrier screening be offered to individuals of Ashkenazi Jewish or white descent and be made available to individuals of other ethnic and racial groups; in one large series, 14% of carrier screening referrals were from Hispanic and African-American individuals, and 12% from individuals with ethnicities other than white or Ashkenazi Jewish. Screening of the siblings of an affected child is also suggested.

Newborn Screening
Newborn screening for CF is mandated in all 50 states. A variety of newborn screening algorithms are in place to identify infants with CF. Most algorithms utilize a combination of immunoreactive trypsinogen results and limited DNA testing on blood spots; all positive screens are followed by a confirmatory sweat analysis. This screening test is ≈95% sensitive. Newborn diagnoses can prevent early nutritional deficiencies and improve long-term growth and may improve cognitive function. Importantly, good nutritional status (50% weight for height or 50% body mass index) is associated with better lung function at 6 yr of age. There is a subset of infants with a positive newborn screen for CF, elevated immunoreactive trypsinogen and 1 or 2 copies of a CFTR mutation, but who have an initial negative sweat test and are asymptomatic. These infants have **CFTR** metabolic syndrome and should be followed in a CF center annually to ensure that they do not develop CF symptoms. Indeed, in some the sweat test becomes abnormal over time; nonetheless if they develop CF the manifestations are mild.

TREATMENT
The treatment plan should be comprehensive and linked to close monitoring and early, aggressive intervention.

General Approach to Care
Initial efforts after diagnosis should be intensive and should include baseline assessment, initiation of treatment, clearing of pulmonary involvement, and education of the patient and parents. Follow-up evaluations are scheduled every 1-3 mo, depending on the age at diagnosis, because many aspects of the condition require careful monitoring. An interval history and physical examination should be obtained at each visit. A sputum sample or, if that is not available, a lower pharyngeal swab taken during or after a forced cough is obtained for culture and antibiotic susceptibility studies. Because irreversible loss of pulmonary function from low-grade infection can occur gradually and without acute symptoms, emphasis is placed on a thorough pulmonary history. Table 403-5 lists symptoms and signs that suggest the need for more intensive antibiotic and physical therapy. Protection against exposure to methicillin-resistant *S. aureus, P. aeruginosa, B. cepacia,* and other resistant Gram-negative organisms is essential, including isolation procedures and careful attention to sterilization of inhalation therapy equipment. A nurse, physical therapist, respiratory therapist, social worker, and dietitian, as members of the multidisciplinary care team, should evaluate children regularly and contribute to the development of a comprehensive daily care plan. Considerable education and programs to empower families and older children to take responsibility for care are likely to result in the best adherence to daily care programs. Standardization of practice, on the part of both caregivers and families, as well as close monitoring and early intervention for new or increasing symptoms appears to result in the best long-term outcomes.

Because secretions of CF patients are not adequately hydrated, attention in early childhood to oral hydration, especially during warm weather or with acute gastroenteritis, may minimize complications

Table 403-5	Symptoms and Signs Associated with Exacerbation of Pulmonary Infection in Patients with Cystic Fibrosis

SYMPTOMS
Increased frequency and duration of cough
Increased sputum production
Change in appearance of sputum
Increased shortness of breath
Decreased exercise tolerance
Decreased appetite
Feeling of increased congestion in the chest

SIGNS
Increased respiratory rate
Use of accessory muscles for breathing
Intercostal retractions
Change in results of auscultatory examination of chest
Decline in measures of pulmonary function consistent with the presence of obstructive airway disease
Fever and leukocytosis
Weight loss
New infiltrate on chest radiograph

From Ramsey B: Management of pulmonary disease in patients with cystic fibrosis, N Engl J Med 335:179, 1996.

Table 403-6	Complications of Therapy for Cystic Fibrosis*

COMPLICATION	AGENT
Gastrointestinal bleeding	Ibuprofen
Hyperglycemia	Corticosteroids (systemic)
Growth retardation	Corticosteroids (systemic, inhaled)
Renal dysfunction:	
Tubular	Aminoglycosides
Interstitial nephritis	Semisynthetic penicillins, nonsteroidal antiinflammatory drugs
Hearing loss, vestibular dysfunction	Aminoglycosides
Peripheral neuropathy or optic atrophy	Chloramphenicol (prolonged course)
Hypomagnesemia	Aminoglycosides
Hyperuricemia, colonic stricture	Pancreatic extracts (very large doses)
Goiter	Iodine-containing expectorants
Gynecomastia	Spironolactone
Enamel hypoplasia or staining	Tetracyclines (used in 1st 8 yr of life)

*Common hypersensitivity reactions to drugs are not included.

associated with impaired mucus clearance. Intravenous therapy for dehydration should be initiated early.

The goal of therapy is to maintain a stable condition for prolonged periods. This can be accomplished for most patients by interval evaluation and adjustments of the home treatment program. Some children have episodic acute or low-grade chronic lung infection that progresses. For these patients, intensive inhalation and airway clearance and intravenous antibiotics are indicated. Improvement is most reliably accomplished in a hospital setting; selected patients have demonstrated successful outcomes while completing these treatments at home. Intravenous antibiotics may be required infrequently or as often as every 2-3 mo. The goal of treatment is to return patients to their previous pulmonary and functional status.

The basic daily care program varies according to the age of the child, the degree of pulmonary involvement, other system involvement, and the time available for therapy. The major components of this care are pulmonary and nutritional therapies. Because therapy is medication-intensive, iatrogenic problems frequently arise. Monitoring for these complications is also an important part of management (Table 403-6).

Pulmonary Therapy

The object of pulmonary therapy is to clear secretions from airways and to control infection. When a child is not doing well, every potentially useful aspect of therapy should be reconsidered.

Inhalation Therapy

Aerosol therapy is used to deliver medications and hydrate the lower respiratory tract. Metered-dose inhalers can deliver some agents, such as bronchodilators and corticosteroids, with a spacer for younger children. Alternately, these medications can be delivered with a compressor that drives a handheld nebulizer. In some patients β-agonists may decrease PaO_2 acutely by increasing ventilation-perfusion mismatch, a concern if the PaO_2 is marginal.

Human recombinant DNase (2.5 mg), given as a single daily aerosol dose, improves pulmonary function, decreases the number of pulmonary exacerbations, and promotes a sense of well-being in patients who have moderate disease and purulent secretions. Benefit for those with normal forced expiratory volume in 1 sec (FEV_1) values or advanced lung disease has also been documented. Improvement is sustained for 12 mo or longer with continuous therapy. Another mucolytic agent, *N*-acetylcysteine, nebulized as a 5-10% solution following β₂-agonist nebulization, is useful for airway clearance and may potentially augment airway levels of the antioxidant, glutathione.

Nebulized hypertonic saline, acting as a hyperosmolar agent, is believed to draw water into the airway and rehydrate mucus and the periciliary fluid layer, resulting in improved mucociliary clearance. A number of studies have reported that 7% hypertonic saline nebulized 2-4 times daily results in increased mucus clearance and improved pulmonary function.

Aerosolized antibiotics are often used when the airways are colonized with *Pseudomonas* as part of daily therapy. Aerosolized tobramycin, TOBI, or aerosolized aztreonam, Cayston, used as a suppressive therapy (on 1 mo, off 1 mo) may reduce symptoms, improve pulmonary function, and alleviate the need for hospitalization (see "Aerosolized Antibiotic Therapy" below).

Airway Clearance Therapy

Airway clearance treatment usually consists of chest percussion combined with postural drainage and derives its rationale from the idea that cough clears mucus from large airways but chest vibrations are required to move secretions from small airways, where expiratory flow rates are low. **Chest physical therapy (PT)** can be particularly useful for patients with CF because they accumulate secretions in small airways first, even before the onset of symptoms. Although immediate improvement of pulmonary function generally cannot be demonstrated after PT, cessation of chest PT in children with mild to moderate airflow limitation results in deterioration of lung function within 3 wk, and prompt improvement of function occurs when therapy is resumed. Chest PT is recommended 1-4 times a day, depending on the severity of lung dysfunction. Cough, huffing, or forced expirations are encouraged after each lung segment is "drained." Vest-type mechanical percussors are also useful. Voluntary coughing, repeated forced expiratory maneuvers with and without positive expiratory pressure, patterned breathing, and use of an array of handheld oscillatory devices are additional aids to clearance of mucus. Routine aerobic exercise appears to slow the rate of decline of pulmonary function, and benefit has also been documented with weight training. No one airway clearance technique is superior to any other, so all modes should be considered in the development of an airway clearance prescription.

Adherence to daily therapy is essential; therefore airway clearance technique plans are individualized for each patient.

Antibiotic Therapy

Antibiotics are the mainstay of therapy designed to control progression of lung infection. The goal is to reduce the intensity of endobronchial infection and to delay progressive lung damage. The usual guidelines for acute chest infections, such as fever, tachypnea, or chest pain, are often absent. Consequently, all aspects of the patient's history and examination, including anorexia, weight loss, and diminished activity, must be used to guide the frequency and duration of therapy. Antibiotic treatment varies from intermittent short courses of 1 antibiotic to nearly continuous treatment with 1 or more antibiotics. Dosages for some antibiotics are often 2-3 times the amount recommended for minor infections because patients with CF have proportionately more lean body mass and higher clearance rates for many antibiotics than other individuals. In addition, it is difficult to achieve effective drug levels of many antimicrobials in respiratory tract secretions.

Oral Antibiotic Therapy

Indications for oral antibiotic therapy in a patient with CF include the presence of respiratory tract symptoms and identification of pathogenic organisms in respiratory tract cultures. Whenever possible, the choice of antibiotics should be guided by in vitro sensitivity testing. Common organisms, including *S. aureus,* nontypeable *Haemophilus influenzae, P. aeruginosa; B. cepacia* and other Gram-negative rods, are encountered with increasing frequency. The first 2 can be eradicated from the respiratory tract in CF with use of oral antibiotics, but *Pseudomonas* is more difficult to treat. The usual course of therapy is ≥2 wk, and maximal doses are recommended. Table 403-7 lists useful oral antibiotics. The quinolones are the only broadly effective oral antibiotics for *Pseudomonas* infection, but resistance against these agents emerges rapidly. Infection with mycoplasma or chlamydial organisms has been documented, providing a rationale for the use of macrolides

on an empirical basis for flare of symptoms. Macrolides may reduce the virulence properties of *P. aeruginosa,* such as biofilm production, and contribute antiinflammatory effects. Long-term therapy with azithromycin 3 times a week improves lung function in patients with chronic *P. aeruginosa* infection.

Aerosolized Antibiotic Therapy

P. aeruginosa and other Gram-negative organisms are frequently resistant to all oral antibiotics. Aerosol delivery of antibiotics has been used as an option for home delivery of additional agents, such as tobramycin, colistin, and gentamicin. Although these therapies are used, the evidence to support aerosolized antibiotics for an acute pulmonary exacerbation is limited. However, there is good evidence to support the use of inhaled tobramycin as a long-term suppressive therapy in a patient colonized with *P. aeruginosa.* When tobramycin is given at a dose of 300 mg twice daily on alternate months for 6 mo, *Pseudomonas* density in sputum decreases, fewer hospitalizations are required, and pulmonary function can improve by ≥10%. Toxicity is negligible. On the basis of available evidence, this therapy is recommended in patients with chronic colonization with *P. aeruginosa,* to lessen symptoms and/or to improve long-term function in patients with moderate to severe disease. Recently, nebulized aztreonam was also approved for 3 times daily therapy on alternate months for patients with chronic *P. aeruginosa.* Another indication for aerosolized antibiotic therapy is to eradicate *P. aeruginosa* in the airways after initial colonization. Early infection may be cleared for months to several years by several protocols, including oral ciprofloxacin and/or aerosolized colistin or tobramycin. However, once chronically established, *P. aeruginosa* infection is rarely eradicated.

Intravenous Antibiotic Therapy

For the patient who has progressive or unrelenting symptoms and signs despite intensive home measures, intravenous antibiotic therapy is indicated. This therapy is usually initiated in the hospital but may be

Table 403-7	Antimicrobial Agents for Cystic Fibrosis Lung Infection			
ROUTE	**ORGANISMS**	**AGENTS**	**DOSAGE (mg/kg/24 hr)**	**NO. DOSES/24 hr**
Oral	*Staphylococcus aureus*	Dicloxacillin	25-50	4
		Linezolid	20	2
		Cephalexin	50	4
		Clindamycin	10-30	3-4
		Amoxicillin-clavulanate	25-45	2-3
	Haemophilus influenzae	Amoxicillin	50-100	2-3
	Pseudomonas aeruginosa	Ciprofloxacin	20-30	2-3
	Burkholderia cepacia	Trimethoprim-sulfamethoxazole	8-10*	2-4
	Empirical	Azithromycin	10, day 1; 5, days 2-5	1
		Erythromycin	30-50	3-4
Intravenous	*S. aureus*	Nafcillin	100-200	4-6
		Vancomycin	40	3-4
	P. aeruginosa	Tobramycin	8-12	1-3
		Amikacin	15-30	2-3
		Ticarcillin	400	4
		Piperacillin	300-400	4
		Ticarcillin-clavulanate	400†	4
		Piperacillin-tazobactam	240-400‡	3
		Meropenem	60-120	3
		Imipenem-cilastatin	45-100	3-4
		Ceftazidime	150	3
		Aztreonam	150-200	4
	B. cepacia	Chloramphenicol	50-100	4
		Meropenem	60-120	3
Aerosol		Tobramycin (inhaled)	300§	2
		Aztreonam (inhaled)	75	3

*Quantity of trimethoprim.
†Quantity of ticarcillin.
‡Quantity of piperacillin.
§In mg per dose.

completed on an ambulatory basis. Although many patients show improvement within 7 days, it is usually advisable to extend the period of treatment to at least 14 days. Permanent intravenous access can be provided for long-term or frequent courses of therapy in the hospital or at home. Thrombophilia screening should be considered before the use of totally implantable intravenous devices or for recurring problems with venous catheters.

Table 403-7 lists commonly used intravenous antibiotics. In general, treatment of *Pseudomonas* infection requires 2-drug therapy. A third agent may be required for optimal coverage of *S. aureus* or other organisms. The aminoglycosides have a relatively short half-life in many patients with CF. The initial parenteral dose, noted in Table 403-7, is generally given every 8 hr. After blood levels have been determined, the total daily dose should be adjusted. Peak levels of 10-15 mg/L are desirable, and trough levels should be kept at <2 mg/L to minimize the risk of ototoxicity and nephrotoxicity. The regimen of once-daily tobramycin dosing has been demonstrated to have equivalent efficacy and the advantage of decreased toxicity over dosing every 8 hr. For once-daily dosing of tobramycin, peak levels should be between 20 and 30 mg/L and trough levels should be 1 mg/L or less. In toddlers, older children, and adults, once-daily intravenous tobramycin therapy is becoming the standard of care. Changes in therapy should be guided by lack of improvement and by culture results. If patients do not show improvement, complications such as heart failure and reactive airways or infection with viruses, *Aspergillus fumigatus* (see Chapter 237), non-tuberculous mycobacteria (see Chapters 217 and 399), or other unusual organisms should be considered. *B. cepacia* complex is the most frequent of a growing list of Gram-negative rods that may be particularly refractory to antimicrobial therapy. Infection control in both the outpatient and inpatient medical setting is critically important to prevent nosocomial spread of resistant bacterial organisms between patients.

Bronchodilator Therapy
Reversible airway obstruction occurs in many children with CF, sometimes in conjunction with frank asthma or acute bronchopulmonary aspergillosis. Reversible obstruction is defined as improvement of ≥12% in flow rates after inhalation of a bronchodilator. In many patients with CF, flow rates may improve by only 5-10%, however. Nevertheless, subjective benefit is claimed by many following use of a β-adrenergic agonist aerosol. Cromolyn sodium and ipratropium hydrochlorides are alternative agents, but there is no evidence to support their use.

Antiinflammatory Agents
Corticosteroids are useful for the treatment of allergic bronchopulmonary aspergillosis and severe reactive airway disease occasionally encountered in children with CF. Prolonged treatment of standard CF lung disease using an alternate-day regimen initially appeared to improve pulmonary function and diminish hospitalization rates. However, a 4-yr double-blind, multicenter study of this regimen for patients with mild to moderate lung disease found only modest efficacy and prohibitive side effects, including growth retardation, cataracts, and abnormalities of glucose tolerance at a dose of 2 mg/kg and growth retardation at 1 mg/kg. Inhaled corticosteroids have theoretical appeal, but there are few data documenting their efficacy and safety; it appears that discontinuing inhaled corticosteroids in patients with CF had no effect on lung function, antibiotic use, or bronchodilator use. Ibuprofen, given long term (dose adjusted to achieve a peak serum concentration of 50-100 μg/mL) for 4 yr, is associated with a slowing of disease progression, particularly in younger patients with mild lung disease. Side effects of nonsteroidal antiinflammatory drugs have been encountered (see Table 403-6); therefore, this therapy has not gained broad acceptance even though ibuprofen is the only antiinflammatory agent with documented efficacy in the patient population.

Endoscopy and Lavage
Treatment of obstructed airways sometimes includes tracheobronchial suctioning or lavage, especially if atelectasis or mucoid impaction is present. Bronchopulmonary lavage can be performed by the instillation of saline or a mucolytic agent through a fiberoptic bronchoscope.

Antibiotics (usually gentamicin or tobramycin) can also be instilled directly at lavage in order to transiently achieve a much higher endobronchial concentration than can be obtained by using intravenous therapy. There is no evidence for sustained benefit from repeated endoscopic or lavage procedures.

Other Therapies
Expectorants such as iodides and guaifenesin do not effectively assist with the removal of secretions from the respiratory tract. Inspiratory muscle training can enhance maximum oxygen consumption during exercise as well as FEV_1.

Emerging Therapies
A major breakthrough in CF therapy is ivacaftor, a small molecule potentiator of the CFTR mutation, G551D (present in ~5% of patients). Ivacaftor activates the CFTR-G551D mutant protein, a class III CFTR mutation that results in protein localized to the plasma membrane but loss of chloride channel function. Ivacaftor therapy resulted in improvement in FEV_1 by an average of 10.6%, decreased the frequency of pulmonary exacerbations by 55%, decreased sweat chloride by an average of 48 mEq/L, and increased weight gain by an average of 2.7 kg. Ivacaftor is approved for CFTR-G551D patients ≥6 yr old, as a 150 mg, twice per day, oral therapy. Additional small molecule correctors are being tested for use in combination with Ivacaftor to correct the processing of the most common CFTR mutation, F508del. The goal of this strategy is to correct the localization of the protein to the apical membrane of the cell and then to potentiate its function.

TREATMENT OF PULMONARY COMPLICATIONS
Atelectasis
Lobar atelectasis occurs relatively infrequently; it may be asymptomatic and noted only at the time of a routine chest radiograph. Aggressive intravenous therapy with antibiotics and increased chest PT directed at the affected lobe may be effective. If there is no improvement in 5-7 days, bronchoscopic examination of the airways may be indicated. If the atelectasis does not resolve, continued intensive home therapy is indicated, because atelectasis may resolve during a period of weeks or months. Lobectomy should be considered only if expansion is not achieved and the patient has progressive difficulty from fever, anorexia, and unrelenting cough (see Chapter 408).

Hemoptysis
Endobronchial bleeding usually reflects airway wall erosion secondary to infection. With increasing numbers of older patients, hemoptysis has become a relatively frequent complication. Blood streaking of sputum is particularly common. Small-volume hemoptysis (<20 mL) should not trigger panic and is usually viewed as a need for intensified antimicrobial therapy and chest PT. When the hemoptysis is persistent or increases in severity, hospital admission is indicated. **Massive hemoptysis,** defined as total blood loss of ≥250 mL in a 24-hr period, is rare in the 1st decade and occurs in <1% of adolescents, but it requires close monitoring and the capability to replace blood losses rapidly. Chest PT is often discontinued until 12-24 hr after the last brisk bleeding episode and is then gradually re-instituted. Patients should receive vitamin K for an abnormal prothrombin time. During brisk hemoptysis, the child and parents require a great deal of reassurance that the bleeding will stop. Blood transfusion is not indicated unless there is hypotension or the hematocrit is significantly reduced. Ticarcillin, salicylates, and nonsteroidal antiinflammatory drugs interfere with platelet function and may aggravate hemoptysis. Bronchoscopy rarely reveals the site of bleeding. Lobectomy is to be avoided, if possible, because functioning lung should be preserved. Bronchial artery embolization can be useful to control persistent, significant hemoptysis.

Pneumothorax
Pneumothorax (see Chapter 411) is encountered in <1% of children and teenagers with CF, although it is more frequently encountered in

older patients and may be life-threatening. The episode may be asymptomatic but is often attended by chest and shoulder pain, shortness of breath, or hemoptysis. A small air collection that does not grow can be observed closely. Chest tube placement with or without pleurodesis is often the initial therapy. Intravenous antibiotics are also begun on admission. An open thoracotomy or video-assisted thoracoscopy with plication of blebs, apical pleural stripping, and basal pleural abrasion should be considered if the air leak persists. Surgical intervention is usually well tolerated even in cases of advanced lung disease. The thoracotomy tube is removed as soon as possible, usually on the 2nd or 3rd postoperative day. The patient can then be mobilized, and full postural drainage therapy resumed. Previous pneumothorax with or without pleurodesis is not a contraindication to subsequent lung transplantation.

Allergic Bronchopulmonary Aspergillosis

Allergic bronchopulmonary aspergillosis occurs in 5-10% of patients with CF and may manifest as wheezing, increased cough, shortness of breath, and marked hyperinflation (see Chapters 237 and 399). In some patients, a chest radiograph shows new, focal infiltrates. The presence of rust-colored sputum, the recovery of *Aspergillus* organisms from the sputum, a positive skin test for *A. fumigatus*, the demonstration of specific immunoglobulin (Ig) E and IgG antibodies against *A. fumigatus,* or the presence of eosinophils in a fresh sputum sample supports the diagnosis. The serum IgE level is usually high. Treatment is directed at controlling the inflammatory reaction with oral corticosteroids. For refractory cases, oral antifungals may be required.

Nontuberculous Mycobacteria Infection

See Chapter 217.

Injured airways with poor clearance may be colonized by *Mycobacterium avium-complex* but also *Mycobacterium abscessus, Mycobacterium chelonae,* and *Mycobacterium kansasii.* Distinguishing endobronchial colonization (frequent) from invasive infection (infrequent) is challenging. Persistent fevers and new infiltrates or cystic lesions coupled with the finding of acid-fast organisms on sputum smear suggest infection. Treatment is prolonged and requires multiple antimicrobial agents. Symptoms may improve, but the nontuberculous mycobacteria are not usually cleared from the lungs.

Bone and Joint Complications

Hypertrophic osteoarthropathy causes elevation of the periosteum over the distal portions of long bones and bone pain, overlying edema, and joint effusions. Acetaminophen or ibuprofen may provide relief. Control of lung infection usually reduces symptoms. Intermittent arthropathy unrelated to other rheumatologic disorders occurs occasionally, has no recognized pathogenesis, and usually responds to nonsteroidal antiinflammatory agents. Back pain or rib fractures from vigorous coughing may require pain management to permit adequate airway clearance. These and other fractures may stem from diminished bone mineralization, the result of reduced vitamin D absorption, corticosteroid therapy, diminished weight-bearing exercises, and, perhaps, other factors. There may be a bone phenotype in CF that is unrelated to therapies or nutritional status and may be due to CFTR dysfunction.

Sleep-Disordered Breathing

Particularly with advanced pulmonary disease and during chest exacerbations, individuals with CF may experience more sleep arousals, less time in rapid eye movement sleep, nocturnal hypoxemia, hypercapnia, and associated neurobehavioral impairment. Nocturnal hypoxemia may hasten the onset of pulmonary hypertension and right-sided heart failure. Efficacy of specific interventions for this complication of CF has not been systematically assessed. Prompt treatment of airway symptoms and nocturnal oxygen supplementation or bilevel positive airway pressure support should be considered in selected cases.

Acute Respiratory Failure

Acute respiratory failure (see Chapter 71) rarely occurs in patients with mild to moderate lung disease and is usually the result of a severe viral or other infectious illness. Because patients with this complication can regain their previous status, intensive therapy is indicated. In addition to aerosol, postural drainage, and intravenous antibiotic treatment, oxygen is required to raise the arterial PaO_2. An increasing PCO_2 may require ventilatory assistance. Endotracheal or bronchoscopic suction may be necessary to clear airway inspissated secretions and can be repeated daily. Right-sided heart failure should be treated vigorously. Recovery is often slow. Intensive intravenous antibiotic therapy and postural drainage should be continued for 1-2 wk after the patient has regained baseline status.

Chronic Respiratory Failure

Patients with CF acquire chronic respiratory failure after prolonged deterioration of lung function. Although this complication can occur at any age, it is now seen most frequently in adult patients. Because a long-standing PaO_2 <50 mm Hg promotes the development of right-sided heart failure, patients usually benefit from low-flow oxygen to raise arterial PO_2 to ≥55 mm Hg. Increasing hypercapnia may prevent the use of optimal fraction of inspired oxygen. Most patients improve somewhat with intensive antibiotic and pulmonary therapy measures and can be discharged from the hospital. Low-flow oxygen therapy is needed at home, especially with sleep. Noninvasive ventilatory support can improve gas exchange and has been documented to enhance quality of life. Ventilatory support may be particularly useful for patients awaiting lung transplantation. These patients usually display cor pulmonale and should reduce their salt intake and be given diuretics. Caution should be exercised to avoid ventilation-suppressing metabolic alkalosis that results from CF-related chloride depletion and, in many cases, from diuretic-induced bicarbonate retention. Chronic pain (headache, chest pain, abdominal pain, and limb pain) is frequent at the end of life and responds to judicious use of analgesics, including opioids. Dyspnea has been ameliorated with nebulized fentanyl.

Lung transplantation is an option for end-stage lung disease (see Chapter 443) but a topic of vigorous debate. Criteria for referral continue to be a subject of investigation and ideally include estimates of longevity with and without transplant based on lung function and exercise tolerance data. Because of bronchiolitis obliterans (see Chapter 394.1) and other complications, transplanted lungs cannot be expected to function for the lifetime of a recipient, and repeat transplantation is increasingly common. The demand for donor lungs exceeds the supply, and waiting lists as well as duration of waits continue to grow. The protocol for matching donor organs with lung transplant recipients has been revised to account for the severity of the patients' lung disease. In a review of lung transplantation in children with CF between 1992 and 2002, pretransplantation colonization with *B. cepacia,* diabetes, and older age decreased posttransplantation survival. The review suggests that transplantation is often associated with many complications and may not prolong life nor significantly improve its quality.

Heart Failure

Some patients experience reversible right-sided heart failure (see Chapter 442) as the result of an acute event such as a viral infection or pneumothorax. Individuals with long-standing, advanced pulmonary disease, especially those with severe hypoxemia (PaO_2 <50 mm Hg), often acquire chronic right-sided heart failure. The mechanisms include hypoxemic pulmonary arterial constriction and loss of the pulmonary vascular bed. Pulmonary arterial wall changes contribute to increased vascular resistance with time. Evidence for concomitant left ventricular dysfunction is often found. Cyanosis, increased shortness of breath, increased liver size with a tender margin, ankle edema, jugular venous distention, an unusual weight gain, increased heart size seen on chest radiograph, or evidence for right-sided heart enlargement on electrocardiogram or echocardiogram helps to confirm the diagnosis. Diuresis induced by furosemide (1 mg/kg administered intravenously) confirms the suspicion of fluid retention. Repeated doses are often required at 24-48 hr intervals to reduce fluid accumulation and accompanying symptoms. Concomitant use of spironolactone may protect against potassium depletion and facilitate long-term diuresis. Hypochloremic alkalosis complicates the long-term use of loop diuretics. Digitalis is not effective in pure right-sided failure but may be useful when there is an associated left-sided dysfunction. The arterial P_{O_2} should be maintained at >50 mm Hg if possible. Intensive pulmonary therapy, including intravenous antibiotics, is most important. Initially, the salt intake should be limited. Volume overload and antibiotics with high sodium content should be avoided. No clear-cut long-term benefit from pulmonary vasodilators has been demonstrated. The prognosis for heart failure is poor, but a number of patients survive for ≥5 yr after the appearance of heart failure. Heart-lung transplantation may be an option (see preceding section).

Nutritional Therapy

Up to 90% of patients with CF have loss of exocrine pancreatic function as well as inadequate digestion and absorption of fats and proteins. They require dietary adjustment, pancreatic enzyme replacement, and supplementary vitamins. In general, children with CF need to exceed the usual required daily caloric intake to grow. Daily supplements of the fat-soluble vitamins are required.

Diet

Historically, at the time of diagnosis many infants presented with nutritional deficits; this situation is changing because of newborn screening. Sometimes young infants with a history of wheezy breathing were often started on soy-protein formulas prior to their evaluation; they did not use this protein well and often acquired hypoproteinemia with anasarca. Although in the past a low-fat, high-protein, high-calorie diet was generally recommended for older children, it resulted in deficiencies of essential fatty acids and poor growth. With the advent of improved pancreatic enzyme products, increased amounts of fat in the diet are well tolerated and preferred.

Most individuals with CF have a higher-than-normal caloric need because of increased work of breathing and perhaps because of increased metabolic activity related to the basic defect. When anorexia of chronic infection supervenes, weight loss occurs. Encouragement to eat high-calorie foods is important, but weight gain is not generally realized unless lung infection is controlled. Weight stabilization or gain sometimes requires nocturnal feeding via nasogastric tube or percutaneous enterostomy or with short-term intravenous hyperalimentation. Not infrequently, parent–child interactions at feeding time are maladaptive, and behavioral interventions can improve caloric intake. Long-term benefits of these interventions include improved quality of life and psychologic well-being. In addition there is good correlation between improved body mass index and maintenance of FEV_1.

Recombinant growth hormone therapy (3 times per week) has improved nutritional outcomes, including positive effects on nitrogen balance and improved height and weight velocities.

Pancreatic Enzyme Replacement

Pancreatic exocrine replacement therapy given with ingested food reduces but does not fully correct stool fat and nitrogen losses. Enzyme dosage and product should be individualized for each patient. Enteric-coated, pH-sensitive enzyme microspheres are most often prescribed. Several strengths up to 25,000 IU of lipase/capsule are available. Administration of excessive doses has been linked to **colonic strictures** requiring surgery. Consequently, enzyme replacement should not exceed 2,500 lipase units/kg/meal in most circumstances. In general, infants need 2,000-4,000 lipase units per feeding, which is most easily given mixed with applesauce on a spoon. Snacks should also be covered. The dose of enzymes required usually increases with age, but some patients have lower requirements as teenagers and young adults. Some individuals require proton pump inhibitor therapy to correct acid pH in the duodenum which is due to lack of exocrine pancreatic secretions; neutralization of duodenal pH permits activation of enteric coated pancreatic exocrine replacement therapy granules.

Vitamin and Mineral Supplements

Because pancreatic insufficiency results in malabsorption of fat-soluble vitamins (A, D, E, K), vitamin supplementation is recommended. Several vitamin preparations containing all 4 vitamins for patients with CF are available. They should be taken daily. Replacement doses may be required when low serum levels are documented or the patient is symptomatic. Infants with zinc deficiency and an acrodermatitis enteropathica–like rash have been described. In addition, attention should be paid to iron status; in one study, almost 30% of children with CF had low serum ferritin concentrations.

TREATMENT OF INTESTINAL COMPLICATIONS

Meconium Ileus

When meconium ileus (see Chapter 102.1) is suspected, a nasogastric tube is placed for suction and the newborn is hydrated. In many cases, diatrizoate (Gastrografin) enemas with reflux of contrast material into the ileum not only confirm the diagnosis but have also resulted in the passage of a meconium plug and clearing of the obstruction. Use of this hypertonic solution requires careful correction of water losses into the bowel. Children in whom this procedure fails require operative intervention. Children who are successfully treated generally have a prognosis similar to that of other patients with severe CF mutations. Infants with meconium ileus should be treated as if they have CF until adequate diagnostic testing can be carried out.

Distal Intestinal Obstruction Syndrome (Meconium Ileus Equivalent) and Other Causes of Abdominal Symptoms

Despite appropriate pancreatic enzyme replacement, 2-5% of patients accumulate fecal material in the terminal portion of the ileum and in the cecum, which may result in partial or complete obstruction. For intermittent symptoms, pancreatic enzyme replacement should be continued or even increased, and stool softeners (polyethylene glycol [MiraLAX] or docusate sodium [Colace]) given. Increased fluid intake is also recommended. Failure to relieve symptoms signals the need for large-volume bowel lavage with a balanced salt solution containing polyethylene glycol taken by mouth or by nasogastric tube. When there is complete obstruction, a diatrizoate enema, accompanied by large amounts of intravenous fluids, can be therapeutic. Intussusception (see Chapter 333.3) and volvulus (see Chapter 329.4) must also be considered in the differential diagnosis. Intussusception, usually ileocolic, occurs at any age and often follows a 1-2 day history of "constipation." It can often be diagnosed and reduced via a diatrizoate enema. If a nonreducible intussusception or a volvulus is present, laparotomy is required. Repeated episodes of intussusception may be an indication for cecectomy.

Chronic appendicitis with or without periappendiceal abscess may manifest as recurrent or persistent abdominal pain, raising the question of need for a laparotomy. A lack of acid buffering in the duodenum appears to promote duodenitis and ulcer formation in some children. Other reasons for surgical procedures include carcinoma of the colon or biliary tract and sclerosing colonopathy.

Gastroesophageal Reflux

See Chapter 323.

Because several factors raise intraabdominal pressure, including cough and obstructed airways, pathologic gastroesophageal reflux is not uncommon and may exacerbate lung disease secondary to reflex wheezing and repeated aspiration. Dietary, positional, and medication therapies should be considered. Cholinergic agonists are contraindicated because they trigger mucus secretion and progressive respiratory difficulty. Reduction of stomach acid secretion can help, with proton pump inhibitors being the most effective agents. Fundoplication is a procedure of last resort.

Rectal Prolapse

See Chapter 344.5.

Though uncommon, rectal prolapse occurs most often in infants with CF, and less frequently in older children with the disease. It is usually related to steatorrhea, malnutrition, and repetitive cough. The prolapsed rectum can usually be replaced manually by continuous gentle pressure with the patient in the knee-chest position. Sedation may be helpful. To prevent an immediate recurrence, the buttocks can be taped closed. Adequate pancreatic enzyme replacement, decreased fat and roughage in the diet, stool softener, and control of pulmonary infection result in improvement. Occasionally, a patient may continue to have rectal prolapse and may require sclerotherapy or surgery.

Hepatobiliary Disease

Liver function abnormalities associated with biliary cirrhosis can be improved by treatment with ursodeoxycholic acid. The ability of bile acids to prevent progression of cirrhosis has not been clearly documented. Portal hypertension with esophageal varices, hypersplenism, or ascites occurs in ≤8% of children with CF (see Chapter 367). The acute management of bleeding esophageal varices includes nasogastric suction and cold saline lavage. Sclerotherapy is recommended after an initial hemorrhage. In the past, significant bleeding has also been treated successfully with portosystemic shunting. Splenorenal anastomosis has been the most effective treatment. Pronounced hypersplenism may require splenectomy. Cholelithiasis should prompt surgical consultation. The management of ascites is discussed in Chapter 370.

Obstructive jaundice in newborns with CF needs no specific therapy. Hepatomegaly with steatosis requires careful attention to nutrition and may respond to carnitine repletion. Rarely, biliary cirrhosis proceeds to hepatocellular failure, which should be treated as in patients without CF (see Chapters 364 and 367). End-stage liver disease is an indication for liver transplantation in children with CF, especially if pulmonary function is good (see Chapter 368).

Pancreatitis

Pancreatitis can be precipitated by fatty meals, alcohol ingestion, or tetracycline therapy. Serum amylase and lipase values may remain elevated for long periods. Treatment of this disorder is discussed in Chapter 351.

Hyperglycemia

Onset of hyperglycemia occurs most frequently after the 1st decade. Approximately 20% of young adults are treated for hyperglycemia, although the incidence of CF-related diabetes may be up to 50% in CF adults. Prevalence is greater in females and in F508del homozygotes. Ketoacidosis is rarely encountered. The pathogenesis includes both impaired insulin secretion and insulin resistance. Routine screening consists of an annual modified 2-hr oral glucose tolerance test after the child reaches age 10 yr. Glucose intolerance without urine glucose losses is usually not treated; glycosylated hemoglobin levels should be followed at least annually. With persistent glucosuria and symptoms, insulin treatment should be instituted. Oral hypoglycemic agents, with or without drugs that reduce insulin resistance, may also be effective. Exocrine pancreatic insufficiency and malabsorption make strict dietary control of hyperglycemia difficult. Corticosteroid therapy should be avoided. The development of significant hyperglycemia favors acquisition of *P. aeruginosa* and *B. cepacia* in the airways and may adversely affect pulmonary function. Thus, careful control of blood glucose level is an important goal. Long-term vascular complications of diabetes can occur, providing an additional rationale for good control of blood glucose levels.

OTHER THERAPY
Nasal Polyps

Nasal polyps (see Chapter 378) occur in 15-20% of patients with CF and are most prevalent in the 2nd decade of life. Local corticosteroids and nasal decongestants occasionally provide some relief. When the polyps completely obstruct the nasal airway, rhinorrhea becomes constant, or widening of the nasal bridge is noticed, surgical removal of the polyps is indicated; polyps may recur promptly or after a symptom-free interval of months to years. Polyps inexplicably stop developing in many adults.

Rhinosinusitis

Opacification of paranasal sinuses is not an indication for intervention. Acute or chronic sinus-related symptoms are treated initially with antimicrobials, with or without maxillary sinus aspiration for culture. Functional endoscopic sinus surgery has anecdotally provided benefit.

Salt Depletion

Salt losses from sweat in patients with CF can be high, especially in warm arid climates. Children should have free access to salt, and precautions against overdressing infants should be observed. Salt supplements are often prescribed to newborns identified through newborn screening and to children who live in hot weather climates. Hypochloremic alkalosis should be suspected in any infant who has had symptoms of gastroenteritis, and prompt fluid and electrolyte therapy should be instituted as needed.

Growth and Maturation

Delayed growth should be vigorously addressed by enhancing nutrition, treating lung disease more vigorously, and, in selected instances, endocrine evaluation and, possibly, growth hormone therapy. The risk:benefit ratio for anabolic steroid therapy does not support its use for undersized children with CF. Delayed sexual maturation, often associated with short stature, occurs fairly frequently in children with CF. Although many patients have severe pulmonary infection or poor nutrition, delayed puberty also occurs in those with otherwise mild disease and is not well explained. Adolescents with CF should receive specific counseling throughout their developing years concerning sexual maturation and reproductive potential.

Surgery

Minor surgical procedures, including dental work, should be performed with the use of local anesthesia if possible in children with CF. Patients with good or excellent pulmonary status can tolerate general anesthesia without any intensive pulmonary measures before the procedure. Those with moderate or severe pulmonary infection usually do better with a 1-2 wk course of intensive antibiotic treatment and increased airway clearance before surgery. If this approach is impossible, prompt intravenous antibiotic therapy is indicated once it is recognized that major surgery is required. The total time of anesthesia should be kept to a minimum. After induction, tracheal suctioning is useful and should be repeated. Patients with severe disease require monitoring of blood gas values and may need ventilatory assistance in the immediate postoperative period.

After major surgery, cough should be encouraged and airway clearance treatments should be re-instituted as soon as possible, usually within 24 hr. Adequate analgesia is important if early effective therapy is to be achieved. For those with significant pulmonary involvement, intravenous antibiotics are continued for 7-14 days postoperatively. Early ambulation and intermittent deep breathing are important; an incentive spirometer can also be helpful. After open thoracotomy for treatment of pneumothorax or lobectomy, the chest tube is the greatest single obstacle to effective pulmonary therapy and should be removed as soon as possible so that full postural drainage therapy can resume.

PROGNOSIS

CF remains a life-limiting disorder, although survival has improved dramatically in the past 30-40 yr. Infants with severe lung disease occasionally succumb, but most children survive this difficult period and are relatively healthy into adolescence or adulthood. The slow progression of lung disease eventually reaches disabling proportions. Life table data now indicate a median cumulative survival of 37 yr. Male survival is somewhat better than female survival for reasons that are not readily apparent. Children in socioeconomically disadvantaged families have, on average, a poorer prognosis.

Children with CF usually have good school attendance records and should not be restricted in their activities. A high percentage eventually attend and graduate from college. Most adults with CF find satisfactory employment, and an increasing number marry. Transitioning care from pediatric to adult care centers by 21 yr of age is an important objective and requires a thoughtful, supportive approach involving both the pediatric and internal medicine specialists.

With increasing life span for patients with CF, a new set of psychosocial considerations has emerged, including dependence-independence issues, self-care, peer relationships, sexuality, reproduction, substance abuse, educational and vocational planning, medical care costs and other financial burdens, and anxiety concerning health and prognosis. Many of these issues are best addressed in an anticipatory fashion, before the onset of psychosocial dysfunction. With appropriate medical and psychosocial support, children and adolescents with CF generally cope well. Achievement of an independent and productive adulthood is a realistic goal for many.

Bibliography is available at Expert Consult.

Chapter 404
Primary Ciliary Dyskinesia (Immotile Cilia Syndrome, Kartagener Syndrome)

Thomas W. Ferkol Jr.

Primary ciliary dyskinesia (PCD) is an inherited disorder characterized by impaired ciliary function leading to diverse clinical manifestations, including chronic sinopulmonary disease, persistent middle ear effusions, laterality defects, and infertility. Although the estimated frequency of PCD is 1 in 12,000 to 1 in 20,000 live births, its prevalence in children with repeated respiratory infections has been estimated to be as high as 5%.

NORMAL CILIARY ULTRASTRUCTURE AND FUNCTION
Three types of cilia exist in the humans: motile cilia; primary (sensory) cilia; and nodal cilia.

Motile cilia are hair-like organelles that move fluids, mucous, and inhaled particulates vectorially from conducting airways, paranasal sinuses, and eustachian tubes. The upper and lower respiratory tracts are continuously exposed to inhaled pathogens, and local defenses have evolved to protect the airway. The respiratory epithelium in the nasopharynx, middle ear, paranasal sinuses, and larger airways are lined by a ciliated, pseudostratified columnar epithelium that is essential for mucociliary clearance (Fig. 404-1). A mature ciliated epithelial cell has approximately 200 uniform motile cilia that are anatomically and functionally oriented in the same direction, moving with intracellular and intercellular synchrony. Anchored by a basal body to the apical cytoplasm and extending from the apical cell surface into the airway lumen, each cilium is a complex, specialized structure, composed of hundreds of proteins. It contains a cylinder of microtubule doublets organized around a central pair of microtubules (Fig. 404-2), leading to the characteristic "9+2" arrangement seen on cross-sectional views on transmission electron microscopy. A membrane continuous

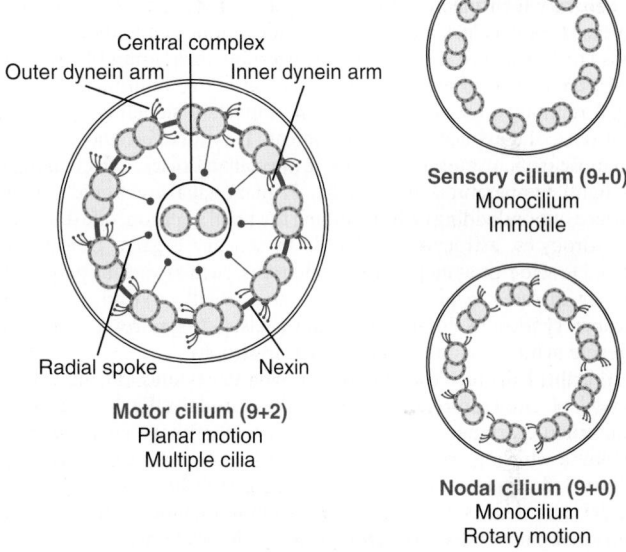

Figure 404-2 Schemata showing the 3 general classes of normal cilia (motile "9+2," motile "9+0," and nonmotile "9+0"), which demonstrate the complex structure and arrangement of the ciliary axoneme.

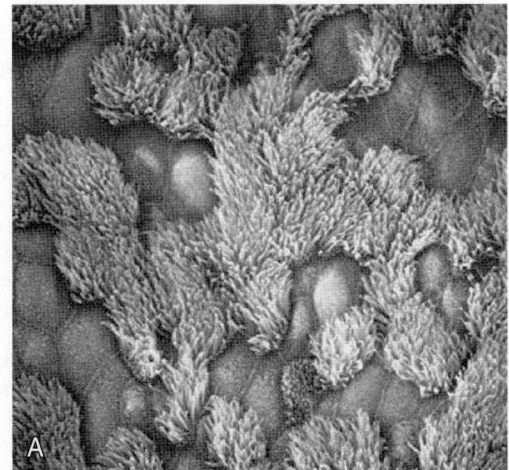
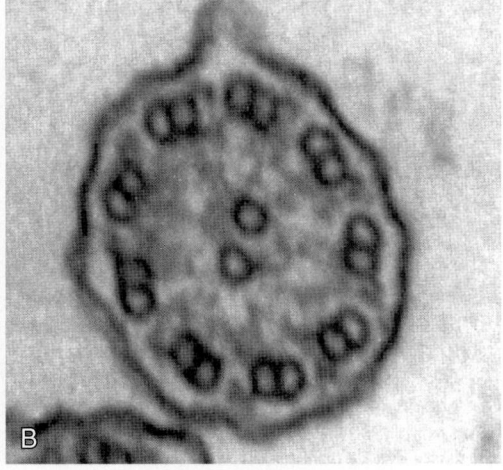

Figure 404-1 Electron photomicrographs showing **(A)** an airway epithelium grown in primary culture, showing ciliated and non-ciliated cells, and **(B)** a normal motor cilium.

with the plasma membrane covers the central fibrillar structure, or axoneme. The ciliary axoneme is highly conserved across species, and the structural elements of simple protozoan flagella and the mammalian cilium are similar. Attached to the A microtubules as distinct inner and outer dynein arms, multiple different adenosine triphosphatases, called **dyneins**, serve as "motors" of the cilium and promote microtubule sliding, which is converted into bending. The inner dynein arm influences the bend shape of the cilium, whereas the outer dynein arm controls beat force and frequency. Nexin links connect adjacent outer microtubular doublets limit the degree of sliding between microtubules, and with the radial spokes are controlled by the dynein regulatory complex. The result is a ciliary stroke and coordinated beating at a frequency constant throughout the airway, 8-20 beats/sec, but can be negatively affected by several factors, such as anesthetics and dehydration. Alternatively, beat frequency may be accelerated by exposure to irritants or bioactive molecules, including β-adrenergic agents, acetylcholine, and serotonin. Cilia beat frequency can be increased through the activity of nitric oxide synthases that are localized in the apical cytoplasm. The coordinated wave-like pattern of ciliary motion has important functions in fluid and cell movement, and any disturbance in the precise, orchestrated movement of the cilia can lead to disease.

Primary (sensory) cilia are present during interphase on most cell types. These cilia lack a central microtubule doublet and dynein arms, thus creating a "9+0" arrangement and leaving them immotile (see Fig. 404-2). For years, these structures were considered nonfunctional vestigial remnants, but primary cilia are important signaling organelles that sense the extracellular environment. They are mechanoreceptors, chemosensors, osmosensors, and, in specialized cases, defect changes in light, temperature, and gravity. Primary cilia are found on the surface of nondividing cells, including the renal nephron, bile ductules, chondrocytes, astrocytes, and cells in sensory organs. Defects are linked to wide-ranging pediatric conditions, such as various polycystic kidney diseases, nephronophthisis, Bardet-Biedl syndrome, Meckel-Gruber syndrome, Joubert syndrome, Alström syndrome, Ellis-van Creveld syndrome, and Jeune thoracic dystrophy.

The third distinct classification of cilia exists only during a brief period of embryonic development. These **nodal cilia** have a "9+0" microtubule arrangement similar to that of primary cilia, but they exhibit a whirling, rotational movement (see Fig. 404-2), resulting in leftward flow of extracellular fluid that establishes body sidedness. Nodal cilia defects result in body orientation abnormalities, such as **situs inversus totalis**, **situs ambiguus**, and **heterotaxy** associated with congenital heart disease, asplenia, and polysplenia (see Chapter 431.11).

GENETICS OF PRIMARY CILIARY DYSKINESIA

PCD is typically has autosomal recessive patterns of inheritance, although rare cases of autosomal dominant and X-linked inheritance have been reported. PCD is a genetically heterogeneous disorder involving multiple genes; mutations in any protein that is involved in ciliary assembly, structure, or function could theoretically cause disease. Early linkage analyses showed substantial locus heterogeneity, which made correlations between ciliary defects and the underlying mutations difficult. Numerous PCD-associated genes have been discovered. The advent of high-throughput sequencing technologies has allowed for even more rapid identification of new mutations in PCD subjects. To date, mutations in 18 different genes have been linked to PCD (Fig. 404-3), including those that encode proteins integral to the outer dynein arm (*DNAH5, DNAI1, DNAL1, DNAI2, TXNDC3,* and *DNAH11*), inner dynein arm and axonemal organization (*CCDC39* and *CCDC40*), and the central apparatus and radial spokes (*RSPH9, RSPH4A,* and *HYDIN*). More recently, mutations in genes that code for cytoplasmic proteins involved in cilia assembly or protein transport (*HEATR2, DNAAF1, DNAAF2, DNAAF3, CCDC103, LRRC6,* and *CCDC114*) have been shown to cause ultrastructural abnormalities. The genetics of PCD has further exposed the gaps in current diagnostic approaches. For instance, *DNAH11* mutations have been shown to cause typical clinical phenotypes without apparent axonemal ultrastructural defects or reduced ciliary beat frequency. Mutations in 2

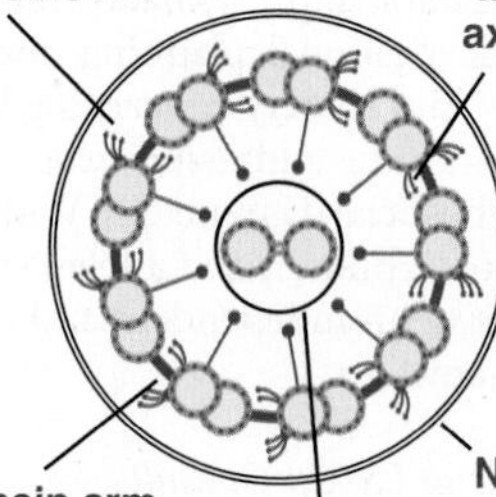

Figure 404-3 Classification of proteins mutated in primary ciliary dyskinesia. *(Adapted from Horani A, Ferkol TW: Molecular genetics of primary ciliary dyskinesia. In Encyclopedia of Life Sciences (eLS), 2014. John Wiley & Sons, Chichester, UK. Available at: http://www.els.net/WileyCDA/ElsArticle/refId-a0024989.html.)*

Table 404-1	Clinical Manifestations of Primary Ciliary Dyskinesia
RESPIRATORY TRACT *Lung* Neonatal respiratory distress Chronic cough Recurrent pneumonia Bronchiectasis *Middle Ear* Chronic otitis media Conductive hearing loss *Paranasal Sinuses* Neonatal rhinitis Chronic mucopurulent rhinitis Chronic pansinusitis Nasal polyposis	**GENITOURINARY TRACT** Male and female infertility **LEFT-RIGHT ORIENTATION DEFECTS** Situs inversus Heterotaxy Congenital heart disease **CENTRAL NERVOUS SYSTEM** Hydrocephalus Retinitis pigmentosa

other genes, *CCDC39* and *CCDC40*, produce inconsistent structural abnormalities characterized by disordered microtubules in some, but not all, cilia, which underscores the observation that current diagnostic testing will miss cases.

CLINICAL MANIFESTATIONS OF PRIMARY CILIARY DYSKINESIA
See Table 404-1.

Most patients with PCD present with **neonatal respiratory distress**, which is manifested as tachypnea, hypoxemia, or even respiratory failure requiring mechanical ventilation. The association of respiratory distress in term neonates with PCD has been underappreciated. The upper respiratory tract is almost universally involved in PCD, and **persistent rhinosinusitis** is common during infancy. Inadequate innate mucus clearance leads to chronic sinusitis (see Chapter 380) and nasal polyposis. Middle ear disease occurs in nearly all children with PCD, with varying degrees of **chronic otitis media** leading to conductive hearing loss and myringotomy tube placement, which is often complicated by intractable otorrhea.

Impaired mucociliary clearance of the lower respiratory tract leads to daily productive cough, often in young children, secondary to chronic bronchitis. Bacterial cultures of sputum or lavage fluid frequently yield nontypeable *Haemophilus influenzae* (see Chapter 194), *Staphylococcus aureus* (see Chapter 181.1), *Streptococcus pneumoniae* (see Chapter 182), and *Pseudomonas aeruginosa* (see Chapter 205.1). Persistent airway infection and inflammation lead to **bronchiectasis**, even in preschool children. Clubbing is a sign of long-standing pulmonary involvement.

Left-right laterality defects (e.g., *situs inversus totalis*) are found in half of all children with PCD. Without functional nodal cilia in the embryonic period, thoracoabdominal orientation is random. These patients have **Kartagener triad**, defined as *situs inversus totalis*, chronic sinusitis, and bronchiectasis. Approximately 25% of patients with *situs inversus totalis* have PCD, so *situs inversus totalis* alone does not establish the diagnosis of PCD. Other laterality defects, such as heterotaxy, are associated with PCD and may coexist with congenital cardiac defects, asplenia, or polysplenia.

Most men with PCD have dysmotile spermatozoa because flagellar and ciliary ultrastructure is similar. Male infertility is typical, but not always found in this disease. Fertility issues in women have also been reported and are likely a result of ciliary dysfunction in the fallopian tubes.

A few case reports have associated **neonatal hydrocephalus** with PCD. The ependyma of the brain ventricles are lined by ciliated epithelium and are important for cerebrospinal fluid flow through the ventricles and aqueduct of Sylvius. The finding of enlarged brain ventricles on sonograms, when linked with *situs inversus totalis*, has been proposed as a prenatal diagnostic marker for PCD. X-linked retinitis pigmentosa has been associated with recurrent respiratory infections in families with *RPGR* gene mutations. Intraflagellar transport proteins are essential for photoreceptor assembly, and when mutated, lead to apoptosis of the retinal pigment epithelium (see Chapter 630).

DIAGNOSIS OF PRIMARY CILIARY DYSKINESIA

The diagnosis of PCD should be suspected in children with chronic or recurring upper and lower respiratory tract symptoms that begin in early infancy and is currently based on the presence of characteristic clinical phenotype and ultrastructural defects of cilia, though this approach will miss affected individuals. The diagnosis is often delayed, even in children who have classic clinical features, such as chronic rhinosinusitis in infancy, persistent otitis media, or even *situs inversus totalis*. The average age at PCD diagnosis is approximately 4 yr; a high index of suspicion is necessary.

Imaging studies show extensive involvement of the paranasal sinuses. Chest radiographs frequently demonstrate bilateral lung overinflation, peribronchial infiltrates, and lobar atelectasis. Computerized x-ray tomography of the chest often reveals bronchiectasis, often involving the anatomic right middle lobe or lingual, even in young children. *Situs inversus totalis* in a child who has chronic respiratory tract symptoms is highly suggestive of PCD, but this configuration occurs in only half of patients with PCD. Pulmonary function testing typically shows progressive intrathoracic airway obstruction.

Transmission electron microscopy is the current gold standard to assess structural defects within the cilium. Curettage from the nasal epithelium or endobronchial brushing can provide an adequate specimen for review. Identification of a discrete, consistent defect in any aspect of the ciliary structure with concurrent phenotypic features is sufficient to make the diagnosis. Shortening or absence of dynein arms is the most common abnormality seen in PCD, accounting for 90% of cases with defined ultrastructural defects (see Fig. 404-3). Other axonemal changes consistent with PCD include microtubular transposition, radial spoke and nexin link defects, and ciliary agenesis. Unfortunately, ultrastructural examination of cilia as a diagnostic test for PCD has significant drawbacks. First, the absence of axonemal defects does not exclude PCD; nearly 30% of all affected individuals have normal ciliary ultrastructure. Careful interpretation of the ultrastructural findings is necessary, because nonspecific changes may be seen in relation to exposure to environmental pollutants or infection. Ciliary defects can be acquired (Table 404-2). Acute airway infection or inflammation can result in structural changes (e.g., compound cilia or blebs). Ciliary disorientation has been proposed as a form of PCD, but this phenomenon is the result of airway injury. Frequently, the diagnosis of PCD can be delayed or missed because of inadequate tissue collection or sample processing as well as the lack of an

Table 404-2	Electron Microscopic Findings in Primary Ciliary Dyskinesia vs Acquired Cilia Abnormality	
	PCD	**ACQUIRED DEFECTS**
EM ultrastructure	Dynein arm deficiency	Compound cilia
	Outer arms	Added peripheral tubules
	Inner arms	Deleted peripheral tubules
	Both	Added central pairs
	Translocation of central tubules	Translocation of central tubules
	Few or absent cilia (generalized)	Few or absent cilia (patchy)
Beat frequency	Hyperkinetic, slow or absent	May be normal or reduced
Wave form	Abnormal	May be normal or abnormal

EM, electron microscopy; PCD, primary ciliary dyskinesia.
From Stillwell PC, Wartchow EP, Sagel SD. Primary ciliary dyskinesia in children: A review for pediatricians, allergists, and pediatric pulmonologists. Pediatr Allergy Immunol Pulmonol 24: 191–196, 2011, Table 1.

experienced pathologist who can distinguish between primary and acquired ciliary defects. Several reviews have advocated culturing of airway epithelial cells and allowing the secondary changes to resolve.

Qualitative tests to assess ciliary function have been used to screen for PCD. Ciliary beat frequency measurements that use conventional microscopic techniques have been used as a screen, but this method alone will miss cases of PCD. Cilia inspection using standard light microscopy is insufficient to support or exclude the diagnosis. High-resolution, high-speed, digital imaging of ciliary motion in multiple planes has permitted comprehensive analysis of abnormal beat patterns. This approach is available only at a limited number of clinical centers and requires sophisticated software and expertise. Immunofluorescence imaging has been used to show mislocalization of dynein arm proteins. Such techniques are research tools and not widely available.

Another promising approach has exploited the observation that nasal nitric oxide concentrations are reduced in subjects with PCD. Because nasal nitric oxide measurements are relatively easy to perform and noninvasive, this method is a promising screen and potentially a diagnostic test for PCD, provided that cystic fibrosis has been excluded (see Chapter 403). Few studies in younger children have been reported, and the accuracy of nasal nitric oxide measurements in infants has not been established.

PCD is highly heterogenic owing to the large number of proteins involved in cilia assembly and function. Recent advances in gene sequencing techniques have led to the identification of a growing number of PCD-associated genes. The pace of new gene discovery has accelerated during the past 2 yr, and new discoveries are forthcoming. Genetic testing for PCD is available, but commercial laboratories offer testing for only some mutations. It is reasonable to expect that genetic testing will become the preferred diagnostic approach for PCD, but disease-causing mutations have only been linked to approximately 60% of known cases.

TREATMENT

No therapies correct ciliary dysfunction in PCD. Many of the treatments applied to PCD patients are similar to those used in other suppurative lung diseases characterized by impaired airway clearance and bronchiectasis, such as cystic fibrosis, but none have been adequately studied to demonstrate their efficacy in PCD.

Strategies to enhance mucociliary clearance are central to PCD therapy, and routine airway clearance techniques using postural drainage, percussion vests, positive expiratory pressure devices, or other techniques should be instituted on a daily basis. Because ciliary function is impaired, cough becomes a critical mechanism for mucus clearance and should not be suppressed. Exercise can enhance airway clearance in patients with PCD and should be encouraged. Inhaled mucolytic agents are often used in cystic fibrosis care, and few case reports have shown improvement in lung function in patients with PCD after treatment.

When children with PCD develop increasing respiratory symptoms consistent with infection, antimicrobial therapy should be instituted on the basis of respiratory culture results and bacterial sensitivities. Early eradication strategies to clear bacteria from the PCD lung have not been studied. Maintenance therapy with inhaled or oral antibiotics can be used cautiously in patients with PCD who have bronchiectasis or frequent exacerbations, although current literature lacks evidence supporting long-term antimicrobial therapy. Immunizations against pertussis, influenza, and pneumococci are cornerstones of care. Additional preventive measures include avoidance of cigarette smoke and other airway irritants.

Although β-adrenergic agonists increase ciliary beat frequency in normal epithelial cells, data is lacking that shows these agents improve function of dyskinetic cilia. Moreover, they do not necessarily provide bronchodilation in patients with PCD and obstructive airway disease.

Surgical resection of bronchiectatic lung has been performed on patients with PCD, typically in cases of localized disease with severe hemoptysis or recurrent febrile illnesses. It is unclear whether surgical interventions provide reduction in symptoms or survival benefit.

Progression to end-stage lung disease and respiratory failure has been reported in patients with PCD. Adult patients have undergone successful heart-lung, double lung, or living donor lobar lung transplantation. *Situs inversus totalis* complicates the procedure owing to anatomic considerations. Otherwise, survival is similar to that for other transplant recipients.

Treatment of chronic otitis media and middle ear effusions in patients with PCD is controversial. Myringotomy tubes are frequently placed in affected children, but they are not without complications, because they may lead to chronic mucoid otorrhea, tympanosclerosis, and permanent membrane perforation. Myringotomy tubes have not measurably improved hearing acuity. Although hearing tends to improve with time, it should be routinely screened and hearing aids used when necessary.

Chronic rhinitis and sinusitis are frequent clinical manifestations of PCD. No treatments have been shown to be effective, although patients are often treated with nasal washes, paranasal sinus lavage, and systemic antibiotics when they are symptomatic. As with any overuse of antimicrobial agents, the development of resistant organisms is a concern. When nasal symptoms are severe or refractory to medical management, endoscopic sinus surgery can be used to promote drainage or local delivery of medications, though the benefit may be short-lived.

PROGNOSIS

Although signs and symptoms related to upper respiratory involvement predominate early in PCD, clinical manifestations of lower respiratory tract disease tend to increase with age and become the leading cause of morbidity and mortality in PCD patients. It is believed that progression and extent of lung disease can be slowed with early diagnosis and therapy. Thus, routine surveillance studies recommended for the care of children with PCD include (1) regular spirometry to monitor pulmonary function, (2) chest imaging, and (3) sputum or oropharyngeal cultures to assess lung respiratory flora.

Patients with PCD typically have slower decline in pulmonary function than those with cystic fibrosis. Its prognosis and long-term survival are better. Many patients with PCD have a normal or near-normal life span, although some do experience progressive bronchiectasis and respiratory deterioration earlier in life.

Bibliography is available at Expert Consult.

Chapter 405
Diffuse Lung Diseases in Childhood

See also Chapter 399.

405.1 Inherited Disorders of Surfactant Metabolism
Lawrence M. Nogee, F. Sessions Cole III, and Aaron Hamvas

Pulmonary surfactant is a mixture of phospholipids and proteins synthesized, packaged, and secreted by alveolar type II pneumocytes (AEC2s) that line the distal air spaces. This mixture forms a monolayer at the air–liquid interface that lowers surface tension at end-expiration of the respiratory cycle, preventing atelectasis and ventilation–perfusion mismatch. Four surfactant-associated proteins have been described: surfactant proteins A and D (SP-A, SP-D) participate in host defense in the lung, whereas surfactant proteins B and C (SP-B, SP-C) contribute to the surface tension–lowering activity of the pulmonary surfactant. The adenosine triphosphate–binding cassette protein member A3, ABCA3, is a transporter located on the limiting membrane of lamellar bodies, the storage organelle for surfactant within alveolar type II cells, and has an essential role in surfactant phospholipid metabolism. The proper expression of the surfactant proteins and ABCA3 is dependent on a number of transcription factors, particularly thyroid transcription factor 1 (TTF-1). Two genes for SP-A (*SFTPA1, SFTPA2*) and 1 gene for SP-D (*SFTPD*) are located on human chromosome 10, whereas single genes encode SP-B (*SFTPB*), SP-C (*SFTPC*), TTF-1 (*NKX2-1*) and ABCA3 (*ABCA3*), which are located on human chromosomes 2, 8, 14, and 16, respectively. Inherited disorders of SP-B, SP-C, ABCA3 and TTF-1 have been identified in humans and are collectively termed **surfactant dysfunction disorders** (Table 405-1).

PATHOLOGY

Histopathologically, these disorders share a unique constellation of features, including AEC2 hyperplasia, alveolar macrophage accumulation, interstitial thickening and inflammation, and alveolar proteinosis. A number of different descriptive terms have historically been applied to these disorders, including ones borrowed from adult forms of interstitial lung disease (**desquamative interstitial pneumonia**, nonspecific interstitial pneumonia) as well as a disorder unique to infancy (**chronic pneumonitis of infancy**). These diagnoses in infants and children are strongly indicative of surfactant dysfunction disorders but do not distinguish which gene is responsible. As the prognosis and inheritance patterns differ depending upon the gene involved, genetic testing should be offered when one of these conditions is reported in the lung biopsy or autopsy of a child.

Deficiency of Surfactant Protein B (Surfactant Metabolism Dysfunction, Pulmonary, 1; SMDP1; OMIM #265120)
Clinical Manifestations
Infants with an inherited deficiency of SP-B present in the immediate neonatal period with respiratory failure. This autosomal recessive disorder is clinically and radiographically similar to the respiratory distress syndrome (RDS) of premature infants (see Chapter 101.3) but typically affects full-term infants. The initial degree of respiratory distress is variable, but the disease is progressive and is refractory to mechanical ventilation, surfactant replacement therapy, glucocorticoid

Table 405-1	Comparison of Surfactant Deficiency Syndromes			
	SP-B DEFICIENCY	**SP-C DISEASE**	**ABCA3 DEFICIENCY**	**TTF-1 DEFICIENCY**
Gene name	*SFTPB*	*SFTPC*	*ABCA3*	*NKX2-1*
Age of onset	Birth	Birth–adulthood	Birth–childhood	Birth–childhood
Inheritance	Recessive	Dominant/sporadic	Recessive	Sporadic/dominant
Mechanism	Loss of function	Gain of toxic function or dominant negative	Loss of function	Loss of function ?Gain of function
Natural history	Lethal	Variable	Generally lethal, may be chronic	Variable
Diagnosis:				
Biochemical *(tracheal aspirate)*	Absence of SP-B and presence of proSP-C	None	None	None
Genetic *(DNA)*	Sequence *SFTPB*	Sequence *SFTPC*	Sequence *ABCA3*	Sequence *NKX2-1*; deletion analysis
Ultrastructural *(lung biopsy–electron microscopy)*	Disorganized lamellar bodies	Not specific; may have dense aggregates	Small dense lamellar bodies with eccentrically placed dense cores	Variable
Treatment	Lung transplantation or compassionate care	Supportive care, lung transplantation if progressing	Consider lung transplantation	Supportive care; treat coexisting conditions (hypothyroidism)

SP, surfactant protein.

administration, and extracorporeal membrane oxygenation. SP-B deficiency is recognized in diverse racial and ethnic groups. Almost all affected patients have died without lung transplantation, but prolonged survival is possible in cases of partial deficiency of SP-B. Although murine lineages heterozygous for SP-B deficiency are susceptible to oxidant injury and pulmonary infection, humans heterozygous for loss-of-function mutations in *SFTPB* are clinically normal as adults but may be at increased risk for obstructive lung disease if they also have a history of smoking.

Genetics

Multiple loss-of-function mutations in *SFTPB* have been identified. The most common is a net 2 base-pair insertion in codon 121 (originally termed 121ins2) that results in a frameshift, an unstable SP-B transcript, and absence of SP-B protein production. This mutation has accounted for 60-70% of the alleles found to date in patients identified with SP-B deficiency. Most other mutations have been family specific. A large deletion encompassing 2 exons of the SP-B gene has also been reported.

Diagnosis

A rapid, definitive diagnosis can be established with sequence analysis of *SFTPB*, which is available through clinical laboratories (http://www.genetests.org). In families in which a mutation was previously identified, antenatal diagnosis can be established by molecular assays of DNA from chorionic villous biopsy or amniocytes, which permits advanced planning of a therapeutic regimen. Other laboratory tests remain investigational, including analysis of tracheal effluent by for the presence or absence of SP-B protein and for incompletely processed precursor proSP-C peptides that have been found in SP-B–deficient human infants and animals. Immunostaining of lung biopsy tissue for the surfactant proteins can also support the diagnosis, although immunohistochemical assays for SP-B and SP-C are also generally available only on a research basis. Staining for SP-B is usually absent, but robust extracellular staining for proSP-C because of incompletely processed proSP-C peptides is observed and is diagnostic for SP-B deficiency. Such studies require a lung biopsy in a critically ill child but may be performed on lung blocks acquired at the time of autopsy, allowing for retrospective diagnosis. With electron microscopy, a lack of tubular myelin, disorganized lamellar bodies, and an accumulation of abnormal-appearing multivesicular bodies, suggest abnormal lipid packaging and secretion.

Surfactant Protein C Gene Abnormalities (Surfactant Metabolism Dysfunction, Pulmonary, 2; SMDP2; OMIM #610913)

SP-C is a very low-molecular-weight, extremely hydrophobic protein that, along with SP-B, enhances the surface tension–lowering properties of surfactant phospholipids. It is derived from proteolytic processing of a larger precursor protein (proSP-C).

Clinical Manifestations

The clinical presentation of patients with *SFTPC* mutations is quite variable. Some patients present at birth with symptoms, signs, and radiographic findings typical of RDS. Others present later in life, ranging from early infancy until well into adulthood, with gradual onset of respiratory insufficiency, hypoxemia, failure to thrive, and chest radiograph demonstration of interstitial lung disease, or, in the 5th or 6th decade of life, as pulmonary fibrosis. The age and severity of disease vary even within families with the same mutation. The natural history is also quite variable, with some patients improving either spontaneously or as the result of therapy, some with persistent respiratory insufficiency, and some progressing to the point of requiring lung transplantation. This variability in severity and course of the disease does not appear to correlate with the specific mutation and also hinders accurate assessment of prognosis.

Genetics

Multiple mutations in *SFTPC* have been identified in association with acute and chronic lung disease in patients ranging in age from newborn to adult. A mutation on only 1 *SFTPC* allele is sufficient to cause disease. Approximately half of these mutations arise spontaneously, resulting in sporadic disease, but the remainder are inherited as a dominant trait. A threonine substitution for isoleucine in codon 73 (termed p.I73T or p.Ile73Thr) accounts for 25-35% of the cases identified to date. Mutations in *SFTPC* are thought to result in production of misfolded proSP-C that accumulates within the alveolar type II cell and causes cellular injury, or alters the normal intracellular routing of proSP-C. The frequency of mutations or disease caused by mutations in *SFTPC* is unknown but is probably low. Mutations have been identified in diverse racial and ethnic groups.

Diagnosis

Sequencing of *SFTPC*, the only definitive diagnostic test, is available in clinical laboratories. The relatively small size of the gene facilitates such analyses, which are quite sensitive, but because most *SFTPC* mutations are missense mutations, distinguishing true disease-causing mutations from rare yet benign sequence variants may be difficult. Immunostaining of lung tissue may demonstrate proSP-C aggregates but is available only on a research basis.

Disease Caused by Mutations in ABCA3 (Surfactant Metabolism Dysfunction, Pulmonary, 3; SMDP3; OMIM #610921)

Clinical Manifestations

Lung disease caused by mutations in *ABCA3* generally presents as either a severe, lethal form that manifests in the immediate newborn period clinically similar to SP-B deficiency, or a chronic form that appears most typically in the 1st yr of life with interstitial lung disease similar to SP-C–associated disease. Infants who are homozygous or compound heterozygous for null mutations, that is, the mutation is predicted to result in absence of protein expression, typically present with lethal neonatal disease, whereas infants with other types of mutations have more variable age of onset and outcomes. Heterozygosity for an *ABCA3* mutation may contribute to the severity of RDS in prematurely born infants, who, in contrast to ABCA3-deficient infants with mutations on both alleles, may eventually completely recover from their initial lung disease.

Genetics

Recessive mutations in *ABCA3* were first described in infants who presented with lethal respiratory distress in the newborn period, but now have been identified in older infants and children with interstitial lung disease. There is considerable allelic heterogeneity: More than 200 mutations scattered throughout the gene have been identified, most of which are family specific. A missense mutation that results in a valine substitution for glutamine in codon 292 (p.E292V or p.Glu292Val) in association with a second *ABCA3* mutation has been found in children with severe neonatal respiratory failure and in older children with interstitial lung disease and is present in approximately 0.4% of the general population. *ABCA3* mutations have been identified in diverse racial and ethnic groups. The precise frequency of disease is unknown, but large-scale sequencing projects indicate that the overall carrier rate for *ABCA3* mutations may be as high as 1 in 50 to 1 in 70 individuals. ABCA3 deficiency may thus contribute to a substantial proportion of **unexplained fatal lung disease** in term infants and of **interstitial lung disease** in older children.

Diagnosis

Sequence analysis of *ABCA3* is available in clinical laboratories and is the most definitive approach for diagnosis. Considerable variation in *ABCA3* necessitates careful interpretation regarding the functionality of an individual variant and its contribution to the clinical presentation. Additionally, sequence analysis is not 100% sensitive as functionally significant mutations may exist in untranslated regions that are not generally analyzed. In these situations, lung biopsy with electron microscopy to examine lamellar body morphology may be a useful adjunct to the diagnostic approach. Small lamellar bodies that contain electron-dense inclusions may be observed in association with *ABCA3* mutations. These findings support the hypothesis that ABCA3 function is necessary for lamellar body biogenesis. There are no biochemical markers to establish the diagnosis.

Disease Caused by Mutations in NKX2-1 (Thyroid Transcription Factor 1, Choreoathetosis, Hypothyroidism, and Neonatal Respiratory Distress, OMIM #600635)

Clinical Manifestations

A large deletion of the region of chromosome 14 (14q13.3) encompassing the *NKX2-1* locus was first recognized in an infant with hypothyroidism and neonatal RDS. Since then, multiple large deletions involving the *NKX2-1* locus and contiguous genes as well as missense, frameshift, nonsense, and small insertion or deletion mutations scattered throughout the gene have been reported in individuals with

hypothyroidism, lung disease, and neurologic symptoms, including benign familial chorea. Manifestation of dysfunction in all 3 organ systems has been referred to as **brain-thyroid-lung syndrome**, but disease may manifest in only 1 or 2 organ systems. The lung disease can range from severe and eventually lethal neonatal respiratory distress to chronic lung disease in childhood and adulthood. Recurrent pulmonary infections have been reported, likely caused by reduced expression of the pulmonary collectins, SP-A and SP-D, but could also result from decreased expression of other proteins. No clear genotype–phenotype correlations have emerged, but children harboring complete gene deletions have tended to have more severe and earlier-onset disease. This observation could also be related to the deletion of other adjacent genes. While limited data are available, the pulmonary phenotype may depend upon the expression of which NKX2-1 target genes are most affected. Children with decreased SP-B or ABCA3 expression may present with acute neonatal respiratory failure whereas those with decreased SP-C or pulmonary collection expression are more likely to have chronic lung disease.

Genetics

The gene is small, spanning <3,000 bases, with only 3 exons. TTF-1 is expressed not only in the lung but also in the thyroid gland, as well as in the central nervous system. In the lung it is important for the expression of a wide variety of proteins, including the surfactant proteins, ABCA3, Clara cell secretory protein, and many others. Two transcripts that differ depending upon whether the transcriptional start site is in the 1st or 2nd exon have been recognized, although the shorter transcript is the predominant one in the lung. Most mutations are thought to result in a loss of function, with the mechanism of disease thus being haploinsufficiency, but discordant effects on different target genes have been reported. The incidence of mutations and incidence and prevalence of disease are unknown; mutations in diverse ethnic groups have been recognized. Most reported mutations and deletions have occurred de novo resulting in sporadic disease, but familial disease transmitted in a dominant manner has been recognized.

Diagnosis

Sequence analysis of the *NKX2-1* gene is available through clinical laboratories and is the preferred method for diagnosis. As deletions comprise a significant fraction of reported mutant alleles, specific methods to look for such deletions should also be performed, such as a comparative genomic hybridization assay or multiplex ligation-dependent probe amplification assay. A mutation on 1 allele is sufficient to cause disease. While isolated pulmonary disease has been recognized, the majority of reported affected individuals have had manifestations in 1 or more other organ systems. Thus the presence of hypothyroidism or neurologic abnormality in a proband or a family history of chorea should prompt consideration of the diagnosis. The most specific neurologic finding is chorea, but hypotonia, developmental delay, ataxia, and dysarthria have been reported. In very young, nonambulatory infants the neurologic symptoms may not be evident, or muscle weakness or hypotonia may be attributed to the severity of lung disease or a result of the hypothyroidism. Affected individuals may not be overtly hypothyroid but have compensated hypothyroidism with borderline low T4 (thyroxine) and high thyroid-stimulating hormone levels. The lung pathology associated with *NKX2-1* mutations may be typical of that of other surfactant dysfunction disorders, but because *NKX2-1* is important for lung development, growth abnormalities and arrested pulmonary development also may be seen. Immunostaining studies of surfactant protein expression have yielded variable results, with decreased expression of 1 or more surfactant-related proteins observed in some patients. No characteristic electron microscopy findings have been identified.

TREATMENT OF SURFACTANT DYSFUNCTION DISORDERS

Virtually all patients with SP-B deficiency die within the 1st yr of life. Conventional neonatal intensive care interventions can maintain extrapulmonary organ function for a limited time (weeks to months).

Replacement therapy with commercially available surfactants is ineffective. Lung transplantation has been successful, but the pretransplantation, transplantation, and posttransplantation medical and surgical care is highly specialized and available only at pediatric pulmonary transplantation centers; prompt recognition is critical if patients are to be considered for lung transplantation. Palliative care consultation is helpful.

No specific treatment is available for patients with lung disease caused by mutations in *SFTPC* or *ABCA3*. Therapeutic approaches used for interstitial lung diseases, such as the use of corticosteroids, quinolones, and macrolide antibiotics have been reported but not systematically evaluated. Infants with severe and progressive respiratory failure attributable to ABCA3 deficiency may be candidates for lung transplantation. The variable natural history of patients with *SFTPC* mutations and older children with ABCA3 deficiency makes predictions of prognosis difficult. Lung transplantation is reserved for patients with progressive and refractory respiratory failure who would otherwise qualify for transplantation irrespective of their diagnosis.

Treatment for patients with *NKX2-1* mutations is largely supportive. Hypothyroidism if present should be treated with thyroid replacement. Corticosteroids and other agents used for other types of surfactant dysfunction have not been formally evaluated. Some individuals have progressive lung disease, and lung transplantation has been performed for some subjects with end-stage lung disease. The variable progression of disease and presence of extrapulmonary disease may make evaluation and selection of subjects for transplantation particularly difficult.

Parents of children with surfactant dysfunction disorders should be offered genetic counseling. This allows for defining the recurrence risks for future pregnancies and the availability of antenatal diagnosis and therapeutic options, as well whether testing should be offered to other family members who may not be symptomatic.

Bibliography is available at Expert Consult.

405.2 Pulmonary Alveolar Proteinosis
Lawrence M. Nogee, F. Sessions Cole III, and Aaron Hamvas

Pulmonary alveolar proteinosis (PAP) is a rare type of diffuse lung disease characterized by the intraalveolar accumulation of pulmonary surfactant. Histopathologic examination shows distal air spaces to be filled with a granular, eosinophilic material that stains positively with periodic acid–Schiff reagent and is diastase resistant. This material contains large amounts of surfactant proteins and lipids and the primary mechanism for its accumulation is impaired catabolism by alveolar macrophages. PAP has historically been classified as either primary (idiopathic) or secondary to a number of different conditions, although this terminology is evolving as specific etiologies for PAP are identified. (A fulminant, usually lethal form manifesting shortly after birth has been termed "congenital alveolar proteinosis," but because this condition is caused by disrupted surfactant metabolism or surfactant dysfunction within alveolar type II cells, the disease is included under "Inherited Disorders of Surfactant Metabolism," above (see Chapter 405.1).

ETIOLOGY AND PATHOPHYSIOLOGY
Disordered signaling of granulocyte-macrophage colony-stimulating factor (GM-CSF) leading to impaired alveolar macrophage maturation is the major underlying cause of primary PAP in children and adults. Most cases of primary PAP in older children and adults are mediated by neutralizing autoantibodies directed against GM-CSF, which can be detected in serum and bronchoalveolar lavage (BAL) fluid. These autoantibodies block binding of GM-CSF to its receptor, thereby inhibiting alveolar macrophage maturation and function and surfactant clearance. Mutations in the genes encoding both the α and β subunits of the GM-CSF receptor *(CSF2RA, CSFR2B)* in children with primary

alveolar proteinosis account for a genetic basis for some cases of primary PAP in childhood. Alveolar proteinosis has also been reported in children, including young infants, with **lysinuric protein intolerance**, a rare autosomal recessive disorder caused by mutations in the cationic amino acid transporter SLC7A7 (see Chapter 85.14). These children generally present with vomiting, hyperammonemia, and failure to thrive, although their pulmonary disease may prove fatal. Defective macrophage function has been demonstrated in lysinuric protein intolerance and a case of recurrence of the disease after lung transplantation also supports a primary role for alveolar macrophage dysfunction in the pathogenesis of PAP associated with lysinuric protein intolerance. PAP is also associated with some subtypes of **Niemann-Pick disease** (see Chapter 86.4).

Secondary alveolar proteinosis also may occur in association with infection, particularly in immunocompromised individuals. However, because the same pathologic process occurs in severely immunodeficient mice raised in a pathogen-free environment, it is not clear whether this phenotype results from a secondary infection or the underlying immunodeficiency. Environmental exposures to dust, silica, and chemicals and chemotherapeutic agents have also been associated with the development of secondary alveolar proteinosis.

CLINICAL MANIFESTATIONS
Infants and children with PAP present with dyspnea, fatigue, cough, weight loss, chest pain, or hemoptysis. In the later stages, cyanosis and digital clubbing may be seen. Pulmonary function changes include decreased diffusing capacity of carbon monoxide, lung volumes with a restrictive abnormality, and arterial blood gas values indicating marked hypoxia and/or chronic respiratory acidosis. Alveolar proteinosis in infants and children is rare. Boys are affected 3 times as often as girls. Usually there is no identifiable etiologic factor (primary), although PAP may occur in association with malignancy or infection, particularly in the setting of systemic immunosuppression or congenital immunodeficiency, or following exposure to several inciting agents, such as dust and chemicals (secondary).

DIAGNOSIS
Histopathologic examination of lung biopsy specimens currently remains the gold standard for diagnosis of PAP in children, although this is likely to change as molecular tests become available. Immunohistochemical staining reveals abundant quantities of alveolar and intracellular surfactant proteins A, B, and D. Latex agglutination tests for the presence of anti–GM-CSF antibodies in BAL fluid or blood are highly sensitive and specific for the autoimmune forms of alveolar proteinosis. Elevations of GM-CSF in peripheral blood suggest a GM-CSF receptor defect, and molecular analysis of these genes should be pursued. The examination of sputum or BAL fluid for surfactant components has been used diagnostically in adults, but these methods have not been validated in children. Examination of peripheral blood and/or bone marrow for clonogenic stimulation of monocyte-macrophage precursors, GM-CSF receptor and ligand expression, and GM-CSF binding and signaling studies are available through research protocols.

TREATMENT
The natural history of primary PAP is highly variable, making prognostic and therapeutic decisions difficult. Total lung lavage has been associated with prolonged remissions of PAP in adults and remains a therapeutic option for patients with childhood PAP (Figs. 405-1 and 405-2). Younger infants with PAP may be more likely to have genetic mechanisms underlying their disease, and the role of repeated BAL in children has not been well studied, nor is it likely to be effective. It may provide a temporizing measure in some circumstances and may benefit patients with autoimmune or secondary PAP. Subcutaneous or inhaled administration of recombinant GM-CSF may improve pulmonary function in some adults with later-onset PAP. The role of exogenous GM-CSF treatment in children has not been well studied, although successful treatment has been reported in an adolescent with autoimmune-mediated PAP. Because children with GM-CSF receptor

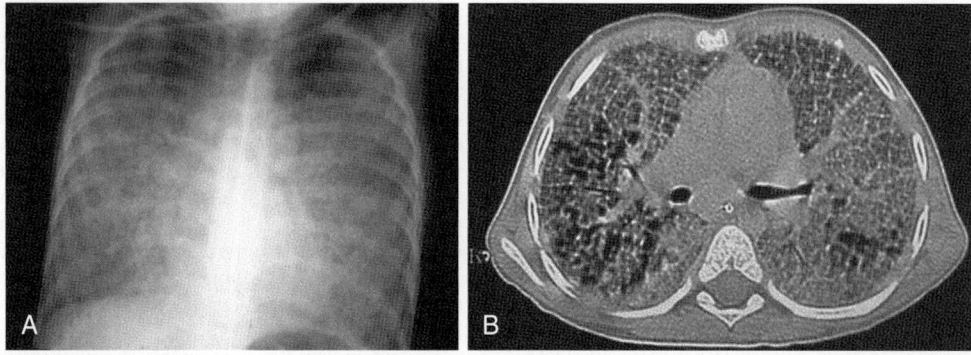

Figure 405-1 Severe pulmonary alveolar proteinosis in a 5 yr old boy before therapeutic lung lavage. **A,** Chest radiograph shows diffuse alveolointerstitial infiltrates. **B,** CT scan demonstrates major air-space opacities and crazy-paving pattern. *(From De Blic J: Pulmonary alveolar proteinosis in children, Paediatr Respir Rev 5:316–322, 2004.)*

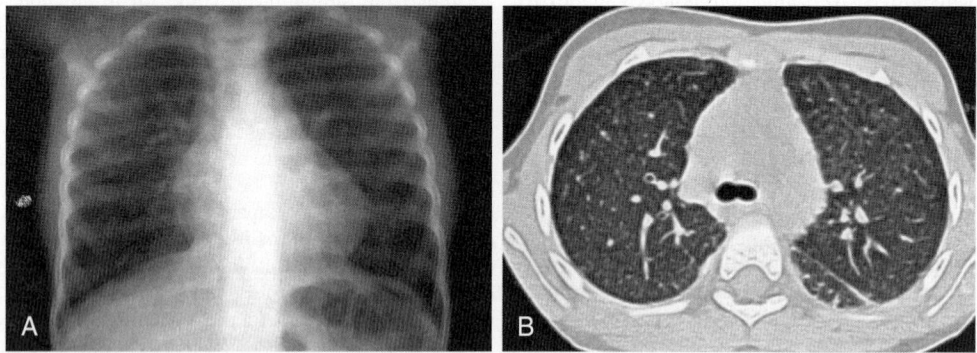

Figure 405-2 Same patient as in Figure 405-1 after 12 therapeutic lung lavages. **A,** Chest radiograph demonstrates improvement of alveolointerstitial infiltrates. **B,** CT scan shows regression of the air-space opacities with a residual micronodular pattern. *(From De Blic J: Pulmonary alveolar proteinosis in children, Paediatr Respir Rev 5:316–322, 2004.)*

defects generally have high serum levels of GM-CSF, exogenous GM-CSF seems unlikely to be effective in most such cases. Depending upon the nature of the mutation(s) responsible for the deficiency, some responsiveness of the receptor may be retained such that a response to exogenous GM-CSF is possible. As the primary defect for PAP resides in the alveolar macrophage, which is a bone marrow–derived cell, lung transplantation would not be expected to correct primary PAP.

Bibliography is available at Expert Consult.

Chapter **406**
Pulmonary Hemosiderosis
Mary A. Nevin

Pulmonary hemorrhage may be characterized as focal or diffuse based on the site(s) of bleeding. A detailed review of pulmonary hemorrhage is in Chapter 407.2. The diagnosis of pulmonary hemosiderosis refers to the subset of patients with **diffuse alveolar hemorrhage (DAH)**. Bleeding in DAH occurs as a result of injury to the microvasculature of the lung and may be slow and insidious due to the low pressure pulmonary circulation. Pulmonary hemosiderosis has classically been characterized by the triad of iron-deficiency anemia, hemoptysis, and multiple alveolar infiltrates on chest radiographs. However, many of those affected, particularly young patients are likely to present

atypically and a high index of suspicion for this condition must be maintained. Pulmonary hemosiderosis can exist in isolation, but more commonly occurs in association with an underlying condition. A precise etiology for hemorrhage may not always be found. A diagnosis of **idiopathic pulmonary hemosiderosis (IPH)** is made when DAH occurs in isolation and an exhaustive evaluation for an underlying pathologic etiology is found to be unrevealing.

ETIOLOGY
Current classification schemes organize the etiologies of pulmonary hemosiderosis on the basis of the presence of absence of pulmonary capillaritis; a pathologic process that is characterized by inflammation and cellular disruption of the alveolar interstitium and capillary bed. Although the finding of pulmonary capillaritis is nonspecific with regard to underlying diagnosis, its presence appears to be an important negative prognostic factor in DAH and may indicate an underlying systemic vasculitic process or collagen vascular disease.

Disorders associated with pulmonary capillaritis may include systemic lupus erythematosus (SLE; see Chapter 158), drug-induced capillaritis, granulomatosis with polyangiitis (previously Wegener granulomatosis), Goodpasture syndrome, and Henoch-Schönlein purpura (see Chapter 167). The finding of DAH in patients with granulomatosis with polyangiitis and microscopic polyangiitis (MPA) (see Chapter 167) is frequently associated with pathologic evidence of pulmonary capillaritis. In patients with Goodpasture syndrome or SLE, DAH has been reported both with and without the associated finding of capillaritis. A number of systemic autoimmune and inflammatory disorders may predispose a host to DAH with pulmonary capillaritis. Similarly, a variety of drugs are associated with pulmonary capillaritis but the mechanisms here have not been identified.

These disorders are distinguished from those without pulmonary capillaritis. Those disorders in which the pathologic finding of capillary

Table 406-1	Diffuse Alveolar Hemorrhage Syndromes
CLASSIFICATION	**SYNDROME**
Disorders with pulmonary capillaritis	Idiopathic pulmonary capillaritis Granulomatosis with polyangiitis (Wegener granulomatosis) Microscopic polyangiitis Systemic lupus erythematosus Goodpasture syndrome Antiphospholipid antibody syndrome Henoch-Schönlein purpura Immunoglobulin A nephropathy Behçet syndrome Cryoglobulinemia Drug-induced capillaritis (hypersensitivity) Idiopathic pulmonary-renal syndrome Eosinophilic granulomatosis angiitis (Churg-Strauss syndrome)
Disorders without pulmonary capillaritis: Noncardiovascular causes	Idiopathic pulmonary hemosiderosis Heiner syndrome Acute idiopathic pulmonary hemorrhage of infancy Bone marrow transplantation Immunodeficiency Coagulation disorders Hemolytic uremic syndromes Celiac disease (Lane-Hamilton syndrome) Infanticide (child abuse) Infection (HIV, cryptococcosis, Legionnaires disease)
Cardiovascular causes	Mitral stenosis Pulmonary venoocclusive disease Arteriovenous malformations Pulmonary lymphangioleiomyomatosis Pulmonary hypertension Pulmonary capillary hemangiomatosis Chronic heart failure Vascular thrombosis with infarction

From Susarla SC, Fan LL: Diffuse alveolar hemorrhage syndromes in children, Curr Opin Pediatr 19:314–320, 2007.

network disruption is absent are further divided into cardiac (pulmonary hypertension, mitral stenosis) and noncardiac (immunodeficiency, Heiner syndrome, coagulopathies, IPH) etiologies. A summary of the diagnoses that may manifest as recurrent or chronic pulmonary bleeding; Table 406-1 lists their classification.

EPIDEMIOLOGY

Disorders that present as DAH are highly variable in their severity, as well as in their associated symptomatology and identifiable abnormalities in laboratory testing; the diagnosis may be significantly delayed, making frequency estimates unreliable. Similarly, the prevalence of IPH is largely unknown. Among many children and young adults who were diagnosed with IPH in the past, the etiology of the hemorrhage might have been discovered if they had been studied with the newer and more advanced diagnostics available today; specific serologic testing has vastly improved our ability to appreciate immune mediated disease. Estimates of prevalence obtained from Swedish and Japanese retrospective case analyses vary from 0.24-1.23 cases per million. In nearly 80% of diagnosed cases the manifestations of IPH are seen before age 10 yr. The remaining 20% of cases are typically diagnosed before age 30 yr. The ratio of affected males:females is 1:1 in the childhood diagnosis group, and men are only slightly more affected in the group diagnosed as young adults.

PATHOLOGY

In pulmonary capillaritis, key histologic features include (1) fibrin thrombi, which occlude capillaries, (2) fibrin clots adherent to interal-

veolar septae, (3) fibrinoid necrosis of capillary walls, and (4) interstitial erythrocytes and **hemosiderin**. Illustrative but nonspecific pathologic findings, such as vascular smooth muscle hypertrophy (pulmonary hypertension), edema (mitral stenosis), or thrombosis (vascular thrombosis with infarction), may be found in those disorders that cause DAH without pulmonary capillaritis. The finding of blood in the airways or alveoli is representative of a recent hemorrhage. With repeated episodes of pulmonary hemorrhage, lung tissue appears brown secondary to this presence of hemosiderin. **Hemosiderin-laden macrophages (HLMs)** are seen with recovering, recurrent, or chronic pulmonary hemorrhage and are identifiable both in bronchoalveolar lavage fluid and in pathologic specimens of lung tissue. It takes 48-72 hr for the alveolar macrophages to convert iron from erythrocytes into hemosiderin. In a murine model, HLMs appear 3 days after a single episode of pulmonary hemorrhage and peak at 7-10 days. HLMs may be detectable for weeks to months after a hemorrhagic event. Other nonspecific pathologic findings include thickening of alveolar septa, goblet cell hyperplasia, and hypertrophy of type II pneumocytes. Fibrosis may be seen with chronic disease.

PATHOPHYSIOLOGY
Diffuse Alveolar Hemorrhage Associated with Pulmonary Capillaritis

Granulomatosis with polyangiitis is a recognized etiology for DAH in children. This disease is classically characterized by necrotizing granuloma formation (with or without cavitation) of the upper and lower respiratory tract and by a necrotizing glomerulonephritis and small vessel vasculitis. In children, presentations attributable to the upper airway, including subglottic stenosis, may suggest the diagnosis. The presence of **antineutrophil cytoplasmic antibodies (ANCAs)** may be helpful in diagnosis and management, but the clinician must be aware that other ANCA-positive vasculitides, such as MPA and Churg-Strauss syndrome, may share this nonspecific laboratory finding. In small-vessel vasculitides, ANCAs cause an inflammatory reaction that results in injury to the microvasculature. **Antiproteinase-3 antibodies (cANCA)** are classically associated with granulomatosis with polyangiitis whereas **antimyeloperoxidase antibodies (pANCA)** are typically found in patients with MPA.

Patients with **MPA** (previously the microscopic variant of polyarteritis nodosa) demonstrate a systemic necrotizing vasculitis with a predilection for small vessels (venules, arterioles, capillaries) but without necrotizing granuloma formation. This diagnosis is precluded by the finding of immune complex deposition in order to differentiate MPA from other diseases (Henoch-Schönlein purpura, cryoglobulinemic vasculitis) that are associated with immune complex–mediated small-vessel vasculitis.

Goodpasture syndrome is an immune complex–mediated disease in which anti–glomerular basement membrane (GBM) antibody binds to the basement membrane of both the alveolus and the glomerulus. GBM antibodies attach to type IV collagen contained in the vascular endothelium. At the alveolar level, immunoglobulin (Ig) G, IgM, and complement are deposited at alveolar septa. Electron microscopy shows disruption of basement membranes and vascular integrity, which allows blood to escape into alveolar spaces.

Although alveolar hemorrhage is not commonly encountered in association with SLE, its occurrence is often severe and potentially life-threatening; mortality rates exceed 50%. Pathologic vasculitic features may be absent. Some immunofluorescent studies have revealed IgG and C3 deposits at the alveolar septa. However, a clear link between immune complex formation and alveolar hemorrhage has not been established.

In **Henoch-Schönlein purpura**, pulmonary hemorrhage is a rare but recognized complication. Pathologic findings have included transmural neutrophilic infiltration of small vessels, alveolar septal inflammation, and intra-alveolar hemorrhage. Vasculitis is the proposed mechanism for hemorrhage.

Pulmonary renal syndromes are defined as those where pulmonary and renal disease manifestations are predominant. These include the aforementioned granulomatosis with polyangiitis, Goodpasture syndrome, SLE, and MPA. As Henoch-Schönlein purpura may also have renal involvement, it has been suggested for inclusion as a pulmonary renal syndrome.

Diffuse Alveolar Hemorrhage Not Associated with Pulmonary Capillaritis

A premature infant's neonatal course can be complicated by pulmonary hemorrhage. The alveolar and vascular networks are immature and particularly prone to inflammation and damage by ventilator mechanics, oxidative stress, and infection. Pulmonary hemorrhage may be unrecognized if the volume of blood is insufficient to reach the proximal airways. The chest radiographic findings in pulmonary hemorrhage may be appreciated instead as a worsening picture of respiratory distress syndrome, edema, or infection.

Pulmonary hemosiderosis in association with **cow's milk hypersensitivity** was first reported by Heiner in 1962. This condition is characterized by variable symptoms of milk intolerance. Symptoms can include grossly bloody or occult heme-positive stools, vomiting, failure to thrive, symptoms of gastroesophageal reflux, and/or upper airway congestion. Pathologic findings have included elevations of IgE and peripheral eosinophilia, as well as alveolar deposits of IgG, IgA, and C3. High titers to cow's milk protein are also typically found in cow's milk hypersensitivity. Association with pulmonary hemorrhage has remained controversial but multiple case series have provided support for the anecdotal association. In one series, infants presenting with recurrent respiratory symptoms and iron-deficiency anemia; all infants improved with elimination of cow's milk from their diets and a subset thereafter had a recurrence of pulmonary disease with a cow's milk challenge. However, many patients with milk precipitins did not have symptoms of hemosiderosis and patients with hemosiderosis did not always have milk precipitins; the relationship may be an association rather than causal in nature.

A number of case reports and case series have suggested an association between **celiac disease** (see Chapter 338.2) and DAH. In these reports, a resolution of intestinal and pulmonary symptoms along with resolution of radiographic disease has been seen after the adoption of a gluten-free diet. Consideration of testing for celiac disease in those patients with pulmonary hemorrhage and suggestive gastrointestinal symptomatology is suggested.

A number of additional associated conditions and exposures exist as causes for DAH. These are typically noninflammatory in nature and may be diversely attributable to cardiac, vascular, lymphatic or hematologic etiologies. **Graft-versus-host disease** has been implicated in transplant recipients and DAH may rarely be attributable to nonaccidental trauma. These etiologies for DAH occur relatively infrequently in the pediatric population, and suggested mechanisms for hemorrhage are variable.

The diagnosis of IPH is a diagnosis of exclusion and is only made when there is evidence of chronic or recurrent DAH and when exhaustive evaluations for primary or secondary etiologies have negative results. Renal and systemic involvement should be absent and a biopsy specimen should not reveal any evidence of granulomatous disease, vasculitis, infection, infarction, immune complex deposition or malignancy. Some patients initially diagnosed with IPH will later be found to have Goodpasture syndrome, SLE, or MPA; therefore, some cases of IPH may represent unrecognized immune-mediated disorders.

CLINICAL MANIFESTATIONS

The clinical presentation of pulmonary hemosiderosis is highly variable. In most symptomatic cases, DAH is heralded by symptoms of hemoptysis and dyspnea with associated hypoxemia and the finding of alveolar infiltration on chest radiograph. The diagnosis may be problematic as young children often lack the ability to effectively expectorate and may not present with hemoptysis. As the presence of blood in the lung is a trigger for airway irritation and inflammation, the patient may present after an episode of hemorrhage with wheezing, cough, dyspnea, and alterations in gas exchange, reflecting bronchospasm, edema, mucus plugging, and inflammation; this presentation may result in an incorrect diagnosis of asthma or bronchiolitis. A lack of pulmonary symptoms does not preclude the diagnosis of DAH and children may present only with chronic fatigue or pallor.

Symptoms may reflect an underlying and associated disease process rather than specifically related to pulmonary hemorrhage. Presentations can vary widely from a relative lack of symptoms to shock or sudden death. Bleeding may occasionally be recognized from the presence of alveolar infiltrates on a chest radiograph alone. It should be noted, however, that the absence of an infiltrate does not rule out an ongoing hemorrhagic process.

On physical examination, the patient may be pale with tachycardia and tachypnea. During an acute exacerbation, children are frequently febrile. Examination of the chest may reveal retractions and differential or decreased aeration, with crackles or wheezes. The patient may present in shock with respiratory failure from massive hemoptysis. Children in particular may present with symptoms of chronic anemia, such as failure to thrive.

LABORATORY FINDINGS AND DIAGNOSIS

Pulmonary hemorrhage is classically associated with a microcytic, hypochromic anemia. Reductions of serum iron levels, decreased or normal total iron-binding capacity and normal to increased ferritin levels may be found with chronic disease. An elevated erythrocyte sedimentation rate is a nonspecific finding. The reticulocyte count is frequently elevated. Patients with pulmonary capillaritis have lower hematocrits and higher erythrocyte sedimentation rates. The anemia of IPH can mimic a hemolytic anemia. Elevations of plasma bilirubin are caused by absorption and breakdown of hemoglobin in the alveoli. Any or all of these hematologic manifestations may be absent in the presence of recent hemorrhage.

White blood cell count and differential should be evaluated for evidence of infection and eosinophilia. A peripheral smear and direct Coombs test may suggest a vasculitic process. A stool specimen positive for occult blood may suggest associated gastrointestinal disease but can also reflect swallowed blood. Renal and liver functions should be reviewed. A urinalysis should be obtained to assess for evidence of a pulmonary–renal syndrome. A coagulation profile, quantitative immunoglobulins (including IgE), and complement studies are recommended. Testing for von Willebrand disease is also indicated.

Testing for ANCA (cANCA, pANCA), antinuclear antibody, double-stranded DNA, rheumatoid factor, antiphospholipid antibody, and GBM antibody evaluates for a number of immune-mediated and vasculitic processes that may be associated with pulmonary capillaritis.

Sputum or pulmonary secretions should be analyzed for significant evidence of blood or HLMs and may provide supportive evidence in a patient who is able to adequately expectorate secretions from the lower airway. Gastric secretions may also reveal HLMs. Flexible bronchoscopy provides visualization of any areas of active bleeding. With bronchoalveolar lavage, pulmonary secretions may be sent for pathologic review and culture analysis. The ability to perform flexible bronchoscopy will be limited if there are large amounts of blood or clots in the airway. Active bleeding may be exacerbated by airway occlusion with a bronchoscope and by installation of fluid. A patient with respiratory failure can be ventilated more effectively through a rigid bronchoscope.

Chest x-rays may reveal evidence of acute or chronic disease. Hyperaeration is frequently seen, especially during an acute hemorrhage. Infiltrates are typically symmetric and may spare the apices of the lung. Atelectasis may also be appreciated. With chronic disease, fibrosis, lymphadenopathy and nodularity may be seen. CT findings may demonstrate a subclinical and contributory disease process. The presence of a cardiac murmur, cardiomegaly on X-ray or a clinical suspicion for left-sided heart lesion suggests the need for a complete cardiac evaluation, including electrocardiogram and echocardiogram

Pulmonary function testing will likely reveal primarily obstructive disease in the acute period. With more chronic disease, fibrosis and restrictive disease tend to predominate. Oxygen saturation levels may be decreased. Lung volumes may reveal air trapping acutely and decreases in total lung capacity chronically. The diffusing capacity of carbon monoxide may be low or normal in the chronic phase but is likely to be elevated in the setting of an acute hemorrhage, because carbon monoxide binds to the hemoglobin in extravasated red blood cells.

Lung biopsy is warranted when DAH occurs without discernible etiology, extrapulmonary disease, or circulating GBM antibodies. When obtained, pulmonary tissue should be evaluated for evidence of vasculitis, immune complex deposition, and granulomatous disease.

Many have supported a diagnosis of IPH without lung biopsy if the patient has a typical presentation with diffuse infiltration on radiography, anemia, HLMs in bronchoalveolar lavage, sputum or gastric aspirate, absence of systemic disease and negative serology for immune-mediated disease. However, a number of patients meeting these criteria have been proven to have pulmonary capillaritis on review of pathologic lung tissue specimens. Therefore, a lung biopsy is recommended in any child presenting with DAH of uncertain etiology.

TREATMENT

Supportive therapy, including volume resuscitation, ventilatory support, supplemental oxygen, and transfusion of blood products, may be warranted in the patient with pulmonary hemosiderosis. Surgical or medical therapy should be directed at any treatable underlying condition. In IPH, systemic corticosteroids are frequently utilized as first-line treatment and are expected to be of particular benefit in the setting of immune-mediated disease. Steroids modulate neutrophil influx and the inflammation associated with hemorrhage; consequently, they may decrease progression toward fibrotic disease.

Treatment may be provided in the form of methylprednisolone 2-4 mg/kg/day divided every 6 hr or in the form of prednisone 0.5-1 mg/kg daily and decreased to every-other-day after resolution of acute symptoms. Successful treatment is also associated with the use of pulse steroid therapy; methylprednisolone may be given at a dose of 10-30 mg/kg (maximum 1 g) infused over 1 hr for 3 consecutive days and repeated monthly. Early treatment with corticosteroids appears to decrease episodes of hemorrhage. Steroid therapy is associated with improved survival and may be tapered as tolerated with disease remission or chronically maintained.

Steroid-sparing agents, including cyclophosphamide, azathioprine, hydroxychloroquine, methotrexate, and intravenous immunoglobulin, have been successfully used as adjunctive therapy in patients with chronic, unremitting or recurrent hemorrhage. Maintenance therapy with 6-mercaptopurine may produce favorable results in achieving long-term remission. The potential adverse effects of these pharmacologic interventions should be recognized and treated patients must be closely monitored for drug-related complications. Cushing syndrome is a well-recognized complication of chronic steroid therapy. Thrombocytopenia in association with low-dose cyclophosphamide has also been reported. Chronically immunosuppressed patients are at risk for opportunistic infection; *Legionella* pneumonia infection has been described in a survivor of IPH.

Plasmapheresis is a recognized therapy for anti-GBM antibody disease. Intravenous immunoglobulin has been used in immune complex–mediated disease.

In chronic disease, progression to debilitating pulmonary fibrosis has been described. Lung transplantation has been performed in patients with IPH refractory to immunosuppressive therapy. In one reported case study, IPH recurred in the transplanted lung.

PROGNOSIS

The outcome of patients suffering from DAH is largely dependent on the underlying disease process. Some conditions respond well to immunosuppressive therapies and remissions of disease are well documented. Other syndromes, especially those associated with pulmonary capillaritis, carry a poorer prognosis. In IPH, mortality is usually attributable to massive hemorrhage or, alternatively, to progressive fibrosis, respiratory insufficiency, and right-sided heart failure.

Long-term prognosis in patients with IPH varies among studies. Initial case study reviews suggested an average survival after symptom onset of only 2.5 yr. In this early review, a minority of patients were treated with steroids. Recent reviews have demonstrated vastly improved 5yr (86%) and 8 yr (93%) survival in association with the use of immunosuppressive therapies. To date, specific immunosuppressive treatment regimens have not been studied in a prospective manner.

Bibliography is available at Expert Consult.

Chapter 407
Pulmonary Embolism, Infarction, and Hemorrhage

407.1 Pulmonary Embolus and Infarction
Mary A. Nevin

Venous thromboembolic disease (VTE) has become an increasingly recognized critical problem in children and adolescents with chronic disease, as well as in those patients without identifiable risk factors (Table 407-1). Improvements in survival with chronic illness have likely contributed to the larger number of children presenting with these thromboembolic events; they are a significant source of morbidity and mortality and may only be recognized on post mortem examination. A high level of clinical suspicion and appropriate identification of at-risk individuals is therefore recommended.

ETIOLOGY

No single classification scheme exists for the etiology of VTE. A number of risk factors may be identified in children and adolescents; the presence of immobility, malignancy, pregnancy, infection, indwelling central venous catheters and a number of inherited and acquired thrombophilic conditions have all been identified as placing an individual at risk. In children, a significantly greater percentage of VTEs are risk associated as compared with their adult counterparts. Children with **deep venous thrombosis (DVT)** and **pulmonary embolism (PE)** are much more likely to have 1 or more identifiable conditions or circumstances placing them at risk. In a retrospective cohort of patients with VTE in U.S. children's hospitals from 2001-2007, the majority (63%) of affected children were found to have 1 or more chronic medical comorbidities. In a large Canadian registry, 96% of pediatric patients were found to have 1 risk factor and 90% had 2 or more risk factors. In contrast, approximately 60% of adults with this disorder have an identifiable risk factor (see Table 407-1).

Embolic disease in children is varied in its origin. An embolus can contain thrombus, air, amniotic fluid, septic material, or metastatic neoplastic tissue. Thromboemboli are the type most commonly encountered. A commonly encountered risk factor for DVT and PE in the pediatric population is the presence of a central venous catheter. More than 50% of DVTs in children and more than 80% in newborns are found in patients with indwelling central venous lines. The presence of a catheter in a vessel lumen, as well as instilled medications, can induce endothelial damage and favor thrombus formation.

Children with malignancies are also at considerable risk. Although PE has been described in children with leukemia, the risk of PE is more significant in children with solid rather than hematologic malignancies. A child with malignancy may have numerous risk factors related to the primary disease process and the therapeutic interventions. Infection from chronic immunosuppression may interact with hypercoagulability of malignancy and chemotherapeutic effects on the endothelium.

Table 407-1	Risk Factors for Pulmonary Embolism

ENVIRONMENTAL
Long-haul air travel
Obesity
Cigarette smoking
Hypertension
Immobility

WOMEN'S HEALTH
Oral contraceptives, including progesterone-only and, especially,
    third-generation pills
Pregnancy
Hormone replacement therapy
Septic abortion

MEDICAL ILLNESS
Previous pulmonary embolism or deep venous thrombosis
Cancer
Heart failure
Chronic obstructive pulmonary disease
Diabetes mellitus
Inflammatory bowel disease
Antipsychotic drug use
Long-term indwelling central venous catheter
Permanent pacemaker
Internal cardiac defibrillator
Stroke with limb paresis
Spinal cord injury
Nursing home confinement or current or repeated hospital
    admission

SURGICAL
Trauma
Orthopedic surgery
General surgery
Neurosurgery, especially craniotomy for brain tumor

THROMBOPHILIA
Factor V Leiden mutation
Prothrombin gene mutation
Hyperhomocysteinanemia (including mutation in
    methylenetetrahydrofolate reductase)
Antiphospholipid antibody syndrome
Deficiency of antithrombin III, protein C, or protein S
High concentrations of factor VIII or XI
Increased lipoprotein (a)

NONTHROMBOTIC
Air
Foreign particles (e.g., hair, talc, as a consequence of intravenous
    drug misuse)
Amniotic fluid
Bone fragments, bone marrow
Fat
Tumors (Wilms tumor)

Modified from Goldhaber SZ: Pulmonary embolism, Lancet 363:1295–1305, 2004.

In a retrospective cohort of patients with VTE from 2001-2007, pediatric malignancy was the medical condition most strongly associated with recurrent VTE.

In the neonatal period, thromboembolic disease and PE may be related to indwelling catheters used for parenteral nutrition and medication delivery. **Pulmonary thromboemboli** in neonates generally occurs as a complication of underlying disease; the most common associated diagnosis is congenital heart disease but sepsis and birth asphyxia are also notable associated conditions. Other risk factors include a relative immaturity of newborn infants' coagulation; plasma concentrations of vitamin K–dependent coagulation factors (II, VII, IX, X); factors XII, XI, and prekallikrein and high-molecular-weight kininogen are only approximately half of adult levels (see Chapter 475). PE in neonates may occasionally reflect maternal risk factors, such as

diabetes and toxemia of pregnancy. Infants with congenitally acquired homozygous deficiencies of antithrombin, protein C, and protein S are also more likely to present with thromboembolic disease in the neonatal period (see Chapter 478).

Pulmonary air embolism is a defined entity in the newborn or young infant and is attributed to the conventional ventilation of critically ill (and generally premature) infants with severe pulmonary disease. In the majority of instances, the pulmonary air embolism is preceded by an air-leak syndrome. Infants may become symptomatic and critically compromised by as little as 0.4 mL/kg of intravascular air; these physiologic derangements are thought to be secondary to the effects of nitrogen.

Prothrombotic disease can also manifest in older infants and children. Disease can be congenital or acquired. **Inherited thrombophilic** conditions include deficiencies of antithrombin, protein C, and protein S, as well as mutations of *factor V Leiden* (G1691A) (see Chapter 478) and *prothrombin (factor II 20210A mutation)* (see Chapter 478), and elevated values of *lipoprotein A. In addition, multiple acquired thrombophilic conditions exist; these include the presence of lupus anticoagulant (may be present without the diagnosis of systemic lupus erythematosus), anticardiolipin antibody, and anti–β_2-glycoprotein 1 antibody.* Finally, conditions such as hyperhomocysteinemia (see Chapter 86) may have both inheritable and dietary determinants. All have all been linked to thromboembolic disease. DVT/PE may be the initial presentation.

Children with sickle cell disease are also at high risk for pulmonary embolus and infarction. Acquired prothrombotic disease is seen in conditions such as *nephrotic syndrome* (see Chapter 527) and *antiphospholipid antibody syndrome.* From one-quarter to one-half of children with *systemic lupus erythematosus* (see Chapter 158) have thromboembolic disease. There is a significant association with VTE onset in children for each inherited thrombophilic trait evaluated, thereby illuminating the importance of screening for thrombophilic conditions for those at risk for VTE.

Other risk factors include infection, cardiac disease, recent surgery, and trauma. Surgical risk is thought to be more significant when immobility will be a prominent feature of the recovery. Use of oral contraceptives confers additional risk, although the level of risk in patients taking these medications appears to be decreasing, perhaps as a result of the lower amounts of estrogen in current formulations.

Septic emboli are rare in children but may be caused by osteomyelitis, jugular vein or umbilical thrombophlebitis, cellulitis, urinary tract infection, and right-sided endocarditis.

EPIDEMIOLOGY

A retrospective cohort study was performed with patients younger than 18 yr of age, discharged from 35-40 children's hospitals across the United States from 2001-2007. During this time, a dramatic increase was noted in the incidence of VTE; the annual rate of VTE increased by 70% from 34 to 58 cases per 10,000 hospital admissions. Although this increased incidence was noted in all age groups, a bimodal distribution of patient ages was found, consistent with prior studies; infants younger than 1 yr of age and adolescents made up the majority of admissions with VTE, but neonates continue to be at greatest risk. The peak incidence for VTE in childhood appears to occur in the 1st mo of life. It is in this neonatal period that thromboembolic events are more problematic, likely as a result of an imbalance between procoagulant factors and fibrinolysis. According to a 2013 update by Nowak-Göttl et al, the yearly incidence of venous events was estimated at 5.3 per 10,000 hospital admissions in children and 24 per 10,000 in the neonatal intensive care.

Pediatric autopsy reviews have estimated the incidence of thromboembolic disease in children as between 1% and 4%, although not all were clinically significant. Thromboembolic pulmonary disease is often unrecognized, and antemortem studies may underestimate the true incidence. Pediatric deaths from isolated pulmonary emboli are rare. Most thromboemboli are related to central venous catheters. The source of the emboli may be lower or upper extremity veins as well as the pelvis and right heart. In adults, the most common location for DVT is the lower leg. However, one of the largest pediatric VTE/PE registries found two-thirds of DVTs occurring in the upper extremity.

PATHOPHYSIOLOGY

Favorable conditions for thrombus formation include injury to the vessel endothelium, hemostasis, and hypercoagulability. In the case of PE, a thrombus is dislodged from a vein, travels through the right atrium and lodges within the pulmonary arteries. In children, emboli that obstruct <50% of the pulmonary circulation are generally clinically silent unless there is significant coexistent cardiopulmonary disease. In severe disease, **right ventricular** afterload is increased with resultant right ventricular dilation and increases in right ventricular and pulmonary arterial pressures. In severe cases, a reduction of cardiac output and hypotension may result from concomitant decreases in left ventricular filling. In rare instances of death from massive pulmonary embolus, marked increases in pulmonary vascular resistance and heart failure are usually present.

Arterial hypoxemia results from unequal ventilation and perfusion; the occlusion of the involved vessel prevents perfusion of distal alveolar units, thereby creating an increase in dead space and hypoxia with an elevated alveolar–arterial oxygen tension difference (see Chapter 373). Most patients are hypocarbic secondary to hyperventilation, which often persists even when oxygenation is optimized. Abnormalities of oxygenation and ventilation are likely to be less significant in the pediatric population, possibly owing to less underlying cardiopulmonary disease and greater reserve. The vascular supply to lung tissue is abundant, and pulmonary infarction is unusual with pulmonary embolus but may result from distal arterial occlusion and alveolar hemorrhage.

CLINICAL MANIFESTATIONS

Presentation is variable, and many pulmonary emboli are silent. Rarely, a massive PE may manifest as cardiopulmonary failure. Children are more likely to have underlying disease processes or risk factors but might still present asymptomatically with small emboli. Common symptoms and signs of PE caused by larger emboli include hypoxia (cyanosis), dyspnea, cough, pleuritic chest pain, and hemoptysis. Pleuritic chest pain is the most common presenting symptom in adolescents (84%), whereas unexplained and persistent tachypnea may suggest PE in all pediatric patients. Localized crackles may occasionally be appreciated on examination. A high level of clinical suspicion is required because a variety of diagnoses may cause similar symptoms; nonspecific complaints may frequently be attributed to an underlying disease process or an unrelated/incorrect diagnosis. Confirmatory testing should follow a clinical suspicion for PE. In adults, clinical prediction rules have been published and are based on risk factors, clinical signs, and symptoms. No such clinical prediction rules have been validated in the pediatric population.

LABORATORY FINDINGS AND DIAGNOSIS

The electrocardiogram, arterial blood gas, and chest radiograph may be utilized to rule out contributing or comorbid disease but are not sensitive or specific in the diagnosis of PE. Electrocardiographs may reveal ST-segment changes or evidence of pulmonary hypertension with right ventricular failure (cor pulmonale); such changes are nonspecific and nondiagnostic. Radiographic images of the chest are often normal in a child with PE and any abnormalities are likely to be nonspecific. Patients with septic emboli may have multiple areas of nodularity and cavitation, which are typically located peripherally in both lung fields. Many patients with PE have hypoxemia. The alveolar–arterial oxygen tension difference gradient is more sensitive in detecting gas exchange derangements.

A review of results of a complete blood count, urinalysis, and coagulation profile is warranted. Prothrombotic diseases should be highly suspected on the basis of past medical or family history; additional laboratory evaluations include fibrinogen assays, protein C, protein S, and antithrombin III studies, and analysis for factor V Leiden mutation, as well as evaluation for lupus anticoagulant and anticardiolipin antibodies.

Echocardiograms may be warranted to assess ventricular size and function. An echocardiogram is required if there is any suspicion of intracardiac thrombi or endocarditis.

Noninvasive venous ultrasound testing with Doppler flow can be used to confirm DVT in the lower extremities; ultrasonography may not detect thrombi in the upper extremities or pelvis (Fig. 407-1A). In patients with significant venous thrombosis, D dimers are usually elevated. It is a sensitive but nonspecific test for venous thrombosis. The D dimer may not be clinically relevant in the children with PE as this group is more likely to have an underlying comorbid condition that is also associated with an increased level of D dimers. When a high level of suspicion exists, confirmatory testing with venography should be pursued. DVT can be recurrent and multifocal and may lead to repeated episodes of PE.

Although a ventilation–perfusion (V̇-Q̇) radionuclide scan is a noninvasive and potentially sensitive method of pulmonary embolus detection, the interpretation of V̇-Q̇ scans can be problematic. Helical or spiral CT with an intravenous contrast agent is valuable and the diagnostic test of choice to detect a PE (see Fig. 407-1B). CT studies detect emboli in lobar and segmental vessels with acceptable sensitivities. Poorer sensitivities may be encountered in the evaluation of the subsegmental pulmonary vasculature. Pulmonary angiography is the

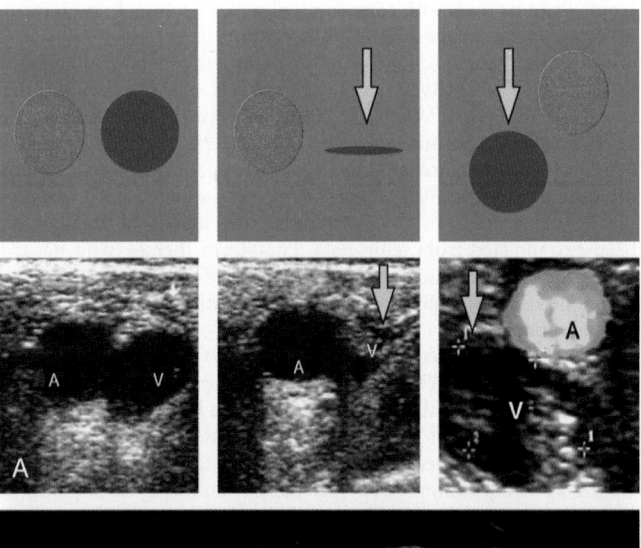

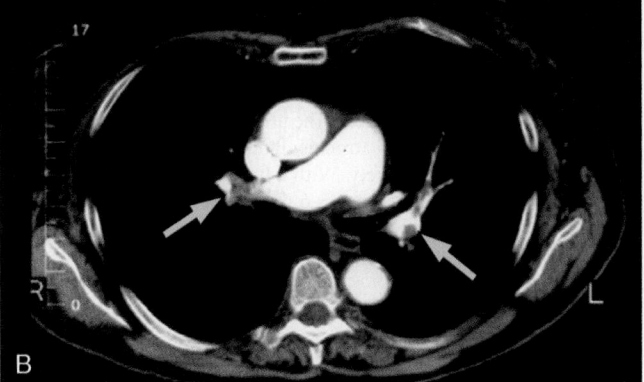

Figure 407-1 A, Compression ultrasound. Upper series, from left to right, representation of vein and artery without and with *(arrow)* gentle compression with the echocardiographic probe; lower series, corresponding echocardiographic findings. The third image from the left show a thrombus in the vein (vein not compressible by the probe). **B,** CT angiography. CT angiography showing several emboli (arrows) in the main right pulmonary artery and in left lobar and segmental arteries. A, artery; V, vein. *(From Goldhaber SZ, Bounameaux H: Pulmonary embolism and deep vein thrombosis. Lancet 379:1835–1844, 2012, Fig. 2, p. 1838.)*

gold standard for diagnosis of PE, but with current availability of multidetector spiral CT angiography, it is not necessary except in unusual cases.

MRI may be emerging as a diagnostic option for patients with VTE. The accuracy of this method is similar to that of multidetector CT. It may be preferable in patients with allergic reactions to contrast material and in pediatric patients in whom the risk of early exposure to ionizing radiation has been established.

TREATMENT

Initial treatment should always be directed toward stabilization of the patient. Careful approaches to ventilation, fluid resuscitation, and inotropic support are always indicated, because improvement in 1 area of decompensation can often exacerbate coexisting pathology.

After the patient with a PE has been stabilized, the next therapeutic step is anticoagulation. Evaluations for prothrombotic disease must precede anticoagulation. Acute-phase anticoagulation therapy may be provided with **unfractionated heparin (UFH)** or **low-molecular-weight heparin (LMWH)**. Heparins act by enhancing the activity of antithrombin. LMWH is generally preferred in children; this drug can be administered subcutaneously and the need for serum monitoring is decreased. The risk of **heparin-induced thrombocytopenia** is also decreased with LMWH as compared to UFH. Alternatively, UFH is preferred with patients who have an elevated risk of bleeding as UFH has a shorter half-life than LMWH. UFH is also used preferentially in patients with compromised renal function. In monitoring of drug levels, laboratories must be aware of the drug chosen in order to use the appropriate assay. For UFH, the therapeutic range is 0.3-0.7 anti-Xa activity units/mL. In LMWH, the therapeutic range is 0.5-1.0 units/mL. When the anti-Xa assay is not available, the activated **partial thromboplastin time** may be used with a goal of 60-85 sec or approximately 1.5-2 times the upper limit of age appropriate normal values. The recommended duration of heparinization during acute treatment is 5-10 days; this length of therapy has been extrapolated from adult data. Long-term therapy with heparin should be avoided whenever possible. Side effects include the aforementioned heparin-induced thrombocytopenia as well as bleeding and osteoporosis.

Extension of anticoagulation therapy occurs in the subacute phase and may utilize LMWH or warfarin. Warfarin is generally initiated after establishing effective anticoagulation with heparin because severe congenital deficiencies of protein C may be associated with warfarin skin necrosis. The starting dose for warfarin in children is generally 0.1 mg/kg orally administered once daily. Monitoring is via the international normalized ratio (INR) and the therapeutic INR range for warfarin therapy in VTE is 2.0-3.0. The INR is generally monitored 5 days after initiating therapy or a similar period after dose changes and weekly thereafter until stable. The INR should be obtained with any evidence of abnormal bleeding and should be discontinued at least 5 days prior to invasive procedures. The utilization of an anticoagulation team and/or established treatment algorithms is recommended in order to optimize patient safety. With a first occurrence of VTE, anticoagulation is recommended for 3-6 mo in the setting of an identifiable, reversible, and resolved risk factor (e.g., postoperative state). Longer treatment is indicated in patients with idiopathic VTE (6-12 mo) and in those with chronic clinical risk factors (12 mo-lifelong). In the setting of a congenital thrombophilic condition, the duration of therapy is often indefinite.

Inhibitors of factor Xa (rivaroxaban, etc.) may become an alternate therapy for both acute PE and long-term treatment.

Thrombolytic agents such as recombinant tissue plasminogen activator, may be utilized in combination with anticoagulants in the early stages of treatment; their use is most likely to be considered in children with hemodynamically significant PE (echocardiogram evidence of right ventricular dysfunction) or other severe potential clinical sequelae of VTE. Combined therapy may reduce the incidences of progressive thromboembolism, pulmonary embolus, and post-thrombotic syndrome. Mortality rate appears to be unaffected by additional therapies;

nonetheless, the additional theoretic risk of hemorrhage limits the use of combination therapy in all but the most compromised patients. The use of thrombolytic agents in patients with active bleeding, recent cerebrovascular accidents, or trauma is contraindicated.

Surgical embolectomy is invasive and is associated with significant mortality. Its application should be limited to those with persistent hemodynamic compromise refractory to standard therapy.

PROGNOSIS

Mortality in pediatric patients with PE is likely to be attributable to an underlying disease process rather than to the embolus itself. Short-term complications include major hemorrhage (either due to the thrombosis or secondary to anticoagulation). Conditions associated with a poorer prognosis include malignancy, infection, and cardiac disease. The mortality rate in children from PE is 2.2%. Recurrent thromboembolic disease may complicate recovery. The practitioner must conduct an extensive evaluation for underlying pathology so as to prevent progressive disease. Postthrombotic syndrome is another recognized complication of pediatric thrombotic disease. Venous valvular damage can be initiated by the presence of DVT, leading to persistent venous hypertension with ambulation and valvular reflux. Symptoms include edema, pain, increases in pigmentation, and ulcerations. Affected pediatric patients may suffer lifelong disability.

Bibliography is available at Expert Consult.

407.2 Pulmonary Hemorrhage and Hemoptysis

Mary A. Nevin

Pulmonary hemorrhage is relatively uncommon but a potentially fatal occurrence in children. The patient with suspected hemoptysis may present acutely or subacutely and to a variety of different practitioners with distinct areas of specialty. Diffuse, slow bleeding in the lower airways may become severe and manifest as anemia, fatigue, or respiratory compromise without the patient ever experiencing episodes of hemoptysis. Hemoptysis must also be separated from episodes of hematemesis or epistaxis, each of which may have indistinguishable presentations in the young patient.

ETIOLOGY

Tables 407-2 and 406-1 (in Chapter 406) present conditions that can manifest as pulmonary hemorrhage or hemoptysis in children. The chronic (opposed to an acute) presence of a foreign body can lead to inflammation and/or infection, thereby inducing hemorrhage. Bleeding is more likely to occur in association with a chronically retained foreign body of vegetable origin.

Hemorrhage most commonly reflects chronic inflammation and infection such as that seen with bronchiectasis due to cystic fibrosis or with cavitary disease in association with infectious tuberculosis. Hemoptysis may occasionally reflect an acute and intense infectious condition such as bronchitis or bronchopneumonia.

Other relatively common etiologies are congenital heart disease and trauma. Pulmonary hypertension secondary to cardiac disease is a prominent etiology for hemoptysis in those patients without cystic fibrosis. Traumatic irritation or damage in the airway may be accidental in nature. Traumatic injury to the airway and pulmonary contusion may result from motor vehicle crashes or other direct force injuries. Bleeding can also be related to instrumentation or iatrogenic irritation of the airway as is commonly seen in a child with a tracheostomy or a child with repeated suction trauma to the upper airway. Children who have been victims of nonaccidental trauma or deliberate suffocation can also be found to have blood in the mouth or airway (see Chapter 40). Fictitious hemoptysis may rarely be encountered in the setting of Factitious Disorder by Proxy (formerly Munchausen's by proxy; see Chapter 40.2).

Table 407-2	Etiology of Pulmonary Hemorrhage (Hemoptysis)*

FOCAL HEMORRHAGE
Bronchitis and bronchiectasis (especially cystic fibrosis–related)
Infection (acute or chronic), pneumonia, abscess
Tuberculosis
Trauma
Pulmonary arteriovenous malformation
Foreign body (chronic)
Neoplasm including hemangioma
Pulmonary embolus with or without infarction
Bronchogenic cysts

DIFFUSE HEMORRHAGE
Idiopathic of infancy
Congenital heart disease (including pulmonary hypertension, venoocclusive disease, congestive heart failure)
Prematurity
Cow's milk hyperreactivity (Heiner syndrome)
Goodpasture syndrome
Collagen vascular diseases (systemic lupus erythematosus, rheumatoid arthritis)
Henoch-Schönlein purpura and vasculitic disorders
Granulomatous disease (granulomatosis with polyangiitis)
Celiac disease
Coagulopathy (congenital or acquired)
Malignancy
Immunodeficiency
Exogenous toxins
Hyperammonemia
Pulmonary hypertension
Pulmonary alveolar proteinosis
Idiopathic pulmonary hemosiderosis
Tuberous sclerosis
Lymphangiomyomatosis or lymphangioleiomyomatosis
Physical injury or abuse
Catamenial

*See also Table 406-1.

Rare causes for hemoptysis include tumors and vascular anomalies such as arteriovenous malformations (Fig. 407-2). Congenital vascular malformations in the lung may also be associated with **hereditary hemorrhagic telangiectasia**. Tumors must be cautiously investigated when encountered with a flexible fiberoptic bronchoscope as bleeding may be massive and difficult to control.

Syndromes associated with vasculitic, autoimmune, and idiopathic disorders can be associated with diffuse alveolar hemorrhage (see Chapter 406).

Acute idiopathic pulmonary hemorrhage of infancy is a distinct entity and is described as an episode of pulmonary hemorrhage in a previously healthy infant born at greater than 32 wk of gestation and whose age is less than 1 yr with the following: (1) abrupt or sudden onset of overt bleeding or frank evidence of blood in the airway, (2) severe presentation leading to acute respiratory distress or failure and requiring intensive care and invasive ventilatory support, and (3) diffuse bilateral infiltration on chest radiographs or computed tomography. Prior suggestions of an association between acute idiopathic pulmonary hemorrhage of infancy and toxic mold exposure have not been supported on subsequent review.

EPIDEMIOLOGY

The frequency with which pulmonary hemorrhage occurs in the pediatric population is difficult to define. This difficulty is largely related to the variability in disease presentation. Chronic bronchiectasis as seen in cystic fibrosis (see Chapter 403) or ciliary dyskinesia (see Chapter 404) can cause hemoptysis, but usually occurs in children older than 10 yr of age. The incidence of pulmonary hemorrhage may be

significantly underestimated because many children and young adults swallow rather than expectorate mucus, a behavior that may prevent recognition of hemoptysis, the primary presenting symptom of the disorder.

PATHOPHYSIOLOGY

Pulmonary hemorrhage can be localized or diffuse. Focal hemorrhage from an isolated bronchial lesion is often secondary to infection or chronic inflammation. Erosion through a chronically inflamed airway into the adjacent bronchial artery is a mechanism for potentially massive hemorrhage. Bleeding from such a lesion is more likely to be bright red, brisk, and secondary to enlarged bronchial arteries and systemic arterial pressures. The severity of more diffuse hemorrhage can be difficult to ascertain. The rate of blood loss may be insufficient to reach the proximal airways. Therefore, the patient may present without hemoptysis. The diagnosis of pulmonary hemorrhage is generally achieved by finding evidence of blood or hemosiderin in the lung. Within 48-72 hr of an episode of bleeding, alveolar macrophages convert the iron from erythrocytes into hemosiderin. It may take weeks to clear these hemosiderin-laden macrophages completely from the alveolar spaces. This fact may allow differentiation between acute and chronic hemorrhage. Hemorrhage is often followed by the influx of neutrophils and other proinflammatory mediators. With repeated or chronic hemorrhage, pulmonary fibrosis can become a prominent pathologic finding.

CLINICAL MANIFESTATIONS

The severity of presentation in patients with hemoptysis and pulmonary hemorrhage is highly variable. Older children and young adults with a focal hemorrhage may complain of warmth or a "bubbling" sensation in the chest wall. This can occasionally aid the clinician in locating the area involved. Rapid and large-volume blood loss manifests as symptoms of cyanosis, respiratory distress, and shock. Chronic, subclinical blood loss may manifest as anemia, fatigue, dyspnea, or altered activity tolerance. Less commonly, patients present with persistent infiltrates on chest radiograph or symptoms of chronic illness such as failure to thrive.

Pulmonary arteriovenous malformations may present with hemoptysis, hemothorax, a round localized mass on x-ray or CT, clubbing, cyanosis, or embolic phenomenon.

LABORATORY FINDINGS AND DIAGNOSIS

A patient with suspected hemorrhage should have a laboratory evaluation with complete blood count and coagulation studies. The complete blood count result may demonstrate a microcytic, hypochromic anemia but may be normal early in an acute bleeding episode. If iron stores are sufficient, a reticulocytosis may be present. Other laboratory findings are highly dependent on the underlying diagnosis. A urinalysis may show evidence of nephritis in patients with a comorbid pulmonary renal syndrome. The classic and definitive finding in pulmonary hemorrhage is that of **hemosiderin-laden macrophages** in pulmonary secretions. Hemosiderin-laden macrophages may be detected by sputum analysis with Prussian blue staining when a patient is able to successfully expectorate sputum from the lower airways. In younger children, or in weak or neurodevelopmentally compromised patients unable to expectorate sputum, induced sputum may provide an acceptable specimen; alternatively, a flexible bronchoscopy with **bronchoalveolar lavage** may be required for specimen retrieval.

Chest radiographs may demonstrate fluffy bilateral densities, as seen in acute idiopathic pulmonary hemorrhage of infancy (Fig. 407-3) or the patchy consolidation seen in idiopathic pulmonary hemosiderosis (Fig. 407-4). Alveolar infiltrates seen on chest radiograph may be regarded as a representation of recent bleeding, but their absence does not rule out the occurrence of pulmonary hemorrhage. Infiltrates, when present, are often symmetric and diffuse and may be preferentially located in the perihilar regions and lower lobes. The costophrenic angles and lung apices are frequently spared. CT may be indicated to assess for underlying disease processes.

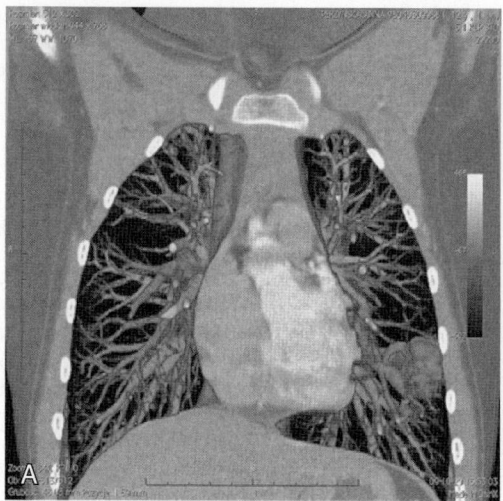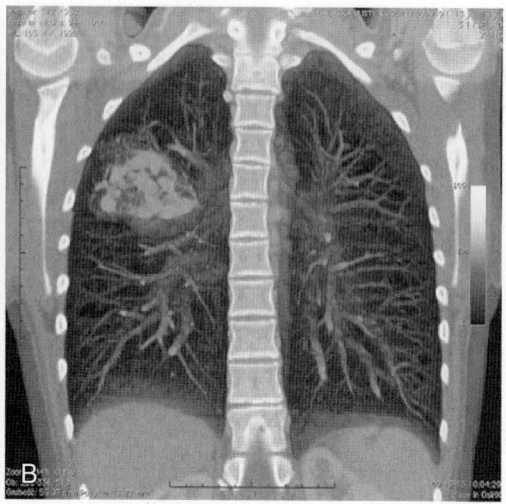

Figure 407-2 A, Volume-rendering reconstruction of the contrast-enhanced spiral CT showing a large arteriovenous fistula in the left upper lobe (lingula). **B,** Volume-rendering reconstruction of the contrast-enhanced spiral CT showing an arteriovenous fistula in the right upper lobe. *(From Grzela K, Krenke K, Kulus M: Pulmonary arteriovenous malformations: clinical and radiological presentation. J Pediatr 158:856, 2011, Figs. 1 and 2, p. 856.)*

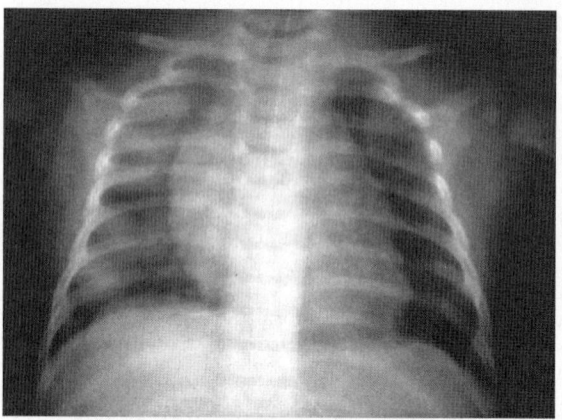

Figure 407-3 Radiographic appearance of acute idiopathic pulmonary hemorrhage in infancy. *(From Brown CM, Redd SC, Damon SA; Centers for Disease Control and Prevention [CDC]: Acute idiopathic pulmonary hemorrhage among infants: recommendations from the Working Group for Investigation and Surveillance, MMWR Recomm Rep 53:1–12, 2004.)*

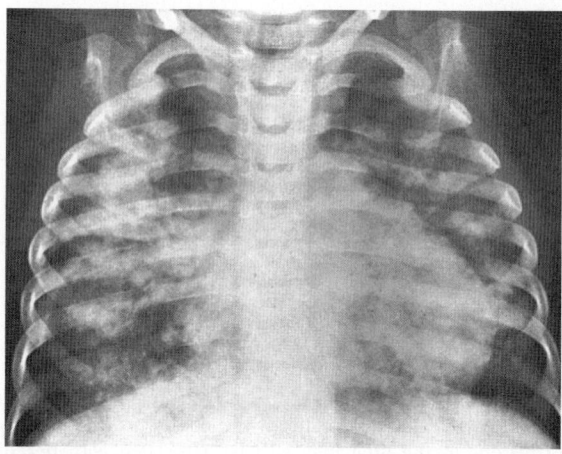

Figure 407-4 Diffuse pulmonary hemorrhage that was thought to be the result of idiopathic pulmonary hemosiderosis in a 3 yr old boy. Frontal radiograph reveals bilateral airspace consolidation that is patchy. Tracheal washing contained large numbers of macrophages filled with hemosiderin. Ten days later, most of the consolidative changes in the lungs had cleared. The patient's anemia was successfully treated with blood transfusion. *(From Slovis T, editor: Caffey's pediatric diagnostic imaging, ed 11, Philadelphia, 2008, Mosby/Elsevier; courtesy of Bertram Girdany, MD, Pittsburgh, PA.)*

Lung biopsy is rarely necessary unless bleeding is chronic or an etiology cannot be determined with other methods. Pulmonary function testing, including a determination of gas exchange, is important to assess the severity of the ventilatory defect. In older children, spirometry may demonstrate evidence of predominantly obstructive disease in the acute period. Restrictive disease secondary to fibrosis is typically seen with more chronic disease. Diffusion capacity of carbon monoxide measurements are typically elevated in the setting of pulmonary hemorrhage because of the strong affinity of the intra-alveolar hemoglobin for carbon monoxide.

TREATMENT

In the setting of massive blood loss, volume resuscitation and transfusion of blood products are necessary. Maintenance of adequate ventilation and circulatory function is crucial. Rigid bronchoscopy may be utilized for localization of bleeding and for removal of debris but active bleeding may be exacerbated by airway manipulation. Flexible bronchoscopy and bronchoalveolar lavage may be required for diagnosis. Ideally, treatment is directed at the specific pathologic process responsible for the hemorrhage. When bronchiectasis is a known entity and a damaged artery can be localized, bronchial artery embolization is often the therapy of choice. If embolization fails, total or partial lobectomy may be required. Embolization is the initial treatment of choice for an arteriovenous malformation. In circumstances of diffuse hemorrhage, corticosteroids and other immunosuppressive agents have been shown to be of benefit. Prognosis depends largely on the underlying disease process and the chronicity of bleeding.

Bibliography is available at Expert Consult.

Chapter **408**
Atelectasis
Ranna A. Rozenfeld

Atelectasis is the incomplete expansion or complete collapse of air-bearing tissue, resulting from obstruction of air intake into the alveolar sacs. Segmental, lobar, or whole lung collapse is associated with the absorption of air contained in the alveoli, which are no longer ventilated.

PATHOPHYSIOLOGY
The causes of atelectasis can be divided into 5 groups (Table 408-1). Respiratory syncytial virus (see Chapter 260) and other viral infections, including influenza viruses in young children can cause multiple areas of atelectasis. Mucous plugs are a common predisposing factor to atelectasis. Massive collapse of 1 or both lungs is most often a postoperative complication but occasionally results from other causes, such as trauma, asthma, pneumonia, tension pneumothorax (see Chapter 411), aspiration of foreign material (see Chapters 387 and 397), and paralysis, or after extubation. Massive atelectasis is usually produced by a combination of factors, including immobilization or decreased use of the diaphragm and the respiratory muscles, obstruction of the bronchial tree, and abolition of the cough reflex.

CLINICAL MANIFESTATIONS
Symptoms vary with the cause and extent of the atelectasis. A small area is likely to be asymptomatic. When a large area of previously normal lung becomes atelectatic, especially when it does so suddenly, dyspnea accompanied by rapid shallow respirations, tachycardia, cough, and often cyanosis occurs. If the obstruction is removed, the symptoms disappear rapidly. Although it was once believed that atelectasis alone can cause fever, studies have shown no association between atelectasis and fever. Physical findings include limitation of chest excursion, decreased breath sound intensity, and coarse crackles. Breath sounds are decreased or absent over extensive atelectatic areas.

Table 408-1	Anatomic Causes of Atelectasis
CAUSE	**CLINICAL EXAMPLES**
External compression on the pulmonary parenchyma	Pleural effusion, pneumothorax, intrathoracic tumors, diaphragmatic hernia
Endobronchial obstruction completely obstructing the ingress of air	Enlarged lymph node, tumor, cardiac enlargement, foreign body, mucoid plug, broncholithiasis
Intraluminal obstruction of a bronchus	Foreign body, asthma, granulomatous tissue, tumor, secretions including mucous plugs, bronchiectasis, pulmonary abscess, chronic bronchitis, acute laryngotracheobronchitis, plastic bronchitis
Intrabronchiolar obstruction	Bronchiolitis, interstitial pneumonitis, asthma
Respiratory compromise or paralysis	Neuromuscular abnormalities, osseous deformities, overly restrictive casts and surgical dressings, defective movement of the diaphragm, or restriction of respiratory effort

Massive pulmonary atelectasis usually presents with dyspnea, cyanosis, and tachycardia. An affected child is extremely anxious and, if old enough, complains of chest pain. The chest appears flat on the affected side, where decreased respiratory excursion, dullness to percussion, and feeble or absent breath sounds are also noted. Postoperative atelectasis usually manifests within 24 hr of operation but may not occur for several days.

Acute lobar collapse is a frequent occurrence in patients receiving intensive care. If undetected, it can lead to impaired gas exchange, secondary infection, and subsequent pulmonary fibrosis. Initially, hypoxemia may result from ventilation-perfusion mismatch. In contrast to atelectasis in adult patients, in whom the lower lobes and, in particular, the left lower lobe are most often involved, 90% of cases in children involve the upper lobes and 63% involve the right upper lobe. There is also a high incidence of upper lobe atelectasis and, especially, right upper lobe collapse in patients with atelectasis being treated in neonatal intensive care units. This high incidence may be a result of movement of the endotracheal tube into the right mainstem bronchus, where it obstructs or causes inflammation of the bronchus to the right upper lobe.

DIAGNOSIS
The diagnosis of atelectasis can usually be established by chest radiographic examination. Typical findings include volume loss and displacement of fissures. Atypical presentations include atelectasis manifesting as a mass like opacity and atelectasis in an unusual location. Lobar atelectasis may be associated with pneumothorax.

In asthmatic children, chest radiography demonstrates an abnormality rate of 44%, compared with a thorax high-resolution CT scan abnormality rate of 75%. Children with asthma and atelectasis have an increased incidence of right middle lobe syndrome, acute asthma exacerbations, pneumonia, and upper airway infections.

In foreign-body aspiration, atelectasis is one of the most common radiographic findings. The site of atelectasis usually indicates the site of the foreign body (see Chapter 377.1). Atelectasis is more common when diagnosis of foreign-body aspiration is delayed for greater than 2 wk.

Bronchoscopic examination reveals a collapsed main bronchus when the obstruction is at the tracheobronchial junction and may also disclose the nature of the obstruction.

Massive pulmonary atelectasis is generally diagnosed on chest radiograph. Typical findings include elevation of the diaphragm, narrowing of the intercostal spaces, and displacement of the mediastinal structures and heart toward the affected side (Fig. 408-1).

TREATMENT
Treatment depends on the cause of the collapse. If effusion or pneumothorax is responsible, the external compression must first be removed. Often vigorous efforts at cough, deep breathing, and percussion will facilitate expansion. Aspiration with sterile tracheal catheters may facilitate removal of mucous plugs. Continuous positive airway pressure may improve atelectasis.

Bronchoscopic examination is immediately indicated if atelectasis is the result of a foreign body or any other bronchial obstruction that can be relieved. For bilateral atelectasis, bronchoscopic aspiration should also be performed immediately. It is also indicated when an isolated area of atelectasis persists for several weeks. If no anatomic basis for atelectasis is found and no material can be obtained by suctioning, the introduction of a small amount of saline followed by suctioning allows recovery of bronchial secretions for culture and, possibly, for cytologic examination. Frequent changes in the child's position, deep breathing, and chest physiotherapy may be beneficial. Intrapulmonary percussive ventilation is a chest physiotherapy technique that is safe and effective. Oxygen therapy is indicated when there is dyspnea or desaturation. Intermittent positive-pressure breathing and incentive spirometry are recommended when atelectasis does not improve after chest physiotherapy.

In some conditions, such as asthma, bronchodilator and corticosteroid treatment may accelerate atelectasis clearance. Recombinant

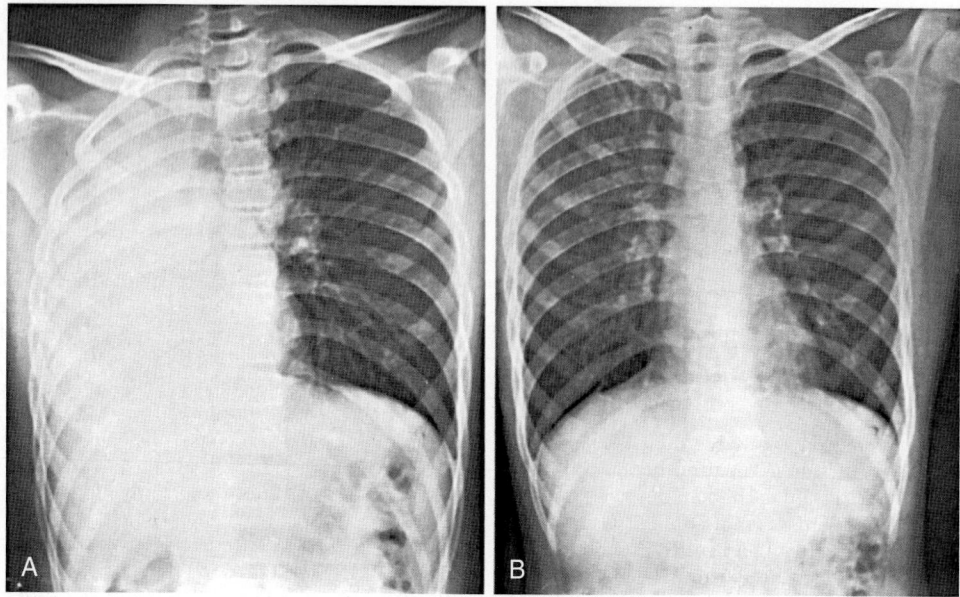

Figure 408-1 A, Massive atelectasis of the right lung. The patient has asthma. The heart and other mediastinal structures shift to the right during the atelectatic phase. **B,** Comparison study after reaeration subsequent to bronchoscopic removal of a mucous plug from the right mainstem bronchus.

human deoxyribonuclease, which is approved only for the treatment of cystic fibrosis, has been used off-label for patients without cystic fibrosis who have persistent atelectasis. This product reduces the viscosity of purulent bronchial debris. In patients with acute severe asthma, diffuse airway plugging with thick viscous secretions frequently occurs, with the resulting atelectasis often refractory to conventional therapy. Recombinant human deoxyribonuclease is used in both nebulized form for nonintubated patients with acute asthma as well as intratracheally for atelectasis in intubated asthmatics, with resolution of atelectasis unresponsive to conventional asthma therapies. Recombinant human deoxyribonuclease is also utilized in ventilated infants and children with atelectasis not caused by asthma.

Hypertonic saline solution increases mucociliary clearance in patients with asthma, bronchiectasis, and cystic fibrosis and infants with acute bronchiolitis. It is delivered via nebulization either via face mask or endotracheal tube. It can be delivered alone or in combination with a bronchodilator. This therapy is being utilized in the outpatient and inpatient setting, as well as in both the neonatal intensive care unit and the pediatric intensive care unit, to help facilitate airway clearance.

Lobar atelectasis in cystic fibrosis is discussed in Chapter 403.

Atelectasis can occur in patients with neuromuscular diseases. These patients tend to have ineffective cough and difficulty expelling respiratory tract secretions, which lead to pneumonia and atelectasis. Several devices and treatments are available to assist these patients, including intermittent positive-pressure breathing, a mechanical insufflator-exsufflator, and noninvasive bilevel positive-pressure ventilation via nasal mask or full-face mask. Patients with neuromuscular disease who have undergone surgery are at substantial risk for postoperative atelectasis and subsequent pneumonia. Migrating atelectasis in the newborn infant, a rare and unique presentation, may be secondary to neuromuscular disease.

There is an association between the development of lobar collapse and the requirement for mechanical ventilation. Although lobar collapse is rarely a cause of long-term morbidity, its occurrence may necessitate the prolongation of mechanical ventilation or re-intubation.

Table 408-2	Benefit of Airway Clearance Therapies in Pediatric Conditions

CLEAR AND PROVEN BENEFIT
Cystic fibrosis

PROBABLE BENEFIT
Neuromuscular disease
Cerebral palsy
Atelectasis in children undergoing mechanical ventilation

POSSIBLE BENEFIT
Prevention of postextubation atelectasis in neonates

MINIMAL TO NO BENEFIT
Acute asthma
Bronchiolitis
Hyaline membrane disease
Respiratory failure without atelectasis
Prevention of atelectasis immediately following surgery

From Schechter MS: Airway clearance applications in infants and children, Respir Care 52:1382–1390, 2007.

In ventilated patients, positive end-expiratory pressure or continuous positive airway pressure is generally indicated.

Airway clearance therapies utilized for adults are often recommended and/or utilized in pediatric populations. However, given the differences in respiratory physiology and anatomy between children and adults, practices applicable to one may or may not apply to the other. Atelectasis caused by cystic fibrosis is the only pediatric entity that clearly benefits from airway clearance therapy, although atelectasis caused by neuromuscular disease, cerebral palsy, or mechanical ventilation probably benefits from such therapy (Table 408-2). Thus far no specific airway clearance therapy has been demonstrated to be superior.

Bibliography is available at Expert Consult.

Chapter 409
Pulmonary Tumors
Susanna A. McColley

ETIOLOGY
Primary tumors of the lung are rare in children and adolescents. An accurate estimate of frequency is currently not possible because the literature is composed of case reports and case series. A high incidence of "inflammatory pseudotumors" further clouds the statistics. **Bronchial adenomas (including bronchial carcinoid, adenoid cystic carcinoma and mucoepidermoid carcinomas)** are the most common primary tumors; bronchial carcinoid tumors represent ≈80%. Carcinoids are low-grade malignancies; carcinoid syndrome is rare in children. Metastatic lesions are the most common forms of pulmonary malignancy in children; primary processes include Wilms tumor, osteogenic sarcoma, and hepatoblastoma (see Part XXII: Cancer and Benign Tumors). Adenocarcinoma and undifferentiated histology are the most common pathologic findings in primary lung cancer; pulmonary blastoma is rarer and frequently occurs in the setting of cystic lung disease. Mediastinal involvement with lymphoma is more common than primary pulmonary malignancies.

CLINICAL MANIFESTATIONS AND EVALUATION
Pulmonary tumors may manifest as fever, hemoptysis, wheezing, cough, pleural effusion, chest pain, dyspnea, or recurrent or persistent pneumonia or atelectasis. Localized wheezing, and wheezing unresponsive to bronchodilators, can occur with bronchial tumors. Tumors may be suspected from plain chest radiographs; CT scanning of the chest is necessary for precise anatomic definition (Fig. 409-1). Depending on the tumor size and location, pulmonary function tests may be normal or show an obstructive, restrictive, or mixed pattern; as with the physical exam, there is no responsiveness to bronchodilators. Bronchial tumors are occasionally diagnosed during fiberoptic bronchoscopy performed for persistent or recurrent pulmonary infiltrates or for hemoptysis.

Patients with symptoms or with radiographic or other laboratory findings suggesting pulmonary malignancy should be evaluated carefully for a tumor at another site before surgical excision is carried out. Isolated primary lesions and isolated metastatic lesions discovered long after the primary tumor has been removed are best treated by excision. The prognosis varies and depends on the type of tumor involved; outcomes for inflammatory pseudotumors and primary pulmonary carcinoid tumors treated with resection are good.

Bibliography is available at Expert Consult.

Chapter 410
Pleurisy, Pleural Effusions, and Empyema
Glenna B. Winnie and Steven V. Lossef

Pleurisy is the inflammation of the pleura; it may be accompanied by an effusion. The most common cause of pleural effusion in children is bacterial pneumonia (see Chapter 400); heart failure (see Chapter 442), rheumatologic causes, and metastatic intrathoracic malignancy are the next most common causes. A variety of other diseases account for the remaining cases, including tuberculosis (see Chapter 215), lupus erythematosus (see Chapter 158), aspiration pneumonitis (see Chapter 397), uremia, pancreatitis, subdiaphragmatic abscess, and rheumatoid arthritis. Males and females are affected equally.

Inflammatory processes in the pleura are usually divided into 3 types: dry or plastic, serofibrinous or serosanguineous, and purulent pleurisy or empyema.

410.1 Dry or Plastic Pleurisy (Pleural Effusion)
Glenna B. Winnie and Steven V. Lossef

ETIOLOGY
Plastic pleurisy may be associated with acute bacterial or viral pulmonary infections or may develop during the course of an acute upper respiratory tract illness. The condition is also associated with tuberculosis and connective tissue diseases such as rheumatic fever.

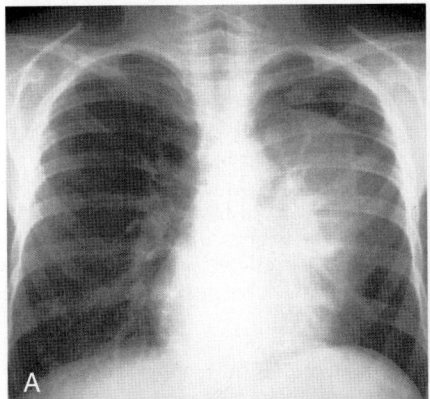
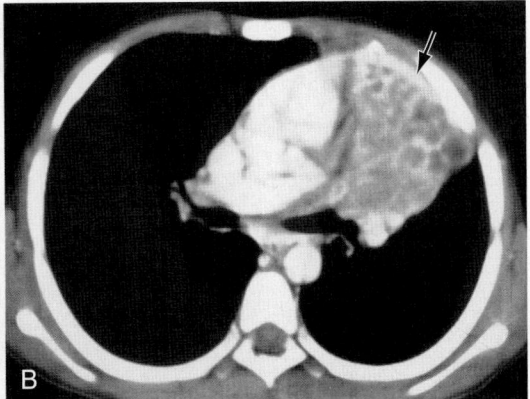

Figure 409-1 Endobronchial mucoepidermoid carcinoma in a 10 yr old boy who presented with cough and fever. **A,** The chest radiograph shows a left upper lobe mass, a hyperinflated left lower lobe, and a prominent left hilum. **B,** The CT scan shows complete obstruction of the left upper lobe bronchus by a low-attenuation mass that extends into the left mainstem bronchus. *(From Slovis TL, editor: Caffey's pediatric diagnostic imaging, ed 11, Philadelphia, 2008, Mosby, Fig. 78-20.)*

PATHOLOGY AND PATHOGENESIS

The process is usually limited to the visceral pleura, with small amounts of yellow serous fluid and adhesions between the pleural surfaces. In tuberculosis, the adhesions develop rapidly and the pleura are often thickened. Occasionally, fibrin deposition and adhesions are severe enough to produce a fibrothorax that markedly inhibits the excursions of the lung.

CLINICAL MANIFESTATIONS

The primary disease often overshadows signs and symptoms. Pain, the principal symptom, is exaggerated by deep breathing, coughing, and straining. Occasionally, pleural pain is described as a dull ache, which is less likely to vary with breathing. The pain is often localized over the chest wall and is referred to the shoulder or the back. Pain with breathing is responsible for grunting and guarding of respirations, and the child often lies on the affected side in an attempt to decrease respiratory excursions. Early in the illness, a leathery, rough, inspiratory and expiratory friction rub may be audible, but it usually disappears rapidly. If the layer of exudate is thick, increased dullness to percussion and decreased breath sounds may be heard. Pleurisy may be asymptomatic. Chronic pleurisy is occasionally encountered with conditions such as atelectasis, pulmonary abscess, connective tissue diseases, and tuberculosis.

LABORATORY FINDINGS

Plastic pleurisy may be detected on radiographs as a diffuse haziness at the pleural surface or a dense, sharply demarcated shadow (Figs. 410-1 and 410-2). The latter finding may be indistinguishable from small amounts of pleural exudate. Chest radiographic findings may be normal, but ultrasonography or CT findings will be positive.

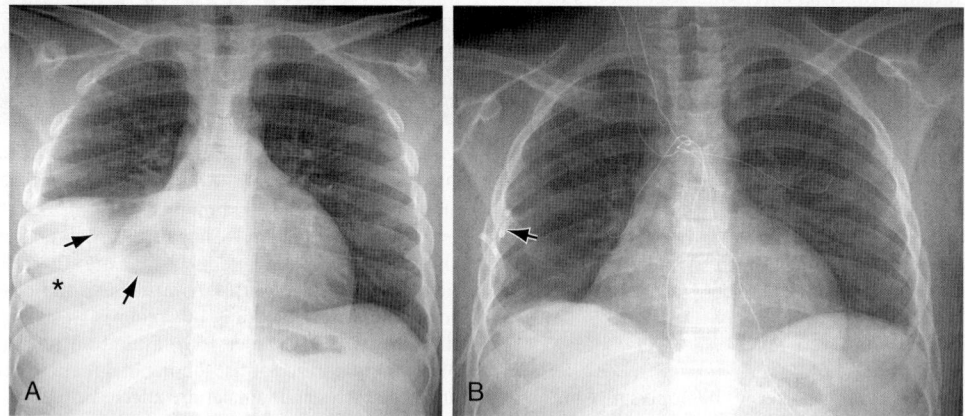

Figure 410-1 A, Right pleural effusion *(asterisk)* caused by lupus erythematosus in a 12 yr old child. Note compressed middle and lower lobes of the right lung *(arrows)*. **B,** The effusion was evacuated and the right lung was completely reexpanded after insertion of the pigtail chest tube *(arrow)*.

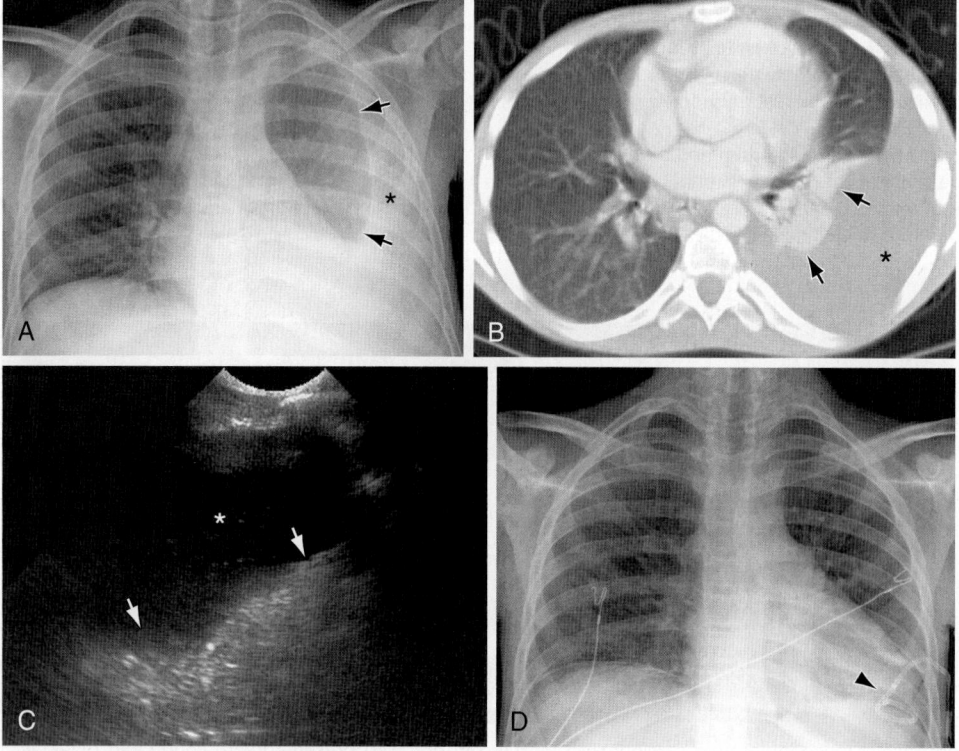

Figure 410-2 Left pleural effusion in a teenager with AIDS and *Mycobacterium avium-intracellulare* infection. The pleural effusion *(asterisk)* is clearly seen on the chest radiograph **(A)**, CT scan **(B)**, and ultrasonogram **(C)** of the left chest. *Arrows* point to the compressed and atelectatic left lung. **D,** A pigtail chest tube *(arrowhead)* was inserted, resulting in reexpansion of the left lung.

DIFFERENTIAL DIAGNOSIS

Plastic pleurisy must be distinguished from other diseases, such as epidemic pleurodynia, trauma to the rib cage (rib fracture), lesions of the dorsal root ganglia, tumors of the spinal cord, herpes zoster, gallbladder disease, and trichinosis. Even if evidence of pleural fluid is not found on physical or radiographic examination, a CT- or ultrasound-guided pleural tap in suspected cases often results in the recovery of a small amount of exudate, which when cultured may reveal the underlying bacterial cause in patients with an acute pneumonia. Patients with pleurisy and pneumonia should always be screened for tuberculosis.

TREATMENT

Therapy should be aimed at the underlying disease. When pneumonia is present, neither immobilization of the chest with adhesive plaster nor therapy with drugs capable of suppressing the cough reflex is indicated. If pneumonia is not present or is under good therapeutic control, strapping of the chest to restrict expansion may afford relief from pain. Analgesia with nonsteroidal antiinflammatory agents may be helpful.

Bibliography is available at Expert Consult.

410.2 Serofibrinous or Serosanguineous Pleurisy (Pleural Effusion)
Glenna B. Winnie

ETIOLOGY

Serofibrinous pleurisy is defined by a fibrinous exudate on the pleural surface and an exudative effusion of serous fluid into the pleural cavity. Generally it is associated with infections of the lung or with inflammatory conditions of the abdomen or mediastinum; occasionally, it is found with connective tissue diseases such as lupus erythematosus, periarteritis, and rheumatoid, arthritis, and it may be seen with primary or metastatic neoplasms of the lung, pleura, or mediastinum; tumors are commonly associated with a hemorrhagic pleurisy.

PATHOGENESIS

Pleural fluid originates from the capillaries of the parietal pleura and is absorbed from the pleural space via pleural stomas and the lymphatics of the parietal pleura. The rate of fluid formation is dictated by the Starling law, by which fluid movement is determined by the balance of hydrostatic and osmotic pressures in the pleural space and pulmonary capillary bed, and the permeability of the pleural membrane. Normally, only 4-12 mL of fluid is present in the pleural space, but if formation exceeds clearance, fluid accumulates. Pleural inflammation increases the permeability of the plural surface, with increased proteinaceous fluid formation; there may also be some obstruction to lymphatic absorption.

CLINICAL MANIFESTATIONS

Because serofibrinous pleurisy is often preceded by the plastic type, early signs and symptoms may be those of plastic pleurisy. As fluid accumulates, pleuritic pain may disappear. The patient may become asymptomatic if the effusion remains small, or there may be only signs and symptoms of the underlying disease. Large fluid collections can produce cough, dyspnea, retractions, tachypnea, orthopnea, or cyanosis.

Physical findings depend on the amount of effusion. Dullness to flatness may be found on percussion. Breath sounds are decreased or absent, and there are a diminution in tactile fremitus, a shift of the mediastinum away from the affected side, and, occasionally, fullness of the intercostal spaces. If the fluid is not loculated, these signs may shift with changes in position. If extensive pneumonia is present, crackles and rhonchi may also be audible. Friction rubs are usually detected only during the early or late plastic stage. In infants, physical signs are less definite, and bronchial breathing may be heard instead of decreased breath sounds.

LABORATORY FINDINGS

Radiographic examination shows a generally homogeneous density obliterating the normal markings of the underlying lung. Small effusions may cause obliteration of only the costophrenic or cardiophrenic angles or a widening of the interlobar septa. Examinations should be performed with the patient both supine and upright, to demonstrate a shift of the effusion with a change in position; the decubitus position may be helpful. **Ultrasonographic** examinations are useful and may guide thoracentesis if the effusion is loculated. Examination of the fluid is essential to differentiate exudates from transudates and to determine the type of exudate. Depending on the clinical scenario, pleural fluid is sent for culture for bacterial, fungal, and mycobacterial cultures; antigen testing; Gram staining; and chemical evaluation of content, including protein, lactic dehydrogenase and glucose, amylase, specific gravity, total cell count and differential, cytologic examination, and pH. Complete blood count and serum chemistry analysis should be obtained; hypoalbuminemia is often present. **Exudates** usually have at least 1 of the following features: protein level >3.0 g/dL, with pleural fluid:serum protein ratio >0.5; pleural fluid lactic dehydrogenase values >200 IU/L; or fluid:serum lactic dehydrogenase ratio >0.6. Although systemic acidosis reduces the usefulness of pleural fluid pH measurements, pH <7.20 suggests an exudate (see Chapter 400). Glucose is usually <60 mg/dL in malignancy, rheumatoid disease, and tuberculosis; the finding of many small lymphocytes and a pH <7.20 suggest tuberculosis. The fluid of serofibrinous pleurisy is clear or slightly cloudy and contains relatively few leukocytes and, occasionally, some erythrocytes. Gram staining may occasionally show bacteria; however, acid-fast staining rarely demonstrates tubercle bacilli.

DIAGNOSIS AND DIFFERENTIAL DIAGNOSIS

Thoracentesis should be performed when pleural fluid is present or is suggested, unless the effusion is small and the patient has a classic-appearing lobar pneumococcal pneumonia. Thoracentesis can differentiate serofibrinous pleurisy, empyema, hydrothorax, hemothorax, and chylothorax. Exudates are usually associated with an infectious process. In hydrothorax, the fluid has a specific gravity <1.015, and evaluation reveals only a few mesothelial cells rather than leukocytes. Chylothorax and hemothorax usually have fluid with a distinctive appearance, but differentiating serofibrinous from purulent pleurisy is impossible without microscopic examination of the fluid. Cytologic examination may reveal malignant cells. Serofibrinous fluid may rapidly become purulent.

COMPLICATIONS

Unless the fluid becomes purulent, it usually disappears relatively rapidly, particularly with appropriate treatment of bacterial pneumonia. It persists somewhat longer if a result of tuberculosis or a connective tissue disease and may recur or remain for a long time if caused by a neoplasm. As the effusion is absorbed, adhesions often develop between the 2 layers of the pleura, but usually little or no functional impairment results. Pleural thickening may develop and is occasionally mistaken for small quantities of fluid or for persistent pulmonary infiltrates. Pleural thickening may persist for months, but the process usually disappears, leaving no residua.

TREATMENT

Therapy should address the underlying disease. With a large effusion, draining the fluid makes the patient more comfortable. When a diagnostic thoracentesis is performed, as much fluid as possible should be removed for therapeutic purposes. Rapid removal of ≥1 L of pleural fluid may be associated with the development of reexpansion pulmonary edema (see Chapter 396). If the underlying disease is adequately treated, further drainage is usually unnecessary, but if sufficient fluid reaccumulates to cause respiratory embarrassment, chest tube drainage should be performed. In older children with suspected parapneumonic effusion, tube thoracostomy is considered necessary if the pleural fluid pH is <7.20 or the pleural fluid glucose level is <50 mg/dL. If the fluid is clearly purulent, tube drainage with **thrombolytic therapy** or less often video-assisted thoracoscopic surgery (VATS) is indicated.

Patients with pleural effusions may need analgesia, particularly after thoracentesis or insertion of a chest tube. Those with acute pneumonia may need supplemental oxygen in addition to specific antibiotic treatment.

Bibliography is available at Expert Consult.

410.3 Purulent Pleurisy or Empyema
Glenna B. Winnie and Steven V. Lossef

ETIOLOGY
Empyema is an accumulation of pus in the pleural space. It is most often associated with pneumonia (see Chapter 400) caused by *Streptococcus pneumoniae* (see Chapter 182), although *Staphylococcus aureus* (see Chapter 181.1) is most common in developing nations and Asia, as well as in posttraumatic empyema. The relative incidence of *Haemophilus influenzae* (see Chapter 194) empyema has decreased since the introduction of the *H. influenzae* type b vaccination. Group A streptococcus, Gram-negative organisms, tuberculosis, fungi, and malignancy are less common causes. The disease can also be produced by rupture of a lung abscess into the pleural space, by contamination introduced from trauma or thoracic surgery, or, rarely, by mediastinitis or the extension of intraabdominal abscesses.

EPIDEMIOLOGY
Empyema is most frequently encountered in infants and preschool children. It is increasing in frequency. It occurs in 5-10% of children with bacterial pneumonia and in up to 86% of children with necrotizing pneumonia.

PATHOLOGY
Empyema has 3 stages: exudative, fibrinopurulent, and organizational. During the **exudative stage**, fibrinous exudate forms on the pleural surfaces. In the **fibrinopurulent stage**, fibrinous septa form, causing loculation of the fluid and thickening of the parietal pleura. If the pus is not drained, it may dissect through the pleura into lung parenchyma, producing bronchopleural fistulas and pyopneumothorax, or into the abdominal cavity. Rarely, the pus dissects through the chest wall (i.e., empyema necessitatis). During the **organizational stage**, there is fibroblast proliferation; pockets of loculated pus may develop into thick-walled abscess cavities or the lung may collapse and become surrounded by a thick, inelastic envelope (peel).

CLINICAL MANIFESTATIONS
The initial signs and symptoms are primarily those of bacterial pneumonia. Children treated with antibiotic agents may have an interval of a few days between the clinical pneumonia phase and the evidence of empyema. Most patients are febrile, develop increased work of breathing or respiratory distress, and often appear more ill. Physical findings are identical to those described for serofibrinous pleurisy, and the 2 conditions are differentiated only by thoracentesis, which should always be performed when empyema is suspected.

LABORATORY FINDINGS
Radiographically, all pleural effusions appear similar, but the absence of a shift of the fluid with a change of position indicates a loculated empyema (Figs. 410-3 to 410-5). Septa may be confirmed by ultrasonography or CT. The maximal amount of fluid obtainable should be withdrawn by thoracentesis and studied as described in Chapter 410.2. The effusion is empyema if bacteria are present on Gram staining, the pH is <7.20, and there are >100,000 neutrophils/μL (see Chapter 400). The appearance of pus produced by different organisms is not distinctive; cultures of the fluid must always be performed. In pneumococcal empyema, the culture is positive in 58% of cases. In patients with negative culture results for pneumococcus, the pneumococcal polymerase chain reaction analysis is most helpful to making a diagnosis. Blood cultures may be positive and have a higher yield than cultures of the

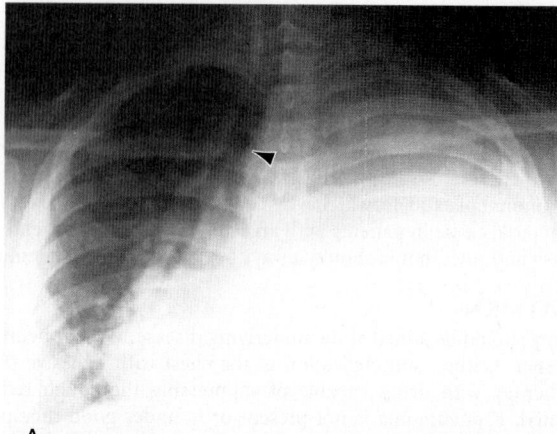

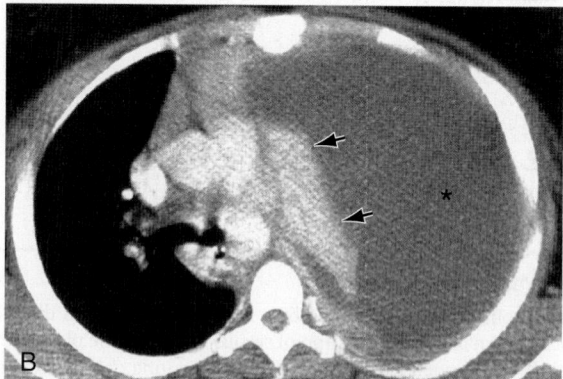

Figure 410-3 Empyema and pneumonia in a teenager. **A,** Chest radiograph shows opacification of the left thorax. Note shift of mediastinum and trachea *(arrowhead)* to right. **B,** Thoracic CT scan shows massive left pleural effusion *(asterisk)*. Note the compression and atelectasis of the left lung *(arrows)* and shift of the mediastinum to the right.

pleural fluid. Leukocytosis and an elevated sedimentation rate may be found.

COMPLICATIONS
With staphylococcal infections, bronchopleural fistulas and pyopneumothorax commonly develop. Other local complications include purulent pericarditis, pulmonary abscesses, peritonitis from extension through the diaphragm, and osteomyelitis of the ribs. Septic complications such as meningitis, arthritis, and osteomyelitis may also occur. Septicemia is often encountered in *H. influenzae* and pneumococcal infections. The effusion may organize into a thick "peel," which may restrict lung expansion and may be associated with persistent fever and temporary scoliosis.

TREATMENT
The aim of empyema treatment is to sterilize pleural fluid and restore normal lung function. Treatment includes systemic antibiotics and thoracentesis and chest tube drainage initially with a fibrinolytic agent; if no improvement occurs, VATS is indicated. Open decortication is indicated if fibrinolysis and VATS are ineffective (see Chapter 411). If empyema is diagnosed early, antibiotic treatment plus thoracentesis achieves a complete cure. The selection of antibiotic should be based on the in vitro sensitivities of the responsible organism. See Chapters 181, 182, and 194 for treatment of infections by *Staphylococcus*, *S. pneumoniae*, and *H. influenzae*, respectively. Clinical response in empyema is slow; even with optimal treatment, there may be little improvement for as long as 2 wk. With staphylococcal infections, resolution is very slow, and systemic antibiotic therapy is required for 3-4 wk. Instillation of antibiotics into the pleural cavity does not improve results.

When pus is obtained by thoracentesis, closed-chest tube drainage with fibrolytics is the initial procedure followed by VATS if there is no improvement. Multiple aspirations of the pleural cavity should not be attempted. If pleural fluid septa are detected on ultrasound, fibrinolysis is attempted followed by VATS if no improvement is noted. Closed-

chest tube drainage is controlled by an underwater seal or continuous suction; sometimes more than 1 tube is required to drain loculated areas. Closed drainage is usually continued for 5-7 days. Chest tubes that are no longer draining are removed.

Instillation of fibrinolytic agents into the pleural cavity via the chest tube may promote drainage, decrease fever, lessen need for surgical intervention, and shorten hospitalization; it does not shorten the course of disease when used after VATS. The optimal drug and dosage have not been determined. Streptokinase 15,000 units/kg in 50 mL of 0.9% saline daily for 3-5 days and urokinase 40,000 units in 40 mL saline every 12 hr for 6 doses have been evaluated in randomized trials in children. Alteplase (tissue plasminogen activator) has also been used. There is a risk of anaphylaxis with streptokinase, and all 3 drugs can be associated with hemorrhage and other complications.

Extensive fibrinous changes may take place over the surface of the lungs owing to empyema, but they eventually resolve. In the child who remains febrile and dyspneic for more than 72 hr after initiation of therapy with intravenous antibiotics and thoracostomy tube drainage, surgical decortication via VATS or, less often, open thoracotomy may speed recovery. If pneumatoceles form, no attempt should be made to treat them surgically or by aspiration, unless they reach sufficient size to cause respiratory embarrassment or become secondarily infected. Pneumatoceles usually resolve spontaneously with time. The long-term clinical prognosis for adequately treated empyema is excellent, and follow-up pulmonary function studies suggest that residual restrictive disease is uncommon, with or without surgical intervention.

Bibliography is available at Expert Consult.

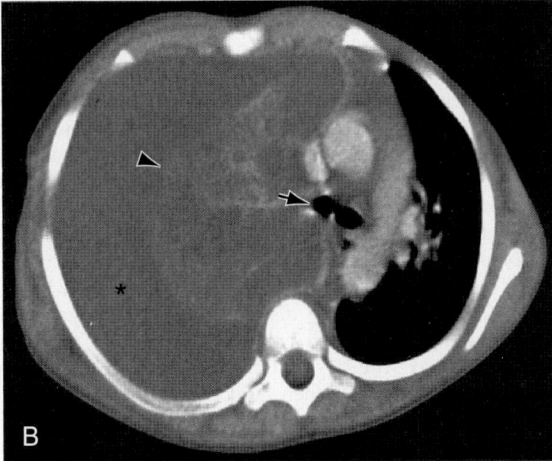

Figure 410-4 Pneumonia and parapneumonic effusion in a 4 yr old child. **A,** Chest radiograph shows complete opacification of the right thorax as a result of a large pleural effusion. Note the shift of the mediastinum and trachea *(arrow)* to the left. **B,** Thoracic CT scan shows a large right pleural effusion *(asterisk)* surrounding and compressing the consolidated right lung *(arrowhead)*. Note the shift of the mediastinum and tracheal carina *(arrow)* to the left.

Chapter **411**
Pneumothorax
Glenna B. Winnie and Steven V. Lossef

Pneumothorax is the accumulation of extrapulmonary air within the chest, most commonly from leakage of air from within the lung. Air leaks can be primary or secondary and can be spontaneous, traumatic, iatrogenic, or catamenial (Table 411-1). Pneumothorax in the neonatal period is also discussed in Chapter 101.12.

ETIOLOGY AND EPIDEMIOLOGY
A **primary spontaneous pneumothorax** occurs without trauma or underlying lung disease. Spontaneous pneumothorax with or without

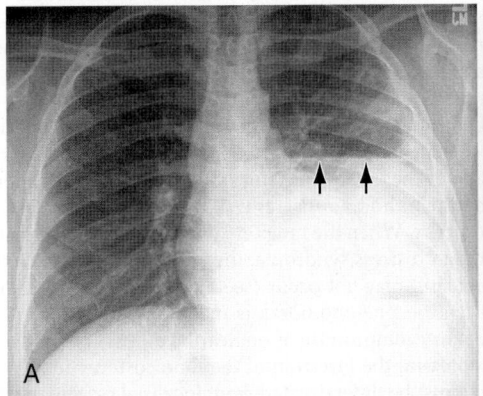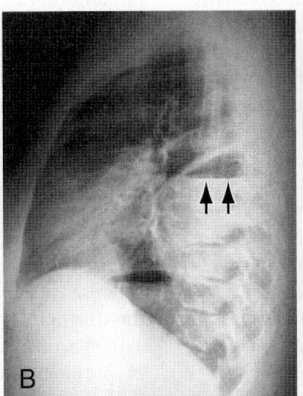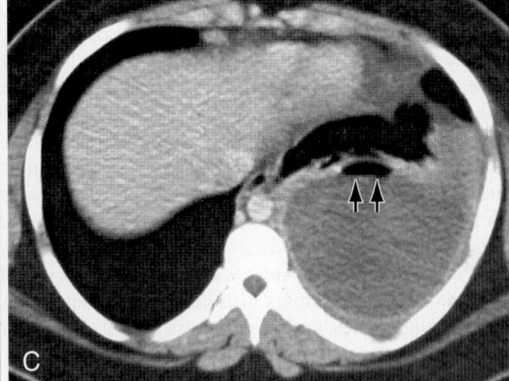

Figure 410-5 Loculated hydropneumothorax. Frontal **(A)** and lateral **(B)** chest radiographs show loculated hydropneumothorax that complicated pneumonia in a 14 yr old child. *Arrows* point to the horizontal air–fluid level at the interface between the intrapleural effusion and air. **C,** Thoracic CT scan helps to localize the loculated hydropneumothorax, with its air–fluid level *(arrows)*.

Table 411-1	Causes of Pneumothorax in Children

SPONTANEOUS
Primary idiopathic—usually resulting from ruptured subpleural blebs
Secondary blebs
Congenital lung disease:
   Congenital cystic adenomatoid malformation
   Bronchogenic cysts
   Pulmonary hypoplasia*
   Birt-Hogg-Dube syndrome
Conditions associated with increased intrathoracic pressure:
   Asthma
   Bronchiolitis
   Air-block syndrome in neonates
   Cystic fibrosis
   Airway foreign body
   Smoking (cigarettes, marijuana, crack cocaine)
Infection:
   Pneumatocele
   Lung abscess
   Echinococcosis
   Bronchopleural fistula
Diffuse lung disease:
   Langerhans cell histiocytosis
   Tuberous sclerosis
   Marfan syndrome
   Ehlers-Danlos syndrome
   Metastatic neoplasm—usually osteosarcoma (rare)
   Pulmonary blastoma

TRAUMATIC
Noniatrogenic
Penetrating trauma
Blunt trauma
High-flow therapy
Loud music (air pressure)
Iatrogenic
Thoracotomy
Thoracoscopy, thoracentesis
Tracheostomy
Tube or needle puncture
Mechanical ventilation

*Associated with renal agenesis, diaphragmatic hernia, amniotic fluid leaks.
From Kuhn JP, Slovis TL, Haller JO, editors: Caffey's pediatric diagnostic imaging, ed 10, Philadelphia, 2004, Mosby.

exertion occurs occasionally in teenagers and young adults, most frequently in males who are tall, thin, and thought to have subpleural blebs. Familial cases of spontaneous pneumothorax occur and have been associated with mutations in the folliculin gene (*FCLN*). *FCLN* mutations may be seen in the Birt-Hogg-Dube syndrome (skin fibrofolliculomas, multiple basal lung cysts, renal malignancies) or in patients with familial or recurrent spontaneous pneumothoraces. Patients with collagen synthesis defects, such as Ehlers-Danlos disease (see Chapter 659) and Marfan syndrome (see Chapter 702) are unusually prone to the development of pneumothorax.

A pneumothorax arising as a complication of an underlying lung disorder but without trauma is a **secondary spontaneous pneumothorax.** Pneumothorax can occur in pneumonia, usually with empyema; it can also be secondary to pulmonary abscess, gangrene, infarct, rupture of a cyst or an emphysematous bleb (in asthma), or foreign bodies in the lung. In infants with staphylococcal pneumonia, the incidence of pneumothorax is relatively high. It is found in ≈5% of hospitalized asthmatic children and usually resolves without treatment. Pneumothorax is a serious complication in cystic fibrosis (see Chapter 403). Pneumothorax also occurs in patients with lymphoma or other malignancies, and in graft-versus-host disease with bronchiolitis obliterans.

External chest or abdominal blunt or penetrating trauma can tear a bronchus or abdominal viscus, with leakage of air into the pleural space. Ecstasy (methylenedioxymethamphetamine), crack cocaine, and marijuana abuse are associated with pneumothorax.

Iatrogenic pneumothorax can complicate transthoracic needle aspiration, tracheotomy, subclavian line placement, thoracentesis, or transbronchial biopsy. It may occur during mechanical or noninvasive ventilation, high-flow nasal cannula therapy, acupuncture, and other diagnostic or therapeutic procedures.

Catamenial pneumothorax, an unusual condition that is related to menses, is associated with diaphragmatic defects and pleural blebs.

Pneumothorax can be associated with a serous effusion (hydropneumothorax), a purulent effusion (pyopneumothorax), or blood (hemopneumothorax). Bilateral pneumothorax is rare after the neonatal period but has been reported after lung transplantation and with *Mycoplasma pneumoniae* infection and tuberculosis.

PATHOGENESIS
The tendency of the lung to collapse, or elastic recoil, is balanced in the normal resting state by the inherent tendency of the chest wall to expand outward, creating negative pressure in the intrapleural space. When air enters the pleural space, the lung collapses. Hypoxemia occurs because of alveolar hypoventilation, ventilation–perfusion mismatch, and intrapulmonary shunt. In simple pneumothorax, intrapleural pressure is atmospheric, and the lung collapses up to 30%. In complicated, or tension, pneumothorax, continuing leak causes increasing positive pressure in the pleural space, with further compression of the lung, shift of mediastinal structures toward the contralateral side, and decreases in venous return and cardiac output.

CLINICAL MANIFESTATIONS
The onset of pneumothorax is usually abrupt, and the severity of symptoms depends on the extent of the lung collapse and on the amount of preexisting lung disease. Pneumothorax may cause dyspnea, pain, and cyanosis. When it occurs in infancy, symptoms and physical signs may be difficult to recognize. Moderate pneumothorax may cause little displacement of the intrathoracic organs and few or no symptoms. The severity of pain usually does not directly reflect the extent of the collapse.

Usually, there is respiratory distress, with retractions, markedly decreased breath sounds, and a tympanitic percussion note over the involved hemithorax. The larynx, trachea, and heart may be shifted toward the unaffected side. When fluid is present, there is usually a sharply limited area of tympany above a level of flatness to percussion. The presence of amphoric breathing or, when fluid is present in the pleural cavity, of gurgling sounds synchronous with respirations suggests an open fistula connecting with air-containing tissues.

DIAGNOSIS AND DIFFERENTIAL DIAGNOSIS
The diagnosis of pneumothorax is usually established by radiographic examination (Figs. 411-1 to 411-6). The amount of air outside the lung varies with time. A radiograph that is taken early shows less lung collapse than one taken later if the leak continues. Expiratory views accentuate the contrast between lung markings and the clear area of the pneumothorax (see Fig. 411-1). When the possibility of diaphragmatic hernia is being considered, a small amount of barium may be necessary to demonstrate that it is not free air but is a portion of the gastrointestinal tract that is in the thoracic cavity. Ultrasound can also be used to establish the diagnosis.

It may be difficult to determine whether a pneumothorax is under tension. **Evidence of tension** includes shift of mediastinal structures away from the side of the air leak. A shift may be absent in situations in which the other hemithorax resists the shift, such as in the case of bilateral pneumothorax. When the lungs are both stiff, such as in cystic fibrosis or respiratory distress syndrome, the unaffected lung may not collapse easily and shift may not occur (see Fig. 411-3). On occasion, the diagnosis of tension pneumothorax is made only on the basis of evidence of circulatory compromise or on hearing a "hiss" of rapid exit of air under tension with the insertion of the thoracostomy tube.

Pneumothorax must be differentiated from localized or generalized emphysema, an extensive emphysematous bleb, large pulmonary cavities or other cystic formations, diaphragmatic hernia, compensatory overexpansion with contralateral atelectasis, and gaseous distention of

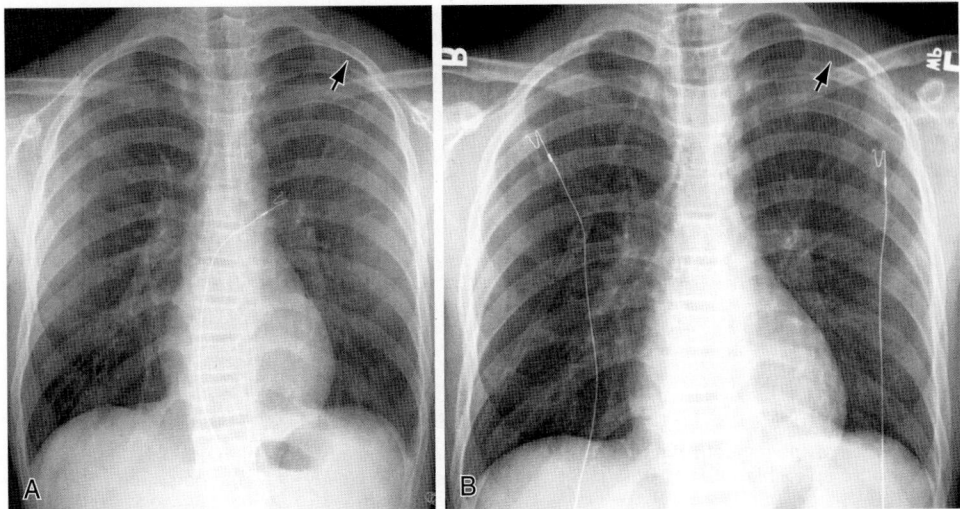

Figure 411-1 Utility of an expiratory film in detection of a small pneumothorax. **A,** Teenage boy with stab wound and subtle radiolucency in the left apical region *(arrow)* on inspiratory chest radiograph. The margin of the visceral pleura is very faintly visible. **B,** On an expiratory film, the pneumothorax *(arrow)* is more obvious as the right lung has deflated and become more opaque, providing better contrast with the air in the pleural space.

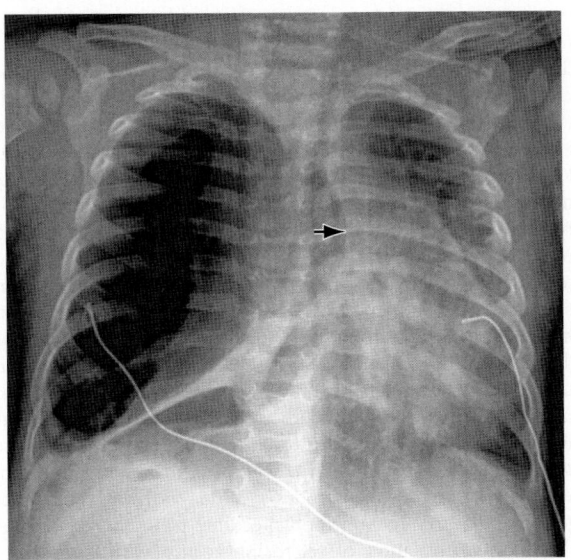

Figure 411-2 Right pneumothorax, with lung collapse of a compliant lung. Shift of the mediastinum to the left *(arrow)* indicates that this is a tension pneumothorax.

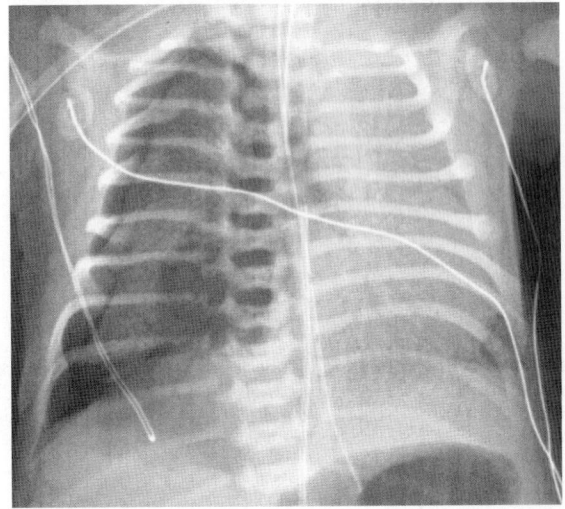

Figure 411-3 Right pneumothorax, with only limited collapse of a poorly compliant lung.

the stomach. In most cases, chest radiography or CT differentiates among these possibilities. In addition, CT may identify underlying pathology such as blebs (Fig. 411-7).

TREATMENT
Therapy varies with the extent of the collapse and the nature and severity of the underlying disease. A small (<5%) or even moderate-sized pneumothorax in an otherwise normal child may resolve without specific treatment, usually within 1 wk. A small pneumothorax complicating asthma may also resolve spontaneously. Administering 100% oxygen may hasten resolution, but patients with chronic hypoxemia should be monitored closely during administration of supplemental oxygen. Pleural pain deserves analgesic treatment. Needle aspiration may be required on an emergency basis for tension pneumothorax and is as effective as tube thoracostomy in the emergency room management of primary spontaneous pneumothorax. If the pneumothorax is recurrent, secondary, or under tension, or there is >5% collapse, chest tube drainage is necessary. Pneumothorax-complicating cystic fibrosis

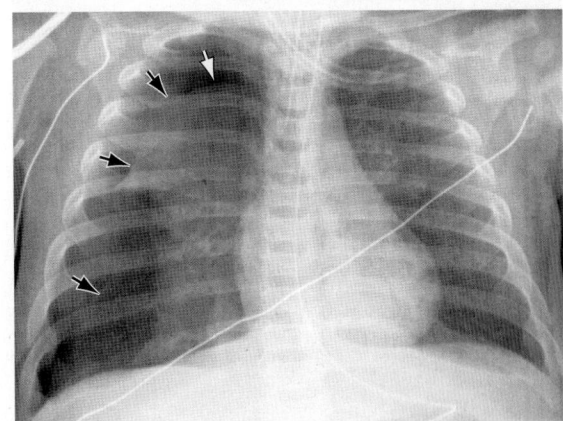

Figure 411-4 Pneumothorax, with collapse of right lung *(arrows)* caused by barotrauma in a 7 mo old child who was intubated for respiratory failure.

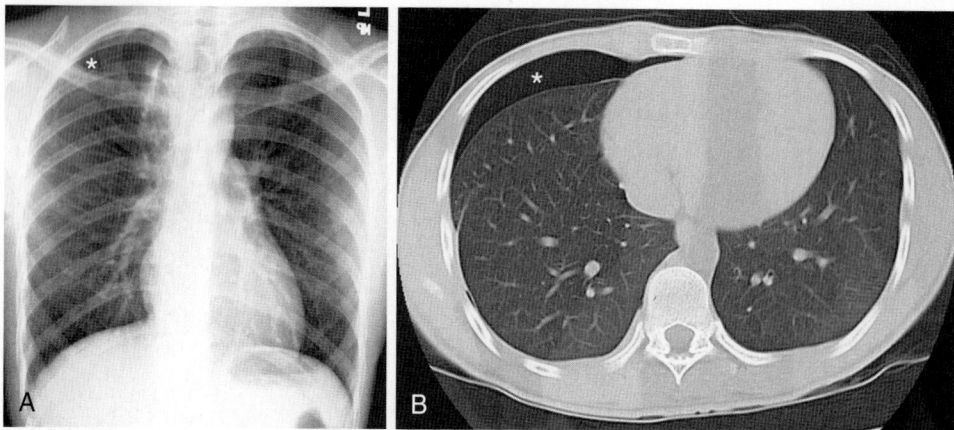

Figure 411-5 Teenager in whom a spontaneous right pneumothorax developed because of a bleb. He had a persistent air leak despite recent surgical resection of the causative apical bleb. Chest radiograph **(A)** and CT scan **(B)** clearly show the persistent pneumothorax *(asterisk)*.

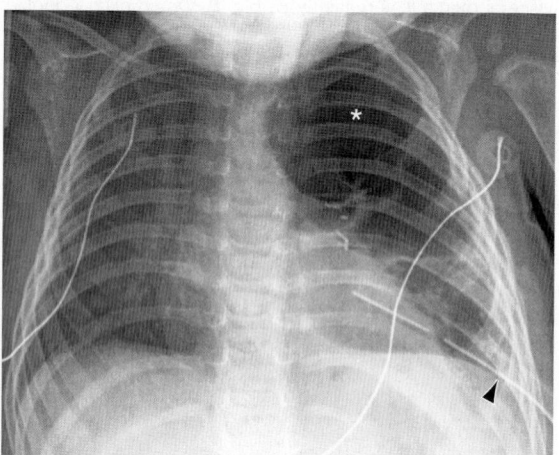

Figure 411-6 Bronchopleural fistula following surgical resection of the left upper lobe as a result of congenital lobar emphysema. Chest radiograph shows localized pneumothorax *(asterisk)* that persisted despite prior insertion of a large-bore chest tube *(arrowhead)*.

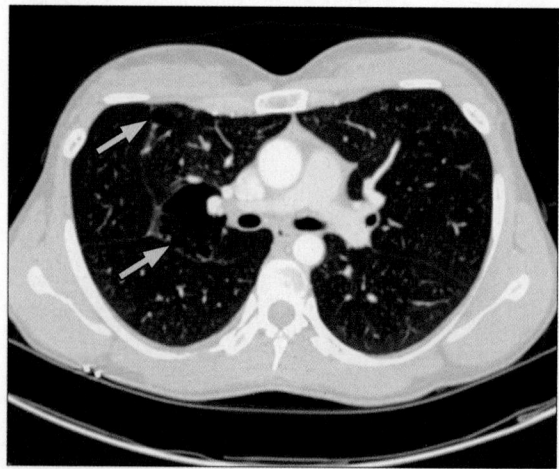

Figure 411-7 High-resolution CT thorax showing multiple basal cysts. *(From Hopkins TG, Maher ER, Reid E, Marciniak S: Recurrent pneumothorax. Lancet 377:1624, 2011, Fig. 1, p. 1624.)*

frequently recurs, and definitive treatment may be justified with the first episode. Similarly, if pneumothorax complicating malignancy does not improve rapidly with observation, chemical pleurodesis or surgical thoracotomy is often necessary. In cases with severe air leak or bronchopleural fistula, occlusion with an endobronchial balloon has been successful.

Closed thoracotomy (simple insertion of a chest tube) and drainage of the trapped air through a catheter, the external opening of which is kept in a dependent position under water, is adequate to reexpand the lung in most patients; pigtail catheters are frequently used. When there have been previous pneumothoraces, it may be indicated to induce the formation of strong adhesions between the lung and chest wall by a sclerosing procedure to prevent recurrence. This can be carried out by the introduction of talc, doxycycline, or iodopovidone into the pleural space (**chemical pleurodesis**). Open thoracotomy through a limited incision, with plication of blebs, closure of fistula, stripping of the pleura (usually in the apical lung, where the surgeon has direct vision), and basilar pleural abrasion is also an effective treatment for recurring pneumothorax. Stripping and abrading the pleura leaves raw, inflamed surfaces that heal with sealing adhesions. Postoperative pain is comparable to that with chemical pleurodesis, but the chest tube can usually be removed in 24-48 hr, compared with the usual 72 hr minimum for closed thoracotomy and pleurodesis. **Video-assisted thoracoscopic surgery** is a preferred therapy for blebectomy, pleural stripping, pleural brushing, and instillation of sclerosing agents, with somewhat less morbidity than occurs with traditional open thoracotomy. There is risk of recurrence after video-assisted thoracoscopic surgery in the pediatric population, although this is often not related to surgical failure, but rather associated with the formation of new bullae.

Pleural adhesions help prevent recurrent pneumothorax, but they also make subsequent thoracic surgery difficult. When lung transplantation may be a future consideration (e.g., in cystic fibrosis), a stepwise approach to treatment of pneumothorax has been proposed. This approach begins with observation and progresses through chest tube drainage and thoracoscopic and then open surgery, and finally to chemical or mechanical pleurodesis. At any step during this approach, the patient and family are given the option of the definitive procedure if they understand that its performance may make lung transplantation difficult or impossible. It should also be kept in mind that the longer a chest tube is in place, the greater the chance of pulmonary deterioration, particularly in a patient with cystic fibrosis, in whom strong coughing, deep breathing, and postural drainage are important. These are all difficult to accomplish with a chest tube in place.

Treatment of the underlying pulmonary disease should begin on admission and should be continued throughout the course of treatment directed at the air leak.

Bibliography is available at Expert Consult.

Chapter 412
Pneumomediastinum
Glenna B. Winnie

Air or gas in the mediastinum is called **pneumomediastinum.**

ETIOLOGY

Typically, pneumomediastinum is caused by alveolar rupture during acute or chronic pulmonary disease. A diverse group of nonrespiratory entities can also cause it, and the lung is not always the source of the air. Lower respiratory tract infection is a common etiology for pneumomediastinum in children younger than age 7 yr, while acute asthma is the most common cause in older children and teenagers. Simultaneous pneumothorax is unusual in these patients. Pneumomediastinum has been reported after vomiting, dental extractions, adenotonsillectomy, high-flow nasal cannula therapy, normal menses, obstetric delivery, diabetes mellitus with ketoacidosis, acupuncture, anorexia nervosa, and inhalation of helium gas. It can also result from esophageal perforation (Boerhaave syndrome), penetrating chest trauma, or inhaled foreign body. Occasionally, no underlying cause is found.

PATHOGENESIS

After intrapulmonary alveolar rupture, air dissects through the perivascular sheaths and other soft tissue, planes toward the hilum, and enters the mediastinum.

CLINICAL MANIFESTATIONS

Dyspnea and transient stabbing chest pain that may radiate to the neck are the principal features of pneumomediastinum. Isolated abdominal pain, cough, and sore throat also occur. Pneumomediastinum is difficult to detect by physical examination alone. Subcutaneous emphysema, if present, is diagnostic. Cardiac dullness to percussion may be decreased, but the chests of many patients with pneumomediastinum are chronically overinflated, and it is unlikely that the clinician can be sure of this finding. A mediastinal "crunch" (Hamman sign) is occasionally heard but is easily confused with a friction rub.

LABORATORY FINDINGS

Chest radiography reveals mediastinal air, with a more distinct cardiac border than normal (Figs. 412-1 to 412-3). On the lateral projection, the posterior mediastinal structures are clearly defined, there may be a lucent ring around the right pulmonary artery, and retrosternal air can usually be seen (see Fig. 412-2). Vertical streaks of air in the mediastinum and subcutaneous air are often observed (see Fig. 412-1).

COMPLICATIONS

Pneumomediastinum is rarely a major problem in older children because the mediastinum can be depressurized by escape of air into the neck or abdomen. In the newborn, however, the rate at which air can leave the mediastinum is limited, and pneumomediastinum can lead to dangerous cardiovascular compromise or pneumothorax (see Chapters 101.12 and 411).

TREATMENT

Treatment is directed primarily at the underlying obstructive pulmonary disease or other precipitating condition. Analgesics are occasionally needed for chest pain. Rarely, subcutaneous emphysema can cause sufficient tracheal compression to justify tracheotomy; the tracheotomy also decompresses the mediastinum. Collar mediastinotomy and percutaneous drainage catheter placement are other treatment modalities.

Bibliography is available at Expert Consult.

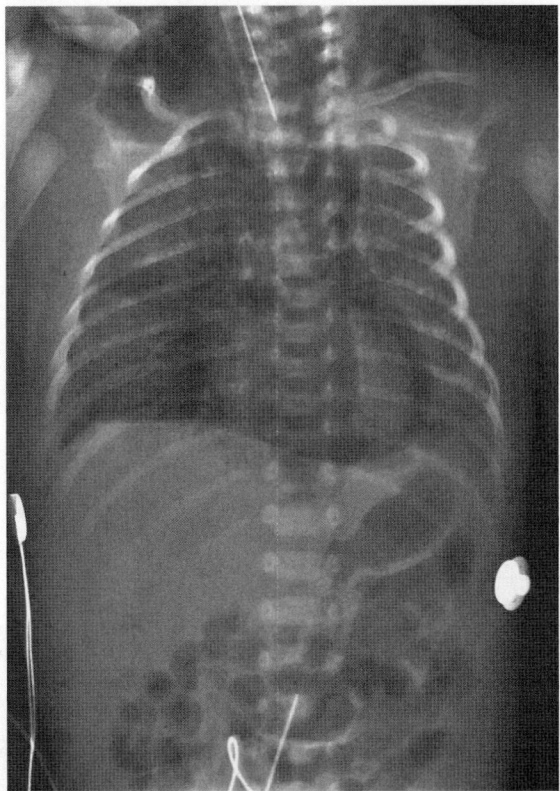

Figure 412-1 Large pneumomediastinum surrounding the heart and dissecting into the neck. *(From Clark DA: Atlas of neonatology, ed 7, Philadelphia, 2000, WB Saunders.)*

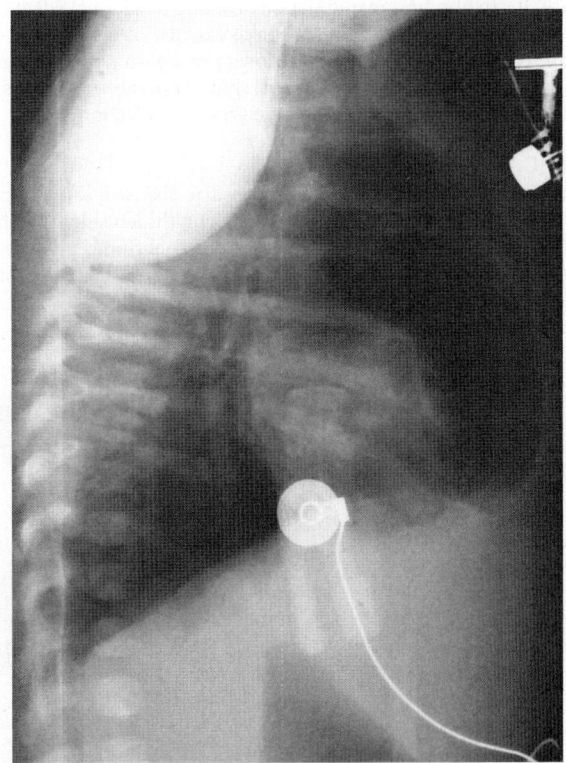

Figure 412-2 Lateral radiograph: upper mediastinal air. *(From Clark DA: Atlas of neonatology, ed 7, Philadelphia, 2000, WB Saunders, p. 94.)*

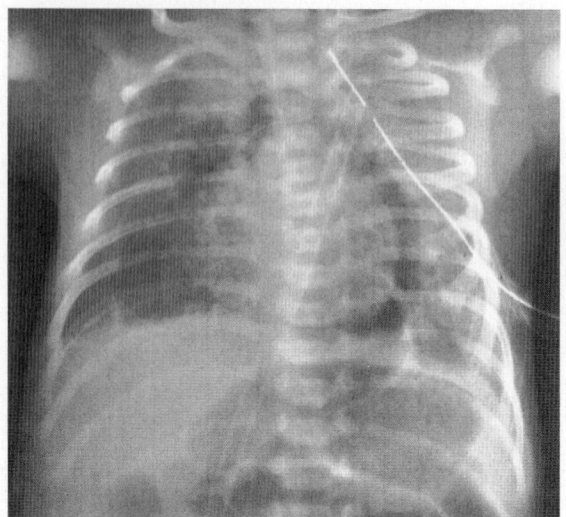

Figure 412-3 Sail sign—thymic elevation. *(From Clark DA: Atlas of neonatology, ed 7, Philadelphia, 2000, WB Saunders, p. 94.)*

Chapter **413**
Hydrothorax
Glenna B. Winnie

Hydrothorax is a transudative pleural effusion; typically, it is caused by abnormal pressure gradients in the lung.

ETIOLOGY
Hydrothorax is most often associated with cardiac, renal, or hepatic disease. It can also be a manifestation of severe nutritional edema and hypoalbuminemia. Rarely, it results from vascular obstruction by neoplasms, enlarged lymph nodes, pulmonary embolism, or adhesions. It may occur from a ventriculoperitoneal shunt or peritoneal dialysis and has been reported in congenital parvovirus B19 infection.

CLINICAL MANIFESTATIONS
Hydrothorax is usually bilateral, but in cardiac disease it can be limited to the right side or greater on the right than on the left side. The physical signs are the same as those described for serofibrinous pleurisy (see Chapter 410.2), but in hydrothorax, there is more rapid shifting of the level of dullness with changes of position. It is usually associated with an accumulation of fluid in other parts of the body.

LABORATORY FINDINGS
The fluid is noninflammatory, has few cells, and has a lower specific gravity (<1.015) than that of a serofibrinous exudate. The ratio of pleural fluid to serum total protein is <0.5, the ratio of pleural fluid to serum lactic dehydrogenase is <0.6, and the pleural fluid lactic dehydrogenase value is less than 66% of the upper limit of the normal serum lactic dehydrogenase range.

TREATMENT
Therapy is directed at the underlying disorder; aspiration may be necessary when pressure symptoms are notable.

Bibliography is available at Expert Consult.

Chapter **414**
Hemothorax
Glenna B. Winnie and Steven V. Lossef

Hemothorax, an accumulation of blood in the pleural cavity, is rare in children.

ETIOLOGY
Bleeding into the chest cavity most commonly occurs after chest trauma, either blunt or penetrating. It can be the result of iatrogenic trauma, including surgical procedures and venous line insertion. Hemothorax can also result from erosion of a blood vessel in association with inflammatory processes such as tuberculosis and empyema. It may complicate a variety of congenital anomalies including sequestration, patent ductus arteriosus, and pulmonary arteriovenous malformation (see Fig. 407-2 in Chapter 407). It is also an occasional manifestation of intrathoracic neoplasms, costal exostoses, blood dyscrasias, bleeding diatheses, or thrombolytic therapy. Rupture of an aneurysm is unlikely during childhood. Hemothorax may occur spontaneously in neonates and older children. A pleural hemorrhage associated with a pneumothorax is a *hemopneumothorax;* it is usually the result of a ruptured bulla with lung volume loss causing a torn pleural adhesion.

CLINICAL MANIFESTATIONS
In addition to the symptoms and signs of pleural effusion (see Chapter 410.2), hemothorax is associated with hemodynamic compromise related to the amount and rapidity of bleeding.

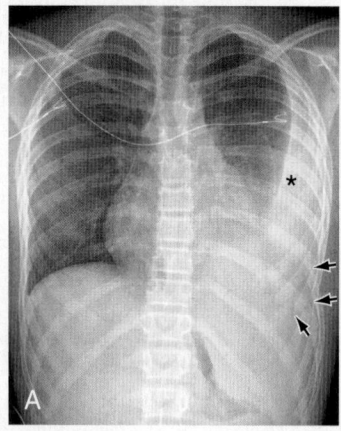
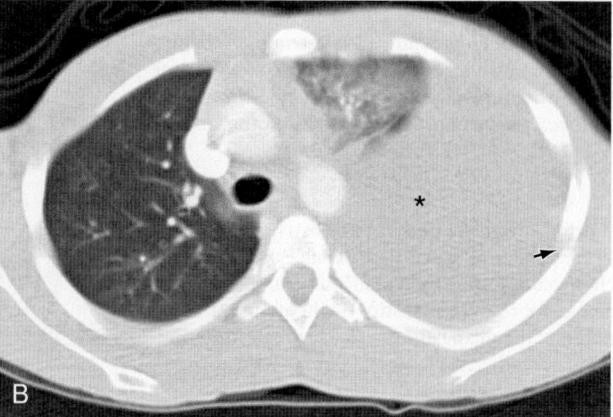

Figure 414-1 Hemothorax *(asterisk)* and associated rib fractures *(arrows)* in a teenager involved in a motor vehicle accident. **A,** Chest radiograph. **B,** CT scan.

DIAGNOSIS
The diagnosis of a hemothorax is initially suspected from radiographs or CT scans but can be made only with thoracentesis (Fig. 414-1). In every case, an effort must be made to determine and treat the cause.

TREATMENT
Initial therapy is tube thoracostomy. Surgical intervention may be required to control active bleeding, and transfusion may be indicated. Inadequate removal of blood in extensive hemothorax may lead to substantial restrictive disease secondary to organization of fibrin; fibrinolytic therapy or a decortication procedure may then be necessary. Embolization is the treatment of choice for an arteriovenous malformation.

Bibliography is available at Expert Consult.

Chapter **415**
Chylothorax
Glenna B. Winnie and Steven V. Lossef

Chylothorax is a pleural collection of fluid formed by the escape of chyle from the thoracic duct or lymphatics into the thoracic cavity.

ETIOLOGY
Chylothorax in children occurs most frequently because of thoracic duct injury as a complication of cardiothoracic surgery (Fig. 415-1). Other cases are associated with chest injury (Fig. 415-2), extracorporeal membrane oxygenation, or with primary or metastatic intrathoracic malignancy (Fig. 415-3), particularly lymphoma. In newborns, rapidly increased venous pressure during delivery may lead to thoracic duct rupture. Less common causes include lymphangiomatosis; restrictive pulmonary diseases; thrombosis of the duct, superior vena cava, or subclavian vein; tuberculosis or histoplasmosis; and congenital anomalies of the lymphatic system (Fig. 415-4). Refractory chylothorax in the fetus has been associated with a missense mutation in integrin aα9 gene. Chylothorax can occur in trauma and child abuse (see Chapter 40). It is important to establish the etiology, because treatment varies with the cause. In some patients, no specific cause is identified.

CLINICAL MANIFESTATIONS
The signs and symptoms of chylothorax are the same as those from pleural effusion of similar size. Chyle is not irritating, so pleuritic pain is uncommon. Onset is often gradual. However, after trauma to the thoracic duct chyle may accumulate in the posterior mediastinum for days and then rupture into the pleural space with sudden onset of dyspnea, hypotension, and hypoxemia. Approximately 50% of newborns with chylothorax present with respiratory distress in the 1st day of life. Chylothorax is rarely bilateral and usually occurs on the right side.

LABORATORY FINDINGS
Thoracentesis demonstrates a chylous effusion, a milky fluid containing fat, protein, lymphocytes, and other constituents of chyle; fluid may be yellow or bloody. In newborn infants or those who are not ingesting food, the fluid may be clear. A pseudochylous milky fluid may be

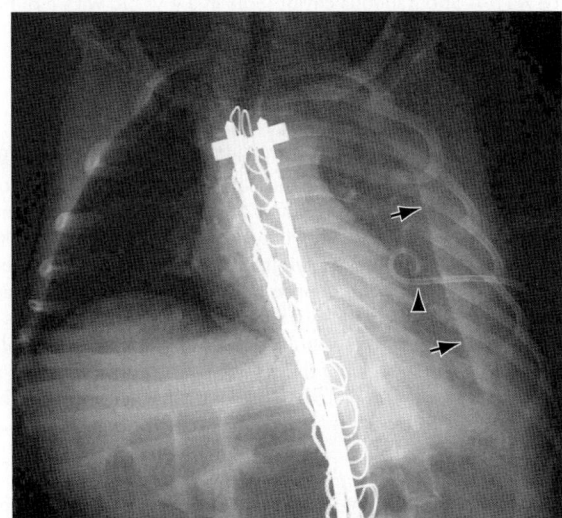
Figure 415-2 Left chylothorax *(arrows)* following spinal fusion with Harrington rods. It is postulated that the thoracic duct was injured during spine surgery. The pigtail chest tube *(arrowhead)* needed to be retracted to better drain the effusion.

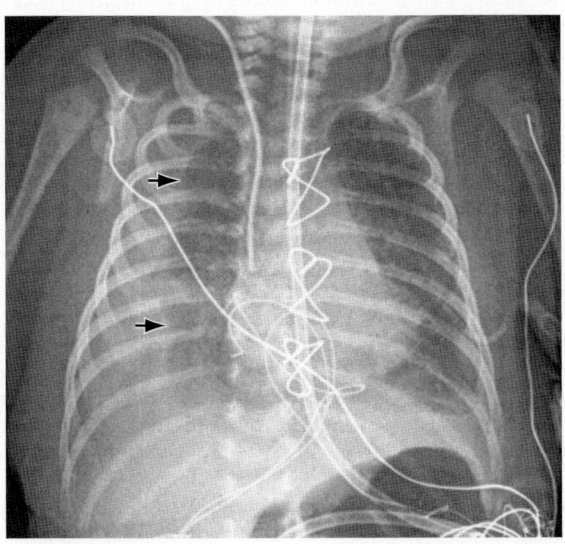
Figure 415-1 Chylothorax *(arrows)* following cardiac surgery in a 2 wk old infant.

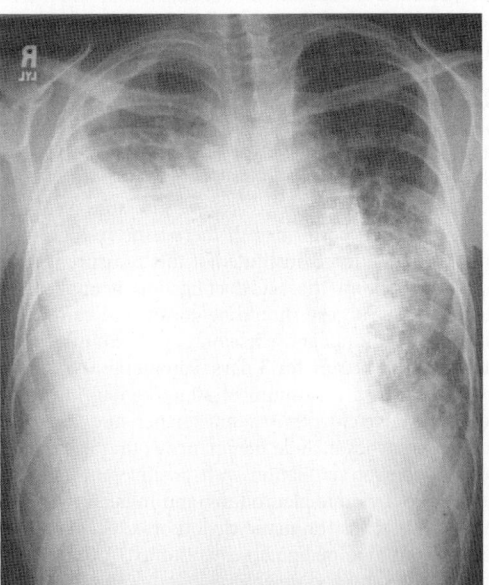
Figure 415-3 Large right chylous effusion opacifying much of the right thorax in a teenager with pulmonary lymphangiomatosis and hemangiomatosis. Note the associated interstitial lung disease.

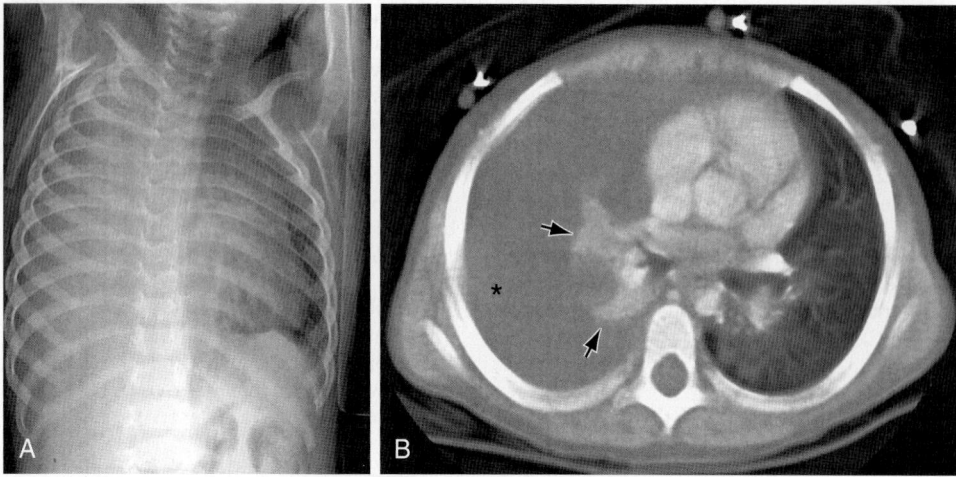

Figure 415-4 Spontaneous chylothorax in a 4 yr old with a duplication of chromosome 6. **A,** Chest radiograph shows opacification of the right thorax. **B,** CT scan shows the chylous pleural effusion *(asterisk)* compressing the atelectatic right lung *(arrows)*.

present in chronic serous effusion, in which fatty material arises from degenerative changes in the fluid and not from lymph. In chylothorax, the fluid triglyceride level is >110 mg/dL, the pleural fluid:serum triglyceride ratio is >1.0, and pleural fluid:serum cholesterol ratio is <1.0; lipoprotein analysis reveals chylomicrons. Fluid immunoglobulin levels are elevated. The cells are primarily T lymphocytes. Chest radiographs show an effusion; CT scans show normal pleural thickness and may reveal a lymphoma as the etiology of the chylothorax. A lymphangiogram can localize the site of the leak, and lymphoscintigraphy may demonstrate abnormalities of the lymphatic trunks and peripheral lymphatics.

COMPLICATIONS
Repeated aspirations may be required to relieve the symptoms of pressure. Chyle reaccumulates quickly, and repeated thoracentesis may cause malnutrition with significant loss of calories, protein, and electrolytes. Immunodeficiencies, including hypogammaglobulinemia and abnormal cell-mediated immune responses, have been associated with repeated and chronic thoracenteses for chylothorax. The loss of T lymphocytes is associated with increased risk of infection in neonates; otherwise, infection is uncommon, but patients should not receive live virus vaccines. Lack of resolution of chylothorax can lead to inanition, infection, and death.

TREATMENT
Spontaneous recovery occurs in >50% of cases of neonatal chylothorax. Initial therapy includes enteral feedings with a low-fat or medium-chain triglyceride, high-protein diet or parenteral nutrition. Thoracentesis is repeated as needed to relieve pressure symptoms; tube thoracostomy is often performed. If there is no resolution in 1-2 wk, total parenteral nutrition is instituted; if this measure is unsuccessful, a pleuroperitoneal shunt, thoracic duct ligation, or application of fibrin glue is considered. Surgery should be considered earlier in neonates with massive chylothorax and chyle output of >50 mL/kg/day despite maximum medical therapy for 3 days. Parenteral octreotide at a dose of 0.5-1 μg/kg/hr to a maximum of 10 μg/kg/day intravenously has been used to manage chylothorax, but further study is needed. Other therapeutic approaches include percutaneous thoracic duct embolization, pressure control ventilation with positive end-expiratory pressure, talc or iodopovidone pleurodesis, and inhalation of nitric oxide. Treatment is similar for traumatic chylothorax. Chemical pleurodesis or irradiation is used in malignant chylothorax. OK432 (picibanil) has been used to treat fetal and newborn chylothorax.

Bibliography is available at Expert Consult.

Chapter 416
Bronchopulmonary Dysplasia
Steven O. Lestrud

Bronchopulmonary dysplasia (BPD) is a pathologic process leading to signs and symptoms of chronic lung disease that originates in the neonatal period (see Chapter 101). The pathogenesis of lung disease in the population of neonates weighing <1,000 g includes the contribution of immature development of airway and vascular structures of the lung. The currently accepted definition includes an oxygen requirement for 28 days postnatally, and the disorder is graded as mild, moderate, or severe on the basis of supplemental oxygen requirement and gestational age (Table 416-1).

CLINICAL MANIFESTATIONS
Physical findings of the pulmonary exam vary with the severity of disease. Tachypnea is a common finding. Mouth breathing because of narrowed nasal passages and high arched palate is noted on upper airway exam. The chest demonstrates an increased anteroposterior diameter that suggests air trapping. Intercostal retractions are frequently present. Although breath sounds are frequently clear when the patient is well and abnormal only during an acute exacerbation, many patients have baseline wheeze or coarse crackles. A persistent fixed wheeze or stridor suggests subglottic stenosis (see Chapter 388) or large airway malacia. Fine crackles may be present in patients prone to fluid overload.

The most severely affected patients require prolonged mechanical ventilation to achieve acceptable gas exchange. Supplemental oxygen may be required to maintain acceptable oxygen saturation and often is needed to minimize the work of breathing. Infants with significant lung disease exhibit growth failure from the elevated energy expenditure essential to maintain the increased metabolic demands of respiration. Chronic respiratory insufficiency may be evident as elevation of serum bicarbonate, elevation of pressure of carbon dioxide on blood gas analysis, or polycythemia.

Patients must be monitored for the development of cor pulmonale, especially if they require supplemental oxygen and have chronic respiratory insufficiency.

Table 416-1	Forms of Bronchopulmonary Dysplasia		
FEATURES OF ALL BPD	**ADDITIONAL FEATURES OF MILD BPD**	**ADDITIONAL FEATURES OF MODERATE BPD**	**ADDITIONAL FEATURES OF SEVERE BPD**
<32 wk PMA Oxygen requirement 1st 28 days	Breathing room air at 36 wk PMA	<30% Supplemental oxygen at 36 wk PMA	>30% Supplemental oxygen at 36 wk PMA and mechanical support, CPAP, or ventilation
>32 wk PMA Oxygen requirement 1st 28 days of life	Breathing room air at 56 days of life	<30% Supplemental oxygen at 56 days of life	>30% Supplemental oxygen at 56 days of life and mechanical support, CPAP, or ventilation

BPD, bronchopulmonary dysplasia; CPAP, continuous positive airway pressure; PMA, postmenstrual age.

Gastroesophageal reflux disease (GERD) (see Chapter 323) and pulmonary aspiration complicate pulmonary status, particularly during an exacerbation when the infant is most tachypneic and when pulmonary mechanics increase the risk of GERD. Other conditions resulting from premature birth–complicating BPD include upper airway obstruction leading to hypoxia, neurodevelopmental delay with increased risk of aspiration, systemic hypertension with left ventricular hypertrophy, poor growth, and electrolyte disturbances.

In severely affected patients and patients with disease disproportionate to their risk for development of chronic lung disease, other pulmonary disease must be suspected, such as asthma (see Chapter 144), cystic fibrosis (see Chapter 403), and chronic aspiration pneumonitis (see Chapter 398). Recurrent episodes of respiratory distress are common, but anatomic airway abnormalities, such as subglottic stenosis (see Chapter 388) and airway malacia (see Chapter 386), must also be considered.

A **pulmonary exacerbation** of BPD is typically triggered during viral upper respiratory infections. Other frequent triggers include viral lower respiratory infections, sinusitis, otitis media, weather changes, exposure to cigarette smoke, and exacerbations of gastroesophageal reflux. During an exacerbation, the infant exhibits increased work of breathing, with tachypnea and retractions becoming more prominent. Chest wall configuration may change, with an increased anteroposterior diameter. If wheezing is a prominent baseline finding, poor air entry during an exacerbation may result in less wheezing, signifying a significant deterioration of respiratory status.

TREATMENT

Treatment is directed toward decreasing the work of breathing and normalizing gas exchange, to allow for optimal growth and neurodevelopment. Infants requiring supplemental oxygen past 35 wk postmenstrual age have a higher incidence of lower airway obstruction and bronchodilator responsiveness and are more likely to be hospitalized during the toddler years than their peers. The etiology of wheezing in BPD may be lower airway inflammation, bronchial smooth muscle irritation, bronchial smooth muscle hypertrophy, and airway malacia. The administration of an inhaled bronchodilator is frequently undertaken to evaluate an individual's response. Most commonly, inhaled β-agonists initially increase air movement and improve comfort of breathing, resulting in short-term improvement in pulmonary function values. For patients whose symptoms respond, the medication should be continued, especially during high-risk periods when triggers are present, such as an upper respiratory infection or hot humid days.

β-Agonists may worsen the air exchange, particularly in infants with BPD and concomitant airway malacia. Bronchial smooth muscle may maintain airway caliber in the affected airway; smooth muscle relaxation after administration of a β-agonist results in increased small airway collapse. Patients in whom β-agonists have these effects may benefit from alternative bronchodilators, such as inhaled ipratropium and oral methylxanthines. The administration of preventive anti-inflammatory medications, such as inhaled glucocorticoids and leukotriene-modifying agents, may be considered in patients with frequent inflammatory triggers.

Targeted goals for supplemental oxygen therapy after discharge from the nursery are to improve oxygen saturation values and decrease likelihood of desaturation, reduce the risk of cor pulmonale, diminish the work of breathing, and improve growth. This therapy likely improves neurodevelopmental outcome and may decrease exacerbations caused by hypoxia. Oxygen saturation values should exceed 90%, but the optimal goal above this level is unknown. The addition of diuretic therapy with furosemide or thiazides may improve pulmonary mechanics by decreasing lung water and allow tapering of supplemental oxygen. Therapy beyond several weeks, however, is not known to improve outcome and places the child at risk for electrolyte disorders.

Adequate caloric intake can be difficult for many reasons, including oral aversion, discoordinated suck and swallow, GERD, aspiration, and aspiration with GERD. In addition, tachypnea, episodic respiratory distress, increased work of breathing, and requirement for supplement oxygen place the infant at risk for growth failure. A high caloric intake is necessary, with ranges of 120-160 kcal/kg/day required, frequently in combination with fluid restriction. To provide such high caloric intake in the compromised infant, supplemental feedings through a nasogastric or gastrostomy tube may be considered. Careful attention is necessary to maintain fluid balance.

Gastroesophageal reflux is common and must be suspected in patients not showing response to therapy and in patients with frequent exacerbations, especially exacerbations without clear triggers. Definitive diagnosis is necessary because these patients will be subject to prolonged promotility and antacid medications. Appropriate antireflux therapy in infants with GERD decreases respiratory complications. Gastroesophageal reflux with pulmonary aspiration or aspiration alone may manifest as chronic chest congestion, wheezing, and episodic hypoxic spells. Fundoplication with a gastrostomy tube is performed in patients showing no response to medical therapy. Evaluation and treatment by a speech therapist, pediatric pulmonologist, or otolaryngologist may decrease the risk for development of chronic lung disease associated with aspiration.

Prevention of respiratory viral illness is vitally important; frequent handwashing by caregivers, especially before they handle the baby and avoidance of contact with children and adults with current respiratory symptoms are essential. Respiratory syncytial virus (see Chapter 260) immunoprophylaxis should be considered on the basis of the severity of lung disease, as well as the patient's gestational age and current age.

The prognosis for infants with BPD is generally good. Through school age, the family can expect frequent medical interactions for episodes of respiratory distress, commonly triggered by simple upper respiratory tract infections and weather changes. Pulmonary function in severely affected patients remains decreased, and exercise limitation may be present because of dyspnea. The most severely affected patients benefit from care administered by a multidisciplinary team of caregivers, including the pediatrician, pulmonologist, speech therapist, nutritionist, and developmental specialists.

Bibliography is available at Expert Consult.

Chapter **417**
Skeletal Diseases Influencing Pulmonary Function

Steven R. Boas

Pulmonary function is influenced by the structure of the chest wall (see Chapter 373). Chest wall abnormalities can lead to restrictive or obstructive pulmonary disease, impaired respiratory muscle strength, and decreased ventilatory performance in response to physical stress. The congenital chest wall deformities include *pectus excavatum, pectus carinatum, sternal clefts, Poland syndrome,* and skeletal and *cartilage dysplasias.* Vertebral anomalies such as kyphoscoliosis can alter pulmonary function in children and adolescents.

417.1 Pectus Excavatum (Funnel Chest)
Steven R. Boas

ETIOLOGY
Pectus excavatum, midline narrowing of the thoracic cavity is usually an isolated skeletal abnormality. The cause is unknown. Pectus excavatum can occur in isolation or it may be associated with a connective tissue disorder (Marfan [see Chapter 702] or Ehlers-Danlos syndrome [see Chapter 659]). It may be acquired secondarily to chronic lung disease, neuromuscular disease, or trauma.

EPIDEMIOLOGY
Pectus excavatum occurs in 1 in 400 births with a 9:1 male preponderance and accounts for >90% of congenital chest wall anomalies. There is a positive family history in one-third of cases.

CLINICAL MANIFESTATIONS
The deformity is present at or shortly after birth in one-third of cases but is usually not associated with any symptoms at that time. In time, fatigue, chest pain, palpitations, recurrent respiratory infections, wheezing, stridor, and cough may be present. Decreased exercise tolerance is one of the most common symptoms. Because of the cosmetic nature of this deformity, children may experience significant psychologic stress. Physical examination may reveal sternal depression, protracted shoulders, kyphoscoliosis, dorsal lordosis, inferior rib flares, rib cage rigidity, forward head tilt, scapular winging, and loss of vertebral contours (Fig. 417-1). Patients exhibit paroxysmal sternal motion and a shift of point of maximal impulse to the left. Innocent systolic murmurs may be heard.

LABORATORY FINDINGS
Lateral chest radiograms demonstrate the sternal depression. Use of the Haller index on chest CT (maximal internal transverse diameter of the chest divided by the minimal anteroposterior diameter at the same level) in comparison with age- and gender-appropriate normative values for determining the extent of depression of the chest wall anomaly has become useful in determining the extent of the anatomic abnormality. An electrocardiogram may show a right-axis deviation or Wolff-Parkinson-White syndrome (see Chapter 436); an echocardiogram may demonstrate mitral valve prolapse (see Chapter 428.3) and ventricular compression. Results of static pulmonary function tests may be normal but commonly show an obstructive defect in the lower airways and, less commonly, a restrictive defect as the result of

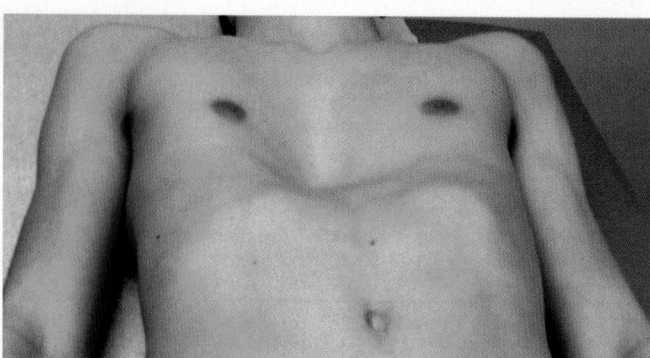

Figure 417-1 Pectus excavatum in a 15 year old male. Note the presence of protracted shoulders, inferior rib flares, and sternal depression.

abnormal chest wall mechanics. Exercise testing may demonstrate either normal tolerance or limitations from underlying cardiopulmonary dysfunction that are associated with the severity of the defect. Ventilatory limitations are commonly seen in younger children and adolescents, whereas cardiac limitations secondary to stroke volume impairments are more commonly seen in older adolescents and young adults.

TREATMENT
Treatment is based on the severity of the deformity and the extent of physiologic compromise as defined by physical examination and physiologic assessment of cardiopulmonary function (lung function and exercise tolerance assessment). Therapeutic options include careful observation, use of physical therapy to address musculoskeletal compromise, and corrective surgery. For patients with significant physiologic compromise, surgical correction may improve the cosmetic deformity and may help minimize or even improve the cardiopulmonary compromise. The 2 main surgical interventions are the Ravitch and Nuss procedures. Although superiority of 1 approach has not been established, there is now more than 20 yr of successful experience with the minimally invasive Nuss procedure. For teenagers with exercise limitations, surgical repair may result in improved exercise tolerance. Normalization of lung perfusion scans and maximal voluntary ventilation have also been observed after surgery. Utilization of a magnetic brace with gradual remodeling of the pectus deformity is under clinical investigation. Ongoing treatment to address the secondary musculoskeletal findings is commonly employed before and after the operation.

Bibliography is available at Expert Consult.

417.2 Pectus Carinatum and Sternal Clefts
Steven R. Boas

PECTUS CARINATUM
Etiology and Epidemiology
Pectus carinatum is a sternal deformity accounting for 5-15% of congenital chest wall anomalies. Anterior displacements of the mid and lower sternum and adjacent costal cartilages are the most common types. They are most commonly associated with protrusion of the upper sternum; depression of the lower sternum occurs in only 15% of patients. Asymmetry of the sternum is common, and localized depression of the lower anterolateral chest is also often observed. Males are affected 4 times more often than females. There is a high familial occurrence and a common association of mild to moderate scoliosis. Mitral valve disease and coarctation of the aorta are associated with this anomaly. Three types of anatomic deformity occur (upper, lower, and lateral pectus carinatum), with corresponding physiologic changes and treatment algorithms.

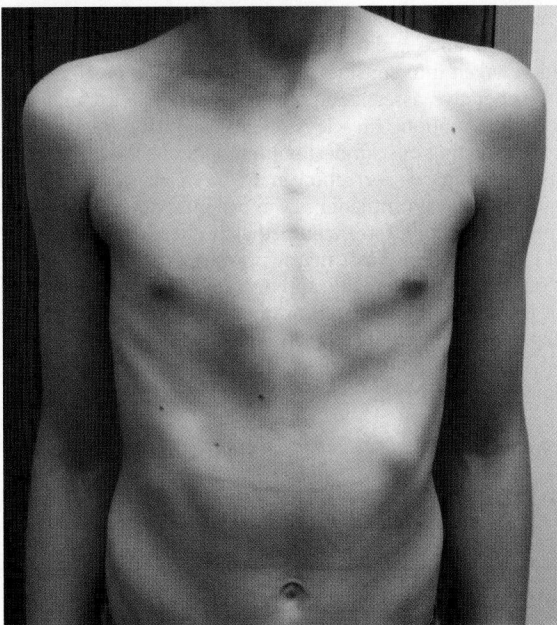

Figure 417-2 Pectus carinatum in a 13 year old male. Note the central sternal prominence.

Clinical Manifestations

In early childhood, symptoms appear minimal. School-age children and adolescents commonly complain of dyspnea with mild exertion, decreased endurance with exercise, and exercise-induced wheezing. The incidence of increased respiratory infections and use of asthma medication is higher than in nonaffected individuals. On physical examination, a marked increase in the anteroposterior chest diameter is seen, with resultant reduction in chest excursion and expansion (Fig. 417-2). Spirometry has demonstrated both restrictive and obstructive patterns, although the majority of individuals have normal values. Increases in residual volume are often present and results in tachypnea and diaphragmatic respirations. Exercise testing shows variable results. Chest radiographs show an increased anteroposterior diameter of the chest wall, emphysematous-appearing lungs, and a narrow cardiac shadow. The pectus severity score (width of chest divided by distance between sternum and spine; analogous to the Haller index) is reduced.

Treatment

For symptomatic patients with pectus carinatum, minimally invasive surgical correction procedures may result in improvement of the clinical symptoms. Many surgeons prefer to utilize bracing techniques as a first-line treatment although prospective outcome data is limited. Although surgery is performed for some individuals who are symptomatic, it is often performed for cosmetic and psychologic reasons.

STERNAL CLEFTS

Sternal clefts are rare congenital malformations that result from the failure of the fusion of the sternum during the 8th wk of gestation. No familial predisposition has been described. Sternal clefts occur in less than 1% of all chest wall deformities. Sternal clefts are classified as partial or complete. Partial sternal clefts are more common and may involve the superior sternum in association with other lesions, such as vascular dysplasias and supraumbilical raphe, or the inferior sternal clefts, which are often associated with other midline defects (pentalogy of Cantrell). Complete sternal clefts with complete failure of sternal fusion are rare. These disorders may also occur in isolation. The paradoxic movement of thoracic organs with respiration may alter pulmonary mechanics. Rarely, respiratory infections and even significant compromise result. Surgery is required early in life, before fixation and immobility occur.

Bibliography is available at Expert Consult.

417.3 Asphyxiating Thoracic Dystrophy (Thoracic-Pelvic-Phalangeal Dystrophy)

Steven R. Boas

ETIOLOGY

A multisystem autosomal recessive disorder, asphyxiating thoracic dystrophy results in a constricted and narrow rib cage. Also known as *Jeune syndrome*, the disorder is associated with a characteristic skeletal abnormalities as well as variable involvement of other systems, including renal, hepatic, neurologic, pancreatic, and retinal abnormalities (see Chapter 700).

CLINICAL MANIFESTATIONS

Most patients with this disorder die shortly after birth from respiratory failure, although less-aggressive forms have been reported in older children. For those who survive the neonatal period, progressive respiratory failure often ensues, owing to impaired lung growth, recurrent pneumonia, and atelectasis originating from the rigid chest wall.

DIAGNOSIS

Physical examination reveals a narrowed thorax that, at birth, is much smaller than the head circumference. The ribs are horizontal, and the child has short extremities. Chest radiographs demonstrate a bell-shaped chest cage with short, horizontal, flaring ribs and high clavicles.

TREATMENT

No specific treatment exists, although thoracoplasty to enlarge the chest wall and long-term mechanical ventilation has been tried. Rib-expanding procedures have resulted in improved survival.

PROGNOSIS

For some children with asphyxiating thoracic dystrophy, improvement in the bony abnormalities occurs with age. However, children younger than age 1 yr often succumb to respiratory infection and failure. Progressive renal disease often occurs with older children. Use of vaccines for influenza and other respiratory pathogens is warranted, as is aggressive use of antibiotics for respiratory infections.

Bibliography is available at Expert Consult.

417.4 Achondroplasia

Steven R. Boas

ETIOLOGY

Achondroplasia is the most common condition characterized by disproportionate short stature (see Chapter 696). This condition is inherited as an autosomal dominant disorder that results in disordered growth. Much has been learned about this disorder, including its genetic origins (95% of cases caused by mutations in the gene coding for fibroblast growth factor receptor type 3) and how to minimize its serious complications.

CLINICAL MANIFESTATIONS

Restrictive pulmonary disease, affecting <5% of children with achondroplasia who are younger than 3 yr, is more likely at high elevation. Recurrent infections, cor pulmonale, and dyspnea are commonly associated. There is an increased risk of obstructive sleep apnea or hypopneas. Hypoxemia during sleep is a common feature. Onset of restrictive lung disease can begin at a very young age. On examination, the breathing pattern is rapid and shallow, with associated abdominal breathing. The anteroposterior diameter of the thorax is reduced. Special growth curves for chest circumference of patients with achondroplasia from birth to 7 yr are available. Three distinct phenotypes exist: phenotypic group 1 patients possess relative adenotonsillar hypertrophy, group 2 patients have muscular upper airway obstruction and progressive hydrocephalus, and group 3 patients have upper airway obstruction without hydrocephalus. Kyphoscoliosis may develop during infancy.

DIAGNOSIS

Pulmonary function tests reveal a reduced vital capacity that is more pronounced in males. The lungs are small but functionally normal. Sleep studies are recommended due to the high prevalence of sleep-disordered breathing. Chest radiographs demonstrate the decreased anteroposterior diameter along with anterior cupping of the ribs. The degree of foramen magnum involvement correlates with the extent of respiratory dysfunction.

TREATMENT

Treatment of sleep apnea, if present, is supportive (see Chapter 19). Physiotherapy and bracing may minimize the complications of both kyphosis and severe lordosis. Aggressive treatment of respiratory infections and scoliosis is warranted.

PROGNOSIS

The life span is normal for most children with this condition, except for the phenotypic groups with hydrocephalus or with severe cervical or lumbar spinal compression.

Bibliography is available at Expert Consult.

417.5 Kyphoscoliosis: Adolescent Idiopathic Scoliosis and Congenital Scoliosis
Steven R. Boas

ETIOLOGY

Adolescent idiopathic scoliosis (AIS) is characterized by lateral bending of the spine (see Chapter 679). It commonly affects children during their teen years, as well as during periods of rapid growth. The cause is unknown. Congenital scoliosis is uncommon, affecting girls more than boys, and is apparent in the 1st yr of life (see Chapter 679.2).

CLINICAL MANIFESTATIONS

The pulmonary manifestations of scoliosis may include chest wall restriction, leading to a reduction in total lung capacity, abnormal gas exchange, and airway obstruction. The angle of scoliosis deformity has been correlated with the degree of lung impairment only for patients with thoracic curves. Vital capacity, forced expiratory volume in 1 sec (FEV_1), work capacity, oxygen consumption, diffusion capacity, chest wall compliance, and partial pressure of arterial oxygen decrease as the severity of thoracic curve increases. These findings can be seen in even mild to moderate AIS (Cobb angle <30 degrees) but generally do not occur in other, nonthoracic curves. Respiratory compromise is often more severe in children younger than 5 yr of age with large scoliotic curves. Reduction in peripheral muscle function is associated with AIS through either intrinsic mechanisms or deconditioning. Severe impairment can lead to cor pulmonale or respiratory failure and can occur before age 20 yr. Children with severe scoliosis, especially boys, may have abnormalities of breathing during sleep, and the resultant periods of hypoxemia may contribute to the eventual development of pulmonary hypertension.

DIAGNOSIS

Physical examination and an upright, posteroanterior radiograph with subsequent measurement of the angle of curvature (Cobb technique) remain the gold standard for assessment of scoliosis. Curves >10 degrees define the presence of scoliosis. Lung volume, respiratory muscle strength, and exercise capacity determination are essential in assessing the degree of respiratory compromise associated with scoliosis.

TREATMENT

Depending on the extent of the curve and the degree of skeletal maturation, treatment options include reassurance, observation, bracing, and surgery (spinal fusion). Influenza vaccine should be administered, given the extent of pulmonary compromise that may coexist. Because vital capacity is a strong predictor for the development of respiratory failure in untreated AIS, surgical goals are to diminish the scoliotic curve, maintain the correction, and prevent deterioration in pulmonary function. Abnormalities of vital capacity and total lung capacity, exercise intolerance, and the rate of change of these variables over time should be taken into consideration for the timing of surgical correction. Preoperative assessment of lung function (i.e., lung volumes, oxygen consumption, muscle strength, ventilation/perfusion) may assist in predicting postsurgical pulmonary difficulties. Many patients undergoing surgical correction may be managed postoperatively without mechanical ventilation. Even patients with mild scoliosis may have pulmonary compromise immediately after spinal fusion, secondary to pain and a body cast that may restrict breathing and interfere with coughing. Children with a preoperative FEV_1 <40% predicted are at risk for requiring prolonged postoperative mechanical ventilation. Rib-expanding procedures have been successful in severe cases of congenital scoliosis. Choice of surgical approach may also impact lung function postoperatively.

Bibliography is available at Expert Consult.

417.6 Congenital Rib Anomalies
Steven R. Boas

CLINICAL MANIFESTATIONS

Isolated defects of the highest and lowest ribs have minimal clinical pulmonary consequences. Missing midthoracic ribs are associated with the absence of the pectoralis muscle (Poland syndrome), and lung function can become compromised. Associated kyphoscoliosis and hemivertebrae may accompany this defect. If the rib defect is small, no significant sequelae ensue. When the 2nd to 5th ribs are absent anteriorly, lung herniation and significant abnormal respiration ensue. The lung is soft and nontender and may be easily reducible on examination. Complicating sequelae include severe lung restriction (secondary to scoliosis), cor pulmonale, and congestive heart failure. Symptoms are often minimal but can cause dyspnea. Respiratory distress is rare in infancy.

DIAGNOSIS

Chest radiographs demonstrate the deformation and absence of ribs with secondary scoliosis. Most rib abnormalities are discovered as incidental findings on a chest film.

TREATMENT

If symptoms are severe enough to cause clinical compromise or significant lung herniation, then homologous rib grafting can be performed. Rib-expanding procedures are also of great value. A modified Nuss procedure has been utilized to correct associated chest wall anomalies with rib abnormalities. Adolescent girls with congenital rib anomalies may require cosmetic breast surgery.

Bibliography is available at Expert Consult.

Chapter 418
Chronic Severe Respiratory Insufficiency
Zehava L. Noah and Cynthia Etzler Budek

The population of pediatric patients receiving long-term mechanical ventilatory support has increased in the United States and many other nations because of improvements in the treatment of acute respiratory failure and advancements in invasive (e.g., tracheostomy with mechanical ventilator) and noninvasive (e.g., mask continuous positive airway pressure [CPAP] or bilevel positive airway pressure [BiPAP]) ventilation. Despite the growing population, less than 1% of patients admitted to pediatric intensive care units require long-term mechanical ventilation. Infants, children, and adolescents with disorders of central control of breathing, disease of the airways, residual lung disease after severe respiratory illness, persistent pulmonary hypertension, and neuromuscular disorders may experience hypercarbic and/or hypoxemic chronic respiratory failure. Generally, the respiratory failure can be attributed to a primary cause, although many children have multiple causative factors. **Chronic respiratory failure** can be defined as pulmonary insufficiency for a protracted period, usually 28 days or longer.

Patients are maintained on long-term ventilation for varying periods of time depending on the underlying pathology. Patients with reversible neuropathies (Guillain-Barré syndrome, neuropathy of critical illness), bronchopulmonary dysplasia, pulmonary hypertension, airway abnormalities, and congenital heart disease before or after surgical intervention require long-term ventilation as a bridge for full recovery. Patients with conditions such as central hypoventilation, progressive neuromuscular disease, and high quadriplegia may need ventilatory support indefinitely. The goals of long-term mechanical ventilation are to sustain and extend life, enhance the quality of life, reduce morbidity, improve physical and psychologic function, and enhance growth and development. These goals are often optimized in the home setting, which is the preferred site of discharge for children who are ventilator dependent. When social circumstances do not allow for a safe discharge to home, patients may be transferred to a highly skilled nursing facility for long-term care.

In an observational cohort analysis of 228 children enrolled in a home ventilation program 52% had chronic pulmonary disease, many with multiple comorbidities. Eventually 30% of children with chronic pulmonary disease were successfully weaned off ventilation and 19% died. Twenty-seven percent of the total population had neuromuscular disease, of which 6% were weaned off ventilation and 21% died. Twenty percent of the total population had central hypoventilation, of which 4% were weaned from ventilation and 24% died. Causes of death included progression of underlying chronic respiratory failure (34%), cardiac failure (21%), acute respiratory failure, tracheal bleeding and tracheal obstruction (8.5% each), and tracheostomy accident (2%). Regression analysis suggested that children with chronic pulmonary disease were more likely to successfully wean off mechanical ventilation than those children in the other two groups.

418.1 Neuromuscular Diseases

Zehava L. Noah and Cynthia Etzler Budek

Neuromuscular diseases (NMDs) of childhood include muscular dystrophies, metabolic and congenital myopathies, anterior horn cell disorders, peripheral neuropathies, and diseases that affect the neuromuscular junction. Decreased muscle strength and endurance resulting from neuromuscular disorders can affect any skeletal muscle, including muscles involved in respiratory function. Of particular concern are those muscles mediating upper airway patency, generation of cough, and lung inflation. Acute respiratory insufficiency is typically the most prominent clinical manifestation of several acute neuromuscular disorders, including high-level spinal cord injury, poliomyelitis, Guillain-Barré syndrome (see Chapter 616), and botulism (see Chapter 210). Respiratory dysfunction constitutes the leading cause of morbidity and mortality in progressive neuromuscular disorders (e.g., Duchenne muscular dystrophy [see Chapter 609], spinal muscular atrophy, congenital myotonic dystrophy, myasthenia gravis [see Chapter 612], and Charcot-Marie-Tooth disease [see Chapter 613]).

PATHOGENESIS

Early onset of NMD can lead to chest wall deformity and lung disease as a consequence of developmental factors. In infancy, the chest wall is very compliant with relatively stiff lungs and small airways. With

progressive weakness of the intercostal muscles, the chest wall becomes even more compliant. Small airways have a tendency to become obstructed, leading to microatelectasis and decreased functional residual capacity. The compliant chest wall with initial sparing of diaphragm function leads to development of a small bell-shaped chest with depressed sternum, protruding abdomen, and paradoxical breathing, typically seen in spinal muscular atrophy (SMA) type 1. As the disease progresses, severe hypotonia develops, chest wall muscles shorten and lose elasticity, costosternal and costovertebral joints contract, and lung volumes decrease. Inspiratory and expiratory pressures subsequently decrease, expiratory pressures more so than inspiratory, causing ineffective cough and poor airway clearance. As the child with NMD ages, kyphoscoliosis commonly develops, increasing the severity of restrictive lung disease. Although central control of breathing remains normal, response to central chemoreceptors may decrease because of chronic hypercapnia.

TREATMENT

Even though gene-targeted therapies are being developed for some NMDs, current interventions are primarily supportive rather than curative. Close surveillance through periodic review of the history and physical examination is critical. The development of personality and behavioral changes, such as irritability, decreased attention span, fatigue, and somnolence, may point to the presence of sleep-associated gas exchange abnormalities and sleep fragmentation. Changes in speech and voice characteristics, nasal flaring, and the use of accessory muscles at rest may indicate progressive muscle dysfunction and respiratory compromise. Although the frequency of periodic reevaluation needs to be tailored to the individual child, guidelines were developed for the Duchenne muscular dystrophy population; an abbreviated summary of such recommendations, applicable to all children with NMDs, is provided in Table 418-1.

Guidelines for evaluation and management of patients with SMA were developed on the basis of expert consensus. Four classifications of SMA, based on age of onset and level of function, are recognized (Table 418-2). Treatment of SMA is focused on level of function (nonsitter, sitter, or walker) rather than SMA type. Unlike patients with Duchenne muscular dystrophy, patients with SMA do not demonstrate correlation between pulmonary function and need for mechanical

Table 418-1	Proposed Guidelines for Initial Evaluation and Follow-Up of Patients with Neuromuscular Disease
INITIAL EVALUATION	**BASIC INTERVENTION/ TRAINING**
History/physical/anthropometrics	Nutritional consultation and guidance
Lung function and maximal respiratory pressures (PFTs)	Regular chest physiotherapy
Arterial blood gases	Use of percussive devices
Polysomnography*	Respiratory muscle training
Exercise testing (in selected cases)	Annual influenza vaccine
If vital capacity >60% predicted or maximal respiratory pressures >60 cm H_2O	Evaluate PFTs every 6 mo CXR and polysomnography every year
If vital capacity <60% predicted or maximal respiratory pressures <60 cm H_2O	Evaluate PFTs every 3-4 mo CXR, MIP/MEP every 6 mo Polysomnography every 6 mo to year

*Please note that if polysomnography is not readily available, multichannel recordings including oronasal airflow, nocturnal oximetry, and end-tidal carbon dioxide levels may provide an adequate alternative.

CXR, chest x-ray; MEP, maximal expiratory pressure; MIP, maximal inspiratory pressure; PFT, pulmonary function test.

Table 418-2	Clinical Classification of Spinal Muscular Atrophy		
SMA TYPE	**AGE OF ONSET**	**HIGHEST FUNCTION**	**NATURAL AGE OF DEATH**
Type 1 (severe)	0-6 mo	Never sits	<2 yr
Type 2 (intermediate)	7-18 mo	Never stands	<2 yr
Type 3 (mild)	Older than 18 mo	Stands and walks	Adult
Type 4 (adult)	Second or third decade	Walks during adult years	Adult

From Wang CH, Finkel RS, Bertini ES, et al: Consensus statement for standard of care in spinal muscular atrophy, J Child Neurol 22:1027–1049, 2007.

ventilatory support. Longitudinal monitoring for signs and symptoms of sleep-disordered breathing and ineffective airway clearance should be utilized to direct patient care.

Bibliography is available at Expert Consult.

418.2 Congenital Central Hypoventilation Syndrome

Zehava L. Noah, Cynthia Etzler Budek, and Debra E. Weese-Mayer

Congenital central hypoventilation syndrome (CCHS) is a clinically complex disorder of respiratory and autonomic regulation. In the classic case of CCHS, symptoms of alveolar hypoventilation are manifest in the newborn period and during sleep only—with diminished tidal volume and a typically monotonous respiratory rate with cyanosis and hypercarbia. In more severe cases of CCHS, the hypoventilation is manifest during wakefulness and sleep. And in the cases of later-onset CCHS (LO-CCHS), symptoms are manifest after 1 mo of age (and often into childhood and adulthood) but hypoventilation is typically during sleep only. CCHS and LO-CCHS are further characterized by ventilatory failure to properly respond to hypercarbia and hypoxemia during wakefulness and sleep coupled with physiologic and/or anatomic autonomic nervous system (ANS) dysregulation (ANSD). Physiologic ANSD may include all organ systems affected by the ANS, specifically the respiratory, cardiac (sinus node pauses, asystole), sudomotor, vasomotor, ophthalmologic, neurologic, and enteric systems. The anatomic or structural ANSD includes Hirschsprung disease and tumors of neural crest origin (neuroblastoma, ganglioneuroma, or ganglioneuroblastoma). Diagnosis and management of individuals with CCHS and LO-CCHS have improved considerably, owing to greater knowledge in genetic testing, comprehensive care, and availability of monitoring technology for the home.

GENETICS

Mutations in the paired-like homeobox 2B (*PHOX2B*) gene are the cause of CCHS. *PHOX2B* is essential to the embryologic development of the ANS from the neural crest, and is expressed in key regions that explain much of the CCHS phenotype. Individuals with CCHS are heterozygous for either a polyalanine repeat expansion mutation (PARM) in exon 3 of the *PHOX2B* gene (normal number of alanines is 20 with normal genotype 20/20), such that individuals with CCHS have 24-33 alanines on the affected allele (genotype range is 20/24-20/33), or a non–PARM (NPARM) resulting from a missense, nonsense, frameshift, or stop codon mutation. Roughly 90-92% of the cases of CCHS have PARMs and the remaining 8-10% of cases have NPARMs. LO-CCHS cases have consistently had the 20/24 or 20/25 genotypes, or, occasionally, a very small NPARM. The specific type of *PHOX2B* mutation is clinically significant as it can help with anticipatory guidance in patient management. Less than 1% of CCHS cases will have a deletion of most of exon 3 or the entire *PHOX2B* gene, although the specific phenotype related to these large deletion mutations is not entirely clear. Stepwise clinical *PHOX2B* testing for probands with the CCHS phenotype is advised (step 1: fragment analysis (screening test); then if negative, step 2: sequel sequencing; then if

negative, step 3: muliplex ligation-dependent probe amplification) to minimize expense and expedite confirmation of the diagnosis.

The majority of CCHS cases occur because of a de novo *PHOX2B* mutation, but up to 25% of children with CCHS inherit the mutation in an autosomal dominant manner from a seemingly asymptomatic parent who is mosaic for the *PHOX2B* mutation. Therefore, an individual with CCHS has a 50% chance of transmitting the mutation and resulting disease phenotype, to each offspring. Mosaic parents have up to a 50% chance of transmitting the *PHOX2B* mutation to each successive offspring. Genetic counseling is essential for family planning and for delivery room preparedness in anticipation of a CCHS birth. *PHOX2B* testing is advised for both parents of a child with CCHS to anticipate risk of recurrence in subsequent pregnancies and to determine if a parent has yet undiagnosed LO-CCHS. However, only fragment analysis *PHOX2B* testing (also known as the screening test) will identify low level somatic mosaicism (it will be missed by sequencing testing). At present, no clinical testing is available to determine germline mosaicism, but prenatal testing for *PHOX2B* mutation is clinically available (http://www.genetests.org) for families with a known *PHOX2B* mutation.

Ventilator Dependence

A correlation between the *PHOX2B* genotype and ventilator dependence is reported. The greater the number of extra alanines, the more likely the need for continuous ventilatory support, at least among the most common *PHOX2B* PARM genotypes (20/25, 20/26, 20/27). Thus patients with the 20/25 genotype seldom require awake ventilatory support, although they do require support during sleep. Patients with the 20/26 genotype have variable awake support needs, and patients with the 20/27 genotype and those with NPARMs are likely to need continuous ventilatory support.

Hirschsprung Disease

See Chapter 332.3.

Overall, 20% of children with CCHS also have Hirschsprung disease, and any infant or child with CCHS or LO-CCHS who presents with constipation should undergo rectal biopsy to screen for absence of ganglion cells. The type of *PHOX2B* mutation can help the primary physician anticipate which individuals are at higher risk. The frequency of Hirschsprung disease seems to increase with the longer polyalanine tracts (genotypes 20/27-20/33) and in those with NPARMs. Thus far only 1 infant with the 20/25 genotype has been reported to have Hirschsprung disease.

Tumors of Neural Crest Origin

Tumors of neural crest origin are more frequent in patients with NPARMs (50%) than in those with PARMs (1%). These extracranial tumors are more often neuroblastomas in individuals with NPARMs, rather than ganglioneuromas and ganglioneuroblastomas, which have been described in patients with longer PARMs (20/29, 20/30, and 20/33 genotype only). Thus far only 1 infant with a PARM (20/33 genotype) has been reported to have a neuroblastoma.

Cardiac Asystole

Transient, abrupt, and prolonged sinus pauses have been identified in patients with CCHS, necessitating implantation of cardiac pacemakers when the pauses are 3 sec or longer. Among patients with the *PHOX2B* genotypes, 19% of those with the 20/26 genotype and 83% of those with the 20/27 genotype have heart beat pauses of 3 sec or longer. Children with the 20/25 genotype are not noted to have prolonged asystole, although 2 adults diagnosed with LO-CCHS demonstrated prolonged asystoles of 4-8 sec duration. Risk for sinus pauses among children with NPARMs is unknown at present.

Autonomic Nervous System Dysregulation
A higher number of polyalanine repeats among the PARMs is associated with an increased number of physiologic symptoms of ANSD. A higher frequency of anatomic ANSD findings is seen in individuals with CCHS who have NPARMs than in those who have PARMs. In addition, there is a spectrum of physiologic ANSD symptoms, including decreased heart rate variability, esophageal/gastric/colonic dysmotility, decreased pupillary response to light, reduced basal body temperature, altered distribution and amount of diaphoresis, and altered perception of anxiety.

Facial Phenotype
Children with CCHS and PARMs have a characteristic facies that is boxy in appearance, flattened on profile, and short relative to its width. The following five variables correctly predict 86% of CCHS cases: upper lip height, binocular width, upper facial height, nasal tip protrusion, and inferior inflection of the lateral one-third of the upper lip vermillion border (lip trait).

Neuropathology
Anatomic findings in the brains of individuals with CCHS from early MRI studies were unremarkable, and those from autopsies were inconsistent before 2003 when *PHOX2B* testing became clinically available. In a small cohort of adolescents with suspected CCHS, although without consistent *PHOX2B* mutation confirmation, neuropathologic brainstem changes were identified by diffusion tensor imaging in structures known to mediate central chemosensitivity and to link a network of cardiovascular, respiratory, and affective responses. The neuroanatomic defects in CCHS are likely the result of focal *PHOX2B* (mis) expression coupled with sequelae of recurrent hypoxemia/hypercarbia in the subset of suboptimally managed patients. On the basis of rodent studies and functional MRI in humans, the following regions pertinent to respiratory control show *PHOX2B* expression in the pons and medulla of the brainstem: locus coeruleus, dorsal respiratory group, nucleus ambiguus, parafacial respiratory group, among other areas. Physiologic evidence suggests that the respiratory failure in these children is mostly based on defects in central mechanisms, but peripheral mechanisms (mainly carotid bodies) may also be important.

Patients with CCHS have deficient carbon dioxide sensitivity during wakefulness and sleep such that they do not respond with a normal increase in ventilation in either state nor do they arouse in response to hypercarbia and/or hypoxemia during sleep. During wakefulness, a subset of patients may respond sufficiently to avoid significant hypercarbia, but most individuals with CCHS have hypoventilation that is severe enough that hypercarbia is apparent in the resting awake state. Children with CCHS also have altered sensitivity to hypoxia while awake and asleep. A key feature of CCHS is the lack of respiratory distress or sense of asphyxia with physiologic compromise (hypercarbia and/or hypoxemia). This lack of responsiveness to hypercarbia and/or hypoxemia with subsequent respiratory failure does not seem to consistently improve with age. A subset of older children with CCHS may show an increase in ventilation (specifically increase in respiratory rate rather than increase in tidal volume) when they are exercised at various work rates, a response that is possibly secondary to neural reflexes from rhythmic limb movements—although the increase in minute ventilation is often insufficient to avoid physiologic compromise.

CLINICAL MANIFESTATIONS
Patients with CCHS usually present in the 1st few hr after birth. Most children are the products of uneventful pregnancies and are term infants with appropriate weight for gestational age; Apgar scores have been variable. The affected infants do not show signs of respiratory

distress, but their shallow respirations and respiratory pauses (apnea) evolve to respiratory failure with apparent cyanosis in the 1st day of life. In neonates with CCHS, the $Paco_2$ accumulates during sleep to very high levels, sometimes >90 mm Hg, and may decline to normal levels after the infants awaken. This problem becomes most apparent with failure of multiple attempts at extubation in an intubated neonate (who appears well with ventilatory support but in whom respiratory failure develops after removal of the support). However, the more severely affected infants hypoventilate awake and asleep; thus the previously described difference in $Paco_2$ between states is not apparent. Often, the respiratory rate is higher in rapid eye movement sleep than in nonrapid eye movement sleep in individuals with CCHS.

LO-CCHS should be suspected in infants, children, and adults who have unexplained hypoventilation, especially subsequent to the use of anesthetic agents, sedation, acute respiratory illness, and potentially treated obstructive sleep apnea. These individuals may have other evidence of chronic hypoventilation, including pulmonary hypertension, polycythemia, elevated bicarbonate concentration, difficulty concentrating, and mild unexplained neurocognitive impairment.

Besides treatment for the alveolar hypoventilation, children with CCHS require comprehensive physiologic evaluation and coordinated care to optimally manage associated abnormalities such as Hirschsprung disease, tumors of neural crest origin, symptoms of physiologic ANSD including cardiac asystole, among other findings (details provided in American Thoracic Society 2010 Statement on CCHS).

DIFFERENTIAL DIAGNOSIS
Testing should be performed to rule out primary neuromuscular, lung, and cardiac disease as well as an identifiable brainstem lesion that could account for the full constellation of symptoms characteristic of CCHS. Introduction of clinically available *PHOX2B* genetic testing allows for early and definitive diagnosis of CCHS. Because CCHS mimics many treatable and/or genetic diseases, the following disorders should be considered: X-linked myotubular myopathy, multiminicore disease, congenital myasthenic syndrome, altered airway or intrathoracic anatomy (diagnosis made with bronchoscopy and chest CT), diaphragm dysfunction (diagnosis made with diaphragm fluoroscopy), congenital cardiac disease, a structural hindbrain or brainstem abnormality (diagnosis made with MRI of the brain and brainstem), Möbius syndrome (diagnosis made with MRI of the brain and brainstem and neurologic examination), and specific metabolic diseases, such as Leigh syndrome, pyruvate dehydrogenase deficiency, and discrete carnitine deficiency. However the profound hypercarbia without respiratory distress during sleep will quickly lead the clinician to consider the diagnosis of CCHS or LO-CCHS.

Rapid-Onset Obesity with Hypothalamic Dysfunction, Hypoventilation, and Autonomic Dysregulation
Previously referred to as LO-CHS with hypothalamic dysfunction, **ROHHAD** (rapid-onset obesity with hypothalamic dysfunction, hypoventilation, and autonomic dysregulation) is a very rare disorder that was renamed to clarify that it is distinct from LO-CCHS (Chapter 47). The acronym describes the general sequence or "unfolding" of presenting symptoms, which can evolve over several years. The most dramatic and sentinel feature of ROHHAD is the rapid-onset weight gain (often >20 lb), which occurs over a 6-12 mo period in a seemingly normal young child. The diagnosis is based on clinical criteria that include onset of obesity and alveolar hypoventilation after the age of 1.5 yr (typically between 2 and 7 yr of age) and evidence of hypothalamic dysfunction as defined by 1 or more of the following findings: rapid-onset obesity, hyperprolactinemia, central hypothyroidism, disordered water balance, failure of response to growth hormone stimulation, corticotropin deficiency, and delayed/precocious puberty. Although it may not be apparent early in the course, all children with ROHHAD will develop hypoventilation. Considering the high prevalence of cardiorespiratory arrest and multisystem involvement, children with this disorder require coordinated comprehensive care with attention to development of hypoventilation (such as with repeated

physiologic recordings awake and asleep), initiation of supported ventilation, bradycardia (via Holter monitor), treatment of hypothalamic dysfunction (with involvement of an pediatric endocrinologist), tumors of neural crest origin (often ganglioneuromas or ganglioneuroblastomas; with involvement of an oncologist), and behavioral/intellectual decline (with annual neurocognitive testing and aggressive educational intervention). With meticulous management of the airway, breathing, and circulation, children with ROHHAD seem to stabilize and begin improvement in awake spontaneous breathing—though longitudinal studies are in a preliminary stage at present. Because of the high incidence of neural crest tumors, ROHHAD may be a paraneoplastic disorder.

Children with ROHHAD may present with **obstructive sleep apnea (OSA)** after development of obesity, but ROHHAD is distinct from **OSA hypoventilation syndrome** and **obesity hypoventilation syndrome**. The child with ROHHAD will go onto to severe hypoventilation despite intervention for the OSA. In children with exogenous obesity, the existence of obesity hypoventilation syndrome is controversial and is often referred to as OSA hypoventilation syndrome because it describes chronic OSA with resulting overnight hypercarbia, hypoxemia, and frequent arousals that lead to an altered set point of the central control of breathing (insensitivity to hypercarbia), awake hypoventilation, and daytime sleepiness. In children with OSA hypoventilation syndrome, treatment of the upper airway obstruction would be expected to result in complete resolution of hypoventilation and daytime sleepiness. In contrast, among children with ROHHAD the relief of upper airway obstruction unveils the central alveolar hypoventilation that requires lifelong ventilatory support. Both are distinguished from LO-CCHS by the absence of a CCHS-related *PHOX2B* mutation and the presence of (often morbid) obesity.

MANAGEMENT
Supported Ventilation—Diaphragm Pacing
Depending on the severity of respiratory control deficit, the individual with CCHS can have various means of artificial ventilation: noninvasive positive pressure ventilation or mechanical ventilation via tracheostomy (see Chapter 418.4). Diaphragm pacing offers another mode of supported ventilation; it involves bilateral surgical implantation of electrodes beneath the phrenic nerves, with connecting wires to subcutaneously implanted receivers. The external transmitter, which is much smaller and lighter in weight than a ventilator, sends a signal to flat donut-shaped antennae that are placed on the skin, over the subcutaneously implanted receivers. A signal travels from the external transmitter, ultimately, to the phrenic nerve to stimulate contraction of the diaphragm. A tracheostomy is typically required, at least initially, because the pacers induce a negative pressure on inspiration as a result of the contraction of the diaphragm being unopposed by pharyngeal dilation. Individuals with CCHS who are ventilator-dependent 24 hr/day are ideal candidates for diaphragm pacing to provide increased ambulatory freedom (without the "ventilator tether") while they are awake; however, they still require mechanical ventilator support while they are asleep. This balance between awake pacing and asleep mechanical ventilation allows for a rest from phrenic nerve stimulation at night. A growing number of children and adults who require artificial ventilatory support during sleep only are now using diaphragm pacing, a more acceptable option since the introduction of thoracoscopic diaphragm pacer implantation and shortened recovery time postoperatively.

Monitoring in the Home
Home monitoring for individuals with CCHS and LO-CCHS is distinctly different from and more conservative than that for other children requiring long-term ventilation because those with CCHS lack innate ventilatory and arousal responses to hypoxemia and hypercarbia. In the event of physiologic compromise, other children are more likely to show clinical signs of respiratory distress. For children and adults with CCHS and LO-CCHS, the only means of determining adequate ventilation and oxygenation is with objective measures from a pulse oximeter, end-tidal carbon dioxide monitor, and close supervision of these values by a trained registered nurse in the home and at

school. At a minimum, it is essential that individuals with CCHS have continuous monitoring with pulse oximetry and end-tidal carbon dioxide with registered nurse supervision during all sleep time. Ideally, this such monitoring should be present 24 hr per day because, even while awake, they are not able to sense or adequately respond to a respiratory challenge as may occur with ensuing respiratory illness, increased activity, or even the simple activity of eating. These recommendations apply to all CCHS and LO-CCHS patients regardless of the nature of their artificial ventilatory support—but especially those with diaphragm pacers as they have no intrinsic alarms in the diaphragm pacer device.

Bibliography is available at Expert Consult.

418.3 Other Conditions
Zehava L. Noah and Cynthia Etzler Budek

MYELOMENINGOCELE WITH ARNOLD-CHIARI TYPE II MALFORMATION
Arnold-Chiari type II malformation (see Chapter 591.11) is associated with myelomeningocele, hydrocephalus, and herniation of the cerebellar tonsils, caudal brainstem, and the fourth ventricle through the foramen magnum. Sleep-disordered breathing, including OSA and hypoventilation, has been reported. Direct pressure on the respiratory centers or brainstem nuclei, or increased intracranial pressure because of the hydrocephalus may be responsible. Vocal cord paralysis, apnea, hypoventilation, and bradyarrhythmias have also been reported. Patients with Arnold-Chiari type II malformation have blunted responses to hypercapnia, and to a lesser degree, hypoxia.

Management
An acute change in the ventilatory state of a patient with this malformation requires immediate evaluation. Consideration must be given to posterior fossa decompression and/or treatment of the hydrocephalus. If this treatment is unsuccessful in resolving central hypoventilation or apnea, tracheostomy and long-term mechanical ventilation should be considered.

RAPID-ONSET OBESITY, HYPOTHALAMIC DYSFUNCTION, AND AUTONOMIC DYSREGULATION
See Chapter 418.2.

Obesity Hypoventilation Syndrome
As its name implies, obesity hypoventilation syndrome is a syndrome of central hypoventilation during wakefulness in obese patients with sleep-disordered breathing. Although it was initially described mainly in adult obese patients, obese children have also demonstrated the syndrome. Sleep-disordered breathing is a combination of OSA, hypopnea, and/or sleep hypoventilation syndrome. Patients are hypercapnic with cognitive impairment, morning headache, and hypersomnolence during the day. Chronic hypoxemia may lead to pulmonary hypertension and cor pulmonale.

Obesity is associated with reduced respiratory system compliance, increased airway resistance, reduced functional residual capacity, and increased work of breathing. Affected patients are unable to increase their respiratory drive in response to hypercapnia. Leptin may have a role in this syndrome. The sleep-disordered breathing leads to compensatory metabolic alkalosis. Because of the long half-life of bicarbonate, its elevation causes compensatory respiratory acidosis during wakefulness with elevated $Paco_2$.

Management
The use of **CPAP** during sleep may be sufficient for many patients. Patients with hypoxemia may require **BiPAP** and supplemental oxygen. Tracheostomy may be considered for patients who do not tolerate mask ventilation.

ACQUIRED ALVEOLAR HYPOVENTILATION

Traumatic, ischemic, and inflammatory injuries to the brainstem, brainstem infarction, brain tumors, bulbar polio, and viral paraneoplastic encephalitis may also result in central hypoventilation.

OBSTRUCTIVE SLEEP APNEA

Epidemiology

Habitual snoring during sleep is extremely common during childhood. As many as 27% of children who snore are affected by **OSA.** The current obesity epidemic has affected the epidemiology of this condition. Peak prevalence is at 2-8 yr of age. The ratio between habitual snoring and OSA is 4:1 to 6:1.

Pathophysiology

OSA occurs when the luminal cross-sectional area of the upper airway is significantly reduced during inspiration. With increased airway resistance and reduced activation of pharyngeal dilators, negative pressure leads to upper airway collapse. The site of upper airway closure in children with OSA is at the level of tonsils and adenoids. The size of tonsils and adenoids increases throughout childhood up to 12 yr of age. Environmental irritants such as cigarette smoke or allergic rhinitis may accelerate the process. Reports now suggest that early viral infections may affect adenotonsillar proliferation.

Clinical Presentation

Snoring during sleep, behavioral disturbances, learning difficulties, excessive daytime sleepiness, metabolic issues, and cardiovascular morbidity may alert the parent or physician to the presence of OSA. Diagnosis is made with the help of airway radiograms and a polysomnogram.

Treatment

When adenotonsillar hypertrophy is suspected, a consultation with an ear, nose, and throat specialist for adenoidectomy and/or tonsillectomy may be indicated. For patients who are not candidates for surgical intervention or persist with OSA despite adenoidectomy and/or tonsillectomy, CPAP or BiPAP during sleep may alleviate the obstruction (see Chapter 19).

SPINAL CORD INJURY

Epidemiology

There are an estimated 11,000 new spinal cord injuries (**SCIs**) annually in the United States, with more than 50% resulting in quadriplegia. SCI is relatively rare in pediatric patients, with an incidence of 1-13% of all SCI patients. The incidence in infancy and early childhood is similar for boys and girls. The preponderance of SCI in adolescents is in males. Motor vehicle accidents, falls, sports injuries, and assaults are the main causes. SCI usually leads to lifelong disability.

Pathophysiology

Children with SCI have a disproportionately higher involvement of the upper cervical spine, high frequency of spinal cord injury without radiographic abnormality, delayed onset of neurologic deficits, and higher proportion of complete injury. Thus, there is a high likelihood in pediatric SCI of quadriplegia with intercostal muscle and/or diaphragmatic paralysis leading to respiratory failure.

Management

Immobilization and stabilization of the spine must be accomplished simultaneously with initial patient resuscitation. Children with high SCI typically require lifelong ventilation, so the decision to place a tracheostomy for chronic ventilatory support is usually made early in their course of treatment. Depending on the child's age and general condition, diaphragmatic pacing may be considered. Often patients with diaphragmatic pacing need tracheostomy placement if there is dyscoordination between pacing and glottal opening. Muscle spasms occur frequently in the SCI patient and are treated with muscle relaxants. Occasionally the muscle spasms involve the chest and present a serious impediment to ventilation. Continuous intrathecal infusion of muscle relaxant via an implanted subcutaneous pump may be indicated (see Chapter 606.5).

METABOLIC DISEASE

Mucopolysaccharidoses

See Chapter 88.

Mucopolysaccharidoses are a group of progressive hereditary disorders that lack the lysosomal enzymes that degrade glycosaminoglycans. Incompletely catabolized mucopolysaccharides accumulate in connective tissue throughout the body. The inheritance is autosomal recessive except for Hunt syndrome, which is X-linked. The diagnosis is suggested by the presence of glycosaminuria and is confirmed by a lysosomal enzyme assay. I-cell disease mucolipidosis type II is an inherited lysosomal disorder with accumulation of mucolipids. Phenotypically, it is similar to mucopolysaccharidoses, but the age of onset is earlier and there is no mucopolysacchariduria. Mucopolysaccharide deposits are frequently found in the head and neck and cause airway obstruction. Typically, the affected child has a coarse face and large tongue. Significant deposits are found in the adenoids, tonsils, and cartilage. Airway radiograms and a polysomnogram may help define the severity of the upper airway obstruction.

Treatment options have included enzyme replacement therapy and stem cell transplantation with limited success. Adenoidectomy and/or tonsillectomy may be indicated but surgery alone seldom solves the problem of airway obstruction. Noninvasive CPAP or BiPAP, or tracheostomy with ventilatory support may be helpful

Dysplasias

Campomelic dysplasia (see Chapter 698) and thanatophoric dysplasia (see Chapter 696) affect rib cage size, shape, and compliance, leading to respiratory failure. Most patients with these disorders do not survive beyond early infancy. Tracheostomy and ventilation may prolong life.

Glycogenosis Type Ii

See Chapter 87.1.

Glycogenosis type II is an autosomal recessive disorder. Clinical manifestations include cardiomyopathy and generalized muscle weakness. Cardiac issues may include heart failure and arrhythmias. Muscle weakness leads to respiratory insufficiency and sleep-disordered breathing. Treatment includes emerging therapies such as enzyme replacement therapy, chaperone molecules, and gene therapy. Supportive therapy may consist of either noninvasive ventilation, or tracheostomy and mechanical ventilation. Cardiac medications, protein-rich nutrition, and judicious physical therapy are additional measures that can be utilized.

Severe Tracheomalacia and/or Bronchomalacia (Airway Malacia)

Conditions associated with airway malacia include tracheoesophageal fistula, innominate artery compression, and pulmonary artery sling after surgical repair (see Chapter 389). Patients with tracheobronchomalacia present with cough, lower airway obstruction, and wheezing. Diagnosis is made via bronchoscopy, preferably with the patient breathing spontaneously in order to evaluate dynamic airway function. Positive end-expiratory pressure titration during the bronchoscopy helps identify the ideal airway pressure required to maintain airway patency and prevent tracheobronchial collapse.

Neuropathy of Severe Illness

Children recuperating from severe illness in the intensive care unit often have neuromuscular weakness from suboptimal nutrition. This neuromuscular weakness can be devastating when coupled with the catabolic effects of severe illness and the residual effects of sedatives, analgesics, and muscle relaxants, particularly if corticosteroids were administered. Children with neuromuscular compromise have limited ability to increase ventilation and usually do so by increasing respiratory rate. Because of weakness, costal and sternal retractions may not be observed. Children with severe neuromyopathy may respond to increased respiratory load by becoming apneic. A look of panic, a change in vital signs such as significant tachycardia or bradycardia, and cyanosis may be the only signs of impending respiratory failure.

HEMATOLOGIC STEM-CELL TRANSPLANTATION

Hematologic stem cell transplant (HSCT) is a life-saving therapy for patients with hematologic, oncologic, and immunologic conditions. Historically, outcomes for these patients have been poor. Lung dysfunction after HSCT is a serious and often fatal complication. Common causes of HSCT lung dysfunction include bacterial, viral, and/or fungal infections, posttransplant lymphoproliferative disorder, idiopathic pneumonia syndrome, diffuse alveolar hemorrhage, pulmonary cytolytic thrombi, engraftment syndrome, and bronchiolitis obliterans. Improvements in the management of HSCT have resulted in decreased graft-versus-host disease severity. Improved critical care practices, such as more in-depth diagnostic evaluation and lung-sparing ventilator strategies, have resulted in improved outcomes. Despite improved outcomes, a subset of HSCT patients will require chronic respiratory support for prolonged periods of time. In addition to post HSCT therapy, ongoing care may include noninvasive or invasive home ventilation, tracheostomy placement, diuretics, and supplemental nutrition.

MITOCHONDRIAL DISEASES
See Chapter 86.

Mitochondria are primarily responsible for the production of adenosine triphosphate. Mitochondrial diseases are a heterogeneous group of diseases in which adenosine triphosphate production is disrupted. Mitochondrial diseases are increasingly recognized and diagnosed in the pediatric population. Organs with high-energy requirements such as the neurons, and skeletal and cardiac muscles are particularly vulnerable. Although myopathy is the most frequently recognized presentation of mitochondrial disease, it is often part of a multisystem disease process. Neurologic complications include progressive proximal myopathy, kyphoscoliosis, dyskinesia, dystonia and spasticity, stroke, epilepsy, and visual and hearing impairment. Nonneurologic manifestations include cardiomyopathy, gastrointestinal dysmotility, gastroesophageal reflux, delayed gastric emptying, and pseudoobstruction.

Respiratory complications of mitochondrial disease are multifactorial. Muscle weakness, kyphoscoliosis, muscle spasms, and movement disorders may result in a restrictive pattern, and respiratory compromise. Additionally, dyscoordinated swallow and reflux may result in aspiration. In some mitochondrial diseases such as Leigh syndrome (see Chapter 86), central hypoventilation is an integral part of the disease. Supportive care for these patients may include noninvasive or invasive ventilation, tracheostomy placement, diuretics, appropriate nutrition, and dietary supplements.

Bibliography is available at Expert Consult.

418.4 Long-Term Mechanical Ventilation
Zehava L. Noah and Cynthia Etzler Budek

Many children with chronic severe respiratory insufficiency will benefit from long-term ventilatory support. The goals of chronic ventilation are to maintain normal oxygenation and ventilation, and to minimize the work of breathing. Caring for a child on long-term ventilatory support in the home is a complex, physically demanding, emotionally taxing, and expensive process for the family. It changes the family routines, priorities, and overall lifestyle, and may adversely affect intrafamilial and extrafamilial relationships. The discharge process for a child likely to require long-term ventilatory support should start early in the hospitalization, before the child is medically stable and prior to transition to a portable ventilator that can be maintained in the home.

The child's disease prognosis is a critical factor to consider when deciding to initiate long-term ventilation. Children with degenerative

neuromuscular disease, such as SMA type I, suffer from respiratory failure very early in life, often triggered by the first respiratory illness. Although some parents of children with SMA decide to provide only palliative end-of-life care (see Chapter 43), others choose long-term invasive or noninvasive ventilatory support. Young children with chronic lung disease and airway malacia have the potential to improve their pulmonary function and to wean successfully off the ventilator if provided with adequate ventilation, good nutrition, and measures to promote development and prevent further lung injury.

Successful home discharge depends on whether there are adequate resources in the community to support the family. Some hospital programs that transition children home on ventilators utilize professional nurses in the home to assist with round-the-clock care. This level of care depends on adequate funding as well as availability of nursing agencies with skilled nurses. Housing can be a significant barrier to discharge if the home lacks adequate space for the child and caretakers, equipment, and supplies, presents environmental safety issues, including building and electrical code violations, and/or requires extensive home modifications for mobility, including ramping and lifts.

Funding for home care is typically a challenge for this pediatric population. Even if they have private insurance, coverage for home care benefits is often very limited. In the United States, most states have public aid funds available to support the special needs of eligible children who are ventilator dependent, although the extent of coverage varies considerably across the country.

RESPIRATORY EQUIPMENT FOR HOME CARE
Modes of mechanical ventilation support are discussed in Chapter 71.1.

Noninvasive Equipment
Supplemental oxygen and positive pressure support can be administered by nasal cannula. The nasal cannula system has the ability to deliver heated, supersaturated, high-flow gases. There are a number of mechanical devices available for the delivery of CPAP and BiPAP. These devices attach to nasal and full-face masks or nasal pillows and are best suited for the treatment of OSA where ventilatory support is required for only a portion of the day, typically during sleep. Long-term use of mask ventilation in small children may result in mid-face dysplasia or pressure wounds. This type of ventilation has also been used in children with mild forms of respiratory insufficiency due to recurrent atelectasis and/or nocturnal hypoventilation, as well as for palliation in more severely affected patients.

Rocker Bed
A rocker bed moves in a longitudinal seesaw motion at a set cycle rate. The child is secured to the bed with a strap across the body. Movement of the bed and gravitational pull promotes diaphragm movement. The rocker bed may be an option for children with mild neuromuscular weakness such as children recuperating from Guillain-Barré syndrome. For safety reasons this device should not be placed in a home with toddlers or young children, who may get trapped in its rotating mechanism.

Cuirasse
The cuirasse is a negative-pressure device that resembles a hard turtle shell. It is a fiberglass piece that is custom fit over the child's anterior chest and provides a tight seal. A hose attached to the cuirasse applies cycled negative pressure that lifts and releases the anterior chest wall. The cuirasse is suitable only for infants and children with mild neuromuscular weakness and pliable chest walls. A similar negative-pressure device utilizes a plastic bag that fits snugly around the chest and operates under the same principle as the cuirasse to lift and release the chest wall.

Iron Lung
The iron lung is a device that also applies negative pressure to the child's body. The child is placed in the iron lung cylinder with his head

extending outside of the device. A cuff is placed around the neck to minimize air leaks. Negative pressure is cycled within the iron lung, facilitating chest wall movement. Ventilation is disrupted whenever the device is opened for patient care. The iron lung is suitable for children with muscular weakness who require ventilation for part of the day. Its main advantage is that it does not require a tracheostomy. However, upper airway obstruction may occur, and this risk requires ongoing evaluation. A smaller, lightweight version of this device is available for travel.

Diaphragmatic Pacing
Detailed in the management section of Ch. 418.2, diaphragm pacers may also be considered in children with spinal cord injury above C3, though the immediate advantages are less apparent than in CCHS.

Positive-Pressure Ventilators
Ideally, a ventilator intended for home use is lightweight and small, quiet so it doesn't interfere with activities of daily living or sleep, able to entrain room air, preferably has continuous flow, and has a wide range of settings (particularly for pressure, volume, pressure support, and rate) that allows ventilatory support from infancy to adulthood. Battery power for the ventilator, both internal and external, should be sufficient to permit unrestricted portability in the home and community. The equipment must also be impervious to electromagnetic interference and must be relatively easy to understand and troubleshoot. A variety of ventilators that are approved for home use are available, and familiarity with these devices is necessary to choose the best option for the individual child.

Children who are chronically ventilated via positive-pressure ventilation will require surgical placement of a tracheostomy tube. The tracheostomy tube provides stable access to the airway, a standardized interface for attaching the ventilator circuit to the patient, and the ability to easily remove airway secretions or deliver inhaled medications. Pediatric tracheostomy tubes typically have a single lumen and may have an inflatable cuff. Tracheostomy tubes with/without cuff inflation should be sized to control the air leak around the tube and promote adequate gas exchange, yet allow enough space around the tube to facilitate vocalization and prevent tracheal irritation and erosion from the tube.

When a tracheostomy tube is surgically placed, a slit opening is made in the trachea between the cartilaginous rings. Stay sutures are attached to the margins of the incision to facilitate emergent tube replacement prior to healing of the stoma tract. The tracheostomy tube is often electively changed by an otolaryngologist approximately 1 wk after initial placement, and the child is subsequently cleared for tracheostomy tube changes by the nursing staff. The child's caregivers, usually parents or family members and home nursing staff, are instructed in all aspects of tracheostomy care: stoma care, elective and emergent tracheostomy change, proper securing of the tracheostomy tube, suctioning of secretions, and recognition of tube obstruction or decannulation. The child's caregivers have to demonstrate competency with all the tasks prior to home discharge.

AIRWAY CLEARANCE
Thick, copious secretions may contribute to increased airway resistance and provide substrate for bacterial and fungal growth. Respiratory infections in turn lead to an increase in the amount of secretions and may increase viscosity, contributing to problems in airway clearance. Patients with neuromuscular weakness often have dyscoordination or absence of swallow, putting them at risk for aspiration of oral secretions or food. Reflux resulting in aspiration is also common. Additionally, many patients have poor or nonexistent cough, and some of them may have ciliary dysfunction.

Common modalities that help with clearance of secretions include postural drainage, manual or mechanical percussion or vibration, and vest or wrap percussion therapy. Force of cough may be enhanced with a cough assist device and/or abdominal binder. In addition, oropharyngeal or tracheal suctioning to remove secretions may promote airway clearance. In rare cases where airway clearance is not amenable

to these measures, intermittent positive ventilation devices may be a useful adjunct.

Control of oral secretions can be achieved pharmacologically with anticholinergic drugs, localized injection of botulinum toxin (Botox), or surgical ligation of selected salivary ducts. In extreme cases, surgical tracheolaryngeal separation may be indicated. If thick, tenacious secretions are problematic, patient hydration and dosing of anticholinergic medication should be reviewed. Administration of nebulized dornase alfa or N-acetylcysteine, hypertonic saline, and/or sodium bicarbonate may be considered to thin secretions. In selected cases, bronchoscopy may be indicated for the removal of inspissated secretions and/or reexpansion of atelectatic pulmonary lobe or segment.

PHYSICAL THERAPY, OCCUPATIONAL THERAPY, AND SPEECH THERAPY
Therapies are very important in management of chronic respiratory failure. Potential goals for physical therapy are mobilization of the patient and strengthening of muscles, particularly truncal and abdominal muscles that are essential to pulmonary rehabilitation. Occupational therapy goals revolve around achieving or maintaining developmental milestones. Child life/developmental therapy focuses on provision of developmentally appropriate environmental stimulation and age-appropriate play. Speech therapy goals deal with oromotor skills for feeding and communication. Evaluation of swallow is a key component of therapy for children with chronic respiratory failure. Sign language is frequently utilized for communication because of delayed speech or hearing loss. Audiology specialists should be involved in the assessment of hearing, as there is a higher incidence of hearing loss in patients undergoing long-term ventilation.

INFECTIONS
Infections—tracheitis (see Chapter 385.2), bronchitis (see Chapter 391.2), and pneumonia (see Chapter 400)—are common in patients with chronic respiratory failure. Infections may be caused by community-acquired viruses (adenovirus, influenza, respiratory syncytial virus, parainfluenza, rhinovirus) or community- or hospital-acquired bacteria. Common pathogens are Gram-negative, highly antimicrobial-resistant pathogens that may cause further deterioration in pulmonary function. Bacterial infection is most likely in the presence of fever, deteriorating lung function (hypoxia, hypercarbia, tachypnea, and retractions), leukocytosis, and mucopurulent sputum. The presence of leukocytes and organisms on Gram stain of tracheal aspirate, as well as the visualization of new infiltrates on radiographs, may be consistent with bacterial infection.

Infection must be distinguished from tracheal colonization of bacteria, which is asymptomatic and associated with normal amounts of clear tracheal secretions. If infection is suspected, it must be treated with antibiotics, based on the culture and sensitivities of organisms recovered from the tracheal aspirate. Starting inhaled tobramycin and polymyxin E early may avert more serious infection. Antibiotics should be used judiciously to prevent further colonization with drug-resistant organisms. However, some patients who have recurrent infections may benefit from prophylaxis with inhaled antibiotics. Preventive measures are essential and include immunizations (influenza, pneumococcus, Haemophilus influenzae type b), passive immunity (respiratory syncytial virus), and good tracheostomy care.

MONITORING
A patient who is ventilated in the home must be electronically and/or physically monitored at all times. Infants and young children, children who are cognitively impaired, and children who are completely tracheostomy dependent for airway patency because of suprastomal obstruction must be under direct observation of the caregivers at all times. Caregivers should also closely monitor children whose pulmonary status is fragile or fluctuant. Continuous monitoring of O_2 saturation and heart rate is recommended during sleep, and either continuous or intermittent monitoring during the daytime, depending on patient stability. Patients with CCHS or pulmonary hypertension are particularly vulnerable to episodes of hypoxemia and/or hypercarbia, and

those with pulmonary hypertension are particularly susceptible to rapid drops in O_2 saturation.

Patients evaluated in pulmonary clinic for follow up should be monitored at each visit for heart rate, O_2 saturation, and transcutaneous and/or end-tidal CO_2 levels. Pulmonary function tests should be considered for those patients who are old enough and able to cooperate, usually after 5 yr of age. Serial echocardiograms should be obtained to monitor progression of pulmonary hypertension. Increased frequency of monitoring and surveillance are recommended for patients whose pulmonary status has improved and are in the process of weaning completely off ventilator support. A polysomnogram performed off the ventilator may be useful when total liberation from mechanical ventilation is being contemplated. In addition to physiologic parameters, patients must be monitored for signs of stress, agitation, and fatigue. Often these signs appear one or more days after the ventilator parameter changes.

WEANING OFF VENTILATOR SUPPORT
Patients recuperating from pulmonary disease, who are on stable ventilator settings with low positive end-expiratory pressure and minimal or no O_2 support, should be evaluated periodically for readiness to begin weaning from mechanical ventilation. Barriers to weaning may include residual lung disease, pulmonary hypertension, impaired central control of breathing, and muscle weakness. Weakness often has a multifactorial etiology. Factors such as underlying neuromuscular disease, use of sedatives, analgesics, steroids and muscle relaxants, and prolonged immobility, as well as utilization of mechanical ventilation, may downregulate mitochondrial activity in the respiratory muscles, and more so the diaphragm, and produce muscular changes resulting in weakness. Consequently, it is important to avoid 24 hr/day patient synchrony with ventilation and titrate the amount of ventilator support to prevent fatigue, yet facilitate spontaneous breathing.

When transitioning from full mechanical ventilatory support to spontaneous breathing, conditioning of the respiratory muscles can be achieved by several methods: gradual decrease of mechanical support by decreasing the ventilator pressures and/or rate, sprints of pressure support ventilation, retraining of the respiratory muscles with breathing exercises against an obstructed airway, and spontaneous breathing sprints off the ventilator. The weaning program may be initiated prior to initial hospital discharge or during follow up clinic visits. An initial weaning schedule may consist of 15 min sprints of free breathing off the ventilator up to 3 times/day while directly observed by caregiver and monitoring of respiratory parameters. The sprints are lengthened gradually with continued monitoring in the home and during frequent clinic visits. Additional factors that reflect tolerance of increased work of breathing, including weight gain, energy levels, general behavior and sleep patterns, are also monitored carefully. When the child has completely weaned off ventilator support while awake and is only on the ventilator approximately 6 hr nightly during sleep, a polysomnogram study performed off the ventilator may be considered prior to complete liberation from the mechanical ventilation device.

DISCHARGE PROCESS
The discharge process for a child going home for the first time on a ventilator is complex. A multidisciplinary, coordinated team approach is needed to develop an individualized, comprehensive plan that addresses medical, psychosocial, developmental, educational, and safety issues. The child should be transitioned to a ventilator suitable for home use that allows portability as well as adequate ventilation. Depending on the type of ventilation employed, a tracheostomy is typically placed to promote comfort and provide a stable airway as soon as the decision for long-term ventilation is made. Medical management should also focus on transitioning oxygen and ventilator parameters to settings appropriate for home care. The ventilated child must demonstrate medical stability at a level that can be safely managed at home; interventions to maintain patient stability should be minimal 1-2 wk before discharge.

Nutrition should be optimized to promote growth yet minimize excessive weight gain and carbon dioxide production. The nutritional

requirements of a ventilated child are frequently decreased due to the supported work of breathing. The ventilated child often has problems with uncoordinated swallowing and oral aversion secondary to intubation. Speech therapy should be introduced early to begin oromotor therapy and return of swallow. Many children require gastrostomy tube placement to replace or supplement oral intake. Evaluation and management of reflux and the risk of aspiration should also be considered. Some children with severe reflux may require jejunal feedings. Communication devices to augment speech and introduction of sign language for speech and hearing impaired should be part of the planning.

Training of family caregivers should be initiated early in the discharge process and should be provided by nurses, respiratory care practitioners, and physical, occupational, and speech therapists knowledgeable in the individual child's care. Home caregivers, typically the parents or family members and home nursing staff, are instructed in all aspects of the child's care, including tracheostomy tube changes and care, tube feedings and care, medication administration, ventilator management and troubleshooting, emergency response, and cardiopulmonary resuscitation. Caregiver independence in delivery of care at the bedside and while transporting the child should be emphasized. Special emphasis should be placed on safety and the appropriate response in the event of an emergency. A standardized emergency bag containing critical tracheostomy and ventilator supplies should accompany the child at all times. A minimum of 2 family members should complete instruction and demonstrate their competency by independently providing their child's care for a 24-48 hr period prior to discharge.

Community agencies are identified for provision of home support services, typically including a nursing agency and equipment vendor. The nursing agency may provide private duty nursing services. Home care nurses should have pediatric tracheostomy and ventilator experience and be well versed in the individual child's care before home discharge. An equipment vendor who can provide the ventilator, medical equipment and supplies, and maintenance/repair service should be selected. A care conference involving the hospital team, funding agency, home nursing agency, equipment vendor, and family caregivers should take place before discharge. The conference is critical for coordination of last-minute details and facilitation of a smooth transition to home.

OUTPATIENT FOLLOW UP
Provision of ongoing medical support to the child and family after discharge is essential. The primary care provider in the community has the central role in coordination of care, and provision of well-child, acute, and chronic care, with the exception of ventilatory management. Equally important is the establishment of lines of communication between the primary care provider and the pulmonary/critical care specialists managing ventilator care, and the provision of timely access for advice and troubleshooting during the intervals between respiratory multidisciplinary clinic visits.

The purpose of the respiratory multidisciplinary clinic is to monitor the patient's progress, ensure that the ventilatory support is sufficient to promote growth and development and, when appropriate, to initiate or continue the ventilator weaning process. Physicians and/or advanced practice nurses who are well versed in ventilator care, typically pulmonary or critical care specialists, as well as respiratory care practitioners, evaluate the patient in clinic. Clinical nutrition, social work, and case management services should also be readily available.

The frequency of the clinic visits depends on the stability of the patient and the frequency of medical interventions needed to maintain clinical stability. A patient discharged from the hospital for the first time on a ventilator is typically evaluated in clinic within a month and may require monthly follow-up visits. Once the child is stable, the frequency decreases to every 3-6 mo. Older long-term patients who are no longer having major growth spurts are typically scheduled for annual visits. Patients who are actively weaning from the ventilator are seen more frequently. During the clinic visit respiratory monitoring is obtained while the child is on the ventilator and, if medically indicated, off the ventilator, and repeated whenever ventilator adjustments are made. Whenever possible, readings obtained from home monitoring devices are compared with clinic monitoring to determine correlation. Recommendations regarding the child's ventilator management are communicated to the primary care provider by letter or phone call after each clinic visit.

TRANSITION OF CARE

The pulmonary team initiates ongoing discussions regarding self-care responsibilities and transitioning of medical care to adult providers with the adolescent and his parents when the patient reaches the early teens. Discussion about self-care should take into consideration realistic expectations about the adolescent's physical and cognitive capabilities. The actual transition of care occurs for most young adults at age 18-21 yr, and includes referral to an internist as well as an adult pulmonologist. Transition of medical care also includes transition from pediatric to adult support services for funding sources and nursing care. Ideally, an outpatient visit that includes current and future adult medical providers together is completed to facilitate communication and formally transition care.

Bibliography is available at Expert Consult.

Chapter **419**

Extrapulmonary Diseases with Pulmonary Manifestations

Susanna A. McColley

Respiratory symptoms commonly originate from extrapulmonary processes. The respiratory system adapts to metabolic demands and is exquisitely responsive to cortical input; therefore, **tachypnea** is common in the presence of metabolic stress such as fever, whereas dyspnea may be related to anxiety. **Cough** most commonly arises from upper or lower respiratory tract disorders, but it can originate from the central nervous system, as with cough tic or psychogenic cough, and it can be a prominent symptom in children with gastroesophageal reflux disease. **Chest pain** does not commonly arise from pulmonary processes in otherwise healthy children but more often has a neuromuscular or inflammatory etiology. **Cyanosis** can be caused by cardiac or hematologic disorders, and **dyspnea** and **exercise intolerance** can have a number of extrapulmonary causes. These disorders may be suspected on the basis of the history and physical examination, or they may be considered in children in whom diagnostic studies have atypical findings or who show poor response to usual therapy. Table 419-1 lists more common causes of such symptoms.

EVALUATION

In the evaluation of a child or adolescent with respiratory symptoms, it is important to obtain a detailed past medical history, family history, and review of systems to evaluate the possibility of extrapulmonary origin. A comprehensive physical examination is also essential in obtaining clues to extrapulmonary disease.

Disorders of other organ systems, and many systemic diseases, can have significant respiratory system involvement. Although it is most common to encounter these complications in patients with known diagnoses, respiratory system disease is sometimes the sole or most prominent symptom at the time of presentation. Acute aspiration during feeding can be the presentation of neuromuscular disease in an infant who initially appears to have normal muscle tone and development. Complications can be life-threatening, particularly in immunocompromised patients. The onset of respiratory findings may be insidious; for example, pulmonary vascular involvement in patients with systemic vasculitis may appear as an abnormality in diffusing capacity of the lung for carbon monoxide before the onset of symptoms. Table 419-2 lists disorders that commonly have respiratory complications.

Bibliography is available at Expert Consult.

Table 419-1	Respiratory Signs and Symptoms Originating from Outside the Respiratory Tract		
SIGN OR SYMPTOM	**NONRESPIRATORY CAUSE(S)**	**PATHOPHYSIOLOGY**	**CLUES TO DIAGNOSIS**
Chest pain	Cardiac disease	Inflammation (pericarditis), ischemia (anomalous coronary artery, vascular disease)	Precordial pain, friction rub on examination; exertional pain, radiation to arm or neck
Chest pain	Gastroesophageal reflux disease	Esophageal inflammation and/or spasm	Heartburn, abdominal pain
Cyanosis	Congenital heart disease Methemoglobinemia	Right-to-left shunt Increased levels of methemoglobin interfere with delivery of oxygen to tissues	Neonatal onset, lack of response to oxygen Drug or toxin exposure, lack of response to oxygen
Dyspnea	Toxin exposure, drug side effect, or overdose	Variable, but often metabolic acidosis	Drug or toxin exposure confirmed by history or toxicology screen, normal oxygen saturation measured by pulse oximetry
	Anxiety, panic disorder	Increased respiratory drive and increased perception of respiratory efforts	Occurs during stressful situation, other symptoms of anxiety or depression

Continued

| Table 419-1 | Respiratory Signs and Symptoms Originating from Outside the Respiratory Tract—cont'd |

SIGN OR SYMPTOM	NONRESPIRATORY CAUSE(S)	PATHOPHYSIOLOGY	CLUES TO DIAGNOSIS
Exercise intolerance	Anemia	Inadequate oxygen delivery to tissues	Pallor, tachycardia, history of bleeding, history of inadequate diet
Exercise intolerance	Deconditioning	Self-explanatory	History of inactivity, obesity
Hemoptysis	Nasal bleeding	Posterior flow of bleeding causes appearance of pulmonary origin	History and physical findings suggest nasal source; normal chest examination, and chest radiography
	Upper gastrointestinal tract bleeding	Hematemesis mimics hemoptysis	History and physical examination suggest gastrointestinal source, normal chest examination and chest radiography
Wheezing, cough, dyspnea	Congenital or acquired cardiac disease	Pulmonary overcirculation (atrioseptal defect, ventriculoseptal defect, patent ductus arteriosus), left ventricular dysfunction	Murmur Refractory to bronchodilators Radiographic changes (prominent pulmonary vasculature, pulmonary edema)
Wheezing, cough	Gastroesophageal reflux disease	Laryngeal and bronchial response to stomach contents Vagally mediated bronchoconstriction	Emesis, pain, heartburn Refractory to bronchodilators

| Table 419-2 | Disorders with Frequent Respiratory Tract Complications |

UNDERLYING DISORDER(S)	RESPIRATORY COMPLICATIONS	DIAGNOSTIC TESTS
Autoimmune disorders	Pulmonary vascular disease, restrictive lung disease, pleural effusion (especially systemic lupus erythematosus), upper airway disease (Wegener granulomatosis)	Spirometry, lung volume determination, oximetry, diffusing capacity of the lung for carbon monoxide, chest radiography, upper airway endoscopy, and/or CT
Central nervous system disease (static or progressive)	Aspiration of oral or gastric contents	Chest radiography, videofluoroscopic swallowing study, esophageal pH probe, fiberoptic bronchoscopy
Immunodeficiency	Infection, bronchiectasis	Chest radiography, fiberoptic bronchoscopy, chest CT
Liver disease	Pleural effusion, hepatopulmonary syndrome	Chest radiography, assessment of orthodeoxia
Malignancy and its therapies	Infiltration, metastasis, malignant or infectious effusion, parenchymal infection, graft-versus-host disease (bone marrow transplant)	Chest radiography, chest CT, fiberoptic bronchoscopy, lung biopsy
Neuromuscular disease	Hypoventilation, atelectasis, pneumonia	Spirometry, lung volume determination, respiratory muscle force measurements
Obesity	Restrictive lung disease, obstructive sleep apnea syndrome, asthma	Spirometry, lung volume determination, nocturnal polysomnography

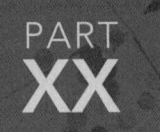

The Cardiovascular System

PART XX

Section 1
Developmental Biology of the Cardiovascular System

Chapter 420
Cardiac Development
Daniel Bernstein

Knowledge of the cellular and molecular mechanisms of cardiac development is necessary for understanding congenital heart defects and will be even more important in developing strategies for prevention, whether cell or molecular therapies or fetal cardiac interventional procedures. Cardiac defects have traditionally been grouped by common morphologic patterns: for example, abnormalities of the outflow tracts (conotruncal lesions such as tetralogy of Fallot and truncus arteriosus) and abnormalities of atrioventricular septation (primum atrial septal defect, complete atrioventricular canal defect). These morphologic categories may be revised or eventually supplanted by new categories as our understanding of the genetic basis of congenital heart disease progresses.

Bibliography is available at Expert Consult.

420.1 Early Cardiac Morphogenesis
Daniel Bernstein

In the early presomite embryo, the first identifiable cardiac progenitor cell clusters are arranged in the anterior lateral plate mesoderm on both sides of the embryo's central axis; these clusters form paired cardiac tubes by 18 days of gestation. The paired tubes fuse in the midline on the ventral surface of the embryo to form the primitive heart tube by 22 days. This straight heart tube is composed of an outer myocardial layer, an inner endocardium, and a middle layer of extracellular matrix known as the cardiac jelly. There are 2 distinct cell lineages: the primary heart field provides precursor cells for the left ventricle, whereas the secondary heart field provides precursors for the atria and right ventricle. Premyocardial cells, including epicardial cells and cells derived from the neural crest, continue their migration into the region of the heart tube. Regulation of this early phase of cardiac morphogenesis is controlled in part by the interaction of specific signaling molecules or ligands, usually expressed by 1 cell type, with specific receptors, usually expressed by another cell type. Positional information is conveyed to the developing cardiac mesoderm by factors such as retinoids (isoforms of vitamin A), which bind to specific nuclear receptors and regulate gene transcription. Migration of epithelial cells into the developing heart tube is directed by extracellular matrix proteins (such as fibronectin) interacting with cell surface receptors (the integrins). Other important regulatory molecules include bone morphogenetic protein 2 (BMP2); fibroblast growth factor 4 (FGF4); the transcription factors Nkx2.5, GATA4, Mesp1, and Mesp2; and members of the Wnt/β-catenin signaling pathway. The clinical importance of these ligands is revealed by the spectrum of **cardiac teratogenic** effects caused by the retinoid-like drug isotretinoin.

As early as 20-22 days, before cardiac looping, the embryonic heart begins to contract and exhibit phases of the cardiac cycle that are surprisingly similar to those in the mature heart. Morphologists initially identified segments of the heart tube that were believed to correspond to structures in the mature heart (Fig. 420-1): the sinus venosus and atrium (right and left atria), the primitive ventricle (left ventricle), the bulbus cordis (right ventricle), and the truncus arteriosus (aorta and pulmonary artery). However, this model is oversimplified. Only the trabecular (most heavily muscularized) portions of the left ventricular myocardium are present in the early cardiac tube; the cells that will become the inlet portion of the left ventricle migrate into the cardiac tube at a later stage (after looping is initiated). Even later to appear are the primordial cells that give rise to the great arteries (truncus arteriosus), including cells derived from the neural crest, which are not present until after cardiac looping is complete. Chamber-specific transcription factors participate in the differentiation of the right and left ventricles. The basic helix-loop-helix (bHLH) transcription factor dHAND is expressed in the developing right ventricle; disruption of this gene or of other transcriptional factors such as myocyte enhancer factors 2C (MEF2C) in mice leads to hypoplasia of the right ventricle. The transcription factor eHAND is expressed in the developing left ventricle and conotruncus and is also critical to their development. How regulation of developmentally coordinated groups of genes is achieved has been the focus of recent research. One mechanism is through the expression of small noncoding RNAs known as microRNAs, each of which regulate the expression of multiple target genes. Another is through modifications in chromatin, the DNA scaffolding which acts as a controller of gene expression. Chromatin remodeling mediated by factors such as Brg1, Chd7, histone demethylases, and methyltransferases is associated with cardiac developmental defects.

420.2 Cardiac Looping
Daniel Bernstein

At approximately 22-24 days, the heart tube begins to bend ventrally and toward the right (see Fig. 420-1). The heart is the first organ to escape from the bilateral symmetry of the early embryo. Looping brings the future left ventricle leftward and in continuity with the sinus venosus (future left and right atria), whereas the future right ventricle is shifted rightward and in continuity with the truncus arteriosus (future aorta and pulmonary artery). This pattern of development explains the relatively common occurrence of the cardiac anomalies double-outlet right ventricle and double-inlet left ventricle and the extreme rarity of double-outlet left ventricle and double-inlet right ventricle (see Chapter 430.5). When cardiac looping is abnormal (situs inversus, heterotaxia), the incidence of serious cardiac malformations is high and there are usually associated abnormalities in the left-right (L-R) patterning of the lungs and abdominal viscera.

Potential mechanisms of cardiac looping include differential growth rates for myocytes on the convex vs the concave surface of the curve, differential rates of programmed cell death (apoptosis), and mechanical forces generated within myocardial cells via their actin cytoskeleton. The signal for this directionality is contained in a concentration gradient between the right and left sides of the embryo in the expression of critical signaling molecules. A number of signaling

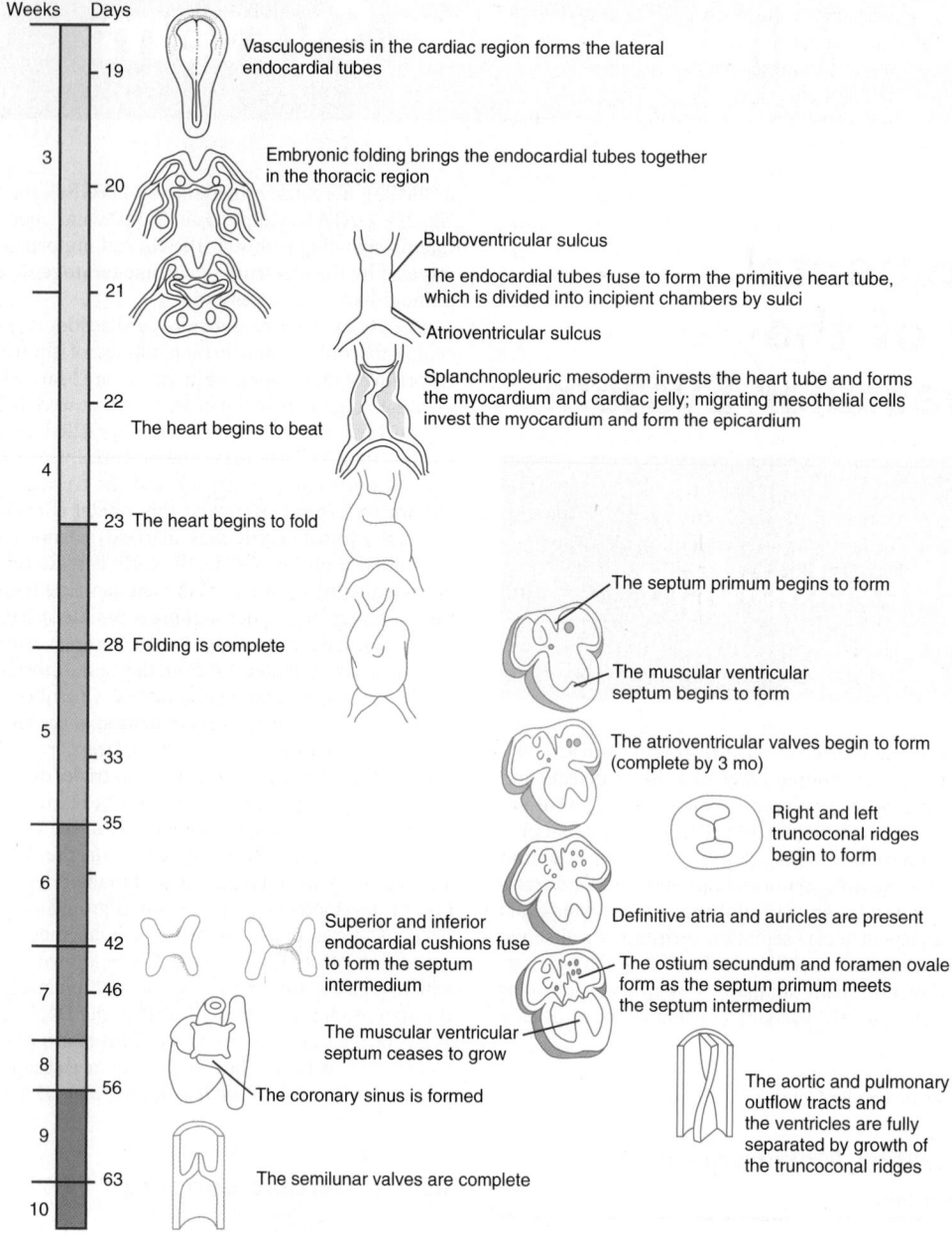

Weeks   Days

19   Vasculogenesis in the cardiac region forms the lateral endocardial tubes

3

20   Embryonic folding brings the endocardial tubes together in the thoracic region

21   Bulboventricular sulcus
The endocardial tubes fuse to form the primitive heart tube, which is divided into incipient chambers by sulci
Atrioventricular sulcus

22   Splanchnopleuric mesoderm invests the heart tube and forms the myocardium and cardiac jelly; migrating mesothelial cells invest the myocardium and form the epicardium
The heart begins to beat

4

23   The heart begins to fold

The septum primum begins to form

28   Folding is complete
The muscular ventricular septum begins to form

5

33   The atrioventricular valves begin to form (complete by 3 mo)

35   Right and left truncoconal ridges begin to form

6

Definitive atria and auricles are present

42   Superior and inferior endocardial cushions fuse to form the septum intermedium
The ostium secundum and foramen ovale form as the septum primum meets the septum intermedium

7   46

The muscular ventricular septum ceases to grow

8

56   The coronary sinus is formed
The aortic and pulmonary outflow tracts and the ventricles are fully separated by growth of the truncoconal ridges

9

63   The semilunar valves are complete

10

TIMELINE. FORMATION OF THE HEART.

Figure 420-1 Timeline of cardiac morphogenesis. *(From Larsen WJ: Essentials of human embryology, New York, 1998, Churchill Livingstone.)*

pathways have been identified as regulators of this L-R asymmetry, including sonic hedgehog (SHH), transforming growth factor-β, nodal, and LR dynein. Interestingly, mice in which the LR dynein gene has been inactivated display random L-R orientation of the heart and abdominal viscera, with 50% of their hearts looping to the right and 50% looping to the left.

420.3 Cardiac Septation
Daniel Bernstein

When looping is complete, the external appearance of the heart is similar to that of a mature heart; internally, the structure resembles a single tube, although it now has several bulges resulting in the appearance of primitive chambers. The common atrium (comprising both the right and left atria) is connected to the primitive ventricle (future left

ventricle) via the atrioventricular canal. The primitive ventricle is connected to the bulbus cordis (future right ventricle) via the bulboventricular foramen. The distal portion of the bulbus cordis is connected to the truncus arteriosus via an outlet segment (the conus).

The heart tube now consists of several layers of myocardium and a single layer of endocardium separated by cardiac jelly, an acellular extracellular matrix secreted by the myocardium. Septation of the heart begins at approximately day 26 with the ingrowth of large tissue masses, the endocardial cushions, at both the atrioventricular and conotruncal junctions (see Fig. 420-1). These cushions consist of protrusions of cardiac jelly, which, in addition to their role in development, also serve a physiologic function as primitive heart valves. Endocardial cells dedifferentiate and migrate into the cardiac jelly in the region of the endocardial cushions, eventually becoming mesenchymal cells that will form part of the atrioventricular valves.

Complete septation of the atrioventricular canal occurs with fusion of the endocardial cushions. Most of the atrioventricular valve tissue is derived from the ventricular myocardium in a process involving undermining of the ventricular walls. Because this process occurs asymmetrically, the tricuspid valve annulus sits closer to the apex of the heart than the mitral valve annulus does. Physical separation of these 2 valves produces the atrioventricular septum, the absence of which is the primary common defect in patients with **atrioventricular canal defects** (see Chapter 426.5). If the process of undermining is incomplete, the right atrioventricular valve may not separate normally from the ventricular myocardium, a possible cause of **Ebstein anomaly** (see Chapter 430.7).

Septation of the atria begins at ≈30 days with growth of the septum primum downward toward the endocardial cushions (see Fig. 420-1). The orifice that remains is the ostium primum. The endocardial cushions then fuse and, together with the completed septum primum, divide the atrioventricular canal into right and left segments. A 2nd opening appears in the posterior portion of the septum primum, the ostium secundum, and it allows a portion of the fetal venous return to the right atrium to pass across to the left atrium. Finally, the septum secundum grows downward, just to the right of the septum primum. Together with a flap of the septum primum, the ostium secundum forms the foramen ovale, through which fetal blood passes from the inferior vena cava to the left atrium (see Chapter 421).

Septation of the ventricles begins at about embryonic day 25 with protrusions of endocardium in both the inlet (primitive ventricle) and outlet (bulbus cordis) segments of the heart. The inlet protrusions fuse into the bulboventricular septum and extend posteriorly toward the inferior endocardial cushion, where they give rise to the inlet and trabecular portions of the interventricular septum. **Ventricular septal defects** can occur in any portion of the developing interventricular septum (see Chapter 426.6). The outlet or conotruncal septum develops from ridges of cardiac jelly, similar to the atrioventricular cushions. These ridges fuse to form a spiral septum that brings the future pulmonary artery into communication with the anterior and rightward right ventricle and the future aorta into communication with the posterior and leftward left ventricle. Differences in cell growth of the outlet

septum lead to lengthening of the segment of smooth muscle beneath the pulmonary valve (conus), a process that separates the tricuspid and pulmonary valves. In contrast, disappearance of the segment beneath the aortic valve leads to fibrous continuity of the mitral and aortic valves. Defects in these processes are responsible for **conotruncal** and **aortic arch defects** (truncus arteriosus, tetralogy of Fallot, pulmonary atresia, double-outlet right ventricle, interrupted aortic arch), a group of cardiac anomalies often associated with deletions of the DiGeorge critical region of chromosome 22q11 (see Chapters 423 and 424). The transcription factor Tbx1 has been implicated as a candidate gene, which may be responsible for DiGeorge syndrome. Several genes have been implicated in valve formation, including *Ptpn11*, which encodes the tyrosine phosphatase Shp-2, and when present in a mutated from is one of the genes responsible for **Noonan syndrome**, associated with pulmonary valve stenosis; and NOTCH1, a regulator of cell differentiation that has been associated with aortic valve disease.

420.4 Aortic Arch Development
Daniel Bernstein

The aortic arch, head and neck vessels, proximal pulmonary arteries, and ductus arteriosus develop from the aortic sac, arterial arches, and dorsal aortae. When the straight heart tube develops, the distal outflow portion bifurcates into the right and left 1st aortic arches, which join the paired dorsal aortae (Fig. 420-2). The dorsal aortae will fuse to form the descending aorta. The proximal aorta from the aortic valve to the left carotid artery arises from the aortic sac. The 1st and 2nd arches largely regress by about 22 days, with the 1st aortic arch giving rise to the maxillary artery and the 2nd to the stapedial and hyoid arteries. The 3rd arches participate in the formation of the innominate artery and the common and internal carotid arteries. The right 4th arch gives rise to the innominate and right subclavian arteries, and the left 4th arch participates in formation of the segment of the aortic arch between

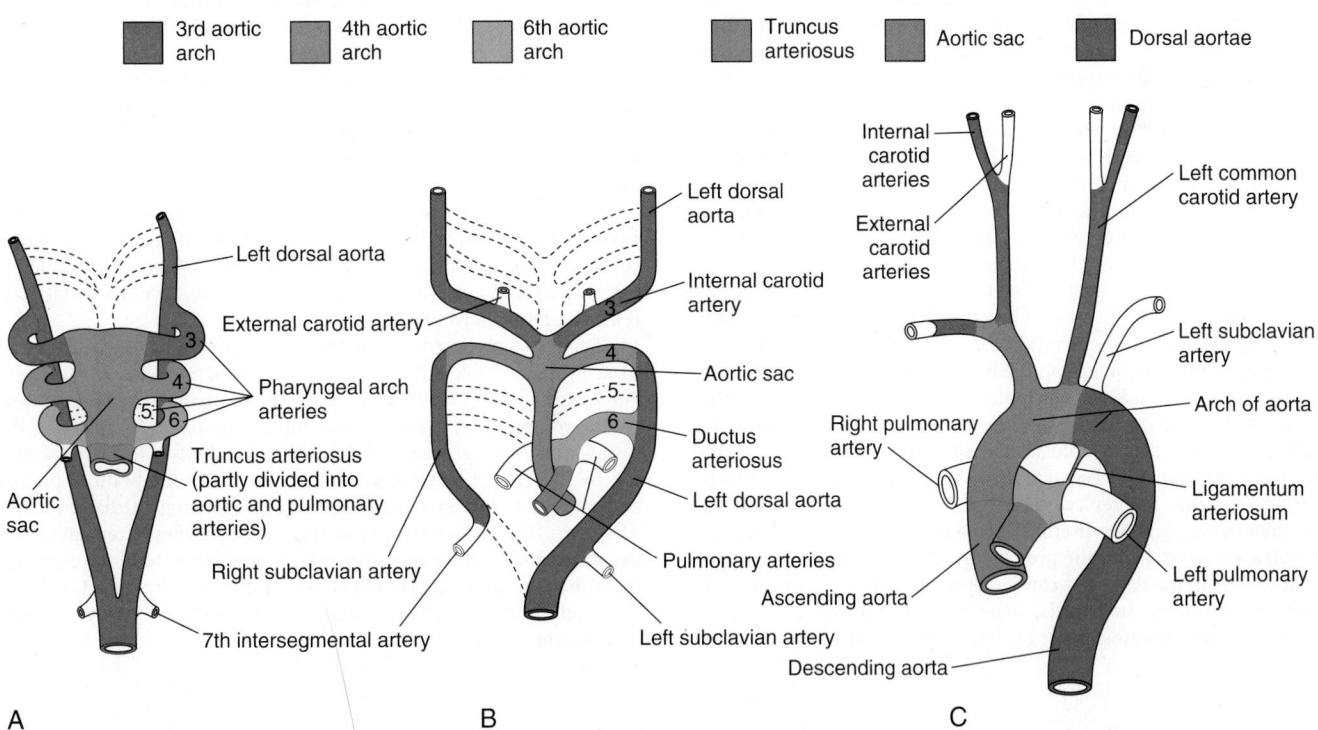

Figure 420-2 Schematic drawings illustrating the changes that result during transformation of the truncus arteriosus, aortic sac, aortic arches, and dorsal aortae into the adult arterial pattern. The vessels that are not shaded or colored are not derived from these structures. **A,** Aortic arches at 6 wk; by this stage the 1st 2 pairs of aortic arches have largely disappeared. **B,** Aortic arches at 7 wk; the parts of the dorsal aortae and aortic arches that normally disappear are indicated by broken lines. **C,** Arterial vessels of a 6 mo old infant. (*From Moore KL, Persaud TVN, Torchia M: The developing human, Philadelphia, 2007, Elsevier.*)

the left carotid artery and the ductus arteriosus. The 5th arch does not persist as a major structure in the mature circulation. The 6th arches join the more distal pulmonary arteries, with the right 6th arch giving rise to a portion of the proximal right pulmonary artery and the left 6th arch giving rise to the ductus arteriosus. The aortic arch between the ductus arteriosus and the left subclavian artery is derived from the left-sided dorsal aorta, whereas the aortic arch distal to the left subclavian artery is derived from the fused right and left dorsal aortae. Abnormalities in development of the paired aortic arches are responsible for **right aortic arch, double aortic arch,** and **vascular rings** (see Chapter 432.1).

420.5 Cardiac Differentiation
Daniel Bernstein

The process by which the totipotential cells of the early embryo become committed to specific cell lineages is differentiation. Precardiac mesodermal cells differentiate into mature cardiac muscle cells with an appropriate complement of cardiac-specific contractile elements, regulatory proteins, receptors, and ion channels. Expression of the contractile protein myosin occurs at an early stage of cardiac development, even before fusion of the bilateral heart primordia. Differentiation in these early mesodermal cells is regulated by signals from the anterior endoderm, a process known as *induction*. Several putative early signaling molecules include fibroblast growth factor, activin, and insulin. Signaling molecules interact with receptors on the cell surface; these receptors activate 2nd messengers, which, in turn, activate specific nuclear transcription factors (GATA-4, MEF2, Nkx, bHLH, and the retinoic acid receptor family) that induce the expression of specific gene products to regulate cardiac differentiation. Some of the primary disorders of cardiac muscle, the **cardiomyopathies,** may be related to defects in some of these signaling molecules (see Chapter 439).

Developmental processes are chamber specific. Early in development, ventricular myocytes express both ventricular and atrial isoforms of several proteins, such as atrial natriuretic peptide (ANP) and myosin light chain (MLC). Mature ventricular myocytes do not express ANP and express only a ventricular-specific MLC 2v isoform, whereas mature atrial myocytes express ANP and an atrial-specific MLC 2a isoform. Heart failure (see Chapter 442), volume overload (see Chapters 426 and 428), and pressure overload hypertrophy (see Chapter 427) are associated with a recapitulation of fetal cell phenotypes in which mature myocytes reexpress fetal proteins. Because different isoforms have different contractile behavior (fast vs. slow activation, high vs. low adenosine triphosphatase activity), expression of different isoforms may have important functional consequences.

The extent to which stem cells can be made to differentiate into cardiac muscle cells is the focus of investigation in the field of regenerative cardiology. The demonstration that fully differentiated adult cells (e.g., skin fibroblasts or peripheral blood mononuclear cells) can be *reprogrammed* into induced pluripotential stem cells and then *differentiated* into beating cardiomyocytes in vitro, has opened up many new avenues to study cardiovascular disease. Some investigators believe that there are precursor cells (cardiac stem cells) resident within the myocardium that can replace damaged myocytes, although at a rate too slow to be clinically useful. Scientists are working on trying to stimulate these cells with the proper regulatory factors, thus inducing them to regenerate damaged cardiac muscle. Others are investigating whether circulating stem cells, bone marrow–derived cells, or the factors they secrete can support cardiac regeneration. Eventually, stem

cells grown on biomechanical scaffolds may be used to build a replacement ventricle for patients with hypoplastic left or right heart.

420.6 Developmental Changes in Cardiac Function
Daniel Bernstein

During development, the composition of the myocardium undergoes profound changes that result in an increase in the number and size of myocytes. During prenatal life, this process involves myocyte division (hyperplasia), whereas after the 1st few postnatal weeks, subsequent cardiac growth occurs mostly by an increase in myocyte size (hypertrophy). The myocytes themselves change shape from round to cylindrical, the proportion of myofibrils (which contain the contractile apparatus) increases, and the myofibrils become more regular in their orientation.

The plasma membrane (known as the *sarcolemma* in myocytes) is the location of the ion channels and transmembrane receptors that regulate the exchange of chemical information from the cell surface to the cell interior. Ion fluxes through these channels control the processes of depolarization and repolarization. Developmental changes have been described for the sodium-potassium pump, the sodium-hydrogen exchanger, and voltage-dependent calcium channels. As the myocyte matures, extensions of the sarcolemma develop toward the interior of the cell (the t-tubule system), which dramatically increases its surface area and enhances rapid activation of the myocyte. Regulation of the membrane's α- and β-adrenergic receptors with development enhances the ability of the sympathetic nervous system to control cardiac function as the heart matures.

The sarcoplasmic reticulum (SR), a series of tubules surrounding the myofibrils, controls the intracellular calcium concentration. A series of pumps regulate calcium release to the myofibrils for initiation of contraction (ryanodine-sensitive calcium channel) and calcium uptake for initiation of relaxation (adenosine triphosphate–dependent SR calcium pump). In immature hearts, this SR calcium transport system is less well developed, and such hearts consequently have an increased dependence on transport of calcium from outside the cell for contraction. In a mature heart, the majority of the calcium to activate contraction comes from the SR. This developmental phenomenon may explain the sensitivity of the infant heart to sarcolemmal calcium channel blockers such as verapamil, which can result in a marked depression in contractility (see Chapter 435).

The major contractile proteins (myosin, actin, tropomyosin, and troponin) are organized into the functional unit of cardiac contraction, the sarcomere. Each has several isoforms that are expressed differentially by location (atrium vs. ventricle) and by developmental stage (embryo, fetus, newborn, adult).

Changes in myocardial structure and myocyte biochemistry result in easily quantifiable differences in cardiac function with development. Fetal cardiac function is less responsive to changes in both preload (filling volume) and afterload (systemic resistance). The most effective means of increasing ventricular function in a fetus is through increasing the heart rate. After birth and with further maturation, preload and afterload play an increasing role in regulating cardiac function. The rate of cardiac relaxation is also developmentally regulated. The decreased ability of the immature SR calcium pump to remove calcium from the contractile apparatus is manifested as a decreased ability of the fetal heart to enhance relaxation in response to sympathetic stimulation.

Chapter **421**
The Fetal to Neonatal Circulatory Transition

421.1 The Fetal Circulation

Daniel Bernstein

The human fetal circulation and its adjustments after birth are similar to those of other large mammals, although rates of maturation differ. In the fetal circulation, the right and left ventricles exist in a parallel circuit, as opposed to the series circuit of a newborn or adult (Fig. 421-1A). In the fetus, the placenta provides for gas and metabolite exchange. Because the lungs do not provide gas exchange, the pulmonary vessels are vasoconstricted, diverting blood away from the pulmonary circulation. Three cardiovascular structures unique to the fetus are important for maintaining this parallel circulation: the ductus venosus, foramen ovale, and ductus arteriosus.

The placenta is not as efficient an oxygen exchange organ as the lungs, so that umbilical venous Po_2 (the highest level of oxygen provided to the fetus) is only about 30-35 mm Hg. Approximately 50% of the umbilical venous blood enters the hepatic circulation, whereas the rest bypasses the liver and joins the inferior vena cava via the ductus venosus, where it partially mixes with poorly oxygenated inferior vena cava blood derived from the lower part of the fetal body. This combined lower body plus umbilical venous blood flow (Po_2 of ≈26-28 mm Hg) enters the right atrium and is preferentially directed

by a flap of tissue at the right atrial–inferior vena caval junction, the eustachian valve, across the foramen ovale to the left atrium (see Fig. 421-1B). This is the major source of left ventricular blood flow, as pulmonary venous return is minimal. Left ventricular blood is then ejected into the ascending aorta where it supplies predominantly the fetal upper body and brain.

Fetal superior vena cava blood, which is considerably less oxygenated (Po_2 of 12-14 mm Hg), enters the right atrium and preferentially flows across the tricuspid valve, rather than the foramen ovale, into the right ventricle. From the right ventricle, the blood is ejected into the pulmonary artery. Because the pulmonary arterial circulation is vasoconstricted, only approximately 5% of right ventricular outflow enters the lungs. The major portion of this blood bypasses the lungs and flows right-to-left through the ductus arteriosus into the descending aorta to perfuse the lower part of the fetal body, including providing flow to the placenta via the 2 umbilical arteries. Thus, the upper part of the fetal body (including the coronary and cerebral arteries and those to the upper extremities) is perfused exclusively from the left ventricle with blood that has a slightly higher Po_2 than the blood perfusing the lower part of the fetal body, which is derived mostly from the right ventricle. Only a small volume of blood from the ascending aorta (10% of fetal cardiac output) flows all the way around the aortic arch (aortic isthmus) to the descending aorta.

The **total fetal cardiac output**—the combined output of both the left and right ventricles—is ≈450 mL/kg/min. Approximately 65% of descending aortic blood flow returns to the placenta; the remaining 35% perfuses the fetal organs and tissues. In the sheep fetus, where most of these circulatory pathways were studied, right ventricular output is approximately 2 times that of the left ventricle. In the human fetus, which has a larger percentage of blood flow going to the brain, right ventricular output is probably closer to 1.3 times left ventricular flow. Thus, during fetal life the right ventricle is not only pumping against systemic blood pressure but is also performing a greater volume of work than the left ventricle.

It has been postulated that blood flow is an important determinant of growth of fetal cardiac chambers, valves, and blood vessels. Thus, in

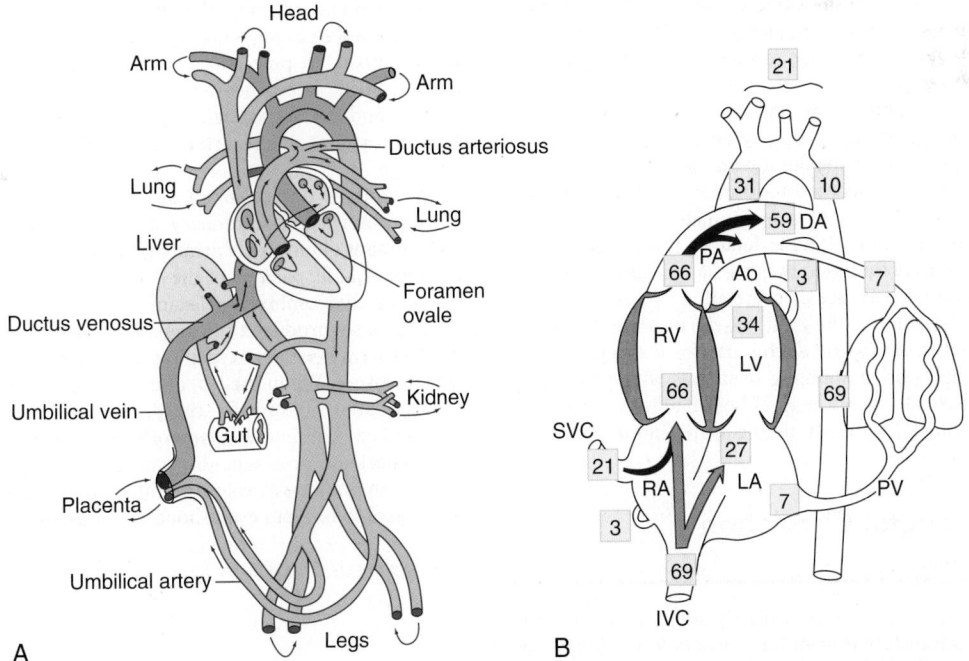

Figure 421-1 A, The human circulation before birth (partly after Dawes). Red indicates more highly oxygenated blood, and arrows indicate the direction of flow. More highly oxygenated blood from the placenta passes through the foramen ovale from the right to the left atrium, thus bypassing the lungs. **B,** Percentages of combined ventricular output that return to the fetal heart, that are ejected by each ventricle, and that flow through the main vascular channels. Figures are those obtained from studies of late-gestation fetal lambs. Ao, aorta; DA, ductus arteriosus; IVC, inferior vena cava; LA, left atrium; LV, left ventricle; PA, pulmonary artery; PV, pulmonary veins; RA, right atrium; RV, right ventricle; SVC, superior vena cava. *(From Rudolph AM: Congenital diseases of the heart, Chicago, 1974, Year Book.)*

the presence of a narrowing (stenosis) of an upstream structure such as the mitral valve, flow downstream into the left ventricle is limited and left ventricular growth may be compromised, leading to hypoplastic left heart syndrome (see Chapter 431.10). Similarly, stenosis of a downstream structure such as the aortic valve can similarly disrupt flow into the left ventricle and lead to hypoplastic left-heart syndrome. Fetal cardiac interventional treatments, currently experimental, are aimed at opening stenotic aortic valves in mid-gestation fetuses, and allowing more normal left ventricular growth.

421.2 The Transitional Circulation
Daniel Bernstein

At birth, mechanical expansion of the lungs and an increase in arterial Po_2 result in a rapid decrease in pulmonary vascular resistance. Concomitantly, removal of the low-resistance placental circulation leads to an increase in systemic vascular resistance. The output from the right ventricle now flows entirely into the pulmonary circulation, and because pulmonary vascular resistance becomes lower than systemic vascular resistance, the shunt through the ductus arteriosus reverses and becomes left to right. In the course of several days, the high arterial Po_2 constricts and eventually closes the ductus arteriosus, which eventually becomes the ligamentum arteriosum. The increased volume of pulmonary blood flow returning to the left atrium from the lungs increases left atrial volume and pressure sufficiently to close the flap of the foramen ovale functionally, although the foramen may remain probe patent for several years.

Removal of the placenta from the circulation also results in closure of the ductus venosus. The left ventricle is now coupled to the high-resistance systemic circulation, and its wall thickness and mass begin to increase. In contrast, the right ventricle is now coupled to the low-resistance pulmonary circulation, and its wall thickness and mass decrease. The left ventricle, which in the fetus pumped blood only to the upper part of the body and brain, must now deliver the entire systemic cardiac output (≈350 mL/kg/min), an almost 200% increase in output. This marked increase in left ventricular performance is achieved through a combination of hormonal and metabolic signals, including an increase in the level of circulating catecholamines and in the density of myocardial β-adrenergic receptors through which catecholamines have their effect.

When congenital structural cardiac defects are superimposed on these dramatic physiologic changes, they often impede this smooth transition and markedly increase the burden on the newborn myocardium. In addition, because the ductus arteriosus and foramen ovale do not close completely at birth, they may remain patent in certain congenital cardiac lesions. Patency of these fetal pathways may either provide a lifesaving pathway for blood to bypass a congenital defect (a patent ductus in pulmonary atresia or coarctation of the aorta or a foramen ovale in transposition of the great vessels) or present an additional stress to the circulation (patent ductus arteriosus in a premature infant, pathway for right-to-left shunting in infants with pulmonary hypertension). Therapeutic agents may either maintain these fetal pathways (prostaglandin E_1) or hasten their closure (indomethacin).

421.3 The Neonatal Circulation
Daniel Bernstein

At birth, the fetal circulation must immediately adapt to extrauterine life as gas exchange is transferred from the placenta to the lungs (see Chapter 101.1). Some of these changes are virtually instantaneous with the first breath, whereas others develop over a period of hours or weeks. With the onset of ventilation, pulmonary vascular resistance is markedly decreased as a consequence of both active (Po_2-related) and passive (mechanical related) pulmonary vasodilation. In a normal neonate, closure of the ductus arteriosus and the fall in pulmonary

vascular resistance decreases pulmonary arterial and right ventricular pressures. The largest decline in pulmonary resistance from the high fetal levels to the low "adult" levels in the human infant at sea level usually occurs within the 1st 2-3 days but may be prolonged for 7 days or more. Over the next several weeks of life, pulmonary vascular resistance decreases even further, secondary to a remodeling of the pulmonary vasculature, including thinning of the vascular smooth muscle and recruitment of new vessels. This decrease in pulmonary vascular resistance significantly influences the timing of the clinical appearance of many congenital heart lesions that are dependent on the relative levels of systemic and pulmonary vascular resistances. The left-to-right shunt through an large ventricular septal defect may be minimal in the 1st wk after birth when pulmonary vascular resistance is still high. As pulmonary resistance decreases in the next week or 2, the volume of the left-to-right shunt through the ventricular septal defect increases and eventually leads to symptoms of heart failure within the 1st mo or 2 of life.

Significant differences between the neonatal circulation and that of older infants include: (1) right-to-left or left-to-right shunting may persist across the patent foramen ovale; (2) in the presence of cardiopulmonary disease, continued patency of the ductus arteriosus may allow left-to-right, right-to-left, or bidirectional shunting; (3) the neonatal pulmonary vasculature constricts more vigorously in response to hypoxemia, hypercapnia, and acidosis; (4) the wall thickness and muscle mass of the neonatal left and right ventricles are almost equal; and (5) newborn infants at rest have relatively high oxygen consumption, which is associated with relatively high cardiac output. The newborn cardiac output (approximately 350 mL/kg/min) falls in the 1st 2 mo of life to approximately 150 mL/kg/min and then more gradually to the normal adult cardiac output of approximately 75 mL/kg/min. Although fetal hemoglobin is beneficial to delivery of oxygen in the low Po_2 fetal circulation, the high percentage of fetal hemoglobin present in the newborn may actually interfere with delivery of oxygen to tissues in the high systemic Po_2 neonatal circulation (see Chapter 101.1).

The foramen ovale is usually functionally closed by the 3rd mo of life, although it is possible to pass a probe through the overlapping flaps in a large percentage of children and in 15-25% of adults. Functional closure of the ductus arteriosus is usually complete by 10-15 hr in a normal neonate, although the ductus may remain patent much longer in the presence of congenital heart disease, especially when associated with cyanosis. In premature newborn infants, an evanescent systolic murmur with late accentuation or a continuous murmur may be audible, and in the context of respiratory distress syndrome, the presence of a patent ductus arteriosus should be suspected (see Chapter 101.3).

The normal ductus arteriosus differs morphologically from the adjoining aorta and pulmonary artery in that the ductus has a significant amount of circularly arranged smooth muscle in its medial layer. During fetal life, patency of the ductus arteriosus appears to be maintained by the combined relaxant effects of low oxygen tension and endogenously produced prostaglandins, specifically prostaglandin E_2. In a full-term neonate, oxygen is the most important factor controlling ductal closure. When the Po_2 of the blood passing through the ductus reaches about 50 mm Hg, the ductal wall begins to constrict. The effects of oxygen on ductal smooth muscle may be direct or mediated by its effects on prostaglandin synthesis. Gestational age also appears to play an important role; the ductus of a premature infant is less responsive to oxygen, even though its musculature is developed.

Bibliography is available at Expert Consult.

421.4 Persistent Pulmonary Hypertension of the Neonate (Persistence of Fetal Circulatory Pathways)

See Chapter 101.7.

Section **2**
Evaluation of the Cardiovascular System

Chapter **422**
History and Physical Examination
Daniel Bernstein

The importance of the history and physical examination cannot be overemphasized in the evaluation of infants and children with suspected cardiovascular disorders. Patients may require further laboratory evaluation and eventual treatment, or the family may be reassured that no significant problem exists. Although the ready availability of echocardiography may entice the clinician to skip these preliminary steps, an initial evaluation by a skilled cardiologist is preferred for several reasons: (1) a cardiac examination allows the cardiologist to guide the echocardiographic evaluation toward confirming or eliminating specific diagnoses, thereby increasing its accuracy; (2) because most childhood murmurs are innocent, evaluation by a pediatric cardiologist can eliminate unnecessary and expensive laboratory tests; and (3) the cardiologist's knowledge and experience are important in reassuring the patient's family and preventing unnecessary restrictions on healthy physical activity. An experienced pediatric cardiologist can differentiate an innocent murmur from serious congenital heart disease by history and physical alone with a high sensitivity and specificity.

HISTORY

A comprehensive cardiac history starts with details of the perinatal period including the presence of cyanosis, respiratory distress, or prematurity. Maternal complications such as gestational diabetes, teratogenic medications, systemic lupus erythematosus, or substance abuse can be associated with cardiac problems. If cardiac symptoms began during infancy, the timing of the initial symptoms should be noted to provide important clues about the specific cardiac condition.

Many of the symptoms of **heart failure** in infants and children are age specific. In infants, feeding difficulties are common. Inquiry should be made about the frequency of feeding and either the volume of each feeding or the time spent on each breast. An infant with heart failure often takes less volume per feeding and becomes dyspneic or diaphoretic while sucking. After falling asleep exhausted, the baby, inadequately fed, will awaken for the next feeding after a brief time. This cycle continues around the clock and must be carefully differentiated from colic or other feeding disorders. Additional symptoms and signs include those of respiratory distress: rapid breathing, nasal flaring, cyanosis, and chest retractions. In older children, heart failure may be manifested as exercise intolerance, difficulty keeping up with peers during sports or the need for a nap after coming home from school, poor growth, or chronic abdominal complaints. Eliciting a history of fatigue in an older child requires questions about age-specific activities, including stair climbing, walking, bicycle riding, physical education class, and competitive sports; information should be obtained regarding more severe manifestations such as orthopnea and nocturnal dyspnea.

Cyanosis at rest is often overlooked by parents; it may be mistaken for a normal individual variation in color. Cyanosis during crying or exercise, however, is more often noted as abnormal by observant

parents. Many infants and toddlers turn "blue around the lips" when crying vigorously or during breath-holding spells; this condition must be carefully differentiated from cyanotic heart disease by inquiring about inciting factors, the length of episodes, and whether the tongue and mucous membranes also appear cyanotic. Newborns often have cyanosis of their extremities (acrocyanosis) when undressed and cold; this response to cold must be carefully differentiated from true cyanosis, where the mucous membranes are also blue.

Chest pain is an unusual manifestation of cardiac disease in pediatric patients, although it is a frequent cause for referral to a pediatric cardiologist, especially in adolescents. Nonetheless, a careful history, physical examination, and, if indicated, laboratory or imaging tests will assist in identifying the cause of chest pain (Table 422-1). For patients with some forms of repaired congenital heart disease or those with a

Table 422-1	Differential Diagnosis of Chest Pain in Pediatric Patients

MUSCULOSKELETAL (COMMON)
Trauma (accidental, abuse)
Exercise, overuse injury (strain, bursitis)
Costochondritis (Tietze syndrome)
Herpes zoster (cutaneous)
Pleurodynia
Fibrositis
Slipping rib
Precordial catch
Sickle cell anemia vasoocclusive crisis
Osteomyelitis (rare)
Primary or metastatic tumor (rare)

PULMONARY (COMMON)
Pneumonia
Pleurisy
Asthma
Chronic cough
Pneumothorax
Infarction (sickle cell anemia)
Foreign body
Embolism (rare)
Pulmonary hypertension (rare)
Tumor (rare)
Bronchiectasis

GASTROINTESTINAL (LESS COMMON)
Esophagitis (gastroesophageal reflux, infectious, pill)
Esophageal foreign body
Esophageal spasm
Cholecystitis
Subdiaphragmatic abscess
Perihepatitis (Fitz-Hugh-Curtis syndrome)
Peptic ulcer disease
Pancreatitis

CARDIAC (LESS COMMON)
Pericarditis
Postpericardiotomy syndrome
Endocarditis
Cardiomyopathy
Mitral valve prolapse
Aortic or subaortic stenosis
Arrhythmias
Marfan syndrome (dissecting aortic aneurysm)
Kawasaki disease
Cocaine, sympathomimetic ingestion
Angina (familial hypercholesterolemia, anomalous coronary artery)

IDIOPATHIC (COMMON)
Anxiety, hyperventilation
Panic disorder

OTHER (LESS COMMON)
Spinal cord or nerve root compression
Breast-related pathologic condition (mastalgia)
Castleman disease (lymph node neoplasm)

history of Kawasaki disease (see Chapter 444.1), however, chest pain should be evaluated carefully for a coronary etiology.

Cardiac disease may be a manifestation of a known congenital malformation syndrome with typical physical findings (Table 422-2) or a manifestation of a generalized disorder affecting the heart and other organ systems (Table 422-3). Extracardiac malformations may be noted in 20-45% of infants with congenital heart disease. Between 5% and 10% of patients have a known chromosomal abnormality; the importance of genetic evaluation will increase as our knowledge of specific gene defects linked to congenital heart disease increases.

A careful family history may also reveal early (at age <50 yr) coronary artery disease or stroke (suggestive of familial hypercholesterolemia or thrombophilia), sudden death (suggestive of cardiomyopathy or familial arrhythmic disorder), generalized muscle disease (suggestive of 1 of the muscular dystrophies, dermatomyositis, or familial or metabolic cardiomyopathy), or 1st-degree relatives with congenital heart disease.

GENERAL PHYSICAL EXAMINATION

A general assessment of the patient is always the first part of the examination, with specific attention directed toward the presence of cyanosis, abnormalities in growth, chest wall abnormalities, and any evidence of respiratory distress. Although the murmur may be the most prominent part of the overall examination, any murmur must be placed in context of other physical findings. Frequently, associated findings, such as the quality of the pulses, the presence of a ventricular heave or thrill, or the splitting of the second heart sound, provide important clues to a specific cardiac diagnosis.

Accurate measurement of height and weight and plotting on a standard growth chart are important because both cardiac failure and chronic cyanosis can result in **failure to thrive.** Growth failure is manifested predominantly by poor weight gain; if length or head circumference is also affected, additional congenital malformations or metabolic disorders should be suspected.

Mild cyanosis may be too subtle for early detection, and clubbing of the fingers and toes is not usually manifested until late in the 1st yr of life, even in the presence of severe arterial oxygen desaturation. **Cyanosis** is best observed over the nail beds, lips, tongue, and mucous membranes. Differential cyanosis, manifested as blue lower extremities and pink upper extremities (usually the right arm), is seen with right-to-left shunting across a ductus arteriosus in the presence of coarctation or an interrupted aortic arch. Circumoral cyanosis or blueness around the forehead may be the result of prominent venous plexuses in these areas, rather than decreased arterial oxygen saturation. The extremities of infants often turn blue when the infant is unwrapped and cold (acrocyanosis), and this condition can be distinguished from central cyanosis by examination of the tongue and mucous membranes.

Heart failure in infants and children usually results in some degree of hepatomegaly and occasionally splenomegaly. The sites of **peripheral** edema are age dependent. In infants, edema is usually seen around the eyes and over the flanks, especially on initially waking. Older children and teenagers manifest both periorbital edema and pedal edema. A not uncommon initial complaint in these older patients is that their clothes no longer fit.

The heart rate of newborn infants is rapid and subject to wide fluctuations (Table 422-4). The average rate ranges from 120-140 beats/min and may increase to 170+ beats/min during crying and activity or drop to 70-90 beats/min during sleep. As the child grows older, the average pulse rate decreases and may be as low as 40 beats/min at rest in athletic adolescents. Persistent tachycardia (>200 beats/min in neonates, 150 beats/min in infants, or 120 beats/min in older children), bradycardia, or an irregular heartbeat other than sinus arrhythmia requires investigation to exclude pathologic arrhythmias (see Chapter 435). Sinus arrhythmia can usually be distinguished by the rhythmic nature of the heart rate variations, occurring in concert with the respiratory cycle, and with a P wave before every QRS complex.

Careful evaluation of the character of the **pulses** is an important early step in the physical diagnosis of congenital heart disease. A wide pulse pressure with bounding pulses may suggest an aortic runoff lesion such as patent ductus arteriosus, aortic insufficiency, an arterial-venous communication, or increased cardiac output secondary to anemia, anxiety, or conditions associated with increased catecholamine or thyroid hormone secretion. The presence of diminished pulses in all extremities is associated with pericardial tamponade, left ventricular outflow obstruction, or cardiomyopathy. The radial and femoral pulses should always be palpated simultaneously. Normally, the femoral pulse should be appreciated immediately before the radial pulse. In infants with coarctation of the aorta, the femoral pulses may be decreased. However, in older children with coarctation of the aorta, blood flow to the descending aorta may channel through collateral vessels and results in the femoral pulse being palpable but delayed until after the radial pulse (**radial-femoral delay**).

Blood pressure should be measured in the legs as well as in the arms to be certain that coarctation of the aorta is not overlooked. Palpation of the femoral or dorsalis pedis pulse, or both, is not reliable alone to exclude coarctation. In older children, a mercury sphygmomanometer with a cuff that covers approximately two-thirds of the upper part of the arm or leg may be used for blood pressure measurement. A cuff that is too small results in falsely high readings, whereas a cuff that is too large records slightly decreased pressure. Pediatric clinical facilities should be equipped with 3, 5, 7, 12, and 18 cm cuffs to accommodate the large spectrum of pediatric patient sizes. The 1st Korotkoff sounds indicate systolic pressure. As cuff pressure is slowly decreased, the sounds usually become muffled before they disappear. Diastolic pressure may be recorded when the sounds become muffled (preferred) or when they disappear altogether; the former is usually slightly higher and the latter slightly lower than true diastolic pressure. For lower-extremity blood pressure determination, the stethoscope is placed over the popliteal artery. Ordinarily, the pressure recorded in the legs with the cuff technique is approximately 10 mm Hg higher than that in the arms.

In infants, blood pressure can be determined by auscultation, palpation, or an oscillometric (Dinamap) device that, when properly used, provides accurate measurements in infants as well as older children.

Blood pressure varies with the age of the child and is closely related to height and weight. Significant increases occur during adolescence, and many temporary variations take place before the more stable levels of adult life are attained. Exercise, excitement, coughing, crying, and struggling may raise the systolic pressure of infants and children as much as 40-50 mm Hg greater than their usual levels. Variability in blood pressure in children of approximately the same age and body build should be expected, and serial measurements should always be obtained when evaluating a patient with hypertension (Figs. 422-1 and 422-2).

Although of little use in infants, in cooperative older children, inspection of the **jugular venous pulse** wave provides information about central venous and right atrial pressure. The neck veins should be inspected with the patient sitting at a 90-degree angle. The external jugular vein should not be visible above the clavicles unless central venous pressure is elevated. Increased venous pressure transmitted to the internal jugular vein may appear as venous pulsations without visible distention; such pulsation is not seen in normal children reclining at an angle of 45 degrees. Because the great veins are in direct communication with the right atrium, changes in pressure and the volume of this chamber are also transmitted to the veins. The 1 exception occurs in superior vena cava obstruction, in which venous pulsatility is lost.

CARDIAC EXAMINATION

The heart should be examined in a systematic manner, starting with inspection and palpation. A **precordial bulge** to the left of the sternum with increased precordial activity suggests cardiac enlargement; such bulges can often best be appreciated by having the child lay supine with the examiner looking up from the child's feet. A **substernal thrust** indicates the presence of right ventricular enlargement, whereas an apical heave is noted with left ventricular enlargement. A hyperdynamic precordium suggests a volume load such as that found with a large left-to-right shunt, although it may be normal in a thin patient.

Table 422-2 | Congenital Malformation Syndromes Associated with Congenital Heart Disease

SYNDROME	FEATURES
CHROMOSOMAL DISORDERS	
Trisomy 21 (Down syndrome)	Endocardial cushion defect, VSD, ASD
Trisomy 21p (cat eye syndrome)	Miscellaneous, total anomalous pulmonary venous return
Trisomy 18	VSD, ASD, PDA, coarctation of aorta, bicuspid aortic or pulmonary valve
Trisomy 13	VSD, ASD, PDA, coarctation of aorta, bicuspid aortic or pulmonary valve
Trisomy 9	Miscellaneous
XXXXY	PDA, ASD
Penta X	PDA, VSD
Triploidy	VSD, ASD, PDA
XO (Turner syndrome)	Bicuspid aortic valve, coarctation of aorta
Fragile X	Mitral valve prolapse, aortic root dilatation
Duplication 3q2	Miscellaneous
Deletion 4p	VSD, PDA, aortic stenosis
Deletion 9p	Miscellaneous
Deletion 5p (cri du chat syndrome)	VSD, PDA, ASD
Deletion 10q	VSD, TOF, conotruncal lesions*
Deletion 13q	VSD
Deletion 18q	VSD
SYNDROME COMPLEXES	
CHARGE association (coloboma, heart, atresia choanae, retardation, genital, and ear anomalies)	VSD, ASD, PDA, TOF, endocardial cushion defect
DiGeorge sequence, CATCH 22 (cardiac defects, abnormal facies, thymic aplasia, cleft palate, and hypocalcemia)	Aortic arch anomalies, conotruncal anomalies
Alagille syndrome (arteriohepatic dysplasia)	Peripheral pulmonic stenosis, PS, TOF
VATER association (vertebral, anal, tracheoesophageal, radial, and renal anomalies)	VSD, TOF, ASD, PDA
FAVS (facioauriculovertebral spectrum)	TOF, VSD
CHILD (congenital hemidysplasia with ichthyosiform erythroderma, limb defects)	Miscellaneous
Mulibrey nanism (muscle, liver, brain, eye)	Pericardial thickening, constrictive pericarditis
Asplenia syndrome	Complex cyanotic heart lesions with decreased pulmonary blood flow, transposition of great arteries, anomalous pulmonary venous return, dextrocardia, single ventricle, single atrioventricular valve
Polysplenia syndrome	Acyanotic lesions with increased pulmonary blood flow, azygos continuation of inferior vena cava, partial anomalous pulmonary venous return, dextrocardia, single ventricle, common atrioventricular valve
PHACE syndrome (posterior brain fossa anomalies, facial hemangiomas, arterial anomalies, cardiac anomalies and aortic coarctation, eye anomalies)	VSD, PDA, coarctation of aorta, arterial aneurysms
TERATOGENIC AGENTS	
Congenital rubella	PDA, peripheral pulmonic stenosis
Fetal hydantoin syndrome	VSD, ASD, coarctation of aorta, PDA
Fetal alcohol syndrome	ASD, VSD
Fetal valproate effects	Coarctation of aorta, hypoplastic left side of heart, aortic stenosis, pulmonary atresia, VSD
Maternal phenylketonuria	VSD, ASD, PDA, coarctation of aorta
Retinoic acid embryopathy	Conotruncal anomalies
OTHERS	
Apert syndrome	VSD
Autosomal dominant polycystic kidney disease	Mitral valve prolapse
Carpenter syndrome	PDA
Conradi syndrome	VSD, PDA
Crouzon disease	PDA, coarctation of aorta
Cutis laxa	Pulmonary hypertension, pulmonic stenosis
de Lange syndrome	VSD
Ellis–van Creveld syndrome	Single atrium, VSD
Holt-Oram syndrome	ASD, VSD, 1st-degree heart block
Infant of diabetic mother	Hypertrophic cardiomyopathy, VSD, conotruncal anomalies
Kartagener syndrome	Dextrocardia
Meckel-Gruber syndrome	ASD, VSD
Noonan syndrome	Pulmonic stenosis, ASD, cardiomyopathy
Pallister-Hall syndrome	Endocardial cushion defect
Rubinstein-Taybi syndrome	VSD
Scimitar syndrome	Hypoplasia of right lung, anomalous pulmonary venous return to inferior vena cava
Smith-Lemli-Opitz syndrome	VSD, PDA
TAR syndrome (thrombocytopenia and absent radius)	ASD, TOF
Treacher Collins syndrome	VSD, ASD, PDA
Williams syndrome	Supravalvular aortic stenosis, peripheral pulmonic stenosis

ASD, atrial septal defect; AV, aortic valve; PDA, patent ductus arteriosus; PS, pulmonary stenosis; TOF, tetralogy of Fallot; VSD, ventricular septal defect.
*Conotruncal includes TOF, pulmonary atresia, truncus arteriosus, and transposition of great arteries.

Table 422-3	Cardiac Manifestations of Systemic Diseases

SYSTEMIC DISEASE	CARDIAC COMPLICATIONS
INFLAMMATORY DISORDERS	
Sepsis	Hypotension, myocardial dysfunction, pericardial effusion, pulmonary hypertension
Juvenile idiopathic arthritis	Pericarditis, rarely myocarditis
Systemic lupus erythematosus	Pericarditis, Libman-Sacks endocarditis, coronary arteritis, coronary atherosclerosis (with steroids), congenital heart block
Scleroderma	Pulmonary hypertension, myocardial fibrosis, cardiomyopathy
Dermatomyositis	Cardiomyopathy, arrhythmias, heart block
Kawasaki disease	Coronary artery aneurysm and thrombosis, myocardial infarction, myocarditis, valvular insufficiency
Sarcoidosis	Granuloma, fibrosis, amyloidosis, biventricular hypertrophy, arrhythmias
Lyme disease	Arrhythmias, myocarditis
Löffler hypereosinophilic syndrome	Endomyocardial disease
INBORN ERRORS OF METABOLISM	
Refsum disease	Arrhythmia, sudden death
Hunter or Hurler syndrome	Valvular insufficiency, heart failure, hypertension
Fabry disease	Mitral insufficiency, coronary artery disease with myocardial infarction
Glycogen storage disease IIa (Pompe disease)	Short P-R interval, cardiomegaly, heart failure, arrhythmias
Carnitine deficiency	Heart failure, cardiomyopathy
Gaucher disease	Pericarditis
Homocystinuria	Coronary thrombosis
Alkaptonuria	Atherosclerosis, valvular disease
Morquio-Ullrich syndrome	Aortic incompetence
Scheie syndrome	Aortic incompetence
CONNECTIVE TISSUE DISORDERS	
Arterial calcification of infancy	Calcinosis of coronary arteries, aorta
Marfan syndrome	Aortic and mitral insufficiency, dissecting aortic aneurysm, mitral valve prolapse
Congenital contractural arachnodactyly	Mitral insufficiency or prolapse
Ehlers-Danlos syndrome	Mitral valve prolapse, dilated aortic root
Osteogenesis imperfecta	Aortic incompetence
Pseudoxanthoma elasticum	Peripheral arterial disease
NEUROMUSCULAR DISORDERS	
Friedreich ataxia	Cardiomyopathy
Duchenne dystrophy	Cardiomyopathy, heart failure
Tuberous sclerosis	Cardiac rhabdomyoma
Familial deafness	Occasionally arrhythmia, sudden death
Neurofibromatosis	Pulmonic stenosis, pheochromocytoma, coarctation of aorta
Riley-Day syndrome	Episodic hypertension, postural hypotension
Von Hippel–Lindau disease	Hemangiomas, pheochromocytomas
ENDOCRINE-METABOLIC DISORDERS	
Graves disease	Tachycardia, arrhythmias, heart failure
Hypothyroidism	Bradycardia, pericardial effusion, cardiomyopathy, low-voltage electrocardiogram
Pheochromocytoma	Hypertension, myocardial ischemia, myocardial fibrosis, cardiomyopathy
Carcinoid	Right-sided endocardial fibrosis
HEMATOLOGIC DISORDERS	
Sickle cell anemia	High-output heart failure, cardiomyopathy, pulmonary hypertension
Thalassemia major	High-output heart failure, hemochromatosis
Hemochromatosis (1° or 2°)	Cardiomyopathy
OTHERS	
Appetite suppressants (fenfluramine and dexfenfluramine)	Cardiac valvulopathy, pulmonary hypertension
Cockayne syndrome	Atherosclerosis
Familial dwarfism and nevi	Cardiomyopathy
Jervell and Lange-Nielsen syndrome	Prolonged QT interval, sudden death
Kearns-Sayre syndrome	Heart block
LEOPARD syndrome (lentiginosis)	Pulmonic stenosis, prolonged Q-T interval
Progeria	Accelerated atherosclerosis
Osler-Weber-Rendu disease	Arteriovenous fistula (lung, liver, mucous membrane)
Romano-Ward syndrome	Prolonged Q-T interval, sudden death
Weill-Marchesani syndrome	Patent ductus arteriosus
Werner syndrome	Vascular sclerosis, cardiomyopathy

LEOPARD, multiple *lentigines*, electrocardiographic conduction abnormalities, ocular hypertelorism, pulmonary stenosis, abnormal genitals, retardation of growth, sensorineural deafness.

Table 422-4	Pulse Rates at Rest		
AGE	**LOWER LIMITS OF NORMAL (beats/min)**	**AVERAGE (beats/min)**	**UPPER LIMITS OF NORMAL (beats/min)**
Newborn	70	125	190
1–11 mo	80	120	160
2 yr	80	110	130
4 yr	80	100	120
6 yr	75	100	115
8 yr	70	90	110
10 yr	70	90	110

	GIRLS	**BOYS**	**GIRLS**	**BOYS**	**GIRLS**	**BOYS**
12 yr	70	65	90	85	110	105
14 yr	65	60	85	80	105	100
16 yr	60	55	80	75	100	95
18 yr	55	50	75	70	95	90

An overly silent precordium with a barely detectable apical impulse suggests pericardial effusion or severe cardiomyopathy but may be normal in an obese patient.

The relationship of the **apical impulse** to the midclavicular line is also helpful in the estimation of cardiac size: the apical impulse moves laterally and inferiorly with enlargement of the left ventricle. Right-sided apical impulses signify dextrocardia, tension pneumothorax, or left-sided thoracic space-occupying lesions (e.g., diaphragmatic hernia).

Thrills are the palpable equivalent of murmurs and correlate with the area of maximal auscultatory intensity of the murmur. It is important to palpate the suprasternal notch and neck for aortic bruits, which may indicate the presence of aortic stenosis or, when faint, pulmonary stenosis. Right lower sternal border and apical systolic thrills are characteristic of ventricular septal defect and mitral insufficiency, respectively. Diastolic thrills are occasionally palpable in the presence of atrioventricular valve stenosis. The timing and localization of thrills should be carefully noted.

Auscultation is an art that improves with practice. The diaphragm of the stethoscope is placed firmly on the chest for high-pitched sounds; a lightly placed bell is optimal for low-pitched sounds. The physician should initially concentrate on the characteristics of the individual heart sounds and their variation with respirations and later concentrate on murmurs. The patient should be supine, lying quietly, and breathing normally. The **1st heart sound** is best heard at the apex, whereas the **2nd heart sound** should be evaluated at the upper left and right sternal borders. The 1st heart sound is caused by closure of the atrioventricular valves (mitral and tricuspid); the 2nd is caused by closure of the semilunar valves (aortic and pulmonary) (Fig. 422-3). During inspiration, the decrease in intrathoracic pressure results in increased filling of the right side of the heart, which leads to an increased right ventricular ejection time and thus delayed closure of the pulmonary valve; consequently, **splitting of the 2nd heart sound** increases during inspiration and decreases during expiration.

Often, the 2nd heart sound seems to be single during expiration. The presence of a normally split 2nd sound is strong evidence against the diagnosis of atrial septal defect, defects associated with pulmonary arterial hypertension, severe pulmonary valve stenosis, aortic and pulmonary atresia, and truncus arteriosus. Wide splitting is noted in atrial septal defect, pulmonary stenosis, Ebstein anomaly, total anomalous pulmonary venous return, and right bundle branch block. An accentuated pulmonic component of the 2nd sound with narrow splitting is a sign of pulmonary hypertension. A single 2nd sound occurs in pulmonary or aortic atresia or severe stenosis, truncus arteriosus, and, often, transposition of the great arteries.

A **3rd heart sound** is best heard with the bell at the apex in mid-diastole. A **4th sound** occurring in conjunction with atrial contraction may be heard just before the 1st heart sound in late diastole. The 3rd sound may be normal in an adolescent with a relatively slow heart rate, but in a patient with the clinical signs of heart failure and tachycardia, it may be heard as a gallop rhythm and may merge with a 4th heart sound, a finding known as a summation gallop. A gallop rhythm is attributed to poor compliance of the ventricle, and exaggeration of the normal 3rd sound is associated with ventricular filling.

Ejection clicks, which are heard in early systole, are usually caused by a mildly to moderately stenotic aortic or pulmonary valve or to a dilated ascending aorta or pulmonary artery. They are heard so close to the 1st heart sound that they may be mistaken for a split 1st sound. Aortic ejection clicks are best heard at the left middle to right upper sternal border and are constant in intensity. They occur in conditions in which the aortic valve is stenotic or the aorta is dilated (tetralogy of Fallot, truncus arteriosus). Pulmonary ejection clicks, which are associated with mild to moderate pulmonary stenosis, are best heard at the left middle to upper sternal border and vary with respirations, often disappearing with inspiration. Split 1st heart sounds are usually heard best at the lower left sternal border. A midsystolic click heard at the apex, often preceding a late systolic murmur, suggests mitral valve prolapse.

Murmurs should be described according to their intensity, pitch, timing (systolic or diastolic), variation in intensity, time to peak intensity, area of maximal intensity, and radiation to other areas. Auscultation for murmurs should be carried out across the upper precordium, down the left or right sternal border, and out to the apex and left axilla. Auscultation should also always be performed in the right axilla and over both sides of the back. Systolic murmurs are classified as ejection, pansystolic, or late systolic according to the timing of the murmur in relation to the 1st and 2nd heart sounds. The intensity of systolic murmurs is graded from I to VI: I, barely audible; II, medium intensity; III, loud but no thrill; IV, loud with a thrill; V, very loud but still requiring positioning of the stethoscope at least partly on the chest; and VI, so loud that the murmur can be heard with the stethoscope off the chest. In patients who have undergone prior heart surgery, a murmur of grade IV or greater may be heard in the absence of a thrill.

Systolic ejection murmurs start a short time after a well-heard 1st heart sound, increase in intensity, peak, and then decrease in intensity; they usually end before the 2nd sound. In patients with severe pulmonary stenosis, however, the murmur may extend beyond the 1st component of the 2nd sound, thus obscuring it. **Pansystolic or holosystolic murmurs** begin almost simultaneously with the 1st heart sound and continue throughout systole, on occasion becoming gradually decrescendo. It is helpful to remember that after closure of the atrioventricular valves (the 1st heart sound), a brief period occurs during which ventricular pressure increases but the semilunar valves remain closed (isovolumic contraction; see Fig. 422-3). Thus, pansystolic murmurs (heard during both isovolumic contraction and the ejection phases of systole) cannot be caused by flow across the semilunar valves because these valves are closed during isovolumic contraction. Pansystolic murmurs must therefore be related to blood exiting the contracting ventricle via either an abnormal opening (a ventricular septal defect) or atrioventricular (mitral or tricuspid) valve insufficiency. Systolic ejection murmurs usually imply increased flow or stenosis across one of the ventricular outflow tracts (aortic or pulmonic). In infants with rapid heart rates, it is often difficult to distinguish between ejection and pansystolic murmurs. If a clear and distinct 1st heart sound can be appreciated, the murmur is most likely ejection in nature.

A **continuous murmur** is a systolic murmur that continues or "spills" into diastole and indicates continuous flow, such as in the presence of a patent ductus arteriosus or other aortopulmonary communication. This murmur should be differentiated from a to-and-fro murmur, where the systolic component of the murmur ends at or before the 2nd sound and the diastolic murmur begins after semilunar valve closure (aortic or pulmonary stenosis combined with insufficiency). A late systolic murmur begins well beyond the 1st heart sound and continues until the end of systole. Such murmurs may be heard

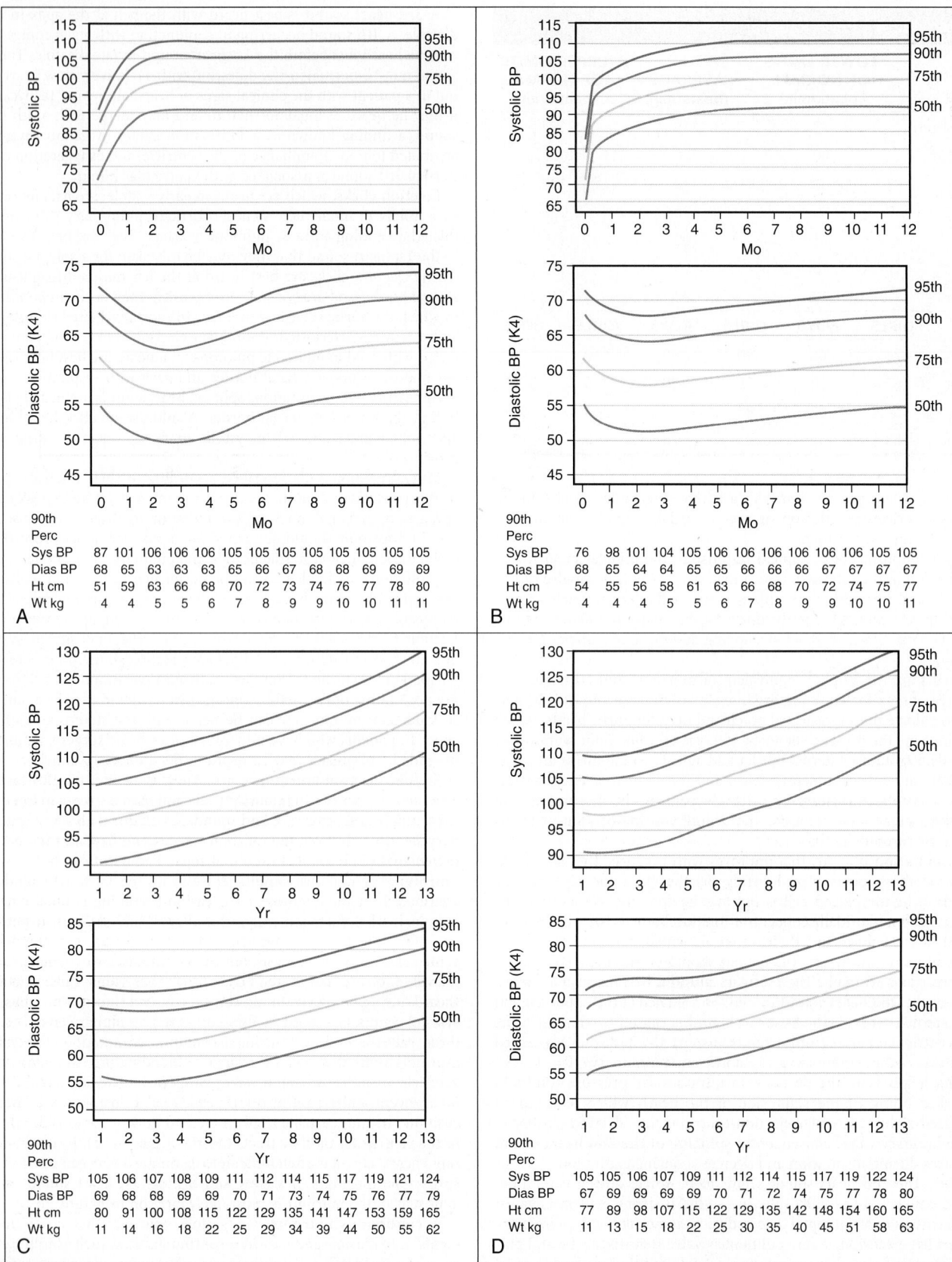

Figure 422-1 A, Age-specific percentiles of blood pressure (BP) measurements in boys from birth to 12 mo of age. **B,** Age-specific percentiles of BP measurements in girls from birth to 12 mo of age. **C,** Age-specific percentiles of BP measurements in boys 1-13 yr of age. **D,** Age-specific percentiles of BP measurements in girls 1-13 yr of age; Korotkoff phase IV (K4) used for diastolic BP. Dias, diastolic; Ht, height; Perc, percentile; Sys, systolic; Wt, weight. *(From Report of the Second Task Force on Blood Pressure Control in Children—1987. National Heart, Lung, and Blood Institute, Bethesda, MD, Pediatrics 79:1–25, 1987. Copyright 1987 by the American Academy of Pediatrics.)*

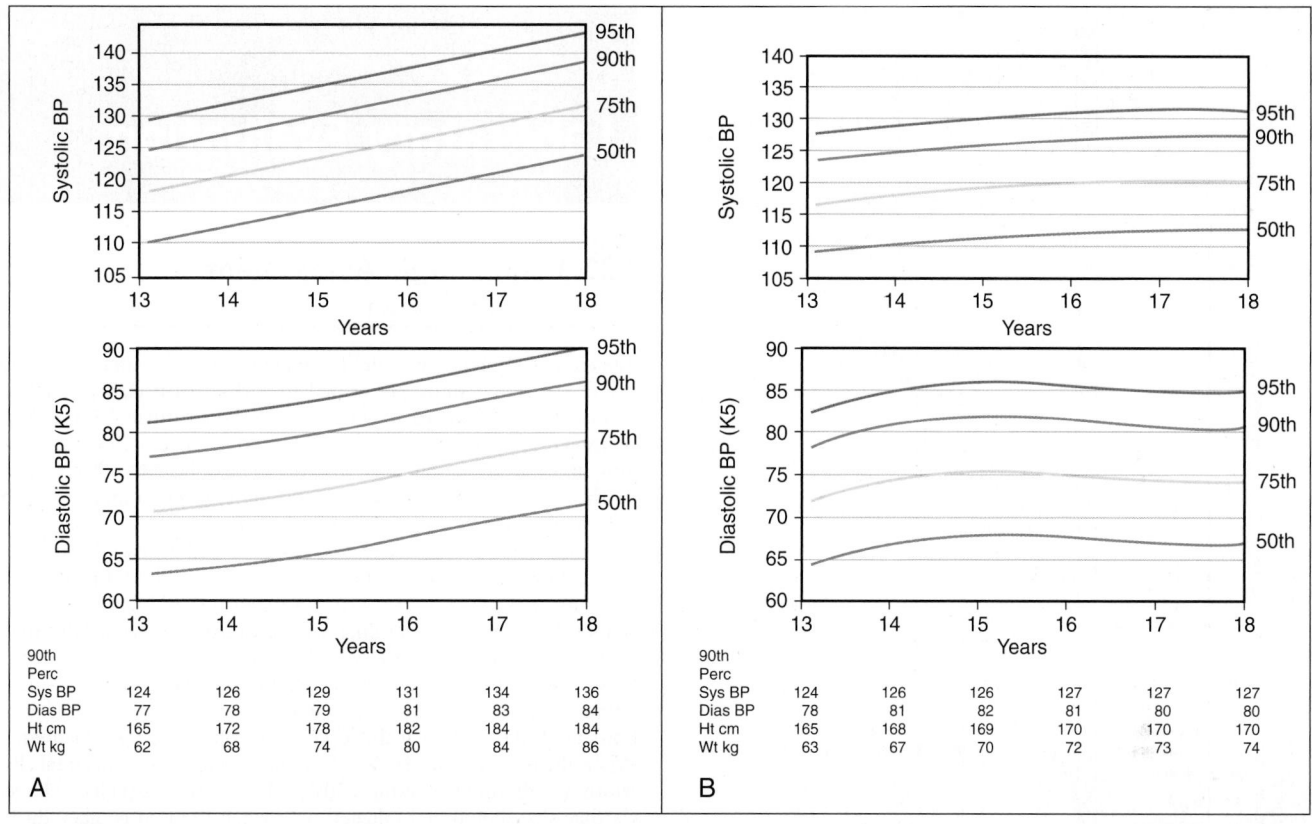

90th Perc						
Sys BP	124	126	129	131	134	136
Dias BP	77	78	79	81	83	84
Ht cm	165	172	178	182	184	184
Wt kg	62	68	74	80	84	86

A

90th Perc						
Sys BP	124	126	126	127	127	127
Dias BP	78	81	82	81	80	80
Ht cm	165	168	169	170	170	170
Wt kg	63	67	70	72	73	74

B

Figure 422-2 **A,** Age-specific percentiles of blood pressure (BP) measurements in boys 13-18 yr of age. **B,** Age-specific percentiles of BP measurements in girls 13-18 yr of age; Korotkoff phase V (K5) used for diastolic BP. Dias, diastolic; Ht, height; Perc, percentile; Sys, systolic; Wt, weight. *(From Report of the Second Task Force on Blood Pressure Control in Children—1987, National Heart, Lung, and Blood Institute, Bethesda, MD, Pediatrics 79:1–25, 1987. Copyright 1987 by the American Academy of Pediatrics.)*

after a midsystolic click in patients with mitral valve prolapse and insufficiency.

Several types of **diastolic murmurs** (graded I-IV) can be identified. A decrescendo diastolic murmur is a blowing murmur along the left sternal border that begins with S_2 and diminishes toward mid-diastole. When high-pitched, this murmur is associated with aortic valve insufficiency or pulmonary insufficiency related to pulmonary hypertension. When low-pitched, this murmur is associated with pulmonary valve insufficiency in the absence of pulmonary hypertension. A low-pitched decrescendo diastolic murmur is typically noted after surgical repair of the pulmonary outflow tract in defects such as tetralogy of Fallot or in patients with absent pulmonary valves. A rumbling mid-diastolic murmur at the left middle and lower sternal border may be due to increased blood flow across the tricuspid valve, such as occurs with an atrial septal defect or, less often, because of actual stenosis of this valve. When this murmur is heard at the apex, it is caused by increased flow across the mitral valve, such as occurs with large left-to-right shunts at the ventricular level (ventricular septal defects), at the great vessel level (patent ductus arteriosus, aortopulmonary shunts), or with increased flow because of mitral insufficiency. When an apical diastolic rumbling murmur is longer and is accentuated at the end of diastole (presystolic), it usually indicates anatomic mitral valve stenosis.

The absence of a precordial murmur does not rule out significant congenital or acquired heart disease. Congenital heart defects, some of which are ductal dependent, may not demonstrate a murmur if the ductus arteriosus closes. These lesions include pulmonary or tricuspid valve atresia and transposition of the great arteries. Murmurs may seem insignificant in patients with severe aortic stenosis, atrial septal defects, anomalous pulmonary venous return, atrioventricular septal defects, coarctation of the aorta, or anomalous insertion of a coronary artery. Careful attention to other components of the physical examination (growth failure, cyanosis, peripheral pulses, precordial impulse, heart sounds) increases the index of suspicion of congenital heart defects in these cases. In contrast, loud murmurs may be present in the absence of structural heart disease, for example, in patients with a large noncardiac arteriovenous malformation, myocarditis, severe anemia, or hypertension.

Many murmurs are not associated with significant hemodynamic abnormalities. These murmurs are referred to as functional, normal, insignificant, or innocent (the preferred term). During routine random auscultation, more than 30% of children may have an innocent murmur at one time in their lives; this percentage increases when auscultation is carried out under nonbasal circumstances (high cardiac output because of fever, infection, anxiety). The most **common innocent murmur** is a medium-pitched, vibratory or "musical," relatively short systolic ejection murmur, which is heard best along the left lower and midsternal border and has no significant radiation to the apex, base, or back. It is heard most frequently in children between 3 and 7 yr of age. The intensity of the murmur often changes with respiration and position and may be attenuated in the sitting or prone position. Innocent pulmonic murmurs are also common in children and adolescents and originate from normal turbulence during ejection into the pulmonary artery. They are higher pitched, blowing, brief early systolic murmurs of grades I-II in intensity and are best detected in the 2nd left parasternal space with the patient in the supine position. Features suggestive of heart disease include murmurs that are pansystolic, grade III or higher, harsh, located at the left upper sternal border, and associated with an early or midsystolic click or an abnormal 2nd heart sound.

A **venous hum** is another example of a common innocent murmur heard during childhood. Such hums are produced by turbulence of blood in the jugular venous system; they have no pathologic significance and may be heard in the neck or anterior portion of the upper part of the chest. A venous hum consists of a soft humming sound

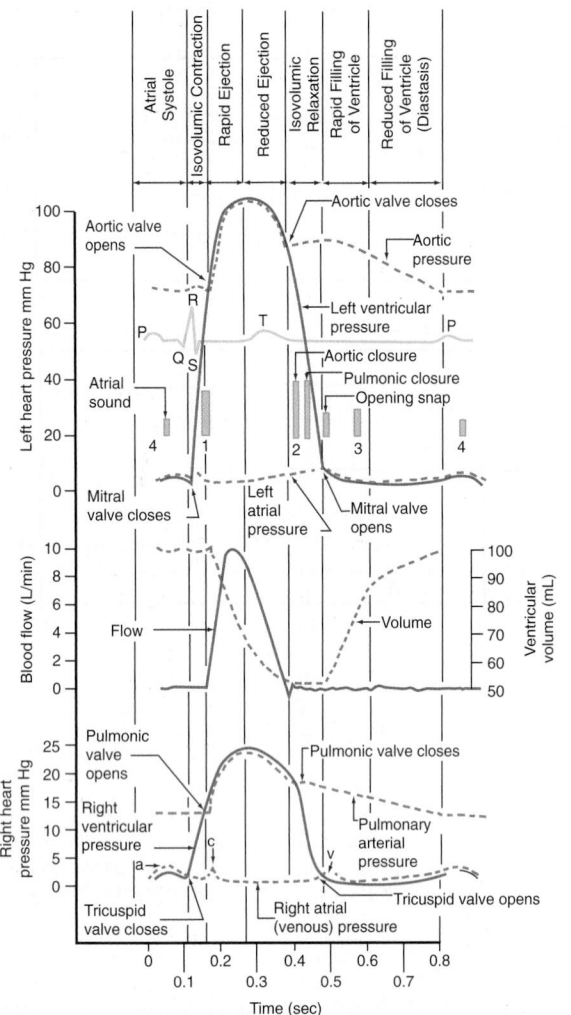

Figure 422-3 Idealized diagram of the temporal events of a cardiac cycle.

heard in both systole and diastole; it can be exaggerated or made to disappear by varying the position of the head, or it can be decreased by lightly compressing the jugular venous system in the neck. These simple maneuvers are sufficient to differentiate a venous hum from the murmurs produced by organic cardiovascular disease, particularly a patent ductus arteriosus.

The lack of significance of an innocent murmur should be discussed with the child's parents. It is important to offer complete reassurance because lingering doubts about the importance of a cardiac murmur may have profound effects on child-rearing practices, most often in the form of overprotectiveness. An underlying fear that a cardiac abnormality is present may negatively affect a child's self-image and subtly influence personality development. The physician should explain that an innocent murmur is simply a "noise" and does not indicate the presence of a significant cardiac defect. When asked, "Will it go away?," the best response is to state that because the murmur has no clinical significance, it does not matter whether it "goes away." Parents should be warned that the intensity of the murmur might increase during febrile illnesses, a time when, typically, another physician examines the child. With growth, however, innocent murmurs are less well heard and often disappear completely. At times, additional studies may be indicated to rule out a congenital heart defect, but "routine" electrocardiographic, chest roentgenographic, and echocardiographic examinations should be avoided in well children with innocent murmurs.

Bibliography is available at Expert Consult.

Chapter 423
Laboratory Evaluation

423.1 Radiologic Assessment
Daniel Bernstein

The chest x-ray remains a highly valuable diagnostic tool and is often the first imaging study performed in a child suspected of having a cardiac defect. It can provide information about cardiac size and shape, pulmonary blood flow (vascularity), pulmonary edema, and associated lung and thoracic anomalies that may be associated with congenital syndromes (skeletal dysplasias, extra or deficient number of ribs, abnormal vertebrae, previous cardiac surgery).

The most frequently used measurement of cardiac size is the maximal width of the cardiac shadow in a posteroanterior chest film taken mid-inspiration. A vertical line is drawn down the middle of the sternal shadow, and perpendicular lines are drawn from the sternal line to the extreme right and left borders of the heart; the sum of the lengths of these lines is the maximal cardiac width. The maximal chest width is obtained by drawing a horizontal line between the right and left inner borders of the rib cage at the level of the top of the right diaphragm. When the maximal cardiac width is more than half the maximal chest width (cardiothoracic ratio >50%), the heart is usually enlarged. Cardiac size should be evaluated only when the film is taken during inspiration with the patient in an upright position. A diagnosis of "cardiac enlargement" on expiratory or prone films is a common cause of unnecessary referrals and laboratory studies.

The cardiothoracic ratio is a less useful index of cardiac enlargement in infants than in older children because the horizontal position of the heart may increase the ratio to >50% in the absence of true enlargement. Furthermore, the thymus may overlap not only the base of the heart but also virtually the entire mediastinum, thus obscuring the true cardiac silhouette.

A lateral chest roentgenogram may be helpful in infants as well as in older children with pectus excavatum or other conditions that result in a narrow anteroposterior chest dimension. In these situations, the heart may appear small in the lateral view and suggest that the apparent enlargement in the posteroanterior projection was due to either the thymic image (anterior mediastinum only) or flattening of the cardiac chambers as a result of a structural chest abnormality.

In the posteroanterior view, the left border of the cardiac shadow consists of 3 convex shadows produced, from above downward, by the aortic knob, the main and left pulmonary arteries, and the left ventricle (Fig. 423-1). In cases of moderate to marked left atrial enlargement, the atrium may project between the pulmonary artery and the left ventricle. The outflow tract of the right ventricle does not contribute to the shadows formed by the left border of the heart. The aortic knob is not as easily seen in infants and children as in adults. The side of the aortic arch (left or right) can often be inferred as being opposite the side of the midline from which the air-filled trachea is visualized. This observation is important because a right-sided aortic arch is often present in cyanotic congenital heart disease, particularly in tetralogy of Fallot. Three structures contribute to the right border of the cardiac silhouette. In the view from above, they are the superior vena cava, the ascending aorta, and the right atrium.

Enlargement of cardiac chambers or major arteries and veins results in prominence of the areas in which these structures are normally outlined on the chest x-ray. In contrast, the electrocardiogram (ECG) is a more sensitive and accurate index of **ventricular hypertrophy.**

The chest roentgenogram is also an important tool for assessing the degree of pulmonary vascularity. Pulmonary overcirculation is usually

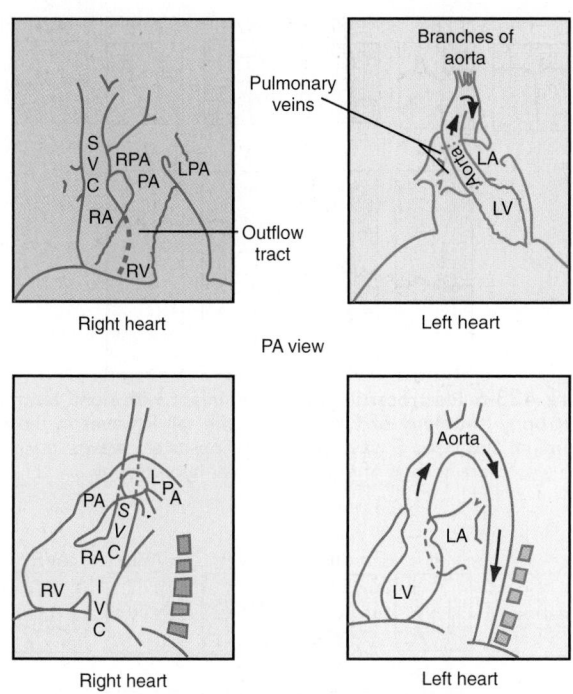

Figure 423-1 Idealized diagrams showing normal position of the cardiac chambers and great blood vessels. IVC, inferior vena cava; LA, left atrium; LPA, left pulmonary artery; LV, left ventricle; PA, pulmonary artery; RA, right atrium; RPA, right pulmonary artery; RV, right ventricle; SVC, superior vena cava. *(Adapted and redrawn from Dotter CT, Steinberg I: Angiocardiographic interpretation, Radiology 153:513, 1949.)*

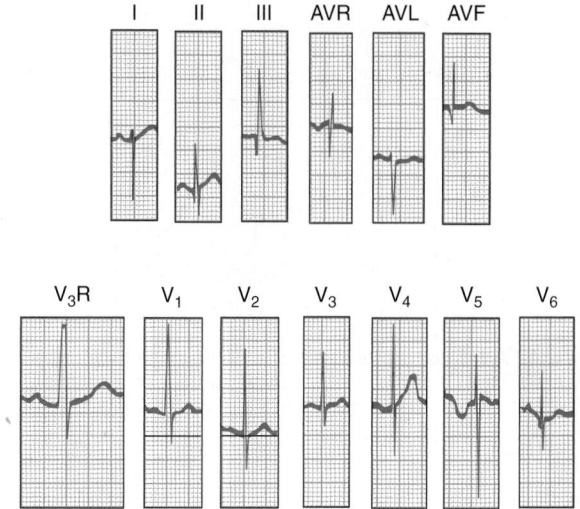

Figure 423-2 Electrocardiogram in a normal neonate <24 hr of age. Note the dominant R wave and upright T waves in leads V_3R and V_1 (V_3R paper speed = 50 mm/sec).

associated with left-to-right shunt lesions, whereas pulmonary undercirculation is associated with obstruction of the outflow tract of the right ventricle. The esophagus is closely related to the great vessels, and a barium esophagogram can help delineate these structures in the initial evaluation of suspected vascular rings, although this has largely been supplanted by CT. Echocardiographic examination best defines the morphologic features of intracardiac chambers, cardiac valves, and intracardiac shunts. CT is used as an adjunct to echo to evaluate extracardiac vascular morphology. MRI is used to quantitate ventricular volumes, cardiac function, and shunt and regurgitant fractions.

423.2 Electrocardiography

Daniel Bernstein

DEVELOPMENTAL CHANGES

The marked changes that occur in cardiac physiology and chamber dominance during the perinatal transition (see Chapter 421) are reflected in the evolution of the ECG during the neonatal period. Because vascular resistance in the pulmonary and systemic circulations is nearly equal in a term fetus, the intrauterine work of the heart results in an equal mass of both the right and left ventricles. After birth, systemic vascular resistance rises when the placental circulation is eliminated, and pulmonary vascular resistance falls when the lungs expand. These changes are reflected in the ECG as the right ventricular wall begins to thin.

The ECG demonstrates these anatomic and hemodynamic features principally by changes in QRS and T-wave morphologic features. Commonly, a 13-lead ECG is performed in pediatric patients, including either lead V_3R or V_4R, which are important in the evaluation of right ventricular hypertrophy. On occasion, lead V_1 is positioned too far leftward to reflect right ventricular forces accurately. This problem is

present particularly in premature infants, in whom the electrocardiographic electrode gel may produce contact among all the precordial leads.

During the 1st days of life, right axis deviation, large R waves, and upright T waves in the right precordial leads (V_3R or V_4R and V_1) are the norm (Fig. 423-2). As pulmonary vascular resistance decreases in the 1st few days after birth, the right precordial T waves become negative. In the great majority of instances, this change occurs within the 1st 48 hr of life. Upright T waves that persist in leads V_3R, V_4R, or V_1 beyond 1 wk of life are an abnormal finding indicating right ventricular hypertrophy or strain, even in the absence of QRS voltage criteria. The T wave in V_1 should never be positive before 6 yr of age and may remain negative into adolescence. This finding represents one of the most important, yet subtle differences between pediatric and adult ECGs and is a common source of error when adult cardiologists interpret pediatric ECGs.

In a newborn, the mean **QRS frontal-plane axis** normally lies in the range of +110 to +180 degrees. The right-sided chest leads reveal a larger positive (R) than negative (S) wave and may do so for months because the right ventricle remains relatively thick throughout infancy. Left-sided leads (V_5 and V_6) also reflect right-sided dominance in the early neonatal period, when the R:S ratio in these leads may be <1. A dominant R wave in V_5 and V_6, reflecting left ventricular forces, quickly becomes evident within the 1st few days of life (Fig. 423-3). Over the years, the QRS axis gradually shifts leftward, and the right ventricular forces slowly regress. Leads V_1, V_3R, and V_4R display a prominent R wave until 6 mo to 8 yr of age. Most children have an R:S ratio >1 in lead V_4R until they are 4 yr of age. The T waves are inverted in leads V_4R, V_1, V_2, and V_3 during infancy and may remain so into the middle of the 2nd decade of life and beyond. The processes of right ventricular thinning and left ventricular growth are best reflected in the QRS-T pattern over the right precordial leads. The diagnosis of right or left ventricular hypertrophy in a pediatric patient can be made only with an understanding of the normal developmental physiology of these chambers at various ages until adulthood is reached. As the left ventricle becomes dominant, the ECG evolves to the characteristic pattern of older children (Fig. 423-4) and adults (Fig. 423-5).

Ventricular hypertrophy may result in increased voltage in the R and S waves in the chest leads. The height of these deflections is governed by the proximity of the specific electrode to the surface of the heart; by the sequence of electrical activation through the ventricles, which can result in variable degrees of cancellation of forces; and by hypertrophy of the myocardium. Because the chest wall in infants and children, as

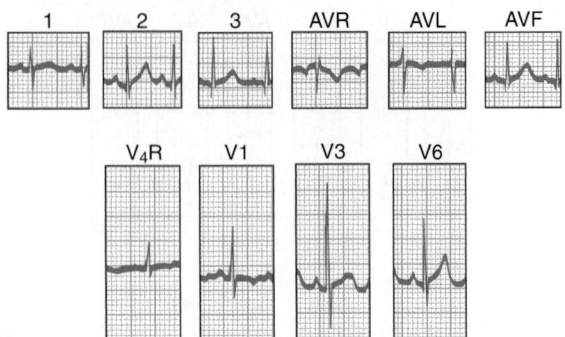

Figure 423-3 Electrocardiogram of a normal infant. Note the tall R and small S waves in V₄R and V₁ and the inverted T wave in these leads. A dominant R wave is also present in V₆.

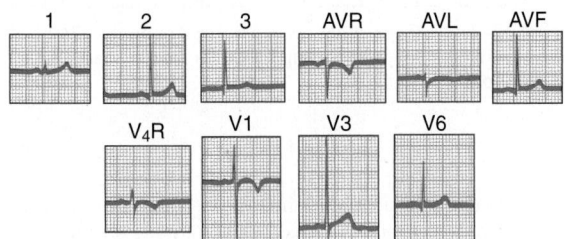

Figure 423-4 Electrocardiogram of a normal child. Note the relatively tall R waves and inversion of the T waves in V₄R and V₁.

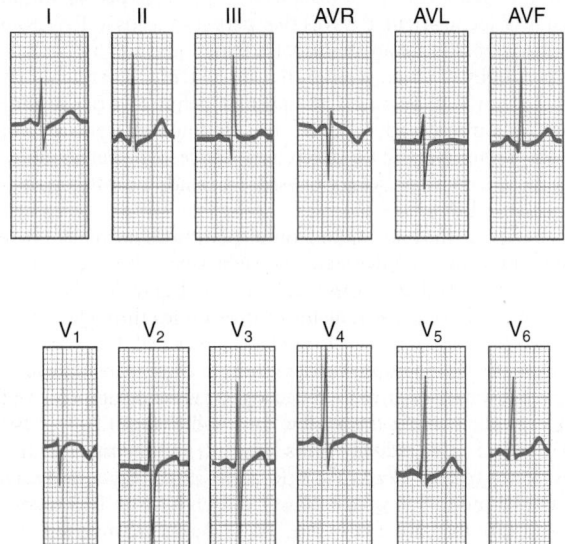

Figure 423-5 Normal adult electrocardiogram. Note the dominant S wave in lead V₁. This pattern in an infant would indicate the presence of left ventricular hypertrophy.

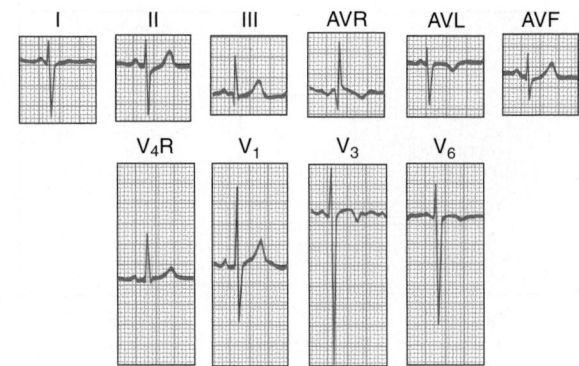

Figure 423-6 Electrocardiogram of an infant with right ventricular hypertrophy (tetralogy of Fallot). Note the tall R waves in the right precordium and deep S waves in V₆. The positive T waves in V₄R and V₁ are also characteristic of right ventricular hypertrophy.

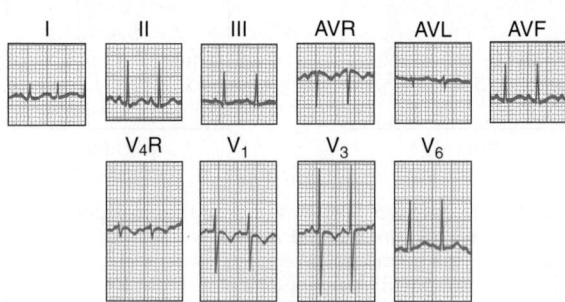

Figure 423-7 Electrocardiogram of a premature infant (weight 2 kg and age 5 wk at the time of the tracing). The cardiovascular system was clinically normal. Left ventricular dominance is manifested by R-wave progression across the chest, similar to tracings obtained from older children. Compare with the tracing from a normal full-term infant (see Fig. 423-3).

well as in adolescents, may be relatively thin, the diagnosis of ventricular hypertrophy should not be based on voltage changes alone.

The diagnosis of pathologic right ventricular hypertrophy is difficult in the 1st wk of life because physiologic right ventricular hypertrophy is a normal finding. Serial tracings are often necessary to determine whether marked right axis deviation and potentially abnormal right precordial forces or T waves, or both, will persist beyond the neonatal period (Fig. 423-6). In contrast, an adult electrocardiographic pattern

(see Fig. 423-5) seen in a neonate suggests left ventricular hypertrophy. The exception is a premature infant, who may display a more "mature" ECG than a full-term infant (Fig. 423-7) as a result of lower pulmonary vascular resistance secondary to underdevelopment of the medial muscular layer of the pulmonary arterioles. Some premature infants display a pattern of generalized low voltage across the precordium.

The ECG should always be evaluated systematically to avoid the possibility of overlooking a minor, but important, abnormality. One approach is to begin with an assessment of rate and rhythm, followed by a calculation of the mean frontal-plane QRS axis, measurements of segment intervals, assessment of voltages, and, finally, assessment of ST and T-wave abnormalities.

RATE AND RHYTHM

A brief rhythm strip should be examined to assess whether a P wave always precedes each QRS complex. The P-wave axis should then be estimated as an indication of whether the rhythm is originating from the sinus node. If the atria are situated normally in the chest, the P wave should be upright in leads I and aVF and inverted in lead aVR. With atrial inversion (situs inversus), the P wave may be inverted in lead I. Inverted P waves in leads II and aVF are seen in low atrial, nodal, or junctional rhythms. The absence of P waves indicates a rhythm originating more distally in the conduction system. In this case, the morphologic features of the QRS complexes are important in differentiating a junctional (usually a narrow QRS complex) from a ventricular (usually a wide QRS complex) rhythm.

P WAVES

Tall (>2.5 mm), narrow, and spiked P waves are indicative of **right atrial enlargement** and are seen in congenital pulmonary stenosis,

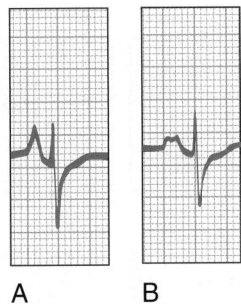

Figure 423-8 Atrial enlargement. **A,** Peaked narrow P waves characteristic of right atrial enlargement. **B,** Wide bifid M-shaped P waves typical of left atrial enlargement.

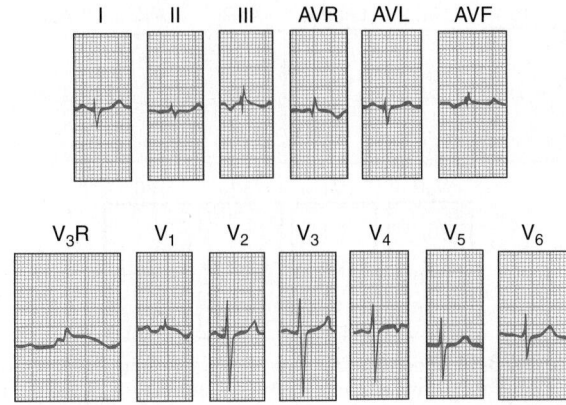

Figure 423-9 Electrocardiogram showing right ventricular conduction delay characterized by an rsR′ pattern in V₁ and a deep S wave in V₆ (V₃R paper speed = 50 mm/sec).

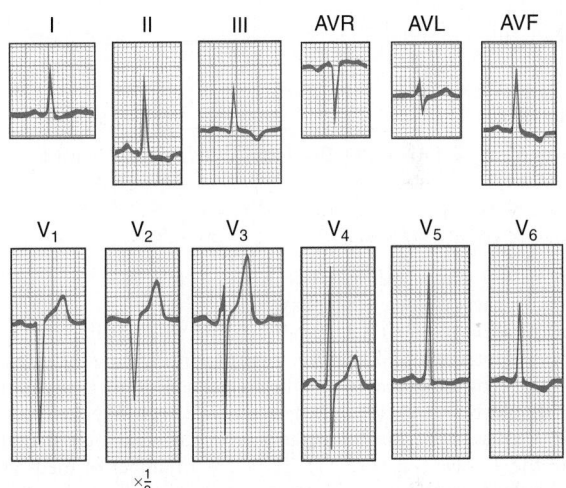

Figure 423-10 Electrocardiogram showing left ventricular hypertrophy in a 12 yr old child with aortic stenosis. Note the deep S wave in V₁-V₃ and tall R in V₅. In addition, T-wave inversion is present in leads II, III, aVF, and V₆.

Ebstein anomaly of the tricuspid valve, tricuspid atresia, and sometimes cor pulmonale. These abnormal waves are most obvious in leads II, V₃R, and V₁ (Fig. 423-8A). Similar waves are sometimes seen in thyrotoxicosis. **Broad P waves,** commonly **bifid** and sometimes **biphasic,** are indicative of left atrial enlargement (Fig. 423-8B). They are seen in some patients with large left-to-right shunts (ventricular septal defect [VSD], patent ductus arteriosus [PDA]) and with severe mitral stenosis or regurgitation. Flat P waves may be encountered in hyperkalemia.

QRS COMPLEX
Right Ventricular Hypertrophy
For the most accurate assessment of ventricular hypertrophy, pediatric ECGs should include the right precordial lead V₃R or V₄R, or both. The diagnosis of right ventricular hypertrophy depends on demonstration of the following changes (see Fig. 423-6): (1) a qR pattern in the right ventricular surface leads; (2) a positive T wave in leads V₃R-V₄R and V₁-V₃ between the ages of 6 days and 6 yr; (3) a monophasic R wave in V₃R, V₄R, or V₁; (4) an rsR′ pattern in the right precordial leads with the 2nd R wave taller than the initial one; (5) age-corrected increased voltage of the R wave in leads V₃R-V₄R or the S wave in leads V₆-V₇, or both; (6) marked right axis deviation (>120 degrees in patients beyond the newborn period); and (7) complete reversal of the normal adult precordial RS pattern. At least 2 of these changes should be present to support a diagnosis of right ventricular hypertrophy.

Abnormal ventricular loading can be characterized as either systolic (as a result of obstruction of the right ventricular outflow tract, as in pulmonic stenosis) or diastolic (as a result of increased volume load, as in atrial septal defects [ASDs]). These 2 types of abnormal loads result in distinct electrocardiographic patterns. The **systolic overload pattern** is characterized by tall, pure R waves in the right precordial leads. In older children, the T waves in these leads are initially upright and later become inverted. In infants and children <6 yr, the T waves in V₃R-V₄R and V₁ are abnormally upright. The **diastolic overload pattern** (typically seen in patients with ASDs) is characterized by an rsR′ pattern (Fig. 423-9) and a slightly increased QRS duration (minor right ventricular conduction delay). Patients with mild to moderate pulmonary stenosis may also exhibit an rsR′ pattern in the right precordial leads.

Left Ventricular Hypertrophy
The following features indicate the presence of left ventricular hypertrophy (Fig. 423-10): (1) depression of the ST segments and inversion of the T waves in the left precordial leads (V₅, V₆, and V₇), known as a *left ventricular strain* pattern—these findings suggest the presence of a severe lesion; (2) a deep Q wave in the left precordial leads; and (3) increased voltage of the S wave in V₃R and V₁ or the R wave in V₆-V₇, or both. It is important to emphasize that evaluation of left ventricular hypertrophy should not be based on voltage criteria alone. The concepts of systolic and diastolic overload, though not always consistent,

are also useful in evaluating left ventricular enlargement. Severe systolic overload of the left ventricle is suggested by straightening of the ST segments and inverted T waves over the left precordial leads; diastolic overload may result in tall R waves, a large Q wave, and normal T waves over the left precordium. Finally, an infant with an ECG that would be considered "normal" for an older child may, in fact, have left ventricular hypertrophy.

Bundle Branch Block
A complete right bundle-branch block may be congenital or may be acquired after surgery for congenital heart disease, especially when a right ventriculotomy has been performed, as in repair of the tetralogy of Fallot. Congenital left bundle-branch block is rare; this pattern is occasionally seen with cardiomyopathy. A bundle-branch block pattern may be indicative of a bypass tract associated with one of the preexcitation syndromes (see Chapter 435).

P-R AND Q-T INTERVALS
The duration of the P-R interval shortens with increasing heart rate; thus, assessment of this interval should be based on age- and rate-corrected nomograms. A long P-R interval is diagnostic of a **1st-degree heart block,** the cause of which may be congenital, postoperative,

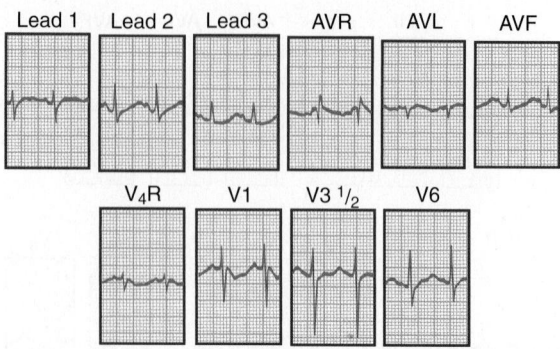

Figure 423-11 Electrocardiogram in hypokalemia (serum potassium, 2.7 mEq/L; serum calcium, 4.8 mEq/L at the time of the tracing). Note the prolongation of electrical systole as evidenced by a widened TU wave, as well as depression of the ST segment in V_4R, V_1, and V_6.

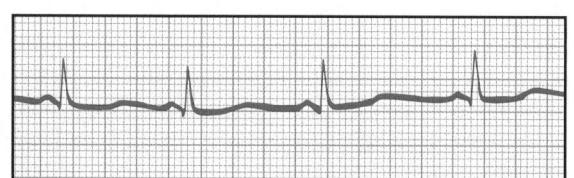

Figure 423-12 Prolonged Q-T interval in a patient with long Q-T syndrome.

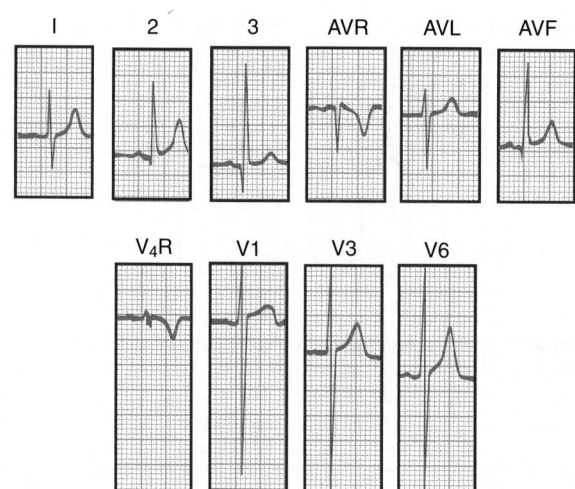

Figure 423-13 Electrocardiogram in hyperkalemia (serum potassium, 6.5 mEq/L; serum calcium, 5.1 mEq/L). Note the tall, tent-shaped T waves, especially in leads I, II, and V_6.

with generalized low voltage. In hyperkalemia, the T waves are commonly of high voltage and are tent-shaped (Fig. 423-13).

Bibliography is available at Expert Consult.

423.3 Hematologic Data
Daniel Bernstein

In acyanotic infants with large left-to-right shunts, the onset of heart failure often coincides with the nadir of the normal physiologic anemia of infancy. Increasing the hematocrit in these patients to >40% may decrease shunt volume and result in an improvement in symptoms; however, this form of treatment is generally reserved for infants who are not otherwise surgical candidates (extremely premature infants or those with exceedingly complex congenital heart disease for whom only palliative surgery is possible). In these select infants, regular evaluation of the hematocrit and booster transfusions when appropriate may be helpful in improving growth.

Polycythemia is frequently noted in cyanotic patients with right-to-left shunts. Patients with severe polycythemia are in a delicate balance between the risks of intravascular thrombosis and a bleeding diathesis. The most frequent abnormalities include accelerated fibrinolysis, thrombocytopenia, abnormal clot retraction, hypofibrinogenemia, prolonged prothrombin time, and prolonged partial thromboplastin time. The preparation of cyanotic, polycythemic patients for elective noncardiac surgery, such as dental extraction, includes evaluation and treatment of abnormal coagulation.

Because of the high viscosity of polycythemic blood (hematocrit >65%), patients with cyanotic congenital heart disease are at risk for the development of vascular thromboses, especially of cerebral veins. Dehydration increases the risk of thrombosis, and thus adequate fluid intake must be maintained during hot weather or intercurrent gastrointestinal illnesses. Diuretics should be used with caution in these patients and may need to be decreased if fluid intake is a concern. Polycythemic infants with concomitant **iron deficiency** are at even greater risk for cerebrovascular accidents, probably because of the decreased deformability of microcytic red blood cells. Iron therapy may reduce this risk somewhat, but surgical treatment of the cardiac anomaly is the best therapy.

Severely cyanotic patients should have periodic determinations of hemoglobin and hematocrit. Increasing polycythemia, often associated with headache, fatigue, dyspnea, or a combination of these conditions, is one indication for palliative or corrective surgical intervention. In cyanotic patients with inoperable conditions, partial exchange

inflammatory (myocarditis, pericarditis, Lyme disease, rheumatic fever), or pharmacologic (digitalis).

The duration of the Q-T interval varies with the cardiac rate; a corrected Q-T interval (Q-Tc) can be calculated by dividing the measured Q-T interval by the square root of the preceding R-R interval. A normal Q-Tc should be <0.45. It is often lengthened with hypokalemia and hypocalcemia; in the former instance, a U wave may be noted at the end of the T wave (Fig. 423-11). There are a number of medications that can also lengthen the Q-T interval. A congenitally prolonged Q-T interval (Fig. 423-12) may also be seen in children with one of the long Q-T syndromes. These patients are at high risk for ventricular arrhythmias, including a form of ventricular tachycardia known as torsades de pointes, and sudden death (see Chapter 435.5).

ST SEGMENT AND T-WAVE ABNORMALITIES
A slight elevation of the ST segment may occur in normal teenagers and is attributed to early repolarization of the heart. In pericarditis, irritation of the epicardium may cause elevation of the ST segment followed by abnormal T-wave inversion as healing progresses. Administration of digitalis is sometimes associated with sagging of the ST segment and abnormal inversion of the T wave.

Depression of the ST segment may also occur in any condition that produces myocardial damage or ischemia, including severe anemia, carbon monoxide poisoning, aberrant origin of the left coronary artery from the pulmonary artery, glycogen storage disease of the heart, myocardial tumors, and mucopolysaccharidoses. An aberrant origin of the left coronary artery from the pulmonary artery may lead to changes indistinguishable from those of acute myocardial infarction in adults. Similar changes may occur in patients with other rare abnormalities of the coronary arteries and in those with cardiomyopathy, even in the presence of normal coronary arteries. These patterns are often misread in young infants because of the unfamiliarity of pediatricians with this "infarct" pattern, and thus a high index of suspicion must be maintained in infants with dilated cardiomyopathy or with symptoms compatible with coronary ischemia (e.g., inconsolable crying).

T-wave inversion may occur in myocarditis and pericarditis, or it may be a sign of either right or left ventricular hypertrophy and strain. Hypothyroidism may produce flat or inverted T waves in association transfusion may be required to treat symptomatic individuals whose hematocrit has risen to the 65-70% level. This procedure is not without risk, especially in patients with an extreme elevation in pulmonary vascular resistance. Because these patients do not tolerate wide fluctuations in circulating blood volume, blood should be replaced with fresh-frozen plasma or albumin.

423.4 Echocardiography

Daniel Bernstein

Transthoracic echocardiography has replaced invasive studies such as cardiac catheterization for the *initial diagnosis* of most forms of congenital heart disease. The echocardiographic examination can be used to evaluate cardiac structure in congenital heart lesions, estimate intracardiac pressures and gradients across stenotic valves and vessels, quantitate cardiac contractile function (both systolic and diastolic), determine the direction of flow across a defect, examine the integrity of the coronary arteries, and detect the presence of vegetations from endocarditis, as well as the presence of pericardial fluid, cardiac tumors, and chamber thrombi. Echocardiography may also be used to assist in the performance of interventional procedures, including pericardiocentesis, balloon atrial septostomy (see Chapter 431.2), atrial or VSD closure and endocardial biopsy, and in the placement of flow-directed pulmonary artery (Swan-Ganz) monitoring catheters. **Transesophageal echocardiography** is used routinely to monitor ventricular function in patients during surgical procedures and can provide an immediate assessment of the results of surgical repair of congenital heart lesions. A complete transthoracic echocardiographic examination usually entails a combination of M-mode and 2-dimensional (2D) imaging, as well as pulsed, continuous, and color Doppler flow studies. Doppler tissue imaging provides a more quantitative assessments of ventricular function. Three-dimensional (3D) echocardiography provides valuable information regarding cardiac morphology.

M-MODE ECHOCARDIOGRAPHY

M-mode echocardiography displays a 1-dimensional slice of cardiac structure varying over time (Fig. 423-14). It is used mostly for the measurement of cardiac dimensions (wall thickness and chamber size) and cardiac function (fractional shortening, wall thickening). M-mode echocardiography is also useful for assessing the motion of intracardiac structures (opening and closing of valves, movement of free walls and septa) and the anatomy of valves (Fig. 423-15). The most frequently used index of cardiac function in children is percent fractional shortening (%FS), which is calculated as (LVED − LVES)/LVED, where LVED is left ventricular (LV) dimension at end-diastole and LVES is

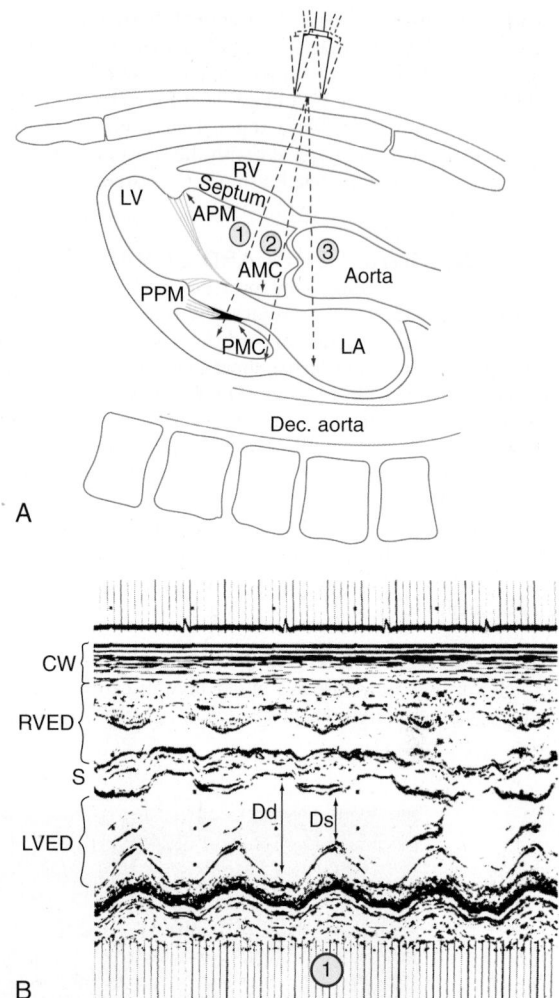

Figure 423-14 M-mode echocardiogram. **A,** Diagram of a sagittal section of a heart showing the structures traversed by the echo beam as it is moved superiorly to positions (1), (2), and (3). AMC, anterior mitral cusp; APM, anterior papillary muscle; Dec. aorta, descending aorta; LA, left atrium; LV, left ventricle; PMC, posterior mitral cusp; PPM, posterior papillary muscle; RV, right ventricle. **B,** Echocardiogram from transducer position (1); this view is the best one for measuring cardiac dimensions and fractional shortening. Fractional shortening is calculated as (LVED − LVES)/LVED. CW, chest wall; Ds, LV dimension in systole; LVED, LV dimension at end-diastole (Dd); RVED, RV dimension at end-diastole.

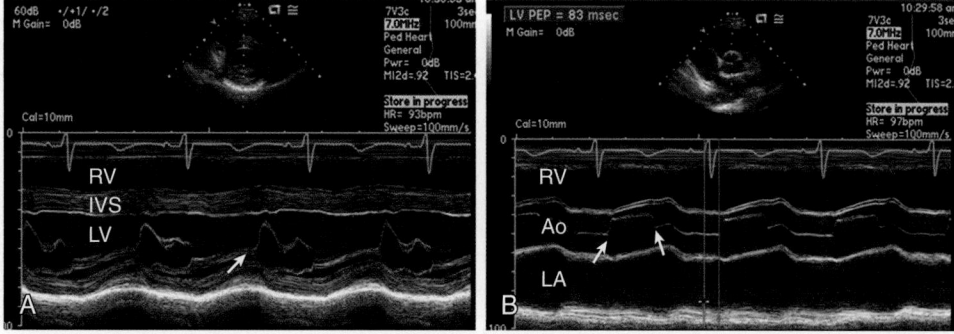

Figure 423-15 M-mode echocardiograms. The small figure at the top of each panel shows the 2D parasternal short axis echo image from which the M-modes are derived. The cursor can be seen midway through the image, indicating the one-dimensional line through which the M-mode is being sampled. **A,** M-mode echocardiogram of a normal mitral valve. *Arrow* shows the opening of the anterior leaflet in early diastole (see ECG tracing above for reference). **B,** M-mode echocardiogram of a normal aortic valve. The opening and closing of the aortic leaflets in systole are outlined by the 2 *arrows*. Ao, aorta; IVS, interventricular septum; LV, left ventricle; RV, right ventricle.

LV dimension at end-systole. Normal fractional shortening is approximately 28-40%. Other M-mode indices of cardiac function include the mean velocity of fiber shortening (mean V_{CF}), systolic time intervals (LVPEP = LV preejection period, LVET = LV ejection time), and isovolemic contraction time. More sophisticated indices of cardiac function can be derived noninvasively with the assistance of echocardiography (pressure–volume relationship, end-systolic wall stress–strain relationship).

TWO-DIMENSIONAL ECHOCARDIOGRAPHY

Two-dimensional echocardiography provides a real-time image of cardiac structures. With 2D echocardiography, the contracting heart is imaged in real time using several standard views, including parasternal long axis (Fig. 423-16), parasternal short axis (Fig. 423-17), apical four chamber (Fig. 423-18), subcostal (Fig. 423-19), and suprasternal (Fig. 423-20) windows, each of which emphasizes specific structures. Two-dimensional echocardiography has replaced cardiac angiography for the preoperative diagnosis of most, but not all congenital heart lesions. When information from the cardiac examination or other studies is not consistent with the echocardiogram (e.g., the size of a left-to-right shunt), cardiac catheterization remains an important tool to confirm the anatomic diagnosis and evaluate the degree of physiologic derangement.

DOPPLER ECHOCARDIOGRAPHY

Doppler echocardiography displays blood flow in cardiac chambers and vascular channels based on the change in frequency imparted to

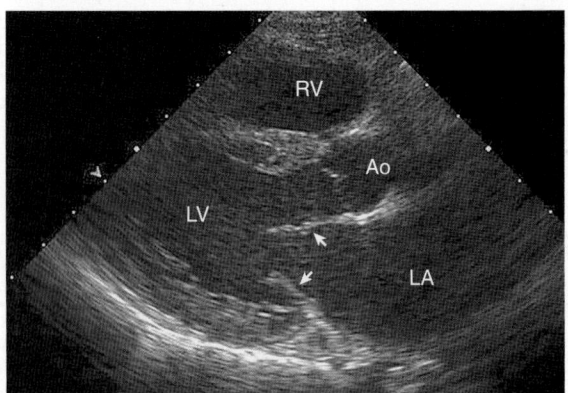

Figure 423-16 Normal parasternal long axis echocardiographic window. The transducer is angulated slightly posteriorly, imaging the left-sided cardiac structures. If the transducer were to be angulated more anteriorly, the right ventricular structures would be imaged. The mitral valve leaflets can be seen in partially open position in early diastole *(arrowheads)*. The closed aortic valve leaflets can be seen just below the label Ao. Ao, aorta; LA, left atrium; LV, left ventricle; RV, right ventricle.

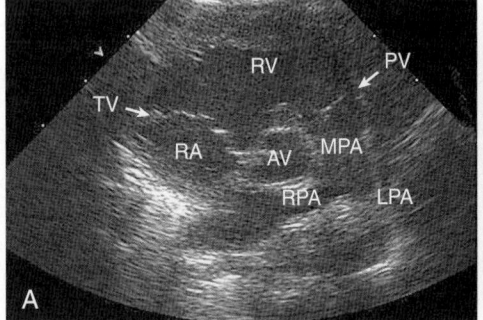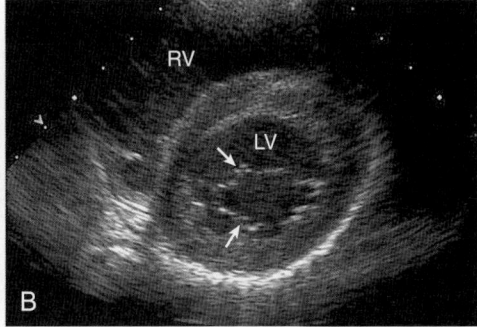

Figure 423-17 Normal parasternal short axis echocardiographic windows. **A,** With the transducer angled superiorly and rightwards, the aortic valve (AV) is imaged, surrounded by both inflow and outflow portions of the right ventricle (RV). LPA, left pulmonary artery; MPA, main pulmonary artery; PV, pulmonary valve; RA, right atrium; RPA, right pulmonary artery; TV, tricuspid valve. **B,** With the transducer angled inferiorly and leftward, the left ventricular chamber is imaged along with cross-sectional view of the mitral valve *(arrows)*. LV, left ventricle; RV, right ventricle.

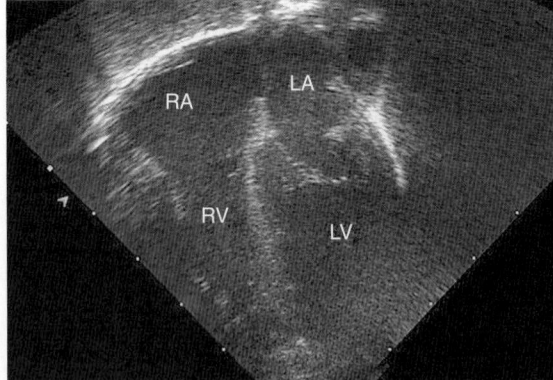

Figure 423-18 Normal apical four chamber echocardiographic window showing all 4 cardiac chambers and both atrioventricular valves opened in diastole. LA, left atrium; LV, left ventricle; RA, right atrium; RV, right ventricle.

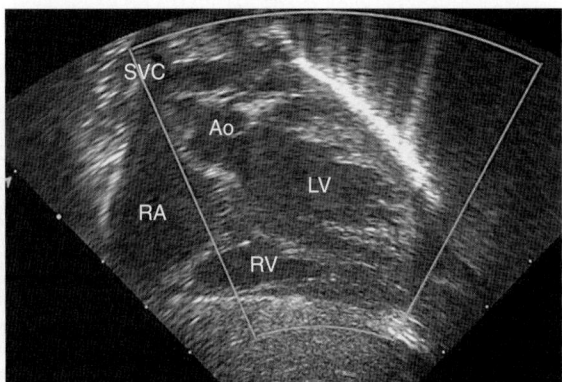

Figure 423-19 Normal subcostal echocardiographic window showing the left ventricular outflow tract. The right-sided structures are not fully imaged in this view. Ao, ascending aorta; LV, left ventricle; RA, right atrium; RV, right ventricle; SVC, superior vena cava.

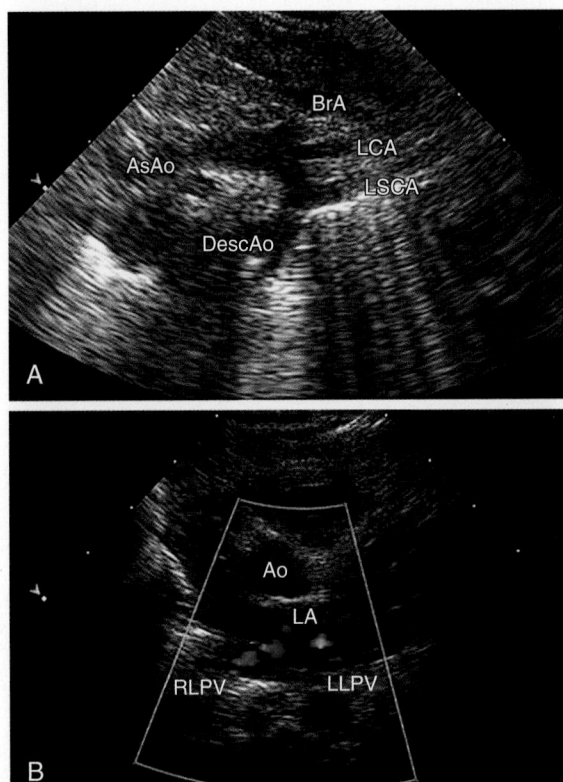

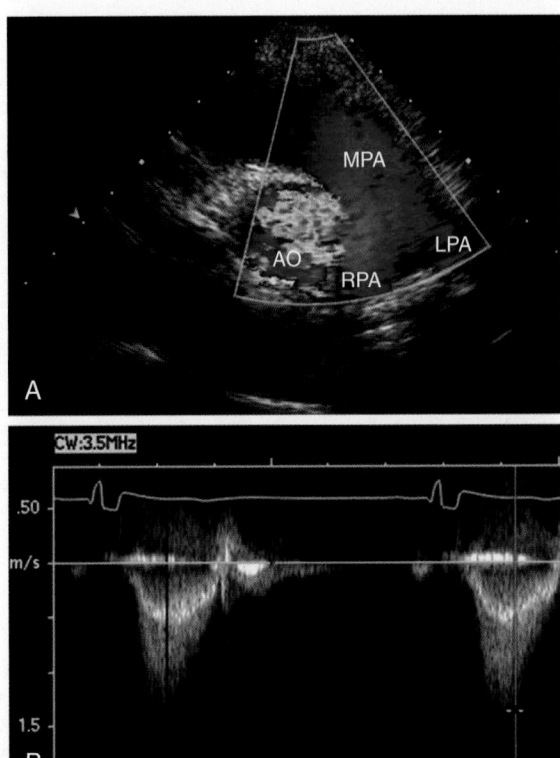

Figure 423-20 A, Normal suprasternal echocardiographic window showing the aortic arch and its major branches. AsAo, ascending aorta; BrA, brachiocephalic artery; DescAo, descending aorta; LCA, left carotid artery; LSCA, left subclavian artery. **B,** Normal high parasternal window showing color Doppler imaging of normal pulmonary venous return to the left atrium (LA) of both right (RLPV) and left (LLPV) lower pulmonary veins.

Figure 423-21 Color and pulsed Doppler evaluation of pulmonary arterial flow. **A,** Color Doppler evaluation of a parasternal short axis view showing normal flow through the pulmonary valve to the main and branch pulmonary arteries. The color of the Doppler flow is blue, indicating that the flow is moving away from the transducer (which is located at the top of the figure, at the apex of the triangular ultrasound window). Note that the color assigned to the Doppler signal does not indicate the oxygen saturation of the blood. AO, aorta; LPA, left pulmonary artery; MPA, main pulmonary artery; RPA, right pulmonary artery. **B,** Pulsed wave Doppler flow pattern through the pulmonary valve showing a low velocity of flow (<1.5 m/sec), indicating the absence of a pressure gradient across the valve. The envelope of the flow signal is below the line, indicating that the flow is moving away from the transducer.

a sound wave by the movement of erythrocytes. In pulsed Doppler and continuous wave Doppler, the speed and direction of blood flow in the line of the echo beam change the transducer's reference frequency. This frequency change can be translated into volumetric flow (L/min) data for estimating systemic or pulmonary blood flow and into pressure (mm Hg) data for estimating gradients across the semilunar or atrioventricular valves or across septal defects or vascular communications such as shunts. Color Doppler permits highly accurate assessment of the presence and direction of intracardiac shunts and allows identification of small or multiple left-to-right or right-to-left shunts (Fig. 423-21). The severity of valvular insufficiency can be evaluated with both pulsed and color Doppler (Fig. 423-22). Alterations in venous Doppler flow patterns can be used to detect abnormalities of systemic and pulmonary veins and alterations of atrioventricular valve Doppler flow patterns can be used to assess ventricular diastolic functional abnormalities.

M-mode, 2D, and Doppler echocardiographic methods of assessing LV systolic and diastolic function (e.g., end-systolic wall stress, dobutamine stress echocardiography, and Doppler tissue imaging) have proved useful in the serial assessment of patients at risk for the development of both systolic and diastolic ventricular dysfunction and ventricular dyssynchrony (where the coordination of left and right ventricular contraction is abnormal). Such patients include those with cardiomyopathies, those receiving anthracycline drugs for cancer chemotherapy, those at risk for iron overload, and those being monitored for rejection or coronary artery disease after heart transplantation.

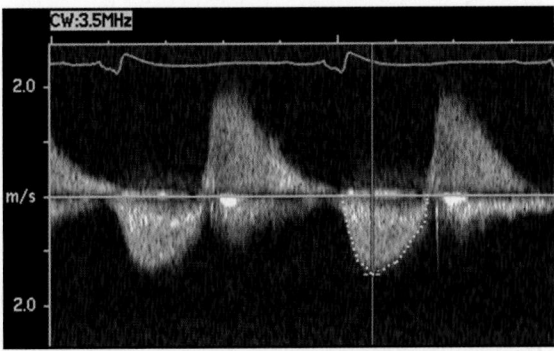

Figure 423-22 Doppler evaluation of a patient who had previously undergone repair of tetralogy of Fallot and who has mild pulmonary stenosis and moderate pulmonary regurgitation. The tracing shows the to-and-fro flow across the pulmonary valve with the signal below the line representing forward flow in systole (see ECG tracing for reference) and the signal above the line representing regurgitation during diastole.

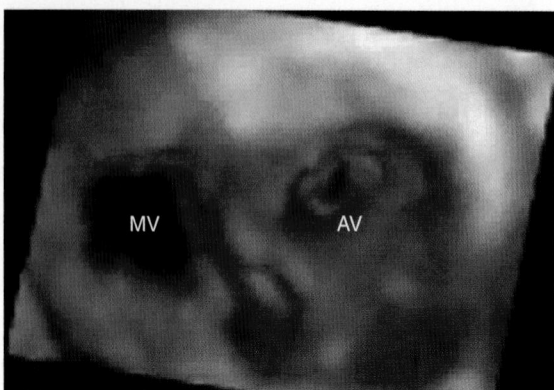

Figure 423-23 Three-dimensional echocardiogram showing a short axis view of the left ventricle. AV, aortic valve; MV, mitral valve. *(Courtesy of Dr. Norman Silverman, Stanford University, Stanford, CA.)*

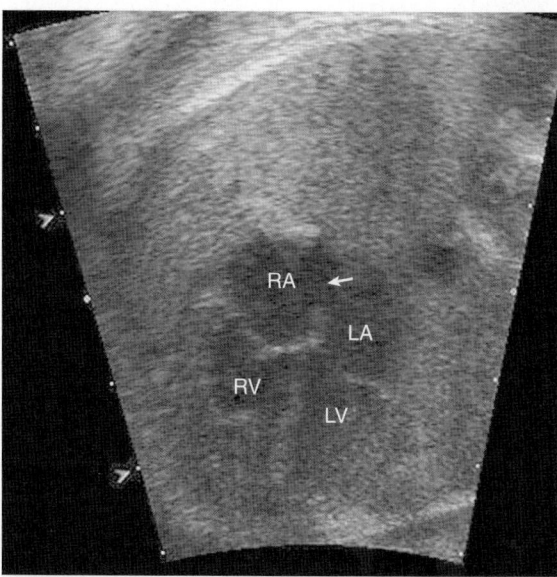

Figure 423-24 Normal 4-chamber view echocardiogram on a fetus at 20 wk of gestation. The foramen ovale *(arrow)* can be seen between the right and left atria. LA, left atrium; LV, left ventricle; RA, right atrium; RV, right ventricle.

THREE-DIMENSIONAL ECHOCARDIOGRAPHY

Real-time 3D echocardiographic reconstruction is valuable for the assessment of cardiac morphology (Fig. 423-23). Details of valve structure, the size and location of septal defects, abnormalities of the ventricular myocardium, and details of the great vessels, which may not be as readily apparent using 2D imaging, can often be appreciated on 3D echocardiography. Reconstruction of the view that the surgeon will encounter in the operating room makes this technique a valuable adjunct for preoperative imaging.

TRANSESOPHAGEAL ECHOCARDIOGRAPHY

Transesophageal echocardiography is an extremely sensitive imaging technique that produces a clearer view of smaller lesions such as vegetations in endocarditis, especially in larger patients. It is useful in visualizing posteriorly located structures such as the atria, aortic root, and atrioventricular valves. Transesophageal echocardiography is extremely useful as an intraoperative technique for monitoring cardiac function during both cardiac and noncardiac surgery and for screening for residual cardiac defects after the patient in initially weaned from cardiopulmonary bypass but before they are disconnected from the bypass circuit. This technique has been especially helpful in evaluating the degree of residual regurgitation or stenosis after valve repairs and in searching for small muscular VSDs that may have been missed during the closure of larger defects.

FETAL ECHOCARDIOGRAPHY

Fetal echocardiography can be used to evaluate cardiac structures or disturbances in cardiac rhythm (Fig. 423-24). Perinatologists often detect gross abnormalities in cardiac structure on routine obstetric ultrasonography or may refer the patient because of unexplained hydrops fetalis, a family history of congenital heart disease, or a maternal condition associated with fetal cardiac pathology such as gestational diabetes. Fetal echocardiography is capable of diagnosing most significant congenital heart lesions as early as 17-19 wk of gestation; accuracy at this early stage is limited and families should understand that these studies cannot totally eliminate the possibility of congenital heart disease. Serial fetal echocardiograms have also demonstrated the importance of flow disturbance in the pathogenesis of congenital heart disease; such studies can show the intrauterine progression of a moderate lesion, such as aortic stenosis, into a more severe lesion, such as hypoplastic left heart syndrome. M-mode echocardiography can diagnose rhythm disturbances in the fetus and can determine the success of antiarrhythmic therapy administered to the mother. A screening fetal echocardiogram is recommended for women with a previous child or 1st-degree relative with congenital heart disease, for those who are at higher risk of having a child with cardiac disease (insulin-dependent diabetics, patients with exposure to teratogenic drugs

during early pregnancy), and in any fetus in which a chromosomal abnormality is suspected or confirmed.

Early detection provides the opportunity to counsel and educate the parents about the severity of the cardiac lesion and potential therapeutic or palliative care options. Referral to a high-risk perinatal service is then performed, for further ultrasound screening for associated anomalies of other organs and potential amniocentesis for karyotyping. For those fetuses with ductal dependent lesions, delivery can be planned at a tertiary care center, avoiding the requirement for postnatal transport of an unstable infant. For those fetuses with complex congenital heart disease at high risk for complications immediately at birth (e.g., hypoplastic left heart syndrome with intact atrial septum), delivery can be arranged with an operating room and surgeon standing by.

Bibliography is available at Expert Consult.

423.5 Exercise Testing
Daniel Bernstein

The normal cardiorespiratory system adapts to the extensive demands of exercise with a several-fold increase in oxygen consumption and cardiac output. Because of the large reserve capacity for exercise, significant abnormalities in cardiovascular performance may be present without symptoms at rest or during ordinary activities. When patients are evaluated in a resting state, significant abnormalities in cardiac function may not be appreciated, or if detected, their implications for quality of life may not be recognized. Permission for children with cardiovascular disease to participate in various forms of physical activity is frequently based on totally subjective criteria. As the importance of aerobic exercise is increasingly recognized, even for children with complex congenital heart lesions, exercise testing can provide a quantitative evaluation of the child's ability to safely participate in both competitive and noncompetitive sports. Exercise testing can also play an important role in evaluating symptoms and quantitating the severity of cardiac abnormalities.

In older children, exercise studies are generally performed on a graded treadmill apparatus with timed intervals of increasing grade and speed. In younger children, exercise studies are often performed on a bicycle ergometer. Many laboratories have the capacity to measure both cardiac and pulmonary function noninvasively during exercise. This allows measurement of both resting and maximal oxygen consumption (Vo_{2max}) and the point at which anaerobic threshold is reached, important indicators of cardiovascular fitness.

As a child grows, the capacity for work is enhanced with increased body size and skeletal muscle mass. All indices of cardiopulmonary function do not increase in a uniform manner. A major response to exercise is an increase in cardiac output, principally achieved through an increase in heart rate, but stroke volume, systemic venous return, and pulse pressure are also increased. Systemic vascular resistance is greatly decreased as the blood vessels in working muscle dilate in response to increasing metabolic demands. As the child becomes older and larger, the response of the heart rate to exercise remains prominent, but cardiac output increases because of growing cardiac volume capacity and, hence, stroke volume. Responses to dynamic exercise are not dependent solely on age. For any given body surface area, boys have a larger stroke volume than size-matched girls. This increase is also mediated by posture. Augmentation of stroke volume with upright, dynamic exercise is facilitated by the pumping action of working muscles, which overcomes the static effect of gravity and increases systemic venous return.

Dynamic exercise testing defines not only endurance and exercise capacity but also the effect of such exercise on myocardial blood flow and cardiac rhythm. Significant ST segment depression reflects abnormalities in myocardial perfusion, for example, the subendocardial ischemia that commonly occurs during exercise in children with hypertrophied left ventricles. The **exercise ECG** is considered abnormal if the ST segment depression is >2 mm and extends for at least 0.06 sec after the J point (onset of the ST segment) in conjunction with a horizontal-, upward-, or downward-sloping ST segment. Provocation of rhythm disturbances during an exercise study is an important method of evaluating selected patients with known or suspected rhythm disorders. The effect of pharmacologic management can also be tested in this manner.

Bibliography is available at Expert Consult.

423.6 MRI, MRA, CT, and Radionuclide Studies

Daniel Bernstein

Magnetic resonance imaging (MRI) and **magnetic resonance angiography (MRA)** are extremely helpful in the diagnosis and management of patients with congenital heart disease. These techniques produce tomographic images of the heart in any projection (Fig. 423-25), with excellent contrast resolution of fat, myocardium, and lung, as well as moving blood from blood vessel walls. MRI is useful in evaluating areas that are less well visualized by echocardiography, such as distal branch pulmonary artery anatomy and anomalies in systemic and pulmonary venous return.

MRA allows the acquisition of images in several tomographic planes. Within each plane, images are obtained at different phases of the cardiac cycle. Thus, when displayed in a dynamic "cine" format, changes in wall thickening, chamber volume, and valve function can be displayed and analyzed. Blood flow velocity and blood flow volume can be calculated. MRA is an excellent technique for following patients serially after repair of complex congenital heart disease, such as tetralogy of Fallot. In these patients, MRA can be used to assess right ventricular volume and mass as well as quantify the amount of regurgitation through either the pulmonary or tricuspid valve. Other MRI techniques, such as myocardial delayed enhancement, can be used to quantify areas of myocardial scar in patients with cardiomyopathy or in patients after congenital heart disease repair, especially tetralogy of Fallot. **Magnetic resonance spectroscopy,** predominantly a research tool at present, provides a means of demonstrating relative

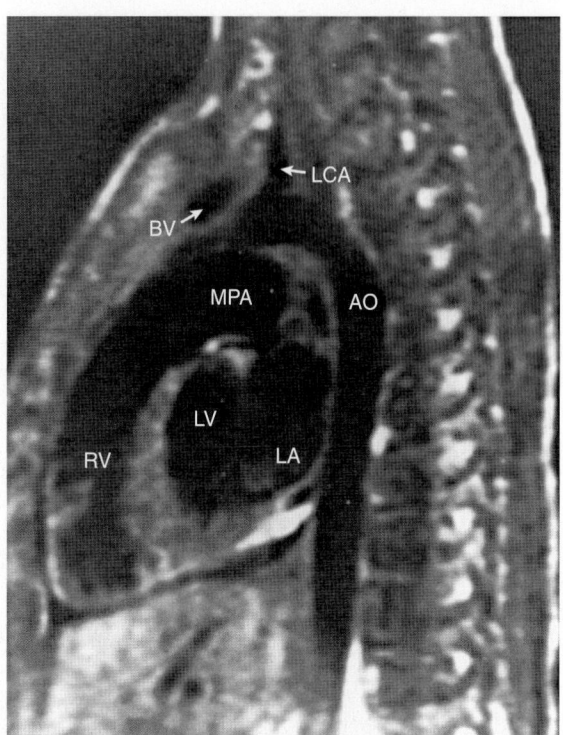

Figure 423-25 Sagittal normal MRI. AO, aorta; BV, brachiocephalic vein; LA, left atrium; LCA, left coronary artery; LV, left ventricle; MPA, main pulmonary artery; RV, right ventricle. *(From Bisset GS III: Cardiac and great vessel anatomy. In El-Khoury GY, Bergman RA, Montgomery WJ, editors: Sectional anatomy by MRI/CT, New York, 1990, Churchill Livingstone.)*

concentrations of high-energy metabolites (adenosine triphosphate, adenosine diphosphate, inorganic phosphate, and phosphocreatine) within regions of the working myocardium.

Computer processing of MRA images allows the noninvasive visualization of the cardiovascular system from inside of the heart or vessels, a technique known as *fly-through imaging.* These images allow the cardiologist to image the interiors of various cardiovascular structures (Fig. 423-26). These imaging techniques are especially helpful in imaging complex peripheral arterial stenoses, especially after balloon angioplasty.

CT scanning can now be used to perform rapid, respiration-gated cardiac imaging in children with resolutions down to 0.5 mm. Three-dimensional reconstruction of CT images (Fig. 423-27) are especially useful in evaluating branch pulmonary arteries, anomalies in systemic and pulmonary venous return, and great vessel anomalies such as coarctation of the aorta.

Radionuclide angiography may be used to detect and quantify shunts and to analyze the distribution of blood flow to each lung. This technique is particularly useful in quantifying the volume of blood flow distribution between the 2 lungs in patients with abnormalities of the pulmonary vascular tree or after a shunt operation (Blalock-Taussig or Glenn), or to quantify the success of balloon angioplasty and intravascular stenting procedures. Gated blood pool scanning can be used to calculate hemodynamic measurements, quantify valvular regurgitation, and detect regional wall motion abnormalities. Thallium imaging can be performed to evaluate cardiac muscle perfusion. These methods can be used at the bedside of seriously ill children and can be performed serially, with minimal discomfort and low radiation exposure.

Bibliography is available at Expert Consult.

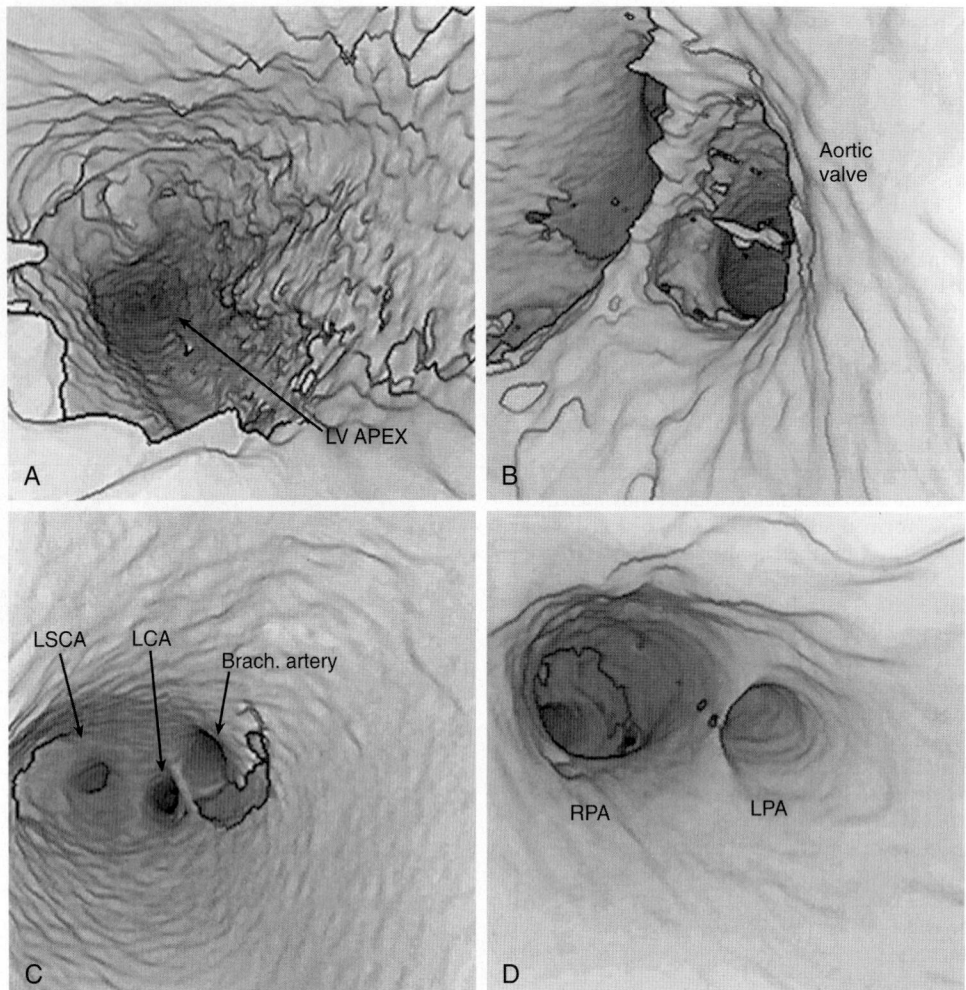

Figure 423-26 Fly-through imaging in a patient with an aortopulmonary window. This series of still frames shows the progression from the left ventricular (LV) chamber **(A),** through the aortic valve **(B),** out to the ascending aorta **(C),** and then through the defect to the branch pulmonary arteries **(D).** Brach., brachiocephalic artery; LCA, left carotid artery; LPA, left pulmonary artery; LSCA, left subclavian artery; RPA, right pulmonary artery.

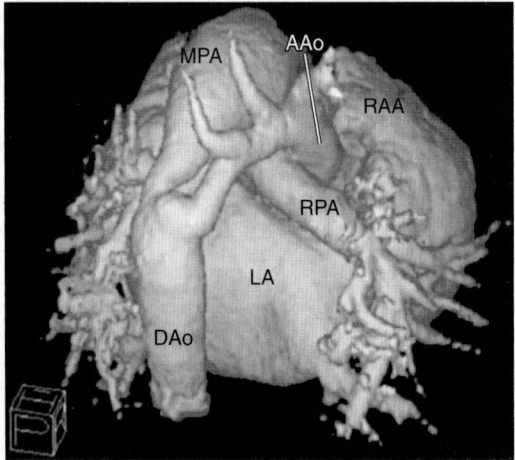

Figure 423-27 Three-dimensional reconstruction of electron-beam CT images from a neonate with severe coarctation of the aorta. The patent ductus arteriosus can be seen toward the left leading from the main pulmonary artery to the descending aorta. The tortuous and narrow coarctated segment is just to the right of the ductus. The transverse aorta is hypoplastic as well. AAo, ascending aorta; DAo, descending aorta; LA, left atrium; MPA, main pulmonary artery; RAA, right atrial appendage; RPA, right pulmonary artery. (*Image courtesy of Dr. Paul Pitlick, Stanford University, Stanford, CA.*)

423.7 Diagnostic and Interventional Cardiac Catheterization

Daniel Bernstein

The catheterization laboratory has become the site of high-technology interventional procedures, allowing for the nonsurgical repair or palliation of heart defects that once required open heart surgery. Some centers have developed hybrid catheterization laboratories, combining standard fluoroscopic imaging with an operating suite, allowing combined approaches to treat complex congenital heart lesions.

DIAGNOSTIC CARDIAC CATHETERIZATION

Diagnostic catheterization is still performed: (1) to assist in the initial diagnosis of some complex congenital heart lesions (e.g., tetralogy of Fallot with pulmonary atresia and major aortopulmonary collateral arteries, pulmonary atresia with intact ventricular septum and coronary sinusoids, hypoplastic left-heart syndrome with mitral stenosis); (2) in cases in which other imaging studies are equivocal; (3) in patients for whom hemodynamic assessment is critical (to determine the size of a left-to-right shunt in borderline cases, or to determine the presence or absence of pulmonary vascular disease in an older patient with a left-to-right shunt); (4) between stages of repair of complex congenital heart disease (e.g., hypoplastic left- or right-heart syndromes); (5) for myocardial biopsy in the diagnosis of cardiomyopathy or in screening for cardiac rejection after cardiac transplantation; and (6) for electrophysiologic study in the evaluation of cardiac arrhythmias (see Chapter 435).

Cardiac catheterization should be performed with the patient in as close to a basal state as possible. Conscious sedation is routine; if a deeper level of general anesthesia is required, careful choice of an anesthetic agent is warranted to avoid depression of cardiovascular function and subsequent distortion of the calculations of cardiac output, pulmonary and systemic vascular resistance, and shunt ratios.

Cardiac catheterization in critically ill infants with congenital heart disease should be performed in a center where a pediatric cardiovascular surgical team is available in the event that an operation is required immediately afterward. The complication rate of cardiac catheterization and angiography is greatest in critically ill infants; they must be studied in a thermally neutral environment and treated quickly for hypothermia, hypoglycemia, acidosis, or excessive blood loss.

Catheterization may be limited to the right-sided cardiac structures, the left-sided structures, or both the right and left sides of the heart. The catheter is passed into the heart under fluoroscopic guidance through a percutaneous entry point in a femoral or jugular vein. In infants and in a number of older children, the left side of the heart can be accessed by passing the catheter across a patent foramen ovale to the left atrium and left ventricle. If the foramen is closed, the left side of the heart can be catheterized by passing the catheter retrograde via a percutaneous entry site in the femoral artery, or if necessary, via a transatrial septal puncture. The catheter can be manipulated through abnormal intracardiac defects (ASDs, VSDs). Blood samples are obtained for measuring oxygen saturation and calculating shunt volumes, pressures are measured for calculating gradients and valve areas, and radiopaque contrast is injected to delineate cardiac and vascular structures. A catheter with a thermosensor tip can be used to measure cardiac output by thermodilution. Specialized catheters can be used to measure more sophisticated indices of cardiac function: Those with pressure-transducer tips can be utilized to measure the first derivative of LV pressure (dP/dt); and conductance catheters can be used to generate pressure-volume loops, from which indices of both contractility (end-systolic elastance) and relaxation can be derived. Complete hemodynamics can be calculated, including cardiac output, intracardiac left-to-right and right-to-left shunts, and systemic and pulmonary vascular resistances. Figure 423-28 depicts normal circulatory dynamics.

THERMODILUTION MEASUREMENT OF CARDIAC OUTPUT

The thermodilution method for measuring cardiac output is performed with a flow-directed, thermistor-tipped, pulmonary artery (Swan-Ganz) catheter. A known change in the heat content of the blood is induced at one point in the circulation (usually the right atrium or inferior vena cava) by injecting room temperature saline, and the resultant change in temperature is detected at a point downstream (usually the pulmonary artery). This method is used to measure cardiac output in the catheterization laboratory in patients without shunts. Monitoring cardiac output by the thermodilution method can occasionally be useful in managing critically ill infants and children in an intensive care setting after cardiac surgery or in the presence of shock. In this case, a triple-lumen catheter is used for both cardiac output determination and measurement of pulmonary artery and pulmonary capillary wedge pressure.

ANGIOCARDIOGRAPHY

The major blood vessels and individual cardiac chambers may be visualized by selective angiocardiography, the injection of contrast material into specific chambers or great vessels. This method allows identification of structural abnormalities without interference from the superimposed shadows of normal chambers. Fluoroscopy is used to visualize the catheter as it passes through the various heart chambers. After the cardiac catheter is properly placed in the chamber to be studied, a small amount of contrast medium is injected with a power injector, and cineangiograms are exposed at rates ranging from 15-60 frames/sec.

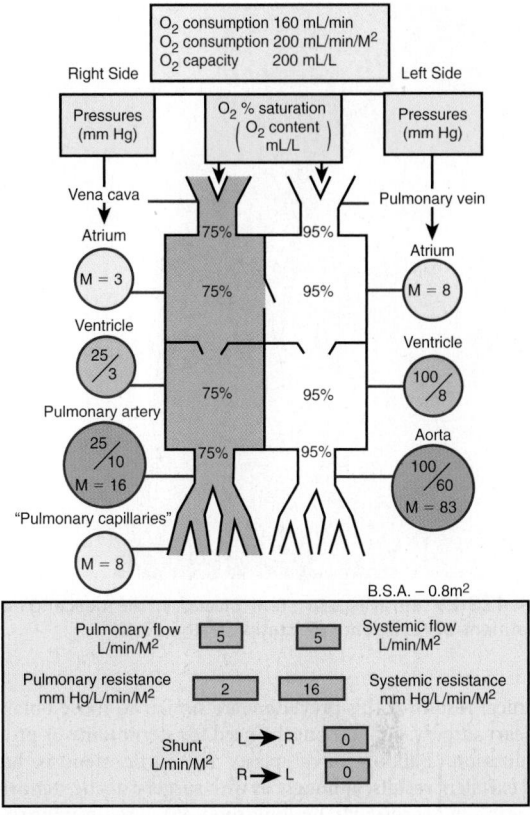

Figure 423-28 Diagram of normal circulatory dynamics with pressure readings, oxygen content, and percent saturation. B.S.A., body surface area. *(Modified from Nadas AS, Fyler DC: Pediatric cardiology, ed 3, Philadelphia, 1972, WB Saunders.)*

Modern catheterization labs utilize digital imaging technology, allowing for a significant reduction in radiation exposure. Biplane cineangiocardiography allows detailed evaluation of specific cardiac chambers and blood vessels in 2 planes simultaneously with the injection of a single bolus of contrast material. This technique is standard in pediatric cardiac catheterization laboratories and allows one to minimize the volume of contrast material used, which is safer for the patient. Various angled views (e.g., left anterior oblique, cranial angulation) are used to display specific anatomic features best in individual lesions.

Rapid injection of contrast medium under pressure into the circulation is not without risk, and each injection should be carefully planned. Contrast agents consist of hypertonic solutions, with some containing organic iodides, which can cause complications, including nausea, a generalized burning sensation, central nervous system symptoms, renal insufficiency, and allergic reactions. Intramyocardial injection is generally avoided by careful placement of the catheter before injection. Hypertonicity of the contrast medium may result in transient myocardial depression and a drop in blood pressure, followed soon afterward by tachycardia, an increase in cardiac output, and a shift of interstitial fluid into the circulation. This shift can transiently increase the symptoms of heart failure in critically ill patients.

INTERVENTIONAL CARDIAC CATHETERIZATION

Catheter treatment is the standard of practice for most cases of isolated pulmonary or aortic valve stenosis (see Fig. 421-4) as well as for re-coarctation of the aorta. A special catheter with a sausage-shaped balloon at the distal end is passed through the obstructed valve. Rapid filling of the balloon with a mixture of contrast material and saline solution results in tearing of the stenotic valve tissue, usually at the site of inappropriately fused raphe. Valvular pulmonary stenosis can be treated successfully by balloon angioplasty; in most patients, angioplasty has replaced surgical repair as the initial procedure of choice.

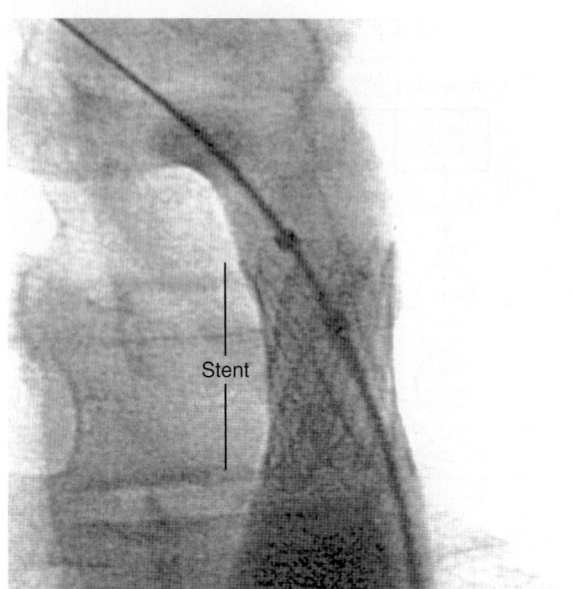

Figure 423-29 Intravascular stent placed in the descending aorta for treatment of recurrent coarctation of the aorta.

The clinical results of this procedure are similar to those obtained by open heart surgery, but without the need for sternotomy or prolonged hospitalization. Balloon valvuloplasty for aortic stenosis has also yielded excellent results, although, as with surgery, aortic stenosis often recurs as the child grows and multiple procedures may thus be required. One complication of both valvuloplasty and surgery is the creation of valvular insufficiency. This complication has more serious implications when it occurs on the aortic vs the pulmonary side of the circulation because regurgitation is less-well tolerated at systemic arterial pressures. Balloon angioplasty is the procedure of choice for patients with restenosis of coarctation of the aorta after earlier surgery. It is controversial whether angioplasty is the best procedure for native (unoperated) coarctation of the aorta because of reports of later aneurysm formation and most centers still refer primary coarctation in infants and young children for surgical repair. However, in older patients with previously undiagnosed coarctation, especially those with decreased LV function, primary angioplasty with possible stent placement may be considered. Other applications of the balloon angioplasty technique include amelioration of mitral stenosis, dilation of surgical conduits (Mustard or Senning atrial baffles), relief of branch pulmonary artery narrowing, dilation of systemic or pulmonary venous obstructions, and the long-used balloon atrial septostomy (Rashkind procedure) for transposition of the great arteries (see Chapter 431.2).

Interventional catheterization techniques are being adapted for use in the **fetus** with lesions such as aortic stenosis in an attempt to prevent their progression to more complex lesions such as hypoplastic left heart syndrome. In these procedures, after administration of appropriate anesthesia, a needle is passed through the maternal abdominal wall, the uterine wall, and the fetal chest wall and directly into the fetal left ventricle (see Fig. 425-13). A coronary angioplasty balloon catheter is passed through the needle and across the stenotic aortic valve, which is then dilated. With the restoration of normal LV blood flow, it is to be hoped that normal LV growth potential is restored. Midterm results with this technique in a growing number of patients show mixed results with good ventricular growth leading to a 2-ventricle circulation in approximately 25% of patients.

In patients with branch pulmonary artery stenoses, the previously mixed results with balloon angioplasty alone have been enhanced with the use of **intravascular stents** (Fig. 423-29) delivered over a balloon catheter and expanded within the vessel lumen. Once placed, they can often be dilated to successively greater sizes as the patient grows, although their use in younger infants and children is limited by the extent to which they can be further expanded. Research into

biodissolvable stents may solve this problem in the future. Stents are also being used in adolescents and young adults with coarctation of the aorta.

Closure of a small PDA is routinely achieved with catheter-delivered coils (see Fig. 420-11), whereas a larger PDA can be closed with a variety of sandwich-type devices. Closure of anomalous vascular connections (coronary fistulas, venovenous collaterals in cyanotic heart lesions) can also be achieved using coils. Secundum ASDs are now routinely closed with a double-disc occluder device (see Fig. 420-3). Versions of these devices are currently in clinical trials for closure of surgically hard-to-reach muscular VSDs and even for the more common perimembranous VSD. Catheter-delivered devices may also be used as an adjunct to complex surgical repairs (dilation or stenting of branch pulmonary artery or pulmonary vein stenosis or closure of a difficult to reach muscular VSD). High-risk patients undergoing the Fontan operation (see Chapter 430.4) often have a small fenestration created between the right and left sides of the circulation to serve as a "popoff valve" for high right-sided pressure in the early surgical period. Patients with these "fenestrated Fontans" are usually candidates for subsequent closure of the fenestration with a catheter-delivered device.

Bibliography is available at Expert Consult.

Section 3
Congenital Heart Disease

Chapter 424
Epidemiology and Genetic Basis of Congenital Heart Disease
Daniel Bernstein

PREVALENCE

Congenital heart disease occurs in approximately 0.8% of live births. The incidence is higher in stillborns (3-4%), spontaneous abortuses (10-25%), and premature infants (approximately 2% excluding patent ductus arteriosus [PDA]). This overall incidence does not include mitral valve prolapse, PDA of preterm infants, and bicuspid aortic valves (present in 1-2% of adults). Congenital cardiac defects have a wide spectrum of severity in infants: approximately 2-3 in 1,000 newborn infants will be symptomatic with heart disease in the 1st yr of life. The diagnosis is established by 1 wk of age in 40-50% of patients with congenital heart disease and by 1 mo of age in 50-60% of patients. With advances in both palliative and corrective surgery, the number of children with congenital heart disease surviving to adulthood has increased dramatically. Despite these advances, congenital heart disease remains the leading cause of death in children with congenital malformations. Table 424-1 summarizes the relative frequency of the most common congenital cardiac lesions.

Most congenital defects are well tolerated in the fetus because of the parallel nature of the fetal circulation. Even the most severe cardiac defects (e.g., hypoplastic left-heart syndrome) can usually be well compensated for by the fetal circulation. In this example, the entire fetal

Table 424-1	Relative Frequency of Major Congenital Heart Lesions*	
LESION		**% OF ALL LESIONS**
Ventricular septal defect		35-30
Atrial septal defect (secundum)		6-8
Patent ductus arteriosus		6-8
Coarctation of aorta		5-7
Tetralogy of Fallot		5-7
Pulmonary valve stenosis		5-7
Aortic valve stenosis		4-7
D-Transposition of great arteries		3-5
Hypoplastic left ventricle		1-3
Hypoplastic right ventricle		1-3
Truncus arteriosus		1-2
Total anomalous pulmonary venous return		1-2
Tricuspid atresia		1-2
Single ventricle		1-2
Double-outlet right ventricle		1-2
Others		5-10

*Excluding patent ductus arteriosus in preterm neonates, bicuspid aortic valve, physiologic peripheral pulmonic stenosis, and mitral valve prolapse.

cardiac output would be ejected by the right ventricle via the ductus arteriosus into both the descending and ascending aortae (the latter filling in a retrograde fashion), so that fetal organ blood flow would be minimally perturbed. Because the placenta provides for gas exchange and the normal fetal circulation has mixing between more highly and more poorly oxygenated blood, fetal organ oxygen delivery is also not dramatically affected. It is only after birth when the fetal pathways (ductus arteriosus and foramen ovale) begin to close that the full hemodynamic impact of an anatomic abnormality becomes apparent. One notable exception is the case of severe regurgitant lesions, most commonly of the tricuspid valve. In these lesions (e.g., Ebstein anomaly or severe right ventricular outflow obstruction [see Chapter 430.7]), the parallel fetal circulation cannot compensate for the volume load imposed on the right side of the heart. In utero heart failure, often with fetal pleural and pericardial effusions, and generalized ascites (nonimmune hydrops fetalis) may occur.

Although the most significant transitions in circulation occur in the immediate perinatal period, the circulation continues to undergo changes after birth, and these later changes may also have a hemodynamic impact on cardiac lesions and their apparent incidence. As pulmonary vascular resistance falls in the 1st several weeks of life, left-to-right shunting through intracardiac defects increases and symptoms become more apparent. Thus, in patients with a ventricular septal defect (VSD), heart failure is often first noticed between 1 and 3 mo of age (see Chapter 426.6). The severity of various defects can also change dramatically with growth; some VSDs may become smaller and even close as the child ages. Alternatively, stenosis of the aortic or pulmonary valve, which may be only moderate in the newborn period, may become worse if valve orifice growth does not keep pace with patient growth (see Chapter 427.5). The physician should always be alert for associated congenital malformations, which can adversely affect the patient's prognosis (see Table 422-2 in Chapter 422).

ETIOLOGY
The cause of most congenital heart defects is still unknown. Many cases of congenital heart disease are multifactorial and result from a combination of genetic predisposition and an as-yet-to-be-determined environmental stimulus. A small percentage of congenital heart lesions are related

to known chromosomal abnormalities, in particular, trisomy 21, 13, and 18 and Turner syndrome; heart disease is found in more than 90% of patients with trisomy 18, 50% of patients with trisomy 21, and 40% of those with Turner syndrome. Other genetic factors may have a role in congenital heart disease; e.g., certain types of VSDs (supracristal) are more common in Asian children. The risk of occurrence of congenital heart disease increases if a 1st-degree relative (parent or sibling) is affected.

A growing list of congenital heart lesions has been associated with specific chromosomal abnormalities, and several have even been linked to specific gene defects. Fluorescent in situ hybridization analysis allows clinicians rapid screening of suspected cases once a specific chromosomal abnormality has been identified, although clinical laboratory tests for specific gene defects are still uncommon. In addition, microarray genomic hybridization has identified previously unknown copy number variations (microdeletions or microduplications) in many patients with congenital heart disease and suspicion of a congenital anomaly syndrome. These variants are submicroscopic and thus not visible on routine chromosome analysis.

A well-characterized genetic cause of congenital heart disease is the deletion of a large region (1.5-3 Mb) of chromosome 22q11.2, known as the **DiGeorge critical region.** At least 30 genes have been mapped to the deleted region; *Tbx1*, a transcription factor involved in early outflow tract development is one gene that has been implicated as a possible cause of DiGeorge syndrome. The estimated prevalence of 22q11.2 deletions is 1/4,000 live births. Cardiac lesions associated with 22q11.2 deletions are most often seen in association with either the DiGeorge syndrome or the **Shprintzen (velocardiofacial) syndrome.** The acronym *CATCH 22* has been used to summarize the major components of these syndromes (cardiac defects, abnormal facies, thymic aplasia, cleft palate, and hypocalcemia). The specific cardiac anomalies are conotruncal defects (tetralogy of Fallot, truncus arteriosus, double-outlet right ventricle, subarterial VSD) and branchial arch defects (coarctation of the aorta, interrupted aortic arch, right aortic arch). Congenital airway anomalies such as tracheomalacia and bronchomalacia are sometimes present. Although the risk of recurrence is extremely low in the absence of a parental 22q11.2 deletion, it is 50% if 1 parent carries the deletion. More than 90% of patients with the clinical features of DiGeorge syndrome have a deletion at 22q11.2. A second genetic locus on the short arm of chromosome 10 (10p13p14) has also been identified, the deletion of which shares some, but not all, phenotypic characteristics with the 22q11.2 deletion; patients with del(10p) have an increased incidence of sensorineural hearing loss.

Other structural heart lesions that have been associated with specific chromosomal abnormalities include **familial secundum atrial septal defect** associated with **heart block** (the transcription factor Nkx2.5 on chromosome 5q35), familial atrial septal defect without heart block (the transcription factor GATA4), Alagille syndrome (Jagged1 on chromosome 20p12), and Williams syndrome (elastin on chromosome 7q11). Of interest, patients with VSDs and atrioventricular septal defects have been found to have multiple Nkx2.5 mutations in cells isolated from diseased heart tissues, but not from normal heart tissues or from circulating lymphocytes, indicating a potential role for somatic mutations leading to mosaicism in the pathogenesis of congenital heart defects. Tables 424-2 and 424-3 are a compilation of known genetic causes of congenital heart disease.

The most progress in identifying the genetic origin of cardiovascular disease has been made in the genetic cardiomyopathies, and in particular, **hypertrophic cardiomyopathy.** Mutations in several genes have been implicated, most of which encode protein components of the cardiac sarcomere, either components of the thick or thin fibers or associated regulatory subunits, although mutations in mitochondrial genes are increasingly recognized and play a larger role in those presenting with hypertrophic cardiomyopathy as young infants than in older children and adults. Mutations of the cardiac β-myosin heavy-chain gene (chromosome 14q1) and the myosin-binding protein C gene (chromosome 11q11) are the most common (see Table 424-4), with less-common mutations including the cardiac troponin T and I genes, α-tropomyosin, regulatory and essential myosin light chains, titin, and the α-myosin heavy chain. More than 200 mutations have

Table 424-2	Genetics of Congenital Heart Disease: Defects Associated with Syndromes		
CARDIOVASCULAR DISEASE	**CHROMOSOMAL LOCATION**	**GENE(S) IMPLICATED***	**COMMON CARDIAC DEFECTS**
DiGeorge syndrome, velocardiofacial syndrome	22q11.2, 11p13p14	*TBX1*	TOF, IAA, TA, VSD
Familial ASD with heart block	5q35	*NKX2.5*	ASD, heart block
Familial ASD without heart block	8p22-23	*GATA4*	ASD
Alagille syndrome (bile duct hypoplasia, right-sided cardiac lesions)	20p12, 1p12	*JAGGED1, NOTCH2*	Peripheral pulmonary hypoplasia, PS, TOF
Holt-Oram syndrome (limb defects, ASD)	12q24	*TBX5*	ASD, VSD, PDA
Trisomy 21 (Down syndrome)	21q22	Not known	AVSD
Isolated familial AV septal defect (without trisomy 21)	1p31-p21, 3p25	*CRELD1*	AVSD
Familial TAPVR	4p13-q12	Not known	TAPVR
Noonan syndrome (PS, ASD, hypertrophic cardiomyopathy)	12q24, 12p1.21, 2p212, 3p25.2, 7q34, 15q22.31, 11p15.5, 1p13.2, 10q25.2, 11q23.3,17q11.2	*PTPN11, KRAS, SOS1, RAF1, BRAF, MEK1, HRAS, NRAS, SHOC2, CBL, NF1*	PS, ASD, VSD, PDA, cardiomyopathy
Ellis–van Creveld syndrome (polydactyly, ASD)	4p16	*EVC, EVC2*	ASD, common atrium
Char syndrome (craniofacial, limb defects, PDA)	6p12-21.1	*TFAP2B*	PDA
Williams-Beuren syndrome (supravalvular AS, branch PS, hypercalcemia)	7q11.23	*ELN* (Elastin)	Supravalvar AS, peripheral PS
Marfan syndrome (connective tissue weakness, aortic root dilation)	15q21	Fibrillin	Aortic aneurysm, mitral valve disease
Familial laterality abnormalities	Xq24-2q7, 1q42, 9p13-21	*ZIC3, DNAI1*	Situs inversus, complex congenital heart disease
Turner	X	Not known	Coarctation of the aorta, Aortic stenosis
Trisomy 13 (Patau syndrome)	13	Not known	ASD, VSD, PDA, valve abnormalities
Trisomy 18 (Edwards syndrome)	18	Not known	ASD, VSD, PDA, Valve abnormalities
Cri du chat	5p15.2	*CTNND2*	ASD, VSD, PDA, TOF
Cat eye	22q11	Not known	TAPVR, TOF
Jacobsen	11q23	*JAM-3*	HLHS
Costello	11p15.5	*HRAS*	PS, hypertrophic cardiomyopathy, arrhythmias
CHARGE	8p12, 7q21.11	*CHD7, SEMA3E*	ASD, VSD, TOF
Kabuki syndrome	12q13.12	*MLL2*	ASD, VSD, TOF, coarctation, TGA
Carney syndrome	2p16	*PRKAR1A*	Atrial and ventricular myxomas

AS, aortic stenosis; ASD, atrial septal defect; AV, atrioventricular; AVSD, atrioventricular septal defect; HLHS, hypoplastic left-heart syndrome; IAA, interrupted aortic arch; PDA, patent ductus arteriosus; PS, pulmonic stenosis; TA, truncus arteriosus; TAPVR, total anomalous pulmonary venous return; TGA, transposition of great arteries; TOF, tetralogy of Fallot; VSD, ventricular septal defect.
*In many cases, mutation of a single gene has been closely linked to a specific cardiovascular disease, for example, by finding a high incidence of mutations or deletions of that gene in a large group of patients. These findings are often confirmed by studies in mice in which deletion or alteration of the gene induces a similar cardiac phenotype to the human disease. In others, mutation of a gene may increase the risk of cardiovascular disease, but with decreased penetrance, suggesting that modifier genes or environmental factors play a role. Finally, in some cases, gene mutations have only been identified in a small number of pedigrees, and confirmation awaits screening of larger numbers of patients.

been identified in these genes, and some patients may carry mutations in more than 1 gene. Routine clinical laboratory tests are now available for most of these mutations.

Progress has also been made in identifying the genetic basis of **dilated cardiomyopathy,** which is familial in 20-50% of cases. Autosomal dominant inheritance is most commonly encountered and, similar to hypertrophic cardiomyopathy, multiple genes have been identified (see Table 424-2). X-linked inheritance accounts for 5-10% of cases of familial dilated cardiomyopathy. Mutations in the dystrophin gene (chromosome Xp21) are the most common in this group. Mutations in the gene encoding *tafazzin* are associated with Barth syndrome and some cases of isolated non-compaction of the

Table 424-3	Genetics of Isolated Congenital Heart Disease (Nonsyndromic)	
GENE IMPLICATED*	**PROTEIN ENCODED**	**CARDIAC DEFECTS**
GENES ENCODING TRANSCRIPTION FACTORS		
ANKRD1	Ankyrin repeat domain	TAPVR
CITED2	cAMP responsive element-binding protein	ASD, VSD
FOG2/ZFPM2	Friend of GATA	TOF
GATA6	GATA6 transcription factor	ASD, VSD, TOF, PS, AVSD, PDA
HAND2	Helix-loop-helix transcription factor	TOF
IRX4	Iroquois homeobox 4	VSD
MED13L	Mediator complex subunit 13-like	TGA
NKX2-5/NKX2.5	Homeobox containing transcription factor	ASD, VSD, TOF, HLHS, CoA, TGA, IAA
TBX20	T-Box 20 transcription factor	ASD, VSD, mitral stenosis
ZIC3	Zinc finger transcription factor	TGA, PS, TAPVR, HLHS, ASD, VSD
GENES ENCODING RECEPTORS AND SIGNALING MOLECULES		
ACVR1/ALK2	BMP receptor	AVSD
ACVR2B	Activin receptor	PS, DORV, TGA
ALDH1A2	Retinaldehyde dehydrogenase	TOF
CFC1/CRYPTIC	Cryptic protein	TOF, TGA, AVSD, ASD, VSD, IAA, DORV
CRELD1	Epidermal growth factor-related proteins	ASD; AVSD
FOXH1	Forkhead activin signal transducer	TOF, TGA
GDF1	Growth differentiation factor-1	TOF, TGA, DORV, heterotaxy
GJA1	Connexin 43	ASD, HLHS, TAPVR
LEFTY2	Left-right determination factor	TGA, AVSD, IAA, CoA
NODAL	Nodal homolog (TGF-β superfamily)	TGA, PA, TOF, DORV, TAPVR, AVSD
NOTCH1	NOTCH1 (Ligand of JAG1)	Bicuspid aortic valve, AS, CoA, HLHS
PDGFRA	Platelet-derived growth factor receptor α	TAPVR
SMAD6	MAD-related protein	Bicuspid aortic valve, CoA, AS
TAB2	TGF-β activated kinase	Outflow tract defects
TDGF1	Teratocarcinoma-derived growth factor 1	TOF, VSD
VEGF	Vascular endothelial growth factor	CoA, outflow tract defects
GENES ENCODING STRUCTURAL PROTEINS		
ACTC	α Cardiac actin	ASD
MYH11	Myosin heavy chain 11	PDA, aortic aneurysm
MYH6	α-Myosin heavy chain	ASD, TA, AS, TGA
MYH7	β-Myosin heavy chain	Ebstein anomaly, ASD

AS, aortic stenosis; ASD, atrial septal defect; AVSD, atrioventricular septal defect; cAMP, cyclic adenosine monophosphate; CoA, coarctation of the aorta; DORV, double-outlet right ventricle; HLHS, hypoplastic left heart syndrome; IAA, interrupted aortic arch; PA, pulmonary artery; PDA, patent ductus arteriosus; PS, pulmonic stenosis; TA, truncus arteriosus; TAPVR, total anomalous pulmonary venous return; TGA, transposition of the great arteries; TGF, transforming growth factor; TOF, tetralogy of Fallot; VSD, ventricular septal defect.

*In many cases, mutation of a single gene has been closely linked to a specific cardiovascular disease, for example, by finding a high incidence of mutations or deletions of that gene in a large group of patients. These findings are often confirmed by studies in mice in which deletion or alteration of the gene induces a similar cardiac phenotype to the human disease. In others, mutation of a gene may increase the risk of cardiovascular disease, but with decreased penetrance, suggesting that modifier genes or environmental factors play a role. Finally, in some cases, gene mutations have only been identified in a small number of pedigrees, and confirmation awaits screening of larger numbers of patients.

Partially adapted from Fahed AC, Gelb BD, Seidman JG, Seidman CE: Genetics of congenital heart disease: the glass half empty. Circ Res 112:707–720, 2013.

left ventricle. Autosomal recessive inheritance is associated with a mutation in cardiac troponin I. Mitochondrial myopathies may be caused by mutations of enzymes of the electron transport chain encoded by nuclear DNA (in which inheritance will follow mendelian genetic patterns) or enzymes of fatty acid oxidation encoded by mitochondrial DNA (which is inherited solely from the mother). Table 424-4 is a compilation of the most common genetic causes of cardiomyopathy.

The genetic basis of **heritable arrhythmias,** most notably the **long Q-T syndromes,** has been linked to mutations of genes coding for subunits of cardiac potassium and sodium channels (see Table 424-2). Other heritable arrhythmias include arrhythmogenic right ventricular dysplasia, familial atrial fibrillation, familial complete heart block, and Brugada syndrome. Table 424-5 is a compilation of the most common genetic causes of arrhythmias.

Of all cases of congenital heart disease, 2-4% are associated with known environmental or adverse maternal conditions and teratogenic influences, including maternal diabetes mellitus, phenylketonuria, or systemic lupus erythematosus; congenital rubella syndrome; and maternal ingestion of drugs (lithium, ethanol, warfarin, thalidomide, antimetabolites, vitamin A derivatives, anticonvulsant agents) (see Table 422-2 in Chapter 422). Associated noncardiac malformations noted in identifiable syndromes may be seen in as many as 25% of patients with congenital heart disease.

Gender differences in the occurrence of specific cardiac lesions have been identified. Transposition of the great arteries and left-sided obstructive lesions are slightly more common in boys (≈65%), whereas atrial septal defect, VSD, PDA, and pulmonic stenosis are more common in girls. No racial differences in the occurrence of congenital heart lesions as a whole have been noted; for specific lesions such as transposition of the great arteries, a higher occurrence is seen in white infants.

GENETIC COUNSELING
Parents who have a child with congenital heart disease require counseling regarding the probability of a cardiac malformation occurring in subsequent children (see Chapter 77). With the exception of syndromes known to be caused by mutation of a single gene, most congenital heart disease is still relegated to a multifactorial inheritance pattern, which should result in a low risk of recurrence. As more genetic etiologies are identified, however, these risks will need constant updating. The incidence of congenital heart disease in the normal population is ≈0.8%, and this incidence increases to 2-6% for a second pregnancy after the birth of a child with congenital heart disease or if a parent is affected. This recurrence risk is highly dependent on the type of lesion in the first child. When two 1st-degree relatives have congenital heart disease, the risk for a subsequent child may reach 20-30%. When a second child is found to have congenital heart disease, it will tend to be of a similar

Table 424-4	Genetics of Cardiomyopathies		
Hypertrophic cardiomyopathy		14q1	β-Myosin heavy chain
		15q2	α-Tropomyosin
		1q31	Troponin T
		19p13.2-19q13.2	Troponin I
		11p13-q13	Myosin-binding protein C
		12q23	Cardiac slow myosin regulatory light chain
		13p21	Ventricular slow myosin essential light chain
		2q31	Titin
		3p25	Caveolin-3
		Mitochondrial DNA	tRNA-glycine
		Mitochondrial DNA	tRNA-isoleucine
Hypertrophic cardiomyopathy with Wolff-Parkinson-White syndrome		7q36.1	AMP-activated protein kinase
Other genetic diseases causing cardiac hypertrophy			
Familial amyloid disease		18q12.1	Transthyretin (TTR)
Noonan syndrome		12q24.1, 2p22.1, 3p25,12p12.1	Protein tyrosine phosphatase 11 (PTPN11), son of sevenless homologue 1 (SOS1), RAF1 protooncogene, GTPase KRAS
Fabry disease		Xq22	α-Galactoside A (GLA)
Danon disease		Xq24	Lysosomal-associated membrane protein 2 (LAMP2)
Hereditary hemochromatosis		6p21.3	Hereditary hemochromatosis protein (HFE)
Pompe disease		17q25	Acid α-glucosidase (GAA)
Dilated cardiomyopathy			
X-linked		Xp21	Dystrophin
		Xp28	Tafazzin
Autosomal recessive		19p13.2-19q13.2	Troponin I

Autosomal dominant: genes encoding multiple proteins have been identified, including cardiac actin; desmin; δ-sarcoglycan; β-myosin heavy chain; cardiac troponin C and T; α-tropomyosin; titin; metavinculin; myosin-binding protein C; muscle LIM protein; α-actinin-2; phospholamban; Cypher/LIM binding domain 3; α-myosin heavy chain; SUR2A (regulatory subunit of K$_{ATP}$ channel); and lamin A/C.
Isolated noncompaction of the left ventricle: autosomal dominant, autosomal recessive, X-linked, and mitochondrial inheritance patterns have been reported. Genes that have been implicated include: α-dystrobrevin, Cypher/ZASP, lamin A/C, Tafazzin, MIB1, and LIM domain-binding protein 3 (LDB3).
Partially adapted from Dunn KE, Caleshu C, Cirino AL, et al. A clinical approach to inherited hypertrophy: the use of family history in diagnosis, risk assessment, and management. Circ Cardiovasc Genet 6:118-131, 2013.

Table 424-5	Genetics of Arrhythmias		
Complete heart block		19q13	Not known
Long Q-T syndrome			
LQT1 (autosomal dominant)		11p15.5	KVLQT1 (K+ channel)
LQT2 (autosomal dominant)		7q35	HERG (K+ channel)
LQT3 (autosomal dominant)		3p21	SCN5A (Na+ channel)
LQT4 (autosomal dominant)		4q25-27	Not known
LQT5 (autosomal dominant)		21q22-q22	KCNE1 (K+ channel)
LQT6		21q22.1	KCNE2 (K+ channel)
Jervell and Lange-Nielsen syndrome (autosomal recessive, congenital deafness)		11p15.5	KVLQT1 (K+ channel)
LQT8-13		Unknown	Private mutations (rare)

Arrhythmogenic RV dysplasia: There are now 11 genes associated with arrhythmogenic right ventricular dysplasia (ARVD1 through 11) usually with autosomal dominant inheritance, but with variable penetrance. These genes are: *TGF-β$_3$* (transforming growth factor β), *RyR2* (ryanodine receptor), *LAMR1* (laminin receptor-1), *PTPLA* (protein tyrosine phosphatase), *DSP* (desmoplakin), *PKP2* (plakophilin-2), *DSG2* (desmoglein), and *DSC2* (desmocollin).

Familial atrial fibrillation (autosomal dominant)		10q22-q24, 6q14-16	Not known
		11p15.5	KVLQT1 (K+ channel)
		11p15.5	KCNQ1 (K+ channel)
		21q22	KCNE2 (K+ channel)
		17q23.1-q24.2	KCNJ2 (K+ channel)
		7q35-q36	KCNH2 (K+ channel)
Brugada syndrome (right bundle-branch block, ST segment elevation, unexpected sudden death)		3p21-p24	SCN5A (Na+ channel)
		3p22-p24	GPD-1L (glycerol-3-phosphate dehydrogenase)
Catecholaminergic polymorphic ventricular tachycardia		–	RYR2 (autosomal dominant)
		–	CASQ2 (autosomal recessive)

class as the lesion in their 1st-degree relative (conotruncal lesions, left-sided obstructive lesions, right-sided obstructive lesions, atrioventricular septation defects). The degree of severity may be variable, as is the presence of associated defects. Careful echocardiographic screening of 1st-degree relatives will often uncover mild forms of congenital heart disease that were clinically silent. For example, the incidence of bicuspid aortic valve is more than double (5% vs. 2% in the general population) in the relatives of children with left ventricular outflow obstructions (aortic stenosis, coarctation of the aorta, or hypoplastic left heart syndrome). Given the rapid advancements in the field of cardiovascular genetics, consultation with a knowledgeable genetic counselor is the most reliable way of providing the family with up-to-date information regarding the risk of recurrence.

Fetal echocardiography improves the rate of detection of congenital heart lesions in high-risk patients (see Chapter 423). The resolution and accuracy of fetal echocardiography are excellent, but not perfect; families should be counseled that a normal fetal echocardiogram does not guarantee the absence of congenital heart disease. Congenital heart lesions may evolve in the course of the pregnancy; moderate aortic stenosis with a normal-sized left ventricle at 18 wk of gestation may evolve into aortic atresia with a hypoplastic left ventricle by 34 wk because of decreased flow through the atria, ventricle, and aorta in the latter half of gestation. This progression has prompted initial clinical trials of interventional treatment, such as fetal aortic balloon valvuloplasty, for the prevention of hypoplastic left heart syndrome (see Chapter 423.7).

The major factor in determining whether a **woman with congenital heart disease,** either unoperated or operated, will be able to carry a fetus to term is the mother's cardiovascular status. In the presence of a mild congenital heart defect or after successful repair of a more complex lesion, normal childbearing is likely. In a woman with palliated congenital heart disease or with poor cardiac function, however, the increased hemodynamic burden imposed by pregnancy may result in a significantly increased risk to both the mother and fetus. The incidence of spontaneous abortion in the presence of severe congenital heart disease is high, especially when the mother is cyanotic. The maternal risk in these situations is also high, and these pregnancies should be managed by an experienced perinatologist in conjunction with a cardiologist with expertise in adult congenital heart disease (see Chapter 434.1). It is important to discuss these risks, as well as various methods of birth control, with young women who have repaired or palliated congenital heart lesions. Antibiotic prophylaxis against endocarditis may also be indicated at the time of delivery.

Bibliography is available at Expert Consult.

Chapter 425
Evaluation and Screening of the Infant or Child with Congenital Heart Disease

Daniel Bernstein

The initial evaluation for suspected congenital heart disease involves a systematic approach with 3 major components. First, congenital cardiac defects can be divided into 2 major groups based on the presence or absence of cyanosis, which can be determined by physical examination aided by pulse oximetry. Second, these 2 groups can usually be further subdivided according to whether the chest radiograph shows evidence of increased, normal, or decreased pulmonary vascular markings. Finally, the electrocardiogram can be used to determine whether right, left, or biventricular hypertrophy exists. The character of the heart sounds and the presence and character of any murmurs further narrow the differential diagnosis. The final diagnosis is then confirmed by echocardiography, CT or MRI, or cardiac catheterization.

Multiple studies demonstrate the benefit of routine pulse oximetry screening for all newborns to detect unsuspected critical cyanotic congenital heart disease; lesions include hypoplastic left-heart syndrome,

pulmonary atresia, tetralogy of Fallot, total anomalous pulmonary venous return, transposition of the great arteries, tricuspid atresia, truncus arteriosus, as well as neonatal coarctation of the aorta, and aortic arch hypoplasia/atresia. Many of these lesions are ductal dependent, and if the ductus arteriosus closes, severe cardiac decompensation will ensue. Such screening has been endorsed by the American Academy of Pediatrics, the American Heart Association, the American College of Cardiology and the March of Dimes, and recommended, although not mandated, by federal agencies such as Health and Human Services. Screening is performed between 24 and 48 hr of life and before discharge in asymptomatic newborns. A pulse oximetry saturation <90% in the right hand or either foot requires urgent echocardiography. A pulse oximetry saturation <95% in either location or a saturation difference >3% between the right hand and either foot is considered a positive test and should be repeated in an hour; if positive again, it should be repeated in another hour. If it remains positive, echocardiography is indicated. In addition, a careful reexamination of the pulses and blood pressure in the upper and lower extremity as well as a cardiac exam are indicated in children with an initial positive exam.

ACYANOTIC CONGENITAL HEART LESIONS

Acyanotic congenital heart lesions can be classified according to the predominant physiologic load that they place on the heart. Although many congenital heart lesions induce more than one physiologic disturbance, it is helpful to focus on the primary load abnormality for purposes of classification. The most common lesions are those that produce a volume load, and the most common of these are left-to-right shunt lesions. Atrioventricular (AV) valve regurgitation and some of the cardiomyopathies are other causes of increased volume load. The second major class of lesions causes an increase in pressure load, most commonly secondary to ventricular outflow obstruction (pulmonic or aortic valve stenosis) or narrowing of 1 of the great vessels (coarctation of the aorta). The chest radiograph and electrocardiogram are useful tools for differentiating between these major classes of volume and pressure overload lesions.

Lesions Resulting in Increased Volume Load

The most common lesions in this group are those that cause left-to-right shunting (see Chapter 426): atrial septal defect, ventricular septal defect (VSD), AV septal defects (AV canal), and patent ductus arteriosus. The pathophysiologic common denominator in this group is communication between the systemic and pulmonary sides of the circulation, which results in shunting of fully oxygenated blood back into the lungs. This shunt can be quantitated by calculating the ratio of pulmonary to systemic blood flow, or Qp:Qs. Thus, a 3:1 shunt implies 3 times the normal pulmonary blood flow.

The direction and magnitude of the shunt across such a communication depend on the size of the defect, the relative pulmonary and systemic pressure and vascular resistances, and the compliances of the 2 chambers connected by the defect. These factors are dynamic and may change dramatically with age: Intracardiac defects may grow smaller with time; pulmonary vascular resistance, which is high in the immediate newborn period, decreases to normal adult levels by several weeks of life; and chronic exposure of the pulmonary circulation to high pressure and blood flow results in a gradual increase in pulmonary vascular resistance (Eisenmenger physiology; see Chapter 433.2). Thus, a lesion such as a large VSD may be associated with little shunting and few symptoms during the initial weeks of life. When pulmonary vascular resistance declines in the next several weeks, the volume of the left-to-right shunt increases, and symptoms begin to appear.

The increased volume of blood in the lungs decreases pulmonary compliance and increases the work of breathing. Fluid leaks into the interstitial space and alveoli and causes pulmonary edema. The infant develops the symptoms we refer to as **heart failure,** such as tachypnea, tachycardia, sweating, chest retractions, nasal flaring, and wheezing. For children with large left-to-right shunts, the term *heart failure* is a misnomer, however; total left ventricular output is not decreased but is actually several times greater than normal, although much of this output is ineffective because it returns directly to the lungs. To maintain this high level of left ventricular output, heart rate and stroke volume are increased, mediated by an increase in sympathetic nervous system activity. The increase in circulating catecholamines, combined with the increased work of breathing, results in an elevation in total body oxygen consumption, often beyond the oxygen transport ability of the circulation. Sympathetic activation leads to the additional symptoms of sweating and irritability and the imbalance between oxygen supply and demand lead to failure to thrive. Remodeling of the heart occurs, with predominantly chamber dilation and a lesser degree of hypertrophy. If left untreated, pulmonary vascular resistance eventually begins to rise and, by several years of age, the shunt volume will decrease and eventually reverse to right-to-left (Eisenmenger physiology; see Chapter 433.2).

Additional lesions that impose a volume load on the heart include regurgitant lesions (see Chapter 428) and the cardiomyopathies (see Chapter 439). Regurgitation through the AV valves is most commonly encountered in patients with partial or complete AV septal defects (AV canal, endocardial cushion defects). In these lesions, the combination of a left-to-right shunt with AV valve regurgitation increases the volume load on the heart and often leads to more severe symptoms. Isolated regurgitation through the tricuspid valve is seen in mild, moderate and severe forms of Ebstein anomaly (see Chapter 430.7). Regurgitation involving 1 of the semilunar (aortic or pulmonary) valves is usually also associated with some degree of stenosis; however, aortic regurgitation may be encountered in patients with a VSD directly under the aortic valve (supracristal VSD) and in patients with membranous subaortic stenosis.

In contrast to left-to-right shunts, in which intrinsic cardiac muscle function is generally either normal or increased, heart muscle function is decreased in the cardiomyopathies. **Cardiomyopathies** may affect systolic contractility or diastolic relaxation, or both. Decreased cardiac function results in increased atrial and ventricular filling pressure, and pulmonary edema occurs secondary to increased capillary pressure. Poor cardiac output leads to decreased organ blood flow, sympathetic activation, and the symptoms of poor perfusion and decreased urine output. The major causes of cardiomyopathy in infants and children include viral myocarditis, metabolic disorders, and genetic defects (see Chapter 439).

Lesions Resulting in Increased Pressure Load

The pathophysiologic common denominator of these lesions is an obstruction to normal blood flow. The most frequent are obstructions to ventricular outflow: valvular pulmonic stenosis, valvular aortic stenosis, and coarctation of the aorta (see Chapter 427). Less common are obstruction to ventricular inflow: tricuspid or mitral stenosis, cor triatriatum and obstruction of the pulmonary veins. Ventricular outflow obstruction can occur at the valve, below the valve (double-chambered right ventricle, subaortic membrane), or above it (branch pulmonary stenosis or supravalvular aortic stenosis). Unless the obstruction is severe, cardiac output will be maintained and the clinical symptoms of heart failure will be either subtle or absent. This compensation predominantly involves an increase in cardiac wall thickness (hypertrophy), but in later stages the affected chamber will begin to dilate and can progress to ventricular failure.

The clinical picture is different when obstruction to outflow is severe, which is usually encountered in the immediate newborn period. The infant may become critically ill within several hours of birth. Severe pulmonic stenosis in the newborn period (critical pulmonic stenosis) results in signs of right-sided heart failure (hepatomegaly, peripheral edema) as well as cyanosis from right-to-left shunting across the foramen ovale. Severe aortic stenosis in the newborn period (critical aortic stenosis) is characterized by signs of left-sided heart failure (pulmonary edema, poor perfusion) and right-sided failure (hepatomegaly, peripheral edema), and it may progress rapidly to total circulatory collapse. In older children, severe pulmonic stenosis leads to symptoms of right-sided heart failure, but usually not to cyanosis unless a pathway persists for right-to-left shunting (e.g., patency of the foramen ovale).

Coarctation of the aorta in older children and adolescents is usually manifested as upper body hypertension and diminished pulses in the lower extremities. In the immediate newborn period, the presentation of coarctation can range from decreased pulses in the lower extremities to total circulatory collapse, depending on the severity of the narrowing. However, the clinical presentation of coarctation may be delayed because of the presence of a patent ductus arteriosus. In these patients, the open aortic end of the ductus may serve as a conduit for blood flow to partially bypass the obstruction or for blood leaving the right ventricle to directly supply the descending aorta (as it did in the fetus). These infants then become symptomatic, often dramatically, when the ductus finally closes, usually within the 1st few wk of life.

CYANOTIC CONGENITAL HEART LESIONS

This group of congenital heart lesions can also be further divided according to pathophysiology: whether pulmonary blood flow is decreased (tetralogy of Fallot, pulmonary atresia with an intact septum, tricuspid atresia, total anomalous pulmonary venous return with obstruction) or increased (transposition of the great vessels, single ventricle, truncus arteriosus, total anomalous pulmonary venous return without obstruction). The chest radiograph is a valuable tool for initial differentiation between these 2 categories.

Cyanotic Lesions with Decreased Pulmonary Blood Flow

These lesions must include both an obstruction to pulmonary blood flow (at the tricuspid valve or right ventricular or pulmonary valve level) and a pathway by which systemic venous blood can shunt from right to left and enter the systemic circulation (via a patent foramen ovale, atrial septal defect, or VSD). Common lesions in this group include tricuspid atresia, tetralogy of Fallot, and various forms of single ventricle with pulmonary stenosis (see Chapter 430). In these lesions, the degree of cyanosis depends on the degree of obstruction to pulmonary blood flow. If the obstruction is mild, cyanosis may be absent at rest. These patients may have hypercyanotic ("tet") spells during conditions of stress. In contrast, if the obstruction is severe, pulmonary blood flow may be totally dependent on patency of the ductus arteriosus. When the ductus closes in the 1st few days of life, the neonate experiences profound hypoxemia and shock.

Cyanotic Lesions with Increased Pulmonary Blood Flow

This group of lesions is not associated with obstruction to pulmonary blood flow. Cyanosis is caused by either abnormal ventricular–arterial connections or total mixing of systemic venous and pulmonary venous blood within the heart (see Chapter 431). Transposition of the great vessels is the most common of the former group of lesions. In this condition, the aorta arises from the right ventricle and the pulmonary artery arises from the left ventricle. Systemic venous blood returning to the right atrium is pumped directly back to the body and oxygenated blood returning from the lungs to the left atrium is pumped back into the lungs. The persistence of fetal pathways (foramen ovale and ductus arteriosus) allows for a small degree of mixing in the immediate newborn period; when the ductus begins to close, these infants can become extremely cyanotic.

Total mixing lesions include cardiac defects with a common atrium or ventricle, total anomalous pulmonary venous return, and truncus arteriosus (see Chapter 431). In this group, deoxygenated systemic venous blood and oxygenated pulmonary venous blood mix completely in the heart and, as a result, oxygen saturation is equal in the pulmonary artery and aorta. If pulmonary blood flow is not obstructed, these infants have a combination of cyanosis and pulmonary overcirculation leading to heart failure. In contrast, if pulmonary stenosis is present, these infants may have cyanosis alone, similar to patients with tetralogy of Fallot.

Bibliography is available at Expert Consult.

Chapter **426**
Acyanotic Congenital Heart Disease: Left-to-Right Shunt Lesions

426.1 Atrial Septal Defect

Daniel Bernstein

Atrial septal defects (ASDs) can occur in any portion of the atrial septum (secundum, primum, or sinus venosus), depending on which embryonic septal structure has failed to develop normally (see Chapter 420). Less commonly, the atrial septum may be nearly absent, with the creation of a functional single atrium. Isolated secundum ASDs account for ≈7% of congenital heart defects. The majority of cases of ASD are sporadic; autosomal dominant inheritance does occur as part of the Holt-Oram syndrome (hypoplastic or absent thumbs, radii, triphalangism, phocomelia, 1st-degree heart block, ASD) or in families with secundum ASD and heart block (see Table 424-2 in Chapter 424).

An isolated valve-incompetent patent foramen ovale (PFO) is a common echocardiographic finding during infancy. It is usually of no hemodynamic significance and is not considered an ASD; a PFO may play an important role if other structural heart defects are present. If another cardiac anomaly is causing increased right atrial pressure (pulmonary stenosis or atresia, tricuspid valve abnormalities, right ventricular dysfunction), venous blood may shunt across the PFO into the left atrium with resultant cyanosis. Because of the anatomic structure of the PFO, left-to-right shunting is unusual outside the immediate newborn period. In the presence of a large volume load or a hypertensive left atrium (secondary to mitral stenosis), the foramen ovale may be sufficiently dilated to result in a significant atrial left-to-right shunt. A valve-competent but probe-PFO may be present in 15-30% of adults. An isolated PFO does not require surgical treatment, although it may be a risk for paradoxical (right to left) systemic embolization. Device closure of these defects has been considered in young adults with a history of thromboembolic stroke.

Bibliography is available at Expert Consult.

426.2 Ostium Secundum Defect

Daniel Bernstein

An ostium secundum defect in the region of the fossa ovalis is the most common form of ASD and is associated with structurally normal atrioventricular (AV) valves. Mitral valve prolapse has been described in association with this defect but is rarely an important clinical consideration. Secundum ASDs may be single or multiple (fenestrated atrial septum), and openings ≥2 cm in diameter are common in symptomatic older children. Large defects may extend inferiorly toward the inferior vena cava and ostium of the coronary sinus, superiorly toward the superior vena cava, or posteriorly. Females outnumber males 3:1 in incidence. Partial anomalous pulmonary venous return, most commonly of the right upper pulmonary vein, may be an associated lesion.

PATHOPHYSIOLOGY

The degree of left-to-right shunting is dependent on the size of the defect, the relative compliance of the right and left ventricles, and the

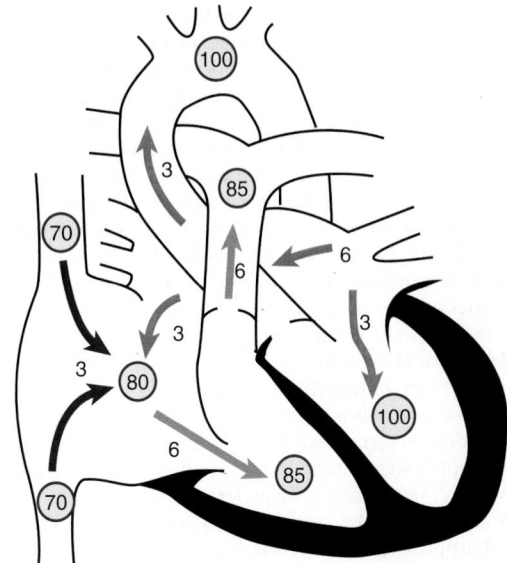

Figure 426-1 Physiology of atrial septal defect. *Circled numbers* represent oxygen saturation values. The *numbers next to the arrows* represent volumes of blood flow (in L/min/m²). This illustration shows a hypothetical patient with a pulmonary-to-systemic blood flow ratio (Qp:Qs) of 2:1. Desaturated blood enters the right atrium from the vena cavae at a volume of 3 L/min/m² and mixes with an additional 3 L of fully saturated blood shunting left to right across the ASD; the result is an increase in oxygen saturation in the right atrium. Six liters of blood flows through the tricuspid valve and causes a mid-diastolic flow rumble. Oxygen saturation may be slightly higher in the right ventricle because of incomplete mixing at the atrial level. The full 6 L flows across the right ventricular outflow tract and causes a systolic ejection flow murmur. Six liters returns to the left atrium, with 3 L shunting left to right across the defect and 3 L crossing the mitral valve to be ejected by the left ventricle into the ascending aorta (normal cardiac output).

relative vascular resistance in the pulmonary and systemic circulations. In large defects, a considerable shunt of oxygenated blood flows from the left to the right atrium (Fig. 426-1). This blood is added to the usual venous return to the right atrium and is pumped by the right ventricle to the lungs. With large defects, the ratio of pulmonary to systemic blood flow (Qp:Qs) is usually between 2:1 and 4:1. The paucity of symptoms in infants with ASDs is related to the structure of the right ventricle in early life when its muscular wall is thick and less compliant, thus limiting the left-to-right shunt. As the infant becomes older and pulmonary vascular resistance drops, the right ventricular wall becomes thinner and the left-to-right shunt across the ASD increases. The increased blood flow through the right side of the heart results in enlargement of the right atrium and ventricle and dilation of the pulmonary artery. The left atrium may also be enlarged, but the left ventricle and aorta are normal in size. Despite the large pulmonary blood flow, pulmonary arterial pressure is usually normal because of the absence of a high-pressure communication between the pulmonary and systemic circulations. Pulmonary vascular resistance remains low throughout childhood, although it may begin to increase in adulthood and may eventually result in reversal of the shunt and clinical cyanosis.

CLINICAL MANIFESTATIONS

A child with an ostium secundum ASD is most often asymptomatic; the lesion is often discovered inadvertently during physical examination. Even an extremely large secundum ASD rarely produces clinically evident heart failure in childhood. However, on closer evaluation, in younger children, subtle failure to thrive may be present; in older children varying degrees of exercise intolerance may be noted. Often, the degree of limitation may go unnoticed by the family until after surgical repair, when the child's growth or activity level increases markedly. Platypnea (dyspnea on standing, relieved when supine) and orthodeoxia (desaturation on standing, relieved when supine) may occur when right to left shunting occurs through on ASD.

The physical findings of an ASD are usually characteristic but fairly subtle and require careful examination of the heart, with special attention to the heart sounds. Examination of the chest may reveal a mild left precordial bulge. A right ventricular systolic lift may be palpable at the left sternal border. Sometimes a pulmonic ejection click can be heard. In most patients with an ASD, the characteristic finding is that the 2nd heart sound is **widely split and fixed in its splitting** during all phases of respiration. Normally, the duration of right ventricular ejection varies with respiration, with inspiration increasing right ventricular volume and delaying closure of the pulmonary valve. With an ASD, right ventricular diastolic volume is constantly increased and the ejection time is prolonged throughout all phases of respiration. A systolic ejection murmur is heard; it is medium pitched, without harsh qualities, seldom accompanied by a thrill, and best heard at the left middle and upper sternal border. It is produced by the increased flow across the right ventricular outflow tract into the pulmonary artery, not by low-pressure flow across the ASD. A short, rumbling mid-diastolic murmur produced by the increased volume of blood flow across the tricuspid valve is often audible at the lower left sternal border. This finding, which may be subtle and is heard best with the bell of the stethoscope, usually indicates a Qp:Qs ratio of at least 2:1.

DIAGNOSIS

The chest roentgenogram shows varying degrees of enlargement of the right ventricle and atrium, depending on the size of the shunt. The pulmonary artery is enlarged, and pulmonary vascularity is increased. These signs vary and may not be conspicuous in mild cases. Cardiac enlargement is often best appreciated on the lateral view because the right ventricle protrudes anteriorly as its volume increases. The electrocardiogram shows volume overload of the right ventricle; the QRS axis may be normal or exhibit right axis deviation, and a minor right ventricular conduction delay (rsR′ pattern in the right precordial leads) may be present.

The echocardiogram shows findings characteristic of right ventricular volume overload, including an increased right ventricular end-diastolic dimension and flattening and abnormal motion of the ventricular septum (Fig. 426-2). A normal septum moves posteriorly during systole and anteriorly during diastole. With right ventricular overload and normal pulmonary vascular resistance, septal motion is either flattened or reversed—that is, anterior movement in systole. The location and size of the atrial defect are readily appreciated by 2-dimensional scanning, with a characteristic brightening of the echo image seen at the edge of the defect (T-artifact). The shunt is confirmed by pulsed and color flow Doppler. The normal entry of all pulmonary veins into the left atrium should be confirmed.

Patients with the classic features of a hemodynamically significant ASD on physical examination and chest radiography, in whom echocardiographic identification of an isolated secundum ASD is made, need not undergo diagnostic catheterization before repair, with the exception of an older patient, in whom pulmonary vascular resistance may be a concern. If pulmonary vascular disease is suspected, cardiac catheterization confirms the presence of the defect and allows measurement of the shunt ratio and pulmonary pressure and resistance.

If catheterization is performed, usually at the time of device closure (see below), the oxygen content of blood from the right atrium will be much higher than that from the superior vena cava. This feature is not specifically diagnostic because it may occur with partial anomalous pulmonary venous return to the right atrium, with a ventricular septal defect (VSD) in the presence of tricuspid insufficiency, with AV septal defects associated with left ventricular to right atrial shunts, and with aorta to right atrial communications (ruptured sinus of Valsalva aneurysm). Pressure in the right side of the heart is usually normal, but small to moderate pressure gradients (<25 mm Hg) may be measured across the right ventricular outflow tract because of functional stenosis related to excessive blood flow. In children and adolescents, the pulmonary vascular resistance is almost always normal. The shunt is

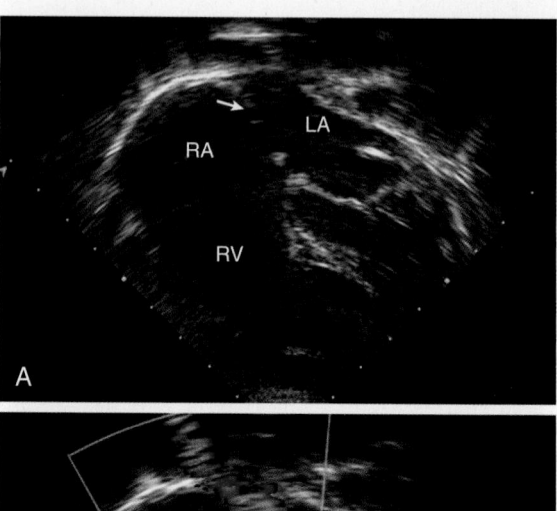

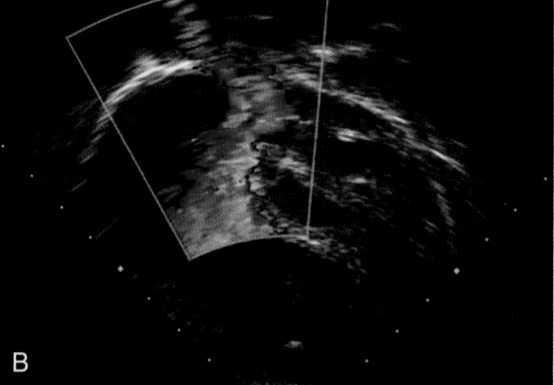

Figure 426-2 Echocardiographic findings in a secundum atrial septal defect. **A,** Two-dimensional echocardiogram (apical 4-chamber view) shows a moderate-sized secundum ASD (arrow). **B,** Color flow Doppler imaging shows left-to-right shunting (the red color represents blood moving toward the ultrasound transducer and does not indicate the level of oxygenation of the blood). LA, left atrium; RA, right atrium; RV, right ventricle.

variable and depends on the size of the defect, but it may be of considerable volume (as high as 20 L/min/m²). Cineangiography, performed with the catheter through the defect and in the right upper pulmonary vein, demonstrates the defect and the location of the right upper pulmonary venous drainage. Alternatively, pulmonary angiography demonstrates the defect on the levophase (return of contrast to the left side of the heart after passing through the lungs).

COMPLICATIONS

Secundum ASDs are usually isolated, although they may be associated with partial anomalous pulmonary venous return, pulmonary valvular stenosis, VSD, pulmonary artery branch stenosis, and persistent left superior vena cava, as well as mitral valve prolapse and insufficiency. Secundum ASDs are associated with the autosomal dominant Holt-Oram syndrome. The gene responsible for this syndrome, situated in the region 12q21-q22 of chromosome 12, is *TBX5*, a member of the T-box transcriptional family. A familial form of secundum ASD associated with AV conduction delay has been linked to mutations in another transcription factor, Nkx2.5. Patients with familial ASD without heart block may carry a mutation in the transcription factor GATA4, located on chromosome 8p22-23 (see Table 424-2 in Chapter 424).

TREATMENT

Transcatheter or surgical device closure is advised for all symptomatic patients and also for asymptomatic patients with a Qp:Qs ratio of at least 2:1 or those with right ventricular enlargement. The timing for elective closure is usually after the 1st yr and before entry into school. Closure carried out at open heart surgery is associated with a mortality rate of <1%. Repair is preferred during early childhood because surgical mortality and morbidity are significantly greater in adulthood; the long-term risk of arrhythmia is also greater after ASD repair in adults. For most patients, the *procedure of choice* is percutaneous catheter device closure using an atrial septal occlusion device, implanted transvenously in the cardiac catheterization laboratory (Fig. 426-3). The results are excellent and patients are discharged the following day. With the latest generation of devices, the incidence of serious complications such as device erosion is 0.1% and can be decreased by identifying high-risk patients such as those with a deficient rim of septum around the device. Echocardiography can usually determine whether a patient is a good candidate for device closure. In patients with small secundum ASDs and minimal left-to-right shunts without right ventricular enlargement, the consensus is that closure is not required. It is unclear at present whether the persistence of a small ASD into adulthood increases the risk for stroke enough to warrant prophylactic closure of all these defects.

PROGNOSIS

Small- to moderate-sized ASDs detected in term infants may close spontaneously. Secundum ASDs are well tolerated during childhood, and symptoms do not usually appear until the 3rd decade or later. Pulmonary hypertension, atrial dysrhythmias, tricuspid or mitral insufficiency, and heart failure are late manifestations; these symptoms

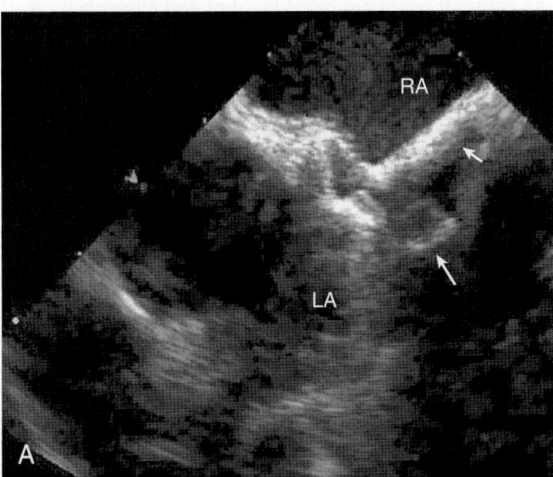

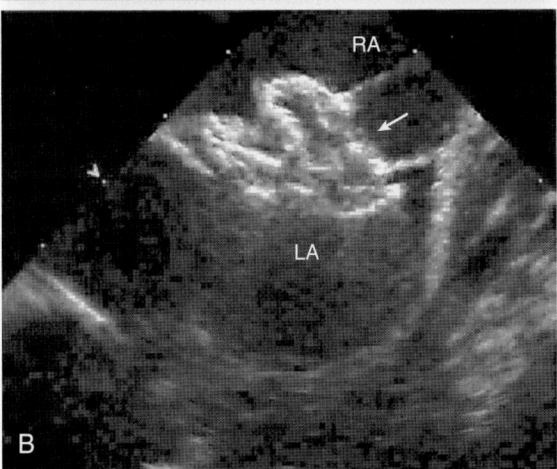

Figure 426-3 Intravascular ultrasound imaging of transcatheter occlusion of an atrial septal defect. **A,** A catheter *(small arrow)* has been advanced across the atrial defect, and the left-sided disk of the device *(large arrow)* has been extruded from the sheath into the left atrium *(LA)*. **B,** The right atrial disk *(arrow)* has now been extruded into the right atrium *(RA)*. The 2 halves of the device are then locked together and the catheter detached from the occluder device and removed.

may initially appear during the increased volume load of pregnancy. Infective endocarditis is extremely rare, and antibiotic prophylaxis for isolated secundum ASDs is not recommended.

The results after surgical or device closure in children with moderate to large shunts are excellent. Symptoms disappear rapidly, and growth is frequently enhanced. Heart size decreases to normal, and the electrocardiogram shows decreased right ventricular forces. Late right-heart failure and arrhythmias are less frequent in patients who have had early repair, becoming more common in patients who undergo surgery after 20 yr of age. Although early and midterm results with device closure are excellent, the long-term effects are not yet known. Reports of resolution of migraine headaches in patients after device closure of ASD or PFO are intriguing, suggesting a possible thromboembolic etiology; there are also paradoxical reports of patients whose migraines began or worsened after placement of one of these devices.

426.3 Sinus Venosus Atrial Septal Defect
Daniel Bernstein

A sinus venosus ASD is situated in the upper part of the atrial septum in close relation to the entry of the superior vena cava. Often, 1 or more pulmonary veins (usually from the right lung) drain anomalously into the superior vena cava. The superior vena cava sometimes straddles the defect; in this case, some systemic venous blood enters the left atrium, but only rarely does it cause clinically evident cyanosis. The hemodynamic disturbance, clinical picture, electrocardiogram, and roentgenogram are similar to those seen in secundum ASD. The diagnosis can usually be made by 2-dimensional echocardiography. If there are questions regarding pulmonary venous drainage, cardiac CT or MRI is usually diagnostic. Cardiac catheterization is rarely required, with the exception being in adult patients where assessment of pulmonary vascular resistance may be important. Anatomic correction generally requires the insertion of a patch to close the defect while incorporating the entry of anomalous veins into the left atrium. If the anomalous vein drains high in the superior vena cava, the vein can be left intact and the ASD closed to incorporate the mouth of the superior vena cava into the left atrium. The superior vena cava proximal to the venous entrance is then detached and anastomosed directly to the right atrium. This procedure avoids direct suturing of the pulmonary vein with less chance of future stenosis. Surgical results are generally excellent. Rarely, sinus venosus defects involve the inferior vena cava.

426.4 Partial Anomalous Pulmonary Venous Return
Daniel Bernstein

One or several pulmonary veins may return anomalously to the superior or inferior vena cava, the right atrium, or the coronary sinus and produce a left-to-right shunt of oxygenated blood. Partial anomalous pulmonary venous return usually involves some or all of the veins from only 1 lung, more often the right one. When an associated ASD is present, it is generally of the sinus venosus type, although can be of the secundum type (see Chapters 426.2 and 426.3). When an ASD is detected by echocardiography, one must always search for associated partial anomalous pulmonary venous return. The history, physical signs, and electrocardiographic and radiologic findings are indistinguishable from those of an isolated ostium secundum ASD. Occasionally, an anomalous vein draining into the inferior vena cava is visible on chest radiography as a crescentic shadow of vascular density along the right border of the cardiac silhouette (**scimitar syndrome**); in these cases, an ASD is not usually present, but **pulmonary sequestration or ipsilateral lung hypoplasia** and anomalous arterial supply to that lobe are common findings. Total anomalous pulmonary venous return is a cyanotic lesion and is discussed in Chapter 431.7. Echocardiography generally confirms the diagnosis. MRI and CT are also useful if there is a question regarding pulmonary venous drainage or in cases of scimitar syndrome. If cardiac catheterization is performed, the presence of anomalous pulmonary veins is demonstrated by selective pulmonary arteriography and anomalous pulmonary arterial supply to the right lung is demonstrated by descending aortography.

The prognosis is excellent, similar to that for ostium secundum ASDs. When a large left-to-right shunt is present, surgical repair is performed. The associated ASD should be closed in such a way that pulmonary venous return is directed to the left atrium. A single anomalous pulmonary vein without an atrial communication may be difficult to redirect to the left atrium; if the shunt is small, it may be left unoperated.

426.5 Atrioventricular Septal Defects (Ostium Primum and Atrioventricular Canal or Endocardial Cushion Defects)

Daniel Bernstein

The abnormalities encompassed by AV septal defects are grouped together because they represent a spectrum of a basic embryologic abnormality, a deficiency of the AV septum. An **ostium primum** defect is situated in the lower portion of the atrial septum and overlies the mitral and tricuspid valves. In most instances, a **cleft** in the **anterior leaflet** of the **mitral valve** is also noted. The tricuspid valve is usually functionally normal, although some anatomic abnormality of the septal leaflet is present. The ventricular septum is intact.

An **AV septal defect,** also known as an **AV canal defect** or an **endocardial cushion defect,** consists of contiguous atrial and VSDs with markedly abnormal AV valves. The severity of the valve abnormalities varies considerably; in the complete form of AV septal defect, a single AV valve is common to both ventricles and consists of an anterior and a posterior bridging leaflet related to the ventricular septum, with a lateral leaflet in each ventricle. The lesion is common in children with **Down syndrome**.

Transitional varieties of these defects also occur and include ostium primum defects with clefts in the anterior mitral and septal tricuspid valve leaflets and small VSDs, and, less commonly, ostium primum defects with normal AV valves. In some patients, the atrial septum is intact, but an inlet VSD is similar to that found in the full AV septal defect. Sometimes AV septal defects are associated with varying degrees of hypoplasia of one of the ventricles, known as either *left-* or *right-dominant atrioventricular septal defect.* If the affected ventricular chamber is too small to establish a 2-ventricle circulation, then surgical palliation, aiming for an eventual Fontan procedure, is performed (see Chapters 430.4 and 431.10).

PATHOPHYSIOLOGY

The basic abnormality in patients with ostium primum defects is the combination of a left-to-right shunt across the atrial defect and mitral (or occasionally tricuspid) insufficiency. The shunt is usually moderate to large, the degree of mitral insufficiency is generally mild to moderate, and pulmonary arterial pressure is typically normal or only mildly increased. The physiology of this lesion is, therefore, similar to that of an ostium secundum ASD.

In complete AV septal defects, the left-to-right shunt occurs at both the atrial and ventricular levels (Fig. 426-4). Additional shunting may occur directly from the left ventricle to the right atrium because of absence of the AV septum. Pulmonary hypertension and an early tendency to increase pulmonary vascular resistance are common. AV valvular insufficiency increases the volume load on one or both ventricles. If the defect is large enough, some right-to-left shunting may also occur at both the atrial and ventricular levels and lead to mild arterial desaturation. With time, progressive pulmonary vascular disease increases the right-to-left shunt so that clinical cyanosis develops (Eisenmenger physiology; see Chapter 433.2).

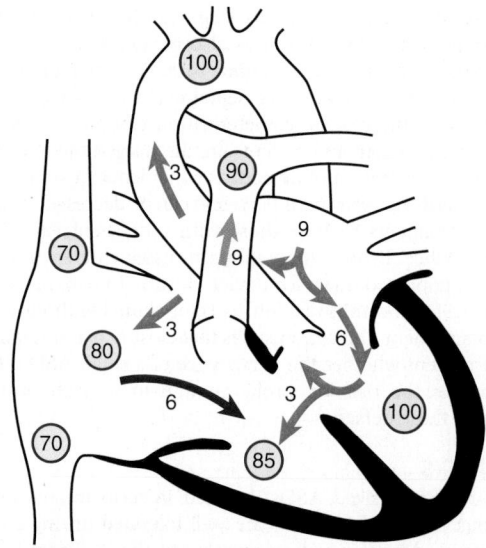

Figure 426-4 Physiology of atrioventricular septal defect. *Circled numbers* represent oxygen saturation values. The *numbers next to the arrows* represent volumes of blood flow (in L/min/m²). This illustration shows a hypothetical patient with a pulmonary-to-systemic blood flow ratio (Qp:Qs) of 3:1. Desaturated blood enters the right atrium from the vena cavae at a volume of 3 L/min/m² and mixes with 3 L of fully saturated blood shunting left to right across the atrial septal defect; the result is an increase in oxygen saturation in the right atrium. Six liters of blood flows through the right side of the common AV valve, joined by an additional 3 L of saturated blood shunting left to right at the ventricular level, further increasing oxygen saturation in the right ventricle. The full 9 L flows across the right ventricular outflow tract into the lungs. Nine liters returns to the left atrium, with 3 L shunting left to right across the defect and 6 L crossing the left side of the common AV valve and causing a mid-diastolic flow rumble. Three liters of this volume shunts left to right across the VSD, and 3 L is ejected into the ascending aorta (normal cardiac output).

CLINICAL MANIFESTATIONS

Many children with ostium primum defects are asymptomatic, and the anomaly is discovered during a general physical examination. In patients with moderate shunts and mild mitral insufficiency, the physical signs are similar to those of the secundum ASD, but with an additional apical holosystolic murmur caused by mitral insufficiency.

A history of exercise intolerance, easy fatigability, and recurrent pneumonia may be obtained, especially in infants with large left-to-right shunts and severe mitral insufficiency. In these patients, cardiac enlargement is moderate or marked, and the precordium is hyperdynamic. Auscultatory signs produced by the left-to-right shunt include a normal or accentuated 1st heart sound; wide, fixed splitting of the 2nd sound; a pulmonary systolic ejection murmur sometimes preceded by a click; and a low-pitched, mid-diastolic rumbling murmur at the lower left sternal edge or apex, or both, as a result of increased flow through the AV valves. Mitral insufficiency may be manifested by a harsh (occasionally very high pitched) apical holosystolic murmur that radiates to the left axilla.

With complete AV septal defects, heart failure and intercurrent pulmonary infection usually appear in infancy. The liver is enlarged and the infant shows signs of failure to thrive. Cardiac enlargement is moderate to marked, and a systolic thrill is frequently palpable at the lower left sternal border. A precordial bulge and lift may be present as well. The 1st heart sound is normal or accentuated. The 2nd heart sound is widely split if the pulmonary flow is massive. A low-pitched, mid-diastolic rumbling murmur is audible at the lower left sternal border, and a pulmonary systolic ejection murmur is produced by the large pulmonary flow. The harsh apical holosystolic murmur of mitral insufficiency may also be present.

DIAGNOSIS

Chest radiographs of children with complete AV septal defects often show moderate to severe cardiac enlargement caused by the prominence of both ventricles and atria. The pulmonary artery is large, and pulmonary vascularity is increased.

The electrocardiogram in patients with a complete AV septal defect is distinctive. The principal abnormalities are (1) superior orientation of the mean frontal QRS axis with left axis deviation to the left upper or right upper quadrant, (2) counterclockwise inscription of the superiorly oriented QRS vector loop (often manifest by a Q wave in leads I and aVL), (3) signs of biventricular hypertrophy or isolated right ventricular hypertrophy, (4) right ventricular conduction delay (rSR' pattern in leads V_3R and V_1), (5) normal or tall P waves, and (6) occasional prolongation of the P-R interval (Fig. 426-5).

The echocardiogram (Fig. 426-6) is diagnostic and shows signs of right ventricular enlargement with encroachment of the mitral valve echo on the left ventricular outflow tract; the abnormally low position of the AV valves results in a "gooseneck" deformity of the left ventricular outflow tract. In normal hearts, the tricuspid valve inserts slightly more toward the apex than the mitral valve does. In AV septal defects, both valves insert at the same level because of absence of the AV septum. In complete AV septal defects, the ventricular septum is also deficient and the common AV valve is readily appreciated. Pulsed and color flow Doppler echocardiography will demonstrate left-to-right shunting at the atrial, ventricular, or left ventricular to right atrial levels and can be used to semiquantitate the degree of AV valve insufficiency. Echocardiography is useful for determining the insertion points of the chordae of the common AV valve and for evaluating the presence of associated lesions such as patent ductus arteriosus (PDA) or coarctation of the aorta.

Cardiac catheterization and angiocardiography is rarely required to confirm the diagnosis unless pulmonary vascular disease is suspected, such as in a patient in whom diagnosis has been delayed beyond early infancy, especially in those with Down syndrome in whom the development of pulmonary vascular disease may be more rapid. Catheterization demonstrates the magnitude of the left-to-right shunt, the degree of elevation of pulmonary vascular resistance, and the severity of insufficiency of the common AV valve. By oximetry, the shunt is usually demonstrable at both the atrial and ventricular levels. Arterial oxygen saturation is normal or only mildly reduced unless severe pulmonary vascular disease is present. Children with ostium primum defects generally have normal or only moderately elevated pulmonary arterial pressure. Conversely, complete AV septal defects are associated with right ventricular and pulmonary hypertension and, in older patients, with increased pulmonary vascular resistance (see Chapter 433.2).

Selective left ventriculography will demonstrate deformity of the mitral or common AV valve and the distortion of the left ventricular outflow tract caused by this valve (gooseneck deformity). The abnormal anterior leaflet of the mitral valve is serrated, and mitral insufficiency is noted, usually with regurgitation of blood into both the left and right atria. Direct shunting of blood from the left ventricle to the right atrium may also be demonstrated.

TREATMENT

Ostium primum defects are approached surgically from an incision in the right atrium. The cleft in the mitral valve is located through the atrial defect and is repaired by direct suture. The defect in the atrial septum is usually closed by insertion of a patch prosthesis. The surgical mortality rate for ostium primum defects is very low.

Surgical treatment of complete AV septal defects is more difficult, although still highly successful. The postoperative course may be prolonged in infants with severe cardiac failure and in those with pulmonary hypertension. Because of the risk of **pulmonary vascular disease** developing as early as 6-12 mo of age, surgical intervention must be performed during infancy. Full correction of these defects can be readily accomplished in infancy; palliation with pulmonary arterial banding, once more common, is reserved for the small subset of patients who have other associated lesions that make early corrective surgery too risky. The atrial and ventricular defects are patched and the AV valves reconstructed. Complications include surgically induced heart block requiring placement of a permanent pacemaker, excessive narrowing of the left ventricular outflow tract requiring surgical revision, and residual tricuspid or mitral regurgitation, which long-term can require replacement with a prosthetic valve.

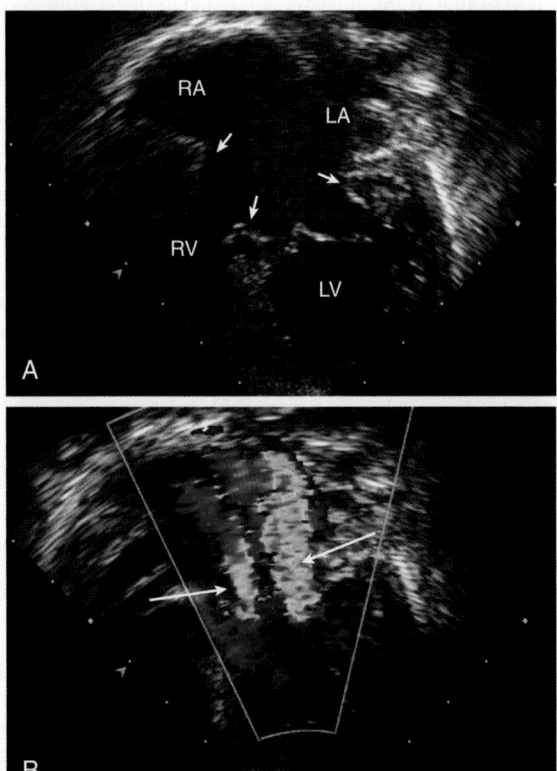

Figure 426-6 Echocardiogram of an atrioventricular septal defect. **A,** Subcostal 4-chamber view demonstrating the common atrioventricular valve *(arrows)* spanning the atrial and ventricular septal defects. **B,** Doppler imaging shows 2 jets of regurgitation through the left side of the common atrioventricular valve *(arrows)*. LA, left atrium; LV, left ventricle; RA, right atrium; RV, right ventricle.

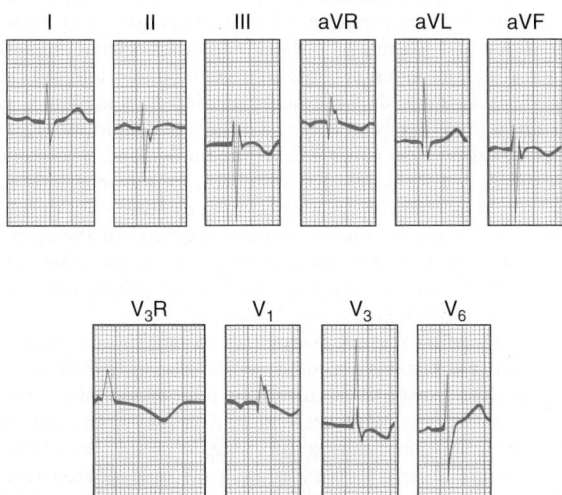

Figure 426-5 Electrocardiogram from a child with an atrioventricular septal defect. Note the QRS axis of −60 degrees and the right ventricular conduction delay with an RSR' pattern in V_1 and V_3R (V_3R paper speed = 50 mm/sec).

PROGNOSIS

The prognosis for unrepaired complete AV septal defects depends on the magnitude of the left-to-right shunt, the degree of elevation of pulmonary vascular resistance, and the severity of AV valve insufficiency. Death from cardiac failure during infancy used to be frequent before the advent of early corrective surgery. In patients who survived without surgery, pulmonary vascular obstructive disease usually developed. Most patients with ostium primum defects and minimal AV valve involvement are asymptomatic or have only minor, nonprogressive symptoms until they reach the 3rd-4th decade of life, similar to the course of patients with secundum ASDs. Late postoperative complications include atrial arrhythmias and heart block, progressive narrowing of the left ventricular outflow tract requiring surgical revision, and eventual worsening of AV valve regurgitation (usually on the left side) requiring replacement with a prosthetic valve.

Bibliography is available at Expert Consult.

426.6 Ventricular Septal Defect

Daniel Bernstein

VSD is the most common cardiac malformation and accounts for 25% of congenital heart disease. Defects may occur in any portion of the ventricular septum, but most are of the membranous type. These defects are in a posteroinferior position, anterior to the septal leaflet of the tricuspid valve. VSDs between the crista supraventricularis and the papillary muscle of the conus may be associated with pulmonary stenosis and other manifestations of tetralogy of Fallot (see Chapter 430.1). VSDs superior to the crista supraventricularis (supracristal) are less common; they are found just beneath the pulmonary valve and may impinge on an aortic sinus and cause aortic insufficiency. VSDs in the midportion or apical region of the ventricular septum are muscular in type and may be single or multiple (Swiss cheese septum).

PATHOPHYSIOLOGY

The physical size of the VSD is a major, but not the only, determinant of the size of the left-to-right shunt. The level of pulmonary vascular resistance in relation to systemic vascular resistance also determines the shunt's magnitude. When a small communication is present (usually <5 mm), the VSD is pressure **restrictive**, meaning that right ventricular pressure is normal. The higher pressure in the left ventricle drives the shunt left to right and the size of the defect limits the magnitude of the shunt. In large **nonrestrictive VSDs** (usually >10 mm), right and left ventricular pressures are equalized. In these defects, the direction of shunting and the shunt magnitude are determined by the ratio of pulmonary to systemic vascular resistance (Fig. 426-7).

After birth in patients with a large VSD, pulmonary vascular resistance may remain elevated, delaying the normal postnatal decrease, and thus the size of the left-to-right shunt may initially be limited. Because of normal involution of the media of small pulmonary arterioles, pulmonary vascular resistance begins to fall in the 1st few wk after birth and the size of the left-to-right shunt increases. Eventually, a large left-to-right shunt develops, and clinical symptoms become apparent. In most cases during early infancy, pulmonary vascular resistance is only slightly elevated, and the major contribution to pulmonary hypertension is the large communication allowing exposure of the pulmonary circulation to systemic pressure and the large pulmonary blood flow. With continued exposure of the pulmonary vascular bed to high systolic pressure and high flow, pulmonary vascular obstructive disease eventually develops. When the ratio of pulmonary to systemic resistance approaches 1:1, the shunt becomes bidirectional, signs of heart failure abate, and the patient begins to show signs of cyanosis (Eisenmenger physiology; see Chapter 433.2). In rare infants with a large VSD, usually those with Down syndrome, pulmonary vascular resistance never decreases, and symptoms may remain minimal until Eisenmenger physiology becomes evident.

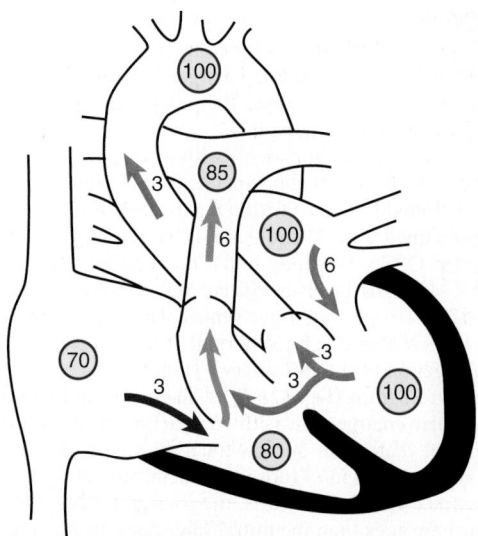

Figure 426-7 Physiology of a large ventricular septal defect. *Circled numbers* represent oxygen saturation values. The *numbers next to the arrows* represent volumes of blood flow (in L/min/m²). This illustration shows a hypothetical patient with a pulmonary-to-systemic blood flow ratio (Qp:Qs) of 2:1. Desaturated blood enters the right atrium from the vena cava at a volume of 3 L/min/m² and flows across the tricuspid valve. An additional 3 L of blood shunts left to right across the VSD, the result being an increase in oxygen saturation in the right ventricle. Six liters of blood is ejected into the lungs. Pulmonary arterial saturation may be further increased because of incomplete mixing at right ventricular level. Six liters returns to the left atrium, crosses the mitral valve, and causes a mid-diastolic flow rumble. Three liters of this volume shunts left to right across the VSD, and 3 L is ejected into the ascending aorta (normal cardiac output).

The magnitude of intracardiac shunts is usually described by the Qp:Qs ratio. If the left-to-right shunt is small (Qp:Qs < 1.5:1), the cardiac chambers are not appreciably enlarged and the pulmonary vascular bed is probably normal. If the shunt is large (Qp:Qs > 2:1), left atrial and ventricular volume overload occurs, as does right ventricular and pulmonary arterial hypertension. The main pulmonary artery, left atrium, and left ventricle are enlarged.

CLINICAL MANIFESTATIONS

The clinical findings of patients with a VSD vary according to the size of the defect and pulmonary blood flow and pressure. Small VSDs with trivial left-to-right shunts and normal pulmonary arterial pressure are the most common. These patients are asymptomatic, and the cardiac lesion is usually found during routine physical examination. Characteristically, a loud, harsh, or blowing holosystolic murmur is present and heard best over the lower left sternal border, and it is frequently accompanied by a thrill. In a few instances, the murmur ends before the 2nd sound, presumably because of closure of the defect during late systole. A short, harsh systolic murmur localized to the apex in a neonate is often a sign of a tiny VSD in the apical muscular septum. In premature infants, the murmur may be heard early because pulmonary vascular resistance decreases more rapidly.

Large VSDs with excessive pulmonary blood flow and pulmonary hypertension are responsible for dyspnea, feeding difficulties, poor growth, profuse perspiration, recurrent pulmonary infections, and cardiac failure in early infancy. Cyanosis is usually absent, but duskiness is sometimes noted during infections or crying. Prominence of the left precordium is common, as are a palpable parasternal lift, a laterally displaced apical impulse and apical thrust, and a systolic thrill. The holosystolic murmur of a large VSD is generally less harsh than that of a small VSD and more blowing in nature because of the absence of a significant pressure gradient across the defect. It is even less likely to be prominent in the newborn period. The pulmonic component of the 2nd heart sound may be increased as a result of pulmonary hypertension. The presence of a mid-diastolic, low-pitched rumble at the apex is caused by increased blood flow across the mitral valve and usually indicates a Qp:Qs ratio of ≥2:1. This murmur is best appreciated with the bell of the stethoscope.

DIAGNOSIS

In patients with small VSDs, the chest x-ray is usually normal, although minimal cardiomegaly and a borderline increase in pulmonary vasculature may be observed. The electrocardiogram is generally normal but may suggest left ventricular hypertrophy. The presence of right ventricular hypertrophy is a warning that the defect is not small and that the patient has pulmonary hypertension or an associated lesion such as pulmonic stenosis. In large VSDs, the chest x-ray shows gross cardiomegaly with prominence of both ventricles, the left atrium, and the pulmonary artery (Fig. 426-8). Pulmonary vascular markings are increased, and frank pulmonary edema, including pleural effusions, may be present. The electrocardiogram shows biventricular hypertrophy; P waves may be notched or peaked.

The 2-dimensional echocardiogram (Fig. 426-9) shows the position and size of the VSD. In small defects, especially those of the muscular septum, the defect itself may be difficult to image and is visualized only by color Doppler examination. In defects of the **membranous septum,** a thin membrane (called a **ventricular septal aneurysm** but consisting of tricuspid valve tissue) can partially cover the defect and limit the volume of the left-to-right shunt. Echocardiography is also useful for estimating shunt size by examining the degree of volume overload of the left atrium and left ventricle; in the absence of associated lesions, the extent of their increased dimensions is a good reflection of the size of the left-to-right shunt. Pulsed Doppler examination shows whether the VSD is pressure restrictive by calculating the pressure gradient across the defect. Such calculation allows an estimation of right ventricular pressure and helps determine whether the patient is at risk for the development of early pulmonary vascular disease. The echocardiogram can also be useful to determine the presence of aortic valve insufficiency or aortic leaflet prolapse in the case of supracristal VSDs.

The hemodynamics of a VSD can also be demonstrated by cardiac catheterization, although catheterization is today performed only when laboratory data do not fit well with the clinical findings or when pulmonary vascular disease is suspected. Oximetry demonstrates increased oxygen content in the right ventricle; because some defects eject blood almost directly into the pulmonary artery (streaming), the full magnitude of the oxygen saturation increase is occasionally apparent only when pulmonary arterial blood is sampled. Small, restrictive VSDs are associated with normal right-heart pressures and pulmonary vascular resistance. Large, nonrestrictive VSDs are associated with equal or nearly equal pulmonary and systemic systolic pressure and

variable elevations in pulmonary vascular resistance. Pulmonary blood flow may be 2-4 times systemic blood flow. In patients with such **"hyperdynamic pulmonary hypertension,"** pulmonary vascular resistance is only minimally elevated because resistance is equal to pressure divided by flow. However, if left untreated until Eisenmenger syndrome is present, pulmonary artery systolic and diastolic pressure will be elevated but the degree of left-to-right shunting minimal. In these cases, desaturation of blood in the left ventricle is usually encountered.

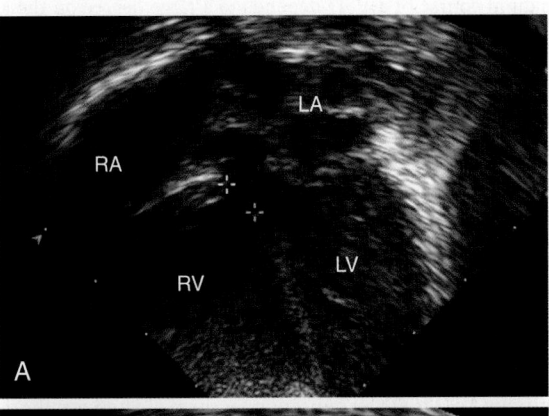

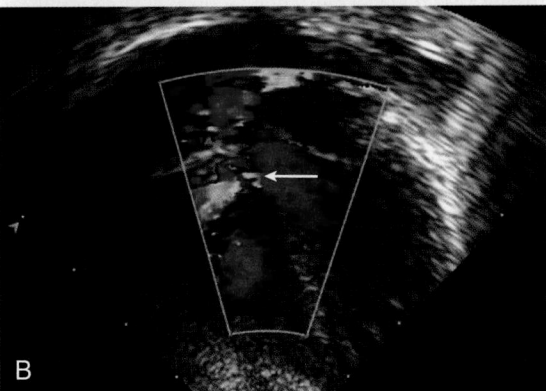

Figure 426-9 Echocardiogram in a patient with a perimembranous ventricular septal defect. **A,** Apical 4-chamber view showing the location of the defect (outlined between 2 *crosshatches*) beneath the aortic valve. **B,** Color Doppler imaging shows the left-to-right shunt *(arrow)* through the defect (the red color represents blood moving toward the ultrasound transducer and does not indicate the level of oxygenation of the blood). LA, left atrium; LV, left ventricle; RA, right atrium; RV, right ventricle.

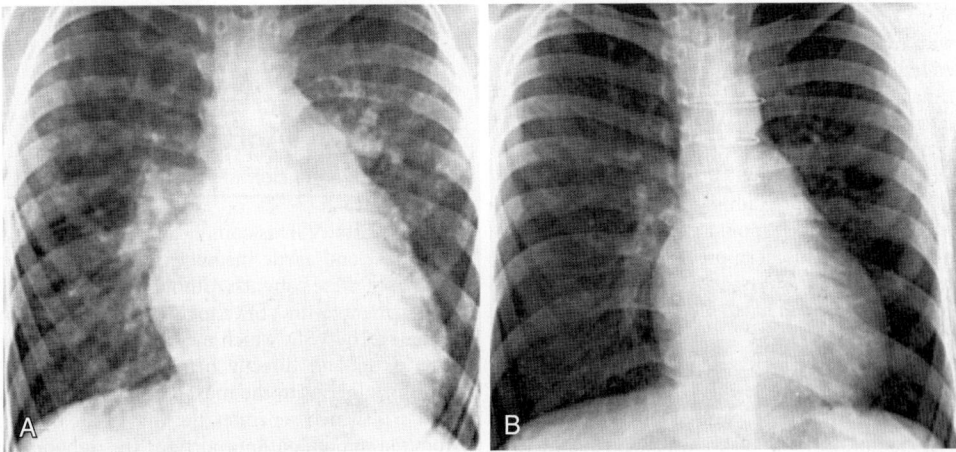

Figure 426-8 A, Preoperative radiograph in a patient with a ventricular septal defect with a large left-to-right shunt and pulmonary hypertension. Significant cardiomegaly, prominence of the pulmonary arterial trunk, and pulmonary overcirculation are evident. **B,** Three years after surgical closure of the defect, heart size is markedly decreased, and the pulmonary vasculature is normal.

The size, location, and number of ventricular defects can be demonstrated by left ventriculography. Contrast medium passes across the defect or defects to opacify the right ventricle and pulmonary artery. Administration of 100% oxygen with and without nitric oxide can be used to determine whether the pulmonary vascular resistance, if elevated, is still reactive and therefore more likely to drop after surgical repair.

TREATMENT

The natural course of a VSD depends to a large degree on the size of the defect. A significant number (30-50%) of small defects close spontaneously, most frequently during the 1st 2 yr of life. Small muscular VSDs are more likely to close (up to 80%) than membranous VSDs (up to 35%). The vast majority of defects that close do so before the age of 4 yr, although spontaneous closure has been reported in adults. VSDs that close often have ventricular septal aneurysm (accessory tricuspid valve) tissue that limits the magnitude of the shunt. Most children with small restrictive defects remain asymptomatic, without evidence of an increase in heart size, pulmonary arterial pressure, or resistance; a long-term risk is infective endocarditis. Some long-term studies of adults with unoperated small VSDs show an increased incidence of arrhythmia, subaortic stenosis, and exercise intolerance. Guidelines from the Council on Cardiovascular Disease in the Young of the American Heart Association state that an isolated, small, hemodynamically insignificant VSD is not an indication for surgery. However, the declining risk of open heart surgery has led some to suggest that all VSDs be closed electively by mid-childhood.

It is less common for moderate or large VSDs to close spontaneously, although even defects large enough to result in heart failure may become smaller and up to 8% may close completely. More commonly, infants with large defects have repeated episodes of respiratory infection and heart failure despite optimal medical management. Heart failure may be manifested in many of these infants primarily as failure to thrive. Pulmonary hypertension occurs as a result of high pulmonary blood flow. These patients are at risk for pulmonary vascular disease if the defect is not repaired during early infancy.

Patients with VSD are also at risk for the development of aortic valve regurgitation, the greatest risk occurring in patients with a supracristal VSD (see Chapter 426.7). A small number of patients with VSD develop **acquired infundibular pulmonary stenosis,** which then protects the pulmonary circulation from the short-term effects of pulmonary overcirculation and the long-term effects of pulmonary vascular disease. In these patients, the clinical picture changes from that of a VSD with a large left-to-right shunt to a VSD with pulmonary stenosis. The shunt may diminish in size, become balanced, or even become a net right-to-left shunt. These patients must be carefully distinguished from those in whom an Eisenmenger physiology develops (see Chapter 433.2).

In patients with small VSDs, parents should be reassured of the relatively benign nature of the lesion, and the child should be encouraged to live a normal life, with no restrictions on physical activity. Surgical repair is not recommended. As protection against infective endocarditis, the integrity of primary and permanent teeth should be carefully maintained; with the latest revision of the American Heart Association guidelines, antibiotic prophylaxis is no longer recommended for dental visits or surgical procedures (see Chapter 437). These patients can be monitored by a combination of clinical examination and noninvasive laboratory tests until the VSD has closed spontaneously. Echocardiography is used to estimate pulmonary artery pressure, screen for the development of left ventricular outflow tract pathology (subaortic membrane or aortic regurgitation), and to confirm spontaneous closure.

In infants with a large VSD, management has 2 aims: to get the symptoms of heart failure under control (see Chapter 442) and prevent the development of pulmonary vascular disease. If early treatment is successful, sometimes the shunt may diminish in size with spontaneous improvement, especially during the 1st yr of life. The clinician must be alert not to confuse clinical improvement caused by a decrease in defect size with clinical changes caused by the development of

Eisenmenger physiology. Because catheter or surgical closure can be carried out at low risk in most infants, medical management should not be pursued in symptomatic infants after an initial unsuccessful trial. Because pulmonary vascular disease can usually be prevented when surgery is performed within the 1st yr of life, even infants with well-controlled heart failure should not have surgery delayed inordinately unless there is evidence that the defect is becoming pressure restrictive.

Indications for surgical closure of a VSD include patients at any age with large defects in whom clinical symptoms and failure to thrive cannot be controlled medically; infants between 6 and 12 mo of age with large defects associated with pulmonary hypertension, even if the symptoms are controlled by medication; and patients older than 24 mo with a Qp:Qs ratio greater than 2:1. Patients with a supracristal VSD of any size are usually referred for surgery because of the high risk for aortic valve regurgitation (see Chapter 426.7). Severe pulmonary vascular disease nonresponsive to pulmonary vasodilators is a contraindication to closure of a VSD.

Transcatheter occlusion closure is most successful in treating muscular VSDs, which may be difficult to access by surgery. Perimembranous VSD catheter closure has a high risk of postprocedure heart block and is not recommended. Hybrid methods employing a sternotomy with device placement through the anterior wall of the right ventricle under transesophageal echo and fluoroscopic visualization has been performed in difficult to approach muscular defects.

PROGNOSIS

The results of primary surgical repair are excellent, and complications leading to long-term problems (residual ventricular shunts requiring reoperation or heart block requiring a pacemaker) are rare. Pulmonary arterial palliative banding with repair in later childhood, once the standard of care, is now reserved for extremely complicated cases or very premature infants. Surgical risks are somewhat higher for defects in the muscular septum, particularly apical defects and multiple (Swiss cheese–type) VSDs. These patients may require pulmonary arterial banding if symptomatic, with subsequent debanding and repair of multiple VSDs at an older age.

After surgical obliteration of the left-to-right shunt, the hyperdynamic heart becomes quiet, cardiac size decreases toward normal (see Fig. 426-8), thrills and murmurs are abolished, and pulmonary artery hypertension regresses. The patient's clinical status improves markedly. Most infants begin to thrive, and cardiac medications are no longer required. Catch-up growth occurs in most patients within the next 1-2 yr. In some instances after successful surgery, systolic ejection murmurs of low intensity persist for months. The long-term prognosis after surgery is excellent. Patients with a small VSD and those who have undergone surgical closure without residua are considered to be at standard risk for health and life insurance.

Bibliography is available at Expert Consult.

426.7 Supracristal Ventricular Septal Defect with Aortic Insufficiency

Daniel Bernstein

A supracristal VSD is complicated by prolapse of the aortic valve into the defect and aortic insufficiency, which may eventually develop in 50-90% of these patients. Although supracristal VSD accounts for ≈5% of all patients with VSD, the incidence is higher in Asian children and in males. The VSD, which may be small or moderate in size, is located anterior to and directly below the pulmonary valve in the outlet septum, superior to the muscular ridge known as the *crista supraventricularis,* which separates the trabecular body of the right ventricle from the smooth outflow portion. The right or, less often, the noncoronary aortic cusp prolapses into the defect and may partially or even completely occlude it. Such occlusion may limit the amount of left-to-right shunting and give the false impression that the defect is not large.

Aortic insufficiency is most often not recognized until 5-9 yr life or beyond. Of note, aortic insufficiency is occasionally associated with VSDs located in the membranous septum.

Early heart failure secondary to a large left-to-right shunt rarely occurs, but without surgery, severe aortic insufficiency and left ventricular failure may ensue. The murmur of a supracristal VSD is usually heard at the mid to upper left sternal border, as opposed to the lower left sternal border, and it is sometimes confused with that of pulmonic stenosis. A decrescendo diastolic murmur will be appreciated at the upper right or mid left sternal borders if there is aortic insufficiency. More advanced degrees of aortic insufficiency will be associated with a wide pulse pressure and a hyperdynamic precordium. These clinical findings must be distinguished from PDA or other defects associated with aortic runoff.

The clinical manifestations vary widely from trivial aortic regurgitation and small left-to-right shunts in asymptomatic children to florid aortic insufficiency and massive cardiomegaly in symptomatic adolescents. Closure of all supracristal ventricular VSDs at the time of diagnosis is commonly recommended to prevent the development of aortic regurgitation, even in an asymptomatic child. Patients who already have significant aortic insufficiency require surgical intervention to prevent irreversible left ventricular dysfunction. Surgical options depend on the degree of damage to the valve. If the insufficiency is mild, they may include simple closure of the defect to bolster the valve apparatus without touching the valve itself, valvuloplasty for more significant degrees of involvement, and replacement with a prosthesis or homograft or aortopulmonary translocation for severe involvement.

426.8 Patent Ductus Arteriosus
Daniel Bernstein

During fetal life, most of the pulmonary arterial blood is shunted right-to-left through the ductus arteriosus into the aorta (see Chapter 421). Functional closure of the ductus normally occurs soon after birth, but if the ductus remains patent when pulmonary vascular resistance falls, aortic blood then is shunted left-to-right into the pulmonary artery. The aortic end of the ductus is just distal to the origin of the left subclavian artery, and the ductus enters the pulmonary artery at its bifurcation. Female patients with PDA outnumber males 2:1. PDA is also associated with maternal rubella infection during early pregnancy, an uncommon occurrence. PDA is a common problem in premature infants, as the smooth muscle in the wall of the preterm ductus is less responsive to high PO_2 and therefore less likely to constrict after birth. In these infants, it can cause severe hemodynamic derangements and several major sequelae (see Chapter 101.3).

When a term infant is found to have a PDA, the wall of the ductus is deficient in both the mucoid endothelial layer and the muscular media, whereas in the premature infant, the PDA usually has a normal structure. Thus, a PDA persisting beyond the 1st few wk of life in a term infant rarely closes spontaneously or with pharmacologic intervention, whereas if early pharmacologic or surgical intervention is not required in a premature infant, spontaneous closure occurs in most instances. A PDA is seen in 10% of patients with other congenital heart lesions and often plays a critical role in providing a source of pulmonary blood flow when the right ventricular outflow tract is stenotic or atretic (see Chapter 430) or in providing systemic blood flow in the presence of aortic coarctation or interruption (see Chapters 426.6 to 427.8).

PATHOPHYSIOLOGY
As a result of the higher aortic pressure postnatally, blood shunts left to right through the ductus, from the aorta to the pulmonary artery. The extent of the shunt depends on the size of the ductus and on the ratio of pulmonary to systemic vascular resistance. If the PDA is small, pressures within the pulmonary artery, the right ventricle, and the right atrium are normal. If the PDA is large, pulmonary artery pressure may be elevated to systemic levels during both systole and diastole. Thus,

patients with a large PDA are at high risk for the development of pulmonary vascular disease if left unoperated.

CLINICAL MANIFESTATIONS
A small PDA is usually asymptomatic. A large PDA will result in heart failure similar to that encountered in infants with a large VSD. Retardation of physical growth may be a major manifestation in infants with large shunts. A small PDA is associated with normal peripheral pulses, and a large PDA results in bounding peripheral arterial pulses and a wide pulse pressure, due to runoff of blood into the pulmonary artery during diastole. The heart is normal in size when the ductus is small, but moderately or grossly enlarged in cases with a large communication. In these cases, the apical impulse is prominent and, with cardiac enlargement, is heaving. A thrill, maximal in the 2nd left interspace, is often present and may radiate toward the left clavicle, down the left sternal border, or toward the apex. It is usually systolic but may also be palpated throughout the cardiac cycle. The classic continuous murmur is described as being like machinery in quality. It begins soon after onset of the 1st sound, reaches maximal intensity at the end of systole, and wanes in late diastole. It may be localized to the 2nd left intercostal space or radiate down the left sternal border or to the left clavicle. When pulmonary vascular resistance is increased, the diastolic component of the murmur may be less prominent or absent. In patients with a large left-to-right shunt, a low-pitched mitral mid-diastolic murmur may be audible at the apex as a result of the increased volume of blood flow across the mitral valve.

DIAGNOSIS
If the left-to-right shunt is small, the electrocardiogram is normal; if the ductus is large, left ventricular or biventricular hypertrophy is present. The diagnosis of an isolated, uncomplicated PDA is untenable when right ventricular hypertrophy is present.

Radiographic studies in patients with a large PDA show a prominent pulmonary artery with increased pulmonary vascular markings. Cardiac size depends on the degree of left-to-right shunting; it may be normal or moderately to markedly enlarged. The chambers involved are the left atrium and left ventricle. The aortic knob may be normal or prominent.

On echocardiogram, the cardiac chambers will be normal in size if the ductus is small. With large shunts, left atrial and left ventricular dimensions are increased. The ductus can easily be visualized directly and its size estimated. Color and pulsed Doppler examinations demonstrate systolic or diastolic (or both) retrograde turbulent flow in the pulmonary artery, and aortic retrograde flow in diastole (Fig. 426-10) in the presence of a large shunt.

The clinical signs and echocardiographic findings are sufficiently distinctive to allow an accurate diagnosis by noninvasive methods in most patients. In rare patients with atypical findings, cardiac catheterization may be indicated for confirmation of diagnosis. Cardiac catheterization will demonstrate either normal or increased pressure in the right ventricle and pulmonary artery, depending on the size of the ductus. The presence of oxygenated blood shunting into the pulmonary artery confirms the left-to-right shunt. The catheter may pass from the pulmonary artery through the ductus into the descending aorta. Injection of contrast medium into the ascending aorta shows opacification of the pulmonary artery from the aorta and identifies the ductus.

Other conditions can produce systolic and diastolic murmurs in the pulmonic area in an acyanotic patient and are described in Chapter 422. An **aorticopulmonary window** defect may rarely be clinically indistinguishable from a patent ductus, although, in most cases, the murmur is only systolic and is loudest at the right rather than the left upper sternal border. A sinus of Valsalva aneurysm that has ruptured into the right side of the heart or pulmonary artery, coronary arteriovenous fistulas, and an aberrant left coronary artery with massive collaterals from the right coronary display dynamics similar to that of a PDA with a continuous murmur and a wide pulse pressure. Truncus arteriosus with torrential pulmonary flow also has an aortic runoff physiology. A peripheral arteriovenous fistula also results in a wide pulse pressure, but the distinctive precordial murmur of a PDA is not present. VSD with aortic insufficiency, repaired tetralogy of Fallot, and combined aortic and mitral insufficiency (usually due to rheumatic fever) may be confused with a PDA, but the murmurs should be differentiated by their to-and-fro rather than continuous nature. The combination of a large VSD and a PDA results in findings more like those of an isolated VSD. Echocardiography should be able to eliminate these other diagnostic possibilities.

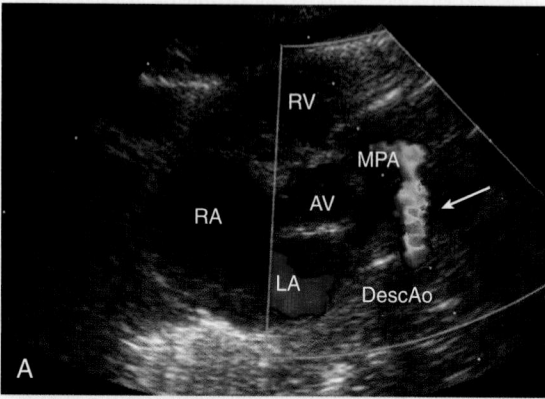

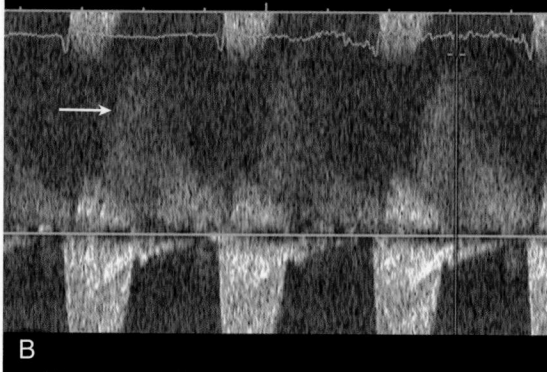

Figure 426-10 Echocardiogram in a newborn with a small- to moderate-size patent ductus arteriosus. **A,** Color Doppler performed in a parasternal short axis view shows flow (*arrow*) from the aorta into the main pulmonary artery. **B,** Doppler evaluation demonstrates retrograde diastolic flow into the pulmonary artery. AV, aortic valve; DescAo, descending aorta; LA, left atrium; MPA, main pulmonary artery; RA, right atrium; RV, right ventricle.

PROGNOSIS AND COMPLICATIONS

Spontaneous closure of the ductus after infancy is extremely rare. Patients with a small PDA may live a normal span with few or no cardiac symptoms, but late manifestations may occur. In patients with a large PDA, cardiac failure most often occurs in early infancy but may occur later in life, even with a moderate-sized communication.

Infective endarteritis may be seen at any age. Pulmonary or systemic emboli may occur. Rare complications include aneurysmal dilation of the pulmonary artery or the ductus, calcification of the ductus, noninfective thrombosis of the ductus with embolization, and paradoxical emboli. Pulmonary hypertension (Eisenmenger syndrome) usually develops in patients with a large PDA who do not undergo ductal closure (see Chapter 433.2).

TREATMENT

Irrespective of age, patients with PDA require catheter or surgical closure. In patients with a small PDA, the rationale for closure is prevention of bacterial endarteritis or other late complications. In patients with a moderate to large PDA, closure is accomplished to treat heart failure or prevent the development of pulmonary vascular disease, or both. Once the diagnosis of a moderate to large PDA is made, treatment should not be unduly postponed after adequate medical therapy for cardiac failure has been instituted.

Transcatheter PDA closure is routinely performed in the cardiac catheterization laboratory (Fig. 426-11). Small PDAs are generally closed with intravascular coils. Moderate to large PDAs may be closed with an umbrella-like device or with a catheter-introduced sac into which several coils are released. Surgical closure of a PDA can be accomplished by a standard left thoracotomy or using thoracoscopic minimally invasive techniques. Because the case fatality rate with interventional or surgical treatment is considerably less than 1% and the risk without it is greater, closure of the ductus is indicated in asymptomatic patients, preferably before 1 yr of age. Pulmonary hypertension is not a contraindication to surgery at any age if it can be demonstrated at cardiac catheterization that the shunt flow is still predominantly left to right and that severe pulmonary vascular disease is not present. After closure, symptoms of cardiac failure rapidly disappear. Infants who had failed to thrive usually have immediate improvement in physical development. The pulse and blood pressure return to normal, and the machinery-like murmur disappears. A functional systolic murmur over the pulmonary area may persist; it may represent turbulence in a persistently dilated pulmonary artery. The radiographic signs of cardiac enlargement and pulmonary overcirculation disappear over a period of several months, and the electrocardiogram becomes normal.

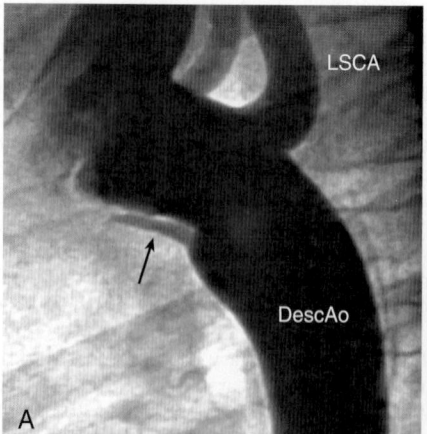
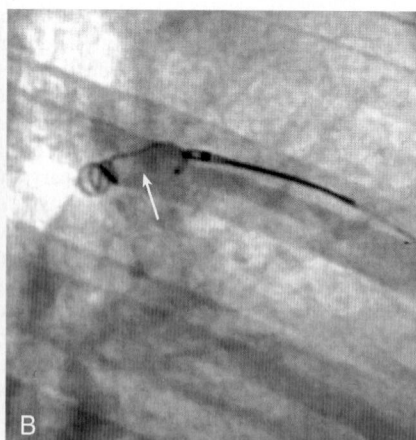
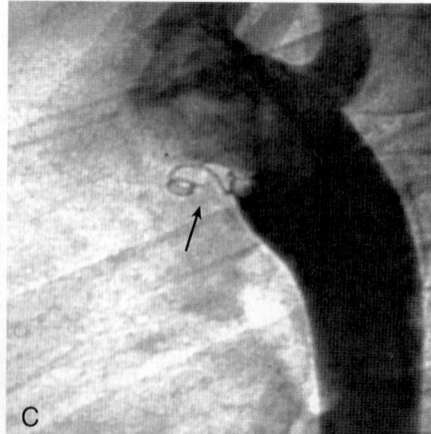

Figure 426-11 Transcatheter closure of a small patent ductus arteriosus using a coil. **A,** Angiogram of transverse and descending aorta shows small PDA (*arrow*). **B,** Coil (*arrow*) has been extruded from sheath and is being positioned in ductal lumen. **C,** Angiogram demonstrating total occlusion of PDA by coil (*arrow*). DescAo, descending aorta; LSCA, left subclavian artery.

PATENT DUCTUS ARTERIOSUS IN LOW BIRTHWEIGHT INFANTS

See Chapter 101.

Bibliography is available at Expert Consult.

426.9 Aortopulmonary Window Defect
Daniel Bernstein

An aortopulmonary window defect consists of a communication between the ascending aorta and the main pulmonary artery. The presence of pulmonary and aortic valves and an intact ventricular septum distinguishes this anomaly from truncus arteriosus (see Chapter 431.8). Symptoms of heart failure appear during early infancy; occasionally, minimal cyanosis is present. The defect is usually large, and the cardiac murmur is usually systolic with an apical mid-diastolic rumble as a result of the increased blood flow across the mitral valve. In the rare instance when the communication is smaller and pulmonary hypertension is absent, the findings on examination can mimic those of a PDA (wide pulse pressure and a continuous murmur at the upper sternal borders). The electrocardiogram shows either left ventricular or biventricular hypertrophy. Radiographic studies demonstrate cardiac enlargement and prominence of the pulmonary artery and intrapulmonary vasculature. The echocardiogram shows enlarged left-sided heart chambers; the window defect can best be delineated with color flow Doppler. CT or MRI angiography can also be used to visualize the defect (see Fig. 423-26 in Chapter 423).

Cardiac catheterization, usually performed in older children to evaluate pulmonary vascular resistance, reveals a left-to-right shunt at the level of the pulmonary artery, as well as hyperkinetic pulmonary hypertension, because the defect is almost always large. Selective aortography with injection of contrast medium into the ascending aorta demonstrates the lesion, and manipulation of the catheter from the main pulmonary artery directly to the ascending aorta is also diagnostic.

An aortopulmonary window defect is surgically corrected during infancy. If surgery is not carried out in infancy, survivors carry the risk of progressive pulmonary vascular obstructive disease, similar to that of other patients who have large intracardiac or great vessel communications.

426.10 Coronary Artery Fistula
Daniel Bernstein

A congenital fistula may exist between a coronary artery and an atrium, ventricle (especially the right), or pulmonary artery. Sometimes, multiple fistulas exist. Regardless of the recipient chamber, the clinical signs are similar to those of PDA, although the machinery-like murmur may be more diffuse. If the flow is substantial, the involved coronary artery may be dilated or aneurysmal. The anatomic abnormality is usually demonstrable by color flow Doppler echocardiography and, during catheterization, by injection of contrast medium into the ascending aorta. Small fistulas may be hemodynamically insignificant and may even close spontaneously. If the shunt is large, treatment consists of either transcatheter coil embolization or, for lesions not amenable to catheter intervention, surgical closure of the fistula.

426.11 Ruptured Sinus of Valsalva Aneurysm
Daniel Bernstein

When 1 of the sinuses of Valsalva of the aorta is weakened by congenital or acquired disease, an aneurysm may form and eventually rupture, usually into the right atrium or ventricle. This condition is extremely rare in childhood. The onset is usually sudden. The diagnosis should be suspected in a patient in whom symptoms of acute heart failure develop in association with a new loud to-and-fro murmur. Color Doppler echocardiography and cardiac catheterization demonstrate the left-to-right shunt at the atrial or ventricular level. Urgent surgical repair is generally required. This condition is often associated with infective endocarditis of the aortic valve.

Chapter **427**
Acyanotic Congenital Heart Disease: Obstructive Lesions

427.1 Pulmonary Valve Stenosis with Intact Ventricular Septum
Daniel Bernstein

Of the various forms of right ventricular outflow obstruction with an intact ventricular septum, the most common is isolated valvular pulmonary stenosis, which accounts for 7-10% of all congenital heart defects. The valve cusps are deformed to various degrees and, as a result, the valve opens incompletely during systole. The valve may be bicuspid or tricuspid and the leaflets partially fused together with an eccentric outlet. This fusion may be so severe that only a pinhole central opening remains. If the valve is not severely thickened, it produces a dome-like obstruction to right ventricular outflow during systole. Isolated infundibular or subvalvular stenosis, supravalvular pulmonary stenosis, and branch pulmonary artery stenosis are also encountered. In cases where pulmonary valve stenosis is associated with a ventricular septal defect (VSD) but without anterior deviation of the infundibular septum and overriding aorta, this condition is better classified as pulmonary stenosis with VSD rather than as tetralogy of Fallot (see Chapter 430.1). Pulmonary stenosis and an atrial septal defect (ASD) are also occasionally seen as associated defects. The clinical and laboratory findings reflect the dominant lesion, but it is important to rule out any associated anomalies. Pulmonary stenosis as a result of valve dysplasia is the most common cardiac abnormality in **Noonan syndrome** (see Chapter 81), and is associated, in approximately 50% of cases, with a mutation in the gene *PTPN11*, encoding the protein tyrosine phosphatase SHP-2 on chromosome 12. The mechanism for pulmonic stenosis is unknown, although maldevelopment of the distal portion of the bulbus cordis and the sequelae of fetal endocarditis have been suggested as etiologies. Pulmonary stenosis can also be a component of **LEOPARD syndrome** (lentigines, electrocardiographic abnormalities, ocular hypertelorism, pulmonary stenosis, abnormalities of genitalia, retardation of growth, deafness syndrome), often associated with hypertrophic cardiomyopathy. Mutations in the genes PTPN11, RAF1 and BRAF have been implicated in LEOPARD syndrome. Pulmonary stenosis, either of the valve or the branch pulmonary arteries, is a common finding in patients with arteriohepatic dysplasia, also known as **Alagille syndrome** (see Chapter 356). In this syndrome and in some patients with isolated pulmonic stenosis, a mutation is present in the *Jagged1* gene.

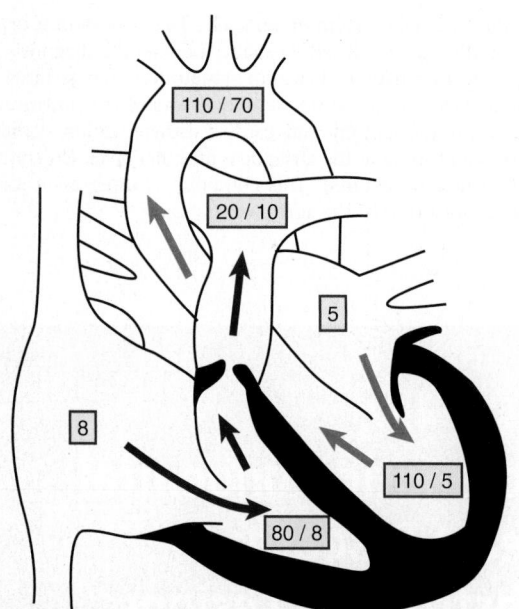

Figure 427-1 Physiology of valvular pulmonary stenosis. Boxed numbers represent pressure in mm Hg. Because of the absence of right-to-left or left-to-right shunting, blood flow through all cardiac chambers is normal at 3 L/min/m². The pulmonary-to-systemic blood flow ratio (Qp : Qs) is 1 : 1. Right atrial pressure is increased slightly as a result of decreased right ventricular compliance. The right ventricle is hypertrophied, and systolic and diastolic pressure is increased. The pressure gradient across the thickened pulmonary valve is 60 mm Hg. The main pulmonary artery pressure is slightly low, and poststenotic dilation is present. Left-heart pressure is normal. Unless right-to-left shunting is occurring through a foramen ovale, the patient's systemic oxygen saturation will be normal.

PATHOPHYSIOLOGY

The obstruction to outflow from the right ventricle to the pulmonary artery results in increased right ventricular systolic pressure and wall stress, which leads to hypertrophy of the right ventricle (Fig. 427-1). The severity of these abnormalities depends on the size of the restricted valve opening. In severe cases, right ventricular pressure may be higher than systemic arterial systolic pressure, whereas with milder obstruction, right ventricular pressure is only mildly or moderately elevated. Pulmonary artery pressure (distal to the obstruction) is normal or decreased. Arterial oxygen saturation will be normal even in cases of severe stenosis, unless an intracardiac communication such as a VSD or ASD is allowing blood to shunt from right to left. When severe pulmonic stenosis occurs in a neonate, decreased right ventricular compliance often leads to cyanosis as a result of right-to-left shunting through a patent foramen ovale, a condition termed *critical pulmonic stenosis*.

CLINICAL MANIFESTATIONS AND LABORATORY FINDINGS

Patients with mild or moderate stenosis usually do not have any symptoms. Growth and development are most often normal. If the stenosis is severe, signs of right ventricular failure such as hepatomegaly, peripheral edema, and exercise intolerance may be present. In a neonate or young infant with critical pulmonic stenosis, signs of right ventricular failure may be more prominent, and cyanosis is often present because of right-to-left shunting at the foramen ovale.

With **mild pulmonary stenosis,** venous pressure and pulse are normal. The heart is not enlarged, the apical impulse is normal, and the right ventricular impulse is not palpable. A sharp pulmonic ejection click immediately after the 1st heart sound is heard at the left upper sternal border during expiration. The 2nd heart sound is split, with a pulmonary component of normal intensity that may be slightly

delayed. A relatively short, low- or medium-pitched systolic ejection murmur is maximally audible over the pulmonic area and radiates minimally to the lung fields bilaterally. The electrocardiogram is normal or characteristic of mild right ventricular hypertrophy; inversion of the T waves in the right precordial leads may be seen. Remember that the T wave in lead V_1 should normally be inverted until at least 6-8 yr of age. Therefore, a positive T wave in V_1 in a young child is a sign of right ventricular hypertrophy. The only abnormality demonstrable radiographically is usually poststenotic dilation of the pulmonary artery. Two-dimensional echocardiography shows right ventricular hypertrophy and a slightly thickened pulmonic valve, which domes in systole; Doppler studies demonstrate a right ventricle to pulmonary artery gradient of ≤30 mm Hg.

In **moderate pulmonic stenosis,** venous pressure may be slightly elevated; in older children, a prominent *a* wave may be noted in the jugular pulse. A right ventricular lift may be palpable at the lower left sternal border. The 2nd heart sound is split, with a delayed and soft pulmonary component. As valve motion becomes more limited with more severe degrees of stenosis, both the pulmonic ejection click and the pulmonic 2nd sound may become inaudible. With increasing degrees of stenosis, the peak of the systolic ejection murmur is prolonged later into systole, and its quality becomes louder and harsher (higher frequency). The murmur radiates more prominently to both lung fields.

The electrocardiogram reveals right ventricular hypertrophy, sometimes with a prominent spiked P wave. Radiographically, the heart can vary from normal size to mildly enlarged with uptilting of the apex because of the prominence of the right ventricle; pulmonary vascularity may be normal or slightly decreased. The echocardiogram shows a thickened pulmonic valve with restricted systolic motion. Doppler examination demonstrates a right ventricle to pulmonary artery pressure gradient in the 30-60 mm Hg range. Mild tricuspid regurgitation may be present and allows Doppler confirmation of right ventricular systolic pressure.

In **severe stenosis,** mild to moderate cyanosis may be noted in patients with an interatrial communication (ASD or patent foramen ovale). In the absence of any intracardiac shunt, cyanosis is absent. If hepatic enlargement and peripheral edema are present, they are an indication of right ventricular failure. Elevation of venous pressure is common and is caused by a large presystolic jugular *a* wave. The heart is moderately or greatly enlarged, and a conspicuous parasternal right ventricular lift is present and frequently extends to the left midclavicular line. The pulmonary component of the 2nd sound is usually inaudible. A loud, long, and harsh systolic ejection murmur, usually accompanied by a thrill, is maximally audible in the pulmonic area and may radiate over the entire precordium, to both lung fields, into the neck, and to the back. The peak of the murmur occurs later in systole as valve opening becomes more restricted. The murmur frequently encompasses the aortic component of the 2nd sound but is not preceded by an ejection click.

The electrocardiogram shows gross right ventricular hypertrophy, frequently accompanied by a tall, spiked P wave. Radiographic studies confirm the presence of cardiac enlargement with prominence of the right ventricle and right atrium. Prominence of the main pulmonary artery segment may be seen due to poststenotic dilation (Fig. 427-2). Intrapulmonary vascularity is decreased. The 2-dimensional echocardiogram shows severe deformity of the pulmonary valve and right ventricular hypertrophy (Fig. 427-3). In the late stages of the disease, systolic dysfunction of the right ventricle may be seen, and in these cases the ventricle may become dilated, with prominent tricuspid regurgitation. Doppler studies demonstrate a high gradient (>60 mm Hg) across the pulmonary valve. The classic findings of severe pulmonary stenosis in older children are rarely seen because of early intervention. Signs of critical pulmonic stenosis, with all of the features of severe pulmonic stenosis plus cyanosis, are usually encountered in the neonatal period.

Cardiac catheterization is not generally required for diagnostic purposes but is undertaken as part of a **balloon valvuloplasty** procedure. Catheterization demonstrates an abrupt pressure gradient across the

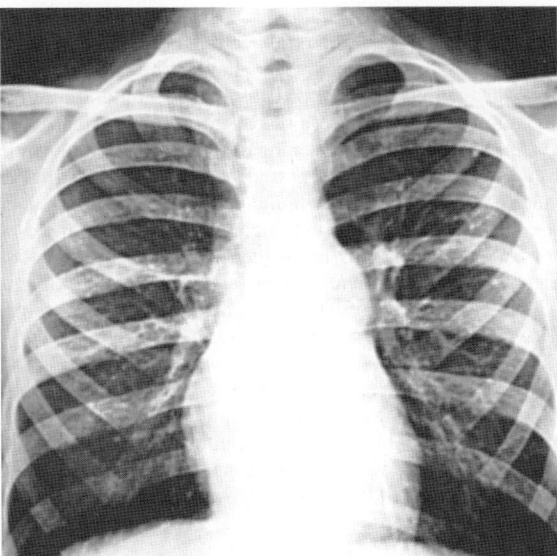

Figure 427-2 X-ray of a patient with valvular pulmonary stenosis and a normal aortic root. The heart size is within normal limits, but post-stenotic dilation of the pulmonary artery is present.

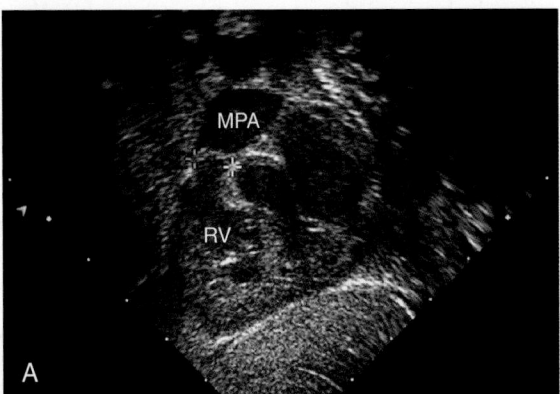

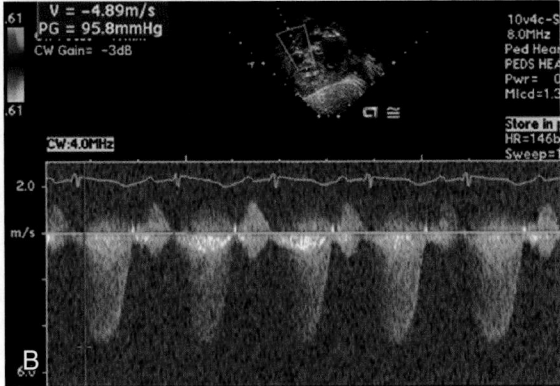

Figure 427-3 Echocardiogram demonstrating valvar pulmonic stenosis. **A,** Subcostal view showing thickened pulmonary valve leaflets (between crosshatches). **B,** Doppler study indicating a 95 mm Hg peak pressure gradient across the stenotic valve. MPA, main pulmonary artery; RV, right ventricle.

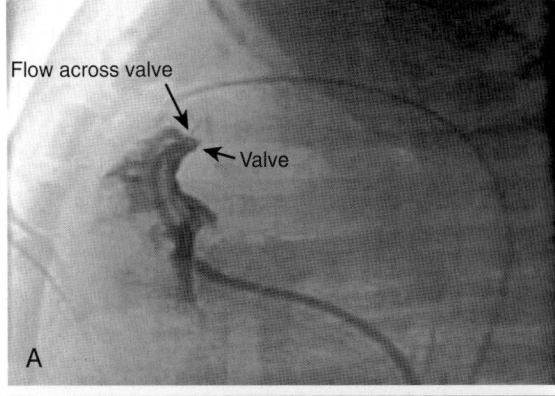

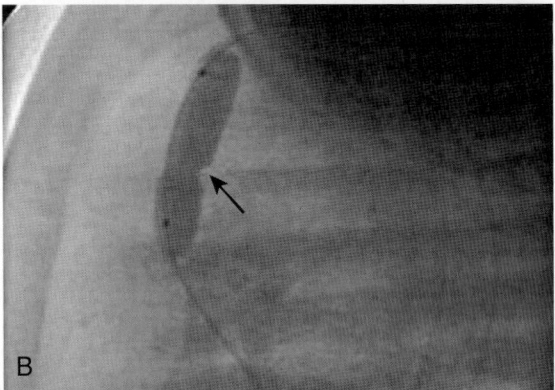

Figure 427-4 Valvar pulmonary stenosis and balloon valvuloplasty. **A,** Right ventricular angiogram showing severely stenotic pulmonary valve with narrow jet of blood flowing across. **B,** Inflation of the balloon catheter showing the indentation *(arrow)* made on the balloon from the stenotic valve. *(Photos courtesy of Dr. Jeffrey Feinstein, Stanford University, Stanford, CA.)*

pulmonary valve. Pulmonary artery pressure is either normal or low. The severity of the stenosis is graded based on the ratio of right ventricular systolic pressure to systemic systolic pressure or the right ventricle to pulmonary artery pressure gradient: a gradient of 10-30 mm Hg in mild cases, 30-60 mm Hg in moderate cases, and >60 mm Hg or with right ventricular pressure greater than systemic pressure in severe cases. If cardiac output is low or a significant right-to-left shunt exists across the atrial septum, the pressure gradient may underestimate the degree of valve stenosis. Selective right ventriculography demonstrates the thickened, poorly mobile valve. In mild to moderate stenosis, doming of the valve in systole is readily seen. Flow of contrast medium through the stenotic valve in ventricular systole produces a narrow jet of dye that fills the dilated main pulmonary artery. Subvalvular hypertrophy that may intensify the obstruction may be present.

TREATMENT

Patients with moderate or severe isolated pulmonary stenosis require relief of the obstruction. Balloon valvuloplasty is the initial treatment of choice for the majority of patients (Fig. 427-4). Patients with severely thickened pulmonic valves, especially common in those with Noonan syndrome, may require surgical intervention. In a neonate with critical pulmonic stenosis, urgent treatment by either balloon valvuloplasty or surgical valvotomy is warranted.

Excellent results are obtained in most instances. The gradient across the pulmonary valve is markedly reduced or abolished. In the early period after balloon valvuloplasty, a small to moderate residual gradient may remain because of muscular infundibular narrowing; it usually resolves with time. A short, early decrescendo diastolic murmur may be heard at the mid to upper left sternal border as a result of pulmonary valvular insufficiency. The degree of insufficiency is not usually clinically significant. No difference in patient status after valvuloplasty or surgery is noted at late follow-up; recurrence is unusual after successful treatment except in those patients with extremely dysplastic valves. In the small minority of patients where the degree of pulmonary regurgitation is more severe, right ventricular dilation may ensue, and these patients require careful follow-up and may require surgical intervention.

PROGNOSIS AND COMPLICATIONS

Heart failure occurs only in severe cases and most often during the 1st mo of life. The development of cyanosis from a right-to-left shunt across a foramen ovale is almost exclusively seen in the neonatal period when the stenosis is severe. Infective endocarditis is a risk, but is not common in childhood.

Children with mild stenosis can lead a normal life, but their progress should be evaluated at regular intervals. Patients who have small gradients rarely show progression and do not need intervention, but a significant gradient is more likely to develop in children with moderate stenosis as they grow older. Worsening of obstruction may also be due to the development of secondary subvalvular muscular and fibrous tissue hypertrophy. In untreated severe stenosis, the course may abruptly worsen with the development of right ventricular dysfunction and cardiac failure. Infants with critical pulmonic stenosis require urgent catheter balloon valvuloplasty or surgical valvotomy. Development of right ventricular failure many years after pulmonary balloon valvuloplasty is uncommon. Nonetheless, patients should be followed serially for worsening pulmonary insufficiency and right ventricular dilation.

Bibliography is available at Expert Consult.

427.2 Infundibular Pulmonary Stenosis and Double-Chamber Right Ventricle
Daniel Bernstein

Infundibular pulmonary stenosis is caused by muscular or fibrous obstruction in the outflow tract of the right ventricle. The site of obstruction may be close to the pulmonary valve or well below it; an infundibular chamber may be present between the right ventricular cavity and the pulmonary valve. In many cases, a VSD may have been present initially and later closed spontaneously. When the pulmonary valve is also stenotic, the combined defect is primarily classified as valvular stenosis with secondary infundibular hypertrophy. The hemodynamics and clinical manifestations of patients with isolated infundibular pulmonary stenosis are similar, for the most part, to those described in the discussion of isolated valvular pulmonary stenosis (see Chapter 427.1).

A common variation in right ventricular outflow obstruction below the pulmonary valve is that of a double-chambered right ventricle. In this condition, a muscular band is present in the mid-right ventricular region; the band divides the chamber into 2 parts and creates obstruction between the inlet and outlet portions. An associated VSD that may close spontaneously is often noted. Obstruction is not usually seen early in life but may progress rapidly in a similar manner to the progressive infundibular obstruction observed with tetralogy of Fallot (see Chapter 430.1).

The diagnosis of isolated right ventricular infundibular stenosis or double-chambered right ventricle is usually made by echocardiography. The ventricular septum must be evaluated carefully to determine whether an associated VSD is present. The prognosis for untreated cases of severe right ventricular outflow obstruction is similar to that for valvular pulmonary stenosis. When the obstruction is moderate to severe, surgery is indicated. After surgery, the pressure gradient is abolished or markedly reduced and the long-term outlook is excellent.

427.3 Pulmonary Stenosis in Combination with an Intracardiac Shunt
Daniel Bernstein

Valvular or infundibular pulmonary stenosis, or both, may be associated with either an ASD or a VSD. In these patients, the clinical features depend on the degree of pulmonary stenosis, which determines whether the net shunt is from left to right or from right to left.

The presence of a large left-to-right shunt at the atrial or ventricular level is evidence that the pulmonary stenosis is mild. These patients have symptoms similar to those of patients with an isolated ASD or VSD. With increasing age, worsening of the obstruction may limit the shunt and result in a gradual improvement in symptoms. Eventually, particularly in patients with pulmonary stenosis and VSD, a further increase in obstruction may lead to right-to-left shunting and cyanosis. When a patient with a VSD has evidence of decreasing heart failure and increased right ventricular forces on the electrocardiogram, one must differentiate between the development of increasing pulmonary stenosis versus the onset of pulmonary vascular disease (Eisenmenger syndrome, Chapter 433.2).

These anomalies are readily repaired surgically. Defects in the atrial or ventricular septum are closed, and the pulmonary stenosis is relieved by resection of infundibular muscle or pulmonary valvotomy, or both, as indicated. Patients with a predominant right-to-left shunt have symptoms similar to those of patients with **tetralogy of Fallot** (see Chapter 430.1).

427.4 Peripheral Pulmonary Stenosis
Daniel Bernstein

Single or multiple constrictions may occur anywhere along the major branches of the pulmonary arteries and may range from mild to severe and from localized to extensive. Frequently, these defects are associated with other types of congenital heart disease, including valvular pulmonic stenosis, tetralogy of Fallot, patent ductus arteriosus (PDA), VSD, ASD, and supravalvular aortic stenosis. A familial tendency has been recognized in some patients with peripheral pulmonic stenosis. A high incidence is found in infants with congenital rubella syndrome. The combination of supravalvular aortic stenosis with pulmonary arterial branch stenosis, idiopathic hypercalcemia of infancy, elfin facies, and mental retardation is known as **Williams syndrome,** a condition associated with deletion of the elastin gene in region 7q11.23 on chromosome 7. Peripheral pulmonary stenosis is also associated with the **Alagille syndrome,** which may be associated with a mutation in the *Jagged1* gene.

A mild constriction has little effect on the pulmonary circulation. With multiple severe constrictions, pressure is increased in the right ventricle and in the pulmonary artery proximal to the site of obstruction. When the anomaly is isolated, the diagnosis is suspected by the presence of murmurs in widespread locations over the chest, either anteriorly or posteriorly. These murmurs are usually systolic ejection in quality but may be continuous. Most often, the physical signs are dominated by the associated anomaly, such as tetralogy of Fallot (see Chapter 430.1).

In the immediate newborn period, a mild and transient form of peripheral pulmonic stenosis may be present. Physical findings are generally limited to a soft systolic ejection murmur, which can be heard over either or both lung fields. It is the absence of other physical findings of valvular pulmonic stenosis (right ventricular lift, soft pulmonic 2nd sound, systolic ejection click, murmur loudest at the upper left sternal border) that supports this diagnosis. This murmur usually disappears by 1-2 mo.

If the stenosis is severe, the electrocardiogram shows evidence of right ventricular and right atrial hypertrophy, and the chest radiograph shows cardiomegaly and prominence of the main pulmonary artery. The pulmonary vasculature is usually normal; in some cases, however, small intrapulmonary vascular shadows are seen that represent areas of poststenotic dilation. Echocardiography is limited in its ability to visualize the distal branch pulmonary arteries. Doppler examination demonstrates the acceleration of blood flow through the stenoses and, if tricuspid regurgitation is present, allows an estimation of right ventricular systolic pressure. MRI and CT are extremely helpful in delineating distal obstructions; if moderate to severe disease is suspected, the diagnosis is usually confirmed by cardiac catheterization.

Severe obstruction of the main pulmonary artery and its primary branches can be relieved during corrective surgery for associated lesions such as the tetralogy of Fallot or valvular pulmonary stenosis. If peripheral pulmonic stenosis is isolated, it may be treated by catheter balloon dilation, sometimes with placement of an intravascular stent (see Fig. 423-29 in Chapter 423).

427.5 Aortic Stenosis
Daniel Bernstein

PATHOPHYSIOLOGY
Congenital aortic stenosis accounts for ≈5% of cardiac malformations recognized in childhood; a bicuspid aortic valve, one of the most common congenital heart lesions overall, is identified in up to 1.5% of adults and may be asymptomatic in childhood. Aortic stenosis is more frequent in males (3:1). There are families with multiple individuals affected with bicuspid aortic valve, and several genes have been implicated, including *NOTCH1* on chromosome 9q34.3.

In the most common form, valvular aortic stenosis, the leaflets are thickened and the commissures are fused to varying degrees. Left ventricular systolic pressure is increased as a result of the obstruction to outflow. The left ventricular wall hypertrophies in compensation; as its compliance decreases, end-diastolic pressure increases as well.

Subvalvular (subaortic) stenosis with a discrete fibromuscular shelf below the aortic valve is also an important form of left ventricular outflow tract obstruction. This lesion is frequently associated with other forms of congenital heart disease such as mitral stenosis and coarctation of the aorta (**Shone syndrome**) and may progress rapidly in severity. It is less commonly diagnosed during early infancy and may develop despite previous documentation of no left ventricular outflow tract obstruction. Subvalvular aortic stenosis may become apparent after successful surgery for other congenital heart defects (coarctation of the aorta, PDA, VSD), may develop in association with mild lesions that have not been surgically repaired, or may occur as an isolated abnormality. Subvalvular aortic stenosis may also be caused by a markedly hypertrophied ventricular septum in association with hypertrophic cardiomyopathy (see Chapter 439.2).

Supravalvular aortic stenosis, the least-common type, may be sporadic, familial, or associated with **Williams syndrome,** which includes mental retardation (IQ range: 41-80), elfin facies (full face, broad forehead, flattened bridge of the nose, long upper lip, and rounded cheeks) (Fig. 427-5), and idiopathic hypercalcemia of infancy. Additional features include loquacious personality, hypersensitivity to sound, spasticity, hypoplastic nails, dental anomalies (partial anodontia, microdontia enamel hypoplasia), joint hypermobility, nephrocalcinosis, hypothyroidism, and poor weight gain. Narrowing of the coronary artery ostia can occur in patients with supravalvar aortic stenosis and should be carefully evaluated. Stenosis of other arteries, in particular, the branch pulmonary arteries, may also be present. Williams syndrome has been shown to be due to a deletion involving the elastin gene on chromosome 7q11.23.

CLINICAL MANIFESTATIONS
Symptoms in patients with aortic stenosis depend on the severity of the obstruction. Severe aortic stenosis that occurs in early infancy is termed **critical aortic stenosis** and is associated with left ventricular failure and signs of low cardiac output. Heart failure, cardiomegaly, and pulmonary edema are severe, the pulses are weak in all extremities, and the skin may be pale or grayish. Urine output may be diminished. If cardiac output is significantly decreased, the intensity of the murmur at the right upper sternal border may be minimal. Most children with less-severe forms of aortic stenosis remain asymptomatic and display normal growth and development. The murmur is usually discovered during routine physical examination. Rarely, fatigue, angina, dizziness, or syncope may develop in an older child with previously undiagnosed severe obstruction to left ventricular outflow. Sudden death has been

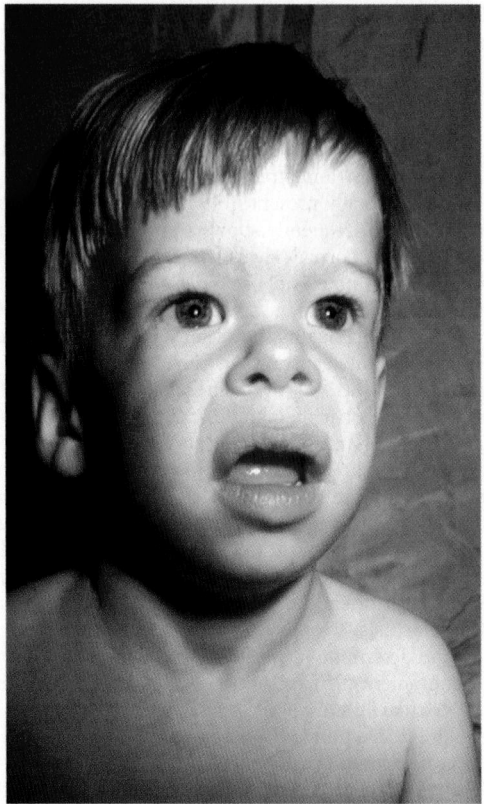

Figure 427-5 Williams syndrome. *(From Jones KL, Smith DW: The Williams elfin facies syndrome: a new perspective, J Pediatr 86:718, 1975.)*

reported with aortic stenosis but usually occurs in patients with severe left ventricular outflow obstruction in whom surgical relief has been delayed.

The physical findings are dependent on the degree of obstruction to left ventricular outflow. In mild stenosis, the pulses, heart size, and apical impulse are all normal. With increasing degrees of severity, the pulses become diminished in intensity and the heart may be enlarged, with a left ventricular apical thrust. Mild to moderate valvular aortic stenosis is usually associated with an early systolic ejection click, best heard at the apex and left sternal edge. Unlike the click in pulmonic stenosis, its intensity does not vary with respiration. Clicks are unusual in more-severe aortic stenosis or in discrete subaortic stenosis. If the stenosis is severe, the 1st heart sound may be diminished because of decreased compliance of the thickened left ventricle. Normal splitting of the 2nd heart sound is present in mild to moderate obstruction. In patients with severe obstruction, the intensity of aortic valve closure is diminished, and, rarely in children, the 2nd sound may be split paradoxically (becoming wider in expiration). A 4th heart sound may be audible when the obstruction is severe as a result of decreased left ventricular compliance.

The intensity, pitch, and duration of the systolic ejection murmur are other indications of severity. The louder, harsher (higher pitch), and longer the murmur, the greater the degree of obstruction is. The typical murmur is audible maximally at the right upper sternal border and radiates to the neck and the left midsternal border. It is usually accompanied by a thrill in the suprasternal notch. In patients with subvalvular aortic stenosis, the murmur may be maximal along the left sternal border or even at the apex. A soft decrescendo diastolic murmur indicative of aortic insufficiency is often present when the obstruction is subvalvular or in patients with a bicuspid aortic valve. Occasionally, an apical short mid-diastolic rumbling murmur is audible; this murmur should raise suspicion of associated mitral valve stenosis.

LABORATORY FINDINGS AND DIAGNOSIS

The diagnosis can usually be made on the basis of the physical examination and the severity of obstruction confirmed by laboratory tests. If the pressure gradient across the aortic valve is mild, the electrocardiogram is likely to be normal. The electrocardiogram may occasionally be normal even with more severe obstruction, but evidence of left ventricular hypertrophy and strain (inverted T waves in the left precordial leads) is generally present if severe stenosis is long-standing. The chest radiograph frequently shows a prominent ascending aorta, but the aortic knob is normal. Heart size is typically normal. Valvular calcification has been noted only in older children and adults. Echocardiography identifies both the site and the severity of the obstruction. Two-dimensional imaging shows left ventricular hypertrophy and the thickened and domed aortic valve (Fig. 427-6). The echo will also demonstrate the number of valve leaflets and their morphology, and the presence of a subaortic membrane or supravalvar stenosis. Associated anomalies of the mitral valve or aortic arch or a VSD or PDA are present in up to 20% of cases. In the absence of left ventricular failure, the shortening fraction of the left ventricle may be increased because the ventricle is hypercontractile. In infants with critical aortic stenosis, the left ventricular shortening fraction is usually decreased and may be quite poor. The endocardium may appear bright, indicative of the development of endocardial fibrous scarring, known as **endocardial fibroelastosis.** Doppler studies show the specific site of obstruction and determine the peak and mean systolic left ventricular outflow tract gradients. When severe aortic obstruction is associated with left ventricular dysfunction, the Doppler-derived valve gradient may markedly underestimate the severity of the obstruction because of the low cardiac output across the valve.

Left-heart catheterization, usually performed in conjunction with aortic balloon valvuloplasty, demonstrates the magnitude of the pressure gradient from the left ventricle to the aorta. The aortic pressure curve is abnormal if the obstruction is severe. In patients with severe obstruction and decreased left ventricular compliance, left atrial pressure is increased and pulmonary hypertension may be present. When a critically ill infant with left ventricular outflow tract obstruction undergoes cardiac catheterization, left ventricular function is often markedly decreased. As with the echocardiogram, the gradient measured across the stenotic aortic valve may underestimate the degree of obstruction because of low cardiac output. Actual measurement of cardiac output by thermodilution and calculation of the aortic valve area may be helpful.

TREATMENT

Balloon valvuloplasty is indicated for children with moderate to severe valvular aortic stenosis to prevent progressive left ventricular dysfunction and the risk of syncope and sudden death. Valvuloplasty should be advised when the peak-to-peak systolic gradient between the left ventricle and aorta exceeds 60-70 mm Hg at rest, assuming normal cardiac output, or for lesser gradients when symptoms or electrocardiographic changes are present. For more rapidly progressive subaortic obstructive lesions, a gradient of 40-50 mm Hg or the presence of aortic insufficiency is considered an indication for surgery. Balloon valvuloplasty is the procedure of choice even in the neonatal period. Surgical treatment is usually reserved for extremely dysplastic aortic valves that are not amenable to balloon therapy or in patients who also have subvalvar or valvar (also known as *supravalvar*) stenosis.

Discrete subaortic stenosis can be resected without damage to the aortic valve, the anterior leaflet of the mitral valve, or the conduction system. This type of obstruction is not usually amenable to catheter treatment. Relief of supravalvular stenosis is also achieved surgically, and the results are excellent if the area of obstruction is discrete and not associated with a hypoplastic aorta. In association with supravalvular aortic stenosis, one or both coronary arteries may be stenotic at their origins because of a thick supra-aortic fibrous ridge. For patients who have aortic stenosis in association with severe tunnel-like subaortic obstruction, the left ventricular outflow tract can be enlarged by "borrowing" space anteriorly from the right ventricular outflow tract (the Konno procedure).

Regardless of whether surgical or catheter treatment has been carried out, aortic insufficiency or calcification with re-stenosis is likely to occur years or even decades later and eventually require reoperation and often aortic valve replacement. When recurrence develops, it may not be associated with early symptoms. Signs of recurrent stenosis include electrocardiographic signs of left ventricular hypertrophy, an increase in the Doppler echocardiographic gradient, deterioration in echocardiographic indices of left ventricular function, and recurrence of signs or symptoms during graded treadmill exercise. Evidence of significant aortic regurgitation includes symptoms of heart failure, cardiac enlargement on roentgenogram, and left ventricular dilation on echocardiogram. The choice of reparative procedure depends on the relative degree of stenosis and regurgitation.

When **aortic valve replacement** is necessary, the choice of procedure often depends on the age of the patient. Homograft valves tend to calcify more rapidly in younger children, but they do not require chronic anticoagulation. Mechanical prosthetic valves are much longer lasting, yet they require anticoagulation, which can be difficult to manage in young children. In adolescent girls who are nearing childbearing age, consideration of the teratogenic effects of warfarin may warrant the use of a homograft valve. None of these options are perfect for a younger child who requires valve replacement because neither homograft nor mechanical valves grow with the patient. An alternative operation is **aortopulmonary translocation (Ross procedure);** it involves removing the patient's own pulmonary valve and using it to replace the abnormal aortic valve. A homograft is then placed in the pulmonary position. The potential advantage of this procedure is the possibility for growth of the translocated living "neoaortic" valve and the increased longevity of the homograft valve when placed in the lower pressure pulmonary circulation. The long-term success of this operation, especially in young children, is still being investigated. Transcatheter stent valves, which are tissue valves sewn into the inside

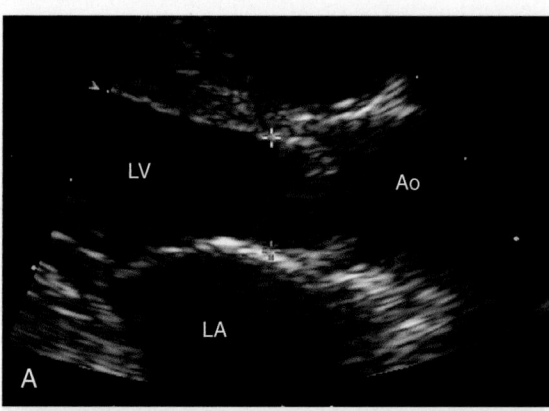

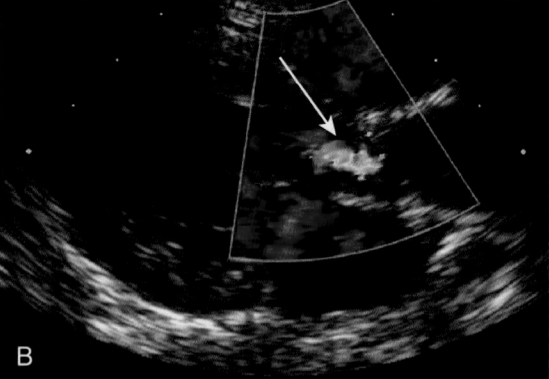

Figure 427-6 Echocardiogram showing valvar aortic stenosis with regurgitation. **A,** In this parasternal long axis view, the stenotic aortic valve can be seen doming in systole. The *crosshatch* marks delineate the aortic annulus. **B,** Doppler study shows the presence of aortic regurgitation *(arrow).* Ao, aorta; LA, left atrium; LV, left ventricle.

of an expandable metal stent, are currently in clinical trials in adults, mainly in those who are not good candidates for standard surgical replacement. These can be implanted in the cardiac catheterization laboratory using a percutaneous approach. Tissue-engineered replacement valves grown in the laboratory from the patient's own arterial endothelial cells are another prospect for long-term palliation and are currently under development in animal models.

PROGNOSIS

Neonates with critical aortic stenosis may have severe heart failure and deteriorate rapidly to a low-output shock state. Emergency surgery or balloon valvuloplasty is lifesaving, but the mortality risk is not trivial. Neonates who die of critical aortic stenosis frequently have significant left ventricular endocardial fibroelastosis. Those who survive may develop signs of left ventricular diastolic muscle dysfunction (restrictive cardiomyopathy) and require cardiac transplantation (see Chapter 443).

In older infants and children with mild to moderate aortic stenosis, the prognosis is reasonably good, although disease progression over a period of 5-10 yr is common. Patients with aortic valve gradients <40-50 mm Hg are considered to have mild disease; those with gradients of 40-70 mm Hg have moderate disease. These patients usually respond well to treatment (either surgery or valvuloplasty), although reoperations on the aortic valve are often required later in childhood or in adult life, and many patients eventually require valve replacement. In unoperated patients with severe obstruction, sudden death is a significant risk and often occurs during or immediately after exercise. Aortic stenosis is one of the causes of sudden cardiac death in the pediatric age group.

Patients with moderate to severe degrees of aortic stenosis should not participate in active competitive sports. In those with milder disease, sports participation is less severely restricted. The status of each patient should be reviewed at least annually and intervention advised if progression of signs or symptoms occurs. Prophylaxis against infective endocarditis is no longer recommended unless a prosthetic valve has been inserted.

Older children and adults with isolated bicuspid aortic valve are at increased risk for developing dilation of their ascending aorta, even in the absence of significant stenosis. This risk increases with age, and the rate of increase is greatest in those with the largest aortic roots. In children, this dilation is usually mild and remains stable over many years of observation, but in older patients the aorta can dilate substantially and progressively. Whether these patients have some undiagnosed form of connective tissue disorder remains to be determined (as this form of dilation is similar to that seen in Marfan syndrome). Patients with Turner syndrome and bicuspid aortic valve do have an increased risk of aortic dilation. Although dissection and rupture are described complications of severe aortic root dilation in adults, there is not yet sufficient data to determine these risks in children. Only isolated cases have been reported.

Bibliography is available at Expert Consult.

427.6 Coarctation of the Aorta
Daniel Bernstein

Constrictions of the aorta of varying degrees may occur at any point from the transverse arch to the iliac bifurcation, but 98% occur just below the origin of the left subclavian artery at the origin of the ductus arteriosus (juxtaductal coarctation). The anomaly occurs twice as often in males as in females. Coarctation of the aorta may be a feature of **Turner syndrome** (see Chapters 81 and 586.1) and is associated with a bicuspid aortic valve in more than 70% of patients. Mitral valve abnormalities (a supravalvular mitral ring or parachute mitral valve) and subaortic stenosis are potential associated lesions. When this group of left-sided obstructive lesions occurs together, they are referred to as the **Shone complex.**

PATHOPHYSIOLOGY

Coarctation of the aorta can occur as a discrete juxtaductal obstruction or as tubular hypoplasia of the transverse aorta starting at one of the head or neck vessels and extending to the ductal area (previously referred to as *preductal* or *infantile-type coarctation;* Fig. 427-7). Often, both components are present. It is postulated that coarctation may be initiated in fetal life by the presence of a cardiac abnormality that results in decreased blood flow anterograde through the aortic valve (e.g., bicuspid aortic valve, VSD). Alternatively, coarctation may be caused by abnormal extension of contractile ductal tissue into the aortic wall.

In patients with discrete juxtaductal coarctation, ascending aortic blood flows through the narrowed segment to reach the descending aorta, although left ventricular hypertension and hypertrophy result. In the 1st few days of life, the PDA may serve to widen the juxtaductal area of the aorta and provide temporary relief from the obstruction. Net left-to-right ductal shunting occurs in these acyanotic infants. With more-severe juxtaductal coarctation or in the presence of transverse arch hypoplasia, right ventricular blood is ejected through the ductus to supply the descending aorta. Perfusion of the lower part of the body is then dependent on right ventricular output (see Fig. 427-7). In this situation, the femoral pulses are palpable, and differential blood pressures may not be helpful in making the diagnosis. The ductal right-to-left shunting is manifested as differential cyanosis, with the upper extremities being pink and the lower extremities blue.

Such infants may have severe pulmonary hypertension and high pulmonary vascular resistance. Signs of heart failure are prominent. Occasionally, severely hypoplastic segments of the aortic isthmus may become completely atretic and result in an interrupted aortic arch, with the left subclavian artery arising either proximal or distal to the interruption. Coarctation associated with arch hypoplasia was once referred to as infantile type because its severity usually led to recognition of the

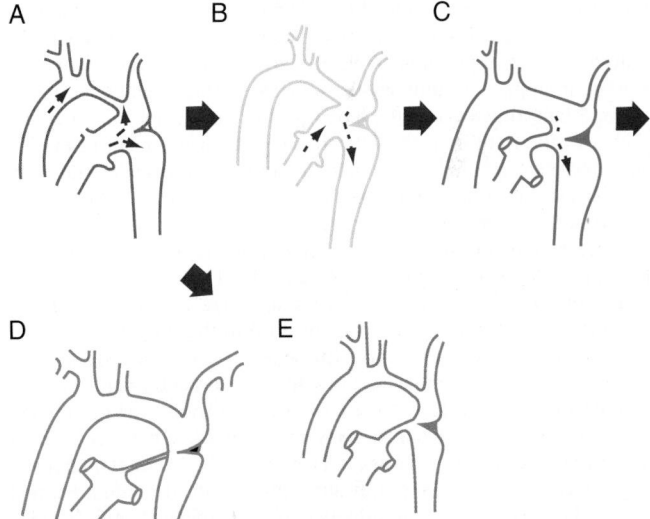

Figure 427-7 Metamorphosis of coarctation. **A,** Fetal prototype with no flow obstruction. **B,** Late gestation. The aortic ventricle increases its output and dilates the hypoplastic segment. Antegrade aortic flow bypasses the shelf via the ductal orifice. **C,** Neonate. Ductal constriction initiates the obstruction by removing the bypass and increasing antegrade arch flow. **D,** Mature juxtaductal stenosis. The bypass is completely obliterated, and intimal hypoplasia on the edge of the shelf is aggravating the stenosis. Collaterals develop. **E,** Persistence of the infantile-type fetal prototype. An intracardiac left-sided heart obstruction precludes an increase in antegrade aortic flow before or after birth. Both isthmus hypoplasia and a contraductal shelf are present. Lower body flow often depends on patency of the ductus. *(From Gersony WM: Coarctation of the aorta. In Adams FH, Emmanouilides GC, Riemenshneider T, editors: Moss heart disease in infants, children, and adolescents, ed 4, Baltimore, 1989, Williams & Wilkins.)*

condition in early infancy. Adult type referred to isolated juxtaductal coarctation, which, if mild, was not usually recognized until later childhood. These terms have been replaced with the more accurate anatomic terms describing the location and severity of the defect.

Blood pressure is elevated in the vessels that arise proximal to the coarctation; blood pressure as well as pulse pressure is lower below the constriction. The hypertension is not caused by the mechanical obstruction alone, but also involves neurohumoral mechanisms. Unless operated on in infancy, coarctation of the aorta usually results in the development of an extensive collateral circulation, chiefly from branches of the subclavian, superior intercostal, and internal mammary arteries, to create channels for arterial blood to bypass the area of coarctation. The vessels contributing to the collateral circulation may become markedly enlarged and tortuous by early adulthood.

CLINICAL MANIFESTATIONS

Coarctation of the aorta recognized after infancy is not usually associated with significant symptoms. Some children or adolescents complain about weakness or pain (or both) in the legs after exercise, but in many instances, even patients with severe coarctation are asymptomatic. Older children are frequently brought to the cardiologist's attention when they are found to be hypertensive on routine physical examination.

The classic sign of coarctation of the aorta is a disparity in pulsation and blood pressure in the arms and legs. The femoral, popliteal, posterior tibial, and dorsalis pedis pulses are weak (or absent in up to 40% of patients), in contrast to the bounding pulses of the arms and carotid vessels. The radial and femoral pulses should always be palpated simultaneously for the presence of a radial-femoral delay. Normally, the femoral pulse occurs slightly before the radial pulse. A radial-femoral delay occurs when blood flow to the descending aorta is dependent on collaterals, in which case the femoral pulse is felt after the radial pulse. In normal persons (except neonates), systolic blood pressure in the legs obtained by the cuff method is 10-20 mm Hg higher than that in the arms. In coarctation of the aorta, blood pressure in the legs is lower than that in the arms; frequently, it is difficult to obtain. This differential in blood pressures is common in patients with coarctation who are older than 1 yr, approximately 90% of whom have systolic hypertension in an upper extremity greater than the 95th percentile for age. It is important to determine the blood pressure in each arm; a pressure higher in the right than the left arm suggests involvement of the left subclavian artery in the area of coarctation. Occasionally, the right subclavian may arise anomalously from below the area of coarctation and result in a left arm pressure that is higher than the right. With exercise, a more prominent rise in systemic blood pressure occurs, and the upper-to-lower extremity pressure gradient will increase.

The precordial impulse and heart sounds are usually normal; the presence of a systolic ejection click or thrill in the suprasternal notch suggests a bicuspid aortic valve (present in 70% of cases). A short systolic murmur is often heard along the left sternal border at the 3rd and 4th intercostal spaces. The murmur is well transmitted to the left infrascapular area and occasionally to the neck. Often, the typical murmur of mild aortic stenosis can be heard in the 3rd right intercostal space. Occasionally, more significant degrees of obstruction are noted across the aortic valve. The presence of a low-pitched mid-diastolic murmur at the apex suggests mitral valve stenosis. In older patients with well-developed collateral blood flow, systolic or continuous murmurs may be heard over the left and right sides of the chest laterally and posteriorly. In these patients, a palpable thrill can occasionally be appreciated in the intercostal spaces on the back.

Neonates or infants with more severe coarctation, usually including some degree of transverse arch hypoplasia, initially have signs of lower body hypoperfusion, acidosis, and severe heart failure. These signs may be delayed days or weeks until after closure of the ductus arteriosus. If detected before ductal closure, patients may exhibit differential cyanosis, best demonstrated by simultaneous oximetry of the upper and lower extremities. On physical examination, the heart is large, and a systolic murmur is heard along the left sternal border with a loud 2nd heart sound.

DIAGNOSIS

Findings on roentgenographic examination depend on the age of the patient and on the effects of hypertension and the collateral circulation. Cardiac enlargement and pulmonary congestion are noted in infants with severe coarctation. During childhood, the findings are not striking until after the 1st decade, when the heart tends to be mildly or moderately enlarged because of left ventricular prominence. The enlarged left subclavian artery commonly produces a prominent shadow in the left superior mediastinum. **Notching** of the **inferior border of the ribs** from pressure erosion by enlarged collateral vessels is common by late childhood. In most instances, the descending aorta has an area of poststenotic dilation.

The electrocardiogram is usually normal in young children but reveals evidence of left ventricular hypertrophy in older patients. Neonates and young infants display right or biventricular hypertrophy. The segment of coarctation can generally be visualized by 2-dimensional echocardiography (Fig. 427-8); associated anomalies of the mitral and aortic valve can also be demonstrated. The descending aorta is hypopulsatile. Color Doppler is useful for demonstrating the specific site of the obstruction. Pulsed and continuous wave Doppler studies determine the pressure gradient directly at the area of coarctation; in the presence of a PDA, however, the severity of the narrowing may be underestimated. CT and MRI are valuable noninvasive tools for evaluation of coarctation when the echocardiogram is equivocal. Cardiac catheterization with selective left ventriculography and aortography is useful in occasional patients with additional anomalies and as a means of visualizing collateral blood flow. In cases that are well defined by echocardiography, CT, or MRI, diagnostic catheterization is not usually required before surgery.

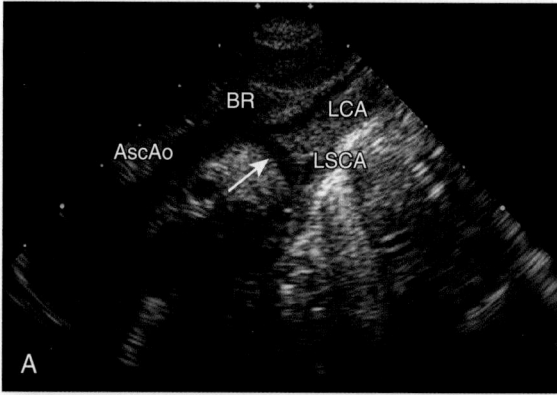

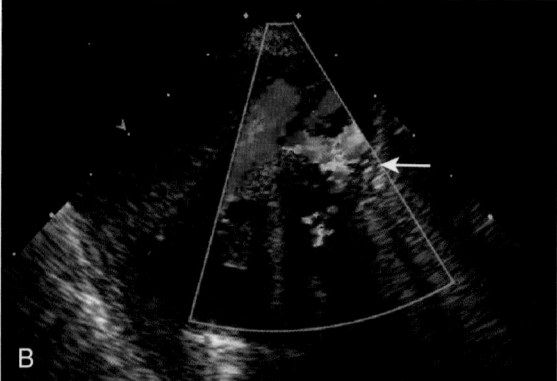

Figure 427-8 Echocardiogram demonstrating coarctation of the aorta with hypoplastic transverse arch. **A,** Suprasternal notch 2-dimensional echocardiogram showing marked narrowing beginning just distal to the brachiocephalic artery. **B,** Color Doppler demonstrates turbulent flow in the juxtaductal area (*arrow*). AscAo, ascending aorta; BR, brachiocephalic artery; LCA, left carotid artery; LSCA, left subclavian artery.

TREATMENT

In neonates with severe coarctation of the aorta, closure of the ductus often results in hypoperfusion, acidosis, and rapid deterioration. These patients should be given an infusion of **prostaglandin E₁** to reopen the ductus and reestablish adequate lower extremity blood flow. Once a diagnosis has been confirmed and the patient stabilized, surgical repair should be performed. Older infants with heart failure but good perfusion should be managed with anticongestive measures to improve their clinical status before surgical intervention. There is usually no reason to delay surgical repair waiting for patient growth; successful repairs have been performed in small premature infants.

Older children with significant coarctation of the aorta should be treated relatively soon after diagnosis. Delay is unwarranted, especially after the 2nd decade of life, when the operation may be less successful because of decreased left ventricular function and degenerative changes in the aortic wall. Nevertheless, if cardiac reserve is sufficient, satisfactory repair is possible well into mid-adult life.

The procedure of choice for isolated juxtaductal coarctation of the aorta is controversial. Surgery remains the treatment of choice at most centers, and several surgical techniques are used. The area of coarctation can be excised and a primary re-anastomosis performed. Most often, the transverse aorta is splayed open and an "extended end-to-end" anastomosis performed to increase the effective cross-sectional area of the repair. The subclavian flap procedure, which involves division of the left subclavian artery and incorporation of it into the wall of the repaired coarctation has grown out of favor because of a higher degree of residual stenosis. Some centers favor a patch aortoplasty, in which the area of coarctation is enlarged with a roof of prosthetic material. The use of **primary angioplasty** for native coarctation remains controversial due to concern over subsequent recoarctation and aneurysm development. The use of **primary stent placement** is currently under evaluation in clinical trials and is most useful in conditions where surgical intervention may be associated with increased risk in patients with severe left ventricular dysfunction.

After surgery, a striking increase in the amplitude of pulsations in the lower extremities is noted. In the immediate postoperative course, **"rebound" hypertension** is common and requires medical management. This exaggerated acute hypertension gradually subsides and, in most patients, antihypertensive medications can be discontinued. Residual murmurs are common and may be the result of associated cardiac anomalies, of a residual flow disturbance across the repaired area, or of collateral blood flow. Rare operative problems include spinal cord injury from aortic cross-clamping if the collaterals are poorly developed, chylothorax, diaphragm injury, and laryngeal nerve injury. If a left subclavian flap approach is used, the radial pulse and blood pressure in the left arm are diminished or absent.

POSTCOARCTECTOMY SYNDROME

Postoperative **mesenteric arteritis** may be associated with acute hypertension and abdominal pain in the immediate postoperative period. The pain varies in severity and may occur in conjunction with anorexia, nausea, vomiting, leukocytosis, intestinal hemorrhage, bowel necrosis, and small bowel obstruction. Relief is usually obtained with antihypertensive drugs (nitroprusside, esmolol, captopril) and intestinal decompression; surgical exploration is rarely required for bowel obstruction or infarction.

PROGNOSIS

Although restenosis in older patients after coarctectomy is rare, a significant number of infants operated on before 1 yr of age require revision later in childhood. All patients should be monitored carefully for the development of recoarctation and an aortic anastomotic aneurysm. Should recoarctation occur, **balloon angioplasty** is the procedure of choice. In these patients, scar tissue from previous surgery may make reoperation more difficult yet makes balloon angioplasty safer because of the lower incidence of aneurysm formation. Relief of obstruction with this technique is usually excellent. **Intravascular stents** are commonly used, especially in adolescents and young adults, with generally excellent results.

Repair of coarctation in the 2nd decade of life or beyond may be associated with a higher incidence of premature cardiovascular disease, even in the absence of residual cardiac abnormalities. Early onset of adult chronic hypertension may occur, even in patients with adequately resected coarctation.

Abnormalities of the aortic valve are present in most patients. Bicuspid aortic valves are common but do not generally produce clinical signs unless the stenosis is significant. The association of a PDA and coarctation of the aorta is also common. VSDs and ASDs may be suspected by signs of a left-to-right shunt; they are exacerbated by the increased resistance to flow through the left side of the heart. Mitral valve abnormalities are also occasionally seen, as is subvalvular aortic stenosis.

Severe neurologic damage or even death may rarely occur from associated cerebrovascular disease. Subarachnoid or intracerebral hemorrhage may result from rupture of congenital aneurysms in the circle of Willis, rupture of other vessels with defective elastic and medial tissue, or rupture of normal vessels; these accidents are secondary to hypertension. Children with **PHACE syndrome** (posterior brain fossa anomalies, facial hemangiomas, arterial anomalies, cardiac anomalies and aortic coarctation, eye anomalies syndrome) may have strokes (see Table 422-2 in Chapter 422). Abnormalities of the subclavian arteries may include involvement of the left subclavian artery in the area of coarctation, stenosis of the orifice of the left subclavian artery, and anomalous origin of the right subclavian artery.

Untreated, the great majority of older patients with coarctation of the aorta would succumb between the ages of 20 and 40 yr; some live well into middle life without serious disability. The common serious complications are related to systemic hypertension, which may result in premature coronary artery disease, heart failure, hypertensive encephalopathy, or intracranial hemorrhage. Heart failure may be worsened by associated anomalies. Infective endocarditis or endarteritis is a significant complication in adults. Aneurysms of the descending aorta or the enlarged collateral vessels may develop.

Bibliography is available at Expert Consult.

427.7 Coarctation with Ventricular Septal Defect

Daniel Bernstein

Coarctation in the presence of a VSD results in both increased preload and afterload on the left ventricle, and patients with this combination of defects will be recognized either at birth or in the 1st mo of life and often have intractable cardiac failure. The magnitude of the left-to-right shunt through a VSD is dependent on the ratio of pulmonary to systemic vascular resistance. In the presence of coarctation, resistance to systemic outflow is enhanced by the obstruction, and the volume of the shunt is markedly increased. The clinical picture is that of a seriously ill infant with tachypnea, failure to thrive, and typical findings of heart failure. Often, the difference in blood pressure between the upper and lower extremities is not very marked because cardiac output may be low. Medical management should be used to stabilize the patient initially; however, it should not be used to delay corrective surgery inordinately.

In most cases, coarctation is the major anomaly causing the severe symptoms, and resection of the coarcted segment results in striking improvement. Many centers routinely repair both the VSD and coarctation at the same operation through a midline sternotomy using cardiopulmonary bypass. Some centers repair the coarctation through a left lateral thoracotomy and, at the same time, place a pulmonary artery band to decrease the ventricular-level shunt. This may be performed when a complicated VSD is present (multiple VSDs, apical muscular VSD), to avoid open heart surgery during infancy for these complex ventricular septal abnormalities.

427.8 Coarctation with Other Cardiac Anomalies and Interrupted Aortic Arch

Daniel Bernstein

Coarctation often occurs in infancy in association with other major cardiovascular anomalies, including hypoplastic left heart, severe mitral or aortic valve disease, transposition of the great arteries, and variations of double-outlet or single ventricle. The clinical manifestations depend on the effects of the associated malformations, as well as on the coarctation itself.

Coarctation of the aorta associated with severe mitral and aortic valve disease may have to be treated within the context of the hypoplastic left heart syndrome (see Chapter 431.10), even if the left ventricular chamber is not severely hypoplastic. Such patients usually have a long segment of narrow transverse aortic arch in addition to an isolated coarctation at the site of the ductus arteriosus. Coarctation of the aorta with transposition of the great arteries or single ventricle may be repaired alone or in combination with other corrective or palliative measures.

Complete interruption of the aortic arch is the most severe form of coarctation and is usually associated with other intracardiac pathology. Interruption may occur at any level, although it is most commonly seen between the left subclavian artery and the insertion of the ductus arteriosus (type A), followed in frequency by those between the left subclavian and left carotid arteries (type B), or between the left carotid and brachiocephalic arteries (type C). In newborns with an interrupted aortic arch, the ductus arteriosus provides the sole source of blood flow to the descending aorta, and differential oxygen saturations between the right arm (normal saturation) and the legs (decreased saturation) is noted. When the ductus begins to close, severe congestive heart failure, lower extremity hypoperfusion, anuria, and shock usually develop. Patients with an interrupted aortic arch can be supported with prostaglandin E$_1$ to keep the ductus patent before surgical repair. As one of the conotruncal malformations, an interrupted aortic arch, especially type B, can be associated with DiGeorge syndrome (cardiac defects, abnormal facies, thymic hypoplasia, cleft palate, hypocalcemia). Cytogenetic analysis using fluorescence in situ hybridization demonstrates deletion of a segment of chromosome 22q11, known as the DiGeorge critical region.

427.9 Congenital Mitral Stenosis

Daniel Bernstein

Congenital mitral stenosis is a rare anomaly that can be isolated or associated with other defects, the most common being subvalvar and valvar aortic stenosis and coarctation of the aorta (**Shone complex**). The mitral valve may be funnel-shaped, with thickened leaflets and chordae tendineae that are shortened and deformed. Other mitral valve anomalies associated with stenosis include parachute mitral valve, caused by a single papillary muscle, and double-orifice mitral valve.

If the stenosis is moderate to severe, symptoms usually appear within the 1st yr or 2 of life. These infants have failure to thrive and various degrees of dyspnea and pallor. In some patients, wheezing may be a dominant symptom, and a misdiagnosis of bronchiolitis or reactive airway disease may have been made. Heart enlargement as a result of dilation and hypertrophy of the right ventricle and left atrium is common. Most patients have rumbling apical diastolic murmurs, but the auscultatory findings may be relatively obscure. The 2nd heart sound is loud and split. An opening snap of the mitral valve may be present. The electrocardiogram reveals right ventricular hypertrophy and may show bifid or spiked P waves indicative of left atrial enlargement. Roentgenograms usually show left atrial and right ventricular enlargement and pulmonary congestion in a perihilar or venous pattern. The echocardiogram is characteristic and shows thickened mitral valve leaflets a significant reduction of the mitral valve orifice, abnormal papillary muscle structure (or a single papillary muscle), and an enlarged left atrium with a normal or small left ventricle. A double orifice may also be visualized. Doppler studies demonstrate a mean pressure gradient across the mitral orifice. Associated anomalies such as aortic stenosis and coarctation can be evaluated. Cardiac catheterization is usually performed to confirm the transmitral pressure gradient before surgery. An increase in right ventricular, pulmonary arterial, and pulmonary capillary wedge pressure can be noted. Angiocardiography shows delayed emptying of the left atrium and the small mitral orifice.

The results of surgical treatment depend on the anatomy of the valve, but if the mitral orifice is significantly hypoplastic, reduction of the gradient may be difficult. In some patients, a mitral valve prosthesis is required, and if the valve orifice is too small, the prosthesis may be placed in the supramitral position. However, whatever prosthesis is used, it must be replaced serially as the child grows. These patients must be managed by anticoagulation with warfarin, and complications of excessive and insufficient anticoagulation are fairly common in infancy. Transcatheter balloon valvuloplasty has been used as a palliative procedure with disappointing results, except in the situation of rheumatic mitral stenosis.

Bibliography is available at Expert Consult.

427.10 Pulmonary Venous Hypertension

Daniel Bernstein

A variety of lesions may give rise to chronic pulmonary venous hypertension, which when extreme may result in pulmonary arterial hypertension and right-sided heart failure. These lesions include congenital mitral stenosis, mitral insufficiency, total anomalous pulmonary venous return with obstruction, left atrial myxomas, cor triatriatum (stenosis of a common pulmonary vein), individual pulmonary vein stenosis, and supravalvular mitral rings. Early symptoms can be confused with chronic pulmonary disease such as asthma because of a lack of specific cardiac findings on physical examination. Subtle signs of pulmonary hypertension may be present. The electrocardiogram shows right ventricular hypertrophy with spiked P waves. Roentgenographic studies reveal cardiac enlargement and prominence of the pulmonary veins in the hilar region, the right ventricle and atrium, and the main pulmonary artery; the left atrium is normal in size or only slightly enlarged.

The echocardiogram may demonstrate left atrial myxoma, cor triatriatum, stenosis of one or more pulmonary veins, or a mitral valve abnormality, especially supravalvar mitral ring. Cardiac catheterization excludes the presence of a shunt and demonstrates pulmonary hypertension with elevated pulmonary arterial wedge pressure. Left atrial pressure is normal if the lesion is at the level of the pulmonary veins, but it is elevated if the lesion is at the level of the mitral valve. Selective pulmonary arteriography usually delineates the anatomic lesion. Cor triatriatum, left atrial myxoma, and supravalvular mitral rings can all be successfully managed surgically.

The **differential diagnosis** includes pulmonary venoocclusive disease, an idiopathic process that produces obstructive lesions in 1 or more pulmonary veins. The cause is uncertain and disease that begins in 1 vein can spread to others. Although it is usually encountered in patients after repair of obstructed total anomalous pulmonary venous return (see Chapter 431.7), it can occur in the absence of congenital heart disease. The patient initially presents with left-sided heart failure on the basis of congested lungs with apparent pulmonary edema. Dyspnea, fatigue, and pleural effusions are common. Left atrial pressure is normal, but pulmonary arterial wedge pressure is usually elevated. A normal wedge pressure may be encountered if collaterals have formed or the wedge recording is performed in an uninvolved segment. Angiographically, the pulmonary veins return normally to the left atrium, but 1 or more pulmonary veins are narrowed, either focally or diffusely.

Studies using lung biopsy have demonstrated pulmonary venous and, occasionally, arterial involvement. Pulmonary veins and venules demonstrate fibrous narrowing or occlusion, and pulmonary artery thrombi may be present. Attempts at surgical repair, balloon dilation, and transcatheter stenting have not significantly improved the generally poor prognosis of these patients. Clinical trials of antiproliferative chemotherapy are currently in progress. Combined heart-lung transplantation (see Chapter 443.2) is often the only alternative therapeutic option.

Chapter **428**
Acyanotic Congenital Heart Disease: Regurgitant Lesions

428.1 Pulmonary Valvular Insufficiency and Congenital Absence of the Pulmonary Valve
Daniel Bernstein

Pulmonary valvular insufficiency most often accompanies other cardiovascular diseases or may be secondary to severe pulmonary hypertension. Incompetence of the valve is an expected result after surgery for right ventricular outflow tract obstruction, for example, pulmonary valvotomy in patients with valvular pulmonic stenosis or valvotomy with infundibular resection in patients with tetralogy of Fallot. Isolated congenital insufficiency of the pulmonary valve is rare. These patients are usually asymptomatic because the insufficiency is generally mild.

The prominent physical sign is a decrescendo diastolic murmur at the upper and midleft sternal border, which has a lower pitch than the murmur of aortic insufficiency because of the lower pressure involved. Radiographs of the chest show prominence of the main pulmonary artery and, if the insufficiency is severe, right ventricular enlargement. The electrocardiogram is normal or shows minimal right ventricular hypertrophy. Pulsed and color Doppler studies demonstrate retrograde flow from the pulmonary artery to the right ventricle during diastole. Cardiac magnetic resonance angiography is useful for quantifying both right ventricular volume and the regurgitant fraction. Isolated pulmonary valvular insufficiency is generally well tolerated and does not require surgical treatment. When pulmonary insufficiency is severe, especially if significant tricuspid insufficiency has begun to develop, replacement with a homograft valve may become necessary to preserve right ventricular function.

Congenital absence of the pulmonary valve is usually associated with a ventricular septal defect, often in the context of tetralogy of Fallot (see Chapter 430.1). In many of these neonates, the pulmonary arteries become widely dilated and compress the bronchi, with subsequent recurrent episodes of wheezing, pulmonary collapse, and pneumonitis. The presence and degree of cyanosis are variable. Florid pulmonary valvular incompetence may not be well tolerated, and death may occur from a combination of bronchial compression, hypoxemia, and heart failure. Correction involves plication of the massively dilated pulmonary arteries, closure of the ventricular septal defect, and placement of a homograft across the right ventricular outflow tract.

Bibliography is available at Expert Consult.

428.2 Congenital Mitral Insufficiency
Daniel Bernstein

Congenital mitral insufficiency is rare as an isolated lesion and is more often associated with other anomalies. It is most commonly encountered in combination with an atrioventricular septal defect, either an ostium primum defect, or a complete atrioventricular septal defect (see Chapter 426.5). Mitral insufficiency is also seen in patients with dilated cardiomyopathy (see Chapter 439.1) as their left ventricular function deteriorates, secondary to dilation of the valve ring. Mitral insufficiency may also be encountered in conjunction with coarctation of the aorta, ventricular septal defect, corrected transposition of the great vessels, anomalous origin of the left coronary artery from the pulmonary artery, or Marfan syndrome. In the absence of other congenital heart disease, endocarditis or rheumatic fever should be suspected in a patient with isolated severe mitral insufficiency (Table 428-1).

In isolated mitral insufficiency, the mitral valve annulus is usually dilated, the chordae tendineae are short and may insert anomalously, and the valve leaflets are deformed. When mitral insufficiency is severe enough to cause clinical symptoms, the left atrium enlarges as a result of the regurgitant flow, and the left ventricle becomes hypertrophied and dilated. Pulmonary venous pressure is increased, and the increased pressure ultimately results in pulmonary hypertension and right ventricular hypertrophy and dilation. Mild lesions produce no symptoms;

Table 428-1	Causes and Mechanisms of Mitral Regurgitation			
	Organic			**Functional**
	TYPE I*	TYPE II†	TYPE IIIA‡	TYPE I*/TYPE IIIB‡
Nonischemic	Endocarditis (perforation); degenerative (annular calcification); congenital (cleft leaflet)	Degenerative (billowing/flail leaflets); endocarditis (ruptured chordae); traumatic (ruptured chord/PM); rheumatic (acute RF)	Rheumatic (chronic RF); iatrogenic (radiation/drug); inflammatory (lupus/anticardiolipin), eosinophilic (endocardial disease, endomyocardial fibrosis)	Cardiomyopathy; myocarditis; left-ventricular dysfunction (any cause)

MR, mitral regurgitation; PM, papillary muscle; RF, rheumatic fever.
*Mechanism involves normal leaflet movement.
†Mechanism involves excessive valve movement.
‡Restricted valve movement, IIIa in diastole, IIIb in systole.
Modified from Sarano ME, Akins CW, Vahanian A: Mitral regurgitation, Lancet 373:1382–1394, 2009, p. 1383, Table 1.

the only abnormal sign is the apical holosystolic murmur of mitral regurgitation. Severe regurgitation results in symptoms that can appear at any age, including poor physical development, frequent respiratory infections, fatigue on exertion, and episodes of pulmonary edema or congestive heart failure. Often, a diagnosis of reactive airway disease will have been made because of the similarity in pulmonary symptoms, including wheezing, which may be a dominant finding in infants and young children.

The typical murmur of mitral insufficiency is a high-pitched, apical holosystolic murmur. If the insufficiency is moderate to severe, it is usually associated with a low-pitched, apical mid-diastolic rumbling murmur indicative of increased diastolic flow across the mitral valve. The pulmonary component of the 2nd heart sound will be accentuated in the presence of pulmonary hypertension. The electrocardiogram usually shows bifid P waves consistent with left atrial enlargement, signs of left ventricular hypertrophy, and sometimes signs of right ventricular hypertrophy. Radiographic examination shows enlargement of the left atrium, which at times is massive. The left ventricle is prominent, and pulmonary vascularity is normal or prominent. The echocardiogram demonstrates the enlarged left atrium and ventricle. Color Doppler demonstrates the extent of the insufficiency, and pulsed Doppler of the pulmonary veins detects retrograde flow when mitral insufficiency is severe. Cardiac catheterization shows elevated left atrial pressure. Pulmonary artery hypertension of varying severity may be present. Selective left ventriculography reveals the severity of mitral regurgitation.

Mitral valvuloplasty can result in striking improvement in symptoms and heart size, but in some patients, installation of a prosthetic mechanical mitral valve may be necessary. Before surgery, associated anomalies must be identified.

428.3 Mitral Valve Prolapse
Daniel Bernstein

Mitral valve prolapse results from an abnormal mitral valve mechanism that causes billowing of one or both mitral leaflets, especially the posterior cusp, into the left atrium toward the end of systole. The abnormality is predominantly congenital but may not be recognized until adolescence or adulthood. Mitral valve prolapse is usually sporadic, is more common in girls, and may be inherited as an autosomal dominant trait with variable expression. It is common in patients with Marfan syndrome, straight back syndrome, pectus excavatum, scoliosis, Ehlers-Danlos syndrome, osteogenesis imperfecta, and pseudoxanthoma elasticum. The dominant abnormal signs are auscultatory, although occasional patients may have chest pain or palpitations. The apical murmur is late systolic and may be preceded by a click, but these signs may vary in the same patient and, at times, only the click is audible. In the standing or sitting position, the click may occur earlier in systole, and the murmur may be more prominent in late systole. Arrhythmias may occur and are primarily unifocal or multifocal premature ventricular contractions.

The electrocardiogram is usually normal but may show biphasic T waves, especially in leads II, III, aVF, and V_6; the T-wave abnormalities may vary at different times in the same patient. The chest roentgenogram is normal. The echocardiogram shows a characteristic posterior movement of the posterior mitral leaflet during mid- or late systole or demonstrates pansystolic prolapse of both the anterior and posterior mitral leaflets. These echocardiographic findings must be interpreted cautiously because the appearance of minimal mitral prolapse may be a normal variant. Prolapse is more precisely defined by single or bileaflet prolapse of >2 mm beyond the long axis annular plane with or without leaflet thickening. Prolapse with valve thickening >5 mm is "classic"; a lesser degree is "nonclassic." Two-dimensional real-time echocardiography shows that both the free edge and the body of the mitral leaflets move posteriorly in systole toward the left atrium. Doppler can assess the presence and severity of mitral regurgitation.

This lesion is not progressive in childhood, and specific therapy is not indicated. Antibiotic prophylaxis is no longer recommended during surgery and dental procedures (see Chapter 437).

Adults (men more often than women) with mitral valve prolapse are at increased risk for cardiovascular complications (sudden death, arrhythmia, cerebrovascular accidents, progressive valve dilation, heart failure, and endocarditis) in the presence of **thickened** (>5 mm) and **redundant** mitral valve leaflets. Risk factors for morbidity also include poor left ventricular function, moderate to severe mitral regurgitation, and left atrial enlargement.

Often, confusion exists concerning the diagnosis of mitral valve prolapse. The high frequency of mild prolapse on the echocardiogram in the absence of clinical findings suggests that, in these cases, true mitral valve prolapse syndrome is not present. These patients and their parents should be reassured of this fact, and no special recommendations should be made regarding management or frequent laboratory studies.

Bibliography is available at Expert Consult.

428.4 Tricuspid Regurgitation
Daniel Bernstein

Isolated tricuspid regurgitation is generally associated with Ebstein anomaly of the tricuspid valve. Ebstein anomaly may occur either without cyanosis or with varying degrees of cyanosis, depending on the severity of the tricuspid regurgitation and the presence of an atrial-level communication (patent foramen ovale or atrial septal defect). Older children tend to have the acyanotic form, whereas if detected in the newborn period, Ebstein anomaly is usually associated with severe cyanosis (see Chapter 430.7).

Tricuspid regurgitation often accompanies right ventricular dysfunction. When the right ventricle becomes dilated because of volume overload or intrinsic myocardial disease, or both, the tricuspid annulus also enlarges, with resultant valve insufficiency. This form of regurgitation may improve if the cause of the right ventricular dilation is corrected, or it may require surgical plication of the valve annulus. Tricuspid regurgitation is also encountered in newborns with perinatal asphyxia. The cause may be related to an increased susceptibility of the papillary muscles to ischemic damage and subsequent transient papillary muscle dysfunction. Finally, tricuspid regurgitation is seen in up to 30% of children after heart transplantation, which can be a risk factor for graft dysfunction but is also seen as a consequence of valve injury as a result of endomyocardial biopsy.

Bibliography is available at Expert Consult.

Chapter **429**
Cyanotic Congenital Heart Disease: Evaluation of the Critically Ill Neonate with Cyanosis and Respiratory Distress

Daniel Bernstein

See also Chapter 101.

A severely ill neonate with cardiorespiratory distress and cyanosis is a diagnostic challenge. The clinician must perform a rapid evaluation to determine whether congenital heart disease is a cause so that potentially lifesaving measures can be instituted. The differential diagnosis of neonatal cyanosis is presented in Table 101-1 in Chapter 101.

CARDIAC DISEASE LEADING TO CYANOSIS

Congenital heart disease produces cyanosis when obstruction to right ventricular outflow causes intracardiac right-to-left shunting or when complex anatomic defects, many unassociated with pulmonary stenosis, cause an admixture of pulmonary and systemic venous return in the heart. Cyanosis from pulmonary edema may also develop in patients with heart failure caused by left-to-right shunts, although the degree is usually less severe. Cyanosis may be caused by persistence of fetal pathways, for example, right-to-left shunting across the foramen ovale and ductus arteriosus in the presence of pulmonary outflow tract obstruction or persistent pulmonary hypertension of the newborn (PPHN) (see Chapter 101.7).

DIFFERENTIAL DIAGNOSIS

The **hyperoxia test** is 1 method of distinguishing cyanotic congenital heart disease from pulmonary disease. Neonates with cyanotic congenital heart disease are usually not able to significantly raise their arterial PaO_2 during administration of 100% oxygen. If the PaO_2 rises above 150 mm Hg during 100% oxygen administration, an intracardiac right-to-left shunt can usually be excluded, although this is not 100% confirmative, as some patients with cyanotic congenital heart lesions may be able to increase their PaO_2 to >150 mm Hg because of favorable intracardiac streaming patterns. In patients with pulmonary disease, PaO_2 generally increases significantly with 100% oxygen as ventilation-perfusion inequalities are overcome. In infants with cyanosis from a central nervous system disorder, the PaO_2 usually normalizes completely during artificial ventilation. Hypoxia in many heart lesions is profound and constant, whereas in respiratory disorders and in PPHN, arterial oxygen tension often varies with time or changes in ventilator management. Hyperventilation may improve the hypoxia in neonates with PPHN and only occasionally in those with cyanotic congenital heart disease.

Although a significant heart murmur usually suggests a cardiac basis for the cyanosis, several of the more severe cardiac defects (transposition of the great vessels) may not initially be associated with a murmur.

The chest roentgenogram may be helpful in the differentiation of pulmonary and cardiac disease; in the latter, it indicates whether pulmonary blood flow is increased, normal, or decreased.

Two-dimensional echocardiography is the definitive noninvasive test to determine the presence of congenital heart disease. Cardiac catheterization is less often used for diagnostic purposes, and is usually performed to examine structures that are sometime less well visualized by echocardiography, such as distal branch pulmonary arteries or aortopulmonary collateral arteries in patients with tetralogy of Fallot with pulmonary atresia (see Chapter 430.2), coronary arteries and right ventricular sinusoids in patients with pulmonary atresia and intact ventricular septum (see Chapter 430.3). If echocardiography is not immediately available, the clinician caring for a newborn with possible cyanotic heart disease should not hesitate to start a prostaglandin infusion (for a possible ductal-dependent lesion). Because of the risk of hypoventilation associated with prostaglandins, a practitioner skilled in neonatal endotracheal intubation must be available.

Chapter **430**
Cyanotic Congenital Heart Lesions: Lesions Associated with Decreased Pulmonary Blood Flow

430.1 Tetralogy of Fallot
Daniel Bernstein

Tetralogy of Fallot is one of the conotruncal family of heart lesions in which the primary defect is an anterior deviation of the infundibular septum (the muscular septum that separates the aortic and pulmonary outflows). The consequences of this deviation are the 4 components: (1) obstruction to right ventricular outflow (pulmonary stenosis), (2) a malalignment type of ventricular septal defect (VSD), (3) dextroposition of the aorta so that it overrides the ventricular septum, and (4) right ventricular hypertrophy (Fig. 430-1). Obstruction to pulmonary arterial blood flow is usually at both the right ventricular infundibulum (subpulmonic area) and the pulmonary valve. The main pulmonary artery may be small, and various degrees of branch pulmonary artery stenosis may be present. Complete obstruction of right ventricular outflow (tetralogy with pulmonary atresia) is classified as an extreme form of tetralogy of Fallot (see Chapter 430.2). The degree of pulmonary outflow obstruction determines the degree of the patient's cyanosis and the age of first presentation.

PATHOPHYSIOLOGY

The pulmonary valve annulus may range from being nearly normal in size to being severely hypoplastic. The valve itself is often bicuspid or unicuspid and, occasionally, is the only site of stenosis. More commonly, the subpulmonic or infundibular muscle, known as the *crista supraventricularis,* is hypertrophic, which contributes to the subvalvar stenosis and results in an infundibular chamber of variable size and contour. When the right ventricular outflow tract is completely

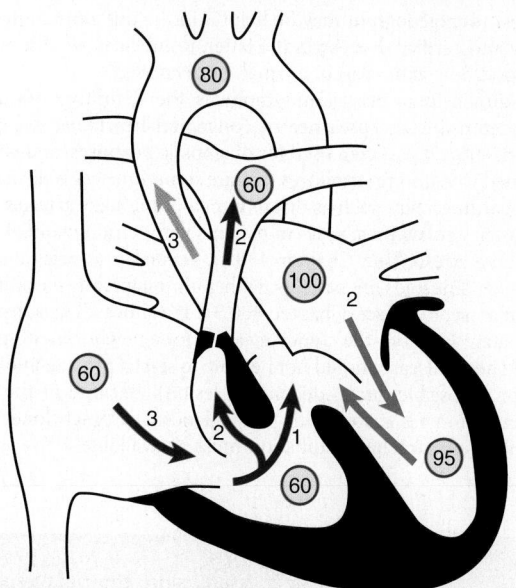

Figure 430-1 Physiology of the tetralogy of Fallot. *Circled numbers* represent oxygen saturation values. The *numbers next to the arrows* represent volumes of blood flow (in L/min/m²). Atrial (mixed venous) oxygen saturation is decreased because of the systemic hypoxemia. A volume of 3 L/min/m² of desaturated blood enters the right atrium and traverses the tricuspid valve. Two liters flows through the right ventricular outflow tract into the lungs, whereas 1 L shunts right to left through the ventricular septal defect (VSD) into the ascending aorta. Thus, pulmonary blood flow is two-thirds normal (Qp:Qs [pulmonary-to-systemic blood flow ratio] of 0.7:1). Blood returning to the left atrium is fully saturated. Only 2 L of blood flows across the mitral valve. Oxygen saturation in the left ventricle may be slightly decreased because of right-to-left shunting across the VSD. Two liters of saturated left ventricular blood mixing with 1 L of desaturated right ventricular blood is ejected into the ascending aorta. Aortic saturation is decreased, and cardiac output is normal.

obstructed **(pulmonary atresia),** the anatomy of the branch pulmonary arteries is extremely variable. A main pulmonary artery segment may be in continuity with right ventricular outflow, separated by a fibrous but imperforate pulmonary valve; the main pulmonary artery may be moderately or severely hypoplastic but still supply part or all of the pulmonary bed; or the entire main pulmonary artery segment may be absent. Occasionally, the branch pulmonary arteries may be discontinuous. Pulmonary blood flow may be supplied by a patent ductus arteriosus (PDA) or by multiple **major aortopulmonary collateral arteries (MAPCAs)** arising from the ascending and/or descending aorta and supplying various lung segments.

The VSD is usually nonrestrictive and large, is located just below the aortic valve, and is related to the posterior and right aortic cusps. Rarely, the VSD may be in the inlet portion of the ventricular septum (atrioventricular septal defect). The normal fibrous continuity of the mitral and aortic valves is usually maintained, and if not (because of the presence of a subaortic muscular conus) the classification is usually that of double-outlet right ventricle (see Chapter 430.5). The aortic arch is right sided in 20% of cases, and the aortic root is usually large and overrides the VSD to varying degrees. When the aorta overrides the VSD by more than 50% and if there is a subaortic conus, this defect is classified as a form of double-outlet right ventricle; however, the circulatory dynamics are the same as that of tetralogy of Fallot.

Systemic venous return to the right atrium and right ventricle is normal. When the right ventricle contracts in the presence of marked pulmonary stenosis, blood is shunted across the VSD into the aorta. Persistent arterial desaturation and cyanosis result, the degree dependent on the severity of the pulmonary obstruction. Pulmonary blood flow, when severely restricted by the obstruction to right ventricular outflow, may be supplemented by a PDA. Peak systolic and diastolic

pressures in each ventricle are similar and at systemic level. A large pressure gradient occurs across the obstructed right ventricular outflow tract, and pulmonary arterial pressure is either normal or lower than normal. The degree of right ventricular outflow obstruction determines the timing of the onset of symptoms, the severity of cyanosis, and the degree of right ventricular hypertrophy. When obstruction to right ventricular outflow is mild to moderate and a balanced shunt is present across the VSD, the patient may not be visibly cyanotic (**acyanotic** or "**pink**" tetralogy of Fallot). When obstruction is severe, cyanosis will be present from birth and worsen when the ductus arteriosus begins to close.

CLINICAL MANIFESTATIONS

Infants with mild degrees of right ventricular outflow obstruction may initially be seen with heart failure caused by a ventricular-level left-to-right shunt. Often, cyanosis is not present at birth; but with increasing hypertrophy of the right ventricular infundibulum as the patient grows, cyanosis occurs later in the 1st yr of life. In infants with severe degrees of right ventricular outflow obstruction, neonatal cyanosis is noted immediately. In these infants, pulmonary blood flow may be partially or nearly totally dependent on flow through the ductus arteriosus. When the ductus begins to close in the 1st few hr or days of life, severe cyanosis and circulatory collapse may occur. Older children with long-standing cyanosis who have not undergone surgery may have dusky blue skin, gray sclerae with engorged blood vessels, and marked clubbing of the fingers and toes. Chapter 434 describes the extracardiac manifestations of long-standing cyanotic congenital heart disease.

In older children with unrepaired tetralogy, dyspnea occurs on exertion. They may play actively for a short time and then sit or lie down. Older children may be able to walk a block or so before stopping to rest. Characteristically, children assume a squatting position for the relief of dyspnea caused by physical effort; the child is usually able to resume physical activity after a few minutes of squatting. These findings occur most often in patients with significant cyanosis at rest.

Paroxysmal hypercyanotic attacks (hypoxic, "**blue**," or "**tet**" spells) are a particular problem during the 1st 2 yr of life. The infant becomes hyperpneic and restless, cyanosis increases, gasping respirations ensue, and syncope may follow. The spells occur most frequently in the morning on initially awakening or after episodes of vigorous crying. Temporary disappearance or a decrease in intensity of the systolic murmur is usual as flow across the right ventricular outflow tract diminishes. The spells may last from a few minutes to a few hours. Short episodes are followed by generalized weakness and sleep. Severe spells may progress to unconsciousness and, occasionally, to convulsions or hemiparesis. The onset is usually spontaneous and unpredictable. Spells are associated with reduction of an already compromised pulmonary blood flow, which, when prolonged, results in severe systemic hypoxia and metabolic acidosis. Infants who are only mildly cyanotic at rest are often more prone to the development of hypoxic spells because they have not acquired the homeostatic mechanisms to tolerate rapid lowering of arterial oxygen saturation, such as polycythemia.

Depending on the frequency and severity of hypercyanotic attacks, 1 or more of the following procedures should be instituted in sequence: (1) placement of the infant on the abdomen in the knee-chest position while making certain that the infant's clothing is not constrictive, (2) administration of oxygen (although increasing inspired oxygen will not reverse cyanosis caused by intracardiac shunting), and (3) injection of morphine subcutaneously in a dose not in excess of 0.2 mg/kg. Calming and holding the infant in a knee-chest position may abort progression of an early spell. Premature attempts to obtain blood samples may cause further agitation and be counterproductive.

Because metabolic acidosis develops when arterial Po_2 is <40 mm Hg, rapid correction (within several minutes) with intravenous administration of sodium bicarbonate is necessary if the spell is unusually severe and the child shows a lack of response to the foregoing therapy. Recovery from the spell is usually rapid once the pH has returned to normal. Repeated blood pH measurements may be necessary because rapid recurrence of acidosis may ensue. For spells that are resistant to this therapy, intubation and sedation are often sufficient to break the spell. Drugs that increase systemic vascular resistance, such as intravenous phenylephrine, can improve right ventricular outflow, decrease the right-to-left shunt, and improve the symptoms. β-Adrenergic blockade by the intravenous administration of propranolol (0.1 mg/kg given slowly to a maximum of 0.2 mg/kg) has also been used. Growth and development may be delayed in patients with severe untreated tetralogy of Fallot, particularly when their oxygen saturation is chronically <70%. Puberty may also be delayed in patients who have not undergone surgery.

The pulse is usually normal, as are venous and arterial pressures. In older infants and children, the left anterior hemithorax may bulge anteriorly because of long-standing right ventricular hypertrophy. A substantial right ventricular impulse can usually be detected. A systolic thrill may be felt along the left sternal border in the 3rd and 4th parasternal spaces. The systolic murmur is usually loud and harsh; it may be transmitted widely, especially to the lungs, but is most intense at the left sternal border. The murmur is generally ejection in quality at the upper sternal border, but it may sound more holosystolic toward the lower sternal border. It may be preceded by a click. The murmur is caused by turbulence through the right ventricular outflow tract. It tends to become louder, longer, and harsher as the severity of pulmonary stenosis increases from mild to moderate; however, it can actually become less prominent with severe obstruction, especially during a hypercyanotic spell due to shunting of blood away from the right ventricular outflow through the aortic valve. Either the 2nd heart sound is single, or the pulmonic component is soft. Infrequently, a continuous murmur may be audible, especially if prominent collaterals are present.

DIAGNOSIS

The typical radiologic configuration as seen in the anteroposterior view consists of a narrow base, concavity of the left heart border in the area usually occupied by the pulmonary artery, and normal overall heart size. The hypertrophied right ventricle causes the rounded apical shadow to be uptilted so that it is situated higher above the diaphragm than normal and pointing horizontally to the left chest wall. The cardiac silhouette has been likened to that of a boot ("coeur en sabot") (Fig. 430-2). The hilar areas and lung fields are relatively clear because of diminished pulmonary blood flow or the small size of the pulmonary arteries, or both. The aorta is usually large, and in approximately 20% of patients it arches to the right, which results in an indentation of the leftward-positioned air-filled tracheobronchial shadow in the anteroposterior view.

The electrocardiogram demonstrates right axis deviation and evidence of right ventricular hypertrophy. A dominant R wave appears in the right precordial chest leads (Rs, R, qR, qRs) or an RSR′ pattern. In some cases, the only sign of right ventricular hypertrophy may initially be a positive T wave in leads V_3R and V_1. The P wave is tall and peaked suggesting right atrial enlargement (see Fig. 423-6 in Chapter 423).

Two-dimensional echocardiography establishes the diagnosis (Fig. 430-3) and provides information about the extent of aortic override of the septum, the location and degree of the right ventricular outflow tract obstruction, the size of the pulmonary valve annulus and main and proximal branch pulmonary arteries, and the side of the aortic arch. The echocardiogram is also useful in determining whether a PDA is supplying a portion of the pulmonary blood flow. In a patient without pulmonary atresia, echocardiography usually obviates the need for catheterization before surgical repair. However, in patients with pulmonary atresia, catheterization is necessary to image the source of blood supply to and size of each lung segment.

Cardiac catheterization demonstrates a systolic pressure in the right ventricle equal to the systemic pressure, since the right ventricle is connected directly to the overriding aorta. If the pulmonary artery is entered, the pressure is markedly decreased, although crossing the right ventricular outflow tract, especially in severe cases, may precipitate a tet spell. Pulmonary arterial pressure is usually lower than normal, in the range of 5-10 mm Hg. The level of arterial oxygen saturation depends on the magnitude of the right-to-left shunt; in "pink tets," the systemic oxygen saturation may be normal, whereas in a moderately cyanotic patient at rest, it is usually 75-85%.

Selective right ventriculography will demonstrate all of the anatomical features. Contrast medium outlines the heavily trabeculated right ventricle. The infundibular stenosis varies in length, width, contour, and distensibility (Fig. 430-4). The pulmonary valve is usually thickened, and the annulus may be small. In patients with pulmonary atresia and VSD, echocardiography alone is not adequate to assess the anatomy of the pulmonary arteries and MAPCAs. Cardiac CT is extremely helpful, and cardiac catheterization with injection into each arterial collateral is indicated. Complete and accurate information regarding the size and peripheral distribution of the main pulmonary arteries and any collateral vessels (MAPCAs) is important when evaluating these children as surgical candidates.

Aortography or coronary arteriography outlines the course of the coronary arteries. In 5-10% of patients with the tetralogy of Fallot, coronary artery abnormalities may be present, most commonly an aberrant coronary artery crossing over the right ventricular outflow

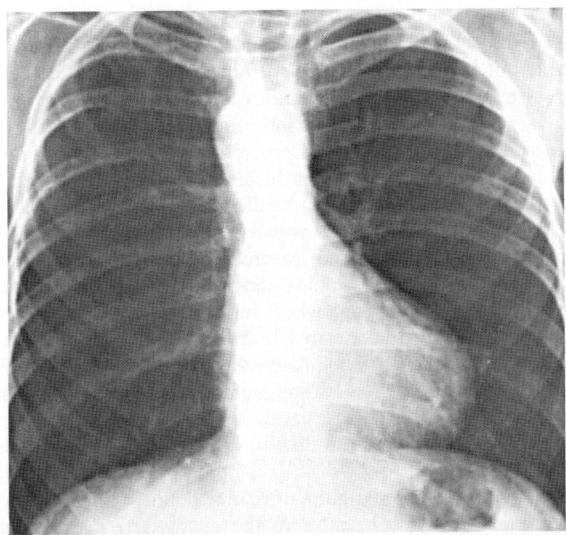

Figure 430-2 Chest x-ray of an 8 yr old boy with the tetralogy of Fallot. Note the normal heart size, some elevation of the cardiac apex, concavity in the region of the main pulmonary artery, right-sided aortic arch, and diminished pulmonary vascularity.

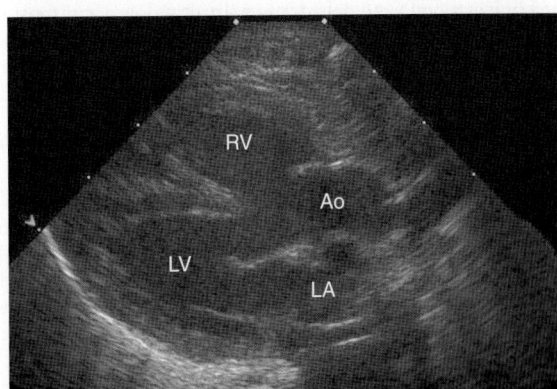

Figure 430-3 Echocardiogram in a patient with the tetralogy of Fallot. This parasternal long-axis 2-dimensional view demonstrates anterior displacement of the outflow ventricular septum that resulted in stenosis of the subpulmonic right ventricular outflow tract, overriding of the aorta, and an associated ventricular septal defect. Ao, overriding aorta; LA, left atrium; LV, left ventricle; RV, right ventricle.

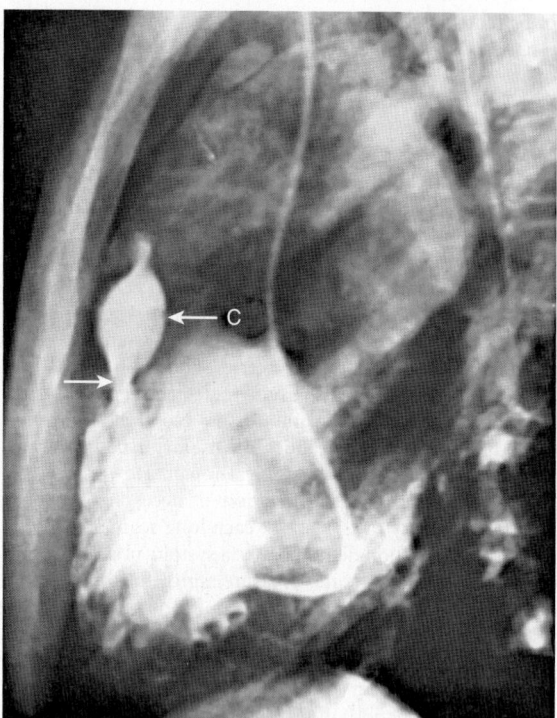

Figure 430-4 Lateral view of a selective right ventriculogram in a patient with the tetralogy of Fallot. The *arrow* points to an infundibular stenosis that is below the infundibular chamber *(C)*. The narrowed pulmonary valve orifice is seen at the distal end of the infundibular chamber.

tract; this artery must not be cut during surgical repair. Verification of normal coronary arteries is important when considering surgery in young infants who may need a patch across the pulmonary valve annulus. Echocardiography can usually delineate the coronary artery anatomy; angiography is reserved for cases in which questions remain.

COMPLICATIONS

Before the age of corrective surgery, patients with tetralogy of Fallot were susceptible to several serious complications. For this reason, most children undergo complete repair (or in some cases palliation) in the 1st few mo of life; consequently, these complications are now rare. **Cerebral thromboses,** usually occurring in the cerebral veins or dural sinuses and occasionally in the cerebral arteries, are a sequelae of extreme polycythemia and dehydration. Thromboses occur most often in patients younger than 2 yr. These patients may have iron-deficiency anemia, frequently with hemoglobin and hematocrit levels in the normal range (but too low for cyanotic heart disease). Therapy consists of adequate hydration and supportive measures. Phlebotomy and volume replacement with albumin or saline are indicated in extremely **polycythemic** patients who are symptomatic.

Brain abscess is less common than cerebral vascular events and extremely rare today. Patients with a brain abscess are usually older than 2 yr. The onset of the illness is often insidious and consists of low-grade fever or a gradual change in behavior, or both. Some patients have an acute onset of symptoms that may develop after a recent history of headache, nausea, and vomiting. Seizures may occur; localized neurologic signs depend on the site and size of the abscess and the presence of increased intracranial pressure. CT or MRI confirms the diagnosis. Antibiotic therapy may help keep the infection localized, but surgical drainage of the abscess is usually necessary (see Chapter 604).

Bacterial endocarditis may occur in the right ventricular infundibulum or on the pulmonic, aortic, or, rarely, tricuspid valves. Endocarditis may complicate palliative shunts or, in patients with corrective

surgery, any residual pulmonic stenosis or VSD. Heart failure is not a usual feature in patients with tetralogy of Fallot, with the exception of some young infants with "pink" or acyanotic tetralogy of Fallot. As the degree of pulmonary obstruction worsens with age, the symptoms of heart failure resolve and eventually the patient experiences cyanosis often by 6-12 mo of age. These patients are at increased risk for hypercyanotic spells at this time.

ASSOCIATED ANOMALIES

A PDA may be present, and defects in the atrial septum are occasionally seen. A right aortic arch occurs in ≈20% of patients, and other anomalies of the pulmonary arteries and aortic arch may also be seen. Persistence of a left superior vena cava draining into the coronary sinus is common but not a concern. Multiple VSDs are occasionally present and must be diagnosed before corrective surgery. Coronary artery anomalies are present in 5-10% and can complicate surgical repair. Tetralogy of Fallot may also occur with an atrioventricular septal defect, often associated with Down syndrome.

Congenital absence of the pulmonary valve produces a distinct syndrome that is usually marked by signs of upper airway obstruction (see Chapter 428.1). Cyanosis may be absent, mild, or moderate; the heart is large and hyperdynamic; and a loud to-and-fro murmur is present. Marked aneurysmal dilation of the main and branch pulmonary arteries results in compression of the bronchi and then produces stridulous or wheezing respirations and recurrent pneumonia. If the airway obstruction is severe, reconstruction of the trachea at the time of corrective cardiac surgery may be required to alleviate the symptoms.

Absence of a branch pulmonary artery, most often the left, should be suspected if the roentgenographic appearance of the pulmonary vasculature differs on the 2 sides; absence of a pulmonary artery is often associated with hypoplasia of the affected lung. It is important to recognize the absence of a pulmonary artery because occlusion of the remaining pulmonary artery during surgery seriously compromises the already reduced pulmonary blood flow.

As 1 of the conotruncal malformations, tetralogy of Fallot can be associated with **DiGeorge syndrome** or **Shprintzen velocardiofacial syndrome,** also known by the acronym **CATCH 22** (cardiac defects, abnormal facies, thymic hypoplasia, cleft palate, hypocalcemia). Cytogenetic analysis using fluorescence in situ hybridization demonstrates deletions of a large segment of chromosome 22q11.2 known as the *DiGeorge critical region.* Deletion or mutation of the gene encoding the transcription factor *Tbx1* has been implicated as a possible cause of DiGeorge syndrome, although several other genes have been identified as possible candidates or modifier genes.

TREATMENT

Treatment of tetralogy of Fallot depends on the severity of the right ventricular outflow tract obstruction. Infants with severe tetralogy require urgent medical treatment and surgical intervention in the neonatal period. Therapy is aimed at providing an immediate increase in pulmonary blood flow to prevent the sequelae of severe hypoxia. The infant should be transported to a medical center adequately equipped to evaluate and treat neonates with congenital heart disease under optimal conditions. Prolonged, severe hypoxia may lead to shock, respiratory failure, and intractable acidosis and will significantly reduce the chance of survival, even when surgically amenable lesions are present. It is critical that normal body temperature be maintained during the transfer because cold increases oxygen consumption, which places additional stress on a cyanotic infant, whose oxygen delivery is already limited. Blood glucose levels should be monitored because hypoglycemia is more likely to develop in infants with cyanotic heart disease.

Neonates with marked right ventricular outflow tract obstruction may deteriorate rapidly because, as the ductus arteriosus begins to close, pulmonary blood flow is further compromised. The intravenous administration of prostaglandin E_1 (0.01-0.20 µg/kg/min), a potent and specific relaxant of ductal smooth muscle, causes dilation of the ductus arteriosus and usually provides adequate pulmonary blood flow until a surgical procedure can be performed. This agent should be administered intravenously as soon as cyanotic congenital heart disease is clinically suspected and continued through the preoperative period and during cardiac catheterization. Because prostaglandin can cause apnea, an individual skilled in neonatal intubation should be readily available.

Infants with less-severe right ventricular outflow tract obstruction who are stable and awaiting surgical intervention require careful observation. Acyanotic patients can fairly quickly progress to having cyanotic episodes. Prevention or prompt treatment of dehydration is important to avoid hemoconcentration and possible thrombotic episodes. Oral propranolol (0.5-1 mg/kg every 6 hr) had been used in the past to decrease the frequency and severity of hypercyanotic spells, but with the excellent surgical results available today, surgical treatment is now indicated as soon as spells begin.

Infants with symptoms and severe cyanosis in the 1st mo of life usually have marked obstruction of the right ventricular outflow tract. Two options are available in these infants. The first is corrective open heart surgery performed in early infancy and even in the newborn period in critically ill infants. This approach has widespread acceptance today with excellent short- and long-term results and has supplanted palliative shunts (see later) for most cases. Early total repair carries the theoretical advantage that early physiologic correction allows for improved growth of the branch pulmonary arteries. In infants with less-severe cyanosis who can be maintained with good growth and absence of hypercyanotic spells, primary repair is performed electively at between 4 and 6 mo of age.

Corrective surgical therapy consists of relief of the right ventricular outflow tract obstruction by resecting obstructive muscle bundles and by patch closure of the VSD. If the pulmonary valve is stenotic, as it usually is, a valvotomy is performed. If the pulmonary valve annulus is too small or the valve is extremely thickened, a valvectomy may be performed, the pulmonary valve annulus split open, and a transannular patch placed across the pulmonary valve ring. The surgical risk of total correction in major centers is <5%. A right ventriculotomy was once the standard approach; a transatrial–transpulmonary approach is routinely performed to reduce the long-term risks of a large right ventriculotomy. In patients in whom repair has been delayed to childhood, increased bleeding in the immediate postoperative period may be a complicating factor because of their extreme polycythemia.

The second option, more common in previous years, is a palliative systemic-to-pulmonary artery shunt (**Blalock-Taussig shunt**) performed to augment pulmonary artery blood flow. The rationale for this surgery, previously the only option for these patients, is to augment pulmonary blood flow to decrease the amount of hypoxia and improve linear growth, as well as augment growth of the branch pulmonary arteries. The modified Blalock-Taussig shunt is currently the most common aortopulmonary shunt procedure and consists of a Gore-Tex conduit anastomosed side to side from the subclavian artery to the homolateral branch of the pulmonary artery (Fig. 430-5). Sometimes the shunt is brought directly from the ascending aorta to the main pulmonary artery; in this case, it is called a central shunt. Postoperative complications after a Blalock-Taussig shunt include chylothorax, diaphragmatic paralysis, and Horner syndrome. Postoperative pulmonary overcirculation leading to symptoms of cardiac failure may be caused by too large a shunt; Chapter 442 describes its treatment. Vascular problems other than a diminished radial pulse and occasional long-term arm length discrepancy are rarely seen in the upper extremity supplied by the subclavian artery used for the anastomosis.

After a successful shunt procedure, cyanosis diminishes. The development of a continuous murmur over the lung fields after the operation indicates a functioning anastomosis. A good continuous shunt murmur may not be heard until several days after surgery. The duration of symptomatic relief is variable. As the child grows, more pulmonary blood flow is needed and the shunt eventually becomes inadequate. When increasing cyanosis develops rapidly, thrombosis of the shunt should be suspected, often requiring emergent surgery.

Currently, Blalock-Taussig shunts are usually reserved for patients with comorbidities, such as other major congenital anomalies or

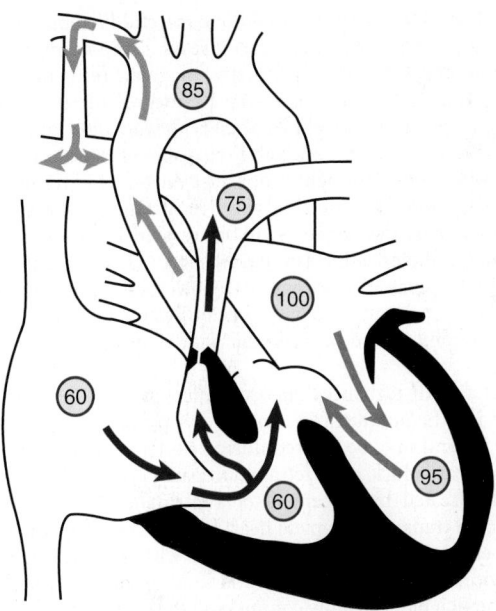

Figure 430-5 Physiology of a Blalock-Taussig shunt in a patient with tetralogy of Fallot. *Circled numbers* represent oxygen saturation values. The intracardiac shunting pattern is as described for Figure 430-1. Blood shunting left to right across the shunt from the right subclavian artery to the right pulmonary artery increases total pulmonary blood flow and results in a higher oxygen saturation than would exist without the shunt (see Fig. 430-1).

prematurity, that would make full repair a higher risk option. However, many surgeons still recommend full repair in these situations, being preferable to the combined risks of a staged procedure, and successful repairs have been done even in small premature infants.

PROGNOSIS

After successful total correction, patients are generally asymptomatic and are able to lead unrestricted lives. Uncommon immediate postoperative problems include right ventricular failure, transient heart block, residual VSD with left-to-right shunting, and myocardial infarction from interruption of an aberrant coronary artery. Postoperative heart failure (particularly in patients with a large transannular outflow patch) may require anticongestive therapy. The long-term effects of isolated, surgically induced pulmonary valvular insufficiency are still being defined as more patients with repaired tetralogy of Fallot reach middle age, but insufficiency is generally well-tolerated through adolescence. Many patients after tetralogy repair and all of those with transannular patch repairs have a to-and-fro murmur at the left sternal border, usually indicative of mild outflow obstruction and mild to moderate pulmonary insufficiency. Patients with more marked pulmonary valve insufficiency may also have moderate to more severe degrees of right ventricular enlargement and may develop tricuspid regurgitation as the tricuspid valve annulus dilates. These patients will develop a holosystolic murmur at the lower left sternal border. Patients with a severe residual gradient across the right ventricular outflow tract may require reoperation, but mild to moderate degrees of residual obstruction usually do not require reintervention.

Follow-up of patients 5-20 yr after surgery indicates that the marked improvement in symptoms is generally maintained. Asymptomatic patients nonetheless have lower than normal exercise capacity, maximal heart rate, and cardiac output. These abnormal findings are more common in patients who underwent placement of a transannular outflow tract patch and may be less frequent when surgery is performed at an early age. As these children move into adolescence and adulthood, some (more commonly those with transannular patches) will develop right ventricular dilation as a result of severe pulmonary

2216 Part XX ◆ The Cardiovascular System

regurgitation. After reaching adulthood, careful lifelong follow-up by a specialist in adult congenital heart disease is important. Serial echocardiography and the more quantitative magnetic resonance angiography are valuable tools for assessing the degree of right ventricular dilation, the presence of right ventricular dysfunction, and for quantifying the regurgitant fraction. Valve replacement is indicated for those patients with increasing right ventricular dilation and tricuspid regurgitation. For patients requiring valve replacement, new nonsurgical options are being developed. Stent valves, which can be delivered in the cardiac catheterization lab, have been used successfully in many patients with repaired tetralogy of Fallot. These are being used predominantly in patients who have previously had a homograft or other artificial conduit placed between the right ventricular and pulmonary arteries.

Conduction disturbances can occur after surgery. The atrioventricular node and the bundle of His and its divisions are in close proximity to the VSD and may be injured during surgery; however, permanent complete heart block after tetralogy repair is rare. When present, it should be treated by placement of a permanently implanted pacemaker. Even transient complete heart block in the immediate postoperative period is rare; it may be associated with an increased incidence of late-onset complete heart block and sudden death. In contrast, right bundle-branch block is quite common on the postoperative electrocardiogram. The duration of the QRS interval has been shown to predict both the presence of residual hemodynamic derangement and the long-term risk of arrhythmia and sudden death. Research is ongoing to determine the effectiveness of biventricular pacing (in which a pacemaker is used to resynchronize the activation of the right and left ventricles) in improving hemodynamics in those patients with long ventricular conduction delays.

A number of children have premature ventricular beats after repair of the tetralogy of Fallot. These beats are of concern in patients with residual hemodynamic abnormalities; 24 hr electrocardiographic (Holter) monitoring studies should be performed to be certain that occult short episodes of ventricular tachycardia are not occurring. Exercise studies may be useful in provoking cardiac arrhythmias that are not apparent at rest. In the presence of complex ventricular arrhythmias or severe residual hemodynamic abnormalities, prophylactic antiarrhythmic therapy, catheter ablation, or implantation of an implantable defibrillator is warranted. Rerepair is indicated if significant residual right ventricular outflow obstruction or severe pulmonary insufficiency is present because arrhythmias may improve after hemodynamics is restored to a more normal level.

Bibliography is available at Expert Consult.

430.2 Tetralogy of Fallot with Pulmonary Atresia
Daniel Bernstein

PATHOPHYSIOLOGY

Tetralogy of a Fallot with pulmonary atresia is the most extreme form of the tetralogy of Fallot. The pulmonary valve is atretic (absent), and the pulmonary trunk may be hypoplastic or atretic as well. The entire right ventricular output is ejected into the aorta. Pulmonary blood flow is then dependent on collateral vessels or MAPCAs, or, rarely, on a PDA. The ultimate prognosis depends on the degree of development of the branch pulmonary arteries, which needs to be assessed by cardiac catheterization. If the pulmonary arteries are severely hypoplastic and fail to grow after palliative shunt procedures, heart-lung transplantation may be the only therapy (see Chapter 443.2). Pulmonary atresia with VSD is also associated with the 22q11.2 deletion and DiGeorge syndrome. The association of severe **tracheomalacia** or **bronchomalacia** with these severe forms of tetralogy/pulmonary atresia may complicate postoperative recovery.

CLINICAL MANIFESTATIONS

Patients with pulmonary atresia and VSD have findings similar to those in patients with severe tetralogy of Fallot. Cyanosis usually appears within the 1st few hr or days after birth; however, the prominent systolic murmur associated with the tetralogy is usually absent. The 1st heart sound may be followed by an ejection click caused by the enlarged aortic root, the 2nd heart sound is single and loud, and continuous murmurs of collateral flow may be heard over the entire precordium, both anteriorly and posteriorly. Most patients are moderately cyanotic and are initially stabilized with a prostaglandin E_1 infusion pending cardiac catheterization or CT scan to further delineate the anatomy. Patients with several large MAPCAs may be less cyanotic and, once the diagnosis is confirmed, can be taken off prostaglandin while awaiting palliative surgical intervention. Some patients may even develop symptoms of heart failure caused by increased pulmonary blood flow via these collateral vessels.

DIAGNOSIS

The chest roentgenogram demonstrates a varying heart size, depending on the amount of pulmonary blood flow, a concavity at the position of the pulmonary arterial segment, and often the reticular pattern of bronchial collateral flow. The electrocardiogram shows right ventricular hypertrophy. The echocardiogram identifies aortic override, a thick right ventricular wall, and atresia of the pulmonary valve. Pulsed and color Doppler echocardiographic studies show an absence of forward flow through the pulmonary valve, with pulmonary blood flow being supplied by MAPCAs, which can usually be seen arising from the descending aorta. At cardiac catheterization, right ventriculography reveals a large aorta, opacified immediately by passage of contrast medium through the VSD, but with no dye entering the lungs through the right ventricular outflow tract. Careful delineation of the native pulmonary arteries, if present, to determine whether they are continuous or discontinuous and whether they arborize to all lung segments is important in planning surgical repair. The location and arborization of all MAPCAs and the presence of any localized stenosis are determined by selective contrast injection. CT angiography has recently been utilized to assist in mapping the extent of MAPCA arborization.

TREATMENT

The surgical procedure of choice depends on whether the main pulmonary artery segment is present and, if so, on the size and branching pattern of the branch pulmonary arteries. If these arteries are well developed, a one-stage surgical repair with a homograft conduit between the right ventricle and pulmonary arteries and closure of the VSD is feasible. If the pulmonary arteries are hypoplastic, extensive reconstruction may be required. This usually involves several staged surgical procedures. If the native pulmonary artery is present but small, a connection made between the aorta and the hypoplastic native pulmonary artery (aortopulmonary window) in the newborn period induces growth. At 3-4 mo of age, the multiple MAPCAs are gathered together (unifocalization procedure) and eventually incorporated into the final repair along with the native pulmonary arteries. This may be accomplished through successive lateral thoracotomies, or through a single midline sternotomy if the anatomy is more favorable.

To be a candidate for full repair, the pulmonary arteries must be of adequate size to accept the full volume of right ventricular output. Complete repair includes closure of the VSD and placement of a homograft conduit from the right ventricle to the pulmonary artery. At the time of reparative surgery, previous shunts are taken down. Because of patient growth as well as homograft narrowing due to proliferation of intimal tissue and calcification, replacement of the homograft conduit replacement is usually required in later life, and multiple replacements may be needed. Many of these patients are candidates for placement of a transcatheter stent valve in the pulmonary position. Patients with obstruction of the very distal branches of the pulmonary arteries may undergo repeat surgical procedures or transcatheter balloon dilation of the multiple branch pulmonary arterial stenosis. Careful follow-up is warranted for these patients to ensure maximal chance of growth of all pulmonary artery segments.

Bibliography is available at Expert Consult.

430.3 Pulmonary Atresia with Intact Ventricular Septum
Daniel Bernstein

PATHOPHYSIOLOGY
In pulmonary atresia with an intact ventricular septum, the pulmonary valve leaflets are completely fused to form a membrane and the right ventricular outflow tract is atretic. Because no VSD is present, no egress of blood from the right ventricle can occur. Any blood that enters the right ventricle will regurgitate back across the tricuspid valve into the right atrium. Right atrial pressure increases, and blood shunts via the foramen ovale into the left atrium, where it mixes with pulmonary venous blood and enters the left ventricle (Fig. 430-6). The combined left and right ventricular output is pumped solely by the left ventricle into the aorta. In a newborn with pulmonary atresia, the only source of pulmonary blood flow occurs via a **PDA.** The right ventricle and tricuspid valve are usually hypoplastic, although the degree of hypoplasia varies considerably. Patients who have a small right ventricular cavity also tend to be those with the smallest tricuspid valve annulus, which limits right ventricular inflow. Patients with pulmonary atresia and intact ventricular septum may have **coronary sinusoidal channels** within the right ventricular wall that communicate directly with the coronary arterial circulation. The high right ventricular

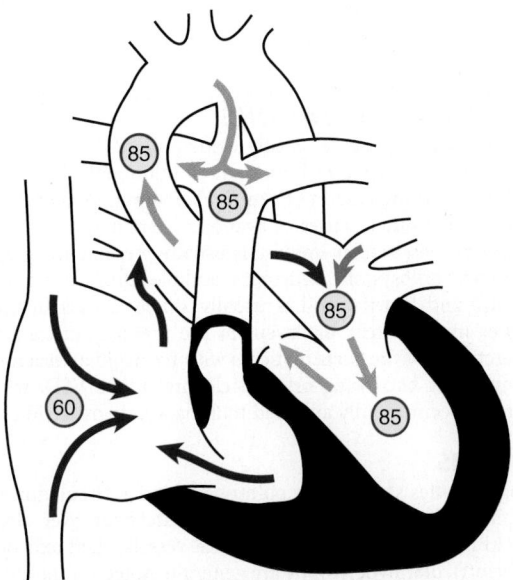

Figure 430-6 Physiology of pulmonary atresia with an intact ventricular septum. *Circled numbers* represent oxygen saturation values. Right atrial (mixed venous) oxygen saturation is decreased secondary to systemic hypoxemia. A small amount of the blood entering the right atrium may cross the tricuspid valve, which is often stenotic as well. The right ventricular cavity is hypertrophied and may be hypoplastic. No outlet from the right ventricle exists because of the atretic pulmonary valve; thus, any blood entering the right ventricle returns to the right atrium via tricuspid regurgitation. Most of the desaturated blood shunts right to left via the foramen ovale into the left atrium, where it mixes with fully saturated blood returning from the lungs. The only source of pulmonary blood flow is via the patent ductus arteriosus. Aortic and pulmonary arterial oxygen saturation will be identical (definition of a total mixing lesion).

pressure results in desaturated blood flowing retrograde via these channels into the coronary arteries. Sometimes there are also stenoses of the coronary arteries proximal to where the sinusoids enter, so that distal coronary artery flow is dependent on flow from the right ventricle (known as *right ventricle–dependent coronary circulation*). The prognosis in patients with these sinusoids and proximal stenosis of the coronary arteries is more guarded than in those patients without sinusoids or with sinusoids but no coronary stenoses. Rarely, the proximal coronary artery may be totally absent.

CLINICAL MANIFESTATIONS
As the ductus arteriosus closes in the 1st hr and days of life, infants with pulmonary atresia and an intact ventricular septum become markedly cyanotic because their only source of pulmonary blood flow is removed. Untreated, most patients die within the 1st wk of life. Physical examination reveals severe cyanosis and respiratory distress. The 2nd heart sound, representing only aortic closure, is single and loud. Often, no murmurs are audible; sometimes a systolic or continuous murmur can be heard secondary to ductal blood flow. A harsh holosystolic murmur may be heard at the lower left sternal border if there is significant tricuspid regurgitation.

DIAGNOSIS
The electrocardiogram shows a frontal QRS axis between 0 and +90 degrees, the amount of leftward shift reflecting the degree of hypoplasia of the right ventricle. Tall, spiked P waves indicate right atrial enlargement. QRS voltages are consistent with left ventricular dominance or hypertrophy; right ventricular forces are decreased in proportion to the decreased size of the right ventricular cavity. Most patients with small right ventricles have decreased right ventricular forces, but, occasionally, patients with larger, thickened right ventricular cavities may have evidence of right ventricular hypertrophy. The chest roentgenogram shows decreased pulmonary vascularity, the degree depending on the size of the branch pulmonary arteries and the patency of the ductus. Unlike in patients with pulmonary atresia and tetralogy of Fallot, the presence of major collateral vessels (MAPCAs) is rare.

The 2-dimensional echocardiogram is useful in estimating right ventricular dimensions and the size of the tricuspid valve annulus, which have been shown to be of prognostic value. Echocardiography can often suggest the presence of sinusoidal channels but cannot be used to evaluate coronary stenoses. Thus, cardiac catheterization is necessary for complete evaluation. Pressure measurements reveal right atrial and right ventricular hypertension. Ventriculography demonstrates the size of the right ventricular cavity, the atretic right ventricular outflow tract, the degree of tricuspid regurgitation, and the presence or absence of intramyocardial sinusoids filling the coronary vessels. Aortography shows filling of the pulmonary arteries via the PDA and is helpful in determining the size and branching patterns of the pulmonary arterial bed. An aortogram, or if necessary selective coronary angiography is performed to evaluate for the presence of proximal coronary artery stenosis (right ventricular dependent coronary circulation).

TREATMENT
Infusion of prostaglandin E$_1$ (0.01-0.20 μg/kg/min) is usually effective in keeping the ductus arteriosus open before intervention, thus reducing hypoxemia and acidemia before surgery. The choice of surgical procedure depends on whether there is an RV dependent coronary circulation and on the size of the right ventricular cavity. In patients with only mild to moderate right ventricular hypoplasia without sinusoids, or in patients with sinusoids but no evidence of coronary stenoses, a surgical pulmonary valvotomy is carried out to relieve outflow obstruction. Often, the right ventricular outflow tract is widened with a patch. To preserve adequate pulmonary blood flow, an aortopulmonary shunt may also be performed during the same procedure. An alternative approach uses interventional catheterization, in which the imperforate pulmonary valve is first punctured either with a wire or a radiofrequency ablation catheter, followed by a balloon valvuloplasty.

If this course is taken, it may take days to weeks before the right ventricular muscle regresses enough for the patient to be weaned from prostaglandin, and many of these patients will still require surgical intervention. The aim of surgery or interventional catheterization is to encourage growth of the right ventricular chamber by allowing some forward flow through the pulmonary valve while using the shunt to ensure adequate pulmonary blood flow. Later, if the tricuspid valve annulus and right ventricular chamber grow to adequate size, the shunt is taken down and any remaining atrial level shunt can be closed. If the right ventricular chamber remains too small for use as a pulmonary ventricle, then the patient is treated as a single ventricle circulation, with a **Glenn procedure** followed by a modified **Fontan procedure** (see Chapter 430.4), allowing blood to bypass the hypoplastic right ventricle by flowing to the pulmonary arteries directly from the venae cavae. When coronary artery stenoses are present and retrograde coronary perfusion occurs from the right ventricle via myocardial sinusoids, the prognosis is more guarded because of a higher risk of arrhythmias, coronary ischemia, and sudden death. It is important for these patients not to try to open the right ventricular outflow tract, as dropping the right ventricular pressure will reduce coronary perfusion, leading to ischemia. These patients are usually treated with an aortopulmonary shunt, followed by the Glenn and Fontan procedure. Although at higher risk than those without coronary stenoses, recent reports show good success with this approach. A small number of these infants, especially those with total atresia of a proximal coronary artery, are referred instead for heart transplantation.

Bibliography is available at Expert Consult.

430.4 Tricuspid Atresia
Daniel Bernstein

PATHOPHYSIOLOGY

In tricuspid atresia, no outlet from the right atrium to the right ventricle is present; the entire systemic venous return leaves the right atrium and enters the left side of the heart by means of the foramen ovale or, most often, through an atrial septal defect (Fig. 430-7). The physiology of the circulation and the clinical presentation will depend on the presence of other congenital heart defects, most notably on whether the great vessels are normally related or are transposed (aorta arising from the right ventricle, pulmonary artery from the left ventricle). In patients with normally related great vessels, left ventricular blood supplies the systemic circulation via the aorta. Blood also usually flows into the right ventricle via a VSD (if the ventricular septum is intact, the right ventricle will be completely hypoplastic and pulmonary atresia will be present [see Chapter 430.3]). *Pulmonary blood flow (and thus the degree of cyanosis) depends on the size of the VSD and the presence and severity of any associated pulmonic stenosis.* Pulmonary blood flow may be augmented by or be totally dependent on a PDA. The inflow portion of the right ventricle is always missing in these patients, but the outflow portion is of variable size. The clinical presentation of patients with tricuspid atresia and normally related great vessels will depend on the degree of pulmonary obstruction. Patients with at least moderate degrees of pulmonary stenosis are recognized in the early days or weeks of life by decreased pulmonary blood flow and cyanosis. Alternatively, in those with a large VSD and minimal or no right ventricular outflow obstruction, pulmonary blood flow may be high; these patients have only mild cyanosis and present with signs of pulmonary overcirculation and heart failure.

In patients with tricuspid atresia and transposition of the great arteries, left ventricular blood flows directly into the pulmonary artery, whereas systemic blood must traverse the VSD and right ventricle to reach the aorta. In these patients, pulmonary blood flow is usually massively increased and heart failure develops early. If the VSD is restrictive, aortic blood flow may be compromised. Coarctation of the aorta is not uncommon in this setting.

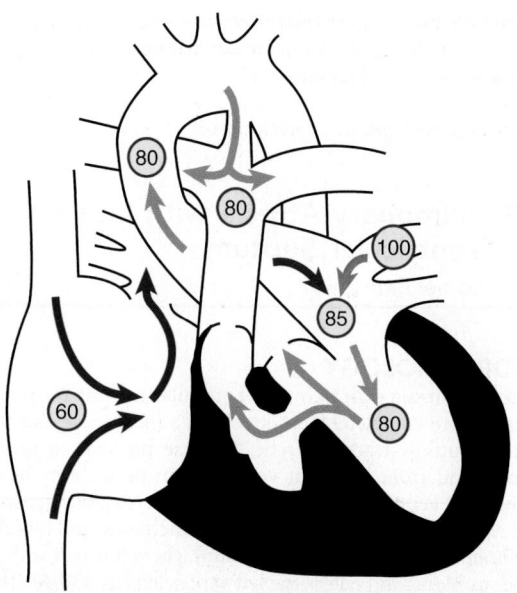

Figure 430-7 Physiology of tricuspid atresia with normally related great vessels. *Circled numbers* represent oxygen saturation values. Right atrial (mixed venous) oxygen saturation is decreased secondary to systemic hypoxemia. The tricuspid valve is nonpatent, and the right ventricle may manifest varying degrees of hypoplasia. The only outlet from the right atrium involves shunting right to left across an atrial septal defect or patent foramen ovale to the left atrium. There, desaturated blood mixes with saturated pulmonary venous return. Blood enters the left ventricle and is ejected either through the aorta or via a ventricular septal defect (VSD) into the right ventricle. In this example, some pulmonary blood flow is derived from the right ventricle, the rest from a patent ductus arteriosus (PDA). In patients with tricuspid atresia, the PDA may close or the VSD may grow smaller and result in a marked decrease in systemic oxygen saturation.

CLINICAL MANIFESTATIONS

Some degree of cyanosis is usually evident at birth, with the extent depending on the degree of limitation to pulmonary blood flow (as noted above). An increased left ventricular impulse may be noted, in contrast to most other causes of cyanotic heart disease, in which an increased right ventricular impulse is usually present. The majority of patients have holosystolic murmurs audible along the left sternal border; the 2nd heart sound is usually single. Pulses in the lower extremities may be weak or absent in the presence of transposition with coarctation of the aorta. Patients with tricuspid atresia are at risk for spontaneous narrowing or even closure of the VSD, which can occasionally occur rapidly and lead to a marked increase in cyanosis.

DIAGNOSIS

Radiologic studies show either pulmonary under circulation (usually in patients with normally related great vessels) or over circulation (usually in patients with transposed great vessels). Left axis deviation and left ventricular hypertrophy are generally noted on the electrocardiogram (except in those patients with transposition of the great arteries), and these features distinguish tricuspid atresia from most other cyanotic heart lesions. Thus the combination of cyanosis and left axis deviation on the electrocardiogram is highly suggestive of tricuspid atresia. In the right precordial leads, the normally prominent R wave is replaced by an rS complex. The left precordial leads show a qR complex, followed by a normal, flat, biphasic, or inverted T wave. RV_6 is normal or tall, and SV_1 is generally deep. The P waves are usually biphasic, with the initial component tall and spiked in lead II. Two-dimensional echocardiography reveals the presence of a fibromuscular membrane in place of a tricuspid valve, a variably small right ventricle, VSD, and the large left ventricle (Fig. 430-8). The relationship of the great vessels (normal or transposed) can be determined. The degree of obstruction at the level of the VSD or at the right ventricular outflow tract can be determined by Doppler examination. Blood flow through a patent ductus can be evaluated by color flow and pulsed Doppler.

Cardiac catheterization, indicated usually only if questions remain after echocardiography, shows normal or slightly elevated right atrial pressure with a prominent *a* wave. If the right ventricle is entered through the VSD, the pressure may be lower than on the left if the VSD is restrictive in size. Right atrial angiography shows immediate opacification of the left atrium from the right atrium followed by left ventricular filling and visualization of the aorta. Absence of direct flow to the right ventricle results in an angiographic filling defect between the right atrium and the left ventricle.

TREATMENT
Management of patients with tricuspid atresia depends on the adequacy of pulmonary blood flow. Severely cyanotic neonates should be

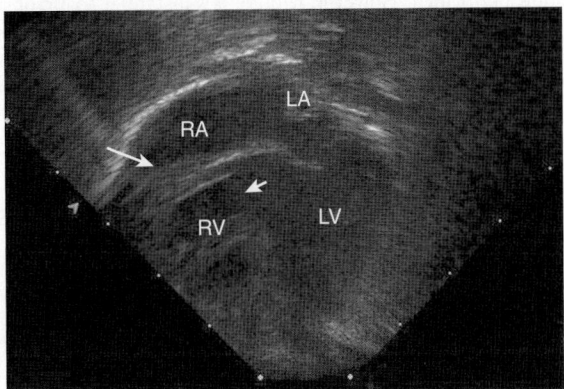

Figure 430-8 Echocardiogram demonstrating tricuspid atresia. The floor of the right atrium consists of a fibromuscular membrane *(large arrow)* instead of the normal tricuspid valve apparatus. The large secundum atrial septal defect can be seen between the right and left atria. The *small arrow* shows the ventricular septal defect. LA, left atrium; LV, left ventricle; RA, right atrium; RV, right ventricle.

maintained on an intravenous infusion of prostaglandin E_1 (0.01-0.20 µg/kg/min) until a surgical aortopulmonary shunt procedure can be performed to increase pulmonary blood flow. The Blalock-Taussig procedure (see Chapter 430.1) or a variation is the preferred anastomosis. Rare patients with restrictive atrial-level communications also benefit from a Rashkind balloon atrial septostomy (see Chapter 431.2) or surgical septectomy.

Infants with increased pulmonary blood flow because of an unobstructed pulmonary outflow tract (more often patients with aortopulmonary transposition) may require pulmonary arterial banding to decrease the symptoms of heart failure and protect the pulmonary bed from the development of pulmonary vascular disease. Infants with just adequate pulmonary blood flow who are well balanced between cyanosis and pulmonary overcirculation can be watched closely for the development of increasing cyanosis, which may occur as the VSD begins to get smaller or the pulmonary outflow becomes narrower and is an indication for surgery.

The next stage of palliation for patients with tricuspid atresia involves the creation of an anastomosis between the superior vena cava and the pulmonary arteries (**bidirectional Glenn shunt;** Fig. 430-9A). This procedure is performed at usually between 3 and 6 mo of age. The benefit of the Glenn shunt is that it reduces the volume load on the left ventricle and may lessen the chance of left ventricular dysfunction developing later in life.

The **modified Fontan operation** is the preferred approach to later surgical management. It is usually performed between 1.5 and 3 yr of age, usually after the patient is ambulatory. Initially, this procedure was performed by anastomosing the right atrium or atrial appendage directly to the pulmonary artery. The most commonly used procedure today is a modification of the Fontan procedure, known as a *cavopulmonary isolation procedure*, which involves anastomosing the inferior vena cava to the pulmonary arteries, either via a baffle that runs along the lateral wall of the right atrium (lateral tunnel Fontan; see Fig. 430-9B) or via a homograft or Gore-Tex tube running outside the heart (external conduit Fontan). The advantage of these later approaches is that blood flows by a more direct route into the pulmonary arteries, thereby decreasing the possibility of right atrial dilation and markedly reducing the incidence of postoperative pleural effusions, which were

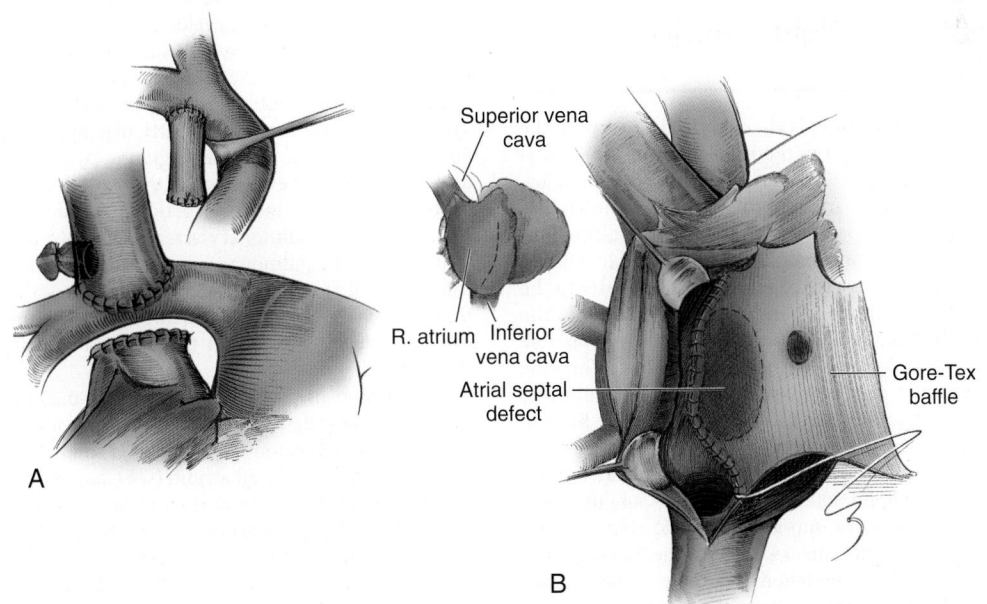

Superior vena cava

R. atrium   Inferior vena cava

Atrial septal defect

Gore-Tex baffle

A

B

Figure 430-9 A, Bidirectional Glenn shunt showing the superior vena cava–right pulmonary anastomosis. **B,** A modified Fontan procedure (cavopulmonary isolation) is completed with placement of a baffle to convey inferior vena cava blood along the lateral wall of the right atrium to the superior vena cava orifice. A 4-mm fenestration is sometimes made on the medial aspect of the polytetrafluoroethylene baffle. *(From Castañeda AR, Jonas RA, Mayer JE Jr, et al: Single-ventricle tricuspid atresia. In Cardiac surgery of the neonate and infant, Philadelphia, 1994, WB Saunders.)*

common with the earlier method. In a completed Fontan repair, desaturated blood flows from both venae cavae directly into the pulmonary arteries. Oxygenated blood returns to the left atrium, enters the left ventricle, and is ejected into the systemic circulation. The volume load is completely removed from the left ventricle, and the right-to-left shunt is abolished. Because of the reliance on passive filling of the pulmonary circulation, the Fontan procedure is contraindicated in patients with elevated pulmonary vascular resistance, in those with pulmonary artery hypoplasia, and in patients with left ventricular dysfunction. The patient must also not have significant mitral insufficiency. Patients who are not in normal sinus rhythm are at increased risk and if a pacemaker is required in these patients, dual chamber pacing is the preferred approach.

Postoperative problems after the Fontan procedure include marked elevation of systemic venous pressure, fluid retention, and pleural or pericardial effusions. In the past, pleural effusions were a problem in 30-40% of patients using the standard Fontan procedure, but the cavopulmonary isolation procedure now in use reduces this risk to approximately 5%. Some centers use a fenestration at the time of the Fontan, consisting of a small communication between the inferior vena cava and the pulmonary artery conduit and the left atrium. This serves as a "pop-off" during early postoperative recovery and may hasten hospital discharge. The fenestration will result in some amount of right-to-left shunting, and is therefore usually closed with a catheter closure device after the immediate postoperative period.

Late complications of the Fontan procedure include baffle obstruction causing superior or inferior vena cava syndrome, vena cava or pulmonary artery thromboembolism, protein-losing enteropathy, plastic bronchitis, supraventricular arrhythmias (atrial flutter, paroxysmal atrial tachycardia), and hepatic cirrhosis (and possibly hepatic carcinoma) as a result of persistently elevated central venous pressures. Oral budesonide or sildenafil has been used with varying success to treat protein losing enteropathy associated with the Fontan procedure. Left ventricular dysfunction may be a late occurrence, usually not until adolescence or young adulthood. Heart transplantation is a successful treatment option for pediatric patients with "failed" Fontan circuits but is a somewhat riskier procedure in adults.

Bibliography is available at Expert Consult.

430.5 Double-Outlet Right Ventricle

Daniel Bernstein

Double-outlet right ventricle (DORV) is characterized when both the aorta and pulmonary artery arise from the right ventricle. The outlet from the left ventricle is through VSD into the right ventricle. Normally, the aortic and mitral valves are in fibrous continuity; in DORV, the aortic and mitral valves are separated by a smooth muscular conus, similar to that seen under the normal pulmonary valve. In DORV, the great arteries may be normally related, with the aorta closer to the VSD, or malposed, with the pulmonary artery closer to the VSD. The great artery closest to the VSD may override the defect by a variable amount but is at least 50% committed to the right ventricle. When the VSD is subaortic, the defect may be viewed as part of a continuum with the tetralogy of Fallot, and the physiology as well as the history, physical examination, electrocardiogram, and roentgenograms are depending on the degree of pulmonary stenosis, similar to the situation in tetralogy of Fallot (see Chapter 430.1). If the VSD is subpulmonic, there may be subvalvar, valvar, or supravalvar aortic stenosis, and coarctation is a possibility as well. This is known as the **Taussig-Bing malformation.** The clinical presentation of these patients will be dependent on the degree of aortic obstruction, but because the pulmonary artery is usually wide open, the presentation will usually include some degree of pulmonary overcirculation and heart failure. If the aortic obstruction is severe or there is a coarctation, poor pulses, hypoperfusion, and cardiovascular collapse are possible presenting signs.

The 2-dimensional echocardiogram demonstrates both great vessels arising from the right ventricle and mitral-aortic valve discontinuity. The relationships between the aorta and pulmonary artery to the VSD can be delineated, and the presence of either pulmonary obstruction or aortic obstruction can be evaluated. Cardiac catheterization is not necessarily required if the echocardiogram is straightforward. Angiography will show that the aortic and pulmonary valves lie in the same horizontal plane and that both arise predominantly or exclusively from the right ventricle.

Surgical correction depends on the relationship of the great vessels to the VSD. If the VSD is subaortic, the repair may be similar to that used for tetralogy of Fallot, or consist of creating an intraventricular tunnel so that the left ventricle ejects blood through the VSD, into the tunnel, and into the aorta. The pulmonary obstruction is relieved either with an outflow patch or with a right ventricular to pulmonary artery homograft conduit (**Rastelli operation**). If the VSD is subpulmonic, the great vessels can be switched (see Chapter 430.6) and the Rastelli operation performed. However, if there is substantial aortic obstruction, or if 1 of the ventricles is hypoplastic, then a Norwood-style single-ventricle repair may be necessary (see Chapter 431.10). In small infants, palliation with an aortopulmonary shunt provides symptomatic improvement and allows for adequate growth before corrective surgery is performed.

430.6 Transposition of the Great Arteries with Ventricular Septal Defect and Pulmonary Stenosis

Daniel Bernstein

This combination of anomalies may mimic tetralogy of Fallot in its clinical features (see Chapter 430.1). However, because of the transposed great vessels, the site of obstruction is in the left as opposed to the right ventricle. The obstruction can be either valvular or subvalvular; the latter type may be dynamic, related to the interventricular septum or atrioventricular valve tissue, or acquired, as in patients with transposition and VSD after pulmonary arterial banding.

The age at which clinical manifestations initially appear varies from soon after birth to later infancy, depending on the degree of pulmonic stenosis. Clinical findings include cyanosis, decreased exercise tolerance, and poor physical development, similar to those described for tetralogy of Fallot; the heart is usually more enlarged. The pulmonary vasculature as seen on the roentgenogram is dependent on the degree of pulmonary obstruction. The electrocardiogram usually shows right axis deviation, right and left ventricular hypertrophy, and sometimes tall, spiked P waves. Echocardiography confirms the diagnosis and is useful in sequential evaluation of the degree and progression of the left ventricular outflow tract obstruction. Cardiac catheterization, if necessary, shows that pulmonary arterial pressure is low and that oxygen saturation in the pulmonary artery exceeds that in the aorta. Selective right and left ventriculography demonstrates the origin of the aorta from the right ventricle, the origin of the pulmonary artery from the left ventricle, the VSD, and the site and severity of the pulmonary stenosis.

An infusion of prostaglandin E_1 (0.01-0.20 µg/kg/min) should be started in neonates who present with cyanosis. When necessary, balloon atrial septostomy is performed to improve atrial-level mixing and to decompress the left atrium (see Chapter 431.2). Cyanotic infants may be palliated with an aortopulmonary shunt (see Chapter 430.1) followed by a Rastelli operation when older as the preferred corrective procedure. The Rastelli procedure achieves physiologic and anatomic correction by (1) closure of the VSD using an interventricular tunnel so that left ventricular blood flow is directed to the aorta, and (2) connection of the right ventricle to the pulmonary artery via an extracardiac homograft conduit between the right ventricle and the distal pulmonary artery (Fig. 430-10). These conduits will eventually become stenotic or functionally restrictive with growth of the patient and require replacement. Patients with milder degrees of pulmonary

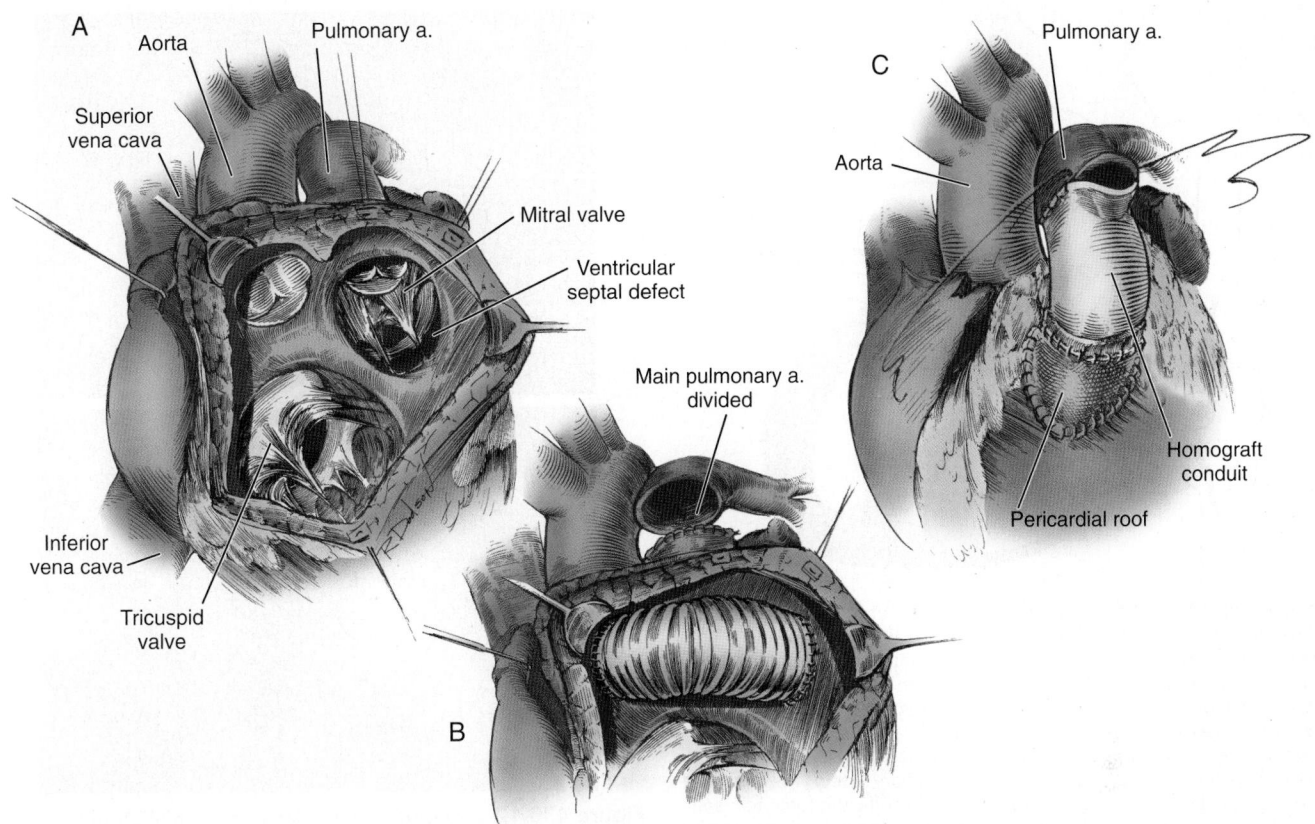

Figure 430-10 A, Taussig-Bing type of double-outlet right ventricle with subpulmonary stenosis necessitating repair by the Rastelli technique. **B,** The main pulmonary artery is divided and oversewn proximally. The pulmonary valve lies within the baffle pathway. **C,** Completion of the Rastelli repair with a right ventricle-pulmonary artery allograft conduit. *(From Castañeda AR, Jonas RA, Mayer JE Jr, et al: Single-ventricle tricuspid atresia. In Cardiac surgery of the neonate and infant, Philadelphia, 1994, WB Saunders.)*

stenosis amenable to simple valvotomy may be able to undergo complete correction with an arterial switch procedure (see Chapter 431.2) and closure of the VSD. Surgical correction by the Mustard operation (see Chapter 431.2) with simultaneous closure of the VSD and relief of left ventricular outflow obstruction may be an alternative when the position of the VSD is not suitable for a Rastelli operation; however, this procedure leaves the right ventricle as the systemic pumping chamber and has fallen out of favor.

430.7 Ebstein Anomaly of the Tricuspid Valve

Daniel Bernstein

PATHOPHYSIOLOGY

Ebstein anomaly consists of downward displacement of an abnormal tricuspid valve into the right ventricle. The defect arises from failure of the normal process by which the tricuspid valve is separated from the right ventricular myocardium (see Chapter 420). The anterior cusp of the valve retains some attachment to the valve ring, but the other leaflets are adherent to the wall of the right ventricle. The right ventricle is thus divided into 2 parts by the abnormal tricuspid valve: the first, a thin-walled "atrialized" portion, is continuous with the cavity of the right atrium; the second, often smaller portion consists of normal ventricular myocardium. The right atrium is enlarged as a result of tricuspid valve regurgitation, although the degree is extremely variable. In more severe forms of Ebstein anomaly, the effective output from the right side of the heart is decreased because of a combination of the poorly functioning small right ventricle, tricuspid valve regurgitation,

and obstruction of the right ventricular outflow tract produced by the large, sail-like, anterior tricuspid valve leaflet. In newborns, right ventricular function may be so compromised that it is unable to generate enough force to open the pulmonary valve in systole, thus producing "functional" pulmonary atresia. Some infants have true anatomic pulmonary atresia. The increased volume of right atrial blood shunts through the foramen ovale (or through an associated atrial septal defect) to the left atrium and produces cyanosis (Fig. 430-11).

CLINICAL MANIFESTATIONS

The severity of symptoms and the degree of cyanosis are highly variable and depend on the extent of displacement of the tricuspid valve and the severity of right ventricular outflow tract obstruction. In many patients, symptoms are mild and may be delayed until the teenage years or young adult life; the patient may initially have fatigue or palpitations as a result of cardiac dysrhythmias. The atrial right-to-left shunt is responsible for cyanosis and polycythemia. Jugular venous pulsations, a index of central venous pressure, may be normal or increased in those with tricuspid insufficiency. On palpation, the precordium is quiet. A holosystolic murmur caused by tricuspid regurgitation is audible over most of the anterior left side of the chest. A gallop rhythm is common and often associated with multiple clicks at the lower left sternal border. A scratchy diastolic murmur may also be heard at the left sternal border. This murmur may mimic a pericardial friction rub.

Newborns with severe forms of Ebstein anomaly have marked cyanosis, massive cardiomegaly, and long holosystolic murmurs. Death may result from cardiac failure, hypoxemia, and pulmonary hypoplasia, the result of severe long-standing intrauterine right atrial enlargement. Spontaneous improvement may occur in some neonates as pulmonary vascular resistance falls and improves the ability of the right ventricle to provide pulmonary blood flow. The majority are

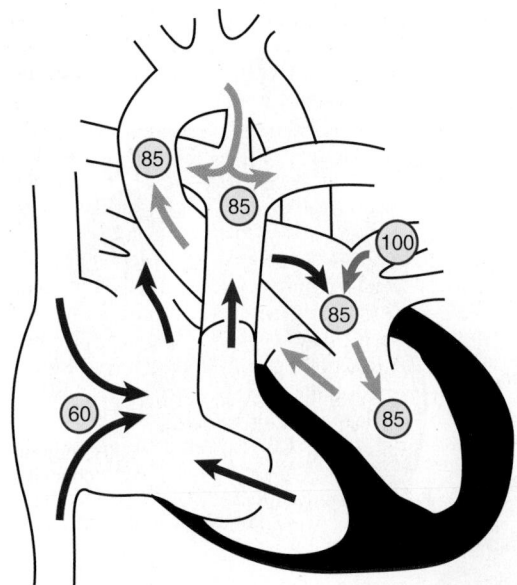

Figure 430-11 Physiology of Ebstein anomaly of the tricuspid valve. *Circled numbers* represent oxygen saturation values. Inferior displacement of the tricuspid valve leaflets into the right ventricle has resulted in a thin-walled, low-pressure "atrialized" segment of right ventricle. The tricuspid valve is grossly insufficient *(clear arrow)*. Right atrial blood flow is shunted right to left across an atrial septal defect or patent foramen ovale into the left atrium. Some blood may cross the right ventricular outflow tract and enter the pulmonary artery; however, in severe cases, the right ventricle may generate insufficient force to open the pulmonary valve, and "functional pulmonary atresia" results. In the left atrium, desaturated blood mixes with saturated pulmonary venous return. Blood enters the left ventricle and is ejected via the aorta. In this example, some pulmonary blood flow is derived from the right ventricle, the rest from a patent ductus arteriosus (PDA). Severe cyanosis will develop in neonates with a severe Ebstein anomaly when the PDA closes.

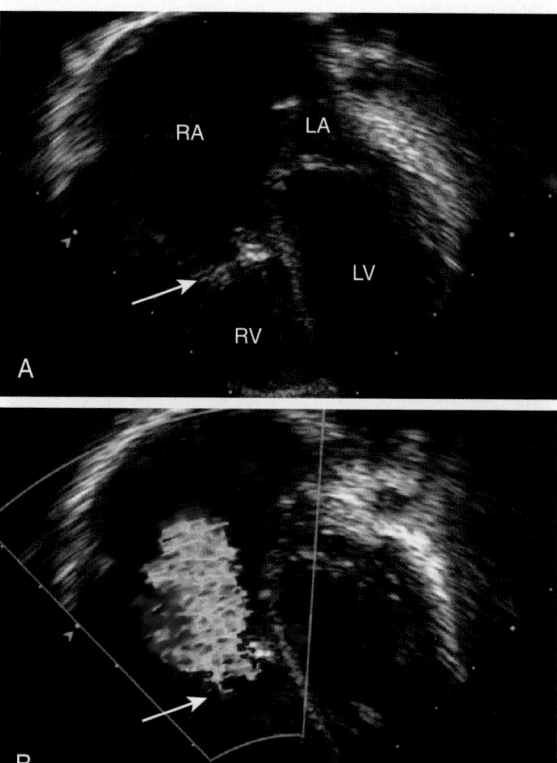

Figure 430-12 Echocardiographic demonstration of Ebstein anomaly of the tricuspid valve. **A,** Subcostal, 4-chamber, 2-dimensional view showing severe displacement of the tricuspid valve leaflets *(large arrow)* inferiorly into the right ventricle. The location of the tricuspid valve annulus is outlined by the 2 *arrowheads*. The portion of the right ventricle between the valve annulus and the valve leaflets is the "atrialized" component. **B,** Color Doppler examination showing severe regurgitation of the dysplastic tricuspid valve. Note that the regurgitant turbulent flow *(arrow)* begins halfway into the right ventricular chamber, at the location of the displaced valve leaflets. LA, left atrium; LV, left ventricle; RA, right atrium; RV, right ventricle.

dependent on a PDA, and thus on a prostaglandin infusion, for pulmonary blood flow.

DIAGNOSIS

The electrocardiogram usually shows a right bundle-branch block without increased right precordial voltage, normal or tall and broad P waves, and a normal or prolonged P-R interval. **Wolff-Parkinson-White syndrome** (see Chapter 435) may be present and these patients may have episodes of supraventricular tachycardia. On radiographic examination, heart size varies from slightly enlarged to massive box-shaped cardiomegaly caused by enlargement of the right atrium. *In newborns with severe Ebstein anomaly, the heart may totally obscure the pulmonary fields.* Echocardiography is diagnostic and shows the degree of displacement of the tricuspid valve leaflets, a dilated right atrium, and any right ventricular outflow tract obstruction (Fig. 430-12). Pulsed and color Doppler examination demonstrates the degree of tricuspid regurgitation. In severe cases, the pulmonary valve may appear immobile and pulmonary blood flow may come solely from the ductus arteriosus. It may be difficult to distinguish true from functional pulmonary valve atresia. Cardiac catheterization, which is not usually necessary, confirms the presence of a large right atrium, an abnormal tricuspid valve, and any right-to-left shunt at the atrial level. The risk of arrhythmia is significant during catheterization and angiographic studies.

PROGNOSIS AND COMPLICATIONS

The prognosis in Ebstein anomaly is extremely variable and depends on the severity of the defect. The prognosis is more guarded for neonates or infants with intractable symptoms and cyanosis. Patients with milder degrees of Ebstein anomaly usually survive well into adult life.

There is an association of a form of left ventricular cardiomyopathy, isolated left ventricular noncompaction, in 18% of patients with Ebstein anomaly, and the severity of the left ventricular dysfunction directly impacts the prognosis.

TREATMENT

Neonates with severe hypoxia who are prostaglandin dependent have been treated with an aortopulmonary shunt alone, by repair of the tricuspid valve, or by surgical patch closure of the tricuspid valve, atrial septectomy, and placement of an aortopulmonary shunt (with eventual single ventricle repair using the Fontan procedure [see Chapter 430.4]). Many infants with Ebstein anomaly who have undergone valve repair will still have enough regurgitation that a Glenn shunt is performed to reduce the volume load on the right ventricle (see Chapter 430.4). In older children with mild or moderate disease, control of supraventricular dysrhythmias is of primary importance; surgical treatment may not be necessary until adolescence or young adulthood. In patients with severe tricuspid regurgitation, repair or replacement of the abnormal tricuspid valve along with closure of the atrial septal defect is carried out. In some older patients, a bidirectional Glenn shunt is also performed, with the superior vena cava anastomosed to the pulmonary arteries. This procedure reduces the volume of blood that the dysfunctional right side of the heart has to pump, thus creating a "one-and-one-half ventricle repair."

Bibliography is available at Expert Consult.

Chapter 431

Cyanotic Congenital Heart Disease: Lesions Associated with Increased Pulmonary Blood Flow

431.1 D-Transposition of the Great Arteries

Daniel Bernstein

Transposition of the great vessels, a common cyanotic congenital anomaly, accounts for ≈5% of all congenital heart disease. In this anomaly, the systemic veins return normally to the right atrium and the pulmonary veins return to the left atrium. The connections between the atria and ventricles are also normal (atrioventricular concordance). The aorta arises from the right ventricle and the pulmonary artery from the left ventricle (Fig. 431-1). In normally related great vessels,

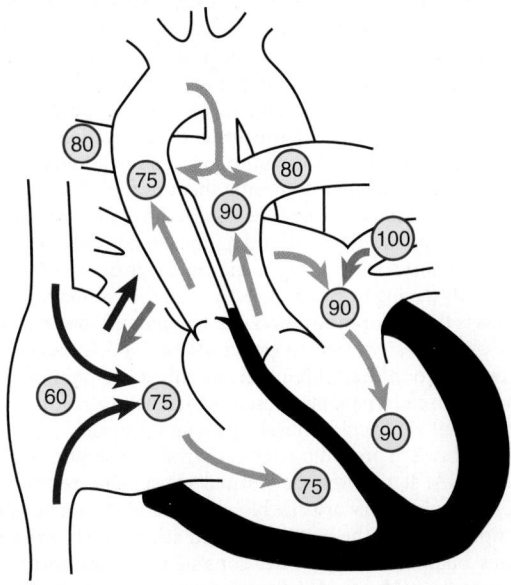

Figure 431-1 Physiology of d-transposition of the great arteries (d-TGA). *Circled numbers* represent oxygen saturation values. Right atrial (mixed venous) oxygen saturation is decreased secondary to systemic hypoxemia. Desaturated blood enters the right atrium, flows through the tricuspid valve into the right ventricle, and is ejected into the transposed aorta with resultant severe aortic desaturation. Fully saturated pulmonary venous blood flows into the left atrium, across the mitral valve into the left ventricle, and across the transposed pulmonary artery into the lungs. Pulmonary arterial oxygen saturation is thus increased. This lesion would not be compatible with life were it not for the ability of blood to shunt via 2 fetal pathways: the patent foramen ovale (PFO) and patent ductus arteriosus (PDA). Blood may shunt left to right or bidirectionally at the PFO. Because systemic vascular resistance tends to be higher than pulmonary vascular resistance, blood tends to shunt across the PDA mostly from the aorta to the pulmonary artery. As pulmonary resistance drops in the 1st few wk of life, pulmonary blood flow will gradually increase in patients with d-TGA.

the aorta is posterior and to the right of the pulmonary artery; in d-transposition of the great arteries (d-TGA), the aorta is anterior and to the right of the pulmonary artery (the *d* indicates a dextropositioned aorta, *transposition* indicates that it arises from the anterior right ventricle). Desaturated blood returning from the body to the right side of the heart goes inappropriately out the aorta and back to the body again, whereas oxygenated pulmonary venous blood returning to the left side of the heart is returned directly to the lungs. Thus, the systemic and pulmonary circulations exist as 2 parallel circuits. Survival in the immediate newborn period is provided by the foramen ovale and the ductus arteriosus, which permit some mixture of oxygenated and deoxygenated blood. Approximately 50% of patients with d-TGA also have a ventricular septal defect (VSD), which usually provides for better mixing. The clinical findings and hemodynamics vary in relation to the presence or absence of associated defects (e.g., VSD or pulmonary stenosis). d-TGA is more common in infants of diabetic mothers and in males (3:1). d-TGA, especially when accompanied by other cardiac defects such as pulmonic stenosis or right aortic arch, can be associated with deletion of chromosome 22q11.2 (DiGeorge syndrome [see Chapter 424]). Before the modern era of corrective or palliative surgery, mortality was >90% in the 1st yr of life.

431.2 D-Transposition of the Great Arteries with Intact Ventricular Septum

Daniel Bernstein

D-TGA with an intact ventricular septum is also referred to as simple TGA or isolated TGA. Before birth, oxygenation of the fetus is only slightly abnormal, but after birth, once the ductus arteriosus begins to close, the minimal mixing of systemic and pulmonary blood via the patent foramen ovale is usually insufficient and severe hypoxemia ensues, generally within the 1st few days of life.

CLINICAL MANIFESTATIONS

Cyanosis and tachypnea are most often recognized within the 1st hr or days of life. Untreated, the vast majority of these infants would not survive the neonatal period. Hypoxemia is usually moderate to severe, depending on the degree of atrial level shunting and whether the ductus is partially open or totally closed. This condition is a medical emergency, and only early diagnosis and appropriate intervention can avert the development of prolonged severe hypoxemia and acidosis, which lead to death. Physical findings, other than cyanosis, may be remarkably nonspecific. The precordial impulse may be normal, or a parasternal heave may be present. The 2nd heart sound is usually single and loud, although it may be split. Murmurs may be absent, or a soft systolic ejection murmur may be noted at the midleft sternal border.

DIAGNOSIS

The electrocardiogram is usually normal, showing the expected neonatal right-sided dominant pattern. Chest x-rays may show mild cardiomegaly, a narrow mediastinum (the classic "egg-shaped heart"), and normal to increased pulmonary blood flow. In the early newborn period, the chest roentgenogram is generally normal. As pulmonary vascular resistance drops during the 1st several wk of life, evidence of increased pulmonary blood flow becomes apparent. Arterial Po_2 is low and does not rise appreciably after the patient breathes 100% oxygen (hyperoxia test), although this test may not be totally reliable. Echocardiography is diagnostic and confirms the transposed ventricular-arterial connections (Fig. 431-2). The size of the interatrial communication and the ductus arteriosus can be visualized and the degree of mixing assessed by pulsed and color Doppler examination. The presence of any associated lesion, such as left ventricular outflow tract obstruction or a VSD, can also be assessed. The origins of the coronary arteries can be imaged, although echocardiography is generally not as accurate as catheterization for this purpose. Cardiac

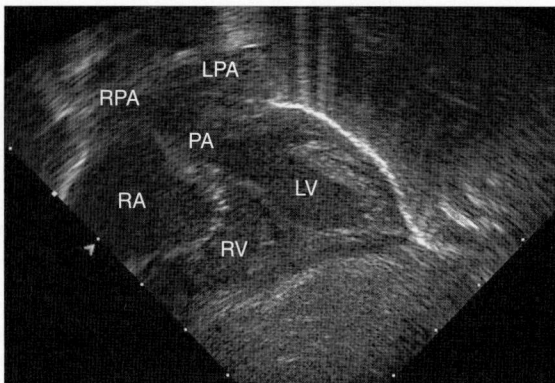

Figure 431-2 Subcostal 4-chamber 2-dimensional echocardiographic demonstration of d-transposition of the great arteries. The pulmonary artery (PA) can be seen arising directly from the left ventricle (LV). The immediate bifurcation of this great vessel into the branch pulmonary arteries differentiates it from the aorta, which branches more distally from the heart. LPA, left pulmonary artery; RA, right atrium; RPA, right pulmonary artery; RV, right ventricle.

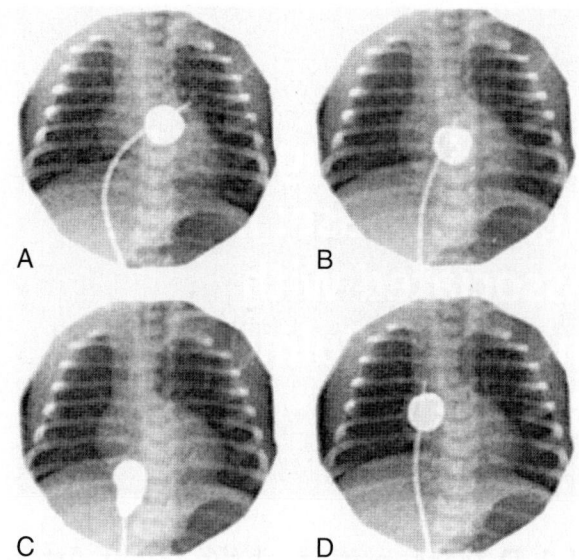

Figure 431-3 Rashkind balloon atrial septostomy. Four frames from a continuous cineangiogram show the creation of an atrial septal defect in a hypoxemic newborn infant with transposition of the great arteries and an intact ventricular septum. **A,** Balloon inflated in the left atrium. **B,** The catheter is jerked suddenly so that the balloon ruptures the foramen ovale. **C,** Balloon in the inferior vena cava. **D,** Catheter advanced to the right atrium to deflate the balloon. The time from **A** to **C** is <1 sec.

catheterization may be performed in patients for whom noninvasive imaging is diagnostically inconclusive, where an unusual coronary artery anomaly is suspected, or in patients who require emergency balloon atrial septostomy (Rashkind procedure). Catheterization will show right ventricular pressure to be systemic because this ventricle is supporting the systemic circulation. The blood in the left ventricle and pulmonary artery has a higher oxygen saturation than that in the aorta. Depending on the age at catheterization, left ventricular and pulmonary arterial pressure can vary from systemic level to <50% of systemic-level pressure. Right ventriculography demonstrates the anterior and rightward aorta originating from the right ventricle, as well as the intact ventricular septum. Left ventriculography shows that the pulmonary artery arises exclusively from the left ventricle.

Anomalous coronary arteries are noted in 10-15% of patients and defined by an aortic root injection or by selective coronary arteriography.

TREATMENT

When transposition is suspected, an infusion of prostaglandin E_1 should be initiated immediately to maintain patency of the ductus arteriosus and improve oxygenation (dosage: 0.01-0.20 μg/kg/min). Because of the risk of apnea associated with prostaglandin infusion, an individual skilled in neonatal endotracheal intubation should be available. Hypothermia intensifies the metabolic acidosis resulting from hypoxemia, and thus the patient should be kept warm. Prompt correction of acidosis and hypoglycemia is essential.

Infants who remain severely hypoxic or acidotic despite prostaglandin infusion should undergo **Rashkind balloon atrial septostomy** (Fig. 431-3). A Rashkind atrial septostomy is also usually performed in all patients in whom any significant delay in surgery is necessary. If surgery is planned during the 1st 2 wk of life, and the patient is stable, catheterization and atrial septostomy may be avoided.

A successful Rashkind atrial septostomy should result in a rise in Pao_2 to 35-50 mm Hg and elimination of any pressure gradient across the atrial septum. Some patients with TGA and VSD (see Chapter 431.3) may require balloon atrial septostomy because of poor mixing, even though the VSD is large. Others may benefit from decompression of the left atrium to alleviate the symptoms of increased pulmonary blood flow and left-sided heart failure.

The **arterial switch (Jatene) procedure** is the surgical **treatment of choice** for neonates with d-TGA and an intact ventricular septum and is usually performed within the 1st 2 wk of life. The reason for this time frame is that as pulmonary vascular resistance declines after birth,

pressure in the left ventricle (connected to the pulmonary vascular bed) also declines. This drop in pressure results in a decrease in left ventricular mass over the 1st few wk of life. If the arterial switch operation is attempted after left ventricular pressure (and mass) has declined too far, the left ventricle will be unable to generate adequate pressure to pump blood to the high pressure systemic circulation. The arterial switch operation involves dividing the aorta and pulmonary artery just above the sinuses and reanastomosing them in their correct anatomic positions. The coronary arteries are removed from the old aortic root along with a button of aortic wall and reimplanted in the old pulmonary root (the "neoaorta"). By using a button of great vessel tissue, the surgeon avoids having to suture directly onto the coronary artery (Fig. 431-4); this is the major innovation that has allowed the arterial switch to replace previous atrial switch operations for d-TGA. Rarely, a 2-stage arterial switch procedure, with initial placement of a pulmonary artery band, may be used in patients presenting late who already have had a reduction in left ventricular muscle mass and pressure.

The arterial switch procedure has a survival rate of >95% for uncomplicated d-TGA. It restores the normal physiologic relationships of systemic and pulmonary arterial blood flow and eliminates the long-term complications of the previously used atrial switch procedure.

Previous operations for d-TGA consisted of some form of **atrial switch procedure** (**Mustard** or **Senning** operation). These procedures produced excellent early survival (≈85-90%), but had significant long-term morbidities. Atrial switch procedures reverse blood flow at the atrial level by the creation of an interatrial baffle that directs systemic venous blood returning from the vena cavae to the left atrium, where it will enter the left ventricle and then, via the pulmonary artery, the lungs. The same baffle also permits oxygenated pulmonary venous blood to cross over to the right atrium, right ventricle, and aorta. Atrial switch procedures involve significant atrial surgery and have been associated with the late development of atrial conduction disturbances, sick sinus syndrome with bradyarrhythmia and tachyarrhythmia, atrial flutter, sudden death, superior or inferior vena cava syndrome, edema, ascites, and protein-losing enteropathy. The atrial switch procedure also leaves the right ventricle as the systemic pumping chamber and these "systemic" right ventricles often begin to fail in young adulthood. Atrial

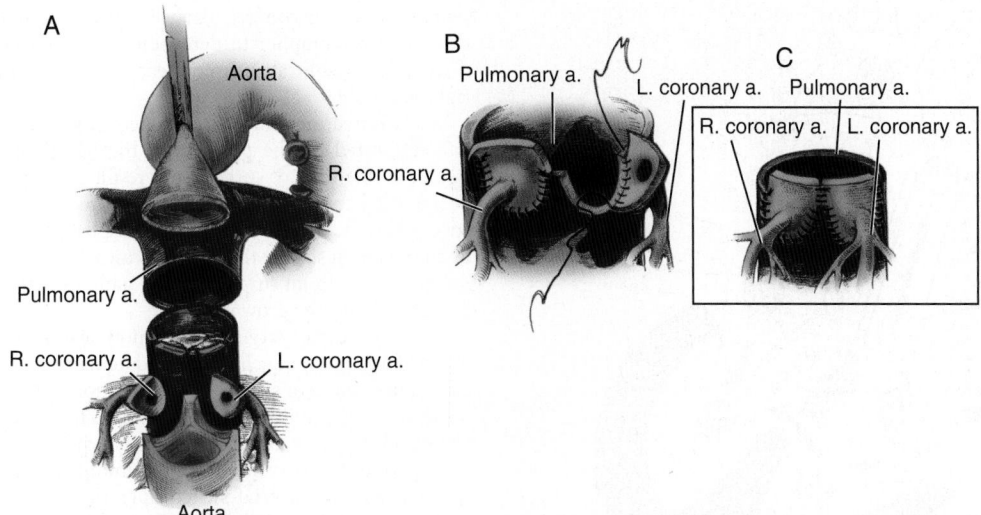

Figure 431-4 Method for translocating the coronary arteries in the arterial switch (Jatene) procedure. **A,** The aorta (anterior) and the pulmonary artery (posterior) have been transected to allow visualization of the left and right coronary arteries. The coronaries have been excised from their respective sinuses, including a large flap (button) of arterial wall. Equivalent segments of the wall of the pulmonary artery (which will become the neoaorta) are also removed. **B,** The aortocoronary buttons are sutured into the proximal portion of the neoaorta. With this technique all sutures are placed in the button of aortic wall rather than directly on the coronary arteries. **C,** Completed anastomosis of the left and right coronary arteries to the neoaorta. *(Adapted from Castañeda AR, Jonas RA, Mayer JE Jr, et al:* Cardiac surgery of the neonate and infant, *Philadelphia, 1994, WB Saunders.)*

switch operations are currently reserved for patients whose anatomy is such that they are not candidates for the arterial switch procedure.

431.3 Transposition of the Great Arteries with Ventricular Septal Defect
Daniel Bernstein

If the VSD associated with d-TGA is small, the clinical manifestations, laboratory findings, and treatment are similar to those described previously for transposition with an intact ventricular septum. A harsh systolic murmur is audible at the lower left sternal border, resulting from flow through the defect. Many of these small defects eventually close spontaneously and may not be addressed at the time of surgery.

When the VSD is large and not restrictive to ventricular ejection, significant mixing of oxygenated and deoxygenated blood usually occurs and clinical manifestations of cardiac failure are seen. The degree of cyanosis may be subtle and sometimes may not be recognized until an oxygen saturation measurement is performed. The murmur is holosystolic and generally indistinguishable from that produced by a large VSD in patients with normally related great arteries. The heart is usually significantly enlarged.

Cardiomegaly, a narrow mediastinal waist, and increased pulmonary vascularity are demonstrated on the chest x-ray. The electrocardiogram shows prominent P waves and isolated right ventricular hypertrophy or biventricular hypertrophy. Occasionally, dominance of the left ventricle is present. Usually, the QRS axis is to the right, but it can be normal or even to the left. The diagnosis is confirmed by echocardiography, and the extent of pulmonary blood flow can also be assessed by the degree of enlargement of the left atrium and ventricle. In equivocal cases, the diagnosis can be confirmed by cardiac catheterization. Right and left ventriculography indicate the presence of arterial transposition and demonstrate the site and size of the VSD. Systolic pressure is equal in the 2 ventricles, the aorta, and the pulmonary artery. Left atrial pressure may be much higher than right atrial pressure, a finding indicative of a restrictive communication at the atrial level. At the time of cardiac catheterization, Rashkind balloon atrial septostomy may be performed to decompress the left atrium, even when adequate mixing is occurring at the ventricular level.

Surgical treatment is advised soon after diagnosis, because heart failure and failure to thrive are difficult to manage and pulmonary vascular disease can develop unusually rapidly in these patients. Preoperative management with diuretics lessens the symptoms of heart failure and stabilizes the patient prior to surgery.

Patients with d-TGA and a VSD without pulmonic stenosis can be treated with an arterial switch procedure combined with VSD closure. In these patients, the arterial switch operation can be safely performed after the 1st 2 wk of life because the VSD results in equal pressure in both ventricles and prevents regression of left ventricular muscle mass. At major centers, however, there is no reason to delay repair, as results are excellent whether the surgery is performed in the neonatal period or later.

431.4 L-Transposition of the Great Arteries (Corrected Transposition)
Daniel Bernstein

In l-transposition (l-TGA), the atrioventricular relationships are discordant: the right atrium is connected to the left ventricle and the left atrium to the right ventricle (also known as *ventricular inversion*). The great arteries are also transposed, with the aorta arising from the right ventricle and the pulmonary artery from the left. In contrast to d-TGA, the aorta arises to the left of the pulmonary artery (hence the designation *l* for levo-transposition). The aorta may be anterior to the pulmonary artery, although often they are nearly side by side.

The physiology of l-TGA is quite different from that of d-TGA. Desaturated systemic venous blood returns via the vena cavae to a normal right atrium, from which it passes through a bicuspid atrioventricular (mitral) valve into a right-sided ventricle that has the architecture and smooth wall morphologic features of the normal left ventricle (Fig. 431-5). Because transposition is also present, however, the desaturated blood ejected from this left ventricle enters the transposed pulmonary artery and flows into the lungs, as it would in the normal circulation. Oxygenated pulmonary venous blood returns to a normal left atrium, passes through a tricuspid atrioventricular valve into a left-sided ventricle, which has the trabeculated morphologic features of a normal right ventricle, and is then ejected into the

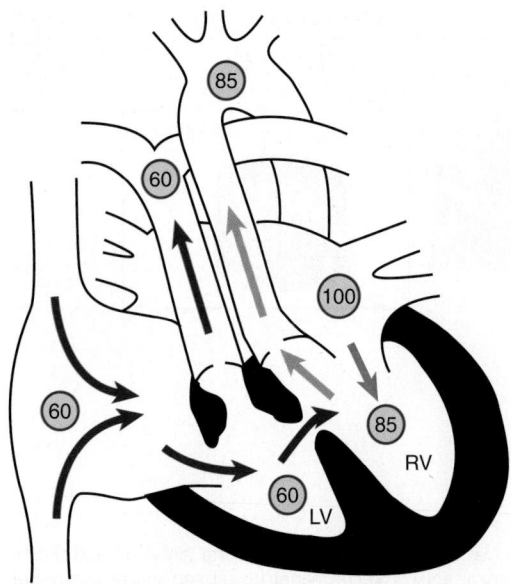

Figure 431-5 Physiology of l- or corrected transposition of the great arteries (l-TGA) with a ventricular septal defect and pulmonic stenosis (VSD + PS). *Circled numbers* represent oxygen saturation values. Right atrial (mixed venous) oxygen saturation is decreased secondary to systemic hypoxemia. Blood from the right atrium flows through the mitral valve into the "inverted" left ventricle (LV). The left ventricle is, however, attached to the transposed pulmonary artery. Therefore, despite the anomalies, desaturated blood still winds up in the pulmonary circulation. Saturated blood returns to the left atrium, traverses the tricuspid valve into the "inverted" right ventricle (RV), and is pumped into the transposed aorta. This circulation would be totally "corrected" were it not for the frequent association of other congenital anomalies, in this case, VSD + PS. Because of the stenotic pulmonary valve, some left ventricular blood flow crosses the VSD and into the right ventricle and the ascending aorta, and systemic desaturation results.

transposed aorta. The double inversion of the atrioventricular and ventriculoarterial relationships result in desaturated right atrial blood appropriately flowing to the lungs and oxygenated pulmonary venous blood appropriately flowing to the aorta. The circulation is thus physiologically "**corrected.**" Without other defects, the hemodynamics would be nearly normal. In most patients, however, associated anomalies coexist: VSD, Ebstein-like abnormalities of the left-sided atrioventricular (tricuspid) valve, pulmonary valvular or subvalvular stenosis (or both), and atrioventricular conduction disturbances (complete heart block, accessory pathways such as Wolff-Parkinson-White syndrome).

CLINICAL MANIFESTATIONS
Symptoms and signs are widely variable and are determined by the associated lesions. If pulmonary outflow is unobstructed, the clinical signs are similar to those of an isolated VSD. If l-TGA is associated with pulmonary stenosis and a VSD, the clinical signs are more similar to those of tetralogy of Fallot.

DIAGNOSIS
The chest x-ray may suggest the abnormal position of the great arteries; the ascending aorta occupies the upper left border of the cardiac silhouette and has a straight profile. The electrocardiogram, in addition to any atrioventricular conduction disturbances, may show abnormal P waves; absent Q waves in V_6; abnormal Q waves in leads III, aVR, aVF, and V_1; and upright T waves across the precordium. The echocardiogram is diagnostic. The characteristic echocardiographic features of the right ventricle (moderator band, coarser trabeculations, tricuspid valve that sits more inferiorly compared to the bicuspid mitral valve, and a smooth muscular conus or infundibulum

separating the atrioventricular valve from the semilunar valve) allow the echocardiographer to determine the presence of atrioventricular discordance (right atrium connected to left ventricle; left atrium to right ventricle).

Surgical treatment of the associated anomalies, most often the VSD, is complicated by the position of the bundle of His, which can be injured at the time of surgery and result in heart block. Identification of the usual course of the bundle in corrected transposition (running superior to the defect) has been accomplished by mapping of the conduction system so that the surgeon can avoid the bundle of His during repair. Even without surgical injury, patients with l-TGA are at risk for heart block as they grow older.

Because simple surgical correction leaves the right ventricle as the systemic pumping chamber, and hence vulnerable to late ventricular failure, surgeons have become more aggressive about trying operations that utilize the left ventricle as the systemic pumping chamber. This is accomplished by performing an atrial switch operation, to reroute the systemic and pulmonary venous returns, in combination with an arterial switch operation to reroute the ventricular outflows (**double switch procedure**). The long-term benefit of this approach in preserving systemic ventricular function is still under investigation.

Bibliography is available at Expert Consult.

431.5 Double-Outlet Right Ventricle Without Pulmonary Stenosis
Daniel Bernstein

In double-outlet right ventricle without pulmonary stenosis, both the aorta and the pulmonary artery arise from the right ventricle (see Chapter 430.5). The only outlet from the left ventricle is through a VSD. In the absence of obstruction to pulmonary blood flow, clinical manifestations are similar to those of an uncomplicated VSD with a large left-to-right shunt, although mild systemic desaturation may be present because of mixing of oxygenated and deoxygenated blood in the right ventricle. The electrocardiogram usually shows biventricular hypertrophy. Echocardiography is diagnostic and shows the right ventricular origin of both great arteries, their anteroposterior relationship, as well as the relationship of the VSD to each of the great arteries. Surgical correction is dependent on these relationships. If the VSD is subaortic, it is accomplished by creation of an intracardiac tunnel. Blood is then ejected from the left ventricle via the VSD into the aorta. If the VSD is subpulmonic, an arterial switch may be performed in combination with an intracardiac tunnel. If pulmonary blood flow is excessive enough to cause congestive heart failure, pulmonary arterial banding may be required in infancy, followed by surgical correction when the child is bigger. When associated pulmonary stenosis is present, cyanosis is more marked, pulmonary blood flow is decreased, and clinical presentation may be similar to that of tetralogy of Fallot (see Chapter 430.5).

431.6 Double-Outlet Right Ventricle with Malposition of the Great Arteries (Taussig-Bing Anomaly)
Daniel Bernstein

In double-outlet right ventricle with malposed great arteries, the VSD is usually directly subpulmonary and the aorta distant from the left ventricle. Sometimes both the pulmonary and aortic valves may be located close to the VSD (doubly committed VSD) and sometimes neither is (doubly uncommitted VSD). The term *malposition* is used instead of *transposition* because both great arteries arise from the right ventricle. Aortic obstructive lesions are common, including valvular and subvalvular aortic stenosis, coarctation of the aorta, and interruption of the aortic arch. Because pulmonary blood flow is unobstructed, patients experience cardiac failure early in infancy and are at risk for the development of pulmonary vascular disease and cyanosis. If aortic obstructive lesions are a component, patients can present with poor systemic output and cardiovascular collapse, particularly after the ductus begins to close. Cardiomegaly is usual, and a parasternal systolic ejection murmur is audible, sometimes preceded by an ejection click and loud closure of the pulmonary valve. The electrocardiogram shows right axis deviation and right, left, or biventricular hypertrophy. The chest x-ray shows cardiomegaly and prominence of the pulmonary vasculature. The anatomic features of the anomaly and associated abnormalities are usually demonstrated by echocardiography, augmented if necessary by either cardiac catheterization, MRI, or CT. Palliation may be achieved by pulmonary arterial banding in infancy and surgical correction at a later age, which may be accomplished by an arterial switch procedure (see Chapter 431.2) combined with an intracardiac baffle, or some modification of the Rastelli procedure (see Chapter 430.5).

431.7 Total Anomalous Pulmonary Venous Return
Daniel Bernstein

PATHOPHYSIOLOGY
Abnormal development of the pulmonary veins may result in either partial or complete anomalous drainage into the systemic venous circulation. Partial anomalous pulmonary venous return is usually an acyanotic lesion (see Chapter 426.4). Total anomalous pulmonary venous return (TAPVR) is associated with total mixing of systemic venous and pulmonary venous blood flow within the heart and thus produces cyanosis.

In TAPVR, the heart has no direct pulmonary venous connection into the left atrium. The pulmonary veins may drain above the diaphragm into the right atrium directly, into the coronary sinus, or into the superior vena cava via a "vertical vein," or they may drain below the diaphragm and join into a "descending vein" that enters into the inferior vena cava or one of its major tributaries, often via the ductus venosus. This latter form of anomalous venous drainage is most commonly associated with obstruction to venous flow, usually as the ductus venosus closes soon after birth, although supracardiac anomalous veins may also become obstructed. Occasionally, the drainage may be mixed, with some veins draining above and others below the diaphragm.

All forms of TAPVR involve mixing of oxygenated and deoxygenated blood before or at the level of the right atrium (total mixing lesion). This mixed right atrial blood either passes into the right ventricle and pulmonary artery or passes through an atrial septal defect (ASD) or patent foramen ovale into the left atrium, which will be the only source of systemic blood flow. The right atrium and ventricle and the pulmonary artery are generally enlarged, whereas the left atrium and ventricle may be normal or small. The clinical manifestations of TAPVR depend on the presence or absence of obstruction of the venous channels (Table 431-1). If pulmonary venous return is obstructed, severe pulmonary congestion and pulmonary hypertension develop; rapid deterioration occurs without surgical intervention. Obstructed TAPVR is a pediatric cardiac surgical emergency because prostaglandin therapy is usually not effective.

CLINICAL MANIFESTATIONS
Two major clinical patterns of TAPVR are seen, depending on the presence or absence of obstruction. Those neonates with severe obstruction to pulmonary venous return, most prevalent in the infracardiac group (see Table 431-1), present with severe cyanosis and respiratory distress. Murmurs may not be present. These infants are severely ill and fail to respond to mechanical ventilation. Rapid diagnosis and surgical correction are necessary for survival. In contrast, those with

Table 431-1	Total Anomalous Pulmonary Venous Return	
SITE OF CONNECTION (% OF CASES)		**% WITH SIGNIFICANT OBSTRUCTION**
Supracardiac (50)		
Left superior vena cava (40)		40
Right superior vena cava (10)		75
Cardiac (25)		
Coronary sinus (20)		10
Right atrium (5)		5
Infracardiac (20)		95-100
Mixed (5)		

mild or no obstruction to pulmonary venous return are usually characterized by the development of heart failure as the pulmonary vascular resistance falls, with mild to moderate degrees of desaturation. Systolic murmurs may be audible along the left sternal border, and a gallop rhythm may be present. Some infants may have mild obstruction in the neonatal period and develop worsening obstruction as time passes.

DIAGNOSIS
The electrocardiogram demonstrates right ventricular hypertrophy (usually a qR pattern in V_3R and V_1, and the P waves are frequently tall and spiked). In neonates with marked pulmonary venous obstruction, the chest x-ray demonstrates a very dramatic perihilar pattern of pulmonary edema and a small heart. This appearance can sometimes be confused with primary pulmonary disease and the differential diagnosis includes persistent pulmonary hypertension of the newborn, respiratory distress syndrome, pneumonia (bacterial, meconium aspiration), pulmonary lymphangiectasia, and other heart defects (hypoplastic left heart syndrome). In older children, if the anomalous pulmonary veins enter the innominate vein and persistent left superior vena cava (Fig. 431-6), a large supracardiac shadow can be seen, which together with the normal cardiac shadow forms a **"snowman"** appearance. In most cases without obstruction, the heart is enlarged, the pulmonary artery and right ventricle are prominent, and pulmonary vascularity is increased.

The echocardiogram demonstrates a large right ventricle and usually identifies the pattern of abnormal pulmonary venous connections (Fig. 431-7). The demonstration of any vein with Doppler flow away from the heart is pathognomonic of TAPVR as normal venous flow is usually toward the heart. Shunting occurs from right to left at the atrial level. The size of the left atrium and left ventricle can be measured and the presence of any associated cardiac defects determined.

Echocardiography should be adequate to demonstrate TAPVR in most cases; however, if there is question about the drainage of 1 or more pulmonary veins, cardiac catheterization, MRI, or CT is performed. Catheterization shows that the oxygen saturation of blood in both atria, both ventricles, and the aorta is similar, indicative of a total mixing lesion. An increase in systemic venous saturation occurs at the site of entry of the abnormal pulmonary venous channel, either above or below the diaphragm. In older patients, pulmonary arterial and right ventricular pressure may be only moderately elevated, but in infants with pulmonary venous obstruction, pulmonary hypertension is usual. Selective pulmonary arteriography shows the anatomy of the pulmonary veins and their point of entry into the systemic venous circulation.

TREATMENT
Surgical correction of TAPVR is indicated during infancy, with emergent repair performed for those patients with venous obstruction. If

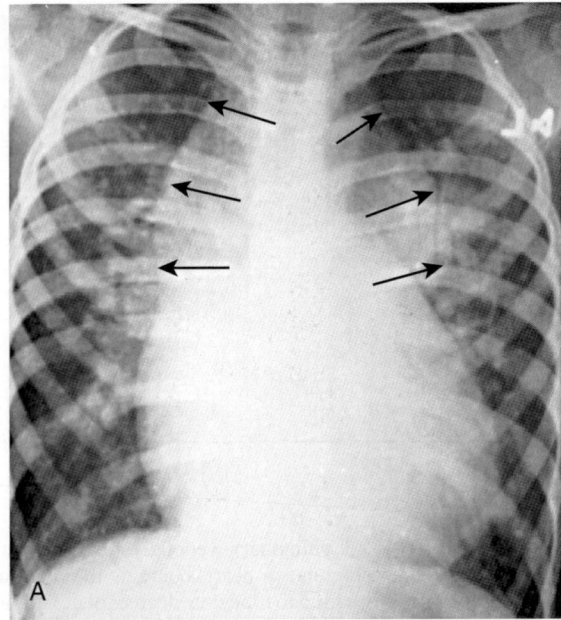

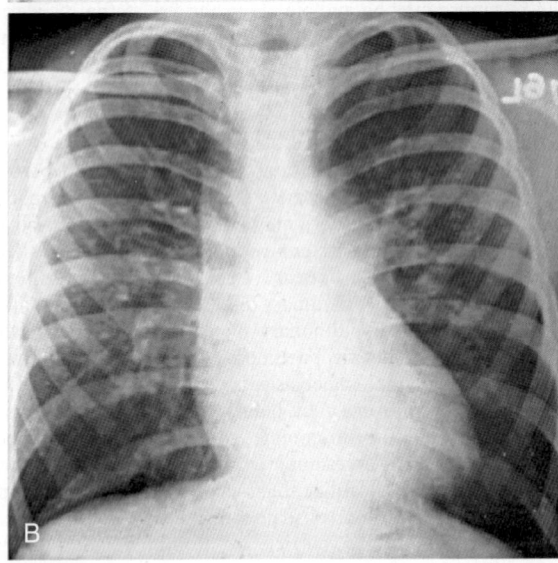

Figure 431-6 Chest x-ray of total anomalous pulmonary venous return to the left superior vena cava. **A,** Preoperative image. *Arrows* point to the supracardiac shadow, which produces the snowman or figure-8 configuration. Cardiomegaly and increased pulmonary vascularity are evident. **B,** Postoperative image showing a decrease in the size of the heart and the supracardiac shadow.

surgery cannot be performed urgently, extracorporeal membrane oxygenation may be required to maintain oxygenation. Surgically, the pulmonary venous confluence is anastomosed directly to the left atrium, the ASD is closed, and any connection to the systemic venous circuit is interrupted. Early results are generally good, even for critically ill neonates. The postoperative period may be complicated by pulmonary vascular hypertensive crises. In some patients, especially those in whom the diagnosis was delayed or the obstruction was severe, recurrent stenosis and development of pulmonary veno-occlusive disease may occur. Attempts have been made to treat recurrent stenosis with surgery, balloon angioplasty, stents, and antiproliferative chemotherapy. To date, the long-term prognosis in these patients is very guarded and in those with aggressive veno-occlusive disease, **heart-lung transplantation** may be the only option (see Chapter 443.2).

Bibliography is available at Expert Consult.

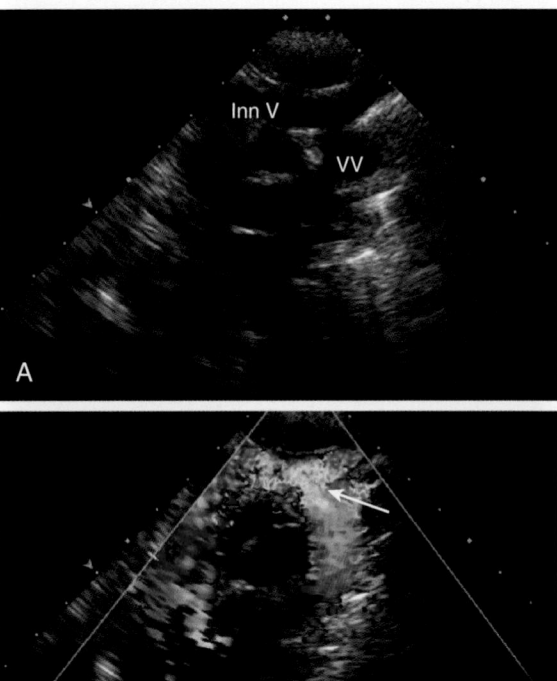

Figure 431-7 Suprasternal 2-dimensional echocardiographic views demonstrating supracardiac total anomalous pulmonary venous return (type I). **A,** The large vertical ascending vein can be seen entering the innominate vein. There is a moderate narrowing where the anomalous vein enters the upper body venous system. **B,** Color Doppler examination shows a venous flow signal (*red color*) indicating that blood is moving away toward the transducer and thus from the heart (all venous flow should normally return toward the heart), diagnostic of anomalous pulmonary venous return. The turbulent acceleration of flow can be seen (*arrow*) where the vertical vein enters the innominate. Inn V, innominate vein; VV, vertical vein.

431.8 Truncus Arteriosus
Daniel Bernstein

PATHOPHYSIOLOGY
In truncus arteriosus, a single arterial trunk (truncus arteriosus) arises from the heart and supplies the systemic, pulmonary, and coronary circulations. A VSD is always present, with the truncus overriding the defect and receiving blood from both the right and left ventricles (Fig. 431-8). The number of truncal valve cusps varies from 2 to as many as 6 and the valve may be stenotic, regurgitant, or both. The pulmonary arteries can arise together from the posterior left side of the persistent truncus arteriosus and then divide into left and right pulmonary arteries **(type I)**. In **types II** and **III** truncus arteriosus, no main pulmonary artery is present, and the right and left pulmonary arteries arise from separate orifices on the posterior **(type II)** or lateral **(type III)** aspects of the truncus arteriosus. **Type IV** truncus is a term no longer used because, in this case, there is no identifiable connection between the heart and pulmonary arteries, and pulmonary blood flow is derived from major aortopulmonary collateral arteries arising from the transverse or descending aorta; this is essentially a form of pulmonary atresia (see Chapter 430.2).

Both ventricles are at systemic pressure and both eject blood into the truncus. When pulmonary vascular resistance is relatively high immediately after birth, pulmonary blood flow may be normal; as pulmonary resistance drops in the 1st mo of life, blood flow to the lungs is greatly increased and heart failure ensues. Truncus arteriosus is a total mixing lesion with complete admixture of pulmonary and systemic venous return. Because of the large volume of pulmonary

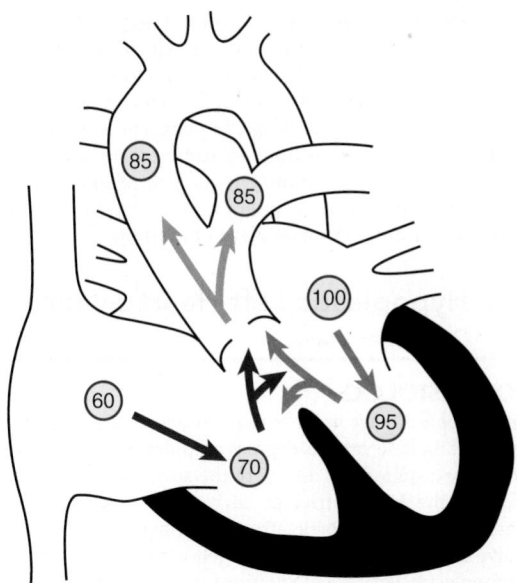

Figure 431-8 Physiology of truncus arteriosus. *Circled numbers* represent oxygen saturation values. Right atrial (mixed venous) oxygen saturation is decreased secondary to systemic hypoxemia. Desaturated blood enters the right atrium, flows through the tricuspid valve into the right ventricle, and is ejected into the truncus. Saturated blood returning from the left atrium enters the left ventricle and is also ejected into the truncus. The common aortopulmonary trunk gives rise to the ascending aorta and to the main or branch pulmonary arteries. Oxygen saturation in the aorta and pulmonary arteries is usually the same (definition of a total mixing lesion). As pulmonary vascular resistance decreases in the 1st few wk of life, pulmonary blood flow increases dramatically and mild cyanosis and congestive heart failure result.

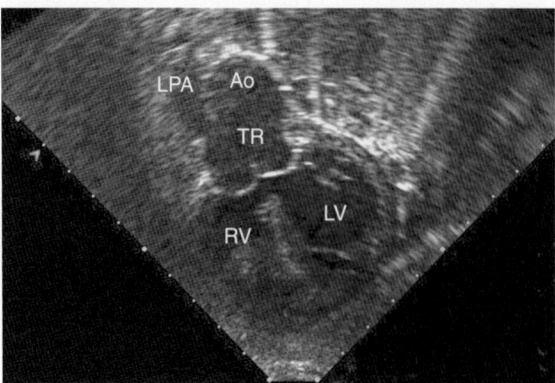

Figure 431-9 Subcostal 2-dimensional echocardiographic demonstration of truncus arteriosus. The large truncal valve can be seen overriding the ventricular septal defect. In this case, only the left pulmonary artery (*LPA*) arises from the truncus (*TR*). The pulmonary arteries are discontinuous and the right pulmonary artery arises from the descending aorta via the ductus arteriosus (not shown). Ao, aorta; LV, left ventricle; RV, right ventricle.

blood flow, clinical cyanosis is usually mild. If the lesion is left untreated, pulmonary resistance eventually increases, pulmonary blood flow decreases, and cyanosis becomes more prominent (Eisenmenger physiology; see Chapter 433.2).

CLINICAL MANIFESTATIONS

The clinical signs of truncus arteriosus vary with age and depend on the level of pulmonary vascular resistance. In the immediate newborn period, signs of heart failure are usually absent; a murmur and minimal cyanosis may be the only initial findings. Over the next 1-2 mo of life, pulmonary blood flow begins to become torrential and the clinical picture is dominated by heart failure, with still mild cyanosis. Runoff of blood from the truncus to the pulmonary circulation may result in a wide pulse pressure and bounding pulses. These findings will be further exaggerated if truncal valve insufficiency is present. The heart is usually enlarged, and the precordium is hyperdynamic. The 2nd heart sound is loud and single. A systolic ejection murmur, sometimes accompanied by a thrill, is generally audible along the left sternal border. The murmur is frequently preceded by an early systolic ejection click due to the abnormal truncal valve. In the presence of truncal valve insufficiency, a high-pitched early diastolic decrescendo murmur is heard at the mid-left sternal border. An apical mid-diastolic rumbling murmur caused by increased flow through the mitral valve is often audible with the bell of the stethoscope, especially as heart failure develops. Truncus arteriosus is a conotruncal malformation and may be associated with **DiGeorge syndrome,** linked to a deletion of a large region of chromosome 22q11 (see Chapter 424).

DIAGNOSIS

The electrocardiogram shows right, left, or combined ventricular hypertrophy. The chest x-ray also shows considerable variation. Cardiac enlargement will develop over the 1st several wk of life, and is a result of the prominence of both ventricles. The truncus may produce a prominent shadow that follows the normal course of the ascending aorta and aortic knob; the aortic arch is right-sided in 50% of patients. Sometimes

a high bulge left of the aortic knob is produced by the main or left pulmonary artery. Pulmonary vascularity is increased after the 1st few wk of life. Echocardiography is diagnostic and demonstrates the large truncal artery overriding the VSD and the pattern of origin of the branch pulmonary arteries (Fig. 431-9). Associated anomalies such as an interrupted aortic arch may be noted. Pulsed and color Doppler studies are used to evaluate truncal valve regurgitation. If required, cardiac catheterization shows a left-to-right shunt at the ventricular level, with right-to-left shunting into the truncus. Systolic pressure in both ventricles and the truncus is similar. Angiography reveals the large truncus arteriosus and more defines the origin of the pulmonary arteries.

PROGNOSIS AND COMPLICATIONS

Surgical results have been excellent, and many patients with repaired truncus are now entering adulthood. The need to replace the right ventricular to pulmonary artery conduit as the child grows means that these patients will need to undergo multiple operations by the time they reach adulthood. When truncus arteriosus is associated with DiGeorge syndrome, the associated endocrine, immunologic, craniofacial, and airway abnormalities may complicate recovery.

TREATMENT

In the 1st few wk of life, many of these infants can be managed with anticongestive medications; as pulmonary vascular resistance falls, heart failure symptoms worsen and surgery is indicated, usually within the 1st few mo. Delay of surgery much beyond this time period may increase the likelihood of pulmonary vascular disease; many centers now perform routine neonatal repair at the time of diagnosis. At surgery, the VSD is closed, the pulmonary arteries are separated from the truncus, and continuity is established between the right ventricle and the pulmonary arteries with a homograft conduit. Immediate surgical results are excellent, but these conduits will develop either regurgitation or stenosis over time, and must be replaced, often several times, as the child grows. If regurgitation is the primary problem, patients can now be treated with a transcatheter stent-valve.

Bibliography is available at Expert Consult.

431.9 Single Ventricle (Double-Inlet Ventricle, Univentricular Heart)

Daniel Bernstein

PATHOPHYSIOLOGY

With a single ventricle, both atria empty through a common atrioventricular valve or via 2 separate valves into a single ventricular chamber, with total mixing of systemic and pulmonary venous return. This chamber may have left, right, or indeterminate ventricular anatomic characteristics. The aorta and pulmonary artery both arise from this single chamber, although one of the great vessels may originate from a rudimentary outflow chamber. The aorta may be posterior, anterior (malposition), or side by side with the pulmonary artery and either to the right or to the left. Pulmonary stenosis or atresia is common.

CLINICAL MANIFESTATIONS

The clinical picture is variable and depends on the associated intracardiac anomalies. If pulmonary outflow is obstructed, the findings are usually similar to those of tetralogy of Fallot: marked cyanosis without heart failure. If pulmonary outflow is unobstructed, the findings are similar to those of transposition with VSD: minimal cyanosis with increasing heart failure.

In patients with **pulmonary stenosis**, cyanosis is present in early infancy. Cardiomegaly is mild or moderate, a left parasternal lift is palpable, and a systolic thrill is common. The systolic ejection murmur is usually loud; an ejection click may be audible, and the 2nd heart sound is single and loud. In patients with **unobstructed pulmonary flow**, as pulmonary vascular resistance drops, torrential pulmonary blood flow develops, and these patients present with tachypnea, dyspnea, failure to thrive, and recurrent pulmonary infections. Cyanosis is only mild or moderate. Cardiomegaly is generally marked, and a left parasternal lift is palpable. A systolic ejection murmur is present but is not usually loud or harsh, and the 2nd heart sound is loud and closely split. A 3rd heart sound is common and may be followed by a short mid-diastolic rumbling murmur caused by increased flow through the atrioventricular valves. The eventual development of pulmonary vascular disease reduces pulmonary blood flow so that the cyanosis increases and signs of cardiac failure appear to improve (Eisenmenger physiology; see Chapter 433.2).

DIAGNOSIS

Findings on the electrocardiogram are nonspecific. P waves are normal, spiked, or bifid. The precordial lead pattern suggests right ventricular hypertrophy, combined ventricular hypertrophy, or sometimes left ventricular dominance. The initial QRS forces are usually to the left and anterior. Radiographic examination confirms the degree of cardiomegaly. If present, a rudimentary outflow chamber may produce a bulge on the upper left border of the cardiac silhouette in the posteroanterior projection. In the absence of pulmonary stenosis, pulmonary vasculature is increased, whereas in the presence of pulmonary stenosis, pulmonary vasculature is diminished. Echocardiography will confirm the absence or near absence of the ventricular septum and can usually determine whether the single ventricle has right, left, or mixed morphologic features. The presence of a rudimentary outflow chamber under one of the great vessels can be identified, and pulsed Doppler can be used to determine whether flow through this communication (known as a *bulboventricular foramen*) is obstructed.

If cardiac catheterization is performed, the pressure in the single ventricular chamber is at systemic level; however, a gradient may be demonstrated across the entrance to a rudimentary outflow chamber. Pressure measurements and angiography demonstrate whether pulmonary stenosis is present.

PROGNOSIS AND COMPLICATIONS

Unoperated, some patients succumb during infancy from heart failure. Others may survive to adolescence and early adult life but finally succumb to the effects of chronic hypoxemia or, in the absence of pulmonary stenosis, to the effects of pulmonary vascular disease. Patients with moderate pulmonary stenosis have the best prognosis because pulmonary blood flow, though restricted, is still adequate. Surgical palliation, eventually leading to Fontan-type circulatory physiology (see Chapter 430.4), has very good short- and intermediate-term results.

TREATMENT

If pulmonary stenosis is severe, a **Blalock-Taussig aortopulmonary shunt** is performed to provide a reliable source of pulmonary blood flow (see Chapter 430.1). If pulmonary blood flow is unrestricted,

pulmonary arterial banding is used to control heart failure and prevent progressive pulmonary vascular disease. The **bidirectional Glenn shunt** is usually performed at between 2 and 6 mo of age, followed by a **modified Fontan operation** (cavopulmonary isolation procedure; see Chapter 430.4) at 2-3 yr of age. If subaortic stenosis is present because of a restrictive connection to a rudimentary outflow chamber, (restrictive bulboventricular foramen) surgical relief can be provided by anastomosing the proximal pulmonary artery to the side of the ascending aorta (**Damus-Stansel-Kaye operation**).

431.10 Hypoplastic Left-Heart Syndrome
Daniel Bernstein

PATHOPHYSIOLOGY

The term *hypoplastic left heart* is used to describe a related group of anomalies that include various degrees of underdevelopment of the left side of the heart: stenosis or atresia of the aortic and mitral valves and hypoplasia of the left ventricular cavity and ascending aorta. Two broad categories include aortic atresia with hypoplastic but perforate mitral valve or with mitral atresia. The left ventricle may be only moderately hypoplastic, very small and nonfunctional, or totally atretic; in the immediate neonatal period the right ventricle maintains both the pulmonary circulation and the systemic circulation via the ductus arteriosus (Fig. 431-10). Pulmonary venous blood passes through an ASD or dilated foramen ovale from the left to the right side of the heart, where it mixes with systemic venous blood (**total mixing lesion**).

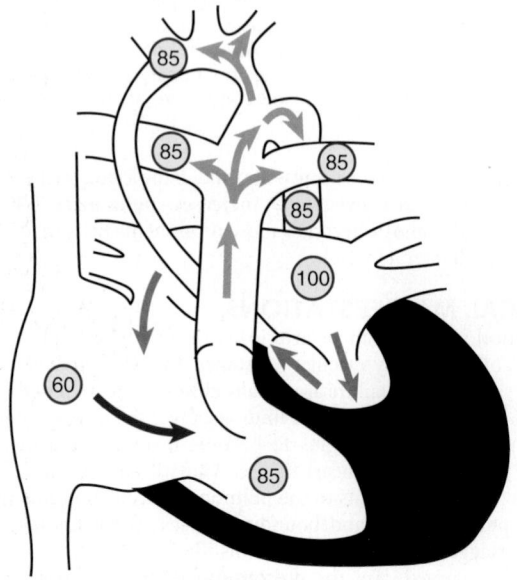

Figure 431-10 Physiology of hypoplastic left-heart syndrome (HLHS). *Circled numbers* represent oxygen saturation values. HLHS is not a single lesion but a constellation of different degrees of hypoplasia of the left-sided heart structures. This drawing shows a patent mitral valve, a small left ventricular cavity, and a diminutive ascending aorta. Right atrial (mixed venous) oxygen saturation is decreased secondary to systemic hypoxemia. Desaturated blood enters the right atrium, flows through the tricuspid valve into the right ventricle, and is ejected into the pulmonary artery. Because of the markedly decreased left ventricular compliance, most of the pulmonary venous blood returning to the left atrium shunts left to right at the atrial level. A small amount of left atrial blood will cross the mitral valve and be ejected into the tiny ascending aorta. The right ventricular oxygen saturation represents a mixing of desaturated systemic venous blood and saturated pulmonary venous blood. Pulmonary artery blood flows into the pulmonary arteries as well as right to left across the patent ductus arteriosus (PDA) into the aorta. Ductal blood flows prograde to the descending aorta as well as retrograde to the ascending aorta, where it supplies the head and neck vessels in addition to the coronary arteries (which arise off the small ascending aorta). Closure of the PDA results in profound hypoxia and circulatory collapse.

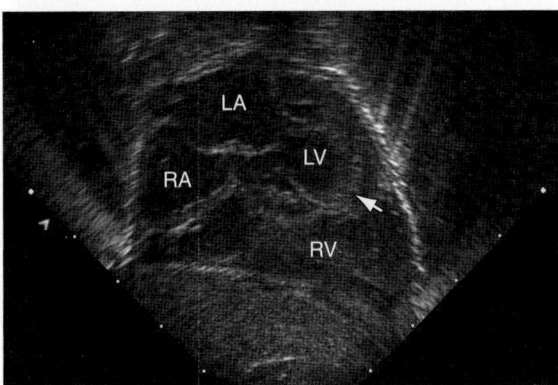

Figure 431-11 Subcostal 2-dimensional echocardiographic diagnosis of hypoplastic left-heart syndrome. The small left ventricular chamber can be seen, the apex of which *(arrowhead)* does not form the apex of the heart. The atrial septum can be seen bowing from the left to the right, indicating that the communication between the 2 atria is pressure restrictive. LA, left atrium; LV, left ventricle; RA, right atrium; RV, right ventricle.

When the ventricular septum is intact, which is usually the case, all the right ventricular blood is ejected into the main pulmonary artery; the descending aorta is supplied via the ductus arteriosus, and flow from the ductus also fills the ascending aorta and coronary arteries in a retrograde fashion. The major hemodynamic abnormalities are inadequate maintenance of the systemic circulation and, depending on the size of the atrial-level communication, either pulmonary venous hypertension (restrictive foramen ovale) or pulmonary overcirculation (moderate or large ASD).

CLINICAL MANIFESTATIONS

Although cyanosis may not always be obvious in the 1st 48 hr of life, a grayish-blue color of the skin is soon apparent and denotes a mix of cyanosis and poor perfusion. The condition is diagnosed in most infants in the 1st few hr or days of life. Once the ductus arteriosus begins to closes, signs of poor systemic perfusion and shock predominate. All of the peripheral pulses may be weak or absent. A palpable right ventricular parasternal lift may be present along with a nondescript systolic murmur.

This lesion may be isolated or associated in 5-15% of patients with known genetic syndromes, such as Turner syndrome, trisomy 13, 18, or 21, Jacobsen syndrome (11q deletion), Holt-Oram syndrome, and Rubinstein-Taybi syndrome. In these circumstances, noncardiac manifestations of the syndrome may be evident and influence the clinical outcomes. Occasionally it is familial and inherited as an autosomal recessive trait.

DIAGNOSIS

On the chest x-ray, the heart is variable in size in the 1st days of life, but cardiomegaly develops rapidly and is associated with increased pulmonary vascularity. The initial electrocardiogram may show only the normal neonatal pattern of right ventricular dominance, but later, P waves become prominent and right ventricular hypertrophy is usual with reduced left ventricular forces. The echocardiogram is diagnostic and demonstrates absence or hypoplasia of the mitral valve and aortic root, a variably small left atrium and left ventricle, and a large right atrium and right ventricle (Fig. 431-11). The size of the atrial communication, by which pulmonary venous blood leaves the left atrium, can be assessed directly and by pulsed and color flow Doppler studies. The small ascending aorta and transverse aortic arch are identified and a discrete coarctation of the aorta in the juxtaductal area may be present, although in the presence of a large ductus, it may be difficult to identify. Doppler echocardiography demonstrates whether the mitral and aortic valves are severely stenotic or totally atretic. The presence of left ventricular coronary sinusoids can be identified. The diagnosis of hypoplastic left-heart syndrome can usually be made without need for

cardiac catheterization. If catheterization is necessary, the hypoplastic ascending aorta is demonstrated by angiography.

PROGNOSIS AND COMPLICATIONS

Untreated patients most often succumb during the 1st few mo of life, usually during the 1st or 2nd wk. Occasionally, unoperated patients may live for months or, rarely, years. Up to 30% of infants with hypoplastic left-heart syndrome have evidence of either a major or minor central nervous system abnormality. Other dysmorphic features may be found in up to 40% of patients. Thus, careful preoperative evaluation (genetic, neurologic, ophthalmologic) should be performed in patients being considered for surgical therapy.

Intermediate-term follow up after completion of all 3 stages of the Norwood procedure demonstrates generally good exercise capacity, and complications equivalent to other patients who have had the Fontan palliation (see Chapter 430.4). Some studies show that patients with hypoplastic left-heart syndrome have a higher risk of neurodevelopmental problems than those with other complex congenital heart lesions. Whether the poor neurodevelopmental outcome is due to prenatal associated central nervous system injury or malformation, the alterations of cerebral hemodynamics during bypass surgery, or poor postoperative perfusion is unknown. In addition, poor outcome is associated with prematurity, chromosome syndromes, and poverty.

TREATMENT

Surgical therapy for hypoplastic left-heart syndrome is associated with improving survival rates, reported as high as 90-95% for the 1st-stage palliation in experienced centers. The 1st-stage repair is designed to construct a reliable source of systemic blood flow arising from the single right ventricle using a combination of aortic and pulmonary arterial tissue, and to limit pulmonary blood flow to avoid heart failure and prevent the development of pulmonary vascular disease. The 2 surgical procedures most commonly utilized are the **Norwood procedure** (Fig. 431-12) and the **Sano procedure.** Primary heart transplantation, previously advocated by a few centers, is much less common because of the substantially improved survival rates with standard surgery and the limited supply of donor organs in this age group.

If a Norwood or Sano procedure is to be performed, preoperative medical management includes correction of acidosis and hypoglycemia, maintenance of ductus arteriosus patency with prostaglandin E_1 (0.01-0.20 µg/kg/min) to support systemic blood flow, and prevention of hypothermia. Preoperative management should avoid excessive pulmonary blood flow; either through management of ventilator settings, increasing the concentration of inspired CO_2, or decreasing the concentration of inspired O_2. Balloon dilation of the atrial septum may be indicated.

The Norwood procedure is usually performed in 3 stages. **Stage I** (see Fig. 431-12) includes an atrial septectomy and transection and ligation of the distal main pulmonary artery; the proximal pulmonary artery is then connected to the transversely opened hypoplastic aortic arch to form a neoaorta, extending through the coarcted segment of the juxtaductal aortic arch. A synthetic aortopulmonary (Blalock-Taussig) shunt connects the aorta to the main pulmonary artery to provide controlled pulmonary blood flow. In the Sano modification, a right ventricle to pulmonary artery conduit is used instead of an aortopulmonary shunt to provide pulmonary blood flow, temporarily creating a double-outlet right ventricle. The operative risk for these 1st-stage procedures has improved dramatically in the past 2 decades and the best reported results demonstrate a 90-95% survival rate.

Stage II consists of a Glenn anastomosis to connect the superior vena cava to the pulmonary arteries (see Chapter 431.4), at between 2 and 6 mo of age. **Stage III**, usually performed at 2-3 yr of age, consists of a modified Fontan procedure (cavopulmonary isolation) to connect the inferior vena cava to the pulmonary arteries via either an intraatrial or external baffle. After **stage III**, all systemic venous return enters the pulmonary circulation directly. Pulmonary venous flow enters the left atrium and is directed across the atrial septum to the tricuspid valve and subsequently to the right (now the systemic) ventricle. Blood leaves the right ventricle via the neoaorta, which supplies the systemic

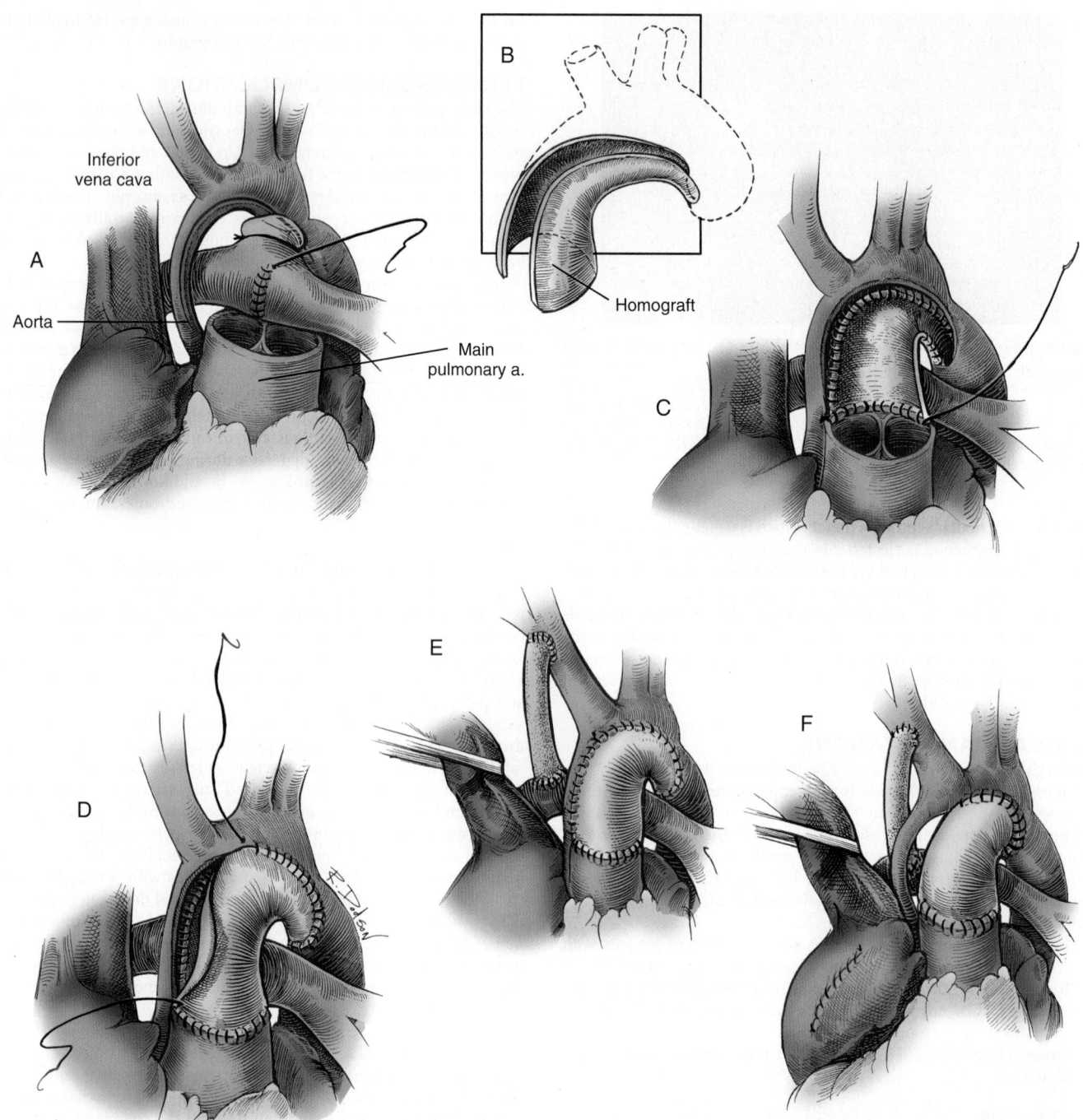

Figure 431-12 The Norwood procedure, 1 of the 2 current techniques for 1st-stage palliation of hypoplastic left-heart syndrome. **A,** Incisions used for the procedure incorporate a cuff of arterial wall allograft. The distal divided main pulmonary artery may be closed by direct suture or with a patch. **B,** Dimensions of the cuff of the arterial wall allograft. **C,** The arterial wall allograft is used to supplement the anastomosis between the proximal divided main pulmonary artery and the ascending aorta, aortic arch, and proximal descending aorta. **D** and **E,** The procedure is completed by an atrial septectomy and a 3.5-mm modified right Blalock shunt. **F,** When the ascending aorta is particularly small, an alternative procedure involves placement of a complete tube of arterial allograft. The tiny ascending aorta may be left in situ, as indicated, or implanted into the side of the neoaorta. *(From Castañeda AR, Jonas RA, Mayer JE Jr, et al: Single-ventricle tricuspid atresia. In Cardiac surgery of the neonate and infant, Philadelphia, 1994, WB Saunders.)*

circulation. The old aortic root now attached to the neoaorta provides coronary blood flow. The risks associated with stages II and III are even less than those of stage I; interstage mortality (usually between stages I and II) has been reduced with the use of home monitoring programs. The short- and long-term benefits of using the Norwood versus the Sano procedure remain to be demonstrated.

An alternative therapeutic approach is to perform a **hybrid procedure** for the 1st stage. This involves performing a Rashkind balloon atrial septostomy, catheter placement of a stent in the ductus arteriosus, and surgical placement of bilateral pulmonary artery bands. After the hybrid procedure, patients can be weaned off prostaglandin and discharged from hospital. After the hybrid procedure, patients need to undergo a more extensive 2nd-stage procedure involving construction of a neoaorta and removal of the pulmonary artery bands.

Another alternative therapy is **cardiac transplantation,** either in the immediate neonatal period, thereby obviating stage I of the Norwood procedure, or after a successful stage I Norwood procedure is performed as a bridge to transplantation. After transplantation, patients usually have normal cardiac function and no symptoms of heart failure; however, these patients have the chronic risk of organ rejection and lifelong immunosuppressive therapy (see Chapter 443.1). The combination of donor shortage and improved results with standard surgical and hybrid procedures has caused most centers to stop recommending transplantation except when associated lesions make the Norwood operation an exceptionally high-risk procedure, or for patients who develop poor ventricular function at some time after the standard surgical approach.

There are some subgroups of patients with hypoplastic left-heart syndrome that may be at increased surgical risk, particularly those with mitral stenosis plus aortic atresia. These data need confirmation in larger studies, and alternative approaches to remain to be developed.

PREVENTION

Serial fetal echocardiographic studies demonstrate that in some fetuses, hypoplastic left-heart syndrome may be a progressive lesion, beginning with simple valvar aortic stenosis in midgestation. The decreased flow through the stenotic aortic valve reduces flow through the left ventricle during development, resulting in gradual ventricular chamber hypoplasia. The potential for preventing this hypoplasia has been demonstrated by performing in utero aortic balloon valvuloplasty in midgestation fetuses (Fig. 431-13). Early results are encouraging,

although even if the aortic valve is successfully opened, adequate ventricular growth occurs in only about 30% of patients. At present, this procedure is regarded as experimental.

Bibliography is available at Expert Consult.

431.11 Abnormal Positions of the Heart and the Heterotaxy Syndromes (Asplenia, Polysplenia)

Daniel Bernstein

Classification and diagnosis of abnormal cardiac position are best performed via a segmental approach, with the position of the viscera and atria defined first, and then the ventricles, followed by the great vessels (Fig. 431-14). Determination of **visceroatrial situs** can be made by radiography demonstration of the position of the abdominal organs and the tracheal bifurcation for recognition of the right and left bronchi and by echocardiography. The atrial situs is usually similar to the situs of the viscera and lungs. In **situs solitus,** the viscera are in their normal positions (stomach and spleen on the left, liver on the right), the

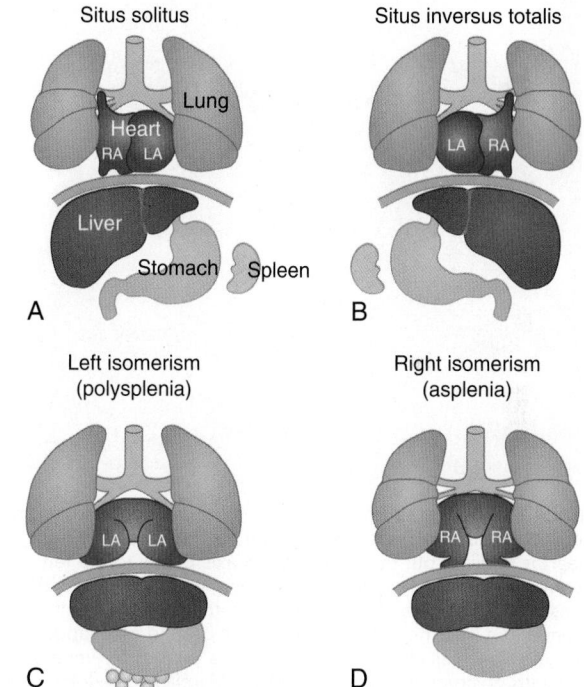

Figure 431-14 Variations in thoracoabdominal situs in congenital heart disease. A, *Situs solitus:* on the right side there is a three-lobed lung, a right atrium (with superior and inferior vena cava entering), and the liver; on the left side there is a two-lobed lung, a left atrium (with pulmonary veins entering), the stomach and the spleen. B, *Situs inversus totalis:* all of the structures are mirror image reversed: on the right side there is a two-lobed lung, a left atrium, the stomach, and the spleen; on the left side there is a three-lobed lung, a right atrium, and the liver. C, *Left isomerism (polysplenia):* there are two left sides: on the right side there is a two-lobed lung and a structure that resembles the left atrium; on the left side there is also a two-lobed lung and a structure that resembles the left atrium; there is usually a midline liver and stomach, and multiple small spleens. D, *Right isomerism (asplenia):* there are two right sides: on the right side there is a three-lobed lung and a structure that resembles the right atrium; on the left side there is also a three-lobed lung and a structure that resembles the right atrium; there is usually a midline liver and stomach, and absent spleen. *(Modified from Fliegauf M, Benzing T, Omran H: When cilia go bad: cilia defects and ciliopathies. Nat Rev Mol Cell Biol 8:880-893, 2007. Fig 2.)*

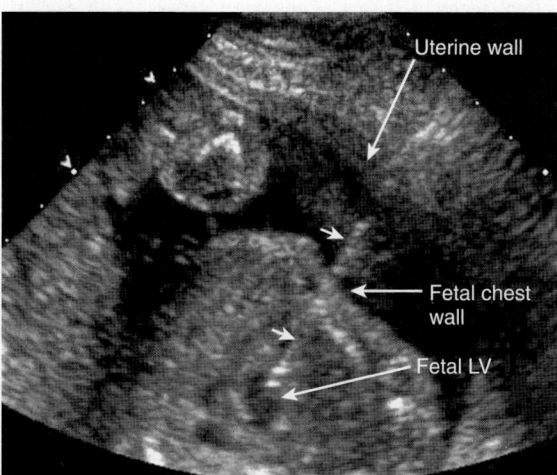

Figure 431-13 Fetal treatment of critical aortic stenosis to prevent development of hypoplastic left-heart syndrome. Fetal ultrasound showing insertion of a needle *(arrowheads)* via the maternal abdominal wall, through the uterus and the fetal chest wall, and into the fetal left ventricle (LV). A balloon catheter is next inserted via the needle into the left ventricular chamber and across the stenotic aortic valve. The balloon is inflated to dilate the valve, the catheter and needle are removed. *(Courtesy of Dr. Stanton Perry, Stanford University, Stanford, CA.)*

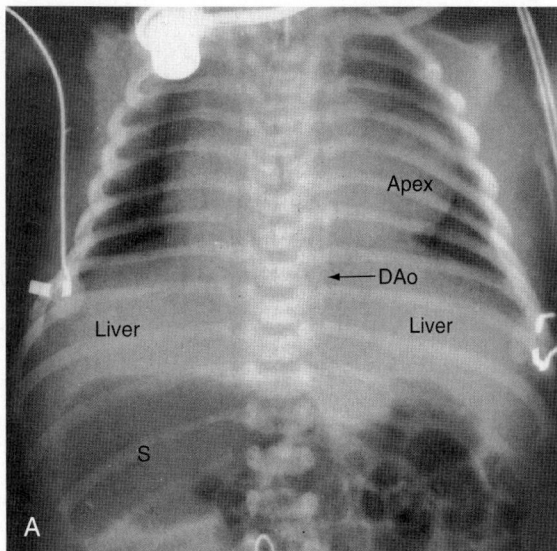

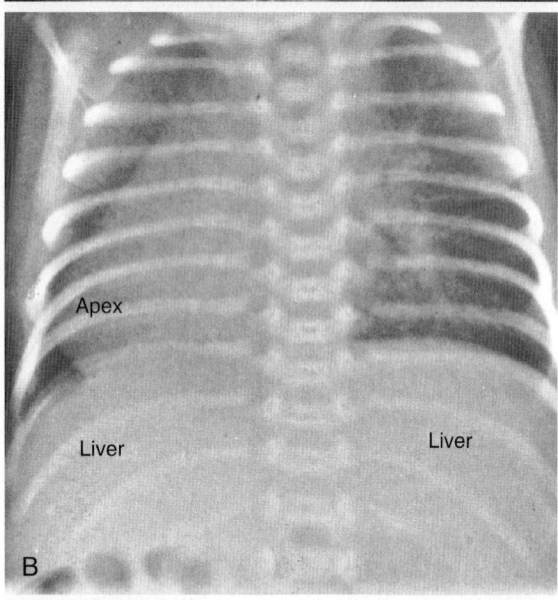

Figure 431-15 A, X-ray from an asplenic male neonate with right isomerism. The liver is transverse, the stomach *(S)* is on the right, and the heart is midline, but the base to apex axis points to the left. DAo, descending aorta. **B,** X-ray from an asplenic male neonate with right isomerism. The liver is transverse, the base to apex axis points to the right, and heart is to the right of midline. The ground-glass appearance of the lungs was caused by total anomalous pulmonary venous connection with obstruction. *(From Perloff JK, Marelli AJ: Perloff's clinical recognition of congenital heart disease, ed 6, Philadelphia, 2012, Elsevier/Saunders, Fig. 3-31, p 32.)*

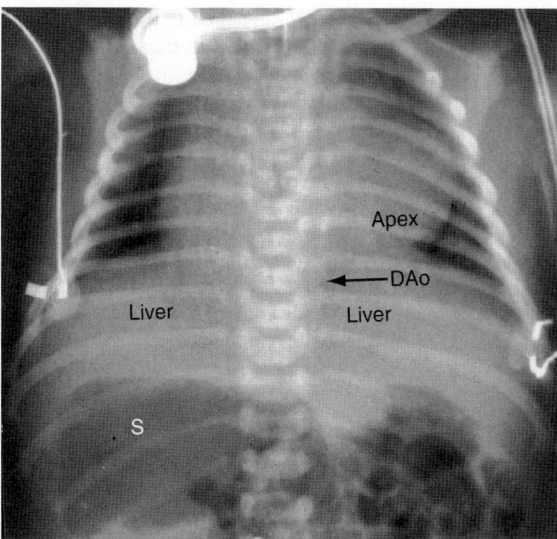

Figure 431-16 X-ray from a polysplenic female neonate with left isomerism. The liver is transverse, the apex is on the left, the stomach *(S)* is on the right, and the descending aorta *(DAo)* is on the left. This opposite-sided arrangement tends to occur in left isomerism. *(From Perloff JK, Marelli AJ: Perloff's clinical recognition of congenital heart disease, ed 6, Philadelphia, 2012, Elsevier/Saunders, Fig. 3-40, p 38.)*

3-lobed right lung is on the right, and the 2-lobed left lung on the left; the right atrium is on the right, and the left atrium is on the left. When the abdominal organs and lung lobation are reversed, an arrangement known as **situs inversus** occur, the left atrium is on the right and the right atrium on the left. If the visceroatrial situs cannot be readily determined, a condition known as **situs indeterminus** or **heterotaxia** exists. The 2 major variations are (1) **asplenia syndrome** (right isomerism or bilateral right-sidedness), which is associated with a centrally located liver, absent spleen, and 2 morphologic right lungs (Fig. 431-15); and (2) **polysplenia syndrome** (left isomerism or bilateral left-sidedness), which is associated with multiple small spleens, absence of the intrahepatic portion of the inferior vena cava, and 2 morphologic left lungs (Fig. 431-16). The heterotaxia syndromes are usually associated with severe congenital heart lesions: ASD, VSD,

atrioventricular septal defect, hypoplasia of 1 of the ventricles, pulmonary stenosis or atresia, and anomalous systemic venous or pulmonary venous return (Table 431-2).

The next segment is localization of the ventricles, which depends on the direction of development of the embryonic cardiac loop. Initial protrusion of the loop to the right (d-loop) carries the future right ventricle anteriorly and to the right, whereas the left ventricle remains posterior and on the left. With situs solitus, a d-loop yields normal atrioventricular connections (right atrium connecting to the right ventricle, left atrium to the left ventricle). Protrusion of the loop to the left (l-loop) carries the future right ventricle to the left and the left ventricle to the right. In this case, in the presence of situs solitus, the right atrium connects with the left ventricle and the left atrium with the right ventricle (**ventricular inversion**).

The final segment is that of the great vessels. With each type of cardiac loop, the ventricular-arterial relationships may be regarded as either normal (right ventricle to the pulmonary artery, left ventricle to the aorta) or transposed (right ventricle to the aorta, left ventricle to the pulmonary artery). A further classification can be based on the position of the aorta (normally to the right and posterior) relative to the pulmonary artery. In transposition, the aorta is usually anterior and either to the right of the pulmonary artery (**d-transposition**) or to the left (**l-transposition**). These segmental relationships can usually be determined by echocardiographic studies demonstrating both atrioventricular and ventriculoarterial relationships. The clinical manifestations of these syndromes of abnormal cardiac position are determined primarily by their associated cardiovascular anomalies.

Dextrocardia occurs when the heart is in the right side of the chest; **levocardia** (the normal situation) is present when the heart is in the left side of the chest. Dextrocardia without associated situs inversus and levocardia in the presence of situs inversus are most often complicated by other severe cardiac malformations. Surveys of older children and adults indicate that dextrocardia with situs inversus and normally related great arteries ("mirror-image" dextrocardia) is often associated with a functionally normal heart, although congenital heart disease of a less severe nature is common.

Anatomic or functional abnormalities of the lungs, diaphragm, and thoracic cage may result in displacement of the heart to the right (**dextroposition**). In this case, however, the cardiac apex is pointed

Table 431-2	Comparison of Cardiosplenic Heterotaxy Syndromes	
FEATURE	**ASPLENIA (RIGHT ISOMERISM)**	**POLYSPLENIA (LEFT ISOMERISM)**
Spleen	Absent	Multiple
Sidedness (isomerism)	Bilateral right	Bilateral left
Lungs	Bilateral trilobar with eparterial bronchi	Bilateral bilobar with hyparterial bronchi
Sex	Male (65%)	Female ≥ male
Right-sided stomach	Yes	Less common
Symmetric liver	Yes	Yes
Partial intestinal rotation	Yes	Yes
Dextrocardia (%)	30-40	30-40
Pulmonary blood flow	Decreased (usually)	Increased (usually)
Severe cyanosis	Yes	No
Transposition of great arteries (%)	60-75	15
Total anomalous pulmonary venous return (%)	70-80	Rare
Common atrioventricular valve (%)	80-90	20-40
Single ventricle (%)	40-50	10-15
Absent inferior vena cava with azygos continuation	No	Characteristic
Bilateral superior vena cava	Yes	Yes
Other common defects	PA, PS	Partial anomalous pulmonary venous return, ventricular septal defect, double-outlet right ventricle
Risk of pneumococcal sepsis	Yes	Yes
Howell-Jolly and Heinz bodies, pitted erythrocytes	Yes	No
Risk of nosocomial infection	Yes	Yes
Absent gallbladder; biliary atresia	No	Yes

PA, pulmonary atresia; PS, pulmonary stenosis.

normally to the left. This anatomic position is less often associated with congenital heart lesions, although hypoplasia of a lung may be accompanied by anomalous pulmonary venous return from that lung (**scimitar syndrome** [see Chapter 426.4]).

The electrocardiogram is difficult to interpret in the presence of lesions with discordant atrial, ventricular, and great vessel anatomy. Diagnosis usually requires detailed echocardiographic and sometimes MRI, CT, or cardiac catheterization studies. The prognosis and treatment of patients with 1 of the cardiac positional anomalies are determined by the underlying defects and are covered in their respective chapters. Asplenia increases the risk of serious infections such as bacterial sepsis and thus requires daily antibiotic prophylaxis. Patients with polysplenia frequently have poor splenic function and may also require prophylaxis against pneumococcal sepsis. Patients with heterotaxia are also at increased risk of intestinal malrotation and volvulus.

Bibliography is available at Expert Consult.

Chapter **432**
Other Congenital Heart and Vascular Malformations

432.1 Anomalies of the Aortic Arch
Daniel Bernstein

RIGHT AORTIC ARCH
In this abnormality, the aorta curves to the right and, if it descends on the right side of the vertebral column, is usually associated with other cardiac malformations. It is found in 20% of cases of tetralogy of Fallot and is also common in truncus arteriosus. A right aortic arch without other cardiac anomalies is not associated with symptoms. It can often be visualized on the chest roentgenogram. The trachea is deviated slightly to the left of the midline rather than to the right, as in the presence of a normal left arch. On a barium esophagogram, the esophagus is indented on its right border at the level of the aortic arch.

VASCULAR RINGS

Congenital abnormalities of the aortic arch and its major branches result in the formation of vascular rings around the trachea and esophagus with varying degrees of compression (Table 432-1). The origin of these lesions can best be appreciated by reviewing the embryology of the aortic arch (see Fig. 420-1 in Chapter 420). The most common anomalies include (1) double aortic arch (Fig. 432-1A), (2) right aortic arch with a left ligamentum arteriosum, (3) anomalous innominate artery arising farther to the left on the arch than usual, (4) anomalous left carotid artery arising farther to the right than usual and passing anterior to the trachea, and (5) anomalous left pulmonary artery (vascular sling). In the latter anomaly, the abnormal vessel arises from an elongated main pulmonary artery or from the right pulmonary artery. It courses between and compresses the trachea and the esophagus. Associated congenital heart disease may be present in 5-50% of patients, depending on the vascular anomaly.

Clinical Manifestations

If the vascular ring produces compression of the trachea and esophagus, symptoms are frequently present during infancy. Chronic wheezing is exacerbated by crying, feeding, and flexion of the neck. Extension of the neck tends to relieve the noisy respiration. Vomiting may also be a component. Affected infants may have a brassy cough, pneumonia, or rarely, sudden death from aspiration.

Diagnosis

Standard roentgenographic examination is not usually helpful. In the past, performing a barium esophagogram was the standard method of diagnosis (Fig. 432-2), replaced today by echocardiography in combination with either MRI or CT. Cardiac catheterization is reserved for cases with associated anomalies or in rare cases where these other modalities are not diagnostic. Bronchoscopy may be helpful in more severe cases to determine the extent of airway narrowing.

Treatment

Surgery is advised for symptomatic patients who have evidence of tracheal compression. The anterior vessel is usually divided in patients with a double aortic arch (see Fig. 432-1B). Compression produced by a right aortic arch and left ligamentum arteriosum is relieved by division of the latter. Anomalous innominate or carotid arteries cannot be

Table 432-1	Vascular Rings					
LESION	SYMPTOMS	PLAIN FILM	BARIUM SWALLOW	BRONCHOSCOPY	MRI ECHOCARDIOGRAPHY	TREATMENT
DOUBLE ARCH	Stridor Respiratory distress Swallowing dysfunction Reflex apnea	AP—wider base of heart Lat.—narrowed trachea displaced forward at C3-C4	Bilateral indentation of esophagus	Bilateral tracheal compression—both pulsatile	Diagnostic	Ligate and divide smaller arch (usually left)
RIGHT ARCH AND LIGAMENTUM/DUCTUS	Respiratory distress Swallowing dysfunction	AP—tracheal deviation to left (right arch)	Bilateral indentation of esophagus R > L	Bilateral tracheal compression—r. pulsatile	Diagnostic	Ligate ligamentum or ductus
ANOMALOUS INNOMINATE	Cough Stridor Reflex apnea	AP—normal Lat.—anterior tracheal compression	Normal	Pulsatile anterior tracheal compression	Unnecessary	Conservative apnea, then suspend
ABERRANT RIGHT SUBCLAVIAN	Occasional swallowing dysfunction	Normal	AP—oblique defect upward to right Lat.—small defect on right posterior wall	Usually normal	Diagnostic	Ligate artery
PULMONARY SLING	Expiratory stridor Respiratory distress	AP—low L. hilum, r. emphysema/atelectasis Lat.—anterior bowing of right bronchus and trachea	±Anterior indentation above carina between esophagus and trachea	Tracheal displacement to left Compression of right main bronchus	Diagnostic	Detach and reanastomose to main pulmonary artery in front of trachea

AP, anteroposterior; L and l., left; Lat., lateral; MRI, magnetic resonance imaging; R and r., right.
From Kliegman RM, Greenbaum LA, Lye PS: Practical strategies in pediatric diagnosis and therapy, ed 2, Philadelphia, 2004, Elsevier, p. 88.

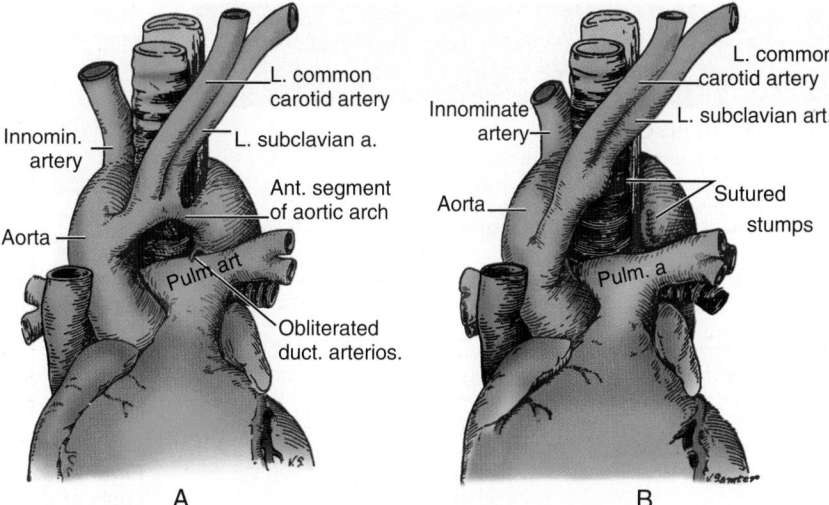

Figure 432-1 Double aortic arch. **A,** Small anterior segment of the double aortic arch (most common type). **B,** Operative procedure for release of the vascular ring.

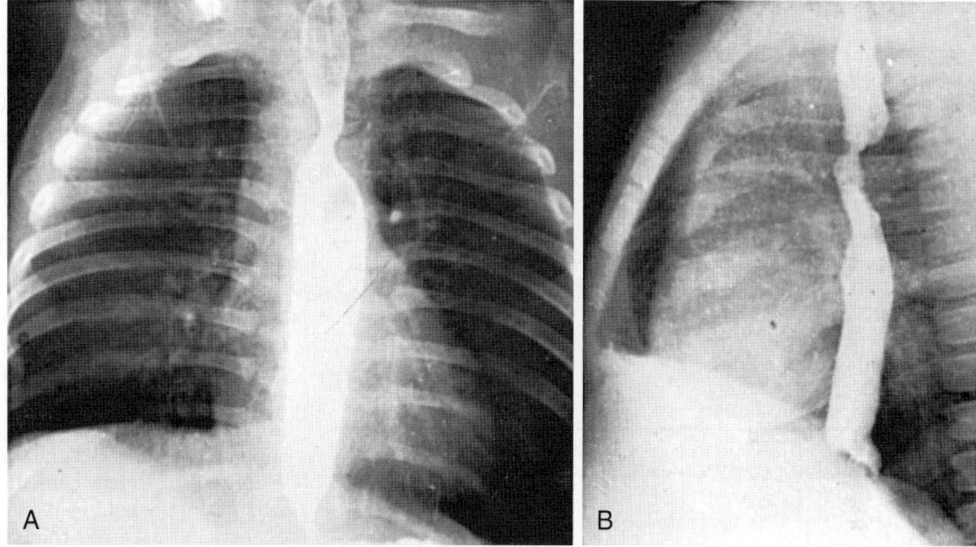

Figure 432-2 Double aortic arch in an infant age 5 mo. **A,** Anteroposterior view. The barium-filled esophagus is constricted on both sides. **B,** Lateral view. The esophagus is displaced forward. The anterior arch was the smaller and was divided at surgery.

divided; attaching the adventitia of these vessels to the sternum usually relieves the tracheal compression. An anomalous left pulmonary artery is corrected by division at its origin and re-anastomosis to the main pulmonary artery after it has been brought in front of the trachea. Severe tracheomalacia, if present, may require reconstruction of the trachea as well.

Bibliography is available at Expert Consult.

432.2 Anomalous Origin of the Coronary Arteries
Daniel Bernstein

Table 432-2 provides a classification system for coronary artery anomalies. Many of these anomalies are isolated. Nonetheless congenital anomalies of the coronary arteries may also be seen in patients with congenital heart disease (tetralogy of Fallot, transposition of the great arteries, congenitally corrected transposition of the great arteries, single ventricle, tricuspid atresia, truncus arteriosus, quadricuspid or bicuspid aortic valves, double-outlet ventricle). In addition, acquired lesions of the coronary arteries caused by existing congenital heart disease may develop as a consequence of hypertension or alterations

in blood flow; congenital heart diseases include coarctation of the aorta, supravalvular aortic stenosis, aortic regurgitation, pulmonary atresia with intact ventricular septum, hypoplastic left-heart syndrome, and coronary ectasia secondary to cyanotic heart disease.

ANOMALOUS ORIGIN OF THE LEFT CORONARY ARTERY FROM THE PULMONARY ARTERY

In anomalous origin of the left coronary artery from the pulmonary artery, the blood supply to the left ventricular myocardium is severely compromised. Soon after birth, as pulmonary arterial pressure falls, perfusion pressure to the left coronary artery becomes inadequate; myocardial ischemia, infarction, and fibrosis result. In some cases, interarterial collateral anastomoses develop between the right and left coronary arteries. Blood flow in the left coronary artery is then reversed, and it empties into the pulmonary artery, a condition known as the "myocardial steal" syndrome. The left ventricle becomes dilated, and its performance is decreased. Mitral insufficiency is a frequent complication secondary to a dilated valve ring or infarction of a papillary muscle. Localized aneurysms may also develop in the left ventricular free wall. Occasional patients have adequate myocardial blood flow during childhood and, later in life, a continuous murmur and a small left-to-right shunt via the dilated coronary system (aorta to right coronary to left coronary to pulmonary artery).

Table 432-2	Congenital Anomalies of Coronary Arteries Unassociated with Congenital Heart Disease

Anomalous Aortic Origin

- Eccentric ostium within an aortic sinus
- Ectopic ostium above an aortic sinus
- Conus artery from the right aortic sinus
- Circumflex coronary artery from the right aortic sinus or from the right coronary artery
- Origin of left anterior descending and circumflex coronary arteries from separate ostia in the left aortic sinus (absence of left main coronary artery)
- Atresia of the left main coronary artery
- Origin of the left anterior descending coronary artery from the right aortic sinus or from the right coronary artery
- Origin of the right coronary artery from the left aortic sinus, from posterior aortic sinus, or from left coronary artery
- Origin of a single coronary artery from the right or left aortic sinus
- Anomalous origin from a noncardiac systemic artery

Anomalous Aortic Origin with Anomalous Proximal Course

- Acute proximal angulation
- Ectopic right coronary artery passing between aorta and pulmonary trunk
  - Ectopic left main coronary artery:
  - Between aorta and pulmonary trunk
  - Anterior to the pulmonary trunk
  - Posterior to the aorta
- Within the ventricular septum (intramyocardial)
- Ectopic left anterior descending coronary artery that is anterior, posterior, or between the aorta and pulmonary trunk

Anomalous Origin of a Coronary Artery from the Pulmonary Trunk

- Left main coronary artery
- Left anterior descending coronary artery
- Right coronary artery
- Both right and left coronary arteries
- Circumflex coronary artery
- Accessory coronary artery

From Perloff JK, Marelli J: Perloff's clinical recognition of congenital heart disease, ed 6, Philadelphia, 2012, Elsevier/Saunders, Table 32-3, p. 532.

Clinical Manifestations

Evidence of heart failure becomes apparent within the 1st few mo of life, and may be exacerbated by respiratory infection. Recurrent attacks of discomfort, restlessness, irritability, sweating, dyspnea, and pallor occur and probably represent **angina pectoris**. Cardiac enlargement is moderate to massive. A gallop rhythm is common. Murmurs may be of the nonspecific ejection type or may be holosystolic due to mitral insufficiency. Older patients with abundant intercoronary anastomoses may have continuous murmurs and minimal left ventricular dysfunction. During adolescence, they may experience angina during exercise. Rare patients with an anomalous right coronary artery may also have such clinical findings.

Diagnosis

Roentgenographic examination confirms the cardiomegaly. The electrocardiogram resembles the pattern described in lateral wall myocardial infarction in adults. A QR pattern followed by inverted T waves is seen in leads I and aVL. The left ventricular surface leads (V_5 and V_6) may also show deep Q waves and exhibit elevated ST segments and inverted T waves (Fig. 432-3). Two-dimensional echocardiography can usually suggest the diagnosis; however, echocardiography is not always reliable in diagnosing this condition. On 2-dimensional imaging alone, the left coronary artery may appear as though it is arising from the aorta. Color Doppler ultrasound examination has improved the accuracy of diagnosis of this lesion, demonstrating the presence of retrograde flow in the left coronary artery. CT or MRI may be helpful in confirming the origin of the coronary arteries. Cardiac catheterization

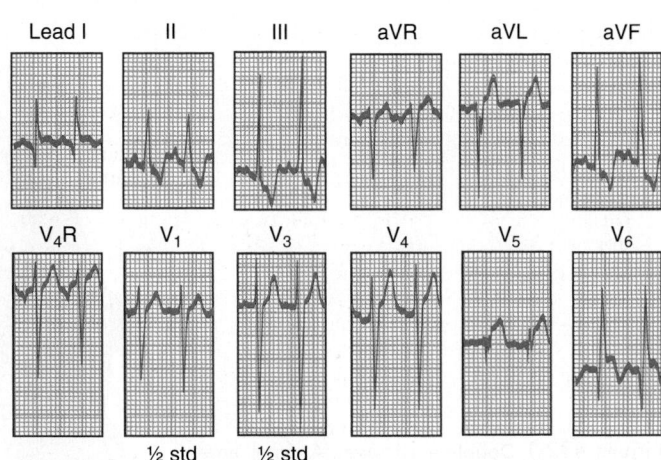

Figure 432-3 Electrocardiogram of a 3 mo old child with anomalous origin of the left coronary artery from the pulmonary artery. Lateral myocardial infarction is present as evidenced by abnormally large and wide Q waves in leads I, V_5, and V_6; an elevated ST segment in V_5 and V_6; and inversion of TV_6.

is diagnostic; aortography shows immediate opacification of the right coronary artery only. This vessel is large and tortuous. After filling of the intercoronary anastomoses, the left coronary artery is opacified, and contrast can be seen to enter the pulmonary artery. Pulmonary arteriography may also opacify the origin of the anomalous left coronary artery. Selective left ventriculography usually demonstrates a dilated left ventricle that empties poorly and mitral regurgitation.

Treatment and Prognosis

Untreated, death often occurs from heart failure within the 1st 6 mo of life. Those who survive generally have abundant intercoronary collateral anastomoses. Medical management includes standard therapy for heart failure (diuretics, angiotensin-converting enzyme inhibitors) and for controlling ischemia (nitrates, β-blocking agents).

Surgical treatment consists of detaching the anomalous coronary artery from the pulmonary artery and anastomosing it to the aorta to establish normal myocardial perfusion. A seriously ill infant with a tiny left coronary artery may present a difficult technical problem. In patients who have already sustained a significant myocardial infarction, cardiac transplantation may be the best option (see Chapter 441.1).

ANOMALOUS ORIGIN OF THE RIGHT CORONARY ARTERY FROM THE PULMONARY ARTERY

Anomalous origin of the right coronary artery from the pulmonary artery is rarely manifested in infancy or early childhood. The left coronary artery is enlarged, whereas the right is thin-walled and mildly enlarged. In early infancy, perfusion of the right coronary artery is from the pulmonary artery, whereas later, perfusion is from collaterals of the left coronary vessels. Angina and sudden death can occur in adolescence or adulthood. When recognized, this anomaly should be repaired by re-anastomosis of the right coronary artery to the aorta.

ECTOPIC ORIGIN OF THE CORONARY ARTERY FROM THE AORTA WITH ABERRANT PROXIMAL COURSE

In ectopic origin of the coronary artery from the aorta with an aberrant proximal course, the aberrant artery may be a left, right, or major branch coronary artery. The site of origin may be the wrong sinus of Valsalva or a proximal coronary artery. The ostium may be hypoplastic, slitlike, or of normal caliber. The aberrant vessel may pass anteriorly, posteriorly, or between the aorta and right ventricular outflow tract; it may tunnel in the conal or interventricular septal tissue. Obstruction resulting from hypoplasia of the ostia, tunneling between the aorta and right ventricular outflow tract or interventricular septum, and acute angulation produces myocardial infarction. Unobstructed vessels produce no symptoms. Patients with this extremely rare abnormality are often initially seen with severe myocardial infarction, ventricular arrhythmias, angina pectoris, or syncope; sudden death may occur, especially in young athletes.

Diagnostic modalities include an electrocardiogram, stress testing, 2-dimensional echocardiography, CT or MRI, radionuclide perfusion scan, and cardiac catheterization with selective coronary angiography.

Treatment is indicated for obstructed vessels and consists of aortoplasty with reanastomosis of the aberrant vessel or, occasionally, coronary artery bypass grafting. The management of asymptomatic infants with these forms of ectopic coronary origin remains controversial.

Bibliography is available at Expert Consult.

432.3 Pulmonary Arteriovenous Fistula
Daniel Bernstein

Fistulous vascular communications in the lungs may be large and localized or multiple, scattered, and small. The most common form of this unusual condition is the **Osler-Weber-Rendu syndrome** (hereditary hemorrhagic telangiectasia type I), which is also associated with angiomas of the nasal and buccal mucous membranes, gastrointestinal tract, or liver. Mutations in the endoglin gene, a cell surface component of the transforming growth factor-β receptor complex causes this syndrome. The usual communication is between the pulmonary artery and pulmonary vein; direct communication between the pulmonary artery and left atrium is extremely rare. Desaturated blood in the pulmonary artery is shunted through the fistula into the pulmonary vein, thus bypassing the lungs, and then enters the left side of the heart resulting in systemic arterial desaturation and, sometimes, clinically detectable cyanosis. The shunt across the fistula is at low pressure and resistance, so pulmonary arterial pressure is normal; cardiomegaly and heart failure are not present.

The clinical manifestations depend on the magnitude of the shunt. Large fistulas are associated with dyspnea, cyanosis, clubbing, a continuous murmur, and polycythemia. Hemoptysis is rare, but when it occurs, it may be massive. Features of the Osler-Weber-Rendu syndrome are seen in ≈50% of patients (or other family members) and include recurrent epistaxis and gastrointestinal tract bleeding. Transitory dizziness, diplopia, aphasia, motor weakness, or convulsions may result from cerebral thrombosis, abscess, or paradoxical emboli. Soft systolic or continuous murmurs may be audible over the site of the fistula. The electrocardiogram is normal. Roentgenographic examination of the chest may show opacities produced by large fistulas; multiple small fistulas may be visualized by fluoroscopy (as abnormal pulsations), MRI, or CT. Selective pulmonary arteriography demonstrates the site, extent, and distribution of the fistulas.

Treatment consisting of excision of solitary or localized lesions by lobectomy or wedge resection results in complete disappearance of symptoms. In most instances, fistulas are so widespread that surgery is not possible. Any direct communication between the pulmonary artery and the left atrium can be obliterated.

Patients who have undergone a **Glenn cavopulmonary** anastomosis for cyanotic congenital heart disease (see Chapter 430.4) are also at risk for the development of pulmonary arteriovenous malformations. In these patients, the arteriovenous malformations are usually multiple and the risk increases over time after the Glenn procedure. These malformations rarely occur after the heart disease is fully palliated by completion of the Fontan operation. This finding suggests that the pulmonary circulation requires an as yet undetermined hepatic factor to suppress the development of arteriovenous malformations. The hallmark of the development of these malformations is a decrease in the patient's oxygen saturation. The diagnosis can often be made with contrast echocardiography; cardiac catheterization is the definitive

test. Completion of the Fontan circuit, so that inferior vena cava blood flow (containing hepatic venous drainage) is routed through the lungs, usually results in improvement or resolution of the malformations.

Bibliography is available at Expert Consult.

432.4 Ectopia Cordis
Daniel Bernstein

In the most common thoracic form of ectopia cordis, the sternum is split and the heart protrudes outside the chest. In other forms, the heart protrudes through the diaphragm into the abdominal cavity or may be situated in the neck. Associated intracardiac anomalies are common. **Pentalogy of Cantrell** consists of ectopia cordis, midline supraumbilical abdominal defect, deficiency of the anterior diaphragm, defect of the lower sternum, and an intracardiac defect (either a ventricular septal defect, tetralogy of Fallot, or diverticulum of the left ventricle). Death may occur early in life, usually from infection, cardiac failure, or hypoxemia. Surgical therapy for neonates without overwhelmingly severe cardiac anomalies consists of covering the heart with skin without compromising venous return or ventricular ejection. Repair or palliation of associated defects is also necessary.

432.5 Diverticulum of the Left Ventricle
Daniel Bernstein

Left ventricular diverticulum is a rare anomaly, where the diverticulum protrudes into the epigastrium. The lesion may be isolated or associated with complex cardiovascular anomalies. A pulsating mass is usually visible and palpable in the epigastrium. Systolic or systolic-diastolic murmurs produced by blood flow into and out of the diverticulum may be audible over the lower part of the sternum and the mass. The electrocardiogram shows a pattern of complete or incomplete left bundle branch block. Roentgenograms of the chest may or may not show the mass. Associated abnormalities include defects of the sternum, abdominal wall, diaphragm, and pericardium (see earlier). Surgical treatment of the diverticulum and associated cardiac defects can be performed in selected cases. Occasionally, a diverticulum may be small and not associated with clinical signs or symptoms. These small diverticula are diagnosed at the time of echocardiographic examination for other indications.

Chapter **433**
Pulmonary Hypertension

433.1 Primary Pulmonary Hypertension
Daniel Bernstein

PATHOPHYSIOLOGY
Primary pulmonary hypertension is characterized by pulmonary vascular obstructive disease and right-sided heart failure. It occurs at any age, although in pediatric patients the mean age at diagnosis is 7-10 yr. In patients with idiopathic or familial disease, females outnumber males 1.7:1; in other patients, both genders are represented equally. Some patients have evidence of either an immunologic disorder or a hypercoagulable state. Mutations in the gene for bone morphogenetic protein receptor-2 (*BMPR-2*, a member of the transforming growth factor-β receptor family) on chromosome 2q33 have been identified in 70% of patients with familial primary pulmonary hypertension (known as *PPH1*) and in 10-20% with idiopathic sporadic pulmonary

hypertension. Other potential disease causing genes include *PPH2*, *ALK1*, *ENG*, *SMAD9*, *CAV1*, and *KCNK3*, which causes a channelopathy in familial and sporadic cases of primary pulmonary hypertension. Viral infection, such as with the vasculotropic human herpesvirus 8, has been suggested as a trigger factor in many patients. Diet pills, particularly fenfluramine, have also been implicated. Pulmonary hypertension is a common complication of sickle cell anemia and other hemolytic anemias. Pulmonary hypertension is associated with precapillary obstruction of the pulmonary vascular bed as a result of hyperplasia of the muscular and elastic tissues and a thickened intima of the small pulmonary arteries and arterioles (Fig. 433-1). Secondary atherosclerotic changes may be found in the larger pulmonary arteries as well. In children, **pulmonary venoocclusive disease** may account for some cases of primary pulmonary hypertension. Before a diagnosis of primary pulmonary hypertension can be made, other causes of elevated pulmonary arterial pressure must be eliminated (chronic pulmonary parenchymal disease, persistent obstruction of the upper airway, congenital cardiac malformations, recurrent pulmonary emboli, alveolar capillary dysplasia, liver disease, autoimmune disease,

and moyamoya disease). Table 433-1 provides a classification system. Idiopathic or familial disease is the most common in pediatric patients (~55%), followed by pulmonary hypertension secondary to congenital heart disease (~35%) and chronic respiratory disorders (~15%).

Pulmonary hypertension places an afterload burden on the right ventricle, which results in right ventricular hypertrophy. Dilation of the pulmonary artery is present, and pulmonary valve insufficiency may occur. In the later stages of the disease, the right ventricle dilates, tricuspid insufficiency develops, and cardiac output is decreased. Arrhythmias, syncope, and sudden death are common.

CLINICAL MANIFESTATIONS

The predominant symptoms include exercise intolerance (dyspnea) and fatigability; occasionally, precordial chest pain, dizziness, or headaches are noted. Syncope may be noted in ~30% of pediatric patients. Peripheral cyanosis may be present, especially during exercise or in patients with a patent foramen ovale through which blood can shunt from right to left; in the late stages of disease, patients may have cold extremities and a gray appearance associated with low cardiac output. Arterial oxygen saturation is usually normal unless there is an associated intracardiac shunt. If right-sided heart failure has supervened, jugular venous pressure is elevated, and hepatomegaly and edema are present. Jugular venous *a* waves are present, and in those with functional tricuspid insufficiency, a conspicuous jugular *cv* wave and systolic hepatic pulsations are manifested. The heart is moderately enlarged, and a right ventricular heave can be noted. The 1st heart sound is often followed

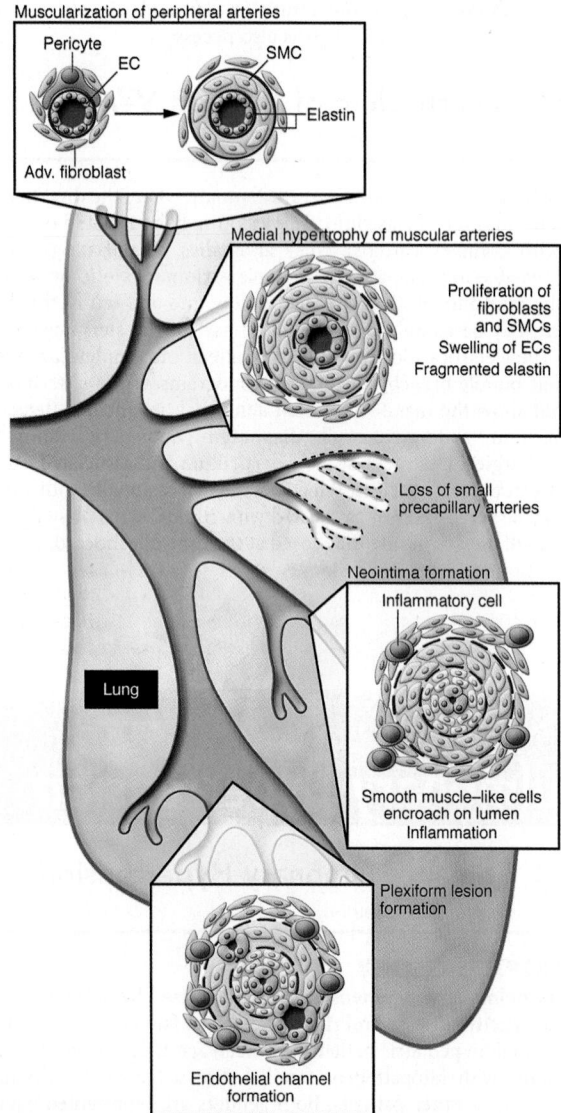

Figure 433-1 Vascular abnormalities associated with pulmonary arterial hypertension: abnormal muscularization of distal and medial precapillary arteries, loss of precapillary arteries, thickening of large pulmonary arterioles, and neointimal formation that is occlusive in vessels <500-100 μM and in plexiform lesions therein. (*From Rabinovitch M: Molecular pathogenesis of pulmonary arterial hypertension. J Clin Invest 122:4306-4313, 2012, Fig. 1.*)

Table 433-1	Revised World Health Organization Classification of Pulmonary Hypertension

1. Pulmonary arterial hypertension (PAH)
  1.1. Idiopathic (IPAH)
  1.2. Familial (FPAH)
  1.3. Associated with (APAH):
    1.3.1. Connective tissue disorder
    1.3.2. Congenital systemic-to-pulmonary shunts
    1.3.3. Portal hypertension
    1.3.4. HIV infection
    1.3.5. Drugs and toxins
    1.3.6. Other (thyroid disorders, glycogen storage disease, Gaucher disease, hereditary hemorrhagic telangiectasia, hemoglobinopathies, chronic myeloproliferative disorders, splenectomy)
  1.4. Associated with significant venous or capillary involvement
    1.4.1. Pulmonary venoocclusive disease (PVOD)
    1.4.2. Pulmonary capillary hemangiomatosis (PCH)
  1.5. Persistent pulmonary hypertension of the newborn
2. Pulmonary hypertension with left-heart disease
  2.1. Left-sided atrial or ventricular heart disease
  2.2. Left-sided valvular heart disease
3. Pulmonary hypertension associated with lung diseases and/or hypoxemia
  3.1. Chronic obstructive pulmonary disease
  3.2. Interstitial lung disease
  3.3. Sleep disordered breathing
  3.4. Alveolar hypoventilation disorders
  3.5. Chronic exposure to high altitude
  3.6. Developmental abnormalities
4. Pulmonary hypertension due to chronic thrombotic and/or embolic disease (CTEPH)
  4.1. Thromboembolic obstruction of proximal pulmonary arteries
  4.2. Thromboembolic obstruction of distal pulmonary arteries
  4.3. Nonthrombotic pulmonary embolism (tumor, parasites, foreign material)
5. Miscellaneous: sarcoidosis, histiocytosis X, lymphangiomatosis, compression of pulmonary vessels (adenopathy, tumor, fibrosing mediastinitis)

From ACCF/AHA: 2009 Expert consensus document on pulmonary hypertension: a report of the American College of Cardiology Foundation Task Force on Expert Consensus Documents and the American Heart Association developed in collaboration with the American College of Chest Physicians; American Thoracic Society, Inc; and the Pulmonary Hypertension Association, J Am Coll Cardiol 53:1573–1619, 2009.

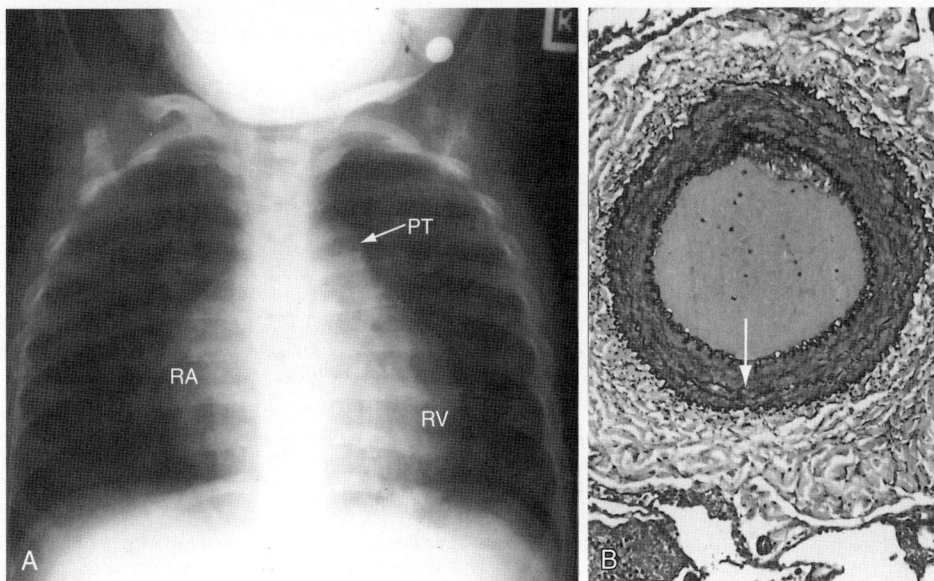

Figure 433-2 A, X-ray from a 3 yr old girl with primary pulmonary hypertension. Pulmonary vascularity is reduced. The pulmonary trunk (PT), right atrium (RA), and right ventricle (RV) are considerably enlarged. **B,** Histology of an intrapulmonary artery at necropsy shows medial hypertrophy *(arrow). (From Perloff JK, Marelli AJ: Perloff's clinical recognition of congenital heart disease, ed 6, Philadelphia, 2012, Elsevier/Saunders, Fig. 14-17, p. 207.)*

by an ejection click emanating from the dilated pulmonary artery. The 2nd heart sound is narrowly split, loud, and sometimes booming in quality; it is frequently palpable at the upper left sternal border. A presystolic gallop rhythm may be audible at the lower left sternal border. The systolic murmur is soft and short and is sometimes followed by a blowing decrescendo diastolic murmur caused by pulmonary insufficiency. In later stages, a holosystolic murmur of tricuspid insufficiency is appreciated at the lower left sternal border.

DIAGNOSIS

Chest radiographs reveal a prominent pulmonary artery and right ventricle (Fig. 433-2). The pulmonary vascularity in the hilar areas may be prominent, in contrast to the peripheral lung fields in which pulmonary markings are decreased. The electrocardiogram shows right ventricular hypertrophy, often with spiked P waves. Echocardiography is used to screen for any congenital cardiac malformations. Doppler evaluation of the tricuspid valve, if insufficiency is present, will allow estimation of the right ventricular (and hence pulmonary arterial) systolic pressure.

At cardiac catheterization, the presence of left-sided obstructive lesions (pulmonary venous stenosis, mitral stenosis, restrictive cardiomyopathy) that result in pulmonary venous hypertension can be evaluated (see Chapters 427.9, 431.7, and 439.3). The presence of pulmonary arterial hypertension with a normal pulmonary capillary wedge pressure is diagnostic of primary pulmonary hypertension. If the wedge pressure is elevated and left ventricular end-diastolic pressure is normal, obstruction at the level of the pulmonary veins, left atrium, or mitral valve should be suspected. If left ventricular end-diastolic pressure is also elevated, the diagnosis of restrictive cardiomyopathy should be entertained. The risks associated with cardiac catheterization are increased in severely ill patients with primary pulmonary hypertension.

PROGNOSIS AND TREATMENT

Primary pulmonary hypertension is progressive, and no cure is currently available. Some success has been reported with oral calcium channel blocking agents such as nifedipine in children who demonstrate pulmonary vasoreactivity when these agents are administered during catheterization. Continuous intravenous infusion of the arachidonic acid metabolite, prostacyclin (epoprostenol), provides relief as long as the infusion is continued. Despite the success of prostacyclin in reducing symptoms and improving quality of life, it slows but does not stop

the progression of the disease. Treprostinil, a prostacyclin analog with a longer half-life has also been shown to be effective. Continuous administration of nitric oxide via nasal cannula, nebulized forms of prostacyclin (iloprost), and orally administered pulmonary vasodilators (bosentan, an antagonist of endothelin receptors; or sildenafil, a phosphodiesterase type 5 inhibitor) have been used with success in adults and in preliminary clinical studies in children (Table 433-2). Anticoagulation may be of value in patients with previous pulmonary thromboemboli; some of these patients may respond to balloon angioplasty of narrowed pulmonary artery segments. Riociguat, a soluble guanylate cyclase stimulator, with vasorelaxation, antiproliferation, and antifibrotic properties, has proven effective in adults with chronic thromboembolic or idiopathic pulmonary hypertension. Despite many advances, definitive therapy is still heart-lung or lung transplantation (see Chapter 443.2). In patients with severe pulmonary hypertension and low cardiac output, the terminal event is often sudden and related to a lethal arrhythmia. Patients with primary pulmonary hypertension diagnosed in infancy often have rapid progression and high mortality.

433.2 Pulmonary Vascular Disease (Eisenmenger Syndrome)

Daniel Bernstein

PATHOPHYSIOLOGY

The term *Eisenmenger syndrome* refers to patients with a ventricular septal defect in which blood is shunted partially or totally from right to left as a result of the development of pulmonary vascular disease. This physiologic abnormality can also occur with atrioventricular septal defect, ventricular septal defect, patent ductus arteriosus or any other communication between the aorta and pulmonary artery, and in many forms of complex congenital heart disease with unrestricted pulmonary blood flow. Pulmonary vascular disease with an isolated atrial septal defect can occur, but is less common and does not occur until late in adulthood.

In Eisenmenger syndrome, pulmonary vascular resistance after birth either remains high or, after having decreased during early infancy, rises thereafter because of increased shear stress on pulmonary arterioles. Factors playing a role in the rapidity of development of pulmonary vascular disease include increased pulmonary arterial pressure, increased pulmonary blood flow, and the presence of hypoxia or hypercapnia. Early

Table 433-2	Summary of Drugs Used to Treat Pulmonary Hypertension*	
DRUG AND MECHANISM OF ACTION	**DOSES USED IN PEDIATRIC STUDIES**	**COMMON SIDE EFFECTS**
Epoprostenol (prostacyclin [PGI₂], a potent vasodilator; also inhibits platelet aggregation)	1 ng/kg/min initially. Increase based on clinical course and tolerance to 5-50 ng/kg/min. Some patients may require even higher doses. Must be given by continuous infusion that is not interrupted	Flushing, headache, nausea, diarrhea, hypotension, chest pain, jaw pain
Iloprost (synthetic analog of PGI₂)	2.5-5.0 μg 6-9 times daily (not more frequently than every 2 hr) via inhalation	Flushing, headache, diarrhea, hypotension, jaw pain, exacerbation of pulmonary symptoms (cough, wheezing)
Treprostinil (synthetic analog of PGI₂)	1 ng/kg/min initially. Target dose ranges from 20-80 ng/kg/min. Given either IV or SC via continuous infusion. Longer half-life than epoprostenol	Flushing, headache, diarrhea, hypotension, jaw pain. Pain at infusion site when given SC
Bosentan, ambrisentan, (endothelin receptor EtA and EtB antagonist)	2 mg/kg/dose bid. Use ½ dose for 1st mo and check for liver function test abnormalities prior to up-titrating	Flushing, headache, diarrhea, hypotension, fluid retention, exacerbation of heart failure, anemia, elevated liver function tests, palpitations
Sildenafil (inhibitor of cyclic guanosine monophosphate-specific phosphodiesterase 5)	1 mg/kg/dose given 3-4 times daily. Initial dosing should be ½ final target dose to evaluate for hypotension	Flushing, headache, diarrhea, myalgia, hypotension, priapism, visual disturbance (blue coloration)
Calcium channel blockers (amlodipine, diltiazem, nifedipine)	Previously widely used. Now indicated only for patients who show a strong response to nitric oxide during cardiac catheterization	Flushing, headache, edema, arrhythmia, headache, hypotension, rash, nausea, constipation, elevated liver function tests

*These medications should only be administered under the direction of a specialist in pulmonary hypertension.

in the course of disease, pulmonary hypertension (elevated pressure in the pulmonary arteries) is the result of markedly increased pulmonary blood flow (hyperkinetic pulmonary hypertension). This form of pulmonary hypertension decreases with the administration of pulmonary vasodilators such as nitric oxide, or oxygen, or both. With the development of Eisenmenger syndrome, pulmonary hypertension is the result of pulmonary vascular disease (obstructive pathologic changes in the pulmonary vessels). This form of pulmonary hypertension is usually only minimally responsive to pulmonary vasodilators or oxygen or not at all.

PATHOLOGY AND PATHOPHYSIOLOGY

The pathologic changes of Eisenmenger syndrome occur in the small pulmonary arterioles and muscular arteries (<300 μm) and are graded on the basis of histologic characteristics (Heath-Edwards classification): **Grade I** changes involve medial hypertrophy alone, **grade II** consists of medial hypertrophy and intimal hyperplasia, **grade III** involves near obliteration of the vessel lumen, **grade IV** includes arterial dilation, and **grades V and VI** include plexiform lesions, angiomatoid formation, and fibrinoid necrosis. Grades IV-VI indicate irreversible pulmonary vascular obstructive disease. Eisenmenger physiology is usually defined by an absolute elevation in pulmonary arterial resistance to greater than 12 Wood units (resistance units indexed to body surface area) or by a ratio of pulmonary to systemic vascular resistance of ≥1.0.

Pulmonary vascular disease occurs more rapidly in patients with trisomy 21 who have left-to-right shunts. It also complicates the natural history of patients with elevated pulmonary venous pressure secondary to mitral stenosis or left ventricular dysfunction, especially in those patients with restrictive cardiomyopathy (see Chapter 445.3). Pulmonary vascular disease can also occur in any patient with transmission of systemic pressure to the pulmonary circulation via a shunt at the interventricular or great vessel level, and in patients chronically exposed to low Po_2 (because of high altitude). Patients with cyanotic congenital heart lesions associated with unrestricted pulmonary blood flow are at particularly high risk.

CLINICAL MANIFESTATIONS

Symptoms do not usually develop until the 2nd or 3rd decade of life, although a more fulminant course may occur. Intracardiac or extracardiac communications that would normally shunt from left to right are converted to right-to-left shunting as pulmonary vascular resistance exceeds systemic vascular resistance. Cyanosis becomes apparent, and dyspnea, fatigue, and a tendency toward dysrhythmias begin to occur. In the late stages of the disease, heart failure, chest pain, headaches, syncope, and hemoptysis may be seen. Physical examination reveals a right ventricular heave and a narrowly split 2nd heart sound with a loud pulmonic component. Palpable pulmonary artery pulsation may be present at the left upper sternal border. A holosystolic murmur of tricuspid regurgitation may be audible along the left sternal border. An early decrescendo diastolic murmur of pulmonary insufficiency may also be heard along the left sternal border. The degree of cyanosis depends on the stage of the disease.

DIAGNOSIS

Roentgenographically, the heart varies in size from normal to greatly enlarged; the latter usually occurs late in the course of the disease. The main pulmonary artery is generally prominent, similar to primary pulmonary hypertension (see Fig. 433-2). The pulmonary vessels are enlarged in the hilar areas and taper rapidly in caliber in the peripheral branches. The right ventricle and atrium are prominent. The electrocardiogram shows marked right ventricular hypertrophy. The P wave may be tall and spiked. Cyanotic patients have various degrees of polycythemia that depend on the severity and duration of hypoxemia.

The echocardiogram shows a thick-walled right ventricle and demonstrates the underlying congenital heart lesion. Two-dimensional echocardiography assists in eliminating from consideration lesions such as obstructed pulmonary veins, supramitral membrane, mitral stenosis, and restrictive cardiomyopathy. Doppler studies demonstrate the direction of the intracardiac shunt and the presence of a typical hypertension waveform in the main pulmonary artery. Tricuspid and pulmonary regurgitation can be used in the Doppler examination to estimate pulmonary arterial systolic and diastolic pressures.

Cardiac catheterization usually shows a bidirectional shunt at the site of the defect. Systolic pressure is generally equal in the systemic and pulmonary circulations. Pulmonary capillary wedge pressure is normal unless a left-sided heart obstructive lesion or left ventricular failure is the cause of the pulmonary arterial hypertension. Arterial oxygen saturation is decreased depending on the magnitude of the right-to-left shunt. The response to vasodilator therapy (oxygen, prostacyclin, nitric oxide) may identify patients with hyperdynamic pulmonary hypertension. Selective pulmonary artery injections may be necessary if pulmonary venous obstruction is suspected because of high wedge pressure and low left ventricular end-diastolic pressure.

TREATMENT

The best management for patients who are at risk for the development of late pulmonary vascular disease is prevention by early surgical elimination of large intracardiac or great vessel communications during infancy. Some patients may be missed because they have not shown early clinical manifestations. Rarely, pulmonary vascular resistance never decreases at birth in these infants, and therefore they never acquire enough left-to-right shunting to become clinically apparent. Such delayed recognition is a particular risk in patients with congenital heart disease who live at high altitude. It is also a risk in infants with trisomy 21, who have a propensity for earlier development of pulmonary vascular disease. Because of the high incidence of congenital heart disease associated with trisomy 21, routine echocardiography is recommended at the time of initial diagnosis, even in the absence of other clinical findings.

Medical treatment of Eisenmenger syndrome is primarily symptomatic. Many patients benefit substantially from either oral (calcium channel blocker, endothelin antagonist, phosphodiesterase inhibitors) or chronic intravenous (prostacyclin) therapy. Combined heart-lung or bilateral lung transplantation is the only surgical option for many of these patients (see Chapter 443.2).

Bibliography is available at Expert Consult.

Chapter **434**

General Principles of Treatment of Congenital Heart Disease

Daniel Bernstein

Most patients who have mild congenital heart disease require no treatment. The parents and child should be made aware that a normal life is expected and that no restriction of the child's activities is necessary. Overprotective parents may use the presence of a mild congenital heart lesion or even a functional heart murmur as a means to exert excessive control over their child's activities. Although fears may not be expressed overtly, the child may become anxious regarding early death or debilitation, especially when an adult member of the family acquires unrelated symptomatic heart disease. The family may have an unexpressed fear of sudden death, and the rarity of this manifestation should be emphasized in discussions directed at improving their understanding of the child's congenital heart defect. The difference between congenital heart disease and degenerative coronary disease in adults should be emphasized. General health maintenance, including a well-balanced, "heart-healthy" diet; aerobic exercise; and avoidance of smoking, should be encouraged.

Even patients with moderate to severe heart disease need not be restricted from all physical activity, although many will tend to limit their own activities. **Physical education** should be modified appropriately to the child's capacity to participate; the extent of such modification can often be guided by formal exercise testing. Although

competitive sports for some patients may need to be discouraged, decisions are made on an individual basis. The influence of coach and peer pressure should be taken into account when recommending competitive versus noncompetitive athletics. Many cardiologists will also prohibit certain high-impact activities ("collision sports") such as tackle football or contact martial arts in patients with some forms of prior open heart surgery.

Routine immunizations should be given, with the inclusion of influenza vaccine during the appropriate season. Prophylaxis against the respiratory syncytial virus is recommended during respiratory syncytial virus season in young infants with unrepaired congenital heart disease and significant hemodynamic abnormalities. However, careful consideration for timing of administration of live-virus vaccination is required in patients who are potential candidates for heart or heart-lung transplantation.

Bacterial infections should be treated vigorously, but the presence of congenital heart disease is not an appropriate reason to use antibiotics indiscriminately. Prophylaxis against bacterial endocarditis should be carried out during dental procedures for appropriate patients. The American Heart Association has recently significantly revised these recommendations, with most patients no longer requiring routine prophylaxis (see Chapter 437). Endocarditis prophylaxis is generally no longer recommended for gastrointestinal or genitourinary procedures.

Cyanotic patients need to be monitored for noncardiac manifestations of oxygen deficiency (Table 434-1). Treatment of iron-deficiency anemia is important in cyanotic patients, who will show improved exercise tolerance and general well-being with adequate hemoglobin levels. These patients should also be carefully observed for excessive polycythemia. Cyanotic patients should avoid situations in which dehydration may occur, which leads to increased viscosity and increases the risk of stroke. Diuretics may need to be decreased or temporarily discontinued during episodes of acute gastroenteritis. High altitudes and sudden changes in the thermal environment should also be avoided. Phlebotomy with partial exchange transfusion is carried out only in symptomatic patients with severe **polycythemia** (usually those whose hematocrit is >65%).

Patients with moderate to severe forms of congenital heart disease or a history of rhythm disturbance should be carefully monitored during anesthesia for even routine surgical procedures. Consultation with an anesthesiologist experienced in the care of children with congenital heart disease is recommended. Women with nonrepaired severe congenital heart disease should be counseled on the risks associated with childbearing and on the use of contraceptives and tubal ligation. Pregnancy may be dangerous to both mother and fetus for patients with chronic cyanosis or pulmonary arterial hypertension. Women with mild to moderate heart disease and many of those who have had corrective surgery can have normal pregnancies, although those with residual hemodynamic derangements or with systemic right ventricles should be followed by a high-risk perinatologist and a cardiologist with expertise in caring for adults with congenital heart disease.

POSTOPERATIVE MANAGEMENT

After successful open heart surgery, the severity of the congenital heart defect, the age and condition (nutritional status) of the patient before surgery, the events in the operating room, and the quality of the postoperative care influence the patient's course. Intraoperative factors that influence survival and that should be noted when a patient returns from the operating room include the duration of cardiopulmonary bypass, the duration of aortic cross-clamping (the time during which the heart is not being perfused), and the duration of profound hypothermia (used in some newborns: the period during which the entire body is not being perfused).

Immediate postoperative care should be provided in an intensive care unit staffed by a team of physicians, nurses, and technicians experienced with the unique problems encountered after open heart surgery in childhood. In most major centers, this occurs in a dedicated pediatric cardiovascular intensive care unit. Preparation for postoperative monitoring begins in the operating room, where the anesthesiologist

Table 434-1	Extracardiac Complications of Cyanotic Congenital Heart Disease and Eisenmenger Physiology	
PROBLEM	**ETIOLOGY**	**THERAPY**
Polycythemia	Persistent hypoxia	Phlebotomy
Relative anemia	Nutritional deficiency	Iron replacement
CNS abscess	Right-to-left shunting	Antibiotics, drainage
CNS thromboembolic stroke	Right-to-left shunting or polycythemia	Phlebotomy
Low-grade DIC, thrombocytopenia	Polycythemia	None for DIC unless bleeding, then phlebotomy
Hemoptysis	Pulmonary infarct, thrombosis, or rupture of pulmonary artery plexiform lesion	Embolization
Gum disease	Polycythemia, gingivitis, bleeding	Dental hygiene
Gout	Polycythemia, diuretic agent	Allopurinol
Arthritis, clubbing	Hypoxic arthropathy	None
Pregnancy complications: abortion, fetal growth retardation, prematurity increase, maternal illness	Poor placental perfusion, poor ability to increase cardiac output	Bed rest, pregnancy prevention counseling
Infections	Associated asplenia, DiGeorge syndrome, endocarditis	Antibiotics
	Fatal RSV pneumonia with pulmonary hypertension	Ribavirin; RSV immunoglobulin (prevention)
Failure to thrive	Increased oxygen consumption, decreased nutrient intake	Treat heart failure; correct defect early; increase caloric intake
Protein-losing enteropathy	S/P Fontan; high right-sided pressures	Oral budesonide or sildenafil
Chylothorax	Injury to thoracic duct	Medium chain triglyceride diet Octreotide Surgical ligation of thoracic duct
Psychosocial adjustment	Limited activity, cyanotic appearance, chronic disease, multiple hospitalizations	Counseling

CNS, central nervous system; DIC, disseminated intravascular coagulation; RSV, respiratory syncytial virus; S/P, status post (after).

or surgeon places an arterial catheter to allow direct arterial pressure measurements and arterial sampling for blood gas determination. A central venous catheter is also placed for measuring central venous pressure and for infusions of cardioactive medications. In more complex cases, right or left atrial or pulmonary artery catheters may be inserted directly into these cardiac structures and used for pressure monitoring purposes. Temporary pacing wires are placed on the atrium or ventricle, or both, in case temporary postoperative heart block occurs. Transcutaneous oximetry provides for continuous monitoring of arterial oxygen saturation. Near-infrared spectroscopy has been used to monitor cerebral and other end-organ perfusion in the perioperative period.

Functional failure of 1 organ system may cause profound physiologic and biochemical changes in another. Respiratory insufficiency, for example, leads to hypoxia, hypercapnia, and acidosis, which, in turn, compromise cardiac, vascular, and renal function. The latter problems cannot be managed successfully until adequate ventilation is reestablished. Thus, it is essential that the primary source of each postoperative problem be identified and treated.

Respiratory failure is a serious postoperative complication encountered after open heart surgery. Cardiopulmonary bypass carried out in the presence of pulmonary congestion results in decreased lung compliance, copious tracheal and bronchial secretions, atelectasis, and increased breathing effort. Because fatigue and, subsequently, hypoventilation and acidosis may rapidly ensue, mechanical positive pressure endotracheal ventilation is usually continued after open heart surgery for a minimum of several hours in relatively stable patients and for up to 2-3 days or longer in severely ill patients, especially infants. Patients with certain congenital heart lesions, particularly those with DiGeorge syndrome, may also have airway abnormalities (micrognathia, tracheomalacia, bronchomalacia) that can make both ventilation and extubation more difficult.

The electrocardiogram should be monitored continuously during the postoperative period. A change in heart rate, even without arrhythmia, may be the first indication of a serious complication such as hemorrhage, hypothermia, hypoventilation, or heart failure. **Cardiac rhythm disorders** must be diagnosed quickly because a prolonged untreated arrhythmia may add a severe hemodynamic burden to the heart in the critical early postoperative period (see Chapter 435). Injury to the heart's conduction system during surgery can result in postoperative complete heart block. This complication is usually temporary and is treated with surgically placed pacing wires that can later be removed. Occasionally, complete heart block is permanent. If heart block persists beyond 10-14 days postoperatively, insertion of a permanent pacemaker is required. Tachyarrhythmias are a common problem in postoperative patients. Junctional ectopic tachycardia can be a particularly troublesome rhythm to manage (see Chapter 435), although it usually responds to antiarrhythmic medications such as intravenous amiodarone.

Heart failure with poor cardiac output after cardiac surgery may be secondary to respiratory failure, serious arrhythmias, myocardial injury, blood loss, hypovolemia, a significant residual hemodynamic abnormality, or any combination of these factors. Treatment specific to the cause should be instituted. Catecholamines, phosphodiesterase inhibitors, nitroprusside and other afterload-reducing agents, and diuretics are the cardioactive agents most often used in patients with myocardial dysfunction in the early postoperative period (see Chapter 442). Postoperative pulmonary hypertension can be managed with hyperventilation and inhaled nitric oxide. In the rare patients who are unresponsive to standard pharmacologic treatment, various ventricular assist devices are available, depending on the patient's size. If pulmonary function is adequate, a left ventricular assist device may be used. If pulmonary function is inadequate, extracorporeal membrane oxygenation may be used. These extraordinary measures are helpful in maintaining the circulation until cardiac function improves, usually within 2-5 days. They have also been used as a bridge to transplantation in patients with severe nonremitting postoperative cardiac failure.

Acidosis secondary to low cardiac output, renal failure, or hypovolemia must be prevented, or if present, promptly corrected. Serial monitoring of arterial blood gases and lactate concentrations is performed. A low arterial pH may not only be a sign of decreased perfusion, but also worsen cardiac function and may be the forerunner of arrhythmias or cardiac arrest.

Renal function may be compromised by congestive heart failure and further impaired by prolonged cardiopulmonary bypass. Blood and fluid replacement, cardiac inotropic agents, and vasodilators will usually reestablish normal urine flow in patients with hypovolemia or cardiac failure. Renal failure secondary to tubular injury may require temporary peritoneal or hemodialysis or hemofiltration.

Neurologic abnormalities can develop after cardiopulmonary bypass, especially in the neonatal period. Seizures may occur when the patient awakens from sedation and can usually be controlled with anticonvulsant medications. In the absence of other neurologic signs, self-limited isolated seizures in the immediate postoperative period usually carry a good long-term prognosis. Thromboembolism and stroke are rarer but serious complications of open heart surgery. In the long-term, both subtle and more substantial learning disabilities may develop. Patients who have undergone surgery entailing the use of cardiopulmonary bypass, especially in the newborn period, should be watched carefully during their early school years for signs of mild to moderate learning disabilities or attention deficit disorders, which are often amenable to early remedial intervention. The risk is higher in patients who have undergone repair using hypothermic total circulatory arrest than in those where systemic blood flow is maintained using cardiopulmonary bypass.

The **postpericardiotomy syndrome** may occur toward the end of the 1st postoperative wk or may sometimes be delayed until weeks or months after surgery. This febrile illness is characterized by fever, decreased appetite, listlessness, nausea, and vomiting. Chest pain is not always present, so a high index of suspicion should be maintained in any recently postoperative patient. Echocardiography is diagnostic. In most instances, the postpericardiotomy syndrome is self-limited; however, when pericardial fluid accumulates rapidly, the potential danger of cardiac tamponade should be recognized (see Chapter 440). Rarely, arrhythmias may also occur. Symptomatic patients usually respond to salicylates or indomethacin and bed rest. Occasionally, steroid therapy or pericardiocentesis is required. Late recurrences are rare and can lead to chronic pericarditis.

Hemolysis of mechanical origin is seen, although rarely, after repair of certain cardiac defects, for example, atrioventricular septal defects (AVSDs), or after the insertion of a mechanical prosthetic valve. It is caused by unusual turbulence of blood at increased pressure. Reoperation may be necessary in rare patients with severe and progressive hemolysis who require frequent blood transfusions, but in most instances, the problem slowly regresses.

Infection is another potentially serious postoperative problem. Patients usually receive a broad-spectrum antibiotic for the initial postoperative period. Potential sites of infection include the lungs (generally related to postoperative atelectasis), the subcutaneous tissues at the incision site, the sternum, and the urinary tract (especially after an indwelling catheter has been in place). Sepsis with infective endocarditis is an infrequent complication, and can be difficult to manage, especially if prosthetic material was placed at the time of surgery (see Chapter 437).

LONG-TERM MANAGEMENT

Patients who have undergone surgery for congenital heart disease can be divided into several major categories: (1) lesions for which total repair has been achieved; (2) lesions for which both anatomic and physiologic correction have been achieved; and (3) lesions for which only palliation, albeit potentially long-term, has been achieved. There is some disagreement among cardiologists as to exactly which categories a particular congenital heart lesion might fall, and to some degree every case should be considered individually. Many argue that only for isolated patent ductus arteriosus is total repair really achieved, with no requirement for long-term follow-up. Patients who are able to undergo

anatomic and physiologic correction include many of the left-to-right shunt lesions (atrial and ventricular septal defects) and milder forms of obstructive lesions (e.g., valvar pulmonic stenosis, some forms of valvar aortic stenosis, and coarctation of the aorta), and some forms of cyanotic heart disease, for example, uncomplicated tetralogy of Fallot and simple transposition of the great arteries. These patients usually have achieved total or near-total physiologic correction of their lesion; however, they are still at some risk of long-term sequelae, including late heart failure or arrhythmia, or recurrence of a significant physiologic abnormality (e.g., recoarctation of the aorta, worsening mitral regurgitation in patients with AVSDs, or long-standing pulmonary regurgitation in patients with tetralogy of Fallot repaired with a transannular patch). These patients require regular follow-up with a pediatric cardiologist (and when old enough, with an **adult congenital heart disease specialist** [see Chapter 434.1]); however, their long-term prognosis is generally very good, although some will require repeat surgeries. Patients with more complex lesions, such as those with single-ventricle physiology, are at much higher risk of long-term sequelae and require even closer follow-up. These patients, particularly those who have undergone the Fontan procedure, are at risk long-term for arrhythmia, thrombosis, protein losing enteropathy, end-organ (especially hepatic) dysfunction, and heart failure. Some may eventually require cardiac transplantation.

Physical limitations are variable, ranging from minimal to none in patients with physiologic correction, to mild to moderate in patients with palliative procedures. The extent to which a patient should be allowed to participate in athletics, both recreational and competitive, can best be determined by the cardiologist, often with the assistance of the data that can be derived from cardiopulmonary exercise testing (see Chapter 423.5).

Long-term morbidities affecting neurologic function and behavior are influenced by many factors, including the effects of any genetic alterations on the developing central nervous system. Data suggest a greater role for prenatal central nervous system abnormalities (anatomic or secondary to alterations in cerebral blood flow or oxygenation) than previously suspected; these include microcephaly, cerebral atrophy, and altered cerebral biochemistry. Chronic hypoxemia and failure to thrive also may influence the developing brain, and there is evidence that the type of intervention required (cardiopulmonary bypass, hypothermic total circulatory arrest, catheter-based therapy) plays a substantial role. In general, in the absence of a significant genetic syndrome or major perioperative complication, most children function at a fairly high level after repair of congenital heart defects and are able to attend regular school. Group mean scores on standard cognitive tests are not different from the general population; however, some areas appear to be more at risk than others, including certain aspects of motor function, speech, visual-motor tracking, and phonologic awareness. Awareness of these potential issues is critical to obtaining prompt remedial assistance if a child is found to be struggling in school.

Bibliography is available at Expert Consult.

434.1 Congenital Heart Disease in Adults
Salil Ginde and Michael G. Earing

The advent of cardiac surgical procedures such as ligation of patent ductus arteriosus, resection of coarctation of aorta, and the Blalock-Taussig shunt, as well as advances in diagnostic, interventional, and critical care skills have resulted in survival of approximately 90% of children with congenital heart disease to adulthood. More adults than children are living with congenital heart disease in the United States, with a 5% increase every year. In the last decade, 35% of hospitalizations for congenital heart disease were patients over the age of 18 yr (mean age: 55 yr).

LONG-TERM MEDICAL CONSIDERATIONS
Approximately 25% of adults with congenital heart disease have a mild form that has allowed them to survive into adulthood without surgical

or interventional cardiac catheterization. The most common lesions in this category include mild aortic valve stenosis (usually in setting of bicuspid aortic valve), small restrictive ventricular septal defects, mild pulmonary valve stenosis, and mitral valve prolapse (Table 434-2). These patients need less-frequent follow-up to assess for progression of disease and to identify associated complications. The majority of adults with congenital heart disease living in the United States are patients who have had previous intervention (Table 434-3). Although most children who undergo surgical intervention will survive to adulthood, with few exceptions, total correction is not the rule. The few exceptions include patent ductus arteriosus, ventricular septal defects, and atrial septal defects; this is true only if they are closed early before the development of irreversible pulmonary vascular changes, and no residual lesions exist.

Because adult patients with congenital heart disease (CHD) are surviving longer than ever, it is becoming increasingly apparent that even the simplest lesions can be associated with long-term complications. These long-term complications include both cardiac and noncardiac problems (Tables 434-4 and 434-5, Fig. 434-1). Cardiac complications include arrhythmias and conduction defects, ventricular dysfunction, residual shunts, valvular lesions (regurgitation and stenosis), hypertension, and aneurysms. Noncardiac sequelae (comorbidities) include pulmonary, renal, and hepatic dysfunction that is caused either directly or indirectly by the underlying CHD. Abnormal pulmonary function most commonly presents as restrictive lung physiology, and likely results from prior sternotomy or thoracotomy, scoliosis, diaphragmatic dysfunction, or parenchymal lung disease. Reduced pulmonary function contributes to reduced exercise tolerance and is a risk factor for mortality in adults with CHD. Renal dysfunction may result from chronic cyanosis, multiple surgeries requiring cardiopulmonary bypass, or from other comorbid conditions, such as hypertension and diabetes mellitus. Hepatic injury from chronic liver congestion in patients with elevated central venous pressures, particularly patients palliated with the Fontan procedure, can result in hepatic fibrosis, cirrhosis, hepatic dysfunction and rarely hepatocellular carcinoma.

Table 434-2	Congenital Heart Defects Associated with Survival into Adulthood Without Surgery or Interventional Cardiac Catheterization

Mild pulmonary valve stenosis
Bicuspid aortic valve
Small to moderate size atrial septal defect
Small ventricular septal defect
Small patent ductus arteriosus
Mitral valve prolapse
Partial atrioventricular canal (ostium primum atrial septal defect and cleft mitral valve)
Marfan syndrome
Ebstein anomaly
Congenitally corrected transposition (atrioventricular and ventriculoarterial discordance)

Table 434-3	Most Common Congenital Heart Defects Surviving to Adulthood After Surgery or Interventional Catheterization

Aortic valve disease following balloon valvuloplasty or surgical valvotomy
Pulmonary valve stenosis following balloon valvuloplasty or surgical valvotomy
Tetralogy of Fallot
Ventricular septal defect
Complete atrioventricular canal defect
Transposition of the great arteries
Coarctation of the aorta
Complex single ventricles after the modified Fontan procedure

Adults with CHD are at risk for developmental abnormalities such as intellectual impairment, somatic abnormalities such as facial dysmorphism (cleft palate/lip), central nervous abnormalities such as seizure disorders from previous thromboembolic events or cerebrovascular accidents, and impairments of hearing or vision loss. Psychosocial problems involving employment, life and health insurance, participation in sports, sexual activity, and contraception are common. As a result of these long-term complications, the majority of adults with CHD need lifelong follow-up. When adults with CHD are hospitalized, it is usually for heart failure or an arrhythmia; others may require catheterization or another cardiac surgical procedure.

SPECIFIC LESIONS
Left-to-Right Shunts
If the initial lesion has a shunt that is large and nonrestrictive (allowing transmission of near systemic pressure to the pulmonary arteries), irreversible pulmonary vascular changes can occur, resulting in pulmonary hypertension at systemic levels with reversed or bidirectional shunting at the level of the defect (Eisenmenger syndrome) (see Chapter 433.2).

Atrial Septal Defects
See Chapter 426.1.

Although, most individuals with an atrial septal defect are diagnosed during childhood after a murmur is noted, a minority of patients

Table 434-4	Risks in Adults Who Have Congenital Heart Disease

Rhythm disorder	Ventral septal defect
Supraventricular tachycardia	Atrial septal defect
Right bundle branch block	Patent ductus arteriosus
Heart block	**Acquired lesions**
Ventricular tachycardia	Subacute bacterial endocarditis
Sudden death	Subvalvular stenosis
Coarctation of aorta	Supravalvular stenosis
Essential hypertension	Valvular insufficiency
Recoarctation	Valvular restenosis
Aneurysm formation	Eisenmenger complex
Residual lesions (shunts)	**Pregnancy risk (see Table 434-5)**

Table 434-5	Lesion Specific Risks of Maternal and Neonatal Complications of Pregnancy

No additional risk	Small septal defects Surgically closed ASD, VSD, PDA Mild to moderate aortic regurgitation Mild to moderate pulmonary stenosis
Slightly increased risk	Postoperative repair of tetralogy of Fallot Transposition of the great arteries, s/p arterial switch procedure
Moderate risk	Transposition of the great arteries, s/p atrial switch procedure Congenitally corrected transposition of the great arteries Single ventricle physiology, s/p Fontan procedure
Severe risk	Cyanotic congenital heart disease, unoperated or palliated Marfan syndrome Prosthetic valves Obstructive lesions including coarctation
Pregnancy contraindicated	Severe pulmonary hypertension Severe obstructive lesions Marfan syndrome, aortic root >40 mm

ASD, atrial septal defect; PDA, patent ductus arteriosus; s/p, status post (after); VSD, ventricular septal defect.

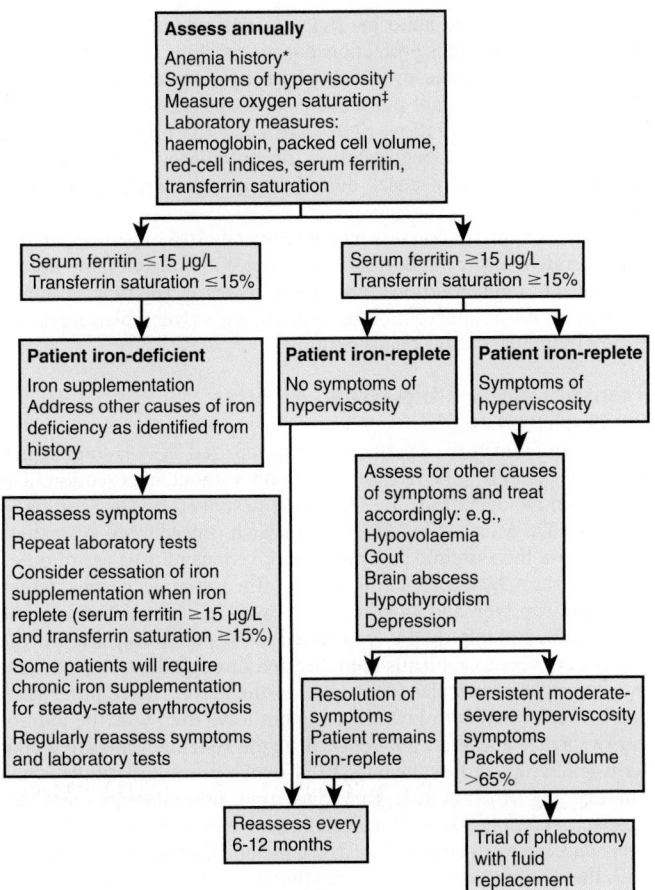

Assess annually

Anemia history*
Symptoms of hyperviscosity†
Measure oxygen saturation‡
Laboratory measures:
haemoglobin, packed cell volume,
red-cell indices, serum ferritin,
transferrin saturation

Serum ferritin ≤15 µg/L
Transferrin saturation ≤15%

Serum ferritin ≥15 µg/L
Transferrin saturation ≥15%

Patient iron-deficient

Iron supplementation
Address other causes of iron
deficiency as identified from
history

Patient iron-replete

No symptoms of
hyperviscosity

Patient iron-replete

Symptoms of
hyperviscosity

Reassess symptoms

Repeat laboratory tests

Consider cessation of iron
supplementation when iron
replete (serum ferritin ≥15 µg/L
and transferrin saturation ≥15%)

Some patients will require
chronic iron supplementation
for steady-state erythrocytosis

Regularly reassess symptoms
and laboratory tests

Assess for other causes
of symptoms and treat
accordingly: e.g.,
Hypovolaemia
Gout
Brain abscess
Hypothyroidism
Depression

Resolution of
symptoms
Patient remains
iron-replete

Persistent moderate-
severe hyperviscosity
symptoms
Packed cell volume
>65%

Reassess every
6-12 months

Trial of phlebotomy
with fluid
replacement

Figure 434-1 Important issues that are crucial to address at time of transition. *(From Spence MS, Balaratnam MS, Gatzoulis MA: Clinical update: cyanotic adult congenital heart disease, Lancet 370:1530–1532, 2007, p. 1531.)*

present with symptoms for the 1st time as adults. Most patients are asymptomatic during the 1st and 2nd decades of life. In the 3rd decade, an increasing number of patients then develop exercise intolerance, palpitations from atrial arrhythmias, and cardiac enlargement. If untreated, survival into adulthood is the rule; life expectancy, however, is not normal and there is significant long-term morbidity. After the age of 40 yr, the mortality rate increases by 6% per year, and more than 20% of patients will have developed atrial fibrillation. By age 60 yr, the number of patients with atrial fibrillation increases to more than 60%.

Late Outcome Following Closure of Atrial Septal Defect

Most patients who have undergone early closure of a defect will have excellent long-term survival with low morbidity if repair is undertaken before age 25 yr. Older age of repair is associated with decreased late survival with an associated increased risk for the development of atrial arrhythmias, thromboembolic event, and pulmonary hypertension. Long-term late complications and survival following transcatheter device closure remain unknown; early and intermediate results are excellent with a high rate of atrial septal defect closure and few major complications.

Ventricular Septal Defects

See Chapter 426.6.

Although isolated ventricular septal defects (VSDs) are 1 of the most common forms of CHD, the diagnosis of a VSD in an adult is rare. The primary reason for this is that most patients with a hemodynamically significant VSD will have undergone repair in childhood or will have

died earlier in life. As result, the spectrum of isolated VSD in adults is limited to (1) those with small restrictive defects, (2) those with Eisenmenger syndrome, and (3) those who had their defects closed in childhood.

For patients with small restrictive VSD, the long-term survival is excellent with estimated 25-yr survival of 96%. In addition, the long-term morbidity for patients with a restrictive VSD also appears to be low. Their clinical course is not completely benign. Reported long-term complications include endocarditis, progressive aortic regurgitation secondary to prolapse of aortic valve into the defect (highest risk is with supracristal type, but also can occur in setting of perimembranous defect), and the development of both right and left outflow tract obstruction from a double-chamber right ventricle or a subaortic membrane. For those patients who develop Eisenmenger syndrome, survival into the 3rd decade is common. With increasing age, the long-term complications of right-heart failure, paradoxical emboli, and polycythemia, usually result in progressive decline in survival, with an average age of death of 37 yr.

Adults with previous VSD closure, without pulmonary hypertension or residual defects, live a normal life expectancy. Because patients with small VSDs are asymptomatic, these patients should be managed conservatively. Given the long-term risks, they do need intermittent follow-up for life to monitor for the development of late complications. The exception to this rule is patients with small supracristal or perimembranous VSD with associated prolapse of the aortic cusp into the defect resulting in progressive aortic regurgitation. These patients should be considered for surgical repair at the time of diagnosis to prevent progressive aortic valve damage.

Complete Atrioventricular Canal
See Chapter 426.5.

The natural history for patients with complete AVSD is characterized by the early development of pulmonary vascular disease, leading to irreversible damage often by age 1 yr (especially in children with Down syndrome). Thus, patients who present in adulthood can be categorized into 2 groups: (1) those with Eisenmenger syndrome and (2) those who had their defects closed in childhood.

Overall, for those patients who underwent early repair before the development of pulmonary vascular disease, the long-term prognosis is good. The most common long-term complication is left atrioventricular valve regurgitation, with approximately 5-10% of patients requiring surgical revision for left atrioventricular valve repair or replacement during follow-up. The second most common long-term complication for this patient group is subaortic stenosis, occurring in up to 5% of patients after repair. Other long-term complications include residual atrial or ventricular level shunts, complete heart block, atrial and ventricular arrhythmias, and endocarditis.

For those patients who have developed Eisenmenger syndrome, all are symptomatic with exertional dyspnea, fatigue, palpitations, edema, and syncope. Survival is similar to other forms of Eisenmenger syndrome, with a mean age of death of 37 yr. Strong predictors for death include syncope, age at presentation of symptoms, poor functional class, low oxygen saturation (<85%), elevated serum creatinine and serum uric acid concentrations, and Down syndrome.

Patients who underwent previous repair and develop significant left atrioventricular valve regurgitation causing symptoms, atrial arrhythmias, or deterioration in ventricular function should undergo elective valve repair or replacement. Those previously repaired patients who develop significant subaortic stenosis (defined as a peak cardiac catheterization or echo gradient of >50 mm Hg) should undergo surgical repair.

Patent Ductus Arteriosus
See Chapter 426.8.

A patent ductus arteriosus (PDA) is usually an isolated lesion in the adult patient. The size of the defect is the primary determinant of clinical course in the adult patient. These clinical courses can be grouped into 5 main categories: (1) silent PDAs; (2) small, hemodynamically insignificant PDAs; (3) moderate size PDAs; (4) large PDAs; and (5) previously repaired PDAs.

A silent PDA is a tiny defect that cannot be heard by auscultation and is only detected by other nonclinical means such as echocardiography. Life expectancy is always normal in this population and the risk for endocarditis is extremely low.

Patients with a small PDA have an audible long-ejection or continuous murmur heard best at the left upper sternal border that radiates to the back. In addition, they have normal peripheral pulses. Because there is negligible left to right shunting these patients have normal left aorta and left ventricle (LV) size and normal pulmonary artery pressure by echocardiography and chest x-ray. These patients like those with silent PDAs are asymptomatic and live a normal life expectancy. They have a higher risk for endocarditis.

Patients with moderate size PDAs may present during adulthood. These patients often will have wide, bounding peripheral pulses and an audible continuous murmur. These patients all have significant volume overload and develop some degree of left aorta and LV enlargement and some degree of pulmonary hypertension. These patients are symptomatic with dyspnea, palpitations, and heart failure.

Patients with large PDAs typically present with signs of severe pulmonary hypertension and Eisenmenger syndrome. By adulthood, the continuous murmur is typically absent and there is differential cyanosis (lower extremity saturations lower than the right arm saturation). These patients have a similar prognosis as other patients with Eisenmenger syndrome.

Patients who underwent repair of a PDA prior to the development of pulmonary hypertension have a normal life expectancy without restrictions.

All patients with *clinical evidence* of a PDA are at increased risk for endocarditis. As result, all PDAs except for small silent PDAs and those patients with severe irreversible pulmonary hypertension should be considered for closure. Catheter device closure is the preferred method in most centers today. Surgical closure is reserved for patients with PDAs too large for device closure or when the anatomy is distorted, such as in the setting of a large ductal aneurysm.

Cyanotic Heart Disease
See Chapters 429, 430, and 431.

Unlike the acyanotic forms of CHD, the majority of patients with cyanotic CHD will have had at least 1 and often several previous interventions prior to adulthood. The most frequent defects seen in the outpatient adult congenital setting is tetralogy of Fallot, complete transposition of the great arteries (TGA, also known as d-transposition), pulmonary valve stenosis, and various forms of single ventricles. Other defects include total anomalous pulmonary venous return, truncus arteriosus, and double-outlet right ventricle.

Tetralogy of Fallot
See Chapter 430.1.

In the developed world, the unoperated adult patient with tetralogy of Fallot has become a rarity because the majority of patients will have undergone palliation or, more often, repair in childhood. Survival in the unoperated patient to the 7th decade has been described but is rare. In general, only 11% of unoperated patients are alive by age 20 yr and only 3% by age 40 yr.

Late survival following repair of tetralogy of Fallot is excellent. Repair is typically performed at 3-12 mo of age and consists of patch closure of the VSD and relief of the pulmonary outflow tract obstruction by patch augmentation of the right ventricular outflow tract, pulmonary valve annulus, or both. Survival rates at 32 and 35 yr have been reported to be 86% and 85%, respectively, compared to 95% in age- and sex-matched controls. Most patients lived an unrestricted life. Many patients do develop late symptoms that include exertional dyspnea, palpitations, syncope, and sudden cardiac death. Late complications include endocarditis, aortic regurgitation with or without aortic root dilation (typically caused by damage of the aortic valve during VSD closure or secondary to an

intrinsic aortic root abnormality), LV dysfunction (secondary to inadequate myocardial protection during previous repair or chronic left ventricular volume overload caused by long-standing palliative arterial shunts), residual pulmonary valve obstruction, residual pulmonary valve regurgitation, right ventricular (RV) dysfunction (as a result of pulmonary regurgitation or pulmonary stenosis), atrial arrhythmias (typically atrial flutter), ventricular arrhythmias, and heart block.

Reintervention is necessary in approximately 10% of patients following reparative surgery at 20-year follow-up. With longer follow-up, the incidence of reintervention continues to increase. The most common indication for reintervention is pulmonary valve replacement for severe pulmonary valve regurgitation.

Transposition of the Great Arteries
See Chapter 431.1.

The natural history of patients with unrepaired TGA is so poor that very few patients survive past childhood without intervention. The first definitive operations for TGA were described by Dr. Senning in 1959 and Dr. Mustard in 1964 (atrial switch procedures). With these procedures, the systemic and pulmonary venous returns are rerouted in the atrium by constructing baffles. The systemic venous return from the superior and inferior vena cavae is directed through the mitral valve and into the LV (connected to the pulmonary artery). The pulmonary venous return is then directed through the tricuspid valve into the right ventricular (connected to the aorta). These procedures can be performed with low mortality but leave the LV as the pulmonary ventricle and the right ventricle as the systemic ventricle. Long-term follow-up studies after the atrial switch procedure show a small but ongoing attrition rate with numerous other intermediate and long-term complications. Two specific problems after the atrial switch procedure are most concerning. These include the loss of sinus rhythm with the development of atrial arrhythmias, occurring at an incidence of 50% by age 25 yr, and the development of systemic ventricular dysfunction, occurring at an incidence of 50% by age 35 yr. Other long-term complications include endocarditis, baffle leaks, baffle obstruction, tricuspid valve regurgitation, and sinus node dysfunction requiring pacemaker placement.

As result of these long-term complications, the arterial switch operation has become the procedure of choice to treat these patients since 1985. During the arterial switch procedure, the great arteries are transected and reanastomosed to the correct ventricle (LV to the aorta and the right ventricle to the pulmonary artery) with coronary artery transfer. Operative survival after the arterial switch procedure in the current surgical era is very good, with a surgical mortality rate of 2-5%. Long-term data on survival and complications does not exist, but intermediate results are promising. Reported intermediate complications include endocarditis, pulmonary outflow tract obstruction (at the supravalvular level or at the takeoff of the peripheral pulmonary arteries), aortic valve regurgitation, and coronary artery compromise (ranging from minor stenosis to complete occlusion).

Because of the high incidence of observed and potential medical problems, all patients who have had both atrial and arterial repair of TGA should have lifelong follow-up by a cardiologist at a center specializing in adult CHD.

Pulmonary Valve Stenosis
See Chapter 427.1.

Most patients with pulmonary valve stenosis are asymptomatic and present with a cardiac murmur. Survival into adult life and the need for intervention however is directly correlated to the degree of obstruction. Patients with trivial stenosis (defined as a peak gradient <25 mm Hg) followed for 25 yr remain asymptomatic and have no significant progression of obstruction over time. For those patients with moderate pulmonary valve stenosis (defined as a peak gradient of 25-49 mm Hg), there is an approximately 20% chance of requiring intervention by age 25 yr. For those patients with severe stenosis (defined as a peak gradient of >50 mm Hg), the majority ultimately require an intervention, either surgery or balloon valvuloplasty by age 25 yr.

Following surgical valvotomy for isolated pulmonary stenosis, long-term survival is excellent. With longer follow-up the incidence of late complications and the need for reintervention do increase. The most common indication for reintervention is pulmonary valve replacement for severe pulmonary regurgitation. Other long-term complications include recurrent atrial arrhythmias, endocarditis, and residual RV outflow tract obstruction.

Patients with moderate to severe pulmonary stenosis (defined as a peak gradient of >50 mm Hg) should be considered for intervention even in the absence of symptoms. Since 1985, percutaneous balloon valvuloplasty has been the accepted treatment for patients of all ages. Prior to 1985, surgical valvotomy had been the gold standard. Surgical valvotomy is reserved for those patients who are unlikely to have successful results from balloon valvuloplasty, such as those with an extremely dysplastic or calcified valve.

Left-Sided Obstructive Lesions
Coarctation of the Aorta
See Chapter 427.6.

The clinical presentation of coarctation of the aorta depends on the severity of obstruction and the associated anomalies. Unrepaired coarctation of the aorta typically presents with symptoms prior to adulthood. These symptoms include headaches related to hypertension, leg fatigue or cramps, exercise intolerance, and systemic hypertension. Those untreated patients surviving to adulthood thus typically have only mild coarctation of the aorta. In the era prior to surgery, without treatment the mean age of death was 32 yr. Causes of death included left ventricular failure, intracranial hemorrhage, endocarditis, aortic rupture/dissection, and premature coronary artery disease.

Following surgical repair, long-term survival is good but is directly correlated with the age at repair, with those repaired after age 14 yr having a lower 20 yr survival than those who were repaired earlier, 91% compared to 79%. With longer follow-up the incidence of long-term complications continues to rise. The most common long-term complication is persistent or new systemic hypertension at rest or during exercise. Other long-term complications include aneurysms of the ascending or descending aorta, recoarctation at the site of previous repair, coronary artery disease, aortic stenosis or regurgitation (in setting of bicuspid aortic valve), rupture of an intracranial aneurysm, and endocarditis.

Patients with significant native or residual coarctation of the aorta (symptomatic patients with a peak gradient across the coarctation of >20 mm Hg) should be considered for intervention, either surgery or catheter intervention with balloon angioplasty with or without stent placement. Surgical repair in the adult patient is technically difficult and is associated with high morbidity. Catheter based intervention has become the preferred method in most experienced adult CHD centers.

Aortic Valve Stenosis
See Chapter 427.5.

The natural history of aortic valve stenosis in adults is quite variable but is characterized by progressive stenosis over time. By age 45 yr, approximately 50% of bicuspid aortic valves will have some degree of stenosis.

Most patients with aortic valve stenosis are asymptomatic and are diagnosed after a murmur is detected. The severity of obstruction at the time of diagnosis correlates with the pattern of progression. Symptoms are rare until patients have severe aortic valve stenosis (mean gradient by echocardiography of >40 mm Hg). Symptoms include chest pain, exertional dyspnea, near syncope, and syncope. When any of these symptoms are present, the risk of sudden cardiac death is very high and as result, surgical intervention is mandated. For patients requiring surgical valvotomy to relieve the stenosis prior to adulthood, the majority of patients do well. However, at 25 yr follow-up, up to 40% of patients will have required a second operation for residual stenosis or regurgitation.

Patients with symptoms and severe aortic valve stenosis should be considered for intervention. Treatment involves manipulating the valve to reduce stenosis. This can be accomplished by transvenous balloon dilation of the valve, open surgical valvotomy, or valve replacement. In absence of significant aortic regurgitation, most centers favor balloon dilation or surgical valvotomy for children and young adults who have pliable valves with fusion of commissures. In older adults, aortic valve replacement is the treatment of choice.

Endocarditis Prophylaxis
See Chapter 437.

The American Heart Association found that very few cases of endocarditis are prevented with antibiotic prophylaxis. Only patients with cardiac conditions associated with the highest risk for adverse outcomes should continue follow antibiotic prophylaxis before surgery: patients with previous endocarditis, unrepaired cyanotic CHD, including palliative shunts and conduits; completely repaired congenital heart defects with prosthetic material or device, whether placed by surgery or by catheter intervention, during the 1st 6 mo after the procedure; and repaired CHD with residual defects at the site or adjacent to the site of a prosthetic patch or prosthetic device (which inhibit endothelialization). Except for the conditions just listed, antibiotic prophylaxis is no longer recommended for other forms of CHD.

PREGNANCY AND CONGENITAL HEART DISEASE
CHD is the most common form of heart disease encountered during pregnancy in developed countries. Heart disease does not preclude a successful pregnancy but increases the risk to both the mother and the baby. During pregnancy there are substantial hemodynamic changes that occur. The hemodynamic changes in pregnancy result in a steady increase in cardiac output during pregnancy until the 32nd wk of gestation, at which time, the cardiac output reaches a plateau at 30-50% above the prepregnancy level. At time of delivery, with uterine contractions an additional 300-500 mL of blood enters the circulation. This in conjunction with increased blood pressure and heart rate during labor increases the cardiac output at delivery to 80% the prepregnancy level.

Despite these hemodynamic changes, the outcome of pregnancy is favorable in most women with CHD provided that functional class and systemic ventricular function are good (see Table 434-5). Pulmonary artery hypertension presents a serious risk during pregnancy, particularly when the pulmonary pressure exceeds 70% of systemic pressure, regardless of functional class. Other contraindications to pregnancy include severe obstructive left-sided lesions (coarctation of the aorta, aortic valve stenosis, mitral valve stenosis, hypertrophic cardiomyopathy), Marfan syndrome with coexisting dilated ascending aorta (defined as >4 cm), persistent cyanosis, and systemic ventricular dysfunction (ejection fraction of ≤40%). The need for full anticoagulation during pregnancy, although not a contraindication, poses an increased risk to both mother and fetus. The relative risks and benefits of the different anticoagulant approaches need to be discussed fully with the prospective mother.

Pregnancy counseling should begin early in adolescence and should be part of the routine cardiac follow-up visit. During counseling, a discussion about the risk of CHD in the offspring should take place. In the general population, the incidence of CHD is 1%. In the offspring of a mother with CHD, the risk increases to 5-6%. Often the cardiac lesion in the offspring is not the same as that in the mother, except for in the case of a syndrome with autosomal dominant inheritance (Marfan syndrome, hypertrophic cardiomyopathy). Risk stratification should include the specific CHD lesion but also needs to take in account the maternal functional class. Although the specific CHD lesion is important, multiple studies demonstrate that the maternal functional class prior to pregnancy is highly predictive of both maternal and fetal outcomes, with those having the best functional class having the best outcomes.

CONTRACEPTION
A critical part of caring for adults with CHD is to provide or make available advice on contraception. Unfortunately, there are limited data on the safety of various contraceptive techniques in adult CHD patients. The estrogen-containing oral contraceptive pill can be used in many adult CHD patients but is not recommended in adult CHD patients at risk of thromboembolism, such as those with cyanosis, prior

Table 434-6	Issues That Require Coordination of Care Between the Cardiologist and the Primary Care Physician

Antibiotic prophylaxis for endocarditis
Medications and drug interactions
Anticoagulation with prosthetic valves
Exercise and sports participation
Educational and vocational planning
Contraception and pregnancy
Drug, alcohol, and tobacco use
Noncardiac surgical planning
Anesthetic issues
New symptoms or acute illnesses
Coexistent medical conditions
Travel

Fontan procedure, atrial fibrillation, or pulmonary artery hypertension. In addition, this form of contraceptive therapy may upset anticoagulation control. Although slightly less effective than contraceptive pills containing combined estrogen/progesterone, medroxyprogesterone, the progesterone-only pills, and levonorgestrel are good options for most adult CHD patients. Medroxyprogesterone and levonorgestrel, however, can cause fluid retention and thus need to be used with caution in patients with heart failure. These medications are also associated with depression and often breakthrough bleeding. Tubal ligation, although the most secure method of contraception, can be a high-risk procedure in patients with complex CHD or those with pulmonary hypertension. Hysteroscopic sterilization (Essure) may be reasonable for high-risk patients. In the past, intrauterine devices were seldom used in cardiac patients because of the associated risk of bacteremia, pelvic inflammatory disease, and endocarditis. Intrauterine devices such as the Mirena, appear to be safe and effective, and are rapidly becoming one of the most commonly used form of contraception in the adult CHD population.

ADOLESCENT TRANSITION

It is well recognized that, as part of the process of obtaining independence, adolescents or young adults must develop a forward-looking, independent approach to their medical care. For children with heart disease, the transition process must begin during early adolescence and should be encouraged by both the primary care provider and the pediatric cardiologist, who must identify an appropriate adult congenital heart program to which transition and transfer will be made at an appropriate time (Table 434-6).

A successful transition program includes the following elements:
◆ Development of a written transition plan that should begin by the age of 14 yr
◆ Because adolescents and young adults are frequently unaware of the details of their cardiac diagnosis and history, a complete, concise, portable medical record, including all pertinent aspects of cardiac care, should be shared with adolescents and their families and prepared for transmittal to the eventual adult care destination.
◆ The primary care provider and cardiologist must address unique adolescent medical issues as they impact the cardiovascular system. In addition to medical problems, education, vocational planning, psychosocial issues, and access to medical care are all topics that should be discussed with adolescents and their families.

There is a tendency for young adults to avoid medical care because of lack of education, denial, or difficulty with access to the medical care system. Thus, a critical goal of the adolescent transition process is to identify an appropriate site for ongoing medical care and ensure maintenance of the medical record and continuity of care for the young adult. The site of care for a young adult with CHD may be a pediatric program or facility, or may be a specialized center or program for the adult with CHD. The critical issues are the continuity of care, the preparation of the patient, and the patient's participation in the process.

Bibliography is available at Expert Consult.

Cardiac Arrhythmias

Chapter **435**
Disturbances of Rate and Rhythm of the Heart
George F. Van Hare

The term *arrhythmia* refers to a disturbance in heart rate or rhythm. Such disturbances can lead to heart rates that are abnormally fast, slow, or irregular. They may be transient or incessant, congenital or acquired, or caused by a toxin or by drugs. They may be associated with particular forms of congenital heart disease, may be a complication of surgical repair of congenital heart disease, may be a result of certain genetic causes, or may be a result of fetal inflammation such as in maternal connective tissue disease. Arrhythmias, either slow or fast, may lead to acutely decreased cardiac output, degeneration into a more dangerous arrhythmia such as ventricular fibrillation, or if incessant may lead to cardiomyopathy. Arrhythmias may lead to syncope or to sudden death. When a patient has an arrhythmia, it is important to determine whether the particular rhythm is likely to lead to severe symptoms or to deteriorate into a life-threatening condition. Rhythm abnormalities, such as single premature atrial and ventricular beats, are common and in children without heart disease, in most instances do not pose a risk to the patient.

A number of pharmacologic agents are available for treating arrhythmias; many have not been studied extensively in children. Insufficient data are available regarding pharmacokinetics, pharmacodynamics, and efficacy in the pediatric population, and therefore the selection of an appropriate agent is necessarily empirical. Fortunately, the majority of rhythm disturbances in children can be reliably controlled with a single agent (Table 435-1). Increasingly, transcatheter ablation is acceptable therapy not only for life-threatening or drug-resistant arrhythmias, but also for the cure of arrhythmias. For patients with bradycardia, implantable pacemakers are small enough for use in all ages, and even in premature infants. Implantable cardioverter-defibrillators (ICDs) are available for use in high-risk patients with malignant ventricular arrhythmias and an increased risk of sudden death.

435.1 Principles of Antiarrhythmic Therapy
George F. Van Hare

When considering drug therapy in the pediatric population, it is important to recognize that there may be marked differences in pharmacokinetics by age and in comparison with adults. Infants may have slower absorption, slow gastric emptying, and differing sizes of drug tissue compartments affecting the volume of distribution. Hepatic metabolism and renal excretion may vary within the pediatric age group as well as in comparison to adults. When considering antiarrhythmic therapy, it is important to recognize that the likely arrhythmia mechanism may be different for the pediatric vs. adult population.

There are many antiarrhythmic agents available for rhythm control. The majority have not been approved by the FDA for use in children; their use is therefore considered "off-label." Pediatric cardiologists have experience with these drugs, and there are well-recognized standards regarding dosing.

With the availability of potentially curative ablation procedures, medical therapy has become less important. Clinicians and patients accept fewer drug side effects. Intolerable side effects, as well as the potential for a proarrhythmia induced by an antiarrhythmic drug, can seriously limit medical therapy and will lead the physician and family toward a potentially curative ablation procedure.

Antiarrhythmic drugs are commonly categorized using the Vaughan Williams classification system. This system comprises 4 classes: Class I includes agents that primarily block the sodium channel, class II includes the β-blockers, class III includes those agents that prolong repolarization, and class IV are the calcium channel blockers. Class I is further divided by the strength of the sodium channel blockade (see Table 435-1).

Table 435-1	Antiarrhythmic Drugs Commonly Used in Pediatric Patients, by Class				
DRUG	INDICATIONS	DOSING	SIDE EFFECTS	DRUG INTERACTIONS	DRUG LEVEL
CLASS IA: INHIBITS NA⁺ FAST CHANNEL, PROLONGS REPOLARIZATION					
Quinidine	SVT, atrial fibrillation, atrial flutter, VT. In atrial flutter, an AV node blocking drug (digoxin, verapamil, propranolol) must be given first to prevent 1:1 conduction	Oral: 30-60 mg/kg/24 hr divided q6h (sulfate) or q8h (gluconate) In adults, 10 mg/kg/day divided q6h Max dose: 2.4g/24 hr	Nausea, vomiting, diarrhea, fever, cinchonism, QRS and QT prolongation, AV nodal block, asystole syncope, thrombocytopenia, hemolytic anemia, SLE, blurred vision, convulsions, allergic reactions, exacerbation of periodic paralysis	Enhances digoxin, may increase PTT when given with warfarin	2-6 µg/mL
Procainamide	SVT, atrial fibrillation, atrial flutter, VT	Oral: 15-50 mg/kg/24 hr divided q4h Max dose: 4 g/24 hr IV: 10-15 mg/kg over 30-45 min load followed by 20-80 µg/kg/min Max dose: 2 g/24 hr	PR, QRS, QT interval prolongation, anorexia, nausea, vomiting, rash, fever, agranulocytosis, thrombocytopenia, Coombs-positive hemolytic anemia, SLE, hypotension, exacerbation of periodic paralysis, proarrhythmia	Toxicity increased by amiodarone and cimetidine	4-8 µg/mL With NAPA <40 µg/mL
Disopyramide	SVT, atrial fibrillation, atrial flutter	Oral: <2 yr: 20-30 mg/kg/24 hr divided q6h or q12h (long-acting form); 2-10 yr: 9-24 mg/kg/24 hr divide q6h or q12h (long-acting form); 11 yr: 5-13 mg/kg/24 hr divided q6h or q12h (long-acting) Max dose: 1.2 g/24 hr	Anticholinergic effects, urinary retention, blurred vision, dry mouth, QT and QRS prolongation, hepatic toxicity, negative inotropic effects, agranulocytosis, psychosis, hypoglycemia, proarrhythmia		2-5 µg/ml
CLASS IB: INHIBITS NA⁺ FAST CHANNEL, SHORTENS REPOLARIZATION					
Lidocaine	VT, VF	IV: 1 mg/kg repeat q 5 min 2 times followed by 20-50 µg/kg/min (max dose: 3 mg/kg)	CNS effects, confusion, convulsions, high grade AV block, asystole, coma, paresthesias, respiratory failure	Propranolol, cimetidine, increases toxicity	1-5 µg/mL
Mexiletine	VT	Oral: 6-15 mg/kg/24 hr divided q8h	GI upset, skin rash, neurologic	Cimetidine	0.8-2 µg/mL
Phenytoin	Digitalis intoxication	Oral: 3-6 mg/kg/24 hr divided q12h Max dose: 600 mg IV: 10-15 mg/kg over 1 hr load	Rash, gingival hyperplasia, ataxia, lethargy, vertigo, tremor, macrocytic anemia, bradycardia with rapid push	Amiodarone, oral anticoagulants, cimetidine, nifedipine, disopyramide, increase toxicity	10-20 µg/mL
CLASS IC: INHIBITS NA⁺ CHANNEL					
Flecainide	SVT, atrial tachycardia, VT	Oral: 6.7-9.5 mg/kg/24 hr divided q8h In older children, 50-200 mg/m²/day divided q12h	Blurred vision, nausea, decrease in contractility, proarrhythmia	Amiodarone increases toxicity	0.2-1 µg/mL
Propafenone	SVT, atrial tachycardia, atrial fibrillation, VT	Oral: 150-300 mg/m²/24 hr divided q6h	Hypotension, decreased contractility, hepatic toxicity, paresthesia, headache, proarrhythmia	Increases digoxin levels	0.2-1 µg/mL

Continued

| **Table 435-1** | Antiarrhythmic Drugs Commonly Used in Pediatric Patients, by Class—cont'd |

DRUG	INDICATIONS	DOSING	SIDE EFFECTS	DRUG INTERACTIONS	DRUG LEVEL
CLASS II: β-BLOCKERS					
Propranolol	SVT, long QT	Oral: 1-4 mg/kg/24 hr divided q6h; Max dose 60 mg/24 hr; IV: 0.1-0.15 mg/kg over 5 min; Max IV dose: 10 mg	Bradycardia, loss of concentration, school performance problems, bronchospasm, hypoglycemia, hypotension, heart block, CHF	Coadministration with disopyramide, flecainide or verapamil may decrease ventricular function	
Atenolol	SVT	Oral: 0.5-1 mg/kg/24 hr once daily or divided q12h	Bradycardia, loss of concentration, school performance problems	Coadministration with disopyramide, flecainide or verapamil may decrease ventricular function	
Nadolol	SVT, long QT	Oral: 1-2 mg/kg/24 hr given once daily	Bradycardia, loss of concentration, school performance problems, bronchospasm, hypoglycemia, hypotension, heart block, CHF	Coadministration with disopyramide, flecainide or verapamil may decrease ventricular function	
CLASS III: PROLONGS REPOLARIZATION					
Amiodarone	SVT, JET, VT	Oral: 10 mg/kg/24 hr in 1-2 divided doses for 4-14 days; reduce to 5 mg/kg/24 hr for several weeks; if no recurrence, reduce to 2.5 mg/kg/24 hr; IV: 2.5-5 mg/kg over 30-60 min, may repeat 3 times, then 2-10 mg/kg/24 hr continuous infusion	Hypothyroidism or hyperthyroidism, elevated triglycerides, hepatic toxicity, pulmonary fibrosis	Digoxin (increases levels), flecainide, procainamide, quinidine, warfarin, phenytoin	0.5-2.5 mg/L
CLASS IV AND MISCELLANEOUS MEDICATIONS					
Digoxin	SVT (not WPW), atrial flutter, atrial fibrillation	Oral/load instructions: Premature: 20 μg/kg; Newborn: 30 μg/kg; >6 mo: 40 μg/kg; Give ½ total dose followed by ¼ q8-12h × 2 doses; Maintenance: 10 μg/kg/24 hr divide q12h; Max dose: 0.5 mg; IV: ¾ PO dose; Max dose: 0.5 mg	PAC, PVC, bradycardia, AV block, nausea, vomiting, anorexia, prolongs PR interval	Quinidine Amiodarone, verapamil, increase digoxin levels	1-2 mg/mL
Verapamil	SVT (not WPW)	Oral: 2-7 mg/kg/24 hr divided q8h; Max dose: 480 mg; IV: 0.1-0.2 mg/kg q 20 min × 2 doses; Max dose: 5-10 mg	Bradycardia, asystole, high degree AV block, PR prolongation, hypotension, CHF	Use with β-blocker or disopyramide exacerbates CHF, increases digoxin level and toxicity	
Adenosine	SVT	IV: 50-300 μg/kg by need rapid IV push; Begin with 50 μg/kg and increase by 50-100 μg/kg/dose; Max dose: 18 mg	Chest pain, flushing, dyspnea, bronchospasm, atrial fibrillation, bradycardia, asystole		

AV, atrioventricular; CHF, congestive heart failure; CNS, central nervous systems; GI, gastrointestinal; IV, intravenous; JET, junctional ectopic tachycardia; NAPA, N-acetyl procainamide; PAC, premature atrial contraction; PTT, partial thromboplastin time; PVC, premature ventricular contraction; SLE, systemic lupus erythematosus–like illness; SVT, supraventricular tachycardia; VF, ventricular fibrillation; VT, ventricular tachycardia; WPW, Wolff-Parkinson-White syndrome.

435.2 Sinus Arrhythmias and Extrasystoles
George F. Van Hare

Phasic sinus arrhythmia represents a normal physiologic variation in impulse discharges from the sinus node related to respirations. The heart rate slows during expiration and accelerates during inspiration. Occasionally, if the sinus rate becomes slow enough, an escape beat arises from the atrioventricular (AV) junction region (Fig. 435-1). Normal phasic sinus arrhythmia is caused by the activity of the parasympathetic nervous system and can be quite prominent in healthy children. It may mimic frequent premature contractions, but the relationship to the phases of respiration can be appreciated with careful auscultation. Drugs that increase vagal tone, such as digoxin, may exaggerate sinus arrhythmia; it is usually abolished by exercise. Other irregularities in sinus rhythm, especially bradycardia associated with periodic apnea are commonly seen in premature infants.

Sinus bradycardia is a result of slow discharge of impulses from the sinus node, the heart's natural pacemaker. A sinus rate <90 beats/min in neonates and <60 beats/min in older children is considered to be sinus bradycardia. It is commonly seen in well-trained athletes; in healthy individuals, it is generally without significance. Sinus bradycardia may occur in systemic disease (hypothyroidism or anorexia nervosa), and it resolves when the disorder is under control. It may also be seen in association with conditions in which there is high vagal tone, such as gastrointestinal obstruction or intracranial processes. Low birthweight infants display great variation in sinus rate. Sinus bradycardia is common in these infants in conjunction with apnea, and may be associated with junctional escape beats. Premature atrial contractions are also frequent. These rhythm changes, especially bradycardia, appear more commonly during sleep and are not associated with symptoms. Usually, no therapy is necessary.

Wandering atrial pacemaker (Fig. 435-2) is defined as an intermittent shift in the pacemaker of the heart from the sinus node to another part of the atrium. It is not uncommon in childhood and usually represents a normal variant; it may also be seen in association with sinus bradycardia in which the shift in atrial focus is an escape phenomenon.

Extrasystoles are produced by the premature discharge of an ectopic focus that may be situated in the atrium, the AV junction, or the ventricle. Usually, isolated extrasystoles are of no clinical or prognostic significance. Under certain circumstances, however, premature beats may be caused by organic heart disease (inflammation, ischemia, fibrosis) or drug toxicity.

Premature atrial contractions are common in childhood, usually in the absence of cardiac disease. Depending on the degree of prematurity of the beat (coupling interval) and the preceding R-R interval (cycle length), premature atrial complexes may result in a normal, a prolonged (aberrancy), or an absent (blocked premature atrial complex) QRS complex. The last occurs when the premature impulse cannot conduct to the ventricle due to refractoriness of the AV node or distal conducting system (Fig. 435-3). Atrial extrasystoles must be distinguished from premature ventricular contractions (PVCs). Careful scrutiny of the electrocardiogram for a premature P wave preceding the QRS will either show a premature P wave superimposed on, and deforming, the preceding T wave, or a P wave that is premature and has a different contour from that of the other sinus P waves. Atrial premature complexes usually reset the sinus node pacemaker, leading to an incomplete compensatory pause, but this feature is not regarded as a reliable means of differentiating atrial from ventricular premature complexes in children.

PVCs may arise in any region of the ventricles. They are characterized by premature, widened, bizarre QRS complexes that are not preceded by a premature P wave (Fig. 435-4). When all premature beats have identical contours, they are classified as uniform, suggesting origin from a common site. When PVCs vary in contour, they are designated as multiform, suggesting origin from more than one ventricular site. Ventricular extrasystoles are often, but not always, followed by a full compensatory pause. The presence of fusion beats, that is, complexes with morphologic features that are intermediate between those of normal sinus beats and those of PVCs, proves the ventricular origin of the premature beat. Extrasystoles produce a smaller stroke and pulse volume than normal and, if quite premature, may not be audible with a stethoscope or palpable at the radial pulse. When frequent, extrasystoles may assume a definite rhythm, for example, alternating with normal beats (**bigeminy**) or occurring after 2 normal beats (**trigeminy**). Most patients are unaware of single PVCs, although some may be aware of a "skipped beat" over the precordium. This sensation is caused by the increased stroke volume of the normal beat after a compensatory pause. Anxiety, a febrile illness, or ingestion of various drugs or stimulants may exacerbate PVCs.

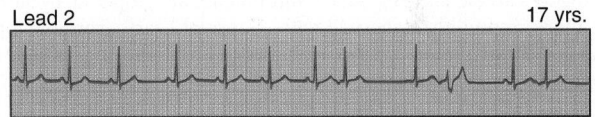

Figure 435-3 Premature atrial contraction (PAC). QRS complexes—the 8th, 10th, and final—in this strip are preceded by a P wave that is inverted, indicative of an ectopic origin of atrial depolarization. Note that the 8th and final QRS complexes resemble those of sinus origin, whereas the 10th is aberrantly conducted. This shift in origin is a function of the preceding cycle length, which influences the refractory period of the bundle branches. The fact that the pause after the PAC is longer than 2 P-P intervals implies that the premature atrial depolarization has invaded and discharged the sinus node and then reset it so that it fires later.

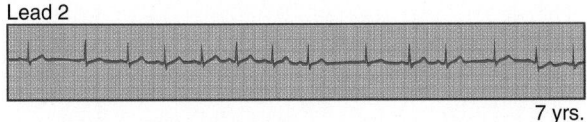

Figure 435-1 Phasic sinus arrhythmia with a junctional escape beat. Note the variation in P-P interval with no significant change in P-wave morphology or PR interval. When the sinus rate is slow enough, the atrioventricular junction takes over and produces escape beats. This rhythm is normal.

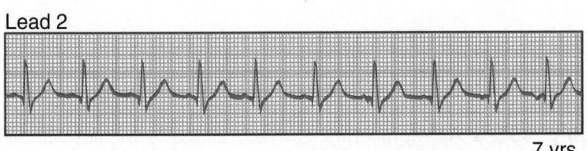

Figure 435-2 Wandering atrial pacemaker. Note the change in P-wave configuration in the 7th, 9th, and 10th beats. The 7th P wave may represent a fusion between the sinus P and the ectopic atrial pacemaker seen in the 10th beat.

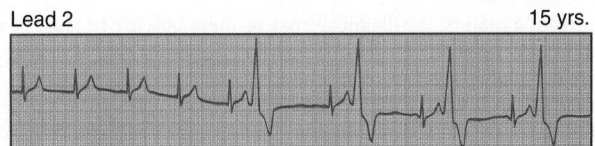

Figure 435-4 Premature ventricular contractions in a bigeminal rhythm, in a patient who is hyperventilating. Note that the premature beat is wide and has a completely different morphology from that of the sinus beat. The premature beat is not preceded by a discernable premature P wave or any appreciable deformation of the preceding T wave.

It is important to distinguish PVCs that are benign from those that are likely to lead to more severe arrhythmias. The former usually disappear during the tachycardia of exercise. If they persist or become more frequent during exercise, the arrhythmia may have greater significance. The following criteria are indications for further investigation of PVCs that could require **suppressive therapy:** (1) 2 or more ventricular premature beats in a row; (2) multiform PVCs; (3) increased ventricular ectopic activity with exercise; (4) R-on-T phenomenon (premature ventricular depolarization occurs on the T wave of the preceding beat); (5) extreme frequency of beats (e.g., >20% of total beats on Holter monitoring); and (6) most importantly, the presence of underlying heart disease, a history of heart surgery, or both. The best therapy for benign PVCs is reassurance that the arrhythmia is not life threatening, although very symptomatic individuals may benefit from suppressive therapy. Malignant PVCs are usually secondary to another medical problem (electrolyte imbalance, hypoxia, drug toxicity, or cardiac injury). Successful treatment includes correction of the underlying abnormality. An intravenous lidocaine bolus and drip is the first line of therapy, with more effective drugs such as amiodarone reserved for refractory cases or for patients underlying ventricular dysfunction or hemodynamic compromise.

435.3 Supraventricular Tachycardia
George F. Van Hare

Supraventricular tachycardia (SVT) is a general term that includes essentially all forms of paroxysmal or incessant tachycardia except ventricular tachycardia. The category of SVT can be divided into 3 major subcategories: reentrant tachycardias using an accessory pathway, reentrant tachycardias without an accessory pathway, and ectopic or automatic tachycardias. Atrioventricular reciprocating tachycardia (AVRT) involves an accessory pathway and is the most common mechanism of SVT in infants. Atrioventricular node reentry tachycardia (AVNRT) is rare in infancy but there is an increasing incidence of AVNRT in childhood and into adolescence. Atrial flutter is rarely seen in children with normal hearts, whereas intraatrial reentry tachycardia also known as atrial flutter, is common in patients following cardiac surgery. Atrial and junctional ectopic tachycardias are more commonly associated with abnormal hearts (cardiomyopathy) and in the immediate postoperative period following surgery for congenital heart disease.

CLINICAL MANIFESTATIONS
Reentrant SVT is characterized by an abrupt onset and cessation; it may occur when the patient is at rest or exercising, and in infants it may be precipitated by an acute infection. Attacks may last only a few seconds or may persist for hours. The heart rate usually exceeds 180 beats/min and may occasionally be as rapid as 300 beats/min. The only complaint may be awareness of the rapid heart rate. Many children tolerate these episodes extremely well, and it is unlikely that short paroxysms are a danger to life. If the rate is exceptionally rapid or if the attack is prolonged, precordial discomfort and heart failure may occur. In children, SVT may be exacerbated by exposure to nonprescription decongestants or by bronchodilators.

In young infants, the diagnosis may be more obscure because of the inability to communicate their symptoms. The heart rate at this age is normally higher than in older children and it increases greatly with crying. Infants with SVT on occasion initially present with heart failure, because the tachycardia may go unrecognized for a long time. The heart rate during episodes is frequently in the range of 240-300 beats/min. If the attack lasts 6-24 hr or more, heart failure may be recognized, and the infant will have an ashen color, and be restless and irritable, with tachypnea, poor pulses and hepatomegaly. When tachycardia occurs in the fetus, it can cause hydrops fetalis, which is the in utero manifestation of heart failure.

In neonates, SVT is usually manifested as a narrow QRS complex (<0.08 sec). The P wave is visible on a standard electrocardiogram in only 50-60% of neonates with SVT, but it is detectable with a transesophageal lead in most patients. **Differentiation from sinus tachycardia** may be difficult, but is important, as sinus tachycardia requires treatment of the underlying problem (e.g., sepsis, hypovolemia) rather than antiarrhythmic medication. If the rate is >230 beats/min with an abnormal P-wave axis (a normal P wave is positive in leads I and aVF), sinus tachycardia is not likely. The heart rate in SVT also tends to be *relatively unvarying*, whereas in sinus tachycardia the heart rate *varies* with changes in vagal and sympathetic tone. AV reciprocating tachycardia uses a bypass tract that may either be able to conduct bidirectionally **(Wolff-Parkinson-White [WPW] syndrome)** or retrograde only **(concealed accessory pathway)**. Patients with WPW syndrome have a small, but real risk of sudden death. If the accessory pathway rapidly conducts in antegrade fashion, the patient is at risk for atrial fibrillation begetting ventricular fibrillation. Risk stratification, including 24 hr Holter monitoring and exercise study, may help differentiate patients at higher risk for sudden death from WPW. Syncope is an ominous symptom in WPW and any patient with syncope and WPW syndrome should have an electrophysiology study and likely catheter ablation.

The typical electrocardiographic features of the WPW syndrome are seen when the patient is not having tachycardia. These features include a short P-R interval and slow upstroke of the QRS (delta wave) (Fig. 435-5). Although most often present in patients with a normal heart, this syndrome may also be associated with Ebstein anomaly of the tricuspid valve, or hypertrophic cardiomyopathy. The critical anatomic structure is an accessory pathway consisting of a muscular bridge connecting atrium to ventricle on either the right or the left side of the AV ring (Fig. 435-6). During sinus rhythm, the impulse is carried over both the AV node and the accessory pathway; it produces some degree of fusion of the 2 depolarization fronts that results in an abnormal QRS. During AVRT, an impulse is carried in antegrade fashion through the AV node **(orthodromic tachycardia)**, which results in a normal QRS complex, and in retrograde fashion

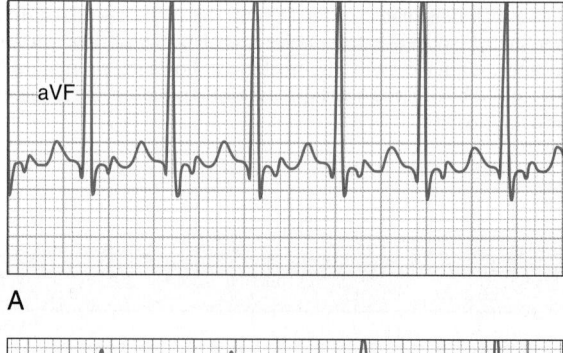

A

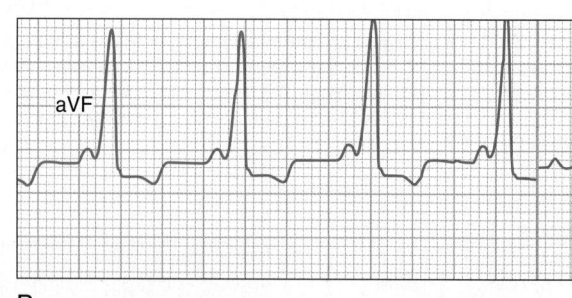

B

Figure 435-5 A, Supraventricular tachycardia in a child with Wolff-Parkinson-White (WPW) syndrome. Note the normal QRS complexes during the tachycardia, as well as clear retrograde P waves seen on the upstroke of the T waves. **B,** Later, the typical features of WPW syndrome are apparent (short P-R interval, delta wave, and wide QRS).

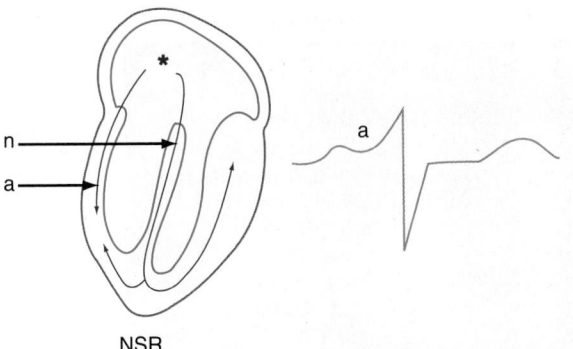

NSR

Figure 435-6 Schematic representation of the heart with a right-sided accessory pathway (Wolff-Parkinson-White syndrome). The *asterisk* indicates initiation of the sinus beat. The *arrows* indicate the direction and spread of excitation. The electrocardiographic complex shown represents a fusion beat that combines activation over the normal *(n)* and accessory *(a)* pathways. The latter inscribes the delta wave. NSR, normal sinus rhythm.

through the accessory pathway to the atrium, thereby perpetuating the tachycardia. In these cases, only after cessation of the tachycardia is the typical ECG features of WPW syndrome recognized (see Fig. 435-5). When rapid antegrade conduction occurs through the accessory pathway during tachycardia and the retrograde re-entry pathway to the atrium is via the AV node (**antidromic tachycardia**), the QRS complexes are wide and the potential for more serious arrhythmias (ventricular fibrillation) is greater, especially if atrial fibrillation occurs.

AVNRT involves the use of 2 pathways within the AV node, so-called *slow* and *fast* AV node pathways. This arrhythmia is more commonly seen in adolescence. It is one of the few forms of SVT that is occasionally associated with syncope. This arrhythmia is often seen in association with exercise.

TREATMENT

Vagal stimulation by placing of the face in ice water (in older children) or by placing an ice bag over the face (in infants) may abort the attack. To terminate the attack, older children may be taught vagal maneuvers such as the Valsalva maneuver, straining, breath holding, or standing on their head. Ocular pressure must never be performed, and carotid sinus massage is very rarely effective. When these measures fail, several pharmacologic alternatives are available (see Table 435-1). In stable patients, adenosine by rapid intravenous push is the **treatment of choice** because of its rapid onset of action and minimal effects on cardiac contractility. The dose may need to be increased if no effect on the tachycardia is seen. Because of the potential for adenosine to initiate atrial fibrillation, it should never be administered without a means for direct current (DC) cardioversion near at hand. Calcium channel blockers such as verapamil have also been used in the initial treatment of SVT in older children. Verapamil may reduce cardiac output and produce hypotension and cardiac arrest in infants younger than 1 yr; it is, therefore, contraindicated in this age group. In urgent situations when symptoms of severe heart failure have already occurred, synchronized DC cardioversion (0.5-2 J/kg) is recommended as the initial management (see Chapter 67).

Once the patient has been converted to sinus rhythm, a longer-acting agent may is selected for maintenance therapy. In patients without an antegrade accessory pathway (non-WPW), the β-blockers are the mainstay of drug therapy. Digoxin is also popular and may be effective in infants, but less so in older children. In children with WPW, digoxin or calcium channel blockers may increase the rate of antegrade conduction of impulses through the bypass tract, with the possibility of ventricular fibrillation, and are therefore contraindicated. These patients are usually managed with β-blockers. In patients with resistant

tachycardias, flecainide, propafenone, sotalol, and amiodarone have all been used. Most antiarrhythmic agents have the potential of causing new dangerous arrhythmias (**proarrhythmia**) and decreasing heart function. Flecainide and propafenone in particular should be limited to use in patients with otherwise normal hearts.

If cardiac failure occurs because of prolonged tachycardia in an infant with a normal heart, cardiac function usually returns to normal after sinus rhythm is reinstituted, although it may take days to weeks. Infants with SVT diagnosed within the 1st 3-4 mo of life have a lower incidence of recurrence than do those in whom it is initially diagnosed at a later age. These patients have an 80% chance of resolution by the 1st yr of life, although approximately 30% will have recurrences later in childhood; if medical therapy is required, it can be tapered within a year and the patient watched for signs of recurrence. Parents should be taught to measure the heart rate in their infants, so that prolonged unapparent episodes of SVT may be detected before heart failure occurs.

Twenty-four hour electrocardiographic (Holter) recordings are useful in monitoring the course of therapy and in detecting brief runs of asymptomatic tachycardia, particularly in younger children and infants. Some centers use **transesophageal pacing** to evaluate the effects of therapy in infants. More detailed electrophysiologic studies performed in the cardiac catheterization laboratory are often indicated in patients with refractory SVTs who are candidates for **catheter ablation**. During an electrophysiologic study, multiple electrode catheters are placed transvenously in different locations in the heart. Pacing is performed to evaluate the conduction characteristics of the accessory pathway and to initiate the tachyarrhythmia, and mapping is performed to locate the accessory pathway. **Catheter ablation** of an accessory pathway is frequently used in children and teenagers, as well as in patients who require multiple agents or find drug side effects intolerable or for whom arrhythmia control is poor. Ablation may be performed either by radiofrequency ablation, which creates tissue heating, or cryoablation, in which tissue is frozen (Fig. 435-7). The overall initial success rate for catheter ablation ranges from approximately 90-98%, depending on the location of the accessory pathway. Surgical ablation of bypass tracts is only rarely done, and is proposed only in carefully selected patients.

The management of SVT caused by **AVNRT** is nearly identical to that for AVRT. Children with AVNRT are not at increased risk of sudden death, as they do not have a manifest accessory pathway. In practice, their episodes are more likely to be brought on by exercise or other forms of stress, and the heart rates can be quite fast, leading to chest pain, dizziness, and, occasionally, syncope. If chronic antiarrhythmic medication is desired, β-blockers are the drugs of choice; acutely, AVNRT responds to adenosine. Less is known about the natural history, but patients with AVNRT are seen quite commonly in adulthood, so spontaneous resolution seems unlikely. Patients are quite amenable to catheter ablation, either using radiofrequency energy or cryoablation, with high success rates and low complication rates.

Atrial ectopic tachycardia is an uncommon tachycardia in childhood. It is characterized by a variable rate (seldom >200 beats/min), identifiable P waves with an abnormal axis, and either a sustained or incessant nonsustained tachycardia. This form of atrial tachycardia has a single automatic focus. Identification of this mechanism is aided by monitoring the electrocardiogram while initiating vagal or pharmacologic therapy. Reentry tachycardias "break" suddenly, whereas automatic tachycardias gradually slow down and then gradually speed up again. Atrial ectopic tachycardias are usually more difficult to control pharmacologically than are the more common reentrant tachycardias. If pharmacologic therapy with a single agent is unsuccessful, catheter ablation is suggested and has a success rate >90%.

Chaotic or multifocal atrial tachycardia is defined as atrial tachycardia with ≥3 ectopic P waves, frequent blocked P waves, and varying P-R intervals of conducted beats. This arrhythmia occurs most often in infants younger than 1 yr, usually without cardiac disease, although some evidence suggests an association with viral myocarditis or pulmonary disease. The goal of drug treatment is slowing of

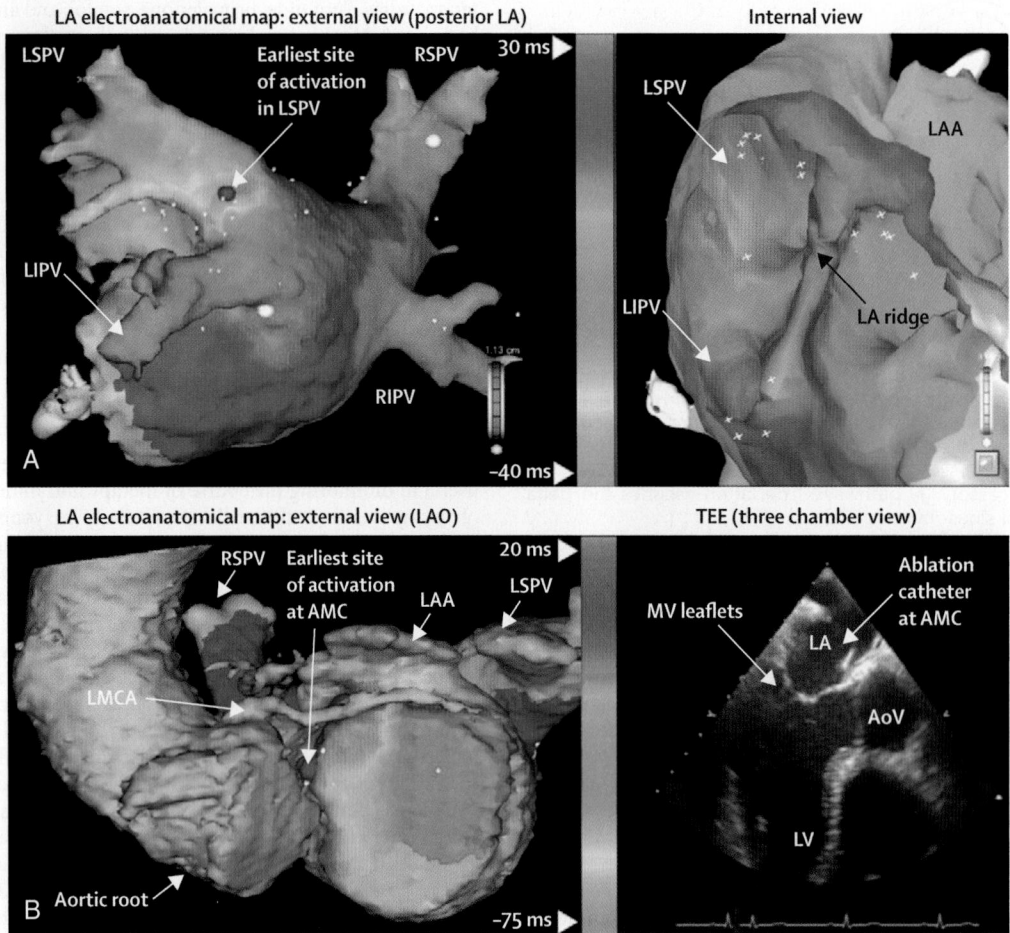

Figure 435-7 Three-dimensional electroanatomical mapping of focal atrial tachycardias. Focal site of early activation *(red)* is shown, with radial propagation away from that central site. The activation map was superimposed onto the patient's cardiac CT scan, taken the day before the procedure and imported into the mapping system. **A,** Earliest site of activation, mapped to the posterior aspect of the LSPV ostium. Posterior external view *(left side)* and endoluminal or internal view looking from within the left atrium into the mouth of the LSPV *(right side)* are shown. **B,** Earliest site mapped to the aortomitral continuity. The anatomic relation between the mitral annulus and the aortic root can be clearly appreciated *(left side)*. The location of the ablation catheter at the site of earliest atrial activation during atrial tachycardia is shown on the TEE image *(right side)*. AMC, aortomitral continuity; AoV, aortic valve; LA, left atrium; LAA, left atrial appendage; LAO, left anterior oblique; LIPV, left inferior pulmonary veins; LMCA, left main coronary artery; LSPV, left superior pulmonary vein; LV, left ventricle; MV, mitral valve; RIPV, right inferior pulmonary veins; RSPV, right superior pulmonary vein; TEE, transesophageal echocardiogram. *(From Lee G, Sanders P, Kalman JM: Catheter ablation of atrial arrhythmias: state of the art. Lancet 380:1509–1518, 2012, Fig 3.)*

the ventricular rate, as conversion to sinus may not be possible, and multiple agents are often required. When this arrhythmia occurs in infancy, it usually terminates spontaneously by 3 yr of age.

Accelerated junctional ectopic tachycardia (JET) is an automatic (non-reentry) arrhythmia in which the junctional rate exceeds that of the sinus node and AV dissociation results. This arrhythmia is most often recognized in the early postoperative period after cardiac surgery and may be extremely difficult to control. Reduction of the infusion rate of catecholamines and control of fever are important adjuncts to management. Congenital JET may be seen in the absence of surgery. It is incessant, and can lead to dilated cardiomyopathy. Intravenous amiodarone is effective in the treatment of postoperative JET. Patients who require chronic therapy may respond to amiodarone or sotalol. Congenital JET can be cured by catheter ablation, but long-term AV block requiring a pacemaker is a prominent complication.

Atrial flutter, also known as *intraatrial reentrant tachycardia,* is an atrial tachycardia characterized by atrial activity at a rate of 250-300 beats/min in children and adolescents, and 400-600 beats/min in neonates. The mechanism of common atrial flutter consists of a reentrant or rhythm originating in the right atrium circling the tricuspid valve annulus. Because the AV node cannot transmit such rapid impulses,

some degree of **AV block** is virtually always present, and the ventricles respond to every 2nd to 4th atrial beat (Fig. 435-8). Occasionally, the response is variable and the rhythm appears irregular.

In older children, atrial flutter usually occurs in the setting of congenital heart disease; neonates with atrial flutter frequently have normal hearts. Atrial flutter may occur during acute infectious illnesses but is most often seen in patients with large stretched atria, such as those associated with long-standing mitral or tricuspid insufficiency, tricuspid atresia, Ebstein anomaly, or rheumatic mitral stenosis. Atrial flutter can also occur after palliative or corrective intra-atrial surgery. Uncontrolled atrial flutter may precipitate heart failure. Vagal maneuvers or adenosine may produce a temporary slowing of the heart rate as a result of increased AV block, allowing a diagnosis to be made. The **diagnosis** is confirmed by electrocardiography, which demonstrates the rapid and regular atrial sawtoothed flutter waves. Atrial flutter usually converts immediately to sinus rhythm by **synchronized DC cardioversion,** which is most often the **treatment of choice.** Patients with chronic atrial flutter in the setting of congenital heart disease may be at increased risk for **thromboembolism** and stroke and should thus undergo anticoagulation before elective cardioversion. β-blockers or calcium channel blockers may be used to slow the ventricular response in atrial flutter by prolonging the AV node refractory period. Other agents may be used to maintain sinus rhythm, and choices include Class I agents such as procainamide or propafenone, Class III agents such as amiodarone and sotalol. Catheter ablation has been used in patients with normal hearts and those with congenital heart disease with moderate success. Following cardioversion, neonates with normal hearts may be followed or may be treated with digoxin or propranolol for 6-12 mo, after which the medication can usually be discontinued, as neonatal atrial flutter generally does not recur.

Atrial fibrillation is uncommon in children and is rare in infants. The atrial excitation is chaotic and more rapid (400-700 beats/min) and produces an irregularly irregular ventricular response and pulse (Fig. 435-9). This rhythm disorder is often associated with atrial enlargement or disease. Atrial fibrillation may be seen in older children with rheumatic mitral valve stenosis. It is also seen rarely as a complication of atrial surgery, in patients with left atrial enlargement secondary to left AV valve insufficiency, and in patients with WPW syndrome. Thyrotoxicosis, pulmonary embolism, pericarditis, or cardiomyopathy may be suspected in a previously normal older child or adolescent with atrial fibrillation. Very rarely, atrial fibrillation may be familial. The best initial treatment is **rate control,** most effectively with calcium channel blockers, to limit the ventricular rate during atrial fibrillation. Digoxin is not given if WPW syndrome is present. Normal sinus rhythm may be restored with intravenous procainamide, ibutilide or amiodarone, or by DC cardioversion, and DC cardioversion is the first choice in hemodynamically unstable patients. Patients with chronic atrial fibrillation are at risk for the development of thromboembolism and stroke and should undergo anticoagulation with warfarin. Patients being treated by elective cardioversion should also undergo anticoagulation.

435.4 Ventricular Tachyarrhythmias
George F. Van Hare

Ventricular tachycardia (VT) is less common than SVT in pediatric patients. VT is defined as at least 3 PVCs at >120 beats/min (Fig. 435-10). It may be paroxysmal or incessant. VT may be associated with myocarditis, anomalous origin of a coronary artery, arrhythmogenic right ventricular dysplasia, mitral valve prolapse, primary cardiac tumors, and dilated or hypertrophic cardiomyopathy. It is seen with prolonged QT interval of either congenital or acquired (proarrhythmic drugs) causation, WPW syndrome, and drug use (cocaine, amphetamines). It may develop years after intraventricular surgery (especially tetralogy of Fallot and related defects) or occur without obvious organic heart disease. VT must be distinguished from SVT with aberrancy or rapid conduction over an accessory pathway (Table 435-2). The presence of clear capture and fusion beats confirms the diagnosis of VT. Although some children tolerate rapid ventricular rates for many hours, this arrhythmia should be promptly treated because hypotension and degeneration into ventricular fibrillation may result. For patients who are hemodynamically stable, intravenous amiodarone, lidocaine, or procainamide are the initial drugs of choice. If treatment is to be successful, it is critical to search for and correct any underlying abnormalities such as electrolyte imbalance, hypoxia, or drug toxicity. Amiodarone is the **treatment of choice** during cardiac arrest (see Chapter 67). Hemodynamically unstable patients with VT should be immediately treated with DC cardioversion. Overdrive ventricular pacing, through temporary pacing wires or a permanent pacemaker, may also be effective, although it may cause the arrhythmia to deteriorate into ventricular fibrillation. In the neonatal period, VT may be associated with an anomalous left coronary artery (see Chapter 432.2) or a myocardial tumor.

Unless a clearly reversible cause is identified, electrophysiologic study is usually indicated for patients in whom VT has developed, and depending on the findings, catheter ablation and/or ICD implantation may be indicated.

A related arrhythmia, **ventricular accelerated rhythm**, is occasionally seen in infants. It is defined the same way as VT, but the rate is only slightly faster than the coexisting sinus rate (within 10%). It is generally benign and resolves spontaneously.

Ventricular fibrillation is a chaotic rhythm that results in death unless an effective ventricular beat is rapidly re-established (see Fig. 435-10). Usually, cardiopulmonary resuscitation and DC defibrillation are necessary. If defibrillation is ineffective or fibrillation recurs, amiodarone or lidocaine may be given intravenously and defibrillation repeated (see Chapter 67). After recovery from ventricular fibrillation, a search should be made for the underlying cause. **Electrophysiologic study** is indicated for patients who have survived

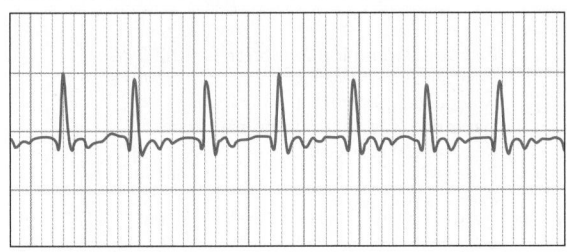

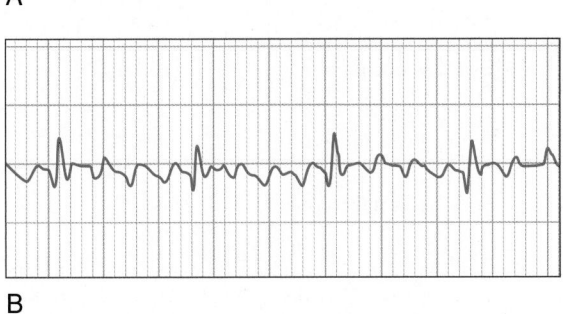

Figure 435-8 Neonatal atrial flutter. Note that the flutter waves are not obvious in the first tracing **(A)** but once a dose of adenosine is given, flutter waves at a rate of about 450 beats/min emerge **(B)**.

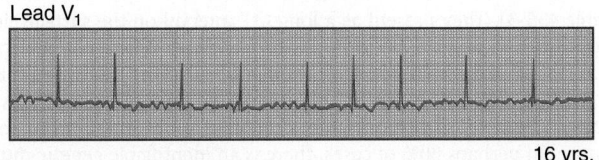

Figure 435-9 Atrial fibrillation, characterized by the absence of clear P waves and an irregularly irregular ventricular response. One can appreciate the irregular, rapid undulations (F waves). Fibrillatory waves may not be visible in all leads and should be carefully sought in every tracing with irregular R-R intervals. Note that no 2 R-R intervals are the same.

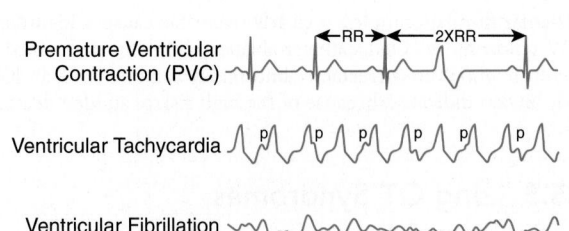

Figure 435-10 Ventricular arrhythmias. *(From Park MY: Pediatric cardiology for practitioners, ed 5, Philadelphia, 2008, Mosby/Elsevier, p. 429, Fig. 24-6.)*

Table 435-2	Diagnosis of Tachyarrhythmias: Electrocardiographic Findings			
	HEART RATE (BEATS/MIN)	**P WAVE**	**QRS DURATION**	**REGULARITY**
Sinus tachycardia	<230	Always present, normal axis	Normal	Rate varies with respiration
Atrial tachycardia	180-320	Present Abnormal P wave morphology and axis	Normal or prolonged (with aberration)	Usually regular but ventricular response may be variable because of Wenckebach conduction
Atrial fibrillation	120-180	Fibrillatory waves	Normal or prolonged (with aberration)	Irregularly irregular (no 2 R-R intervals alike)
Atrial flutter	Atrial: 250-400 Ventricular response variable: 100-320	Sawtoothed flutter waves	Normal or prolonged (with aberration)	Regular ventricular response (e.g., 2:1, 3:1, 3:2, and so on)
Junctional tachycardia	120-280	Atrioventricular dissociation with no fusion, and normal QRS capture beats	Normal or prolonged (with aberration)	Regular (except with capture beats)
Ventricular tachycardia	120-300	Atrioventricular dissociation with capture beats and fusion beats	Prolonged for age	Regular (except with capture beats)

Table 435-3	Inherited Channel Mutations in Long and Short QT Syndromes				
CHROMOSOME	**GENE**	**PROTEIN**	**ION CURRENT AFFECTED**	**TRIGGER**	**SPECIAL FEATURES/ OCCURRENCE**
LQTS TYPE					
1 11p15.5	KCNQ1	KvLQT1 (Kv7.1)	I_{Ks}	Exercise (swimming), emotion	42-54%
2 7q35-36	KCNH2	HERG, (Kv11.1)	I_{Kr}	Rest, emotion, exercise (acoustic, postpartum), surprise (sudden loud noise)	35-45%
3 3p24-21	SCN5A	Nav1.5	I_{Na}	Rest, sleep, emotion	1.7-8%; high lethality
4 4q24-27	ANK2	Ankyrin-B	I_{Na-K}, I_{Na-Ca}, I_{Na}	Exercise	<1%
5 21q22	KCNE1	MinK	I_{Ks}	Exercise, emotion	<1%
6 21q22	KCNE2	MiRP1	I_{Kr}	Rest, exercise	<1%
7 17q23	KCNJ2	Kir2.1	I_{K1}	Rest, exercise	Periodic paralysis, dysmorphic feature
8 12p13.3	CACNA1C	Cav1.2	I_{Ca}	Exercise, emotion	Rare, syndactyly
9 3p25.3	CAV3	Caveolin-3	I_{Na}	Nonexertional, sleep	Rare
10 11q23.3	SCN4B	NaVβ4	I_{Na}	Exercise, postpartum	<0.1%
11 7q21-22	AKAP9	Yotiao	I_{Ks}	Poorly characterized	<1%
12 2q11.2	SNTA1	Syntrophin α1	I_{Na}	Poorly characterized	<1%
13 11q24	KCNJ5	Kir3.4	K_{Ir}	Poorly characterized	<1%
SHORT QT SYNDROME TYPE					
1 7q35-36	KCNH2	HERG (Kv11.1)	I_{Kr}	Exercise, rest (acoustic)	—
2 11p15.5	KCNQ1	KvLQT1 (Kv7.1)	I_{Ks}	—	—
3 17q23	KCNJ2	Kir2.1	I_{K1}	Sleep	—
4 12p13.3	CACNA1C	Cav1.2	I_{Ca}	—	—
5 10p12.33	CACNB2b	CaV β2b	I_{Ca}	—	—
JERVELL AND LANGE-NIELSEN SYNDROME TYPE					
1 11p15.5	KCNQ1	KvLQT1 (Kv7.1)	I_{Ks}	Exercise (swimming), emotion	1-7%; deafness
2 21q22	KCNE1	MinK	I_{Ks}	Exercise (swimming), emotion	<1%; deafness

From Morita H, Wu J, Zipes DP: The QT syndromes: long and short, Lancet 372:750–762, 2008, p. 751, Table 1.

ventricular fibrillation unless a clearly reversible cause is identified. If WPW syndrome is noted, catheter ablation should be performed. For patients in whom no correctable abnormality can be found, an ICD is nearly always indicated, because of the high risk of sudden death.

435.5 Long QT Syndromes
George F. Van Hare

Long QT syndromes (LQTS) are genetic abnormalities of ventricular repolarization, with an estimated incidence of about 1 per 10,000 births

(Table 435-3). They present as a long QT interval on the surface electrocardiogram and are associated with malignant ventricular arrhythmias (torsades de pointes and ventricular fibrillation). They are a cause of syncope and sudden death and may be the cause of some cases of sudden infant death syndrome, drowning, and intrauterine fetal demise. In perhaps 80% of cases, there is an identifiable genetic mutation. The old distinction between dominant and recessive forms of the disease (Romano-Ward syndrome vs. Jervell-Lange-Nielsen syndrome) is no longer made, as the latter recessive condition is known to be a result of the homozygous state. Jervell-Lange-Nielsen syndrome is associated with congenital sensorineural deafness. Asymptomatic but at-risk patients carrying the gene mutation may not all have a

Table 435-4	Acquired Causes of QT Prolongation*

DRUGS

Antibiotics—erythromycin, clarithromycin, azithromycin, telithromycin, trimethoprim/sulfamethoxazole, fluoroquinolones[†]
Antifungal agents[†]—fluconazole, itraconazole, ketoconazole
Antiprotozoal agents—pentamidine isethionate
Antihistamines—astemizole, terfenadine (Seldane; Seldane has been removed from the market for this reason)
Antidepressants—tricyclics such as imipramine (Tofranil), amitriptyline (Elavil), desipramine (Norpramin), and doxepin (Sinequan)
Antipsychotics—haloperidol, risperidone, phenothiazines such as thioridazine (Mellaril) and chlorpromazine (Thorazine), selective serotonin
 uptake inhibitors
Antiarrhythmic agents
Class 1A (sodium channel blockers)—quinidine, procainamide, disopyramide
Class III (prolong depolarization)—amiodarone (rare), bretylium, dofetilide, N-acetyl-procainamide, sotalol
Lipid-lowering agents—probucol
Antianginals—bepridil
Diuretics (through K+ loss)—furosemide (Lasix), ethacrynic acid (bumetanide [Bumex])
Opiates—methadone, oxycodone
Oral hypoglycemic agents—glibenclamide, glyburide
Organophosphate insecticides
Motility agents—cisapride, domperidone
Vasodilators—prenylamine
Other drugs—Ondansetron, HIV protease inhibitors, Chinese herbs

ELECTROLYTE DISTURBANCES

Hypokalemia—diuretics, hyperventilation
Hypocalcemia
Hypomagnesemia

UNDERLYING MEDICAL CONDITIONS

Bradycardia—complete atrioventricular block, severe bradycardia, sick sinus syndrome
Myocardial dysfunction—anthracycline cardiotoxicity, congestive heart failure, myocarditis, cardiac tumors
Endocrinopathy—hyperparathyroidism, hypothyroidism, pheochromocytoma
Neurologic—encephalitis, head trauma, stroke, subarachnoid hemorrhage
Nutritional—alcoholism, anorexia nervosa, starvation

*A more exhaustive updated list of medications that can prolong the QTc interval is available at the University of Arizona Center for Education and Research of Therapeutics website (www.azcert.org).
[†]Combinations of quinolones plus azoles increase the risk of prolonged QT intervals.
From Park MY: Pediatric cardiology for practitioners, ed 5, Philadelphia, 2008, Mosby/Elsevier, p. 433, Box 24-1.

prolonged QT duration. QT interval prolongation may become apparent with exercise or during catecholamine infusions.

Genetic studies have identified mutations in cardiac potassium and sodium channels (see Table 435-3). Additional forms (up to 13 variants) of LQTS have been described, but these are much more uncommon. Genotype may predict clinical manifestations; for example, **LQT1 events are usually stress induced,** whereas events in **LQT3 often occur during sleep.** LQT2 events have an intermediate pattern. LQT3 has the highest probability for sudden death, followed by LQT2 and then LQT1. Drugs may prolong the QT interval directly but more often do so when drugs such as erythromycin or ketoconazole inhibit their metabolism (Table 435-4).

The **clinical manifestation** of LQTS in children is most often a syncopal episode brought on by exercise, fright, or a sudden startle; some events occur during sleep (LQT3). Patients can initially be seen with seizures, presyncope, or palpitations; approximately 10% are initially in cardiac arrest. The diagnosis is based on electrocardiographic and clinical criteria. Not all patients with long QT intervals have LQTS, and patients with normal QT intervals on a resting electrocardiogram may have LQTS. A heart rate–corrected QT interval of >0.47 sec is highly indicative, whereas a QT interval of >0.44 sec is suggestive. Other features include notched T waves in 3 leads, T-wave alternans, a low heart rate for age, a history of syncope (especially with stress), and a familial history of either LQTS or unexplained sudden death. Twenty-four hour Holter monitoring and exercise testing are adjuncts to the diagnosis. Genotyping is available and can identify the mutation is approximately 80% of patients known to have LQTS by clinical criteria. Genotyping is not useful in ruling out the diagnosis in individuals suspected of having the disease, but when positive is very useful in identifying asymptomatic affected relatives of the index case.

Short QT syndromes (see Table 435-3) manifest with atrial or ventricular fibrillation and are associated with syncope and sudden death. They are often caused by a gain-of-function mutation in cardiac potassium channels.

Treatment of LQTS includes the use of β-**blocking agents** at doses that blunt the heart rate response to exercise. Propranolol and nadolol may be more effective than atenolol and metoprolol. Some patients require a **pacemaker** because of drug-induced bradycardia. In patients with continued syncope despite treatment, an implantable cardiac defibrillator is indicated for those who do not respond to β-blocking drugs and those who have experienced cardiac arrest. Genotype-phenotype correlative studies have suggested that β-blocking agents are not effective in patients with LQT3, and in those individuals, an ICD is usually indicated.

435.6 Sinus Node Dysfunction
George F. Van Hare

Sinus arrest and **sinoatrial block** may cause a sudden pause in the heartbeat. The former is presumably caused by failure of impulse formation within the sinus node and the latter by a block between the sinus pacemaker complex and the surrounding atrium. These arrhythmias are rare in childhood except in patients who have had extensive atrial surgery.

Sick sinus syndrome is the result of abnormalities in the sinus node or atrial conduction pathways, or both. This syndrome may occur in the absence of congenital heart disease and has been reported in siblings, but it is most commonly seen after surgical correction of congenital heart defects, especially the Fontan procedure and the atrial switch (Mustard or Senning) operation for transposition of the great

Continuous monitor lead

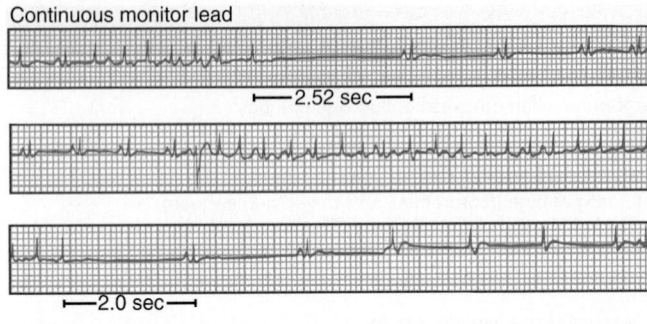

Figure 435-11 The "tachy-brady" syndrome with sinus node dysfunction. Note the bursts of supraventricular tachycardia, probably multifocal atrial in origin, followed by long periods of sinus arrest and by sinus bradycardia. Often, symptoms are caused by the long sinus pauses following termination of tachycardia, rather than by the tachycardia itself.

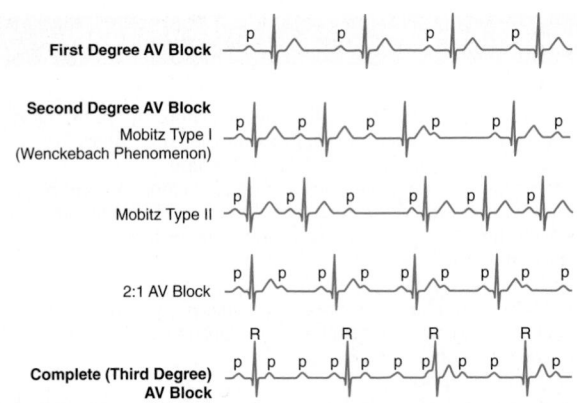

Figure 435-12 Atrioventricular block. *(From Park MY: Pediatric cardiology for practitioners, ed 5, Philadelphia, 2008, Mosby/Elsevier, p. 446, Fig. 25-1.)*

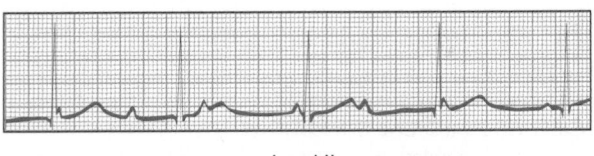

Lead II

Figure 435-13 Congenital complete atrioventricular (AV) block. The ventricular rate is regular at 53 beats/min. The atrial rate is somewhat variable, from 65-95 beats/min, and completely dissociated from the ventricle. The QRS morphology is normal, which is common in congenital complete AV block.

arteries. Clinical manifestations depend on the heart rate. Most patients remain asymptomatic without treatment, but dizziness and syncope can occur during periods of marked sinus slowing with failure of junctional escape (Fig. 435-11). Pacemaker therapy is indicated in patients who experience symptoms such as exercise intolerance or syncope.

Patients with sinus node dysfunction may also have episodes of SVT (**"tachy-brady syndrome"**) with symptoms of palpitations, exercise intolerance, or dizziness. Treatment must be individualized. Drug therapy to control tachyarrhythmias (propranolol, sotalol, amiodarone) may suppress sinus and AV node function to such a degree that further symptomatic bradycardia may be produced. Therefore, insertion of a pacemaker in conjunction with drug therapy is usually necessary for such patients, even in the absence of symptoms ascribable to low heart rate.

435.7 AV Block
George F. Van Hare

AV block may be divided into 3 forms. In **1st-degree AV block,** the PR interval is prolonged, but all the atrial impulses are conducted to the ventricle (Fig. 435-12). In **2nd-degree AV block,** not every atrial impulse is conducted to the ventricle. In the variant of 2nd-degree block known as the **Wenckebach type** (also called **Mobitz type I**), the PR interval increases progressively until a P wave is not conducted. In the cycle following the dropped beat, the PR interval normalizes (see Fig. 435-12). In **Mobitz type II,** there is no progressive conduction delay or subsequent shortening of the PR interval after a blocked beat. This conduction defect is less common but has more potential to cause syncope and may be progressive. A related condition is **high-grade 2nd-degree AV block,** in which 2 or more P waves in a row fail to conduct. This is even more dangerous. In **3rd-degree AV block (complete heart block),** no impulses from the atria reach the ventricles (see Fig. 435-12). An independent escape rhythm is usually present, but may not be reliable, leading to symptoms such as syncope.

Congenital complete AV block in children is presumed to be caused by autoimmune injury of the fetal conduction system by maternally derived immunoglobulin G antibodies (anti-SSA/Ro, anti-SSB/La) in a mother with overt or, more often, asymptomatic systemic lupus erythematosus or Sjögren syndrome. Autoimmune disease accounts for 60-70% of all cases of congenital complete heart block and ≈80% of cases in which the heart is structurally normal (Fig. 435-13). A mutation of the homeobox gene Nkx2-5 is described in which congenital AV block is seen most commonly in association with atrial septal defects. Complete AV block is also seen in patients with complex congenital heart disease and abnormal embryonic development of the

conduction system. It has been associated with myocardial tumors and myocarditis. It is a known complication of myocardial abscess secondary to endocarditis. It is also seen in genetic abnormalities including LQTS and Kearn-Sayre syndrome. It is also a complication of congenital heart disease repair and, in particular, repairs involving ventricular septal defect closure.

The incidence of congenital complete heart block is 1 per 20,000-25,000 live births; a high fetal loss rate may cause an underestimation of its true incidence. In some infants of mothers with systemic lupus erythematosus, complete heart block is not present at birth but develops within the 1st 3-6 mo after birth. The arrhythmia is often diagnosed in the fetus (secondary to the dissociation between atrial and ventricular contractions seen on fetal echocardiography) and may produce hydrops fetalis. Maternal treatment with steroids to halt progression or reverse AV block is controversial. Infants with associated congenital heart disease and heart failure have a high mortality rate.

In older children with otherwise normal hearts, the condition is often asymptomatic, although syncope and sudden death may occur. Infants and toddlers may have night terrors, tiredness with frequent naps, and irritability. The peripheral pulse is prominent as a result of the compensatory large ventricular stroke volume and peripheral vasodilation; systolic blood pressure is elevated. Jugular venous pulsations occur irregularly and may be large when the atrium contracts against a closed tricuspid valve (cannon wave). Exercise and atropine may produce an acceleration of ≥10-20 beats/min. Systolic murmurs are frequently audible along the left sternal border, and apical mid-diastolic murmurs are not unusual. The 1st heart sound is variable, as a result of variable ventricular filing with AV dissociation. AV block results in enlargement of the heart on the basis of increased diastolic ventricular filling.

The **diagnosis** is confirmed by electrocardiography; the P waves and QRS complexes have no constant relationship (see Fig. 435-13). The

QRS duration may be prolonged, or it may be normal if the heartbeat is initiated high in the AV node or bundle of His.

The **prognosis** for congenital complete heart block is usually favorable; patients who have been observed to the age of 30-40 yr have lived normal, active lives. Some patients have episodes of exercise intolerance, dizziness, and syncope (Stokes-Adams attacks); this symptom requires the implantation of a permanent cardiac pacemaker. Pacemaker implantation should be considered for patients who develop symptoms such as progressive cardiac enlargement, prolonged pauses, or daytime average heart rates of ≤50 beats/min. In addition, prophylactic pacemaker implantation in adolescents is reasonable considering the low risk of the implant procedure and the difficulty in predicting who will develop sudden severe symptoms.

Cardiac pacing is recommended in neonates with low ventricular rates (≤50 beats/min), evidence of heart failure, wide complex rhythms, or congenital heart disease. Isoproterenol, atropine, or epinephrine may be used to try to increase the heart rate temporarily until pacemaker placement can be arranged. Transthoracic epicardial pacemaker implants have traditionally been used in infants; transvenous placement of pacemaker leads is available for young children. Postsurgical complete AV block can occur after any open heart procedure requiring suturing near the AV valves or crest of the ventricular septum. Postoperative heart block is initially managed with temporary pacing wires. The likelihood of a return to sinus rhythm after 10-14 days is low; a permanent pacemaker is recommended after that time.

Bibliography is available at Expert Consult.

Chapter **436**
Sudden Death
George F. Van Hare

Sudden death other than sudden infant death syndrome (see Chapter 375) is rare in children younger than 18 yr. Sudden death can be divided into either traumatic or nontraumatic origin. Traumatic causes of sudden death are the most common in children; these include motor vehicle crashes, violent deaths, recreational deaths, and occupational deaths. Nontraumatic sudden deaths are often the result of specific cardiac causes. The incidence of sudden death varies from 0.8-6.2 per 100,000 per year in children and adolescents as opposed to the higher incidence of sudden cardiac death in adults of 1 per 1,000. Approximately 65% of sudden deaths are a result of heart-related problems in patients with either normal or congenitally (corrected, palliated, or unoperated) abnormal hearts. Competitive high-school sports (basketball, football) are high-risk environmental factors. The most common cause of death in competitive athletes is hypertrophic cardiomyopathy, with or without obstruction to left ventricular outflow. Table 436-1 lists other potential causes. These can be classified as structural abnormalities, including aortic stenosis and coronary artery abnormalities; myocardial disease, such as myocarditis; conduction system disease, including long QT syndrome; and miscellaneous causes, including pulmonary hypertension and commotio cordis. Symptoms may be absent before the event but, if present, include syncope, chest pain, dyspnea, and palpitations. Patients may have a family history of heart disease (dilated or hypertrophic cardiomyopathy, long QT interval, arrhythmogenic right ventricular dysplasia, Brugada or Marfan syndromes) or sudden death. Death often follows exertion or exercise.

MECHANISM OF SUDDEN DEATH
There are 3 mechanisms of sudden death: arrhythmic, nonarrhythmic cardiac (circulatory and vascular causes), and noncardiac. Ventricular fibrillation, while the most common final cause of sudden death in adults, is only the final cause in 10-20% of children with sudden cardiac death. More commonly, bradycardia leads either to ventricular fibrillation or asystole (see Chapter 435).

CONGENITAL HEART DISEASE
Valvar aortic stenosis is the congenital defect most commonly associated with sudden death in children. Historically, approximately 5% of children with this disease die, although this has become quite rare in the modern era. A history of syncope, chest pain, and evidence of severe obstruction and left ventricular hypertrophy are risk factors (see Chapter 434.5).

Coronary artery anomalies are also commonly associated with sudden death in children and adolescents. The most common abnormality associated with sudden death is the origin of the left main coronary artery from the right sinus of Valsalva. The coronary artery therefore courses between the aorta and pulmonary artery, and may also be intramural in course. Exercise results in a rise in pulmonary and aortic pressure, and this is thought to compress the left main coronary artery and results in ischemia due to compression or kinking. Anomalous origin of the right coronary artery from the left sinus of Valsalva is much more common, but only rarely is a cause of sudden death.

CARDIOMYOPATHY
All 3 major types of cardiomyopathy (hypertrophic, dilated, and restrictive) are associated with sudden death in the pediatric population; sudden death may be the initial manifestation of the cardiomyopathy (see Chapter 439).

Hypertrophic cardiomyopathy (HCM) is the most common cause of sudden death in the athletic adolescent. The annual risk of sudden death in young patients with HCM is 2% per year. Risk factors for sudden death include a family history of sudden death, symptoms, ventricular arrhythmias, and presentation at an early age. Many patients with HCM have obstruction to the left ventricular outflow tract. The mechanism of sudden death is arrhythmic and may be secondary to development of dynamic obstruction with exercise and resultant loss of cardiac output, or may be related to cardiac ischemia. Thus, patients without left ventricular outflow tract obstruction are also at risk of sudden death. The **dilated cardiomyopathies** are also associated with sudden cardiac death in children, although the risk is clearly lower than in adults.

Arrhythmogenic right ventricular dysplasia is a specific form of cardiomyopathy associated with exercise-induced ventricular arrhythmias and sudden death. The diagnosis can be difficult; MRI, electrophysiology study, or endomyocardial biopsy is used with limited reliability. Pathology includes transmural fatty replacement of right ventricular myocardium, with patchy areas of fibrosis.

Myocarditis has been found commonly on pathology of patients with sudden death of unknown etiology. Symptoms prior to sudden death may be absent, or may include overt heart failure or subtle findings such as a high heart rate. Pediatric patients may have complete heart block or ventricular arrhythmias with this disease.

CARDIAC ARRHYTHMIA
A primary conduction system abnormality may result in sudden death. Causes include Wolff-Parkinson-White (WPW) syndrome, long QT syndrome, and Brugada syndrome. Besides causing supraventricular tachycardia, WPW syndrome can result in atrial fibrillation with rapid conduction across the accessory pathway leading to ventricular fibrillation and sudden death (Fig. 436-1). This is unusual in pediatric patients but has an increasing incidence in adolescence. In adults, there is an incidence of sudden death in asymptomatic patients of 1 per 1,000 patient-years, but this rate may well be higher in children, who by definition have not survived to adulthood. As digoxin and verapamil can augment conduction down accessory pathways, these drugs are contraindicated in WPW syndrome.

Long QT syndrome (see Chapter 435), a group of channelopathies that affect ventricular repolarization, is also associated with sudden

Table 436-1	Potential Causes of Sudden Death in Infants, Children, and Adolescents

SIDS AND SIDS "MIMICS"
SIDS
Long QT syndromes*
Inborn errors of metabolism
Child abuse
Myocarditis
Ductal-dependent congenital heart disease

CORRECTED OR UNOPERATED CONGENITAL HEART DISEASE
Aortic stenosis
Tetralogy of Fallot
Transposition of great vessels (postoperative atrial switch)
Mitral valve prolapse
Hypoplastic left-heart syndrome
Eisenmenger syndrome

CORONARY ARTERIAL DISEASE
Anomalous origin*
Anomalous tract (tunneled)
Kawasaki disease
Periarteritis
Arterial dissection
Marfan syndrome (rupture of aorta)
Myocardial infarction

MYOCARDIAL DISEASE
Myocarditis
Hypertrophic cardiomyopathy*
Dilated cardiomyopathy
Arrhythmogenic right ventricular dysplasia
Lyme carditis

CONDUCTION SYSTEM ABNORMALITY/ARRHYTHMIA
Long QT syndromes*
Brugada syndrome
Proarrhythmic drugs
Preexcitation syndromes
Heart block
Commotio cordis
Idiopathic ventricular fibrillation
Arrhythmogenic right ventricular dysplasia
Catecholaminergic polymorphic ventricular tachycardia
Heart tumor

MISCELLANEOUS
Pulmonary hypertension
Pulmonary embolism
Heat stroke
Cocaine and other stimulant drugs or medications
Anorexia nervosa
Electrolyte disturbances

SIDS, sudden infant death syndrome.
*Common.

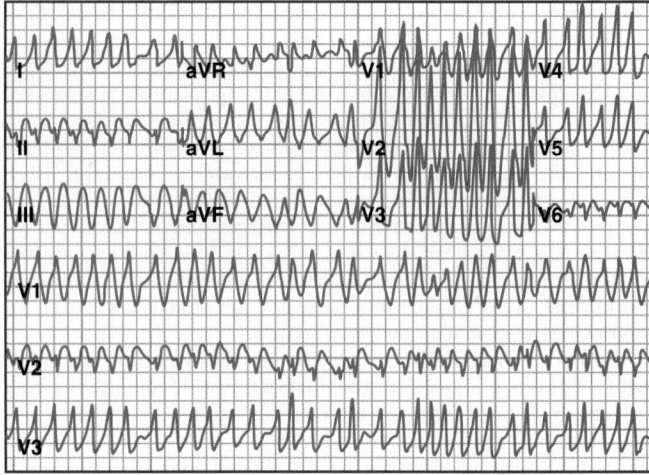

Figure 436-1 Atrial fibrillation in a patient with Wolff-Parkinson-White syndrome and rapid conduction to the ventricle. Note the wide QRS complexes, a result of full preexcitation, and the irregularly irregular ventricular response, caused by the atrial fibrillation.

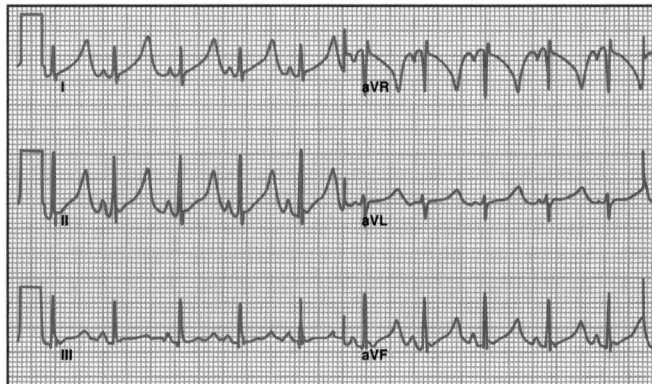

Figure 436-2 Long QT syndrome in a neonate. QTc is markedly prolonged. T waves are also peaked and abnormal in appearance.

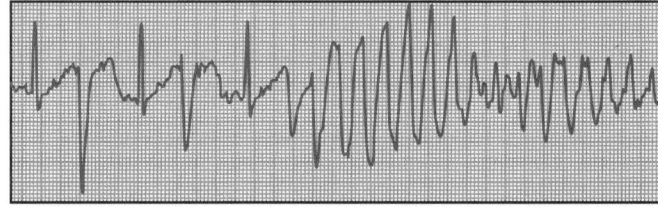

Figure 436-3 Episode of torsades de pointes in a patient with long QT syndrome.

death (Fig. 436-2). The mechanism of sudden death is polymorphic ventricular tachycardia (torsades de pointes) (Fig. 436-3). An initial presentation of sudden cardiac death is found in 9% of patients. Thus, treatment of asymptomatic patients with a long QT interval on electrocardiogram (ECG) and positive family history is advised.

Acquired long QT intervals may be seen in patients with marked electrolyte abnormalities, central nervous system injury, or starvation (including bulimia and anorexia nervosa). Medications can also result in prolongation of the QT interval (see Table 435-4 in Chapter 435). These patients are also at risk of malignant ventricular arrhythmias, and correction of the underlying problem may be necessary to reduce the risk of sudden death.

Brugada syndrome, an autosomal dominant disorder, caused in approximately 30% of patients to a mutation in the *SCN5A* gene, is associated with sudden cardiac death, often associated with fever, drugs, nighttime electrolyte disorders, or after a large meal (see Fig. 436-4). Typical ECG findings include coved ST segment elevations in

leads V_1-V_3; death results from either ventricular fibrillation or tachycardia.

MISCELLANEOUS CAUSES

Commotio cordis is a nearly universally fatal condition that follows blunt nonpenetrating trauma to the chest (e.g., from a baseball or hockey puck). Occasionally, innocent-appearing chest blows incurred at home or at a playground may be fatal. Patients experience immediate ventricular fibrillation in the absence of identifiable cardiac trauma (contusion, hematoma, lacerated coronary artery). Historically death results from ventricular fibrillation that is unresponsive to resuscitative efforts in 85-90% of children. Immediate direct current defibrillation may be

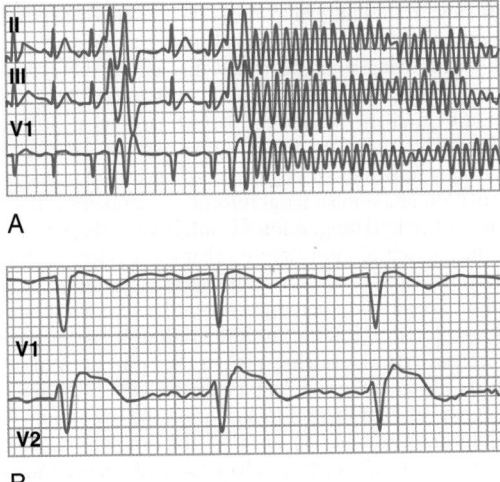

Figure 436-4 Brugada syndrome. **A,** Frequent ventricular ectopy and sustained polymorphic ventricular tachycardia. **B,** Persistent coved type ST segment elevation in lead V₁ and V₂ characteristic for Brugada type I. *From Talib S, van de Poll SE: Brugada syndrome diagnosed after Ramadan. Lancet 382:100, 2013.*

effective, if available, particularly if employed immediately; however, it is reported to be successful in only approximately 25% of cases.

EVALUATION AND THERAPY FOR RESUSCITATED PATIENTS

It is important to focus therapy on potentially reversible causes of sudden death. These include correction of major hemodynamic defects, pacing therapy for a patient with bradycardia, or supportive therapy for myocarditis. Unfortunately, reversible causes are not always found in young cardiac arrest survivors. Added to this dilemma is the fact that there is a limited ability to predict antiarrhythmic drug response or risk of recurrence. Thus, the implantable cardioverter defibrillator is the **therapy of choice** for survivors of arrhythmic sudden death.

MEDICATION FOR ATTENTION-DEFICIT DISORDER

There has been some concern about the possibility that stimulant medications prescribed for the treatment of children with attention-deficit disorder could potentially increase the risk of sudden death. The concern arises from a limited number of reports to the U.S. Food and Drug Administration of sudden death of unknown etiology in individuals taking stimulant medications, most of whom are adults. In a few cases, left ventricular hypertrophy caused by hypertension, coarctation of the aorta, or HCM has been identified at postmortem examination. There are no prospective studies to support the notion that these medications increase the risk, and little or no evidence that electrocardiographic screening will reliably identify a subgroup at risk. Some suggest ECG screening of children prior to starting these medications, but there is no consensus that such an approach is effective.

PREVENTION OF SUDDEN DEATH

The probability of survival to hospital discharge for a young patient who experiences an out-of-hospital cardiac arrest is <20%. The presence of immediate automatic external defibrillators, when combined with standard cardiopulmonary resuscitation at the site of exercise (gym, track, basketball, or football arena), may improve survival substantially. Thus, identifying patients at risk is extremely important.

Many of the more common causes of sudden death in children and adolescents can be identified from the patient's history (prodromal symptoms), the family history, and physical examination. The American Academy of Pediatrics makes available a downloadable "Preparticipation Physical Evaluation" form that is useful for this

purpose (http://www.aap.org). Of paramount importance is the careful evaluation of any child who experiences syncope in association with exercise, as this may be the last opportunity to diagnose a life-threatening condition in such a patient.

Patient avoidance of high-risk behavior (cocaine use, anorexia nervosa) and knowledge of drug side effects or drug interactions and contraindications is critical. Chest-protecting equipment has not been shown to prevent commotio cordis. Prompt bystander cardiopulmonary resuscitation and rapid defibrillation by an automatic external defibrillator has the best chance of leading to survival. Family survivors of victims of sudden death should be evaluated for genetic causes such as long QT syndrome and HCM.

The use of a preparticipation ECG for the detection of those athletes at risk for sudden death is controversial. Because many athletes either have no pre-event symptoms or are unwilling to admit to symptoms for fear of not being able to play, some have proposed that the ECG may identify a small but at-risk group with HCM or the prolonged QT, Brugada, or WPW syndromes. Preparticipation ECG testing is mandatory in several European countries but not in the United States. If the ECG is positive, echocardiography is performed. Cost-effectiveness studies suggest that the cost for implementation of a national program in the United States would be prohibitive because of the low incidence of sudden death in the pediatric population, the high rate of false-positive ECGs, and the difficulty in definitively excluding cardiac disease in patients with borderline ECG findings. Although studies of regional or national screening programs have suggested some benefit (e.g., the Veneto region of Italy) others have failed to demonstrate any effect of screening on the background incidence of sudden death in young individuals.

Bibliography is available at Expert Consult.

Section 5
Acquired Heart Disease

Chapter 437
Infective Endocarditis
Daniel Bernstein

Infective endocarditis includes acute and subacute bacterial endocarditis, as well as nonbacterial endocarditis caused by viruses, fungi, and other microbiologic agents. It is a significant cause of morbidity and mortality in children and adolescents despite advances in the management and prophylaxis of the disease with antimicrobial agents. The inability to eradicate infective endocarditis by prevention or early treatment stems from several factors. The disease represents a complex interplay between a pathogen and host factors such as endothelial disruption and immune function that is still not completely understood; the nature of the infecting organism has changed over time; diagnosis may be difficult during early stages and is thus often delayed until a more serious infection has set in; and special risk groups have emerged, including intravenous drug users; survivors of cardiac surgery, especially those with mechanical prosthesis; patients taking immunosuppressant medications; and patients who require chronic intravascular catheters. Some patients get endocarditis on what was thought to be a previously healthy native valve, although on surgical inspection is found to have mild structural abnormalities.

ETIOLOGY

Viridans-type streptococci (α-hemolytic streptococci) and *Staphylococcus aureus* remain the leading causative agents for endocarditis in pediatric patients. Other organisms cause endocarditis less frequently and, in ≈6% of cases, blood cultures are negative for any organisms (Table 437-1). No relationship exists between the infecting organism and the type of congenital defect, the duration of illness, or the age of the child. Staphylococcal endocarditis is more common in patients with no underlying heart disease; viridans group streptococcal infection is more common after dental procedures; group D enterococci are seen more often after lower bowel or genitourinary manipulation; *Pseudomonas aeruginosa* or *Serratia marcescens* is seen more frequently in intravenous drug users; and fungal organisms are encountered after open heart surgery. Coagulase-negative staphylococci are common in the presence of an indwelling central venous catheter.

EPIDEMIOLOGY

Infective endocarditis is often a complication of congenital or rheumatic heart disease but can also occur in children without any abnormal valves or cardiac malformations. In developed countries, congenital heart disease is the overwhelming predisposing factor. Endocarditis is rare in infancy; in this age group, it usually follows open heart surgery or is associated with a central venous line.

Patients with congenital heart lesions where there is turbulent blood flow because of a hole or stenotic orifice, especially if there is a high-pressure gradient across the defect, are most susceptible to endocarditis. This turbulent flow traumatizes the vascular endothelium, creating a substrate for deposition of fibrin and platelets, leading to the formation of a nonbacterial thrombotic embolus (NBTE) that is thought to be the initiating lesion for infective endocarditis. Biofilms form on the surface of implanted mechanical devices such as valves, catheters, or pacemaker wires that also serve as the adhesive substrate for infection. The development of transient bacteremia then colonizes this NBTE or biofilm, leading to proliferation of bacteria within the lesion. Bacterial surface proteins, such as the FimA antigen in viridans streptococci, act as adhesion factors to the NBTE or biofilm, after which bacteria can rapidly proliferate within the vegetation. Given the heavy colonization of mucosal surfaces (the oropharynx, or gastrointestinal, vaginal, or urinary tracts) by potentially pathogenic bacteria, these surfaces are thought to be the origin of this transient bacteremia. There is controversy over the extent to which daily activities (such as brushing or flossing the teeth) versus invasive procedures (such as dental cleanings or surgery) contribute to this bacteremia. Transient bacteremia is reported to occur in 20-68% of patients after tooth brushing and flossing, and even in 7-51% of patients after chewing food. The magnitude of this bacteremia is also similar to that resulting from dental procedures. Maintenance of good oral hygiene may be a more important factor in decreasing the frequency and magnitude of bacteremia.

Children at **highest risk** of adverse outcome after infective endocarditis include those with prosthetic cardiac valves or other prosthetic material used for cardiac valve repair, unrepaired cyanotic congenital heart disease (including those palliated with shunts and conduits), completely repaired defects with prosthetic material or device during the 1st 6 mo after repair, repaired congenital heart disease with residual defects at or adjacent to the site of a prosthetic patch or device, valve stenosis or insufficiency occurring after heart transplantation, permanent valve disease from rheumatic fever (mitral stenosis, aortic regurgitation), and previous infective endocarditis. Patients with high velocity blood flow lesions such as ventricular septal defects and aortic stenosis are also at high risk. In older patients, congenital bicuspid aortic valves and mitral valve prolapse with regurgitation pose additional risks for endocarditis. Surgical correction of congenital heart disease may reduce but does not eliminate the risk of endocarditis, with the exception of repair of a simple atrial septal defect or patent ductus arteriosus without prosthetic material.

In ≈30% of patients with infective endocarditis, a predisposing factor is presumably recognized. Although a preceding dental procedure may be identified in 10-20% of patients, the time of the procedure may range from 1 to 6 mo prior to the onset of symptoms, hence the continued controversy over the absolute risk of infective endocarditis after dental procedures. Primary bacteremia with *S. aureus* is thought to be another risk for endocarditis. The occurrence of endocarditis directly after most routine heart surgery is relatively low, but it can be an antecedent event, especially if prosthetic material is utilized.

CLINICAL MANIFESTATIONS

Table 437-2 outlines the manifestations of infective endocarditis.

Early manifestations are usually mild, especially when viridans group streptococci are the infecting organisms. Prolonged fever without other manifestations (except, occasionally, weight loss) that persists for as long as several months may be the only symptom. Alternatively, the onset may be acute and severe, with high, intermittent fever and prostration. Usually, the onset and course vary between these 2 extremes. The symptoms are often nonspecific and consist of low-grade fever with afternoon elevations, fatigue, myalgia, arthralgia, headache, and, at times, chills, nausea, and vomiting. **New or changing heart murmurs** are common, particularly with associated heart failure. Splenomegaly and petechiae are relatively common.

Table 437-1	Bacterial Agents in Pediatric Infective Endocarditis

COMMON: NATIVE VALVE OR OTHER CARDIAC LESIONS
Viridans group streptococci (*Streptococcus mutans, Streptococcus sanguinis, Streptococcus mitis*)
Staphylococcus aureus
Group D streptococcus (enterococcus) (*Streptococcus bovis, Streptococcus faecalis*)

UNCOMMON: NATIVE VALVE OR OTHER CARDIAC LESIONS
Streptococcus pneumoniae
Haemophilus influenzae
Coagulase-negative staphylococci
Abiotrophia defectiva (nutritionally variant streptococcus)
Coxiella burnetii (Q fever)*
Neisseria gonorrhoeae
*Brucella**
*Chlamydia psittaci**
*Chlamydia trachomatis**
*Chlamydia pneumoniae**
*Legionella**
*Bartonella**
*Tropheryma whipplei** (Whipple disease)
HACEK group†
*Streptobacillus moniliformis**
*Pasteurella multocida**
Campylobacter fetus
Culture negative (6% of cases)

PROSTHETIC VALVE
Staphylococcus epidermidis
Staphylococcus aureus
Viridans group streptococcus
Pseudomonas aeruginosa
Serratia marcescens
Diphtheroids
Legionella species*
HACEK group†
Fungi‡

*These fastidious bacteria plus some fungi may produce culture-negative endocarditis. Detection may require special media, incubation for more than 7 days, polymerase chain reaction on blood or valve for 16SrRNA (bacteria) or 18SrRNA (fungi), or serologic tests.
†The HACEK group includes *Haemophilus* species (*H. paraphrophilus, H. parainfluenzae, H. aphrophilus*), *Actinobacillus actinomycetemcomitans, Cardiobacterium hominis, Eikenella corrodens,* and *Kingella* species.
‡*Candida* species, *Aspergillus* species, *Pseudallescheria boydii, Histoplasma capsulatum.*

Table 437-2	Manifestations of Infective Endocarditis

HISTORY
Prior congenital or rheumatic heart disease
Preceding dental, urinary tract, or intestinal procedure
Intravenous drug use
Central venous catheter
Prosthetic heart valve

SYMPTOMS
Fever
Chills
Chest and abdominal pain
Arthralgia, myalgia
Dyspnea
Malaise, weakness
Night sweats
Weight loss
CNS manifestations (stroke, seizures, headache)

SIGNS
Elevated temperature
Tachycardia
Embolic phenomena (Roth spots, petechiae, splinter nail bed
  hemorrhages, Osler nodes, CNS or ocular lesions)
Janeway lesions
New or changing murmur
Splenomegaly
Arthritis
Heart failure
Arrhythmias
Metastatic infection (arthritis, meningitis, mycotic arterial aneurysm,
  pericarditis, abscesses, septic pulmonary emboli)
Clubbing

LABORATORY
Positive blood culture
Elevated erythrocyte sedimentation rate; may be low with heart or
  renal failure
Elevated C-reactive protein
Anemia
Leukocytosis
Immune complexes
Hypergammaglobulinemia
Hypocomplementemia
Cryoglobulinemia
Rheumatoid factor
Hematuria
Renal failure: azotemia, high creatinine (glomerulonephritis)
Chest radiograph: bilateral infiltrates, nodules, pleural effusions
Echocardiographic evidence of valve vegetations, prosthetic valve
  dysfunction or leak, myocardial abscess, new-onset valve
  insufficiency

CNS, central nervous system.

Serious neurologic complications such as embolic strokes, cerebral abscesses, mycotic aneurysms, and hemorrhage are most often associated with staphylococcal disease and may be late manifestations. Meningismus, increased intracranial pressure, altered sensorium, and focal neurologic signs are manifestations of these complications. Myocardial abscesses may occur with staphylococcal disease and may damage the cardiac conducting system, causing heart block, or may rupture into the pericardium and produce purulent pericarditis. Pulmonary and other systemic emboli are infrequent, except with fungal disease. Many of the classic skin findings develop late in the course of the disease; they are seldom seen in appropriately treated patients. Such manifestations include **Osler nodes** (tender, pea-size intradermal nodules in the pads of the fingers and toes), **Janeway lesions** (painless small erythematous or hemorrhagic lesions on the palms and soles), and **splinter hemorrhages** (linear lesions beneath the nails). These lesions may represent vasculitis produced by circulating antigen–antibody complexes.

Table 437-3	Diagnostic Approach to Uncommon Pathogens Causing Endocarditis

PATHOGEN	DIAGNOSTIC PROCEDURE
Brucella spp.	Blood cultures; serology; culture, immunohistology, and PCR of surgical material
Coxiella burnetii	Serology (IgG phase I >1 in 800); tissue culture, immunohistology, and PCR of surgical material
Bartonella spp.	Blood cultures; serology; culture, immunohistology, and PCR of surgical material
Chlamydia spp.	Serology; culture, immunohistology, and PCR of surgical material
Mycoplasma spp.	Serology; culture, immunohistology, and PCR of surgical material
Legionella spp.	Blood cultures; serology; culture, immunohistology, and PCR of surgical material
Tropheryma whipplei	Histology and PCR of surgical material

IgG, immunoglobulin G; PCR, polymerase chain reaction.
From Moreillon P, Que YA: Infective endocarditis, Lancet *363:139–148, 2004.*

Identification of infective endocarditis is most often based on a high index of suspicion during evaluation of an infection in a child with an underlying risk factor.

DIAGNOSIS

The critical information for appropriate treatment of infective endocarditis is obtained from blood cultures. All other laboratory data are secondary in importance (see Table 437-2). Blood specimens for culture should be obtained as promptly as possible, even if the child feels well and has no other physical findings. Three to 5 separate blood collections should be obtained after careful preparation of the phlebotomy site. Contamination presents a special problem inasmuch as bacteria found on the skin may themselves cause infective endocarditis. The timing of collections is not important because bacteremia can be expected to be relatively constant. In 90% of cases of endocarditis, the causative agent is recovered from the first 2 blood cultures. Bacteremia is low grade in 80% (<100 colony-forming units [CFU]/mL or blood). The laboratory should be notified that endocarditis is suspected so that, if necessary, the blood can be cultured on enriched media for longer than usual (>7 days) to detect nutritionally deficient and fastidious bacteria or fungi. Although bacteremia may occur in the absence of endocarditis, bacteremia secondary to *Streptococcus mutans, Streptococcus bovis I, Streptococcus mitior, Streptococcus sanguis,* and *S. aureus* (in the absence of focal musculoskeletal infection) is highly concerning for endocarditis. Antimicrobial pretreatment of the patient reduces the yield of blood cultures to 50-60%. The microbiology laboratory should be notified if the patient has received antibiotics so that more sophisticated methods can be used to recover the offending agent. Other specimens that may be cultured include scrapings from cutaneous lesions, urine, synovial fluid, abscesses, and, in the presence of manifestations of meningitis, cerebrospinal fluid. Serologic diagnosis or polymerase chain reaction of resected valve tissues is necessary in patients with unusual or fastidious microorganisms (Table 437-3; Fig. 437-1).

The index of suspicion should be high when evaluating infection in a child with an underlying contributing factor. The combination of transthoracic and transesophageal echocardiography enhances the ability to diagnose endocarditis. Two-dimensional echocardiography can identify the size, shape, location, and mobility of the lesion; when combined with Doppler studies, the presence of valve dysfunction

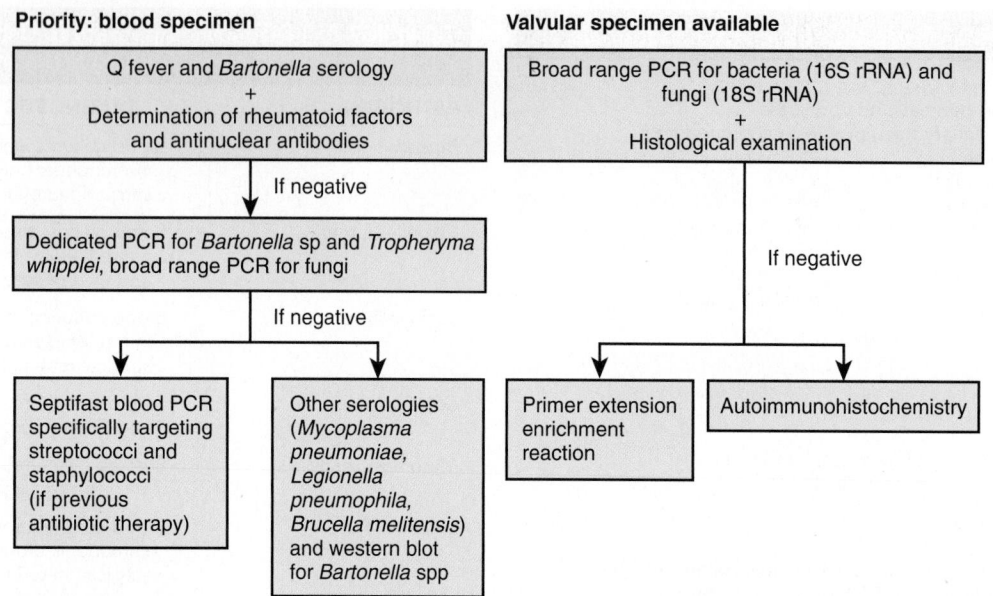

Figure 437-1 Diagnostic tests applied to clinical specimens for the identification of the causative agents of blood culture–negative endocarditis. Septifast, LightCycler SeptiFast (Roche). Serum should be considered a priority specimen, with Q fever and *Bartonella* serologic analysis being routinely done. We also suggest that detection of antinuclear antibodies and rheumatoid factor should be routinely done for diagnosis of noninfective endocarditis. (*From Thuny F, Grisoli D, Collart F, et al. Management of infective endocarditis: challenges and perspectives. Lancet 379:965–975, 2012, Fig. 2, p. 969.*)

(regurgitation, obstruction) can be determined and its effect on left ventricular performance quantified. Echocardiography may also be helpful in predicting embolic complications, given that lesions >1 cm and fungating masses are at greatest risk for embolization. The absence of vegetations does not exclude endocarditis, and vegetations are often not visualized in the early phases of the disease or in patients with complex congenital heart lesions.

The **Duke criteria** help in the diagnosis of endocarditis. **Major criteria** include (1) positive blood cultures (2 separate cultures for a usual pathogen, 2 or more for less-typical pathogens), and (2) evidence of endocarditis on echocardiography (intracardiac mass on a valve or other site, regurgitant flow near a prosthesis, abscess, partial dehiscence of prosthetic valves, or new valve regurgitant flow). **Minor criteria** include predisposing conditions, fever, embolic-vascular signs, immune complex phenomena (glomerulonephritis, arthritis, rheumatoid factor, Osler nodes, Roth spots), a single, positive blood culture or serologic evidence of infection, and echocardiographic signs not meeting the major criteria. Two major criteria, 1 major and 3 minor, or 5 minor criteria suggest definite endocarditis. A modification of the Duke criteria may increase sensitivity while maintaining specificity. The following minor criteria are added to those already listed: the presence of newly diagnosed clubbing, splenomegaly, splinter hemorrhages, and petechiae; a high erythrocyte sedimentation rate; a high C-reactive protein level; and the presence of central nonfeeding lines, peripheral lines, and microscopic hematuria.

PROGNOSIS AND COMPLICATIONS

Despite the use of antibiotic agents, mortality remains high, in the range of 20-25%. Serious morbidity occurs in 50-60% of children with documented infective endocarditis; the most common is heart failure caused by vegetations involving the aortic or mitral valve. Myocardial abscesses and toxic myocarditis may also lead to heart failure without characteristic changes in auscultatory findings and, occasionally, to life-threatening arrhythmias. Systemic emboli, often with central nervous system manifestations, are a major threat. Pulmonary emboli may occur in children with ventricular septal defect or the tetralogy of Fallot, although massive life-threatening pulmonary embolization is rare. Other complications include mycotic aneurysms, rupture of a sinus of Valsalva, obstruction of a valve secondary to large vegetations,

acquired ventricular septal defect, and heart block as a result of involvement (abscess) of the conduction system. Additional complications include meningitis, osteomyelitis, arthritis, renal abscess, purulent pericarditis, and immune complex-mediated glomerulonephritis.

TREATMENT

Antibiotic therapy should be instituted immediately once a definitive diagnosis is made. When virulent organisms are responsible, small delays may result in progressive endocardial damage and are associated with a greater likelihood of severe complications. The choice of antibiotics, method of administration, and length of treatment should be coordinated with consultants from both cardiology and infectious diseases (Tables 437-4 and 437-5). Empirical therapy before the identifiable agent is recovered may be initiated with vancomycin plus gentamicin in patients without a prosthetic valve and when there is a high risk of *S. aureus*, enterococcus, or viridans streptococci (the 3 most common organisms). High serum bactericidal levels must be maintained long enough to eradicate organisms that are growing in relatively inaccessible avascular vegetations. Between 5 and 20 times the minimal in vitro inhibiting concentration must be produced at the site of infection to destroy bacteria growing at the core of these lesions. Several weeks are required for a vegetation to organize completely; therapy must be continued through this period so that recrudescence can be avoided. A total of 4-6 wk of treatment is usually recommended. Depending on the clinical and laboratory responses, antibiotic therapy may require modification and, in some instances, more prolonged treatment is required. With highly sensitive viridans group streptococcal infections, shortened regimens that include oral penicillin for some portion have been recommended. In nonstaphylococcal disease, bacteremia usually resolves in 24-48 hr, whereas fever resolves in 5-6 days with appropriate antibiotic therapy. Resolution with staphylococcal disease takes longer.

If the infection occurs on a valve and induces or increases symptoms and signs of heart failure, appropriate therapy should be instituted, including diuretics, afterload reducing agents, and in some cases, digitalis. Surgical intervention for infective endocarditis is indicated for severe aortic, mitral or prosthetic valve involvement with intractable heart failure. Severe heart failure may be associated with acute valve regurgitation, obstruction, or fistula formation. Rarely, a

Table 437-4	Therapy of Native Valve Endocarditis Caused by Highly Penicillin-Susceptible Viridans Group Streptococci and *Streptococcus bovis*

REGIMEN	DOSAGE* AND ROUTE	DURATION, WK	COMMENTS
Aqueous crystalline penicillin G sodium	12-18 million U/24 hr IV either continuously or in 4 or 6 equally divided doses	4	Preferred in patients with impairment of 8th cranial nerve function or renal function
or			
Ceftriaxone sodium	2 g/24 hr IV/IM in 1 dose	4	
	Pediatric dose†: penicillin 200,000 U/kg per 24 hr IV in 4-6 equally divided doses; ceftriaxone 100 mg/kg per 24 hr IV/IM in 1 dose		
Aqueous crystalline penicillin G sodium	12-18 million U/24 hr IV either continuously or in 6 equally divided doses	2	2 wk regimen not intended for patients with known cardiac or extracardiac abscess or for those with creatinine clearance of <20 mL/min, impaired 8th cranial nerve function, or *Abiotrophia*, *Granulicatella*, or *Gemella* spp. infection; gentamicin dosage should be adjusted to achieve peak serum concentration of 3-4 μg/mL and trough serum concentration of <1 μg/mL when 3 divided doses are used; nomogram used for single daily dosing
or			
Ceftriaxone sodium	2 g/24 hr IV/IM in 1 dose	2	
plus			
Gentamicin sulfate‡	3 mg/kg per 24 hr IV/IM in 1 dose, or 3 equally divided doses	2	
	Pediatric dose: penicillin 200,000 U/kg per 24 hr IV in 4-6 equally divided doses; ceftriaxone 100 mg/kg per 24 hr IV/IM in 1 dose; gentamicin 3 mg/kg per 24 hr IV/IM in 1 dose or 3 equally divided doses§		
Vancomycin hydrochloride¶	30 mg/kg per 24 hr IV in 2 equally divided doses not to exceed 2 g/24 hr unless concentrations in serum are inappropriately low	4	Vancomycin therapy recommended only for patients unable to tolerate penicillin or ceftriaxone; vancomycin dosage should be adjusted to obtain peak (1 hr after infusion completed) serum concentration of 30-45 μg/mL and a trough concentration range of 10-15 μg/mL
	Pediatric dose: 40 mg/kg per 24 hr IV in 2-3 equally divided doses		

Minimum inhibitory concentration ≤0.12 μg/mL.
*Dosages recommended are for patients with normal renal function.
†Pediatric dose should not exceed that of a normal adult.
‡Other potentially nephrotoxic drugs (e.g., nonsteroidal antiinflammatory drugs) should be used with caution in patients receiving gentamicin therapy.
§Data for once-daily dosing of aminoglycosides for children exist, but no data for treatment of infective endocarditis exist.
¶Vancomycin dosages should be infused during course of at least 1 hr to reduce risk of histamine-release "red man" syndrome.
From Baddour LM, Wilson WR, Bayer AS, et al: Infective endocarditis: diagnosis, antimicrobial therapy, and management of complications, Circulation 111:e394–e433, 2005; correction: Circulation 112:2373, 2005.

mycotic aneurysm, rupture of an aortic sinus, intraseptal abscess causing complete heart block, or dehiscence of an intracardiac patch requires an emergency operation. Other surgical indications include failure to sterilize the blood despite adequate antibiotic levels in 7-10 days in the absence of extracardiac infection, myocardial abscess, recurrent emboli, and increasing size of vegetations while receiving therapy. Vegetations (aortic, mitral, prosthetic valve) >10-15 mm are at high risk of embolism. Although antibiotic therapy should be administered for as long as possible before surgical intervention, active infection is not a contraindication if the patient is critically ill as a result of severe hemodynamic deterioration from infective endocarditis. Removal of vegetations and, in some instances, valve replacement may be lifesaving, and sustained antibiotic administration will most often prevent reinfection. Replacement of infected prosthetic valves carries a higher risk.

Fungal endocarditis is difficult to manage and has a poorer prognosis. It has been encountered after cardiac surgery, in severely debilitated or immunosuppressed patients, and in patients on prolonged courses of antibiotics. The drugs of choice are amphotericin B (liposomal or standard preparation) and 5-fluorocytosine. Surgery to excise infected tissue is occasionally attempted, though often with limited success. Recombinant tissue plasminogen activation may help lyse intracardiac vegetations and avoid surgery in some high-risk patients.

PREVENTION

Recommendations by the American Heart Association for antimicrobial prophylaxis before dental and other surgical procedures received a major revision in 2007. A substantial reduction in the number of patients who require prophylactic treatment and the procedures requiring coverage was recommended. The primary reasons for these revised recommendations were that (1) infective endocarditis is much more likely to result from exposure to the more frequent random bacteremias associated with daily activities than from a dental or surgical procedure; (2) routine prophylaxis may prevent "an exceedingly

Table 437-5	Therapy for Endocarditis Caused by Staphylococci in the Absence of Prosthetic Materials		
REGIMEN	**DOSAGE* AND ROUTE**	**DURATION**	**COMMENTS**
OXACILLIN-SUSCEPTIBLE STRAINS			
Nafcillin or oxacillin[†]	12 g/24 hr IV in 4-6 equally divided doses	6 wk	For complicated right-sided IE and for left-sided IE; for uncomplicated right-sided IE, 2 wk
with			
Optional addition of gentamicin sulfate[‡]	3 mg/kg per 24 hr IV/IM in 2 or 3 equally divided doses	3-5 day	
	Pediatric dose[§]: Nafcillin or oxacillin 200 mg/kg per 24 hr IV in 4-6 equally divided doses; gentamicin 3 mg/kg per 24 hr IV/IM in 3 equally divided doses		Clinical benefit of aminoglycosides has not been established
For penicillin-allergic (nonanaphylactoid-type) patients:			Consider skin testing for oxacillin-susceptible staphylococci and questionable history of immediate-type hypersensitivity to penicillin
Cefazolin	6 g/24 hr IV in 3 equally divided doses	6 wk	Cephalosporins should be avoided in patients with anaphylactoid-type hypersensitivity to β-lactams; vancomycin should be used in these cases[§]
with			
Optional addition of gentamicin sulfate	3 mg/kg per 24 hr IV/IM in 2 or 3 equally divided doses	3-5 day	Clinical benefit of aminoglycosides has not been established
	Pediatric dose: cefazolin 100 mg/kg per 24 hr IV in 3 equally divided doses; gentamicin 3 mg/kg per 24 hr IV/IM in 3 equally divided doses		
OXACILLIN-RESISTANT STRAINS			
Vancomycin[¶]	30 mg/kg per 24 hr IV in 2 equally divided doses	6 wk	Adjust vancomycin dosage to achieve 1 hr serum concentration of 30-45 μg/mL and trough concentration of 10-15 μg/mL
	Pediatric dose: 40 mg/kg per 24 hr IV in 2 or 3 equally divided doses		

IE, infective endocarditis.

*Dosages recommended are for patients with normal renal function.

[†]Penicillin G 24 million U/24 hr IV in 4-6 equally divided doses may be used in place of nafcillin or oxacillin if strain is penicillin susceptible (minimum inhibitory concentration ≤0.1 μg/mL) and does not produce β-lactamase.

[‡]Gentamicin should be administered in close temporal proximity to vancomycin, nafcillin, or oxacillin dosing.

[§]Pediatric dose should not exceed that of a normal adult.

[¶]For specific dosing adjustment and issues concerning vancomycin, see Table 437-4 footnotes.

From Baddour LM, Wilson WR, Bayer AS, et al: Infective endocarditis: diagnosis, antimicrobial therapy, and management of complications, Circulation 111:e394–e433, 2005; corrections Circulation 112:2373, 2005.

small" number of cases; and (3) the risk of antibiotic-related adverse events exceeds the benefits of prophylactic therapy. Improving general dental hygiene was felt to be a more important factor in reducing the risk of infective endocarditis resulting from routine daily bacteremias. The current recommendations limit the use of prophylaxis to those patients with cardiac conditions associated with the greatest risk of an adverse outcome from infective endocarditis (Table 437-6). Patients with permanently damaged valves from rheumatic heart disease should also be considered for prophylaxis. Prophylaxis for these patients is recommended for "all dental procedures that involve manipulation of gingival tissue or the periapical region of teeth or perforation of the oral mucosa." Furthermore, "placement of removable prosthodontic or endodontic appliances, adjustment of orthodontic appliances, placement of orthodontic brackets, shedding of deciduous teeth and bleeding from trauma to the lips or oral mucosa" are not indications for prophylaxis. Given that many invasive respiratory tract procedures do cause bacteremia, prophylaxis for many of these procedures is considered reasonable. In contrast to prior recommendations, prophylaxis for gastrointestinal or genitourinary procedures is no longer recommended in the majority of cases. Prophylaxis for patients undergoing cardiac surgery with placement of prosthetic material is still recommended. Given the highly individual nature of these recommendations and the continued concern amongst some cardiologists over their adoption, direct consultation with the child's cardiologist is still the best method for determining a specific patient's ongoing need for prophylaxis (Table 437-7).

Continuing education regarding both oral hygiene and, in appropriate cases, the need for prophylaxis is important, especially in teenagers

Table 437-6	2007 Statement of the American Heart Association (AHA): Cardiac Conditions Associated with the Highest Risk of an Adverse Outcome from Infective Endocarditis for Which Prophylaxis with Dental Procedures Is Reasonable

Prosthetic cardiac valve or prosthetic material used for cardiac valve repair

Previous infective endocarditis

CONGENITAL HEART DISEASE (CHD)*

Unrepaired cyanotic CHD, including palliative shunts and conduits

Completely repaired CHD with prosthetic material or device, whether placed by surgery or catheter intervention, during the 1st 6 mo after the procedure[†]

Repaired CHD with residual defects at the site or adjacent to the site of a prosthetic patch, or prosthetic device (which inhibit endothelialization)

Cardiac transplantation recipients who develop cardiac valvulopathy

*Except for the conditions listed here, antibiotic prophylaxis is no longer recommended by the AHA for any other form of CHD.

[†]Prophylaxis is reasonable because endothelialization of prosthetic material occurs within 6 mo after the procedure.

From Wilson W, Taubert KA, Gewitz M, et al: Prevention of infective endocarditis. Guidelines from the American Heart Association, Circulation 116:1736–1754, 2007.

Table 437-7	2007 Statement of the American Heart Association (AHA): Prophylactic Antibiotic Regimens for a Dental Procedure		
SITUATION	**AGENT**	**ADULTS**	**CHILDREN**
Oral	Amoxicillin	2 g	50 mg/kg
Unable to take oral medication	Ampicillin *or* cefazolin or ceftriaxone	2 g IM or IV 1 g IM or IV	50 mg/kg IM or IV 50 mg/kg IM or IV
Allergic to penicillins or ampicillin—oral	Cephalexin*† *or* Clindamycin *or* Azithromycin or clarithromycin	2 g 600 mg 500 mg	50 mg/kg 20 mg/kg 15 mg/kg
Allergic to penicillins or ampicillin and unable to take oral medication	Cefazolin or ceftriaxone† *or* clindamycin	1 g IM or IV 600 mg IM or IV	50 mg/kg IM or IV 20 mg/kg IM or IV

IM, intramuscular; IV, intravenous.
*Or other first- or second-generation oral cephalosporin in equivalent adult or pediatric dosage.
†Cephalosporins should not be used in an individual with a history of anaphylaxis, angioedema, urticaria with penicillins or ampicillin.
From Wilson W, Taubert KA, Gewitz M, et al: Prevention of infective endocarditis. Guidelines from the American Heart Association, Circulation 116:1736–1754, 2007.

and young adults. Vigorous treatment of sepsis and local infections and careful asepsis during heart surgery and catheterization reduce the incidence of infective endocarditis.

Bibliography is available at Expert Consult.

Chapter 438
Rheumatic Heart Disease
Daniel Bernstein

Rheumatic involvement of the valves is the most important sequelae of acute rheumatic fever (see Chapter 183.1). The valvular lesions begin as small verrucae composed of fibrin and blood cells along the borders of one or more of the heart valves. The mitral valve is affected most often, followed in frequency by the aortic valve; right-sided heart manifestations are rare. As the inflammation subsides, the verrucae tend to disappear and leave scar tissue. With repeated attacks of rheumatic fever, new verrucae form near the previous ones, and the mural endocardium and chordae tendineae become involved.

A single episode of acute rheumatic fever usually results in complete healing of valvular lesions while repeated episodes, especially on previously affected valves result in rheumatic heart disease. Diagnosing acute rheumatic fever requires the fulfillment of the Jones criteria (see Chapter 183.1), while the diagnosis of rheumatic heart disease is based on cardiac auscultation signs of mitral or aortic valve involvement, which may not detect early valve injury. Screening large populations at risk for rheumatic heart disease with echocardiography has demonstrated a substantially greater number of patients with rheumatic heart disease than those detected by auscultation (Fig. 438-1). If this is confirmed, it has important public health significance in that many more patients will need to receive prophylaxis to prevent further episodes of acute rheumatic fever and worsening of valve injury.

PATTERNS OF VALVULAR DISEASE
Mitral Insufficiency
Pathophysiology
Mitral insufficiency is the result of structural changes that usually include some loss of valvular substance and shortening and thickening of the chordae tendineae. During acute rheumatic fever with severe cardiac involvement, heart failure is caused by a combination of mitral insufficiency coupled with inflammatory disease of the pericardium, myocardium, endocardium, and epicardium. Because of the high volume load and inflammatory process, the left ventricle becomes enlarged. The left atrium dilates as blood regurgitates into this chamber. Increased left atrial pressure results in pulmonary congestion and symptoms of left-sided heart failure. Spontaneous improvement usually occurs with time, even in patients in whom mitral insufficiency is severe at the onset. The resultant chronic lesion is most often mild or moderate in severity, and the patient is asymptomatic. More than half of patients with acute mitral insufficiency no longer have the mitral murmur 1 yr later. In patients with severe chronic mitral insufficiency, pulmonary arterial pressure becomes elevated, the right ventricle and atrium become enlarged, and right-sided heart failure subsequently develops.

Clinical Manifestations
The physical signs of mitral insufficiency depend on its severity. With mild disease, signs of heart failure are not present, the precordium is quiet, and auscultation reveals a high-pitched holosystolic murmur at the apex that radiates to the axilla. With severe mitral insufficiency, signs of chronic heart failure may be noted. The heart is enlarged, with a heaving apical left ventricular impulse and often an apical systolic thrill. The 2nd heart sound may be accentuated if pulmonary hypertension is present. A 3rd heart sound is generally prominent. A holosystolic murmur is heard at the apex with radiation to the axilla. A short mid-diastolic rumbling murmur is caused by increased blood flow across the mitral valve as a result of the insufficiency. Auscultation of a diastolic murmur does not necessarily mean that mitral stenosis is present. The latter lesion takes many years to develop and is characterized by a diastolic murmur of greater length, usually with presystolic accentuation.

The electrocardiogram and chest x-rays are normal if the lesion is mild. With more severe insufficiency, the electrocardiogram shows prominent bifid P waves, signs of left ventricular hypertrophy, and associated right ventricular hypertrophy if pulmonary hypertension is present. Roentgenographically, prominence of the left atrium and ventricle can be seen. Congestion of perihilar vessels, a sign of pulmonary venous hypertension, may also be evident. Calcification of the mitral valve is rare in children. Echocardiography shows enlargement of the

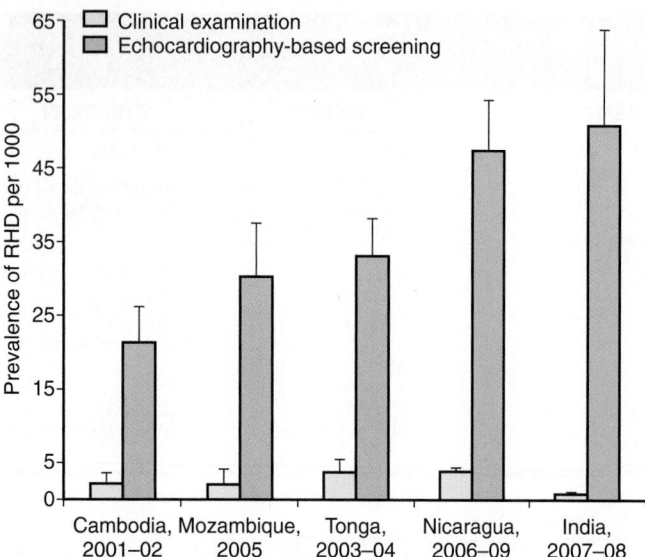

Figure 438-1 Rheumatic heart disease (RHD) prevalence rates in children: echocardiography-based screening versus clinical examination. Results of the first 4 studies to investigate differences in RHD detection methods are shown. In Cambodia and Mozambique, echocardiography-based RHD was defined as regurgitant jet seen in at least 2 planes and morphologic features suggestive of the disease, such as restricted leaflet mobility, focal or generalized valvular thickening, and abnormal subvalvular thickening. In Tonga, echocardiography-based RHD was defined by a combination of World Health Organization criteria (regurgitant jet >1 cm in length in at least 2 planes, mosaic color jet with a peak velocity >2.5 m/sec, persistence of jet throughout systole [mitral valve] and diastole [aortic valve], and morphologic criteria such as valvular thickening and elbow deformity of the anterior mitral valve leaflet). If only mitral regurgitation with no morphologic changes was seen, the case was considered as definite only if mitral regurgitation was graded at least as mild. Mitral or aortic stenoses were a sign of definite RHD, defined by a transmitral mean pressure gradient greater than 4 mm Hg and a transaortic peak velocity greater than 2 m/sec, respectively. If only very mild mitral regurgitation and no morphologic changes were seen, the child was classified as having borderline RHD (not reported here). In Nicaragua, echocardiography-based RHD, including possible cases, was defined by morphologic mitral changes (thickened mitral valve leaflets or dogleg deformity of the anterior mitral valve leaflet or both), and substantial left-side regurgitation (holosystolic mitral regurgitation jet ≥2 cm and ≥1 cm for aortic regurgitation, in 2 planes, of high velocity). In India, echocardiography-based RHD was defined by regurgitant jet greater than 1 cm in length in at least 2 planes, mosaic color jet with a peak velocity greater than 2.5 m/sec, and persistence of jet throughout systole (mitral valve) and diastole (aortic valve). Prevalence would only be 14.1 per 1000 with more stringent criteria combining Doppler echocardiography and pronounced mitral valve thickening (>6 mm). *(From Marijon E, Mirabel M, Celermajer DS, Jouven X: Rheumatic heart disease. Lancet 379:953-964, 2012, Fig. 5.)*

left atrium and ventricle, an abnormally thickened mitral valve, and Doppler studies demonstrate the severity of the mitral regurgitation. Heart catheterization and left ventriculography are considered only if diagnostic questions are not totally resolved by noninvasive assessment.

Complications
Severe mitral insufficiency may result in cardiac failure that may be precipitated by progression of the rheumatic process, the onset of atrial fibrillation, or infective endocarditis. The effects of chronic mitral insufficiency may become manifest after many years and include right ventricular failure and atrial and ventricular arrhythmias.

Treatment
In patients with mild mitral insufficiency, prophylaxis against recurrences of rheumatic fever is all that is required. Treatment of

complicating heart failure (see Chapter 442), arrhythmias (see Chapter 435), and infective endocarditis (see Chapter 437) is described elsewhere. Afterload-reducing agents (angiotensin-converting enzyme inhibitors or angiotensin receptor blockers) may reduce the regurgitant volume and preserve left ventricular function. Surgical treatment is indicated for patients who despite adequate medical therapy have persistent heart failure, dyspnea with moderate activity, and progressive cardiomegaly, often with pulmonary hypertension. Although annuloplasty provides good results in some children and adolescents, valve replacement may be required. In patients with a prosthetic mitral valve replacement, prophylaxis against bacterial endocarditis is warranted for dental procedures, as the routine antibiotics taken by these patients for rheumatic fever prophylaxis are insufficient to prevent endocarditis.

Mitral Stenosis
Pathophysiology
Mitral stenosis of rheumatic origin results from fibrosis of the mitral ring, commissural adhesions, and contracture of the valve leaflets, chordae, and papillary muscles over time. It usually takes 10 yr or more for the lesion to become fully established, although the process may occasionally be accelerated. Rheumatic mitral stenosis is seldom encountered before adolescence and is not usually recognized until adult life. Significant mitral stenosis results in increased pressure and enlargement and hypertrophy of the left atrium, pulmonary venous hypertension, increased pulmonary vascular resistance, and pulmonary hypertension. Right ventricular hypertrophy and right atrial dilation ensue and are followed by right ventricular dilation, tricuspid regurgitation, and clinical signs of right-sided heart failure.

Clinical Manifestations
Generally, the correlation between symptoms and the severity of obstruction is good. Patients with mild lesions are asymptomatic. More severe degrees of obstruction are associated with exercise intolerance and dyspnea. Critical lesions can result in orthopnea, paroxysmal nocturnal dyspnea, and overt pulmonary edema, as well as atrial arrhythmias. When pulmonary hypertension has developed, right ventricular dilation may result in functional tricuspid insufficiency, hepatomegaly, ascites, and edema. Hemoptysis caused by rupture of bronchial or pleurohilar veins and, occasionally, by pulmonary infarction may occur.

Jugular venous pressure is increased in severe disease with heart failure, tricuspid valve disease, or severe pulmonary hypertension. In mild disease, heart size is normal; however, moderate cardiomegaly is usual with severe mitral stenosis. Cardiac enlargement can be massive when atrial fibrillation and heart failure supervene. A parasternal right ventricular lift is palpable when pulmonary pressure is high. The principal auscultatory findings are a loud 1st heart sound, an opening snap of the mitral valve, and a long, low-pitched, rumbling mitral diastolic murmur with presystolic accentuation at the apex. The mitral diastolic murmur may be virtually absent in patients who are in significant heart failure. A holosystolic murmur secondary to tricuspid insufficiency may be audible. In the presence of pulmonary hypertension, the pulmonic component of the 2nd heart sound is accentuated. An early diastolic murmur may be caused by associated rheumatic aortic insufficiency or pulmonary valvular insufficiency secondary to pulmonary hypertension.

Electrocardiograms and roentgenograms are normal if the lesion is mild; as the severity increases, prominent and notched P waves and varying degrees of right ventricular hypertrophy become evident. Atrial fibrillation is a common late manifestation. Moderate or severe lesions are associated with roentgenographic signs of left atrial enlargement and prominence of the pulmonary artery and right-sided heart chambers; calcifications may be noted in the region of the mitral valve. Severe obstruction is associated with a redistribution of pulmonary blood flow so that the apices of the lung have greater perfusion (the reverse of normal). Echocardiography shows thickening of the mitral valve, distinct narrowing of the mitral orifice during diastole and left atrial enlargement. Doppler can estimate the transmitral pressure gradient. Cardiac catheterization quantitates the diastolic gradient across the mitral valve, allows for the calculation of valve area, and assesses the degree of elevation of pulmonary arterial pressure.

Treatment

Intervention is indicated in patients with clinical signs and hemodynamic evidence of severe obstruction but before the severe manifestations outlined earlier. Surgical valvotomy or balloon catheter mitral valvuloplasty generally yields good results; valve replacement is avoided unless absolutely necessary. Balloon valvuloplasty is indicated for symptomatic, stenotic, pliable, noncalcified valves of patients without atrial arrhythmias or thrombi.

Aortic Insufficiency

In chronic rheumatic aortic insufficiency, sclerosis of the aortic valve results in distortion and retraction of the cusps. Regurgitation of blood leads to volume overload with dilation and hypertrophy of the left ventricle. Combined mitral and aortic insufficiency is more common than aortic involvement alone.

Clinical Manifestations

Symptoms are unusual except in severe aortic insufficiency. The large stroke volume and forceful left ventricular contractions may result in palpitations. Sweating and heat intolerance are related to excessive vasodilation. Dyspnea on exertion can progress to orthopnea and pulmonary edema; angina may be precipitated by heavy exercise. Nocturnal attacks with sweating, tachycardia, chest pain, and hypertension may occur.

The pulse pressure is wide with bounding peripheral pulses. Systolic blood pressure is elevated, and diastolic pressure is lowered. In severe aortic insufficiency, the heart is enlarged, with a left ventricular apical heave. A diastolic thrill may be present. The typical murmur begins immediately with the 2nd heart sound and continues until late in diastole. The murmur is heard over the upper and midleft sternal border with radiation to the apex and upper right sternal border. Characteristically, it has a high-pitched blowing quality and is easily audible in full expiration with the diaphragm of the stethoscope placed firmly on the chest and the patient leaning forward. An aortic systolic ejection murmur is frequent because of the increased stroke volume. An apical presystolic murmur (**Austin Flint murmur**) resembling that of mitral stenosis is sometimes heard and is a result of the large regurgitant aortic flow in diastole preventing the mitral valve from opening fully.

Chest x-rays show enlargement of the left ventricle and aorta. The electrocardiogram may be normal, but in advanced cases it reveals signs of left ventricular hypertrophy and strain with prominent P waves. The echocardiogram shows a large left ventricle and diastolic mitral valve flutter or oscillation caused by regurgitant flow hitting the valve leaflets. Doppler studies demonstrate the degree of aortic runoff into the left ventricle. Magnetic resonance angiography (MRA) can be useful in quantitating regurgitant volume. Cardiac catheterization is necessary only when the echocardiographic data are equivocal.

Prognosis and Treatment

Mild and moderate lesions are well tolerated. Unlike mitral insufficiency, aortic insufficiency does not regress. Patients with combined lesions during the episode of acute rheumatic fever may have only aortic involvement 1-2 yr later. Treatment consists of afterload reducers (angiotensin-converting enzyme inhibitors or angiotensin receptor blockers) and prophylaxis against recurrence of acute rheumatic fever. Surgical intervention (valve replacement) should be carried out well in advance of the onset of heart failure, pulmonary edema, or angina, when signs of decreasing myocardial performance become evident as manifested by increasing left ventricular dimensions on the echocardiogram. Surgery is considered when early symptoms are present, ST-T wave changes are seen on the electrocardiogram, or evidence of decreasing left ventricular ejection fraction is noted.

Tricuspid Valve Disease

Primary tricuspid involvement is rare after rheumatic fever. Tricuspid insufficiency is more common secondary to right ventricular dilation resulting from unrepaired left-sided lesions. The signs produced by tricuspid insufficiency include prominent pulsations of the jugular veins, systolic pulsations of the liver, and a blowing holosystolic murmur at the lower left sternal border that increases in intensity during inspiration. Concomitant signs of mitral or aortic valve disease, with or without atrial fibrillation, are frequent. In these cases, signs of tricuspid insufficiency decrease or disappear when heart failure produced by the left-sided lesions is successfully treated. Tricuspid valvuloplasty may be required in rare cases.

Pulmonary Valve Disease

Pulmonary insufficiency usually occurs on a functional basis secondary to pulmonary hypertension and is a late finding with severe mitral stenosis. The murmur (**Graham Steell murmur**) is similar to that of aortic insufficiency, but peripheral arterial signs (bounding pulses) are absent. The correct diagnosis is confirmed by two-dimensional echocardiography and Doppler studies.

Bibliography is available at Expert Consult.

Section **6**

Diseases of the Myocardium and Pericardium

Chapter **439**

Diseases of the Myocardium

Robert L. Spicer and Stephanie M. Ware

The extremely heterogeneous heart muscle diseases associated with structural remodeling and/or abnormalities of cardiac function (cardiomyopathy) are important causes of morbidity and mortality in the pediatric population. Several classification schemes have been formulated in an effort to provide logical, useful, and scientifically based etiologies for the cardiomyopathies. Insight into the molecular genetic basis of cardiomyopathies has increased exponentially and etiologic classification schemes continue to evolve.

Table 439-1 classifies the cardiomyopathies based on their anatomic (ventricular morphology) and functional pathophysiology. Dilated cardiomyopathy, the most common form of cardiomyopathy, is characterized predominantly by left ventricular dilation and decreased left ventricular systolic function (Fig. 439-1). Hypertrophic cardiomyopathy demonstrates increased ventricular myocardial wall thickness, normal or increased systolic function, and often, diastolic (relaxation) abnormalities (Table 439-2; Figs. 439-2 and 439-3). Restrictive cardiomyopathy is characterized by nearly normal ventricular chamber size and wall thickness with preserved systolic function, but dramatically impaired diastolic function leading to elevated filling pressures and atrial enlargement (Fig. 439-4). Arrhythmogenic right ventricular cardiomyopathy and left ventricular noncompaction are characterized by specific morphologic abnormalities and heterogeneous functional disturbances.

Bibliography is available at Expert Consult.

Table 439-1	Etiology of Pediatric Myocardial Disease

CARDIOMYOPATHY

Dilated Cardiomyopathy (DCM)

Neuromuscular diseases	Muscular dystrophies (Duchenne, Becker, limb girdle, Emery-Dreifuss, congenital muscular dystrophy, etc.), myotonic dystrophy, myofibrillar myopathy
Inborn errors of metabolism	Fatty acid oxidation disorders (trifunctional protein, VLCAD), carnitine abnormalities (carnitine transport, CPTI, CPTII), mitochondrial disorders (including Kearns-Sayre syndrome), organic acidemias (propionic acidemia)
Genetic mutations in cardiomyocyte structural apparatus	Familial or sporadic DCM
Genetic syndromes	Alstrom syndrome, Barth syndrome (phospholipid disorders)
Ischemic	Most common in adults
Chronic tachyarrhythmias	

Hypertrophic Cardiomyopathy (HCM)

Inborn errors of metabolism	Mitochondrial disorders (including Friedreich ataxia, mutations in nuclear or mitochondrial genome), storage disorders (glycogen storage disorders, especially Pompe; mucopolysaccharidoses; Fabry disease; sphingolipidoses; hemochromatosis; Danon disease)
Genetic mutations in cardiomyocyte structural apparatus	Familial or sporadic HCM
Genetic syndromes	Noonan, Costello, cardiofaciocutaneous, Beckwith-Wiedemann syndrome
Infant of a diabetic mother	Transient hypertrophy

Restrictive Cardiomyopathy (RCM)

Neuromuscular disease	Myofibrillar myopathies
Metabolic	Storage disorders
Genetic mutations in cardiomyocyte structural apparatus	Familial or sporadic RCM

Arrhythmogenic Right Ventricular Cardiomyopathy (ARVC)

Genetic mutations in cardiomyocyte structural apparatus	Familial or sporadic ARVC
LVNC	X-linked (Barth syndrome), autosomal dominant, autosomal recessive, mitochondrial inheritance, or sporadic LVNC

SECONDARY OR ACQUIRED MYOCARDIAL DISEASE

Myocarditis (see also Table 439-3)	**Viral:** parvovirus B19, adenovirus, coxsackievirus A and B, echovirus, rubella, varicella, influenza, mumps, Epstein-Barr virus, cytomegalovirus, measles, poliomyelitis, smallpox vaccine, hepatitis C virus, human herpesvirus 6, HIV virus, or opportunistic infections **Rickettsial:** psittacosis, *Coxiella*, Rocky Mountain spotted fever, typhus **Bacterial:** diphtheria, mycoplasma, meningococcus, leptospirosis, Lyme disease, typhoid fever, tuberculosis, streptococcus, listeriosis **Parasitic:** Chagas disease, toxoplasmosis, *Loa loa, Toxocara canis,* schistosomiasis, cysticercosis, echinococcus, trichinosis **Fungal:** histoplasmosis, coccidioidomycosis, actinomycosis
Systemic inflammatory disease	SLE, infant of mother with SLE, scleroderma, Churg-Strauss vasculitis, rheumatoid arthritis, rheumatic fever, sarcoidosis, dermatomyositis, periarteritis nodosa, hypereosinophilic syndrome (Löffler syndrome), acute eosinophilic necrotizing myocarditis, giant cell myocarditis, Kawasaki disease
Nutritional deficiency	Beriberi (thiamine deficiency), kwashiorkor, Keshan disease (selenium deficiency)
Drugs, toxins	Doxorubicin (Adriamycin), cyclophosphamide, chloroquine, ipecac (emetine), sulfonamides, mesalazine, chloramphenicol, alcohol, hypersensitivity reaction, envenomations, irradiation, herbal remedy (blue cohosh)
Coronary artery disease	Kawasaki disease, medial necrosis, anomalous left coronary artery from the pulmonary artery, other congenital coronary anomalies (anomalous right coronary, coronary ostial stenosis), familial hypercholesterolemia
Hematology-oncology	Anemia, sickle cell disease, leukemia
Endocrine-neuroendocrine	Hyperthyroidism, carcinoid tumor, pheochromocytoma

CPTI/CPTII, carnitine palmitoyltransferase 1/2; LVNC, left ventricular noncompaction; SLE, systemic lupus erythematosus; VLCAD, very long chain acyl coenzyme A dehydrogenase.

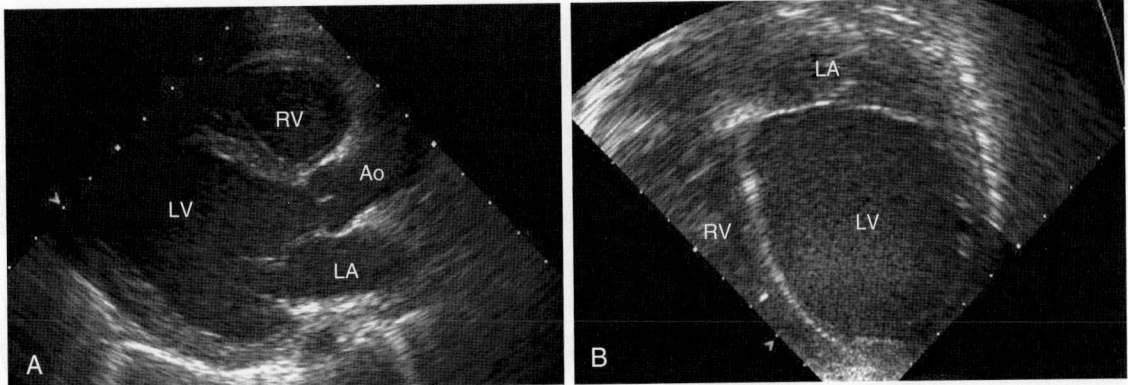

Figure 439-1 Echocardiogram of a patient with dilated cardiomyopathy. **A,** Parasternal long-axis view showing the enlarged left ventricle. **B,** Apical 4-chamber view showing the large left ventricle compressing the right ventricle. Ao, ascending aorta; LA, left atrium; LV, left ventricle; RV, right ventricle.

Table 439-2	Cardiomyopathies				
	DCM	**HCM**	**RCM**	**LVNC**	**ARVC**
Prevalence	50/100,000	1/500	Unknown	Unknown	1/2,000
Familial	30-50% AD, AR, X-L, Mt	50% AD, Mt	AD, % unknown	AD, X-L, Mt, % unknown	30-50% AD, rare AR (Naxos disease; Carvajal syndrome)
Genes*	Sarcomere: *MYH7, MYBPC3, TNNI3, TNNT2, TNNC1, MYH6, TPM1, ACTC1* Cytoskeleton or Z-disc: *DMD, TTN, CSRP3, TCAP, VCL, ACTN2, DES, LDB3, SGCD, MYPN, ANKRD1, BAG3, NEBL, NEXN* Nuclear envelope: *LMNA, EMD, TMPO* Cardiolipin metabolism: *TAZ* Mitochondrial function: mt DNA depletion; Mt genome mutations/deletions Other: *CRYAB, SCN5A, EYA4, ABCC9, PLN, PSEN1, PSEN2, FCMD, ALMS1, CAV3, LAMA4, LAMP2, RBM20*	Sarcomere: *MYH7, MYBPC3, MYL2, MYL3, TNNT2, TNNI3, TNNC1, MYH6, TPM1, ACTC1* Cytoskeleton or Z-disc: *TTN, CSRP3, LDB3, TCAP, VCL, ACTN2, MYOZ2, ANKRD1, BAG3* Storage: *PRKAG2, LAMP2, GLA, GAA, AGL* Mitochondrial function: *FRDA, SCO2, SURF1, COX* genes, *ANT1*, Mt genome mutations/deletions Cell signaling: *PTPN11, RAF1, SOS1, KRAS, HRAS, BRAF, MEK1, MEK2, MYLK2* Other: *PLN, JPH2, CALR3*	Sarcomere: *MYH7, TNNT2, TNNI3, ACTC1* Cytoskeleton or Z-disc: *DES*	Cytoskeletal or Z-disc: *DTNA, LDB3* Cardiolipin metabolism: *TAZ* Sarcomere: *MYH7, MYBPC3, ACTC1* Mitochondrial function: see HCM and DCM Other: *CASQ2, DTNA*	Desmosome: *DSP, PKP2, DSG2, DSC2, JUP* Other: *TMEM43, TGFB3, RYR2*
Sudden death	Yes	Yes	Yes	Yes	Yes
Arrhythmias	Atrial, ventricular, and conduction disturbances	Atrial and ventricular	Atrial fibrillation		Ventricular and conduction disturbances
Ventricular function	Systolic and diastolic dysfunction	Diastolic dysfunction Dynamic systolic outflow obstruction	Diastolic dysfunction Normal systolic function	Systolic or diastolic dysfunction	Normal-reduced systolic and diastolic function

ACE, angiotensin-converting enzyme; AD, autosomal dominant inheritance; AR, autosomal recessive inheritance; ARVC, arrhythmogenic right ventricular cardiomyopathy; DCM, dilated cardiomyopathy; HCM, hypertrophic cardiomyopathy; ICD, implantable cardioverter-defibrillator; LVNC, left ventricular noncompaction; Mt, mitochondrial inheritance; RCM, restrictive cardiomyopathy; X-L, X-linked inheritance.
*Genes are listed using the human gene symbol.

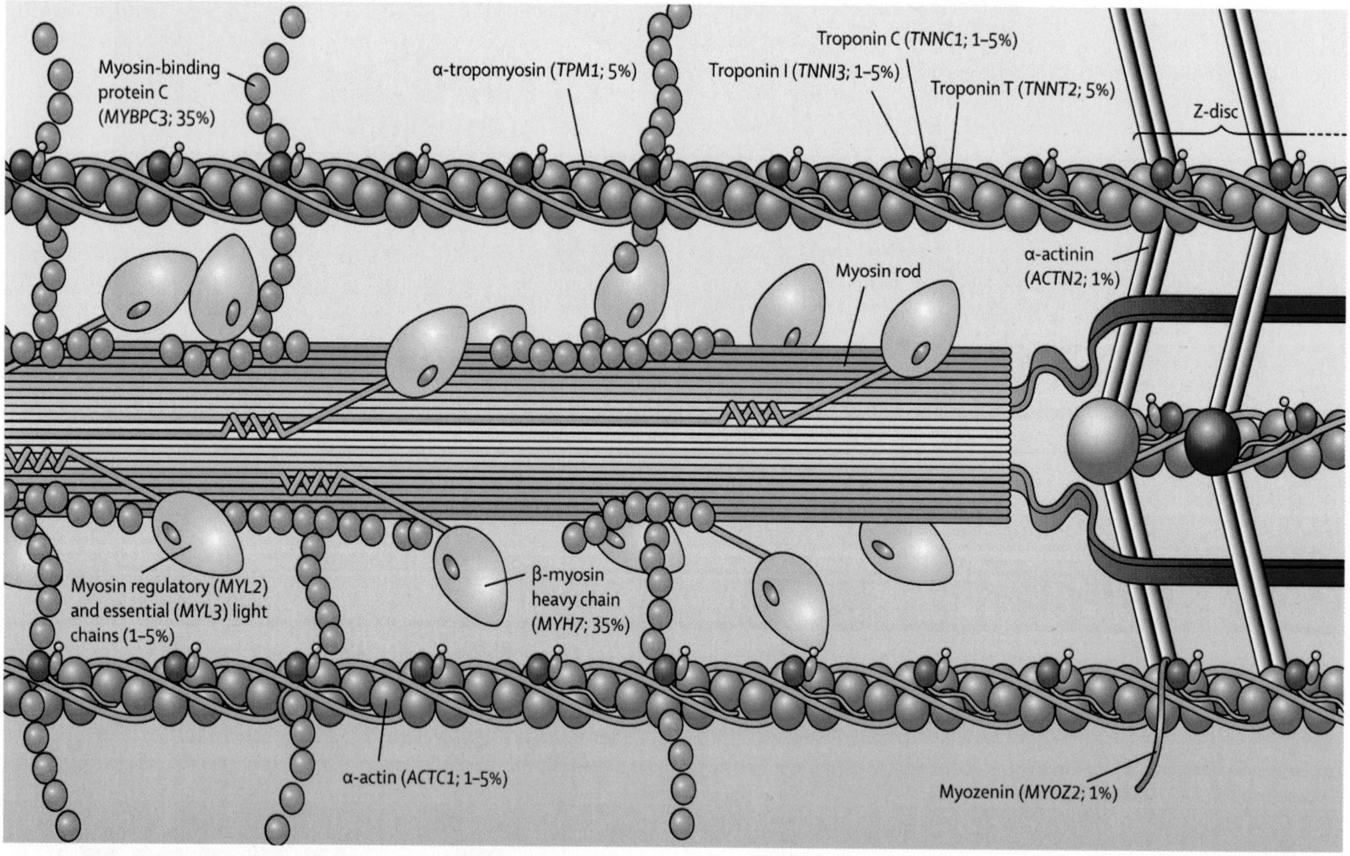

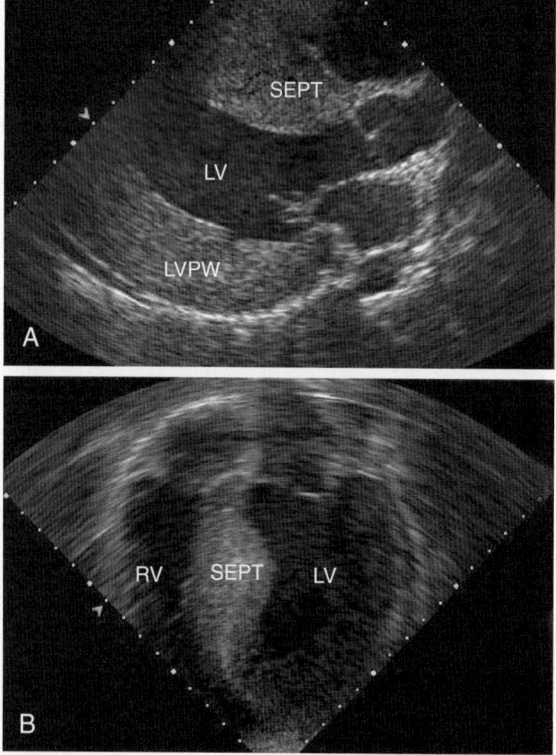

Figure 439-2 Locations of genes within the cardiac sarcomere known to cause hypertrophic cardiomyopathy. Prevalence of every gene (derived from data of unrelated hypertrophic cardiomyopathy probands with positive genotyping) is shown in parentheses. (From Maron BJ, Maron MS: Hypertrophic cardiomyopathy. Lancet 381:242–252, 2013, Fig. 1, p 243.)

Figure 439-3 Echocardiograms demonstrating hypertrophic cardiomyopathy. A, Parasternal long-axis view of a patient with severe concentric left ventricular hypertrophy. B, Four-chamber view of a patient with asymmetric septal hypertrophy. LV, left ventricle; LVPW, left ventricular posterior wall; RV, right ventricle; SEPT, septum.

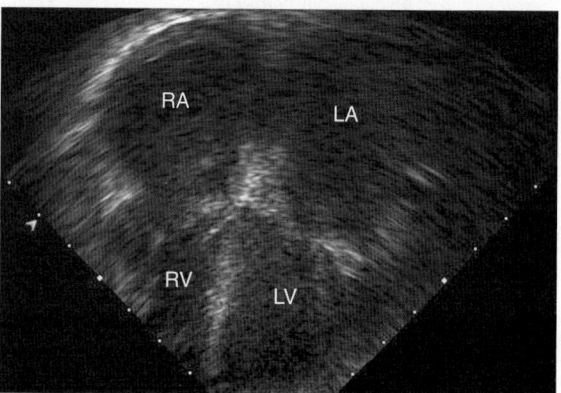

Figure 439-4 Echocardiogram of a patient with restrictive cardiomyopathy. The apical 4-chamber view shows the markedly enlarged right and left atria, compared to the normal size left and right ventricular chambers. LA, left atrium; LV, left ventricle; RA, right atrium; RV, right ventricle.

439.1 Dilated Cardiomyopathy

Robert L. Spicer and Stephanie M. Ware

ETIOLOGY AND EPIDEMIOLOGY

Dilated cardiomyopathy (DCM), the most common form of cardiomyopathy in children, is the cause of significant morbidity and mortality as well as a common indication for cardiac transplantation. The etiologies are diverse. Unlike adult patients with DCM, ischemic etiologies are rare in children, although these include anomalous origin of the left coronary artery from the pulmonary artery, premature coronary atherosclerosis (homozygous type II hypercholesterolemia), and coronary inflammatory diseases, such as Kawasaki disease. It is estimated that up to 50% of cases are genetic (usually autosomal dominant; some are autosomal recessive or X-linked), including some with metabolic causes (see Table 439-1). Although the most common etiology of DCM remains idiopathic, it is likely that undiagnosed familial/genetic conditions and myocarditis predominate. Associate features may include conduction defects or sensorineural hearing loss. The annual incidence of DCM in children younger than 18 yr is 0.57 cases per 100,000 per year. Incidence is higher in males, African-Americans, and in infants less than 1 yr old.

PATHOGENESIS

The pathogenesis of the ventricular dilation and altered contractility seen in DCM varies depending on the underlying etiology; systolic dysfunction and myocyte injury are common. Genetic abnormalities of several components of the cardiac muscle including sarcomere protein, the cytoskeleton, and the proteins that bridge the contractile apparatus to the cytoskeleton, have been identified in autosomal dominant and X-linked inherited disorders. DCM can occur following viral myocarditis and, although the primary pathogenesis varies from direct myocardial injury to viral-induced inflammatory injury, the resulting myocardial damage, ventricular enlargement, and poor function likely occur by a final common pathway similar to that which occurs in genetic disorders.

In 20-50% of cases, the DCM is familial with autosomal dominant inheritance most common (see Table 439-2). **Duchenne and Becker muscular dystrophies** (see Chapter 609.1) are X-linked cardiomyopathies that account for 5-10% of familial DCM cases. These dystrophinopathies result in an abnormal sarcomere–cytoskeleton connection, causing impaired myocardial force generation, myocyte damage/scarring, chamber enlargement, and altered function.

Mitochondrial myopathies, like the muscular dystrophies, may present clinically with a predominance of extracardiac findings and are inherited in a recessive or mitochondrial pattern. Disorders of **fatty acid oxidation** present with systemic derangements of metabolism (hypoketotic hypoglycemia, acidosis, and hepatic dysfunction), some with peripheral myopathy and neuropathy, and others with sudden death or life-threatening cardiac arrhythmias.

Anthracycline cardiotoxicity (doxorubicin [Adriamycin]) on rare occasion causes acute inflammatory myocardial injury, but more classically results in DCM and occurs in up to 30% of patients given a cumulative dose of doxorubicin exceeding 550 mg/m^2. The risk of toxicity appears to be exacerbated by concomitant radiation therapy.

CLINICAL MANIFESTATIONS

Although more prevalent in patients less than 1 yr of age, all age groups may be affected. Clinical manifestations of DCM are most commonly those of heart failure, but can also include palpitations, syncope, and sudden death. Irritability or lethargy can be accompanied by additional nonspecific complaints of failure to thrive, nausea, vomiting, or abdominal pain. Respiratory symptoms (tachypnea, wheezing, cough, or dyspnea on exertion) are often present. Uncommonly, patients may present acutely with pallor, altered mentation, hypotension, and shock. Patients can be tachycardic with narrow pulse pressure and have hepatic enlargement, and rales or wheezing. The precordial cardiac impulse is increased and the heart may be enlarged to palpation or percussion. Auscultation may reveal a gallop rhythm in addition to tachycardia and occasionally murmurs of mitral or, less commonly, tricuspid insufficiency may be present. The presence of hypoglycemia, acidosis, hypotonia, or signs of liver dysfunction suggests an inborn error of metabolism. Neurologic or skeletal muscle deficits are associated with mitochondrial disorders or muscular dystrophies.

LABORATORY FINDINGS

Electrocardiographic screening reveals atrial or ventricular hypertrophy, nonspecific T-wave abnormalities, and, occasionally, atrial or ventricular arrhythmias. The chest x-ray may demonstrate cardiomegaly and pulmonary vascular prominence or pleural effusions. The echocardiogram is often diagnostic, demonstrating the characteristic findings of left ventricular enlargement, decreased ventricular contractility, and occasionally a globular (remodeled) left ventricular contour (see Fig. 439-1). Right ventricular enlargement and depressed function are

occasionally noted. Echo Doppler studies can reveal evidence of pulmonary hypertension, mitral regurgitation, or other structural cardiac or coronary abnormalities.

Additional testing should include complete blood count, renal and liver function tests, creatine phosphokinase, cardiac troponin I, lactate, brain natriuretic peptide, plasma amino acids, urine organic acids, and an acylcarnitine profile. Additional genetic and enzymatic testing may be useful (see Table 439-2). Cardiac catheterization and endomyocardial biopsy are not routine but may be useful in patients with acute DCM. Biopsy samples can be examined histologically for the presence of mononuclear cell infiltrates, myocardial damage, storage abnormalities, and for evidence of infection. It is considered standard of care to screen 1st-degree family members utilizing echocardiography and electrocardiogram (ECG) in idiopathic and familial cases of DCM.

PROGNOSIS AND MANAGEMENT

The 1 and 5 yr freedom from death or transplantation in patients diagnosed with DCM is 61% and 47%, respectively. Independent risk factors at DCM diagnosis for subsequent death or transplantation include older age, congestive heart failure, lower left ventricular fractional shortening z score, and underlying etiology. DCM is the most common cause for cardiac transplantation in pediatric and adult studies.

The therapeutic approach to patients with DCM includes a careful assessment to uncover possible treatable etiologies, screening of family members, and rigorous pharmacologic therapy. Decongestive therapy may improve symptoms of heart failure, prolong survival, and occasionally results in complete resolution of dysfunction. Patients are often treated with diuretics and angiotensin-converting enzyme inhibitors. The use of digitalis and angiotensin receptor blockers may be of additional benefit. β-Adrenergic blockade with carvedilol or metoprolol is often used in patients with chronic heart failure although pediatric specific outcome data have failed to show effectiveness. In patients presenting with extreme degrees of heart failure or circulatory collapse, intensive care measures are often required, including intravenous inotropes and diuretics, mechanic ventilatory support, and on occasion, mechanical circulatory support, which may include ventricular assist devices, extracorporeal membrane oxygenation, and ultimately cardiac transplantation. In patients with DCM and atrial or ventricular arrhythmias, specific antiarrhythmic therapy should be instituted.

Bibliography is available at Expert Consult.

439.2 Hypertrophic Cardiomyopathy
Robert L. Spicer and Stephanie M. Ware

ETIOLOGY AND EPIDEMIOLOGY

Hypertrophic cardiomyopathy (HCM) is a heterogeneous, relatively common, and potentially life-threatening form of cardiomyopathy. The causes of HCM are heterogeneous and include inborn errors of metabolism, neuromuscular disorders, syndromic conditions, and genetic abnormalities of the structural components of the cardiomyocyte (see Table 439-1). Both the age of onset and associated features are helpful in identifying the underlying etiology.

HCM is a genetic disorder and frequently occurs as a result of mutations in sarcomere or cytoskeletal components of the cardiomyocyte (see Fig. 439-2). Mutations of the genes encoding cardiac β-myosin heavy-chain (*MYH7*) and myosin-binding protein C (*MYBPC3*) are the most common (see Table 439-2). Mutations are inherited in an autosomal dominant pattern with widely variable penetrance; many cases represent de novo mutations. Some patients have mutations in more than 1 sarcomere or cytoskeletal gene and may manifest disease earlier and with more-severe symptoms. Additional genetic causes for HCM include nonsarcomeric protein mutations, such as the γ$_2$-regulatory subunit of adenosine monophosphate–activated protein kinase (*PRKAG2*) and the lysosome-associated membrane protein 2α-galactosidase (Danon disease, a form of glycogen storage disease). Syndromic conditions, such as Noonan syndrome, may present with

HCM at birth and recognition of extracardiac manifestations is important in making the diagnosis.

Glycogen storage disorders such as Pompe disease often present in infancy with a heart murmur, abnormal ECG, systemic signs and symptoms, and occasionally heart failure. The characteristic ECG in Pompe disease demonstrates prominent P waves, a short P-R interval, and massive QRS voltages; the echocardiogram confirms severe, often concentric, left ventricular hypertrophy.

PATHOGENESIS

HCM is characterized by the presence of increased left ventricular wall thickness in the absence of structural heart disease or hypertension. Often the interventricular septum is disproportionately involved, leading to the previous designation of idiopathic hypertrophic subaortic stenosis or the current term of asymmetric septal hypertrophy. In the presence of a resting or provokable outflow tract gradient, the term hypertrophic obstructive cardiomyopathy is used. Although the left ventricle is predominantly affected, the right ventricle may be involved, particularly in infancy. The mitral valve can demonstrate systolic anterior motion and mitral insufficiency. Left ventricular outflow tract obstruction occurs in 25% of patients, is dynamic in nature, and may in part be secondary to the abnormal position of the mitral valve as well as the obstructing subaortic hypertrophic cardiac muscle. The cardiac myofibrils and myofilaments demonstrate disarray and myocardial fibrosis.

Typically, systolic pump function is preserved or even hyperdynamic, though systolic dysfunction may occur late. Outflow tract obstruction with or without mitral insufficiency may be provoked by physiologic manipulations such as the Valsalva maneuver, positional changes, and physical activity. Frequently, the hypertrophic and fibrosed cardiac muscle demonstrates relaxation abnormalities (diminished compliance) and left ventricular filling may be impaired (diastolic dysfunction).

CLINICAL MANIFESTATIONS

Many patients are asymptomatic, and 50% of cases present with a heart murmur or during screening when another family member has been diagnosed with HCM. Symptoms of HCM may include palpitations, chest pain, easy fatigability, dyspnea, dizziness, and syncope. Sudden death is a well-recognized but uncommon manifestation that often occurs during physical exertion.

Characteristic physical examination findings include an overactive precordial impulse with a lift or heave, abnormal peripheral pulses (hyperdynamic or diminished), a systolic ejection murmur in the aortic region *not* associated with an ejection click, and an apical blowing murmur of mitral insufficiency.

DIAGNOSIS

The ECG typically demonstrates left ventricular hypertrophy with ST segment and T-wave abnormalities. Intraventricular conduction delays and signs of ventricular preexcitation (Wolff-Parkinson-White syndrome) may be present and should raise the possibility of Danon disease or Pompe disease. Chest radiography demonstrates normal or mildly increased heart size with a prominence of the left ventricle. Echocardiography is diagnostic in identifying, localizing, and quantifying the degree of myocardial hypertrophy (see Fig. 439-3). Doppler interrogation defines, localizes, and quantifies the degree of ventricular outflow tract obstruction and also demonstrates and quantifies the degree of mitral insufficiency. Diastolic dysfunction can be confirmed by M-mode, flow, and tissue Doppler techniques.

Cardiac catheterization may be indicated in some cases of HCM to define the left ventricular outflow gradient with and without pharmacologic provocation, to measure left ventricular diastolic pressures, to perform electrophysiologic testing of assessment of arrhythmia risk, or in rare cases, endomyocardial biopsy.

Additional diagnostic studies include metabolic testing, genetic testing for specific syndromes, or genetic testing for mutations in genes known to cause isolated HCM (see Table 439-2). The clinical availability of these tests is expanding. In adults, where isolated HCM is a common genetic diagnosis, it has been possible to identify a subset of mutations that confer an increased risk for arrhythmia or sudden death. As identification of the molecular basis of disease in children increases, similar correlations are expected to emerge. In addition, genetic diagnosis is useful to identify at-risk family members who require ongoing surveillance.

PROGNOSIS AND MANAGEMENT

Children under 1 yr of age or with inborn errors of metabolism or malformation syndromes or those with a mixed HCM/DCM have a significantly poorer prognosis. The risk of sudden death in older patients is greater in those with a history of cardiac arrest, ventricular tachycardia, exercise hypotension, syncope, excessive (>3 cm) ventricular wall thickness, and a ventricular obstruction gradient greater than 30 mm Hg. Although intrafamilial variability in symptoms occurs, a family history of sudden death is a highly significant predictor of risk.

Competitive sports and strenuous physical activity should be prohibited as most sudden deaths in patients with HCM occur during or immediately after vigorous physical exertion. β-adrenergic blocking agents (propranolol, atenolol) or calcium channel blocking agents (verapamil) may be useful in diminishing ventricular outflow tract obstruction, modifying ventricular hypertrophy, and improving ventricular filling. Although significant symptomatic improvement occurs in some patients, the risk for development of heart failure or sudden death has not been lessened. In patients with atrial or ventricular arrhythmias, specific antiarrhythmic therapy should be used. Patients with documented ventricular arrhythmias, strong family histories of arrhythmias or sudden death, or patients with syncope should be treated with an implantable cardioverter defibrillator.

Innovative interventional procedures to anatomically or physiologically reduce the degree of left ventricular outflow tract obstruction have been used. Dual-chamber pacing, alcohol septal ablation, surgical septal myomectomy, and mitral valve replacement have all met with some success.

First-degree relatives of patients identified as having HCM should be screened with electrocardiography and echocardiography. Genetic testing is available clinically. It is important to first test the affected individual in the family rather than "at-risk" individuals because 20-40% of cases of HCM will not demonstrate mutations in currently available panels of genes. If a causative mutation is identified, "at-risk" members of the family can be effectively tested. In families with HCM without demonstrable gene mutations, repeat noninvasive cardiac screening with ECG and echo should be undertaken in at risk individuals every 3-5 yr for patients younger than 12 yr of age and yearly throughout the teenage years and young adulthood. The clinical course of other affected family members and the results of genetic testing may be of some use in stratifying risk in an affected child.

Bibliography is available at Expert Consult.

439.3 Restrictive Cardiomyopathy
Robert L. Spicer and Stephanie M. Ware

ETIOLOGY AND EPIDEMIOLOGY

Restrictive cardiomyopathy (RCM) accounts for <5% of cardiomyopathy cases. Incidence increases with age, and is more common in females. In equatorial Africa, RCM accounts for a large number of deaths. Infiltrative myocardial causes and storage disorders frequently result in associated left ventricular hypertrophy and may represent HCM with restrictive physiology. Noninfiltrative causes include mutations in genes encoding sarcomeric or cytoskeletal proteins. Although there has been significant success in discovering new gene mutations causing RCM, the majority of are considered idiopathic.

PATHOGENESIS

RCM is characterized by normal ventricular chamber dimensions, normal myocardial wall thickness, and preserved systolic function. Dramatic atrial dilation can occur as a result of the abnormal myocardial compliance and high ventricular diastolic pressure. Autosomal dominant inheritance has been demonstrated for families with mutations in sarcomeric and cytoskeletal genes.

CLINICAL MANIFESTATIONS

Abnormal ventricular filling, sometimes referred to as *diastolic heart failure*, is manifest in the systemic venous circulation with edema, hepatomegaly, or ascites. Elevation of left-sided filling pressures result in cough, dyspnea, or pulmonary edema. With activity, patients may experience chest pain, shortness of breath, syncope/near syncope, or even sudden death. Pulmonary hypertension and pulmonary vascular disease develop and may progress rapidly. Heart murmurs are typically absent, but a gallop rhythm may be prominent. In the presence of pulmonary hypertension, an overactive right ventricular impulse and pronounced pulmonary component of the second heart sound are present.

DIAGNOSIS

The characteristic electrocardiographic finding of prominent P waves is usually associated with normal QRS voltages and nonspecific ST and T-wave changes. Right ventricular hypertrophy occurs in patients with pulmonary hypertension. The chest x-ray may be normal or demonstrate a prominent atrial shadow and pulmonary vascular redistribution. The echocardiogram is often diagnostic, demonstrating normal-sized ventricles with preserved systolic function and dramatic enlargement of the atria (see Fig. 439-4). Flow and tissue Doppler interrogation reveal abnormal filling parameters. Differential diagnosis from constrictive pericarditis is critical, as the latter can be treated surgically. Magnetic resonance imaging may be necessary to demonstrate the thickened or calcified pericardium often present in constrictive pericardial disease.

PROGNOSIS AND MANAGEMENT

Pharmacologic treatment modalities are of limited use and the prognosis of patients with RCM is generally poor with often progressive clinical deterioration. Sudden death is a significant risk, with a 2-yr survival of 50%. When signs of heart failure exist, judicious use of diuretics can result in clinical improvement. As a result of the dramatic atrial enlargement, these patients are predisposed to the development of atrial tachyarrhythmias and thromboemboli. Antiarrhythmic agents may be necessary and anticoagulation with platelet inhibitors or Coumadin is indicated.

Cardiac transplantation is the treatment of choice in many centers for patients with RCM, and the results are excellent in patients without pulmonary hypertension, pulmonary vascular disease, or severe congestive heart failure.

Bibliography is available at Expert Consult.

439.4 Left Ventricular Noncompaction, Arrhythmogenic Right Ventricular Cardiomyopathy, and Endocardial Fibroelastosis
Robert L. Spicer and Stephanie M. Ware

Left ventricular noncompaction (LVNC) was initially believed to be a rare disorder found only in children, but is now known to affect individuals of all ages. LVNC is characterized by a distinctive trabeculated or spongy-appearing left ventricle (Fig. 439-5) commonly associated with left ventricular hypertrophy and/or dilation, and at times, systolic or diastolic dysfunction. LVNC may be isolated or associated with structural congenital cardiac defects. Patients may present with signs of heart failure, arrhythmias, syncope, sudden death, or as an asymptomatic finding during screening of family members.

Imaging studies using ultrasound or magnetic resonance can demonstrate the characteristic pattern of deeply trabeculated left ventricle myocardium, most characteristically within the apex of the left ventricle. ECG findings are nonspecific and include chamber hypertrophy, ST and T-wave changes, or arrhythmias. In some patients, preexcitation is

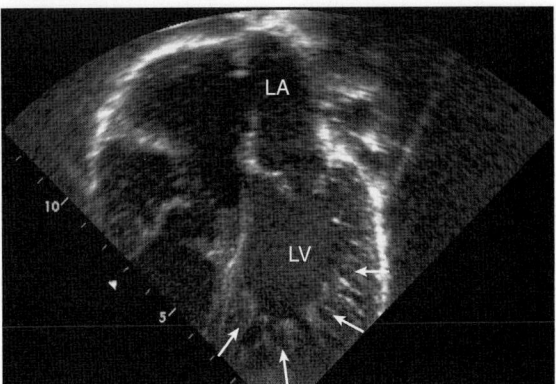

Figure 439-5 Echocardiogram of a patient with left ventricular noncompaction cardiomyopathy. Apical view showing the abnormal trabeculations of the left ventricle at the apex *(arrows)*. For comparison, see the smooth walled LV in Figure 439-1. LA, left atrium; LV, left ventricle.

notable and giant QRS voltages occur in approximately 30% of younger children. Metabolic screening should be considered, especially in young children. Elevated serum lactate and urine 3-methylglutaconic acid may be seen in Barth syndrome, an X-linked disorder of phospholipid metabolism caused by a mutation in the tafazzin (*TAZ*) gene. Clinical testing for *TAZ* mutations is available and should be considered, especially in males. Patients with mitochondrial disorders frequently demonstrate signs of LVNC. These children are at risk for atrial or ventricular arrhythmias and thromboembolic complications. Treatment includes anticoagulation, antiarrhythmic therapy if needed, and treatment of heart failure if present. In patients refractory to medical therapy, cardiac transplantation has been used successfully.

Arrhythmogenic right ventricular cardiomyopathy (ARVC) is thought to be uncommon in North America but is among the most common forms of cardiomyopathy in Europe, especially Italy. Autosomal dominant inheritance is common. In addition, recessive forms associated with severe ARVC and skin manifestations are known. Comprehensive genetic screening has been reported to identify a cause in up to 50% of cases. ARVC is typically characterized by a dilated right ventricle with fibrofatty infiltration of the right ventricle wall; increasingly, left ventricle involvement is being recognized. Global and regional right and left ventricular dysfunction and ventricular tachyarrhythmias are the major clinical findings. Syncope or aborted sudden death can occur and should be treated with antiarrhythmic medications and placement of a defibrillator. In patients with ventricular dysfunction, heart failure management as indicated for patients with DCM may be of use.

Endocardial fibroelastosis (EFE), at one time an important cause of heart failure in children, is uncommon. The decline in primary EFE is likely related to the abolition of mumps virus infections by immunization practices. Rare familial cases exist, but the causative genes are unknown. Secondary EFE can occur with severe left-sided obstructive lesions such as aortic stenosis or atresia, hypoplastic left heart syndrome, or coarctation of the aorta. EFE is characterized by an opaque, white, fibroelastic thickening on the endocardial surface of the ventricle, which leads to systolic and/or diastolic dysfunction. Surgical removal of the endocardial fibrosis has been successfully utilized to improve cardiac function. Standard heart failure management including transplantation has been utilized in the management of EFE.

Bibliography is available at Expert Consult.

439.5 Myocarditis
Robert L. Spicer and Stephanie M. Ware

Acute or chronic inflammation of the myocardium is characterized by inflammatory cell infiltrates, myocyte necrosis, or myocyte

Table 439-3	Causes of Myocarditis			
INFECTIOUS			**IMMUNE-MEDIATED**	**TOXIC**

Viral	Adenovirus
	 Parvovirus
	 Coxsackie B virus Epstein-Barr
	   virus
	 Hepatitis C virus
	 Measles virus
	 Human herpes virus
	 Varicella-zoster virus
	 Human immunodeficiency virus
	 Influenza viruses
		Autoantigens	Churg-Strauss syndrome
			 Inflammatory bowel disease
			 Giant cell myocarditis
			 Diabetes mellitus
			 Sarcoidosis
			 Systemic lupus
			   erythematosus
			 Thyrotoxicosis
			 Takayasu arteritis
			 Kawasaki syndrome
			 Celiac disease
			 Whipple disease
				Anthracyclines
				 Cocaine
				 Interleukin-2
				 Ethanol
				 Heavy metals
				 Spider bite
				 Snake bite
				 Scorpion bite
				 Electric shock

Bacterial	*Mycobacteria* *Streptococcus* spp. *Mycoplasma pneumoniae* *Treponema pallidum* *Corynebacterium diphtheriae* *Borrelia burgdorferi* *Ehrlichia*			
Fungal	*Aspergillus* *Candida* *Coccidioides* *Cryptococcus* *Histoplasma*	Hypersensitivity	Granulomatosis with polyangiitis Sulfonamides Cephalosporins Diuretics	
Protozoal	*Trypanosoma cruzi* *Toxoplasma gondii* *Babesia*		Tricyclic antidepressants Dobutamine	
Parasitic	Schistosomiasis Larva migrans (visceral)			

Data from Feldman AM, McNamara D: Myocarditis, N Engl J Med 343:1388–1398, 2000; Magnani JW, Dec GW: Myocarditis: current trends in diagnosis and treatment, Circulation 113:876–990, 2006.

degeneration and may be caused by infectious, connective tissue, granulomatous, toxic, or idiopathic processes. There may be associated systemic manifestations of the disease and on occasion the endocardium or pericardium is involved, though coronary pathology is uniformly absent. Patients may be asymptomatic, have nonspecific prodromal symptoms, or present with overt congestive heart failure, compromising arrhythmias, or sudden death. It is thought that viral infections are the most common etiology though myocardial toxins, drug exposures, hypersensitivity reactions, and immune disorders may also lead to myocarditis (Table 439-3).

ETIOLOGY AND EPIDEMIOLOGY
Viral Infections
Coxsackievirus and other enteroviruses, adenovirus, parvovirus, Epstein-Barr virus, parechovirus, influenza virus, and cytomegalovirus are the most common causative agents in children, though most known viral agents have been reported. In Asia, hepatitis C virus appears to be significant as well. The true incidence of viral myocarditis is unknown as mild cases probably go undetected. The disease is typically sporadic but may be epidemic. Manifestations are, to some degree, age dependent: in neonates and young infants, viral myocarditis can be fulminant; in children, it often will occur as an acute, myopericarditis with heart failure; and in older children and adolescents, it may present with signs and symptoms of acute or chronic heart failure or chest pain.

Bacterial Infections
Bacterial myocarditis has become far less common with the advent of advanced public health measures, which have minimized infectious causes such as diphtheria. Diphtheritic myocarditis (see Chapter 187) is unique as bacterial toxin may produce circulatory collapse and toxic myocarditis characterized by atrioventricular block, bundle-branch block, or ventricular ectopy. Any overwhelming systemic bacterial infection can manifest with circulatory collapse and shock with evidence of myocardial dysfunction characterized by tachycardia, gallop

rhythm, and low cardiac output. Additional nonviral infectious causes of myocarditis include rickettsia, protozoa, parasitic infections, and fungal disease.

PATHOPHYSIOLOGY
Myocarditis is characterized by myocardial inflammation, injury or necrosis, and ultimately fibrosis. Cardiac enlargement and diminished systolic function occur as a direct result of the myocardial damage. Typical signs of congestive heart failure occur and may progress rapidly to shock, atrial or ventricular arrhythmias, and sudden death. Viral myocarditis may also become a chronic process with persistence of viral nucleic acid in the myocardium, and the perpetuation of chronic inflammation secondary to altered host immune response including activated T lymphocytes (cytotoxic and natural killer cells) and antibody-dependent cell mediated damage. Additionally, persistent viral infection may alter the expression of major histocompatibility complex antigens with resultant exposure of neoantigens to the immune system. Some viral proteins share antigenic epitopes with host cells, resulting in autoimmune damage to the antigenically related myocyte. Cytokines such as tumor necrosis factor-α and interleukin-1 are inhibitors of myocyte response to adrenergic stimuli and result in diminished cardiac function. The final result of viral-associated inflammation can be DCM.

CLINICAL MANIFESTATIONS
Manifestations of myocarditis range from asymptomatic or nonspecific generalized illness to acute cardiogenic shock and sudden death. Infants and young children more often have a fulminant presentation with fever, respiratory distress, tachycardia, hypotension, gallop rhythm, and cardiac murmur. Associated findings may include a rash or evidence of end organ involvement such as hepatitis or aseptic meningitis.

Patients with acute or chronic myocarditis may present with chest discomfort, fever, palpitations, easy fatigability, or syncope/near syncope. Cardiac findings include overactive precordial impulse, gallop rhythm, and an apical systolic murmur of mitral insufficiency.

In patients with associated pericardial disease, a rub may be noted. Hepatic enlargement, peripheral edema, and pulmonary findings such as wheezes or rales may be present in patients with decompensated heart failure.

DIAGNOSIS

Electrocardiographic changes are nonspecific and may include sinus tachycardia, atrial or ventricular arrhythmias, heart block, diminished QRS voltages, and nonspecific ST and T-wave changes, often suggestive of acute ischemia. Chest x-rays in severe, symptomatic cases reveal cardiomegaly, pulmonary vascular prominence, overt pulmonary edema, or pleural effusions. Echocardiography often shows diminished ventricular systolic function, cardiac chamber enlargement, mitral insufficiency, and occasionally, evidence of pericardial infusion.

Cardiac MRI is a standard imaging modality for the diagnosis of myocarditis; information on the presence and extent of edema, gadolinium-enhanced hyperemic capillary leak, myocyte necrosis, left ventricular dysfunction, and evidence of an associated pericardial effusion assist in the cardiac MRI diagnosis of myocarditis.

Endomyocardial biopsy may be useful in identifying inflammatory cell infiltrates or myocyte damage and performing molecular viral analysis using polymerase chain reaction techniques. Catheterization and biopsy, although not without risk (perforation and arrhythmias), should be performed by experienced personnel in patients suspected to have myocarditis or if there is strong suspicion for unusual forms of cardiomyopathy such as storage diseases or mitochondrial defects. Nonspecific tests include sedimentation rate, creatine phosphokinase isoenzymes, cardiac troponin I, and brain natriuretic peptide levels.

DIFFERENTIAL DIAGNOSIS

The predominant diseases mimicking acute myocarditis include carnitine deficiency, other metabolic disorders of energy generation, hereditary mitochondrial defects, idiopathic DCM, pericarditis, EFE, and anomalies of the coronary arteries (see Table 439-1).

TREATMENT

Primary therapy for acute myocarditis is supportive (see Chapter 442). Acutely, the use of inotropic agents, preferably milrinone, should be entertained but used with caution because of their proarrhythmic potential. Diuretics are often required as well. If in extremis, mechanical ventilatory support and mechanical circulatory support with ventricular assist device implantation or extracorporeal membrane oxygenation may be needed to stabilize the patient's hemodynamic status and serve as a bridge to recovery or cardiac transplantation. Diuretics, angiotensin-converting enzyme inhibitors, and angiotensin receptor blockers are of use in patients with compensated congestive heart failure in the outpatient setting but may be contraindicated in those presenting with fulminant heart failure and cardiovascular collapse. In patients manifesting with significant atrial or ventricular arrhythmias, specific antiarrhythmic agents (for example, amiodarone) should be administered and implantable cardioverter defibrillator placement considered.

Immunomodulation of patients with myocarditis is controversial. **Intravenous immune globulin** may have a role in the treatment of acute or fulminant myocarditis and **corticosteroids** have been reported to improve cardiac function, but the data are not convincing in children. Relapse has been noted in patients receiving immunosuppression who have been weaned from support. There are no studies to recommend specific antiviral therapies for myocarditis.

PROGNOSIS

The prognosis of symptomatic acute myocarditis in newborns is poor, and a 75% mortality has been reported. The prognosis is better for children and adolescents, although patients who have persistent evidence of DCM often progress to need for cardiac transplantation. Recovery of ventricular function has been reported in 10-50% of patients, however.

Bibliography is available at Expert Consult.

Chapter **440**
Diseases of the Pericardium
Robert L. Spicer and Stephanie M. Ware

The heart is enveloped in a bilayer membrane, the pericardium, which normally contains a small amount of serous fluid. The pericardium is not vital to normal function of the heart, and primary diseases of the pericardium are uncommon. However, the pericardium may be affected by a variety of conditions (Table 440-1), often as a manifestation of a systemic illness and can result in serious, even life-threatening, cardiac compromise.

440.1 Acute Pericarditis
Robert L. Spicer and Stephanie M. Ware

PATHOGENESIS

Inflammation of the pericardium may have only minor pathophysiologic consequences in the absence of significant fluid accumulation in the pericardial space. When the amount of fluid in the nondistensible pericardial space becomes excessive, pressure within the pericardium increases and is transmitted to the heart resulting in impaired filling. Although small to moderate amounts of pericardial effusion can be well tolerated and clinically silent, once the noncompliant pericardium has been distended maximally, any further fluid accumulation causes abrupt impairment of cardiac filling and is termed cardiac tamponade. When untreated, tamponade can lead to shock and death. Pericardial effusions may be serous/transudative, exudative/purulent, fibrinous, or hemorrhagic.

Table 440-1	Etiology of Pericardial Disease

CONGENITAL
Absence (partial, complete)
Cysts
Mulibrey nanism (*TRIM 37* gene mutation)
Camptodactyly-arthropathy-coxa vara-pericarditis syndrome (*PRG4* gene mutation)

INFECTIOUS
Viral (coxsackievirus B, Epstein-Barr virus, influenza, adenovirus, parvovirus, HIV, mumps)
Bacterial (*Haemophilus influenzae*, streptococcus, pneumococcus, staphylococcus, meningococcus, mycoplasma, tularemia, listeria, leptospirosis, tuberculosis, Q-fever, salmonella)
Immune complex (meningococcus, *H. influenzae*)
Fungal (actinomycosis, histoplasmosis)
Parasitic (toxoplasmosis, echinococcosis)

NONINFECTIOUS
Idiopathic
Systemic inflammatory diseases (acute rheumatic fever, juvenile idiopathic arthritis, systemic lupus erythematosus, mixed connective tissue disorders, systemic sclerosis, Kawasaki disease, Churg-Strauss syndrome, Behçet syndrome, sarcoidosis, familial Mediterranean fever and other recurrent fever syndromes, pancreatitis, granulomatosis with polyangiitis)
Metabolic (uremia, hypothyroidism, Gaucher disease, very-long-chain acyl-CoA dehydrogenase deficiency)
Traumatic (surgical, catheter, blunt)
Lymphomas, leukemia, radiation therapy
Primary pericardial tumors

CLINICAL MANIFESTATIONS

The most common symptom of acute pericarditis is chest pain, typically described as sharp/stabbing, positional, radiating, worse with inspiration, and relieved by sitting upright or prone. Cough, fever, dyspnea, abdominal pain, and vomiting are nonspecific symptoms associated with pericarditis. Additionally, signs and symptoms of organ system involvement may occur in the presence of generalized systemic disease.

Muffled or distant heart sounds, tachycardia, narrow pulse pressure, jugular venous distention, and a pericardial friction rub provide clues to the diagnosis of acute pericarditis. Cardiac tamponade is recognized by the excessive fall of systolic blood pressure (>10 mm Hg) with inspiration. This pulsus paradoxus can be assessed by careful auscultatory blood pressure determination (automated blood pressure cuffs are inadequate), arterial pressure line wave form, or pulse oximeter tracing inspection. Conditions other than cardiac tamponade, which may result in pulsus paradoxus include severe dyspnea, obesity, and positive pressure ventilator support.

DIAGNOSIS

The electrocardiogram is often abnormal in acute pericarditis although the findings are nonspecific. Low voltage QRS amplitude may be seen as a result of pericardial fluid accumulation. Tachycardia and abnormalities of the ST segments, PR segments, and T waves may be present as well.

Although the chest x-ray findings in a patient with pericarditis without effusion are usually normal, in the presence of a significant effusion, cardiac enlargement will be seen and cardiac contour may be unusual (Erlenmeyer flask or water bottle appearance) (Fig. 440-1). Echocardiography is the most sensitive technique for identifying the size and location of a pericardial effusion. Compression and collapse of the right atrium and/or right ventricle are present with cardiac tamponade (Fig. 440-2). Abnormal diastolic filling parameters have also been described in cases of tamponade.

DIFFERENTIAL DIAGNOSIS

Chest pain similar to that present in pericarditis can occur with lung diseases, especially pleuritis, and with gastroesophageal reflux. Pain related to myocardial ischemia is usually more severe, more prolonged, and occurs with exercise, allowing distinction from pericarditis-induced pain. The presence of a pericardial effusion by echocardiography is virtually diagnostic of pericarditis.

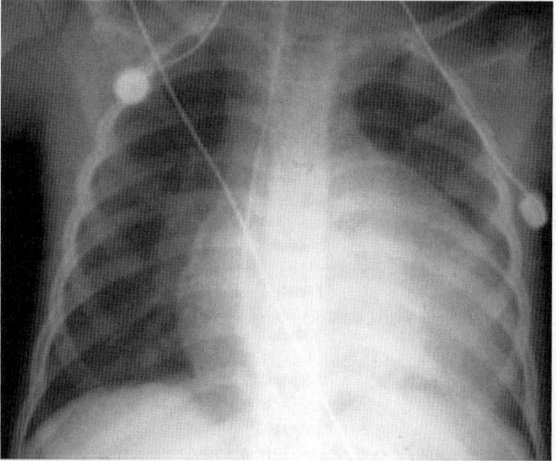

Figure 440-1 Water bottle silhouette. This chest radiograph shows marked cardiomegaly, also known as a water bottle silhouette, which is seen in the presence of large pericardial effusions. Also note the associated pulmonary edema from associated high left atrial and left ventricular filling pressures. *(Courtesy of Dr. Steven M. Selbst, Wilmington, DE; from Durani Y, Giordani K, Goudie BW: Myocarditis and pericarditis in children. Pediatr Clin North Am 57:1281–1303, 2010, Fig 7.)*

Infectious Pericarditis

A number of viral agents are known to cause pericarditis, and the clinical course of the majority of these infections is mild and spontaneously resolving. The term acute benign pericarditis is synonymous for viral pericarditis. Agents identified as causing pericarditis include the enteroviruses, influenza, adenovirus, respiratory syncytial virus, and parvovirus. As the course of this illness is usually benign, symptomatic treatment with nonsteroidal antiinflammatory agents is often sufficient. Patients with large effusions and tamponade may require pericardiocentesis. Presumed viral but often idiopathic pericarditis may have an autoimmune component. In up to 30%, there may be recurrences of pericarditis. Treatment and/or prevention of recurrences with colchicine improve symptoms and avoid recurrences in most of these patients. Patients with idiopathic recurrent pericarditis may also respond to treatment with anakinra. If the condition becomes chronic or relapsing, surgical pericardiectomy or creation of a pericardial window may be necessary.

Echocardiography is useful in differentiating pericarditis from myocarditis, the latter of which will show evidence of diminished myocardial contractility or valvular dysfunction. Pericarditis and myocarditis may occur together in some cases of viral infection.

Purulent pericarditis, often caused by bacterial infections, has become much less common with the advent of new immunizations for haemophilus and pneumococcal disease. Historically, purulent pericarditis was seen in association with severe pneumonias, epiglottitis, meningitis, or osteomyelitis. Patients with purulent pericarditis are acutely ill. Unless the infection is recognized and treated expeditiously, the course can be fulminant, leading to tamponade and death. Tuberculous pericarditis is rare in developed countries, but can be seen as a relatively common complication of HIV infection in regions where tuberculosis is endemic and access to antiretroviral therapy is limited. Immune-complex mediated pericarditis is a rare complication that may result in a nonpurulent (sterile) effusion following systemic bacterial infections such as meningococcus or haemophilus.

Noninfectious Pericarditis

Systemic inflammatory diseases including autoimmune, rheumatologic, and connective tissue disorders may involve the pericardium and result in serous pericardial effusions. Pericardial inflammation may be a component of the type II hypersensitivity reaction seen in patients with acute rheumatic fever. It is often associated with rheumatic valvulitis and responds quickly to antiinflammatory agents including steroids. Tamponade is very uncommon (see Chapters 183.1 and 438).

Juvenile idiopathic arthritis, usually systemic onset disease, can manifest with pericarditis. Differentiating rheumatoid pericardial inflammation from that seen with systemic lupus erythematosus is difficult and requires careful rheumatologic evaluation. Aspirin and/or corticosteroids can result in rapid resolution of a pericardial effusion but may be needed on a chronic basis to prevent relapse. Many of the autoinflammatory recurrent fever syndromes present with pericarditis, usually with other manifestations of those disorders (Chapter 163).

Patients with chronic renal failure or hypothyroidism may have pericardial effusions and should be carefully screened with physical exam, and, if indicated, imaging studies, during the course of their illness should clinical suspicion arise.

Especially common in referral centers with hematology/oncology units is the presence of pericardial effusion related to neoplastic disease. Conditions resulting in effusion include Hodgkin disease, lymphomas, and leukemia. Radiation therapy directed to the mediastinum of patients with malignancy can result in pericarditis and later constrictive pericardial disease.

The postpericardiotomy syndrome occurs in patients having undergone cardiac surgery and is characterized by fever, lethargy, anorexia, irritability, and chest/abdominal discomfort beginning 7-14 days postoperatively. There can be associated pleural effusions and serologic evidence of elevated antiheart antibodies. Postpericardiotomy syndrome is effectively treated with aspirin, nonsteroidal inflammatory

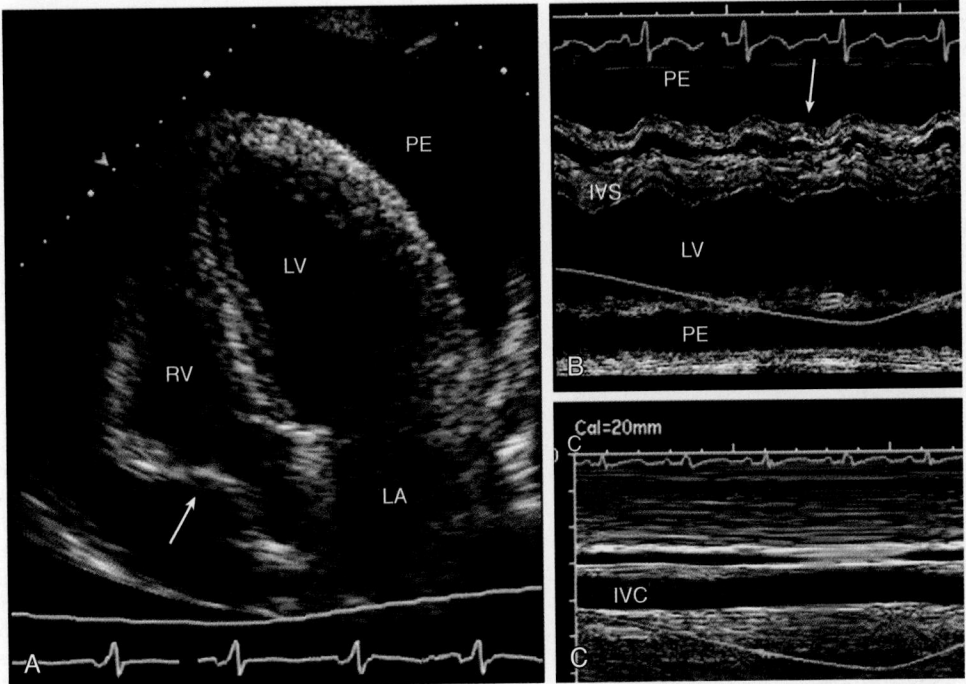

Figure 440-2 Echocardiographic images of large pericardial effusion with features of tamponade. **A,** Apical 4-chamber view of LV, LA, and RV that shows large PE with diastolic right-atrial collapse *(arrow).* **B,** M-mode image with cursor placed through RV, IVS, and LV in parasternal long axis. The view shows circumferential PE with diastolic collapse of RV free wall *(arrow)* during expiration. **C,** M-mode image from subcostal window in same patient that shows IVC plethora without inspiratory collapse. IVC, inferior vena cava; IVS, interventricular septum; LA, left atrium; LV, left ventricle; PE, pericardial effusion; RV, right ventricle. *(From Troughton RW, Asher CR, Klein AL: Pericarditis,* Lancet *363:717–727, 2004.)*

agents, and in severe cases, corticosteroids. Pericardial drainage is necessary in those patients with cardiac tamponade.

440.2 Constrictive Pericarditis
Robert L. Spicer and Stephanie M. Ware

Rarely, chronic pericardial inflammation can result in fibrosis, calcification, and thickening of the pericardium. Pericardial scarring may lead to impaired cardiac distensibility and filling and is termed constrictive pericarditis. Constrictive pericarditis can occur following recurrent or chronic pericarditis, cardiac surgery, or radiation to the mediastinum as a treatment for malignancies, most commonly Hodgkin disease or lymphoma.

Clinical manifestations of systemic venous hypertension predominate in cases of restrictive pericarditis. Jugular venous distention, peripheral edema, hepatomegaly, and ascites may precede signs of more significant cardiac compromise such as tachycardia, hypotension, and pulsus paradoxus. A pericardial knock, rub, and distant heart sounds might be present on auscultation. Abnormalities of liver function tests, hypoalbuminemia, hypoproteinemia, and lymphopenia may be present. On occasion, x-rays of the chest demonstrate calcifications of the pericardium.

Constrictive pericarditis may be difficult to distinguish clinically from restrictive cardiomyopathy as both conditions result in impaired myocardial filling (see Chapter 439.3). Echocardiography may be helpful in distinguishing constrictive pericardial disease from restrictive cardiomyopathy, but magnetic resonance imaging and computed tomographic imaging are more sensitive in detecting abnormalities of the pericardium. In rare instances, exploratory thoracotomy with direct examination of the pericardium may be required to confirm the diagnosis.

Although acute pericardial constriction is reported to respond to antiinflammatory agents, the more typical chronic constrictive pericarditis will respond only to surgical pericardiectomy with extensive resection of the pericardium.

Bibliography is available at Expert Consult.

Chapter 441
Tumors of the Heart
Robert L. Spicer and Stephanie M. Ware

Although cardiac tumors occur rarely in pediatric patients, they may result in serious hemodynamic or electrophysiologic abnormalities depending on tumor type and location.

The vast majority of tumors originating from the heart are benign. **Rhabdomyomas** are the most common pediatric cardiac tumors and are associated with tuberous sclerosis in 70-95% of cases (see Chapter 596.2). Rhabdomyomas may occur at any age, from fetal life through late adolescence. They are often multiple, can occur in any cardiac chamber, and originate within the myocardium extending, often, into the atrial or ventricular cavities (Fig. 441-1). Depending on their location and size, they can result in inflow or outflow obstruction leading to cyanosis or cardiac failure; many are asymptomatic. Atrial and ventricular arrhythmias have been reported with rhabdomyomas, and on occasion, ventricular preexcitation (Wolff-Parkinson-White) is present on electrocardiogram.

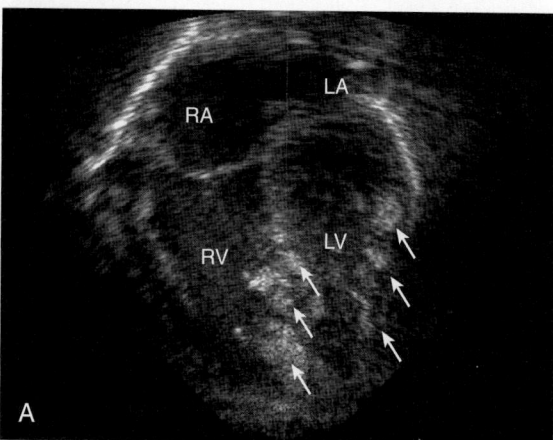

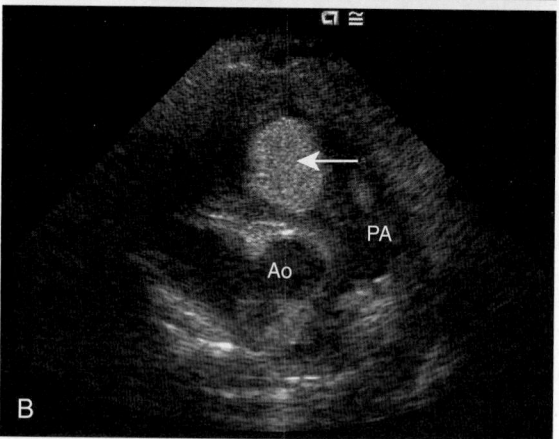

Figure 441-1 Echocardiograms demonstrating rhabdomyomas. **A,** Apical 4-chamber view showing multiple rhabdomyomas *(arrows)* within the septum and left ventricular myocardium. **B,** Short-axis view showing a large rhabdomyoma *(arrow)* extending into the right ventricular outflow tract. Ao, ascending aorta; LA, left atrium; LV, left ventricle; PA, pulmonary artery; RA, right atrium; RV, right ventricle.

Fibromas are the second most common pediatric cardiac tumor, and in contrast to rhabdomyomas, are usually solitary and intramyocardial. They can, by size and location, lead to heart failure, cyanosis, or rhythm disturbances. Loss of the tumor suppressor *PTCH1* is associated with the development of cardiac fibromas in sporadic cases. There is an increased incidence in patients with **Gorlin syndrome** (3%).

Myxomas, the most common cardiac tumor seen in adults, are infrequent in the pediatric population. Myxomas are predominantly intraatrial, appear pedunculated, and are rather mobile. They may cause obstruction to inflow or outflow and may present with a murmur, heart failure, or syncope. On occasion, atrial myxomas are associated with systemic symptoms of fever, malaise, and arthralgia. **Carney complex** is a familial autosomal dominant multiple neoplasia (often endocrine: pituitary adenoma, thyroid, testis, ovarian) and lentiginosis syndrome in which cardiac myxomas can occur at a young age in any or all cardiac chambers. *PRKAR1A* is the gene mutation in some families.

Other benign tumors include hemangiomas, Purkinje cell tumors, papillomas, lipomas, and mesotheliomas. Depending on their location, these benign tumors can result in valvular function abnormalities, myocardial dysfunction, or heart block and other arrhythmias.

Malignant pediatric cardiac tumors are far less common than benign tumors (75% vs. 25%), and the vast majority of such malignancies are sarcomas including angiosarcomas, rhabdosarcomas, or fibrosarcomas. Lymphomas and pheochromocytomas are reported but rare. Tumors originating from noncardiac sources that invade, extend, or metastasize to the heart are more commonly seen than primary malignant cardiac tumors. In pediatric patients, Wilms tumor and lymphoma/leukemia are the most common causes of such secondary tumors.

Although the manifestations of cardiac tumors in pediatric patients are protean, when a tumor is suspected, noninvasive imaging with echocardiography and/or magnetic resonance imaging may be diagnostic and can determine tumor type, location, extent, and hemodynamic impact. Electrocardiogram and Holter studies are valuable adjuncts when rhythm abnormalities are suspected. Cardiac catheterization is rarely indicated, but may be utilized to confirm tumor location, assess intracardiac hemodynamics, and perform biopsy for histologic assessment. Risks including blood loss, perforation, arrhythmia, and vessel injury should be considered when discussing catheterization and biopsy.

Because the natural history of rhabdomyomas is one of spontaneous diminution or complete resolution, treatment of the majority of cardiac tumors in pediatric patients is usually unnecessary. Everolimus, an inhibitor of the mammalian target of rapamycin, may enhance resolution in symptomatic patients with cardiac rhabdomyomas. Careful clinical follow-up and imaging are important. Antiarrhythmic medications may be prescribed to control rhythm disorders. Surgical removal of a cardiac tumor may be indicated to relieve obstruction, improve myocardial or valve function, or control arrhythmias. Heart transplantation has been performed in cases of unresectable tumors with significant hemodynamic compromise. Wilms tumors extending from the inferior vena cava into the atrium may require cardiopulmonary bypass support during the course of primary resection of the renal tumor. Radiation or chemotherapy can improve cardiac function in rare cases of lymphoma or leukemia compressing the heart with hemodynamic compromise.

Bibliography is available at Expert Consult.

Section 7
Cardiac Therapeutics

Chapter 442
Heart Failure
Daniel Bernstein

Heart failure occurs when the heart cannot deliver adequate cardiac output to meet the metabolic needs of the body. In the early stages of heart failure, various compensatory mechanisms are evoked to maintain normal metabolic function. When these mechanisms become ineffective, increasingly severe clinical manifestations result (see Chapter 70).

PATHOPHYSIOLOGY

The heart can be viewed as a pump with an output proportional to its filling volume and inversely proportional to the resistance against which it pumps. As ventricular end-diastolic volume increases, a healthy heart increases cardiac output until a maximum is reached and cardiac output can no longer be augmented (the Frank-Starling principle; Fig. 442-1). The increased stroke volume obtained in this manner is a result of stretching of myocardial fibers, but it also results in increased wall tension, which elevates myocardial oxygen consumption. Hearts working under various types of stress function along different Frank-Starling curves. Cardiac muscle with compromised intrinsic contractility requires a greater degree of dilation to produce increased stroke volume and does not achieve the same maximal

Frank-Starling Curve

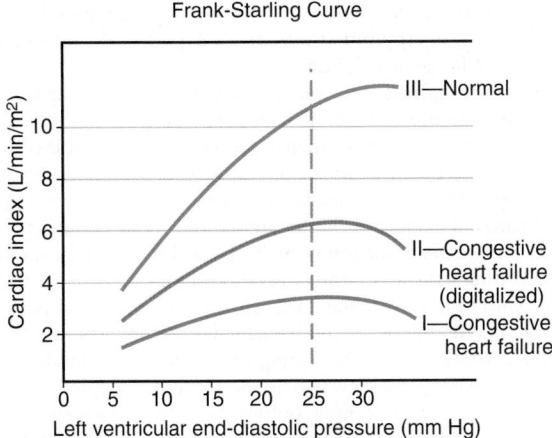

Figure 442-1 The Frank-Starling relationship. As left ventricular end-diastolic (LVED) pressure increases, the cardiac index increases, even in the presence of congestive heart failure, until a critical level of LVED pressure is reached. Adding an inotropic agent (digoxin) shifts the curve from I to II. *(From Gersony WM, Steep CN. In Dickerman JD, Lucey JF, editors: Smith's The critically ill child: diagnosis and medical management, ed 3, Philadelphia, 1984, WB Saunders.)*

cardiac output as normal myocardium does. If a cardiac chamber is already dilated because of a lesion causing increased preload (e.g., a left-to-right shunt or valvular insufficiency), there is little room for further dilation as a means of augmenting cardiac output. The presence of lesions that result in increased afterload to the ventricle (aortic or pulmonic stenosis, coarctation of the aorta) decreases cardiac performance, thereby resulting in a depressed Frank-Starling relationship.

Systemic oxygen transport is calculated as the product of cardiac output and systemic oxygen content. **Cardiac output** can be calculated as the product of heart rate and stroke volume. The primary determinants of stroke volume are the afterload (pressure work), preload (volume work), and contractility (intrinsic myocardial function). Abnormalities in heart rate can also compromise cardiac output; for example, tachyarrhythmias shorten the diastolic time interval for ventricular filling. Alterations in the oxygen-carrying capacity of blood (e.g., anemia or hypoxemia) also lead to a decrease in systemic oxygen transport and, if compensatory mechanisms are inadequate, can result in decreased delivery of substrate to tissues.

In some cases of heart failure, cardiac output is normal or increased, yet because of decreased systemic oxygen content (secondary to anemia) or increased oxygen demands (secondary to hyperventilation, hyperthyroidism, or hypermetabolism), an inadequate amount of oxygen is delivered to meet the body's needs. This condition, high-output failure, results in the development of signs and symptoms of heart failure when there is no basic abnormality in myocardial function and cardiac output is greater than normal. It is also seen with large systemic arteriovenous fistulas. These conditions reduce peripheral vascular resistance and cardiac afterload and increase myocardial contractility. Heart "failure" results when the demand for cardiac output exceeds the ability of the heart to respond. Chronic severe high-output failure may eventually result in a decrease in myocardial performance as the metabolic requirements of the myocardium are not met.

There are multiple systemic compensatory mechanisms used by the body to adapt to chronic heart failure. Some are mediated at the molecular/cellular level, such as upregulation or downregulation of various metabolic pathway components leading to changes in efficiency of oxygen and other substrate utilization. Others are mediated by neurohormones such as the renin–angiotensin system and the sympathoadrenal axis. One of the principal mechanisms for increasing cardiac output is an increase in sympathetic tone secondary to increased secretion of circulating epinephrine by the adrenals and increased release of norepinephrine at the neuromuscular junction. The initial beneficial effects of sympathetic stimulation include an increase in

heart rate and myocardial contractility, mediated by these hormones' action on cardiac β-adrenergic receptors, increasing cardiac output. These hormones also cause vasoconstriction, mediated by their action on peripheral arterial α-adrenergic receptors. Some vascular beds may constrict more readily than others, so that blood flow is redistributed from the cutaneous, visceral, and renal beds to the heart and brain. Whereas these acute effects are beneficial, chronically increased sympathetic stimulation can have deleterious effects, including hypermetabolism, increased afterload, arrhythmogenesis, and increased myocardial oxygen requirements. Peripheral vasoconstriction can result in decreased renal, hepatic, and gastrointestinal tract function. Chronic exposure to circulating catecholamines leads to a decrease in the number of cardiac β-adrenergic receptors (downregulation) and also causes direct myocardial cell damage. Thus, therapeutic agents for heart failure are directed at restoring balance to these neuroendocrine systems.

CLINICAL MANIFESTATIONS

The clinical manifestations of heart failure depend in part on the degree of the child's cardiac reserve. A critically ill infant or child who has exhausted the compensatory mechanisms to the point that cardiac output is no longer sufficient to meet the basal metabolic needs of the body will be symptomatic at rest. Other patients may be comfortable when quiet but are incapable of increasing cardiac output in response to even mild activity without experiencing significant symptoms. Conversely, it may take rather vigorous exercise to compromise cardiac function in children who have less severe heart disease. A thorough history is extremely important in making the diagnosis of heart failure and in evaluating the possible causes. Parents who observe their child on a daily basis may not recognize subtle changes that have occurred over the course of days or weeks. Gradually worsening perfusion or increasing respiratory effort may not be recognized as an abnormal finding. Edema may be passed off as normal weight gain, and exercise intolerance as lack of interest in an activity. The history of a young infant should also focus on feeding (see Chapter 416). An infant with heart failure often takes less volume per feeding, becomes dyspneic while sucking, and may perspire profusely. Eliciting a history of fatigue in an older child requires detailed questions about activity level and its course over several months.

In children, the signs and symptoms of heart failure may be similar to those in adults and include fatigue, effort intolerance, anorexia, dyspnea, and cough. Many children, however, especially adolescents, may have primarily abdominal symptoms (abdominal pain, nausea, anorexia) and a surprising lack of respiratory complaints. Attention to the cardiovascular system may come only after an abdominal roentgenogram unexpectedly catches the lower end of an enlarged heart. The elevation in systemic venous pressure may be gauged by clinical assessment of jugular venous pressure and liver enlargement. Orthopnea and basilar rales are variably present; edema is usually discernible in dependent portions of the body, or anasarca may be present. Cardiomegaly is invariably noted. A gallop rhythm is common; when ventricular dilation is advanced, the holosystolic murmur of mitral or tricuspid valve regurgitation may be heard.

In infants, heart failure may be difficult to distinguish from other causes of respiratory distress. Prominent manifestations include tachypnea, feeding difficulties, poor weight gain, excessive perspiration, irritability, weak cry, and noisy, labored respirations with intercostal and subcostal retractions, as well as flaring of the alae nasi. The signs of cardiac-induced pulmonary congestion may be indistinguishable from those of bronchiolitis; wheezing is often a more prominent finding in young infants with heart failure than rales. Pneumonitis with or without atelectasis is common, especially in the right middle and lower lobes, a result of bronchial compression by the enlarged heart. Hepatomegaly usually occurs, and cardiomegaly is invariably present. In spite of pronounced tachycardia, a gallop rhythm can frequently be recognized. The other auscultatory signs are those produced by the underlying cardiac lesion. Clinical assessment of jugular venous pressure in infants may be difficult because of the shortness of the neck and the difficulty of observing a relaxed state; palpation of an enlarged

Table 442-1	Etiology of Heart Failure

FETAL
Severe anemia (hemolysis, fetal-maternal transfusion, parvovirus B19–induced anemia, hypoplastic anemia)
Supraventricular tachycardia
Ventricular tachycardia
Complete heart block
Severe Ebstein anomaly or other severe right-sided lesions
Myocarditis

PREMATURE NEONATE
Fluid overload
Patent ductus arteriosus
Ventricular septal defect
Cor pulmonale (bronchopulmonary dysplasia)
Hypertension
Myocarditis
Genetic cardiomyopathy

FULL-TERM NEONATE
Asphyxial cardiomyopathy
Arteriovenous malformation (vein of Galen, hepatic)
Left-sided obstructive lesions (coarctation of aorta, hypoplastic left heart syndrome)
Large mixing cardiac defects (single ventricle, truncus arteriosus)
Myocarditis
Genetic cardiomyopathy

INFANT-TODDLER
Left-to-right cardiac shunts (ventricular septal defect)
Hemangioma (arteriovenous malformation)
Anomalous left coronary artery
Genetic or metabolic cardiomyopathy
Acute hypertension (hemolytic-uremic syndrome)
Supraventricular tachycardia
Kawasaki disease
Myocarditis

CHILD-ADOLESCENT
Rheumatic fever
Acute hypertension (glomerulonephritis)
Myocarditis
Thyrotoxicosis
Hemochromatosis-hemosiderosis
Cancer therapy (radiation, doxorubicin)
Sickle cell anemia
Endocarditis
Cor pulmonale (cystic fibrosis)
Genetic or metabolic cardiomyopathy (hypertrophic, dilated)

liver is a more reliable sign. Edema may be generalized and usually involves the eyelids as well as the sacrum and less often the legs and feet. The differential diagnosis is age dependent (Table 442-1).

DIAGNOSIS

X-rays of the chest show cardiac enlargement. Pulmonary vascularity is variable and depends on the cause of the heart failure. Infants and children with large left-to-right shunts have exaggeration of the pulmonary arterial vessels to the periphery of the lung fields, whereas patients with cardiomyopathy may have a relatively normal pulmonary vascular bed early in the course of disease. Fluffy perihilar pulmonary markings suggestive of venous congestion and acute pulmonary edema are seen only with more severe degrees of heart failure. Cardiac enlargement is often noted as an unexpected finding on a chest roentgenogram performed to evaluate for a possible pulmonary infection, bronchiolitis, or asthma.

Chamber hypertrophy noted by electrocardiography may be helpful in assessing the cause of heart failure but does not establish the diagnosis. In cardiomyopathies, left or right ventricular ischemic changes may correlate with other noninvasive parameters of ventricular function. Low-voltage QRS morphologic characteristics with ST-T–wave abnormalities may also suggest myocardial inflammatory disease, but

can be seen with pericarditis as well. The electrocardiogram is the best tool for evaluating rhythm disorders as a potential cause of heart failure, especially tachyarrhythmias.

Echocardiography is the standard technique for assessing ventricular function. The most commonly used parameter in children is fractional shortening (a single dimensional variable), determined as the difference between end-systolic and end-diastolic diameter divided by end-diastolic diameter. Normal fractional shortening is between approximately 28% and 42%. In adults, the most commonly used parameter is ejection fraction (which uses 2-dimensional data to calculate a 3-dimensional volume) and the normal range is 55-65%. In children with right ventricular enlargement or other cardiac pathology resulting in flattening of the interventricular septum, ejection fraction is used because fractional shortening measured in the standard echocardiographic short-axis view will not be accurate. Doppler studies can also be used to estimate cardiac output. Doppler assessment of transmitral flow can also be used as a noninvasive assessment of diastolic function. Doppler tissue imaging can assess not only cardiac function, but wall motion abnormalities that can interfere with normal synchronous cardiac contraction. Magnetic resonance angiography is also very useful in quantifying left and right ventricular function, volume and mass as well as coronary artery anatomy. If valvar regurgitation is present, magnetic resonance angiography can quantify the regurgitant fraction.

Arterial oxygen levels may be decreased when ventilation–perfusion inequalities occurs secondary to pulmonary edema. When heart failure is severe, respiratory or metabolic acidosis, or both, may be present. Infants with heart failure often display hyponatremia as a result of renal water retention. Chronic diuretic treatment can decrease serum sodium levels further. **Serum B-type natriuretic peptide,** a cardiac neurohormone released in response to increased ventricular wall tension, is elevated in adult patients with congestive heart failure. In children, B-type natriuretic peptide may be elevated in patients with heart failure as a result of systolic dysfunction (cardiomyopathy), as well as in children with volume overload (left-to-right shunts such as ventricular septal defect).

TREATMENT

The underlying cause of cardiac failure must be removed or alleviated if possible. If the cause is a congenital cardiac anomaly amenable to surgery, medical treatment of the heart failure is indicated to prepare the patient for surgery. With today's excellent outcomes of primary surgical repair of congenital heart defects, even in the neonatal period, few children require aggressive heart failure management to "grow big enough for surgery." In contrast, if the cause of heart failure is cardiomyopathy, medical management provides temporary relief from symptoms and may allow the patient to recover if the insult is reversible (e.g., myocarditis). If the lesion is not reversible, heart failure management usually allows the child to return to normal activities for some period and delay, sometimes for months or years, the need for heart transplantation.

General Measures

Strict bed rest is rarely necessary except in extreme cases, but it is important that the child be allowed to rest during the day as needed and sleep adequately at night. Some older patients feel better sleeping in a semi-upright position, using several pillows (orthopnea). For infants with heart failure, an infant chair may be advisable. After patients begin to respond to treatment, restrictions on activities can often be modified within the context of the specific diagnosis and the patient's ability. Formal cardiopulmonary exercise testing can be used to assess the patient's ability to perform exercise in a controlled environment and is useful for recommending rational exercise restrictions. For patients with pulmonary edema, positive pressure ventilation may be required along with other drug therapy. For those in low-output heart failure, positive pressure ventilation can significantly reduce total body oxygen consumption by eliminating the work of breathing, and help to reverse metabolic acidosis. β-Adrenergic agonists such as dopamine, dobutamine, and epinephrine are usually used in combination with phosphodiesterase inhibitors such as milrinone. If the blood pressure will allow, afterload-reducing agents (nitroprusside, angiotensin-converting enzyme inhibitors [ACEIs] or angiotensin receptor blockers [ARBs]) may be beneficial. These agents are initiated in an intensive care setting with proper invasive monitoring of central venous and arterial blood pressure.

Diet

Infants with heart failure usually fail to thrive because of a combination of increased metabolic demands and decreased caloric intake. Increasing daily calories is an important aspect of their management. Increasing the number of calories per ounce of infant formula (or supplementing breastfeeding) may be beneficial. Many infants do not tolerate an increase beyond 24 calories/oz because of diarrhea or because these formulas provide too large a solute load for compromised kidneys.

Severely ill infants and children may lack sufficient strength for effective sucking because of extreme fatigue, rapid respirations, and generalized weakness. In these circumstances, nasogastric feedings may be helpful. In many patients with cardiac enlargement, gastroesophageal reflux is a major problem. The use of continuous drip nasogastric feedings at night, administered by pump, may improve caloric intake while decreasing problems with reflux. Occasionally, especially in infants with heart failure caused by complex congenital heart disease, medical or surgical intervention to correct reflux is necessary (Nissen fundoplication). Continued malnutrition may be an important factor in the decision to undertake earlier surgical intervention in patients who have an operable congenital heart lesion or for listing for transplantation in patients with cardiomyopathy.

The use of low-sodium formulas in the routine management of infants with heart failure is not recommended because these preparations are often poorly tolerated and may exacerbate diuretic-induced hyponatremia. Human breast milk is the ideal low-sodium nutritional source. The use of more potent diuretic agents allows more palatable standard formulas to be used for nutrition while controlling salt and water balance by chronic diuretic administration. Most older children can be managed with "no added salt" diets and abstinence from foods containing large amounts of sodium. A strict, extremely-low-sodium diet is rarely required, and rarely adhered to.

Diuretics

These agents interfere with reabsorption of water and sodium by the kidneys, which results in a reduction in circulating blood volume and thereby reduces pulmonary fluid overload and ventricular filling pressure. Diuretics are usually the first mode of therapy initiated in patients with congestive heart failure.

Furosemide is the most commonly used diuretic in pediatric patients with heart failure. It inhibits the reabsorption of sodium and chloride in the distal tubules and the loop of Henle. Patients requiring acute diuresis should be given intravenous or intramuscular furosemide at an initial dose of 1-2 mg/kg, which usually results in rapid diuresis and prompt improvement in clinical status, particularly if symptoms of pulmonary congestion are present. Chronic furosemide therapy is then prescribed at a dose of 1-4 mg/kg/24 hr given between 1 and 4 times a day. Careful monitoring of electrolytes is necessary with long-term furosemide therapy because of the potential for significant loss of potassium. Potassium chloride supplementation is usually required unless the potassium-sparing diuretic spironolactone is given concomitantly. Chronic administration of furosemide may cause contraction of the extracellular fluid compartment and result in "contraction alkalosis" (see Chapter 55.7). Diuretic-induced hyponatremia may become difficult to manage in patients with severe heart failure.

Spironolactone is an inhibitor of aldosterone and enhances potassium retention, often eliminating the need for oral potassium supplementation, which is frequently poorly tolerated. This drug is usually given orally in 2 divided doses of 2 mg/kg/24 hr. Combinations of spironolactone and chlorothiazide are sometimes used for convenience. Adults with heart failure have improved survival when an aldosterone inhibitor is included in the diuretic regimen.

Chlorothiazide is also used for diuresis in children with heart failure. It is less immediate in action and less potent than furosemide, and it affects the reabsorption of electrolytes in the renal tubules only. The usual dose is 10-40 mg/kg/24 hr in 2 divided doses. Potassium supplementation is often required if this agent is used alone.

Afterload Reducers, Including Angiotensin-Converting Enzyme Inhibitors and Angiotensin II Receptor Blockers

These 2 groups of drugs reduce ventricular afterload by decreasing peripheral vascular resistance and thereby improving myocardial performance. Some of these agents also decrease systemic venous tone, which significantly reduces preload. Afterload reducers are especially useful in children with heart failure secondary to cardiomyopathy and in patients with severe mitral or aortic insufficiency. They may also be effective in patients with heart failure caused by left-to-right shunts. They are not generally used in the presence of stenotic lesions of the left ventricular outflow tract because of concern over coronary perfusion. ACEIs and ARBs may have additional beneficial effects on cardiac remodeling independent of their influence on afterload by directly influencing cardiac intracellular signaling pathways. In adult patients with dilated cardiomyopathy, the addition of an ACEI to standard medical therapy reduces both morbidity and mortality. Afterload-reducing agents are most often used in conjunction with other anticongestive drugs such as diuretics and, in some patients, digoxin.

Intravenously administered agents such as nitroprusside should be administered only in an intensive care setting and for as short a time as possible. Nitroprusside's short intravenous half-life makes it ideal for titrating the dose in critically ill patients. Peripheral arterial vasodilation and afterload reduction are the major effects, but venodilation causing a decrease in venous return to the heart may also be beneficial. Blood pressure must be continuously monitored because sudden hypotension can occur. Consequently, nitroprusside is contraindicated in patients with preexisting hypotension. As the drug is metabolized, small amounts of circulating cyanide are produced and detoxified in the liver to thiocyanate, which is excreted in urine. When high doses of nitroprusside are administered for several days, toxic symptoms related to thiocyanate poisoning may occur (fatigue, nausea, disorientation, acidosis, and muscular spasm). If nitroprusside use is prolonged, blood thiocyanate levels should be monitored. Phosphodiesterase inhibitors (see later) are also excellent, although somewhat less-potent afterload-reducing agents, without the toxicity of nitroprusside.

The orally active ACEIs captopril and enalapril produce arterial dilation by blocking the production of angiotensin II, thereby resulting in significant afterload reduction. Venodilation and consequent preload reduction also have been reported. In addition, these agents interfere with aldosterone production and therefore also help control salt and water retention. ACEIs have additional beneficial effects on cardiac structure and function that may be independent of their effect on afterload. The oral dose for captopril is 0.3-6 mg/kg/24 hr given in 3 divided doses; for enalapril the oral dose is 0.05-0.5 mg/kg/24 hr given in 1 or 2 daily doses. Adverse reactions to ACEIs include hypotension and its sequelae (weakness, dizziness, syncope) and hyperkalemia. A maculopapular pruritic rash is encountered in a small number of patients, but the drug may be continued because the rash often disappears spontaneously with time. Neutropenia, renal toxicity, and chronic cough also occur.

Digitalis Glycosides

Digoxin, once the mainstay of heart failure management in both children and adults, is currently used less frequently, as a result of the introduction of newer therapies and the recognition of its potential toxicities. Many cardiologists will use digitalis as an adjunct to ACEIs and diuretics in patients with symptomatic heart failure, whereas others have moved away from its use altogether. Despite multiple clinical studies, predominantly in adults, the controversy over digitalis remains.

Digoxin is the digitalis glycoside used most often in pediatric patients. It has a half-life of 36 hr and it is absorbed well by the gastrointestinal tract (60-85%), even in infants. An initial effect can be seen as early as 30 min after administration, and the peak effect for oral digoxin occurs at ≈2-6 hr. When the drug is administered intravenously, the initial effect is seen in 15-30 min, and the peak effect occurs at 1-4 hr. The kidney eliminates digoxin, so dosing must be adjusted according to the patient's renal function. The half-life of digoxin may be up to 6 days in patients with anuria because slower hepatic excretion pathways are used in these patients.

Rapid digitalization of infants and children in heart failure may be carried out intravenously. The dose depends on the patient's age (Table 442-2). The recommended digitalization schedule is to give half the total digitalizing dose immediately and the succeeding 2 one-quarter doses at 12-hr intervals later. The electrocardiogram must be closely monitored and rhythm strips obtained before each of the 3 digitalizing doses. Digoxin should be discontinued if a new rhythm disturbance is noted. Prolongation of the P-R interval is not necessarily an indication to withhold digitalis, but a delay in administering the next dose or a reduction in the dosage should be considered, depending on the patient's clinical status. Minor ST segment or T-wave changes are commonly noted with digitalis administration and should not affect the digitalization regimen. Baseline serum electrolyte levels should be measured before and after digitalization. Hypokalemia and hypercalcemia exacerbate digitalis toxicity. Because hypokalemia is relatively common in patients receiving diuretics, potassium levels should be monitored closely in those receiving a potassium-wasting diuretic in combination with digitalis. In patients with active myocarditis, some cardiologists recommend avoiding digitalis altogether and if used, maintenance digitalis should be started at half the normal dose without digitalization due to the increased risk of arrhythmia in these patients.

Patients who are not critically ill may be given digitalis initially by the oral route, and in most instances digitalization is completed within 24 hr. When slow digitalization is desirable, for example, in the

Table 442-2	Dosage of Drugs Commonly Used for the Treatment of Congestive Heart Failure
DRUG	**DOSAGE**
DIGOXIN	
Digitalization (½ initially, followed by ¼ q12h × 2)	Premature: 20 µg/kg Full-term neonate (up to 1 mo): 20-30 µg/kg Infant or child: 25-40 µg/kg Adolescent or adult: 0.5-1 mg in divided doses NOTE: These doses are PO; IV dose is 75% of PO dose
Maintenance digoxin	5-10 µg/kg/day, divided q12h Trough serum level: 1.5-3.0 ng/mL <6 mo old; 1-2 ng/mL >6 mo old NOTE: These doses are PO; IV dose is 75% of PO dose
DIURETICS	
Furosemide (Lasix)	IV: 0.5-2 mg/kg/dose PO: 1-4 mg/kg/day, divided qd-qid
Bumetanide (Bumex)	IV: 0.01-0.1 mg/kg/dose PO: 0.01-0.1 mg/kg/day q24-48h
Chlorothiazide (Diuril)	PO: 20-40 mg/kg/day, divided bid or tid
Spironolactone (Aldactone)	PO: 1-3 mg/kg/day, divided bid or tid
Nesiritide (B-type natriuretic peptide)	IV: 0.001-0.03 µg/kg/min
ADRENERGIC AGONISTS (ALL IV)	
Dobutamine	2-20 µg/kg/min
Dopamine	2-30 µg/kg/min
Isoproterenol	0.01-0.5 µg/kg/min
Epinephrine	0.1-1.0 µg/kg/min
Norepinephrine	0.1-2.0 µg/kg/min
PHOSPHODIESTERASE INHIBITORS (ALL IV)	
Milrinone	0.25-1.0 µg/kg/min
AFTERLOAD-REDUCING AGENTS	
Captopril (Capoten), all PO	Prematures: start at 0.01 mg/kg/dose; 0.1-0.4 mg/kg/day, divided q6-24h Infants: 1.5-6 mg/kg/day, divided q6-12h Children: 2.5-6 mg/kg/day, divided q6-12h
Enalapril (Vasotec), all PO	0.08-0.5 mg/kg/day, divided q12-24h
Hydralazine (Apresoline)	IV: 0.1-0.5 mg/kg/dose (maximum: 20 mg) PO: 0.75-5 mg/kg/day, divided q6-12h
Nitroglycerin	IV: 0.25-0.5 µg/kg/min start; increase to 20 µg/kg/min maximum
Nitroprusside (Nipride)	IV: 0.5-8 µg/kg/min
β-ADRENERGIC BLOCKERS	
Carvedilol (Coreg)	PO: initial dose 0.1 mg/kg/day (maximum: 6.25 mg) divided bid, increase gradually (usually 2 wk intervals) to maximum of 0.5-1 mg/kg/day over 8-12 wk as tolerated; adult maximal dose: 50-100 mg/day
Metoprolol (Lopressor, Toprol-XL)	PO, nonextended release form: 0.2 mg/kg/day divided bid, increase gradually (usually 2 wk intervals) to maximum dose of 1-2 mg/kg/day PO, extended release form (Toprol-XL) is given once daily; adult initial dose 25 mg/day, maximum dose is 200 mg/day

Note: Pediatric doses based on weight should not exceed adult doses. Because recommendations may change, these doses should always be double-checked. Doses may also need to be modified in any patient with renal or hepatic dysfunction.

Maintenance digitalis therapy is started ≈12 hr after full digitalization. The daily dosage, one quarter of the total digitalizing dose, is divided in 2 and given at 12-hr intervals. The oral maintenance dose is usually 20-25% higher than when digoxin is used parenterally (see Table 442-2). The normal daily dose of digoxin for older children (>5 yr of age) calculated by body weight should not exceed the usual adult dose of 0.125-0.5 mg/24 hr.

immediate postoperative period, initiation of a maintenance digoxin schedule without a previous loading dose achieves full digitalization in 7-10 days.

Measurement of **serum digoxin levels** is useful under several circumstances: (1) when an unknown amount of digoxin has been administered or ingested accidentally, (2) when renal function is impaired or if drug interactions are possible, (3) when questions regarding compliance are raised, and (4) when a toxic response is suspected. Therapeutic trough blood levels are usually 2-4 ng/mL in infants and 1-2 ng/mL in older children. Exceeding these levels does not generally add significantly to the management of heart failure and only increases the risk of toxicity. In suspected toxicity, elevated serum digoxin levels are not in themselves diagnostic of toxicity but must be interpreted as an adjunct to other clinical and electrocardiographic findings (rhythm and conduction disturbances). Hypokalemia, hypomagnesemia, hypercalcemia, cardiac inflammation secondary to myocarditis, and prematurity may all potentiate digitalis toxicity. A cardiac arrhythmia that develops in a child who is taking digitalis may also be related to the primary cardiac disease rather than the drug, however, any arrhythmia occurring after the institution of digitalis therapy must be considered to be drug related until proven otherwise. There are many drugs that interact with digoxin and may increase levels or risk of toxicity, so care should be taken when a patient on digoxin is being considered for additional pharmacologic therapy of any kind.

α- and β-Adrenergic Agonists

These drugs are usually administered in an intensive care setting, where the dose can be carefully titrated to hemodynamic response. Continuous determinations of arterial blood pressure and heart rate are performed; measuring serial mixed venous oxygen saturations or cardiac output directly with a pulmonary thermodilution (Swan-Ganz) catheter may be helpful in assessing drug efficacy, although this technique is much less commonly used in children compared to adults. Though extremely efficacious in the acute intensive care setting, long-term administration of adrenergic agonists has been shown to increase morbidity and mortality in adults with heart failure and is usually avoided unless the patient is totally dependent on these agents.

Dopamine is a predominantly β-adrenergic receptor agonist, but it has α-adrenergic effects at higher doses. Dopamine has less chronotropic and arrhythmogenic effect than the pure β-agonist isoproterenol does. In addition, it results in selective renal vasodilation because of its interaction with renal dopamine receptors, which is particularly useful in patients with the compromised kidney function that is often associated with low cardiac output, although some recent studies in adults question the efficacy of dopamine for this indication. At a dose of 2-10 μg/kg/min, dopamine results in increased contractility with little peripheral vasoconstrictive effect. If the dose is increased beyond 15 μg/kg/min, however, its peripheral α-adrenergic effects may result in vasoconstriction. Fenoldopam is a dopamine DA1 receptor agonist and is used at a low dose (0.03 μg/kg/min) to increase renal blood flow and urine output. It can cause hypotension, so blood pressure should be carefully monitored.

Dobutamine, a derivative of dopamine, is also useful in treating low cardiac output. It has direct inotropic effects and causes a moderate reduction in peripheral vascular resistance. Dobutamine can be used alone or as an adjunct to dopamine therapy to avoid the vasoconstrictive effects of higher-dose dopamine. Dobutamine is also less likely to cause cardiac rhythm disturbances than isoproterenol is. The usual dose is 2-20 μg/kg/min.

Isoproterenol is a pure β-adrenergic agonist that has a marked chronotropic effect; it is most effective in patients with slow heart rates and is less commonly used in patients with heart failure and normal or increased heart rates, because of the increased risk of arrhythmias.

Epinephrine is a mixed α- and β-adrenergic receptor agonist that is usually reserved for patients with cardiogenic shock and low arterial blood pressure. Although epinephrine can raise blood pressure effectively, it also increases systemic vascular resistance, and therefore increases the afterload against which the heart has to work and is associated with an increased risk of arrhythmia.

Phosphodiesterase Inhibitors

Milrinone is useful in treating patients with low cardiac output who are refractory to standard therapy and has been shown to be highly effective in managing the low-output state present in children after open heart surgery. It works by inhibition of phosphodiesterase, which prevents the degradation of intracellular cyclic adenosine monophosphate. Milrinone has both positive inotropic effects on the heart and peripheral vasodilatory effects and has generally been used as an adjunct to dopamine or dobutamine therapy in the intensive care unit. It is given by intravenous infusion at 0.25-1 μg/kg/min, sometimes with an initial loading dose of 50 μg/kg. A major side effect is hypotension secondary to peripheral vasodilation, especially when a loading dose is used. The hypotension can generally be managed by the administration of intravenous fluids to restore adequate intravascular volume.

Chronic Treatment with β-Blockers

Studies in adults with dilated cardiomyopathy show that β-adrenergic blocking agents, introduced gradually as part of a comprehensive heart failure treatment program, improve exercise tolerance, decrease hospitalizations, and reduce overall mortality. The agents most often used are carvedilol, an agent with both α- and β-adrenergic receptor blocking as well as free radical scavenging effects and metoprolol, a β1-adrenergic receptor selective antagonist. β-Blockers are used for the chronic treatment of patients with heart failure and should not be administered when patients are still in the acute phase of heart failure (i.e., receiving intravenous adrenergic agonist infusions). Although very efficacious in adults, clinical studies in children have shown mixed results, potentially due to the significant heterogeneity of the populations being studied and differences in the types of β-blocking agents.

ELECTROPHYSIOLOGIC APPROACHES TO HEART FAILURE MANAGEMENT

Significant improvements in symptomatology and functional capacity have been achieved in selected adult patients with cardiomyopathy using biventricular resynchronization pacing. This technique improves cardiac output by restoring normal synchrony between right and left ventricular contraction, which is often lost in patients with dilated cardiomyopathy (these patients usually manifest a left bundle branch block on electrocardiogram). There is growing experience with resynchronization pacing in children and reports show early success in patients with left ventricular failure (in the setting of cardiomyopathy), right ventricular failure (in the setting of previously repaired tetralogy of Fallot), and somewhat less so in patients with single ventricular failure (in the setting of complex congenital heart disease).

Arrhythmia is a leading cause of sudden death in patients with severe cardiomyopathy (both dilated and hypertrophic). Although antiarrhythmic medications can sometimes reduce this risk, for patients at particularly high risk (e.g., those with a condition known to be associated with a high risk of ventricular arrhythmia or those who have already experienced a "missed sudden death" episode), use of an implantable cardioverter-defibrillator can be lifesaving (see Chapter 429).

442.1 Cardiogenic Shock

Daniel Bernstein

Cardiogenic shock (see Chapter 70) may occur as a complication of (1) severe cardiac dysfunction before or after cardiac surgery, (2) septicemia, (3) severe burns, (4) anaphylaxis, (5) cardiomyopathy, (6) myocarditis, (7) myocardial infarction or stunning, and (8) acute central nervous system disorders. It is characterized by low cardiac output and hypotension, and therefore results in inadequate tissue perfusion.

Treatment is aimed at reinstitution of adequate cardiac output to prevent the untoward effects of prolonged ischemia on vital organs, as

Table 442-3	Treatment of Cardiogenic Shock*		
	DETERMINANTS OF STROKE VOLUME		
	Preload	**Contractility**	**Afterload**
Parameters measured	CVP, PCWP, LAP, cardiac chamber size on echocardiography	CO, BP, fractional shortening or ejection fraction on echocardiography, MV O₂ saturation	BP, peripheral perfusion, SVR
Treatment to improve cardiac output	Volume expansion (crystalloid, colloid, blood)	β-Adrenergic agonists, phosphodiesterase inhibitors	Afterload-reducing agents: milrinone, nitroprusside, ACE inhibitors

ACE, angiotensin-converting enzyme; BP, blood pressure; CO, cardiac output (measured with a thermodilation catheter); CVP, central venous pressure; LAP, left atrial pressure (measured with an indwelling LA line); MV O₂ saturation, mixed venous oxygen saturation (measured with a central venous catheter); PCWP, pulmonary capillary wedge pressure (measured with a thermodilation catheter); SVR, systemic vascular resistance (calculated from CO and mean BP).

*The goal is to improve peripheral perfusion by increasing cardiac output, where: cardiac output = heart rate × stroke volume.

well as management of the underlying cause. Under normal physiologic conditions, cardiac output is increased as a result of sympathetic stimulation, which increases both contractility and heart rate. If contractility is depressed, cardiac output can be improved by increasing heart rate, increasing ventricular filling pressure (preload) through the Frank-Starling mechanism, or by decreasing systemic vascular resistance (afterload). Optimal filling pressure is variable and depends on a number of extracardiac factors, including ventilatory support and intra-abdominal pressure. The increased pressure necessary to fill a relatively noncompliant ventricle should also be considered, particularly after open heart surgery, or in patients with restrictive or hypertrophic cardiomyopathies. If carefully administered incremental fluid does not result in improved cardiac output, abnormal myocardial contractility or an abnormally high afterload, or both, must be implicated as the cause of the low cardiac output. Although tachycardia is one mechanism to increase cardiac output, an excessive increase in heart rate may reduce cardiac output because of decreased time for diastolic filling.

Myocardial contractility usually improves when treatment of the basic cause of shock is instituted, hypoxia is eliminated, and acidosis is corrected. β-Adrenergic agonists such as dopamine, epinephrine, and dobutamine improve cardiac contractility, increase heart rate, and ultimately increase cardiac output. However, some of these agents also have α-adrenergic effects, which cause peripheral vasoconstriction and increase afterload, so careful consideration of the balance of these effects in an individual patient is important. The use of cardiac glycosides to treat acute low cardiac output states should be avoided.

Patients in cardiogenic shock may have a marked increase in systemic vascular resistance resulting in high afterload and poor peripheral perfusion. If the increased systemic vascular resistance is persistent and the administration of positive inotropic agents alone does not improve tissue perfusion, the use of afterload-reducing agents may be appropriate, for example, nitroprusside or milrinone in combination with a β-adrenergic agonist. Milrinone, which acts through inhibition of phosphodiesterase is also a positive inotropic agent, and combined with a β-adrenergic agonist, works synergistically to increase levels of myocardial cyclic adenosine monophosphate.

Sequential evaluation and management of cardiovascular shock are mandatory (see Chapter 70). Table 442-3 outlines the general treatment principles for acute cardiac circulatory failure under most circumstances. Treatment of infants and children with low cardiac output after cardiac surgery also depends on the nature of the operative procedure, any intraoperative complications, and the physiology of the circulation after repair or palliation (see Chapter 428). If cardiogenic shock does not respond rapidly to medical therapy, consideration of mechanical support is warranted. Modalities available for pediatric patients include extracorporeal membrane oxygenation for short-term support, and left and right ventricular assist devices for longer-term support.

Bibliography is available at Expert Consult.

Chapter **443**
Pediatric Heart and Heart-Lung Transplantation

443.1 Pediatric Heart Transplantation
Daniel Bernstein

Pediatric heart transplantation is standard therapy for children with end-stage cardiomyopathy and other lesions not amenable to surgical repair. As of 2010, >7,500 heart transplants had been performed on children in the United States and Europe, with ≈500 transplants annually; a quarter of these being performed on children <1 yr of age. Survival rates among children compare favorably with those of adults. For children transplanted in the 1980s and early 1990s, 1 yr survival has been 75-80%, whereas for those transplanted after 2000, 1 yr survival is now in the range of 90%; during the same time periods, 5 yr survival has improved from 60-65% to 75% (Fig. 443-1). A growing number of children are now reaching their 15, 20, and 30 yr posttransplant anniversaries.

INDICATIONS
Heart transplantation is performed in infants and children with end-stage cardiomyopathy who have become refractory to medical therapy, in patients with previously repaired or palliated congenital heart disease who have developed ventricular dysfunction or other nonoperable late-term complications, and (less frequently) in patients with complex congenital heart disease (pulmonary atresia with intact septum and coronary arterial stenoses, some forms of hypoplastic left-heart syndrome) for whom standard surgical procedures are extremely high risk. Cardiomyopathies account for >50% of heart transplants in pediatric patients older than 1 yr, with the percentage of patients with previously repaired complex congenital heart lesions at ~30%. In infants younger than 1 yr, congenital heart lesions used to represent >80% of transplants; this fraction has dropped to ~60% as standard surgical results for complex congenital heart disease (hypoplastic left heart syndrome) have improved.

RECIPIENT AND DONOR SELECTION
Potential heart transplant recipients must be free of serious noncardiac medical problems such as neurologic disease, active systemic infection, severe hepatic or renal disease, and severe malnutrition. Many children with ventricular dysfunction are at risk for the development of pulmonary vascular disease, which if severe enough would preclude heart transplantation. Therefore, pulmonary vascular resistance is measured

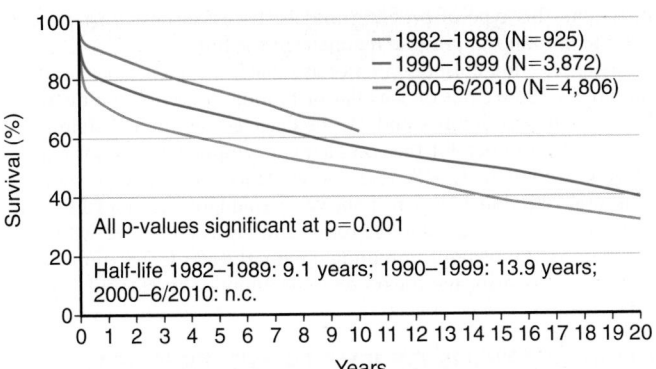

Figure 443-1 Survival after pediatric heart transplantation comparing current and past eras, based on >9,600 patients who received heart transplants in the United States and Europe from 1982 through 2010, as listed with the Registry of the International Society for Heart and Lung Transplantation. Survival has significantly improved over each successive time period. *(From Kirk R, Edwards LB, Kucheryavaya AY, et al. The Registry of the International Society for Heart and Lung Transplantation: thirteenth official pediatric heart transplantation report—2010. J Heart Lung Transplant 29:1119–1128, 2010, Fig. 7.)*

at cardiac catheterization in heart transplant candidates, both at rest and, if elevated, in response to vasodilators. Patients with fixed elevated pulmonary vascular resistance are at higher risk for heart transplantation and may be considered candidates for either heterotopic heart transplantation (see later) or heart-lung transplantation (see Chapter 443.2). However, with recent advances in postoperative management of pulmonary hypertension (e.g., inhaled nitric oxide), many patients with moderate elevations in pulmonary vascular resistance can undergo heart transplant alone. A comprehensive social services evaluation is an important component of the recipient evaluation. Because of the complex posttransplantation medical regimen, the family must have a history of compliance. Detailed informed consent indicating that the family (and if old enough, the patient) understand the lifelong commitment to immunosuppressive medication and careful monitoring, must be obtained.

Donor shortage is a serious problem for both adults and children. At the national registry of transplant recipients in the United States (the United Network for Organ Sharing [UNOS]), allografts are matched by ABO blood group and body weight. HLA matching is not currently performed unless the recipient has preformed antibodies against a particular HLA antigen, in which case a prospective crossmatch can be obtained. ABO matching may not be required for young infants; the exact age under which ABO tolerance develops has not yet been determined. Contraindications to organ donation include prolonged cardiac arrest with persistent moderate to severe cardiac dysfunction, ongoing systemic illness or infection, and preexisting severe cardiac disease. Physicians caring for a patient who may be a potential donor should always contact the organ donor coordinator at their institution, who can best judge the appropriateness of organ donation and has experience in interacting with potential donor families. A history of resuscitation alone or reparable congenital heart disease is not an automatic exclusion for donation.

The decision of when to place a patient on the transplant waiting list is based on a combination of many factors, including poor ventricular function, markedly decreased exercise tolerance as determined by cardiopulmonary exercise testing (see Chapter 423.5), poor response to medical anticongestive therapy, multiple hospitalizations for heart failure, arrhythmia, progressive deterioration in renal or hepatic function, early stages of pulmonary vascular disease, and poor nutritional status. In patients awaiting transplantation, those with poor left ventricular function are usually started on a regimen of anticoagulation to reduce the risk of mural thrombosis and thromboembolism. Patients with low cardiac output resulting in decreases in end-organ (renal or hepatic) function unresponsive to standard pharmacologic treatment,

or those that require chronic assisted ventilation or high-dose inotropic agents are now considered candidates for placement of left ventricular or biventricular assist devices, which can stabilize hemodynamics, improve renal and hepatic function, allow for extubation, and serve as a bridge to transplantation (see Chapter 442). The more recent availability of ventricular assist devices (e.g., the Berlin Heart EXCOR) that are small enough to support young infants has revolutionized the approach to supporting pediatric patients awaiting cardiac transplantation. The role of extracorporeal membrane oxygenation (ECMO) for these patients has been reduced; the need for ECMO support is still a risk factor for poorer outcomes after transplant. There is now limited but growing experience with totally implantable artificial heart devices in older children and adolescents, used either as a bridge to transplant, or in cases (e.g., children with peripheral muscular disorders) where transplantation would be a much higher risk.

PERIOPERATIVE MANAGEMENT

In the classic operation, both donor and recipient hearts were excised so that the posterior portions of the atria containing the venae cavae and pulmonary veins are left intact. The aorta and pulmonary artery are divided above the level of the semilunar valves. The anterior portion of the donor's atria was then connected to the remaining posterior portion of the recipient's atria, thereby avoiding the need for delicate suturing of the venae cavae or pulmonary veins. The donor and recipient great vessels were connected via end-to-end anastomoses. This has largely been supplanted by the bicaval anastomosis, with the donor right atrium (and sinus node) left intact and the suture lines at the superior and inferior vena cavae; the left atrial connection is still performed as in the classic procedure. **Heterotopic heart transplantation** has been used occasionally for patients with left ventricular cardiomyopathy and elevated pulmonary vascular resistance. In this operation, the donor and recipient hearts are connected in parallel so that the recipient right ventricle (which has hypertrophied over time as a result of the elevated pulmonary pressures) pumps mostly to the lungs, and the donor left ventricle pumps mostly to the body. This operation may be preferable to heart-lung transplant for appropriate candidates (patients with pulmonary hypertension but without parenchymal lung disease, without evidence of right ventricular failure, and without serious congenital heart disease), as it is associated with a greater survival at all posttransplant time points.

In the immediate postoperative period, **immunosuppression** is achieved with either a triple- or double-drug regimen, with more centers adopting a minimal steroid or steroid-free regimen. The most common combinations are a calcineurin inhibitor (either cyclosporine or tacrolimus) plus a white blood cell enzyme inhibitor (mycophenolate mofetil or azathioprine), plus or minus prednisone. In many centers, induction therapy (usually an antilymphocyte preparation) is added in the 1st wk, either antithymocyte globulin (ATG) or the humanized anti–interleukin 2 receptor antibodies (basiliximab). In children who do not experience significant graft rejection, steroids can be gradually eliminated after the 1st 6-12 mo. Some centers do not use steroids as part of maintenance immunosuppression, but do use them as bolus treatment for acute rejection episodes.

Most pediatric heart transplant recipients can be extubated within the 1st 48 hr after transplantation and are out of bed within 3-4 days. These patients are often discharged within the 1st 2 wk after transplantation. In patients with preexisting high-risk factors, postoperative recovery may be considerably prolonged. For those with preoperative pulmonary hypertension, the use of nitric oxide in the postoperative period can buy time to allow the donor right ventricle to hypertrophy in response to elevated pulmonary artery pressures. Occasionally, these patients will require right ventricular assist device support.

DIAGNOSIS AND MANAGEMENT OF ACUTE GRAFT REJECTION

Posttransplantation management consists of adjusting medications to maintain a balance between the risk of rejection and the side effects of over-immunosuppression. Along with infection, acute graft rejection is a leading cause of death in pediatric heart transplant recipients. The incidence of acute rejection is greatest in the 1st 3 mo after transplantation and decreases considerably thereafter. Many pediatric patients experience at least 1 episode of acute rejection in the 1st 2 yr after transplantation, although modern immunosuppressive regimens have decreased the frequency of serious rejection episodes. Because the symptoms of rejection can mimic many routine pediatric illnesses (pneumonia, gastroenteritis), *it is mandatory that the transplant center be notified whenever a heart transplant recipient is seen in the pediatrician's office or emergency room for any acute illness.*

Clinical manifestations of **acute rejection** may include fatigue, fluid retention, fever, diaphoresis, abdominal symptoms, and a gallop rhythm. The electrocardiogram may show reduced voltage, atrial or ventricular arrhythmias, or heart block but is usually nondiagnostic. Roentgenographic examination may show an enlarged heart, effusions, or pulmonary edema, but usually only in the more advanced stages of rejection. Most rejection episodes occur without any detectable clinical symptoms. On echocardiography, indices of systolic left ventricular function may be decreased; however, these usually do not deteriorate until rejection is at least moderately severe. Techniques to evaluate wall thickening and left ventricular diastolic function have not fulfilled their promise as predictors of early rejection. Most transplant centers do not rely on echocardiography alone for rejection surveillance.

Myocardial biopsy is the most reliable method of monitoring patients for rejection. Biopsy specimens are taken from the right ventricular side of the interventricular septum and can be harvested relatively safely, even in small infants. In older children, myocardial biopsies may be performed as often as every 1-4 wk during the 1st 3-6 mo after transplantation. The frequency is then reduced over the next 2 yr to between 2 and 4 biopsies per year unless the patient has an episode of rejection. In infants, surveillance biopsies are usually performed less often and may be as infrequent as once or twice per year. Children may have clinically unsuspected rejection episodes even 5-10 yr after transplantation; most pediatric transplant centers continue routine surveillance biopsies, albeit at less-frequent intervals (every 6-12 mo).

Criteria for **grading cardiac rejection** are based on a system developed by the International Society for Heart and Lung Transplantation (ISHLT); these criteria take into account the degree of cellular infiltration and whether myocyte necrosis is present. ISHLT rejection grade 1R (former grades 1A, 1B, and 2) is usually mild enough that it is often not treated with bolus steroids, and many of these episodes resolve spontaneously. A repeat biopsy specimen is often obtained within a shorter time frame. For patients with ISHLT grade 2R (formerly grade 3A) rejection, treatment is instituted with either intravenous methylprednisolone or a "bump and taper" of oral prednisone. Asymptomatic patients >3 mo posttransplant and with normal echocardiograms are often treated as outpatients. Patients with grade 3R (formerly grades 3B or 4), or anyone with hemodynamic instability, are admitted to the hospital for intravenous steroid and potentially more aggressive antirejection therapy. For rejection episodes resistant to steroid therapy, additional therapeutic regimens include a repeat course of an antilymphocyte preparation (antithymocyte globulin), methotrexate, or total lymphoid irradiation. Patients with repeated episodes of rejection may also benefit from being switched from cyclosporine to tacrolimus (or vice versa). Refractory rejection is not considered a good indication for retransplantation because of the relatively poor outcomes compared with other indications for retransplantation.

Gene expression profiling of peripheral blood mononuclear cells has been validated in adults as a highly sensitive, and moderately selective, method of rejection surveillance. These results have not been confirmed in children. Other current techniques which may hold promise include the profiling of donor cell free DNA released in the serum of patients during episodes of graft injury. Progress has also been made in genetic profiling as a means to determine which patients are most at risk for rejection. Children who have single-nucleotide polymorphisms leading to greater activity of inflammatory cytokines or decreased activity of regulatory cytokines are at increased risk of

rejection. This type of profiling may be useful in designing patient-specific immunosuppressive regimens in the future.

Some rejection episodes are not associated with a cellular infiltrate on biopsy. These cases of acellular or humoral rejection are mediated by circulating antibodies and can be detected by immunostaining of the biopsy specimen for the complement component C4d, for macrophages expressing CD68, and for evidence of histologic damage. Humoral rejection is less responsive to standard therapies for acute cellular rejection (e.g., bolus steroids) and has been treated with plasmapheresis, intravenous immunoglobulin, the anti-CD20 monoclonal antibody rituximab, and the proteasome inhibitor bortezomib, all with mixed results.

COMPLICATIONS OF IMMUNOSUPPRESSION
Infection
Infection is 1 of the 2 leading causes of death in pediatric transplant patients (Fig. 443-2). The incidence of infection is greatest in the 1st 3 mo after transplantation when immunosuppressive doses are highest. Viral infections are the most common, which accounts for as many as 25% of infectious episodes. Cytomegalovirus (CMV) infection used to be 1 of the leading causes of morbidity and mortality and may occur as a primary infection in patients without previous exposure to the virus or as a reactivation. Severe CMV infection can be disseminated or associated with pneumonitis or gastroenteritis and may provoke an episode of acute graft rejection or graft coronary disease. Most centers use intravenous ganciclovir or CMV immune globulin (CytoGam), or both, as prophylaxis in any patient receiving a heart from a donor who is positive for CMV or in any recipient who has serologic evidence of previous CMV disease. Oral preparations of ganciclovir with improved absorption profiles are available for chronic therapy and have largely replaced intravenous preparations for prophylaxis. These regimens have significantly reduced the burden of CMV disease in heart transplant patients. Polymerase chain reaction enhances the ability to diagnose CMV infection and to monitor the efficacy of therapy serially.

Most normal childhood viral illnesses are well tolerated and do not usually require special treatment. Otitis media and routine upper respiratory tract infections can be treated in the outpatient setting, although fever or symptoms that last beyond the usual course require further investigation. Gastroenteritis, especially with vomiting, can result in markedly reduced absorption of immunosuppressive medications and provoke a rejection episode. In this setting, drug levels should be closely monitored and the use of intravenous medications considered. Gastroenteritis can also be a sign of rejection, so a high index of suspicion must always be maintained. Varicella is another childhood illness of some concern for immunosuppressed patients. If a heart transplant recipient acquires clinical varicella infection, treatment with intravenous acyclovir usually attenuates the illness.

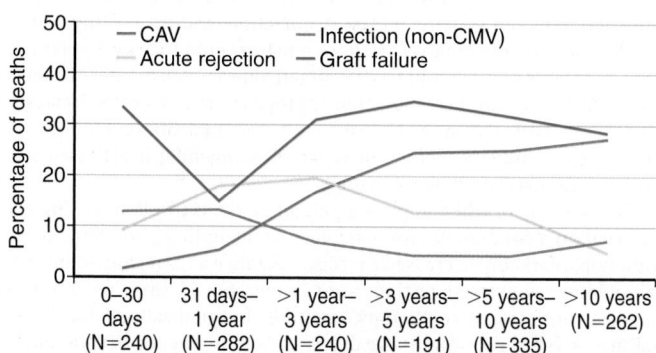

Figure 443-2 Major causes of death after pediatric heart transplantation by time since transplant. CAV, coronary artery vasculopathy; CMV, cytomegalovirus. *(From Kirk R, Edwards LB, Kucheryavaya AY, et al. The Registry of the International Society for Heart and Lung Transplantation: thirteenth official pediatric heart transplantation report—2010. J Heart Lung Transplant 29:1119–1128, 2010, Fig. 9.)*

Bacterial infections are the next most frequent, with the lung being the most common site of infection (35%), followed by the blood, the urinary tract, and, less commonly, the sternotomy site. Other sources of posttransplantation infection include fungi (14%) and protozoa (6%). Many centers use nystatin mouthwash to decrease fungal colonization and trimethoprim/sulfamethoxazole (Bactrim, Septra) during the time a patient is on steroids as prophylaxis to prevent *Pneumocystis carinii* infection.

Growth Retardation
Patients requiring chronic steroid administration usually have decreased linear growth, thus most pediatric transplant programs aim for steroid-free immunosuppression within the 1st yr posttransplant. In those patients who experience rejection when steroids are withdrawn, alternate-day steroid regimens result in improved linear growth. Total lymphoid irradiation has shown promise as a steroid-sparing protocol. Despite these concerns, 75% of long-term survivors of pediatric heart transplantation have normal growth.

Hypertension
Hypertension is common in patients treated with cyclosporine, caused by a combination of plasma volume expansion and defective renal sodium excretion. Corticosteroids usually potentiate cyclosporine-induced hypertension. Patients are typically managed with a combination of a diuretic and a vasodilator. Agents that work via calcium channel blockade have the additional advantage of possibly attenuating graft coronary disease. The incidence of hypertension is slightly lower in patients treated with tacrolimus.

Renal Function
Chronic administration of cyclosporine or tacrolimus can lead to a tubulointerstitial nephropathy in adults, but severe renal dysfunction is less common in children. Most pediatric patients gradually have an increase in serum creatinine in the 1st yr after transplantation; if renal dysfunction occurs, it usually responds to a decrease in calcineurin inhibitor dosage. The addition of sirolimus, a target of rapamycin inhibitor, instead of mycophenolate allows a reduction in the dose of calcineurin inhibitor in patients with renal dysfunction. Infection with BK virus, a growing problem in renal transplant patients, has been described as a source of renal dysfunction in heart transplant patients. Fortunately, pediatric heart transplant patients infrequently require renal transplantation long-term.

Neurologic Complications
Neurologic side effects of cyclosporine and tacrolimus include tremor, myalgias, paresthesias, and, rarely, seizures. These complications can be treated with reduced doses of medication and occasionally with oral magnesium supplementation. Intracranial infections pose a significant risk, especially because some of the more frequent signs (nuchal rigidity) may be absent in immunosuppressed patients. Potential organisms include *Aspergillus*, *Cryptococcus neoformans*, and *Listeria monocytogenes*. A rare form of encephalopathy, known as PRES (posterior reversible encephalopathy syndrome) can occur in patients on calcineurin inhibitors (either cyclosporine or tacrolimus). PRES presents with hypertension, headaches and seizures, requires MRI for diagnosis, and is usually managed by changing calcineurin inhibitor or in rare cases eliminating calcineurin inhibitors totally in favor of other immunosuppressive agents (e.g., sirolimus/mycophenolate).

Tumors
One of the serious complications limiting long-term survival in pediatric heart transplant patients is the risk of neoplastic disease. The most common is posttransplant lymphoproliferative disease (PTLD), a condition associated with Epstein-Barr virus infection. Patients who are Epstein-Barr virus seronegative at the time of transplant (usually infants and young children) are at increased risk of developing PTLD if they subsequently seroconvert, acquiring the virus either from the donor organ or from primary infection (mononucleosis). Unlike true

cancer, many cases of PTLD respond to a reduction in immunosuppression plus antiviral therapy with acyclovir. A monoclonal antibody directed against the CD20 antigen on activated lymphocytes (rituximab) has been effective against some forms of PTLD. However, PTLD can behave more aggressively and many cases eventually require chemotherapy. An increased risk of skin cancer requires that children use appropriate precautions when exposed to sunlight.

Chronic Rejection
Graft coronary artery disease (GCAD) is a manifestation of chronic graft rejection that occurs in ≈20% of children 5 yr after transplant. The cause is still unclear, although it is thought to be a form of immunologically mediated vessel injury (chronic rejection). Hypercholesterolemia and hyperglycemia are thought to increase the risk of this disease. Unlike native coronary atherosclerosis, GCAD is a diffuse process with a high degree of distal vessel involvement. Because the transplanted heart has been denervated, patients may not experience symptoms such as angina pectoris during ischemic episodes, and the initial manifestation may be cardiovascular collapse or sudden death. Most centers perform coronary angiography annually to screen for coronary abnormalities; some also perform coronary intravascular ultrasound on adolescents. Standard coronary artery bypass procedures are usually not helpful because of the diffuse nature of the process, although transcatheter stenting can sometimes be effective for isolated lesions. For severe cases, repeat heart transplantation has been the only effective treatment. Thus, prevention has been the focus of most current research. The cell-cycle inhibitors sirolimus and everolimus have been shown to decrease coronary arterial intimal thickening in adult transplant patients. Other drugs that have been shown to reduce the risk of GCAD include the calcium channel blockers (such as diltiazem) and the cholesterol-lowering HMG-CoA (3-hydroxy-3-methyl-coenzyme A) reductase inhibitors (such as pravastatin or atorvastatin).

Other Complications
Corticosteroids usually result in cushingoid facies, steroid acne, and striae. Cyclosporine can cause a subtle change in facial features such as hypertrichosis and gingival hyperplasia. These cosmetic features can be particularly disturbing to adolescents and may be the motivation for noncompliance, one of the leading risks for late morbidity and mortality. Most of these cosmetic complications are dose related and improve as immunosuppressive medications are weaned. Osteoporosis and aseptic necrosis are additional reasons for reducing the steroid dosage as soon as possible. Diabetes and pancreatitis are rare but serious complications.

Rehabilitation
Despite the potential risks of immunosuppression, the prospect for rehabilitation in pediatric heart transplant recipients is excellent. More than 95% of pediatric heart transplant recipients have no functional limitations in their daily lives. The majority of patients do not require rehospitalization for transplant-related problems.

Pediatric heart transplant recipients can attend daycare or school and participate in non-collision competitive sports (no tackle football or martial arts) and other age-appropriate activities. Standardized measurements of ventricular function are close to normal. Because the transplanted heart is denervated, the increase in heart rate and cardiac output during exercise is slower in transplant recipients, and maximal heart rate and cardiac output responses are mildly attenuated. These subtle abnormalities are rarely noticeable by the patient.

Growth of the transplanted heart is excellent, although a mild degree of ventricular hypertrophy is commonly seen, even years after transplantation. The sites of atrial and great vessel anastomoses usually grow without the development of obstruction. In neonates who undergo transplantation for hypoplastic left heart syndrome, however, juxtaductal aortic coarctation may recur.

As assessed by standardized testing, the psychologic adjustment to heart transplantation in children is usually good. However, a serious problem with noncompliance often occurs once patients reach adolescence, and life-threatening rejection may result. Early intervention by social workers, counselors, and psychologists may be able to reduce this risk.

Bibliography is available at Expert Consult.

443.2 Heart-Lung and Lung Transplantation
Daniel Bernstein

More than 670 heart-lung and 1,700 lung (single or double) transplants have been performed in children in the United States and Europe, with ≈140 procedures performed annually. Primary indications for heart-lung transplantation include cystic fibrosis, primary pulmonary hypertension, complex congenital heart disease with pulmonary hypoplasia or Eisenmenger syndrome, congenital lung abnormalities, and end-stage parenchymal lung disease (bronchopulmonary dysplasia, chronic lung disease, and interstitial fibrosis). Many of these patients with normal hearts are candidates for single- or double-lung transplantation if right ventricular function is preserved and there has been a trend towards decreasing combined heart-lung transplant for this reason. In some patients with Eisenmenger physiology, double-lung transplantation can be performed in combination with repair of intracardiac defects. Patients with cystic fibrosis are not candidates for single-lung grafts because of the risk of infection from the diseased contralateral lung. Patients are selected according to many of the same criteria as for heart transplant recipients (see Chapter 443.1).

Posttransplant immunosuppression is usually achieved with a triple-drug regimen, combining a calcineurin inhibitor (cyclosporine or tacrolimus) with a white blood cell enzyme inhibitor (mycophenolate or azathioprine) and prednisone. Most patients receive induction therapy with an antithymocyte or anti-T cell preparation. Unlike patients with isolated heart transplants, patients with heart or heart-lung transplants cannot be weaned totally off steroids. Prophylaxis against *P. carinii* infection is achieved with trimethoprim-sulfamethoxazole or aerosolized pentamidine. Ganciclovir and CMV immune globulin prophylaxis are used as in heart transplant recipients (see Chapter 443.1).

Pulmonary rejection is common in lung or heart-lung transplant recipients, whereas heart rejection is encountered much less often than in patients with isolated heart transplants. Symptoms of lung rejection may include fever and fatigue, although many episodes are minimally symptomatic. Surveillance for rejection is performed by monitoring pulmonary function (forced vital capacity; forced expiratory volume in 1 sec [FEV_1]; forced expiratory flow, midexpiratory phase [$FEF_{25-75\%}$]), systemic arterial oxygen tension, and chest roentgenograms and by transbronchial biopsy.

Actuarial survival rates after lung or heart-lung or lung transplantation in children are currently 75% at 1 yr and 50% at 5 yr; improved patient selection and postoperative management are continually improving these survival statistics from prior eras. Graft failure and infection are the leading cause of early death, whereas a form of chronic rejection known as **bronchiolitis obliterans** accounts for nearly 50% of late mortality. Other causes of early morbidity and mortality include tracheal complications, pulmonary venous obstruction, donor lung dysfunction, bleeding, and acute rejection. Additional late complications include the development of airway stenosis, late graft failure, PTLD, and other side effects of chronic immunosuppression.

Postoperative indices of cardiopulmonary function and exercise capacity show significant improvement. Nearly 90% of patients are without activity limitations at 3 yr follow-up and more than 80% at 5 yr follow-up. Problems of donor availability are even more severe with lung transplantation than with isolated heart transplantation. Living related lung transplantation, in which a lobe from a parent is transplanted into a child, has been used to partially alleviate this problem.

Bibliography is available at Expert Consult.

Section 8
Diseases of the Peripheral Vascular System

Chapter 444
Diseases of the Blood Vessels (Aneurysms and Fistulas)

444.1 Kawasaki Disease
Daniel Bernstein

See also Chapter 166.

Aneurysms of the coronary and occasionally the systemic arteries may complicate Kawasaki disease and are the leading cause of morbidity in this disease (Figs. 444-1 and 444-2). Other than in Kawasaki disease, aneurysms are not common in children and occur most frequently in the aorta in association with coarctation of the aorta, patent ductus arteriosus, Ehlers-Danlos type IV (arterial ecchymotic form), hyperimmunoglobulin E syndrome, and Marfan syndrome and in intracranial vessels (see Chapter 601). They may also occur secondary to an infected embolus; infection contiguous to a blood vessel; trauma; congenital abnormalities of vessel structure, especially the medial wall; and arteritis, for example, polyarteritis nodosa, Behçet syndrome, and Takayasu arteritis (see Chapter 167.2).

444.2 Arteriovenous Fistulas
Daniel Bernstein

Arteriovenous fistulas may be limited and small or may be extensive producing systemic complications (see Chapters 505 and 650). The most common sites in infants and children are within the cranium, in the liver, in the lung, in the extremities, and in vessels in or near the thoracic wall. These fistulas, though usually congenital, may follow trauma or be a manifestation of hereditary hemorrhagic telangiectasia (Osler-Weber-Rendu disease). Femoral arteriovenous fistulas are a rare complication of percutaneous femoral catheterization.

CLINICAL MANIFESTATIONS
Clinical symptoms occur only in association with large arteriovenous communications when arterial blood flows into a low-pressure venous system without the resistance of the capillary bed; local venous pressure is increased, and arterial flow distal to the fistula is decreased. Systemic arterial resistance falls because of the runoff of blood through the fistula. Compensatory mechanisms include tachycardia and increased stroke volume so that cardiac output rises. Total blood volume is also increased. In large fistulas, left ventricular dilation, a widened pulse pressure, and high output heart failure occur. CT, MRI, or injection of contrast material into an artery proximal to the fistula confirms the diagnosis.

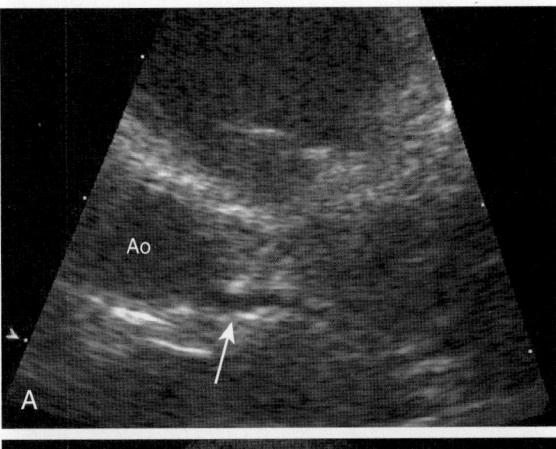

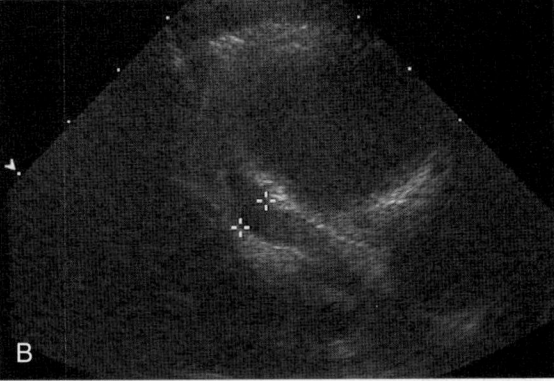

Figure 444-1 Two-dimensional echocardiogram comparing a normal left main coronary artery (*arrow* in **A**) with a giant coronary artery aneurysm (outlined by *cross marks* in **B**) in a patient with Kawasaki disease. Ao, aorta.

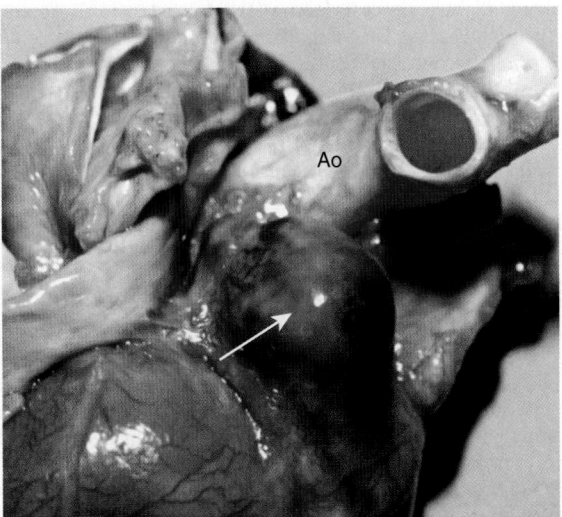

Figure 444-2 Pathologic specimen showing giant aneurysm of left main coronary artery (*arrow*). Ao, ascending aorta.

Large intracranial arteriovenous fistulas most often occur in newborn infants in association with a **vein of Galen malformation.** The large intracranial left-to-right shunt results in heart failure secondary to the demand for high cardiac output. Patients with smaller communications may not have cardiovascular manifestations but may later be disposed to hydrocephalus (see Chapter 591.11) or seizure disorders. The diagnosis can often be made by auscultation of a continuous murmur over the cranium. Older children with more diffuse intracranial arteriovenous malformations may be recognized on the basis of intracranial calcification and high cardiac output without cardiac failure.

Hepatic arteriovenous fistulas may be generalized or localized in the liver and may be hemangioendotheliomas or cavernous hemangiomas. The fistula may be located between the hepatic artery and the ductus venosus or portal vein. Congenital hemorrhagic telangiectasia may also be present. Large arteriovenous fistulas are associated with increased cardiac output and heart failure. Hepatomegaly is usual, and systolic or continuous murmurs may be audible over the liver.

Peripheral arteriovenous fistulas generally involve the extremities and are associated with disfigurement, swelling of the extremity, and visible hemangiomas. Some are located in areas that result in upper airway obstruction. Because only a small minority results in large arterial runoff, cardiac failure is uncommon.

TREATMENT

Medical management of heart failure is initially helpful in neonates with these conditions; with time, the size of the shunt may diminish and symptoms spontaneously regress. Hemangiomas of the liver often eventually disappear completely. Large liver hemangiomas have been treated with steroids, ε-aminocaproic acid, interferon, local compression, embolization, or local irradiation; the beneficial effects of these management options are not firmly established because individual patients display marked variation in clinical course without treatment. Catheter embolization is becoming the treatment of choice for many patients with a symptomatic arteriovenous fistula. Embolic agents that have been used include detachable balloons, steel (Gianturco) coils, and liquid tissue adhesives (cyanoacrylate). Often, multiple procedures are necessary before flow is significantly reduced. Gamma knife radiosurgery has been used successfully in patients with cerebral arteriovenous malformations. Surgical removal of a large fistula may be attempted in patients with severe cardiac failure and lack of improvement with medical treatment. Surgical treatment may be contraindicated or unsuccessful when the lesion is extensive and diffuse or is located in a position where adjoining tissue may be injured during the surgery or related procedures.

444.3 Generalized Arterial Calcification of Infancy/Idiopathic Infantile Arterial Calcification

Robert M. Kliegman

Generalized arterial calcification of infancy (GACI) is a rare and often lethal autosomal recessive disorder characterized by calcification of muscular arteries with fibrotic myointimal proliferation and subsequent vascular stenosis leading to tissue ischemia, poor function or infarction. Diffuse arterial calcification may begin in utero leading to hydrops fetalis; in the neonate diffuse arterial calcification leads to respiratory distress and heart failure or myocardial infarction (coronary, pulmonary arteries), hypertension (renal arteries), and poor femoral pulses (aorta, femoral arteries).

Mutations in the ectonucleotide pyrophosphatase 1gene (*ENPP1*) are noted in 75% of patients. Serum calcium, phosphate and alkaline phosphatase levels are normal and although the vascular calcification may be seen on plain x-rays (Fig. 444-3), ultrasonography (Fig. 444-4), or CT scans may reveal calcifications not visible on plain films.

A subset of patients with GACI have monoallelic or biallelic mutations in the adenosine triphosphate–binding cassette subfamily C number 6 gene (*ABCC6*), which is the gene responsible for pseudoxanthoma elasticum (PXE). PXE, an autosomal recessive disorder, is classically associated with a later onset of ectopic mineralization of elastic fibers in the skin, eyes and arteries. In addition, some surviving infants with *ENPP1* mutation develop PXE symptoms involving skin and retina (angioid streaking).

Infants with GACI have been treated with bisphosphonates with variable success. In addition, some survivors have developed hypophosphatemic rickets.

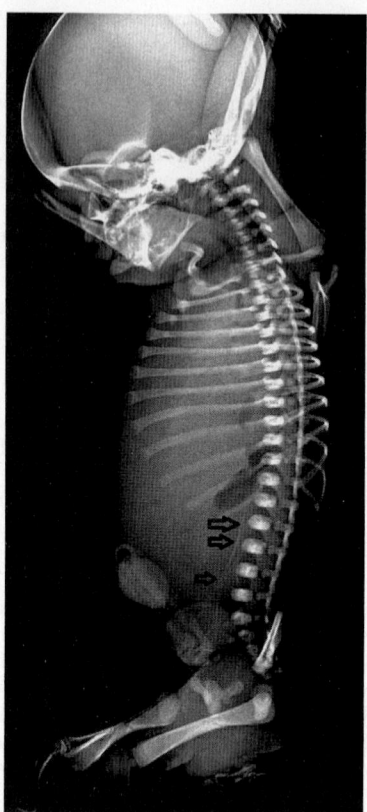

Figure 444-3 Lateral radiograph of the neonate showing calcification of descending aorta and its bifurcation *(arrows)*. *(From Karthikeyan G: Generalized arterial calcification of infancy. J Pediatr 162:1074, 2013, Fig. 3, p. 1074).*

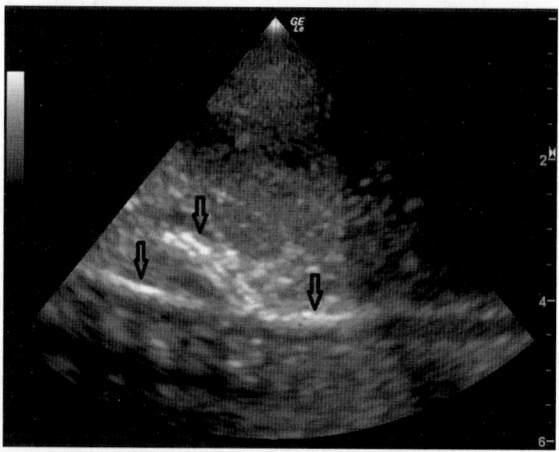

Figure 444-4 Ultrasonography of abdominal aorta showing calcification of descending aorta and its branches *(arrows)*. *(From Karthikeyan G: Generalized arterial calcification of infancy. J Pediatr 162:1074, 2013, Fig. 1, p. 1074).*

444.4 Arterial Calcifications Caused by Deficiency of CD73

Robert M. Kliegman

This rare autosomal recessive disorder, due to mutations in the 5 exonucleotidase CD73 *(NT5E)* results in joint and arterial (lower extremity) calcification in adults. Patients present with intermittent claudication and joint pain. Onset is probably before adulthood, as patients may be undiagnosed with nonspecific findings during adolescence.

Bibliography is available at Expert Consult.

Chapter 445

Systemic Hypertension

Marc B. Lande

Primary (essential) hypertension occurs commonly in adults and, if untreated, is a major risk factor for myocardial infarction, stroke, and renal failure. In adults with hypertension, a 5 mm Hg increase in diastolic blood pressure (BP) increased the risk of coronary artery disease by 20% and the risk of stroke by 35%. Furthermore, hypertension is implicated in the etiology of nearly 50% of adults with end-stage renal disease. The prevalence of adult hypertension increases with age, ranging from 15% in young adults to 60% in individuals older than 65 yr.

Hypertensive children, although usually asymptomatic, already manifest evidence of target organ damage. Up to 40% of hypertensive children have left ventricular hypertrophy and hypertensive children have increased carotid intima–media thickness, a marker of early atherosclerosis. Primary hypertension during childhood often tracks into adulthood. Children with BP >90th percentile have a 2.4-fold greater risk of having hypertension as adults. Similarly, nearly half of hypertensive adults had a BP >90th percentile as children. There is also an association between childhood hypertension and early atherosclerosis in young adulthood.

PREVALENCE OF HYPERTENSION IN CHILDREN

In infants and young children, systemic hypertension is uncommon, with a prevalence of <1%, but when present, it is often indicative of an underlying disease process **(secondary hypertension)**. *Severe and symptomatic hypertension in children is usually caused by secondary hypertension.* In contrast, the prevalence of primary essential hypertension, mostly in older school-age children and adolescents, has increased in prevalence in parallel with the obesity epidemic. School screening studies show that approximately 10% of U.S. youth overall have prehypertension and 2.5% have hypertension. The influence of obesity on elevated BP is evident in children as young as 2-5 yr old. Approximately 20% of American youth are obese, and up to 10% of obese youth have hypertension.

DEFINITION OF HYPERTENSION

The definition of hypertension in adults is BP ≥140/90 mm Hg, regardless of body size, sex, or age. This is a functional definition that relates level of BP elevation with the likelihood of subsequent cardiovascular events. Because hypertension-associated cardiovascular events, such as myocardial infarction or stroke, usually do not occur in childhood, the definition of hypertension in children is statistical rather than functional. The National High Blood Pressure Education Program Working Group on High Blood Pressure in Children and Adolescents published the *Fourth Report on the Diagnosis, Evaluation, and Treatment of High Blood Pressure in Children and Adolescents* (Fourth Report) in 2004. This report established normal values based on the normative distribution of BP in healthy children and included tables with systolic and diastolic values for the 50th, 90th, 95th, and 99th percentile by age, sex, and height percentile. These normative tables can be obtained online at www.nhlbi.nih.gov/guidelines/hypertension/child_tbl.htm. The Fourth Report defined hypertension as average systolic blood pressure (SBP) and/or diastolic BP that is ≥95th percentile for age, sex, and height on ≥3 occasions. **Prehypertension** was defined as average SBP or diastolic BP that are ≥90th percentile but <95th percentile. In adolescents beginning at age 12 yr, prehypertension is defined as BP between 120/80 mm Hg and the 95th percentile. A child with BP levels

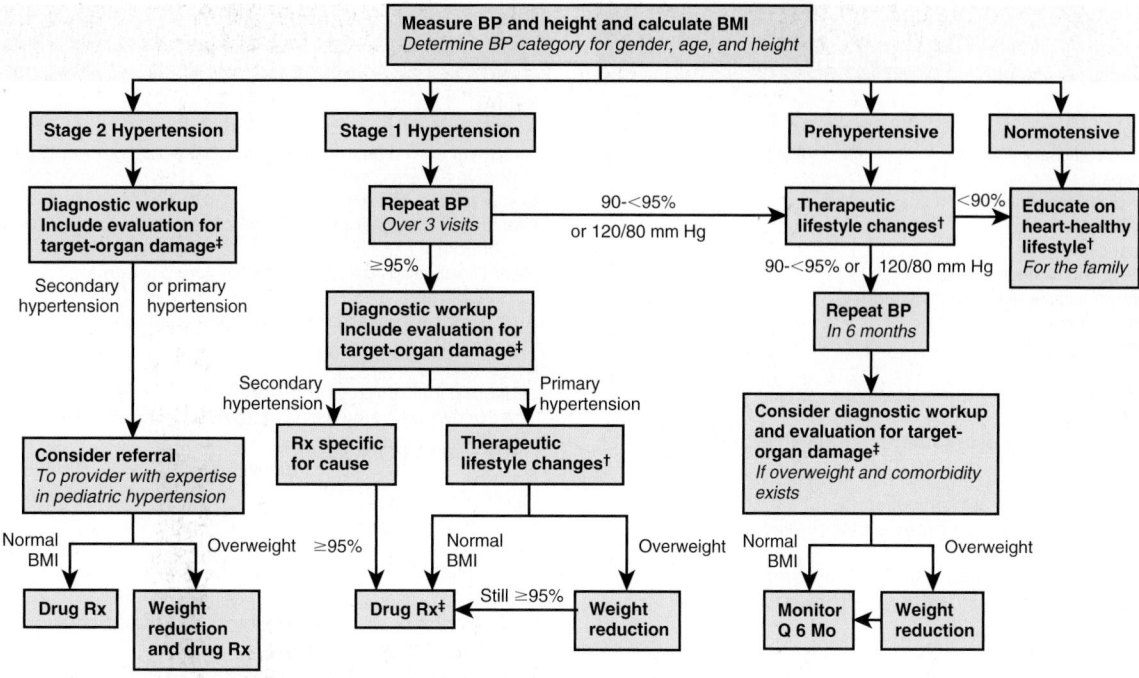

Figure 445-1 Management algorithm. BMI, body mass index; BP, blood pressure; Q, every; Rx, prescription; † diet modification and physical activity; ‡ especially if younger, very high BP, little or no family history, diabetic, or other risk factors. (*From National High Blood Pressure Education Program Working Group on High Blood Pressure in Children and Adolescents. The fourth report on the diagnosis, evaluation, and treatment of high blood pressure in children and adolescents, Pediatrics 114[2 Suppl 4th Report]:571, 2004.*)

≥95th percentile in a medical setting but normal BP outside of the office has **white coat hypertension.**

The Fourth Report further recommended that if BP is ≥95th percentile, then the hypertension should be staged. Children with BP between the 95th and 99th percentile plus 5 mm Hg are categorized as **stage 1 hypertension,** and children with BP above the 99th percentile plus 5 mm Hg have **stage 2 hypertension**. Stage 1 hypertension, if asymptomatic and without target organ damage, allows time for evaluation before starting treatment, whereas stage 2 hypertension calls for more prompt evaluation and pharmacologic therapy (Fig. 445-1).

MEASUREMENT OF BP IN CHILDREN

The Fourth Report and the American Heart Association recommends that children 3 yr or older should have their BP checked during every healthcare episode (the AHA recommends annual BP checks). Selected children <3 yr old should also have their BP checked, including those with a history of prematurity, congenital heart disease, renal disease, solid-organ transplant, cancer, treatment with drugs known to raise BP, other illnesses associated with hypertension (neurofibromatosis, tuberous sclerosis, others), or evidence of increased intracranial pressure. The preferred method is by auscultation and a BP cuff appropriate for the size of the child's arm should be used. Elevated readings should be confirmed on repeat visits before determining that a child is hypertensive. The BP should be measured with the child in the sitting position after a period of quiet for at least 5 min. Careful attention to cuff size is necessary to avoid over diagnosis, as a cuff that is too short or narrow artificially increases BP readings. A wide variety of bladder sizes should be available in any medical office where children are routinely seen. An appropriate sized cuff has an inflatable bladder that is at least 40% of the arm circumference at a point midway along the upper arm. The inflatable bladder should cover at least two thirds of the upper arm length and 80-100% of its circumference.

Systolic pressure is indicated by appearance of the 1st Korotkoff sound. Diastolic pressure has been defined by consensus as the 5th Korotkoff sound. Palpation is useful for rapid assessment of SBP, although the palpated pressure is generally about 10 mm Hg less than that obtained via auscultation. Oscillometric techniques are used frequently in infants and young children, but they are susceptible to artifacts and are best for measuring mean BP.

Ambulatory blood pressure monitoring (ABPM) is a procedure where the child wears a device that records BP frequently, usually every 20-30 min, throughout a 24 hr period while the child goes about usual daily activities, including sleep. This allows calculation of the mean daytime BP, sleep BP, and mean BP over 24 hr. The physician can also determine the proportion of BP measurements that are in the hypertensive range (BP load) and whether there is an appropriate decrease in BP during sleep (nocturnal dip). ABPM is particularly useful in the evaluation for white coat hypertension and may also be useful for determining risk of hypertensive target organ damage, evaluating resistance to pharmacologic therapy, and evaluating patients with hypotensive episodes on antihypertensive medication. ABPM is also useful for certain special populations, such as children with chronic kidney disease, kidney transplant, and diabetes mellitus where it may provide important information on cardiovascular risk that cannot be determined as well by office measurements.

ETIOLOGY AND PATHOPHYSIOLOGY

BP is the product of cardiac output and peripheral vascular resistance. An increase in either cardiac output or peripheral resistance results in an increase in BP; if 1 of these factors increases while the other decreases, BP may not increase. When hypertension is the result of another disease process, it is referred to as secondary hypertension. When no identifiable cause can be found, it is referred to as primary (essential) hypertension. Many factors, including heredity, diet, stress, and obesity, may play a role in the development of primary hypertension. Secondary hypertension is most common in infants and younger children. The younger the child, the higher the BP and the presence of symptoms related to hypertension, the more likely there will be an underlying secondary cause of hypertension. Many childhood diseases can be responsible for chronic hypertension (Table 445-1) or acute/intermittent hypertension (Table 445-2). The most likely cause varies with age. Hypertension in the premature infant is sometimes associated with umbilical artery catheterization and renal artery thrombosis. Hypertension during early childhood may be caused by renal disease,

Table 445-1	Conditions Associated with Chronic Hypertension in Children

RENAL
Chronic pyelonephritis
Chronic glomerulonephritis
Hydronephrosis
Congenital dysplastic kidney
Multicystic kidney
Solitary renal cyst
Vesicoureteral reflux nephropathy
Segmental hypoplasia (Ask-Upmark kidney)
Ureteral obstruction
Renal tumors
Renal trauma
Rejection damage following transplantation
Postirradiation damage
Systemic lupus erythematosus (other connective tissue diseases)

VASCULAR
Coarctation of thoracic or abdominal aorta
Renal artery lesions (stenosis, fibromuscular dysplasia, thrombosis, aneurysm)
Umbilical artery catheterization with thrombus formation
Neurofibromatosis (intrinsic or extrinsic narrowing for vascular lumen)
Renal vein thrombosis
Vasculitis
Arteriovenous shunt
Williams-Beuren syndrome
Moyamoya disease
Takayasu arteritis

ENDOCRINE
Hyperthyroidism
Hyperparathyroidism
Congenital adrenal hyperplasia (11β-hydroxylase and 17-hydroxylase defect)
Cushing syndrome
Primary aldosteronism
Apparent mineralcorticoid excess
Glucocorticoid remedial aldosteronism (familial aldosteronism type 1)
Glucocorticoid resistance (Chrousos syndrome)
Pseudohypoaldosteronism type 2 (Gordon syndrome)
Pheochromocytoma
Other neural crest tumors (neuroblastoma, ganglioneuroblastoma, ganglioneuroma)
Liddle syndrome
Geller syndrome

CENTRAL NERVOUS SYSTEM
Intracranial mass
Hemorrhage
Residual following brain injury
Quadriplegia

Table 445-2	Conditions Associated with Transient or Intermittent Hypertension in Children

RENAL
Acute postinfectious glomerulonephritis
Anaphylactoid (Henoch-Schönlein) purpura with nephritis
Hemolytic-uremic syndrome
Acute tubular necrosis
After renal transplantation (immediately and during episodes of rejection)
After blood transfusion in patients with azotemia
Hypervolemia
After surgical procedures on the genitourinary tract
Pyelonephritis
Renal trauma
Leukemic infiltration of the kidney
Obstructive uropathy associated with Crohn disease

DRUGS AND POISONS
Cocaine
Oral contraceptives
Sympathomimetic agents
Amphetamines
Phencyclidine
Corticosteroids and adrenocorticotropic hormone
Cyclosporine or sirolimus treatment posttransplantation
Licorice (glycyrrhizic acid)
Lead, mercury, cadmium, thallium
Antihypertensive withdrawal (clonidine, methyldopa, propranolol)
Vitamin D intoxication

CENTRAL AND AUTONOMIC NERVOUS SYSTEM
Increased intracranial pressure
Guillain-Barré syndrome
Burns
Familial dysautonomia
Stevens-Johnson syndrome
Posterior fossa lesions
Porphyria
Poliomyelitis
Encephalitis
Spinal cord injury (autonomic storm)

MISCELLANEOUS
Preeclampsia
Fractures of long bones
Hypercalcemia
After coarctation repair
White cell transfusion
Extracorporeal membrane oxygenation
Chronic upper airway obstruction

coarctation of the aorta, endocrine disorders, or medications. In older school-age children and adolescents, primary hypertension becomes increasingly common.

Secondary hypertension in children is most commonly caused by renal abnormalities; cardiovascular disease or endocrinopathies are additional etiologies. Renal (chronic glomerulonephritis, reflux or obstructive nephropathy, hemolytic uremic syndrome, polycystic or dysplastic renal diseases), or renovascular hypertension, account for approximately 90% of children with secondary hypertension. Renal parenchymal disease and renal artery stenosis lead to water and sodium retention thought to be, in part, secondary to increased renin secretion. Coarctation of the aorta should always be considered. Several endocrinopathies are associated with hypertension, usually those involving the thyroid, parathyroid, and adrenal glands. Systolic hypertension and tachycardia are common in hyperthyroidism; diastolic pressure is not usually elevated. Hypercalcemia, whether secondary to hyperparathyroidism or other causes, often results in mild elevation in BP because of an increase in vascular tone. Adrenocortical disorders (aldosterone-

secreting tumors, sodium retaining congenital adrenal hyperplasia, Cushing syndrome) may produce hypertension in patients with increased mineralocorticoid secretion. It is important to consider conditions associated with real or apparent mineralocorticoid excess (Table 445-3) and thus a suppressed renin level form of secondary hypertension. Pheochromocytomas are catecholamine-secreting tumors that give rise to hypertension because of the cardiac and peripheral vascular effects of epinephrine and norepinephrine. Children with pheochromocytoma usually have sustained rather than intermittent or exercise-induced hypertension. Pheochromocytoma develops in approximately 5% of patients with neurofibromatosis. Rarely, secondary hypertension can be caused by pseudohyperaldosteronism, which leads to elevated BP in the face of a suppressed renin level. Such disorders include Liddle syndrome, apparent mineralocorticoid excess, and dexamethasone suppressible aldosteronism. Altered sympathetic tone can be responsible for acute or intermittent elevation of BP in children with Guillain-Barré syndrome, poliomyelitis, burns, and Stevens-Johnson syndrome. Sympathetic outflow from the central nervous system is also affected by intracranial lesions.

A number of drugs of abuse, therapeutic agents, and toxins may cause hypertension. Cocaine may provoke a rapid increase in BP and can

Table 445-3	Clinical Findings in Patients with Mineralocorticoid Excess
CONDITION	**CLINICAL PRESENTATION**
CAH: 11β-hydroxylase deficiency	Early growth spurt initially, then short adult stature, advanced bone age, premature adrenarche, acne, precocious puberty in males, amenorrhea/hirsutism/virilism in females
CAH: 17α-hydroxylase deficiency	Pseudohermaphroditism (male), sexual infantilism (female)
Apparent mineralocorticoid excess	Growth retardation/short stature, nephrocalcinosis
Liddle syndrome	Severe hypertension, hypokalemia, and metabolic alkalosis, muscle weakness
Geller syndrome	Early onset of hypertension (before age 20 years), exacerbated in pregnancy
Glucocorticoid remediable aldosteronism (GRA) (familial aldosteronism type 1)	Early onset of hypertension, presence of family history of mortality or morbidity from early hemorrhagic stroke
Pseudohypaldosteronism type 2 (Gordon syndrome)	Short stature, hyperkalemic and hyperchloremic metabolic acidosis, borderline blood pressure
Glucocorticoid resistance (children) (Chrousos syndrome)	Ambiguous genitalia, precocious puberty; women may have acne, excessive hair, oligo/anovulation, infertility

From Melcescu E, Phillips J, Moll G, et al: 11 Beta-hydroxylase deficiency and other syndromes of mineralcorticoid excess as a rare cause of endocrine hypertension. Horm Metab Res 44:867-878, 2012 (Table 1, p. 869).

result in seizures or intracranial hemorrhage. Phencyclidine causes transient hypertension that may become persistent in chronic abusers. Tobacco use may also increase BP. Sympathomimetic agents used as nasal decongestants, appetite suppressants, and stimulants for attention deficit disorder produce peripheral vasoconstriction and varying degrees of cardiac stimulation. Individuals vary in their susceptibility to these effects. Oral contraceptives should be suspected as a cause of hypertension in adolescent girls, although the incidence is lower with the use of low-estrogen preparations. Immunosuppressant agents such as cyclosporine and tacrolimus cause hypertension in organ transplant recipients, and the effect is exacerbated by the co-administration of steroids. BP may be elevated in patients with poisoning by a heavy metal.

Children and adolescents with primary (essential) hypertension are commonly overweight, often have a strong family history of hypertension, and usually have BP values at or only slightly above the 95th percentile for age. Primary hypertension is the most common form of hypertension in adults, and it is recognized more often in adolescents than in young children. The cause of primary hypertension is likely to be multifactorial; obesity, genetic alterations in calcium and sodium transport, vascular smooth muscle reactivity, the renin–angiotensin system, sympathetic nervous system overactivity, and insulin resistance have been implicated in this disorder. Elevated uric acid levels may play a role in the pathophysiology of primary hypertension and proof-of-concept studies have confirmed that lowering of uric acid levels results in lower BP in overweight youth with hypertension or prehypertension. Some children and adolescents demonstrate salt-sensitive hypertension, a factor that is ameliorated with weight loss and sodium restriction.

Normotensive children of hypertensive parents may show abnormal physiologic responses that are similar to those of their parents. When subjected to stress or competitive tasks, the offspring of hypertensive adults, as a group, respond with greater increases in heart rate and BP than do children of normotensive parents. Similarly, some children of hypertensive parents may excrete higher levels of urinary catecholamine metabolites or may respond to sodium loading with greater weight gain and increases in BP than do those without a family history of hypertension. The abnormal responses in children with affected parents tend to be greater in the black population than among white individuals.

CLINICAL MANIFESTATIONS

Children and adolescents with primary hypertension are usually asymptomatic; the BP elevation is usually mild and is detected during a routine examination or evaluation before athletic participation. These children may also be obese. Children with secondary hypertension can have BP elevations ranging from mild to severe. Unless the pressure

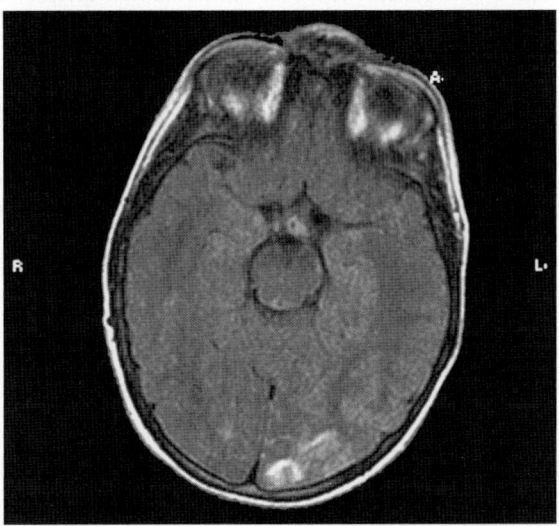

Figure 445-2 Magnetic resonance image of brain of a 6 yr old boy with end-stage renal disease and hypertensive encephalopathy (i.e., posterior reversible leukoencephalopathy syndrome). Bilateral occipital high signal intensity is more pronounced on the left side. (From Daroff RB, Fenichel GM, Jankovic J, Mazziotta JC, editors, Bradley's neurology in clinical practice, ed 6, vol 2, Philadelphia, 2012, Elsevier/Saunders, Fig. 49B.4, p. 924.)

has been sustained or is rising rapidly, hypertension does not usually produce symptoms. Therefore, clinical manifestations may instead reflect the underlying disease process, such as growth failure in children with chronic kidney disease. With substantial hypertension, headache, dizziness, epistaxis, anorexia, visual changes, and seizures may occur. **Hypertensive encephalopathy** (generalized or posterior reversible encephalopathy syndrome) is suggested by the presence of headache, vomiting, temperature elevation, visual disturbances, ataxia, depressed level of consciousness, CT abnormalities, and seizures (Fig. 445-2). Cardiac failure, pulmonary edema, and renal dysfunction (malignant hypertension) may occur in the face of marked hypertension. Bell palsy may be seen in asymptomatic or symptomatic patients. **Hypertensive crisis** may manifest with decreased vision (retinal hemorrhages of hypertensive retinopathy) and papilledema, encephalopathy (headache, seizures, depressed level of consciousness), heart failure, or accelerated deterioration of renal function.

Subclinical hypertensive target-organ injury is a common clinical manifestation in children with essential hypertension. With the use of echocardiography using pediatric normative data, left ventricular hypertrophy is detected in up to 40% of hypertensive children. Other markers of target organ damage that have been demonstrated in hypertensive children include increased carotid intima–media thickness, hypertensive retinopathy, and microalbuminuria. Children with prehypertension also have evidence of target organ damage, often at a magnitude intermediate between that of normotensive and hypertensive children.

DIAGNOSIS

The evaluation of the child with chronic hypertension should be directed toward uncovering potential underlying causes of the hypertension, evaluating for comorbidities, and screening for evidence of target organ damage. The extent of the evaluation for underlying causes of hypertension depends on the type of hypertension that is suspected. When secondary hypertension is a strong consideration, as in younger children with severe and symptomatic hypertension, an extensive evaluation may be necessary (Fig. 445-3). Alternatively, overweight adolescents with a family history of hypertension who have mild elevations of BP may need only a limited number of tests.

In all cases, a careful history and physical examination are warranted. A family history for early cardiovascular events should be obtained. Growth parameters should be determined to detect evidence of chronic disease. BP should be obtained in all 4 extremities to detect coarctation (thoracic or abdominal) of the aorta. Table 445-4 identifies other features of the physical examination that may provide evidence of an underlying cause of hypertension. Unless the history and physical examination suggest another cause, children with confirmed hypertension should have an evaluation to detect renal disease, including urinalysis, electrolytes, blood urea nitrogen, creatinine, complete blood count, urine culture, and renal ultrasound. Table 445-5 provides a more complete list of tests to consider in the clinical evaluation of a child with confirmed hypertension. Measuring serum potassium is essential because hypokalemia may be present in Liddle syndrome, glucocorticoid remedial aldosteronism, and apparent mineralcorticoid excess syndrome, while hyperkalemia may be seen in Gordon syndrome.

Renovascular hypertension is often associated with other diseases (Table 445-6) but may be isolated. Magnetic resonance or CT angiography can reveal renal artery stenosis, but fluoroscopic angiography may be needed, especially to detect intrarenal arterial stenosis (Fig. 445-4).

Primary hypertension often clusters with other risk factors. All hypertensive children should be screened for comorbidities that may increase cardiovascular risk, including hyperlipidemia and glucose intolerance. A fasting lipid panel and fasting glucose level should be obtained. In addition, a sleep history should be obtained in children with confirmed hypertension to screen for sleep disordered breathing, an entity that is associated with high BP, particularly in overweight children.

Left ventricular hypertrophy (LVH) is the most common manifestation of target-organ damage in hypertensive children. All children with confirmed hypertension should have echocardiography to evaluate for the presence of LVH. Left ventricular mass measurements should be indexed to height ($m^{2.7}$) to account for the effect of body size. The presence of LVH is an indication to treat the hypertension with pharmacologic therapy.

PREVENTION

Prevention of high BP may be viewed as part of the prevention of cardiovascular disease and stroke, the leading cause of death in adults in the United States. Other risk factors for cardiovascular disease include obesity, elevated serum cholesterol levels, high dietary sodium intake, and a sedentary lifestyle, as well as alcohol and tobacco use. The

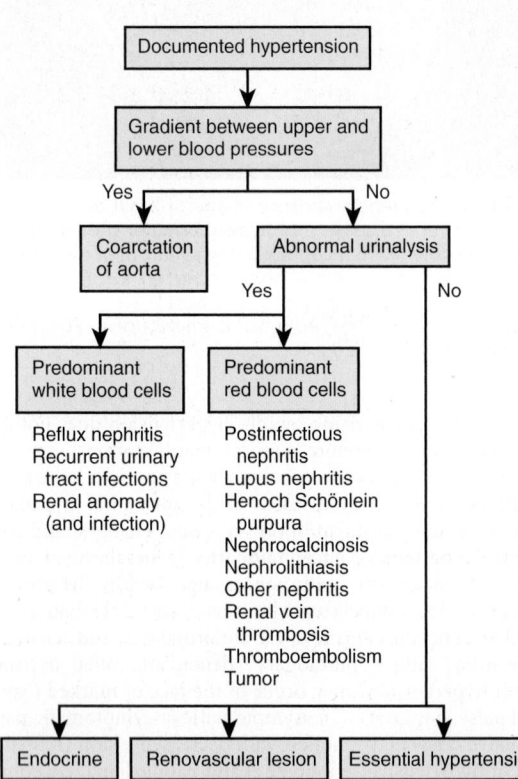

Figure 445-3 Initial diagnostic algorithm in the evaluation of hypertension. *(From Kliegman RM, Greenbaum LA, Lye PS: Practical strategies in pediatric diagnosis and therapy, ed 2, Philadelphia, 2004, Elsevier, p. 222.)*

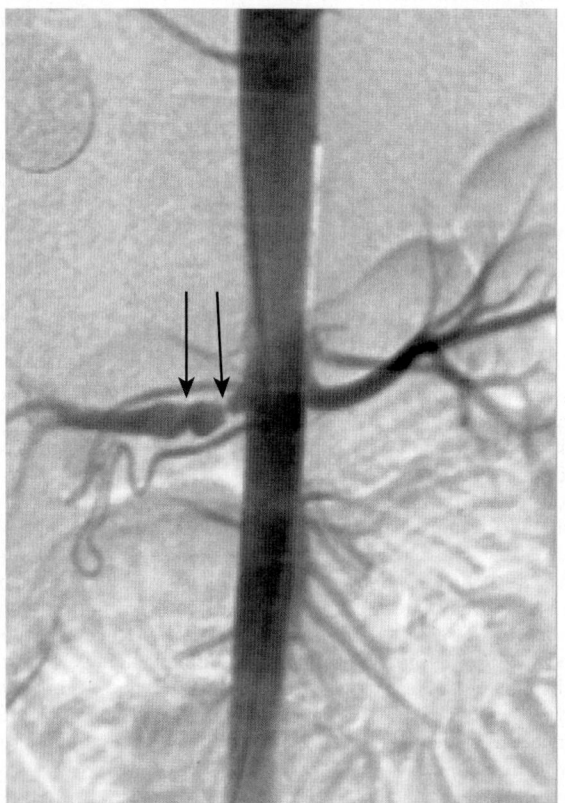

Figure 445-4 Renal angiogram in 7 yr old boy with hypertension. Right renal artery is visible with a string-of-beads appearance characteristic of fibromuscular dysplasia *(arrows)*. The aorta and left renal artery appear normal. *(From Tullus K, Brennan E, Hamilton G, et al: Renovascular hypertension in children, Lancet 371:1453–1463, 2008, p. 1454, Fig. 1.)*

Table 445-4	Findings to Look for on Physical Examination in Patients with Hypertension

PHYSICAL FINDINGS	POTENTIAL RELEVANCE
GENERAL	
Pale mucous membranes, edema, growth retardation	Chronic renal disease
Elfin facies, poor growth, retardation	Williams syndrome
Webbing of neck, low hairline, widespread nipples, wide carrying angle	Turner syndrome
Moon face, buffalo hump, hirsutism, truncal obesity, striae, acne	Cushing syndrome
HABITUS	
Thinness	Pheochromocytoma, renal disease, hyperthyroidism
Virilization	Congenital adrenal hyperplasia
Rickets	Chronic renal disease
SKIN	
Café-au-lait spots, neurofibromas	Neurofibromatosis, pheochromocytoma
Tubers, "ash-leaf" spots	Tuberous sclerosis
Rashes	Systemic lupus erythematosus, vasculitis (Henoch-Schönlein purpura), impetigo with acute nephritis
Pallor, evanescent flushing, sweating	Pheochromocytoma
Needle tracks	Illicit drug use
Bruises, striae	Cushing syndrome
Acanthosis nigricans	Type 2 diabetes, insulin resistance
EYES	
Extraocular muscle palsy	Nonspecific, chronic, severe
Fundal changes	Nonspecific, chronic, severe
Proptosis	Hyperthyroidism
HEAD AND NECK	
Goiter	Thyroid disease
Adenotonsillar hypertrophy	Sleep disordered breathing
CARDIOVASCULAR SIGNS	
Absent of diminished femoral pulses, low leg pressure relative to arm pressure	Aortic coarctation
Heart size, rate, rhythm; murmurs; respiratory difficulty, hepatomegaly	Aortic coarctation, congestive heart failure
Bruits over great vessels	Arteritis or arteriopathy
Rub	Pericardial effusion secondary to chronic renal disease
PULMONARY SIGNS	
Pulmonary edema	Congestive heart failure, acute nephritis
Picture of bronchopulmonary dysplasia	Bronchopulmonary dysplasia-associated hypertension
ABDOMEN	
Epigastric bruit	Primary renovascular disease or in association with Williams syndrome, neurofibromatosis, fibromuscular dysplasia, or arteritis
Abdominal masses	Wilms tumor, neuroblastoma, pheochromocytoma, polycystic kidneys, hydronephrosis, dysplastic kidneys
NEUROLOGIC SIGNS	
Neurologic deficits	Chronic or severe acute hypertension with stroke
Muscle weakness	Hyperaldosteronism, Liddle syndrome
GENITALIA	
Ambiguous, virilized	Congenital adrenal hyperplasia

increase in arterial wall rigidity and blood viscosity that is associated with exposure to the components of tobacco may exacerbate hypertension. Population approaches to prevention of primary hypertension include a reduction in obesity, reduced sodium intake, and an increase in physical activity through school- and community-based programs.

TREATMENT

The Fourth Report recommended a management algorithm for children with confirmed hypertension according to whether the child has prehypertension, stage 1 hypertension, or stage 2 hypertension (see Figs. 445-1 and 445-5). The mainstay of therapy for children with asymptomatic mild hypertension without evidence of target-organ damage is therapeutic lifestyle modification with dietary changes and regular exercise. Weight loss is the primary therapy in obesity-related hypertension. It is recommended that all hypertensive children have a diet increased in fresh fruits, fresh vegetables, fiber, and nonfat dairy, and reduced in sodium. In addition, regular aerobic physical activity for at least 30-60 min on most days along with a reduction of sedentary activities to less than 2 hr per day is recommended. Indications for pharmacologic therapy include symptomatic hypertension, secondary hypertension, hypertensive target organ damage, diabetes (types 1 and 2), and persistent hypertension despite nonpharmacologic measures (Table 445-7). When indicated, antihypertensive medication should be initiated as a single agent at low dose (see Fig. 445-5). The dose can then be increased until the goal BP is achieved. Once the highest recommended dose is reached or if the child develops side effects, then a second drug from a different class can be added. Acceptable drug classes for use in children include angiotensin-converting enzyme inhibitors, angiotensin receptor blockers, β-blockers, calcium channel blockers, and diuretics. Details on recommended doses of different

Table 445-5	Clinical Evaluation of Confirmed Hypertension	
STUDY OR PROCEDURE	**PURPOSE**	**TARGET POPULATION**
EVALUATION FOR IDENTIFIABLE CAUSES		
History, including sleep history, family history, risk factors, diet, and habits such as smoking and drinking alcohol; physical examination	History and physical examination help focus subsequent evaluation	All children with persistent BP ≥95th percentile
Blood urea nitrogen, creatinine, electrolytes, urinalysis, and urine culture	R/O renal disease and chronic pyelonephritis, mineralocorticoid excess states	All children with persistent BP ≥95th percentile
Complete blood count	R/O anemia, consistent with chronic renal disease	All children with persistent BP ≥95th percentile
Renal ultrasound	R/O renal scar, congenital anomaly, or disparate renal size	All children with persistent BP ≥95th percentile
EVALUATION FOR COMORBIDITY		
Fasting lipid panel, fasting glucose	Identify hyperlipidemia, identify metabolic abnormalities	Overweight patients with BP at 90th-94th percentile; all patients with BP ≥95th percentile; family history of hypertension or cardiovascular disease; child with chronic renal disease
Drug screen	Identify substances that might cause hypertension	History suggestive of possible contribution by substances or drugs.
Polysomnography	Identify sleep disorder in association with hypertension	History of loud, frequent snoring
EVALUATION FOR TARGET-ORGAN DAMAGE		
Echocardiogram	Identify left ventricular hypertrophy and other indications of cardiac involvement	Patients with comorbid risk factors* and BP 90th-94th percentile; all patients with BP ≥95th percentile
Retinal exam	Identify retinal vascular changes	Patients with comorbid risk factors and BP 90th-94th percentile; all patients with BP ≥95th percentile
ADDITIONAL EVALUATION AS INDICATED		
Ambulatory blood pressure monitoring	Identify white coat hypertension, abnormal diurnal BP pattern, BP load	Patients in whom white coat hypertension is suspected, and when other information on BP pattern is needed
Plasma renin determination	Identify low renin, suggesting mineralocorticoid-related disease	Young children with stage 1 hypertension and any child or adolescent with stage 2 hypertension Positive family history of severe hypertension
Renovascular imaging Isotopic scintigraphy (renal scan) Magnetic resonance angiography Duplex Doppler flow studies 3-Dimensional CT Arteriography: digital subtraction arteriography or classic	Identify renovascular disease	Young children with stage 1 hypertension and any child or adolescent with stage 2 hypertension
Plasma and urine steroid levels	Identify steroid-mediated hypertension	Young children with stage 1 hypertension and any child or adolescent with stage 2 hypertension
Plasma and urine catecholamines	Identify catecholamine-mediated hypertension	Young children with stage 1 hypertension and any child or adolescent with stage 2 hypertension

R/O, rule out.

*Comorbid risk factors also include diabetes mellitus and kidney disease.

From National High Blood Pressure Education Program Working Group on High Blood Pressure in Children and Adolescents. The fourth report on the diagnosis, evaluation, and treatment of high blood pressure in children and adolescents, Pediatrics 114(2 Suppl 4th Report):562, 2004.

Table 445-6	Causes of Renovascular Hypertension in Children

Fibromuscular dysplasia
Syndromic
  • Neurofibromatosis type 1
  • Tuberous sclerosis
  • Williams syndrome
  • Marfan syndrome
  • Other syndromes
Vasculitis
  • Takayasu disease
  • Polyarteritis nodosa
  • Kawasaki disease
  • Other systemic vasculitides
	Extrinsic compression
	  • Neuroblastoma
	  • Wilms tumor
	  • Other tumors
	Other causes
	  • Radiation
	  • Umbilical artery catheterization
	  • Trauma
	  • Congenital rubella syndrome
	  • Transplant renal artery stenosis

From Tullus K, Brennan E, Hamilton G, et al: Renovascular hypertension in children, Lancet 371:1453–1463, 2008, p. 1454, Panel 1.

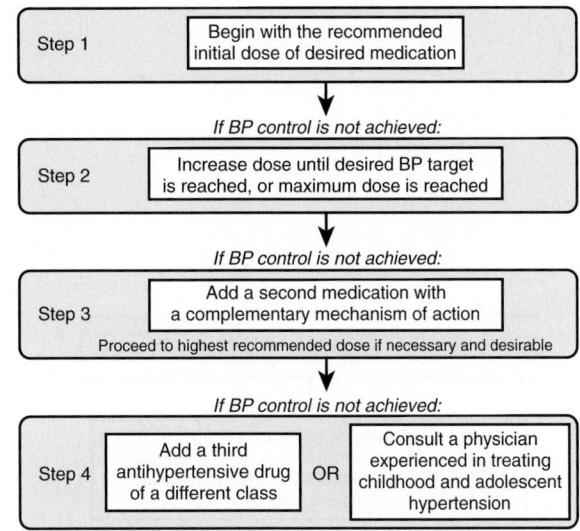

Figure 445-5 Stepped-care approach to antihypertensive therapy in children and adolescents. BP, blood pressure. *(From Flynn JT, Daniels SR: Pharmacologic treatment of hypertension in children and adolescents, J Pediatr 149:746–754, 2006, p. 751, Fig. 2.)*

Table 445-7	Recommended Doses for Selected Antihypertensive Agents for Use in Hypertensive Children and Adolescents			
CLASS	**DRUG**	**STARTING DOSE**	**INTERVAL**	**MAXIMUM DOSE***
Aldosterone receptor antagonist	Eplerenone	25 mg/day	qd-bid	100 mg/day
	Spironolactone†	1 mg·kg⁻¹·day⁻¹	qd-bid	3.3 mg·kg⁻¹·day⁻¹ up to 100 mg/day
Angiotensin-converting enzyme inhibitors	Benazepril†	0.2 mg·kg⁻¹·day⁻¹ up to 10 mg/day	qd	0.6 mg·kg⁻¹·day⁻¹ up to 40 mg/day
	Captopril†	0.3-0.5 mg/kg/dose	bid-tid	6 mg·kg⁻¹·day⁻¹ up to 450 mg/day
	Enalapril†	0.08 mg·kg⁻¹·day⁻¹	qd	0.6 mg·kg⁻¹·day⁻¹ up to 40 mg/day
	Fosinopril	0.1 mg·kg⁻¹·day⁻¹ up to 10 mg/day	qd	0.6 mg/kg/day up to 40 mg/day
	Lisinopril†	0.07 mg·kg⁻¹·day⁻¹ up to 5 mg/day	qd	0.6 mg/kg/day up to 40 mg/day
	Quinapril	5-10 mg/day	qd	80 mg/day
Angiotensin receptor blockers	Candesartan	1-6 yr, 0.2 mg·kg⁻¹·day⁻¹ 6-17 yr, <50 kg 4-8 mg once daily >50 kg 8-16 mg qdqd	qd	1-6 yr, 0.4 mg/kg; 6-17 yr, <50 kg 16 mg qd; >50 kg 32 mg qd
	Losartan†	0.75 mg·kg⁻¹·day⁻¹ up to 50 mg/day	qd	1.4 mg·kg⁻¹·day⁻¹ up to 100 mg/day
	Olmesartan	20 to <35 kg 10 mg qd; ≥35 kg 20 mg qd	qd	20 to <35 kg 20 mg qd ≥35 kg 40 mg qd
	Valsartan†	6-17 yr, 1.3 mg/kg/day up to 40 mg/day; <6 yr: 5-10 mg/day	qd	6-17 yr, 2.7 mg·kg⁻¹·day⁻¹ up to 160 mg/day; <6 yr: 80 mg/day
α- and β-Adrenergic antagonists	Labetalol†	2-3 mg·kg⁻¹·day⁻¹	bid	10-12 mg·kg⁻¹·day⁻¹ up to 1.2 g/day
	Carvedilol	0.1 mg/kg/dose up to 12.5 mg bid	bid	0.5 mg/kg/dose up to 25 mg bid
β-adrenergic antagonists	Atenolol†	0.5-1 mg·kg⁻¹·day⁻¹	qd-bid	2 mg·kg⁻¹·day⁻¹ up to 100 mg/day
	Bisoprolol/ HCTZ	0.04 mg·kg⁻¹·day⁻¹ up to 2.5/6.25 mg/day	qd	10/6.25 mg/day
	Metoprolol	1-2 mg·kg⁻¹·day⁻¹	bid	6 mg·kg⁻¹·day⁻¹ up to 200 mg/day
	Propranolol	1 mg·kg⁻¹·day⁻¹	bid-tid	16 mg·kg⁻¹·day⁻¹ up to 640 mg/day
Calcium channel blockers	Amlodipine†	0.06 mg·kg⁻¹·day⁻¹	qd	0.3 mg·kg⁻¹·day⁻¹ up to 10 mg/day
	Felodipine	2.5 mg/day	qd	10 mg/day
	Isradipine†	0.05-0.15 mg/kg/dose	tid-qid	0.8 mg·kg⁻¹·day⁻¹ up to 20 mg/day
	Extended-release nifedipine	0.25-0.5 mg·kg⁻¹·day⁻¹	qd-bid	3 mg·kg⁻¹·day⁻¹ up to 120 mg/day
Central α-agonist	Clonidine†	5-10 µg/kg/day	bid-tid	25 µg/kg/day up to 0.9 mg/day
Diuretics	Amiloride	5-10 mg/day	qd	20 mg/day
	Chlorthalidone	0.3 mg·kg⁻¹·day⁻¹	qd	2 mg·kg⁻¹·day⁻¹ up to 50 mg/day
	Furosemide	0.5-2.0 mg/kg/dose	qd-bid	6 mg·kg⁻¹·day⁻¹
	HCTZ	0.5-1 mg·kg⁻¹·day⁻¹	qd	3 mg·kg⁻¹·day⁻¹ up to 50 mg/day
Vasodilators	Hydralazine	0.25 mg/kg/dose	tid-qid	7.5 mg·kg⁻¹·day⁻¹ up to 200 mg/day
	Minoxidil	0.1-0.2 mg·kg⁻¹·day⁻¹	bid-tid	1 mg·kg⁻¹·day⁻¹ up to 50 mg/day

bid, Twice-daily; HCTZ, hydrochlorothiazide; qd, once daily; qid, 4 times daily; tid, 3 times daily.
*The maximum recommended adult dose should never be exceeded.
†Information on preparation of a stable extemporaneous suspension is available for these agents.
From Flynn JT. Management of hypertension in the young: role of antihypertensive medications. J Cardiovasc Pharmacol 2011:58(2)111–120.

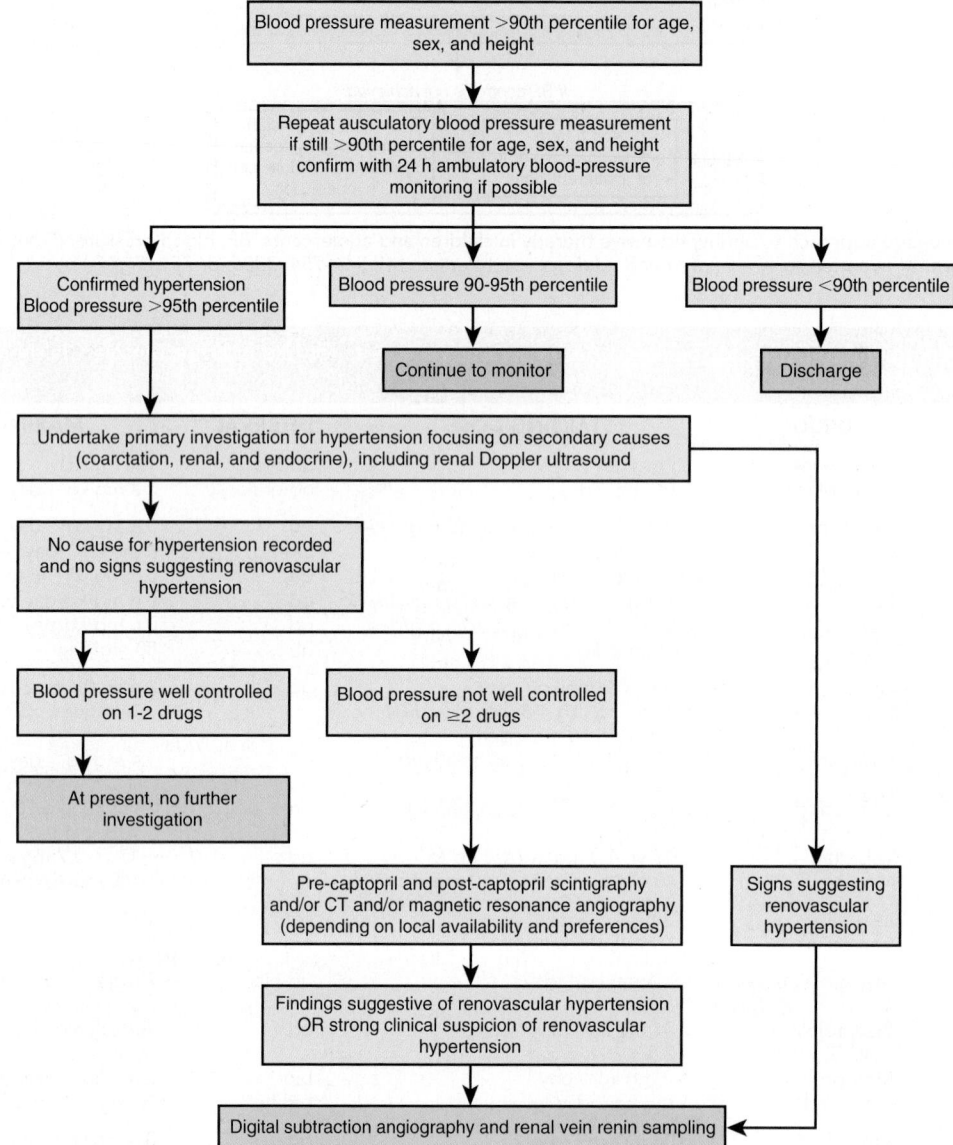

Figure 445-6 Diagnostic pathway for renovascular hypertension. *(From Tullus K, Brennan E, Hamilton G, et al: Renovascular hypertension in children, Lancet 371:1453–1463, 2008, p. 1458, Fig. 6.)*

Table 445-8	Antihypertensive Drugs for Management of Severe Hypertension in Children 1–17 Yr			
DRUG	**CLASS**	**DOSE**	**ROUTE**	**COMMENTS**
USEFUL FOR SEVERELY HYPERTENSIVE PATIENTS WITH LIFE-THREATENING SYMPTOMS				
Esmolol	β-Adrenergic blocker	100-500 µg/kg/min	IV infusion	Very short acting—constant infusion preferred. May cause profound bradycardia
Hydralazine	Direct vasodilator	0.2-0.6 mg/kg/dose	IV, IM	Should be given q4h when given IV bolus
Labetalol	α- and β-adrenergic blocker	bolus: 0.20-1.0 mg/kg/dose, up to 40 mg/dose infusion: 0.25-3.0 mg/kg/hr	IV bolus or infusion	Asthma and overt heart failure are relative contraindications
Nicardipine	Calcium channel blocker	Bolus: 30 mcg/kg up to 2 mg/dose Infusion: 0.5-4 µg/kg/min	IV bolus or infusion	May cause reflex tachycardia
Sodium nitroprusside	Direct vasodilator	0.5-10 µg/kg/min	IV infusion	Monitor cyanide levels with prolonged (>72 hr) use or in renal failure; or coadminister with sodium thiosulfate
USEFUL FOR SEVERELY HYPERTENSIVE PATIENTS WITH LESS-SIGNIFICANT SYMPTOMS				
Clonidine	Central α-agonist	0.05-0.1 mg/dose, may be repeated up to 0.8 mg total dose	PO	Side effects include dry mouth and drowsiness
Enalaprilat	ACE inhibitor	5-10 µg/kg/dose up to 1.25 mg/dose	IV bolus	May cause prolonged hypotension and acute renal failure, especially in neonates
Fenoldopam	Dopamine receptor agonist	0.2-0.8 µg/kg/min	IV infusion	Produced modest reductions in BP in a pediatric clinical trial in patients up to 12 yr
Hydralazine	Direct vasodilator	0.25 mg/kg/dose up to 25 mg/dose	PO	Extemporaneous suspension stable for only 1 wk
Isradipine	Calcium channel blocker	0.05-0.1 mg/kg/dose up to 5 mg/dose	PO	Stable suspension can be compounded
Minoxidil	Direct vasodilator	0.1-0.2 mg/kg/dose up to 10 mg/dose	PO	Most potent oral vasodilator; long acting

ACE, angiotensin-converting enzyme, IM, intramuscular, IV, intravenous, PO, oral.
From Flynn JT: Correction to severe hypertension in children and adolescents: pathophysiology and treatment, Pediatr Nephrol 27(3):503–504, 2012.

classes of antihypertensive medications for children can be found in the Fourth Report available free online at www.nhlbi.nih.gov/health/prof/heart/hbp/hbp_ped.pdf.

The goal of therapy for hypertension should be to reduce BP below the 95th percentile, except in the presence of chronic kidney disease, diabetes, or target-organ damage, when the goal should be to reduce BP to less than the 90th percentile. Angiotensin-converting enzyme inhibitors or angiotensin receptor blockers should be used for children with diabetes and microalbuminuria or proteinuric renal disease. β-Blockers or calcium channel blockers should be considered for hypertensive children with migraine headaches.

Severe, symptomatic hypertension is a hypertensive emergency that is often accompanied by cardiac failure, retinopathy, renal failure, encephalopathy, and seizures. Intravenous administration is often preferred so that the fall in BP can be carefully titrated (Table 445-8). Drug choices include labetalol, nicardipine, and sodium nitroprusside. Because too rapid a reduction in BP may interfere with adequate organ perfusion, a stepwise reduction in pressure should be planned. In general, the pressure should be reduced by 10% in the 1st hr, and 15% more in the next 3-12 hr, but not to normal during the acute phase of treatment. Hypertensive urgencies, usually accompanied by few serious symptoms such as severe headache or vomiting, can be treated either orally or intravenously. The Fourth Report also includes detailed information on antihypertensive drugs used for the management of severe hypertension in children.

Treatment of secondary hypertension must also focus on the underlying disease such as chronic renal disease, hyperthyroidism, adrenal–genital syndrome, pheochromocytoma, coarctation of the aorta, or renovascular hypertension. The treatment of renovascular stenosis includes antihypertensive medications, angioplasty, or surgery (Fig. 445-6). If bilateral renovascular hypertension or renovascular disease in a solitary kidney is suspected, drugs acting on the renin-angiotensin axis are usually contraindicated because they may reduce glomerular filtration rates and produce renal failure.

Bibliography is available at Expert Consult.

Diseases of the Blood

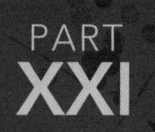

PART XXI

Section 1

The Hematopoietic System

Chapter 446

Development of the Hematopoietic System

Robert D. Christensen and Robin K. Ohls

HEMATOPOIESIS IN THE HUMAN EMBRYO AND FETUS

Hematopoiesis is the process by which the cellular elements of blood are formed. In the developing human embryo and fetus, hematopoiesis is conceptually divided into 3 anatomic stages: mesoblastic, hepatic, and myeloid. Mesoblastic hematopoiesis occurs in extraembryonic structures, principally in the yolk sac, and begins between the 10th and 14th days of gestation. By 6-8 wk of gestation the liver replaces the yolk sac as the primary site of blood cell production, and during this time the placenta also contributes as a hematopoietic site. By 10-12 wk extraembryonic hematopoiesis has essentially ceased. Hepatic hematopoiesis occurs through the remainder of gestation, although hepatic production diminishes during the second trimester while bone marrow (myeloid) hematopoiesis increases. The liver remains the predominant erythropoietic organ (few if any neutrophils are produced in the human fetal liver) through 20-24 wk of gestation.

Each hematopoietic organ houses distinct populations of cells. At 18-20 wk the fetal liver is predominantly an erythropoietic organ, while the marrow produces both erythrocytes and neutrophils. The types of leukocytes present in the fetal liver and marrow differ with gestation. Macrophages precede neutrophils in the marrow, and the ratio of macrophages to neutrophils decreases as gestation progresses. Regardless of gestational age or anatomic location, production of all hematopoietic tissues begins with pluripotent stem cells capable of both self-renewal and clonal maturation into all blood cell lineages. Progenitor cells differentiate under the influence of hematopoietic growth factors (Table 446-1). Fetal hematopoietic growth factor production is independent of maternal growth factor production (Fig. 446-1).

Erythrocytes in the fetus are larger than in adults, and at 22-23 wk gestation the mean corpuscular volume can be as high as 135 fL (Fig. 446-2, *upper panel*). Similarly, the mean corpuscular hemoglobin is very high at 22-23 wk, and falls relatively linearly with advancing gestation (Fig. 446-2, *lower panel*). In contrast, the mean corpuscular hemoglobin concentration is constant throughout gestation at 34±1 g/dL. While the size and quantity of hemoglobin in erythrocytes diminish during gestation, the hematocrit and blood hemoglobin concentration gradually increase (Fig. 446-3, *upper* and *lower panels*, respectively).

Concentrations of platelets in the blood increase gradually between 22 and 40 wk gestation (Fig. 446-4) but the platelet size, assessed by mean platelet volume, remains constant at 8±1 fL. No differences are observed between males and females in fetal and neonatal reference ranges for erythrocyte indices, hematocrit, hemoglobin, platelet counts, or mean platelet volume measurements.

FETAL GRANULOCYTOPOIESIS

Neutrophils are first observed in the human fetus about 5 wk postconception as small clusters of cells around the aorta. The fetal bone marrow space begins to develop around the 8th wk postconception, and from 8-10 wk the marrow space enlarges, but no neutrophils appear there until 10.5 wk. From 14 wk through term, the most common granulocytic cell type in the fetal bone marrow space is the neutrophil. Neutrophils and macrophages originate from a common progenitor cell but macrophages appear prior to neutrophils in the fetus, first in the yolk sac, liver, lung, and brain, all before the bone marrow cavity is formed.

Granulocyte colony-stimulating factor (G-CSF) and macrophage colony-stimulating factor (M-CSF) are expressed in developing fetal bone as early as 6 wk postconception and both are expressed in the fetal liver as early as 8 wk. Granulocyte-macrophage colony-stimulating factor (GM-CSF) and stem cell factor also are distributed widely in human fetal tissues. However, no changes in expression of any of these factors, or of their specific receptors, appear to be the signal for fetal production of neutrophils or macrophages, as those signals have not yet been identified.

Fetal blood contains few neutrophils until the third trimester. At 20 wk gestation the blood neutrophil count is 0-500/mm³. Although mature neutrophils are scarce, progenitor cells with the capacity to generate neutrophil clones are abundant in fetal blood. When cultured in vitro in the presence of recombinant G-CSF, they mature into large colonies of neutrophils. The physiologic role of G-CSF includes upregulating neutrophil production, and this appears to be the case for the fetus and neonate, as well as for adults. Thus, the low quantities of circulating neutrophils the mid-trimester human fetus may be partly a result of low production of G-CSF. Monocytes isolated from the blood of adults produce G-CSF when stimulated with a variety of inflammatory mediators such as bacterial lipopolysaccharide (LPS) or interleukin (IL)-1. In contrast, monocytes isolated from the blood or organs of fetuses up to 24 wk gestation generate only small quantities of G-CSF protein and messenger RNA (mRNA) after lipopolysaccharide or IL-1 stimulation. Despite this, G-CSF receptors on the surface of neutrophils of newborn infants are equal in number and affinity to those on adult neutrophils.

In the fetus, actions of the granulocytopoietic factors (G-CSF, M-CSF, GM-CSF, and stem cell factor) are not limited to hematopoiesis. Receptors for each of these are located in areas of the fetal central nervous system and gastrointestinal tract, where their patterns of expression change with development. Important developmental roles exist for these factors beyond hematopoiesis.

FETAL THROMBOPOIESIS

Platelet production occurs from 2 pools of cells: megakaryocyte progenitors and megakaryocytes. Megakaryocyte progenitors are categorized as *burst-forming unit–megakaryocytes* (BFU-MK), which are primitive megakaryocyte progenitors, and *colony-forming unit–megakaryocytes* (CFU-MK), which are more differentiated. BFU-MK produce large multifocal colonies containing ≥50 megakaryocytes, whereas CFU-MK generate smaller (3-50 cells/colony) unifocal colonies. The colonies generated by BFU-MK of fetal origin contain significantly more megakaryocytes than do those of adult origin and on that basis are thought to represent somewhat more primitive cells. Megakaryocytes are identified by their morphologic characteristics, as they undergo endoreduplication, which results in large cells with

| Table 446-1 | Characteristics of Hematopoietic Growth Factors |

GROWTH FACTOR	MOLECULAR MASS (kDa)	CHROMOSOMAL LOCATION	PRINCIPAL TARGET CELL
ERYTHROPOIETIN	30-39	7q11-12	CFU-E, fetal BFU-E, endothelial cells, neurons, astrocytes, oligodendrocytes
COLONY-STIMULATING FACTORS			
G-CSF	18-22	17q11.2-21	CFU-G, CFU-MIX, mature neutrophils
GM-CSF	18-30	5q23-31	CFU-MIX, CFU-GM, BFU-E, monocytes, mature neutrophils
M-CSF	45-70 (Dimer of 2 subunits)	5q33.1	CFU-M, macrophages
SCF	36	12q21.32	CFU-MIX, BFU-E, CFU-GM, mast cells
TGF-β	25 Homodimeric protein	19q13.2	BL-CFC
CSF-1	192 Amino acid protein	1p13.3	Monocytes, macrophages, dendritic cells, Langerhans cells
INTERLEUKINS			
IL-1	17	Alpha 2q13 Beta 2q13-21	Hepatocytes, macrophages, lymphocytes
IL-2	15-20	4q26-27	T cells, cytotoxic lymphocytes
IL-3	14-30	5q23-31	CFU-MIX, CFU-Meg, CFU-GM, BFU-E, macrophage
IL-4	16-20	5q23-31	T cells, B cells, dendritic cells
IL-5	46 (Dimer of 2 subunits)	5q23-31	CFU-Eo, B cells
IL-6	19-26	7p21-24	CFU-MIX, CFU-GM, BFU-E, monocytes, B cells, T cells, cytotoxic lymphocytes
IL-7	35	8q12-13	B cells
IL-8	8-10	4q13.3	Neutrophils, endothelial cells, T cells
IL-9	16	5q31-32	BFU-E, CFU-MIX
IL-10	18.7	1q32.1	Macrophages, lymphocytes
IL-11	23	19q13	CFU-Meg, B cells, keratinocytes
IL-12	70-75 (Dimer of 2 subunits)	p35/p40	3 (p35) and 11 (p40) T cells, NK cells, macrophages
IL-13	9	5q23-31	Pre-B lymphocytes, macrophages
IL-14	53	5q31	B cells
IL-15	14-15	4q25-35	B cells, T cells
IL-16	12-14	15q23-26	T cells
IL-17	20-30	2q31	Marrow stromal cells
IL-18	24	9p13	CD4+ T cells, NK cells
IL-21		4q26-q27	T cells
IL-23	Dimer of subunits	p19/IL-12p40	CD4+ T cells
IL-25		14q11.2	T cells, monocytes, marrow stromal cells
IL-31	4-Helix bundle	12q24.31	T cells, hematopoietic progenitors
IL-34	222 Amino acid protein	16q22.1	Monocytes, macrophages
THROMBOPOIETIN	35-38	3q27–28	Megakaryocyte progenitors, megakaryocytes

BFU-E, burst-forming units–erythroid; BL-CFU, blast colony-forming cell; CFU-E, colony-forming units–erythroid; CFU-Eo, colony-forming units–eosinophil; CFU-G, colony-forming units–granulocyte; CFU-GM, colony-forming units–granulocyte macrophage; CFU-M, colony-forming units–macrophage; CFU-Meg, colony-forming units–megakaryocyte; CFU-MIX, colony-forming units–mixed; CSF-1, colony-stimulating factor-1; G-CSF, granulocyte colony-stimulating factor; GM-CSF, granulocyte-macrophage colony-stimulating factor; IL, interleukin; M-CSF, macrophage colony-stimulating factor; NK, natural killer; SCF, stem cell factor; TGF-β, transforming growth factor-beta.

polyploid nuclei. Megakaryocytes, unlike megakaryocyte progenitors, do not have the capacity to generate clones. Rather, they undergo maturation, progressing from small mononuclear cells to large polyploid cells. The modal megakaryocyte ploidy (the number of sets of complete chromosomes) in normal adult marrow is 16N. In the fetus and neonate, ploidy is lower and megakaryocyte size is smaller. However, umbilical cord blood has a higher concentration of megakaryocytes than adult blood. Large megakaryocytes generate more platelets than do small megakaryocytes; thus, it is assumed that megakaryocytes of neonates produce fewer platelets than do their adult counterparts.

The processes of platelet production and release from megakaryocytes are not well understood. It has been speculated that small buds, proplatelets, are formed on megakaryocytes and that these are released from the marrow as platelets. An alternate possibility is that platelets are principally released from megakaryocytes in the lungs, as a consequence of shear forces.

Thrombopoietin (TPO) is the physiologic regulator of platelet production and acts as a stimulator of all stages of megakaryocyte growth and development (see Table 446-1). The gene encoding TPO is located on the long arm of chromosome 3. TPO-mRNA is expressed primarily in liver and kidney and, to a lesser extent, in marrow stroma. TPO is

a primary, but not exclusive, regulator of platelet production and stimulates the proliferation and survival not only of megakaryotic progenitors but also of erythroid, myeloid, and multipotent progenitors. Recombinant TPO supports the growth of megakaryocytic colonies of neonates and children and progenitors of preterm neonates are more sensitive to recombinant TPO than are progenitors of term neonates.

FETAL ERYTHROPOIESIS
Similar to hematopoietic production of other cell lines, fetal erythropoiesis is regulated by growth factors produced by the fetus, not by the mother. Erythropoietin (EPO) does not cross the human placenta. Stimulating maternal EPO production does not stimulate fetal erythropoiesis, and suppressing maternal erythropoiesis by hypertransfusion does not suppress fetal erythropoiesis.

It is unclear to what extent the mechanisms regulating erythropoiesis in adults are operative in the fetus. Of all the factors known to be involved in stimulating erythropoiesis, none plays a more central regulatory role than does EPO, a 30-39 kDa glycoprotein that binds to specific receptors on the surface of erythroid precursors and stimulates their differentiation and clonal maturation into mature

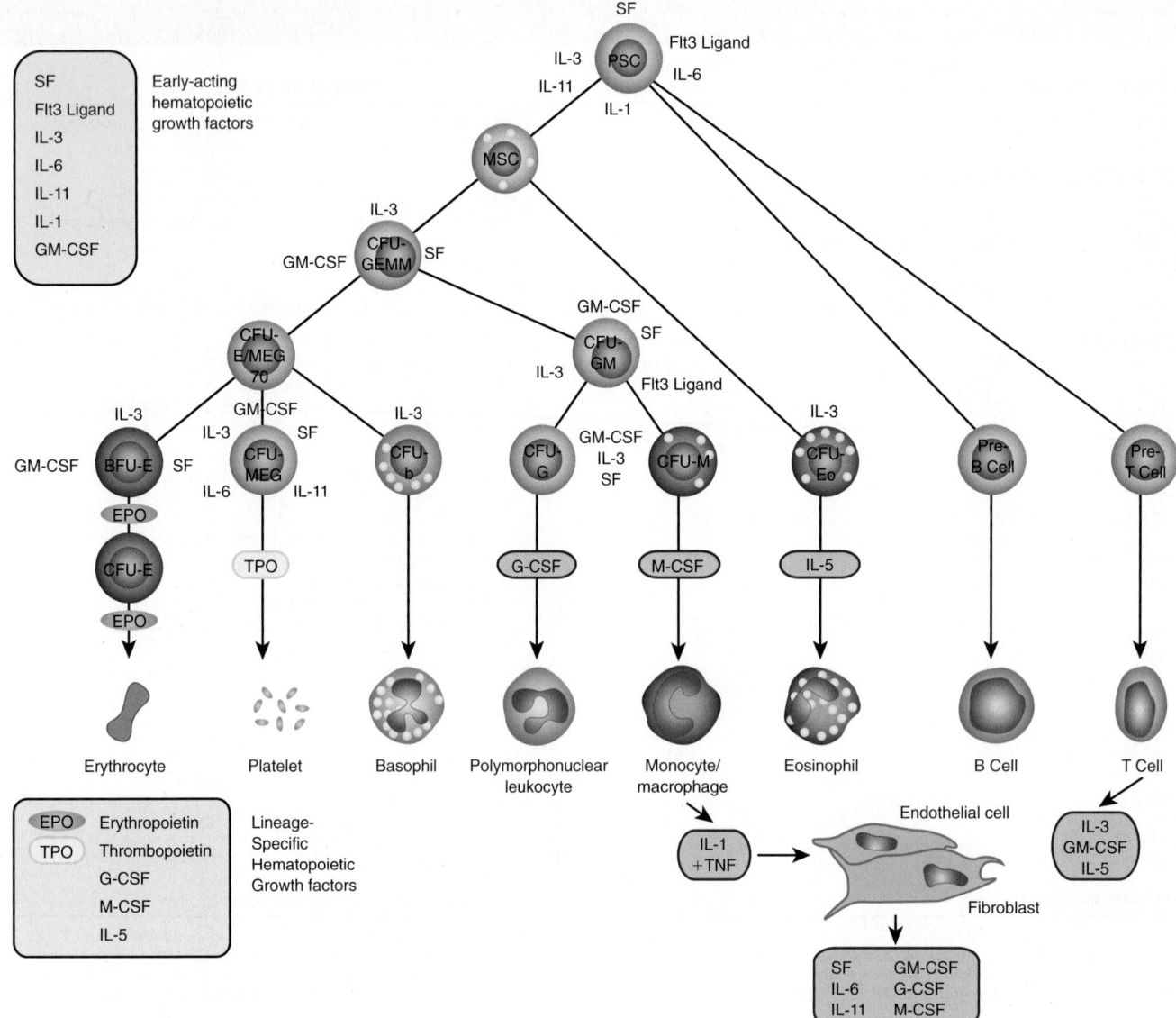

Figure 446-1 Major cytokine sources and actions to promote hematopoiesis. Cells of the bone marrow microenvironment, such as macrophages, endothelial cells, and reticular fibroblasts, produce macrophage colony-stimulating factor (M-CSF), granulocyte-macrophage colony-stimulating factor (GM-CSF), and granulocyte colony-stimulating factor (G-CSF) after stimulation. These cytokines and others listed in the text have overlapping interactions during hematopoietic differentiation, as indicated; for all lineages, optimal development requires a combination of early- and late-acting factors. BFU, burst-forming unit; CFU, colony-forming unit; EPO, erythropoietin; MSC, myeloid stem cells; PSC, pluripotent stem cell. *(From Sieff CA, Nathan DG, Clark SC: The anatomy and physiology of hematopoiesis. In Orkin SH, Nathan DG, editors: Hematology of infancy and childhood, ed 5, Philadelphia, 1998, WB Saunders, p. 168.)*

erythrocytes. Regulating EPO gene expression involves an oxygen-sensing mechanism. EPO mRNA production is regulated by *cis*-acting elements in the promoter and 3′ enhancer regions that are responsive to hypoxia. Two factors, hepatic nuclear factor 4 and hypoxia inducible factor (HIF-1), exhibit transcriptional activation for EPO and other hypoxia-inducible genes. Hepatic nuclear factor 4 binds to the EPO promoter and enhancer regions of the gene. HIF-1 is a basic helix-loop-helix transcription factor composed of HIF-1α and HIF-1β subunits that bind to *cis*-acting hypoxia-response elements and induce EPO transcription. HIF-1 is expressed in many cells and is involved in upregulating a variety of oxygen-regulated proteins, including vascular endothelial growth factor. HIF-1α appears to be constitutively expressed and rapidly degraded under normoxic conditions. RNA stability depends on the ubiquitin proteasome degradation system; inhibition of this system leads to increased HIF-1 and increased EPO, even under normoxic conditions.

EPO is produced in fetal liver during the first and second trimesters, principally by cells of monocyte/macrophage origin. After birth, the anatomic site of EPO production shifts to the kidney. The specific stimulus for this shift is unknown but may involve the increase in arterial oxygen tension that occurs at birth. Epigenetic modification of gene expression may also play a role, as it appears that renal and hepatic EPO genes are methylated to different degrees. Although EPO mRNA and protein can be found in the human fetal kidney, it is not known whether this production is biologically relevant. However, it appears that renal production of EPO is not essential for normal fetal erythropoiesis, as evidenced by the normal serum EPO concentrations and normal hematocrits of anephric fetuses.

Hemoglobins in the Fetus and Neonate

The evolutionary development of oxygen-carrying proteins, the **hemoglobins,** increased the ability of blood to transport oxygen. The

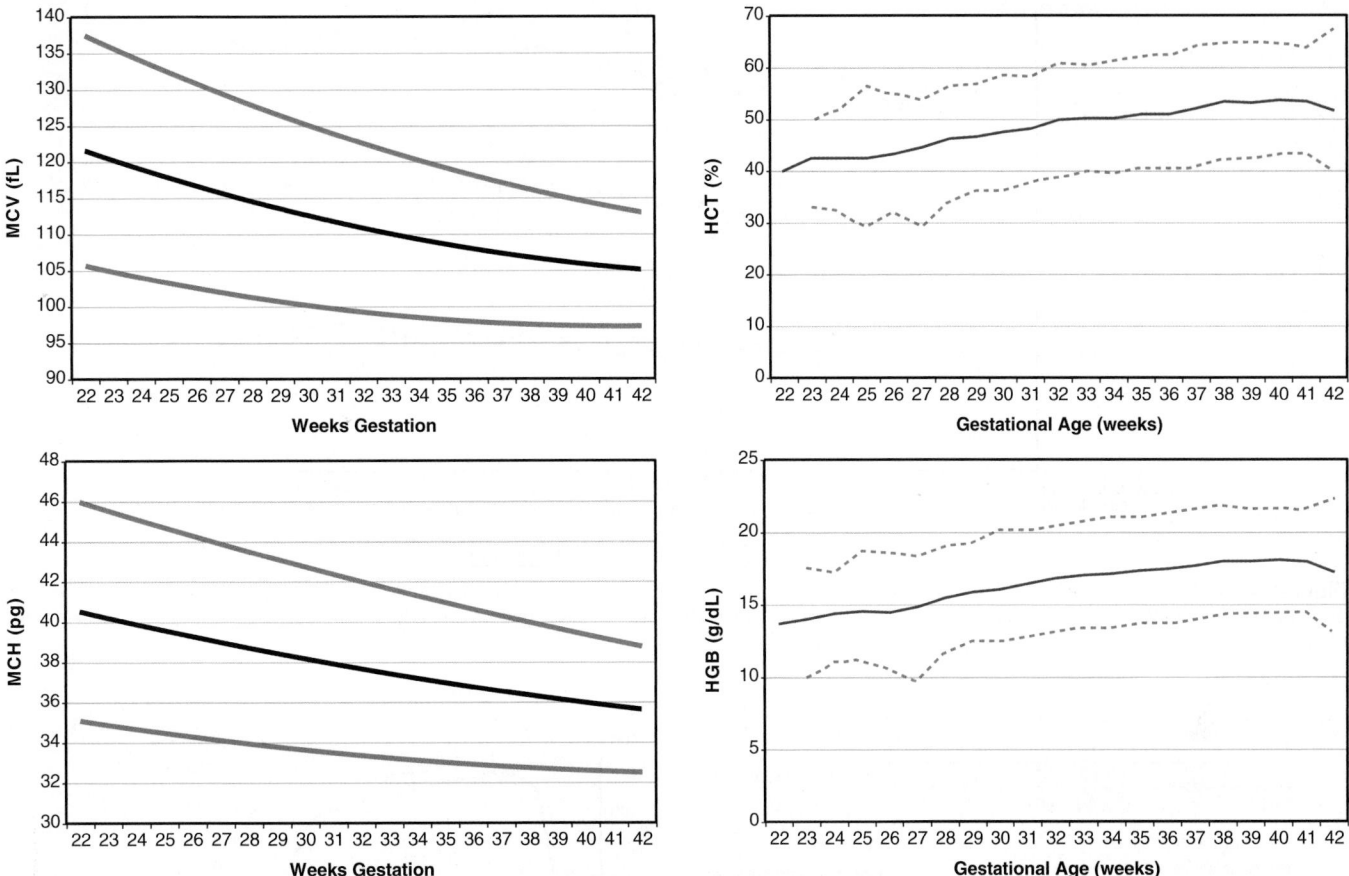

Figure 446-2 Erythrocyte mean corpuscular volume (MCV) and mean corpuscular hemoglobin (MCH) from 22 wk gestation through term. The lines represent the 5th percentile, the mean, and the 95th percentile reference range. *(From Christensen RD, Jopling J, Henry E, et al: The erythrocyte indices of neonates, defined using data from over 12,000 patients in a multihospital healthcare system, J Perinatol 28:24–28, 2008.)*

Figure 446-3 Hematocrit (HCT) and blood hemoglobin concentration (HGB) from 22 wk gestation through term. The lines represent the 5th percentile, the mean, and the 95th percentile reference range. *(From Jopling J, Henry E, Wiedmeier SE, et al: Reference ranges for hematocrit and blood hemoglobin concentration during the neonatal period: data from a multihospital healthcare system, Pediatrics 123:e333–e337, 2009.)*

combination of oxygen with hemoglobin and its dissociation from hemoglobin are accomplished without expenditure of metabolic energy.

Hemoglobin is a complex protein consisting of iron-containing heme groups and the protein moiety globin. A dynamic interaction between heme and globin gives hemoglobin its unique properties in the reversible transport of oxygen. The hemoglobin molecule is a tetramer made up of 2 pairs of polypeptide chains, with each chain having a heme group attached. The polypeptide chains of various hemoglobins are of chemically different types. The major hemoglobin of a normal adult (HbA) is made up of 1 pair of alpha (α) and 1 pair of beta (β) polypeptide chains, represented as $\alpha_2\beta_2$. The major hemoglobin in the fetus (HbF), which is made up of 2 α- and 2 γ-globin chains, is represented by $\alpha_2\gamma_2$.

The various globin chains differ in both the number and sequence of amino acids, and their synthesis is directed by separate genes (Fig. 446-5). Two sets of genes for the α chains are located on human chromosome 16. Two pairs of alleles provide the genetic information for the structure of the α chain. The β, γ, and δ genes are closely linked on chromosome 11.

Within the red blood cell (RBC) mass of an embryo, fetus, child, and adult, 6 different hemoglobins may normally be detected (Fig. 446-6): the **embryonic hemoglobins,** Gower-1, Gower-2, and Portland; **fetal hemoglobin,** HbF; and the **adult hemoglobins,** HbA and HbA₂. The electrophoretic mobilities of hemoglobins vary with their chemical structures. The time of appearance and quantitative relationships

among the hemoglobins are determined by complex developmental processes.

Embryonic Hemoglobins
The blood of early human embryos contains 2 slowly migrating hemoglobins, *Gower-1* and *Gower-2,* and *Hb Portland,* which has HbF-like mobility. The zeta (ζ) chains of Hb Portland and Gower-1 are structurally quite similar to α chains. Both Gower hemoglobins contain a unique type of polypeptide chain, the epsilon (ε) chain. Hb Gower-1 has the structure $\zeta_2\varepsilon_2$, while Gower-2 has the structure $\alpha_2\varepsilon_2$. Hb Portland has the structure $\zeta_2\gamma_2$. In embryos of 4-8 wk gestation, the Gower hemoglobins predominate, but by the 3rd mo they have disappeared.

Fetal Hemoglobin
HbF contains γ polypeptide chains in place of the β chains of HbA. Its resistance to denaturation by strong alkali is the basis for determining the presence of fetal RBCs in the maternal circulation (the **Kleihauer-Betke test**). After the 8th wk, HbF is the predominant hemoglobin; at 24 wk gestation it constitutes 90% of the total hemoglobin. During the 3rd trimester, a gradual decline occurs, so that at birth HbF averages 70% of the total hemoglobin. Synthesis of HbF decreases rapidly postnatally (Fig. 446-7), and by 6-12 mo of age only a trace is present. Less than 2.0% can be detected by alkali denaturation in older children and adults.

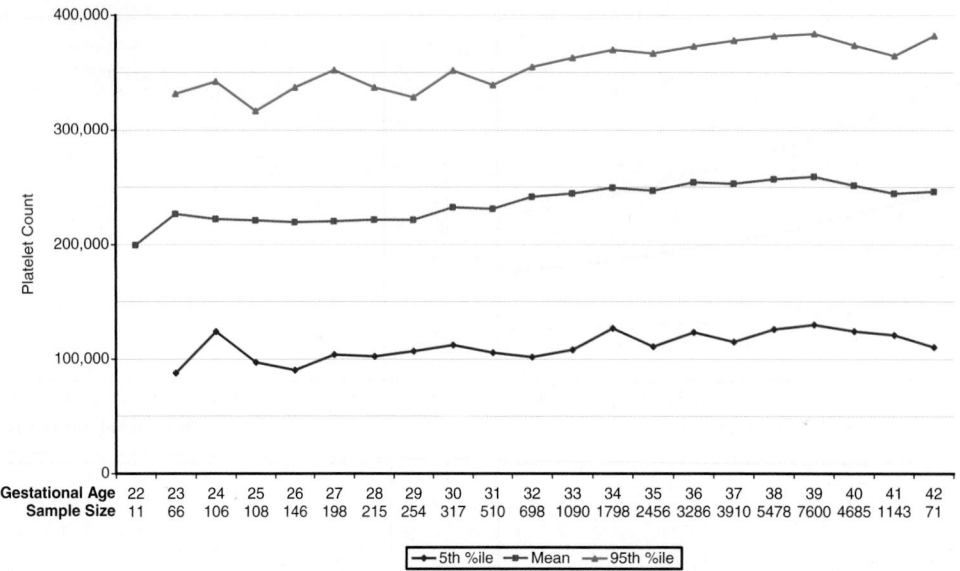

Figure 446-4 Platelet count from 22 wk gestation through term. The lines represent the 5th percentile, the mean, and the 95th percentile reference range. *(From Wiedmeier SE, Henry E, Sola-Visner MC, et al: Platelet reference ranges for neonates, defined using data from over 47,000 patients in a multihospital healthcare system,* J Perinatol *29:130–136, 2009.)*

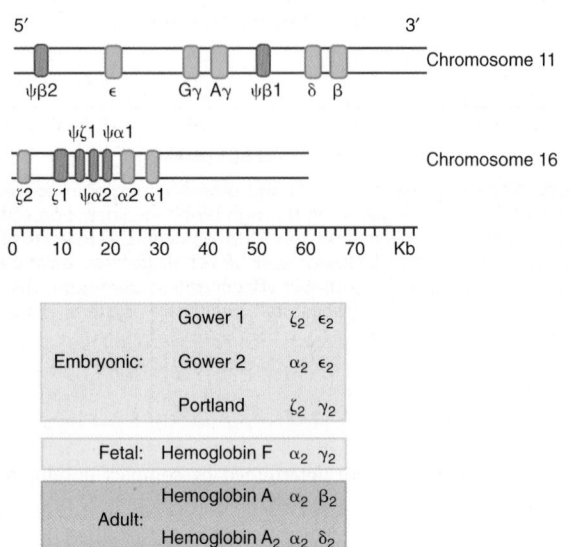

Figure 446-5 Organization of the globin genes. The bottom line reflects the scale in kilobases. The upper segment represents the beta-like globin genes on chromosome 11, and the lower segment the alpha-like genes on chromosome 16. Regions of the gene that code for primary globin proteins are shown as blue segments, and regions that code for pseudogenes ("ψ," nonexpressed remnants) are shown as pink segments. The composition of embryonic, fetal, and adult hemoglobins is listed. α, alpha; β, beta; γ, gamma; δ, delta; ε, epsilon; ζ, zeta.

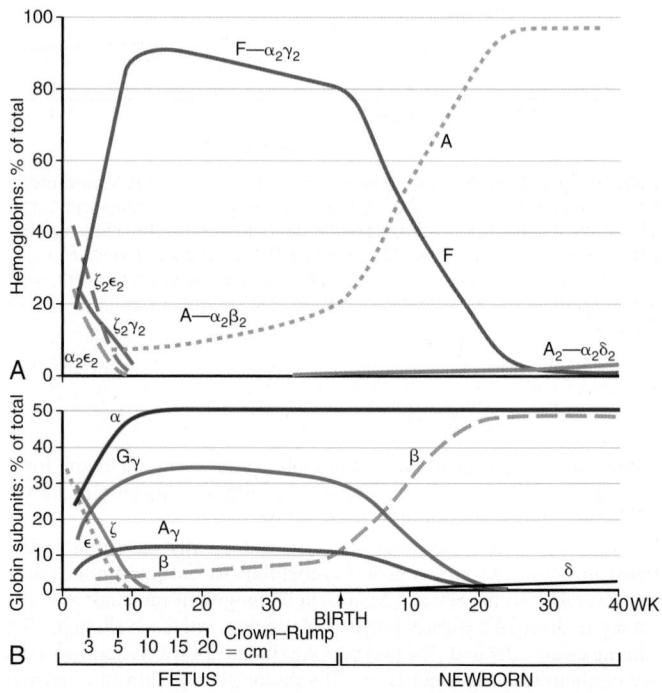

Figure 446-6 Changes in hemoglobin tetramers (**A**) and in globin subunits (**B**) during human development from embryo to early infancy. *(From Polin RA, Fox WW:* Fetal and neonatal physiology, *ed 2, Philadelphia, 1998, WB Saunders, p. 1769.)*

Adult Hemoglobins

By the 24th wk of gestation, HbA constitutes 5-10% of total hemoglobin. A steady increase follows, so that at term, HbA averages 30%. By 6-12 mo of age, the normal HbA pattern appears. The minor HbA component, HbA$_2$, contains δ chains and has the structure α$_2$δ$_2$. It is seen only when significant amounts of HbA are also present. At birth, <1.0% of HbA$_2$ is seen, but by 12 mo of age the normal level of 2.0-3.4% is attained. Throughout life, the normal ratio of HbA to HbA$_2$ is about 30:1.

Normal Relationships Among the Hemoglobins

During fetal life and early childhood, the rates of synthesis of γ and β chains and the amounts of HbA and HbF are inversely related. This relationship has been attributed to a "switch mechanism" similar to genetic regulatory mechanisms in bacteria, but the genetic, biologic, and developmental processes that direct a switchover from predominantly γ-chain synthesis in utero to predominantly β-chain synthesis after birth are unclear. It is not certain whether the mechanisms involve selective genetic inhibition or facilitation. The increase in the α$_1$-globin

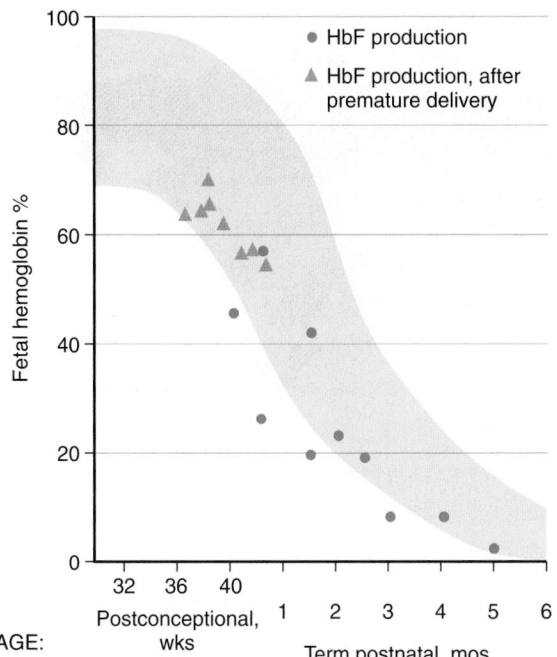

Figure 446-7 Pre- and postnatal changes in the percentage of total hemoglobin represented by fetal hemoglobin (HbF) (yellow). The triangles represent postnatal production by reticulocytes in premature infants, and the circles represent cord blood and postnatal reticulocyte production in term infants. *(From Brown MS: Fetal and neonatal erythropoiesis. In Stockman JA, Pochedly C, editors: Developmental and neonatal hematology, New York, 1988, Raven Press.)*

to α_2-globin ratio occurring after 36 wk gestation corresponds with a rapid decline in γ-globin synthesis, suggesting that these changes could be regulated by a coordinated molecular mechanism. Differential selection and amplified production of RBC precursors derived from burst-forming unit erythroid cells result in considerable HbF production. This may be the basis for the increased levels of HbF that occur in many hypoproliferative or hemolytic anemias. Alternative explanations involve more basic epigenetic regulation through processes such as methylation and deacetylation in the DNA sequences that flank the hemoglobin gene complexes.

Alterations of the Hemoglobins by Disease

Because hemoglobins containing ε chains normally are present only very early in intrauterine life, in the past they were largely of theoretical interest. Interest has been renewed by the growing method of isolation of free fetal DNA in the maternal circulation, allowing for noninvasive fetal diagnosis of a variety of genetic traits, such as RhD (rhesus antigen D) positivity in the fetus of an RhD negative mother. In addition, small amounts of the Gower hemoglobins have been detectable in a few newborns with trisomy 13. Increased levels of Hb Portland have been found in cord blood of stillborn infants with homozygous α-thalassemia.

HbF levels may be influenced by various factors. Because the HbF level is elevated during the 1st yr of life, knowledge of its normal decline is important (see Figs. 446-6 and 446-7). In persons heterozygous for β-thalassemia (β-thalassemia trait), postpartum decrease of HbF is delayed; approximately 50% of such persons have elevated levels of HbF (>2%) in later life. In homozygous thalassemia (Cooley anemia) and in hereditary persistence of HbF, large amounts of HbF characteristically are found. In patients with major β-chain hemoglobinopathies (HbSS [homozygous hemoglobin S], HbSC [sickle cell hemoglobin C]), HbF usually is increased, particularly during childhood. Preterm infants treated with human recombinant EPO increase HbF production during active erythropoiesis. Moderate elevations of HbF may

occur in many diseases accompanied by hematologic stress, such as hemolytic anemias, leukemia, and aplastic anemia, because of a minor population of RBCs that contain increased amounts of HbF. Tetramers of γ chains (γ_4 or Hb Barts) or β chains (β_4, HbH) may be found in α-thalassemia syndromes.

The normal adult level of HbA_2 (2.0-3.4%) is seldom altered. Levels of HbA_2 >3.4% are found in most persons with the β-thalassemia trait and in those with megaloblastic anemias secondary to vitamin B_{12} and folic acid deficiency. Decreased HbA_2 levels are found in those with iron-deficiency anemia (see Chapter 455) and α-thalassemia (see Chapter 462).

RED CELL LIFE SPAN OF THE FETUS AND NEONATE

In general, the highest hematocrit during a person's lifetime occurs at birth, and the lowest occurs about 10 wk later. The reasons for this rapid fall are complex, but a shortened life-span of fetal/neonatal RBC has been suggested as an important component. Specifically, the RBC life span during the fetal and neonatal period is generally thought to be considerably less than the 120 day erythrocyte life span found in normal adults. Estimates of an average 60-90 day life span were derived in the 1960s from studies of chromium (^{51}Cr)-labeled RBC. The "extinction time" is the number of days after transfusing labeled RBC when the label is completely gone from the circulating RBC, thus it estimates the maximal RBC life span. Recent studies indicate that the extinction time of fetal/neonatal RBC is similar to that of adults. For instance, fetal RBC transfused into an ABO-compatible mother, by a fetomaternal transfusion, have an extinction time of 120 days. Moreover, erythrocytes drawn from neonates, labeled with biotin, and transfused back to the neonate, have a half-disappearance time similar to adult donor erythrocytes.

It is possible that some fraction of fetal RBC survive 120 days and are then removed in the spleen by senescence, just as occurs case in healthy adults, while other RBC are removed prematurely by an active process. Neocytolysis is one possibility explaining the active process. Neocytolysis is the active removal of young erythrocytes that were generated in relatively hypoxic conditions, following normoxic or hyperoxic conditions. Neocytolysis is the process whereby the high hematocrit of persons acclimated to high altitude falls rapidly after descent to sea level (a process somewhat analogous to the change from fetal to postbirth oxygen saturations). It will be instructive to determine whether neocytolysis is, indeed, an important regulator of erythrocyte life span and bilirubin production after birth, and whether this process explains the marked fall in hematocrit but a normal RBC "extinction time" in human neonatal physiology.

Bibliography is available at Expert Consult.

Chapter 447
The Anemias
Norma B. Lerner

Anemia is defined as a reduction of the hemoglobin concentration or red blood cell (RBC) volume below the range of values occurring in healthy persons. "Normal" hemoglobin and hematocrit (packed red cell volume) vary substantially with age and sex (Table 447-1). There are also racial differences, with significantly lower hemoglobin levels in African-American children than in white non-Hispanic children of comparable age (Table 447-2). Anemia is a significant global health problem affecting children and reproductive age women (Figs. 447-1 and 447-2).

Physiologic adjustments to anemia include increased cardiac output, augmented oxygen extraction (increased arteriovenous oxygen difference), and a shunting of blood flow toward vital organs and tissues. In

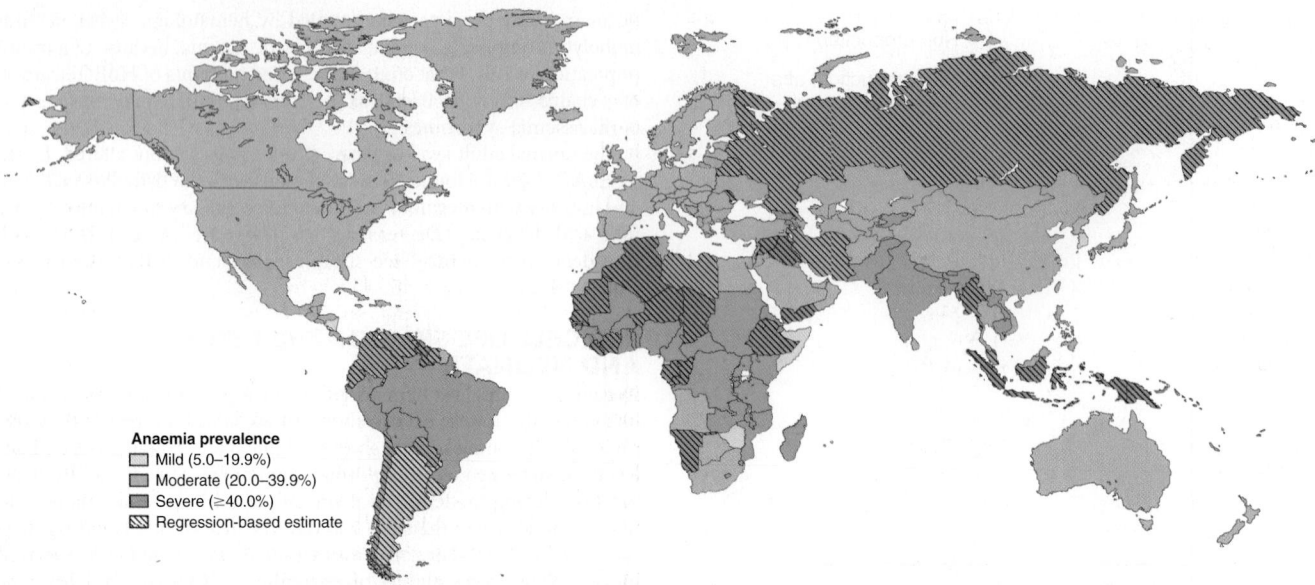

Figure 447-1 Global prevalence of anaemia in children of preschool age (0–5 yr). *(Adapted from* Worldwide prevalence of anaemia 1993–2005: WHO global database on anaemia. *Geneva, Switzerland, 2008, World Health Organization.)*

Table 447-1	Normal Mean and Lower Limits of Normal for Hemoglobin, Hematocrit, and Mean Corpuscular Volume					
	HEMOGLOBIN (g/dL)		**HEMATOCRIT (%)**		**MEAN CORPUSCULAR VOLUME (μM³)**	
Age (yr)	**Mean**	**Lower Limit**	**Mean**	**Lower Limit**	**Mean**	**Lower Limit**
0.5-1.9	12.5	11.0	37	33	77	70
2-4	12.5	11.0	38	34	79	73
5-7	13.0	11.5	39	35	81	75
8-11	13.5	12.0	40	36	83	76
12-14 female	13.5	12.0	41	36	85	78
12-14 male	14.0	12.5	43	37	84	77
15-17 female	14.0	12.0	41	36	87	79
15-17 male	15.0	13.0	46	38	86	78
18-49 female	14.0	12.0	42	37	90	80
18-49 male	16.0	14.0	47	40	90	80

From Brugnara C, Oski FJ, Nathan DG: Nathan and Oski's hematology of infancy and childhood, ed 7, Philadelphia, 2009, WB Saunders, p. 456.

Table 447-2	NHANES III Hemoglobin Values for Non-Hispanic Whites and African-Americans Ages 2-18 Yr			
	WHITE NON-HISPANIC		**AFRICAN-AMERICAN**	
Age (yr)	**Mean**	**−2 SD**	**Mean**	**−2 SD**
2-5	12.21	10.8	11.95	10.37
6-10	12.87	11.31	12.40	10.74
11-15 male	13.76	11.76	13.06	10.88
11-15 female	13.32	11.5	12.61	10.85
16-18 male	15.00	13.24	14.18	12.42
16-18 female	13.39	11.61	12.37	10.37

Sample size is 5,142 (white, 2,264; African-American, 2,878).
Modified from Robbins EB, Blum S: Hematologic reference values for African American children and adolescents, Am J Hematol 82:611–614, 2007.

addition, the concentration of 2,3-diphosphoglycerate increases within the RBC. The resultant "shift to the right" of the oxygen dissociation curve reduces the affinity of hemoglobin for oxygen and results in more complete transfer of oxygen to the tissues. The same shift in the oxygen dissociation curve can also occur at high altitude. Higher levels of erythropoietin (EPO) and consequent increased red cell production by the bone marrow further assist the body to adapt.

HISTORY AND PHYSICAL EXAMINATION

As with any medical condition, a detailed history and thorough physical exam are essential when evaluating an anemic child. Important historical facts should include age, sex, race and ethnicity, diet, medications, chronic diseases, infections, travel, and exposures. A family history of anemia and/or associated difficulties such as splenomegaly, jaundice, or early age onset of gallstones is also of consequence. There often are few physical symptoms or signs that result solely from a low hemoglobin, particularly when the anemia develops slowly. Clinical findings generally do not become apparent until the hemoglobin level falls to <7-8 g/dL. Clinical features can include pallor, sleepiness, irritability, and decreased exercise tolerance. Pallor can involve the tongue, nail beds, palms, or palmar creases. A flow murmur is often present. Ultimately, weakness, tachypnea, shortness of breath on exertion, tachycardia, cardiac dilation, and high-output heart failure will result from increasingly severe anemia, regardless of its cause. Unusual physical findings linked to particular underlying disease etiologies are discussed in detail in sections describing the associated disorders.

LABORATORY STUDIES
Initial laboratory testing should include hemoglobin, hematocrit, and red cell indices as well as a white blood cell count and differential, platelet count, reticulocyte count, and examination of the peripheral blood smear. The need for additional laboratory studies is dictated by the history, the physical, and the results of this initial testing.

DIFFERENTIAL DIAGNOSIS
Anemia is not a specific entity but rather can result from any of number of underlying pathologic processes. To narrow the diagnostic possibilities, anemias may be classified on the basis of their morphology and/or physiology (Fig. 447-3).

Anemias may be morphologically categorized on the basis of RBC size (mean corpuscular volume [MCV]), and microscopic appearance. They can be classified as microcytic, normocytic, or macrocytic based on whether the MCV is low, normal, or high, respectively. RBC size also changes with age, and normal developmental changes in MCV should be recognized before a designation is made (see Table 447-1). Examination of a peripheral blood smear often reveals changes in RBC appearance that will help to further narrow the diagnostic categories (Fig. 447-4). Details regarding morphologic changes associated with particular disorders are described in subsequent sections.

Anemias may also be further divided on the basis of underlying physiology. The 2 major categories are decreased production and increased destruction or loss. The 2 groups are not always mutually exclusive. Decreased RBC production may be a consequence of ineffective erythropoiesis or a complete or relative failure of erythropoiesis. Increased destruction or loss may be secondary to hemolysis, sequestration, or bleeding. The peripheral blood reticulocyte percentage or absolute number will help to make a distinction between the 2 physiologic categories. The normal reticulocyte percentage of total RBCs during most of childhood is approximately 1%, with an absolute reticulocyte count of 25,000-75,000/mm^3. In the presence of anemia, EPO production and the absolute number of reticulocytes should rise. Low or normal numbers of reticulocytes generally represent an inadequate response to anemia that is associated with relative bone marrow failure or ineffective erythropoiesis. Increased numbers of reticulocytes represent a normal bone marrow response to ongoing RBC destruction (hemolysis), sequestration, or loss (bleeding).

Figure 447-3 presents a useful approach to assessing the common causes of anemia in the pediatric age group. Children with microcytic anemia and low or normal reticulocyte counts most often have defects in erythroid maturation or ineffective erythropoiesis. *Iron deficiency* (see Chapter 455) is the most common cause. *Thalassemia trait* (see Chapter 462) constitutes the primary differential diagnosis when iron deficiency is suspected. Distinctions between these entities are presented in Table 455-1 (see Chapter 455). *Chronic disease or inflammation (more often normocytic), lead poisoning, and sideroblastic anemias* should also be considered and are discussed in other chapters. Microcytosis and elevated reticulocyte counts are associated with thalassemia syndromes and hemoglobins C and E (see Chapter 462). Notably, thalassemias and hemoglobinopathies are most commonly seen in patients of Mediterranean, Middle Eastern, African, or Asian descent.

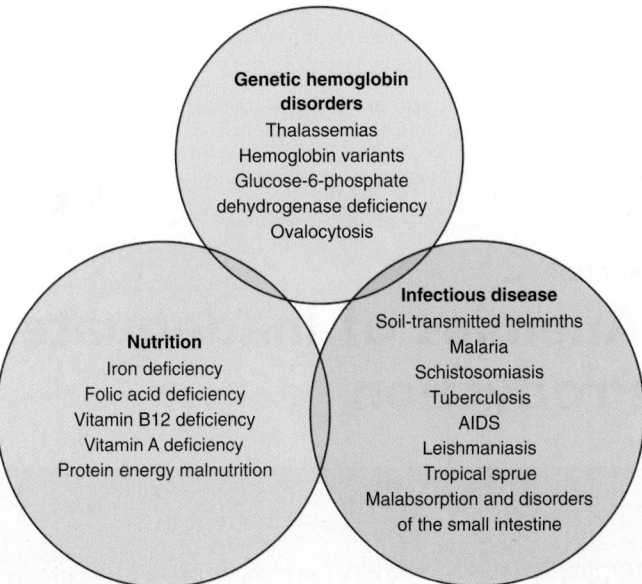

Figure 447-2 Causes of anaemia in countries with low or middle incomes. *(From Balarajan Y, Ramakrishnan U, Özaltin E, et al: Anaemia in low-income and middle-income countries. Lancet 378:2123–2134, 2011, Fig. 3.)*

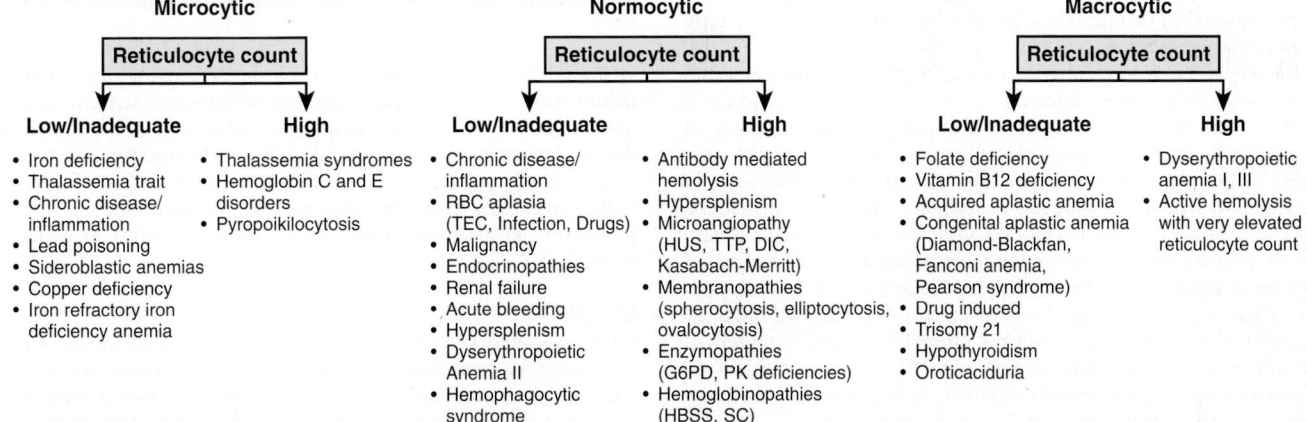

Figure 447-3 Use of the mean corpuscular volume (MCV) and reticulocyte count in the diagnosis of anemia. *(Adapted from Brunetti M, Cohen J: The Harriet Lane handbook, ed 17, Philadelphia, 2005, Elsevier Mosby, p 338.)*

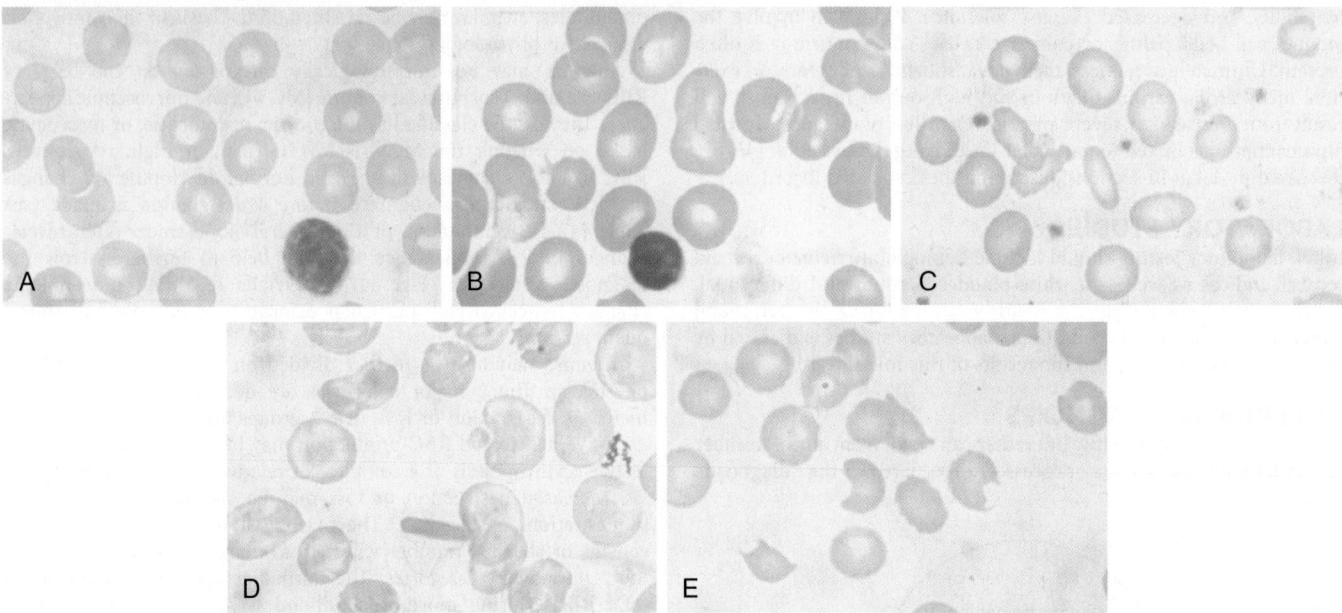

Figure 447-4 Morphologic abnormalities of the red blood cell. **A,** Normal. **B,** Macrocytes (folic acid or vitamin B_{12} deficiency). **C,** Hypochromic microcytes (iron deficiency). **D,** Target cells (HbCC disease). **E,** Schizocytes (hemolytic-uremic syndrome). *(Courtesy of Dr. E. Schwartz.)*

Normocytic anemia and low reticulocyte count characterize a large number of anemias. The *anemia of chronic disease/inflammation* (see Chapter 455) is usually normocytic. The anemia associated with renal failure, primarily a result of reduced EPO production, will invariably be associated with clinical and laboratory evidence of significant kidney disease. Decreased or absent red cell production secondary to transient erythroblastopenia of childhood, infection, drugs, or endocrinopathy usually results in a normocytic anemia, as does bone marrow infiltration by malignancy. In the case of invading leukemia or malignancy, abnormal leukocytes or tumor cells in association with thrombocytopenia or reduced or elevated white cell counts may be seen. Acute bleeding, hypersplenism, and congenital dyserythropoietic anemia type II (see Chapter 452) are also normocytic.

In children with normocytic anemia and an appropriate (high) reticulocyte response, the anemia is usually a consequence of bleeding, hypersplenism, or ongoing hemolysis. In hemolytic conditions, reticulocytosis, indirect hyperbilirubinemia, and increased serum lactate dehydrogenase are indicators of accelerated erythrocyte destruction. There are many causes of hemolysis, resulting from conditions that are extrinsic (usually acquired) or intrinsic (usually congenital) to the red cell. Abnormal RBC morphology (e.g., spherocytes, sickle forms, microangiopathy) identified on the peripheral smear is often helpful in ascertaining the cause.

The anemia seen in children with macrocytic blood cells is sometimes megaloblastic (see Chapter 454), resulting from impaired DNA synthesis and nuclear development. The peripheral blood smear in megaloblastic anemias contains large macroovalocytes, and the neutrophils often show nuclear hypersegmentation. The major causes of megaloblastic anemia include folate deficiency, vitamin B_{12} deficiency, and rare inborn errors of metabolism. Other macrocytic anemias with low or normal reticulocyte counts include acquired and congenital (Diamond-Blackfan and Fanconi) aplastic anemias and hypothyroidism. Patients with trisomy 21 have macrocytic cells, although an accompanying anemia is generally not present. High MCV and reticulocytosis is seen in congenital dyserythropoietic anemias I and III, and in situations wherein hemolysis results in such a large outpouring of young red cells that the mean MCV is abnormally high.

Bibliography is available at Expert Consult.

Section 2
Anemias of Inadequate Production

Chapter **448**
Congenital Hypoplastic Anemia (Diamond-Blackfan Anemia)
Norma B. Lerner

Diamond-Blackfan anemia (DBA) is a rare, congenital bone marrow failure syndrome that usually becomes symptomatic in early infancy. More than 90% of cases are recognized in the 1st yr of life. The disorder is characterized by anemia, usually normochromic and macrocytic, reticulocytopenia, and insufficient or absent of red blood cell (RBC) precursors in an otherwise normally cellular bone marrow. Up to 50% of affected individuals have additional, extrahematopoietic anomalies.

ETIOLOGY

DBA associated mutations were initially identified in *RPS19*, a gene that encodes a component protein of the small 40S ribosomal subunit. Such *RPS19* mutations, all dominantly inherited, were found to be present in approximately 25% of patients. Nine other DBA genes were subsequently recognized, each encoding a different small (40S) or large (60S) ribosomal subunit protein. Mutations in 1 of the 10 ribosomal protein (RP) genes were ultimately identified in 50-70% of cases. Although the disorder is often referred to as a **ribosomopathy**, the mechanism by which RP haploinsufficiency leads to DBA has not been fully elucidated. One hypothesis is that unaffected RPs pile up and then bind and inhibit the p53 regulator, MDM_2. This process allows p53 to accumulate, causing cell-cycle arrest and apoptosis of erythroid precursors.

Two distinct mutations in the hematopoietic transcription factor GATA-1 were identified in 2 siblings and 1 unrelated patient with corticosteroid-dependent DBA. It remains unclear whether two pathways, one related to ribosomal dysfunction and one to impaired GATA-1 production, independently cause the same phenotype, or, alternatively that DBA results from problems in a single pathway involving functional links between ribosomes and GATA-1.

EPIDEMIOLOGY

DBA affects about 7 individuals per 1 million live births. It is primarily an autosomal dominant disease, although other inheritance patterns may yet be demonstrated. Notably, there is substantial phenotypic diversity in DBA, even in families whose members share the same mutation, suggesting that additional genetic modifiers affect phenotypic expression of the disease. International consensus recommendations suggest that a diagnosis of "nonclassical" DBA be applied to family members harboring an established mutation or those without a known mutation but with an associated anomaly or laboratory abnormality.

CLINICAL MANIFESTATIONS

Profound anemia usually becomes evident by 2-6 mo of age, occasionally somewhat later. Approximately 25% of patients are anemic at birth and hydrops fetalis occurs rarely; 92% are diagnosed within the first year of life. Approximately 50% of patients have congenital anomalies and more than 1 anomaly is found in 21% of individuals with DBA (Table 448-1). Craniofacial abnormalities are the most common (50% of patients) and include hypertelorism, snub nose, and high arched palate. Skeletal anomalies, mostly upper limb and hand, affect 30% of patients. Thumb abnormalities, including flattening of the thenar eminence and triphalangeal thumb, may be bilateral or unilateral. The radial pulse may be absent. Genitourinary (38% of patients), cardiac (30% of patients), ophthalmologic, and musculoskeletal anomalies have also been identified. Short stature is common, but it is often unclear whether this characteristic results from the disease itself, related therapies, or both.

LABORATORY FINDINGS

The RBCs are usually macrocytic for age, but no hypersegmented neutrophils or other characteristics of megaloblastic anemia are appreciated on the peripheral blood smear. Red cell enzyme patterns are similar to those of a "fetal" RBC population with increased expression of "i" antigen and elevated fetal hemoglobin. Erythrocyte adenosine deaminase (ADA) activity is increased in most patients with this disorder, a finding that helps distinguish congenital RBC aplasia from acquired *transient erythroblastopenia of childhood* (see Chapter 450). Because elevated ADA activity is not a fetal RBC feature, measurement of this enzyme may be particularly helpful when diagnosing DBA in very young infants. Thrombocytosis or, rarely, thrombocytopenia, and occasionally neutropenia, may also be present. Reticulocyte percentages are characteristically very low despite severe anemia. Bone marrow erythrocyte precursors are markedly reduced in most patients; other marrow elements are usually normal. Serum iron levels are elevated. Unlike Fanconi anemia, there is no increase in chromosomal breaks when lymphocytes are exposed to alkylating agents.

DIFFERENTIAL DIAGNOSIS

DBA must be differentiated from other anemias associated with low reticulocyte counts. The syndrome of **transient erythroblastopenia of childhood (TEC)** is often the primary alternative diagnosis. Table 450-1 in Chapter 450 shows a useful comparison of findings in these

Table 448-1	Range of Congenital Anomalies Observed in Diamond-Blackfan Anemia
Craniofacial	Hypertelorism Broad, flat nasal bridge Cleft palate High arched palate Microcephaly Micrognathia Microtia Low-set ears Low hair line Epicanthus Ptosis
Ophthalmologic	Congenital glaucoma Strabismus Congenital cataract
Neck	Short neck Webbed neck Sprengel deformity Klippel-Feil deformity
Thumbs	Triphalangeal Duplex or bifid Hypoplastic Flat thenar eminence Absent radial artery
Urogenital	Absent kidney Horseshoe kidney Hypospadias
Cardiac	Ventricular septal defect Atrial septal defect Coarctation of the aorta Complex cardiac anomalies
Other musculoskeletal	Growth retardation Syndactyly
Neuromotor	Learning difficulties

The list includes the anomalies that are most characteristic of DBA but is not exhaustive. Multiple anomalies, most commonly including craniofacial, are present in up to 25% of affected individuals.
From Vlachos A, Ball S, Dahl N, et al: Diagnosing and treating Diamond Blackfan anaemia: results of an international clinical consensus conference. Br J Haematol 142:859–876, 2008 (Table IV, p. 862).

two disorders. TEC often is differentiated from DBA by its relatively late onset, although it occasionally develops in infants <6 mo of age (see Chapter 450). Macrocytosis, congenital anomalies, fetal red cell characteristics, and elevated erythrocyte ADA are generally associated with DBA and not with TEC.

Other inherited macrocytic bone marrow failure syndromes, particularly Fanconi anemia and Shwachman-Diamond syndrome, should also be considered in the differential as should myelodysplastic syndrome. Hemolytic disease of the newborn can also mimic features of DBA because it can have a protracted course and can be coupled with markedly reduced erythropoiesis. The anemia in this disorder usually resolves spontaneously at 5-8 wk of age. Several types of chronic hemolytic disease may be complicated by an **aplastic crisis**, characterized by reticulocytopenia and decreased numbers of RBC precursors. This event usually occurs after the first several mo of life and is often caused by parvovirus B19 infection (see Chapter 450). Infection with parvovirus B19 (see Chapter 251) in utero also may be associated with pure RBC aplasia in infancy, and even with hydrops fetalis at birth. When diagnosing DBA in young infants, it is important to rule out parvovirus B19 infection using the polymerase chain reaction. Other infections, including HIV, as well as drugs, immune processes, and Pearson syndrome (see Chapter 449) should also be ruled out.

TREATMENT

Corticosteroids are a mainstay of therapy, and approximately 80% of patients initially respond. Because corticosteroids impair linear growth as well as physical and neurocognitive development, many hematologists maintain infants on chronic transfusion therapy and delay the start of steroids until after age 1 yr. Prednisone or prednisolone in doses totaling 2 mg/kg/day is used as an initial trial. An increase in RBC precursors is usually seen in the bone marrow 1-3 wk after therapy is begun and is followed by peripheral reticulocytosis. The hemoglobin can reach normal levels in 4-6 wk, although the rate of response is quite variable. Once it is established that the hemoglobin concentration is increasing, the dose of corticosteroid may be reduced gradually by tapering and then by eliminating all except a single, lowest effective daily dose. This dose may then be doubled, used on alternate days, and tapered still further while maintaining the hemoglobin level at ≥9 g/dL. The target maintenance dose should not exceed 0.5 mg/kg/day or 1 mg/kg every other day. In some patients, very small amounts of prednisone, as low as 2.5 mg twice a wk, may be sufficient to sustain adequate erythropoiesis. Scheduled surveillance examinations and testing for corticosteroid side effects should be pursued in all patients, regardless of dose. Appropriate *Pneumocystis* prophylaxis should be used after the first month of high-dose steroids and continued until the patient is on low-dose alternate-day therapy. Many children with DBA stop taking corticosteroids, usually because of unacceptable side effects or the evolution of corticosteroid refractoriness. Only 37% of patients in the Diamond-Blackfan Anemia Registry (DBAR) (http://www.dbar.org/) remained on corticosteroids.

Patients who are nonresponders or who fail to tolerate corticosteroid therapy require transfusions at intervals of 3-5 wk to maintain a hemoglobin level greater than 8 g/dL. Some younger children may require hemoglobin levels greater than 9 g/dL in order to sustain normal growth and activities. Appropriate screening and, ultimately, the initiation of chelation therapy will be required as excess iron accumulates secondary to repeated transfusions. In one case report, a patient with DBA who was treated with L-leucine became transfusion independent and remained in remission at >5 mo.

Spontaneous remission of anemia with independence from steroid or red cell transfusion therapy has been reported. The likelihood of remission is 25% by age 25 yr, with the majority of patients experiencing remission during the first decade. Mild macrocytic anemia and increased erythrocyte ADA levels persist in these circumstances.

Hematopoietic stem cell transplantation (HSCT) can be curative. As the best outcomes occur using human leukocyte antigen (HLA)-matched sibling donors in patients 9 yr of age or younger. HLA-matched sibling HSCT is recommended in affected, transfusion dependent children between the ages of 3 and 9 yr. It is important that sibling donors be carefully screened, including genotype if known, to ensure that the donor does not carry the patient's DBA gene. Improvements in alternative donor HSCT suggests that this modality may also provide an important option for select patients.

PROGNOSIS

DBA has been identified as a cancer predisposition syndrome. The risk is increased for myelodysplastic syndrome, acute myeloid leukemia, colon carcinoma, osteogenic sarcoma, and female genital cancers. The overall actuarial survival of all patients with DBA is approximately 75% at age 40 yr, with approximately 87% for those maintained on steroids, and approximately 57% for transfusion-dependent patients. Of reported deaths, 67% were treatment related and 22% were DBA-related (malignancy and severe aplastic anemia).

Bibliography is available at Expert Consult.

Chapter 449
Pearson Syndrome
Norma B. Lerner

Pearson marrow-pancreas syndrome is a rare mitochondrial disorder that presents with a hypoplastic anemia that may be initially confused with Diamond-Blackfan syndrome or transient erythroblastopenia of childhood. The marrow failure usually appears in the neonatal period and is characterized by a macrocytic anemia and, occasionally, neutropenia and thrombocytopenia. There are vacuolated erythroblasts and myeloblasts in the bone marrow. This disorder is considered a unique variant of **congenital sideroblastic anemia** as the marrow also contains ringed sideroblasts. The hemoglobin F level is elevated. There is multiorgan involvement manifested by failure to thrive and symptoms of exocrine pancreas dysfunction, liver and renal tubular defects, malabsorption, and myopathy. Endocrine dysfunction has also been reported. In rare cases, when the disease is not fatal in early childhood, the disorder may evolve to include symptoms consistent with Kearns-Sayre syndrome.

This disorder is caused by a mitochondrial DNA deletion of variable size and location that is similar to the mitochondrial DNA (mtDNA) deletion found in Kearns-Sayre syndrome. There is heterogeneity in different tissues and between patients, accounting for the variable clinical picture. The proportion of deleted mtDNA in the bone marrow correlates with the severity of the hematologic picture, and a change in the percentage of tissue mtDNA types over time may be associated with spontaneous improvement of red blood cell hypoproliferation. Therapy for the hematologic manifestations of the disease is primarily supportive and includes red cell transfusions to correct anemia and granulocyte colony-stimulating factor to reverse episodes of severe neutropenia.

Bibliography is available at Expert Consult.

Chapter 450
Acquired Pure Red Blood Cell Anemia
Norma B. Lerner

TRANSIENT ERYTHROBLASTOPENIA OF CHILDHOOD

Transient erythroblastopenia of childhood (TEC) is the most common *acquired red cell aplasia* occurring in children. It is more prevalent than congenital hypoplastic (Diamond-Blackfan) anemia. This syndrome of severe, transient hypoplastic anemia occurs mainly in previously healthy children between 6 mo and 3 yr of age; most of the children are older than 12 mo at onset. Only 10% of affected patients are >3 yr of age. The annual incidence is estimated to be 4.3 cases per 100,000 children, although it is likely higher, because many cases might go undiagnosed and resolve spontaneously. The suppression of erythropoiesis has been linked to immunoglobulin (Ig) G, IgM, and cell-mediated mechanisms. Familial cases have been reported, suggesting a hereditary component. TEC often follows a viral illness, although no specific virus has been consistently implicated.

The temporary suppression of erythropoiesis results in reticulocytopenia and moderate to severe normocytic anemia. Some degree of neutropenia occurs in up to 20% of cases. Platelet numbers are normal or elevated. Similar to the situation observed in iron-deficiency anemia and other red blood cell (RBC) hypoplasias, thrombocytosis is presumably caused by increased erythropoietin, which has some homology with thrombopoietin. Mean corpuscular volume (MCV) is characteristically normal for age, and fetal hemoglobin (HbF) levels are normal before the recovery phase. RBC adenosine deaminase levels are normal in this disorder, thus contrasting with the elevation noted in most cases of congenital hypoplastic anemia (Table 450-1). Differentiation from the latter disease is sometimes difficult, but differences in age at onset and in age-related MCV, HbF, and adenosine deaminase are usually helpful. The peak occurrence of TEC coincides with that of iron-deficiency anemia in infants receiving milk as their main caloric source; differences in MCV should help to distinguish between these 2 disorders.

Virtually all children recover within 1-2 mo. RBC transfusions may be necessary for severe anemia in the absence of signs of early recovery. The anemia develops slowly, and significant symptoms usually develop only with severe anemia. Corticosteroid therapy is of no value in this disorder. Any child with presumed TEC who requires >1 transfusion should be reevaluated for another possible diagnosis. In rare instances, a prolonged case of apparent TEC may be caused by parvovirus-induced RBC aplasia, occurring in children with *hemolytic anemia* or *congenital* or *acquired immunodeficiencies.*

RED CELL APLASIA ASSOCIATED WITH PARVOVIRUS B19 INFECTION

Parvovirus B19 is a common infectious agent that causes erythema infectiosum (fifth disease) (see Chapter 251). It is also the best-documented viral cause of RBC aplasia in patients with chronic hemolysis, patients who are immunocompromised, and fetuses in utero. This small, nonenveloped single-stranded virus is particularly infective and cytotoxic to marrow erythroid progenitor cells, interacting specifically via binding to the red cell P antigen. In addition to decreased or absent erythroid precursors, characteristic nuclear inclusions in erythroblasts and giant pronormoblasts may be seen under the light microscope in bone marrow specimens. The virus does not cause significant anemia in immunocompetent individuals with normal red cell life spans.

CHRONIC HEMOLYSIS

Because parvovirus infection is usually transient, with recovery occurring in <2 wk, anemia is either not present or not appreciated in otherwise normal children whose peripheral RBC life span is 100-120 days. The RBC life span is much shorter in patients with hemolysis secondary to conditions such as hereditary spherocytosis, immune hemolytic anemia, or sickle cell disease. In these children, a brief cessation of erythropoiesis can cause severe anemia, a condition known as an **aplastic crisis**. When a definitive diagnosis is required, the work-up should include serum parvovirus IgM and IgG titers and, if needed, viral detection using polymerase chain reaction (PCR) techniques. Recovery from moderate to severe anemia is usually spontaneous, heralded by a wave of nucleated RBCs and subsequent reticulocytosis in the peripheral blood. A RBC transfusion may be necessary if the anemia is associated with significant symptoms. Notably, parvovirus-induced aplastic crisis usually occurs only once in children with chronic hemolysis. In families with >1 child affected with a hemolytic disorder, parents should be warned that a similar aplastic episode can occur in the other children if they have not been previously infected.

IMMUNODEFICIENCY

Persistent parvovirus infection may occur in children with congenital immunodeficiency diseases, lymphoproliferative disorders, those being treated with immunosuppressive agents, and those with HIV/AIDS, because these children may be unable to mount an adequate antibody response. The resultant pure RBC aplasia may be severe, and affected children may be thought to have TEC. This type of RBC aplasia differs from TEC in that there is no spontaneous recovery and >1 transfusion is often needed. The diagnosis of parvovirus infection is made by PCR of peripheral blood or bone marrow DNA because the usual serologic responses, reflected by parvovirus serum IgM or IgG titers, are impaired in immunodeficient children. In chronically infected patients, the disease may be treated with high doses of intravenous immunoglobulin, which contains neutralizing antibody to parvovirus and is effective in the short term.

MISCARRIAGE AND HYDROPS FETALIS

Parvovirus infection and destruction of erythroid precursors can also occur in utero. Such events are associated with increased fetal wastage in the first and second trimesters. Infants may be born with hydrops fetalis (see Chapter 103) and anemia. The presence of persistent congenital parvovirus infection is detected by PCR of peripheral blood and/or bone marrow DNA, because immunologic tolerance to the virus can prevent the usual development of specific antibodies.

OTHER RED CELL APLASIAS IN CHILDREN

Acquired red cell aplasia in adults is usually mediated by a chronic antibody and often associated with disorders such as chronic lymphocytic leukemia, lymphoma, thymoma, lymphoproliferative disorders, and systemic lupus erythematosus. This chronic antibody-mediated type of RBC aplasia, often responsive to immunosuppressive therapy,

Table 450-1	Comparison of Diamond-Blackfan Anemia and Transient Erythroblastopenia of Childhood	
FEATURE	**DBA**	**TEC**
Male:female	1.1	1.3
AGE AT DIAGNOSIS, MALE (MO)		
Mean	10	26
Median	2	23
Range	0-408	1-120
AGE AT DIAGNOSIS, FEMALE (MO)		
Mean	14	26
Median	3	23
Range	0-768	1-192
Boys >1 yr	9%	82%
Girls >1 yr	12%	80%
Etiology	Genetic	Acquired
Antecedent history	None	Viral illness
Physical examination abnormal (congenital anomalies present)	25%	0%
LABORATORY		
Hemoglobin (g/dL)	1.2-14.8	2.2-12.5
WBCs <5,000/µL	15%	20%
Platelets >400,000/µL	20%	45%
Adenosine deaminase	Increased	Normal
MCV increased at diagnosis	80%	5%
MCV increased during recovery	100%	90%
MCV increased in remission	100%	0%
HbF increased at diagnosis	100%	20%
HbF increased during recovery	100%	100%
HbF increased in remission	85%	0%
i Antigen increased	100%	20%
i Antigen increased during recovery	100%	60%
i Antigen increased in remission	90%	0%

DBA, Diamond-Blackfan anemia; HbF, fetal hemoglobin; MCV, mean cell volume; TEC, transient erythroblastopenia of childhood; WBC, white blood cell.
From Nathan DG, Orkin SH, Ginsburg D, et al, editors: Nathan and Oski's hematology of infancy and childhood, ed 6, vol 1, Philadelphia, 2003, WB Saunders, p. 329. Adapted from Alter BP: The bone marrow failure syndromes. In Nathan DG, Oski FA, editors: Hematology of infancy and childhood, ed 3, Philadelphia, 1987, WB Saunders, p. 159; and Link MP, Alter BP: Fetal erythropoiesis during recovery from transient erythroblastopenia of childhood (TEC), Pediatr Res 15:1036–1039, 1981.

is quite rare in childhood. Cases of acquired pure red cell aplasia, attributable to T-cell suppression, have also been described.

Certain drugs, such as chloramphenicol, also can inhibit erythropoiesis in a dose-dependent manner. Reticulocytopenia, erythroid hypoplasia, and vacuolated pronormoblasts in the bone marrow are reversible effects of this drug. These effects are distinct from the idiosyncratic and rare development of severe aplastic anemia in chloramphenicol recipients. Acquired antibody-mediated pure red cell aplasia has also been found to be a rare complication in chronic kidney disease patients treated with erythropoiesis-stimulating agents. In addition to discontinuing erythropoiesis-stimulating agents therapy and addressing anemia with red cell transfusions, further treatment may include immunosuppression and renal transplantation.

Bibliography is available at Expert Consult.

Chapter 451
Anemia of Chronic Disease and Renal Disease

451.1 Anemia of Chronic Disease
Norma B. Lerner

The anemia of chronic disease (ACD), also referred to as **anemia of inflammation**, is found in conditions where there is ongoing immune activation. It occurs in a wide a range of disorders including infections, malignancies, autoimmunity, and graft-versus-host disease. A similar anemia is associated with chronic kidney disease. ACD is typically a mild to moderate normocytic, normochromic, hypoproliferative anemia associated with a decreased serum iron and low transferrin saturation.

ETIOLOGY
Decreased red cell life span, impaired erythropoiesis, and an increased uptake of iron in the reticuloendothelial system are important mechanisms contributing to the anemia. The modest reduction in erythrocyte longevity is perhaps the least well understood part of the pathophysiology of ACD. Elevated levels of cytokines such as interleukin-1 may increase the macrophage's ability to ingest and destroy erythrocytes. Defective erythropoiesis, both proliferation and differentiation of precursors, has been attributed to immune cell/cytokine-driven inhibition of erythropoietin production and suppression of the bone marrow.

ACD associated alterations in iron recycling is characterized by an accumulation of iron in reticuloendothelial macrophages despite low levels of serum iron. The diversion of iron from the circulation into the reticuloendothelial system results in functional iron deficiency, which results in the impaired heme synthesis and iron-restricted erythropoiesis that contribute to anemia. These alterations in iron metabolism have been attributed to inflammation-associated excess synthesis of **hepcidin**, a key regulatory protein that controls intestinal iron absorption and tissue distribution. Hepcidin, although mainly synthesized by hepatocytes, is also expressed in other cells, including monocytes and macrophages. It functions by binding to and initiating the degradation of the iron exporter, ferroportin.

CLINICAL MANIFESTATIONS
Although the important symptoms and signs associated with ACD are those of the underlying disease, the mild to moderate anemia can affect the patient's quality of life.

LABORATORY FINDINGS
Hemoglobin concentrations are generally 6-9 g/dL. The anemia is usually normochromic and normocytic, although some patients have modest hypochromia and microcytosis, particularly if there is concomitant iron deficiency. Absolute reticulocyte counts are normal or low, and leukocytosis is common. The serum iron level is low, without the increase in serum transferrin that occurs in iron deficiency. This pattern of low serum iron and low-to-normal iron-binding protein (serum transferrin) is a regular and valuable diagnostic feature. *The serum ferritin level may be elevated.* The bone marrow has normal cellularity; the red blood cell precursors are decreased or adequate, marrow hemosiderin may be increased, and granulocytic hyperplasia may be present.

TREATMENT
The best approach to ACD is the treatment, when possible, of the underlying disorder. If the associated systemic disease can be controlled, the anemia will improve or resolve. Transfusions raise the hemoglobin concentration temporarily but are rarely indicated. Erythropoietic stimulating agents (ESAs), such as recombinant human erythropoietin (EPO) or related extended half-life formulations, increase the hemoglobin level and improve activity and the sense of well-being. When using ESAs, treatment with iron is usually necessary to produce optimal effect. Response to these agents is highly variable and poorly responsive patients may require high doses to reach target hemoglobin levels. In adults, such high doses are associated with a higher incidence of adverse events, such as stroke, cardiovascular events, cancer progression, and death, leading the FDA to require a black box warning on labels.

ACD does not respond to iron alone unless there is concomitant deficiency. Unfortunately it is a common clinical challenge to identify iron deficiency in patients with an inflammatory disease (see Chapters 447 and 455). In this circumstance, a trial of iron therapy might be helpful, although there may be no response as persistent inflammation impairs iron absorption and utilization; intravenous iron may further increase hepcidin production. Therapeutic agents that target the hepcidin–ferroportin axis are under investigation.

Bibliography is available at Expert Consult.

451.2 Anemia of Renal Disease
Norma B. Lerner

Anemia is common in children with chronic kidney disease (CKD). The anemia is usually normocytic, and the absolute reticulocyte count is normal or low. While most patients with end-stage renal disease (ESRD) are anemic, earlier stages of CKD are associated with a lower prevalence. In adults, lower glomerular filtration rate (GFR) has been correlated with lower hemoglobin concentration, and hemoglobin has been reported to decline below a GFR threshold of 40-60 mL/min/1.73 m². In children with CKD, hemoglobin levels decline as the GFR decreases below 43 mL/min/1.73 m².

Decreased hemoglobin values are linked to increased incidence of left ventricular hypertrophy, impaired physical activity, and a reduced quality of life in pediatric patients with CKD. In those with ESRD who are on dialysis, anemia is also associated with increased risk of hospitalization and mortality.

ETIOLOGY
Although the anemia of CKD shares many features with the ACD, its predominant cause is decreased EPO production by diseased kidneys. Other important causes include absolute and/or functional iron deficiency as a result of chronic blood loss (from blood sampling, surgeries, and dialysis) and disturbances in the iron metabolic pathway. Higher hepcidin levels have also been implicated in the anemia of CKD. Hepcidin is filtered by the glomerulus and excreted by the kidney; serum concentrations are increased in patients with decreased

GFR. Inflammation may also be a contributing factor in pediatric dialysis patients who have elevated levels of proinflammatory cytokines. Hyperparathyroidism and deficiencies of vitamin B_{12}, folate, and carnitine may also have a role in anemia of CKD.

LABORATORY FINDINGS
Anemia in children with CKD is defined by age: hemoglobin (Hb) <11.0 g/dL (0.5-5 yr), <11.5 g/dL (5-12 yr), <12 g/dL (12-15 yr), <13.0 g/dL (males older than 15 yr), and <12.0 g/dL (females older than 15 yr). The anemia of CKD is hypoproliferative and usually normocytic and normochromic, unless there is concomitant iron deficiency or vitamin deficiency. The EPO level and absolute reticulocyte count are usually low. White cell and platelet counts are generally normal. Ferritin will be low if there is accompanying iron deficiency, and high if there is associated inflammation.

TREATMENT
Oral iron therapy is recommended for all pediatric CKD patients with anemia. Consideration of IV iron therapy may be given for those receiving maintenance hemodialysis. Oral iron at 3-6 mg of elemental iron/kg of target dry weight once daily for 3 mo and possibly IV iron if transferrin saturation (serum iron × 100/total iron-binding capacity) and/or ferritin fail to improve is recommended.

ESAs are the mainstay of therapy and, particularly for children with ESRD, these medications have greatly reduced the need for frequent transfusions, decreasing the incidence of associated iron overload and alloimmunization. It is suggested to start ESA in all children with CKD when Hb concentrations are at 9-10 g/dL, with a goal of 11-12 g/dL (some recommend 11-13 g/dL) for children on maintenance ESA therapy. Dosing varies with age and dialysis modality. Darbepoetin, a synthetic form of EPO, appears to be equally effective as recombinant human EPO and has the benefit of less-frequent dosing as a consequence of a longer half-life. Iron therapy should be continued when using ESAs as treatment demands additional iron for hemoglobin synthesis.

A subset of patients is hyporesponsive to ESAs. In the past, pediatric nephrologists often responded to EPO resistance by further escalating the dose. The increased incidence of adverse events associated with dose escalation in the adult nondialysis CKD patients has prompted some concern about this approach. Several pediatric studies have demonstrated the value of IV iron supplementation in the setting of ESA hyporesponsiveness. In the rare case in which antibody-mediated (to EPO) pure red cell aplasia develops, ESA therapy should be stopped. A study including pediatric hemodialysis patients showed a nearly 50% decrease in hepcidin levels during treatment, suggesting that for those with ESA hyporesponsiveness and iron-restricted erythropoiesis, more frequent or longer duration sessions might be of benefit.

Bibliography is available at Expert Consult.

Chapter **452**
Congenital Dyserythropoietic Anemias
Norma B. Lerner

The congenital dyserythropoietic anemias (CDAs) are a heterogeneous class of inherited disorders resulting from abnormalities of late erythropoiesis. These rare conditions are characterized by variable degrees of anemia, ineffective erythropoiesis, and secondary hemochromatosis. Dyserythropoiesis is the major cause of anemia but a

shortened half-life of circulating red cells may also contribute. The CDAs have historically been classified into 3 major types (I, II, and III) based upon distinctive bone marrow morphology and clinical features, although additional subgroups and variants have also been identified.

TYPE I CONGENITAL DYSERYTHROPOIETIC ANEMIA
Pathogenesis
Type I CDA is an autosomal recessive disorder. The causative gene (*CDAN1*) was mapped to chromosome 15 between q15.1 and q15.3 and then successfully cloned. The gene encodes codanin-1, which is a ubiquitously expressed protein that may expedite histone assembly into chromatin and regulate the cell cycle. Although the majority of patients with bone marrow characteristics indicative of CDA1 have mutations within *CDAN1*, such mutations have not been detected in approximately 20% of families. Two distinctive mutations in the gene *C15ORF4*, predicted to encode an endonuclease, have been identified in 3 different CDA I pedigrees.

Clinical Manifestations
As of 2011, there were 169 cases from 143 families recorded in the literature. Most families were from Europe and the Middle East. Although CDA I may be diagnosed at any age, most cases are recognized during childhood or adolescence. CDA I is rarely diagnosed in utero. In addition to anemia-related symptoms, other findings often include splenomegaly, jaundice, and hepatomegaly. In more severe cases, evidence of extramedullary hematopoiesis in frontal or parietal bones of the skull and in paravertebral tumors may be present. Cholelithiasis and iron overload develop over time. Type I CDA has been associated with dysmorphic features in 4-14% of cases, primarily involving the digits (syndactyly, absence of nails, supernumerary toes). Retinal angioid streaks and macular abnormalities also have been reported.

Laboratory Findings
Hemoglobin concentrations generally range between 7 and 11 g/dL. The anemia is usually macrocytic (mean corpuscular volume 100-120 fL), but normocytic indices may be seen during childhood. Anisopoikilocytosis is appreciated on the peripheral blood smear. In some cases, normoblasts and basophilic stippling of red blood cells (RBCs) may be seen. The reticulocyte count is inadequate for the degree of anemia. Laboratory evidence of iron overload may be present. The bone marrow aspirate shows erythroid hyperplasia, megaloblastosis, and basophilic stippling. Binucleated and, more rarely, multinucleated polychromatophilic erythroblasts are also appreciated. Incompletely divided cells with thin chromatin bridges between nuclei of pairs of erythrocytes are highly specific for type I CDA. Electron microscopy is the gold standard for diagnosis, revealing erythroblasts with a characteristic "Swiss cheese" heterochromatin pattern.

Treatment
Treatment of this disorder is primarily supportive. Approximately 50% of neonates with CDA I will need at least 1 red cell transfusion and some may remain transfusion dependent over subsequent years. Adolescents and adults may only require episodic transfusions during aplastic crises, infection or pregnancy. If anemia is further exacerbated by coinherited disorders, such as thalassemia or RBC enzymopathy, the patient may become transfusion dependent. The most important long-term complication is **hemosiderosis,** which is caused by increased intestinal absorption of iron and ineffective erythropoiesis; consequently, transfusions should be avoided when possible to prevent further iron loading. Regular phlebotomies result in normal ferritin concentrations but if this approach is untenable oral chelation therapy should be employed when repeated ferritin levels exceed 1000 µg/L. In many cases of documented CDA type I, **interferon-α** has effectively raised the hemoglobin concentration, reduced splenomegaly, and reduced iron overload. *Patients do not respond to erythropoietin.* Splenectomy is generally not

recommended. Cholecystectomy is often required. Allogeneic bone marrow transplantation from a human-leukocyte-antigen-identical sibling has been successful in a few severe cases.

TYPE II CONGENITAL DYSERYTHROPOIETIC ANEMIA

Pathogenesis
CDA II is also an autosomal recessive disorder. Genome-wide linkage analysis identified a region of chromosome 20p11.2 as the location of the candidate *CDAN2* gene that was later identified to be the *SEC23B* gene. This gene is known to encode the cytoplasmic coat protein (COP) II component SEC23B that is involved in endoplasmic reticulum vesicle trafficking. *SEC23B* gene mutations have been associated with the majority of CDA II cases.

Clinical Manifestations
As of 2011, there were 454 cases from 356 families with CDA II recorded, making it the most common form of CDA. Families were mostly from Europe and the Middle East. In contrast to CDA I, this diagnosis is usually made later in life, often because symptoms may be milder. Also, CDA II may be initially misdiagnosed as hereditary spherocytosis. Characteristic findings can include anemia, jaundice, splenomegaly, or hepatomegaly. Posterior mediastinal or paravertebral masses of extramedullary hematopoietic tissue may be noted and signs of iron overload may also be present.

Laboratory Findings
The anemia is normocytic and is generally mild. Hemoglobin levels are lower in children than adults and range between 8 and 11 g/dL. The reticulocyte count, although inadequate, may appear to be normal or increased. Anisopoikilocytosis is noted and occasional basophilic stippling, as well as a few, sometimes binucleate, mature erythroblasts may be found on the peripheral smear. The bone marrow aspirate is normoblastic but hypercellular, with erythroid hyperplasia. In contrast to CDA I, there are many binucleate late polychromatic erythroblasts (10-35%) as well as a few that are multinucleate. Pseudo-Gaucher cells may be present. Electron micrographs show vesicles that are laden with endoplasmic reticulum proteins running beneath the plasma membrane. The pathognomonic finding in type II CDA is that the patient's RBCs lyse in acidified serum because of an immunoglobulin M antibody that recognizes an antigen present on CDA II cells but absent on normal cells. Type II CDA is also known by the acronym **HEMPAS** (*h*ereditary *e*rythroblastic *m*ultinuclearity with a *p*ositive *a*cidified *s*erum test) because it features both erythroblast multinuclearity and circulating RBCs that are sensitive to lysis by acidified normal serum. As this test is technically difficult, the diagnosis is usually made by analyzing red cell membrane proteins via sodium dodecyl sulfate-polyacrylamide gel electrophoresis (SDS-PAGE). In CDAII there is a thinner band size and faster migration of erythrocyte anion transporter (EA1), or band 3, and band 4.5 proteins.

Treatment
Approximately 10% of patients will require red cell transfusions in infancy and childhood but rarely during adulthood. In contrast to type I CDA, splenectomy may provide hematologic improvement. Splenectomy does not prevent further iron overloading, even in those patients whose hemoglobin is normalized, presumably because of persistent ineffective erythropoiesis in the bone marrow. Like CDA I, secondary hemochromatosis is the most prominent long-term complication and should be approached as outlined above. Allogeneic bone marrow transplantation was successful when pursued in an adult with CDA II and β-thalassemia trait. Most patients can lead a normal life and have a normal life expectancy if complications and consequences are managed appropriately.

TYPE III CONGENITAL DYSERYTHROPOIETIC ANEMIA
Type III CDA is an extremely rare, ill-defined entity, manifested by a mild-to-moderate macrocytic anemia. It is inherited in an autosomal dominant fashion, although there have been cases that might represent de novo mutations or other inheritance patterns. The gene for type III CDA is *KIF23*, which encodes a ubiquitous protein that regulates daughter cell separation during mitosis. In contrast to other CDA types, iron overload is not clinically significant (probably because hemolysis is predominantly intravascular) and spleen size is generally normal. Patients can present with angioid streaks with macular degeneration. The blood smear shows macrocytes, anisopoikilocytosis, and occasional basophilic stippling. The bone marrow is notable for giant erythroid precursors that are often multinucleated, containing up to 12 nuclei per cell. Such multinucleated erythroblasts can also be seen in myelodysplasia and erythroleukemia. Transfusions are usually not required.

Bibliography is available at Expert Consult.

Chapter 453
Physiologic Anemia of Infancy
Norma B. Lerner

At birth, normal full-term infants have higher hemoglobin (Hb) levels and larger red blood cells (RBCs) than do older children and adults. However, within the 1st wk of life, a progressive decline in Hb level begins and then persists for 6-8 wk. The resulting anemia is known as the **physiologic anemia of infancy.**

With the onset of respiration at birth, considerably more oxygen becomes available for binding to Hb, and, as a consequence, the Hb–oxygen saturation increases from 50% to 95% or more. There is also a gradual, normal developmental switch from fetal to adult Hb synthesis after birth that results in the replacement of high-oxygen-affinity fetal Hb with lower-affinity adult Hb, capable of delivering more oxygen to tissues. The increase in blood oxygen content and delivery results in the downregulation of erythropoietin (EPO) production, leading to suppression of erythropoiesis. Because there is no erythropoiesis, aged RBCs that are removed from the circulation are not replaced and the Hb level decreases. The Hb concentration continues to decline until tissue oxygen needs become greater than oxygen delivery. Normally, this point is reached between 8 and 12 wk of age, when the Hb concentration is about 11 g/dL. In healthy term infants, the nadir rarely falls below 10 g/dL. At this juncture, EPO production increases and erythropoiesis resumes. The supply of stored reticuloendothelial iron, derived from previously degraded RBCs, remains sufficient for this renewed Hb synthesis, even in the absence of dietary iron intake, until approximately 20 wk of age. In all, this "anemia" should be viewed as a physiologic adaptation to extrauterine life, reflecting the excess oxygen delivery relative to tissue oxygen requirements. There is no hematologic problem, and no therapy is required unless physiologic anemia of infancy is exacerbated by other ongoing processes.

A late **hyporegenerative anemia**, with absence of reticulocytes, can occur in infants with mild hemolytic disease of the newborn. The persistence of maternally derived anti-RBC antibodies in the infant's circulation can lead to an ongoing low-grade hemolytic anemia that can exaggerate the physiologic anemia. Lower-than-expected Hb at the "physiologic" nadir has also been seen in infants after intrauterine or neonatal RBC transfusions. When infants are transfused with adult blood containing HbA, the associated shift of the oxygen dissociation curve facilitates oxygen delivery to the tissues. Accordingly, the definition of anemia and the need for transfusion should be based not only on the infant's Hb level, but also on oxygen requirements and the ability of circulating RBCs to release oxygen to the tissues.

Premature infants also develop a physiologic anemia, known as *physiologic anemia of prematurity*. The Hb decline is both more extreme and more rapid. Minimal Hb levels of 7-9 g/dL commonly are reached by 3-6 wk of age, and levels may be even lower in very small premature infants (see Chapter 103). The same physiologic factors at play in term infants are operative in preterm infants but are exaggerated. In premature infants, the physiologic Hb decline may be intensified by blood loss from repeated phlebotomies obtained to monitor ill neonates. Demands on erythropoiesis are further heightened by the premature infant's shortened RBC life span (40-60 days) and the accelerated expansion of RBC mass that accompanies the premature baby's rapid rate of growth. Nonetheless, plasma EPO levels are lower than would be expected for the degree of anemia, resulting in a suboptimal erythropoietic response. The reason for diminished EPO levels is not fully understood. During fetal life, EPO synthesis is handled primarily by the liver, whose oxygen sensor is relatively insensitive to hypoxia when compared to the oxygen sensor of the kidney. The developmental switch from liver to kidney EPO production is not accelerated by early birth, and thus the preterm infant must rely on the liver as the primary site for synthesis, leading to diminished responsiveness to anemia. An additional mechanism thought to contribute to diminished EPO levels may be accelerated EPO metabolism. As the pronounced decline in Hb that occurs in many very low birthweight infants is associated with abnormal clinical signs, this "anemia of prematurity" is not considered to be benign and usually requires transfusions.

Some dietary factors, such as folic acid deficiency, can aggravate physiologic anemia. Unless there has been significant blood loss, iron stores should be sufficient to maintain erythropoiesis early on. Vitamin E deficiency does not play a role in anemia of prematurity. Breast milk and infant formulas provide adequate vitamin E.

TREATMENT

In the full-term infant, physiologic anemia requires no therapy beyond ensuring that the infant's diet contains essential nutrients for normal hematopoiesis. In premature infants, an optimal Hb has not been established and is usually dictated by the infant's overall clinical condition. Transfusions may be needed to maintain the Hb at what is considered safe for that child. Premature infants who are feeding well and growing normally rarely need transfusion unless iatrogenic blood loss has been significant. Although factors such as poor weight gain, respiratory difficulties, and abnormal heart rate have prompted transfusion, the beneficial effect has not been documented. Laboratory tests such as blood lactate, EPO, and mixed venous oxygen saturation have poor predictive value. Liberal and restrictive transfusion strategies have been compared in this population. A restrictive strategy does not increase infant morbidity or mortality. In addition, long-term neurodevelopmental outcomes have been found to be poorer in liberally transfused neonates. Late exposure to packed RBC may be related to the development of necrotizing enterocolitis, and early transfusions may be associated with the risk of intraventricular hemorrhage.

When transfusions are necessary, an RBC volume of 10-15 mL/kg is recommended. It is good practice to split units derived from a single donor so that sequential transfusions can be given as required and donor exposure can be minimized. In early preterm infants (weighing <1,250 g), the half-life of transfused RBCs is about 30 days. Delayed cord clamping or umbilical cord milking at birth results in fewer transfusions and a reduction in both intraventricular hemorrhage and necrotizing enterocolitis in preterm infants. Given the impact of phlebotomy losses during monitoring in the neonatal ICU, attention to reducing unnecessary blood draws also has been advocated.

Because premature infants are known to have low plasma EPO levels, recombinant human EPO may be an alternative to transfusion for the treatment of symptomatic preterm infants with anemia of prematurity. In early studies, it was unclear whether EPO reliably reduced donor exposures and reports of adverse effects, such as a possible increase in retinopathy of prematurity, further limited a willingness to use this expensive treatment. One study of preterm infants compared the weekly use of the long-acting agent darbepoetin to triweekly EPO or placebo. Supplemental iron, folate, and vitamin E were provided and the infants were transfused according to an established protocol. Those receiving either EPO or darbepoetin received half the number of transfusions and about half the donors compared with the placebo group. The incidence of mortality, retinopathy, and intracranial hemorrhage was no different between the groups. Nonetheless, this remains an area of controversy.

Bibliography is available at Expert Consult.

Chapter 454
Megaloblastic Anemias
Norma B. Lerner

Megaloblastic anemia describes a group of disorders that are caused by impaired DNA synthesis. Red blood cells (RBCs) are larger than normal at every developmental stage, and there is maturational asynchrony between the nucleus and cytoplasm of erythrocytes. The delayed nuclear development becomes increasingly evident as cell divisions proceed. Myeloid and platelet precursors are also affected, and giant metamyelocytes and neutrophil bands are often present in the bone marrow. *There is often an associated thrombocytopenia and leukopenia.* The peripheral blood smear is notable for large, often oval, RBCs with increased mean corpuscular volume. Neutrophils are characteristically hypersegmented, with many having >5 lobes. Most cases of childhood megaloblastic anemia result from a deficiency of folic acid or vitamin B_{12} (cobalamin), vitamins essential for DNA synthesis. Rarely, these anemias may be caused by inborn errors of metabolism. Megaloblastic anemias resulting from malnutrition are relatively uncommon in the United States, but are important worldwide (see Chapters 46 and 447).

454.1 Folic Acid Deficiency
Norma B. Lerner

Folic acid, or pteroylglutamic acid, consists of pteroic acid conjugated to glutamic acid. Biologically active folates are derived from folic acid and serve as 1-carbon donors and acceptors in many biosynthetic pathways. To form functional compounds, folates must be reduced to tetrahydrofolates in a process catalyzed by the enzyme dihydrofolate reductase. As such, they are essential for DNA replication and cellular proliferation. Like other mammals, humans cannot synthesize folate and depend on dietary sources, including green vegetables, fruits, and animal organs (e.g., liver, kidney). Folates are heat labile and water soluble; consequently, boiling or heating folate sources leads to decreased amounts of vitamin. Naturally occurring folates are in a polyglutamated form that is less efficiently absorbed than the monoglutamate species (i.e., folic acid). Dietary folate polyglutamates are hydrolyzed to simple folates that are absorbed primarily in the proximal small intestine by a specific carrier-mediated system. Folates travel in the bloodstream and are taken up in cells primarily in the form of unconjugated methyltetrahydrofolate, which is subsequently reconjugated (polyglutamated) in the cell. There is an active enterohepatic circulation. Although rare, megaloblastic anemia as a consequence of folate deficiency has its peak incidence at 4-7 mo of age, somewhat earlier than iron-deficiency anemia, although both conditions may be present concomitantly in infants with poor nutrition.

ETIOLOGY

Folic acid deficiency can occur as a consequence of inadequate folate intake, decreased folate absorption, or acquired and congenital disorders of folate metabolism or transport.

Inadequate Folate Intake

In the United States, anemia caused by insufficient folate intake usually occurs in the context of increased vitamin requirements associated with pregnancy, periods of accelerated growth, and/or chronic hemolysis. Folate requirements increase markedly during pregnancy, in part to meet fetal needs, and deficiencies are common in mothers, particularly those who are poor or malnourished. Folate supplementation is recommended from the start of pregnancy to prevent neural tube defects and to meet the needs of the developing fetus. Fortunately, folate-deficient mothers generally do not give birth to infants with clinical folate deficiency because there is selective transfer of folate to the fetus via placental folate receptors. Rapid growth after birth increases demands for folic acid and infants who are premature or ill and those with certain hemolytic disorders will have particularly high folate requirements. Human breast milk, infant formulas, and pasteurized cow's milk provide adequate amounts of folic acid. *Goat's milk is deficient*, and supplementation must be given when it is the child's main food. Unless supplemented, powdered milk may also be a poor source of folic acid.

Malnutrition is the most common cause of folate deficiency in older children, and those with hemoglobinopathies, infections, and/or malabsorption are at increased risk. Because body stores of folate are limited, deficiency can develop quickly in malnourished individuals. On a folate-free diet, megaloblastic anemia will occur after 2-3 mo.

Decreased Folate Absorption

Malabsorption caused by chronic diarrheal states or diffuse inflammatory disease can lead to folate deficiency. In both situations, some of the decreased folate absorption may be caused by impaired folate conjugase activity. Chronic diarrhea also interferes with the enterohepatic circulation of folate, thereby enhancing folate losses because of rapid intestinal passage. Megaloblastic anemia because of folic acid deficiency can occur in celiac disease or chronic infectious enteritis and in association with enteroenteric fistulas. Previous intestinal surgery is another potential cause of decreased folate absorption.

Certain anticonvulsant drugs (e.g., phenytoin, primidone, phenobarbital) can impair folic acid absorption, and many patients treated with these drugs have low serum levels. Frank megaloblastic anemia is rare and readily responds to folic acid therapy, even when administration of the offending drug is continued. Alcohol overuse also is associated with folate malabsorption.

Congenital Abnormalities in Folate Transport and Metabolism

Inborn errors of folate transport or metabolism are rare but can be life-threatening. Those associated with megaloblastic anemia include hereditary folate malabsorption and certain extremely uncommon enzyme deficiencies.

Hereditary folate malabsorption (HFM) is an autosomal recessive disorder that is linked to several loss-of-function mutations in the *SLC46A1* gene encoding the protein-coupled folate transporter. HFM is associated with an inability to absorb folic acid, 5-tetrahydrofolate, 5-methyltetrahydrofolate, or 5-formyltetrahydrofolate (folinic acid). It can become apparent at 2-6 mo of age with megaloblastic anemia and other deficits, including infections and diarrhea. Neurologic abnormalities, attributable to folate deficiency in the central nervous system, include seizures, developmental delay, and mental retardation. Folate transport is impaired in both the intestine and at the brain's choroid plexus. Serum and cerebrospinal fluid (CSF) folate levels are very low, with a loss of the normal 3:1 ratio of CSF to serum folate.

Treatment, specifically in the context of HFM, usually involves parenteral folate, although oral administration has been useful in some cases. Reduced folates are more effective than folic acid. Folate sufficiency should be maintained in both the blood and the CSF so as to avoid important complications. The megaloblastic anemia in HFM can be reversed with relatively low levels of serum folate, but adequate CSF levels may be quite difficult to achieve, and very large folate doses may be needed.

Functional methionine synthase deficiency may result from mutations affecting the function of methionine synthase reductase or methionine synthase. These disorders are autosomal recessive and are characterized not only by megaloblastic anemia, but also by cerebral atrophy, nystagmus, blindness, and altered muscle tone. Both respond to hydroxocobalamin plus betaine with variable clinical success. Dihydrofolate reductase deficiency is extremely rare and is associated with homozygous mutations in the DHFR gene. Clinical symptoms include megaloblastic anemia and neurologic manifestations. Although **methylenetetrahydrofolate (MTHFR) deficiency** is the most common inborn error of folate metabolism and severe cases can produce a number of neurologic and vascular complications, there is no associated megaloblastic anemia.

Drug-Induced Abnormalities in Folate Metabolism

A number of drugs have anti–folic acid activity as their primary pharmacologic effect and regularly produce megaloblastic anemia. Methotrexate binds to dihydrofolate reductase and prevents formation of tetrahydrofolate, the active form of folate. Pyrimethamine, used in the therapy of toxoplasmosis, and trimethoprim, used for treatment of various infections, can induce folic acid deficiency and, occasionally, megaloblastic anemia. Therapy with folinic acid (5-formyltetrahydrofolate) is usually beneficial.

CLINICAL MANIFESTATIONS

Besides the clinical features associated with anemia, folate-deficient infants and children may manifest irritability, chronic diarrhea, and/or poor weight gain. Hemorrhages from thrombocytopenia may occur in advanced cases. Congenital folate malabsorption and other rare etiologies of folate deficiency may be further associated with hypogammaglobulinemia, severe infections, failure to thrive, neurologic abnormalities, and cognitive delays.

LABORATORY FINDINGS

The anemia is macrocytic (mean corpuscular volume >100 fL). Variations in RBC shape and size are common (see Fig. 447-4B in Chapter 447). The reticulocyte count is low, and nucleated RBCs with megaloblastic morphology are often seen in the peripheral blood. Neutropenia and thrombocytopenia may be present, particularly in patients with long-standing and severe deficiencies. The neutrophils are large, some with hypersegmented nuclei. The bone marrow is hypercellular because of erythroid hyperplasia, and megaloblastic changes are prominent. Large, abnormal neutrophilic forms (giant metamyelocytes) with cytoplasmic vacuolation are also seen.

Normal serum folic acid levels are 5-20 ng/mL; with deficiency, levels are <3 ng/mL. Levels of RBC folate are a better indicator of chronic deficiency. The normal RBC folate level is 150-600 ng/mL of packed cells. Levels of iron and vitamin B_{12} in serum usually are normal or elevated. Serum activity of lactate dehydrogenase, a marker of ineffective erythropoiesis, is markedly elevated.

TREATMENT

When the diagnosis of folate deficiency is established, folic acid may be administered orally or parenterally at 0.5-1.0 mg/day. If the specific diagnosis is in doubt, smaller doses of folate (0.1 mg/day) may be used for 1 wk as a diagnostic test, because a hematologic response can be expected within 72 hr. Doses of folate >0.1 mg can correct the anemia of vitamin B_{12} deficiency but might aggravate any associated neurologic abnormalities. In most medical settings in developed countries, this therapeutic trial to distinguish the different causes of megaloblastic anemia is rarely necessary because vitamin B_{12} and folate blood levels are usually readily available. Folic acid therapy (0.5-1.0 mg/day) should be continued for 3-4 wk until a definite hematologic response has occurred. Maintenance therapy with a multivitamin (containing 0.2 mg of folate) is adequate. As described above, very high doses of folate may be required in the setting of HFM. Transfusions are indicated only when the anemia is severe or the child is very ill.

Bibliography is available at Expert Consult.

454.2 Vitamin B₁₂ (Cobalamin) Deficiency

Norma B. Lerner

Vitamin B_{12}, a generic term encompassing all biologically active cobalamins, is a water-soluble vitamin with a central, functional cobalt atom and a planar corrin ring. Methylcobalamin and adenosylcobalamin are the metabolically active derivatives, serving as cofactors in 2 essential metabolic reactions, namely methylation of homocysteine to methionine (via methionine synthase) and conversion of methyl-malonyl-coenzyme A (CoA) to succinyl CoA (via L-methyl-malonyl-CoA mutase). The products and by-products of these enzymatic reactions are critical to DNA, RNA, and protein synthesis.

Cobalamin is synthesized exclusively by microorganisms and humans must rely on dietary sources (animal products including meat, eggs, fish, and milk) for their needs. Unlike folate, older children and adults have sufficient vitamin B_{12} stores to last 3-5 yr. In young infants born to mothers with low vitamin B_{12} stores, clinical signs of cobalamin deficiency can become apparent in the first 6-18 mo of life.

METABOLISM

Under normal circumstances, cobalamin is released from food protein in the stomach via peptic digestion. Cobalamin then binds to haptocorrin (HC), a salivary glycoprotein. This complex moves into the duodenum, where HC is digested by pancreatic proteases and cobalamin is liberated. Cobalamin then binds to intrinsic factor (IF), another glycoprotein that is produced by gastric parietal cells. The cobalamin-IF complex subsequently enters mucosal cells of the distal ilium by receptor-mediated endocytosis. The IF-cobalamin receptors are composed of a complex of 2 proteins, cubilin (CUBN) and amnionless (AMN), collectively known as cubam. Following internalization into enterocytes, IF is degraded in the lysosome and cobalamin is released. The transporter ABCC1 (also known as MRP1) exports cobalamin bound to the transport protein transcobalamin (TC), out of the cell. In the bloodstream, cobalamin is associated with either TC (approximately 20%) or HC. TC mediates B_{12}'s transport across cells after complexing with the TC receptor, which is internalized in the lysosome. Lysosomal degradation of TC releases cobalamin which remains in the cell where it is further processed. Two distinct membrane proteins transport cobalamin across the lysosomal membrane into the cytoplasm. There cobalamins are processed to a common intermediate that can be allocated to the methylcobalamin and adenosylcobalamin synthesis pathways to meet cellular needs. It is postulated that the MMACHC protein, a product of the cobalamin (Cbl) C locus, accepts the cobalamins exiting the lysosome. A definitive role for HC is yet to be established, but it has been suggested that it plays a role in B_{12} storage.

ETIOLOGY

Vitamin B_{12} deficiency can result from inadequate dietary intake of Cbl, lack of IF, impaired intestinal absorption of IF-Cbl, or absence of vitamin B_{12} transport protein

Inadequate Vitamin B₁₂ Intake

B_{12} deficiency in infants is most often nutritional, resulting from low Cbl levels in the breast milk of B_{12}-deficient mothers. Associated megaloblastic anemia often appears during the 1st yr of life. Maternal deficiency may be caused by pernicious anemia or gastrointestinal disorders such as *Helicobacter pylori* infection, celiac disease, Crohn disease, or pancreatic insufficiency. Previous gastric bypass surgery, treatment with proton pump inhibitors, or inadequate intake from a strict vegetarian diet has also been implicated. Fortunately, as a result of active placental Cbl transport in utero, most children of deficient

mothers maintain Cbl levels sufficient to support adequate prenatal development. Such infants are born with low stores, the depletion of which is associated with a gradual onset of clinical manifestations. B_{12} replacement often results in rapid improvement, but the longer the deficient period, the greater the likelihood of permanent disabilities. Neonatal screening programs may detect maternal–neonatal nutritional B_{12} deficiency as a result of an increase in propionyl carnitine, but there is higher sensitivity using a measurement of methylmalonic acid. In high-income countries, dietary deficiency during childhood or adolescence is infrequent but can result, as in adults, from strict vegetarian or vegan diet. Daily requirements range from 0.4-2.4 μg.

Impaired Absorption

Gastric surgery or medications that impair gastric acid secretion may result in IF deficiency, leading to decreased vitamin B_{12} absorption. Pancreatic insufficiency can also lead to Cbl deficiency as a consequence of impaired cleavage and IF complex formation. Patients with neonatal necrotizing enterocolitis, inflammatory bowel disease, celiac disease, or surgical removal of the terminal ileum, may also have impaired absorption of vitamin B_{12}. An overgrowth of intestinal bacteria within diverticula or duplications of the small intestine can cause vitamin B_{12} deficiency by consumption of (or competition for) the vitamin or by splitting of its complex with IF. In these cases, hematologic response can follow appropriate antibiotic therapy. In endemic areas, when the fish tapeworm *Diphyllobothrium latum* infests the upper small intestine, similar mechanisms may be operative. When megaloblastic anemia occurs in such situations, the serum vitamin B_{12} level is low and the gastric fluid contains IF.

Hereditary intrinsic factor deficiency (HIFD) is a rare autosomal recessive disorder caused by a variety of mutations in the IF gene that produce a lack of gastric IF or a functionally abnormal IF. It differs from typical adult pernicious anemia in that gastric acid is secreted normally and the stomach is histologically normal. It is not associated with antibodies or endocrine abnormalities. Unlike Imerslund-Grasbeck syndrome (described below), hereditary IF deficiency is only occasionally associated with proteinuria. Symptoms become prominent at an early age (6-24 mo), consistent with exhaustion of vitamin B_{12} stores acquired in utero. As the anemia becomes severe, weakness, irritability, anorexia, and listlessness occur. The tongue is smooth, red, and painful. Neurologic manifestations include ataxia, paresthesias, hyporeflexia, Babinski responses, and clonus. Oral vitamin B_{12} is usually ineffective and lifelong parenteral (IM) Cbl should be used to bypass the absorption defect. The natural form, hydroxocobalamin (OHCbl) is believed to be more effective than the synthetic form, cyanocobalamin (CNCbl). In one retrospective study involving patients with HIFD and Imerslund-Grasbeck syndrome, patients with acute and severe anemia were initially treated with 1 mg of IM OHCbl daily until reticulocyte recovery after which dosing was spaced to once a week. Those without severe anemia were treated with weekly IM OHCbl or CNCbl. With cautious monitoring, all patients were ultimately safely maintained on a schedule of 1 mg of IM OHCbl or CNCbl every 6 mo.

Imerslund-Grasbeck syndrome is a rare, recessively inherited pediatric disorder resulting in selective vitamin B_{12} malabsorption in the ileum, and consequent vitamin B_{12} deficiency. It usually becomes clinically apparent within the first 6 yr of life. In addition to megaloblastic anemia, the patient may also have neurologic defects (such as hypotonia, developmental delay, brain atrophy, movement disorders, and dementia) and/or proteinuria. Patients carry mutations in either CUBN or AMN, proteins that form the cubam receptor for the ileal IF-Cbl complex. Because CUBN is also a key receptor for protein reabsorption in the kidney, impaired expression at this site results in associated proteinuria. The disease can be fatal if it remains untreated. Early diagnosis and treatment with IM Cbl (see treatment for HIFD above) will reverse the hematologic and neurologic abnormalities. Proteinuria does not respond to therapy.

Classic pernicious anemia (autoimmune gastritis) usually occurs in older adults but can rarely affect children. This disorder (juvenile pernicious anemia) usually presents during adolescence. In such cases, the disease is associated with various detectable antibodies, including those against IF and the hydrogen potassium adenosine triphosphatase proton pump in gastric parietal cells. These children can have additional immunologic abnormalities, cutaneous candidiasis, hypoparathyroidism, and other endocrine deficiencies. There may be atrophy of the gastric mucosa and achlorhydria. Parenteral vitamin B_{12} should be administered regularly.

Absence of Vitamin B_{12} Transport Protein

TC deficiency is a rare cause of megaloblastic anemia. A congenital deficiency is inherited as an autosomal recessive condition resulting in a failure to absorb and transport vitamin B_{12}. Most patients lack TC but some have functionally defective forms. This disorder usually manifests in the first weeks of life. Characteristically, there is failure to thrive, diarrhea, vomiting, glossitis, neurologic abnormalities, and megaloblastic anemia. The diagnosis can be difficult given that total serum vitamin B_{12} levels are often normal because approximately 80% of serum Cbl is bound to HC. The diagnosis is suggested by the presence of severe megaloblastic anemia in the face of normal folate levels and no evidence of any other inborn errors of metabolism. Plasma homocysteine and/or methylmalonic acid levels are elevated. A definitive diagnosis is made by measuring plasma TC. The serum vitamin B_{12} levels must be kept high in order to force enough Cbl into cells to allow normal function. Oral Cbl (CNCbl or OHCbl) 500-1,000 μg twice a wk, or IM OHCbl 1,000 μg per wk, may be used for initial therapy. Symptoms and laboratory studies should be monitored and doses adjusted as needed.

Inborn Errors of Cobalamin Metabolism

The conversion of Cbl to methylcobalamin (MeCbl) and adenosylcobalamin (AdoCbl) involves a number of steps, abnormalities of which have been tied to several distinct alphabetically labeled disorders. In CblE and CblG, defective N5-methyltetrahydrofolate-homocysteine methyltransferase fails to produce MeCbl. Patients present in infancy with megaloblastic anemia, vomiting, and mental retardation, and are found to have homocystinuria and hyperhomocysteinemia. They do not have methylmalonic aciduria or methylmalonic acidemia. They show good response to CNCbl. AdoCbl and MeCbl are both affected by CblC (the most common of the Cbl inborn errors), CblD, and CblF. Patients can present in early infancy through adolescence. Newborns have lethargy, failure to thrive, and neurologic problems. Older patients may present with neurologic difficulties, dementia, and psychological problems. Megaloblastic anemia occurs in about half the cases. Patients have elevations of homocysteine and methylmalonic acid in both urine and blood. Affected individuals respond partially to OHCbl or CNCbl. CblA, CblB, and CblH are associated with methylmalonic aciduria and a variety of serious symptoms, but megaloblastic anemia is absent.

CLINICAL MANIFESTATIONS

Children with Cbl deficiency often present with nonspecific manifestations such as weakness, lethargy, feeding difficulties, failure to thrive, and irritability. Other common findings include pallor, glossitis, vomiting, diarrhea, and icterus. Neurologic symptoms can include paresthesia, sensory deficits, hypotonia, seizures, developmental delay, developmental regression, and neuropsychiatric changes. Neurologic problems from vitamin B_{12} deficiency may occur in the absence of any hematologic abnormalities.

LABORATORY FINDINGS

The hematologic manifestations of folate and Cbl deficiency are identical. The anemia resulting from Cbl deficiency is macrocytic, with prominent macro-ovalocytosis of the RBCs (see Fig. 447-2 in Chapter 447). The neutrophils may be large and hypersegmented. In advanced cases, neutropenia and thrombocytopenia can occur, simulating aplastic anemia or leukemia. Serum vitamin B_{12} levels are low, and the serum concentrations of methylmalonic acid and homocysteine are usually elevated. Concentrations of serum iron and serum folic acid are normal or elevated. Serum lactate dehydrogenase activity is markedly increased, a reflection of ineffective erythropoiesis. Moderate elevations of serum bilirubin levels (2-3 mg/dL) also may be found.

Excessive excretion of methylmalonic acid in the urine (normal, 0-3.5 mg/24 hr) is a reliable and sensitive index of vitamin B_{12} deficiency.

DIAGNOSIS

A comprehensive medical history is essential to the clinical recognition of possible Cbl deficiency. Information regarding clinical symptoms, dietary history, diseases, surgeries, or medications are likely to provide important clues. The physical exam may reveal relevant findings such as irritability, pallor, or specific neurologic symptoms. Screening laboratory findings (described above) offer important information but more focused testing will be required to confirm a diagnosis of vitamin B_{12} deficiency and its cause. Cbl deficiency is usually identified by measuring total or TC bound vitamin B_{12} in the blood. Although an extremely low level is generally diagnostic, this may not be the case, and false negatives and positives are reportedly common using currently available assays. As a result, it is wise not to discount vitamin B deficiency, particularly in the face of clinical symptoms, macrocytic anemia, an abnormal blood smear, and a normal folate level. In nontreated patients, methylmalonic acid and total homocystine levels are often helpful as they are markedly elevated in the majority of those with clinical signs of B_{12} deficiency. Excessive excretion of methylmalonic acid in the urine (normal: 0-3.5 mg/24 hr) is also a sensitive index of vitamin B_{12} deficiency. Although modest increases occur with renal failure, elevated methylmalonic acid is otherwise quite specific for vitamin B_{12} deficiency. Notably, however, serum homocystine is also elevated in folate deficiency, homocystinuria, and renal failure.

If B_{12} deficiency has been confirmed and there is no evidence of inadequate dietary intake or, in the case of an infant, inadequate maternal B_{12}, malabsorption should be investigated. In the past, the Schilling test, a measure of Cbl absorption, was the gold standard. The test is no longer available and there is currently no comparable replacement for it. Anti–IF antibodies and anti–parietal cell antibodies are useful for the diagnosis of pernicious anemia. Measurement of IF and help from more specialized laboratories may be required for less common disorders.

TREATMENT

Treatment regimens in children have not been well studied. The cause of vitamin B_{12} deficiency should ultimately dictate treatment dosage as well as the duration of therapy. Dose adjustments should be made in response to clinical status and laboratory values. The physiologic requirement for vitamin B_{12} is about 1-3 μg/day. Hematologic responses have been observed with small doses, indicating that administration of a minidose may be used as a therapeutic test when the diagnosis of vitamin B_{12} deficiency is in doubt or in circumstances where the anemia is severe and higher initial doses might result in severe metabolic disturbances.

Bibliography is available at Expert Consult.

454.3 Other Rare Megaloblastic Anemias
Norma B. Lerner

Orotic aciduria is a rare autosomal recessive disorder that usually appears in the 1st yr of life and is characterized by growth failure, developmental retardation, megaloblastic anemia, and increased urinary excretion of orotic acid (see Chapter 89). This defect is the most common metabolic error in the de novo synthesis of pyrimidines and therefore affects nucleic acid synthesis. The usual form of hereditary orotic aciduria is caused by a deficiency (in all body tissues) of orotic phosphoribosyl transferase and orotidine-5-phosphate decarboxylase, 2 sequential enzymatic steps in pyrimidine nucleotide synthesis. The diagnosis is suggested by the presence of severe megaloblastic anemia with normal serum B_{12} and folate levels and no evidence of TC deficiency. A presumptive diagnosis is made by finding increased urinary orotic acid. However, confirmation of the diagnosis requires assay of the transferase and decarboxylase enzymes in the patient's erythrocytes. Physical and mental retardation often accompany this condition. The anemia is refractory to vitamin B_{12} or folic acid, but responds promptly to administration of uridine.

Thiamine-responsive megaloblastic anemia (Rogers syndrome) is a very rare autosomal recessive disorder characterized by megaloblastic anemia, sensorineural deafness, and diabetes mellitus. Congenital heart defects, arrhythmias, visual problems, short stature, tri-lineage myelodysplasia, and strokes are also described. Thiamine-responsive megaloblastic anemia usually presents in infancy but may occasionally develop in childhood and adolescence and occurs in several ethnically distinct populations. The bone marrow is characterized not only by megaloblastic changes but also by ringed sideroblasts. The defect is caused by mutations in the *SCL19A2* gene on chromosome 1, which encodes a high-affinity plasma membrane thiamine transporter. Continuous thiamine supplementation usually reverses the anemia and diabetes but not existing hearing defects.

Bibliography is available at Expert Consult.

Chapter **455**
Iron-Deficiency Anemia
Richard Sills

Iron deficiency is the most widespread and common nutritional disorder in the world. It is estimated that 30% of the global population has iron-deficiency anemia, and most of them live in developing countries. In the United States, 9% of children ages 12-36 mo are *iron deficient*, and 30% of this group progresses to iron-deficiency *anemia*.

A full-term newborn infant contains about 0.5 g of iron, compared to 5 g of iron in adults. This change in quantity of iron from birth to adulthood means that an average of 0.8 mg of iron must be absorbed each day during the first 15 yr of life. A small additional amount is necessary to balance normal losses of iron by shedding of cells. It is therefore necessary to absorb approximately 1 mg daily to maintain positive iron balance in childhood. Because <10% of dietary iron usually is absorbed, a dietary intake of 8-10 mg of iron daily is necessary to maintain iron levels. During infancy, when growth is most rapid, the approximately 1 mg/L of iron in cow's and breast milk makes it difficult to maintain body iron. Breastfed infants have an advantage because they absorb iron 2-3 times more efficiently than infants fed cow's milk.

ETIOLOGY

Most iron in neonates is in circulating hemoglobin. As the relatively high hemoglobin concentration of the newborn infant falls during the first 2-3 mo of life, considerable iron is recycled. These iron stores are usually sufficient for blood formation in the first 6-9 mo of life in term infants. Stores are depleted sooner in low-birthweight infants or infants with perinatal blood loss because their iron stores are smaller. Delayed (1-3 min) clamping of the umbilical cord can improve iron status and reduce the risk of iron deficiency, whereas early clamping (<30 sec) puts the infant at risk for iron deficiency. Dietary sources of iron are especially important in these infants. In term infants, anemia caused solely by inadequate dietary iron usually occurs at 9-24 mo of age and is relatively uncommon thereafter. The usual dietary pattern observed in infants and toddlers with nutritional iron-deficiency anemia in developed countries is excessive consumption of cow's milk (low iron content, blood loss from milk protein colitis) in a child who is often overweight. Worldwide, undernutrition is usually responsible for iron deficiency.

Blood loss must be considered as a possible cause in every case of iron-deficiency anemia, particularly in older children and adolescents.

Chronic iron-deficiency anemia from occult bleeding may be caused by a lesion of the gastrointestinal (GI) tract, such as peptic ulcer, Meckel diverticulum, polyp, hemangioma, or inflammatory bowel disease. Infants can have chronic intestinal blood loss induced by exposure to whole cow's milk protein. This GI reaction is not related to enzymatic abnormalities in the mucosa, such as lactase deficiency, or to an immunoglobulin E–associated milk allergy. Involved infants characteristically develop anemia that is more severe and occurs earlier than would be expected simply from an inadequate intake of iron. The ongoing loss of blood in the stools can be prevented either by breastfeeding or by delaying the introduction of whole cow's milk in the 1st yr of life and then limiting the quantity to <24 oz/24 hr. Unrecognized blood loss also can be associated with chronic diarrhea and, rarely, with pulmonary hemosiderosis. In developing countries, infections with hookworm, *Trichuris trichiura*, *Plasmodium*, and *Helicobacter pylori* often contribute to iron deficiency. Celiac disease and giardiasis may interfere with iron absorption.

Approximately 2% of adolescent girls have iron-deficiency anemia, largely as a result of their adolescent growth spurt and menstrual blood loss. The highest risk of iron-deficiency anemia (>30%) is among teenagers who are or have been pregnant.

CLINICAL MANIFESTATIONS

Most children with iron deficiency are asymptomatic and are identified by recommended laboratory screening at 12 mo of age, or sooner if at high risk. Pallor is the most important clinical sign of iron deficiency but is not usually visible until the hemoglobin falls to 7-8 g/dL. It is most readily noted as pallor of the palms, palmar creases, nail beds, or conjunctivae. Parents often fail to note the pallor because of the typical slow decline of hemoglobin over time. Often a visiting friend or relative is the first to notice. In mild to moderate iron deficiency (i.e., hemoglobin levels of 6-10 g/dL), compensatory mechanisms, including increased levels of 2,3-diphosphoglycerate and a shift of the oxygen dissociation curve, may be so effective that few symptoms of anemia aside from mild irritability are noted. When the hemoglobin level falls to <5 g/dL, irritability, anorexia, and lethargy develop, and systolic flow murmurs are often heard. As the hemoglobin continues to fall, tachycardia and high output cardiac failure can occur.

Iron deficiency has nonhematologic systemic effects. Both iron deficiency and iron-deficiency anemia are associated with impaired neurocognitive function in infancy. There is also an association of iron-deficiency anemia and later, possibly irreversible, cognitive defects. Although there is support for iron deficiency with or without anemia causing these defects, it has not been established unequivocally. Some studies suggest an increased risk of seizures, strokes, breathholding spells in children, and exacerbations of restless leg syndrome in adults. Given the frequency of iron deficiency and iron-deficiency anemia and the potential for adverse neurodevelopmental outcomes, minimizing the incidence of iron deficiency is an important goal.

Other nonhematologic consequences of iron deficiency include pica, the desire to ingest nonnutritive substances, and **pagophagia,** the desire to ingest ice. The pica can result in the ingestion of lead-containing substances and result in concomitant **plumbism** (see Chapter 721).

LABORATORY FINDINGS

In progressive iron deficiency, a sequence of biochemical and hematologic events occurs (Tables 455-1 and 455-2). First, tissue iron stores are depleted. This depletion is reflected by reduced serum ferritin, an iron-storage protein, which provides an estimate of body iron stores in the absence of inflammatory disease. Next, serum iron levels decrease, the iron-binding capacity of the serum (serum transferrin) increases, and the transferrin saturation falls below normal. As iron stores decrease, iron becomes unavailable to complex with protoporphyrin to form heme. Free erythrocyte protoporphyrins accumulate, and hemoglobin synthesis is impaired. At this point, iron deficiency progresses to iron-deficiency anemia. With less available hemoglobin in each cell, the red cells become smaller and varied in size. The variation in red cell size is measured by an increasing red cell distribution width. This is followed by a decrease in mean corpuscular volume and mean corpuscular hemoglobin. Developmental changes in mean corpuscular

| Table 455-1 | Indicators of Iron-Deficiency Anemia |

INDICATOR	SELECTED CUTOFF VALUES TO DEFINE IRON DEFICIENCY	COMMENTS
Hemoglobin (g/dL)	<11.0 for non-Hispanic whites ages 0.5-4 yr	When used alone, it has low specificity and sensitivity. Use appropriate age specific normal values found in Table 447-1. Normal values for African-Americans are found in Table 447-2.
Mean corpuscular volume (MCV) (μm³)	<70 from 6-24 months	A reliable, but late indicator of iron deficiency (ID) Low values can also be a result of thalassemia and other causes of microcytosis. Normal values are found in Table 447-1.
Serum ferritin (SF) (μg/L)	≤5 yr <12 Children >5 yr <15 In all age groups in the presence of infection <30	It is probably the most useful laboratory measure of iron stores and helps identify ID; a low value of SF is diagnostic of iron-deficiency anemia (IDA) in a patient with anemia. SF is an acute phase reactant that increases in many acute or chronic inflammatory conditions independent of iron status. Combining SF with a measurement of C-reactive protein (CRP) helps to identify these false-negative SF results.
Reticulocyte hemoglobin content (CHr) (pg)	In infants and young children <27.5 In adults ≤28.0	A sensitive indicator that falls within days of onset of iron-deficient erythropoiesis and is unaffected by inflammation. It is an excellent tool to recognize ID as well as IDA. False normal values can occur when MCV is increased and in thalassemia. It is not yet widely available on hematology analyzers.
Serum transferrin receptor (sTfR)	Cutoff varies with assay and with patient's age and ethnic origin	This soluble receptor is upregulated in ID and is found in increased amounts in serum. It also increased during enhanced erythropoiesis. sTfR is not substantially affected by the acute-phase response, but it might be affected by malaria, age, and ethnicity. Its application is limited by high cost of commercial assays and lack of an international standard, but it has great promise as an indicator of ID.
Transferrin saturation	<16%	It is inexpensive, but its use is limited by diurnal variation in serum iron and by many clinical disorders that affect transferrin concentrations including in inflammatory conditions.
Erythrocyte zinc protoporphyrin (ZPP) (μmol/mol heme)	≤5 yr >70 Children >5 yr >80 Children >5 yr on washed red cells >40	It can be measured directly on a drop of blood with a portable hematofluorometer. A useful screening test in field surveys, particularly in children, in whom uncomplicated ID is the primary cause of anemia. Lead poisoning can increase values, particularly in urban and industrial settings.
Hepcidin	To be defined; usually ≤10 ng/mL	Extremely elevated in anemia of inflammation and suppressed in iron deficiency anemia

Modified from Zimmermann MB, Hurrell RF: Nutritional iron deficiency, Lancet 370:511–520, 2007.

| Table 455-2 | Laboratory Studies Differentiating the Most Common Microcytic Anemias |

STUDY	IRON-DEFICIENCY ANEMIA	α- OR β-THALASSEMIA	ANEMIA OF CHRONIC DISEASE
Hemoglobin	Decreased	Decreased	Decreased
MCV	Decreased	Decreased	Normal-decreased
RDW	Increased	Normal or minimally increased	Normal-increased
RBC	Decreased	Normal-increased	Normal-decreased
Serum ferritin	Decreased	Normal	Increased
Total Fe binding capacity	Increased	Normal	Decreased
Transferrin saturation	Decreased	Normal	Decreased
FEP	Increased	Normal	Increased
Transferrin receptor	Increased	Normal	Increased
Reticulocyte hemoglobin concentration	Decreased	Normal	Normal-decreased

FEP, free erythrocyte protoporphyrin; MCV, mean corpuscular volume; RBC, red blood cell count; RDW, red cell distribution width.
Modified from Zimmermann MB, Hurrell RF: Nutritional iron deficiency, Lancet 370:511–520, 2007.

volume require the use of age-related standards for recognizing microcytosis (see Table 447-1). The red blood cell count also decreases. The reticulocyte percentage may be normal or moderately elevated, but absolute reticulocyte counts indicate an insufficient response to the degree of anemia. The blood smear reveals hypochromic, microcytic red cells with substantial variation in cell size. Elliptocytic or cigar-shaped red cells are often seen (Fig. 455-1). Detection of increased soluble transferrin receptor and decreased reticulocyte hemoglobin concentration provide very useful and early indicators of iron deficiency, but their availability is more limited.

White blood cell count is normal, and thrombocytosis is often present. Thrombocytopenia is occasionally seen with iron deficiency,

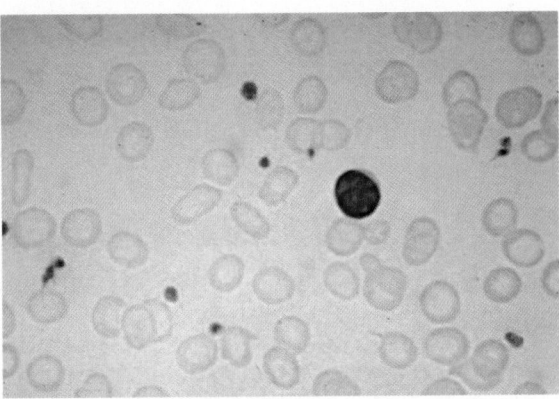

Figure 455-1 Peripheral blood smear from a patient with severe iron-deficiency anemia. The hypochromia is marked. The nucleus of a normal lymphocyte that is comparable in size to a normocytic red cell serves to document many microcytic erythrocytes. The elliptocytic ("cigar-forms") red cells are typical of iron deficiency. Note the variation in red cell size. (*Courtesy of the University of Washington/American Society of Hematology Slide Bank.*)

Table 455-3	Differential Diagnosis of Microcytic Anemia That Fails to Respond to Oral Iron

Poor compliance (true intolerance of Fe is uncommon)
Incorrect dose or medication
Malabsorption of administered iron
Ongoing blood loss, including gastrointestinal, menstrual, and pulmonary
Concurrent infection or inflammatory disorder inhibiting the response to iron
Concurrent vitamin B_{12} or folate deficiency
Diagnosis other than iron deficiency
    Thalassemias
    Hemoglobins C and E disorders
    Anemia of chronic disease
    Lead poisoning
    Sickle thalassemias, hemoglobin SC disease
    Iron refractory iron deficiency anemia (IRIDA)
    Rare microcytic anemias (see Chapter 456)

Table 455-4	Responses to Iron Therapy in Iron-Deficiency Anemia

TIME AFTER IRON ADMINISTRATION	RESPONSE
12-24 hr	Replacement of intracellular iron enzymes; subjective improvement; decreased irritability; increased appetite
36-48 hr	Initial bone marrow response; erythroid hyperplasia
48-72 hr	Reticulocytosis, peaking at 5-7 days
4-30 days	Increase in hemoglobin level
1-3 mo	Repletion of stores

potentially confusing the diagnosis with bone marrow failure disorders. Stool for occult blood should be checked to exclude blood loss as the cause of iron deficiency.

A presumptive diagnosis of iron-deficiency anemia is most often made by a complete blood count demonstrating a microcytic anemia with a high red cell distribution width, reduced red blood cell count, normal white blood cell count, and normal or elevated platelet count. Other laboratory studies, such as reduced serum ferritin, reduced serum iron, and increased total iron-binding capacity, are not usually necessary unless severe anemia requires a more rapid diagnosis, other complicating clinical factors are present, or the anemia does not respond to iron therapy. An increase in hemoglobin ≥1 g/dL after a month of iron therapy is usually the most practical means to establish the diagnosis.

A diagnosis of iron deficiency in the absence of anemia is more challenging. Serum ferritin is a useful measure whose value is increased by also measuring C-reactive protein to help identify false negative results because of concomitant inflammation. Detection of increased soluble transferrin receptor and decreased reticulocyte hemoglobin concentration may find increasing use as they become more available.

DIFFERENTIAL DIAGNOSIS

The most common alternative causes of microcytic anemia are α- or β-thalassemia and other hemoglobinopathies, including hemoglobins E and C (see Chapter 462.9). The anemia of inflammation is usually normocytic but can be microcytic in a minority of cases (see Chapter 451.1). Lead poisoning can cause microcytic anemia, but more often the microcytic anemia is due to iron deficiency causing pica and secondary lead intoxication (see Chapter 721). Table 455-2 compares the use of laboratory studies in the diagnosis of the most common microcytic anemias. Other etiologies of microcytic anemia are found in Table 455-3. Although the platelet count can be abnormal, the white blood cell count and neutrophil count should be normal.

When anemia is identified solely by hemoglobin or hematocrit, 60% of children in developed countries have anemia not because of iron deficiency. Caution should be used in treating these children with iron without the benefit of a complete blood and differential count to ensure that a more serious diagnosis is not missed.

PREVENTION

Iron deficiency is best prevented to avoid both its systemic manifestations and the anemia. Breastfeeding should be encouraged, with the addition of supplemental iron at 4 mo of age. Infants who are not breastfed should only receive iron-fortified formula (12 mg of iron per liter) for the first year, and thereafter cow's milk should be limited to <20-24 oz daily. This approach encourages the ingestion of foods richer in iron and prevents blood loss as a result of cow's milk–induced enteropathy.

When these preventive measures fail, routine screening helps prevent the development of severe anemia. Routine screening using hemoglobin or hematocrit is done at 12 mo of age, or earlier if at 4 mo of age the child is assessed to be at high risk for iron deficiency. Thereafter screening should continue if risk factors are identified.

TREATMENT

The regular response of iron-deficiency anemia to adequate amounts of iron is a critical diagnostic and therapeutic feature (Table 455-4). Oral administration of simple ferrous salts (most often ferrous sulfate) provides inexpensive and effective therapy. There is no evidence that the addition of any trace metal, vitamin, or other hematinic substance significantly increases the response to simple ferrous salts. Aside from the unpleasant taste of iron, intolerance to oral iron is uncommon in young children. In contrast, older children and adolescents sometimes have GI complaints.

The therapeutic dose should be calculated in terms of elemental iron. A daily total dose of 3-6 mg/kg of elemental iron in 3 divided doses is adequate, with the higher dose used in more severe cases. The maximum dose would be 150-200 mg of elemental iron daily. Ferrous sulfate is 20% elemental iron by weight and is ideally given between meals with juice, although this timing is usually not critical with a therapeutic dose. Parenteral iron preparations are only used when malabsorption is present or when compliance is poor, because oral therapy is otherwise as fast, as effective, much less expensive and less toxic. When necessary, parenteral iron sucrose, ferric carboxymaltose, and ferric gluconate complex have a lower risk of serious reactions than iron dextran, although only the latter is FDA approved for use in children.

Iron therapy may increase the virulence of malaria and certain Gram-negative bacteria, particularly in developing countries. Iron overdose is associated with *Yersinia* infection.

In addition to iron therapy, dietary counseling is usually necessary. Excessive intake of milk, particularly cow's milk, should be limited. Iron deficiency in adolescent girls secondary to menorrhagia is treated with iron and menstrual control with hormone therapy (see Chapter 116.2).

If the anemia is mild, the only additional study is to repeat the blood count approximately 4 wk after initiating therapy. At this point, the hemoglobin has usually risen by at least 1-2 g/dL and has often normalized. If the anemia is more severe, earlier confirmation of the diagnosis can be made by the appearance of a reticulocytosis usually within 48-96 hr of instituting treatment. The hemoglobin will then begin to increase 0.1-0.4 g/dL per day depending on the severity of the anemia. Iron medication should be continued for 2-3 mo after blood values normalize to reestablish iron stores. Good follow-up is essential to ensure a response to therapy. When the anemia responds poorly or not at all to iron therapy, there are multiple considerations, including diagnoses other than iron deficiency (see Table 455-3).

Because a rapid hematologic response can be confidently predicted in typical iron deficiency, blood transfusion is rarely necessary. It should only be used when heart failure is imminent or if the anemia is severe with evidence of substantial ongoing blood loss. Unless there is active bleeding, transfusions must be given slowly to avoid precipitating or exacerbating congestive heart failure.

Bibliography is available at Expert Consult.

Chapter **456**
Other Microcytic Anemias
Richard Sills

There are a number of rare microcytic anemias that need to be considered when children with microcytic anemia fail to respond to oral iron and more common diagnoses (see Chapter 462) are eliminated. In addition, although the anemia of chronic inflammation is usually normocytic, it can also be microcytic.

INFANTILE POIKILOCYTOSIS AND HEREDITARY PYROPOIKILOCYTOSIS
Infants with common hereditary elliptocytosis (see Chapter 459) may initially present with hemolytic anemia characterized by marked poikilocytosis with budding and fragmentation of the red blood cells. These small red blood cell fragments reduce the overall mean corpuscular volume, resulting in microcytosis. By 2 yr of age, the findings become typical of hereditary elliptocytosis. Hereditary pyropoikilocytosis is a much less common variant of hereditary elliptocytosis, in which the hemolytic anemia and red cell changes are more severe.

COPPER DEFICIENCY
Copper deficiency is a rare cause of microcytic anemia. It is associated with malabsorption, severe malnutrition often with feeding of milk alone, or parenteral nutrition with inadvertent omission of supplemental copper.

DEFECTS OF IRON METABOLISM
Rare microcytic anemias may be associated with defects in iron trafficking and regulation. Most are inherited and usually identified in childhood. They include defects of iron absorption, transport, utilization, and recycling. A *defect of iron absorption* is **iron refractory iron deficiency anemia**. This defect of transmembrane proteins causes a

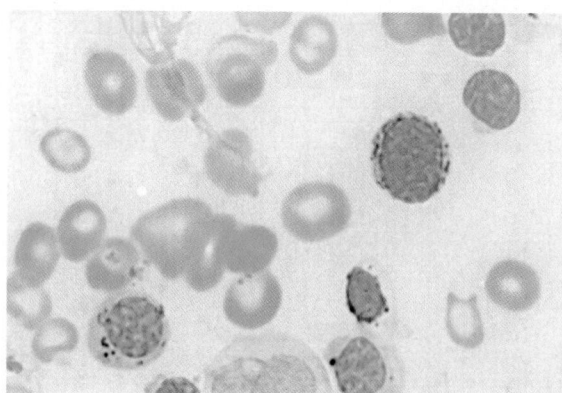

Figure 456-1 Ring sideroblast in myelodysplastic syndrome (refractory anemia with ring sideroblasts)—iron stain. *(From Ryan DH, Cohen HJ: Bone marrow examination. In Hoffman R, Benz EJ Jr, Shattil SJ, et al, editors: Hematology, ed 4, Philadelphia, 2005, Churchill Livingstone.)*

remarkably severe microcytosis out of proportion to the degree of anemia. This is an autosomal recessive disease due to loss of function mutations in *TMPRSS6*. In most cases, it is unresponsive to oral iron and partially responsive to intravenous iron. *Defects of iron recycling* include **aceruloplasminemia,** in which iron cannot be appropriately transported from macrophages to plasma.

Defects of mitochondrial iron utilization are a diverse group of acquired and inherited defects known as **sideroblastic anemias**. Impaired heme synthesis leads to retention of iron within the mitochondria of marrow red blood cells (RBCs). The perinuclear distribution of mitochondria results in a pattern of iron staining surrounding the nucleus. These are ringed sideroblasts (Fig. 456-1), which are distinct from the more diffuse cytoplasmic distribution of iron in normal RBC precursors. The anemia is characterized by hypochromic microcytic RBCs mixed with normal RBCs, so the complete blood cell count indicates a very high RBC distribution width. The serum iron concentration usually is elevated, and the transferrin saturation of iron is increased.

Congenital sideroblastic anemia is usually an X-linked disorder and is most commonly a result of mutations in erythrocytic isozyme 5-aminolevulinic acid synthetase, the rate-limiting enzyme reaction in heme synthesis. An important cofactor for 5-aminolevulinic acid synthetase is pyridoxal phosphate. Several of these mutations occur near the binding site for pyridoxal phosphate. Severe anemia is recognized in infancy or early childhood, whereas milder cases might not become apparent until early adulthood or later. **Clinical findings** include pallor, icterus, and moderate splenomegaly and/or hepatomegaly. The severity of the anemia varies such that some patients require no therapy and others need regular RBC transfusions. A subset of patients with hereditary sideroblastic anemia manifests a hematologic response to pharmacologic doses of pyridoxine. Iron overload as manifested by elevated serum ferritin, elevated serum iron, and increased transferrin saturation is a major complication of this disorder. Clinical evidence of iron overload (e.g., diabetes mellitus, liver dysfunction) may be found in some patients who have little or no anemia. Stem cell transplantation has been used to treat affected children who are dependent on RBC transfusions.

A unique variant of congenital sideroblastic anemia is **Pearson syndrome** (see Chapter 449), but the anemia is usually macrocytic and not microcytic. Another rare variant of sideroblastic anemia is due to mutations in *TRNT1* and manifests with developmental delay, recurrent fevers, and immunodeficiency in addition to anemia.

Acquired sideroblastic anemias can be triggered by drugs and toxins that disturb mitochondrial iron metabolism, including lead and isoniazid. The acquired neoplastic sideroblastic syndromes seen in adults are very rare in children.

Bibliography is available at Expert Consult.

Section **3**
Hemolytic Anemias

Chapter **457**
Definitions and Classification of Hemolytic Anemias

George B. Segel

Hemolysis is defined as the premature destruction of red blood cells (RBCs) (a shortened RBC life span). Anemia results when the rate of destruction exceeds the capacity of the marrow to produce RBCs. Normal RBC survival time is 110-120 days (half-life: 55-60 days), and thus, approximately 0.85% of the most senescent RBCs are removed and replaced each day. During hemolysis, RBC survival is shortened, the RBC count falls, erythropoietin is increased, and the stimulation of marrow activity results in heightened RBC production, reflected in an increased percentage of reticulocytes in the blood. Thus, hemolysis should be suspected as a cause of anemia if an elevated reticulocyte count is present. The reticulocyte count may also be elevated as a response to acute blood loss or for a short period after replacement therapy for iron, vitamin B$_{12}$, or folate deficiency. The marrow can increase its output 2-3–fold acutely, with a maximum of 6-8–fold in long-standing hemolysis. The reticulocyte percentage can be corrected to measure the magnitude of marrow production in response to hemolysis as follows:

$$\text{Reticulocyte index} = \text{reticulocyte\%} \times \frac{\text{Observed hematocrit}}{\text{Normal hematocrit}} \times \frac{1}{\mu}$$

where μ is a maturation factor of 1-3 related to the severity of the anemia (Fig. 457-1). The normal reticulocyte index is 1.0; therefore, the index measures the fold increase in erythropoiesis (e.g., 2-fold, 3-fold).

As anemia becomes more severe, the erythropoietin concentration increases and reticulocytes are released from the marrow earlier; they are identifiable as reticulocytes in the blood that last for >1 day. Because the reticulocyte index is essentially a measure of RBC production per day, the maturation factor, μ, provides this correction (see Fig. 457-1).

The erythroid hyperplasia resulting from chronic hemolytic anemia in children, especially thalassemia, may be so extensive that the medullary spaces expand at the expense of the cortical bone. These changes may be evident on physical examination or on radiographs of the skull and long bones (see Fig. 462-7). A propensity to fracture long bones can also occur.

Direct assessment of the severity of hemolysis requires measurement of RBC survival time using RBCs tagged with the radioisotope Na$_2$^{51}CrO$_4$. The normal half-life of chromium 51–labeled RBCs is 25-35 days. This value is less than the expected half-life of 55-60 days because of the elution of chromium 51 from the labeled RBCs at the rate of approximately 1% day. Techniques to measure RBC survival using RBC biotin labeling do not require the use of isotopes.

The exaggerated degradation rate of hemoglobin results in increased biliary excretion of heme pigment derivatives and increased urinary and fecal urobilinogen (Fig. 457-2). Gallstones composed of calcium bilirubinate may be formed in children with chronic hemolysis as young as 4 yr of age. Elevations of serum unconjugated bilirubin and lactate dehydrogenase also can accompany hemolysis.

Three heme-binding proteins in the plasma are altered during hemolysis (see Fig. 457-2). Hemoglobin binds to haptoglobin and hemopexin, both of which are cleared more rapidly as conjugates, resulting in a reduced plasma concentration. Oxidized heme binds to albumin to form methemalbumin, which is increased in the plasma. When the capacity of these binding molecules is exceeded, free hemoglobin appears in the plasma, and the pink color can be seen if the plasma is partitioned after centrifugation in a capillary hematocrit tube. If present, free hemoglobin in the plasma is prima facie evidence of intravascular hemolysis. Free hemoglobin dissociates into dimers and is filtered by the kidneys. When the tubular reabsorptive capacity of the kidneys for hemoglobin is exceeded, free hemoglobin appears in the urine. Even in the absence of hemoglobinuria, iron loss can result from reabsorbed hemoglobin and the shedding of renal epithelial cells in which the iron from hemoglobin is stored as hemosiderin. This iron loss can lead to iron deficiency during chronic intravascular hemolysis. When hemoglobin is degraded, an α-methene bridge is broken in the cyclic tetrapyrrole of the heme moiety, with

MATURATION TIME - DAYS

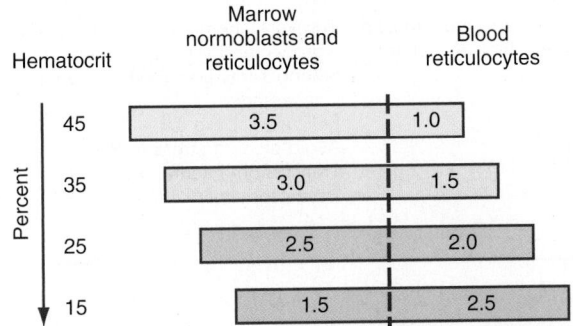

Figure 457-1 Number of days for maturation of reticulocytes to mature erythrocytes in the marrow and blood. The duration of maturation as blood reticulocytes is taken as μ, which is used in the correction equation in this chapter. (*Modified from Hillman RS, Finch CA: Red cell manual, Philadelphia, 1983, FA Davis.*)

RED CELL DESTRUCTION

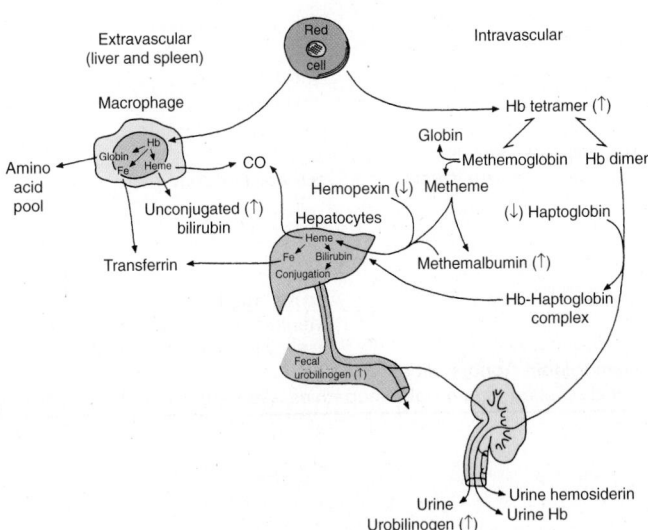

Figure 457-2 Red cell destruction and catabolism of hemoglobin (Hb) based on the description by Hillman and Finch. Fe, iron. (*From Hillman RS, Finch CA: Red cell manual, Philadelphia, 1983, FA Davis.*)

release of carbon monoxide (CO) (see Fig. 457-2). The amount of CO in the blood or expired air provides a dynamic measure of the hemolytic rate; end-tidal CO is not available in most clinical laboratories to measure hemolysis.

The hematocrit level depends on the severity of hemolysis and on the erythropoietic response. The shortened RBC life span and heightened RBC production result in a marked susceptibility to aplastic or hypoplastic crises, characterized by erythroid marrow failure and reticulocytopenia, accompanied by a rapid reduction in hemoglobin and hematocrit to extremely low levels. The most common cause of aplastic crisis is infection with parvovirus B19, which is erythrocytotropic (see Chapters 251 and 450). An aplastic crisis can produce a precipitous and life-threatening decline in hematocrit that usually lasts 10-14 days. Such transient erythroid marrow failure has only a mild effect in persons with a normal RBC life span, but it has a proportionately greater effect if the RBC life span is shortened by hemolysis. A second infection with parvovirus B19 is uncommon, but other infections can compromise erythroid marrow output, resulting in various degrees of hypoplasia or hypoplastic crises.

Hemolytic anemias may be classified as either cellular, resulting from intrinsic abnormalities of the membrane, enzymes, or hemoglobin; or extracellular, resulting from antibodies, mechanical factors, or plasma factors. Most cellular defects are inherited (paroxysmal nocturnal hemoglobinuria is acquired), and most extracellular defects are acquired (abetalipoproteinemia with acanthocytosis is inherited). Table 457-1 shows the most common hemolytic anemias, their underlying defects, the diagnostic laboratory tests, and recommendations for treatment.

Table 457-1	Hemolytic Anemias and Their Treatment		
DIAGNOSIS	**DEFECT**	**LABORATORY TESTS**	**TREATMENT**
CELLULAR DEFECTS			
Membrane Defects			
Hereditary spherocytosis	Cytoskeletal protein defects Often involve vertical interactions of spectrin ankyrin, protein 3	Spherocytes on blood film Negative Coombs test eliminates immune hemolysis Increased incubated osmotic fragility Abnormal cytoskeletal protein analysis	If Hb >10 g/dL and reticulocyte count <10%: none If severe anemia, poor growth, aplastic crises, and age <2 yr: transfusion Folic acid, 1 mg qd Splenectomy (see text)
Hereditary elliptocytosis	Cytoskeletal protein defects Often involve horizontal interactions of spectrin, protein 4.1, and glycophorin c	Elliptocytes on blood film RBCs mildly heat-sensitive Abnormal cytoskeletal protein analysis	Mild types: no treatment Chronic hemolysis: transfusion and splenectomy as recommended for spherocytosis (see above) Folic acid, 1 mg qd
Hereditary pyropoikilocytosis	Cytoskeletal protein defects Homozygous or double heterozygous abnormality in horizontal interactions of α-spectrin	Extreme variation in RBC size and shape on blood film Thermal sensitivity- fragmentation at 45°C (113°F) for 15 min	Transfusion and splenectomy as recommended for spherocytosis (see above) Folic acid, 1 mg qd
Hereditary stomatocytosis	Cytoskeletal protein defects Decreased protein 7.2b (1 subset) Abnormal RBC cation and water content	Stomatocytes on blood film	Splenectomy should be avoided (see text) Folic acid, 1 mg qd
Paroxysmal nocturnal hemoglobinuria	Primary acquired marrow disorder RBCs unusually sensitive to complement-mediated lysis	Decreased WBC CD55 and CD59 or decreased RBC CD59 by flow cytometry Marrow aspirate and biopsy to assess cellularity Decreased decay-accelerating factor	Folic acid, 1 mg qd Mild cytopenias: no treatment Chronic hemolysis and other cytopenias: prednisone, qd initially, and then qod for maintenance therapy Iron for secondary iron deficiency Eculizumab (inhibits C5) Anticoagulation Marrow transplant for pancytopenia
Enzyme Deficiencies			
Pyruvate kinase deficiency	Decreased or abnormal enzyme	Pyruvate kinase assay: decreased V_{max} or, rarely, high K_m variant	In severe anemia with symptoms, poor growth and age <2 yr: transfusion Splenectomy age >6 yr, but earlier if necessary Folic acid, 1 mg qd
G6PD deficiency	A⁻ type: age-labile enzyme Mediterranean type: no enzyme activity in circulating RBCs	G6PD assay	Avoid oxidant stress to RBCs Transfusion if acute anemia is symptomatic
Hemoglobin Abnormalities			
For discussion of hemoglobinopathies, see sections on these topics.			

Table 457-1	Hemolytic Anemias and Their Treatment—cont'd		
DIAGNOSIS	**DEFECT**	**LABORATORY TESTS**	**TREATMENT**
EXTRACELLULAR DEFECTS			
Autoimmune			
"Warm" antibody	Alteration in membrane surface antigen (Rh) or abnormal response of B lymphocytes, causing autoantibody formation "Molecular mimicry" to viral antigen	Spherocytes on blood film Positive direct antiglobulin (Coombs) test to IgG "warm" antibody or anti-C3d directed against RBCs Positive indirect Coombs test and antibody detectable in plasma Thermal amplitude 35-40°C (95-104°F) Some complement (C3b) may be detected on RBCs Tests for underlying disease	If Hb >10 g/dL and reticulocyte count <10%—none Severe anemia may require transfusion; prednisone, 2 mg/kg/24 hr IVIG *Rituximab* Splenectomy Immunosuppressives Folic acid, 1 mg/24 hr if chronic
"Cold" antibody	"Cold" or IgM autoantibody directed against I/i antigen system	Agglutination or rouleaux on blood film Positive direct Coombs test to complement (C3b) Tests for underlying disease Serology for infectious mononucleosis; anti-i present Serology for *Mycoplasma pneumoniae*; anti-I present	If Hb >10 g/dL and reticulocyte count <10%: none Severe anemia might require transfusion Avoid exposure to cold If severe: *Rituximab* Immunosuppressives and plasmapheresis Prednisone is less effective Splenectomy is not useful Folic acid, 1 mg/24 hr if chronic
Fragmentation Hemolysis			
DIC, TTP, HUS, aHUS, pneumococcal-induced HUS See Table 465-1	Direct damage to RBC membrane	Fragments on blood film	Treat underlying condition Transfusion, but transfused cells also will have shortened life span
Extracorporeal membrane oxygenation	Direct damage to RBC membrane	Fragments on blood film	Supportive Transfusion until ECMO is discontinued
Prosthetic heart valve	Direct damage to RBC membrane	Fragments on blood film	Folic acid, 1 mg/24 hr Iron for secondary iron deficiency
Burns, thermal injury	Direct damage to RBC membrane	Spherocytes on blood film	Supportive Transfusion
Hypersplenism	Effects of sequestration, ↓ pH, lipases and other enzymes, and macrophages on RBCs	Thrombocytopenia and neutropenia	Treat underlying condition: cytopenias all usually mild Splenectomy if complicating other anemia (e.g., thalassemia major) Folic acid, 1 mg/24 hr
Plasma Factors			
Liver disease	Alteration in plasma cholesterol and phospholipids	Target cells or spiculated RBCs on blood film Abnormal liver function tests	Treat underlying condition Transfusion, but transfused cells also will have shortened life span Folic acid, 1 mg/24 hr
Abetalipoproteinemia	Absence of apolipoprotein β Vitamin E deficiency and heightened sensitivity to oxidative damage	Acanthocytes on blood film Absent chylomicrons, VLDL, and LDL	Vitamin E (A, K, and D) Folic acid, 1 mg/24 hr Dietary restriction of triglycerides
Infections	Toxic effects on RBCs	Associated symptoms and signs Cultures	Antibiotics Supportive
Wilson disease	Effect of copper on RBC membrane, usually self-limited	Spherocytes on blood film Copper, ceruloplasmin Kaiser Fleischer rings Penicillamine challenge and urine copper excretion Liver biopsy for Cu content Gene analysis for mutation of ATP7B	Penicillamine Supportive Transfusion if acute anemia is symptomatic

aHUS, atypical hemolytic uremic syndrome; Cu, copper; DIC, disseminated intravascular coagulation; ECMO, extracorporeal membrane oxygenation; G6PD, glucose-6-phosphate dehydrogenase; Hb, hemoglobin; HUS, hemolytic uremic syndrome; Ig, immunoglobulin; IVIG, intravenous immunoglobulin; LDL, low-density lipoprotein; K_m, Michaelis constant; RBC, red blood cell; TTP, thrombotic thrombocytopenic purpura; VLDL, very-low-density lipoprotein; V_{max}, maximal velocity; WBC, white blood cell.

Modified from Asselin BL, Segel GB: In Rakel R, editor: Conn's current therapy, Philadelphia, 1994, Saunders, pp 338–339.

Chapter 458

Hereditary Spherocytosis

George B. Segel and Denise Casey

Hereditary spherocytosis (HS) is a common cause of hemolysis and hemolytic anemia, with a prevalence of approximately 1 in 5,000 persons. It is the most common inherited abnormality of the red blood cell (RBC) membrane. Although common among persons of Northern European origin, HS has been described in most ethnic groups. The more rare defects found in the United States and in Europe are the more common mutations described in the Japanese population. The clinical spectrum varies widely. Affected patients may be asymptomatic, without anemia and with minimal hemolysis, or they may have severe hemolytic anemia requiring regular blood transfusions and a splenectomy.

ETIOLOGY

Hereditary spherocytosis usually is transmitted as an autosomal dominant or, less commonly, as an autosomal recessive disorder. As many as 25% of patients have no previous family history. Of these patients, most represent new mutations, and a few cases result from recessive inheritance or represent nonpaternity. The pathophysiology underlying HS involves 5 proteins, which are key components of the cytoskeleton responsible for RBC shape (Table 458-1). Abnormalities of spectrin or ankyrin are the most common molecular defects. Dominant defects have been described in β-spectrin and band 3. Recessive defects have been described in α-spectrin and protein 4.2. Both dominant and recessive defects have been described in ankyrin (Table 458-1). A deficiency in spectrin, band 3, ankyrin, or protein 4.2 results in uncoupling in the "vertical" interactions of the lipid bilayer skeleton and subsequent release of membrane microvesicles. The loss of membrane surface area without a proportional loss of cell volume causes sphering of the RBCs, and an associated increase in cation permeability, cation transport, adenosine triphosphate use, and glycolysis. The decreased deformability of the spherocytic RBCs impairs cell passage from the splenic cords to the splenic sinuses, and the spherocytic RBCs are destroyed prematurely in the spleen (Figs. 458-1 and 458-2). Splenectomy markedly improves RBC life span and may be indicated in some patients with HS.

CLINICAL MANIFESTATIONS

In the neonatal period, HS is a significant cause of hemolytic disease and can be manifest as anemia and hyperbilirubinemia sufficiently severe to require phototherapy or exchange transfusions. Hemolysis may be more prominent in the newborn because hemoglobin F binds 2,3-diphosphoglycerate poorly, and the increased level of free 2,3-diphosphoglycerate destabilizes interactions among spectrin, actin, and protein 4.1 in the RBC membrane (see Fig. 458-1). The need for exchange transfusion at birth or transfusions in infancy is not indicative of more severe disease later in life because infants do not mount an adequate reticulocyte response until several months after birth.

Some patients remain asymptomatic into adulthood, but others have severe anemia with pallor, jaundice, fatigue, and exercise intolerance. Severe cases may be marked by expansion of the diploë of the skull as a result of marrow hyperplasia (frontal bossing), but to a lesser extent than in thalassemia major. Depending on the severity of the anemia and the comorbidities associated with severe anemia, some patients benefit from a splenectomy (Table 458-2).

After infancy, splenomegaly is common; there is no correlation between spleen size and disease severity. Bilirubin gallstone formation is a function of age; they can form as early as age 4-5 yr and are present in the majority of adult patients.

Children with HS are also susceptible to aplastic crises, primarily as a result of parvovirus B19 infection, and to hypoplastic crises associated with various other infections (Fig. 458-3). High RBC turnover in the setting of erythroid marrow failure can result in profound anemia (hematocrit <10%), high-output heart failure, cardiovascular collapse, and death. White blood cell and platelet counts can also fall (Fig. 458-3). Rare complications associated with HS include splenic sequestration crisis, gout, cardiomyopathy, priapism, leg ulcers, and spinocerebellar degeneration.

DIAGNOSIS

Evidence of hemolysis includes reticulocytosis and indirect hyperbilirubinemia. The hemoglobin level usually is 6-10 g/dL, but it can be in the normal range. The reticulocyte percentage often is increased to 6-20%, with a mean of approximately 10%. The mean corpuscular

Table 458-1	Common Gene Mutations in Hereditary Spherocytosis				
PROTEIN	**GENE**	**COMMON MUTATIONS***	**PREVALENCE**	**INHERITANCE**	**DISEASE SEVERITY**
Ankyrin-1	ANK1	Frameshift Nonsense Splicing Missense Promoter region	50-67% 5-10% in Japan	Dominant and recessive	Mild to moderate
Band 3	AE1 (SLC4A1)	Missense Nonsense Polymorphism Mutant protein	15-20%	Mostly dominant	Mild to moderate
β-Spectrin	SPTB	Null Nonsense Missense Polymorphism	15-20%	Dominant	Mild to moderate
α-Spectrin	SPTA1	Splicing αLEPRA allele	<5%	Recessive	Severe
Protein 4.2	EPB42	Missense Nonsense Splicing	<5% 45-50% in Japan	Recessive	Mild to moderate

*Detected mutations in order of frequency
Modified from Bolton-Maggs PHB, Langer JC, Iolascon A, et al: Guidelines for the diagnosis and management of hereditary spherocytosis–2011 update, Br J Haematol 156:37–49, 2011.

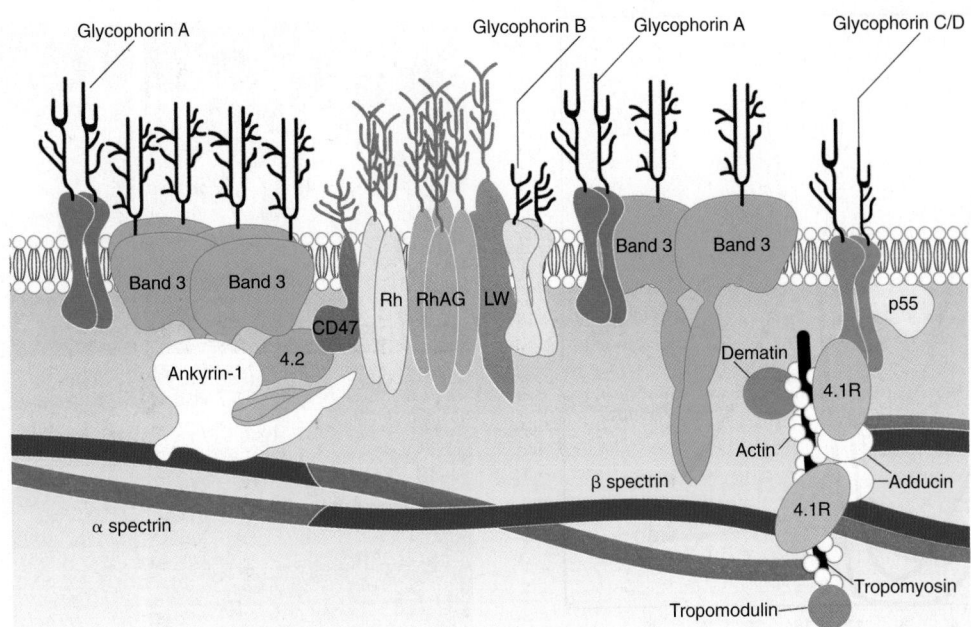

Figure 458-1 A simplified cross-section of the red blood cell (erythrocyte) membrane. The lipid bilayer forms the equator of the cross-section with its polar heads (small circles) turned outward. 4.1 R, protein; 4.2, protein 4.2; LW, Landsteiner-Wiener glycoprotein; Rh, Rhesus polypeptide; RhAG, Rh-associated glycoprotein. *(From Perrotta S, Gallagher PG, Mohandas N: Hereditary spherocytosis, Lancet 372:1411–1426, 2008.)*

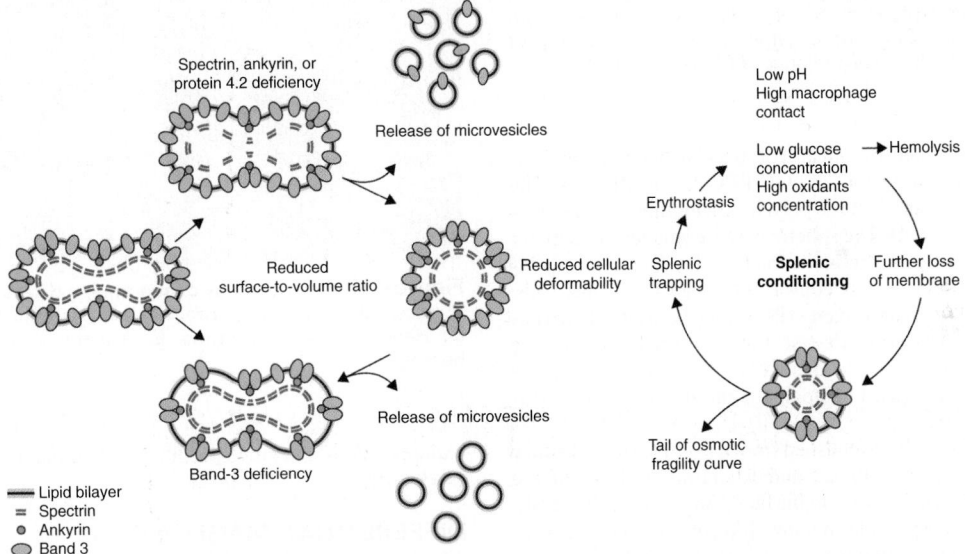

Figure 458-2 Pathophysiologic effects of hereditary spherocytosis. *(From Perrotta S, Gallagher PG, Mohandas N: Hereditary spherocytosis, Lancet 372:1411–1426, 2008.)*

Table 458-2	Hereditary Spherocytosis Disease Classification			
	TRAIT	**MILD**	**MODERATE**	**SEVERE**
Hemoglobin (g/dL)	Normal	11-15	8-12	<6-8
Reticulocytes (%)	Normal (<3)	3-6	>6	>10
Bilirubin	<17	17-34	>34	>51
Transfusions	0	0	0-2	Regular
Typical heredity	AD	AD	AD or de novo mutation	AR
Splenectomy	Not indicated	Not indicated	May be indicated*	Indicated

*Splenectomy indicated if patient requires frequent transfusions for hypoplastic crises or shows poor growth or cardiomegaly.
  AD, autodominant; AR, autorecessive.
  Modified from Bolton-Maggs PHB, Langer JC, Iolascon A, et al: Guidelines for the diagnosis and management of hereditary spherocytosis–2011 update, Br J Haematol 156:37–49, 2011.

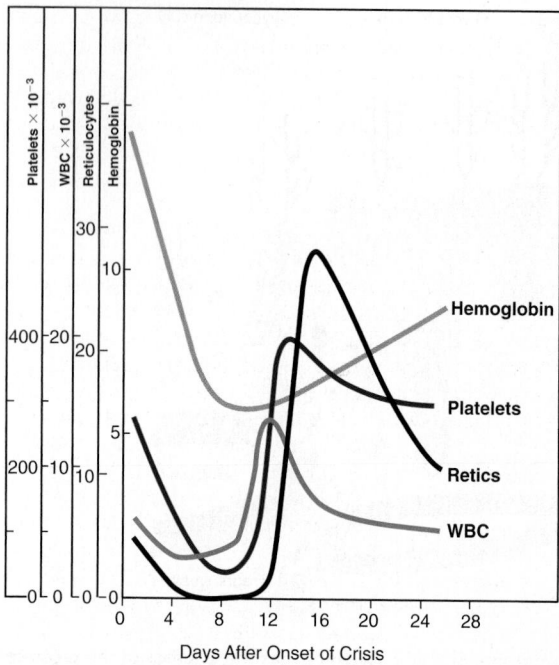

Figure 458-3 Parvovirus-induced aplastic crisis. Progression of the changes in blood count is shown for a patient with hereditary spherocytosis and infection with parvovirus. Note that the fall in baseline reticulocytosis is associated with a rapid fall in hemoglobin. White blood cells (WBC) and platelets are also affected. *(Modified from Nathan DG, Orkin SH, Ginsburg D, et al, editors: Hematology of infancy and childhood, ed 6, Philadelphia, 2003, WB Saunders.)*

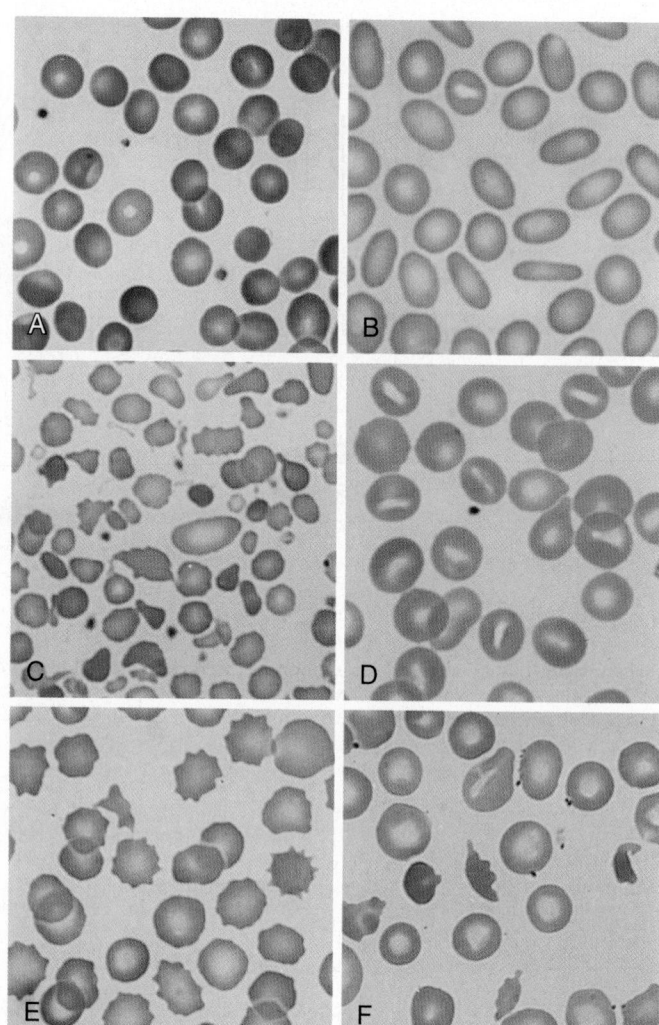

Figure 458-4 Morphology of abnormal red cells. **A,** Hereditary spherocytosis. **B,** Hereditary elliptocytosis. **C,** Hereditary pyropoikilocytosis. **D,** Hereditary stomatocytosis. **E,** Acanthocytosis. **F,** Fragmentation hemolysis.

volume is normal, although the mean corpuscular hemoglobin concentration often is increased (36-38 g/dL RBCs). The RBCs on the blood smear vary in size and include polychromatophilic reticulocytes and spherocytes (Fig. 458-4). The spherocytes are smaller in diameter and appear hyperchromic as a result of the high hemoglobin concentration. The central pallor is less conspicuous than in normal cells. Spherocytes may be the predominant cells or may be relatively sparse, depending on the severity of the disease, but they usually account for >15% of the cells when hemolytic anemia is present. Other evidence of hemolysis includes decreased haptoglobin and the presence of gallstones on ultrasonography.

The diagnosis of HS can be established from a positive family history and the presence of typical clinical and laboratory features of the disease: splenomegaly, spherocytes on the blood smear, reticulocytosis, and an elevated mean corpuscular hemoglobin concentration. If these are present, no additional testing is necessary to confirm the diagnosis. If the diagnosis is less certain, the recommended tests that have a high predictive value for HS are the flow cytometric EMA (eosin-5-maleimide) binding test and the cryohemolysis test. Although no test for HS is 100% reliable, the EMA binding test had a diagnostic sensitivity and specificity of 93% and 98%, respectively, in a recent large study. Other assays, such as the acidified glycerol lysis test and osmotic gradient ektacytometry, also have increased sensitivity for HS. The classic incubated osmotic fragility test can detect the presence of spherocytes in the blood; however, it is not specific to HS and may be abnormal in other hemolytic anemias. The RBCs are incubated in progressive dilutions of sodium chloride causing the RBCs to swell and eventually lyse. Spherocytes lyse at a higher sodium chloride concentration than biconcave cells in hypotonic solutions because they have a lower surface area:volume ratio. Unfortunately, this test has poor sensitivity relative to other screening assays and can miss up to 20% of mild HS cases.

As a research tool and for atypical cases, the specific membrane abnormality can be established by gel electrophoresis analysis of RBC membrane proteins. Molecular diagnosis also is possible because most patients having a family-specific private mutation can be detected by DNA analysis.

DIFFERENTIAL DIAGNOSIS

The major alternative considerations when large numbers of spherocytes are seen on the blood smear are isoimmune and autoimmune hemolysis. Isoimmune hemolytic disease of the newborn, particularly when a result of ABO incompatibility, mimics the cell appearance of HS. The detection of antibody on an infant's RBCs using a direct antiglobulin (Coombs) test should establish the diagnosis of immune hemolysis. Autoimmune hemolytic anemias also are characterized by spherocytes; however, there may be evidence of previously normal values for hemoglobin, hematocrit, and reticulocyte count. Rare causes of spherocytosis include thermal injury, clostridial septicemia, and Wilson disease, each of which can manifest as transient hemolytic anemia (see Table 457-1 in Chapter 457).

TREATMENT
General Supportive Care

Parents should be advised of the risk of newborn jaundice and the potential need for phototherapy and exchange transfusion after birth to decrease bilirubin levels. Infants born to parents with known HS should be monitored carefully as hyperbilirubinemia may peak several days after birth. A minority of infants will be transfusion-dependent until development of adequate erythropoiesis to compensate for the ongoing hemolysis. Continued transfusion-dependence is not common after 6-12 mo of age.

Once the baseline level of disease severity is reached, an annual visit to the hematologist usually is sufficient. Growth should be monitored, exercise tolerance and spleen size documented, and parents should receive anticipatory guidance regarding the risk of aplastic crisis secondary to parvovirus, and hypoplastic crises with other infections. Parents and patients should be informed of an increased risk for gallstone development. The degree of splenomegaly does not correlate with disease severity. Folic acid supplementation is recommended in moderate and severe HS because of an enhanced requirement with increased erythropoiesis.

Guidelines for Splenectomy

Because the spherocytes are destroyed almost exclusively in the spleen, splenectomy eliminates most of the hemolysis. After splenectomy, the anemia, hyperbilirubinemia, and incidence of gallstones are significantly lessened, if not completely eradicated. However, splenectomy is associated with immediate surgical morbidities in addition to a lifelong increased risk for sepsis, particularly that caused by pneumococcal species. This risk is not completely eliminated with the requisite preoperative and postoperative vaccination against pneumococcus, meningococcus, and *Haemophilus influenzae type b*.

Splenectomy is recommended for patients with severe HS. It should be considered for patients with moderate HS and frequent hypoplastic or aplastic crises, poor growth, or cardiomegaly. It is generally not recommended for patients with mild HS. When splenectomy is indicated, it should be performed after the age of 6 yr, if possible, to avoid the heightened risk of postsplenectomy sepsis in younger children. The laparoscopic approach has less surgical morbidity and is recommended if the surgeon is adequately trained in this approach. Partial splenectomy may be beneficial but needs further study. In children undergoing splenectomy, a concomitant cholecystectomy should be performed if there are gallstones. It is controversial whether to perform a concomitant splenectomy in less-severely ill patients who are undergoing cholecystectomy for gallstone disease. Postsplenectomy thrombocytosis is commonly observed, but requires no treatment and usually resolves spontaneously. Vaccines for encapsulated organisms, such as pneumococcus, meningococcus, and *H. influenzae type b*, should be administered at least 14 days before splenectomy, and prophylactic oral penicillin VK prescribed indefinitely.

Bibliography is available at Expert Consult.

Chapter 459
Hereditary Elliptocytosis
George B. Segel

Hereditary elliptocytosis is a less common disorder than spherocytosis and also varies markedly in severity. Mild hereditary elliptocytosis produces no symptoms; more severe varieties can result in neonatal poikilocytosis (shape variation) and hemolysis, chronic or sporadic hemolytic anemia, or **hereditary pyropoikilocytosis (HPP)**, which is a severe disorder with microspherocytosis and poikilocytosis. Hereditary elliptocytosis is rare in Western populations and is more common among West Africans.

ETIOLOGY
Hereditary elliptocytosis is inherited as a dominant disorder. In the rare instances, when 2 abnormal alleles are inherited (HPP), the patient exhibits particularly severe hemolytic anemia. Various molecular defects have been described in hereditary elliptocytosis; these produce abnormalities of α- and β-spectrin and defective spectrin heterodimer self-association (see Fig. 458-1). The abnormalities (spectrin mutations) can provide resistance to malarial infection. Such defects in horizontal protein interactions result in gross membrane fragmentation, particularly in homozygous HPP. Less commonly, mutations in protein 4.1 and glycophorin C can produce elliptocytosis.

CLINICAL MANIFESTATIONS
Elliptocytosis may be an incidental finding on a blood film examination and might not be associated with clinically significant hemolysis (see Fig. 458-4B). The diagnosis of hereditary elliptocytosis is established by the findings on the blood film, the autosomal dominant inheritance pattern, and the absence of other causes of elliptocytosis, such as deficiencies of iron, folic acid, or vitamin B_{12}. Hemolytic elliptocytosis can produce neonatal jaundice, even though characteristic elliptocytosis might not be evident at that time. The blood of the affected newborn can show bizarre poikilocytes and pyknocytes. Transient augmented fragmentation and hemolysis in the newborn can result from the presence of hemoglobin F that binds poorly to the glycolytic intermediate 2,3-diphosphoglycerate. The increased 2,3-diphosphoglycerate tends to destabilize the spectrin–actin–protein 4.1 complex, leading to membrane instability (see Fig. 458-1).

The usual features of a chronic hemolytic process with elliptocytosis are manifested later as anemia, jaundice, splenomegaly, and osseous changes. Cholelithiasis can occur in later childhood; aplastic crises have been reported. The most severe form is HPP, which is characterized by extreme microcytosis (mean corpuscular volume, 50-60 fL/cell), extraordinary variation in cell size and shape, and primarily microspherocytic rather than elliptocytic cells (see Fig. 458-4C). The red blood cells (RBCs) have heightened sensitivity to heat, hence the "pyro" designation. These patients usually inherit a mutant spectrin from one parent, who has mild or no elliptocytosis (silent carrier), and a partial spectrin deficiency from the other parent, who is hematologically normal.

Ovalocytes, in contrast to elliptocytes, are less elongated and might reflect a condition known as *Southeast Asian ovalocytosis* (SAO). SAO is associated with an abnormal protein 3, which functions as an anion exchanger. This disorder can produce neonatal hyperbilirubinemia, but it causes little hemolysis later. It might offer protection against *Plasmodium falciparum* malaria because normal protein 3 is one of the malarial receptors. Protein 3 as an anion exchanger is also expressed in renal tubular cells and can cause distal renal tubular acidosis in association with SAO.

LABORATORY FINDINGS
The blood film is the most important test to establish hereditary elliptocytosis (see Fig. 458-4B). The RBCs show various degrees of elongation and can actually be rod shaped. In hereditary elliptocytosis, other abnormal RBC shapes may be present, depending on the severity of hemolysis. They include microcytes, spherocytes, and other poikilocytes. The increase in the reticulocyte percentage reflects the severity of hemolysis; erythroid hyperplasia and indirect hyperbilirubinemia may be present. Increased thermal instability is characteristic of HPP. The abnormal spectrin denatures and the cells lyse at 45-46°C (113-114.8°F) instead of the usual 49-50°C (120.2-122°F). The specific protein abnormality can be established by protein separation and analysis techniques. The eosin-5-maleimide binding test, which detects binding to protein band 3 by flow cytometry, may be useful in conjunction with the mean corpuscular volume in diagnosing hereditary elliptocytosis and hereditary spherocytosis. Molecular defects are defined only in research laboratories.

TREATMENT
If hereditary elliptocytosis represents a morphologic abnormality on the blood film without evident hemolysis, no treatment is necessary. Patients with chronic hemolysis should receive folic acid, 1 mg daily, to prevent secondary folic acid deficiency. Splenectomy decreases the

hemolysis and should be considered if the hemoglobin is <10 g/dL and the reticulocyte count is >10%. The RBCs on the blood film may be more abnormal after splenectomy, even though hemoglobin increases and reticulocytes decrease. The hematologic features of SAO do not require treatment beyond the newborn period.

Bibliography is available at Expert Consult.

Chapter **460**
Hereditary Stomatocytosis
George B. Segel and Lisa R. Hackney

Hereditary stomatocytosis includes a rare group of dominantly inherited hemolytic anemias in which there are characteristic morphologic changes in the red blood cells (RBCs) and increased red cell cation permeability. The RBCs are cup-shaped, creating a mouth-shaped area (stoma) of central pallor instead of the usual circular area of central pallor. Hereditary stomatocytosis is classified by the RBC hydration status. The 2 major varieties are either overhydrated (hydrocytosis) or dehydrated (xerocytosis).

HYDROCYTOSIS
Pathophysiology
Stomatocytes of the hydrocytic variant have excess intracellular sodium and water content and decreased intracellular potassium content. The principal defect in this variant is an increase in Na^+ and K^+ permeability, caused by mutations in rhesus-associated glycoproteins. However, the amount of Na^+ influx exceeds the K^+ efflux, and the cells subsequently develop increased cation content and water, and thus swell. These hydrocytic cells have increased osmotic fragility. Additionally, the integral membrane protein, stomatin or band 7.2 b, is decreased or absent from the erythrocyte membrane. The function of stomatin is not fully understood, although it might act as a switch that influences the function of GLUT1, the glucose transporter. It has been found that stomatin in the hydrocytic variant is synthesized early in RBC development but is lost as the cell matures. The mechanism for this loss of stomatin is not yet determined. It also is unclear how the loss of stomatin expression contributes to the cation leak, which is characteristic of this variant.

Clinical Features
The hydrocytic variant is the most severe form of hereditary stomatocytosis and is characterized by moderate to severe hemolysis, macrocytosis, and large numbers of stomatocytes on the blood smear. Patients commonly develop jaundice, splenomegaly, and cholelithiasis.

XEROCYTOSIS
Pathophysiology
The xerocytic variant is the more common form of hereditary stomatocytosis and usually results in a milder anemia in affected patients. The underlying cation defect is a net loss of RBC potassium that is not accompanied by an increase in sodium. Subsequently, the erythrocyte develops decreased intracellular water content and becomes dehydrated. It may be associated with a syndrome of perinatal edema and ascites. These findings are transient and remain unexplained.

Clinical Features
Patients affected by the xerocytic variant have a mild compensated macrocytic hemolytic anemia, variable numbers of stomatocytes and/or target cells on peripheral smear, increased mean corpuscular hemoglobin concentration as a result of the cellular dehydration, and, typically, jaundice and splenomegaly.

INTERMEDIATE SYNDROMES
The **Rh deficiency syndrome** is characterized by an absence or profound decrease in the Rh antigen on the RBC membrane. Affected RBCs in this disorder are dehydrated and have decreased cell cation and water content. This decreased cell cation content may be the result of increased potassium leak in spite of increased Na^+-K^+ pump activity. This syndrome is associated with mild to moderate hemolytic anemia, reticulocytosis, and stomatocytes and spherocytes on the blood smear.

Cryohydrocytosis is a mild form of stomatocytosis, typically caused by mutations in *SLC4A1* coding for the band 3 anion exchanger, in which the RBCs lyse on cooling in vitro and may be associated with "pseudohyperkalemia."

Absence of high-density lipoproteins (an α-lipoproteinemia or **Tangier disease**) can lead to hematologic manifestations such as a moderate hemolytic anemia, stomatocytosis, and thrombocytopenia. Affected patients can also have large orange tonsils, hepatosplenomegaly, lymphadenopathy, cloudy corneas, and peripheral neuropathy.

One of the most flagrant forms of stomatocytosis is seen in **phytosterolemia**, another metabolic disorder, in which the absorption of sterols, both cholesterol and its plant-derived relatives (e.g., sitosterol), is unlimited and unselective. The cells are not leaky to cations; there is macrothrombocytopenia and a degree of short stature. The plasma cholesterol may or may not be abnormal, but mass spectrography always shows a massive increase in plant sterol levels.

OTHER DISORDERS ASSOCIATED WITH STOMATOCYTOSIS
Acquired stomatocytosis may be seen with liver disease but also in alcoholism, malignancy, and cardiovascular disease. Stomatocytes can be seen on the blood smears of normal patients as a result of drying artifact.

TREATMENT
For severe hemolysis, patients might require RBC transfusion. Splenectomy is not recommended as a treatment for cation-leaky hereditary stomatocytosis. It is not effective and predisposes patients to in situ thrombosis after splenectomy. The thrombosis appears related to abnormal adherence of stomatocytic erythrocytes to the vascular endothelium.

Bibliography is available at Expert Consult.

Chapter **461**
Paroxysmal Nocturnal Hemoglobinuria and Acanthocytosis
George B. Segel

PAROXYSMAL NOCTURNAL HEMOGLOBINURIA
Etiology
Paroxysmal nocturnal hemoglobinuria (PNH) reflects an abnormality of marrow stem cells that affects each blood cell lineage. The disease is

Alternative pathway of complement

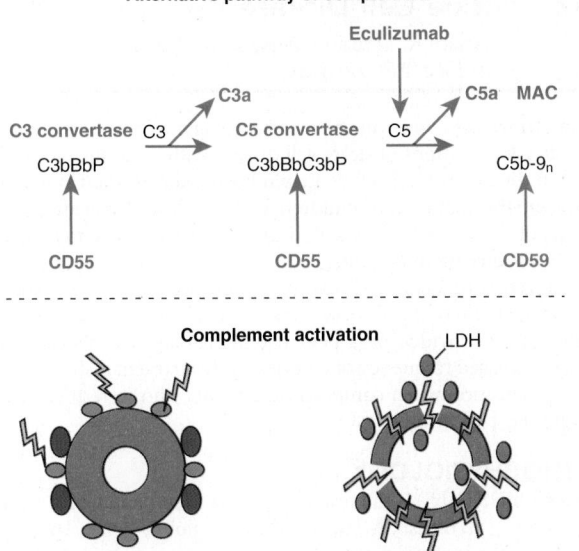

Figure 461-1 Complement-mediated lysis in PNH. Red circles are hemoglobin. Blue circles are decay accelerating factor (CD55). Green circles are membrane inhibitor of reactive lysis (CD59). Bb, activated factor B; C3b, activated C3; C5b, activated C5; GPI, glycosyl phosphatidylinositol; MAC, membrane attack complex (consisting of C5b, C6, C7, C8, and several molecules of C9 [9n]); RBC, red blood cell. *(From Parker C: Eculizumab for paroxysmal nocturnal haemoglobinuria,* Lancet *373:759–767, 2009.)*

an acquired somatic mutation that results in a defect in proteins of the cell membrane that renders the red blood cells (RBCs) and other cells susceptible to damage by normal plasma complement proteins (Fig. 461-1). The deficient membrane-associated proteins include decay-accelerating factor (CD55), the membrane inhibitor of reactive lysis (CD59), the C8 binding protein, and other proteins that normally impede complement lysis at various steps, specifically, the alternative pathway, which is constitutively activated. The underlying defect involves the glycolipid anchor that maintains these protective proteins on the cell surface. Various mutations in the *PIGA* gene that is involved in glycosylphosphatidylinositol anchor protein biosynthesis have been identified in patients with PNH. Glycosylphosphatidylinositol-deficient cells are found at low frequency in normal persons, suggesting that injury to the normal marrow stem cells provides a selective advantage to the progeny of PNH clones in the genesis of this disease.

Clinical Manifestations
PNH is a rare disorder in children. Approximately 60% of pediatric patients have marrow failure, and the remainder have either intermittent or chronic anemia, often with prominent intravascular hemolysis. Nocturnal and morning hemoglobinuria is a classic finding in adults when hemolysis is worse during sleep; chronic hemolysis is more common. In addition to chronic hemolysis, thrombocytopenia and leukopenia are often characteristic. Hemoglobinuria is rarely seen in children compared to adults with PNH. *Thrombosis and thromboembolic phenomena* are serious complications that may be related to altered glycoproteins on the platelet surface and resultant platelet activation and production of procoagulant microparticles. Abdominal venous thrombosis presents as recurrent episodes of abdominal pain, Budd-Chiari syndrome (hepatic veins), or splenomegaly (splenic vein). Furthermore, released free hemoglobin results in depletion of nitric oxide, fostering vasoconstriction, thrombosis, and pain. Back and head pain may also be prominent. Hypoplastic or aplastic pancytopenia can precede or follow the diagnosis of PNH; rarely, PNH may progress to acute myelogenous leukemia. At the time of presentation, more than 90% of patients with PNH have some blood abnormality (including

~35% with anemia alone, ~15% with anemia and thrombocytopenia, ~7% with anemia and neutropenia, and ~30% with pancytopenia), >10% have abdominal pain, and >5% have thrombosis. The mortality in PNH is related primarily to the development of aplastic anemia or thrombotic complications. The predicted survival rate for children before the development of eculizumab (see Treatment below) was 80% at 5 yr, 60% at 10 yr, and 28% at 20 yr.

Laboratory Findings
Hemosiderinuria, an elevated reticulocyte percentage, a low serum haptoglobin, and increased lactic dehydrogenase are common and reflect chronic intravascular hemolysis. Initially, the anemia is normocytic, but if iron deficiency develops, it becomes microcytic. Markedly reduced levels of RBC acetylcholinesterase activity and decay-accelerating factor also are found. Flow cytometry is the diagnostic test of choice for PNH. With the use of anti-CD59 for RBCs and anti-CD55 and anti-CD59 for granulocytes, flow cytometry is more sensitive than the classic RBC lysis (ham or sucrose) tests in detecting these reduced glycolipid-bound membrane proteins. Fluorescent-labeled aerolysin testing can heighten the sensitivity of detection by binding selectively to glycosylphosphatidylinositol anchors.

Treatment
Glucocorticoids such as prednisone (2 mg/kg/24 hr) have been used to treat acute hemolytic episodes; the dosage should be tapered as soon as the hemolysis abates. Prolonged anticoagulation (heparin or low-molecular-weight heparin) therapy may be of benefit when thromboses occur. Because of chronic urinary loss of iron as hemosiderin, iron therapy may be necessary. Androgens (e.g., fluoxymesterone [Halotestin]), antithymocyte globulin, cyclosporine, and growth factors (e.g., erythropoietin and granulocyte colony-stimulating factor) have been used to treat marrow failure. Bone marrow transplantation is successful in treating some cases; nonmyeloablative transplantation can reduce transplant-related mortality and morbidity.

Marrow failure and severe thrombosis are the most serious complications in children. Treatment has included hematopoietic stem cell transplantation if a suitable donor exists. Eculizumab has also resulted in sustained survival in the majority of patients. Eculizumab is an approved and effective treatment for PNH in adults. It is a monoclonal antibody against complement component C5, and it interrupts the excessive complement destruction of RBC and activation of platelets. It decreases the rate of hemolysis, stabilizes hemoglobin levels, reduces the number of transfusions, and reduces the risk of thrombosis. Survival in adults with PNH treated with eculizumab may not be different from sex- and age-matched control patients from the general population. However, the medication does not improve the hematopoietic clonal expansion or prevent marrow failure. Because of the cost and length of treatment required, particularly in children, it may be most useful in preventing thrombosis, anemia, and other symptoms while stem cell transplant is considered. Before beginning eculizumab, it is recommended to immunize patients with the meningococcal vaccine if the patient hasn't already received this vaccine. A poor response to eculizumab may be due to polymorphisms in the C5 gene that produce resistance to eculizumab blockades.

ACANTHOCYTOSIS
Acanthocytosis is characterized by RBCs with irregular circumferential pointed projections (see Fig. 458-4*E*). This morphologic finding is seen with alterations in the cholesterol:phospholipid ratio in some patients with liver disease or vitamin E deficiency, and in congenital abetalipoproteinemia or hypoprebetalipoproteinemia, associated with fat malabsorption, neuromuscular abnormalities, and retinitis pigmentosa (see Chapters 86.3 and 630). Normoproteinemic **neuroacanthocytosis** is also associated with 4 genetically diverse conditions (Table 461-1). These include chorea-acanthocytosis and the rare X-linked McLeod syndrome, which has absence of the KX (Kell) antigen, late-onset myopathy, peripheral neuropathy, chorea, splenomegaly, and hemolysis with acanthocytosis. There is usually >3% acanthocytes on peripheral smear and caudate atrophy noted on MRI. Acanthocytes

Table 461-1	Neuroacanthocytosis	
DISEASE	**INHERITANCE**	**MUTATION**
Chorea acanthocytosis	Autosomal recessive	VPS13A (CHAC gene)
McLeod syndrome	X-linked recessive	XK gene
Huntington disease–like 2	Autosomal dominant	JPH3
Pantothenate kinase-associated neurodegeneration	Autosomal recessive	PANK2

also are seen in pantothenate kinase-associated neurodegeneration (dystonia, rigidity, chorea, dysarthria, spasticity, retinopathy) and Huntington disease–like 2. The production of acanthocytes in chorea-acanthocytosis appears related to altered Lyn kinase activity with increased tyrosine phosphorylation and altered linkage of band 3 to other RBC membrane proteins.

In contrast, echinocytes or "burr cells" have a more regular distribution of projections or serrations along the surface of the RBCs. They often are seen as artifact, and less often in end-stage renal disease, and in some patients with liver disease.

Bibliography is available at Expert Consult.

Chapter **462**

Hemoglobinopathies

Michael R. DeBaun, Melissa J. Frei-Jones, and Elliott P. Vichinsky

HEMOGLOBIN DISORDERS

Hemoglobin is a tetramer consisting of 2 pairs of globin chains. Abnormalities in these proteins are referred to as *hemoglobinopathies*.

More than 800 variant hemoglobins have been described. The most common and useful clinical classification of hemoglobinopathies is based on nomenclature associated with alteration of the involved globin chain. Two hemoglobin gene clusters are involved in the production of hemoglobin and are located at the end of the short arms of chromosomes 16 and 11. Their control is complex, including an upstream locus control region on each respective chromosome and an X-linked control site. On chromosome 16, there are 3 genes within the alpha (α) gene cluster, namely zeta (ζ), alpha 1 (α_1), and alpha 2 (α_2). On chromosome 11, there are 5 genes within the beta (β) gene cluster, namely epsilon (ε), 2 gamma genes (γ), a delta gene (δ), and a beta gene (β).

The order of gene expression within each cluster roughly follows the order of expression during the embryonic period, fetal period, and eventually childhood. After 8 wk of fetal life, the embryonic hemoglobins, Gower-1 ($\zeta_2\varepsilon_2$), Gower-2 ($\alpha_2\varepsilon_2$), and Portland ($\zeta_2\gamma_2$), are formed. At 9 wk of fetal life, the major hemoglobin (Hb) is HbF ($\alpha_2\gamma_2$). HbA ($\alpha_2\beta_2$) first appears at approximately 1 mo of fetal life, but does not become the dominant hemoglobin until after birth, when HbF levels start to decline. HbA$_2$ ($\alpha_2\delta_2$) is a minor hemoglobin that appears shortly before birth and remains at a low level after birth. The final hemoglobin distribution pattern that occurs in childhood is not achieved until at least 6 mo of age and sometimes later. The normal hemoglobin pattern is ≥95% HbA, ≤3.5 HbA$_2$, and <2.5% HbF.

462.1 Sickle Cell Disease

Michael R. DeBaun, Melissa J. Frei-Jones, and Elliott P. Vichinsky

Great strides have been made in the management of both acute and chronic complications of sickle cell disease with a significant improvement in the life expectancy of a child born today in the United States. However, the majority of children with sickle cell disease are born outside of the United States with limited access to preventive care and disease-modifying treatments.

Children with sickle cell disease should be followed by experts in the management of this disease, most often by pediatric hematologists. Medical care provided by a pediatric hematologist is also associated with a decreased frequency of emergency department visits and length of hospitalization when compared to patients who were not seen by a hematologist within the last year.

PATHOPHYSIOLOGY

Hemoglobin S (HbS) is the result of a single base-pair change, thymine for adenine, at the sixth codon of the β-globin gene. This change encodes valine instead of glutamine in the 6th position in the β-globin molecule. Sickle cell anemia (HbSS), homozygous HbSS, occurs when both β-globin alleles have the sickle cell mutation (βs). Sickle cell disease refers to not only patients with sickle cell anemia, but also to compound heterozygotes where one β-globin allele includes the sickle cell mutation and the second β-globin allele includes a gene mutation other than the sickle cell mutation, such as HbC, β-thalassemia, HbD, and HbO^{Arab}. In sickle cell anemia, HbS is commonly as high as 90% of the total hemoglobin; whereas as in sickle cell disease, HbS is >50% of all hemoglobin.

In red blood cells, the hemoglobin molecule has a highly-specified conformation allowing for the transport of oxygen in the body. In the absence of globin-chain mutations, hemoglobin molecules do not interact with one another. However, the presence of HbS results in a conformational change in the hemoglobin tetramer and, in the deoxygenated state, HbS molecules can now interact with each other forming rigid polymers that give the red blood cell its characteristic "sickled" shape. The lung is the only organ capable of reversing the polymers, and any disease of the lung can be expected to compromise the degree of reversibility.

Intravascular sickling primarily occurs in the postcapillary venules and is a function of both mechanical obstruction by sickled red blood cells and increased adhesion between red blood cells, leukocytes and the vascular endothelium. Sickle cell disease is also an inflammatory disease based on nonspecific markers of inflammation, including, but not limited to, elevated baseline white blood cell count and cytokines.

DIAGNOSIS AND EPIDEMIOLOGY

Every state in the United States has instituted a mandatory newborn screening program for sickle cell disease. Such programs identify newborns with the disease and provide prompt diagnosis and referral to providers with expertise in sickle cell disease for anticipatory guidance and the initiation of penicillin before 4 mo of age.

The most commonly used procedures for newborn diagnosis include thin layer/isoelectric focusing and high-performance liquid chromatography (HPLC). A confirmatory step is recommended, with all patients who have initial abnormal screens being retested during the first clinical visit and after 6 mo of age to determine the final hemoglobin phenotype. In addition, a complete blood cell count (CBC) and hemoglobin phenotype determination is recommended for both parents to confirm the diagnosis and to provide an opportunity for genetic counseling. Table 462-1 correlates the initial hemoglobin phenotype at birth with the type of hemoglobinopathy, baseline hemoglobin range, and requirement for a hematologist.

In newborn screening programs, the hemoglobin with the greatest quantity is reported first, followed by other hemoglobins in order of decreasing quantity. In newborns with a hemoglobin analysis result

| Table 462-1 | Various Newborn Sickle Cell Disease Screening Results with Baseline Hemoglobin |

NEWBORN SCREENING RESULTS: SICKLE CELL DISEASE*	POSSIBLE HEMOGLOBIN PHENOTYPE[†]	BASELINE HEMOGLOBIN RANGE	EXPERTISE IN HEMATOLOGY CARE REQUIRED
FS	SCD-SS	6-11 g/dL	Yes
	SCD-S β^0 thal	6-10 g/dL	Yes
	SCD-S β^+ thal	9-12 g/dL	Yes
	SCD-S $\delta\beta^-$ thal	10-12 g/dL	Yes
	S HPFH	12-14 g/dL	Yes
FSC	SCD-SC	10-15 g/dL	Yes
FSA	SCD-S β^+ thal	9-12 g/dL	Yes
FS other	SCD-S β^0 thal	6-10 g/dL	Yes
	SCD-SD, SO^{Arab}, SC^{Harlem}, S^{Lepore}	Variable	Yes
AFS	SCD-SS	6-10 g/dL	Yes
	SCD-S β^+ thal	6-9 g/dL	Yes
	SCD-S β^0 thal[‡]	7-13 g/dL variable	Yes

*Hemoglobins are reported in order of quantity.
[†]Requires confirmatory hemoglobin analysis after at least 6 mo of age and, if possible, hemoglobin analysis from both parents for accurate diagnosis of hemoglobin phenotype.
[‡]Impossible to determine the diagnosis because the infant received a blood transfusion before testing.
A, normal hemoglobin; C, hemoglobin C; F, fetal hemoglobin; HPFH, hereditary persistence of fetal hemoglobin; O^{Arab}, hemoglobin O^{Arab}; S, sickle hemoglobin; SC, sickle-hemoglobin C; SCD, sickle cell disease; SS, homozygous sickle cell disease; thal, thalassemia.

of FS, the pattern supports HbSS, HbS hereditary persistent fetal hemoglobin (HPFH), or HbSβ-thalassemia zero. In a newborn with a hemoglobin analysis of FSA, the pattern is supportive of diagnosis HbSβ-thalassemia+. The diagnosis of HbSβ-thalassemia+ is confirmed if at least 50% of the hemoglobin is HbS, HbA is present, and the amount of HbA$_2$ is elevated (typically >3.5%); although, HbA$_2$ is not elevated in the newborn period. In newborns with a hemoglobin analysis of FSC, the pattern supports a diagnosis of HbSC. In newborns with a hemoglobin analysis of FAS, the pattern supports a diagnosis of HbAS (sickle cell trait).

A newborn with a hemoglobin analysis of AFS has been transfused with red blood cells prior to collection of the newborn screen because the amount of HbA is greater than the amount of HbF or there has been an error. The patient may have either sickle cell disease or sickle cell trait and should be started on penicillin prophylaxis until the final diagnosis can be determined.

Given the implications of a diagnosis of sickle cell disease versus sickle cell trait in a newborn, repeating the hemoglobin analysis in the patient and obtaining a hemoglobin analysis and CBC to evaluate the smear and red blood cell parameters in the parents for genetic counseling cannot be overemphasized. Unintended mistakes do occur in state newborn screening programs. Newborns who have the initial phenotype of HbFS but whose final true phenotype included HbSβ-thalassemia+ have been described as one of the more common errors identified in newborn screening hemoglobinopathy programs. Determining an accurate phenotype is important for appropriate genetic counseling for the parents.

In the event that the parents are tested for sickle cell trait or hemoglobinopathy trait testing, full disclosure must be provided that in some circumstances, the issue of paternity may be disclosed. For this reason and because of healthcare privacy, we always seek permission for the genetic testing and to ensure confidentiality, we report the hemoglobinopathy trait results back separately to each parent during separate visits.

In the United States, sickle cell disease is the most common genetic disorder identified through the state-mandated newborn screening program, occurring in 1:2,647. In regard to race in the United States, sickle cell disease occurs in African-Americans at a rate of 1:396 births, and in Hispanics at a rate of 1:36,000 births. In the United States, an estimated 90,000 people are affected by sickle cell disease, with an ethnic distribution of 90% African-American and 10% Hispanic. The United States sickle cell disease population represents a fraction of the worldwide burden of the disease, with global estimates of 312,000 neonates born annually with HbSS disease.

CLINICAL MANIFESTATIONS AND TREATMENT OF SICKLE CELL ANEMIA (HB SS)
Fever and Bacteremia

Fever in a child with sickle cell anemia is a medical emergency, requiring prompt medical evaluation and delivery of antibiotics because of the increased risk of bacterial infection and subsequent high mortality rate. Infants with sickle cell anemia, as early as 6 mo of age, develop abnormal immune function due to splenic infarction. By 5 yr of age, most children with sickle cell anemia have complete functional asplenia. Regardless of age, all patients with sickle cell anemia are at increased risk of infection and death from bacterial infection, particularly encapsulated organisms such as *Streptococcus pneumoniae*, *Haemophilus influenzae type b*, and *Neisseria meningitidis*.

The rate of bacteremia in children with sickle cell disease, presenting with fever in busy pediatric emergency department is less than 1%. Several clinical strategies have been developed to manage children with sickle cell anemia who present with fever. These vary from hospital admission for intravenous (IV) antimicrobial therapy to administering a 3rd-generation cephalosporin in an emergency department or outpatient setting to patients without established risk factors for occult bacteremia (Table 462-2). Given the observation that the average time for a positive blood culture is <20 hr in children with sickle cell anemia, admission for 24 hr is probably the most prudent strategy for children and families who live out of town or who are identified as high risk for poor follow-up.

Outpatient management of fever without a source should be considered in children with the lowest risk of bacteremia and after intravenous ceftriaxone or other cephalosporin is given. Observation after antibiotic administration is important as children who have sickle cell anemia treated with ceftriaxone can develop severe, rapid, and life-threatening immune hemolysis. In the event that *Salmonella* spp. or *Staphylococcus aureus* bacteremia occurs, strong consideration should be given to an evaluation for osteomyelitis with a bone scan given the increased risk of osteomyelitis in children with sickle cell anemia when compared to the general population.

Aplastic Crisis

Human parvovirus B19 poses a unique threat for patients with sickle cell anemia because such infections result in temporary **red cell aplasia**, limiting the production of reticulocytes and causing profound anemia. Any child with sickle cell disease, fever, and reticulocytopenia should be considered to have parvovirus B19 until proven otherwise. The acute anemia of an aplastic crisis is treated conservatively using

Table 462-2	Clinical Factors Associated with Increased Risk of Bacteremia Requiring Admission in Febrile Children with Sickle Cell Disease

Seriously ill appearance

Hypotension: systolic blood pressure <70 mm Hg at 1 yr of age or <70 mm Hg + 2 × the age in yr for older children

Poor perfusion: capillary-refill time >4 sec

Temperature >40.0°C (104°F)

A corrected white-cell count >30,000/mm³ or <5000/mm³

Platelet count <100,000/mm³

History of pneumococcal sepsis

Severe pain

Dehydration: poor skin turgor, dry mucous membranes, history of poor fluid intake, or decreased output of urine

Infiltration of a segment or a larger portion of the lung

Hemoglobin level <5.0 g/dL

From Wilimas JA, Flynn PM, Harris S et al: A randomized study of outpatient treatment with ceftriaxone for selected febrile children with sickle cell disease, N Engl J Med 329:472–476, 1993.

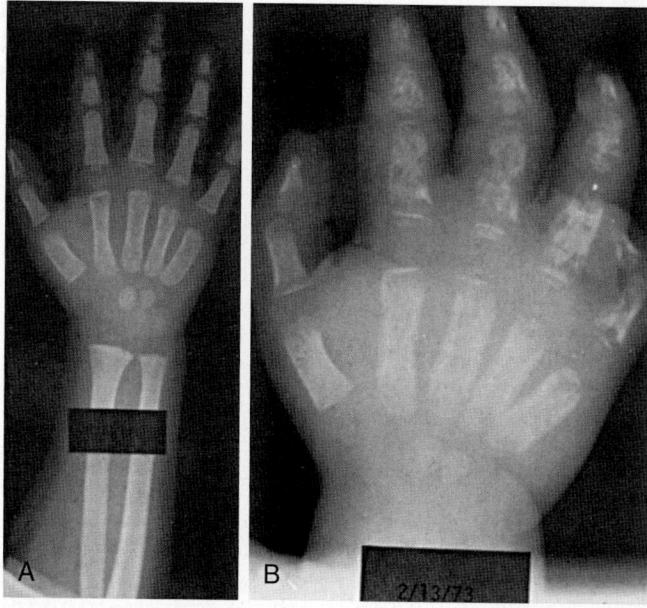

Figure 462-1 Roentgenograms of an infant with sickle cell anemia and acute dactylitis. **A,** The bones appear normal at the onset of the episode. **B,** Destructive changes and periosteal reaction are evident 2 wk later.

red blood cell transfusion when the patient becomes hemodynamically symptomatic or has a concurrent illness, such as acute chest syndrome. In addition, acute infection with parvovirus B19 is associated with pain, splenic sequestration, acute chest syndrome (ACS), glomerulo-nephritis, and stroke. Patients with parvovirus-associated aplastic crisis are contagious and infection precautions should be taken to avoid nosocomial spread of the infection.

Splenic Sequestration

Acute splenic sequestration is a life-threatening complication occurring primarily in infants and young children with sickle cell anemia. The incidence of splenic sequestration has declined from an estimated 30% to 12.6% with early identification by newborn screening and parental education. Sequestration can occur as early as 5 wk of age, but most often occurs in children between the ages of 6 mo and 2 yr.

Splenic sequestration is associated with rapid spleen enlargement causing left-sided abdominal pain and a decline in hemoglobin of at least 2 g/dL from the patient's baseline. Sequestration may lead to signs of hypovolemia as a result of the trapping of blood in the spleen; profound anemia, with total hemoglobin falling below 3 g/dL, has been reported. Reticulocytosis and a decrease in the platelet count may also be present. Sequestration may be triggered by fever, bacteremia, or viral infections.

Treatment includes early intervention and maintenance of hemodynamic stability using isotonic fluid or blood transfusions. Careful blood transfusions with red blood cells are recommended to treat both the sequestration and the resultant anemia. Blood transfusion aborts the red blood cell sickling in the spleen and allows release of the patient's blood cells that have become sequestered, often raising the hemoglobin above baseline values. We typically recommend only 5 mL/kg of red blood cells because the goal is to prevent hypovolemia. Blood transfusion that results in hemoglobin levels above 10 g/dL may put the patient at risk for hyperviscosity syndrome because of the risk that that patient may release the blood within the spleen.

Repeated episodes of splenic sequestration are common, occurring in two-thirds of patients. Most recurrent episodes develop within 6 mo of the previous episode. Prophylactic splenectomy performed after an acute episode has resolved is the only effective strategy for preventing future life-threatening episodes. Although blood transfusion therapy has been used with the goal of preventing subsequent episodes, evidence strongly suggests this strategy does not reduce the risk of recurrent splenic sequestration when compared to no transfusion therapy.

Furthermore, prophylactic blood transfusion therapy may put the patient at risk for autotransfusion (the phenomenon when the blood sequestered in the spleen is released and dramatically increases the hemoglobin concentration, putting the patient at risk for hyperviscosity syndrome).

Hepatic and Gallbladder Involvement
See Chapters 360 and 366.

Sickle Cell Pain
Dactylitis, referred to as **hand-foot syndrome**, is often the first manifestation of pain in infants and young children with sickle cell anemia, occurring in 50% of children by their 2nd yr of life (Fig. 462-1). Dactylitis often manifests with symmetric or unilateral swelling of the hands and/or feet. Unilateral dactylitis can be confused with osteomyelitis, and careful evaluation to distinguish between the two is important because treatment differs significantly. Dactylitis requires palliation with pain medications, such as hydrocodone, whereas osteomyelitis requires at least 4-6 wk of IV antibiotics. Given the recent association between genotype and metabolism of codeine, a subgroup of children may not get pain relief from codeine. Hence, feedback from the parents is needed to determine if therapy was successful in relieving pain.

The cardinal clinical feature of sickle cell anemia is **acute vasoocclusive pain**. No written definition can describe the visual picture of a child with sickle cell anemia experiencing pain. Acute sickle cell pain is characterized as unremitting discomfort that can occur in any part of the body but most often occurs in the chest, abdomen, or extremities. These painful episodes are often abrupt and cause disruption of daily life activities and anguish for children and their caregivers. A patient with sickle cell anemia has approximately 1 painful episode per year that requires medical attention.

The exact etiology of pain is unknown, but the pathogenesis is initiated when blood flow is disrupted in the microvasculature by sickled cells, resulting in tissue ischemia. Acute sickle cell pain may be precipitated by physical stress, infection, dehydration, hypoxia, local or systemic acidosis, exposure to cold, and swimming for prolonged periods. Successful treatment of painful episodes requires education of both the caregivers and patients regarding the recognition of symptoms and the optimal management strategy. Given the absence of any reliable objective laboratory or clinical parameter associated with pain, trust between the patient and the treating physician is paramount to successful clinical management. Specific therapy for pain varies greatly but generally includes the use of acetaminophen or a nonsteroidal antiinflammatory agent early in the course of pain, followed by escalation to a combination analgesic such as hydrocodone, or to a single-agent short- or long-acting oral opioid.

Some patients require hospitalization for administration of intravenous morphine or derivatives of morphine. The incremental increase and decrease in the use of the medication to relieve pain roughly parallels the 8 phases associated with a chronology of pain and comfort (Table 462-3). The average hospital length of stay for children admitted in pain is 4.4 days. The American Pain Society has published clinical guidelines for treating acute and chronic pain in patients with sickle cell disease of any type. These recommendations are comprehensive and represent a starting point for treating pain (http://www.ampainsoc.org/pub/sc.htm).

The only measure for degree of pain is the patient. Healthcare providers working with children in pain should use a consistent, validated pain scale, such as the Wong-Baker FACES Scale for assessing pain. Although pain scales have proved useful for some children, others require prenegotiated activities to determine when opioid therapy should be initiated and decreased. For instance, sleeping through the night might be an indication for decreasing pain medication by 20% the following morning. The majority of painful episodes in patients with sickle cell anemia are managed at home with comfort measures, such as heating blanket, relaxation techniques, massage, and oral pain medication.

Several myths have been propagated regarding the treatment of pain in sickle cell anemia. The concept that painful episodes in children should be managed without opioids is without foundation and results in unwarranted suffering on the part of the patient. Blood transfusion therapy during an existing painful episode does not decrease the intensity or duration of the painful episode as tissue necrosis occurs well before the ability to administer the transfusion. Intravenous hydration does not relieve or prevent pain and is appropriate when the patient is dehydrated or unable to drink as a result of the severe pain. *Opioid dependency in children with sickle cell anemia is rare and should never be used as a reason to withhold pain medication.* However, patients with multiple painful episodes requiring hospitalization within a year or with pain episodes that require hospitalization for more than 7 days should be evaluated for comorbidities and environmental stressors that are contributing to the frequency or duration of pain. Children with chronic pain should be evaluated for other reasons associated with vasoocclusive pain episodes, including, but not limited to, overexertion with physical activities, such as participating in the school band, sports, or heavy lifting of backpacks to and from school and up and down steps. A careful history is warranted to distinguish chronic pain that often is not relieved by opioids alone versus acute unremitting vasoocclusive pain episodes.

Skeletal pain (bone or bone marrow infarction) with or without fever must be differentiated from osteomyelitis. Both *Salmonella* spp. and *S. aureus* cause osteomyelitis in children with sickle cell anemia, which is often in the diaphysis of long bones (in contrast to children without sickle cell anemia where osteomyelitis is in the metaphyseal region of the bone). Differentiating osteonecrosis from a vasoocclusive

Table 462-3	Summary of the Chronology of Pain in Children with Sickle Cell Disease	
PHASE	**PAIN CHARACTERISTICS**	**SUGGESTED COMFORT MEASURES USED**
1 (Baseline)	No vasoocclusive pain; pain of complications may be present, such as that connected with avascular necrosis of the hip	No comfort measures used
2 (Prepain)	No vasoocclusive pain; pain of complications may be present; prodromal signs of impending vasoocclusive episode may appear, e.g., "yellow eyes" and/or fatigue	No comfort measures used; caregivers may encourage child to increase fluids to prevent pain event from occurring
3 (Pain start point)	First signs of vasoocclusive pain appear, usually in mild form	Mild oral analgesic often given; fluids increased; child usually maintains normal activities
4 (Pain acceleration)	Intensive of pain increases from mild to moderate Some children skip this level or move quickly from phase 3 to phase 5	Stronger oral analgesic are given; rubbing, heat, or other activities are often used; child usually stays in school until the pain becomes more severe, then stays home and limits activities; is usually in bed; family searches for ways to control the pain
5 (Peak pain experience)	Pain accelerates to high moderate or severe levels and plateaus; pain can remain elevated for extended period Child's appearance, behavior, and mood are significantly different from normal	Oral analgesics are given around the clock at home; combination of comfort measures is used; family might avoid going to the hospital; if pain is very distressing to the child, parent takes the child to the emergency department After child enters the hospital, families often turn over comforting activities to healthcare providers and wait to see if the analgesics work Family caregivers are often exhausted from caring for the child for several days with little or no rest
6 (Pain decrease start point)	Pain finally begins to decrease in intensity from the peak pain level	Family caregivers again become active in comforting the child but not as intensely as during phases 4 and 5
7 (Steady pain decline)	Pain decreases more rapidly, become more tolerable for the child Child and family are more relaxed	Healthcare providers begin to wean the child from the IV analgesic; oral opioids given; discharge planning is started Children may be discharged before they are pain free
8 (Pain resolution)	Pain intensity is at a tolerable level, and discharge is imminent Child looks and acts like "normal" self; mood improves	May receive oral analgesics

Adapted from Beyer JE, Simmons LE, Woods GM, et al: A chronology of pain and comfort in children with sickle cell disease, Arch Pediatr Adolesc Med 153:913–920, 1999.

crisis and osteomyelitis is often difficult; patients with osteomyelitis often have a longer duration of fever and pain, swelling of the affected area, fewer or only 1 location of pain *and* tenderness, higher white blood cell counts, and an elevated C-reactive protein. Blood cultures, when positive, are helpful.

Imaging studies, which must include MRI with contrast, are helpful in distinguishing osteomyelitis from bone or marrow infarction, although rarely an osteomyelitis may initially appear "cold" (infarctive osteomyelitis), whereas an infarct, over time, may appear hyperemic as it heals. Both lesions may demonstrate marrow signal intensity abnormalities, periosteal elevation, and bone, periosteal, or extraosseous fluid collections. MRI findings suggestive of osteomyelitis include localized medullary fluid, sequestrum, and cortical defects. Ultimately, aspiration with or with or without biopsy and culture will be needed to differentiate the 2 processes (see Chapter 684).

Avascular Necrosis

Avascular necrosis (AVN) occurs at a higher rate among children with sickle cell anemia than in the general population, and is a source of both acute and chronic pain. Most commonly, the femoral head is affected and AVN. Unfortunately, the AVN of the hip may cause limp and leg-length discrepancy. Other sites affected include the humeral head and mandible. Risk factors for AVN include HbSS disease with α-thalassemia trait, frequent vasoocclusive episodes, and elevated hematocrit (for patients with sickle cell anemia). Optimal treatment of AVN has not been determined and individual management requires consultation with the disease-specific specialist, orthopedic surgeon, physical therapist, hematologist and primary care physician. Initial management may include referral to a physical therapist to address strategies to increase strength and decrease weight bearing daily activities that may exacerbate the pain associated with AVN. Opioids are often used, but usually can be tapered after the acute pain has subsided with AVN. Regular blood transfusion therapy has not been demonstrated as an effective therapy to abate the acute and chronic pain associated AVN.

Priapism

Priapism is defined as an unwanted painful erection of the penis and most commonly affects males with sickle cell anemia. The mean age of first episode is 15 yr, although priapism has been reported in children as young as 3 yr. The actuarial probability of a patient experiencing priapism is approximately 90% by 20 yr of age.

Priapism occurs in 2 patterns: prolonged, lasting more than 4 hr, or stuttering, with brief episodes that resolve spontaneously but may occur in clusters and herald a prolonged event. Both types occur from early childhood to adulthood. Most episodes occur between 3 A.M. and 9 A.M. Priapism in sickle cell disease represents a low flow state caused by venous stasis from sickling of red blood cells in the corpora cavernosa. Recurrent prolonged episodes of priapism are associated with impotence.

The optimal treatment for acute priapism is unknown. Acutely, supportive therapy, such as a hot shower, short aerobic exercise, or pain medication, is commonly used by patients at home. A prolonged episode lasting >4 hr should be treated by aspiration of blood from the corpora cavernosa followed by irrigation with dilute epinephrine to produce immediate and sustained detumescence. Urology consultation is required to initiate this procedure, with appropriate input from a hematologist. Simple blood transfusion and exchange transfusion has been proposed for the acute treatment of priapism, but limited evidence supports this strategy as the initial management. We typically refer a patient to the urology service first, and if no benefit is obtained from surgical management, consider transfusion therapy. However, detumescence may not occur for up to 24 hr (far longer than with urologic aspiration) after transfusion and transfusion for priapism has been associated with acute neurologic events.

Neurologic Complications

Neurologic complications associated with sickle cell anemia are varied and complex, ranging from *acute* ischemic stroke with focal neurologic deficit to clinically *silent* abnormalities found on radiologic imaging. Prior to the development of transcranial Doppler to screen for stroke risk among children with sickle cell anemia, approximately 11% experienced an overt stroke and 20% a silent stroke before their 18th birthday. A functional definition of overt stroke is the presence of a focal neurologic deficit lasting for >24 hr and/or abnormal neuroimaging of the brain indicating a cerebral infarct on T2-weighted magnetic resonance imaging (MRI) corresponding to the focal neurologic deficit (Figs. 462-2 and 462-3). A silent cerebral infarct, as its name indicates, lacks focal neurologic findings lasting >24 hr and is diagnosed by abnormal imaging on T2-weighted MRI. Children with other

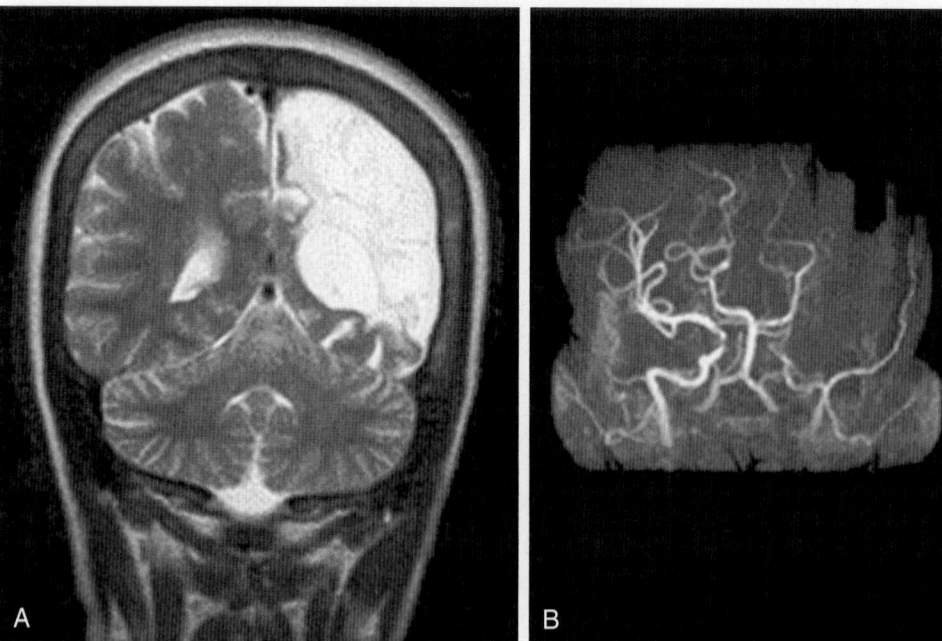

Figure 462-2 T2-weighted MRI and magnetic resonance angiography of the brain. **A,** T2-weighted MRI shows remote infarction of the territories of the left anterior cerebral artery and middle cerebral artery. **B,** Magnetic resonance angiography shows occlusion of the left internal carotid artery siphon distal to the takeoff of the ophthalmic artery.

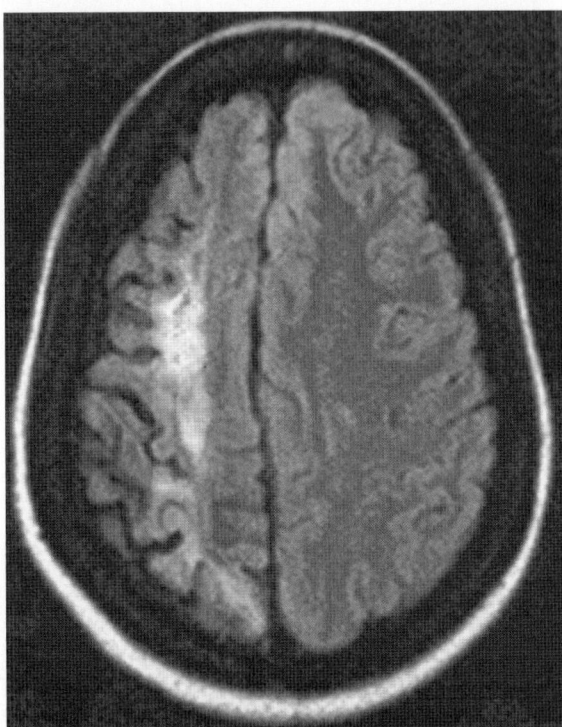

Figure 462-3 Fast fluid-attenuated inversion recovery sequence MRI of the brain showing a right hemisphere border-zone cerebral infarction in a child with sickle cell anemia. *(From Switzer JA, Hess DC, Nichols F, et al: Pathophysiology and treatment of stroke in sickle-cell disease: present and future. Lancet Neurol 5:501–512, 2006.)*

types of sickle cell disease, such as HbSC or HbSβ-thalassemia+, develop overt or silent cerebral infarcts as well, but at a lower frequency than children with HbSS and HbSβ-thalassemia zero. Other neurologic complications include headaches that may or may not correlate to degree of anemia, seizures, cerebral venous thrombosis and reversible posterior leukoencephalopathy syndrome, also referred to as posterior reversible encephalopathy syndrome (PRES).

For patients presenting with acute focal neurologic deficit, a prompt pediatric neurologic evaluation is recommended, as well as consultation with a pediatric hematologist. In addition, oxygen administration to keep oxygen saturations >96% and simple blood transfusion within 1 hr of presentation with a goal of increasing the hemoglobin to a maximum of 10 g/dL is warranted. A timely simple blood transfusion is important because this is the most efficient strategy to dramatically increase oxygen content of the blood, if the oxygen saturation is above 96%. To exceed this hemoglobin threshold limits oxygen delivery to the brain as a result of hyperviscosity by increasing the hemoglobin significantly over the patient's baseline values. Subsequently, prompt treatment with an exchange transfusion should be considered, either manually or with automated erythrocytapheresis, to reduce the HbS percentage to at least <50%, and ideally to <30%. Exchange transfusion at the time of acute stroke is associated with a decreased risk of second stroke when compared to simple transfusion alone. Computed tomography (CT) of the head to exclude cerebral hemorrhage should be performed as soon as possible, and if available, MRI of the brain with diffusion-weighted imaging to distinguish between ischemic infarcts and PRES. Magnetic resonance (MR) venography is useful to evaluate the possibility of cerebral venous thrombosis, a rare but potential cause of focal neurologic deficit in children with sickle cell disease. MR angiography may identify evidence of cerebral vasculopathy; these images are not critical in the initial time management of a child with sickle cell disease presenting with a focal neurologic deficit.

The clinical presentation of PRES or central venous thrombosis can mimic a stroke but would require a different treatment course. For both PRES and cerebral venous thrombosis, the optimal management has not been defined in patients with sickle cell disease, resulting in the need for consultation with both a pediatric neurologist and a pediatric hematologist.

Transcranial Doppler Ultrasonography

Primary prevention of overt stroke can be accomplished using **transcranial Doppler ultrasonography** (TCD) assessment of the blood velocity in the terminal portion of the internal carotid and the proximal portion of the middle cerebral artery. Children with sickle cell anemia with an elevated time-averaged mean maximum (TAMM) blood-flow velocity >200 cm/sec are at increased risk for a cerebrovascular event. A TAMM measurement of <200 cm/sec but ≥180 cm/sec represents a conditional threshold. A repeat measurement is suggested within a few months because of the high rate of conversion to a TCD velocity >200 cm/sec in this group of patients.

Two distinct methods of measuring TCD velocity exist: a nonimaging and an imaging technique. The nonimaging technique was the method used in the TCD trial sponsored by the National Institutes of Health, whereas most pediatric radiologists in practice use the imaging technique. When compared to each other, the imaging technique produces values that are 10-15% below that of the nonimaging technique. The imaging technique uses the time-averaged mean of the maximum velocity (TAMX), and this measure is believed to be equivalent to the nonimaging calculation of TAMM. A downward adjustment for the transfusion threshold is appropriate for centers using the imaging method to assess TCD velocity. The magnitude of the transfusion threshold in the imaging technique has not been settled, but a transfusion threshold of a TAMX of 185 cm/sec and a conditional threshold of TAMX of 165 cm/sec, seems reasonable.

The primary approach for prevention of recurrent overt stroke is blood transfusion therapy aimed at keeping the maximum HbS concentration <30%. Despite regular blood transfusion therapy, around 20% of patients will have a second stroke and 30% of this group will have a third stroke. Children with TCD values above defined thresholds should begin chronic blood transfusion therapy to maintain HbS levels <30% to decrease the risk of first stroke. This strategy results in an 85% reduction in the rate of overt strokes. Once transfusion therapy is initiated, patients are expected to continue it indefinitely as discontinuation of blood transfusion therapy is associated with an increase in the development of silent infarcts.

Pulmonary Complications

Lung disease in children with sickle cell anemia is the second most common reason for hospital admission and is associated with significant mortality. ACS refers to a life-threatening pulmonary complication of sickle cell disease defined as a new radiodensity on chest radiography plus any 2 of the following: fever, respiratory distress, hypoxia, cough, or chest pain (Fig. 462-4). Even in the absence of respiratory symptoms, all patients with fever should receive a chest radiograph to identify evolving ACS because clinical examination alone is insufficient to identify patients with a new radiographic density and early detection of ACS will alter clinical management. The radiographic findings in ACS are variable but may include single lobe involvement, predominantly left lower lobe; multiple lobes, most often both lower lobes; and pleural effusions, either unilateral or bilateral. ACS may progress rapidly from a simple infiltrate to extensive infiltrates and a pleural effusion. Therefore, continued pulse oximetry and frequent clinical exams are required, and repeat chest x-rays are indicated for progressive hypoxia, dyspnea, tachypnea, and other signs of respiratory distress.

The majority of patients with ACS do not have a single identifiable cause. Infection is the most well-known etiology, yet only 30% of ACS episodes will have positive sputum or bronchoalveolar culture, and the most common pathogens are *S. pneumoniae*, *Mycoplasma pneumoniae*, and *Chlamydia* sp. The most frequent event preceding ACS is a painful episode requiring systemic opioid treatment. Fat emboli has also been implicated as a cause of ACS, arising from infarcted bone marrow, and can be life-threatening if large amounts are released to the lungs. Fat

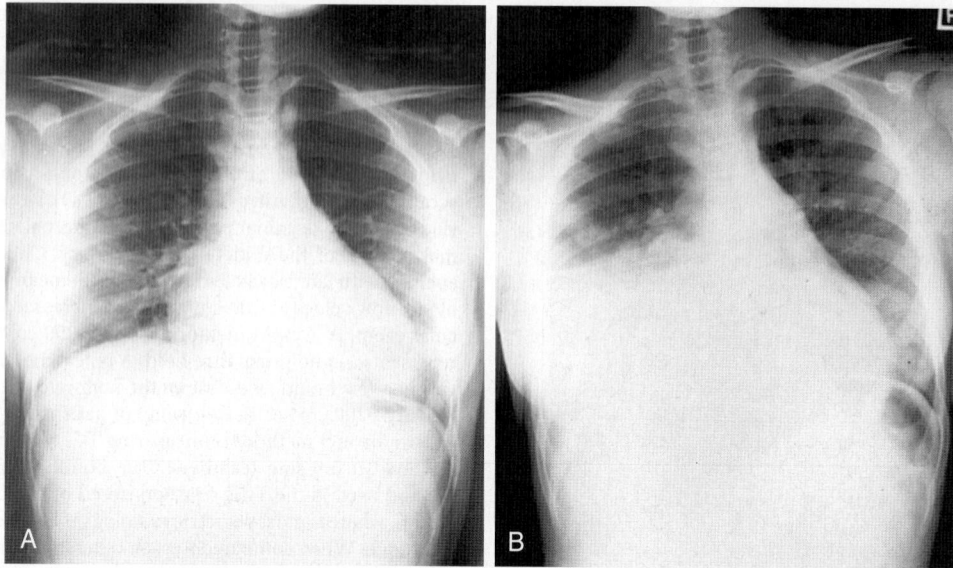

Figure 462-4 Probable pulmonary infarction in a 15 yr old patient with Hb-SS. **A,** Frontal radiograph shows consolidation and a small pleural effusion posteriorly in the right lower lobe. **B,** Radiograph obtained <24 hr later shows massive right middle and lower lobe consolidation and effusion. No organisms could be cultured. The diagnosis of "probably pulmonary infarction" was established clinically. *(Courtesy of Dr. Thomas L. Stovis, Children's Hospital of Michigan, Detroit, MI. From Kuhn JP, Slovis TL, Haller JO: Caffey's pediatric diagnostic imaging, vol 1, ed 10, Philadelphia, 2004, Mosby, p. 1087.)*

emboli can be difficult to diagnose but should be considered in any patient with sickle cell disease, presenting with rapid onset of respiratory distress and altered mental status changes. Petechial rash, may also occur, but may be difficult to detect if not looked for carefully.

Given that the causes of ACS are varied, recommended management is also multimodal (Table 462-4). The type of opioid, with morphine being more likely to cause ACS than nalbuphine hydrochloride, is associated with an increase in the risk of ACS in part because of hypoventilation. However, under no circumstance should opioid administration be limited to prevent ACS; rather, care must be taken to prevent ACS from developing. In patients with chest pain, regular use of an incentive spirometer at 10-12 breaths every 2 hr can significantly reduce the frequency of subsequent acute chest pain episodes. As a result of the clinical overlap between pneumonia and ACS, all episodes should be treated promptly with antimicrobial therapy, including at least a macrolide and possibly a third-generation cephalosporin. A previous diagnosis of asthma or airway hyperresponsiveness should prompt treatment following standard of care for an asthma exacerbation with corticosteroids and bronchodilators. The diagnosis of ACS does not negate the recommended management of a patient with asthma exacerbation. Oxygen should be administered for patients who demonstrate hypoxia. Blood transfusion therapy using either simple or exchange (manual or automated) transfusion is the only method to abort a rapidly progressing episode of ACS. The decision when to give blood and whether the transfusion should be a simple or exchange transfusion is less clearly defined. Commonly blood transfusions are given when at least 1 of the following clinical features are present: decreasing oxygen saturation, increasing work of breathing, rapid change in respiratory effort either with or without a worsening chest radiograph, a drop in hemoglobin of 2 g/dL below their baseline, or previous history of severe ACS requiring admission to the intensive care unit.

Pulmonary hypertension has been identified as a major risk factor for death in adults with sickle cell anemia. The natural history of pulmonary hypertension in children with sickle cell anemia is unknown. Optimal strategies for screening at risk patients have not been identified (echocardiogram results are not supported by right heart catheterization results demonstrating elevated pulmonary artery pressures) and the best diagnostic methodology carries significant risk of harm. Attempts to identify targeted therapeutic interventions to

Table 462-4	Overall Strategies for the Management of Acute Chest Syndrome

PREVENTION
Incentive spirometry and periodic ambulation in patients admitted for sickle cell pain, surgery, or febrile episodes
Watchful waiting in any hospitalized child or adult with sickle cell disease (pulse oximetry monitoring and frequent respiratory assessments)
Cautious use of intravenous fluids
Intense education and optimum care of patients who have sickle cell anemia and asthma

DIAGNOSTIC TESTING AND LABORATORY MONITORING
Blood cultures
Nasopharyngeal samples for viral culture (respiratory syncytial virus, influenza)
Blood counts every day and appropriate chemistries
Continuous pulse oximetry
Chest radiographs

TREATMENT
Blood transfusion (simple or exchange)
Supplemental O_2 for drop in pulse oximetry by 4% over baseline, or values <90%
Empirical antibiotics (third-generation cephalosporin and macrolide)
Continued respiratory therapy (incentive spirometry and chest physiotherapy as necessary)
Bronchodilators and steroids for patients with asthma
Optimum pain control and fluid management

alter the natural history of pulmonary hypertension in adults have been unsuccessful.

Renal Disease and Enuresis

Renal disease among patients with sickle cell disease is a major comorbid condition that can lead to premature death. Seven sickle cell disease nephropathies have been identified: (1) gross hematuria, (2) papillary necrosis, (3) nephrotic syndrome, (4) renal infarction, (5) hyposthenuria, (6) pyelonephritis, and (7) renal medullary carcinoma. As expected, the presentation of these entities is varied but may include hematuria, proteinuria, renal insufficiency, concentrating defects, or hypertension.

The common presence of nocturnal enuresis occurring in children with sickle cell anemia is not well defined but is troublesome to affected children and their parents. The overall prevalence of enuresis was 33% in the Cooperative Study of Sickle Cell Disease with the highest prevalence (42%) among children ages 6-8 yr. Furthermore, enuresis may still occur in approximately 9% of the older adolescent group. As would be the case in all children with nocturnal enuresis, we would systematically evaluate the children for recurrent urinary tract infections, kidney function, and possibly obstructive sleep apnea syndrome with a supportive history. Unfortunately, most children with nocturnal enuresis do not have an etiology and targeted therapeutic interventions have been of limited success.

Cognitive and Psychological Complications
As with any child with a chronic illness, good health maintenance must include routine psychological and social assessment. Ongoing evaluation of the family unit and identification of the resources available to cope with a chronic illness are critical for optimal management. Children and adolescents with sickle cell disease also have decreased quality of life, as measured on standardized assessments, compared to their siblings and children with other chronic diseases. Furthermore, children with sickle cell disease are at great risk for academic failure and have a 20% high school graduation rate. One reason behind the low high school graduation rate is that approximately a third of children with sickle cell anemia have had a cerebral infarct—either silent cerebral infarcts or overt strokes. Children with cerebral infarcts require ongoing cognitive and school performance assessment so that education resources can be focused to optimize educational attainment. Relevant support groups and attendance in group activities, such as camps for children with sickle cell disease, may be of direct benefit by improving self-esteem and establishing peer relationships.

Other Complications
In addition to the previously mentioned organ dysfunctions, patients with sickle cell anemia can have other significant complications. These complications include, but are not limited to sickle cell retinopathy, delayed onset of puberty, and leg ulcers. Optimal treatment for each of these entities has not been determined and individual management requires consultation with the disease-specific specialist, a hematologist, and primary care physician.

THERAPEUTIC CONSIDERATIONS
Hydroxyurea
Hydroxyurea, a myelosuppressive agent, is the only drug proven effective in reducing the frequency of painful episodes. In a large clinical trial of adults with sickle cell anemia, hydroxyurea was found to decrease the rate of hospitalization for painful episodes by 50% and the rate of ACS and blood transfusion by almost 50%. Follow-up of the original trial found that adults taking hydroxyurea had shorter hospital stays and required less pain medication during hospitalization. In children with sickle cell anemia, a safety feasibility trial of hydroxyurea demonstrated that hydroxyurea was safe and well tolerated in children >5 yr of age. No clinical adverse events were identified in this study; the primary toxicities were limited to myelosuppression that reversed upon cessation of the drug. Infants treated with hydroxyurea also experienced fewer episodes of pain, dactylitis, and ACS, and were less-often hospitalized or received a blood transfusion. Despite being a myelosuppressive agent, the infants treated with hydroxyurea did not experience increased rates of bacteremia or serious infection.

Hydroxyurea may be indicated for other sickle cell–related complications, especially in patients who are unable to tolerate other treatments. For patients who either will not or cannot continue blood transfusion therapy to prevent recurrent stroke, hydroxyurea therapy may be a reasonable alternative. The trial assessing the efficacy of hydroxyurea as an alternative to transfusions to prevent second stroke was terminated early after the data safety and monitoring found an increased stroke rate in the hydroxyurea arm compared to the transfu-

sion arm (0 vs. 7 [10%]). Hydroxyurea alone is inferior to transfusion therapy for secondary stroke prevention in patients who do not have contraindications to ongoing transfusions. Although not investigated as a primary outcome, hydroxyurea appears to have promise for the prevention of recurrent priapism. One study found hydroxyurea decreased glomerular hyperfiltration in young children with sickle cell anemia.

The long-term toxicity associated with initiating hydroxyurea in very young children has not yet been established. However, all evidence to date suggests that the benefits far outweigh the risks. For these reasons, children >2 yr of age receiving hydroxyurea require well-informed parents and medical care by pediatric hematologists, or at least comanagement by a physician with expertise in immunosuppressive medications. The typical starting dose of hydroxyurea is 15-20 mg/kg given once daily, with an incremental dosage increase every 8 wk of 5 mg/kg, and if no toxicities occur, up to a maximum of 35 mg/kg per dose. The infant hydroxyurea study found young children could safely be started at 20 mg/kg/day without increased toxicity. Achievement of the therapeutic effect of hydroxyurea can require several months, and for this reason, inpatient initiating of hydroxyurea is not optimal. We prefer to introduce the concept to parents within the first year of life, provide literature that describes both the pros and cons of starting hydroxyurea in children with severe symptoms of sickle cell disease, and educate parents on starting hydroxyurea in asymptomatic children as a preventative therapy for repetitive pain and ACS events. Other effects of hydroxyurea that may vary include an increase in the total hemoglobin level and a decrease in the TCD velocity.

Hematopoietic Stem Cell Transplantation
The only cure for sickle cell anemia is transplantation with human leukocyte antigen (HLA)–matched **hematopoietic stem cells** from a sibling or unrelated donor. The most common indications for transplant are recurrent ACS, stroke and abnormal TCD. Sibling-matched stem cell transplantation has a lower risk for graft-versus-host disease than unrelated donors. However, few children have suitable sibling donors. Stem cell transplantation using an unrelated but well-matched donor is the subject of an open clinical trial. The decision to consider unrelated transplantation should involve appropriate consultation and counseling from physicians with expertise in sickle cell transplantation.

Stem cell transplantation for children with sickle cell disease with a genetically matched sibling is not routinely done, in part because of the known risk of transplantation-related mortality and morbidity in a short period of time, commonly less than 2 yr after the transplantation versus the high probability that patients will live to and through adulthood. The use of hydroxyurea has dramatically decreased the disease burden for the patient and family, with associated far fewer hospitalizations for pain or ACS episodes and less use of blood transfusions. Furthermore, the field of stem cell transplantation is progressing so rapidly that in a decade or less haplo-identical transplantation will be considered a viable option for not only individuals with severe disease, but also those with less-severe manifestations. Haplo-identical transplantations in adults with severe manifestations of sickle cell disease resulted in no deaths, and approximately 60% of the participants were cured of the disease. Low intensity, nonmyeloablative HLA-matched sibling allogenic stem cell transplantation has been employed in patients ≥16 years of age.

Red Blood Cell Transfusions
Red blood cell transfusions are frequently used in the management of children with sickle cell anemia, both in the treatment of acute complications such as ACS, aplastic crisis, splenic sequestration, and acute stroke, and to prevent surgery-related ACS and first stroke in patients with abnormal TCD or MRI findings (silent stroke). Patients with sickle cell disease are at increased risk of developing alloantibodies to less-common red cell surface antigens after receiving even a single transfusion. In addition to standard cross-matching for major blood group antigens (A, B, O, RhD), more extended matching should be performed to identify donor units that are C-, E-, and Kell-antigen

negative. Some centers have begun to perform full red blood cell phenotyping for patients receiving chronic blood transfusions.

Three methods of blood transfusion therapy are used in the management of acute and chronic complications associated with sickle cell anemia: automated erythrocytapheresis, manual exchange transfusion (phlebotomy of a set amount of patient's blood followed by rapid administration of donated packed red blood cells), and simple transfusion. Automated erythrocytapheresis is the preferred method for patients requiring chronic blood transfusion therapy because there is a minimum net iron balance after the procedure, followed by manual exchange transfusion. Simple transfusion therapy is the least-preferable method for regular blood transfusion therapy because this strategy results in the highest net-positive iron balance after the procedure. Despite being the preferred method, erythrocytapheresis is less-frequently performed because of the requirement of technical expertise, large venous access, multiple units of matched red blood cells, and an available cytapheresis machine.

Preparation for surgery for children with sickle cell disease requires a coordinated effort between the hematologist, surgeon, and primary care provider. ACS and pain are the 2 most common postoperative complications, with ACS being a significant risk factor for postoperative death. Blood transfusion prior to surgery for children with sickle cell anemia is recommended to raise the hemoglobin level preoperatively to no more than 10 g/dL, although benefit also may be seen at lower hemoglobin values. The rate of serious complications, including a higher rate of ACS in patients who do not receive blood transfusion when compared to those who do. When available, blood transfusion therapy prior to surgery should be the standard approach. When preparing a child with sickle cell anemia for surgery with a simple blood transfusion, caution must be used not to elevate the hemoglobin beyond 10 g/dL because of the risk of hyperviscosity syndrome. For children with sickle cell anemia, exchange transfusion prior to surgery is of no greater benefit than simple blood transfusion and carries significantly higher risk of red blood cell alloimmunization. For children with milder forms of sickle cell disease, such as HbSC or HbSβ-thalassemia, a decision must be made on a case-by-case basis as to whether an exchange transfusion is warranted, because a simple transfusion may raise the hemoglobin to an unacceptable level.

Excessive Iron Stores

The primary toxic effect of blood transfusion therapy relates to **excessive iron stores**, which can result in organ damage and premature death. Excessive iron stores develop after 100 mL/kg of red cell transfusion or about 10 transfusions. The assessment of iron overload in children receiving regular blood transfusions is difficult. The most commonly used and least-invasive method of estimating total-body iron involves serum ferritin levels. Ferritin measurements have significant limitations in their ability to estimate iron stores for several reasons, including, but not limited to, elevation during acute inflammation and poor correlation with excessive iron in specific organs after 2 yr of regular blood transfusion therapy. Advances in technology have improved the assessment of iron stores among children with sickle cell disease receiving regular blood transfusion therapy. MRI of the liver has proven to the most effective and common approach for assessment of iron stores. The imaging strategy is more accurate than serum ferritin in measuring heart and liver iron content. MRI T2* and MRI R2 and R2* sequences are now being used to estimate iron levels in the heart and liver. The standard for iron assessment previously was biopsy of the liver, which is an invasive procedure exposing children to the risk of general anesthesia, bleeding, and pain. Liver biopsy alone does not accurately estimate total-body iron, as iron deposition in the liver is not homogenous and varies among the affected organs; that is, the amount of iron found in the liver is not equivalent to cardiac tissues. The major advantage of a liver biopsy is that histologic assessment of the parenchyma can be ascertained along with appropriate staging of suspected pathology, particularly cirrhosis.

The primary treatment of excessive iron stores resulting from red blood cell transfusion requires iron chelation using medical therapy. In the United States, 3 chelating agents are commercially available and

approved for use in transfusional iron overload. Deferoxamine is administered subcutaneously 5 of 7 nights/wk for 10 hr a night. Deferasirox is an effervescent tablet that is dissolved in liquid and taken by mouth daily, and deferiprone is available in tablets taken orally twice a day. The FDA approved deferasirox, the newest orally administered chelator, in 2005 for use in patients age ≥2 yr. Deferiprone is an older oral chelator that has been widely used outside of the United States for many years and was approved by the FDA in 2011, but requires weekly monitoring of complete blood counts because of a risk of neutropenia throughout therapy. Transfusion-related excessive iron stores in children with sickle cell disease should be managed by a physician with expertise in chelation therapy owing to the risk of significant toxicity from available chelation therapies.

OTHER SICKLE CELL SYNDROMES

The most commonly occurring sickle cell syndromes besides HbSS are HbSC, HbSβ-thalassemia zero, and HbSβ-thalassemia+. The other syndromes—HbSD, HbSO^Arab^, HbS HPFH, and other variants—are much less common. Patients with HbSβ-thalassemia zero have a clinical phenotype similar to those with HbSS. HbSC does not polymerize like HbSS, but crystals of HbC interact with membrane ion transport, dehydrating red cells and inducing sickling. Children who have HbSC disease can experience the same symptoms and complications as those with severe HbSS disease, but the frequency of such experience is less. Children with HbSC also have increased incidence of retinopathy, chronic hypersplenism, splenic sequestration, and renal medullary carcinoma. The natural history of the other sickle cell syndromes is variable and difficult to predict because of the lack of systematic evaluation.

There is no validated model that can predict the clinical course of an individual with sickle cell disease. A patient with HbSC can have a more-severe clinical course than a patient with HbSS. Management of end-organ dysfunction in children with sickle cell syndromes requires the same general principles as managing patients with sickle cell anemia; however, each situation should be managed on a case-by-case basis and requires consultation with a pediatric hematologist.

ANTICIPATORY GUIDANCE

The 2 primary goals of pediatric care are to promote health and prevent disease. Children with sickle cell disease should receive general health maintenance as recommended for all children with special attention to the following disease specific guidance.

Spleen Palpation

Splenomegaly is a common complication of sickle cell anemia and splenic sequestration can be life-threatening. Parents and primary caregivers should be taught how to palpate the spleen to determine if the spleen is enlarging starting at the first visit with reinforcement at subsequent visits. Parents should also demonstrate spleen palpation to the provider.

Prophylactic Penicillin

Children with sickle cell anemia should receive prophylactic oral penicillin VK until at least 5 yr of age (125 mg twice a day up to age 3 yr, and then 250 mg twice a day thereafter). No established guidelines exist for penicillin prophylaxis beyond 5 yr of age, and some clinicians continue penicillin prophylaxis, whereas others recommend discontinuation. Continuation of penicillin prophylaxis should be continued beyond 5 yr of age in children with history of pneumococcal infection because of the increased risk of a recurrent infection. An alternative for children who are allergic to penicillin is erythromycin ethyl succinate 10 mg/kg twice a day.

Immunizations

In addition to penicillin prophylaxis, routine childhood immunizations, as well as the annual administration of influenza vaccine, are highly recommended. Children with sickle cell anemia develop functional asplenia and also require immunizations to protect against encapsulated organisms including additional pneumococcal and meningococcal vaccinations. Vaccination guidelines can be found at the Centers for Disease Control and Prevention website: http://www.immunize.org/catg.d/p2010.pdf.

Transcranial Doppler Ultrasound

Primary stroke prevention using TCD has resulted in a decrease in the prevalence of overt stroke among children with sickle cell anemia. Children with HbSS or HbSβ-thalassemia zero should be screened annually with TCD starting at age 2 yr. TCD is best performed when the child is quietly awake and in their usual state of health. TCD measurements may be falsely elevated in the setting of acute anemia or falsely low immediately after blood transfusions or if procedural sedation is used. Screening should occur annually from age 2-16 yr. Abnormal values should be repeated within 2-4 wk to identify patients at greatest risk of overt stroke. Conditional values should be repeated within 3 mo, and normal values repeated annually. Routine neuroimaging with MRI in asymptomatic patients is not currently recommended.

Hydroxyurea

Monitoring children on hydroxyurea is labor intensive. Hydroxyurea is a chemotherapeutic agent that requires the same level of nursing and physician oversight as any child with cancer receiving chemotherapy. The parents must be educated about the consequences of therapy, and when ill, children should be promptly evaluated. Complete blood count should be checked at least every 4 wk after initiation of therapy or any dose change to monitor for hematologic toxicity and then every 8 wk.

Hydroxyurea should be temporarily discontinued and dose adjusted if the absolute neutrophil count falls below 2,000/µL or platelets fall below 80,000/µL. Hydroxyurea is a pregnancy class D medication and adolescents should be counseled regarding methods to prevent pregnancy while taking hydroxyurea. Close monitoring of the patient requires a commitment by the parents and patient, as well as diligence by a physician, to identify toxicity early.

Regular Blood Transfusion Therapy

At the initiation of blood transfusion therapy, children with sickle cell anemia should have testing to identify the presence of alloantibodies and red blood cell phenotyping, which is performed to identify the best matched blood. Children meeting criteria for chronic transfusion therapy should receive annual evaluation for transfusion transmitted infections including hepatitis B, hepatitis C, and human immunodeficiency virus (HIV). After receiving 100 mg/kg of red blood cell transfusions, regular assessments of iron overload should begin; usually periodic measurements of serum ferritin. For children requiring chelation therapy, an audiogram should be performed annually, as well as monitoring for organ toxicity, including liver function tests and endocrine evaluation of pituitary dysfunction because of iron deposition.

Pulmonary and Asthma Screening

Pulmonary complications of sickle cell disease are common and life-threatening. Asthma is common particularly in African-American children. As would be the case in all children, good clinical practice necessitates evaluation for asthma symptoms and asthma risk factors in children with sickle cell disease, particularly in light of the insurmountable evidence that asthma is associated with increased rate of sickle cell disease morbidity and mortality. All children should receive annual screening for signs and symptoms of lower airway disease, such as nighttime cough and exercise-induced cough. In children with symptoms consistent with lower airway disease, consider consultation with an asthma specialist. Pulse oximetry readings should be performed during well visits to identify children with abnormally low daytime oxygen saturations. For children with snoring and daytime somnolence, and symptoms associated with obstructive sleep apnea syndrome, referral to a sleep specialist should be considered.

Retinopathy

Effective therapy for retinopathy associated with sickle cell disease exists. Patients at highest risk for the development of retinopathy should receive annual screening by an ophthalmologist to identify vascular changes that would benefit from laser therapy. Although changes may occur earlier, children with sickle cell disease should begin annual screening at age 10 yr.

Renal

Sickle cell–associated renal disease, starts in infancy and may not become clinically manifested until adulthood. Screening for early signs of sickle nephropathy using urinalysis to identify proteinuria is recommended with annual albumin:creatinine ratios. The age to begin screening for proteinuria has not been defined, but some experts recommend screening annually after at least 10 yr of age if not sooner. If the albumin:creatinine ratio is elevated (>30 mg/g), it should be repeated with an early morning urine collection, and if still elevated, the patient should be referred to a pediatric nephrologist. Males with sickle cell disease should also receive counseling regarding the diagnosis and treatment of priapism. Because of the high frequency of enuresis beyond early childhood, approximately 9% of adolescents between 18 and 20 yr of age, parents and caregivers should be educated about the prolonged nature of enuresis in this disease. As is the case in the general population, obstructive sleep apnea syndrome is associated with an increased prevalence of enuresis in sickle cell disease. Unfortunately, no evidence-based therapies have been developed to treat enuresis in children and young adults with sickle cell disease. In children with enuresis who have symptoms and clinical features of obstructive sleep apnea syndrome, referral to sleep specialists for evaluation is recommended.

Echocardiography

Echocardiography has gained popularity as a screening tool to identify individuals with sickle cell disease who have pulmonary artery hypertension. No evidence currently exists that children with sickle cell disease and elevated tricuspid jet velocity above 2.5 cm/sec have an increased rate of mortality. Subsequent studies in adults with sickle cell disease have found the echocardiography to be insensitive at identifying individuals truly at risk for pulmonary hypertension, although an elevated tricuspid velocity measurement may still be a risk factor for premature death in adults with sickle cell disease. The current recommendation is to refer those with severe cardiopulmonary symptoms from associated pulmonary artery hypertension to pediatric cardiologist for a more formal evaluation.

Bibliography is available at Expert Consult.

462.2 Sickle Cell Trait (Hemoglobin AS)

Michael R. DeBaun, Melissa J. Frei-Jones, and Elliott P. Vichinsky

The prevalence of sickle cell trait varies throughout the world; in the United States, the incidence is 7-10% of African-Americans. Because all state newborn screening programs include sickle cell disease, for most children, sickle cell trait is first identified on their newborn screen. Communication of sickle cell trait status from infancy to young adulthood for the affected individual, family, and healthcare providers is often inconsistent and many young adults are unaware of their sickle cell trait status.

The production of HbS is influenced by the number of α-thalassemia genes present, and the amount of HbS. By definition among individuals with sickle cell trait, the HbS level is <50%. The life span of people with sickle cell trait is normal, and serious complications are extremely rare. The CBC is within the normal range (Fig. 462-5B). Hemoglobin analysis is diagnostic, revealing a predominance of HbA, typically >50%, and HbS <50%. Rare complications of sickle cell trait are associated with sudden death during rigorous exercise, splenic infarction at high altitude, hematuria, hyposthenuria, deep vein thrombosis, and susceptibility to eye injury with formation of a hyphema (Table 462-5). Renal

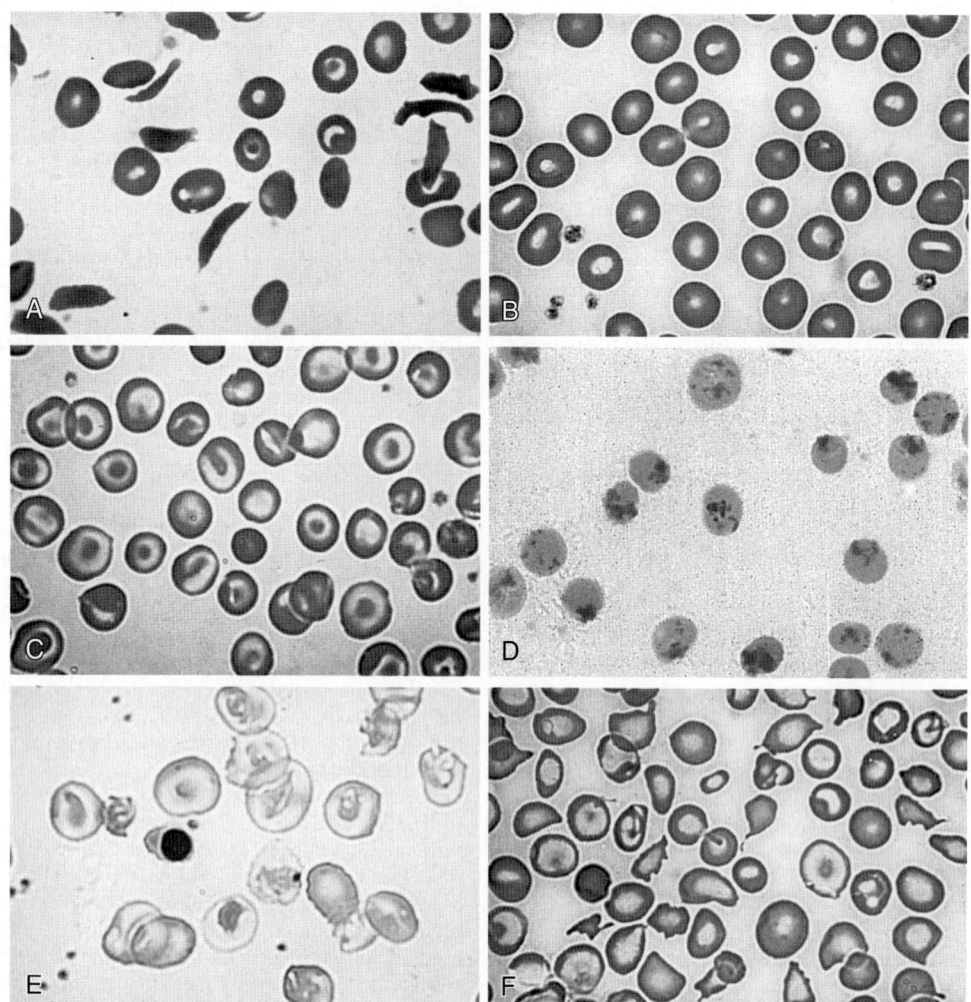

Figure 462-5 Red blood cell morphology associated with hemoglobin disorders. **A,** Sickle cell anemia (HbSS): target cells and fixed (irreversibly sickled) cells. **B,** Sickle cell trait (HbAS): normal red blood cell (RBC) morphology. **C,** Hemoglobin CC: target cells and occasional spherocytes. **D,** Congenital Heinz body anemia (unstable hemoglobin): RBCs stained with supravital stain (brilliant cresyl blue) reveal intracellular inclusions. **E,** Homozygous β0-thalassemia: severe hypochromia with deformed RBCs and normoblasts. **F,** Hemoglobin H disease (α-thalassemia): anisopoikilocytosis with target cells. *(Courtesy of Dr. John Bolles, The ASH Collection, University of Washington, Seattle.)*

Table 462-5	Complications Associated with Sickle Cell Trait

DEFINITE ASSOCIATIONS
Renal medullary cancer
Hematuria
Renal papillary necrosis
Hyposthenuria
Splenic infarction
Exertional rhabdomyolysis
Exercise-related sudden death
Protection against severe falciparum malaria
Microalbuminuria (adults)

From Tsaras G, Owusu-Ansah A, Boateng O, et al: Complications associated with sickle cell trait: a brief narrative review, Am J Med 122:507–512, 2009.

medullary carcinoma is also associated with sickle cell trait and occurs predominantly in young adults and children.

Children with sickle cell trait do not require limitations on physical activities. Sudden death in persons with sickle cell trait while exercising under extreme conditions is most likely associated with a second genetic factor and/or environmental factors, and not the presence of sickle cell trait itself. No causal pathway has been implicated for the presence of sickle cell trait and sudden death. All patients with sickle cell trait who participate in rigorous athletic activities should receive maximum hydration and appropriate rest during exertion, as would be the precautionary steps for all athletes, particularly when participating in hot humid conditions. The presence of sickle cell trait should never be a reason to exclude a person from athletic participation but rather should serve as an indication that prudent surveillance is necessary to ensure appropriate hydration and prevention of exhaustion from heat or other strenuous exercise. If athletes are to be screened for sickle cell trait, then appropriate genetic counseling should be provided, along with the knowledge that genetic information may provide opportunities to challenge paternity. Such situations are typically handled by a pediatrician or hematologist accustomed to providing both a balanced approach to genetic counseling and addressing the challenges about paternity.

462.3 Other Hemoglobinopathies

Michael R. DeBaun, Melissa J. Frei-Jones, and Elliott P. Vichinsky

HEMOGLOBIN C

The mutation for HbC is at the same site as HbS, with substitution of lysine instead of valine for glutamine. In the United States, hemoglobin C trait (HbAC) occurs in 1:40 and homozygous hemoglobin C disease (HbCC) occurs in 1:5,000 African-Americans. HbAC is asymptomatic. HbCC can result in mild anemia, splenomegaly, and cholelithiasis; rare cases of spontaneous splenic rupture have been reported. Sickling does not occur. This condition is usually diagnosed through newborn screening programs. HbC crystallizes, disrupting the red cell membrane, and HbC crystals may be visible on peripheral smear (see Fig. 462-5C).

HEMOGLOBIN E

HbE is an abnormal hemoglobin resulting from a qualitative mutation in the β-globin gene and is the second most common globin mutation worldwide. Patients may have asymptomatic hemoglobin E trait (HbAE) or benign homozygous hemoglobin E disease (HbEE). Compound heterozygous hemoglobin E/β-thalassemia produces clinical phenotypes ranging from moderate to severe anemia depending on the β-thalassemia mutation. In California, HbE/β-thalassemia is found almost exclusively in persons of Southeast Asian descent, with a prevalence of 1:2,600 births.

HEMOGLOBIN D

At least 16 variants of HbD exist. HbD-Punjab (Los Angeles) is a rare hemoglobin that is seen in 1-3% of Western Indians and in some Europeans with Asian-Indian ancestry and produces symptoms of sickle cell disease when present in combination with HbS. Heterozygous HbD or hemoglobin D trait (HbAD) is clinically silent. Homozygous HbDD or HbD disease produces a mild to moderate anemia with splenomegaly.

462.4 Unstable Hemoglobin Disorders
Michael R. DeBaun, Melissa J. Frei-Jones, and Elliott P. Vichinsky

At least 200 rare unstable hemoglobins have been identified; the most common is Hb Köln. Most patients seem to have de novo mutations rather than inherited hemoglobin disorders. The best studied unstable hemoglobins are the ones leading to hemoglobin denaturation from mutations affecting heme binding. The denatured hemoglobin can be visualized during severe hemolysis or after splenectomy as Heinz bodies. Unlike the Heinz bodies seen after toxic exposure, in unstable hemoglobins, Heinz bodies are present in reticulocytes and older red cells (see Fig. 462-5D). Heterozygotes are asymptomatic.

Children with homozygous gene mutations can present in early childhood with anemia and splenomegaly or with unexplained hemolytic anemia. Hemolysis is increased with febrile illness and with the ingestion of oxidant medications (similar to glucose-6-phosphate dehydrogenase [G6PD] deficiency) with some unstable hemoglobins. If the spleen is functional, the blood smear can appear almost normal or have only hypochromasia and basophilic stippling. A diagnosis may be made by demonstrating Heinz bodies, hemoglobin instability, or an abnormal hemoglobin analysis (although some unstable hemoglobins have normal mobility and are not detected on hemoglobin analysis).

Treatment is supportive. Transfusion may be required during hemolytic episodes in severe cases. Oxidative drugs should be avoided, and folate supplementation may be helpful if dietary deficiency is a concern. Splenectomy may be considered in patients requiring recurrent transfusion or demonstrating poor growth, but the complications of splenectomy, including bacterial sepsis, risk of thrombosis, and the possibility of developing pulmonary hypertension, should be considered before surgery.

462.5 Abnormal Hemoglobins with Increased Oxygen Affinity
Michael R. DeBaun, Melissa J. Frei-Jones, and Elliott P. Vichinsky

More than 110 high-affinity hemoglobins have been characterized. These mutations affect the state of hemoglobin configuration during oxygenation and deoxygenation. Hemoglobin changes structure when in the oxygenated versus the deoxygenated state. The deoxygenated state is termed the T (tense) state and is stabilized by 2,3-diphosphoglycerate. When fully oxygenated, hemoglobin assumes the R (relaxed) state. The exact molecular interactions between these 2 states are unknown. High-affinity hemoglobins contain mutations that either stabilize the R form or destabilize the T form. The interactions between the R and T forms are complex, and the mechanisms of the mutations are not known. In most cases, the high-affinity hemoglobins can be identified by hemoglobin analysis; approximately 20% must be characterized under controlled conditions where measurements are obtained with the P_{50} lowered to 9-21 mm Hg (normal: 23-29 mm Hg). The decreased P_{50} in these hemoglobins leads to an erythrocytosis with hemoglobin levels of 17-20 g/dL. Levels of erythropoietin and 2,3-diphosphoglycerate are normal. Patients are usually asymptomatic and do not need phlebotomy. If phlebotomy is performed, oxygen delivery could be problematic owing to the reduced number of hemoglobin molecules to carry oxygen.

462.6 Abnormal Hemoglobins Causing Cyanosis
Michael R. DeBaun, Allison Grimes, Melissa J. Frei-Jones, and Elliott P. Vichinsky

Abnormal hemoglobins causing cyanosis, also called structural methemoglobinemias, are rare. They are referred to as "M-hemoglobins" and represent a group of hemoglobin variants which result from point mutations in one of the globin chains, α, β, or γ located in the heme pocket. Thirteen known variants exist. These unstable hemoglobins lead to hemolytic anemia, most pronounced when the β-globin gene is affected. Clinically, these children are cyanotic from birth, without other signs or symptoms of disease, if the mutation is in the α-globin gene (HbM Boston, HbM Iwate, Hb Auckland). Infants with β-globin mutations become cyanotic later in infancy after the fetal hemoglobin switch (HbM Saskatoon, HbM Chile, HbM Milwaukee 1 and 2). γ-Chain mutations (HbF-M Fort Ripley, HbF-M Osaka, HbF Cincinnati, HbF Circleville, HbF Toms River, HbF Viseu) are all transient, presenting with cyanosis at birth, which resolves during the neonatal period after HbF production discontinues. The abnormal M hemoglobins exhibit autosomal dominant inheritance and are diagnosed by hemoglobin analysis. HbM variants may be not be isolated reliably using hemoglobin analysis (HPLC or isoelectric focusing [IEF]), consequently diagnostic confirmation may require DNA sequencing or mass spectrometry. There is no specific treatment and affected patients do not respond to treatments used for enzyme-deficient methemoglobinemia. Beyond cyanosis, individuals are otherwise asymptomatic and do not require additional monitoring. Children with the β-globin form should avoid oxidant drugs. Individuals with all forms have a normal life expectancy and pregnancy course.

Low-affinity hemoglobins have less cyanosis than the M hemoglobins. The amino acid substitutions destabilize the oxyhemoglobin and lead to decreased oxygen saturation. The best characterized are Hb Kansas, Hb Beth Israel, and Hb Denver. Hemoglobin analysis (IEF and HPLC techniques) may be normal in affected individuals. When clinically suspected, oxygen affinity studies reveal a right-shifted dissociation curve and heat testing demonstrates unstable hemoglobin. Children present with mild cyanosis only.

462.7 Hereditary Methemoglobinemia
Michael R. DeBaun, Allison Grimes, Melissa J. Frei-Jones, and Elliott P. Vichinsky

Hereditary methemoglobinemia is a clinical syndrome caused by an increase in the serum concentration of methemoglobin either as a result of congenital changes in hemoglobin synthesis or of metabolism leading to imbalances in reduction and oxidation of hemoglobin. The iron molecule in hemoglobin is normally in the ferrous state (Fe^{2+}), which is essential for oxygen transport. Under physiologic conditions there is a slow, constant loss of electrons to released oxygen, and the ferric (Fe^{3+}) form combines with water, producing methemoglobin (MetHb). The newly formed MetHb has a reduced ability to bind oxygen.

Two pathways for MetHb reduction exist. The physiologic and predominant pathway is a reduced form of nicotinamide adenine dinucleotide (NADH)-dependent reaction catalyzed by cytochrome b5 reductase. This mechanism is >100-fold more efficient than the production of MetHb. The alternate pathway utilizes nicotinamide adenine dinucleotide phosphate generated by G6PD in the hexose monophosphate shunt and requires an extrinsic electron acceptor to be activated (i.e., methylene blue, ascorbic acid, riboflavin). In normal individuals, oxidation of hemoglobin to MetHb occurs at a slow rate, 0.5-3%, which is countered by MetHb reduction to maintain a steady state of 1% MetHb.

MetHb may be increased in the red cell owing to exposure to toxic substances or to absence of reductive pathways, such as NADH-cytochrome b5 reductase deficiency. Toxic methemoglobinemia is much more common than hereditary methemoglobinemia (Table 462-6). Infants are exceptionally vulnerable to hemoglobin oxidation because their erythrocytes have half the amount of cytochrome b5 reductase seen in adults, fetal hemoglobin is more susceptible to oxidation than hemoglobin A, and the more alkaline infant gastrointestinal tract promotes the growth of nitrite-producing Gram-negative bacteria. When MetHb levels are >1.5 g/24 hr, cyanosis is visible (15% MetHb); a level of 70% MetHb is lethal. The MetHb level is usually reported as a percentage of normal hemoglobin, and the toxic level is lower at a lower hemoglobin level. Methemoglobinemia has been described in infants who ingested foods and water high in nitrates, who were exposed to aniline teething gels or other chemicals, and in some infants with severe gastroenteritis and acidosis. Methemoglobin can color the blood brown (Fig. 462-6).

462.8 Hereditary Methemoglobinemia with Deficiency of NADH Cytochrome b5 Reductase

Michael R. DeBaun, Allison Grimes, Melissa J. Frei-Jones, and Elliott P. Vichinsky

The first reported inherited disorder causing methemoglobinemia resulted from an enzymatic deficiency of NADH cytochrome b5 reductase, which was classified into 2 distinct phenotypes. In type I, the most common form, the deficiency of NADH cytochrome b5 activity is found only in erythrocytes, with other cell types unaffected. In type II, the enzyme deficiency is present in all tissues and results in more significant symptoms beginning in infancy with encephalopathy, mental retardation, spasticity, microcephaly, and growth retardation with death most often by 2 yr of age. Both types exhibit an autosomal recessive inheritance pattern.

Clinically, cyanosis varies in intensity with season and diet. The time of cyanosis onset also varies; in some patients it appears at birth, in others as late as adolescence. Although as much as 50% of the total circulating hemoglobin may be in the form of nonfunctional MetHb, little or no cardiorespiratory distress occurs in these patients, except on exertion.

Daily oral treatment with ascorbic acid (200-500 mg/day in divided doses) gradually reduces the MetHb to approximately 10% of the total

Table 462-6	Known Etiologies of Acquired Methemoglobinemia

MEDICATIONS
Benzocaine
Chloroquine
Dapsone
EMLA (eutectic mixture of local anesthetics) topical anesthetic
  (lidocaine 2.5% and prilocaine 2.5%)
Flutamide
Lidocaine
Metoclopramide
Nitrates
Nitric oxide
Nitroglycerin
Nitroprusside
Nitrous oxide
Phenazopyridine
Prilocaine
Primaquine
Riluzole
Silver nitrate
Sodium nitrate
Sulfonamides

MEDICAL CONDITIONS
Pediatric gastrointestinal infection, sepsis
Recreational drug overdose with amyl nitrate ("poppers")
Sickle cell disease–related painful episode

MISCELLANEOUS
Aniline dyes
Fume inhalation (automobile exhaust, burning of wood and plastics)
Herbicides
Industrial chemicals: nitrobenzene, nitroethane (found in nail polish,
  resins, rubber adhesives)
Pesticides
Gasoline octane booster

From Ash-Bernal R, Wise R, Wright SM: Acquired methemoglobinemia, Medicine (Baltimore) *83:265–273, 2004.*

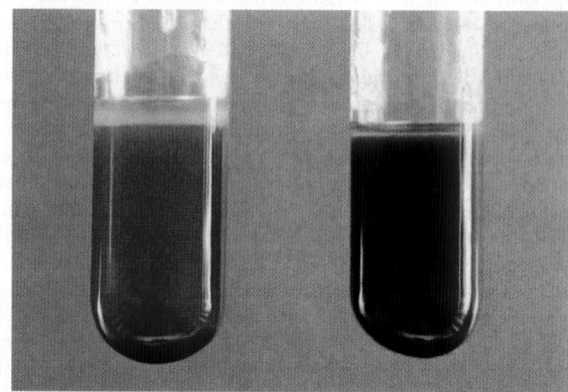

Figure 462-6 Normal arterial blood versus methemoglobinemia. Arterial whole blood with 1% methemoglobin *(left)* versus arterial whole blood with 72% methemoglobin *(right)*. Note the characteristic chocolate-brown color of the sample with an elevated methemoglobin level. Both samples were briefly exposed to 100% oxygen and shaken. This quick analysis is a good bedside test for methemoglobinemia. The sample on the *left* turned bright red, whereas the sample on the *right* remained chocolate-brown. Methods: Whole blood samples were drawn at the same time from the same person. The measured hemoglobin concentration was 11.7 g/dL. Calculated concentration of methemoglobin: 11.7 g/dL × 0.01 = 0.117 g/dL *(left)* and 11.7 g/dL × 0.72 = 8.42 g/dL *(right)*. An elevated methemoglobin level was made in vitro by adding 0.1 mL of a 0.144 molar solution of sodium nitrate *(right)*, and 0.1 mL of normal saline was added as a control *(left)*. Cooximetry measurements were taken on both samples shortly after the blood was drawn and 20 min after the addition of sodium nitrate solution. Both blood samples were exposed to 100% oxygen before the second measurement. *(Protocol based on personal communication with Dr. Ali Mansouri, December 2002.)*

pigment and alleviates the cyanosis as long as therapy is continued. Chronic high doses of ascorbic acid have been associated with hyperoxaluria and renal stone formation. Ascorbic acid should not be used to treat toxic methemoglobinemia. When immediately available, poison control should be contacted to verify the most up-to-date therapeutic strategies. Like ascorbic acid, riboflavin utilizes the alternate pathway of MetHb reduction and is most effective when given in high doses (400 mg once daily). Methylene blue, administered intravenously (1-2 mg/kg initially), is used to treat toxic methemoglobinemia. An oral dose can be administered (100-300 mg PO per day) as maintenance therapy.

Methylene blue should not be used in patients with G6PD deficiency. This treatment is ineffective and can cause severe oxidative hemolysis. In the event that methylene blue is given to a patient with G6PD deficiency, there will be no improvement in symptoms and marked hemolysis has been reported within 24 hr of administration. Because G6PD deficiency status is rarely known at the time of treatment, a careful history should be elicited. When the history is negative for symptoms of G6PD deficiency, treatment with methylene blue should be initiated judiciously, and the patient should be closely monitored for improvement.

462.9 Syndromes of Hereditary Persistence of Fetal Hemoglobin

Michael R. DeBaun, Melissa J. Frei-Jones, and Elliott P. Vichinsky

HPFH syndromes are a form of thalassemia; mutations are associated with a decrease in the production of either or both β- and δ-globins. There is an imbalance in the α:non-α synthetic ratio (see Chapter 462.9) characteristic of thalassemia. More than 20 variants of HPFH have been described. They are deletional, $\delta\beta^0$ (Black, Ghanaian, Italian), nondeletional (Tunisian, Japanese, Australian), linked to the β-globin–gene cluster (British, Italian-Chinese, Black), or unlinked to the β-globin–gene cluster (Atlanta, Czech, Seattle). The $\delta\beta^0$ forms have deletions of the entire δ- and β-globin gene sequences, and the most common form in the United States is the Black (HPFH 1) variant. As a result of the δ and β gene deletions, there is production only of γ-globin and formation of HbF. In the homozygous form, no manifestations of thalassemia are present. There is only HbF with very mild anemia and slight microcytosis. When inherited with other variant hemoglobins, HbF is elevated into the 20-30% range; when inherited with HbS, there is an amelioration of sickle cell disease with fewer complications.

462.10 Thalassemia Syndromes

Michael R. DeBaun, Melissa J. Frei-Jones, and Elliott P. Vichinsky

Thalassemia refers to a group of genetic disorders of globin chain production in which there is an imbalance between the α-globin and β-globin chain production. β-Thalassemia syndromes result from a decrease in β-globin chains, which results in a relative excess of α-globin chains. β^0-Thalassemia refers to the absence of production of the β-globin. When patients are homozygous for the β-thalassemia gene, they cannot make any normal β chains (HbA). β^+-Thalassemia indicates a mutation that makes decreased amounts of normal β-globin, but it is still present (HbA). β^0-Thalassemia syndromes are more severe than β^+-thalassemia syndromes, but there is significant variability between the genotype and phenotype. β-Thalassemia major refers to the severe β-thalassemia patient who requires early transfusion therapy and often is homozygous for β^0 mutations. β-Thalassemia intermedia is a clinical diagnosis of a patient with a less-severe clinical phenotype that usually does not require transfusion therapy in childhood. Many of these patients have at least 1 β^+-thalassemia mutation. β-Thalassemia

syndromes usually require a β-thalassemia mutation in both β-globin genes. Carriers with a single β-globin mutation are generally asymptomatic, except for microcytosis and mild anemia. In α-thalassemia, there is an absence or reduction in α-globin production. Normal individuals have 4 α-globin genes. The more genes affected, the more severe the disease. An α^0-mutation indicates no α-chains produced from that gene. An α^+ mutation produces a decreased amount of α-globin chain. The primary pathology in the thalassemia syndromes stems from the quantity of globin produced, whereas the primary pathology in sickle cell disease is related to the quality of β-globin produced.

EPIDEMIOLOGY

There are >200 different mutations resulting in absent or decreased globin production. Although most are rare, the 20 most common abnormal alleles constitute 80% of the known thalassemias worldwide; 3% of the world's population carries alleles for β-thalassemia, and in Southeast Asia 5-10% of the population carry alleles for α-thalassemia. In a particular region, there are fewer common alleles. In the United States, an estimated 2,000 persons have β-thalassemia major.

PATHOPHYSIOLOGY

Two related features contribute to the sequelae of β-thalassemia major: inadequate β-globin gene production leading to decreased levels of normal hemoglobin (HbA) and unbalanced α- and β-globin chain production. In β-thalassemia major, α-globin chains are in excess to non–α-globin chains, and α-globin tetramers (α_4) are formed and appear as red cell inclusions. The free α-globin chains and inclusions are very unstable, precipitate in red cell precursors, damage the red cell membrane, and shorten red cell survival leading to anemia and increased erythroid production. Table 462-7 shows selected features of thalassemia. This results in a marked increase in erythropoiesis with early erythroid precursor death in the bone marrow. Clinically, this is characterized by a lack of maturation of erythrocytes and an inappropriately low reticulocyte count. This ineffective erythropoiesis and the compensatory massive marrow expansion with erythroid hyperactivity characterize β-thalassemia. Because the β^0-thalassemia patient cannot make HbA, the α-chains combine with γ-chains, resulting in HbF ($\alpha_2\gamma_2$) being the dominant hemoglobin. In addition to the natural survival effect, the γ-globin chains may be produced in increased amounts, which is regulated by genetic polymorphisms. δ-Chain synthesis is not usually affected in β-thalassemia or β-thalassemia trait, and, therefore, patients have a relative or absolute increase in HbA_2 production ($\alpha_2\delta_2$).

In the α-thalassemia syndromes, 2 genes with 2 maternal and 2 paternal alleles control α-globin production, which varies from complete absence (hydrops fetalis) to only slightly reduced (α-thalassemia silent carrier). In the α-thalassemia syndromes, an excess of β- and γ-globin chains are produced. These excess chains form Bart hemoglobin (γ_4) in fetal life and HbH (β_4) after birth. These abnormal tetramers are nonfunctional hemoglobins with very high oxygen affinity. They do not transport oxygen and result in extravascular hemolysis. A fetus with the most severe form of α-thalassemia (hydrops fetalis) develops in utero anemia and fetal loss because HbF production requires sufficient amounts of α-globin. In contrast, infants with β-thalassemia major become symptomatic only after birth when HbA predominates and insufficient β-globin production manifests in clinical symptoms.

HOMOZYGOUS β-THALASSEMIA (THALASSEMIA MAJOR, COOLEY ANEMIA)
Clinical Manifestations

If not treated, children with homozygous β^0-thalassemia usually become symptomatic from progressive hemolytic anemia, with profound weakness and cardiac decompensation during the 2nd 6 mo of life. Depending on the mutation and degree of fetal hemoglobin production, transfusions in β-thalassemia major are necessary beginning in the 2nd mo to 2nd yr of life, but rarely later. The decision to transfuse is multifactorial but is not determined solely by the degree of anemia. The developing signs of ineffective erythropoiesis such as growth

Table 462-7	The Thalassemias

THALASSEMIA	GLOBIN GENOTYPE	FEATURES	EXPRESSION	HEMOGLOBIN ANALYSIS
α-THALASSEMIA				
1 Gene allele deletion	$-,\alpha/\alpha,\alpha$	Normal	Normal	Newborn: Bart 1-2%
2 Gene allele deletion trait	$-,\alpha/-,\alpha -, -/\alpha,\alpha$	Microcytosis, mild hypochromasia	Normal, mild anemia	Newborn: Bart: 5-10%
3 Gene allele deletion hemoglobin H	$-,-/-,\alpha$	Microcytosis, hypochromic	Mild anemia, transfusions not required	Newborn: Bart: 20-30%
2 Gene allele deletion + Constant Spring	$-,-/\alpha,\alpha^{Constant\ Spring}$	Microcytosis, hypochromic	Moderate to severe anemia, transfusion, splenectomy.	2-3% Constant Spring, 10-15% HbH
4 Gene allele deletion	$-,-/-,-$	Anisocytosis, poikilocytosis	Hydrops fetalis	Newborn: 89-90% Bart with Gower 1 and 2 and Portland
Nondeletional	$\alpha,\alpha/\alpha,\alpha^{variant}$	Microcytosis, mild anemia	Normal	1-2% variant hemoglobin
β-THALASSEMIA				
β^0 or β^+ heterozygote: trait	$\beta^0/A, \beta^+/A$	Variable microcytosis	Normal	Elevated A_2, variable elevation of F
β^0-Thalassemia	$\beta^0/\beta^0, \beta^+/\beta^0, E/\beta^0$	Microcytosis, nucleated RBC	Transfusion dependent	F 98% and A_2 2%, E 30-40%
β^+-Thalassemia severe	β^+/β^+	Microcytosis nucleated RBC	Transfusion dependent/ thalassemia intermedia	F 70-95%, A_2 2%, trace A
Silent	β^+/A	Microcytosis	Normal with only microcytosis	A_2 3.3-3.5%
β^+/β^+		Hypochromic, microcytosis	Mild to moderate anemia	A_2 2-5%, F 10-30%
Dominant (rare)	B^0/A	Microcytosis, abnormal RBCs	Moderately severe anemia, splenomegaly	Elevated F and A_2
δ-Thalassemia	A/A	Normal	Normal	A_2 absent
$(\delta\beta)^0$-Thalassemia	$(\delta\beta)^0/A$	Hypochromic	Mild anemia	F 5-20%
$(\delta\beta)^+$-Thalassemia Lepore	β^{Lepore}/A	Microcytosis	Mild anemia	Lepore 8-20%
Lepore	$\beta^{Lepore}/\beta^{Lepore}$	Microcytic, hypochromic	Thalassemia intermedia	F 80%, Lepore 20%
γδβ-Thalassemia	$(\gamma^A\delta\beta)^0/A$	Microcytosis, microcytic, hypochromic	Moderate anemia, splenomegaly, homozygote: thalassemia intermedia	Decreased F and A2 compared with δβ-thalassemia
γ-Thalassemia	$(\gamma^A\gamma^G)^0/A$	Microcytosis	Insignificant unless homozygote	Decreased F
HEREDITARY PERSISTENCE OF FETAL HEMOGLOBIN				
Deletional	A/A	Microcytic	Mild anemia	F 100% homozygotes
Nondeletional	A/A	Normal	Normal	F 20-40%

failure, bone deformities secondary to marrow expansion, hepatosplenomegaly are important variables in determining transfusion initiation.

The classic presentation of children with severe disease includes thalassemic facies (maxilla hyperplasia, flat nasal bridge, frontal bossing), pathologic bone fractures, marked hepatosplenomegaly, and cachexia and is now primarily seen in countries without access to chronic transfusion therapy. Occasionally, patients with moderate anemia develop these features because of severe compensatory ineffective erythropoiesis.

In nontransfused patients with severe ineffective erythropoiesis, marked splenomegaly can develop with hypersplenism and abdominal symptoms. The features of ineffective erythropoiesis include expanded medullary spaces (with massive expansion of the marrow of the face and skull producing the characteristic thalassemic facies), extramedullary hematopoiesis, and higher metabolic needs (Fig. 462-7). The chronic anemia without transfusion exposure produces an increase in iron absorption from the gastrointestinal tract and secondary hemosiderosis-induced organ injury.

Chronic transfusion therapy dramatically improves the quality of life and reduces the complications of severe thalassemia. Transfusion-induced hemosiderosis becomes the major clinical complication of transfusion-dependent thalassemia. Each mL of packed red cells contains 1 mg of iron. Physiologically, there is no mechanism to eliminate excess body iron. Iron is initially deposited in the liver. Liver hemosiderosis develops after 1 yr of chronic transfusion therapy and is followed by iron deposition in the endocrine system. This leads to a high rate of hypothyroidism, hypogonadotrophic gonadism, growth hormone deficiency, hypoparathyroidism, and diabetes mellitus. After 10 yr of transfusion, cardiac dysfunction secondary to hemosiderosis begins. Eventually, most patients not receiving adequate iron chelation therapy die from cardiac failure and/or cardiac arrhythmias secondary to hemosiderosis. Hemosiderosis induced morbidity can be prevented by adequate iron chelation therapy.

Laboratory Findings

In the United States, some children with β-thalassemia major will be identified on newborn screening as a result of the detection of only HbF on hemoglobin electrophoresis. However, the ethnicity and the mutations associated with transfusion-dependent thalassemia in United States have dramatically changed. Many of the patients have diverse mutations, such as HbE thalassemia, which may not be identified or followed up by a newborn screening program. HbFE in the newborn may be a very common benign mutation caused by homozygous HbEE or an uncommon severe HbE β⁰-thalassemia. The lack of standardized neonatal diagnosis of thalassemia disorders requires close follow-up of newborns with unclear thalassemia mutations and/or babies from high-risk ethnic groups.

Infants with serious β-thalassemia disorders have a progressive anemia after the newborn period. Microcytosis (MCV), hypochromia (MCH), and targeting characterize the red cells. Nucleated red cells, marked anisopoikilocytosis, and a relative reticulocytopenia are typically seen (see Fig. 462-5E). The hemoglobin level falls progressively to <6 g/dL unless transfusions are given. The reticulocyte count is

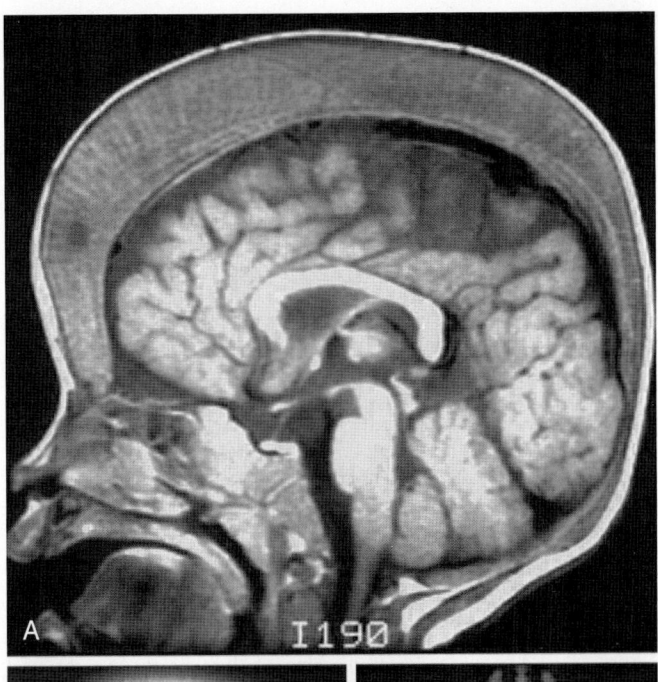

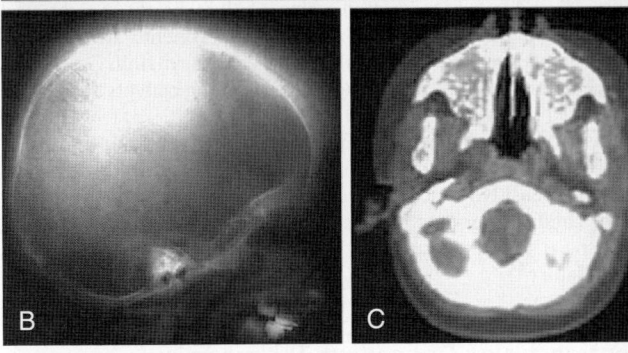

Figure 462-7 Ineffective erythropoiesis in a 3 yr old patient who has β-thalassemia major and has not received a transfusion. **A,** Massive widening of the diploic spaces of the skull as seen on MRI. **B,** Radiographic appearance of the trabeculae as seen on plain radiograph. **C,** Obliteration of the maxillary sinuses with hematopoietic tissue as seen on CT scan.

commonly <8% and is inappropriately low when compared to the degree of anemia as a result of ineffective erythropoiesis. The unconjugated serum bilirubin level is usually elevated, but other chemistries may be normal early on. Even if the child does not receive transfusions, iron eventually accumulates with elevated serum ferritin and transferrin saturation. Bone marrow hyperplasia can be seen on radiographs (see Fig. 462-7).

Early definitive diagnosis is recommended. Newborn screening techniques such as hemoglobin electrophoresis is not definitive. DNA diagnosis of the β-thalassemia mutation, along with testing for common genetic modifiers of the clinical phenotype, is recommended. Coinheritance of an α-thalassemia mutation is common, and it decreases the severity of the β-thalassemia disease. Some patients' mutations cannot be diagnosed by standard electrophoresis or common DNA probes. Referral of the samples to a tertiary laboratory along with parental and family testing are indicated. Following the definitive diagnosis, families should undergo detailed counseling.

Management and Treatment of Thalassemia
Transfusion Therapy
Before initiating chronic transfusions, the diagnosis of transfusion dependent β-thalassemia should be confirmed by both clinical and

laboratory parameters. β-Thalassemia major is a clinical diagnosis that requires the integration of laboratory findings and the clinical course. Of patients with homozygous β^0-thalassemia (the most severe mutations), 15-20% may have a clinical course that is phenotypically consistent with thalassemia intermedia. In contrast, 25% of patients with homozygous β^+-thalassemia, typically a more benign genotype, may become transfusion-dependent thalassemia major. Transient clinical events, such as a sudden fall in hemoglobin secondary to an episode of parvovirus requiring transfusion, do not necessarily indicate the patient is a transfusion-dependent patient. The long-term observation of the clinical characteristics, such as growth, bony changes, and hemoglobin, are necessary to determine chronic transfusion therapy.

Guidelines for Transfusion Therapy. Patients at risk for transfusion therapy should have an extended red cell phenotype and/or genotype. Patients should receive red cells depleted of leukocytes and matched for, at least, D, C, c, E, e, and Kell antigens. Cytomegalovirus-negative units are indicated in stem cell transplantation candidates. Transfusions should generally be given at intervals of 3-4 wk, with the goal being to maintain a pretransfusion hemoglobin level of 9.5-10.5 g/dL. Ongoing monitoring for transfusion-associated transmitted infections (hepatitis A, hepatitis B, hepatitis C, HIV), alloimmunization, annual blood transfusion requirements, and transfusion reactions is essential.

Iron Overload Monitoring
Excessive iron stores from transfusion cause many of the complications of β-thalassemia major. Accurate assessment of excessive iron stores is essential to optimal therapy. Serial serum ferritin levels are a useful screening technique in assessing iron balance trends, but results may not accurately predict quantitative iron stores. Undertreatment or overtreatment of presumed excessive iron stores can occur in managing a patient based on serum ferritin alone. Noninvasive measurement of quantitative organ injury is rapidly improving the treatment of iron overload. Quantitative measurement of liver iron and cardiac iron are standard and measurement of pancreatic and gonadal iron may be available soon. This technology, in collaboration with access to multiple chelators, will enable targeted chelation therapy for patients with organ specific hemosiderosis before the onset of overt organ failure. Available data suggests integration of these imaging technologies with chelation therapy may prevent heart failure, diabetes, and other pending organ dysfunction.

Quantitative liver iron by approved MRI technology is the best indicator of total-body iron stores and should be obtained in chronically transfused patients after chronic transfusion therapy has initiated. The liver iron results will help guide the chelation regimen.. Quantitative cardiac iron, determined by T2* MRI cardiac software, should be obtained after 7 yr of transfusion therapy. It is not uncommon to have a discrepancy between the liver iron and the heart iron because of different rates of tissue loading and cardiac chelation efficacy.

Chelation Therapy
Iron-chelation therapy should start as soon as the patient becomes significantly iron overloaded. In general, this occurs after 1 yr of transfusion therapy and correlates with the serum ferritin >1,000 ng/mL and/or a liver iron concentration of >2,500 μg/g dry weight.

There are 3 available iron chelators (deferoxamine, deferasirox, and deferiprone); each varies in its route of administration, pharmacokinetics, adverse events, and efficacy. Many patients require combination chelation therapy at various points in their illness. The overall goal is to prevent hemosiderosis-induced tissue injury and avoid chelation toxicity. This requires close monitoring of the patients. In general, chelation toxicity increases as iron stores decrease.

Deferoxamine (Desferal) is the most studied iron chelator; it has an excellent safety and efficacy profile. It requires subcutaneous, or intravenous, administration because of a half-life of less than 30 min, necessitating administration of at least 8 hr daily, 5-7 days/wk. Deferoxamine is initially started at 20 mg/kg and can be increased to 60 mg/kg in heavily iron-overloaded patients. The major problem with deferoxamine is noncompliance because of the route of administration.

Adverse side effects include ototoxicity, retinal changes, and bone dysplasia with truncal shortening.

The oral iron chelator deferasirox (Exjade) is commercially available in the United States. Of patients on Desferal, 70% have switched to deferasirox because it is orally available. Deferasirox has a half-life of more than 16 hr and requires once-a-day administration of a dispersible tablet in water. Initial dose is 20 mg/kg with gradual escalation to 30 mg/kg. The most common side effects are gastrointestinal symptoms. The most serious side effect of deferasirox is potential kidney damage. Up to 30% of patients have transient increases in creatinine that requires temporary modifications of dosing. All patients require monthly chemistry panels and ongoing monitoring for proteinuria. Long-term studies in thousands of patients have not demonstrated progressive renal dysfunction, but isolated cases of renal failure in patients have occurred.

Deferiprone (Ferriprox), an oral iron chelator previously only available in Europe, is approved in the United States. Deferiprone has a half-life of approximately 3 hr and requires 25 mg/kg 3 times a day. Deferiprone, a small molecule, effectively enters cardiac tissue and may be more effective than other chelators in reducing cardiac hemosiderosis. The most serious side effect of deferiprone is transient agranulocytosis, which occurs in 1% of patients. It is associated with rare deaths where patients were not adequately monitored. The use of deferiprone requires weekly white blood cell counts.

As thalassemia patients are living longer, the iron-chelation goals have changed. Aggressive treatment with combination chelation therapy is often used in heavily iron-overloaded patients to prevent or reverse organ dysfunction. Deferoxamine, in combination with deferiprone, is routinely used in patients with increased cardiac iron. Combination therapy of deferoxamine and deferasirox may also be efficacious in similar patients.

Hydroxyurea

Hydroxyurea, a DNA antimetabolite, increases stress erythropoiesis, which results in increased HbF production. It has been most successfully used in sickle cell disease and in some patients with β-thalassemia intermedia. Studies in β-thalassemia major are limited. In many parts of the world, hydroxyurea therapy is used in thalassemia intermedia patients. Even though increases in HbF levels are observed, they do not predictively correlate with increase in total hemoglobin in these patients. In general, there appears to be a mean increase in hemoglobin of 1 g (range: 0.1-2.5 g). Hydroxyurea therapy in thalassemia intermedia may have other benefits including decreasing the vascular disease associated with thalassemia intermedia. The initial starting dose for thalassemia intermedia is 10 mg/kg and because these patients are more sensitive to toxicity than sickle cell disease, higher doses are used with great caution.

Hematopoietic Stem Cell Transplantation

Hematopoietic stem cell transplantation has cured >3,000 patients who had β-thalassemia major. In low-risk HLA-matched sibling patients, there is at least a 90% survival and an 80% event-free survival. In general, myeloablative conditioning regimens are required in order to prevent graft rejection and thalassemia recurrence. Most success has been in children younger than 15 yr of age without excessive iron stores and hepatomegaly who undergo sibling HLA-matched allogeneic transplantation. All children who have an HLA-matched sibling should be offered the option of bone marrow transplantation. Alternative transplantation regimens for patients without donors are experimental and have variable success.

Splenectomy
Surgical Asplenia

Splenectomy may be required in thalassemia patients who develop hypersplenism. These patients have a falling steady state hemoglobin and/or a rising transfusion requirement. Overall, splenectomy is less frequently used as a therapeutic option. There is an increased recognition of serious adverse effects of splenectomy beyond infection risk. In thalassemia intermedia, splenectomized patients have a marked increased risk of venous thrombosis, pulmonary hypertension, leg ulcers, and silent cerebral infarction compared to nonsplenectomized patients. All patients should be fully immunized against encapsulated bacteria and should be on long-term penicillin prophylaxis with appropriate instructions regarding fever management. Prophylactic penicillin should be administered postsplenectomy to prevent sepsis, and families need to be educated on the risk of fever and sepsis.

Preventative Monitoring of Thalassemia Patients

Cardiac. Cardiac disease is the major cause of death in thalassemia. Serial echocardiograms should be monitored to evaluate cardiac function and pulmonary artery pressure. Pulmonary hypertension frequently occurs in non-transfused thalassemia patients and may be an indication for transfusion therapy. After 8 yr of chronic transfusion therapy, cardiac hemosiderosis may occur; consequently, cardiac T2* MRI imaging studies are recommended. Patients with cardiac hemosiderosis and decreasing cardiac ejection fraction require intensive combination chelation therapy.

Endocrine. Endocrine function progressively declines with age secondary to hemosiderosis and nutritional deficiencies. Iron deposition in the pituitary and endocrine organs can result in multiple endocrinopathies, including hypothyroidism, growth hormone deficiency, delayed puberty, and hypoparathyroidism, diabetes mellitus, osteoporosis, and adrenal insufficiency. Monitoring for endocrine dysfunction starts early, around 5 yr of age, or after at least 3 yr of chronic transfusions. All children require monitoring of their height, weight, and sitting height semi-annually. Nutritional assessments are required. Most patients need vitamin D, calcium, vitamin B, vitamin C, and zinc replacement. Fertility is a growing concern among patients and should be assessed routinely.

Psychosocial Support. Thalassemia imposes major disruption in the family unit and significant obstacles to normal development. Culturally sensitive anticipatory counseling is necessary, and the early use of child life services decreases psychological trauma of therapy. Early social service consultation to address financial and social issues is mandatory.

OTHER β-THALASSEMIA SYNDROMES
Nontransfusion-Dependent Thalassemia: β-Thalassemia Intermedia

The β-thalassemia syndromes are characterized by decreased production of β-globin chains of HbA. There are 200-300 β-thalassemia alleles that have now been characterized. These mutations can affect any step in the transcription of β-globin genes. As discussed, β⁰-thalassemia is absent production of normal β-chains, and production of β⁺ is decreased. Some β-thalassemia mutations have structural mutations such as HbE. Others, such as δβ-thalassemia or HPFH, are variants of β-thalassemia that have decreased production of β-globin gene with increased compensation of HbF. Because phenotypic correlation with genotype is variable, β-thalassemia patients are largely classified by their clinical spectrum. Transfusion-dependent thalassemia, or thalassemia major, is the most severe group. Nontransfusion-dependent thalassemia intermedia include a spectrum of patients who initially are not chronically transfused in infancy but may be sporadically transfused throughout their lifetime. The major determining characteristic of these patients is less α–β-globin chain imbalance than observed in thalassemia major. Sometimes, genetic modifiers alter the primary mutation severity and improve the globin chain imbalance. Coinheritance of α-thalassemia trait or polymorphisms of globin promoters such as BCL11 may convert a thalassemia major patient to a nontransfusion-dependent thalassemia intermedia patient. HbEβ-thalassemia is a common cause of both transfusion-dependent and nontransfusion-dependent thalassemia. These secondary genetic modifiers play a role in altering the severity of this disorder. Occasionally, patients with a single β-thalassemia mutation or autosomal dominant β-thalassemia trait have clinical features of thalassemia intermedia, or nontransfusion-dependent thalassemia. Genetic studies of these patients often uncover a coinheritance of genetic modifiers that worsen the condition such as α-gene triplication or an unstable β-globin mutation.

Thalassemia intermedia patients have significant ineffective erythropoiesis that leads to microcytic anemia with hemoglobin of approximately 7 g/dL (range: 6-10 g/dL). These patients have some of the complications characterized in untransfused thalassemia major patients, but the severity varies depending on the degree of ineffective erythropoiesis. They can develop medullary hyperplasia, hepatosplenomegaly, hematopoietic pseudotumors, pulmonary hypertension, thrombotic events, and growth failure. Many patients develop hemosiderosis secondary to increased gastrointestinal absorption of iron requiring chelation. Extramedullary hematopoiesis can occur in the vertebral canal, compressing the spinal cord and causing neurologic symptoms; the latter is a medical emergency requiring immediate local radiation therapy to halt erythropoiesis. Transfusions are indicated in thalassemia intermedia patients with significant clinical morbidity.

Thalassemia trait is often misdiagnosed as iron deficiency in children because the two produce similar hematologic abnormalities on CBC, and iron deficiency is much more prevalent. A short course of iron and reevaluation is all that is required to identify children who will need further evaluation. Children who have β-thalassemia trait have a persistently normal red cell distribution width and low mean corpuscular volume (MCV), whereas patients with iron deficiency develop an elevated red cell distribution width with treatment. On hemoglobin analysis, they have an elevated HbF and usually increased levels of HbA$_2$. There are "silent" forms of β-thalassemia trait, and if the family history is suggestive, further studies may be indicated.

α-THALASSEMIA SYNDROMES

The same evolutionary pressures that produced β-thalassemia and sickle cell disease produced α-thalassemia. Infants are identified in the newborn period by the increased production of Bart hemoglobin (γ$_4$) during fetal life and its presence at birth. The α-thalassemia syndromes occur most commonly in Southeast Asia. Deletion mutations are common in α-thalassemia. In addition to deletional mutations, there are nondeletional α-globin gene mutations, the most common being Constant Spring ($\alpha^{CS}\alpha$); these mutations cause a more severe anemia and clinical course than the deletional mutations. There are 4 α-globin gene alleles and 4 deletional α-thalassemia phenotypes. The different phenotypes in α-thalassemia largely result from whether one (α^+-thalassemia) or both (α^0-thalassemia) α-globin genes are deleted in each of the 2 loci.

The deletion of 1 α-globin gene allele (silent trait) is not identifiable hematologically. Specifically, no alterations are noted in the MCV and mean corpuscular hemoglobin. Persons with this deletion are usually diagnosed after the birth of a child with a 2-gene deletion or HbH (β$_4$), but some newborn screening programs report even low concentrations of Hb Bart. During the newborn period, <3% Hb Bart is observed. The deletion of 1 α-globin gene allele is common in African-Americans.

The deletion of 2 α-globin gene alleles results in α-thalassemia trait. The α-globin alleles can be lost in a *trans*-($-\alpha/-\alpha$) or *cis*- ($\alpha,\alpha/^{-SEA}$) configuration. The *trans* or *cis* mutations can combine with other mutations and lead to HbH or α-thalassemia major. In persons from Africa or of African descent, the most common α-globin deletions are in the *trans* configuration; whereas, in persons from or descended from Asia or the Mediterranean region, *cis* deletions are most common.

α-Thalassemia trait manifest as a microcytic anemia that can be mistaken for iron-deficiency anemia (see Fig. 462-5F). The hemoglobin analysis is normal, except during the newborn period, when Hb Bart is commonly <8% but >3%. Children with a deletion of 2 α-globin alleles are commonly thought to have iron deficiency, given the presence of both low MCV and mean corpuscular hemoglobin. The simplest approach to distinguish between iron deficiency and α-thalassemia trait is with a good dietary history. Children with iron-deficiency anemia often have a diet that is low in iron and drink significant amount of cow's milk. Alternatively, a brief course of iron supplementation along with monitoring of erythrocyte parameters might confirm the diagnosis of iron deficiency. If both parents of a child diagnosed with α-thalassemia trait are carriers, they are at risk for a future hydrops fetalis pregnancy. Thus, family screening and genetic counseling are indicated.

The deletion of 3 α-globin gene alleles leads to the diagnosis of HbH disease. A more severe form of HbH disease may be caused by a nondeletional α-globin mutation with 2 allele deletions. HbH Constant Spring ($-\alpha/\alpha,\alpha^{CS}$) is the most common type of nondeletional HbH disease.

In California, where a large population of persons of Asian descent resides, approximately 1:10,000 of all newborns have HbH disease. The simplest manner of diagnosing HbH disease is during the newborn period, when excess in γ-tetramers are present and Hb Bart is commonly >25%. Obtaining supporting evidence from the parents is also necessary. Later in childhood, there is an excess of β-globin chain tetramers that results in HbH. A definitive diagnosis of HbH disease requires DNA analysis with supporting evidence. Brilliant cresyl blue can stain HbH, but it is rarely used for diagnosis. Patients with HbH disease have a marked microcytosis, anemia, mild splenomegaly, and, occasionally, scleral icterus or cholelithiasis. Chronic transfusion is not commonly required for therapy because the range of hemoglobin is 7-11 g/dL, with MCV 51-73 fL but intermittent transfusions for worsening anemia may be needed.

The deletion of all 4 α-globin gene alleles causes profound anemia during fetal life, resulting in hydrops fetalis; the ζ-globin gene must be present for fetal survival. There are no normal hemoglobins present at birth (primarily Hb Bart, with Hb Gower 1, Gower 2, and Portland). If the fetus survives, immediate exchange transfusion is indicated. These infants with severe α-thalassemia are transfusion dependent, and hematopoietic stem cell transplantation is the only cure.

Treatment of HbH disease requires ongoing monitoring of growth and organ dysfunction. Dietary supplement with folate and multivitamins without iron is indicated. Older patients may develop decreased bone density with calcium and vitamin D deficiency. Iron supplementation should be avoided. Intermittent transfusion requirements during child development and infection may occur, particularly in nondeletional HbH. Splenectomy is occasionally indicated and because of the high risk of postsplenectomy thrombosis, aspirin or other anticoagulant therapy following splenectomy should be considered. Hemosiderosis, secondary to gastrointestinal iron absorption and/or transfusion exposure, may develop in older patients and require therapy. Because HbH is an unstable hemoglobin sensitive to oxidative injury, oxidative medications should be avoided. At-risk couples for hydrops fetalis should be identified and offered molecular diagnosis on fetal tissue obtained early in pregnancy. Later in pregnancy, intrauterine transfusion can improve fetal survival, but chronic transfusion therapy or bone marrow transplantation for survivors will be required.

Bibliography is available at Expert Consult.

Chapter 463
Enzymatic Defects

463.1 Pyruvate Kinase Deficiency
George B. Segel

Congenital hemolytic anemia occurs in persons homozygous or compound heterozygous for autosomal recessive genes that cause either a marked reduction in red blood cell (RBC) pyruvate kinase (PK) or production of an abnormal enzyme with decreased activity resulting in impaired conversion of phosphoenolpyruvate to pyruvate. Generation of adenosine triphosphate (ATP) within RBCs at this step is impaired, and low levels of ATP, pyruvate, and the oxidized form

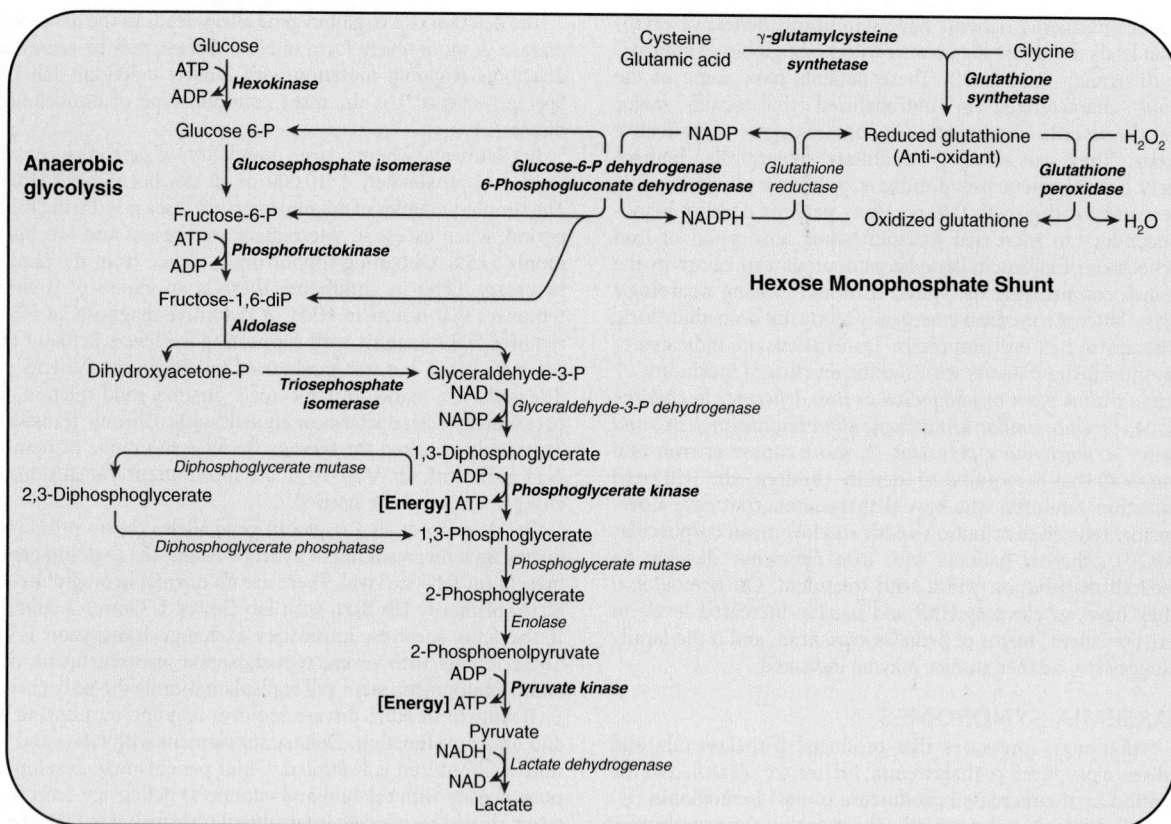

Figure 463-1 Red blood cell metabolism. Glycolysis and the hexose monophosphate pathway. The enzyme deficiencies clearly associated with hemolysis are shown in bold type. ATP, adenosine triphosphate; ADP, adenosine diphosphate; NADP, nicotinamide adenine dinucleotide phosphate; NADPH, reduced form of NADP.

of nicotinamide adenine dinucleotide (NAD^+) are found (Fig. 463-1). The concentration of 2,3-diphosphoglycerate is increased; this isomer is beneficial in facilitating oxygen release from hemoglobin but detrimental in inhibiting hexokinase and enzymes of the hexose monophosphate shunt. In addition, an unexplained decrease occurs in the sum of the adenine (ATP, adenosine diphosphate, and adenosine monophosphate) and pyridine (NAD^+ and the reduced form of NAD) nucleotides, further impairing glycolysis. As a consequence of decreased ATP, RBCs cannot maintain their potassium and water content; the cells become rigid, and their life span is considerably reduced.

ETIOLOGY

There are 2 mammalian PK genes, but only the *PKLR* gene is expressed in red cells. The human *PKLR* gene is located on chromosome 1q21. More than 180 mutations are reported in this structural gene, which codes for a 574–amino-acid protein that forms a functional tetramer. These mutations include missense, splice site, and insertion–deletion alterations, and there is some correlation of the type, location, and amino acid substitution with disease severity. Most affected patients are compound heterozygotes for 2 different PK gene defects. The many possible combinations likely account for the variability in clinical severity. The mutations 1456 C to T and 1529 G to A are the most common mutations in the white population.

CLINICAL MANIFESTATIONS AND LABORATORY FINDINGS

The clinical manifestations of PK deficiency vary from severe neonatal hemolytic anemia to mild, well-compensated hemolysis first noted in adulthood. Severe jaundice and anemia may occur in the neonatal period, and kernicterus has been reported. The hemolysis in older children and adults varies in severity, with hemoglobin values ranging from 8-12 g/dL associated with some pallor, jaundice, and splenomegaly. Patients with these findings usually do not require transfusion. A severe form of the disease has a relatively high incidence among the Amish of the midwestern United States. PK deficiency may possibly provide protection against falciparum malaria.

Polychromatophilia and mild macrocytosis reflect the elevated reticulocyte count. Spherocytes are uncommon, but a few spiculated pyknocytes may be found. Diagnosis relies on demonstration of a marked reduction of RBC PK activity or an increase in the Michaelis-Menten dissociation constant (K_m) for its substrate, phosphoenolpyruvate (high K_m variant). Other RBC enzyme activity is normal or elevated, reflecting the reticulocytosis. No abnormalities of hemoglobin are noted. The white cells have normal PK activity and must be rigorously excluded from the red cell hemolysates used to measure PK activity. Heterozygous carriers usually have moderately reduced levels of PK activity.

TREATMENT

Phototherapy and exchange transfusions may be indicated for hyperbilirubinemia in newborns. Transfusions of packed RBCs are necessary for severe anemia or for aplastic crises. If the anemia is consistently severe and frequent transfusions are required, iron chelation may be necessary, and splenectomy should be performed after the child is 5-6 yr of age. Although it is not curative, splenectomy may be followed by higher hemoglobin levels and by strikingly high (30-60%) reticulocyte counts. Death resulting from overwhelming pneumococcal sepsis has followed splenectomy; thus, immunization with vaccines for encapsulated organisms should be given before splenectomy, and prophylactic penicillin should be administered after the procedure.

463.2 Other Glycolytic Enzyme Deficiencies
George B. Segel

Chronic nonspherocytic hemolytic anemias of varying severity have been associated with deficiencies of other enzymes in the glycolytic pathway, including hexokinase, glucose phosphate isomerase, and aldolase, which are inherited as autosomal recessive disorders. **Phosphofructokinase deficiency,** which occurs primarily in Ashkenazi Jews in the United States, results in hemolysis associated with a myopathy classified as glycogen storage disease type VII (see Chapter 87.1). Clinically, hemolytic anemia is complicated by muscle weakness, exercise intolerance, cramps, and possibly myoglobinuria. Enzyme assays for phosphofructokinase yield low values for RBCs and muscle.

Triose phosphate isomerase deficiency is an autosomal recessive disorder affecting many systems. Affected patients have hemolytic anemia, cardiac abnormalities, and lower motor neuron and pyramidal tract impairment, with or without evidence of cerebral impairment. They usually die in early childhood. The gene for triose phosphate isomerase has been cloned and sequenced and is located on chromosome 12.

Phosphoglycerate kinase (PGK) is the first ATP-generating step in glycolysis. At least 23 kindreds with PGK deficiency have been described. PGK is the only glycolytic enzyme inherited on the X chromosome. Affected males may have progressive extrapyramidal disease, myopathy, seizures, and variable mental retardation in conjunction with hemolytic anemia. Nine Japanese patients had neural or myopathic symptoms with hemolysis; 6 had hemolysis alone; 7 had neural or myopathic symptoms alone; and 1 had no symptoms. The gene for PGK is particularly large, spanning 23 kb, and various genetic abnormalities, including nucleotide substitutions, gene deletions, missense, and splicing mutations, result in PGK deficiency.

DEFICIENCIES OF ENZYMES OF THE HEXOSE MONOPHOSPHATE PATHWAY

The most important function of the hexose monophosphate pathway is to maintain glutathione (GSH) in its reduced state as protection against the oxidation of RBCs (see Fig. 463-1). Approximately 10% of the glucose taken up by RBCs passes through this pathway to provide the reduced form of NAD phosphate (NADPH) necessary for the conversion of oxidized GSH to reduced GSH. Maintenance of reduced GSH is essential for the physiologic inactivation of oxidant compounds, such as hydrogen peroxide, that are generated within RBCs. If glutathione, or any compound or enzyme necessary for maintaining it in the reduced state, is decreased, the SH groups of the RBC membrane are oxidized and the hemoglobin becomes denatured and may precipitate into RBC inclusions called **Heinz bodies.** Once Heinz bodies have formed, an acute hemolytic process results from damage to the RBC membrane by the precipitated hemoglobin, the oxidant agent, and the action of the spleen. The damaged RBCs then are rapidly removed from the circulation.

463.3 Glucose-6-Phosphate Dehydrogenase Deficiency and Related Deficiencies
George B. Segel and Lisa R. Hackney

Glucose-6-phosphate dehydrogenase (G6PD) deficiency, the most frequent disease involving enzymes of the hexose monophosphate pathway, is responsible for 2 clinical syndromes, episodic hemolytic anemia and chronic nonspherocytic hemolytic anemia. The most common manifestations of this disorder are neonatal jaundice and episodic acute hemolytic anemia, which is induced by infections, certain drugs, and, rarely, fava beans. This X-linked deficiency affects more than 400 million people worldwide, representing an overall 4.9% global prevalence. The global distribution of this disorder parallels that of malaria, representing an example of "balanced polymorphism," in

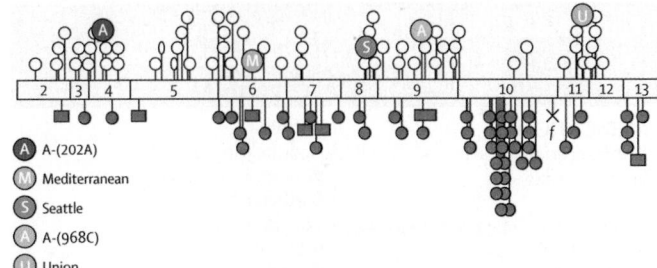

Figure 463-2 Most common mutations along coding sequence of G6PD gene. Exons are shown as *open numbered boxes. Open circles* are mutations causing classes II and III variants. *Filled circles* represent sporadic mutations giving rise to severe variants (class I). *Open ellipses* are mutations causing class IV variants. X a nonsense mutation; *f*, a splice site mutation; *filled square*, small deletion. 202A and 968C are the two sites of base substitution in G6PD-A. *(From Cappellini MD, Fiorelli G: Glucose-6-phosphate dehydrogenase deficiency,* Lancet *371:64–74, 2008.)*

which there is an evolutionary advantage of resistance to falciparum malaria in heterozygous females that outweighs the small negative effect of affected hemizygous males.

The deficiency is caused by inheritance of any of a large number of abnormal alleles of the gene responsible for the synthesis of the G6PD protein. About 140 mutations have been described in the gene responsible for the synthesis of the G6PD protein. Many of these mutations are single base changes leading to amino acid substitutions and destabilization of the G6PD enzyme. A web-accessible database catalogs G6PD mutations (http://www.bioinf.org.uk/g6pd). Figure 463-2 shows some of the mutations that cause episodic versus chronic hemolysis. Milder disease is associated with mutations near the amino terminus of the G6PD molecule, and chronic nonspherocytic hemolytic anemia is associated with mutations clustered near the carboxyl terminus. The normal enzyme found in most populations is designated G6PD B+. A normal variant, designated G6PD A+, is common in Americans of African descent.

EPISODIC OR INDUCED HEMOLYTIC ANEMIA
Etiology

G6PD catalyzes the conversion of glucose 6-phosphate to 6-phosphogluconic acid. This reaction produces NADPH, which maintains GSH in the reduced, functional state (see Fig. 463-1). Reduced GSH provides protection against oxidant threats from certain drugs and infections that would otherwise cause precipitation of hemoglobin (Heinz bodies) or damage the RBC membrane.

Synthesis of RBC G6PD is determined by a gene on the X chromosome. Thus, heterozygous females have intermediate enzymatic activity and have 2 populations of RBCs: one is normal, and the other is deficient in G6PD activity. Because they have fewer susceptible cells, most heterozygous females do not have evident clinical hemolysis after exposure to oxidant drugs. Rarely, the majority of RBCs is G6PD deficient in heterozygous females because the inactivation of the normal X chromosome is random and sometimes exaggerated (Lyon-Beutler hypothesis).

Disease involving this enzyme therefore occurs more frequently in males than in females. Approximately 13% of male Americans of African descent have a mutant enzyme **(G6PD A−)** that results in a deficiency of RBC G6PD activity (5-15% of normal). Italians, Greeks, and other Mediterranean, Middle Eastern, African, and Asian ethnic groups also have a high incidence, ranging from 5% to 40%, of a variant designated **G6PD B−** (**G6PD Mediterranean**). In these variants, the G6PD activity of homozygous females or hemizygous males is <5% of normal. Therefore, the defect in Americans of African descent is less severe than that in Americans of European descent. A third mutant enzyme with markedly reduced activity (**G6PD Canton**) occurs in approximately 5% of the Chinese population.

Table 463-1	Agents Precipitating Hemolysis in Glucose-6-Phosphate Dehydrogenase Deficiency
MEDICATIONS *Antibacterials* Sulfonamides Dapsone Trimethoprim-sulfamethoxazole Nalidixic acid Chloramphenicol Nitrofurantoin *Antimalarials* Primaquine Pamaquine Chloroquine Quinacrine *Antihelminths* β-Naphthol Stibophen Niridazole	*Others* Acetanilide Vitamin K analogs Methylene blue Toluidine blue Probenecid Dimercaprol Acetylsalicylic acid Phenazopyridine Rasburicase **CHEMICALS** Phenylhydrazine Benzene Naphthalene (moth balls) 2,4,6-Trinitrotoluene **ILLNESS** Diabetic acidosis Hepatitis Sepsis

From Asselin BL, Segel GB: In Rakel R, editor: Conn's current therapy, Philadelphia, 1994, WB Saunders, p. 341.

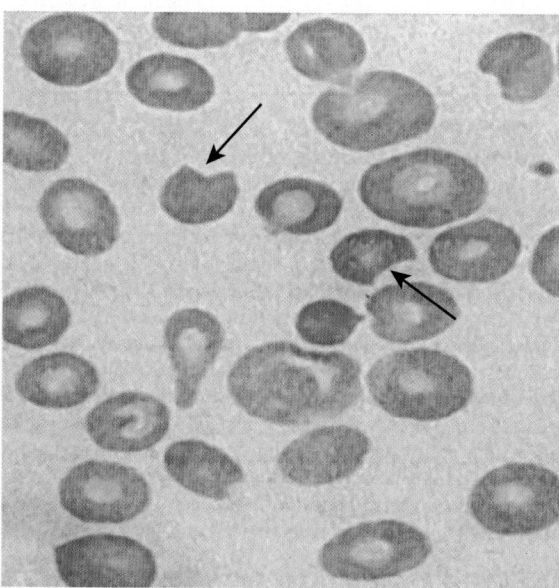

Figure 463-3 Morphologic erythrocyte changes (anisopoikilocytosis, bite cells) during acute hemolysis in a G6PD-deficient patient. *Arrows show bite cells. Anisopoikilocytosis is abnormality in the shape or size of erythrocytes. (From Cappellini MD, Fiorelli G: Glucose-6-phosphate dehydrogenase deficiency, Lancet 371:64–74, 2008.)*

Clinical Manifestations

Most individuals with G6PD deficiency are asymptomatic, with no clinical manifestations of illness unless triggered by infection, drugs, or ingestion of fava beans. Typically, hemolysis ensues in about 24-48 hr after a patient has ingested a substance with oxidant properties. In severe cases, hemoglobinuria and jaundice result, and the hemoglobin concentration may fall precipitously. Drugs that elicit hemolysis in these individuals include aspirin, sulfonamides, rasburicase, and antimalarials, such as primaquine (Table 463-1). The degree of hemolysis varies with the inciting agent, amount ingested, and severity of the enzyme deficiency. In some individuals, ingestion of fava beans also produces an acute, severe hemolytic syndrome, known as *favism*. Fava beans contain divicine, isouramil, and convicine, which ultimately lead to production of hydrogen peroxide and other reactive oxygen products. Favism is thought to be more frequently associated with the G6PD B− variant.

In the G6PD A− variant, the stability of the folded protein dimer is impaired, and this defect is accentuated as the RBCs age. Thus, hemolysis decreases as older red cells are destroyed, even if administration of the drug is continued. This recovery results from the age-labile enzyme, which is abundant and more stable in younger RBCs. The associated reticulocytosis produces a compensated hemolytic process in which the blood hemoglobin may be only slightly decreased, despite continued exposure to the offending agent.

G6PD deficiency can produce hemolysis in the neonatal period. In G6PD A−, spontaneous hemolysis and hyperbilirubinemia have been observed in preterm infants. In newborns with the G6PD B− and G6PD Canton varieties, hyperbilirubinemia and even kernicterus may occur. Neonates with coinheritance of G6PD deficiency and a mutation of the promoter of uridine-diphosphate-glucuronyl transferase (UGT1A1), seen in Gilbert syndrome, have more severe neonatal jaundice. When a pregnant woman ingests oxidant drugs, they may be transmitted to her G6PD-deficient fetus, and hemolytic anemia and jaundice may be apparent at birth.

Laboratory Findings

The onset of acute hemolysis usually results in a precipitous fall in hemoglobin and hematocrit. If the episode is severe, the hemoglobin binding proteins, such as haptoglobin, are saturated, and free hemoglobin may appear in the plasma and subsequently in the urine. Unstained or supravital preparations of RBCs reveal precipitated

hemoglobin, known as Heinz bodies. The RBC inclusions are not visible on the Wright-stained blood film. Cells that contain these inclusions are seen only within the first 3-4 days of illness because they are rapidly cleared from the blood. Also, the blood film may contain red cells with what appears to be a bite taken from their periphery and polychromasia (evidence of bluish, larger RBCs), representing reticulocytosis (Fig. 463-3).

Diagnosis

The diagnosis depends on direct or indirect demonstration of reduced G6PD activity in RBCs. By direct measurement, enzyme activity in affected persons is ≤10% of normal, and the reduction of enzyme activity is more extreme in Americans of European descent and in Asians than in Americans of African descent. Satisfactory screening tests are based on decoloration of methylene blue, reduction of methemoglobin, or fluorescence of NADPH. Immediately after a hemolytic episode, reticulocytes and young RBCs predominate. These young cells have significantly higher enzyme activity than do older cells in the A− variety (African). Testing may therefore have to be deferred for a few weeks before a diagnostically low level of enzyme can be shown. The diagnosis can be suspected when G6PD activity is within the low-normal range in the presence of a high reticulocyte count. G6PD variants also can be detected by electrophoretic and molecular analysis. G6PD deficiency should be considered in any neonatal patients with hyperbilirubinemia and borderline low G6PD activity.

Prevention and Treatment

Prevention of hemolysis constitutes the most important therapeutic measure. When possible, males belonging to ethnic groups with a significant incidence of G6PD deficiency (e.g., Greeks, southern Italians, Sephardic Jews, Filipinos, southern Chinese, Americans of African descent, and Thais) should be tested for the defect before known oxidant drugs are given. The usual doses of aspirin and trimethoprim-sulfamethoxazole do not cause clinically relevant hemolysis in the A− variety. Aspirin administered in doses used for acute rheumatic fever (60-100 mg/kg/24 hr) may produce a severe hemolytic episode. Infants with severe neonatal jaundice who belong to these ethnic groups also require testing for G6PD deficiency because of their heightened risk for this defect. If severe hemolysis has occurred, supportive therapy may require blood transfusions, although recovery is the rule when the oxidant agent is discontinued.

CHRONIC HEMOLYTIC ANEMIAS ASSOCIATED WITH DEFICIENCY OF G6PD OR RELATED FACTORS

Chronic nonspherocytic hemolytic anemia has been associated with profound deficiency of G6PD caused by enzyme variants, particularly those defective in quantity, activity, or stability. The gene defects leading to chronic hemolysis are located primarily in the region of the NADP binding site near the carboxyl terminus of the protein (see Fig. 463-2). These include the Loma Linda, Tomah, Iowa, Beverly Hills, Nashville, Riverside, Santiago de Cuba, and Andalus variants. Persons with G6PD B–enzyme deficiency occasionally have chronic hemolysis, and the hemolytic process may worsen after ingestion of oxidant drugs. Splenectomy is of little value in these types of chronic hemolysis.

Other enzyme defects may impair the regeneration of GSH as an oxidant "sump" (see Fig. 463-1). Mild, chronic nonspherocytic anemia has been reported in association with decreased RBC GSH, resulting from γ-glutamylcysteine or GSH synthetase deficiencies. Deficiency of 6-phosphogluconate dehydrogenase has been associated primarily with drug-induced hemolysis, and hemolysis with hyperbilirubinemia has been related to a deficiency of GSH peroxidase in newborn infants.

Bibliography is available at Expert Consult.

Chapter **464**

Hemolytic Anemias Resulting from Extracellular Factors— Immune Hemolytic Anemias

Charles H. Packman and George B. Segel

AUTOIMMUNE HEMOLYTIC ANEMIAS

A number of extrinsic agents and disorders may lead to premature destruction of red blood cells (RBCs). Among the most clearly defined are antibodies associated with immune hemolytic anemias. The hallmark of this group of diseases is the positive result of the direct antiglobulin (Coombs) test, which detects a coating of immunoglobulin or components of complement on the RBC surface. The most important immune hemolytic disorder in pediatric practice is hemolytic disease of the newborn (erythroblastosis fetalis), caused by transplacental transfer of maternal antibody active against the RBCs of the fetus, that is, isoimmune hemolytic anemia (see Chapter 103.2). Various other immune hemolytic anemias are autoimmune (Table 464-1) and may be idiopathic or related to various infections (Epstein-Barr virus, and rarely HIV, cytomegalovirus, and mycoplasma), immunologic diseases (systemic lupus erythematosus [SLE], rheumatoid arthritis), immunodeficiency diseases (agammaglobulinemia, autoimmune lymphoproliferative disorder, dysgammaglobulinemias), neoplasms (lymphoma, leukemia, and Hodgkin disease), or drugs (methyldopa, ʟ-dopa). Other drugs (penicillins, cephalosporins) cause hemolysis by means of "drug-dependent antibodies"—that is antibodies directed toward the drug and in some cases toward an RBC membrane antigen as well.

Table 464-1	Diseases Characterized by Immune-Mediated Red Blood Cell Destruction

AUTOIMMUNE HEMOLYTIC ANEMIA CAUSED BY WARM REACTIVE AUTOANTIBODIES
Primary (idiopathic)
Secondary
  Lymphoproliferative disorders
  Connective tissue disorders (especially systemic lupus erythematosus)
  Nonlymphoid neoplasms (e.g., ovarian tumors)
  Chronic inflammatory diseases (e.g., ulcerative colitis)
  Immunodeficiency disorders

AUTOIMMUNE HEMOLYTIC ANEMIA CAUSED BY COLD REACTIVE AUTOANTIBODIES (CRYOPATHIC HEMOLYTIC SYNDROMES)
Primary (idiopathic) cold agglutinin disease
Secondary cold agglutinin disease
  Lymphoproliferative disorders
  Infections (*Mycoplasma pneumoniae*, Epstein-Barr virus)
  Paroxysmal cold hemoglobinuria
  Primary (idiopathic)
  Viral syndromes (most common)
  Congenital or tertiary syphilis

DRUG-INDUCED IMMUNE HEMOLYTIC ANEMIA (see Table 464-2)
Hapten/drug adsorption (e.g., penicillin)
Ternary (immune) complex (e.g., quinine or quinidine)
True autoantibody induction (e.g., methyldopa)

Modified from Packman CH: Autoimmune hemolytic anemias. In Rakel R, editor: Conn's current therapy, Philadelphia, 1995, WB Saunders, p. 305.

AUTOIMMUNE HEMOLYTIC ANEMIAS ASSOCIATED WITH "WARM" ANTIBODIES
Etiology

In the autoimmune hemolytic anemias, autoantibodies are directed against RBC membrane antigens, but the pathogenesis of antibody induction is uncertain. The autoantibody may be produced as an inappropriate immune response to an RBC antigen or to another antigenic epitope similar to an RBC antigen, known as *molecular mimicry*. Alternatively, an infectious agent may alter the RBC membrane so that it becomes "foreign" or antigenic to the host. The antibodies usually react to epitopes (antigens) that are "public" or common to all human RBCs, such as Rh proteins.

In most instances of warm antibody hemolysis, no underlying cause can be found; this is the primary or idiopathic type (see Table 464-1). If the autoimmune hemolysis is associated with an underlying disease, such as a lymphoproliferative disorder, SLE, Evans syndrome, or immunodeficiency, it is secondary. In as many as 20% of cases of immune hemolysis, drugs may be implicated (Table 464-2).

Drugs (penicillin or sometimes cephalosporins) that cause hemolysis via the "hapten" mechanism (immune but not autoimmune) bind tightly to the RBC membrane (see Table 464-1). Antibodies to the drug, either newly or previously formed, bind to the drug molecules on RBCs, mediating their destruction in the spleen. In other cases, certain drugs, such as quinine and quinidine, do not bind to RBCs but, rather, form part of a "ternary complex," consisting of the drug, an RBC membrane antigen, and an antibody that recognizes both (see Table 464-1). Methyldopa and sometimes cephalosporins may, by unknown mechanisms, incite true autoantibodies to RBC membrane antigens, so that the presence of the drug is not required to cause hemolysis. Cephalosporins are the most common cause of drug-immune hemolytic anemia.

Clinical Manifestations

Autoimmune hemolytic anemias may occur in either of 2 general clinical patterns. The first, an acute transient type lasting 3-6 mo and occurring predominantly in children ages 2-12 yr, accounts for 70-80% of patients. It is frequently preceded by an infection, usually respiratory.

Table 464-2	Selected Drugs That Cause Immune-Mediated Hemolysis		
MECHANISM	**DRUG ADSORPTION (HAPTEN)**	**TERNARY (IMMUNE) COMPLEX**	**AUTOANTIBODY INDUCTION**
Direct antiglobulin test	Positive (anti-IgG)	Positive (anti-C3)	Positive (anti-IgG)
Site of hemolysis	Extravascular	Intravascular	Extravascular
Medications	Penicillins Cephalosporins 6-mercaptopurine Tetracycline Oxaliplatin Hydrocortisone	Cephalosporins Quinidine Amphotericin B Hydrocortisone Rifampin (Rifadin) Metformin Quinine Probenecid Chlorpromazine Oxaliplatin	α-Methyldopa Cephalosporins Oxaliplatin L-Dopa Procainamide Ibuprofen Diclofenac (Voltaren) Interferon alfa

Ig, immunoglobulin.

Adapted from Packman CH: Hemolytic anemia resulting from immune injury. In Kaushansky K, Lichtman MA, Beutler E, et al, editors: Williams Hematology, ed 8, New York, 2010, McGraw-Hill, pp. 777–798.

Onset may be acute, with prostration, pallor, jaundice, fever, and hemoglobinuria, or more gradual, with primarily fatigue and pallor. The spleen is usually enlarged and is the primary site of destruction of immunoglobulin (Ig) G–coated RBCs. Underlying systemic disorders are unusual. A consistent response to glucocorticoid therapy, a low mortality rate, and full recovery are characteristic of the acute form. The other clinical pattern involves a prolonged and chronic course, which is more frequent in infants and in children >12 yr old. Hemolysis may continue for many months or years. Abnormalities involving other blood elements are common, and the response to glucocorticoids is variable and inconsistent. The mortality rate is approximately 10%, and death is often attributable to an underlying systemic disease.

Laboratory Findings
In many cases, anemia is profound, with hemoglobin levels <6 g/dL. Considerable spherocytosis and polychromasia (reflecting the reticulocyte response) are present. More than 50% of the circulating RBCs may be reticulocytes, and nucleated RBCs usually are present. In some cases, a low reticulocyte count may be found, particularly early in the episode. Leukocytosis is common. The platelet count is usually normal, but concomitant immune thrombocytopenic purpura sometimes occurs (**Evans syndrome**). The prognosis for patients with Evans syndrome is guarded, because many have or eventually have a chronic disease, including SLE, an immunodeficiency syndrome, or the autoimmune lymphoproliferative syndrome.

Results of the direct antiglobulin test are strongly positive, and free antibody can sometimes be demonstrated in the serum (indirect Coombs test). These antibodies are active at 35-40°C (95-104°F) ("warm" antibodies) and most often belong to the IgG class. They do not require complement for activity and are usually *incomplete* antibodies that do not produce agglutination in vitro. Antibodies from the serum and those eluted from the RBCs react with the RBCs of many persons in addition to those of the patient. They often have been regarded as nonspecific panagglutinins, but careful studies have revealed specificity for RBC antigens of the Rh system in 70% of patients (≈50% of adult patients). Complement, particularly fragments of C3b, may be detected on the RBCs in conjunction with IgG. The Coombs test result is *rarely* negative *because of* the limited sensitivity of the Coombs reaction. A minimum of 260-400 molecules of IgG per cell is necessary on the RBC membrane to produce a positive reaction. Special tests are required to detect the antibody in cases of "Coombs-negative" autoimmune hemolytic anemia. In warm antibody hemolytic anemia, the direct Coombs test may detect IgG alone, both IgG– and complement fragments, or solely complement fragments if the level of RBC-bound IgG is below the detection limit of the anti-IgG Coombs reagent.

Treatment
Transfusions may provide only transient benefit but may be lifesaving in cases of severe anemia by providing delivery of oxygen until the effect of other treatment is observed. All tested units for transfusion are serologically incompatible. It is important to identify the patient's ABO blood group to avoid a hemolytic transfusion reaction mediated by anti-A or anti-B. The blood bank should also test for the presence of an underlying alloantibody, which could cause rapid hemolysis of transfused red cells. Patients who have neither been previously transfused nor pregnant are unlikely to harbor an alloantibody. Early consultation between the clinician and the blood bank physician is essential. Failure to transfuse a profoundly anemic infant or child may lead to serious morbidity and even death.

Patients with mild disease and compensated hemolysis may not require any treatment. If the hemolysis is severe and results in significant anemia or symptoms, treatment with glucocorticoids is initiated. Glucocorticoids decrease the rate of hemolysis by blocking macrophage function by downregulating Fcγ receptor expression, decreasing the production of the autoantibody, and perhaps enhancing the elution of antibody from the RBCs. Prednisone or its equivalent is administered at a dose of 2 mg/kg/24 hr. In some patients with severe hemolysis, doses of prednisone of up to 6 mg/kg/24 hr may be required to reduce the rate of hemolysis. Treatment should be continued until the rate of hemolysis decreases, and then the dose gradually reduced. If relapse occurs, resumption of the full dosage may be necessary. The disease tends to remit spontaneously within a few weeks or months. The Coombs test result may remain positive even after the hemoglobin level returns to normal. It is usually safe to discontinue prednisone once the direct Coombs test result becomes negative. When hemolytic anemia remains severe despite glucocorticoid therapy, or if very large doses are necessary to maintain a reasonable hemoglobin level, IV immunoglobulin may be tried. Rituximab, a monoclonal antibody that targets B lymphocytes, the source of antibody production, is useful in chronic cases refractory to conventional therapy. Plasmapheresis has been used in refractory cases but generally is not helpful. Splenectomy may be beneficial but is complicated by a heightened risk of infection with encapsulated organisms, particularly in patients <6 yr. Prophylaxis with appropriate vaccines (pneumococcal, meningococcal, and *Haemophilus influenzae* type b) before splenectomy and with oral penicillin after splenectomy are indicated.

Course and Prognosis
Acute idiopathic autoimmune hemolytic disease in childhood varies in severity but is self-limited; death from untreatable anemia is rare. Approximately 30% of patients have chronic hemolysis, often associated with an underlying disease, such as SLE, lymphoma, or leukemia.

The presence of antiphospholipid antibodies in adult patients with immune hemolysis predisposes to thrombosis. Mortality in chronic cases depends on the primary disorder.

AUTOIMMUNE HEMOLYTIC ANEMIAS ASSOCIATED WITH "COLD" ANTIBODIES

"Cold" antibodies agglutinate RBCs at temperatures <37°C (98.6°F). They are primarily of the IgM class and require complement for hemolytic activity. The highest temperature at which RBC agglutination occurs is called the *thermal amplitude*. A higher thermal amplitude antibody—that is, one that can bind to RBCs at temperatures achievable in the body—results in hemolysis with exposure to a cold environment. High antibody titers are associated with a high thermal amplitude.

Cold Agglutinin Disease

Cold antibodies usually have specificity for the oligosaccharide antigens of the I/i system. They may occur in primary or idiopathic cold agglutinin disease, secondary to infections such as those from *Mycoplasma pneumoniae* and Epstein-Barr virus, or secondary to lymphoproliferative disorders. After *M. pneumoniae* infection, the anti-I levels may increase considerably, and occasionally, enormous increases may occur to titers ≥1/30,000. The antibody has specificity for the I antigen and thus reacts poorly with human cord RBCs, which possess the i antigen but exhibit low levels of I. Patients with infectious mononucleosis occasionally have cold agglutinin disease, and the antibodies in these patients often have anti-i specificity. This antibody causes less hemolysis in adults than in children because adults have fewer i molecules on their RBCs. Spontaneous RBC agglutination is observed in the cold and in vitro, and RBC aggregates are seen on the blood film. Mean corpuscular volume may be spuriously elevated because of RBC agglutination. The severity of the hemolysis is related to the thermal amplitude of the antibody, which itself partly depends on the IgM antibody titer.

When very high titers of cold antibodies are present and active near body temperature, severe intravascular hemolysis with hemoglobinemia and hemoglobinuria may occur and may be heightened on a patient's exposure to cold (external temperature or ingested foods). Each IgM molecule has the potential to activate a C1 molecule so that large amounts of complement are found on the RBCs in cold agglutinin disease. These sensitized RBCs may undergo intravascular complement-mediated lysis or may be destroyed in the liver and spleen. Only complement, not IgM, is detected on RBCs because the IgM is removed during the washing steps of the direct antiglobulin test.

Cold agglutinin disease is less common in children than in adults and more frequently results in an acute, self-limited episode of hemolysis. Glucocorticoids are much less effective in cold agglutinin disease than in disease with warm antibodies. Patients should avoid exposure to cold and should be treated for underlying disease. In the uncommon patients with severe hemolytic disease, treatment includes immunosuppression and plasmapheresis. Successful treatment of cold agglutinin disease has been reported with the monoclonal antibody rituximab, which effectively depletes B lymphocytes. Splenectomy is not useful in cold agglutinin disease.

Paroxysmal Cold Hemoglobinuria

Paroxysmal cold hemoglobinuria is mediated by the Donath-Landsteiner (D-L) hemolysin, which is an IgG cold-reactive autoantibody with anti-P specificity. In vitro, the D-L antibody binds to RBCs in the cold and the RBCs are lysed by complement as the temperature is increased to 37 degrees C. A similar sequence is thought to occur in vivo as RBCs move from the cooler extremities to warmer parts of the circulation. Most reported cases are self-limited; many patients experience only one paroxysm of hemolysis. Congenital or acquired syphilis used to be the most common underlying cause of paroxysmal cold hemoglobinuria, but today, most cases are associated with nonspecific viral infections. This disorder accounts for 30% of immune hemolytic episodes among children. Treatment includes transfusion for severe anemia and avoidance of cold ambient temperatures.

Bibliography is available at Expert Consult.

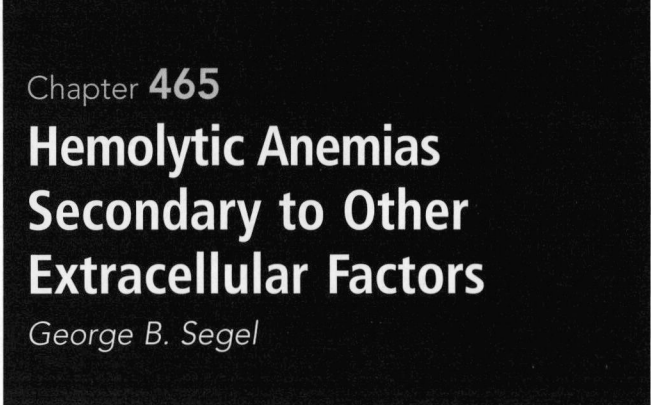

Chapter 465
Hemolytic Anemias Secondary to Other Extracellular Factors

George B. Segel

FRAGMENTATION HEMOLYSIS

(See Table 457-1 in Chapter 457.)

Red blood cell (RBC) destruction may occur in hemolytic anemias because of mechanical injury as the cells traverse a damaged vascular bed. Damage may be microvascular when RBCs are sheared by fibrin in the capillaries during intravascular coagulation or when renovascular disease accompanies the hemolytic-uremic syndrome (HUS) (see Chapter 518) or thrombotic thrombocytopenic purpura (see Chapter 484.5). Larger vessels may be involved in Kasabach-Merritt syndrome (giant hemangioma and thrombocytopenia; see Chapter 505) or when a replacement heart valve is poorly epithelialized. The blood film shows many "schistocytes," or fragmented cells, as well as polychromatophilia, reflecting the reticulocytosis (see Fig. 458-4F in Chapter 458). Secondary iron deficiency may complicate the intravascular hemolysis because of urinary hemoglobin and hemosiderin iron loss (see Fig. 457-2 in Chapter 457). Treatment should be directed toward the underlying condition, and the prognosis depends on the effectiveness of this treatment. The benefit of transfusion may be transient because the transfused cells are destroyed as quickly as those produced by the patient.

It is critical to determine the precise etiology of the fragmentation hemolysis because the treatment depends on the underlying problem (Table 465-1). Thrombotic thrombocytopenic purpura results from an antibody to an enzyme (AdamTS13) that regulates the size of von Willebrand multimers. The lack of this enzyme results in a marked increase in multimer size and a resultant thrombotic microangiopathy. The treatment involves plasmapheresis (PLEX) to remove the antibody and replace the AdamTS13. In contrast, HUS results from *Shiga* toxin produced by *Escherichia coli* 0157 and may not be helped by PLEX. Atypical HUS involves activation of the alternative complement pathway and is currently treated with eculizumab (anti C5), an inhibitor of the complement pathway. PLEX may reduce the RBC fragmentation and improve the platelet count but has little effect on the tissue (kidney) vasculopathy and thus is not usually recommended. Pneumococcal-induced HUS results from neuraminidase produced by the bacteria, which damages the membranes of the RBCs and the kidney, exposing the T-antigen. Plasma contains natural antibody to the T-antigen producing hemolysis, renal damage, and a thrombotic microangiopathy.

THERMAL INJURY

Extensive burns may directly damage the RBCs and cause hemolysis that results in the formation of spherocytes. Blood loss and marrow suppression may contribute to anemia and require blood transfusion. Erythropoietin (EPO) has been used as treatment for diminished RBC production.

RENAL DISEASE

The anemia of uremia is multifactorial in origin. EPO production may be decreased and the marrow suppressed by toxic metabolites. Furthermore, the RBC life span often is shortened owing to retention of

Table 465-1	Thrombotic Microangiopathies			
DISEASE*	**PATHOPHYSIOLOGY**	**LAB FINDINGS**	**MANAGEMENT**	
TTP	Ab to AdamTS13	AdamTS13 <10%[†] Ab to AdamTS13	PLEX with plasma	
HUS	E. coli 0157, Shiga toxin	E. coli 0157, Shiga toxin	Supportive ? value of PLEX	
aHUS	Complement-mediated alternative pathway	AdamTS13 >10% Decreased factors H and I (inhibitors of complement)[‡]	Eculizumab (ab to C5) PLEX not indicated	
Pneumococcal-induced HUS	Neuraminidase-induced RBC, platelet, and kidney damage Exposure of T-antigen on RBC and kidney	Pneumococcal infection AdamTS13 >10%	PLEX with albumin for neuraminidase and endogenous T ab removal	
DIC	Sepsis, shock, endotoxin	Decreased fibrinogen, increased fibrin split products, decreased clotting factors and platelets	Treat underlying condition; replace factors and platelets if bleeding	

*All show fragmentation hemolytic anemia, thrombocytopenia and potential renal and other organ damage. An elevated lactate dehydrogenase and reduced haptoglobin usually are present secondary to hemolysis.
  [†]Rarely a congenital defect in AdamTS13.
  [‡]May be related to inherited defect in factor H or I.
  Ab/ab, antibody; aHUS, atypical hemolytic uremic syndrome; DIC, disseminated intravascular coagulation; E. coli, Escherichia coli; HUS, hemolytic uremic syndrome; PLEX, plasmapheresis; RBC, red blood cell; TTP, thrombotic thrombocytopenic purpura.

metabolites and organic acidemia. The use of EPO in chronic renal disease has markedly decreased the need for blood transfusion.

LIVER DISEASE

A change in the ratio of cholesterol to phospholipids in the plasma may result in changes in the composition of the RBC membrane and shortening of the RBC life span. Some patients with liver disease have many target RBCs on the blood film, whereas others have a preponderance of spiculated cells. These morphologic changes reflect the alterations in the plasma lipid composition.

TOXINS AND VENOMS

Bacterial sepsis caused by *Haemophilus influenzae*, staphylococci, or streptococci may be complicated by accompanying hemolysis. Particularly severe hemolytic anemia has been observed in clostridial infections and results from a hemolytic clostridial toxin. Large numbers of spherocytes may be seen on the blood film. Spherocytic hemolysis also may be noted after bites by various snakes, including cobras, vipers, and rattlesnakes, which have phospholipases in their venom. Large numbers of bites by insects, such as bees, wasps, and yellow jackets, also may cause spherocytic hemolysis by a similar mechanism (see Chapter 725).

WILSON DISEASE

(See Chapter 357.2.)

An acute and self-limited episode of hemolytic anemia may precede by years the onset of hepatic or neurologic symptoms in Wilson disease. This event appears to result from the toxic effects of free copper on the RBC membrane. The blood film often (but not always) shows large numbers of spherocytes, and the Coombs test result is negative. Because early diagnosis of Wilson disease permits prophylactic treatment with penicillamine and prevention of hepatic and neurologic disease, correct assessment of this rare type of hemolysis is important.

Bibliography is available at Expert Consult.

Section 4
Polycythemia (Erythrocytosis)

Chapter 466
Polycythemia
Amanda M. Brandow and
Bruce M. Camitta

Polycythemia exists when the red blood cell (RBC) count, hemoglobin level, and total RBC volume all exceed the upper limits of normal. In postpubertal individuals, an RBC mass >25% above the mean normal value (based on body surface area) or a hemoglobin >18.5 g/dL (in males) or >16.5 g/dL (in females) indicate absolute erythrocytosis. A decrease in plasma volume, such as occurs in acute dehydration and burns, may result in a high hemoglobin value. These situations are more accurately designated as *hemoconcentration* or *relative polycythemia* because the RBC mass is not increased and normalization of the plasma volume restores hemoglobin to normal levels. Once the diagnosis of true polycythemia is made, sequential studies should be done to determine the underlying etiology (Fig. 466-1).

CLONAL (PRIMARY) POLYCYTHEMIA (POLYCYTHEMIA RUBRA VERA)
Pathogenesis

Polycythemia vera is an acquired clonal myeloproliferative disorder. Although primarily manifesting as erythrocytosis, thrombocytosis and leukocytosis can also be seen. When isolated severe thrombocytosis exists in the absence of erythrocytosis, the myeloproliferative disorder is called *essential thrombocythemia*. Polycythemia vera is rare in children. A gain-of-function mutation of *JAK2*, a cytoplasmic tyrosine kinase, is found in more than 90% of adult patients with polycythemia vera, but in <30% of children with this condition. The erythropoietin

Table 466-1	WHO Diagnostic Criteria for Polycythemia Vera

MAJOR CRITERIA

1. Hb >18.5 g/dL (men) or Hb >16.5 g/dL (women)
or
Hb or Hct >99th percentile of reference range for age, sex, or altitude of residence
or
Hb >17 g/dL (men) or Hb >15 g/dL (women) if associated with a sustained increase of ≥2 g/dL from baseline that cannot be attributed to correction of iron deficiency
or
elevated red cell mass >25% above mean normal predicted value
2. Presence of *JAK2* or similar mutation

MINOR CRITERIA

1. Bone marrow trilineage myeloproliferation
2. Subnormal serum erythropoietin level
3. Endogenous erythroid colony growth

DIAGNOSIS

Both major criteria and one minor criteria *or* first major criteria and 2 minor criteria.

Hb, hemoglobin; Hct, hematocrit.
From Tefferi A, Vardiman JW: Classification and diagnosis of myeloproliferative neoplasms: the 2008 World Health Organization criteria and point-of-care diagnostic algorithms. Leukemia 22:14–22, 2008.

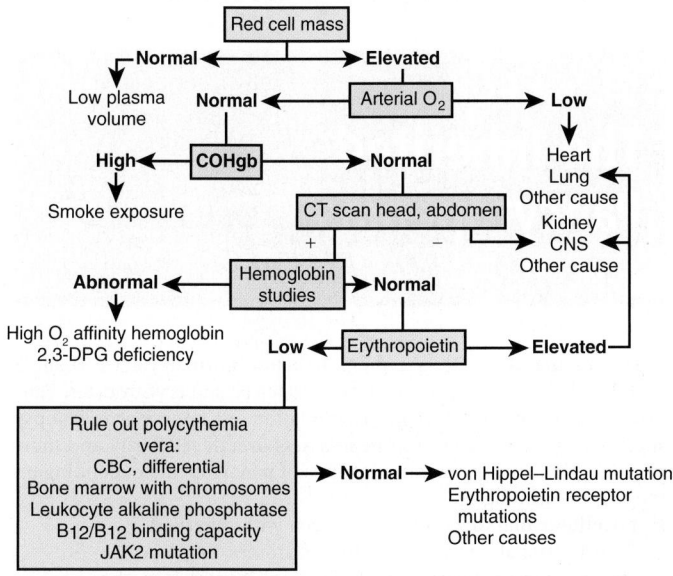

Figure 466-1 Sequential studies to evaluate polycythemia. CBC, complete blood count; CNS, central nervous system; COHgb, carboxy-hemoglobin; 2,3-DPG, 2,3-diphosphoglycerate.

receptor is normal, and serum erythropoietin levels are normal or low. In vitro cultures do not require added erythropoietin to stimulate growth of erythroid precursors. Risk factors for development of polycythemia vera include a family history of polycythemia vera and presence of an autoimmune disorder such as Crohn disease.

Clinical Manifestations

Patients with polycythemia vera usually have hepatosplenomegaly. Erythrocytosis may cause hypertension, headache, shortness of breath, or neurologic symptoms and increases the risk of thrombosis. Granulocytosis may cause diarrhea or pruritus from histamine release. Thrombocytosis (with or without platelet dysfunction) may cause thrombosis or hemorrhage. Table 466-1 lists the diagnostic criteria for polycythemia vera.

Treatment

Phlebotomy is the initial treatment of choice to alleviate symptoms of hyperviscosity and decrease the risk of thrombosis. Iron supplementa-

tion should be given to prevent viscosity problems from iron-deficient microcytosis or thrombocytosis. In patients with marked thrombocytosis, antiplatelet agents (e.g., aspirin) may reduce the risks of thrombosis and bleeding. If these treatments are unsuccessful or the patient has progressive hepatosplenomegaly, antiproliferative treatments (hydroxyurea, anagrelide, interferon-α) may be helpful. The use of JAK2 inhibitors is an active area of investigation. Transformation of the disease into myelofibrosis or acute leukemia is rare in children. Prolonged survival is not unusual.

Bibliography is available at Expert Consult.

Chapter 467
Non-Clonal Polycythemia
Amanda M. Brandow and Bruce M. Camitta

PATHOGENESIS

Nonclonal polycythemia is diagnosed when polycythemia is caused by a physiologic process that is not derived from a single cell (Table 467-1). Nonclonal polycythemia can be congenital or acquired (secondary).

Congenital Polycythemia

Lifelong or familial polycythemia should trigger a search for a congenital problem. These inherited conditions may be transmitted as dominant or recessive disorders. Autosomal dominant causes include hemoglobins that have increased oxygen affinity (P_{50} [partial pressure of oxygen in the blood at which the hemoglobin is 50% saturated] <20 mm Hg), erythropoietin receptor mutations resulting in an enhanced effect of erythropoietin or mutations in the von Hippel–Lindau gene that result in altered intracellular oxygen sensing. Another rare cause is autosomal recessive 2,3-ddiphosphoglyceric acid deficiency, which leads to a left shift of the oxygen dissociation curve, increased oxygen affinity, and consequent polycythemia.

Table 467-1	Differential Diagnosis of Polycythemia

CLONAL (PRIMARY)
Polycythemia vera

NONCLONAL
Congenital
High-oxygen affinity hemoglobinopathy (e.g., hemoglobin
  Chesapeake, Malmo, San Diego)
Erythropoietin receptor mutations (primary familial and congenital
  polycythemia [PFCP])
Methemoglobin reductase deficiency
Hemoglobin M disease
2,3-Diphosphoglycerate deficiency
Acquired
Hormonal
  Adrenal disease
    Virilizing hyperplasia, Cushing syndrome
  Anabolic steroid therapy
  Malignant tumors
    Adrenal, cerebellar, hepatic, other
  Renal disease
    Cysts, hydronephrosis, renal artery stenosis
Hypoxia
  Altitude
  Cardiac disease
  Lung disease
  Central hypoventilation
  Chronic carbon monoxide exposure
Neonatal
Delayed cord clamping (placental-fetal transfusion)
  Normal intrauterine environment
  Placental insufficiency (preeclampsia, maternal chronic
    hypertension, placental abruption)
  Twin–twin or maternal–fetal hemorrhage
  Perinatal asphyxia
  Infants of diabetic mothers
  Intrauterine growth retardation
  Trisomy 13, 18, or 21
  Adrenal hyperplasia
  Thyrotoxicosis
Spurious
Plasma volume decrease

Subtle decreases in oxygen delivery to tissues may cause polycythemia. Congenital methemoglobinemia resulting from an autosomal recessive deficiency of cytochrome b5 reductase may cause cyanosis and polycythemia (see Chapter 462.7). Most affected individuals are asymptomatic. Neurologic abnormalities may be present in patients whose enzyme deficits are not limited to hematopoietic cells. Hemoglobin M disease (autosomal dominant) causes methemoglobinemia and can lead to polycythemia. Cyanosis may occur in the presence of as little as 1.5 g/dL of methemoglobin but is uncommon in other hemoglobin variants unless hyperviscosity results in localized hypoxemia.

Acquired Polycythemia
Polycythemia may be present in clinical situations associated with chronic arterial oxygen desaturation. Cardiovascular defects involving right-to-left shunts and pulmonary diseases interfering with proper oxygenation are the most common causes of hypoxic polycythemia. Clinical findings usually include cyanosis, hyperemia of the sclerae and mucous membranes, and clubbing of the fingers. As the hematocrit rises to >65%, clinical manifestations of hyperviscosity, such as headache and hypertension, may require phlebotomy. Living at high altitudes also causes hypoxic polycythemia; the hemoglobin level increases approximately 4% for each rise of 1,000 m in altitude. Partial obstruction of a renal artery rarely results in polycythemia. Polycythemia has also been associated with benign and malignant tumors that secrete erythropoietin. Exogenous or endogenous excess of anabolic steroids also may cause polycythemia. A common spurious cause is a decrease in plasma volume such as in moderate to severe dehydration.

DIAGNOSIS
Figure 466-1 outlines sequential studies to evaluate polycythemia.

TREATMENT
For mild disease, observation is sufficient. When the hematocrit is >65-70% (hemoglobin >23 g/dL), blood viscosity markedly increases. Periodic phlebotomy may prevent or decrease symptoms such as headache, dizziness, or exertional dyspnea. Apheresed blood should be replaced with plasma or saline to prevent hypovolemia in patients accustomed to a chronically elevated total blood volume. Increased demand for red blood cell production may cause iron deficiency. Iron-deficient microcytic red cells are more rigid, further increasing the risk of intracranial and other thromboses in patients with polycythemia. Periodic assessment of iron status, with treatment of iron deficiency, should be performed.

Bibliography is available at Expert Consult.

Section 5
The Pancytopenias

Chapter 468
The Inherited Pancytopenias
Yigal Dror and Melvin H. Freedman

Pancytopenia refers to a reduction below normal values of all 3 peripheral blood lineages: leukocytes, platelets, and erythrocytes. Pancytopenia requires microscopic examination of a bone marrow biopsy specimen and a marrow aspirate to assess overall cellularity and morphology. There are 3 general categories of pancytopenia depending on the marrow findings.

Hypocellular marrow on biopsy is seen with inherited ("constitutional") marrow failure syndromes, acquired aplastic anemia of varied etiologies (see Chapter 469), the hypoplastic variant of myelodysplastic syndrome (MDS), and some cases of paroxysmal nocturnal hemoglobinuria with pancytopenia.

Cellular marrow is seen (a) with primary bone marrow disease, such as acute leukemia (see Chapter 494), and MDS, and (b) secondary to systemic disease, such as autoimmune disorders (systemic lupus erythematosus; Chapter 158), vitamin B_{12} or folate deficiency (see Chapters 49.6 and 49.7), storage disease (Gaucher and Niemann-Pick diseases; see Chapter 86.4), overwhelming infection, sarcoidosis, and hypersplenism.

Bone marrow infiltration can cause pancytopenia in metastatic solid tumors, myelofibrosis, hemophagocytic lymphohistiocytosis (see Chapter 507) and osteopetrosis (see Chapter 699).

Inherited ("constitutional") pancytopenia is defined as a decrease in marrow production of the 3 major hematopoietic lineages that occurs on an inherited basis, resulting in anemia, neutropenia, and thrombocytopenia. Any of these conditions (Tables 468-1 and 468-2) can be transmitted as a simple mendelian disorder by mutant genes with inherited patterns of autosomal dominant, autosomal recessive, or X-linked types. Modifying genes and acquired factors may also be operative. Inherited pancytopenias account for approximately 30% of cases of pediatric marrow failure. Fanconi anemia is the most common of these disorders.

FANCONI ANEMIA

Etiology and Epidemiology

Fanconi anemia (FA) is primarily inherited in an autosomal recessive manner (one uncommon form is X-linked recessive). It occurs in all racial and ethnic groups. At presentation, patients with FA may have: (1) typical physical anomalies and abnormal hematologic findings (majority of the patients); (2) normal physical features but abnormal hematologic findings (about one-third of patients); or (3) physical anomalies and normal hematologic findings (unknown percentage). There can be sibling discordance in clinical and hematologic findings, even in affected monozygotic twins. Approximately 75% of patients are 3-14 yr of age at the time of diagnosis.

Pathology

Patients have abnormal chromosome fragility, which is seen in metaphase preparations of peripheral blood lymphocytes cultured with phytohemagglutinin and enhanced by adding clastogenic agents such as diepoxybutane (DEB) and mitomycin C. Cell fusion of FA cells with normal cells or with cells from some unrelated patients with FA produces a corrective effect on chromosomal fragility, a process called *complementation*. This phenomenon allows subtyping of cases of FA into discrete complementation groups. Fifteen different complementation groups have been identified with different FA (*FANC*) genes that are mutated in each of them: A, B, C, D1/BRCA2, D2, E, F, G, I, J, L, M, N, O, P). An additional 2 genes, *XRCC2* and *ECCR4*, have been published and need further studies. After their discovery, the genes are prefixed with *FANC* (*FANCA*, *FANCB*, and so on). *FANCD1* is identical to the breast cancer susceptibility gene, *BRCA2*. The protein products of wild-type *FANC* genes are involved in the DNA damage recognition and repair biochemical pathways. Therefore, mutant gene proteins lead to genomic instability and chromosome fragility. An inability of FA cells to remove oxygen-free radicals, resulting in oxidative damage, is an additional mechanism that may contribute to the disease pathogenesis. Leukocyte telomere length is significantly shortened but telomerase activity is increased, suggesting a high proliferative rate of marrow progenitors that ultimately leads to their premature senescence. Increased marrow cell apoptosis occurs and is

Table 468-1	Inherited Pancytopenia Syndromes

Fanconi anemia
Shwachman-Diamond syndrome
Dyskeratosis congenita
Congenital amegakaryocytic thrombocytopenia
Reticular dysgenesis
Unclassified inherited bone marrow failure syndromes
Other genetic syndromes
  Down syndrome
  Dubowitz syndrome
  Seckel syndrome
  Schimke immunoosseous dysplasia
  Cartilage-hair hypoplasia
  Noonan syndrome

Table 468-2	Distinguishing Clinical Features of the Inherited Bone Marrow Failure Syndromes That May Be Initially Diagnosed in Adulthood

Distinguishing Features	DISEASES		
	Fanconi Anemia	Dyskeratosis Congenita	Schwachman-Diamond Anemia
History	Skeletal and renal malformations, low birthweight, pancytopenia, family member with bone marrow failure, MDS, acute myelogenous leukemia (AML), or squamous cell carcinoma at an early age; family member with Fanconi anemia	Intrauterine growth retardation, developmental delay, and short stature. Family history of MDS, AML, marrow failure, abnormal fingernails or toenails, leukoplakia, head and neck cancer, or pulmonary fibrosis	Pancreatic insufficiency, low birth weight, metaphyseal dysostosis, initial neutropenia, delayed development
Physical findings	Thumb and radial malformations, hyperpigmented skin lesions (café-au-lait spots), short stature, MDS, AML, squamous cell carcinoma at young age, renal and cardiac malformations, microcephaly, hypogonadism	Lacy reticular pigmentation of skin, dystrophic fingernails and toenails, premature graying of hair, hair loss, short stature, oral leukoplakia, squamous cell cancer of head and neck, pulmonary fibrosis, osteopenia, hypogonadism	Short stature, abnormal thorax
Genes inactivated	*FANCA, FANCB, FANCC, FANCD1 (aka BRCA2), FANCD2, FANCE, FANCF, FANCG (aka XRCC9), FANCI, FANCJ (aka BACH1 and BRIP1), FANCL (aka PHF9 and POG), FANCM (aka Hef), and FANCN (aka PALB2)*. These genes encode proteins known to protect the genome from excessive damage induced by chemical crosslinking agents. These genes account for most cases of Fanconi anemia	*DKC1, TERC, TERT, TINF2, NOLA2,* and *NOLA3*. These genes encode proteins known to participate in maintenance of telomeres. They account for only half of dyskeratosis cases, so there are additional genes to be discovered	*SBDS* autosomal recessive marrow clonal expansion in ~15%
Screening and diagnostic tests	1. Chromosomal breakage test (in response to mitomycin C or diepoxybutane) 2. Complementation analysis (flow cytometric analysis of G_2 arrest in melphalan-exposed cells after transduction with retroviral vectors expressing normal Fanconi anemia genes) 3. Gene sequencing	1. Quantitative analysis of telomere length ("flow FISH") 2. Gene sequencing	CT demonstrates fatty infiltration of pancreas Gene testing May evolve to myelodysplasia or leukemia Absence of pancreatic lipomatosis, fecal fat, or dysostosis does not rule out diagnosis

ADA, adenosine deaminase; FISH, fluorescent in situ hybridization.

Modified from Bagby GC: Aplastic anemia and related bone marrow failure states. In Goldman L, Schafer AI, editors, Goldman's Cecil medicine, *ed 24, Philadelphia, 2012, WB Saunders, Table 168-3, p. 1086.*

mediated by Fas, a membrane glycoprotein receptor containing an integral death domain. A consistent finding is diminished cellular interleukin-6 production along with markedly heightened tumor necrosis factor-α generation.

Clinical Manifestations

The most common anomaly in FA is hyperpigmentation of the trunk, neck, and intertriginous areas, as well as café-au-lait spots and vitiligo, alone or in combination (Fig. 468-1 and Table 468-3). Half the patients have short stature. In some patients, growth failure is aggravated by abnormal growth hormone secretion or with hypothyroidism. Absence of radii and thumbs that are hypoplastic, supernumerary, bifid, or absent are common. The "r" radial pulse may be weak or absent. Anomalies of the feet, congenital hip dislocation, and leg abnormalities are seen. A male patient with FA may have an underdeveloped penis; undescended, atrophic, or absence of the testes; and hypospadias or phimosis. Females can have malformations of the vagina, uterus, and ovary. Many patients have a FA "facies," including microcephaly, small eyes, epicanthal folds, and abnormal shape, size, or positioning of the ears (Fig. 468-1). Ectopic, pelvic, or horseshoe kidneys are detected by imaging and may show other organs as duplicated, hypoplastic, dysplastic, or absent kidneys. Cardiovascular and gastrointestinal malformations also occur. Approximately 10% of patients with FA are cognitively delayed.

Table 468-3	Characteristic Physical Anomalies in Fanconi Anemia	
ANOMALY		**APPROXIMATE FREQUENCY (% OF PATIENTS)**
Skin pigment changes ± café-au-lait spots		55
Short stature		51
Upper limb abnormalities (thumbs, hands, radii, ulnas)		43
Hypogonadal and genital changes (mostly male)		35
Other skeletal findings (head/face, neck, spine)		30
Eye/lid/epicanthal fold anomalies		23
Renal malformations		21
Gastrointestinal/cardiopulmonary malformations		11
Hip, leg, foot, toe abnormalities		10
Ear anomalies (external and internal), deafness		9

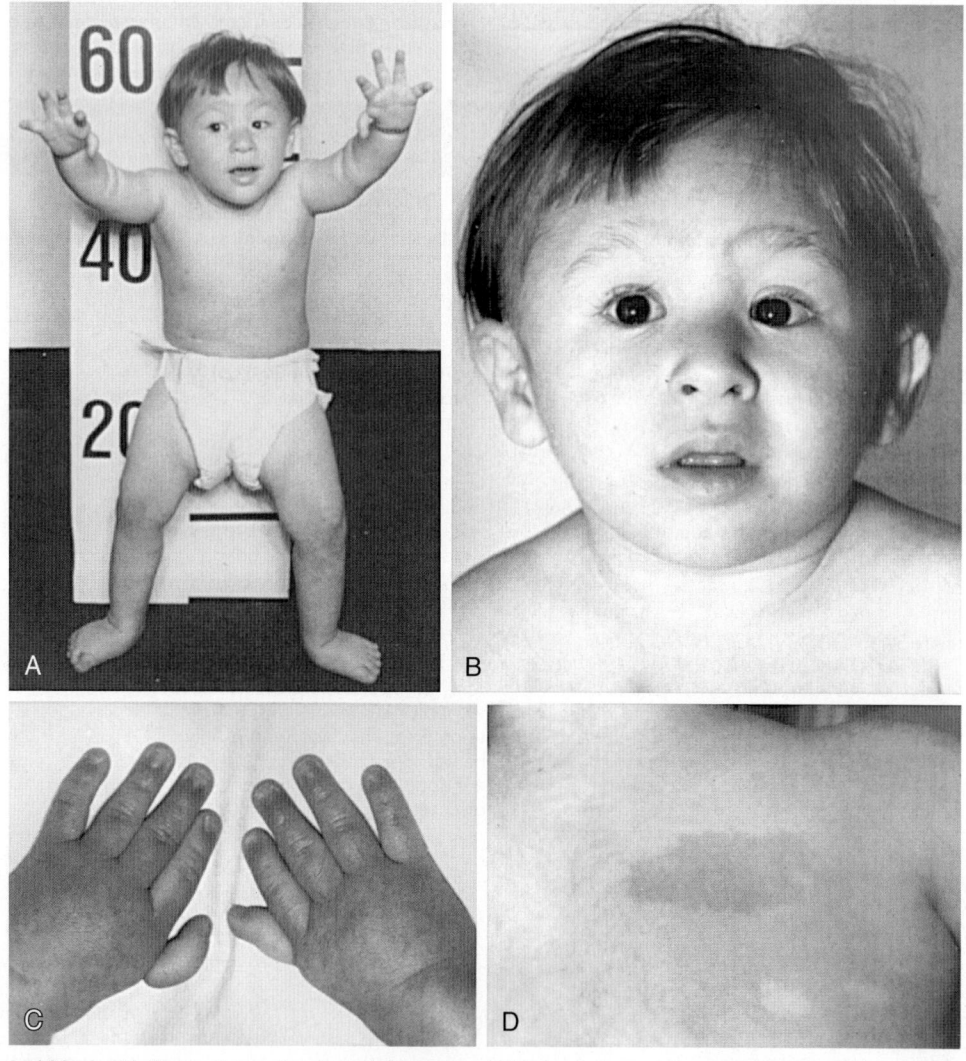

Figure 468-1 A 3 yr old boy with Fanconi anemia who exhibits several classic phenotype features. **A,** Front view. **B,** Face. **C,** Hands. **D,** Back right shoulder. The features to be noted include short stature, dislocated hips, microcephaly, a broad nasal base, epicanthal folds, micrognathia, thumbs attached by a thread, and café-au-lait spots with hypopigmented areas beneath. *(From Nathan DC, Orkin SH, Ginsburg D, et al, editors: Nathan and Oski's hematology of infancy and childhood, ed 6, vol I, Philadelphia, 2003, WB Saunders, p. 285.)*

Laboratory Findings

Marrow failure usually ensues in the 1st decade of life. Thrombocytopenia and red blood cell macrocytosis often appears initially, with subsequent onset of granulocytopenia and then anemia. Severe aplasia develops in most cases, but its full expression is variable and evolves over a period of months to years. The marrow becomes progressively hypocellular and fatty, like that in severe acquired aplastic anemia. Chromosome fragility is indicated by spontaneously occurring chromatid breaks, rearrangements, gaps, endoreduplications, and chromatid exchanges in blood lymphocytes cultured with phytohemagglutinin as well as in cultured skin fibroblasts, underscoring the constitutional nature of the disorder. With addition of DEB or mitomycin C, fragility is strikingly enhanced in lymphocyte cultures of patients with FA in comparison with those of controls. For prenatal diagnosis, abnormal chromosome breakage analysis and genetic testing can be performed in amniotic fluid cells or in tissue from a chorionic villus biopsy.

Complications

In addition to the low blood counts and physical anomalies, a major feature of the phenotype of FA is the propensity for cancer. The most frequent solid tumors are squamous cell carcinomas of the head, neck, and upper esophagus, followed by carcinomas of the vulva and/or anus, cervix, and lower esophagus. Human papilloma virus is suspected in the pathogenesis. Some patients experience oral cancer after bone marrow transplantation; it is unclear whether this treatment has an effect on the incidence. Benign and malignant liver tumors occur (adenomas, hepatomas) are usually associated with androgen therapy for aplastic anemia. Androgens are also implicated in the etiology of peliosis hepatis (blood-filled hepatic sinusoids). Peliosis hepatis is reversible when androgen therapy is discontinued, and tumors may regress. Clonal marrow cytogenetic abnormalities are common in FA, and at follow-up can either be stable, intermittently detected, or progressive and develop to advanced MDS and acute myelogenous leukemia. Approximately 15% of patients with FA are at risk for acute leukemia by the age of 35 yr.

Diagnosis

FA should be considered in all children and young adults with unexplained cytopenias. Abnormal hematologic findings and characteristic physical anomalies suggest the diagnosis, which is confirmed with a lymphocyte chromosomal breakage study using DEB. No other inherited pancytopenia is associated with a prominent in vitro hypersensitivity to DEB or mitomycin C by the chromosomal breakage study. Ten percent to 15% of patients with suspected FA have "somatic mosaicism" and their lymphocytes may not show characteristic high level of chromosomal fragility because of mixed populations of somatic cells, some with 2 abnormal alleles and some with 1 (caused by spontaneous somatic gene correction in a portion of the cells). Testing of skin fibroblasts instead of lymphocytes confirms the diagnosis.

Most patients have stable elevations of serum α-fetoprotein expressed constitutively, independent of liver complications or androgen therapy. Because of its low specificity compared to the chromosomal fragility and molecular tests the laboratory measurement of serum α-fetoprotein has not been widely used as a screening test.

As a result of the large number of *FANC* genes, genetic diagnosis has traditionally been commenced with complementation testing. This is done by determining whether cellular hypersensitivity to crosslinking agents (e.g., mitomycin C or radiation) or immunoblotting for *FANCD2* is restored after generating hybridoma of the patient cells with known genetic complementation cells or after transducing the cells with a known *FANC* gene. The mutant gene or the complementation group is deduced when a specific wild-type *FANC* gene corrects the abnormal chromosome fragility.

Treatment

A hematologist and a multidisciplinary team should supervise patients with FA. If the hematologic findings are stable and there are no transfusion requirements, observation is indicated. Subspecialty consultations for anomalies and disabilities can be arranged during this interval. If growth velocity is below expectations, endocrine evaluation is needed to identify growth hormone deficiency or hypothyroidism. Screening for glucose intolerance and hyperinsulinemia should be performed annually or biannually, depending on the degree of hyperglycemia found on initial testing. Blood counts should be performed every 1-3 mo; bone marrow aspiration and biopsy are indicated annually for leukemia and MDS surveillance by means of morphology and cytogenetics. Patients should be assessed for solid tumors at least annually. Beginning at menarche, female patients should be screened annually for gynecologic cancer. Administration of human papilloma virus quadrivalent vaccine to prevent squamous cell carcinoma is currently advised.

Hematopoietic stem cell transplantation (HSCT; see Chapter 135) is the only curative therapy for the hematologic abnormalities. Patients <10 yr old with FA who undergo transplantation using an human leukocyte antigen (HLA)–identical sibling donor have a survival rate >80%. Survival rates are lower for patients >10 yr old who are undergoing the procedure. Preparative regimens are continuously evaluated, refined, and improved worldwide. For patients who do not have an HLA–matched sibling donor, a search for a matched unrelated donor (including a search of umbilical cord blood banks) might be initiated. Because of the need for more intensive preparation regimen and the heightened graft-versus-host response in patients with FA, the survival and cure rates have not been as good as those for matched sibling donor HSCT (≈50% survival). Molecular technology has led to preimplantation genetic diagnosis on parent-derived blastomeres to find an HLA-matched sibling donor without FA.

Androgens produce a response in 50% of patients, heralded by reticulocytosis and a rise in hemoglobin within 1-2 mo. White blood cell counts may increase next, followed by platelet counts, but it may take many months to achieve the maximum response. When the response plateaus, androgen dosage can be slowly tapered but not stopped entirely. Oral oxymetholone is used most frequently once a day. The beneficial effect of adding low-dose prednisone to androgens is controversial, but when administered orally every second day, they may counter androgen-induced growth acceleration and prevent thrombocytopenic bleeding by promoting vascular stability. In many patients who are taking androgens, the disease becomes refractory as marrow failure progresses. Potential side effects include masculinization, elevated hepatic enzymes, cholestasis, peliosis hepatis, and liver tumors. Screening for these changes should be performed serially.

The potential for recombinant growth factor (cytokine) therapy for FA has not been defined. Granulocyte colony-stimulating factor (G-CSF) can usually induce an increase in the absolute neutrophil count and occasionally may boost platelet counts and hemoglobin levels. There may be a heightened risk of expansion of marrow cells with clonal cytogenetic abnormalities such as monosomy 7. Combination therapy consisting of G-CSF given subcutaneously daily or every 2 days along with erythropoietin given subcutaneously or IV 3 times/wk results in improved neutrophil counts in almost all patients and a sustained rise in platelets and hemoglobin levels in approximately one-third of patients, although most patients lose the response after 1 yr owing to progression of marrow failure.

The premise for gene therapy in FA is based on the assumption that corrected hematopoietic cells offer a growth advantage. Attempts at gene therapy have been disappointing, possibly because of the type of vector but also because of the chromosomal fragility and impaired proliferative function of the hematopoietic progenitors. Encouraging preclinical data from studies using lentiviral vectors offer hope that gene therapy will be a safe and effective treatment for FA.

Prognosis

From FA cases reported in the 1990s, the projected median survival was >30 yr of age, an improvement over that in the previous decade. Successes with HSCT have dramatically improved the outlook. Careful surveillance for known complications, especially cancer, and prompt intervention on their detection has also contributed to the improved survival.

SHWACHMAN-DIAMOND SYNDROME
Etiology and Epidemiology

Shwachman-Diamond syndrome (SDS) is inherited in an autosomal recessive manner; it occurs in all racial and ethnic groups. As FA, SDS is also a multisystem disorder. The nonhematologic manifestations are different and usually include exocrine pancreatic insufficiency and skeletal abnormalities such as metaphyseal dysplasia. There is no increased chromosomal breakage after DEB testing of SDS lymphocytes.

Pathology

The mutant gene *SBDS* maps to chromosome 7q11 and in 90% of cases is responsible for the multisystem, pleiotropic phenotype. The wild-type gene protein product is involved in ribosomal biogenesis. Pancreatic insufficiency is a result of failure of pancreatic acinar development. Fatty replacement of pancreatic tissue is prominent. Bone marrow failure is characterized by dysfunctional hematopoietic stem cells, accelerated apoptosis of marrow progenitors and a defective marrow microenvironment that does not support and maintain normal hematopoiesis.

Clinical Manifestations

Most patients with SDS have symptoms of fat malabsorption from birth that are caused by pancreatic insufficiency, but steatorrhea is not always obvious. Approximately 50% of patients appear to exhibit an improvement in pancreatic enzyme secretion as they age. The clinical picture can be dominated by complications from anemia, neutropenia, or thrombocytopenia. Bacterial and fungal infections secondary to neutropenia, neutrophil dysfunction, and immune deficiency can occur. Short stature is a consistent feature of the syndrome; most patients show normal growth velocity yet remain consistently below the 3rd percentile for height and weight. The occasional SDS adult achieves the 25th percentile for height. Although skeletal abnormalities are variable, classic findings are delayed bone maturation, metaphyseal dysplasia, short or flared ribs, and thoracic dystrophy. Some patients have hepatomegaly and elevations of liver enzymes. Most patients have dental abnormalities and poor oral health. Many have neurocognitive problems and poor social skills.

Laboratory Findings

Fatty replacement of pancreatic tissue can be visualized by CT scan or ultrasound. Fat malabsorption is proven by assay on a 72-hr stool collection. Pancreatic function tests show markedly impaired enzyme secretion, but with preservation of ductal function. Age-adjusted serum trypsinogen and isoamylase levels are reduced. Neutropenia is present in 100% of patients with SDS on at least 1 occasion. It can be chronic persistent or intermittent. It has been identified in some neonates during an episode of sepsis. Neutrophils may have a defect in mobility, migration, and chemotaxis owing to alterations in neutrophil cytoskeletal or microtubular function. Anemia, thrombocytopenia, and pancytopenia are seen in 66%, 60%, and up to 44% of cases, respectively. Pancytopenia can be severe as a result of full-blown aplastic anemia. Bone marrow biopsy specimens and aspirates usually show varying degrees of marrow hypoplasia and fat infiltration. Patients may also have B-cell defects with 1 or more of the following: low immunoglobulin G or immunoglobulin G subclasses, low percentage of circulating B lymphocytes, decreased in vitro B-cell proliferation, and lack of specific antibody production. Patients may have a low percentage of circulating T cells, subsets, or natural killer cells, and decreased in vitro T-cell proliferation.

Diagnosis

The clinical diagnosis of SDS relies on having an evidence of bone marrow dysfunction and exocrine pancreatic dysfunction. However, up to 20% of the patients may lack clear evidence of exocrine pancreatic defects at the time of diagnosis. Mutational analysis for *SBDS* is definitive in 90% of cases. Pearson syndrome (see Chapter 450), consisting of refractory sideroblastic anemia, cytoplasmic vacuolization of bone marrow precursors, lactic acidosis, exocrine pancreatic insufficiency, and a diagnostic mitochondrial DNA mutation is similar to SDS, but the clinical course, morphologic features of the bone marrow, and gene mutation are different. Also, severe anemia requiring transfusion, rather than neutropenia, is present from birth to 1 yr of age. SDS shares some manifestations with FA, such as marrow dysfunction and growth failure, but patients with SDS are readily distinguished because of pancreatic insufficiency with fat malabsorption, fatty changes within the pancreatic body that can be visualized by imaging, characteristic skeletal abnormalities not seen in FA, and a normal chromosomal breakage study with DEB.

Complications

Patients with SDS are predisposed to MDS and leukemic transformation. The crude rate of MDS or acute leukemia in patients with SDS is 8-33%. Marrow cell clonal cytogenetic abnormalities are an isolated finding, occurring in up to 41% of patients. Isochromosome 7 [i(7q)] is particularly common, suggesting that it is a fairly specific clonal marker of SDS and probably related to the presence of mutant *SBDS* on 7q11. Other clonal chromosome abnormalities include monosomy 7, i(7q) combined with monosomy 7, deletions or translocations involving part of 7q, and deletions of 20q [Del(20q)]. Although i(7q) and Del(20q) are rarely related to leukemic transformation or MDS, the prognostic significance of all marrow clonal changes requires prospective monitoring.

Treatment

Fat malabsorption responds to oral pancreatic enzyme replacement and supplemental fat-soluble vitamins, administered according to guidelines similar to those for cystic fibrosis (see Chapter 403). A long-term plan should be initiated to monitor changes in peripheral blood counts that require corrective action and to look for early evidence of malignant myeloid transformation. The latter requires serial bone marrow aspirations for smears and cytogenetics and marrow biopsy. One recommendation is to perform marrow testing every 1-2 yr and complete blood counts every 3 mo.

Daily subcutaneous G-CSF for profound neutropenia is effective in inducing a sustained increase in neutrophils. Some patients require transfusion support for management of severe anemia or thrombocytopenia. Experience with erythropoietin is limited. In some patients who received androgens plus steroids, blood counts have improved. The only curative option for severe marrow failure in SDS is allogeneic HSCT, although experience has been limited. Traditional myeloblastic HSCT resulted in treatment-related mortality in 35-50% of the patients. The risk of cardiotoxicity has been noted. Fludarabine-based protocols using reduced-intensity conditioning appear to be safer and effective for SDS HSCT.

Prognosis

The accurate life expectancy of SDS patients is unknown. Analysis of published cases revealed a median survival of 35 yr. Because the number of undiagnosed patients with mild or asymptomatic disease is unknown, the overall prognosis may be better than previously thought. Approximately 50% of patients experience spontaneous conversion from pancreatic insufficiency to pancreatic sufficiency as a result of improvement in pancreatic enzyme secretion. Enzyme replacement therapy is then no longer needed. Although all patients have some degree of hematologic cytopenia, the changes in most patients are mild to moderate and do not require therapeutic intervention. Severe neutropenia responds well to G-CSF, but there is concern that the predisposition to MDS and acute leukemia can be heightened by the agent's powerful growth stimulus on marrow cells. HSCT for severe marrow failure has produced a 50-70% survival rate, but safer protocols are being introduced. Malignant marrow transformation remains ominous.

DYSKERATOSIS CONGENITA
Etiology and Epidemiology

Dyskeratosis congenita (DC) is an inherited multisystem disorder characterized by mucocutaneous abnormalities, bone marrow failure,

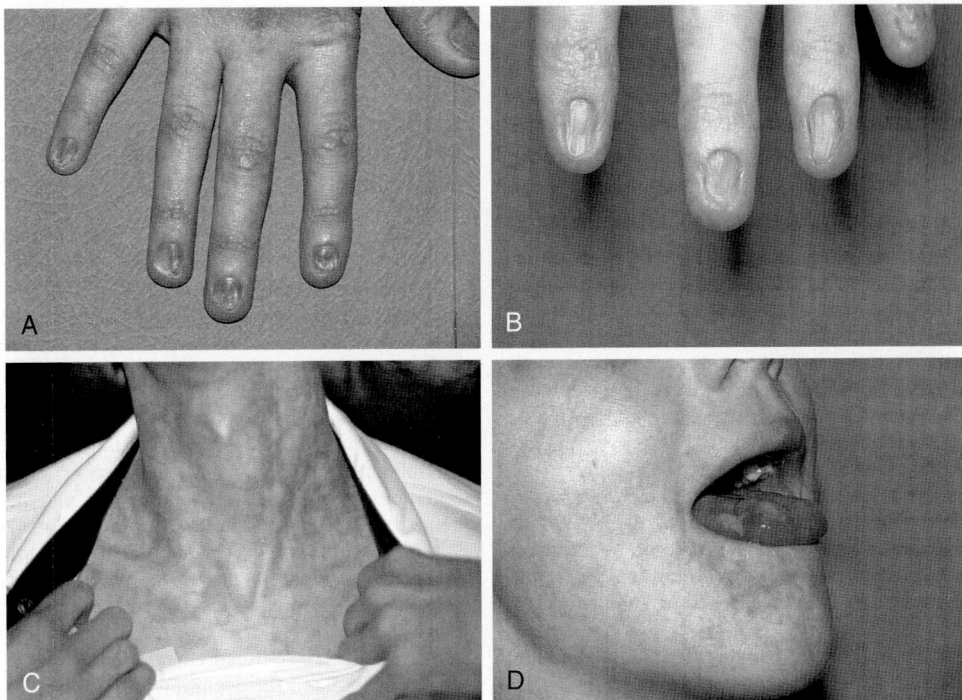

Figure 468-2 Physical findings in patients with dyskeratosis congenita. **A** and **B,** Dystrophic fingernails in 2 different patients. **C,** Lacy reticular pigmentation. **D,** Leukoplakia on the tongue. *(From Nathan DG, Orkin SH, Ginsburg D, et al, editors: Nathan and Oski's hematology of infancy and childhood, ed 6, vol I, Philadelphia, 2003, WB Saunders, p. 300.)*

and a predisposition to cancer and MDS. The diagnostic **mucocutaneous (ectodermal) triad** is reticulate skin pigmentation of the upper body, mucosal leukoplakia, and nail dystrophy (Fig. 468-2). Skin and nail findings usually become apparent in the 1st 10 yr of life, whereas oral leukoplakia is seen later. These manifestations tend to progress as patients get older. Varying degrees of bone marrow failure are seen in about 90% of the patients. Severe aplastic anemia occurs in approximately 50% of cases, usually in the 2nd decade of life. Many patients with DC are male, a finding compatible with the high frequency of the X-linked recessive form of the disease. The remainder have either an autosomal dominant or autosomal recessive mode of inheritance.

Pathology

DC is genetically heterogeneous, and patients have mutations in genes that encode components of the telomerase complex (*DKC1, TERT, TERC, NOP10,* and *NHP2*), T-loop disassembly protein (*RTEL1*), telomere capping (*CTC1*), the telomere shelterin complex (*TINF2*), and the telomerase trafficking protein (*TCAB1*), all components critical for telomere maintenance. The **X-linked recessive form** of DC maps to Xq28, and many mutations have been identified in the *DKC1* gene, which codes for the nuclear protein dyskerin. The **autosomal dominant form** is due to mutations in *TINF2,* or in *TERC* or *TERT,* the RNA and enzymatic components of telomerase, respectively. **Autosomal recessive** DC is linked to mutations in *NOP10, NHP2, RTEL1, TCAB1,* and *CTC1.* Because of impaired telomere maintenance in all 3 inherited forms of DC, short telomeres are demonstrated in the peripheral blood cells of all patients and are a cardinal marker for DC and for marrow failure. The failure is likely a result of progressive attrition and depletion of hematopoietic stem cells because of premature senescence, which manifests as pancytopenia.

Clinical Manifestations

Skin pigmentation and nail changes typically appear first, mucosal leukoplakia and excessive ocular tearing appear later, and by the mid-teens, patients with DC have bone marrow failure and malignancy. Many female patients have the same features as male patients. In males, cutaneous findings are the most consistent feature. Lacy reticulated

skin pigmentation affecting the face, neck, chest, and arms is a common finding (89%). The degree of pigmentation increases with age and can involve the entire skin surface. There may also be a telangiectatic erythematous component. Nail dystrophy of both hands and feet is the next most common finding (88%). It usually starts with longitudinal ridging, splitting, or pterygium formation and may progress to complete nail loss. Leukoplakia usually involves the oral mucosa (78%), especially the tongue but may also be seen in the conjunctiva and the anal, urethral, or genital mucosa. Hyperhidrosis of the palms and soles is common, and hair loss is sometimes seen. Eye abnormalities are observed in approximately 50% of cases. Excessive tearing (epiphora) secondary to nasolacrimal duct obstruction is common. Other ophthalmologic manifestations include conjunctivitis, blepharitis, loss of eyelashes, strabismus, cataracts, and optic atrophy. An increased rate of dental decay and early loss of teeth are common. Skeletal abnormalities, such as osteoporosis, avascular necrosis, abnormal bone trabeculation, scoliosis, and mandibular hypoplasia, are seen in approximately 20% of cases. Genitourinary abnormalities include hypoplastic testes, hypospadias, phimosis, urethral stenosis, and horseshoe kidney. Gastrointestinal findings, such as esophageal strictures, vascular lesions causing bleeding, hepatomegaly, and fibrosis are seen in 10% of cases. A subset of patients has pulmonary complications, with reduced diffusion capacity and/or a restrictive defect. In fatal cases, lung tissue shows pulmonary fibrosis and abnormalities of the pulmonary vasculature.

Laboratory Findings

The initial hematologic change in DC is usually thrombocytopenia, anemia, or both, followed by full-blown pancytopenia and aplastic anemia. The red cells are often macrocytic, and the fetal hemoglobin value can be elevated initially. Initial bone marrow specimens may be hypercellular, but with time, a symmetric depletion of all hematopoietic lineages ensues. Some patients have immunologic abnormalities, including reduced or elevated immunoglobulin values, decreased B- and/or T-lymphocyte count, and reduction of or absence of lymphocyte proliferative responses to phytohemagglutinin. This is particularly common and severe in the DKC1-associated disease. Primary skin fibroblasts in culture have abnormal morphologic features and doubling rate and show numerous unbalanced chromosome rearrangements, such as dicentrics, tricentrics, and translocations, in the absence of DEB. These findings provide evidence of a defect that predisposes patient cells to chromosomal rearrangements and possibly to DNA damage.

Diagnosis

The following abnormalities are seen in patients with DC but not in those with FA: nail dystrophy, leukoplakia, and tooth abnormalities, hyperhidrosis of the palms and soles, and hair loss (see Table 468-2). There are overlap syndromes that share some of the features of DC. **Hoyeraal-Hreidarsson syndrome** is a multisystem disorder comprising aplastic anemia, immunodeficiency, microcephaly, growth retardation, and cerebellar hypoplasia. The syndrome is genetically heterogeneous; some cases are X-linked recessive and caused by mutations in *DKC1*, and others are autosomal recessive owing to homozygous *TERT* mutations. **Revesz syndrome** consists of dystrophic nails, leukoplakia, aplastic anemia, cerebellar hypoplasia, growth retardation, microcephaly, and bilateral exudative retinopathy. *TINF2* is mutated in Revesz syndrome, which hence is an autosomal dominant variant of DC. Coats' plus syndrome is caused by mutations in the *CTC1* gene. It is characterized by retinal telangiectasia and exudates, intracranial calcification, leukodystrophy, brain cysts, osteopenia, gastrointestinal bleeding and portal hypertension caused by the development of vasculature ectasias in the stomach, small intestine and liver. Some patients with this disease has the additional manifestations of DC, which include sparse and graying hair, dystrophic nails, and anemia. Telomeres are short.

Complications

Cancer develops in approximately 10-15% of patients with DC, usually in the 3rd and 4th decades of life. Patients with DC are predisposed to MDS as well as to solid tumors. Forty percent of the cancers in such patients are squamous cell carcinomas of the head and neck (tongue, mouth, pharynx). Cancer of the skin and gastrointestinal tract (esophagus, stomach, colon, and especially the anorectal site) is also common. Other life-threatening complications include pulmonary fibrosis and severe gastrointestinal bleeding.

Treatment

Androgens (with or without low-dose prednisone) can induce improvement of marrow function in approximately 50% of patients. When the response is maximal, the androgen dose can be slowly tapered but not stopped. DC can become refractory to androgens as the aplastic anemia progresses. There is no published information on the use of immunosuppressive therapy for this disorder, but the authors are aware of several patients who were misdiagnosed with acquired aplastic anemia and treated with immunosuppressive therapy without response. Although reports are scanty, cytokine therapy with granulocyte-macrophage colony-stimulating factor or with G-CSF alone or combined with erythropoietin appears to offer potential benefit, at least in the short term, especially for improving neutrophil numbers.

Allogeneic HSCT has been used to correct marrow failure in patients with DC, long-term survival is only 50%. Vascular lesions and fibrosis involving various organs are not prevented by HSCT and can occur early and late after transplantation; carrying a high mortality rate. Patients with DC may be more susceptible to endothelial damage that occurs after HSCT as a result of various factors, including the conditioning regimen, infectious disease, and graft-versus-host disease. Up to 40% of patients with DC experience fatal pulmonary complications after transplantation.

Prognosis

Considerable heterogeneity exists in DC. Patients with certain genetic groups (e.g., *TERC* and *TERT*) have milder clinical manifestations. Patients with other genetic groups (e.g., *DKC1*, *TINF2* and *RTEL1*) appear to have more physical anomalies and a higher incidence of aplastic anemia and cancer. The mean age of death for patients with DC who are diagnosed in childhood is approximately 30 yr. The main causes of death are bone marrow failure, complications of HSCT, cancer, fatal pulmonary problems, and gastrointestinal bleeding.

CONGENITAL AMEGAKARYOCYTIC THROMBOCYTOPENIA
Etiology and Epidemiology

Congenital amegakaryocytic thrombocytopenia (CAMT) is the rarest of the 4 major inherited pancytopenias. It is transmitted in an autosomal recessive manner. CAMT manifests in infancy as isolated thrombocytopenia as a result of reduction of marrow megakaryocytes with initial preservation of granulopoietic and erythroid lineages. Pancytopenia caused by aplastic anemia often ensues in the first few years of life. The defect in CAMT is directly related to mutations in *MPL*, the gene for the receptor of thrombopoietin, the growth factor that promotes hematopoietic stem cell survival and stimulates megakaryocyte proliferation and maturation. Carriers of the mutant gene have normal hematology; affected individuals have mutations in both alleles. Genotype–phenotype correlations predict disease course and prognosis. **Nonsense mutations** cause a complete loss of function of the thrombopoietin receptor, causing persistently low platelet counts because of the absence of megakaryocytes and a fast progression to pancytopenia and aplastic anemia (CAMT type I). Because thrombopoietin also has an antiapoptotic and cell survival effect on stem cells, impaired stem cell survival with *MPL* nonsense mutations explains the evolution of CAMT into aplastic anemia. **Missense mutations** of *MPL* are associated with a milder course, a transient increase in platelets during the 1st yr of life, and delayed onset, if any, of pancytopenia, indicating residual receptor function (CAMT type II). Biologically active plasma thrombopoietin is consistently elevated in all patients with CAMT.

Clinical Manifestations

Patients with CAMT have petechial rash, bruising, or bleeding at birth or in the 1st yr of life. Most, but not all, patients with proven *MPL* mutations have normal physical and imaging features. Approximately 20% of published phenotypic CAMT cases involved physical anomalies, but *MPL* mutation analyses were not available in all cases. The most common anomalies in the published cases are neurologic and cardiac. Findings related to cerebellar and cerebral atrophy are frequent, and developmental delay is a prominent feature. Congenital heart disease includes atrial septal defects, ventricular septal defects, patent ductus arteriosus, tetralogy of Fallot, and coarctation of the aorta. Some of these occur in combinations. Other anomalies include abnormal hips or feet, kidney malformations, eye anomalies, and cleft or high-arched palate. Some patients have microcephaly and an abnormal facies.

Laboratory Findings

Thrombocytopenia is the major laboratory finding in CAMT, with normal hemoglobin levels and white blood cell counts initially. Peripheral blood platelets are reduced or totally absent. As in other inherited bone marrow failure syndromes, red blood cells may be macrocytic. Hemoglobin F may be elevated, and there may be increased expression of i antigen. Initial bone marrow aspirates and biopsy specimens show normal cellularity with marked reduction or absence of megakaryocytes. In patients in whom aplastic anemia develops, marrow cellularity is decreased, with fatty replacement; erythropoietic and granulopoietic lineages are also symmetrically reduced.

Diagnosis

If thrombocytopenia persists beyond the neonatal period or is associated with adequate platelet transfusion response and no obvious precipitating cause such as infections or immunologic reactions, a marrow aspirate and biopsy is indicated. Deficient megakaryocytes in such cases suggest the diagnosis, and mutational analysis will confirm it. If CAMT occurs at birth or shortly after, it must be distinguished from other causes of inherited and acquired neonatal thrombocytopenia (see Chapter 484.8). Thrombocytopenia with absent radii (TAR syndrome) is distinguished from CAMT because in TAR syndrome the radii are absent. The distinction from DC may be evident by mucocutaneous, neurologic, and immunologic findings that are characteristic to the early onset DC. CAMT blood lymphocytes do not show increased chromosomal breakage when exposed to DEB, distinguishing the disease it from FA.

Complications
In some patients, clonal marrow cell cytogenetic abnormalities appear such as monosomy 7 and trisomy 8. CAMT can evolve into MDS and also acute leukemia, but the true risk cannot be defined because of the rarity of the disease and the paucity of published data.

Therapy and Prognosis
The mortality rate in patients with *MPL* **nonsense** mutations from thrombocytopenic bleeding, complications of aplastic anemia, or leukemic transformation has been very close to 100%. Patients with **missense** mutations have a milder course but may still have serious complications. HSCT is the only curative option. The majority of patients with CAMT who undergo HSCT are cured, especially if the procedure is performed with HLA-matched sibling donors. Before transplantation, platelet transfusion should be used discretely. Platelet count should not always be the sole indication; clinical bleeding is an appropriate trigger. Single-donor filtered platelets are preferred to minimize sensitization. Leukodepleted platelet units might be adequate, but further studies are necessary to support such an alternative. In a patient for whom HSCT is a possibility, all blood products should be free of cytomegalovirus. Corticosteroids are not effective for treatment of the thrombocytopenia. For aplastic anemia, androgens may induce a temporary partial improvement. Interleukin-3 may be an important adjunct to the medical management of CAMT, but it was not adopted broadly and is no longer available. The role of thrombomimetic agents has to be studied; however, the induction of fibrosis by these agents and the risk of MDS/leukemia in CAMT render HSCT the preferred treatment for patients with severe cytopenia.

OTHER INHERITED SYNDROMES
Pancytopenia and bone marrow failure can occur in the context of several non-hematologic syndromes and familial settings that do not exactly correspond to the entities already described.

Down Syndrome
Down syndrome (trisomy 21; see Chapter 81.2) has a unique association with aberrant hematologic findings. In addition to the propensity for acute lymphoblastic and myeloblastic leukemias, especially acute megakaryoblastic leukemia, at least 6 patients with Down syndrome have been reported as having pancytopenia caused by aplastic anemia.

Dubowitz Syndrome
Dubowitz syndrome is an autosomal recessive disorder characterized by a peculiar facies, infantile eczema, small stature, and mild microcephaly. The face is small, with a shallow supraorbital ridge, a nasal bridge at the same level as the forehead, short palpebral fissures, variable ptosis, and micrognathia. There is a predilection to cancer as well as to bone marrow dysfunction in these patients. Approximately 10% of patients have hematopoietic disorders including moderate pancytopenia, hypoplastic anemia, bone marrow hypoplasia, and full-blown aplastic anemia. No gene mutation has been identified.

Seckel Syndrome
Seckel (SCKL) syndrome, sometimes called "bird-headed dwarfism," is an autosomal recessive developmental disorder characterized by marked growth failure and mental deficiency, microcephaly, a hypoplastic face with a prominent nose, and low-set and/or malformed ears. Approximately 25% of patients have aplastic anemia or malignancies. There is broad genetic heterogeneity comprising 7 classifiable types: SCKL1, *ATR* mutation; SCKL2, *RBBP8* mutation; SCKL3, maps to 14q21-q22; SCKL4, *CENPJ* mutation; SCKL5, *CEP152* mutation; SCKL6, *CEP63* mutation; and, SCKL7, *NIN* mutation.

Reticular Dysgenesis
Reticular dysgenesis (see Chapter 126) is an immunologic deficiency syndrome coupled with congenital agranulocytosis. The mode of inheritance autosomal recessive in some cases; there is evidence that reticular dysgenesis is caused by homozygous or compound heterozygous mutation in the mitochondrial adenylate kinase-2 gene *AK2* on chromosome 1p35 but an X-linked mode is also possible in some cases. The disorder is a variant of severe combined immune deficiency in which cellular and humoral immunity are absent and severe lymphopenia and neutropenia are also seen. Anemia and thrombocytopenia may also be present. Bone marrow specimens are hypocellular, with markedly reduced myeloid and lymphoid elements. The only curative therapy is HSCT.

Schimke Immunoosseous Dysplasia
Schimke immunoosseous dysplasia is an autosomal recessive disorder caused by mutations in the chromatin remodeling protein *SMARCAL1*. Patients have spondyloepiphyseal dysplasia with exaggerated lumbar lordosis and a protruding abdomen. There are pigmentary skin changes and abnormally discolored and configured teeth. Renal dysfunction can be problematic, with proteinuria and nephrotic syndrome. Approximately 50% of patients have hypothyroidism, 50% have cerebral ischemia, and 10% have bone marrow failure with neutropenia, thrombocytopenia, and anemia, and about 5% are predisposed to non-Hodgkin lymphoma. Lymphopenia and altered cellular immunity are present in almost all patients. In 2 published case reports, 2 patients underwent successful bone marrow transplantation.

Noonan Syndrome
Noonan syndrome is a developmental disorder characterized by the "Noonan facies" (hypertelorism, ptosis, short neck, low-set ears), short stature, congenital heart disease, and multiple skeletal and hematologic abnormalities. It is primarily an autosomal dominant disorder composed of at least 7 genetic types. Heterozygous mutations in *PTPN11* cause approximately 50% of cases of the syndrome; others are caused by mutations in *NF1, KRAS, SOS1, RAF1, NRAS,* or *BRAF*. Autosomal recessive forms have also been identified due to a mutation of *SHOC2* or of *CBL*. In addition to an association with juvenile myelomonocytic leukemia, Noonan syndrome patients can develop amegakaryocytic thrombocytopenia as well as pancytopenia with a hypocellular marrow.

Cartilage-Hair Hypoplasia
Cartilage-hair hypoplasia, an autosomal recessive syndrome seen mostly in Finnish or Amish populations, is characterized by metaphyseal dysostosis, short-limbed dwarfism, and fine, sparse hair. Additional skeletal findings are scoliosis, lordosis, chest deformity, and varus lower limbs. Gastrointestinal abnormalities also occur. Mutations in the *RMRP* gene cause cartilage-hair hypoplasia. Macrocytic anemia is seen in most patients and is sometimes severe and persistent. Neutropenia, lymphopenia, and a predisposition to lymphoma and other cancers are also features.

UNCLASSIFIED INHERITED BONE MARROW FAILURE SYNDROMES
Unclassified inherited bone marrow failure syndromes are heterogeneous disorders that may be either atypical presentations of identifiable diseases or new syndromes. Characterized by various cytopenias because of underproductive bone marrow with or without physical manifestations, they do not fit into a classic genetic bone marrow failure disease because all features may not be evident at the time of presentation. Compared with classic disorders (presentation ≈1 mo of age), infants with unclassified disorders present later (≈9 mo) and manifest single or multilineage cytopenia, aplastic anemia, myelodysplasia, or malignancy with variable expression of malformations. Table 468-4 lists the criteria for the diagnosis. With follow-up, some may demonstrate typical physical features of known syndromes, such as SDS, although without obvious mutations in the *SBDS* gene.

Table 468-4	Canadian Inherited Marrow Failure Registry Criteria for Unclassified Inherited Bone Marrow Failure Syndromes

FULFILLS CRITERIA 1 AND 2:
1. Does not fulfill criteria for any categorized inherited bone marrow failure syndrome*
2. Fulfills both of the following

FULFILLS AT LEAST 2 OF THE FOLLOWING:
a. Chronic cytopenia(s) detected on at least 2 occasions over at least 3 mo[†]
b. Reduced marrow progenitors or reduced clonogenic potential of hematopoietic progenitor cells or evidence of ineffective hematopoiesis[‡]
c. High fetal hemoglobin for age[‡]
d. Red blood cell macrocytosis (not caused by hemolysis or a nutritional deficiency)

FULFILLS AT LEAST 1 OF THE FOLLOWING:
a. Family history of bone marrow failure
b. Presentation at age <1 yr
c. Anomalies involving multiple systems to suggest an inherited syndrome

*The Canadian Inherited Marrow Failure Registry diagnostic guidelines for selected syndromes were adapted from the literature and are available at http://www.sickkids.ca/cimfr.
[†]Cytopenia was defined as follows: neutropenia, neutrophil count of <1.5 × 10⁹/L; thrombocytopenia, platelet count of <150 × 10⁹/L; anemia, hemoglobin concentration of <2 standard deviations below mean, adjusted for age.
[‡]Hemoglobinopathies with ineffective erythropoiesis and high hemoglobin F should be excluded by clinical or laboratory testing.

Familial cases with aplastic anemia that cannot be readily classified into discrete diagnostic entities such as FA have been reported. When the patients present not early after birth and without physical malformations an acquired etiology cannot be ruled out. Detailed genetic testing for known inherited bone marrow failure syndrome genes or by whole exome or genome sequencing may identify an inherited etiology.

Bibliography is available at Expert Consult.

Chapter 469
The Acquired Pancytopenias
Jeffrey D. Hord

ETIOLOGY AND EPIDEMIOLOGY
Drugs, chemicals, toxins, infectious agents, radiation, and immune disorders can result in pancytopenia by direct destruction of hematopoietic progenitors, disruption of the marrow microenvironment, or immune-mediated suppression of marrow elements (Table 469-1). A careful history of exposure to known risk factors should be obtained for every child presenting with pancytopenia. Even in the absence of the classic associated physical findings, the possibility of a genetic predisposition to bone marrow failure should always be considered (see Chapter 468). The majority of cases of acquired marrow failure in childhood are "idiopathic," in that no causative agent is identified. Many are probably immune-mediated through activated T lymphocytes and cytokine destruction of marrow progenitor cells. The overall

Table 469-1	Etiology of Acquired Aplastic Anemia

Radiation, drugs, and chemicals:
  Predictable: chemotherapy, benzene
  Idiosyncratic: chloramphenicol, antiepileptics, gold; 3,4-methylenedioxymethamphetamine
Viruses:
  Cytomegalovirus
  Epstein-Barr
  Hepatitis B
  Hepatitis C
  Hepatitis non-A, non-B, non-C (seronegative hepatitis)
  HIV
Immune diseases:
  Eosinophilic fasciitis
  Hypoimmunoglobulinemia
  Thymoma
Pregnancy
Paroxysmal nocturnal hemoglobinuria
Marrow replacement:
  Leukemia
  Myelodysplasia
  Myelofibrosis
Autoimmune
Other:
  Cryptic dyskeratosis congenita (no physical stigmata)
  Telomerase reverse transcriptase haploinsufficiency

incidence of acquired aplastic anemia is relatively low, with an approximate incidence in both children and adults in the United States and Europe of 2-6 cases/million population/yr. The incidence is higher in Asia, with as many as 14 cases/million population/yr in Japan.

Severe bone marrow suppression can develop after exposure to many different drugs and chemicals, including certain chemotherapeutic agents, insecticides, antibiotics, anticonvulsants, nonsteroidal antiinflammatory agents, and recreational drugs. Some of the most notable agents are benzene, chloramphenicol, gold, and, 3,4,-methylenedioxymethamphetamine (Ecstasy).

A number of viruses can either directly or indirectly result in bone marrow failure. Parvovirus B19 is classically associated with isolated red blood cell aplasia, but in patients with sickle cell disease or immunodeficiency, it can result in transient pancytopenia (see Chapter 251). Prolonged pancytopenia can occur after infection with many of the hepatitis viruses, herpes viruses, Epstein-Barr virus (see Chapter 254), cytomegalovirus (see Chapter 255), and HIV (see Chapter 276).

Patients with evidence of bone marrow failure should also be evaluated for inherited forms of marrow failure, paroxysmal nocturnal hemoglobinuria (PNH; see Chapter 464), and collagen vascular diseases. Pancytopenia without peripheral blasts may be caused by bone marrow replacement by leukemic blasts or neuroblastoma cells.

PATHOLOGY AND PATHOGENESIS
The hallmark of aplastic anemia is peripheral pancytopenia, coupled with hypoplastic or aplastic bone marrow. The severity of the clinical course is related to the degree of myelosuppression. **Severe aplastic anemia** is defined as a condition in which 2 or more cell components have become seriously compromised (absolute neutrophil count <500/mm³, platelet count <20,000/mm³, reticulocyte count <1% after correction for hematocrit) in a patient whose bone marrow biopsy material is moderately or severely hypocellular. Approximately 65% of patients who first present with **moderate aplastic anemia** (absolute neutrophil count 500-1,500/mm³, platelet count 20,000-100,000/mm³, reticulocyte count <1%) eventually progress to meet the criteria for severe disease, if they are simply observed. Bone marrow failure may be a consequence of a direct cytotoxic effect on hematopoietic stem cells from a drug or chemical or may result from either cell-mediated or antibody-dependent cytotoxicity. There is strong evidence that many cases of idiopathic aplastic anemia are caused by an immune-mediated process, with increased circulating activated T lymphocytes producing cytokines (interferon-γ) that suppress hematopoiesis. Abnormal telomere

length and telomerase activity in granulocytic precursors and increased expression of cell surface Flt3 ligand (a member of the class III receptor tyrosine kinase family) in the lymphocytes of patients with aplastic anemia suggest that early apoptosis of hematopoietic progenitors may play a role in the pathogenesis of this disease.

CLINICAL MANIFESTATIONS, LABORATORY FINDINGS, AND DIFFERENTIAL DIAGNOSIS

Pancytopenia results in increased risks of cardiac failure, infection, bleeding, and fatigue. Acquired pancytopenia is typically characterized by anemia, leukopenia, and thrombocytopenia in the setting of elevated serum cytokine values. Other treatable disorders, such as cancer, collagen vascular disorders, PNH, and infections that may respond to specific therapies (IV immune globulin for parvovirus), should be considered in the differential diagnosis. Careful examination of the peripheral blood smear for red blood cell, leukocyte, and platelet morphologic features is important. A reticulocyte count should be performed to assess erythropoietic activity. In children, the possibility of congenital pancytopenia must always be considered, and chromosomal breakage analysis should be performed to evaluate for Fanconi anemia (see Chapter 468). The presence of fetal hemoglobin suggests congenital pancytopenia but is not diagnostic. To assess for the possibility of PNH, flow cytometric analysis of erythrocytes for CD55 and CD59 is the most sensitive test. Bone marrow examination should include both aspiration and a biopsy, and the marrow should be carefully evaluated for morphologic features, cellularity, and cytogenetic abnormalities.

TREATMENT

The treatment of children with acquired pancytopenia requires comprehensive supportive care coupled with an attempt to treat the underlying marrow failure. For patients with an human leukocyte antigen–identical family member donor, allogeneic hematopoietic stem cell transplantation (HSCT) offers a 90% chance of long-term survival. The typical preparative regimen today consists of cyclophosphamide, fludarabine, and horse antithymocyte globulin (ATG). The risks associated with this approach include the immediate complications of transplantation, graft failure, and graft versus host disease. Late adverse effects associated with transplantation may include secondary cancers, cataracts, short stature, hypothyroidism, and gonadal dysfunction (see Chapters 136-139). Only 1 in 5 patients has a human leukocyte antigen–matched sibling donor, so matched-related HSCT is not an option for the majority of patients.

For patients without a sibling donor, the major form of therapy is immunosuppression with horse ATG and cyclosporine, with a response rate of 70-80%. The median time to response is 6 mo. As many as 30% of responders experience relapse after discontinuation of immunosuppression, and some patients must continue cyclosporine for several years to maintain a hematologic response. Among those who relapse after immunosuppression, approximately 50% show response to a second course of ATG and cyclosporine. There is an increased risk (<10%) of clonal bone marrow disease, such as leukemia, myelodysplasia (MDS), or PNH after immunosuppression with karyotypic abnormalities most frequently involving chromosomes 6, 7, and 8. To accelerate neutrophil recovery, a hematopoietic colony-stimulating factor (e.g., granulocyte colony-stimulating factor, granulocyte-macrophage colony-stimulating factor) is sometimes added to ATG and cyclosporine for treatment of patients with very severe neutropenia (absolute neutrophil count <200/mm^3), but there is no clear evidence that this treatment influences response rate or survival. In a few cases, tacrolimus has been given successfully with ATG for treatment of aplastic anemia in patients unable to tolerate cyclosporine. Higher baseline reticulocyte count correlates with a higher probability of response to immunosuppression and survival. There is an inverse correlation between telomere length and the probability of relapse post-immunosuppression.

For patients who show no response to immunosuppression or who experience relapse after immunosuppression, matched unrelated HSCT and T-cell depleted haploidentical family member donor HSCT

are treatment options, with a response rate approaching 90%. Cord blood transplants have been carried out in this refractory group of patients but there is a significant incidence of non-engraftment. High-dose cyclophosphamide has been used successfully in the treatment of patients with newly diagnosed aplastic anemia and in patients without adequate response to immunosuppression. This therapy leads to prolonged severe pancytopenia, increasing the risk of life-threatening infection, especially fungal. Other therapies that have been used in the past with inconsistent results include androgens, corticosteroids, and plasmapheresis. However, preliminary studies with eltrombopag (an oral thrombopoietin mimetic agent) have resulted in a hematologic response with improvements in platelet and neutrophil counts and hemoglobin levels in some patients. In patients who responded, bone marrow biopsies demonstrated trilineage normalization of hematopoiesis; some who were dependent on platelet or erythrocyte transfusions no longer needed transfusions.

COMPLICATIONS

The major complications of severe pancytopenia are predominantly related to the risk of life-threatening bleeding from prolonged thrombocytopenia or to infection secondary to protracted neutropenia. Patients with protracted neutropenia as a result of bone marrow failure are at risk not only for serious bacterial infections but also for invasive mycoses. Patients who have been transfused with red blood cells regularly over a long period are at increased risk of developing alloantibodies to red cell antigens and may require iron chelation therapy for transfusional iron overload. The general principles of supportive care that have evolved from the use of chemotherapy-related myelosuppression to treat patients with cancer should be fully extended to the care of patients with acquired pancytopenia.

PROGNOSIS

Spontaneous recovery from pancytopenia rarely occurs. If left untreated, severe pancytopenia has an overall mortality rate of approximately 50% within 6 mo of diagnosis and of >75% overall, with infection and hemorrhage being the major causes of morbidity and mortality. The majority of children with acquired severe aplastic anemia show response to allogeneic marrow transplantation or immunosuppression, leaving them with normal or near-normal blood cell counts.

PANCYTOPENIA CAUSED BY MARROW REPLACEMENT

Processes that either infiltrate or replace the bone marrow can manifest as acquired pancytopenia. Infiltration can be caused by malignancy (classically, neuroblastoma or leukemia) or occur as a consequence of myelofibrosis, MDS, or osteoporosis. Although uncommon, evidence of hypoplastic anemia can precede the onset of acute leukemia, generally by a few months. This relationship is important to appreciate in evaluating and monitoring children who present with what appears to be acquired aplastic anemia. Morphologic examination of the peripheral blood and bone marrow and marrow cytogenetic studies are critically important in making the diagnoses of leukemia, myelofibrosis, and MDS.

MDS is very rare in children, but when it occurs, its clinical course is more aggressive than the same category of MDS in adults. Pediatric MDS can be subdivided into refractory cytopenia of childhood (peripheral blasts <2% and marrow blasts <5%), refractory anemia with excess blasts (peripheral blasts 2-19% and/or marrow blasts 5-19%), and refractory anemia with excess blasts in transformation (peripheral and/or marrow blasts 20-29%). Disease in children with >30% blasts is usually defined as acute myelocytic leukemia.

A number of inherited conditions are associated with an increased risk for development of MDS, including Down syndrome, severe congenital neutropenia, Noonan syndrome, Fanconi anemia, trisomy 8 mosaicism, neurofibromatosis, and Shwachman syndrome. Significant clonal abnormalities are found within the marrow of approximately 50% of patients with MDS, with monosomy 7 and being most common but prognostically neutral. Those with a structurally complex karyotype have a very poor outcome.

The transition time from pediatric MDS to acute leukemia is relatively short, at 14-26 mo, so aggressive treatment, such as HSCT, must be considered shortly after diagnosis. With allogeneic HSCT, the survival rate is approximately 60%. One exception to such an aggressive therapeutic approach is MDS and acute myelocytic leukemia in children with Down syndrome, because this disease in this specific population is very responsive to conventional chemotherapy, with long-term survival rates >80%.

The decision on how to treat a child with MDS who lacks a suitable hematopoietic stem cell donor should be made with the specific clonal abnormality found within the child's marrow taken into consideration. Lenalidomide produces the best responses among patients who have the chromosomal abnormality, 5q–. Immunosuppressive therapy with ATG and cyclosporine is most effective in patients with trisomy 8, especially in the presence of a PNH clone. Imatinib mesylate targets mutations in the tyrosine kinase receptor family of genes found in patients with t(5;12) and del(4q12). The DNA hypomethylating agents azacitidine and decitabine have also been used in treating MDS without a known molecular target and have some effect.

Bibliography is available at Expert Consult.

Section 6
Blood Component Transfusions

Chapter 470
Red Blood Cell Transfusions and Erythropoietin Therapy
Ronald G. Strauss

Red blood cells (RBCs) are transfused to increase the oxygen-carrying capacity of the blood, with the goal to increase or maintain satisfactory tissue oxygenation; this goal may not be achieved simply by increasing the blood hemoglobin concentration or hematocrit by an RBC transfusion because tissue oxygenation depends on several additional factors including oxygen off-loading from RBCs, microvascular blood flow, and diffusion of oxygen into tissue cells. Although some attempts have been made to accurately relate posttransfusion blood hemoglobin concentration or hematocrit values to changes in posttransfusion tissue oxygenation (e.g., improvements in the ratio of cerebral versus mesenteric oxygenation patterns assessed by serial near-infrared spectroscopy measurements), decisions to transfuse RBCs per physiologic indications, rather than degree of anemia, remain investigational.

Because neonates, especially extremely low birthweight preterms are not "small" children (i.e., RBC physiology and the pathophysiology of the anemia of prematurity are unique), RBC transfusions for neonates and older children will be considered separately. Guidelines for RBC transfusions in children and adolescents are based on maintaining a specified hemoglobin or hematocrit level considered to be optimal (per the best evidence available) for the clinical condition present at the time of the transfusion. The guidelines are similar to those for adults (Table 470-1). Transfusions may be given more stringently to children,

Table 470-1	Guidelines for Pediatric Red Blood Cell Transfusions*†

CHILDREN AND ADOLESCENTS
1. Maintain stable status with acute loss of >25% of circulating blood volume
2. Maintain hemoglobin >7.0 g/dL† in the perioperative period
3. Maintain hemoglobin >12.0 g/dL with *severe* cardiopulmonary disease
4. Maintain hemoglobin >12.0 g/dL during extracorporeal membrane oxygenation
5. Maintain hemoglobin >7.0 g/dL and *symptomatic* chronic anemia
6. Maintain hemoglobin >7.0 g/dL and *marrow failure*

INFANTS ≤4 MO OLD
1. Maintain hemoglobin >12.0 g/dL and *severe* pulmonary disease
2. Maintain hemoglobin >12.0 g/dL during extracorporeal membrane oxygenation
3. Maintain hemoglobin >10.0 g/dL and *moderate* pulmonary disease
4. Maintain hemoglobin >12.0 g/dL and *severe* cardiac disease
5. Maintain hemoglobin >10.0 g/dL preoperatively and during *major* surgery
6. Maintain hemoglobin >7.0 g/dL postoperatively
7. Maintain hemoglobin >7.0 g/dL and *symptomatic* anemia

*Words in *italics* must be defined for local transfusion guidelines.
†Pretransfusion blood hemoglobin level (convert to hematocrit values if preferred by multiplying hemoglobin values by 3) "triggering" an RBC transfusion. Hemoglobin values to maintain vary among published reports, and the guideline values to maintain should be determined locally to fit the practices judged to be optimal by local MDs.

because normal hemoglobin levels are lower in healthy children than in adults and, as is often the case, children do not have the underlying multiorgan, cardiorespiratory, and vascular diseases that develop with aging in adults to suggest a need for RBC transfusions Thus, children may compensate better for RBC loss than elderly adults and, as is true for patients of all ages, there is increasing enthusiasm for applying conservative practices (i.e., accept lower pretransfusion hematocrit values to "trigger" a RBC transfusion).

In the perioperative period, it is unnecessary for most children to maintain hemoglobin levels of 8 g/dL or greater, a level frequently desired for adults. The desired preoperative hemoglobin level should take into account the estimated blood loss for the surgical procedure planned and the rate of bleeding. There should be a compelling reason to prescribe any postoperative RBC transfusion, such as continued bleeding with hemodynamic instability, because most children (without continued bleeding) can, in a relatively short time, restore their RBC mass with iron therapy. The most important measures in the treatments of acute hemorrhage are to control the hemorrhage and, if blood loss is modest, to restore the circulating blood volume and tissue perfusion with crystalloid or, less often, colloid solutions. If the estimated blood loss is >25% of the circulating blood volume (>15 mL/kg of an estimated 60 mL/kg total estimated blood volume) *and* the patient's condition is unstable despite intravenous fluids, RBC transfusions may be indicated; given with plasma transfusions at a 1:1 ratio of RBC:plasma volumes. Details of combined RBC and plasma transfusions, the volume ratio transfused, and considerations for adding platelet transfusions to treat bleeding patients are controversial. Accordingly, each hospital should develop and follow a "massive transfusion" protocol to ensure consistent practices.

In critically ill children with severe cardiac or pulmonary disease requiring assisted ventilation, it is common practice to maintain the hemoglobin level close to the normal range, although the efficacy of this practice has not been well documented. A similar approach is used for children with acute cardiac, pulmonary, or cardiopulmonary disorders managed with extracorporeal membrane oxygenation.

The pretransfusion blood hemoglobin level or hematocrit that should "trigger" a RBC transfusion is controversial (i.e., restrictive or a low pretransfusion level vs. liberal or a high pretransfusion level) despite a substantial amount of published information, including randomized clinical trials. The current trend in critical care settings is to transfuse RBCs quite conservatively, following restrictive guidelines, and to permit modest anemia because there appears to be no disadvantage to conservative/restrictive transfusion practices, and some patients with hemoglobin levels maintained close to the normal range by RBC transfusions (i.e., liberal guidelines) have poorer outcomes. Studies in critically ill adults demonstrated better outcomes when the hemoglobin level was maintained at 7-9 g/dL versus 10-12 g/dL. Anemic adults with significant cardiac disease did better with hemoglobin levels maintained at 13 g/dL than at 10 g/dL. Similar studies in children admitted to intensive care units found no inferiority when RBC transfusions were given by restrictive guidelines (transfusion threshold of 7 g/dL). It must be remembered that the children studied were in stable clinical status and needed few transfusions. Therefore, results of the trial cannot be automatically extended to all patients admitted to intensive care units, as unstable critically ill children, who were not studied, may need more liberal RBC transfusions.

With chronic anemia, the decision to transfuse RBCs should not be based solely on blood hemoglobin levels, because children compensate well and may be asymptomatic despite low hemoglobin levels. Patients with iron-deficiency anemia are often treated successfully with oral iron alone, even at hemoglobin levels <5 g/dL. Factors other than hemoglobin concentration to be considered in the decision to transfuse RBCs include: (1) the patient's symptoms, signs, and compensatory capacities; (2) the presence of underlying cardiorespiratory, vascular, and central nervous system disease; (3) the cause and anticipated course of the anemia; and (4) alternative therapies, such as recombinant human erythropoietin (EPO) therapy, which is known to reduce the need for RBC transfusions and to improve the overall condition of children with chronic renal insufficiency (see Chapter 535.2). In anemias that are likely to be permanent, it is also important to balance the detrimental effects of the degree of long-standing anemia on growth and development against the potential toxicity associated with repeated transfusions given to maintain the blood hemoglobin concentration at a specified level. RBC transfusions for disorders such as sickle cell anemia and thalassemia are discussed in Chapters 462.1 and 462.9.

For neonates, nearly all aspects of RBC transfusions remain controversial (i.e., the accepted indications for RBC transfusions; restrictive vs. liberal pretransfusion hemoglobin/hematocrit levels; optimal RBC product to be transfused; fresh vs. stored RBC units), and clinical practices vary greatly. Generally, RBCs are given to maintain a hemoglobin value believed to be the most desirable for each neonate's clinical status (see Table 470-1). Restrictive guidelines (i.e., lower pretransfusion hemoglobin/hematocrit levels) have been compared to more liberal transfusion practices, but both short-term and long-term results/outcomes have been inconsistent and controversial, particularly as to neurodevelopmental status, with poorer outcomes seen in both the restrictive and liberal study arms. Accordingly, conventional guidelines are recommended to avoid problems caused by either undertransfusion or overtransfusion, until more definitive data are published (see Table 470-1).

This clinical approach is imprecise, but more physiologic guidelines/indications such as measurement of RBC mass, calculations of oxygen delivery and tissue extraction, imaging of microcirculatory flow, and comparative measures of tissue perfusion (e.g., ratio of cerebral:mesenteric oxygenation patterns), are too cumbersome for day-to-day clinical practice.

During the first few weeks of life, all neonates experience a decline in circulating RBC mass caused both by physiologic factors and, in sick premature infants, by phlebotomy blood losses. In healthy term infants, the nadir hemoglobin value rarely falls to <11 g/dL at an age of 10-12 wk. This benign *physiologic anemia of infancy* does not require transfusions. In contrast, the decline occurs earlier and is more pronounced in premature infants, in whom the mean hemoglobin concentration falls to approximately 7 g/dL in infants weighing <1 kg at birth, resulting in the *anemia of prematurity*, for which there often is need for RBC transfusions.

A key reason that the nadir hemoglobin values of premature infants are lower than those of term infants is the former group's relatively diminished plasma EPO level in response to anemia (see Chapters 103.1 and 446). Another factor is the rapid disappearance of EPO from infant plasma (i.e., accelerated metabolism).

Low plasma EPO levels provide a rationale for the possible use of recombinant EPO in the treatment of anemia of prematurity; treatment with EPO and iron effectively stimulate neonatal erythropoiesis. Despite its erythropoietic effect, the efficacy of EPO therapy to substantially diminish the need for RBC transfusions has not been convincingly demonstrated, particularly for sick, extremely premature neonates, and recombinant EPO has not been widely accepted as a treatment for anemia of prematurity (see Chapter 103.1).

Because of the controversies over recombinant EPO therapy, many low birthweight preterm infants need RBC transfusions (see Table 470-1). Although the practice to maintain a very high hemoglobin level (hemoglobin >13 g/dL or hematocrit >40%) was once widely recommended, currently more restrictive guidelines have been suggested. Consistent with the rationale for oxygen delivery in neonates with severe respiratory disease, it seems appropriate to keep the hemoglobin value relatively high in neonates with *severe cardiac disease* leading to either cyanosis or congestive heart failure, but convincing and consistent data are lacking.

The optimal hemoglobin level for neonates facing major surgery has not been established. However, it seems reasonable to begin surgery in neonates with the hemoglobin level no lower than 10 g/dL (hematocrit >30%) and to maintain that value during major surgery because even modest blood loss will have a relatively large effect on the small blood volume of the neonate; neonates with underlying pulmonary problems have limited ability to compensate for anemia, and the inferior offloading of oxygen because of the diminished interaction between fetal hemoglobin and 2,3-diphosphoglycerate. Postoperatively, a lower pretransfusion hemoglobin value should be followed to "trigger" a transfusion.

Stable neonates do not require RBC transfusion, regardless of their blood hemoglobin levels, unless they exhibit clinical symptoms attributable to anemia. Proponents of RBC transfusions for symptomatic anemia in preterm neonates believe that the low RBC mass contributes to tachypnea, dyspnea, tachycardia, apnea and bradycardia, feeding difficulties, and lethargy, which can be alleviated by transfusion of RBCs. However, anemia is only one of several possible causes of these problems, and RBC transfusions should only be given when clinical benefit seems likely.

The RBC product of choice to transfuse neonates, infants, children, and adolescents is prestorage leukocyte-reduced RBCs suspended in an anticoagulant/preservative storage solution at a hematocrit value of approximately 60% for storage up to 42 days. The usual dose is 10-15 mL/kg, but transfusion volumes vary greatly, depending on clinical circumstances (continued vs. arrested bleeding, hemolysis). For neonates, some prefer a centrifuged RBC concentrate (hematocrit 70-90%). Unless transfusions are being given to treat rapid bleeding, RBCs are infused slowly (over 2-4 hr) at a dose of approximately 15 mL/kg. In this small-volume transfusion, because of the small quantity of extracellular fluid transfused and the slow rate of infusion, the type of RBC anticoagulant/preservative solution does not pose any risk for premature infants; there are no data to justify separate inventories of different RBC products for neonates and infants (e.g., citrate-phosphate-dextrose or citrate-phosphate-dextrose-adenine) versus older children (e.g., AS-1, AS-3, or AS-5).

The historical practice of transfusing fresh RBCs (<7 days of storage) for the small-volume (15 mL/kg) transfusions commonly given was supplanted several years ago in most centers by reserving a single unit of RBCs for an infant, from which multiple aliquots were obtained for transfusions as needed throughout the 42 days of storage. Concerns about high concentrations of extracellular potassium, loss of 2,3-diphosphoglycerate, altered RBC shape and deformability, and nitric oxide quenching were found not to pose clinically significant problems. Preterm neonates allocated to "fresh RBC" (<7 day storage) transfusions versus "stored RBC" (up to 42 day storage) transfusions, have no advantage for fresh RBC transfusions in altering either the composite clinical outcome of mortality plus necrotizing enterocolitis, retinopathy of prematurity, bronchopulmonary dysplasia, and intraventricular hemorrhage or of the individual disorders.

For children weighing >30 kg who are to undergo elective surgery for which RBC transfusions are likely to be needed, autologous RBC transfusions offer an alternative to donor allogeneic RBCs. **Preoperative autologous** blood collections from the patient occur up to 6 wk before the surgery and require careful considerations for the volume to be drawn, vascular access, and use of EPO and iron to help restore the donated RBCs. **Acute normovolemic hemodilution** occurs in the preoperative period, in which blood is withdrawn from the patient and replaced with saline, a task often difficult in centers without experience in the process. **Salvaged autologous blood** is collected from blood loss during the operation but is impractical unless the volume of blood salvaged is fairly large to permit washing and transfusion of a significant number of RBCs. Because of all of these difficulties plus the relative safety of the usual allogeneic blood supply, autologous RBC transfusions are not commonly used in the pediatric setting.

Bibliography is available at Expert Consult.

Chapter **471**
Platelet Transfusions
Ronald G. Strauss

Guidelines for platelet (PLT) support of children and adolescents with quantitative and qualitative PLT disorders are similar to those for adults (Table 471-1), in whom the risk of life-threatening bleeding after injury or occurring spontaneously can be related somewhat imprecisely, particularly for the occurrence of spontaneous bleeding to the severity of thrombocytopenia.

For children and adolescents with overt bleeding, therapeutic PLT transfusions should be given when the blood PLT count falls below 50 × 10⁹/L and repeated as needed to maintain the PLT count >50 × 10⁹/L

Table 471-1 | Guidelines for Pediatric Platelet Transfusion*

CHILDREN AND ADOLESCENTS
1. Maintain PLT count >50 × 10⁹/L with bleeding
2. Maintain PLT count >50 × 10⁹/L with *major invasive* procedure; >25 × 10⁹/L with minor
3. Maintain PLT count >20 × 10⁹/L and *marrow failure* WITH hemorrhagic risk factors
4. Maintain PLT count >10 × 10⁹/L and *marrow failure* WITHOUT hemorrhagic risk factors
5. Maintain PLT count at any level with PLT dysfunction PLUS bleeding or invasive procedure

INFANTS ≤4 MO OLD
1. Maintain PLT count >100 × 10⁹/L with bleeding or during extracorporeal membrane oxygenation
2. Maintain PLT count >50 × 10⁹/L and an invasive procedure
3. Maintain PLT count >20 × 10⁹/L and *clinically stable*
4. Maintain PLT count >50 × 10⁹/L and *clinically unstable and/or bleeding* or not when on indomethacin, nitric oxide, antibiotics, etc. affecting PLT function
5. Maintain PLT count at any level with PLT dysfunction PLUS bleeding invasive procedure

*Words in italics must be defined for local transfusion guidelines.
PLT, platelet.

during bleeding and for 48 hr after bleeding ceases to allow the clot to "stabilize." Similarly, for a major invasive procedure (e.g., surgical procedure), the PLT count should be maintained >50 × 10⁹/L until any bleeding that occurs ceases and the patient is stable. For minor invasive procedures (e.g., lumbar puncture or placing an intravascular catheter) practices vary, but it is reasonable to maintain the PLT count >25 × 10⁹/L.

Historical studies of patients with thrombocytopenia resulting from bone marrow failure suggest that the risk of spontaneous bleeding increases when blood PLT levels fall to <20 × 10⁹/L particularly when hemorrhagic risk factors (infection, organ failure, clotting abnormalities, minor skin/mucosal bleeding, mucosal lesions, severe graft-versus-host disease, or anemia) are present. In this high-risk setting, prophylactic PLT transfusions are given to maintain a PLT count >20 × 10⁹/L. This threshold has been challenged by several studies of adult patients, who, in many instances, were carefully selected to be in relatively good clinical condition *without* hemorrhagic risk factors. Consequently, a higher PLT transfusion trigger of 50×10⁹/L is recommended for stable (i.e., low-risk) patients.

In practice, severe thrombocytopenia that is prolonged beyond 1 wk commonly becomes complicated by the development of risk factors including fever, antimicrobial therapy, graft-versus-host disease, active bleeding, need for an invasive procedure, disseminated intravascular coagulation, and liver or kidney dysfunction with clotting abnormalities. In these situations, prophylactic PLT transfusions are given to maintain relatively high PLT counts (e.g., at least >30 × 10⁹/L). Despite the desire by some physicians to elevate the blood PLT count to 80 × 10⁹/L or 100 × 10⁹/L, there are no definitive data to justify a true benefit of PLT transfusions given at a PLT count >50 × 10⁹/L, unless bleeding is ongoing with a PLT count between 50 and 100 × 10⁹/L *and* thrombocytopenia seems to be the only cause for the bleeding.

Qualitative PLT disorders may be inherited or acquired (in advanced hepatic or renal insufficiency or when blood flows through an extracorporeal circuit, such as during extracorporeal membrane oxygenation or cardiopulmonary bypass). In patients with inherited disorders, PLT transfusions are justified only if the risk of significant bleeding is quite high or if bleeding is overt because inherited PLT dysfunction often is lifelong and repeated transfusions may lead to alloimmunization and refractoriness (i.e., poor response to PLT transfusions). Accordingly, prophylactic PLT transfusions are rarely justified, unless an invasive procedure is planned, and therapeutic PLT transfusions must be given judiciously.

When managing patients with PLT dysfunction, it is important to remember that, an abnormal test result with a modern PLT function device or, historically, a bleeding time more than twice the upper limit of normal provides diagnostic evidence of PLT dysfunction. However, an abnormal bleeding time or any other abnormal laboratory test is poorly predictive of hemorrhagic risk and/or the need to transfuse PLTs. Alternative therapies, particularly desmopressin acetate, should be considered to avoid PLT transfusions. Antiplatelet medications (nonsteroidal antiinflammatory drugs) should also be avoided.

In neonates, thrombopoiesis and the risks of bleeding are substantially different from that in older children; the approach to thrombocytopenia and PLT transfusions likewise differs (see Table 471-1). Thrombopoietin (TPO) levels are higher in healthy neonates than in older individuals. Megakaryocyte progenitors of neonates are more sensitive to TPO, have higher proliferative potential, and give rise to larger megakaryocyte colonies than do adult PLT progenitors. Fetal/neonatal megakaryocytes are smaller in size and have lower ploidy than do their adult counterparts; this is an important factor because small megakaryocytes of low ploidy produce fewer PLTs than larger megakaryocytes of higher ploidy. Presumably, this allows the expanding marrow of the growing fetus and neonate to be supplied with sufficient numbers of megakaryocytes, yet not allowing blood PLT counts to become excessively high during proliferation, because of the lower numbers of PLTs produced by each megakaryocyte.

An important contrasting point is that older children and adults respond to situations of increased demand for PLTs by first increasing megakaryocyte size and ploidy, which is followed in 3-5 days by increased megakaryocyte number. In thrombocytopenic neonates, megakaryocyte numbers increase, but not their size. Moreover, although cytoplasmic maturation is achieved per TPO stimulation, increases in ploidy are relatively diminished and actually appear to be inhibited by TPO, resulting in large numbers of small megakaryocytes that are cytoplasmically mature, but with low ploidy and, consequently, lower PLT production.

Blood PLT counts $\geq 150 \times 10^9$/L are present after 17 wk gestational age, and it is accepted that neonates have blood PLT counts in the same range as older children and adults (150,000-450,000/μL). However, recent data suggest a lower limit of 120,000/μL for extremely small preterm infants. Approximately 1% of term infants demonstrate PLT counts $<150 \times 10^9$/L, but bleeding in such infants is rare. In contrast, 25-35% of preterm of neonates treated in intensive care units exhibit blood PLT counts $<150 \times 10^9$/L at some time during admission, with approximately 4% overall receiving PLT transfusions. Notably, when only extremely low birthweight preterm infants (<1 kg birthweight) were considered in one report, 73% had PLT counts $<150 \times 10^9$/L and 62% of thrombocytopenic neonates received PLT transfusions. Multiple pathogenetic mechanisms underlie thrombocytopenia in these sick neonates; predominantly accelerated PLT destruction plus diminished PLT production, as evidenced by decreased numbers of megakaryocyte progenitors and relatively low upregulation of TPO levels during thrombocytopenia, compared with thrombocytopenic children and adults.

Blood PLT counts $<100 \times 10^9$/L pose significant clinical risks for premature neonates. Bleeding time may be prolonged at PLT counts $<100 \times 10^9$/L in infants with a birthweight <1.5 kg, and PLT dysfunction is suggested by bleeding times (a test no longer performed) that are disproportionately long for the degree of thrombocytopenia. The risk of hemorrhage may be increased in thrombocytopenic infants. However, in a randomized trial, transfusing PLTs prophylactically whenever the PLT count fell to $<150 \times 10^9$/L (i.e., at the lower limit of the normal range) to maintain the average PLT count at $>200 \times 10^9$/L, compared to not transfusing PLTs until the PLT count fell to $<50 \times 10^9$/L to maintain the average PLT count at approximately 100×10^9/L, did not result in a lower incidence of intracranial hemorrhage (28% vs. 26%, respectively). Thus, there is no documented benefit for prophylactic PLT transfusions to maintain PLT counts within the normal range or to correct modest thrombocytopenia (PLT count $>50 \times 10^9$/L). As an exception, infants with inherited PLT dysfunction disorders *and* bleeding, and those at high risk of bleeding owing to acquired PLT dysfunction, such as during extracorporeal membrane oxygenation, commonly receive transfusions to keep their PLT counts $>100 \times 10^9$/L.

Table 471-1 lists guidelines that are acceptable to many neonatologists. One particularly contentious issue is how to manage critically ill neonates receiving drugs/agents known to adversely affect PLT function (e.g., indomethacin, nitric oxide, antibiotics). Some reports suggest increased risk of bleeding for these neonates, but the efficacy of PLT transfusions has not been convincingly proven, particularly when given prophylactically. For optimal PLT transfusion practices, each hospital should modify the guidelines to comply with local practices, and audits/reviews should be performed to avoid violations of the recommended practices. The posttransfusion goal of most PLT transfusions is to raise the PLT count well above 50×10^9/L, hopefully to $\geq 100 \times 10^9$/L. These increases can be achieved consistently in children weighing up to 30 kg by infusion of 5-10 mL/kg of standard (unmodified) PLT concentrates, obtained either from processing whole blood units or by plateletpheresis. For larger children, the appropriate dose is 3-4 pooled whole blood–derived PLT units or 1 apheresis unit. Because PLT concentration/quantity varies in different PLT products made available for transfusion, each hospital should monitor posttransfusion PLT counts to determine the dose that works best locally. PLT concentrates should be transfused as rapidly as the patient's overall condition permits, certainly within 2 hr. Neonates/infants requiring repeated PLT transfusions should receive leukocyte-reduced blood products, including PLT concentrates, to diminish alloimmunization and PLT refractoriness and to reduce the risk of transfusion-transmitted cytomegalovirus infection.

Routinely reducing the volume of PLT concentrates for infants and small children by additional centrifugation steps is both unnecessary and unwise. Transfusion of 10 mL/kg of an unmodified PLT concentrate is adequate because it adds approximately 10×10^9 PLTs to 70 mL of blood (the estimated intravascular blood volume of a 1 kg neonate), a dose/volume calculated to increase the PLT count by 100×10^9/L. This calculated increment is consistent with actual posttransfusion increment reported in patients. Moreover, 10 mL/kg is not an excessive transfusion volume, provided that the intake of other IV fluids, medications, and nutrients is monitored and adjusted.

It is important to select PLT units for transfusion with the donor ABO group identical to that of the neonate/infant and to avoid repeated transfusion of group O PLTs to group A or B recipients because passive transfusion anti-A or anti-B in group O plasma, can occasionally lead to hemolysis.

Bibliography is available at Expert Consult.

Chapter **472**
Neutrophil (Granulocyte) Transfusions
Ronald G. Strauss

Table 472-1 lists guidelines for granulocyte transfusion (GTX). GTX has been used sparingly in older infants and children. The current ability to collect markedly higher numbers of neutrophils from donors stimulated with combined recombinant granulocyte colony-stimulating factor (G-CSF) plus dexamethasone has led to renewed interest for patients with neutropenic infections, particularly when severe neutropenia is prolonged (e.g., in the setting of placental/cord blood hematopoietic progenitor cell transplantation). Because of the higher neutrophil yields with this collection approach, adding GTX to antibiotics should be considered at institutions where neutropenic patients continue either to die of progressive bacterial and fungal infections or to suffer substantial morbidity despite optimal antiinfection measures, including antibiotics and recombinant myeloid growth factors.

The use of GTX added to antibiotics for children with severe neutropenia (blood neutrophil count $<0.5 \times 10^9$/L) because of bone marrow failure is similar to that for adults. Unfortunately, two randomized clinical trials comparing antibiotics plus GTX from donors stimulated with G-CSF plus dexamethasone versus antibiotics without GTX

Table 472-1	Guidelines for Pediatric Granulocyte Transfusions*

CHILDREN AND ADOLESCENTS
1. Severe neutropenia (blood neutrophil count $<0.5 \times 10^9$/L) and infection (bacterial, yeast, or fungal) *unresponsive or progressive* despite appropriate antimicrobial therapy
2. Qualitative neutrophil defect, neutropenia not required, and infection (bacterial or fungal) *unresponsive or progressive* to appropriate antimicrobial therapy

INFANTS ≤4 MO OLD†
Blood neutrophil count $<3.0 \times 10^9$/L in 1st wk of life or $<1.0 \times 10^9$/L thereafter and *fulminant* bacterial infection.

*Words in italics must be defined for local transfusion guidelines.
†No longer commonly used.

to treat neutropenic infections in children have not provided definitive guidelines. However in practice, neutropenic patients with bacterial infections usually show response to antibiotics alone, provided bone marrow function recovers within the 1st 7-10 days of infection onset so that severe neutropenia is relatively brief. Children with newly diagnosed acute lymphoblastic leukemia show rapid response to induction chemotherapy, and they rarely are candidates for GTX. In contrast, infected children with more sustained bone marrow failure and consequent severe neutropenia (e.g., acute myeloblastic leukemia, malignant neoplasms resistant to treatment, severe aplastic anemia, and placental/cord blood hematopoietic progenitor cell transplant recipients) may benefit when GTX is added to antibiotics.

Currently, the efficacy of GTX obtained from G-CSF plus dexamethasone-stimulated donors for bacterial sepsis unresponsive to antibiotics in patients with severe neutropenia (blood neutrophil count $<0.5 \times 10^9$/L) is not well supported by trials in children. In contrast, GTX efficacy for yeast and fungal infections remains unproven despite transfusing GTX with relatively large numbers of neutrophils.

Children with qualitative neutrophil defects (**neutrophil dysfunction**) usually have adequate or even increased numbers of blood neutrophils but suffer serious infections, because their neutrophils kill pathogenic microorganisms inefficiently. Neutrophil dysfunction syndromes are rare; accordingly, no definitive studies have established GTX efficacy. However, several patients with progressive life-threatening infections have shown striking improvement with the addition of GTX, often given for long periods of time, to antimicrobial therapy. These disorders are chronic, and because of the risk of inducing alloimmunization to leukocyte antigens, and in some patients with chronic granulomatous disease, to antigens of the Kell system of red blood cells, GTX is recommended only when serious infections are clearly unresponsive to antimicrobial drugs.

Neonates are unusually susceptible to severe bacterial infections, and a number of defects of neonatal body defenses contribute, including actual or "relative" neutropenia. Neonates with fulminant sepsis who exhibit relative neutropenia (blood neutrophil count $<3.0 \times 10^9$/L during the 1st wk of life and $<1.0 \times 10^9$/L thereafter) and a severely diminished neutrophil marrow storage pool (with <10% of nucleated marrow cells being postmitotic neutrophils) are at risk of dying if treated only with antibiotics. GTX is rarely used because results of clinical trials are mixed and not uniformly convincing, and it is difficult to obtain neutrophil apheresis concentrates in timely fashion.

Current data are insufficient to determine whether recombinant myeloid growth factors have a role in treating septic neonates, despite the fact that both G-CSF and granulocyte-macrophage colony-stimulating factor have been demonstrated to enhance myelopoiesis and raise neutrophil counts in infants. Importantly, G-CSF is efficacious for the long-term treatment of several types of severe congenital neutropenia.

If the decision to provide a GTX has been made, an adequate dose of neutrophils/granulocytes collected by leukapheresis must be transfused as shortly after collection as possible. To facilitate this, experienced donors with required infectious disease (HIV, hepatitis) tests having been done recently (usually within the past 30 days) are selected, and the collected neutrophils are transfused before results of current infectious disease tests are known (i.e., infectious disease test results are "waived").

Neonates and infants weighing <10 kg should receive $1\text{-}2 \times 10^9$/kg neutrophils per each GTX. Larger infants and small children should receive a minimal total dose of 1×10^{10} neutrophils per each GTX. The preferred dose for adolescents is $5\text{-}8 \times 10^{10}$ neutrophils per each GTX, a dose requiring donors to be stimulated with G-CSF plus dexamethasone. GTX should be given daily until either the infection resolves or the blood neutrophil count is sustained above 1.5×10^9/L for a few days. Because neutrophils transfused per the GTX often passively increase the blood neutrophil count, it may be necessary to skip 1-2 days of GTXs to be certain severe neutropenia does not recur, as would be seen if endogenous myelopoiesis had not recovered.

Bibliography is available at Expert Consult.

Chapter **473**
Plasma Transfusions
Ronald G. Strauss

Guidelines for plasma transfusion in pediatric patients (Table 473-1) are similar to those for adults but with the understanding that plasma levels of coagulant and anticoagulant proteins can be developmentally quite low in preterm infants so that transfusions of plasma and plasma-derived commercial concentrates should be determined by actual bleeding or a significant risk of bleeding, not simply prolonged clotting time results. Plasma is transfused to replace clinically significant deficiencies of plasma proteins for which more highly purified protein concentrates that have been treated to reduce infectious disease risks are not available nearly always to provide clotting proteins when bleeding is occurring or in settings when prevention of bleeding is deemed critical.

Two interchangeable plasma products are available for transfusion, plasma frozen within 8 hr of collection (**fresh-frozen plasma**) and plasma frozen within 24 hr of collection. Although levels of factors V and VIII are modestly reduced in the latter plasma product (generally, not more than 25% lower), they are equally efficacious for all indications for which plasma is transfused (see Table 473-1). Recommendations for the volume of plasma to be transfused vary with the specific protein being replaced and the severity of the deficiency, but a starting dose of 15 mL/kg is usually sufficient to elevate plasma levels satisfactorily.

Transfusion of plasma is efficacious for the treatment of deficiencies of clotting factors II, V, X, and XI. Deficiencies of factor XIII and fibrinogen are treated either with cryoprecipitate or specific commercial concentrates; although for patients being given large doses of plasma (e.g., in massive transfusion settings or to treat bleeding in liver failure), additional sources of fibrinogen may not be necessary, as plasma contains large amounts of fibrinogen. It is always useful to include a measurement of plasma fibrinogen when performing clotting assays (e.g., prothrombin time [PT]/international normalized ratio [INR] and activated partial thromboplastin time [aPTT]). *Transfusion of plasma is not recommended for the treatment of patients with severe hemophilia A or B, von Willebrand disease, or factor VII deficiency, because safer factors VII, VIII, IX, and von Willebrand factor concentrates are available.* Moreover, mild to moderate hemophilia A and certain types of von Willebrand disease can be treated with intranasal or intravenous desmopressin (see Chapter 477). An important use of plasma is for rapid reversal of the effects of warfarin in patients who are actively bleeding or who require emergency surgery (in whom

Table 473-1	Guidelines for Pediatric Plasma Transfusions*

1. *Severe* clotting factor deficiency AND bleeding
2. *Severe* clotting factor deficiency AND an invasive procedure
3. *Emergency reversal* of warfarin effects
4. Dilutional coagulopathy and bleeding (e.g., massive transfusion)
5. Anticoagulant protein (antithrombin III, proteins C and S) replacement
6. Plasma exchange replacement fluid for thrombotic thrombocytopenic purpura or for disorders with overt bleeding or in which there is risk of bleeding because of clotting protein abnormalities (e.g., liver failure)

*Words in *italics* must be defined for local transfusion guidelines.

functional deficiencies of factors II, VII, IX, and X cannot be rapidly reversed by vitamin K). Prothrombin "complex" concentrates can also be used for this purpose.

Results of screening coagulation tests (PT/INR, aPTT, and thrombin times, and plasma fibrinogen levels) should not be assumed by themselves to reflect the integrity of the coagulation system or be regarded as indications for plasma transfusions. This is particularly true for neonates. To justify plasma transfusions, coagulation test results must be related to the patient's clinical condition pertaining to bleeding and/or the risk of bleeding. Transfusion of plasma in patients with chronic liver disease and prolonged clotting times is not recommended unless bleeding is present or an invasive procedure is planned, because correction of the clotting factor deficiencies is brief and of questionable benefit.

Plasma also contains several anticoagulant proteins (antithrombin III, protein C, and protein S) whose deficiencies have been associated with **thrombosis**. In selected situations, plasma may be appropriate as replacement therapy, along with anticoagulant treatment, in patients with these disorders; when available, purified concentrates are preferred. Other indications for plasma include replacement fluid during plasma exchange in patients with thrombotic thrombocytopenic purpura (i.e., thrombotic microangiopathies) or other disorders for which plasma is likely to be beneficial (plasma exchange in a patient with overt bleeding due to the underlying disorder such as Goodpasture syndrome or vasculitis or disorders with significant severe coagulopathy that would be made substantially more severe by replacement using albumin solutions only). Plasma is not indicated for correction of hypovolemia or as immunoglobulin replacement therapy, because safer alternatives exist (albumin or crystalloid solutions and IV immunoglobulin, respectively).

In neonates, clotting times are "physiologically" prolonged owing to developmental deficiency of clotting proteins; plasma should be transfused only after reference to normal values adjusted for the birthweight and age of the infant (i.e., not to normal ranges for older children and adults). The indications for plasma in neonates include: (1) reconstitution of red blood cell (RBC) concentrates to simulate whole blood for use in massive transfusions (exchange transfusion, cardiac bypass surgery, and extracorporeal membrane oxygenation); (2) hemorrhage secondary to vitamin K deficiency; (3) disseminated intravascular coagulation *with* bleeding; and (4) bleeding in congenital coagulation factor deficiency when more specific treatment is either unavailable or inappropriate. The use of prophylactic plasma transfusion to prevent intraventricular hemorrhage in premature infants is not recommended. Plasma should not be used as a suspending agent to adjust the hematocrit values of RBC concentrates before small-volume RBC transfusions to neonates because it offers no apparent medical benefit over the use of sterile solutions such as crystalloid and albumin. Similarly, the use of plasma in partial exchange transfusion for the treatment of neonatal hyperviscosity syndrome is unnecessary, because safer crystalloid or colloid solutions are available.

In the treatment of bleeding infants, cryoprecipitate is often considered because of its small infusion volume. However, cryoprecipitate contains significant quantities of only fibrinogen, von Willebrand factor, and factors VIII and XIII. Thus, it is not effective for treating the usual clinical situation in bleeding infants in which multiple clotting factor deficiencies exist.

In preliminary studies, infusions of very small volumes of recombinant activated factor VII have been lifesaving in patients with hemorrhage caused by several mechanisms. Because the efficacy and toxicity of factor VIIa have not been fully defined in these "off-label" uses (not approved by the U.S. Food and Drug Administration), it must be considered experimental therapy at this time.

Bibliography is available at Expert Consult.

Chapter 474
Risks of Blood Transfusions
Ronald G. Strauss

The greatest risk of a blood transfusion is receiving a transfusion intended for another patient; misidentification usually as a result of mistakes made labeling the patient's blood sample sent to the blood bank or not accurately matching the unit with the patient at the time the blood is transfused. This risk is particularly high for infants because identification bands may not be attached directly to their bodies, difficulties in drawing blood samples for pretransfusion compatibility testing may lead to deviations from usual policies, and infants cannot speak to identify themselves. Thus, particular care must be taken to ensure accurate patient and blood sample identification.

Although the infectious disease risks of allogeneic blood transfusions are extremely low, transfusions must be given judiciously because "emerging infections" are a constant threat, and testing is not done for every microorganism possibly transmitted by blood transfusions (Table 474-1, Fig. 474-1). Taking nucleic acid amplification testing

Table 474-1	Estimated Risks in Transfusion Per Unit Transfused in the United States
ADVERSE EFFECT	**ESTIMATED RISK**
Febrile reaction	1/300
Urticaria or other cutaneous reaction	1/50-100
Red blood cell alloimmunization	1/100
Mistransfusion	1/14,000-19,000
Hemolytic reaction	1/6,000
Fatal hemolysis	1/1,000,000
Transfusion-related acute lung injury (TRALI)	1/5,000
HIV1 and HIV2	1/2,000,000-3,000,000
Hepatitis B	1/100,000-200,000
Hepatitis C	1/1,000,000-2,000,000
Human T-cell lymphotrophic virus (HTLV) I and II	1/641,000
Bacterial contamination (usually platelets)	1/5,000,000
Malaria	1/4,000,000
Anaphylaxis	1/20,000-50,000
Graft-versus-host disease	Uncommon
Immunomodulation	Unknown
Hepatitis A	Unknown
Parvovirus	Unknown
Dengue fever	Unknown
Babesiosis	Unknown
West Nile virus	Unknown
Trypanosoma cruzi	Unknown
Leishmania spp.	Unknown
Variant Creutzfeldt-Jakob prion disease	Unknown

From Klein HG, Spahn DR, Carson JL: Red blood cell transfusion in clinical practice, Lancet 370:415–426, 2007.

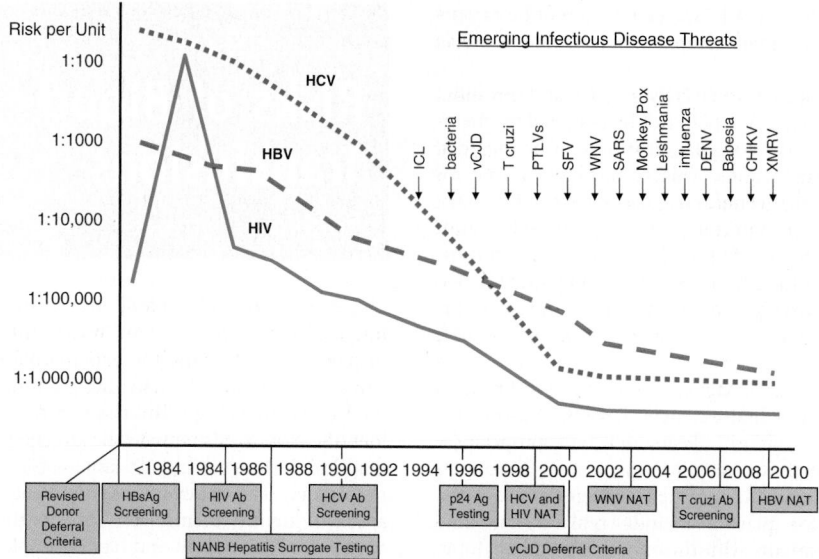

Figure 474-1 Risks of major transfusion-transmitted viruses related to interventions, and accelerating rate of emerging infectious diseases of concern to blood safety. Evolution of the risks of transmission by blood transfusion for HIV, hepatitis B virus, and hepatitis C virus. Major interventions to reduce risks are shown below the time line on the x axis. Emerging infectious disease threats in the past 20 yr are shown above in the top right quadrant of the figure. Ab, antibody; Ag, antigen; CHIKV, chikungunya virus; DENV, dengue virus; HBsAg, hepatitis B surface antigen; HBV, hepatitis B virus; HCV, hepatitis C virus; ICL, idiopathic CD4 T-lymphocytopenia; NANB, non-A, non-B hepatitis; NAT, nucleic acid testing; PTLVs, primate T lymphotropic viruses; SARS, severe acute respiratory syndrome; SFV, simian foamy virus; vCJD, variant Creutzfeldt-Jakob disease; WNV, West Nile virus; XMRV, xenotropic murine leukemia virus-related virus. *(From Busch MP. Transfusion-transmitted viral infections: building bridges to transfusion medicine to reduce risks and understand epidemiology and pathogenesis. 2005 Emily Cooley Award Lecture,* Transfusion *46:1624-1640, 2006.)*

(NAT) and all other donor-screening activities (antibody and epidemiology screening) into account, a current estimate of the risk of transfusion-associated HIV is approximately 1 per every 2,000,000 donor exposures. Similarly, with NAT, the risk of viral hepatitis C is 1 per every 1,500,000-2,000,000 donor exposures (Table 474-1). NAT identifies circulating viral nucleic acids that appear in the window period before antibodies develop, and NAT is used routinely to detect HIV, hepatitis C, and West Nile virus. NAT is also available for hepatitis B, but its use for this purpose is variable and controversial.

Transfusion-associated cytomegalovirus (CMV) has been nearly eliminated by transfusion of leukocyte-reduced cellular blood products or by selection of blood collected from donors who are seronegative for antibody to CMV. Although it is logical to hypothesize that first collecting blood components from CMV-seronegative donors and then removing the white blood cells might further improve safety, no data are available to document the superior efficacy of this combined approach. Importantly, considerable care must be taken not to place children at risk of delayed or missed transfusions while awaiting/searching for blood from CMV-seronegative donors to, then, leukocyte-reduce (i.e., risks must not be taken for practices with no established benefits).

Another consideration is that emerging data suggest that this combined approach using CMV-seronegative blood, surprisingly, may be incorrect. Large quantities of CMV viral material are present "free" in the plasma of healthy-appearing donors during the early phase of primary infection (while CMV antibodies are either absent ["window" phase] or are newly emerging and are at low inconsistently detected levels in plasma), rather than being leukocyte-associated as occurs with CMV as substantial quantities of immunoglobulin G antibodies appear. As a result of this biology of CMV primary infection, plasma "free" virus will not be removed by leukocyte-reduction during early infection, and CMV-seronegative donors who may be asymptomatic or deny symptoms of infection during blood donor screening will be misclassified as being CMV safe. They are not safe because antibody is below the limits of detection, while plasma "free" CMV is plentiful during early infection. Because nearly all plasma "free" CMV disappears and becomes almost exclusively cell-associated, once donors are

CMV-seropositive with antibody present for several months, it has been proposed that the best method to reduce CMV risk may be to effectively perform leukocyte reduction of blood from donors known to be CMV-seropositive for at least 1 year. However, data to prove the efficacy of this proposal are lacking, and in practice, several studies have shown that the most efficacious method currently available to prevent transfusion-transmitted CMV is to perform leukocyte-reduction in the blood center/bank without regard for the CMV-antibody status of the donor/unit (i.e., leukocyte-reduction alone performed by the blood center/bank is sufficient).

Additional infectious risks include other types of hepatitis (A, B, E) and retroviruses (human T-cell lymphotropic virus types I and II, and HIV-2), syphilis, parvovirus B19, Epstein-Barr virus, human herpesvirus 8, West Nile virus, yellow fever vaccine virus, malaria, babesiosis, *Anaplasma phagocytophilum,* and Chagas disease. Variant Creutzfeldt-Jacob disease has also been transmitted by blood transfusions in humans. All are reported very uncommonly, but nonetheless, provide the rationale to transfuse only when true benefits are likely.

Transfusion-associated risks of a noninfectious nature that may occur include hemolytic and nonhemolytic transfusion reactions, fluid overload, graft versus host disease, electrolyte and acid-base imbalances, iron overload if repeated transfusions are needed long term, increased susceptibility to oxidant damage, exposure to plasticizers, hemolysis with T-antigen activation of red blood cells, posttransfusion purpura, transfusion-related acute lung injury, post-transfusion immunosuppression and immunomodulation, and alloimmunization (see Table 474-1). The risk of transfusion-related acute lung injury may be reduced by reducing the use of plasma or platelets from female donors who were possibly sensitized during pregnancy or are negative for human leukocyte antigen (HLA) antibodies.

Immunologic adverse effects, including immunosuppression, immunomodulation, and alloimmunization may be reduced by leukocyte-reduction. Transfusion reactions and alloimmunization to red blood cell and leukocyte antigens seem to be uncommon in infants, perhaps because of developmental immaturity of the immune system or deficient cytokine production. When they do occur, adverse effects are seen primarily in massive transfusion settings, such as exchange transfusions and trauma or surgery, in which relatively large quantities of blood are needed but are rare with the small-volume transfusions usually given.

Premature infants are known to have immune dysfunction, but their relative risk of posttransfusion graft-versus-host disease is controversial. The postnatal age of the infant, the number of immunocompetent lymphocytes in the transfusion product, the degree of HLA compatibility between donor and recipient, and other poorly described phenomena determine which infants are truly at risk for graft-versus-host disease. Regardless, many centers caring for preterm infants transfuse exclusively irradiated cellular products. Directed donations with blood drawn from blood relatives must always be irradiated because of the risk of engraftment with transfused HLA-homozygous, haploidentical lymphocytes. Cellular blood products given as intrauterine and/or exchange transfusions should be irradiated, as are transfusions for patients with severe congenital immunodeficiency disorders (severe combined immunodeficiency syndrome and DiGeorge syndrome requiring heart surgery) and transfusions for recipients of hematopoietic progenitor cell transplants. Other groups who are potentially at risk but for whom no conclusive data are available include patients given T-cell antibody therapy (antithymocyte globulin or OKT3), those with organ allografts, those receiving immunosuppressive drug regimens, and those infected with HIV.

Current practice uses irradiation from a cesium, cobalt, or linear acceleration source at doses ranging from 2,500-5,000 cGy; a minimum dose of 2,500 cGy is required. All cellular blood components should be irradiated, but frozen "acellular" products, such as plasma and cryoprecipitate, do not require it. Leukocyte reduction cannot be substituted for irradiation to prevent graft versus host disease.

Bibliography is available at Expert Consult.

Section 7
Hemorrhagic and Thrombotic Diseases

Chapter 475
Hemostasis
J. Paul Scott and Leslie J. Raffini

Hemostasis is the active process that clots blood in areas of blood vessel injury yet simultaneously limits the clot size only to the areas of injury. Over time, the clot is lysed by the fibrinolytic system, and normal blood flow is restored. If clotting is impaired, hemorrhage occurs. If clotting is excessive, thrombotic complications ensue. The hemostatic response needs to be rapid and regulated such that trauma does not trigger a systemic reaction but must initiate a rapid, localized response. Key to the speed and coordination of response is that when a platelet adheres to a site of vascular injury, the platelet surface provides a reaction surface where clotting factors bind. The active enzyme is brought together with its substrate and a catalytic cofactor on a reaction surface, accelerating reaction rates and providing activated products for reaction with clotting factors further down the coagulation cascade. Active clotting is controlled by negative feedback loops that inhibit the clotting process when the procoagulant process comes in contact with intact endothelium. The main components of the hemostatic process are the **vessel wall, platelets, coagulation proteins, anticoagulant proteins,** and **fibrinolytic system.** Most components of hemostasis are multifunctional; fibrinogen serves as the ligand between platelets

during platelet aggregation and also serves as the substrate for thrombin that forms the fibrin clot. Platelets provide the reaction surface on which clotting reactions occur, form the plug at the site of vessel injury, and contract to constrict and limit clot size.

THE PROCESS
The intact vascular endothelium is the primary barrier against hemorrhage. The endothelial cells that line the vessel wall normally inhibit coagulation and provide a smooth surface that permits rapid blood flow.

After vascular injury, vasoconstriction occurs and flowing blood comes in contact with the subendothelial matrix (Fig. 475-1). In flowing blood, when exposed to subendothelial matrix proteins, von Willebrand factor (VWF) changes conformation and provides the glue to which the platelet VWF receptor, the glycoprotein Ib complex, binds, tethering platelets to sites of injury. When the VWF receptor binds its ligand, complex signaling occurs from the outside membrane receptor to intracellular pathways, activating the platelets and triggering secretion of storage granules containing adenosine diphosphate (ADP), serotonin, and stored plasma and platelet membrane proteins. Upon activation, the platelet receptor for fibrinogen, $\alpha IIb\beta_3$, is switched on ("inside out" signaling) to bind fibrinogen and triggers the aggregation and recruitment of other platelets to form the platelet plug. Multiple physiologic agonists can trigger platelet activation and aggregation, including ADP, collagen, thrombin, and arachidonic acid. Aggregation involves the interaction of specific receptors on the platelet surface with plasma hemostatic proteins, primarily fibrinogen.

One of the subendothelial matrix proteins that are exposed after vascular injury is tissue factor. Just as exposed subendothelial matrix proteins bind VWF, exposed tissue factor binds to factor VII and

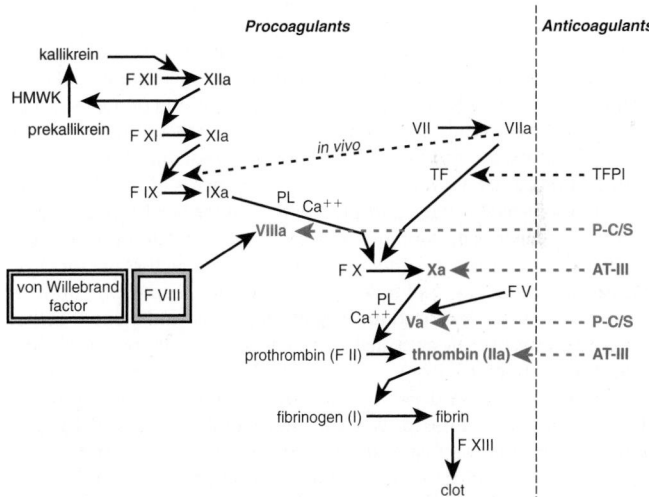

Figure 475-1 The clotting cascade, with sequential activation and amplification of clot formation. Many of the factors (F) are activated by the clotting factors shown above them in the cascade. The activated factors are designated by the addition of an *a*. On the right side, the major anticoagulants and the sites that they regulate are shown: Tissue factor pathway inhibitor (TFPI) regulates tissue factor [TF]); factor VIIa, protein C, and protein S (P-C/S) regulate factors VIII and V; and antithrombin III (AT-III) regulates factor Xa and thrombin (factor IIa). The *dotted line* shows that, in vivo, TF and factor VIIa activate both factors IX and X, but that, in vitro, only the activation of factor X is measured. Unactivated factor VIII, when bound to its carrier protein, von Willebrand factor, is protected from protein C inactivation. When thrombin, or factor Xa activates factor VIII, it becomes unbound from von Willebrand factor, whereupon it can participate with factor IXa in the activation of factor X in the presence of phospholipid (PL) and Ca^{2+} (the "tenase" complex). Factor XIIIa crosslinks the fibrin clot and thereby makes it more stable. Prekallikrein, high-molecular-weight kininogen (HMWK), and factor XII are shown in *blue* because they do not have a physiologic role in coagulation, although they contribute to the clotting time in partial thromboplastin time (PTT).

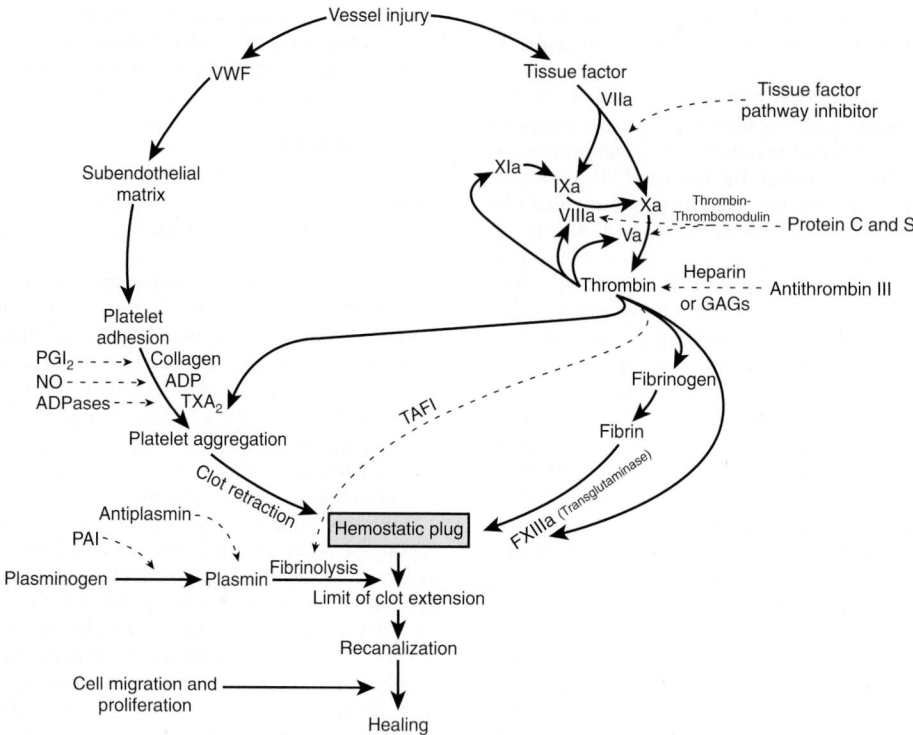

Figure 475-2 The hemostatic mechanism. ADP, adenosine diphosphate; GAGs, glycosaminoglycans; NO, nitric oxide; PGI₂, prostacyclin; PAI, plasminogen activator inhibitor; TAFI, thrombin-activated fibrinolytic inhibitor; TXA₂, thromboxane A₂; VWF, von Willebrand factor.

activates the clotting cascade, as shown in Figure 475-2. The activated clotting factor then initiates the activation of the next sequential clotting factor in a systematic manner. Our understanding of the sequence of steps in the cascade followed assignment of the numerals for the clotting factors for the participant proteins, and thus the sequence seems "out of numerical order." During the process of platelet activation, internalized platelet phospholipids (primarily phosphatidylserine) become externalized and interact at 2 specific, rate-limiting steps in the clotting process—those involving the cofactors factor VIII (X-ase complex) and factor V (prothrombinase complex). Both of these reactions are localized to the platelet surface and bring together the active enzyme, an activated cofactor, and the zymogen that will form the next active enzyme in the cascade. This sequence results in amplification of the process, which supplies a burst of clotting where it is physiologically needed. In vivo, autocatalysis of factor VII generates small amounts of VIIa continuously, so the system is always poised to act. Near the bottom of the cascade, the multipotent enzyme thrombin is formed. Thrombin converts fibrinogen into fibrin, activates factors V, VIII, and XI, and aggregates platelets. Activation of factor XI by thrombin amplifies further thrombin generation and contributes to inhibition of fibrinolysis. Thrombin also activates factor XIII. The stable fibrin-platelet plug is ultimately formed through clot retraction and cross linking of the fibrin clot by factor XIIIa.

Virtually all procoagulant proteins are balanced by an anticoagulant protein that regulates or inhibits procoagulant function. Four clinically important, naturally occurring anticoagulants regulate the extension of the clotting process: antithrombin III (AT-III), protein C, protein S, and tissue factor pathway inhibitor. AT-III is a serine protease inhibitor that regulates factor Xa and thrombin primarily and factors IXa, XIa, and XIIa to a lesser extent. When thrombin in flowing blood encounters intact endothelium, thrombin binds to thrombomodulin, its endothelial receptor. The thrombin–thrombomodulin complex then converts protein C into activated protein C. In the presence of the cofactor protein S, activated protein C proteolyses and inactivates factor Va and factor VIIIa. Inactivated factor Va is, in fact, a functional anticoagulant that inhibits clotting. Tissue factor pathway inhibitor

limits activation of factor X by factor VIIa and tissue factor and shifts the activation site of tissue factor and factor VIIa to that of factor IX (see Figs. 475-1 and 475-2).

Once a stable fibrin-platelet plug is formed, the fibrinolytic system limits its extension and also lyses the clot (fibrinolysis) to reestablish vascular integrity. Plasmin, generated from plasminogen by either urokinase-like or tissue-type plasminogen activator, degrades the fibrin clot. In the process of dissolving the fibrin clot, fibrin degradation products are produced. The fibrinolytic pathway is regulated by plasminogen activator inhibitors and α₂-antiplasmin, as well as by the thrombin-activatable fibrinolysis inhibitor. Finally, the flow of blood in and around the clot is crucial, because flowing blood returns to the liver, where activated clotting factor complexes are removed and new procoagulant and anticoagulant proteins are synthesized to maintain homeostasis of the hemostatic system.

PATHOLOGY

Congenital deficiency of an individual procoagulant protein leads to a bleeding disorder, whereas deficiency of an anticoagulant (clotting factor inhibitor) predisposes the patient to thrombosis. In acquired hemostatic disorders, there are frequently multiple problems with homeostasis that perturb and dysregulate hemostasis. A primary illness (sepsis) and its secondary effects (shock and acidosis) activate coagulation and fibrinolysis and impair the host's ability to restore normal hemostatic function. When sepsis triggers **disseminated intravascular coagulation,** platelets, procoagulant clotting factors, and anticoagulant proteins are consumed, leaving the hemostatic system unbalanced and prone to bleeding or clotting. Similarly, newborn infants and patients with severe liver disease have synthetic deficiencies of both procoagulant and anticoagulant proteins. Such dysregulation causes the patient to be predisposed to both hemorrhage and thrombosis with mild or moderate triggers that result in major alterations in the hemostatic process.

In the laboratory evaluation of hemostasis, parameters are manipulated to allow assessment of isolated aspects of hemostasis and limit the multifunctionality of some of its components. The coagulation process is studied in plasma anticoagulated with citrate to bind calcium, with added phospholipid to mimic the reaction surface normally provided by the platelet membrane and with a stimulus to trigger clotting. Calcium is added to restart the clotting process. This results in anomalies such that the in vivo physiologic pathway of clotting in which factor VIIa activates factor IX is bypassed; instead, in prothrombin time (PT), factor VIIa activates factor X. If this were truly the physiologic situation, then there would be an in vivo bypass mechanism that would ameliorate severe factor VIII and factor IX deficiencies, the 2 most common severe bleeding disorders.

475.1 Clinical and Laboratory Evaluation of Hemostasis

J. Paul Scott, Leslie J. Raffini, and Robert R. Montgomery

HISTORY

For most hemostatic disorders, the clinical history provides the most useful information. To evaluate for a bleeding disorder, the history should determine the site or sites of bleeding, the severity and duration of hemorrhage, and the age at onset. Was the bleeding spontaneous, or did it occur after trauma? Was there a previous personal or family history of similar problems? Did the symptoms correlate with the degree of injury or trauma? Does bruising occur spontaneously? Are there lumps with bruises for which there is minimal trauma? If the patient had previous surgery or significant dental procedures, was there any increased bleeding? If a child or adolescent has had surgery that affects the mucosal surfaces, such as a tonsillectomy or major dental extractions, the absence of bleeding usually rules out a hereditary bleeding disorder. Delayed or slow healing of superficial injuries may suggest a hereditary bleeding disorder. In postpubertal females, it is important to take a careful menstrual history. Because some common bleeding disorders, such as von Willebrand disease (VWD), have a fairly high prevalence, mothers and family members may have the same mild bleeding disorder and may not be cognizant that the child's menstrual history is abnormal. Women with mild VWD who have a moderate history of bruising frequently have a reduction of that bruising during pregnancy or after administration of oral contraceptives. Some medications, such as aspirin and other nonsteroidal antiinflammatory drugs, inhibit platelet function and increase bleeding symptoms in patients with a low platelet count or abnormal hemostasis. Standardized bleeding scores have been developed and are undergoing investigation for their sensitivity and specificity in children.

Outside the neonatal period, thrombotic disorders are relatively rare until adulthood. In the neonate, physiologic deficiencies of procoagulants and anticoagulants cause the hemostatic mechanism to be dysregulated, and clinical events can lead to either hemorrhage or thrombosis. If a child or teenager presents with deep venous thrombosis or pulmonary emboli, a detailed family history must be obtained to evaluate for deep venous thrombosis, pulmonary emboli, myocardial infarction, or stroke in other family members. The presence of thrombosis, especially in the absence of a provoking agent in the child or teenager, should induce the clinician to take a careful family history and consideration of evaluation for a hereditary or acquired predisposition to thrombosis.

PHYSICAL EXAMINATION

The physical examination should focus on whether bleeding symptoms are associated primarily with the mucous membranes or skin (mucocutaneous bleeding) or with the muscles and joints (deep bleeding). The examination should determine the presence of petechiae, ecchymoses, hematomas, hemarthroses, or mucous membrane bleeding. Patients with defects in platelet-blood vessel wall interaction (VWD or platelet function defects) usually have mucocutaneous bleeding, which may include epistaxis, menorrhagia, petechiae, ecchymoses, occasional hematomas and, less commonly, hematuria and gastrointestinal

bleeding. Individuals with a clotting factor deficiency of factor VIII or IX (hemophilia A or B) have symptoms of deep bleeding into muscles and joints, with much more extensive ecchymoses and hematoma formation. Patients with mild VWD or other mild bleeding disorders may have no abnormal findings on physical examination. Individuals with disorders of the collagen matrix and vessel wall may have loose joints and lax skin associated with easy bruising (**Ehlers-Danlos syndrome**).

Patients undergoing evaluation for thrombotic disorders should be asked about swollen, warm, tender extremities or internal organs (venous thrombosis), unexplained dyspnea or persistent "pneumonia," especially in the absence of fever (pulmonary emboli), and varicosities and postphlebitic changes. Arterial thrombi usually cause an acute, dramatic impairment of organ function, such as stroke, myocardial infarction, or a painful, white, cold extremity.

LABORATORY TESTS

In patients who have a positive bleeding history or who are actively hemorrhaging, a platelet count, PT, and partial thromboplastin time (PTT) should be performed as screening tests. In individuals with abnormal screening tests, further evaluation should be based upon those results. In a patient with an abnormal bleeding history and a positive family history, normal screening tests should not preclude further laboratory evaluation, which may include a thrombin time, VWF testing, and platelet function studies.

There are no useful routine screening tests for hereditary thrombotic disorders. If the family history is positive or clinical thrombosis is unexplained, specific thrombophilia assays should be performed. Thrombosis is rare in children, and when it is present, the possibility of a hereditary predisposition should be considered (see Chapter 478).

Platelet Count

Platelet count is essential in the evaluation of the child with a positive bleeding history because thrombocytopenia is the most common acquired cause of a bleeding diathesis in children. Patients with a platelet count of >50,000/mm³ rarely have significant clinical bleeding. Thrombocytosis in children is usually reactive and is not associated with bleeding or thrombotic complications. Persistent, severe thrombocytosis in the absence of an underlying illness may require evaluation for the very rare pediatric presentation of essential thrombocythemia or polycythemia vera.

Prothrombin Time and Activated Partial Thromboplastin Time

Because clotting factors were named in the order of discovery, they do not necessarily reflect the sequential order of activation (Table 475-1). In fact, factors III, IV, and VI were not subsequently found to be independent proteins; thus, these terms are no longer used. Only 2 factors have commonly used names: fibrinogen (factor I) and prothrombin (factor II). The dual mechanisms of activating clotting have been termed the **intrinsic** (surface activation) and **extrinsic** (tissue factor–mediated) pathways. Study of the hemostatic mechanism is further complicated in that the interactions in vivo may use different pathways from those studied in clinical laboratory testing. PT measures the activation of clotting by tissue factor (thromboplastin) in the presence of calcium. Addition of tissue factor causes a burst of factor VIIa generation. The tissue factor–factor VIIa complex activates factor X. Whether factor X is activated by the intrinsic or the extrinsic pathway, factor Xa on the platelet phospholipid surface complexes with factor V and calcium (the "prothrombinase" complex) to activate prothrombin to thrombin (also referred to as *factor IIa*). Once thrombin is generated, fibrinogen is converted to a fibrin clot, the end point of the reaction (see Fig. 475-2). PT is not prolonged with deficiencies of factors VIII, IX, XI, and XII. In most laboratories, the normal PT value is 10-13 sec. PT has been standardized using the **international normalized ratio (INR)** so that values can be compared from one laboratory or instrument to another. This ratio is used to determine similar degrees of anticoagulation with warfarin (Coumadin)–like medications.

Table 475-1	Coagulation Factors	
CLOTTING FACTOR	**SYNONYM**	**DISORDER**
I	Fibrinogen	Congenital deficiency (afibrinogenemia) or dysfunction (dysfibrinogenemia)
II	Prothrombin	Congenital deficiency or dysfunction
V	Labile factor, proaccelerin	Congenital deficiency (parahemophilia)
VII	Stable factor or proconvertin	Congenital deficiency
VIII	Antihemophilic factor	Congenital deficiency is hemophilia A (classic hemophilia)
IX	Christmas factor	Congenital deficiency is hemophilia B (sometimes referred to as Christmas disease)
X	Stuart-Prower factor	Congenital deficiency
XI	Plasma thromboplastin antecedent	Congenital deficiency (sometimes referred to as hemophilia C)
XII	Hageman factor	Congenital deficiency is not associated with clinical symptoms
XIII	Fibrin-stabilizing factor	Congenital deficiency

Partial Thromboplastin Time

The intrinsic pathway involves the initial activation of factor XII, which is accelerated by 2 other plasma proteins, prekallikrein and high-molecular-weight kininogen. In the clinical laboratory, factor XII is activated using a surface (silica or glass) or a contact activator, such as ellagic acid. Factor XIIa, in turn, activates factor XI to factor XIa, which then catalyzes factor IX to factor IXa. On the platelet phospholipid surface, factor IXa complexes with factor VIII and calcium to activate factor X ("tenase" complex).

This process is accelerated by interaction with phospholipid and calcium at the steps involving factors V and VIII. An isolated deficiency of a single clotting factor may result in isolated prolongation of PT, PTT, or both, depending on the location of the factor in the clotting cascade. This approach is useful in determining hereditary clotting factor deficiencies; however, in acquired hemostatic disorders encountered in clinical practice, >1 clotting factor is frequently deficient, so the relative prolongation of PT and PTT must be assessed.

Measurement of PTT as performed in the clinical laboratory is actually "activated" PTT; however, most refer to it as *PTT*. This test measures the initiation of clotting at the level of factor XII through sequential steps to the final clot end point. It does not measure factor VII, factor XIII, or anticoagulants. PTT uses a contact activator (silica, kaolin, or ellagic acid) in the presence of calcium and phospholipid. Because of differences in reagents and laboratory instruments, the normal range for PTT varies among hospital laboratories. Normal ranges for PTT are much more variable from laboratory to laboratory than those for PT.

Thus, the mechanisms studied by PT and PTT allow the evaluation of clotting factor deficiencies, even though these pathways may not be the same as those occurring physiologically. In vivo, factor VIIa activates factors IX and X, but as routinely studied in the clinical laboratory, the pathway through which factor VIIa activates factor IX is not evaluated. If the tissue factor–factor VIIa complex activated only factor X, it would be difficult to explain why the most severe bleeding disorders are deficiencies of factor VIII (hemophilia A) and factor IX (hemophilia B). In vivo, thrombin is generated and feeds back to activate factor XI and accelerate the clotting process. Clotting in PTT can be prolonged by deficiencies of factor XII, prekallikrein, and high-molecular-weight kininogen, yet these deficiencies are asymptomatic conditions.

Thrombin Time

Thrombin time measures the final step in the clotting cascade, in which fibrinogen is converted to fibrin. The normal thrombin time varies between laboratories but is usually 11-15 sec. Prolongation of thrombin time occurs with reduced fibrinogen levels (*hypofibrinogenemia* or *afibrinogenemia*), with dysfunctional fibrinogen (*dysfibrinogenemia*), or in the presence of substances that interfere with fibrin polymeriza-

tion, such as heparin and fibrin split products. If heparin contamination is a potential cause of prolonged thrombin time, a reptilase time is usually ordered. Alternatively, heparanase can be added to the sample and the thrombin time repeated.

Reptilase Time

Reptilase time uses snake venom to clot fibrinogen. Unlike thrombin time, reptilase time is not sensitive to heparin and is prolonged only by reduced or dysfunctional fibrinogen and fibrin split products. Therefore, if thrombin time is prolonged but reptilase time is normal, the prolonged thrombin time is due to heparin and does not indicate the presence of fibrin split products or reduced concentration or function of fibrinogen.

Mixing Studies

If there is unexplained prolongation of PT or PTT, a mixing study is usually performed. Normal plasma is added to the patient's plasma, and the PT or PTT is repeated. Correction of PT or PTT by 1 : 1 mixing with normal plasma suggests deficiency of a clotting factor, because a 50% level of individual clotting proteins is sufficient to produce normal PT or PTT. If the clotting time is not corrected or only partially corrected, an inhibitor is usually present. An inhibitor of clotting may be either a chemical similar to heparin that delays coagulation or an antibody directed against a specific clotting factor or the phospholipid used in clotting tests. In the inpatient setting, the most common cause of this finding is heparin contamination of the sample. The presence of heparin in the sample can be ruled in or out either by addition of heparinase to the sample and repeating the thrombin time. If the mixing study is not corrected or if its result becomes more prolonged and the patient has clinical bleeding, an inhibitor of a specific clotting factor (antibody directed against the factor), most commonly factor VIII, factor IX, or factor XI, may be present. If the patient has no bleeding symptoms and both PTT and the mixing study are prolonged, a lupus-like anticoagulant (see Chapter 476) is often present. Patients with these findings usually have a long PTT, do not bleed, and may have a clinical predisposition to excessive clotting.

Bleeding Time

Bleeding time assesses the function of platelets and their interaction with the vascular wall. Disposable standardized devices have been developed that control the length and depth of the skin incision. A blood pressure cuff is applied to the upper arm and inflated to 40 mm Hg for children and adults. In term newborns and younger children, a modified device has been developed that is used with a lower blood pressure cuff pressure. Bleeding time is a difficult laboratory test to standardize, and there is much interlaboratory and interindividual variation. Although platelet counts of <100,000/mm³ are associated with prolonged bleeding time, disproportionate prolongation of bleeding time may suggest a qualitative platelet defect or VWD. Use of the bleeding time is declining in many centers.

Platelet Function Analyzer

In an attempt to evaluate the early stages of hemostasis (platelet function and VWF interaction under high shear), several in vitro platelet analyzers have been developed. The greatest experience has been with the platelet function analyzer (PFA-100, Siemens Healthcare Diagnostics, Inc., Deerfield, IL). The PFA-100 measures platelet adhesion-aggregation in whole blood at high shear when exposed to either collagen-epinephrine or collagen-ADP. Results are reported as the closure time measured in sec. The PFA-100 appears to be sensitive to severe forms of VWD and platelet dysfunction. The PFA-100 has variable sensitivity, particularly in the detection of mild VWD and some platelet function defects. Its use as a preoperative screening tool has been disappointing in some studies.

D-Dimer

D-dimer is formed by plasmin degradation of crosslinked fibrin, produced when fibrinogen is clotted by thrombin and cross-linked by factor XIIIa and is more specific for fibrinolysis than fibrin degradation products. D-dimer is elevated in patients with disseminated intravascular coagulation or acute deep vein thrombosis but is relatively nonspecific in that other ill hospitalized patients often have elevated levels of D-dimer. Adult studies show that the D-dimer can be useful to help exclude venous thrombosis and pulmonary embolus because of its high negative predictive value; for example, a patient with a normal D-dimer value is unlikely to have an acute thrombosis.

Clotting Factor Assays

Each of the clotting factors can be measured in the clinical laboratory using individual factor–deficient plasmas. For most clotting factors, activity is measured against pooled normal plasma or against a standard, by which 100% activity is expressed as 100 IU/dL. By definition, 1 IU of each factor is defined as that amount in 1 mL of normal plasma referenced against a standard established by the World Health Organization. For most clotting factors, the normal range is 50-150 IU/dL (50-150%) (Table 475-2).

In patients with hemophilia A or hemophilia B, inhibitors of factor VIII or factor IX may develop after exposure to replacement therapy.

Table 475-2	Reference Values for Coagulation Tests in Healthy Children*						
TEST	**28-31 Wk GESTATION**	**30-36 Wk GESTATION**	**FULL TERM**	**1-5 Yr**	**6-10 Yr**	**11-18 Yr**	**ADULT**
SCREENING TESTS							
Prothrombin time (sec)	15.4 (14.6-16.9)	13.0 (10.6-16.2)	13.0 (10.1-15.9)	11 (10.6-11.4)	11.1 (10.1-12.0)	11.2 (10.2-12.0)	12 (11.0-14.0)
Activated partial thromboplastin time (sec)	108 (80-168)	53.6 (27.5-79.4)[‡§]	42.9 (31.3-54.3)[‡]	30 (24-36)	31 (26-36)	32 (26-37)	33 (27-40)
Bleeding time (min)				6 (2.5-10)[‡]	7 (2.5-13)[‡]	5 (3-8)[‡]	4 (1-7)
PROCOAGULANTS							
Fibrinogen	256 (160-550)	243 (150-373)[‡§]	283 (167-399)	276 (170-405)	279 (157-400)	300 (154-448)	278 (156-40)
Factor II	31 (19-54)	45 (20-77)[‡]	48 (26-70)[‡]	94 (71-116)[‡]	88 (67-107)[‡]	83 (61-104)[‡]	108 (70-146)
Factor V	65 (43-80)	88 (41-144)[§]	72 (34-108)[‡]	103 (79-127)	90 (63-116)[‡]	77 (55-99)[‡]	106 (62-150)
Factor VII	37 (24-76)	67 (21-113)[‡]	66 (28-104)[‡]	82 (55-116)[‡]	86 (52-120)[‡]	83 (58-115)[‡]	105 (67-143)
Factor VIII procoagulant	79 (37-126)	111 (5-213)	100 (50-178)	90 (59-142)	95 (58-132)	92 (53-131)	99 (50-149)
von Willebrand factor	141 (83-223)	136 (78-210)	153 (50-287)	82 (60-120)	95 (44-144)	100 (46-153)	92 (50-158)
Factor IX	18 (17-20)	35 (19-65)[‡§]	53 (15-91)[†‡]	73 (47-104)[‡]	75 (63-89)[‡]	82 (59-122)[‡]	109 (55-163)
Factor X	36 (25-64)	41 (11-71)[‡]	40 (12-68)[‡]	88 (58-116)[‡]	75 (55-101)[‡]	79 (50-117)	106 (70-152)
Factor XI	23 (11-33)	30 (8-52)[‡§]	38 (40-66)[‡]	30 (8-52)[‡]	38 (10-66)	74 (50-97)[‡]	97 (56-150)
Factor XII	25 (5-35)	38 (10-66)[‡§]	53 (13-93)[‡]	93 (64-129)	92 (60-140)	81 (34-137)[‡]	108 (52-164)
Prekallikrein	26 (15-32)	33 (9-89)[‡]	37 (18-69)[‡]	95 (65-130)	99 (66-131)	99 (53-145)	112 (62-162)
High-molecular-weight kininogen	32 (19-52)	49 (9-89)[‡]	54 (6-102)[‡]	98 (64-132)	93 (60-130)	91 (63-119)	92 (50-136)
Factor XIIIaⁱ		70 (32-108)[‡]	79 (27-131)[‡]	108 (72-143)	109 (65-151)	99 (57-140)	105 (55-155)
Factor XIIIbⁱ		81 (35-127)[‡]	76 (30-122)[‡]	113 (69-156)[‡]	116 (77-154)[‡]	102 (60-143)	98 (57-137)
ANTICOAGULANTS							
Antithrombin-III	28 (20-38)	38 (14-62)[‡§]	63 (39-87)[‡]	111 (82-139)	111 (90-131)	106 (77-132)	100 (74-126)
Protein C		28 (12-44)[‡§]	35 (17-53)[‡]	66 (40-92)[‡]	69 (45-93)[‡]	83 (55-111)[‡]	96 (64-128)
Protein S:							
Total (units/mL)		26 (14-38)[‡§]	36 (12-60)[‡]	86 (54-118)	78 (41-114)	72 (52-92)	81 (61-113)
Free (units/mL)				45 (21-69)	42 (22-62)	38 (26-55)	45 (27-61)
Plasminogen (units/mL)		170 (112-248)	195 (125-265)	98 (78-118)	92 (75-108)	86 (68-103)	99 (77-122)
Tissue-type plasminogen activator (ng/mL)		8.48 (3.00-16.70)	9.6 (5.0-18.9)	2.15 (1.0-4.5)[‡]	2.42 (1.0-5.0)[‡]	2.16 (1.0-4.0)[‡]	1.02 (0.68-1.36)
Antiplasmin (units/mL)		78 (40-116)	85 (55-115)	105 (93-117)	99 (89-110)	98 (78-118)	102 (68-136)
Plasminogen activator inhibitor-I		5.4 (0.0-12.2)[‡]	6.4 (2.0-15.1)	5.42 (1.0-10.0)	6.79 (2.0-12.0)[‡]	6.07 (2.0-10.0)[‡]	3.60 (0.0-11.0)

*All factors except fibrinogen are expressed as units/mL (fibrinogen in mg/mL), in which pooled normal plasma contains 1 unit/mL. All data are expressed as the mean, followed by the upper and lower boundaries encompassing 95% of the normal population (shown in parentheses). Normal ranges above vary based on the reagents and instruments used.

[†]Levels for 19-27 wk and 28-31 wk gestation are from multiple sources and cannot be analyzed statistically.

[‡]Values are significantly different from those of adults.

[§]Values are significantly different from those of full-term infants.

ⁱValue given as CTA (Committee on Thrombolytic Agents) units/mL. Normal ranges above vary based on the reagents and instruments used.

Data from Andrew M, Paes B, Johnston M: Development of the hemostatic system in the neonate and young infant, Am J Pediatr Hematol Oncol 12:95, 1990; and Andrew M, Vegh P, Johnston M, et al: Maturation of the hemostatic system during childhood, Blood 80:1998, 1992.

To quantitate the amount of inhibitor present, the standardized clinical assay of these clotting inhibitors is the Bethesda assay. One Bethesda unit is defined as the amount that will inhibit 50% of the clotting factor in normal plasma.

Platelet Aggregation

When a qualitative platelet function defect is suspected, platelet aggregation testing is usually ordered. Platelet-rich plasma from the patient is activated with 1 of a series of agonists (ADP, epinephrine, collagen, thrombin or thrombin-receptor peptide, and ristocetin). Some platelet aggregometers measure specific adenosine triphosphate release from the platelets, as reflected in generating luminescence (lumiaggregometer), and are more sensitive in detecting abnormalities of the platelet release reaction from storage granules. Repeat testing or testing of other symptomatic family members can help to determine the hereditary nature of the defect. Many medications, especially aspirin, other nonsteroidal antiinflammatory drugs, and valproic acid, alter platelet function testing. Figure 475-1 provides an approach to the differential diagnosis of many common bleeding disorders based on screening tests.

Testing for Thrombotic Predisposition

Hereditary predisposition to thrombosis is associated with a reduction of anticoagulant function (protein C, protein S, AT-III); the presence of a factor V molecule that is resistant to inactivation by protein C (factor V Leiden); elevated levels of procoagulants (a mutation of the prothrombin gene); or a deficiency of fibrinolysis (plasminogen deficiency); and the rare metabolic disease homocystinuria. When patients are being screened for prothrombotic tendencies, specific tests of the natural anticoagulants and polymerase chain reaction analysis for common prothrombotic mutations are warranted. Although both immunologic and functional tests are usually available, functional assays of protein C, protein S, and AT-III are clinically more useful.

Factor V Leiden is a common mutation in factor V that is associated with an increased risk of thrombosis. A point mutation in the factor V molecule prevents the inactivation of factor Va by activated protein C and, thereby, the persistence of factor Va. This defect, also known as *activated protein C resistance,* is easily diagnosed with DNA testing.

The **prothrombin gene mutation (G20210A)** is a mutation in the noncoding portion of the prothrombin gene, with a glycine (G) at position 20210 being replaced by an alanine (A). This mutation increases the amount of prothrombin messenger RNA, is associated with elevations of prothrombin, and causes a predisposition to thrombosis. This abnormality is easily identified with molecular diagnostic (DNA) testing.

Elevated Homocysteine

Levels of homocysteine may be increased as a result of genetic mutations, causing homocystinuria. Patients with homocysteine elevation are predisposed to arterial and venous thrombosis as well as to an increase in arteriosclerosis.

Tests of the Fibrinolytic System

Euglobulin clot lysis time is a screening test used in some laboratories to assess fibrinolysis. More specific tests are available in most laboratories to determine the levels of plasminogen, plasminogen activator, and inhibitors of fibrinolysis. An increase in fibrinolysis may be associated with hemorrhagic symptoms, and a delay in fibrinolysis is associated with thrombosis.

DEVELOPMENTAL HEMOSTASIS

The normal newborn infant has reduced levels of most procoagulants and anticoagulants (see Table 475-1). In general, there is a more marked abnormality in the preterm infant. Although major differences exist in the normal ranges for newborn and preterm infants, these ranges vary greatly among laboratories based upon the instruments and reagents used. During gestation, there is progressive maturation and increase of the clotting factors synthesized by the liver. The extremely premature infant has prolonged PT and PTT values as well

as a marked reduction in anticoagulant protein levels (protein C, protein S, and AT-III). Levels of fibrinogen, factors V and VIII, VWF, and platelets are near-normal throughout the later stages of gestation (see Chapter 103.4). Because protein C and protein S are physiologically reduced, the normal factors V and VIII are not balanced with their regulatory proteins. In contrast, the physiologic deficiency of vitamin K–dependent procoagulant proteins (factors II, VII, IX, and X) is partially balanced by the physiologic reduction of AT-III. The net effect is that newborns (especially premature infants) are at increased risk for complications of bleeding, clotting, or both.

Bibliography is available at Expert Consult.

Chapter **476**

Hereditary Clotting Factor Deficiencies (Bleeding Disorders)

J. Paul Scott and Veronica H. Flood

Hemophilia A (factor VIII deficiency) and **hemophilia B** (factor IX deficiency) are the most common and serious congenital coagulation factor deficiencies. The clinical findings in hemophilia A and hemophilia B are virtually identical. **Hemophilia C** is the bleeding disorder associated with reduced levels of factor XI (see Chapter 476.2). Reduced levels of the *contact factors* (factor XII, high-molecular-weight kininogen, and prekallikrein) are associated with significant prolongation of activated partial thromboplastin time (aPTT; also referred to as *PTT*), but are not associated with hemorrhage, as discussed in Chapter 476.3. Other coagulation factor deficiencies that are less common are briefly discussed in subsequent subchapters.

476.1 Factor VIII or Factor IX Deficiency (Hemophilia A or B)

J. Paul Scott

Deficiencies of factors VIII and IX are the most common severe inherited bleeding disorders. Recombinant factor VIII and factor IX concentrates are available to treat patients with hemophilia and thereby avoid the infectious risk of plasma-derived transfusion-transmitted diseases.

PATHOPHYSIOLOGY

Factors VIII and IX participate in a complex required for the activation of factor X. Together with phospholipid and calcium, they form the "tenase," or factor X–activating, complex. Figure 475-1 in Chapter 475 shows the clotting process as it occurs in the test tube, with factor X being activated by either the complex of factors VIII and IX or the complex of tissue factor and factor VII. In vivo, the complex of factor VIIa and tissue factor activates factor IX to initiate clotting. In the laboratory, prothrombin time (PT) measures the activation of factor X by factor VII and is therefore normal in patients with factor VIII or factor IX deficiency.

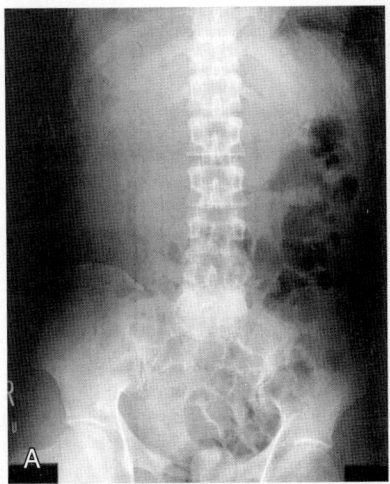
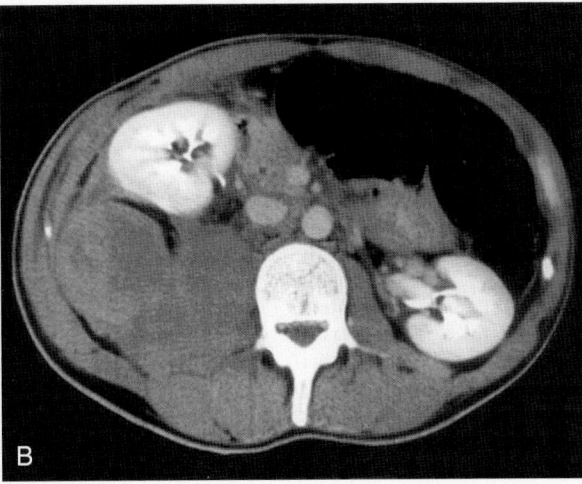
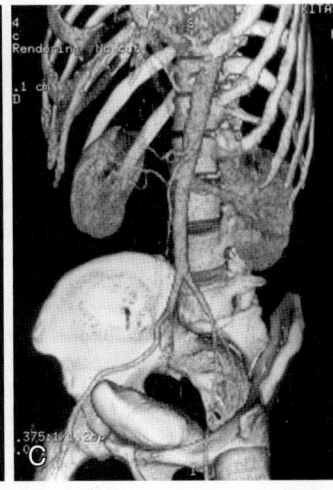

Figure 476-1 Massive hematoma into the iliopsoas muscle in a patient with hemophilia B. A 38 yr old man with severe deficiency of factor IX (hemophilia B) was admitted for right lower abdominal pain of progressively increasing severity and tenderness. He had had a common cold with severe cough and loss of appetite for approximately 1 wk. **A,** Abdominal radiograph shows presence of the psoas sign on the right side and left-shifted colon gas. **B,** CT scan shows massive hematoma in the right iliopsoas muscle, resulting in anterior translocation of the right kidney. **C,** Reconstructed 3-dimensional image shows more clearly the kidney translocation and the extended, but intact, large vessels. These are useful findings for the diagnostic procedures, because progressive right lower abdominal pain may closely simulate acute appendicitis. The hemorrhage was successfully managed by replacement of factor IX for 1 wk without any recurrence. The patient did not have any inhibitors to factor IX. *(From Miyazaki K, Higashihara M: Massive hemorrhage into the iliopsoas muscle,* Intern Med *44:158, 2005.)*

After injury, the initial hemostatic event is formation of the platelet plug, together with the generation of the fibrin clot that prevents further hemorrhage. In hemophilia A or B, clot formation is delayed and is not robust. Inadequate thrombin generation leads to failure to form a tightly crosslinked fibrin clot to support the platelet plug. Patients with hemophilia slowly form a soft, friable clot. When untreated bleeding occurs in a closed space, such as a joint, cessation of bleeding may be the result of tamponade. With open wounds, in which tamponade cannot occur, profuse bleeding may result in significant blood loss. The clot that is formed may be friable, and rebleeding occurs during the physiologic lysis of clots or with minimal new trauma.

CLINICAL MANIFESTATIONS

Neither factor VIII nor factor IX crosses the placenta; bleeding symptoms may be present from birth or may occur in the fetus. Only 2% of neonates with hemophilia sustain intracranial hemorrhages, and 30% of male infants with hemophilia bleed with circumcision. Thus, in the absence of a positive family history (hemophilia has a high rate of spontaneous mutation), hemophilia may go undiagnosed in the newborn. Obvious symptoms such as easy bruising, intramuscular hematomas, and hemarthroses begin when the child begins to cruise. Bleeding from minor traumatic lacerations of the mouth (a torn frenulum) may persist for hours or days and may cause the parents to seek medical evaluation. Even in patients with severe hemophilia, only 90% have evidence of increased bleeding by 1 yr of age. Although bleeding may occur in any area of the body, the hallmark of hemophilic bleeding is **hemarthrosis.** Bleeding into the joints may be induced by minor trauma; many hemarthroses are spontaneous. The earliest joint hemorrhages appear most commonly in the ankle. In the older child and adolescent, hemarthroses of the knees and elbows are also common. Whereas the child's early joint hemorrhages are recognized only after major swelling and fluid accumulation in the joint space, older children are frequently able to recognize bleeding before the physician does. They complain of a warm, tingling sensation in the joint as the first sign of an early joint hemorrhage. Repeated bleeding episodes into the same joint in a patient with severe hemophilia may become a "target" joint. Recurrent bleeding may then become spontaneous because of the underlying pathologic changes in the joint.

Although most muscular hemorrhages are clinically evident owing to localized pain or swelling, bleeding into the iliopsoas muscle requires

specific mention. A patient may lose large volumes of blood into the **iliopsoas muscle,** verging on hypovolemic shock, with only a vague area of referred pain in the groin. The hip is held in a flexed, internally rotated position owing to irritation of the iliopsoas. The diagnosis is made clinically from the inability to extend the hip but must be confirmed with ultrasonography or CT (Fig. 476-1). Life-threatening bleeding in the patient with hemophilia is caused by bleeding into vital structures (central nervous system, upper airway) or by exsanguination (external trauma, gastrointestinal or iliopsoas hemorrhage). Prompt treatment with clotting factor concentrate for these life-threatening hemorrhages is imperative. If head trauma is of sufficient concern to suggest radiologic evaluation, factor replacement should precede radiologic evaluation. Simply put: "Treat first, image second!" Life-threatening hemorrhages require replacement therapy to achieve a level equal to that of normal plasma (100 IU/dL, or 100%).

Patients with mild hemophilia who have factor VIII or factor IX levels >5 IU/dL usually do not have spontaneous hemorrhages. These individuals may experience prolonged bleeding after dental work, surgery, or injuries from moderate trauma and may not be diagnosed until they are older.

LABORATORY FINDINGS AND DIAGNOSIS

The laboratory screening test that is affected by a reduced level of factor VIII or factor IX is PTT. In severe hemophilia, the PTT value is usually 2-3 times the upper limit of normal. Results of the other screening tests of the hemostatic mechanism (platelet count, bleeding time, prothrombin time, and thrombin time) are normal. Unless the patient has an inhibitor to factor VIII or IX, the mixing of normal plasma with patient plasma results in correction of PTT value. The specific assay for factors VIII and IX will confirm the diagnosis of hemophilia. If correction does not occur on mixing, an inhibitor may be present. In 25-35% of patients with hemophilia who receive infusions of factor VIII or factor IX, a factor-specific antibody may develop. These antibodies are directed against the active clotting site and are termed *inhibitors.* In such patients, the quantitative Bethesda assay for inhibitors should be performed to measure the antibody titer.

DIFFERENTIAL DIAGNOSIS

In young infants with severe bleeding manifestations, the differential diagnosis includes severe thrombocytopenia; severe platelet function disorders, such as Bernard-Soulier syndrome and Glanzmann thrombasthenia; type 3 (severe) von Willebrand disease; and vitamin K deficiency. Hemostatic screening tests should differentiate these entities from hemophilia.

GENETICS AND CLASSIFICATION

Hemophilia occurs in approximately 1:5,000 males, with 85% having factor VIII deficiency and 10-15% having factor IX deficiency. Hemophilia shows no apparent racial predilection, appearing in all ethnic groups. The severity of hemophilia is classified on the basis of the patient's baseline level of factor VIII or factor IX, because factor levels usually correlate with the severity of bleeding symptoms. By definition, 1 IU of each factor is defined as that amount in 1 mL of normal plasma referenced against a standard established by the World Health Organization (WHO); thus, 100 mL of normal plasma has 100 IU/dL (100% activity) of each factor. For ease of discussion, henceforth in this chapter, we use the term % *activity* to refer to the percentage found in normal plasma (100% activity). Factor concentrates are also referenced against an international WHO standard, so treatment doses are usually referred to in IU. **Severe hemophilia** is characterized as having <1% activity of the specific clotting factor, and bleeding is often spontaneous. Patients with **moderate hemophilia** have factor levels of 1-5% and usually require mild trauma to induce bleeding. Individuals with **mild hemophilia** have levels >5%, may go many years before the condition is diagnosed, and frequently require significant trauma to cause bleeding. The hemostatic level for factor VIII is >30-40%, and for factor IX, it is >25-30%. The lower limit of levels for factors VIII and IX in normal individuals is approximately 50%.

The genes for factors VIII and IX are carried near the terminus of the long arm of the X chromosome and are therefore X-linked traits. The majority of patients with hemophilia have reduced clotting factor protein; 5-10% of those with hemophilia A and 40-50% of those with hemophilia B make a dysfunctional protein. Approximately 45-50% of patients with severe hemophilia A have the same mutation, in which there is an internal inversion within the factor VIII gene that results in production of no protein. This mutation can be detected in the blood of patients or carriers and in the amniotic fluid by molecular techniques. African-Americans often have a different factor VIII haplotype, and this difference may be the reason that African-Americans have higher inhibitor formation (see later). Because of the multiple genetic causes of either factor VIII or factor IX deficiency, most cases of hemophilia are classified according to the amount of factor VIII or factor IX clotting activity. In the newborn, factor VIII values may be artificially elevated because of the acute-phase response elicited by the birth process. This artificial elevation may cause a mildly affected patient to have normal or near-normal levels of factor VIII. Patients with severe hemophilia do not have detectable levels of factor VIII. In contrast, factor IX levels are physiologically low in the newborn. If severe hemophilia is present in the family, an undetectable level of factor IX is diagnostic of severe hemophilia B. In some patients with mild factor IX deficiency, the presence of hemophilia can be confirmed only after several weeks of life.

Through lyonization of the X chromosome, some **female carriers** of hemophilia A or B have sufficient reduction of factor VIII or factor IX to produce mild bleeding disorders. Levels of these factors should be determined in all known or potential carriers to assess the need for treatment in the event of surgery or clinical bleeding.

Because factor VIII is carried in plasma by von Willebrand factor, the ratio of factor VIII to von Willebrand factor is sometimes used to diagnose carriers of hemophilia. When possible, specific genetic mutations should be identified in the propositus and used to test other family members who are at risk of either having hemophilia or being carriers.

TREATMENT

Early, appropriate therapy is the hallmark of excellent hemophilia care. When mild to moderate bleeding occurs, values of factor VIII or factor IX must be raised to hemostatic levels, in the 35-50% range. For life-threatening or major hemorrhages, the dose should aim to achieve levels of 100% activity.

Calculation of the dose of recombinant factor VIII (FVIII) or recombinant factor IX (FIX) is as follows:

Dose of rFVIII (IU)

$$= \% \text{ desired (rise in rFVIII)} \times \text{Body weight (kg)} \times 0.5$$

Dose of rFIX (IU)

$$= \% \text{ desired (rise in plasma FIX)} \times \text{Body weight (kg)} \times 1.4$$

For factor VIII, the correction factor is based on the volume of distribution of factor VIII. For factor IX, the correction factor is based on the volume of distribution and the observed rise in plasma level after infusion of recombinant factor IX.

Table 476-1 summarizes the treatment of some common types of hemorrhage in a patient with hemophilia.

With the availability of recombinant replacement products, **prophylaxis is the standard of care** for most children with severe hemophilia, to prevent spontaneous bleeding and early joint deformities. In addition to currently available recombinant factors, products are being developed to increase the plasma half-life and reduce the immunogenicity of hemostatic factors. A study comparing prophylaxis with aggressive episodic treatment provides evidence for the superiority of prophylaxis in preventing debilitating joint disease. If target joints develop, "secondary" prophylaxis is often initiated.

With mild factor VIII hemophilia, the patient's endogenously produced factor VIII can be released by the administration of desmopressin acetate. In patients with moderate or severe factor VIII deficiency, the stored levels of factor VIII in the body are inadequate, and desmopressin treatment is ineffective. The risk of exposing the patient with mild hemophilia to transfusion-transmitted diseases and the cost of recombinant products warrant the use of desmopressin, if it is effective. A concentrated intranasal form of **desmopressin acetate**, not the enuresis or pituitary replacement dose, can also be used to treat patients with mild hemophilia A. The dose is 150 μg (1 puff) for children weighing <50 kg and 300 μg (2 puffs) for children and young adults weighing >50 kg. Most centers administer a trial of desmopressin to determine the level of factor VIII achieved after its infusion. Desmopressin is not effective in the treatment of factor IX–deficient hemophilia.

Preliminary trials of an adeno-associated virus vector containing the factor IX gene are underway with some encouraging initial results.

PROPHYLAXIS

Many patients are now given lifelong prophylaxis to prevent spontaneous joint bleeding. The National Hemophilia Foundation recommends that prophylaxis be considered optimal therapy for children with severe hemophilia. Usually, such programs are initiated with the first joint hemorrhage. Young children often require the insertion of a central catheter to ensure venous access. Such programs are expensive but are highly effective in preventing or greatly limiting the degree of joint pathology; however, complications include central line infection and thrombosis. Treatment is usually provided every 2-3 days to maintain a measurable plasma level of clotting factor (1-2%) when assayed just before the next infusion (trough level). Whether prophylaxis should be continued into adulthood has not yet been adequately studied. If moderate arthropathy develops, prevention of future bleeding will require higher plasma levels of clotting factors. In the older child who is not given primary prophylaxis, secondary prophylaxis is frequently initiated if a target joint develops.

SUPPORTIVE CARE

Although it is easy to tell parents that their child should avoid trauma, this advice is not practical in active children and adolescents. Toddlers are active, are curious about everything, and injure themselves easily. Effective measures include anticipatory guidance, including the use of car seats, seatbelts, and bike helmets, and the importance of avoiding high-risk behaviors. Older boys should be counseled to avoid violent contact sports, but this issue is a challenge. Boys with severe hemophilia often sustain hemorrhages in the absence of known trauma. Early psychosocial intervention helps the family achieve a balance

Table 476-1	Treatment of Hemophilia	
TYPE OF HEMORRHAGE	**HEMOPHILIA A**	**HEMOPHILIA B**
Hemarthrosis*	50-60 IU/kg factor VIII concentrate[†] on day 1; then 20-30 IU/kg on days 2, 3, 5 until joint function is normal or back to baseline. Consider additional treatment every other day for 7-10 days. Consider prophylaxis.	80-100 IU/kg on day 1; then 40 IU/kg on days 2, 4. Consider additional treatment every other day for 7-10 days. Consider prophylaxis.
Muscle or significant subcutaneous hematoma	50 IU/kg factor VIII concentrate; 20 IU/kg every-other-day treatment may be needed until resolved	80 IU/kg factor IX concentrate[‡]; treatment every 2-3 days may be needed until resolved
Mouth, deciduous tooth, or tooth extraction	20 IU/kg factor VIII concentrate; antifibrinolytic therapy; remove loose deciduous tooth	40 IU/kg factor IX concentrate[‡]; antifibrinolytic therapy[§]; remove loose deciduous tooth
Epistaxis	Apply pressure for 15-20 min; pack with petrolatum gauze; give antifibrinolytic therapy; 20 IU/kg factor VIII concentrate if this treatment fails[∣]	Apply pressure for 15-20 min; pack with petrolatum gauze; antifibrinolytic therapy; 30 IU/kg factor IX concentrate[‡] if this treatment fails
Major surgery, life-threatening hemorrhage	50-75 IU/kg factor VIII concentrate, then initiate 25 IU/kg q8-12h to maintain trough level >50 IU/dL for 5-7 days, then 50 IU/kg q24h to maintain trough >25 IU/dL for 7 days	120 IU/kg factor IX concentrate[‡], then 50-60 IU/kg every 12-24 hr to maintain factor IX at >40 IU/dL for 5-7 days, and then at >30 IU/dL for 7 days
Iliopsoas hemorrhage	50 IU/kg factor VIII concentrate, then 25 IU/kg every 12 hr until asymptomatic, then 20 IU/kg every other day for a total of 10-14 days**	120 IU/kg factor IX concentrate[‡]; then 50-60 IU/kg every 12-24 hr to maintain factor IX at >40 IU/dL until patient is asymptomatic; then 40-50 IU every other day for a total of 10-14 days**[††]
Hematuria	Bed rest; 1.5× maintenance fluids; if not controlled in 1-2 days, 20 IU/kg factor VIII concentrate; if not controlled, give prednisone (unless patient is HIV-infected)	Bed rest; 1.5× maintenance fluids; if not controlled in 1-2 days, 40 IU/kg factor IX concentrate[‡]; if not controlled, give prednisone (unless patient is HIV-infected)
Prophylaxis	20-40 IU/kg factor VIII concentrate every other day to achieve a trough level ≥1%	30-50 IU/kg factor IX concentrate[‡] every 2-3 days to achieve a trough level ≥1%

*For hip hemarthrosis, orthopedic evaluation for possible aspiration is advisable to prevent avascular necrosis of the femoral head.
[†]For mild or moderate hemophilia, desmopressin, 0.3 µg/kg, should be used instead of factor VIII concentrate, if the patient is known to respond with a hemostatic level of factor VIII; if repeated doses are given, monitor factor VIII levels for tachyphylaxis.
[‡]Stated doses apply for recombinant factor IX concentrate; for plasma-derived factor IX concentrate, use 70% of the stated dose.
[§]Do not give antifibrinolytic therapy until 4-6 hr after a dose of prothrombin complex concentrate.
[∣]Nonprescription coagulation-promoting products may be helpful.
**Repeat radiologic assessment should be performed before discontinuation of therapy.
[††]If repeated doses of factor IX concentrate are required, use highly purified, specific factor IX concentrate.
Adapted from Montgomery RR, Gill JC, Scott JP: Hemophilia and von Willebrand disease. In Nathan DG, Orkin SH, editors: Nathan and Oski's hematology of infancy and childhood, ed 5, Philadelphia, 1998, WB Saunders.

between overprotection and permissiveness. Patients with hemophilia should avoid aspirin and other nonsteroidal antiinflammatory drugs that affect platelet function. The child with a bleeding disorder should receive the appropriate vaccinations against hepatitis B, even though recombinant products may avoid exposure to transfusion-transmitted diseases. Patients exposed to plasma-derived products should be screened periodically for hepatitis B and C, HIV, and abnormalities in liver function.

CHRONIC COMPLICATIONS

Long-term complications of hemophilia A and B include chronic arthropathy, the development of an inhibitor to either factor VIII or factor IX, and the risk of transfusion-transmitted infectious diseases. Although an aggressive, or prophylactic, approach to treatment has reduced the problems of chronic arthropathy, these problems have not been eliminated.

Historically, chronic arthropathy has been the major long-term disability associated with hemophilia. The natural history of untreated hemophilia is one of cyclic recurrent hemorrhages into specific joints, including hemorrhages into the same (target) joint. In young children, the joint distends easily and a large volume of blood may fill the joint until tamponade ensues or therapy intervenes. After joint hemorrhage, proteolytic enzymes are released by white blood cells into the joint space, and heme iron induces macrophage proliferation, leading to inflammation of the synovium. The synovium thickens and develops frondlike projections into the joint that are susceptible to being pinched and may induce further hemorrhage. The cartilaginous surface becomes eroded and ultimately may even expose raw bone, leaving the

joint susceptible to articular fusion. In the older patient with advanced arthropathy, bleeding into the target joint, with its thickened synovium, causes severe pain, because the joint may have little space to accommodate blood. Once a target joint is seen to be developing, the patient is usually given short- or long-term prophylaxis to prevent progression of the arthropathy and reduce inflammation.

Inhibitor Formation

Infusion of the deficient clotting factor may initiate an immune response in patients with either factor VIII or factor IX deficiency. Inhibitors are antibodies directed against factor VIII or factor IX that block the clotting activity. Failure of a bleeding episode to respond to appropriate replacement therapy is usually the first sign of an inhibitor. Less often, inhibitors are identified during routine follow-up screening for inhibitors. Inhibitors develop in approximately 25-35% of patients with hemophilia A; the percentage is somewhat lower in patients with hemophilia B, many of whom make an inactive dysfunctional protein that renders them less susceptible to an immune response. Highly purified factor IX or recombinant factor IX seems to increase the frequency of inhibitor development, and some anti–factor IX inhibitors induce anaphylaxis. Many patients who have an inhibitor lose it with continued regular infusions. Others have a higher titer of antibody with subsequent infusions and may need to go through **desensitization** (immune tolerance induction) programs, in which high doses of factor VIII for hemophilia A or factor IX for hemophilia B are infused in an attempt to saturate the antibody and permit the body to develop tolerance. Factor IX immune tolerance programs have resulted in nephrotic syndrome in some patients. Rituximab has been used, off-label (i.e., in a use not approved by the FDA), as an alternate therapy for patients with high inhibitor titers in whom immune tolerance programs have failed. Some centers first begin with prednisone with or without cyclophosphamide; others add cyclosporine if there is a poor response. If desensitization fails, bleeding episodes are treated with either recombinant factor VIIa or activated prothrombin complex concentrates (factor VIII inhibitor bypassing activity). The use of these products bypasses the inhibitor in many instances but may increase the risk of thrombosis. Some patients with low titers of inhibitor can be treated with high-dose factor VIII during a bleeding episode. Patients with inhibitors require referral to a center that cares for many such patients and has a comprehensive hemophilia program.

In the past, plasma-derived treatment products transmitted hepatitis B and C as well as HIV to large numbers of patients with hemophilia. In the era of recombinant products, the risk of acquiring such infections should be minimal, but patients should receive appropriate immunizations against hepatitis B. Those who are exposed to blood products should be monitored for transfusion-related infections. Reports have also identified the transmission of variant Creutzfeldt-Jakob disease to patients receiving therapeutic plasma and may warrant study of patients with hemophilia for prion transmission from plasma-derived factor concentrates.

COMPREHENSIVE CARE

Patients with hemophilia are best managed through comprehensive hemophilia care centers. Such centers are dedicated to patient and family education as well as to the prevention and/or treatment of the complications of hemophilia, including chronic joint disease and inhibitor development as well as infection, such as hepatitis B and C or HIV. Such centers involve a team of physicians, nurses, orthopedists, physical therapists, and psychosocial workers, among others. Education remains crucial in hemophilia care, because patients who are receiving prophylaxis may be less "experienced" in recognizing bleeding episodes than affected children from previous eras.

Bibliography is available at Expert Consult.

476.2 Factor XI Deficiency (Hemophilia C)
J. Paul Scott

Factor XI deficiency is an autosomal deficiency associated with mild to moderate bleeding symptoms. It is frequently encountered in Ashkenazi Jews but has been found in many other ethnic groups. In Israel, 1-3/1,000 individuals are homozygous for this deficiency.

The bleeding tendency is not as severe as in factor VIII or factor IX deficiency. The bleeding associated with factor XI deficiency is not correlated with the amount of factor XI. Some patients with severe deficiency may have minimal or no symptoms at the time of major surgery. Because factor XI augments thrombin generation and leads to activation of the fibrinolytic inhibitor thrombin-activatable fibrinolysis inhibitor, surgical bleeding is more prominent in sites of high fibrinolytic activity like the oral cavity. Unless the patient previously had surgery without bleeding, replacement therapy should be considered and given preoperatively, depending on the nature of the surgical procedure. No approved concentrate of factor XI is available in the United States; therefore, the physician must use fresh-frozen plasma (FFP).

Bleeding during minor surgery can be controlled with local pressure. Patients undergoing dental extractions can be monitored closely and may benefit from treatment with fibrinolytic inhibitors like aminocaproic acid, with plasma replacement therapy used only if hemorrhage occurs. In a patient with homozygous deficiency of factor XI, PTT is often longer than it is in patients with either severe factor VIII or factor IX deficiency. The paradox of fewer clinical symptoms in combination with longer PTT is surprising, but it occurs because factor VIIa can activate factor IX in vivo. The deficiency of factor XI can be confirmed by specific factor XI assays. Plasma infusions of 1 IU/kg usually increase the plasma concentration by 2%. Thus, infusion of plasma at 10-15 mL/kg will result in a plasma level of 20-30%, which is usually sufficient to control moderate hemorrhage. Frequent infusions of plasma would be necessary to achieve higher levels of factor XI. Because the half-life of factor XI is usually ≥48 hr, maintaining adequate levels of factor XI commonly is not difficult.

Chronic joint bleeding is rarely a problem in factor XI deficiency, and for most patients, the deficiency is a concern only at the time of major surgery unless there is a second underlying hemostatic defect (e.g., von Willebrand disease).

Bibliography is available at Expert Consult.

476.3 Deficiencies of the Contact Factors (Nonbleeding Disorders)
J. Paul Scott

Deficiency of the "contact factors" (factor XII, prekallikrein, and high-molecular-weight kininogen) causes prolonged PTT but no bleeding symptoms. Because these contact factors function at the step of initiation of the intrinsic clotting system by the reagent used to determine PTT, the PTT is markedly prolonged when these factors are absent. Thus, there is the paradoxical situation in which PTT is extremely prolonged with no evidence of clinical bleeding. It is important that individuals with these findings be well informed about the meaning of their clotting factor deficiency because they do not need treatment, even for major surgery.

476.4 Factor VII Deficiency
J. Paul Scott

Factor VII deficiency is a rare autosomal bleeding disorder that is usually detected only in the homozygous state. Severity of bleeding varies from mild to severe with hemarthroses, spontaneous intracranial hemorrhage, and mucocutaneous bleeding, especially nosebleeds and menorrhagia. Patients with this deficiency have markedly prolonged PT but normal PTT. Factor VII assays show a marked reduction in factor VII. Because the plasma half-life of factor VII is 2-4 hr, therapy with FFP is difficult and is often complicated by fluid overload. A commercial concentrate of recombinant factor VIIa is effective in treating patients with factor VII deficiency.

Bibliography is available at Expert Consult.

476.5 Factor X Deficiency
J. Paul Scott

Factor X deficiency is a rare (estimated 1/1,000,000) autosomal disorder with variable severity. Mild deficiency results in mucocutaneous and posttraumatic bleeding, whereas severe deficiency results in spontaneous hemarthroses and intracranial hemorrhages. Factor X deficiency is the result of either a quantitative deficiency or a dysfunctional molecule. A reduced factor X level is associated with prolongation of both PT and PTT. In patients with hereditary factor X deficiency, factor X levels can be increased with use of either FFP or prothrombin complex concentrate. The half-life of factor X is approximately 30 hr, and its volume of distribution is similar to that of factor IX. Thus, 1 unit/kg will increase the plasma level of factor X by 1%.

Although it is rarely a problem in pediatric patients, **systemic amyloidosis** may be associated with factor X deficiency, owing to the adsorption of factor X on the amyloid protein. In the setting of amyloidosis, transfusion therapy often is not successful because of the rapid clearance of factor X.

476.6 Prothrombin (Factor II) Deficiency
J. Paul Scott

Prothrombin deficiency is caused either by a markedly reduced prothrombin level (hypoprothrombinemia) or by functionally abnormal prothrombin (dysprothrombinemia). Laboratory testing in homozygous patients shows prolonged PT and PTT. Factor II, or prothrombin, assays show a markedly reduced prothrombin level. Mucocutaneous bleeding in infancy and posttraumatic bleeding later are common. Patients are treated with either FFP or, rarely, prothrombin complex concentrates. In prothrombin deficiency, FFP is useful, because the half-life of prothrombin is 3.5 days. Administration of 1 IU/kg of prothrombin will increase the plasma activity by 1%.

Bibliography is available at Expert Consult.

476.7 Factor V Deficiency
J. Paul Scott

Deficiency of factor V is an autosomal recessive, mild to moderate bleeding disorder that has also been termed **parahemophilia.** Hemarthroses occur rarely; mucocutaneous bleeding and hematomas are the most common symptoms. Severe menorrhagia is a frequent symptom in women. Laboratory evaluation shows prolonged PTT and PT. Specific assays for factor V show a reduction in factor V levels. FFP is the only currently available therapeutic product that contains factor V. Factor V is lost rapidly from stored FFP. Patients with severe factor V deficiency are treated with infusions of FFP at 10 mL/kg every 12 hr. Rarely, a patient with a negative family history of bleeding has an acquired antibody to factor V. Often, such a patient does not bleed because the factor V in platelets prevents excessive bleeding.

Bibliography is available at Expert Consult.

476.8 Combined Deficiency of Factors V and VIII
J. Paul Scott

Combined deficiency of factors V and VIII occurs secondary to the absence of an intracellular transport protein that is responsible for transporting factors V and VIII from the endoplasmic reticulum to the Golgi compartments. This explains the paradoxical deficiency of 2 factors, one encoded on chromosome 1 and the other on the X chromosome. Bleeding symptoms are often milder than for hemophilia A and are treated with FFP to replace both factors V and VIII.

476.9 Fibrinogen (Factor I) Deficiency
J. Paul Scott

Congenital afibrinogenemia is a rare autosomal recessive disorder in which there is an absence of fibrinogen. Patients with this disorder do not bleed as frequently as patients with hemophilia and rarely have hemarthroses. Affected patients may present in the neonatal period with gastrointestinal hemorrhage or hematomas after vaginal delivery. In addition to marked prolongation of PT and PTT, thrombin time is prolonged. In the absence of consumptive coagulopathy, an unmeasur-

able fibrinogen level is diagnostic. In addition to the quantitative deficiency of fibrinogen, a number of dysfunctional fibrinogens have been reported (**dysfibrinogenemia**). Rarely patients with dysfibrinogenemia present with thrombosis. A human fibrinogen concentrate is commercially available for therapy of bleeding episodes in afibrinogenemic patients. Because the plasma half-life of fibrinogen is 2-4 days, treatment with either FFP or cryoprecipitate is also effective. The hemostatic level of fibrinogen is >60 mg/dL. Each bag of cryoprecipitate contains 100-150 mg of fibrinogen. Some clinical assays for fibrinogen are inhibited by high doses of heparin. Thus, a markedly prolonged thrombin time associated with a low fibrinogen level should be evaluated with determination of reptilase time. Prolonged reptilase time confirms that functional levels of fibrinogen are low and that heparin is not present.

476.10 Factor XIII Deficiency (Fibrin-Stabilizing Factor or Transglutaminase Deficiency)
J. Paul Scott

Because factor XIII is responsible for the crosslinking of fibrin to stabilize the fibrin clot, symptoms of delayed hemorrhage are secondary to instability of the clot. Typically, patients have trauma 1 day and then have a bruise or hematoma the next day. Clinical symptoms include mild bruising, delayed separation of the umbilical stump beyond 4 wk in neonates, poor wound healing, and recurrent spontaneous abortions in women. Rare kindreds with XIII deficiency with hemarthroses and intracranial hemorrhage have been described. Results of the usual screening tests for hemostasis are normal in patients with factor XIII deficiency. Screening tests for factor XIII deficiency are based on the observation that there is increased solubility of the clot because of the failure of crosslinking. The normal clot remains insoluble in the presence of 5M urea, whereas in a patient with XIII deficiency, the clot dissolves. More specific assays for factor XIII are immunologic. The half-life of factor XIII is 5-7 days and the hemostatic level is 2-3% activity. There is a heat-treated, lyophilized concentrate of coagulation factor XIII available to treat bleeding episodes or for prophylaxis.

Bibliography is available at Expert Consult.

476.11 Antiplasmin or Plasminogen Activator Inhibitor Deficiency
J. Paul Scott

Deficiency of either antiplasmin or plasminogen activator inhibitor, both of which are antifibrinolytic proteins, results in increased plasmin generation and premature lysis of fibrin clots. Affected patients have a mild bleeding disorder characterized by mucocutaneous bleeding but rarely have joint hemorrhages. Because results of the usual hemostatic tests are normal, further work-up of a patient with a positive bleeding history should include euglobulin clot lysis time (if available), which measures fibrinolytic activity and yields a shortened result in the presence of these deficiencies. Specific assays for α_2-antiplasmin and plasminogen activator inhibitor are available. Bleeding episodes are treated with FFP; bleeding in the oral cavity may respond to aminocaproic acid.

Bibliography is available at Expert Consult.

Chapter **477**

Von Willebrand Disease

Veronica H. Flood and J. Paul Scott

von Willebrand disease (VWD) is the most common inherited bleeding disorder, with an estimated prevalence cited at 1 : 100 to 1 : 10,000 depending on the criteria used for diagnosis. Patients with VWD typically present with mucosal bleeding. A family history of either VWD or bleeding symptoms and confirmatory laboratory testing are also required for the diagnosis of VWD.

PATHOPHYSIOLOGY

VWD is caused by a defect in von Willebrand factor (VWF). VWF has several functions in coagulation. First, VWF serves to tether platelets to injured subendothelium via binding sites for platelets and for collagen. Second, VWF serves as a carrier protein for factor VIII (FVIII), protecting FVIII from degradation in plasma. VWF is stored in endothelial cells and in platelet Weibel-Palade bodies and circulates as a large multimeric glycoprotein. Shear stress induces a conformational change in VWF that facilitates its ability to bind platelets through a binding site on platelet glycoprotein Ib (GPIb). This enables VWF to recruit platelets to the site of clot formation, a function that is dependent on the high-molecular-weight multimer forms of VWF.

VWD typically presents with mucosal bleeding, similar to that seen with other platelet defects. Epistaxis, easy bruising, and menorrhagia in women are common complaints. Symptoms, however, are variable, and do not necessarily correlate well with VWF levels. Surgical bleeding, particularly with dental extractions or adenotonsillectomy, is another common presentation. Severe type 3 VWD may present with joint bleeds. Most patients will have a family history of bleeding. Women are more likely to be diagnosed with VWD because of the potential for symptoms with menorrhagia, but men and women are equally likely to have VWD. Diagnosis based on symptoms may be difficult, however, as minor bruising and epistaxis are not uncommon in childhood. Significant unexplained bruising is more often from nonaccidental trauma than from an underlying bleeding disorder.

CLASSIFICATION

VWD may be caused by quantitative or qualitative defects in VWF. Mild to moderate quantitative defects are classified as type 1 VWD, while severe quantitative defects, in which there is no detectable VWF protein, are classified as type 3 VWD. The qualitative defects are grouped together as type 2 VWD.

Type 1 VWD is by far the most common type, accounting for 60-80% of all VWD patients. Typical symptoms include mucosal bleeding, such as epistaxis and menorrhagia as well as easy bruising and potentially surgical bleeding. Guidelines from the National Heart, Lung, and Blood Institute of the National Institutes of Health use a VWF level, as measured by the VWF antigen assay (VWF : Ag), of <30 IU/dL for diagnosis of VWD. Patients with VWF : Ag <20-30 IU/dL are most likely to have a genetic defect in VWF. Patients with VWF : Ag between 30 and 50 IU/dL are said to have "low VWF." Whether or not this category truly represents VWD is a subject of some debate. Because some patients with VWF levels in this range do experience bleeding, many physicians elect to treat them, especially for surgeries such as tonsillectomy.

Patients with low VWF may have VWD as a result of increased clearance of their VWF, or type 1C VWD. Diagnosis of this subtype is important because treatment of these patients with desmopressin is likely to be ineffective, necessitating administration of VWF-containing products.

VWF levels can be influenced by external factors. Blood type has long been known to affect VWF, with lower VWF levels seen in people with blood group O. Stress, exercise, and pregnancy all increase VWF levels; therefore, a single normal VWF level does not necessarily rule out the presence of VWD. Certain diseases, such as *hypothyroidism*, and medications, such as *valproic acid*, can lower VWF levels in affected patients. Repeat testing may be required to rule out or confirm a diagnosis of VWD.

Type 3 VWD is the most severe form and presents with symptoms similar to those seen in mild hemophilia. In type 3 VWD, the VWF protein is completely absent. Type 3 VWD is seen at a frequency of approximately 1 in 1,000,000. In addition to mucosal bleeding, patients may experience joint bleeds or central nervous system hemorrhage. Some physicians elect to treat patients with prophylaxis, or modified prophylaxis following injury, given that these patients typically have very low FVIII (<10 IU/dL). Because type 3 VWD is caused by a lack of VWF, treatment with VWF-containing concentrates is required.

Type 2A VWD is characterized by a defect in VWF multimerization and decreased VWF activity in terms of platelet binding. It is the most common of the type 2 variants, accounting for approximately 10% of VWD cases. Type 2A VWD can result from mutations that affect multimer assembly and processing, or mutations that result in increased proteolysis of secreted VWF. Some mutations affect both secretion and clearance of the VWF. Regardless of the mechanism, all type 2A VWD patients lack the high-molecular-weight multimers, and therefore have reduced VWF activity which results in bleeding. Symptoms are typically more severe than those seen in type 1 VWD. Desmopressin may have clinical efficacy for treatment of minor bleeding, but significant surgical challenges or major bleeding symptoms generally require a VWF-containing concentrate for treatment.

Type 2B VWD results from gain-of-function mutations that increase the ability of VWF to bind platelets. This leads to increased clearance of both VWF and platelets from circulation and results in the loss of high-molecular-weight multimers and decreased VWF activity, similar to that seen in type 2A VWD. Special testing is, therefore, required to diagnose type 2B VWD, either by direct measurement of the increased platelet binding or by an increased response to low-dose ristocetin on platelet aggregation testing. Thrombocytopenia is not always present and may be more prominent during times of stress such as surgery or pregnancy. Desmopressin is relatively contraindicated in type 2B VWD as it may accelerate VWF-platelet binding and clearance.

Platelet-type, pseudo-VWD occurs when a mutation in platelet GPIb causes spontaneous binding to VWF and also presents with decreased VWF activity, loss of high-molecular-weight multimers, and thrombocytopenia similar to type 2B VWD. Specific testing is required to distinguish the 2 conditions. Because the defect involves platelets, treatment generally requires platelet transfusion.

Type 2M VWD includes those patients with decreased VWF activity but normal (or near-normal) multimer distribution. This is generally caused by a defect in the ability of VWF to bind platelet GPIb, but this category also includes patients with defects in VWF-collagen interactions. Some minor bleeding in type 2M VWD may respond to desmopressin, but because type 2M VWD is a functional defect, treatment with VWF-containing concentrates is usually required.

Type 2N VWD is characterized by a defect in the ability of VWF to bind FVIII. Some patients with type 2N VWD may be misdiagnosed as mild hemophilia, therefore a high index of suspicion for this diagnosis is required in patients with low FVIII and an absent family history of FVIII deficiency.

LABORATORY DIAGNOSIS

There are no reliable screening tests for VWD. Patients with significant bleeding may present with anemia, and some patients with type 2B VWD or platelet-type, pseudo-VWD may have thrombocytopenia. The partial thromboplastin time may be prolonged if FVIII is low, but especially in mild type 1 VWD it is often normal, precluding use of the partial thromboplastin time as a screening test. Platelet function analysis has been considered as a screening test for VWD, but suboptimal

	Normal	Type 1	Type 1C (Vicenza)	Type 3	Type 2A	Type 2B	Type 2N	Type 2M	PT-VWD
VWF:Ag	N	↓	↓↓	absent	↓	↓	N or ↓	↓ or N	↓
VWF:RCo	N	↓	↓↓	absent	↓↓↓	↓↓	N or ↓	↓↓	↓↓
FVIII:C	N	N or ↓	↓	2-10 IU/dL	N or ↓	N or ↓	↓↓	N	N or ↓
VWFpp/VWF:Ag ratio	N	N	↑↑	absent	N or ↑	↑	N	N	↑
RIPA	N	often N	↓	absent	↓	often N	N	N or ↓	often N
LD-RIPA	absent	absent	absent	absent	absent	↑↑↑	absent	absent	↑↑↑
PFA'	N	N or ↑	↑	↑↑↑	↑	↑	N	↑	↑
BT'	N	N or ↑	↑	↑↑↑	↑	↑	N	↑	↑
Platelet count	N	N	N	N	N	↓ or N	N	N	↓
VWF multimers	N	N but ↓	N but ↓	absent	abnormal	abnormal	N but ↓	N but ↓	abnormal

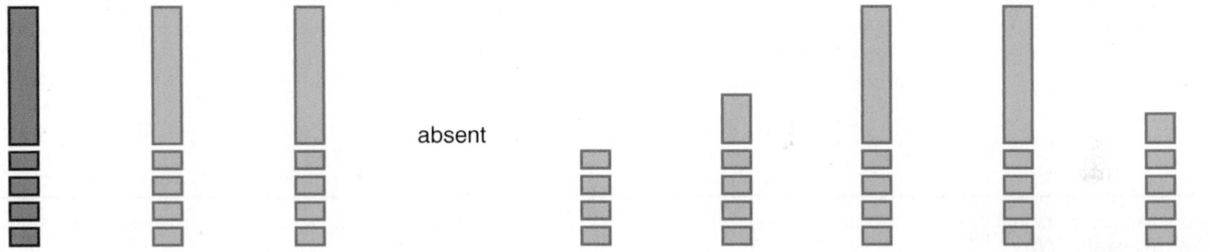

Figure 477-1 Specialized laboratory testing for VWD. ↓,↓↓,↓↓↓, Relative decrease; ↑,↑↑,↑↑↑, relative increase; BT, bleeding time; FVIII:C, factor VIII coagulant activity; LD-RIPA, low-dose ristocetin-induced platelet aggregation; N, normal; N but ↓, normal but decreased in intensity; PT-VWD, platelet-type VWD; RIPA, ristocetin-induced platelet aggregation; VWF:Ag, VWF antigen; VWF:RCo, VWF activity by ristocetin cofactor; VWFpp, VWF propeptide. *(Courtesy of Dr. Robert R. Montgomery.)*

Table 477-1	Laboratory Testing for VWD	
TEST	**ABBREVIATION**	**PURPOSE**
VWF antigen	VWF:Ag	Measures total amount of VWF protein present
VWF activity	VWF:RCo	Assess interaction of VWF and platelets as mediated by ristocetin
VWF activity/antigen ratio	VWF:RCo/VWF:Ag	A decreased ratio (<0.7) is found in type 2A, type 2B, and type 2M VWD
Factor VIII activity	FVIII	Measures circulating FVIII, which will be very low in type 2N and type 3 VWD
Multimer distribution	VWF multimers	Allows visualization of VWF multimers, used to identify high-molecular-weight multimers, which will be absent in types 2A and 2B VWD

sensitivity and specificity render results difficult to interpret. Bleeding times are similarly unreliable in diagnosis of VWD.

Unfortunately there is no single test that can reliably diagnose VWD. Therefore a panel of tests is usually required. Table 477-1 lists the laboratory tests commonly used in diagnosis of VWD. These include VWF antigen (VWF:Ag), which measures the total amount of VWF protein present, and VWF activity, which is typically performed using the ristocetin cofactor activity assay (VWF:RCo) and provides a measure of the amount of functional VWF. FVIII activity is also usually included in the workup. Another important test is the VWF multimer distribution, although this is not routinely performed by all laboratories. Table 477-2 summarizes the expected laboratory findings for each type of VWD. Figure 477-1 provides more detailed analysis.

Additional specialized testing may be employed to help ascertain the correct diagnosis. Specific testing for type 1C (clearance defects), type 2B, and type 2N VWD can confirm these diagnoses. Genetic diagnosis is not typically performed, partly as a result of the large size of the VWF gene and the large number of benign sequence variations. Large gene

deletions are responsible for some cases of VWD and will not be picked up on routine DNA sequencing. Use of genetic diagnosis is increasing, however, particularly for types 2A, 2B, 2M, and 2N VWD.

TREATMENT
Treatment of VWD depends on the type of VWD present and on the reason for treatment. Table 477-3 outlines the options for treatment. In general, type 1 VWD patients may be treated with desmopressin, which increases the amount of circulating VWF by release from storage. The exceptions are the rare type 1 patient who lacks a response to desmopressin, and patients with type 1C VWD who do respond with an increase in VWF levels, but whose rapid clearance of circulating endogenous VWF results in a rapid return to baseline levels. Treatment of types 2 and 3 VWD requires VWF-containing concentrates similar to the treatment of hemophilia. Dosing depends on the type of VWD, and reason for treatment. Careful monitoring of VWF and FVIII levels is recommended to tailor treatment for surgeries and major trauma. For all types of VWD, adjunct therapy should be

| Table 477-2 | VWD Classification |

	TYPE 1	TYPE 3	TYPE 2A	TYPE 2B*	TYPE 2M	TYPE 2N
VWF:Ag	↓	Absent	↓	↓	↓	Normal or ↓
VWF:RCo	↓	Absent	↓↓	↓↓	↓↓	Normal or ↓
FVIII	Normal	↓↓	Normal or ↓	Normal or ↓	Normal or ↓	↓↓
Multimer distribution	Normal	Absent	Loss of HMWM	Loss of HMWM	Normal	Normal

*Platelet count is also usually decreased in type 2B VWD.
FVIII, factor VIII; HMWM, high-molecular-weight multimers; VWF:Ag, VWF antigen; VWF:RCo, VWF ristocetin cofactor activity.

| Table 477-3 | VWD Treatment |

TREATMENT	VWD TYPES	ADMINISTRATION	DOSING
Desmopressin*	Type 1 VWD Some type 2 VWD (use with caution)	IV or IN	0.3 µg/kg IV† 1 spray IN (<50 kg) 2 sprays IN (>50 kg)
von Willebrand factor concentrates‡	Type 3 VWD Type 2 VWD Severe type 1 VWD (or type 1 clearance defects)	IV	40-60 ristocetin cofactor activity units/kg (adjust dose depending on baseline VWF level and desired peak VWF level)
Antifibrinolytics	Mucosal bleeding, all types of VWD	PO or IV	Aminocaproic acid: 100 mg/kg PO loading dose followed by 50 mg/kg q 6 hours§ Tranexamic acid: 1300 mg PO tid × 5 days

*Recommended treatment with Stimate brand nasal spray, as this form is concentrated to give 150 µg/spray. Other forms are much more dilute and will not result in desired increase in VWF.
†Maximum recommended dose is 20-30 µg/day.
‡Currently both Humate-P and Wilate are approved for treatment of VWD. A recombinant VWF preparation is currently undergoing clinical trials.
§Maximum recommended dose is 24 g/day.
IN, intranasal; IV, intravenous; PO, oral administration.

considered when possible, such as the use of antifibrinolytics for oral surgery or hormonal treatment for menorrhagia.

Alternate treatment strategies should also be considered, particularly for difficult symptoms or severe VWD. Hormonal therapy for women with menorrhagia, although not specific to VWD, can be very helpful in managing symptoms and improving quality of life. Local treatment of epistaxis, such as nasal cautery or packing, may be helpful in some circumstances. Iron therapy for patients with iron-deficiency anemia may also be required.

Bibliography is available at Expert Consult.

Chapter 478
Hereditary Predisposition to Thrombosis
Leslie J. Raffini and J. Paul Scott

Pediatricians are frequently asked to evaluate children for inherited risk factors for thrombosis with symptomatic thrombosis or asymptomatic children who have relatives affected with either thrombosis or thrombophilia. The clinical utility of thrombophilia testing is debated, both in adults and children.

Thrombophilia testing rarely influences the acute management of a child with a thrombotic event. The association between inherited thrombophilia and pediatric thrombosis varies based on the clinical scenario: children with unprovoked thrombotic events have a high prevalence of inherited defects, while the role of thrombophilic defects in children with catheter-related thrombotic events is questionable. Although some thrombophilic defects are associated with a higher risk of recurrent venous thromboembolism in children, how to use these results to guide the duration of therapy has not been determined. Prospective longitudinal analyses of such patients to determine outcome and response to treatment as well as the impact of known thrombophilic states on these outcomes are clearly needed.

The decision to perform thrombophilia testing in an otherwise healthy child with a family history of thrombosis or thrombophilia should be carefully considered, weighing the potential advantages and limitations of such an approach. Given that the absolute risk of thrombosis in children is extremely low (0.07/100,000), it is unlikely that an inherited thrombophilia will have any impact on clinical decision-making for a young child. The risk of thrombosis increases with age, so identification of a thrombophilic defect in an adolescent may guide thromboprophylaxis in high-risk situations (lower extremity casting or prolonged immobility), inform the discussion about estrogen-based contraceptives, and promote lifestyle modification to avoid behavioral prothrombotic risk factors (sedentary lifestyle, dehydration, obesity, and smoking). Limitations of such testing include the cost as well as the potential for causing unnecessary anxiety or false reassurance.

Table 478-1 lists the most common inherited thrombophilias and their prevalence in the general population. The inherited defects in which the pathogenic link is best understood include the factor V Leiden mutation, the prothrombin gene mutation, and deficiencies of

Table 478-1	Common Inherited Thrombophilias and Accompanying Diagnostic Laboratory Studies		
THROMBOPHILIA	**PREVALENCE IN WHITE POPULATION %**	**ODDS RATIO FOR FIRST EPISODE VTE IN CHILDHOOD***	**LABORATORY STUDIES**
Factor V Leiden mutation			DNA-based PCR assay (or screen with activated protein C resistance)
Heterozygote	3-7	3.8	
Homozygote	0.06-0.25	80-100	
Prothrombin 20210 mutation			DNA-based PCR assay
Heterozygote	1-3	2.6	
Homozygote	–	–	
Antithrombin deficiency	0.02-0.04	9.4	Antithrombin activity via chromogenic or clotting assay
Protein S deficiency	0.03-0.13	5.8	Protein S activity via assay or immunologic assay of free and total protein S antigen
Protein C deficiency	0.2	7.7	Protein C activity via chromogenic or clotting assay
Hyperhomocystinemia	–	–	Fasting homocysteine
Elevated VIII	–	–	Factor VIII activity via one-stage clotting or chromogenic assay

*Data from Young G, Albisetti M, Bonduel M, et al: Impact of inherited thrombophilia on venous thromboembolism in children. *Circulation* 118:1373–1382, 2008.
PCR, polymerase chain reaction; VTE, venous thromboembolism.

protein C, protein S, and antithrombin (AT). Elevated levels of factor VIII and homocysteine are associated with thrombosis, though these are less-well characterized and not necessarily genetically determined. Although there are additional alterations in coagulation that have been associated with thrombotic risk, including elevated concentrations of factors IX and XI, heparin cofactor II deficiency, elevated lipoprotein (a), and dysfibrinogenemia, none has gained widespread acceptance in routine testing of children for inherited thrombophilia.

The **factor V Leiden mutation** is the result of a single nucleotide change at nucleotide 1765 within the factor V gene. This mutation causes factor Va to become resistant to inactivation by activated protein C and is the most common inherited risk factor for thrombosis. This defect is also known as *activated protein C resistance*. Approximately 5% of the U.S. white population is heterozygous for this mutation, and it is less prevalent in other ethnic groups. Individuals who are heterozygous have a 5-7–fold increase in risk of venous thrombosis, while homozygotes have a relative risk of 80-100. The baseline annual risk of thrombosis for young women of reproductive age is 1 per 12,500 and increases to 1 per 3,500 for those on oral contraceptives. For young women who are heterozygous for the factor V Leiden mutation and are taking oral contraceptives, this baseline annual risk is increased 20-30–fold (relative risk) to approximately to 1 per 500 women.

The **prothrombin 20210 gene mutation** is a G-to-A transition in the 3′ untranslated region of the gene that results in increased levels of prothrombin messenger RNA. This variant is present in approximately 2% of U.S. whites. It is a weaker risk factor for venous thrombosis than factor V Leiden, with a relative risk of 2-3.

Deficiencies of protein C, protein S, and AT, the natural anticoagulant proteins, are more rare than the common genetic mutations described previously but are associated with a stronger risk of thrombosis. Although heterozygous deficiencies do not often present during childhood, homozygous defects may result in significant symptoms in infancy. Neonates with homozygous deficiencies of AT, protein C, or protein S may present with purpura fulminans. This condition is characterized by rapidly spreading purpuric skin lesions resulting from thromboses of the small dermal vessels followed by bleeding into the skin. In addition, these infants may also develop cerebral thrombosis, ophthalmic thrombosis, disseminated intravascular coagulation, and large vessel thrombosis. An infant with purpuric skin lesions of

unknown cause should receive initial replacement with fresh-frozen plasma. Definitive diagnosis can be difficult in the sick premature neonate who may have undetectable levels of these factors but not have a true genetic deficiency. Protein C and AT concentrates are also available and have been demonstrated to be effective.

Both venous and arterial thromboses are common in young patients with **homocystinuria,** an inborn error of metabolism caused by deficiency of cystathione β-synthase. In this very rare condition, plasma levels of homocysteine exceed 100 μmol/L. Much more common are mild to moderate elevations of homocysteine, which may be acquired or associated with a polymorphism in the methylenetetrahydrofolate reductase (*MTHFR*) gene. Although moderate elevations of homocysteine have been associated with both venous and arterial thrombotic events, testing for polymorphisms in the *MTHFR* gene are not indicated, because these polymorphisms are not associated with venous thromboembolism. The pathogenic mechanisms for thrombosis in homocystinemia are not well understood.

Increased plasma concentrations of **factor VIII** (>150 IU/dL) appear to be regulated by both genetic and environmental factors and are associated with an increased risk of thrombosis. Although there is a strong component of heritability contributing to factor VIII levels, the molecular mechanisms responsible for elevated factor VIII are not well understood. Factor VIII is also considered to be an acute-phase reactant, and may increase transiently during periods of inflammation.

Although interpretation of genetic studies (Factor V Leiden and Prothrombin gene mutations) are fairly straightforward, there are several **challenges in interpretation of thrombophilia studies** that are unique to pediatric patients. Neonates have decreased concentrations of protein C, protein S, and AT that increase rapidly over the first 6 mo of life; protein C concentrations remain below adult levels throughout much of childhood. It is important to use pediatric normal ranges when evaluating these values, and recognize that often the normal range overlaps with heterozygous defects and retesting may be required, particularly in young children. There are several nongenetic factors that many also influence the results of inherited thrombophilia testing, including acute thrombosis, infection, inflammation, hepatic dysfunction, nephrotic syndrome, medication and vitamin K deficiency. In some cases, the hereditary nature may be confirmed by testing the parents.

Bibliography is available at Expert Consult.

Chapter 479
Thrombotic Disorders in Children

Leslie J. Raffini and J. Paul Scott

Compared to adults, children are generally protected from venous and arterial thromboses. Advancements in the treatment and supportive care of critically ill children, coupled with a heightened awareness of genetic risk factors for thrombosis, have led to an increase in the diagnosis of thromboembolic events (TEs) in children. As a result, TEs are not infrequent in pediatric tertiary care centers and may result in significant acute and chronic morbidity. Despite the fact that TEs in children are increasing in relative terms, they are still rare. This rarity has been the major impediment to prospective clinical trials, resulting in a deficit of evidence-based medicine. Diagnosis and treatment is often extrapolated from adult data.

EPIDEMIOLOGY
Studies have confirmed a significant increase in the diagnosis of venous thromboembolism (VTE) in pediatric tertiary hospitals across the United States. Although the overall incidence of thrombosis in the general pediatric population is quite low (0.07/100,000), the rate of VTE in hospitalized children is 60/10,000 admissions. Infants <1 yr old account for the largest proportion of pediatric VTEs, with a second peak during adolescence.

The majority of children who develop a TE have multiple risk factors that may be acquired, inherited, and/or anatomic (Table 479-1). The presence of a central venous catheter (CVC and peripherally inserted central venous catheter) is the single most important risk factor for VTE in pediatric patients, associated with approximately 90% of neonatal VTE and 60% of childhood VTE. These catheters are often necessary for the care of premature neonates and children with acute and chronic diseases and are used for intravenous hyperalimentation, chemotherapy, dialysis, antibiotics, or supportive therapy. CVCs may damage the endothelial lining and/or cause blood flow disruption, increasing the risk of thrombosis. There are multiple other acquired risk factors that are associated with thrombosis, including trauma, infection, chronic medical illnesses, and medications. Cancer, congenital heart disease, and prematurity are the most common medical conditions associated with TEs.

Antiphospholipid antibody syndrome (APS) is a well-described syndrome in adults characterized by recurrent fetal loss and/or thrombosis. Antiphospholipid antibodies are associated with both venous and arterial thrombosis. The mechanism by which these antibodies cause thrombosis is not well understood. A diagnosis of APS requires the presence of both clinical and laboratory abnormalities (see "Laboratory Testing" below). The laboratory abnormalities must be persistent for 12 wk. Because of the high risk of recurrence, patients with APS often require long-term anticoagulation. It is important to note that healthy children may have a transient lupus anticoagulant, often diagnosed because of a prolonged partial thromboplastin time on routine preoperative testing. These antibodies may be associated with a recent viral infection and are not a risk factor for thrombosis.

Anatomic abnormalities that impede blood flow also predispose patients to thrombosis at an earlier age. Atresia of the inferior vena cava has been described in association with acute and chronic lower extremity deep venous thrombosis (DVT). **May-Thurner syndrome** (compression of the left iliac vein by the overlying right iliac artery) should be considered in patients who present spontaneously with left iliofemoral thrombosis, and **thoracic outlet obstruction (Paget-**

Table 479-1	Risk Factors for Thrombosis
General	Indwelling catheter including PICC (peripherally inserted central venous catheter) lines Infection Trauma Surgery Cancer Immobility Cardiac disease/prosthetic valve Systemic lupus Rheumatoid arthritis Inflammatory bowel disease Polycythemia/dehydration Nephrotic syndrome Diabetes Pregnancy Obesity Prematurity Paroxysmal nocturnal hemoglobinuria Antiphospholipid antibody syndrome Thrombotic thrombocytopenic purpura
Inherited thrombophilia	Factor V Leiden mutation Prothrombin mutation Antithrombin deficiency Protein C deficiency Protein S deficiency Homocystinuria Elevated factor VIII Dysfibrinogenemia
Anatomic	Thoracic outlet obstruction (Paget-Schroetter syndrome) May-Thurner syndrome Absence of the inferior vena cava
Medications	Estrogen-containing contraceptives Asparaginase Heparin (heparin-induced thrombocytopenia) Corticosteroids

Schroetter syndrome) frequently presents with effort-related axillary-subclavian vein thrombosis.

CLINICAL MANIFESTATIONS
Extremity Deep Vein Thrombosis
Children with acute DVT often present with extremity pain, swelling, and discoloration. A history of a current or recent CVC in that extremity should be very suggestive. Many times, symptoms of CVC-associated thrombosis are more subtle and chronic, including repeated CVC occlusion or sepsis, or prominent venous collaterals on the chest, face, and neck.

Pulmonary Embolism
Symptoms of pulmonary embolism (PE) include shortness of breath, pleuritic chest pain, cough, hemoptysis, fever, and, in the case of massive PE, hypotension and right-heart failure. Based on autopsy studies, PE is often not diagnosed, perhaps because young children are unable to accurately describe their symptoms and their respiratory deterioration may be masked by other conditions (see Chapter 407.1).

Cerebral Sinovenous Thrombosis
Symptoms may be subtle and may develop over many hours or days. Neonates often present with seizures, whereas older children often complain of headache, vomiting, seizures, and focal signs. They may also have papilledema and abducens palsy. Some patients may have a concurrent sinusitis or mastoiditis that has contributed to the thrombosis.

Renal Vein Thrombosis

Renal vein thrombosis is the most common spontaneous TE in neonates. Affected infants may present with hematuria, an abdominal mass, and/or thrombocytopenia. Infants of diabetic mothers are at increased risk, although the mechanism for this increased risk is unknown. Approximately 25% of cases are bilateral.

Peripheral Arterial Thrombosis

With the exception of stroke, the majority of arterial TEs in children are secondary to catheters, often in neonates related to umbilical artery lines or in patients with cardiac defects undergoing cardiac catheterization. Patients with an arterial thrombosis affecting blood flow to an extremity will present with a cold, pale, blue extremity with poor or absent pulses.

Stroke

Ischemic stroke commonly presents with hemiparesis, loss of consciousness, or seizures. This condition may occur secondary to pathology that affects the intracranial arteries (e.g., sickle cell disease, vasculopathy, or traumatic arterial dissection) or may be a result of venous thrombi that embolize to the arterial circulation (placental thrombi, children with congenital heart disease or patent foramen ovale).

Rapidly Progressive Thrombosis/Thrombotic Storm

Rapid progression or multifocal thrombosis is a rare complication of the APS, heparin-induced thrombocytopenia with thrombosis or thrombotic thrombocytopenia purpura while on appropriate antithrombotic therapy. Multiple organ dysfunctions develop in the presence of small vessel occlusion and elevated D-dimer levels. Recurrences may occur as well as postthrombotic syndrome (PTS). Treatment includes aggressive anticoagulation, often with direct thrombin inhibitors or fondaparinux followed by prolonged warfarin therapy.

DIAGNOSIS

Ultrasound with Doppler flow is the most commonly employed imaging study for the diagnosis of upper, or more often lower, extremity VTE. Spiral CT is used most frequently for the diagnosis of PE (Fig. 479-1). Other diagnostic imaging options include CT and MR venography, which are noninvasive, although the sensitivity and specificity of these studies is not known. They may be particularly helpful in evaluating proximal thrombosis. For the diagnosis of cerebral sinovenous thrombosis and acute ischemic stroke, the most sensitive imaging study is brain magnetic resonance imaging with venography or diffusion weighted imaging.

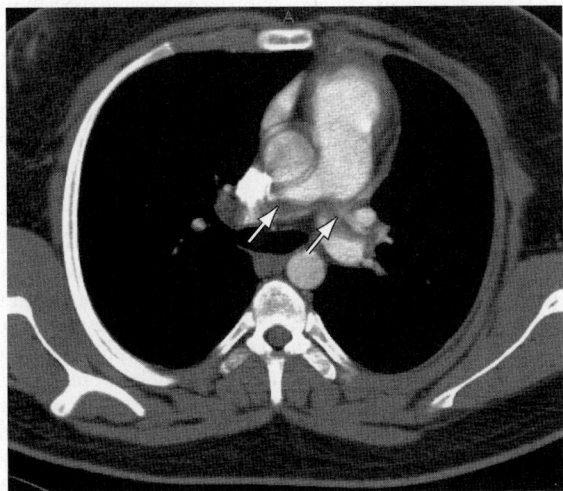

Figure 479-1 Chest CT from a 15 yr old male with a large pulmonary embolism. There are large filling defects in both the right and left main pulmonary arteries.

LABORATORY TESTING

All children with a TE should have a complete blood count and a baseline prothrombin time (PT) and activated partial thromboplastin time (aPTT) to assess their coagulation status. In adults suspected to have a DVT, the D-dimer level has a high negative predictive value. The D-dimer is a fragment produced when fibrin is degraded by plasmin and is a measure of fibrinolysis. Based on the clinical scenario, other laboratory studies, such as renal and hepatic function, may be indicated. Testing for APS includes evaluation for the lupus anticoagulant as well as anticardiolipin and anti–β_2-glycoprotein antibodies.

There is some debate regarding which patients should have testing for inherited risk factors. Thrombophilia testing rarely influences the acute management of a child with a thrombotic event. Identification of an inherited thrombophilia may influence the duration of treatment, particularly for those with combined defects, and may aid in counseling the patient about their risk of recurrence.

The evaluation of coagulation studies in pediatric patients is often complicated the developing hemostatic system and the differences in normal ranges between infants and adults In addition, there is often significant variation in the laboratory assays used to test anticoagulant levels. It is important to refer to the age-related normal ranges when interpreting pediatric coagulation studies. One limitation of these normal ranges is that they were performed many years ago, using assays that may not be equivalent to those used today. Molecular assays are not age dependent.

TREATMENT

Therapeutic options for children with thrombosis include anticoagulation, thrombolysis, surgery, and observation. The goal of **anticoagulation** is to reduce the risk of embolism, halt clot extension, and prevent recurrence. In premature neonates and critically ill children who may have an increased risk of bleeding, the potential benefits must be weighed against the risks. Anticoagulants and thrombolysis are discussed in greater detail in Chapter 479.1. Surgery may be necessary for life- or limb-threatening thrombosis when there is a contraindication to thrombolysis. The optimal treatment for a child with acute ischemic stroke depends on the likely etiology and the size of the infarct. Children with sickle cell disease who develop stroke are treated with chronic red blood cell transfusions to reduce recurrence.

COMPLICATIONS

Complications of VTE include recurrent thrombosis (either local or distant), and development of PTS. A thrombosed blood vessel may partially or fully recanalize or may remain occluded. Over time, an occluded deep vein may cause venous hypertension, resulting in blood flow being directed from the deep system into the superficial veins and potentially producing pain, swelling, edema, discoloration, and ulceration. This clinical picture is known as PTS and may be chronically disabling. Several prospective studies in adults have shown PTS to be present in 17-50% of patients with a history of thrombosis. The likelihood of developing PTS is highest in the first 2 yr but continues to increase over time.

479.1 Anticoagulant and Thrombolytic Therapy

Leslie J. Raffini and J. Paul Scott

Initial options for anticoagulation in children include unfractionated heparin (UFH) or low-molecular-weight heparin (LMWH) (Table 479-2). Although there are additional agents, including target specific oral anticoagulants, none have been carefully investigated in children. Both UFH and LMWH act by catalyzing the action of antithrombin (AT)- III. UFH consists of large-molecular-weight polysaccharide chains that interact with AT, catalyzing the inhibition of factor Xa and thrombin, as well as other serine proteases. In contrast, LMWH contains smaller-molecular-weight polysaccharide chains. The interaction of the smaller chains with AT-III results primarily in the inhibition of

		UNFRACTIONATED		LMW HEPARIN
	rTPA	HEPARIN*	WARFARIN	(ENOXAPARIN)
Indication	Recent onset of life- or limb-threatening thrombus	Acute or chronic thrombus, prophylaxis	Subacute or chronic thrombosis, thromboprophylaxis for cardiac valves	Acute or chronic thrombus, prophylaxis
Administration	IV, Continuous infusion	IV, Continuous infusion	PO, once daily	SC injection, twice daily
Monitoring	"Lytic state": FDP or D-dimer	PTT	INR	Anti-Xa activity
Other	Higher risk of bleeding	Difficult to titrate, requires frequent dose adjustments	Heavily influenced by drug and diet	More stable and easy to titrate; concern of osteopenia with long-term use

Table 479-2 Comparison of Antithrombotic Agents

FDP, fibrin degradation product; INR, international normalized ratio; LMW, low-molecular-weight; PTT, partial thromboplastin time; rTPA, recombinant tissue-type plasminogen activator.

*Higher dose is required in newborns.

Xa, with less of an effect on thrombin. There are several LMWHs available, and they have variable inhibitory effects on thrombin. For this reason, the PTT is not a reliable measure of the anticoagulant effect of LMWH, and the anti–factor Xa activity is used instead.

The optimal **duration of anticoagulation** for children with TEs is not well established. Current guidelines recommend that neonates receive 6 wk-3mo of therapy for VTE, and older children receive 3-6 mo of therapy. Patients with strong inherited thrombophilia, recurrent thrombosis, and APS may require indefinite anticoagulation.

UNFRACTIONATED HEPARIN
Heparin Dosing
Based on adult data, a therapeutic heparin dose achieves a prolongation of the aPTT of 1.5-2.5 the upper limit of normal. A bolus dose of 75-100 units/kg results in a therapeutic PTT in the majority of children. This bolus should be followed by a continuous infusion. Initial dosing is based on age, with infants having the highest requirements. It is important to continue to monitor the PTT closely. In some situations, such as patients with a lupus anticoagulant, elevated factor VIII, or neonates, the partial thromboplastin time may not accurately reflect the degree of anticoagulation, and heparin can be monitored using a heparin anti-Xa level of 0.35-0.7 units/mL.

Heparin Complications
Maintaining the aPTT in the therapeutic range can be difficult in young children for several reasons. The bioavailability of heparin is difficult to predict and may be influenced by plasma proteins. In many patients, this results in multiple dose adjustments requiring close monitoring with frequent venipuncture. UFH also requires continuous intravenous access, which may be difficult to maintain in young children.

The most common adverse effect related to heparin therapy is bleeding. This is well documented in the adult medical literature, and there are case reports of serious life-threatening bleeding in children treated with heparin. The true frequency of bleeding in pediatric patients on heparin has not been well established and is reported as 1-24%. If the anticoagulant effect of heparin must be reversed immediately, protamine sulfate may be administered to neutralize the heparin.

Other adverse effects include osteoporosis and heparin-induced thrombocytopenia (HIT). Although rare in pediatric populations, HIT is a prothrombotic, immune-mediated complication in which antibodies develop to a complex of heparin and platelet factor 4. These antibodies result in platelet activation, stimulation of coagulation, thrombocytopenia, and in some cases, life-threatening thrombosis. If HIT is strongly suspected, heparin must be discontinued immediately. There are several alternative parenteral anticoagulants (argatroban, lepirudin, or bivalirudin) that may be used in this situation.

LOW-MOLECULAR-WEIGHT HEPARIN
Because of the ease of dosing and need for less monitoring, **LMWH** is being used more frequently in pediatric patients. Unlike UFH, which is monitored using the aPTT, LMWH is monitored via the anti-Xa activity. The LMWH formulation that has been used most often in pediatric patients is enoxaparin

Enoxaparin Dosing
The recommended standard starting dose of enoxaparin for infants <2 mo is 1.5 mg/kg/dose SQ every 12 hr; for patients >2 mo it is 1 mg/kg SQ every 12 hr. In general, peak levels are achieved 2-6 hr following an injection. A therapeutic anti–factor Xa level, drawn 4 hr after the 2nd or 3rd dose, should be between 0.5 and 1.0 IU/mL. The dose can be titrated to achieve this range. The elimination half-life of enoxaparin is 4-6 hr. Enoxaparin is cleared by the kidney and should be used with caution in patients with renal insufficiency. It should be avoided in patients with renal failure.

After an initial period of anticoagulation with heparin or LMWH, patients may continue to receive LMWH as an outpatient for the duration of therapy, or may be transitioned to an oral anticoagulant, such as warfarin.

WARFARIN
Warfarin is an oral anticoagulant that competitively interferes with vitamin K metabolism, exerting its action by decreasing concentrations of the vitamin K–dependent coagulation factors II, VII, IX, and X, as well as protein C and protein S. Therapy should be started while a patient is anticoagulated with heparin or LMWH because of the risk of warfarin-induced skin necrosis. This transient hypercoagulable condition may occur when levels of protein C drop more rapidly than the procoagulant factors.

Warfarin Dosing
Warfarin therapy is often initiated with a loading dose, with subsequent dose adjustments made according to a nomogram. When initiating a patient on warfarin, UFH or LMWH should be continued until the international normalized ratio (INR) is therapeutic for 2 days. In most cases, this takes 5-7 days. The PT is used to monitor the anticoagulant effect of warfarin. Because the thromboplastin reagents used in PT assays have widely varying sensitivities, it is not possible to compare the PT performed in one laboratory to that performed in another laboratory. As a result, the INR was developed as a mechanism to standardize the variation in the thromboplastin reagent. The target INR range depends on the clinical situation. In general, a range of 2.0-3.0 is the target for the treatment of VTE. High-risk patients, such as those with mechanical heart valves, APS, and recurrent thrombosis, may require a higher target range.

Warfarin Complications

As with the other anticoagulants, bleeding is the most common adverse effect. The risk of serious bleeding in children receiving warfarin for the treatment of VTE has been reported at 1.7%. Children who have supratherapeutic INRs are at higher risk. There is considerable interpatient variation in dose. Diet, medications, and illness may influence the metabolism of warfarin, requiring frequent dose adjustments and laboratory studies. Numerous medications can affect the pharmacokinetics of warfarin by altering its clearance or rate of absorption. This can have a profound effect on the INR, and must be considered when monitoring a patient on warfarin.

The strategies used to reverse warfarin therapy depend on the clinical situation and whether or not there is bleeding. Vitamin K can be administered to reverse the effect of warfarin but takes some time to have effect. If the patient is having significant bleeding, fresh-frozen plasma (15 mL/kg) should be given along with the vitamin K.

Nonhemorrhagic complications are uncommon in children. Warfarin is a teratogen, particularly in the first trimester. Warfarin embryopathy is characterized by bone and cartilage abnormalities known as chondrodysplasia punctata. Affected infants may have nasal hypoplasia and excessive calcifications in the epiphyses and vertebrae.

DIRECT THROMBIN OR FACTOR XA INHIBITORS

Direct thrombin inhibitors (dabigatran) or inhibitors of factor Xa (apixaban, rivaroxaban) have been tested as agents to prevent or treat venous thrombosis in adult populations with increased risk of thrombosis (surgery, immobilization, atrial fibrillation). Fixed dosing, oral administration, no dietary interference with vitamin K, and no need to monitor laboratory tests, as well as initial results suggesting noninferiority to warfarin and fewer bleeding episodes, have favored the use of these agents. Currently there is a paucity of evidence of their utility in children.

THROMBOLYTIC THERAPY

Although anticoagulation alone is often effective at managing thrombosis, there are times when more rapid clot resolution is necessary or desirable. In these situations, thrombolytic agents that activate the fibrinolytic system are of potential benefit. The pharmacologic activity of thrombolytic agents is dependent on the conversion of endogenous plasminogen to plasmin. Plasmin is then able to degrade several plasma proteins including fibrin and fibrinogen. Because of the high risk of bleeding, thrombolytic therapy is generally reserved for patients with life or limb-threatening thrombosis.

Tissue plasminogen activator (TPA) is available as a recombinant product and has become the primary agent used for thrombolysis in children, although proper dose finding studies have not been performed in a pediatric population.

Dosing

There is an extremely wide range of doses of TPA that have been used for systemic therapy, and there is no consensus as to the optimal dose. Previously recommended doses of systemic TPA were 0.1-0.6 mg/kg/hr; however there are recent reports of successful therapy with fewer bleeding complications using prolonged infusions with very low doses—0.01-0.06 mg/kg/hr.

Monitoring

There is no specific laboratory test to document a "therapeutic range" for thrombolytic therapy. It is important to maintain the fibrinogen >100 mg/dL and the platelet count >75,000/mm^3 during treatment. Supplementation of plasminogen using fresh-frozen plasma is generally recommended in neonates prior to initiating thrombolysis because of their low baseline levels.

The clinical and radiologic response to thrombolysis should be closely monitored. The duration of therapy depends on the clinical response. Invasive procedures including urinary catheterization, arterial puncture and rectal temperatures should be avoided.

The role of adjuvant UFH during thrombolytic therapy is controversial. Animal models have demonstrated that thrombolytic therapy can induce a procoagulant state with activation of the coagulation system, generation of thrombin, and extension or reocclusion of the thrombosis. In pediatric patients thought to be at low risk for bleeding, adjuvant UFH should be considered using doses of 10-20 units/kg/hr.

Complications

The most serious complication from thrombolysis is bleeding, which has been reported in 0-40% of patients. Absolute contraindications to thrombolysis include major surgery within 7 days, history of significant bleeding (intracranial, pulmonary or gastrointestinal), peripartum asphyxia with brain damage, uncontrolled hypertension and severe thrombocytopenia. In the event of serious bleeding, thrombolysis should be stopped and cryoprecipitate may be given to replace fibrinogen.

THROMBOPROPHYLAXIS

There have been no formal trials of prevention of venous thromboembolic disease in children. Hospitalized adolescents with multiple risk factors for thrombosis who are immobilized for a protracted time may benefit from prophylactic treatment with enoxaparin 0.5 mg/kg q12hr (maximum: 30 mg).

ANTIPLATELET THERAPY

Inhibition of platelet function using agents such as **aspirin** is more likely to be protective against arterial TEs than VTEs. Aspirin, also known as acetylsalicylic acid, exerts its antiplatelet effect by irreversibly inhibiting cyclooxygenase, preventing platelet thromboxane A$_2$ production. Aspirin is used routinely in children with Kawasaki disease and may also be useful in children with stroke, ventricular assist devices, and those with single-ventricle cardiac defects. The recommended dose of aspirin to achieve an antiplatelet effect in children is 1-5 mg/kg/day.

Bibliography is available at Expert Consult.

Chapter 480
Postneonatal Vitamin K Deficiency
J. Paul Scott

Although "late" hemorrhagic disease has been reported in breastfed children, vitamin K deficiency occurring after the neonatal period is usually secondary to a lack of oral intake of vitamin K, alterations in the gut flora as a consequence of the long-term use of broad-spectrum antibiotics, liver disease, or malabsorption of vitamin K. Intestinal malabsorption of fats may accompany cystic fibrosis or biliary atresia and result in a deficiency of fat-soluble dietary vitamins, with reduced synthesis of vitamin K–dependent clotting factors (factors II, VII, IX, and X, and proteins C and S). Prophylactic administration of water-soluble vitamin K orally is indicated in these cases (2-3 mg/24 hr for children and 5-10 mg/24 hr for adolescents and adults), or vitamin K may be administered at 1-2 mg IV. In patients with advanced cirrhosis, synthesis of many of the clotting factors may be reduced because of hepatocellular damage. In these patients, vitamin K may be ineffective. The anticoagulant properties of warfarin (Coumadin) and related anticoagulants depend on interference with vitamin K, with a concomitant reduction of factors II, VII, IX, and X. Rat poison (superwarfarin) produces a similar deficiency; vitamin K is a specific antidote.

Bibliography is available at Expert Consult.

Chapter 481
Liver Disease
J. Paul Scott

Because all of the clotting factors, except factor VIII, are produced exclusively in the liver, coagulation abnormalities are very common in patients with severe liver disease. Only 15% of such patients have significant clinical bleeding states. The severity of the coagulation abnormality appears to be directly proportional to the extent of hepatocellular damage. The most common mechanism causing the defect is decreased synthesis of coagulation factors. Patients with severe liver disease characteristically have normal to increased (not reduced) levels of factor VIII activity in plasma. In some instances, disseminated intravascular coagulation (see Chapter 483) or hyperfibrinolysis may complicate liver disease, making laboratory differentiation of severe liver disease from disseminated intravascular coagulation difficult.

Treatment of the coagulopathy of liver disease should be reserved for patients with clinical bleeding. Because a reduction in vitamin K–dependent coagulation factors is common in those with acute or chronic liver disease, vitamin K therapy can be given as a trial. Vitamin K can be given orally, subcutaneously, or intravenously (not intramuscularly) at a dose of 1 mg/24 hr for infants, 2-3 mg/24 hr for children, and 5-10 mg/24 hr for adolescents and adults. Inability to correct coagulopathy with vitamin K indicates that the coagulopathy may be caused by reduced levels of clotting factors that are not vitamin K–dependent and/or by inadequate production of precursor vitamin K proteins. Treatment for bleeding consists of factor replacement with fresh-frozen plasma (FFP) or cryoprecipitate. FFP (10-15 mL/kg) contains all clotting factors, but replacement of fibrinogen for severe hypofibrinogenemia may require cryoprecipitate at a dose of 1 bag/5 kg body weight. In severe liver disease, it is often difficult to attain correction of abnormal clotting studies despite vigorous therapy with FFP and cryoprecipitate. Some patients with bleeding as a result of liver disease have responded to therapy with desmopressin, and others have responded to treatment with recombinant factor VIIa.

Frequently, severe liver disease is associated with moderate prolongation of bleeding time that is not corrected by either vitamin K or plasma replacement. Desmopressin (0.3 μg/kg IV) is effective in shortening bleeding time and is used effectively to augment hemostasis before liver biopsy. In clinical trials of adults, recombinant factor VIIa has not been shown to be effective for the treatment of bleeding caused by severe liver disease.

Bibliography is available at Expert Consult.

Chapter 482
Acquired Inhibitors of Coagulation
J. Paul Scott

Acquired circulating anticoagulants (inhibitors) are antibodies that react or crossreact with clotting factors or components used in coagulation screening tests (phospholipids), thereby prolonging screening tests, such as prothrombin time and partial thromboplastin time. Some of these anticoagulants are autoantibodies that react with phospholipid and thereby interfere with clotting in vitro but not in vivo. The most common form of these antiphospholipid antibodies has been referred to as the *lupus anticoagulant* (see Chapter 476.1). This anticoagulant is found in patients with systemic lupus erythematosus (see Chapter 158), in those with other collagen-vascular diseases, and in association with HIV. In otherwise healthy children, spontaneous lupus-like inhibitors have developed transiently after incidental viral infection. These transient inhibitors are usually not associated with either bleeding or thrombosis.

Although the classic lupus anticoagulant is more often associated with a predisposition to thrombosis than with bleeding symptoms, bleeding symptoms in a patient with the lupus anticoagulant may be caused by thrombocytopenia, as a manifestation of the antiphospholipid syndrome or of lupus itself, or, rarely, by a coexistent specific autoantibody against prothrombin (factor II). This antiprothrombin antibody does not inactivate prothrombin, but causes accelerated clearance of the protein, resulting in low levels of prothrombin.

Rarely, antibodies may arise spontaneously against a specific clotting factor, such as factor VIII or von Willebrand factor, similar to those seen more frequently in elderly patients. These patients are prone to excessive hemorrhage and may require specific treatment. In patients with a hereditary deficiency of a clotting factor (factor VIII or factor IX), antibodies may develop after exposure to transfused factor concentrates. These hemophilic inhibitory antibodies are discussed in Chapter 479.1.

LABORATORY FINDINGS
Inhibitors against specific coagulation factors usually affect factors VIII, IX, and XI, or, rarely, prothrombin. Depending on the target of the antibody, prothrombin time, partial thromboplastin time, or both may be prolonged. The mechanism by which the inhibitory antibody functions determines whether mixing patient plasma with normal plasma will normalize (correct) the clotting time. Patient plasma containing antibodies directed against the active site of the clotting factor (factor VIII or factor IX) will not correct on 1:1 mixing with normal plasma, whereas antibodies that lead to increased clearance of the factor (prothrombin) will correct on 1:1 mixing. Specific factor assays are used to determine which factor is involved.

TREATMENT
Management of the bleeding patient with an inhibitor against factor VIII or IX is the same as for the patient with hemophilia who has an alloantibody against factor VIII or factor IX. Infusions of recombinant factor VIIa or activated prothrombin complex concentrate may be needed to control significant bleeding. Immunosuppressive agents have used off-label to treat the inhibitor or reduce titers. Acute bleeding caused by an antiprothrombin antibody can often be treated with a plasma infusion and may benefit from a short course of corticosteroid therapy.

Asymptomatic spontaneous inhibitors that arise after a viral infection tend to disappear within a few weeks to months. Inhibitors seen with an underlying disease, such as systemic lupus erythematosus, often disappear when the primary disease is effectively treated.

Bibliography is available at Expert Consult.

Chapter **483**
Disseminated Intravascular Coagulation
J. Paul Scott and Leslie J. Raffini

Thrombotic microangiopathy refers to a heterogeneous group of conditions, including disseminated intravascular coagulation (DIC), that result in consumption of clotting factors, platelets, and anticoagulant proteins. Consequences of this process include widespread intravascular deposition of fibrin, leading to tissue ischemia and necrosis, a generalized hemorrhagic state, and hemolytic anemia.

ETIOLOGY
Any life-threatening severe systemic disease (Table 483-1) associated with hypoxia, acidosis, tissue necrosis, shock, and/or endothelial damage may trigger DIC. Better understanding of the pathophysiology of hemostasis has lead to an appreciation of the critical interaction of the coagulation pathways with the innate immune system and inflammatory response that likely contributes to the widespread dysregulation present in DIC. Activation and release of cytokines and chemokines alter endothelial function to a more prothrombotic state, enhancing the formation of microvascular thromboses, with resultant consumption of pro- and anticoagulant proteins. Excessive activation of clotting consumes both the physiologic anticoagulants (protein C, protein S, and antithrombin III) and procoagulants, resulting in a deficiency of factor V, factor VIII, prothrombin, fibrinogen, and platelets. Commonly, the clinical result of this sequence of events is hemorrhage. The hemostatic dysregulation may also result in thromboses in the skin, kidneys, and other organs.

CLINICAL MANIFESTATIONS
DIC accompanies a severe systemic disease process, usually with shock. Bleeding frequently first occurs from sites of venipuncture or surgical incision. The skin may show petechiae and ecchymoses. Tissue necrosis may involve many organs and can be most spectacularly seen as infarction of large areas of skin, subcutaneous tissue, or kidneys. Anemia caused by hemolysis may develop rapidly, owing to microangiopathic hemolytic anemia.

LABORATORY FINDINGS
There is no well-defined sequence of events. Certain coagulation factors (factors II, V, and VIII, and fibrinogen) and platelets may be consumed by the ongoing intravascular clotting process, with resultant prolongation of the prothrombin, partial thromboplastin, and thrombin times. Platelet counts may be profoundly depressed. The blood smear may contain fragmented, burr- and helmet-shaped red blood cells (schistocytes). In addition, because the fibrinolytic mechanism is activated, fibrinogen degradation products (D-dimers) appear in the blood. The D-dimer is formed by fibrinolysis of a crosslinked fibrin clot. The D-dimer assay is as sensitive as the fibrinogen degradation product test and more specific for activation of coagulation and fibrinolysis.

TREATMENT
The first 2 steps in the treatment of DIC are the most critical: (a) treat the trigger that caused DIC and (b) restore normal homeostasis by correcting the shock, acidosis, and hypoxia that usually complicate DIC. If the underlying problem can be controlled and the patient stabilized, bleeding quickly ceases, and there is improvement of the abnormal laboratory findings. Blood components are used for replacement therapy in patients with hemorrhage and may consist of platelet

Table 483-1	Causes of Disseminated Intravascular Coagulation

INFECTIOUS
Meningococcemia (purpura fulminans)
Bacterial sepsis (staphylococcal, streptococcal, *Escherichia coli*, *Salmonella*)
Rickettsia (Rocky Mountain spotted fever)
Virus (cytomegalovirus, herpes simplex, hemorrhagic fevers)
Malaria
Fungus

TISSUE INJURY
Central nervous system trauma (massive head injury)
Multiple fractures with fat emboli
Crush injury
Profound shock or asphyxia
Hypothermia or hyperthermia
Massive burns

MALIGNANCY
Acute promyelocytic leukemia
Acute monoblastic or promyelocytic leukemia
Widespread malignancies (neuroblastoma)

VENOM OR TOXIN
Snake bites
Insect bites

MICROANGIOPATHIC DISORDERS
"Severe" thrombotic thrombocytopenic purpura or hemolytic-uremic syndrome
Giant hemangioma (Kasabach-Merritt syndrome)

GASTROINTESTINAL DISORDERS
Fulminant hepatitis
Ischemic bowel
Pancreatitis

HEREDITARY THROMBOTIC DISORDERS
Antithrombin III deficiency
Homozygous protein C deficiency

NEWBORN
Maternal toxemia
Bacterial or viral sepsis (group B streptococcus, herpes simplex)
Abruptio placenta
Severe respiratory distress syndrome
Necrotizing enterocolitis
Erythroblastosis fetalis
Fetal demise of a twin

MISCELLLANEOUS
Severe acute graft rejection
Acute hemolytic transfusion reaction
Severe collagen-vascular disease
Kawasaki disease
Heparin-induced thrombosis
Infusion of "activated" prothrombin complex concentrates
Hyperpyrexia/encephalopathy, hemorrhagic shock syndrome

Modified from Montgomery RR, Scott IP: Hemostasis: diseases of the fluid phase. In Nathan DG, Oski FA, editors: Hematology of infancy and childhood, vol 2, ed 4, Philadelphia, 1993, WB Saunders.

infusions (for thrombocytopenia), cryoprecipitate (for hypofibrinogenemia), and/or fresh-frozen plasma (for replacement of other coagulation factors and natural inhibitors).

The role of heparin in DIC is limited to patients who have vascular thrombosis in association with DIC or who require prophylaxis because they are at high risk for venous thromboembolism. Such individuals should be treated as outlined in Chapter 479, with careful attention to replacement therapy to maintain an adequate platelet count and thus limit bleeding complications.

The prognosis of patients with DIC is primarily dependent on the outcome of the treatment of the primary disease and prevention of end-organ damage.

Bibliography is available at Expert Consult.

Chapter **484**
Platelet and Blood Vessel Disorders
J. Paul Scott

MEGAKARYOPOIESIS

Platelets are nonnucleated cellular fragments produced by megakaryocytes within the bone marrow and other tissues. Megakaryocytes are large polyploid cells. When the megakaryocyte approaches maturity, budding of the cytoplasm occurs and large numbers of platelets are liberated. Platelets circulate with a life span of 10-14 days. **Thrombopoietin** (TPO) is the primary growth factor that controls platelet production (Fig. 484-1). Levels of TPO appear to correlate inversely with platelet number and megakaryocyte mass. Levels of TPO are highest in the thrombocytopenic states associated with decreased marrow megakaryopoiesis and may be variable in states of increased platelet production.

The platelet plays multiple hemostatic roles. The platelet surface possesses a number of important receptors for adhesive proteins, including von Willebrand factor (VWF) and fibrinogen, as well as receptors for agonists that trigger platelet aggregation, such as thrombin, collagen, and adenosine diphosphate (ADP). After injury to the blood vessel wall, the extracellular matrix containing adhesive and procoagulant proteins is exposed. Subendothelial collagen binds VWF. VWF undergoes a conformational change that induces binding of the platelet glycoprotein Ib (GPIb) complex, the VWF receptor. This process is called *platelet adhesion*. Platelets then undergo activation. During the process of activation, the platelets generate thromboxane A_2 from arachidonic acid via the enzyme cyclooxygenase. After activation, platelets release agonists, such as ADP, adenosine triphosphate (ATP), Ca^{2+}, serotonin, and coagulation factors, into the surrounding milieu. Binding of VWF to the GPIb complex triggers a complex signaling cascade that results in activation of the fibrinogen receptor, the major platelet integrin glycoprotein αIIb-β_3 (GPIIb-IIIa). Circulating fibrinogen binds to its receptor on the activated platelets, complex linking platelets together in a process called *aggregation*. This series of events forms a hemostatic plug at the site of vascular injury. The serotonin and histamine that are liberated during activation increase local vasoconstriction. In addition to acting in concert with the vessel wall to form the platelet plug, the platelet provides the catalytic surface on which coagulation factors assemble and eventually generate thrombin through a sequential series of enzymatic cleavages. Last, the platelet contractile proteins and cytoskeleton mediate clot retraction.

THROMBOCYTOPENIA

The normal platelet count is $150\text{-}450 \times 10^9/L$. *Thrombocytopenia* refers to a reduction in platelet count to $<150 \times 10^9/L$. Causes of thrombocytopenia include decreased production on either a congenital or an acquired basis, sequestration of the platelets within an enlarged spleen or other organ, and increased destruction of normally synthesized platelets on either an immune or a nonimmune basis (see Chapter 475; Tables 484-1 and 484-2 and Fig. 484-2).

Bibliography is available at Expert Consult.

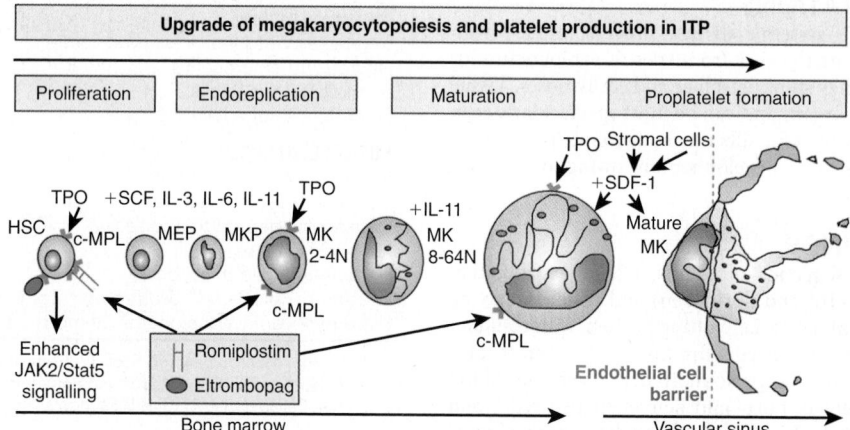

Figure 484-1 Scheme of megakaryocytopoiesis and platelet production in idiopathic thrombocytopenic purpura. Hematopoietic stem cells (HSC) are mobilized and megakaryocyte (MK) and erythroid progenitors (MEP) accumulate with MK-committed progenitors (MKP) giving rise to mature MKs under control of thrombopoietin (TPO) working with chemokines, cytokines, and growth factors, including stem cell factor (SCF) and interleukin (IL)-3, IL-6, and IL-11. Endoreplication results in ploidy changes in MKs and increased chromosome number (up to 64N). Mature MKs migrate to the endothelial cell barrier delimiting the vascular sinus and, under the influence of stromal-derived factor-1 (SDF-1), give rise to proplatelets that protrude into the circulation and produce large numbers of platelets under hemodynamic determinants. Therapeutically given romiplostim and eltrombopag enter the marrow and join with TPO to stimulate megakaryocytopoiesis and platelet production. *(From Nurden AT, Viallard JF, Nurden P: New-generation drugs that stimulate platelet production in chronic immune thrombocytopenic purpura, Lancet 373:1562–1568, 2009, p. 1563.)*

| **Table 484-1** | Differential Diagnosis of Thrombocytopenia in Children and Adolescents |

DESTRUCTIVE THROMBOCYTOPENIAS
Primary Platelet Consumption Syndromes
Immune thrombocytopenias
  Acute and chronic ITP
  Autoimmune diseases with chronic ITP as a manifestation
    Cyclic thrombocytopenia
    Autoimmune lymphoproliferative syndrome and its variants
    Systemic lupus erythematosus
    Evans syndrome
    Antiphospholipid antibody syndrome
    Neoplasia-associated immune thrombocytopenia
  Thrombocytopenia associated with HIV
  Neonatal immune thrombocytopenia
    Alloimmune
    Autoimmune (e.g., maternal ITP)
  Drug-induced immune thrombocytopenia (including heparin-induced thrombocytopenia)
  Posttransfusion purpura
  Allergy and anaphylaxis
  Posttransplant thrombocytopenia
Nonimmune thrombocytopenias
  Thrombocytopenia of infection
    Bacteremia or fungemia
    Viral infection
    Protozoan
  Thrombotic microangiopathic disorders
    Hemolytic-uremic syndrome
    Eclampsia, HELLP syndrome
    Thrombotic thrombocytopenic purpura
    Bone marrow transplantation-associated microangiopathy
    Drug-induced

Platelets in contact with foreign material
Congenital heart disease
Drug-induced via direct platelet effects (ristocetin, protamine)
Type 2B VWD or platelet-type VWD

Combined Platelet and Fibrinogen Consumption Syndromes
Disseminated intravascular coagulation
Kasabach-Merritt syndrome
Virus-associated hemophagocytic syndrome

IMPAIRED PLATELET PRODUCTION
Hereditary disorders
Acquired disorders
  Aplastic anemia
  Myelodysplastic syndrome
  Marrow infiltrative process—neoplasia
  Osteopetrosis
  Nutritional deficiency states (iron, folate, vitamin B_{12}, anorexia nervosa)
  Drug- or radiation-induced thrombocytopenia
  Neonatal hypoxia or placental insufficiency

SEQUESTRATION
Hypersplenism
Hypothermia
Burns

HELLP, hemolysis, elevated liver enzymes, and low platelets; HIV, human immunodeficiency virus; ITP, immune thrombocytopenic purpura; VWD, von Willebrand disease.
   From Wilson DB: Acquired platelet defects. In Orkin SH, Nathan DG, Ginsburg D, et al, editors: Nathan and Oski's hematology of infancy and childhood, ed 7, Philadelphia, 2009, WB Saunders, p. 1555, Box 33-1.

| **Table 484-2** | Classification of Fetal and Neonatal Thrombocytopenias* |

	CONDITION		**CONDITION**
Fetal	Alloimmune thrombocytopenia **Congenital infection** (e.g., CMV, toxoplasma, rubella, HIV) Aneuploidy (e.g., trisomy 18, 13, or 21, or triploidy) Autoimmune condition (e.g., ITP, SLE) Severe Rh hemolytic disease Congenital/inherited (e.g., Wiskott-Aldrich syndrome)		Thrombosis (e.g., aortic, renal vein) Bone marrow replacement (e.g., congenital leukemia) Kasabach-Merritt syndrome Metabolic disease (e.g., proprionic and methylmalonic acidemia) Congenital/inherited (e.g., TAR, CAMT)
Early-onset neonatal (<72 hr)	**Placental insufficiency** (e.g., PET, IUGR, diabetes) **Perinatal asphyxia** **Perinatal infection** (e.g., *Escherichia coli*, GBS, herpes simplex) DIC Alloimmune thrombocytopenia Autoimmune condition (e.g., ITP, SLE) Congenital infection (e.g., CMV, toxoplasma, rubella, HIV)	Late-onset neonatal (>72 hr)	**Late-onset sepsis** **NEC** Congenital infection (e.g., CMV, toxoplasma, rubella, HIV) Autoimmune Kasabach-Merritt syndrome Metabolic disease (e.g., proprionic and methylmalonic acidemia) Congenital/inherited (e.g., TAR, CAMT)

*The most common conditions are shown in bold.
  CAMT, congenital amegakaryocytic thrombocytopenia; CMV, cytomegalovirus; DIC, disseminated intravascular coagulation; GBS, group B streptococcus; ITP, idiopathic thrombocytopenic purpura; IUGR, intrauterine growth restriction; NEC, necrotizing enterocolitis; PET, preeclampsia; SLE, systemic lupus erythematosus; TAR, thrombocytopenia with absent radii.
  From Roberts I, Murray NA: Neonatal thrombocytopenia: causes and management, Arch Dis Child Fetal Neonatal Ed 88:F359–F364, 2003.

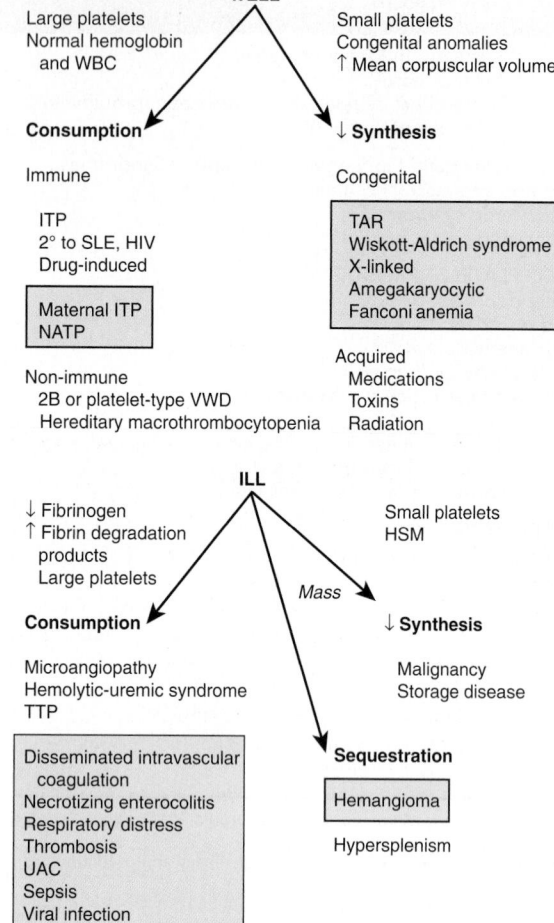

Figure 484-2 Differential diagnosis of childhood thrombocytopenic syndromes. The syndromes initially are separated by their clinical appearance. Clues leading to the diagnosis are shown in *italics*. The mechanisms and common disorders leading to these findings are shown in the *lower part* of the figure. Disorders that commonly affect neonates are listed in the *shaded boxes*. HSM, hepatosplenomegaly; ITP, idiopathic immune thrombocytopenic purpura; NATP, neonatal alloimmune thrombocytopenic purpura; SLE, systemic lupus erythematosus; TAR, thrombocytopenia-absent radius; TTP, thrombotic thrombocytopenic purpura; UAC, umbilical artery catheter; VWD, von Willebrand disease; WBC, white blood cell. (*From Scott JP: Bleeding and thrombosis. In Kliegman RM, editor:* Practical strategies in pediatric diagnosis and therapy, *Philadelphia, 1996, WB Saunders, p. 849; Kliegman RM, Marcdante KJ, Jenson HB, et al, editors:* Nelson essentials of pediatrics, *ed 5, Philadelphia, 2006, Elsevier/Saunders, p. 716.*)

484.1 Idiopathic (Autoimmune) Thrombocytopenic Purpura

J. Paul Scott

The most common cause of acute onset of thrombocytopenia in an otherwise well child is (autoimmune) idiopathic thrombocytopenic purpura (ITP).

EPIDEMIOLOGY

In a small number of children, estimated at 1 in 20,000, 1-4 wk after exposure to a common viral infection, an autoantibody directed against the platelet surface develops with resultant sudden onset of thrombocytopenia. A recent history of viral illness is described in 50-65% of cases of childhood ITP. The peak age is 1-4 yr, although the age ranges from early in infancy to the elderly. In childhood, males and females are equally affected. ITP seems to occur more often in late winter and spring after the peak season of viral respiratory illness.

PATHOGENESIS

Why some children develop the acute presentation of an autoimmune disease is unknown. The exact antigenic target for most such antibodies in most cases of childhood acute ITP remains undetermined. Although in chronic ITP, many patients demonstrate antibodies against the platelet glycoprotein complexes, αIIb-β$_3$ and GPIb. After binding of the antibody to the platelet surface, circulating antibody-coated platelets are recognized by the Fc receptor on splenic macrophages, ingested, and destroyed. Most common viruses have been described in association with ITP, including Epstein-Barr virus (see Chapter 254) and HIV (see Chapter 276). Epstein-Barr virus-related ITP is usually of short duration and follows the course of infectious mononucleosis. HIV-associated ITP is usually chronic. In some patients ITP appears to arise in children infected with *Helicobacter pylori* or rarely following vaccines.

CLINICAL MANIFESTATIONS

The classic presentation of ITP is a previously healthy 1-4 yr old child who has sudden onset of generalized petechiae and purpura. The parents often state that the child was fine yesterday and now is covered with bruises and purple dots. There may be bleeding from the gums and mucous membranes, particularly with profound thrombocytopenia (platelet count <10 × 10^9/L). There is a history of a preceding viral infection 1-4 wk before the onset of thrombocytopenia. Findings on physical examination are normal, other than the finding of petechiae and purpura. Splenomegaly, lymphadenopathy, bone pain, and pallor are rare. An easy to use classification system has been proposed from the United Kingdom to characterize the severity of bleeding in ITP on the basis of symptoms and signs, but not platelet count:

1. No symptoms
2. Mild symptoms: bruising and petechiae, occasional minor epistaxis, very little interference with daily living
3. Moderate: more severe skin and mucosal lesions, more troublesome epistaxis and menorrhagia
4. Severe: bleeding episodes—menorrhagia, epistaxis, melena—requiring transfusion or hospitalization, symptoms interfering seriously with the quality of life

The presence of abnormal findings such as hepatosplenomegaly, bone or joint pain, remarkable lymphadenopathy other cytopenias, or congenital anomalies suggests other diagnoses (leukemia, syndromes). When the onset is insidious, especially in an adolescent, chronic ITP or the possibility of a systemic illness, such as systemic lupus erythematosus (SLE), is more likely.

OUTCOME

Severe bleeding is rare (<3% of cases in 1 large international study). In 70-80% of children who present with acute ITP, spontaneous resolution occurs within 6 mo. Therapy does not appear to affect the natural history of the illness. Fewer than 1% of patients develop an intracranial hemorrhage. Those who favor interventional therapy argue that the objective of early therapy is to raise the platelet count to >20 × 10^9/L and prevent the rare development of intracranial hemorrhage. There is no evidence that therapy prevents serious bleeding. Approximately 20% of children who present with acute ITP go on to have chronic ITP. The outcome/prognosis may be related more to age, as ITP in younger children is more likely to resolve whereas the development of chronic ITP in adolescents approaches 50%.

LABORATORY FINDINGS

Severe thrombocytopenia (platelet count <20 × 10^9/L) is common, and platelet size is normal or increased, reflective of increased platelet turnover (Fig. 484-3). In acute ITP, the hemoglobin value, white blood cell (WBC) count, and differential count should be normal. Hemoglobin may be decreased if there have been profuse nosebleeds or menorrhagia. Bone marrow examination shows normal granulocytic and erythrocytic series, with characteristically normal or increased

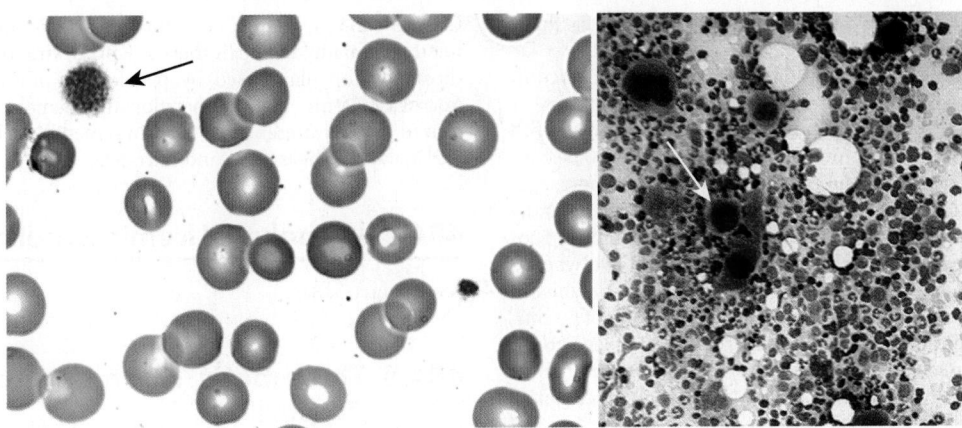

Figure 484-3 Blood smear and bone marrow aspirate from a child who had ITP showing large platelets (blood smear *[left]*) and increased numbers of megakaryocytes, many of which appear immature (bone marrow aspirate *[right]*). *(From Blanchette V, Bolton-Maggs P: Childhood immune thrombocytopenic purpura: diagnosis and management, Pediatr Clin North Am 55:393–420, 2008, p. 400, Fig. 4.)*

numbers of megakaryocytes. Some of the megakaryocytes may appear to be immature and are reflective of increased platelet turnover. **Indications for bone marrow** aspiration/biopsy include an abnormal WBC count or differential or unexplained anemia as well as findings on history and physical examination suggestive of a bone marrow failure syndrome or malignancy. Other laboratory tests should be performed as indicated by the history and physical examination. HIV studies should be done in at-risk populations, especially sexually active teens. Platelet antibody testing is seldom useful in acute ITP. A direct antiglobulin test (Coombs) should be done if there is unexplained anemia to rule out Evans syndrome (autoimmune hemolytic anemia and thrombocytopenia) (see Chapter 458) or before instituting therapy with IV anti-D.

DIAGNOSIS/DIFFERENTIAL DIAGNOSIS

The well-appearing child with moderate to severe thrombocytopenia, an otherwise normal complete blood cell count (CBC), and normal findings on physical examination has a limited differential diagnosis that includes exposure to medication that induces drug-dependent antibodies, splenic sequestration because of previously unappreciated portal hypertension, and, rarely, early aplastic processes, such as Fanconi anemia (see Chapter 468). Other than congenital thrombocytopenia syndromes (see Chapter 484.8), such as thrombocytopenia-absent radius (TAR) syndrome and MYH9-related thrombocytopenia, most marrow processes that interfere with platelet production eventually cause abnormal synthesis of red blood cells (RBCs) and WBCs, and therefore manifest diverse abnormalities on the CBC. Disorders that cause increased platelet destruction on a nonimmune basis are usually serious systemic illnesses with obvious clinical findings (e.g., hemolytic-uremic syndrome [HUS], disseminated intravascular coagulation [DIC]) (see Table 483-1 in Chapter 483, and Fig. 484-2). Patients on heparin may develop heparin-induced thrombocytopenia. Isolated enlargement of the spleen suggests the potential for hypersplenism owing to either liver disease or portal vein thrombosis. Autoimmune thrombocytopenia may be an initial manifestation of SLE, HIV infection, common variable immunodeficiency, and, rarely, lymphoma or autoimmune lymphoproliferative syndrome. Wiskott-Aldrich syndrome (WAS; Chapter 126.2) must be considered in young males found to have thrombocytopenia with small platelets, particularly if there is a history of eczema and recurrent infection.

TREATMENT

There are no data showing that treatment affects either short- or long-term clinical outcome of ITP. Many patients with new-onset ITP have mild symptoms, with findings limited to petechiae and purpura on the skin, despite severe thrombocytopenia. Compared with untreated control subjects, treatment appears to be capable of inducing a more rapid rise in platelet count to the theoretically safe level of >20 × 10⁹/L,

although there are no data indicating that early therapy prevents intracranial hemorrhage. Antiplatelet antibodies bind to transfused platelets as well as they do to autologous platelets. Thus, platelet transfusion in ITP is usually contraindicated unless life-threatening bleeding is present. Initial approaches to the management of ITP include the following:

1. No therapy other than education and counseling of the family and patient for patients with minimal, mild, and moderate symptoms, as defined earlier. This approach emphasizes the usually benign nature of ITP and avoids the therapeutic roller coaster that ensues once interventional therapy is begun. This approach is far less costly, and side effects are minimal.

2. Per the American Society of Hematology Guidelines: "A single dose of IVIG [intravenous immunoglobulin] (0.8-1.0 g/kg) or a short course of corticosteroids should be used as first-line treatment." IVIG at a dose of 0.8-1.0 g/kg/day for 1-2 days induces a rapid rise in platelet count (usually >20 × 10⁹/L) in 95% of patients within 48 hr. IVIG appears to induce a response by downregulating Fc-mediated phagocytosis of antibody-coated platelets. IVIG therapy is both expensive and time-consuming to administer. Additionally, after infusion, there is a high frequency of headaches and vomiting, suggestive of IVIG-induced aseptic meningitis.

3. Prednisone. Corticosteroid therapy has been used for many years to treat acute and chronic ITP in adults and children. Doses of prednisone of 1-4 mg/kg/24 hr appear to induce a more rapid rise in platelet count than in untreated patients with ITP. Corticosteroid therapy is usually continued for short course until a rise in platelet count to >20 × 10⁹/L has been achieved to avoid the long-term side effects of corticosteroid therapy, especially growth failure, diabetes mellitus, and osteoporosis.

4. Intravenous anti-D therapy. For Rh-positive patients, IV anti-D at a dose of 50-75 μg/kg causes a rise in platelet count to >20 × 10⁹/L in 80-90% of patients within 48-72 hr. When given to Rh-positive individuals, IV anti-D induces mild hemolytic anemia. RBC-antibody complexes bind to macrophage Fc receptors and interfere with platelet destruction, thereby causing a rise in platelet count. IV anti-D is ineffective in Rh-negative patients. Rare life-threatening episodes of intravascular hemolysis have occurred in children and adults following infusion of IV anti-D.

Each of these medications may be used to treat ITP exacerbations, which commonly occur several weeks after an initial course of therapy. In the special case of intracranial hemorrhage, multiple modalities should be used, including platelet transfusion, IVIG, high-dose corticosteroids, and prompt consultation by neurosurgery and surgery.

There is no consensus regarding the management of acute childhood ITP, except that patients who are bleeding significantly (less than 5% of children with ITP) should be treated. Intracranial hemorrhage remains rare, and there are no data showing that treatment actually reduces its incidence.

The role of splenectomy in ITP should be reserved for 1 of 2 circumstances. The older child (≥4 yr) with severe ITP that has lasted >1 yr (chronic ITP) and whose symptoms are not easily controlled with therapy is a candidate for splenectomy. Splenectomy must also be considered when life-threatening hemorrhage (intracranial hemorrhage) complicates acute ITP, if the platelet count cannot be corrected rapidly with transfusion of platelets and administration of IVIG and corticosteroids. Splenectomy is associated with a lifelong risk of overwhelming postsplenectomy infection caused by encapsulated organisms, increased risk of thrombosis, and the potential development of pulmonary hypertension in adulthood. As an alternative to splenectomy, rituximab has been used off-label in children to treat chronic ITP. In 30-40% of children, rituximab has induced a partial or complete remission.

CHRONIC AUTOIMMUNE THROMBOCYTOPENIC PURPURA

Approximately 20% of patients who present with acute ITP have persistent thrombocytopenia for **>12 mo** and are said to have chronic ITP. At that time, a careful reevaluation for associated disorders should be performed, especially for autoimmune disease, such as SLE; chronic infectious disorders, such as HIV; and nonimmune causes of chronic thrombocytopenia, such as type 2B and platelet-type von Willebrand disease, X-linked thrombocytopenia, autoimmune lymphoproliferative syndrome, common variable immunodeficiency syndrome, autosomal macrothrombocytopenia, and WAS (also X-linked). The presence of coexisting *H. pylori* infection should be considered and, if found, treated. Therapy should be aimed at controlling symptoms and preventing serious bleeding. In ITP, the spleen is the primary site of both antiplatelet antibody synthesis and platelet destruction. Splenectomy is successful in inducing complete remission in 64-88% of children with chronic ITP. This effect must be balanced against the lifelong risk of overwhelming postsplenectomy infection. This decision is often affected by quality of life issues, as well as the ease with which the child can be managed using medical therapy, such as IVIG, corticosteroids, IV anti-D, or rituximab. Two effective agents that act to stimulate thrombopoiesis, romiplastin and eltrombopag (see Fig. 484-1), are approved by the FDA to treat adults with chronic ITP. Preliminary data using thrombopoietic agents in children are encouraging.

Bibliography is available at Expert Consult.

484.2 Drug-Induced Thrombocytopenia
J. Paul Scott

A number of drugs are associated with immune thrombocytopenia as the result of either an immune process or megakaryocyte injury. Some common drugs used in pediatrics that cause thrombocytopenia include valproic acid, phenytoin, carbamazepine, sulfonamides, vancomycin, and trimethoprim-sulfamethoxazole. Heparin-induced thrombocytopenia (and, rarely, an associated thrombosis) is seldom seen in pediatrics, but it occurs when, after exposure to heparin, the patient has an antibody directed against the heparin–platelet factor 4 complex. Recommended treatment for heparin-induced thrombocytopenia in adults includes argatroban, lepirudin, or danaparoid.

Bibliography is available at Expert Consult.

484.3 Nonimmune Platelet Destruction
J. Paul Scott

The syndromes of DIC (see Chapter 483), HUS (see Chapters 484.4 and 518), and thrombotic thrombocytopenic purpura (TTP) (see

Chapter 484.5) share the hematologic picture of a thrombotic microangiopathy in which there is RBC destruction and consumptive thrombocytopenia caused by platelet and fibrin deposition in the microvasculature. The microangiopathic hemolytic anemia is characterized by the presence of RBC fragments, including helmet cells, schistocytes, spherocytes, and burr cells.

484.4 Hemolytic-Uremic Syndrome

See Chapter 518.

484.5 Thrombotic Thrombocytopenic Purpura
J. Paul Scott

TTP is a rare pentad of **fever, microangiopathic hemolytic anemia, thrombocytopenia, abnormal renal function,** and **central nervous system changes** that is clinically similar to HUS, although TTP can be congenital, it usually presents in adults and occasionally in adolescents. Microvascular thrombi within the central nervous system cause subtle, shifting neurologic signs that vary from changes in affect and orientation to aphasia, blindness, and seizures. Initial manifestations are often nonspecific (weakness, pain, emesis); prompt recognition of this disorder is critical. Laboratory findings provide important clues to the diagnosis and show microangiopathic hemolytic anemia characterized by morphologically abnormal RBCs, with schistocytes, spherocytes, helmet cells, and an elevated reticulocyte count in association with thrombocytopenia. Coagulation studies are usually nondiagnostic. Blood urea nitrogen and creatinine are sometimes elevated. The treatment of TTP is plasmapheresis (plasma exchange), which is effective in 80-95% of cases. Treatment with plasmapheresis should be instituted on the basis of thrombocytopenia and microangiopathic hemolytic anemia even if other symptoms are not yet present. Rituximab, corticosteroids, and splenectomy are reserved for refractory cases.

The majority of cases of TTP are caused by an autoantibody–mediated deficiency of a metalloproteinase (ADAMTS-13) that is responsible for cleaving the high-molecular-weight multimers of VWF and appears to play a pivotal role in the evolution of the thrombotic microangiopathy. In contrast, levels of the metalloproteinase in HUS are usually normal. **Congenital deficiency** of the metalloproteinase causes rare familial cases of TTP/HUS, usually manifested as recurrent episodes of thrombocytopenia, hemolytic anemia, and renal involvement, with or without neurologic changes, that often present in infancy after an intercurrent illness. Abnormalities of the complement system have now also been implicated in rare cases of familial TTP. ADAMTS-13 deficiency can be treated by repeated infusions of fresh-frozen plasma.

Bibliography is available at Expert Consult.

484.6 Kasabach-Merritt Syndrome
J. Paul Scott

See also Chapter 650.

The association of a giant hemangioma with localized intravascular coagulation causing thrombocytopenia and hypofibrinogenemia is called *Kasabach-Merritt syndrome.* In most patients, the site of the hemangioma is obvious, but retroperitoneal and intraabdominal hemangiomas may require body imaging for detection. Inside the hemangioma there is platelet trapping and activation of coagulation, with fibrinogen consumption and generation of fibrin(ogen) degradation products. Arteriovenous malformation within the lesions can cause heart failure. Pathologically, Kasabach-Merritt syndrome appears to develop more often as a result of a kaposiform hemangioendothelioma or tufted hemangioma rather than a simple hemangioma. The peripheral blood smear shows microangiopathic changes. Multiple modalities have been used to treat Kasabach-Merritt syndrome, including propranolol, surgical excision (if possible), laser photocoagulation, high-dose corticosteroids, local radiation therapy, antiangiogenic agents, such as interferon-α_2, and vincristine. Over time, most patients who present in infancy have regression of the hemangioma. Treatment of the associated coagulopathy may benefit from a trial of antifibrinolytic therapy with ε-aminocaproic acid (Amicar).

484.7 Sequestration
J. Paul Scott

Thrombocytopenia develops in individuals with massive splenomegaly because the spleen acts as a sponge for platelets and sequesters large numbers. Most such patients also have mild leukopenia and anemia on CBC. Individuals who have thrombocytopenia caused by splenic sequestration should undergo a work-up to diagnose the etiology of splenomegaly, including infectious, inflammatory, infiltrative, neoplastic, obstructive, and hemolytic causes.

484.8 Congenital Thrombocytopenic Syndromes
J. Paul Scott

See Table 484-2.

Congenital amegakaryocytic thrombocytopenia (CAMT) usually manifests within the 1st few days to week of life, when the child presents with petechiae and purpura caused by profound thrombocytopenia. CAMT is caused by a rare defect in hematopoiesis as a result of a mutation in the stem cell TPO receptor (MPL). Other than skin and mucous membrane abnormalities, findings on physical examination are normal. Examination of the bone marrow shows an absence of megakaryocytes. These patients often progress to marrow failure (aplasia) over time. Hematopoietic stem cell transplantation is curative.

TAR syndrome consists of thrombocytopenia (absence or hypoplasia of megakaryocytes) that presents in early infancy with bilateral radial anomalies of variable severity, ranging from mild changes to marked limb shortening (Fig. 484-4). Many such individuals also have other skeletal abnormalities of the ulna, radius, and lower extremities. Thumbs are present. Intolerance to cow's milk formula (present in 50%) may complicate management by triggering gastrointestinal bleeding, increased thrombocytopenia, eosinophilia, and a leukemoid reaction. The thrombocytopenia of TAR syndrome frequently remits over the 1st few yrs of life. The molecular basis of TAR syndrome remains to be defined. A few patients have been reported to have a syndrome of **amegakaryocytic thrombocytopenia with radioulnar synostosis** caused by a mutation in the *HOXA11* gene. Different from TAR syndrome, this mutation causes marrow aplasia.

WAS is characterized by thrombocytopenia, with tiny platelets, eczema, and recurrent infection as a consequence of immune deficiency (see Chapter 126.2). WAS is inherited as an X-linked disorder, and the gene for WAS has been sequenced. The WAS protein appears to play an integral role in regulating the cytoskeletal architecture of both platelets and T lymphocytes in response to receptor-mediated cell signaling. The WAS protein is common to all cells of hematopoietic lineage. Molecular analysis of families with X-linked thrombocytopenia has shown that many affected members have a point mutation within the WAS gene, whereas individuals with the full manifestation of WAS have large gene deletions. Examination of the bone marrow in WAS shows the normal number of megakaryocytes, although they may have bizarre morphologic features. Transfused platelets have a normal life span. Splenectomy often corrects the thrombocytopenia, suggesting that the platelets formed in WAS have accelerated destruction. After splenectomy, these patients are at increased risk for overwhelm-

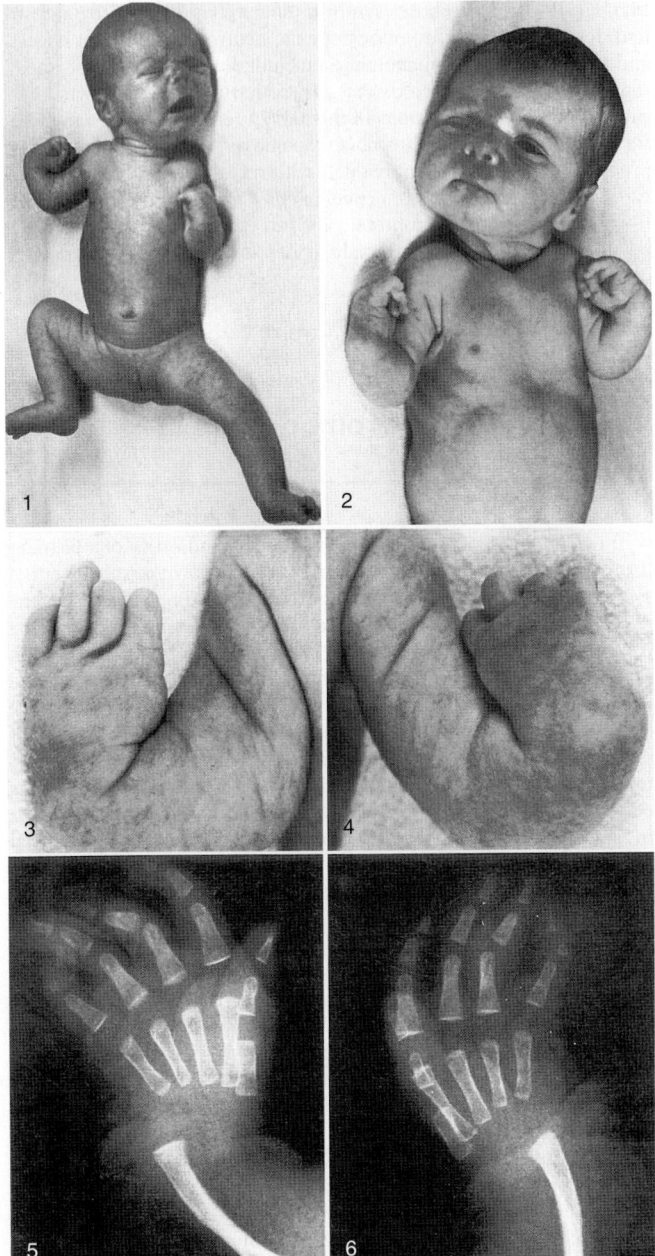

Figure 484-4 A newborn, the first child of young, healthy parents, with fully expressed TAR syndrome, including thrombocytopenia, hypereosinophilia, and anemia. Hypoplasia of the distal humeri and the shoulder girdles, bilateral hip dysplasia, mild talipes calcaneus, and clinodactyly of both little fingers are seen. This patient had a pronounced allergy to cow's milk, with exposure followed by diarrhea, vomiting, and decreased weight and platelet count, making a cow's milk–free diet mandatory. A persistent depressed nasal bridge and development of pronounced bowed legs are seen. *(From Wiedemann H-R, Kunze J, Grosse F-R, editors: Clinical syndromes, ed 3, [English translation], London, 1997, Mosby-Wolfe, p. 430.)*

ing infection and require lifelong antibiotic prophylaxis against encapsulated organisms. Approximately 5-15% of patients with WAS develop lymphoreticular malignancies. Successful hematopoietic stem cell transplantation cures WAS. **X-linked macrothrombocytopenia** and **dyserythropoiesis** have been linked to mutations in the *GATA-1* gene, an erythroid and megakaryocytic transcription factor.

MYH9-related thrombocytopenia: A diverse number of hereditary thrombocytopenia syndromes, given names such as Sebastian, Epstein,

May-Hegglin, and Fechtner syndromes, are characterized by autosomal dominant macrothrombocytopenia, neutrophil inclusion bodies, and a variety of physical anomalies, including sensorineural deafness, renal disease, and/or eye disease. These have all been shown to be caused by different mutations in the *MYH9* gene (nonmuscle myosin-IIa heavy chain). The thrombocytopenia is usually mild and not progressive. Some other individuals with recessively inherited macrothrombocytopenia have abnormalities in chromosome 22q11. Mutations in the gene for glycoprotein Ibβ, an essential component of the platelet VWF receptor, can result in Bernard-Soulier syndrome (see Chapter 484.13).

Bibliography is available at Expert Consult.

484.9 Neonatal Thrombocytopenia

J. Paul Scott

See also Chapter 103.4.

Thrombocytopenia in the newborn rarely is indicative of a primary disorder of megakaryopoiesis but more often is the result of either systemic illness or transfer of maternal antibodies directed against fetal platelets (see Table 484-2). Neonatal thrombocytopenia often occurs in association with congenital viral infection, especially rubella; cytomegalovirus; protozoal infection, such as toxoplasmosis; syphilis; and perinatal bacterial infection, especially those caused by Gram-negative bacilli. Thrombocytopenia associated with DIC may be responsible for severe spontaneous bleeding. The constellation of marked thrombocytopenia and abnormal abdominal findings is common in necrotizing enterocolitis and other causes of necrotic bowel. Thrombocytopenia in an ill child requires a prompt search for viral and bacterial pathogens.

Antibody-mediated thrombocytopenia in the newborn occurs because of transplacental transfer of maternal antibodies directed against fetal platelets. Neonatal alloimmune thrombocytopenic purpura (NATP) is caused by the development of maternal antibodies against antigens present on fetal platelets that are shared with the father and recognized as foreign by the maternal immune system. This is the platelet equivalent of Rh disease of the newborn. The incidence of NATP is 1/4,000-5,000 live births. The clinical manifestations of NATP are those of an apparently well child who, within the 1st few days after delivery, has generalized petechiae and purpura. Laboratory studies show a normal maternal platelet count, yet moderate to severe thrombocytopenia in the newborn. Detailed review of the history should show no evidence of maternal thrombocytopenia. Up to 30% of infants with severe NATP may have intracranial hemorrhage, either prenatally or in the perinatal period. Unlike Rh disease, first pregnancies may be severely affected. Subsequent pregnancies are often more severely affected than the first.

The **diagnosis** of NATP is made by checking for the presence of maternal alloantibodies directed against the father's platelets. Specific studies can be done to identify the target alloantigen. The most common cause is incompatibility for the platelet alloantigen HPA-1a. Specific DNA sequence polymorphisms have been identified that permit informative prenatal testing to identify at-risk pregnancies. The differential diagnosis of NATP includes transplacental transfer of maternal antiplatelet autoantibodies (maternal ITP), and, more commonly, viral or bacterial infection.

Treatment of NATP requires the administration of IVIG prenatally to the mother. Therapy usually begins in the 2nd trimester and is continued throughout the pregnancy. Fetal platelet count can be monitored by percutaneous umbilical blood sampling. Delivery should be performed by cesarean section. After delivery, if severe thrombocytopenia persists, transfusion of 1 unit of platelets that share the maternal alloantigens (e.g., washed maternal platelets) will cause a rise in platelet counts to provide effective hemostasis. After there has been 1 affected child, genetic counseling is critical to inform the parents of the high risk of thrombocytopenia in subsequent pregnancies.

Children born to mothers with ITP (**maternal ITP**) appear to have a lower risk of serious hemorrhage than infants born with NATP, although severe thrombocytopenia may occur. The mother's preexisting platelet count may have some predictive value in that severe maternal thrombocytopenia before delivery appears to predict a higher risk of fetal thrombocytopenia. In mothers who have had splenectomy for ITP, the maternal platelet count may be normal and is not predictive of fetal thrombocytopenia.

Treatment includes prenatal administration of corticosteroids to the mother and administration of IVIG and sometimes corticosteroids to the infant after delivery. Thrombocytopenia in an infant, whether a result of NATP or maternal ITP, usually resolves within 2-4 mo after delivery. The period of highest risk is the immediate perinatal period.

Two syndromes of congenital failure of platelet production often present in the newborn period. In **CAMT,** the newborn manifests petechiae and purpura shortly after birth. Findings on physical examination are otherwise normal. Megakaryocytes are absent from the bone marrow. This syndrome is caused by a mutation in the megakaryocyte TPO receptor that is essential for development of all hematopoietic cell lines. Pancytopenia eventually develops, and hematopoietic stem cell transplantation is curative. **TAR syndrome** consists of thrombocytopenia that presents in early infancy, with bilateral radial anomalies of variable severity, ranging from mild changes to marked limb shortening. Thumbs are present. In many such individuals, there are also other skeletal abnormalities of the lower extremities. Intolerance to cow's milk formula is present in 50% of patients. TAR syndrome frequently remits over the 1st few yr of life (see Chapter 484.8) (see Fig. 484-4).

Bibliography is available at Expert Consult.

484.10 Thrombocytopenia from Acquired Disorders Causing Decreased Production

J. Paul Scott and Veronica Flood

Disorders of the bone marrow that inhibit megakaryopoiesis usually affect RBC and WBC production. Infiltrative disorders, including malignancies, such as acute lymphocytic leukemia, histiocytosis, lymphomas, and storage disease, usually cause either abnormalities on physical examination (lymphadenopathy, hepatosplenomegaly, or masses) or abnormalities of the WBC count, or anemia. Aplastic processes may present as isolated thrombocytopenia, although there are usually clues on the CBC (leukopenia, neutropenia, anemia, or macrocytosis). Children with constitutional aplastic anemia (Fanconi anemia) often have abnormalities on examination, including radial anomalies, other skeletal anomalies, short stature, microcephaly, and hyperpigmentation. Bone marrow examination should be performed when thrombocytopenia is associated with abnormalities found on physical examination or on examination of the other blood cell lines.

484.11 Platelet Function Disorders

J. Paul Scott

Bleeding time and the platelet function analyzer (PFA-100) are the only commonly available tests to screen for abnormal platelet function. Bleeding time measures the interaction of platelets with the blood vessel wall and thus is affected by both platelet count and platelet function. The predictive value of bleeding time is problematic because bleeding time is dependent on a number of other factors, including the skill of the technician and the cooperation of the patient, often a challenge in the infant or young child. A normal bleeding time does not rule out a mild platelet function defect in a clinically symptomatic individual. The PFA-100 measures platelet adhesion and aggregation in whole blood at high shear when the blood is exposed to either collagen-epinephrine or collagen-ADP. Results are reported as the closure time measured in sec. Many clinical laboratories have replaced bleeding time with the use of the PFA-100. Both the PFA-100 and bleeding time are sensitive to moderate/severe von Willebrand disease and platelet dysfunction. Both are variably insensitive to mild platelet function abnormalities and mild von Willebrand disease. The use of the PFA-100 as a screening test remains controversial and, like the bleeding time, lacks specificity. Bleeding time is the only commonly available test to assess platelet–vessel wall interaction. For patients with a positive history of bleeding suggestive of von Willebrand disease or platelet dysfunction, specific VWF testing and platelet function studies should be done, irrespective of the results of the bleeding time or PFA-100.

Platelet function in the clinical laboratory is currently measured using platelet aggregometry. In the aggregometer, agonists, such as collagen, ADP, ristocetin, epinephrine, arachidonic acid, and thrombin (or the thrombin receptor peptide), are added to platelet-rich plasma, and the clumping of platelets over time is measured by an automated machine. At the same time, other instruments measure the release of granular contents, such as ATP, from the platelets after activation. The ability of platelets to aggregate and their metabolic activity can be assessed simultaneously. When a patient is being evaluated for possible platelet dysfunction, it is critically important to exclude the presence of other exogenous agents and to study the patient, if possible, off all medications for 2 wk. Further evaluation using flow cytometric analysis or molecular testing are often necessary to make a more definitive diagnosis.

484.12 Acquired Disorders of Platelet Function
J. Paul Scott

A number of systemic illnesses are associated with platelet dysfunction, most commonly, liver disease, kidney disease (uremia), and disorders that trigger increased amounts of fibrin degradation products. These disorders frequently cause prolonged bleeding time and are often associated with other abnormalities of the coagulation mechanism. The most important element of management is to treat the primary illness. If treatment of the primary process is not feasible, infusions of desmopressin have been helpful in augmenting hemostasis and correcting bleeding time. In some patients, transfusions of platelets and/or cryoprecipitate have also been helpful in improving hemostasis.

Many drugs alter platelet function. The most commonly used drug in adults that alters platelet function is acetylsalicylic acid (aspirin). Aspirin irreversibly acetylates the enzyme cyclo-oxygenase, which is critical in the formation of thromboxane A_2. Aspirin usually causes moderate platelet dysfunction that becomes more prominent if there is another abnormality of the hemostatic mechanism. In children, commonly used drugs that affect platelet function include other nonsteroidal antiinflammatory drugs, valproic acid, and high-dose penicillin. Specific agents to inhibit platelet function therapeutically include those that block the platelet ADP receptor (clopidogrel) and αIIb-β₃ receptor antagonists, as well as aspirin.

484.13 Congenital Abnormalities of Platelet Function
J. Paul Scott

Severe platelet function defects usually present with petechiae and purpura shortly after birth, especially after vaginal delivery. Defects in the platelet GPIb complex (the VWF receptor) or the αIIb-β₃ complex (the fibrinogen receptor) cause severe congenital platelet dysfunction.

Bernard-Soulier syndrome, a severe congenital platelet function disorder, is caused by absence or severe deficiency of the VWF receptor (GPIb complex) on the platelet membrane. This syndrome is characterized by thrombocytopenia, with giant platelets and markedly

prolonged bleeding time (>20 min) or PFA-100 closure time. Platelet aggregation tests show absent ristocetin-induced platelet aggregation, but normal aggregation to all other agonists. Ristocetin induces the binding of VWF to platelets and agglutinates platelets. Results of studies of VWF are normal. The GPIb complex interacts with the platelet cytoskeleton; a defect in this interaction is believed to be the cause of the large platelet size. Bernard-Soulier syndrome is inherited as an autosomal recessive disorder. Genetic mutations causing Bernard-Soulier syndrome are usually identified in the genes forming the GPIb complex of glycoproteins Ibα, Ibβ, V, and IX.

Glanzmann thrombasthenia is a congenital disorder associated with severe platelet dysfunction that yields prolonged bleeding time and a normal platelet count. Platelets have normal size and morphologic features on the peripheral blood smear, and closure times for PFA-100 or bleeding time are markedly abnormal. Aggregation studies show abnormal or absent aggregation with all agonists used except ristocetin, because ristocetin agglutinates platelets and does not require a metabolically active platelet. This disorder is caused by deficiency of the platelet fibrinogen receptor αIIb-β₃, the major integrin complex on the platelet surface that undergoes conformational changes by inside out signaling when platelets are activated. Fibrinogen binds to this complex when the platelet is activated and causes platelets to aggregate. Caused by identifiable mutations in the genes for αIIb or β₃, this disorder is inherited in an autosomal recessive manner. For both Bernard-Soulier syndrome and Glanzmann thrombasthenia, the diagnosis is confirmed by flow cytometric analysis of the patient's platelet glycoproteins.

Hereditary deficiency of platelet storage granules occurs in 2 well-characterized but rare syndromes that involve deficiency of intracytoplasmic granules. **Dense body deficiency** is characterized by absence of the granules that contain ADP, ATP, Ca^{2+}, and serotonin. This disorder is diagnosed by the finding that ATP is not released on platelet aggregation studies and ideally is characterized by electron microscopic studies. **Gray platelet syndrome** is caused by the absence of platelet α granules, resulting in large platelets that are large and appear gray on Wright stain of peripheral blood. In this rare syndrome, aggregation and release are absent with most agonists other than thrombin and ristocetin. Electron microscopic studies are diagnostic.

OTHER HEREDITARY DISORDERS OF PLATELET FUNCTION
Abnormalities in the pathways of platelet signaling/activation and release of granular contents cause a heterogeneous group of platelet function defects that are usually manifested as increased bruising, epistaxis, and/or menorrhagia. Symptoms may be subtle and are often made more obvious by high-risk surgery, such as tonsillectomy or adenoidectomy, or by administration of nonsteroidal antiinflammatory drugs. In the laboratory, bleeding time is variable and closure time as measured by the PFA-100 is frequently, but not always, prolonged. Platelet aggregation studies show deficient aggregation with 1 or 2 agonists and/or abnormal release of granular contents.

The formation of thromboxane from arachidonic acid after the activation of phospholipase is critical to normal platelet function. Deficiency or dysfunction of enzymes, such as cyclo-oxygenase and thromboxane synthase, which metabolize arachidonic acid, causes abnormal platelet function. In the aggregometer, platelets from such patients do not aggregate in response to arachidonic acid.

The most common platelet function defects are those characterized by variable bleeding time/PFA closure times and abnormal aggregation with 1 or 2 agonists, usually ADP and/or collagen. These patients have normal aggregation with thrombin receptor peptide. Some of these individuals have only decreased release of ATP from intracytoplasmic granules; the significance of this finding is debated.

TREATMENT OF PATIENTS WITH PLATELET DYSFUNCTION
Successful treatment depends on the severity of both the diagnosis and the hemorrhagic event. In all but severe platelet function defects, desmopressin 0.3 μg/kg IV may be used for mild to moderate bleeding

episodes. In addition to its effect on stimulating levels of VWF and factor VIII, desmopressin corrects bleeding time and augments hemostasis in many individuals with mild to moderate platelet function defects. For individuals with Bernard-Soulier syndrome or Glanzmann thrombasthenia, platelet transfusions of 1 unit/5-10 kg corrects the defect in hemostasis and may be lifesaving. Rarely, antibodies develop to the deficient platelet protein, rendering the patient refractory to the transfused platelets. In such patients, the off-label use of recombinant factor VIIa has been effective, and this treatment is undergoing clinical trials. In both conditions, hematopoietic stem cell transplantation has been curative.

Bibliography is available at Expert Consult.

484.14 Disorders of the Blood Vessels
J. Paul Scott

Disorders of the vessel walls or supporting structures mimic the findings of a bleeding disorder although coagulation studies are usually normal. The findings of petechiae and purpuric lesions in such patients are often attributable to an underlying vasculitis/vasculopathy. Skin biopsy can be particularly helpful in elucidating the type of vascular pathology.

HENOCH-SCHÖNLEIN PURPURA
See Chapter 167.1.

EHLERS-DANLOS SYNDROME
See Chapter 659.

OTHER ACQUIRED DISORDERS
Scurvy, chronic corticosteroid therapy, and severe malnutrition are associated with "weakening" of the collagen matrix that supports the blood vessels. Therefore, these factors are associated with easy bruising, and particularly in the case of scurvy, bleeding gums and loosening of the teeth. Lesions of the skin that initially appear to be petechiae and purpura may be seen in vasculitic syndromes, such as SLE.

Bibliography is available at Expert Consult.

Section 8
The Spleen

Chapter 485
Anatomy and Function of the Spleen
Amanda M. Brandow and Bruce M. Camitta

ANATOMY
The splenic precursor is recognizable by 5 wk of gestation. At birth, the spleen weighs approximately 11 g. Thereafter, it enlarges until puberty, reaching an average weight of 135 g, and then diminishes in size during adulthood. Approximately 15% of patients will have an accessory spleen. The major splenic components are a lymphoid compartment (*white pulp*) and a filtering system (*red pulp*). The white pulp consists of periarterial lymphatic sheaths of T lymphocytes with embedded germinal centers containing B lymphocytes. The red pulp has a skeleton of fixed reticular cells, mobile macrophages, partially collapsed endothelial passages (cords of Billroth), and splenic sinuses. A *marginal zone* rich in dendritic (antigen-presenting) cells separates the red pulp from the white pulp. The splenic capsule contains smooth muscle and contracts in response to epinephrine. Approximately 10% of the blood delivered to the spleen flows rapidly through a closed vascular network. The other 90% flows more slowly through an open system (the *splenic cords*), where it is filtered through 1-5 μm slits before entering the splenic sinuses.

FUNCTION
The unique anatomy and blood flow of the spleen enable it to perform reservoir, filtering, and immunologic functions. The spleen receives 5-6% of the cardiac output, but normally contains only 25 mL of blood. It can retain much more when it enlarges leading to cytopenias. Hematopoiesis is a major splenic function at 3-6 mo of fetal life but then disappears. Splenic hematopoiesis can be resumed in patients with myelofibrosis or severe hemolytic anemia. Factor VIII and one-third of the circulating platelet mass are sequestered in the spleen and can be released by stress or epinephrine injection. Thrombocytosis and leukocytosis occur with loss of the splenic reservoir function. A high platelet count after the loss of splenic function or splenectomy is not associated with an increased risk of thrombosis in children.

Slow blood flow past macrophages and through small openings in the sinus walls facilitates the filtering functions of the spleen. Excess membrane is removed from young red blood cells (RBCs); loss of this function is characterized by target cells, poikilocytosis, and decreased osmotic fragility. The spleen is the primary site for destruction of old RBCs; this function is assumed by other reticuloendothelial cells after splenectomy. The spleen also removes damaged/abnormal red cells (such as spherocytes and antibody-coated RBCs) and damaged/senescent platelets. Intracytoplasmic inclusions may be removed from RBCs without cell lysis. Functional or anatomic hyposplenia is characterized by continued circulation of cells containing nuclear remnants (**Howell-Jolly bodies**), denatured hemoglobin (**Heinz bodies**), and other debris in RBCs. This debris may appear as "**pits**" on indirect microscopy.

The spleen plays a large role in host defense against infection. The spleen is the largest lymphoid organ in the body and contains nearly half of the body's total immunoglobulin-producing B lymphocytes. The spleen processes foreign material to stimulate production of opsonizing antibody. Properdin and tuftsin are also produced in the spleen. Thus, young (nonimmune) or hyposplenic individuals are at increased risk for **sepsis** caused by pneumococci and other encapsulated bacteria. The spleen can also use phagocytosis to trap and destroy intracellular parasites. The spleen has a minor role in antibody response to intramuscularly or subcutaneously injected antigens but is required for early antibody production after exposure to intravenous antigens. The spleen may be an important site of antibody production in immune thrombocytopenia purpura.

Bibliography is available at Expert Consult.

Chapter 486
Splenomegaly
Amanda M. Brandow and Bruce M. Camitta

CLINICAL MANIFESTATIONS
A soft, thin spleen is palpable in 15% of neonates, 10% of normal children, and 5% of adolescents. In most individuals, the spleen must be 2-3 times its normal size before it is palpable. The spleen is best examined when standing on the right side of a supine patient by

Table 486-1	Differential Diagnosis of Splenomegaly by Pathophysiology

ANATOMIC LESIONS
Cysts, pseudocysts
Hamartomas
Polysplenia syndrome
Hemangiomas and lymphangiomas
Hematoma or rupture (traumatic)
Peliosis

HYPERPLASIA CAUSED BY HEMATOLOGIC DISORDERS
Acute and Chronic Hemolysis*
Hemoglobinopathies (sickle cell disease in infancy with or without sequestration crisis and sickle variants, thalassemia major, unstable hemoglobins)
Erythrocyte membrane disorders (hereditary spherocytosis, elliptocytosis, pyropoikilocytosis)
Erythrocyte enzyme deficiencies (severe G6PD deficiency, pyruvate kinase deficiency)
Immune hemolysis (autoimmune and isoimmune hemolysis)
Paroxysmal nocturnal hemoglobinuria
Chronic Iron Deficiency
Extramedullary Hematopoiesis
Myeloproliferative diseases: CML, juvenile CML, myelofibrosis with myeloid metaplasia, polycythemia vera
Osteopetrosis
Patients receiving granulocyte and granulocyte-macrophage colony-stimulating factors

INFECTIONS†
Bacterial
Acute sepsis: *Salmonella typhi, Streptococcus pneumoniae, Haemophilus influenzae* type b, *Staphylococcus aureus*
Chronic infections: infective endocarditis, chronic meningococcemia, brucellosis, tularemia, cat-scratch disease
Local infections: splenic abscess (*S. aureus*, streptococci, less often *Salmonella* species, polymicrobial infection), pyogenic liver abscess (anaerobic bacteria, Gram-negative enteric bacteria), cholangitis
Viral*
Acute viral infections, especially in children
Congenital CMV, herpes simplex, rubella
Hepatitides A, B, and C; CMV
EBV
Viral hemophagocytic syndromes: CMV, EBV, HHV-6
HIV
Spirochetal
Syphilis, especially congenital syphilis
Leptospirosis
Rickettsial
Rocky Mountain spotted fever
Q fever
Typhus
Fungal/Mycobacterial
Miliary tuberculosis
Disseminated histoplasmosis
South American blastomycosis
Systemic candidiasis (in immunosuppressed patients)

Parasitic
Malaria
Toxoplasmosis, especially congenital
Toxocara canis, Toxocara cati (visceral larva migrans)
Leishmaniasis (kala-azar)
Schistosomiasis (hepatic-portal involvement)
Trypanosomiasis
Fascioliasis
Babesiosis

IMMUNOLOGIC AND INFLAMMATORY PROCESSES*
Systemic lupus erythematosus
Rheumatoid arthritis
Mixed connective tissue disease
Systemic vasculitis
Serum sickness
Drug hypersensitivity, especially to phenytoin
Graft-versus-host disease
Sjögren syndrome
Cryoglobulinemia
Amyloidosis
Sarcoidosis
Autoimmune lymphoproliferative syndrome
Posttransplant lymphoproliferative disease
Large granular lymphocytosis and neutropenia
Histiocytosis syndromes
Hemophagocytic syndromes (nonviral, familial)

MALIGNANCIES
Primary: leukemia (acute, chronic), lymphoma, angiosarcoma, Hodgkin disease, mastocytosis
Metastatic

STORAGE DISEASES
Lipidosis (Gaucher disease, Niemann-Pick disease, infantile GM1 gangliosidosis)
Mucopolysaccharidoses (Hurler, Hunter-type)
Mucolipidosis (I-cell disease, sialidosis, multiple sulfatase deficiency, fucosidosis)
Defects in carbohydrate metabolism: galactosemia, fructose intolerance, glycogen storage disease IV
Sea-blue histiocyte syndrome
Tangier disease
Wolman disease
Hyperchylomicronemia type I, IV

CONGESTIVE*
Heart failure
Intrahepatic cirrhosis or fibrosis
Extrahepatic portal (thrombosis), splenic, and hepatic vein obstruction (thrombosis, Budd-Chiari syndrome)

*Common.
†Chronic or recurrent infection suggests underlying immunodeficiency.
   CML, chronic myelogenous leukemia; CMV, cytomegalovirus; EBV, Epstein-Barr virus; G6PD, glucose-6-phosphate dehydrogenase; HHV-6, human herpesvirus 6; HIV, human immunodeficiency virus.

palpating across the abdomen as the patient inspires deeply or with the patient in the right lateral decubitus position. A splenic edge felt more than 2 cm below the left costal margin is abnormal. An enlarged spleen might descend into the pelvis; when splenomegaly is suspected, the abdominal examination should begin at a lower starting point. Superficial abdominal venous distention may be present when splenomegaly is a result of portal hypertension. Patients may also complain of left upper quadrant pain as the spleen enlarges. Radiologic detection or confirmation of splenic enlargement is done with ultrasonography, CT, or technetium-99 sulfur colloid scan. The latter also assesses splenic function.

DIFFERENTIAL DIAGNOSIS

Table 486-1 lists specific causes of splenomegaly. A thorough history with a focus on systemic complaints (fever, night sweats, malaise, weight loss) and a complete physical exam (with special attention to adenopathy), in combination with a complete blood count and careful review of the peripheral smear can help guide diagnosis.

Pseudosplenomegaly

Abnormally long mesenteric connections may produce a wandering or ptotic spleen. An enlarged left lobe of the liver, a left upper quadrant mass, or a splenic hematoma may be mistaken for splenomegaly.

Splenic cysts may contribute to splenomegaly or mimic it; these may be congenital (epidermoid) or acquired (pseudocyst) after trauma or infarction. Cysts are usually asymptomatic and are found on radiologic evaluation. Splenosis after splenic rupture or an accessory spleen (present in 15% of normal individuals) may also mimic splenomegaly; most are not palpable. The syndrome of congenital polysplenism includes cardiac defects, left-sided organ anomalies, bilobed lungs, biliary atresia, and pseudosplenomegaly (see Chapter 431.11).

Hypersplenism

Increased splenic function (sequestration or destruction of circulating cells) can result in peripheral blood cytopenias (thrombocytopenia, neutropenia, anemia), increased bone marrow activity, and splenomegaly. It is usually secondary to another disease and may be cured by treatment of the underlying condition or, if absolutely necessary, moderated by splenectomy.

Congestive Splenomegaly (Banti Syndrome)

Splenomegaly may result from obstruction in the hepatic, portal, or splenic veins leading to hypersplenism. Wilson disease (see Chapter 357.2), galactosemia (see Chapter 87.2), biliary atresia (see Chapter 356.1), and α_1-antitrypsin deficiency (see Chapter 357) may result in hepatic inflammation, fibrosis, and vascular obstruction. Congenital abnormalities (absence or hypoplasia) of the portal or splenic veins may cause vascular obstruction. Septic omphalitis or thrombophlebitis (spontaneous or as a result of umbilical venous catheterization in neonates) may result in secondary obliteration of these vessels. Splenic venous flow may be obstructed by masses of sickled erythrocytes leading to infarction. When the spleen is the site of vascular obstruction, splenectomy cures hypersplenism. However, since obstruction usually is in the hepatic or portal systems, portacaval shunting may be more helpful, because both portal hypertension and thrombocytopenia contribute to variceal bleeding.

Bibliography is available at Expert Consult.

Chapter 487

Hyposplenism, Splenic Trauma, and Splenectomy

*Amanda M. Brandow and
Bruce M. Camitta*

HYPOSPLENISM

Congenital absence of the spleen is associated with complex cyanotic heart defects, dextrocardia, bilateral trilobed lungs, and heterotopic abdominal organs (Ivemark syndrome; see Chapter 431.11). Splenic function is usually normal in children with **congenital polysplenia.** **Functional hyposplenism** may occur in normal neonates, especially premature infants. Children with sickle cell hemoglobinopathies (see Chapter 462.1) may have splenic hypofunction as early as 6 mo of age. Initially, this is caused by vascular obstruction, which can be reversed with red blood cell (RBC) transfusion or hydroxyurea. The spleen eventually autoinfarcts and becomes fibrotic and permanently nonfunctional. Functional hyposplenism may also occur in malaria (see Chapter 288), after irradiation to the left upper quadrant, and when the reticuloendothelial function of the spleen is overwhelmed (as in severe hemolytic anemia or metabolic storage disease). Splenic hypofunction has been reported occasionally in patients with autoimmune diseases

Table 487-1	Diseases Associated with Hyposplenism or Splenic Atropy

CONGENITAL FORMS	AUTOIMMUNE DISORDERS
Normal and premature neonates	Systematic lupus erythematosus
Isolated congenital hypoplasia	Rheumatoid arthritis
Ivemark syndrome	Glomerulonephritis
Autoimmune polyendocrinopathy-candidiasis-ectodermal dystrophy (APECED) syndrome	Wegener granulomatosis
	Goodpasture syndrome
Hypoparathyroidism syndrome	Sjögren syndrome
Stormorken syndrome	Nodous polyarteritis
Heterotaxia syndromes	Thyroiditis
	Sarcoidosis
GASTROINTESTINAL DISORDERS	**INFECTIOUS DISEASES**
Coeliac disease	HIV/AIDS
Inflammatory bowel disease	Pneumococcal meningitis
Whipple disease	Malaria
Dermatitis herpetiformis	
Intestinal lymphangiectasia	
Idiopathic chronic ulcerative enteritis	
HEPATIC DISORDERS	**IATROGENIC FORMS**
Active chronic hepatitis	Exposure to methyldopa
Primary biliary cirrhosis	High-dose steroids
Hepatic cirrhosis and portal hypertension	Total parenteral nutrition
	Splenic irradiation
Alcoholism and alcoholic hepatopathy	
ONCOHEMATOLOGIC DISORDERS	**ALTERATION IN SPLENIC CIRCULATION**
Hemoglobin S diseases	Thrombosis of splenic artery
Bone marrow transplantation	Thrombosis of splenic vein
Chronic graft-versus-host disease	Thrombosis of coeliac artery
Acute leukemia	**MISCELLANEOUS**
Chronic myeloproliferative disorders	Amyloidosis
Fanconi syndrome	
Splenic tumors	
Mastocytosis	

From Di Sabatino A, Carsetti R, Corazza GR. Post-splenectomy and hyposplenic states, Lancet 378(9785):86-97, 2011.

(i.e., rheumatoid arthritis, lupus, sarcoidosis), nephritis, inflammatory bowel disease, celiac disease, chronic hepatitis, Pearson syndrome, Fanconi anemia, and graft-versus-host disease) (Table 487-1).

Splenic hypofunction is characterized by RBC inclusions in peripheral blood smears (Howell-Jolly bodies or Heinz bodies), **"pits"** on interference microscopy, and poor uptake of technetium or other spleen scans (Table 487-2, Fig. 487-1). Reduced immunoglobulin M memory B cells may also be detected and is a risk factor for overwhelming sepsis. Patients with functional hyposplenism or asplenia are at increased risk for sepsis from encapsulated bacteria and benefit from antibiotic prophylaxis.

SPLENIC TRAUMA

Injury to the spleen may occur with abdominal trauma. Small splenic capsular tears may cause abdominal or referred left shoulder pain as a result of diaphragmatic irritation by blood. Larger tears result in more severe blood loss, with similar pain and signs of hypovolemic shock. Previously enlarged spleens (as in patients with infectious mononucleosis) are more likely to rupture with minor trauma. Patients with splenomegaly should avoid contact sports and other activities that increase the risk of splenic trauma. CT scan with IV contrast is the best imaging modality to assess splenic trauma.

Treatment of a small capsular injury should include careful observation with attention to changes in vital signs or abdominal findings, serial hemoglobin determinations, and the availability of prompt surgical intervention if a patient's condition deteriorates (see Chapter 72).

Table 487-2	Diagnostic Techniques for and Features of Spleen Dysfunction	
	DESCRIPTION	**COMMENTS**
Immunoglobulin M memory B cells	Cells dependent on spleen for survival. Produced in marginal zone	Special tests required
Technetium-99m–labeled sulphur colloidal scintiscan	Quantitation of splenic uptake of colloidal sulphur particles enables a fairly accurate static assessment of spleen function	Hypertrophy of the left hepatic lobe might be a limiting factor (this technique does not clearly show whether the mass originated in the liver or the spleen in the presence of an overlapping hypertropic left hepatic lobe)
Technetium-99m–labeled or rubidium-81–labeled heat-damaged autologous erythrocyte clearance	Measurement of clearance time allows a dynamic evaluation of spleen function	Preexisting erythrocyte defects, difficult erythrocyte incorporation of the radioisotope, false-positive or false-negative results in relation to excessive or insufficient heat damage make the test not suitable for clinical practice
Detection of Howell-Jolly bodies by staining	Erythrocytes with nuclear remnants Flow cytometry	No need for special equipment; inaccurate in the quantitation of splenic hypofunction
Detection of pitted erythrocytes by phase-interference microscopy	Erythrocytes with membrane indentations (4% upper limit of the normal range)	Need for phase-interference microscopy; counts enable a wide range of measurements and correlate with radioisotopic methods

From Di Sabatino A, Carsetti R, Corazza GR. Post-splenectomy and hyposplenic states, Lancet 378(9785):86-97, 2011, Table 1.

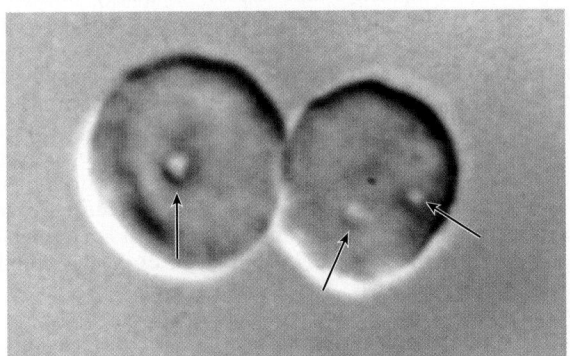

Figure 487-1 Characteristic pitted erythrocytes. A pitted erythrocyte is recognizable on phase-interference microscopy by the characteristic "pit" on the cell membrane (arrows). (From Di Sabatino A, Carsetti R, Corazza GR. Post-splenectomy and hyposplenic states, Lancet 378[9785]:86-97, 2011, Fig. 2.)

RBC transfusion requirements should be minimal (<25 mL/kg/48 hr). These patients are usually hospitalized for 10-14 days and have their activities restricted for months. Laparotomy, with or without splenectomy, is indicated for more marked abdominal bleeding, in patients who have clinical instability or deterioration, or when other organ damage is suspected. Partial splenectomy and splenic repair should be substituted for total splenectomy when feasible to maintain some splenic immune function.

SPLENECTOMY

Splenectomy should be limited to specific indications where medical therapy is (or has been) ineffective. These include traumatic splenic rupture, anatomic defects, severe transfusion dependent hemolytic anemia, immune cytopenias, metabolic storage diseases, and secondary hypersplenism. The major long-term risk of splenectomy is sudden, overwhelming postsplenectomy infections (sepsis or meningitis). This risk is especially high in children younger than 5 yr at the time of surgery. The risk of sepsis is less when splenectomy is performed for trauma, RBC membrane defects, and immune thrombocytopenia (2-4%) than when there is sickle cell anemia, thalassemia, or a preexisting immune deficiency (Wiskott-Aldrich syndrome, Hodgkin disease) or reticuloendothelial blockade (storage disease, severe hemolytic anemia) (8-30%). The overall risk is 2-5 per 1,000 asplenic patient years, with a lifelong risk of overwhelming postsplenectomy infections of 5%; more than half occur within 2 yr after splenectomy, although

the risk remains lifelong. The use of laparoscopic splenectomy has decreased surgical morbidity and hospitalization time.

Encapsulated bacteria, such as *Streptococcus pneumoniae* (>60% of cases), *Haemophilus influenzae,* and *Neisseria meningitidis,* account for >80% of cases of postsplenectomy sepsis. Because the spleen is responsible for filtering the blood and for early antibody responses, sepsis (with or without meningitis) can progress rapidly, leading to death within 12-24 hr of onset. Febrile splenectomized patients should be evaluated and treated promptly with antibiotics to cover the organisms previously mentioned. This treatment should be initiated at home if access to definitive medical care will be delayed. A broad-spectrum cephalosporin (cefotaxime or ceftriaxone) is recommended until specific antibiotic susceptibility and presence or absence of meningitis is known. Vancomycin (to cover penicillin-resistant pneumococci) should be initiated, depending on the illness severity and susceptibilities of pneumococci at the institution. Splenectomized patients are also at increased risk for contracting protozoal infections, such as malaria and babesiosis. Serious infection may occur after an animal bite (particularly dogs) and is due to *Capnocytophaga canimorsus* or *C. cynodegmi.* Prophylactic antibiotics should be given after a bite to potentially prevent sepsis caused by these organisms (see Chapter 724).

Preoperative, intraoperative, and **postoperative** management may decrease the risk of postsplenectomy infection. It is important to be certain of the need for splenectomy and, if possible, to postpone the operation until the patient is 5 yr of age or older. Pneumococcal, meningococcal, and *H. influenzae* conjugate vaccines given at least 14 days before splenectomy may reduce postsplenectomy sepsis. The 7-valent pneumococcal polysaccharide-protein conjugate vaccine (PCV7) was replaced with the 13-valent pneumococcal polysaccharide-protein conjugate vaccine (PCV13). Thus, depending on what primary pneumococcal vaccine was given, a single dose of PCV13 may be recommended. In addition, the 23-valent pneumococcal polysaccharide vaccine (Pneumovax) should be given at age ≥2 yr and a second dose 5 yr later. Yearly influenza vaccine should also be given as influenza infection is a risk factor for secondary pneumococcal infections. Prophylaxis with oral penicillin VK (125 mg twice daily for children younger than 5 yr; 250 mg twice daily for children 5 yr or older) should be given until at least 5 yr of age and for at least 2 yr after splenectomy. Although the greatest risk is in the immediate postoperative period, reports of deaths occurring years after splenectomy suggest that the risk (and the need for prophylaxis) may be lifelong. Lifelong prophylaxis should be strongly considered in patients who have had an invasive pneumococcal infection or who have an underlying immune deficiency. In children with sickle cell disease, penicillin prophylaxis should be started as soon as the diagnosis is made.

Prophylaxis may be continued into adulthood for higher-risk patients, including those with a history of pneumococcal sepsis, but effectiveness in this older group has not been well documented.

In patients with traumatic injury, splenic repair or partial splenectomy should be considered in an attempt to preserve splenic function. Partial splenectomy or partial splenic embolization may be sufficient to ameliorate some forms of hemolytic anemia. Up to 50% of children whose spleen is removed because of trauma have spontaneous **splenosis**; surgical splenosis (distributing small pieces of spleen throughout the abdomen) may decrease the risk of sepsis in patients whose splenectomy is necessitated by trauma. However, in both of these settings, the splenic tissue that regrows frequently has poor function.

In addition to postsplenectomy sepsis, splenectomized patients may be at risk for **thromboembolic** complications, including arterial and venous thrombosis and **pulmonary hypertension**. These findings have been reported regardless of the underlying reason for splenectomy and the postsplenectomy platelet count. Proposed mechanisms include loss of filtering function of the spleen, allowing abnormal RBCs to remain in the circulation and activate the coagulation cascade. Portal vein thrombosis has been reported as a complication of laparoscopic splenectomy.

Bibliography is available at Expert Consult.

Section 9
The Lymphatic System

Chapter 488
Anatomy and Function of the Lymphatic System
Richard L. Tower and Bruce M. Camitta

The lymphatic system participates in many biologic processes, including fluid homeostasis, absorption of dietary fat, and initiation of specific immune responses. This system includes circulating lymphocytes, lymphatic vessels, lymph nodes, spleen, tonsils, adenoids, Peyer patches, and thymus. Lymph, an ultrafiltrate of blood, is collected by lymphatic capillaries that are present in all organs except the brain, bone marrow, retina, cartilage, epidermis, hair, and nails. These join to form progressively larger vessels that drain regions of the body. The lymphatic vessels carry lymph to the lymph nodes, where it is filtered through sinuses, particulate matter and infectious organisms are phagocytosed, and antigens are presented to surrounding lymphocytes. These actions stimulate antibody production, T-cell responses, and cytokine secretion (see Chapter 123). Lymph is ultimately returned to the intravascular circulation.

The composition of lymph can vary with the site of lymph drainage. It is usually clear, but lymph drained from the intestinal tract may be milky (chylous) because of the presence of fats. The protein content is intermediate between that of an exudate and a transudate. The protein level may be increased with inflammation and in lymph drained from the liver or intestines. Lymph also contains variable numbers of lymphocytes and antigen-presenting cells.

Embryonic lymphatic development (primary lymphangiogenesis) proceeds from the stage of lymphatic competence, through lymphatic commitment, specification, coalescence, and maturation. Secondary lymphangiogenesis occurs in the settings of wound healing and inflammation. Many genes are crucial to normal lymphatic development and function, including *Prox1*, vascular endothelial growth factor–C (*VEGF-C*), and vascular endothelial growth factor receptor–3 (*VEGFR-3*).

Bibliography is available at Expert Consult.

Chapter 489
Abnormalities of Lymphatic Vessels
Richard L. Tower and Bruce M. Camitta

Abnormalities of the lymph vessels may be congenital or acquired. Signs and symptoms result from increased lymphatic tissue mass or from leakage of lymph. **Lymphangiectasia** is dilation of the lymphatics. Pulmonary lymphangiectasia causes respiratory distress (see Chapter 395.6). Involvement of the intestinal lymphatics causes hypoproteinemia and lymphocytopenia secondary to loss of lymph into the intestines (see Chapter 338). Therapy includes minimizing the hydrostatic pressure in the lymphatic system. Reducing dietary intake of long-chain fatty acids and substituting medium-chain triglycerides may accomplish this goal. If unsuccessful, octreotide or propanolol may be tried. **Lymphangioma** is a congenital lymphatic malformation, usually detected by age 2 yr. **Lymphangioma circumscriptum** is defined as the presence of many small, superficial lymphangiomas. Deeper lymphangiomas are classified as either **cavernous lymphangiomas** or **cystic hygromas**.

Lymphangiomatosis is the presence of multiple or disseminated malformations. Some of these lesions also have a hemangiomatous component (see Chapter 505). Thoracic lymphangiomatosis presents with chylothorax, a mass, or with pulmonary infiltrates. Associated features include bone, skin, and splenic lesions. The disorder is either diffuse or multifocal and is differentiated from lymphangiectasia by the presence of complex anastomosis of vessels with dilation rather than simple dilation of preexisting lymphatic capillaries. Emergent surgical treatment is infrequently necessary due to mass effects. Most lesions may be observed for 18-24 mo to assess for involution. Surgery is effective for superficial lesions, but there is a high incidence of recurrence when used for deeper lesions. Intralesional sclerosing with OK-432, a streptococcal derivative, has been used successfully in selected patients. Other sclerotherapy agents include pure ethanol and bleomycin. Macrocystic lesions appear to respond better than microcystic lymphangiomas to sclerotherapy. Radiofrequency ablation has been used for lymphatic lesions of the tongue. **Lymphatic dysplasia** may cause multisystem problems. These include lymphedema, chylous ascites, chylothorax, and lymphangiomas of the bone, lung, or other sites.

Lymphangioleiomyomatosis is characterized by proliferation of lymphatic endothelial cells and smooth muscle cells in the lungs, leading to airway and lymphatic obstruction, cyst formation, pneumothorax, and respiratory failure. It may initially be mistaken for asthma. Lymphangioleiomyomatosis occurs in young women and is also associated with mutations in the tuberous sclerosis tumor-suppressor gene *TSC2* in one-third of cases. Sirolimus (rapamycin) stabilizes lung function, reduces symptoms, and improves life quality; lung transplantation may be required.

Lymphedema, a localized swelling caused by impaired lymphatic flow, can be congenital or acquired. Congenital lymphedema may be found in Turner syndrome, Noonan syndrome, and the autosomal dominantly inherited Milroy disease, among other chromosomal abnormalities. Several families with Milroy disease have mutations in the vascular endothelial growth factor receptor–3 gene (*VEGFR-3*).

Autosomal recessive and X-linked inheritance has also been reported. Mutations in *GJC2* are associated with hereditary lymphedema. **Lymphedema praecox** (Meige disease) causes progressive lower extremity edema, usually in females during the peripubertal period or pregnancy. **Hypotrichosis-lymphedema-telangiectasia syndrome**, which has dominant and recessive inheritance patterns, has been linked to mutations in *SOX18*. Lymphedema has also been found in association with intestinal lymphangiectasia, cerebrovascular malformation, ptosis, yellow dystrophic nails, distichiasis, and cholestasis. Mutations in *FOXC2* are associated with lymphedema-distichiasis syndrome, which has a pubertal onset of lymphedema. Mutations in *CCBE1*, *PTPN14*, and *GATA2* are associated with Hennekam lymphangiectasia-lymphedema syndrome (lymphedema of the extremities, intestinal lymphangiectasia, mental retardation), lymphedema-choanal atresia syndrome, and Emberger syndrome (lymphedema of the lower extremities and genitalia, deafness, immune dysfunction, and warts), respectively.

Acquired obstruction of the lymphatics can result from tumor, postirradiation fibrosis, and postinflammatory scarring. **Filariasis** is an important cause of lymphedema in Africa, Asia, and Latin America; of the estimated 120 million infected persons, approximately 40 million (primarily older adolescents and adults) are believed to have lymphedema or hydrocele. Injury to the major lymphatic vessels can cause collection of lymph fluid in the abdomen (chylous ascites) or chest (chylothorax). Untreated lymphedema can be disabling and is associated with immune dysfunction, inflammation, fibrosis, adipose tissue overgrowth, and **lymphangiosarcoma**. Current treatment modalities attempt to reduce localized swelling through massage, exercise, and compression. No drugs have been proven efficacious. Diuretic use should be avoided. The recently discovered gene mutations provide potential for targeted therapy, including gene therapy. Autologous lymph node transplantation and use of growth factors to stimulate lymphangiogenesis may also be on the horizon for treatment of lymphedema.

Lymphangitis is an inflammation of the lymphatics that drain an area of infection. Tender, erythematous streaks extend proximally from the infected area. Regional nodes may also be tender. Group A streptococci and *Staphylococcus aureus* are the most frequent pathogens and therapy should include antibiotics that treat these organisms.

Bibliography is available at Expert Consult.

Chapter 490
Lymphadenopathy
Richard L. Tower and Bruce M. Camitta

Palpable lymph nodes are common in pediatrics. Lymph node enlargement is caused by proliferation of normal lymphoid elements or by infiltration with malignant or phagocytic cells. In most patients, a careful history and a complete physical examination suggest the proper diagnosis.

DIAGNOSIS

Is the mass a lymph node? Nonlymphoid masses (cervical rib, thyroglossal cyst, branchial cleft cyst or infected sinus, cystic hygroma, goiter, sternomastoid muscle tumor, thyroiditis, thyroid abscess, neurofibroma) occur frequently in the neck and less often in other areas. **Is the node enlarged?** Lymph nodes are not usually palpable in the newborn. With antigenic exposure, lymphoid tissue increases in volume. They are not considered enlarged until their diameter exceeds 1 cm for cervical and axillary nodes and 1.5 cm for inguinal nodes. Other lymph nodes usually are not palpable or visualized with plain radiographs. **What are the characteristics of the node?** Acutely infected nodes are usually

Table 490-1	Differential Diagnosis of Systemic Generalized Lymphadenopathy	
INFANT	**CHILD**	**ADOLESCENT**
COMMON CAUSES		
Syphilis	Viral infection	Viral infection
Toxoplasmosis	EBV	EBV
CMV	CMV	CMV
HIV	HIV	HIV
	Toxoplasmosis	Toxoplasmosis
		Syphilis
RARE CAUSES		
Chagas disease (congenital)	Serum sickness	Serum sickness
Leukemia	SLE, JIA	SLE, JIA
Tuberculosis	Leukemia/ lymphoma	Leukemia/lymphoma/ Hodgkin disease
Reticuloendotheliosis	Tuberculosis	Lymphoproliferative disease
Lymphoproliferative disease	Measles	Tuberculosis
Metabolic storage disease	Sarcoidosis	Histoplasmosis
Histiocytic disorders	Fungal infection	Sarcoidosis
	Plague	Fungal infection
	Langerhans cell histiocytosis	Plague
	Chronic granulomatous disease	Drug reaction
	Sinus histiocytosis	Castleman disease
	Drug reaction	

CMV, cytomegalovirus; EBV, Epstein-Barr virus; HIV, human immunodeficiency virus; JIA, juvenile idiopathic arthritis (as Still disease); SLE, systemic lupus erythematosus.
From Kliegman RM, Greenbaum LA, Lye PS: Practical strategies in pediatric diagnosis and therapy, ed 2, Philadelphia, 2004, Elsevier, p. 863.

tender. There may also be erythema and warmth of the overlying skin. Fluctuance suggests abscess formation. Tuberculous nodes may be matted. With chronic infection, many of these signs are not present. Tumor-bearing nodes are usually firm and nontender and may be matted or fixed to the skin or underlying structures.

Is the lymphadenopathy localized or generalized? Generalized adenopathy (enlargement of >2 noncontiguous node regions) is caused by systemic disease (Table 490-1) and is often accompanied by abnormal physical findings in other systems. In contrast, regional adenopathy is most frequently the result of infection in the involved node and/or its drainage area (Table 490-2). When caused by infectious agents other than bacteria, adenopathy may be characterized by atypical anatomic areas, a prolonged course, a draining sinus, lack of prior pyogenic infection, and unusual clues in the history (cat scratches, tuberculosis exposure, venereal disease). A firm, fixed node should always raise the question of malignancy, regardless of the presence or absence of systemic symptoms or other abnormal physical findings.

TREATMENT

Evaluation and treatment of lymphadenopathy is guided by the probable etiologic factor, as determined from the history and physical examination. Many patients with cervical adenopathy have a history compatible with viral infection and need no intervention. If bacterial infection is suspected, antibiotic treatment covering at least streptococci and staphylococci is indicated. Those who do not respond to oral antibiotics, as demonstrated by persistent swelling and fever, require IV antistaphylococcal antibiotics. If there is no response in 1-2 days, or if there are signs of airway obstruction or significant toxicity, ultrasound, CT, or MRI of the neck should be obtained. If pus is present, it may be aspirated, with CT or ultrasound guidance, or if it is extensive, may require incision and drainage. Gram stain and culture of the pus should be obtained. The sizes of involved nodes should be documented before treatment. Failure to decrease in size within 10-14 days also suggests the need for further evaluation. This may include a complete blood cell

Table 490-2	Sites of Local Lymphadenopathy and Associated Diseases

CERVICAL
Oropharyngeal infection (viral or group A streptococcal, staphylococcal)
Scalp infection/infestation (head lice)
Mycobacterial lymphadenitis (tuberculosis and nontuberculous mycobacteria)
Viral infection (EBV, CMV, HHV-6)
Cat-scratch disease
Toxoplasmosis
Kawasaki disease
Thyroid disease
Kikuchi disease
Sinus histiocytosis (Rosai-Dorfman disease)
Autoimmune lymphoproliferative disease
Periodic fever, aphthous stomatitis, pharyngitis, cervical adenopathy (PFAPA) syndrome

ANTERIOR AURICULAR
Conjunctivitis
Other eye infection
Oculoglandular tularemia
Facial cellulitis
Otitis media
Viral infection (especially rubella, parvovirus)

SUPRACLAVICULAR
Malignancy or infection in the mediastinum (right)
Metastatic malignancy from the abdomen (left)
Lymphoma
Tuberculosis

EPITROCHLEAR
Hand infection, arm infection*
Lymphoma[†]
Sarcoid
Syphilis

INGUINAL
Urinary tract infection
Venereal disease (especially syphilis or lymphogranuloma venereum)
Other perineal infections
Lower extremity suppurative infection
Plague

HILAR (NOT PALPABLE, FOUND ON CHEST RADIOGRAPH OR CT)
Tuberculosis[†]
Histoplasmosis[†]
Blastomycosis[†]
Coccidioidomycosis[†]
Leukemia/lymphoma[†]
Hodgkin disease[†]
Metastatic malignancy*
Sarcoidosis[†]
Castleman disease

AXILLARY
Cat-scratch disease
Arm or chest wall infection
Malignancy of chest wall
Leukemia/lymphoma
Brucellosis

ABDOMINAL
Malignancies
Mesenteric adenitis (measles, tuberculosis, *Yersinia*, group A streptococcus)

*Unilateral.
[†]Bilateral.
CMV, cytomegalovirus; CT, computed tomography; EBV, Epstein-Barr virus; HHV-6, human herpesvirus 6.
From Kliegman RM, Greenbaum LA, Lye PS: Practical strategies in pediatric diagnosis and therapy, ed 2, Philadelphia, 2004, Elsevier, p. 864.

count with differential; Epstein-Barr virus, cytomegalovirus, *Toxoplasma,* and cat-scratch disease titers; antistreptolysin O or anti-DNAse serologic tests; tuberculin skin test; and chest radiograph. If these are not diagnostic, consultation with an infectious disease or oncology specialist may be helpful. Biopsy should be considered if there is persistent or unexplained fever, weight loss, night sweats, supraclavicular location, mediastinal mass, hard nodes, or fixation of the nodes to surrounding tissues. Biopsy may also be indicated if there is an increase in size over baseline in 2 wk, no decrease in size in 4-6 wk, no regression to "normal" in 8-12 wk, or if new signs and symptoms develop.

Differentiating benign disorders from a malignancy may initially be difficult. Hard, nontender, nonerythematous nodes involving multiple regions (including mediastinum and abdomen), hepatic or splenic enlargement, fever, night sweats, and weight loss suggest malignancy or a granulomatous process. Persistence of symptoms and lymphadenopathy greater than 2 wk and certain locations (supraclavicular, mediastinal, abdomen) also suggest malignancy. Cytopenias and elevated blood lactate dehydrogenase are associated with malignancy and certain inflammatory disorders. CT imaging is helpful in identifying other affected nodes and organs; CT or ultrasonographic guided biopsy is helpful in determining the etiology. Fine needle aspiration or excisional biopsy may be needed for superficial nodes to determine a diagnosis.

Bibliography is available at Expert Consult.

490.1 Kikuchi-Fujimoto Disease (Histiocytic Necrotizing Lymphadenitis)
Richard L. Tower and Bruce M. Camitta

Kikuchi-Fujimoto disease is a rare, usually self-limiting disease that was originally reported in patients of Asian heritage. Cases are now described in all ethnic groups. Familial cases have been reported. Presentation is varied and may include fever of unknown origin, but more often, it occurs in children 8-16 yr of age as firm unilateral posterior cervical adenitis, fever, malaise, elevated erythrocyte sedimentation rate, atypical lymphocytosis, and leukopenia. Nodes range in size from only 0.5-6.0 cm, are painful or tender in only 50% of cases, may be multiple, and must be differentiated from lymphoma. Node involvement may occasionally be bilateral or present in axillary or supraclavicular nodes.

The etiology is unknown, although viral and bacterial causes have been suggested. Growing evidence supports an abnormal immune response; the diagnosis is made by lymph node biopsy. Histologic features include necrosis with karyorrhexis, a histiocytic infiltrate, crescentic plasmacytoid monocytes and an absence of neutrophils. The disease is self-limiting and usually spontaneously resolves within 6 mo, although relapses have occurred up to 16 yr later. Therapy with systemic steroids is reserved for cases with severe symptoms. Rarely, the disease has been fatal. Many autoimmune diseases have been associated with Kikuchi-Fujimoto disease, most commonly systemic lupus erythematosus. The differential diagnosis includes lymphoma, tuberculosis, and systemic lupus erythematosus.

Bibliography is available at Expert Consult.

490.2 Sinus Histiocytosis with Massive Lymphadenopathy (Rosai-Dorfman Disease)
Richard L. Tower and Bruce M. Camitta

This uncommon, benign, and usually self-limited disease has a worldwide distribution but is more common in Africa and the Caribbean. The etiology is unknown, but immune dysfunction is suspected. Patients present with massive bilateral, painless, mobile cervical adenopathy, along with fever, leukocytosis, high erythrocyte sedimentation rate, and polyclonal elevation of immunoglobulin G (hypergamma-globulinemia). Night sweats and weight loss are common. Autoimmune hemolytic anemia is an uncommon associated finding. It rarely occurs at birth or in siblings, and males are affected more often than females.

Other nodal chains may be involved. Extranodal involvement occurs in 40% of cases. Soft-tissue involvement of all organ systems has been reported. The most common sites are the skin, followed by the nasal cavity and sinuses, palate, orbit, bone, and central nervous system. Occasionally autoantibodies to erythrocytes or synovium may be present. A biopsy that demonstrates pale histiocytes containing engulfed lymphocytes (**emperipolesis**), and immunoreactivity to S100 protein in large histiocytes, in conjunction with expected clinical features, is diagnostic. The differential diagnosis includes Langerhans cell histiocytosis, myeloproliferative disorders, and lymphoma.

Therapy is usually not needed for this self-limited disease. However, the disease may recur frequently for many years. Life- or organ-threatening disease or exacerbations may respond to prednisone. Refractory cases have been treated with surgical excision or radiation. Rare patients have been treated with immune-modulating therapy, including interferon-α, 2-chlorodeoxyadenosine, imatinib, and rituximab. Therapy with antibiotics and chemotherapy has been unsuccessful.

Bibliography is available at Expert Consult.

490.3 Castleman Disease
Richard L. Tower and Bruce M. Camitta

Castleman disease is an uncommon lymphoproliferative disease and is also called *angiofollicular lymph node hyperplasia*. The underlying etiology is unknown, although an association with human herpesvirus 8 has been identified. Human herpesvirus 8 may stimulate excessive production of interleukin 6 (IL-6). The disease usually presents in adolescents or young adults. Enlargement of a single node, most often in the mediastinum or abdomen, is the most common localized presentation. Some patients may have fever, night sweats, weight loss, and fatigue. Management includes surgery and/or radiation therapy.

Multicentric Castleman disease is a systemic lymphoproliferative disorder that causes lymphadenopathy, hepatosplenomegaly, fever, anemia, overexpression of IL-6, and polyclonal hypergammaglobulinemia. Multicentric Castleman disease may be associated with HIV infection, autoimmune disease–associated lymphadenopathy, and POEMS syndrome (polyneuropathy, organomegaly, endocrinopathy, M-proteins, and skin lesions). Non-Hodgkin lymphoma may be concurrent or may develop as a result of disease progression. There is no standard treatment for multicentric Castleman disease. Therapeutic options include chemotherapy, steroids, monoclonal antibodies to CD20 (rituximab), monoclonal antibodies (siltuximab) to IL-6, anti-IL-6–receptor antibodies (tocilizumab), antiviral agents, and interferon-α. Chemotherapy regimens used for diffuse large B-cell lymphoma and/or rituximab is currently the most common frontline therapies and has achieved durable remissions. Ganciclovir is the most active antiviral agent. Steroids and anti-IL-6 therapies provide symptomatic relief, but symptoms return after stopping therapy.

Bibliography is available at Expert Consult.

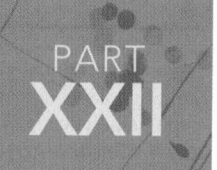

Chapter 491

Epidemiology of Childhood and Adolescent Cancer

Barbara L. Asselin

Cancer in patients younger than 20 yr of age is uncommon, with an age-adjusted annual incidence of 18.7 per 100,000 children ages 0-19 yr, representing only approximately 1% of all new cancer cases in a year in the United States or an estimated 16,600 new cases/yr in 2014. This translates to nearly a 1 in 300 chance of developing cancer by age 20 yr. Although the relative 5 yr survival rates have improved from 61% in 1977 to 83.6% in 2010 in all age groups 0-19 yr (Fig. 491-1), malignant neoplasms remain the leading cause of disease-related (noninjury) mortality (12%) among persons 1-19 yr of age with 1,800-1,900 cancer-related deaths annually in the United States among children and adolescents 0-19 yr of age. The relative contribution of cancer to the overall mortality in infants 0-1 yr old and adolescents 15-19 yr old is lower than for children ages 1-14 yr. The impressive improvements in survival over the past 3.5 decades are attributed primarily to advances in treatment and enrollment in clinical trials for the majority of patients. Multiinstitutional cooperative clinical trials investigating novel therapies and investigating ways to improve survival rates even further and to decrease treatment-related long-term complications are ongoing. Because increasingly more patients survive their disease, clinical investigations also are focusing on the quality of life among survivors and the late outcomes of therapy for pediatric and adult survivors of childhood cancer. The National Cancer Institute estimates that in 2010 there were 380,000 persons alive (in all age groups) who had survived childhood cancer, corresponding to 1 in 810 of persons younger than 20 yr of age and 1 in 1,000 persons 20-39 yr of age in the U.S. population.

Pediatric malignancies differ markedly from adult malignancies in both prognosis and distribution by histology and tumor site. Lymphohematopoietic cancers (i.e., acute lymphoblastic leukemia, myeloid leukemia, Hodgkin and non-Hodgkin lymphomas) account for approximately 40%, central nervous system cancers for approximately 30%, and embryonal tumors and sarcomas for approximately 10% among the broad categories of childhood cancers (Table 491-1). In contrast, epithelial tumors of organs such as lung, colon, breast, and prostate, which are commonly seen among adults, are rare malignancies in children. Incidence patterns in the pediatric age group show 2 peaks: the first in early childhood and the second in adolescence (Fig. 491-2). During the 1st yr of life, *embryonal tumors* such as neuroblastoma, nephroblastoma (Wilms tumor), retinoblastoma, rhabdomyosarcoma, hepatoblastoma, and medulloblastoma are most common (Figs. 491-3 and 491-4). These tumors are much less common in older children and adults after cell differentiation processes have slowed considerably. Embryonal tumors, acute leukemias, non-Hodgkin lymphomas, and gliomas peak in incidence from 2-5 yr of age. As children age, bone malignancies, Hodgkin disease, gonadal germ cell malignancies (testicular and ovarian carcinomas), and other carcinomas increase in incidence. Adolescence is a transitional period between the common early childhood malignancies and characteristic carcinomas

of adulthood (Fig. 491-4). Incidence rates also vary by gender (generally higher in boys vs girls), race/ethnicity (more common in whites), and between countries (data assembled by the International Agency for Research in Cancer in Lyon, France, http://www.iarc.fr/). Over the past 35 yr, 1975-2010, there has been some increase in the incidence of children and adolescents diagnosed with cancer particularly in occurrence of leukemia and among adolescents. These variations are not fully understood but likely reflect differences in genetic susceptibility and environmental exposures related to both known and unknown causes and risk factors for cancer (Table 491-2).

Childhood cancer includes a diverse array of malignant tumors, termed "cancers," and nonmalignant tumors arising from disorders of genetic processes involved in control of cellular growth and development. Although many genetic conditions are associated with increased risks for childhood cancer, such conditions are believed to account for <5% of all occurrences (see Chapter 492). The most notable genetic conditions that impart susceptibility to childhood cancer are neurofibromatosis types 1 and 2, Down syndrome, Beckwith-Wiedemann syndrome, tuberous sclerosis, von Hippel-Lindau disease, xeroderma pigmentosum, ataxia-telangiectasia, nevus basal cell carcinoma syndrome, and Li-Fraumeni (*P53*) syndrome. The varying incidence patterns of individual childhood cancers around the world imply additional genetic and epidemiologic risk factors that remain uncharacterized.

Compared with adult epithelial tumors, an extremely small fraction of pediatric cancers appear to be explained by known environmental exposures (see Table 491-2). Ionizing radiation exposure and several chemotherapeutic agents explain only a small number of pediatric cases (see Chapter 718). The association between fetal exposures and pediatric cancer is largely not established, with the exception of maternal diethylstilbestrol intake during pregnancy and subsequent vaginal adenocarcinoma in adolescent daughters. Environmental exposures that have been studied without convincing evidence for a causal role include nonionizing power frequency electromagnetic fields, pesticides, parental occupational chemical exposures, dietary factors, in vitro fertilization, and environmental cigarette smoke. Viruses have been associated with certain pediatric cancers, such as polyomaviruses (BK, JC, SV40) associated with brain cancer and Epstein-Barr virus with non-Hodgkin lymphoma, but the etiologic importance remains unclear. The etiology of cancer in children still is poorly understood, and epidemiology studies demonstrate that the likely mechanisms are multifactorial, possibly resulting from potential interactions between genetic susceptibility traits and environmental exposures. Ongoing studies are investigating the role of polymorphisms of genes encoding enzymes, which function in the activation or metabolism of xenobiotics, protection of cells against oxidative stress, DNA repair, and/or immune modulation.

Curative therapy with chemotherapy, radiation, and/or surgery can adversely affect a child's development and result in serious long-term medical and psychosocial effects in childhood and adulthood. Potential adverse late effects include subsequent second malignancy, early mortality, infertility, reduced stature, cardiomyopathy, pulmonary fibrosis, osteoporosis, neurocognitive impairment, affective disorders, and altered social functioning. Much has been learned about the incidence of late effects from large multisite cohort studies such as the Childhood Cancer Survivor Study, an ongoing study of medical and psychosocial outcomes in survivors, which has provided data for the development of clinical care guidelines for survivors (http://www.survivorshipguidelines.org).

Given the relative rarity of specific types of childhood cancer and the sophisticated technology and expertise required for diagnosis, treatment, and monitoring of late effects, all children with cancer

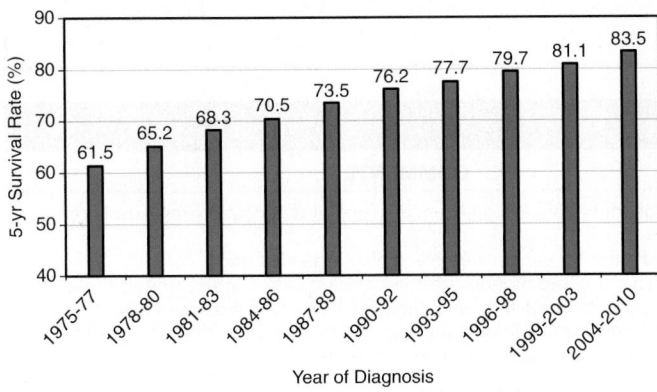

Figure 491-1 Five yr relative survival rates (%) by year of diagnosis of all cancers in children 19 yr of age or younger. The difference between the periods 1975-1977 and 2004-2010 is statistically significant (p < 0.05). Rates based on follow-up of patients into 2011 from Surveillance, Epidemiology, and End Results (SEER) database. *(Data compiled from Howlader N, Noone AM, Krapcho M, et al, editors: SEER Cancer Statistics Review, 1975-2011, Section 28. Bethesda, MD, National Cancer Institute. Available at http://seer.cancer.gov/csr/1975_2011/, posted to the SEER website, April 2014.)*

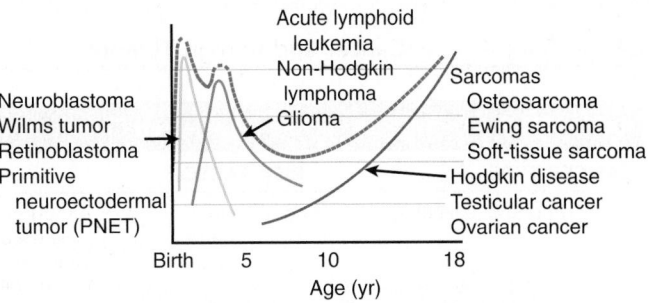

Figure 491-3 Generalized incidence of the most common types of cancer in children by age. The cumulative incidence of all cancers is shown as a dashed line. *(Courtesy of Archie Bleyer, MD.)*

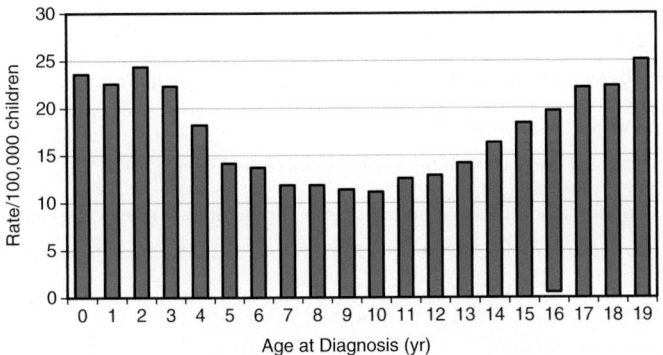

Figure 491-2 Age-specific cancer incidence rates per 100,000 children within the United States. Rates based on data from 2007-2011 from Surveillance, Epidemiology, and End Results (SEER) database. *(Data compiled from Howlader N, Noone AM, Krapcho M, et al, editors: SEER Cancer Statistics Review, 1975-2011, Section 28. Bethesda, MD, National Cancer Institute. Available at http://seer.cancer.gov/csr/1975_2011/, posted to the SEER website, April 2014.)*

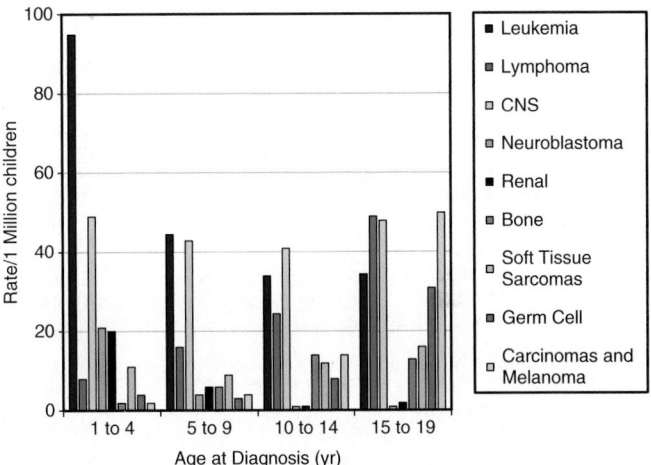

Figure 491-4 Surveillance, Epidemiology, and End Results (SEER) incidence rates by International Classification of Childhood Cancer (ICCC) and age group <20 yr. CNS, central nervous system. *(Data compiled from Howlader N, Noone AM, Krapcho M, et al, editors: SEER Cancer Statistics Review, 1975-2011, Section 29. Bethesda, MD, National Cancer Institute. Available at http://seer.cancer.gov/csr/1975_2011/, posted to the SEER website, April 2014.)*

Table 491-1	Age-Adjusted Incidence and Survival Rates of Malignant Neoplasms By Tumor Type Among U.S. Children					
	ANNUAL INCIDENCE RATES PER 1 MILLION CHILDREN, 2007-2011					**5-YR SURVIVAL (%) AGE ≤19 YR AT DIAGNOSIS, 2004-2011**
	Age <1 Yr	**Age 1-4 Yr**	**Age 5-9 Yr**	**Age 10-14 Yr**	**Age 15-19 Yr**	
All malignancies combined	242	221	128	136	219	82.5
Leukemia (ALL/AML)	52 (20/19)	95 (80/11)	44 (37/4.5)	34 (22/7)	34 (18/10)	82 (87/62)
Lymphoma (Hodgkin)	5.5 (—)	8 (1)	16 (5.4)	24.5 (12)	49 (32)	92 (96)
CNS tumors	49	49	43	41	48	73
Neuroblastoma	51	21	4	1	0.9	78
Nephroblastoma/Wilms (renal cell carcinoma)	15 (—)	20 (—)	5 (—)	0.7 (—)	— (1.5)	90
Bone	—	2	6	14	13	69.5
Soft tissue sarcomas	20	11	9	12	16	71
Retinoblastoma	28	9	—	—	—	97
Hepatoblastoma (hepatic carcinoma)	10 (—)	6 (—)	— (—)	— (0.8)	— (1.4)	80 (70)
Germ cell tumors	19	4	3	8	31	92
Malignant epithelial cancer	—	1.8	4	14	50	92 (99.5*/95†)

Based on the International Classification of Childhood Cancer (ICCC). Rates are per 1,000,000 children and are age-adjusted to the 2000 U.S. standard population.
*Thyroid carcinoma.
†Malignant melanoma.
—, Indicates that the rate could not be calculated with <16 cases for the time interval; ALL, acute lymphoid leukemia; AML, acute myeloid leukemia; CNS, central nervous system.
Data compiled From Howlader N, Noone AM, Krapcho M, et al, editors: SEER Cancer Statistics Review, 1975-2011, Section 29. Bethesda, MD, National Cancer Institute. Available at http://seer.cancer.gov/csr/1975_2011/, posted to the SEER website, April 2014.

Table 491-2	Known Risk Factors for Selected Childhood Cancers	
CANCER TYPE	**RISK FACTOR**	**COMMENTS**
Acute lymphoid leukemia	Ionizing radiation	Although primarily of historical significance, prenatal diagnostic x-ray exposure increases risk.
		Therapeutic irradiation for cancer treatment also increases risk.
	Race	White children have a 2-fold higher rate than black children in the United States.
	Genetic factors*	Down syndrome is associated with an estimated 10-20–fold increased risk.
		NF1, Bloom syndrome, ataxia-telangiectasia, and Langerhans cell histiocytosis, among others, are associated with an elevated risk.
Acute myeloid leukemias	Chemotherapeutic agents	Alkylating agents and epipodophyllotoxins increase risk.
	Genetic factors*	Down syndrome and NF1 are strongly associated.
		Familial monosomy 7 and several other genetic syndromes are also associated with increased risk.
Brain cancers	Therapeutic ionizing radiation to the head	With the exception of cancer radiation therapy, higher risk from radiation treatment is essentially of historical importance.
	Genetic factors*	NF1 is strongly associated with optic gliomas, and, to a lesser extent, with other central nervous system tumors.
		Tuberous sclerosis and several other genetic syndromes are associated with increased risk.
Hodgkin disease	Family history	Monozygotic twins and siblings are at increased risk.
	Infections	EBV is associated with increased risk.
Non-Hodgkin lymphoma	Immunodeficiency	Acquired and congenital immunodeficiency disorders and immunosuppressive therapy increase risk.
	Infections	EBV is associated with Burkitt lymphoma in Africa.
Osteosarcoma	Ionizing radiation	Cancer radiation therapy and high radium exposure increase risk.
	Chemotherapy	Alkylating agents increase risk.
	Genetic factors*	Increased risk is apparent with Li-Fraumeni syndrome and hereditary retinoblastoma.
Ewing sarcoma	Race	White children have about a 9-fold higher incidence rate than black children in the United States.
Neuroblastoma		Neurocristopathies.
Retinoblastoma	Genetic factors*	No established other risk factors.
Wilms tumor	Congenital anomalies	Aniridia, Beckwith-Wiedemann syndrome, and other congenital and genetic conditions are associated with increased risk.
	Race	Asian children reportedly have about half the rates of white and black children.
Renal medullary carcinoma	Sickle cell trait	Etiology unknown.
Rhabdomyosarcoma	Congenital anomalies and genetic conditions	Li-Fraumeni syndrome and NF1 are believed to be associated with increased risk. There is some concordance with major birth defects.
Hepatoblastoma	Genetic factors*	Beckwith-Wiedemann syndrome, hemihypertrophy, Gardner syndrome, and family history of adenomatous polyposis are associated with increased risk.
Leiomyosarcoma	Immunosuppression and EBV infection	EBV is associated with leiomyosarcoma for all forms of congenital and acquired immunosuppression but not leiomyosarcoma among immunocompetent persons.
Malignant germ cell tumors	Cryptorchidism	Cryptorchidism is a risk factor for testicular germ cell tumors.

*See Chapter 492, Table 492-2.
EBV, Epstein-Barr virus; NF1, neurofibromatosis type 1.
Scheurer ME, Bondy ML, Gurney JG: Epidemiology of childhood cancer. In Pizzo PA, Poplack DG, editors: Principles and practice of pediatric oncology, ed 6, Philadelphia, 2011, Lippincott Williams & Wilkins, p. 15.

should be treated with standardized clinical protocols in pediatric clinical research settings whenever possible. Promoting such treatment, the Children's Oncology Group is a multiinstitutional research consortium that facilitates cooperative clinical, biologic, and epidemiologic research in more than 200 affiliated institutions in the United States, Canada, and other countries (http://childrensoncologygroup .org/). Coordinated participation in such research trials has been a major factor in the increased survival for many children with cancer. Such ongoing efforts are critical to better understand the etiology of childhood cancers, improve survival for malignancies with a poor prognosis, and maximize the quality of life for survivors.

INFLUENCING THE INCIDENCE OF CANCER
Pediatricians have a unique opportunity to educate children and adolescents, and their parents, regarding means of preventing cancer. There are only a few recognized environmental causes of childhood cancer that can be avoided or counteracted. One example is immunization against hepatitis B, which does decrease the risk of hepatocellular carcinoma in adolescence and adulthood; another is human papillomavirus vaccination, which prevents cervical cancer. Associations between cumulative radiation exposure from common diagnostic radiologic tests such as CT scans and an increased risk of malignancy later in life are of great concern for pediatricians. Guidelines to ensure the safe clinical use of diagnostic imaging are being evaluated (http://www.imagegently.org/). An objective of pediatric medicine is to teach children how to adopt healthy lifestyles to reduce their risk of cancer during adulthood, such as avoiding tobacco, alcohol, high-fat diets, and obesity. The earlier these habits are instilled, the greater the lifelong benefit and the more likely it is to be present and sustained during adulthood.

Bibliography is available at Expert Consult.

Chapter **492**
Molecular and Cellular Biology of Cancer
Laura L. Worth

Cancer is a complex of diseases arising from alterations that can occur in a wide variety of genes. Alterations in normal cellular processes such as signal transduction, cell-cycle control, DNA repair, cellular growth and differentiation, translational regulation, senescence, and apoptosis (programmed cell death) can result in a malignant phenotype.

GENES INVOLVED IN ONCOGENESIS

Two major classes of genes are implicated in the development of cancer: oncogenes and tumor-suppressor genes. **Protooncogenes** are cellular genes that are important for normal cellular function and code for various proteins, including transcriptional factors, growth factors, and growth factor receptors. These proteins are vital components in the network of signal transduction that regulate cell growth, division, and differentiation. Protooncogenes can be altered to form **oncogenes**—genes that, when translated, can result in the malignant transformation of a cell.

Oncogenes can be divided into 5 different classes based on their mechanisms of action. Changes in any of these normal cellular components can result in unchecked cell growth. Some oncogenes code for **growth factors** that bind to a receptor and stimulate the production of a protein. Other oncogenes code for **growth factor receptors.** These are proteins on the cell surface. When growth factors bind to a growth factor receptor, they can turn the receptor on or off. Mutational or posttranslational modifications of the receptor can result in a receptor being permanently turned on with consequent unregulated growth. **Signal transducers** or effectors make up another class. Signal transducers are responsible for taking the signal from the cell surface receptor to the cell nucleus. *NRAS*, as described below, is an example of this class of protein. **Transcription factors** are molecules that bind to specific areas of the DNA and control transcription. *MYC*, described below, is an example of a transcription factor that results in overstimulation of cell division. The final class of oncogenes interferes with apoptosis. Cells that no longer respond to the signal to die can continue to proliferate.

The 3 main mechanisms by which protooncogenes can be activated include amplification, point mutations, and translocation (Table 492-1). *MYC*, which codes for a protein that regulates transcription, is an example of a protooncogene that is activated by amplification. Patients with neuroblastoma in which the *MYC* gene is amplified 10-300–fold have a poorer outcome. Point mutations can also activate protooncogenes. The *NRAS* protooncogene codes for a guanine nucleotide–binding protein with guanosine triphosphatase activity that is important in signal transduction and is mutated in 25-30% of acute nonmyelogenous leukemias, resulting in a constitutively active protein. The RET protein is a transmembrane tyrosine kinase receptor that is important in signal transduction. A point mutation in the *RET* gene results in the constitutive activation of a tyrosine kinase, as found in multiple neoplasia syndromes and familial thyroid carcinoma.

The third mechanism by which protooncogenes become activated is by chromosomal translocation. In some leukemias and lymphomas, transcription factor controlling sequences are relocated in front of T-cell receptors or immunoglobulin genes, resulting in unregulated transcription of the genes and leukemogenesis. Chromosomal translocations can also result in **fusion genes**; transcription of the fusion gene can result in the production of a chimeric protein with new and potentially oncogenic activity. Examples of cancers associated with fusion genes include the childhood solid tumors like Ewing sarcoma [t(11;22)] and alveolar rhabdomyosarcoma [t(2;13) or t(1;13)]. The translocations result in novel proteins that are useful as diagnostic markers. The best-described translocation in leukemia is the **Philadelphia chromosome's t(9;22)**, which results in the BCR/ABL protein found in chronic myelogenous leukemia. This translocation results in a tyrosine kinase protein that is constitutively activated. In addition, the protein is localized to the cytoplasm instead of the nucleus, exposing the kinase to a new spectrum of substrates.

Alteration in the regulation of tumor-suppressor genes is another mechanism involved in oncogenesis. Tumor-suppressor genes are important regulators of cellular growth and apoptosis. They have been called recessive oncogenes because the inactivation of both alleles of a tumor-suppressor gene is required for expression of a malignant phenotype.

Knudson's **"2-hit" model of cancer development** was based on the observation of the behavior of the *RB* tumor-suppressor gene. In sporadic cases of retinoblastoma, both alleles of the *RB* gene must be inactivated. However, in familial cases, children inherit an inactivated allele from 1 parent and consequently require the inactivation of the only remaining normal allele. This helps explain why familial cases of retinoblastoma occur earlier in childhood than sporadic cases, because only 1 "hit" is required.

Another major tumor-suppressor protein is P53, which is known as the "guardian of the genome" because it detects the presence of

Table 492-1	Oncogene Activators of Pediatric Tumors			
MECHANISM	**CHROMOSOME**	**GENES**	**PROTEIN FUNCTION**	**TUMOR**
Chromosomal translocation	t(9;22)	BCR-ABL	Chimeric tyrosine kinase	CML, ALL
	t(1;19)	E2A-PBX1	Chimeric transcription factor	Pre-B ALL
	t(14;18)	CMYC	Transcription factor	Burkitt lymphoma
	t(15;17)	APL-RARα	Chimeric transcription factor	APL
	11:q23 and others	MLL	Methyl transferase activity	ALL AML Biphenotypic
	t(12;q21)	TEL-AML 1	Chimeric protein	ALL
	t(2;13)(q35;q14) or t(1,13)(p36q14)	FKHF-PAX3	Transcription factor	Rhabdomyosarcoma
	t(11;q22) or t(7;q22)	EWS-FLI1	Transcription factor	Wilms
Gene amplification	Amplicon	NMYC	Transcription factor	Neuroblastoma
	Amplicon	EGFR	Growth factor kinase, tyrosine kinase	Glioblastoma
	Amplicon	Flt3	Tyrosine kinase receptor	AML
Point mutation	1p	NRAS	Guanosine triphosphatase	AML
	10q	RET	Tyrosine kinase	MEN2

ALL, acute lymphocytic leukemia; AML, acute myelocytic leukemia; APL, acute promyelocytic leukemia; CML, chronic myelogenous leukemia; MEN2, multiple endocrine neoplasia, type 2.

chromosomal damage and prevents the cell from dividing until repairs have been made. In the presence of damage beyond repair, P53 initiates apoptosis and the cell dies. More than 50% of all tumors have abnormal P53 proteins. Mutations in the *P53* gene are important in many cancers, including breast, colorectal, lung, esophageal, stomach, ovarian, and prostatic carcinomas as well as gliomas, sarcomas, and some leukemias.

PTEN (phosphatase and tensin homolog) is one of the most commonly lost tumor suppressors in human cancer. PTEN is a phosphatase that regulates cell-cycle progression. The dephosphorylation of proteins disrupts the Akt/PKB signaling pathway that moderates cell-cycle progression. Loss of PTEN enzyme activity is seen in Proteus, Cowden, and Bannayan-Riley-Ruvalcaba syndromes and in glioblastoma, endometrial carcinoma, and prostate cancer. Decreased phosphatase activity is found in lung and breast cancer. More than 170 putative tumor-suppressor genes are identified.

SYNDROMES PREDISPOSING TO CANCER

Several syndromes are associated with an increased risk of developing malignancies, which can be characterized by different mechanisms (Table 492-2). One mechanism involves the inactivation of tumor-suppressor genes such as *RB* in **familial retinoblastoma**. Interestingly, patients with retinoblastoma in which 1 of the alleles is inactivated

throughout all of the patient's cells are also at a very high risk for developing osteosarcoma. A familial syndrome, **Li-Fraumeni syndrome**, in which 1 mutant *P53* allele is inherited, also has been described in patients who develop sarcomas, leukemias, and cancers of the breast, bone, lung, and brain. **Neurofibromatosis** is a condition characterized by the proliferation of cells of neural crest origin, leading to neurofibromas. These patients are at a higher risk of developing malignant schwannomas and pheochromocytomas. Neurofibromatosis is often inherited in an autosomal dominant fashion, although 50% of the cases present without a family history and occur secondary to the high rate of spontaneous mutations of the *NF1* gene.

A second mechanism responsible for an inherited predisposition to develop cancer involves defects in DNA repair. Syndromes associated with an excessive number of broken chromosomes due to repair defects include **Bloom syndrome** (short stature, photosensitive telangiectatic erythema), ataxia-telangiectasia (childhood ataxia with progressive neuromotor degeneration), and **Fanconi anemia** (short stature, skeletal and renal anomalies, pancytopenia). As a result of the decreased ability to repair chromosomal defects, cells accumulate abnormal DNA that results in significantly increased rates of cancer, especially leukemia. **Xeroderma pigmentosum** likewise increases the risk of skin cancer, owing to defects in repair to DNA damaged by ultraviolet light. These disorders display an autosomal recessive pattern.

Table 492-2	Familial or Genetic Susceptibility to Malignancy	
DISORDER	**TUMOR/CANCER**	**COMMENT**
CHROMOSOMAL SYNDROMES		
Chromosome 11p deletion syndrome with sporadic aniridia	Wilms tumor	Associated with genitourinary anomalies, mental retardation, *WT1* gene
Chromosome 13q deletion syndrome	Retinoblastoma, sarcoma	Associated with intellectual disability, skeletal malformations; autosomal dominant (bilateral) or sporadic new mutations, *RB1* gene
Trisomy 21	Lymphocytic or nonlymphocytic leukemia, especially megakaryocytic leukemia; transient leukemoid reaction	Risk of ALL is increased 20%; risk of AML is increased 400%; patients have an increased sensitivity to chemotherapy
Klinefelter syndrome (47,XXY)	Breast cancer, extragonadal germ cell tumors	
Trisomy 8	Preleukemia	
Noonan syndrome	JMML	Autosomal dominant; mutations in *PTPN11* gene
Monosomy 5 or 7	Myelodysplastic syndrome	Recurrent infections may precede neoplasia
CHROMOSOMAL INSTABILITY		
Xeroderma pigmentosum	Basal cell and squamous cell carcinomas; melanoma	Autosomal recessive; failure to repair UV-damaged DNA. Mutations in *XP* gene on chromosome 3p25
Fanconi anemia	Leukemia, myelodysplastic syndrome, liver neoplasias, rare head and neck tumors, GI and GU cancers	Autosomal recessive; chromosome fragility; positive diepoxybutane test result. Mutations in *FANCX* gene family
Bloom syndrome	Leukemia, lymphoma, and solid tumors	Autosomal recessive; increase sister chromatid exchange; mutations in *BLM* gene; member of the RecQ helicase gene
Ataxia-telangiectasia	Lymphoma, leukemia, less commonly central nervous system and nonneural solid tumors	Autosomal recessive; sensitive to X-irradiation, radiomimetic drugs; mutation in *ATM* tumor-suppressor gene
Dysplastic nevus syndrome	Melanoma	Autosomal dominant; some cases associated with mutations in *CDKN2A* gene
Rothmund-Thompson syndrome	Osteosarcoma; skin cancers	Autosomal recessive; mutation in RecQ helicase gene family
Werner syndrome (premature aging)	Soft tissue sarcomas	Autosomal recessive; mutation in the *WRN* gene; member of the RecQ helicase gene family
IMMUNODEFICIENCY SYNDROMES		
Wiskott-Aldrich syndrome	Lymphoma, leukemia	X-linked recessive; *WAS* gene mutation (Xp11.22-23); WASP protein functions in signal transduction associated with cytoskeletal actin filament rearrangement
X-linked immunodeficiency (Duncan syndrome)	Lymphoproliferative disorder	X-linked; Epstein-Barr viral infection can result in fatal outcome; mutation in *SH2D1A* gene locus
X-linked agammaglobulinemia (Bruton disease)	Lymphoma, leukemia	X-linked; mutation in *BKT* gene resulting in absence of mature B cells
Severe combined immunodeficiency	Leukemia, lymphoma	X-linked; mutations in *ADA* gene

Table 492-2	Familial or Genetic Susceptibility to Malignancy—cont'd	
DISORDER	**TUMOR/CANCER**	**COMMENT**
OTHERS		
Neurofibromatosis 1	Neurofibroma, optic glioma, acoustic neuroma, astrocytoma, meningioma, pheochromocytoma, sarcoma	Autosomal dominant; mutation in tumor-suppressor gene, *NF1*
Neurofibromatosis 2	Bilateral acoustic neuromas, meningiomas	Autosomal dominant; mutation in tumor-suppressor gene, *NF2*
Tuberous sclerosis	Fibroangiomatous nevi, myocardial rhabdomyoma	Autosomal dominant
Gorlin-Goltz syndrome (nevus basal cell carcinoma syndrome)	Multiple basal cell carcinomas; medulloblastoma	Autosomal dominant; mutation in *PTCH* gene
Li-Fraumeni syndrome	Bone, soft tissue sarcoma, breast	Mutation of *P53* tumor-suppressor gene, autosomal dominant
Retinoblastoma	Sarcoma	Autosomal recessive; increased risk of secondary malignancy 10-20 yr later; mutation in *RB* tumor-suppressor gene
Hemihypertrophy ± Beckwith syndrome	Wilms tumor, hepatoblastoma, adrenal carcinoma	*WT1* gene; 25% develop tumor, most in 1st 5 yr of life
von Hippel-Landau disease	Hemangioblastoma of the cerebellum and retina, pheochromocytoma, renal cancer	Autosomal dominant; mutation of tumor-suppressor gene, *VHL* gene
Multiple endocrine neoplasia syndrome, type 1 (Wermer syndrome)	Parathyroid, pancreatic islet, and pituitary tumors	Autosomal dominant; mutation in *PYGM* tumor-suppressor gene
Multiple endocrine neoplasia syndrome, type 2A (Sipple syndrome)	Medullary carcinoma of the thyroid, hyperparathyroidism, pheochromocytoma	Autosomal dominant; mutations in CYS-rich regions of the *RET* gene activate this protooncogene; *RET* codes for a tyrosine kinase; monitor calcitonin and calcium levels
Multiple endocrine neoplasia type 2B (multiple mucosal neuroma syndrome)	Mucosal neuroma, pheochromocytoma, medullary thyroid carcinoma, Marfan habitus; neuropathy	Autosomal dominant; mutation in catalytic site (codon 883 or 914) activates protooncogene; *RET* codes for a tyrosine kinase
Familial adenomatous polyposis	Colorectal, thyroid carcinoma, duodenal and periampullar carcinomas; pediatric hepatoblastoma	Autosomal dominant; mutation in *APC* gene
Familial juvenile polyposis	Colorectal carcinoma	Autosomal dominant; mutation in *SMAD4* gene
Hereditary nonpolyposis colon cancer (Lynch syndrome, NHPCC)	Colon cancer	Autosomal dominant; mutation in mismatch repair genes; *hMSH2, hMLH1, PMS1, PMS2, hMSH6, hMSG3*
Turcot syndrome	Pediatric brain tumors and increased risk of colon carcinoma and polyps	Mutation in *APC* gene
Familial adenomatous polyposis coli	Adenocarcinoma of colon	Autosomal dominant, *APC* gene
Gardner syndrome	Adenocarcinoma of colon, skull and soft tissue tumors	Autosomal dominant, *APC* gene
Peutz-Jeghers syndrome	Gastrointestinal carcinoma, ovarian neoplasia	Autosomal dominant, *LKB1* gene codes for a Ser/Thr kinase that regulates cell cycle, metabolism, cell polarity
Hemochromatosis	Hepatocellular carcinoma	Autosomal dominant; malignancy associated with cirrhotic liver
Glycogen storage disease 1 (von Gierke disease)	Hepatocellular carcinoma	Autosomal recessive; malignancy associated with cirrhotic liver Mutation in glucose-6-phosphatase or glucose-6-phosphatase translocase genes
Tyrosinemia, galactosemia	Hepatocellular carcinoma	Autosomal recessive; tumor associated with cirrhotic liver
BRCA1 and *BRCA2*	Breast, ovarian	DNA repair defect
Diamond-Blackfan anemia	AML, myelodysplastic syndrome, osteogenic sarcoma	Autosomal dominant; family 9 genes encoding ribosomal proteins
Shwachman-Diamond syndrome	AML, myelodysplasia	Autosomal recessive; *SBDS* gene; chromosome 7q11.21
Hereditary diffuse gastric cancer	Gastric cancer	Autosomal dominant; *CDH1* gene
Pleuropulmonary blastoma family tumor and dysplasia syndrome (DICER1)	Pulmonary blastoma	Encoded protein is a ribonuclease required for microRNA processing
Hereditary neuroblastoma	Neuroblastoma	Two genes have been identified: • Anaplastic lymphoma kinase (*ALK*) at chromosome 2p23 • Paired-like homeobox 2b (*PHOX2B*) at chromosome 4q12
Hereditary paraganglioma–pheochromocytoma syndrome	Paraganglioma Pheochromocytomas	Mutation in the mitochondrial enzyme succinate dehydrogenase protein (SDH)
Congenital or cyclic neutropenia	Myelodysplastic syndrome AML	*ELANE* mutation at 19p13.3; elastase; neutrophil expressed

ALL, acute lymphocytic leukemia; AML, acute myelocytic leukemia; GI, gastrointestinal; GU, genitourinary; JMML, juvenile myelomonocytic leukemia; NHPCC, nonhereditary polyposis colon cancer.

The third category of inherited cancer predisposition is characterized by **defects in immune surveillance**. This group includes patients with Wiskott-Aldrich syndrome, severe combined immunodeficiency, common variable immunodeficiency, and the X-linked lymphoproliferative syndrome. The most common types of malignancy in these patients are lymphoma and leukemia. Cure rates for immunodeficient children with cancer are much poorer than for nonimmunodeficient children with similar malignancies, suggesting a role for the immune system in cancer treatment as well as in cancer prevention.

OTHER FACTORS ASSOCIATED WITH ONCOGENESIS
Viruses
Several viruses have been implicated in the pathogenesis of malignancy. The association of the Epstein-Barr virus (EBV) with Burkitt lymphoma and nasopharyngeal carcinoma was identified more than 30 yr ago, but EBV infection alone is not sufficient for malignant transformation. EBV is also associated with mixed cellularity and lymphocyte-depleted Hodgkin disease, as well as some T-cell lymphomas, which is particularly intriguing because EBV normally does not infect T lymphocytes. The most conclusive evidence for a role of EBV in lymphogenesis is the direct causal role of EBV for B-cell lymphoproliferative disease in immunocompromised persons, especially those with AIDS.

Children who are chronically infected with hepatitis B (hepatitis B surface antigen–positive) have a >200-fold increased risk of developing hepatocellular carcinoma. In adults, the latency period between viral infection and the development of hepatocellular carcinoma approaches 20 yr. However, in children who acquire the viral infection through perinatal transmission, the latency period can be as short as 6-7 yr. The additional factors that are required for the malignant transformation of the virally infected hepatocytes are not clear. Hepatitis C virus infection is another risk factor for hepatocellular carcinoma and is also associated with splenic lymphoma.

Nearly all cervical carcinomas contain human papillomavirus (HPV). High-risk HPVs include types 16 and 18 but also types 31, 33, 35, 45, and 56, which are also commonly found in women without lesions. The low-risk HPVs, including 6 and 11 that are commonly found in genital warts, are almost never associated with malignancies. Like other virus-associated cancers, the presence of HPV alone is not sufficient to cause malignant transformation. The mechanism by which HPV 19 induces malignant transformation is thought to involve *P53* and *RB* tumor-suppressor genes, which regulate the cell cycle by acting as gatekeepers of the G1/S and G2/M checkpoints. By interfering with these proteins, HPV alters the regulation of cell growth.

Human herpesvirus 8 is associated with Kaposi sarcoma, primary effusion B-cell lymphoma, and the plasma cell variant of Castleman disease, all of which occur primarily in persons with AIDS. Human T-cell leukemia virus 1 is associated with adult T-cell leukemia and lymphoma.

Genomic Imprinting
The development of cancer has also been linked to genomic imprinting, which is the selective inactivation of 1 of 2 alleles of a certain gene. The inactivated gene is determined by whether the gene is inherited from the mother or father. For example, normally the maternal *IGF2* (insulin-like growth factor receptor 2) gene is inactivated. The inactivation is thought to be secondary to methylation of specific CpG sequences upstream of the *IGF2* promoter, which interferes with the transcription of the *IGF2* gene. In some Wilms tumors, there is loss of methylation in the upstream area of the maternal gene, which, in turn, allows transcript expression of the maternal *IGF2* gene. At the same time the *H19* gene (whose function is not yet clear), a previously actively transcribed maternal gene, is silenced by methylation. Beckwith-Wiedemann syndrome, an overgrowth syndrome characterized by macrosomia, macroglossia, hemihypertrophy, omphalocele, and renal anomalies, is associated with an increased risk of Wilms tumor, hepatoblastoma, rhabdomyosarcoma, neuroblastoma, and adrenal cortical carcinoma. The increased risk in developing cancer is

associated with changes in the methylation pattern of genes on the 11p15 chromosome. Studies indicate that methylation patterns in a given individual change over time and that specific groups of methylation changes tend to cluster within families, suggesting heritability of the pattern of changes.

Telomerase
Telomeres are a series of tens to thousands of TTAGGG repeats at the ends of chromosomes that are important for stabilizing the chromosomal ends and limiting breakage, translocation, and loss of DNA material. With DNA replication there is a progressive shortening of telomere length, which is a hallmark of cellular aging and may be a senescence signal. In some instances telomerase, an enzyme that adds telomeres to the ends of chromosomes, becomes active. The addition of telomeres can be found in immortalized cell lines and most tumor types, and as a consequence, these cells might have a survival advantage, allowing them to undergo additional cell divisions. Therapy aimed at inhibiting telomerase activity can result in cell death.

Bibliography is available at Expert Consult.

Chapter **493**
Principles of Diagnosis
A. Kim Ritchey and Erika Friehling

Childhood cancer is uncommon and can manifest with symptoms seen with benign illnesses. The challenge for the pediatrician is to be alert to the clues suggesting a diagnosis of cancer. In addition to the classic manifestations, any persistent, unexplained symptom or sign should be evaluated as potentially emanating from a cancerous or precancerous condition. As part of the diagnostic evaluation, the pediatrician and pediatric oncologist must convey the possible diagnosis to the patient and family in a sensitive and informative manner.

SIGNS AND SYMPTOMS
The symptoms and signs of cancer are variable and nonspecific in pediatric patients. The types of cancer that occur during the 1st 20 yr of life vary dramatically as a function of age—more so than at any other comparable age range (see Chapter 491). Unlike cancers in adults, childhood cancers usually originate from the deeper, visceral structures and from the parenchyma of organs rather than from the epithelial layers that line the ducts and glands of organs and compose the skin. In children, dissemination of disease at diagnosis is common, and presenting symptoms or signs are often caused by systemic involvement. Pain was one of the initial presenting symptoms in more than 50% of children with cancer in one study. Infants and young children cannot express or localize their symptoms well. Another factor is the variability in the physiology and biology of the host that are related to growth and development during infancy, childhood, and adolescence.

The signs of cancer in children are often attributed to other causes before the malignancy is recognized. Delays in diagnosis are particularly problematic during late adolescence and are the result of a variety of factors prominent in this age group, including loss of health insurance coverage.

Although there is no clearly established set of warning signs of cancer in young people, the most common cancers in children suggest some guidelines that may be helpful in early recognition of signs and symptoms of cancer (Table 493-1). Most of the symptoms and signs are not specific and might represent other possibilities in a differential diagnosis. Nonetheless, these hints encompass the common cancers of childhood and have been very useful in early detection.

Table 493-1	Common Manifestations of Childhood Malignancies		
	SIGNS AND SYMPTOMS	**POTENTIAL ETIOLOGY**	**POSSIBLE ONCOLOGIC DIAGNOSIS**
Constitutional/Systemic	Fever, persistent or recurrent infection, neutropenia	Bone marrow infiltration	Leukemia, neuroblastoma
	Fever of unknown origin, weight loss, night sweats	Lymphoma	Hodgkin and non-Hodgkin lymphoma
	Painless lymphadenopathy	Lymphoma, metastatic solid tumor	Leukemia, Hodgkin lymphoma, non-Hodgkin lymphoma, Burkitt lymphoma, thyroid carcinoma
	Hypertension	Renal or adrenal tumor	Neuroblastoma, pheochromocytoma, Wilms tumor
	Soft tissue mass	Local or metastatic tumor	Ewing sarcoma, osteosarcoma, neuroblastoma, thyroid carcinoma, rhabdomyosarcoma, Langerhans cell histiocytosis
Neurologic/Ophthalmologic	Headache with emesis, visual disturbances, ataxia, papilledema, cranial nerve palsies	Increased intracranial pressure	Primary brain tumor; metastasis
	Leukokoria (white pupil)	Retinal mass	Retinoblastoma
	Periorbital ecchymosis	Metastasis	Neuroblastoma
	Miosis, ptosis, heterochromia	Horner syndrome: compression of cervical sympathetic nerves	Neuroblastoma
	Opsoclonus myoclonus, ataxia	Neurotransmitters? Autoimmunity?	Neuroblastoma
	Exophthalmos, proptosis	Orbital tumor	Rhabdomyosarcoma, lymphoma, Langerhans cell histiocytosis
Respiratory/Thoracic	Cough, stridor, pneumonia, tracheal-bronchial compression; superior vena cava syndrome	Anterior mediastinal mass	Germ cell tumor, non-Hodgkin lymphoma, Hodgkin lymphoma
	Vertebral or nerve root compression; dysphagia	Posterior mediastinal mass	Neuroblastoma, neuroenteric cyst
Gastrointestinal	Abdominal mass	Adrenal, renal, or lymphoid tumor	Neuroblastoma, Wilms tumor, lymphoma
	Diarrhea	Vasoactive intestinal polypeptide	Neuroblastoma, ganglioneuroma
Hematologic	Pallor, anemia	Bone marrow infiltration	Leukemia, neuroblastoma
	Petechiae, thrombocytopenia	Bone marrow infiltration	Leukemia, neuroblastoma
Musculoskeletal	Bone pain, limp, arthralgia	Primary bone tumor, metastasis to bone	Osteosarcoma, Ewing sarcoma, leukemia, neuroblastoma
Endocrine	Diabetes insipidus, galactorrhea, poor growth	Neuroendocrine involvement of hypothalamus or pituitary gland	Adenoma, craniopharyngioma, prolactinoma, Langerhans cell histiocytosis

Modified from Marcdante KJ, Kliegman RM, Jenson HB, et al, editors: Nelson essentials of pediatrics, ed 6, Philadelphia, 2011, WB Saunders, p. 588.

PHYSICAL EXAMINATION

Physical examination findings in a child with malignancy are dependent on whether the cancer is systemic (see Table 493-1) or localized. The cancers most common in children involve the lymphohematopoietic system. When the bone marrow is compromised by malignancy (e.g., leukemia, disseminated neuroblastoma), typical findings include pallor from anemia; bleeding, petechiae, or purpura from thrombocytopenia or coagulopathy; cellulitis or other localized infection from leukopenia; skin nodules (especially in infants) and hepatosplenomegaly from malignant leukocytosis. Abnormalities found in lymphatic malignancies include peripheral adenopathy (Fig. 493-1) and signs of superior vena cava syndrome from an anterior mediastinal mass (Fig. 493-2), including respiratory distress, and facial and neck plethora and edema. Enlargement of cervical lymph nodes is common in children, but when persistent, progressive, and painless it often suggests lymphoma. In particular, supraclavicular adenopathy suggests underlying malignancy.

Abnormalities of the central nervous system that can indicate cancer include decreased level of consciousness, cranial nerve palsies, ataxia, afebrile seizures, ptosis, decreased visual activity, neuroendocrine deficits, and increased intracranial pressure, which may be diagnosed by the presence of papilledema (Fig. 493-3). Any focal neurologic deficit in the motor or sensory system, especially a decrease in cranial nerve function, should prompt further investigation for malignancy.

Abdominal masses can be divided into upper, middle, and lower locations. Malignancies in the upper abdomen include Wilms tumor, neuroblastoma, hepatoblastoma, germ cell tumors, and sarcomas. Enlargement of the liver or spleen from leukemia can be mistaken for an upper abdominal mass. Midabdominal masses include non-Hodgkin lymphoma, neuroblastoma, germ cell tumors, and sarcomas. Lower abdominal masses include ovarian tumors, germ cell tumors, and sarcomas.

Rhabdomyosarcoma commonly appears as an extremity mass, particularly in adolescents. These tumors can be deceptively benign in appearance, but as with all unexplained masses they require immediate attention. Sacrococcygeal masses in neonates are usually teratomas, which are usually benign but can undergo malignant transformation if not removed promptly. Neuroblastoma can present as "blueberry muffin" spots on the skin of neonates or as periorbital ecchymosis in older children.

Ophthalmologic presentation of malignancy includes a white pupillary reflex (Fig. 493-4) rather than the usual red reflection from

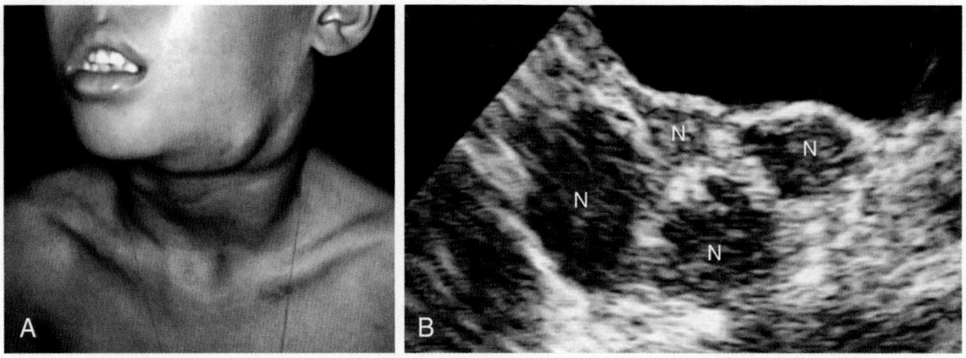

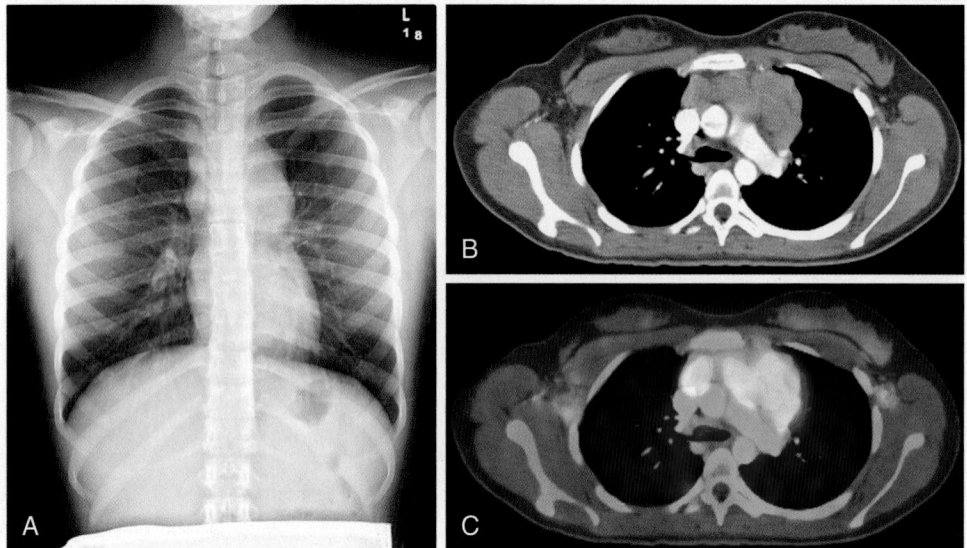

Figure 493-1 Cervical lymphadenopathy. Manifestations on physical examination **(A)** and on ultrasound examination **(B)**. *N,* Abnormally enlarged lymph nodes. *(From Sinniah D, D'Angio GJ, Chatten J, et al: Atlas of pediatric oncology, London, 1996, Arnold.)*

Figure 493-2 Anterior upper mediastinal mass from non-Hodgkin lymphoma. **A,** Plain chest X-ray. **B,** CT scan. **C,** Positron emission tomography (PET) scan.

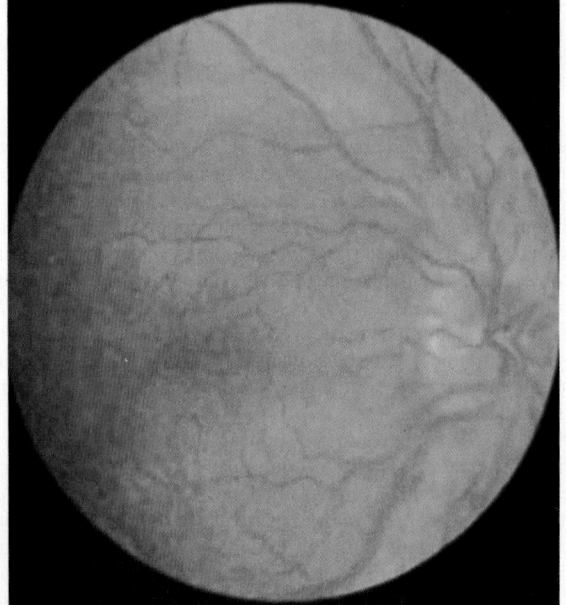

Figure 493-3 Papilledema on funduscopic examination. *(From Sinniah D, D'Angio GJ, Chatten J, et al: Atlas of pediatric oncology, London, 1996, Arnold.)*

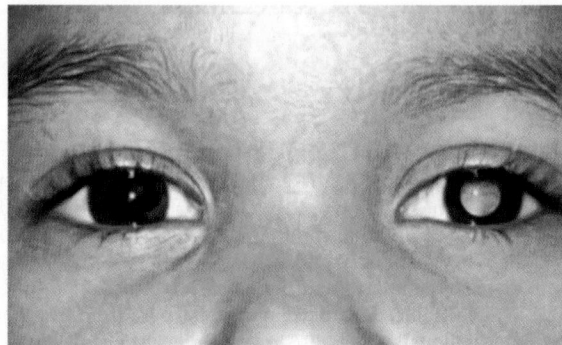

Figure 493-4 White pupillary reflex in the left eye. *(From Sinniah D, D'Angio GJ, Chatten J, et al: Atlas of pediatric oncology, London, 1996, Arnold.)*

incident light. A white pupillary reflex is essentially pathognomonic for retinoblastoma, although some benign conditions can mimic this finding. Proptosis can be produced by rhabdomyosarcoma, neuroblastoma, lymphoma, and Langerhans cell histiocytosis. Horner syndrome, iris heterochromia, and opsoclonus-myoclonus all suggest a diagnosis of neuroblastoma.

AGE-RELATED MANIFESTATIONS

Because various types of cancer in children occur at specific ages, the physician should tailor the history and physical examination based on the age of the child. The embryonal tumors, including neuroblastoma, Wilms tumor, retinoblastoma, hepatoblastoma, and rhabdomyosarcoma, usually occur during the 1st 2 yr of life (see Fig. 491-4). From 1-4 yr of age, acute lymphoblastic leukemia peaks in incidence. Brain tumors have a peak incidence in the 1st decade of life. Non-Hodgkin lymphomas are uncommon earlier than 5 yr of age but steadily increase thereafter. During adolescence, bone tumors, Hodgkin disease, and the gonadal and soft tissue sarcomas predominate. Hence, for infants and toddlers, special attention should be paid to the possibility of embryonal and intraabdominal tumors. Preschool-age and early school-age children showing compatible signs and symptoms should be specifically evaluated for leukemia. School-age children might present with lymphoma or with brain tumors. Adolescents require assessment for bone and soft tissue sarcomas and gonadal malignancies, as well as for Hodgkin lymphoma.

EARLY DETECTION

The prognosis of malignancy in children depends primarily on tumor type, extent of disease at diagnosis, and rapidity of response to treatment. Early diagnosis helps to ensure that appropriate therapy is given in a timely fashion and hence optimizes the chances of cure. Because most physicians in general practice rarely encounter children with undiagnosed cancer, they should remember to investigate the possibility of malignancy, especially when they encounter an atypical course of a common childhood condition, unusual manifestations that do not fit common conditions, and any persistent symptom that defies diagnosis.

Delays in diagnosis are particularly likely in certain clinical situations. The cardinal symptom of both osteosarcoma and Ewing sarcoma is localized and usually persistent pain. Because these tumors occur during the 2nd decade of life, a time of increased physical activity, patients often assume the pain results from trauma. Prompt radiologic evaluation can help confirm the diagnosis. Lymphoma, especially during adolescence, often manifests as an anterior mediastinal mass. Symptoms such as chronic cough, unexplained shortness of breath, or "new-onset asthma" are typical with this presentation and are often overlooked. Tumors of the nasopharynx or middle ear can mimic infection. Prolonged, unexplained ear pain, nasal discharge, retropharyngeal swelling, and trismus should be investigated as possible signs of malignancy.

Early symptoms of leukemia may be limited to prolonged or unexplained low-grade fever or bone and joint pain. Blood counts with abnormalities in two or more cell lines might indicate the need for bone marrow examination, even when leukemic blast cells are not seen in the blood smear (see Table 493-1).

Mass screening for children with malignancy is not feasible. A screening program to detect early-stage neuroblastoma was successful in documenting more cases of the disease, but it had no impact on overall outcome. However, certain children are at increased risk for cancer and require an individualized plan to ensure early detection of malignancy. Selected examples include children with certain chromosome abnormalities, such as Down syndrome, Klinefelter syndrome, WAGR syndrome (Wilms tumor, aniridia, genital abnormalities, and mental retardation); children with overgrowth syndromes, such as Beckwith-Wiedemann syndrome, and hemihypertrophy; children with certain inherited single-gene disorders, including retinoblastoma, P53 mutations (Li-Fraumeni syndrome), familial adenomatous polyposis, and neurofibromatosis (see Table 492-2).

ENSURING THE DIAGNOSIS

When a malignant neoplasm is suspected, the immediate goal is to confirm the diagnosis. A tentative diagnosis can often be established on the basis of the patient's age, symptoms, and location of masses. Selected imaging techniques and tumor markers can facilitate the diagnostic approach (Table 493-2). Especially when a solid tumor is present,

Table 493-2	Work-up of Common Pediatric Malignancies to Assess Primary Tumor and Potential Metastases								
MALIGNANCY	BONE MARROW ASPIRATE OR BIOPSY	CHEST X-RAY	CT SCAN	MRI	PET SCAN	BONE SCAN	CSF ANALYSIS	SPECIFIC MARKERS	OTHER TESTS
Leukemia	Yes (includes flow cytometry, cytogenetics, molecular studies)	Yes	—	—	—	—	Yes	—	—
Non-Hodgkin lymphoma	Yes (includes flow cytometry, cytogenetics, molecular studies)	Yes	Yes	—	Yes	Yes (selected cases)	Yes	—	—
Hodgkin lymphoma	Yes (in advanced stage)	Yes	Yes	—	Yes	Yes (selected cases)	—	—	—
CNS tumors	—	—	—	Yes	—	—	Yes (selected tumors)	—	—
Neuroblastoma	Yes (includes cytogenetics, molecular studies)	—	Yes	—	—	Yes	—	VMA, HVA	MIBG scan; bone x-rays
Wilms tumor	—	Yes	Yes	—	—	—	—	—	—

Continued

Table 493-2	Work-up of Common Pediatric Malignancies to Assess Primary Tumor and Potential Metastases—cont'd

MALIGNANCY	BONE MARROW ASPIRATE OR BIOPSY	CHEST X-RAY	CT SCAN	MRI	PET SCAN	BONE SCAN	CSF ANALYSIS	SPECIFIC MARKERS	OTHER TESTS
Rhabdomyosarcoma	Yes	Yes	Yes	Yes (selected sites)	—	Yes	Yes (for parameningeal tumors only)	—	—
Osteosarcoma	—	Yes	Yes (of chest)	Yes (for primary tumors)	—	Yes	—	—	—
Ewing sarcoma	Yes	Yes	Yes (of chest)	Yes (for primary tumors)	—	Yes	—	—	—
Germ cell tumors	—	Yes	Yes	Consider MRI of brain	—	—	—	AFP, HCG	—
Liver tumors	—	Yes	Yes	—	—	—	—	AFP	—
Retinoblastoma	Selected cases	—	Yes	Yes (includes brain)	—	Selected cases	Selected cases	—	—

AFP, α-Fetoprotein; CNS, central nervous system; CSF, cerebrospinal fluid; HCG, human chorionic gonadotropin; HVA, homovanillic acid; MIBG, metaiodobenzylguanidine; PET, positron emission tomography; VMA, vanillylmandelic acid.

Modified from Marcdante KJ, Kliegman RM, Jenson HB, et al, editors: Nelson essentials of pediatrics, *ed 6, Philadelphia, 2011, WB Saunders, p. 589.*

the pediatric oncologist, surgeon, and pathologist should work as a team to determine the site of biopsy, amount of tissue required, and whether fine-needle aspiration, percutaneous image-guided biopsy, incisional biopsy, or excisional biopsy and tumor resection are indicated. For selected situations, at the time of the initial diagnostic procedure, plans for bone marrow aspiration and biopsy and placement of central venous access may be appropriate.

Pathologic evaluation of pediatric malignancies requires appropriate handling of tissue so that multiple different techniques can be used. It is important that fresh tissue not be placed in formalin. Besides routine light microscopy, pathologic evaluation may include immunochemistry, flow cytometry, cytogenetics, and molecular genetic studies (fluorescence in situ hybridization, reverse-transcriptase polymerase chain reaction). Emerging technologies include DNA microarray analysis and cancer genome sequencing that can identify specific gene expression patterns and sequences in tumors. In time, these technologies might ensure more accurate classification and treatment.

STAGING

Once a specific diagnosis is confirmed, studies to define the extent of the malignancy are necessary to determine prognosis and treatment. Table 493-2 outlines the minimum evaluation required for common pediatric malignancies. In addition, for many tumors (e.g., Wilms tumor, neuroblastoma, rhabdomyosarcoma) a surgical staging system is used. Surgical stage can be determined at the time of the initial diagnostic procedure or subsequently. For example, a patient who has abdominal surgery for possible Wilms tumor or neuroblastoma should have careful evaluation and biopsy of all adjacent lymph nodes. A child with rhabdomyosarcoma can require a subsequent biopsy of sentinel lymph nodes as determined by scintigraphy or dye injection adjacent to the primary tumor. The pathologist facilitates staging by examining margins of the specimen to determine residual tumor.

Bibliography is available at Expert Consult.

Chapter 494
Principles of Treatment
Archie Bleyer, A. Kim Ritchey, and Erika Friehling

Treatment of children with cancer begins with an absolute requirement for the correct diagnosis (including subtype), proceeds through accurate and thorough staging of the extent of disease and determination of prognostic subgroup, provides appropriate multidisciplinary and usually multimodal therapy, and requires assiduous evaluation of the possibilities of recurrent disease and of adverse late effects of the disease and the therapies rendered. Throughout treatment, every child with cancer should have the benefit of the expertise of specialized teams of providers of pediatric cancer care, including pediatric oncologists, pathologists, radiologists, surgeons, radiotherapists, nurses, and support staff, including nutritionists, social workers, psychologists, pharmacists, other medical specialists, and teachers trained to work with seriously ill children.

The best chance for cure of cancer is during the initial course of treatment; the cure rates for patients with recurrent disease are much lower than those for patients with primary disease. All patients with cancer should be referred to an appropriate specialized center as soon as possible when the diagnosis of cancer is suspected. All such centers in North America are identified on the Children's Oncology Group website (http://www.childrensoncologygroup.org) and on the National Cancer Institute cancer trials website (http://www.clinicaltrials.gov). The remarkable increases in cure rates for childhood malignancies since the 1970s would not have occurred without the collective participation of patients and their physicians in clinical research programs at these centers. In the United States, the National Cancer Institute's Clinical Trials Cooperative Groups Program is associated with a >80% reduction in the incidence of mortality from childhood cancer despite an overall increase in cancer incidence during this interval (Fig. 494-1). After what appeared to be a plateau in the rate of decline in mortality in the early 2000s, there is now evidence that the mortality rate

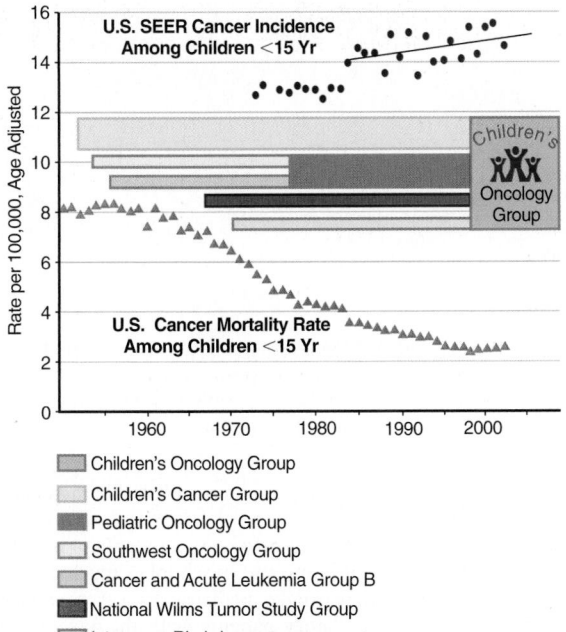

Figure 494-1 Reduction in the national cancer mortality rate among children younger than 15 yr of age *(triangles)* in the United States as a direct consequence of the National Cooperative Group Program sponsored by the National Cancer Institute, and in comparison to the rising incidence of cancer before age 15 yr *(circles)*. The *horizontal bars* indicate the duration of the existence of the national pediatric cancer cooperative groups, beginning with the Children's Cancer Group in 1955. Other groups are the Pediatric Oncology Group, which was derived from the Pediatrics Divisions of the Southwest Oncology Group and the Cancer and Acute Leukemia Group B, the National Wilms Tumor Study Group, and the Intergroup Rhabdomyosarcoma Study Group. In 2000, the 4 pediatric cooperative groups merged into the Children's Oncology Group. *(Incidence and mortality rate data from Ries LAG, Eisner MP, Kosary CL, et al, editors: SEER Cancer Statistics Review, 1975-2002, Bethesda, MD, National Cancer Institute; http:// seer.cancer.gov/csr/1975_2002/, based on November 2004 SEER [Surveillance Epidemiology and End Results] data submission. The mortality rate data are national rates, and the incidence data are derived from the SEER program, representing approximately 15% of the United States. The most current information on treatment of all types of childhood cancer is available in the PDQ [Physician Data Query] on the National Cancer Institute website [http://www.cancer.gov/cancertopics/ pdq/pediatrictreatment].)*

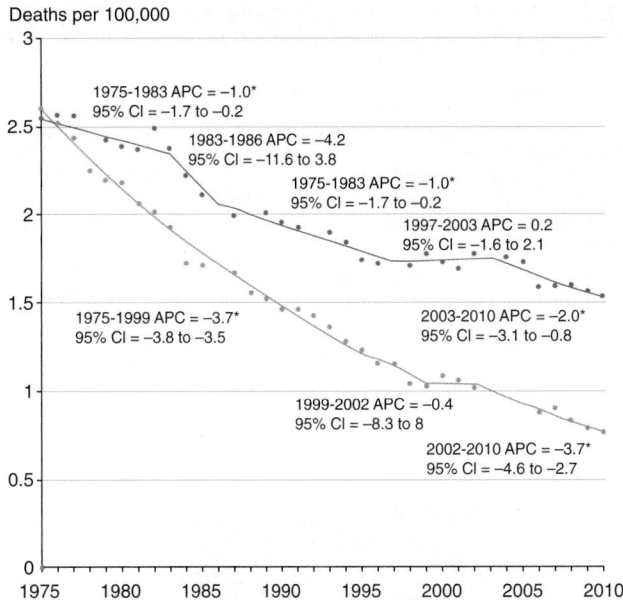

Figure 494-2 Age-adjusted mortality trends for all malignant cancers among children age <20 years in the United States from 1975 through 2010 along with annual percentage changes (APCs) for joinpoint segments. Asterisk indicates that the slope of the joinpoint segment is statistically different from zero (P<.05). The green line indicates leukemias and lymphomas, and the blue line indicates all other cancer sites. CI indicates confidence interval. *(From Smith MA, Altekruse SF, Adamson PC, et al: Declining childhood and adolescent cancer mortality,* Cancer *120:2497-2506, 2014.)*

continues to decline. Notably, a greater decline in mortality has been seen in the adolescent and young adult population when compared to children <15 yr old, reversing prior trends (Fig. 494-2). The most current information on treatment of all types of childhood cancer is available in the PDQ (Physician Data Query) on the National Cancer Institute website (http://www.cancer.gov/cancertopics/pdq/ pediatrictreatment).

DIAGNOSIS AND STAGING
Accurate diagnosis and staging of the extent of disease are imperative, especially for childhood cancers that have high cure rates, because the nature of therapy depends strongly on the type of cancer. In addition, **prognostic subgroups** based on the stage of disease have been established for most cancers that occur in children. Accordingly, children with a better prognosis are treated with less-intensive therapy, including lower doses of chemotherapy or radiation therapy, a shorter duration of treatment, or elimination of at least one treatment modality (radiation therapy, chemotherapy, surgery). Accurate staging thus reduces the risk of excessive acute adverse effects and long-term complications of therapy in patients whose prognosis indicates that less therapy is required for cure. Overtreatment of patients with a more favorable prognosis is a definite risk if the patient is not referred to a

cancer treatment center for management of adverse effects of such treatment. Conversely, undertreatment also is a clear risk if the diagnosis and stage are not correct, resulting in a compromise of an otherwise high potential for cure.

Diagnostic imaging is a critical phase of evaluation in most children with solid tumors (i.e., cancers other than leukemia). MRI, CT, ultrasonography, scintigraphy (nuclear medicine scans), positron emission tomography, and spectroscopy, as appropriate, all serve a clear purpose in the evaluation of children with cancer, not only before treatment to determine the extent of disease and the appropriate therapy but also during follow-up to determine whether the therapy was effective. In addition, response to treatment as determined by imaging techniques is being increasingly used to guide changes in the therapy.

Expertise in pathology and laboratory medicine provides critical diagnostic support and guides therapy in most children with cancer. Relatively noninvasive methods of obtaining tumor tissue (such as fine-needle aspiration and percutaneous image-guided biopsies) can be performed in pediatric centers with appropriate expertise in diagnostic imaging, interventional radiology, cytology, and anesthesia support. Sentinel node mapping is increasingly being applied in the staging of children's cancers. Determining the adequacy of surgery by evaluating frozen sections of the surgical margins for tumor cells is essential in many tumor operations.

A MULTIMODAL, MULTIDISCIPLINARY APPROACH
Many pediatric subspecialties are involved in the evaluation, treatment, and management of children with cancer, including provision of primary therapy and supportive care services (Fig. 494-3). More than two of the primary modalities are often used together, with chemotherapy being the most widely used, followed, in order of use, by surgery, radiation therapy, and biologic agent therapy (Fig. 494-4).

The leukemias that occur in childhood usually are managed with chemotherapy alone, with a small proportion of patients receiving cranial or craniospinal radiation therapy to prevent or treat overt central nervous system (CNS) leukemia. Children with non-Hodgkin

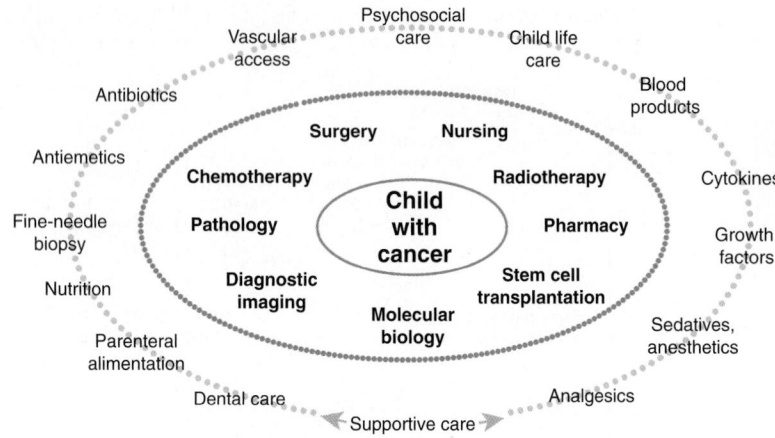

Figure 494-3 Multidisciplinary care of children with cancer. The *inner circle* designates primary modalities, and the *outer ring* identifies supportive care elements to which all children with cancer have access.

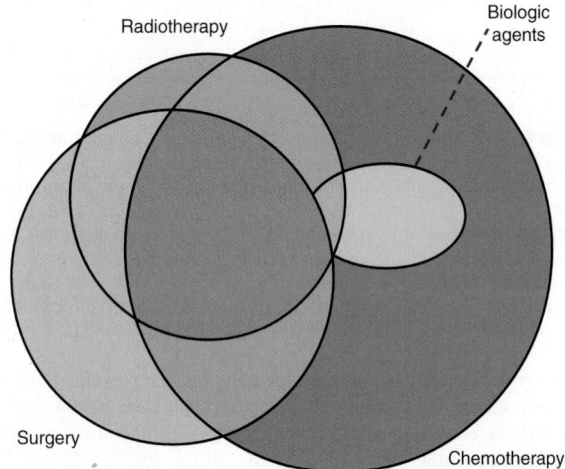

Figure 494-4 The primary modalities of therapy used in the treatment of children with cancer. The relative sizes of the circles designate the approximate proportion of overall role in the management of pediatric cancers.

lymphoma also are treated with chemotherapy alone, with the exception of radiation therapy for CNS involvement. Localized therapy with surgery or irradiation, or both, is an important component of treatment of most solid tumors, including Hodgkin lymphoma, but systemic multiagent chemotherapy usually is necessary because tumor dissemination generally is present even if it is undetectable. Chemotherapy alone usually is not adequate to eradicate gross residual tumors. Hence, it is not unusual for children with malignant tumors to require treatment with all 3 modalities (see Fig. 494-3). Unfortunately, most treatments that are effective in children with cancer have a narrow therapeutic index (a low ratio of efficacy to toxicity). The acute and chronic adverse effects of these treatments can be minimized but not entirely avoided.

Biologic agent therapy has become an important modality in a few childhood cancers (see Fig. 494-4). This type of treatment generally refers to immunotherapy, biologic response modifiers, or endogenously occurring molecules that have therapeutic effects in supraphysiologic doses. Examples are retinoic acid therapy in acute promyelocytic leukemia, monoclonal antibody therapy for neuroblastoma and certain non-Hodgkin lymphomas, tyrosine kinase inhibitors such as imatinib mesylate for chronic myelogenous and Philadelphia chromosome–positive leukemias, and radioactive metaiodobenzylguanidine therapy for neuroblastoma.

Chemotherapy is used more widely in children than in adults because children better tolerate the acute adverse effects and the malignant diseases that occur in childhood are more responsive to chemotherapy than are malignant diseases of adults. Radiation therapy is used

sparingly in children because they are more vulnerable than adults to its late adverse effects.

Whenever possible, treatment is given on an outpatient basis. Children should remain living at home and in school as much as possible throughout treatment. Increasingly, pediatric cancer therapies are being administered to ambulatory patients, with the advent of such innovations as programmable infusion pumps, oral chemotherapeutic regimens, early discharge from hospital with intensive outpatient supportive care, and home healthcare services. Some patients miss a considerable amount of school in the 1st yr after diagnosis because of the intensity of therapy or its adverse effects and of the ensuing complications of the disease or therapy. Tutoring should be encouraged so that children do not fall behind in their schooling; counseling should be provided as appropriate. In-hospital school services should be provided for patients who must spend much of their time as inpatients receiving therapy for disease or for managing adverse effects.

Development of selective, highly effective therapy for cancer in both children and adults had been hindered by a lack of understanding of the molecular mechanisms that underlie malignant transformation. De novo or acquired resistance to chemotherapy and radiation therapy remains an obstacle to cure. Ongoing discoveries of molecular and cellular mechanisms that explain the cancer process have led to increasingly specific antineoplastic therapies, generally referred to as **molecularly targeted therapies**. Their most prominent feature is a relative lack of normal tissue toxicity, such that the additional therapeutic benefit occurs with minimum additional toxicity. Many of the new biologic agent therapies, such as imatinib and rituximab, fall into this category (Table 494-1). **Complementary** and **alternative remedies** are increasingly being provided by parents to their children with cancer, with or without knowledge of the medical professionals entrusted with the child's care (see Chapter 64). Many of these have not been evaluated by rigorous testing and most are ineffective; some are toxic or interfere with the metabolism of other drugs.

DISCUSSING THE TREATMENT PLAN WITH THE PATIENT AND FAMILY

The diagnostic and treatment plan must be carefully explained to parents and, if the child is old enough to understand, to the patient. An honest discussion of the facts is the best policy. Children should be given as much information as they can understand and would find useful or that information they express a desire or wish to know. Effects of treatment, such as the possible need to amputate a limb, loss of hair during chemotherapy, and possible temporary or permanent functional impairment must be anticipated and fully discussed. The possibility and probability of death from cancer should be covered in an age-appropriate manner. It usually is necessary to repeat explanations several times before distraught family members fully understand. Throughout treatment, parents, patients, siblings, and medical staff will need help in expressing feelings of anxiety, depression, guilt, and anger. The pediatrician, pediatric oncologist, and nurses should call on experienced professionals, including pediatric social workers, child

Table 494-1	Protein Tyrosine Kinase Inhibitors and Monoclonal Antibodies	
AGENT	**TARGET**	**MALIGNANCY**
Imatinib	BCR-ABL	CML Philadelphia chromosome–positive ALL
	PDGFRα	Hypereosinophilic syndrome Systemic mastocytosis
	PDGFRβ	CMML
	cKIT	Systemic mastocytosis Gastrointestinal stromal tumor
Dasatinib, Nilotinib	BCR-ABL	CML Philadelphia chromosome–positive ALL
Gefitinib, Erlotinib, Cetuximab	EGFR	Non–small cell lung cancer
Rituximab	CD20	Non-Hodgkin lymphoma
Trastuzumab	ERBB2/HER-2	Breast cancer
Bevacizumab	VEGFR-1, -2	Non–small cell lung cancer Breast cancer Renal cell carcinoma Colorectal cancer Glioblastoma

ALL, Acute lymphoblastic leukemia; CML, chronic myelogenous leukemia; CMML, chronic myelomonocytic leukemia.

psychologists and psychiatrists, child-life specialists, and schoolteachers with special expertise in managing students with cancer to assist when needed.

TREATMENTS
Chemotherapy

The most widely used modality in pediatric cancer therapy is chemotherapy (see Fig. 494-3). Therapy nearly always involves combinations of drugs, such as VAC (vincristine, dactinomycin [Actinomycin D], and cyclophosphamide) and CHOP (cyclophosphamide, doxorubicin [hydroxydaunorubicin/Adriamycin], vincristine [Oncovin], and prednisone). Sequential single-drug therapy rarely results in complete responses, and partial responses usually are infrequent and transient and grow progressively shorter in duration with each drug used. Combination chemotherapy is the standard when combinations of drugs with different mechanisms of action and non-overlapping toxicities were first demonstrated to be effective in childhood leukemia. Most of the cytotoxic drugs for childhood cancer are selected from several classes of agents, including alkylating agents, antimetabolites, antibiotics, hormones, plant alkaloids, and topoisomerase inhibitors (Table 494-2). The increased metabolic and cell-cycle activity of malignant cells makes them more susceptible to the cytotoxic effects of these types of agents (Fig. 494-5).

Because most antineoplastic agents are cell-cycle dependent, their adverse effects usually are related to the proliferation kinetics of individual cell populations. Most susceptible are tissues or organs with high rates of cell turnover: bone marrow, oral and intestinal mucosa, epidermis, liver, and spermatogonia. The most common acute adverse

Table 494-2	Common Chemotherapeutic Agents Used in Children			
DRUG	**MECHANISM OF ACTION OR CLASSIFICATION**	**INDICATION(S)**	**ADVERSE REACTIONS (PARTIAL LIST)**	**COMMENTS**
Methotrexate	Folic acid antagonist; inhibits dihydrofolate reductase	ALL, non-Hodgkin lymphoma, osteosarcoma, Hodgkin lymphoma, medulloblastoma	Myelosuppression, mucositis, stomatitis, dermatitis, hepatitis With long-term administration; osteopenia and bone fractures With high-dose administration; renal and CNS toxicity With intrathecal administration; arachnoiditis, leukoencephalopathy, leukomyelopathy	Systemic administration may be PO, IM, or IV; also may be administered intrathecally Plasma methotrexate levels must be monitored with high-dose therapy and when low doses are administered to patients with renal dysfunction, and leucovorin rescue applied accordingly
6-Mercaptopurine (Purinethol)	Purine analog; inhibits purine synthesis	ALL	Myelosuppression, hepatic necrosis, mucositis; allopurinol increases toxicity	Allopurinol inhibits metabolism
Cytarabine (cytosine arabinoside; Ara-C)	Pyrimidine analog; inhibits DNA polymerase	ALL, AML, non-Hodgkin lymphoma, Hodgkin lymphoma	Nausea, vomiting, myelosuppression, conjunctivitis, mucositis, CNS dysfunction With intrathecal administration; arachnoiditis, leukoencephalopathy, leukomyelopathy	Systemic administration may be PO, IM, or IV; may also be administered intrathecally
Cyclophosphamide (Cytoxan)	Alkylates guanine; inhibits DNA synthesis	ALL, non-Hodgkin lymphoma, Hodgkin lymphoma, soft tissue sarcoma, Ewing sarcoma, Wilms tumor, neuroblastoma	Nausea, vomiting, myelosuppression, hemorrhagic cystitis, pulmonary fibrosis, inappropriate ADH secretion, bladder cancer, anaphylaxis	Requires hepatic activation and thus is less effective in presence of liver dysfunction. Mesna prevents hemorrhagic cystitis
Ifosfamide (Ifex)	Alkylates guanine; inhibits DNA synthesis	Non-Hodgkin lymphoma, Wilms tumor, soft tissue sarcoma	Nausea, vomiting, myelosuppression, hemorrhagic cystitis, pulmonary fibrosis, inappropriate ADH secretion, CNS dysfunction, cardiac toxicity, anaphylaxis	Mesna prevents hemorrhagic cystitis

Continued

Table 494-2	Common Chemotherapeutic Agents Used in Children—cont'd			
DRUG	**MECHANISM OF ACTION OR CLASSIFICATION**	**INDICATION(S)**	**ADVERSE REACTIONS (PARTIAL LIST)**	**COMMENTS**
Doxorubicin (Adriamycin), daunorubicin (Cerubidine), and idarubicin (Idamycin)	Binds to DNA, intercalation	ALL, AML, osteosarcoma, Ewing sarcoma, Hodgkin lymphoma, non-Hodgkin lymphoma, neuroblastoma	Nausea, vomiting, cardiomyopathy, red urine, tissue necrosis on extravasation, myelosuppression, conjunctivitis, radiation dermatitis, arrhythmia	Dexrazoxane reduces risk of cardiotoxicity
Dactinomycin	Binds to DNA, inhibits transcription	Wilms tumor, rhabdomyosarcoma, Ewing sarcoma	Nausea, vomiting tissue necrosis on extravasation, myelosuppression, radiosensitizer, mucosal ulceration	
Bleomycin (Blenoxane)	Binds to DNA, cleaves DNA strands	Hodgkin disease, non-Hodgkin lymphoma, germ cell tumors	Nausea, vomiting, pneumonitis, stomatitis, Raynaud phenomenon, pulmonary fibrosis, dermatitis	
Vincristine (Oncovin)	Inhibits microtubule formation	ALL, non-Hodgkin lymphoma, Hodgkin disease, Wilms tumor, Ewing sarcoma, neuroblastoma, rhabdomyosarcoma	Local cellulitis, peripheral neuropathy, constipation, ileus, jaw pain, inappropriate ADH secretion, seizures, ptosis, minimal myelosuppression	IV administration only; must not be allowed to extravasate
Vinblastine (Velban)	Inhibits microtubule formation	Hodgkin lymphoma, non-Hodgkin lymphoma, Langerhans cell histiocytosis, CNS tumors	Local cellulitis, leukopenia	IV administration only; must not be allowed to extravasate
L-Asparaginase	Depletion of L-asparagine	ALL; AML, when used in combination with cytarabine	Allergic reaction pancreatitis, hyperglycemia, platelet dysfunction and coagulopathy, encephalopathy	PEG-asparaginase now preferred to L-asparaginase
Pegaspargase (Oncaspar)	Polyethylene glycol conjugate of L-asparagine	ALL	Indicated for prolonged asparagine depletion and for patients with allergy to L-asparaginase	
Prednisone and dexamethasone (Decadron)	Lymphatic cell lysis	ALL; Hodgkin lymphoma, non-Hodgkin lymphoma	Cushing syndrome, cataracts, diabetes, hypertension, myopathy, osteoporosis, avascular necrosis, infection, peptic ulceration, psychosis	
Carmustine (BiCNU)	Carbamylation of DNA; inhibits DNA synthesis	CNS tumors, non-Hodgkin lymphoma, Hodgkin lymphoma	Nausea, vomiting, delayed myelosuppression (4-6 wk); pulmonary fibrosis, carcinogenic stomatitis	Phenobarbital increases metabolism, decreases activity
Carboplatin and cisplatin (Platinol)	Inhibits DNA synthesis	Osteosarcoma, neuroblastoma, CNS tumors, germ cell tumors	Nausea, vomiting, renal dysfunction, myelosuppression, ototoxicity, tetany, neurotoxicity, hemolytic-uremic syndrome, anaphylaxis	Aminoglycosides may increase nephrotoxicity
Etoposide (VePesid)	Topoisomerase inhibitor	ALL, non-Hodgkin lymphoma, germ cell tumor, Ewing sarcoma	Nausea, vomiting, myelosuppression, secondary leukemia	
Tretinoin (all *trans*-retinoic acid); and isotretinoin (cis-retinoic acid; Accutane)	Enhances normal differentiation	Acute promyelocytic leukemia; neuroblastoma	Dry mouth, hair loss, pseudotumor cerebri, premature epiphyseal closure, birth defects	

ADH, antidiuretic hormone; ALL, acute lymphoblastic leukemia; AML, acute myelogenous leukemia; CNS, central nervous system; PEG, polyethylene glycol.

effects are myelosuppression (with neutropenia and thrombocytopenia being the most problematic), immunosuppression, nausea and vomiting, hepatic dysfunction, upper and lower gastrointestinal mucositis, dermatitis, and alopecia. Fortunately, the tissues affected also recover relatively quickly, so that the acute adverse effects are nearly always reversible. Life-threatening effects of many chemotherapy agents include severe neutropenia with infection, fungemia or fungal pneumonia as a result of immunosuppression, and septicemia, not infrequently linked to indwelling intravascular devices (Table 494-3; see Chapters 178 and 179). Cardiomyopathy caused by anthracyclines (e.g., doxorubicin and daunorubicin) and renal failure from platinum-containing agents also may be life-threatening or disabling.

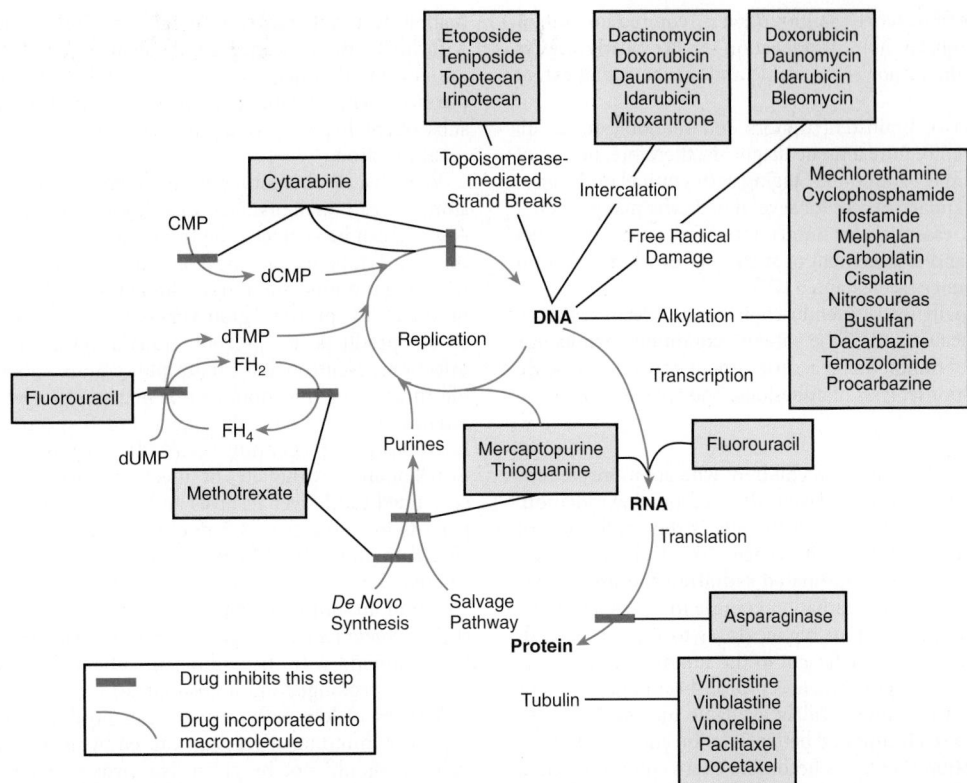

Figure 494-5 Site of action of the commonly used anticancer drugs. *CMP,* Cytidine monophosphate; *dCMP,* deoxycytidine monophosphate; *dTMP,* deoxythymidine monophosphate; *dUMP,* deoxyuridine monophosphate; *FH2,* dihydrofolate; *FH4,* tetrahydrofolate. (*Redrawn from Adamson PC, Balis FM, Blaney SM: General principles of chemotherapy. In Pizzo PA, Poplack DG, editors: Principles and practice of pediatric oncology, ed 6, Philadelphia, 2011, Lippincott Williams & Wilkins, p. 283.*)

Table 494-3	Infectious Complications of Malignancy		
PREDISPOSING FACTOR	**ETIOLOGY**	**SITE OF INFECTION**	**INFECTIOUS AGENTS**
Neutropenia	Chemotherapy, bone marrow infiltration	Sepsis, shock, pneumonia, soft tissue, proctitis, mucositis	*Streptococcus viridans, Staphylococcus aureus, Staphylococcus epidermidis, Escherichia coli, Pseudomonas aeruginosa, Candida, Aspergillus,* anaerobic oral and rectal bacteria
Immunosuppression, lymphopenia, lymphocyte-monocyte dysfunction	Chemotherapy, corticosteroid	Pneumonia, meningitis, disseminated viral infection	*Pneumocystis jiroveci, Cryptococcus neoformans, Mycobacterium, Nocardia, Listeria monocytogenes, Candida, Aspergillus, Strongyloides, Toxoplasma,* varicella-zoster virus, cytomegalovirus, herpes simplex
Indwelling central venous catheter	Nutrition, administration of chemotherapy	Line sepsis, tract of tunnel, exit site	*S. epidermidis, S. aureus, Candida albicans, P. aeruginosa, Aspergillus, Corynebacterium, Streptococcus faecalis, Mycobacterium fortuitum, Propionibacterium acnes*

Modified from Kliegman RM, Marcdante KJ, Jenson HB, et al, editors: Nelson essentials of pediatrics, ed 6, Philadelphia, 2011, WB Saunders, Chapter 121.

Least susceptible to chemotherapy and radiation therapy are cells that do not replicate or that replicate slowly, such as neurons, muscle cells, connective tissue, and bone. However, children are not exempt from toxicities of these tissues, probably because they are still undergoing proliferation, albeit at a slower pace than other tissues, during growth and growth spurts.

Physically, children can endure the acute adverse effects of chemotherapy better than adults can in many ways. The maximum tolerated dosage in children, when expressed on the basis of body surface area or body weight, commonly is greater than that in adults. A comparison of anticancer drugs tested in phase I trials in both adult and pediatric patients showed that the maximum tolerated dosage in children was greater than that in adults for 70% of the agents, equal to that in adults for 15% of the agents, and less than the adult dose for

only 15% of the agents. For all the drugs that were compared, the mean pediatric maximum tolerated dosage was greater than the adult mean.

Tumor-directed therapies are evolving in the field of pediatric oncology. Tumor antigen–specific monoclonal antibodies have been incorporated into the standard therapy of neuroblastoma (anti–ganglioside GD$_2$). The antiangiogenic agent bevacizumab (monoclonal antibody against vascular endothelial growth factor A) shows promise in the treatment of CNS tumors, especially low-grade gliomas.

Surgery
Superb pediatric surgical and anesthesia services are indispensable for children with cancer. The pediatric surgeon's role varies, depending on the type of tumor. For solid tumors, complete resection with

documented evidence of negative margins often is required for cure or long-term control. Considerable prolongation of life nearly always depends on whether the tumor is resectable and on the actual extent of resection.

With the exception of brainstem tumors and retinoblastoma, all solid tumors in children require a tissue diagnosis; therefore, biopsy of the suspected neoplasm is paramount. Staging with sentinel node biopsies has become the standard of care for several pediatric malignancies. Surgical expertise is essential for implantation of vascular access devices and removal and replacement of such devices when infection or thrombosis supervenes (see Chapter 179).

Increasingly, minimally invasive endoscopic surgical techniques are being used when indicated and, if the patient's condition permits, for biopsy and resection of tumor, direct ascertainment of residual disease and assessment of response, lysis of adhesions, and splenectomy.

Radiation Therapy

Radiation therapy is used sparingly in children, who are more susceptible than are adults to the adverse delayed effects of ionizing radiation. A major advance in pediatric radiation therapy is the application of **conformal irradiation** to children with cancer. This technique, most commonly applied as **intensity-modulated radiation therapy,** spares normal tissue by conforming the radiation volume to the shape of the tumor, thereby enabling delivery of higher doses to the tumor with lower exposure of normal tissue adjacent to the tumor or in the path of the radiation beam. Another example is proton-beam radiotherapy, which has just begun to be more widely available for children with cancer. With more focused beams and better sedation and immobilization techniques, radiation therapy is becoming more commonly used in children. Acute adverse effects from radiation therapy are less severe than those from chemotherapy and depend on which part of the body is irradiated and the means of administration. Dermatitis is the most common general adverse effect, because skin is always in the treatment field. Nausea and diarrhea are common subacute adverse effects with abdominal radiation therapy. Mucositis nearly always occurs to some extent whenever oral or intestinal mucosa is in the treatment volume. Somnolence is common with cranial irradiation. Alopecia occurs where hair is in the radiation field.

Most radiation therapy schedules require treatment 5 days per week for 4-7 wk, depending on the dose needed to control the tumor and on the amount and nature of normal tissue in the field. Most adverse effects are not noted until the second half of the course of irradiation. Late effects can occur months to years after radiation therapy and usually are dose-limiting manifestations. The type of delayed toxicity also depends on the site of irradiation. Examples are impaired growth resulting from cranial or vertebral irradiation, endocrine dysfunction from midbrain irradiation, pulmonary or cardiac insufficiency from chest irradiation, strictures and adhesions from abdominal irradiation, and infertility from pelvic irradiation. Second malignancy can also develop in the radiation field, for example, breast cancer from chest irradiation and brain tumors from CNS irradiation.

ACUTE TOXIC EFFECTS AND SUPPORTIVE CARE

Adverse treatment effects that occur early in therapy can result in oncologic emergencies. These include metabolic disorders, bone marrow suppression, and compression by tumors on vital structures (Table 494-4). In tumor lysis syndrome (TLS), uric acid, phosphates, and potassium are released in the circulation in large quantities from death of tumor cells. Hyperuricemia can lead to impairment of renal function, which further exacerbates the metabolic abnormalities. TLS can occur before therapy in patients with a large tumor burden (e.g., Burkitt lymphoma, lymphoblastic lymphoma, and high white blood cell count leukemia), but it is usually seen within 12-48 hr of initiating chemotherapy. TLS is infrequently reported in other tumors (Hodgkin lymphoma, neuroblastoma, hepatoblastoma). Before therapy is initiated, the serum levels of uric acid, electrolytes, calcium, phosphorus, and creatinine should be measured and adequate hydration ensured. Allopurinol (a xanthine oxidase inhibitor) should be started to prevent

further accumulation of uric acid. In patients with established TLS with high uric acid levels or those at high risk for TLS, rasburicase (an enzyme that degrades uric acid) should be given instead of allopurinol. Symptomatic hyperkalemia and hyperphosphatemia with subsequent hypocalcemia can develop in the setting of inadequate renal function.

Virtually all chemotherapy regimens can produce **myelosuppression,** as can malignancies that invade and replace bone marrow. Anemia can be corrected by transfusions of packed erythrocytes, and thrombocytopenia can be corrected by platelet infusions. Patients receiving immunosuppressive therapy should receive irradiated blood products to prevent graft-versus-host disease and leukoreduced blood products to prevent transfusion-associated reactions and infections. Neutropenia (neutrophil counts <500/μL) poses a risk of life-threatening infection. Febrile neutropenic patients should be hospitalized and treated with empiric broad-spectrum intravenous antimicrobial therapy pending the results of appropriate cultures of blood, urine, or any obvious sites of infection (see Chapter 178). Treatment is continued until fever resolves and the neutrophil count rises. If fever persists for more than 3-5 days while the patient is receiving broad-spectrum antibiotics, the possibility of fungal infection must be considered. Fungal infections caused by *Candida* and *Aspergillus* are common in immunosuppressed patients. Opportunistic organisms such as *Pneumocystis jiroveci* can produce fatal pneumonia. Prophylactic treatment with trimethoprim-sulfamethoxazole is given when severe or prolonged immunosuppression is anticipated.

Viruses of low pathogenicity can produce serious disease in the setting of immunosuppression caused by malignancy or its treatment. Patients should not be given live virus vaccines. Children who are receiving chemotherapy and who are exposed to chickenpox should receive varicella-zoster immunoglobulin, or, if varicella-zoster immunoglobulin is not available, oral acyclovir should be considered. If clinical disease develops, the child should be hospitalized and treated with intravenous acyclovir.

Adequate **pain management** is critical. The World Health Organization (WHO) guidelines are particularly useful in the management of pain associated with cancer and cancer therapy (see Chapter 62).

Depending on the type of cancer therapy, patients can lose more than 10% of body weight. Patients sometimes reduce their food intake because of temporary, treatment-associated nausea, stomatitis, and vomiting. Appetite loss is not a cause for alarm. Malnutrition is a particular risk in patients receiving radiation therapy involving the abdomen or the head and neck, intensive chemotherapy, or total-body irradiation and high-dose chemotherapy before marrow transplantation. If oral supplementation proves inadequate, such patients can require enteral tube feedings or parenteral hyperalimentation.

LATE ADVERSE EFFECTS

Injury to tissues with low repair potential often results in long-lasting or permanent deficit. These effects can be either from the tumor or its treatment. For example, a brain or spinal tumor can leave the child with a permanent paresis or autonomic dysfunction, anthracycline-induced cardiomyopathy usually produces refractory cardiac dysfunction, and the leukoencephalopathy caused by intrathecal methotrexate and by CNS radiation therapy often is only partially reversible. The potential types of late adverse effects depend on the child's age at the time of treatment, the location(s) of the cancer, and the therapy administered. A good resource for the pediatrician, patient, and family who have to anticipate the possibilities is available at http://www.survivorshipguidelines.org.

Late adverse effects of therapy can cause substantial morbidity (Table 494-5). Successful surgical resection can result in loss of important functional structures. Irradiation can produce irreversible organ damage, with symptoms and functional limitations depending on the organ involved and the severity of the damage. Many problems related to radiation therapy do not become obvious until the patient is fully grown, such as asymmetry between irradiated and nonirradiated areas or extremities. Irradiation of fields that include endocrine organs can cause hypothyroidism, pituitary dysfunction, or infertility. In sufficient

Table 494-4	Oncologic Emergencies			
CONDITION	**MANIFESTATIONS**	**ETIOLOGY**	**MALIGNANCY**	**TREATMENT**
METABOLIC				
Hyperuricemia	Uric acid nephropathy	Tumor lysis syndrome	Lymphoma, leukemia	Allopurinol, alkalinize urine; hydration and diuresis, rasburicase
Hyperkalemia	Arrhythmias, cardiac arrest	Tumor lysis syndrome	Lymphoma, leukemia	Kayexalate, sodium bicarbonate, glucose, and insulin; check for pseudohyperkalemia from leukemic cell lysis in test tube
Hyperphosphatemia	Hypocalcemic tetany; metastatic calcification, photophobia, pruritus	Tumor lysis syndrome	Lymphoma, leukemia	Hydration, forced diuresis; stop alkalinization; oral aluminum hydroxide to bind phosphate
Hyponatremia	Seizure, lethargy (may also be asymptomatic)	SIADH; fluid, sodium losses in vomiting	Leukemia, CNS tumor	Restrict free water for SIADH; replace sodium if depleted
Hypercalcemia	Anorexia, nausea, polyuria, pancreatitis, gastric ulcers; prolonged PR, shortened QT interval	Bone resorption; ectopic parathormone, vitamin D, or prostaglandins	Metastasis to bone, rhabdomyosarcoma, leukemia	Hydration and furosemide diuresis; corticosteroids; calcitonin, bisphosphonates
HEMATOLOGIC				
Anemia	Pallor, weakness, heart failure	Bone marrow suppression or infiltration; blood loss	Any with chemotherapy	Packed red blood cell transfusion
Thrombocytopenia	Petechiae, hemorrhage	Bone marrow suppression or infiltration	Any with chemotherapy	Platelet transfusion
Disseminated intravascular coagulation	Shock, hemorrhage	Sepsis, hypotension, tumor factors	Promyelocytic leukemia, others	Fresh-frozen plasma; platelets, cryoprecipitate, treat underlying disorder
Neutropenia	Infection	Bone marrow suppression or infiltration	Any with chemotherapy	If febrile, administer broad-spectrum antibiotics, and filgrastim (G-CSF) if appropriate
Hyperleukocytosis (>100,000/mm³)	Hemorrhage, thrombosis; pulmonary infiltrates, hypoxia; tumor lysis syndrome	Leukostasis; vascular occlusion	Leukemia	Leukapheresis; chemotherapy; hydroxyurea
Graft-versus-host disease	Dermatitis, diarrhea, hepatitis	Immunosuppression and nonirradiated blood products; bone marrow transplantation	Any with immunosuppression	Corticosteroids; cyclosporine; tacrolimus; antithymocyte globulin
SPACE-OCCUPYING LESIONS				
Spinal cord compression	Back pain ± radicular *Cord above T10:* symmetric weakness, increased deep tendon reflex; sensory level present; toes up *Conus medullaris (T10-L2):* symmetric weakness, increased knee reflexes; decreased ankle reflexes; saddle sensory loss; toes up or down *Cauda equina (below L2):* asymmetric weakness; loss of deep tendon reflex and sensory deficit; toes down	Metastasis to vertebra and extramedullary space	Neuroblastoma; medulloblastoma	MRI or myelography for diagnosis; corticosteroids; radiotherapy; laminectomy; chemotherapy
Increased intracranial pressure	Confusion, coma, emesis, headache, hypertension, bradycardia, seizures, papilledema, hydrocephalus; cranial nerves III and VI palsies	Primary or metastatic brain tumor	Neuroblastoma, astrocytoma; glioma	CT or MRI for diagnosis; corticosteroids; phenytoin; ventriculostomy tube; radiotherapy; chemotherapy
Superior vena cava syndrome	Distended neck veins plethora, edema of head and neck, cyanosis, proptosis, Horner syndrome	Superior mediastinal mass	Lymphoma	Chemotherapy; radiotherapy
Tracheal compression	Respiratory distress	Mediastinal mass compressing trachea	Lymphoma	Radiation, corticosteroids

CNS, Central nervous system; G-CSF, granulocyte colony-stimulating factor; SIADH, syndrome of inappropriate antidiuretic hormone secretion.
Modified from Kliegman RM, Marcdante KJ, Jenson HB, et al, editors: Nelson essentials of pediatrics, ed 6, Philadelphia, 2011, WB Saunders, p. 590.

| Table 494-5 | Late Effects and High-Risk Features of Childhood Cancer and Its Treatment |

LATE EFFECTS	EXPOSURE	SELECTED HIGH-RISK FACTORS	AT-RISK DIAGNOSTIC GROUPS
NEUROCOGNITIVE			
Neurocognitive deficits	Chemotherapy:	Age <3 yr at time of treatment	Acute lymphoblastic
Functional deficits in:	• Methotrexate	Female sex	leukemia
• Executive function	Radiation affecting brain:	Supratentorial tumor	Brain tumor
• Sustained attention	• Cranial	Premorbid or family history of	Sarcoma (head and neck or
• Memory	• Ear/infratemporal	learning or attention problems	osteosarcoma)
• Processing speed	• Total-body irradiation (TBI)	Radiation doses >24 Gy	
• Visual-motor integration		Whole-brain irradiation	
Learning deficits			
Diminished IQ			
Behavioral change			
NEUROSENSORY			
Hearing loss, sensorineural	Chemotherapy:	Higher cisplatin dose (360 mg/m^2)	Brain tumor
	• Cisplatin	Higher radiation dose impacting ear	Germ cell tumor
	• Carboplatin	(>30 Gy)	Sarcoma (head and neck)
	Radiation affecting hearing:	Concurrent radiation and cisplatin	Neuroblastoma
	• Cranial		Hepatoblastoma
	• Infratemporal		
	• Nasopharyngeal		
Hearing loss, conductive	Radiation affecting hearing:	Higher radiation dose affecting ear	Brain tumor
Tympanosclerosis	• Cranial	(>30 Gy)	Sarcoma (head and neck)
Otosclerosis	• Infratemporal		
Eustachian tube dysfunction	• Nasopharyngeal		
Visual impairment	Chemotherapy:	Higher radiation dose impacting eye	Brain tumor
Cataracts	• Busulfan	(≥15 Gy for cataracts; >45 Gy for	Acute lymphoblastic
Lacrimal duct atrophy	• Glucocorticoids	retinopathy and visual impairment)	leukemia
Xerophthalmia	Radiation affecting eye:		Retinoblastoma
Retinopathy	• Cranial		Rhabdomyosarcoma (orbital)
Glaucoma	• Orbital/eye		Allogeneic HSCT
	• TBI		
Peripheral neuropathy,	Chemotherapy:	Higher cisplatin dose (≥300 mg/m^2)	Acute lymphoblastic
sensory	• Vincristine		leukemia
	• Vinblastine		Brain tumor
	• Cisplatin		Hodgkin lymphoma
	• Carboplatin		Germ cell tumor
			Non-Hodgkin lymphoma
			Sarcoma
			Neuroblastoma
			Wilms tumor
			Carcinoma
NEUROMOTOR			
Peripheral neuropathy,	Chemotherapy:		Acute lymphoblastic
motor	• Vincristine		leukemia
	• Vinblastine		Hodgkin lymphoma
			Non-Hodgkin lymphoma
			Sarcoma
			Brain tumor
			Neuroblastoma
			Wilms tumor
ENDOCRINE			
GH deficiency	Radiation affecting HPA:	Female sex	Acute lymphoblastic
Precocious puberty	• Cranial	Radiation dose to HPA >18 Gy	leukemia
	• Orbital/eye		Sarcoma (facial)
			Carcinoma (nasopharyngeal)
Obesity	Ear/infratemporal	Female sex	Acute lymphoblastic
	Nasopharyngeal	Younger age (<4 yr)	leukemia
Hypothyroidism, central	TBI	Radiation dose to HPA >18 Gy	Brain tumor
Gonadotropin deficiency			Sarcoma (facial)
Adrenal insufficiency, central			Carcinoma (nasopharyngeal)
Hypothyroidism, primary	Neck, mantle irradiation	Radiation dose to thyroid >20 Gy	Hodgkin lymphoma

| Table 494-5 | Late Effects and High-Risk Features of Childhood Cancer and Its Treatment—cont'd |

LATE EFFECTS	EXPOSURE	SELECTED HIGH-RISK FACTORS	AT-RISK DIAGNOSTIC GROUPS
REPRODUCTIVE			
Gonadal dysfunction Delayed or arrested puberty Premature menopause Germ cell dysfunction or failure Infertility	Chemotherapy, alkylating: • Busulfan • Carmustine (BCNU) • Chlorambucil • Cyclophosphamide • Ifosfamide • Lomustine (CCNU) • Mechlorethamine • Melphalan • Procarbazine Radiation affecting reproductive system: • Whole abdomen (girls) • Pelvic • Lumbar/sacral spine (girls) • Testicular (boys) • TBI	Higher alkylating agent dose Alkylating agent conditioning for HSCT Radiation dose ≥15 Gy in prepubertal girls Radiation dose ≥10 Gy in pubertal girls For germ cell failure in boys, any pelvic irradiation For androgen insufficiency, gonadal irradiation, ≥20-30 Gy in boys	Acute lymphoblastic leukemia, high risk Brain tumor Hodgkin lymphoma, advanced or unfavorable Non-Hodgkin lymphoma, advanced or unfavorable Sarcoma Neuroblastoma Wilms tumor, advanced Autologous or allogeneic HSCT
CARDIAC			
Cardiomyopathy Arrhythmias	Chemotherapy: • Daunorubicin • Doxorubicin • Idarubicin	Female sex Age <5 yr at time of treatment Higher doses of chemotherapy (≥300 mg/m²) Higher doses of cardiac radiation (≥30 Gy) Combined-modality therapy with cardiotoxic chemotherapy and irradiation	Hodgkin lymphoma Leukemia Non-Hodgkin lymphoma Sarcoma Wilms tumor Neuroblastoma
Cardiomyopathy Arrhythmias Pericardial fibrosis Valvular disease Myocardial infarction Atherosclerotic heart disease	Radiation affecting heart: • Chest • Mantle • Mediastinum • Axilla • Spine • Upper abdomen		
PULMONARY			
Pulmonary fibrosis Interstitial pneumonitis Restrictive lung disease Obstructive lung disease	Chemotherapy: • Bleomycin • Busulfan • Carmustine (BCNU) • Lomustine (CCNU) Radiation impacting lungs: • Mantle • Mediastinum • Whole lung • TBI	Higher doses of chemotherapy Combined modality therapy with pulmonary toxic chemotherapy and irradiation	Brain tumor Germ cell tumor Hodgkin lymphoma Sarcoma (chest wall or intrathoracic) Autologous or allogeneic HCST
GASTROINTESTINAL			
Chronic enterocolitis Strictures Bowel obstruction	Radiation affecting gastrointestinal tract (≥30 Gy) Abdominal surgery	Higher radiation dose to bowel (≥45 Gy) Combined modality therapy with abdominal irradiation and radiomimetic chemotherapy (dactinomycin or anthracyclines) Combined modality therapy with abdominal surgery and irradiation	Sarcoma (retroperitoneal or pelvic primary)
HEPATIC			
Hepatic fibrosis Cirrhosis	Radiation affecting liver	Higher radiation dose or treatment volume (20-30 Gy to entire liver or ≥40 Gy to at least one third of liver)	Sarcoma Neuroblastoma
RENAL			
Renal insufficiency Hypertension Glomerular injury Tubular injury	Chemotherapy: • Ifosfamide • Cisplatin • Carboplatin Radiation affecting kidneys: • Whole abdomen • Upper abdominal fields • TBI		

GH, Growth hormone; HPA, hypothalamic–pituitary–adrenal axis; HSCT, hematopoietic stem cell transplantation; TBI, total-body irradiation.
From Kurt BA, Arnstrong GT, Cash DK, et al: Primary care management of the childhood cancer survivor, J Pediatr 152:458–466, 2008.

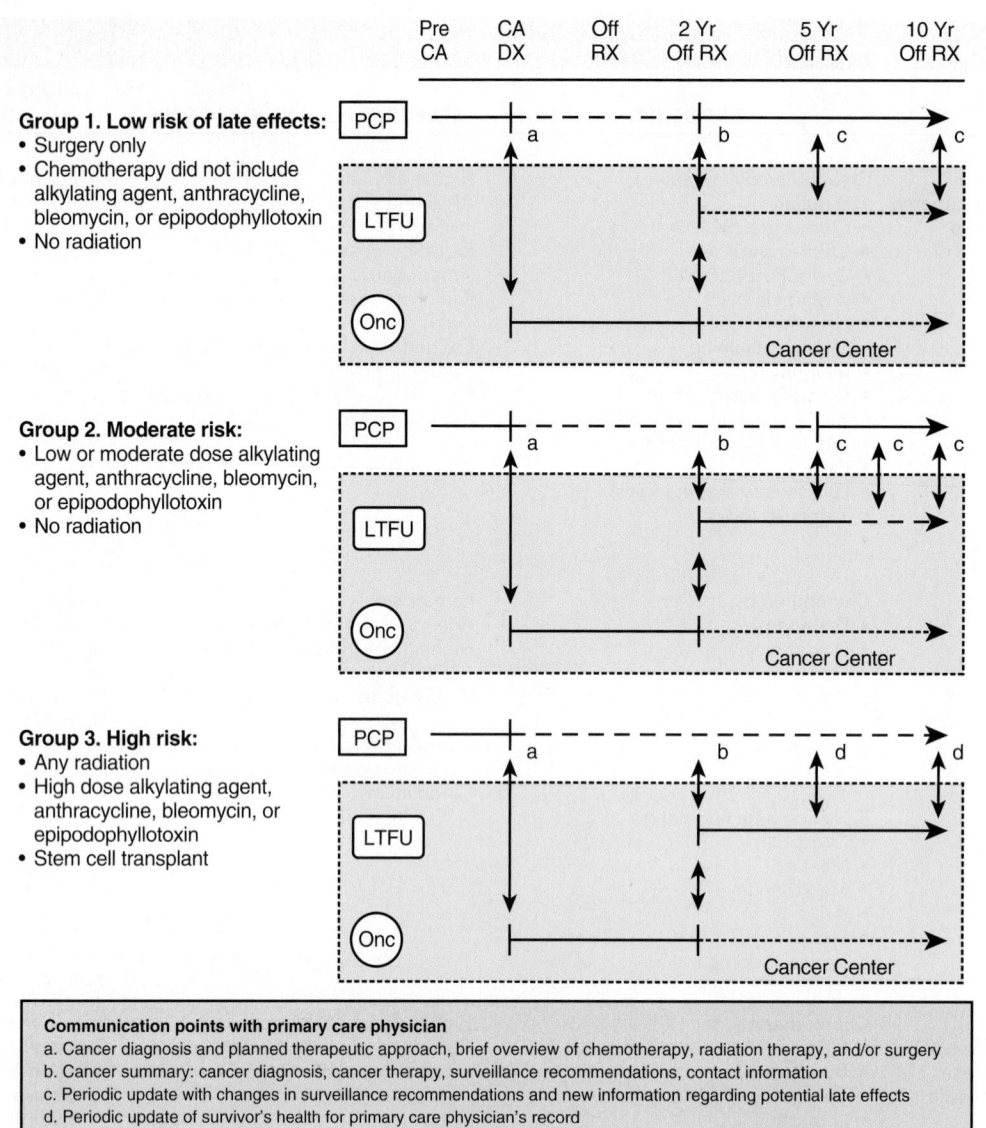

Figure 494-6 Proposed risk-stratified shared care model for childhood cancer survivors. *Solid line* denotes primary responsibility for risk-based care; risk stratification based upon determination of the long-term follow-up staff. *CA*, Cancer; *DX*, diagnosis; *Onc*, oncologist; *PCP*, primary care provider; *RX*, therapy. (*Adapted from Oeffinger KC, McCabe MS. Models for delivering survivorship care, J Clin Oncol 24(32):5119, 2006; with permission from the American Society of Clinical Oncology. From Oeffinger KC, Nathan PC, Kremer LCM: Challenges after curative treatment for childhood cancer and long-term follow up of survivors, Pediatr Clin North Am 55:251–273, 2008.)*

doses, cranial irradiation can produce neurologic dysfunction and spinal irradiation can produce growth retardation.

Chemotherapy also carries the risk of long-lasting organ damage. Of particular concern are leukoencephalopathy after high-dose methotrexate therapy; infertility in male patients treated with alkylating agents (e.g., cyclophosphamide); myocardial damage caused by anthracyclines; pulmonary fibrosis caused by bleomycin; renal dysfunction caused by ifosfamide, nitrosourea, or platinum agents; and hearing loss from cisplatin. Development of these sequelae may be dose-related and usually is irreversible. Appropriate baseline and intermittent testing should be performed before these drugs are administered to ensure that there is no preexisting damage to the organs likely to be affected and to permit monitoring of the adverse effects of treatment-induced changes.

Perhaps the most serious late adverse effect is the occurrence of **second cancers** in patients successfully cured of a first malignancy. The risk appears to be cumulative, increasing by approximately 0.5% per year, resulting in approximately a 12% incidence at 25 yr after treatment. Patients who have been treated for childhood cancer should be examined annually, with particular attention to possible late adverse effects of therapy, including second malignancies (Fig. 494-6).

PALLIATIVE CARE

At all stages of caring for children with cancer, principles of palliative care should be applied to relieve pain and suffering and to provide comfort (see Chapter 43). Pain is a serious cause of suffering among patients with cancer. It may be the result of organ obstruction or compression or bone metastasis, or it may be neuropathic. Pain should be managed in a stepwise manner, as recommended by the WHO, in accordance with the principles of selecting the appropriate analgesic, prescribing the appropriate dosage, administering the drug by the appropriate route, and choosing an appropriate dosing schedule to prevent persistent pain and to relieve breakthrough pain (see Chapter 62). In addition, the dosage should be titrated aggressively while attempts are made to prevent, anticipate, and manage side effects. Adjuvant drugs and sequential trials of analgesic drugs should be considered.

The goals in the care of dying patients are to avoid distress for the patient, family, and caregivers; to provide care consistent with the patient's and family's wishes; and to comply with and advocate for clinical, cultural, and ethical standards.

Bibliography is available at Expert Consult.

Chapter **495**
The Leukemias

David G. Tubergen, Archie Bleyer,
A. Kim Ritchey, and Erika Friehling

The leukemias are the most common malignant neoplasms in childhood, accounting for approximately 31% of all malignancies that occur in children younger than 15 yr of age. Each year leukemia is diagnosed in approximately 3,250 children younger than 15 yr of age in the United States, an annual incidence of 4.5 cases per 100,000 children. Acute lymphoblastic leukemia (ALL) accounts for approximately 77% of cases of childhood leukemia, acute myelogenous leukemia (AML) for approximately 11%, chronic myelogenous leukemia (CML) for 2-3%, and juvenile myelomonocytic leukemia (JMML) for 1-2%. The remaining cases consist of a variety of acute and chronic leukemias that do not fit classic definitions for ALL, AML, CML, or JMML.

The leukemias may be defined as a group of malignant diseases in which genetic abnormalities in a hematopoietic cell give rise to an unregulated clonal proliferation of cells. The progeny of these cells have a growth advantage over normal cellular elements, because of their increased rate of proliferation and a decreased rate of spontaneous apoptosis. The result is a disruption of normal marrow function and, ultimately, marrow failure. The clinical features, laboratory findings, and responses to therapy vary depending on the type of leukemia.

495.1 Acute Lymphoblastic Leukemia

Erika Friehling, A. Kim Ritchey, David G. Tubergen, and Archie Bleyer

Childhood ALL was the first disseminated cancer shown to be curable. It actually is a heterogeneous group of malignancies with a number of distinctive genetic abnormalities that result in varying clinical behaviors and responses to therapy.

EPIDEMIOLOGY

ALL is diagnosed in approximately 2,400 children younger than 15 yr of age in the United States each year. ALL has a striking peak incidence at 2-3 yr of age and occurs more in boys than in girls at all ages. This peak age incidence was apparent decades ago in white populations in advanced socioeconomic countries, but it has since been confirmed in the black population of the United States as well. The disease is more common in children with certain chromosomal abnormalities, such as Down syndrome, Bloom syndrome, ataxia-telangiectasia, and Fanconi anemia. Among identical twins, the risk to the second twin if 1 twin develops leukemia is greater than that in the general population. The risk is >70% if ALL is diagnosed in the first twin during the 1st yr of life and the twins shared the same (monochorionic) placenta. If the first twin develops ALL by 5-7 yr of age, the risk to the second twin is at least twice that of the general population, regardless of zygosity.

ETIOLOGY

In virtually all cases, the etiology of ALL is unknown, although several genetic and environmental factors are associated with childhood leukemia (Table 495-1). Most cases of ALL are thought to be caused by postconception somatic mutations in lymphoid cells. However, the identification of the leukemia-specific fusion-gene sequences in archived neonatal blood spots of some children who develop ALL at a later date indicates the importance of in utero events in the initiation of the malignant process in some cases. The long lag period before the onset of the disease in some children, reported to be as long as 14 yr, supports the concept that additional genetic modifications are required for disease expression. Moreover, those same mutations have been

Table 495-1	Factors Predisposing to Childhood Leukemia

GENETIC CONDITIONS
Down syndrome
Fanconi anemia
Bloom syndrome
Diamond-Blackfan anemia
Shwachman-Diamond syndrome
Kostmann syndrome
Neurofibromatosis type 1
Ataxia-telangiectasia
Severe combined immune deficiency
Paroxysmal nocturnal hemoglobinuria
Li-Fraumeni syndrome

ENVIRONMENTAL FACTORS
Ionizing radiation
Drugs
Alkylating agents
Epipodophyllotoxin
Benzene exposure

found in neonatal blood spots of children who never go on to develop leukemia.

Exposure to medical diagnostic radiation both in utero and in childhood is associated with an increased incidence of ALL. In addition, published descriptions and investigations of geographic clusters of cases have raised concern that environmental factors can increase the incidence of ALL. Thus far, no such factors other than radiation have been identified in the United States. In certain developing countries, there is an association between B-cell ALL (B-ALL) and Epstein-Barr viral infections.

CELLULAR CLASSIFICATION

The classification of ALL depends on characterizing the malignant cells in the bone marrow to determine the morphology, phenotype as measured by cell membrane markers, and cytogenetic and molecular genetic features. **Morphology** is usually adequate alone to establish a diagnosis, but the other studies are essential for disease classification, which can have a major influence on the prognosis and the choice of appropriate therapy. The current system used is the World Health Organization (WHO) classification of leukemias. Phenotypically, surface markers show that approximately 85% of cases of ALL are classified as B lymphoblastic leukemia (previously termed precursor B-ALL or pre–B-ALL), approximately 15% are T-lymphoblastic leukemia, and approximately 1% are derived from mature B cells. The rare leukemia of mature B cells is termed *Burkitt leukemia* and is one of the most rapidly growing cancers in humans, requiring a different therapeutic approach than other subtypes of ALL. A small percentage of children with leukemia have a disease characterized by surface markers of both lymphoid and myeloid derivation.

Chromosomal abnormalities are used to subclassify ALL into prognostic groups (Table 495-2). Many genetic alterations, including inactivation of tumor-suppressor genes and mutations that activate the *NOTCH1* or *RAS* pathways, have been discovered and might one day be incorporated into clinical practice (Fig. 495-1).

The polymerase chain reaction and fluorescence in situ hybridization techniques offer the ability to pinpoint molecular genetic abnormalities and can be used to detect small numbers of malignant cells at diagnosis as well as during follow-up (**minimal residual disease [MRD]**, see below) and are of proven clinical utility. The development of DNA microanalysis makes it possible to analyze the expression of thousands of genes in the leukemic cell. This technique promises to further enhance the understanding of the fundamental biology and to provide clues to the therapeutic approach of ALL.

CLINICAL MANIFESTATIONS

The initial presentation of ALL usually is nonspecific and relatively brief. Anorexia, fatigue, malaise, and irritability often are present, as is

Table 495-2	Common Chromosomal Abnormalities in Acute Lymphoblastic Leukemia of Childhood			
SUBTYPE	**CHROMOSOMAL ABNORMALITY**	**GENETIC ALTERATION**	**PROGNOSIS**	**INCIDENCE**
B-ALL	Trisomies 4, 10, and 17	—	Favorable	25%
B-ALL	t(12;21)	ETV6-RUNX1	Favorable	20-25%
B-ALL	t(1;19)	E2A-PBX	None	5-6%
B-ALL	t(4;11)	MLL-AF4	Unfavorable	2%
B-ALL	t(9;22)	BCR-ABL	Unfavorable	3%
Mature B-cell leukemia (Burkitt)	t(8;14)	IGH-MYC	None	1-2%
B-ALL	Hyperdiploidy	—	Favorable	20-25%
B-ALL	Hypodiploidy	—	Unfavorable	1%
T-ALL	t(10;14)	TLX1/HOX11	Favorable	5-10%
Infant	11q23	MLL rearrangements	Unfavorable	2-10%

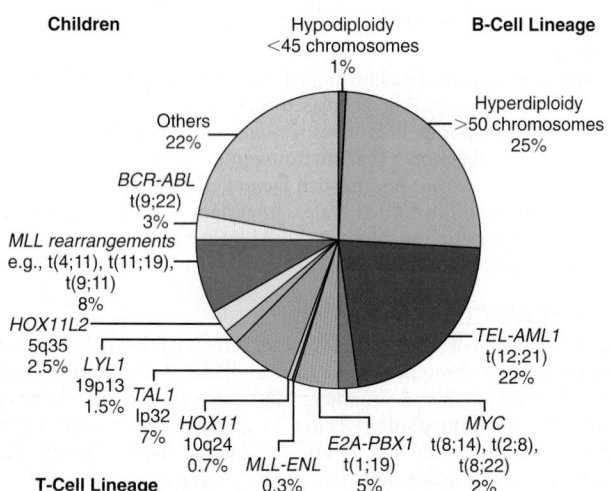

Figure 495-1 Estimated frequency of specific genotypes in childhood ALL. The genetic lesions that are exclusively seen in cases of T-cell ALL are indicated in *gold* and those commonly associated with B-cell ALL in *blue*. The *darker gold* or *blue* color indicates those subtypes generally associated with poor prognosis. (*From Pui CH, Mulligan CG, Evans WE: Pediatric acute lymphoblastic leukemia: where are we going and how do we get there? Blood 120:1165–1174, 2012.*)

an intermittent, low-grade fever. Bone or joint pain, particularly in the lower extremities, may be present. Less commonly, symptoms may be of several months' duration, may be localized predominantly to the bones or joints, and can include joint swelling. Bone pain is severe and can wake the patient at night. As the disease progresses, signs and symptoms of bone marrow failure become more obvious with the occurrence of pallor, fatigue, exercise intolerance, bruising, or epistaxis, as well as fever, which may be caused by infection or the disease. Organ infiltration can cause lymphadenopathy, hepatosplenomegaly, testicular enlargement, or central nervous system (CNS) involvement (cranial neuropathies, headache, seizures). Respiratory distress may be due to severe anemia or mediastinal node compression of the airways.

On **physical examination,** findings of pallor, listlessness, purpuric and petechial skin lesions, or mucous membrane hemorrhage can reflect bone marrow failure (see Chapter 493). The proliferative nature of the disease may be manifested as lymphadenopathy, splenomegaly, or, less commonly, hepatomegaly. In patients with bone or joint pain, there may be exquisite tenderness over the bone or objective evidence

of joint swelling and effusion. Nonetheless, with marrow involvement, deep bone pain may be present but tenderness will not be elicited. Rarely, patients show signs of increased intracranial pressure that indicate leukemic involvement of the CNS. These include papilledema (see Fig. 493-3), retinal hemorrhages, and cranial nerve palsies. Respiratory distress usually is related to anemia but can occur in patients with an obstructive airway problem (wheezing) as the result of a large anterior mediastinal mass (e.g., in the thymus or nodes). This problem is most typically seen in adolescent boys with T-cell ALL (T-ALL). T-ALL also usually has a higher leukocyte count.

B-lymphoblastic leukemia is the most common immunophenotype, with onset at 1-10 yr of age. The median leukocyte count at presentation is 33,000/μL, although 75% of patients have counts <20,000/μL; thrombocytopenia is seen in 75% of patients, and hepatosplenomegaly is seen in 30-40% of patients. In all types of leukemia, CNS symptoms are seen at presentation in 5% of patients (5-10% have blasts in the cerebrospinal fluid [CSF]). Testicular involvement is rarely evident at diagnosis, but prior studies indicate occult involvement in 25% of boys. There is no indication for testicular biopsy.

DIAGNOSIS

The diagnosis of ALL is strongly suggested by peripheral blood findings that indicate bone marrow failure. Anemia and thrombocytopenia are seen in most patients. Leukemic cells might not be reported in the peripheral blood in routine laboratory examinations. Many patients with ALL present with total leukocyte counts of <10,000/μL. In such cases, the leukemic cells often are reported initially to be atypical lymphocytes, and it is only on further evaluation that the cells are found to be part of a malignant clone. When the results of an analysis of peripheral blood suggest the possibility of leukemia, the bone marrow should be examined promptly to establish the diagnosis. It is important that all studies necessary to confirm a diagnosis and adequately classify the type of leukemia be performed, including bone marrow aspiration and biopsy, flow cytometry, cytogenetics, and molecular studies.

ALL is diagnosed by a bone marrow evaluation that demonstrates >25% of the bone marrow cells as a homogeneous population of lymphoblasts. Initial evaluation also includes CSF examination. If lymphoblasts are found and the CSF leukocyte count is elevated, overt CNS or meningeal leukemia is present. This finding reflects a worse stage and indicates the need for additional CNS and systemic therapies. The staging lumbar puncture may be performed in conjunction with the first dose of intrathecal chemotherapy, if the diagnosis of leukemia was previously established from bone marrow evaluation. An experienced proceduralist should perform the initial lumbar puncture, because a traumatic lumbar puncture is associated with an increased risk of CNS relapse.

DIFFERENTIAL DIAGNOSIS

The diagnosis of leukemia is readily made in the patient with typical signs and symptoms, anemia, thrombocytopenia, and elevated white blood count with blasts present on smear. Elevation of the lactate dehydrogenase is often a clue to the diagnosis of ALL. When only pancytopenia is present, aplastic anemia (congenital or acquired) and myelofibrosis should be considered. Failure of a single cell line, as seen in transient erythroblastopenia of childhood, immune thrombocytopenia, and congenital or acquired neutropenia, is rarely the presenting feature of ALL. A high index of suspicion is required to differentiate ALL from infectious mononucleosis in patients with acute onset of fever and lymphadenopathy and from juvenile idiopathic arthritis in patients with fever, bone pain but often no tenderness, and joint swelling. These presentations also can require bone marrow examination.

ALL must be differentiated from AML and other malignant diseases that invade the bone marrow and can have clinical and laboratory findings similar to ALL, including neuroblastoma, rhabdomyosarcoma, Ewing sarcoma, and retinoblastoma.

TREATMENT

The single most important prognostic factor in ALL is the treatment: without effective therapy, the disease is fatal. Considerable progress has been made in event-free survival for children with ALL since the 1970s through use of multiagent chemotherapeutic regimens, intensification of therapy, and selection of treatment based upon relapse risk (Fig. 495-2). Survival is also related to age (Fig. 495-3) and subtype (Fig. 495-4).

Risk-directed therapy has become the standard of current ALL treatment and takes into account age at diagnosis, initial white blood cell count, immunophenotypic and cytogenetic characteristics of blast populations, rapidity of early treatment response (i.e., how quickly the leukemic cells can be cleared from the marrow or peripheral blood),

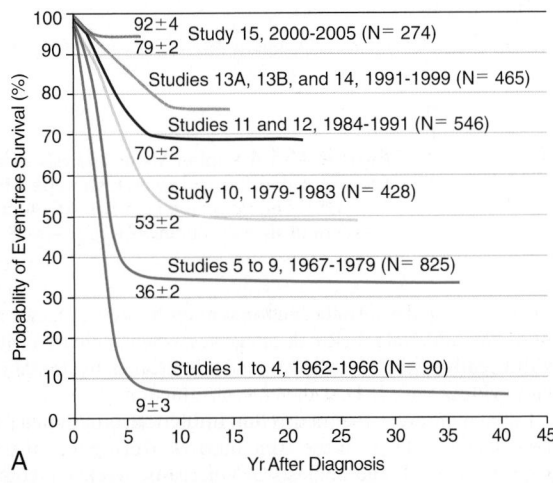
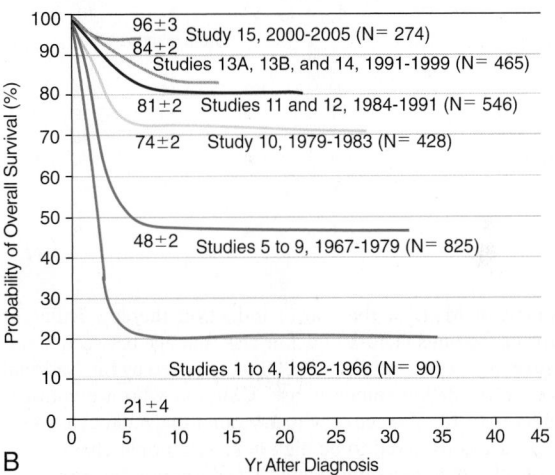

Figure 495-2 Kaplan-Meier analyses of event-free survival **(A)** and overall survival **(B)** in 2,628 children with newly diagnosed ALL. The patients participated in 15 consecutive studies conducted at St. Jude Children's Research Hospital from 1962-2005. The 5 yr event-free and overall survival estimates (±SE) are shown, except for Study 15, for which preliminary results at 4 yr are provided. The results demonstrate steady improvement in clinical outcome over the past 4 decades. The difference in event-free and overall survival rates has narrowed in the more recent periods, suggesting that relapses or second cancers that occur after contemporary therapy are more refractory to treatment. *(From Pui CH, Evans WE: Treatment of acute lymphoblastic leukemia,* N Engl J Med *354:166–178, 2006.)*

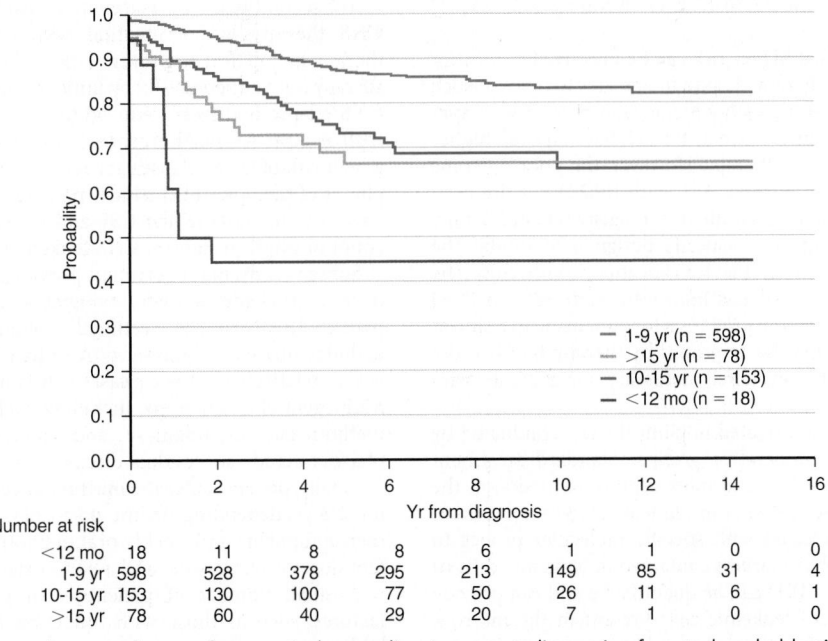

Figure 495-3 Kaplan-Meier estimates of event-free survival according to age at diagnosis of acute lymphoblastic leukemia. *(From Pui CH, Robinson LL, Look AT: Acute lymphoblastic leukaemia,* Lancet *371:1030–1042, 2008.)*

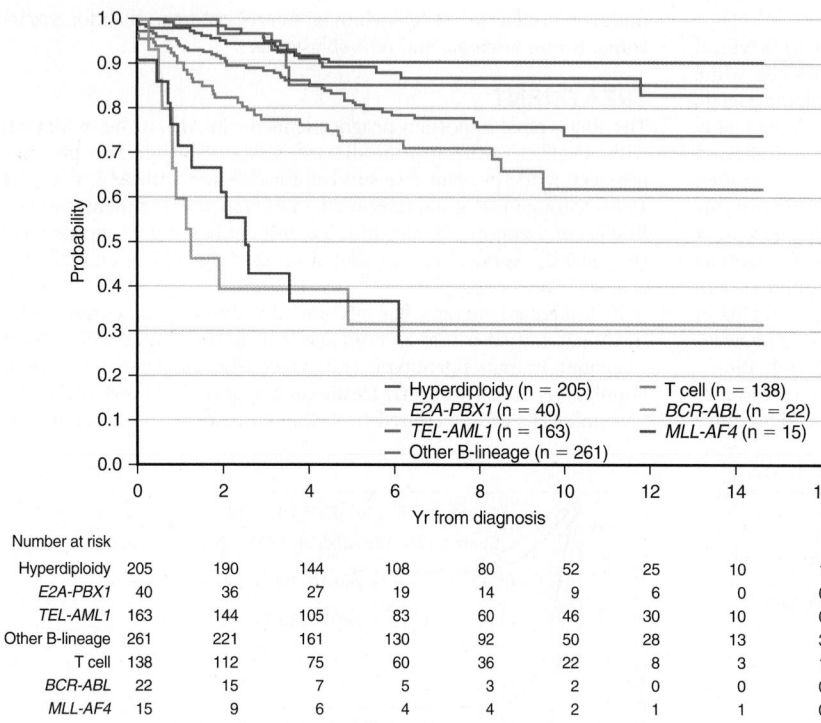

Number at risk

Hyperdiploidy	205	190	144	108	80	52	25	10	1
E2A-PBX1	40	36	27	19	14	9	6	0	0
TEL-AML1	163	144	105	83	60	46	30	10	0
Other B-lineage	261	221	161	130	92	50	28	13	3
T cell	138	112	75	60	36	22	8	3	1
BCR-ABL	22	15	7	5	3	2	0	0	0
MLL-AF4	15	9	6	4	4	2	1	1	0

Figure 495-4 Kaplan-Meier analysis of event-free survival according to biologic subtype of leukemia. *(From Pui CH, Robinson LL, Look AT: Acute lymphoblastic leukaemia, Lancet 371:1030–1042, 2008.)*

and assessment of MRD at the end of induction therapy. Different study groups use various factors to define risk, but age between 1 and 10 yr old and a leukocyte count of <50,000/μL are used by the National Cancer Institute to define standard risk. Children who are younger than 1 or older than 10 yr of age or who have an initial leukocyte count of >50,000/μL are considered to be high risk. Additional characteristics that adversely affect outcome include T-cell immunophenotype or a slow response to initial therapy. Chromosomal abnormalities, including hypodiploidy, the Philadelphia chromosome, and *MLL* gene rearrangements, portend a poorer outcome. Other mutations, such as in the *IKZF1* gene, have been shown to be associated with a poor prognosis and may become important in treatment algorithms in the future. More favorable characteristics include a rapid response to therapy, hyperdiploidy, trisomy of specific chromosomes (4, 10, and 17), and rearrangements of the *ETV6-RUNX1* (formerly *TEL-AML1*) genes.

The outcome for patients at higher risk can be improved by administration of more intensive therapy despite the greater toxicity of such therapy. Infants with ALL, along with patients who present with specific chromosomal abnormalities, such as t(4;11), have an even higher risk of relapse despite intensive therapy. However, the poor outcome of Philadelphia chromosome positive ALL with t(9;22) has dramatically changed by the addition of imatinib to an intensive chemotherapy backbone. Imatinib is an agent specifically designed to inhibit the BCR-ABL kinase resulting from the translocation. With this new approach, the event-free survival has improved from 30% to 70%. Clinical trials demonstrate that the prognosis for patients with a slower response to initial therapy may be improved by therapy that is more intensive than the therapy considered necessary for patients who respond more rapidly.

Most children with ALL are treated in clinical trials conducted by national or international cooperative groups. Standard treatment involves chemotherapy for 2-3 yr and most achieve remission at the end of the induction phase. Patients in clinical remission can have **MRD** that can only be detected with specific molecular probes to translocations and other DNA markers contained in leukemic cells or specialized flow cytometry. MRD can be quantitative and can provide an estimate of the burden of leukemic cells present in the marrow. Higher levels of MRD present at the end of induction suggest a poorer prognosis and higher risk of subsequent relapse. MRD of >0.01% on

the marrow on day 29 of induction is a significant risk factor for shorter event-free survival for all risk categories, when compared with patients with negative MRD. Therapy for ALL intensifies treatment in patients with evidence of MRD at the end of induction.

Initial therapy, termed **remission induction**, is designed to eradicate the leukemic cells from the bone marrow. During this phase, therapy is given for 4 wk and consists of vincristine weekly, a corticosteroid such as dexamethasone or prednisone, and usually a single dose of a long-acting, pegylated asparaginase preparation. Patients at higher risk also receive daunomycin at weekly intervals. With this approach, 98% of patients are in **remission**, as defined by <5% blasts in the marrow and a return of neutrophil and platelet counts to near-normal levels after 4-5 wk of treatment. Intrathecal chemotherapy is always given at the start of treatment and at least once more during induction.

The second phase of treatment, **consolidation**, focuses on intensive **CNS therapy** in combination with continued intensive systemic therapy in an effort to prevent later CNS relapses. Intrathecal chemotherapy is given repeatedly by lumbar puncture. The likelihood of later CNS relapse is thereby reduced to <5%, from historical incidence as high as 60%. A small percentage of patients with features that predict a high risk of CNS relapse may receive irradiation to the brain in later phases of therapy. This includes patients who, at the time of diagnosis, have lymphoblasts in the CSF and either an elevated CSF leukocyte count or physical signs of CNS leukemia, such as cranial nerve palsy.

Subsequently, many regimens provide 14-28 wk of therapy, with the drugs and schedules used varying depending on the risk group of the patient. This period of treatment is often termed **intensification** and includes phases of aggressive treatment (**delayed intensification**) as well as relatively nontoxic phases of treatment (**interim maintenance**). Multiagent chemotherapy, including such medications as cytarabine, methotrexate, asparaginase, and vincristine, is used during these phases to eradicate residual disease.

Finally, patients enter the **maintenance** phase of therapy, which lasts for 2-3 yr, depending on the protocol used. Patients are given daily mercaptopurine and weekly oral methotrexate, usually with intermittent doses of vincristine and a corticosteroid.

A small number of patients with particularly poor prognostic features, such as those with induction failure or extreme hypodiploidy, may undergo bone marrow transplantation during the first remission.

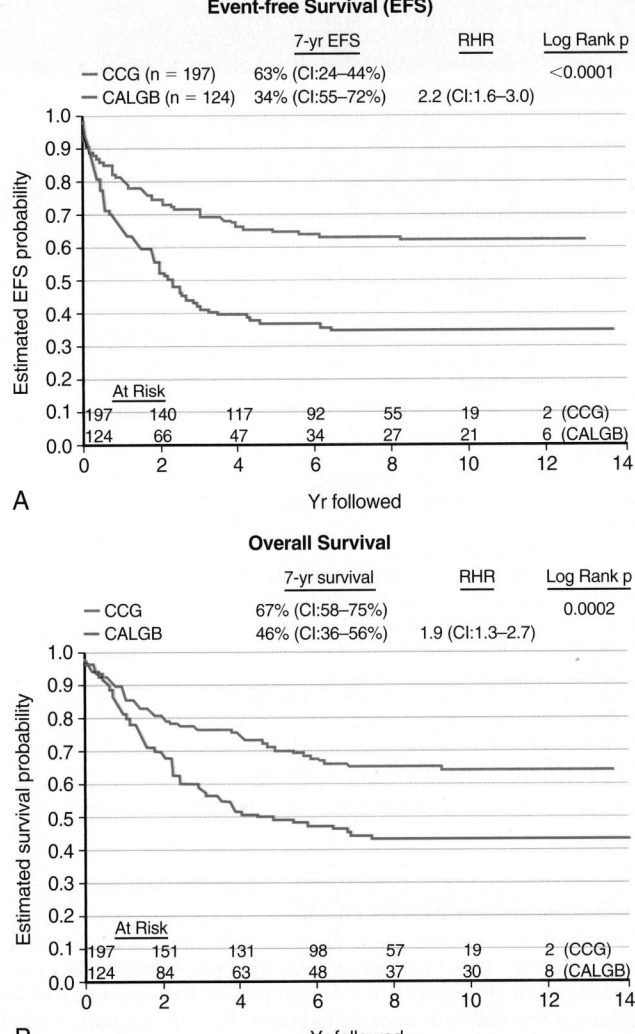

Figure 495-5 Comparison of event-free survival among Cancer and Leukemia Group B (CALGB) (adult protocol, *green line*) and Children's Cancer Group (CCG) (pediatric protocol, *red line*) patients. *(From Stock W, La M, Sanford B, et al: What determines the outcomes for adolescents and young adults with acute lymphoblastic leukemia treated on cooperative group protocols? A comparison of Children's Cancer Group and Cancer and Leukemia Group B studies, Blood 112: 1646–1654, 2008.)*

Adolescents and young adults with ALL have an inferior prognosis compared to children younger than 15 yr old. They often have adverse prognostic factors and require more intensive therapy. Patients in this age group have a superior outcome when treated with pediatric as opposed to adult treatment protocols (Fig. 495-5). Although the explanation for these findings may be multifactorial, it is important that these patients be treated with pediatric treatment protocols, ideally in a pediatric cancer center.

There are genetic polymorphisms of enzymes important in drug metabolism, which may impact both the efficacy and toxicity of chemotherapeutic medications. **Pharmacogenetic testing** of the thiopurine *S*-methyltransferase *(TPMT)* gene, which encodes one of the metabolizing enzymes of mercaptopurine, can identify patients who are wild type (normal TPMT enzyme activity), heterozygous (slightly decreased TPMT enzyme activity), or homozygous (low or absent enzyme activity). Decreased TPMT enzyme activity results in an accumulation of a toxic metabolite of mercaptopurine and results in severe myelosuppression, requiring dose reductions of the chemotherapy (see Chapter 59). In the future, treatment also may be stratified by gene expression profiles of leukemic cells. In particular, gene expression

arrays induced by exposure to a chemotherapeutic agent can predict which patients have drug-resistant ALL.

Treatment of Relapse

The major impediment to a successful outcome is relapse of the disease. Outcomes remain poor among those that relapse, with the most important prognostic indicators being time from diagnosis and the site of relapsed disease. In addition, other factors, such as immunophenotype (T-ALL worse than B-ALL) and age at initial diagnosis, have prognostic significance.

Relapse occurs in the bone marrow in 15-20% of patients with ALL and carries the most serious implications, especially if it occurs during or shortly after completion of therapy. Intensive chemotherapy with agents not previously used in the patient followed by allogeneic stem cell transplantation can result in long-term survival for some patients with bone marrow relapse (see Chapter 135).

The incidence of CNS relapse has decreased to <5% since introduction of preventive CNS therapy. CNS relapse may be discovered at the time of a routine lumbar puncture in the asymptomatic patient. Symptomatic patients with relapse in the CNS usually present with signs and symptoms of increased intracranial pressure and can present with isolated cranial nerve palsies. The diagnosis is confirmed by demonstrating the presence of leukemic cells in the CSF. The treatment includes intrathecal medication and cranial or craniospinal irradiation. Systemic chemotherapy also must be used, because these patients are at high risk for subsequent bone marrow relapse. Most patients with leukemic relapse confined to the CNS do well, especially those in whom the CNS relapse occurs longer than 18 mo after initiation of chemotherapy.

Testicular relapse occurs in less than 2% of boys with ALL, usually after completion of therapy. Such relapse occurs as painless swelling of 1 or both testes. The diagnosis is confirmed by biopsy of the affected testis. Treatment includes systemic chemotherapy and possibly local irradiation. A high proportion of boys with a testicular relapse can be successfully retreated, and the survival rate of these patients is good.

The most current information on treatment of childhood ALL is available in the PDQ (Physician Data Query) on the National Cancer Institute website (http://www.cancer.gov/cancertopics/pdq/treatment/childALL/healthprofessional/).

SUPPORTIVE CARE

Close attention to the medical supportive care needs of the patients is essential in successfully administering aggressive chemotherapeutic programs. Patients with high white blood counts are especially prone to tumor lysis syndrome as therapy is initiated. The kidney failure associated with very high levels of serum uric acid can be prevented or treated with allopurinol or urate oxidase. Chemotherapy often produces severe myelosuppression, which can require erythrocyte and platelet transfusion and which always requires a high index of suspicion and aggressive empiric antimicrobial therapy for sepsis in febrile children with neutropenia. Patients must receive prophylactic treatment for *Pneumocystis jiroveci* pneumonia during chemotherapy and for several months after completing treatment.

The successful therapy of ALL is a direct result of intensive and often toxic treatment. However, such intensive therapy can incur substantial academic, developmental, and psychosocial costs for children with ALL and considerable financial costs and stress for their families. Both long-term and acute toxicity effects can occur. An array of cancer care professionals with training and experience in addressing the myriad of problems that can arise is essential to minimize the complications and achieve an optimal outcome.

PROGNOSIS

Improvements in therapy and risk stratification have resulted in significant increases in survival rates, with current data showing overall 5 yr survival around 90% (Fig. 495-6). However, survivors are more likely to experience significant chronic medical conditions compared to siblings, including musculoskeletal, cardiac, and neurologic conditions. Overall, long-term management following ALL should be

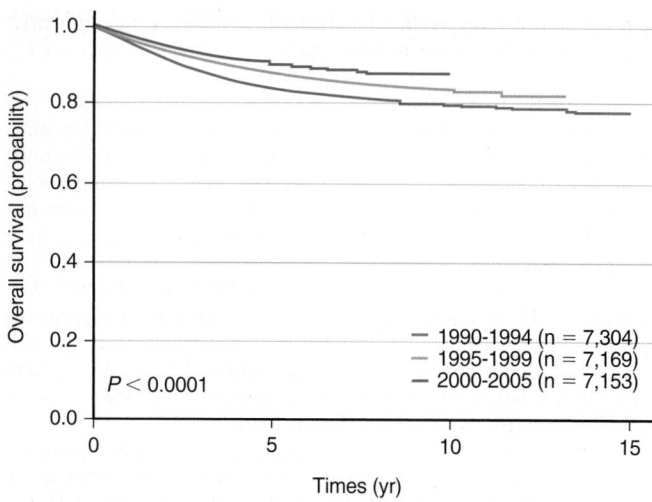

Figure 495-6 Overall survival probabilities by treatment era for patients with ALL enrolled in Children's Oncology Group trials in 1990-1994, 1995-1999, and 2000-2005. (*From Hunger SP, Lu X, Devidas M, et al: Improved survival for children and adolescents with acute lymphoblastic leukemia between 1990 and 2005: A report from the Children's Oncology Group, J Clin Oncol 30:1663–1669, 2012.*)

conducted in a clinic where children and adolescents can be followed by a variety of specialists to address the challenges of these unique patients.

Bibliography is available at Expert Consult.

495.2 Acute Myelogenous Leukemia

David G. Tubergen, Archie Bleyer, Erika Friehling, and A. Kim Ritchey

EPIDEMIOLOGY

AML accounts for 11% of the cases of childhood leukemia in the United States; it is diagnosed in approximately 370 children annually. The relative frequency of AML increases in adolescence, representing 36% of cases of leukemia in 15-19 yr olds. One subtype, acute promyelocytic leukemia (APL), is more common in certain regions of the world, but the incidence of the other types is generally uniform. Several chromosomal abnormalities associated with AML have been identified, but no predisposing genetic or environmental factors can be identified in most patients (see Table 495-1). Nonetheless, a number of risk factors have been identified, including ionizing radiation, chemotherapeutic agents (e.g., alkylating agents, epipodophyllotoxin), organic solvents, paroxysmal nocturnal hemoglobinuria, and certain syndromes: Down syndrome, Fanconi anemia, Bloom syndrome, Kostmann syndrome, Shwachman-Diamond syndrome, Diamond-Blackfan syndrome, Li-Fraumeni syndrome, and neurofibromatosis type 1.

CELLULAR CLASSIFICATION

The characteristic feature of AML is that >20% of bone marrow cells on bone marrow aspiration or biopsy touch preparations constitute a fairly homogeneous population of blast cells, with features similar to those that characterize early differentiation states of the myeloid-monocyte-megakaryocyte series of blood cells. Current practice requires the use of flow cytometry to identify cell surface antigens and use of chromosomal and molecular genetic techniques for additional diagnostic precision and to aid the choice of therapy. The WHO has proposed a new classification system that incorporates morphology, chromosome abnormalities, and specific gene mutations. This system provides significant biologic and prognostic information (Table 495-3).

Table 495-3	WHO Classification of Acute Myeloid Neoplasms

Acute myeloid leukemia with recurrent genetic abnormalities
- AML with t(8;21)(q22;q22); *RUNX1-RUNX1T1*
- AML with inv(16)(p13.1q22) or t(16;16)(p13.1;q22); *CBFB-MYH11*
- APL with t(15;17)(q22;q12); *PML-RARA*
- AML with t(9;11)(p22;q23); *MLLT3-MLL*
- AML with t(6;9)(p23;q34); *DEK-NUP214*
- AML with inv(3)(q21q26.2) or t(3;3)(q21;q26.2); *RPN1-EVI1*
- AML (megakaryoblastic) with t(1;22)(p13;q13); *RBM15-MKL1*
- *Provisional entity: AML with mutated NPM1*
- *Provisional entity: AML with mutated CEBPA*

Acute myeloid leukemia with myelodysplasia-related changes
Therapy-related myeloid neoplasms
Acute myeloid leukemia, not otherwise specified
- AML with minimal differentiation
- AML without maturation
- AML with maturation
- Acute myelomonocytic leukemia
- Acute monoblastic/monocytic leukemia
- Acute erythroid leukemia
  - Pure erythroid leukemia
  - Erythroleukemia, erythroid/myeloid
- Acute megakaryoblastic leukemia
- Acute basophilic leukemia
- Acute panmyelosis with myelofibrosis

Myeloid sarcoma
Myeloid proliferations related to Down syndrome
- Transient abnormal myelopoiesis
- Myeloid leukemia associated with Down syndrome

Blastic plasmacytoid dendritic cell neoplasm

AML, acute myelogenous leukemia; APL, acute promyelocytic leukemia.

CLINICAL MANIFESTATIONS

The production of symptoms and signs of AML is a result of replacement of bone marrow by malignant cells and caused by secondary bone marrow failure. Patients with AML can present with any or all of the findings associated with **marrow failure** in ALL. In addition, patients with AML present with signs and symptoms that are uncommon in ALL, including **subcutaneous nodules** or "blueberry muffin" lesions (especially in infants), infiltration of the gingiva (especially in monocytic subtypes), signs and laboratory findings of **disseminated intravascular coagulation** (especially indicative of APL), and discrete masses, known as **chloromas** or **granulocytic sarcomas.** These masses can occur in the absence of apparent bone marrow involvement and typically are associated with a t(8;21) translocation. Chloromas also may be seen in the orbit and epidural space.

DIAGNOSIS

Analysis of bone marrow aspiration and biopsy specimens of patients with AML typically reveals the features of a hypercellular marrow consisting of a monotonous pattern of cells. Flow cytometry and special stains assist in identifying myeloperoxidase-containing cells, thus confirming both the myelogenous origin of the leukemia and the diagnosis. Some chromosomal abnormalities and molecular genetic markers are characteristic of specific subtypes of disease (Table 495-4).

PROGNOSIS AND TREATMENT

Aggressive multiagent chemotherapy is successful in inducing remission in approximately 85-90% of patients. Survival has increased dramatically since the 1970s, when only 15% of newly diagnosed patients survived, compared to a current survival rate of 60-70% with modern therapy (Fig. 495-7). Targeting therapy to genetic markers may be beneficial (see Table 495-4). Up to 5% of patients die of either infection or bleeding before a remission can be achieved. Matched-sibling bone marrow or stem cell transplantation after remission achieves long-term disease-free survival in about two thirds of patients. Continued chemotherapy for patients who do not have a matched sibling donor is

Table 495-4	Prognostic Implications of Common Chromosomal Abnormalities in Pediatric Acute Myelogenous Leukemia		
CHROMOSOMAL ABNORMALITY	**GENETIC ALTERATION**	**USUAL MORPHOLOGY**	**PROGNOSIS**
t(8;21)	AML1-ETO	Myeloblasts with differentiation	Favorable
inv(16)	CBFB-MYHII	Myeloblasts plus abnormal eosinophils with dysplastic basophilic granules	Favorable
t(15;17)	PML-RARA	Promyelocytic	Favorable
11q23 abnormalities	MLL rearrangements	Monocytic	Unfavorable
FLT3 mutation	FLT3-ITD	Any	Unfavorable
del(7q), −7	Unknown	Myeloblasts without differentiation	Unfavorable

Modified from Nathan DG, Orkin SH, Ginsburg D, et al, editors: Nathan and Oski's hematology of infancy and childhood, ed 6, Philadelphia, 2003, WB Saunders, p. 1177.

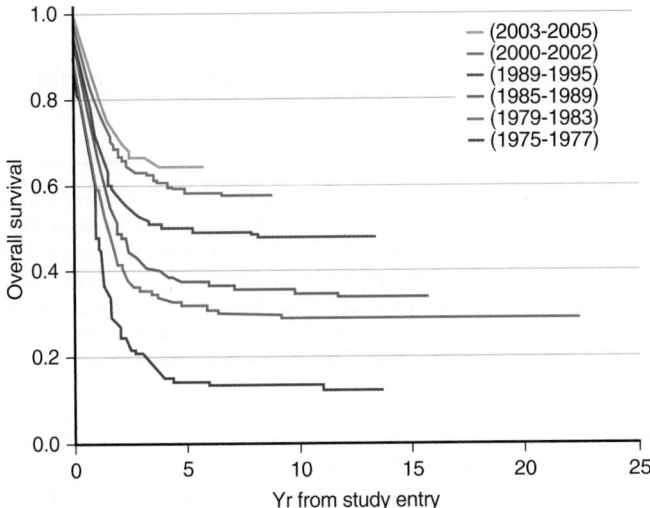

Figure 495-7 Overall survival showing incremental improvements over the last 40 yr in Children's Oncology Group and legacy trials in childhood AML. (From Gamis AS, Alonzo TA, Perentesis JP, Meshinchi S, on behalf of the COG Acute Myeloid Leukemia Committee: Children's Oncology Group's 2013 blueprint for research: acute myeloid leukemia, Pediatr Blood Cancer 60:964–971, 2013.)

generally less effective than marrow transplantation, but nevertheless is curative in about half of patients. However, for selected patients with favorable prognostic features [t(8;21); t(15;17); inv(16); APL] and improved outcome with chemotherapy, matched sibling stem cell transplantation is recommended only after a relapse. Matched unrelated donor stem cell transplants may be effective therapy, but they carry the risk of significant graft-vs-host disease as well as the complications associated with intensive myeloablative therapy. Matched unrelated donor transplants are usually reserved for patients who have a relapse. However, patients with unfavorable prognostic features (e.g., monosomies 7 and 5, 5q−, and 11q23 abnormalities) who have inferior outcome with chemotherapy might benefit from matched unrelated donor stem cell transplant in first remission.

APL, characterized by a gene rearrangement involving the retinoic acid receptor [t(15;17); PML-RARA], is very responsive to **all-*trans*-retinoic acid (ATRA, tretinoin)** combined with anthracyclines and cytarabine. The success of this therapy makes marrow transplantation in first remission unnecessary for patients with this disease. Arsenic trioxide is an effective noncytotoxic therapy for APL. Data from trials in adults show promising results with the use of combined ATRA/arsenic without cytotoxic drugs as initial therapy for APL and would support a new trial of this regimen in children.

Increased supportive care is needed in patients with AML because the intensive therapy they receive produces prolonged bone marrow suppression with a very high incidence of serious infections, especially *Streptococcal viridans* sepsis and fungal infection. These patients may require prolonged hospitalization, filgrastim (granulocyte colony-stimulating factor), and prophylactic antimicrobials.

The most current information on treatment of AML is available in the PDQ (Physician Data Query) on the National Cancer Institute website (http://www.cancer.gov/cancertopics/pdq/treatment/childAML/healthprofessional/).

Bibliography is available at Expert Consult.

495.3 Down Syndrome and Acute Leukemia and Transient Myeloproliferative Disorder

David G. Tubergen, Archie Bleyer, Erika Friehling, and A. Kim Ritchey

Acute leukemia occurs about 15-20 times more frequently in children with Down syndrome than in the general population (see Chapters 81 and 492). The ratio of ALL to AML in patients with Down syndrome is the same as that in the general population. The exception is during the 1st 3 yr of life, when AML is more common. In children with Down syndrome who have ALL, the expected outcome of treatment is slightly inferior to that for other children, which can be partially explained by a lack of good prognostic characteristics, such as *ETV6-RUNX1* and trisomies, as well as genetic abnormalities that are associated with an inferior prognosis, such as *IKZF1*. Patients with Down syndrome demonstrate a remarkable sensitivity to methotrexate and other antimetabolites, which can result in substantial toxicity if standard doses are administered. In AML, however, patients with Down syndrome have much better outcomes than non–Down syndrome children, with a >80% long-term survival rate. After induction therapy, these patients receive therapy that is less intensive to achieve better results.

Approximately 10% of neonates with Down syndrome develop a transient leukemia or **myeloproliferative disorder** characterized by high leukocyte counts, blast cells in the peripheral blood, and associated anemia, thrombocytopenia, and hepatosplenomegaly. These features usually resolve within the 1st 3 mo of life. Although these neonates can require temporary transfusion support, they do not require chemotherapy unless there is evidence of life-threatening complications. However, patients who have Down syndrome and who develop this transient leukemia or myeloproliferative disorder require close follow-up, because 20-30% will develop typical leukemia (often acute megakaryocytic leukemia) by 3 yr of life (mean onset, 16 mo). *GATA1* mutations (a transcription factor that controls megakaryopoiesis) are present in blasts from patients with Down syndrome who have

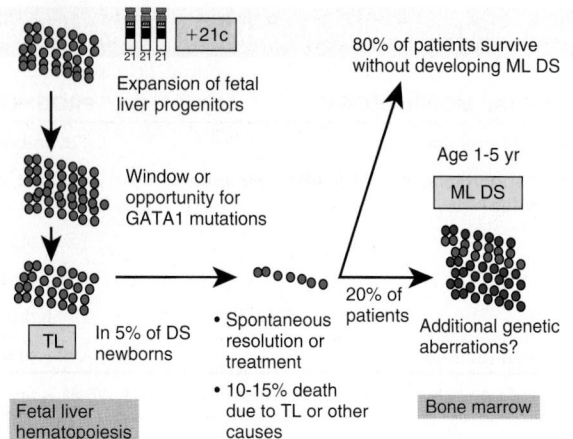

Figure 495-8 Stepwise development of myeloid leukemia in Down syndrome (ML DS) following transient leukemia (TL). TL arises from expanded fetal liver progenitors as a result of constitutional trisomy 21, providing a window of opportunity for the occurrence of acquired mutations in the hematopoietic transcription factor GATA1. In most cases TL spontaneously disappears, but some children need treatment because of severe TL-related symptoms. Approximately 20% of children with TL subsequently develop ML DS, which requires additional hits. *(From Zwaan MC, Reinhardt D, Hitzler J, Vyas P: Acute leukemias in children with Down syndrome, Pediatr Clin North Am 55:53–70, 2008.)*

transient myeloproliferative disease and also in those with leukemia (Fig. 495-8). Transient myeloproliferative disease also can occur in patients who do not have phenotypic features of Down syndrome. Blasts from these patients might have trisomy 21, suggesting a mosaic state.

Bibliography is available at Expert Consult.

495.4 Chronic Myelogenous Leukemia

David G. Tubergen, Archie Bleyer, Erika Friehling, and A. Kim Ritchey

CML is a clonal disorder of the hematopoietic tissue that accounts for 2-3% of all cases of childhood leukemia. Approximately 99% of the cases are characterized by a specific translocation, t(9;22)(q34;q11), known as the **Philadelphia chromosome,** resulting in a *BCR-ABL* fusion protein.

The presenting symptoms of CML are nonspecific and can include fever, fatigue, weight loss, and anorexia. Splenomegaly also may be present, resulting in pain in the left upper quadrant of the abdomen. The diagnosis is suggested by a high white blood cell count with myeloid cells at all stages of differentiation in the peripheral blood and bone marrow and is confirmed by cytogenetic and molecular studies that demonstrate the presence of the characteristic Philadelphia chromosome and the *BCR-ABL* gene rearrangement. This translocation, although characteristic of CML, is also found in a small percentage of patients with ALL.

The disease is characterized by an initial chronic phase in which the malignant clone produces an elevated leukocyte count with a predominance of mature forms but with increased numbers of immature granulocytes. In addition to leukocytosis, blood counts can reveal mild anemia and thrombocytosis. Typically, the chronic phase terminates 3-4 yr after onset, when the CML moves into the accelerated or "blast crisis" phase. At this point, the blood counts rise dramatically and the clinical picture is indistinguishable from acute leukemia. Additional manifestations can occur, including neurologic symptoms from hyperleukocytosis, which causes increased blood viscosity with decreased CNS perfusion.

Imatinib (Gleevec), an agent designed specifically to inhibit the *BCR-ABL* tyrosine kinase, has been used in adults and children and has shown an ability to produce major cytogenetic responses in >70% of patients (see Table 494-1). Experience in children suggests it can be used safely with results comparable to those seen in adults. Second-generation tyrosine kinase inhibitors, such as **dasatinib,** have improved remission rates in adults and are now included in the first-line therapy in that population while they are being studied in children. While waiting for a response to the tyrosine kinase inhibitor, disabling or threatening signs and symptoms of CML can be controlled during the chronic phase with hydroxyurea, which gradually returns the leukocyte count to normal. Prolonged morphologic and cytogenetic responses are expected, but the opportunity for cure is enhanced by human leukocyte antigen–matched family donor allogeneic stem cell transplant, with up to 80% of children achieving a cure.

Bibliography is available at Expert Consult.

495.5 Juvenile Myelomonocytic Leukemia

David G. Tubergen, Archie Bleyer, Erika Friehling, and A. Kim Ritchey

JMML, formerly termed **juvenile CML,** is a clonal proliferation of hematopoietic stem cells that typically affects children younger than 2 yr of age. JMML is rare, constituting <1% of all cases of childhood leukemia. Patients with this disease do not have the Philadelphia chromosome that is characteristic of CML. Patients with JMML present with rashes, lymphadenopathy, splenomegaly, and hemorrhagic manifestations. Analysis of the peripheral blood often shows an elevated leukocyte count with increased monocytes, thrombocytopenia, and anemia with the presence of erythroblasts. The bone marrow shows a myelodysplastic pattern, with blasts accounting for <20% of cells. Most patients with JMML have been found to have mutations that lead to activation of the *RAS* oncogene pathway including *NF1* and *PTPN11*. Patients with neurofibromatosis type 1 and Noonan syndrome have a predilection for this type of leukemia, since they have germline mutations involved in *RAS* signaling. Therapeutic reports are largely anecdotal. Stem cell transplantation offers the best opportunity for cure but much less so than for classic CML.

Bibliography is available at Expert Consult.

495.6 Infant Leukemia

David G. Tubergen, Archie Bleyer, Erika Friehling, and A. Kim Ritchey

Approximately 2% of cases of leukemia during childhood occur before the age of 1 year. In contrast to older children, the ratio of ALL to AML is 2 : 1. Leukemic clones have been noted in cord blood at birth before symptoms appear, and in 1 case the same clone was noted in maternal cells (maternal to fetal transmission). Chromosome translocations can also occur in utero during fetal hematopoiesis, thus leading to malignant clone formation.

Several unique biologic features and a particularly poor prognosis are characteristic of ALL during infancy. More than 80% of the cases demonstrate rearrangements of the *MLL* gene, found at the site of the 11q23 band translocation, the majority of which are the t(4;11). This subset of patients largely accounts for the very high relapse rate. These patients often present with hyperleukocytosis and extensive tissue infiltration producing organomegaly, including CNS disease. Subcutaneous nodules, known as **leukemia cutis,** and tachypnea caused by diffuse pulmonary infiltration by leukemic cells are observed more often in infants than in older children. The leukemic cell morphology is usually that of large irregular lymphoblasts, with a phenotype negative for the CD10 (common ALL antigen) marker (pro-B) unlike most older children with B-ALL who are CD10+.

Very intensive chemotherapy programs, including stem cell transplantation, are being explored in infants with *MLL* gene rearrangements, but none has yet proved satisfactory. Infants with leukemia who lack the 11q23 rearrangements have a prognosis similar to that of older children with ALL.

Infants with AML often present with CNS or skin involvement and have a subtype known as **acute myelomonocytic leukemia.** The treatment may be the same as that for older children with AML, with similar outcome. Meticulous supportive care is necessary because of the young age and aggressive therapy needed in these patients.

Bibliography is available at Expert Consult.

Chapter **496**
Lymphoma
Jessica Hochberg, Lisa Giulino-Roth, and Mitchell S. Cairo

Lymphoma is the third most common cancer among U.S. children (age 14 yr or younger), with an annual incidence of 15 cases per 1 million children. It is the most common cancer in adolescents, accounting for >25% of newly diagnosed cancers in persons 15-19 yr old. The 2 broad categories of lymphoma, Hodgkin lymphoma (HL) and non-Hodgkin lymphoma (NHL), have different clinical manifestations and treatments.*

496.1 Hodgkin Lymphoma
Jessica Hochberg, Lisa Giulino-Roth, and Mitchell S. Cairo

Hodgkin lymphoma (HL) is a malignant process involving the lymphoreticular system that accounts for 6% of childhood cancers. In the United States, HL accounts for approximately 5% of cancers in persons 14 yr of age or younger; it accounts for approximately 15% of cancers in adolescents (15-19 yr of age), making HL the most common malignancy in this age group.

EPIDEMIOLOGY
The worldwide incidence of HL is approximately 2-4 new cases/100,000 population/yr; there is a bimodal age distribution, with peaks at 15-35 yr of age and again after 50 yr. It is the most common cancer seen in adolescents and young adults, and the third most common in children younger than the age of 15 yr. In developing countries, the early peak tends to occur prior to adolescence. A male:female predominance is found among young children, but lessens with age. Infectious agents may be involved, such as human herpesvirus 6, cytomegalovirus, and **Epstein-Barr virus (EBV)**. The role of EBV is supported by prospective serologic studies. Infection with EBV confers a 4-fold higher risk of developing HL and may precede the diagnosis by years. EBV antigens have been demonstrated in HL tissues, particularly type II latent membrane proteins 1 and 2, although EBV status is not thought to be prognostic of outcome.

PATHOGENESIS
The **Reed-Sternberg (RS) cell,** a pathognomonic feature of HL, is a large cell (15-45 μm in diameter) with multiple or multilobulated nuclei. This cell type is considered the hallmark of HL, although similar cells are seen in infectious mononucleosis, NHL, and other conditions. The RS cell is clonal in origin and arises from the germinal center B cells but typically has lost most B-cell gene expression and function. There is no single simple genetic aberration that leads to malignant transformation of the RS cell, but rather a combination of somatic mutations, chromosomal instability, and complex chromosomal rearrangements have been reported with no particular pattern or frequency. This typically leads to cell regulation defects such as constitutive activation of the nuclear factor-κB pathway or abnormal regulation of the Bcl-2 family of proteins. HL is characterized by a variable number of RS cells surrounded by an inflammatory infiltrate of lymphocytes, plasma cells, and eosinophils in different proportions, depending on the HL histologic subtype. The interaction between the RS cell and these background inflammatory cells with their associated cytokine release is important in the development and progression of HL. Reactive infiltration of eosinophils and CD68+ macrophages, and increased concentrations of cytokines, such as interleukins 1 and 6 and tumor necrosis factor, are all associated with an unfavorable prognosis, including advanced stage, the presence of "B" symptoms, decreased response to therapy, and reduced survival. In addition, evidence of CD8+ T cells surrounding the RS cell offers evidence of an important role in T-cell promotion of malignant cell survival, perhaps through the CD30 and CD40 ligands found on RS cells. Other features that distinguish the histologic subtypes include various degrees of fibrosis and the presence of collagen bands, necrosis, or malignant reticular cells (Fig. 496-1). The distribution of subtypes varies with age.

The **Revised World Health Organization Classification of Lymphoid Neoplasms** (Table 496-1) includes 2 modifications of the older Rye system. HL appears to arise in lymphoid tissue and spread to adjacent lymph node areas in a relatively orderly fashion. Hematogenous spread also occurs, leading to involvement of the liver, spleen, bone, bone marrow, or brain, and is usually associated with systemic symptoms.

CLINICAL MANIFESTATIONS
Patients commonly present with painless, nontender, firm, rubbery, cervical or supraclavicular lymphadenopathy and usually some degree of mediastinal involvement. Clinically detectable hepatosplenomegaly is rarely encountered. Depending on the extent and location of nodal and extranodal disease, patients may present with symptoms and signs of airway obstruction (dyspnea, hypoxia, cough), pleural or pericardial effusion, hepatocellular dysfunction, or bone marrow infiltration (anemia, neutropenia, or thrombocytopenia). Disease manifesting below the diaphragm is rare and occurs in approximately 3% of all cases. Systemic symptoms, classified as **B symptoms** that are considered important in staging, are unexplained fever >38°C (100.4°F), weight loss >10% total body weight over 6 mo, and drenching night sweats. Less common and not considered of prognostic significance are symptoms of pruritus, lethargy, anorexia, or pain that worsens after ingestion of alcohol. Patients also exhibit immune system abnormalities that often persist during and after therapy.

DIAGNOSIS
Any patient with persistent, unexplained lymphadenopathy unassociated with an obvious underlying inflammatory or infectious process should undergo chest radiography to identify the presence of a large mediastinal mass before undergoing lymph node biopsy. Formal excisional biopsy is preferred over needle biopsy to ensure that adequate tissue is obtained, both for light microscopy and for appropriate immunohistochemical and molecular studies. Once the diagnosis of HL is established, extent of disease (stage) should be determined to allow selection of appropriate therapy (Table 496-2). Evaluation includes history, physical examination, and imaging studies, including chest radiograph; CT scans of the neck, chest, abdomen, and pelvis; and positron emission tomography (PET) scan. Laboratory studies should include a complete blood cell count to identify abnormalities that might suggest marrow involvement; erythrocyte sedimentation rate; and measurement of serum ferritin, which is of some prognostic

---

*The views expressed are the result of independent work and do not necessarily represent the views or findings of the U.S. Food and Drug Administration or the United States.

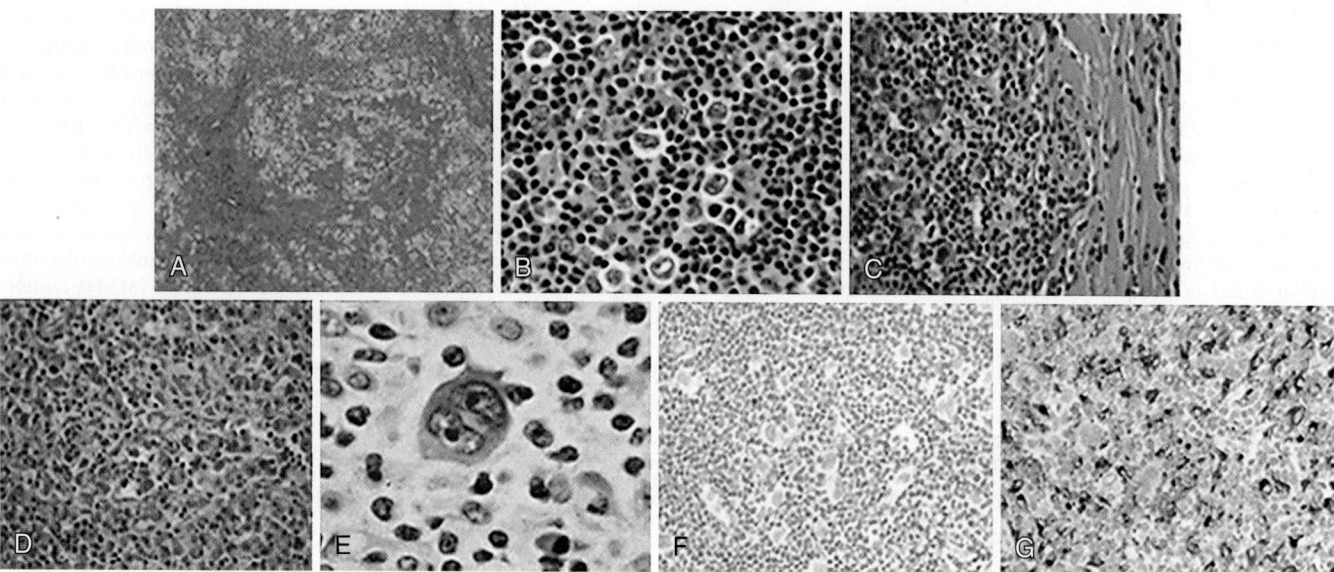

Figure 496-1 Histologic subtypes of Hodgkin lymphoma. **A,** Hematoxylin & eosin stains of nodular lymphocyte–predominant Hodgkin lymphoma (NLPHL) demonstrating a nodular proliferation with a moth-eaten appearance. **B,** High-power view demonstrating the neoplastic L and H cells found in NLPHL. **C,** Classic Hodgkin lymphoma, nodular sclerosis subtype. Large mononuclear and binucleate Reed-Sternberg cells are seen admixed in the inflammatory cell background. **D,** Classic Hodgkin lymphoma, mixed cellularity subtype, demonstrating increased numbers of Reed-Sternberg cells in a mixed inflammatory background without sclerotic changes. **E,** High-power view of a classic Reed-Sternberg cell showing binucleate cells with prominent eosinophilic nucleoli and relatively abundant cytoplasm. **F,** Few CD68+ macrophages in a treatment success patient. **G,** Many CD68+ macrophages in a treatment failure patient.

Table 496-1	New World Health Organization/Revised European–American Classification of Lymphoid Neoplasms Classification System for Hodgkin Lymphoma

Nodular lymphocyte predominance
Classical Hodgkin lymphoma
Lymphocyte rich
Mixed cellularity
Nodular sclerosis
Lymphocyte depletion

From Harris NL, Jaffe ES, Diebold J, et al: The World Health Organization classification of neoplastic diseases of the haematopoietic and lymphoid tissues: report of the Clinical Advisory Committee Meeting, Airlie House, Virginia, November 1997, Histopathology 36:69–87, 2000.

Table 496-2	Ann Arbor Staging Classification for Hodgkin Lymphoma*

STAGE	DEFINITION
I	Involvement of a single lymph node (I) or of a single extralymphatic organ or site (IE)
II	Involvement of 2 or more lymph node regions on the same side of the diaphragm (II) or localized involvement of an extralymphatic organ or site and 1 or more lymph node regions on the same side of the diaphragm (IIE)
III	Involvement of lymph node regions on both sides of the diaphragm (III), which may be accompanied by involvement of the spleen (IIIS) or by localized involvement of an extralymphatic organ or site (IIIE) or both (IIISE)
IV	Diffuse or disseminated involvement of 1 or more extralymphatic organs or tissues with or without associated lymph node involvement

*The absence or presence of fever >38°C (100.4°F) for 3 consecutive days, drenching night sweats, or unexplained loss of >10% of body weight in the 6 mo preceding admission are to be denoted in all cases by the suffix letter A or B, respectively.
From Lister TA, Crowther D, Sutcliffe SB, et al: Report of a committee convened to discuss the evaluation and staging of patients with Hodgkin's disease: Cotswolds meeting, J Clin Oncol 7:1630–1636, 1989.

significance and, if abnormal at diagnosis, serves as a baseline to evaluate the effects of treatment. A chest radiograph is particularly important for measuring the size of the mediastinal mass in relation to the maximal diameter of the thorax (Fig. 496-2). This determines "bulk" disease and becomes prognostically significant. Chest CT more clearly defines the extent of a mediastinal mass if present and identifies hilar nodes and pulmonary parenchymal involvement, which may not be evident on chest radiographs. Bone marrow aspiration and biopsy should be performed to rule out advanced disease. Bone scans are performed in patients with bone pain and/or elevation of alkaline phosphatase. Gallium scan can be particularly helpful in identifying areas of increased uptake, which can then be reevaluated at the end of treatment. Fluorodeoxyglucose PET imaging has advantages over gallium scanning, as it is a 1-day procedure with higher resolution, better dosimetry, less intestinal activity, and the potential to quantify disease. PET scans are being evaluated as a prognostic tool in HL, enabling therapy to be reduced in those predicted to have a good outcome.

The staging classification currently used for HL was adopted at the **Ann Arbor Conference** in 1971 and was revised in 1989 (see Table 496-2). HL can be subclassified into A or B categories: *A* is used to

identify asymptomatic patients and *B* is for patients who exhibit any B symptoms. Extralymphatic disease resulting from direct extension of an involved lymph node region is designated by category E. A complete response in HL is defined as the complete resolution of disease on clinical examination and imaging studies or at least 70-80% reduction of disease and a change from initial positivity to negativity on either gallium or PET scanning because residual fibrosis is common.

TREATMENT

Multiple agents allow different mechanisms of action to have non-overlapping toxicities so that full doses can be given to each patient.

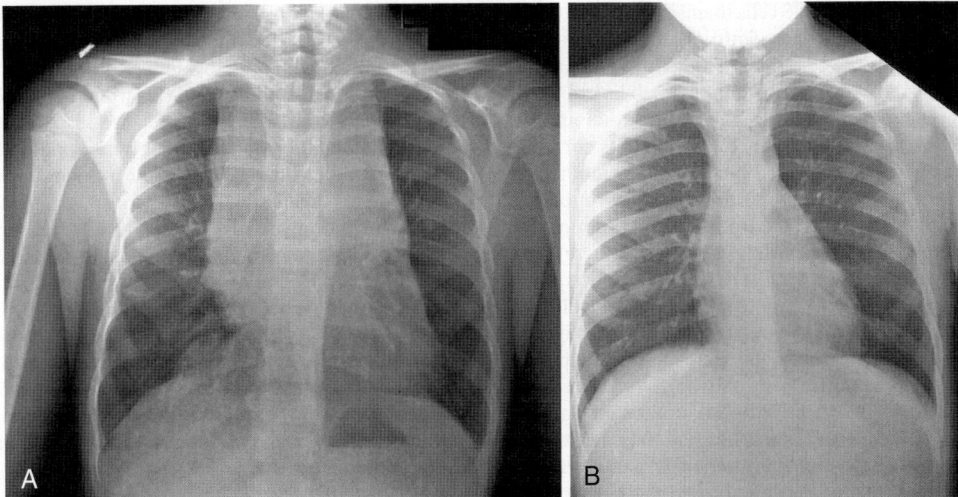

Figure 496-2 A, Anterior mediastinal mass in a patient with Hodgkin disease before therapy. **B,** After 2 mo of chemotherapy, the mediastinal mass has disappeared.

Chemotherapy and radiation therapy are both effective in the treatment of HL. Treatment of HL in pediatric patients is risk adapted and involves the use of combined chemotherapy with or without low-dose involved-field radiation therapy based on response. Treatment is determined largely by disease stage, presence or absence of B symptoms, and the presence of bulky nodal disease. Radiation therapy alone, once given at higher doses, initially resulted in prolonged remission and cure rates in patients with low-stage HL. However, this treatment also caused significant long-term morbidity in pediatric patients, including growth retardation, thyroid dysfunction, and cardiac and pulmonary toxicity. The development of effective multiagent combination chemotherapy was a major milestone in the treatment of HL resulting in a complete response rate of 70-80% and cure rate of 40-50% in patients with advanced-stage disease. However, this regimen also led to significant acute and long-term toxicity. The desire to reduce side effects and morbidity has stimulated attempts to reduce the intensity of chemotherapy as well as radiation dose and volume. Newer combinations of chemotherapy have reduced the risk of secondary cancers. Also, current radiation therapy utilizes lower amounts of overall radiation in addition to narrowing the radiation treatment field to either involved-field or even involved-node irradiation. The current Children's Oncology Group trials are investigating whether radiation therapy can be eliminated altogether in patients who have a very good rapid early response to pre-radiation induction chemotherapy.

Chemotherapy agents commonly used to treat children and adolescents with HL include cyclophosphamide, procarbazine, vincristine or vinblastine, prednisone or dexamethasone, doxorubicin, bleomycin, dacarbazine, etoposide, methotrexate, and cytosine arabinoside. The combination chemotherapy regimens in current use are based on **COPP** (cyclophosphamide, vincristine [Oncovin], procarbazine, and prednisone) or **ABVD** (doxorubicin [Adriamycin], bleomycin, vinblastine, and dacarbazine), with the addition of prednisone, cyclophosphamide, and etoposide (**ABVE-PC** and **BEACOPP**) or **BAVD** (brentuximab vedotin, doxorubicin [Adriamycin], vincristine, dacarbazine) in various combinations for intermediate- and high-risk groups (Table 496-3). "Risk-adapted" protocols are based on both staging criteria and rapidity of response to initial chemotherapy. The aim is to reduce total drug doses and treatment duration and to eliminate radiation therapy if possible.

Agents such as those that disrupt the nuclear factor-κB pathway or monoclonal antibodies that target RS tumor cells as well as the benign reactive cells that surround them are currently being investigated. Ongoing clinical trials report encouraging results with the use of anti-CD20 antibody (rituximab), particularly in nodular lymphocyte-predominant Hodgkin lymphoma where trials in relapsed disease have shown an overall response rate of 94%. In addition, anti-CD30 agents

Table 496-3	Chemotherapy Regimens Commonly Used for Children, Adolescents, and Young Adults with Hodgkin Lymphoma
CHEMOTHERAPY REGIMEN	**CORRESPONDING AGENTS**
ABVD	Doxorubicin (Adriamycin), bleomycin, vinblastine, dacarbazine
ABVD-Rituxan	Doxorubicin (Adriamycin), bleomycin, vinblastine, dacarbazine, rituximab
ABVD	Doxorubicin (Adriamycin), brentuximab, vinblastine, dacarbazine
ABVE (DBVE)	Doxorubicin (Adriamycin), bleomycin, vincristine, etoposide
VAMP	Vincristine, doxorubicin (Adriamycin), methotrexate, prednisone
OPPA ± COPP (females)	Vincristine (Oncovin), prednisone, procarbazine, doxorubicin (Adriamycin), cyclophosphamide, vincristine (Oncovin), prednisone, procarbazine
OEPA ± COPP (males)	Vincristine (Oncovin), etoposide, prednisone, doxorubicin (Adriamycin), cyclophosphamide, vincristine (Oncovin), prednisone, procarbazine
COPP/ABV	Cyclophosphamide, vincristine (Oncovin), prednisone, procarbazine, doxorubicin (Adriamycin), bleomycin, vinblastine
BEACOPP (advanced stage)	Bleomycin, etoposide, doxorubicin (Adriamycin), cyclophosphamide, vincristine (Oncovin), prednisone, procarbazine
COPP	Cyclophosphamide, vincristine (Oncovin), prednisone, procarbazine
CHOP	Cyclophosphamide, doxorubicin (Adriamycin), vincristine (Oncovin), prednisone
ABVE-PC (DBVE-PC)	Doxorubicin (Adriamycin), bleomycin, vincristine, etoposide, prednisone, cyclophosphamide
ICE ± (Brentuximab)	Ifosfamide, carboplatin, etoposide ± brentuximab
Ifos/Vino ± (Brentuximab)	Ifosfamide, vinorelbine ± brentuximab

are being used that are targeted to the RS cells themselves, where CD30 is abundantly expressed. Brentuximab vedotin is an antibody–drug conjugate that is now FDA approved to treat Hodgkin lymphoma. It combines the chimeric anti-CD30 antibody brentuximab linked to the antimitotic agent monomethyl auristatin E. This agent shows impressive efficacy as single-agent therapy in refractory HL and is currently being tested as part of upfront therapy combined with chemotherapy in patients with newly diagnosed disease. EBV-specific cytotoxic T lymphocytes (CTLs) can also be generated from allogeneic donors for patients with advanced HL (Fig. 496-3). In clinical trials, these show promising results, with enhanced antiviral activity and stabilization of disease even though all patients continue to have persistent disease. EBV-CTLs have been developed and are currently being investigated. These enhanced EBV-CTLs are designed to be latent membrane protein 1/2 specific and can be generated from second (in the case of bone marrow transplant recipients) or even third-party donors for patients with refractory disease. These newer approaches represent an exciting new direction in adoptive cellular tumor immunology, and it remains to be determined whether CTLs will have improved cytotoxicity that can overcome inhibitory signals.

RELAPSE

Most relapses occur within the 1st 3 yr after diagnosis, but relapses as late as 10 yr have been reported. Relapse cannot be predicted accurately with this disease. Poor prognostic features include tumor bulk, stage at diagnosis, extralymphatic disease, and presence of B symptoms. Patients who achieve an initial chemosensitive response but relapse or progress less than 12 mo from diagnosis are candidates for myeloablative chemotherapy and autologous stem cell transplantation with or without the addition of radiation therapy. Retrospective studies show a significant decrease in relapse in patients with HL following allogeneic vs autologous stem cell transplant (18% vs 41%). Although in earlier studies there was no improvement in overall survival owing to a high transplantation-related mortality, reduced-intensity conditioning or nonmyeloablative regimens are successful at reducing regimen-related morbidity and mortality associated with myeloablative allogeneic stem cell transplantation while still achieving a strong graft-versus-HL effect. For more difficult-to-treat refractory cases, agents such as Zevalin or Bexxar are being trialed, often in combination with stem cell transplantation strategies. Both are monoclonal anti-CD20 antibodies to which a radioactive isotope is directly linked. Clinical trials show each to be more effective than rituximab in NHL patients, and there is some interest in studying their use in the CD20 subpopulation of HL patients.

PROGNOSIS

With the use of current therapeutic regimens, patients with favorable prognostic factors and early-stage disease have an event-free survival (EFS) of 85-90% and an overall survival (OS) at 5 yr of >95%. Patients with advanced-stage disease have slightly lower EFS (80-85%) and OS (90%), respectively, although OS has approached 100% with dose-intense chemotherapy (Table 496-4). Prognosis after relapse depends

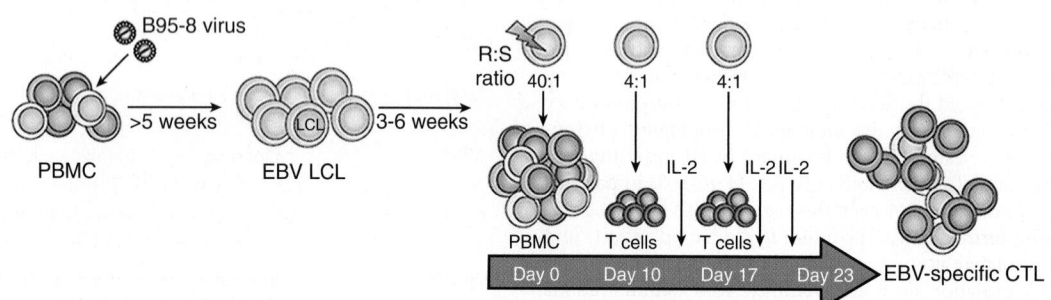

Figure 496-3 Epstein-Barr virus (EBV)–specific cytotoxic T lymphocyte (CTL) production. EBV-transformed B-cell lymphoblastoid cell line (LCLs) are prepared from the CTL donor by infection of peripheral blood mononuclear cells (PBMCs) with a clinical-grade laboratory strain of EBV (B95-8) in the presence of cyclosporine. Once the LCL is established (about 6 wk), it is irradiated and used to stimulate PBMCs from the same donor at a 40:1 ratio of PBMC:LCL. From 9-12 days later and weekly thereafter, the T cells are restimulated with the LCL at a 4:1 ratio. Interleukin 2 is added 3 days after the second stimulation and twice weekly thereafter. The CTLs should kill autologous LCLs but not autologous phytohemagglutinin blasts. Their specificity is donor dependent and they may have specificity for any of the 10 latency-associated antigens and/or for early lytic cycle proteins that are expressed by a small fraction of the LCLs, which are grown in acyclovir to prevent the production of infectious virus by blocking the viral thymidine kinase. *(Adapted from Bollard CM, Rooney CM, Heslop HE. T-cell therapy in the treatment of post-transplant lymphoproliferative disease. Nat Rev Clin Oncol 9:510–519, 2012, Fig. 2.)*

Table 496-4		Treatment Regimens and Outcome by Disease Staging		
		LOCALIZED/LOW STAGE	**INTERMEDIATE**	**ADVANCED**
Hodgkin lymphoma	Treatment	*POG study 9426/GPOH-HD 95:* ABVD-type therapy ± IFRT (risk adapted based on early response to chemotherapy)	*Stanford/DAL-HD-90:* COPP-based or dose-intense multiagent chemotherapy + low-dose RT *POG 9426/CCG 5942:* ABVD-type therapy ± IFRT (risk adapted)	*POG 8725/DAL-HD-90:* Dose-intense multiagent chemotherapy + low-dose RT *HD9/HD12/CCG 59704:* Dose-intense BEACOPP ± IFRT
	Prognosis	5 yr EFS: 85-90% 5 yr OS: 95%	*Stanford/DAL-HD-90:* 5 yr EFS: 89-92% *POG 9426/CCG 5942:* 5 yr EFS: 84% 5 yr OS: 91%	*POG 8725:* 5-yr EFS: 72-89% (age based) *DAL-HD-90:* 5 yr EFS: 86% 5 yr OS: 85-90% *HD9/HD12/CCG 59704:* 5 yr EFS/OS: 88-93/~100%

Table 496-4		Treatment Regimens and Outcome by Disease Staging—cont'd		
		LOCALIZED/LOW STAGE	**INTERMEDIATE**	**ADVANCED**
Burkitt lymphoma and diffuse large B-cell lymphoma	Treatment	*FAB/LMB 96 Group A therapy:* Complete surgical resection followed by 2 cycles of chemotherapy	*FAB/LMB 96 Group B therapy* with reduced cyclophosphamide and no maintenance therapy; *COG ANHL01P1:* FAB/LMB Group B therapy + rituximab	*FAB/LMB 96:* standard-intensity Group C therapy: Reduction, induction, intensification, and maintenance therapy *COG ANHL01P1:* FAB/LMB Group C therapy + rituximab
	Prognosis	4 yr EFS: 98% (CI$_{95}$ 94-99.5%) 4 yr OS: 99% (CI$_{95}$ 96-99.9%)	*FAB/LMB96:* 4 yr EFS: 92% (CI$_{95}$ 90-94%) 4 yr OS: 95% (CI$_{95}$ 93-96%) *PMB DLBCL has worse prognosis (EFS/OS: 66/73%) COG ANHL01P1:* 3 yr EFS 93% (CI$_{95}$ 79-98%) 3 yr OS 95% (CI$_{95}$ 83-99%)	*FAB/LMB96:* 4 yr EFS: BM+/CNS−: 91% ± 3% BM−/CNS+: 85% ± 6% BM+/CNS+: 66% ± 7% *COG ANHL01P1:* 3 yr EFS/OS: BM+ or CNS+: 90% (CI$_{95}$ 75-96%) CNS+: 93% (CI$_{95}$ 61-99%)
Lymphoblastic lymphoma	Treatment	*NHL-BFM86/90/95: COG A5971:* ALL-type therapy × 2 yr without prophylactic cranial RT	No intermediate group; disease classified as localized (stages I/II) or advanced (stages III/IV)	*NHL-BFM86/90/95:* ALL-type therapy × 2 yr ± px CRT *CCG 5941:* Intensive chemotherapy × 1 yr + cranial RT if CNS + at diagnosis *NHL-BFM95:* 5 yr EFS: 90% ± 3% (III), 95 ± 5% (IV) *CCG 5941:* 5 yr EFS/OS: 78% ± 5%/85% ± 4%
	Prognosis	*COG A5971:* 5 yr EFS: 90 (CI$_{95}$ 78-96%) 5 yr OS: 96 (CI$_{95}$ 84-99%)	No intermediate group; see above	
Anaplastic large cell lymphoma	Treatment	*EICHNL ALCL 99:* Short intensive chemotherapy + HD MTX Completely resected stage I disease may be treated with surgery alone	No intermediate group; disease classified as standard risk (no skin, visceral, or mediastinal involvement) or high risk (presence of skin, mediastinal, or visceral involvement)	*ALCL 99, CCG 5941:* Short intensive chemotherapy + HD MTX *COG ANHL0131:* APO (doxorubicin, prednisone, vincristine) ± vinblastine
	Prognosis	*EICHNL database:* 5 yr PFS: 89% (CI$_{95}$ 82-96%) 5 yr OS: 94% (CI$_{95}$ 89-99%)	No intermediate group; see above	*ALCL99:* 2 yr EFS: 71% (CI$_{95}$ 75-77%) 2 yr OS: 94% (CI$_{95}$ 89-95%) *COG5941:* 5 yr EFS 68% (CI$_{95}$ 57-78%) 5 yr OS: 80% (CI$_{95}$ 69-87%) *COH ANHL0131:* 2 yr EFS 79% (CI$_{95}$ 71-88%) 2 yr OS 89% (CI$_{95}$ 83-95%)

ABVD, doxorubicin (Adriamycin), bleomycin, vinblastine, dacarbazine; ALCL, anaplastic large cell lymphoma; ALL, acute lymphoblastic leukemia; BEACOPP, bleomycin, etoposide, doxorubicin (Adriamycin), cyclophosphamide, vincristine (Oncovin), prednisone, procarbazine; BM, bone marrow (involvement); CCG, Children's Cancer Group; CI$_{95}$, 95% confidence interval; CNS, central nervous system (involvement); COG, Children's Oncology Group; COPP, cyclophosphamide, vincristine (Oncovin), prednisone, procarbazine; CRT, chemoradiotherapy; EFS, event-free survival; EICHNL, European Intergroup for Childhood Non-Hodgkin Lymphoma; FAB, French-American-British; HD MTX, high-dose methotrexate; IFRT, involved field radiation therapy; LMB, Lymphome Malins de Burkit; MTX, methotrexate; NHL-BFM, non-Hodgkin lymphoma Berlin-Frankfurt-Munster; OS, overall survival; PFS, progression-free survival; PMB DLBCL, primary mediastinal B-cell diffuse large B-cell lymphoma; POG, Pediatric Oncology Group; px, prophylactic; RT, radiation therapy.

on the time from completion of treatment to recurrence, site of relapse (nodal vs extranodal), and presence of B symptoms at relapse. Patients whose disease relapses >12 mo after chemotherapy alone or combined-modality therapy have the best prognosis, and their relapses usually respond to additional standard therapy, resulting in a long-term survival of 60-70%. A myeloablative autologous stem cell transplantation in patients with refractory disease or relapse within 12 mo of therapy results in a long-term survival rate of only 40-50%. Allogeneic stem cell transplantation has shown promise in patients with poor risk features at relapse/progression.

Bibliography is available at Expert Consult.

496.2 Non-Hodgkin Lymphoma

Jessica Hochberg, Lisa Giulino-Roth, and Mitchell S. Cairo

Non-Hodgkin lymphoma (NHL) accounts for approximately 60% of lymphomas in children and is the second most common malignancy in patients age 15-35 yr. The annual incidence of pediatric NHL in the United States is 750-800 cases/yr. In contrast to adult NHL, which is typically indolent, pediatric NHL is usually high grade and aggressive. Although more than 70% of patients present with advanced disease, the prognosis has improved dramatically, with survival rates of 90-95% for localized disease and 70-95% with advanced disease.

EPIDEMIOLOGY
Although most children and adolescents with NHL present with de novo disease, a small number of patients have NHL secondary to specific etiologies, including inherited or acquired immune deficiencies (e.g., severe combined immunodeficiency syndrome, Wiskott-Aldrich syndrome), viruses (e.g., HIV, EBV), and as part of genetic syndromes (e.g., ataxia-telangiectasia, Bloom syndrome). However most children in North America and Europe in whom NHL develops have no obvious genetic or environmental etiology.

PATHOGENESIS
The 4 major pathologic subtypes of childhood and adolescent NHL are **lymphoblastic lymphoma (LBL)**, **Burkitt lymphoma (BL)**, **diffuse large B-cell lymphoma (DLBCL)**, and **anaplastic large cell**

lymphoma (ALCL; Figs. 496-4 and 496-5). LBL arises from immature B or T lymphocytes whereas BL, DLBCL, and ALCL are mature B- or T-cell neoplasms. DLBCL is further divided into several subtypes: the germinal center B-cell–like, which carries a favorable prognosis and accounts for the vast majority of pediatric cases of DLBCL, and the subtypes with poorer prognosis, activated B-cell–like and primary mediastinal B-cell subtypes. The cell of origin varies among NHL histologic subtypes. Almost all BLs and DLBCLs are of B-cell origin; 90% cases of LBL are of T-cell origin and 10% of B-cell origin; and 70% of cases of ALCL are of T-cell origin, 20% are of null-cell origin, and 10% are of B-cell origin. Cellular surface markers can aid in differentiating NHL subtypes and also present opportunities for targeted treatments. BL and DLBCL frequently express the B-cell antigens CD19, CD20, and CD22. ALCL, in contrast, expresses the CD30 antigen. Some pathologic subtypes have specific cytogenetic aberrations. Children with BL commonly have a t(8;14) translocation (90%) or, less commonly, a t(2;8) or t(8;22) translocation (10%). Children with BL who have a 13q deletion or complex karyotype have a poor prognosis. Those with DLBCL may have a t(8;14) translocation (30%) and often have a complex (80%) and aneuploid (80%) karyotype. Patients with ALCL commonly have a t(2;5) translocation (90%), which results in the formation of a fusion gene encoding the constitutively active nucleophosmin-anaplastic lymphoma kinase tyrosine kinase. Variant anaplastic lymphoma kinase (ALK) translocations, all with a breakpoint at 2p23, have also been reported. T-cell LBL harbors many of the same cytogenetic abnormalities as T-cell acute lymphoblastic leukemia (T-ALL), including rearrangements with breakpoints at 14q11.2 involving the T-cell receptor, and t(5;14) translocation (20%), which does not involve the 14q11.2 breakpoint.

Genomic studies have offered insights into NHL pathogenesis as well as elucidated potential targets for novel therapies. Gene expression profiling of T-LBL and T-ALL has implicated the activation of oncogenic transcription factors as a result of aberrant T-cell receptor gene rearrangement. One of the most frequently activated signaling pathways is NOTCH1, which may be amenable to therapeutic targeting with γ-secretase inhibitors. In BL and DLBCL, extensive genomic work has identified unique gene expression signatures that differentiate these 2 mature B-cell neoplasms. In addition, next-generation sequencing of BL has identified genetic lesions in *TCF3* and *ID3*, which lead to activation of the AKT/PI3 kinase pathway. Other genetic lesions that have been described in BL include loss of function of the chromatin remodeling genes *ARID1A* and *SMARCA4*. Importantly, many of these alterations are potentially targetable by agents that are currently in development.

CLINICAL MANIFESTATIONS

The clinical manifestations of childhood and adolescent NHL depend primarily on pathologic subtype and sites of involvement. The staging system used for NHL is the St. Jude/Murphy classification (Table 496-5), although this classification schema is currently under an

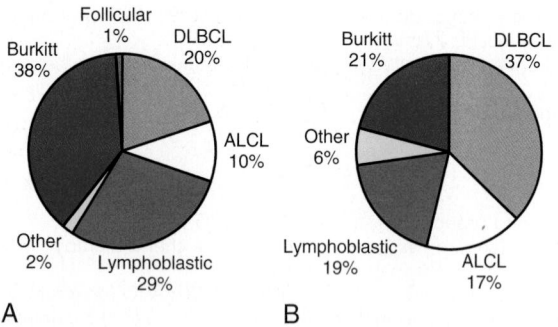

Figure 496-4 Incidence of non-Hodgkin lymphoma subtypes in **(A)** 0-14 yr age group and **(B)** 15-19 yr age group. *ALCL,* anaplastic large cell lymphoma; *DLBCL,* diffuse large B-cell lymphoma. *(Adapted from Hochberg J, Waxman IM, Kelly KM, et al: Adolescent non-Hodgkin lymphoma and Hodgkin lymphoma: state of the science, Br J Haematol 144:24–40, 2008.)*

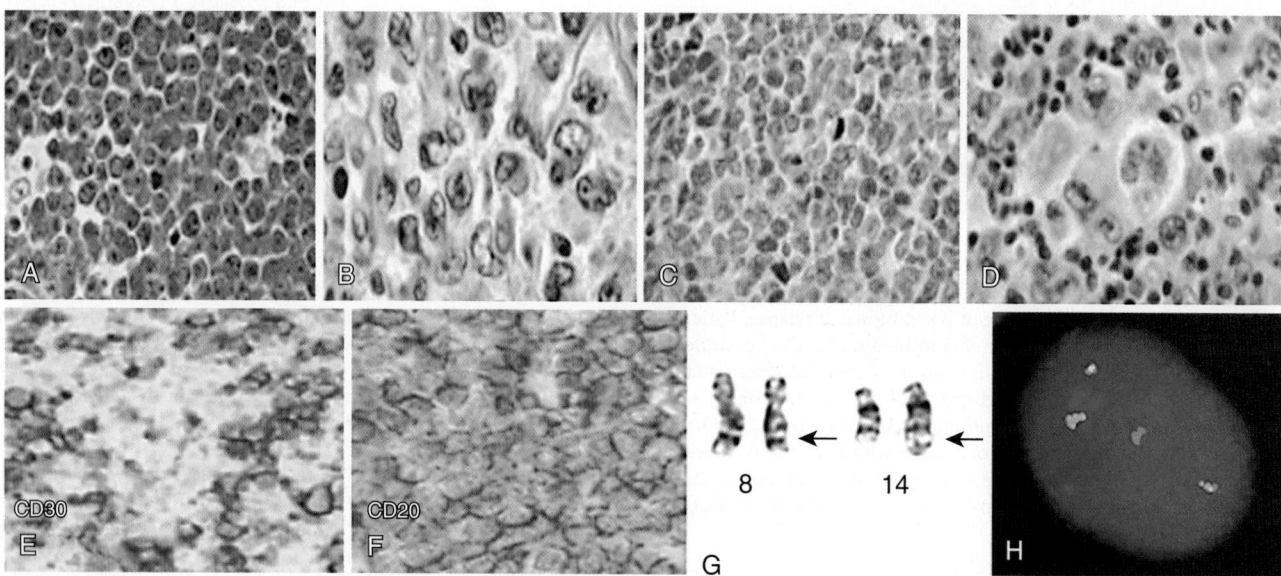

Figure 496-5 Histologic subtypes of childhood and adolescent non-Hodgkin lymphoma. **A-D:** Hematoxylin & eosin stains showing morphology of Burkitt lymphoma (**A,** high power), diffuse large B-cell lymphoma (**B,** high power), precursor T-lymphoblastic lymphoma (**C,** high power), and anaplastic large cell lymphoma (**D,** high power). **E-F:** Characteristic surface markers for ALCL (CD30; **E**) and BL (CD20; **F**). **G-H:** Cytogenetic analysis of BL demonstrating t(8;14). **G:** Karyotype showing the conventional t(8;14)(q24;q32). **H:** Interphase fluorescence in situ hybridization showing a balanced translocation involving MYC and immunoglobulin (Ig) H loci. The chromosome 8 centromere is labeled with spectrum aqua, MYC probe is labeled with spectrum orange, and IgH is labeled with spectrum green. Two fusion signals are seen as well as one red and one green representing the normal chromosomes. *(**A-D** from Cairo MS, Raetz E, Lim MS, et al: Childhood and adolescent non-Hodgkin lymphoma: new insights in biology and critical challenges for the future, Pediatr Blood Cancer 45:753–769, 2005. **E-H** from Giulino-Roth, Cesarman E: Molecular biology of Burkitt lymphoma. In Robertson ES, editor, Burkitt's lymphoma. New York, 2012, Springer.)*

Table 496-5	St. Jude Staging System for Childhood Non-Hodgkin Lymphoma

STAGE	DESCRIPTION
I	A single tumor (extranodal) or single anatomic area (nodal), with the exclusion of mediastinum or abdomen
II	A single tumor (extranodal) with regional node involvement
Two or more nodal areas on the same side of the diaphragm
Two single (extranodal) tumors with or without regional node involvement on the same side of the diaphragm
A primary gastrointestinal tract tumor, usually in the ileocecal area, with or without involvement of associated mesenteric nodes only, which must be grossly (>90%) resected
III	Two single tumors (extranodal) on opposite sides of the diaphragm
Two or more nodal areas above and below the diaphragm
Any primary intrathoracic tumor (mediastinal, pleural, or thymic)
Any extensive primary intraabdominal disease
IV	Any of the above, with initial involvement of central nervous system or bone marrow at time of diagnosis

From Murphy SB: Classification, staging and end results of treatment of childhood non-Hodgkin's lymphomas: dissimilarities from lymphomas in adults, Semin Oncol 7:332–339, 1980.

Table 496-6	Risk Stratification Groups for Pediatric B-Cell NHL	
Low Risk	Berlin-Frankfurt-Munster (BFM)	French-American-British (FAB)
	R1
Stage I or II, completely resected	**Group A**
Resected stage I and abdominal completely resected stage II
	R2
Stage I or II, not resected
Stage III with LDH <500 U/L	
	R3
Stage III with LDH ≥500 to <1000 U/L or
Stage IV with LDH <1000 U/L and CNS-negative	**Group B**
All patients not in Group A or C
	R4
Stage III or IV with LDH ≥1000 U/L and/or CNS-positive	**Group C**
Bone marrow disease (≥25% L3 blasts) and/or CNS-positive
High Risk		

CNS, central nervous system; LDH, lactate dehydrogenase.

international revision. Patients are further classified based on risk categories according to pediatric international cooperative group trials (Table 496-6). Approximately 70% of patients with NHL present with advanced disease (stage III or IV), including extranodal disease with bone marrow and central nervous system (CNS) involvement. B symptoms of fever, weight loss, and night sweats can be seen, particularly in ALCL, but are not prognostic. Capillary leak syndrome may be seen in ALK+ ALCLs.

The primary site of tumor involvement and metastasis pattern varies by pathologic subtype. LBL commonly manifests as an intrathoracic or mediastinal supradiaphragmatic mass and also has a pre-

dilection for spreading to the bone marrow and CNS. BL commonly manifests as abdominal (sporadic type) or head and neck (endemic type) tumor and can metastasize to the bone marrow or CNS. DLBCL commonly manifests as either an abdominal or mediastinal primary and, rarely, disseminates to the bone marrow or CNS. ALCL manifests either as a primary cutaneous manifestation (10%) or as systemic disease (90%) with dissemination to liver, spleen, lung, or mediastinum. Bone marrow or CNS disease is rare in ALCL. Site-specific manifestations of NHL include painless, rapid lymph node enlargement; cough or dyspnea with thoracic involvement; superior mediastinal syndrome; ascites, increased abdominal girth or intestinal obstruction with an abdominal mass; nasal congestion, earache, hearing loss, or tonsil enlargement with Waldeyer ring involvement; and localized bone pain.

NHL can present as a life-threatening oncologic emergency. These manifestations are important to recognize as they require intensive supportive care and, in some cases, alterative treatment. Superior mediastinal syndrome can occur as a consequence of a large mediastinal mass causing obstruction of blood flow or respiratory airways. Spinal cord tumors can cause cord compression and acute paraplegias requiring emergent radiation therapy. Lastly, tumor lysis syndrome (TLS) can occur from rapid cell turnover, which is especially common in BL. TLS can result in severe metabolic abnormalities including hyperuricemia, hyperphosphatemia, hyperkalemia, and hypocalcemia. This can rapidly lead to renal insufficiency/failure as well as cardiac abnormalities if not aggressively treated.

LABORATORY FINDINGS
Recommended laboratory and radiologic testing includes complete blood cell count; measurements of electrolytes, lactate dehydrogenase, uric acid, calcium, phosphorus, blood urea nitrogen, creatinine, bilirubin, alanine aminotransferase, and aspartate aminotransferase; bone marrow aspiration and biopsy; lumbar puncture with cerebrospinal fluid cytology, cell count and protein; chest radiographs; and neck, chest, abdominal, and pelvic CT scans (head CT for suspicion of CNS disease), and PET scan. Tumor tissue (i.e., biopsy, bone marrow, cerebrospinal fluid, or pleurocentesis/paracentesis fluid) should be tested by flow cytometry for immunophenotypic origin (T, B, or null) and cytogenetics (karyotype). Additional tests might include fluorescent in situ hybridization or quantitative reverse transcription polymerase chain reaction for specific genetic translocations, T- and B-cell gene rearrangement studies, and molecular profiling by oligonucleotide microarray.

TREATMENT
The primary modality of treatment for childhood and adolescent NHL is **multiagent systemic chemotherapy with intrathecal chemotherapy** (see Table 496-4). Surgery is used mainly for diagnosis. Radiation therapy is used only in special circumstances, such as CNS involvement in LBL or, in the presence of acute superior mediastinal syndrome or paraplegias. Newly diagnosed patients, especially those with BL and LBL, are at high risk for TLS. These patients require vigorous hydration, frequent electrolyte monitoring, and either a xanthine oxidase inhibitor (allopurinol, 10 mg/kg/day PO divided into 3 doses daily) or recombinant urate oxidase (rasburicase, 0.2 mg/kg/day IV once daily for up to 5 days). Recombinant urate oxidase is preferred in patients with a high risk of tumor lysis. Frequently, only a single dose is needed; however, repeat doses can be given if a subsequent rise in uric acid is seen.

Burkitt Lymphoma and Diffuse Large B-cell Lymphoma
Pediatric BL and DLBCL are treated with similar chemotherapy regimens, which are designed for mature B-NHL. Regimens vary based on stage and risk stratification. For patients with localized disease, multiagent chemotherapy is given over a 6 wk to 6 mo period and the prognosis is excellent. In the international FAB/LMB 96 (French-American-British Lymphoma, mature B cell) trial, patients with

localized, completely resected disease received 2 cycles of COPAD (cyclophosphamide, vincristine, prednisone, and doxorubicin) resulting in a 4 yr OS of 99%. Advanced disease is usually treated with a 4-6 mo regimen of multiagent chemotherapy, such as FAB/LMB 96 protocol therapy or NHL-BFM (Berlin-Frankfurt-Munich) 95 protocol therapy with an OS of 79-90%. A subset of patients that likely require a different treatment approach are those with primary mediastinal B-cell lymphoma (PMBCL). PMBCL is a histologic subtype that represents 2% of mature B-NHLs. Pediatric patients with PMBCL have an inferior outcome when treated with standard mature B-NHL protocols (EFS of only 66%). Alternative treatment strategies, including rituximab and other novel agents, may be of benefit to this group.

Rituximab is a monoclonal antibody directed at CD20 that improves outcomes in adult patients with B-NHL. As nearly all pediatric BLs and DLBCLs express CD20, rituximab has been examined in pediatric B-NHL; however, the efficacy in this setting is not yet known. A window study of rituximab given to pediatric patients with newly diagnosed BL and DLBCL demonstrated its activity as a single agent with a response rate of 41%. Additionally, a Children's Oncology Group study examined the safety and pharmacokinetics of rituximab when added to standard chemotherapy for intermediate-risk patients. Rituximab was found to be safe, and survival in this cohort was the best reported to date (3 yr OS of 95%). In a similar cohort of CNS-positive patients, the addition of rituximab to the chemotherapy backbone resulted in a 93% EFS.

Lymphoblastic Lymphoma

Localized or advanced LBL requires 12-24 mo of therapy including chemotherapy, intrathecal therapy, and cranial radiation in some cases. The best results in advanced LBL have been obtained using the NHL-BFM 90 protocol, which uses therapeutic approaches similar to those for childhood acute leukemia, including induction, consolidation, interim maintenance, and reinduction (advanced disease only) phases as well as a year-long maintenance phase with 6-mercaptopurine and methotrexate. Studies have attempted to determine whether cranial radiation can be omitted, with promising results; however, the sample size in these studies is small. For patients with relapsed disease, the outcome is poor (OS of 10%) and novel treatments are needed. Nelarabine is a purine analog with significant T-lymphocyte toxicity; nelarabine has been investigated in T-LBL. Nelarabine is currently undergoing investigation in high-risk patients with T-ALL and T-LBL.

Anaplastic Large Cell Lymphoma

For patients who present with localized disease, surgical resection alone is sufficient. The majority of patients, however, have advanced disease, which requires multiagent chemotherapy. Various chemotherapy regimens have been studied with similar outcomes and survival ranging from 70-79%. CNS prophylaxis consists of intrathecal chemotherapy; however, it may be possible to omit this with the substitution of high-dose methotrexate. CNS disease, although rare, can be seen and is treated with intrathecal chemotherapy and cranial radiation.

Two novel targeted agents have shown substantial promise in early-phase trials in ALCL. The CD30 antibody–drug conjugate brentuximab and the ALK inhibitor crizotinib both have impressive activity and minimal toxicity in patients with relapsed ALCL. Given the high efficacy and low toxicity profile, it may be possible to use these agents in newly diagnosed patients to eliminate the reliance on and toxicity of conventional chemotherapy.

Relapsed Non-Hodgkin Lymphoma

Patients with NHL in whom progressive or relapsed disease develops require reinduction chemotherapy and either allogeneic or autologous stem cell transplantation (SCT). The specific reinduction regimen or transplantation type depends on the pathologic subtype, previous therapy, site of reoccurrence, and stem cell donor availability. Although there are no randomized trials examining autologous vs allogeneic

SCT for relapsed NHL, data from retrospective studies suggest that outcomes are similar with the exception of LBL and ALCL where allogeneic SCT is superior, perhaps because of a graft-vs-lymphoma effect.

As relapsed NHL can be difficult to treat, efforts have been made to identify those patients at higher risk of relapse to tailor the initial therapy. The measurement of minimal residual disease may serve as a prognostic marker and aid in risk stratification. Minimal residual disease is prognostic in ALCL and LBL. In ALCL, there is also evidence that a humoral response to the ALK kinase can be used to predict outcome with a superior outcome in patients who mount an antibody titer to ALK. Minimal residual disease measurement in intermediate-risk B-NHL is feasible and is currently being evaluated in an international trial.

COMPLICATIONS

Patients receiving multiagent chemotherapy for advanced disease are at acute risk for serious mucositis, infections, cytopenias that require red blood cell and platelet blood product transfusions, electrolyte imbalances, and poor nutrition. Long-term complications include the risk of growth retardation, cardiac toxicity, gonadal toxicity with infertility, and secondary malignancies.

PROGNOSIS

The prognosis is excellent for most forms of childhood and adolescent NHL (see Table 496-4). Patients with localized disease have a 90-100% chance of survival, and those with advanced disease have a 70-95% chance of survival. As outcomes for pediatric patients with NHL have improved substantially, the focus has now shifted to minimizing the long-term toxicity of therapy. Novel targeted agents are desirable as they have the potential to improve outcomes and decrease the reliance on toxic conventional chemotherapy.

Bibliography is available at Expert Consult.

496.3 Late Effects in Children and Adolescents with Lymphoma

Jessica Hochberg, Lisa Giulino-Roth, and Mitchell S. Cairo

The majority of patients with newly diagnosed HL and NHL have OS rates above 90%. There are approximately 270,000 survivors of childhood cancer in the United States, which equates to about 1 of every 640 adults between the ages of 20 and 40 yr. However, this survival has often been achieved at the expense of an increased relative risk of long-term complications, including solid tumors, leukemia, cardiac disease, pulmonary complications, thyroid disease, and infertility. An analysis of more than 1,000 long-term childhood NHL survivors found increased rates of death >20 yr after treatment. A review of Surveillance, Epidemiology and End Results data over a 25 yr follow-up period demonstrates that the relative survival curves do not plateau after 10 yr following diagnosis of HL but, rather, accelerate. This finding highlights the importance of late morbidity and mortality among survivors of lymphoma. The first Childhood Cancer Survivor Study, a retrospective cohort study of 10,397 cancer survivors, shows that 62.3% of survivors report at least 1 chronic condition, with 27.5% reporting severe or life-threatening conditions. The survivor's adjusted relative risk of a severe or life-threatening chronic condition, compared with that of a sibling, was 8.2 (95% confidence interval, 6.9-9.7). When disease-specific health outcomes were looked at, both HL and NHL were found to be associated with a cumulative incidence of chronic health conditions approaching 70-80%, with severe conditions being reported in close to 50% of HL survivors (Fig. 496-6).

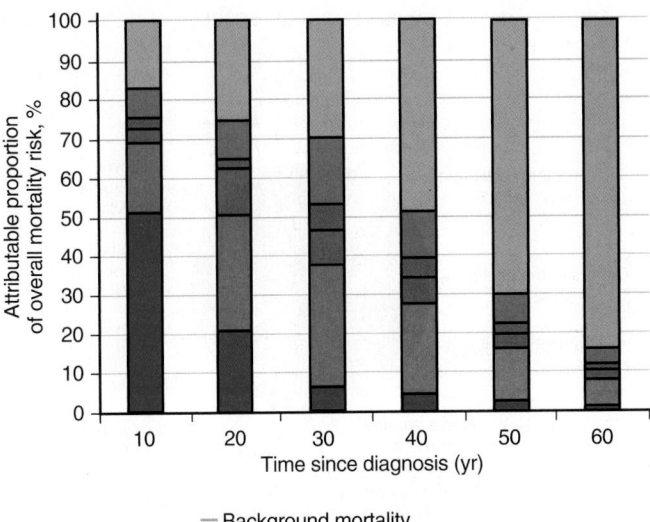

Figure 496-6 Percentage of attributable proportions of overall mortality risk in survivors of childhood cancer. *(Adapted from Yeh JM, Nekhlyudov L, Goldie SJ, et al: A model-based estimate of cumulative excess mortality in survivors of childhood cancer, Ann Intern Med 152[7]:409–417, 2010.)*

Chapter 497
Brain Tumors in Childhood
Joann L. Ater and John F. Kuttesch Jr.

Primary central nervous system (CNS) tumors are a heterogeneous group of diseases that are, collectively, the second most common malignancy in childhood and adolescence. The overall mortality among this group approaches 30%. Patients with CNS tumors have the highest morbidity—primarily neurologic—of all children with malignancies. Outcomes have improved over time with innovations in neurosurgery and radiation therapy as well as the introduction of chemotherapy as a therapeutic modality. The treatment approach for these tumors is multimodal. Surgery with complete resection, if feasible, is the foundation, with radiation therapy and chemotherapy utilized according to the diagnosis, patient age, and other factors.

ETIOLOGY
The etiology of pediatric brain tumors is not well defined. A male predominance is noted in the incidence of medulloblastoma and ependymoma. Familial and hereditary syndromes associated with an increased incidence of brain tumors account for approximately 5% of cases (Table 497-1). Cranial exposure to ionizing radiation also is associated with a higher incidence of brain tumors. There are sporadic reports of brain tumors within families without evidence of a heritable syndrome. The molecular events associated with tumorigenesis of pediatric brain tumors are not known.

EPIDEMIOLOGY
Approximately 4,600 primary brain tumors are diagnosed each year in children and adolescents in the United States, with an overall annual incidence of approximately 47 cases/1 million children younger than

20 yr of age. The incidence of CNS tumors is highest in infants and children 5 yr of age or younger (approximately 52 cases/1 million children).

PATHOGENESIS
More than 100 histologic categories and subtypes of primary brain tumors are described in the World Health Organization (WHO) classification of tumors of the CNS. In children 0-14 yr of age, the most common tumors are pilocytic astrocytomas (PAs) and medulloblastoma/primitive neuroectodermal tumors (PNETs). In adolescents (15-19 yr), the most common tumors are pituitary tumors and PAs (Fig. 497-1).

The Surveillance, Epidemiology, and End Results program reported a slight predominance of infratentorial tumor location (43.2%), followed by the supratentorial region (40.9%), spinal cord (4.9%), and multiple sites (11%) (Fig. 497-2, Table 497-2). There are age-related differences in primary location of tumor. During the 1st yr of life, supratentorial tumors predominate and include, most commonly, choroid plexus complex tumors and teratomas. In children 1-10 yr of age, infratentorial tumors predominate, owing to the high incidence of juvenile PA and medulloblastoma. After 10 yr of age, supratentorial tumors again predominate, with diffuse astrocytomas most common. Tumors of the optic pathway and hypothalamus region, the brainstem, and the pineal–midbrain region are more common in children and adolescents than in adults.

CLINICAL MANIFESTATIONS
The clinical presentation of the patient with a brain tumor depends on the tumor location, the tumor type, and the age of the child. Signs and symptoms are related to obstruction of cerebrospinal fluid (CSF) drainage paths by the tumor, leading to **increased intracranial pressure (ICP)** or causing focal brain dysfunction. Subtle changes in personality, mentation, and speech may precede these classic signs and symptoms; such changes often occur with supratentorial (cortical) lesions. In young children, the diagnosis of a brain tumor may be delayed because the symptoms are similar to those of more common illnesses, such as gastrointestinal disorders, with associated vomiting. Infants with open cranial sutures may present with signs of increased ICP, such as vomiting, lethargy, and irritability, as well as the later finding of macrocephaly. The **classic triad** of headache, nausea, and vomiting as well as papilledema is associated with midline or infratentorial tumors. Disorders of equilibrium, gait, and coordination occur with infratentorial tumors. **Torticollis** may occur in cases of cerebellar tonsil herniation. Blurred vision, diplopia, and nystagmus also are associated with infratentorial tumors. Tumors of the brainstem region may be associated with gaze palsy, multiple cranial nerve palsies, and upper motor neuron deficits (e.g., hemiparesis, hyperreflexia, clonus). **Supratentorial tumors** are more commonly associated with lateralized deficits, such as focal motor weakness, focal sensory changes, language disorders, focal seizures, and reflex asymmetry. Infants with supratentorial tumors may present with premature hand preference. Optic pathway tumors manifest as visual and/or afferent oculomotor disturbances, such as decreased visual acuity, Marcus Gunn pupil (afferent pupillary defect), nystagmus, and/or visual field defects. Suprasellar region tumors and third ventricular region tumors may manifest initially as **neuroendocrine deficits,** such as subacute development of obesity, abnormal linear growth velocity, diabetes insipidus, galactorrhea, precocious puberty, delayed puberty, and hypothyroidism. In fact, signs of endocrine dysfunction preceded symptoms of neuroophthalmologic dysfunction by an average of 1.9 yr, and their recognition as a possible sign of hypothalamic or pituitary neoplasm can hasten diagnosis and improve outcome. The **diencephalic syndrome,** which manifests as failure to thrive, emaciation despite normal caloric intake, and inappropriately normal or happy affect, occurs in infants and young children with tumors in these regions. **Parinaud syndrome** is seen with pineal region tumors and is manifested by paresis of upward gaze, pupillary caliber reactive to accommodation but not to light (pseudo-Argyll Robertson pupil), nystagmus to convergence or retraction, and eyelid retraction. Spinal cord tumors and spinal cord dissemination of brain tumors may manifest as long nerve tract motor and/or sensory

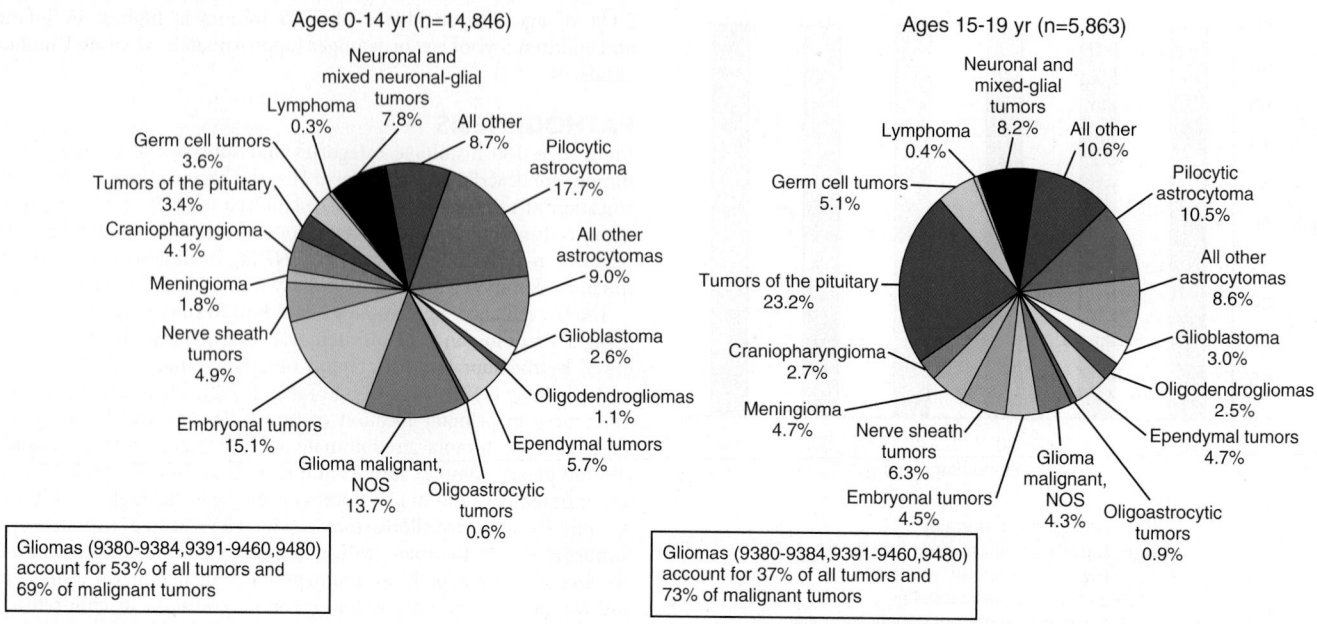

Figure 497-1 Distribution of childhood primary brain and CNS tumors by histology. *(From Dolecek TA, Propp JM, Stroup NE, Kruchko C: CBTRUS statistical report: primary brain and central nervous system tumors diagnosed in the United States in 2005-2009, Neuro Oncol 14:v1-v49, 2012.)*

Table 497-1	Familial Syndromes Associated with Pediatric Brain Tumors		
SYNDROME	**CENTRAL NERVOUS SYSTEM MANIFESTATIONS**	**CHROMOSOME**	**GENE**
Neurofibromatosis type 1 (autosomal dominant)	Optic pathway gliomas, astrocytoma, malignant peripheral nerve sheath tumors, neurofibromas	17q11	*NF1*
Neurofibromatosis type 2 (autosomal dominant)	Vestibular schwannomas, meningiomas, spinal cord ependymoma, spinal cord astrocytoma, hamartomas	22q12	*NF2*
von Hippel–Lindau (autosomal dominant)	Hemangioblastoma	3p25-26	*VHL*
Tuberous sclerosis (autosomal dominant)	Subependymal giant cell astrocytoma, cortical tubers	9q34 16q13	*TSC1* *TSC2*
Li-Fraumeni (autosomal dominant)	Astrocytoma, primitive neuroectodermal tumor	17q13	*TP53*
Cowden (autosomal dominant)	Dysplastic gangliocytoma of the cerebellum (Lhermitte-Duclos disease)	10q23	*PTEN*
Turcot (autosomal dominant)	Medulloblastoma Glioblastoma	5q21 3p21 7p22	*APC* *hMLH1* *hPSM2*
Nevoid basal cell carcinoma Gorlin (autosomal dominant)	Medulloblastoma	9q31	*PTCH1*

Modified from Kleihues P, Cavenee WK: World Health Organization classification of tumors: pathology and genetics of tumors of the nervous system, Lyon, 2000, IARC Press.

deficits often localized to below a specific spinal level, bowel and bladder deficits, and back or radicular pain. The signs and symptoms of meningeal metastatic disease from brain tumors or leukemia include head or back pain and symptoms referable to compression of cranial nerves or spinal nerve roots.

DIAGNOSIS

The evaluation of a patient in whom a brain tumor is suspected is an emergency. Initial evaluation should include a complete history, physical (including ophthalmic) examination, and neurologic assessment with neuroimaging. For primary brain tumors, **MRI** with and without gadolinium is the neuroimaging standard. Tumors in the pituitary/suprasellar region, optic path, and infratentorium are better delineated with MRI than with CT. Patients with tumors of the midline and the

pituitary/suprasellar/optic chiasmal region should undergo evaluation for **neuroendocrine dysfunction.** Formal ophthalmologic examination is beneficial in patients with optic path region tumors to document the impact of the disease on oculomotor function, visual acuity, and fields of vision. The suprasellar and pineal regions are preferential sites for germ cell tumors (Fig. 497-3). Both serum and CSF measurements of **β-human chorionic gonadotropin** and **α-fetoprotein** can assist in the diagnosis of germ cell tumors. In tumors with a propensity for spreading to the leptomeninges, such as medulloblastoma/PNET, ependymoma, and germ cell tumors, lumbar puncture with cytologic analysis of the CSF is indicated; lumbar puncture is contraindicated in individuals with newly diagnosed hydrocephalus secondary to CSF flow obstruction, in tumors that cause supratentorial midline shift, and in individuals with infratentorial tumors. Lumbar puncture in these individuals may lead to brain herniation, resulting in neurologic compromise and death. Therefore, in children with newly diagnosed intracranial tumors and signs of increased ICP, the lumbar puncture usually is delayed until surgery or shunt placement.

SPECIFIC TUMORS
Astrocytomas

Astrocytomas are a heterogeneous group of tumors that account for approximately 40% of pediatric CNS malignancies. These tumors occur throughout the CNS.

Low-grade astrocytomas (LGAs), the predominant group of astrocytomas in childhood, are characterized by an indolent clinical course. **PA** is the most common astrocytoma in children, accounting for approximately 20% of all brain tumors. On the basis of clinicopathologic features using the WHO Classification System, PA is classified as

a WHO grade I tumor. Although PA can occur anywhere in the CNS, the classic site is the **cerebellum** (Fig. 497-4A). Other common sites include the hypothalamic/third ventricular region and the optic nerve and chiasmal region (Fig. 497-4B). The classic but not exclusive neuroradiologic finding in PA is the presence of a contrast medium–enhancing nodule within the wall of a cystic mass (Fig. 497-4A). The microscopic findings include the biphasic appearance of bundles of compact fibrillary tissue interspersed with loose microcystic, spongy areas. The presence of **Rosenthal fibers,** which are condensed masses of glial filaments occurring in the compact areas, helps establish the diagnosis. PA has a low metastatic potential and is rarely invasive. A

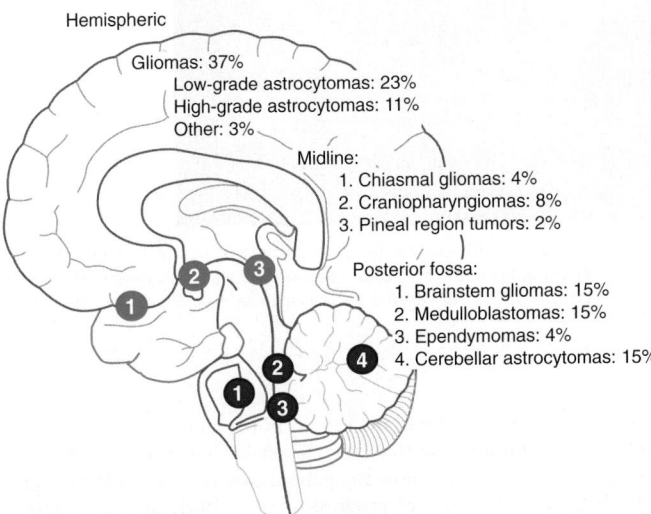

Figure 497-2 Childhood brain tumors occur at any location within the central nervous system. The relative frequency of brain tumor histologic types and the anatomic distribution are shown. (*Redrawn from Albright AL: Pediatric brain tumors, CA Cancer J Clin 43:272–288, 1993.*)

Labels in figure:
Hemispheric
Gliomas: 37%
 Low-grade astrocytomas: 23%
 High-grade astrocytomas: 11%
 Other: 3%
Midline:
 1. Chiasmal gliomas: 4%
 2. Craniopharyngiomas: 8%
 3. Pineal region tumors: 2%
Posterior fossa:
 1. Brainstem gliomas: 15%
 2. Medulloblastomas: 15%
 3. Ependymomas: 4%
 4. Cerebellar astrocytomas: 15%

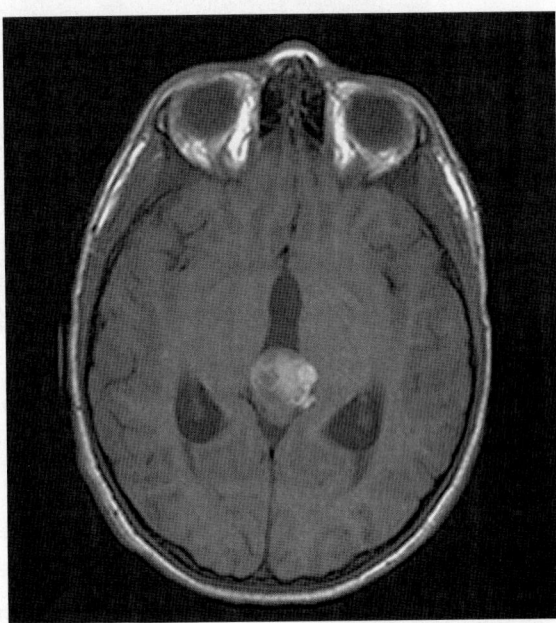

Figure 497-3 Axillary T1-weighted MR image with gadolinium of a 10 yr old boy presenting with mixed germ cell tumor of the pineal region, with early onset of puberty, headaches, and elevated α-fetoprotein and β–human chorionic gonadotropin in the spinal fluid and serum.

Table 497-2	Posterior Fossa Tumors of Childhood			
TUMOR	**RELATIVE INCIDENCE (%)**	**PRESENTATION**	**DIAGNOSIS**	**PROGNOSIS**
Medulloblastoma	35-40	2-3 mo of headaches, vomiting, truncal ataxia	Heterogeneously or homogeneously enhancing fourth ventricular mass; may be disseminated	65-85% survival; dependent on stage/type; poorer (20-70%) in infants
Cerebellar astrocytoma	35-40	3-6 mo of limb ataxia; secondary headaches, vomiting	Cerebellar hemisphere mass, usually with cystic and solid (mural nodule) components	90-100% survival in totally resected pilocytic type
Brainstem glioma	10-15	1-4 mo of double vision, unsteadiness, weakness, and cranial nerve dysfunction, including facial weakness, swallowing dysfunction, and oculomotor abnormalities	Diffusely expanded, minimally or partially enhancing mass in 80%; 20% more focal tectal or cervicomedullary lesion	>90% mortality in diffuse tumors; better in localized
Ependymoma	10-15	2-5 mo of unsteadiness, headaches, double vision, and facial asymmetry	Usually enhancing, fourth ventricular mass with cerebellopontine predilection	>75% survival in totally resected lesions
Atypical teratoid/ rhabdoid	>5 (10-15% of infantile malignant tumors)	As in medulloblastoma, but primarily in infants; often associated facial weakness and strabismus	As in medulloblastoma, but often more laterally extended	≤20% survival in infants

Modified from Packer RJ, MacDonald T, Vezina G: Central nervous system tumors, Pediatr Clin North Am 55:121–145, 2008.

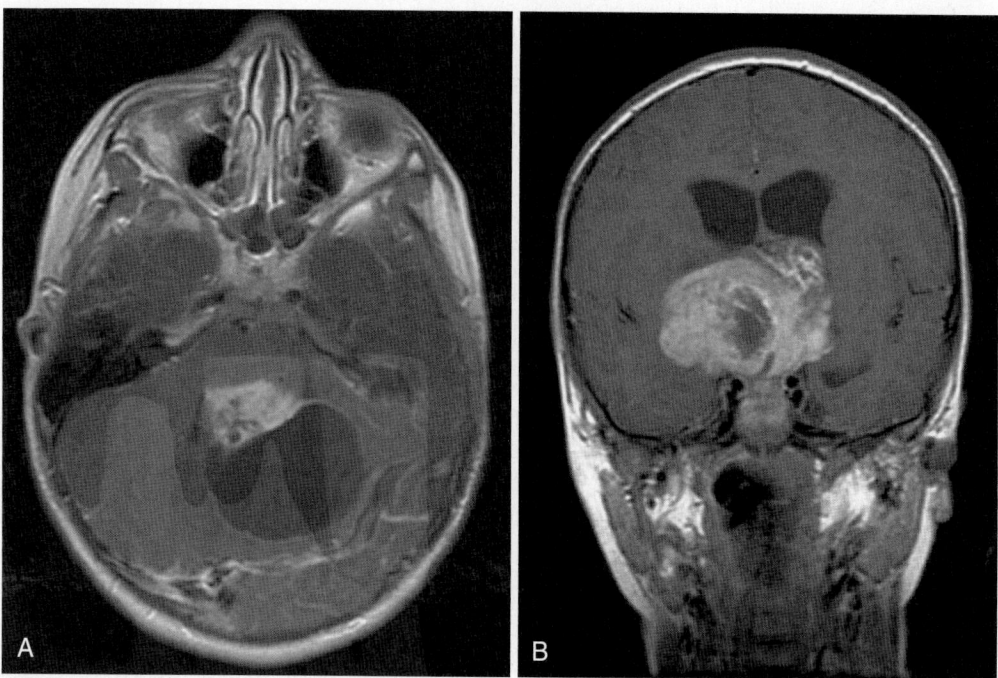

Figure 497-4 A, Gadolinium-enhanced axial T1-weighted MR image in a 4 yr old child with cerebellar pilocytic astrocytoma presenting with headaches, emesis, and ataxia demonstrates a predominantly cystic mass with enhancement of the solid component and enhancement of the capsule. **B,** Gadolinium-enhanced coronal view of a cystic juvenile pilocytic astrocytoma of the suprasellar region from a 4 yr old child presenting with visual loss and headaches.

small proportion of these tumors can progress and develop lepto-meningeal spread, particularly when they occur in the optic path region. A PA very rarely undergoes malignant transformation to a more aggressive tumor. A PA of the optic nerve and chiasmal region is a relatively common finding in patients with neurofibromatosis type 1 (15% incidence). Unlike in diffuse fibrillary astrocytomas, there are no characteristic cytogenetic abnormalities in PA. Other tumors occurring in the pediatric age group with clinicopathologic characteristics similar to those of PA include pleomorphic xanthoastrocytoma, desmoplastic cerebral astrocytoma of infancy, and subependymal giant cell astrocytoma.

The second most common astrocytoma is **fibrillary infiltrating astrocytoma,** which consists of a group of tumors characterized by a pattern of diffuse infiltration of tumor cells amidst normal neural tissue and potential for anaplastic progression. On the basis of their clinico-pathologic characteristics, they are grouped as LGAs (WHO grade II), malignant astrocytomas (anaplastic astrocytoma; WHO grade III), and glioblastoma multiforme (WHO grade IV). Fibrillary LGA accounts for 15% of brain tumors. Histologically, these low-grade tumors demonstrate greater cellularity than normal brain parenchyma, with few mitotic figures, nuclear pleomorphism, and microcysts. The characteristic MRI finding is a lack of enhancement after contrast agent infusion. Molecular genetic abnormalities found among low-grade diffuse infiltrating astrocytomas include mutations of *P53* and overexpression of platelet-derived growth factor α-chain and platelet-derived growth factor receptor-α. **Evolution of fibrillary infiltrating astrocytoma** into malignant astrocytoma is associated with cumulative acquisition of multiple molecular abnormalities.

Pilomyxoid astrocytoma occurs most commonly in the hypothalamic/optic chiasmic region and carries a high risk of local as well as cerebrospinal spread. This astrocytoma affects young children and infants. It is classified as a WHO grade II tumor.

The **clinical management** of LGAs focuses on a multimodal approach incorporating surgery as the primary treatment as well as radiation therapy and chemotherapy. With complete surgical resection the overall survival approaches 80-100%. In patients with partial resection (<80% resection), overall survival varies from 50-95%, depending

on the anatomic location of the tumor. In the patient who has undergone partial tumor resection and has stable neurologic status, the current approach is to follow the patient closely by examination and imaging. With evidence of progression, a second surgical resection should be considered. In patients in whom a second procedure was less than complete or is not feasible, radiation therapy is beneficial. Radiation therapy is delivered to the tumor bed at a total cumulative dose ranging from 50-55 Gy given on a daily schedule over 6 wk. Historically, patients with deep midline tumors have been treated empirically with radiation therapy and without surgery or biopsy, with variable survival rates from 33-75%. Modern surgical techniques and innovative radiation therapy methodology, including proton-beam radiation, may have a positive impact on the survival and clinical outcome of these patients. The role of chemotherapy in the management of LGAs is evolving. Because of concerns regarding morbidity from radiation therapy in young children, several chemotherapy approaches have been evaluated, especially in children younger than 10 yr of age. Complete response to chemotherapy is uncommon; however, these approaches have yielded durable control of disease in 70-100% of patients. Patients with midline tumors in the hypothalamic/optic chiasmatic region (see Fig. 497-4B) have tended to do less well. Taken together, the chemotherapy approaches have permitted delay and, potentially, avoidance of radiation therapy. Chemotherapy agents given singly or in combination for LGA include carboplatin, vincristine, lomustine, procarbazine, temozolomide, and vinblastine. Observation is the primary approach in clinical management of selected patients with LGAs that are biologically indolent. One such group includes patients with neurofibromatosis type 1, in whom an LGA of the optic chiasm/optic pathway or brainstem may be found incidentally. Another group includes patients with midbrain astrocytoma who have resolution of clinical symptoms after ventricular shunting and do not require further intervention. Astrocytomas associated with tuberous sclerosis have responded to everolimus, a mammalian target of rapamycin inhibitor.

Malignant astrocytomas are much less common in children and adolescents than in adults, accounting for 7-10% of all childhood tumors. Among this group, **anaplastic astrocytoma** (WHO grade III,

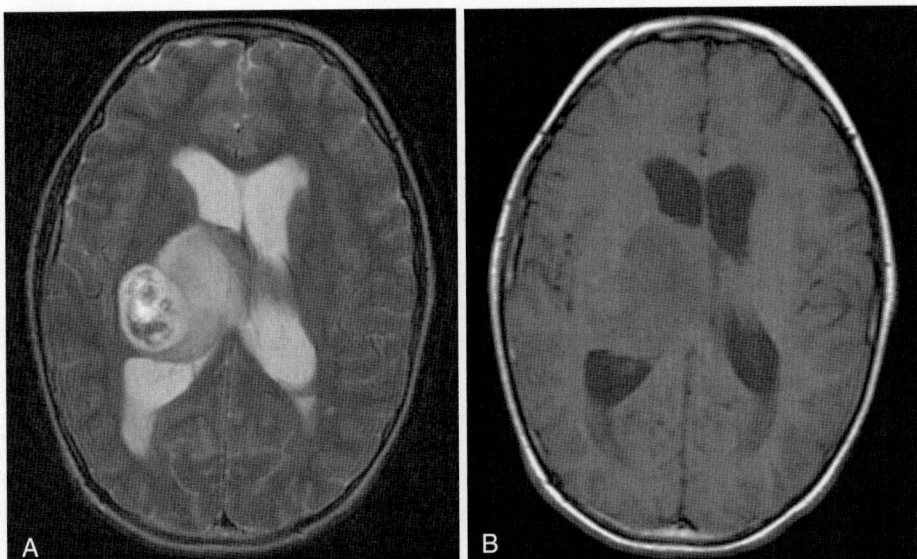

Figure 497-5 A, Nonenhanced axial T2-weighted MR image of grade III astrocytoma of the right thalamus demonstrating diffuse hyperintensity and area of necrotic cyst formation. **B,** Gadolinium-enhanced sagittal T1-weighted MR image showing slight enhancement and hypodensity of grade III astrocytoma of the thalamus. This 14 yr old child presented with left arm and leg numbness and weakness and right-sided headaches.

Fig. 497-5) is more common than **glioblastoma multiforme** (WHO grade IV). The histopathology of anaplastic astrocytomas demonstrates greater cellularity than that of low-grade diffuse astrocytomas, with cellular and nuclear atypia, presence of mitoses, and, variably, microvascular proliferation. Characteristic histopathologic findings in glioblastoma multiforme include dense cellularity, high mitotic index, microvascular proliferation, and foci of tumor necrosis. Limited information is available regarding the molecular abnormalities in malignant astrocytomas in children. Overexpression of *P53* in malignant astrocytoma in a child is an adverse prognostic factor. The frequency of mutations in *P53* and of the loss of heterozygosity at 19q and 22q in childhood malignant astrocytomas are similar to that noted in adults, although the frequency of such mutations in malignant astrocytomas of children younger than 3 yr of age is lower. This finding suggests differing mechanisms of oncogenesis in younger and older children, respectively. Optimal therapeutic approaches for malignant astrocytomas have yet to be defined. Standard therapy continues to be surgical resection followed by involved-field radiation therapy. A study of adult glioblastoma showed significantly better survival with temozolomide during and after irradiation than with irradiation alone. Current therapeutic approaches incorporate novel chemotherapeutic agents with radiation therapy. Enrollment in a clinical trial may be the best therapeutic option in these tumors where standard therapy is suboptimal.

Oligodendrogliomas are uncommon tumors of childhood. These infiltrating tumors occur predominantly in the cerebral cortex and originate in the white matter. Histologically, oligodendrogliomas consist of rounded cells with little cytoplasm and microcalcifications. Observation of a **calcified cortical mass** on CT in a patient presenting with a seizure is suggestive of oligodendroglioma. Treatment approaches are similar to those for infiltrating astrocytomas.

Ependymal Tumors

Ependymal tumors are derived from the ependymal lining of the ventricular system. Ependymoma (WHO grade II) is the most common of these neoplasms, occurring predominantly in childhood and accounting for 10% of childhood tumors. Approximately 70% of ependymomas in childhood occur in the posterior fossa. The mean age of patients is 6 yr, with approximately 40% of cases occurring in children younger than 4 yr of age. The incidence of leptomeningeal spread approaches 10% overall. Clinical presentation can be insidious and often depends on the anatomic location of the tumor. MRI demon-

strates a well-circumscribed tumor with variable and complex patterns of gadolinium enhancement, with or without cystic structures (Fig. 497-6). These tumors usually are noninvasive, extending into the ventricular lumen and/or displacing normal structures, sometimes leading to significant obstructive hydrocephalus. Histologic characteristics include perivascular pseudorosettes, ependymal rosettes, monomorphic nuclear morphology, and occasional nonpalisading foci of necrosis. Other histologic subtypes include anaplastic ependymoma (WHO grade III), which is much less common in childhood and is characterized by a high mitotic index and histologic features of microvascular proliferation and pseudopalisading necrosis. Myxopapillary ependymoma (WHO grade I) is a slow-growing tumor arising from the filum terminale and conus medullaris and appears to be a biologically different subtype. There are no well-defined characteristic cytogenetic or molecular genetic alterations in ependymoma, largely owing to their heterogeneous nature, although association of various genotypes with susceptibility to ependymoma have been implicated. Preliminary studies suggest that there are genetically distinct subtypes of ependymoma, exemplified by an association between alterations in the *NF2* gene and spinal ependymoma. Surgery is the primary treatment modality, with extent of surgical resection a major prognostic factor. Two other major prognostic factors are age, with younger children having poorer outcomes, and tumor location, with localization in the posterior fossa, which often is seen in young children, associated with poorer outcomes. Surgery alone is rarely curative. Multimodal therapy incorporating irradiation with surgery has resulted in long-term survival in approximately 40% of patients with ependymoma undergoing gross total resection. Recurrence is predominantly local. Ependymoma is sensitive to a spectrum of chemotherapeutic agents; the role of chemotherapy in multimodal therapy of ependymoma is still unclear. Current investigations are directed toward identification of optimal radiation dose, surgical questions addressing the use of second-look procedures after chemotherapy, and further evaluation of classic as well as novel chemotherapeutic agents.

Choroid Plexus Tumors

Choroid plexus tumors account for 2-4% of childhood CNS tumors. They are the most common CNS tumor in children younger than 1 yr of age and account for 10-20% of CNS tumors in infants. These tumors are intraventricular epithelial neoplasms arising from the choroid plexus. Children present with signs and symptoms of increased ICP.

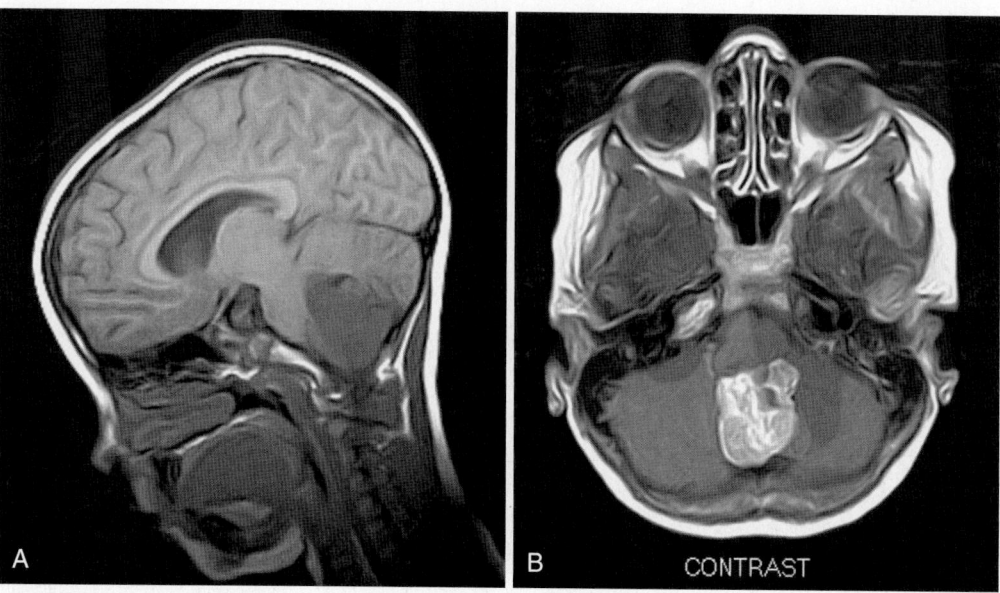

Figure 497-6 A, Sagittal T1-weighted MR image of a 6 yr old patient with ependymoma, demonstrating a hypointense mass within the fourth ventricle compressing the brainstem. **B,** Gadolinium-enhanced axial T1-weighted image of an ependymoma showing an enhancing mass within the fourth ventricle.

Infants may present with macrocephaly and focal neurologic deficits. In children, these tumors predominantly occur supratentorially in the lateral ventricles. **Choroid plexus papilloma** (WHO grade I), the most common of this group, is a well-circumscribed lesion on neuroimaging and closely resembles normal choroid plexus histologically. **Choroid plexus carcinoma** (WHO grade III) is a malignant tumor with metastatic potential to seed into the CSF pathways. This malignancy has the following histologic characteristics: nuclear pleomorphism, high mitotic index, and increased cell density. Immunopositivity for transthyretin (prealbumin) is useful in confirming the diagnosis of choroid plexus tumors. These tumors are associated with the **Li-Fraumeni syndrome. Simian virus 40** may also play an etiologic role in choroid plexus tumors. After complete surgical resection, the frequency of cure for choroid plexus papilloma approaches 100%, whereas the frequency of cure for choroid plexus carcinoma approaches 20-40%. Reports suggest that radiation therapy and/or chemotherapy may lead to better disease control for choroid plexus carcinoma.

Embryonal Tumors
Embryonal tumors or **PNETs** are the most common group of *malignant* CNS tumors of childhood, accounting for approximately 20% of pediatric CNS tumors. They have the potential to metastasize to the neuraxis and beyond. The group includes medulloblastoma, supratentorial PNET, ependymoblastoma, medulloepithelioblastoma, and atypical teratoid/rhabdoid tumor, all of which are histologically classified as WHO grade IV tumors.

Medulloblastoma, which accounts for 90% of embryonal CNS tumors, is a cerebellar tumor occurring predominantly in males and at a median age of 5-7 yr. Most of these tumors occur in the midline cerebellar vermis; however, older patients may present with tumors in the cerebellar hemisphere. CT and MRI demonstrate a solid, homogeneous, contrast medium–enhancing mass in the posterior fossa causing fourth ventricular obstruction and hydrocephalus (Fig. 497-7). Up to 30% of patients with medulloblastoma present with neuroimaging evidence of leptomeningeal spread. Among a variety of diverse histologic patterns of this tumor, the most common is a monomorphic sheet of undifferentiated cells classically noted as small, blue, round cells. Neuronal differentiation is more common among these tumors and is characterized histologically by the presence of Homer Wright rosettes and by immunopositivity for synaptophysin. An anaplastic variant is often more aggressive and may be associated with worse prognosis.

Patients present with signs and symptoms of increased ICP (i.e., headache, nausea, vomiting, mental status changes, and hypertension) and cerebellar dysfunction (i.e., ataxia, poor balance, dysmetria). Standard clinical staging evaluation includes MRI of the brain and spine, both preoperatively and postoperatively, as well as lumbar puncture after the increased ICP has resolved. The Chang staging system, originally based on surgical information, has been modified to incorporate information from neuroimaging to identify risk categories. Clinical features that have consistently demonstrated prognostic significance include age at diagnosis, extent of disease, and extent of surgical resection. Patients younger than 4 yr of age have a poor outcome, partly as the result of a higher incidence of disseminated disease on presentation and past therapeutic approaches that have used less intense therapies. Patients with disseminated disease at diagnosis (M >0), including positive CSF cytologic result alone (M1), have a markedly worse outcome than those patients with no dissemination (M0). Similarly, patients with gross residual disease after surgery have worse outcomes than those in whom surgery achieved gross total resection of disease.

Cytogenetic and molecular genetic studies have demonstrated multiple abnormalities in medulloblastoma. The most common abnormality involves chromosome 17p deletions, which occur in 30-40% of all cases. These deletions are not associated with *P53* mutations. Several signaling pathways have been shown to be active in medulloblastomas, including the sonic hedgehog (SHH) pathway, predominately associated with the desmoplastic variants, and the WNT pathway, which can occur in up to 15% of cases and has been associated with improved survival. Integrative genomic studies have recently identified at least 4 distinct molecular subgroups of medulloblastoma—WNT, SHH, group 3, and group 4—which exhibit highly discriminate transcriptional, cytogenetic, and mutational spectra, in addition to divergent patient demographics and clinical behavior. These prognostic groups still must be validated in larger prospective studies. With the evolution of gene array technology, preliminary studies have identified clusters of genes/ gene expression that appear to be associated with metastatic medulloblastoma and outcome.

A multimodal treatment approach is pursued in medulloblastoma, with surgery as the starting point of treatment. Medulloblastoma is sensitive to both chemotherapy and radiation therapy. With technologic advances in neurosurgery, neuroradiology, and radiation therapy, as well as identification of chemotherapy as an effective modality, the overall outcome among all patients approaches 60-70%. Standard

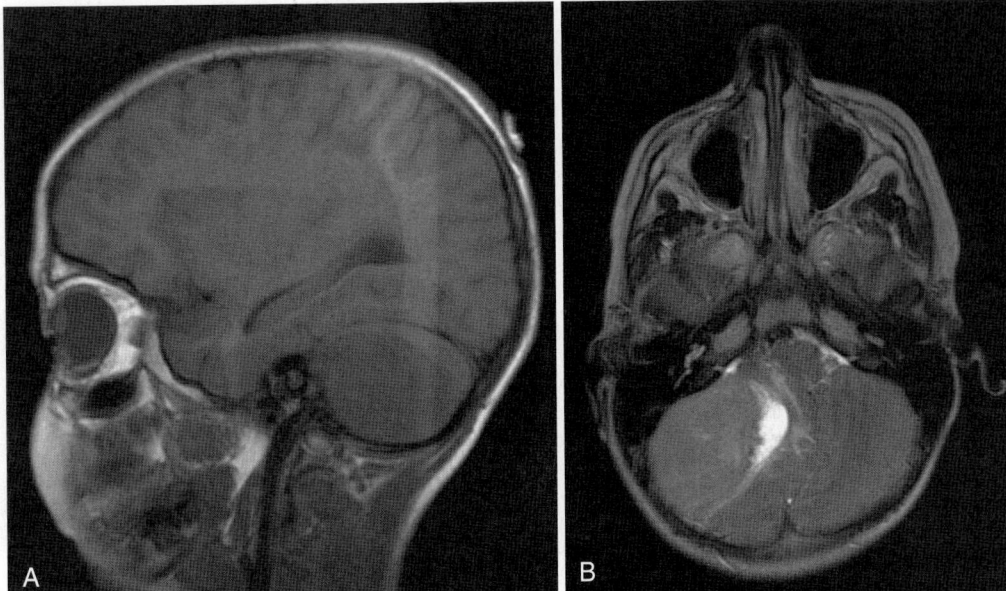

Figure 497-7 A, Sagittal T1-weighted MR image shows hypointense mass involving the cerebellar hemisphere in a 6 yr old child with desmoplastic variant of medulloblastoma. **B,** Axial T2-weighted image of the same child shows hyperintense mass involving the cerebellar hemisphere.

radiation treatment in standard risk medulloblastoma incorporates craniospinal radiation at a total cumulative dose of 24 Gy, with a cumulative dose of 50-55 Gy to the tumor bed. Craniospinal radiation at this dose in children younger than 3 yr of age results in severe late neurologic sequelae, including microcephaly, learning disabilities, cognitive impairment, neuroendocrine dysfunction (growth failure, hypothyroidism, hypogonadism, and absence/delay of puberty), and/or second malignancies. Similarly, in older children, late sequelae, such as learning disabilities, neuroendocrine dysfunction, and/or second malignancies, can occur. These observations have resulted in stratification of treatment approaches into the following 3 strata: (1) patients younger than 3 yr of age; (2) standard-risk patients older than 3 yr of age with surgical total resection and no disease dissemination (M0); and (3) high-risk patients older than 3 yr of age with disease dissemination (M >0) and/or bulky residual disease after surgery. With the risk-based approach to treatment, children with high-risk medulloblastoma receive high-dose cranial–spinal radiation (36 Gy) with chemotherapy during and after radiation therapy, and those with standard-risk (nonmetastatic) disease receive lower-dose craniospinal radiation (24 Gy) with chemotherapy during and after radiation therapy. Because the dose of radiation depends on the risk stratification, complete staging with MRI of the spine before starting treatment is essential for the best chance of survival. Approaches in young children (younger than 4 yr of age) incorporate high-dose chemotherapy with peripheral stem cell reinfusion and exclude radiation therapy. Overall survival in children with nonmetastatic medulloblastoma and gross total tumor resection approaches 85%. The presence of bulky residual tumor (56% survival) or metastases (38% survival) confers a poor prognosis.

Supratentorial primitive neuroectodermal tumors (SPNETs) account for 2-3% of childhood brain tumors, primarily in children within the 1st decade of life. These tumors are similar histologically to medulloblastoma and are composed of undifferentiated or poorly differentiated neuroepithelial cells. Historically, patients with SPNETs have had poorer outcomes than those with medulloblastoma after combined-modality therapy. In current clinical trials, children with SPNETs are considered among the high-risk group and receive dose-intense chemotherapy with craniospinal radiation therapy.

Atypical teratoid/rhabdoid tumor is a very aggressive embryonal malignancy that occurs predominantly in children younger than 5 yr of age and can occur at any location in the neuraxis. The histology demonstrates a heterogeneous pattern of cells, including rhabdoid cells that express epithelial membrane antigen and neurofilament antigen. The characteristic cytogenetic pattern is partial or complete deletion of chromosome 22q11.2 that is associated with mutation in the *INI1* gene. The relation between this mutation and tumorigenesis is unclear. Outcome after combined-modality therapy with intensive chemotherapy is very poor and there is no standard chemotherapy. However, long-term survival is reported for some children, primarily with complete resection and focal radiotherapy.

Pineal Parenchymal Tumors

The pineal parenchymal tumors are the most common malignancies after germ cell tumors that occur in the pineal region. These include pineoblastoma, occurring predominantly in childhood, pineocytoma, and the mixed pineal parenchymal tumors. The therapeutic approach in this group of diseases is multimodal. There was significant concern regarding the location of these masses and the potential complications of surgical intervention. With developments in neurosurgical technique and surgical technology, the morbidity and mortality associated with these approaches have markedly decreased. Stereotactic biopsy of these tumors may be adequate to establish diagnosis; however, consideration should be given to total resection of the lesion before institution of additional therapy. Pineoblastoma, the more malignant variant, is considered a subgroup of childhood PNETs. Chemotherapy regimens incorporate cisplatin, cyclophosphamide (Cytoxan), etoposide (VP-16), and vincristine and/or lomustine. Data have shown that survival outcome of combined chemotherapy and radiation therapy in pineal-region PNETs approaches 70% at 5 yr, similar to that noted for medulloblastoma. Pineocytoma usually is approached with surgical resection.

Craniopharyngioma

Craniopharyngioma (WHO grade I) is a common tumor of childhood, accounting for 7-10% of all childhood tumors. The adamantinomatous variant of craniopharyngioma predominates in childhood. Children with craniopharyngioma often present with endocrinologic abnormalities such as growth failure and delayed sexual maturation. Visual changes can occur and may include decreased acuity or visual field abnormalities. These tumors are often quite large and heterogeneous, displaying both solid and cystic components, and occur within the suprasellar region. They are minimally invasive, adhere to adjacent brain parenchyma, and engulf normal brain structures. MRI demonstrates the solid tumor with cystic structures containing fluid of intermediate density. CT may show calcifications associated with the solid and cystic wall components. Surgery is the primary treatment modality, with gross total resection curative in small lesions. Controversy exists regarding the relative roles of surgery and radiation therapy in large, complex tumors. Significant morbidity (panhypopituitarism, growth failure, visual loss) is associated with these tumors and their therapy, owing to the anatomic location. There is no role for chemotherapy in craniopharyngioma.

Germ Cell Tumors

Germ cell tumors of the CNS are a heterogeneous group of tumors that are primarily tumors of childhood, arising predominantly in midline structures of the pineal and suprasellar regions (see Fig. 497-3). They account for 3-5% of pediatric brain tumors. The peak incidence of these tumors is in children 10-12 yr of age. Overall, there is a male preponderance, although there is a female preponderance for suprasellar tumors. Germ cell tumors occur multifocally in 5-10% of cases. This group of tumors is much more prevalent in Asian populations than European populations. Delays in diagnosis can occur because these tumors have a particularly insidious course; the initial presenting symptoms may be subtle, including poor school performance and behavior problems. As in peripheral germ cell tumors, the analysis of protein markers, α-fetoprotein, and β-human chorionic gonadotropin may be useful in establishing the diagnosis and monitoring treatment response. Surgical biopsy is recommended to establish the diagnosis; however, nongerminomatous germ cell tumors may be diagnosed on the basis of protein marker elevations. Therapeutic approaches to germinomas and mixed germ cell tumors are different. The survival proportion among patients with pure germinoma exceeds 90%. The postsurgical treatment of pure germinomas is somewhat controversial in defining the relative roles of chemotherapy and radiation therapy. Clinical trials have investigated the use of chemotherapy and reduced-dose radiation after surgery in pure germinomas. The therapeutic approach to nongerminomatous germ cell tumors is more aggressive, combining more intense chemotherapy regimens with craniospinal radiation therapy. Survival rates among patients with these tumors are markedly lower than those noted in patients with germinoma, ranging from 40-70% at 5 yr. Trials have shown the benefit of the use of high doses of chemotherapy with peripheral blood stem cell rescue.

Tumors of the Brainstem

Tumors of the brainstem are a heterogeneous group of tumors that account for 10-15% of childhood primary CNS tumors. Outcome depends on tumor location, imaging characteristics, and the patient's clinical status. Patients with these tumors may present with motor weakness, cranial nerve dysfunction, cerebellar dysfunction, and/or signs of increased ICP. On the basis of MRI evaluation and clinical findings, tumors of the brainstem can be classified into 4 types: focal (5-10% of patients); dorsally exophytic (5-10%); cervicomedullary (5-10%); and diffuse intrinsic (70-85%) (Fig. 497-8). Surgical resection is the primary treatment approach for focal and dorsally exophytic tumors and leads to a favorable outcome. Histologically, these 2 groups usually are low-grade gliomas. Cervicomedullary tumors, owing to their location, may not be amenable to surgical resection but are sensitive to radiation therapy. Diffuse intrinsic tumors, characterized by the diffuse infiltrating pontine glioma, are associated with a very poor outcome independent of histologic diagnosis. These tumors are not amenable to surgical resection. Biopsy in children in whom MRI shows a diffuse intrinsic tumor is controversial and is not recommended unless there is suspicion of another diagnosis, such as infection, vascular malformation, multiple sclerosis or other disorder of myelination, or metastatic tumor. These diagnoses are much more common in adults. The standard approach for treatment of diffuse infiltrating pontine gliomas has been radiation therapy, and median survival with this treatment is 12 mo, at best. Use of chemotherapy, including high-dose chemotherapy with peripheral blood stem cell rescue, has not yet

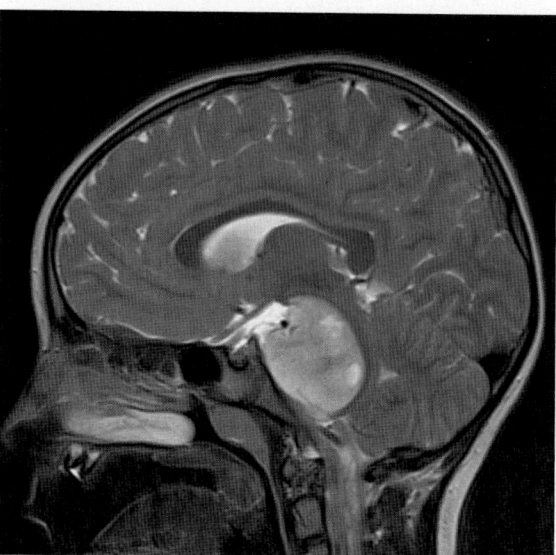

Figure 497-8 T2-weighted sagittal MR image of a diffuse infiltrating pontine glioma in a 5 yr old girl presenting with headaches, left facial droop, and lethargy.

been of survival benefit in this group of patients. Current approaches include evaluation of investigational agents alone or in combination with radiation therapy, similar to approaches being pursued in patients with malignant gliomas.

Metastatic Tumors

Metastatic spread of other childhood malignancies to the brain is uncommon. Childhood acute lymphoblastic leukemia and non-Hodgkin lymphoma can spread to the leptomeninges, causing symptoms of communicating hydrocephalus. **Chloromas,** which are collections of myeloid leukemia cells, can occur throughout the neuraxis. Rarely, brain parenchymal metastases occur from lymphoma, neuroblastoma, rhabdomyosarcoma, Ewing sarcoma, osteosarcoma, and clear cell sarcoma of the kidney. Therapeutic approaches are based on the specific histologic diagnosis and may incorporate radiation therapy, intrathecal administration of chemotherapy, and/or systemic administration of chemotherapy. Medulloblastoma is the childhood brain tumor that most commonly metastasizes extraneurally. Less commonly, extraneural metastases from malignant glioma, PNET, and ependymoma can occur. Ventriculoperitoneal shunts have been known to allow extraneural metastases, primarily within the peritoneal cavity but also systemically.

COMPLICATIONS AND LONG-TERM MANAGEMENT

Data from the National Cancer Institute Surveillance, Epidemiology and End Results Program indicate that more than 70% of patients with childhood brain tumors will be long-term survivors. At least 50% of these survivors will experience chronic problems as a direct result of their tumors and treatment. These problems include chronic neurologic deficits such as focal motor and sensory abnormalities, seizure disorders, neurocognitive deficits (e.g., developmental delays, learning disabilities), and neuroendocrine deficiencies (e.g., hypothyroidism, growth failure, delay or absence of puberty). These patients are also at significant risk for secondary malignancies. Supportive multidisciplinary interventions for children with brain tumors both during and after therapy may help improve the ultimate outcome. Optimal seizure management, physical therapy, endocrine management with timely growth hormone and thyroid replacement therapy, tailored educational programs, and vocational interventions may enhance the childhood brain tumor survivor's quality of life.

Bibliography is available at Expert Consult.

Chapter 498
Neuroblastoma
Peter E. Zage and Joann L. Ater

Neuroblastomas are embryonal cancers of the peripheral sympathetic nervous system with heterogeneous clinical presentation and course, ranging from tumors that undergo spontaneous regression to very aggressive tumors unresponsive to very intensive multimodal therapy. The causes of most cases remain unknown, and although significant advances have been made in the treatment of children with these tumors, the outcomes for aggressive forms of neuroblastoma remain poor.

EPIDEMIOLOGY
Neuroblastoma is the most common extracranial solid tumor in children and the most commonly diagnosed malignancy in infants. Approximately 600 new cases are diagnosed each year in the United States, accounting for 8-10% of childhood malignancies and one third of cancers in infants. Neuroblastoma accounts for >15% of the mortality from cancer in children. The median age of children at diagnosis of neuroblastoma is 22 mo, and 90% of cases are diagnosed by 5 yr of age. The incidence is slightly higher in boys and in whites.

PATHOLOGY
Neuroblastoma tumors, which are derived from primordial neural crest cells, form a spectrum with variable degrees of neural differentiation, ranging from tumors with primarily undifferentiated small round cells (neuroblastoma) to tumors consisting of mature and maturing Schwannian stroma with ganglion cells (ganglioneuroblastoma or ganglioneuroma). The tumors may resemble other **small round blue cell tumors,** such as rhabdomyosarcoma, Ewing sarcoma, and non-Hodgkin lymphoma. The prognosis of children with neuroblastoma varies with the histologic features of the tumor, and prognostic factors include the presence and amount of Schwannian stroma, the degree of tumor cell differentiation, and the mitosis-karyorrhexis index.

PATHOGENESIS
The etiology of neuroblastoma in most cases remains unknown. Familial neuroblastoma accounts for 1-2% of all cases, is associated with a younger age at diagnosis, and is linked to mutations in the *PHOX2B* and *ALK* genes. The *BARD1* gene has also been identified as a major

genetic contributor to neuroblastoma risk. Neuroblastoma is associated with other neural crest disorders, including Hirschsprung disease, central hypoventilation syndrome, and neurofibromatosis type I, and potentially congenital cardiovascular malformations (Table 498-1). Children with Beckwith-Wiedemann syndrome and hemihypertrophy also have a higher incidence of neuroblastoma. Increased incidence of neuroblastoma is associated with some maternal and paternal occupational chemical exposures, farming, and work related to electronics, although no single environmental exposure has been shown to directly cause neuroblastoma.

Genetic characteristics of neuroblastoma tumors that are of prognostic importance include amplification of the *MYCN* (*N-myc*) protooncogene and tumor cell DNA content, or ploidy (Tables 498-2 to 498-4). Amplification of *MYCN* is strongly associated with advanced tumor stage and poor outcomes. Hyperdiploidy confers better prognosis if the child is younger than 1 yr of age at diagnosis. Other chromosomal abnormalities, including loss of heterozygosity of 1p, 11q, and 14q, and gain of 17q, are commonly found in neuroblastoma tumors and are also associated with worse outcomes. In addition, many other biologic factors are associated with neuroblastoma outcomes, including tumor vascularity and the expression levels of nerve growth factor receptors (TrkA, TrkB), ferritin, lactate dehydrogenase, ganglioside GD2, neuropeptide Y, chromogranin A, CD44, multidrug resistance–associated protein, and telomerase. These factors and many others are under investigation in clinical trials to determine whether they can be used to reduce therapy for children predicted to fare well with minimal therapy and to intensify therapy for those predicted to be at high risk for relapse.

CLINICAL MANIFESTATIONS
Neuroblastoma may develop at any site of sympathetic nervous system tissue. Approximately half of neuroblastoma tumors arise in the adrenal glands, and most of the remainder originate in the paraspinal sympathetic ganglia. Metastatic spread, which is more common in children older than 1 yr of age at diagnosis, occurs via local invasion or distant hematogenous or lymphatic routes. The most common sites of metastasis are the regional or distant lymph nodes, long bones and skull, bone marrow, liver, and skin. Lung and brain metastases are rare, occurring in >3% of cases.

The signs and symptoms of neuroblastoma reflect the tumor site and extent of disease, and the symptoms of neuroblastoma can mimic many other disorders, a fact that can result in a delayed diagnosis. Metastatic disease can cause a variety of signs and symptoms, including fever, irritability, failure to thrive, bone pain, cytopenias, bluish subcutaneous nodules, orbital proptosis, and periorbital ecchymoses (Fig. 498-1). Localized disease can manifest as an asymptomatic mass or can cause

Table 498-1	Syndromes Associated with Neuroblastoma
EPONYM	**FEATURES**
Pepper syndrome	Massive involvement of the liver with metastatic disease with or without respiratory distress.
Horner syndrome	Unilateral ptosis, myosis, and anhidrosis associated with a thoracic or cervical primary tumor. Symptoms do not resolve with tumor resection.
Hutchinson syndrome	Limping and irritability in young child associated with bone and bone marrow metastases.
Opsoclonus-myoclonus-ataxia syndrome	Myoclonic jerking and random conjugate eye movements with or without cerebellar ataxia. Often associated with a biologically favorable and differentiated tumor. The condition is likely immune mediated, may not resolve with tumor removal, and often exhibits progressive neuropsychologic sequelae.
Kerner-Morrison syndrome	Intractable secretory diarrhea due to tumor secretion of vasointestinal peptides. Tumors are generally biologically favorable.
Neurocristopathy syndrome	Neuroblastoma associated with other neural crest disorders, including congenital hypoventilation syndrome or Hirschsprung disease. Germline mutations in the paired homeobox gene *PHOX2B* have been identified in a subset of patients with this disease.
ROHHAD	Approximately 40% may have neural crest-derived tumors. Obesity and neurologic issues may be part of a paraneoplastic syndrome.

ROHHAD, rapid-onset obesity, hypothalamic dysfunction, hypoventilation, autonomic dysregulation.
From Park JR, Eggert A, Caron H: Neuroblastoma: biology, prognosis, and treatment, Pediatr Clin North Am 55:97–120, 2008.

Table 498-2	Children's Oncology Group Neuroblastoma Risk Stratification				
RISK GROUP	**STAGE**	**AGE**	**MYCN AMPLIFICATION STATUS**	**PLOIDY**	**SHIMADA**
Low risk	1	Any	Any	Any	Any
Low risk	2A/2B	Any	Not amplified	Any	Any
High risk	2A/2B	Any	Amplified	Any	Any
Intermediate risk	3	<547 days	Not amplified	Any	Any
Intermediate risk	3	≥547 days	Not amplified	Any	FH
High risk	3	Any	Amplified	Any	Any
High risk	3	≥547 days	Not amplified	Any	UH
High risk	4	<365 days	Amplified	Any	Any
Intermediate risk	4	<365 days	Not amplified	Any	Any
High risk	4	365 to <547 days	Amplified	Any	Any
High risk	4	365 to <547 days	Any	DNA index = 1	Any
High risk	4	365 to <547 days	Any	Any	UH
Intermediate risk	4	365 to <547 days	Not amplified	DNA index > 1	FH
High risk	4	≥547 days	Any	Any	Any
Low risk	4S	<365 days	Not amplified	DNA index > 1	FH
Intermediate risk	4S	<365 days	Not amplified	DNA index = 1	Any
Intermediate risk	4S	<365 days	Not amplified	Any	UH
High risk	4S	<365 days	Amplified	Any	Any

FH, Favorable histology; UH, unfavorable histology.
   Courtesy of Children's Oncology Group; from Park JR, Eggert A, Caron H: Neuroblastoma: biology, prognosis, and treatment, Pediatr Clin North Am 55:97–120, 2008.

Table 498-3	International Neuroblastoma Staging System		
STAGE	**DEFINITION**	**INCIDENCE (%)**	**SURVIVAL AT 5 YR* (%)**
1	Localized tumor with complete gross excision, with or without microscopic residual disease; representative ipsilateral lymph nodes negative for tumor microscopically (nodes attached to and removed with the primary tumor may be positive)	5	≥90
2A	Localized tumor with incomplete gross excision; representative ipsilateral nonadherent lymph nodes negative for tumor microscopically	10	70-80
2B	Localized tumor with or without complete gross excision, with ipsilateral nonadherent lymph nodes positive for tumor; enlarged contralateral lymph nodes must be negative microscopically	10	70-80
3	Unresectable unilateral tumor infiltrating across the midline,[†] with or without regional lymph node involvement; or localized unilateral tumor with contralateral regional lymph node involvement; or midline tumor with bilateral extension by infiltration (resectable) or by lymph node involvement	25	40-70
4	Any primary tumor with dissemination to distant lymph nodes; bone, bone marrow, liver, skin, and other organs (except as defined for stage 4S)	60	85-90 if age at diagnosis is <18 mo 30-40 if age at diagnosis is >18 mo
4S	Localized primary tumor (as defined for stage 1, 2A, or 2B), with dissemination limited to skin, liver, and bone marrow[‡] (limited to infants <1 yr of age)	5	>80

*Survival is influenced by other characteristics, such as MYCN amplification. Percentages are approximate.
   [†]The *midline* is defined as the vertebral column. Tumors originating on one side and crossing the midline must infiltrate to or beyond the other side of the vertebral column.
   [‡]Marrow involvement in stage 4S should be minimal (i.e., <10% of total nucleated cells identified as malignant on bone marrow biopsy or on marrow aspirate). More extensive marrow involvement would be considered stage 4. Results of the metaiodobenzylguanidine (MIBG) scan (if performed) should be negative in the marrow.
   Modified from Kliegman RM, Marcdante KJ, Jenson HB, et al, editors: Nelson essentials of pediatrics, ed 5, Philadelphia, 2006, WB Saunders, p. 746; and Brodeur GM, Pritchard J, Berthold F, et al: Revisions of the international criteria for neuroblastoma diagnosis, staging, and response to treatment, J Clin Oncol 11:1466–1477, 1993.

symptoms because of the mass itself, including spinal cord compression, bowel obstruction, and superior vena cava syndrome.

Children with neuroblastoma can also present with neurologic signs and symptoms. Neuroblastoma originating in the superior cervical ganglion can result in **Horner syndrome.** Paraspinal neuroblastoma

tumors can invade the neural foramina, causing spinal cord and nerve root compression. Neuroblastoma can also be associated with a paraneoplastic syndrome of autoimmune origin, termed *opsoclonus–myoclonus–ataxia syndrome*, in which patients experience rapid, uncontrollable jerking eye and body movements, poor coordination,

| Table 498-4 | Phenotypic and Genetic Features of Neuroblastoma, Treatment, and Survival According to Prognostic Category |

	PROGNOSTIC CATEGORY*			
VARIABLE	Low Risk	Intermediate Risk	High Risk	Tumor Stage 4S
Pattern of disease	Localized tumor	Localized tumor with locoregional lymph node extension; metastases to bone marrow and bone in infants	Metastases to bone marrow and bone (except in infants)	Metastases to liver and skin (with minimal bone marrow involvement) in infants
Tumor genomics	Whole-chromosome gains	Whole-chromosome gains	Segmental chromosomal aberrations	Whole-chromosome gains
Treatment	Surgery†	Moderate-intensity chemotherapy; surgery†	Dose-intensive chemotherapy, surgery, and external-beam radiotherapy to primary tumor and resistant metastatic sites; myeloablative chemotherapy with autologous hematopoietic stem cell rescue; isotretinoin with anti–ganglioside GD2 immunotherapy	Supportive care‡
Survival rate	>98%	90-95%	40-50%	>90%

*Patients are assigned to prognostic groups according to risk, as described by the Children's Oncology Group, with the level of risk defining the likelihood of death from disease. Stage 4S disease is considered separately here because of the unique phenotype of favorable biologic features and relentless early progression but ultimately full and complete regression of the disease.
†The goal of surgery is to safely debulk the tumor mass and avoid damage to surrounding normal structures while also obtaining sufficient material for molecular diagnostic studies. Some localized tumors may spontaneously regress without surgery.
‡Low-dose chemotherapy or radiation therapy, or both, is used in patients with life-threatening hepatic involvement, especially in infants <2 mo of age, who are at much higher risk for life-threatening complications from massive hepatomegaly.
From Maris JM: Recent advances in neuroblastoma, N Engl J Med 362:2202–2210, 2010.

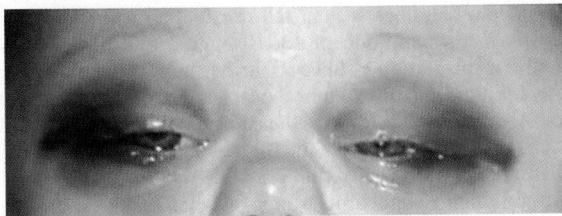

Figure 498-1 Periorbital metastases of neuroblastoma with ecchymoses and proptosis.

and cognitive dysfunction. Some tumors produce catecholamines that can cause increased sweating and hypertension, and some release vasoactive intestinal peptide, causing a profound secretory diarrhea. Children with extensive tumors can also experience tumor lysis syndrome and disseminated intravascular coagulation. Infants younger than 1 yr of age also can present in unique fashion, termed *stage 4S*, with widespread subcutaneous tumor nodules, massive liver involvement, limited bone marrow disease, and a small primary tumor without bone involvement or other metastases.

DIAGNOSIS

Neuroblastoma is usually discovered as a mass or multiple masses on plain radiography, CT, or MRI (Fig. 498-2A). The mass often contains calcification and hemorrhage that can be appreciated on plain radiography or CT. Prenatal diagnosis of neuroblastoma on maternal ultrasound scans is sometimes possible. Tumor markers, including catecholamine metabolites homovanillic acid and vanillylmandelic acid, are elevated in the urine of approximately 95% of cases and help to confirm the diagnosis. A pathologic diagnosis is established from tumor tissue obtained by biopsy. Neuroblastoma can be diagnosed without a primary tumor biopsy if small round blue tumor cells are observed in bone marrow samples (Fig. 498-3) and the levels of vanillylmandelic acid or homovanillic acid are elevated in the urine.

Evaluations for metastatic disease should include CT or MRI of the chest and abdomen, bone scans to detect cortical bone involvement, and at least 2 independent bone marrow aspirations and biopsies to evaluate for marrow disease. **Iodine-123 metaiodobenzylguanidine (¹²³I-MIBG)** studies should be used when available to better define the extent of disease (see Fig. 498-2B and C). MRI of the spine should be performed in cases with suspected or potential spinal cord compression, but imaging of the brain with either CT or MRI is not routinely performed unless dictated by the clinical presentation.

The **International Neuroblastoma Staging System (INSS)** is currently used to stage patients with neuroblastoma after initial surgical resection (see Table 498-3). INSS stage 1 tumors are confined to the organ or structure of origin and are completely resected. INSS stage 2 tumors extend beyond the structure of origin but not across the midline, either with (stage 2B) or without (stage 2A) ipsilateral lymph node involvement. INSS stage 3 tumors extend beyond the midline, with or without bilateral lymph node involvement, whereas INSS stage 4 tumors are disseminated, with metastases to bones, bone marrow, liver, distant lymph nodes, and other organs. INSS stage 4S refers to neuroblastoma in children younger than 1 yr of age with dissemination to liver, skin, and/or bone marrow without bone involvement and with a primary tumor that would otherwise be staged as INSS stage 1 or 2. A new International Neuroblastoma Risk Group Staging System was recently developed to allow for more effective comparisons of treatments and outcomes worldwide.

TREATMENT

Treatment strategies for neuroblastoma have changed dramatically over the past 20 yr, with significant reduction in treatment intensity for children who have localized low-risk tumors and with continued increased treatment intensity and addition of new agents for treatment of children who have high-risk neuroblastoma. The patient's age and tumor stage are combined with cytogenetic and molecular features of the tumor to determine the treatment risk group and estimated prognosis for each patient (see Tables 498-2 to 498-4). The usual treatment for children with low-risk neuroblastoma is surgery for stages 1 and 2 and observation for stage 4S with cure rates generally >90% without further therapy. Treatment with chemotherapy or radiation for the rare child with local recurrence can still be curative. Children with spinal cord compression at diagnosis also may require urgent treatment with chemotherapy, surgery, or radiation to avoid neurologic

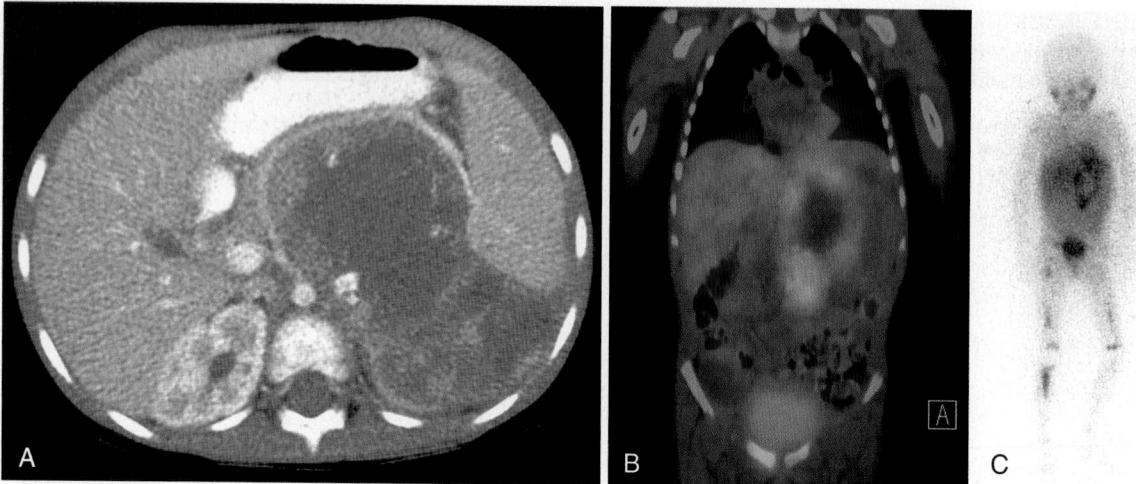

Figure 498-2 A, CT scan of an abdominal neuroblastoma with central necrosis at diagnosis. **B,** Coronal fused CT and metaiodobenzylguanidine (MIBG) image of same child with extensive retroperitoneal mass and central necrosis, probably an adrenal primary with extensive lymph node involvement. **C,** MIBG avid neuroblastoma with increased uptake of radiolabeled tracer can be detected in multiple sites of disease, including bone and soft tissue.

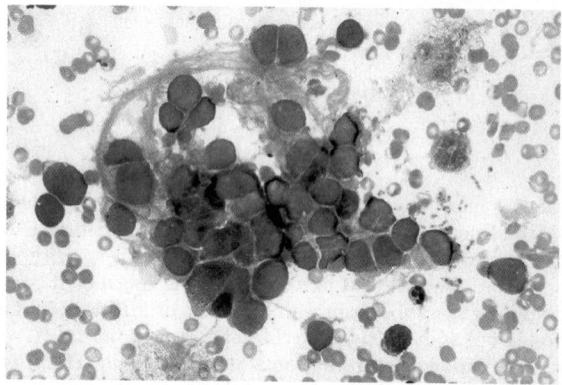

Figure 498-3 Neuroblastoma cells aspirated from the bone marrow. Clumps of cells often contain ≥3 cells with or without evidence of rosette formation. Rosettes of cells surrounding an inner mass of fibrillary material are characteristic of neuroblastoma.

damage. Stage 4S neuroblastomas have a very favorable prognosis, and many regress spontaneously without therapy. Chemotherapy or resection of the primary tumor does not improve survival rates, but for infants with massive liver involvement and respiratory compromise, small doses of cyclophosphamide or low-dose hepatic irradiation may alleviate symptoms. For children with stage 4S neuroblastoma who require treatment for symptoms, the survival rate is 81%.

Treatment of intermediate-risk neuroblastoma includes surgery, chemotherapy, and, in some cases, radiation therapy. The chemotherapy usually includes moderate doses of cisplatin or carboplatin, cyclophosphamide, etoposide, and doxorubicin given for several months. Radiation therapy is used for tumors with incomplete response to chemotherapy. Children with intermediate-risk neuroblastoma, including children with stage 3 disease and infants with stage 4 disease and favorable characteristics, have an excellent prognosis and >90% survival with this moderate treatment. In this intermediate-risk group, obtaining adequate diagnostic material for determination of the underlying biologic features of the tumor, such as the Shimada pathologic classification and *MYCN* gene amplification, is critical, so that children with unfavorable characteristics can receive more-aggressive treatment and those with favorable features can be spared excessive toxic therapy.

Children with high-risk neuroblastoma have long-term survival rates between 25% and 35% with current treatment that consists of intensive chemotherapy, high-dose chemotherapy with autologous stem cell rescue, surgery, radiation, and 13-*cis*-retinoic acid (isotreti-

noin, Accutane). Induction chemotherapy for children with high-risk neuroblastoma includes combinations of cyclophosphamide, topotecan, doxorubicin, vincristine, cisplatin, and etoposide. After completion of induction chemotherapy, resection of the residual primary tumor is followed by high-dose chemotherapy with autologous stem cell rescue and focal radiation therapy to tumor sites. A national cooperative group trial demonstrated significantly better survival with chemotherapy plus autologous stem cell rescue than with chemotherapy alone. The further addition of 13-*cis*-retinoic acid after autologous stem cell transplantation resulted in further improvements in survival rates. In addition, a national clinical trial has demonstrated an increase in short-term survival rates with the addition of the monoclonal antibody ch14.18, interleukin 2, and granulocyte-macrophage colony-stimulating factor to 13-*cis*-retinoic acid therapy.

Cases of high-risk neuroblastoma are associated with frequent relapses, and children with recurrent neuroblastoma have a <50% response rate to alternative chemotherapy regimens. New treatment strategies and agents are needed for children with both high-risk and recurrent neuroblastoma. Therapies currently under investigation include new chemotherapeutic agents and other novel therapies directed against critical intracellular signaling pathways, radiolabeled targeted agents (such as ^{131}I-MIBG), immunotherapy, and antitumor vaccines. Ongoing biologic studies of neuroblastoma will also hopefully lead to the identification of new molecular and genetic targets for therapy.

Bibliography is available at Expert Consult.

Chapter **499**
Neoplasms of the Kidney

499.1 Wilms Tumor
Najat C. Daw, Vicki Huff, and Peter M. Anderson

Wilms tumor (WT), also known as nephroblastoma, is the most common primary malignant renal tumor of childhood; other renal tumors are very rare. It is the second most common malignant abdominal tumor in childhood. The most common sites of metastases are the lungs, regional lymph nodes, and liver. Histologically, the classic WT is made up of varying proportions of blastemal, stromal, and epithelial cells, recapitulating stages of normal renal development. The treatment includes surgery and chemotherapy with or without radiotherapy. The use of multimodality treatment and multiinstitutional cooperative group trials has dramatically improved the cure rate of WT from <30% to approximately 90% (Table 499-1).

EPIDEMIOLOGY

WT accounts for 6% of pediatric malignancies and more than 95% of kidney tumors in children. In the United States, the incidence of WT is approximately 8 cases per 1 million children younger than 15 yr of age per year, and about 650 new cases are diagnosed each year. Approximately 75% of the cases occur in children younger than 5 yr with a peak incidence at 2-3 yr of age. It can arise in 1 or both kidneys; the incidence of bilateral WTs is 7%. Most cases are sporadic, but approximately 2% of patients have a family history. In 8-10% of patients, WT is observed in the context of hemihypertrophy, aniridia, genitourinary anomalies, and a variety of rare syndromes, including **Beckwith-Wiedemann syndrome** and **Denys-Drash syndrome** (Table 499-2). An earlier age of diagnosis and an increased incidence of bilateral disease are generally observed in syndromic and familial cases.

Table 499-1	Ten Yr Outcomes for Patients with Wilms Tumor Treated in the National Wilms Tumor Study IV	
HISTOLOGY	**STAGE**	**RECURRENCE-FREE SURVIVAL (%)**	**OVERALL SURVIVAL (%)**
Favorable	I	91	96
Favorable	II	85	93
Favorable	III	84	89
Favorable	IV	75	81
Favorable	V	65	78
Anaplastic	I	69	82
Anaplastic	II-III	43	49
Anaplastic	IV	18	18

Table 499-2	Syndromes Associated with Wilms Tumor	
SYNDROME	**CLINICAL CHARACTERISTICS**	**GENETIC ANOMALIES**
Wilms tumor, aniridia, genitourinary abnormalities, and mental retardation (WAGR)	Aniridia, genitourinary abnormalities, mental retardation	Del 11p13 (*WT1* and *PAX6*)
Denys-Drash	Early-onset renal failure with renal mesangial sclerosis, male pseudohermaphroditism	*WT1* missense mutation
Beckwith-Wiedemann	Organomegaly (liver, kidney, adrenal, pancreas) macroglossia, omphalocele, hemihypertrophy	Unilateral paternal disomy, duplication of 11p15.5, loss of imprinting, mutation of *p57KIP57* Del 11p15.5 *IGF2* and *H19* imprinting control region

ETIOLOGY: GENETICS AND MOLECULAR BIOLOGY

WT is thought to be derived from incompletely differentiated renal mesenchyme, and tumors are typically composed of cells reminiscent of the undifferentiated and partially differentiated cells that normally arise from renal mesenchyme. Foci of benign, undifferentiated mesenchyme (nephrogenic rests) that persist abnormally in the kidney into postnatal life are observed in approximately 1% of children in the general population, but are present in up to 90% of children who have a family history of WT, develop bilateral tumors, or display features of WT-related syndromes. Nephrogenic rests usually regress or differentiate, but those that persist can become malignant.

To date genetic mutations have been detected, either individually or in combination, in a third of WTs. Mutations in *WT1*, a gene located at 11p13 and encoding a zinc finger transcription factor, are observed in 15-20% of tumors. These are homozygous and result in loss of *WT1* function. The majority of *WT1* mutations are somatic, result in loss of *WT1* function, and are present homozygously. However, germline *WT1* mutations are also observed, primarily in patients with WT-associated syndromes, or sometimes in patients with bilateral disease. In these instances, the wild-type allele present in the germline is mutated or lost in the tumor, resulting in loss of *WT1* function. Interestingly, nephrogenic rests assessed from patients heterozygous for a germline *WT1* mutation are homozygous for the *WT1* mutation, with additional somatic mutations being observed in the autologous tumors. The vast majority of *WT1* mutations are deletion/truncating mutations or missense mutations that affect amino acid residues critical for *WT1* function. Germline truncating mutations are usually associated with WT in the context of genitourinary anomalies or the WAGR (Wilms, aniridia, genitourinary anomalies, mental retardation) syndrome. Missense germline mutations are usually observed in children with Denys-Drash syndrome in which early-onset renal failure is observed.

Mutations in *CTNNB1*, encoding β-catenin, which acts as a major regulatory point in the wnt signaling pathway and also acts at the cytoplasmic membrane, are observed in approximately 15% of WTs, very often those that have sustained *WT1* mutations. *WTX*, a gene located on the X chromosome that encodes a protein that also plays a role in wnt pathway regulation, is mutated in approximately 20% of tumors. *CTNNB1* and *WTX* mutations are somatic. Somatic mutation of the p53 gene, *TP53*, is observed in approximately 5% of tumors and is associated with anaplastic tumor histology, a poor prognostic feature of WT.

In approximately 70% of tumors, loss of heterozygosity (usually copy number neutral) or loss of imprinting at imprinted loci at 11p15 is observed. This epigenetic alteration (the observation of which led to the designation of a "WT2" gene) occurs in tumors both with and without *WT1*, *CTNNB1*, or *WTX* mutations, and often results in biallelic expression of *IGF2*, a normally imprinted gene that encodes insulin-like growth factor 2, in addition to the loss of imprinting of other 11p15 genes. Families with Beckwith-Wiedemann syndrome, a somatic overgrowth syndrome in which predisposition to embryonal tumors (including WT) is observed, have been genetically linked to 11p15, and microdeletions within the *IGF2* imprinting control region are present in Beckwith-Wiedemann syndrome families in which WT is observed.

WT is occasionally observed in families with a predisposition to **pleuropulmonary blastoma**, and mutations in the *DICER1* gene, located at 14q31 and encoding a key protein in the generation of microRNAs, are observed in these families. However, outside the context of these families, *DICER1* mutations are rare in WTs.

A family history of WT is noted in approximately 2% of WT patients, and predisposition is inherited as an autosomal dominant trait with incomplete penetrance. Predisposition to other tumor types or other phenotypes are not observed in the vast majority of these families. *WT1* mutations are detected in <5% of families, and these *WT1*-related families are small, with only 2 affected individuals. Genetic linkage analyses of large WT families have localized predisposition genes to 19q and 17q, but neither gene has been identified yet. However, some

Table 499-3	Differential Diagnosis of Abdominal and Pelvic Tumors in Children		
TUMOR	**PATIENT AGE**	**CLINICAL SIGNS**	**LABORATORY FINDINGS**
Wilms	Preschool	Unilateral flank mass, aniridia, hemihypertrophy	Hematuria, polycythemia, thrombocytosis, elevated partial thromboplastin time value
Neuroblastoma	Preschool	Gastrointestinal/genitourinary obstruction, raccoon eyes, myoclonus opsoclonus, diarrhea, skin nodules	Increased urinary vanillylmandelic acid, or homovanillic acid, or ferritin, stippled calcification in the mass
Non-Hodgkin lymphoma	>1 yr	Intussusception in patients >2 yr old	Increased lactic dehydrogenase, blood cytopenia from bone marrow involvement
Rhabdomyosarcoma	All	Gastrointestinal/genitourinary obstruction, abdominal pain, vaginal bleeding, paratesticular mass	Hypercalcemia, blood cytopenia from bone marrow involvement
Germ cell tumor/teratoma	Preschool, teenage	Girls: abdominal pain, vaginal bleeding Boys: testicular mass, new-onset hydrocele, sacrococcygeal mass/dimple	Increased human chorionic gonadotropin, increased α-fetoprotein
Hepatoblastoma	Birth-3 yr	Large firm liver	Increased α-fetoprotein
Hepatoma	School age, teenage	Large firm nodule, hepatitis B, cirrhosis	Increased α-fetoprotein

families carry neither of these mutations, suggesting that additional WT loci exist. Some families are not linked to either of these genomic regions, indicating that additional WT predisposition genes exist. Similarly, somatic alterations at 1q, 7p, 16q, chromosome 12, and other genomic regions are observed in some WTs and are thought to harbor genes important in WT development.

CLINICAL PRESENTATION

The most common initial clinical presentation for WT is the incidental discovery of an asymptomatic **abdominal mass** by parents while bathing or clothing an affected child or by a physician during a routine physical examination (Table 499-3). At presentation the mass can be quite large because retroperitoneal masses can grow unhampered by strict anatomic boundaries. Functional defects in paired organs like the kidney, with good functional reserve, are also unlikely to be detected early. **Hypertension** is present in approximately 25% of tumors at presentation and has been attributed to increased renin activity. **Abdominal pain, gross painless hematuria, and fever** are other frequent findings at diagnosis. Occasionally, rapid **abdominal enlargement and anemia** occur as a result of bleeding into the renal parenchyma or pelvis. WT thrombus extends into the inferior vena cava in 4-10% of patients, and rarely into the right atrium. Patients might also have microcytic anemia from iron deficiency or anemia of chronic disease, polycythemia, elevated platelet count, and acquired deficiency of von Willebrand factor or factor VII deficiency.

DIAGNOSIS AND DIFFERENTIAL DIAGNOSIS

An abdominal mass in a child should be considered malignant until diagnostic imaging, laboratory findings, and pathology can define its true nature (see Table 499-3). Imaging studies include plain abdominal radiography, abdominal ultrasonography, and CT of the abdomen to define the intrarenal origin of the mass and differentiate it from adrenal masses (e.g., neuroblastoma) and other masses in the abdomen. Abdominal ultrasonography helps differentiate solid from cystic masses. WT might show focal areas of necrosis or hemorrhage and hydronephrosis caused by obstruction of the renal pelvis by the tumor. Ultrasonography with Doppler imaging of renal veins and the inferior vena cava is a useful first study that not only can look for WT but also can evaluate the collecting system and demonstrate tumor thrombi in the renal veins and inferior vena cava.

CT (Fig. 499-1) is useful to define the extent of the disease, integrity of the contralateral kidney, and metastasis. MRI requires sedation in young children and is not routinely used; it may be helpful in defining an extensive tumor thrombus that extends up to the level of the hepatic veins or even into the right atrium, and to distinguish WT from nephrogenic rests. Chest CT is more sensitive than chest radiography to

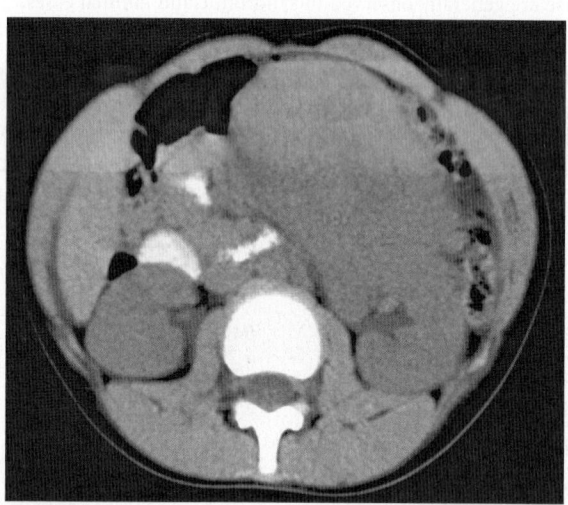

Figure 499-1 Abdominal CT scan showing a Wilms tumor arising from the left kidney. Because of their retroperitoneal location, such tumors can become very large (>10 cm) before clinical symptoms occur.

screen for pulmonary metastasis, and is preferably performed before surgery because effusions and atelectasis can confound the interpretation of postoperative imaging studies. A bone scan is performed if the histologic diagnosis confirms clear cell sarcoma of the kidney to look for bone metastasis. Brain imaging with CT or MRI is obtained in cases of clear cell sarcoma of the kidney or rhabdoid tumor of the kidney as these tumors can spread to the brain.

WT lesions are metabolically active and concentrate fluorodeoxyglucose. Regional spread and metastatic lesions can be visualized on positron emission tomography/CT scanning. The diagnosis is usually made by imaging studies and confirmed by histology at the time of nephrectomy. Although biopsy is a reliable diagnostic tool, it is discouraged as it results in disease upstaging. A core needle biopsy obtained via a posterior approach should be performed in cases of unusual presentation (older age, signs of infection, inflammation) or unusual imaging findings (significant adenopathy, no renal parenchyma seen, intratumoral calcification).

TREATMENT

There are 2 major schools of thought in the management of WT. The Children's Oncology Group, formerly National Wilms Tumor Study Group, advocates upfront surgery prior to initiating treatment. On the

Table 499-4	Staging of Wilms Tumor
Stage I	Tumor *confined to the kidney* and completely resected. Renal capsule or sinus vessels not involved. Tumor not ruptured or biopsied. Regional lymph nodes examined and negative.
Stage II	Tumor extends *beyond the kidney* but is completely resected with negative margins and lymph nodes. At least 1 of the following has occurred: (a) penetration of renal capsule, (b) invasion of renal sinus vessels.
Stage III	*Residual tumor* present following surgery confined to the abdomen, including gross or microscopic tumor; spillage of tumor preoperatively or intraoperatively; biopsy prior to nephrectomy, regional lymph node metastases; tumor implants on the peritoneal surface; extension of tumor thrombus into the inferior vena cava including thoracic vena cava and heart.
Stage IV	*Hematogenous metastases* (lung, liver, bone, brain, etc.) or lymph node metastases outside the abdominopelvic region.
Stage V	*Bilateral* renal involvement by tumor.

other hand, the International Society of Pediatric Oncology recommends preoperative chemotherapy. Each approach has advantages and limitations but they have similar outcomes. Early surgery provides accurate diagnosis and staging, and can facilitate risk-adapted therapy. Preoperative chemotherapy can make surgery easier and reduces the risk of intraoperative tumor rupture and hemorrhage. Surgery entails a radical nephrectomy with meticulous dissection to avoid rupture of the tumor capsule and lymph node sampling despite the absence of abnormal nodes on preoperative imaging studies or intraoperative assessment. Partial nephrectomy is performed in patients with bilateral disease or with unilateral WT and a predisposing syndrome such as Denys-Drash and WAGR, so as to minimize the risk of future renal failure.

Prognostic factors for risk-adapted therapy include age, stage, tumor weight, and loss of heterozygosity at chromosomes 1p and 16q (Table 499-4). Histology plays a major role in risk stratification of WT. Absence of anaplasia is considered a favorable histologic finding. Presence of anaplasia is further classified as focal or diffuse, both of which are unfavorable histologic findings.

The Children's Oncology Group has specific drug dose and schedule recommendations for risk-adapted treatment of WT. Patients with favorable histologic findings of WT have a good outcome and are generally treated in the outpatient setting. Nephrectomy alone may be sufficient for patients younger than 2 yr of age with stage I disease and a tumor weighing <550 g. Patients with stages I and II disease receive chemotherapy with 2 drugs, vincristine and actinomycin D (also called dactinomycin), every 1-3 wk for a total of 18 wk (regimen EE4A). Patients with stage III or IV disease receive chemotherapy with 3 drugs (vincristine, doxorubicin, and actinomycin D) every 1-3 wk for a total of 24 wk (regimen DD4A) and radiation therapy. Patients with regional lymph node metastases, residual disease after surgery, or tumor rupture receive radiation therapy to the flank or abdomen, and those with lung metastases receive radiation therapy to the lungs. The presence of loss of heterozygosity at 1p and 16q confers an adverse prognosis, and deserves treatment intensification.

Anaplastic histology (focal and diffuse) accounts for approximately 11% of WT cases. Patients with diffuse anaplasia, in particular, have a poor outcome. They are treated with intensive chemotherapy regimens that include vincristine, cyclophosphamide, doxorubicin, etoposide, carboplatin, and ifosfamide, in addition to radiation therapy.

RECURRENT DISEASE
Approximately 15% of WT patients with favorable histology and 50% of those with anaplastic histology suffer relapse; most relapses occur early (within 2 yr of diagnosis). Factors associated with a favorable outcome after relapse include low stage (I/II) at diagnosis, treatment with vincristine and actinomycin D only, no prior radiotherapy, favorable histology, relapse to lung only, and interval from nephrectomy to relapse 12 mo or longer. Patients with recurrent WT who previously received only vincristine and actinomycin D had a 4 yr survival of approximately 80%, whereas those who previously received the 3 drug regimen of vincristine, actinomycin D, and doxorubicin had a 4 yr survival of only 50%. Other agents used to treat recurrent WT include doxorubicin, carboplatin, cyclophosphamide, ifosfamide, etoposide, and topotecan. Metachronous WT may not represent tumor relapse but instead may indicate development of a new tumor in the opposite kidney.

PROGNOSIS
Despite some adverse risk factors that decrease prognosis (metastases, unfavorable histology, recurrent disease, and loss of heterozygosity of both 1p and 16q), most children with WT have a very favorable prognosis. Overall, the survival of children with WT approaches 90%, with some prognostic factors (low stage, favorable histology, young age, low tumor weight) conferring even better outcomes.

LATE EFFECTS
Current strategies are successful with relatively few long-term effects of therapy. Late complications are a consequence of treatment type and intensity; the use of radiotherapy and anthracyclines increases the risk of these complications. Clinically significant late sequelae include musculoskeletal effects, cardiac toxicity, pulmonary disease, reproductive problems, renal dysfunction, and the development of second malignant neoplasms.

499.2 Other Pediatric Renal Tumors
Najat C. Daw, Vicki Huff, and Peter M. Anderson

MESOBLASTIC NEPHROMA
Mesoblastic nephroma is the most common solid renal tumor identified in the **neonatal period** and the most frequent benign renal tumor in childhood. It represents 3-10% of all pediatric renal tumors. Many cases are diagnosed with prenatal ultrasound and can manifest as polyhydramnios, hydrops, and premature delivery. Most of the patients are diagnosed before 3 mo of age, whereas WT is rarely diagnosed before 6 mo of age. Radical nephrectomy is the treatment of choice and may be sufficient by itself. Local recurrence is uncommon. Although rare, malignant variants do occur, marked by metastases to the lung, liver, heart, and brain.

CLEAR CELL SARCOMA OF THE KIDNEY
Clear cell sarcoma of the kidney is an uncommon renal neoplasm of childhood with approximately 20 new cases diagnosed each year in North America. Peak incidence is between 1 and 4 yr of age, usually presenting as an abdominal mass. Gene expression profiles of clear cell sarcoma of the kidney suggest the cell of origin to be a renal mesenchymal cell with neural markers. Bone is the most common site of distant metastasis followed by lung, abdomen, retroperitoneum, brain, and liver. Therefore, the staging work-up should include a bone scan. Early-stage disease has an excellent prognosis, especially with the addition of doxorubicin.

RHABDOID TUMOR OF THE KIDNEY
Malignant rhabdoid tumor of the kidney has rhabdomyoblast-like morphology. It is a rare but aggressive cancer. Hematuria is a common presenting feature. Both rhabdoid tumor of the kidney and central nervous system atypical teratoid rhabdoid tumors have deletions and mutations of the *hSNF5/INI1* gene and are considered to be related. Prognosis is poor with current therapeutic protocols. The 5 yr overall survival rate is <30%.

RENAL CELL CARCINOMA

Renal cell carcinoma (RCC) is rare in children, accounting for <5% of all renal tumors of childhood. Patients may present with frank hematuria, flank pain, and/or a palpable mass, although RCC can be asymptomatic and detected incidentally. It has a propensity to metastasize to the lungs, bone, liver, and brain. RCC can be associated with von Hippel–Lindau disease. Unlike the case for adult RCC, local lymph node involvement is not a poor prognostic indicator in pediatric RCC. Nephrectomy alone may be adequate for early-stage RCC.

Bibliography is available at Expert Consult.

Chapter 500
Soft Tissue Sarcomas
Carola A.S. Arndt

The annual incidence of soft tissue sarcomas is 8.4 cases per 1 million white children younger than 14 yr of age. Rhabdomyosarcoma accounts for more than 50% of soft tissue sarcomas. The prognosis most strongly correlates with age and extent of disease at diagnosis, primary tumor site and histology, and expression of the fusion protein, PAX-FOXO1.

RHABDOMYOSARCOMA
Epidemiology

The most common pediatric soft tissue sarcoma, rhabdomyosarcoma, accounts for approximately 3.5% of childhood cancers. These tumors may occur at virtually any anatomic site but are usually found in the head and neck (25%), orbit (9%), genitourinary tract (24%), and extremities (19%); retroperitoneal and other sites account for the remainder of primary sites. The incidence at each anatomic site is related to both patient age and tumor type. Extremity lesions are more likely to occur in older children and to have alveolar histology. Rhabdomyosarcoma occurs with increased frequency in patients with neurofibromatosis and other family cancer predisposition syndromes such as Li-Fraumeni syndrome.

Pathogenesis

Rhabdomyosarcoma is thought to arise from the same embryonic mesenchyme as striated skeletal muscle although a large percentage of these tumors arise in areas lacking skeletal muscle (e.g., bladder, prostate, vagina). On the basis of light microscopic appearance, it belongs to the general category of small round cell tumors that includes Ewing sarcoma, neuroblastoma, and non-Hodgkin lymphoma. Definitive diagnosis of a pathologic specimen requires immunohistochemical studies using antibodies to skeletal muscle (desmin, muscle-specific

actin, myogenin) and reverse transcription polymerase chain reaction or, in the case of alveolar tumors, fluorescent in situ hybridization for PAX-FOXO1 transcript.

Determination of the specific histologic subtype is important in treatment planning and assessment of prognosis. There are 3 recognized histologic subtypes. The **embryonal type** accounts for approximately 60% of all cases and has an intermediate prognosis. The **botryoid type,** a variant of the embryonal form in which tumor cells and an edematous stroma project into a body cavity like a bunch of grapes, is found most often in the vagina, uterus, bladder, nasopharynx, and middle ear. The **alveolar type** accounts for approximately 25-40% of cases and often is characterized by the presence of PAX-FOXO1 fusion transcript. The tumor cells tend to grow in nests that often have cleft-like spaces resembling alveoli. Alveolar tumors occur most often in the trunk and extremities and carry the poorest prognosis. The **pleomorphic type** (adult form) is rare in childhood, accounting for <1% of cases.

Clinical Manifestations

The most common presenting feature of rhabdomyosarcoma is a mass that may or may not be painful. Symptoms are caused by displacement or obstruction of normal structures (Table 500-1). Origin in the nasopharynx may be associated with nasal congestion, mouth breathing, epistaxis, and difficulty with swallowing and chewing. Regional extension into the cranium can produce cranial nerve paralysis, blindness, and signs of increased intracranial pressure with headache and vomiting. When the tumor develops in the face or cheek, there may be swelling, pain, trismus, and, as extension occurs, paralysis of cranial nerves. Tumors in the neck can produce progressive swelling with neurologic symptoms after regional extension. Orbital primary tumors are usually diagnosed early in their course because of associated proptosis, periorbital edema, ptosis, change in visual acuity, and local pain. When the tumor arises in the middle ear, the most common early signs are pain, hearing loss, chronic otorrhea, or a mass in the ear canal; extensions of tumor produce cranial nerve paralysis and signs of an intracranial mass on the involved side. An unremitting croupy cough and progressive stridor can accompany rhabdomyosarcoma of the larynx. Because most of these signs and symptoms also are associated with common childhood conditions, clinicians must be alert to the possibility of tumor.

Rhabdomyosarcoma of the trunk or extremities often is first noticed after trauma and initially may be regarded as a hematoma. If the swelling does not resolve or increases, malignancy should be suspected. Involvement of the genitourinary tract can produce hematuria, obstruction of the lower urinary tract, recurrent urinary tract infections, incontinence, or a mass detectable on abdominal or rectal examination. Paratesticular tumor usually manifests as a painless, rapidly growing mass in the scrotum. Vaginal rhabdomyosarcoma may manifest as a grape-like mass of tumor tissue bulging through the vaginal orifice, known as **sarcoma botryoides,** and can cause urinary tract or large bowel symptoms. Vaginal bleeding or obstruction of the urethra or rectum may occur. Similar findings can be noted with uterine primaries.

Table 500-1	Staging System for Rhabdomyosarcoma				
STAGE	**SITE**	**T STAGE**	**SIZE**	**NODE STATUS**	**METASTASIS**
1	Favorable	T1 or T2	a or b	N0 or N1 or Nx	M0
2	Unfavorable	T1 or T2	a	N0 or Nx	M0
3	Unfavorable	T1 or T2	a	N1	M0
			b	N0 or N1 or Nx	
4	Any	T1 or T2	a or b	N0 or N1 or Nx	M1

T1, confined to anatomic site of origin; T2, extension and/or fixative to surrounding tissue.
Size: a, <5 cm in diameter; b, ≥5 cm in diameter.
Nodes: N0, regional nodes not involved; N1, regional nodes involved; Nx, regional node status unknown.
Metastases: M0, no distant metastases; M1, metastases present (includes positive cytology in CSF, pleural, or peritoneal fluid).

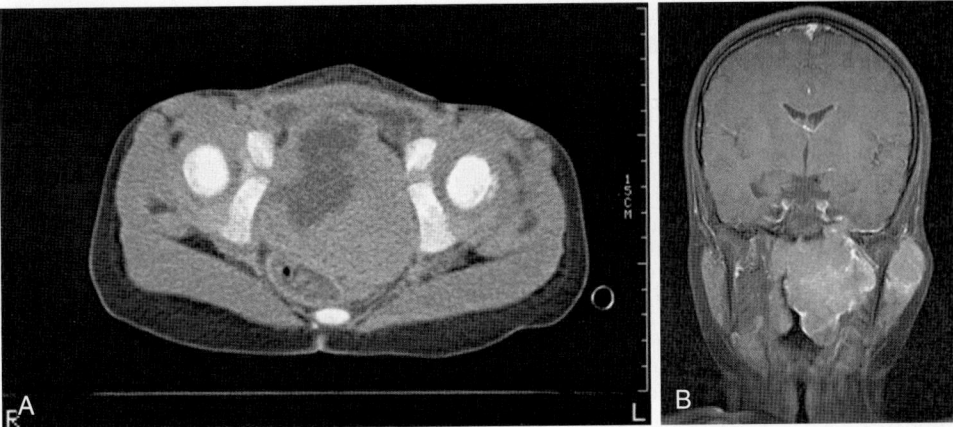

Figure 500-1 A, Pelvic CT scan of a child with a bladder rhabdomyosarcoma. **B,** MR image of a child with a parameningeal rhabdomyosarcoma.

Table 500-2	Risk Groups and Outcome for Rhabdomyosarcoma, Children's Oncology Group		
RISK GROUP	**STAGE/GROUP**	**HISTOLOGY**	**LONG-TERM EFS**
Low, subset 1	Stage 1, Groups I-II Stage 1, Group III (orbit) Stage 2, Groups I-II	Embryonal	85-95%
Low, subset 2	Stage 1, Group III (nonorbit) Stage 3, Groups I-II	Embryonal	70-85%
Intermediate	Stage 2-3, Group III Stage 1-3, Groups I-III	Embryonal Alveolar	73% 65%
High	Stage 4, Group IV Stage 4, Group IV	Embryonal Alveolar	35% 15%

From Hawkins DS, Spunt SL, Skapek SX: Children's Oncology Group's 2013 blueprint for research: soft tissue sarcomas. Pediatr Blood Cancer 60:1001–1008, 2013, Table I, p. 1002.

Tumors in any location may disseminate early and cause symptoms of pain or respiratory distress associated with pulmonary metastases. Extensive bone involvement can produce symptomatic hypercalcemia. In such cases, it may be difficult to identify the primary lesion.

Diagnosis

Early diagnosis of rhabdomyosarcoma requires a high index of suspicion. The microscopic appearance is that of a small, round, blue cell tumor. Neuroblastoma, lymphoma, and Ewing sarcoma also are **small, round, blue cell tumors** from which suspected rhabdomyosarcomas must be differentiated. The differential diagnosis depends on the site of presentation. Definitive diagnosis is established by biopsy, microscopic appearance, and results of immunohistochemical stains and analysis of PAX/FOXO1 expression. A lesion in an extremity may be thought to be a hematoma or hemangioma; an orbital lesion resulting in proptosis may be treated as an orbital cellulitis; or bladder-obstructive symptoms may be missed. Adolescents may ignore or be embarrassed to mention paratesticular lesions for a long time. Unfortunately, several months often elapse between the initial symptoms and biopsy. Diagnostic procedures are determined mainly by the area of involvement. CT or MRI is necessary for evaluation of the primary tumor site. With signs and symptoms in the head and neck area, radiographs should be examined for evidence of a tumor mass and for indications of bony erosion. MRI should be performed to identify intracranial extension or meningeal involvement and also to reveal bony involvement or erosion at the base of the skull. For abdominal and pelvic tumors, CT with a contrast agent or MRI can help delineate the tumor (Fig. 500-1). A radionuclide bone scan, chest CT, and bilateral bone marrow aspiration and biopsy should be performed to evaluate the patient for the presence of metastatic disease and to plan treatment. Fluorodeoxyglucose positron emission tomography is being used more frequently to enhance staging. The most critical element of the diagnostic work-up is examination of tumor tissue, which includes the use of special histochemical stains and immunostains. Molecular genetics is important to detect fusion transcripts present in alveolar rhabdomyosarcoma (PAX-FOX1). Lymph nodes also should be sampled for the presence of disease spread, especially in tumors of the extremities and in boys older than 10 yr of age with paratesticular tumors.

Treatment

Treatment is multidisciplinary and includes the pediatric oncologist, pediatric surgeon or other surgical subspecialist, and most often radiation oncologist. Only if the tumor is able to be completely resected, with negative margins, without loss of function or major cosmetic deformity should this be attempted initially. Unfortunately, most rhabdomyosarcomas are not completely resectable at initial diagnosis. Treatment is based on risk classification of the tumor, which is determined by the stage of tumor, the tumor histology, and the amount of tumor that was surgically resected prior to chemotherapy ("surgical group"). Stage is dependent on primary site (favorable vs unfavorable), tumor invasiveness (T1 or T2), lymph node status, tumor size, and presence of metastasis. Favorable sites include female genital, paratesticular, and head and neck (nonparameningeal) regions; all other sites are considered unfavorable. Table 500-1 shows the Children's Oncology Group staging system for rhabdomyosarcoma.

Patients should be offered enrollment in clinical trials. Table 500-2 shows current risk stratification and outcome based on results of recent studies. Patients with low-risk disease can be cured with minimal therapy consisting of vincristine and of actinomycin with or without lower doses of cyclophosphamide; radiation therapy can be used in the case of residual disease after initial surgery. Treatment for patients with intermediate-risk disease consists of vincristine, actinomycin, and cyclophosphamide along with radiation. Clinical trials in North

Table 500-3	Features of Most Common Types of Nonrhabdomyosarcoma Soft Tissue Sarcomas	
TISSUE TYPE	**TUMOR**	**NATURAL HISTORY AND BIOLOGY**
Adipose	Liposarcoma	A very rare tumor. Usually arises in the extremities or retroperitoneum; associated with a nonrandom translocation, t(12;16)(q13;p11). Tends to be locally invasive and rarely metastasizes; wide local excision is the treatment of choice. The role of radiation therapy and chemotherapy in treating gross residual or metastatic disease is not established.
Fibrous	Fibrosarcoma	Most common soft tissue sarcoma in children younger than 1 yr. Congenital fibrosarcoma is a low-grade malignancy that commonly arises in the extremities or trunk and rarely metastasizes. Surgical excision is treatment of choice; dramatic responses to preoperative chemotherapy may occur. In children older than 4 yr, the natural history is similar to that in adults (a 5 yr survival rate of 60%); wide surgical excision and preoperative chemotherapy are commonly used. Associated with t(12;15)(p13;q25) or trisomy 11, also +8, +17, +20.
	Malignant fibrous histiocytoma	Most commonly arises in the trunk and extremities, deep in the subcutaneous layer. Histologically subdivided into storiform, giant cell, myxoid, and angiomatoid variants. The angiomatoid type tends to affect younger patients and is curable with surgical resection alone. Wide surgical excision is the treatment of choice. Chemotherapy has produced objective tumor regressions.
Vascular	Hemangiopericytoma	Often arises in the lower extremities or retroperitoneum; may manifest as hypoglycemia and hypophosphatemic rickets. Both benign and malignant histology. Nonrandom translocations t(12;19)(q13;q13) and t(13;22)(q22;q13.3) have been described. Complete surgical excision is the treatment of choice. Chemotherapy and radiation therapy may produce responses.
	Angiosarcoma	Rare in children; 33% arise in skin, 25% in soft tissue, and 25% in liver, breast, or bone. Associated with chronic lymphedema and exposure to vinyl chloride in adults. Survival rate is poor (12% at 5 yr) despite some responses to chemotherapy/radiation therapy.
	Hemangioendothelioma	Can occur in soft tissue, liver, and lung. Localized lesions have a favorable outcome; lesions in lung and liver often are multifocal and have a poor prognosis.
Peripheral nerves	Neurofibrosarcoma	Also known as the malignant peripheral nerve sheath tumor. Develops in up to 16% of patients with neurofibromatosis type 1 (NF1); almost 50% occur in patients with NF1. Deletions of chromosome 22q11-q13 or 17q11 and p53 mutations have been reported. Commonly arises in trunk and extremities and is usually locally invasive. Complete surgical excision is necessary for survival; response to chemotherapy is suboptimal.
Synovium	Synovial sarcoma	The most common nonrhabdomyosarcoma soft tissue sarcoma in some series. Often manifesting in the 3rd decade, but 33% of patients are younger than age 20 yr. Typically arises around the knee or thigh and is characterized by a nonrandom translocation t(X;18)(p11;q11). Wide surgical excision is necessary. Radiation therapy is effective in microscopic residual disease, and ifosfamide-based therapy is active in advanced disease.
Unknown	Alveolar soft part sarcoma	Slow-growing tumor; tends to recur or to metastasize to lung and brain years after diagnosis. Often arises in the extremities and head and neck.
Smooth muscle	Leiomyosarcoma	Often arises in the gastrointestinal tract and may be associated with a t(12;14)(q14;q23) translocation. Associated with Epstein-Barr virus in immunodeficiency syndromes (including AIDS). Complete surgical excision is the treatment of choice.

America are investigating the role of topoisomerase inhibitors in this group of patients. For patients with high-risk disease, newer approaches using intensive multiagent chemotherapy along with biologic agents are being investigated.

Prognosis

Prognostic factors include age, stage, histology, and primary site. Among patients with resectable tumor and favorable histology, 80-90% have prolonged disease-free survival. Unresectable tumor localized to certain favorable sites, such as the orbit, also has a high likelihood of cure. Approximately 65-70% of patients with incompletely resected tumor also achieve long-term disease-free survival. Patients with disseminated disease have a poor prognosis; only approximately 50% achieve remission, and fewer than 50% of these are cured. Older children have a poorer prognosis than younger children. For all patients, surveillance for late effects of cancer treatment is extremely important. Some examples of late effects include infertility from cyclophosphamide, late effects in the radiation field such as bladder dysfunction, infertility, cataracts, impaired bone growth, and secondary malignancies.

OTHER SOFT TISSUE SARCOMAS

The nonrhabdomyosarcoma soft tissue sarcomas constitute a heterogeneous group of tumors that account for 3% of all childhood

malignancies (Table 500-3). Because they are relatively rare in children, much of the information about their natural history and treatment has been derived from studies in adult patients. In children, the median age at diagnosis is 12 yr, with a male:female ratio of 2.3:1. These tumors commonly arise in the trunk or lower extremities. The most common histologic types are synovial sarcoma (42%), fibrosarcoma (13%), malignant fibrous histiocytoma (12%), and neurogenic tumors (10%). Molecular genetic studies often prove useful in diagnosis, because several of these tumors have characteristic chromosomal translocations. Tumor size, stage (clinical group), invasiveness, and histologic grade correlate with survival.

Surgery remains the mainstay of therapy, but a careful search for lung and bone metastases should be undertaken before surgical excision. Chemotherapy and radiation therapy should be considered for large, high-grade, and unresectable tumors. The role of chemotherapy for nonrhabdomyosarcoma soft tissue sarcomas is not as well defined as for rhabdomyosarcoma. Patients with unresectable or metastatic disease are treated with multiagent chemotherapy in addition to irradiation and/or surgery. Patients with completely resected small (<5 cm) tumors are generally treated with surgery alone and can be expected to have an excellent outcome regardless of whether the tumor is high or low grade.

Bibliography is available at Expert Consult.

Chapter 501
Neoplasms of Bone

501.1 Malignant Tumors of Bone
Carola A.S. Arndt

The annual incidence of malignant bone tumors in the United States is approximately 7 cases per 1 million white children younger than 14 yr of age, with a slightly lower incidence in African-American children. Osteosarcoma is the most common primary malignant bone tumor in children and adolescents, followed by Ewing sarcoma (Table 501-1; Fig. 501-1). In children younger than 10 yr of age, Ewing sarcoma is more common than osteosarcoma. Both tumor types are most likely to occur in the second decade of life.

OSTEOSARCOMA
Epidemiology
The annual incidence of osteosarcoma in the United States is 5.6 cases per 1 million children younger than 15 yr of age. The highest risk period for development of osteosarcoma is during the adolescent growth spurt, suggesting an association between rapid bone growth and malignant transformation. Patients with osteosarcoma are taller than their peers of similar age.

Pathogenesis
Although the cause of osteosarcoma is unknown, certain genetic or acquired conditions predispose patients to development of osteosarcoma. Patients with **hereditary retinoblastoma** have a significantly increased risk for development of osteosarcoma. The sites of osteosarcoma in these patients were initially thought to be only in previously irradiated areas, but later studies show them to arise in sites far from the original retinoblastoma radiation field. Predisposition to development of osteosarcoma in these patients may be related to loss of heterozygosity of the *RB* gene. Osteosarcoma also occurs in the **Li-Fraumeni syndrome**, which is a familial cancer syndrome associated with germline mutations of the *P53* gene. Kindreds with

Table 501-1	Comparison of Features of Osteosarcoma and the Ewing Family of Tumors	
FEATURE	**OSTEOSARCOMA**	**EWING FAMILY OF TUMORS**
Age	Second decade	Second decade
Race	All races	Primarily whites
Sex (M:F)	1.5:1	1.5:1
Cell	Spindle cell–producing osteoid	Undifferentiated small round cell, probably of neural origin
Predisposition	Retinoblastoma, Li-Fraumeni syndrome, Paget disease, radiotherapy	None known
Site	Metaphyses of long bones	Diaphyses of long bones, flat bones
Presentation	Local pain and swelling; often, history of injury	Local pain and swelling; fever
Radiographic findings	Sclerotic destruction (less commonly lytic); sunburst pattern	Primarily lytic, multilaminar periosteal reaction ("onion-skinning")
Differential diagnosis	Ewing sarcoma, osteomyelitis	Osteomyelitis, eosinophilic granuloma, lymphoma, neuroblastoma, rhabdomyosarcoma
Metastasis	Lungs, bones	Lungs, bones
Treatment	Chemotherapy Ablative surgery of primary tumor	Chemotherapy Radiotherapy and/or surgery of primary tumor
Outcome	Without metastases, 70% cured; with metastases at diagnosis, ≤20% survival	Without metastases, 60% cured; with metastases at diagnosis, 20-30% survival

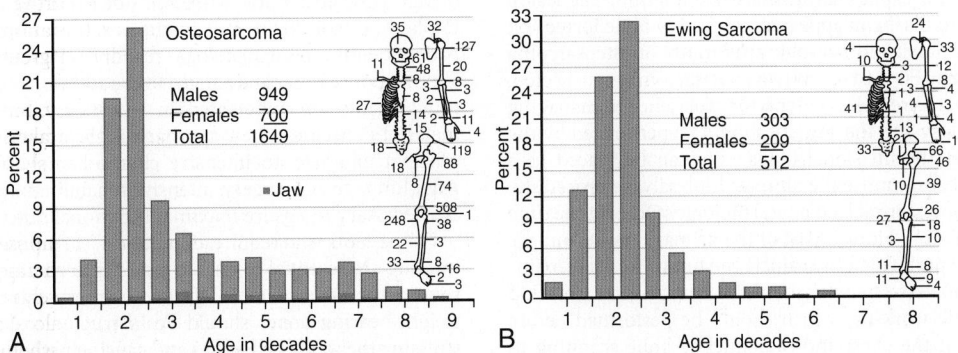

Figure 501-1 A, Age and skeletal distribution of 1,649 cases of osteosarcoma in the Mayo Clinic files. **B,** Age and skeletal distribution of 512 cases of Ewing sarcoma in the Mayo Clinic files. *(From Unni KK, editor: Dahlin's bone tumors: general aspects and data on 11,087 cases, ed 5, Philadelphia, 1996, Lippincott-Raven. Reprinted by permission of the Mayo Foundation.)*

Li-Fraumeni syndrome have a spectrum of malignancies in 1st-degree relatives, including carcinoma of the breast, soft tissue sarcomas, brain tumors, leukemia, adrenal cortical carcinoma, and other malignancies. **Rothmund-Thomson syndrome** is a rare syndrome associated with short stature, skin telangiectasia, small hands and feet, hypoplasticity or absence of the thumbs, and a high risk of osteosarcoma. Osteosarcoma also can be induced by irradiation for Ewing sarcoma, craniospinal irradiation for brain tumors, or high-dose irradiation for other malignancies. Other benign conditions that can be associated with malignant transformation to osteosarcoma include Paget disease, enchondromatosis, multiple hereditary exostoses, and fibrous dysplasia.

The pathologic diagnosis of osteosarcoma is made by demonstration of a highly malignant, pleomorphic, spindle cell neoplasm associated with the formation of malignant osteoid and bone. There are 4 pathologic subtypes of conventional high-grade osteosarcoma: osteoblastic, fibroblastic, chondroblastic, and telangiectatic. No significant differences in outcome are associated with the various subtypes, although the chondroblastic component of that subtype may not respond as well to chemotherapy. The role in prognosis of various genes such as drug resistance–related genes, tumor-suppressor genes, and genes related to apoptosis is being evaluated.

Telangiectatic osteosarcoma may be confused with aneurysmal bone cyst because of its lytic appearance on radiography. High-grade osteosarcoma typically arises in the diaphyseal region of long bones and invades the medullary cavity. It also may be associated with a soft tissue mass. Two variants of osteosarcoma, parosteal and periosteal osteosarcoma, should be distinguished from conventional osteosarcoma because of their characteristic clinical features. **Parosteal osteosarcoma** is a low-grade, well-differentiated tumor that does not invade the medullary cavity and most commonly is found in the posterior aspect of the distal femur. Surgical resection alone often is curative in this lesion, which has a low propensity for metastatic spread. **Periosteal osteosarcoma** is a rare variant that arises on the surface of the bone but has a higher rate of metastatic spread than the parosteal type and an intermediate prognosis.

Clinical Manifestations
Pain, limp, and swelling are the most common presenting manifestations of osteosarcoma. Because these tumors occur most often in active adolescents, initial complaints may be attributed to a sports injury or sprain; any bone or joint pain not responding to conservative therapy within a reasonable time should be investigated thoroughly. Additional clinical findings may include limitation of motion, joint effusion, tenderness, and warmth. Results of routine laboratory tests, such as a complete blood cell count and chemistry panel, are usually normal, although alkaline phosphatase or lactate dehydrogenase values may be elevated.

Diagnosis
Bone tumor should be suspected in a patient who presents with deep bone pain, often causing nighttime awakening, in whom there is a palpable mass and radiographs that demonstrate a lesion. The lesion may be mixed lytic and blastic in appearance, but new bone formation is usually visible. The classic radiographic appearance of osteosarcoma is the **sunburst pattern** (Fig. 501-2). When osteosarcoma is suspected, the patient should be referred to a center with experience in managing bone tumors. The biopsy and the surgery should be performed by the same surgeon so that the incisional biopsy site can be placed in a manner that will not compromise the ultimate limb salvage procedure. Tissue usually is obtained for molecular and biologic studies at the time of the initial biopsy. Before biopsy, MRI of the primary lesion and the entire bone should be performed to evaluate the tumor for its proximity to nerves and blood vessels, soft tissue and joint extension, and skip lesions. The metastatic work-up, which should be performed before biopsy, includes CT of the chest and radionuclide bone scanning to evaluate for lung and bone metastases, respectively. The **differential diagnosis** of a lytic bone lesion includes histiocytosis, Ewing sarcoma, lymphoma, and bone cyst.

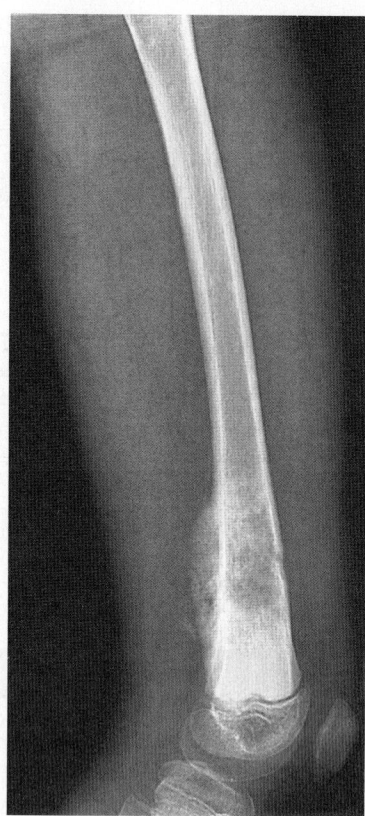

Figure 501-2 Radiograph of an osteosarcoma of the femur with typical "sunburst" appearance of bone formation.

Treatment
With chemotherapy and surgery, the 5-yr disease-free survival rate of patients with nonmetastatic extremity osteosarcoma is 65-75%. Complete surgical resection of the tumor is important for cure. The current approach is to treat patients with preoperative chemotherapy in an attempt to facilitate limb salvage operations and to treat micrometastatic disease immediately. Up to 80% of patients are able to undergo limb salvage operations after initial chemotherapy. It is important to resume chemotherapy as soon as possible after surgery. Lung metastases present at diagnosis should be resected by thoracotomies at some time during the course of treatment. Active agents currently in use in multidrug chemotherapy regimens for conventional osteosarcoma include doxorubicin, cisplatin, methotrexate, and ifosfamide.

One of the most important prognostic factors in osteosarcoma is the histologic response to chemotherapy. An international cooperative group is performing a randomized trial of the postoperative addition of high-dose ifosfamide with etoposide to standard 3 drug therapy with cisplatin, doxorubicin, and methotrexate to improve the outcome of patients with a poor histologic response. Patients with a good histologic response were randomized to the addition of pegylated interferon-α2b. Results are anticipated in the near future. For patients with metastatic disease, a new approach is the addition of zoledronic acid, a bisphosphonate, to intensive chemotherapy, with results pending. After limb salvage surgery, intensive rehabilitation and physical therapy are necessary to ensure maximal functional outcome.

For patients who require amputation, early prosthetic fitting and gait training are essential to enable patients to resume normal activities as soon as possible. Before definitive surgery, patients with tumors on weight-bearing bones should be instructed to use crutches to avoid stressing the weakened bones and causing pathologic fracture. The role of chemotherapy in parosteal and periosteal osteosarcomas is not well defined, and chemotherapy is generally reserved for use in patients with tumors which have a high-grade microscopic appearance.

Prognosis

Surgical resection alone is curative only for patients with parosteal osteosarcoma. Conventional osteosarcoma requires multiagent chemotherapy. Up to 75% of patients with nonmetastatic extremity osteosarcoma are cured with current multiagent treatment protocols. The prognosis is not as favorable for patients with pelvic tumors as for those with primary tumors in the extremities. Twenty percent to 30% of patients who have limited numbers of pulmonary metastases also can be cured with aggressive chemotherapy and resection of lung nodules. Patients with bone metastases and those with widespread lung metastases have an extremely poor prognosis. Long-term follow-up of patients with osteosarcoma is important to monitor for late effects of chemotherapy, such as cardiotoxicity from anthracycline and hearing loss from cisplatin. Patients in whom late, isolated lung metastases develop may be cured with surgical resection of the metastatic lesions alone.

EWING SARCOMA
Epidemiology

The incidence of Ewing sarcoma in the United States is 2.1 cases per 1 million children. It is rare among African-American children. Ewing sarcoma, an undifferentiated sarcoma of bone, also may arise from soft tissue. The term **Ewing sarcoma family of tumors** refers to a group of small, round cell, undifferentiated tumors thought to be of neural crest origin that generally carry the same chromosomal translocation. This family of tumors includes Ewing sarcoma of bone and soft tissue and peripheral **primitive neuroectodermal tumor**. Treatment protocols for these tumors are the same whether the tumors arise in bone or soft tissue. Anatomic sites of primary tumors arising in bone are distributed evenly between the extremities and the central axis (pelvis, spine, and chest wall). Primary tumors arising in the chest wall are often referred to as **Askin tumors**.

Pathogenesis

Immunohistochemical staining assists in the diagnosis of Ewing sarcoma to differentiate it from **small, round, blue cell tumors** such as lymphoma, rhabdomyosarcoma, and neuroblastoma. Histochemical stains may react positively with certain neural markers on tumor cells (neuron-specific enolase and S-100), especially in peripheral primitive neuroectodermal tumors. Reactivity with muscle markers (e.g., desmin, actin) is absent. Additionally, MIC-2 (CD99) staining is usually positive. A specific chromosomal translocation, t(11;22), or a variant thereof is found in most of the Ewing sarcoma family of tumors. Analysis for the translocation by FISH (fluorescent in situ hybridization) or polymerase chain reaction analysis for the chimeric fusion gene products EWS/FLI1 or EWS/ERG is utilized routinely in diagnosis.

Clinical Manifestations

Symptoms of Ewing sarcoma are similar to those of osteosarcoma. Pain, swelling, limitation of motion, and tenderness over the involved bone or soft tissue are common presenting symptoms. Patients with huge chest wall primary tumors may present with respiratory distress. Patients with paraspinal or vertebral primary tumors may present with symptoms of cord compression. Ewing sarcoma often is associated with **systemic manifestations**, such as fever and weight loss; patients may have undergone treatment for a presumptive diagnosis of osteomyelitis or a fever of unknown origin. Patients also may have a delay in diagnosis when their pain or swelling is attributed to a sports injury.

Diagnosis

The diagnosis of Ewing sarcoma should be suspected in a patient who presents with pain and swelling, with or without systemic symptoms, and with a radiographic appearance of a primarily lytic bone lesion with periosteal reaction, the characteristic **onion-skinning** (Fig. 501-3). A large, associated, soft tissue mass often is visualized on MRI or CT (Fig. 501-4). The **differential diagnosis** includes osteosarcoma, osteomyelitis, Langerhans cell histiocytosis, primary lymphoma of bone, metastatic neuroblastoma, or rhabdomyosarcoma in the case of a pure soft tissue lesion. Patients should be referred to a center with

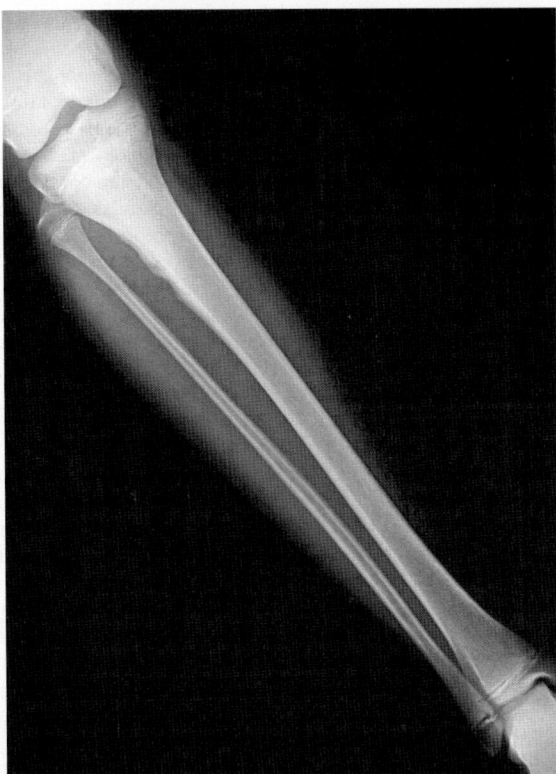

Figure 501-3 Radiograph of tibial Ewing sarcoma showing periosteal elevation or "onion-skinning."

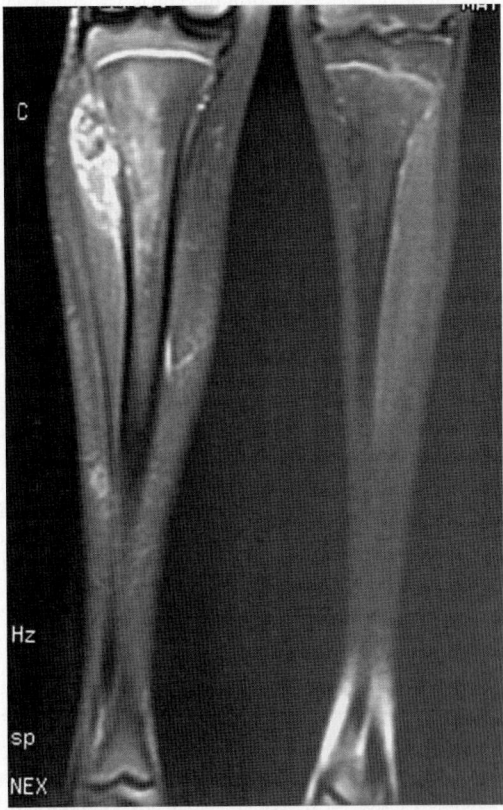

Figure 501-4 MR image of tibial Ewing sarcoma showing a large associated soft tissue mass.

experience in managing bone tumors for evaluation and biopsy. Thorough evaluation for metastatic disease includes CT of the chest, radionuclide bone scan, and bone marrow aspiration and biopsy specimens from at least 2 sites. MRI of the tumor and the entire length of involved bone should be performed to determine the exact extension of the soft tissue and bony mass and the proximity of tumor to neurovascular structures. Fluorodeoxyglucose positron emission tomography scanning is being incorporated to enhance staging. Studies are also using fluorodeoxyglucose positron emission tomography to evaluate response to therapy.

To avoid compromising an ultimate potential for limb salvage by a poorly planned biopsy incision, the same surgeon should perform the biopsy and the surgical procedure. CT-guided biopsy of the lesion often provides diagnostic tissue. It is important to obtain adequate tissue for special stains and molecular studies.

Treatment

Tumors of the Ewing sarcoma family are best managed with a comprehensive multidisciplinary approach in which the surgeon, chemotherapist, and radiation oncologist plan therapy. Multiagent chemotherapy is important because it can shrink the tumor rapidly and is usually given before local control is attempted. In North America, standard chemotherapy for nonmetastatic Ewing sarcoma includes vincristine, doxorubicin, cyclophosphamide, etoposide, and ifosfamide. Chemotherapy usually causes dramatic shrinkage of the soft tissue mass and rapid, significant pain relief. The most recent published randomized study for patients with nonmetastatic Ewing sarcoma showed a statistically significantly better outcome when patients were treated on a 14 day schedule than on a 21 day schedule. Current studies are evaluating the addition of topoisomerase inhibitors to standard chemotherapy, and plans are under way to investigate the role of insulin-like growth factor receptor inhibitors for certain groups of patients. An international cooperative group trial is evaluating whether myeloablative chemotherapy and stem cell rescue is superior to chemotherapy with lung irradiation for patients with pulmonary metastases. Ewing sarcoma is considered a radiosensitive tumor, and local control may be achieved with irradiation or surgery. Radiation therapy is associated with a risk of radiation-induced second malignancies, especially osteosarcoma, as well as failure of bone growth in skeletally immature patients. Many centers prefer surgical resection, if possible, to achieve local control. It is important to provide the patient with crutches if the tumor is in a weight-bearing bone, to avoid a pathologic fracture before definitive local control. Chemotherapy should be resumed as soon as possible after surgery.

Prognosis

Patients with small, nonmetastatic, distally located extremity tumors have the best prognosis, with a cure rate of up to 75%. Patients with pelvic tumors have, until recently, had a much worse outcome. Patients with metastatic disease at diagnosis, especially bone or bone marrow metastases, have a poor prognosis, with <30% surviving long term. New approaches, such as very intensive chemotherapy with peripheral blood stem cell rescue, are being investigated in these patients.

Long-term follow-up of patients with Ewing sarcoma is important because of the potential for late effects of treatment, such as anthracycline cardiotoxicity; second malignancies, especially in the radiation field; and late relapses, even as long as 10 yr after initial diagnosis.

501.2 Benign Tumors and Tumor-Like Processes of Bone

Carola A.S. Arndt

Benign bone lesions in children are common in comparison with the relatively rare malignant neoplasms of bone. They present diagnostic challenges. Some, although histologically benign, can be life-threatening. No single element in the history or diagnostic test is sufficient to rule out malignancies or suggest the existence of non-neoplastic conditions. A broad range of diagnostic possibilities must be considered when the physician is confronted with an undiagnosed bone lesion. Benign lesions may be painless or painful, especially if a pathologic fracture is impending. Night pain that awakens a child suggests malignancy, but relief of such pain with aspirin is common with benign lesions such as osteoid osteomas. Rapidly enlarging lesions usually are associated with malignancy, but several benign lesions, such as aneurysmal bone cysts, can enlarge faster than most malignancies. Several conditions, such as osteomyelitis, can simulate the appearance of benign bone tumors.

Many benign bone tumors are diagnosed incidentally or after pathologic fracture. Management of these fractures is similar to that of nonpathologic fractures in the same location. It is unusual for benign bone tumors to interfere with fracture healing. Likewise, the fractures rarely result in changes or healing of these tumors, which usually are treated after the fracture has healed.

Radiographs of any suspected bone lesion should always be obtained in 2 planes. Additional studies may be necessary to help arrive at the correct diagnosis and to guide treatment. Although these lesions are benign, many do require intervention.

Osteochondroma (exostosis) is one of the most common benign bone tumors in children. Because many are completely asymptomatic and unrecognized, the true incidence of this lesion is unknown. Most osteochondromas develop in childhood, arising from the metaphysis of a long bone, particularly the distal femur, proximal humerus, and proximal tibia. The lesion enlarges with the child until skeletal maturity. Most are discovered at 5-15 yr of age, when the child or parent notices a bony, nonpainful mass. Some are discovered because they are irritated by pressure during athletic or other activities. Osteochondromas appear radiographically as stalks or broad-based projections from the surface of the bone, usually in a direction away from the adjacent joint. Invariably, the lesion is radiographically smaller than suggested by palpation because the cartilage cap covering the lesion is not seen. This cartilage cap may be up to 1 cm thick. Both the cortex of the bone and the marrow space of the involved bone are continuous with the lesion. Malignant degeneration of a chondrosarcoma is rare in children but occurs in as many as 1% of adults. Routine removal is not performed unless the lesion is large enough to cause symptoms or grows rapidly.

Multiple hereditary exostoses is a related but rare condition characterized by the presence of multiple osteochondromas. Severely involved children can have short stature, limb-length inequality, premature partial physeal arrests, and deformity of both the upper and lower extremities. These children must be monitored carefully during growth.

Enchondroma is a benign lesion of hyaline cartilage that occurs centrally in the bone. Most of these lesions are asymptomatic and occur in the hands. Most are discovered incidentally, although pathologic fractures often lead to the diagnosis. Radiographically, the lesions occupy the medullary canal, are radiolucent, and are sharply marginated. Punctate or stippled calcification may be present within the lesion, but this is much more common in adults than in children. Almost all enchondromas are solitary. Most can simply be observed, with curettage and bone grafting reserved for lesions that are symptomatic or large enough to weaken the bone structurally. Multifocal involvement is referred to as **Ollier disease** and can result in bone dysplasia, short stature, limb-length inequality, and joint deformity. Surgery may be necessary to correct or prevent such deformities. When multiple enchondromas are associated with angiomas of the soft tissue, the condition is referred to as **Maffucci syndrome**. A high rate of malignant transformation has been reported in both of these multifocal conditions.

Chondroblastoma is a rare lesion usually found in the epiphysis of long bones. Most patients present in the 2nd decade with complaints of mild to moderate pain in the adjacent joint. Common sites include the hip, shoulder, and knee. Muscle atrophy and local tenderness may be the only clinical findings. The lesion appears radiographically as a sharply marginated radiolucency within the epiphysis or apophysis, occasionally with metaphyseal extension across the physis. Proximity to the joint can cause deformity of the subchondral bone, an effusion, or erosion into the joint. Recognition is important because most lesions can be cured with curettage and bone grafting before joint destruction occurs.

Chondromyxoid fibroma is an uncommon benign bone tumor in children. This metaphyseal lesion usually causes pain and local tenderness. The lesion occasionally is asymptomatic. Chondromyxoid fibroma appears radiographically as eccentric, lobular, metaphyseal radiolucency with sharp, sclerotic, and scalloped margins. The lower extremity is involved most often. Treatment usually consists of curettage and bone grafting or en bloc resection.

Osteoid osteoma is a small benign bone tumor. Most of these tumors are diagnosed between 5 and 20 yr of age. The clinical pattern is characteristic, consisting of unremitting and gradually increasing pain that often is worst at night and is relieved by aspirin. Boys are affected more often than girls. Any bone can be involved, but the most common sites are the proximal femur and tibia. Vertebral lesions can cause scoliosis or symptoms that mimic a neurologic disorder. Examination can reveal a limp, atrophy, and weakness when the lower extremity is involved. Palpation and range of motion do not alter the discomfort. Radiographs are distinctive, showing a round or oval metaphyseal or diaphyseal lucency (0.5-1.0 cm in diameter) surrounded by sclerotic bone. The central lucency, or nidus, shows intense uptake on bone scan. Approximately 25% of osteoid osteomas are not visualized on plain radiographs but can be identified with CT. Because of the small size of the lesion and its location adjacent to thick cortical bone, MRI is poor at detecting osteoid osteomas. Treatment is directed at removing the lesion. This can involve en bloc excision, curettage, or percutaneous CT-guided ablation of the nidus. Patients with mild pain may be treated with salicylates. Some lesions resolve spontaneously after skeletal maturity.

Osteoblastoma is a locally destructive, progressively growing lesion of bone with a predilection for the vertebrae, although almost any bone may be involved. Most patients note the insidious onset of dull aching pain, which may be present for months before patients seek medical attention. Spinal lesions can cause neurologic symptoms or deficits. The radiographic appearance is variable and less distinctive than that of other benign bone tumors. Approximately 25% show features suggesting a malignant neoplasm, making biopsy necessary in many cases. Expansile spinal lesions often involve the posterior elements. Treatment involves curettage and bone grafting or en bloc excision; care must be taken to preserve nerve roots when treating spinal lesions. Surgical stabilization of the spine may be necessary.

Fibromas (nonossifying fibroma, fibrous cortical defect, metaphyseal fibrous defect) are fibrous lesions of bone that occur in 40% of children older than 2 yr of age. They most likely represent a defect in ossification rather than a neoplasm and usually are asymptomatic. Most are discovered incidentally when radiographs are taken for other reasons, usually to rule out a fracture after trauma. Occasional pathologic fractures can occur through rare large lesions. Physical examination usually is unrevealing. Radiographs show a sharply marginated eccentric lucency in the metaphyseal cortex. Lesions may be multilocular and expansile, with extension from the cortex into the medullary bone. The long axis of the lesion runs parallel to that of the bone. Approximately 50% are bilateral or multiple. Because of the characteristic radiographic appearance, most lesions do not require biopsy or treatment. Spontaneous regression can be expected after skeletal maturity. Curettage and bone grafting may be recommended for lesions occupying >50% of the bone diameter because of the risk of a pathologic fracture.

Unicameral bone cysts can occur at any age in childhood but are rare in children younger than 3 yr of age and after skeletal maturity. The cause of these fluid-filled lesions is unknown. Some resolve spontaneously after skeletal maturity is reached. Most are asymptomatic until diagnosis, which usually follows a pathologic fracture. Such fractures can occur with relatively minor trauma, such as with throwing or catching a ball. Unicameral bone cysts appear radiographically as solitary, centrally located lesions within the medullary portion of the bone. These cysts are most common in the proximal humerus or femur. They often extend to (but not through) the physis and are sharply marginated. The cortex expands, but that does not exceed the width of the adjacent physis. Treatment involves allowing the pathologic fracture to heal, followed by aspiration and injection with methylprednisolone or bone marrow. Repeat injections, curettage, and bone grafting occasionally are necessary to treat recurrent lesions.

Aneurysmal bone cyst is a reactive lesion of bone seen in persons younger than 20 yr of age. The lesion is characterized by cavernous spaces filled with blood and solid aggregates of tissue. Although the femur, tibia, and spine are most commonly involved, this progressively growing, expansile lesion develops in any bone. Pain and swelling are common. Spinal involvement can lead to cord or nerve root compression and associated neurologic symptoms, including paralysis. Radiographs show eccentric lytic destruction and expansion of the metaphysis surrounded by a thin sclerotic rim of bone. Posterior elements of the spine are involved more commonly than the vertebral body. Unlike most other benign bone tumors, which usually are confined to a single bone, aneurysmal bone cysts can involve adjacent vertebrae. Rapid growth is characteristic and can lead to confusion with malignant neoplasms. Treatment consists of curettage and bone grafting or excision. Spinal lesions can require stabilization after excision. As with other benign tumors, attempts are made to preserve nerve roots and other vital structures. Recurrence after surgical treatment occurs in 20-30% of patients, is more common in younger than older children, and usually occurs in the 1st 1-2 yr after treatment.

Fibrous dysplasia is a developmental abnormality characterized by fibrous replacement of cancellous bone. Lesions may be solitary or multifocal (polyostotic), relatively stable, or progressively more severe. Most children are asymptomatic, although those with skull involvement might have swelling or exophthalmos. Pain and limp are characteristic of proximal femoral involvement. Limb-length discrepancy, bowing of the tibia or femur, and pathologic fractures may be presenting complaints. The triad of polyostotic disease, precocious puberty, and cutaneous pigmentation is known as Albright syndrome. Radiographic features of fibrous dysplasia include a lytic or ground-glass expansile lesion of the metaphysis or diaphysis. The lesion is sharply marginated and often is surrounded by a thick rim of sclerotic bone. Bowing, especially of the proximal femur, may be present. Treatment usually involves observation. Surgery is indicated for patients with progressive deformity, pain, or impending pathologic fractures. Bone grafting is not as successful in the treatment of fibrous dysplasia as with other benign tumors, because the lesion often recurs within the grafted bone. Reconstructive surgical techniques often are necessary to provide stability.

Osteofibrous dysplasia affects children 1-10 yr of age. This lesion usually involves the tibia. It is clinically, radiographically, and histologically distinct from fibrous dysplasia. Most children present with anterior swelling or enlargement of the leg. Progression is unlikely after 10 yr of age. Radiographs show solitary or multiple lucent cortical diaphyseal lesions surrounded by sclerosis. Anterior bowing of the tibia often is present. The radiographic appearance closely resembles that of adamantinoma, a malignant neoplasm, making biopsy more common than with other benign bone tumors. Treatment involves observation. Some lesions heal spontaneously. Excision and bone grafting should be delayed until the child is older than 10 yr of age because of a high recurrence rate before this age. Pathologic fractures heal with immobilization.

Langerhans cell histiocytosis is a monostotic or polyostotic disease that can also involve the skin, liver, or other organs. Single-site disease should be distinguished from the other forms of Langerhans cell histiocytosis (Hand-Schüller-Christian or Letterer-Siwe variants), which can have a less favorable prognosis (see Chapter 507). Langerhans cell histiocytosis usually occurs during the 1st 3 decades of life and is most common in boys 5-10 yr of age. The skull is most commonly affected, but any bone may be involved. Patients usually present with local pain and swelling. Marked tenderness and warmth often are present in the area of the involved bone. Spinal lesions can cause pain, stiffness, and occasional neurologic symptoms. The radiographic appearance of the skeletal lesions is similar in all forms of Langerhans cell histiocytosis but is variable enough to mimic many other benign and malignant lesions of bone. The radiolucent lesions have well-defined or irregular margins with expansion of the involved bone and periosteal new bone formation. Spine involvement can cause uniform compression or flattening of the vertebral body. A skeletal survey is warranted because polyostotic involvement and the typical skull lesions strongly suggest the diagnosis of eosinophilic granuloma. Biopsy often is necessary to confirm the diagnosis because of the broad radiographic differential diagnosis. Treatment includes curettage and bone grafting, low-dose radiation therapy, or corticosteroid injection. Observation for symptomatic lesions is reasonable because most osseous lesions heal spontaneously and do not recur. Children with bone lesions should be evaluated for visceral involvement because treatment of Hand-Schüller-Christian disease and Letterer-Siwe disease is more complex and often systemic.

Bibliography is available at Expert Consult.

Chapter 502
Retinoblastoma
Nidale Tarek and Cynthia E. Herzog

Retinoblastoma is an embryonal malignancy of the retina and the most common intraocular tumor in children. Although the survival rate of children in the United States and developed countries with retinoblastoma is extremely high, retinoblastoma progresses to metastatic disease and death in over 50% of children worldwide. Furthermore, the associated loss of vision and side effects of therapy are significant problems that remain to be addressed.

EPIDEMIOLOGY
Approximately 250-350 new cases of retinoblastoma are diagnosed each year in the United States, with no known racial or gender predilection. The cumulative lifetime incidence of retinoblastoma is approximately 1:20,000 live births, and retinoblastoma accounts for 4% of all pediatric malignancies. The median age at diagnosis is approximately 2 yr, and more than 90% of cases are diagnosed in children younger than 5 yr of age. Overall, about 66-75% of children with retinoblastoma have unilateral tumors, with the remainder having bilateral retinoblastoma. Bilateral involvement is more common in younger children, particularly in those diagnosed younger than the age of 1 yr, and is always heritable. There is a possible increased risk of retinoblastoma in children conceived by in vitro fertilization.

Retinoblastoma can be either hereditary or sporadic. Hereditary cases usually are diagnosed at a younger age and are multifocal and bilateral, whereas sporadic cases are usually diagnosed in older children who tend to have unilateral, unifocal involvement. The hereditary form is associated with loss of function of the **retinoblastoma gene (RB1)** via gene mutation or deletion. The *RB1* gene is located on chromosome 13q14 and encodes the **retinoblastoma protein,** a tumor-suppressor protein that controls cell-cycle phase transition and has roles in apoptosis and cell differentiation. Many different causative mutations have been identified, including translocations, deletions, insertions, point mutations, and epigenetic modifications such as gene methylation. The nature of the predisposing mutation can affect the penetrance and expressivity of retinoblastoma development.

According to Knudson's "two-hit" model of oncogenesis, 2 mutational events are required for retinoblastoma tumor development (see Chapter 492). In the hereditary form of retinoblastoma, the first mutation in the *RB1* gene is inherited through germinal cells and a second mutation occurs subsequently in somatic retinal cells. Second mutations that lead to retinoblastoma often result in the loss of the normal allele and concomitant loss of heterozygosity. Parents and siblings of a child with a germline mutation should be referred to a genetic specialist for testing; most children with hereditary retinoblastoma have spontaneous new germinal mutations, and both parents have wild-type retinoblastoma genes. All 1st-degree relatives of children with known or suspected hereditary retinoblastoma should have retinal examinations to identify retinomas or retinal scars, which may suggest hereditary retinoblastoma even though malignant retinoblastoma did not develop. In the sporadic form of retinoblastoma, the 2 mutations occur in somatic retinal cells. Heterozygous carriers of oncogenic *RB1* mutations demonstrate variable phenotypic expression.

PATHOGENESIS
Histologically, retinoblastoma appears as a small round blue cell tumor with rosette formation (Flexner-Wintersteiner rosettes). It may arise in any of the nucleated layers of the retina and exhibit various degrees of differentiation. Retinoblastoma tumors tend to outgrow their blood supply, resulting in necrosis and calcification.

Endophytic tumors arise from the inner surface of the retina and grow into the vitreous, and can also grow as tumors suspended within the vitreous itself, known as **vitreous seeding.** Exophytic tumors grow from the outer retinal layer and can cause retinal detachment. Diffuse infiltrating tumors grow intraretinally and remain flat; these are less common and can cause iris neovascularization. Tumors can also be both endophytic and exophytic. These tumors can also spread by direct extension to the choroid or along the optic nerve beyond the lamina cribrosa to the central nervous system, or by hematogenous or lymphatic spread to distant sites, including bones, bone marrow, and lungs.

CLINICAL MANIFESTATIONS
Retinoblastoma classically presents with **leukocoria,** a white pupillary reflex (Fig. 502-1), which often is first noticed when a red reflex is not present at a routine newborn or well-child examination or in a flash photograph of the child. Strabismus often is an initial presenting complaint. Decreased vision, orbital inflammation, hyphema, and pupil irregularity can occur with advancing disease. Pain can occur if secondary glaucoma is present. Only approximately 10% of retinoblastoma cases are detected by routine ophthalmologic screening in the context of a positive family history.

DIAGNOSIS
The diagnosis is established by the characteristic ophthalmologic findings of a chalky, white-gray retinal mass with a soft, friable consistency.

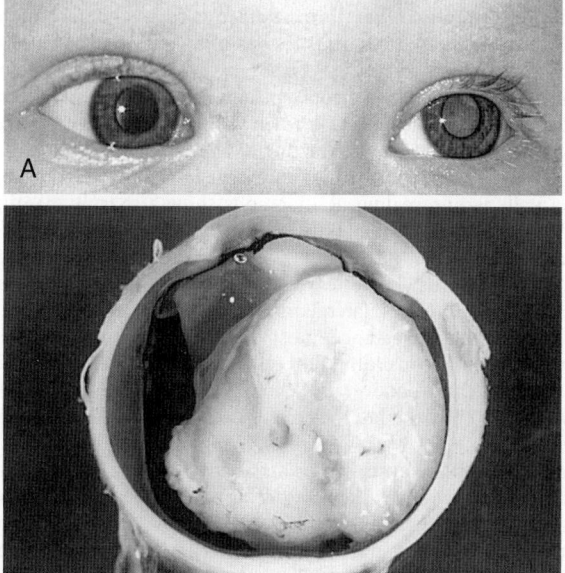

Figure 502-1 A, Leukocoria noted in the left eye of a child presenting with retinoblastoma. **B,** A large white tumor mass noted within the posterior chamber of the enucleated eye. *(From Shields JA, Shields CL: Current management of retinoblastoma, Mayo Clin Proc 69:50–56, 1994.)*

Imaging studies are not diagnostic, and biopsies are contraindicated. Indirect ophthalmoscopy with slit-lamp evaluation can detect retinoblastoma tumors, but a complete evaluation requires an examination under general anesthesia by an experienced ophthalmologist to obtain complete visualization of both eyes, which also facilitates photographing and mapping of the tumors. Retinal detachment or vitreous hemorrhage can complicate the evaluation.

Orbital ultrasonography, CT, or MRI is used to evaluate the extent of intraocular disease and extraocular spread. Occasionally (~60%), a pineal area (primitive neuroectodermal) tumor is detected in a child with hereditary and bilateral retinoblastoma, a phenomenon known as **trilateral retinoblastoma.** MRI allows for better evaluation of optic nerve involvement. Metastatic disease is rarely present at diagnosis; evaluation of the cerebrospinal fluid and bone marrow for tumor metastasis and radionuclide bone scan are required only if indicated by other clinical, laboratory, or imaging findings.

The **differential diagnosis** of retinoblastoma includes other causes of leukocoria, including persistent hyperplastic primary vitreous, Coats disease, vitreous hemorrhage, cataract, endophthalmitis from *Toxocara canis*, choroidal coloboma, retinopathy of prematurity, and familial exudative vitreoretinopathy.

TREATMENT

Treatment is determined by the size and location of the tumors, if the disease is localized to the eye or has spread either to the brain or to the rest of the body, and whether the child has hereditary or sporadic disease. The primary goal of treatment is always cure; the secondary goals include preserving vision and the eye itself and decreasing the risk of late side effects, mainly secondary malignancies. As newer modalities for local control of intraocular tumors and more effective systemic chemotherapy have emerged, primary enucleation is being performed less often.

Most unilateral disease presents with a solitary, large tumor. Enucleation is performed if there is no potential for the salvage of useful vision. With bilateral disease, chemoreduction in combination with **focal therapy** (laser photocoagulation or cryotherapy) has replaced the traditional approach of enucleation of the more severely affected eye and irradiation of the remaining eye. If feasible, small tumors can be treated with focal therapy with careful follow-up for recurrence or new tumor growth. Larger tumors often respond to multiagent chemotherapy, including carboplatin, vincristine, and etoposide. If this approach fails, external-beam irradiation should be considered, although this approach may result in significant orbital deformity and increased incidence of second malignancies in patients with germline *RB1* mutations. Brachytherapy, or episcleral plaque radiotherapy, is an alternative with less morbidity. Enucleation may be required for unresponsive or recurrent tumors. Alternative treatment options currently under investigation include other systemic chemotherapy agents such as topotecan, other methods of chemotherapy administration, including periocular, intravitreal, and ophthalmic artery infusions, and intense multiagent chemotherapy with autologous stem cell rescue for patients with metastatic disease.

PROGNOSIS

Approximately 95% of children in the United States with retinoblastoma are cured with modern treatment. Current efforts using chemotherapy in combination with focal therapy are intended to preserve useful vision and avoid external-beam radiation or enucleation. Routine ophthalmologic examinations should continue until children are older than age 7 yr. Unfortunately, the diagnosis of retinoblastoma in many children from 3rd-world countries is delayed, resulting in spread of the tumor outside of the orbit. The prognosis for children with retinoblastoma that has spread outside of the eye is poor. Trilateral retinoblastoma, disease involving both eyes and the pineal region, is almost universally fatal.

Children with germline *RB1* mutations are at significant risk for development of second malignancies, especially osteosarcoma and also soft tissue sarcomas and malignant melanoma. The risk of second malignancies is further increased by the use of radiation therapy.

Other radiation-related late adverse effects include cataracts, orbital growth deformities, lacrimal dysfunction, and late retinal vascular injury.

Bibliography is available at Expert Consult.

Chapter **503**
Gonadal and Germ Cell Neoplasms
Cynthia E. Herzog and Winston W. Huh

EPIDEMIOLOGY

Malignant germ cell tumors (GCTs) and gonadal tumors are rare, with an incidence of 12 cases per 1 million persons younger than 20 yr of age. Most malignant tumors of the gonads in children are GCTs. The incidence varies according to age and sex, although the incidence of GCTs in adolescent males has increased over time. Sacrococcygeal tumors occur predominantly in infant girls. Testicular GCTs occur predominantly before age 4 yr and after puberty. Klinefelter syndrome is associated with an increased risk of mediastinal GCTs; Down syndrome, undescended testes, infertility, testicular atrophy, testicular microlithiasis, testicular dysgenesis syndrome, and inguinal hernias are associated with an increased risk of testicular cancer. The risk of testicular cancer in patients with cryptorchidism is reduced but not eliminated if orchiopexy is performed before 13 yr of age. The risk of testicular GCT is increased in 1st-degree relatives and is highest among monozygotic twins.

PATHOGENESIS

The GCTs and non-GCTs arise from primordial germ cells and coelomic epithelium, respectively. Testicular and sacrococcygeal GCTs arising during early childhood characteristically have deletions at chromosome arms 1p and 6q and gains at 1q, and lack the isochromosome 12p that is highly characteristic of malignant GCTs of adults. Testicular GCT also may demonstrate loss of imprinting. Ovarian GCTs from older girls characteristically have deletions at 1p and gains at 1q and 21. Because GCTs may contain benign and mixed malignant elements in different areas of the tumor, extensive sectioning is essential to confirm the correct diagnosis. The many histologically distinct subtypes of GCTs include teratoma (mature and immature), endodermal sinus tumor, and embryonal carcinoma (Fig. 503-1). Non-GCTs of the ovary include epithelial (serous and mucinous) and sex cord–stromal tumors; non-GCTs of the testicle include sex cord/stromal (e.g., Leydig cell, Sertoli cell) tumors. *DICER1* mutations have been observed in nonepithelial ovarian cancers, especially in Sertoli-Leydig tumors.

CLINICAL MANIFESTATIONS AND DIAGNOSIS

The clinical presentation of germ cell neoplasms depends on location. Ovarian tumors often are quite large by the time they are diagnosed (Fig. 503-2). Extragonadal GCTs occur in the midline, including the suprasellar region, pineal region, neck, mediastinum, and retroperitoneal and sacrococcygeal areas (Fig. 503-3). Symptoms relate to mass effect, but the intracranial GCTs often present with anterior and posterior pituitary deficits (see Chapter 497).

The **serum α-fetoprotein (AFP)** level is elevated with endodermal sinus tumors and may be minimally elevated with teratomas. Infants normally have higher levels of AFP, which fall to normal adult levels by about age 8 mo; consequently, high AFP levels must be interpreted with caution in this age group. Elevation of the β subunit of **human chorionic gonadotropin,** which is secreted by syncytiotrophoblasts, is seen with choriocarcinoma and germinomas. Lactate dehydrogenase,

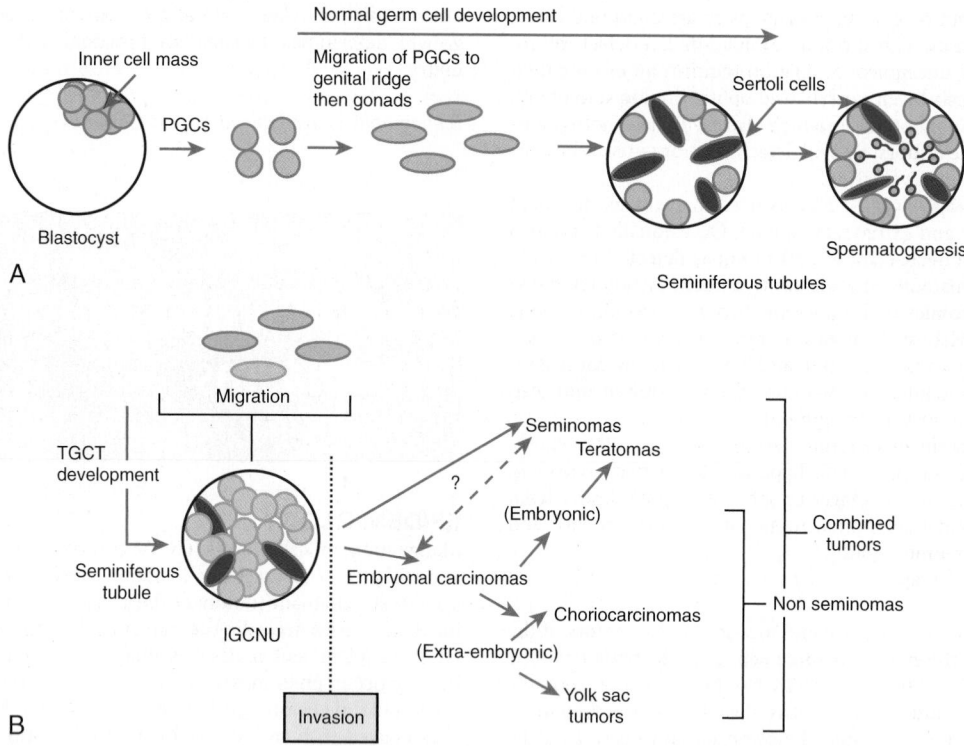

Figure 503-1 A, Normal germ cell development. **B,** Model for the origin and histogenesis of different subtypes of testicular germ cell tumors. *IGCNU,* intratubular germ cell neoplasia unclassified; *PGC,* primary germ cell; *TGCT,* testicular germ cell tumor(s).

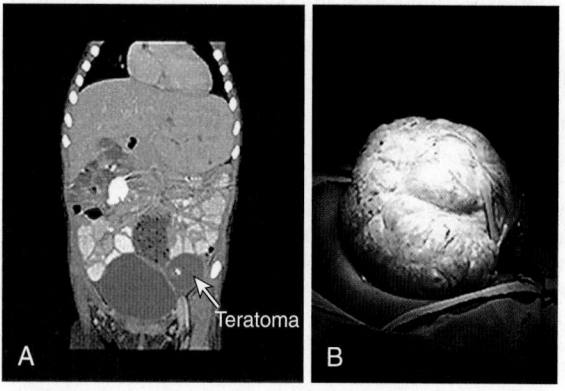

Figure 503-2 A, Postnatal MRI showing a left ovarian teratoma with bony calcification. **B,** Massive ovarian teratoma. *(From Lakhoo K. Neonatal teratomas. Early Hum Dev 86(10):643–647, 2010.)*

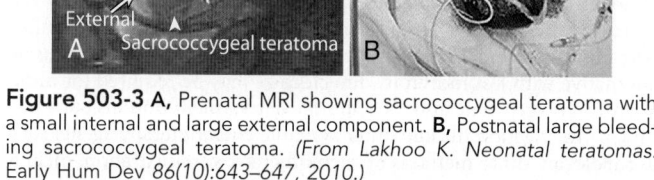

Figure 503-3 A, Prenatal MRI showing sacrococcygeal teratoma with a small internal and large external component. **B,** Postnatal large bleeding sacrococcygeal teratoma. *(From Lakhoo K. Neonatal teratomas. Early Hum Dev 86(10):643–647, 2010.)*

although nonspecific, may be a useful marker. If elevated, these markers provide important confirmation of the diagnosis and provide a means to monitor the patient for tumor response and recurrence. Both serum and cerebrospinal fluid should be assayed for these markers in patients with intracranial lesions.

Diagnosis begins with physical examination and imaging studies, including plain radiographs of the chest and ultrasonography of the abdomen. CT or MRI can further delineate the primary tumor. If germ cell malignancy is strongly suggested, preoperative staging with CT of the chest and bone scan is appropriate. Primary surgical resection is indicated for tumors deemed resectable. For older patients with testicular tumors, ipsilateral retroperitoneal lymph node sampling may be required to determine extent of disease and aid in treatment planning. Ovarian tumors also require detailed surgical evaluation including lymph node removal and pelvic washings for cytologic analysis for peritoneal spread. Diagnosis of intracranial lesions can be established with imaging and AFP or β-human chorionic gonadotropin determinations of serum and cerebrospinal fluid.

Gonadoblastomas often occur in patients with gonadal dysgenesis and all or parts of a Y chromosome. Gonadal dysgenesis is characterized by failure to fully masculinize the external genitalia. If this syndrome is diagnosed, imaging of the gonad with ultrasonography or CT is performed, and surgical resection of the tumor usually is curative. Prophylactic resection of dysgenetic gonads at the time of diagnosis is recommended, because gonadoblastomas, some of which contain malignant GCT elements, often develop. Gonadoblastomas may produce abnormal amounts of estrogen.

Teratomas occur in many locations, presenting as masses. They are not associated with elevated markers unless malignancy is present. The sacrococcygeal region is the most common site for teratomas. Sacrococcygeal teratomas occur most commonly in infants and may be diagnosed in utero or at birth, with most found in girls. The rate of malignancy in this location varies, ranging from <10% in children younger than 2 mo of age to >50% in children older than 4 mo of age.

Germinomas occur intracranially, in the mediastinum, and in the gonads. In the ovary, they are called **dysgerminomas;** in the testis, seminomas. They usually are tumor-marker–negative masses despite being malignant. Endodermal sinus or yolk sac tumor and choriocarcinoma appear highly malignant by histologic criteria. Both occur at gonadal and extragonadal sites. Embryonal carcinoma most often occurs in the testes. Choriocarcinoma and embryonal carcinoma rarely occur in the pure form and are usually found as part of a mixed malignant GCT.

Non–germ cell gonadal tumors are very uncommon in pediatrics and occur predominantly in the ovary. Epithelial carcinomas (usually an adult tumor), Sertoli-Leydig cell tumors, and granulosa cell tumors may occur in children. Carcinomas account for about one third of ovarian tumors in females younger than 20 yr of age; most of these occur in older teens and are of the serous or mucinous subtype. Sertoli-Leydig cell tumors and granulosa cell tumors produce hormones that can cause virilization, feminization, or precocious puberty, depending on pubertal stage and the balance between Sertoli cells (estrogen production) and Leydig cells (androgen production). Diagnostic evaluation usually focuses on the chief complaint of inappropriate sex steroid effect and includes hormone measurements, which reflect gonadotropin-independent sex steroid production. Appropriate imaging also is performed to rule out a functioning gonadal tumor. Surgery usually is curative. No effective therapy for nonresectable disease has been found.

TREATMENT
Complete surgical excision of the tumor usually is indicated, except for patients with intracranial tumors, where the primary therapy consists of radiation therapy and chemotherapy. For testicular tumors, an inguinal approach is indicated, and complete resection should include the entire spermatic cord. When complete excision cannot be accomplished, preoperative chemotherapy is indicated, with second-look surgery. For completely resected nonseminomatous testicular tumors, there is debate on whether patients can be clinically observed following surgery. For teratomas, both mature and immature, and completely resected malignant tumors of the testes, surgery alone is the treatment. For ovarian tumors, unless the contralateral ovary is obviously also involved by tumor, a fertility-sparing surgery should be performed. Cisplatin-based chemotherapy regimens usually are curative in GCTs that cannot be completely resected, even if metastases are present. However, sex cord–stromal tumors tend to be refractory to chemotherapy. Except for GCTs of the central nervous system, radiation therapy is limited to those tumors that are not amenable to complete excision and are refractory to chemotherapy.

PROGNOSIS
The overall cure rate for children with GCTs is >80%. Age is the most predictive factor of survival for extragonadal GCTs. Children older than 12 yr of age have a 4-fold higher risk of death, and a 6-fold higher risk if the tumor is thoracic. Histology has little effect on prognosis. Nonresected extragonadal GCTs have a slightly worse prognosis.

Bibliography is available at Expert Consult.

Chapter **504**
Neoplasms of the Liver
Nidale Tarek and Cynthia E. Herzog

Hepatic tumors are rare in children. Primary tumors of the liver account for approximately 1% of malignancies in children younger than 15 yr of age, with an annual incidence of 1.6 cases per 1 million children in the United States. Between 50% and 60% of hepatic tumors in children are malignant, with >65% of these malignancies being hepatoblastomas and most of the remainder being hepatocellular

carcinomas. Rare hepatic malignancies include embryonal sarcoma, angiosarcoma, malignant germ cell tumor, rhabdomyosarcoma of the liver, and undifferentiated sarcoma. More common childhood malignancies, such as neuroblastoma, Wilms tumor, and lymphoma, can metastasize to the liver. Benign liver tumors, which usually present in the 1st 6 mo of life, include hemangiomas, hamartomas, and hemangioendotheliomas.

HEPATOBLASTOMA
Epidemiology
Approximately 100 new cases of hepatoblastoma are diagnosed each yr in the United States. Hepatoblastoma occurs predominantly in children younger than 3 yr of age and the median age of diagnosis is 1 yr. The etiology is unknown. Hepatoblastomas are associated with familial adenomatous polyposis. Alterations in the antigen-presenting cell/β-catenin pathway have been found in most of the tumors evaluated. Hepatoblastomas are also associated with Beckwith-Wiedemann syndrome, hemihyperplasia, and other somatic overgrowth syndromes. Increased expression of insulin-like growth factor 2 secondary to genetic mutations or epigenetic changes is implicated in hepatoblastoma development in patients with Beckwith-Wiedemann syndrome. All children with Beckwith-Wiedemann syndrome or hemihyperplasia should be routinely screened with α-fetoprotein (AFP) levels and abdominal ultrasounds. Prematurity and low birthweight is associated with increased incidence of hepatoblastoma, with the risk increasing as birthweight decreases.

Pathogenesis
Hepatoblastoma arises from precursors of hepatocytes and is histologically classified as whole epithelial type, containing fetal or embryonal malignant cells (either as a mixture or as pure elements), and mixed type, containing both epithelial and mesenchymal elements. Histologic classification has a direct correlation with clinical outcome. The pure fetal histology subtype predicts a more favorable outcome and the small cell undifferentiated subtype is associated with normal AFP levels and predicts a worse outcome.

Clinical Manifestations
Hepatoblastoma usually presents as a large, asymptomatic abdominal mass. It arises from the right lobe 3 times more often than the left and usually is unifocal. As the disease progresses, fatigue, fever, weight loss, anorexia, vomiting, and abdominal pain may ensue. Rarely, hepatoblastoma presents with hemorrhage secondary to trauma or spontaneous rupture. Metastatic spread of hepatoblastoma most commonly involves regional lymph nodes and the lungs.

Diagnosis
A biopsy of liver tumors is necessary to establish the diagnosis. A valuable serum tumor marker, **AFP,** is used in the diagnosis and monitoring of hepatic tumors. The AFP levels are elevated in almost all hepatoblastomas. Bilirubin and liver enzymes usually are normal. Anemia is common, and thrombocytosis occurs in approximately 30% of patients. Serologic testing for hepatitides B and C should be performed, but the results usually are negative in hepatoblastoma.

Diagnostic imaging should include plain radiographs and ultrasonography of the abdomen to characterize the hepatic mass. Ultrasonography can differentiate malignant hepatic masses from benign vascular lesions. Either CT or MRI is an accurate method of defining the extent of intrahepatic tumor involvement and the potential for surgical resection. Evaluation for metastatic disease should include CT of the chest.

Treatment
In general, the cure of malignant hepatic tumors in children depends on complete resection of the primary tumor (Fig. 504-1); as much as 85% of the liver can be resected, with hepatic regeneration noted within 3-4 mo after surgery. Treatment of hepatoblastoma is based on surgery and systemic chemotherapy using cisplatin in combination with vincristine and 5-fluorouracil or doxorubicin. In 30% of cases,

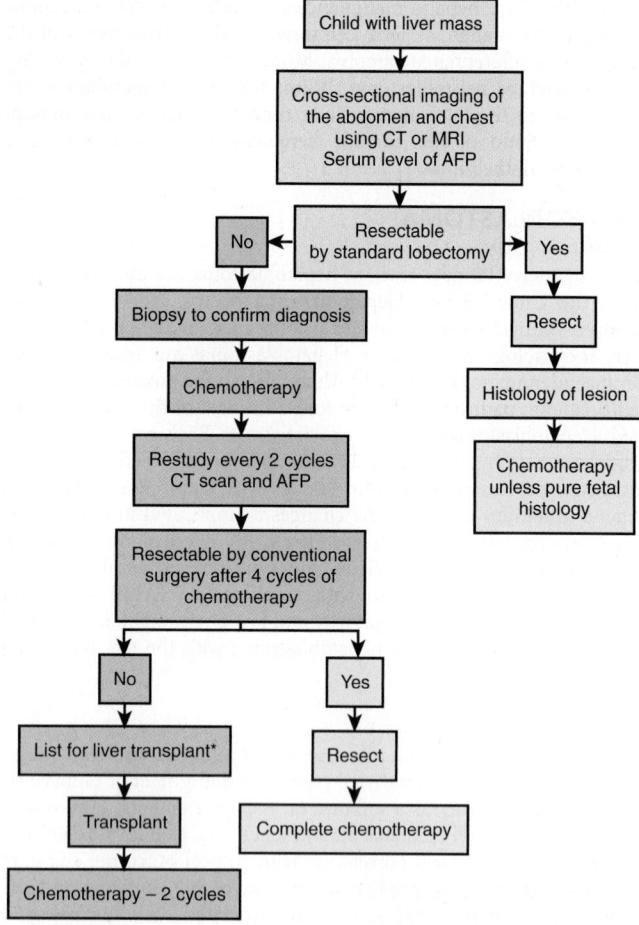

Figure 504-1 Algorithm for the management of a child who presents with a hepatoblastoma. AFP, α-fetoprotein. (*From Tiao GM, Bobey N, Allen S, et al: The current management of hepatoblastoma: a combination of chemotherapy, conventional resection, and liver transplantation, J Pediatr 146:204–211, 2005.*)

tumors are resectable at diagnosis; a safe attempt for initial gross total resection should be made followed by adjuvant chemotherapy. Unresectable tumors with or without metastatic disease, at presentation, usually respond to chemotherapy; preresection chemotherapy is indicated, and excision of the primary tumor and extrahepatic disease should be attempted as soon as it becomes feasible, followed by additional chemotherapy. Liver transplant is a viable option for unresectable primary hepatic malignancies and results in good long-term survival. The pretransplant medical condition is an important predictor of outcome, and thus transplant is much more effective as the primary surgery than as salvage therapy. Alternative treatment options currently under investigation include other systemic chemotherapy agents such as carboplatin, ifosfamide, etoposide, and irinotecan. Other treatment approaches include transarterial chemoembolization, cryoablation, and radiofrequency ablation.

Prognosis

In low-stage tumors, survival rates >90% can be achieved with multimodal treatment, including surgery and adjuvant chemotherapy. With tumors unresectable at diagnosis, survival rates of approximately 60%

can be obtained. Metastatic disease further reduces survival, but complete regression of disease often can be obtained with chemotherapy and surgical resection of the primary tumor and isolated pulmonary metastatic disease, resulting in survival rates of approximately 25%. Treatment-related long-term adverse effects include cardiac toxicity with doxorubicin and renal and ototoxicity with cisplatin.

HEPATOCELLULAR CARCINOMA
Epidemiology

Hepatocellular carcinoma occurs mostly in adolescents and often is associated with hepatitis B or C infection. It is more common in East Asia and other areas where hepatitis B is endemic; the incidence has decreased following the introduction of hepatitis B vaccination. In these areas it also tends to occur in a bimodal pattern, with the younger age peak overlapping the age of hepatoblastoma presentation. It also occurs in the chronic form of hereditary tyrosinemia, galactosemia, glycogen storage disease, α_1-antitrypsin deficiency, and biliary cirrhosis. Aflatoxin B contamination of food is another risk factor.

Pathogenesis

Hepatocellular carcinoma usually arises in an abnormal or cirrhotic liver and presents as a multicentric, invasive tumor consisting of large pleomorphic cells of epithelial origin. Compared to adults, cirrhosis in children is less common and congenital liver disorders are more common. Hepatocellular carcinomas are classified as classical or fibrolamellar. The fibrolamellar variant occurs more often in adolescent and young adult patients and is not associated with cirrhosis. Although previous reports have suggested that the fibrolamellar type has a better prognosis, more recent data analysis refutes this.

Clinical Manifestations

Hepatocellular carcinoma usually presents as a hepatic mass with abdominal distention and symptoms of anorexia, weight loss, and abdominal pain. Hepatocellular carcinoma can present as an acute abdominal crisis with rupture of the tumor and hemoperitoneum. Metastatic spread usually involves regional lymph nodes and the lungs. The AFP level is elevated in approximately 60% of children. Evidence of hepatitides B and C infection usually is found in endemic areas but not in Western countries or with the fibrolamellar type. Bilirubin usually is normal, but liver enzymes may be abnormal.

Diagnostic imaging should include plain radiographs and ultrasonography of the abdomen to characterize the hepatic mass. Ultrasonography can differentiate malignant hepatic masses from benign vascular lesions. Either CT or MRI is an accurate method of defining the extent of intrahepatic tumor involvement and the potential for surgical resection. Evaluation for metastatic disease should include CT of the chest.

Treatment

Complete tumor resection is crucial for curative treatment. Because of the multicentric origin of hepatocellular carcinoma and underlying liver disease, complete resection is accomplished in only 30-40% of cases. A gross total resection should be attempted at diagnosis when possible; combination chemotherapy following surgery is necessary. For unresectable tumors, chemotherapy followed by surgical assessment is essential; liver transplant is an option for unresectable tumors. Even with complete surgical resection, only 30% of children are long-term survivors. Chemotherapy, including cisplatin, doxorubicin, etoposide, and 5-fluorouracil, has shown some activity against this tumor, but improved long-term outcome has been difficult to achieve. Other techniques, such as cryosurgery, radiofrequency ablation, transarterial chemoembolization, and ethanol injection, are under study as therapy for hepatocellular carcinomas.

Bibliography is available at Expert Consult.

Chapter 505
Benign Vascular Tumors

505.1 Hemangiomas
Cynthia E. Herzog

Hemangiomas, the most common benign tumors of infancy, occur in approximately 5-10% of term infants (see Chapter 650). The risk of hemangioma is 3-5 times higher in girls than boys. The risk is doubled in premature infants and 10 times higher in offspring of women who had chorionic villus sampling. Hemangiomas can be present at birth but usually arise shortly after birth and grow rapidly during the 1st yr of life, with slowing of growth in the next 5 yr and involution by 10-15 yr of age.

CLINICAL MANIFESTATIONS
More than 50% of all hemangiomas are located in the head and neck region. Most are solitary lesions, but the presence of more than 1 cutaneous lesion increases the likelihood of visceral hemangiomas. The liver is the primary site of visceral involvement; other involved organs include the brain, intestines, and lung. Infantile hemangiomas can be differentiated from other lesions with which they may be confused by the expression of GLUT1. Most hemangiomas require no therapy, but approximately 10% of hemangiomas cause significant impairment and 1% are life-threatening because of their location. Hemangiomas around the airway can cause airway obstruction, and those around the eyes can result in loss of vision. Ulceration is a common complication and can lead to secondary infection. With or without treatment, after involution of a hemangioma, residual skin abnormalities remain. Large hepatic hemangiomas or hemangioendotheliomas may result in hepatomegaly, anemia, thrombocytopenia, and high-output heart failure.

Kasabach-Merritt syndrome (see Chapter 650) is characterized by a rapidly enlarging lesion, thrombocytopenia, microangiopathic hemolytic anemia, and coagulopathy as a result of platelet and red blood cell trapping and activation of the clotting system within the vasculature of the hemangioma. This syndrome is associated with kaposiform hemangioendotheliomas or tufted angiomas but not with infantile hemangiomas.

Cutaneous lesions usually can be diagnosed by typical appearance and rapid proliferation. Segmental hemangiomas, or those with geographic localization and some plaque-like features, recently have been shown to have a higher risk of complications and association with developmental abnormalities. A deep lesion may require imaging studies to help differentiate it from a lymphangioma. The presence of a midline hemangioma in the lumbosacral area indicates the need for an MRI to search for underlying asymptomatic neurologic abnormalities. Location also may dictate the need for an ophthalmologic or surgical consultation. An ultrasonographic scan or MRI of the liver should be performed if multiple cutaneous lesions are present.

TREATMENT
See Chapter 650.

Bibliography is available at Expert Consult.

505.2 Lymphangiomas and Cystic Hygromas
Cynthia E. Herzog

Lymphatic malformations, including lymphangiomas and cystic hygromas, which arise in the embryonic lymph sac, are the second most common benign vascular tumors in children. About half are located in the head and neck area. Approximately 50% are present at birth, with most presenting by 2 yr of age. There is no gender predisposition. Spontaneous regression has been reported but is not typical.

Lymphatic malformations present as soft, painless masses that transilluminate if superficial. Intrathoracic lymphatic malformation can present as symptoms related to a mediastinal mass or pericardial or pleural effusion. Rapid enlargement can occur with infection or hemorrhage. Localized lesions may be surgically resected, but this can be difficult, owing to their infiltrative nature. Recurrence is common with incompletely resected lesions. Aspiration can provide temporary relief in an emergency, such as in the presence of dyspnea, but reaccumulation will occur. Treatment by injection of sclerosing agents, laser therapy, and systemic interferon therapy also has been used. The streptococcal immunotherapeutic agent OK-432 (Picibanil) is the sclerosing agent of choice; its use will prevent the need for surgery in most cases. Bleomycin is also an effective sclerosing agent but has a risk of pulmonary toxicity. It appears to be especially effective for the treatment of macrocystic lymphangiomas of the head and neck.

Bibliography is available at Expert Consult.

Chapter 506
Rare Tumors

506.1 Thyroid Tumors
Steven G. Waguespack

See Chapter 569.

BENIGN THYROID TUMORS
Benign thyroid tumors represent approximately 75% of all thyroid nodules presenting in the pediatric population. The work-up of a suspected thyroid nodule includes the laboratory assessment of thyroid function, ultrasound to assess the nodule and regional lymph node characteristics, and fine-needle aspiration biopsy under ultrasound guidance for definitive pathologic diagnosis. Nuclear scintigraphy using radioactive iodine (^{123}I) or ^{99m}Tc-pertechnetate is not recommended in the initial diagnostic evaluation, except in the event of a suppressed thyroid-stimulating hormone (TSH) level.

MALIGNANT THYROID TUMORS
Pediatric thyroid malignancies are rare tumors that include medullary thyroid carcinoma (MTC) and the differentiated thyroid carcinomas (DTCs): papillary thyroid carcinoma (PTC) and follicular thyroid carcinoma. PTC represents the vast majority of thyroid cancers in children, who have an excellent overall prognosis with anticipated survival over decades, even in the presence of metastatic disease at diagnosis. The major established environmental risk factor for the development of PTC is exposure to ionizing radiation.

MTC is a very uncommon disease in childhood that almost always occurs in the context of an autosomal dominant, hereditary endocrine tumor syndrome that arises secondary to activating mutations in the *RET* (*RE*arranged during *T*ransfection) protooncogene: multiple endocrine neoplasia type 2a (MEN2A) or type 2b (MEN2B). In addition to the almost complete penetrance of MTC in the most common *RET* mutations, patients with MEN2A and MEN2B have up to a 50% lifetime risk of developing pheochromocytomas. Up to 20% of MEN2A patients will develop primary hyperparathyroidism. Patients with MEN2B do not develop hyperparathyroidism but have a distinct phenotype with a characteristic facial appearance, marfanoid body habitus, and a generalized ganglioneuromatosis, manifested most obviously by the presence of oral mucosal neuromas (Fig. 506-1). The

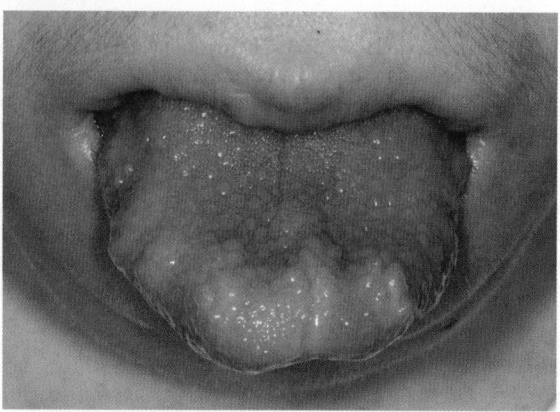

Figure 506-1 Classic appearance of oral mucosal neuromas on the tongue in a boy with MEN2B secondary to the typical M918T mutation in the *RET* protooncogene.

pathognomonic phenotype of MEN2B is not apparent in very early childhood, although an inability to cry tears and constipation represent early clues to diagnosis in these patients.

Children with thyroid cancer usually present with an asymptomatic thyroid mass and/or cervical lymphadenopathy, although children with MEN2 are often diagnosed only after a positive genetic test result or, in the case of MEN2B, after the clinical phenotype is recognized. Lymph node metastases are present in the majority of PTC cases and lung metastases are identified in up to 20% of patients, primarily in those children with a high burden of neck disease.

The primary therapy for thyroid cancer is a total thyroidectomy and a compartment-oriented lymph node dissection, as indicated, performed by a highly experienced thyroid cancer surgeon. In DTC, ^{131}I is used postoperatively to treat distant metastasis and unresectable residual neck disease. In PTC, the routine use of ^{131}I is limited to those children who are most likely to benefit from treatment. Children with MTC do not require ^{131}I therapy. The TSH level is initially suppressed by giving supraphysiologic levothyroxine in the case of DTC, as TSH stimulates DTC tumor growth; the TSH is kept normal in the case of MTC. Long-term follow-up involves monitoring of tumor markers (thyroglobulin in DTC and calcitonin/carcinogenic embryonic antigen in MTC), as well as routine imaging, primarily neck ultrasound.

In MEN2, there are well-documented genotype-phenotype correlations, and the biologic aggressiveness of MTC depends on the hereditary setting in which it develops. With the advent of genetic testing for *RET* mutations, MTC has become one of the few malignancies that can be cured via early thyroidectomy before the cancer becomes metastatic. Recommendations regarding the age at surgery of children who are carriers of a *RET* mutation are evolving and incorporate clinical testing (ultrasound and calcitonin levels) in addition to knowledge regarding the genotype. Novel oral tyrosine kinase inhibitors are approved by the FDA for the treatment of advanced MTC and DTC in adults.

Bibliography is available at Expert Consult.

506.2 Melanoma
Dennis P.M. Hughes and Cynthia E. Herzog

See Chapter 651.

The incidence of melanoma in persons younger than 20 yr of age in the United States is 4.2 cases per 1 million, with 73% occurring in 15-19 year olds, 17% in 10-14 year olds, and 10% occurring in children younger than 10 yr of age (see Chapter 651). Melanoma is more common among adolescent females than males. In the United States, incident rates of melanoma in younger age groups are increasing, although at a slower rate than in adults. UV light, especially sun

exposure, is a well-known risk factor for melanoma in adults, and also contributes to teenage melanoma, as shown by the tendency of lesions to develop on sun-exposed areas in this age group. In younger patients, melanoma does not appear to be associated with sun exposure and often occurs in skin that is not frequently exposed to the sun. Pediatricians should counsel patients regarding avoidance of sun exposure and the use of tanning beds to decrease the risk of later development of melanoma. Patients with fair skin and a family history of melanoma are at particularly high risk. Known risk factors for children are a giant hairy nevus (>10 cm), dysplastic nevus syndrome, and xeroderma pigmentosum. These conditions merit total skin examination at least annually.

Findings of a rapidly enlarging nevus that is dark, has changed colors, has irregular borders, or bleeds easily should raise a concern of melanoma. However, more than half of pediatric melanomas are nonpigmented, and can easily be confused with a wart or other benign finding. Diagnosis is based on pathology, and a punch biopsy is preferred. However, extra care must be taken in the diagnosis of melanoma in children because making the distinction from other lesions, particularly Spitz nevus, can be difficult. Management in a center with expertise in pediatric melanoma may be advisable, especially for anything other than thin melanomas (Breslow thickness of 1 mm or greater).

Prognosis and treatment recommendations have previously been extrapolated from adult data; however, specific prognostic factors for pediatric melanoma are starting to accrue. The initial diagnosis is best made with a punch biopsy. Shave biopsy is specifically discouraged, as this method tends to leave the base of the lesion behind, and specific information about the depth of invasion is lost. Biopsy sites that test positive for melanoma should be reexcised with appropriate margins based on thickness. Lymph node mapping and sentinel node biopsy should also be performed for all melanomas with a Breslow thickness >0.5-1 mm, or any lesions in which the tumor base was not resected. If the sentinel node is positive, a formal lymph node dissection is essential for ensuring the best probability of survival. To date, the treatment of childhood melanoma still mirrors treatment of adult melanoma. High-dose adjuvant interferon shows some efficacy in the treatment of adult melanoma, whereas chemotherapy in combination with biologic agents and vaccine therapy has been used for treatment of distant metastases. Although novel therapies such as targeted B-Raf inhibitors and immune-modulating agents have received regulatory approval for treatment of adult melanoma, their use in children is still investigational.

Bibliography is available at Expert Consult.

506.3 Nasopharyngeal Carcinoma
Cynthia E. Herzog

Nasopharyngeal carcinoma is rare in the pediatric population but is one of the most common nasopharyngeal tumors in pediatric patients. In adults, the incidence is highest in South China, but it is also high among the Inuit people and in North Africa and Northeast India. In China, it is rare in the pediatric population, but in other populations a substantial proportion of cases occur in the pediatric age group, primarily in adolescents. It occurs in males twice as often as in females and is more common in blacks. In the pediatric population the tumors are more commonly of undifferentiated histology and associated with Epstein-Barr virus. Nasopharyngeal carcinoma is associated with specific human leukocyte antigen types, and other genetic factors may play a role, especially in low-incidence populations.

Most pediatric patients present with advanced locoregional disease manifesting as cervical lymphadenopathy. Epistaxis, trismus, and cranial nerve deficits also may be present. The diagnosis is established from biopsy of the nasopharynx or cervical lymph nodes. In most cases the lactate dehydrogenase level is elevated, but this finding is nonspecific. CT or MRI evaluation of the head and neck is performed to determine the extent of locoregional disease. Chest radiography, CT, bone scan, and liver scan are used to evaluate for metastatic disease. Positron emission tomography scans appear to be useful for monitoring both primary disease and looking for metastases. Epstein-Barr virus DNA levels correlate with disease stage, have prognostic value, and can be used to monitor for recurrence.

Treatment is a combination of chemotherapy and irradiation. Cisplatin given concurrently with radiation, with or without neoadjuvant cisplatin-based chemotherapy, is the standard treatment. The outcome depends on the extent of disease; patients with distant metastases have a very poor prognosis. Using intensity-modulated radiation therapy improves local control and reduces the late adverse effects associated with radiation therapy, including hormonal dysfunction, dental caries, fibrosis, and second malignancies. Use of proton therapy may result in further reduction of adverse effects.

Bibliography is available at Expert Consult.

506.4 Adenocarcinoma of the Colon and Rectum
Cynthia E. Herzog and Winston W. Huh

Colorectal carcinoma (CRC) is rare in the pediatric population with an estimated incidence rate of approximately 1 case per 1 million. Even in patients with predisposing conditions, CRC usually does not present until late adolescence or adulthood. Hereditary nonpolyposis colon cancer (HNPCC) is an autosomal dominant disorder, with germline mutations in DNA mismatch repair genes *(MMR)* causing DNA repair errors and microsatellite instability. Familial adenomatous polyposis (FAP) and attenuated FAP are autosomal disorders, with germline mutations in the *APC* gene. In addition to CRC, patients with HNPCC, FAP, and attenuated FAP are predisposed to a number of extracolonic cancers. Desmoid tumors can occur in patients with FAP, whereas patients with HNPCC have an increased risk for tumors involving the genitourinary tract, stomach, and small intestine. *MYH*-associated polyposis, Peutz-Jeghers syndrome, and juvenile polyposis also predispose to CRC.

Genetic testing is available, and screening for cancer in HNPCC and FAP should begin during childhood or adolescence. Likewise, genetic evaluation for these conditions should be pursued in young patients presenting with colon cancer, even when there is no history of predisposing genetic conditions.

Presenting symptoms include bloody stools or melena, abdominal pain, weight loss, and changes in bowel patterns. In many cases, signs are vague, often resulting in a delay in diagnosis, sometimes not until the disease has reached an advanced stage. The histologic subtype differs from that seen in adults, with the majority of pediatric tumors being either mucinous adenocarcinoma or signet ring cell carcinoma. Treatment consists of surgical resection when possible, with chemotherapy for unresectable tumors. Adequate lymph node removal should be performed at the time of surgical resection of primary tumor. Radiation therapy is useful in the treatment of rectal carcinomas.

Bibliography is available at Expert Consult.

506.5 Adrenal Tumors
Steven G. Waguespack

See Chapters 579 to 581.

Adrenocortical tumors (ACTs) arise from the outer adrenal cortex, whereas pheochromocytomas (PHEOs) derive from the catecholamine-producing chromaffin cells of the adrenal medulla. When catecholamine-producing tumors arise outside of the adrenal medulla, they are called paragangliomas (PGLs). The pathologic categorization of these tumors

as benign or malignant does not always correlate well with the clinical behavior, making it difficult to differentiate malignant from benign disease based upon pathology alone. Hence, long-term follow-up is warranted. Because of the greater association with genetic disease, genetic counseling is also advised for all children diagnosed with an ACT or PHEO/PGL.

ACTs are very rare and tend to present before age 5 yr. They have a female predominance and are functional tumors in >90% of cases, primarily producing androgens and causing clinically apparent virilization. ACT may also present as an abdominal mass or pain. In children, ACTs are associated with Li-Fraumeni syndrome (germline inactivating mutations in the *TP53* tumor-suppressor gene), Beckwith-Wiedemann syndrome, hemihyperplasia other than that seen as part of Beckwith-Wiedemann syndrome, and, very rarely, congenital adrenal hyperplasia. Other unusual causes of nodular adrenocortical disease, which usually present with Cushing syndrome, include the Carney complex and macronodular adrenal hyperplasia.

PHEOs/PGLs are rare tumors that are more likely to be bilateral, malignant, and secondary to a heritable tumor syndrome when diagnosed in children. von Hippel–Lindau disease is the most common genetic cause of PHEOs/PGLs in the pediatric population, followed by the familial PGL syndromes caused by mutations in the succinate dehydrogenase gene. MEN2 (types 2A and 2B) and neurofibromatosis type 1 are also in the differential diagnosis, but are mostly associated with a PHEO diagnosis during adulthood. Although hypertension is usually paroxysmal in adults with PHEO, hypertension is usually sustained in children, who may also lack the typical triad of headache, palpitations, and diaphoresis seen commonly in adults. The best screening test for PHEO/PGL is measurement of plasma and/or urine metanephrine levels.

The initial treatment of ACT and PHEO/PGL is surgery. Children with PHEO/PGL require **preoperative medical management**, typically with α and β blockade. First-line medical therapy for metastatic ACT includes mitotane and chemotherapy with cisplatin, etoposide, and doxorubicin. Metastatic PHEO/PGL has historically been treated with cyclophosphamide, vincristine, and dacarbazine. In cases of both ACT and PHEO/PGL, novel targeted agents are being studied for the treatment of advanced metastatic disease, which is typically nonresponsive to standard chemotherapeutic approaches. Endocrine therapy targeting hormonal overproduction may also be needed to palliate symptoms and improve quality of life.

Bibliography is available at Expert Consult.

506.6 Desmoplastic Small Round Cell Tumor
Nidale Tarek and Cynthia E. Herzog

Desmoplastic small round cell tumor is a very rare and aggressive mesenchymal tumor that occurs predominantly in adolescent and young adult males. It is associated with a diagnostic chromosomal translocation between the Ewing tumor gene and the Wilms tumor gene, t(11;22)(p13;q12). Patients typically present with a bulky abdominal mass, multiple peritoneal and omental implants, and symptoms of abdominal sarcomatosis, including pain, ascites, intestinal obstruction, hydronephrosis, and weight loss. Desmoplastic small round cell tumor mainly involves the abdominal cavity but can spread to the lymph nodes, liver, lungs, and bones. Aggressive treatment with combination chemotherapy, debulking surgery, and whole abdominopelvic irradiation results almost universally in a poor outcome. Median survival ranges between 17 and 25 mo, and the 5 yr overall survival remains less than 20%. Alternative treatment options currently under investigation include hyperthermic intraperitoneal chemotherapy and radioimmunotherapy with monoclonal antibodies targeting different surface antigens on tumor cells.

Bibliography is available at Expert Consult.

Chapter **507**

Histiocytosis Syndromes of Childhood

Stephan Ladisch

The childhood histiocytoses constitute a diverse group of disorders, which, although individually rare, are frequently severe in their clinical expression. These disorders are grouped together because they have in common a prominent proliferation or accumulation of cells of the monocyte–macrophage system of bone marrow origin. Although these disorders sometimes are difficult to distinguish clinically, accurate diagnosis is essential nevertheless for facilitating progress in treatment. A systematic classification of the childhood histiocytoses is based on histopathologic findings (Table 507-1). A thorough, comprehensive evaluation of a biopsy specimen obtained at the time of diagnosis is essential. This evaluation includes studies such as electron microscopy and immunostaining that may require special sample processing.

CLASSIFICATION AND PATHOLOGY

Three classes of childhood histiocytosis are defined, based on histopathologic findings. The most well-known childhood histiocytosis, **Langerhans cell histiocytosis (LCH),** previously known as **histiocytosis X,** includes the clinical entities of eosinophilic granuloma, **Hand-Schüller-Christian disease,** and **Letterer-Siwe disease.** The normal Langerhans cell is an antigen-presenting cell of the skin. The hallmark of LCH in all forms is the presence of a clonal proliferation of cells of the monocyte lineage containing the characteristic electron microscopic findings of a Langerhans cell. This is the **Birbeck granule,** a tennis racket–shaped bilamellar granule that, when seen in the cytoplasm of lesional cells in LCH, is diagnostic of the disease. The Birbeck granule expresses a newly characterized antigen, langerin (CD207),

which is involved in antigen presentation to T lymphocytes. CD207 expression has been established to be uniformly present in LCH lesions and thus becomes an additional reliable diagnostic marker. It appears more likely that the LCH cell is not actually a (differentiated) Langerhans cell but rather an immature cell of myeloid origin, possibly in an arrested state of development. Nevertheless, the definitive diagnosis of LCH is established by demonstrating CD1a-positivity of lesional cells, which is done using fixed tissue (Fig. 507-1). Lesional cells must be distinguished from normal Langerhans cells of the skin, which are also CD1a-positive but are not diagnostic of LCH. The lesions may contain various proportions of these Langerhans granule-containing CD1a-positive cells, lymphocytes, granulocytes, monocytes, and eosinophils.

In contrast to the prominence of an antigen-presenting cell in LCH, the other common group of histiocytoses are nonmalignant proliferative disorders that are characterized by accumulation of activated antigen-processing cells (macrophages and lymphocytes). These are known as the **hemophagocytic lymphohistiocytoses (HLHs).** They are the result of uncontrolled hemophagocytosis and uncontrolled activation (upregulation) of inflammatory cytokines with some similarities to the macrophage activation syndrome (see Table 155-5). Tissue infiltration by activated CD8 T lymphocytes, activated macrophages, and hypercytokinemia are classic features (Fig. 507-2). With the characteristic morphology of normal macrophages by light microscopy, these phagocytic cells (Fig. 507-1) are negative for the markers (Birbeck granules, CD1a-positivity, CD207-positivity) characteristic of LCH cells but are CD163-positive.

The 2 major forms of hemophagocytic lymphohistiocytosis have indistinguishable pathologic findings but are very important to distinguish from one another because of implications for both treatment and for prognosis. One is **familial hemophagocytic lymphohistiocytosis (FHLH),** originally named **familial erythrophagocytic lymphohistiocytosis,** which is an autosomal recessive disorder and represents approximately 25% of patients with HLH. Genes are known for 4 of the 5 FHLH syndromes; these mutations affect the ability of T lymphocytes and natural killer cells to synthesize and release perforin and granzymes, thus reducing cytotoxic granule formation. The other is the **infection-associated hemophagocytic syndrome,** also called secondary hemophagocytic lymphohistiocytosis (Table 507-2). Both

	Table 507-1	Classification of the Childhood Histiocytoses		
	DISEASE	**CELLULAR CHARACTERISTICS OF LESIONS**	**TREATMENT**	
LCH	Langerhans cell histiocytosis	Langerhans-like cells (CD1a-positive, CD207-positive) with Birbeck granules (LCH cells)	Local therapy for isolated lesions; chemotherapy for disseminated disease	
HLH	Familial hemophagocytic lymphohistiocytosis Infection-associated hemophagocytic syndrome[†] Associated with albinism syndromes[*] Associated with immunocompromised states Associated with autoimmune/autoinflammatory states	Morphologically normal reactive macrophages with prominent erythrophagocytosis, and CD8-positive T cells	Chemotherapy; allogeneic bone marrow transplantation	
Other	Juvenile xanthogranuloma	Characteristic vacuolated lesional histiocytes with foamy cytoplasm	None or excisional biopsy for localized disease; chemotherapy, radiotherapy for disseminated disease	
	Rosai-Dorfman disease	Hemophagocytic histiocytes	None if localized; surgery for bulk reduction; chemotherapy if organ systems involvement	
	Malignant histiocytosis	Neoplastic proliferation of cells with characteristics of monocytes/macrophages or their precursors	Antineoplastic chemotherapy, including anthracyclines	
Other	Acute monocytic leukemia[‡]	M5 by FAB classification	Antineoplastic chemotherapy	

*Chediak-Higashi and Hermansky-Pudlak syndromes.
[†]Also called secondary hemophagocytic lymphohistiocytosis.
[‡]See Chapter 495.2.
FAB, French-American-British; LCH, Langerhans cell histiocytosis; HLH, hemophagocytic lymphohistiocytosis.

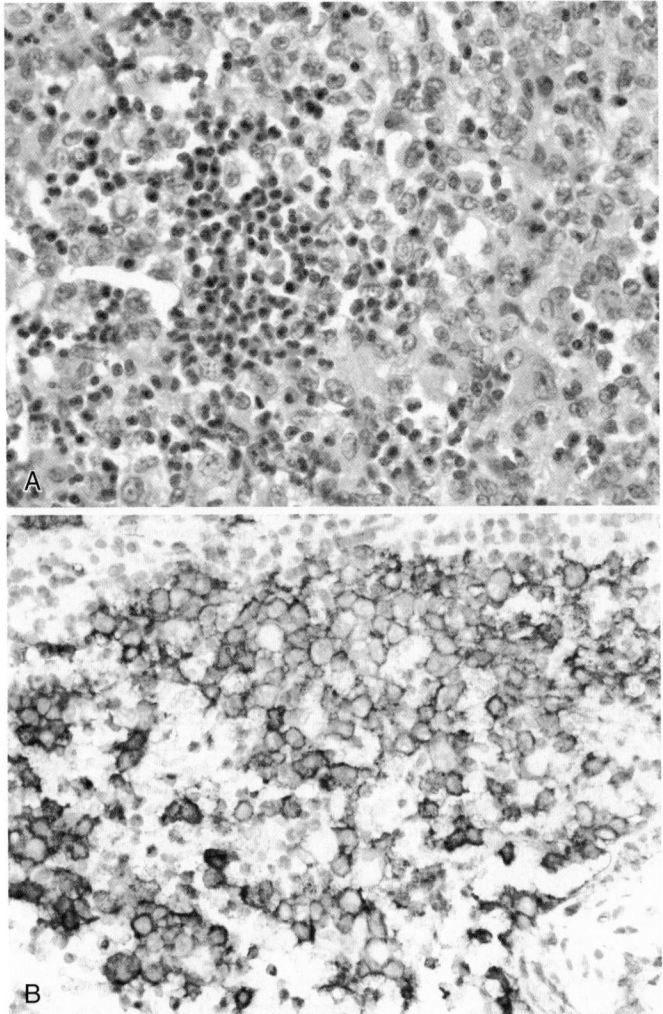

Figure 507-1 A, Histopathology of Langerhans cell histiocytosis (LCH). Shown is the eosinophilic granuloma of a lytic bone lesion of the femoral head. Multiple LCH cells with characteristic grooved nuclei, as well as numerous eosinophils, are visible in this mixed infiltrate. **B,** CD1a staining, characteristic and diagnostic of lesions with LCH cells.

Table 507-2	Infections Associated with Hemophagocytic Syndrome

VIRAL
Adenovirus
Cytomegalovirus
Dengue virus
Epstein-Barr virus
Enteroviruses
Herpes simplex viruses (HSV1, HSV2)
Human herpesviruses (HHV6, HHV8)
Human immunodeficiency virus
Influenza viruses
Parvovirus B19
Varicella-zoster virus
Hepatitis viruses
Measles
Parechovirus

BACTERIAL
Babesia microti
Brucella abortus
Enteric Gram-negative rods
Haemophilus influenzae
Mycoplasma pneumoniae
Staphylococcus aureus
Streptococcus pneumoniae

FUNGAL
Candida albicans
Cryptococcus neoformans
Histoplasma capsulatum
Fusarium

MYCOBACTERIAL
Mycobacterium tuberculosis

RICKETTSIAL
Coxiella burnetii
Other rickettsial diseases

PARASITIC
Leishmania donovani
Plasmodium

From Nathan DG, Orkin SH, Ginsburg D, et al, editors: Nathan and Oski's hematology of infancy and childhood, ed 6, Philadelphia, 2003, WB Saunders, p. 1381.

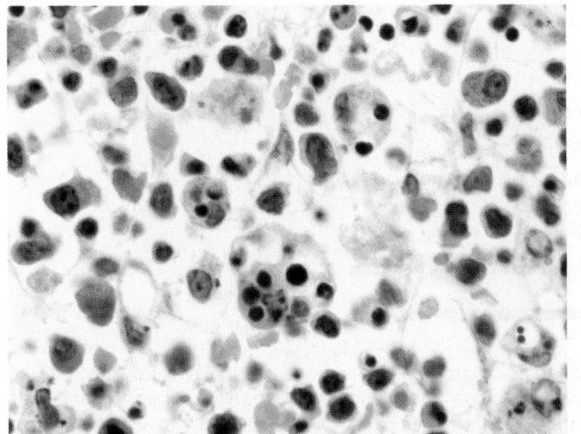

Figure 507-2 Bone marrow aspirate of a child with familial (genetically confirmed) hemophagocytic lymphohistiocytosis. Numerous characteristic hemophagocytic cells (which are CD163-positive macrophages) ingesting various blood elements are visualized.

diseases are characterized by disseminated lesions that involve many organ systems. The lesions are characterized by infiltration of the involved organ with activated phagocytic macrophages and lymphocytes, in which the lymphocyte defects (cytolytic pathway) are considered to be the primary abnormality.

Noninfectious causes that may trigger secondary HLH include drugs (phenytoin, highly active antiretroviral therapy), bone marrow transplantation, chemotherapy, autoimmune diseases, inflammatory bowel disease, and immunodeficiency states (DiGeorge syndrome, Bruton agammaglobulinemia, severe combined immunodeficiency syndrome, chronic granulomatous disease, cancer).

These diseases together comprise **HLH** (Table 507-3 and Fig. 507-3). Multiple different steps in granule formation and release by cytotoxic T cells, when inhibited by genetic mutation, can result in primary HLH (Fig. 507-3, bottom). In an analogous way, a trigger (e.g., infection) can result in secondary HLH (Fig. 507-3, top).

The mixed cellular lesions of both LCH and HLH are increasingly believed to point to these being disorders of immune regulation resulting from either an unusual and unidentified antigenic stimulation and/or an abnormal and defective cellular immune response. Mutations in the perforin (*PRF1*) gene or the *MUNC13-4* gene are the most common causes of defective function of the cytotoxic lymphocytes whose activity is inhibited in FHLH. Some cases of LCH demonstrate clonality of individual lesions. In LCH, a mutated form of the *BRAF* gene has been identified in many patients; its pathophysiologic significance is being

	DEFECTIVE GENE	FUNCTION	NOTABLE CLINICAL FINDINGS	RAPID DIAGNOSIS BY FLOW CYTOMETRY
Table 507-3	**Classification of Primary HLH, Notable Clinical Findings, and Rapid Diagnostic Results**			

	DEFECTIVE GENE	FUNCTION	NOTABLE CLINICAL FINDINGS	RAPID DIAGNOSIS BY FLOW CYTOMETRY
HLH TYPE				
FHLH-1	*Unknown*	Unknown		
FHLH-2	*PRF1*	Pore formation		Decreased/absent perforin expression
FHLH-3	*Munc 13.4*	Vesicle priming	Increased incidence of CNS HLH	Decreased CD107a expression
FHLH-4	*STX11*	Vesicle fusion	Mild, recurrent HLH, colitis	Decreased CD107a expression
FHLH-5	*STXBP2*	Vesicle fusion	Colitis, bleeding, hypogammaglobulinemia	Decreased CD107a expression
SYNDROMES				
Griscelli syndrome type II	*RAB27A*	Vesicle docking	Partial albinism and silvery-gray hair	Decreased CD107a expression, abnormal hair shaft examination*
Chediak-Higashi syndrome	*LYST*	Vesicle trafficking	Partial albinism, bleeding tendency, and recurrent pyogenic infection	Decreased CD107a expression, abnormal neutrophil granules†
Hermansky-Pudlak syndrome type II	*AP3B1*	Vesicle trafficking	Partial albinism, bleeding tendency, and immunodeficiency	Decreased CD107a expression
EPSTEIN-BARR VIRUS–DRIVEN				
XLP-1	*SAP/SH2D1A*	Signaling in T, NK, and NK T cells	Hypogammaglobulinemia and lymphoma	Decreased/absent SAP expression
XLP-2/XIAP‡	*BIRC4*	Signaling pathways involving NF-κB	Mild, recurrent HLH and colitis	Decreased/absent XIAP expression
IL-2–inducible T-cell kinase deficiency	*ITK*	Signaling in T cell	AR, Hodgkin lymphoma	NA (gene sequencing required)
CD27 deficiency	*CD27*	Lymphocyte costimulatory molecule	AR, combined immunodeficiency	Absent CD27 expression on B cells
XMEN	*MAGT1*	T-cell activation via T-cell receptor	Combined immunodeficiency, chronic viral infections, and lymphoma	Decreased CD4 cells and defects in T-cell receptor signaling

*Light microscopy examination of a hair shaft shows a characteristic abnormal clumping of pigment.
†Light microscopy examination of peripheral blood smear shows giant granules in neutrophils and other leukocytes.
‡Defect is present in all tissues.
AR, autosomal recessive; CNS, central nervous system; FHLH, familial hemophagocytic lymphohistiocytosis; HLH, hemophagocytic lymphohistiocytosis; IL, interleukin; NA, not available; NF-κB, nuclear factor kappa light chain enhancer of activated B cells; NK, natural killer; SAP, signaling lymphocyte-activating molecule–associated protein; XIAP, X-linked inhibitor of apoptosis protein; XLP, X-linked lymphoproliferative; XMEN, X-linked immunodeficiency with Mg²⁺ defect, Epstein-Barr virus infection, and neoplasia.

(From Chandrakasan S, Filipovich AH. Hemophagocytic lymphohistiocytosis: advances in pathophysiology, diagnosis, and treatment. J Pediatr 163(5):1253-1259, 2013.)

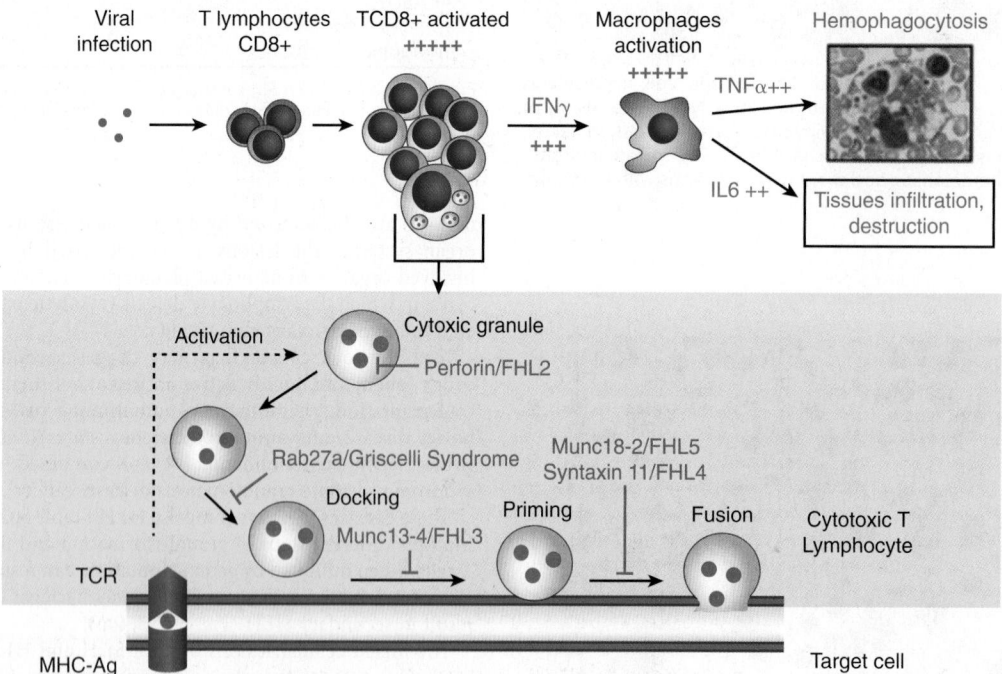

Figure 507-3 Inborn errors in the cytotoxic activity of lymphocytes. *Top:* Schematic diagram of the immune mechanisms leading to the occurrence of a hemophagocytic syndrome. Following a viral infection, antigen-specific CD8⁺ T lymphocytes undergo massive expansion and activation and secrete high levels of interferon (IFN)-γ. The overwhelming activated effector cells induce excessive macrophage activation and proinflammatory cytokine production including tumor necrosis factor (TNF)-α and interleukin-6 (IL-6). Macrophages spontaneously phagocytose blood elements (here shown: platelets, red blood cells, and a polymorphonuclear cell). Activated lymphocytes and macrophages infiltrate various organs, resulting in massive tissue necrosis and organ failure. *Bottom:* The genetic defects causing hemophagocytic lymphohistiocytic syndrome (HLH) affect a precise step of the cytotoxic machinery, i.e. granule content, docking, priming, or fusion. Only the defects causing Griscelli syndrome (GS) and familial hemophagocytic lymphohistiocytosis (FHL) are shown. *(From Pachlopnik Schmid J, Cote M, Menager MM, et al: Inherited defects in cytotoxic lymphocyte activity. Immunol Rev 235:10–23, 2010.)*

assessed. The *BRAF* mutation suggests both that there is an autonomous proliferative element to the disease and that there may potentially be a new avenue for therapeutic approaches.

In addition to these two most common forms of childhood histiocytosis, LCH and HLH, a number of rarer diseases are also included under this rubric, because they have in common various abnormalities of these cell populations of myeloid origin. These other diseases include **juvenile xanthogranuloma**, in which the lesional histiocytes are vacuolated, with foamy cytoplasm, and the lesions evolve into mixed granulomas also containing eosinophils, lymphocytes, and other cells. Another rare histiocytosis is **Rosai-Dorfman disease**, also known as **sinus histiocytosis** with massive lymphadenopathy. Packing of sinusoids of the lymph nodes with histiocytes that are hemophagocytic characterizes Rosai-Dorfman disease, although extranodal involvement is not uncommon. The etiology of these 2 diseases is unknown. Finally, there is also a group of unequivocal malignancies of cells of monocyte–macrophage lineage. By this definition, acute monocytic leukemia and true malignant histiocytosis are included among the class III histiocytoses (see Chapter 495). True neoplasms of Langerhans cells, while extremely rare, have been reported.

507.1 Langerhans Cell Histiocytosis
Stephan Ladisch

CLINICAL MANIFESTATIONS
LCH has an extremely variable presentation. The skeleton is involved in 80% of patients and may be the only affected site, especially in children older than 5 yr of age. Bone lesions may be single or multiple and are seen most commonly in the skull (Fig. 507-4). Other sites include the pelvis, femur, vertebra, maxilla, and mandible. They may be asymptomatic or associated with pain and local swelling. Involvement of the spine may result in collapse of the vertebral body, which can be seen radiographically, and may cause secondary compression of the spinal cord. In flat and long bones, osteolytic lesions with sharp borders occur and no evidence exists of reactive new bone formation until the lesions begin to heal. Lesions that involve weight-bearing long bones may result in pathologic fractures. Chronically draining, infected ears are commonly associated with destruction in the mastoid area. Bone destruction in the mandible and maxilla may result in teeth that, on radiographs, appear to be free floating. With response to therapy, healing may be complete.

Approximately 50% of patients experience skin involvement at some time during the course of disease, usually as a hard-to-treat scaly, papular, seborrheic dermatitis of the scalp, diaper, axillary, or posterior auricular regions. The lesions may spread to involve the back, palms, and soles. The exanthem may be petechial or hemorrhagic, even in the absence of thrombocytopenia. Localized or disseminated lymphadenopathy is present in approximately 33% of patients. Hepatosplenomegaly occurs in approximately 20% of patients. Various degrees of hepatic malfunction may occur, including jaundice and ascites.

Exophthalmos, when present, often is bilateral and is caused by retroorbital accumulation of granulomatous tissue. Gingival mucous membranes may be involved with infiltrative lesions that appear superficially like candidiasis. Otitis media is present in 30-40% of patients; deafness may follow destructive lesions of the middle ear. In 10-15% of patients, pulmonary infiltrates are found on radiography. The lesions may range from diffuse fibrosis and disseminated nodular infiltrates to diffuse cystic changes. Rarely, pneumothorax may be a complication. If the lungs are severely involved, tachypnea and progressive respiratory failure may result.

Pituitary dysfunction or hypothalamic involvement may result in growth retardation. In addition, patients may have diabetes insipidus; patients suspected of having LCH should demonstrate the ability to concentrate their urine before going to the operating room for a biopsy. Rarely, panhypopituitarism may occur. Primary hypothyroidism as a result of thyroid gland infiltration also may occur.

Patients with multisystem disease who are affected more severely are those who have systemic manifestations, including fever, weight loss, malaise, irritability, and failure to thrive. These systemic manifestations will distinguish between patients who are at high risk of mortality (i.e., "risk organ"-positive patients), and those without, who are at low risk (i.e., "risk organ"-negative patients). The risk organs are liver, spleen hematopoietic system, and lung. The distinction is important for deciding the intensity of the treatment approach and has been incorporated into standard treatment approaches for LCH, as delineated in the Histiocyte Society protocols. Bone marrow involvement may cause anemia and thrombocytopenia. Two uncommon but serious manifestations of LCH are hepatic involvement (leading to fibrosis and cirrhosis) and a peculiar central nervous system (CNS) involvement characterized by ataxia, dysarthria, and other neurologic symptoms. Hepatic involvement is associated with multisystem disease that is often already present at the time of diagnosis. In contrast, the CNS involvement, which is progressive and histopathologically characterized by gliosis, and for which no treatment is known, may be observed only many years after the initial diagnosis of LCH, which itself may have consisted only of mild bone disease. Neither of these manifestations evidences Langerhans cells or Birbeck granules, and both are suspected to be driven initially by cytokine abnormalities.

After tissue biopsy, which is diagnostic and is easiest to perform on skin or bone lesions, a thorough clinical and laboratory evaluation should be undertaken. This should include a series of studies in all patients (complete blood cell count, liver function tests, coagulation studies, skeletal survey, chest radiograph, and measurement of urine osmolality). In addition, detailed evaluation of any organ system that has been shown to be involved by physical examination or by these studies should be performed to establish the extent of disease before initiation of treatment.

TREATMENT AND PROGNOSIS
The clinical course of single-system disease (usually bone, lymph node, or skin) generally is benign, with a high chance of spontaneous remission. Therefore, treatment should be minimal and should be directed at arresting the progression of a bone lesion that could result in permanent damage before it resolves spontaneously. Curettage or, less often, steroid injection or low-dose local radiation therapy (5-6 Gy) may accomplish this goal. Multisystem disease, in contrast, should be treated with systemic multiagent chemotherapy. Several different regimens have been proposed, but central elements are the inclusion of vinblastine and steroids, both of which have been found to be very effective in treating LCH. Etoposide has more recently been excluded from standard treatment of multisystem LCH, while treatment of multisystem LCH includes therapy with multiple agents, designed to reduce mortality, reactivation of disease, and long-term consequences.

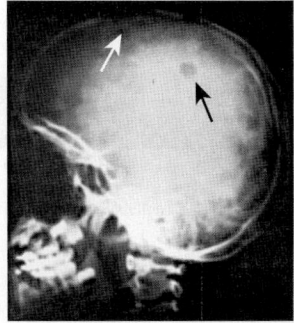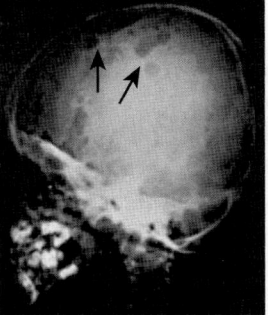

Figure 507-4 Two skull radiographs from patients with Langerhans cell histiocytosis (LCH). *Left,* The patient was older than 2 yr of age and had involvement limited to isolated bone lesions *(arrows)*. She had a good recovery. *Right,* The patient was younger than 2 yr of age and had extensive bone disease *(arrows)*, a febrile course, anemia, severe skin eruption, generalized lymphadenopathy, hepatosplenomegaly, pulmonary infiltrates, and a fatal outcome despite antitumor chemotherapy. These patients represent opposite ends of the clinical spectrum of LCH.

The response rate to therapy is now quite high, and mortality in severe LCH has been substantially reduced by multiagent chemotherapy, especially if the diagnosis is made accurately and expeditiously. The most recent treatment results, employing lengthened continuation therapy, show a greater than 85% survival rate in severe multisystem disease and a reduced rate of reactivation. Experimental therapies, suggested only for unresponsive disease (often in very young children with multisystem disease and organ dysfunction who have not responded to multiagent initial treatment), include immunosuppressive therapy with cyclosporine/antithymocyte globulin and possibly imatinib, 2-chlorodeoxyadenosine, and stem cell transplantation. Late (fibrotic) complications, whether hepatic or pulmonary, are irreversible and require organ transplantation to be definitively treated. Current treatment approaches and experimental protocols for both LCH and HLH can be obtained at the website for the Histiocyte Society (http://www.histiocytesociety.org). An unresolved problem is treatment of the (usually late-onset) severe, progressive, and intractable LCH-associated neurodegenerative syndrome.

Bibliography is available at Expert Consult.

507.2 Hemophagocytic Lymphohistiocytosis
Stephan Ladisch

(See "Classification and Pathology" above.)

CLINICAL MANIFESTATIONS
The major forms of HLH, FHLF and secondary HLH, have a remarkably similar presentation consisting of a generalized disease process, most often with fever (90-100%), maculopapular and/or petechial rash (10-60%), weight loss, and irritability (see Tables 507-4 and 507-5). FHLH also is characterized by severe immunodeficiency. Children with FHLH generally are younger than 4 yr of age, and children with secondary HLH may present at an older age, but both forms are recognized as presenting at any age. **Physical examination** often reveals hepatosplenomegaly (70-100%), lymphadenopathy (20-50%), respiratory distress (40-90%), jaundice, and symptoms of CNS involvement (~50%) that are not unlike those of aseptic meningitis or acute demyelinating encephalomyelitis (see Chapter 600.3). MRI may demonstrate systemic T2-weighted/FLAIR hyperintensities in gray and white matter and in supratentorial and infratentorial regions. The cerebrospinal fluid pleocytosis (50-90%) in CNS involvement of FHLH is

characterized by cells that are the same phagocytic macrophages found in the peripheral blood or bone marrow. The **diagnosis** can be made either on the basis of a molecular (genetic) defect (see "Treatment and Prognosis" below) or on the pathologic findings of hemophagocytosis in bone marrow biopsy, and is suggested by clinical findings of fever, splenomegaly, and associated laboratory findings (in both forms of HLH), including hypertriglyceridemia (80-100%), hypofibrinogenemia (65-85%), elevated levels of hepatic enzymes (30-90%), extremely elevated levels of circulating soluble interleukin-2 receptors released by the activated lymphocytes, very high levels of serum ferritin (often >10,000), and cytopenias (in ~90-100%; especially pancytopenia from hemophagocytosis in the marrow). Hemophagocytosis is not specific for HLH without other features. In addition, in some subgroups of HLH perforin assays may be normal. In the absence of genetic mutations, the diagnosis of HLH is based on a set of specific criteria formulated by the Histiocyte Society, the presence of 5 of 8 of which is considered diagnostic of HLH (see Table 507-4): fever, splenomegaly, cytopenia of 2 cell lines, hypertriglyceridemia or hypofibrinogenemia, hyperferritinemia, elevated soluble CD25 (interleukin-2 receptor), reduced or absent natural killer cells, and bone marrow, cerebrospinal fluid, or lymph node evidence of hemophagocytosis. There are patients with FHLH who have no known identifiable gene mutation. No absolute clinical or laboratory distinction can be made between FHLH and secondary HLH, although genetic markers for FHLH can complement a positive family history for other affected children.

In the absence of either (1) documented genetic defect coupled with defective NK cell cytotoxicity or (2) frank hemophagocytosis, great care should be taken in making the diagnosis of (secondary) HLH, with its implication of the use of cytotoxic chemotherapy. This is because the otherwise nonspecific criteria (indicative of inflammation) used to diagnose HLH can also be seen in diseases that are not always associated with hemophagocytosis (such as an overwhelming acute viral infection without T cell overactivation) in which the cytotoxic and immunosuppressive therapy used in treating HLH might be contraindicated.

TREATMENT AND PROGNOSIS
The diagnostic distinction between FHLH and secondary HLH sometimes can be based on the acute onset of secondary HLH in the presence of a documented infection. In this case, treatment of the underlying infection, coupled with supportive care, is critical. If the diagnosis is made in a setting of iatrogenic immunodeficiency, immunosuppressive treatment should be withdrawn and supportive care should be instituted along with specific therapy for underlying infection. When FHLH (gene mutations in perforin or Munc13-4 proteins) is diagnosed or is suspected together with no documentation of an infection, therapy currently includes etoposide, corticosteroids, and intrathecal methotrexate. It should be stressed that pancytopenia is not a

Table 507-4	Diagnostic Guidelines for Hemophagocytic Lymphohistiocytosis

The diagnosis of HLH is established by fulfilling one of the following two criteria:
1. A molecular diagnosis consistent with HLH (e.g., PRF mutations, SAP mutations)

or

2. Having 5 of the following 8 signs or symptoms:
   a. Fever
   b. Splenomegaly
   c. Cytopenia (affecting ≥2 cell lineages; hemoglobin ≤9 g/dL [or ≤10 g/dL for infants <4 wk of age], platelets <100,000/μL, neutrophils <1,000/μL)
   d. Hypertriglyceridemia (≥265 mg/dL) and/or hypofibrinogenemia (≤150 mg/dL)
   e. Hemophagocytosis in the bone marrow, spleen, or lymph nodes without evidence of malignancy
   f. Low or absent natural killer cell cytotoxicity
   g. Hyperferritinemia (≥500 ng/mL)
   h. Elevated soluble CD25 (interleukin-2Rα chain; ≥2,400 U/mL)

Adapted from Verbsky JW, Grossman WJ: Hemophagocytic lymphohistiocytosis: diagnosis, pathophysiology, treatment, and future perspectives, Ann Med 38:20–31, 2006, p. 21, Table 1.

Table 507-5	Spectrum of Diseases Characterized By Hemophagocytosis

PRIMARY HLH (see Table 507-3)

HLH WITH IMMUNODEFICIENCY, AUTOINFLAMMATORY STATES (see Table 507-3)

INFECTION-ASSOCIATED HLH (see Table 507-2)

MALIGNANCY-ASSOCIATED HLH
Lymphoma
Leukemia

MACROPHAGE ACTIVATION SYNDROME (MAS) ASSOCIATED WITH AUTOIMMUNE DISEASE

Systemic-onset juvenile idiopathic arthritis
Systemic lupus erythematosus
Enthesitis-related arthritis
Inflammatory bowel disease

contraindication to cytotoxic therapy in FHLH. Some recommend antithymocyte globulin and cyclosporine for maintenance therapy. Nevertheless, even with chemotherapy, FHLH remains ultimately fatal, often after a relapse of the disease. Allogeneic **stem cell transplantation** is effective in curing approximately 60% of patients with FHLH.

In contrast, in secondary HLH, it is critical that the underlying disease (e.g., infection, malignancy, or other) be identified and successfully treated. In many cases, such as when an infection can be documented and effectively treated, the prognosis may be excellent without any other specific treatment. However, when a treatable infection or other cause cannot be documented, which is the case in many patients presumed to have secondary HLH, the prognosis may be as poor as that of FHLH, and an identical chemotherapeutic approach, including etoposide, is recommended, even in the face of cytopenias. It is theorized that in both cases, by its cytotoxic effect on macrophages, etoposide interrupts cytokine production, the hemophagocytic process, and the accumulation of macrophages, all of which may contribute to the pathogenesis of infection-associated hemophagocytic syndrome. A broad spectrum of infectious agents, including viruses (e.g., cytomegalovirus, Epstein-Barr virus, human herpesvirus 6), fungi, protozoa, and bacteria, may trigger secondary HLH, often in the setting of immunodeficiency (see Table 507-2). A thorough evaluation for infection should be undertaken in immunodeficient patients with hemophagocytosis. The same syndrome may be identified in conjunction with a rheumatologic disorder (e.g., systemic lupus erythematosus, Kawasaki

disease) or a neoplasm (leukemia); in these cases, effective treatment of the underlying disease may cause resolution of the hemophagocytosis. In some patients, interferon and intravenous immunoglobulin have been effective.

Bibliography is available at Expert Consult.

507.3 Other Histiocytoses
Stephan Ladisch

Other rare histiocytoses are appropriately named for their clinical presentation. Examples include xanthogranuloma in juvenile xanthogranuloma and striking lymphadenopathy in Rosai-Dorfman disease (sinus histiocytosis with massive lymphadenopathy). Juvenile xanthogranuloma may require systemic treatment with cytotoxic chemotherapy if the disease is disseminated. Rosai-Dorfman disease is usually not treated, although the massive lymphadenopathy may require treatment because of its tendency to cause physical obstruction. Acute monocytic leukemia and true malignant histiocytosis are included because they are unequivocal malignancies of the monocyte-macrophage lineage; they are discussed in Chapter 490.

Bibliography is available at Expert Consult.

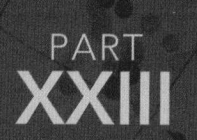
Section 1
Glomerular Disease

Chapter 508
Introduction to Glomerular Diseases

508.1 Anatomy of the Glomerulus

Cynthia G. Pan and Ellis D. Avner

The kidneys lie in the retroperitoneal space slightly above the level of the umbilicus. They range in length and weight, respectively, from approximately 6 cm and 24 g in a full-term newborn to ≥12 cm and 150 g in an adult. The kidney (Fig. 508-1) has an outer layer, **the cortex**, which contains the glomeruli, proximal and distal convoluted tubules, and collecting ducts; and an inner layer, **the medulla**, that contains the straight portions of the tubules, the loops of Henle, the vasa recta, and the terminal collecting ducts (Fig. 508-2).

The blood supply to each kidney usually consists of a main renal artery that arises from the aorta; multiple renal arteries can occur. The main artery divides into segmental branches within the medulla, becoming the interlobar arteries that pass through the medulla to the corticomedullary junction. At this point, the interlobar arteries branch to form the arcuate arteries, which run parallel to the surface of the kidney. Interlobular arteries originate from the arcuate arteries and give rise to the afferent arterioles of the glomeruli. Specialized muscle cells in the wall of the afferent arteriole and specialized distal tubular cells adjacent to the glomerulus (macula densa) form the juxtaglomerular apparatus that controls the secretion of renin. The afferent arteriole divides into the glomerular capillary network, which then recombines into the efferent arteriole (see Fig. 508-2). The juxtamedullary efferent arterioles are larger than those in the outer cortex and provide the blood supply, as the vasa recta, to the tubules and medulla.

Each kidney contains approximately 1 million nephrons (each consisting of a glomerulus and associated tubules). There is a large distribution of "normal nephron number" in humans, with the mean ±2 SD ranging from 200,000 to 2 million nephrons/kidney. This variation can have major pathophysiologic significance as a risk factor for the later development of hypertension and progressive renal dysfunction. In humans, formation of nephrons is complete at 36-40 wk of gestation, but functional maturation with tubular growth and elongation continues during the 1st decade of life. Because new nephrons cannot be formed after birth, any disease that results in progressive loss of nephrons can lead to renal insufficiency. A decreased number of nephrons secondary to low birthweight, prematurity, and/or unknown genetic or environmental factors has been implicated as a significant risk factor for the development of primary hypertension and progressive renal dysfunction in adulthood. Low nephron number presumably results in hyperfiltration and eventual sclerosis of "overworked" nephron units.

The glomerular network of specialized capillaries serves as the filtering mechanism of the kidney. The glomerular capillaries are lined by endothelial cells (Fig. 508-3) and have very thin cytoplasm that contains many holes (fenestrations). The glomerular basement membrane (GBM) forms a continuous layer between the endothelial and mesangial cells on one side and the epithelial cells on the other. The membrane has 3 layers: a central electron-dense lamina densa; the lamina rara interna, which lies between the lamina densa and the endothelial cells; and the lamina rara externa, which lies between the lamina densa and the epithelial cells. The visceral epithelial cells cover the capillary and project cytoplasmic foot processes, which attach to the lamina rara externa. Between the foot processes are spaces or filtration slits. The

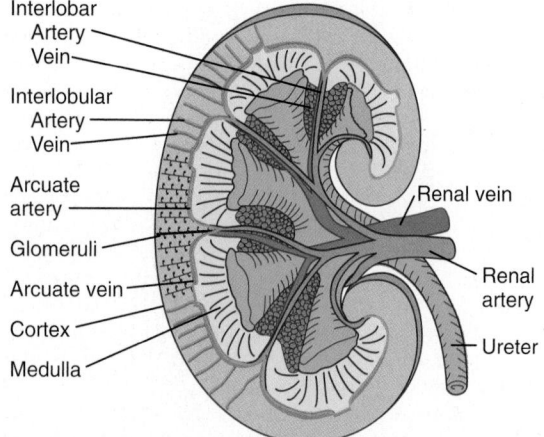

Figure 508-1 Gross morphology of the renal circulation. *(From Pitts RF: Physiology of the kidney and body fluids, ed 3, Chicago, 1974, Year Book Medical Publishers.)*

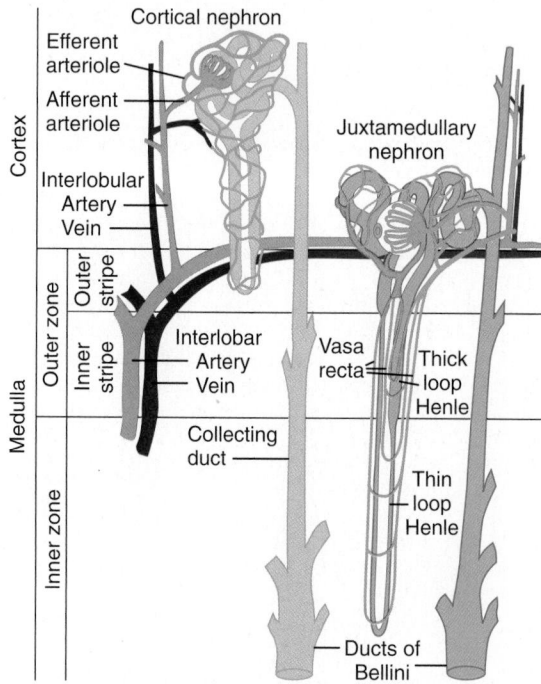

Figure 508-2 Comparison of the blood supplies of cortical and juxtamedullary nephrons. *(From Pitts RF: Physiology of the kidney and body fluids, ed 3, Chicago, 1974, Year Book Medical Publishers.)*

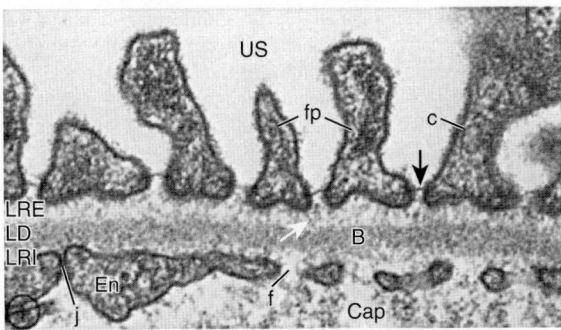

Figure 508-3 Electron micrograph of the normal glomerular capillary (Cap) wall demonstrating the endothelium (En) with its fenestrations (f), the glomerular basement membrane (B) with its central dense layer, the lamina densa (LD), and adjoining lamina rara interna (LRI) and externa (LRE) (*white arrow*), and the epithelial cell foot processes (fp) with their thick cell coat (c). The glomerular filtrate passes through the endothelial fenestrae, crosses the basement membrane, and passes through the filtration slits (*black arrow*) between the epithelial cell foot processes to reach the urinary space (US) (×60,000). J is the junction between 2 endothelial cells. (*From Farquhar MG, Kanwar YS: Functional organization of the glomerulus: state of the science in 1979. In Cummings NB, Michael AF, Wilson CB, editors:* Immune mechanisms in renal disease, *New York, 1982, Plenum.*)

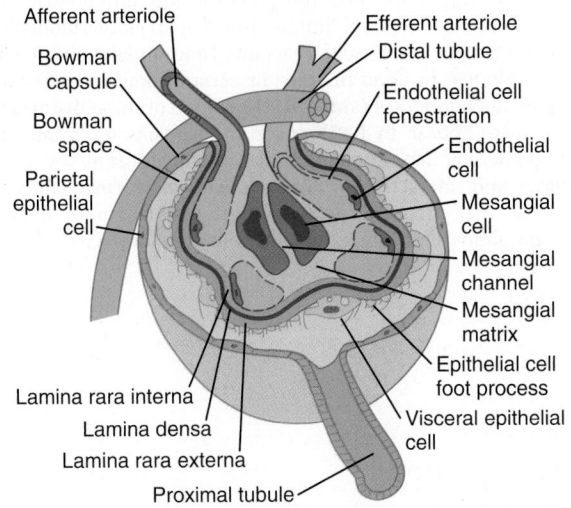

Figure 508-4 Schematic depiction of the glomerulus and surrounding structures.

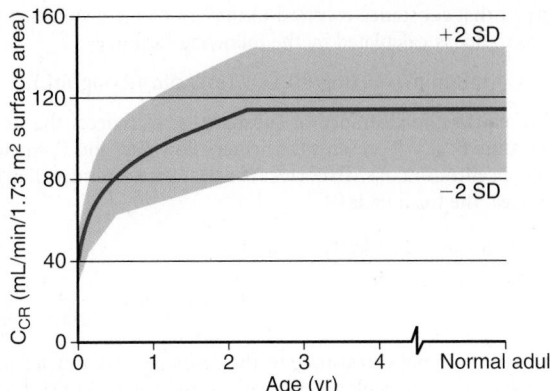

Figure 508-5 Changes in the normal value of the glomerular filtration rate, as measured by the creatinine clearance (Ccr), when standardized to mL/min/1.73 m² of body surface area. The *solid line* depicts the mean, and the *shaded area* includes 2 SD. (*From McCrory W:* Developmental nephrology, *Cambridge, MA, 1972, Harvard University Press.*)

mesangium (mesangial cells and matrix) lies between the glomerular capillaries on the endothelial cell side of the GBM and forms the medial part of the capillary wall. The mesangium may serve as a supporting, stalk-like structure for the glomerular capillaries and probably has a role in the regulation of glomerular blood flow, filtration, and the removal of macromolecules (such as immune complexes) from the glomerulus. Bowman's capsule, which surrounds the glomerulus, is composed of a basement membrane, which is continuous with the basement membranes of the glomerular capillaries and the proximal tubules, and the parietal epithelial cells, which are adjacent to the visceral epithelium (Fig. 508-4).

Bibliography is available at Expert Consult.

508.2 Glomerular Filtration
Cynthia G. Pan and Ellis D. Avner

Kidney function is best measured as glomerular filtration rate (GFR). As the blood passes through the glomerular capillaries, the plasma is filtered through the glomerular capillary walls. The ultrafiltrate, which is cell free, contains all of the substances in plasma (electrolytes, glucose, phosphate, urea, creatinine, peptides, low-molecular-weight proteins) except proteins having a molecular weight of ≥68 kDa (such as albumin and globulins). The filtrate is collected in Bowman's space and enters the tubules. There its composition is modified by tightly regulated secretion and absorption of solute and fluid by the multiple tubular segments of the nephron and the ductal system, until it exits the kidney, via the ureter, as urine.

Glomerular filtration is the net result of opposing forces applied across the capillary wall. The force for ultrafiltration (glomerular capillary hydrostatic pressure) is a result of systemic arterial pressure, modified by the tone of the afferent and efferent arterioles. The major force opposing ultrafiltration is glomerular capillary oncotic pressure, created by the gradient between the high concentration of plasma proteins within the capillary and the almost protein-free ultrafiltrate in Bowman's space. Filtration may be modified by the rate of glomerular plasma flow, the hydrostatic pressure within Bowman's space, and/or the permeability of the glomerular capillary wall.

Although glomerular filtration begins at approximately the 6th wk of fetal life, kidney function is not necessary for normal intrauterine homeostasis because the placenta serves as the major fetal excretory organ. After birth, the GFR increases until renal growth ceases (by age ~18-20 yr in most people). To compare GFRs of children and adults, the GFR is standardized to the body surface area (1.73 m²) of an "ideal" 70-kg adult. Even after correction for surface area, the GFR of a child does not approximate adult values until the 3rd yr of life (Fig. 508-5). The GFR may be estimated by measurement of the serum creatinine level. Creatinine is derived from muscle metabolism. Its production is relatively constant, and its excretion is primarily through glomerular filtration, although tubular secretion can become important as serum creatinine rises in renal insufficiency. In contrast to the concentration of blood urea nitrogen, which is affected by state of hydration and nitrogen balance, the serum creatinine level is primarily influenced by muscle mass and the level of glomerular function. The serum creatinine is of value only in estimating the GFR under steady-state conditions. A patient can have a normal serum creatinine level without effective renal function very shortly after the onset of acute renal failure with anuria. In this clinical setting, serum creatinine is an insensitive measure of decreased renal function because its level does not rise above normal until GFR falls by 30-40%.

The precise measurement of the GFR is accomplished by quantitating the clearance of a substance that is freely filtered across the capillary wall and is neither reabsorbed nor secreted by the tubules. The clearance (C_s) of such a substance is the volume of plasma that, when completely cleared of the contained substance, would yield an equal quantity of that substance excreted in the urine over a specified time. Renal clearance is calculated by the following formula:

$$C_s\,(mL/min) = U_s(mg/mL) \times V\,(mL/min)/P_s(mg/mL)$$

where C_s equals the clearance of substance s, U_s reflects the urinary concentration of s, V represents the urinary flow rate, and P_s equals the plasma concentration of s. To correct the clearance for individual body surface area, the formula is:

Corrected clearance $(mL/min/1.73\,m^2)$

$$= C_s(mL/min) \times \frac{1.73}{Surface\ area\ (m^2)}$$

The GFR is optimally measured by the clearance of inulin, a fructose polymer having a molecular weight of approximately 5 kDa. Because the inulin clearance technique is cumbersome for use in clinical practice, the GFR is commonly estimated by the clearance of endogenous creatinine. Formulas that estimate creatinine clearance accurately in clinical settings have been useful tools in patient care. The "bedside" Schwartz formula is the most widely used pediatric formula and is based on the serum creatinine, patient height, and an empirical constant. The accuracy of this equation is further improved utilizing an additional endogenous marker, cystatin C, in addition to serum creatinine. Cystatin C is a 13.6 kDa protease inhibitor produced by nucleated cells. It continues to be tested as a clinical tool to completely replace creatinine-based formulas, as it has distinct advantages in estimating GFR. Unlike creatinine, cystatin C is unaffected by sex, height, muscle mass, bilirubin, or red blood cell hemolysis, and is not secreted by the renal tubules under any conditions.

The absence of plasma proteins larger than the size of albumin from the glomerular filtrate confirms the effectiveness of the glomerular capillary wall as a filtration barrier. Major factors restricting the filtration of these and other macromolecules include their size and their ionic charge. Morphologic studies suggest that the size-selective filtration barrier resides within the GBM. The endothelial cell, basement membrane, and epithelial cell of the glomerular capillary wall all possess strong negative ionic charges (heparan sulfate and glycoproteins containing sialic acid). Proteins in the blood have a relatively low isoelectric point, carry a net negative charge, and are repelled by the negatively charged sites of the glomerular capillary wall, thus restricting filtration.

Bibliography is available at Expert Consult.

508.3 Glomerular Diseases
Cynthia G. Pan and Ellis D. Avner

PATHOGENESIS
Glomerular injury may be a result of genetic, immunologic, perfusion, or coagulation disorders. Genetic disorders of the glomerulus may result from mutations in DNA exons encoding proteins located within the glomerulus, interstitium, or tubular epithelium; mutations in regulatory genes controlling DNA transcription; abnormal posttranscriptional modification of RNA transcripts; or abnormal posttranslational modification of proteins. Immunologic injury to the glomerulus results in **glomerulonephritis,** which is a generic term for several diseases, but more precisely a histopathologic term defining inflammation of the glomerular capillaries. Evidence that glomerulonephritis is caused by immunologic injury includes morphologic and immunopathologic similarities to experimental immune-mediated glomerulonephritis; the demonstration of immune reactants (immunoglobulin, complement) in glomeruli; abnormalities in serum complement; and the finding of autoantibodies (anti-GBM) in some of these diseases (Fig. 508-6). There appear to be 2 major mechanisms of immunologic injury: glomerular deposition of circulating antigen–antibody immune complexes and interaction of antibody with glomerular antigens in situ. In the latter circumstance, the antigen may be a normal component of the glomerulus (the noncollagenous domain [NC-1] of type IV

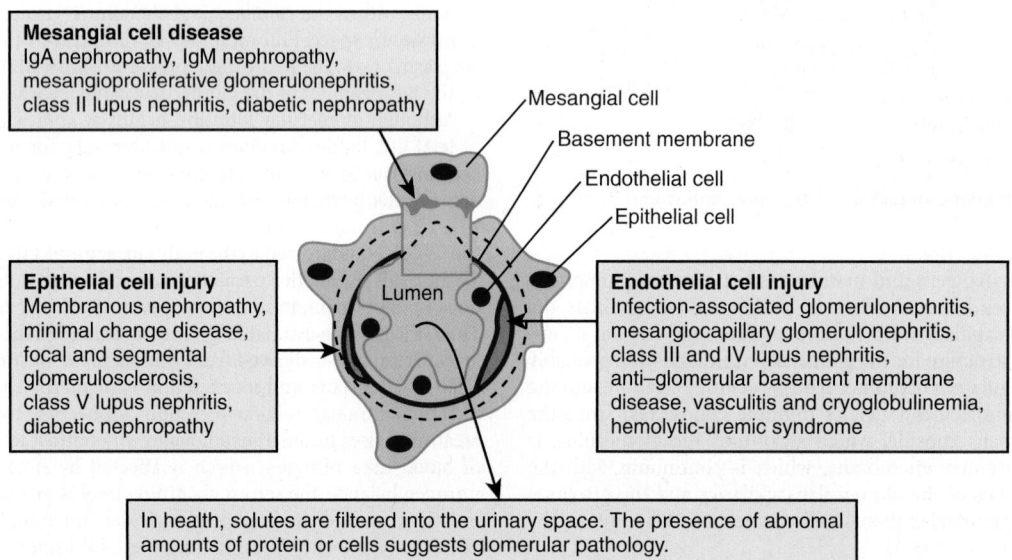

Figure 508-6 Cellular location of injury during glomerulonephritis. Mesangial cells are directly exposed to the circulation. Deposition of immune complexes within these cells is typically seen in disorders such as immunoglobulin A (IgA) nephropathy; it results in proliferation and expansion of the cells, leading to hematuria, proteinuria, and renal impairment. Epithelial cells, in conjunction with basement membrane, allow filtration of plasma solutes but retard passage of cells and plasma proteins. Disease related to these cells is typified by the presence of subepithelial deposits and flattening of the foot processes that engage the basement membrane, resulting in disruption of the filtration barrier and proteinuria. Endothelial cell disease can result from deposition of immune complex (as occurs in mesangiocapillary glomerulonephritis), attachment of antibody to the basement membrane (Goodpasture disease), or trauma and activation of coagulation (hemolytic-uremic syndrome). Endothelial cell proliferation and necrosis are accompanied by leukocyte accumulation, and rupture of the basement membrane, crescent formation, and disruption of glomerular architecture can develop. A nephritic or rapidly progressive presentation ensues. *(From Chadban SJ, Atkins RC: Glomerulonephritis,* Lancet *365:1797–1806, 2005.)*

collagen, a putative antigen in human anti-GBM nephritis) or an antigen that has been deposited in the glomerulus.

In **immune complex–mediated** diseases, antibody is produced against, and combines with, a circulating antigen that is usually unrelated to the kidney (see Fig. 508-6). The immune complexes accumulate in GBMs and activate the complement system, leading to immune injury. Acute serum sickness in rabbits is produced by a single intravenous injection of bovine albumin. Within 1 wk after injection, a rabbit produces antibody against bovine albumin, and the antigen remains in the blood in high concentration. As antibody enters the circulation, it forms immune complexes with antigen. Although the amount of antigen in the circulation exceeds that of antibody (antigen excess), the complexes formed are small, remain soluble in the circulation, and are deposited in glomeruli. The processes involved in glomerular localization are not well understood but include characteristics of the complex (concentration, charge, size) and/or the glomerulus (mesangial trapping, negatively charged capillary wall); hydrodynamic forces; and the influence of various chemical mediators (angiotensin II, prostaglandins).

With deposition of immune complexes in glomeruli, rabbits develop an acute proliferative glomerulonephritis. Immunofluorescence microscopy demonstrates granular (**"lumpy-bumpy"**) deposits containing immunoglobulin and complement in the glomerular capillary wall. Electron microscopic studies show these deposits to be on the epithelial side of the GBM and in the mesangium. For the next few days, as additional antibody enters the circulation, the antigen is ultimately removed from the circulation and the glomerulonephritis subsides.

An example of in situ antigen–antibody interaction is **anti–GBM antibody disease,** in which antibody reacts with antigen(s) of the GBM. Immunopathologic studies reveal linear deposition of immunoglobulin and complement along the GBM in Goodpasture syndrome (see Chapter 517) and certain types of rapidly progressive glomerulonephritis (see Chapter 516).

The inflammatory reaction that follows immunologic injury results from activation of 1 or more mediator pathways. The most important of these is the complement system, which has 2 initiating sequences: the classic pathway, which is activated by antigen–antibody immune complexes, and the alternative or properdin pathway, which is activated by polysaccharides and endotoxin. These pathways converge at C3; from that point on, the same sequence leads to lysis of cell membranes (see Chapter 133). The major noxious products of complement activation are produced after activation of C3 and include anaphylatoxin (which stimulates contractile proteins within vascular walls and increases vascular permeability) and chemotactic factors (C5a) that recruit neutrophils and perhaps macrophages to the site of complement activation, leading to consequent damage to vascular cells and basement membranes. Therapeutic agents to block the antibody production and components of the complement cascade are available and may provide additional tools to treat immune-mediated kidney injury (see Chapters 514 and 518).

The coagulation system may be activated **directly,** after endothelial cell injury that exposes the thrombogenic subendothelial layer (thereby initiating the coagulation cascade), or it may be activated **indirectly,** after complement activation. Consequently, fibrin is deposited within glomerular capillaries or within Bowman's space as crescents. Activation of the coagulation cascade can also activate the kinin system, which produces additional chemotactic and anaphylatoxin-like factors.

PATHOLOGY

The glomerulus may be injured by several mechanisms, but it has only a limited number of histopathologic responses; different disease states can produce similar microscopic changes.

Proliferation of glomerular cells occurs in most forms of glomerulonephritis and may be generalized (involving all glomeruli) or focal (involving only some glomeruli and sparing others). Within a single glomerulus, proliferation may be diffuse (involving all parts of the glomerulus) or segmental (involving only 1 or more tufts, but not others). Proliferation commonly involves the endothelial and mesangial cells and is often associated with an increase in the mesangial matrix (see Fig. 508-6). Mesangial proliferation can result from deposition of immune complex within the mesangium. The resultant increase in cell size and number, and production of mesangial matrix, can increase glomerular size and narrow the lumens of glomerular capillaries, leading to renal insufficiency.

Crescent formation in Bowman's space (capsule) is a result of proliferation of parietal epithelial cells and is often associated with clinical signs of renal dysfunction. Crescents develop in several forms of glomerulonephritis (termed **rapidly progressive** or **crescentic**; see Chapter 516) and are a characteristic response to deposition of fibrin in Bowman's space. Newly formed crescents contain fibrin, the proliferating epithelial cells of Bowman's space, basement membrane–like material produced by these cells, and macrophages that might have a role in the genesis of glomerular injury. Over the subsequent days to weeks, the crescent is invaded by connective tissue and becomes a fibroepithelial crescent. This process generally results in glomerular obsolescence and the clinical development of chronic renal failure. Crescent formation is often associated with glomerular cell death. The necrotic glomerulus has a characteristic eosinophilic appearance and usually contains nuclear remnants. Crescent formation is usually associated with generalized proliferation of the mesangial cells and with either immune complex or anti-GBM antibody deposition in the glomerular capillary wall.

Certain forms of acute glomerulonephritis show glomerular exudation of blood cells, including neutrophils, eosinophils, basophils, and mononuclear cells. The thickened appearance of GBM can result from a true increase in the width of the membrane (as seen in membranous glomerulopathy; see Chapter 512), from massive deposition of immune complexes that have staining characteristics similar to the membrane (as seen in systemic lupus erythematosus; see Chapter 514), or from the interposition of mesangial cells and matrix into the subendothelial space between the endothelial cells and the GBM. The last can give the basement membrane a split appearance, as seen in type I membranoproliferative glomerulonephritis (see Chapter 513) and other diseases.

Sclerosis refers to the presence of scar tissue within the glomerulus. Occasionally, pathologists use this term to refer to an increase in mesangial matrix.

Tubulointerstitial fibrosis is present in all patients who have glomerular disease and who develop progressive renal injury. This fibrosis is initiated by injury to either the glomeruli, which, if severe, may secondarily involve the tubules, or direct injury to the tubules themselves. Tubular injury recruits mononuclear cell infiltrate, which releases a variety of soluble factors that have fibrosis-promoting effects. Matrix proteins of the renal interstitium begin to accumulate, leading to eventual destruction of renal tubules and peritubular capillaries. The actual transformation of tubular epithelium to mesenchymal tissue can contribute to progressive tubulointerstitial fibrosis, a process termed *epithelial-mesenchymal transformation.*

Bibliography is available at Expert Consult.

Section 2
Conditions Particularly Associated with Hematuria

Chapter 509
Clinical Evaluation of the Child with Hematuria

Cynthia G. Pan and Ellis D. Avner

Hematuria is defined as the presence of at least 5 red blood cells (RBCs) per microliter of urine and occurs with a prevalence of 0.5-2.0% among school-age children. Quantitative studies demonstrate that normal children can excrete more than 500,000 RBCs per 12 hr period; this increases with fever and/or exercise. In the clinical setting, qualitative estimates are provided by a urinary dipstick that uses a very sensitive peroxidase chemical reaction between hemoglobin (or myoglobin) and a colorimetric chemical indicator impregnated on the dipstick. Chemstrip (Boehringer Mannheim), a common commercially available dipstick, is capable of detecting 3-5 RBCs/µL of unspun urine. The presence of 10-50 RBCs/µL may suggest underlying pathology, but significant hematuria is generally considered as >50 RBCs/µL. False-negative results can occur in the presence of formalin (used as a urine preservative) or high urinary concentrations of ascorbic acid (i.e., in patients with vitamin C intake >2000 mg/day). False-positive results may be seen in a child with an alkaline urine (pH > 8), or more commonly following contamination with oxidizing agents such as hydrogen peroxide used to clean the perineum before obtaining a specimen. Microscopic analysis of 10-15 mL of freshly voided and centrifuged urine is essential in confirming the presence of RBCs suggested by >10 RBCs/µL, or a 1+ positive urinary dipstick reading.

Red urine **without** RBCs is seen in a number of conditions (Table 509-1). Clinically significant heme-positive urine without RBCs may

Table 509-1	Other Causes of Red Urine
HEME POSITIVE Hemoglobin Myoglobin **HEME NEGATIVE** **Drugs** Chloroquine Deferoxamine Ibuprofen Iron sorbitol Metronidazole Nitrofurantoin Phenazopyridine (Pyridium) Phenolphthalein Phenothiazines Rifampin Salicylates Sulfasalazine	**Dyes (Vegetable/Fruit)** Beets Blackberries Food and candy coloring Rhubarb **Metabolites** Homogentisic acid Melanin Methemoglobin Porphyrin Tyrosinosis Urates

be caused by the presence of either hemoglobin or myoglobin. Hemoglobinuria without hematuria can occur in the presence of acute or chronic hemolysis. Myoglobinuria without hematuria occurs in the presence of rhabdomyolysis resulting from skeletal muscle injury and is generally associated with a 5-fold increase in the plasma concentration of creatinine kinase. **Rhabdomyolysis** is always clinically significant as it may lead to acute renal injury. It can occur secondary to viral myositis, crush injury, severe electrolyte abnormalities (hypernatremia, hypophosphatemia), hypotension, disseminated intravascular coagulation, toxins (drugs, venom), metabolic disorders of muscles, and prolonged seizures. Clinically innocuous heme-negative urine can appear red, cola colored, or burgundy, owing to ingestion of various drugs, foods (blackberries, beets), or dyes used in food and candy, whereas dark brown (or black) urine can result from various urinary metabolites.

Evaluation of the child with hematuria begins with a careful history, physical examination, and urinalysis. This information is used to determine the level of hematuria (upper vs lower urinary tract) and to determine the urgency of the evaluation based on symptomatology. Special consideration needs to be given to family history, identification of anatomic abnormalities and malformation syndromes, presence of gross hematuria, and manifestations of hypertension, edema, or heart failure.

Table 509-2 lists causes of hematuria. Upper urinary tract sources of hematuria originate within the nephron (glomerulus, tubular system, or interstitium). Lower urinary tract sources of hematuria originate from the pelvocaliceal system, ureter, bladder, or urethra. Hematuria from within the glomerulus is often associated with brown, cola- or tea-colored, or burgundy urine, proteinuria >100 mg/dL via dipstick, urinary microscopic findings of RBC casts, and deformed urinary RBCs (particularly acanthocytes). Hematuria originating within the tubular system may be associated with the presence of leukocytes or renal tubular casts. Lower urinary tract sources of hematuria may be associated with gross hematuria that is bright red or pink, terminal hematuria (gross hematuria occurring at the end of the urine stream), blood clots, normal urinary RBC morphology, and minimal proteinuria on dipstick (<100 mg/dL).

Patients with hematuria can present with a number of symptoms suggesting specific disorders. Tea- or cola-colored urine, facial or body edema, hypertension, and oliguria are classic symptoms of **glomerulonephritis.** Diseases commonly manifesting as glomerulonephritis include postinfectious glomerulonephritis, immunoglobulin A (IgA) nephropathy, membranoproliferative glomerulonephritis, Henoch-Schönlein purpura (HSP) nephritis, systemic lupus erythematosus (SLE) nephritis, granulomatosis with polyangiitis (formerly Wegener granulomatosis), microscopic polyarteritis nodosa, Goodpasture syndrome, and hemolytic-uremic syndrome. A history of recent upper respiratory, skin, or gastrointestinal infection suggests postinfectious glomerulonephritis, hemolytic-uremic syndrome, or HSP nephritis. Rash and joint complaints suggest HSP or SLE nephritis.

Hematuria associated with glomerulonephritis is typically painless, but can be associated with flank pain when acute or unusually severe. Frequency, dysuria, and unexplained fevers suggest a urinary tract infection, whereas renal colic suggests nephrolithiasis. A flank mass can suggest hydronephrosis, renal cystic diseases, renal vein thrombosis, or tumor. Hematuria associated with headache, mental status changes, visual changes (diplopia), epistaxis, or heart failure suggests significant hypertension. Patients with hematuria and a history of trauma require immediate evaluation (see Chapter 72). Child abuse must always be suspected in the child presenting with unexplained perineal bruising and hematuria.

A careful family history is critical in the initial assessment of the child with hematuria given the numerous genetic causes of renal disorders. Hereditary glomerular diseases include hereditary nephritis (Alport syndrome), thin glomerular basement membrane disease, SLE nephritis, and IgA nephropathy (Berger disease). Other hematuric renal disorders with a hereditary component include both autosomal recessive and autosomal dominant polycystic kidney diseases, atypical hemolytic-uremic syndrome, urolithiasis, and sickle cell disease/trait.

A complete physical examination is critical to assess the cause of hematuria. Hypertension, edema, or signs of heart failure suggest acute glomerulonephritis. Several malformation syndromes are associated with renal disease including VATER (*v*ertebral body anomalies, *a*nal atresia, *t*racheo*e*sophageal fistula, and *r*enal dysplasia) syndrome. Abdominal masses may be caused by bladder distention in posterior urethral valves, hydronephrosis in ureteropelvic junction obstruction, polycystic kidney disease, or Wilms tumor. Hematuria seen in patients with neurologic or cutaneous abnormalities may be the result of a number of syndromic renal disorders including tuberous sclerosis, von Hippel-Lindau syndrome, and Zellweger (cerebrohepatorenal) syndrome. Anatomic abnormalities of the external genitalia may be associated with hematuria and/or renal disease.

Patients with gross hematuria present additional challenges because of the associated parental anxiety. The most common cause of gross hematuria is bacterial urinary tract infection. **Urethrorrhagia**, which is urethral bleeding in the absence of urine, is associated with dysuria and blood spots on underwear after voiding. This condition, which often occurs in prepubertal boys at intervals several months apart, has a benign self-limited course. Less than 10% of patients have evidence of glomerulonephritis. Recurrent episodes of gross hematuria suggest IgA nephropathy, Alport syndrome, or thin glomerular basement membrane disease. Dysuria and abdominal or flank pain are symptoms of idiopathic hypercalciuria, or urolithiasis. Table 509-3 lists common causes of gross hematuria; Figure 509-1 outlines a general approach to the laboratory and radiologic evaluation of the patient with glomerular or extraglomerular hematuria. Asymptomatic patients with isolated microscopic hematuria should not undergo extensive diagnostic evaluation, because such hematuria is often transient and benign.

Table 509-2	Causes of Hematuria in Children

UPPER URINARY TRACT DISEASE
Isolated renal disease
Immunoglobulin (Ig) A nephropathy (Berger disease)
Alport syndrome (hereditary nephritis)
Thin glomerular basement membrane nephropathy
Postinfectious GN (poststreptococcal GN)*
Membranous nephropathy
Membranoproliferative GN*
Rapidly progressive GN
Focal segmental glomerulosclerosis
Anti–glomerular basement membrane disease
Multisystem disease
Systemic lupus erythematosus nephritis*
Henoch-Schönlein purpura nephritis
Granulomatosis with polyangiitis (formerly Wegener granulomatosis)
Polyarteritis nodosa
Goodpasture syndrome
Hemolytic-uremic syndrome
Sickle cell glomerulopathy
HIV nephropathy
Tubulointerstitial disease
Pyelonephritis
Interstitial nephritis
Papillary necrosis
Acute tubular necrosis
Vascular
Arterial or venous thrombosis
Malformations (aneurysms, hemangiomas)
Nutcracker syndrome
Hemoglobinopathy (sickle cell trait/disease)
Crystalluria
Anatomic
Hydronephrosis
Cystic-syndromic kidney disease
Polycystic kidney disease
Multicystic dysplasia
Tumor (Wilms tumor, rhabdomyosarcoma, angiomyolipoma, medullary carcinoma)
Trauma

LOWER URINARY TRACT DISEASE
Inflammation (infectious and noninfectious)
Cystitis
Urethritis
Urolithiasis
Trauma
Coagulopathy
Heavy exercise
Bladder tumor
Factitious syndrome, factitious syndrome by proxy†

*Denotes glomerulonephritides presenting with hypocomplementemia.
†Formerly Munchausen syndrome and Munchausen syndrome by proxy.
GN, glomerulonephritis.

Table 509-3	Common Causes of Gross Hematuria

Urinary tract infection
Meatal stenosis
Perineal irritation
Trauma
Urolithiasis
Hypercalciuria
Coagulopathy
Tumor
Glomerular
Postinfectious glomerulonephritis
Henoch-Schönlein purpura nephritis
IgA nephropathy
Alport syndrome (hereditary nephritis)
Thin glomerular basement membrane disease
Systemic lupus erythematosus nephritis

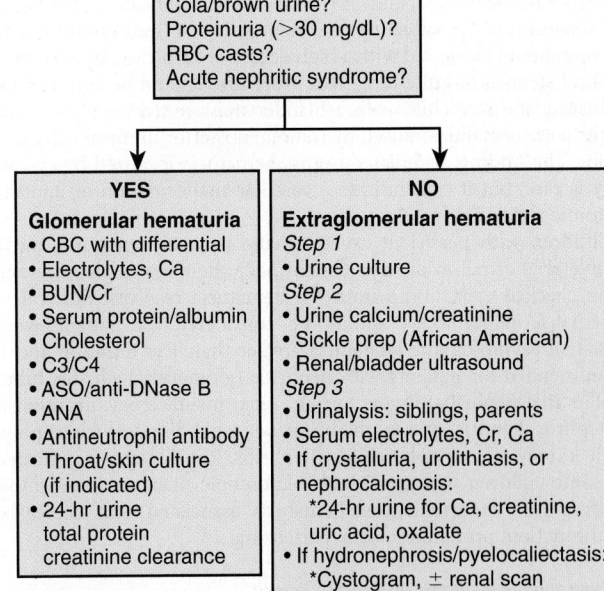

Figure 509-1 Algorithm of the general approach to the laboratory and radiologic evaluation of the patient with glomerular or extraglomerular hematuria. ANA, antinuclear antibody; ASO, antistreptolysin O; BUN, blood urea nitrogen; C3/C4, complement; CBC, complete blood cell count; Cr, creatinine; RBC, red blood cell.

The child with completely asymptomatic isolated microscopic hematuria that persists on at least 3 urinalyses observed over a minimum of a 2 wk period poses a dilemma in regard to the degree of further diagnostic testing that should be performed. Significant disease of the urinary tract is uncommon with this clinical presentation. The initial evaluation of these children should include a urine culture followed by a spot urine for hypercalciuria with a calcium : creatinine ratio in culture-negative patients. In African-American patients, a sickle cell screen should be included. If these studies are normal, urinalysis of all first-degree relatives is indicated. Renal and bladder ultrasonography should be considered to rule out structural lesions such as tumor, cystic disease, hydronephrosis, or urolithiasis. Ultrasonography of the urinary tract is most informative in patients presenting with gross hematuria, abdominal pain, flank pain, or trauma. If these initial studies are normal, assessment of serum creatinine and electrolytes is recommended.

The finding of certain hematologic abnormalities can narrow the differential diagnosis. Anemia in this setting may be caused by hypervolemia with dilution associated with acute renal failure; decreased RBC production in chronic renal failure; hemolysis from hemolytic-uremic syndrome, a chronic hemolytic anemia, or SLE; blood loss from pulmonary hemorrhage, as seen in Goodpasture syndrome; or melena in patients with HSP or hemolytic-uremic syndrome. Inspection of the peripheral blood smear might reveal a microangiopathic process consistent with the hemolytic-uremic syndrome. The presence of autoantibodies in SLE can result in a positive Coombs test, the presence of antinuclear antibody, leukopenia, and multisystem disease. Thrombocytopenia can result from decreased platelet production (malignancies) or increased platelet consumption (SLE, idiopathic thrombocytopenic purpura, hemolytic-uremic syndrome, renal vein thrombosis, or congenital hepatic fibrosis with portal hypertension secondary to autosomal recessive polycystic kidney disease). Although urinary RBC morphology may be normal with lower tract bleeding and dysmorphic from glomerular bleeding, it is not sensitive enough to unequivocally delineate the site of hematuria. A bleeding diathesis is an unusual cause of hematuria. Coagulation studies are not routinely obtained unless personal or family history suggests a bleeding tendency.

A voiding cystourethrogram is only required in patients with a urinary tract infection, renal scarring, hydroureter, or pyelocaliectasis. Cystoscopy is an unnecessary and costly procedure in most pediatric patients with hematuria, and carries the associated risks of anesthesia. The diagnosis of "possible urethral stenosis" as an indication for cystoscopy should be viewed with a high degree of suspicion, because true urethral stenosis is quite rare. This procedure should be reserved for evaluating the rare child with a bladder mass noted on ultrasound, urethral abnormalities caused by trauma, posterior urethral valves, or tumor. The finding of unilateral gross hematuria localized by cystoscopy is rare, but it can indicate a vascular malformation or another anatomic abnormality.

Children with persistent asymptomatic isolated hematuria and a completely normal evaluation should have their blood pressure and urine checked every 3 mo until the hematuria resolves. Referral to a pediatric nephrologist should be considered for patients with persistent asymptomatic hematuria greater than 1 yr duration and is recommended for patients with nephritis (glomerulonephritis, tubulointerstitial nephritis), hypertension, renal insufficiency, urolithiasis or nephrocalcinosis, or a family history of renal disease such as polycystic kidney disease or hereditary nephritis. Renal biopsy is indicated for some children with persistent microscopic hematuria, and most children with recurrent gross hematuria associated with decreased renal function, proteinuria, or hypertension.

Bibliography is available at Expert Consult.

Chapter 510
Isolated Glomerular Diseases with Recurrent Gross Hematuria
Cynthia G. Pan and Ellis D. Avner

Approximately 10% of children with gross hematuria have an acute or a chronic form of glomerulonephritis that may be associated with a systemic illness. The gross hematuria, which is usually characterized by brown or cola-colored urine, may be painless or associated with vague flank or abdominal pain. Presentation with gross hematuria is common within 1-2 days after the onset of an apparent viral upper respiratory tract infection in immunoglobulin (Ig) A nephropathy, and typically resolves within 5 days. This relatively short period contrasts to a latency period of 7-21 days occurring between the onset of a streptococcal pharyngitis or impetiginous skin infection and the development of poststreptococcal acute glomerulonephritis. Gross hematuria in these circumstances can last as long as 4-6 wk. Gross hematuria can also be seen in children with glomerular basement membrane (GBM) disorders such as hereditary nephritis (Alport syndrome [AS]) and thin GBM disease. These glomerular diseases can also manifest as microscopic hematuria and/or proteinuria without gross hematuria.

510.1 Immunoglobulin A Nephropathy (Berger Nephropathy)
Cynthia G. Pan and Ellis D. Avner

IgA nephropathy is the most common chronic glomerular disease in children. It is characterized by a predominance of IgA within mesangial glomerular deposits in the absence of systemic disease. Diagnosis requires renal biopsy, which is performed when clinical features warrant confirmation of the diagnosis or characterization of the histologic severity, which might affect therapeutic decisions.

PATHOLOGY AND PATHOLOGIC DIAGNOSIS
Focal and segmental mesangial proliferation and increased mesangial matrix are seen in the glomerulus (Fig. 510-1). Renal histology

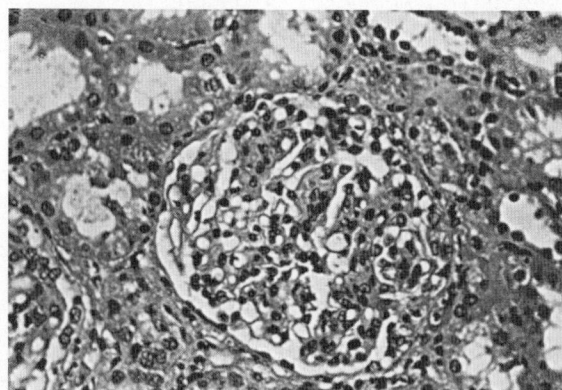

Figure 510-1 Light microscopy of IgA nephropathy demonstrating segmental mesangial proliferation and increased matrix (×180).

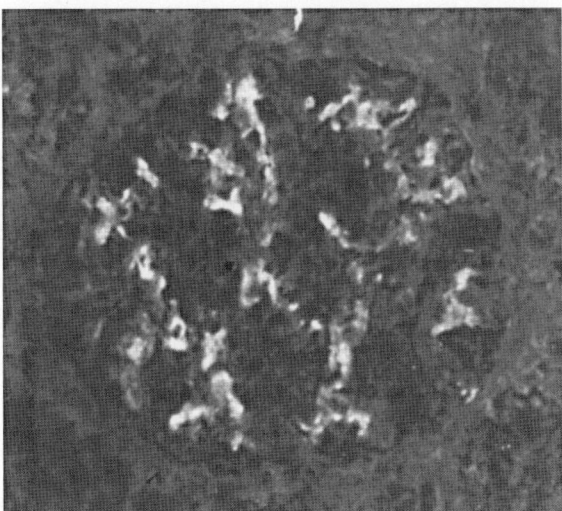

Figure 510-2 Immunofluorescence microscopy of the biopsy specimen from a child with episodes of gross hematuria demonstrating mesangial deposition of IgA (×150).

demonstrates mesangial proliferation that may be associated with epithelial cell crescent formation and sclerosis. IgA deposits in the mesangium are often accompanied by C3 complement (Fig. 510-2).

IgA nephropathy is an immune complex disease initiated by excessive amounts of poorly galactosylated IgA_1 in the serum causing the production of IgG and IgA autoantibodies. The abnormalities identified in the IgA system have also been observed in patients with Henoch-Schönlein purpura, and this finding lends support to the hypothesis that these 2 diseases are part of the same disease spectrum. Familial clustering of IgA nephropathy cases suggests the importance of genetic factors. Genome-wide linkage analysis suggests the linkage of IgA nephropathy to 6q22-23 in multiplex IgA nephropathy kindreds.

CLINICAL AND LABORATORY MANIFESTATIONS

IgA nephropathy is seen more often in male than in female patients. Although there are rare cases of rapidly progressive forms of the disease, the clinical presentation of childhood IgA nephropathy is often benign in comparison to that of adults. IgA nephropathy is an uncommon cause of end-stage renal failure during childhood. A majority of children with IgA nephropathy in the United States and Europe present with gross hematuria, whereas microscopic hematuria and/or proteinuria is a more common presentation in Japan. Other presentations include acute nephritic syndrome, nephrotic syndrome, or a combined nephritic-nephrotic picture. Gross hematuria often occurs within 1-2 days of onset of an upper respiratory or gastrointestinal infection, in contrast to the longer latency period observed in acute postinfectious glomerulonephritis, and may be associated with loin pain. Proteinuria is often <1000 mg/24 hr in patients with asymptomatic microscopic hematuria. Mild to moderate hypertension is most often seen in patients with nephritic or nephrotic syndrome, but is rarely severe enough to result in hypertensive emergencies. Normal serum levels of C3 in IgA nephropathy help to distinguish this disorder from poststreptococcal glomerulonephritis. Serum IgA levels have no diagnostic value because they are elevated in only 15% of pediatric patients.

PROGNOSIS AND TREATMENT

Although IgA nephropathy does not lead to significant kidney damage in most children, progressive disease develops in 20-30% of patients 15-20 yr after disease onset. Therefore, most children with IgA nephropathy do not display progressive renal dysfunction until adulthood, prompting the need for careful long-term follow-up. Poor prognostic indicators at presentation or follow-up include persistent

hypertension, diminished renal function, and significant, increasing, or prolonged proteinuria. A more severe prognosis is correlated with histologic evidence of diffuse mesangial proliferation, extensive glomerular crescents, glomerulosclerosis, and diffuse tubulointerstitial changes, including inflammation and fibrosis.

The primary treatment of IgA nephropathy is appropriate blood pressure control and management of significant proteinuria. Angiotensin-converting enzyme inhibitors and angiotensin II receptor antagonists are effective in reducing proteinuria and retarding the rate of disease progression when used individually or in combination. Fish oil, which contains antiinflammatory omega-3 polyunsaturated fatty acids, may decrease the rate of disease progression in adults. If renin-angiotensin blockade proves ineffective and significant proteinuria persists, then addition of immunosuppressive therapy with corticosteroids is recommended. Corticosteroids reduce proteinuria and improve renal function in those patients with a glomerular filtration rate >60 mL/min/m². It remains unclear if the effects of glucocorticoids deter progression to end-stage renal failure to a degree to offset their significant side effects. To date, additional immunosuppression with cyclophosphamide or azathioprine has not appeared to be effective, but further randomized clinical trials are in progress. Tonsillectomy has been used as treatment for IgA nephropathy in many countries including Japan. Performing a tonsillectomy in the absence of significant tonsillitis in association with IgA nephropathy is currently not recommended until appropriate prospective, controlled trials have been performed and demonstrate efficacy. Patients with IgA nephropathy may undergo successful kidney transplantation. Although recurrent disease is frequent, allograft loss caused by IgA nephropathy occurs in only 15-30% of patients.

Bibliography is available at Expert Consult.

510.2 Alport Syndrome
Cynthia G. Pan and Ellis D. Avner

AS, or hereditary nephritis, is a genetically heterogeneous disease caused by mutations in the genes coding for type IV collagen, a major component of basement membranes. These genetic alterations are associated with marked variability in clinical presentation, natural history, and histologic abnormalities.

GENETICS

Approximately 85% of patients have X-linked inheritance caused by a mutation in the *COL4A5* gene encoding the α5 chain of type IV collagen. Patients with a subtype of X-linked AS and diffuse leiomyomatosis demonstrate a contiguous mutation within the *COL4A5* and *COL4A6* genes that encodes the α5 and α6 chains, respectively, of type IV collagen. Autosomal recessive forms of AS are caused by mutations in the *COL4A3* and *COL4A4* genes on chromosome 2 encoding the α3 and α4 chains, respectively, of type IV collagen. An autosomal dominant form of AS linked to the *COL4A3-COL4A4* gene locus occurs in 5% of cases.

PATHOLOGY

Kidney biopsy specimens during the 1st decade of life show few changes on light microscopy. Later, the glomeruli may develop mesangial proliferation and capillary wall thickening, leading to progressive glomerular sclerosis. Tubular atrophy, interstitial inflammation and fibrosis, and lipid-containing tubular or interstitial cells, called *foam cells,* develop as the disease progresses. Immunopathologic studies are usually nondiagnostic.

In most patients, electron microscopy reveals diffuse thickening, thinning, splitting, and layering of the glomerular and tubular basement membranes (Fig. 510-3). To confound diagnosis, ultrastructural analysis of the GBM in all genetic forms of AS may be completely normal, display nonspecific alterations, or demonstrate only uniform thinning.

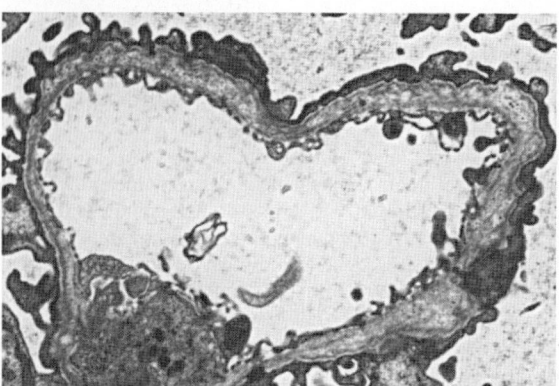

Figure 510-3 Electron micrograph of a biopsy specimen from a child with AS depicting thickening, thinning, splitting, and layering of the GBM (×1,650). *(From Yum M, Bergstein JM: Basement membrane nephropathy, Hum Pathol 14:996–1003, 1983.)*

CLINICAL MANIFESTATIONS

All patients with AS have asymptomatic microscopic hematuria, which may be intermittent in girls and younger boys. Single or recurrent episodes of gross hematuria commonly occurring 1-2 days after an upper respiratory infection are seen in approximately 50% of patients. Proteinuria is often seen in boys but may be absent, mild, or intermittent in girls. Progressive proteinuria, often exceeding 1 g/24 hr, is common by the 2nd decade of life and can be severe enough to cause nephrotic syndrome.

Bilateral sensorineural hearing loss, which is never congenital, develops in 90% of hemizygous males with X-linked AS, 10% of heterozygous females with X-linked AS, and 67% of patients with autosomal recessive AS. This deficit begins in the high-frequency range, but progresses to involve hearing associated with normal speech, prompting the need for hearing aids. Ocular abnormalities, which occur in 30-40% of patients with X-linked AS, include anterior lenticonus (extrusion of the central portion of the lens into the anterior chamber), macular flecks, and corneal erosions. Leiomyomatosis of the esophagus, tracheobronchial tree, and female genitals in association with platelet abnormalities has been reported, but is rare.

DIAGNOSIS

A combination of careful family history, a screening urinalysis of 1st-degree relatives, an audiogram, and an ophthalmologic examination are critical in making the diagnosis of AS. The presence of anterior lenticonus is pathognomonic. AS is highly likely in the patient who has hematuria and at least 2 of the following characteristic clinical features: macular flecks, recurrent corneal erosions, GBM thickening and thinning, or sensorineural deafness. Absence of epidermal basement membrane staining for the α5 chain of type IV collagen in male hemizygotes and discontinuous epidermal basement membrane staining in female heterozygotes on skin biopsy is pathognomonic for X-linked AS and can preclude diagnostic renal biopsy. Genetic testing is clinically available for X-linked AS and COL4A5 mutations. Prenatal diagnosis is available for families with members who have X-linked AS and who carry an identified mutation.

PROGNOSIS AND TREATMENT

The risk of progressive renal dysfunction leading to end-stage renal disease (ESRD) is highest among hemizygotes and autosomal recessive homozygotes. ESRD occurs before age 30 yr in approximately 75% of hemizygotes with X-linked AS. The risk of ESRD in X-linked heterozygotes is 12% by age 40 yr and 30% by age 60 yr. Risk factors for progression are gross hematuria during childhood, nephrotic syndrome, and prominent GBM thickening. Intrafamilial variation in phenotypic expression results in significant differences in the age of ESRD among family members. No specific therapy is available to treat AS, although angiotensin-converting enzyme inhibitors (and possibly

angiotensin-2 receptor inhibitors) can slow the rate of progression. Careful management of renal failure complications such as hypertension, anemia, and electrolyte imbalance is critical. Patients with ESRD are treated with dialysis and kidney transplantation (see Chapter 535). Approximately 5% of kidney transplantation recipients develop anti-GBM nephritis, which occurs primarily in males with X-linked AS who develop ESRD before age 30 yr.

Pharmacologic treatment of proteinuria with angiotensin-converting enzyme inhibition or angiotensin II receptor blockade has proven effective in other glomerular diseases and has also shown promise in AS. Screening of heterozygote carriers for significant renal disease in later adulthood and possible treatment of significant proteinuria is also recommended.

Bibliography is available at Expert Consult.

510.3 Thin Basement Membrane Disease
Cynthia G. Pan and Ellis D. Avner

Thin basement membrane disease (TBMD) is defined by the presence of persistent microscopic hematuria and isolated thinning of the GBM (and, occasionally, tubular basement membranes) on electron microscopy. Microscopic hematuria is often initially observed during childhood and may be intermittent. Episodic gross hematuria can also be present, particularly after a respiratory illness. Isolated hematuria in multiple family members without renal dysfunction is referred to as **benign familial hematuria**. Although most of these patients will not undergo renal biopsy, it is often presumed that the underlying pathology is TBMD. TBMD may be sporadic or transmitted as an autosomal dominant trait. Heterozygous mutations in the COL4A3 and COL4A4 genes, which encode the α3 and α4 chains of type IV collagen present in the GBM, result in TBMD. Rare cases of TBMD progress, and such patients develop significant proteinuria, hypertension, or renal insufficiency. Homozygous mutations in these same genes result in autosomal recessive AS. Therefore, in these rare cases, the absence of a positive family history for renal insufficiency or deafness would not necessarily predict a benign outcome. Consequently, monitoring patients with benign familial hematuria for progressive proteinuria, hypertension, or renal insufficiency is important through childhood and young adulthood.

Bibliography is available at Expert Consult.

Chapter 511
Glomerulonephritis Associated with Infections

511.1 Acute Poststreptococcal Glomerulonephritis
Cynthia G. Pan and Ellis D. Avner

Group A β-hemolytic streptococcal infections are common in children and can lead to the postinfectious complication of acute glomerulonephritis (GN). Acute poststreptococcal glomerulonephritis (APSGN) is a classic example of the **acute nephritic syndrome** characterized by the sudden onset of gross hematuria, edema, hypertension, and renal insufficiency. It is one of the most common glomerular causes of gross

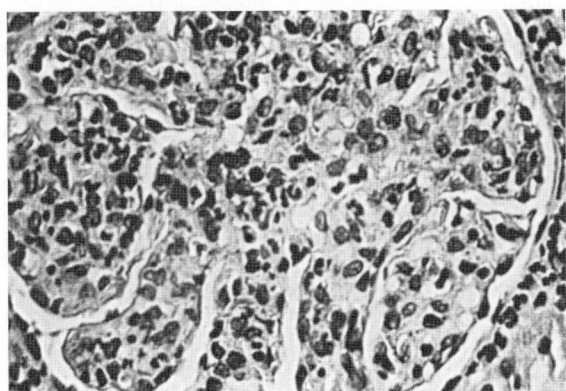

Figure 511-1 Glomerulus from a patient with poststreptococcal glomerulonephritis appears enlarged and relatively bloodless and shows mesangial proliferation and exudation of neutrophils (×400).

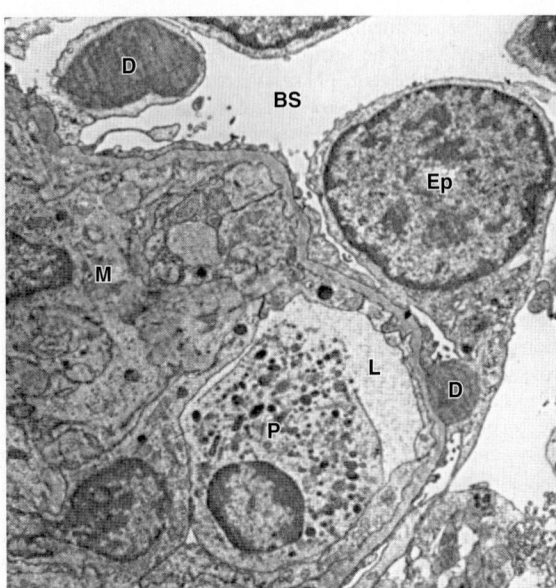

Figure 511-2 Electron micrograph in poststreptococcal glomerulonephritis demonstrating electron-dense deposits (D) on the epithelial cell (Ep) side of the glomerular basement membrane. A polymorphonuclear leukocyte (P) is present within the lumen (L) of the capillary. BS, Bowman space; M, mesangium.

hematuria in children and is a major cause of morbidity in group A β-hemolytic streptococcal infections.

ETIOLOGY AND EPIDEMIOLOGY

APSGN follows infection of the throat or skin by certain "nephritogenic" strains of group A β-hemolytic streptococci. Epidemics and clusters of household (camps, military) cases occur throughout the world, and 97% of cases occur in less-developed countries. The overall incidence has decreased in industrialized nations, presumably as a result of improved hygienic conditions and the near eradication of streptococcal pyoderma. Poststreptococcal GN commonly follows streptococcal pharyngitis during cold-weather months and streptococcal skin infections or pyoderma during warm-weather months. Although epidemics of nephritis have been described in association with throat (serotypes M1, M4, M25, and some strains of M12) and skin (serotype M49) infections, this disease is most commonly sporadic.

PATHOLOGY

Glomeruli appear enlarged and relatively bloodless and show diffuse mesangial cell proliferation, with an increase in mesangial matrix (Fig. 511-1). Polymorphonuclear leukocyte infiltration is common in glomeruli during the early stage of the disease. Crescents and interstitial inflammation may be seen in severe cases, but these changes are not specific for poststreptococcal GN. Immunofluorescence microscopy reveals a pattern of "lumpy-bumpy" deposits of immunoglobulin and complement on the glomerular basement membrane and in the mesangium. On electron microscopy, electron-dense deposits, or "humps," are observed on the epithelial side of the glomerular basement membrane (Fig. 511-2).

PATHOGENESIS

Morphologic studies and a depression in the serum complement (C3) level provide strong evidence that ASPGN is mediated by immune complexes. Circulating immune complex formation with streptococcal antigens and subsequent glomerular deposition is thought less likely to be a pathogenic mechanism. Molecular mimicry whereby circulating antibodies elicited by streptococcal antigens react with normal glomerular antigens, in situ immune complex formation of antistreptococcal antibodies with glomerular deposited antigen, and complement activation by directly deposited streptococcal antigens continue to be considered as probable mechanisms of immunologic injury.

Group A streptococci possess M proteins, and nephritogenic strains are related to the M protein serotype. The search for the precise nephritogenic antigen(s) that cause disease suggests that streptococcal pyogenic exotoxin (SPE) B and nephritis-associated streptococcal plasmin receptor are promising candidates. Both have been identified in glomeruli of affected patients, and in 1 study, circulating antibodies to SPE

B were found in all patients. Cross-reactivity of SPE B and other M proteins with various components of the glomerular basement membrane also give evidence for molecular mimicry.

CLINICAL MANIFESTATIONS

Poststreptococcal GN is most common in children ages 5-12 yr and uncommon before the age of 3 yr. The typical patient develops an acute nephritic syndrome 1-2 wk after an antecedent streptococcal pharyngitis or 3-6 wk after a streptococcal pyoderma. The history of a specific infection may be absent, because symptoms may have been mild or have resolved without patients receiving specific treatment or seeking the care of a medical provider.

The severity of kidney involvement varies from asymptomatic microscopic hematuria with normal renal function to gross hematuria with acute renal failure. Depending on the severity of renal involvement, patients can develop various degrees of edema, hypertension, and oliguria. Patients are at risk for developing encephalopathy and/or heart failure secondary to hypertension or hypervolemia. Hypertensive encephalopathy must be considered in patients with blurred vision, severe headaches, altered mental status, or new seizures. The effects of acute hypertension not only depend on the severity of hypertension but also the absolute change in comparison to the patient's baseline blood pressure and the rate at which it has risen. Respiratory distress, orthopnea, and cough may be symptoms of pulmonary edema and heart failure. Peripheral edema typically results from salt and water retention and is common; nephrotic syndrome develops in a minority (<5%) of childhood cases. Nonspecific symptoms such as malaise, lethargy, abdominal pain, or flank pain are common. Atypical presentations of APSGN include those with subclinical disease and those with severe symptoms but an absence of initial urinary abnormalities; in individuals who present with a purpuric rash, it is difficult to distinguish APSGN from Henoch-Schönlein purpura without a renal biopsy.

The acute phase generally resolves within 6-8 wk. Although urinary protein excretion and hypertension usually normalize by 4-6 wk after onset, persistent microscopic hematuria can persist for 1-2 yr after the initial presentation.

DIAGNOSIS

Urinalysis demonstrates red blood cells, often in association with red blood cell casts, proteinuria, and polymorphonuclear leukocytes. A mild normochromic anemia may be present from hemodilution and low-grade hemolysis. The serum C3 level is significantly reduced in >90% of patients in the acute phase, and returns to normal 6-8 wk after onset. Although serum CH_{50} is commonly depressed, C4 is most often normal in APSGN, or only mildly depressed.

Confirmation of the diagnosis requires clear evidence of a prior streptococcal infection. A positive throat culture report might support the diagnosis or might represent the carrier state. A rising antibody titer to streptococcal antigen(s) confirms a recent streptococcal infection. The antistreptolysin O titer is commonly elevated after a pharyngeal infection but rarely increases after streptococcal skin infections. The best single antibody titer to document cutaneous streptococcal infection is the antideoxyribonuclease B level. If available, a positive streptozyme screen (which measures multiple antibodies to different streptococcal antigens) is a valuable diagnostic tool. Serologic evidence for streptococcal infections is more sensitive than the history of recent infections and far more sensitive than positive bacterial cultures obtained at the time of onset of acute nephritis.

Magnetic resonance imaging of the brain is indicated in patients with severe neurologic symptoms and can demonstrate **posterior reversible encephalopathy syndrome** in the parietooccipital areas on T2-weighted images. Chest x-ray is indicated in those with signs of heart failure or respiratory distress, or physical exam findings of a heart gallop, decreased breath sounds, rales, or hypoxemia.

The clinical diagnosis of poststreptococcal GN is quite likely in a child presenting with acute nephritic syndrome, evidence of recent streptococcal infection, and a low C3 level. However, it is important to consider other diagnoses such as systemic lupus erythematosus, endocarditis, membranoproliferative GN, and an acute exacerbation of chronic GN. Renal biopsy should be considered only in the presence of acute renal failure, nephrotic syndrome, absence of evidence of streptococcal infection, or normal complement levels. In addition, renal biopsy is considered when hematuria and proteinuria, diminished renal function, and/or a low C3 level persist more than 2 mo after onset. Persistent hypocomplementemia can indicate a chronic form of postinfectious GN or another disease such as membranoproliferative GN.

The differential diagnosis of poststreptococcal GN includes many of the causes of hematuria listed in Tables 509-2 and 511-1, and an algorithm to help with diagnosis is presented in Figure 511-3. Acute postinfectious GN can also follow other infections with coagulase-positive and coagulase-negative staphylococci, *Streptococcus pneumoniae*, and Gram-negative bacteria. The clinical course, histopathology, and laboratory features are similar to those described for APSGN. For some, the terms APSGN and acute postinfectious GN are used synonymously. Acute GN can occur after certain fungal, rickettsial, protozoan, parasitic, or viral diseases. Among the latter, influenza and parvovirus infections are particularly notable.

COMPLICATIONS

Acute complications result from hypertension and acute renal dysfunction. Hypertension is seen in 60% of patients and is associated

Table 511-1	Summary of Primary Renal Diseases That Manifest as Acute Glomerulonephritis			
DISEASES	**POSTSTREPTOCOCCAL GLOMERULONEPHRITIS**	**IgA NEPHROPATHY**	**GOODPASTURE SYNDROME**	**IDIOPATHIC RAPIDLY PROGRESSIVE GLOMERULONEPHRITIS**
CLINICAL MANIFESTATIONS				
Age and sex	All ages, mean 7 yr, 2:1 male	10-35 yr, 2:1 male	15-30 yr, 6:1 male	Adults, 2:1 male
Acute nephritic syndrome	90%	50%	90%	90%
Asymptomatic hematuria	Occasionally	50%	Rare	Rare
Nephrotic syndrome	10-20%	Rare	Rare	10-20%
Hypertension	70%	30-50%	Rare	25%
Acute renal failure	50% (transient)	Very rare	50%	60%
Other	Latent period of 1-3 wk	Follows viral syndromes	Pulmonary hemorrhage; iron deficiency anemia	None
Laboratory findings	↑ ASO titers (70%) Positive streptozyme (95%) ↓C3-C9; normal C1, C4	↑ Serum IgA (50%) IgA in dermal capillaries	Positive anti-GBM antibody	Positive ANCA in some
Immunogenetics	HLA-B12, D "EN" (9)*	HLA-Bw 35, DR4 (4)*	HLA-DR2 (16)*	None established
RENAL PATHOLOGY				
Light microscopy	Diffuse proliferation	Focal proliferation	Focal → diffuse proliferation with crescents	Crescentic GN
Immunofluorescence	Granular IgG, C3	Diffuse mesangial IgA	Linear IgG, C3	No immune deposits
Electron microscopy	Subepithelial humps	Mesangial deposits	No deposits	No deposits
Prognosis	95% resolve spontaneously 5% RPGN or slowly progressive	Slow progression in 25-50%	75% stabilize or improve if treated early	75% stabilize or improve if treated early
Treatment	Supportive	Uncertain (options include steroids, fish oil, and ACE inhibitors)	Plasma exchange, steroids, cyclophosphamide	Steroid pulse therapy

*Relative risk.
ACE, angiotensin-converting enzyme; ANCA, antineutrophil cytoplasmic antibody; ASO, anti-streptolysin O; GBM, glomerular basement membrane; GN, glomerulonephritis; HLA, human leukocyte antigen; Ig, immunoglobulin; RPGN, idiopathic rapidly progressive glomerulonephritis.
From Kliegman RM, Greenbaum LA, Lye PS: Practical strategies in pediatric diagnosis and therapy, ed 2, Philadelphia, 2004, Elsevier, p. 427.

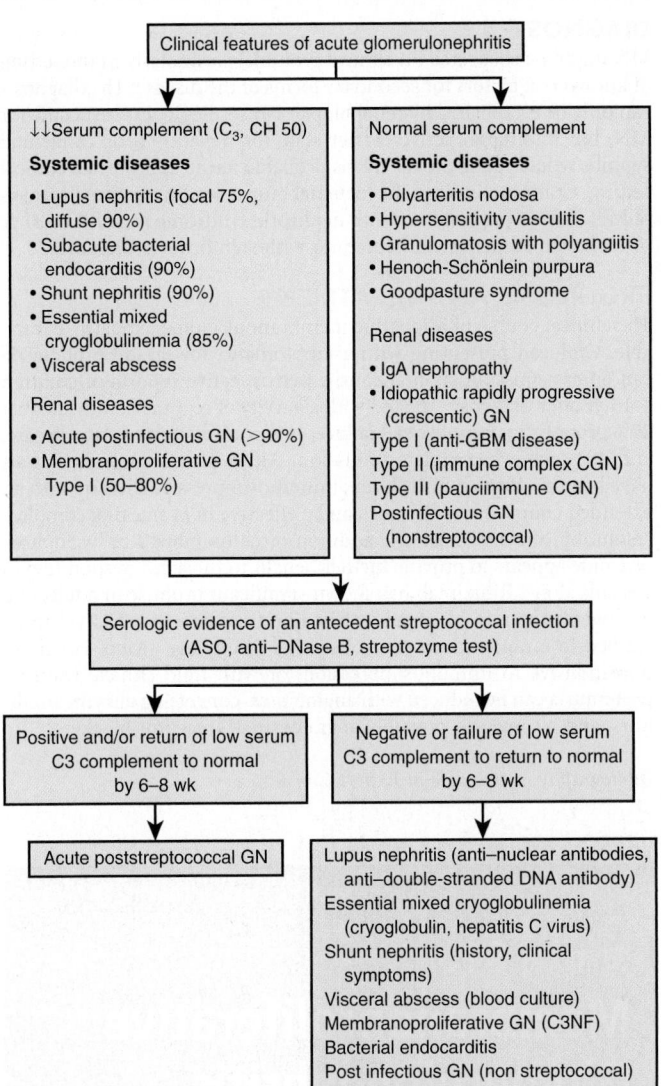

Figure 511-3 Differential diagnosis of acute glomerulonephritis (GN). ASO, anti–streptolysin O; GBM, glomerular basement membrane; NF, nuclear factor. (*Adapted from Sulyok E: Acute proliferative glomerulonephritis. In Avner ED, Harmon WE, Niaudet P, editors: Pediatric nephrology, ed 5, Philadelphia, 2004, Lippincott Williams & Wilkins, Fig. 30-4.*)

with hypertensive encephalopathy in 10% of cases. Although the neurologic sequelae are often reversible with appropriate management, severe prolonged hypertension can lead to intracranial bleeding. Other potential complications include heart failure, hyperkalemia, hyperphosphatemia, hypocalcemia, acidosis, seizures, and uremia. Acute renal failure can require treatment with dialysis.

PREVENTION
Early systemic antibiotic therapy for streptococcal throat and skin infections does not eliminate the risk of GN. Family members of patients with acute GN, especially young children, should be considered at risk and be cultured for group A β-hemolytic streptococci and treated if positive. Family pets, particularly dogs, have also been reported as carriers.

TREATMENT
Management is directed at treating the acute effects of renal insufficiency and hypertension (see Chapter 535.1). Although a 10 day course

of systemic antibiotic therapy with penicillin is recommended to limit the spread of the nephritogenic organisms, antibiotic therapy does not affect the natural history of APSGN. This is unlike the GN seen in the context of ongoing or chronic infections, as noted in Chapter 511.2. Sodium restriction, diuresis (usually with intravenous furosemide), and pharmacotherapy with calcium channel antagonists, vasodilators, or angiotensin-converting enzyme inhibitors, are standard therapies used to treat hypertension.

PROGNOSIS
Complete recovery occurs in >95% of children with APSGN. Recurrences are extremely rare. Mortality in the acute stage can be avoided by appropriate management of acute renal failure, cardiac failure, and hypertension. Infrequently, the acute phase is severe and leads to glomerulosclerosis and chronic renal disease in <2% of affected children.

Bibliography is available at Expert Consult.

511.2 Other Chronic Infections
Cynthia G. Pan and Ellis D. Avner

GN is a recognized complication of various chronic infections. Classic examples include bacterial endocarditis caused by viridans streptococcus and other organisms, and ventriculoatrial shunts infected with *Staphylococcus epidermidis*. Other infections, observed less commonly in children than in adults, include hepatitis B virus, hepatitis C virus, syphilis, and candidiasis. Parasitic infections associated with glomerular disease include malaria, schistosomiasis, leishmaniasis, filariasis, hydatid disease, trypanosomiasis, and toxoplasmosis. In each condition, the infecting organism has low virulence and the host is chronically infected with foreign antigen. In the presence of high levels of circulating antigen, the host's antibody response leads to formation of immune complexes that deposit in the kidneys and initiate glomerular inflammation. Foreign antigens can also stimulate an autoimmune response through the production of antibodies that cross-react with such antigens incorrectly "recognized" as glomerular structural components.

The renal histopathology can resemble poststreptococcal GN, membranous GN, or membranoproliferative GN. The clinical manifestations are generally those of an acute nephritic or nephrotic syndrome. The serum C3 and CH50 complement levels are often decreased.

In HIV-associated nephropathy, direct viral infection of nephrons occurs because renal cells express a variety of lymphocyte chemokine receptors that are essential for and facilitate viral invasion. The renal expression of HIV infection is quite variable and includes an immune complex injury and a direct cytopathic effect. The classic histopathologic lesion of HIV-associated nephropathy is focal segmental glomerulosclerosis, but systemic lupus erythematosus–like glomerulonephritis, immunoglobulin A nephropathy, and membranous nephropathy have been reported. In the era of antiretroviral therapy, the decline in mortality has led to the increased recognition of renal disorders as an important complication to perinatally HIV-infected children.

Prompt eradication of any infection before severe glomerular injury occurs usually results in resolution of the GN. Progression to end-stage renal failure has been described but is uncommon. Spontaneous resolution of hepatitis B infection is common in children (30-50%) and results in remission of the glomerulopathy. Specific antivirals, interferon therapy, plasmapheresis, and immunosuppressive treatment have all been used successfully in adults with hepatitis C disease, but no controlled trials with any of these agents have been performed in pediatric patients.

Bibliography is available at Expert Consult.

Chapter **512**
Membranous Nephropathy
Scott K. Van Why and Ellis D. Avner

Membranous nephropathy (MN), amongst the most common causes of nephrotic syndrome in adults, is a rare cause of nephrotic syndrome in children. MN is classified as the primary, idiopathic form, where there is isolated renal disease, or secondary MN, where nephropathy is associated with other identifiable systemic diseases or medications. In children, secondary MN is far more common than primary, idiopathic MN. The most common etiologies of secondary MN are systemic lupus erythematosus or chronic infections. Among the latter, chronic hepatitis B infection and congenital syphilis are the best characterized and recognized causes of MN. Other chronic infections have also been associated with MN, including malaria, which is likely the most common cause of nephrotic syndrome worldwide. Certain medications, such as penicillamine and gold, or chronic factor replacement in patients with hemophilia can also cause MN. Rare causes associated with MN include tumors, such as neuroblastoma, or other idiopathic systemic diseases. Identification of secondary causes of MN is critical, because removal of the offending agent or treatment of the causative disease often leads to resolution of the associated nephropathy and improves patient outcome.

PATHOLOGY
Glomeruli have diffuse thickening of the glomerular basement membrane (GBM), without significant cell proliferative changes. Immunofluorescence and electron microscopy typically demonstrate granular deposits of immunoglobulin G and C3 located on the epithelial side of the GBM. The GBM thickening presumably results from the production of membrane-like material in response to deposition of immune complexes.

PATHOGENESIS
MN is believed to be caused by in situ immune complex formation. Therefore, antigens from the infectious agents or medications associated with secondary MN directly contribute to the pathogenesis of the renal disease. The causative antigen in idiopathic MN is not established, but the M-type phospholipase A_2 receptor, present on normal podocytes, may be a target antigen in idiopathic MN. Antigen from this receptor is found in immune deposits extracted from glomeruli in patients with idiopathic MN. The majority of idiopathic MN patients have circulating antibody against this podocyte membrane antigen, as well as against several podocyte cytoplasmic antigens. Childhood MN may be associated with anticationic bovine serum albumin antibodies. In addition, neutral endopeptidase antigen may be the antigen in neonatal onset MN.

CLINICAL MANIFESTATIONS
In children, MN is most common in the 2nd decade of life, but it can occur at any age, including infancy. The disease usually manifests as nephrotic syndrome and accounts for 2-6% of all cases of childhood nephrotic syndrome. Most patients also have microscopic hematuria and only rarely present with gross hematuria. Approximately 20% of children have hypertension at presentation. A subset of patients with MN present with a major venous thrombosis, commonly renal vein thrombosis. This well-known complication of nephrotic syndrome (see Chapter 527) is particularly common in patients with MN. Serum C3 and CH_{50} levels are normal, except in cases of systemic lupus erythematosus, where levels may be depressed (see Fig. 511-3 in Chapter 511).

DIAGNOSIS
MN might be suspected on clinical grounds, particularly in the setting of known risk factors for secondary forms of the disease. The diagnosis can only be established by renal biopsy. No serologic test is specific for MN, but finding an active carrier state for hepatitis B or congenital syphilis would make the diagnosis probable in the appropriate clinical setting. Common indications for renal biopsy leading to the diagnosis of MN include presentation with nephrotic syndrome in a child >10 yr or unexplained persistent hematuria with significant proteinuria.

PROGNOSIS AND TREATMENT
The clinical course of idiopathic membranous glomerulopathy is variable. Children presenting with asymptomatic, low-grade proteinuria can enter remission spontaneously. Retrospective reports of children 1-15 yr after diagnosis, treated with a variety of regimens, indicate that 20% progress to chronic renal failure, 40% continue with active disease, and 40% achieve complete remission. Although no controlled trials have been performed in children, immunosuppressive therapy with an extended course of prednisone can be effective in promoting complete resolution of symptoms. The addition of chlorambucil or cyclophosphamide appears to provide further benefit to those not responding to steroids alone. Rituximab has shown significant promise in adults and has been proposed by some as first line treatment but has yet to be studied in a randomized controlled trial in any age group. For those unresponsive to immunosuppression, or with mild clinical features, proteinuria can be reduced with angiotensin-converting enzyme inhibitors, and by analogy, probably angiotensin-II–receptor blockers.

Bibliography is available at Expert Consult.

Chapter **513**
Membranoproliferative Glomerulonephritis
Scott K. Van Why and Ellis D. Avner

Membranoproliferative glomerulonephritis (MPGN), also known as mesangiocapillary glomerulonephritis, most commonly occurs in children or young adults. MPGN can be classified into primary (idiopathic) and secondary forms of glomerular disease. Secondary forms of MPGN are most commonly associated with subacute and chronic infection, including hepatitides B and C, syphilis, subacute bacterial endocarditis, and infected shunts, especially ventriculoatrial shunts (shunt nephritis). MPGN can also be one of the glomerular lesions seen in lupus nephritis (see Chapter 514).

PATHOLOGY
Primary MPGN is defined by the histologic pattern of glomeruli as seen by light, immunofluorescence, and electron microscopy. Two subtypes have been defined on histologic criteria and are associated with different clinical phenotypes. **Type I MPGN** is most common. Glomeruli have an accentuated lobular pattern from diffuse mesangial expansion, endocapillary proliferation, and an increase in mesangial cells and matrix. The glomerular capillary walls are thickened, often with splitting from interposition of the mesangium. Crescents, if present, indicate a poor prognosis. Immunofluorescence microscopy reveals C3 and lesser amounts of immunoglobulin in the mesangium and along the peripheral capillary walls in a lobular pattern. Electron

microscopy confirms numerous deposits in the mesangial and subendothelial regions.

Far less common is **type II MPGN,** also called dense deposit disease, which has similar light microscopic findings as type I MPGN. Differentiation from type I disease is by immunofluorescence and electron microscopy. In type II disease, C3 immunofluorescence typically is prominent, without concomitant immunoglobulin. By electron microscopy, the lamina densa in the glomerular basement membrane undergoes a very dense transformation, without evident immune complex–type deposits.

C3 glomerulonephritis (C3GN) is a related but separate diagnostic category. By light and electron microscopy C3GN usually has features indistinguishable from classical MPGN. Immunofluorescence studies distinguish between the two, with C3GN having only C3 deposition and MPGN having both C3 and immunoglobulin fluorescence.

PATHOGENESIS

Although the histology of **type I MPGN** produced by primary and secondary forms is indistinguishable, it appears that **type I** disease occurs when circulating immune complexes become trapped in the glomerular subendothelial space, which then causes injury, resulting in the characteristic proliferative response and mesangial expansion. Further evidence confirming this pathway to glomerular injury is the finding of complement activation through the classical pathway in as many as 50% of affected patients.

Type II MPGN appears **not** to be mediated by immune complexes. The pathogenesis of the disease is not known, but the characteristic finding of severely depressed serum complement levels suggests that deranged complement regulation might play a major role in the disease. A typical finding is markedly depressed serum C3 complement levels, with normal levels of other complement components. In many patients with type II MPGN, **C3 nephritic factor** (anti–C3 convertase antibody) is present. This factor activates the alternative complement pathway. In unusual cases, patients with type II MPGN demonstrate an associated systemic disease called **partial lipodystrophy,** where there is diffuse loss of adipose tissue and decreased complement in the presence of C3 nephritic factor. Correlation between the presence of C3 nephritic factor, complement levels, and disease presence or severity is not strong, indicating that the complement abnormalities alone are not sufficient to cause the disease.

Type II MPGN (dense deposit disease) is considered part of the broader spectrum of C3GN. The latter, as defined above pathologically, appears to be caused by primary dysregulation of the alternative or terminal cascade complement pathways.

CLINICAL MANIFESTATIONS

MPGN is most common in the 2nd decade of life. Systemic features may provide clues to which type of MPGN may be present, but the two histologic types of idiopathic MPGN are indistinguishable in terms of their renal manifestations. Patients present in equal proportions with nephrotic syndrome, acute nephritic syndrome (hematuria, hypertension, and some level of renal insufficiency), or persistent asymptomatic microscopic hematuria and proteinuria. Serum C3 complement levels are low in the majority of cases (see Fig. 511-3 in Chapter 511).

DIFFERENTIAL DIAGNOSIS

The differential diagnosis includes all forms of acute and chronic glomerulonephritis, including idiopathic and secondary forms, along with postinfectious glomerulonephritis. Postinfectious glomerulonephritis, far more common than MPGN, usually does not have nephrotic features but typically has hematuria, hypertension, renal insufficiency, and transiently low C3 complement, all features that may be seen with MPGN or C3GN. In contrast to MPGN and C3GN, where C3 levels usually remain persistently low, C3 returns to normal within 2 mo after onset of postinfectious glomerulonephritis (see Chapter 511.3). The diagnosis of MPGN is made by renal biopsy. Indications for biopsy include nephrotic syndrome in an older child, significant proteinuria with microscopic hematuria, and hypocomplementemia lasting >2 mo in a child with acute nephritis. If C3 but no immunoglobulin deposi-

tion is found in glomeruli with MPGN, genetic testing and functional assays to define defects of complement cascade regulation should be pursued.

PROGNOSIS AND TREATMENT

It is important to determine whether MPGN is idiopathic or secondary to a systemic disease, particularly lupus or chronic infection, because treatment of the causative disease can result in resolution of MPGN. Untreated, idiopathic MPGN, regardless of type, has a poor prognosis. By 10 yr following onset, 50% of patients with MPGN have progressed to end-stage renal disease. By 20 yr following onset, up to 90% have lost renal function. Those with nephrotic syndrome at the time of presentation progress to renal failure more rapidly. No definitive therapy exists, but several reports, including a randomized controlled trial, indicate that extended courses of alternate-day prednisone (for years) provide benefit. Some patients treated with steroids enter a complete clinical remission of their disease, but many have ongoing disease activity. Nevertheless, an extended course of prednisone is associated with significant preservation of renal function when compared with patients receiving no such treatment.

The prognosis of C3GN, separate from dense deposit disease (considered a part of C3GN by some) and other forms of classically defined MPGN is as yet hard to define, since reports of outcome of such patients previously had been grouped in studies of all forms of MPGN (types I and II, and even a poorly characterized type III form not considered above). The apparent pathophysiology of C3GN promises that treatments targeting the interruption of complement activation pathways, such as complement factor H replacement or shutting down the terminal complement cascade by blocking C5 activation with eculizumab (anti–C5 antibody), could be beneficial in preventing progression of renal disease.

Bibliography is available at Expert Consult.

Chapter **514**
Glomerulonephritis Associated with Systemic Lupus Erythematosus
Cynthia G. Pan and Ellis D. Avner

Systemic lupus erythematosus (SLE) is characterized by fever, weight loss, dermatitis, hematologic abnormalities, arthritis, and involvement of the heart, lungs, central nervous system, and kidneys (see Chapter 158). Glomerulonephritis is the most important cause of morbidity and mortality in SLE. Renal disease in childhood SLE is present in up to 80% of patients and is more active than that seen in adults. Occasionally, renal disease is the only presenting clinical manifestation.

PATHOGENESIS AND PATHOLOGY

The clinical manifestations of SLE are mediated by immune complexes. Autoantibodies are directed predominantly at nuclear antigens which act as immunogens. Binding of autoantibodies to glomerular components rather than the passive "trapping" of circulating immune complexes is central to the development of glomerulonephritis. Other pathogenic mechanisms include alterations in innate immunity that result in amplification of inflammation. Deficiency of the complement component C1q is rare but is the strongest single genetic risk for SLE.

Kidney biopsy and evaluation of renal histopathology remain the gold standard for establishing the diagnosis of SLE nephritis and determining specific therapeutic regimens. The World Health Organization (WHO) classification of lupus nephritis is based on a combination of features including light microscopy, immunofluorescence, and electron microscopy. In patients with **WHO class I nephritis** (minimal mesangial lupus nephritis), no histologic abnormalities are detected on light microscopy but mesangial immune deposits are present on immunofluorescence or electron microscopy. In **WHO class II nephritis** (mesangial proliferative nephritis), light microscopy shows both mesangial hypercellularity and increased matrix along with mesangial deposits containing immunoglobulin and complement.

WHO class III nephritis and **WHO class IV nephritis** are interrelated lesions characterized by both mesangial and endocapillary lesions. Class III nephritis is defined by <50% glomeruli with involvement and class IV has ≥50% glomerular involvement. Immune deposits are present in both the mesangium and subendothelial areas. A subclassification scheme helps grade severity of the proliferative lesion based on whether the glomerular lesions are segmental (<50% glomerular tuft involved) or global (≥50% glomerular tuft involved). The WHO classification scheme also delineates whether there is a predominance of chronic disease versus active disease. Chronic injury results in glomerular sclerosis and is felt to be the consequence of significant proliferative disease seen in classes III and IV. Other signs of active disease include capillary walls that are thickened secondary to subendothelial deposits (creating the wire-loop lesion), necrosis, and crescent formation. WHO class IV nephritis is associated with poorer outcomes but can be successfully treated with aggressive immunosuppressive therapy.

WHO class V nephritis (membranous lupus nephritis) is less commonly seen as an isolated lesion and resembles idiopathic membranous nephropathy with subepithelial immune deposits. This lesion is often seen in combination with class III or IV proliferative nephritis, and if the membranous lesion is present in >50% glomeruli, both classes are noted in designation. This classification scheme also identifies cases with combinations of mixed classes III, IV, and V lesions, directing appropriate treatment for such patients. Another classification scheme by both the International Society of Nephrology and the Renal Pathology Society differs mainly in its subclassification of class IV into diffuse global and diffuse segmental lesions (Table 514-1). The value of utilizing this classification scheme, and more importantly, its impact on therapy and the results of clinical trials is unknown at this time.

Transformation of the histologic lesions of lupus nephritis from one class to another is common. This is more likely to occur among inadequately treated patients and usually results in progression to a more severe histologic lesion.

CLINICAL MANIFESTATIONS

The majority of children with SLE are adolescent females. Lupus nephritis affects most pediatric patients, and although commonly presenting within the first year of diagnosis, may occur at any time during the course of the disease. Ethnicity and socioeconomic factors strongly predict the development of lupus nephritis in adults with SLE but not in children. The clinical findings in patients having milder forms of lupus nephritis (all classes I-II, some class III) include hematuria, normal renal function, and proteinuria <1 g/24 hr. Some patients with class III and all patients with class IV nephritis have hematuria and proteinuria, hypertension, reduced renal function, nephrotic syndrome, or acute renal failure. The urinalysis may be normal on rare occasions in patients with proliferative lupus nephritis. Patients with class V nephritis commonly present with nephrotic syndrome.

DIAGNOSIS

The diagnosis of SLE is confirmed by the detection of circulating antinuclear antibodies and by demonstrating antibodies that react with

Table 514-1	Classification of Lupus Nephritis
CLASS	**CLINICAL FEATURES**
I. Minimal mesangial LN	No renal findings
II. Mesangial proliferative LN	Mild clinical renal disease; minimally active urinary sediment; mild to moderate proteinuria (never nephrotic) but may have active serology
III. Focal proliferative LN <50% glomeruli involved A. Active A/C. Active and chronic C. Chronic	More active sediment changes; often active serology; increased proteinuria (approximately 25% nephrotic); hypertension may be present; some evolve into class IV pattern; active lesions require treatment, chronic do not
IV. Diffuse proliferative LN (>50% glomeruli involved); all may be with segmental or global involvement (S or G) A. Active A/C. Active and chronic C. Chronic	Most severe renal involvement with active sediment, hypertension, heavy proteinuria (frequent nephrotic syndrome), often reduced glomerular filtration rate; serology very active. Active lesions require treatment
V. Membranous LN glomerulonephritis	Significant proteinuria (often nephrotic) with less active lupus serology
VI. Advanced sclerosing LN	More than 90% glomerulosclerosis; no treatment prevents renal failure

LN, lupus nephritis.
From Appel GB, Radhakrishnan J: Glomerular disorders and nephrotic syndromes. In Goldman L, Schafer AI, editors, Goldman's Cecil medicine, ed 24, St. Louis, 2012, Elsevier Saunders, Table 123-7, p. 769.

native double-stranded DNA. In most patients with active disease, C3 and C4 levels are depressed. In view of the lack of a clear correlation between the clinical manifestations and the severity of the renal involvement, renal biopsy should be performed in all patients with SLE. Histopathologic findings are used to determine the selection of specific immunosuppressive therapies.

TREATMENT

Children with SLE should be treated by pediatric specialists in medical centers where medical and psychologic support can be provided for patients and their families. The goal of immunosuppressive therapy in lupus nephritis is to produce both a clinical remission, defined as normalization of renal function and proteinuria, and a serologic remission, defined as normalization of anti-DNA antibody, C3, and C4 levels. Therapy is initiated in all patients with prednisone at a dose of 1-2 mg/kg/day in divided doses followed by a slow steroid taper over 4-6 mo beginning 4-6 wk after achieving a serologic remission. For patients with severe forms of nephritis (WHO classes III and IV), induction therapy consists of 6 consecutive monthly intravenous infusions of cyclophosphamide at a dose of 500-1,000 mg/m². Pulse intravenous methylprednisolone (1000 mg/m²) is also used in addition to oral corticosteroids. In adult clinical trials, mycophenolate mofetil was shown to be equally efficacious for induction therapy and may be considered for use in children using 600 mg/m² per dose twice daily. Maintenance therapy previously consisted of additional Cytoxan infusions every 3 mo for 18 mo, which reduced the risk of progressive renal dysfunction. Maintenance therapy using mycophenolate mofetil or azathioprine may be as efficacious as intravenous cyclophosphamide and result in less-serious side effects, such as infections, hair loss, hemorrhagic cystitis, and gonadal failure. Mycophenolate mofetil is particularly more efficacious than cyclophosphamide in African-Americans. Azathioprine, at a single daily dose of 1.5-2.0 mg/kg, may be used as a steroid-sparing agent in patients with WHO class I or II lupus nephritis. Rituximab, a chimeric monoclonal antibody specific for human CD20, is ineffective for induction therapy for diffuse proliferative disease but may be considered in cases where resistance to conventional treatment is demonstrated. Plasmapheresis is ineffective in lupus nephritis unless there is accompanying thrombotic thrombocytopenic purpura or antineutrophilic cytoplasmic antibody–associated disease. New therapies include belimumab, a fully humanized monoclonal antibody against a type II transmembrane protein that functions in the normal survival and differentiation of B cells, which is FDA-approved for use in SLE. Its role in lupus nephritis, either in combination with current therapies or to replace them, requires extensive further study.

Hydrochloroquine is prescribed in most patients with SLE for extrarenal manifestations, but is thought to have a beneficial effect in maintaining remission in lupus nephritis. It is a rational choice given its low side effect profile. Use of antihypertensive drugs to aggressively treat hypertension as well as the specific use of drugs that block the renin–angiotensin system (angiotensin-converting enzyme inhibitors and angiotensin-receptor blockers) to reduce proteinuria are also important therapies that appear to decrease long-term progression of renal disease.

PROGNOSIS

Overall, renal survival (defined as chronic kidney disease without the need for end-stage renal disease therapy) is seen in 80% of patients 10 yr after the diagnosis of SLE nephritis. Patients with diffuse proliferative WHO class IV lupus nephritis exhibit the highest risk for progression to end-stage renal disease. Concerns regarding the side effects of chronic immunosuppressive therapy and the risk of recurrent disease are lifelong. Close monitoring for relapse of disease is critical to ensure maximally successful renal outcomes. Special care must be taken to minimize the risks of infection, osteoporosis, obesity, poor growth, hypertension, and diabetes mellitus associated with chronic corticosteroid therapy. Patients require counseling regarding the risk of malignancy or infertility, which may be increased in those receiving a cumulative dose of >20 g of cyclophosphamide or other immunosuppressant therapies.

Bibliography is available at Expert Consult.

Chapter **515**
Henoch-Schönlein Purpura Nephritis
Scott K. Van Why and Ellis D. Avner

Henoch-Schönlein purpura (HSP) is the most common small vessel vasculitis in childhood. It is characterized by a purpuric rash and commonly accompanied by arthritis and abdominal pain (see Chapter 167.1). Approximately 50% of patients with HSP develop renal manifestations, which vary from asymptomatic microscopic hematuria to severe, progressive glomerulonephritis.

PATHOGENESIS AND PATHOLOGY

The pathogenesis of HSP nephritis appears to be mediated by the deposition of polymeric immunoglobulin A (IgA) in glomeruli. This is analogous to the same type of IgA deposits seen in systemic small vessels, primarily those of the skin and intestine. The glomerular findings can be indistinguishable from those of IgA nephropathy (see Chapter 510.1). IgA deposits are present by immunofluorescence, and a broad spectrum of glomerular lesions that can range from mild proliferation to necrotic and crescentic changes can be seen.

CLINICAL AND LABORATORY MANIFESTATIONS

The nephritis associated with HSP usually follows onset of the rash, often presenting weeks or even months after the initial presentation of the disease. Nephritis can be manifest at initial presentation, but only rarely before onset of the rash. Patients at presentation rarely display a severe combined acute nephritic and nephrotic picture (hematuria, hypertension, renal insufficiency, significant proteinuria, and nephrotic syndrome). Most patients have only mild renal manifestations, principally isolated microscopic hematuria without significant proteinuria. Initial mild renal involvement can occasionally progress to more severe nephritis despite resolution of all other features of HSP. The severity of the systemic manifestations does not correlate with the severity of the nephritis. Most patients who develop nephritis have urinary abnormalities by 1 mo, and nearly all have abnormalities by 3 mo after onset of HSP. Therefore, a urinalysis should be performed weekly in patients with HSP during the period of active clinical disease. Thereafter, a urinalysis should be performed once a month for up to 6 mo. If all urinalyses are normal during this follow-up interval, nephritis is unlikely to develop. If proteinuria, renal insufficiency, or hypertension develops along with hematuria, consultation with a pediatric nephrologist is indicated.

PROGNOSIS AND TREATMENT

The prognosis of HSP nephritis for most patients is excellent. Spontaneous and complete resolution of the nephritis typically occurs in the majority of patients with mild initial manifestations (isolated hematuria with insignificant proteinuria). However, such patients uncommonly can progress to severe renal involvement, including development of chronic renal failure. Patients with acute nephritic or nephrotic syndrome at presentation have a guarded renal prognosis, particularly if they are found to have concomitant necrosis or substantial crescentic changes on renal biopsy. Untreated, the risk of developing chronic kidney disease, including renal failure, is 2-5% in all patients with HSP, but almost 50% in those with the most severe early renal clinical and histologic features.

No studies have demonstrated any efficacy of short courses (weeks) of oral corticosteroids administered promptly after onset of HSP on either preventing the development of nephritis or decreasing the severity of subsequent HSP nephritis. Tonsillectomy has been proposed as an intervention for HSP nephritis, but it also does not appear to have any measurable effect on renal outcome. Mild HSP nephritis does not require treatment, because it usually resolves spontaneously.

Efficacy of treatment for moderate or severe HSP nephritis, which is far more likely to progress to chronic renal failure, is more difficult to assess. Limited prospective controlled trials for severe HSP nephritis have not shown benefit from any therapy studied. Several uncontrolled studies have reported significant benefit from aggressive immunosuppression (high-dose and extended courses of corticosteroids with cyclophosphamide or azathioprine) in patients with poor prognostic features on renal biopsy; such patients are at high risk of progressing to chronic renal failure based on historic controls. Anecdotal reports of treatment of high-risk patients with either plasmapheresis or rituximab have indicated a potential benefit. Balancing the absence of controlled data with the severe side effects of aggressive therapies in patients with poor renal prognostic factors is difficult. Aggressive therapy with careful monitoring may be reasonable in those with the most severe HSP nephritis (>50% crescents on biopsy).

Bibliography is available at Expert Consult.

Chapter 516

Rapidly Progressive (Crescentic) Glomerulonephritis

Scott K. Van Why and Ellis D. Avner

"Rapidly progressive" describes the clinical course of several forms of glomerulonephritis whose unifying feature is the histopathologic finding of crescents in the majority of glomeruli (Fig. 516-1). The terms *rapidly progressive glomerulonephritis* (RPGN) and *crescentic glomerulonephritis* (CGN) are synonymous. The natural history of most forms of CGN is rapid and relentless progression to end-stage renal failure.

CLASSIFICATION

CGN can be a severe manifestation of essentially every defined primary and secondary glomerulonephritis (GN), but particular forms of GN are more likely to present as, or evolve into, RPGN (Table 516-1). If no underlying cause is identified by systemic features, serologic testing, or histologic examination, the disease is classified as idiopathic CGN. The

Table 516-1	Classification of Rapidly Progressive ("Crescentic") Glomerulonephritis

PRIMARY
Type I: Anti–glomerular basement membrane antibody disease, Goodpasture syndrome (with pulmonary disease)
Type II: Immune complex mediated
Type III: Pauciimmune (usually antineutrophil cytoplasmic antibody-positive)

SECONDARY
Membranoproliferative glomerulonephritis
Immunoglobulin A nephropathy, Henoch-Schönlein purpura
Poststreptococcal glomerulonephritis
Systemic lupus erythematosus
Polyarteritis nodosa, hypersensitivity angiitis

From Appel GB, Radhakrishnan J: Glomerular disorders and nephrotic syndromes. In Goldman L, Schafer AI, editors: Goldman's Cecil medicine, ed 24, St. Louis, 2012, Elsevier Saunders, Table 122-3, p. 758.

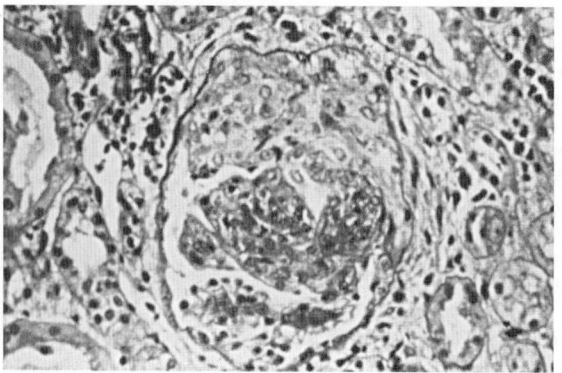

Figure 516-1 Light micrograph of a biopsy specimen from a child with Henoch-Schönlein purpura glomerulonephritis demonstrating a crescent overlying the glomerulus (×180).

incidence of specific etiologies of CGN in children varies widely; certain common themes are shared in all such reports. Patients with systemic vasculitis appear to be particularly prone to develop CGN. Patients with Henoch-Schönlein purpura (HSP), antineutrophil cytoplasmic antibody (ANCA)–mediated GN (microscopic polyangiitis and granulomatosis with polyangiitis), and systemic lupus erythematosus account for the majority of patients with CGN. Postinfectious GN or endocarditis rarely progresses to CGN, but because it is the most common form of GN in childhood it accounts for a significant percentage of patients with CGN in most reports. Membranoproliferative GN and idiopathic disease make up most of the remaining cases of CGN. Immunoglobulin (Ig) A nephropathy, a common GN, only rarely is rapidly progressive. Goodpasture disease often has rapidly progressive GN as a component of the syndrome, but its rarity in childhood results in its making up only a small percentage of children with CGN.

PATHOLOGY AND PATHOGENESIS

The hallmark of CGN is the histopathologic finding of crescents in glomeruli (see Fig. 516-1). Crescent formation, through proliferation of parietal epithelial cells in Bowman's space, may be the final pathway of any severe inflammatory glomerular injury. Podocytes and renal progenitor cells are involved in the pathogenesis of CGN. Fibrous crescents, in which proliferative cellular crescents are replaced by collagen, are a late finding. The immunofluorescence findings, as well as the pattern of any deposits by electron microscopy can delineate the underlying glomerulopathy in CGN secondary to lupus, HSP nephritis, membranoproliferative glomerulonephritis, postinfectious GN, IgA nephropathy, or Goodpasture disease. Rare or absent findings by immunofluorescence and electron microscopy typify pauciimmune GN (Wegener disease and microscopic polyangiitis) and idiopathic crescentic GN.

CLINICAL MANIFESTATIONS

Most children present with acute nephritis (hematuria, some degree of renal insufficiency, and hypertension) and usually have concomitant proteinuria, often with nephrotic syndrome. Occasional patients present late in the course of disease with oliguric renal failure. Extrarenal manifestations, such as pulmonary involvement, joint symptoms, or skin lesions, can help lead to the diagnosis of the underlying systemic disease causing the CGN.

DIAGNOSIS AND DIFFERENTIAL DIAGNOSIS

The diagnosis of CGN is made by biopsy. Delineation of the underlying etiology is reached by a combination of additional biopsy findings (described earlier), extrarenal symptoms and signs, and serologic testing, including evaluation of antinuclear and anti-DNA antibodies, serum complement levels, and ANCA. If the patient has no extrarenal manifestations and a negative serologic evaluation, and if the biopsy has no immune or electron microscopy deposits, the diagnosis is idiopathic, rapidly progressive CGN.

PROGNOSIS AND TREATMENT

Although the outcome is not uniformly positive, children with crescentic postinfectious GN can spontaneously recover. The natural course of CGN is far more severe in the setting of other etiologies, including the idiopathic category, and progression to end-stage renal failure within weeks to months from onset is common. Having a majority of fibrous crescents on a renal biopsy portends a poor prognosis, because the disease usually has progressed to irreversible injury. Although there are few controlled data, the consensus of most nephrologists is that the combination of high-dose corticosteroids and cyclophosphamide may be effective in preventing progressive renal failure in patients with systemic lupus erythematosus, HSP nephritis, Wegener granulomatosis, and IgA nephropathy if given early in the course when acute cellular crescents predominate. Although such therapy can also be effective in the other diseases causing RPGN, renal outcomes in those settings are less favorable. Progression to end-stage renal disease often occurs despite aggressive immunosuppressive therapy. In combination with immunosuppression, plasmapheresis has been reported to benefit patients with Goodpasture disease. Plasmapheresis may also benefit patients with ANCA-associated CGN, in particular those with the most severe renal dysfunction at presentation. The possible benefits of plasmapheresis in other forms of RPGN are unclear.

Bibliography is available at Expert Consult.

Chapter 517
Goodpasture Disease
Scott K. Van Why and Ellis D. Avner

Goodpasture disease is characterized by pulmonary hemorrhage and glomerulonephritis. The disease results from attack on these organs by antibodies directed against certain epitopes of type IV collagen, located within the alveolar basement membrane in the lung and glomerular basement membrane (GBM) in the kidney. The production of pathologic autoantibody against specific domains in type IV collagen is triggered by an acquired conformational change in $\alpha345NC1$ hexamers, central structural elements in type IV collagen. The resulting structural alteration reveals neoepitopes that become the target of the pathogenic Goodpasture autoantibody.

PATHOLOGY
Kidney biopsy shows crescentic glomerulonephritis in most patients. Immunofluorescence microscopy demonstrates continuous linear deposition of immunoglobulin G along the GBM (Fig. 517-1).

CLINICAL MANIFESTATIONS
Goodpasture disease is rare in childhood. Patients usually present with hemoptysis from pulmonary hemorrhage that can be life-threatening. Concomitant renal manifestations include acute glomerulonephritis with hematuria, proteinuria, and hypertension, which usually follows a rapidly progressive course. Renal failure commonly develops within days to weeks of clinical presentation. Uncommonly, patients can have anti-GBM nephritis manifesting as isolated, rapidly progressive glomerulonephritis without pulmonary hemorrhage. In essentially all cases, serum anti-GBM antibody is present and complement C3 level is normal. Antineutrophilic cytoplasmic antibody levels can be found to be elevated along with the anti-GBM antibody; such patients doubly positive for these autoantibodies, who have severe disease at presentation, appear to have a more severe prognosis.

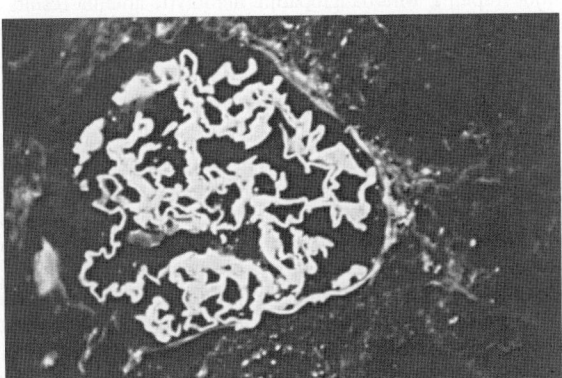

Figure 517-1 Immunofluorescence micrograph demonstrating the continuous linear staining of immunoglobulin G along the glomerular basement membrane in Goodpasture disease ($\times250$).

DIAGNOSIS AND DIFFERENTIAL DIAGNOSIS
The diagnosis is made by a combination of the clinical presentation of pulmonary hemorrhage with acute glomerulonephritis, the presence of serum antibodies directed against GBM (anti–type IV collagen in GBM), and characteristic renal biopsy findings. Other diseases that can cause a pulmonary-renal syndrome need to be considered and include systemic lupus erythematosus, Henoch-Schönlein purpura, granulomatosis with polyangiitis, nephrotic syndrome–associated pulmonary embolism, and microscopic polyangiitis. These diseases are ruled out by the absence of other characteristic clinical features, kidney biopsy findings, and negative serologic studies for antibodies against nuclear (antinuclear antibody), DNA (anti-dsDNA), and neutrophil cytoplasmic components (antineutrophilic cytoplasmic antibody).

PROGNOSIS AND TREATMENT
Untreated, the prognosis of Goodpasture disease is poor. The combination of high-dose intravenous methylprednisolone, cyclophosphamide, and plasmapheresis appears to improve survival. Nevertheless, patients who survive the pulmonary hemorrhage often progress to end-stage renal failure despite ongoing immunosuppressive therapy.

Bibliography is available at Expert Consult.

Chapter 518
Hemolytic-Uremic Syndrome
Scott K. Van Why and Ellis D. Avner

Hemolytic-uremic syndrome (HUS) is a common cause of community-acquired acute kidney injury in young children. It is characterized by the triad of microangiopathic hemolytic anemia, thrombocytopenia, and renal insufficiency. HUS has clinical features in common with thrombotic thrombocytopenic purpura (TTP) (see Chapter 484.5). The etiology and pathophysiology of the more common forms of HUS clearly delineate childhood HUS as separate from idiopathic TTP.

ETIOLOGY
The various etiologies of HUS and other related thrombotic microangiopathies allow classification into infection-induced, genetic, medication-induced, and HUS associated with systemic diseases characterized by microvascular injury (Tables 518-1 and 518-2). The most common form of HUS is caused by toxin-producing *Escherichia coli* that causes prodromal acute enteritis and is commonly termed *diarrhea-associated HUS*. In the subcontinent of Asia and in southern Africa, the toxin of *Shigella dysenteriae* type 1 is causative, whereas in Western countries, verotoxin or Shiga-like toxin producing *E. coli* (STEC) is the usual cause.

Several serotypes of *E. coli* can produce the toxin; O157:H7 is most common in Europe and the Americas. A large epidemic of HUS in Europe was caused by Shiga toxin–producing *E. coli* O104:H4. The reservoir of STEC is the intestinal tract of domestic animals, usually cows. Disease commonly is transmitted by undercooked meat or unpasteurized (raw) milk and apple cider. Local outbreaks have followed ingestion of undercooked, contaminated hamburger or other foods cross-contaminated on unwashed cutting boards at fast food restaurants; contaminated municipal water supplies; petting farms; and swimming in contaminated ponds, lakes, or pools. With broad food distribution, wider epidemics have been traced to lettuce, raw spinach, and bean sprouts contaminated with STEC. Less often, STEC has been spread by person-to-person contact within families or child care centers. A rare but distinct entity of infection-triggered HUS is related

Table 518-1	Thrombotic Microangiopathies Overview and Classification

TMA associated with genetic or immune-mediated abnormalities of the complement system
  Genetically determined factor H deficiency
  Genetic membrane cofactor protein (CD46) abnormalities
  Complement factor 1 deficiency
  Gain-of-function mutations of complement factor B
  Complement C3 mutations
  Acquired anti-C3 autoantibodies
  Immune-mediated factor H deficiency
TTP associated with genetic or immune-mediated ADAMTS13 abnormalities
Infectious disease–associated TMA
  STEC-HUS
  Neuraminidase (pneumococcal)–associated TMA
  HIV infection
Systemic disease–associated TMA
  Antiphospholipid syndrome
  Systemic lupus erythematosus
  Scleroderma
  Malignant hypertension
  Malignancy
Pregnancy-associated TMA
  TTP
  Hemolysis, elevated liver enzymes, and low platelet count syndrome
  Postpartum HUS
Drug-associated TMA (>50 substances reported)
  Mitomycin
  Quinidine
  Ticlopidine
  Clopidogrel
  Calcineurin inhibitors
  Oral contraception
  Gemcitabine
  Anti-VEGF
Metabolic disease–associated TMA
  Deficiency in cobalamin C metabolism HUS
Transplant-associated TMA
  De novo HUS
  Recurrent posttransplantation HUS

ADAMTS13, a disintegrin and metalloproteinase with a thrombospondin type 1 motif, member 13; HIV, human immunodeficiency virus; HUS, hemolytic-uremic syndrome; STEC-HUS, Shiga toxin–producing *Escherichia coli* hemolytic-uremic syndrome; TMA, thrombotic microangiopathy; TTP, thrombotic thrombocytopenic purpura; VEGF, vascular endothelial growth factor.
From Ruggenenti P, Cravedi P, Remuzzi G: Thrombotic microangiopathies including hemolytic uremic syndrome. In Floege J, Johnson R, Feehally J, editors: Comprehensive Clinical Nephrology, vol 1, St. Louis, 2010, Elsevier Saunders, pp. 344–355.

to **neuraminidase-producing** *Streptococcus pneumoniae*. HUS develops during acute infection with this organism, typically manifesting as pneumonia with empyema. A thrombotic microangiopathy, similar to HUS or TTP, also can occur in patients with untreated HIV infection.

Genetic forms of HUS (atypical, nondiarrheal) compose the second major category of the disease (see Tables 518-1 and 518-2). Inherited deficiencies of either von Willebrand factor–cleaving protease (ADAMTS13) or complement factor H, I, or B, and defects in vitamin B_{12} metabolism can cause HUS. A specific genetic defect has not been identified in approximately 50% of familial cases transmitted in classic mendelian autosomal dominant or recessive patterns. A major feature characteristic of genetic forms of HUS is the absence of a preceding diarrhea prodrome. Genetic forms of HUS can be indolent and unremitting once they become manifest, or they can have a relapsing pattern precipitated by an infectious illness. The latter feature likely explains the association of many infectious agents with HUS, particularly in reports published before the recognition of the unique pathophysiology of STEC and neuraminidase-producing pneumococci in causing HUS.

HUS can be superimposed on any disease associated with microvascular injury, including malignant hypertension, systemic lupus erythematosus, and antiphospholipid syndrome (see Chapter 484.4). It can also occur following bone marrow or solid organ transplantation, and may be triggered by the use of the calcineurin inhibitors cyclosporine and tacrolimus in that setting. Several other medications also can induce HUS (see Table 518-1).

PATHOLOGY

Kidney biopsies are only rarely performed in HUS because the diagnosis is usually established by clinical criteria and the risks of biopsy are significant during the active phase of the disease. Early glomerular changes include thickening of the capillary walls caused by swelling of endothelial cells and accumulation of fibrillar material between endothelial cells and the underlying basement membrane, causing narrowing of the capillary lumens. Platelet–fibrin thrombi are often seen in glomerular capillaries. Thrombi are also seen in afferent arterioles and small arteries with fibrinoid necrosis of the arterial wall, leading to renal cortical necrosis from vascular occlusion. Late findings include glomerular sclerosis and obsolescence secondary to either severe direct glomerular involvement or glomerular ischemia from arteriolar involvement.

PATHOGENESIS

Microvascular injury with endothelial cell damage is characteristic of all forms of HUS. In the diarrhea-associated form of HUS, enteropathic organisms produce either Shiga toxin or the highly homologous Shiga-like verotoxin both of which directly cause endothelial cell damage. Shiga toxin can directly activate platelets to promote their aggregation. In pneumococcal-associated HUS, neuraminidase cleaves sialic acid on membranes of endothelial cells, red cells, and platelets to reveal the underlying cryptic Thomsen-Friedenreich (T) antigen. Endogenous immunoglobulin M (IgM) recognizes the T antigen and triggers the microvascular angiopathy.

The familial recessive and dominant forms of HUS, including the inherited deficiencies of ADAMTS13 and regulators of the complement cascade, probably predispose patients to developing HUS but do not cause the disease per se, because these patients might not develop HUS until later childhood or even adulthood. In such cases, HUS is often triggered by an inciting event such as an infectious disease. The absence of ADAMTS13 impairs cleavage of von Willebrand factor multimers, which enhances platelet aggregation. Factor H plays a central role in complement regulation, primarily arresting amplification and propagation of complement activation. It is possible that mild endothelial injury that would normally resolve instead evolves to an aggressive microangiopathy because of the inherited deficiencies of these factors.

In each form of HUS, capillary and arteriolar endothelial injury in the kidney leads to localized thrombosis, particularly in glomeruli, causing a direct decrease in glomerular filtration. Progressive platelet aggregation in the areas of microvascular injury results in consumptive thrombocytopenia. Microangiopathic hemolytic anemia results from mechanical damage to red blood cells as they pass through the damaged and thrombotic microvasculature.

CLINICAL MANIFESTATIONS

HUS is most common in preschool and school-age children, but it can occur in adolescents and adults. In HUS caused by toxigenic *E. coli*, onset of HUS occurs a few days after onset of gastroenteritis with fever, vomiting, abdominal pain, and diarrhea. The prodromal intestinal symptoms may be severe and require hospitalization, but they can also be relatively mild and considered trivial. The diarrhea is often bloody, but not necessarily so. Following the prodromal illness, the sudden onset of pallor, irritability, weakness, and lethargy heralds the onset of HUS. Oliguria can be present in early stages but may be masked by ongoing diarrhea, because the prodromal enteritis often overlaps the onset of HUS, particularly with ingestion of large doses of toxin. Thus, patients with HUS can present with either significant dehydration or volume overload, depending on whether the enteritis or renal

| Table 518-2 | Genetic Abnormalities and Clinical Outcome in Patients with Atypical Hemolytic-Uremic Syndrome |

GENE	PROTEIN AFFECTED	MAIN EFFECT	FREQUENCY (%)	RESPONSE TO SHORT-TERM PLASMA THERAPY*	LONG-TERM OUTCOME†	OUTCOME OF KIDNEY TRANSPLANTATION
CFH	Factor H	No binding to endothelium	20-30	Rate of remission: 60% (dose and timing dependent)	Rate of death or ESRD: 70-80%	Rate of recurrence: 80-90%‡
CFHR1/3	Factor HR1, R3	Anti–factor H antibodies	6	Rate of remission 70-80% (plasma exchange combined with immunosuppression)	Rate of ESRD: 30-40%	Rate of recurrence: 20%§
MCP	Membrane cofactor protein	No surface expression	10-15	No definitive indication for therapy	Rate of death or ESRD: <20%	Rate of recurrence: 15-20%§
CFI	Factor I	Low level or low cofactor activity	4-10	Rate of remission: 30-40%	Rate of death or ESRD: 60-70%	Rate of recurrence: 70-80%‡
CFB	Factor B	C3 convertase stabilization	1-2	Rate of remission: 30%	Rate of death or ESRD: 70%	Recurrence in one case
C3	Complement C3	Resistance to C3b inactivation	5-10	Rate of remission: 40-50%	Rate of death or ESRD: 60%	Rate of recurrence: 40-50%
THBD	Thrombomodulin	Reduced C3b inactivation	5	Rate of remission: 60%	Rate of death or ESRD: 60%	Recurrence in 1 patient

*Remission was defined as either complete remission or partial remission (i.e., hematologic remission with renal sequelae).
†The long-term outcome was defined as the outcome 5-10 yr after onset.
‡Patients in this category were eligible for combined liver and kidney transplantation.
§Patients in this category were eligible for single kidney transplantation.
ESRD, end-stage renal disease.
From Norris M, Remuzzi G: Atypical hemolytic-uremic syndrome, N Engl J Med 361:1676–1687, 2009.

insufficiency from HUS predominates, and the amount of fluid that has been administered.

Patients with pneumococci-associated HUS usually are ill with pneumonia, empyema, and bacteremia when they develop HUS. Onset can be insidious in patients with the genetic forms of HUS, with HUS triggered by a variety of illnesses, including mild, nonspecific gastroenteritis or respiratory tract infections.

HUS can be relatively mild, or can progress to a severe and fatal multisystem disease. Leukocytosis, severe prodromal enteritis, hyponatremia, and antibiotic use portend a severe course, but no presenting features reliably predict the severity of HUS in any given patient. Patients with HUS who appear mildly affected at presentation can rapidly develop severe, multisystem, life-threatening complications. Renal insufficiency can be mild but also can rapidly evolve into severe oliguric or anuric renal failure. The combination of rapidly developing renal failure and severe hemolysis can result in life-threatening hyperkalemia. Volume overload, hypertension, and severe anemia can all develop soon after onset of HUS, and together can precipitate heart failure. Direct cardiac involvement is rare, but pericarditis, myocardial dysfunction, or arrhythmias can occur without predisposing features of hypertension, volume overload, or electrolyte abnormalities.

The majority of patients with HUS have some central nervous system (CNS) involvement. Most have mild manifestations, with significant irritability, lethargy, or nonspecific encephalopathic features. Severe CNS involvement occurs in ≤20% of cases. Seizures and significant encephalopathy are the most common manifestations in those with severe CNS involvement, resulting from focal ischemia secondary to microvascular CNS thrombosis. Small infarctions in the basal ganglion and cerebral cortex have also been reported, but large strokes and intracranial hemorrhage are rare. Hypertension may produce an encephalopathy and seizures. Intestinal complications can be protean and include severe inflammatory colitis, ischemic enteritis, bowel perforation, intussusception, and pancreatitis. Patients can develop petechiae, but significant or severe bleeding is rare despite very low platelet counts.

DIAGNOSIS AND DIFFERENTIAL DIAGNOSIS

The diagnosis is made by the combination of microangiopathic hemolytic anemia with schistocytes, thrombocytopenia, and some degree of

kidney involvement. The anemia can be mild at presentation, but rapidly progresses. Thrombocytopenia is an invariable finding in the acute phase, with platelet counts usually 20,000-100,000/mm³. Partial thromboplastin and prothrombin times are usually normal. The Coombs test is negative, with the exception of pneumococci-induced HUS, where the Coombs test is usually positive. Leukocytosis is often present and significant. Urinalysis typically shows microscopic hematuria and low-grade proteinuria. The renal insufficiency can vary from mild elevations in serum blood urea nitrogen and creatinine to acute, anuric kidney failure.

The etiology of HUS is often clear with the presence of a diarrheal prodrome or pneumococcal infection. The presence or absence of toxigenic organisms on stool culture has little role in making the diagnosis of diarrhea-associated, enteropathic HUS. Only a minority of patients infected with those organisms develops HUS, and the organisms that cause HUS may be rapidly cleared. Therefore, the stool culture is often negative in patients who have diarrhea-associated HUS. If no history of diarrheal prodrome or pneumococcal infection is obtained, then evaluation for genetic forms of HUS should be considered, because those patients are at risk for recurrence, have a severe prognosis, and can benefit from different therapy. Other causes of acute kidney injury associated with a microangiopathic hemolytic anemia and thrombocytopenia should be considered and excluded, such as systemic lupus erythematosus, malignant hypertension, and bilateral renal vein thrombosis (see Table 518-1). A kidney biopsy is rarely indicated to diagnose HUS.

PROGNOSIS AND TREATMENT

With early recognition and intensive supportive care, the mortality for diarrhea-associated HUS is <5% in most major medical centers. Up to half of patients may require dialysis support during the acute phase of the disease. Most recover renal function completely, but of surviving patients, 5% remain dependent on dialysis, and up to 30% are left with some degree of chronic renal insufficiency. The prognosis for HUS not associated with diarrhea is more severe. Pneumococci-associated HUS causes increased patient morbidity, with mortality reported as 20%. The familial, genetic forms of HUS can be insidiously progressive or relapsing diseases and have a poor prognosis (see Table

518-2). Identification of specific factor deficiencies in some of these genetic forms provides opportunity for directed therapy to improve outcome.

The primary approach that has substantially improved acute outcome in HUS is early recognition of the disease, monitoring for potential complications, and meticulous supportive care. Supportive care includes careful management of fluid and electrolytes, including prompt correction of volume deficit, control of hypertension, and early institution of dialysis if the patient becomes significantly oliguric or anuric, particularly with hyperkalemia. Early intravenous volume expansion before the onset of oligo anuria may be nephroprotective in diarrhea-associated HUS. Red cell transfusions are usually required as hemolysis can be brisk and recurrent until the active phase of the disease has resolved. In pneumococci-associated HUS, it is critical that **any administered red cells be washed** before transfusion to remove residual plasma, because endogenous IgM directed against the revealed T antigen can play a role in accelerating the pathogenesis of the disease. Platelets should generally not be administered, regardless of platelet count, to patients with HUS because they are rapidly consumed by the active coagulation and theoretically can worsen the clinical course. Despite low platelet counts, serious bleeding is very rare in patients with HUS.

There is no evidence that any therapy directed at arresting the disease process of the most common, diarrhea-associated form of HUS provides benefit, and some can cause harm. Attempts have been made using anticoagulants, antiplatelet agents, fibrinolytic therapy, plasma therapy, immune globulin, and antibiotics. Anticoagulation, antiplatelet, and fibrinolytic therapies are specifically contraindicated because they increase the risk of serious hemorrhage. Antibiotic therapy to clear enteric toxigenic organisms (STEC) can result in increased toxin release, potentially exacerbating the disease, and therefore is not recommended. However, prompt treatment of causative pneumococcal infection is important. The European experience with *E. coli* O104:H4 in adults who were treated with azithromycin demonstrated more rapid elimination of the organism. Furthermore, in vitro evidence suggests that meropenem, rifaximin, and azithromycin downregulate the release and expression of Shiga toxin. Nonetheless in children with *E. coli* O157:H7–associated HUS, antibiotics are considered contraindicated.

Plasma infusion or plasmapheresis has been proposed for patients suffering severe manifestations of HUS with serious CNS involvement. There are no controlled data demonstrating the effectiveness of this approach, and it is specifically contraindicated in those with pneumococcal-associated HUS as it could exacerbate the disease. The use of plasma therapy in STEC-HUS was one of many treatment strategies during one of the largest reported outbreaks of STEC-HUS, which occurred in Europe in 2011. This outbreak was caused by an uncommon serotype (O104:H4) that had unique virulence factors. Thought initially to cause more severe disease, it differed epidemiologically from other STEC-HUS serotypes by affecting primarily healthy adults, rather than the usual pattern of affecting children and the elderly. Treatment in this epidemic included plasma exchange in most of the adult patients, as well as the use of eculizumab.

Eculizumab is an anti-C5 antibody that inhibits complement activation, a pathway that contributes to active disease in some forms of atypical familial HUS; this pathway may contribute to the process in STEC-HUS. Eculizumab is FDA approved for the treatment of atypical HUS. Because of the risk of meningococcal disease in patients with congenital defects in terminal complement components, it is recommended to give the meningococcal vaccine prior to giving eculizumab (if the patient has not been primarily immunized). While initial reports suggested that eculizumab provided benefit in patients with diarrhea-associated HUS, subsequent systematic analysis showed no benefit from either plasma exchange or eculizumab.

Plasma therapy can be of substantial benefit to patients with identified deficits of ADAMTS13 or factor H. It may also be considered in patients with other genetic forms of HUS, such as the undefined familial (recessive or dominant) form or sporadic but recurrent HUS. In contrast to its use in STEC-HUS, eculizumab shows great promise in treatment of atypical HUS, including HUS occurring following renal transplantation. Whether it should be combined with plasma therapy, or used as a primary treatment of atypical HUS, is still undetermined.

Most patients with diarrhea-associated HUS recover completely with little risk of long-term sequelae. Patients with hypertension, any level of renal insufficiency, or residual urinary abnormalities persisting a year after an episode of diarrhea-positive HUS (particularly significant proteinuria) require careful follow-up. Patients who have recovered completely with no residual urinary abnormalities after a yr are unlikely to manifest long-term sequelae. Because of some reports of late sequelae in such patients, annual examinations with a primary physician are still warranted.

Bibliography is available at Expert Consult.

Chapter 519
Upper Urinary Tract Causes of Hematuria

519.1 Interstitial Nephritis
See Chapter 523.

519.2 Toxic Nephropathy
See Chapter 533.

519.3 Cortical Necrosis
See Chapter 534.

519.4 Pyelonephritis
See Chapter 538.

519.5 Nephrocalcinosis
See Chapter 547.

519.6 Vascular Abnormalities
Craig C. Porter and Ellis D. Avner

Hemangiomas, hemangiolymphangiomas, angiomyomas, and arteriovenous malformations of the kidneys and lower urinary tract are rare causes of hematuria. They can present clinically with microscopic hematuria or gross hematuria with clots. When associated cutaneous vascular malformations are present, they can offer a clue to these underlying causes of hematuria. Renal colic can develop with any upper tract vascular abnormality that obstructs urinary drainage, induces an inflammatory response, or distends the renal capsule. The diagnosis may be confirmed by angiography or endoscopy.

Unilateral bleeding of varicose veins of the left ureter, resulting from compression of the left renal vein between the aorta and superior mesenteric artery (mesoaortic compression), is referred to as the **nutcracker syndrome.** Patients with this syndrome typically present with persistent microscopic hematuria (and occasionally, recurrent gross hematuria) that may be accompanied by proteinuria, left lower abdominal pain, left flank pain, or orthostatic hypotension. Diagnosis requires a high degree of suspicion and is confirmed by Doppler ultrasonography, CT, phlebography of the left renal vein, or magnetic resonance angiography.

Bibliography is available at Expert Consult.

519.7 Renal Vein Thrombosis
Craig C. Porter and Ellis D. Avner

EPIDEMIOLOGY
Renal vein thrombosis (RVT) occurs in 2 distinct clinical settings: (1) In newborns and infants, RVT is commonly associated with asphyxia, dehydration, shock, sepsis, congenital hypercoagulable states, and maternal diabetes; and (2) in older children, RVT is seen in patients with nephrotic syndrome, cyanotic heart disease, inherited hypercoagulable states, sepsis, following kidney transplantation, and following exposure to angiographic contrast agents.

PATHOGENESIS
RVT begins in the intrarenal venous circulation and can then extend to the main renal vein and even the inferior vena cava. Thrombus formation is mediated by endothelial cell injury resulting from hypoxia, endotoxin, or contrast media. Other contributing factors include hypercoagulability from either nephrotic syndrome or mutations in genes that encode clotting factors (i.e., factor V Leiden deficiency); hypovolemia and decreased venous blood flow associated with septic shock, dehydration, or nephrotic syndrome; and intravascular sludging caused by polycythemia.

CLINICAL MANIFESTATIONS
The development of RVT is classically heralded by the sudden onset of gross hematuria and unilateral or bilateral flank masses. However, patients can also present with any combination of microscopic hematuria, flank pain, hypertension, or a microangiopathic hemolytic anemia with thrombocytopenia or oliguria. RVT is usually unilateral. Bilateral RVT results in acute kidney failure.

DIAGNOSIS
The diagnosis of RVT is suggested by the development of hematuria and flank masses in patients seen in the high-risk clinical settings or with the predisposing clinical features noted above. Ultrasonography shows marked renal enlargement, and radionuclide studies reveal little or no renal function in the affected kidney(s). Doppler flow studies of the inferior vena cava and renal vein confirm the diagnosis. Contrast studies should be avoided to minimize the risk of further vascular damage.

DIFFERENTIAL DIAGNOSIS
The differential diagnosis of RVT includes other causes of hematuria that are associated with rapid development of microangiopathic hemolytic anemia or enlargement of the kidney(s). These include hemolytic-uremic syndrome, hydronephrosis, polycystic kidney disease, Wilms tumor, and intrarenal abscess or hematoma. All patients should be evaluated for congenital and acquired hypercoagulable states.

TREATMENT
The primary treatment of RVT starts with aggressive supportive intensive care, including correction of fluid and electrolyte imbalance and treatment of renal insufficiency. The American College of Chest Physicians recommends that the additional initial treatment of bilateral RVT should include tissue plasminogen activator and unfractionated heparin followed by continued anticoagulation with unfractionated or low-molecular-weight heparin. Treatment recommendations for unilateral RVT with inferior vena cava extension include either unfrac-

tionated or low-molecular-weight heparin. There is no consensus as to whether unilateral RVT without extension should be managed with heparin or with supportive therapy alone. Aggressive treatment with thrombolytic agents in all of these clinical settings, as well as antithrombotic prevention of patients with documented thrombotic risk, remains controversial despite such recommendations given the significant risks of bleeding. Evidence-based data, particularly in children, do not exist despite such "best-practice" recommendations. Children with severe hypertension secondary to RVT who are refractory to antihypertensive medications may require nephrectomy.

PROGNOSIS
Perinatal mortality from RVT has decreased significantly over the past 20 yr. Partial or complete renal atrophy is a common sequela of RVT in the neonate, leading to an increased risk of renal insufficiency, renal tubular dysfunction, and systemic hypertension. These complications are also seen in older children. However, recovery of renal function is not uncommon in older children with RVT resulting from nephrotic syndrome or cyanotic heart disease with correction of the underlying etiology.

Bibliography is available at Expert Consult.

519.8 Idiopathic Hypercalciuria
Craig C. Porter and Ellis D. Avner

Idiopathic hypercalciuria, which may be inherited as an autosomal dominant disorder, can clinically present as recurrent gross hematuria, persistent microscopic hematuria, dysuria, or abdominal pain in the absence of stone formation. Hypercalciuria can also accompany conditions resulting in hypercalcemia, such as hyperparathyroidism, vitamin D intoxication, immobilization, and sarcoidosis. Hypercalciuria may be associated with Cushing syndrome, corticosteroid therapy, tubular dysfunction secondary to Fanconi syndrome (Wilson disease, oculocerebrorenal syndrome), Williams syndrome, distal renal tubular acidosis, or Bartter syndrome (see Chapter 531). Hypercalciuria may also be seen in patients with **Dent disease,** which is an X-linked form of nephrolithiasis associated with hypophosphatemic rickets. Although microcrystal formation with consequent tissue irritation is believed to mediate symptoms, the precise mechanism by which hypercalciuria causes hematuria or dysuria is unknown.

DIAGNOSIS
Hypercalciuria is diagnosed by a 24 hr urinary calcium excretion >4 mg/kg. A screening test for hypercalciuria may be performed on a random urine specimen by measuring the calcium and creatinine concentrations. A spot urine calcium : creatinine ratio (mg/dL : mg/dL) >0.2 suggests hypercalciuria in an older child. Normal ratios may be as high as 0.8 in infants <7 mo of age.

TREATMENT
Left untreated, hypercalciuria leads to nephrolithiasis in approximately 15% of cases. Hypercalciuria has also been associated with an increased risk for development of low bone mineral density as well as an increased incidence of urinary tract infections. Idiopathic hypercalciuria has been identified as a risk factor in 40% of children with kidney stones, and a low urinary citrate level has been associated as a risk factor in approximately 38% of this group. Oral thiazide diuretics can normalize urinary calcium excretion by stimulating calcium reabsorption in the proximal and distal tubules. Such therapy can lead to resolution of gross hematuria or dysuria and can prevent nephrolithiasis. The precise indications for thiazide treatment (including its duration if initiated) remain controversial.

In patients with persistent gross hematuria or dysuria, therapy is initiated with hydrochlorothiazide at a dose of 1-2 mg/kg/24 hr as a single morning dose. The dose is titrated upward until the 24 hr urinary calcium excretion is <4 mg/kg and clinical manifestations resolve. After 1 yr of treatment, hydrochlorothiazide is usually discontinued, but may be resumed if gross hematuria, nephrolithiasis, or dysuria recurs. During hydrochlorothiazide therapy, the serum potassium level should be monitored periodically to avoid hypokalemia. **Potassium citrate** at a dose of 1 mEq/kg/24 hr may also be beneficial, particularly in patients with low urinary citrate excretion and symptomatic dysuria.

Sodium restriction is important because urinary calcium excretion parallels sodium excretion. Importantly, *dietary calcium restriction is not recommended* (except in children with massive calcium intake >250% of recommended dietary allowance by dietary history) because calcium is a critical requirement for growth, and no evidence supports a relationship between decreased calcium intake and decreased urinary calcium levels. This is particularly important given the association of hypercalciuria in some patients with reduced bone mineral density. A number of uncontrolled, small-scale studies support a role for bisphosphonate therapy, which leads to a reduction in urinary calcium excretion and improvement in bone mineral density. Controlled studies are necessary to establish a clear role for such therapy in children with hypercalciuria.

Bibliography is available at Expert Consult.

Chapter 520
Hematologic Diseases Causing Hematuria

520.1 Sickle Cell Nephropathy
Craig C. Porter and Ellis D. Avner

Gross or microscopic hematuria may be seen in children with sickle cell disease or sickle trait. Hematuria tends to resolve spontaneously in the majority of children (see Chapters 462.1 and 462.2). With the exception of an association with renal cell carcinoma, clinically apparent renal involvement occurs more commonly in patients with sickle cell disease than in those with sickle cell trait.

ETIOLOGY
The renal manifestations of sickle cell nephropathy (SSN) are generally related to microthrombosis secondary to sickling in the relatively hypoxic, acidic, hypertonic renal medulla where vascular stasis is present. Analgesic use, volume depletion with consequent prerenal failure, infection, and iron-related hepatic disease are independent contributing factors. Glomerular hyperfiltration, mediated by the intrarenal production of prostaglandins and synthesis of nitric oxide, is involved in the pathogenesis of proteinuria and kidney failure in SSN.

PATHOLOGY
Ischemia, papillary necrosis, and interstitial fibrosis are common pathologic findings in SSN. The specific sickle cell glomerular lesion consists of glomerular hypertrophy, with glomerulomegaly and distended capillaries. In addition, a variety of glomerular lesions are also found in SSN; most commonly these include focal segmental glomerulosclerosis, membranoproliferative glomerulonephritis, and thrombotic microangiopathy. The pathophysiology of these specific glomerulonephritic lesions in SSN is poorly understood but is probably

associated with the same factors that produce idiopathic or secondary disease as previously described (see Chapters 511-513).

CLINICAL MANIFESTATIONS
Clinical manifestations of SSN include polyuria caused by a urinary concentrating defect, renal tubular acidosis, and proteinuria associated with the glomerular lesions noted above.

Approximately 20-30% of patients with sickle cell disease develop proteinuria. Nephrotic-range proteinuria with or without clinically apparent nephrotic syndrome occurs in up to 30% of patients with SSN, and when present generally heralds progressive renal failure.

TREATMENT
Tubular manifestations have no specific treatment other than those recommended generally for patients with sickle cell disease. However, angiotensin-converting enzyme inhibitors and/or angiotensin II receptor inhibitors can be used to effect a significant reduction in urine protein excretion in patients with daily urine protein excretion exceeding 500 mg, and may slow progression of renal failure. Gross hematuria secondary to papillary necrosis may respond to treatment with ε-aminocaproic acid or desmopressin acetate. Hydroxyurea and newer treatments for sickle cell disease (see Chapter 462.1) have decreased the manifestations of SSN in proportion to the other complications of the primary hemoglobinopathy.

PROGNOSIS
SSN can eventually lead to hypertension, renal insufficiency, and progressive kidney failure. Dialysis and eventual kidney transplantation are successful treatment modalities when kidney failure is irreversible.

Bibliography is available at Expert Consult.

520.2 Coagulopathies and Thrombocytopenia
Craig C. Porter and Ellis D. Avner

Gross or microscopic hematuria may be associated with inherited or acquired disorders of coagulation (hemophilia, disseminated intravascular coagulation, thrombocytopenia). In these cases, however, hematuria is not usually the presenting complaint or a major factor affecting clinical management of outcome (see Chapters 475-484).

Chapter 521
Anatomic Abnormalities Associated with Hematuria

521.1 Congenital Anomalies
Craig C. Porter and Ellis D. Avner

Gross or microscopic hematuria may be associated with many different types of malformations of the urinary tract. The sudden onset of gross hematuria after minor trauma to the flank is often associated with ureteropelvic junction obstruction, cystic kidneys, or enlarged kidneys from any cause (see Chapter 537).

521.2 Autosomal Recessive Polycystic Kidney Disease

Craig C. Porter and Ellis D. Avner

Also previously referred to as **infantile polycystic disease,** autosomal recessive polycystic kidney disease (ARPKD) is an autosomal recessive disorder occurring with an incidence of 1:10,000 to 1:40,000, and a gene carrier rate in the general population of 1/70. The gene for ARPKD *(PKHD1 [polycystic kidney and hepatic disease])* encodes fibrocystin, a large protein (>4,000 amino acids) with multiple isoforms.

PATHOLOGY

Both kidneys are markedly enlarged and grossly show innumerable cysts throughout the cortex and medulla. Microscopic studies demonstrate dilated, ectatic collecting ducts radiating from the medulla to the cortex, although transient proximal tubule cysts have been reported in the fetus. Development of progressive interstitial fibrosis and tubular atrophy during advanced stages of disease eventually leads to renal failure. ARPKD causes dual-organ disease and should be considered as *ARPKD/congenital hepatic fibrosis.* Liver involvement is characterized by a basic ductal plate abnormality that leads to bile duct proliferation and ectasia, as well as progressive hepatic fibrosis.

PATHOGENESIS

Fibrocystin may form a multimeric complex with proteins of other primary genetic cystic diseases. It appears that altered intracellular signaling from these complexes, located at epithelial apical cell surfaces, intercellular junctions, and basolateral cell surfaces in association with the focal adhesion complex, is a critical feature of disease pathophysiology.

A large number of mutations in *PKHD1* (without identified specific "hot spots") cause disease, and the same mutation can give variable degrees of disease severity in the same family. This clinical observation is consistent with preclinical data demonstrating many environmental and unknown genetic factors affecting disease expression. The false-negative rate for genetic diagnosis is approximately 10%. Limited available information suggests only gross genotype-phenotype correlation: mutations that modify fibrocystin appear to cause less-severe disease than those that truncate fibrocystin.

CLINICAL MANIFESTATIONS

The typical child presents with bilateral flank masses during the neonatal period or in early infancy. ARPKD may be associated with oligohydramnios, pulmonary hypoplasia, respiratory distress, and spontaneous pneumothorax in the neonatal period. Perinatal demise (approximately 25-30%) appears to be associated with truncating mutations. Components of the oligohydramnios complex (Potter syndrome), including low-set ears, micrognathia, flattened nose, limb-positioning defects, and intrauterine growth restriction, may be present at death from pulmonary hypoplasia. Hypertension is usually noted within the first few weeks of life, is often severe, and requires aggressive multidrug therapy for control. Oliguria and acute renal failure are uncommon, but transient hyponatremia, often in the presence of acute renal failure, often responds to diuresis. Renal function is usually impaired but may be initially normal in 20-30% of patients. Approximately 50% of patients with a neonatal-perinatal presentation develop end-stage renal disease (ESRD) by age 10 yr.

ARPKD is increasingly recognized in infants (and, rarely, in adolescents and young adults) with a mixed renal-hepatic clinical picture. Such children and young adults often present with predominantly hepatic manifestations in combination with variable degrees of renal disease. Hepatic disease manifests as portal hypertension, hepatosplenomegaly, gastroesophageal varices, episodes of ascending cholangitis, prominent cutaneous periumbilical veins, reversal of portal vein flow, and thrombocytopenia. Renal findings in patients with a hepatic presentation may range from asymptomatic abnormal renal ultrasonography to systemic hypertension and renal insufficiency. In the newborn, clinical evidence of liver disease by radiologic or clinical laboratory assessment is present in approximately 45% of children and believed to be universal by microscopic evaluation. Natural history studies of ARPKD patients presenting as infants and young children have classified this group in terms of the severity of their dual-organ phenotype: 40% severe renal/severe kidney and 20% of each of the following—severe kidney/mild liver, severe liver/mild kidney, and mild kidney/mild liver.

DIAGNOSIS

The diagnosis of ARPKD is strongly suggested by bilateral palpable flank masses in an infant with pulmonary hypoplasia, oligohydramnios, and hypertension and the absence of renal cysts by sonography of the parents (Fig. 521-1). Markedly enlarged and uniformly hyper-echogenic kidneys with poor corticomedullary differentiation are commonly seen on ultrasonography (Fig. 521-2). The diagnosis is supported by clinical and laboratory signs of hepatic fibrosis, pathologic findings of ductal plate abnormalities seen on liver biopsy, anatomic and pathologic proof of ARPKD in a sibling, or parental consanguinity. The diagnosis can be confirmed by genetic testing. The differential diagnosis includes other causes of bilateral renal enlargement and/or cysts, such as multicystic dysplasia, hydronephrosis, Wilms tumor, and bilateral renal vein thrombosis (Tables 521-1 and 521-2).

Nephronophthisis, an autosomal recessive disorder with renal fibrosis, tubular atrophy, and cyst formation is a common cause of ESRD in children and adolescents (Tables 521-1 and 521-2). Associated external findings include retinal degeneration (Senior-Loken syndrome), cerebellar ataxia (Joubert syndrome), and hepatic fibrosis (Boichis disease). Symptoms include polyuria (salt wasting, poor concentrating ability), failure to thrive, and anemia. Hypertension and edema are seen later when ESRD develops. Prenatal diagnostic testing using genetic linkage analysis or direct mutation analysis is available in families with a previously affected child.

Preimplantation genetic diagnosis with in vitro fertilization may avoid the birth of another affected child with ARPKD.

TREATMENT

The current treatment of ARPKD is supportive. Aggressive ventilatory support is often necessary in the neonatal period secondary to pulmonary hypoplasia, hypoventilation, and the respiratory illnesses of prematurity. Careful management of hypertension (angiotensin-converting enzyme inhibitors), fluid and electrolyte abnormalities, osteopenia, and clinical manifestations of renal insufficiency is essential. Children with severe respiratory failure or feeding intolerance from enlarged kidneys can require unilateral or, more commonly, bilateral nephrectomies, prompting the need for renal replacement therapy. For many children approaching ESRD therapy, significant portal hypertension is present. This in combination with the dramatic improvement in liver transplantation survival has led to consideration of dual renal and hepatic transplantation in a carefully selected group of patients. Dual transplantation thus avoids the later development of end-stage liver disease despite successful renal transplantation.

PROGNOSIS

Mortality has improved dramatically, although approximately 30% of patients die in the neonatal period from complications of pulmonary hypoplasia. Neonatal respiratory support and renal replacement therapies have increased the 10 yr survival of children surviving beyond the 1st yr of life to >80%. Fifteen-year survival is currently estimated at 70-80%. Consideration of dual renal and hepatic transplantation and the development of disease-specific therapies for pediatric clinical trials will further positively impact the natural history of ARPKD. An important resource for families of patients is the ARPKD/CHF Alliance (**www.arpkdchf.org**).

Bibliography is available at Expert Consult.

Table 521-1 Comparison of Clinical Features of Cystic Kidney Diseases

DISEASE	INHERITANCE	FREQUENCY	GENE PRODUCT	AGE OF ONSET	CYST ORIGIN	RENOMEGALY	CAUSE OF ESRD	OTHER MANIFESTATIONS
ADPKD	AD	400-1,000	Polycystin 1 Polycystin 2	20s and 30s; <2% before age 15 Occasional perinatal onset	Anywhere (including the Bowman capsule)	Yes	Yes	Liver cysts Cerebral aneurysms Hypertension Mitral valve prolapse Kidney stones UTIs
ARPKD	AR	6,000-10,000	Fibrocystin/polyductin	First yr of life; perinatal onset	Distal nephron, CD	Yes	Yes	Hepatic fibrosis Pulmonary hypoplasia Hypertension
ACKD	No	90% of ESRD patients at 8 yr	None	Years after onset of ESRD	Proximal and distal tubules	Rarely	No	None
Simple cysts	No	50% in those older than 40 yr	None	Adulthood	Anywhere (usually cortical)	No	No	None
Nephronophthisis	AR	80,000	Nephrocystins (NPHP1-9)	Childhood or adolescence	Medullary DCT	No	Yes	Retinal degeneration; neurologic, skeletal, hepatic, cardiac malformations
MCKD	AD	Rare	Uromodulin, others	Adulthood	Medullary DCT	No	Yes	Hyperuricemia, gout
MSK	No	5,000-20,000	None	30s	Medullary CD	No	No	Kidney stones Hypercalciuria
Tuberous sclerosis	AD	10,000	Hamartin (TSC1) Tuberin (TSC2)	Childhood	Loop of Henle, DCT	Rarely	Rarely	Renal cell carcinoma Tubers, seizures Angiomyolipoma Hypertension
VHL syndrome	AD	40,000	VHL protein	20s	Cortical nephrons	Rarely	Rarely	Retinal angioma, CNS hemangioblastoma, renal cell carcinoma, pheochromocytoma
Oral-facial-digital syndrome	XD	250,000	OFD1 protein	Childhood or adulthood	Renal glomeruli	Rarely	Yes	Malformation of the face, oral cavity, and digits; liver cysts; mental retardation
Bardet-Biedl syndrome	AR	65,000-160,000	BBS 14	Adulthood	Renal calyces	Rarely	Yes	Syndactyly and polydactyly, obesity, retinal dystrophy, male hypogenitalism, hypertension, mental retardation

ACKD, acquired cystic kidney disease; AD, autosomal dominant; ADPKD, autosomal dominant polycystic kidney disease; AR, autosomal recessive; ARPKD, autosomal recessive polycystic kidney disease; CD, collecting duct; CNS, central nervous system; DCT, distal convoluted tubule; ESRD, end-stage renal disease; MCKD, medullary cystic kidney disease; MSK, medullary sponge kidney; UTI, urinary tract infection; VHL, von Hippel-Lindau; XD, X-linked dominant.

From Arnaout MA: Cystic kidney disease. In Goldman L, Schafer AI, editors: Goldman's Cecil medicine, ed 24, Philadelphia, 2012, Elsevier Saunders, Table 129-1, p. 796.

Table 521-2	Autosomal Recessive Polycystic Kidney Disease and Hepatorenal Fibrocystic Disease Phenocopies			
DISEASE	**GENE(S)**	**RENAL DISEASE**	**HEPATIC DISEASE**	**SYSTEMIC FEATURES**
ARPKD	*PKHD1*	Collecting duct dilation	CHF; Caroli disease	No
ADPKD	*PKD1; PKD2*	Cysts along entire nephron	Biliary cysts; CHF (rare)	Yes: adults
NPHP	*NPHP1-NPHP16*	Cysts at the corticomedullary junction	CHF	+/−
Joubert syndrome and related disorders	*JBTS1-JBTS20*	Cystic dysplasia; NPHP	CHF; Caroli disease	Yes
Bardet-Biedel syndrome	*BBS1-BBS18*	Cystic dysplasia; NPHP	CHF	Yes
Meckel-Gruber syndrome	*MKS1-MKS10*	Cystic dysplasia	CHF	Yes
Oral-facial-digital syndrome, type I	*OFD1*	Glomerular cysts	CHF (rare)	Yes
Glomerulocystic disease	*PKD1; HNF1B; UMOD*	Enlarged; normal or hypoplastic kidneys	CHF (with PKD1 mutations)	+/−
Jeune syndrome (asphyxiating thoracic dystrophy)	*IFT80 (ATD2) DYNC2H1 (ADT3) ADT1, ADT4, ADT5*	Cystic dysplasia	CHF; Caroli disease	Yes
Renal-hepatic-pancreatic dysplasia (Ivemark II)	*NPHP3, NEK8*	Cystic dysplasia	Intrahepatic biliary dysgenesis	Yes
Zellweger syndrome	*PEX1-3;5-6;10-11;13;14;16;19;26*	Renal cortical microcysts	Intrahepatic biliary dysgenesis	Yes

NPHP, Nephronophthisis. CHF, congenital hepatic fibrosis.
Modified from Guay-Woodford LM, Bissler JJ, Braun MC, et al: Consensus expert recommendations for the diagnosis and management of autosomal recessive polycystic kidney disease: Report of an international conference. J Pediatr 165:611-617, 2014.

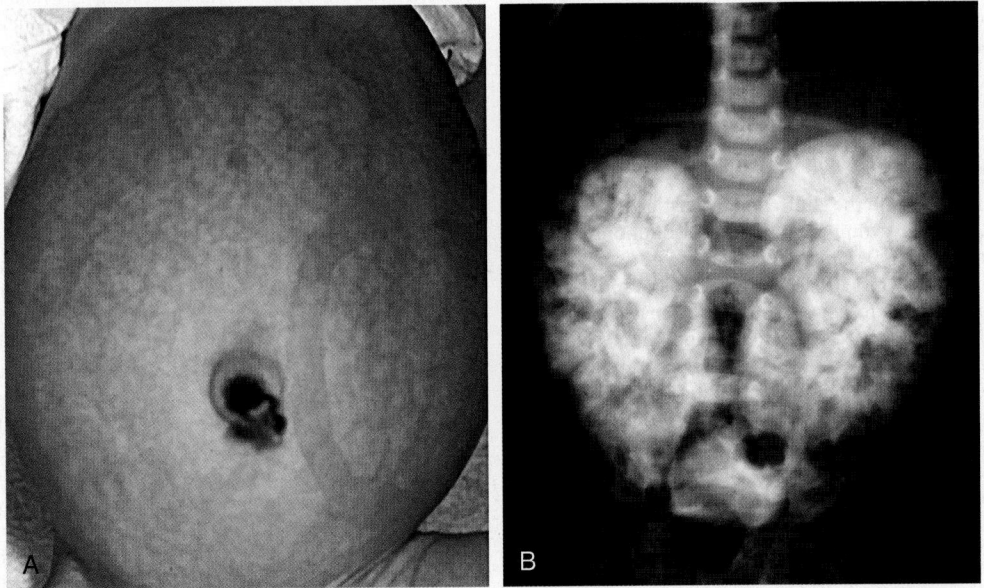

Figure 521-1 Infant with infantile polycystic kidney disease. **A,** This infant shows marked abdominal distention and bilaterally enlarged kidneys, as indicated by the *outlined area*. **B,** Intravenous pyelogram of the same patient shows the characteristic mottled nephrogram with brush-like medullary opacification secondary to retention of contrast material in dilated cortical and medullary collecting ducts. *(From Zitelli BJ, Davis HW, editors: Atlas of pediatric physical diagnosis, ed 4, St. Louis, 2002, Mosby, p. 470.)*

521.3 Autosomal Dominant Polycystic Kidney Disease
Craig C. Porter and Ellis D. Avner

Autosomal dominant polycystic kidney disease (ADPKD) is the most common hereditary human kidney disease, with an incidence of 1/400 to 1/1,000. It is a systemic disorder with possible cyst formation in multiple organs (liver, pancreas, spleen, brain) and the development of saccular cerebral aneurysms.

PATHOLOGY
Both kidneys are enlarged and show cortical and medullary cysts originating from all regions of the nephron.

PATHOGENESIS
Approximately 85% of patients with ADPKD have mutations that map to the *PKD1* gene on the short arm of chromosome 16, which encodes polycystin, a transmembrane glycoprotein. Another 10-15% of ADPKD mutations map to the *PKD2* gene on the long arm of chromosome 4, which encodes polycystin 2, a proposed nonselective cation channel.

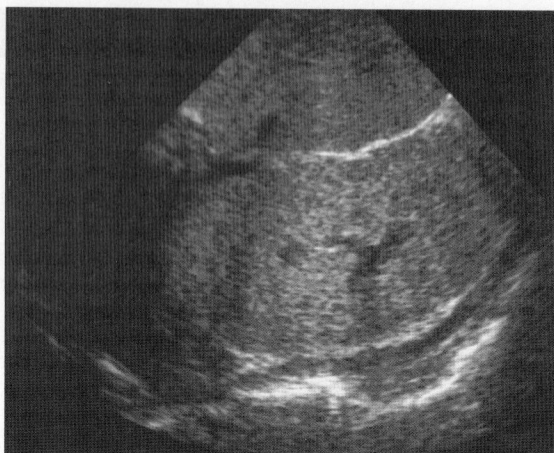

Figure 521-2 Ultrasound examination of a neonate with autosomal recessive polycystic kidney disease demonstrating renal enlargement (9 cm) and increased diffuse echogenicity with complete loss of corticomedullary differentiation resulting from multiple small cystic interfaces.

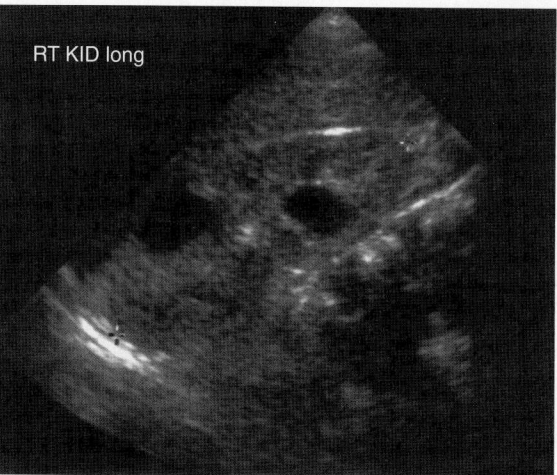

Figure 521-3 Ultrasound examination of an 18 mo old boy with autosomal dominant polycystic kidney disease demonstrating renal enlargement (10 cm) and 2 large cysts.

The majority of mutations appear to be unique to a given family. At present, a mutation can be found in 85% of patients with well-characterized disease. Approximately 8-10% of patients will have de novo, disease-causing mutations. Mutations of *PKD1* are associated with more severe renal disease than mutations of *PKD2*. The pathophysiology of the disease appears to be related to disruption of normal multimeric cystoprotein complexes, with consequent abnormal intracellular signaling resulting in abnormal proliferation, tubular secretion, and cyst formation. Abnormal growth factor expression, coupled with low intracellular calcium and elevated cyclic adenosine monophosphate, appear to be important features leading to formation of cysts and progressive enlargement.

CLINICAL PRESENTATION

The severity of renal disease and the clinical manifestations of ADPKD are highly variable. Although symptomatic ADPKD commonly occurs in the 4th or 5th decade of life, symptoms, including gross or microscopic hematuria, bilateral flank pain, abdominal masses, hypertension, and urinary tract infection, may be seen in neonates, children, and adolescents. With the increased utilization of abdominal sonography in the pediatric population, as well as ADPKD families now requesting possible screening in their asymptomatic, at-risk offspring (with the passage of the Genetic Information Nondiscrimination Act in the United States), most children with ADPKD are diagnosed by abnormal renal sonography in the absence of symptoms. Renal ultrasonography usually demonstrates multiple bilateral macrocysts in enlarged kidneys (Fig. 521-3), although normal kidney size and unilateral disease may be seen in the early phase of the disease in children.

ADPKD is a multiorgan disorder affecting many tissue types. Cysts may be asymptomatic but present within the liver, pancreas, spleen, and ovaries and when present help confirm the diagnosis in childhood. **Intracranial aneurysms,** which appear to segregate within certain families, have an overall prevalence of 15% and are an important cause of mortality in adults, but occasionally occur in children. Mitral valve prolapse is seen in approximately 12% of children; aortic and coronary artery aneurysms and aortic valve insufficiency are noted in affected adults. Hernias, bronchiectasis, and intestinal diverticula can also occur in these children.

DIAGNOSIS

ADPKD is confirmed by the presence of enlarged kidneys with bilateral macrocysts in a patient with an affected 1st-degree relative. De novo mutations occur in 8-10% of patients with newly diagnosed disease. The diagnosis might be made in children before their affected parent, making parental renal sonography an important diagnostic test to be performed in families with no apparent family history. Among patients with genetically defined ADPKD, screening renal ultrasonography results may be normal in ≤20% by 20 yr of age and <5% by 30 yr of age.

Prenatal diagnosis is suggested from the presence of enlarged kidneys with or without cysts on ultrasonography in families with known ADPKD. Prenatal DNA testing is available in families with affected members whose disease is caused by identified mutations in the *PKD1* or *PKD2* genes.

The differential diagnosis includes renal cysts associated with glomerulocystic kidney disease, tuberous sclerosis, and von Hippel-Lindau disease, which may be inherited in an autosomal dominant pattern (see Table 521-1). The neonatal manifestations of ADPKD and ARPKD may rarely be indistinguishable.

TREATMENT AND PROGNOSIS

Treatment of ADPKD is primarily supportive. Control of blood pressure is critical because the rate of disease progression in ADPKD correlates with the presence of hypertension. Angiotensin-converting enzyme inhibitors and/or angiotensin II receptor antagonists are agents of choice. Obesity, caffeine ingestion, smoking, multiple pregnancies, male gender, and possibly the use of calcium channel blockers appear to accelerate disease progression. Older patients with a *family history* of intracranial aneurysm rupture should be screened for cerebral aneurysms.

Although neonatal ADPKD may be fatal, long-term survival of the patient and the kidneys is possible for children surviving the neonatal period. ADPKD that occurs initially in older children has a favorable prognosis, with normal renal function during childhood seen in >80% of children.

Although disease-specific therapy is not yet available, a number of clinical trials are in progress based on promising preclinical laboratory investigation (www.clinicaltrials.gov). A valuable resource for patients and their families is the Polycystic Kidney Disease Foundation (www.pkdcure.org).

Bibliography is available at Expert Consult.

521.4 Trauma

Craig C. Porter and Ellis D. Avner

Infants and children are more susceptible to renal injury following blunt or penetrating injury to the back or abdomen because of their decreased muscle mass "protecting" the kidney. Gross or microscopic hematuria, flank pain, and abdominal rigidity can occur; associated injuries may be present (see Chapter 72). In the absence of hemodynamic instability, most renal trauma can be managed nonoperatively. Urethral trauma can result from crush injury, often associated with a fractured pelvis or from direct injury. Such injury is suspected in the appropriate clinical setting when gross blood appears at the external urethral meatus. Rhabdomyolysis and consequent renal failure is another complication of crush injury that can be ameliorated by vigorous fluid resuscitation. There may be a relationship between microscopic hematuria and recreational accidents in individuals >16 yr of age, none of whom exhibited hypotension or required surgical intervention.

Bibliography is available at Expert Consult.

521.5 Renal Tumors

See Chapters 498 and 499.

Chapter 522
Lower Urinary Tract Causes of Hematuria

522.1 Infectious Causes of Cystitis and Urethritis
Priya Pais and Ellis D. Avner

Gross or microscopic hematuria may be associated with bacterial, mycobacterial, or viral infections of the bladder (see Chapter 538).

522.2 Hemorrhagic Cystitis
Priya Pais and Ellis D. Avner

Hemorrhagic cystitis is defined as the presence of sustained hematuria and lower urinary tract symptoms (e.g., dysuria, frequency, urgency) in the absence of other bleeding conditions such as vaginal bleeding, a generalized bleeding condition, or a bacterial urinary tract infection. Depending on the severity, patients can present with microscopic or gross hematuria, often with clots. In severe forms, bleeding can lead to a significant decrease in blood hemoglobin levels.

Hemorrhagic cystitis can occur in response to chemical toxins (cyclophosphamide, penicillins, busulfan, thiotepa, dyes, insecticides), viruses (adenovirus types 11 and 21 [see Chapter 262] and influenza A), radiation, and amyloidosis. The polyoma BK virus, present latently in immunocompetent hosts, is associated with the development of drug-induced cystitis in immunosuppressed patients. The pediatric bone marrow transplantation population is particularly susceptible to hemorrhagic cystitis.

For chemical irritation related to use of cyclophosphamide, hydration and the use of mesna disulfide, which inactivates urinary cyclophosphamide metabolites, help to protect the bladder. Administration of oral cyclophosphamide in the morning followed by aggressive oral hydration throughout the remainder of the day is very effective in minimizing the risk of hemorrhagic cystitis. Treatment of hemorrhagic cystitis consists of a combination of intensive intravenous hydration, forced diuresis, analgesia, and spasmolytic drugs. Consultation with a urologist is recommended for more invasive measures if the cystitis does not respond to conservative measures. Gross

hematuria associated with viral hemorrhagic cystitis usually resolves within 1 wk.

Bibliography is available at Expert Consult.

522.3 Vigorous Exercise
Priya Pais and Ellis D. Avner

Gross or microscopic hematuria can follow vigorous exercise. Exercise hematuria is less common in females and can be associated with dysuria. Approximately 30-60% of runners completing marathons have dipstick-positive urine for blood. In limited follow-up, none appeared to have any significant urinary tract abnormalities. The color of the urine following vigorous exercise can vary from red to black. Blood clots may be rarely present in the urine. Findings on urine culture, intravenous pyelography, voiding cystourethrography, and cystoscopy are normal in most patients. This seems to be a benign condition, and the hematuria generally resolves within 48 hr after cessation of exercise. The absence of red blood cell casts or evidence of renal disease and the presence of dysuria and blood clots in some patients suggest that the source of bleeding lies in the lower urinary tract. **Rhabdomyolysis** with myoglobinuria or hemoglobinuria must be considered in the differential diagnosis when associated with symptoms in the appropriate clinical context. Hydronephrosis or anatomic abnormalities must be considered in any child who presents with hematuria (particularly gross) after mild exercise or following mild trauma. Appropriate imaging studies are indicated in this setting.

Bibliography is available at Expert Consult.

Section 3
Conditions Particularly Associated with Proteinuria

Chapter 523
Introduction to the Child with Proteinuria
Priya Pais and Ellis D. Avner

NORMAL PHYSIOLOGY
The charge and size selective properties of the glomerular capillary wall prevent significant amounts of albumin, globulin, and other large plasma proteins from entering the urinary space (see Chapter 508). Smaller proteins (low-molecular-weight proteins) do cross the capillary wall but are reabsorbed by the proximal tubule. A very small amount of protein that normally appears in the urine is the result of normal tubular secretion. The normally excreted protein mostly consists of Tamm-Horsfall protein (uromodulin), a protective glycoprotein secreted by the tubules that inactivates cytokines.

PATHOPHYSIOLOGY OF PROTEINURIA
Abnormal amounts of protein may appear in the urine from 3 possible mechanisms: **glomerular proteinuria**, which occurs as a result of

Table 523-1	Methods Available to Test for Proteinuria		
METHOD	**INDICATIONS**	**NORMAL RANGE**	**COMMENTS**
Dipstick testing	Routine screening for proteinuria performed in the office	Negative or trace in a concentrated urine specimen (specific gravity: ≥1.020)	False-positive test can occur if urine is very alkaline (pH > 8.0) or very concentrated (specific gravity: >1.025)
24 hr urine for protein and creatinine* excretion	Quantitation of proteinuria (as well as creatinine clearances)	<100 mg/m^2/24 hr or <150 mg/24 hr in a documented 24 hr collection	More accurate than spot urine analysis; inconvenient for patient; limited use in pediatric practice
Spot urine for protein/creatinine ratio—preferably on first morning urine specimen	Semiquantitative assessment of proteinuria	<0.2 mg protein/mg creatinine in children >2 yr old <0.5 mg protein/mg creatinine in those 6–24 mo old	Simplest method to quantitate proteinuria; less accurate than measuring 24 hr proteinuria
Microalbuminuria	Assess risk of progressive glomerulopathy in patients with diabetes mellitus	<30 mg urine albumin per gram of creatinine on first morning urine	Therapy should be intensified in diabetics with microalbuminuria

*Note that in a 24 hr urine specimen, the creatinine content should be measured to determine whether the specimen is truly a 24 hr collection. The amount of creatinine in a 24 hr specimen can be estimated as follows: females, 15-20 mg/kg; males, 20-25 mg/kg.

Adapted from Hogg RJ, Portman RJ, Milliner D, et al, Evaluation and management of proteinuria and nephrotic syndrome in children: recommendations from a Pediatric Nephrology Panel Established at the National Kidney Foundation Conference on Proteinuria, Albuminuria, Risk Assessment, Detection, and Elimination (PARADE), Pediatrics 105(6):1242–1249, 2000.

disruption of the glomerular capillary wall; **tubular proteinuria,** a tubular injury or dysfunction that leads to ineffective reabsorption of mostly low-molecular-weight proteins; and **increased production of plasma proteins**—in multiple myeloma, rhabdomyolysis, or hemolysis—which may cause the production or release of very large amounts of protein that are filtered at the glomerulus and overwhelm the absorptive capacity of the proximal tubule.

MEASUREMENT OF URINE PROTEIN

Urine protein can be measured in random collected samples or in timed (e.g., 24 hr or overnight) samples. Tests to accurately quantify urine protein concentration rely on precipitation with sulfosalicylic acid and measurement of turbidity (Table 523-1).

Urine Dipstick Measurement of Protein

Total protein concentration in urine can be estimated with chemically impregnated plastic strips that contain a pH-sensitive colorimetric indicator that changes color when negatively charged proteins, such as albumin, bind to it. Dipsticks primarily detect albuminuria and are less sensitive for other forms of proteins (low-molecular-weight proteins, Bence Jones protein, gamma globulins). Visual changes in the color of the dipstick are a semiquantitative measure of urinary protein concentration. The dipstick is reported as negative, trace (10-29 mg/dL), 1+ (30-100 mg/dL), 2+ (100-300 mg/dL), 3+ (300-1000 mg/dL), and 4+ (>1000 mg/dL). **False-positive** results can occur with a very high urine pH (>7.0), a highly concentrated urine specimen, or contamination of the urine with blood. **False-negative** test results can occur in patients with dilute urine or a large volume of urine output or in disease states in which the predominant urinary protein is not albumin.

Positive urine dipstick test for protein is considered to be present if there is more than a trace (10-29 mg/dL) in a urine sample in which the specific gravity is <1.010. If the specific gravity is >1.015, the dipstick must read ≥1+ (>30 mg/dL) to be considered clinically significant.

Because the dipstick reaction offers only a qualitative measurement of urinary protein excretion, children with persistent proteinuria should have proteinuria quantitated more precisely. **Timed (24 hr) urine collections** offer more precise information regarding urine protein excretion than a randomly performed dipstick test. Urinary protein excretion in the normal child is less than 100 mg/m^2/day or a total of 150 mg/day. In neonates, normal urinary protein excretion is higher, up to 300 mg/m^2, because of reduced reabsorption of filtered proteins. A reasonable upper limit of normal protein excretion in healthy children is 150 mg/24 hr. More specifically, normal protein excretion in children is defined as ≤4 mg/m^2/hr; abnormal proteinuria

is defined as excretion of 4-40 mg/m^2/hr; and nephrotic-range protein-uria is defined as >40 mg/m^2/hr.

Timed urine collections are cumbersome to obtain, and the sensitivity and specificity of the test can be influenced by fluid intake, the volume of urine output, and the importance of including a complete collection without missed voids.

Urine Protein-to-Creatinine Ratio Measurement

Urine protein-to-creatinine ratio measurement of an untimed (spot) urine specimen has largely replaced timed urine collection. In children, urine protein-to-creatinine ratios have been shown to significantly correlate with measurements of 24 hr urine protein and are useful to screen for proteinuria and to longitudinally monitor urine protein levels.

This ratio is calculated by dividing the urine protein concentration (mg/dL) by the urine creatinine concentration (mg/dL) to provide a simple measure. It should be ideally performed on a first morning voided urine specimen to eliminate the possibility of orthostatic (postural) proteinuria (see Chapter 525). A ratio of <0.5 in children <2 yr of age and <0.2 in children >2 yr of age suggests normal urinary protein excretion. A ratio greater than 2 suggests nephrotic-range proteinuria.

CLINICAL CONSIDERATIONS

The finding of proteinuria in children and adolescents in a single, non–first morning urine specimen is common, varying between 5% and 15%. The prevalence of persistent proteinuria on repeated testing is much less common. The challenge is to differentiate the child with proteinuria related to renal disease from the otherwise healthy child with transient or other benign forms of proteinuria. When proteinuria is detected it is important to determine if it is transient, orthostatic, or fixed in nature.

Microalbuminuria is defined as the presence of albumin in the urine above the normal level but below the detectable range of conventional urine dipstick methods. In adults, persistent microalbuminuria (defined as a urinary albumin excretion of 30-300 mg/g creatinine on at least 2-3 samples) is accepted as evidence of diabetic nephropathy and also a predictor of cardiovascular and renal disease. The mean level of urinary albumin excretion falls between 8 and 10 mg/g of creatinine in children >6 yr of age. Similar to adults, microalbuminuria in children has been found to be associated with obesity and to predict, with reasonable specificity, the development of diabetic nephropathy in type 1 diabetes mellitus.

Bibliography is available at Expert Consult.

Chapter **524**
Transient Proteinuria
Craig C. Porter and Ellis D. Avner

The majority of children found to have positive tests for protein on urinary dipsticks will have negative evaluations on repeated dipsticks and normal urinary protein if formally quantitated. Approximately 10% of children who undergo random urinalysis have proteinuria by a single dipstick measurement. Across the school-age spectrum, this finding occurs more commonly in adolescents than in younger children. In most cases, serial testing of the patient's urine demonstrates resolution of the abnormality. This phenomenon defines **transient proteinuria,** and its cause remains elusive. Defined contributing factors include a temperature >38.3°C (101°F), exercise, dehydration, cold exposure, heart failure, seizures, or stress. Transient proteinuria usually does not exceed 1-2+ on the dipstick. No evaluation or therapy is needed for children with this benign condition. Persistence of proteinuria, even if low grade, is not consistent with the diagnosis and suggests the need for additional evaluation.

Bibliography is available at Expert Consult.

Chapter **525**
Orthostatic (Postural) Proteinuria
Craig C. Porter and Ellis D. Avner

Orthostatic proteinuria is the most common cause of persistent proteinuria in school-age children and adolescents, occurring in up to 60% of children with persistent proteinuria. Children with this condition are usually asymptomatic, and the condition is discovered by routine urinalysis. Patients with orthostatic proteinuria excrete normal or minimally increased amounts of protein in the supine position. In the upright position, urinary protein excretion may be increased 10-fold, up to 1,000 mg/24 hr (1 g/24 hr). *Hematuria, hypertension, hypoalbuminemia, edema, and renal dysfunction are absent.*

In a child with persistent asymptomatic proteinuria, the initial evaluation should include an assessment for orthostatic proteinuria. It begins with the collection of a first morning urine sample, with subsequent testing of any urinary abnormalities by a complete urinalysis and determination of a spot protein:creatinine (Pr:Cr) ratio. The correct collection of the first morning urine sample is critical. The child must fully empty the bladder before going to bed and then collect the first voided urine sample immediately upon arising in the morning. The absence of proteinuria (dipstick negative or trace for protein; and a normal ratio of urinary protein [mg/dL] to urinary creatinine [mg/dL] = [uPr/uCr] <0.2) on the first morning urine sample for 3 consecutive days confirms the diagnosis of orthostatic proteinuria. No further evaluation is necessary, and the patient and family should be reassured of the benign nature of this condition. However, if there are other abnormalities of the urinalysis (e.g., hematuria), or if the urine uPr:uCr ratio is >0.2, the patient should be referred to a pediatric nephrologist for a complete evaluation.

The cause of orthostatic proteinuria is unknown, although altered renal hemodynamics and partial left renal vein obstruction in the upright, lordotic position have been proposed as possible causes.

Increased body mass index is recognized as a strong correlate of orthostatic proteinuria. Long-term follow-up studies in young adults suggest that orthostatic proteinuria is a benign process, but similar data are not available for children. Therefore, long-term follow-up of children is prudent. Patients should be monitored for the development of nonorthostatic proteinuria, particularly in the presence of hematuria, hypertension, or edema. Such findings may herald underlying kidney disease.

Bibliography is available at Expert Consult.

Chapter **526**
Fixed Proteinuria
Priya Pais and Ellis D. Avner

Children found to have fixed proteinuria on a first morning urine sample on 3 separate occasions should be further investigated. Fixed proteinuria is defined as a first morning urine sample that is ≥1+ on dipstick testing with a urine specific gravity >1.015 or with a protein-to-creatinine ratio of ≥0.2. Fixed proteinuria indicates a potential kidney disease caused by either glomerular or tubular disorders.

526.1 Glomerular Proteinuria
Priya Pais and Ellis D. Avner

The glomerular capillary wall consists of 3 layers: the fenestrated capillary endothelium, the glomerular basement membrane, and the podocytes (with foot processes and intercalated slit diaphragms) (Fig. 526-1). Glomerular proteinuria results from alterations in the permeability of any of the layers of the glomerular capillary wall to normally filtered proteins and occurs in a variety of renal diseases (Table 526-1). Glomerular proteinuria can range widely from <1 g to >30 g of protein in a 24 hr period. The podocyte is the predominant cell of injury in most glomerular diseases characterized by heavy proteinuria.

Glomerular proteinuria should be suspected in any patient with a first morning urine protein:creatinine ratio >1.0, or significant proteinuria of any degree, accompanied by hypertension, hematuria, edema, or renal dysfunction (elevated blood urea nitrogen, creatinine). Disorders characterized primarily by proteinuria include idiopathic (minimal change) nephrotic syndrome, focal segmental glomerulosclerosis, mesangial proliferative glomerulonephritis, membranous nephropathy, membranoproliferative glomerulonephritis, diabetic nephropathy, and obesity-related glomerulopathy. Other renal disorders that can include proteinuria as a prominent feature include acute postinfectious glomerulonephritis, immunoglobulin A nephropathy, lupus nephritis, Henoch-Schönlein purpura nephritis, and Alport syndrome.

Initial evaluation of a child with fixed proteinuria should include measurement of serum creatinine and electrolyte panel, first morning urine protein:creatinine ratio, serum albumin level, and complement levels. The child should be referred to a pediatric nephrologist for further evaluation and management. Renal biopsy is often necessary to establish a diagnosis and guide therapy.

In asymptomatic patients with low-grade proteinuria (protein:creatinine ratio between 0.2 and 1.0) in whom all other findings are normal, renal biopsy might not be indicated because the underlying process may be transient or resolving or because specific pathologic features of a chronic kidney disease might not yet be apparent. Such patients should have periodic reevaluation (ideally every 4-6 mo unless the patient is symptomatic). The evaluation should consist of a physical examination with accurate blood pressure measurement, urinalysis, measurement of serum creatinine and a repeat first morning urine

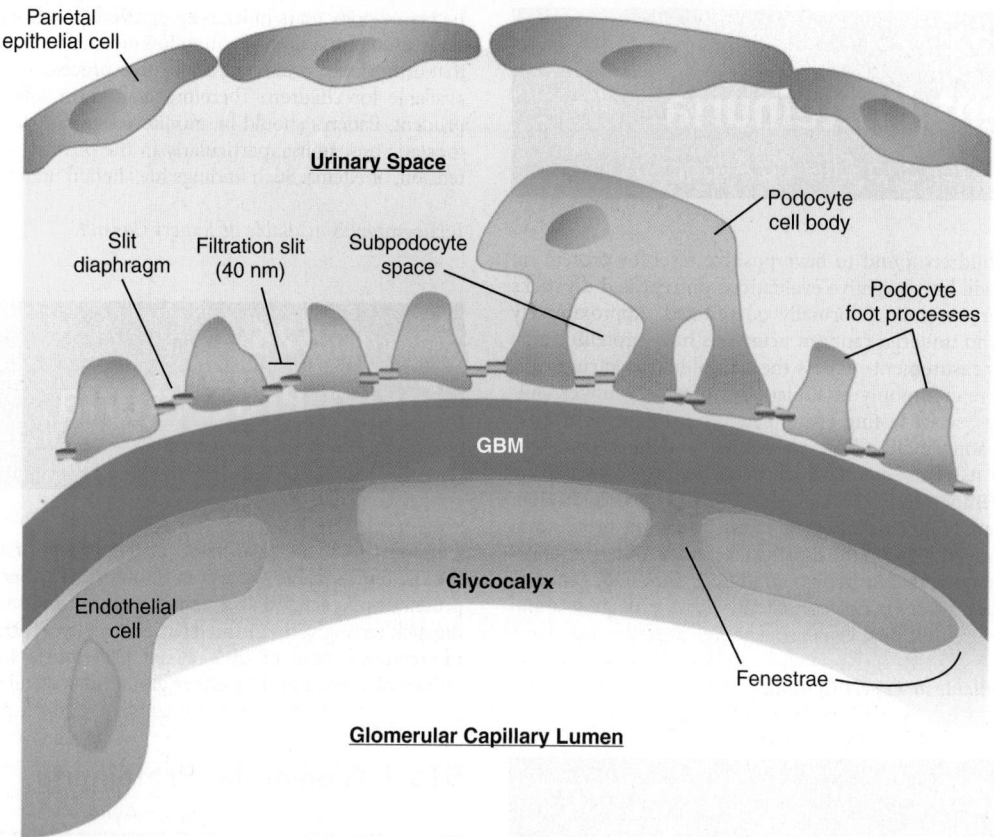

Figure 526-1 Glomerular capillary wall. The 3 layers of the capillary wall (glomerular endothelial cell, glomerular basement membrane [GBM], and podocyte) act as the glomerular filtration barrier (GFB), preventing proteins and large molecules from passing from the capillary lumen into the urinary space. The podocyte cell body lies with in the urinary space, and the cell is attached to the GBM through foot processes. Adjacent foot processes are separated by the filtration slit, bridged by the slit diaphragm. Disruption of the GFB leads the passage of protein across the capillary wall, leading to proteinuria. *(From Jefferson JA, Nelson PJ, Najafian B, Shankland SJ. Podocyte disorders: core curriculum 2011. Am J Kidney Dis 58:666–677, 2011, Fig 1.)*

Table 526-1	Causes of Proteinuria

TRANSIENT PROTEINURIA Fever Exercise Dehydration Cold exposure Congestive heart failure Seizure Stress **ORTHOSTATIC (POSTURAL) PROTEINURIA** **GLOMERULAR DISEASES CHARACTERIZED BY ISOLATED PROTEINURIA** Idiopathic (minimal change) nephrotic syndrome Focal segmental glomerulosclerosis Mesangial proliferative glomerulonephritis Membranous nephropathy Membranoproliferative glomerulonephritis Amyloidosis Diabetic nephropathy Sickle cell nephropathy	**GLOMERULAR DISEASES WITH PROTEINURIA AS A PROMINENT FEATURE** Acute postinfectious glomerulonephritis (streptococcal, endocarditis, hepatitis B or C virus, HIV) Immunoglobulin A nephropathy Henoch-Schönlein purpura nephritis Lupus nephritis Serum sickness Alport syndrome Vasculitic disorders Reflux nephropathy **TUBULAR DISEASES** Cystinosis Wilson disease Lowe syndrome Dent disease (X-linked recessive nephrolithiasis) Galactosemia Tubulointerstitial nephritis Acute tubular necrosis Renal dysplasia Polycystic kidney disease Reflux nephropathy Drugs (penicillamine, lithium, NSAID) Heavy metals (lead, gold, mercury)

NSAID, nonsteroidal antiinflammatory drug.

protein:creatinine ratio. Indications for renal biopsy include increasing proteinuria (protein:creatinine >1.0) or the development of hematuria, hypertension, or diminished renal function.

Bibliography is available at Expert Consult.

526.2 Tubular Proteinuria
Priya Pais and Ellis D. Avner

A variety of renal disorders that primarily involve the tubulointerstitial compartment of the kidney can cause low-grade fixed proteinuria (protein:creatinine ratio 0.2:1.0). In the healthy state, large amounts of proteins of lower molecular weight than albumin are filtered by the glomerulus and reabsorbed in the proximal tubule. Injury to the proximal tubules can result in diminished reabsorptive capacity and the loss of these low-molecular-weight proteins in the urine.

Tubular proteinuria (see Table 526-1) may be seen in acquired and inherited disorders and may be associated with other defects of proximal tubular function, such as the Fanconi syndrome (glycosuria, phosphaturia, bicarbonate wasting, and aminoaciduria). Tubular proteinuria is a consistent finding among patients with the X-linked tubular syndrome, Dent disease, caused by mutations of the renal chloride channel.

Asymptomatic patients having persistent proteinuria generally have glomerular rather than tubular proteinuria. In occult cases, glomerular and tubular proteinuria can be distinguished by electrophoresis of the urine. In tubular proteinuria, little or no albumin is detected, whereas in glomerular proteinuria, the major protein is albumin.

Bibliography is available at Expert Consult.

Chapter 527
Nephrotic Syndrome
Priya Pais and Ellis D. Avner

Nephrotic syndrome is the clinical manifestation of glomerular diseases associated with heavy (nephrotic-range) proteinuria. Nephrotic-range proteinuria is defined as proteinuria >3.5 g/24 hr or a urine protein:creatinine ratio >2. The **triad of clinical findings associated with nephrotic syndrome** arising from the large urinary losses of protein are hypoalbuminemia (≤2.5 g/dL), edema, and hyperlipidemia (cholesterol >200 mg/dL).

Nephrotic syndrome affects 1-3 per 100,000 children <16 yr of age. Without treatment, nephrotic syndrome in children is associated with a high risk of death, most commonly from infections. Fortunately, 80% of children with nephrotic syndrome respond to corticosteroid therapy. Although glucocorticoid therapy is standard therapy for nephrotic syndrome, neither the target cell nor the mechanism of action of steroids has been determined. Early referral to a pediatric nephrologist is recommended for initial management of nephrotic syndrome. However, continued care of these children is always a collaborative effort between the nephrologist and the primary care physician.

ETIOLOGY
Most children with nephrotic syndrome have a form of **primary** or idiopathic nephrotic syndrome (Table 527-1). Glomerular lesions associated with idiopathic nephrotic syndrome include minimal change disease (the most common), focal segmental glomerulosclerosis, membranoproliferative glomerulonephritis, C3 glomerulopathy,

and membranous nephropathy (Table 527-2). These etiologies have different age distributions (Fig. 527-1). Nephrotic syndrome may also be **secondary** to systemic diseases such as systemic lupus erythematosus, Henoch-Schönlein purpura, malignancy (lymphoma and leukemia), and infections (hepatitis, HIV, and malaria) (see Table 527-1). A number of **hereditary** proteinuria syndromes are caused by mutations in genes that encode critical protein components of the glomerular filtration apparatus (Table 527-3).

PATHOGENESIS
Role of the Podocyte
The underlying abnormality in nephrotic syndrome is an increased permeability of the glomerular capillary wall, which leads to massive proteinuria and hypoalbuminemia. The podocyte plays a crucial role in the development of proteinuria and progression of glomerulosclerosis. The podocyte is a highly differentiated epithelial cell located on the outside of the glomerular capillary loop (see Chapter 508.1). Foot processes are extensions of the podocyte that terminate on the glomerular basement membrane. The foot processes of a podocyte interdigitate with those from adjacent podocytes and are connected by a slit called the slit diaphragm. The podocyte functions as structural support of the capillary loop, is a major component of the glomerular filtration barrier to proteins, and is involved in synthesis and repair of the glomerular basement membrane. The slit diaphragm is one of the major impediments to protein permeability across the glomerular capillary wall. Slit diaphragms are not simple passive filters—they consist of numerous proteins that contribute to complex signaling pathways and play an important role in podocyte function. Important component proteins of the slit diaphragm include nephrin, podocin, CD2AP, and α-actinin 4. Podocyte injury or genetic mutations of genes producing podocyte proteins may cause nephrotic-range proteinuria (see Table 527-3).

In idiopathic, hereditary, and secondary forms of nephrotic syndrome, there are immune and nonimmune insults to the podocyte that lead to foot process effacement of the podocyte, a decrease in number of functional podocytes, and altered slit diaphragm integrity. The end result is increased protein "leakiness" across the glomerular capillary wall into the urinary space.

Role of the Immune System
Minimal change nephrotic syndrome (MCNS) may occur after viral infections and allergen challenges. MCNS has also been found to occur in children with Hodgkin lymphoma and T-cell lymphoma. That immunosuppression occurs with drugs such as corticosteroids and cyclosporine provides indirect additional evidence that the immune system contributes to the overall pathogenesis of the nephrotic syndrome.

CLINICAL CONSEQUENCES OF NEPHROTIC SYNDROME
Edema
Edema is the most common presenting symptom of children with nephrotic syndrome. Despite its almost universal presence, there is uncertainty as to the exact mechanism of edema formation. There are 2 opposing theories, the *underfill hypothesis* and the *overfill hypothesis*, that have been proposed as mechanisms causing nephrotic edema.

The *underfill hypothesis* is based on the fact that nephrotic-range proteinuria leads to a fall in the plasma protein level with a corresponding decrease in intravascular oncotic pressure. This leads to leakage of plasma water into the interstitium, generating edema. As a result of reduced intravascular volume, there is increased secretion of vasopressin and atrial natriuretic factor, which, along with aldosterone, result in increased sodium and water retention by the tubules. Sodium and water retention therefore occur as a consequence of intravascular volume depletion.

This hypothesis does not fit the clinical picture of some patients with edema caused by nephrotic syndrome who have clinical signs of intravascular volume overload, not volume depletion. Treating these patients with albumin alone may not be sufficient to induce a diuresis

| Table 527-1 | Causes of Childhood Nephrotic Syndrome |

IDIOPATHIC NEPHROTIC SYNDROME	SECONDARY CAUSES OF NEPHROTIC SYNDROME

Minimal change disease
Focal segmental glomerulosclerosis
Membranous nephropathy
Glomerulonephritis associated with nephrotic syndrome–
  membranoproliferative glomerulonephritis, crescentic
  glomerulonephritis, immunoglobulin A nephropathy
	Infections
	  Endocarditis
	  Hepatitides B, C
	  HIV-1
	  Infectious mononucleosis
	  Malaria
	  Syphilis (congenital and secondary)
	  Toxoplasmosis
	  Schistosomiasis
	  Filariasis

GENETIC DISORDERS ASSOCIATED WITH PROTEINURIA OR NEPHROTIC SYNDROME
Nephrotic Syndrome (Typical)
  Finnish-type congenital nephrotic syndrome (absence of nephrin)
  Focal segmental glomerulosclerosis (mutations in nephrin, podocin,
    MYO1E, α-actinin 4, TRPC6)
  Diffuse mesangial sclerosis (mutations in laminin β_2 chain)
  Denys-Drash syndrome (mutations in WT1 transcription factor)
  Congenital nephrotic syndrome with lung and skin involvement
    (integrin α-3 mutation)
  Mitochondrial disorders)
Proteinuria With or Without Nephrotic Syndrome
  Nail-patella syndrome (mutation in LMX1B transcription factor)
  Alport syndrome (mutation in collagen biosynthesis genes)
Multisystem Syndromes With or Without Nephrotic Syndrome
  Galloway-Mowat syndrome
  Charcot-Marie-Tooth disease
  Jeune syndrome
  Cockayne syndrome
  Laurence-Moon-Biedl-Bardet syndrome
Metabolic Disorders With or Without Nephrotic Syndrome
  Alagille syndrome
  α_1-Antitrypsin deficiency
  Fabry disease
  Glutaric acidemia
  Glycogen storage disease
  Hurler syndrome
  Partial lipodystrophy
  Mitochondrial cytopathies
  Sickle cell disease
	Drugs
	  Captopril
	  Penicillamine
	  Gold
	  Nonsteroidal antiinflammatory drugs
	  Pamidronate
	  Interferon
	  Mercury
	  Heroin
	  Lithium
	Immunologic or Allergic Disorders
	  Vasculitis syndromes
	  Castleman disease
	  Kimura disease
	  Beesting
	  Food allergens
	  Serum sickness
	Associated With Malignant Disease
	  Lymphoma
	  Leukemia
	  Solid tumors
	Glomerular Hyperfiltration
	  Oligomeganephronia
	  Morbid obesity
	  Adaptation to nephron reduction

Adapted from Eddy AA, Symons JM: Nephrotic syndrome in childhood, Lancet 362:629–638, 2003.

without the concomitant use of diuretics. Also, reducing the renin–aldosterone axis with mineralocorticoid receptor antagonists does not result in a marked increase in sodium excretion. With the onset of remission of MCNS, many children will have increased urine output before their urinary protein excretion is measurably reduced.

The *overfill hypothesis* postulates that nephrotic syndrome is associated with primary sodium retention, with subsequent volume expansion and leakage of excess fluid into the interstitium. There is accumulating evidence that the epithelial sodium channel in the distal tubule may play a key role in sodium reabsorption in nephrotic syndrome. The clinical weaknesses of this hypothesis are evidenced by the numerous nephrotic patients who present with an obvious clinical picture of intravascular volume depletion: low blood pressure, tachycardia, and elevated hemoconcentration. Furthermore, amiloride, an epithelial sodium channel blocker, used alone is not sufficient to induce adequate diuresis.

The goal of therapy should be a gradual reduction of edema with judicious use of diuretics, sodium restriction, and cautious use of intravenous albumin infusions, if indicated.

Hyperlipidemia

There are several alterations in the lipid profile in children with nephrotic syndrome, including an increase in cholesterol, triglycerides, low-density lipoprotein, and very-low-density lipoproteins. The high-density lipoprotein level remains unchanged or is low. In adults, this results in an increase in the adverse cardiovascular risk ratio, although the implications for children are not as serious, especially those with steroid-responsive nephrotic syndrome. Hyperlipidemia is thought to be the result of increased synthesis as well as decreased catabolism of

lipids. Although commonplace in adults, the use of lipid-lowering agents in children is uncommon.

Increased Susceptibility to Infections

Children with nephrotic syndrome are especially susceptible to infections such as cellulitis, spontaneous bacterial peritonitis, and bacteremia. This occurs as a result of many factors, particularly hypoglobulinemia as a result of the urinary losses of immunoglobulin (Ig) G. In addition, defects in the complement cascade from urinary loss of complement factors (predominantly C3 and C5), as well as alternative pathway factors B and D, lead to impaired opsonization of microorganisms. Children with nephrotic syndrome are at significantly increased risk for infection with encapsulated bacteria and, in particular, pneumococcal disease. **Spontaneous bacterial peritonitis** presents with fever, abdominal pain, and peritoneal signs. Although *Pneumococcus* is the most frequent cause of peritonitis, Gram-negative bacteria also are associated with a significant number of cases. Children with nephrotic syndrome and fever or other signs of infection must be evaluated aggressively, with appropriate cultures drawn, and should be treated promptly and empirically with antibiotics. Peritoneal leukocyte counts >250 are highly suggestive of spontaneous bacterial peritonitis.

Hypercoagulability

Nephrotic syndrome is a hypercoagulable state resulting from multiple factors: vascular stasis from hemoconcentration and intravascular volume depletion, increased platelet number and aggregability, and changes in coagulation factor levels. There is an increase in hepatic production of fibrinogen along with urinary losses of antithrombotic

| Table 527-2 | Summary of Primary Renal Diseases That Manifest as Idiopathic Nephrotic Syndrome |

FEATURES	MINIMAL CHANGE NEPHROTIC SYNDROME	FOCAL SEGMENTAL GLOMERULOSCLEROSIS	MEMBRANOUS NEPHROPATHY	MEMBRANOPROLIFERATIVE GLOMERULONEPHRITIS Type I	Type II
DEMOGRAPHICS					
Age (yr)	2-6, some adults	2-10, some adults	40-50	5-15	5-15
Sex	2:1 male	1.3:1 male	2:1 male	Male-female	Male-female
CLINICAL MANIFESTATIONS					
Nephrotic syndrome	100%	90%	80%	60%*	60%*
Asymptomatic proteinuria	0	10%	20%	40%	40%
Hematuria (microscopic or gross)	10-20%	60-80%	60%	80%	80%
Hypertension	10%	20% early	Infrequent	35%	35%
Rate of progression to renal failure	Does not progress	10 yr	50% in 10-20 yr	10-20 yr	5-15 yr
Associated conditions	Usually none	HIV, heroin use, sickle cell disease, reflux nephropathy	Renal vein thrombosis; medications; SLE; hepatitides B, C; lymphoma; tumors	None	Partial lipodystrophy
GENETICS	None except in congenital nephrotic syndrome (see Table 527-3)	Podocin, α-actinin 4, TRPC6 channel, INF-2, MYH-9	None	None	None
LABORATORY FINDINGS	Manifestations of nephrotic syndrome ↑ BUN in 15-30% Normal complement levels	Manifestations of nephrotic syndrome ↑ BUN in 20-40% Normal complement levels	Manifestations of nephrotic syndrome Normal complement levels	Low complement levels—C1, C4, C3-C9	Normal complement levels—C1, C4, low C3-C9
RENAL PATHOLOGY					
Light microscopy	Normal	Focal sclerotic lesions	Thickened GBM, spikes	Thickened GBM, proliferation	Lobulation
Immunofluorescence	Negative	IgM, C3 in lesions	Fine granular IgG, C3	Granular IgG, C3	C3 only
Electron microscopy	Foot process fusion	Foot process fusion	Subepithelial deposits	Mesangial and subendothelial deposits	Dense deposits
REMISSION ACHIEVED AFTER 8 WK OF ORAL CORTICOSTEROID THERAPY	90%	15-20%	Resistant	Not established/resistant	Not established/resistant

*Approximate frequency as a cause of idiopathic nephrotic syndrome. Approximately 10% of cases of adult nephrotic syndrome are a result of various diseases that usually manifest as acute glomerulonephritis.
↑, Elevated; BUN, blood urea nitrogen; C, complement; GBM, glomerular basement membrane; Ig, immunoglobulin; SLE, systemic lupus erythematosus.
Modified from Couser WG: Glomerular disorders. In Wyngaarden JB, Smith LH, Bennett JC, editors: Cecil textbook of medicine, ed 19, Philadelphia, 1992, WB Saunders, p. 560.

factors such as antithrombin III and protein S. Deep venous thrombosis may occur in any venous bed, including the cerebral venous sinus, renal vein, and pulmonary veins. The clinical risk is low in children (2-5%) compared to adults, but has the potential for serious consequences.

Bibliography is available at Expert Consult.

527.1 Idiopathic Nephrotic Syndrome

Priya Pais and Ellis D. Avner

Approximately 90% of children with nephrotic syndrome have idiopathic nephrotic syndrome. Idiopathic nephrotic syndrome is associated with primary glomerular disease without an identifiable causative disease or drug. Idiopathic nephrotic syndrome includes multiple histologic types: minimal change disease, mesangial proliferation, focal segmental glomerulosclerosis, membranous nephropathy, and membranoproliferative glomerulonephritis.

PATHOLOGY

In minimal change nephrotic syndrome (**MCNS**) (approximately 85% of total cases of nephrotic syndrome in children), the glomeruli appear normal or show a minimal increase in mesangial cells and matrix. Findings on immunofluorescence microscopy are typically negative, and electron microscopy simply reveals effacement of the epithelial cell foot processes. More than 95% of children with minimal change disease respond to corticosteroid therapy.

Table 527-3	Nephrotic Syndrome in Children Caused by Genetic Disorders of the Podocyte			
GENE	**NAME**	**LOCATION**	**INHERITANCE**	**RENAL DISEASE**
STEROID-RESISTANT NEPHROTIC SYNDROME				
NPHS1	Nephrin	19q13.1	Recessive	Finnish-type congenital nephrotic syndrome
NPHS2	Podocin	1q25	Recessive	FSGS
WT1	Wilms tumor-suppressor gene	11p13	Dominant	Denys-Drash syndrome with diffuse mesangial sclerosis Frasier syndrome with FSGS
LMX1B	LIM-homeodomain protein	9q34	Dominant	Nail-patella syndrome
SMARCAL1	SW1/SNF2-related, matrix-associated, actin-dependent regulator of chromatin, subfamily a-like 1	2q35	Recessive	Schimke immunoosseous dysplasia with FSGS*

*Podocyte expression of SMARCAL1 is presumptive but not yet established. Mutations in another protein, CD2-AP or NEPH1 (a novel protein structurally related to nephrin), cause congenital nephrotic syndrome in mice. A mutational variant in the CD2AP gene has been identified in a few patients with steroid-resistant nephrotic syndrome.
FSGS, focal segmental glomerulosclerosis.
Modified from Eddy AA, Symons JM: Nephrotic syndrome in childhood, Lancet 362:629–638, 2003.

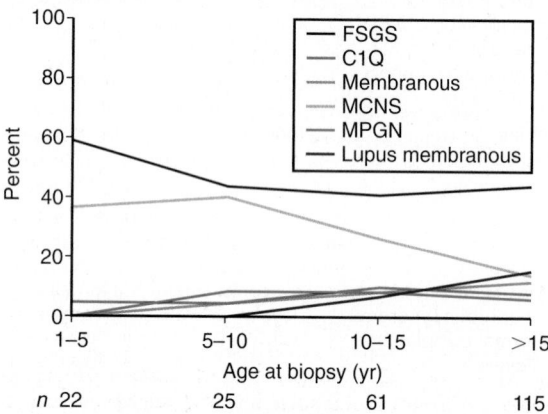

Figure 527-1 Kidney biopsy results from 223 children with proteinuria referred for diagnostic kidney biopsy (Glomerular Disease Collaborative Network, J. Charles Jennette, MD, Hyunsook Chin, MS, and D.S. Gipson, 2007). C1Q, nephropathy; FSGS, focal segmental glomerulosclerosis; MCNS, minimal change nephrotic syndrome; MPGN, membranoproliferative glomerulonephritis; n, number of patients. *(From Gipson DS, Massengill SF, Yao L, et al: Management of childhood onset nephrotic syndrome, Pediatrics 124:747–757, 2009.)*

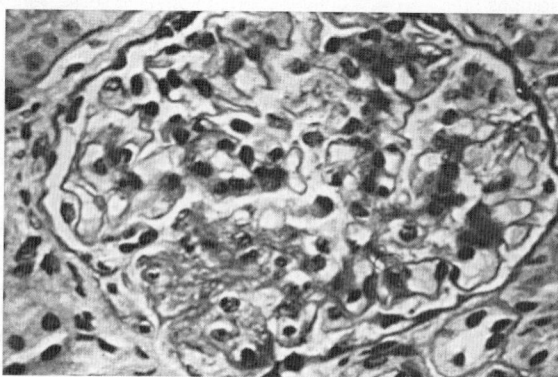

Figure 527-2 Glomerulus from a patient with steroid-resistant nephrotic syndrome showing mesangial hypercellularity and an area of sclerosis in the lower portion (×250).

Mesangial proliferation is characterized by a diffuse increase in mesangial cells and matrix on light microscopy. Immunofluorescence microscopy might reveal trace to 1+ mesangial IgM and/or IgA staining. Electron microscopy reveals increased numbers of mesangial cells and matrix as well as effacement of the epithelial cell foot processes. Approximately 50% of patients with this histologic lesion respond to corticosteroid therapy.

In **focal segmental glomerulosclerosis (FSGS)**, glomeruli show lesions that are both focal (present only in a proportion of glomeruli) and segmental (localized to ≥1 intraglomerular tufts). The lesions consist of mesangial cell proliferation and segmental scarring on light microscopy (Fig. 527-2 and see Table 527-2). Immunofluorescence microscopy is positive for IgM and C3 staining in the areas of segmental sclerosis. Electron microscopy demonstrates segmental scarring of the glomerular tuft with obliteration of the glomerular capillary lumen. Similar lesions may be seen secondary to HIV infection, vesicoureteral reflux, and intravenous use of heroin and other drugs of abuse. Only 20% of patients with FSGS respond to prednisone. The disease is often progressive, ultimately involving all glomeruli, and ultimately leads to end-stage renal disease in most patients.

MINIMAL CHANGE NEPHROTIC SYNDROME
Clinical Manifestations

The idiopathic nephrotic syndrome is more common in boys than in girls (2:1) and most commonly appears between the ages of 2 and 6 yr (see Fig. 527-1). However, it has been reported as early as 6 mo of age and throughout adulthood. MCNS is present in 85-90% of patients <6 yr of age. In contrast, only 20-30% of adolescents who present for the first time with nephrotic syndrome have MCNS. The more common cause of idiopathic nephrotic syndrome in this older age group is FSGS. The incidence of FSGS may be increasing; it may be more common in African-American, Hispanic, and Asian patients.

The initial episode of idiopathic nephrotic syndrome, as well as subsequent relapses, usually follows minor infections and, uncommonly, reactions to insect bites, beestings, or poison ivy.

Children usually present with mild edema, which is initially noted around the eyes and in the lower extremities. Nephrotic syndrome can initially be misdiagnosed as an allergic disorder because of the periorbital swelling that decreases throughout the day. With time, the edema becomes generalized, with the development of ascites, pleural effusions, and genital edema. Anorexia, irritability, abdominal pain, and diarrhea are common. Important features of minimal change idiopathic nephrotic syndrome are the absence of hypertension and gross hematuria (the so-called nephritic features).

The differential diagnosis of the child with marked edema includes protein-losing enteropathy, hepatic failure, heart failure, acute or chronic glomerulonephritis, and protein malnutrition. A diagnosis other than MCNS should be considered in children <1 yr of age, with a positive family history of nephrotic syndrome, and/or the presence of extrarenal findings (e.g., arthritis, rash, anemia), hypertension or pulmonary edema, acute or chronic renal insufficiency, and gross hematuria.

Diagnosis

Recommendations for the Initial Evaluation of Children with Nephrotic Syndrome

Confirming the Diagnosis of Nephrotic Syndrome.

The diagnosis of nephrotic syndrome is confirmed by urinalysis with first morning urine protein:creatinine ratio and serum electrolytes, blood urea nitrogen, creatinine, albumin, and cholesterol levels; evaluation to rule out secondary forms of nephrotic syndrome (children ≥10 yr): complement C3 level, antinuclear antibody, double-stranded DNA and hepatitides B and C, and HIV in high-risk populations; and kidney biopsy (for children ≥12 yr, who are less likely to have MCNS).

The urinalysis reveals 3+ or 4+ proteinuria, and microscopic hematuria is present in 20% of children. A spot urine protein:creatinine ratio should be >2.0. The serum creatinine value is usually normal, but it may be abnormally elevated if there is diminished renal perfusion from contraction of the intravascular volume. The serum albumin level is <2.5 g/dL, and serum cholesterol and triglyceride levels are elevated. Serum complement levels are normal. A renal biopsy is not routinely performed if the patient fits the standard clinical picture of MCNS.

Treatment

Children with their first episode of nephrotic syndrome and mild to moderate edema may be managed as outpatients. Such outpatient management is not practiced in all major centers, because the time required for successful education of the family regarding all aspects of the condition can require a short period of hospitalization. The child's parents must be able to recognize the signs and symptoms of the complications of the disease and may be taught how to use a dipstick and interpret the results to monitor for the degree of proteinuria. Tuberculosis must be ruled out prior to starting immunosuppressive therapy with corticosteroids by placing a purified protein derivative or obtaining an interferon release assay, and confirming a negative result.

Children with onset of uncomplicated nephrotic syndrome between 1 and 8 yr of age are likely to have steroid-responsive MCNS, and steroid therapy may be initiated without a diagnostic renal biopsy. Children with features that make MCNS less likely (gross hematuria, hypertension, renal insufficiency, hypocomplementemia, or age <1 yr or >12 yr) should be considered for renal biopsy before treatment.

Use of Corticosteroids to Treat Minimal Change Nephrotic Syndrome

Corticosteroids are the mainstay of therapy for MCNS. The treatment guidelines for corticosteroid use presented below are adapted from and based on the 2012 Kidney Disease: Improving Global Outcomes (KDIGO) clinical practice guidelines on glomerulonephritis.

Treatment of Initial Episode of Nephrotic Syndrome

In children with presumed MCNS, prednisone or prednisolone should be administered as a single daily dose of 60 mg/m^2/day or 2 mg/kg/day to a maximum of 60 mg daily for 4-6 wk followed by alternate-day prednisone (starting at 40 mg/m^2 qod or 1.5 mg/kg qod) for a period ranging from 8 wk to 5 mo, with tapering of the dose. When planning the duration of steroid therapy, the side effects of prolonged corticosteroid administration must be kept in mind.

Approximately 80-90% of children respond to steroid therapy. **Response** is defined as the attainment of remission within the initial 4 wk of corticosteroid therapy. **Remission** consists of a urine protein:creatinine ratio of <0.2 or <1+ protein on urine dipstick for 3 consecutive days. The vast majority of children who respond to prednisone therapy do so within the first 5 wk of treatment.

Managing the Clinical Sequelae of Nephrotic Syndrome

Edema. Children with severe symptomatic edema, including large pleural effusions, ascites, or severe genital edema, should be hospitalized. In addition to sodium restriction (<1500 mg daily), water/fluid restriction may be necessary if the child is hyponatremic. A swollen scrotum may be elevated with pillows to enhance fluid removal by gravity. Diuresis may be augmented by the administration of loop diuretics (furosemide), orally or intravenously, **although extreme caution should be exercised**. Aggressive diuresis can lead to intravascular volume depletion and an increased risk for acute renal failure and intravascular thrombosis.

When a patient has severe generalized edema with evidence of intravascular volume depletion (e.g., hemoconcentration, hypotension, tachycardia), IV administration of 25% albumin (0.5-1.0 g albumin/kg) as a slow infusion followed by furosemide (1-2 mg/kg/dose IV) is sometimes necessary. Such therapy should be used only in collaboration with a pediatric nephrologist and mandates close monitoring of volume status, blood pressure, serum electrolyte balance, and renal function. Symptomatic volume overload, with hypertension, heart failure, and pulmonary edema, is a potential complication of parenteral albumin therapy, particularly when administered as rapid infusions.

Dyslipidemia. Dyslipidemia should be managed with a low-fat diet. Dietary fat intake should be limited to <30% of calories with saturated fat intake <10% calories. Dietary cholesterol intake should be <300 mg/day. There are insufficient data to recommend the use of 3-hydroxy-3-methylgluataryl coenzyme A (HMG-CoA) reductase inhibitors routinely in children with dyslipidemia.

Infections. Families of children with nephrotic syndrome should be counseled regarding the signs and symptoms of infections such as cellulitis, peritonitis, and bacteremia. If there is suspicion of infection, a blood culture should be drawn prior to starting empiric antibiotic therapy. In the case of spontaneous bacterial peritonitis, peritoneal fluid should be collected if there is sufficient fluid to perform a paracentesis and sent for cell count, Gram stain, and culture. The antibiotic provided must be of broad enough coverage to include *Pneumococcus* and Gram-negative bacteria. A 3rd-generation cephalosporin is a common choice of IV antibiotic.

Thromboembolism. Children who present with the clinical signs of thromboembolism should be evaluated by appropriate imaging studies to confirm the presence of a clot. Studies to delineate a specific underlying hypercoagulable state are recommended. Anticoagulation therapy in children with thrombotic events appears to be effective— heparin, low-molecular-weight heparin, and warfarin are therapeutic options.

Obesity and Growth. Glucocorticoids may increase the body mass index in children who are overweight when steroid therapy is initiated, and these children are more likely to remain overweight. Anticipatory dietary counseling is recommended. Growth may be affected in children who require long-term corticosteroid therapy. Steroid-sparing strategies may improve linear growth in children who require prolonged courses of steroids.

Relapse of Nephrotic Syndrome. Relapse of nephrotic syndrome is defined as a urine protein:creatinine ratio of >2 or ≥3+ protein on urine dipstick testing for 3 consecutive days. Relapses are common, especially in younger children, and are often triggered by upper respiratory or gastrointestinal infections. Relapses are usually treated in a manner similar to the initial episode, except that daily prednisone courses are shortened. Daily high-dose prednisone is given until the child has achieved remission, and the regimen is then switched to alternate-day therapy. The duration of alternate day therapy varies depending on the frequency of relapses of the individual child. Children are classified as infrequent relapsers or frequent relapsers, and as being steroid dependent based on the number of relapses in a 12 mo period or their inability to remain in remission following discontinuation of steroid therapy.

Steroid Resistance. Steroid resistance is defined as the failure to achieve remission after 8 wk of corticosteroid therapy. Children with steroid-resistant nephrotic syndrome require further evaluation, including a diagnostic kidney biopsy, evaluation of kidney function, and quantitation of urine protein excretion (in addition to urine dipstick testing). Steroid-resistant nephrotic syndrome is usually caused by FSGS (80%), MCNS, or membranoproliferative glomerulonephritis.

Implications of Steroid-Resistant Nephrotic Syndrome.
Steroid-resistant nephrotic syndrome, and specifically FSGS, is associated with a 50% risk for end-stage kidney disease within 5 yr of diagnosis if patients do not achieve a partial or complete remission. Persistent nephrotic syndrome is associated with poor patient-reported quality of life, hypertension, serious infections, and thromboembolic events. Children reaching end-stage kidney disease have a greatly reduced life expectancy compared to their peers.

Alternative Therapies to Corticosteroids in the Treatment of Nephrotic Syndrome.
Steroid-dependent patients, frequent relapsers, and steroid-resistant patients are candidates for alternative therapies, particularly if they have severe corticosteroid toxicity (cushingoid appearance, hypertension, cataracts, and/or growth failure). **Cyclophosphamide** prolongs the duration of remission and reduces the number of relapses in children with **frequently relapsing** and **steroid-dependent** nephrotic syndrome. The potential side effects of the drug (neutropenia, disseminated varicella, hemorrhagic cystitis, alopecia, sterility, increased risk of future malignancy) should be carefully reviewed with the family before initiating treatment. Cyclophosphamide (2 mg/kg) is given as a single oral dose for a total duration of 8-12 wk. Alternate-day prednisone therapy is often continued during the course of cyclophosphamide administration. During cyclophosphamide therapy, the white blood cell count must be monitored weekly and the drug should be withheld if the count falls below 5,000/mm^3. The cumulative threshold dose above which oligospermia or azoospermia occurs in boys is >250 mg/kg.

Calcineurin inhibitors (cyclosporine or tacrolimus) are recommended as initial therapy for children with steroid-resistant nephrotic syndrome. Children must be monitored for side effects, including hypertension, nephrotoxicity, hirsutism, and gingival hyperplasia. **Mycophenolate** can maintain remission in children with steroid-dependent or frequently relapsing nephrotic syndrome. **Levamisole,** an antihelmintic agent with immunomodulating effects that has been shown to reduce the risk of relapse in comparison to prednisone, is not available in the United States. There are also uncontrolled preliminary data regarding prolonged remissions achieved with rituximab, the chimeric monoclonal antibody against CD20, in children with steroid-dependent and/or steroid-resistant nephrotic syndrome. There are no data from randomized clinical trials directly comparing the various corticosteroid-sparing agents. Most children who respond to cyclosporine, tacrolimus, or mycophenolate therapy tend to relapse when the medication is discontinued. Angiotensin-converting enzyme inhibitors and angiotensin II receptor blockers may be helpful as adjunct therapy to reduce proteinuria in steroid-resistant patients.

Immunizations in Children with Nephrotic Syndrome.
To reduce the risk of serious infections in children with nephrotic syndrome, give full pneumococcal vaccination (with the 13-valent conjugant vaccine and 23-valent polysaccharide vaccine) and influenza vaccination annually to the child and their household contacts; defer vaccination with live vaccines until the prednisone dose is below either 1 mg/kg daily or 2 mg/kg on alternate days. Live virus vaccines are contraindicated in children receiving corticosteroid-sparing agents such as cyclophosphamide or cyclosporine. Following close contact with varicella infection, give immunocompromised children on immunosuppressive agents varicella-zoster immune globulin if available; immunize healthy household contacts with live vaccines to minimize the risk of transfer of infection to the immunosuppressed child, but avoid direct exposure of the child to gastrointestinal or respiratory secretions of vaccinated contacts for 3-6 wk after vaccination.

Table 527-4 provides monitoring recommendations for children with nephrotic syndrome.

Prognosis
Most children with steroid-responsive nephrotic syndrome have repeated relapses, which generally decrease in frequency as the child grows older. Although there is no proven way to predict an individual child's course, children who respond rapidly to steroids and those who have no relapses during the first 6 mo after diagnosis are likely to follow an infrequently relapsing course. It is important to indicate to the family that the child with steroid-responsive nephrotic syndrome is unlikely to develop chronic kidney disease, that the disease is rarely hereditary, and that the child (in the absence of prolonged cyclophosphamide therapy) will remain fertile. To minimize the psychologic

Table 527-4	Monitoring Recommendations for Children with Nephrotic Syndrome											
DISEASE AND TREATMENT	HOME URINE PROTEIN	WEIGHT, GROWTH, BMI	BLOOD PRESSURE	CREATININE	ELECTROLYTES	SERUM GLUCOSE	CBC	LIPID PROFILE	DRUG LEVELS	LIVER FUNCTION	URINALYSIS	CPK
DISEASE TYPE												
Mild (steroid responsive)	•	•	•								•	
Moderate (frequent relapsing, steroid dependent)	•	•	•					•			•	
Severe (steroid resistant)	•	•	•	•				•			•	
THERAPY												
Corticosteroids		•	•			•		•			•	
Cyclophosphamide				•			•					
Mycophenolate mofetil							•			•		
Calcineurin inhibitors			•	•	•				•			
ACEIs/ARBs			•	•	•							
HMG-CoA reductase inhibitors								•		•		•

ACEI, angiotensin-converting enzyme inhibitor; ARB, angiotensin II receptor blocker; BMI, body mass index; CBC, complete blood count; CPK, creatine phospho kinase; HMG-CoA, 3-hydroxy-3-methylglutaryl coenzyme A.
From Gipson DS, Massengill SF, Yao L, et al: Management of childhood onset nephrotic syndrome, Pediatrics 124:747–757, 2009.

effects of the condition and its therapy, children with idiopathic nephrotic syndrome should not be considered chronically ill and should participate in all age-appropriate childhood activities and maintain an unrestricted diet when in remission.

Children with steroid-resistant nephrotic syndrome, most often caused by FSGS, generally have a much poorer prognosis. These children develop progressive renal insufficiency, ultimately leading to end-stage renal disease requiring dialysis or kidney transplantation. Recurrent nephrotic syndrome develops in 30-50% of transplant recipients with FSGS.

Bibliography is available at Expert Consult.

527.2 Secondary Nephrotic Syndrome

Priya Pais and Ellis D. Avner

Nephrotic syndrome can occur as a secondary feature of many forms of glomerular disease. Membranous nephropathy, membranoproliferative glomerulonephritis, postinfectious glomerulonephritis, lupus nephritis, and Henoch-Schönlein purpura nephritis can all have a nephrotic component (see Tables 527-1 and 527-2). Secondary nephrotic syndrome should be suspected in patients >8 yr and those with hypertension, hematuria, renal dysfunction, extrarenal symptoms (rash, arthralgias, fever), or depressed serum complement levels. In certain areas of the world, malaria and schistosomiasis are the leading causes of nephrotic syndrome. Other infectious agents associated with nephrotic syndrome include hepatitis B virus, hepatitis C virus, filaria, leprosy, and HIV.

Nephrotic syndrome has been associated with malignancy, particularly in the adult population. In patients with solid tumors, such as carcinomas of the lung and gastrointestinal tract, the renal pathology often resembles membranous glomerulopathy. Immune complexes composed of tumor antigens and tumor-specific antibodies presumably mediate the renal involvement. In patients with lymphomas, particularly Hodgkin lymphoma, the renal pathology most often resembles MCNS. The proposed mechanism of the nephrotic syndrome is that the lymphoma produces a lymphokine that increases permeability of the glomerular capillary wall. Nephrotic syndrome can develop before or after the malignancy is detected, resolve as the tumor regresses, and return if the tumor recurs.

Nephrotic syndrome has also developed during therapy with numerous drugs and chemicals. The histologic picture can resemble membranous glomerulopathy (penicillamine, captopril, gold, nonsteroidal antiinflammatory drugs, mercury compounds), MCNS (probenecid, ethosuximide, methimazole, lithium), or proliferative glomerulonephritis (procainamide, chlorpropamide, phenytoin, trimethadione, paramethadione).

Bibliography is available at Expert Consult.

527.3 Congenital Nephrotic Syndrome

Priya Pais and Ellis D. Avner

Nephrotic syndrome (massive proteinuria, hypoalbuminemia, edema, and hypercholesterolemia) has a poorer prognosis when it occurs in the 1st yr of life, when compared to nephrotic syndrome manifesting in childhood. Congenital nephrotic syndrome is defined as nephrotic syndrome manifesting at birth or within the *1st 3 mo of life.* Congenital nephrotic syndrome may be classified as primary or as secondary to a number of etiologies such as in utero infections (cytomegalovirus, toxoplasmosis, syphilis, hepatitides B and C, HIV), infantile systemic lupus erythematosus, or mercury exposure.

Primary congenital nephrotic syndrome is due to a variety of syndromes inherited as autosomal recessive disorders (see Table 527-3). A number of structural and functional abnormalities of the glomerular

Table 527-5	Causes of Nephrotic Syndrome in Infants Younger Than 1 Year

SECONDARY CAUSES

Infections
Syphilis
Cytomegalovirus
Toxoplasmosis
Rubella
Hepatitis B
HIV
Malaria
Drug reactions
Toxins
Mercury
Systemic lupus erythematosus
Syndromes with associated renal disease
Syndromes with associated renal disease
Nail-patella syndrome
Lowe syndrome
Nephropathy associated with congenital brain malformation
Denys-Drash syndrome: Wilms tumor
Hemolytic-uremic syndrome

PRIMARY CAUSES
Congenital nephrotic syndrome
Diffuse mesangial sclerosis
Minimal change disease
Focal segmental sclerosis
Membranous nephropathy

From Kliegman RM, Greenbaum LA, Lye PS: Practical strategies in pediatric diagnosis and therapy, ed 2, Philadelphia, 2004, Saunders, p. 418.

filtration barrier causing congenital nephrotic syndrome have been elucidated. In a large European cohort of children with congenital nephrotic syndrome, 85% carried disease-causing mutations in 4 genes (*NPHS1, NPHS2, WT1,* and *LAMB2*), the first 3 of which encode components of the glomerular filtration barrier. The Finnish type of congenital nephrotic syndrome is caused by mutations in the *NPHS1* or *NPHS2* gene, which encodes nephrin and podocin, critical components of the slit diaphragm. Affected infants most commonly present at birth with edema caused by massive proteinuria, and they are typically delivered with an enlarged placenta (>25% of the infant's weight). Severe hypoalbuminemia, hyperlipidemia, and hypogammaglobulinemia result from loss of filtering selectivity at the glomerular filtration barrier. Prenatal diagnosis can be made by the presence of elevated maternal and amniotic α-fetoprotein levels.

Denys-Drash syndrome is caused by mutations in the *WT1* gene, which results in abnormal podocyte function. Patients present with early-onset nephrotic syndrome, progressive renal insufficiency, ambiguous genitalia, and Wilms tumors.

Mutations in the *LAMB2* gene, seen in **Pierson syndrome,** lead to abnormalities of β$_2$-laminin, a critical component of glomerular and ocular basement membranes. In addition to congenital nephrotic syndrome, affected infants display bilateral microcoria (fixed narrowing of the pupil).

Regardless of the etiology of congenital nephrotic syndrome, diagnosis is made clinically in newborns or infants who demonstrate severe generalized edema, poor growth and nutrition with hypoalbuminemia, increased susceptibility to infections, hypothyroidism (from urinary loss of thyroxin-binding globulin), and increased risk of thrombotic events. Most infants have progressive renal insufficiency.

Secondary congenital nephrotic syndrome can resolve with treatment of the underlying cause, such as syphilis (Table 527-5). The management of primary congenital nephrotic syndrome includes intensive supportive care with intravenous albumin and diuretics, regular administration of intravenous γ-globulin, and aggressive nutritional support (often parenteral), while attempting to pharmacologically decrease urinary protein loss with angiotensin-converting enzyme inhibitors, angiotensin II receptor inhibitors, and prostaglandin synthesis inhibitors, or even unilateral nephrectomy. If conservative management fails and patients suffer from persistent anasarca or repeated severe infections, bilateral nephrectomies are performed and chronic dialysis is initiated. Renal transplantation is the definitive treatment of congenital nephrotic syndrome, though recurrence of the nephrotic syndrome has been reported to occur after transplantation.

Bibliography is available at Expert Consult.

Section 4
Tubular Disorders

Chapter 528
Tubular Function
Rajasree Sreedharan and Ellis D. Avner

Water and electrolytes are freely filtered at the level of the glomerulus. Thus, the electrolyte content of ultrafiltrate at the beginning of the proximal tubule is similar to that of plasma. Carefully regulated processes of tubular reabsorption and/or tubular secretion determine the final water content and electrolyte composition of urine. Bulk movement of solute tends to occur in the proximal portions of the nephron, and fine adjustments tend to occur distally (see Chapter 55).

SODIUM
Sodium is essential in maintaining extracellular fluid balance and, thus, volume status. The kidney is capable of effecting large changes in sodium excretion in a variety of normal and pathologic states.

There are 4 main sites of sodium transport. Approximately 60% of sodium is absorbed in the proximal tubule by coupled transport with glucose or amino acids, 25% in the ascending loop of Henle (mediated by NKCC2, the bumetanide-sensitive sodium-potassium 2 chloride transporter), and 15% in the distal tubule (mediated by NCCT, the thiazide-sensitive sodium chloride cotransporter) and collecting tubule (mediated by ENaC, the epithelial sodium channel).

The urinary excretion of sodium normally approximates the sodium intake of 2-6 mEq/kg/24 hr for a child consuming a typical American diet, minus 1-2 mEq/kg/24 hr required for normal metabolic processes. However, in states of volume depletion (dehydration, blood loss) or decreased effective circulating blood volume (septic shock, hypoalbuminemic states, heart failure), there may be a dramatic decrease in urinary sodium excretion to as low as 1 mEq/L. Changes in systemic volume status are detected by (1) baroreceptors in the atria, afferent arteriole, and carotid sinus and (2) by the macula densa, which detects changes in chloride delivery.

The major hormonal mechanisms mediating sodium balance include the renin–angiotensin–aldosterone axis, atrial natriuretic factor, and norepinephrine. Angiotensin II and aldosterone increase sodium reabsorption in the proximal tubule and distal tubule, respectively. Norepinephrine, released in response to volume depletion, does not directly act on tubular transport mechanisms but affects sodium balance by decreasing renal blood flow, thus decreasing the filtered load of sodium

as well as stimulating renin release. With more severe volume depletion, antidiuretic hormone is also released (see Chapter 530). Sodium excretion is promoted by atrial natriuretic factor and suppression of renin.

POTASSIUM
Extracellular potassium homeostasis is regulated because small changes in plasma potassium concentrations have dramatic effects on cardiac, neural, and neuromuscular function (see Chapter 55.4). Essentially, all filtered potassium is fully reabsorbed in the proximal tubule. Therefore, urinary excretion of potassium is completely dependent on tubular secretion by potassium channels present in the principal cells of the collecting tubule. Factors that promote potassium secretion include aldosterone, increased sodium delivery to the distal nephron, and increased urine flow rate.

CALCIUM
A significant portion of filtered calcium (70%) is reabsorbed in the proximal tubule. Additional calcium is reabsorbed in the ascending loop of Henle (20%) and the distal tubule and collecting duct (5-10%). Calcium is reabsorbed by passive movement between cells (paracellular absorption) in a process driven by sodium chloride reabsorption and potassium recycling into the lumen. In addition, calcium uptake is actively regulated by calcium receptors, specific transporters, and calcium channels. Factors that promote calcium reabsorption include parathyroid hormone (released in response to hypocalcemia), calcitonin, vitamin D, thiazide diuretics, and volume depletion (see Chapter 570). Factors that promote calcium excretion include volume expansion, increased sodium intake, and diuretics such as mannitol and furosemide.

PHOSPHATE
The majority of filtered phosphate is reabsorbed in the proximal tubule by active transport. Reabsorption is increased by dietary phosphorus restriction, volume contraction, and growth hormone. Parathyroid hormone and volume expansion increase phosphate excretion.

MAGNESIUM
Approximately 25% of filtered magnesium is reabsorbed in the proximal tubule. Modulation of renal magnesium excretion occurs primarily in the ascending loop of Henle, with some contribution of the distal convoluted tubule. Although specific magnesium transporters have been identified, the precise mechanisms by which they are regulated remain unclear.

ACIDIFICATION AND CONCENTRATING MECHANISMS
Acidification and concentration are addressed in the sections on renal tubular acidosis and nephrogenic diabetes insipidus, respectively (see Chapters 529 and 530).

DEVELOPMENTAL CONSIDERATIONS
Tubular transport capabilities of neonates (especially premature infants) and young infants are less than those of adults. Although nephrogenesis (the formation of new glomerular/tubular units) is complete by about 36 wk of gestation, significant tubular maturation occurs during infancy. Renal tubular immaturity, reduced glomerular filtration rate, decreased concentrating gradient, and diminished responsiveness to antidiuretic hormone are characteristic of young infants. These factors can contribute to impaired regulation of water, solute, and electrolyte and acid–base homeostasis, particularly during times of acute illness.

Bibliography is available at Expert Consult.

Renal Tubular Acidosis
Rajasree Sreedharan and Ellis D. Avner

Renal tubular acidosis (RTA) is a disease state characterized by a normal anion gap (hyperchloremic) metabolic acidosis in the setting of normal or near-normal glomerular filtration rate. There are 4 main types: proximal (type II) RTA, classic distal (type I) RTA, hyperkalemic (type IV) RTA, and combined proximal and distal (type III). Proximal RTA results from impaired bicarbonate reabsorption and distal RTA from failure to secrete acid. Either of these defects may be inherited and persistent from birth or acquired, as is seen more commonly in clinical practice.

NORMAL URINARY ACIDIFICATION
Kidneys contribute to acid–base balance by reabsorption of filtered bicarbonate (HCO_3^-) and excretion of hydrogen ion (H^+) produced every day. Hydrogen ion secretion from tubule cells into the lumen is key in the reabsorption of HCO_3^-, and the formation of titratable acid (H^+ bound to buffers such as HPO_4^{2-}), and ammonium ions (NH_4^+). Because loss of filtered HCO_3^- is equivalent to addition of H^+ to the body, all filtered bicarbonate should be absorbed before dietary H^+ can be excreted. Approximately 90% of filtered bicarbonate is absorbed in the proximal tubule, and the remaining 10% in the distal segments, mostly the thick ascending limb and outer medullary collecting tubule (Fig. 529-1). In the proximal tubule and thick ascending limb of the loop of Henle, H^+ from water is secreted by the Na^+-H^+ exchanger on the luminal membrane. H^+ combines with filtered bicarbonate resulting in the formation of H_2CO_3, which splits into water and CO_2 in the presence of carbonic anhydrase IV. CO_2 diffuses freely back into the cell, combines with OH^- (from H_2O) to form HCO_3^- in the presence of carbonic anhydrase II, and returns to the systemic circulation via a Na^+-HCO_3^- cotransporter situated at the basolateral membrane of the cell. In the collecting tubule, H^+ is secreted into lumen by H^+ATPase (adenosine triphosphatase) and HCO_3^- is returned to the systemic circulation by the HCO_3^--Cl^- exchanger located on the basolateral

membrane. The H^+ secreted proximally and distally in excess of the filtered HCO_3^- is excreted in the urine either as titratable acid or as NH_4^+.

529.1 Proximal (Type II) Renal Tubular Acidosis
Rajasree Sreedharan and Ellis D. Avner

PATHOGENESIS
Proximal RTA can be inherited and persistent from birth or occur as a transient phenomenon during infancy. Although rare, it may be primary and isolated. Proximal RTA usually occurs as a component of global proximal tubular dysfunction or **Fanconi syndrome,** which is characterized by low-molecular-weight proteinuria, glycosuria, phosphaturia, aminoaciduria, and proximal RTA. Table 529-1 outlines the causes of proximal RTA (pRTA) and Fanconi syndrome. Many of these causes are inherited disorders. In addition to **cystinosis** and **Lowe syndrome,** autosomal recessive and dominant pRTA are addressed further in this section. Other inherited forms of Fanconi syndrome include **galactosemia** (see Chapter 87.2), **hereditary fructose intolerance** (see Chapter 87.3), **tyrosinemia** (see Chapter 85.2), and **Wilson disease** (see Chapter 357.2). **Dent disease** or X-linked nephrolithiasis, is discussed in Chapter 531.3. In children, an important form of secondary Fanconi syndrome is exposure to ifosfamide, a component of many treatment regimens for Wilms tumor and other solid tumors.

Autosomal Recessive Disease
Isolated **autosomal recessive pRTA** is caused by mutations in the gene encoding the sodium bicarbonate cotransporter NBC1. It manifests with ocular abnormalities (band keratopathy, cataracts, and glaucoma, often leading to blindness), short stature, enamel defects of the teeth, intellectual impairment, and occasionally basal ganglia calcification along with pRTA. Autosomal dominant pattern of inheritance has been identified in a single pedigree with 9 members presenting with hyperchloremic metabolic acidosis, normal ability to acidify urine, normal renal function, and growth retardation.

Cystinosis
Cystinosis is a systemic disease caused by a defect in the metabolism of cysteine that results in accumulation of cystine crystals in most of the major organs of the body, notably the kidney, liver, eye, and brain. It occurs at an incidence of $1:100,000$ to $1:200,000$. In certain populations, such as French Canadians, the incidence is much higher. At least 3 clinical patterns have been described. Young children with the most severe form of the disease (*infantile* or *nephropathic cystinosis*) present in the 1st 2 yr of life with severe tubular dysfunction and growth failure. If the disease is not treated, the children develop end-stage renal disease by the end of their 1st decade. A milder form of the disease manifests in adolescents and is characterized by less-severe tubular abnormalities and a slower progression to renal failure. A benign adult form with no renal involvement also exists.

Cystinosis is caused by mutations in the *CTNS* gene, which encodes a novel protein, cystinosin. Cystinosin is thought to be an H^+-driven lysosomal cystine transporter. Genotype–phenotype studies demonstrate that patients with severe nephropathic cystinosis carry mutations that lead to complete loss of cystinosin function. Patients with milder clinical disease have mutations that lead to expression of partially functional protein. Patients with nephropathic cystinosis present with **clinical manifestations** reflecting their pronounced tubular dysfunction and Fanconi syndrome, including polyuria and polydipsia, growth failure, and rickets. Fever, caused by dehydration or diminished sweat production, is common. Patients are typically fair skinned and blond because of diminished pigmentation. Ocular presentations include photophobia, retinopathy, and impaired visual acuity. Patients also can develop hypothyroidism, hepatosplenomegaly, and delayed sexual

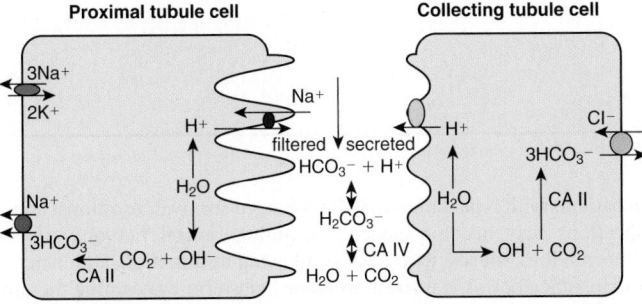

Figure 529-1 Major cellular luminal events in acid–base regulation in the proximal and the collecting tubule cells. In the proximal tubule, H^+, split from H_2O, is secreted into the lumen via Na^+/H^+ exchanger, and HCO_3^-, formed by combination of OH^- (split from H_2O) with CO_2 in the presence of carbonic anhydrase (CA) II, is returned to the systemic circulation by an Na^+-$3HCO_3^-$ cotransporter. Similarly, in the collecting tubule, H^+ is secreted into the lumen by an active H^+ATPase (adenosine triphosphatase), and HCO_3^- is returned to the systemic circulation via an HCO_3^--Cl^- exchanger. H^+ secreted into the lumen combines with filtered HCO_3^- to form carbonic acid (H_2CO_3) and then CO_2 and H_2O in the presence of CA IV, which can be passively reabsorbed. *(Modified from Rose BD, Post TW: Clinical physiology of acid-base and electrolyte disorders, ed 5, New York, 2001, McGraw-Hill.)*

Table 529-1	Common Causes of Renal Tubular Acidosis

PROXIMAL RENAL TUBULAR ACIDOSIS

Primary

Sporadic

Inherited
- Inherited renal disease (idiopathic Fanconi)
  - Sporadic (most common)
  - Autosomal dominant
  - Autosomal recessive
  - X-linked (Dent disease)
- Inherited syndromes
  - Cystinosis
  - Tyrosinemia type 1
  - Galactosemia
  - Oculocerebral dystrophy (Lowe syndrome)
  - Wilson disease
- Hereditary fructose intolerance

Secondary

Intrinsic renal disease
- Autoimmune diseases (Sjögren syndrome)
- Hypokalemic nephropathy
- Renal transplant rejection

Hematologic disease
- Myeloma

Drugs
- Gentamicin
- Cisplatin
- Ifosfamide
- Sodium valproate

Heavy metals
- Lead
- Cadmium
- Mercury

Organic compounds
- Toluene

Nutritional
- Kwashiorkor

Hormonal
- Primary hyperparathyroidism

DISTAL RENAL TUBULAR ACIDOSIS

Primary

Sporadic

Inherited
- Inherited renal diseases
  - Autosomal dominant
  - Autosomal recessive
  - Autosomal recessive with early-onset hearing loss
  - Autosomal recessive with later-onset hearing loss
- Inherited syndromes associated with type I renal tubular acidosis
  - Marfan syndrome
  - Wilson syndrome
  - Ehlers-Danlos syndrome
- Familial hypercalciuria

Secondary

Intrinsic renal
- Interstitial nephritis
- Pyelonephritis
- Transplant rejection
- Sickle cell nephropathy
- Lupus nephritis
- Nephrocalcinosis
- Medullary sponge kidney

Urologic
- Obstructive uropathy
- Vesicoureteral reflux
- Hepatic
- Cirrhosis

Toxins or medications
- Amphotericin B
- Lithium
- Toluene
- Cisplatin

HYPERKALEMIC RENAL TUBULAR ACIDOSIS

Primary

Sporadic

Genetic
- Hypoaldosteronism
- Addison disease
- Congenital adrenal hyperplasia
- Pseudohypoaldosteronism (type I or II)

Secondary

Urologic
- Obstructive uropathy

Intrinsic renal
- Pyelonephritis
- Interstitial nephritis

Systemic
- Diabetes mellitus
- Sickle cell nephropathy

Drugs
- Trimethoprim/sulfamethoxazole
- Angiotensin-converting enzyme inhibitors
- Cyclosporine
- Prolonged heparinization

Addison disease

---

maturation. With progressive tubulointerstitial fibrosis, renal insufficiency is invariant.

The **diagnosis** of cystinosis is suggested by the detection of cystine crystals in the cornea and confirmed by measurement of increased leukocyte cystine content. Prenatal testing is available for at-risk families.

Treatment of cystinosis is directed at correcting the metabolic abnormalities associated with Fanconi syndrome or chronic renal failure. In addition, specific therapy is available with **cysteamine,** which binds to cystine and converts it to cysteine. This facilitates lysosomal transport and decreases tissue cystine. Oral cysteamine does not achieve adequate levels in ocular tissues, so additional therapy with cysteamine eyedrops is required. Early initiation of the drug can prevent or delay deterioration of renal function. Patients with growth failure that does not improve with cysteamine might benefit from treatment with growth hormone. Kidney transplantation is a viable option

in patients with renal failure. With prolonged survival, additional complications may become evident, including central nervous system abnormalities, muscle weakness, swallowing dysfunction, and pancreatic insufficiency. It is unclear whether long-term cysteamine therapy will decrease these complications.

Lowe Syndrome

Lowe syndrome (*oculocerebrorenal syndrome of Lowe*) is a rare X-linked disorder characterized by congenital cataracts, mental retardation, and Fanconi syndrome. The disease is caused by mutations in the *OCRL1* gene, which encodes the phosphatidylinositol polyphosphate 5-phosphatase protein. The abnormalities seen in Lowe syndrome are thought to be caused by abnormal transport of vesicles within the Golgi apparatus. Kidneys show nonspecific tubulointerstitial changes. Thickening of glomerular basement membrane and changes in proximal tubule mitochondria are also seen.

Patients with Lowe syndrome typically present in infancy with cataracts, progressive growth failure, hypotonia, and Fanconi syndrome. Significant proteinuria is common. Blindness and renal insufficiency often develop. Characteristic behavioral abnormalities are also seen, including tantrums, stubbornness, stereotypy (repetitive behaviors), and obsessions. There is no specific therapy for the renal disease or neurologic deficits. Cataract removal is generally required.

CLINICAL MANIFESTATIONS OF PROXIMAL RENAL TUBULAR ACIDOSIS AND FANCONI SYNDROME

Patients with isolated, sporadic, or inherited pRTA present with growth failure in the 1st yr of life. Additional symptoms can include polyuria, dehydration (from sodium loss), anorexia, vomiting, constipation, and hypotonia. Patients with primary Fanconi syndrome have additional symptoms, secondary to phosphate wasting, such as rickets. Those with systemic diseases present with additional signs and symptoms specific to their underlying disease. *A non–anion gap metabolic acidosis is present.* Urinalysis in patients with isolated pRTA is generally unremarkable. The urine pH is acidic (<5.5) because distal acidification mechanisms are intact in these patients. Urinary indices in patients with Fanconi syndrome demonstrate varying degrees of phosphaturia, aminoaciduria, glycosuria, uricosuria, and elevated urinary sodium or potassium. Depending on the nature of the underlying disorder, laboratory evidence of chronic renal insufficiency, including elevated serum creatinine, may be present.

529.2 Distal (Type I) Renal Tubular Acidosis
Rajasree Sreedharan and Ellis D. Avner

PATHOGENESIS
Distal RTA can be sporadic or inherited. It can also occur as a complication of inherited or acquired diseases of the distal tubules. Primary or secondary causes of distal RTA can result in damaged or impaired functioning of one or more transporters or proteins involved in the acidification process, including the H^+/ATPase, the HCO_3^-/Cl^- anion exchangers, or the components of the aldosterone pathway. Because of impaired hydrogen ion excretion, urine pH cannot be reduced to <5.5, despite the presence of severe metabolic acidosis. Loss of sodium bicarbonate distally, owing to lack of H^+ to bind to in the tubular lumen (see Fig. 529-1), results in increased chloride absorption and hyperchloremia. Inability to secrete H^+ is compensated by increased K^+ secretion distally, leading to hypokalemia. **Hypercalciuria** is usually present and can lead to nephrocalcinosis or nephrolithiasis. Chronic metabolic acidosis also impairs urinary citrate excretion. **Hypocitraturia** further increases the risk of calcium deposition in the tubules. Bone disease is common, resulting from mobilization of organic components from bone to serve as buffers to chronic acidosis.

CLINICAL MANIFESTATIONS
Distal RTA shares features with those of pRTA, including non–anion gap metabolic acidosis and growth failure; distinguishing features of distal RTA include nephrocalcinosis and hypercalciuria. The phosphate and massive bicarbonate wasting characteristic of pRTA is generally absent. Table 529-1 lists the causes of primary and secondary distal RTA. Although inherited forms are rare, 3 specific inherited forms of distal RTA have been identified, including an autosomal recessive form associated with sensorineural deafness.

Medullary sponge kidney is a relatively rare sporadic disorder in children, although not uncommon in adults. It is characterized by cystic dilation of the terminal portions of the collecting ducts as they enter the renal pyramids. Ultrasonographically, patients often have medullary nephrocalcinosis. Although patients with this condition typically maintain normal renal function through adulthood, complications include nephrolithiasis, pyelonephritis, hyposthenuria (inability to concentrate urine), and distal RTA. Associations of medullary sponge kidney with Beckwith-Wiedemann syndrome or hemihypertrophy have been reported.

529.3 Hyperkalemic (Type IV) Renal Tubular Acidosis
Rajasree Sreedharan and Ellis D. Avner

PATHOGENESIS
Type IV RTA occurs as the result of impaired aldosterone production *(hypoaldosteronism)* or impaired renal responsiveness to aldosterone *(pseudohypoaldosteronism)*. Acidosis results because aldosterone has a direct effect on the H^+/ATPase responsible for hydrogen secretion. In addition, aldosterone is a potent stimulant for potassium secretion in the collecting tubule; consequently, lack of aldosterone results in hyperkalemia. This further affects acid–base status by inhibiting ammoniagenesis and, thus, H^+ excretion. Aldosterone deficiency typically occurs as a result of adrenal gland disorders such as Addison disease or some forms of congenital adrenal hyperplasia. In children, aldosterone unresponsiveness is a more common cause of type IV RTA. This can occur transiently, during an episode of acute pyelonephritis or acute urinary obstruction, or chronically, particularly in infants and children with a history of obstructive uropathy. The latter patients can have significant hyperkalemia, even in instances when renal function is normal or only mildly impaired. Rare examples of inherited forms of type IV RTA have been identified.

CLINICAL MANIFESTATIONS
Patients with type IV RTA can present with growth failure in the first few years of life. Polyuria and dehydration (from salt wasting) are common. Rarely, patients (especially those with pseudohypoaldosteronism type 1) present with life-threatening hyperkalemia. Patients with obstructive uropathies can present acutely with signs and symptoms of pyelonephritis, such as fever, vomiting, and foul-smelling urine. Laboratory tests reveal a hyperkalemic non–anion gap metabolic acidosis. Urine may be alkaline or acidic. Elevated urinary sodium levels with inappropriately low urinary potassium levels reflect the absence of aldosterone effect.

DIAGNOSTIC APPROACH TO RENAL TUBULAR ACIDOSIS
The first step in the evaluation of a patient with suspected RTA is to confirm the presence of a normal anion gap metabolic acidosis, identify electrolyte abnormalities, assess renal function, and rule out other causes of bicarbonate loss such as diarrhea (see Chapter 55). Metabolic acidosis associated with diarrheal dehydration is extremely common, and acidosis generally improves with correction of volume depletion. Patients with protracted diarrhea can deplete their total-body bicarbonate stores and can have persistent acidosis despite apparent restoration of volume status. In instances where a patient has a recent history of severe diarrhea, full evaluation for RTA should be delayed for several days to permit adequate time for reconstitution of total-body bicarbonate stores. If acidosis persists beyond a few days in this setting, additional studies are indicated.

Serum electrolytes, blood urea nitrogen, calcium, phosphorus, creatinine, and pH should be obtained by venous puncture. Traumatic blood draws (such as heel-stick specimens), small volumes of blood in "adult-size" specimen collection tubes, or prolonged specimen transport time at room temperature can lead to falsely low bicarbonate levels, often in association with an elevated serum potassium value. True hyperkalemic acidosis is consistent with type IV RTA, whereas the finding of normal or low potassium suggests type I or II. The **blood anion gap** should be calculated using the formula $[Na^+] - [Cl^- + HCO_3^-]$. Values of <12 demonstrate the absence of an anion gap. Values of >20 indicate the presence of an anion gap. If such an anion gap is found, then other diagnoses (lactic acidosis, inborn errors of

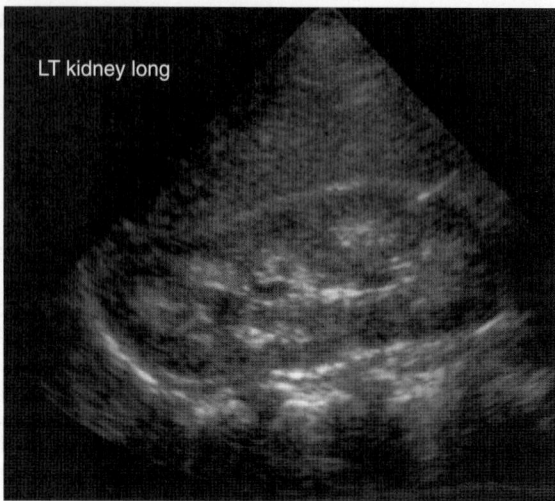

Figure 529-2 Ultrasound examination of a child with distal RTA demonstrating medullary nephrocalcinosis.

metabolism, ingested toxins) should be investigated. If tachypnea is noted, evaluation of an arterial blood gas might help to rule out the possibility of a mixed acid-base disorder primarily involving respiratory and metabolic components. A detailed history, with particular attention to growth and development, recent or recurrent diarrheal illnesses, and a family history of mental retardation, failure to thrive, end-stage renal disease, infant deaths, or miscarriages is essential. Physical examination should determine growth parameters and volume status as well as the presence of any dysmorphic features suggesting an underlying syndrome.

Once the presence of a non–anion gap metabolic acidosis is confirmed, urine pH can help distinguish distal from proximal causes. A urine pH <5.5 in the presence of acidosis suggests pRTA, whereas patients with distal RTA typically have a urine pH >6.0. The **urine anion gap** ([urine Na^+ + urine K^+] − urine Cl^-) is sometimes calculated to confirm the diagnosis of distal RTA. A positive gap suggests a deficiency of ammoniagenesis and, thus, the possibility of a distal RTA. A negative gap is consistent with proximal tubule bicarbonate wasting (gastrointestinal bicarbonate wasting). A urinalysis should also be obtained to determine the presence of glycosuria, proteinuria, or hematuria, suggesting more global tubular damage or dysfunction. Random or 24 hr urine calcium and creatinine measurements will identify hypercalciuria. Renal ultrasonography should be performed to identify underlying structural abnormalities such as obstructive uropathies as well as to determine the presence of nephrocalcinosis (Fig. 529-2).

TREATMENT AND PROGNOSIS

The mainstay of therapy in all forms of RTA is bicarbonate replacement. Patients with pRTA often require large quantities of bicarbonate, up to 20 mEq/kg/24 hr, in the form of sodium bicarbonate or sodium citrate solution (Bicitra or Shohl solution). The base requirement for distal RTAs is generally in the range of 2-4 mEq/kg/24 hr, although patients' requirements can vary. Patients with Fanconi syndrome usually require phosphate supplementation. Patients with distal RTA should be monitored for the development of hypercalciuria. Those with symptomatic hypercalciuria (recurrent episodes of gross hematuria), nephrocalcinosis, or nephrolithiasis can require thiazide diuretics to decrease urine calcium excretion. Patients with type IV RTA can require chronic treatment for hyperkalemia with sodium-potassium exchange resin (Kayexalate).

Prognosis of RTA depends to a large part on the nature of any existing underlying disease. Patients with treated isolated proximal or distal RTA generally demonstrate improvement in growth, provided serum

bicarbonate levels can be maintained in the normal range. Patients with systemic illness and Fanconi syndrome can have ongoing morbidity with growth failure, rickets, and signs and symptoms related to their underlying disease.

Bibliography is available at Expert Consult.

529.4 Rickets Associated with Renal Tubular Acidosis
Russell W. Chesney

Rickets may be present in primary RTA, particularly in type II or pRTA. Hypophosphatemia and phosphaturia are common in the renal tubular acidoses, which are also characterized by hyperchloremic metabolic acidosis, various degrees of bicarbonaturia, and, often, hypercalciuria and hyperkaluria. Bone demineralization without overt rickets usually is detected in type I and distal RTA. This metabolic bone disease may be characterized by bone pain, growth retardation, osteopenia, and, occasionally, pathologic fractures. Although acute metabolic acidosis in vitamin D–deficient animals can impair the conversion of 25-hydroxyvitamin D (25[OH]D) to 1,25-dihydroxyvitamin D (1,25[OH]$_2$D), resulting in reduced levels of this active metabolite, the circulating levels of 1,25(OH)$_2$D in patients with either type of RTA are generally normal. If patients with RTA have chronic renal insufficiency, serum 1,25(OH)$_2$D levels are reduced in relation to the degree of renal impairment.

Bone demineralization in distal RTA probably relates to dissolution of bone because the calcium carbonate in bone serves as a buffer against the metabolic acidosis due to the hydrogen ions retained by patients with RTA.

Administration of sufficient bicarbonate to reverse acidosis reverses bone dissolution and the hypercalciuria that is common in distal RTA. Proximal RTA is treated with both bicarbonate and oral phosphate supplements to heal rickets. Doses of phosphate similar to those used in familial hypophosphatemia or Fanconi syndrome may be indicated. Vitamin D is required to offset the secondary hyperparathyroidism that complicates oral phosphate therapy. Following therapy, growth in patients with type II (proximal) RTA is greater than in patients with primary Fanconi syndrome. In addition, "double osteomalacia" may be evident when patients with either type of RTA also have vitamin D deficiency.

Chapter **530**
Nephrogenic Diabetes Insipidus
Rajasree Sreedharan and Ellis D. Avner

Nephrogenic diabetes insipidus (NDI) is a rare congenital or, more commonly, acquired, disorder of water metabolism characterized by an inability to concentrate urine, even in the presence of antidiuretic hormone (ADH). The most common pattern of inheritance in congenital NDI is as an X-linked recessive disorder. Rarely, affected females are seen, presumably secondary to partial X-chromosome inactivation. Approximately 10% of cases of congenital NDI are inherited as autosomal dominant or recessive disorders, with males and females affected equally. The clinical phenotype of autosomal recessive forms is similar to that of the X-linked form. Secondary (acquired), either partial or complete, forms of NDI are not uncommon. They may be seen in many disorders affecting renal tubular function including obstructive uropathies, acute or chronic renal failure, renal cystic diseases, interstitial nephritis, nephrocalcinosis, or toxic nephropathy caused by hypokalemia, hypercalcemia, lithium, or amphotericin B.

PATHOGENESIS

The ability to concentrate urine (and thus absorb water) requires the delivery of urine to the collecting tubule; an intact concentrating gradient in the renal medulla; and the ability to modulate water permeability in the collecting tubule by ADH. ADH (also called arginine vasopressin [AVP]), is synthesized in the hypothalamus and stored in the posterior pituitary. Under basal situations, the collecting tubule is impermeable to water. However, in response to increased serum osmolarity (as detected by osmoreceptors in the hypothalamus) and/or severe volume depletion, ADH is released into the systemic circulation. It then binds to its receptor, vasopressin V_2 (AVPR2), on the basolateral membrane of the collecting tubule cell. Binding of the hormone to its receptor activates a cyclic adenosine monophosphate–dependent cascade that results in movement of preformed water channels (aquaporin 2 [AQP2]) to the luminal membrane of the collecting duct, rendering it permeable to water.

Defects in the *AVPR2* gene cause the more common X-linked form of NDI. Mutations in the *AQP2* gene have been identified in patients with the rarer autosomal dominant and recessive forms. Prenatal testing is available for families at risk for X-linked NDI. Patients with secondary forms of NDI can have ADH resistance owing to defective aquaporin expression (lithium intoxication). Secondary ADH resistance usually occurs as the result of loss of the hypertonic medullary gradient as a result of solute diuresis or tubular damage, resulting in the inability to absorb sodium or urea.

CLINICAL MANIFESTATIONS

Patients with congenital NDI typically present in the newborn period with massive polyuria, volume depletion, hypernatremia, and hyperthermia. Irritability and crying are common features. Constipation and poor weight gain are also seen. After multiple episodes of hypernatremic dehydration, patients can have developmental delay and mental retardation. Enuresis, caused by large urine volumes, is common. Because of the need to consume large volumes of water during the day, patients often have diminished appetite and poor food intake. However, even with adequate caloric supplementation, patients still exhibit growth abnormalities. Patients with congenital NDI also exhibit behavioral problems, including hyperactivity and short-term memory problems. Patients with the secondary form generally present later in life, primarily with hypernatremia and polyuria. Associated symptoms such as developmental delay and behavioral abnormalities are less common in this latter group.

DIAGNOSIS

The diagnosis is suggested in a male infant with polyuria, hypernatremia, and diluted urine. Simultaneous serum and urine osmolality measurements should be obtained. **If the serum osmolality value is 290 mOsm/kg or higher with a simultaneous urine osmolality value of <290 mOsm/kg, a formal water deprivation test is not necessary.** Because the differential diagnosis includes causes of **central diabetes insipidus,** the inability to respond to ADH (and thus the presence of NDI) should then be confirmed by the administration of vasopressin (10-20 μg intranasally) followed by serial urine and serum osmolality measurements hourly for 4 hr. In patients with possible "partial" or secondary diabetes insipidus, in whom the initial serum osmolality value may be <290 mOsm/kg, a water-deprivation test should be considered. Fluids should be withheld and urine and serum osmolalities measured periodically until the serum osmolality value is >290 mOsm/kg; vasopressin is then given as before. Criteria for premature termination of a water-deprivation test include a decrease in body weight of >3%. If NDI is confirmed or suspected, additional evaluation should include a detailed history to assess possible toxic exposures, determination of renal function by serum creatinine and blood urea nitrogen levels, and renal ultrasonography to identify

obstructive uropathies or cystic disease. Because of massive urine output, patients with congenital NDI can have *nonobstructive hydronephrosis* of varying severity.

TREATMENT AND PROGNOSIS

Treatment of NDI includes maintenance of adequate fluid intake and access to free water, minimizing urine output by limiting solute load with a low-osmolar, low-sodium diet, and administering medications directed at decreasing urine output. For infants, human milk or a low-solute formula, such as Similac PM 60/40, is preferred. Most infants with congenital NDI require gastrostomy or nasogastric feedings to ensure adequate fluid administration throughout the day and night. Sodium intake in older patients should be <0.7 mEq/kg/24 hr. Thiazide diuretics (2-3 mg/kg/24 hr of hydrochlorothiazide) effectively induce sodium loss and stimulate proximal tubule reabsorption of water. Potassium-sparing diuretics, in particular, amiloride (0.3 mg/kg/24 hr in 3 divided doses), are often indicated. Patients who have an inadequate response to diuretics alone might benefit from the addition of indomethacin (2 mg/kg/24 hr), which has an additive effect in reducing water excretion in some patients. Renal function must be monitored closely in such patients because indomethacin can cause deterioration in renal function over time. Patients with secondary NDI might not require medications but should have access to free water. Such patients should have serum electrolytes and volume status monitored closely, particularly during periods of superimposed acute illnesses.

Prevention of recurrent dehydration and hypernatremia in patients with congenital NDI has significantly improved the neurodevelopmental outcome of these patients. However, behavioral issues remain a significant problem. In addition, chronic use of nonsteroidal antiinflammatory drugs can predispose patients to renal insufficiency. Prognosis of patients with secondary NDI generally depends on the nature of the underlying disease.

Bibliography is available at Expert Consult.

Chapter **531**

Bartter and Gitelman Syndromes and Other Inherited Tubular Transport Abnormalities

531.1 Bartter Syndrome

Rajasree Sreedharan and Ellis D. Avner

Bartter syndrome is a group of disorders characterized by hypokalemic metabolic alkalosis with hypercalciuria and salt wasting (see Chapter 55) (Table 531-1). **Antenatal** Bartter syndrome (types I, II, and IV; also called **hyperprostaglandin E syndrome**) typically manifests in infancy and has a more-severe phenotype than **classic** Bartter syndrome (type III); perinatal onset includes maternal polyhydramnios, neonatal salt wasting, and severe episodes of recurrent dehydration. The milder

Table 531-1	Bartter and Gitelman Syndromes					
	TYPE I BARTTER SYNDROME	**TYPE II BARTTER SYNDROME**	**TYPE III BARTTER SYNDROME**	**TYPE IV BARTTER SYNDROME**	**TYPE V BARTTER SYNDROME**	**GITELMAN SYNDROME**
Inheritance	AR	AR	AR	AR	AD	AR
Affected tubular region	TAL	TAL + CCD	TAL + DCT	TAL + DCT	TAL	DCT
Gene	*SLC12A2*	*KCNJ1*	*CLCBRK*	*BSND*	*CASR*	*SLC12A3* Few have *CLCNKB*
Onset	Prenatal, postnatal	Prenatal, postnatal	Variable	Prenatal, postnatal	Variable	Adolescent, adult
Urine PGE2	Very high	Very high	Slightly elevated	Elevated	Elevated	Normal
Hypokalemic metabolic alkalosis	Present	Present	Present	Present	Present	Present
Features	Polyhydramnios, prematurity, nephrocalcinosis, dehydration, hyposthenuria, polyuria, failure to thrive	Same as type I	Failure to thrive, dehydration, salt craving, low serum magnesium in 20%, mildest form	Same as type I, with sensorineural hearing loss and no nephrocalcinosis	Hypocalcemia, low parathyroid hormone levels, hypercalciuria, uncommon cause of Bartter syndrome	Hypomagnesemia in 100%, mild dehydration, occasional growth retardation, tetany

AD, autosomal dominant; AR, autosomal recessive; CCD, cortisol collecting duct; DCT, descending convoluted tubule; PGE₂, prostaglandin E₂; TAL, thick ascending loop of Henle.

phenotype, **classic** Bartter syndrome, manifests in childhood with failure to thrive and a history of recurrent episodes of dehydration. A phenotypically related disease, Gitelman syndrome, has a distinct genetic defect and is discussed in Chapter 531.2 (Table 531-1). One distinct variant of antenatal Bartter syndrome is associated with sensorineural deafness (type IV).

PATHOGENESIS
The biochemical features of Bartter syndrome, including hypokalemic metabolic alkalosis with hypercalciuria, resemble those seen with chronic use of loop diuretics and reflect a defect in sodium, chloride, and potassium transport in the ascending loop of Henle. The loss of sodium and chloride, with resultant volume contraction, stimulates the renin–angiotensin II–aldosterone axis. Aldosterone promotes sodium uptake and potassium secretion, exacerbating the hypokalemia. It also stimulates hydrogen ion secretion distally, worsening the metabolic alkalosis. Hypokalemia stimulates prostaglandin synthesis, which further activates the renin–angiotensin II–aldosterone axis. Bartter syndrome has been associated with 5 distinct genetic defects in loop of Henle transporters (see Table 531-1). Each contributes, in some manner, to sodium and chloride transport. Mutations in the genes that encode the Na⁺/K⁺/2Cl⁻ transporter (NKCC2, the site of action of furosemide), the luminal potassium channel (ROMK), combined chloride channel (CLC-Ka, CLC-Kb), or subunit of chloride channels (barttin) cause neonatal Bartter syndrome. Isolated defects in the genes that produce a specific basolateral chloride channel (ClC-Kb) cause classic Bartter syndrome.

CLINICAL MANIFESTATIONS
A history of maternal polyhydramnios with or without prematurity may be elicited. Dysmorphic features, including triangular facies, protruding ears, large eyes with strabismus, and drooping mouth may be present on physical examination. Consanguinity suggests the presence of an autosomal recessive disorder. Older children can have a history of recurrent episodes of polyuria with dehydration, failure to thrive, nonspecific fatigue, dizziness and chronic constipation. Older children may also present with muscle cramps and weakness secondary to chronic hypokalemia. Blood pressure is usually normal, although patients with the antenatal form can have severe salt wasting, resulting

in dehydration and hypotension. Serum chemistry reveals the classic biochemical abnormalities of a hypokalemic metabolic alkalosis. Renal function is typically normal. Urinary calcium levels are typically elevated, as are urinary potassium and sodium levels. Serum renin, aldosterone, and prostaglandin E levels are often markedly elevated, particularly in the more-severe antenatal form. Nephrocalcinosis, resulting from hypercalciuria, may be seen on ultrasound examination (types I and II).

DIAGNOSIS
The diagnosis is usually made based on clinical presentation and laboratory findings. The diagnosis in the neonate or infant is suggested by severe hypokalemia, usually <2.5 mmol/L, with metabolic alkalosis. Hypercalciuria is typical; hypomagnesemia is seen in a minority of patients but is more common in Gitelman syndrome. Because features of Bartter syndrome resemble chronic use of loop diuretics, diuretic abuse should be considered in the differential diagnosis, even in young children. Chronic vomiting can also give a similar clinical picture but can be distinguished by **measurement** of **urinary chloride,** which is elevated in Bartter syndrome and low in patients with chronic vomiting. Kidneys demonstrate hyperplasia of the juxtaglomerular apparatus. Renal biopsy is rarely performed to diagnose this condition.

TREATMENT AND PROGNOSIS
Treatment of Bartter syndrome is directed at preventing dehydration, maintaining nutritional status, and correcting hypokalemia. Potassium supplementation, often at very high doses, is required; potassium-sparing (aldosterone antagonist) diuretics may be of value. Even with appropriate therapy, serum potassium values might not normalize, particularly in patients with the neonatal form. Infants and young children require a high-sodium diet and at times sodium supplementation. Indomethacin, a prostaglandin inhibitor, can also be effective. If hypomagnesemia is present, magnesium supplementation is required. With close attention to electrolyte balance, volume status, and growth, the long-term prognosis is generally good. In a minority of patients, chronic hypokalemia, nephrocalcinosis, and chronic indomethacin therapy can lead to chronic interstitial nephritis and chronic renal failure.

531.2 Gitelman Syndrome
Rajasree Sreedharan and Ellis D. Avner

Gitelman syndrome (often called a "Bartter syndrome variant") is a rare autosomal recessive cause of hypokalemic metabolic alkalosis, with distinct features of **hypocalciuria** and **hypomagnesemia.** Patients with Gitelman syndrome typically present in late childhood or early adulthood (see Table 531-1).

PATHOGENESIS
The biochemical features of Gitelman syndrome resemble those of chronic use of thiazide diuretics. Thiazides act on the sodium chloride cotransporter NCCT, present in the distal convoluted tubule. Through linkage analysis and mutational studies, defects in the gene encoding NCCT have been demonstrated in patients with Gitelman syndrome.

CLINICAL MANIFESTATIONS
Patients with Gitelman syndrome typically present at a later age than those with Bartter syndrome and may have symptoms similar to older children with Bartter syndrome (see Chapter 531.1). Patients often have a history of recurrent muscle cramps and spasms, presumably caused by low serum magnesium levels, nocturia, polyuria, and occasional hypotension. They usually do not have a history of recurrent episodes of dehydration. Biochemical abnormalities include hypokalemia, metabolic alkalosis, and hypomagnesemia. The urinary calcium level is usually very low (in contrast to the elevated urinary calcium level often seen in Bartter syndrome), and the urinary magnesium level is elevated. Renin and aldosterone levels are usually normal, and prostaglandin E secretion is not elevated. Growth failure is less prominent in Gitelman syndrome than in Bartter syndrome.

DIAGNOSIS
The diagnosis of Gitelman syndrome is suggested in an adolescent or adult presenting with hypokalemic metabolic alkalosis, hypomagnesemia, and hypocalciuria.

TREATMENT
Therapy is directed at correcting hypokalemia and hypomagnesemia with supplemental potassium and magnesium. Sodium supplementation or treatment with prostaglandin inhibitors is generally not necessary because patients typically do not have episodes of volume depletion or elevated prostaglandin E excretion.

531.3 Other Inherited Tubular Transport Abnormalities
Rajasree Sreedharan and Ellis D. Avner

Inherited abnormalities in distinct transporters in each segment of the nephron have now been identified and the molecular defects have been characterized. Renal tubular acidosis and nephrogenic diabetes insipidus are discussed in detail in Chapters 529 and 530, respectively. **Cystinuria** is an autosomal recessive disorder seen primarily in patients of Middle Eastern descent and is characterized by recurrent stone formation. The disease is caused by a defective high-affinity transporter for L-cystine and dibasic amino acids present in the proximal tubule.

Dent disease is an X-linked proximal tubulopathy with characteristic abnormalities that include low-molecular-weight proteinuria, hypercalciuria, and other features of Fanconi syndrome, such as glycosuria, aminoaciduria, and phosphaturia. Although some patients develop nephrocalcinosis, nephrolithiasis, progressive renal failure, and hypophosphatemic rickets, patients with Dent disease typically do not have proximal renal tubular acidosis or extrarenal manifestations. Loss-of-function mutations of the *CLCN5* gene, which is located in Xp11.22 and encodes a renal Cl^-/H^+ antiporter (ClC-5), are reported in patients with Dent disease. Genetic heterogeneity of Dent disease in some patients who exhibit mutations in the gene for OCRL1 (responsible for Lowe syndrome) also meets Dent disease criteria: Dent-2 disease. Dent disease includes X-linked recessive nephrolithiasis with renal failure, X-linked recessive hypophosphatemic rickets, and idiopathic low-molecular-weight proteinuria seen in Japanese children.

Mutations in an extracellular basolateral calcium-sensing receptor, normally present in the loop of Henle, can cause a **dominant Bartter syndrome–like picture.** These patients' predominant symptoms are hypocalcemic and suppressed parathyroid hormone function, which differentiates them from patients with Bartter syndrome.

In the distal convoluted tubule, gain-of-function mutations in *WNK1* and loss-of-function mutations in *WNK4*, both serine threonine kinases, lead to excessive NCCT-mediated salt reabsorption with the clinical picture of pseudohypoaldosteronism type 2 (familial hyperkalemic hypertension, or **Gordon syndrome**).

In the collecting duct, gain-of-function mutations of the gene that encodes the epithelial sodium channel cause an inherited form of hypertension, **Liddle syndrome.** Patients with this disorder have constitutive sodium uptake in the collecting duct, with hypokalemia and suppressed aldosterone. Conversely, loss-of-function mutations cause pseudohypoaldosteronism, characterized by severe sodium wasting and hyperkalemia. A variant of the latter disorder is associated with systemic abnormalities, including defects in sweat chloride, and can resemble cystic fibrosis.

Renal hypouricemia, a defect in the *SLC22A12* gene, presents with low serum uric acid levels and is complicated by exercise-induced acute renal failure. Patients have elevated urine uric acid levels and present with loin pain, nausea, and vomiting after exercise. Treatment is for acute renal failure and reducing the intensity of exercise.

Bibliography is available at Expert Consult.

Chapter 532
Tubulointerstitial Nephritis
Craig C. Porter and Ellis D. Avner

Tubulointerstitial nephritis (TIN, also called interstitial nephritis) is the term applied to conditions characterized by tubulointerstitial inflammation and damage with relative sparing of glomeruli and vessels. Both acute and chronic primary forms exist. Interstitial nephritis can also be present with primary glomerular diseases as well as systemic diseases affecting the kidney.

ACUTE TUBULOINTERSTITIAL NEPHRITIS
Pathogenesis and Pathology
The hallmarks of acute TIN are lymphocytic infiltration of the tubulointerstitium, tubular edema, and varying degrees of tubular damage. Eosinophils may be present, particularly in drug-induced TIN; occasionally, granulomas occur. The pathogenesis is not fully understood, but a T-cell–mediated immune mechanism has been postulated. A large number of medications, especially antimicrobials, anticonvulsants, and analgesics, have been implicated as etiologic agents (Table 532-1). Other causes include infections, primary glomerular diseases, and systemic diseases such as systemic lupus erythematosus.

Table 532-1	Etiology of Interstitial Nephritis

ACUTE	**CHRONIC**
Drugs	Drugs and toxins
• Antimicrobials	• Analgesics
• Penicillin derivatives	• Cyclosporine
• Cephalosporins	• Lithium
• Sulfonamides	• Heavy metals
• Trimethoprim-sulfamethoxazole	Infections (see Acute)
• Ciprofloxacin	Disease-associated
• Tetracyclines	• Metabolic and hereditary
• Vancomycin	• Cystinosis
• Erythromycin derivatives	• Oxalosis
• Rifampin	• Fabry disease
• Amphotericin B	• Wilson disease
• Acyclovir	• Sickle cell nephropathy
• Anticonvulsants	• Alport syndrome
• Carbamazepine	• Juvenile nephronophthisis, medullary cystic disease
• Phenobarbital	Immunologic
• Phenytoin	• Systemic lupus erythematosus
• Sodium valproate	• Crohn disease
• Other drugs	• Chronic allograft rejection
• Allopurinol	• Tubulointerstitial nephritis and uveitis (TINU) syndrome
• All-*trans*-retinoic acid	• Antitubular basement disease
• 5-Aminosalicylic acid	Urologic
• Cimetidine	• Posterior urethral valves
• Cyclosporine	• Eagle-Barrett syndrome
• Diuretics	• Ureteropelvic junction obstruction
• Escitalopram	• Vesicoureteral reflux
• Interferon	Miscellaneous
• Mesalazine	• Balkan nephropathy
• Quetiapine	• Radiation
• Olanzapine	• Sarcoidosis
• Nonsteroidal antiinflammatory drugs	• Neoplasm
• Protease inhibitors	Idiopathic
• Proton pump inhibitors	
• Aristolochic acid (traditional Chinese herb)	
Infections	
• Adenovirus	
• Bacteria associated with acute pyelonephritis	
• BK virus	
• *Brucella*	
• Streptococcal species	
• Cytomegalovirus	
• Epstein-Barr virus	
• Hepatitis B virus	
• Histoplasmosis	
• Human immunodeficiency virus	
• Hantavirus	
• Leptospirosis	
• *Toxoplasma gondii*	
Disease-associated	
• Glomerulonephritis (e.g., systemic lupus erythematosus)	
• Acute allograft rejection	
• Tubulointerstitial nephritis and uveitis (TINU) syndrome	
Idiopathic	

Clinical Manifestations

The classic presentation of acute TIN is fever, rash, and arthralgia in the setting of a rising serum creatinine. Although the full triad may be noted in drug-induced TIN, many patients with acute TIN do not demonstrate all of the typical features. The rash can vary from maculopapular to urticarial and is often transient. Patients often have nonspecific constitutional symptoms of nausea, vomiting, fatigue, and weight loss. Flank pain may be present, presumably secondary to stretching of the renal capsule from acute inflammatory enlargement of the kidney. If acute TIN is caused by a systemic disease such as systemic lupus erythematosus, the clinical presentation will be consistent with specific signs and symptoms of the underlying disease. Unlike the typical presentation of oliguric acute renal failure seen with glomerular diseases, 30-40% of patients with acute TIN are nonoliguric, and hypertension is less common. Peripheral eosinophilia can occur, especially with drug-induced TIN. Some degree of microscopic hematuria

is invariably present, but significant hematuria or proteinuria >1.5 g/day is uncommon. One exception is patients whose TIN is caused by nonsteroidal antiinflammatory drugs (NSAIDs), who can present with the nephrotic syndrome. Urinalysis can reveal white blood cell, granular, or hyaline casts, but red blood cell casts (a characteristic of glomerular disease) are absent. The presence of urine eosinophils is neither sensitive nor specific. *Because of pyuria, the initial diagnosis may be a urinary tract infection.*

Diagnosis

The diagnosis is usually based on clinical presentation and laboratory findings. A renal biopsy will establish the correct diagnosis in cases where the etiology or clinical course confounds the diagnosis. A careful history of the timing of disease onset in relation to drug exposure is essential in suspected drug-induced TIN. Because of the immune-mediated nature of TIN, signs or symptoms generally appear within 1-2 wk following exposure. In children, antimicrobials are a common inciting agent. NSAIDs are an important cause of acute TIN in children, and volume depletion or underlying chronic renal disease can increase the risk of occurrence. Urinalysis and serial measurements of serum creatinine and electrolytes should be monitored. Renal ultrasonography is not diagnostic but can demonstrate enlarged, echogenic kidneys. Removal of a suspected offending agent followed by spontaneous improvement in renal function is highly suggestive of the diagnosis, and additional testing is generally not performed in this setting. In more severe cases, in which the cause is unclear or the patient's renal function deteriorates rapidly, a renal biopsy is indicated.

Treatment and Prognosis
Treatment includes supportive care directed at addressing complications of acute renal failure such as hyperkalemia or volume overload (see Chapter 535.1). Corticosteroid administration within 2 wk of the discontinuation of certain offending agents (e.g., NSAIDs or antibiotics) can hasten recovery and improve the long-term prognosis in drug-induced TIN. Whether such therapy is indicated in other causes on TIN is not clear. For patients with prolonged renal insufficiency, the prognosis remains guarded, and severe acute TIN from any cause can progress to chronic TIN.

CHRONIC TUBULOINTERSTITIAL NEPHRITIS
In children, chronic TIN most commonly occurs in the context of (1) an underlying congenital urologic renal disease, such as obstructive uropathy or vesicoureteral reflux, or (2) an underlying metabolic disorder affecting the kidneys (see Table 532-1) Chronic TIN can occur as an idiopathic disease, although this is more common in adults.

The **juvenile nephronophthisis (JN)–medullary cystic kidney disease complex (MCKD)** is a group of inherited, genetically determined cystic renal diseases that share the common histologic finding of chronic TIN. At least 15 different genes are associated with JN, usually inherited as an autosomal recessive disease. These genes only define 30% of cases, and new genes are being identified at a rapid pace. Although uncommon in the United States, JN causes 10-20% of pediatric end-stage renal disease (ESRD) in Europe. Patients with JN typically present with polyuria, growth failure, unexplained anemia, and chronic renal failure in late childhood or adolescence. As a ciliopathy, JN is often associated with extrarenal features such as retinal degeneration, hepatobiliary disease, cerebellar vermis hypoplasia, laterality defects, intellectual disability, and shortening of bones. These features are represented in a number of syndromes, such as **Senior-Løken syndrome (retinitis pigmentosa), Joubert syndrome (cerebellar vermis hypoplasia), Bardet-Biedel syndrome (intellectual disability, obesity)**, and **Jeune asphyxiating thoracic dystrophy (shortening of the long bones, narrow rib cage)**, and many others. **MCKD** is an autosomal dominant disease that typically manifests in adulthood. **TIN with uveitis** is a rare autoimmune syndrome of chronic TIN with anterior uveitis and bone marrow granulomas that occurs primarily in adolescent girls. Chronic TIN is seen in all forms of progressive renal disease, regardless of the underlying cause, and the severity of interstitial disease is the single most important factor predicting progression to ESRD.

Pathogenesis and Pathology
The pathophysiology of chronic TIN is undefined, but data suggest that, in addition to abnormal cilia structure and function in JN and MCKD, it is immune mediated. Cells making up the interstitial infiltrate appear to be a combination of native interstitial cells, inflammatory cells recruited from the circulation, and resident tubular cells that undergo epithelial-mesenchymal transformation. Grossly, kidneys can appear pale and small for age. Microscopically, tubular atrophy and "dropout" with interstitial fibrosis and a patchy lymphocytic interstitial inflammation are seen. Patients with JN often have characteristic small cysts in the corticomedullary region. In primary chronic TIN, glomeruli are relatively spared until late in the disease course. Patients with chronic TIN secondary to a primary glomerular disease have histologic evidence of the primary disease.

Clinical Manifestations
The clinical features of chronic TIN are often nonspecific and can reflect signs and symptoms of chronic renal insufficiency (see Chapter 535). Fatigue, growth failure, polyuria, polydipsia, and enuresis are often present. Anemia that is seemingly disproportionate to the degree of renal insufficiency is common and is a particularly prominent feature in JN. Because tubular damage often leads to renal salt wasting, significant hypertension is unusual. Fanconi syndrome, proximal renal tubular acidosis, distal renal tubular acidosis, and hyperkalemic distal renal tubular acidosis can occur.

Diagnosis
The diagnosis is suggested by signs or symptoms of renal tubular damage such as polyuria and an elevated serum creatinine value, coupled with a history suggestive of a chronic disease, such as long-standing enuresis or the presence of anemia resistant to iron therapy. Radiographic studies, in particular ultrasonography, can give additional evidence of chronicity, such as small, echogenic kidneys, corticomedullary microcysts suggesting JN, or findings of obstructive uropathy. A vesicocystourethrogram can demonstrate the presence of vesicoureteral reflux or bladder abnormalities. If JN is suspected, molecular diagnosis is available. In instances in which the cause is unclear, a renal biopsy may be performed. In cases of advanced disease, a renal biopsy might not be diagnostic. Many end-stage kidney diseases display a common histologic appearance of tubular fibrosis and inflammation.

Treatment and Prognosis
Therapy is directed at maintaining fluid and electrolyte balance and avoiding further exposure to nephrotoxic agents. Patients with obstructive uropathies can require salt supplementation and treatment with potassium-binding resin (Kayexalate). Prevention of infection by antibiotic prophylaxis can slow progression of renal damage in appropriate patients. Prognosis in patients with chronic TIN depends in large part on the nature of the underlying disease. Patients with obstructive uropathy or vesicoureteral reflux can have a variable degree of renal damage and thus a variable course. ESRD can develop over mo to years. Patients with JN uniformly progress to ESRD by adolescence. Patients with metabolic disorders can benefit from treatment when available.

Bibliography is available at Expert Consult.

Section 5
Acute Kidney Injury and Chronic Kidney Disease

Chapter 533
Toxic Nephropathy
Craig C. Porter and Ellis D. Avner

Aberrant renal function often results from purposeful or accidental exposure to any number of agents that are potential or actual nephrotoxins. Iodinated radiocontrast agents are generally well tolerated by most patients without significant adverse consequences. In volume-depleted patients or patients with underlying chronic kidney

Table 533-1	Renal Syndromes Produced by Nephrotoxins

NEPHROTIC SYNDROME
Angiotensin-converting enzyme inhibitors
Gold salts
Interferon
Mercury compounds
Nonsteroidal antiinflammatory drugs
Penicillamine

NEPHROGENIC DIABETES INSIPIDUS
Amphotericin B
Cisplatin
Colchicine
Demeclocycline
Lithium
Methoxyflurane
Propoxyphene
Vinblastine

RENAL VASCULITIS
Hydralazine
Isoniazid
Penicillins
Propylthiouracil
Sulfonamides
Numerous other drugs that can cause a hypersensitivity reaction

THROMBOTIC MICROANGIOPATHY
Cyclosporine A
Oral contraceptive agents
Mitomycin C

NEPHROCALCINOSIS OR NEPHROLITHIASIS
Allopurinol
Bumetanide
Ethylene glycol
Furosemide
Melamine
Methoxyflurane
Topiramate
Vitamin D

ACUTE RENAL FAILURE
Acetaminophen
Acyclovir
Aminoglycosides
Amphotericin B
Angiotensin-converting enzyme inhibitors
Biologic toxins (snake, spider, bee, wasp)
Cisplatin
Cyclosporine
Ethylene glycol
Halothane
Heavy metals
Ifosfamide
Lithium
Methoxyflurane
Nonsteroidal antiinflammatory drugs
Radiocontrast agents
Tacrolimus
Vancomycin

OBSTRUCTIVE UROPATHY
Sulfonamides
Acyclovir
Methotrexate
Protease inhibitors
Ethylene glycol
Methoxyflurane

FANCONI SYNDROME
Aminoglycosides
Chinese herbs (aristolochic)
Cisplatin
Heavy metals (cadmium, lead, mercury, and uranium)
Ifosfamide
Lysol
Outdated tetracycline

RENAL TUBULAR ACIDOSIS
Amphotericin B
Lead
Lithium
Toluene

INTERSTITIAL NEPHRITIS
Amidopyrine
p-Aminosalicylate
Carbon tetrachloride
Cephalosporins
Cimetidine
Cisplatin
Colistin
Copper
Cyclosporine
Ethylene glycol
Foscarnet
Gentamicin
Gold salts
Indomethacin
Interferon-α
Iron
Kanamycin
Lithium
Mannitol
Mercury salts
Mitomycin C
Neomycin
Nonsteroidal antiinflammatory drugs
Penicillins (especially methicillin)
Pentamidine
Phenacetin
Phenylbutazone
Poisonous mushrooms
Polymyxin B
Radiocontrast agents
Rifampin
Salicylate
Streptomycin
Sulfonamides
Tacrolimus
Tetrachloroethylene
Trimethoprim-sulfamethoxazole

disease, their use poses a serious risk for the development of acute kidney injury with significant attendant morbidity and mortality. Biologic nephrotoxins include venomous exposures from insects, reptiles, amphibians, and a wide variety of sea-dwelling animals. The most common forms of toxic nephropathy unfortunately relate to the exposure of children to pharmacologic agents, accounting for close to 20% of episodes of acute kidney injury occurring in children and adolescents. Age, underlying medical condition, including surgical exposure, genetics, exposure dose, and the concomitant use of other drugs all influence the likelihood of developing acute kidney injury.

Table 533-1 summarizes the agents that commonly cause acute kidney injury and some of their clinical manifestations. Mechanisms of injury often help to explain the presentation; multiple toxic exposures in patients with complicated clinical histories often limit the ability to clearly establish clinical cause and effect. For example, diminished urine output may be the clinical hallmark of tubular obstruction caused by agents such as methotrexate or agents that cause acute tubular necrosis, such as amphotericin B or pentamidine. Alternatively, nephrogenic diabetes insipidus may be the critical clinical manifestation of agents that cause interstitial nephritis, such as lithium or cisplatin. Nephrotoxicity is often reversible if the noxious agent is promptly removed.

Clinical use of potential nephrotoxins should be used judiciously. Necessity of exposure, dosing parameters, and the use of drug levels or pharmacogenomic data, when available, should always be considered. Caution is particularly mandated for patients with complex medical conditions that include preexisting renal disease, cardiac disease, diabetes, and/or complicated surgeries. Alternative approaches to imaging, or use of different pharmacologic options should be considered when possible. Imaging modalities such as ultrasonography, radionuclide scanning, or magnetic resonance imaging may be preferable to contrast studies in some patients. Alternatively, judicious volume expansion with or without the administration of N-acetylcysteine might offer renoprotection when radioiodinated contrast studies are critical. Pharmacologic agents with no known renal effects can often be substituted for known nephrotoxins with equal clinical efficacy. In all cases, simultaneous use of known nephrotoxins should be avoided whenever necessary.

Bibliography is available at Expert Consult.

Chapter 534
Cortical Necrosis
Priya Pais and Ellis D. Avner

Renal cortical necrosis is a rare cause of acute renal failure occurring secondary to extensive ischemic damage of the renal cortex. It occurs most commonly in neonates and in adolescents of childbearing age (see Chapter 535).

ETIOLOGY
In newborns, cortical necrosis is most commonly associated with hypoxic or ischemic insults caused by perinatal asphyxia, placental abruption, and twin–twin or fetal-maternal transfusion. Other causes include renal vascular thrombosis and severe congenital heart disease. After the neonatal period, cortical necrosis is most commonly seen in children with septic shock or severe hemolytic-uremic syndrome. In adolescents and women, cortical necrosis occurs in association with obstetric complications including prolonged intrauterine fetal death, placental abruption, or amniotic fluid embolism.

Less-common causes of cortical necrosis include malaria, extensive burns, snakebites, infectious endocarditis, and medications (e.g., nonsteroidal antiinflammatory agents). Acute renal cortical necrosis has also been reported to occur in systemic lupus erythematosus–associated antiphospholipid antibody syndrome.

CLINICAL MANIFESTATIONS
Cortical necrosis clinically presents as acute renal failure in patients with predisposing causes. Urine output is diminished and gross and/or microscopic hematuria may be present. Hypertension is common, and thrombocytopenia may be present as a result of renal microvascular injury.

LABORATORY AND RADIOLOGIC FINDINGS
Laboratory results are consistent with acute renal failure: an elevated blood urea nitrogen and creatinine, hyperkalemia, and metabolic acidosis. Anemia and thrombocytopenia are common. Urinalysis reveals hematuria and proteinuria.

Ultrasound examination with Doppler flow studies or CT scan demonstrates decreased perfusion to both kidneys. A radionuclide renal scan shows decreased uptake with significantly delayed or absent function.

TREATMENT
It is important to prevent or treat the underlying cause of acute cortical necrosis, when possible. Therapy involves medical management of acute renal failure, often with the initiation of dialysis as indicated. Management is otherwise supportive and involves volume repletion, correction of asphyxia, and treatment of sepsis.

PROGNOSIS
Untreated, renal cortical necrosis has a high mortality rate. Twenty to 40% of patients have partial recovery of renal function, the extent of which depends on the amount of preserved cortical tissue. All patients require long-term follow-up for chronic kidney disease.

Bibliography is available at Expert Consult.

Chapter 535
Renal Failure

535.1 Acute Kidney Injury
Rajasree Sreedharan and Ellis D. Avner

Acute kidney injury (AKI), formerly called acute renal failure, is a clinical syndrome in which a sudden deterioration in renal function results in the inability of the kidneys to maintain fluid and electrolyte homeostasis. AKI occurs in 2-3% of children admitted to pediatric tertiary care centers and in as many as 8% of infants in neonatal intensive care units. A classification system has been proposed to standardize the definition of AKI in adults. These criteria of **risk**, **injury**, **failure**, **loss**, and **end-stage renal disease** were given the acronym of RIFLE. A modified RIFLE criteria (pRIFLE) was developed to characterize the pattern of AKI in critically ill children (Table 535-1). Because RIFLE focuses on the glomerular filtration rate (GFR), a modification (Acute Kidney Injury Network) categorizes severity by rise in serum creatinine: stage 1 >150%, stage II >200%, stage III >300%.

PATHOGENESIS
AKI has been conventionally classified into 3 categories: prerenal, intrinsic renal, and postrenal (Table 535-2 and Fig. 535-1).

Table 535-1	Pediatric-Modified Rifle (pRIFLE) Criteria	
CRITERIA	**ESTIMATED CCL**	**URINE OUTPUT**
Risk	eCCl decrease by 25%	<0.5 mL/kg/hr for 8 hr
Injury	eCCl decrease by 50%	<0.5 mL/kg/hr for 16 hr
Failure	eCCl decrease by 75% or eCCl <35 mL/min/1.73 m²	<0.3 mL/kg/hr for 24 hr or anuric for 12 hr
Loss	Persistent failure >4 wk	
End-stage	End-stage renal disease (persistent failure >3 mo)	

CCl, creatinine clearance; eCCl, estimated creatinine clearance; pRIFLE, pediatric risk, injury, failure, loss, and end-stage renal disease.

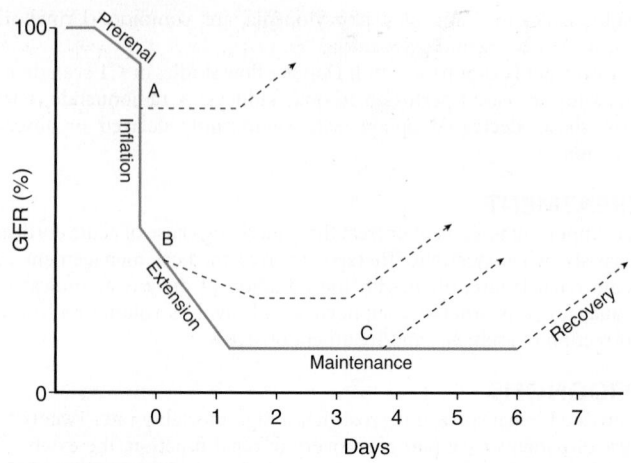

Figure 535-1 Phases of acute kidney injury. GFR, glomerular filtration rate. *(From Sutton TA, Fisher CJ, Molitoris BA. Microvascular endothelial injury and dysfunction during ischemic acute renal failure, Kidney Int 62:1539–1549, 2002.)*

Table 535-2	Common Causes of Acute Kidney Injury

PRERENAL
Dehydration
Hemorrhage
Sepsis
Hypoalbuminemia
Cardiac failure

INTRINSIC RENAL
Glomerulonephritis
- Postinfectious/poststreptococcal
- Lupus erythematosus
- Henoch-Schönlein purpura
- Membranoproliferative
- Anti–glomerular basement membrane
Hemolytic-uremic syndrome
Acute tubular necrosis
Cortical necrosis
Renal vein thrombosis
Rhabdomyolysis
Acute interstitial nephritis
Tumor infiltration
Tumor lysis syndrome

POSTRENAL
Posterior urethral valves
Ureteropelvic junction obstruction
Ureterovesicular junction obstruction
Ureterocele
Tumor
Urolithiasis
Hemorrhagic cystitis
Neurogenic bladder

Prerenal AKI, also called *prerenal azotemia,* is characterized by diminished effective circulating arterial volume, which leads to inadequate renal perfusion and a decreased GFR. Evidence of kidney damage is absent. Common causes of prerenal AKI include dehydration, sepsis, hemorrhage, severe hypoalbuminemia, and cardiac failure. If the underlying cause of the renal hypoperfusion is reversed promptly, renal function returns to normal. If hypoperfusion is sustained, intrinsic renal parenchymal damage can develop.

Intrinsic renal AKI includes a variety of disorders characterized by renal parenchymal damage, including sustained hypoperfusion and ischemia. Many forms of **glomerulonephritis,** including postinfectious glomerulonephritis, lupus nephritis, Henoch-Schönlein purpura nephritis, membranoproliferative glomerulonephritis, and anti–glomerular basement membrane nephritis, can cause AKI. Ischemic/

hypoxic injury and nephrotoxic insults are the most common causes of intrinsic AKI in the United States, and are more common with an underlying comorbid condition; most are associated with cardiac, oncologic, urologic, renal, and genetic disorders or prematurity. Severe and prolonged ischemic/hypoxic injury and nephrotoxic insult lead to **acute tubular necrosis (ATN),** seen most often in critically ill infants and children. Mechanisms leading to ischemic AKI include hypotension/intravascular volume depletion (hemorrhage, third-space fluid losses, diarrhea), decreased effective intravascular volume (heart failure, cirrhosis, hepatorenal syndrome, peritonitis, abdominal compartment syndrome), vasodilation/vasoconstriction (sepsis, hepatorenal syndrome), renal artery obstruction (thrombosis, embolization, stenosis), intrarenal artery disease (vasculitis, hemolytic-uremic syndrome, sickle cell anemia, transplant rejection), and impaired renal blood flow (cyclosporine, tacrolimus, angiotensin-converting enzyme [ACE] inhibitors, angiotensin-receptor blocking agents, radiocontrast agents).

The typical pathologic feature of ATN is tubular cell necrosis, although significant histologic changes are not consistently seen in patients with clinical ATN. The mechanisms of injury in ATN can include alterations in intrarenal hemodynamics, tubular obstruction, and passive backleak of the glomerular filtrate across injured tubular cells into the peritubular capillaries.

Tumor lysis syndrome is a specific form of AKI related to spontaneous or chemotherapy-induced cell lysis in patients with lymphoproliferative malignancies. This disorder is primarily caused by obstruction of the tubules by uric acid crystals (see Chapters 495 and 496). **Acute interstitial nephritis** is another common cause of AKI and is usually a result of a hypersensitivity reaction to a therapeutic agent or various infectious agents (see Chapter 532).

Postrenal AKI includes a variety of disorders characterized by obstruction of the urinary tract. In neonates and infants, congenital conditions, such as posterior urethral valves and bilateral ureteropelvic junction obstruction, account for the majority of cases of AKI. Other conditions, such as urolithiasis, tumor (intraabdominal lesion or within the urinary tract), hemorrhagic cystitis, and neurogenic bladder, can cause AKI in older children and adolescents. In a patient with 2 functioning kidneys, obstruction must be bilateral to result in AKI. Relief of the obstruction usually results in recovery of renal function, except in patients with associated renal dysplasia or prolonged urinary tract obstruction.

CLINICAL MANIFESTATIONS AND DIAGNOSIS

A carefully taken history is critical in defining the cause of AKI. An infant with a 3 day history of vomiting and diarrhea most likely has prerenal AKI caused by volume depletion, but hemolytic-uremic syndrome (HUS) must be a consideration. A 6 yr old child with a recent pharyngitis who presents with periorbital edema, hypertension, and gross hematuria most likely has intrinsic AKI related to acute postinfectious glomerulonephritis. A critically ill child with a history of protracted hypotension or with exposure to nephrotoxic medications most likely has ATN. A neonate with a history of hydronephrosis on prenatal ultrasound and a palpable bladder most likely has congenital urinary tract obstruction, probably related to posterior urethral valves.

The physical examination must be thorough, with careful attention to volume status. Tachycardia, dry mucous membranes, and poor peripheral perfusion suggest an inadequate circulating volume and the possibility of prerenal AKI (see Chapter 57). Hypertension, peripheral edema, rales, and a cardiac gallop suggest volume overload and the possibility of intrinsic AKI from glomerulonephritis or ATN. The presence of a rash and arthritis might indicate systemic lupus erythematosus (SLE) or Henoch-Schönlein purpura nephritis. Palpable flank masses may be seen with renal vein thrombosis, tumors, cystic disease, or urinary tract obstruction.

LABORATORY FINDINGS

Laboratory abnormalities can include anemia (the anemia is usually dilutional or hemolytic, as in SLE, renal vein thrombosis,

| Table 535-3 | Urinalysis, Urine Chemistries, and Osmolality in Acute Kidney Injury |

	HYPOVOLEMIA	ACUTE TUBULAR NECROSIS	ACUTE INTERSTITIAL NEPHRITIS	GLOMERULONEPHRITIS	OBSTRUCTION
Sediment	Bland	Broad, brownish granular casts	White blood cells, eosinophils, cellular casts	Red blood cells, red blood cell casts	Bland or bloody
Protein	None or low	None or low	Minimal but may be increased with NSAIDs	Increased, >100 mg/dL	Low
Urine sodium, mEq/L*	<20	>30	>30	<20	<20 (acute) >40 (few days)
Urine osmolality, mOsm/kg	>400	<350	<350	>400	<350
Fractional excretion of sodium %†	<1	>1	Varies	<1	<1 (acute) >1 (few days)

*The sensitivity and specificity of urine sodium of <20 mEq/L in differentiating prerenal azotemia from acute tubular necrosis are 90% and 82%, respectively.
†Fractional excretion of sodium is the urine:plasma (U:P) ratio of sodium divided by U:P of creatinine ×100. The sensitivity and specificity of fractional excretion of sodium of <1% in differentiating prerenal azotemia from acute tubular necrosis are 96% and 95%, respectively.
NSAIDs, nonsteroidal antiinflammatory drugs.
From Singri N, Ahya SN, Levin ML: Acute renal failure, JAMA 289:747–751, 2003.

HUS); leukopenia (SLE, sepsis); thrombocytopenia (SLE, renal vein thrombosis, sepsis, HUS); hyponatremia (dilutional); metabolic acidosis; elevated serum concentrations of blood urea nitrogen, creatinine, uric acid, potassium, and phosphate (diminished renal function); and hypocalcemia (hyperphosphatemia).

The serum C3 level may be depressed (postinfectious glomerulonephritis, SLE, or membranoproliferative glomerulonephritis), and antibodies may be detected in the serum to streptococcal (poststreptococcal glomerulonephritis), nuclear (SLE), neutrophil cytoplasmic (granulomatosis with polyangiitis, microscopic polyarteritis), or glomerular basement membrane (Goodpasture disease) antigens.

The presence of hematuria, proteinuria, and red blood cell or granular urinary casts suggests intrinsic AKI, in particular glomerular disease and ATN. The presence of white blood cells and white blood cell casts with low-grade hematuria and proteinuria suggests tubulointerstitial disease. Urinary eosinophils may be present in children with drug-induced tubulointerstitial nephritis.

Urinary indices may be useful in differentiating prerenal AKI from intrinsic AKI (Table 535-3). Patients whose urine shows an elevated specific gravity (>1.020), elevated urine osmolality (UOsm > 500 mOsm/kg), low urine sodium (UNa < 20 mEq/L), and fractional excretion of sodium <1% (<2.5% in neonates) most likely have prerenal AKI. Those with a specific gravity of <1.010, low urine osmolality (UOsm < 350 mOsm/kg), high urine sodium (UNa > 40 mEq/L), and fractional excretion of sodium >2% (>10% in neonates) most likely have intrinsic AKI.

Chest radiography may reveal cardiomegaly, pulmonary congestion (fluid overload), or pleural effusions. Renal ultrasonography can reveal hydronephrosis and/or hydroureter, which suggest urinary tract obstruction, or nephromegaly, consistent with intrinsic renal disease. Renal biopsy can ultimately be required to determine the precise cause of AKI in patients who do not have clearly defined prerenal or postrenal AKI.

Although serum creatinine is used to measure kidney function, it is an insensitive and delayed measure of decreased kidney function following AKI. Other biomarkers under investigation include changes in plasma neutrophil gelatinase–associated lipocalin and cystatin C levels and urinary changes in neutrophil gelatinase-associated lipocalin, interleukin 18, and kidney injury molecule-1.

TREATMENT
Medical Management
In infants and children with urinary tract obstruction, such as in a newborn with suspected posterior ureteral valves, a bladder catheter should be placed immediately to ensure adequate drainage of the urinary tract. The placement of a bladder catheter may also

be considered in nonambulatory older children and adolescents to accurately monitor urine output during AKI; however, precautions to prevent iatrogenic infection should be taken.

Determination of the volume status is of critical importance when initially evaluating a patient with AKI. If there is no evidence of volume overload or cardiac failure, intravascular volume should be expanded by intravenous administration of isotonic saline, 20 mL/kg over 30 min. In the absence of blood loss or hypoproteinemia, colloid-containing solutions are not required for volume expansion. Severe hypovolemia may require additional fluid boluses (see Chapters 56, 57, and 70). Determination of the central venous pressure may be helpful if adequacy of the blood volume is difficult to determine. After volume resuscitation, hypovolemic patients generally void within 2 hr; failure to do so suggests intrinsic or postrenal AKI. Hypotension caused by sepsis requires vigorous fluid resuscitation followed by a continuous infusion of norepinephrine.

Diuretic therapy should be considered only after the adequacy of the circulating blood volume has been established. Furosemide (2-4 mg/kg) and mannitol (0.5 g/kg) may be administered as a single IV dose. Bumetanide (0.1 mg/kg) may be given as an alternative to furosemide. If urine output is not improved, then a continuous diuretic infusion may be considered. To increase renal cortical blood flow, many clinicians administer dopamine (2-3 μg/kg/min) in conjunction with diuretic therapy, although no controlled data support this practice. There is little evidence that diuretics or dopamine can prevent AKI or hasten recovery. Mannitol may be effective in prevention of pigment (myoglobin, hemoglobin)-induced renal failure. Atrial natriuretic peptide may be of value in preventing or treating AKI, although there is little pediatric evidence to support its use.

If there is no response to a diuretic challenge, diuretics should be discontinued and fluid restriction is essential. Patients with a relatively normal intravascular volume should initially be limited to 400 mL/m²/24 hr (insensible losses) plus an amount of fluid equal to the urine output for that day. Extrarenal (blood, gastrointestinal tract) fluid losses should be replaced, milliliter for milliliter, with appropriate fluids. Markedly hypervolemic patients can require further fluid restriction, omitting the replacement of insensible fluid losses, urine output, and extrarenal losses to diminish the expanded intravascular volume. Fluid intake, urine and stool output, body weight, and serum chemistries should be monitored on a daily basis.

In AKI, rapid development of **hyperkalemia** (serum potassium level > 6 mEq/L) can lead to cardiac arrhythmia, cardiac arrest, and death. The earliest electrocardiographic change seen in patients with developing hyperkalemia is the appearance of peaked T waves. This may be followed by widening of the QRS intervals, ST segment depression, ventricular arrhythmias, and cardiac arrest (see Chapter 55.4).

Procedures to deplete body potassium stores should be initiated when the serum potassium value rises to >6.0 mEq/L. Exogenous sources of potassium (dietary, intravenous fluids, total parenteral nutrition) should be eliminated. Sodium polystyrene sulfonate resin (Kayexalate), 1 g/kg, should be given orally or by retention enema. This resin exchanges sodium for potassium and can take several hr to take effect. A single dose of 1 g/kg can be expected to lower the serum potassium level by about 1 mEq/L. Resin therapy may be repeated every 2 hr, the frequency being limited primarily by the risk of sodium overload.

More severe elevations in serum potassium (>7 mEq/L), especially if accompanied by electrocardiographic changes, require emergency measures in addition to Kayexalate. The following agents should be administered:

- Calcium gluconate 10% solution, 1.0 mL/kg IV, over 3-5 min
- Sodium bicarbonate, 1-2 mEq/kg IV, over 5-10 min
- Regular insulin, 0.1 units/kg, with glucose 50% solution, 1 mL/kg, over 1 hr

Calcium gluconate counteracts the potassium-induced increase in myocardial irritability but does not lower the serum potassium level. Administration of sodium bicarbonate, insulin, or glucose lowers the serum potassium level by shifting potassium from the extracellular to the intracellular compartment. A similar effect has been reported with the acute administration of β-adrenergic agonists in adults, but there are no controlled data in pediatric patients. Because the duration of action of these emergency measures is just a few hours, persistent hyperkalemia should be managed by dialysis.

Mild **metabolic acidosis** is common in AKI because of retention of hydrogen ions, phosphate, and sulfate, but it rarely requires treatment. If acidosis is severe (arterial pH < 7.15; serum bicarbonate < 8 mEq/L) or contributes to significant hyperkalemia, treatment is indicated. The acidosis should be corrected partially by the intravenous route, generally giving enough bicarbonate to raise the arterial pH to 7.20 (which approximates a serum bicarbonate level of 12 mEq/L). The remainder of the correction may be accomplished by oral administration of sodium bicarbonate after normalization of the serum calcium and phosphorus levels. Correction of metabolic acidosis with intravenous bicarbonate can precipitate tetany in patients with renal failure as rapid correction of acidosis reduces the ionized calcium concentration (see Chapter 55).

Hypocalcemia is primarily treated by lowering the serum phosphorus level. Calcium should not be given intravenously, except in cases of tetany, to avoid deposition of calcium salts into tissues. Patients should be instructed to follow a low-phosphorus diet, and phosphate binders should be orally administered to bind any ingested phosphate and increase GI phosphate excretion. Common agents include sevelamer (Renagel), calcium carbonate (Tums tablets or Titralac suspension), and calcium acetate (PhosLo). Aluminum-based binders, commonly employed in the past, should be avoided because of the risk of aluminum toxicity.

Hyponatremia is most commonly a dilutional disturbance that must be corrected by fluid restriction rather than sodium chloride administration. Administration of hypertonic (3%) saline should be limited to patients with symptomatic hyponatremia (seizures, lethargy) or those with a serum sodium level <120 mEq/L. Acute correction of the serum sodium to 125 mEq/L (mmol/L) should be accomplished using the following formula:

mEq sodium required
$$= 0.6 \times \text{weight in kg} \times (125 - \text{serum sodium in mEq/L}).$$

AKI patients are predisposed to **GI bleeding** because of uremic platelet dysfunction, increased stress, and heparin exposure if treated with hemodialysis or continuous renal replacement therapy. Oral or intravenous H_2 blockers such as ranitidine are commonly administered to prevent this complication.

Hypertension can result from hyperreninemia associated with the primary disease process and/or expansion of the extracellular fluid volume and is most common in AKI patients with acute glomerulonephritis or HUS. Salt and water restriction is critical, and diuretic administration may be useful (see Chapter 445). Isradipine (0.05-0.15 mg/kg/dose, maximum dose 5 mg qid) may be administered for relatively rapid reduction in blood pressure. Longer-acting agents such as calcium channel blockers (amlodipine, 0.1-0.6 mg/kg/24 hr qd or divided bid) or β blockers (propranolol, 0.5-8.0 mg/kg/24 hr divided bid or tid; labetalol, 4-40 mg/kg/24 hr divided bid or tid) may be helpful in maintaining control of blood pressure. Children with severe symptomatic hypertension (hypertensive urgency or emergency) should be treated with continuous infusions of nicardipine (0.5-5.0 μg/kg/min), sodium nitroprusside (0.5-10.0 μg/kg/min), labetalol (0.25-3.0 mg/kg/hr), or esmolol (150-300 μg/kg/min) and converted to intermittently dosed antihypertensives when more stable.

Neurologic symptoms in AKI can include headache, seizures, lethargy, and confusion (encephalopathy). Potential etiologic factors include hypertensive encephalopathy, hyponatremia, hypocalcemia, cerebral hemorrhage, cerebral vasculitis, and the uremic state. Benzodiazepams are the most effective agents in acutely controlling seizures, and subsequent therapy should be directed toward the precipitating cause.

The **anemia** of AKI is generally mild (hemoglobin 9-10 g/dL) and primarily results from volume expansion (hemodilution). Children with HUS, SLE, active bleeding, or prolonged AKI can require transfusion of packed red blood cells if their hemoglobin level falls below 7 g/dL. In hypervolemic patients, blood transfusion carries the risk of further volume expansion, which can precipitate hypertension, heart failure, and pulmonary edema. Slow (4-6 hr) transfusion with packed red blood cells (10 mL/kg) diminishes the risk of hypervolemia. The use of fresh, washed red blood cells minimizes the acute risk of hyperkalemia, and the chronic risk of sensitization if the patient becomes a future candidate for renal replacement therapy. In the presence of severe hypervolemia or hyperkalemia, blood transfusions are most safely administered during dialysis or ultrafiltration.

Nutrition is of critical importance in children who develop AKI. In most cases, sodium, potassium, and phosphorus should be restricted. Protein intake should be moderately restricted while maximizing caloric intake to minimize the accumulation of nitrogenous wastes. In critically ill patients with AKI, parenteral hyperalimentation with essential amino acids should be considered.

Dialysis

Indications for dialysis in AKI include the following:

- Anuria/oliguria
- Volume overload with evidence of hypertension and/or pulmonary edema refractory to diuretic therapy
- Persistent hyperkalemia
- Severe metabolic acidosis unresponsive to medical management
- Uremia (encephalopathy, pericarditis, neuropathy)
- Blood urea nitrogen >100-150 mg/dL (or lower if rapidly rising)
- Calcium:phosphorus imbalance, with hypocalcemic tetany that cannot be controlled by other measures

An additional indication for dialysis is the inability to provide adequate nutritional intake because of the need for severe fluid restriction. In patients with AKI, dialysis support may be necessary for days or for up to 12 wk. Many patients with AKI require dialysis support for 1-3 wk. Table 535-4 lists the advantages and disadvantages of the 3 types of dialysis.

Intermittent hemodialysis is useful in patients with relatively stable hemodynamic status. This highly efficient process accomplishes both fluid and electrolyte removal in 3-4 hr sessions using a pump-driven extracorporeal circuit and large central venous catheter. Intermittent hemodialysis may be performed 3-7 times per week based on the patient's fluid and electrolyte balance.

Peritoneal dialysis is most commonly employed in neonates and infants with AKI, although this modality may be used in children and adolescents of all ages. Hyperosmolar dialysate is infused into the peritoneal cavity via a surgically or percutaneously placed peritoneal dialysis catheter. The fluid is allowed to dwell for 45-60 min and is then drained from the patient by gravity (manually or with the use of machine-driven cycling), accomplishing fluid and electrolyte removal. Cycles are repeated for 8-24 hr/day based on the patient's fluid and electrolyte balance. Anticoagulation is not necessary. Peritoneal dialysis is contraindicated in patients with significant abdominal pathology.

Continuous renal replacement therapy (CRRT) is useful in patients with unstable hemodynamic status, concomitant sepsis, or multiorgan failure in the intensive care setting. CRRT is an extracorporeal therapy in which fluid, electrolytes, and small- and medium-size solutes are continuously removed from the blood (24 hr/day) using a specialized pump-driven machine. Usually, a double-lumen catheter is placed into the subclavian, internal jugular, or femoral vein. The patient is then connected to the pump-driven CRRT circuit, which continuously passes the patient's blood across a highly permeable filter.

CRRT may be performed in 3 basic fashions. In continuous venovenous hemofiltration, a large volume of fluid is driven by systemic or pump-assisted pressure across the filter, bringing with it by convection other molecules such as urea, creatinine, phosphorus, and uric acid. The blood volume is reconstituted by IV infusion of a replacement fluid having a desirable electrolyte composition similar to that of blood. Continuous venovenous hemofiltration dialysis uses the principle of diffusion by circulating dialysate in a countercurrent direction on the ultrafiltrate side of the membrane. No replacement fluid is used. Continuous hemodiafiltration employs both replacement fluid and dialysate, offering the most effective solute removal of all forms of CRRT.

Table 535-4 compares the relative risks and benefits of the various renal replacement therapies.

PROGNOSIS

The mortality rate in children with AKI is variable and depends entirely on the nature of the underlying disease process rather than on the renal failure itself. Children with AKI caused by a renal-limited condition such as postinfectious glomerulonephritis have a very low mortality rate (<1%); those with AKI related to multiorgan failure have a very high mortality rate (>90%).

The prognosis for recovery of renal function depends on the disorder that precipitated AKI. Recovery of renal function is likely after AKI resulting from prerenal causes ATN, acute interstitial nephritis, or tumor lysis syndrome. Recovery of renal function is unusual when AKI results from most types of rapidly progressive glomerulonephritis,

bilateral renal vein thrombosis, or bilateral cortical necrosis. Medical management may be necessary for a prolonged period to treat the sequelae of AKI, including chronic renal insufficiency, hypertension, renal tubular acidosis, and urinary concentrating defect.

Bibliography is available at Expert Consult.

535.2 Chronic Kidney Disease
Rajasree Sreedharan and Ellis D. Avner

Chronic kidney disease (CKD) is determined by the presence of kidney damage and level of kidney function (GFR), irrespective of diagnosis. The stage of the CKD is assigned based on the level of kidney function (Tables 535-5 and 535-6). The prevalence of CKD in the pediatric population is approximately 18 per 1 million. The prognosis for the infant, child, or adolescent with CKD has improved dramatically since the 1970s because of improvements in medical management (aggressive nutritional support, recombinant erythropoietin, recombinant growth hormone), dialysis techniques, and kidney transplantation.

ETIOLOGY
In children, CKD may be the result of congenital, acquired, inherited, or metabolic renal disease, and the underlying cause correlates closely with the age of the patient at the time when CKD is first detected. CKD in children <5 yr old is most commonly a result of congenital abnormalities such as renal hypoplasia, dysplasia, or obstructive uropathy. Additional causes include congenital nephrotic syndrome, prune belly syndrome, cortical necrosis, focal segmental glomerulosclerosis, autosomal recessive polycystic kidney disease, renal vein thrombosis, and HUS.

After 5 yr of age, acquired diseases (various forms of glomerulonephritis including lupus nephritis) and inherited disorders (familial

Table 535-4	Comparison of Peritoneal Dialysis, Intermittent Hemodialysis, and Continual Renal Replacement Therapy		
	PD	**IHD**	**CRRT**
BENEFITS			
Fluid removal	+	++	++
Urea and creatinine clearance	+	++	+
Potassium clearance	++	++	+
Toxin clearance	+	++	+
COMPLICATIONS			
Abdominal pain	+	−	−
Bleeding	−	+	+
Dysequilibrium	−	+	−
Electrolyte imbalance	+	+	+
Need for heparinization	−	+	+/−
Hyperglycemia	+	−	−
Hypotension	+	++	+
Hypothermia	−	−	+
Central line infection	−	+	+
Inguinal or abdominal hernia	+	−	−
Peritonitis	+	−	−
Protein loss	+	−	−
Respiratory compromise	+	−	−
Vessel thrombosis	−	+	+

PD, peritoneal dialysis; IHD, intermittent hemodialysis; CRRT, continual renal replacement therapy.
Adapted from Rogers MC: Textbook of pediatric intensive care, Baltimore, 1992, Williams & Wilkins.

Table 535-5	Criteria for Definition of Chronic Kidney Disease (NKF KDOQI Guidelines)

Patient has CKD if either of the following criteria are present:
1. Kidney damage for ≥3 mo, as defined by structural or functional abnormalities of the kidney, with or without decreased GFR, manifested by 1 or more of the following features:
   - Abnormalities in the composition of the blood or urine
   - Abnormalities in imaging tests
   - Abnormalities on kidney biopsy
2. GFR <60 mL/min/1.73 m² for ≥3 mo, with or without the other signs of kidney damage described above

NKF KDOQI, National Kidney Foundation Kidney Disease Outcomes Quality Initiative.

Table 535-6	Standardized Terminology for Stages of Chronic Kidney Disease (NKF KDOQI Guidelines)	
STAGE	**DESCRIPTION**	**GFR (mL/min/1.73 m²)**
1	Kidney damage with normal or increased GFR	>90
2	Kidney damage with mild decrease in GFR	60-89
3	Moderate decrease in GFR	30-59
4	Severe decrease in GFR	5-29
5	Kidney failure	<15 or on dialysis

GFR, glomerular filtration rate; NKF KDOQI, National Kidney Foundation Kidney Disease Outcomes Quality Initiative.

juvenile nephronophthisis, Alport syndrome) predominate. CKD related to metabolic disorders (cystinosis, hyperoxaluria) and certain inherited disorders (both autosomal dominant and recessive polycystic kidney disease) can occur throughout the childhood years.

PATHOGENESIS

In addition to progressive injury with ongoing structural or metabolic genetic diseases, renal injury can progress despite removal of the original insult.

Hyperfiltration injury may be an important final common pathway of glomerular destruction, independent of the underlying cause of renal injury. As nephrons are lost, the remaining nephrons undergo structural and functional hypertrophy characterized by an increase in glomerular blood flow. The driving force for glomerular filtration is thereby increased in the surviving nephrons. Although this compensatory hyperfiltration temporarily preserves total renal function, it can cause progressive damage to the surviving glomeruli, possibly by a direct effect of the elevated hydrostatic pressure on the integrity of the capillary wall and/or the toxic effect of increased protein traffic across the capillary wall. Over time, as the population of sclerosed nephrons increases, the surviving nephrons suffer an increased excretory burden, resulting in a vicious cycle of increasing glomerular blood flow and hyperfiltration injury.

Proteinuria itself can contribute to renal functional decline. Proteins that traverse the glomerular capillary wall can exert a direct toxic effect on tubular cells and recruit monocytes and macrophages, enhancing the process of glomerular sclerosis and tubulointerstitial fibrosis. Uncontrolled **hypertension** can exacerbate disease progression by causing arteriolar nephrosclerosis and by increasing the hyperfiltration injury.

Hyperphosphatemia can increase progression of disease by leading to calcium phosphate deposition in the renal interstitium and blood vessels. Hyperlipidemia, a common condition in CKD patients, can adversely affect glomerular function through oxidant-mediated injury.

CKD may be viewed as a continuum of disease, with increasing biochemical and clinical manifestations as renal function deteriorates. Regardless of etiology, the progression of tubulointerstitial fibrosis is the primary determinant of progression of CKD. Table 535-7 outlines the pathophysiologic manifestations of CKD. End-stage renal disease (ESRD) is an administrative term in the United States; it is used to define all patients who are treated with dialysis or kidney transplantation. Patients with ESRD are a subset of the patients with stage 5 CKD.

CLINICAL MANIFESTATIONS

The clinical presentation of CKD is varied and depends on the underlying renal disease. Children and adolescents with CKD from chronic glomerulonephritis can present with edema, hypertension, hematuria, and proteinuria. Infants and children with congenital disorders such as renal dysplasia and obstructive uropathy can present in the neonatal period with failure to thrive, polyuria, dehydration, urinary tract infection, or overt renal insufficiency. Congenital kidney disease is diagnosed with prenatal ultrasonography in many infants, allowing early diagnostic and possible therapeutic intervention. Children with familial juvenile nephronophthisis can have a very subtle presentation with nonspecific complaints such as headache, fatigue, lethargy, anorexia, vomiting, polydipsia, polyuria, and growth failure over a number of years.

The physical examination in patients with CKD can reveal pallor and a sallow appearance. Patients with long-standing untreated CKD can have short stature and the bony abnormalities of renal osteodystrophy (see Chapter 529.4). Children with CKD caused by chronic glomerulonephritis (or children with advanced renal failure from any cause) can have edema, hypertension, and other signs of extracellular fluid volume overload.

LABORATORY FINDINGS

Laboratory findings can include elevations in blood urea nitrogen and serum creatinine and can reveal hyperkalemia, hyponatremia (if

Table 535-7	Pathophysiology of Chronic Kidney Disease
MANIFESTATION	**MECHANISMS**
Accumulation of nitrogenous waste products	Decrease in glomerular filtration rate
Acidosis	Decreased ammonia synthesis Impaired bicarbonate reabsorption Decreased net acid excretion
Sodium retention	Excessive renin production Oliguria
Sodium wasting	Solute diuresis Tubular damage
Urinary concentrating defect	Solute diuresis Tubular damage
Hyperkalemia	Decrease in glomerular filtration rate Metabolic acidosis Excessive potassium intake Hyporeninemic hypoaldosteronism
Renal osteodystrophy	Impaired renal production of 1,25-dihydroxycholecalciferol Hyperphosphatemia Hypocalcemia Secondary hyperparathyroidism
Growth retardation	Inadequate caloric intake Renal osteodystrophy Metabolic acidosis Anemia Growth hormone resistance
Anemia	Decreased erythropoietin production Iron deficiency Folate deficiency Vitamin B_{12} deficiency Decreased erythrocyte survival
Bleeding tendency	Defective platelet function
Infection	Defective granulocyte function Impaired cellular immune functions Indwelling dialysis catheters
Neurologic symptoms (fatigue, poor concentration, headache, drowsiness, memory loss, seizures, peripheral neuropathy)	Uremic factor(s) Aluminum toxicity Hypertension
Gastrointestinal symptoms (feeding intolerance, abdominal pain)	Gastroesophageal reflux Decreased gastrointestinal motility Serositis (uremia)
Hypertension	Volume overload Excessive renin production
Hyperlipidemia	Decreased plasma lipoprotein lipase activity
Pericarditis, cardiomyopathy	Uremic factor(s) Hypertension Fluid overload
Glucose intolerance	Tissue insulin resistance

volume overloaded), hypernatremia (loss of free water), acidosis, hypocalcemia, hyperphosphatemia, and an elevation in uric acid. Patients with heavy proteinuria can have hypoalbuminemia. A complete blood cell count may show a normochromic, normocytic anemia. Serum cholesterol and triglyceride levels are often elevated. In children with CKD caused by glomerulonephritis, the urinalysis shows hematuria and proteinuria. In children with CKD from congenital lesions such as renal dysplasia, the urinalysis usually has a low specific gravity and minimal abnormalities by dipstick or microscopy.

Inulin clearance is the gold standard to determine GFR, but it is not easy to measure. Endogenous creatinine clearance is the most widely used marker of GFR, but creatinine secretion falsely elevates the calculated GFR. Several other markers are under investigation to accurately determine GFR in children, such as cystatin C and iohexol. In children age 1-16 yr, the degree of renal dysfunction may be determined by applying a new bedside formula that estimates GFR between 15 and 75 mL/min/1.73 m²: estimated GFR = 0.43 × height in cm/serum creatinine in mg/dL

TREATMENT

The treatment of CKD is aimed at replacing absent or diminished renal functions, which progressively deteriorate in parallel with the progressive loss of GFR, and slowing the progression of renal dysfunction. Children with CKD should be treated at a pediatric center capable of supplying multidisciplinary services, including medical, nursing, social service, nutritional, and psychological support.

The management of CKD requires close monitoring of a patient's clinical and laboratory status. Blood studies to be followed routinely include serum electrolytes, blood urea nitrogen, creatinine, calcium, phosphorus, albumin, alkaline phosphatase, and hemoglobin levels. Periodic measurement of intact parathyroid hormone (PTH) levels and roentgenographic studies of bone may be of value in detecting early evidence of renal osteodystrophy. Echocardiography should be performed periodically to identify left ventricular hypertrophy and cardiac dysfunction that can occur as a consequence of the complications of CKD.

Nutrition

Nutritional management by a dietician experienced in pediatric renal patients is recommended by the National Kidney Foundation Kidney Disease Outcomes Quality Initiative (NKF KDOQI). Counseling based on individualized assessment should be considered for all children and their families with CKD stages 2 to 5 and 5D. Patients should receive 100% of estimated energy requirement for age, individually adjusted for physical activity level, body mass index, and response in rate of weight gain or loss. When oral supplemental nutrition with increased calories or fluid volume is insufficient, tube feeding should be considered. Calories should be balanced between carbohydrate, unsaturated fat in physiological ranges (per dietary reference intake [DRI]), and protein. Protein intake recommendation is 100-140% of the DRI for ideal weight for children with stage 3 CKD, 100-120% of the DRI in stages 4 and 5 CKD, and 100% with allowance for dialysis loss in CKD stage 5D, with use of commercial supplements as needed. Children with CKD stages 2-5 should receive 100% of DRI of vitamins and trace elements; water-soluble vitamin supplements are often required in CKD stage 5D.

Renal Osteodystrophy

The term *renal osteodystrophy* is used to indicate a spectrum of bone disorders seen in patients with CKD. The most common condition seen in children is high-turnover bone disease caused by secondary hyperparathyroidism. The skeletal pathologic finding in this condition is osteitis fibrosa cystica.

The **pathophysiology** of renal osteodystrophy is complex. Early in the course of CKD, when the GFR declines to approximately 50% of normal, the decrease in functional kidney mass leads to a decline in renal 1α-hydroxylase activity, with decreased production of activated vitamin D (1,25-dihydroxycholecalciferol). This deficiency in activated vitamin D results in decreased intestinal calcium absorption, hypocalcemia, and increased parathyroid gland activity. Excessive PTH secretion attempts to correct the hypocalcemia by increasing bone resorption. Later in the course of CKD, when the GFR declines to 20-25% of normal, compensatory mechanisms that have been operative to enhance renal phosphate excretion become inadequate, resulting in hyperphosphatemia, which further promotes hypocalcemia and increased PTH secretion.

Clinical manifestations of renal osteodystrophy include muscle weakness, bone pain, and fractures with minor trauma. In growing children, rachitic changes, varus and valgus deformities of the long bones, and slipped capital femoral epiphyses may be seen. Laboratory studies can demonstrate a decreased serum calcium level and increased serum phosphorus, alkaline phosphatase, and PTH levels. Radiographs of the hands, wrists, and knees show subperiosteal resorption of bone with widening of the metaphyses.

The goals of **treatment** are to prevent bone deformity and normalize growth velocity using both dietary and pharmacologic interventions. The target phosphorus level for adolescents is between 3.5 and 5.5 mg/dL, and for children 1-12 yr of age it is 4-6 mg/dL. Children and adolescents should follow a low-phosphorus diet, and infants should be provided with a low-phosphorus formula such as Similac PM 60/40. It is impossible to fully restrict phosphorus intake, and so phosphate binders are used to enhance GI phosphate excretion. Although calcium-based binders have historically been the most commonly used, non–calcium-based binders such as sevelamer (Renagel) are increasing in use, particularly in older children and adolescent patients who are prone to hypercalcemia. Because aluminum may be absorbed from the GI tract and can lead to aluminum toxicity, aluminum-based binders should be avoided.

The cornerstone of therapy for renal osteodystrophy is vitamin D administration. **Vitamin D therapy** is indicated in patients with 1,25-dihydroxy-vitamin D levels below the established goal range for the child's particular stage of CKD or in patients with PTH levels above the established goal range for CKD stage. Patients with low 1,25-dihydroxy-vitamin D and elevated PTH levels should be treated with 0.01-0.05 µg/kg/24 hr of calcitriol (Rocaltrol, 0.25-µg capsules or 1 µg/mL suspension). Newer activated vitamin D analogs such as paricalcitol and doxercalciferol are increasingly useful, especially in patients who are predisposed to hypercalcemia. Phosphate binders and vitamin D should be adjusted to maintain the PTH level within the designated goal range and the serum calcium and phosphorus levels within the normal range for age. Many nephrologists also attempt to maintain the calcium/phosphorus product (Ca × PO₄) at <55 mg²/dL² in adolescents and <65 mg²/dL² in younger children to minimize the possibility of tissue deposition of calcium phosphorus salts with consequent damage.

Adynamic Bone Disease

Adynamic bone disease (low-turnover bone disease) has been recognized in children and adults with CKD. The pathologic finding is osteomalacia and is associated with oversuppression of PTH, perhaps related to the widespread use of calcium-containing phosphate binders and vitamin D analogs.

Fluid and Electrolyte Management

Most children with CKD maintain normal sodium and water balance, with the sodium intake derived from an appropriate diet. Infants and children whose CKD is a consequence of renal dysplasia may be polyuric, with significant urinary sodium or free water losses. These children may benefit from high-volume, low-caloric-density feedings with sodium supplementation. Children with high blood pressure, edema, or heart failure may require sodium restriction and diuretic therapy. Fluid restriction is rarely necessary in children with CKD until the development of ESRD requires the initiation of dialysis.

In most children with CKD, potassium balance is maintained until renal function deteriorates to the level at which dialysis is initiated. Hyperkalemia can develop, however, in patients with moderate renal insufficiency who have excessive dietary potassium intake, severe acidosis, or hyporeninemic hypoaldosteronism (related to destruction of the renin-secreting juxtaglomerular apparatus). Hyperkalemia may be treated by restriction of dietary potassium intake, administration of oral alkalinizing agents, and/or treatment with Kayexalate.

Acidosis

Metabolic acidosis develops in almost all children with CKD as a result of decreased net acid excretion by the failing kidneys. Either Bicitra

(1 mEq sodium citrate/mL) or sodium bicarbonate tablets (650 mg = 8 mEq of base) may be used to maintain the serum bicarbonate level >22 mEq/L.

Growth

Short stature is a significant long-term sequela of childhood CKD. Children with CKD have an apparent growth hormone–resistant state, with elevated growth hormone levels but decreased insulin-like growth factor 1 levels and major abnormalities of insulin-like growth factor–binding proteins.

Children with CKD who remain less than −2 SD for height despite optimal medical support (adequate caloric intake and effective treatment of renal osteodystrophy, anemia, and metabolic acidosis) might benefit from treatment with pharmacologic doses of recombinant human growth hormone (rHuGH). Treatment may be initiated with rHuGH (0.05 mg/kg/24 hr) subcutaneously, with periodic adjustment in the dose to achieve a goal of normal height velocity for age.

Treatment with rHuGH continues until the patient reaches the 50th percentile for midparental height, achieves a final adult height, or undergoes kidney transplantation. Long-term rHuGH treatment significantly improves final adult height and induces persistent catch-up growth; some patients achieve normal adult height.

Anemia

Anemia in patients with CKD is primarily the result of inadequate erythropoietin production by the failing kidneys and usually becomes manifest in patients with stages 3-4 CKD.

Other possible contributory factors include iron deficiency, folic acid or vitamin B_{12} deficiency, and decreased erythrocyte survival. Recombinant human erythropoietin (rHuEPO) therapy has decreased the need for transfusion in patients with CKD. Erythropoietin is usually initiated when the patient's hemoglobin concentration falls below 10 g/dL, at a dose of 50-150 mg/kg/dose subcutaneously 1-3 times weekly. The dose is adjusted to maintain the hemoglobin concentration between 11 and 12 g/dL. All patients receiving rHuEPO therapy should be provided with either oral or intravenous iron supplementation. Patients who appear to be resistant to rHuEPO should be evaluated for iron deficiency, occult blood loss, a chronic infection or inflammatory state, vitamin B_{12} or folate deficiency, or bone marrow fibrosis related to secondary hyperparathyroidism. An alternative option to rHuEPO is darbepoetin alfa (Aranesp), a longer-acting agent administered at a dose of 0.45 μg/kg/wk. The chief advantage of this agent is that it may be dosed once weekly to once monthly because of its extended duration of action.

Hypertension

Children with CKD can have sustained hypertension related to volume overload and/or excessive renin production related to glomerular disease. Hypertensive children with suspected volume overload should follow a salt-restricted diet (<2 g/24 hr) and may benefit from diuretic therapy. Thiazide diuretics (hydrochlorothiazide 2 mg/kg/24 hr divided bid) are the initial diuretic class of choice for children with mild renal dysfunction (CKD stages 1-3). However, when a patient's estimated GFR falls below this range, thiazides are ineffective and loop diuretics (furosemide 1-2 mg/kg/dose bid or tid) become the diuretic class of choice. **ACE inhibitors** (enalapril, lisinopril) and **angiotensin II receptor blockers** (losartan) are the antihypertensive medications of choice in all children with proteinuric renal disease because of their potential ability to decrease proteinuria and slow the progression to ESRD (by mechanisms still not completely delineated). Extreme care must be used with these agents, however, to monitor renal function and electrolyte balance, particularly in children with advanced CKD. Calcium channel blockers (amlodipine), β-blockers (propranolol, atenolol), and centrally acting agents (clonidine) may be useful as adjunctive agents in children with CKD whose blood pressure cannot be controlled using dietary sodium restriction, diuretics, and ACE inhibitors.

Immunizations

Children with CKD should receive all standard immunizations according to the schedule used for healthy children. An exception must be made in withholding live virus vaccines from children with CKD related to glomerulonephritis, or any disease, during treatment with immunosuppressive medications. It is critical, however, to make every attempt to administer live virus vaccines for measles, mumps, rubella, and varicella before kidney transplantation. These vaccines are not advised for use in immunosuppressed patients. All children with CKD should receive a yearly influenza vaccine. Data from a number of studies suggest that children with CKD might respond suboptimally to immunizations.

Adjustment In Drug Dose

Because many drugs are excreted by the kidneys, their dosing might need to be adjusted in patients with CKD to maximize effectiveness and minimize the risk of toxicity. Strategies in dosage adjustment include lengthening of the interval between doses or decreasing the absolute dose, or both. Such adjustments become even more important as pharmacogenomic profiling of drug metabolism becomes routine.

Progression of Disease

Although there are no definitive treatments to improve renal function in children or adults with CKD other than treatment of a specific underlying disorder when possible, there are several general strategies that may be effective in slowing the rate of progression of renal dysfunction. Optimal control of hypertension (maintaining the blood pressure at lower than the 75th percentile and perhaps even lower) is critical in all patients with CKD. ACE inhibitors or angiotensin II receptor blockers should be the antihypertensive drugs of choice in hypertensive children with chronic proteinuric renal disease as previously noted. Such agents should also be strongly considered in children with CKD who have significant proteinuria, even in the absence of hypertension, although there are no controlled studies to support this approach. Serum phosphorus should be maintained within the normal range for age and the calcium–phosphorus product <55 to minimize renal calcium–phosphorus deposition. Prompt treatment of infectious complications and episodes of dehydration can minimize additional loss of renal parenchyma.

Other potentially beneficial recommendations include correction of anemia with erythropoietin or darbepoetin alfa therapy, control of hyperlipidemia, avoidance of cigarette smoking, prevention of obesity, and avoidance of nonsteroidal antiinflammatory and other potential nephrotoxic medications. This includes a variety of illegal street drugs as well as herbal and/or homeopathic medications or "supplements." Although dietary protein restriction may be useful in adults, this recommendation is generally not suggested for children with CKD because of the concern about adverse effects on growth and development.

Bibliography is available at Expert Consult.

535.3 End-Stage Renal Disease

Rajasree Sreedharan and Ellis D. Avner

ESRD represents the state in which a patient's renal dysfunction has progressed to the point at which homeostasis and survival can no longer be sustained with native kidney function and maximal medical management. At this point, renal replacement therapy (dialysis or renal transplantation) becomes necessary. The ultimate goal for children with ESRD is successful kidney transplantation (see Chapter 536) because it provides the most normal lifestyle and possibility for rehabilitation for the child and family.

In the United States, 75% of children with ESRD require a period of dialysis before transplantation can be performed. It is recommended that plans for renal replacement therapy be initiated when a child reaches stage 4 CKD. The optimal time to actually initiate dialysis, however, is based on a combination of the biochemical and clinical characteristics of the patient including refractory fluid overload, electrolyte imbalance, acidosis, growth failure, or uremic symptoms, including fatigue, nausea, and impaired school performance. In general, most nephrologists attempt to initiate dialysis early enough to prevent the development of severe fluid and electrolyte abnormalities, malnutrition, and uremic symptoms. Preemptive transplantation before initiation of dialysis is increasingly being utilized.

The selection of dialysis modality must be individualized to fit the needs of each child. In the United States, two thirds of children with ESRD are treated with peritoneal dialysis, whereas one third are treated with hemodialysis. Age is a defining factor in dialysis modality selection: 88% of infants and children from birth to 5 yr of age are treated with peritoneal dialysis, and 54% of children >12 yr of age are treated with hemodialysis.

Peritoneal dialysis is a technique that employs the patient's peritoneal membrane as a dialyzer. Excess body water is removed by an osmotic gradient created by the high dextrose concentration in the dialysate; wastes are removed by diffusion from the peritoneal capillaries into the dialysate. Access to the peritoneal cavity is achieved by a surgically inserted, tunneled catheter.

Peritoneal dialysis may be provided either as continuous ambulatory peritoneal dialysis or as an automated therapy using a cycler (continuous cyclic peritoneal dialysis, intermittent peritoneal dialysis, or nocturnal intermittent peritoneal dialysis). The majority of U.S. children treated with peritoneal dialysis use cycler-driven therapy, which allows the child and family to be free of dialysis demands during the waking hours. The exchanges are performed automatically during sleep by machine. This permits an uninterrupted day of activities, a reduction in the number of dialysis catheter connections and disconnections (which decreases the risk of peritonitis), and a reduction in the time required by patients and parents to perform dialysis, reducing the risk of fatigue and burnout. Because peritoneal dialysis is not as efficient as hemodialysis, it must be performed daily rather than 3 times weekly. Table 535-8 outlines the benefits of peritoneal dialysis.

Hemodialysis, unlike peritoneal dialysis, is usually performed in a hospital setting. Children and adolescents typically have 3 treatments (3-4 hr each) per wk during which fluid and solute wastes are removed. Access to the child's circulation is achieved by a surgically created arteriovenous fistula, graft, or indwelling subclavian or internal jugular catheter.

Bibliography is available at Expert Consult.

Chapter 536
Renal Transplantation
Minnie M. Sarwal

Kidney transplantation is the optimal therapy for children with end-stage renal disease (ESRD). Five yr survival rates in children who receive a kidney transplant are greater than survival rates of those who remain on hemodialysis or peritoneal dialysis. Children and adolescents with ESRD have special needs that differ from adults, including the need to achieve normal growth and cognitive development. Successful transplantation leads to improvement in their linear growth and allows them to attend school and be free of dietary restrictions. Immunosuppression protocols that employ steroid minimization or avoidance after transplantation demonstrate dramatic improvements in growth patterns for young children after transplantation. Improvements in surgical techniques and a reduction in the early complications of thrombosis have given young children the best long-term outcomes of all age groups among transplant recipients.

INCIDENCE AND ETIOLOGY
The incidence of ESRD in pediatric patients in the United States varies by age group (Table 536-1). There is an adjusted incident rate of 14.4 per million population for ages 0-19 yr.

The etiology of ESRD in children varies significantly by age (Table 536-2). Congenital, hereditary, and cystic diseases cause ESRD in more than 52% of children 0-4 yr of age, whereas glomerulonephritis and focal segmental glomerulosclerosis (FSGS) account for 38% of cases of ESRD in patients 10-19 yr of age. The most common diagnosis in children with *transplanted kidneys* is structural disease (49%), followed by various forms of glomerulonephritis (14%) and FSGS (12%).

INDICATIONS
Almost all children with ESRD are considered to be candidates for renal transplantation. There are very few absolute contraindications for pediatric kidney transplantation. Relative contraindications include children with preexisting metastatic malignancy or HIV. Patients with remission of malignancy off maintenance treatment for a minimum of 2 yr may be reconsidered on an individual basis for transplantation, with close posttransplantation surveillance. Similarly, patients with autoimmune diseases resulting in ESRD are candidates for transplantation after a period of immunologic quiescence of the primary disease for a period of at least 1 yr before transplantation. Another relative contraindication includes severe neurologic dysfunction, but the wishes of the parents and the potential for rehabilitation must be considered.

Table 535-8	Merits of Peritoneal Dialysis in Pediatric Patients with End-Stage Renal Disease

ADVANTAGES
Ability to perform dialysis treatment at home
Technically easier than hemodialysis, especially in infants
Ability to live a greater distance from medical center
Freedom to attend school and after-school activities
Less-restrictive diet
Less expensive than hemodialysis
Independence (adolescents)

DISADVANTAGES
Catheter malfunction
Catheter-related infections (peritonitis, exit site)
Impaired appetite (due to full peritoneal cavity)
Negative body image
Caregiver burnout

Table 536-1	Incident Rates of Reported ESRD in the United States	
AGE RANGE (YR)		**ADJUSTED INCIDENT RATES* PER MILLION POPULATION**
0-4		9.5
5-9		6.1
10-14		13
15-19		29

*Rates are adjusted for sex and race.
ESRD, end-stage renal disease.
From U.S. Renal Data System, USRDS 2009 Annual data report: atlas of end-stage renal disease in the United States, *National Institutes of Health, National Institute of Diabetes and Digestive and Kidney Diseases, Bethesda, MD, 2009, www.usrds.org.*

Table 536-2	Common Causes of ESRD in Pediatric Transplant Recipients (N = 9854)
CAUSES	**% OF RECIPIENTS**
Aplasia, hypoplasia, dysplasia	15.9
Obstructive uropathy	15.6
Focal segmental glomerulosclerosis	11.7
Reflux nephropathy	5.2
Chronic glomerulonephritis	3.3
Polycystic disease	2.9
Medullary cystic disease	2.8
Hemolytic-uremic syndrome	2.6
Prune belly syndrome	2.6
Congenital nephrotic syndrome	2.6
Familial nephritis	2.3
Cystinosis	2.0
Idiopathic crescentic glomerulonephritis	1.7
MPGN type I	1.7
Berger (IgA) nephritis	1.3
Henoch-Schönlein nephritis	1.1
MPGN type II	0.8

ESRD, end-stage renal disease; MPGN, membranoproliferative glomerulonephritis.

Data from the North American Pediatric Renal Trials and Collaborative Studies, https://web.emmes.com/study/ped/.

Renal transplantation is considered for any child when renal replacement therapy is indicated. In children, dialysis may be required for a period before transplantation to optimize nutritional and metabolic conditions, to achieve an appropriate size in small children, or to keep a patient stable until a suitable donor is available. For young infants, a recipient may need to weigh at least 8-10 kg to minimize the risk for vascular thrombosis and to accommodate an adult-size kidney. This can require a period of dialysis support until the child is at least 12-18 mo of age. Transplantation with an adult-size kidney has been successful in children who weighed <10 kg or were <6 mo of age.

Preemptive transplantation (i.e., transplantation without prior dialysis) continues to account for approximately 25% of all pediatric renal transplants, based mostly on a desire by the child and the family to avoid dialysis. There may be a small benefit in allograft outcome if transplantation occurs without prior dialysis, which might relate to a lower incidence of infections and cardiovascular risk factors. Preemptive renal transplant should be considered when the glomerular filtration rate (GFR) is <10-15 mL/min/1.73 m² and with symptomatic ESRD or rapidly declining GFR and need for dialysis within 6-12 mo. The rates of preemptive transplantation differ moderately for different age groups, being 20% for recipients age ≤2 yr, 24% for age 2-5 yr, 28% for age 6-12 yr, and 22% for age 13-17 yr.

CHARACTERISTICS OF DONORS AND RECIPIENTS

Almost half of all pediatric kidney transplants come from living donors. The highest rates of transplantation are in the 5-9 yr old group, with 40 live donor transplants and 46 cadaver donor transplants performed per 100 dialysis patient-years. The Organ Procurement and Transplantation Network (OPTN) provides preference for children waiting for a deceased-donor renal transplant. Owing to improved outcomes in deceased-donor pediatric transplantation using donors 5-35 yr of age, OPTN in 2005 implemented a pediatric kidney allocation policy that gave priority for kidneys from deceased donors <35 yr of age. These kidneys were assigned to recipients <18 yr, after 0

mismatch transplants, recipients with a panel reactive antibody >80, or candidates receiving a kidney with a nonrenal origin. This policy shortened the wait time for children versus adults and is associated with improved outcomes.

Living-donor kidney transplantation graft survival has improved over the years, and from 2003-2007 the graft survival rate in living-donor renal transplants was 96.1%, unchanged from the 1999-2002 rate of 95.9%. Graft survival rates for deceased donors from 2003-2007 are 94.4%, also improved from 92.7% in 1999-2002. For children awaiting deceased-donor renal transplants the goals are to minimize waiting times, transplanting kidneys into children 0-6 yr of age within 6 mo, children 7-12 yr within 12 mo, and children 12-18 yr within 18 mo.

EVALUATION AND PREPARING FOR TRANSPLANTATION

The team approach includes evaluations by a transplantation surgeon, nephrologist, nutritionist, social worker, psychologist, financial counselor, pretransplantation nurse, and dialysis nurse (if the patient is undergoing dialysis).

Primary renal disease can recur in a number of renal diseases, but it is not a contraindication to transplantation. Recurrent disease in the renal graft accounts for graft loss in almost 7% of primary transplantations and 10% in repeat transplantations.

With FSGS and primary oxalosis, patients are at risk for major renal function impairment with recurrence of disease. Grafts in approximately 20-30% of patients with the diagnosis of FSGS fail because the disease recurs. In patients with the original disease of FSGS whose grafts fail, the mean time to failure is 17 mo. Alport syndrome can recur as an anti–glomerular basement membrane (anti-GBM) glomerulonephritis in approximately 3-4% of patients after transplantation and lead to graft loss. Histologic evidence of recurrence of membranoproliferative glomerulonephritis type I varies widely, from 20% to 70%, and graft loss can occur in ≤30% of cases. Histologic recurrence of membranoproliferative glomerulonephritis type II disease occurs in virtually all cases, with graft loss in ≤50% of cases. Histologic recurrence with mesangial immunoglobulin (Ig) A deposits is common and occurs in about half of the patients with IgA nephropathy and in approximately 30% of patients with Henoch-Schönlein purpura. Congenital nephrotic syndrome rarely recurs after transplantation, although patients can develop antinephrin antibodies and present with nephrotic syndrome. Some cases (~25%) of nephrotic syndrome after transplantation are likely de novo. Membranous nephropathy occurs very rarely in children. The recurrence rate after kidney transplantation for patients who have been treated for Wilms tumor is approximately 13%.

Owing to the high risk of developing Wilms tumor, patients with Denys-Drash syndrome should undergo bilateral nephrectomy before transplantation. Other *indications for bilateral native nephrectomies* include hyposthenuria with polyuria, significant proteinuria, and severe hypertension resistant to medical management. Nephrectomies are also indicated in cases such as polycystic kidney disease, where more room may be needed to place the transplanted kidney and to create space in the abdominal cavity to improve feeding tolerability and the infant's ability to thrive.

Failure to maintain adequate perfusion of the adult-size kidney, secondary to a "perfusion steal" by the native kidneys results in a histologic picture of "chronic" acute tubular necrosis and a negative impact on graft function.

Urologic problems, such as vesicoureteral reflux, posterior urethral valves, abnormal urinary bladders, and/or neurogenic bladders, should be addressed before surgery. Malformations and voiding abnormalities (e.g., neurogenic bladder, bladder dyssynergia, remnant posterior urethral valves, and urethral strictures) should be identified and repaired if possible. Children with urologic disease and renal dysplasia often require multiple operations to optimize urinary tract anatomy and function. Such procedures include ureteric reimplantation to correct vesicoureteral reflux, bladder augmentation or reconstruction, creation of a vesicocutaneous fistula by using the appendix to provide a simple, continent, and cosmetically acceptable way for intermittent catheterization (Mitrofanoff procedure), and excision of duplicated systems or ectopic ureteroceles that could cause recurrent infections. There are reports of excellent outcomes often being achieved in posterior urethral valve bladders by following a staged procedure of initial valve resection to limit any injury to the posterior urethra, and bladder rehabilitation, without the requirement of augmentation, by a process of regimented double voiding.

A comprehensive **nutritional assessment** needs to be done to ensure that optimal nutritional status is achieved before transplant. Many children with ESRD and especially those on dialysis require nutritional supplements to provide them with sufficient protein and calories. Infants and young children on dialysis often require nasogastric or gastric tube feedings to overcome decreased oral intake from nausea and anorexia due to uremia. Optimal outcomes result from transplanting adult-size kidneys from living donors when the child weighs ≥10 kg.

Bone disease needs to be evaluated for and treated before transplantation. Secondary hyperparathyroidism needs to be treated before transplant to avoid posttransplant urinary phosphate wasting and hypercalcemia. High calcium phosphorus product before transplantation leads to vascular stiffness and calcifications, increasing the patient's risk for cardiovascular disease.

In the United States, >25% of the mortality in children on maintenance dialysis is a result of **cardiovascular disease**. Cardiac death is the leading cause of death in young patients after transplant in childhood. Therefore, evaluation of cardiac function is required before a kidney transplant in a pediatric patient to be sure that patient has sufficient cardiac function to tolerate the large fluid load that accompanies kidney transplantation. All patients being evaluated for kidney transplant have at least an echocardiogram and electrocardiogram. Hypertension is common and can result from fluid overload and/or intrinsic native renal disease. Blood pressure needs to be under optimal control before transplant. If blood pressure cannot be controlled with medical management, bilateral nephrectomy may need to be performed before transplant to control the hyperreninemic response from the failing kidneys.

Anemia needs to be treated before transplantation. Most patients are taking erythropoietin, folate, and iron to maintain goals for hemoglobin levels between 11 and 12 g/dL. Blood transfusions should be avoided owing to concerns for sensitizing the patient to human leukocyte antigens before transplant. If a blood transfusion is required, patients should receive cytomegalovirus negative, leukoreduced red blood cells. Blood should not be irradiated owing to concerns for trauma to the cells and potential for increased antigen exposure.

Evaluation for **venous thrombosis** and **hypercoagulable states** is important before renal transplantation. The third leading cause of graft failure is vascular thrombosis; the leading causes are chronic (34.9%) and acute (13.1%) rejection. Risk factors for graft thrombosis include surgical technique, perfusion and reperfusion injury of graft, young donor age (<2 yr), young recipient (<5 yr), cold ischemia time >24 hr, arterial hypotension, prior history of peritoneal dialysis, and/or hypoperfusion of adult kidney transplant in a small child. Particularly in the young recipient, before transplantation, there needs to be evaluation for thrombosis of iliac vessels or inferior vena cava if the patient has had previous surgery or central line placement. Femoral line catheterizations greatly increase the risk for inferior vena cava thrombosis. Children who have large protein losses, such as from nephrotic syndrome and/or peritoneal dialysis, can be at increased risk for thrombosis because of protein loss, such as protein S, protein C, and antithrombin III. Doppler ultrasound, computed tomographic angiography, and magnetic resonance angiography have all been used to evaluate vessels. Magnetic resonance angiography has been used less owing to the concern about exposure to gadolinium and nephrogenic systemic fibrosis. In patients with renal compromise receiving contrast media, intravenous hydration is needed before and after the study for patients with residual renal function, acidosis should be corrected before giving contrast, and N-acetyl cysteine should be administered before and after the CT angiogram to reduce the risk of contrast nephropathy. If the patient is on dialysis, dialysis clearance can be done after contrast administration; hemodialysis is the optimal method for clearance.

Infections need to be identified and treated before transplantation. Infectious disease screening includes a complete history of household contacts with treatment for active or latent tuberculosis, vaccine history for varicella and pertussis, travel history within the past 2 yr and/or if there was significant time spent in another country, history of bacille Calmette-Guérin, animal and/or insect exposure, sexual activity, and consumption of high-risk foods such as unpasteurized products. Screening includes tuberculosis skin test (purified protein derivative), cytomegalovirus IgG, Epstein-Barr virus (EBV) antibody panel, varicella titer, measles antibody, hepatitis B serologies, hepatitis C antibody, HIV, and toxoplasmosis. Additional testing for patients who lived in or visited the central valleys of California, Utah, Nevada, Arizona, and/or New Mexico includes *Coccidioides* immunodiffusion. Patients from the Ohio River valley should also have *Histoplasma* antibody checked. Patients from Mexico should have *Coccidioides* immunodiffusion, *Histoplasma* antibody, and ova and parasite screen to evaluate for *Strongyloides*. Those from South America should have *Coccidioides* immunodiffusion, *Histoplasma* antibody, and *Toxoplasma* antibody. Sexually active patients should also be screened for syphilis, gonorrhea, HIV, and *Chlamydia*.

Immunizations need to be up to date before transplantation. All live vaccines need to be given before transplantation because these vaccines should not be given to immunosuppressed patients. Therefore, measles-mumps-rubella and varicella should be given before transplant and antibody titers should be checked to monitor for response. Measles-mumps-rubella may be given as early as 6 mo of age. Inhaled influenza vaccine should not be given to transplant patients, family members, or healthcare providers.

Psychiatric evaluation should be performed before transplantation to evaluate patients' and their families' ability to cope with the stressors that accompany caring for a child with a kidney transplant. A psychologist should also evaluate the patient and their caregivers for depression, substance abuse, and/or noncompliance so that problems can be identified and managed before kidney transplantation. If noncompliance is identified or anticipated, interventions should be in place before transplantation. These should include social and psychiatric interventions, where possible.

Children need 2 ABO blood types checked before being listed for a kidney transplantation and a donor should be sought who shares HLA-A, HLA-B, and/or HLA-DR antigens. The 2008 North American Pediatric Renal Trials and Collaborative Studies (NAPRTCS) data have shown increased risk for rejection and graft failure with 2-DR mismatch compared to a 0-DR mismatch. The recipient's blood is also checked to see if the patient is sensitized. Patients can become sensitized by prior transplant, blood transfusions, sepsis, and/or pregnancy.

IMMUNOSUPPRESSION

Most pediatric kidney transplant centers employ a combination of drug therapy consisting of a calcineurin inhibitor and corticosteroids with or without an antiproliferative agent. Approximately 80% of transplantation patients receive a 3-drug regimen at 6 mo after transplantation. The rationale for this combination therapy in children is to provide effective immunosuppression and at the same time minimize the toxicity of any single drug.

Induction Therapy

Induction therapy is commonly used in pediatric renal transplant recipients to prevent acute rejection. Graft survival rates are higher in patients treated with antilymphocyte induction therapy. Acute rejection episodes are approximately 30% less frequent and tend to occur later. Induction therapy may consist of T-cell antibodies, interleukin-2 receptor antibodies, and/or therapies that target B cells.

T-Cell Antibodies

Antithymocyte globulin (ATGAM) and Thymoglobulin are polyclonal antibodies that should be given intravenously through a central line to avoid sclerosis and injury to smaller vessels. These medications are used to prevent the development of the first rejection. Thymoglobulin is polyclonal antibodies against human T-lymphocyte antigens resulting in a rapid depletion of T lymphocytes. Some limit the use of Thymoglobulin induction to sensitized high-risk patients or patients who have concerns for delayed graft function and want to avoid high calcineurin inhibitor levels in the early postoperative period. Dosage is 1.5-2.0 mg/kg/dose, with daily monitoring of CD3$^+$ subsets; the dose should not be given if the CD3$^+$ count exceeds 20 cells/mm^3.

OKT3 is a monoclonal antibody that is also given daily for 10-14 days. Studies have not shown a clear advantage using OKT3.

Interleukin-2 Receptor Antibodies

Monoclonal antibodies, such as basiliximab and daclizumab, chimeric or humanized monoclonal anti-CD25 antibodies, prevent T-cell proliferation but do not cause T-cell depletion. Basiliximab is given on day 0 and day 4 of the transplant as 12 mg/m^2/dose in children. Daclizumab is given on day 0 and then every 2 wk for a total of 5 doses at 1 mg/kg/dose in patients with steroid-based immunosuppression. Patients who are steroid free receive a 2 mg/kg dose on day 0 and the remaining doses at 1 mg/kg at wk 2, 4, 6, 8, 11, 15, 19, and 23. This provides the patient with extra immunosuppression for 3 mo for steroid-based patients and 6 mo for steroid-free patients. Patients tend to tolerate IL-2 receptor antagonists well. With the withdrawal of daclizumab from the market because of manufacturing deficits, many pediatric transplantation programs are using basiliximab or a short course (3 days) of Thymoglobulin at 1.5 mg/kg/day for children at low risk of sensitization and the recommended dosing of Thymoglobulin (5-7 days) or alemtuzumab for children at high risk of sensitization (see below).

Alemtuzumab (Campath-1H) is a monoclonal antibody against CD52 antigen present on T and B cells, monocytes, and natural killer cells. The pediatric data on the use of alemtuzumab show promising results.

Other Induction Therapies

Other induction therapies for highly sensitized patients include targeting B cells and/or removing neutralizing antibodies by using rituximab against the CD20 epitope on early-and intermediate-lineage B cells, the proteosome inhibitor bortezomib, and plasmapheresis and/or high-dose intravenous immunoglobulin for removing donor-specific antibodies.

Belatacept is a fusion protein composed of the Fc fragment of a human IgG$_1$ linked to the extracellular domain of CTLA-4, which is a molecule crucial for T-cell costimulation, selectively blocking the process of T-cell activation. Belatacept usage extends from induction to limited maintenance therapy, and is intended to provide optimal immunosuppression and limiting of the toxicity generated by standard immune-suppressing regimens, such as calcineurin inhibitors, thus limiting fibrosing graft injury and improving renal function. Complications include a higher incidence and grade of acute rejection episodes and a higher incidence of posttransplant lymphoproliferative disorders, with greatest risk in EBV seronegative recipients.

Maintenance Immunosuppression

For maintenance immunosuppression, calcineurin inhibitors, mycophenolate mofetil (MMF), steroids, azathioprine, and/or rapamycin may be used. Most pediatric kidney transplant recipients are maintained with a triple-immunosuppressant regimen. Central to many current pediatric immunosuppressive regimens is a calcineurin inhibitor (cyclosporine or tacrolimus) in combination with steroids and an adjunctive antiproliferative agent (azathioprine, sirolimus, or MMF). MMF is used as the adjunctive agent in more than two thirds of the pediatric kidney transplants performed. Sirolimus is used in 10-15%, and azathioprine is used in only approximately 2%. Corticosteroids continue to be used in approximately 80-85% of transplant recipients.

Calcineurin Inhibitors

The side-effect profile of **cyclosporine** in children is similar to that seen in adults, but the impact on children is more pronounced. Hypertrichosis, gingival hyperplasia, and coarsening facial features may be particularly troublesome in children. Hispanic and African-American children appear to be at higher risk for significant hypertrichosis. In the adolescent population, especially girls, these side effects can cause severe emotional distress, possibly leading to noncompliance. Seizures, although uncommon, are observed more commonly in children treated with cyclosporine than in adults. Children are likely to develop hypercholesterolemia and hypertriglyceridemia and may be candidates for lipid-lowering agents. Hyperglycemia occurs in <5% of children treated with cyclosporine.

The hyperlipidemia associated with cyclosporine and other immunosuppressive agents is also absent with **tacrolimus**. On the other hand, posttransplantation glucose intolerance, tremor, alopecia, and mild sleep disturbances are more common with tacrolimus. Historically, **posttransplant lymphoproliferative disease** has been significantly more common in children receiving tacrolimus. The lack of cosmetic side effects makes tacrolimus a very attractive alternative for children. This is especially true for young adolescents and female patients, in whom the cosmetic side effects can lead to noncompliance.

Direct comparative data in pediatrics between cyclosporine and tacrolimus are limited. The published results comparing these 2 agents show that overall acute rejection rates at 6 mo were 59.1% versus 36.9% for cyclosporine and tacrolimus, respectively. In the tacrolimus group, graft function was better at 1 yr after transplantation. The mean total steroid dose from time of transplant to 6 mo posttransplantation was significantly lower in the tacrolimus group. The overall safety profiles of the 2 calcineurin inhibitors were equivalent, with essentially no difference in posttransplant lymphoproliferative disorder or in diabetes requiring insulin treatment. The combination of drugs (tacrolimus and sirolimus) may be the biggest risk factor for PTLD.

Mycophenolate Mofetil

MMF is the morpholinoethylester prodrug of mycophenolic acid, an inhibitor of de novo purine synthesis. MMF is part of the initial maintenance immunosuppression regimen in approximately 66% of U.S. pediatric renal transplant recipients. It has largely replaced azathioprine. Acute rejection rates with MMF are approximately 20-30% when used with cyclosporine and corticosteroids. When MMF is used with tacrolimus and/or humanized monoclonal antibodies to the IL-2 receptor, lower rejection rates are usually seen.

The use of MMF has often facilitated the use of a lower dose of corticosteroids after transplantation. It has also proved useful in calcineurin inhibitor–sparing protocols, in which MMF is combined with sirolimus and corticosteroids. In steroid-avoidance regimens in kidney transplantation, the bioavailability of mycophenolic acid has been found to be greater than when the drug is used with steroids. This has allowed reduced dosing of MMF when combined with steroid avoidance in children. The absence of nephrotoxicity, hyperlipidemia, and hepatotoxicity has also contributed to the usefulness of MMF.

Gastrointestinal and hematologic side effects can be troublesome. Most of these instances can be treated with a dosage reduction and/or brief discontinuation of the drug, with resumption after 7-14 days at a lower dose. Enteric-coated mycophenolic acid has been shown to decrease the upper gastrointestinal side effects of MMF in adult transplant recipients.

Sirolimus

Sirolimus, an inhibitor of the mammalian target of rapamycin, is used primarily as an adjunctive immunosuppressive agent in combination with a calcineurin inhibitor. It is used in approximately 10-15% of pediatric renal transplant recipients. Limited anecdotal experience with sirolimus as a rescue agent in cases of refractory acute rejection, chronic allograft nephropathy, calcineurin inhibitor nephrotoxicity, and PTLD has been promising.

Most early reports in pediatric kidney transplantation appear to describe combinations of sirolimus with either tacrolimus or MMF; usually these are combined with prednisone, although efficacy has also been demonstrated with dual therapy (MMF and sirolimus) with complete steroid avoidance.

Corticosteroids

Corticosteroids remain an integral part of many immunosuppressive protocols despite their multifaceted toxicities. In children, retarded skeletal growth is the most noteworthy side effect of corticosteroids. Concerns remain about side effects, such as hypertension, obesity, diabetes mellitus, hyperlipidemia, osteopenia, and aseptic necrosis of bone (particularly the femoral heads). Cosmetic side effects, such as cushingoid faces and acne, are significant additional problems of chronic steroid use. Such side effects often tempt children and adolescent to stop taking their immunosuppressive drugs.

Steroid withdrawal attempts have led to improvements in blood pressure, lipid profiles, and growth. The benefits of steroid withdrawal have been overshadowed by high rates of acute rejection that occur in 25-70% of children. Studies using tacrolimus maintenance have shown safety in late steroid withdrawal, with low rates of acute rejection and no rebound early rejections. A steroid withdrawal trial using sirolimus had low rates of acute rejection but a high incidence of PTLD, which resulted in premature discontinuation of the study.

Complete steroid avoidance has emerged as an alternative strategy to prevent steroid-associated morbidities in children. The immunologic outcomes of these studies are the lower rates of acute rejection seen in these studies compared with standard of care protocols using steroids, suggesting that steroid avoidance might also have immunologic benefits. Building on such observations, investigators at a single center (Stanford University, Stanford, CA) initiated a steroid-avoidance protocol and demonstrated that complete steroid avoidance can be successfully achieved with excellent long-term outcomes at 8 yr, using tacrolimus in combination with MMF, and an extended 6 mo course of daclizumab. Other centers have had similar experience with complete steroid avoidance, using a similar protocol with tacrolimus and MMF and induction with either extended daclizumab or Thymoglobulin. The Stanford steroid-avoidance protocol has been replicated in a randomized multicenter U.S. trial (NIH/NIAID/CCTPT UO1 AI-55795) across 12 different pediatric kidney transplant programs in the United States, and this seminal trial confirms the safety of steroid avoidance in low-risk pediatric kidney transplant recipients with lower acute rejection rates, and significant benefits for growth, hypertension, and hyperlipidemia. Importantly, this study also confirmed the overall safety of steroid avoidance, with no adverse effects on generation of donor-specific antibody posttransplantation or histologic injury.

FLUID MANAGEMENT IN INFANTS AND SMALL CHILDREN

Maintenance of adequate blood flow to an adult-sized kidney in an infant or small child is crucial to avoid acute tubular necrosis (ATN) and graft loss from vascular thrombosis and primary nonfunction. The recipient aortic blood flow early after transplantation of an adult-size kidney more than doubles from pretransplantation aortic blood flow. The maximum blood flow that can be obtained in an adult-size kidney transplanted into a small child is approximately 65% of what was in the donor. Low blood flow states such as with hypovolemia or hypotension increase the risk for ATN, graft thrombosis, and graft nonfunction. In the postoperative period, patients are maintained on high fluid volumes.

Close attention is paid to blood pressure and hydration status in the operating room in an attempt to reduce the incidence of delayed graft function. Typically, a central venous catheter is inserted to monitor the central venous pressure throughout the operation. To achieve adequate renal perfusion, a central venous pressure of 12-15 cm H_2O should be achieved before removing the vascular clamps; a higher central venous pressure may be desirable in the case of a small infant receiving an adult-size kidney. Dopamine is usually started in the operating room at 2 to 3 µg/kg/min, increased if required, and continued for 24-48 hr postoperatively. It is used to facilitate diuresis and perhaps to affect renal vasodilation. The mean arterial blood pressure is kept >65-70 mm Hg by adequate hydration with a crystalloid solution and 5% albumin, and, if necessary, by using dopamine at higher doses. A blood transfusion with packed red blood cells may be required in very small recipients because the hemoglobin can drop as a result of sequestration

of approximately 150-250 mL of blood in the transplanted kidney. Mannitol and/or furosemide may be given before removing the vascular clamps to increase the effective circulatory volume and facilitate diuresis. Mannitol can also act as a free-radical scavenger, and together with renal dose dopamine it is a critical factor for minimizing the ischemia–reperfusion injury in steroid-avoidance regimens. After the transplanted kidney starts to produce urine, volume replacement should be immediately started with normal saline.

Infants continue to receive aggressive fluid management by nasogastric or gastrostomy tube feedings of at least 2500 mL/m²/day for ≥6 mo after transplant if the child is unable to take in sufficient volume. This aggressive fluid management showed 30 mL/min greater GFR in infants who received adult-size kidneys and who were maintained on this higher fluid requirement than infants who were not.

RENAL BIOPSY

Renal biopsy is the gold standard for diagnosis of acute allograft dysfunction. Protocol biopsies may improve graft outcome by detecting early pathology and help monitor drug nephrotoxicity. The largest serial analysis of protocol biopsies at implantation, 3, 6, 12, and 24 mo posttransplantation (the NIH SNSO1 trial, 2004-9) established that the prime risk factor for chronic histologic injury was discrepancy between recipient size and donor mass and time posttransplantation.

REJECTION

Hyperacute rejection occurs immediately when the kidney is transplanted and is caused by preformed antibodies against the donor HLA, ABO, or other antigens. Hyperacute rejection is rare. The only treatment is removal of the graft.

Acute cellular rejection needs to be identified and treated early. Diagnosis of acute rejection in the very young transplant recipient is often not straightforward. Because most small children receive adult-size kidneys, an elevation in serum creatinine may be a late sign of rejection as a result of the large renal reserve compared with the body mass. Thus, significant allograft dysfunction may be present with little or no increase in the serum creatinine level. One of the earliest and most sensitive signs of rejection is the development of hypertension along with low-grade fever. In children, any increase in serum creatinine, especially if it is accompanied by hypertension, should be considered a symptom of acute rejection until proved otherwise. Late diagnosis and treatment of rejection are associated with a higher incidence of resistant rejections and graft loss. Genomic studies in pediatric kidney transplantation have demonstrated molecular heterogeneity for different acute rejection episodes, not distinguishable by pathologic grading, but with a key established role for B cells as antigen-presenting cells for aggressive T-cell–mediated recalcitrant rejection.

Chronic rejection is the leading cause of graft loss and primarily results from immune and nonimmune injuries such as hypertension, diabetes, and hyperlipidemia. Children often have a gradual decline in their renal function and often have fixed proteinuria and hypertension. Despite initial excitement about the potential of MMF and sirolimus mitigating chronic graft injury, this has not translated readily into observable clinical benefits. Humoral immunity, relating the generation of posttransplant donor-specific anti-HLA antibodies, has been implicated in this injury; attention has also shifted to evaluating the impact of non-HLA antibodies after organ transplantation, as direct mediators of organ injury.

GRAFT SURVIVAL

Five yr graft survival is higher in living-donor recipients compared to grafts from deceased donors. The OPTN/SRTR 2007 annual report gives graft survival at 5 yr (2000-2005) for living-donor kidney transplant as 88.0% for recipients 1-5 yr of age, 84.6% for those 6-10 yr of age, and 74.4% for those 11-17 yr of age. Survival in deceased-donor recipients was 74.4% for those 1-5 yr of age, 72.1% for those 6-10 yr of age, and 63% for those 11-17 yr of age.

From the NAPRTCS data, graft survival rates of pediatric kidney transplants have improved since 1987 with 1 yr survival rates during 2003-2006 of 95.7% for living-donor transplants and 95%

for deceased-donor transplants. Children <10 yr of age have the best long-term graft and patient survival rates of all transplant recipients. Graft survival in adolescent patients is the lowest of all the age groups. It is well known that noncompliance is a difficult problem in this age group. Other risk factors for graft failure are race, previous transplant history, history of multiple blood transfusions, HLA-B matches, sex, and transplant year. Approximately 25% of pediatric kidney transplants are preemptive. Graft survival for living and deceased-donor kidneys is significantly better in the preemptive group compared to patients who are on dialysis first. The 3 most common causes of graft failure are chronic rejection of graft (34.9%), acute rejection of graft (13%), and vascular thrombosis (10.1%). Approximately 6.4% of patients had graft failure as a result of recurrence of primary disease (NAPRTCS 2007). The NAPRTCS 2003-2007 data showed the probability of the first rejection at 12 mo being 8.7% for the living donor and 17.7% for the deceased donor.

Graft survival is significantly worse in the presence of ATN in either donor group. ATN is defined by NAPRTCS as requiring the use of dialysis within the first transplant week. NAPRTCS 2008 data report a 5.1% delay in graft function in living-donor renal transplants compared to the ATN rate of 16.4% in children who received deceased-donor transplants.

COMPLICATIONS WITH IMMUNOSUPPRESSION INFECTIONS

Since the mid-1990s, the incidence of acute rejection has decreased but the incidence of infections after transplantation has been increasing.

Pneumonia and urinary tract infection are the most common post-transplant bacterial infections. Urinary tract infections can progress rapidly to urosepsis and may be confused with episodes of acute rejection. Trimethoprim-sulfamethoxazole is used for urinary tract infection antibiotic prophylaxis as well as *Pneumocystis carinii* pneumonia prophylaxis for at least the first 6 mo after transplant. Opportunistic infections associated with unusual organisms usually do not occur until after the first month after transplantation.

The **herpesviruses** (cytomegalovirus, herpesvirus, varicella-zoster virus, and EBV) pose a special problem in view of their common occurrence in children. Many young children have not yet been exposed to these viruses, and because they lack protective immunity, their predisposition to serious primary infection is high. The incidence of cytomegalovirus seropositivity is approximately 30% in children >5 yr of age and rises to approximately 60% in teenagers. Thus, the younger child is at a greater potential risk for serious infection when a cytomegalovirus-positive donor kidney is transplanted. About half the children are seronegative for EBV, and infection occurs in approximately 75% of these patients. Most EBV infections are clinically silent. PTLD in children may be related to EBV infection in the presence of vigorous immunosuppression. The incidence of these infections is higher in children who receive antibody induction therapy and after treatment of acute rejection. It has also been shown in children that subclinical replication of these viruses is much higher in regimens with maintenance steroids, versus protocols with complete steroid avoidance, and that even subclinical viral replication can have a detrimental effect on the incidence of acute rejection and graft function. Antiviral prophylaxis with ganciclovir and valganciclovir for 3-12 mo after transplantation, especially in the higher-risk groups (recipient-negative, donor-positive), have been effective in reducing the incidence of clinical cytomegalovirus disease. Serial surveillance for these viruses by quantitative polymerase chain reaction for viral load in the peripheral blood has also allowed educated minimization of immunosuppression with resultant reduction in viral burden.

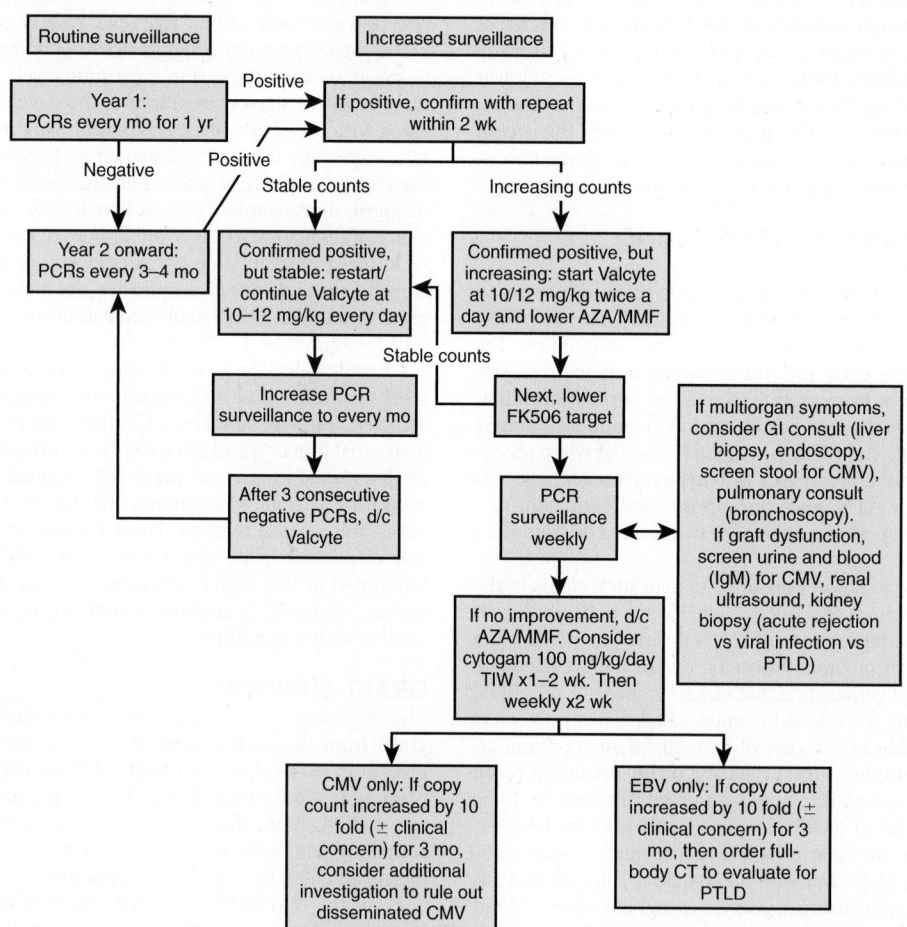

Figure 536-1 Surveillance for cytomegalovirus and Epstein-Barr virus infections after pediatric kidney transplantation.

Polyomavirus nephropathy is an important cause of allograft dysfunction; almost 30% of children have BK viruria, although allograft dysfunction is observed in lower numbers (~5%). The increased incidence of polyomavirus nephropathy is thought to be the result of more-potent immunosuppressive regimens. A renal biopsy, with identification of polyoma by immunoperoxidase staining, may be required to make the diagnosis with certainty. Reducing immunosuppression is the main form of therapy, and cidofovir and leflunomide are used as adjunctive therapies.

It is important to monitor for **PTLD** with routine examinations for lymphadenopathy, hepatosplenomegaly, and EBV screen. Figure 536-1 provides a schematic plan to monitor for EBV, cytomegalovirus, and PTLD.

Hypertension, hyperlipidemia, and posttransplant diabetes mellitus are other potential complications of immunosuppressant medications that need to be monitored for and treated when necessary.

Nonadherence with immunosuppressive medications is one of the most important and most elusive problems facing the medical team. At least half of the pediatric deceased-donor transplant recipients demonstrated significant medication nonadherence in the posttransplantation period by using as an assessment direct reporting to the medical team. This figure exceeded 60% in adolescents. Because direct reporting of nonadherence can significantly underestimate its true incidence, this analysis points out the potential magnitude of the problem. Nonadherence appears to be the principal cause of graft loss in 10-15% of all pediatric kidney transplant recipients; for patients with retransplants, this figure might exceed 25%. Risk factors that suggest an increased propensity toward medication nonadherence include female sex, adolescent age, family instability, insufficient emotional support, lower social economic class, and maladaptive behavior.

Although **growth** improves after transplantation, chronic steroid use does not allow a child to reach full potential height. The precise mechanism by which steroids impair skeletal growth is unknown. Steroids could reduce the release of growth hormone, reduce insulin growth factor activity, impair growth cartilage directly, decrease calcium absorption, or increase renal phosphate wasting. The use of recombinant human growth hormone in pediatric renal transplant recipients significantly improves growth velocity and standard deviation score (SDS). An allograft GFR of <60 mL/min/1.73 m^2 is associated with poor growth and low insulin growth factor levels; optimal growth occurs with a GFR >90 mL/min/1.73 m^2. Graft function is the most important factor after a high corticosteroid dosage in the genesis of posttransplantation growth failure. Steroid minimization and withdrawal protocols have demonstrated growth benefits, and the steroid-avoidance data in children show significant catch-up growth at 5 yr after transplantation. These factors have even greater weight than for age-matched, and gender-matched peers. It is thus likely that with a well-functioning kidney and no maintenance steroids, children might now be able to realize their full height potential.

LONG-TERM OUTCOME

With advances in transplant care and treatment modalities and with diligent attention to the pediatric patient's psychosocial, educational, vocational, and developmental rehabilitation, the social and emotional functioning of the child and the child's family appears to return to preillness levels within 1 yr of successful transplantation. Renal transplantation leads to improvement in linear growth in children. School function tests improve after renal transplantation. Most patients can reenter school and social activities after a short recovery time of 4-6 wk after surgery. A 3 yr follow-up shows that nearly 90% of children are in their appropriate school or job placement positions. Surveys of 10 year survivors of pediatric kidney transplants report that most patients consider their health to be good, and they engage in appropriate social, educational, and sexual activities while experiencing a very good to excellent quality of life.

Bibliography is available at Expert Consult.

Urologic Disorders in Infants and Children

PART
XXIV

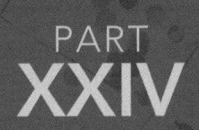

Chapter 537
Congenital Anomalies and Dysgenesis of the Kidneys

Jack S. Elder

EMBRYONIC DEVELOPMENT

The kidney is derived from interaction between the ureteral bud and the metanephric blastema. During the 5th wk of gestation, the ureteral bud arises from the mesonephric (wolffian) duct and penetrates the metanephric blastema, which is an area of undifferentiated mesenchyme on the nephrogenic ridge. The ureteral bud undergoes a series of approximately 15 generations of divisions and by the 20th wk of gestation forms the entire collecting system: the ureter, renal pelvis, calyces, papillary ducts, and collecting tubules. Signals from the mesenchymal cells induce ureteral bud formation from the wolffian duct as well as ureteric bud branching. Reciprocal signals from the ureteric bud and, later, from its branching tips induce mesenchymal cells to condense, proliferate, and convert into epithelial cells. Under the inductive influence of the ureteral bud, nephron differentiation begins during the 7th wk of gestation. By the 20th wk of gestation, when the collecting system is developed, approximately 30% of the nephrons are present. Nephrogenesis continues at a nearly exponential rate and is complete by the 36th wk of gestation. During nephrogenesis, the kidneys ascend to a lumbar site just below the adrenal glands. At least 16 signaling agents have been identified that regulate renal development. Defects in any of the signaling activities could cause a kidney not to form (**renal agenesis**), or to differentiate abnormally (**renal dysgenesis**). Dysgenesis of the kidney includes **aplasia, dysplasia, hypoplasia,** and certain forms of **renal cystic disease**.

The fetal kidneys play a minor role in the maintenance of fetal salt and water homeostasis. The rate of urine production increases throughout gestation; at term, volumes have been reported to be 50 mL/hr. The glomerular filtration rate is 25 mL/min/1.73 m² at term and triples by 3 mo postterm. The increase in glomerular filtration rate is caused by a reduction in intrarenal vascular resistance and redistribution of intrarenal blood flow to the cortex, where more nephrons are located.

RENAL AGENESIS

Renal agenesis, or absent kidney development, can occur secondary to a defect of the wolffian duct, ureteric bud, or metanephric blastema. Unilateral renal agenesis has an incidence of 1 in 450-1,000 births. Unilateral renal agenesis often is discovered during the course of an evaluation for other congenital anomalies (VACTERL [vertebral defects, imperforate anus, congenital heart disease, tracheoesophageal fistula, renal and limb defects] syndrome; e.g., see Chapter 344). Its incidence is increased in newborns with a single umbilical artery. In true agenesis, the ureter and the ipsilateral bladder hemitrigone are absent. The contralateral kidney undergoes compensatory hypertrophy, to some degree prenatally but primarily after birth. Approximately 15% of these children have contralateral vesicoureteral reflux, and most males have an ipsilateral absent vas deferens because the wolffian duct

is absent. Because the wolffian and müllerian ducts are contiguous, müllerian abnormalities in girls also are common. The **Mayer-Rokitansky-Küster-Hauser** syndrome (1 in 4,000-1 in 10,000 female births) is a group of associated findings that may include vaginal aplasia, uterine maldevelopment, and normal ovaries. Two types are described—type I and type II. In type II, renal anomalies, for example, unilateral renal agenesis or a horseshoe kidney, are common, and skeletal anomalies are present in 10% (see Chapter 554).

Renal agenesis is distinguished from aplasia, in which a nubbin of nonfunctioning tissue is seen capping a normal or abnormal ureter. This distinction may be difficult but usually is clinically insignificant. Unilateral renal agenesis is diagnosed in some patients based on the finding of an absent kidney on ultrasonography or renal scintigraphy (renal scan). Some of these patients were born with a hypoplastic kidney or a multicystic dysplastic kidney that underwent complete cyst regression. Although the specific diagnosis is not critical, if the finding of an absent kidney is based on an ultrasonogram, a functional imaging study such as an MR urogram or renal scan should be performed because some of these patients have an ectopic kidney in the pelvis. If there is a normal contralateral kidney, long-term renal function usually remains normal.

Bilateral renal agenesis is incompatible with extrauterine life and produces the **Potter syndrome.** Death occurs shortly after birth from pulmonary hypoplasia. The newborn has a characteristic facial appearance, termed *Potter facies* (Fig. 537-1). The eyes are widely separated with epicanthic folds, the ears are low set, the nose is broad and compressed flat, the chin is receding, and there are limb anomalies. Bilateral renal agenesis should be suspected when maternal ultrasonography demonstrates **oligohydramnios,** nonvisualization of the bladder, and absent kidneys. The incidence of this disorder is 1 in 3,000 births, with a male predominance, and represents 20% of newborns with the Potter phenotype. Other common causes of neonatal renal failure associated with the Potter phenotype include cystic renal dysplasia and obstructive uropathy. Less-common causes are autosomal recessive polycystic kidney disease (infantile), renal hypoplasia, and medullary dysplasia. Neonates with bilateral renal agenesis die of pulmonary insufficiency from pulmonary hypoplasia rather than renal failure (see Chapter 101).

The term **familial renal adysplasia** describes families in which renal agenesis, renal dysplasia, multicystic kidney (dysplasia), or a combination, occurs in a single family. This disorder has an autosomal dominant inheritance pattern with a penetrance of 50-90% and variable expression. Because of this association, some clinicians advise screening 1st-degree relatives of persons who have renal agenesis or dysplasia, but this is not standard practice.

Whether persons with a solitary kidney should avoid contact sports such as football and karate is unresolved. The arguments favoring participation are that there are other solitary organs (spleen, liver, and brain) that do not preclude participation in contact sports, and there have been only a few reports of persons losing a kidney from sports injuries. The arguments against such participation are that the contralateral normal kidney is hypertrophic and not as well protected by the ribs, and a serious renal injury could have serious lifelong consequences. The American Academy of Pediatrics recommends an "individual assessment for contact, collision, and limited-contact sports."

RENAL DYSGENESIS: DYSPLASIA, HYPOPLASIA, AND CYSTIC ANOMALIES

Renal dysgenesis refers to maldevelopment of the kidney that affects its size, shape, or structure. The 3 principal types of dysgenesis are dysplastic, hypoplastic, and cystic. Although dysplasia always is accompanied by a decreased number of nephrons (hypoplasia), the converse is not true: Hypoplasia can occur in isolation. When both conditions are

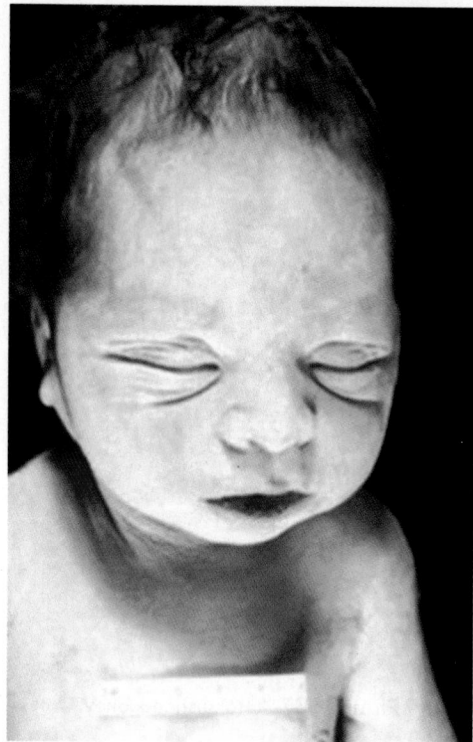

Figure 537-1 Stillborn infant with renal agenesis exhibiting characteristic Potter facies.

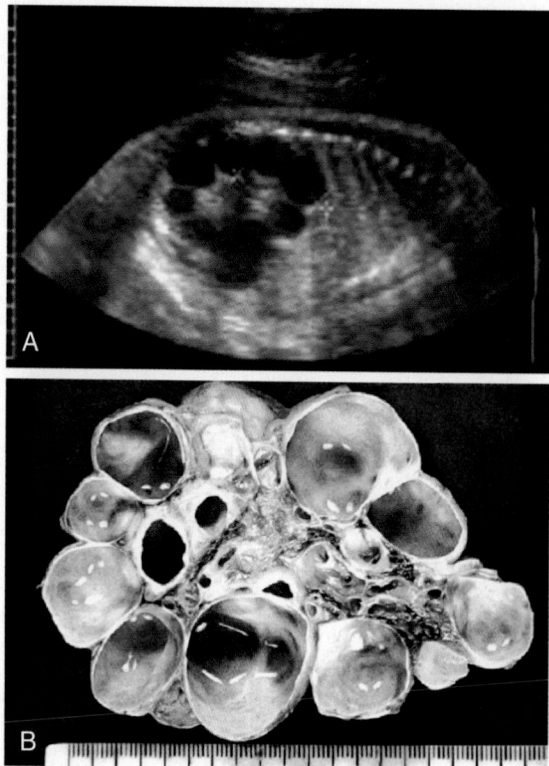

Figure 537-2 A, Prenatal sonogram demonstrating multicystic dysplastic kidney. **B,** Surgical specimen.

present, the term **hypodysplasia** is preferred. The term **dysplasia** is technically a histologic diagnosis and refers to focal, diffuse, or segmentally arranged primitive structures, specifically primitive ductal structures, resulting from abnormal metanephric differentiation. Nonrenal elements, such as cartilage, also may be present. The condition can affect all or only part of the kidney. If cysts are present, the condition is termed **cystic dysplasia.** If the entire kidney is dysplastic with a preponderance of cysts, the kidney is referred to as a **multicystic dysplastic kidney** (MCDK) (Fig. 537-2).

The pathogenesis of dysplasia is multifactorial. The "bud" theory proposes that if the ureteral bud arises in an abnormal location, such as an ectopic ureter, there is abnormal penetration and induction of the metanephric blastema, which causes abnormal kidney differentiation, resulting in dysplasia. Renal dysplasia also can occur with severe obstructive uropathy early in gestation, as with the most severe cases of posterior urethral valves or in an MCDK, in which a portion of the ureter is absent or atretic.

MCDK is a congenital condition in which the kidney is replaced by cysts and does not function; it can result from ureteral atresia. Kidney size is highly variable. The incidence is approximately 1 in 2,000. Some clinicians incorrectly use the terms *multicystic kidney* and *polycystic kidney* interchangeably. However, polycystic kidney disease is an inherited disorder that may be autosomal recessive or autosomal dominant and affects both kidneys (see Chapter 521). MCDK usually is unilateral and generally is not inherited. Bilateral MCDKs are incompatible with life.

MCDK is the most common cause of an abdominal mass in the newborn, but the vast majority are nonpalpable at birth. In most cases, it is discovered incidentally during prenatal sonography. In some patients, the cysts are identified prenatally, but the cysts regress in utero and no kidney is identified on imaging at birth. Contralateral hydronephrosis is present in 5-10% of patients. Sonography shows the characteristic appearance of a kidney replaced by multiple cysts of varying sizes that do not communicate, and no identifiable parenchyma is present. In the past, most cases were confirmed with a renal scan, which should demonstrate nonfunction. However, presently the diag-

nosis of MCDK is usually straightforward based on the renal ultrasound, and a scan generally is unnecessary. In some patients, usually boys, a small nonobstructing ureterocele is present in the bladder (see Chapter 540). Although 15% have contralateral vesicoureteral reflux, it is usually low grade, and obtaining a voiding cystourethrogram also is unnecessary, unless there is significant contralateral hydronephrosis or the child develops an upper urinary tract infection. Management is controversial. Complete cyst regression occurs in nearly half of MCDKs by age 7 yr. The risk of associated hypertension is 0.2-1.2%, and the risk of Wilms tumor arising from an MCDK is approximately 1 in 1,200. Because neoplasms arise from the stromal rather than the cystic component, even if the cysts regress completely, the likelihood that the kidney could develop a neoplasm is not altered.

Because of the occult nature of these potential problems, many clinicians advise annual follow-up with sonography and blood pressure measurement. The most important aspect of follow-up is being certain that the solitary kidney is functioning normally. If there is an abdominal mass, the cysts enlarge, the stromal core increases in size, or hypertension develops, nephrectomy is recommended. In lieu of follow-up screening, laparoscopic nephrectomy may be performed.

Renal hypoplasia refers to a small nondysplastic kidney that has fewer than the normal number of calyces and nephrons. The term encompasses a group of conditions with an abnormally small kidney and should be distinguished from aplasia, in which the kidney is rudimentary. If the condition is unilateral, the diagnosis usually is made incidentally during evaluation for another urinary tract problem or hypertension. Bilateral hypoplasia usually manifests with signs and symptoms of chronic renal failure and is a leading cause of end-stage renal disease during the 1st decade of life. A history of polyuria and polydipsia is common. Urinalysis results may be normal. In a rare form of bilateral hypoplasia called **oligomeganephronia,** the number of nephrons is markedly reduced and those present are markedly hypertrophied.

The **Ask-Upmark kidney,** also termed **segmental hypoplasia,** refers to small kidneys, usually weighing not more than 35 g, with 1 or more

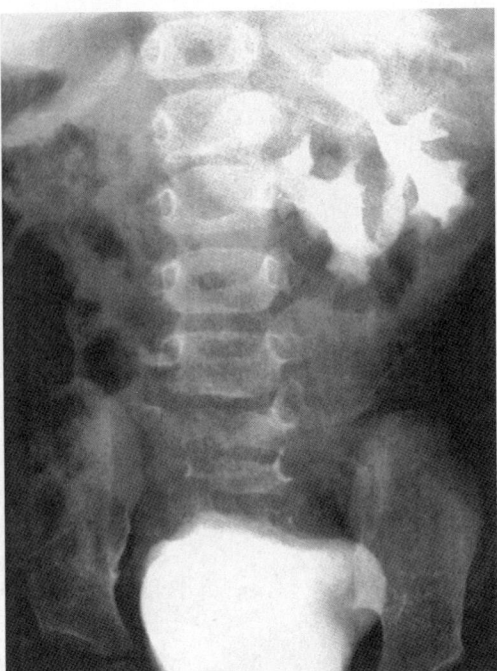

Figure 537-3 Crossed renal ectopia. Intravenous urography shows both renal collecting systems to the left of the spine. Segmentation anomalies of the sacrum, which are subtle in this child, are one of the skeletal anomalies associated with renal ectopia. *(From Slovis T, editor: Caffey's pediatric diagnostic imaging, ed 11, vol 2, Philadelphia, 2008, Mosby, Fig. 145-23A, p. 2244.)*

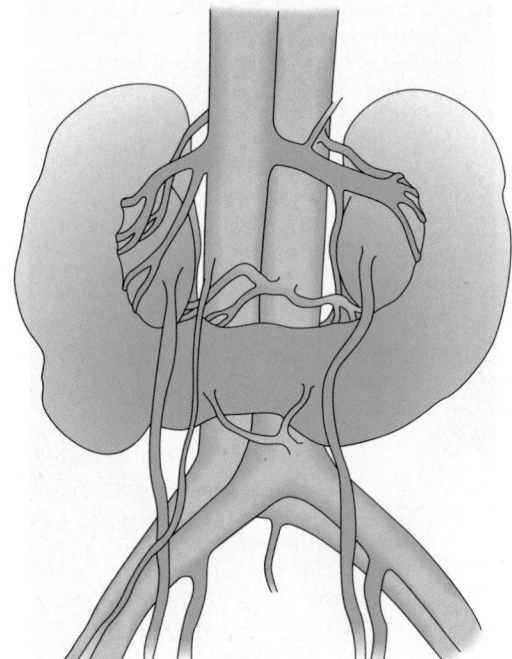

Figure 537-4 Horseshoe kidney.

deep grooves on the lateral convexity, underneath which the parenchyma consists of tubules resembling those in the thyroid gland. It is unclear whether the lesion is congenital or acquired. Most patients are 10 yr or older at diagnosis and have severe hypertension. Nephrectomy usually controls the hypertension.

ANOMALIES IN SHAPE AND POSITION

During renal development the kidneys normally ascend from the pelvis into their normal position behind the ribs. The normal process of ascent and rotation of the kidney may be incomplete, resulting in renal ectopia or nonrotation. The ectopic kidney may be in a pelvic, iliac, thoracic, or contralateral position. If the ectopia is bilateral, in 90% of persons the 2 kidneys fuse. The incidence of renal ectopia is approximately 1 in 900 (Fig. 537-3).

Renal fusion anomalies are more common. The lower poles of the kidneys can fuse in the midline, resulting in a horseshoe kidney (Fig. 537-4); the fused portion is termed the *isthmus* and may be thick functioning parenchyma or a thin fibrous strand. Horseshoe kidneys occur in 1 in 400-500 births but are seen in 7% of patients with Turner syndrome. Horseshoe kidney is one of the many renal anomalies that occur in 30% of patients with Turner syndrome (see Chapter 586). Wilms tumors are 4 times more common in children with horseshoe kidneys than in the general population. Stone disease and hydronephrosis secondary to ureteropelvic junction obstruction are other potential late complications. The incidence of MCDK affecting 1 of the 2 sides of a horseshoe kidney also appears to be increased. With crossed fused ectopia, 1 kidney crosses over to the other side and the parenchyma of the 2 kidneys is fused. Renal function usually is normal. In the most common finding, the left kidney may cross over and fuse with the lower pole of the right kidney. The insertion of the ureter to the bladder does not change, and the adrenal glands remain in their normal positions. The clinical significance of this anomaly is that if renal surgery is necessary, the blood supply is variable and can make partial nephrectomy more difficult.

ASSOCIATED PHYSICAL FINDINGS

Upper urinary tract anomalies are more common in children with certain physical findings. The incidence of renal anomalies is increased if there is a single umbilical artery and an abnormality of another organ system (congenital heart disease). External ear anomalies (particularly if the child has multiple congenital anomalies), imperforate anus, and scoliosis are associated with renal anomalies. Infants with these physical findings should undergo a renal sonogram.

Bibliography is available at Expert Consult.

Chapter **538**
Urinary Tract Infections
Jack S. Elder

PREVALENCE AND ETIOLOGY

Urinary tract infections (UTIs) occur in 1% of boys and 1-3% of girls. The prevalence of UTIs varies with age. During the 1st yr of life, the male : female ratio is 2.8-5.4 : 1. Beyond 1-2 yr, there is a female preponderance, with a male : female ratio of 1 : 10. In boys, most UTIs occur during the 1st yr of life; UTIs are much more common in uncircumcised boys, especially in the 1st yr of life. In girls, the first UTI usually occurs by the age of 5 yr, with peaks during infancy and toilet training.

UTIs are caused primarily by colonic bacteria. In girls, 75-90% of all infections are caused by *Escherichia coli* (see Chapter 200), followed by *Klebsiella* spp. and *Proteus* spp. (see Chapter 109). Although *E. coli* is also the most common organism in males, some series report that in boys older than 1 yr of age, *Proteus* is as common a cause as *E. coli*; others report a preponderance of Gram-positive organisms in boys. *Staphylococcus saprophyticus* and enterococcus are pathogens in both sexes. Adenovirus and other viral infections also can occur, especially as a cause of cystitis with gross hematuria.

UTIs have been considered a risk factor for the development of renal insufficiency or end-stage renal disease in children, although some have questioned the importance of UTI as an isolated risk factor, because only 2% of children with renal insufficiency report a history of UTI. This paradox may be secondary to better recognition of the risks of UTI and prompt diagnosis and therapy. Furthermore, many children receive antibiotics for fever without a specific diagnosis (e.g., treating a questionable otitis media) resulting in a partially treated UTI.

CLINICAL MANIFESTATIONS AND CLASSIFICATION
The 3 basic forms of UTI are **pyelonephritis**, **cystitis**, and **asymptomatic bacteriuria**. Focal pyelonephritis ("nephronia") and renal abscesses are less common.

Clinical Pyelonephritis
Clinical pyelonephritis is characterized by any or all of the following: abdominal, back, or flank pain; fever; malaise; nausea; vomiting; and, occasionally, diarrhea. *Fever may be the only manifestation.* Newborns can show nonspecific symptoms such as poor feeding, irritability, jaundice, and weight loss. Pyelonephritis is the most common serious bacterial infection in infants younger than 24 mo of age who have fever without an obvious focus (see Chapter 177). These symptoms are an indication that there is bacterial involvement of the upper urinary tract. Involvement of the renal parenchyma is termed *acute pyelonephritis,* whereas if there is no parenchymal involvement, the condition may be termed *pyelitis.* Acute pyelonephritis can result in renal injury, termed *pyelonephritic scarring.*

Acute lobar nephronia (acute lobar nephritis) is a renal mass caused by acute focal infection without liquefaction. It may be an early stage in the development of a renal abscess. Manifestations are identical to pyelonephritis; renal imaging demonstrates the abnormality (Fig. 538-1). *Renal abscess* can occur following a pyelonephritic infection caused by the usual uropathogens or may be secondary to hematogenous infection (*Staphylococcus aureus*). *Perinephric abscess* (Fig. 538-2) can occur secondary to contiguous infection in the perirenal area (e.g., vertebral osteomyelitis, psoas abscess) or pyelonephritis that dissects to the renal capsule.

Xanthogranulomatous pyelonephritis is a rare type of renal infection characterized by granulomatous inflammation with giant cells and foamy histiocytes. It can manifest clinically as a renal mass or an acute or chronic infection. Renal calculi, obstruction, and infection with *Proteus* spp. or *E. coli* contribute to the development of this lesion, which usually requires total or partial nephrectomy.

Cystitis
Cystitis indicates that there is bladder involvement; symptoms include dysuria, urgency, frequency, suprapubic pain, incontinence, and mal-

odorous urine. Cystitis does not cause fever and does not result in renal injury. Malodorous urine is not specific for a UTI.

Acute hemorrhagic cystitis often is caused by *E. coli;* it also has been attributed to adenovirus types 11 and 21. Adenovirus cystitis is more common in boys; it is self-limiting, with hematuria lasting approximately 4 days.

Eosinophilic cystitis is a rare form of cystitis of obscure origin that occasionally is found in children. The usual symptoms are those of

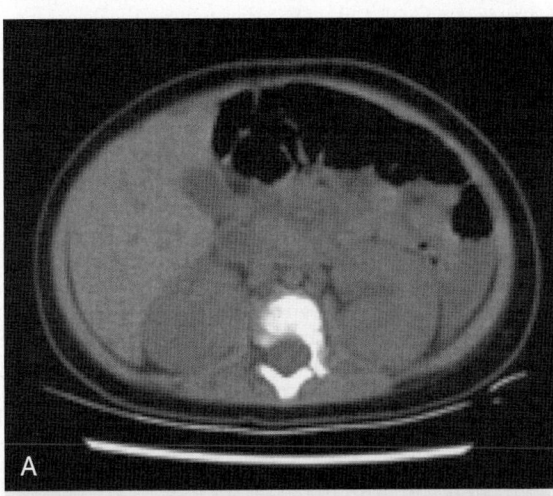
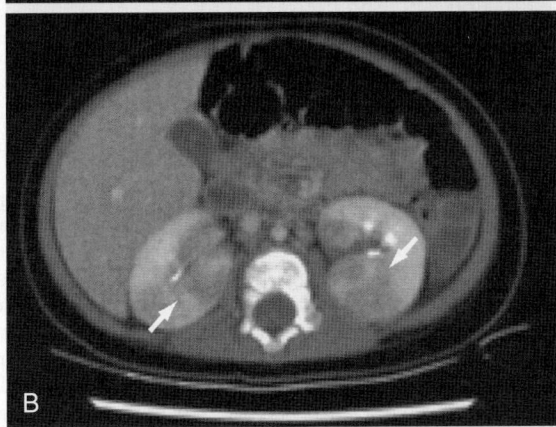

Figure 538-1 Characteristic precontrast **(A)** and contrast-enhanced **(B)** CT scans for an 8 mo old patient who had acute lobar nephronia and presented with severe bilateral nephromegaly but without a focal mass sonographically. No attenuation area is seen in the kidney before enhancement. *(From Cheng CH, Tsau YK, Lin TY: Effective duration of antimicrobial therapy for the treatment of acute lobar nephronia, Pediatrics 117:e84–e89, 2006.)*

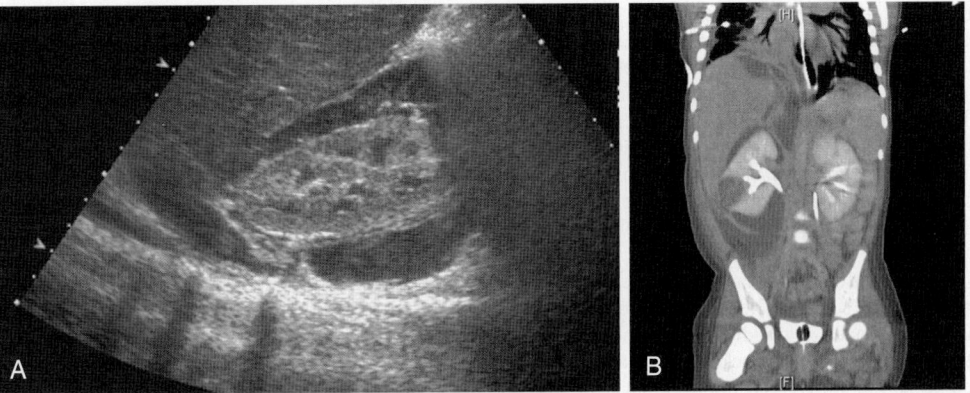

Figure 538-2 A, Renal sonogram, 19 mo old girl with perirenal abscess secondary to methicillin-resistant *Staphylococcus aureus*. **B,** CT scan demonstrates extensive perinephric and focal intrarenal abscess. Patient underwent incision and drainage.

cystitis with hematuria. On imaging, typically there are multiple solid bladder masses that consist histologically of inflammatory infiltrates with eosinophils. Ureteral dilation with hydronephrosis also is common. Children with eosinophilic cystitis may have been exposed to an allergen. Bladder biopsy often is necessary to exclude a neoplastic process. Treatment usually includes antihistamines and nonsteroidal antiinflammatory agents.

Interstitial cystitis is characterized by irritative voiding symptoms such as urgency, frequency, and dysuria, and bladder and pelvic pain relieved by voiding with a negative urine culture. The disorder is most likely to affect adolescent girls and is idiopathic. Diagnosis is made by cystoscopic observation of mucosal ulcers with bladder distention. Treatments have included bladder hydrodistention and laser ablation of ulcerated areas, but no treatment provides sustained relief.

Asymptomatic Bacteriuria

Asymptomatic bacteriuria refers to a condition in which there is a positive urine culture without any manifestations of infection. It is most common in girls. The incidence is <1% in preschool and school-age girls and is rare in boys. This condition is benign and does not cause renal injury, except in pregnant women, in whom asymptomatic bacteriuria, if left untreated, can result in a symptomatic UTI. Some girls are mistakenly identified as having asymptomatic bacteriuria, whereas they actually are experiencing day or night incontinence or perineal discomfort secondary to UTI; these patients should undergo antibiotic therapy.

PATHOGENESIS AND PATHOLOGY

Nearly all UTIs are ascending infections. The bacteria arise from the fecal flora, colonize the perineum, and enter the bladder via the urethra. In uncircumcised boys, the bacterial pathogens arise from the flora beneath the prepuce. In some cases, the bacteria causing cystitis ascend to the kidney to cause pyelonephritis. Rarely, renal infection occurs by hematogenous spread, as in endocarditis or in some neonates.

If bacteria ascend from the bladder to the kidney, acute pyelonephritis can occur. Normally the simple and compound papillae in the kidney have an antireflux mechanism that prevents urine in the renal pelvis from entering the collecting tubules. However, some compound papillae, typically in the upper and lower poles of the kidney, allow intrarenal reflux. Infected urine then stimulates an immunologic and inflammatory response. The result can cause renal injury and scarring (Figs. 538-3 and 538-4). Children of any age with a febrile UTI can have acute pyelonephritis and subsequent renal scarring, but the risk is highest in those younger than 2 yr of age.

Table 538-1 lists the host risk factors for UTI. Vesicoureteral reflux is discussed in Chapter 539. If there is grade III, IV, or V vesicoureteral reflux and a febrile UTI, 90% have evidence of acute pyelonephritis on renal scintigraphy or other imaging studies. In girls, UTIs often occur at the onset of toilet training because of bladder/bowel dysfunction that occurs at that age. The child is trying to retain urine to stay dry, yet the bladder may have uninhibited contractions forcing urine out. The result may be high-pressure, turbulent urine flow or incomplete bladder emptying, both of which increase the likelihood of bacteriuria. Bladder/bowel dysfunction can occur in the toilet-trained child who voids infrequently. Similar problems can arise in school-age children who refuse to use the school bathroom. Obstructive uropathy resulting in hydronephrosis increases the risk of UTI because of urinary stasis. Urethral catheterization for urine output monitoring or during a voiding cystourethrogram or nonsterile catheterization can infect the bladder with a pathogen. Constipation with fecal impaction can increase the risk of UTI because it can cause bladder dysfunction.

The pathogenesis of UTI is based in part on the presence of bacterial pili or fimbriae on the bacterial surface. There are 2 types of fimbriae, type I and type II. Type I fimbriae are found on most strains of *E. coli*. Because attachment to target cells can be blocked by D-mannose, these fimbriae are referred to as *mannose sensitive*. They have no role in pyelonephritis. The attachment of type II fimbriae is not inhibited by mannose, and these are known as *mannose resistant*. These fimbriae

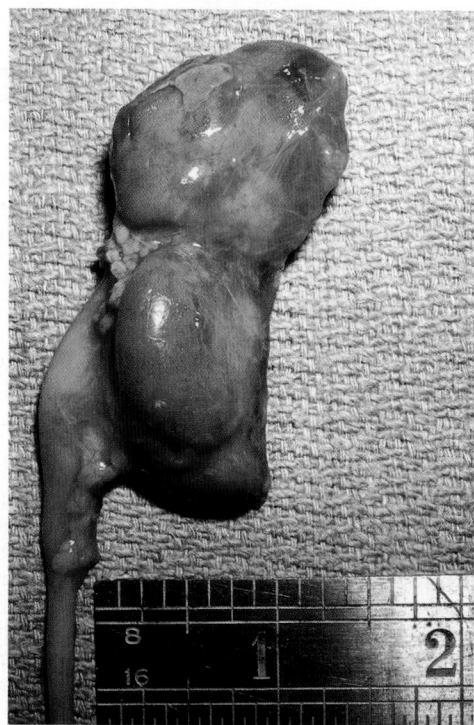

Figure 538-3 Scarred kidney from recurrent pyelonephritis.

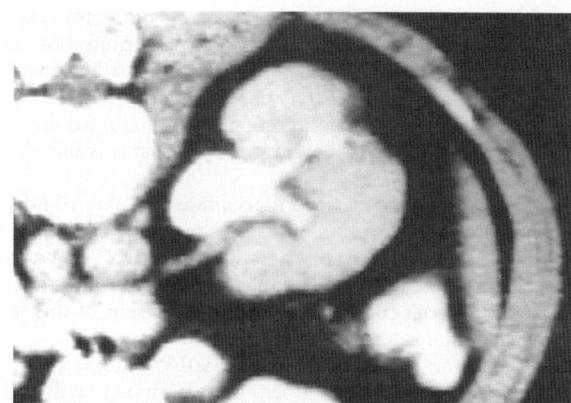

Figure 538-4 CT scan showing an area of parenchymal thinning corresponding to an underlying calyx, characteristic of pyelonephritic scarring or reflux nephropathy.

Table 538-1	Risk Factors for Urinary Tract Infection
Female gender	Tight clothing (underwear)
Uncircumcised male	Pinworm infestation
Vesicoureteral reflux*	Constipation
Toilet training	Bacteria with P fimbriae
Voiding dysfunction	Anatomic abnormality (labial
Obstructive uropathy	adhesion)
Urethral instrumentation	Neuropathic bladder
Wiping from back to front in	Sexual activity
girls	Pregnancy
Bubble bath?	

*Risk increased for clinical pyelonephritis, not cystitis.

are expressed by only certain strains of *E. coli*. The receptor for type II fimbriae is a glycosphingolipid that is present on both the uroepithelial cell membrane and red blood cells. The Gal 1-4 Gal oligosaccharide fraction is the specific receptor. Because these fimbriae can agglutinate by P blood group erythrocytes, they are known as P fimbriae. Bacteria with P fimbriae are more likely to cause pyelonephritis. Between 76% and 94% of pyelonephritogenic strains of *E. coli* have P fimbriae, compared with 19-23% of cystitis strains.

Other host factors for UTI include anatomic abnormalities precluding normal micturition, such as a labial adhesion. This lesion acts as a barrier and causes vaginal voiding. A neuropathic bladder can predispose to UTIs if there is incomplete bladder emptying and/or detrusor–sphincter dyssynergia. Sexual activity is associated with UTIs in girls, in part because of incomplete bladder emptying. From 4-7% of pregnant women have asymptomatic bacteriuria, which can develop into a symptomatic UTI. The incidence of UTI in infants who are breastfed is lower than in those fed with formula.

DIAGNOSIS

UTI may be suspected based on symptoms or findings on urinalysis, or both; *a urine culture is necessary for confirmation and appropriate therapy.* There are several ways to obtain a urine sample; some are more accurate than others. In toilet-trained children, a midstream urine sample usually is satisfactory; the introitus should be cleaned before obtaining the specimen. In uncircumcised boys, the prepuce must be retracted; if the prepuce is not retractable, a voided sample may be unreliable and contaminated with skin flora. According to the 2011 American Academy of Pediatrics (AAP) Clinical Guideline for children 2-24 mo, in children who are not toilet trained, a catheterized or suprapubic aspirate urine sample should be obtained. Alternatively, the application of an adhesive, sealed, sterile collection bag after disinfection of the skin of the genitals can be useful only if the culture is negative or if a single uropathogen is identified. However, a positive culture can result from skin contamination, particularly in girls and uncircumcised boys. If treatment is planned immediately after obtaining the urine culture, a bagged specimen should not be the method because of a high rate of contamination, often with mixed organisms. A suprapubic aspirate generally is unnecessary.

Nitrites and leukocyte esterase usually are positive in infected urine. Microscopic hematuria is common in acute cystitis, but microhematuria alone does not suggest UTI. White blood cell casts in the urinary sediment suggest renal involvement, but in practice these are rarely seen. If the child is asymptomatic and the urinalysis result is normal, it is unlikely that there is a UTI. However, if the child is symptomatic, a UTI is possible, even if the urinalysis result is negative (Table 538-2).

Pyuria (leukocytes on urine microscopy) suggests infection, but infection can occur in the absence of pyuria; this finding is more confirmatory than diagnostic. Conversely, pyuria can be present without UTI. Figure 538-3 shows the predictive value of leukocyte esterase, nitrites, and leukocytes.

Sterile pyuria (positive leukocytes, negative culture) may occur in partially treated bacterial UTIs, viral infections, renal tuberculosis, renal abscess, UTI in the presence of urinary obstruction, urethritis as a consequence of a sexually transmitted infection (see Chapter 120),

inflammation near the ureter or bladder (appendicitis, Crohn disease), or interstitial nephritis (eosinophils). Prompt plating of the urine sample for culture is important, because if the urine sits at room temperature for more than 60 min, overgrowth of a minor contaminant can suggest a UTI when the urine might not be infected. Refrigeration is a reliable method of storing the urine until it can be cultured.

If the culture shows >50,000 colonies of a single pathogen (suprapubic or catheter sample), or if there are 10,000 colonies and the child is symptomatic, the child is considered to have a UTI. In a bag sample, if the urinalysis result is positive, the patient is symptomatic, and there is a single organism cultured with a colony count >100,000, there is a presumed UTI. If any of these criteria are not met, confirmation of infection with a catheterized sample is recommended.

With acute renal infection, leukocytosis, neutrophilia, and elevated serum erythrocyte sedimentation rate, procalcitonin, and C-reactive protein are common. However these are all nonspecific markers of inflammation, and their elevation does not prove that the child has acute pyelonephritis. With a renal abscess, the white blood cell count is markedly elevated to >20,000-25,000/mm^3. An elevated serum procalcitonin level is associated with pyelonephritis and a high risk of renal scarring. Because sepsis is common in pyelonephritis, particularly in infants and in any child with obstructive uropathy, blood cultures should be drawn before starting antibiotics if possible.

According to the 2011 AAP Guidelines for children 2-24 mo, risk factors for girls include white race, age younger than 12 mo, temperature >39°C (102.2°F), fever for longer than 2 days, and absence of another source of infection. Risk factors for boys include nonblack race, temperature >39°C (102.2°F), fever for longer than 24 hr, and absence of another source of infection. Atypical features include failure to respond within 48 hr of appropriate antibiotics, poor urine flow, an abdominal flank or suprapubic mass, non–*E. coli* pathogen, urosepsis, and an elevated creatinine level.

TREATMENT

Acute cystitis should be treated promptly to prevent possible progression to pyelonephritis. If the symptoms are severe, presumptive treatment is started pending results of the culture. If the symptoms are mild or the diagnosis is doubtful, treatment can be delayed until the results of culture are known, and the culture can be repeated if the results are uncertain. If treatment is initiated before the results of a culture and sensitivities are available, a 3- to 5-day course of therapy with trimethoprim-sulfamethoxazole (TMP-SMX) or trimethoprim is effective against many strains of *E. coli*. Nitrofurantoin (5-7 mg/kg/24 hr in 3-4 divided doses) also is effective and has the advantage of being active against *Klebsiella* and *Enterobacter* organisms. Amoxicillin (50 mg/kg/24 hr) also is effective as initial treatment but has a high rate of bacterial resistance.

In acute febrile infections suggesting **clinical pyelonephritis,** a 7-14 day course of broad-spectrum antibiotics capable of reaching significant tissue levels is preferable. Children who are dehydrated, are vomiting, are unable to drink fluids, are 1 mo of age or younger, have complicated infection, or in whom urosepsis is a possibility should be admitted to the hospital for IV rehydration and IV antibiotic therapy. Parenteral treatment with ceftriaxone (50-75 mg/kg/24 hr, not to

Table 538-2	Sensitivity and Specificity of Components of Urinalysis, Alone and in Combination		
TEST		**SENSITIVITY (RANGE) %**	**SPECIFICITY (RANGE) %**
Leukocyte esterase test		83 (67-94)	78 (64-92)
Nitrite test		53 (15-82)	98 (90-100)
Leukocyte esterase or nitrite test positive		93 (90-100)	72 (58-91)
Microscopy (white blood cells)		73 (32-100)	81 (45-98)
Microscopy (bacteria)		81 (16-99)	83 (11-100)
Leukocyte esterase test, nitrite test, or microscopy positive		99.8 (99-100)	70 (60-92)

From Subcommittee on Urinary Tract Infection, Steering Committee on Quality Improvement and Management: Clinical practice guideline. Urinary tract infection: clinical practice guideline for the diagnosis and management of the initial UTI in Febrile infants and children 2 to 24 months. Pediatrics 128:595–610, 2011.

exceed 2 g) or cefotaxime (100 mg/kg/24 hr), or ampicillin (100 mg/kg/24 hr) with an aminoglycoside such as gentamicin (3-5 mg/kg/24 hr in 1-3 divided doses) is preferable. The potential ototoxicity and nephrotoxicity of aminoglycosides should be considered; serum creatinine should be obtained before initiating treatment, and daily trough gentamicin levels should be obtained during therapy. Treatment with aminoglycosides is particularly effective against *Pseudomonas* spp., and alkalinization of urine with sodium bicarbonate increases its effectiveness in the urinary tract.

Oral third-generation cephalosporins such as cefixime are as effective as parenteral ceftriaxone against a variety of Gram-negative organisms other than *Pseudomonas*, and these medications are considered by some authorities to be the treatment of choice for oral outpatient therapy. Nitrofurantoin should not be used routinely in children with a febrile UTI because it does not achieve significant renal tissue levels. The oral fluoroquinolone ciprofloxacin is an alternative agent for resistant microorganisms, particularly *Pseudomonas*, in patients older than age 17 yr. It also has been used on occasion for short-course therapy in younger children with *Pseudomonas* UTI. Levofloxacin is an alternative quinolone with a good safety profile in children. However, the clinical use of fluoroquinolones in children should be used with caution because of potential cartilage damage. In some children with a febrile UTI, intramuscular injection of a loading dose of ceftriaxone followed by oral therapy with a third-generation cephalosporin is effective. A urine culture 1 wk after the termination of treatment of a UTI ensures that the urine is sterile but is not routinely needed. A urine culture during treatment almost invariably is negative.

Children with a renal or perirenal abscess or with infection in obstructed urinary tracts can require surgical or percutaneous drainage in addition to antibiotic therapy and other supportive measures (see Fig. 538-2). Small abscesses may initially be treated without drainage.

In a child with recurrent UTIs, identification of predisposing factors is beneficial. Many school-age girls have **bladder–bowel dysfunction** (see Chapter 543); treatment of this condition often reduces the likelihood of recurrent UTI. Some children with UTIs void infrequently, and many also have severe constipation (see Chapters 306 and 332). Behavioral modification, with treatment of constipation as described in Chapter 543, often is effective. Antimicrobial prophylaxis using trimethoprim or nitrofurantoin at 30% of the normal therapeutic dose once a day is another approach to this problem but is unnecessary in most children with recurrent UTIs in the absence of severe reflux. Prophylaxis with TMP-SMZ, amoxicillin, or cephalexin can also be effective, but the risk of breakthrough UTI may be higher because bacterial resistance may be induced. Urologic conditions for recurrent UTIs that might benefit from long-term prophylaxis include neuropathic bladder, urinary tract stasis and obstruction, severe vesicoureteral reflux (see Chapter 539), and urinary calculi. There is interest in probiotic therapy, which replaces pathologic urogenital flora, and cranberry juice, which prevents bacterial adhesion and biofilm formation, but these agents have not proved beneficial in preventing UTI in children.

The main consequences of chronic renal damage caused by pyelonephritis are arterial hypertension and end-stage renal insufficiency; when they are found they should be treated appropriately (see Chapters 445 and 535).

IMAGING STUDIES IN CHILDREN WITH A FEBRILE UTI

The goal of imaging studies in children with a UTI is to identify anatomic abnormalities that predispose to infection, determine whether there is active renal involvement, and to assess whether renal function is normal or at risk.

There are 2 *historical* approaches to imaging, the traditional "bottom-up" and the "top-down" approaches.

1. The "bottom-up" method was a renal sonogram plus voiding cystourethrogram; this approach will identify upper and lower urinary tract abnormalities, including vesicoureteral reflux, bladder–bowel dysfunction, and bladder abnormalities, such as a paraureteral diverticulum. It is unlikely to detect renal scarring unless it is significant (renal cortical irregularity, small kidney on renal ultrasound). A dimercaptosuccinic acid (DMSA) scan is necessary to provide the best assessment of renal scarring. In some centers, the voiding cystourethrogram (VCUG) is delayed for 2-6 wk to allow inflammation in the bladder to resolve; however, the incidence of reflux is identical, regardless of whether the VCUG is obtained acutely at the time of treatment of the UTI or after 6 wk. Obtaining the VCUG before the child is discharged from the hospital is appropriate and ensures that the evaluation is complete. If available, a radionuclide VCUG rather than a contrast VCUG can be used in girls; this technique causes less radiation exposure to the gonads than does the contrast study. However, the radioisotope VCUG does not provide anatomic definition of the bladder, allow precise grading of reflux, demonstrate a paraureteral diverticulum, or show whether reflux is occurring into a duplicated collecting system or an ectopic ureter. In boys, VCUG definition of the urethra is important to detect posterior urethral valves (see Chapter 504).

2. The "top-down" approach was intended to reduce the number of VCUG examinations. It begins with a DMSA renal scan, to identify areas of acute pyelonephritic involvement, termed **acute pyelonephritis** (Fig. 538-5). The DMSA scan in younger children generally requires sedation. This condition is characterized by fever, malaise, abdominal or flank pain, and occasionally nausea and vomiting, and is a significant risk factor for renal injury and scarring. On DMSA, involved areas of the kidney are photopenic and the kidney is enlarged. Of children with a febrile UTI, approximately 50% have a positive DMSA scan. Of those with a positive scan, approximately 50% develop renal scarring in the areas of acute pyelonephritis, and in the remainder with acutely positive scans, the renal appearance will normalize. In children with dilating grades of reflux (III, IV, V), 80-90% with a febrile UTI have a DMSA scan consistent with acute pyelonephritis. Children with grades I and II reflux and those without reflux can also develop acute pyelonephritis. In longitudinal studies of children with grades I and II reflux and acute pyelonephritis, the reflux usually resolves. If the DMSA scan is normal during a febrile UTI, no scarring will result from that particular infection. CT is another diagnostic tool that can image acute pyelonephritis, but clinical experience with DMSA is much greater, and CT scans have significant radiation. If the DMSA scan is positive, then a VCUG is performed (Fig. 538-6), because 90% of children with dilating reflux have a positive DMSA scan. If reflux is identified, treatment is based on the perceived long-term risk of the reflux to the child (see Chapter 539). One limitation to this approach is that many hospitals caring for children with a febrile UTI might not have facilities for performing a DMSA scan in children. In these cases, a renal sonogram should be performed, after which the clinician decides whether to send the child to a facility with

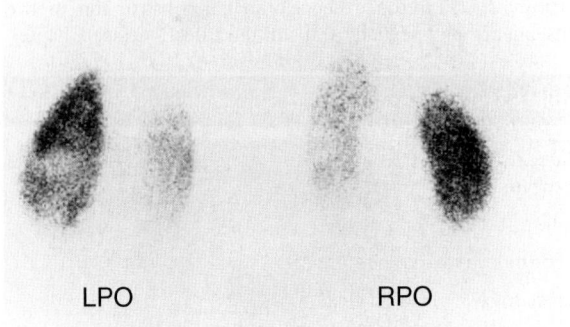

LPO   RPO

Figure 538-5 Dimercaptosuccinic acid renal scan showing bilateral photopenic areas indicating acute pyelonephritis and renal scarring. *LPO*, left posterior oblique; *RPO*, right posterior oblique.

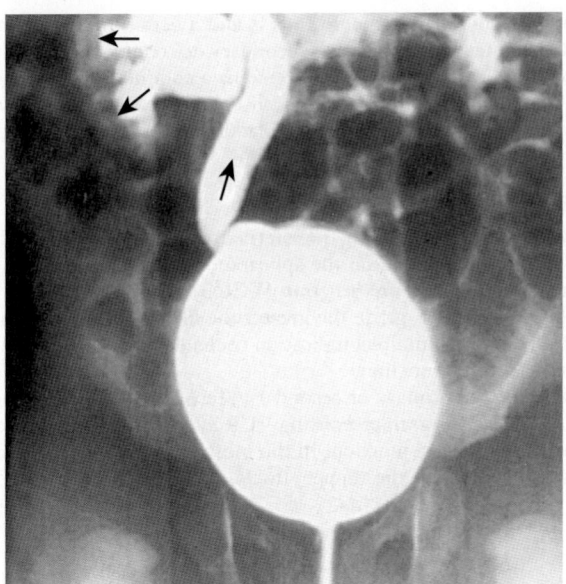

Figure 538-6 Intrarenal reflux. Voiding cystourethrogram in an infant boy with a past history of a urinary tract infection. Note the right vesicoureteral reflux with ureteral dilation, with opacification of the renal parenchyma representing intrarenal reflux.

DMSA capability or instead do a VCUG. In addition, if the DMSA scan is positive, then a follow-up scan is indicated 4-6 mo later to determine whether renal scarring occurred.

The AAP recommends that in a typical first-episode of UTI, initial imaging should be ultrasonography of the kidneys, ureters, and bladder. VCUG is indicated if the ultrasound study is abnormal, the patient has atypical features, or after a recurrent febrile UTI (Table 538-3).

In children with a history of cystitis, (dysuria, urgency, frequency, suprapubic pain), imaging is usually unnecessary. Instead, assessment and treatment of bladder and bowel dysfunction is important. If there are numerous lower UTIs, then a renal sonogram is appropriate, but a VCUG rarely adds useful information.

The AAP recommendation has resulted in a significant decrease in the number of VCUGs ordered. However, the pediatric urologic community has raised numerous concerns regarding the recommendations, and prospective studies will be necessary before determining whether they should be adopted. One consequence is that many primary care physicians have generalized these recommendations, which were intended for children *2-24 mo*, to *all* children.

Similarly, in 2007, the NICE (National Institute for Health and Clinical Excellence, UK) guidelines for diagnosis, management, and imaging after UTI were released (Table 538-4). These recommendations divided children into those younger than 6 mo, 6 mo-3 yr, and older than 3 yr of age. An initial VCUG is recommended only in children younger than age 6 mo. These recommendations are highly controversial

---

Table 538-3 | Guideline Recommendations for Diagnostic Evaluation Following a Febrile Urinary Tract Infection in Infants

GUIDELINE	ULTRASONOGRAPHY	VCUG	LATE DMSA SCAN
National Institute for Health And Care Excellence (NICE)*	(see Table 538-4)		
American Academy of Pediatrics	Yes	If abnormal ultrasonogram	No
Italian Society for Paediatric Nephrology (ISPN)	Yes	If abnormal ultrasonogram or if risk factors are present[†]	If abnormal ultrasonogram or VUR

*Upper urinary tract dilation on ultrasonography, poor urinary flow, infection with organism other than *E. coli*, or family history of vesicoureteral reflux.
[†]Abnormal antenatal ultrasonogram of fetal urinary tract, family history of reflux, septicemia, renal failure, age younger than 6 mo in a male infant, likely family noncompliance, incomplete bladder emptying, no clinical response to appropriate antibiotic therapy within 72 hr, or infection with organism other than *E. coli*.
DMSA, dimercaptosuccinic acid; VCUG, voiding cystourethrogram; VUR, vesicoureteral reflux.

Table 538-4 | Recommended Imaging Schedule for Children with Urinary Tract Infection

	Type of Infection		
CHILD AGE AND TESTS	RESPONDS WELL TO TREATMENT WITHIN 48 HR	ATYPICAL INFECTION	RECURRENT INFECTION
CHILDREN YOUNGER THAN 6 MO OLD			
Ultrasound scan during acute infection	No	Yes	Yes
Ultrasound scan within 6 wk of infection	Yes	No	No
DMSA scan 4-6 mo after acute infection	No	Yes	Yes
Micturating cystograms	Consider if ultrasound scan abnormal	Yes	Yes
CHILDREN 6 MO-3 YR OLD			
Ultrasound scan during acute infection	No	Yes	No
Ultrasound scan within 6 wk of infection	No	No	Yes
DMSA scan 4-6 mo after acute infection	No	Yes	Yes
Micturating cystograms	No	Not routine, consider if dilation on ultrasound, poor urine flow, non–*E. coli* infection, or family history of vesicoureteric reflux	
CHILDREN OLDER THAN AGE 3 YR			
Ultrasound scan during acute infection	No	Yes	No
Ultrasound scan within 6 wk of infection	No	No	Yes
DMSA scan 4-6 mo after acute infection	No	Yes	Yes
Micturating cystograms	No	No	No

DMSA, dimercaptosuccinic acid.
Adapted from National Institute for Health and Clinical Excellence. Urinary tract infection in children: diagnosis, treatment, and long-term management. NICE clinical guidelines, no. 54. London, 2007, RCOG Press, Tables 6-13, 6-14, and 6-15.

because the methodology was not based on evidence but on expert opinion. In addition, there was no retrospective or prospective assessment of the potential of this approach to identify significant uropathology. There is evidence that a significant number of children with uropathology would not have been identified under these guidelines.

PROPHYLAXIS OF RECURRENT URINARY TRACT INFECTION

See Chapter 539.

In children with a first episode of pyelonephritis in an otherwise anatomically normal urinary tract and no evidence of reflux, no antimicrobial prophylaxis is required in an attempt to prevent a recurrence or renal scarring.

Bibliography is available at Expert Consult.

Chapter **539**
Vesicoureteral Reflux
Jack S. Elder

Vesicoureteral reflux (VUR) describes the retrograde flow of urine from the bladder to the ureter and kidney. The ureteral attachment to the bladder normally is oblique, between the bladder mucosa and detrusor muscle, creating a flap-valve mechanism that prevents VUR (Fig. 539-1). VUR occurs when the submucosal tunnel between the mucosa and detrusor muscle is short or absent. Affecting 1-2% of children, VUR usually is congenital and often is familial. VUR is present in approximately 30% of females who had a urinary tract infection and in 5-15% of infants with antenatal hydronephrosis.

VUR predisposes to kidney infection (pyelonephritis) by facilitating the transport of bacteria from the bladder to the upper urinary tract (see Chapter 538). The inflammatory reaction caused by pyelonephritis can result in renal injury or scarring, also termed **reflux-related renal injury** or **reflux nephropathy.** In children with a febrile **urinary tract infection (UTI),** those with VUR are 3 times more likely to develop renal injury compared to those without VUR. Extensive renal scarring impairs renal function and can result in renin-mediated hypertension (see Chapter 445), renal insufficiency or end-stage renal disease (see Chapter 535), impaired somatic growth, and morbidity during pregnancy. Scarring associated with reflux may be present at birth or develop in the absence of infection.

In the past, reflux nephropathy accounted for as much as 15-20% of end-stage renal disease in children and young adults. With greater attention to the management of UTIs and a better understanding of VUR, end-stage renal disease secondary to reflux nephropathy is uncommon. Reflux nephropathy remains a common cause of hypertension in children. VUR in the absence of infection or elevated bladder pressure (e.g., neuropathic bladder, posterior urethral valves) rarely causes renal injury.

CLASSIFICATION

VUR severity is graded using the International Reflux Study Classification of I-V and is based on the appearance of the urinary tract on a contrast *voiding cystourethrogram* **(VCUG)** (Figs. 539-2 and 539-3). The higher the VUR grade the greater the likelihood of renal injury. VUR severity is an indirect indication of the degree of abnormality of the ureterovesical junction.

VUR may be primary or secondary (Table 539-1). Bladder–bowel dysfunction can worsen preexisting VUR if there is a marginally competent ureterovesical junction. In the most severe cases, there is such massive VUR into the upper tracts that the bladder becomes

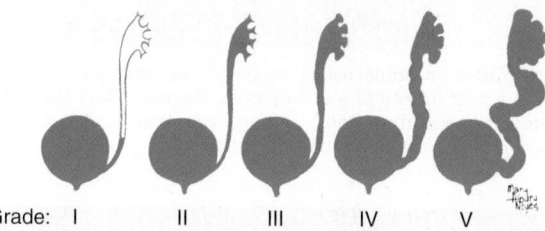

Grade: I   II   III   IV   V

Figure 539-2 Grading of vesicoureteral reflux. Grade I: VUR into a nondilated ureter. Grade II: VUR into the upper collecting system without dilation. Grade III: VUR into dilated ureter and/or blunting of calyceal fornices. Grade IV: VUR into a grossly dilated ureter. Grade V: massive VUR, with significant ureteral dilation and tortuosity and loss of the papillary impression.

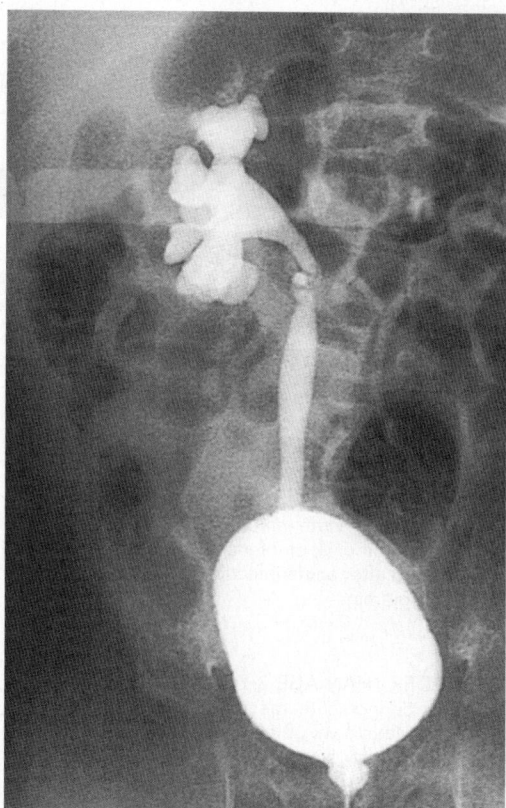

Figure 539-3 Voiding cystourethrogram showing grade IV right vesicoureteral reflux.

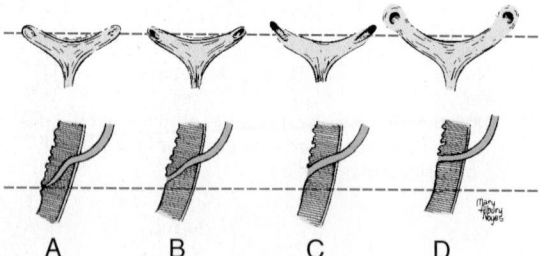

A   B   C   D

Figure 539-1 Normal and abnormal configuration of the ureteral orifices. Shown from *left* to *right*, progressive lateral displacement of the ureteral orifices and shortening of the intramural tunnels. *Top,* Endoscopic appearance. *Bottom,* Sagittal view through the intramural ureter.

overdistended. This condition, the **megacystis-megaureter syndrome,** occurs primarily in boys and may be unilateral or bilateral (Fig. 539-4). Reimplantation of the ureters into the bladder to correct VUR corrects the condition.

Approximately 1 in 125 children have a **duplication** of the upper urinary tract, in which 2 ureters rather than 1 drain the kidney. Duplication may be partial or complete. In partial duplication, the ureters join above the bladder and there is 1 ureteral orifice. In complete duplication, the attachment of the lower pole ureter to the bladder is superior and lateral to the upper pole ureter. The valve-like mechanism for the lower pole ureter often is marginal, and VUR into the lower ureter occurs in as many as 50% of cases (Fig. 539-5). With a duplication anomaly, some patients have an ectopic ureter, in which the upper pole ureter drains outside the bladder (see Chapters 540 and 543 and Figs. 543-6 and 543-7). If the ectopic ureter drains into the bladder neck, typically it is obstructed and refluxes. Duplication anomalies also are common in children with a ureterocele, which is a cystic swelling

of the intramural portion of the distal ureter. These patients often have VUR into the associated lower pole ureter or the contralateral ureter. In addition, generally VUR is present when the ureter enters a bladder diverticulum (Fig. 539-6).

VUR is present at birth in 25% of children with **neuropathic bladder,** as occurs in myelomeningocele (see Chapter 591.4), sacral agenesis, and many cases of high imperforate anus. VUR is seen in 50% of boys with posterior urethral valves. VUR with increased intravesical pressure (as in detrusor–sphincter dyssynergia or bladder outlet obstruction) can result in renal injury because of increased intravesical pressure transmitted to the upper urinary tract, even in the absence of infection.

Primary VUR occurs in association with several congenital urinary tract abnormalities. Of children with a multicystic dysplastic kidney or renal agenesis (see Chapter 537), 15% have VUR into the contralateral kidney, and 10-15% of children with a ureteropelvic junction obstruction have VUR into either the hydronephrotic kidney or the contralateral kidney.

Table 539-1	Classification of Vesicoureteral Reflux	
TYPE	**CAUSE**
Primary	Congenital incompetence of the valvular mechanism of the vesicoureteral junction
Primary associated with other malformations of the ureterovesical junction	Ureteral duplication Ureterocele with duplication Ureteral ectopia Paraureteral diverticula
Secondary to increased intravesical pressure	Neuropathic bladder Nonneuropathic bladder dysfunction Bladder outlet obstruction
Secondary to inflammatory processes	Severe bacterial cystitis Foreign bodies Vesical calculi Clinical cystitis
Secondary to surgical procedures involving the ureterovesical junction	Surgery

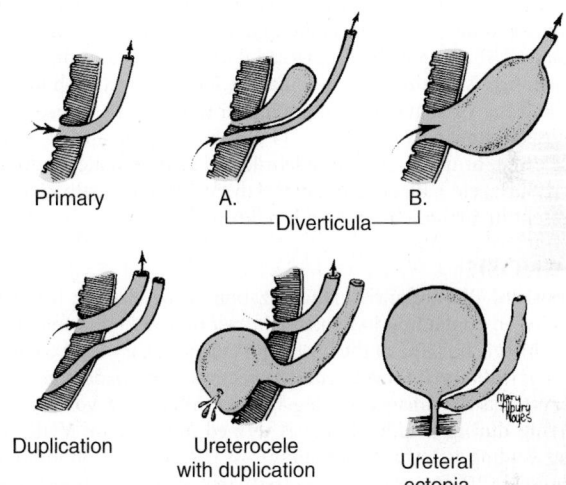

Figure 539-5 Various anatomic defects of the ureterovesical junction associated with vesicoureteral reflux.

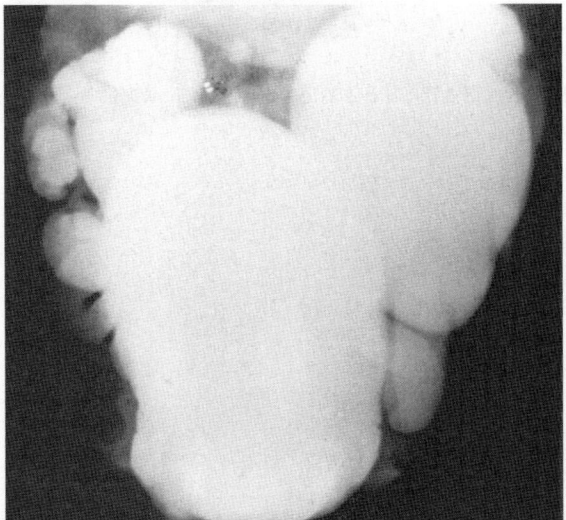

Figure 539-4 Voiding cystourethrogram in newborn boy with megacystis-megaureter syndrome. Note the massive ureteral dilation caused by high-grade vesicoureteral reflux. The bladder is very distended. There was no urethral obstruction or neuropathic dysfunction.

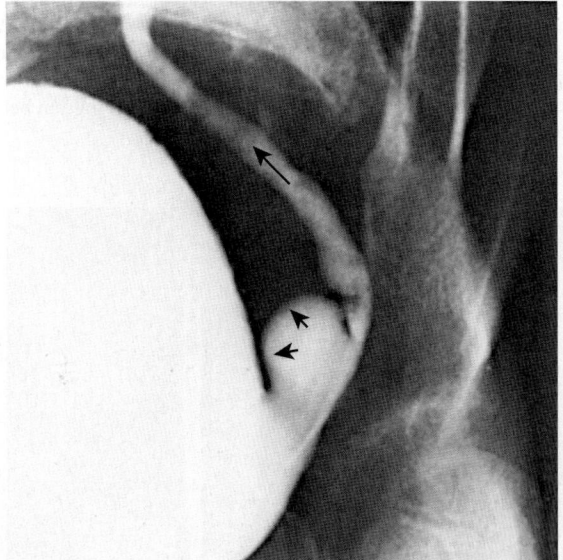

Figure 539-6 VUR and bladder diverticulum. The voiding cystourethrogram demonstrates left vesicoureteral reflux and a paraureteral diverticulum.

VUR (idiopathic) appears to be an autosomal dominant inherited trait with variable penetrance. Approximately 35% of siblings of children with VUR also have VUR, and VUR is found in nearly half of newborn siblings. The likelihood of a sibling having VUR is independent of the grade of VUR or sex of the index child. Approximately 12% of asymptomatic siblings with VUR have evidence of renal scarring. In addition, 50% of children born to women with a history of VUR also have VUR. In 2010 the American Urological Association Vesicoureteral Reflux Guidelines Panel stated that, in siblings of individuals with VUR, a VCUG or radionuclide cystogram is recommended if there is evidence of renal cortical abnormalities or renal size asymmetry on sonography, or if the sibling has a history of UTI. Otherwise, screening is optional. VUR may be suggested on a prenatal ultrasound, which demonstrates dilated renal calyces. Primary VUR is uncommon in African-Americans.

CLINICAL MANIFESTATIONS

VUR usually is discovered during evaluation for a UTI (see Chapter 538). Among these children, 80% are female, and the average age at diagnosis is 2-3 yr. In other children, a VCUG is performed during evaluation of bladder–bowel dysfunction, renal insufficiency, hypertension, or other suspected pathologic process of the urinary tract. Primary VUR also may be discovered during evaluation for antenatal hydronephrosis. In this select population, 80% of affected children are male, and the VUR grade usually is higher than in girls whose VUR is diagnosed following a UTI. The UTI may be symptomatic, an isolated febrile event, or more often both febrile and symptomatic (abdominal pain, dysuria, etc.). Bladder and bowel dysfunction (constipation) may be present in 50% of children with reflux and a UTI.

DIAGNOSIS

Diagnosis of VUR requires catheterization of the bladder, instillation of a solution containing iodinated contrast or a radiopharmaceutical, and radiologic imaging of the lower and upper urinary tract: a contrast VCUG or *radionuclide cystogram*, respectively. The bladder and upper urinary tracts are imaged during bladder filling and voiding. VUR occurring during bladder filling is termed *low-pressure* VUR; VUR during voiding is termed *high-pressure* VUR. VUR in children with low-pressure VUR is significantly less likely to resolve spontaneously than in children who exhibit only high-pressure VUR. Radiation exposure during a radionuclide cystogram is significantly less than that from a contrast VCUG. However, the contrast VCUG provides more anatomic information, such as demonstration of a duplex collecting system, ectopic ureter, paraureteral (bladder) diverticulum, bladder outlet obstruction in boys, upper urinary tract stasis, and signs of voiding dysfunction, such as a "spinning top" urethra in girls. The VUR grading system is based on the appearance on contrast VCUG, and the grade reported is the maximum grade observed during the study. For follow-up evaluation, some prefer the radionuclide cystogram because

of the lower radiation exposure (Fig. 539-7), although it is difficult to determine whether the VUR severity has changed.

Children undergoing cystography may be psychologically traumatized by the catheterization. Careful preparation by caregivers, use of Child Life individuals, or administration of oral or nasal midazolam (for sedation and amnesia) or propofol before the study can result in a less-distressing experience.

Indirect cystography is a technique of detecting VUR without catheterization that involves injecting an intravenous radiopharmaceutical that is excreted by the kidneys, waiting for it to be excreted into the bladder, and imaging the lower urinary tract while the patient voids. This technique detects only 75% of VUR cases. Another technique, which avoids radiation exposure, involves instilling sonographic contrast medium through a urethral catheter. The kidneys are imaged sonographically to determine whether any of the material refluxes. This technique is investigational.

After VUR is diagnosed, assessment of the upper urinary tract is important. The goal of upper tract imaging is to assess whether renal scarring and associated urinary tract anomalies are present. Renal imaging typically is performed with a renal sonogram or renal scintigraphy (Fig. 539-8; see Chapter 538).

The child should be evaluated for bladder–bowel dysfunction, including urgency, frequency, diurnal incontinence, infrequent voiding,

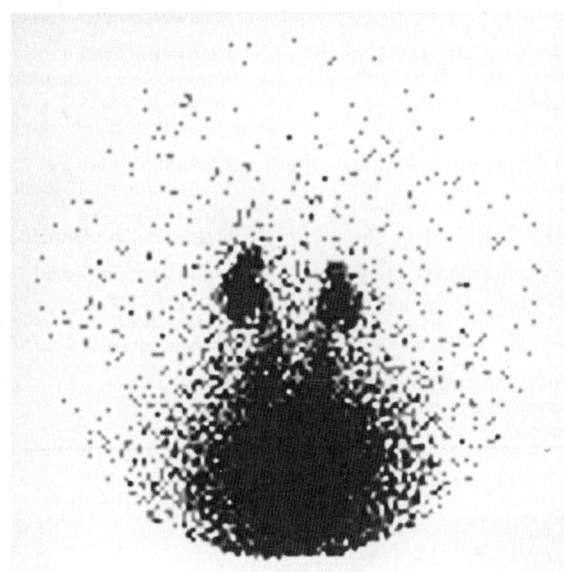

Figure 539-7 Radionuclide cystogram shows bilateral VUR.

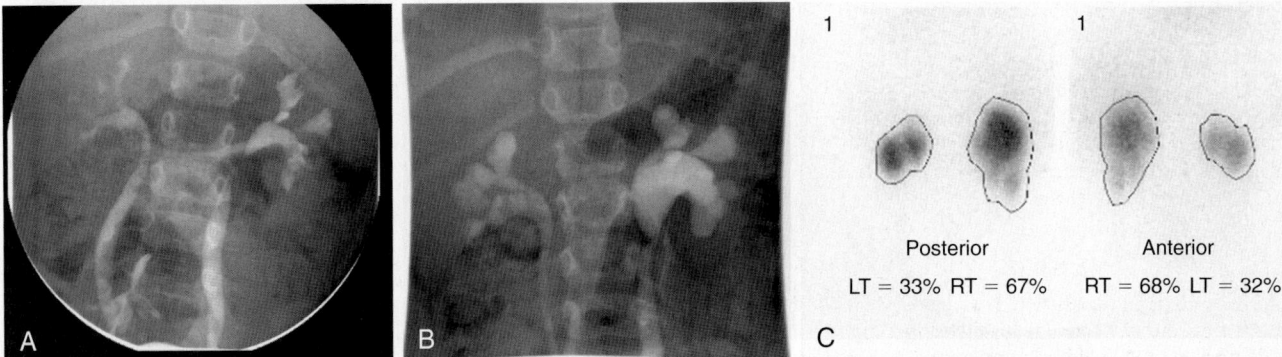

Figure 539-8 A, Voiding cystourethrogram (VCUG) in a 3 yr old girl with 2 febrile urinary tract infections shows bilateral grade III VUR. **B,** At 5 yr, repeat VCUG shows worsening VUR and calyceal clubbing, indicating renal scarring. **C,** At 11 yr, she has developed renin-mediated hypertension. Dimercaptosuccinic acid (DMSA) renal scan shows significant VUR-related renal scarring.

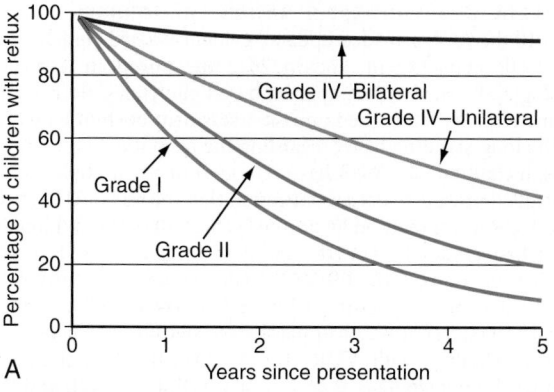
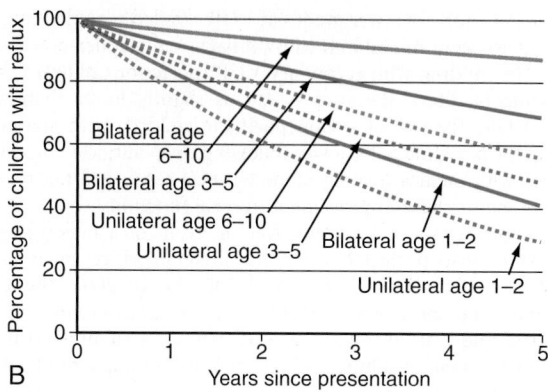

Figure 539-9 A, Percentage chance of VUR persistence, grades I, II, and IV, for 1-5 yr after presentation. **B,** Percentage chance of VUR persistence by age at presentation, grade III, for 1-5 yr after presentation. *(From Elder JS, Peters CA, Arant BS Jr, et al: Pediatric Vesicoureteral Reflux Guidelines Panel summary report on the management of primary vesicoureteral vesicoureteral reflux in children, J Urol 157:1846–1851, 1997.)*

or a combination of these (see Chapter 543). Children with an overactive bladder often undergo a regimen of behavioral modification with timed voiding, and, on occasion, anticholinergic therapy.

After diagnosis, the child's height, weight, and blood pressure should be measured and monitored. If upper tract imaging shows renal scarring, a serum creatinine measurement should be obtained. The urine should be assessed for infection and proteinuria.

NATURAL HISTORY

The incidence of reflux-related renal scarring increases with VUR grade. With bladder growth and maturation, the VUR grade often resolves or improves. Lower grades of VUR are much more likely to resolve than are higher grades. For grades I and II VUR, the likelihood of resolution is similar regardless of age at diagnosis and whether it is unilateral or bilateral. For grade III, a younger age at diagnosis and unilateral VUR usually are associated with a higher rate of spontaneous resolution (Fig. 539-9). Bilateral grade IV VUR is much less likely to resolve than is unilateral grade IV VUR. Grade V VUR rarely resolves. The mean age at VUR resolution is 6 yr.

VUR does not usually cause renal injury in the absence of infection, but in situations with high-pressure VUR, as in children with posterior urethral valves, neuropathic bladder, and nonneurogenic neurogenic bladder (i.e., Hinman syndrome), sterile VUR can cause significant renal damage. Children with high-grade VUR who acquire a UTI are at significant risk for acute and recurrent pyelonephritis and new renal scarring (see Fig. 539-8).

TREATMENT

The goals of treatment are to prevent pyelonephritis, VUR-related renal injury, and other complications of VUR. Medical therapy is based on the principle that VUR often resolves over time and that if UTIs can be prevented, the morbidity or complications of VUR may be avoided without surgery. Medical therapy includes observation with behavioral modification or behavioral modification with antimicrobial prophylaxis in some patients. The basis for surgical therapy is that in selected children, ongoing VUR has caused or has significant potential for causing renal injury or other VUR-related complications, and that elimination of VUR minimizes the risk of these problems. Therapy for VUR should be individualized based on a particular patient's risk factors.

Observation

In children undergoing observation, therapeutic emphasis is directed to minimizing the risk of UTI by behavioral modification. These methods include timed voiding during the day, ensuring regular fecal elimination, increased fluid intake, periodic assessment of satisfactory bladder emptying, and prompt assessment and treatment of UTIs, particularly febrile UTIs. This approach is most appropriate for

children with grades I and II VUR, and perhaps older children with persistent VUR and normal kidneys who have not experienced clinical pyelonephritis.

Antimicrobial Prophylaxis

In the past, based on clinical series demonstrating the effectiveness of antibiotic prophylaxis and the 1997 ***American Urological Association*** (***AUA***) Reflux Guidelines, daily prophylaxis was recommended as initial therapy for most children with VUR. Currently, many families express concern regarding the safety and benefit of prophylaxis. In addition, as a result of several prospective clinical trials, the benefit of prophylaxis has been questioned in children with VUR. The risk of recurrent UTI is highest in patients with grade III or IV reflux, those with bowel and bladder dysfunction, and those whose first reflux associated UTI was febrile rather than just symptomatic without fever. Antibiotic prophylaxis after a reflux associated UTI decreases the risk of recurrent UTI but increases the risk of developing resistant bacteria. In one study, antibiotic prophylaxis reduced the risk of new renal scars in children with grade III or IV reflux; while in another larger study antibiotic prophylaxis did not have an effect on the incidence of new renal scars in those with severe reflux (approximately 10% developed new scars regardless of prophylaxis).

Surgery

The purpose of surgical therapy is to minimize the risks of ongoing VUR and nonsurgical therapy (prophylaxis and follow-up testing). VUR can be corrected through a lower abdominal or inguinal incision (open), laparoscopically (with or without robotic assistance), or endoscopically with subureteral injection.

Open surgical management involves modifying the abnormal ureterovesical attachment to create a 4 : 1 to 5 : 1 ratio of intramural ureter length : ureteral diameter. The operation can be performed from either outside or inside the bladder. When VUR is associated with severe ureteral dilation (i.e., megaureter), the ureter must be tailored or narrowed to a more normal size to allow a smaller length : width ratio for the intramural tunnel, and a corner of the bladder is attached to the psoas tendon, forming a *psoas hitch*. Most children can be discharged 1-2 days following the surgical procedure. If the refluxing kidney is poorly functioning, nephrectomy or nephroureterectomy is indicated. Laparoscopic VUR correction and robotic-assisted laparoscopic ureteral reimplantation have being investigated and have been shown to have similar results to conventional open surgery in older children.

The success rate of conventional open ureteral reimplantation in children with primary VUR is >95-98% for grades I-IV, with 2% experiencing persistent VUR and 1% having ureteral obstruction that requires correction. The success rate is so high that many pediatric urologists do not perform a postoperative VCUG unless the child develops clinical pyelonephritis. For grade V VUR, the success rate is approximately 80%. In lower grades of VUR, a failed reimplantation is most likely to occur in children with undiagnosed bladder-bowel dysfunction. In children with secondary VUR (posterior urethral valves, neuropathic bladder), the success rate is slightly lower than with primary VUR. The risk of pyelonephritis in children with grades III and IV VUR is significantly lower following open surgical correction compared with medical management. Surgical repair will not reverse renal scarring or cause improvement in renal function.

Endoscopic repair of VUR involves injection of a bulking agent through a cystoscope just beneath the ureteral orifice, creating an artificial flap-valve (Figs. 539-10 and 539-11). In 2001, the FDA approved the use of a biodegradable material, dextranomer microspheres suspended in hyaluronic acid (Deflux), for subureteral injection. The advantage of subureteral injection is that it is a noninvasive outpatient procedure (performed under general anesthesia) with no recovery time. The success rate is 70-80% and is highest for lower grades of VUR. If the first injection is unsuccessful, 1 or 2 repeat injections can be performed. The VUR recurrence rate is approximately 10%.

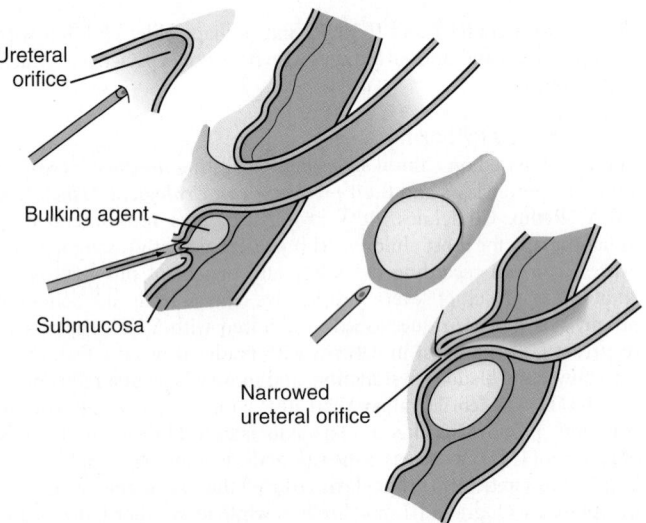

Figure 539-10 Endoscopic correction of VUR. Through a cystoscope, a needle is inserted into the submucosal plane deep to the ureteral orifice and bulking agent is injected, creating a flap-valve to prevent VUR. *(Adapted from Ortenberg J: Endoscopic treatment of vesicoureteral reflux in children,* Urol Clin North Am *25:151–156, 1998.)*

Current Vesicoureteral Reflux Guidelines

In 2010 the AUA provided updated evidence-based guidelines regarding VUR management, and in 2012 the European Association of Urology published expert opinion based guidelines. Both society recommendations were based on risk assessment of children with VUR.

The long-standing belief regarding the benefit of antibiotic prophylaxis in children with VUR has been questioned. Multiple randomized controlled prospective trials suggested that the risk of UTI in children with VUR is not reduced by prophylaxis. Most of the children in these trials had grades I-III VUR, and few younger than 1 yr old were studied. In contrast, the PRIVENT (Prevention of Recurrent Urinary Tract Infection in Children with Vesicoureteric Reflux and Normal Renal Tracts) trial from Australia showed significant benefit to prophylaxis in children with VUR. The Swedish VUR Trial in Children studied children younger than 2 yr of age with grades III and IV VUR; they compared antibiotic prophylaxis to observation and endoscopic injection therapy. Girls in the surveillance group had a significantly higher incidence of febrile UTI and new renal scarring compared to the other treatment groups. The largest randomized trial (RIVUR [Randomized Intervention for Children with Vesicoureteral Reflux]) enrolled more than 600 children and demonstrated a reduction in the recurrence rate of UTIs but no reduction of the occurrence of renal scarring with antibiotic prophylaxis.

Prophylaxis is recommended by the AUA in children at greatest risk for VUR-related renal injury (i.e., those younger than 1 yr of age). In addition, evaluation for *bladder and bowel dysfunction* is considered a standard part of initial and ongoing patient evaluation in children with VUR. Because children with bladder and bowel dysfunction and VUR are much more likely to have recurrent UTIs and renal scarring, prophylaxis is recommended for these children. In children with VUR who are being managed by surveillance, if a febrile UTI occurs, prophylaxis is recommended. The decision whether to recommend observation, medical therapy, or surgery is based on the risk of VUR to the patient, the likelihood of spontaneous resolution, and the parents' and patient's preferences, and the family should understand the risks and benefits of each treatment approach.

Another aspect of VUR management pertains to screening. VUR is known to be a familial disorder with autosomal dominant transmission with variable penetrance. The advantage of early VUR detection is to implement treatment before a potentially damaging episode of clinical pyelonephritis. In siblings of an index patient with VUR, optional management includes screening of asymptomatic siblings or offspring with a renal ultrasound or VCUG. The AUA recommends that a VCUG should be obtained if a screening ultrasound demonstrated a renal abnormality or if the sibling had a UTI.

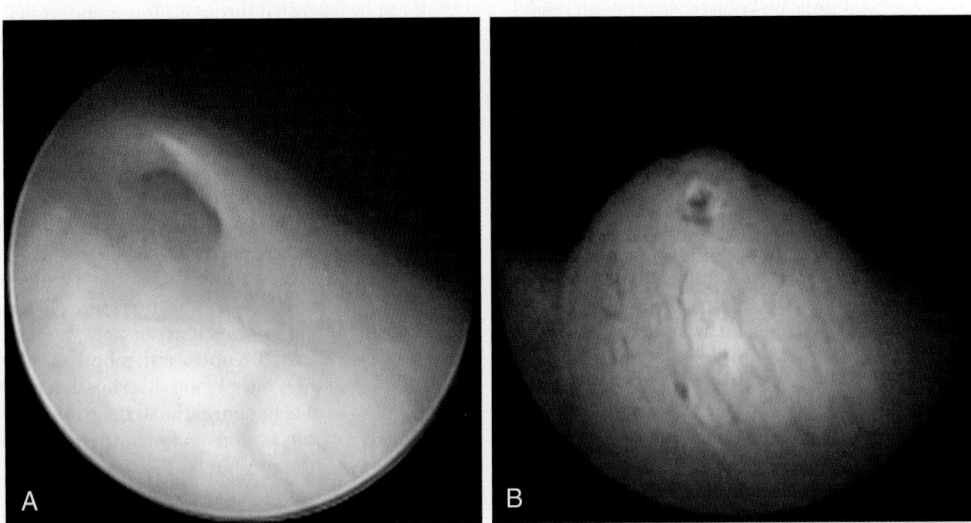

Figure 539-11 A, Endoscopic view of right vesicoureteral refluxing ureter. **B,** The same ureter after subureteral injection of dextranomer microspheres.

The AUA also determined that female newborns with renal pelvic dilation were significantly more likely than male newborns to have VUR. The AUA recommended that a VCUG should be performed in neonates with grade 3-4 antenatal hydronephrosis (moderate to severe pelvocaliceal dilation), hydroureter, or an abnormal bladder. In children with less-severe renal pelvic dilation, an observational approach without screening for VUR, with prompt treatment of any UTI, is appropriate. However, they also indicated that obtaining a VCUG is considered an appropriate option for neonates with lesser grades of hydronephrosis.

Bibliography is available at Expert Consult.

Chapter 540
Obstruction of the Urinary Tract
Jack S. Elder

Most childhood obstructive lesions are congenital, although urinary tract obstruction can be caused by trauma, neoplasia, calculi, inflammatory processes, or surgical procedures. Obstructive lesions occur at any level from the urethral meatus to the calyceal infundibula (Table 540-1). The pathophysiologic effects of obstruction depend on its level, the extent of involvement, the child's age at onset, and whether it is acute or chronic.

ETIOLOGY
Ureteral obstruction occurring early in fetal life results in renal dysplasia, ranging from multicystic kidney, which is associated with ureteral or pelvic atresia (see Fig. 537-2 in Chapter 537), to various degrees of histologic renal cortical dysplasia that are seen with less-severe obstruction. Chronic ureteral obstruction in late fetal life or after birth results in dilation of the ureter, renal pelvis, and calyces, with alterations of renal parenchyma ranging from minimal tubular changes to dilation of Bowman's space, glomerular fibrosis, and interstitial fibrosis. After birth, infections often complicate obstruction and can increase renal damage.

Prenatal screening with ultrasonography may detect antenatal hydronephrosis, which is graded by the trimester and the anterior-posterior diameter of the renal pelvis (Table 540-2); most are mild. Table 540-3 notes the eventual etiology.

CLINICAL MANIFESTATIONS
Obstruction of the urinary tract generally causes **hydronephrosis,** which typically is asymptomatic in its early phases. An obstructed kidney secondary to a **ureteropelvic junction (UPJ)** or **ureterovesical junction** obstruction can manifest as a unilateral mass or cause upper abdominal or flank pain on the affected side. Pyelonephritis can occur because of urinary stasis. An upper urinary tract stone can occur, causing abdominal and flank pain and hematuria. With bladder outlet obstruction, the urinary stream may be weak; urinary tract infection (UTI; see Chapter 538) is common. Many of these lesions are identified by antenatal ultrasonography; an abnormality involving the genitourinary tract is suspected in as many as 1 in 100 fetuses.

Obstructive renal insufficiency can manifest itself by failure to thrive, vomiting, diarrhea, or other nonspecific signs and symptoms. In older children, *infravesical obstruction* can be associated with overflow urinary incontinence or a poor urine stream. *Acute ureteral obstruction* causes flank or abdominal pain; there may be nausea and vomiting. *Chronic ureteral obstruction* can be silent or can cause vague abdominal or typical flank pain with increased fluid intake.

Table 540-1 Types and Causes of Urinary Tract Obstruction

LOCATION	CAUSE
Infundibula	Congenital Calculi Inflammatory (tuberculosis) Traumatic Postsurgical Neoplastic
Renal pelvis	Congenital (infundibulopelvic stenosis) Inflammatory (tuberculosis) Calculi Neoplasia (Wilms tumor, neuroblastoma)
Ureteropelvic junction	Congenital stenosis Calculi Neoplasia Inflammatory Postsurgical Traumatic
Ureter	Congenital obstructive megaureter Midureteral structure Ureteral ectopia Ureterocele Retrocaval ureter Ureteral fibroepithelial polyps Ureteral valves Calculi Postsurgical Extrinsic compression Neoplasia (neuroblastoma, lymphoma, and other retroperitoneal or pelvic tumors) Inflammatory (Crohn disease, chronic granulomatous disease) Hematoma, urinoma Lymphocele Retroperitoneal fibrosis
Bladder outlet and urethra	Neurogenic bladder dysfunction (functional obstruction) Posterior urethral valves Anterior urethral valves Diverticula Urethral strictures (congenital, traumatic, or iatrogenic) Urethral atresia Ectopic ureterocele Meatal stenosis (males) Calculi Foreign bodies Phimosis Extrinsic compression by tumors Urogenital sinus anomalies

Table 540-2 Definition of Antenatal Hydronephrosis by Anterior-Posterior Diameter

DEGREE OF ANTENATAL HYDRONEPHROSIS	SECOND TRIMESTER	THIRD TRIMESTER
Mild	4 to <7 mm	7 to <9 mm
Moderate	7 to ≤10 mm	9 to ≤15 mm
Severe	>10 mm	>15 mm

From Nguyen HT, Herndon CDA, Cooper C, et al: The society for fetal urology consensus statement on the evaluation and management of antenatal hydronephrosis. J Pediatr Urol 6:212–231, 2010, Table 2, p. 215.

DIAGNOSIS

Urinary tract obstruction may be diagnosed prenatally by ultrasonography, which typically shows hydronephrosis and occasionally a distended bladder. More complete evaluation, including imaging studies, should be undertaken in these children in the neonatal period.

Urinary tract obstruction is often silent. In the newborn infant, a palpable abdominal mass most commonly is a hydronephrotic or multicystic dysplastic kidney. With posterior urethral valves, which is an infravesical obstructive lesion in boys, a walnut-sized mass representing the bladder is palpable just above the pubic symphysis. A **patent draining urachus** also can suggest urethral obstruction. **Urinary ascites** in the newborn usually is caused by renal or bladder urinary extravasation secondary to posterior urethral valves. Infection and sepsis may be the first indications of an obstructive lesion of the urinary tract. The combination of infection and obstruction poses a serious threat to infants and children and generally requires parenteral administration of antibiotics and drainage of the obstructed kidney. Renal ultrasonography should be performed in all children during the acute stage of an initial febrile UTI.

Imaging Studies
Renal Ultrasonography

Hydronephrosis is the most common characteristic of obstruction (Fig. 540-1). Upper urinary tract dilation is not diagnostic of obstruction and often persists after surgical correction of a significant obstructive lesion. Dilation can result from vesicoureteral reflux, or it may be a manifestation of abnormal development of the urinary tract, even when there is no obstruction. Renal length, degree of caliectasis and

Table 540-3	The Etiology of Antenatal Hydronephrosis
ETIOLOGY	**INCIDENCE**
Transient hydronephrosis	41-88%
Ureteropelvic junction obstruction	10-30%
Vesicoureteral reflux	10-20%
Ureterovesical junction obstruction/megaureters	5-10%
Multicystic dysplastic kidney	4-6%
Posterior urethral valve/urethral atresia	1-2%
Ureterocele/ectopic ureter/duplex system	5-7%
Others: prune belly syndrome, cystic kidney disease, congenital ureteric strictures, and megalourethra	Uncommon

From Nguyen HT, Herndon CDA, Cooper C, et al: The society for fetal urology consensus statement on the evaluation and management of antenatal hydronephrosis. J Pediatr Urol 6:212–231, 2010, Table 5, p. 217.

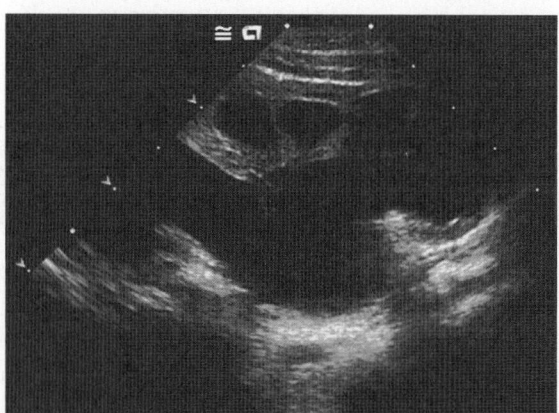

Figure 540-1 Ultrasonographic image of the kidney with marked pelvic and calyceal dilation (grade 4 hydronephrosis) in a newborn with ureteropelvic junction obstruction.

parenchymal thickness, and presence or absence of ureteral dilation should be assessed. Most pediatric urologists grade the severity of hydronephrosis from 1-4 using the Society for Fetal Urology grading scale (Table 540-4), whereas pediatric radiologists generally utilize the adjectives mild, moderate, and severe. The clinician should ascertain that the contralateral kidney is normal, and the bladder should be imaged to see whether the bladder wall is thickened, the lower ureter is dilated, and bladder emptying is complete. In acute or intermittent obstruction, the dilation of the collecting system may be minimal and ultrasonography may be misleading.

Voiding Cystourethrogram

In neonates and infants with congenital grade 3 or 4 hydronephrosis and in any child with ureteral dilation, a **contrast voiding cystourethrogram (VCUG)** should be obtained, because the dilation is secondary to vesicoureteral reflux in 15% of cases. In boys, the VCUG also is performed to rule out urethral obstruction, particularly in cases of suspected posterior urethral valves. In older children, the urinary flow rate can be measured noninvasively with a urinary flowmeter; decreased flow with a normal bladder contraction suggests infravesical obstruction (e.g., posterior urethral valves, urethral stricture). When the urethra cannot be catheterized to obtain a VCUG, the clinician should suspect a urethral stricture or an obstructive urethral lesion. Retrograde urethrography with contrast medium injected into the urethral meatus helps delineate the anatomy of the urethral obstruction.

Radioisotope Studies

Renal scintigraphy is used to assess renal anatomy and function. The 2 most commonly used radiopharmaceuticals are mercaptoacetyl triglycine (MAG-3) and technetium-99m-labeled dimercaptosuccinic acid. MAG-3, which is excreted by renal tubular secretion, is used to assess differential renal function, and when furosemide is administered, drainage also can be measured. An alternative to MAG-3 is diethylene tetrapentaacetic acid, which is cleared by glomerular filtration. The background activity of diethylene tetrapentaacetic acid is much higher than that of MAG-3. Dimercaptosuccinic acid is a renal cortical imaging agent and is used to assess differential renal function and to demonstrate whether renal scarring is present. It is used infrequently in children with obstructive uropathy.

In a MAG-3 diuretic renogram, a small dose of technetium-labeled MAG-3 is injected intravenously (Figs. 540-2 and 540-3). During the 1st 2-3 min, renal parenchymal uptake is analyzed and compared, allowing computation of differential renal function. Subsequently,

Table 540-4	Society for Fetal Urology Grading System for Hydronephrosis	
	Renal Image	
GRADE OF HYDRONEPHROSIS	**CENTRAL RENAL COMPLEX**	**RENAL PARENCHYMAL THICKNESS**
0	Intact	Normal
1	Slight splitting	Normal
2	Evident splitting, complex confined within renal border	Normal
3	Wide splitting pelvis dilated outside renal border, calyces uniformly dilated	Normal
4	Further dilation of pelvis and calyces (calyces may appear convex)	Thin

After Maizels M, Mitchell B, Kass E, et al: Outcome of nonspecific hydronephrosis in the infant: a report from the registry of the Society for Fetal Urology, J Urol 152:2324–2327, 1994.

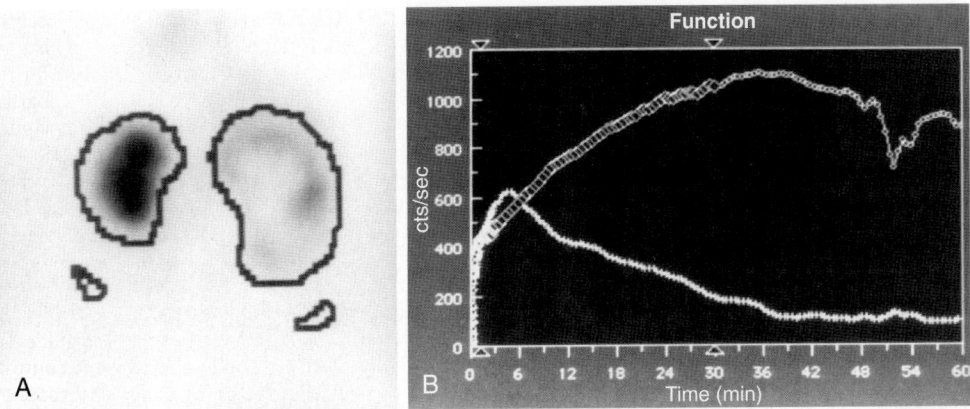

Figure 540-2 Same patient as in Figure 540-1. MAG-3 diuretic renogram of a 6 wk old patient. The right kidney is on the *right* side of the image. **A,** Differential renal function: left kidney 70%, right kidney 30%. **B,** After administration of furosemide, drainage from the left kidney was normal and drainage from the right kidney was slow, consistent with right ureteropelvic junction obstruction. Pyeloplasty was performed on the right kidney.

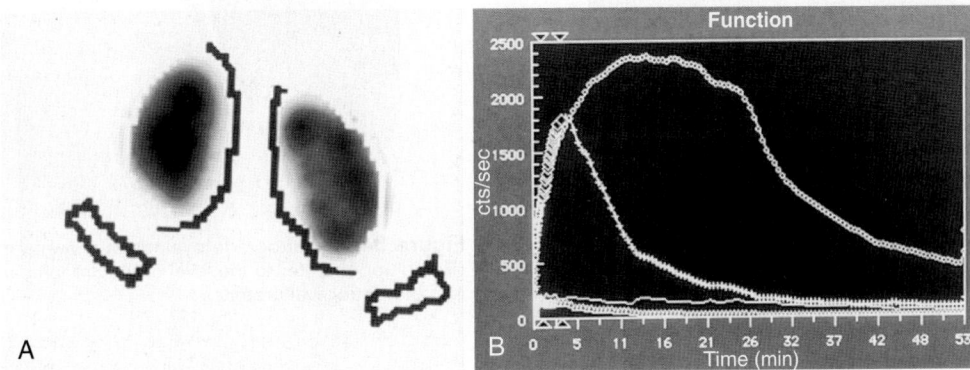

Figure 540-3 Same patient as in Figure 540-1. **A,** MAG-3 diuretic renogram at 14 mo of age shows equal function in the 2 kidneys. **B,** Prompt drainage after the administration of furosemide.

excretion is evaluated. After 20 min, furosemide 1 mg/kg is injected intravenously, and the rapidity and pattern of drainage from the kidneys to the bladder are analyzed. If no obstruction is present, half of the radionuclide should be cleared from the renal pelvis within 10-15 min, termed the half-time ($t_{1/2}$). If there is significant upper tract obstruction, the $t_{1/2}$ usually is longer than 20 min. A $t_{1/2}$ of 15-20 min is indeterminate. An elevated $t_{1/2}$ is suggestive but not diagnostic of obstruction. The images generated usually provide an accurate assessment of the site of obstruction. Numerous variables affect the outcome of the diuretic renogram. For example, newborn kidneys are functionally immature, and, in the 1st mo of life, normal kidneys might not demonstrate normal drainage after diuretic administration. Patient dehydration prolongs parenchymal transit and can blunt the diuretic response. Giving an insufficient dose of furosemide can result in slow drainage. If vesicoureteral reflux is present, continuous bladder drainage is mandatory to prevent the radionuclide from refluxing from the bladder into the dilated upper tract, which would prolong the washout phase..

The MAG-3 diuretic renogram is considered superior to the excretory urogram in infants and children with hydronephrosis, because bowel gas and immaturity of renal function often cause the intravenous pyelogram (IVP) images to be suboptimal. The diuretic renogram provides an objective assessment of the relative function of each kidney.

Excretory Urogram

Excretory urogram is rarely used in assessing the pediatric urinary tract, although it may be useful in selected cases with indeterminate upper urinary tract obstruction or a suspected duplication anomaly.

Magnetic Resonance Urography

MR urography is also used to evaluate suspected upper urinary tract pathology. The child is hydrated and given intravenous furosemide. Gadolinium-diethylene tetrapentaacetic acid is injected and routine T1-weighted and fat-suppressed fast spin-echo T2-weighted imaging is performed through the kidneys, ureters, and bladder. This study provides superb images of the pathology, and methodology permits assessment of differential renal function and drainage (Fig. 540-4). There is no radiation exposure; however, young children need sedation or anesthesia. It is used primarily when renal sonography and nuclear imaging fail to delineate complex pathology.

Computed Tomography

In children with a suspected ureteral calculus, noncontrast spiral CT of the abdomen and pelvis is a standard method of demonstrating whether a calculus is present, its location, and whether there is significant proximal hydronephrosis. This study is the initial study of choice in many of these patients. The disadvantage of CT is the significant radiation exposure, and it should be used only when the results will direct management decisions (see Chapter 718).

Ancillary Studies

In unusual cases, an **antegrade pyelogram** (insertion of a percutaneous nephrostomy tube and injection of contrast agent), can be performed to assess the anatomy of the upper urinary tract. This procedure usually requires general anesthesia. In addition, an **antegrade pressure-perfusion flow study** (Whitaker test) may be performed, in which fluid is infused at a measured rate, usually 10 mL/min. The pressures

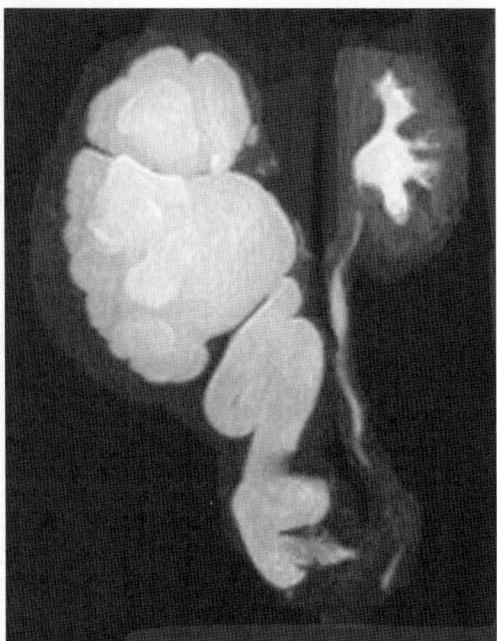

Figure 540-4 MR urogram in boy with distal ureterovesical obstruction.

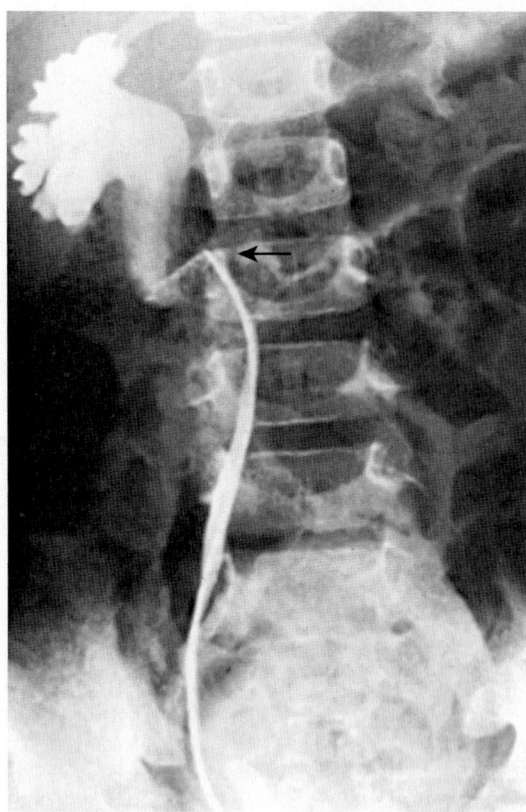

Figure 540-5 Retrograde pyelogram showing medial deviation of a dilated upper ureter to the level of the 3rd lumbar vertebra, characteristic of a retrocaval ureter.

in the renal pelvis and the bladder are monitored during this infusion, and pressure differences exceeding 20 cm H_2O suggest obstruction. In other cases, cystoscopy with retrograde pyelography provides excellent images of the upper urinary tract (Fig. 540-5).

SPECIFIC TYPES OF URINARY TRACT OBSTRUCTION AND THEIR TREATMENT

Hydrocalycosis

The term *hydrocalycosis* refers to a localized dilation of the calyx caused by obstruction of its infundibulum, termed *infundibular stenosis*. This condition can be developmental in origin or secondary to inflammatory processes, such as UTI. It usually is discovered during evaluation for pain or UTI. The diagnosis of infundibular stenosis is usually established by sonograph and CT scan or MR urography.

Ureteropelvic Junction Obstruction

UPJ obstruction is the most common obstructive lesion in childhood and usually is caused by intrinsic stenosis (see Figs. 540-1 to 540-3). An accessory artery to the lower pole of the kidney also can cause extrinsic obstruction. The typical appearance on ultrasonography is grade 3 or 4 hydronephrosis without a dilated ureter. UPJ obstruction most commonly manifests on antenatal sonography revealing fetal hydronephrosis; as a palpable renal mass in a newborn or infant; as abdominal, flank, or back pain; as a febrile UTI; or as hematuria after minimal trauma. Approximately 60% of cases occur on the left side, and the male : female ratio is 2 : 1. *UPJ obstruction is bilateral in only 10% of cases.* In kidneys with UPJ obstruction, renal function may be significantly impaired from pressure atrophy, but approximately half of affected kidneys have relatively normal glomerular function. The anomaly is corrected by performing a pyeloplasty, in which the stenotic segment is excised and the normal ureter and renal pelvis are reattached. Success rates are 91-98%. Pyeloplasty can be performed using laparoscopic techniques, often robotic-assisted using the da Vinci robot.

Lesser degrees of UPJ narrowing might cause mild hydronephrosis, which usually is nonobstructive, and typically these kidneys function normally. The spectrum of UPJ abnormalities has been referred to as *anomalous UPJ.* Another cause of mild hydronephrosis is fetal folds of the upper ureter, which also are nonobstructive.

The diagnosis can be difficult to establish in an asymptomatic infant in whom dilation of the renal pelvis is found incidentally in a prenatal ultrasonogram. After birth, the sonographic study is repeated to confirm the prenatal finding. A VCUG is necessary because 10-15% of patients have ipsilateral vesicoureteral reflux. Because neonatal oliguria can cause temporary decompression of a dilated renal pelvis, it is ideal to perform the first postnatal sonogram after the 3rd day of life. Delaying the sonogram may be impractical. If no dilation is found on the initial sonogram, a repeat study should be performed at 1 mo of age. If the kidney shows grade 1 or 2 hydronephrosis and the renal parenchyma appears normal, a period of observation usually is appropriate, with sequential renal ultrasonograms to monitor the severity of hydronephrosis, and the hydronephrosis usually disappears. **Antibiotic prophylaxis** is not indicated for children with mild hydronephrosis. If the hydronephrosis is grade 3 or 4, spontaneous resolution is less likely and obstruction is more likely to be present, particularly if the renal pelvic diameter is 3 cm. A diuretic renogram with MAG-3 is performed at 4-6 wk of age. If there is poor upper tract drainage or the differential renal function is poor, pyeloplasty is recommended. After pyeloplasty the differential renal function often improves, and improved drainage with furosemide stimulation is expected.

If the differential function on renography is normal, and drainage is satisfactory, the infant can be followed with serial ultrasonograms, even with grade 4 hydronephrosis. If the hydronephrosis remains severe with no improvement, a repeat diuretic renogram after 6-12 mo can help in the decision between continued observation and surgical repair. Prompt surgical repair is indicated in infants with an abdominal mass, bilateral severe hydronephrosis, a solitary kidney, or diminished function in the involved kidney. In unusual cases in which the differential renal function is <10% but the kidney definitely has some function, insertion of a percutaneous nephrostomy tube allows drainage of the hydronephrotic kidney for a few weeks to allow reassessment of renal function. In older children who present with symptoms, the diagnosis of UPJ obstruction usually is established by ultrasonography and diuretic renography.

The following entities should be considered in the **differential diagnosis:** megacalycosis, a congenital nonobstructive dilation of the calyces without pelvic or ureteric dilation; vesicoureteral reflux with marked dilation and kinking of the ureter; midureteral or distal ureteral obstruction when the ureter is not well visualized on the urogram; and retrocaval ureter.

Midureteral Obstruction

Congenital ureteral stenosis or a ureteral valve in the midureter is rare. It is corrected by excision of the strictured segment and reanastomosis of the normal upper and lower ureteral segments. A **retrocaval ureter** is an anomaly in which the upper right ureter travels posterior to the inferior vena cava. In this anomaly, the vena cava can cause extrinsic compression and obstruction. An IVP or MR urogram shows the right ureter to be medially deviated at the level of the 3rd lumbar vertebra. The diagnosis may be confirmed by retrograde pyelography (see Fig. 540-5). Surgical treatment consists of transection of the upper ureter, moving it anterior to the vena cava, and reanastomosing the upper and lower segments. Repair is necessary only when obstruction is present. Retroperitoneal tumors, fibrosis caused by surgical procedures, inflammatory processes (as in chronic granulomatous disease), and radiation therapy can cause acquired midureteral obstruction.

Ectopic Ureter

A ureter that drains outside the bladder is referred to as an **ectopic ureter.** This anomaly is 3 times as common in girls as in boys and usually is detected prenatally. The ectopic ureter typically drains the upper pole of a duplex collecting system (2 ureters).

In girls, approximately 35% of these ureters enter the urethra at the bladder neck, 35% enter the urethrovaginal septum, 25% enter the vagina, and a few drain into the cervix, uterus, Gartner duct, or a urethral diverticulum. Often the terminal aspect of the ureter is narrowed, causing hydroureteronephrosis. With the exception of the ectopic ureter entering the bladder neck, in girls an ectopic ureter causes continuous urinary incontinence from the affected renal moiety. UTI is common because of urinary stasis.

In boys, ectopic ureters enter the posterior urethra (above the external sphincter) in 47%, the prostatic utricle in 10%, the seminal vesicle in 33%, the ejaculatory duct in 5%, and the vas deferens in 5%. Consequently, in boys, an ectopic ureter does not cause incontinence, and most patients present with a UTI or epididymitis.

Evaluation includes a renal sonogram, VCUG, and renal scan, which demonstrates whether the affected segment has significant function. The sonogram shows the affected hydronephrotic kidney or dilated upper pole and ureter down to the bladder (Fig. 540-6). If the ectopic ureter drains into the bladder neck (female), a VCUG usually shows reflux into the ureter. Otherwise, there is no reflux into the ectopic ureter, but there may be reflux into the ipsilateral lower pole ureter or contralateral collecting system.

Treatment depends on the status of the renal unit drained by the ectopic ureter. If there is satisfactory function, ureteral reimplantation into the bladder or ureteroureterostomy (anastomosing the ectopic upper pole ureter into the normally inserting lower pole ureter) is indicated. If function is poor, partial or total nephrectomy is indicated. In many centers this procedure is done laparoscopically and often with robotic assistance using the da Vinci robot.

Ureterocele

A ureterocele is a cystic dilation of the terminal ureter and is obstructive because of a pinpoint ureteral orifice. Ureteroceles are much more common in girls than in boys. Affected children usually are discovered by prenatal ultrasonography, but some present with a febrile UTI. Ureteroceles may be ectopic, in which case the cystic swelling extends through the bladder neck into the urethra, or orthotopic, in which case the ureterocele is entirely within the bladder. Both orthotopic and ectopic ureteroceles can be bilateral.

In girls, ureteroceles nearly always are associated with ureteral duplication (Fig. 540-7), whereas in 50% of affected boys there is only 1

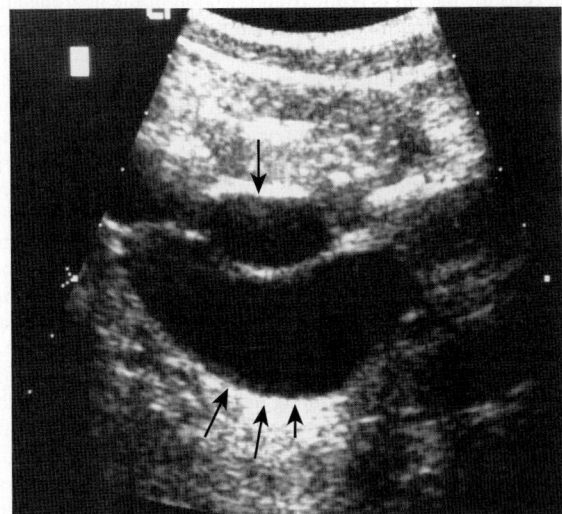

Figure 540-6 Ultrasonographic image of the right dilated ureter *(bottom arrows)* extending behind and caudal to a nearly empty bladder *(top arrow)* in a girl with urinary incontinence and ectopic ureter draining into the vagina.

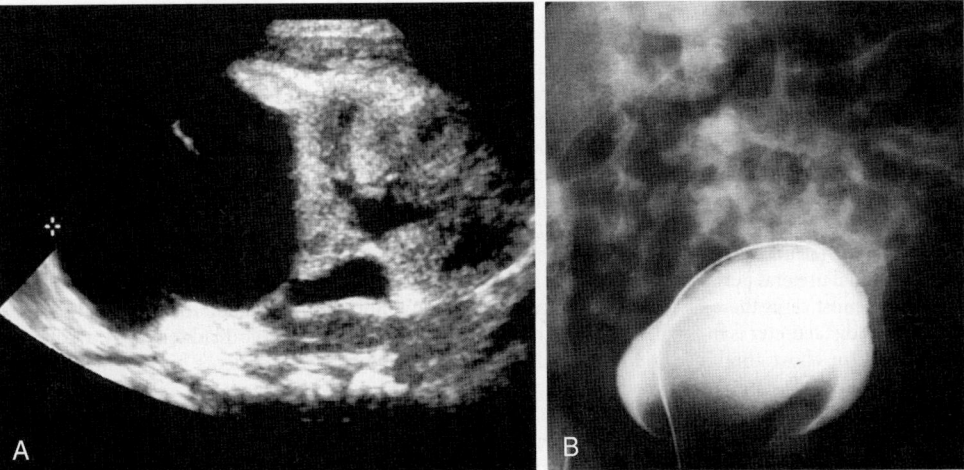

Figure 540-7 A, Infant with ectopic ureterocele. Sonogram of the left kidney shows massive dilation of the upper pole and a normal lower pole. **B,** Voiding cystourethrogram shows large ureterocele, draining the left upper pole, in the bladder. No reflux is present.

ureter. When associated with a duplication anomaly, the ureterocele drains the upper renal moiety, which commonly functions poorly or is dysplastic because of congenital obstruction. The lower pole ureter drains into the bladder superior and lateral to the upper pole ureter and may reflux.

An **ectopic ureterocele** extends submucosally into the urethra. Rarely, large ectopic ureteroceles can cause bladder outlet obstruction and retention of urine with bilateral hydronephrosis. In girls, the ureterocele can prolapse from the urethral meatus. Ultrasonography is effective in demonstrating the ureterocele and whether the associated obstructed system is duplicated or single. VCUG usually shows a filling defect in the bladder, sometimes large, corresponding to the ureterocele, and it often shows reflux into the adjacent lower pole collecting system with typical findings of a "drooping lily" appearance to the kidney. Nuclear renal scintigraphy is most accurate in demonstrating whether the affected renal moiety has significant function.

Treatment of ectopic ureteroceles varies among different medical centers and depends on whether the upper pole functions on renal scan and whether there is reflux into the lower pole ureter. If there is nonfunction of the upper pole of the kidney and there is no reflux, treatment usually involves laparoscopic, robotic, or open excision of the obstructed upper pole and most of the associated ureter. If there is function in the upper pole or significant reflux into the lower pole ureter, or if the patient is septic from infection of the hydronephrotic kidney, then transurethral incision with cautery is appropriate initial therapy to decompress the ureterocele. Reflux into the incised ureterocele is common, and subsequent excision of the ureterocele and ureteral reimplantation usually is necessary. An alternative method is to perform a upper-to-lower ureteroureterostomy, allowing the obstructed upper pole ureter to drain through the normal lower ureter; this procedure often is performed with minimally invasive laparoscopic (robotic) technique or through a small incision.

Orthotopic ureteroceles are associated with duplicated or single collecting systems, and the orifice is in the expected location in the bladder (Fig. 540-8). These anomalies usually are discovered during an investigation for prenatal hydronephrosis or a UTI. Ultrasonography is sensitive for detecting the ureterocele in the bladder and hydroureteronephrosis. IVP reveals varying degrees of ureteral and calyceal dilation, and there is a round filling defect in the bladder. In delayed films, cystic dilation of the ureter may be clearly visible and full of contrast material. Transurethral incision of the ureterocele effectively relieves the obstruction, but it can result in vesicoureteral reflux, necessitating ureteral reimplantation later. Some prefer open excision of the ureterocele and reimplantation as the initial form of treatment. Small, simple ureteroceles discovered incidentally without upper tract dilation generally do not require treatment.

Megaureter

Table 540-5 presents a classification of megaureters (dilated ureter). Numerous disorders can cause ureteral dilation, and many are nonobstructive.

Megaureters usually are discovered during antenatal sonography, postnatal UTI, hematuria, or abdominal pain. A careful history, physical examination, and VCUG identify causes of secondary megaureters and refluxing megaureters as well as the prune-belly syndrome. Primary obstructed megaureters and nonobstructed megaureters probably represent varying degrees of severity of the same anomaly.

The primary obstructed nonrefluxing megaureter results from abnormal development of the distal ureter, with collagenous tissue replacing the muscle layer. Normal ureteral peristalsis is disrupted, and the proximal ureter widens. In most cases there is not a true stricture. On IVP or an MR urogram, the distal ureter is more dilated in its distal segment and tapers abruptly at or above the junction of the bladder (Fig. 540-9). The lesion may be unilateral or bilateral. Significant hydroureteronephrosis suggests obstruction. Megaureter predisposes to UTI, urinary stones, hematuria, and flank pain because of urinary stasis. In most cases, diuretic renography and sequential sonographic studies can reliably differentiate obstructed from nonobstructed megaureters. In most nonobstructed megaureters, the hydroureteronephro-

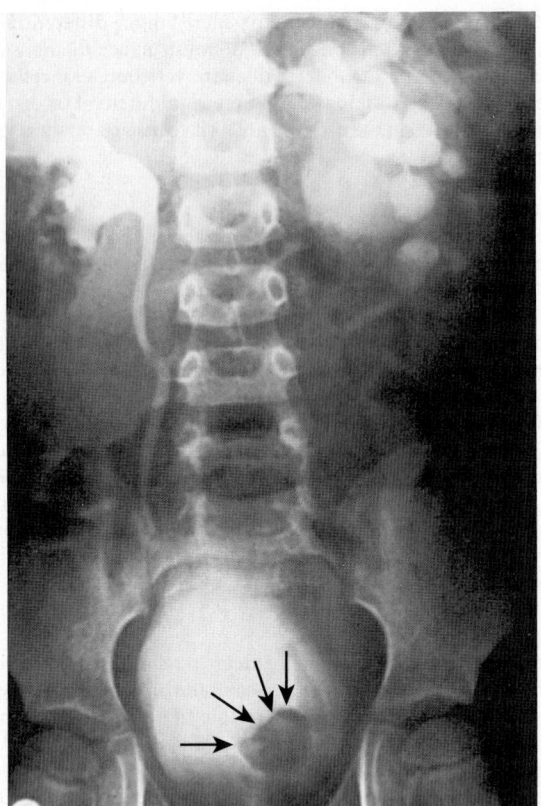

Figure 540-8 Simple intravesical ureterocele. The excretory urogram shows left hydronephrosis and a round filling defect on the left side of the bladder corresponding to a simple ureterocele causing left ureteral obstruction. This lesion was treated by transurethral incision and drainage of the ureterocele.

sis diminishes gradually (Fig. 540-10). Truly obstructed megaureters require surgical treatment, with excision of the narrowed segment, ureteral tapering, and reimplantation of the ureter. The results of surgical reconstruction usually are good, but the prognosis depends on preexisting renal function and whether complications develop.

If differential renal function is normal (>45%) and the child is asymptomatic, it is safe to manage the patient with observation with serial ultrasonography and periodic diuretic renography to monitor renal function and drainage. In children with grade 4 hydroureteronephrosis, prophylactic antimicrobial therapy should be prescribed, as these children are prone to upper UTI. If renal function deteriorates, upper urinary tract drainage slows, or UTI occurs, ureteral reimplantation is recommended. Approximately 15% of children with a nonrefluxing megaureter undergo ureteral reimplantation.

Prune-Belly Syndrome

Prune-belly syndrome, also called **triad syndrome** or **Eagle-Barrett syndrome,** occurs in approximately 1 in 40,000 births; 95% of affected children are male. The characteristic association of deficient abdominal muscles, undescended testes, and urinary tract abnormalities probably results from severe urethral obstruction in fetal life (Fig. 540-11). Oligohydramnios and pulmonary hypoplasia are common complications in the perinatal period. Many affected infants are stillborn. Urinary tract abnormalities include massive dilation of the ureters and upper tracts and a very large bladder, with a patent urachus or a urachal diverticulum. Most patients have vesicoureteral reflux. The prostatic urethra usually is dilated, and the prostate is hypoplastic. The anterior urethra may be dilated, resulting in a megalourethra. Rarely, there is urethral stenosis or atresia. The kidneys usually show various degrees of dysplasia, and the testes usually are intraabdominal. Malrotation of the bowel often is present. Cardiac abnormalities occur in 10% of cases; >50% have abnormalities of the musculoskeletal system, including

Table 540-5	Classification of Megaureter				
Refluxing		**Obstructed**		**Nonrefluxing and Nonobstructed**	
PRIMARY	SECONDARY	PRIMARY	SECONDARY	PRIMARY	SECONDARY
Primary reflux	Neuropathic bladder	Intrinsic (primary obstructed megaureter)	Neuropathic bladder	Nonrefluxing, nonobstructive	Diabetes insipidus
Megacystic-megaureter syndrome	Hinman syndrome	Ureteral valve	Hinman syndrome		Infection
Ectopic ureter	Posterior urethral valves	Ectopic ureter	Posterior urethral valves		Persistent after relief of obstruction
Prune-belly syndrome	Bladder diverticulum Postoperative	Ectopic uterocele	Ureteral calculus Extrinsic Postoperative		

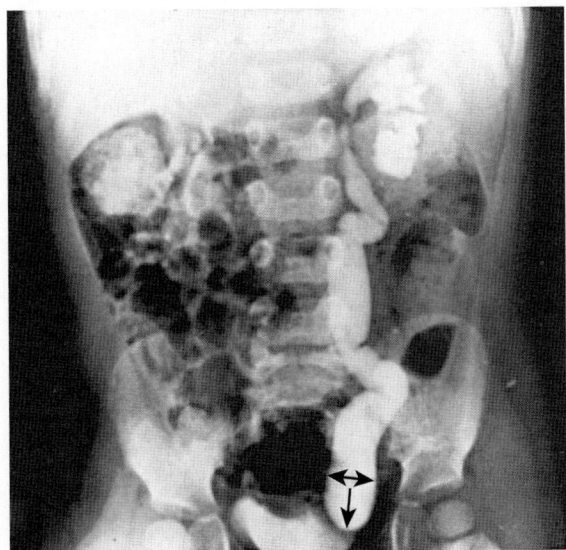

Figure 540-9 Obstructed nonrefluxing megaureter. Excretory urogram in a girl with a history of a febrile urinary tract infection. The right side is normal. The left side reveals hydroureteronephrosis with predominant dilation of the distal ureter. Note the characteristic appearance of the distal ureter. There was no vesicoureteral reflux. The diagnosis of obstruction was confirmed by diuretic renography.

limb abnormalities and scoliosis. In girls, anomalies of the urethra, uterus, and vagina usually are present.

Many neonates with prune-belly syndrome have difficulty with effective bladder emptying because the bladder musculature is poorly developed, and the urethra may be narrowed. When no obstruction is present, the goal of treatment is the prevention of UTI with antibiotic prophylaxis. When obstruction of the ureters or urethra is demonstrated, temporary drainage procedures, such as a vesicostomy, can help to preserve renal function until the child is old enough for surgery. Some children with prune-belly syndrome have been found to have classic or atypical posterior urethral valves. UTIs occur often and should be treated promptly. Correction of the undescended testes by orchidopexy can be difficult in these children because the testes are located high in the abdomen and surgery is best accomplished in the 1st 6 mo of life. Reconstruction of the abdominal wall offers cosmetic and functional benefits.

The prognosis ultimately depends on the degree of pulmonary hypoplasia and renal dysplasia. One third of children with prune-belly syndrome are stillborn or die in the 1st few mo of life because of pulmonary hypoplasia. As many as 30% of the long-term survivors develop end-stage renal disease from dysplasia or complications of

infection or reflux and eventually require renal transplantation. Renal transplantation in these children offers good results.

Bladder Neck Obstruction
Bladder neck obstruction usually is secondary to ectopic ureterocele, bladder calculi, or a tumor of the prostate (rhabdomyosarcoma). The manifestations include difficulty voiding, urinary retention, UTI, and bladder distention with overflow incontinence. Apparent bladder neck obstruction is common in cases of posterior urethral valves, but it seldom has any functional significance. Primary bladder neck obstruction is extremely rare.

Posterior Urethral Valves
The most common cause of severe obstructive uropathy in children is posterior urethral valves, affecting 1 in 8,000 boys. The urethral valves are tissue leaflets fanning distally from the prostatic urethra to the external urinary sphincter. A slit-like opening usually separates the leaflets. Valves are of unclear embryologic origin and cause varying degrees of obstruction. Approximately 30% of patients experience end-stage renal disease or chronic renal insufficiency. The prostatic urethra dilates, and the bladder muscle undergoes hypertrophy. Vesicoureteral reflux occurs in 50% of patients, and distal ureteral obstruction can result from a chronically distended bladder or bladder muscle hypertrophy. The renal changes range from mild hydronephrosis to severe renal dysplasia; their severity probably depends on the severity of the obstruction and its time of onset during fetal development. As in other cases of obstruction or renal dysplasia, there may be oligohydramnios and pulmonary hypoplasia.

Affected boys with posterior urethral valves often are discovered prenatally when maternal ultrasonography reveals bilateral hydronephrosis, a distended bladder, and, if the obstruction is severe, oligohydramnios. Prenatal bladder decompression by percutaneous vesicoamniotic shunt or open fetal surgery has been reported. Experimental and clinical evidence of the possible benefits of fetal intervention is lacking, and few affected fetuses are candidates. Prenatally diagnosed posterior urethral valves, particularly when discovered in the 2nd trimester, carry a poorer prognosis than those detected in the 3rd trimester following a normal second fetal ultrasound. In the male neonate, posterior urethral valves are suspected when there is a palpably **distended bladder** and the **urinary stream is weak.** If the obstruction is severe and goes unrecognized during the neonatal period, infants can present later in life with failure to thrive because of uremia or sepsis caused by infection in the obstructed urinary tract. With lesser degrees of obstruction, children present later in life with difficulty in achieving diurnal urinary continence or with UTI. The diagnosis is established with a VCUG (Fig. 540-12) or by perineal ultrasonography.

After the diagnosis is established, renal function and the anatomy of the upper urinary tract should be carefully evaluated. In the healthy neonate, a small polyethylene feeding tube (No. 5 or No. 8 French) is inserted in the bladder and left for several days. Passing the feeding

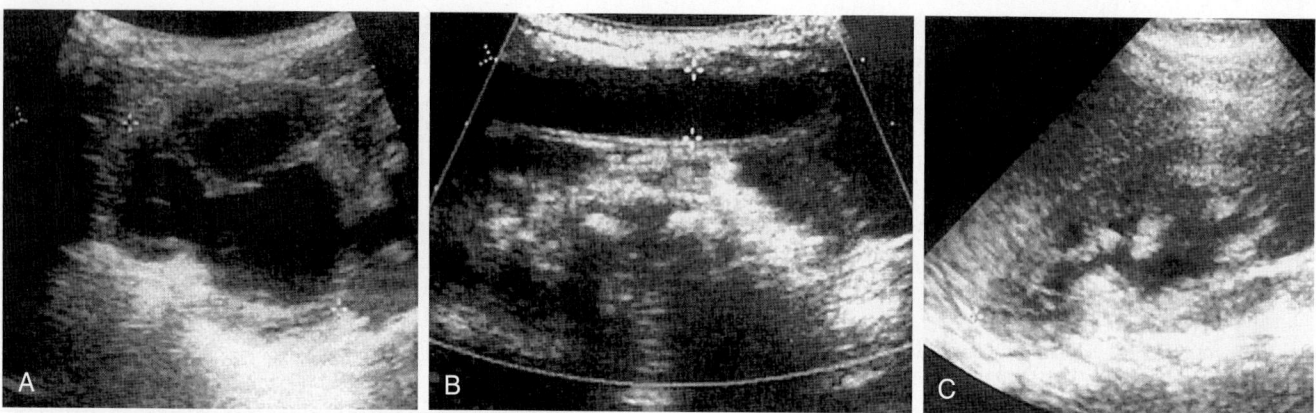

Figure 540-10 Neonate with primary nonrefluxing megaureter. **A,** Renal sonogram shows grade 4 hydronephrosis. **B,** Dilated ureter. Renal scan showed equal function with the contralateral kidney and satisfactory drainage with diuresis stimulation. **C,** Follow-up sonogram at 10 mo shows complete resolution of hydronephrosis.

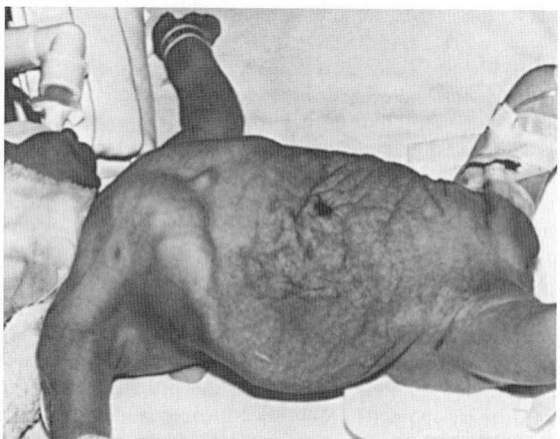

Figure 540-11 Photograph of a 1,600-g newborn with the prune-belly syndrome. Note the lack of tonicity of the abdominal wall and the wrinkled appearance of the skin.

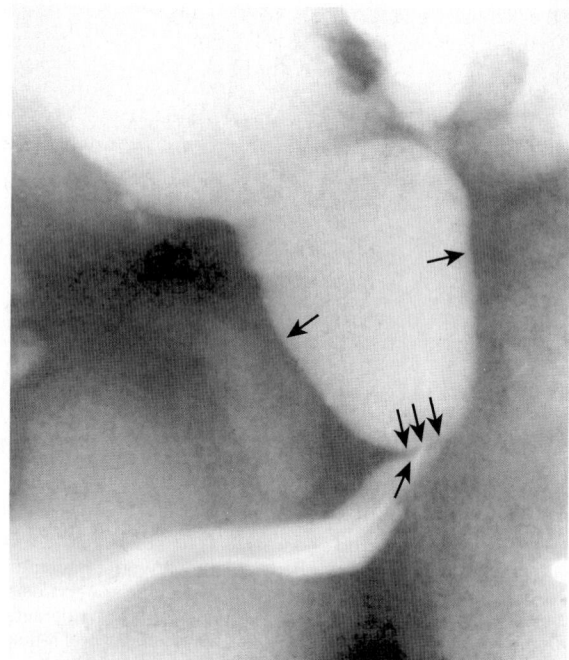

Figure 540-12 Voiding cystourethrogram in an infant with posterior urethral valves. Note the dilation of the prostatic urethra and the transverse linear filling defect corresponding to the valves.

tube may be difficult, because the tip of the tube can coil in the prostatic urethra. A sign of this problem is that urine drains around the catheter rather than through it. A Foley (balloon) catheter **should not be used**, because the balloon can cause severe bladder spasm, which can produce severe ureteral obstruction.

If the serum creatinine level remains normal or returns to normal, treatment consists of transurethral ablation of the valve leaflets, which is performed endoscopically under general anesthesia. If the urethra is too small for transurethral ablation, temporary vesicostomy is preferred, in which the dome of the bladder is exteriorized on the lower abdominal wall. When the child is older, the valves may be ablated and the vesicostomy closed.

If the serum creatinine level remains high or increases despite bladder drainage by a small catheter, secondary ureteral obstruction, irreversible renal damage, or renal dysplasia should be suspected. In such cases, a vesicostomy should be considered. Cutaneous pyelostomy rarely affords better drainage when compared with cutaneous vesicostomy, and the latter also allows continued bladder growth and gradual improvement in bladder wall compliance.

In the septic and uremic infant, lifesaving measures must include prompt correction of the electrolyte imbalance and control of the infection by appropriate antibiotics. Drainage of the upper tracts by percutaneous nephrostomy and hemodialysis may be necessary. After the patient's condition becomes stable, evaluation and treatment may be undertaken. Posterior valves are diagnosed in some older boys because of a poor stream, diurnal incontinence, or a UTI; these boys generally are treated by primary valve ablation.

Favorable prognostic factors include a normal prenatal ultrasonogram between 18 and 24 wk of gestation, a serum creatinine level <0.8-1.0 mg/dL after bladder decompression, and visualization of the corticomedullary junction on renal sonography. In several situations, a "popoff valve" can occur during urinary tract development, which preserves the integrity of 1 or both kidneys. For example, 15% of boys with posterior urethral valves have unilateral reflux into a nonfunctioning dysplastic kidney, termed the **VURD syndrome** (*v*alves, *u*nilateral *r*eflux, *d*ysplasia). In these boys, the high bladder pressure is dissipated into the nonfunctioning kidney, allowing normal development of the contralateral kidney. In newborn boys with urinary ascites, the urine generally leaks out from the obstructed collecting system through the renal fornices, allowing normal development of the kidneys. Unfavorable prognostic factors include the presence of oligohydramnios in utero, identification of hydronephrosis before 24 wk of gestation, a serum creatinine level >1.0 mg/dL after bladder decompression, identification of cortical cysts in both kidneys, and persistence of diurnal incontinence beyond 5 yr of age.

The prognosis in the newborn is related to the child's degree of pulmonary hypoplasia and potential for recovery of renal function. Severely affected infants often are stillborn. Of those who survive the neonatal period, approximately 30% eventually require kidney transplantation and 15% have renal insufficiency. In some series, kidney transplantation in children with posterior urethral valves has a lower success rate than does transplantation in children with normal bladders, presumably because of the adverse influence of altered bladder function on graft function and survival.

After valve ablation, antimicrobial prophylaxis is beneficial in preventing UTI, because hydronephrosis to some degree often persists for many years. These boys should be evaluated annually with a renal ultrasonogram, physical examination including assessment of somatic growth and blood pressure, urinalysis, and determination of serum levels of electrolytes. Many boys have significant polyuria resulting from a concentrating defect secondary to prolonged obstructive uropathy. If these children acquire a systemic illness with vomiting and/or diarrhea, urine output cannot be used to assess their hydration status. They can become dehydrated quickly, and there should be a low threshold for hospital admission for intravenous rehydration. Some of these patients have renal tubular acidosis, requiring oral bicarbonate therapy. If there is any significant degree of renal dysfunction, growth impairment, or hypertension, the child should be followed closely by a pediatric nephrologist. When vesicoureteral reflux is present, expectant treatment and prophylactic doses of antibacterial drugs are advisable. If breakthrough UTI occurs, surgical correction should be undertaken.

After treatment, boys with urethral valves often do not achieve diurnal urinary continence as early as other boys. Incontinence can result from a combination of factors, including uninhibited bladder contractions, poor bladder compliance, bladder atonia, bladder neck dyssynergia, or polyuria. Often these boys require urodynamic evaluation with urodynamics or videourodynamics to plan therapy. Boys with noncompliance are at significant risk for ongoing renal damage, even in the absence of infection. Overnight catheter drainage has been shown to be beneficial in boys with polyuria and can help preserve renal function. Urinary incontinence usually improves with age, particularly after puberty. Meticulous attention to bladder compliance, emptying, and infection can improve results in the future.

Urethral Atresia

The most severe form of obstructive uropathy in boys is urethral atresia, a rare condition. In utero there is a distended bladder, bilateral hydroureteronephrosis, and oligohydramnios. In most cases, these infants are stillborn or succumb to pulmonary hypoplasia. Some boys with prune-belly syndrome also have urethral atresia. If the urachus is patent, oligohydramnios is unlikely and the infant usually survives. Urethral reconstruction is difficult, and most patients are managed with continent urinary diversion.

Urethral Hypoplasia

Urethral hypoplasia is a rare form of obstructive uropathy in boys that is less severe than urethral atresia. In urethral hypoplasia, the urethral lumen is extremely small. Neonates with urethral hypoplasia typically have bilateral hydronephrosis and a distended bladder. Passage of a small pediatric feeding tube through the urethra is difficult or impossible. Usually a cutaneous vesicostomy must be performed to relieve upper urinary tract obstruction, and the severity of renal insufficiency is variable. The most severely affected boys have end-stage renal disease. Treatment includes urethral reconstruction, gradual urethral dilation, or continent urinary diversion.

Urethral Strictures

Urethral strictures in boys usually result from urethral trauma, either iatrogenic (catheterization, endoscopic procedures, previous urethral reconstruction) or accidental (straddle injuries, pelvic fractures). Because these lesions can develop gradually, the decrease in force of the urinary stream is seldom noticed by the child or the parents. More commonly, the obstruction causes symptoms of bladder instability,

hematuria, or dysuria. Catheterization of the bladder usually is impossible. The diagnosis is made by a retrograde urethrogram, in which contrast is injected toward the bladder through a catheter inserted into the distal urethra. Ultrasonography also has been used to diagnose urethral strictures. Endoscopy is confirmatory. Endoscopic treatment of short strictures by direct vision urethrotomy is often successful initially and results in a profoundly improved urinary stream, but often the stricture recurs and is found at long-term follow-up. Longer strictures surrounded by periurethral fibrosis often require urethroplasty. Repeated endoscopic procedures generally should be avoided, because they can cause additional urethral damage. Noninvasive measurement of the urinary flow rate and pattern is useful for diagnosis and follow-up.

In girls, true urethral strictures are rare because the female urethra is protected from trauma, particularly in childhood. In the past it was thought that a distal urethral ring commonly caused obstruction of the female urethra and UTI and that affected girls benefited from urethral dilation. The diagnosis was suspected when a "spinning top" deformity of the urethra was found in the VCUG (see Fig. 543-3 in Chapter 543) and was confirmed by urethral calibration. There is no correlation between the radiologic appearance of the urethra in the VCUG and the urethral caliber and no significant difference in urethral caliber between girls with recurrent cystitis and normal age-matched controls. The finding usually is secondary to detrusor–sphincter dyssynergia. Consequently, urethral dilation in girls rarely is indicated.

Anterior Urethral Valves and Urethral Diverticula in the Male

Anterior urethral valves are rare. The obstruction is not obstructing valve leaflets, as occurs in the posterior urethra. Rather, it is a urethral diverticulum in the penile urethra that expands during voiding. Distal extension of the diverticulum causes extrinsic compression of the distal penile urethra, causing urethral obstruction. Typically there is a soft mass on the ventral surface of the penis at the penoscrotal junction. In addition, the urinary stream often is weak, and the physical findings associated with posterior urethral valves often are present. The diverticulum may be small and minimally obstructive, or, in other cases, may be severely obstructive and cause renal insufficiency. The diagnosis is suspected on physical examination and is confirmed by the VCUG. Treatment involves open excision of the diverticulum or transurethral excision of the distal urethral cusp. Urethral diverticula occasionally occur after extensive hypospadias repair.

Fusiform dilation of the urethra or **megalourethra** can result from underdevelopment of the corpus spongiosum and support structures of the urethra. This condition is commonly associated with the prunebelly syndrome.

Male Urethral Meatal Stenosis

See Chapter 544 for information on urethral meatal stenosis in males.

Bibliography is available at Expert Consult.

Chapter 541
Anomalies of the Bladder
Jack S. Elder

BLADDER EXSTROPHY

Exstrophy of the urinary bladder occurs in approximately 1 in 35,000-40,000 births. The male : female ratio is 2 : 1. The severity ranges from simple **epispadias** (in boys) to complete exstrophy of the cloaca involving exposure of the entire hindgut and the bladder (termed **cloacal exstrophy**).

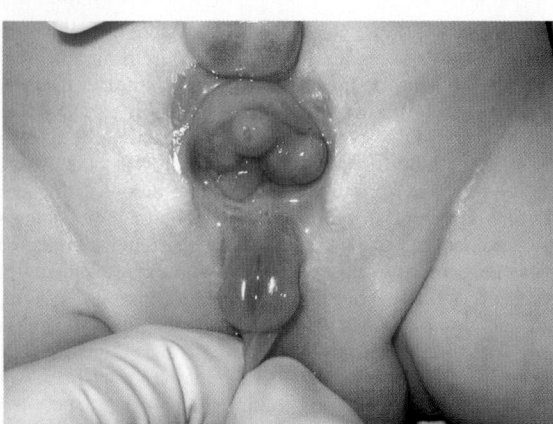

Figure 541-1 Classic bladder exstrophy in a newborn boy. The bladder is exposed in the midline, the umbilical cord is displaced caudad, the penis is epispadiac, and the scrotum is broad.

Clinical Manifestations

Anomalies of the bladder are hypothesized to result when the mesoderm fails to invade the cephalad extension of the cloacal membrane; the extent of this failure determines the degree of the anomaly. In classic bladder exstrophy (Fig. 541-1), the bladder protrudes from the abdominal wall and its mucosa is exposed. The umbilicus is displaced downward, the pubic rami are widely separated in the midline, and the rectus muscles are separated. In boys, there is complete epispadias with dorsal chordee, and the overall penile length is approximately half that of unaffected boys. The scrotum typically is separated slightly from the penis and is wide and shallow. Undescended testes and inguinal hernias are common. Girls also have epispadias, with separation of the 2 halves of the clitoris and wide separation of the labia. The anus is displaced anteriorly in both sexes, and there may be rectal prolapse. The pubic rami are widely separated. Persons with exstrophy tend to be shorter than normal.

The consequences of untreated bladder exstrophy are total urinary incontinence and an increased incidence of bladder cancer, usually adenocarcinoma. The genital deformities can produce sexual disability in both sexes, particularly in males. The wide separation of the pubic rami causes a characteristic broad-based gait but no significant disability. In classic bladder exstrophy, the upper urinary tracts usually are normal.

Treatment

Management of bladder exstrophy should start at birth. The bladder should be covered with plastic wrap to keep the bladder mucosa moist. **Application of gauze or petroleum-gauze to the bladder mucosa should be avoided, because significant inflammation will result.** The infant should be transferred promptly to a center with pediatric urologic and anesthetic support for the treatment of such anomalies. These children are prone to **latex allergy,** so latex precautions should be practiced in their care.

There are 2 surgical approaches: staged reconstruction and total single-stage reconstruction. Most babies also undergo bilateral iliac osteotomy, which allows the pubic symphysis to be approximated, which supports the bladder closure. In a staged reconstruction, the initial stage is bladder closure, the 2nd stage (in boys) is epispadias repair, and the final stage is bladder neck reconstruction. The single-stage reconstruction attempts to reconstruct the entire malformation in a single procedure. When this operation is performed in the newborn, there is an increased risk of intraoperative penile injury and postoperative hydronephrosis, compared with the staged reconstruction. The complication rate is high with both approaches and there is no consensus on which is better.

Although bladder closure within 48 hr has been the standard in the past, more recently, many centers of excellence defer the procedure for 1-2 wk to be certain that the appropriate experienced surgical and anesthetic team is available. During bladder exstrophy closure, the abdominal wall is mobilized and the pubic rami are brought together in the midline following pelvic osteotomy. Early bladder closure can be performed in almost all neonates with classic bladder exstrophy. Treatment should be deferred in selected situations when surgical therapy would be excessively risky or complex, such as in a premature baby or when it would have to be performed by inexperienced surgeons. In the staged approach, in boys, epispadias repair usually is performed at 1-2 yr of age. At this point the child has total urinary incontinence because there is no functional external urinary sphincter. At 3-6 yr, if the bladder is sufficiently large, bladder neck reconstruction is performed to try to create a functional sphincter.

Total single-stage reconstruction includes closure of the bladder, closure of the abdominal wall, and, in boys, correction of epispadias using a technique of penile disassembly, in which the 2 corpora cavernosa and the midline urethra are mobilized separately into 3 parts. Postoperatively, the infant's upper urinary tract is monitored closely for the possible development of hydronephrosis and infection. Most infants with bladder exstrophy have vesicoureteral reflux and should receive antibiotic prophylaxis. The final stage of reconstruction involves creation of a sphincter muscle for bladder control and correction of the vesicoureteral reflux. At this point the child is 3-6 yr old, the bladder capacity should be at least 80-90 mL, and the child must have gained rectal control. Typically, bladder capacity is monitored every 12-24 mo using cystoscopy under anesthesia.

At puberty, often the pubic hair is distributed to the sides of the external genitals. A monsplasty can performed to provide a normal escutcheon.

Long-Term Prognosis

This plan of treatment has yielded a continence rate of 60-70% in a few centers, with <15% deterioration of the upper urinary tract. This continence rate reflects not only the successful reconstruction but also the quality and size of the bladder. The reconstructed bladder neck does not relax during voiding as in a normal child; instead the patient must void by Valsalva. Children who undergo reconstructive surgery as newborns have a greater chance of obtaining a normally functioning bladder.

Children who remain incontinent for more than 1 yr after bladder neck reconstruction or those who are not eligible for bladder neck reconstruction because of a small bladder capacity are candidates for an alternative reconstructive procedure to achieve dryness. In selected cases, cystoscopic injection of dextranomer or polydimethylsiloxane microspheres into the bladder neck can provide sufficient bladder neck coaptation to establish continence. Alternatively, if the child is not a candidate for endoscopic therapy, options include:

* Augmentation cystoplasty, in which the bladder is enlarged with a patch of small or large bowel to increase its capacity.
* Creation of a neobladder out of small and large bowel with placement of a continent abdominal stoma through which clean intermittent catheterization can be performed.
* Placement of an artificial urinary sphincter, with possible augmentation cystoplasty.
* Ureterosigmoidostomy, in which the ureters are detached from the bladder and sutured to the sigmoid colon; individuals void urine and stool from the rectum and rely on their anal sphincter for continence.
* Mainz II procedure, in which the sigmoid colon is reconfigured into a "bladder" into which the ureters are connected, and the patient voids 3-6 times daily through the rectum, and the stool tends to be more solid.

Ureterosigmoidostomy carries a significant risk of chronic pyelonephritis (see Chapter 538), upper urinary tract damage, metabolic acidosis resulting from absorption of hydrogen ion and chloride in the intestine, and at least a 15% long-term risk of colon carcinoma. Patients from less-developed countries often undergo the Mainz II procedure because the continence rate is high and pyelonephritis and upper tract changes are uncommon.

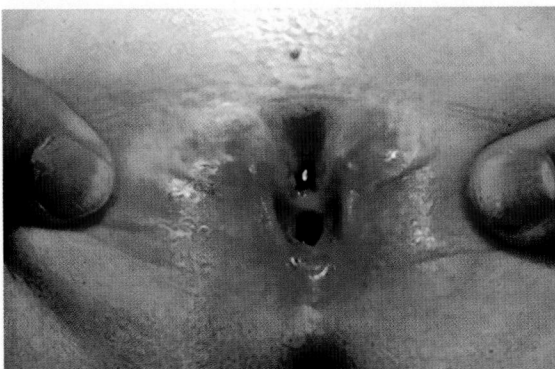

Figure 541-2 Girl with complete epispadias. *(From Gearhart JP, Rink RC, Mouriquand PDE, editors: Pediatric urology, ed 2, Philadelphia, 2010, WB Saunders.)*

Late follow-up has shown that although men with exstrophy have a penis that is half normal length, they usually experience satisfactory sexual function. Fertility has been low, possibly because of iatrogenic injury to the secondary sexual organs during reconstruction. With artificial reproductive technology, nearly all men can be fertile. In women, fertility is not affected, but uterine prolapse during pregnancy is a problem. In women who have undergone a continent urinary diversion, delivery by cesarean section may be necessary.

OTHER EXSTROPHY ANOMALIES

Children with more complex cases of **cloacal exstrophy,** which has an incidence of 1 in 400,000, have an omphalocele and severe abnormalities of the colon and the rectum and often have short bowel syndrome (see Chapter 338.7), the most devastating anomaly managed by pediatric urologists. Approximately 50% of patients have an upper urinary tract anomaly, and 50% have spina bifida (see Chapter 591). Children with cloacal exstrophy do not achieve normal urine or stool continence. Reconstructive techniques result in a satisfactory outcome in most patients with permanent urinary diversion (either ileal conduit or continent urinary diversion) and a colostomy. Because the penis in boys with cloacal exstrophy usually is diminutive, genital reconstruction in boys with cloacal exstrophy has been unsatisfactory. Until recently, most specialists recommended assigning a female gender to such infants, but currently there is debate whether these children, who have a 46,XY karyotype and androgen imprinting in utero, can have a satisfactory female gender identity (see Chapter 110.2). Many assume male gender characteristics by adolescence. Decisions regarding gender assignment should be made jointly by the physicians caring for the infant (surgical team, pediatric endocrinologist, child psychiatrist, and ethicist) and family.

Epispadias is in the spectrum of exstrophy anomalies, affecting approximately 1 in 117,000 boys and 1 in 480,000 girls. In boys, the diagnosis is obvious because the prepuce is distributed primarily on the ventral aspect of the penile shaft and the urethral meatus is on the dorsum of the penis. Distal epispadias in boys usually is associated with normal urinary control and normal upper urinary tracts and should be repaired by 6-12 mo of age. In girls, the clitoris is bifid and the urethra is split dorsally (Fig. 541-2). In more severely affected boys and in all girls with epispadias, there is total urinary incontinence because the sphincter is incompletely formed, and there is wide separation of the pubic rami. These children require surgical reconstruction of the bladder neck, similar to the final management stage in children with classic bladder exstrophy.

BLADDER DIVERTICULA

Bladder diverticula develop as herniations of bladder mucosa between defects of bladder smooth muscle fibers. Primary bladder diverticula usually develop at the ureterovesical junction and may be associated with vesicoureteral reflux, because the diverticulum interferes with the normal flap-valve attachment between the ureter and bladder. In rare

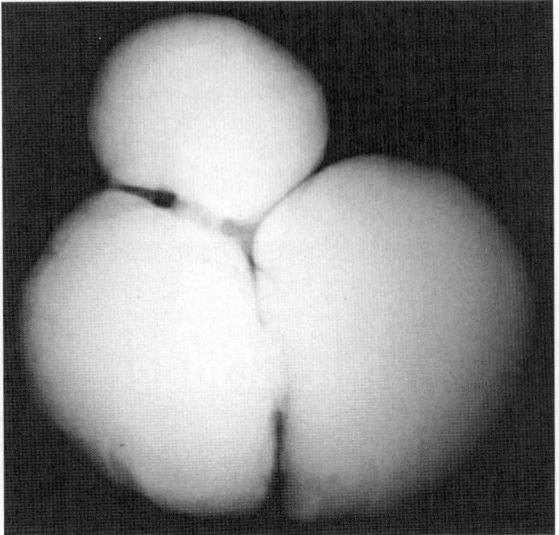

Figure 541-3 Girl with Menkes syndrome with multiple large bladder diverticula causing inability to void and recurrent urinary tract infections. The condition was managed by bladder diverticulectomy.

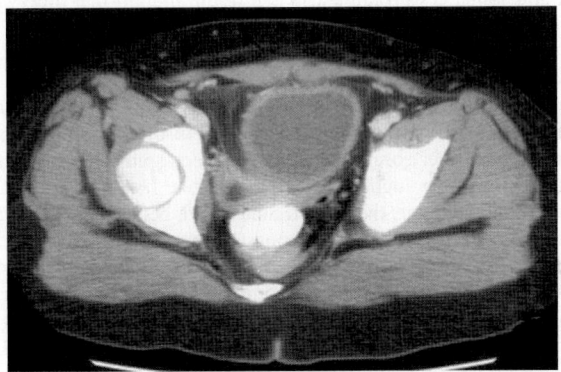

Figure 541-4 CT scan demonstrating infected urachal abscess in an 8 yr old girl. The condition was managed by drainage and excision.

circumstances the diverticulum is so large that it interferes with normal micturition by obstructing the bladder neck. Bladder diverticula also commonly are associated with distal urethral obstruction such as posterior urethral valves or neurogenic bladder dysfunction. They occur commonly in children with connective tissue disorders including Williams syndrome, Ehlers-Danlos syndrome, and Menkes syndrome (Fig. 541-3). Small diverticula require no treatment other than that of the primary disease, whereas large diverticula can contribute to inefficient voiding, residual urine, urinary stasis, and urinary tract infections and should be excised.

URACHAL ANOMALIES

The urachus is an embryologic canal connecting the dome of the fetal bladder with the allantois, a structure that contributes to the formation of the umbilical cord. The lumen of the urachus is normally obliterated during embryonic development, transforming the urachus into a solid cord. Urachal abnormalities are more common in boys than in girls. A **patent urachus** can occur as an isolated anomaly; it may be associated with prune-belly syndrome or posterior urethral valves (see Chapter 540). In this condition there is continuous urinary drainage from the umbilicus. The tract should be excised. Another urachal anomaly is the **urachal cyst,** which can become infected. Typical symptoms and physical findings include suprapubic pain, fever, irritative voiding symptoms, and an infraumbilical mass, which can be erythematous. Diagnosis is made by ultrasonography or CT (Fig. 541-4).

Treatment is intravenous antibiotic therapy and drainage and excision. Other urachal anomalies include the **vesicourachal diverticulum**, which is a diverticulum of the bladder dome, and **umbilical–urachal sinus**, which is a blind external sinus that opens at the umbilicus. These lesions should be excised.

Bibliography is available at Expert Consult.

Chapter 542
Neuropathic Bladder
Jack S. Elder

Neuropathic bladder dysfunction in children usually is congenital, generally resulting from neural tube defects or other spinal abnormalities. Acquired diseases and traumatic lesions of the spinal cord are less common. Central nervous system tumors, sacrococcygeal teratoma, spinal abnormalities associated with imperforate anus (see Chapter 344), and spinal cord trauma also can result in abnormal innervation of the bladder and/or sphincter.

NEURAL TUBE DEFECTS
Neural tube defects, resulting from failure of the neural tube to close spontaneously between the 3rd and 4th wk in utero, result in abnormalities of the vertebral column that affect spinal cord function, including myelomeningocele and meningocele (see Chapter 591). A few medical centers in the United States have been performing antenatal myelomeningocele closure. Long-term results from one large trial (the "MOMS trial"), have not shown a definite improvement in lower urinary tract function, although some children have demonstrated nearly normal bladder function, and overall there has been a significant reduction in the need for ventriculoperitoneal shunting.

CLINICAL MANIFESTATIONS AND DIAGNOSIS
The most important urologic consequences of neuropathic bladder dysfunction associated with neural tube defects are urinary incontinence (see Chapter 543), urinary tract infections (UTIs; see Chapter 538), and hydronephrosis from vesicoureteral reflux (see Chapter 539), or detrusor–sphincter dyssynergia (see Chapter 540). Pyelonephritis and renal functional deterioration (see Chapter 535) are common causes of premature death of affected patients.

In the neonate, renal ultrasonography, assessment of postvoid residual urine volumes, and a voiding cystourethrogram are performed after closure of the myelomeningocele. Approximately 10-15% of newborns with myelomeningocele have hydronephrosis, and renal malformations are common; 25% have vesicoureteral reflux. A urodynamic study also should be performed. This study involves filling the bladder with saline, measuring the bladder volume and pressure, and assessing sphincter tone. During bladder filling, the bladder might show (1) uninhibited (premature) contractions (termed hyperreflexia) at low volumes, (2) normal bladder volume with contraction at an appropriate volume, or (3) atonia (lack of bladder contraction). Bladder compliance or elasticity also may be reduced. The sphincter can show (1) normal tonicity with relaxation during bladder contraction, (2) reduced or absent tonicity, or (3) normal or increased tonicity that increases during a bladder contraction (termed detrusor-sphincter dyssynergia) (Fig. 542-1).

RENAL DAMAGE
Renal damage usually results from detrusor–sphincter dyssynergia. This dyssynergia causes functional obstruction of the bladder outlet, leading to bladder muscle hypertrophy and trabeculation, high

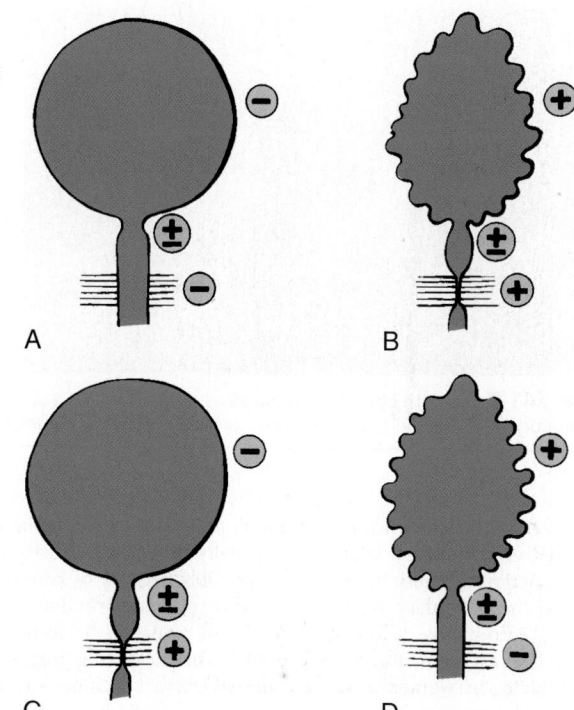

Figure 542-1 Grouping of neurogenic bladder dysfunction according to the innervation, tonicity, and coordination of the detrusor and sphincters described by Guzman. This grouping is based on data from imaging studies, cystometrography, and electromyography of the sphincters. Patients in group B are at risk of developing reflux and hydronephrosis. For guidance in the treatment of incontinence, group A benefits from procedures that increase outlet resistance, group B from anticholinergics or bladder augmentation surgery, and group C from intermittent catheterization. Group D requires both increased outlet resistance and pharmacologic or surgical bladder enlargement. Most patients require intermittent catheterization to empty. *(Modified from Gonzalez R: Urinary incontinence. In Kelalis PK, King LR, Belman AB, editors: Clinical pediatric urology, Philadelphia, 1992, WB Saunders, p. 387.)*

intravesical pressure, and transmission of this high pressure into the upper urinary tracts, causing hydronephrosis (Fig. 542-2). Vesicoureteral reflux and UTI compound the problem. Treatment includes reduction of bladder pressure with anticholinergic drugs (e.g., oxybutynin, 0.2 mg/kg/24 hr in 2 or 3 divided doses) and clean intermittent catheterization every 3-4 hr. If the child has vesicoureteral reflux or UTI, antimicrobial prophylaxis also is prescribed.

Temporary urinary diversion by cutaneous vesicostomy is an alternative in the newborn or infant with severe reflux, if intermittent catheterization is difficult or anticholinergic medications are not well tolerated. Another option to treat the severely trabeculated bladder is transurethral injection of botulinum toxin (Botox) into the detrusor muscle, which reduces bladder hypertonicity for approximately 6 mo. A different approach in these children is to temporarily inactivate the tight sphincter by urethral overdilation or transurethral injection of botulinum toxin into the sphincter. In children with upper tract changes, continuous overnight bladder drainage allows significant bladder relaxation and can reduce bladder wall thickening and lessen hydronephrosis.

Clean intermittent catheterization and anticholinergic therapy cure reflux in up to 80% of children with grade I or II reflux. Children with more severe reflux often require subureteral endoscopic injection therapy (see Chapter 539) or open antireflux surgery followed by intermittent catheterization and anticholinergic drugs. In older children with myelomeningocele with high-grade reflux, UTI, and hydronephrosis, augmentation enterocystoplasty (enlarging the bladder with a

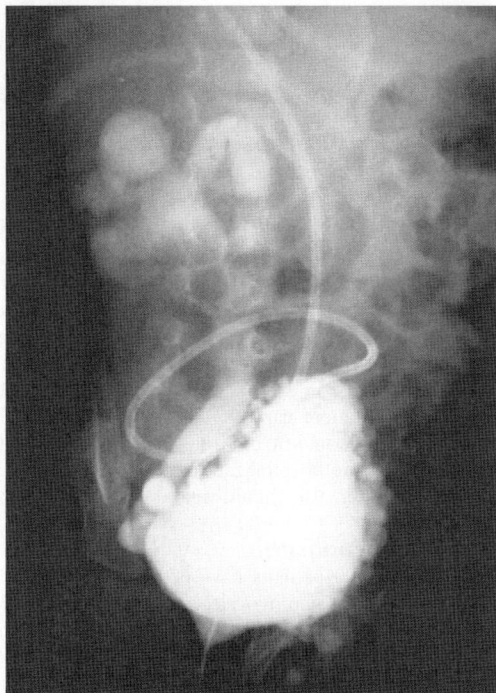

Figure 542-2 Voiding cystourethrogram in an infant with myelodysplasia shows a severely trabeculated bladder with multiple diverticula and grade V (out of V) right vesicoureteral reflux. Evaluation showed severe detrusor–sphincter dyssynergia.

patch of intestine) with intermittent catheterization may be necessary. This intervention allows a normal capacity bladder with low bladder pressure and effective drainage of the bladder.

URINARY INCONTINENCE
Incontinence in the child with neuropathic bladder can result from total or partial denervation of the sphincter, bladder hyperreflexia, poor bladder compliance, chronic urinary retention, or a combination of these factors.

Incontinence often is addressed around 4 yr of age and is tailored to the individual child. Nearly all children require clean intermittent catheterization to stay dry. This technique allows efficient bladder emptying with minimal risk of symptomatic UTI. The urinary tract should be reevaluated with renal ultrasonography, a voiding cystourethrogram, and a urodynamic study, including bladder capacity. If the external sphincter tone is sufficient and the bladder has adequate compliance, intermittent catheterization every 3-4 hr usually is successful in keeping the child dry. If there are unstable bladder contractions, an anticholinergic medication such as oxybutynin chloride, hyoscyamine, or tolterodine is prescribed to increase bladder capacity. If there is sphincter incompetence, α-adrenergic medications are prescribed to enhance outlet resistance. Bacteriuria is seen in up to 50% of children using intermittent self-catheterization, but it seldom causes symptoms. In the absence of reflux, there seems to be little cause for concern. Performing intermittent catheterization with a new catheter (hydrophilic or standard silicone) each time also is quite effective in preventing bacteriuria and avoids the need for antibiotic prophylaxis. With this treatment plan, 40-85% of patients are dry, depending on the definition of continence; some children wear a pad in their underwear or a diaper but feel that they are dry.

If there is persistent incontinence despite medical therapy, reconstructive urinary tract surgery nearly always can provide complete or satisfactory continence. If urethral resistance is low, bladder neck reconstructive procedures such as a periurethral sling often are successful. Alternatively, implantation of an artificial sphincter usually is successful. This sphincter consists of an inflatable cuff that is placed around the bladder neck, a pressure-regulating balloon implanted in the extraperitoneal space, and a pumping mechanism that is implanted in the scrotum of boys and in the labia majora of girls. If the bladder capacity or bladder compliance is low, or if there are persistent uninhibited contractions despite anticholinergic therapy, enlargement of the bladder with a patch of small or large intestine, termed **augmentation cystoplasty** or **enterocystoplasty,** is effective.

These patients still need to perform clean intermittent catheterization. If urethral catheterization is difficult, a continent urinary stoma may be incorporated into the urinary tract reconstruction. A common method is the **Mitrofanoff procedure,** in which the appendix is isolated from the cecum on its vascular pedicle and is interposed between the bladder and abdominal wall to allow intermittent catheterization through a dry stoma. An ileal conduit with a bag on the abdominal wall is rarely used.

Complications of Augmentation Cystoplasty
Urinary Tract Infection
The urine may be colonized with Gram-negative bacteria, and attempts to sterilize the urine for prolonged periods usually fail. There is no evidence that chronic bacteriuria in patients who have had enterocystoplasty is associated with renal damage; therefore, only symptomatic UTIs should be treated.

Metabolic Acidosis
The enteric mucosal surface in contact with the urine absorbs ammonium, chloride, and hydrogen ions and loses potassium. Hyperchloremic metabolic acidosis can result, possibly requiring medical treatment (see Chapter 55). Chronic acidosis can compromise skeletal growth. This condition is common with colocystoplasty but is rare with ileocystoplasty. Metabolic acidosis also is common in patients with compromised renal function. To overcome this limitation of enterocystoplasty in patients with chronic renal insufficiency, a composite augmentation using stomach and small or large bowel gastric segment can be used. The stomach secretes chloride and hydrogen ions; thus, preexisting metabolic acidosis remains stable or improves.

Spontaneous Perforation
Perforation of the augmented bladder is a life-threatening complication that results most often from acute or chronic overdistention of the augmented bladder. Patients with this complication typically present with severe abdominal pain and signs of peritonitis. Prompt diagnosis and treatment with exploratory laparotomy and bladder closure are necessary. Meticulous adherence to the prescribed program of intermittent catheterization to avoid bladder overdistention is important.

Bladder Calculi
Bladder calculi have developed in as many as 70% of children followed for 10 yr after enterocystoplasty. The calculi develop in response to mucus that accumulates in the bladder and act as a nidus for stone formation. This complication can be prevented by daily irrigation of the bladder with sterile saline.

Malignant Neoplasm
Invasive transitional cell carcinoma has been reported in nearly 2% of patients undergoing enterocystoplasty (compared with a 1% risk in spina bifida patients without enterocystoplasty). The pathogenesis is uncertain but is speculated that it is related to bacteriuria and the bowel-bladder contact. The risk seems to be highest following gastrocystoplasty. The risk seems to increase 10 yr following enterocystoplasty. Although these patients probably should undergo screening, there are no guidelines or recommendations regarding this practice. It seems appropriate to advise yearly endoscopic examinations or urine cytologic studies beginning in the 10th postoperative year.

Future Management
The development of a tissue-engineered bladder using a composite scaffold, which could be attached to the dome of the bladder to increase capacity and compliance, might help patients achieve continence

(Fig. 542-3). In addition, there is a nerve-rerouting procedure in which the dorsal nerve root from the lumbar nerve is sutured to the ventral sacral nerve root, allowing the child to scratch the thigh to stimulate a bladder contraction. This procedure is controversial.

ASSOCIATED DISORDERS

Constipation

Many patients with spina bifida also have bowel problems with constipation, and a vigorous bowel regimen is important. Some benefit from the **Malone antegrade continence enema procedure,** in which the appendix is brought out to the skin to allow a catheter to be inserted into the cecum for antegrade enema. The stoma is continent, and an antegrade enema can be performed with tap water each day. This form of management allows the patient to be continent of stool and be more self-sufficient.

Latex Allergy

Latex allergy is a very serious problem encountered by as many as half of patients with spina bifida and other urologic conditions who require clean intermittent catheterization and urinary tract reconstructive procedures. This immunoglobulin E–mediated allergy is acquired and is secondary to repeated exposure to the latex allergen. Latex allergy can manifest as watery eyes, sneezing, itching, hives, or anaphylaxis when blowing up a balloon or if an examiner is using latex gloves. Intraoperatively, a sensitized patient can experience anaphylactic shock. A latex-free environment should be provided for all children with spina bifida in the office, during hospitalization, and during operative procedures. Affected children also should wear a medical alert bracelet.

Occult Spinal Dysraphism

Approximately 1 in 4,000 patients have occult spinal dysraphism, a category that includes lipomeningocele, intradural lipoma, diastematomyelia, tight filum terminale, dermoid cyst-sinus, aberrant nerve roots, anterior sacral meningocele, and cauda equina tumor. More than 90% of patients have a cutaneous abnormality overlying the lower spine, including a small dimple, tuft of hair, dermal vascular malformation, or subcutaneous lipoma (Fig. 542-4). Often these children have high-arched feet, discrepancy in muscle size and strength between the legs, and a gait abnormality. Newborns and young infants often have a normal neurologic examination. Older children often have absent perineal sensation and back pain. Lower urinary tract function is abnormal in 40% of patients, including incontinence, recurrent UTI, and fecal soiling. The likelihood of a normal examination is inversely related to the child's age at surgical correction of the spinal lesion. In infants with abnormal urodynamics, 60% revert to normal; in older children, only 27% become normal. Management of the urinary tract in other children is similar to that described earlier for neural tube defects.

Sacral Agenesis

Sacral agenesis is defined as the absence of part or all of ≥2 lower vertebral bodies. This condition is more common in the offspring of women with diabetes. These children have a flattened buttock and a low, short gluteal cleft but usually have no orthopedic deformity, although some have high-arched feet. Palpation of the coccygeal area detects the absent vertebrae. Approximately 20% of cases are undetected until the age of 3-4 yr; many are diagnosed after unsuccessful

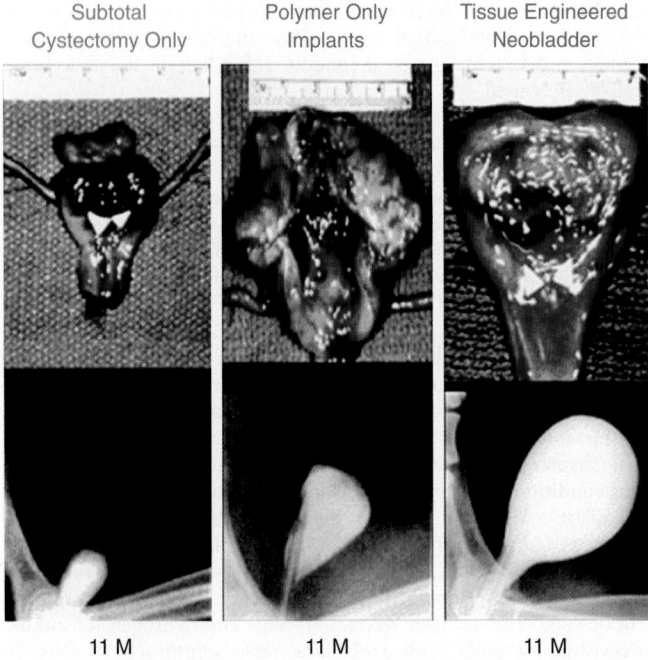

Subtotal Cystectomy Only   **Polymer Only Implants**   **Tissue Engineered Neobladder**

11 M   11 M   11 M

Figure 542-3 Gross specimens and cystograms at 11 mo of the cystectomy-only, nonseeded controls, and cell-seeded tissue engineered bladder replacements in dogs. The cystectomy-only bladder had a capacity of 22% of the preoperative value and a decrease in bladder compliance to 10% of the preoperative value. The nonseeded controls showed significant scarring and had a capacity of 46% of the preoperative value and a decrease in bladder compliance to 42% of the preoperative value. An average bladder capacity of 95% of the original precystectomy volume was achieved in the cell-seeded tissue engineered bladder replacements, and the compliance showed almost no difference from preoperative values that were measured when the native bladder was present (106%). *(From Atala A: Bioengineered tissues for urogenital repair in children, Pediatr Res 63:569–575, 2008.)*

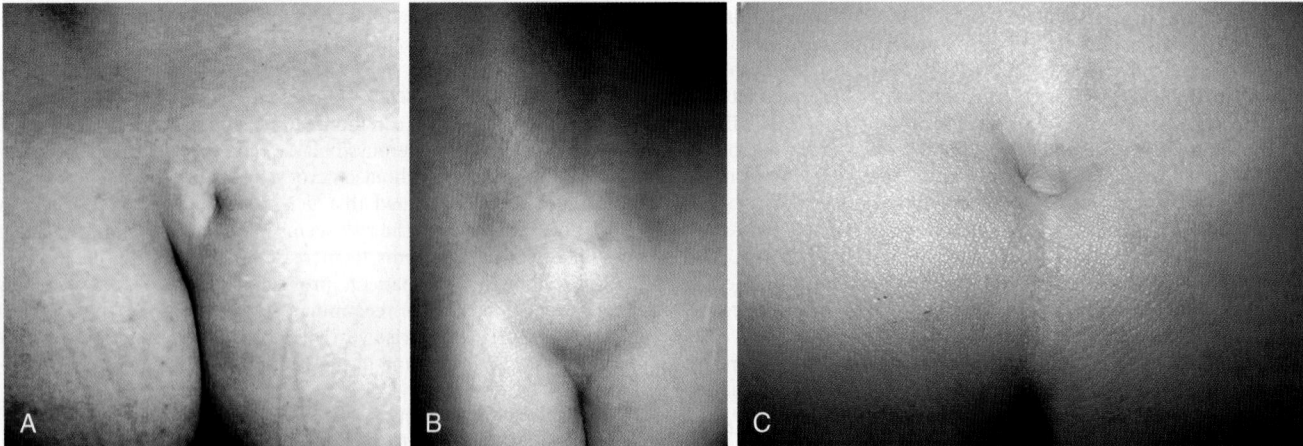

Figure 542-4 A, Buttocks of teenage boy with tethered cord secondary to lipomeningocele. Note sacral dimple and deviation of gluteal fold to the left. **B,** Fat deposit over sacrum in girl with tethered cord secondary to lipomeningocele. **C,** Deep sacral pit in child with neuropathic bladder.

toilet training. Urodynamic studies in these children show a variety of patterns, and most need clean intermittent catheterization and pharmacotherapy to stay dry.

Imperforate Anus

Approximately 30-45% of children with a high imperforate anus have a neuropathic bladder, often because of sacral agenesis. Newborns with imperforate anus should undergo a spinal ultrasound during their initial evaluation, and if these children have difficulty with toilet training, complete urologic evaluation with upper and lower urinary tract imaging and urodynamics should be performed. See Chapter 344 for further details.

Cerebral Palsy

Children with cerebral palsy (see Chapter 598.1) often have reasonable bladder control. However, they achieve continence at a later age than unaffected children. Overall, 25-50% are incontinent, and the risk is directly related to the severity of physical impairment. Their upper urinary tracts usually are normal. Urodynamic studies have shown that most have uninhibited bladder contractions. Timed voiding and anticholinergic therapy are usually effective. Clean intermittent catheterization rarely is necessary.

Bibliography is available at Expert Consult.

Chapter **543**
Enuresis and Voiding Dysfunction
Jack S. Elder

NORMAL VOIDING AND TOILET TRAINING

Fetal voiding occurs by reflex bladder contraction in concert with simultaneous contraction of the bladder and relaxation of the sphincter. Urine storage results from sympathetic and pudendal nerve-mediated inhibition of detrusor contractile activity accompanied by closure of the bladder neck and proximal urethra with increased activity of the external sphincter. The infant has coordinated reflex voiding as often as 15-20 times/day. Over time, bladder capacity increases. In children up to the age of 14 yr, the mean bladder capacity in ounces is equal to the age (in years) plus 2.

At 2-4 yr, the child is developmentally ready to begin toilet training. To achieve conscious bladder control, several conditions must be present: awareness of bladder filling; cortical inhibition (suprapontine modulation) of reflex (unstable) bladder contractions; ability to consciously tighten the external sphincter to prevent incontinence; normal bladder growth; and motivation by the child to stay dry. The transitional phase of voiding refers to the period when children are acquiring bladder control. Girls typically acquire bladder control before boys, and bowel control typically is achieved before bladder control.

A common condition in children is **bladder–bowel dysfunction**. This term was coined by the American Urological Association Vesicoureteral Reflux Guidelines Committee and refers to disorders of bladder and/or bowel function. The previous term for this condition was dysfunctional elimination syndrome.

DIURNAL INCONTINENCE

Daytime incontinence not secondary to neurologic abnormalities is common in children. The most common cause of daytime inconti-

Table 543-1	Causes of Urinary Incontinence in Childhood

Overactive bladder (urge incontinence or diurnal urge syndrome)
Infrequent voiding (underactive bladder)
Voiding postponement
Detrusor–sphincter dyssynergia
Nonneurogenic neurogenic bladder (Hinman syndrome)
Vaginal voiding
Giggle incontinence
Cystitis
Bladder outlet obstruction (posterior urethral valves)
Ectopic ureter and fistula
Sphincter abnormality (epispadias, exstrophy; urogenital sinus abnormality)
Neuropathic
Overflow incontinence
Traumatic
Iatrogenic
Behavioral
Combinations

nence is an **overactive bladder (urge incontinence)**. At age 5 yr, 95% have been dry during the day at some time and 92% are dry. At 7 yr, 96% are dry, although 15% have significant urgency at times. At 12 yr, 99% are dry during the day. Table 543-1 lists the causes of diurnal incontinence in children.

The history should assess the pattern of incontinence, including the frequency, the volume of urine lost during incontinent episodes, whether the incontinence is associated with urgency or giggling, whether it occurs after voiding, and whether the incontinence is continuous. The frequency of voiding and whether there is nocturnal enuresis, a strong, continuous urinary stream, or sensation of incomplete bladder emptying should be assessed. A diary of when the child voids and whether the child was wet or dry is helpful. Other urologic problems such as urinary tract infections (UTIs), vesicoureteral reflux, neurologic disorders, or a family history of duplication anomalies should be assessed. Bowel habits also should be evaluated, because incontinence is common in children with constipation and/or encopresis. Diurnal incontinence can occur in girls with a history of sexual abuse. Physical examination is directed at identifying signs of organic causes of incontinence: short stature, hypertension, enlarged kidneys and/or bladder, constipation, labial adhesion, ureteral ectopy, back or sacral anomalies (see Fig. 542-4 in Chapter 542), and neurologic abnormalities.

Assessment tools include urinalysis, with culture if indicated; bladder diary (recorded times and volumes voided, whether wet or dry); postvoid residual urine volume (generally obtained by bladder scan); and **Dysfunctional Voiding Symptom Score** (Fig. 543-1). An alternative to the Dysfunctional Voiding Symptom Score is the **Vancouver Nonneurogenic Lower Urinary Tract Dysfunction/ Dysfunctional Elimination Syndrome** questionnaire. This questionnaire is a validated tool that consists of 14 questions scored on a 5-point Likert scale to assess lower urinary tract and bowel dysfunction. In most cases, a uroflow with or without electromyography (noninvasive assessment of urinary flow pattern and measurement of external sphincter activity) is indicated. Another item that may be useful in children older than age 5 yr is the **Pediatric Symptom Checklist (PSC)**. The Pediatric Symptom Checklist is a brief screening questionnaire consisting of 35 questions that is used by pediatricians and other health professionals to improve the recognition and treatment of psychosocial problems in children.

Bowel function should be assessed also. The Bristol Stool Form Score (Fig. 543-2) also should be recorded. In addition, the clinician should utilize the Rome III diagnostic criteria, which classify functional gastrointestinal disorders that do not have underlying structural or tissue-based causes. Children 4 yr of age or older are diagnosed as being

Patient name:
Hospital number:
Reason for referral:
Date:

Over the last month	Almost never	Less than half the time	About half the time	Almost every time	Not available
1. I have had wet clothes or wet underwear during the day.	0	1	2	3	NA
2. When I wet myself, my underwear is soaked.	0	1	2	3	NA
3. I miss having a bowel movement every day.	0	1	2	3	NA
4. I have to push for my bowel movements to come out.	0	1	2	3	NA
5. I only go to the bathroom one or two times each day.	0	1	2	3	NA
6. I can hold onto my pee by crossing my legs, squatting or doing the "pee dance."	0	1	2	3	NA
7. When I have to pee, I cannot wait.	0	1	2	3	NA
8. I have to push to pee.	0	1	2	3	NA
9. When I pee it hurts.	0	1	2	3	NA
10. Parents to answer. Has your child experienced something stressful like the example below?	No (0)			Yes (3)	
Total*					

- New baby.
- New home.
- New school.
- School problems.
- Abuse (sexual/physical).
- Home problems (divorce/death).
- Special events (birthday).
- Accident/injury.
- Others.

*Females with a score ≥6 and males with a score ≥9 are most likely to have dysfunctional voiding.

Figure 543-1 Dysfunctional Voiding Symptom Score questionnaire. *(From Farhat W, Bagli DJ, Capolicchio G, et al: The dysfunctional voiding scoring system: quantitative standardization of dysfunctional voiding symptoms in children, J Urol 164:1011–1015, 2000.)*

Bristol Stool Chart

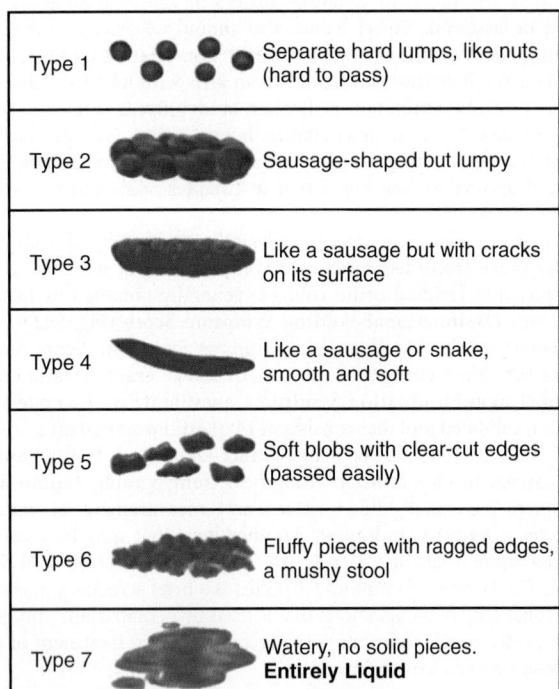

Figure 543-2 Bristol Stool Chart for evaluating bowel function.

constipated if they fulfill 2 or more of the following criteria over a period of 2 mo: 2 or fewer defecations in the toilet per week, at least 1 episode of fecal incontinence per week, a history of retentive posturing or excessive volitional stool retention, history of painful or hard bowel movements, presence of a large fecal mass in the rectum, and history of large-diameter stools that obstruct the toilet.

Imaging is performed in children who have significant physical findings, a family history of urinary tract anomalies or UTIs, and those who do not respond to therapy appropriately. A renal ultrasonogram with or without a **voiding cystourethrogram** is indicated. Urodynamics should be performed if there is evidence of neurologic disease and may be helpful if empirical therapy is ineffective. If there is any evidence of a neurologic disorder, an MRI of the lower spine should be obtained.

OVERACTIVE BLADDER (DIURNAL URGE SYNDROME)

Children with an overactive bladder typically exhibit urinary frequency, urgency, and urge incontinence. Often a girl will squat down on her foot to try to prevent incontinence (termed *Vincent's curtsy*). The bladder in these children is functionally, but not anatomically, smaller than normal and exhibits strong uninhibited contractions. Approximately 25% of children with nocturnal enuresis also have symptoms of an overactive bladder. Many children indicate they do not feel the need to urinate, even just before they are incontinent. In girls, a history of recurrent UTI is common, but incontinence can persist long after infections are brought under control. It is not clear if the voiding dysfunction is a sequela of the UTIs or if the voiding dysfunction predisposes to recurrent UTIs. In girls, voiding cystourethrography often shows a dilated urethra ("spinning-top deformity," Fig. 543-3) and narrowed bladder neck with bladder wall hypertrophy. The urethral finding results from inadequate relaxation of the external

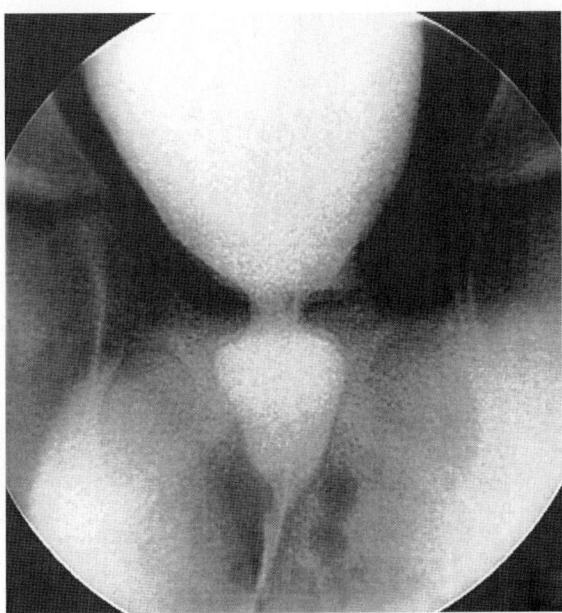

Figure 543-3 Spinning-top deformity. Voiding cystourethrogram demonstrating dilation of the urethra with distal urethral narrowing and contraction of the bladder neck.

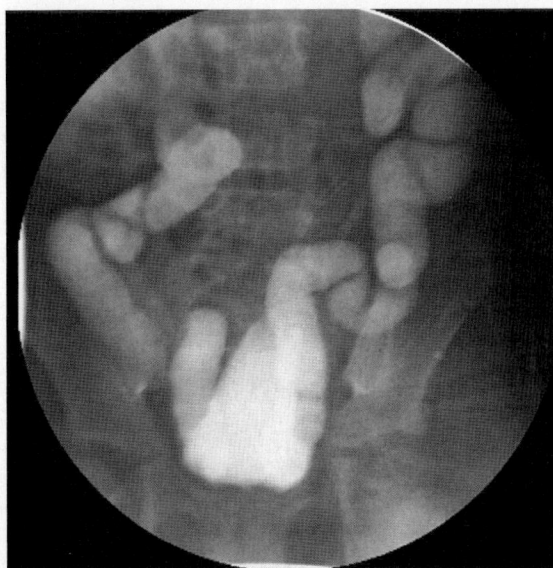

Figure 543-4 Voiding cystourethrogram demonstrating severe bladder trabeculation and vesicoureteral reflux in a 12 yr old boy with Hinman syndrome. The patient presented with day and night incontinence, had chronic renal failure, and underwent kidney transplantation.

urinary sphincter. Constipation is common and should be treated, particularly with any child with Bristol Stool Score 1 or 2.

The overactive bladder nearly always resolves, but the time to resolution is highly variable, sometimes not until the teenage years. Initial therapy is timed voiding, every 1.5-2.0 hr. Treatment of constipation and UTIs is important. Another treatment is biofeedback, in which children are taught pelvic floor exercises (Kegel exercises), because there is evidence that daily performance of these exercises can reduce or eliminate unstable bladder contractions. Biofeedback often includes participation with animated computer games. Biofeedback also may include periodic uroflow studies with sphincter electromyography to be certain that the pelvic floor relaxes during voiding, and assessment of postvoid residual urine volume by sonography. Anticholinergic therapy with oxybutynin chloride, hyoscyamine, or tolterodine reduces bladder overactivity and may help the child achieve dryness. Treatment with an α-adrenergic blocker such as terazosin or doxazosin can aid in bladder emptying by promoting bladder neck relaxation; α-adrenergic blockers also have mild anticholinergic properties. If pharmacologic therapy is successful, the dosage should be tapered periodically to determine its continued need. Children who do not respond to therapy should be evaluated urodynamically to rule out other possible forms of bladder or sphincter dysfunction. In refractory cases, sacral nerve stimulation (InterStim) is a surgical procedure that has shown promise.

If the child has constipation based on the criteria described above, treatment generally is initiated with polyethylene glycol powder, which has been shown to be safe in children and generally more effective than other laxative preparations.

NONNEUROGENIC NEUROGENIC BLADDER (HINMAN SYNDROME)

Hinman syndrome is a very serious but uncommon disorder involving failure of the external sphincter to relax during voiding in children without neurologic abnormalities. Children with this syndrome, also called **nonneurogenic neurogenic bladder**, typically exhibit a staccato stream, day and night wetting, recurrent UTIs, constipation, and encopresis. Evaluation of affected children often reveals vesicoureteral reflux, a trabeculated bladder, and a decreased urinary flow rate with an intermittent pattern (Fig. 543-4). In severe cases, hydronephrosis,

renal insufficiency, and end-stage renal disease can occur. The pathogenesis of this syndrome is thought to involve learning abnormal voiding habits during toilet training; the syndrome is rarely seen in infants. Urodynamic studies and magnetic resonance imaging of the spine are indicated to rule out a neurologic cause for the bladder dysfunction.

The treatment usually is complex and can include anticholinergic and α-adrenergic blocker therapy, timed voiding, treatment of constipation, behavioral modification, and encouragement of relaxation during voiding. Biofeedback has been used successfully in older children to teach relaxation of the external sphincter. In some cases botulinum toxin (Botox) injection into the external sphincter can provide temporary sphincteric paralysis and thereby reduce outlet resistance. In severe cases, intermittent catheterization is necessary to ensure bladder emptying. In selected patients, external urinary diversion is necessary to protect the upper urinary tract. These children require long-term treatment and careful follow-up.

INFREQUENT VOIDING (UNDERACTIVE BLADDER)

Infrequent voiding is a common disorder of micturition, usually associated with UTIs. Affected children, usually girls, void only twice a day rather than the normal 4-7 times. With bladder overdistention and prolonged retention of urine, bacterial growth can lead to recurrent UTIs. Some of these children are constipated. Some also have occasional episodes of incontinence from overflow or urgency. The disorder is behavioral. If the child has UTIs, treatment includes antibacterial prophylaxis and encouragement of frequent voiding and complete emptying of the bladder by double voiding until a normal pattern of micturition is re-established.

VAGINAL VOIDING

In girls with vaginal voiding, incontinence typically occurs after urination after the girl stands up. Usually the volume of urine is 5-10 mL. One of the most common causes is labial adhesion (Fig. 543-5). This lesion, typically seen in young girls, can be managed either by topical application of estrogen cream to the adhesion or lysis in the office. Some girls experience vaginal voiding because they do not separate their legs widely during urination. These girls either are overweight

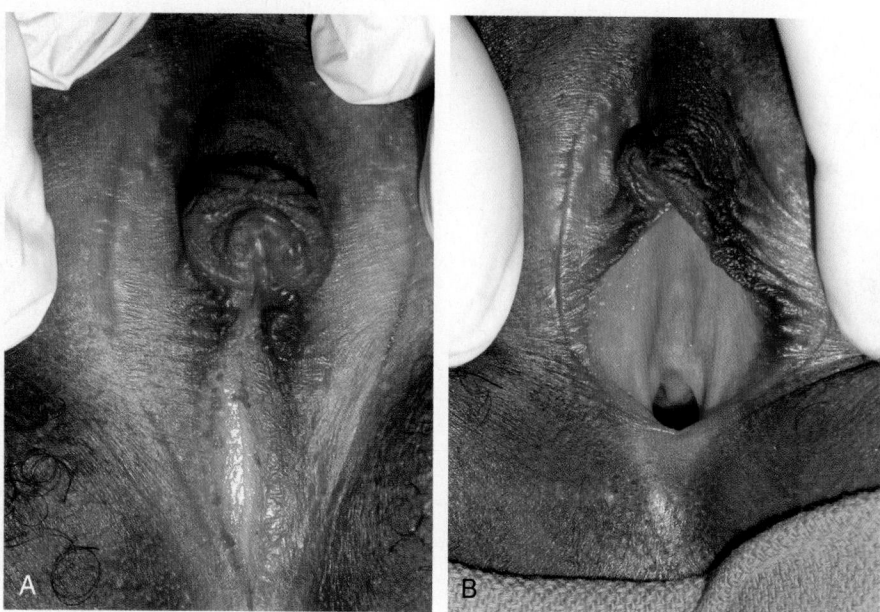

Figure 543-5 A, Labial adhesion. Note the inability to visualize the urethral meatus and vagina. **B,** Normal female external genitalia following lysis of labial adhesion.

or do not pull their underwear down to their ankles when they urinate. Management involves encouraging the girl to separate the legs as widely as possible during urination. The most effective way to do this is to have the child sit backward on the toilet seat during micturition.

OTHER CAUSES OF INCONTINENCE IN GIRLS

Ureteral ectopia, usually associated with a duplicated collecting system in girls, refers to a ureter that drains outside the bladder, often into the vagina or distal urethra. It can produce urinary incontinence characterized by constant urinary dripping all day, even though the child voids regularly. Sometimes the urine production from the renal segment drained by the ectopic ureter is small, and urinary drainage is confused with watery vaginal discharge. Children with a history of vaginal discharge or incontinence and an abnormal voiding pattern require careful study. The ectopic orifice usually is difficult to find. On ultrasonography or intravenous urography, one may suspect duplication of the collecting system (Fig. 543-6), but the upper collecting system drained by the ectopic ureter usually has poor or delayed function. CT scanning of the kidneys or an MR urogram should demonstrate subtle duplication anomalies. Examination under anesthesia for an ectopic ureteral orifice in the vestibule or the vagina may be necessary (Fig. 543-7). The treatment in these cases is either partial nephrectomy, with removal of the upper pole segment of the duplicated kidney and its ureter down to the pelvic brim, or ipsilateral ureteroureterostomy, in which the upper pole ectopic ureter is anastomosed to the normally positioned lower pole ureter. These procedures often are performed by minimally invasive laparoscopy with or without robotic assistance.

Giggle incontinence typically affects girls 7-15 yr of age. The incontinence occurs suddenly during giggling, and the entire bladder volume is lost. The pathogenesis is thought to be sudden relaxation of the urinary sphincter. Anticholinergic medication and timed voiding occasionally are effective. The most effective treatment is low-dose methylphenidate.

Total incontinence in girls may be secondary to **epispadias** (see Fig. 541-2 in Chapter 541). This condition, which affects only 1 in 480,000 females, is characterized by separation of the pubic symphysis, separation of the right and left sides of the clitoris, and a patulous urethra. Treatment is bladder neck reconstruction or placement of an artificial urinary sphincter to repair the incompetent urethra.

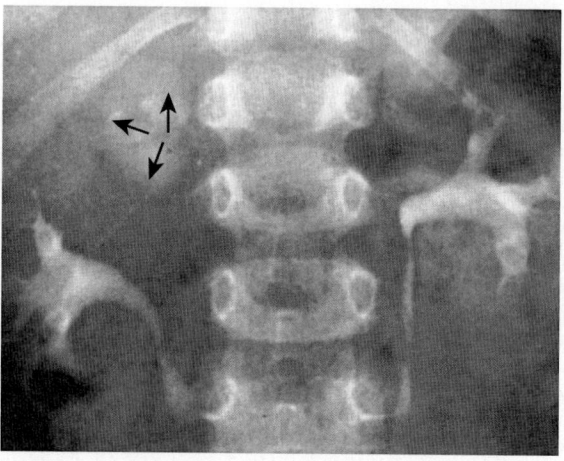

Figure 543-6 Duplication of the right collecting system with ectopic ureter. Excretory urogram in a girl presenting with a normal voiding pattern and constant urinary dribbling. The left kidney is normal, and the right side, well visualized, is the lower collecting system of a duplicated kidney. On the upper pole opposite the 1st and 2nd vertebral bodies, note the accumulation of contrast material corresponding with a poorly functioning upper pole drained by a ureter opening in the vestibule.

A short, incompetent urethra may be associated with certain urogenital sinus malformations. The diagnosis of these malformations requires a high index of suspicion and a careful physical examination of all incontinent girls. In these cases, urethral and vaginal reconstruction often restores continence.

VOIDING DISORDERS WITHOUT INCONTINENCE

Some children have abrupt onset of severe urinary frequency, voiding as often as every 10-15 min during the day, without dysuria, UTI, daytime incontinence, or nocturia. The most common age for these symptoms to occur is 4-6 yr, after the child is toilet trained, and the vast majority are boys. This condition is termed the **daytime frequency syndrome of childhood** or **pollakiuria**. The condition is functional;

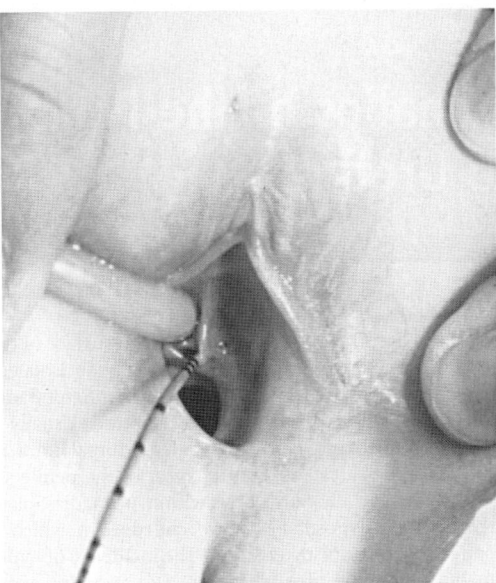

Figure 543-7 This photograph shows an ectopic ureter entering the vestibule next to the urethral meatus. The thin ureteral catheter with transverse marks has been introduced into this ectopic ureter. This girl had a normal voiding pattern and constant urinary dribbling.

Table 543-2	Nocturnal Enuresis

CAUSES

Delayed maturation of the cortical mechanisms that allow voluntary control of the micturition reflex

Defective sleep arousal

Reduced antidiuretic hormone production at night, resulting in an increased urine output (nocturnal polyuria)

Genetic factors, with chromosomes 12 and 13q the likely sites of the gene for enuresis

Bladder factors (lack of inhibition, reduced capacity, overactive)

Constipation

Organic factors, such as urinary tract infection or obstructive uropathy

Sleep disorders

Sleep disordered breathing secondary to enlarged adenoids

Psychologic factors more often implicated in secondary enuresis

OTHER FEATURES

Enuresis can occur in any stage of sleep (but usually non–rapid eye movement sleep)

All children are most difficult to arouse in the first third of the night and easiest to awaken in the last third, but enuretic children are more difficult to arouse than those with normal bladder control

Enuretic children often are described as "soaking the bed"

Family history in enuretic children often positive for enuresis

Risk increased with developmental delay, attention-deficit/hyperactivity disorder, autism spectrum disorders

no anatomic problem is detected. Often the symptoms occur just before a child starts kindergarten or if the child is having emotional family stress-related problems. These children should be checked for UTIs, and the clinician should ascertain that the child is emptying the bladder satisfactorily. Occasionally, pinworms cause these symptoms. The condition is self-limited, and symptoms generally resolve within 2-3 mo. Anticholinergic therapy rarely is effective.

Some children have the **dysuria-hematuria syndrome**, in which the child has dysuria without UTI but with microscopic or gross hematuria. This condition affects children who are toilet-trained and is often secondary to hypercalciuria. A 24-hr urine sample should be obtained and calcium and creatinine excretion assessed. A 24-hr calcium excretion of >4 mg/kg is abnormal and deserves treatment with thiazides, because some of these children are at risk for urolithiasis.

NOCTURNAL ENURESIS

By 5 yr of age, 90-95% of children are nearly completely continent during the day, and 80-85% are continent at night. Nocturnal enuresis refers to the occurrence of involuntary voiding at night after 5 yr, the age when volitional control of micturition is expected. Enuresis may be primary (estimated 75-90% of children with enuresis; nocturnal urinary control never achieved) or secondary (10-25%; the child was dry at night for at least a few months and then enuresis developed). In addition, 75% of children with enuresis are wet only at night, and 25% are incontinent day and night. This distinction is important, because children with both forms are more likely to have an abnormality of the urinary tract. **Monosymptomatic enuresis** is more common than non-monosymptomatic enuresis (associated urgency, hesitancy, frequency, day time incontinence).

Epidemiology

Approximately 60% of children with nocturnal enuresis are boys. Family history is positive in 50% of cases. Although primary nocturnal enuresis may be polygenetic, candidate genes have been localized to chromosomes 12 and 13. If one parent was enuretic, each child has a 44% risk of enuresis; if both parents were enuretic, each child has a 77% likelihood of enuresis. Nocturnal enuresis without overt daytime voiding symptoms affects up to 20% of children at the age of 5 yr; it ceases spontaneously in approximately 15% of involved children every year thereafter. Its frequency among adults is <1%.

Pathogenesis

The pathogenesis of nocturnal enuresis (normal daytime voiding habits) is multifactorial (Table 543-2).

Clinical Manifestations and Diagnosis

A careful history should be obtained, especially with respect to fluid intake at night and pattern of nocturnal enuresis. Children with diabetes insipidus (see Chapter 558), diabetes mellitus (see Chapter 589), and chronic renal disease (see Chapter 535) can have a high obligatory urinary output and a compensatory polydipsia. The family should be asked whether the child snores loudly at night. A complete physical examination should include palpation of the abdomen and rectal examination after voiding to assess the possibility of a chronically distended bladder. The child with nocturnal enuresis should be examined carefully for neurologic and spinal abnormalities. There is an increased incidence of bacteriuria in enuretic girls, and, if found, it should be investigated and treated (see Chapter 538), although this does not always lead to resolution of bedwetting. A urine sample should be obtained after an overnight fast and evaluated for specific gravity or osmolality to exclude polyuria as a cause of frequency and incontinence and to ascertain that the concentrating ability is normal. The absence of glycosuria should be confirmed. If there are no daytime symptoms, the physical examination and urinalysis are normal, and the urine culture is negative, further evaluation for urinary tract pathology generally is not warranted. A renal ultrasonogram is reasonable in an older child with enuresis or in children who do not respond appropriately to therapy.

Treatment

The best approach to treatment is to reassure the child and parents that the condition is self-limited and to avoid punitive measures that can affect the child's psychologic development adversely. Fluid intake should be restricted to 2 oz after 6 or 7 PM. The parents should be certain that the child voids at bedtime. Avoiding extraneous sugar and caffeine after 4 PM also is beneficial. If the child snores and the adenoids are enlarged, referral to an otolaryngologist should be considered, because adenoidectomy can cure the enuresis.

Active treatment should be avoided in children younger than 6 yr of age, because enuresis is extremely common in younger children. Treatment is more likely to be successful in children approaching puberty compared with younger children. In addition, treatment is most likely to be effective in children who are motivated to stay dry. Treatment should be viewed as a facilitator that requires active participation by the child (e.g., a coach and an athlete).

The simplest initial measure is **motivational therapy** and includes a star chart for dry nights. Waking children a few hours after they go to sleep to have them void often allows them to awaken dry, although this measure is not curative. Some have recommended that children try holding their urine for longer periods during the day, but there is no evidence that this approach is beneficial. **Conditioning therapy** involves use of a loud auditory or vibratory alarm attached to a moisture sensor in the underwear. The alarm sounds when voiding occurs and is intended to awaken children and alert them to void. This form of therapy has a reported success of 30-60%, although the relapse rate is significant. Often the auditory alarm wakes up other family members and not the enuretic child; persistent use of the alarm for several months often is necessary to determine whether this treatment is effective. Conditioning therapy tends to be most effective in older children. Another form of therapy to which some children respond is self-hypnosis. The primary role of psychologic therapy is to help the child deal with enuresis psychologically and help motivate the child to void at night if he or she awakens with a full bladder.

Pharmacologic therapy is intended to treat the symptom of enuresis and thus is regarded as second line and is not curative. Direct comparisons of the bell and bed with pharmacologic therapy favor the former because of lower relapse rates, although initial response rates are equivalent.

One form of treatment is **desmopressin acetate**, a synthetic analog of antidiuretic hormone that reduces urine production overnight. This medication is FDA-approved and is available as a tablet, with a dosage of 0.2-0.6 mg at bedtime. In the past a nasal spray was used, but some children experienced hyponatremia and convulsions with this formulation and the nasal spray is no longer recommended for nocturnal enuresis. Hyponatremia has not been reported in children using the oral tablets. Fluid restriction at night is important, and the drug should not be used if the child has a systemic illness with vomiting or diarrhea or if the child has polydipsia. Desmopressin acetate is effective in as many as 40% of children. If effective, it should be used for 3-6 mo, and then an attempt should be made to taper the dosage. If tapering results in recurrent enuresis, the child should return to the higher dosage. Few adverse events have been reported with the long-term use of desmopressin acetate.

For therapy-resistant enuresis or children with symptoms of an overactive bladder, **anticholinergic therapy** is indicated. Oxybutynin 5 mg or tolterodine 2 mg at bedtime often are prescribed. If the medication is ineffective, the dosage may be doubled. The clinician should monitor for constipation as a potential side effect.

A third-line treatment is **imipramine**, which is a tricyclic antidepressant. This medication has mild anticholinergic and α-adrenergic effects, reduces urine output slightly, and also might alter the sleep pattern. The dosage of imipramine is 25 mg in children age 6-8 yr, 50 mg in children age 9-12 yr, and 75 mg in teenagers. Reported success rates are 30-60%. Side effects include anxiety, insomnia, and dry mouth, and heart rhythm may be affected. If there is any history of palpitations or syncope in the child, or sudden cardiac death or unstable arrhythmia in the family, long QT syndrome in the patient needs to be excluded. The drug is one of the most common causes of poisoning by prescription medication in younger siblings.

In unsuccessful cases, combining therapies often is effective. Alarm therapy plus desmopressin is more successful than either alone. The combination of oxybutynin chloride and desmopressin is more successful than either alone. Desmopressin and imipramine also may be combined.

Bibliography is available at Expert Consult.

Chapter **544**
Anomalies of the Penis and Urethra
Jack S. Elder

HYPOSPADIAS

Hypospadias is a urethral opening on the ventral surface of the penile shaft affecting 1 in 250 male newborns. Typically an isolated defect, but its incidence is increased in disorders of sex differentiation, anorectal malformation, and congenital heart disease. Usually there is incomplete development of the prepuce, called a **dorsal hood**, in which the foreskin is on the sides and dorsal aspect of the penile shaft and deficient or absent ventrally. Some boys with hypospadias, particularly those with proximal hypospadias, have **chordee**, in which there is ventral penile curvature during erection. The incidence of hypospadias appears to be increasing, possibly because of in utero exposure to estrogenic or antiandrogenic endocrine-disrupting chemicals (e.g., polychlorobiphenyls, phytoestrogens).

Clinical Manifestations

Hypospadias is classified according to the position of the urethral meatus after taking into account whether chordee is present (Fig. 544-1). The deformity is described as glanular (on the glans penis), coronal, subcoronal, midpenile, penoscrotal, scrotal, or perineal. Approximately 65% of cases are distal, 25% are subcoronal or midpenile, and 10% are proximal. In the most severe cases, the scrotum is bifid and sometimes there is moderate penoscrotal transposition. As many as 10% of affected boys have a **megameatal variant**, in which the foreskin is developed normally (megameatus intact prepuce variant), and there is either glanular or subcoronal hypospadias with a "fish mouth" meatus. These cases might not be diagnosed until after a circumcision is performed.

Approximately 10% of boys with hypospadias have an undescended testis; inguinal hernias also are common. In the newborn, the differential diagnosis of midpenile or proximal hypospadias associated with an undescended testis should include forms of a disorder of sex development, particularly mixed gonadal dysgenesis, partial androgen insensitivity, true hermaphroditism, and congenital adrenal hyperplasia in a female (see Chapter 576). In the latter situation, neither gonad would be palpable. A karyotype should be obtained in patients with midpenile or proximal hypospadias and cryptorchidism (see Chapter 588). In boys with penoscrotal hypospadias, a voiding cystourethrogram should be considered because 5-10% of these children have a dilated prostatic utricle, which is a remnant of the müllerian system (see Chapter 554). The incidence of upper urinary tract abnormalities is low unless there are abnormalities of other organ systems.

Complications of untreated hypospadias include deformity of the urinary stream, typically ventral deflection or severe splaying; sexual dysfunction secondary to penile curvature; infertility if the urethral meatus is proximal; meatal stenosis (congenital), which is uncommon; and cosmetic appearance. The goal of hypospadias surgery is to correct the functional and cosmetic deformities. Whereas hypospadias repair is recommended for all boys with midpenile and proximal hypospadias, some boys with distal hypospadias have no functional abnormality and do not need any surgical correction.

Treatment

Management begins in the newborn period. Circumcision should be avoided, because the foreskin often is used in the repair in most cases. The ideal age for repair in a healthy infant is 6-12 mo, because the risk of general anesthesia at this age is similar to older children; penile growth over the next several years is slow; the child does not remember the surgical procedure; and postoperative analgesic needs are less than

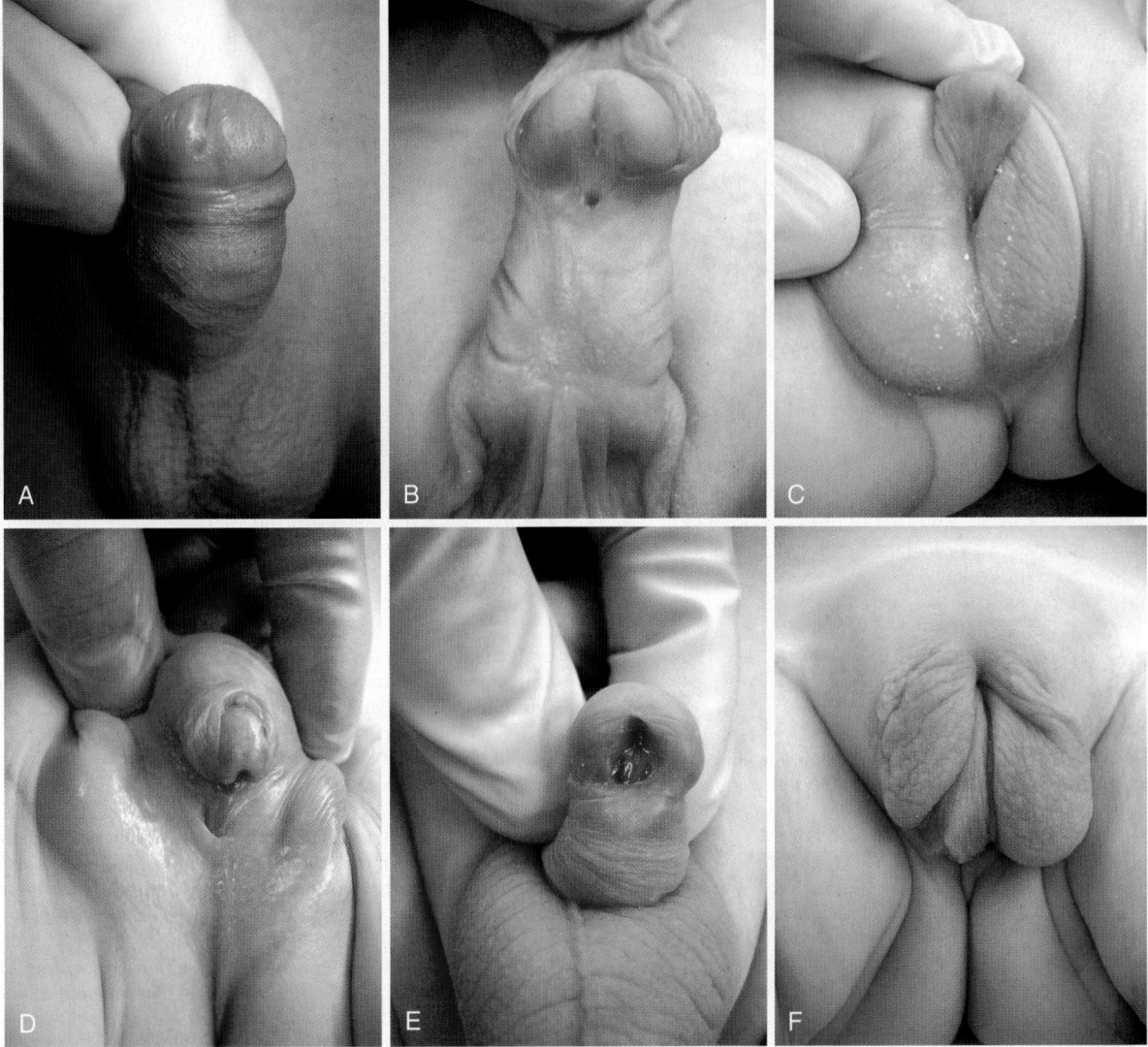

Figure 544-1 Varying forms of hypospadias. **A,** Glanular hypospadias. **B,** Subcoronal hypospadias. Note the dorsal hood of foreskin. **C,** Penoscrotal hypospadias with chordee. **D,** Perineal hypospadias with chordee and partial penoscrotal transposition. **E,** Megameatal variant of hypospadias diagnosed following circumcision; note absence of hooded foreskin. **F,** Complete penoscrotal transposition with scrotal hypospadias.

in older children. With the exception of proximal hypospadias, virtually all cases are repaired in a single operation on an ambulatory basis. The most common repair involves tubularization of the urethral plate distal to the urethral meatus, with coverage by a vascularized flap from the foreskin, termed a *tubularized incised plate* repair. Proximal cases might require a 2-stage repair. The complication rate is low: 5% for distal hypospadias, 10% for midpenile hypospadias, and 20% for proximal hypospadias. The most common complications include urethrocutaneous fistula and meatal stenosis. Other complications include a deformed urinary stream, persistent penile curvature, and dehiscence of the hypospadias repair. Treatment of these complications generally is straightforward. In complex cases, a buccal mucosa graft is used to create urethral mucosa. Repair of hypospadias is a technically demanding operation and should be performed by a surgeon with specialty training in pediatric urology and extensive experience.

CHORDEE WITHOUT HYPOSPADIAS

In some boys there is mild or moderate ventral penile curvature (**chordee**) and incomplete development of the foreskin (**dorsal hood**), but the urethral meatus is at the tip of the glans (Fig. 544-2). In most of these boys, the urethra is normal but there is insufficient ventral penile skin or prominent, inelastic ventral bands of dartos fascia that prevent a straight erection. In some cases, the urethra is hypoplastic,

and a formal urethroplasty is necessary for repair. The only sign of this anomaly in the neonate may be the hooded foreskin, and delayed repair under general anesthesia at 6 mo of age is recommended.

PHIMOSIS AND PARAPHIMOSIS

Phimosis refers to the inability to retract the prepuce. At birth, phimosis is physiologic. Over time, the adhesions between the prepuce and glans lyse and the distal phimotic ring loosens. In 80% of uncircumcised boys the prepuce becomes retractable by 3 yr of age. Accumulation of epithelial debris under the infant's prepuce is physiologic and does not mandate circumcision. In older boys, phimosis may be physiologic, may be pathologic from inflammation and scarring at the tip of the foreskin (Fig. 544-3), or occurs after circumcision. The prepuce might have been retracted forcefully on 1 or 2 occasions in the past, which can result in a cicatricial scar that prevents subsequent retraction of the foreskin. In boys with persistent physiologic or pathologic phimosis, application of corticosteroid cream to the foreskin 3 times daily for 1 mo loosens the phimotic ring in two-thirds of cases. If there is ballooning of the foreskin during voiding or phimosis beyond 10 yr of age and topical corticosteroid therapy is ineffective, circumcision is recommended.

Paraphimosis occurs when the foreskin is retracted proximal to the coronal sulcus and the prepuce cannot be pulled back over the glans

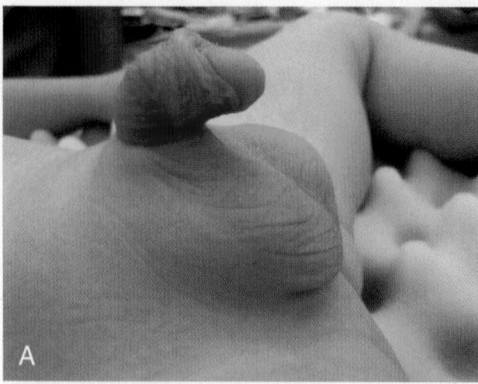
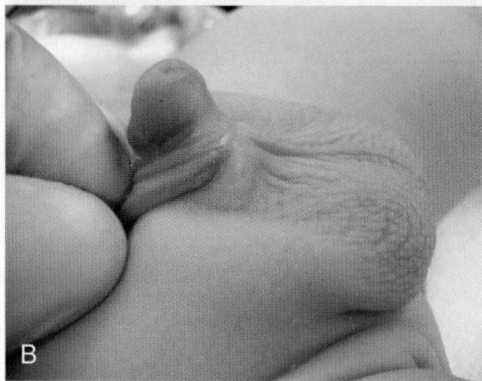

Figure 544-2 A and **B,** Two examples of chordee without hypospadias. Note hooded foreskin and normal location of urethral meatus.

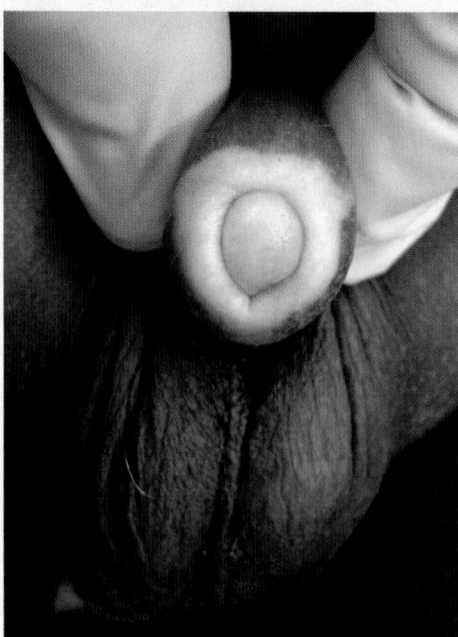

Figure 544-3 Balanitis xerotica obliterans. Note whitish cicatricial plaque.

(Fig. 544-4). Painful venous stasis in the retracted foreskin results, with edema leading to severe pain and inability to reduce the foreskin (pull it back over the glans). Treatment includes lubricating the foreskin and glans and then simultaneously compressing the glans and placing distal traction on the foreskin to try to push the phimotic ring past the coronal sulcus. Topical application of granulated sugar has been reported to aid in reduction of edema by creation of an osmotic gradient, facilitating reduction of paraphimosis. In addition, injection of

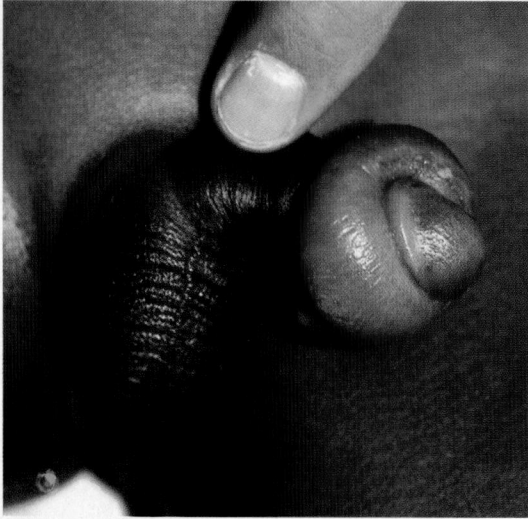

Figure 544-4 Paraphimosis. The foreskin has been retracted proximal to the glans penis and has become markedly swollen secondary to venous congestion.

hyaluronidase into the edematous skin has been reported to result in immediate reduction in swelling. In rare cases, emergency circumcision under general anesthesia is necessary.

CIRCUMCISION

In the United States, circumcision usually is performed for cultural reasons. In 2012, a multidisciplinary task force of the American Academy of Pediatrics stated that evidence indicates that the health benefits of newborn male circumcision outweigh the risks and that the procedure's benefits justify access to this procedure for families who choose it. Specific benefits identified included prevention of urinary tract infections (UTIs), penile cancer, reducing the risk and transmission of some sexually transmitted infections, including HIV. The American College of Obstetricians and Gynecologists endorsed this policy statement. By contrast, European medical professional groups have been less likely to endorse this practice.

When performing a neonatal circumcision, local analgesia, such as a dorsal nerve block or application of EMLA (eutectic mixture of local anesthetics) cream (lidocaine 2.5% and prilocaine 2.5%) is recommended.

UTIs are 10-15 times more common in uncircumcised infant boys than in circumcised infants, with the urinary pathogens arising from bacteria that colonize the space between the prepuce and glans. The risk of febrile UTI (see Chapter 538) is highest between birth and 6 mo, but there is an increased risk of UTI until at least 5 yr of age. Many recommend circumcision in infants who are predisposed to UTI, such as those with congenital hydronephrosis and vesicoureteral reflux. Circumcision reduces the risk of sexually transmitted infections in adults (see Chapter 120), in particular HIV (see Chapter 276). There have been only a handful of reports of men who were circumcised at birth and subsequently acquired penile carcinoma, but in Scandinavian countries, where few men are circumcised and hygiene is good, the incidence of penile cancer is low.

Complications after neonatal circumcision include bleeding, wound infection, meatal stenosis, secondary phimosis, removal of insufficient foreskin, and fibrous penile adhesions (skin bridge; Fig. 544-5); 0.2-3.0% of patients undergo a subsequent operative procedure. Boys with a large hydrocele or hernia are at particular risk for secondary phimosis because the scrotal swelling tends to displace the penile shaft skin over the glans. Potentially serious complications include sepsis, amputation of the distal part of the glans, removal of an excessive amount of foreskin, and urethrocutaneous fistula. Circumcision should not be performed in neonates with hypospadias, chordee without hypospadias, or a dorsal hood deformity (relative contraindication) or in those with

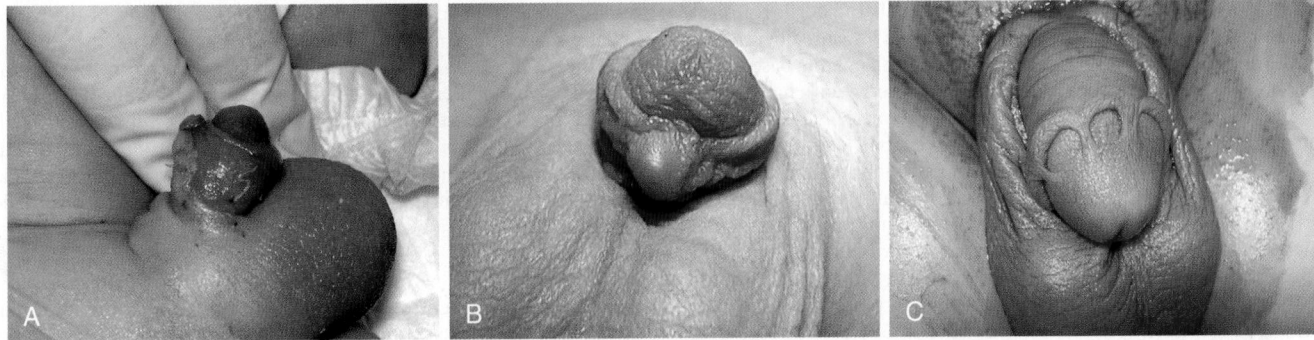

Figure 544-5 Complications of circumcision. **A,** Denuded penile shaft. With local care, the penis healed and appeared normal. **B,** Midline epithelial inclusion cyst. **C,** Fibrous penile skin bridges.

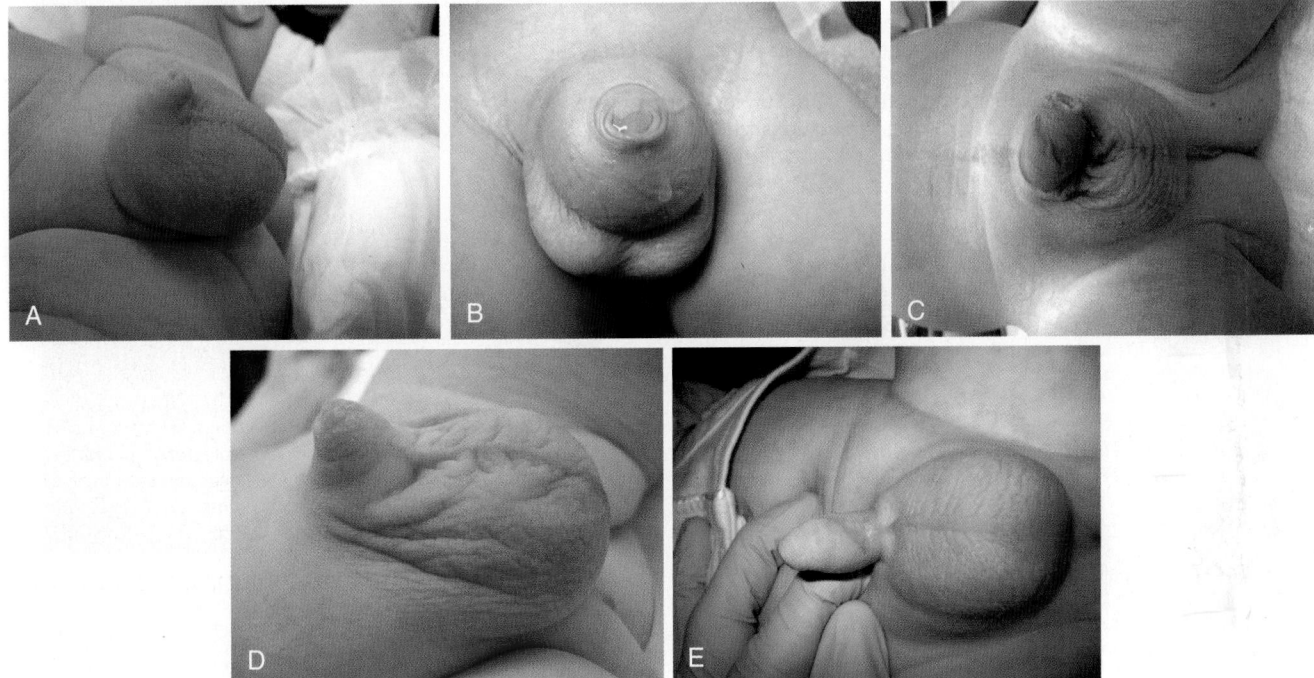

Figure 544-6 Examples of congenital deformities in which neonatal circumcision may be contraindicated. **A,** Hidden penis. **B,** Megaprepuce. **C,** Penile torsion to left side. **D,** Webbed penis; note scrotal attachment to penile shaft. **E,** Example of wandering raphe, with deviation of the median raphe to the left side. This finding may be an indication of penile torsion or hypospadias.

a small penis (Fig. 544-6). In boys with a **wandering raphe** (Fig. 544-6), in which the median raphe deviates to 1 side, there may be underlying penile torsion or hypospadias, and evaluation by a pediatric urologist is suggested before performing a circumcision.

PENILE TORSION

Penile torsion, a rotational defect of the penile shaft, usually occurs in a counterclockwise direction (to the left side: see Fig. 544-6). In most cases, penile development is normal, and the condition is unrecognized until circumcision is performed or the foreskin is retractable. In many cases the midline raphe of the penile shaft is deviated. Penile torsion also occurs in some boys with hypospadias. The defect has primarily cosmetic significance and correction is unnecessary if the rotation is <60 degrees from the midline.

INCONSPICUOUS PENIS

The term *inconspicuous penis* refers to a penis that appears to be small. A **webbed penis** is a condition in which the scrotal skin extends onto the ventral penile shaft. This deformity represents an abnormality of the attachment between the penis and scrotum. Although the deformity

might appear mild, if a routine circumcision is performed, the penis can retract into the scrotum, resulting in secondary phimosis (**trapped penis**). The concealed (**hidden or buried**) penis is a normally developed penis that is camouflaged by the suprapubic fat pad (Fig. 544-7). This anomaly may be congenital, iatrogenic after circumcision, or a result of obesity. Surgical correction is indicated for cosmetic reasons or if there is a functional abnormality with a splayed stream.

A **trapped penis** is an acquired form of inconspicuous penis and refers to a phallus that becomes embedded in the suprapubic fat pad after circumcision (Fig. 544-8). This deformity can occur after neonatal circumcision in an infant who has significant scrotal swelling from a large hydrocele or inguinal hernia or after routine circumcision in an infant with a webbed penis. This complication can predispose to UTIs and can cause urinary retention. Initial treatment of a trapped penis should include topical corticosteroid cream, which often loosens the phimotic ring. In some cases secondary repair is necessary at 6-9 mo.

MICROPENIS

Micropenis is defined as a normally formed penis that is at least 2.5 SD below the mean in size (Fig. 544-9). Typically, the ratio of the length of the penile shaft to its circumference is normal. The pertinent measurement is the **stretched penile length**, which is measured by stretching the penis and measuring the distance from the penile base under the pubic symphysis to the tip of the glans. The mean length of the term newborn penis is 3.5 ± 0.7 cm and the diameter is 1.1 ± 0.2 cm. The diagnosis of micropenis is made if the stretched length is <1.9 cm.

Micropenis usually results from a hormonal abnormality that occurs after 14 wk of gestation. Common causes include hypogonadotropic hypogonadism, hypergonadotropic hypogonadism (primary testicular failure), and idiopathic micropenis. If growth hormone deficiency also is present, neonatal hypoglycemia can occur. The most common cause of micropenis is failure of the hypothalamus to produce an adequate amount of gonadotropin-releasing hormone, as typically occurs in Kallmann syndrome (see Chapter 583), Prader-Willi syndrome (see Chapter 108), and Lawrence-Moon-Bardet-Biedl syndrome. In some cases, there is growth hormone deficiency. Primary testicular failure can result from gonadal dysgenesis or rudimentary testes syndrome and also occurs in **Robinow syndrome** (characterized by hypoplastic genitalia, shortening of the forearms, frontal bossing, hypertelorism, wide palpebral fissures, short broad nose, long philtrum, small chin, brachydactyly, and a normal karyotype).

A pediatric endocrinologist, geneticist, and pediatric urologist should examine all children with these syndromes. **Evaluation** includes a karyotype, assessment of anterior pituitary function and testicular function, and MRI to determine the anatomic integrity of the hypothalamus and the anterior pituitary gland as well as the midline structure of the brain. One of the difficult questions is whether androgen therapy is essential during childhood, because androgenic stimulation of penile growth in a prepubertal boy can limit the growth potential of the penis in puberty. Studies of small groups of men with micropenis suggest that many, although not all, have satisfactory sexual function. Consequently, a decision for gender reassignment is made infrequently.

PRIAPISM

Priapism is a persistent penile erection at least 4 hr in duration that continues beyond, or is unrelated to, sexual stimulation. Typically, only the corpora cavernosa are affected. There are 3 subtypes:

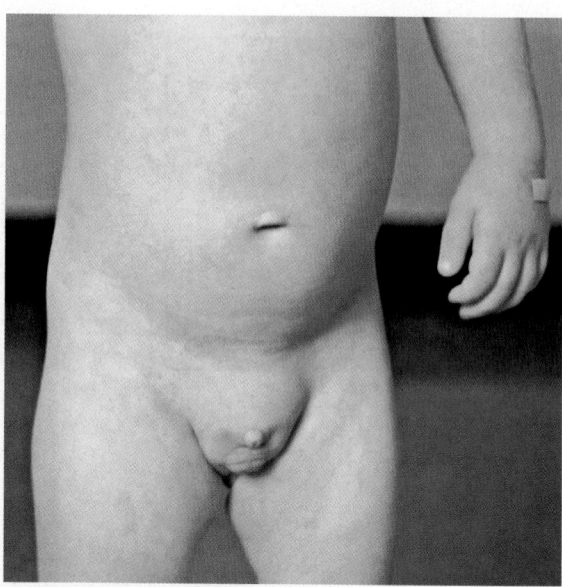

Figure 544-9 Micropenis secondary to hypopituitarism in an 8-year-old boy. (*From Wein AJ, Kavoussi LR, Novick AC, et al, editors: Campbell-Walsh urology, ed 9, Philadelphia, 2007, WB Saunders, Fig. 126-5a, p. 2341.*)

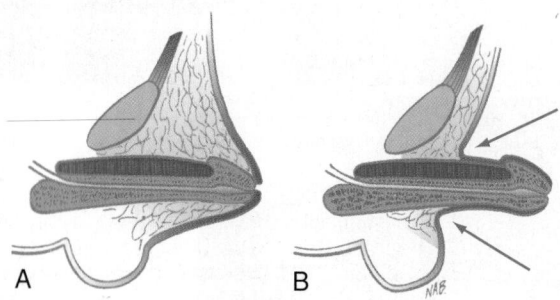

Figure 544-7 Concealed penis **(A)**, which may be visualized by retracting skin lateral to penile shaft **(B)**. (*From Wein AJ, Kavoussi LR, Novick AC, et al, editors: Campbell-Walsh urology, ed 9, Philadelphia, 2007, WB Saunders, Fig. 126-4, p. 2339.*)

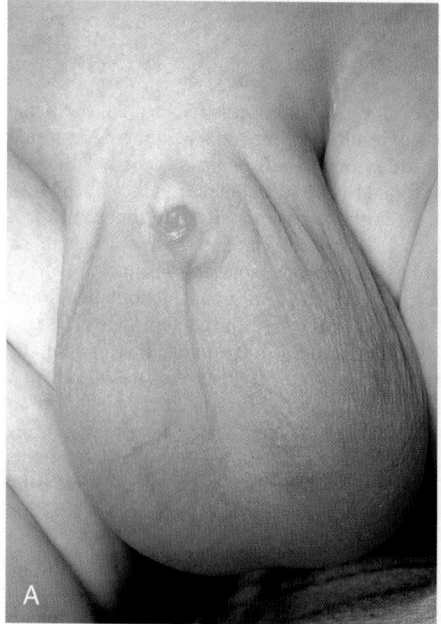
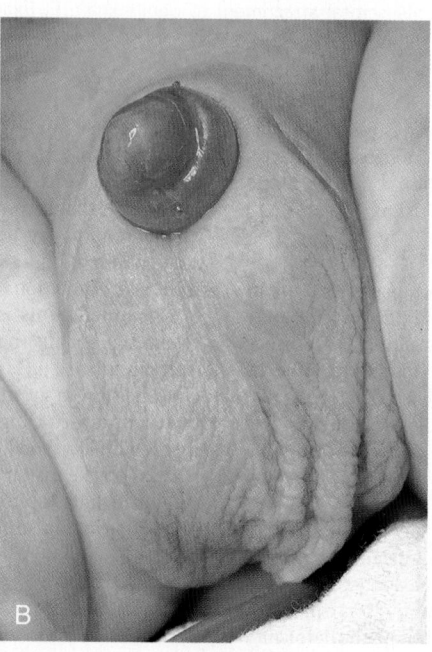

Figure 544-8 A, Trapped (concealed) penis resulting from circumcision. **B,** Same patient after revision of circumcision. (*From Wein AJ, Kavoussi LR, Novick AC, et al, editors: Campbell-Walsh urology, ed 9, Philadelphia, 2007, WB Saunders, Fig. 126-2, p. 2340.*)

◆ Ischemic (venoocclusive, low-flow) priapism is characterized by little or no cavernous blood flow, and cavernous blood gases are hypoxic, hypercapnic, and acidotic. The corpora are rigid and tender to palpation.

◆ Nonischemic (arterial, high-flow) priapism is caused by unregulated cavernous arterial inflow. Typically, the penis is neither fully rigid nor painful. There is often a history of antecedent trauma resulting in a cavernous artery–corpora cavernosa fistula.

◆ Stuttering (intermittent) priapism is a recurrent form of ischemic priapism with painful erections with intervening periods of detumescence.

The most common cause of priapism in children is sickle cell disease, which is characterized by predominance of sickle cell hemoglobin (see Chapter 462.1). As many as 27.5% of children with sickle cell disease develop priapism. The priapism is generally related to a low-flow state, secondary to sickling of red blood cells within the sinusoids of the corpora cavernosa during normal erection, resulting in venous stasis. This situation results in decreased local oxygen tension and pH, which potentiates further stasis and sickling. Priapism typically occurs during sleep, when mild hypoventilatory acidosis depresses oxygen tension and pH in the corpora. There is typically significant corporal engorgement with sparing of the glans penis. If the spongiosum is involved, voiding may be impaired. Evaluation includes complete blood count and serum chemistry. If sickle cell status is unknown, hemoglobin electrophoresis should be performed. In some cases, corporal aspiration is performed to distinguish between a high-flow and low-flow state. Other causes of low-flow priapism include sildenafil ingestion and leukemia.

In priapism secondary to sickle cell disease, medical therapy includes exchange transfusion, intravenous hydration, alkalinization, pain management with morphine, and oxygen. The American Urological Association guideline on priapism also recommends concurrent intracavernous treatment beginning with corporal aspiration and irrigation with a sympathomimetic agent, such as phenylephrine. If priapism has been present >48 hr, ischemia and acidosis impair the intracavernous smooth muscle response to sympathomimetics. If irrigation and medical therapy are unsuccessful, a corporoglanular shunt should be considered. For stuttering priapism, administration of an oral α-adrenergic agent (pseudoephedrine) once or twice daily is first-line therapy. If this treatment is unsuccessful, an oral β-agonist (terbutaline) is recommended; a gonadotropin-releasing hormone analog plus flutamide is recommended as third-line therapy. Long-term follow-up of adults treated for sickle cell disease as children shows that satisfactory erectile function is inversely related to the patient's age at onset of priapism and duration of priapism.

Nonischemic (high-flow) priapism most commonly follows perineal trauma, such as a straddle injury, that results in laceration of the cavernous artery. Typically, the aspirated blood is bright red, and the aspirate is similar to arterial blood. Color Doppler ultrasonography often demonstrates the fistula. The priapism can spontaneously resolve. If it does not, angiographic embolization is indicated.

OTHER PENILE ANOMALIES

Agenesis of the penis affects approximately 1 in 10 million boys. The karyotype is almost always 46,XY, and the usual appearance is that of a well-developed scrotum with descended testes and an absent penile shaft. Upper urinary tract abnormalities are common. In most cases, gender reassignment is recommended in the newborn period. **Diphallia** ranges from a small accessory penis to complete duplication. **Lateral penile curvature** usually is caused by overgrowth or hypoplasia of a corporal (erectile) body and usually is congenital. Surgical repair is recommended at age 6-12 mo.

MEATAL STENOSIS

Meatal stenosis is a condition that almost always is acquired and occurs after neonatal circumcision. It probably results from severe inflammation of the denuded glans, and is difficult to prevent. If the meatus is pinpoint, boys void with a forceful, fine stream that goes a great distance. These boys can experience dysuria, frequency, hematuria, or a combination of these conditions, typically at age 3-8 yr. UTI is uncommon. Other boys have dorsal deflection of the urinary stream. Although the meatus may be small, hydronephrosis or voiding difficulty is extremely rare unless there is associated **balanitis xerotica obliterans** (see Fig. 544-3; chronic dermatitis of unknown etiology, generally involving the glans and prepuce, occasionally extending into the urethra). **Treatment** is meatoplasty, in which the urethral meatus is opened surgically; this procedure can be performed either under anesthesia as an outpatient or in the office using local anesthesia (EMLA cream) with or without sedation. Routine cystoscopy is unnecessary.

OTHER MALE URETHRAL ANOMALIES

Parameatal urethral cyst manifests as an asymptomatic small cyst on one side of the urethral meatus. Treatment is excision under anesthesia. **Congenital urethral fistula** is a rare deformity in which a fistula is present from the penile urethra. It usually is an isolated abnormality. Treatment is fistula closure. **Megalourethra** is a large urethra that usually is associated with abnormal development of the corpus spongiosum. This condition is most commonly associated with prune-belly syndrome (see Chapter 540). **Urethral duplication** is a rare condition in which the 2 urethral channels lie in the same sagittal plane. There are many variations with complete and incomplete urethral duplication. These boys often have a double stream. Most commonly the dorsal urethra is small and the ventral urethra is normal caliber. Treatment involves excision of the small urethra. **Urethral hypoplasia** is a rare condition in which the urethra is extremely small but patent. In some cases, a temporary cutaneous vesicostomy is necessary for satisfactory urinary drainage. Either gradual enlargement of the urethra or major urethroplasty is necessary. **Urethral atresia** refers to maldevelopment of the urethra and nearly always is fatal unless the urachus remains patent throughout gestation.

URETHRAL PROLAPSE (FEMALE)

Urethral prolapse is encountered predominantly in black girls 1-9 yr of age. The most common signs are bloody spotting on the underwear or diaper, although dysuria or perineal discomfort also can occur (Fig. 544-10). An inexperienced examiner can mistake the finding for sexual

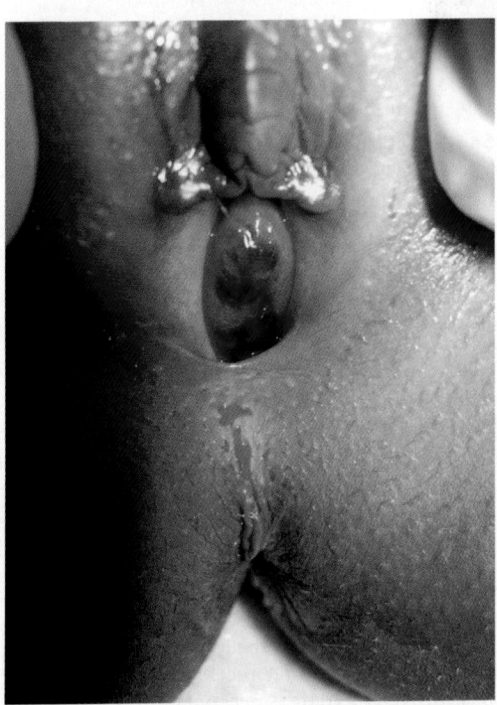

Figure 544-10 Urethral prolapse in a 4 yr old African-American girl who had bloody spotting on her underwear.

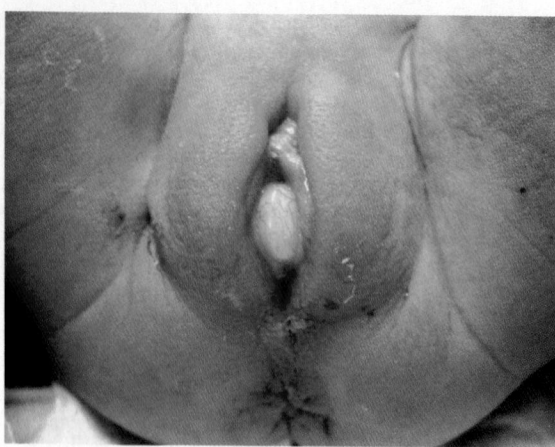

Figure 544-11 Paraurethral cyst in a newborn girl.

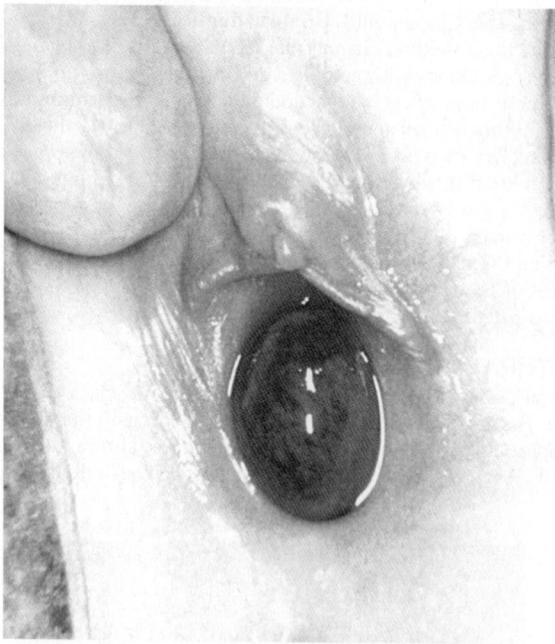

Figure 544-12 Prolapsed ectopic ureterocele in a female infant. She had a nonfunctioning upper pole collecting system connected to the ureterocele.

abuse. The usual therapy consists of application of estrogen cream 2-3 times daily for 3-4 wk and sitz baths. Surgical excision and reapproximation of the mucosal edges is recommended for girls that fail medical therapy and is curative.

OTHER FEMALE URETHRAL LESIONS

Paraurethral cyst results from retained secretions in the Skene glands secondary to ductal obstruction (Fig. 544-11). These lesions are present at birth, and most regress in size during the 1st 4-8 wk, although occasionally incision and drainage is necessary. A **prolapsed ectopic ureterocele** appears as a cystic mass protruding from the urethra and is a presenting symptom in 10% of girls with a ureterocele, which is a cystic swelling of the terminal ureter (Fig. 544-12). Ultrasonography should be performed to visualize the upper urinary tracts to confirm the diagnosis. Usually, either the ureterocele is incised or an upper urinary tract reconstructive procedure is necessary.

Bibliography is available at Expert Consult.

Chapter 545
Disorders and Anomalies of the Scrotal Contents
Jack S. Elder

UNDESCENDED TESTIS (CRYPTORCHIDISM)
The absence of a palpable testis in the scrotum indicates that the testis is undescended, absent, or retractile.

Epidemiology
An undescended (**cryptorchid**) testis is the most common disorder of sexual differentiation in boys. At birth, approximately 4.5% of boys have an undescended testis. Because testicular descent occurs at 7-8 mo of gestation, 30% of premature male infants have an undescended testis; the incidence is 3.4% at term. The majority of congenital undescended testes descend spontaneously during the 1st 3 mo of life, and by 6 mo the incidence decreases to 0.8%. Spontaneous descent occurs secondary to a temporary testosterone surge during the 1st 2 mo, which also results in significant penile growth. If the testis has not descended by 4 mo, it will remain undescended. Cryptorchidism is bilateral in 10% of cases. There is some evidence that the incidence of cryptorchidism is increasing. Although cryptorchidism usually is considered to be congenital, some boys have a scrotal testis that "ascends" to a low inguinal position, and therefore requires an orchiopexy. In addition, 1-2% of neonatal and young boys undergoing hernia repair have secondary cryptorchidism.

Pathogenesis
The process of testicular descent is regulated by an interaction between hormonal and mechanical factors, including testosterone, dihydrotestosterone, müllerian-inhibiting factor, the gubernaculum, intraabdominal pressure, and the genitofemoral nerve. The testis develops at 7-8 wk of gestation. At 10-11 wk, the Leydig cells produce testosterone, which stimulates differentiation of the wolffian (mesonephric) duct into the epididymis, vas deferens, seminal vesicle, and ejaculatory duct. At 32-36 wk, the testis, which is anchored at the internal inguinal ring by the gubernaculum, begins its process of descent. The gubernaculum distends the inguinal canal and guides the testis into the scrotum. Following testicular descent, the patent processus vaginalis (hernia sac) normally involutes. A small percentage have Klinefelter syndrome or mutations in the insulin-like factor 3 receptor.

Clinical Manifestations
Undescended testes are classified as **abdominal** (nonpalpable), **peeping** (abdominal but can be pushed into the upper part of the inguinal canal), **inguinal, gliding** (can be pushed into the scrotum but retracts immediately to the pubic tubercle), and **ectopic** (superficial inguinal pouch or, rarely, perineal). Most undescended testes are palpable just distal to the inguinal canal over the pubic tubercle.

A **disorder of sex development** should be suspected in a newborn phenotypic male with bilateral nonpalpable testes, as the child could be a virilized girl with congenital adrenal hyperplasia (see Chapter 576). In a boy with midpenile or proximal hypospadias and a palpable undescended testis, disorder of sexual development is present in 15%, and the risk is 50% if the testis is nonpalpable.

The **consequences of cryptorchidism** include poor testicular growth, infertility, testicular malignancy, associated hernia, torsion of the cryptorchid testis, and the possible psychologic effects of an empty scrotum.

The undescended testis is normal at birth histologically, but pathologic changes can be demonstrated by 6-12 mo. Delayed germ cell maturation, reduction in germ cell number, hyalinization of the seminiferous tubules, and reduced Leydig cell number are typical; these changes are progressive over time if the testis remains undescended. Similar, although less severe, changes are found in the contralateral descended testis after 4-7 yr. After treatment for a unilateral undescended testis, 85% of patients are fertile, which is slightly less than the 90% rate of fertility in an unselected population of men. In contrast, following bilateral orchiopexy, only 50-65% of patients are fertile.

The risk of a **germ cell malignancy** (see Chapter 503) developing in an undescended testis is 4 times higher than in the general population and is approximately 1 in 80 with a unilateral undescended testis and 1 in 40-50 for bilateral undescended testes. Testicular tumors are less common if the orchiopexy is performed before 10 yr of age, but they still occur, and adolescents should be instructed in testicular self-examination. The peak age for developing a testis tumor is 15-45 yr. The most common tumor developing in an undescended testis in an adolescent or adult is a **seminoma** (65%); after orchiopexy, nonseminomatous tumors represent only 65% of testis tumors. Orchiopexy seems to reduce the risk of seminoma. Whether early orchiopexy reduces the risk of developing cancer of the testis is controversial, but it is uncommon for testis tumors to occur if the orchiopexy performed before the age of 2 yr. The contralateral scrotal testis is not at increased risk for malignancy.

An indirect inguinal hernia usually accompanies a congenital undescended testis but rarely is symptomatic. Torsion and infarction of the cryptorchid testis also are uncommon but can occur because of excessive mobility of undescended testes. Consequently, inguinal pain and/or swelling in a boy with an undescended testis should raise the suspicion of an incarcerated hernia or testicular torsion of the undescended testis.

"Acquired" or **ascending undescended testes** occurs when a boy has a descended testis at birth, but during childhood, usually between 4-10 yr of age, the testis does not remain in the scrotum. Such boys often have a history of a retractile testis. With testicular ascent, on physical examination the testis often can be manipulated into the scrotum, but there is obvious tension on the spermatic cord. This condition is speculated to result from incomplete involution of the processus vaginalis, restricting spermatic cord growth, resulting in the testis gradually moving out of its scrotal position during a boy's somatic growth.

Retractile testes may be misdiagnosed as undescended testes. Boys older than age 1 yr often have a brisk cremasteric reflex, and if the child is anxious or ticklish during scrotal examination, the testis may be difficult to manipulate into the scrotum. Boys should be examined with their legs in a relaxed frogleg position, and if the testis can be manipulated into the scrotum comfortably, it is probably retractile. It should be monitored every 6-12 mo with follow-up physical examinations, because it can become an acquired undescended testis. Overall, as many as one-third of boys with a retractile testis develop an acquired undescended testis, and boys younger than 7 yr of age at diagnosis of a retractile testis are at greatest risk. Although definitive data are not available, it is generally thought that boys with a retractile testis are not at increased risk for infertility or malignancy.

Approximately 10% of undescended testes are **nonpalpable testis**. Of these, 50% are viable testes in the abdomen or high in the inguinal canal, and 50% are atrophic or absent, almost always in the scrotum, secondary to spermatic cord torsion in utero (**vanishing testis**). If the nonpalpable testis is abdominal, it will not descend after 3 mo of age. Although sonography often is performed to try to identify whether the testis is present, it rarely changes clinical management, because the abdominal testis and atrophic testis are not identified on sonography. As part of the ABIM Choosing Wisely campaign, in 2012 the American Urological Association recommended that inguinal/scrotal sonography not be performed routinely in boys with a nonpalpable testis, because it rarely alters the surgical management. However, inguinal/scrotal sonography might be beneficial in obese boys with a nonpalpable testis; in this clinical setting, the undescended testis often is nonpalpable, and an inguinal/scrotal sonogram can be beneficial in surgical planning. CT scanning is relatively accurate in demonstrating the presence of the testis, but the radiation exposure is significant. MRI

is even more accurate, but the disadvantage is that general anesthesia is necessary in most young children. None of these imaging studies are 100% accurate and in general do not add significantly to clinical decision making by the pediatric urologist or pediatric surgeon. Consequently, its routine use is discouraged.

On **physical examination** of the scrotum, the child should be entirely undressed, to help him relax. The examiner should examine the patient's scrotum and inguinal canal using their dominant hand. The nondominant hand is positioned over the pubic tubercle and is pushed inferiorly toward the scrotum. The examiner's dominant hand is used to try to palpate the testis. If the testis is nonpalpable, the "soap test" often is useful; soap is applied to the inguinal canal and the examiner's hand, significantly reducing friction and facilitating identification of an inguinal testis. In addition, pulling on the scrotum can pull a high inguinal testis into a palpable position. One soft sign that a testis is absent is contralateral testicular hypertrophy, but this finding is not 100% diagnostic.

Treatment

The congenital undescended testis should be treated surgically by 9-15 mo of age. With anesthesia by a pediatric anesthesiologist, surgical correction at 6 mo is appropriate, because spontaneous descent of the testis will not occur after 4 mo of age. Most testes can be brought down to the scrotum with an orchiopexy, which involves an inguinal incision, mobilization of the testis and spermatic cord, and correction of an indirect inguinal hernia. The procedure is typically performed on an outpatient basis and has a success rate of 98%. In some boys with a testis that is close to the scrotum, a prescrotal orchiopexy can be performed. In this procedure, the entire operation is performed through an incision along the edge of the scrotum. Often the associated inguinal hernia also can be corrected with this incision. Advantages of this approach over the inguinal approach include shorter operative time and less postoperative discomfort.

In boys with a nonpalpable testis, diagnostic laparoscopy is performed in most centers. This procedure allows safe and rapid assessment of whether the testis is intraabdominal. In most cases, orchiopexy of the intraabdominal testis located immediately inside the internal inguinal ring is successful, but orchiectomy should be considered in more difficult cases or when the testis appears to be atrophic. A 2-stage orchiopexy sometimes is needed in boys with a high abdominal testis. Boys with abdominal testes are managed with laparoscopic techniques at many institutions. Testicular prostheses are available for older children and adolescents when the absence of the gonad in the scrotum might have an undesirable psychologic effect. The FDA has approved a saline testicular implant. Solid silicone "carving block" implants also are used (Fig. 545-1). Placement of testicular prostheses early in childhood is recommended for boys with anorchia (absence of both testes).

The American Urological Association released guidelines for the evaluation and treatment of boys with an undescended testis in 2014. Table 545-1 summarizes the primary statements.

SCROTAL SWELLING

Scrotal swelling may be acute or chronic and painful or painless. Abrupt onset of painful scrotal swelling necessitates prompt evaluation because some conditions, such as testicular torsion and incarcerated inguinal hernia, require emergency surgical management. Tables 545-2 and 545-3 show the differential diagnosis.

Clinical Manifestations

A detailed history is helpful in determining the cause of the swelling and includes onset of pain—with testicular torsion, the pain often is sudden in onset and may be associated with exercise or minor genital trauma; duration of pain; radiation of pain—inguinal discomfort is common with testicular torsion, inguinal hernia, or epididymitis, and associated flank pain can occur with passage of a ureteral calculus; previous episodes of similar pain, which are common in boys with intermittent testicular torsion or inguinal hernia; nausea and vomiting, which are associated with testicular torsion and inguinal hernia; and irritative urinary symptoms, such as dysuria, urgency, and frequency,

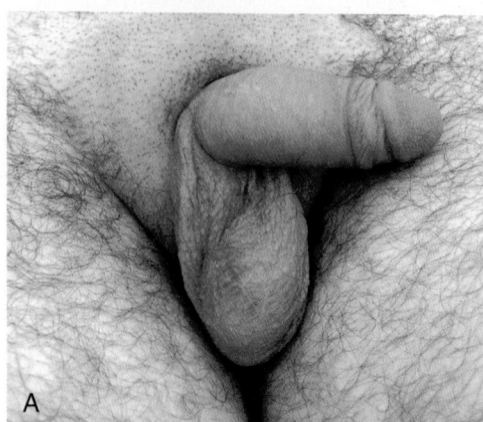
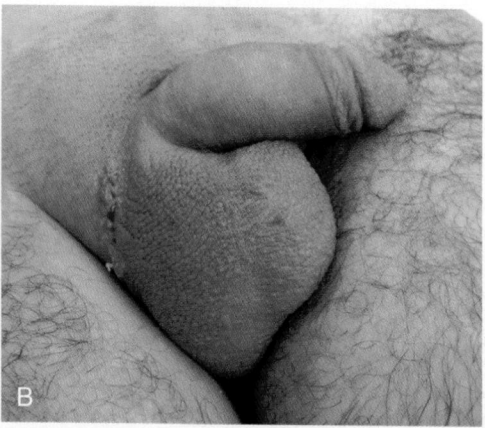

Figure 545-1 A, Adolescent with solitary left testis. **B,** Appearance following implantation of right testicular prosthesis.

Table 545-1	American Urological Association Guidelines for Evaluation and Treatment of Boys with an Undescended Testis

DIAGNOSIS

Primary care providers should palpate testes for quality and position at each recommended well-child visit. (Standard)

Providers should refer infants with a history of cryptorchidism (detected at birth) who do not have spontaneous testicular descent by 6 mo (corrected for gestational age) to an appropriate surgical specialist for timely evaluation. (Standard)

Providers should refer boys with the possibility of newly diagnosed (acquired) cryptorchidism after 6 mo. (Standard)

Providers must immediately consult an appropriate specialist for all phenotypic male newborns with bilateral, nonpalpable testes for evaluation of a possible disorder of sex development (DSD). (Standard)

Providers should not perform ultrasound (US) or other imaging modalities in the evaluation of boys with cryptorchidism before referral because these studies rarely assist in decision making. (Standard)

Providers should assess the possibility of a disorder of sex development (DSD) when there is increasing severity of hypospadias with cryptorchidism. (Recommendation)

In boys with retractile testes, providers should monitor the position of the testes at least annually to monitor for secondary ascent. (Standard)

TREATMENT

Providers should not use hormonal therapy to induce testicular descent, since evidence shows low response rates and lack of evidence for long-term efficacy. (Standard)

In the absence of spontaneous testicular descent by 6 mo (corrected for gestational age), specialists should perform surgery within the next year. (Standard)

In prepubertal boys with nonpalpable testes, surgical specialists should perform examination under anesthesia to reassess for palpability of testes. If nonpalpable, surgical exploration and, if indicated, abdominal orchidopexy should be performed. (Standard)

In boys with a normal contralateral testis, surgical specialists may perform an orchiectomy (removal of the undescended testis) if a boy has a normal contralateral testis and either very short testicular vessels and vas deferens, dysmorphic or very hypoplastic testis, or postpubertal age. (Clinical Principle)

Providers should counsel boys with a history of cryptorchidism and/or monorchidism and their parents regarding potential long-term risks and provide education on infertility and cancer risk. (Clinical Principle)

Adapted from Kolon TF, Herndon CDA, Baker LA, et al: Evaluation and treatment of cryptorchidism: AUA Guideline. http://www.auanet.org/common/pdf/education/clinical-guidance/Cryptorchidism.pdf

Table 545-2	Differential Diagnosis of Scrotal Masses in Boys and Adolescents

PAINFUL	PAINLESS
Testicular torsion	Hydrocele
Torsion of appendix testis	Inguinal hernia*
Epididymitis	Varicocele*
Trauma: ruptured testis, hematocele	Spermatocele*
Inguinal hernia (incarcerated)	Testicular tumor*
Mumps orchitis	Henoch-Schönlein purpura*
Testicular vasculitis	Idiopathic scrotal edema

*May be associated with discomfort.

Table 545-3	Differential Diagnosis of Scrotal Swelling in Newborn Boys

Hydrocele	Scrotal hematoma
Inguinal hernia (reducible)	Testicular tumor
Inguinal hernia (incarcerated)*	Meconium peritonitis
Testicular torsion*	Epididymitis*

*May be associated with discomfort.

which indicate a urinary tract infection that can cause epididymitis. Some boys report a recent history of scrotal trauma. There are multiple reports of familial testicular torsion. Boys with lower urinary tract pathology such as urethral stricture or neuropathic bladder may be prone to epididymitis.

Physical examination may be difficult in boys with a painful scrotum. Some have advocated performing a spermatic cord block or administering intravenous analgesia to facilitate the examination, but such measures usually are unnecessary. Scrotal wall erythema is common in testicular torsion, epididymitis, torsion of the appendix testis, and an incarcerated hernia. In boys with a normal cremasteric reflex, testicular torsion is unlikely. Absence of a cremasteric reflex is nondiagnostic.

Laboratory Findings and Diagnosis

Pertinent laboratory studies include a urinalysis and culture. A positive urinalysis suggests bacterial epididymitis. Serum studies are not helpful in establishing a diagnosis, unless a testicular malignancy is suspected. After initial evaluation, in boys with testicular pain color Doppler ultrasonography often is helpful in establishing the diagnosis, because it assesses whether testicular blood flow is normal, reduced, or increased (Fig. 545-2). If a hydrocele is present and the testis is nonpalpable, or if an abnormality of the testis is found, sonography also is indicated. Imaging studies are not 100% accurate; they should not be used to decide whether a boy with testicular pain should be referred for urologic evaluation.

Color Doppler ultrasonography allows assessment of testicular blood flow and testicular morphologic features. Accuracy is >95% if the ultrasonographer is experienced and the patient is older than 2 yr old. A false-negative study (demonstrates normal testicular blood flow) can occur in a boy with testicular torsion if the degree of torsion is <360 degrees and the duration of torsion is short, because there may be continued testicular perfusion. In young boys, including neonates, blood flow may be difficult to demonstrate in 15% of normal testes.

TESTICULAR (SPERMATIC CORD) TORSION
Etiology
Testicular torsion requires prompt diagnosis and treatment to salvage the testis. Torsion is the most common cause of testicular pain in boys age 12 yr and older, and is uncommon before age 10 yr. It is caused by inadequate fixation of the testis within the scrotum, resulting from a redundant tunica vaginalis, allowing excessive mobility of the testis. The abnormal attachment is termed a *bell clapper deformity* and often is bilateral. Shortly after torsion occurs, venous congestion begins and subsequently arterial flow is interrupted. The likelihood of testis survival depends on the duration and severity of torsion. Following 4-6 hr of absent blood flow to the testis, irreversible loss of spermatogenesis can occur. Torsion may be familial in approximately 10% of males.

Diagnosis
Testicular torsion produces acute pain and swelling of the scrotum. On examination, the scrotum is swollen, and the testis is exquisitely tender and often difficult to examine. The cremasteric reflex nearly always is

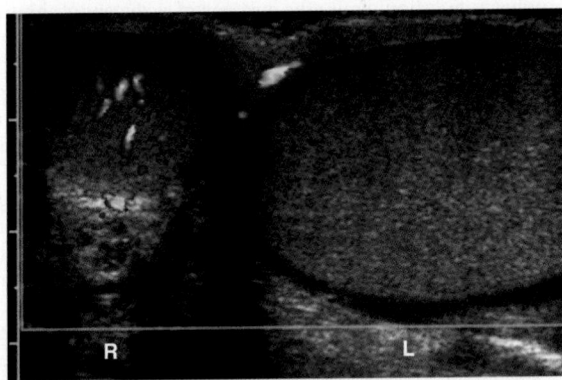

Figure 545-2 Testicular torsion and axis change. A color Doppler ultrasound in the transverse plane shows color flow in the right testicle. The right testicle is oval to circular, because it has been evaluated in the transverse plane. The left testicle is elongated as if it is in longitudinal plane. This axis change is the ultrasound equivalent of the worrisome clinical finding suggestive of torsion when accompanied by a history of sudden pain. Lack of color Doppler flow in the left testicle confirms a left testicular torsion. *(From Coley BD, editor: Caffey's pediatric imaging, ed 12, Philadelphia, Elsevier, 2013, Fig. 126-13, p. 1300).*

absent. The position (lie) of the testis is abnormal and there is often associated nausea and vomiting. The condition can be differentiated from an incarcerated hernia because swelling in the inguinal area typically is absent with torsion. If the pain duration is <4-6 hr, manual detorsion may be attempted. In 65% of cases the torsed testis rotates inward, so detorsion should be attempted in the opposite direction (e.g., the left testis is rotated clockwise). Successful manual detorsion results in dramatic pain relief.

Some adolescents experience *intermittent testicular torsion*. These boys report episodes of severe unilateral testicular pain that resolves spontaneously after 30-60 min. Treatment is elective bilateral scrotal orchiopexy (see Treatment).

Treatment
Treatment is prompt surgical exploration and detorsion. If the testis is explored within 6 hr of torsion, up to 90% of the gonads survive. Testicular salvage decreases rapidly with a delay of >6 hr. If the degree of torsion is 360 degrees or less, the testis might have sufficient arterial flow to allow the gonad to survive, even after 24-48 hr. Following detorsion the testis is fixed in the scrotum with nonabsorbable sutures, termed *scrotal orchiopexy,* to prevent torsion in the future. The contralateral testis also should be fixed in the scrotum because the predisposing anatomic condition often is bilateral. If the testis appears nonviable, orchiectomy is performed (Fig. 545-3A). Some adolescents do not undergo prompt evaluation and treatment and present with "late phase testicular torsion," in which the spermatic cord contracts and the testis is high in the scrotum and nontender (Fig. 545-3B). Fertility is reduced in men who experience spermatic cord torsion in adolescence, irrespective of whether detorsion or orchiectomy is performed.

Spermatic cord torsion also can occur in the fetus or neonate. This condition results from incomplete attachment of the tunica vaginalis to the scrotal wall and is "extravaginal." When torsion occurs in utero, the baby usually is born with a large, firm, nontender testis. Usually the ipsilateral hemiscrotum is ecchymotic (Fig. 545-4). In these cases, the testis rarely is viable because torsion was a remote event. However, the contralateral testis is at increased risk for torsion until 1-2 mo beyond term. The pediatric urology community is divided regarding whether immediate exploration is necessary in a male newborn who has suspected testicular torsion at birth, but if observation is recommended, the family needs to be counseled regarding the risk of contralateral spermatic cord torsion. On the other hand, if the initial exam is normal, and the newborn subsequently develops scrotal swelling and erythema, and imaging is consistent with spermatic cord torsion, emergency scrotal exploration is indicated.

TORSION OF THE APPENDIX TESTIS
Torsion of the appendix testis is the most common cause of testicular pain in boys 2-10 yr but is rare in adolescents. The appendix testis is a stalk-like structure that is a vestigial embryonic remnant of the müllerian (paramesonephric) ductal system that is attached to the upper

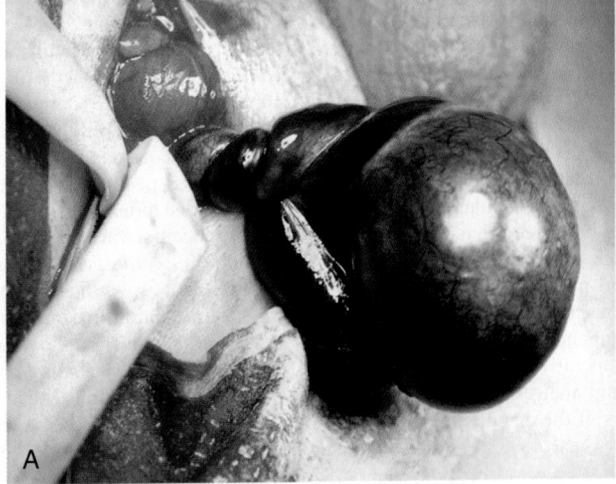
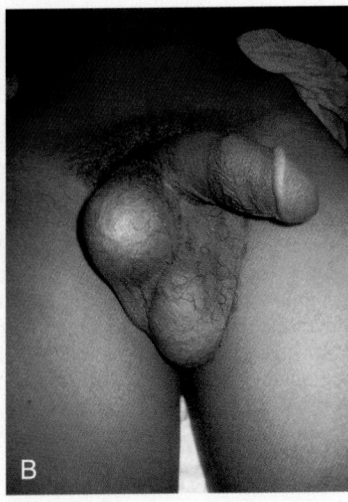

Figure 545-3 A, Left testicular torsion in adolescent with acute scrotum; the testis is necrotic. **B,** "Late-phase torsion" in an adolescent with severe testicular pain 1 mo previously. Note absence of inflammation and high position of testis in scrotum.

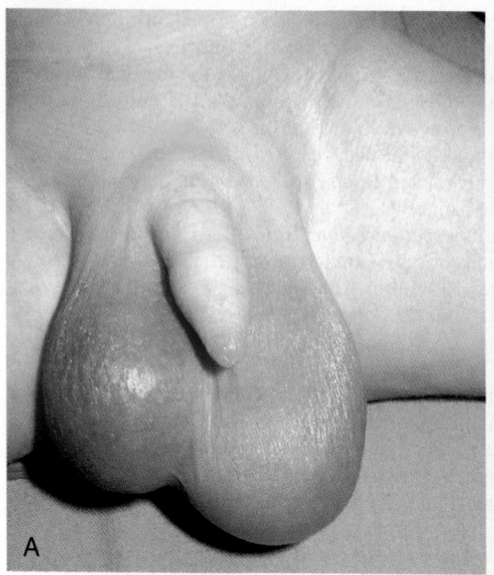

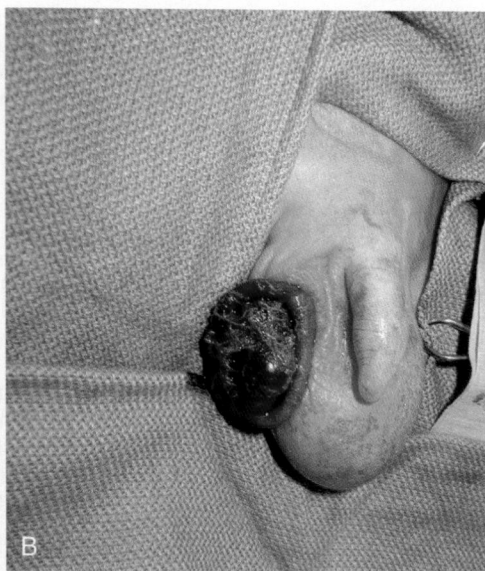

Figure 545-4 **A** and **B,** Right testicular torsion in a newborn. The right hemiscrotum is darker, and the testis was indurated and enlarged.

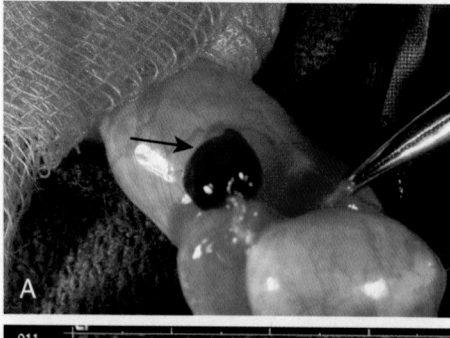

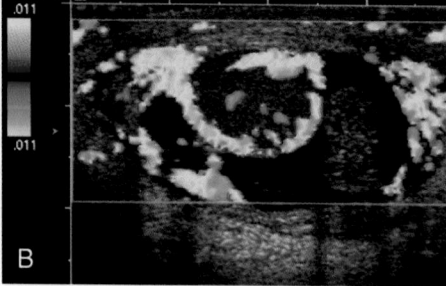

Figure 545-5 **A,** Torsion of the appendix testis; the appendix testis is necrotic (arrow). **B,** Color Doppler scrotal sonogram showing hyperemia to the testis and absent flow to the appendix testis (right side). Symptoms resolved with medical therapy.

pole of the testis. When it undergoes torsion, progressive inflammation and swelling of the testis and epididymis occurs, resulting in testicular pain and scrotal erythema. The onset of pain usually is gradual. Palpation of the testis usually reveals a 3-5 mm tender indurated mass on the upper pole (Fig. 545-5A). In some cases, the appendage that has undergone torsion may be visible through the scrotal skin, in the "blue dot" sign. In some boys, distinguishing torsion of the appendix from testicular torsion is difficult. In such cases, a testicular flow scan or color Doppler ultrasonography is useful because testicular blood flow should be normal or increased. In such cases, the radiologist often recognizes epididymal enlargement and makes the diagnosis of epididymitis, reflecting the inflammatory reaction (Fig. 545-5B).

The natural history of torsion of the appendix testis is for the inflammation to resolve in 3-10 days. Nonoperative treatment is recommended, including bed rest for 24 hr and analgesia with nonsteroidal antiinflammatory medication for 5 days. If the diagnosis is uncertain, scrotal exploration is recommended.

EPIDIDYMITIS

Acute inflammation of the epididymis is an ascending retrograde infection from the urethra, through the vas into the epididymis. This condition causes acute scrotal pain, erythema, and swelling. It is rare before puberty and should raise the question of a congenital abnormality of the wolffian duct, such as an ectopic ureter entering the vas. In younger boys, the responsible organism is often *Escherichia coli* (see Chapter 200). After puberty, bacterial epididymitis becomes progressively more common and is the principal cause of acute painful scrotal swelling in young sexually active men. Urinalysis usually reveals pyuria. Epididymitis can be infectious (usually gonococcus or *Chlamydia*; see Chapters 192 and 226), but often the organism remains undetermined. Additional etiologies include familial Mediterranean fever, enterovirus, and adenoviruses. Treatment consists of bed rest and antibiotics as indicated. Differentiation from torsion can be difficult, and surgical exploration may be required in children.

Henoch-Schönlein purpura (see Chapter 484) is a systemic vasculitis that involves multiple organ systems and that can involve the kidney and spermatic cord. When the spermatic cord is involved, typically there is bilateral painful scrotal swelling with purpuric lesions involving the scrotum. Scrotal sonography should show normal testicular blood flow. Treatment is directed toward systemic treatment of the Henoch-Schönlein purpura. Isolated testicular vasculitis is less common than that in Henoch-Schönlein purpura; polyarteritis nodosa should be suspected.

VARICOCELE

A varicocele is a congenital condition in which there is abnormal dilation of the pampiniform plexus in the scrotum, often described as a "bag of worms" (Fig. 545-6). Dilation of the pampiniform venous plexus results from valvular incompetence of the internal spermatic vein. Approximately 15% of adult men have a varicocele; of these, approximately 10-15% are subfertile. Varicocele is the most common (and virtually the only) surgically correctable cause of subfertility in men. A varicocele is found in 5-15% of adolescent boys, but it rarely is diagnosed in boys younger than 10 yr old, because the varicocele becomes distended only after the increased blood flow associated with puberty occurs. Varicoceles occur predominantly on the left side, are bilateral in 2% of cases, and rarely involve the right side only. A varicocele in a boy younger than age 10 yr or on the right side might indicate an abdominal or retroperitoneal mass; an abdominal sonogram or CT scan should be performed in such cases.

A varicocele typically is a painless paratesticular mass. Occasionally patients describe a dull ache in the affected testis. Usually the varicocele is not apparent when the patient is supine because it is decompressed; in contrast, the varicocele becomes prominent when the patient is

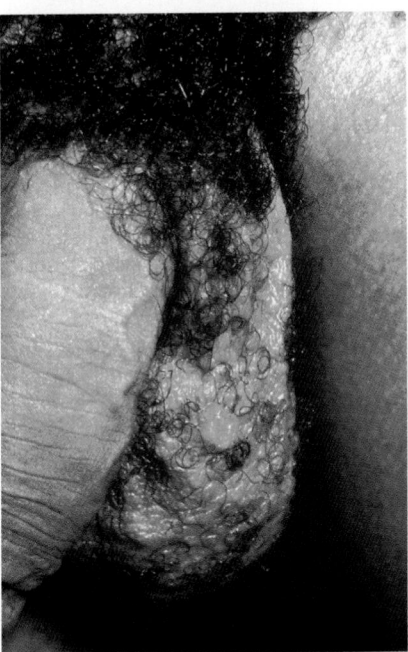

Figure 545-6 Left varicocele in an adolescent boy.

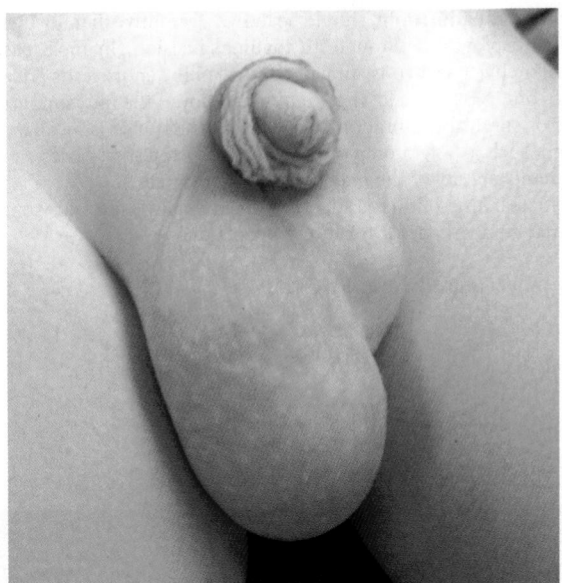

Figure 545-7 Newborn with large right hydrocele.

standing and enlarges with a Valsalva maneuver. Many pediatricians do not routinely screen adolescents for a varicocele. Varicoceles typically are graded from 1-3 with the boy standing: **grade 1** is palpable only with Valsalva; **grade 2** is palpable without Valsalva but is not visible on inspection; and **grade 3** is visible with inspection. Boys with a grade 3 varicocele are at greatest risk for testicular growth arrest. Testicular size should be documented with calipers, an orchidometer, or scrotal sonography, because if the affected left testis is significantly smaller than the right testis, spermatogenesis probably has been adversely affected. A semen analysis should be considered in sexually mature adolescents who are Tanner stage V.

The goal of varicocelectomy is to maximize chances for fertility. Surgical treatment of varicoceles is indicated in boys with a significant disparity in testicular size or pain in the affected testis or if the contralateral testis is diseased or absent. Typically the involved testis enlarges and catches up with the normal testis over the following 1-2 yr. Varicocelectomy should also be considered in boys with a large grade 3 varicocele, even if there is not a disparity in testicular size. Surgical repair is accomplished with a variety of techniques by ligation of the veins of the pampiniform plexus laparoscopically or through an inguinal or subinguinal incision (with or without an operating microscope) or by ligating the internal spermatic vein in the retroperitoneum. The operation is performed on an ambulatory basis.

SPERMATOCELE

A spermatocele is a cystic lesion that contains sperm and is attached to the upper pole of the sexually mature testis. Spermatoceles usually are painless and are incidental findings on physical examination. Enlargement of the spermatocele or significant pain is an indication for removal.

HYDROCELE
Etiology

A hydrocele is an accumulation of fluid in the tunica vaginalis (Fig. 545-7). Between 1% and 2% of neonates have a hydrocele. In most cases, the hydrocele is noncommunicating (the processus vaginalis was obliterated during development). In such cases, the hydrocele fluid disappears by 1 yr of age. If there is a persistently patent processus, the hydrocele persists and becomes progressively larger during the day and is small in the morning. A rare variant of a hydrocele is the abdominoscrotal hydrocele, in which there is a large, tense hydrocele that extends into the lower abdominal cavity. In some older boys, a non-

communicating hydrocele can result from an inflammatory condition within the scrotum, such as testicular torsion, torsion of the appendix testis, epididymitis, or testicular tumor. The long-term risk of a communicating hydrocele is the development of an inguinal hernia. Some older boys and adolescents also develop a hydrocele. In some cases hydrocele develop acutely after an episode of scrotal trauma or epididymoorchitis, whereas others develop more insidiously.

Diagnosis

On examination, hydroceles are smooth and nontender. Transillumination of the scrotum confirms the fluid-filled nature of the mass. It is important to palpate the testis, because some young men develop a hydrocele in association with a testis tumor. If compression of the fluid-filled mass completely reduces the hydrocele, an inguinal hernia/hydrocele is the likely diagnosis.

Treatment

Most congenital hydroceles resolve by 12 mo of age following reabsorption of the hydrocele fluid. If the hydrocele is large and tense, however, early surgical correction should be considered, because it is difficult to verify that the child does not have a hernia, and large hydroceles rarely disappear spontaneously. Hydroceles persisting beyond 12-18 mo usually are communicating and should be repaired. Surgical correction is similar to a herniorrhaphy (see Chapter 346). Through an inguinal incision, the spermatic cord is identified, the hydrocele fluid is drained, and a high ligation of the processus vaginalis is performed. If an older boy has a large hydrocele, often diagnostic laparoscopy can be performed to determine whether there is a patent processus vaginalis, and if the internal ring is closed, then the hydrocele may be corrected with a scrotal incision.

INGUINAL HERNIA

Inguinal hernia is discussed in Chapter 346.

TESTICULAR TUMOR

Testicular and paratesticular tumors can occur at any age, even in the newborn. Approximately 35% of prepubertal testis tumors are malignant; most commonly they are yolk sac tumors, although rhabdomyosarcoma and leukemia also can occur in this age group. In adolescents, 98% of painless solid testicular masses are malignant (see Chapter 503). Most manifest as a painless, hard testicular mass that does not transilluminate. Scrotal ultrasonography should be performed to confirm the finding of a testicular mass and it can help to delineate the type of testis tumor. Serum tumor markers, including α-fetoprotein and β-**human**

chorionic gonadotropin, should be drawn. Definitive therapy includes surgical exploration through an inguinal incision. In most cases, a radical orchiectomy, consisting of removal of the entire testis and spermatic cord, is performed. In a prepubertal boy, if the ultrasonographic study or surgical exploration suggests that the tumor is localized and benign, such as a teratoma or epidermoid cyst, testis-sparing surgery with removal only of the mass may be appropriate.

Testicular microlithiasis identified incidentally with ultrasonography may be a risk factor for future neoplasia.

Bibliography is available at Expert Consult.

Chapter **546**
Trauma to the Genitourinary Tract
Jack S. Elder

ETIOLOGY

Most injuries to the genitourinary tract in children result from blunt trauma during falls, athletic activities, or motor vehicle crashes (see Chapter 72). Children are at greater risk of blunt renal injury than are adults, because they have less body fat and because the kidneys are not located directly behind the ribs. Children with a preexisting renal anomaly, such as hydronephrosis secondary to a ureteropelvic junction obstruction, horseshoe kidney, or renal ectopia, also are at increased risk for renal injury. Blunt abdominal or flank trauma often causes a renal injury. Falling can cause a deceleration injury that results in an injury to the renal pedicle, interrupting blood flow to the kidney. If the bladder is full, blunt lower abdominal trauma can cause a bladder rupture. Rupture of the membranous urethra occurs in 5% of pelvic fractures. Straddle injuries usually are associated with trauma to the bulbous urethra.

Symptoms and signs of urinary tract injury include gross or microscopic hematuria, bleeding from the urethral meatus, abdominal or flank pain, a flank mass, fractured lower ribs or lumbar transverse processes, and a perineal or scrotal hematoma.

In more than 50% of cases there also are major injuries to the brain, spinal cord, skeleton, lungs, or abdominal organs.

DIAGNOSIS

Evaluation of the patient begins after an adequate airway has been established and the patient is hemodynamically stable (see Chapter 67). With significant abdominal injury, gross hematuria or >50 red blood cells per high-power field, or suspicion of renal injury (deceleration injury, flank pain or bruise), renal imaging is indicated. The bladder should be catheterized unless blood is dripping from the urethral meatus, which is an indication of potential urethral injury. Passing the catheter in the presence of a urethral injury can increase the extent of the damage and convert a partial membranous urethral tear into a total disruption. In these patients, a retrograde urethrogram should be performed by injecting radiopaque contrast medium into the urethral meatus under fluoroscopy. Oblique radiographs demonstrate the extent of the injury and whether urethral continuity is preserved or has been disrupted.

A **3-phase spiral CT scan** should be performed to evaluate the kidneys, ureters, and bladder. The delayed images are important to detect renal extravasation of blood or urine. Prompt function of both kidneys without extravasation usually excludes significant renal injury. Renal injuries are classified according to the grading scale presented in Table 546-1. Minor renal injuries are most common; these include contusion of the renal parenchyma and shallow cortical lacerations not involving the collecting system. Major renal injuries include deep lacerations involving the collecting system, the shattered kidney, and renal pedicle injuries (Fig. 546-1). Complete absence of function of 1 kidney without contralateral compensatory hypertrophy (indicating congenital absence) should be regarded as an indication of major injury to the renal pedicle. Renal angiography, once used for further evaluation of renal injuries, particularly if a renal pedicle injury is suspected, now is rarely used because such patients are often hemodynamically unstable, and management is not significantly affected by the findings. In some cases, a preexisting renal anomaly is demonstrated on the study. A ruptured ureteropelvic junction obstruction may be apparent if the kidney is intact but the distal ureter is not visualized.

If there is a pelvic fracture, a urethral transection injury should be suspected. The risk is directly related to the number of broken pubic

Table 546-1	Grading of Renal Injuries
GRADE	**DESCRIPTION**
1	Renal contusion or subcapsular hematoma
2	Nonexpanding perirenal hematoma, <1 cm parenchymal laceration, no urinary extravasation; all renal fragments viable; confined to renal retroperitoneum
3	Nonexpanding perirenal hematoma, >1 cm parenchymal laceration, no urinary extravasation; renal fragments may be viable or devitalized
4	Laceration extending into the collecting system with urinary extravasation; renal fragments may be vital or devitalized *or* Injury to the main renal vasculature with contained hemorrhage
5	Completely shattered kidney; by definition multiple major lacerations >1 cm associated with multiple devitalized fragments *or* Injury to the main renal vasculature with uncontrolled hemorrhage, renal hilar avulsion

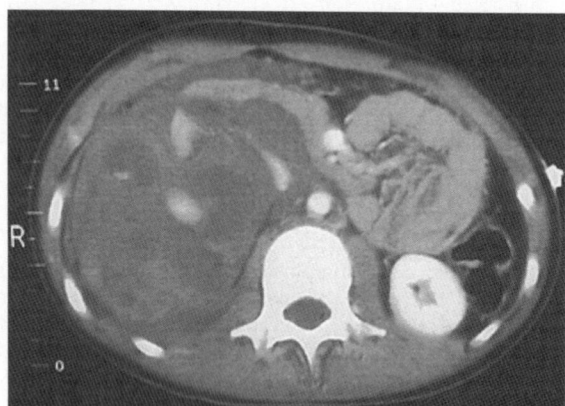

Figure 546-1 CT scan of a girl who sustained major renal injury when she fell off a bicycle. The scan demonstrates a ruptured right kidney with urinary extravasation.

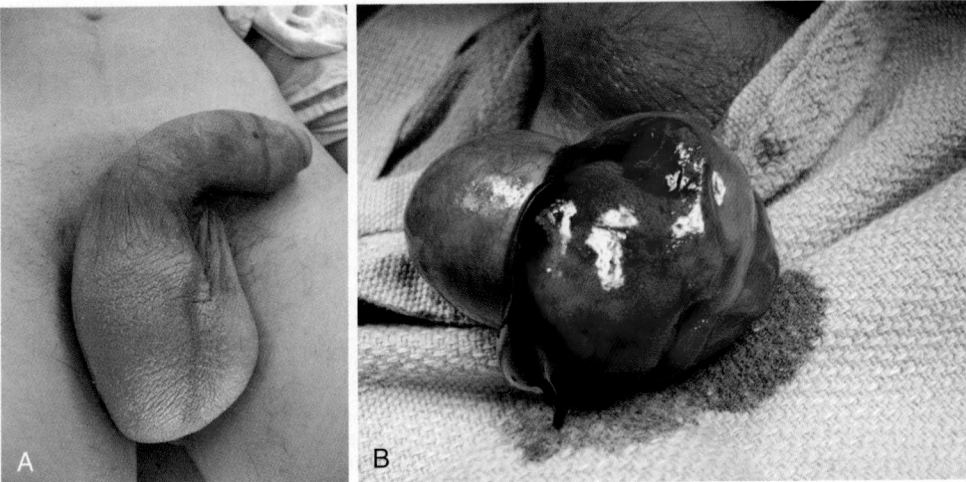

Figure 546-2 A, Adolescent boy with blunt right testicular injury. **B,** Tunica albuginea of testis is ruptured; the patient underwent debridement and closure of testicular capsule.

rami and whether there is separation of the pubic symphysis or displacement of the posterior pubic arch. Radiographic evaluation with retrograde urethrography should be performed if there is blood at the urethral or vaginal meatus, inability to void, and a perineal or penile hematoma.

TREATMENT

Minor renal injuries such as contusions are managed by bed rest and monitoring of vital signs until abdominal or flank discomfort and gross hematuria have resolved. Children with a major renal injury usually are admitted to an intensive care unit for continuous monitoring of vital signs and urine output. Intravenous antibiotics are also administered. These injuries also are managed nonoperatively, because Gerota's fascia often causes tamponade of bleeding from the kidney, and dramatic healing of the injured parenchyma can occur even with significant urinary extravasation.

Approximately 10% of children with a major renal injury undergo surgical exploration because of hemodynamic instability, persistent extravasation, or persistent hematuria or to correct a congenital renal deformity. It can be difficult to identify normal and devitalized parenchyma, and the likelihood of having to remove the kidney is significant. If the child is undergoing exploration for other abdominal injuries, the injured kidney is examined. If there is persistent extravasation because of intermittent ureteral obstruction from a blood clot, passage of a temporary double-J stent endoscopically between the bladder and kidney might allow resolution. If the renal pedicle is injured, nephrectomy is necessary. The kidney can be salvaged by emergency renal revascularization only if the kidney is explored within 2-3 hr of the injury. Virtually all penetrating injuries of the kidneys should be explored.

In addition to loss of renal function, the main long-term complication of renal injury is renin-mediated hypertension. Children who sustain significant renal injuries should have periodic measurement of blood pressure if they have any residual renal abnormality.

Ureteral injuries usually are iatrogenic. Injuries of the ureter by blunt or penetrating trauma require immediate surgical attention.

When the bladder can be catheterized, a static cystogram is obtained, infusing a contrast solution through the catheter by gravity, ideally using fluoroscopy. Flat and oblique views are often obtained; a postvoid film also should be obtained because, in some cases, extravasation may be hidden by the full bladder.

Bladder ruptures can be intraperitoneal or extraperitoneal. All intraperitoneal ruptures require surgical repair. Minor extraperitoneal near-ruptures might be treated by catheter drainage but generally require surgical treatment.

Treatment of a membranous urethral injury is controversial. Erectile dysfunction, urethral stricture, and urinary incontinence are the major late complications of rupture of the membranous urethra, and therapy is directed at minimizing the risk of these problems. A large pelvic hematoma with tamponade often is present, and an immediate attempt to repair the injury can be technically difficult and result in significant hemorrhage. Many such injuries are managed initially by temporary suprapubic cystostomy, with continuous bladder drainage for 3-6 mo. Subsequently, open or endoscopic urethroplasty can be performed. Alternatively, some try to achieve urethral continuity under anesthesia and leave a urethral catheter for several months. These patients typically require subsequent open urethroplasty.

Penile injury is uncommon. A risk of newborn circumcision with a Mogen clamp is partial or complete glans amputation. With immediate surgical repair, often the excised glans tissue can be replaced as a free graft. Some boys who are in the process of toilet training sustain an injury to the glans penis if the lid of the toilet falls while they are urinating. These boys often have a hematoma covering the distal half of the glans. Typically, they have no difficulty urinating and do not need extensive evaluation. Some male infants develop an inadvertent hair coil tourniquet or strangulation injury. Typically a very narrow constriction is noted with severe distal penile swelling and pain. Identification and incision of the hair allows prompt resolution of the edema. The urethra and penile vascularity should be assessed after release of the hair coil. Adolescent boys who indulge in extremely vigorous sexual intercourse may sustain rupture of one of the corporal bodies. These boys have severe swelling of the penile shaft and require emergency exploration and repair. Boys with penetrating injuries of the penis also require emergency debridement and repair.

Testicular injuries are relatively uncommon in children because of the small size of the testes and their mobility within the scrotum. Such injuries usually result from blunt trauma during athletic activity. Typically, these boys have significant scrotal swelling, testicular pain, and tenderness (Fig. 546-2A). Ultrasonography demonstrates rupture of the tunica albuginea, which is the capsule of the testis, and surrounding hemorrhage. Prompt surgical treatment of testicular injuries increases the salvage rate (Fig. 546-2B). An uncommon injury is the zipper injury, which can affect either the scrotum or foreskin. This problem generally occurs in boys who do not wear underwear. The zipper can be cut with bone cutters or metal cutters. Sedation generally is unnecessary.

Bibliography is available at Expert Consult.

Chapter **547**
Urinary Lithiasis

Jack S. Elder

Urinary lithiasis in children is related to genetic, climatic, dietary, and socioeconomic factors. The incidence is increasing: in 1996 the rate of symptomatic nephrolithiasis was 7.9 in 10,000, whereas in 2007 it was 18.5 in 10,000. Adolescents are 10 times more likely to have a symptomatic calculus compared to children 0-3 yr. The increase in stone disease in the United States is attributed to obesity and changes in dietary habits, such as increased sodium and fructose intake, and decreased calcium and water intake.

Urolithiasis is less common in the United States than in other parts of the world. Approximately 7% of urinary calculi occur in children younger than 16 yr of age. In the United States, many children with stone disease have a metabolic abnormality. The exceptions are patients with a neuropathic bladder (see Chapter 542), who are prone to infection-initiated renal stones, and those who have urinary tract reconstruction with small or large intestine, which predisposes to bladder calculi. The incidence of metabolic stones is similar in boys and girls; they are most common in southeastern United States and are uncommon in African-Americans. In Southeast Asia, urinary calculi are endemic and are related to dietary factors. Contamination of infant formula with the organic base and illegally added nitrogen-containing food additive melamine was reported in China in 2008 and is the source of much study in that country.

STONE FORMATION

Nearly 90% of urinary stones contain calcium as a major constituent, and 60% are composed of calcium oxalate. Most "spontaneous" stones are composed of calcium, oxalate, or phosphate crystals; others are caused by uric acid, cystine, ammonium crystals, or phosphate crystals, or a combination of these substances (Table 547-1). The risk of stone formation increases in the presence of increasing concentrations of these crystals and is reduced with increasing concentrations of urinary inhibitors. Renal calculi develop from crystals that form on the calyx and aggregate to form a calculus. Bladder calculi may be stones that formed in the kidney and traveled down the ureter, or they can form primarily in the bladder.

Low urine volume, low urine pH, calcium, sodium, oxalate, and urate are known to promote stone formation. Many inorganic (e.g., citrate, magnesium) and organic (e.g., glycosaminoglycans, osteopontin) substances are known to inhibit stone formation. Organic inhibitory compounds adsorb to the surface of the crystal, thereby inhibiting crystal growth and nucleation.

Stone formation depends on 4 factors: matrix, precipitation–crystallization, epitaxy, and the absence of inhibitors of stone formation in the urine. **Matrix** is a mixture of protein, nonamino sugars, glucosamine, water, and organic ash that makes up 2-9% of the dry weight of urinary stones and is arranged within the stones in organized concentric laminations. **Precipitation–crystallization** refers to supersaturation of the urine with specific ions composing the crystal. Crystals aggregate by chemical and electrical forces. Increasing the saturation of urine with respect to the ions increases the rate of nucleation, crystal growth, and aggregation and increases the likelihood of stone formation and growth. **Epitaxy** refers to the aggregation of crystals of different composition but similar lattice structure, thus forming stones of a heterogeneous nature. The lattice structures of calcium oxalate and monosodium urate have similar structures, and calcium oxalate crystals can aggregate on a nucleus of monosodium urate crystals. Urine also contains **inhibitors of stone formation,** including citrate, diphosphonate, and magnesium ion.

Table 547-1	Classification of Urolithiasis

CALCIUM STONES (CALCIUM OXALATE AND CALCIUM PHOSPHATE)*
Hypercalciuria
Absorptive: increased Ca absorption from gut; types I and II
Renal leak: decreased tubular reabsorption of Ca
Resorptive
Primary hyperparathyroidism (rare in children)
Iatrogenic
Loop diuretics
Ketogenic diet
Corticosteroids
Adrenocorticotropic hormone administration
Methylxanthines (theophylline, aminophylline)
Distal renal tubular acidosis, type 1 (calcium phosphate)
Hypocitraturia—citrate most important inhibitor of Ca crystallization
Vitamin D excess
Immobilization
Sarcoidosis
Cushing disease
Hyperuricosuria
Heterozygous cystinuria
Hyperoxaluria (calcium oxalate)
Primary hyperoxaluria, types 1 and 2
Secondary hyperoxaluria
Enteric hyperoxaluria

CYSTINE STONES
Cystinuria

STRUVITE STONES (MAGNESIUM AMMONIUM PHOSPHATE)
Urinary tract infection (urea-splitting organism)
Foreign body
Urinary stasis

URIC ACID STONES
Hyperuricosuria
Lesch-Nyhan syndrome
Myeloproliferative disorders
After chemotherapy
Inflammatory bowel disease

INDINAVIR STONES

MELAMINE

NEPHROCALCINOSIS

*Most common.

CLINICAL MANIFESTATIONS

Children with urolithiasis usually have gross or microscopic hematuria. If the calculus causes obstruction, then severe flank pain (renal colic) or abdominal pain occurs. The calculus typically causes obstruction at areas of narrowing of the urinary tract—the ureteropelvic junction, where the ureter crosses the iliac vessels, and the ureterovesical junction. The ureter progressively narrows distally, and its most narrow segment is the ureterovesical junction. Typically the pain radiates anteriorly to the scrotum or labia. Often the pain is intermittent, corresponding to periods of obstruction of urine flow, which increases the pressure in the collecting system. If the calculus is in the distal ureter, the child can have irritative symptoms of dysuria, urgency, and frequency. If the stone passes into the bladder, the child usually is asymptomatic. If the stone is in the urethra, dysuria and difficulty voiding can result, particularly in boys. Some children pass small amounts of gravel-like material. Stones can also be asymptomatic, although it is uncommon to pass a ureteral calculus without symptoms.

DIAGNOSIS

Approximately 90% of urinary calculi are calcified to some degree and consequently are radiopaque on a plain abdominal film. However, many calculi are only a few millimeters in diameter and are difficult to

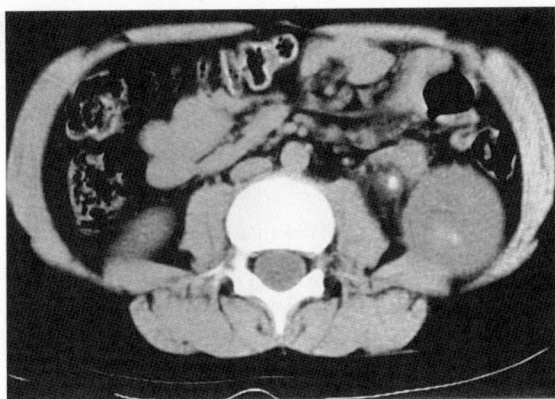

Figure 547-1 Noncontrast CT scan of the midabdomen in a male infant with cystinuria shows a left-sided calculus at the ureteropelvic junction with proximal hydronephrosis.

Table 547-2	Laboratory Tests Suggested for Evaluation of Urolithiasis

SERUM
Calcium
Phosphorus
Uric acid
Electrolytes and anion gap
Creatinine
Alkaline phosphatase
	URINE
	Urinalysis
	Urine culture
	Calcium:creatinine ratio
	Spot test for cystinuria
	24 hr collection for:
	   Creatinine clearance
	   Calcium
	   Phosphate
	   Oxalate
	   Uric acid
	   Dibasic amino acids (if cystine
	      spot test result is positive)

see, particularly if they are in the ureter. Struvite (magnesium ammonium phosphate) stones are radiopaque. Cystine, xanthine, and uric acid calculi may be radiolucent but often are slightly opacified. Some children have **nephrocalcinosis,** which is calcification of the renal tissue itself. Nephrocalcinosis is seen most commonly in premature neonates receiving furosemide, which causes hypercalciuria, and in children with medullary sponge kidney.

In a child with suspected renal colic, there are multiple imaging options. The most accurate study is an **unenhanced spiral CT scan** of the abdomen and pelvis (Fig. 547-1). This study takes only a few minutes to perform, has 96% sensitivity and specificity in delineating the number and location of calculi, and demonstrates whether the involved kidney is hydronephrotic. However, the radiation exposure is high. An alternative is to obtain a plain radiograph of the abdomen and pelvis plus a renal ultrasonogram. These studies can demonstrate hydronephrosis and possibly the calculus on the radiograph; however, the calculus is not visualized on sonography unless it is adjacent to the bladder. In addition, renal calculi <3 mm typically are not seen. Consequently, the clinician needs to carefully balance the risks of CT imaging against the lower sensitivity of the plain abdominal film plus sonography.

In 2008 the Society for Pediatric Radiology initiated the Image Gently initiative to educate providers on the risks of radiologic imaging in children and to encourage the use of limited imaging in children, particularly those with suspected urolithiasis (http://www.pedrad.org/associations/5364/ig/). In a child with an already-diagnosed calculus, serial plain x-rays or renal ultrasonography can be used to follow the status of the calculus, such as whether it has grown or diminished in size or has moved. If a child has a renal pelvic calculus, a ureteropelvic junction obstruction should be suspected. In some cases, it can be difficult to determine whether hydronephrosis in such a child is secondary to an obstructing stone, ureteropelvic junction obstruction, or both.

Any material that resembles a calculus should be sent for analysis by a laboratory that specializes in identifying the components of urinary calculi.

METABOLIC EVALUATION

A metabolic evaluation for the most common predisposing factors should be undertaken in all children with urolithiasis, bearing in mind that structural, infectious, and metabolic factors often coexist. This evaluation should not be undertaken in a child who is in the process of passing a stone, because the altered diet and hydration status, as well as the effect of obstruction on the kidney, can alter the results of the study. Table 547-2 lists the basic laboratory studies required, and Table 547-3 shows the normal values for 24-hr urine collections. In children with hypercalciuria, further studies of calcium excretion with dietary calcium restriction and calcium loading are necessary.

PATHOGENESIS OF SPECIFIC RENAL CALCULI
Calcium Oxalate and Calcium Phosphate Calculi

Most urinary calculi in children in the United States are composed of calcium oxalate and/or calcium phosphate. The most common metabolic abnormality in these patients is normocalcemic **hypercalciuria.** Between 30% and 60% of children with calcium stones have hypercalciuria without hypercalcemia. Other metabolic aberrations that predispose to stone disease include hyperoxaluria, hyperuricosuria, hypocitruria, heterozygous cystinuria, hypomagnesuria, hyperparathyroidism, and renal tubular acidosis (see Chapter 529).

Hypercalciuria may be absorptive, renal, or resorptive. The primary disturbance in absorptive hypercalciuria is intestinal hyperabsorption of calcium. In some children, an increase in 1,25-dihydroxyvitamin D is associated with the increased calcium absorption, whereas in others the process is independent of vitamin D. **Renal hypercalciuria** refers to impaired renal tubular reabsorption of calcium (see Chapter 519.8). Renal leak of calcium causes mild hypocalcemia, which triggers an increased production of parathyroid hormone, with increased intestinal absorption of calcium and increased mobilization of calcium stores. Resorptive hypercalciuria is uncommon and is found in patients with primary hyperparathyroidism. Excess parathyroid hormone secretion stimulates intestinal absorption of calcium and mobilization of calcium stores. Table 547-4 summarizes the metabolic evaluation of children with hypercalciuria.

Hyperoxaluria is another potentially important cause of calcium stones. Oxalate increases the solubility product of calcium oxalate crystallization 7-10 times more than calcium. Consequently, hyperoxaluria significantly increases the likelihood of calcium oxalate precipitation. Oxalate is found in high concentration in tea, coffee, spinach, and rhubarb. Primary hyperoxaluria is a rare autosomal recessive disorder that can be subclassified into glycolic aciduria and L-glyceric aciduria. Most patients with primary hyperoxaluria have glycolic aciduria; oxalic and glycolic acids are increased in the urine of affected persons. Both defects cause increased endogenous production of oxalate, with hyperoxaluria, urolithiasis, nephrocalcinosis, and injury to the kidneys. Death from renal failure occurs by age 20 yr in untreated patients. **Oxalosis,** defined as extrarenal deposition of calcium oxalate, occurs when renal insufficiency is present with elevated plasma oxalate. Calcium oxalate deposits appear first in blood vessels and bone marrow, and with time they appear throughout the body. Secondary hyperoxaluria is more common and can occur in patients with increased intake of oxalate and oxalate precursors such as vitamin C, in those with pyridoxine deficiency, and in children with intestinal malabsorption.

Enteric hyperoxaluria refers to disorders such as inflammatory bowel disease (see Chapter 336), pancreatic insufficiency (see Chapter 350), and biliary disease (see Chapter 356), in which there is gastrointestinal malabsorption of fatty acids, which bind intraluminal calcium and form salts that are excreted in the feces. Normally, calcium forms a complex with oxalate to reduce oxalate absorption, but if calcium is unavailable, there is increased absorption of unbound oxalate.

Table 547-3	Urine Chemistry: Normal Values			
URINE CONSTITUENT	**AGE**	**RANDOM**	**TIMED**	**COMMENTS**
Calcium	0-6 mo 7-12 mo ≥2 yr	<0.8 mg/mg creat <0.6 mg/mg creat <0.21 mg/mg creat	<4 mg/kg/24 hr	Prandial variation Sodium-dependent
Oxalate*	<1 yr 1-<5 yr 5-12 yr >12 yr	0.15-0.26 mmol/mmol creat 0.11-0.12 mmol/mmol creat 0.006-0.15 mmol/mmol creat 0.002-0.083 mmol/mmol creat	≥2 yr: <0.5 mmol/1.73 m^2/24 hr	Random urine mmol/mmol highly age-dependent Excretion rate/1.73 m^2 constant through childhood and adulthood
Uric acid	Term infant >3 yr	3.3 mg/dL GFR† <0.53 mg/dL GFR	<815 mg/1.73 m^2/24 hr	Excretion rate/1.73 m^2 from >1 yr age; constant through childhood
Magnesium	>2 yr	<0.12 mg/mg creat	<88 mg/1.73 m^2/24 hr	Excretion rate/1.73 m^2 constant through childhood
Citrate		>400 mg/g creat		Limited data available for children
Cystine		<75 mg/g creat	<60 mg/1.73 m2/24 hr	Cystine >250 mg/g creat suggests homozygous cystinuria

*Oxalate oxidase assay.
†(mg/dL uric acid) (serum creatinine concentration/urine creatinine concentration).
creat, Creatinine; GFR, glomerular filtration rate.
From Milliner DS: Urolithiasis. In Avner ED, Harmon WE, Naiudet P, editors: Pediatric nephrology, ed 5, Philadelphia, 2004, Lippincott Williams & Wilkins, p. 1103, with permission.

Table 547-4	Metabolic Evaluation of Children with Hypercalciuria			
TYPE	**SERUM CALCIUM**	**RESTRICTED CALCIUM (URINE)**	**FASTING CALCIUM (URINE)**	**CALCIUM LOAD (URINE)**	**PARATHYROID HORMONE (SERUM)**
Absorptive	N	N or I	N	I	I
Renal	N	I	I	I	N
Resorptive	I	I	I	I	I

I, increased; N, normal.

Hypocitraturia refers to a low excretion of citrate, which is an important inhibitor of calcium stone formation. Citrate acts as an inhibitor of calcium urolithiasis by forming complexes with calcium, increasing the solubility of calcium in the urine, and inhibiting the aggregation of calcium phosphate and calcium oxalate crystals. Disorders such as chronic diarrhea, intestinal malabsorption, and renal tubular acidosis (see below) can cause hypocitraturia. It may also be idiopathic.

Renal tubular acidosis (RTA) is a syndrome involving a disturbance of acid–base balance within the kidney that can be classified into 3 types, one of which predisposes to renal calculi that typically are calcium phosphate (see Chapter 529). In type 1 RTA, the distal nephron does not secrete hydrogen ion into the distal tubule. The urine pH is never <5.8, and hyperchloremic hypokalemic acidosis results. Patients acquire nephrolithiasis, nephrocalcinosis, muscle weakness, and osteomalacia. Type 1 RTA can be an autosomal dominant disorder, but more often it is acquired and associated with systemic diseases such as Sjögren syndrome, Wilson disease, primary biliary cirrhosis, and lymphocytic thyroiditis, or it results from amphotericin B, lithium, or toluene (an organic solvent associated with glue sniffing).

From 5-8% of patients with **cystic fibrosis** (see Chapter 403) have urolithiasis. Typically the stones are calcium, and they often become manifest in adolescence or young adulthood. Microscopic nephrocalcinosis also occurs in younger children with the disease. These patients do not have hypercalciuria, and the propensity for urolithiasis has been speculated to result from an inability to excrete a sodium chloride load or from intestinal malabsorption.

Other disorders can play a role in causing calcium stones. **Hyperuricosuria** may be related to the epitactic growth of calcium oxalate crystals around a nucleus of uric acid crystals or to the action of uric acid as a counter inhibitor of urinary mucopolysaccharides, which inhibit calcium oxalate crystallization. **Heterozygous cystinuria** is found in some patients with calcium stones. The mechanism is unknown but may be similar to that of uric acid. Sarcoidosis (see Chapter 165) causes an increased sensitivity to vitamin D$_3$ and thus an increased absorption of calcium from the gastrointestinal tract. In Lesch-Nyhan syndrome (see Chapter 89), there is excessive uric acid synthesis. These patients are more likely to form uric acid stones, but some of these stones may be calcified. **Immobility** can cause hypercalciuria by mobilization of calcium stores. High-dose corticosteroids can cause hypercalciuria and calcium oxalate precipitation. Furosemide, which is administered in the neonatal intensive care unit, also can cause severe hypercalciuria, urolithiasis, and nephrocalcinosis.

In some children, calcium calculi are idiopathic. A complete metabolic evaluation must be performed before this diagnosis is made.

Cystine Calculi

Cystinuria accounts for 1% of renal calculi in children. The condition is a rare autosomal recessive disorder of the epithelial cells of the renal tubule that prevents absorption of the 4 dibasic amino acids (cystine, ornithine, arginine, lysine) and results in excessive urinary excretion of these products. The only known complication of this familial disease is the formation of calculi, because of the low solubility of cystine. The patients usually have acidic urine, which leads to a higher rate of precipitation. In the homozygous patient, the daily excretion of cystine usually exceeds 500 mg, and stone formation occurs at an early age. Heterozygotes excrete 100-300 mg/day and typically do not have clinical urolithiasis. The sulfur content of cystine gives these stones their faint radiopaque appearance.

Struvite Calculi

Urinary tract infections (see Chapter 538) caused by urea-splitting organisms (most often *Proteus* spp., and occasionally *Klebsiella* spp., *Escherichia coli*, *Pseudomonas* spp., and others) result in urinary alkalinization and excessive production of ammonia, which can lead to the precipitation of magnesium ammonium phosphate (struvite) and calcium phosphate. In the kidney, the calculi often have a staghorn configuration, filling the calyces. The calculi act as foreign bodies, causing obstruction, perpetuating infection, and causing gradual kidney damage. Patients with struvite stones also can have metabolic abnormalities that predispose to stone formation. These stones often are seen in children with neuropathic bladder, particularly those who have undergone a urinary tract reconstructive procedure (see Chapter 542). Struvite stones also can form in the reconstructed bladder of children who have undergone augmentation cystoplasty or continent urinary diversion.

Uric Acid Calculi

Calculi containing uric acid represent <5% of all cases of lithiasis in children in the United States but are more common in less-developed areas of the world. Hyperuricosuria with or without hyperuricemia is the common underlying factor in most cases. The stones are radiolucent on x-ray. The diagnosis should be suspected in a patient with persistently acid urine and urate crystalluria.

Hyperuricosuria can result from various inborn errors of purine metabolism that lead to overproduction of uric acid, the end product of purine metabolism in humans. Children with the Lesch-Nyhan syndrome and patients with glucose-6-phosphatase deficiency (see Chapter 87) form urate calculi as well. In children with short-bowel syndrome (see Chapter 338.7), and particularly those with ileostomies, chronic dehydration and acidosis sometimes are complicated by uric acid lithiasis.

One of the most common causes of uric acid lithiasis is the rapid turnover of purine with some tumors and myeloproliferative diseases. The risk of uric acid lithiasis is especially great when treatment of these diseases causes rapid breakdown of nucleoproteins. Uric acid calculi or "sludge" can fill the entire upper collecting system and cause renal failure and even anuria. Urates also are present within calcium-containing stones. In these cases, >1 predisposing factor for stone formation can exist.

Indinavir Calculi

Indinavir sulfate is a protease inhibitor approved for treating HIV infection (see Chapter 276). Up to 4% of patients acquire symptomatic nephrolithiasis. Most of the calculi are radiolucent and are composed of indinavir-based monohydrate, although calcium oxalate and/or phosphate have been present in some. After each dose, 12% of the drug is excreted unchanged in the urine. The urine in these patients often contains crystals of characteristic rectangles and fan-shaped or starburst crystals. Indinavir is soluble at a pH of <5.5. Consequently, dissolution therapy by urinary acidification with ammonium chloride or ascorbic acid should be considered.

Nephrocalcinosis

Nephrocalcinosis refers to calcium deposition within the renal tissue. Often nephrocalcinosis is associated with urolithiasis. The most common causes are furosemide (administered to premature neonates), distal RTA, hyperparathyroidism, medullary sponge kidney, hypophosphatemic rickets, sarcoidosis, cortical necrosis, hyperoxaluria, prolonged immobilization, Cushing syndrome, hyperuricosuria, monogenetic causes of hypertension, and renal candidiasis.

TREATMENT

In a child with a renal or ureteral calculus, the decision whether to remove the stone depends on its location, size, and composition (if known) and whether obstruction and/or infection is present. Pain is managed with nonsteroidal antiinflammatory drugs or opiates. Small ureteral calculi often pass spontaneously, although the child might experience severe renal colic. The narrowest segment of the ureter is the ureterovesical junction. α-Adrenergic blockers, such as tamsulosin, terazosin, and doxazosin, facilitate stone passage in children and adults by decreasing ureteral pressure below the stone and decreasing the frequency of the peristaltic contractions of the obstructed ureter. In many cases, passage of a **ureteral stent** past the stone endoscopically relieves pain and dilates the ureter sufficiently to allow the calculus to pass. In cases such as children with a uric acid calculus or an infant with a furosemide-associated calculus, dissolution alkaline therapy may be effective.

If the calculus does not pass or seems unlikely to pass or if there is associated urinary tract infection, removal is necessary (Table 547-5). **Lithotripsy** of bladder, ureteral, and small renal pelvic calculi using the holmium laser through a flexible or rigid ureteroscope is quite effective. Extracorporeal shock wave lithotripsy has been successfully applied to children with renal and ureteral stones, with a success rate of >75%. Another alternative is percutaneous nephrostolithotomy, in which access to the renal collecting system is obtained percutaneously, and the calculi are broken down by ultrasonic lithotripsy. In cases in which these modalities are unsuccessful, an alternative is laparoscopic removal; this procedure can be performed using the da Vinci robot.

In children with urolithiasis, the underlying metabolic disorder should be addressed (Table 547-6). Because lithiasis results from elevated concentrations of specific substances in the urine, maintaining a continuous high urine output by maintaining a high fluid intake often is an effective method of preventing further stones. The high fluid intake should be continued at night, and usually it is necessary for the child to get up at least once at night to urinate and drink more water.

Table 547-5	Primary Surgical Treatment Options vs Stone Size and Location		
STONES	**SHOCK WAVE LITHOTRIPSY**	**URETEROSCOPY**	**PERCUTANEOUS NEPHROLITHOTOMY**
RENAL			
<1 cm	Most common	Optional	Optional
1-2 cm	Most common	Optional	Optional
>2 cm	Optional	Rare	Most common
LOWER POLE			
<1 cm	Most common	Optional	Optional
>1 cm	Optional	Optional	Most common
URETERAL			
Proximal	Most common	Optional	Occasional
Distal	Optional	Most common	Rare

After Durkee CT, Balcom A: Surgical management of urolithiasis, Pediatr Clin North Am 53:465–477, 2006, with permission.

Table 547-6	Suggested Therapy for Urolithiasis Caused by Metabolic Abnormalities	
METABOLIC ABNORMALITY	**INITIAL TREATMENT**	**SECOND-LINE TREATMENT**
Hypercalciuria	Reduction of dietary Na+	Potassium citrate
	Dietary calcium at RDA Thiazides	Neutral phosphate
Hyperoxaluria	Adjustment of dietary oxalate	Neutral phosphate*
	Potassium citrate	Magnesium Pyridoxine*
Hypocitric aciduria	Potassium citrate Bicarbonate	
Hyperuricosuria	Alkalinization	Allopurinol
Cystinuria	Alkalinization Reduction of dietary Na+	Tiopronin (Thiola) D-Penicillamine
		Captopril

*Initial therapy in primary hyperoxaluria.
RDA, recommended dietary allowance.
From Milliner DS: Urolithiasis. In Avner ED, Harmon WE, Niaudet P, editors: Pediatric nephrology, ed 5, Philadelphia, 2004, Lippincott Williams & Wilkins, p. 1104, with permission.

A daily fluid intake of 2-2.5 L in adolescent stone formers is recommended, with greater intake during summer months.

Dietary sodium intake in children has increased significantly, up to 6.8 g/day as a consequence of increased consumption of salty, processed foods. High sodium intake increases urinary excretion of calcium and may result in hypocitraturia. In addition, increased salt intake induces metabolic acidosis. To compensate for the acid load, the kidneys conserve anions, including urinary citrate, which contributes to hypocitraturia. Reduction in dietary intake of sodium and increased potassium intake is indicated.

Although counterintuitive, low-calcium diets are less effective in the treatment of calcium stones than diets containing normal amounts of calcium and limited amounts of sodium and animal protein. Low-sodium, low-protein diets reduce urinary calcium and oxalate excretion. Children with stone disease should avoid excess calcium intake. However, children require calcium for bone development and recommendations for daily calcium intake vary by age. Consequently, calcium restriction in children should be avoided. Thiazide diuretics also reduce renal calcium excretion. Addition of potassium citrate, an inhibitor of calcium stones, with a dosage of 1-2 mEq/kg/24 hr is beneficial. An excellent source of citrate is lemonade, because 4 oz of lemon juice contains 84 mEq of citric acid. A daily mixture of 4 oz of reconstituted lemon juice in 2 L of water and sweetened to taste should significantly increase the urinary citrate level. In difficult cases, neutral orthophosphate should be given also, although it is poorly tolerated.

In patients with uric acid stones, allopurinol is effective. Allopurinol is an inhibitor of xanthine oxidase and is effective in reducing the production of both uric acid and 2,8-dihydroxyadenine and can help control recurrence of both types of stones. In addition, urinary alkalinization with sodium bicarbonate or sodium citrate is beneficial. The urine pH should be ≥6.5 and can be monitored at home by the family.

Maintaining a high urine pH can also prevent recurrence of cystine calculi. Cystine is much more soluble when the urinary pH is >7.5, and alkalinization of urine with sodium bicarbonate or sodium citrate is effective. Another important medication is D-penicillamine, which is a chelating agent that binds to cysteine or homocysteine, increasing the solubility of the product. Although poorly tolerated by many patients, it has been reported to be effective in dissolving cystine stones and in preventing recurrences when hydration and urinary alkalinization fail. N-Acetylcysteine appears to have low toxicity and may be effective in controlling cystinuria, but long-term experience with it is lacking.

Treatment of type 1 RTA involves correcting the metabolic acidosis and replacing lost potassium and sodium. Sodium or potassium citrate therapy, or both, is necessary. When the metabolic acidosis is corrected, the urinary citrate excretion returns to normal.

Treatment of primary hyperoxaluria involves liver transplantation because the defective enzymes are hepatic. Ideally, this procedure is performed before renal failure occurs. In the most severe cases, kidney transplantation is also necessary.

Bibliography is available at Expert Consult.

Gynecologic Problems of Childhood

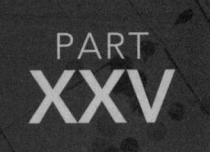

PART XXV

Chapter **548**

History and Physical Examination

*Kathryn C. Stambough and
Diane F. Merritt*

HISTORY

The approach to both the history and physical examination of a child is often a collaborative effort that involves the child, her caregiver, and the provider. With a preverbal or very young patient, clinicians obtain the majority of the history from a parent or caregiver. Even for the very young patient, developmentally appropriate social questions directed to the patient can put her at ease and help to develop cooperation and rapport that will facilitate a subsequent examination. Specific patient, caregiver, or provider concerns about vaginal discharge or bleeding, pruritus, external genital lesions or abnormalities should direct a problem-focused history. In a patient presenting with vaginal bleeding, questions should focus on recent growth and development, signs of pubertal progression, trauma, vaginal discharge, medication exposure, and any history of foreign objects in the vagina. For complaints of vulvovaginal irritation, pruritus, or discharge, questions should concentrate on perineal hygiene, the onset and duration of symptoms, the presence and quality of discharge, exposure to skin irritants, recent antibiotic use, travel, presence of medical comorbidities or infections in the patient and her family members, and other systemic symptoms of illness or skin conditions. Throughout the history, the patient should be encouraged to ask her own questions. Occasionally, the child is brought to the clinician because she or her parents have concerns about anatomic findings, developmental changes, or congenital anomalies. It helps to understand the family's concerns and if a specific reason, event, or family history raised the need for a gynecologic consultation.

GYNECOLOGIC EXAMINATION

The physical examination of the patient should be tailored to the child's age, complaint, and any other concerns elicited in the history. The menstrual period should be included with an assessment of other vital signs as age appropriate.

Neonates

The delivering obstetrician should briefly examine the external genitals of female infants to confirm the patency of the vagina and assess the presence of any obvious genital anomalies. The pediatrician's newborn examination should note any abnormal findings such as ambiguous genitalia, imperforate hymen, urogenital abnormalities, abdominal mass, or inguinal hernia that might herald a gynecologic problem.

Placing the infant in the supine position with thighs flexed against the abdomen allows visualization of the neonate's external genitals. Estrogenic effects commonly notable in neonates include prominence of the labia majora and a white vaginal discharge. The labia minora and hymen may protrude slightly from the vestibule. A small amount of neonatal vaginal bleeding from endometrial sloughing following maternal hormone withdrawal might occur. Bleeding that is excessive or persistent beyond 1 mo of life requires further evaluation. Breast buds may be palpable at the time of the neonatal examination but should regress in the 1st mo of life; occasionally, nipple discharge occurs.

The vaginal orifice may be difficult to see. Gentle lateral traction on the labia majora usually allows complete visualization of the hymen and vaginal orifice. The hymen should be evaluated for patency. Most hymenal variations—imperforate, microperforate, septate—do not require treatment during the neonatal period. Variations should be noted and readdressed in subsequent visits. The hymen originates from the urogenital sinus. The uterus and vagina originate from the müllerian ducts. The concomitant renal malformations seen with müllerian anomalies are not associated with hymenal anomalies. Hymenal polyps seen in newborns typically regress in size as the maternal estrogen effects subside. Cervicovaginal mucus secretions can accumulate behind the blocked outflow tract of an imperforate hymen and manifest as a mucocolpos. *In this instance, correction of the imperforate hymen in the neonatal period is indicated if urinary obstruction occurs.*

The clitoris may appear large in proportion to the other genital structures, especially in premature infants. If the clitoris appears enlarged, the clitoral width should be measured; values >6 mm in a newborn indicate a need for further evaluation. *If clitoromegaly and ambiguous genitals are present, the obstetrician and pediatrician should immediately obtain expert consultation for evaluation of the infant and to counsel the parents.* Congenital adrenal hyperplasia is the most common cause of ambiguous genitals (accounting for more than 90% of cases), and the salt-wasting forms can lead to rapid dehydration with subsequent fluid and electrolyte imbalance (see Chapter 576). Delay in the diagnosis and treatment of congenital adrenal hyperplasia may be life-threatening.

In the neonate, the ovaries are <1 cm in diameter and average 1 cm³ in volume. Antenatal or postnatal abdominopelvic ultrasound might reveal small simple ovarian cysts, which represent normal follicles. Because of the abdominal location of ovaries in the neonate, ovarian enlargement can manifest as a palpable abdominal mass. Large cysts (>4-5 cm) or those of a complex nature pose the risk of ovarian torsion, hemorrhage into the cyst, or, uncommonly, an ovarian tumor. A non-resolving or enlarging neonatal ovarian cyst warrants expert consultation. If the mass causes respiratory compromise or gastrointestinal obstruction, decompression is usually performed. Cyst aspiration can give temporary relief, but it is not recommended as the fluid aspirated is not reliable for diagnosis and fluid may reaccumulate. If a cystectomy is done for appropriate clinical indications the cyst wall should be surgically excised to prevent reaccumulation of fluid and to provide a pathologic diagnosis, the remaining ovarian tissue should be left in situ, and the contralateral ovary should be inspected. Preservation of normal ovarian tissue is recommended for all benign lesions, and salpingo-oophorectomy should not be performed unless clinically indicated.

Infants and Prepubertal Girls

As the maternal estrogen effect subsides, the genitals of the female infant change in appearance. The labia begin to flatten. The hymenal membrane loses its redundancy and becomes translucent. The hypoestrogenic prepubertal vaginal epithelium appears thin, red, and sensitive to the touch. The vaginal mucosa of young children can have longitudinal ridges running along the axis of the vagina at 3 o'clock, 6 o'clock, and 9 o'clock, which can cause small protrusions on the hymen at these locations. The cervix usually appears flat and flush with the vaginal vault. During infancy, the uterus regresses in size and does not return to its birth size until the 5th or 6th year. The prepubertal cervix:fundus ratio is 2:1.

As puberty approaches, the child experiences increasing endocrine activity of the hypothalamus, pituitary gland, adrenal gland, and ovaries (see Chapter 561). The labia majora begin to fill out, and the labia minora thicken and elongate as a result of increased estrogen levels. The hymen thickens and becomes more redundant. Clear or white physiologic secretions may be present. Breast buds begin to appear, either bilateral or initially unilateral with subsequent development of the contralateral breast.

Indications for Genital Examination

Genitourinary complaints or suspected genitourinary pathology warrant assessment of the external and internal genitals of pediatric patients, specifically in cases of vaginal bleeding, vaginal discharge, vulvar trauma, presence of a foreign body, perineal or pelvic masses, vulvovaginal ulcerative or inflammatory lesions, congenital anomalies, or suspected sexual abuse.

Preparation

The genital examination in prepubertal girls requires a gentle, patient approach to maximize cooperation and minimize fear and embarrassment. A clear, simple explanation of what the exam involves can facilitate the child's comfort and cooperation. The presence of a parent or caregiver during the entire examination provides reassurance for most children. For the older prepubertal patient, the physician may discuss whether the patient wishes to have a family member present during the examination. Even in the presence of the caregiver, the examiner should speak directly to the child. Prior to initiating any part of the examination, the provider should explicitly verify with both the patient and her caregiver that the caregiver has given permission for the examination. This provides an opportunity to explain to the child the privacy of body parts and who may examine or touch those areas. It is useful to educate the patient and caregiver about the basic anatomy and hygiene of the external genital area. Before each step of the examination, the physician should explain what will occur. Allowing an older child the option of watching her examination with a handheld mirror may contribute to her comfort and understanding. Forcible restraint is never indicated; if optimal evaluation is not possible, the clinician must assess the acuity of the complaint and pathology and determine the potential need for a multi-visit examination or an examination under anesthesia.

Positioning

A variety of techniques and positions can facilitate the genital examination in prepubertal patients. Children younger than 4 yr of age can be placed on the parent or caregiver's lap with the child's legs straddling the parent's thighs. If the child permits, she may be positioned on the table in the supine position with the hips fully abducted and the feet together in the frogleg (diamond or butterfly) position. Older children may prefer to use the stirrups. The head of the examination table should be raised so that eye contact can be maintained with the patient throughout the examination. When the child is supine, grasping the labia majora along the inferior portion between the thumb and index finger and gently pulling outward and posteriorly (labial traction) allows visualization of the vaginal introitus. Alternatively, the child may be placed in the knee–chest position with elevation of the buttocks and hips. This position provides exposure of the inferior portion of the hymen, the lower vagina, and possibly the upper vagina and cervix but has the disadvantage of having the child face away from the examiner.

Some extremely cooperative children tolerate a vaginoscopic examination in an outpatient office setting for better intravaginal assessment. The endoscope (either a cystoscope or a hysteroscope) is placed in the vagina and the labia are gently opposed, allowing the vagina to distend with water. This technique permits visualization of the vagina and cervix, allowing for the evaluation of an injury, lesion, and anatomic variant or for the presence of a foreign body. Application of 2% lidocaine gel at the introitus makes the insertion easier and less irritating

for the patient. If a more complete examination is indicated or if the child is too young, frightened or unable to cooperate, an examination under anesthesia is recommended.

Documentation

Clinicians should thoroughly and accurately document genital exam findings in the medical record, reserving conclusions and diagnostic terms for the impression and plan portion of the documentation rather than in the description of exam findings. Each structure visualized should be noted (e.g., clitoris, labia majora, labia minora, urethra, vestibule, and rectum) with attention to describing normal appearance and any anatomic variations (e.g., the configuration of the hymen as annular, crescentic, etc.). Describing any findings or lesions using a clock-face method provides a consistent reference point; a sketch or magnified photograph may also be helpful. Future examiners will rely on this documentation as a record with which they compare their findings and note any variances. Changes should be noted in any follow-up examinations.

Adolescents

Some teens prefer to initially meet and discuss the reason for their visit with the provider without their parent or guardian present, and this request should be honored (see Chapter 112). A majority of the time, obtaining a history from an adolescent begins with meeting the patient and her parent or caregiver together to review her history and the reason for the visit and to explain the concepts of confidentiality and privacy. Familiarity with local laws governing limitations to confidential services should guide the protection of the adolescent and her parents' rights to information access and privacy. The Guttmacher Institute provides an up-to-date listing of state and federal laws in the United States affecting access to medical care (http://www.guttmacher.org/statecenter/spibs/index.html). Brief discussions of normal pubertal development and menstruation can reassure both patients and their parents or guardians and provide valuable education on appropriate menstrual flow, menstrual hygiene and the duration and frequency of bleeding. Introducing the menstrual diary as an invaluable tool for the teen can help patients, parents, and clinicians identify abnormal bleeding patterns that might require further evaluation. Many apps are available for tracking menstrual periods on a smart phone or computer.

After the initial interview with the teen and her parent or caregiver, the confidential and sensitive portion of the history, particularly sexual history and alcohol, tobacco, and drug use, is taken with the teen alone. Such a request could be phrased as follows: "I would like to give your daughter an opportunity to ask any questions she might have privately, so would you mind stepping out of the room for a moment?" Concerns for the presence of vaginal discharge, the potential for sexually transmitted infections, pregnancy, or menstrual aberration should be explored. Teens and their parents should be informed of the proper use and accessibility of condoms, all contraceptive methods, and emergency contraception.

A number of resources for educating adolescents regarding their first pelvic examination and in-depth sexual history and psychosocial screening tools are available. These include the North American Society for Pediatric and Adolescent Gynecology (http://www.naspag.org), the American Academy of Pediatrics (http://www.aap.org), the Society for Adolescent Health and Medicine (http://www.adolescenthealth.org), and the American College of Obstetricians and Gynecologists (http://acog.org/Patients).

Pelvic Examination

Table 548-1 presents the indications for the first pelvic examination in adolescents: age older than 21 yr, abnormal uterine bleeding, vulvovaginitis, severe dysmenorrhea, unexplained dysuria or abdominal pain, evaluation and removal of a foreign body, and placement of an intrauterine device. If an adolescent does not meet 1 of the criteria

Table 548-1	Suggested Indications for Pelvic Examination in Adolescents

Age 21 yr for initial Pap test
Unexplained menstrual irregularities, including pubertal aberrations
Severe dysmenorrhea
Unexplained abdominal pain
Unexplained dysuria
Abnormal vaginal discharge
Placement of intrauterine device
Removal of foreign body

Modified from The initial reproductive visit. Committee Opinion No. 460. American College of Obstetricians and Gynecologists. Obstet Gynecol 116:240–243, 2010.

Table 548-2	Recommendations for First Gynecologic Evaluation

Between 13 and 15 yr of age
First gynecologic encounter focuses on patient education; pelvic examination is generally not indicated
First pelvic examination with Pap test at 21 yr of age, unless otherwise indicated by Table 548-1

Modified from Well-woman visit. Committee Opinion No. 534. American College of Obstetricians and Gynecologists. Obstet Gynecol 120:421–424, 2012.

listed in Table 548-1, the American College of Obstetricians and Gynecologists recommends that the first gynecologic encounter occur between the ages of 13 and 15 yr (Table 548-2) with attention toward anticipatory guidance focusing on normal pubertal development and menstruation. Patients should undergo screening for sexually transmitted infection with each new sexual partner. With the availability of urine and vaginal swab nucleic acid amplification testing for chlamydia and gonorrhea, sexually transmitted infection screening does not necessitate a speculum exam.

Prior to the initiation of a physical examination, all young women should be offered the choice of having a medical attendant, family member, or friend present during her examination. At the initial gynecologic exam, the physician should explain the process in understandable terms. A thorough evaluation begins with an assessment of body mass index, blood pressure, menstruation status, thyroid, lymph nodes, breast development, abdominal exam, and skin. The external genitals should be examined with the patient in the dorsal lithotomy position while communication is maintained between the physician and patient. Elevating the head of the examination table allows the teen and her examiner to maintain eye contact. The teen can hold a mirror to follow along with the examination, and she should be encouraged to ask questions. Inspection of the vulva is followed by inspection of the Bartholin, urethral, and Skene glands. The clitoris, normally 2-4 mm in width, is then assessed; a clitoris wider than 10 mm, especially in the presence of other signs of virilization, suggests a need for further evaluation. The hymenal anatomy should also be evaluated. Throughout the examination, the proper nomenclature for genital anatomy should be emphasized with the teen to empower her to use proper wordage with the avoidance of slang when referring to her body.

Because the initial Papanicolaou test is deferred until 21 yr of age and cultures for sexually transmitted infections can be obtained from urine or vaginal swabs, the need for a speculum exam is decreasing in this age group. If a speculum exam is indicated, use an appropriate sized speculum, such as the Huffman ($\frac{1}{2}$ in wide × 4 in long) or Pedersen ($\frac{7}{8}$ in wide × 4 in long). Shorter speculums will not allow visualization of the entire vaginal canal. The adolescent patient should be reassured that the exam may be uncomfortable but should not be painful and that her request to stop or wait will be honored. Encouraging the patient to watch with a hand-held mirror facilitates patient education and can be empowering. She may be told before the insertion of the speculum that she will experience a pressure sensation.

Before touching the introitus, it may be useful to touch the inner thigh with the speculum. Compression of the urethra anteriorly should be avoided. Gentle pressure with a finger for displacement of the fourchette posteriorly further facilitates proper speculum placement. After visualization of the vagina and cervix, specimens should be obtained as indicated. A bimanual examination, sometimes with a single digit, allows palpation of the vaginal walls and cervix and bimanual assessment of the uterus and adnexa. Reassurance of normal findings throughout the examination should be provided, and normal variants to anatomy should be pointed out to the teen as they are encountered (e.g., asymmetric labia minora).

Following the examination, it is appropriate to review the exam findings with the teen (and her parent) and initiate a collaborative discussion of the management plan. Encouraging the adolescent to participate in decision making empowers her to undertake responsibility for her health, may strengthen compliance with the medical plan, and acknowledge her as a unique individual.

Bibliography is available at Expert Consult.

Chapter **549**
Vulvovaginitis
Holly R. Hoefgen and Diane F. Merritt

Vulvovaginitis, the most common gynecologic-based problem for prepubertal children, is typically caused by either inadequate or excessive hygiene or chemical irritants. The condition is usually improved by hygiene measures and education of the caregivers and child.

ETIOLOGY
Vulvitis refers to external genital pruritus, burning, redness, or rash. **Vaginitis** implies inflammation of the vagina, which can manifest as a discharge with or without an odor or bleeding. These may occur simultaneously as vulvovaginitis. When a child presents with vulvovaginitis, the history should include questions on hygiene (wiping from front to back) and information about possible chemical irritants (bath soaps, laundry detergents, swimming pools, or hot tubs). The caregiver can be asked about a history of diarrhea, perianal itching, or nighttime itching. The possibility of foreign objects being placed into the vagina should also be asked, although the young child is unlikely to remember or recall. Children are especially prone to nonspecific vulvovaginitis for a variety of reasons, including their nonestrogenized state, poor perianal hygiene, and the proximity of the anus to the vagina, which is without geographic barriers given the flattened labia and lack of pubic hair (Fig. 549-1 and Table 549-1).

EPIDEMIOLOGY
Infectious vulvovaginitis, where a specific pathogen is isolated as the cause of symptoms, may be caused by fecal or respiratory pathogens and cultures might reveal *Escherichia coli* (see Chapter 200), *Streptococcus pyogenes*, *Staphylococcus aureus* (see Chapter 181), *Haemophilus influenzae* (see Chapter 194), *Enterobius vermicularis*, and, rarely, *Candida* spp. (see Chapter 234). These organisms may be transmitted by the child using improper toilet hygiene and manually from the nasopharynx to the vagina. The children present with perianal redness, an inflamed introitus, and often a yellow-green or mildly bloody discharge. They may be observed to be grabbing their genital area or "digging" in their underwear, which is usually stained with yellow-brown discharge. Attempts to treat these bacterial etiologies with antifungal medication will fail and often the antifungal product will lead to more irritation. Table 549-2 gives specific treatment recommendations based on the bacteria localized.

Neisseria gonorrhoeae or *Chlamydia trachomatis* also are causes of specific infectious vulvovaginitis (see Chapter 120). Management of children who have sexually transmitted infections requires close cooperation between clinicians and child-protection authorities. Official investigations for sexual abuse, when indicated, should be initiated promptly (see Chapter 40). If acquired after the neonatal period, some diseases (e.g., gonorrhea, syphilis, and chlamydia) are virtually 100% indicative of sexual contact. For other diseases (e.g., human papillomavirus infection and herpes simplex virus), the association with

sexual contact is not as clear. Presumptive treatment for children who have been sexually assaulted or abused is not recommended because (1) the incidence of most sexually transmitted infections in children is low after abuse/assault, (2) prepubertal girls appear to be at lower risk for ascending infection than adolescent or adult women, and (3) regular follow-up of children usually can be ensured. Although *Trichomonas vaginalis* can be transmitted vertically and can be seen in children up to 1 yr of age, it is an uncommon cause of specific infectious vulvovaginitis in the unestrogenized prepubertal girl.

Other causes of specific infectious vulvovaginitis include *Shigella* (see Chapter 199), which often manifests with a blood-tinged purulent discharge, and *Yersinia enterocolitica* (see Chapter 203). *Candida* infections (yeast) commonly cause diaper rash, but they are unlikely to cause vaginitis in children because the alkaline pH of the prepubertal vagina does not support fungal infections. Exceptions can occur in diabetic or immunocompromised children or children on prolonged antibiotics. Pinworms are the most common helminthic infestation in the United States, with the highest rates in school-age and preschool children. Perianal itching can lead to excoriation and, rarely, bleeding.

CLINICAL MANIFESTATIONS
Diaper Dermatitis
Diaper dermatitis is the most common dermatologic problem in infancy and occurs in half of all diaper-wearing infants and children. The moisture and contact with urine and feces irritates the skin, and colonization with *Candida* spp. increases the severity of the dermatitis. First-line treatment includes hygiene measures such as increasing the frequency of diaper changes, allowing the infant to be diaper free,

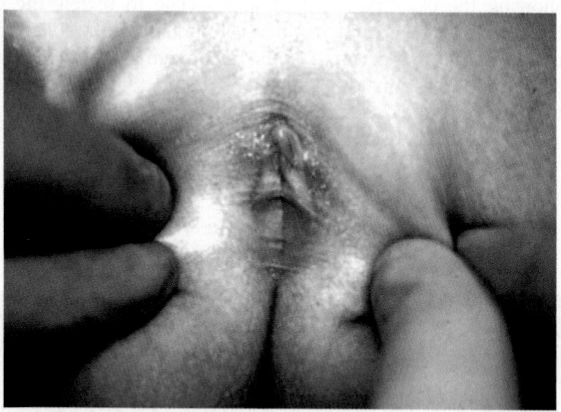
Figure 549-1 Labial adhesions. *(Photo courtesy of Diane F. Merritt, MD.)*

Table 549-1	Specific Vulvar Disorders in Children		
ORGANISM	**PRESENTATION**	**DIAGNOSIS**	**TREATMENT**
Molluscum contagiosum (Fig. 549-7)	1-5 mm discrete, skin-colored, dome-shaped, umbilicated lesions with a central cheesy plug	Diagnosis usually is made by visual inspection	The disease generally is self-limited and the lesions can resolve spontaneously. Treatment choices in children may include cryosurgery, laser, application of topical anesthetic and curettage, podophyllotoxin, and topical silver nitrate. Use of topical 5% imiquimod cream and 10% potassium hydroxide has been reported with similar effects
Condyloma acuminata	Skin-colored papules, some with a shaggy, cauliflower-like appearance	Diagnosis usually is made by visual inspection. Biopsy should be reserved for when the diagnosis is in question. Human papillomavirus DNA testing is not helpful	Many lesions in children resolve spontaneously, "wait and see" often utilized in children (60 days). Topical treatment with imiquimod cream and podophyllotoxin is the most studied (daily qhs 3 times/wk × 16 wk, wash 6-10 hr after application). General anesthesia is usually required for surgical/ablative procedures (cryotherapy, laser therapy, electrocautery)—reserve for symptomatic or large lesions. Other treatments have been utilized in adults, including trichloroacetic acid, 5-fluorouracil, sinecatechins, topical cidofovir, and cimetidine. The efficacy and safety of these treatments in children has not been established
Herpes simplex	Blisters that break, leaving tender ulcers	Visual inspection confirmed by culture from lesion	*Infants:* Acyclovir 20 mg/kg body weight IV q8 hr × 21 days for disseminated and central nervous system disease or × 14 days for disease limited to the skin and mucous membranes. *Genital/mucocutaneous disease:* Age 3 mo–2 yr: 15 mg/kg/day IV divided in q8h × 5-7 days. Age 2-12 yr (1st episode): Same as above or 1,200 mg/day divided in q8h dosing × 7-10 days. Age 2-12 yr (Reoccurrence): 1,200 mg/day in q8h dosing or 1,600 mg/day in bid dosing × 5 days (give 3-5 days for children older than 12 yr)

Table 549-1	Specific Vulvar Disorders in Children—cont'd		
ORGANISM	**PRESENTATION**	**DIAGNOSIS**	**TREATMENT**
Labial agglutination (see Fig. 549-1)	May be asymptomatic or can cause vulvitis, urinary dribbling, urinary tract infection, or urethritis	Diagnosis is made by visual inspection of the adherent labia, often with a central semitranslucent line	Does not require treatment if the patient is asymptomatic *Symptomatic patients:* Topical estrogen cream or betamethasone ointment applied alone or in combination daily for 6 wk directly to the line of adhesion, using a cotton swab while applying gentle labial traction Estrogen should be interrupted if breast budding occurs Mechanical or surgical separation of the adhesions is rarely indicated The adhesions usually resolve in 6-12 wk; unless good hygiene measures are followed, reoccurrence is common To decrease the risk of recurrence, an emollient (petroleum jelly, A and D ointment) should be applied to the inner labia for 1 mo or longer at bedtime
Lichen sclerosus (Fig. 549-4)	A sclerotic, atrophic, parchment-like plaque with an hourglass or keyhole appearance of vulvar, perianal, or perineal skin, subepithelial hemorrhages may be misinterpreted as sexual abuse or trauma The patient can experience perineal itching, soreness, or dysuria	Diagnosis usually is made by visual inspection Biopsy should be reserved for when the diagnosis is in question	Ultrapotent topical corticosteroids are the first-line therapy (clobetasol propionate ointment 0.05%) once or twice a day for 4-8 wk Once symptoms are under control, the patient should be tapered off the drug unless therapy is required for a flare-up In many girls, the condition resolves with puberty; however, this is not always the case and patients may require long-term follow-up
Psoriasis	Children are more likely than adults to have vulvar psoriasis noted as pruritic, well-demarcated, nonscaly, brightly erythematous, symmetrical plaques. The classic extragenital lesion are similar but with a silver scaly appearance	Diagnosis may be confirmed by locating other affected areas on the scalp or in nasolabial folds or behind the ears	Vulvar lesions may be treated with low to medium potency topical corticosteroids, increasing strength as necessary
Atopic dermatitis	Chronic cases can result in crusty, weepy lesions that are accompanied by intense pruritus and erythema Scratching often results in excoriation of the lesions and secondary bacterial or candidal infection	It may be seen in the vulvar area but characteristically affects the face, neck, chest, and extremities	Children with this condition should avoid common irritants and use topical corticosteroids (such as 1% hydrocortisone) for flare-ups If dry skin is present, lotion or bath oil can be used to seal in moisture after bathing
Contact dermatitis	Erythematous, edematous, or weepy vulvar vesicles or pustules can result, but more often the skin appears inflamed	Associated with exposure to an irritant, such as perfumed soaps, bubble bath, talcum powder, lotions, elastic bands of undergarments, or disposable diaper components	Avoidance of irritant Topical corticosteroids for flare-ups
Seborrheic dermatitis	Erythematous and greasy, yellowish scaling on vulva and labial crural folds associated with greasy dandruff-type rash of scalp, behind ears and face	Diagnosis usually is made by visual inspection	Gentle cleaning, topical clotrimazole with 1% hydrocortisone added
Vitiligo (Fig. 549-5)	Sharply demarcated hypopigmented patches, often symmetric in vaginal and anal regions. May be present in periphery at body orifices and extensor surfaces	Clinical. Test for associated illness if clinically warranted (thyroid disease, Addison disease, pernicious anemia, diabetes mellitus)	If desired, treat limited lesions with low-potency corticosteroids or tacrolimus. See dermatologist for extensive lesions.

2610 Part XXV ◆ Gynecologic Problems of Childhood

Table 549-2	Antibiotic Recommendations for Specific Vulvovaginal Infections
ETIOLOGY	**TREATMENT**
Streptococcus pyogenes *Streptococcus pneumoniae*	Penicillin V, 250 mg PO bid-tid ×10 days Amoxicillin 50 mg/kg/day (max: 500 mg/dose) divided into 3 doses daily × 10 days Erythromycin ethyl succinate, 30-50 mg/kg/day (max: 400 mg/dose) divided into 4 doses daily TMP-SMX 6-10 mg/kg/day (TMP component) divided into 2 doses daily × 10 days Clarithromycin 7.5 mg/kg bid (max: 1 g/day) × 5-10 days Reoccurrence most likely from asymptomatic pharyngeal carriage in child or family member. However, failure of penicillin regimens can occur For penicillin resistance: Rifampin 10 mg/kg every 12 hr × 2 days
Staphylococcus aureus	Topical mupirocin 2% 3 times daily to the affected skin area If systemic therapy required: Amoxicillin-clavulanate, 45 mg/kg/day (amoxicillin) PO divided into 2 or 3 doses daily × 7 days (first-line treatment because of high penicillin resistance) Extensive resistance to common antibiotics noted, recommend susceptibility testing for further antibiotic use MRSA: TMP-SMX double-strength 8-10 mg/kg/day; culture abscesses, incision and drainage
Haemophilus influenzae	Amoxicillin, 40 mg/kg/day divided into 3 doses daily × 7 days Cases of treatment failure or non-encapsulated *H. influenzae*, amoxicillin–clavulanate is recommended
Yersinia	TMP-SMX 6 mg/kg (TMP component) daily for 3 days
Shigella	TMP-SMX 10/50 mg/kg/day (max: 160/600) divided into 2 doses daily × 5 days Ampicillin 50-100 mg/kg/day divided into 4 doses daily (adult max: 4 g/day) × 5 days Azithromycin 12 mg/kg (max: 500) × 1 day, then 6 mg/kg/day (max: 250 mg) × 4 days (in areas of high resistance to above regimens or when sensitivities are unknown) For resistant organisms: Ceftriaxone 50-75 mg/kg/day IV or IM divided into 1 or 2 doses (max: 2 g/day) × 2-5 days
Chlamydia trachomatis	*Children weighing <45 kg:* Erythromycin base or ethylsuccinate 50 mg/kg/day PO divided into 4 daily doses × 14 days *Children weighing >45 kg but age younger than 8 yr:* azithromycin 1 g PO in a single dose *Children age older than 8 yr (treat per adult regimens):* *Preferred regimens:* Azithromycin 1 g PO in a single dose *or* Doxycycline 100 mg PO twice daily × 7 days *Alternative regimens:* Erythromycin base 500 mg PO 4 times daily × 7 days Erythromycin ethylsuccinate 800 mg PO 4 times daily × 7 days Levofloxacin 500 mg PO daily × 7 days Ofloxacin 300 mg PO twice daily for 7 days
Neisseria gonorrhoeae	*Children weighing <45 kg:* Ceftriaxone, 125 mg IM in a single dose *Children weighing ≥45 kg:* Treat with adult regimen of 250 mg IM in a single dose *Children with bacteremia or arthritis:* Ceftriaxone, 50 mg/kg (max dose for children weighing <45 kg: 1 g) IM or IV in a single dose daily × 7 days *Dual treatment:* Addition of either azithromycin 1 g PO in a single dose or doxycycline 100 mg PO twice daily × 7 days to the above regimens may assist in hindering the development of antibiotic resistance. *Note:* The CDC removed cefixime 400 mg PO in a single dose from recommended medications because of increasing resistance; however, can be used as part of a dual therapy if ceftriaxone is unavailable
Trichomonas	Metronidazole, 15-30 mg/kg/day tid (max: 250 mg tid) × 5-7 days *or* Tinidazole 50 mg/kg (≤2 g) as a single dose for children older than 3 yr
Pinworms (*Enterobius vermicularis*)	Mebendazole (Vermox), 1 chewable 100 mg tablet, repeated in 2 wk *or* Albendazole, 100 mg for child younger than age 2 yr or 400 mg for older child, repeated in 2 wk Pyrantel pamoate 10 mg/kg in a single administration

MRSA, methicillin-resistant *Staphylococcus aureus*; TMP-SMX, trimethoprim-sulfamethoxazole.

frequent bathing, and application of water-repellant barriers such as zinc oxide. If diaper dermatitis persists after these conservative measures, or if the classic satellite lesions of *Candida* are present, treatment with an antifungal can decrease the inflammation.

Physiologic Leukorrhea
Neonates and peripubertal girls can present with a white or clear or mucus discharge, which is a physiologic effect of estrogen. Some girls complain of the moisture and mucus, but an explanation should reassure the patient and her mother.

Genital Ulcers
Acute genital ulceration of the vulva (Fig. 549-2) is described in young adolescents who are not sexually active and can occur in association with oral aphthous ulcers. Although linked to infectious causes such as Epstein-Barr, cytomegalovirus, mycoplasma, and influenza A, recent data suggest these ulcers may be idiopathic vulvar aphthoses.

Other potential etiologies include inflammatory bowel disease, Behçet disease, pemphigoid, Stevens-Johnson syndrome, drug eruption, or mouth and genital ulcers with inflamed cartilage (MAGIC) syndrome.

These lesions usually appear on the mucosal surfaces of the introitus as painful red or white lesions that evolve into sharply demarcated red-rimmed ulcers with a necrotic or eschar-like base. The time course is generally 10-14 days until remission occurs. The lesions are quite painful and pain management and urinary diversion with a Foley catheter may be necessary. Patients with acute genital ulcers show a fairly consistent picture of flu-like prodromal symptoms, dysuria, and

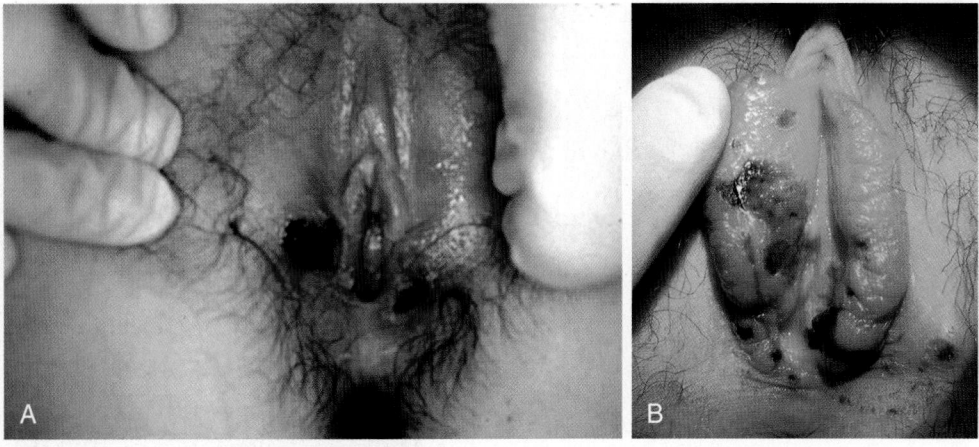

Figure 549-2 Aphthous ulcers. *(Photo courtesy of Diane F. Merritt, MD.)*

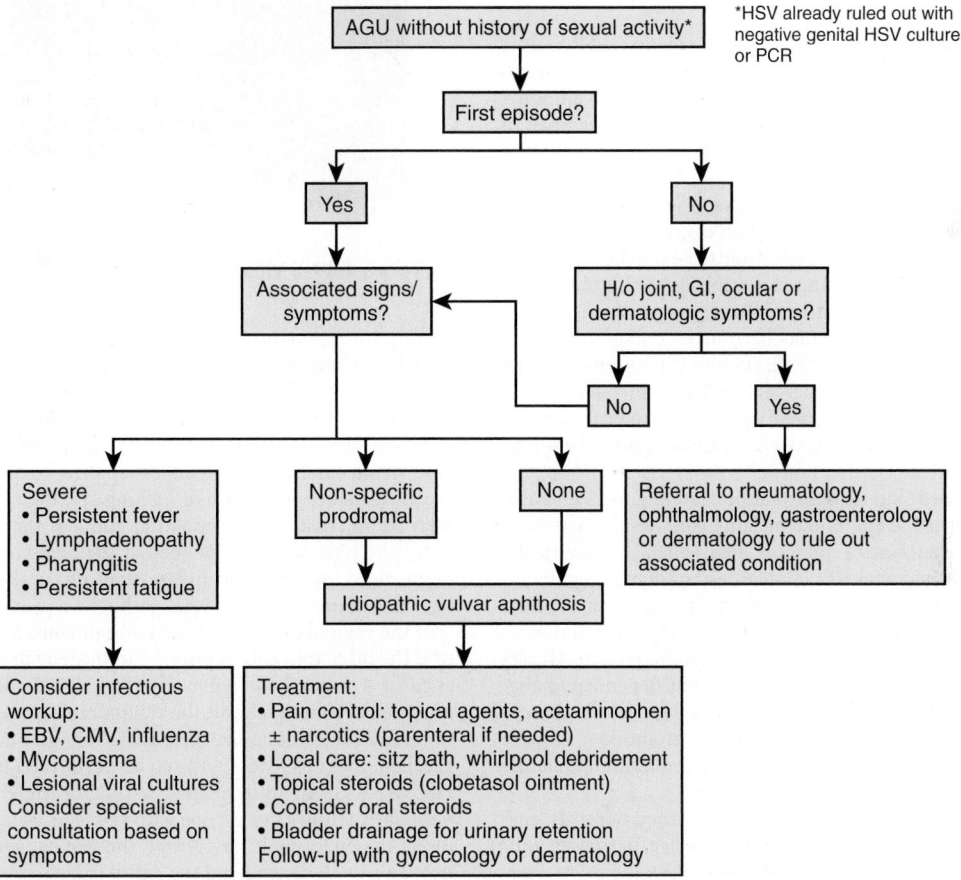

Figure 549-3 Algorithm for evaluation and management of acute genital ulcers in nonsexually active young girls. *(From Rosman IS, Berk DR, Bayliss SJ, et al: Acute genital ulcers in nonsexually active young girls: case series, review of the literature, and evaluation and management recommendations. Pediatr Dermatol 29(2);147–153, 2012.)*

vulvar pain. One-third of patients present with a history of or develop oral ulcerations. Evaluation includes culture for herpes simplex virus to exclude this etiology. Special testing for systemic disease depends on history. Biopsies are usually nondiagnostic as they yield acute and chronic inflammatory changes. Figure 549-3 outlines suggested evaluation and management for initial and recurrent disease. Evaluation for Behçet disease (see Chapter 161) using the International Study Group diagnostic guidelines should be considered with recurrent or severe cases. (See Table 549-1 for other common etiologies.) Treatment of acute genital ulcers should include topical Xylocaine 2% jelly, sitz baths, good hygiene, and acetaminophen. Nonsteroidal

antiinflammatory drug avoidance is suggested because of a possible causative link. Hospitalization may be required for pain management not controlled with oral narcotics, urinary retention requiring Foley catheterization or for whirlpool debridement should hygiene become difficult. Antibiotic treatment is not required unless evidence of bacterial superinfection exists or the patient is immunocompromised. Insufficient evidence exists to recommend whether oral steroid treatment is effective but may be helpful in the setting of recurrent outbreaks. Ultrapotent topical steroids (clobetasol 0.05% ointment), however, are beneficial in oral aphthous ulcers and may prove helpful in acute genital ulcers as well.

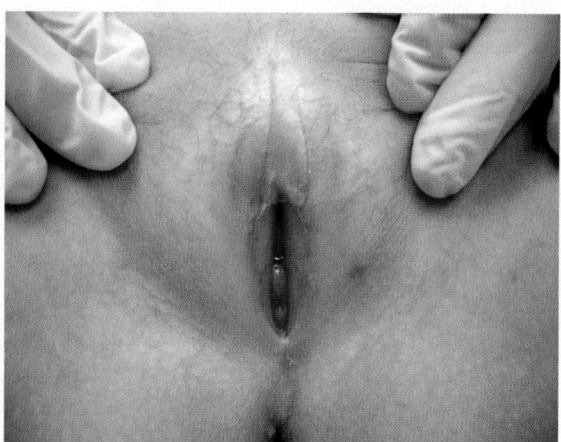

Figure 549-4 Lichen sclerosus. *(Photo courtesy of Diane F. Merritt, MD.)*

Dermatoses

Dermatologic conditions often affect the vulvar area in children; it is important to determine if the girl presenting with vulvar irritation has a skin condition elsewhere on the body. Lichen sclerosus is commonly seen in the anogenital region and has a characteristic appearance of white skin changes associated with areas of erosion, ulceration, and petechia. This disease can cause severe discomfort and most commonly presents with vulvar or perianal pruritus, dysuria, and constipation. Patients may also present without any symptoms, which may lead to underrecognition and under treatment. If untreated, lichen sclerosus can lead to destruction and scarring of normal genital architecture, including labial resorption, obliteration of the clitoris, narrowing of the introitus, and painful fissures that may become secondarily infected. Once thought to resolve with puberty, this theory is now controversial and many postmenarchal adolescents still suffer from disease (Fig. 549-4). Lichen sclerosis may be treated with potent topical steroids, clobetasol propionate 0.05% applied once or twice daily until the symptoms resolve.

Vitiligo is an acquired skin depigmentation resulting from an autoimmune process directed at epidermal melanocytes. Lesions appear as sharply demarcated patches of pigment loss, often symmetrically located around vagina and anal area. Similar lesions of hypopigmentation can be found surrounding body orifices and extensor surfaces (Fig. 549-5). Although diagnosis is clinical, there is an association with other autoimmune or endocrine disorders (hypothyroidism, Graves disease, Addison disease, pernicious anemia, insulin-dependent diabetes mellitus) and workup should include evaluation for at least thyroid dysfunction. Mild topical corticosteroid cream or ointment may be prescribed for children. Dermatologists may offer immunomodulators (tacrolimus), and phototherapy.

Vulvar psoriasis presents as pruritic, well-demarcated nonscaly, erythematous, symmetrical plaques that involve the vulva, perineum and/or gluteal folds. Lesions on the mons pubis may have the more characteristic scaly appearance. The classic signs of psoriasis may also be appreciated with pitting nail beds, posterior auricular erythema or a silvery scaling rash found elsewhere on the body. Many of the treatments used in adults may not be appropriate in children. Psoriasis may be treated with moisturizers, topical steroids, and light therapy. Teens may be treated with coal tar, retinoids, tacrolimus, and calcipotriene, which is a derivative of vitamin D_3.

DIAGNOSIS AND DIFFERENTIAL DIAGNOSIS

Children with symptoms of vulvovaginitis often have had a previous evaluations and treatment failures. Cultures with sensitivities to test for specific pathogens may be obtained with cotton swabs or urethral (Calgiswab) swabs moistened with nonbacteriostatic saline. Use of a swab can cause discomfort or, rarely, minimal bleeding. The premoistened swab can be placed vertically between the labia minora to collect secretions, as it is not necessary to place the swab into the vagina.

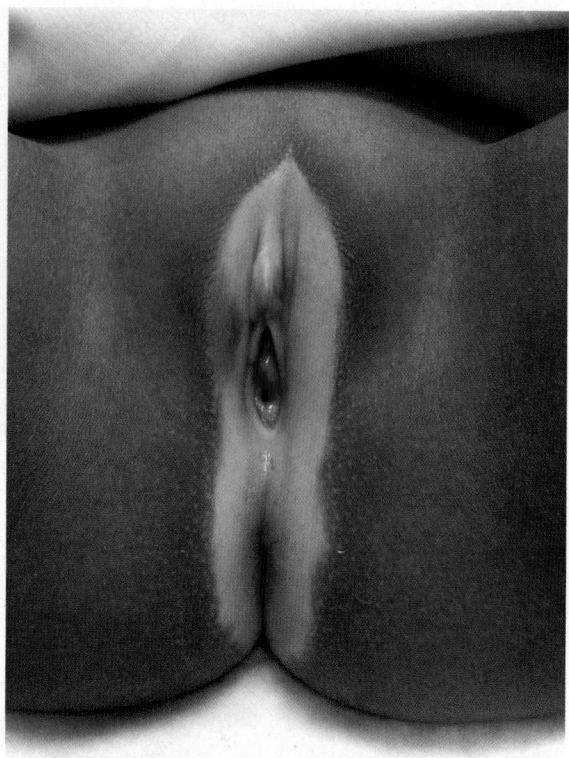

Figure 549-5 Vitiligo. *(Photo courtesy of Diane F. Merritt, MD.)*

Testing for gonorrhea and chlamydia may be done by culture or by nucleic acid amplification testing, depending on institutional or state and Centers for Disease Control guidelines. Tests for *Shigella* and *H. influenzae* might require special media and collection procedures.

If pinworms (see Chapter 294) are suspected, transparent adhesive tape or an anal swab should be applied to the anal region in the morning before defecation or bathing and then placed on a slide. Eggs seen on microscopic examination confirm the diagnosis, and sometimes the pinworms can be seen at the anal verge. Clinical history is often more indicative of disease than physical exam, and a negative tape test does not rule out this pathogen as a cause.

If the vaginal discharge is serosanguineous, if a foul odor is present, or if the discharge fails to respond to hygiene measures, consider presence of a vaginal foreign body (Fig. 549-6). If inspection suggests presence of a foreign body, the vagina can be irrigated, or an examination under anesthesia may reveal the foreign body. Vaginoscopy is an excellent diagnostic tool and can be performed in an unsedated cooperative patient in an outpatient setting, or under general anesthesia if necessary. Using a cystoscope with saline or water irrigation to gravity, insert the endoscopic device into the vagina, gently oppose the labia, the vagina will distend and the entire vaginal cavity and cervix may be easily assessed.

TREATMENT AND PREVENTION

The treatment of specific vulvovaginitis should be directed at the organism causing the symptoms (see Table 549-1). Treatment of nonspecific vulvovaginitis includes sitz baths and avoidance of irritating or harsh soaps and chemicals and tight clothing that abrades the perineum. External application of bland emollient barriers such as nonprescription diaper rash medications and petroleum jelly may be helpful. Proper perineal hygiene is critical for long-term improvement. Younger children need supervised perineal hygiene, and caregivers should be advised to wipe the genital area from front to back. Use of a warm moistened washcloth or diaper wipe is helpful after initially wiping with toilet tissue. Girls should wear cotton underwear and limit time spent in tights, leotards, jeggings, tight jeans, and wet swimsuits. Soaking in warm clean bathwater for 15 min intervals (no shampoo or

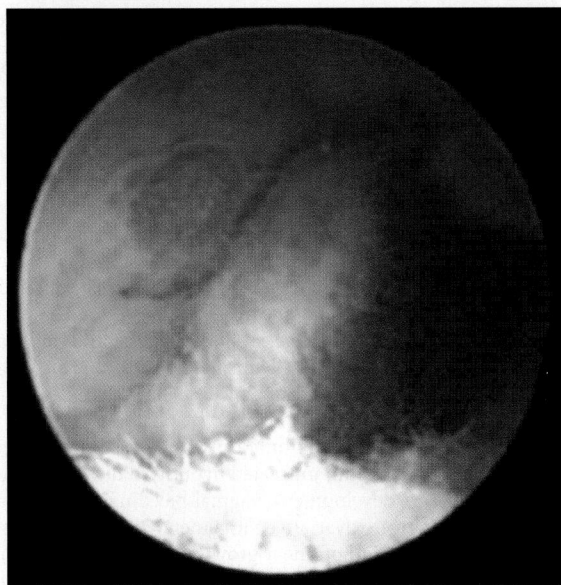

Figure 549-6 Vaginal foreign body as seen through vaginoscope. *(Photo courtesy of Diane F. Merritt, MD.)*

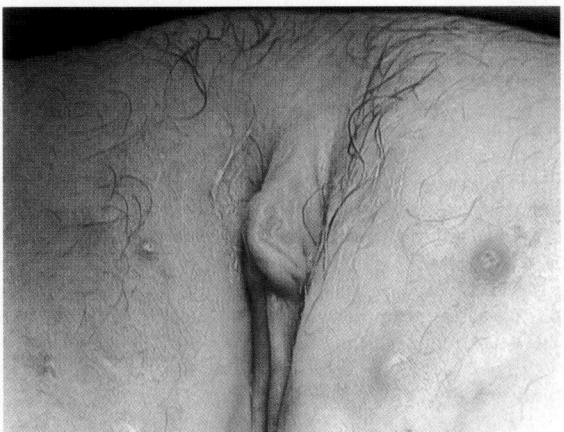

Figure 549-7 Molluscum contagiosum. *(Photo courtesy of Diane F. Merritt, MD.)*

bubble bath) is soothing and helps with cleaning the area. Parents should be counseled to avoid all scented, antiseptic, and deodorant-based soaps, and to eliminate the use of fabric softeners or dryer sheets when laundering undergarments.

Bibliography is available at Expert Consult.

Chapter **550**
Bleeding
Diane F. Merritt

Vaginal bleeding in infants and prepubescent children should always be evaluated. Bleeding can be seen as early as the 1st wk of life, resulting from endometrial sloughing associated with maternal estrogen withdrawal. A thorough history and physical must be obtained as the 1st step in evaluating the problem. Common causes for vaginal bleeding

in children are vulvovaginitis, vaginal foreign bodies, dermatologic conditions, and urethral prolapse; less common causes are endogenous or exogenous estrogenic effects; and the most worrisome causes include neoplasms and trauma.

Vulvovaginitis (see Chapter 549) may be caused by respiratory, oral and fecal pathogens, some of which produce serosanguineous drainage (e.g., *Streptococcus, Shigella*) or cause vulvar bleeding resulting from irritation and excoriation of the skin. Prepubertal girls are at a higher risk for developing these irritations because the protective labia of pubertal girls are not fully developed and thus, the vaginal opening and vagina are easily more exposed to irritants. Further, the hypoestrogenic vaginal mucosa is thin and lacks the protective effects of an acidic pH from lactobacilli. The alkaline vaginal pH noted in prepubertal girls results in an environment more prone to infection. Handwashing, improved perineal hygiene (wiping front to back, use of wet wipes after bowel movement), and avoidance of topical irritants, chemicals, and perfumed or deodorant soaps and bubble baths will reduce nonspecific vulvovaginitis. External application of bland emollient barriers such as over the counter diaper rash ointments or petroleum jelly may helpful (see Table 549-2 in Chapter 549). Antibiotics will help with recurrent or persistent infections if a specific pathogen is identified by culture.

Hematuria is suspected when the urine is red or brown. Gross hematuria may be confused with vaginal bleeding. A positive urinary dipstick can confirm blood, but pigments and metabolites may also cause red or brown urine (see Chapter 509). The cause of gross hematuria in symptomatic children is usually elicited by a complete history, physical examination and urinalysis. Additional diagnostic studies may include ultrasound of the kidneys and bladder, urine culture, measurements of urine calcium/creatinine, and serum C3 and creatinine. Treatment depends on the diagnosis.

Dermatoses may present with bleeding. Lichen sclerosus (see Fig. 549-4 and Table 549-1 in Chapter 549). is characterized by chronic inflammation, intense pruritus, loss of normal architecture, thinning and whitening of the vulvar and perianal skin often in a butterfly or keyhole distribution. Petechiae or blood blisters can arise and be mistaken as a sign of sexual abuse. Diagnosis is based on these classic clinical characteristics, but may be confirmed by a tissue biopsy if necessary. As a first-line treatment, potent topical steroids, such as clobetasol propionate ointment 0.05%,may be applied sparingly to the affected tissue 1-2 times a day under physician supervision; they usually result in improvements in appearance and pruritus. The steroid should be used for the shortest duration necessary then be stopped or tapered. Flare-ups can occur and require retreatment.

Foreign bodies are a common cause of vaginal bleeding, and children present with blood-stained and foul-smelling discharge. The most common object found in prepubertal girls is toilet paper. A physical exam in knee–chest or frogleg position can sometimes reveal the object. Vaginal irrigation may be done in the office setting using a small feeding tube, a syringe, and warm water. If the object is not visible on examination, irrigation is unlikely to remove it and examination under anesthesia and vaginoscopy are often required. Vaginoscopy not only allows removal of a foreign object but also can facilitate diagnosis of other causes of the bleeding.

Trauma to the vulva or vagina is especially concerning. Most of these injuries are accidental, but physical and sexual abuse must be ruled out (see Chapter 40). Straddle injuries such as falling on the cross bar of a bicycle or slipping in the bathtub may result in bruising, hematomas, and lacerations. In general, if the trauma is accidental, the hymen and vagina are spared as most accidental injuries involve the mons and labia. *If there are no eyewitnesses to the injury, if there is no history to explain the clinical findings, and especially if there is a laceration of the hymen, abuse must be considered in the differential diagnosis, and a forensic interview of the patient and family should take place.* If the injury is penetrating, further examination and imaging are necessary to evaluate the urethra, bladder, anus, and intraabdominal structures. General anesthesia may be needed to fully assess injuries and allow adequate repair; while minor lacerations may be repaired in a cooperative child under sedation or local anesthesia. If the patient is able to void spontaneously, nonexpanding hematomas can be observed and treated with ice, pressure, and pain medications. Large expanding hematomas should be carefully evaluated and may require drainage, ligation of the bleeding vessels, and/or placement of a closed suction drain, especially if the overlying skin is showing signs of necrosis. A Foley catheter should be placed for children who are having difficulty with voiding.

Urethral prolapse (see Chapter 544) is another potential cause of bleeding in the prepubertal girl. The patient may present with a circular protrusion of the urethral mucosa through the external meatus forming a friable vulvar mass. Downward traction at the introitus enables visualization of the vaginal orifice separate from the urethral mass and assists with confirming the correct diagnosis. Patients may be asymptomatic or present with bleeding, dysuria, or difficulty with urination. Low estrogen state, trauma, chronic cough, and constipation are believed to be predisposing factors. Treatment is conservative, with application of estrogen cream at the area of prolapse twice daily for 1-2 wk and then, if prolapse is still present, continued use until the prolapse resolves. Surgical excision is very rarely necessary to remove necrotic tissue.

Neoplasms of the vulva and vagina are rare (see Chapter 553). Infantile hemangiomas are the most common benign vascular neoplasm of infancy, affecting 5% of all infants. Most lesions proliferate then involute, and only a few require intervention. Hemangiomas of the perineum may be associated with spinal dysraphism, so a neurologic assessment should be performed. Intralesion and systemic steroids have been used to treat infantile hemangiomas. Propranolol therapy results in a good response rate. Laser therapy and surgical excision are sometimes used.

Like hemangiomas, hymenal polyps are usually benign. If these polyps are noted at birth, they generally regress after maternal levels of estrogen decrease in the infant. If hymenal polyps persist, grow, or cause discomfort they may be removed. Vaginal polyps, especially if they cause bleeding, should be removed (not followed) and sent for pathologic evaluation. Yolk sac (endodermal sinus) tumors of the vagina are rare but may cause vaginal bleeding. Serum α-fetoprotein is a reliable marker. Rhabdomyosarcoma is the most common soft-tissue sarcoma of childhood. In children, the most common sites are the head and neck (35%) and genitourinary region (25%) (see Chapter 500). Rhabdomyosarcoma arising in the genitourinary tract are commonly the sarcoma botryoides variant and are typically seen in the 1st decade, often before age 3 yr, and present with vaginal discharge and bleeding. Treatment consists of a multimodal approach, including surgery, radiation therapy, and chemotherapy. The survival rate is >90% when an early diagnosis is made.

Vaginal bleeding can be a presenting sign of precocious puberty, which is defined as pubertal development that is 2.5-3.0 SD earlier than the average age. Guidelines for the evaluation of premature development state that pubic hair or breast development requires evaluation generally when it occurs before age 7 yr in non–African-American girls and before age 6 yr in African-American girls (see Chapters 561 and 562). Rapidity of pubertal progression, such as Tanner stage 3 breast development before 8 yr of age, may also require evaluation. The most common etiology is gonadotropin-dependent or central precocious puberty (see Chapter 562.1) where there is premature enhancement of pulsatile gonadotropin-releasing hormone release resulting in ovarian follicle growth and estrogen production. Gonadotropin-independent precocious puberty, where estrogen production is not under hypothalamic control and is produced peripherally, such as from an ovarian/adrenal tumor or McCune Albright syndrome, is less common.

A thorough physical exam must be done, looking for secondary sex characteristics and documenting breast and pubic hair development using the Sexual Maturation Index (Tanner Staging; see Chapter 110.1). Documenting height and weight on a growth chart will assist in identifying accelerated growth velocity. Diagnostic tests include a left wrist x-ray to look for advanced bone age. Elevated serum luteinizing hormone levels are highly suggestive of central precocity, but the gold standard is measurement of gonadotropins after gonadotropin-releasing hormone or gonadotropin-releasing hormone–agonist stimulation. In all cases of central precocious puberty, MRI imaging of the brain is needed to determine if a tumor is present. Pelvic ultrasound might show presence of ovarian or adrenal pathology or uterine maturation in response to estrogen. Benign premature ovarian follicles or malignant ovarian germ cell tumors can produce elevated serum estradiol levels >100 pg/mL. If the estradiol is elevated, pelvic imaging by transabdominal ultrasound is mandated. Usually benign ovarian follicles produce short periods of estrogen elevation which is enough to stimulate the endometrial lining and result in endometrial shedding. Usually by the time the pelvic ultrasound is obtained the follicular structure has collapsed and resolved and the estrogen level has dropped to prepubertal range. If indicated central precocious puberty can be suppressed with leuprolide injections or histrelin implants. Germ cell tumors are treated by excision, staging and chemo or radiation therapy by protocols provided by oncologists.

Juvenile hypothyroidism commonly causes pubertal delay. Patients with severe, long-standing and untreated hypothyroidism may present with premature breast development, vaginal bleeding and abdominal distention resulting from ovarian enlargement and possibly ascites associated with deceleration of linear growth. A proposed mechanism is thyroid-releasing hormone–associated elevations of thyroid-stimulating hormone crossreacting with follicle-stimulating hormone resulting in follicle maturation and estradiol production. Treatment of the hypothyroidism results in improvement and reversal of symptoms.

Another etiology for childhood vaginal bleeding is exogenous exposures to estrogens. These exposures can occur from ingestion of birth control pills, foods, beauty products, and plastics that contain estrogen or estrogen-like components. Several other studies have assessed the risk of bisphenol A leaching from plastic cups and bottles. The importance of this is still being studied, but bisphenol A is known to have an estrogenic effect and thus could potentially be a cause for vaginal bleeding if ingested in high levels.

Vaginal bleeding in the prepubertal girl or infant can have many causes, which range from benign to malignant. A thoughtful history and physical examination must be done to identify the source of bleeding so that treatment can occur. The risk benefit of any therapy should be reviewed carefully with the family.

Bibliography is available at Expert Consult.

Chapter **551**
Breast Concerns
Kora N. Felsch and Diane F. Merritt

Presenting concerns of girls with breast disorders typically including the development or appearance of their breasts, breast pain, nipple discharge, or concerns about the presence of a mass. Although children and adolescents are very unlikely to have malignant or life-threatening breast problems, this population of patients should be referred to practitioners who have experience and familiarity with the immature and developing breast to avoid overtreatment with unnecessary diagnostic or surgical procedures.

BREAST DEVELOPMENT

Development of the breast begins around wk 5 of gestation, when the ectoderm on the anterior body wall thickens into 2 ridges known as the *mammary ridges*. They extend from the area of the developing axilla to the area of the developing inguinal canal. The ridge above and below the area of the pectoralis muscle recedes in utero, leaving the mammary primordium, which is the origin of the lactiferous ducts.

The initial lactiferous ducts form between wk 10 and 20 and become interspersed through the developing mesenchyme, which becomes the fibrous and fatty portions of the breast. The breast bud, under the stimulation of maternal estrogen, becomes palpable at wk 34 of gestation. This breast bud regresses within the 1st mo of life, because the estrogen stimulation is no longer present. The areola appears at 5 mo of gestation, and the nipple is seen shortly after birth. It is initially depressed and later becomes elevated.

Thelarche, or the onset of pubertal breast development, is hormonally mediated and normally occurs between the ages of 8 and 13 yr, with an average age of 10.3 yr. The initiation of thelarche and progression in females is affected by race, with normal thelarche occurring earlier in African-American girls than in white or Asian girls. This occurs when the hypothalamus releases gonadotropin-releasing hormone, which stimulates the pituitary gland to produce follicle-stimulating hormone and luteinizing hormone, which then stimulates the ovaries to produce estrogen. The estrogen leads to breast development.

Once thelarche is initiated, normal development of the breast occurs over 2-4 yr and is classified by the **sexual maturity rating** system (also known as Tanner Staging) into 5 stages (Chapter 110.1). Maturation can sometimes occur asymmetrically owing to fluctuation of the hormonal environments and various end organ sensitivities. Lack of development by age 13 yr is considered delayed and warrants endocrinology evaluation. Menarche usually occurs approximately 2 yr after initiation of breast development.

BREAST EXAMINATION
A breast examination should be included in the annual examination of all children and adolescents. Examination of the *newborn* includes assessment of breast size, nipple position, presence of accessory nipples, and nipple discharge. Examination of the *prepubertal girl* includes inspection and palpation of the chest wall for masses, pain, nipple discharge, and signs of premature thelarche. Examination of the *adolescent* is performed with the patient in the supine position; the arm ipsilateral to the breast that is being examined should be placed next to the patient's head. The breast tissue is examined with the flat pads of the middle fingers and the examiner can feel for abnormalities on the breast with a pattern similar to spokes on a wheel, in a circular clockwise pattern with concentric circles or by moving in a rotary fashion around the breast. Whatever the method used, the goal is to palpate all the breast tissue in a uniform fashion. The sexual maturity rating should be noted and axillary, supraclavicular, and infraclavicular nodes evaluated for lymphadenopathy. The areola should be compressed to assess for nipple discharge.

BREAST SELF-EXAMINATION
Controversy exists as to the utility of breast self-examination in the adolescent population. Experts believe that it might be ill advised to encourage breast self-examination in the adolescent because of a potential for unnecessary anxiety and possible unwarranted treatment in a population that is at low risk for malignant disease. The American College of Obstetricians and Gynecologists states that despite a lack of definitive data for or against breast self-examination, breast self-examination may be recommended beginning at age 19 yr. Women with previous exposure to *therapeutic chest radiation* therapy are advised to begin breast self-examination 8 yr after radiation therapy.

ABNORMAL DEVELOPMENT
Neonatal Breast Abnormalities
The condition in which breasts enlarge in the newborn period is *neonatal breast hypertrophy*. This is quite common in term infants of either sex and can occur as a result of elevated circulating maternal endogenous steroid hormones in late gestation. As maternal estrogen levels fall, prolactin levels can increase and the breasts can produce a clear or cloudy (milk-like) nipple discharge ("witch's milk") in male and female infants. Repeated manipulation of the breast can exacerbate the condition. On occasion, the hypertrophy is associated with mastitis

caused by a staphylococcal or streptococcal infection; antibiotics should be administered.

Precocious Puberty
Premature thelarche is usually an isolated condition and is more common than previously thought. In one study, patients with a sexual maturity rating 2 or greater at 7 yr of age were 10.4% of white, 23.4% of black non-Hispanic, and 14.9% of Hispanic girls. However, it may also be the first symptom of precocious puberty. Precocious puberty occurs in 14-18% of girls with premature thelarche (see Chapter 562). Serial examinations, with particular emphasis on growth velocity, secondary sex characters such as pubic hair, pigmentation of the labia or areola, or vaginal bleeding are imperative to identify precocious puberty. Unless there are associated signs of precocious puberty, the parents should be reassured and the child should be followed.

Amastia
Complete absence of the breast, or amastia, is rare and is thought to occur from lack of formation or obliteration of the mammary ridge. Amastia is usually unilateral and can be congenital or associated with systemic disorders (e.g., ectodermal dysplasia, Crohn disease) or endocrine disorders (e.g., congenital adrenal hyperplasia, gonadal dysgenesis, hypogonadotropic hypogonadism). Novel gene mutations have been discovered that may be linked to syndromic amastia, including *PTPRF*, a protein tyrosine receptor type F gene, and ectodysplasin A receptor *(EDAR)*. It can be associated with anomalies of the underlying mesoderm, such as abnormal pectoralis muscles seen in Poland syndrome (aplasia of the pectoralis muscles, rib deformities, webbed fingers, and radial nerve aplasia) (Fig. 551-1). Amastia or hypomastia can also be iatrogenic, resulting from injuries sustained during thoracotomy, chest tube placement, radiotherapy, severe burns, and inappropriate biopsy of the breast bud. Treatment is surgical correction.

Polymastia and Polythelia
Supernumerary breast tissue (polymastia) and accessory nipples (polythelia) occur in approximately 1-6% of the population (Fig. 551-2). The abnormally placed tissue can be seen anywhere along the mammary ridges as a result of incomplete involution but is usually noted on the chest, upper abdomen, or just inferior to the normally positioned breast. There is an association between polythelia and anomalies of the urinary and cardiovascular system. Surgical excision of the accessory breasts or nipple is not usually needed. Resection of accessory tissue may be warranted if the patient has pain or for cosmetic reasons.

Breast Asymmetry and Hypomastia
Some degree of asymmetry is normal in women, and it may be more pronounced during puberty while the breasts are developing.

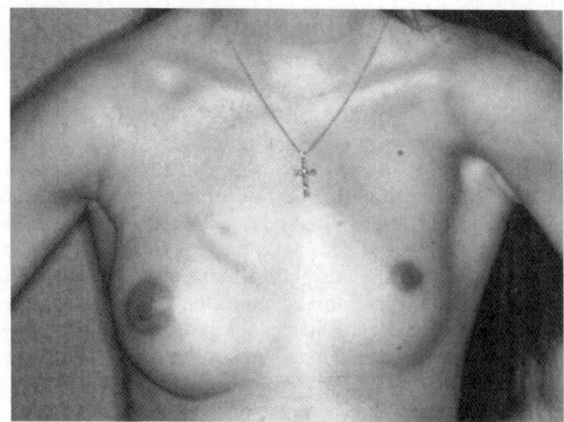

Figure 551-1 Preoperative frontal view of a patient with left breast hypoplasia secondary to Poland syndrome. (*From Sadove AM, van Aalst JA: Congenital and acquired pediatric breast anomalies: a review of 20 years' experience, Plast Reconstr Surg 115:1039–1050, 2005, Fig. 13A.*)

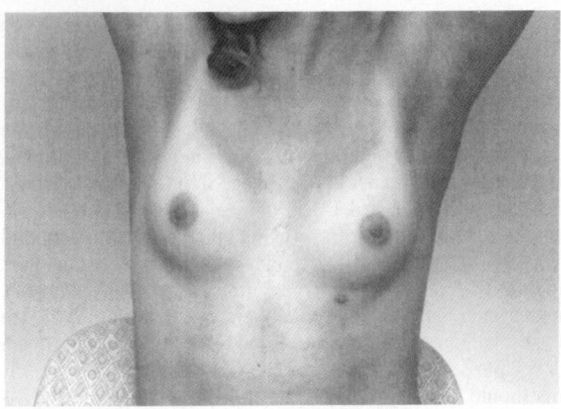

Figure 551-2 Accessory nipple located inferior to the left breast. *(From Sadove AM, van Aalst JA: Congenital and acquired pediatric breast anomalies: a review of 20 years' experience, Plast Reconstr Surg 115:1039–1050, 2005, Fig. 3.)*

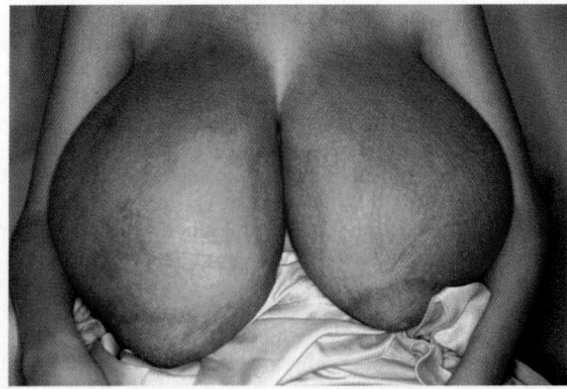

Figure 551-3 Virginal mammary hypertrophy in a 12 yr old female. *(From Al-Saif AA, Al-Yahya GM, Al-Qattan MM: Juvenile mammary hypertrophy: Is reduction mammoplasty always feasible? J Plast Reconstr Aesthet Surg 62:1470–1472, 2009, Fig. 1.)*

Table 551-1	Differential Diagnosis of Macromastia	
Juvenile hypertrophy	Adrenal cortical tumors
Tumors of the breast	Exogenous hormones
Giant fibroadenoma	Estrogen
Hamartoma	Testosterone
Cystosarcoma phyllodes	Gonadotropins
Carcinoma	Corticosterone
Hormonally active tumors	Medications
Ovarian granulosa cell tumor	Cannabis
Ovarian follicular cysts	

From Desilva N, Brandt M: Breast disorders in children and adolescents. In Sanfilippo J, Lara-Torre E, editors: Clinical pediatric and adolescent gynecology, London, 2008, Taylor & Francis.

Hypoplasia of the breasts varies in degree from a nearly total absence of breast tissue to well-formed breasts that are considered by the patient to be too small. There are several causes for poor or absent breast development. The onset of breast development may be delayed with normal secondary sex characters; the breasts develop slowly but are normal in all other respects; a patient's family history might include late breast development. Other causes include ovarian dysfunction, hypothyroidism, and chest wall irradiation or surgery. Hypoplastic breast tissue can also be associated with a tuberous breast anomaly. Treatment depends on the underlying cause. Patients with mild asymmetry and with no other associated pathology should be reassured. Surgical correction is an option for women with marked asymmetry but should be delayed until after puberty.

Juvenile or Virginal Hypertrophy

Spontaneous massive growth of the breasts during puberty and adolescence is thought to be the result of excessive end-organ sensitivity to gonadal hormones, although both the hormone receptors and serum estradiol levels are normal. The underlying cause, if any, should be determined and removed (Table 551-1). When growth is extreme it is termed *macromastia* or *gigantomastia*. It is more commonly bilateral, often occurs over a brief period, and most commonly affects adolescent girls (Fig. 551-3). Physical and psychologic problems can affect posture and quality of life. Strong emotional support should be provided as this can affect an adolescent's self-esteem at a vulnerable time in her psychologic development. Management should be individualized and may range from reassurance or the use of supportive brassieres to reduction mammoplasty or even mastectomy. Medical therapy, such as tamoxifen, is available to slow breast growth in extreme cases until surgery can be performed. Surgical intervention often necessitates relocation of the nipple, which can result in decreased sensation and altered lactation, and it is not uncommon for the lesion to recur.

INFECTIONS

Mastitis is the most common infection of the breast. Although it is most common in lactating mothers, it can occur in young infants and adolescents. Neonatal mastitis is an infection that usually occurs in term or near-term infants. It should be treated aggressively to reduce the risk of forming abscesses. Adolescents can develop nonlactational mastitis or a breast abscess for unknown reasons, as a result of irritation of the skin (through shaving or nipple stimulation), trauma, a foreign body (e.g., piercing), ductal abnormality (such as ductal ectasia), or infection of an epidermal cyst. The initial therapy of all breast infections is antibiotics and analgesics. *Staphylococcus aureus* (see Chapter 181.1) or anaerobic bacilli (*bacteroides*) are the offending organism is almost all cases, and methicillin-resistant *S. aureus* coverage should be considered in communities where prevalence is high. Owing to the potential for breast abscess, the neonatal population should be treated with parenteral antibiotics for methicillin-resistant *S. aureus* or guided by gram stain, when available. Adolescents may be initially treated with warm compresses and oral antibiotics. Abscesses should be surgically evaluated (with ultrasound guidance if necessary) and drained as necessary. If incision and drainage is performed, a small, periareolar incision is indicated.

TRAUMA AND INFLAMMATION

Breast trauma is common in adolescent girls participating in contact sports. The trauma usually takes the form of contusion or hematoma and can resolve spontaneously or may be associated with late cystic changes in the breast or fibrosis with retraction of the skin or the nipple over the injured area.

NIPPLE DISCHARGE

Nipple discharge must be carefully evaluated and a distinction made among galactorrhea (milky white discharge), blood, or other discharge (Table 551-2). A careful history and physical examination directed at the possible etiologies of galactorrhea will help the practitioner determine the etiology. Examination of the discharge assists in diagnosis. Benign conditions are usually associated with a milky, sticky, thick discharge; infection is associated with a purulent discharge; intraductal papilloma and cancer are associated with a serous, serosanguineous, or bloody discharge. Preoperative evaluations by mammography, hemoccult, ductography, and cytology are poor predictors of histologic diagnosis. Therefore, patients with pathologic nipple discharge should undergo biopsy for accurate diagnosis.

Galactorrhea

Cytologic evaluation of nipple discharge is not recommended. Serum pregnancy testing and prolactin and thyroid levels are obtained to rule out the presence of a thyroid abnormality, a pituitary prolactinoma, and pregnancy (in the postpubertal adolescent). If the prolactin level

Table 551-2	Common Causes of Nipple Discharge

Pregnancy
Medicines
Hormones (oral contraceptives, estrogen, progesterone)
Blood pressure drugs (methyldopa, verapamil)
Tricyclic antidepressants
Tranquilizers (antipsychotics)
Antinausea drugs (metoclopramide)
Herbs (nettle, fennel, blessed thistle, anise, fenugreek seed)
Illicit drugs (marijuana, opiates)
Stimulation of the breast (sexual or from exercise)
Thyroid abnormalities
Chronic emotional stress
Hypothalamic tumors
Chest wall conditions
Herpes zoster
Trauma
Burns
Tumors
Breast conditions
Mammary duct ectasia
Chronic cystic mastitis
Intraductal cysts
Intraductal papillomas

Table 551-3	Breast Masses in the Adolescent Girl

BENIGN
Fibroadenoma
Fibrocystic changes or cysts
Unilateral thelarche
Hemangioma
Intramammary lymph node
Fat necrosis
Abscess
Mastitis
Lipoma
Hematoma
Hamartoma
Macromastia (juvenile hypertrophy)
Galactocele
Intraductal papilloma
Juvenile papillomatosis
Lymphangioma

MALIGNANT
Malignant cystosarcoma phyllodes
Breast carcinoma
Metastatic disease
Lymphoma, neuroblastoma, sarcoma, rhabdomyosarcoma, acute
  leukemia

Data from Dehner LP, Hill DA, Deschryver K: Pathology of the breast in children, adolescents, and young adults, Semin Diagn Pathol 16:235–247, 1999; Simmons PS: Diagnostic considerations in breast disorders of children and adolescents, Obstet Gynecol Clin North Am 19:91–102, 1992; and Divasta AD, Weldon C, Labow BI: The breast examination and lesions. In Emans SJ, Laufer MR, Goldstein DP, editors: Pediatric and adolescent gynecology, ed 6, Philadelphia, 2012, Lippincott Williams & Wilkins, pp. 405–420.

is elevated, visual field studies and a head MRI might reveal presence of a pituitary adenoma (see Chapter 560). Treatment is directed by results of history, physical exam, and lab studies. Patients should be instructed to avoid nipple stimulation and stop any offending drugs. Hypothyroidism should be treated and prolactin tumors managed with appropriate medical or surgical care. Treatment of galactorrhea (not thyroid related) consists primarily of dopamine agonists such as bromocriptine or cabergoline. Surgical intervention, usually transsphenoidal hypophysectomy, is rarely required.

Bloody Discharge

In adolescent athletes, bloody discharge may be due to chronic nipple irritation (jogger's nipple), discharge from the ducts of Montgomery (on the edge of the areola, not through the nipple) or duct ectasia. Cytologic assessment should be performed. Surgical consultation for a mass is indicated because intraductal breast papillomas have occurred in adolescents. However, there have been no reported cases of breast cancer in infants. Bloody nipple discharge in infants is most likely from mammary duct ectasia, and if the following studies are normal (prolactin, estradiol, thyrotropin, and ultrasound) then watchful waiting may be appropriate.

MASTALGIA

The most common causes of breast pain in adolescents are exercise and benign breast changes. Physiologic swelling and tenderness occur on a cyclic basis, most commonly during the premenstrual phase, and are secondary to hormonal stimulation and resulting proliferative changes. Hormonal imbalance can cause exaggerated responses in the breast tissue, especially in the upper and outer quadrants. Nodularity, poorly localized tenderness, and a soreness radiating to the axilla and arm are usual accompanying findings. The preferable term for these changes is *benign breast changes* rather than fibrocystic disease. Treatments recommended for this condition and exercise-induced pain include a firm supportive sports-type bra, heat, and analgesics. Oral contraceptives often improve the breast pain. A course of nonsteroidal antiinflammatory drugs is also effective. Methylxanthines (caffeine in coffee, tea, carbonated drinks) and smoking should be eliminated. Evening primrose oil and vitamin E are popular but unproven treatments.

BREAST MASSES
Peripubertal Masses

A mass in the developing breast can be of concern to the adolescent and her family. Initial breast development at the onset of thelarche can be asymmetric and thus mistaken for a "mass." The breast bud is palpable in these cases and should be distinguishable. Such asynchronous

thelarche should be recognized to avoid biopsy and potential injury to the maturing breast. If there is any question, ultrasound can be used to evaluate for a mass. Unilateral thelarche has also been reported as a side effect of cimetidine and is reversible when the medication is stopped.

Common Adolescent Breast Masses

Table 551-3 shows the differential diagnosis for breast masses in the adolescent patient. The patient should be questioned about the variation in symptoms with the menstrual cycle, associated symptoms such as nipple discharge, recent trauma to the breast, family history of breast masses or cancer, and history of chest radiation or malignancy. Because breast cancer in the adolescent is extremely rare, masses can be expectantly managed for extended periods with little concern for malignancy in this population.

The most common solid mass seen in adolescent girls is the **fibroadenoma**. Fibroadenomas are most often located in the upper outer quadrant of the breast. The average size is 2-3 cm, and 10-25% of patients have multiple lesions. The physical examination is usually diagnostic because these lesions are well circumscribed, rubbery, mobile, and not tender. In equivocal cases, an ultrasound may be helpful in making the diagnosis. Mammography is not indicated in the adolescent patient.

Fibroadenomas can develop because of a local exaggerated response to estrogen stimulation, and they can enlarge during the menstrual cycle. These lesions may be safely watched for at least 2 menstrual cycles, and some investigators suggest observation until adulthood. Approximately 10% of fibroadenomas regress spontaneously. The option of expectantly managing the patient until adulthood should be considered because the risk of primary cancer is very low in this population. If expectant management is chosen, serial ultrasounds every 6-12 mo may be done to ensure that the mass does not have malignant characteristics on imaging and that it is not enlarging or changing in contour until it starts regressing at which time the ultrasounds can be done on longer intervals. Approximately 4% of fibroadenomas grow, and so fine-needle aspiration or excision is recommended when a mass is enlarging, grows >5 cm (because of the risk of giant fibroadenoma or **cystosarcoma phyllodes**), or the mass is causing anxiety to the patient or her family. Combined estrogen-progesterone birth control pills have been found to be protective of fibroadenomas.

Cysts are very common masses seen in the pediatric breast. Cysts vary in size over the course of a menstrual cycle, so a patient with a possible cyst should be reexamined a few weeks after the initial evaluation to see if the mass is still present. If a mass persists, then it may be imaged by sonography or aspirated with a needle to evaluate if it truly is a cyst. Aspirated fluid that is clear may be discarded. Bloody fluid and other aspirated material should be sent for cytology. Cystic lesions that resolve with aspiration should be reevaluated in 3 mo. If they recur they should be evaluated with sonography.

Malignant Masses
Primary breast cancer is extremely rare in adolescents. Surveillance Epidemiology and End Results data from 1975-2009 establishes an incidence of invasive breast cancer of 0.2/100,000 for females ages 15-19 yr and 1.6/100,000 for females ages 20-24 yr. Although malignancy is rare, lesions with suspicious imaging findings or progressive growth should undergo cytologic or histologic examination. A small study in Austria noted a 4.7% malignancy rate among palpable masses in teens.

Cystosarcoma phyllodes can occur in adolescents and has been reported in a child as young as 10 yr old. It is characterized by asymmetric breast enlargement in association with a firm, mobile, circumscribed mass. It can mimic a giant fibroadenoma. The tumor often grows rapidly and can become quite large. The majority of these tumors have a favorable prognosis, but malignant cystosarcoma phyllodes has been reported to recur both locally and with metastases. Fatal metastatic cystosarcoma phyllodes in an adolescent has occurred. Excision with 1 cm margins is the preferred initial therapy in adolescent patients, regardless of the histologic classification of the lesion.

Juvenile papillomatosis is a marker for increased breast cancer risk in family members, and in patients with these, up to 15% may have a juvenile secretory carcinoma. Treatment of juvenile papillomatosis is total resection of the lesion with preservation of the breast.

Secondary cancers in adolescents with previous therapeutic radiation to the chest or with malignancies with the potential to metastasize to the breast should be monitored more closely for breast masses. Rhabdomyosarcoma is the most common to metastasize to the breast. Breast tumors also may be the first manifestation of relapse (extramedullary) in acute lymphoblastic leukemia.

Imaging of Breast Masses
Because the dense breast tissue of the adolescent obstructs the visualization of a palpable mass, mammography is not advised for this age group. Ultrasonography is the imaging modality of choice for breast abnormalities in the pediatric population. Color Doppler ultrasound can be useful in evaluating breast abnormalities such as fibroadenomas or abscesses.

Recommendations for Daughters of Women with Breast Cancer
Risk Reduction
There are a limited number of things that young women can do to lower their risk of breast cancer. The American Cancer Society recommends regular physical activity, limiting alcohol, and maintaining a healthy weight. Breastfeeding has a slight effect on breast cancer risk and that effect is only among women who have breastfed for a long time. Breastfeeding seems to be more protective against the most aggressive types of breast cancer, including tumors in women with mutations in the *BRCA-1* gene, hormone-receptor negative, and possibly triple-negative tumors.

Screening Procedures
Breast self-examination is an option for women starting in their 20s. Women should be told about the benefits and limitations of breast self-examination. Women should report any breast changes to their health professional. Women in their 20s and 30s should have a clinical breast exam as part of a periodic (regular) health exam by a health

professional, at least every 3 yr. After age 40 yr, women should have a breast exam by a health professional every year and a screening mammogram every year and should continue to do so for as long as they are in good health.

Genetic Testing in Children
Genetic testing for mutations in cancer susceptibility genes in children is particularly complex. Both parents and providers may request or recommend testing for minor children; however, many experts (including the American Society of Clinical Oncology) recommend that unless there is evidence that the test result will influence the medical management of the child or adolescent, genetic testing should be deferred until legal adulthood (18 yr or older) because of concerns about autonomy, potential discrimination, and possible psychosocial effects.

COSMETIC SURGERY
A dramatic increase in adolescents desiring breast augmentation has occurred since the turn of the century. Breast augmentation in adolescents is discouraged owing to associated psychologic and physical immaturity. The American Society of Plastic Surgeons discourages breast augmentation in girls younger than age 18 yr for purely cosmetic reasons. The FDA also considers breast implants in adolescents younger than age 18 yr for solely cosmetic reasons to be an off-label use.

Breast reduction surgery might be considered when an adolescent is bothered by extremely large breasts that result in neck and back pain and prevent participation in sports. Breast reduction allows these girls to feel less self-conscious, have less pain, and be more active. Also girls with marked asymmetry in breasts from the pathologies noted earlier can feel self-conscious and request breast surgery. Before performing breast-altering surgery, practitioners must ensure proper selection of teens and families who have an appropriate understanding of the risks and benefits of surgery and realistic expectations of the procedure.

Bibliography is available at Expert Consult.

Chapter **552**
Polycystic Ovary Syndrome and Hirsutism
Mark Gibson and Heather G. Huddleston

POLYCYSTIC OVARY SYNDROME
Etiology and Definition
Polycystic ovary syndrome (PCOS) is a common disorder of reproductive hormone function that is characterized by the triad of oligoovulation or anovulation, clinical or biochemical hyperandrogenism, and ovaries with a polycystic morphology on ultrasound examination (≥12 follicles in 1 ovary and/or ovarian volume >10 mm^3). Various expert bodies prioritize these elements differently for establishing the diagnosis, and few require the presence of all 3 (Table 552-1). Hyperandrogenism with ovulatory dysfunction (with exclusion of other causes) is most often considered sufficient for diagnosis in the United States. Abnormalities commonly associated with PCOS include obesity, insulin resistance, and the metabolic syndrome, but the phenotype is variable and affected individuals may display none of these. The disorder, affecting 5-8% of women of reproductive age, typically emerges in adolescence when a normal menstrual pattern is not established and there is clinical evidence of androgen excess.

Pathology Pathogenesis and Genetics

PCOS has a high concordance rate in twins, and in some studies either epigenetic or dominant inheritance patterns are observed. Nonetheless, a consistent hereditary pattern has not been identified.

Gonadotropic dysregulation with increased luteinizing hormone (LH) pulsatility and abnormally high ratios of circulating LH to follicle-stimulating hormone (FSH) are found in many patients with PCOS. Increased *ovarian* production of androgen in response to LH and impaired folliculogenesis owing to lower FSH are attributed to this gonadotropic pattern. Abnormal regulation of gonadotropin-releasing hormone agonist and abnormal gonadotropin secretion more likely reflect the abnormal hormonal milieu of the syndrome than explain its origin (Fig. 552-1). An increased ratio of circulating levels of LH:FSH is *not* a diagnostic criterion for PCOS.

Alterations in activities of steroidogenic enzymes that would explain *ovarian androgenic* hyperfunction are seen in PCOS subjects, but they are not consistently present in all patients and it is unclear whether these alterations are a cause of PCOS or are a consequence of ovarian dysregulation. The mass of ovarian stromal cells responsible for androgen production is increased, and surgery that reduces this ovarian component (ovarian wedge resection, or laparoscopic ablative procedures) reduces circulating androgen levels and often restores ovarian cyclicity. Patients with hyperandrogenic congenital or adult-onset adrenal hyperplasia exhibit PCOS-like ovarian dysfunction that can be reversed by reducing the *adrenal-derived* androgens with glucocorticoid therapy. A primary role for androgen excess in the pathophysiology of all instances of PCOS seems unlikely; many patients have minimal hyperandrogenism, and elimination of androgen excess (with gonadotropin-releasing hormone agonists) does not affect associated insulin resistance.

Measures of insulin resistance are greater and more prevalent among women with PCOS than controls even when accounting for body mass index (BMI). Insulin enhances ovarian androgen production directly and contributes to elevations of free testosterone levels through its suppression of hepatic production of sex steroid–binding globulin. Treatment with insulin sensitivity–enhancing agents that can reduce insulin levels is associated with modest reductions in measures of androgen excess and, in some patients, restoration of regular ovulation. The association of insulin resistance with weight might explain the appearance of features of PCOS among some women who gain weight as well as the resolution of PCOS among affected women who lose weight.

Clinical Manifestations

PCOS, a lifelong disorder, commonly becomes manifest as puberty progresses, but its onset can occur later during young adulthood.

Table 552-1	Diagnostic Criteria for Polycystic Ovary Syndrome	
NATIONAL INSTITUTES OF HEALTH CRITERIA	**ROTTERDAM CRITERIA**	**ANDROGEN EXCESS SOCIETY**
Oligo or anovulation *and* Clinical or biochemical hyperandrogenism	Two of 3 of the following: Oligo or anovulation Polycystic ovaries on ultrasonography (12 or more follicles in a single ovary or ovarian volume of >10 mm³ in 1 ovary) Clinical and/or biochemical hyperandrogenism	Clinical or biochemical hyperandrogenism and at least 1 of the following: Polycystic ovaries *or* Oligo or anovulation

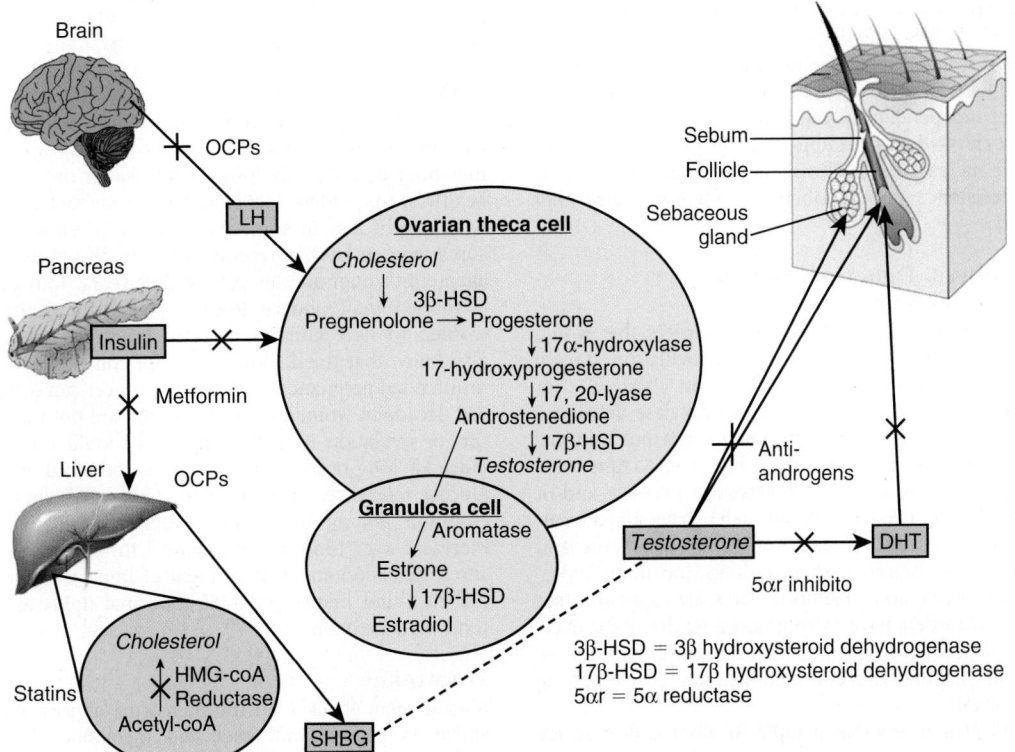

Figure 552-1 Schematic of pathophysiology of polycystic ovary syndrome and mechanism of therapeutic drugs. DHT, dihydrotestosterone; LH, luteinizing hormone; OCPs, oral contraceptive pills; SHBG, sex hormone-binding globulin. (*Adapted from Hassan A, Gordon CM: Polycystic ovary syndrome in adolescence, Curr Opin Pediatr 19[4]:389–397, 2007.*)

Table 552-2	Phenotypes for Polycystic Ovary Syndrome Based on 2003 Rotterdam Criteria			
SIGNS, RISKS, AND PREVALENCE	**SEVERE PCOS**	**HYPERANDROGENISM AND CHRONIC ANOVULATION**	**OVULATORY PCOS**	**MILD PCOS**
Periods	Irregular	Irregular	Normal	Irregular
Ovaries on ultrasonography	Polycystic	Normal	Polycystic	Polycystic
Androgen concentrations	High	High	High	Mildly raised
Insulin concentrations	Increased	Increased	Increased	Normal
Risks	Potential long-term	Potential long-term	Unknown	Unknown
Prevalence in affected women	61%	7%	16%	16%

PCOS, polycystic ovary syndrome.
From Norman RJ, Dewailly D, Legro RS, et al: Polycystic ovary syndrome, Lancet 370:685–696, 2007.

Clinical hallmarks are menstrual abnormalities and manifestations of *hyperandrogenism* but the severity of the disorder is variable (Table 552-2). Ovulation is typically irregular or absent, and menses are consequently irregular or absent. When menstrual bleeding does occur, it may be anovulatory bleeding, which is often heavy and/or protracted as a result of an extended period of unopposed endometrial growth. Alternatively, bleeding can be relatively normal in character as a consequence of a preceding ovulation. Protracted spells of anovulation, with accompanying unopposed estrogen is a risk factor for endometrial hyperplasia, and more severe premalignant and frankly malignant changes may eventuate.

The diagnosis of PCOS in adolescents may be made on the basis of a lack of resolution of the normal pattern of anovulatory menstrual cycles present in the 1st 2 postmenarchal years. Less commonly, the diagnosis is made in the setting of primary amenorrhea. Serum androgen levels may be elevated and clinical findings of androgen excess are common, although distinction of normal androgenic expressions of puberty (acne, mild hirsutism) from early manifestations of PCOS may be difficult and serum hormonal testing may be helpful.

Obesity is common among affected women, and in some patients expression of PCOS features is conditional on elevation of BMI and reversible with weight loss. However, there is a subset of patients present with a "lean" PCOS phenotype and thus absence of excess weight should not preclude consideration of the PCOS diagnosis. PCOS is associated with an increased prevalence of insulin resistance and type 2 diabetes independent of the tendency for many affected patients to have an elevated BMI. Additionally, PCOS confers a substantial and specific increase in risk for metabolic syndrome (hyperlipidemia, insulin resistance, type 2 diabetes) in adolescent girls after accounting for BMI.

Laboratory Findings, Diagnosis, and Differential Diagnosis

The diagnosis of PCOS requires exclusion of disorders that would otherwise account for hyperandrogenism and anovulation. Serum 17-hydroxyprogesterone should be measured when there is clear androgen excess to screen for adult-onset 21-hydroxylase deficiency (see Chapter 576). In the adolescent with amenorrhea but minimal hyperandrogenic findings, consideration should be given to functional hypothalamic suppression as a result of excessive exercise and/or dieting, and a careful history taken to rule out such behavioral patterns. All patients should be clinically evaluated for Cushing syndrome, and biochemical evaluation is indicated when findings, including hypertension and/or characteristic body habitus features, are suggestive (see Chapter 577). The 2 disorders have in common a tendency for overweight and varying degrees of insulin resistance and androgen excess, but they differ in that Cushing syndrome demonstrates muscle wasting as a result of catabolism.

Evidence for androgen excess that is rapid in onset and/or severe especially if masculinizing, warrants measurement of androgens (total testosterone, dehydroepiandrosterone [DHEAS]) to exclude the possibility of an androgen-secreting adrenal or ovarian tumor. The laboratory evaluation is completed with the exclusion of hyperprolactinemia,

premature ovarian failure, and thyroid disease as causes of anovulation: determinations of functional hyperprolactinemia, FSH, and thyroid-stimulating hormone, respectively.

The diagnosis of PCOS is confirmed from the constellation of oligoovulation or anovulation, androgen excess (clinically or with biochemical confirmation), and typical ovarian morphology on ultrasound. Various experts weigh these 3 features differently and do not, as a rule, require the presence of all (see Table 552-1). Young women often exhibit the ovarian appearance of PCOS without any other evidence, and not all patients with PCOS by the criteria of hyperandrogenism and ovulatory disruption exhibit ovarian changes typical of PCOS. Ultrasound study to diagnose PCOS is not always required if oligoovulation and features of androgen excess are present. Clinical androgen excess (particularly acne) often appears in late puberty and does not necessarily signal PCOS. Nevertheless, young women with persistent oligoovulation or anovulation, accompanied by androgen excess, will likely have persistence of these symptoms and should be considered to have PCOS.

Insulin resistance is common among women with PCOS, and although not requisite for diagnosis, should be considered when PCOS is likely. Adolescents with hyperandrogenemia and anovulation should be evaluated for diabetes or impaired glucose tolerance with a 2 hr (75 g glucose load) glucose tolerance test.

Complications and Long-Term Outlook

Fertility management, prevention of endometrial cancer, and reduction in the likelihood and severity of the common accompanying metabolic disorders are long-term tasks for the PCOS patient and her healthcare providers (Table 552-3). Notwithstanding its reversibility with weight loss in some patients and a tendency to ameliorate in some women later in reproductive life, PCOS usually requires management throughout the reproductive years. Young patients should be counseled that modern fertility management allows most affected women to have children without great difficulty, and they should also know that the disorder does not confer reliable protection from unintended pregnancy. Endometrial cancer can develop as early as the 3rd decade in women with PCOS who are not managed with progestins or ovulation induction; patients should understand the importance of long-term strategies for endometrial protection. Impaired glucose tolerance, type 2 diabetes, and metabolic syndrome are more common among obese adolescents with PCOS; their prevalence increases over time. Weight control through diet and lifestyle measures, detection and management of impaired glucose tolerance and diabetes, and management of abnormal lipids are targets for long-term management.

Treatment

Management focuses on the menstrual abnormalities, symptoms of androgen excess, and associated metabolic changes. Weight loss through lifestyle change, use of hormonal contraceptive agents for menstrual regulation as well as androgen suppression, antiandrogens as adjuncts for hirsutism treatment, and insulin-sensitizing agents are common components of treatment.

Table 552-3	Lifelong Health Complications	
PRENATAL OR CHILDHOOD	**ADOLESCENCE, REPRODUCTIVE YEARS**	**POSTMENOPAUSAL**
REPRODUCTIVE		
Premature adrenarche	Menstrual irregularity	Delayed menopause?
Early menarche	Hirsutism	
	Acne	
	Infertility	
	Endometrial cancer	
	Miscarriage	
	Pregnancy complications	
METABOLIC		
Abnormal fetal growth	Obesity	Obesity
	Impaired glucose tolerance	Impaired glucose tolerance
	Insulin resistance	Insulin resistance
	Dyslipidemia	Dyslipidemia
	Type 2 diabetes	Type 2 diabetes
OTHER		
	Sleep apnea	Cardiovascular disease?
	Fatty liver	
	Depression	

From Norman RJ, Dewailly D, Legro RS, et al: Polycystic ovary syndrome, Lancet 370:685–696, 2007.

Lifestyle Changes

Several studies have shown that comprehensive lifestyle programs for overweight and obese *women* with PCOS aimed at fitness and weight loss can yield high rates of restoration of normal menstrual function, reduction of free androgen index, reduction in measures of insulin resistance, and improvements in serum lipids. Limited data show similar benefits from such interventions for obese *adolescents* with PCOS. Successful weight loss programs for adolescents with PCOS using both psychologic and nutritional counseling do result in improved menstrual function.

Hormonal Contraceptives

Combined (estrogen and progestin) hormonal contraceptive medications are considered first-line therapy for adults not desiring fertility and for adolescents (see Chapter 117). Adolescents with PCOS are at risk for unintended pregnancy; their fertility would be expected to be reduced relative to that of their peers, but they are still at risk for pregnancy.

Avoidance of hyperplastic endometrial states resulting from unopposed estrogen and management of abnormal uterine bleeding in anovulatory episodes can be accomplished with the use of combined hormonal contraceptives. The progestational component inhibits endometrial proliferation and the schedule of pill administration predictably regulates menstrual bleeding. The estrogenic component of combined oral contraceptive elevates circulating sex hormone-binding globulin, which reduces free and bioavailable testosterone levels. Both of the hormonal elements in oral contraceptives combine to suppress gonadotropic (particularly LH) stimulation of ovarian androgen production. DHEAS levels, often contributory to hyperandrogenemia in PCOS, are usually decreased by combined contraceptive use. Products with less-androgenic progestational components (drospirenone, desogestrel) may provide better relief from androgenic symptoms.

Using a product that is well tolerated in long-term use is more important than using a product with particular progestational component. Products with reduced frequency and duration of pill-free intervals can provide superior androgen suppression and a welcome decrease in frequency of bleeding episodes. Depot medroxyprogesterone acetate for contraception, endometrial protection, and androgen suppression may be a suitable alternative to combined hormonal contraceptives; it provides even more profound suppression of ovarian

androgen production, but it does not elevate sex hormone-binding globulin. Low-dose progestin-only regimens (oral minipills, implantable progestational contraceptives, and progestin-releasing intrauterine devices) also provide effective endometrial protection but would be expected to provide only partial and/or inconsistent androgen suppression, would not elevate sex hormone-binding globulin, and have not been shown to be consistently helpful in regard to abnormal bleeding patterns.

Patients without the need for management of hyperandrogenic symptoms or contraception are often treated with periodic use of oral progestins to induce predictable menstrual bleeding and prevent endometrial hyperplasia and malignancy. Twelve-day courses of medroxyprogesterone acetate 10 mg daily or norethindrone acetate 5 mg daily are effective and safe for this purpose when taken every 1-2 mo.

Metformin

Metformin is a biguanide medication used to treat type 2 diabetes, its only FDA-approved indication. It has been used in a variety of settings and with differing objectives for patients with PCOS. Metformin exerts its principal effect by reducing hepatic production of glucose and limiting intestinal absorption of glucose. Studies show that a subset of women with PCOS resume regular ovulation and menses when treated with metformin, obviating the need for progestational therapy or ovulation-induction medications to protect endometrial health. For some patients the resulting normal reproductive function is appealing regardless of interest in fertility.

Metformin reduces insulin resistance and the levels of androgens. Its extended use can reduce the likelihood of development of impaired glucose tolerance or the progression of impaired glucose tolerance to type 2 diabetes; these effects are not yet proved for patients with PCOS. It should not be used in the presence of renal or hepatic impairment. Typical dosing is 1,500-2,000 mg/day, achieved through gradual increments because gastrointestinal intolerance is common. Long-acting preparations are helpful when gastrointestinal intolerance is a problem.

The use of metformin in the treatment of PCOS depends on the patient's goals and preference. For the treatment of hyperandrogenic symptoms, metformin effects may be modest compared to other available agents. There are no empiric data supporting the theoretical benefits of long-term use of metformin in adolescents with PCOS and obesity compared to the outcomes achieved with weight loss and oral contraceptive medications. Use of metformin as a first-line agent is favored by some experts, in part for improvement in serum measures of intermediate outcomes, and in part because of evidence in other populations of reduced progression of insulin resistance. There is no evidence for long-term benefit to clinical outcomes of adding metformin to treatment for women managed primarily with oral contraceptives. For adolescents receiving metformin as a first-line medication, progestational management (combined contraceptives or periodic progestins) will still be necessary for those not resuming ovulatory function and oral contraceptives may still be an important adjunct for management of clinical hyperandrogenism and/or contraception.

Antiandrogens

Antiandrogenic medications may be added to other therapies or used alone for the treatment of hirsutism. These agents are usually used integrally or adjunctively with ovarian hormonal suppression, in part because of better reduction in hirsutism when antiandrogens are combined with ovarian suppression but also to reduce the risk of unintended embryonic or fetal exposure. The highly active androgen antagonist and progestin, cyproterone, is available in Europe and in Canada as a single agent for treatment of hirsutism or in combination with ethinyl estradiol as an oral contraceptive with enhanced antiandrogenic profile. In the United States, spironolactone is the most commonly used antiandrogen. Spironolactone antagonizes androgens at their receptor and also impairs androgen synthesis. Doses of 100-200 mg daily are commonly used. Other agents that have been studied are finasteride, a 5α-reductase inhibitor, and flutamide, a nonsteroidal and highly specific androgen receptor antagonist. These are rarely used because of lack of evidence of superior effectiveness, cost, and, in the case of flutamide, the potential for hepatotoxicity.

HIRSUTISM

Hirsutism is defined as abnormally increased terminal (mature, heavy, dark) hair growth in areas of the body where hair growth is normally androgen dependent (see Chapter 662). Its presence is a result of the combination of extent of androgenic stimulation and familial regional follicle sensitivity to androgens, which varies considerably among ethnic groups. Patients' cosmetic concerns generally determine whether findings of hirsutism are a matter for clinical investigation and treatment. Hirsutism as an isolated finding is to be distinguished from masculinization. The latter includes alteration in muscle mass, clitoral enlargement, and voice change, generally manifesting as a rapid evolution (over months). Masculinization mandates a search for neoplastic source of androgen. Elevations of testosterone or DHEAS commonly indicate an ovarian or adrenal androgen source, respectively; specific imaging and occasionally selective catheterization studies are indicated.

Hirsutism without masculinization is common. The potential causes to consider are PCOS (when there is hyperandrogenism and anovulation), benign functional androgen excess (measurable hyperandrogenism without anovulation), idiopathic hirsutism (increased hair in androgen-dependent areas without measurable androgen excess), and adult-onset adrenal hyperplasia (Table 552-4). Patients can be primar-

Table 552-4	Causes of Hirsutism

PERIPHERAL
Idiopathic
Partial androgen insensitivity (5α-reductase deficiency)
HAIR-AN syndrome (hirsutism, androgenization, insulin resistance, and acanthosis nigricans)
Hyperprolactinemia

GONADAL
Polycystic ovary syndrome (polycystic ovaries, chronic anovulation)
Ovarian neoplasm (Sertoli-Leydig cell, granulosa cell, thecoma, gynandroblastoma, lipoid cell, luteoma, hypernephroma, Brenner tumor)
Gonadal dysgenesis (Turner mosaic with XY or H-Y antigen–positive)

ADRENAL
Cushing syndrome
Adrenal hyperresponsiveness
Congenital adrenal hyperplasia (classic, cryptic, adult onset)
21-Hydroxylase deficiency
11-Hydroxylase deficiency
3β-Hydroxysteroid deficiency
17β-Hydroxylase deficiency
Adrenal neoplasm (adenoma, cortical carcinoma)

EXOGENOUS
Minoxidil
Dilantin
Cyclosporine
Anabolic steroids
Acetazolamide (Diamox)
Penicillamine
Oral contraceptives with androgenic progestins
Danazol
Androgenic steroids
Psoralens
Hydrochlorothiazide
Phenothiazines

CONGENITAL ANOMALIES
Trisomy 18 (Edwards syndrome)
Cornelia de Lange syndrome
Hurler syndrome
Juvenile hypothyroidism

Adapted from Bailey-Pridham DD, Sanfilippo JS: Hirsutism in the adolescent female, Pediatr Clin North Am 36:581–599, 1989.

ily distinguished by evidence of ovulatory disorder by menstrual history, and for those with absent or irregular menses, a diagnosis of PCOS can be made. The remainder, for whom adult-onset adrenal hyperplasia and PCOS have been excluded, either have normal androgen levels with enhanced end-organ sensitivity owing to familial or ethnic predisposition or have a functional and benign overproduction of ovarian androgens. Measures of androgens (testosterone, DHEAS) may be normal or mildly elevated in the latter group. Testosterone suppresses circulating sex-steroid binding globulin, so states of testosterone overproduction might not be accompanied by elevated measures of total testosterone, although estimates of "free" or "bioavailable" testosterone reveal hyperandrogenism. Measures of unbound testosterone distinguish idiopathic hirsutism from mild benign hyperandrogenic states; making this distinction contributes little to patient management and adds cost. Idiopathic hirsutism (without evidence of androgen excess) usually responds to antiandrogen or androgen suppression therapy similarly to hirsutism associated with elevated androgens and anovulation (PCOS), and benign hyperandrogenism not associated with PCOS.

If hirsutism is present, and clinical evaluation excludes neoplasm, adult-onset adrenal hyperplasia, and Cushing syndrome, then management for symptoms for hyperandrogenism (regardless of whether measures of circulating androgens are elevated or not) can proceed as for patients with PCOS. Estrogen and progestin suppression of ovarian function, with or without added antiandrogen treatment, is the mainstay of therapy for these patients. Androgen suppression and/or antagonism results in gradual regression of the size and productivity of follicles in androgen-sensitive areas of the face and body, and these changes will evolve over successive and months-long generations of hair growth and shedding. Patients should therefore be advised that the effects of medical therapy accrue slowly, over many months.

Bibliography is available at Expert Consult.

Chapter 553
Neoplasms and Adolescent Screening for Human Papillomavirus
Nora T. MacZura and Diane F. Merritt

GYNECOLOGIC MALIGNANCIES

After injuries, cancer is the second most common cause of death in adolescents. Although rare, gynecologic malignancies can be followed by infertility, depression, and poor self-image, which may be lifelong.

The most common type of gynecologic malignancy found in children and adolescents is of ovarian origin and usually manifests as an abdominal mass, which must be distinguished from other organ-based tumors and ovarian functional, physiologic, inflammatory/infectious, or pregnancy-related processes. Ovarian neoplasms constitute 1% of all childhood malignancies, but account for 60-70% of all gynecologic malignancies in this age group. Approximately 10-30% of all childhood or adolescent ovarian neoplasms are malignant. Less often, the vagina or cervix is a site of malignant lesions in children, with a few specific tumors having their greatest incidence within this population. Cervical dysplasia can occur in adolescents, and healthcare providers need to be aware of current screening guidelines as well as updates on preventive measures. Vulvar malignancies in children and adolescents are exceedingly rare.

IMPACT OF CANCER THERAPY ON FERTILITY

Chemotherapy and radiation therapy are associated with acute ovarian failure and premature menopause (Table 553-1). Risk factors include older age, abdominal or spinal radiation, and certain chemotherapeutic drugs, such as alkylating agents (cyclophosphamide, busulfan). Uterine irradiation is associated with infertility, spontaneous pregnancy loss, and intrauterine growth restriction. Decreased uterine volume has been noted in girls who received abdominal radiation. The vagina, bladder, ureters, urethra, and rectum can also be injured by radiation. Vaginal shortening, vaginal stenosis, urinary tract fistulas, and diarrhea are important side effects of pelvic irradiation for pelvic cancers. Pregnancy outcomes appear to be influenced by prior chemotherapy and radiation treatment; 15% of childhood cancer survivors have infertility. Cancer survivors have an increased rate of spontaneous abortions, premature deliveries, and low birthweight infants compared to their normal healthy siblings. No data support an increased incidence of congenital malformations in offspring.

Childhood cancer survivors require extensive counseling about these specific future health implications. As part of informed consent

Table 553-1	Effect of Cancer Treatment on Development of Amenorrhea			
	CANCER TREATMENT PROTOCOL	**PATIENT AND DOSE FACTORS**	**COMMON USAGE**	**FERTILITY PLANNING CONSIDERATIONS**
High Risk	Any alkylating agent (e.g., busulfan, carmustine, cyclophosphamide, ifosfamide, lomustine, melphalan, procarbazine) + total body irradiation		Conditioning for HSCT for leukemias, lymphomas, myelomas, Ewing's sarcoma, neuroblastoma, choriocarcinoma	>70% of women develop amenorrhea after treatment. Any treatments containing high doses of alkylating agents and/or radiation to the abdomen, pelvis, or hypothalamic axis present the highest level of risk for gonadal impact and immediate amenorrhea. Patients should be counseled about fertility preservation before treatment.
	Any alkylating agent + pelvic radiation		Sarcomas, ovarian	
	Total cyclophosphamide	5 g/m^2 in women age >40 7.5 g/m^2 in women and girls age <20	Multiple cancers: breast cancer, NHL, conditioning for HSCT	
	Protocols containing procarbazine: MOPP BEACOPP	>3 cycles >6 cycles	Hodgkin lymphoma	
Intermediate Risk	Protocols containing temozolomide or BCNU + cranial radiation		Brain tumor	~30-70% of women develop amenorrhea post-treatment. Lower levels of alkylating agents and/or radiation to the abdomen, pelvis or hypothalamic axis reduce risk of immediate amenorrhea but do not eliminate risk of gonadal damage. Patients should be counseled about fertility preservation prior to treatment. For Bevacizumab, risk of amenorrhea is intermediate, yet the outcome of fertility is unknown.
	Whole abdominal or pelvic radiation doses	>6 Gy in adult women >10 Gy in postpubertal girls >15 Gy in prepubertal girls	Wilms' tumor, neuroblastoma, sarcomas, Hodgkin lymphoma, ovarian	
	Total body irradiation (TBI) doses		HSCT	
	Cranial radiation	>40 Gy	Brain tumor	
	Total cyclophosphamide	5 g/m^2 in women age 30-40	Multiple cancers, breast	
	AC for breast cancer	×4 + paclitaxel or Docetaxel in women age <40	Breast	
	Monoclonal antibodies, e.g., bevacizumab (Avastin)		Colon, non-small cell lung, head and neck, breast	
	FOLFOX$_4$		Colon	
	Protocols containing cisplatin		Cervical	
	Abdominal/pelvic radiation	10-15 Gy in prepubertal girls 5-10 Gy in postpubertal girls	Wilms' tumor, neuroblastoma, spinal tumors, brain tumor, relapsed ALL or NHL	
Lower Risk	Protocols containing nonalkylating agents or lower levels of alkylating agents (e.g., ABVD, CHOP, COP; multi-agent therapies for leukemia)		Hodgkin lymphoma, NHL, leukemia	<30% of women develop amenorrhea after treatment. These treatments are unlikely to cause immediate amenorrhea at standard dosage; however, patients should be counseled that they may be at risk for early menopause. Patients may want to consider fertility preservation before or after treatment.
	Protocols for breast cancer containing cyclophosphamide (e.g., CMF, CEF, or CAF)	Women < 30	Breast	
	Anthracycline + cytarabine		AML	
Very Low / No Risk	Multi-agent therapies using vincristine		Leukemia, lymphoma, breast and lung cancer	
	Radioactive iodine		Thyroid	
Unknown	Monoclonal antibodies, e.g., cetuximab (Erbitux), trastuzumab (Herceptin)		Colon, non-small cell lung, head and neck, breast	Negligible to no effects on menses. Patients should be counseled regarding the lack of conclusive data about the reproductive effects of these drugs; fertility preservation options should be discussed.
	Tyrosine kinase inhibitors, e.g., erlotinib (Tarceva), imatinib (Gleevec)		Non-small cell lung, pancreatic, CML, GIST	

for cancer therapy, the possibility of infertility should be discussed with young patients and their families. Counseling and embryo or mature oocyte cryopreservation for postpubertal females before gonadotoxic therapy should be offered as standard of care. Cryopreservation of ovarian tissue for prepubertal children remains experimental and may be offered as part of a research protocol. Premature ovarian insufficiency is associated with an increased risk for cardiovascular complications, osteoporosis, and difficulties with sexual function. Risks and benefits of hormonal therapy need to be addressed.

OVARIES
Neonatal and Pediatric Ovarian Cysts
Normal follicles or physiologic ovarian cysts are seen by ultrasound examination of the ovaries in all healthy prepubertal girls. Most of these are <1 cm in diameter and not pathologic. In the neonatal period, physiologic follicular cysts as a result of maternal estrogen stimulation usually resolve spontaneously and may be followed with serial ultrasounds in the asymptomatic child. Children with an ovarian mass might have no symptoms and the mass may be detected incidentally or during a routine examination. Other children present with abdominal pain that may be accompanied by nausea, vomiting, or urinary frequency or retention. The cyst's most common complication, **ovarian torsion**, can result in loss of the ovary (autoamputation of the ovary has been documented to occur antenatally). Successful reports of antenatal aspiration and postnatal laparoscopic treatment exist. Large cysts (>4-5 cm), those with complex characteristics, or any ovarian cyst in premenarchal girls with associated signs or symptoms of hormonal stimulation deserve prompt evaluation. The incidence of ovarian cysts increases again with puberty.

Functional Cysts
Hemorrhagic cysts are an expected part of follicular development during the menstrual cycle. Normally, a dominant follicle forms and increases in size. Following ovulation, the dominant follicle becomes a corpus luteum that, if it bleeds, is termed a *hemorrhagic corpus luteum*. These can become symptomatic owing to size or peritoneal irritation from blood, and they have a characteristic complex appearance on ultrasound. Expectant management for a presumed functional or hemorrhagic cyst is appropriate. Physiologic cysts are usually ≤5 cm and resolve over the course of 6-8 wk during subsequent ultrasound imaging. Monophasic oral contraceptives can be used to suppress follicular development to prevent formation of additional cysts.

Teratomas
The most common neoplasm in adolescents is the *mature cystic teratoma (dermoid cyst)*. Most are benign and contain mature tissue of ectodermal (skin, hair, sebaceous glands), mesodermal, or endodermal origin. Occasionally, well-formed teeth, cartilage, and bone are found. Calcification on an abdominal radiograph is often a hallmark of a benign teratoma. These tumors may be asymptomatic and found incidentally, or they can manifest as a mass or with abdominal pain (associated with torsion or rupture). If the major component of the dermoid is thyroid tissue (struma ovarii), hyperthyroidism can be the clinical presentation. Benign teratomas should be carefully resected, preserving as much normal ovarian tissue as possible. Oophorectomy (and salpingo-oophorectomy) for this benign lesion is excessive treatment. During surgery, both ovaries should be evaluated, and if there is any question about the nature of the lesion, the specimen should be evaluated by a pathologist. An association of dermoid tumors with neural elements and *anti–N-methyl-D-aspartase receptor encephalitis* has been reported. Excision of the ovarian tumor has led to improvement in neurologic symptoms in some patients.

Immature teratoma of the ovary is an uncommon tumor, accounting for <1% of ovarian teratomas. In contrast to the mature cystic teratoma, which is encountered most often during the reproductive years but occurs at all ages, the immature teratoma has a specific age incidence, occurring most commonly in the 1st 2 decades of life. By definition, an immature teratoma contains immature neural elements. Because

the lesion is rarely bilateral in its ovarian involvement, the present method of therapy consists of unilateral salpingo-oophorectomy with wide sampling of peritoneal implants.

Cystadenomas
Serous and mucinous cystadenomas are the second most common benign ovarian tumor. These cystic lesions can become very large, yet with care, the tumor can be resected, preserving normal ovarian tissue for future reproductive potential.

Endometriomas
Endometriosis is a syndrome defined by the presence of ectopic endometrial tissue usually located within the pelvis and abdomen. The principal clinical symptoms in adolescents consist of severe menstrual pain and pelvic pain. Endometriomas (chocolate cysts) form when the ovaries are involved and are collections of old blood and hemosiderin within an endometrium-lined cyst. They have a typical homogeneous echogenic appearance on ultrasound and are more common in adults than in adolescents. Conservative management (suppressive therapy with ovulation suppression, and nonsteroidal antiinflammatory drugs) and ovarian cystectomy with preservation of as much functioning ovary as possible is recommended for adolescents.

Pelvic Inflammatory Disease and Tuboovarian Abscess
Pelvic inflammatory disease complicated by a tuboovarian abscess should be considered in a sexually active adolescent with an adnexal mass and pain on examination (see Chapter 120). These patients also typically exhibit fever with leukocytosis and cervical motion tenderness. Treatment consists of administration of intravenous antibiotics. If the lesion persists or is refractory to antibiotics, drainage of the pelvic abscess by interventional radiology should be considered.

Adnexal Torsion
Adnexal torsion of the ovary and/or fallopian tube can occur in children or adolescents with normal adnexa or more often those enlarged by cystic (follicular, tubal) changes or ovarian (teratoma, cystadenoma) neoplasms. When torsion occurs, the venous outflow is obstructed first, and the ovary swells and becomes hemorrhagic. Once the arterial flow is interrupted, necrosis begins. It is not known how long torsed adnexa will remain viable. When a female patient presents with acute lower abdominal pain, either episodic or constant, and if imaging studies shows unilateral enlargement of an adnexa, the diagnosis of adnexal torsion must be considered and acted upon. The sonographic presence of Doppler flow does not exclude the diagnosis of torsion. Prompt surgical intervention (laparoscopic detorsion) is warranted if clinical suspicion is high. Detorsion of the adnexa and observation for viability is recommended, with excision only for obviously nonviable necrotic tissues. Recovery of ovarian function after detorsion has been reported with identification of normal follicle development. Oophoropexy (plication) of the affected and the contralateral adnexa remains controversial.

Ovarian Carcinoma
Ovarian cancer is very uncommon in children; only 2% of all ovarian cancers are diagnosed in patients younger than 25 yr old. The Surveillance, Epidemiology, and End Results (SEER) incidence rates are ≤0.8/100,000 at age 0-14 yr and 1.5/100,000 at ages 15-19 yr. Germ cell tumors are the most common and originate from primordial germ cells that then develop into a number of heterogeneous tumor types including dysgerminomas, malignant teratomas, endodermal sinus tumors, embryonal carcinomas, mixed cell neoplasms, and gonadoblastomas. Immature teratomas and endodermal sinus tumors are more aggressive malignancies than dysgerminomas and occur in a significantly higher proportion of younger girls (younger than 10 yr of age). Sex-cord stromal tumors are more common among adolescents (Table 553-2). Tumor markers such as α-fetoprotein, carcinoembryonic antigen, and the antigen CA-125 are also used for diagnosis and treatment surveillance (Table 553-3).

Table 553-2	Malignant Ovarian Tumors in Children and Adolescents	
TUMOR	**OVERALL 5-YR SURVIVAL**	**CLINICAL FEATURES**
GERM CELL TUMORS		
Dysgerminoma	85%	10-20% bilateral
		Most common ovarian malignancy
		Gonadal dysgenesis/androgen insensitivity
		Sensitive to chemotherapy/radiation
Immature teratoma	97-100%	All 3 germ layers present
Endodermal sinus tumor	80%	Almost always large (>15 cm)
		Schiller-Duval bodies
Choriocarcinoma	30%	Rare
		Can mimic ectopic pregnancy
Embryonal carcinoma	25%	Endocrinologic symptoms (precocious puberty)
		Highly malignant
Gonadoblastoma	100%	Primary amenorrhea
		Virilization
		45,X or 45,X/46,XY mosaicism
SEX CORD STROMAL TUMORS		
Juvenile granulosa stroma cell tumor	92%	Produce estrogen
		Menstrual irregularities
		Isosexual precious pseudopuberty
		Call-Exner bodies rare
Sertoli-Leydig cell tumor	70-90%	Virilization in 40%
		Produce testosterone
Lipoid cell tumors	~80%	Rare heterogenous group with lipid-filled parenchyma
Gynandroblastoma	90% or greater	Rare low-grade mixed tumors that produce either estrogen or androgen

Table 553-3	Serum Tumor Markers									
TUMOR	**CA-125**	**AFP**	**hCG**	**LDH**	**E2**	**T**	**INHIBIN**	**MIS**	**VEGF**	**DHEA**
Epithelial tumor	+									
Immature teratoma	+	+			+					+
Dysgerminoma			+	+	+					
Endodermal sinus tumor		+								
Embryonal carcinoma		+	+		+					
Choriocarcinoma			+							
Mixed germ cell		+	+	+						
Granulosa cell tumor	+				+		+	+		
Sertoli-Leydig						+	+			
Gonadoblastoma					+	+	+			+
Theca-fibroma									+	

AFP, α-fetoprotein; CA-125, cancer antigen 125; DHEA, dehydroepiandrostenedione; E2, estradiol; hCG, human chorionic gonadotropin; LDH, lactate dehydrogenase; T, testosterone, MIS, müllerian inhibiting substance; VEGF, vascular endothelial growth factor.

Treatment is surgical excision followed by postoperative chemotherapy that usually consists of bleomycin, etoposide, and cisplatin. Radiotherapy is sometimes administered for disease recurrence in dysgerminomas, but it is otherwise not included in routine treatment. Staging at the beginning of therapy is of the utmost importance. In rare cases, a second-look laparotomy may be indicated for neoplasms with teratomatous elements or for those incompletely resected.

Epithelial ovarian cancers account for 19% of ovarian masses in the pediatric population, with a total of 16% being malignant. These tumors manifest almost exclusively after puberty. Common presenting symptoms include dysmenorrhea, abdominal pain, abdominal distention, nausea and vomiting, and vaginal discharge. Tumors of low malignant potential are common in adolescents and account for 30% of epithelial ovarian cancers in this age group. Given the young age of this population, although not the standard of care for adult patients, consideration may be given to conserving the contralateral ovary and uterus if they appear normal. Data suggest that in patients with early-stage disease, such an approach with appropriate surgical staging results in optimal outcomes. Overall 5 yr survival rates are approxi-

mately 73%. The number of term pregnancies and use of oral contraceptives decrease the risk of invasive epithelial ovarian cancer. Young women with a family history of ovarian cancer should seriously consider using long-term oral contraceptives for the preventive benefits when pregnancy is not being sought.

UTERUS

Rhabdomyosarcomas are the most common type of soft-tissue sarcoma occurring in patients younger than 20 yr of age (see Chapter 500). They can develop in any organ or tissue within the body except bone, and roughly 3% originate from the uterus or vagina. Of the various histologic subtypes, embryonal rhabdomyosarcomas in the female patient most often occur in the genital tract of infants or young children. They are rapidly growing entities that can cause the tumor to be expelled through the cervix, with subsequent complications such as uterine inversion or large cervical polyps. Irregular vaginal bleeding may be another presenting clinical symptom. They are defined histologically by the presence of mesenchymal cells of skeletal muscle in various stages of differentiation intermixed with myxoid stroma.

Treatment recommendations are based on protocols coordinated by the Intergroup Rhabdomyosarcoma Study Group and consist of a multimodal approach including radiation therapy and chemotherapy. Vincristine, Adriamycin, and cyclophosphamide with or without radiation therapy are the first line of treatment. Resection rates are now very low; chemotherapy with restrictive surgery has enabled many patients to retain their uterus while achieving excellent long-term survival rates.

Leiomyosarcomas and **leiomyomas** are extremely rare, occurring in <2 in 10 million individuals within the pediatric/adolescent age group, although their numbers are increasing among pediatric patients with AIDS. They usually involve the spleen, lung, or gastrointestinal tract, but they could also originate from uterine smooth muscle. Pathogenesis is thought to correlate with the Epstein-Barr virus (see Chapter 254). Despite treatment that demands complete surgical resection (and chemotherapy for the sarcomas), they tend to recur frequently.

Endometrial stromal sarcoma and endometrial adenocarcinoma of the uterine corpus are extremely rare in children and adolescents, with only case reports noted in the literature. Vaginal bleeding not associated with sexual precocity is a common presenting sign. Treatment consists of hysterectomy, with removal of the ovaries, followed by adjunctive radiotherapy and/or chemotherapy, depending on the operative findings.

VAGINA

Sarcoma botryoides is a variant of embryonal rhabdomyosarcoma that occurs most commonly in the vagina of pediatric patients. Sarcoma botryoides tends to arise in the anterior wall of the vagina and manifests as a submucosal lesion that is grape-like in appearance; if located at the cervix it could resemble a cervical polyp or polypoid mass. These lesions were formerly treated with exenterative procedures; equal success has occurred with less-radical surgery (polypectomy, conization, and local excision) and adjuvant chemotherapy with or without radiotherapy. A combination of vincristine, dactinomycin, and cyclophosphamide appears to be effective. Outcomes depend on tumor size, extent of disease at time of diagnosis, and histologic subtype. The 5-year survival rates for patients with clinical stages I-IV were 83%, 70%, 52%, and 25%, respectively.

Vaginal adenosis can lead to the development of clear cell adenocarcinoma of the vagina in females exposed to diethylstilbestrol in utero.

Pregnant women at risk for miscarriage are no longer exposed to diethylstilbestrol, and thus fewer adolescent girls and young women are at risk for this unusual tumor.

A rare tumor occurring in the vagina of infants is the **endodermal sinus tumor**. This disease usually occurs in children younger than 2 yr of age, and survival rates are poor. Combination surgery and chemotherapy are appropriate. Benign papillomas can arise in the vagina of children and result in vaginal bleeding. Rarely, vaginal bleeding is secondary to leukemia or a hemangioma.

VULVA

Any questionable vulvar lesion should be biopsied and submitted for histologic examination. Lipoma, liposarcoma, and malignant melanoma of the vulva have been reported in young patients. The most common lesion is likely condyloma acuminata, associated with the human papilloma virus (HPV) (see Chapter 266). Diagnosis is usually made by visual inspection. Treatment consists of observation for spontaneous regression, topical trichloroacetic acid, local cryotherapy, electrocautery, excision, and laser ablation. Some products used to treat skin lesions in adults have not been approved for children, including provider application of podophyllin resin and home application of imiquimod, podofilox, and sinecatechins ointment.

CERVIX

Cervical cancer screening has been cytology based using the Papanicolaou (Pap) test and Bethesda Classification System (Table 553-4). Advances in epidemiologic research and molecular techniques have allowed the identification of the integral role of HPV in development of cervical cancer. HPV has become an important factor in the interpretation of cytologic results and subsequent management. The discovery of HPV presents a unique target for cervical cancer prevention, with the pediatric and adolescent population at the forefront of its implementation. Two HPV vaccines (bivalent HPV2 and quadrivalent HPV4) are currently available to protect against cervical cancer, and the HPV4 vaccine also protects against genital warts and cancers of the anus, vagina, and vulva. HPV vaccines offer the best protection if all three vaccine doses are administered before the patient is ever sexually active. The American Congress of Obstetrics and Gynecology recommends vaccination for all girls and women ages 9-26 yr, and The Advi-

Table 553-4	Management of Cytologic Abnormalities in Adolescents Who Are Screened in Error and Immunocompromised Women <21 Years of Age		
CYTOLOGY RESULT	**MANAGEMENT RECOMMENDATION**	**HPV TESTING?**	**COLPOSCOPY?**
ASCUS	Repeat cytologic testing in 1 year	No	At 1 yr follow-up if HGSIL or greater result At 2 yr follow-up if persistent ASCUS or greater
LGSIL	Repeat cytologic testing in 1 year	No	At 1 yr follow-up if HGSIL or greater result At 2 yr follow-up if ASCUS or greater
HGSIL	If colposcopy is unsatisfactory or if CIN is ungraded: excisional procedure If colposcopy is satisfactory: • If no CIN1-3: Pap and colposcopy q6mo until 2 are negative. **If persistent HGSIL without CIN1-3 identified, then excisional procedure at 2 yr** • If CIN1: (ASCUS/LGSIL protocol) • If CIN2, CIN2-3: Pap or colposcopy q6mo until 2 are negative, or else rebiopsy at 1 yr, treat if persistent at 2 yr • If CIN3: excisional procedure	No	Yes, immediately
ASC-H or AGC	There are no specific recommendations in regard to adolescents; see ASCCP guidelines for adults Endometrial biopsy is not advised in adolescents	No	Yes, immediately

Note: Cryotherapy and laser ablation are acceptable treatment options only for biopsy-proven CIN2+ lesion and satisfactory colposcopic examination.
AGC, atypical glandular cells; ASCCP, American Society for Colposcopy and Cervical Pathology; ASC-H, atypical squamous cell changes, high grade; ASCUS, atypical squamous cell changes of undetermined significance; CIN, cervical dysplasia; HGSIL, high-grade squamous intraepithelial dysplasia; LGSIL, low-grade squamous intraepithelial dysplasia; Pap, Papanicolaou smear.

sory Committee on Immunization Practices (http://www.cdc.gov/vaccines/schedules/hcp/index.html) recommends routine vaccination of girls ages 11-12 yr with 3 doses of quadrivalent HPV vaccine, starting as early as age 9 yr. Catch-up vaccination is indicated for girls and women ages 13-26 yr who have not been fully vaccinated. Female patients should be vaccinated even if sexually exposed; vaccination prior to exposure is ideal. Pap testing and screening for HPV DNA or HPV antibody is not required before vaccination. The American Congress of Obstetrics and Gynecology recommends that cervical cancer screening of women who have been immunized against HPV-16 and HPV-18 should not differ from that of nonimmunized women and should follow the exact same regimen.

The adolescent population presents a unique challenge to cervical cancer screening, because the prevalence of HPV is high. In adolescents ages 15-19 yr, HPV cumulative incidence rates after initiation of sexual activity are reported as 17% at 1 yr and 35.7% at 3 yr. Correlating with the natural history of an HPV infection, >90% of low-grade intraepithelial lesions regress within this age group, giving the presence of HPV in this population little clinical significance. The overall incidence of a high-grade lesion on Pap test in the adolescent population remains low (0.7%); cervical cancer is uncommon in the age group. In the United States, the Surveillance, Epidemiology, and End Results Cancer Statistics Review 1975-2006 published by the National Cancer Institute reports an incidence of invasive cervical cancer as 0.1/100,000 in 15-19 yr olds, with no cases reported before the age of 15 yr; similar rates (≤0.3 cases per 100,000 among women ages 15-19 yr) have been reported by the Canadian Cancer Registry. Therefore, colposcopy for minor cytologic abnormalities within this age group should be highly discouraged, because it will result more often in harm than produce any clinical benefit. The American Society for Colposcopy and Cervical Pathology and the American College of Obstetricians and Gynecologists guidelines recommend that adolescents should be managed conservatively and should not receive Pap smear screening until age 21 yr regardless of age of onset of sexual intercourse. If an HPV test is done, the results should be ignored. However, sexually active immunocompromised (HIV-positive patients or organ transplant recipients) adolescents should undergo screening twice within the 1st yr after diagnosis and annually thereafter. Table 553-4 demonstrates management recommendations for abnormal cytologic results for adolescents who are screened in error and immunocompromised sexually active adolescents who are screened. Routine screening for cervical cancer in the general adolescent population (younger than age 21 yr) is *not* recommended.

Clinic protocols that require teenagers to undergo Pap smears before prescribing contraceptives should be reconsidered in light of these recommendations.

Bibliography is available at Expert Consult.

Chapter 554
Vulvovaginal and Müllerian Anomalies
Natalia M. Grindler and Amber R. Cooper

EMBRYOLOGY

Cellular differentiation, duct elongation, fusion, resorption, canalization, and programmed cell death are all involved in the sequence of events that occur in a developing embryo and early fetus to create a normal reproductive system. Myriad gonadal, müllerian, and/or vulvovaginal anomalies can result from interruption of the intricate sequence or functions of any one of these processes during formation

Table 554-1	Common Müllerian Anomalies
ANOMALY	**DESCRIPTION**
Hydrocolpos	Accumulation of mucus or nonsanguineous fluid in the vagina
Hemihematometra	Atretic segment of vagina with menstrual fluid accumulation
Hydrosalpinx	Accumulation of serous fluid in the fallopian tube, often an end result of pyosalpinx
Didelphic uterus	Two cervices, each associated with 1 uterine horn
Bicornuate uterus	One cervix associated with 2 uterine horns
Unicornuate uterus	Result of failure of 1 müllerian duct to descend

of the reproductive system (Table 554-1). Genetic, epigenetic, enzymatic, and environmental factors all have some role in the process (Table 554-2).

Phenotypic sexual differentiation, especially during formation of the vulvovaginal and müllerian systems, is determined from genetic (46,XX), gonadal, and hormonal influences (see Chapter 582). The genetic sex of the embryo is determined at fertilization when the gamete pronuclei fuse. The primordial germ cells (oogonia or spermatogonia) migrate from the yolk sac to the gonadal ridges. The primitive gonads are indistinguishable until about the 7th wk of development. Gonadal development determines the progression or regression of the genital ducts and subsequent hormonal production and, thus, the external genitalia. Critical areas in the SRY region (sex-determining region on the Y chromosome) are believed to be the factors that drive the development of a testis from a primitive gonad as well as spermatogenesis. The testis begins to develop between 6 and 7 wk of gestation, first with Sertoli cells followed by Leydig cells, and testosterone production begins at approximately 8 wk of gestation. The genital tract begins to differentiate later than the gonads. The differentiation of the wolffian ducts begins with an increase in testosterone, and the local action of testosterone activates development of the epididymis, vas deferens, and seminal vesicle. Further male genital duct and external genital structures depend on the conversion of testosterone to dihydrotestosterone.

In a 46,XX embryo, female sexual differentiation occurs about 2 wk later than gonadal differentiation in the male. Because the ovaries develop prior to and separately from the müllerian ducts, females with müllerian ductal anomalies usually have normal ovaries and steroid hormone production. The regression of the wolffian ducts results from the lack of local gonadal testosterone production, and the persistence of the **müllerian** (or paramesonephric) **ducts** results from the absence of **antimüllerian hormone** (or müllerian-inhibiting substance) production. The müllerian ducts continue to differentiate into the fallopian tubes, uterus, and upper vagina without interference from antimüllerian hormone. There are complex interactions among the mesonephric, paramesonephric, and metanephric ducts early in embryonic development, and normal development of the müllerian system depends on such interaction. If this process is interrupted, coexisting müllerian and renal anomalies are often discovered in the female patient at the time of evaluation. Differentiation along the female pathway is often referred to as the *default pathway*, but it is an extremely intricate process regulated by the absence, presence, or dosage compensation of numerous gene products (i.e., SRY, SF-1, WT1, SOX9, Wnt-4, GATA4, DAX-1, BMP4, HOX genes) and remains not entirely understood.

By 10 wk of gestation, the caudal portions of the müllerian ducts fuse together in the midline to form the uterus, cervix, and upper vagina, in a Y-shaped structure, with the open upper arms of the Y forming the primordial fallopian tubes. Initially the müllerian ducts are solid cords that gradually canalize as they grow along and cross the mesonephric ducts ventrally and fuse in the midline. The mesonephric ducts caudally open into the **urogenital sinus**, and the müllerian ducts contact the dorsal wall of the urogenital sinus, where proliferation of the cells at the point of contact form the müllerian tubercle. Cells between the müllerian tubercle and the urogenital sinus continue to proliferate, forming the vaginal plate. At the same time of the midline fusion of the müllerian ducts, the medial walls begin to degenerate and resorption occurs to form the central cavity of the uterovaginal canal. Uterine septal resorption is thought to occur in a caudal to cephalad direction and to be complete at approximately 20 wk of gestation. This theory has been scrutinized because some anomalies do not fit the standard classification system. It is possible that septal resorption starts at some point in the middle and proceeds in both directions. At approximately 16 wk of gestation the central cells of the vaginal plate desquamate and resorption occurs, forming the vaginal lumen. The lumen of the vagina is initially separated from the urogenital sinus by a thin hymenal membrane. The hymenal membrane undergoes apoptosis and central resorption and is usually perforate before birth.

EPIDEMIOLOGY

Müllerian anomalies can include abnormalities in portions or all of the fallopian tubes, uterus, cervix, and vagina (Fig. 554-1). True estimates of prevalence are difficult because of the varied presentations and asymptomatic nature of some of the anomalies. Imaging techniques have made significant contributions to uterovaginal anomaly diagnoses, which has increased reporting of anomalies and led to additional combinations of anomalies. Most estimate that müllerian anomalies are present in 2-4% of the female population. The incidence increases in women with a history of adverse pregnancy outcomes or infertility: 5-10% of infertile women undergoing hysterosalpingogram, 5-10% of women with recurrent pregnancy loss, and 25% or more of women with late miscarriages and/or preterm delivery have müllerian defects.

CLINICAL MANIFESTATIONS

Vulvovaginal and müllerian anomalies can manifest at a variety of chronological time points during a female's life: from infancy, through childhood and adolescence, and adulthood (see Table 554-1). The majority of external genitalia malformations manifest at birth, and often even subtle deviations from normal in either a male or female newborn warrant evaluation. Structural reproductive tract abnormalities can be seen at birth or can cluster at menarche or any time during a woman's reproductive life. Some müllerian anomalies are asymptomatic, whereas others can cause gynecologic, obstetric, or infertility issues.

Clinical manifestations and treatments depend on the specific type of müllerian anomaly and are varied. There may be a pelvic mass, which may or may not be associated with symptoms. A mass bulging at the introitus or within the vagina indicates complete or partial

Table 554-2	Heritable Disorders Associated with Müllerian Anomalies	
MODE OF INHERITANCE	**DISORDER**	**ASSOCIATED MÜLLERIAN DEFECT**
Autosomal dominant	Camptobrachydactyly	Longitudinal vaginal septa
	Hand-foot-genital	Incomplete müllerian fusion
Autosomal recessive	McKusick-Kaufman	Transverse vaginal septa
	Johanson-Blizzard	Longitudinal vaginal septa
	Renal-genital-middle ear anomalies	Vaginal atresia
	Fraser syndrome	Incomplete müllerian fusion
	Uterine hernia syndrome	Persistent müllerian duct derivatives
Polygenic/multifactorial	Mayer-Rokitansky-Küster-Hauser syndrome	Müllerian aplasia
X-linked	Uterine hernia syndrome	Persistent müllerian duct derivatives

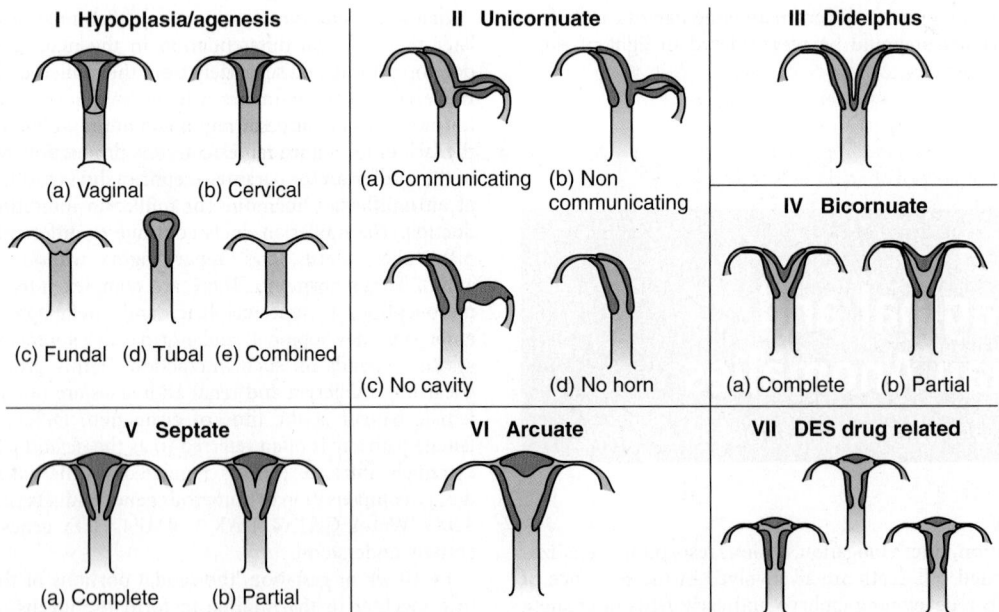

Figure 554-1 Classification system of müllerian duct anomalies developed by the American Fertility Society. *(From Gholoum S, Puligandla PS, Hui T, et al: Management and outcome of patients with combined vaginal septum, bifid uterus, and ipsilateral renal agenesis [Herlyn-Werner-Wunderlich syndrome]. J Pediatr Surg 41:987–992, 2006, Fig. 3.)*

outflow tract obstruction. An adolescent can present with pelvic pain either in association with primary amenorrhea or several months after the onset of menarche. Patients also may be asymptomatic until they present with miscarriage, pregnancy loss, or preterm delivery. When presentation is acutely symptomatic, emergency management may be required. Obstruction can result from a number of distinct anomalies including an **imperforate hymen, transverse vaginal septum,** and **noncommunicating rudimentary horn.** As menstrual fluid accumulates proximal to the obstruction, the resulting **hematocolpos** and **hematometra** cause cyclic pain or a pelvic mass.

Prenatal or neonatal presentation of hydrometrocolpos from distal vaginal obstruction produces fluid accumulation in the vagina and uterus and presents as a lower abdominal mass with or without associated acute urinary tract obstruction. **Hydrometrocolpos with polydactyly** may be a result of 2 disorders: McKusick-Kaufman syndrome (with associated congenital heart disease) and Bardet-Biedl syndrome (with obesity, learning disabilities, retinitis pigmentosa, renal anomalies). Both are autosomal recessive disorders.

Adolescent patients can present with acute obstruction of the outflow tract because of a müllerian anomaly, which requires emergency evaluation and surgical treatment. A small percentage of girls present with concomitant urinary retention caused by an altered urethral angle or pressure on the sacral plexus. Urinary hesitancy and incomplete emptying symptoms may be present before abdominopelvic pain from the obstruction in a patient of any age.

LABORATORY FINDINGS
Several radiographic studies have been used, often in combination, to aid in diagnosis including ultrasound, hysterosalpingogram, sonohysterography (saline-infusion sonography), and MRI. Laparoscopy and hysteroscopy were the gold standard for evaluation of müllerian anomalies, but the new standard may be MRI because of its noninvasive, high-quality capabilities. MRI is the most sensitive and specific imaging technique used for evaluating müllerian anomalies because it can image nearly all reproductive structures, blood flow, external contours, junctional zone resolution on T2-weighted images, and associated renal and other anomalies. MRI also has a high correlation with surgical findings because of its multiplanar capabilities and high spatial resolution. Three-dimensional ultrasound is another useful diagnostic tool and may be superior to traditional pelvic ultrasound and hysterosalpingogram. Three-dimensional ultrasound and MRI results are highly concordant in the diagnosis of uterine malformations. Evaluation of the external contour of the uterus is important for differentiating types of uterine anomalies. This often requires a combination of radiologic modalities for uterine cavity, external contour, and possible tubal patency. Diagnostic laparoscopy or hysteroscopy may be necessary depending on the presentation, but it is used less with the advancement of MRI and other imaging.

Diagnosis of müllerian anomalies should include a physical exam, pelvic ultrasound, possibly MRI, and renal and skeletal inspections for associated anomalies. Renal anomalies are noted in 30-40% and skeletal anomalies are associated in 10-15% of patients with müllerian anomalies. Unilateral renal agenesis occurs in 15% of patients. The most common skeletal anomalies are vertebral. Patients usually have a normal female karyotype (46,XX), but several familial segregations and gene mutations and/or abnormal karyotypes have been reported (see Table 554-2). Approximately 5-8% of patients with congenital müllerian anomalies have abnormal karyotypes. Most malformations are sporadic, with a polygenic mechanism and multifactorial etiology.

UTERINE ANOMALIES
Anomalous development of the uterus may be symmetric or asymmetric and/or obstructed or nonobstructed. Patients can present with primary amenorrhea or have either irregular or regular menstrual cycles. There may be an asymptomatic pelvic mass or dysmenorrhea. In adolescents and adults, pregnancy loss can cause the first suspicion of a uterine anomaly. Treatment is highly specific to the specific anomaly.

SEPTATE UTERUS
A **uterine septum** is the most common of all müllerian anomalies, accounting for just over half of all abnormalities, and it is the most common structural uterine anomaly. After the 2 müllerian ducts fuse in the midline, resorption must occur to unify the endometrial cavities; failure of this process results in some degree of uterine septum. It can vary in length from just below the fundus to beyond the cervix, depending on the amount of caudal resorption. A **septate uterus** has a normal external uterine contour, which is what distinguishes it from a bicornuate or didelphic uterus. An MRI can help delineate between a predominantly fibrous septum and a muscular or myometrial septum. Because the septum may be poorly vascularized, a septate uterus is the most significant anomaly associated with pregnancy loss, as well as other untoward pregnancy outcomes. Hysteroscopic metroplasty (septal excision) is generally recommended in the setting of a previous pregnancy loss. Controversy still exists regarding whether a woman should have such a surgical procedure without a previous pregnancy loss. Correction of uterine septum improves the prognosis in patients with a history of adverse obstetrical outcomes (i.e., spontaneous abortions, preterm delivery). The length of the septum might not correlate with the frequency or occurrence of untoward pregnancy outcomes. Differentiating precisely between bicornuate and septate uteri is extremely important to determine effective and safe treatment plans.

Bicornuate Uterus
Both müllerian ducts develop and elongate in this anomaly, but they do not completely fuse in the midline. The vagina and external cervix are normal, but the extent of division of the 2 endometrial cavities can vary depending on the extent of failed fusion between the cervix and the fundus. Bicornuate uteri are also associated with increased preterm labor and delivery, malpresentation, and miscarriage. This anomaly accounts for approximately 10-20% of müllerian anomalies and a significant percentage of uterine anomalies.

Unicornuate Uterus and Rudimentary Horns
A **unicornuate uterus** results from a normal creation of a fallopian tube, functional uterus, cervix and vagina from 1 müllerian duct. The other side fails to develop, resulting in either absence of the contralateral müllerian duct or a rudimentary horn. There is a 30-40% association of renal anomalies. If a rudimentary horn is identified, it is important to determine whether functional endometrium is present (usually with T2-weighted MRI images). About two-thirds of rudimentary horns are noncommunicating, some with a fibrous band connecting the 2 structures. Rudimentary horns can also communicate with the contralateral uterus. A fertilized ovum can implant and develop within a rudimentary horn. These pregnancies are incompatible with expectant gestation, and rupture of the horn could be life-threatening. Rupture tends to occur at a later gestation than with an ectopic pregnancy, and hemorrhage is severe. Patients with rudimentary horns with functioning endometrium can also present with pain caused by accumulating menses. Because the other horn has a normal outflow pathway, these patients present with pain, not primary amenorrhea. Pregnancies that arise in a unicornuate uterus are associated with increased preterm labor and delivery, malpresentation, and miscarriage.

Uterine Didelphys
A **uterine didelphys** is the result a complete failure of fusion and represents 5% of müllerian anomalies. There are 2 fallopian tubes, 2 completely separate uterine cavities, 2 cervices, and often 2 vaginal canals or 2 partial canals because of an associated longitudinal vaginal septum (75% of the time). Evaluation for renal anomalies should be pursued because they are common as well. At times, the longitudinal septum attaches to 1 sidewall and obstructs 1 side of the vagina (or hemivagina). The combination of uterine didelphys, obstructed hemivagina, and ipsilateral renal agenesis is a variant of the broad spectrum of müllerian anomalies that is referred to as the **Heryln-Werner-Wunderlich syndrome** or **obstructed hemivagina and ipsilateral**

renal anomaly syndrome in the literature. Adolescents with this disorder usually present with abdominal pain shortly after menarche. Although there still may be a risk of adverse pregnancy outcomes with a uterine didelphys (preterm labor, malpresentation), overall pregnancy outcomes are generally good and are associated with less risk than in other uterine anomalies.

Arcuate Uterus

An **arcuate uterus** is a uterine cavity that has a small midline septum, from lack of a small amount of resorption, and sometimes a slight indentation of the uterine fundus. An arcuate uterus might represent a variant of normal rather than a müllerian anomaly. Untoward pregnancy outcomes are rare and surgical correction is not warranted.

Uterine Anomalies in Diethylstilbestrol-Exposed Patients

Intrauterine diethylstilbestrol (DES) exposure is associated with an increased risk for development of uterine anomalies and clear cell adenocarcinoma of the vagina and cervix. DES was used to prevent preterm delivery, but this practice was discontinued in 1971. Commonly observed uterine features associated with DES exposure include the following: T-shaped uterus, cervical hypoplasia, fallopian tube irregularities, scalloped or irregularly shaped endometrial contour, constriction bands, and others. DES suppresses and/or alters *Wnt* and *HOX* genes in mice and thus might work by affecting gene expression in müllerian duct development, causing uterine abnormalities, vaginal adenosis, and potentially carcinoma.

Treatment

Treatment depends on the specific anomaly. Hysteroscopic surgical resection is widely supported for uterine septa. If a septate uterus extends through the cervical canal, many choose to leave this cervical portion of the septum because of concerns for future incompetence, although case reports indicate that incisions have been done with uneventful follow-up. Most would support the incision of a uterine septum in the clinical setting of pregnancy loss, but some would also support prophylactic metroplasty without a history of miscarriage, especially before in vitro fertilization.

A noncommunicating horn with functional endometrium should be resected to improve quality of life or prevent future complications; opinions vary as to whether resection of a communicating horn or one with no functional endometrium is warranted. Any surgical resection of a rudimentary horn requires careful surgical technique to protect the ipsilateral ovarian blood supply and the myometrium of the remaining unicornuate uterus.

Although metroplasty had been advocated with didelphic and bicornuate uteri and a history of poor pregnancy outcomes in the past, currently most clinicians feel there is not enough evidence to support such a complicated procedure. Any obstruction to the outflow tract must also be relieved; this can necessitate creation of a vaginal window or excision of a hemivaginal septum.

VAGINAL ANOMALIES
Abnormalities of the Hymen

An **imperforate hymen** is the most common obstructive anomaly, and familial occurrences have been reported. Its incidence is most often reported as approximately 1 in 1,000. In the newborn period and early infancy, it may be diagnosed by a bulging membrane caused by a mucocolpos from maternal estrogen stimulation of the vaginal mucosa. This can eventually reabsorb if it is not too large or symptomatic. More often it is diagnosed at the time of menarche, when menstrual fluid accumulates. The clinical manifestations often are a bulging blue-black membrane, pain, primary amenorrhea, and normal secondary sex characters. Depending on the circumstance, patients might have cyclic abdominal pain or a pelvic mass. Other hymenal abnormalities have been reported. A normal hymen can have various configurations (annular, crescentic). Some hymenal membranes do not undergo complete resorption or perforation, resulting in microperforate, cribriform, or septate-shaped hymen. Infants and children vary in age as to when

these are recognized, but hymenal anomalies are often discovered after menarche when it is difficult for an adolescent to place a tampon, so resection is indicated.

Congenital Absence of the Vagina and Mayer-Rokitansky-Küster-Hauser Syndrome

Vaginal agenesis or **atresia** results when the vaginal plate fails to canalize. On physical exam it appears as an extremely foreshortened vagina, sometimes referred to as a *vaginal dimple*. Isolated (partial) vaginal agenesis involves an area of aplasia between the distal vaginal portion and a normal upper vagina, cervix, and uterus. On initial presentation it may be confused with a low transverse septum or imperforate hymen, and therefore clear delineation of the anomaly is critical before attempting surgical repair. It can also manifest with cyclic pain and a bulging mass just after menarche. Surgical repair and reconstruction are complicated and individualized and best performed with consultation of specialists.

Uterine and vaginal agenesis often occur together because of their close association during development, when müllerian ductal development fails early in the process. The most common cause of vaginal agenesis is **Mayer-Rokitansky-Küster-Hauser syndrome**, with an incidence reported at 1 in 4,000-10,000 female births. After gonadal dysgenesis, müllerian agenesis is the second most common cause of primary amenorrhea. The cause is unknown and likely has a multigenetic and multifactorial etiology. Mayer-Rokitansky-Küster-Hauser syndrome is characterized by primary amenorrhea, normal vulva, anomalies of the uterus (usually aplasia or agenesis), attenuated fallopian tubes, normal ovaries, normal female karyotype and phenotype, and associated anomalies (most commonly renal and skeletal). The vagina either is completely absent or only has a small dimpled opening. Although most patients with müllerian agenesis have small rudimentary müllerian bulbs, approximately 2-7% of patients can have active endometrium within these uterine structures. These patients will often present with cyclic pelvic pain. MRI imaging is often necessary to determine if any small uterine remnant is present (often located on the pelvic sidewall or near the ovaries and only a small fibromuscular remnant) and to clearly delineate the anomaly. Laparoscopy is not necessary to diagnosis müllerian agenesis but may be useful in the treatment of rudimentary uterine horns, particularly when removal of obstructed uterine structures or associated endometriosis is indicated for pelvic pain. Absence of the vagina and uterus has significant anatomic, physiologic, and psychologic implications for the patient and family. Any diagnosis of müllerian agenesis must be differentiated from androgen insensitivity (testicular feminization) as well; karyotype, serum testosterone levels, and pubic hair distribution usually help distinguish between the two.

Lesions involving other organ systems occur in association with the Mayer-Rokitansky-Küster-Hauser syndrome. The most common are urinary tract anomalies (15-40%) primarily involving unilateral absence of a kidney, a horseshoe or pelvic kidney, and skeletal anomalies (5-10%), which primarily involve vertebral development but can also include hearing impairment.

Longitudinal Vaginal Septa

Longitudinal vaginal septa represent failure of complete canalization of the vagina. These often occur in the presence of uterine anomalies as noted earlier.

Transverse Vaginal Septa (Vertical Fusion Defects)

Vertical fusion defects can result in a transverse septum, which may be imperforate and associated with hematocolpos or hematometra in adolescents or with mucocolpos in infants. These are much less common anomalies, reportedly found in 1 in 80,000 females. Most patients present with amenorrhea and cyclical pain around the time of menarche. Patients who have a small opening in the transverse septa might present with prolonged vaginal drainage and discharge. Transverse vaginal septa vary in location in the vagina (15-20% in the lower third, but most in the middle or upper third of the vagina) and thickness but are generally ≤1 cm thick. High locations, thick septa, and narrow vaginal orifices present challenging surgical cases.

Transverse vaginal septa may be associated with other congenital anomalies, although this occurs less often than with müllerian agenesis. These patients have a functional normal uterus, unlike women with Mayer-Rokitansky-Küster-Hauser syndrome. There is also an increased incidence of endometriosis secondary to retrograde menstruation.

Evaluation of transverse vaginal septa includes careful pelvic examination and often pelvic imaging, usually with MRI and ultrasound, to delineate the anatomic abnormalities. MRI is especially helpful to determine the thickness of the septum and presence of a cervix and for surgical planning. Diagnosis and treatment plans should be made as soon as possible after menarche, because significant accumulation of hematometra and/or hematosalpinx could affect future reproductive success by negatively affecting uterine and/or tubal function.

Treatment

An imperforate hymen requires resection to prevent or relieve the outflow tract obstruction. Many approach it with a horizontal, lunate or cruciate incision, excision of excess tissue, and reanastomosis of the mucosal edges. Repair should be done at time of diagnosis, if the patient is symptomatic. Although the lesion may be repaired any time during infancy, childhood, or adolescence, surgery is facilitated by estrogen stimulation and thus is ideally performed in adolescence, either after puberty or menarche. Variants in the hymen with microperforations or hymenal septa may interfere with tampon use and resection of this tissue is usually electively performed.

Treatment of congenital absence of the vagina is usually delayed until the patient is ready to be sexually active. The nonsurgical approach is the most common first-line therapy owing to the high success rate and extremely low morbidity. It requires dedicated use of dilators to create a functional vagina. The series of dilators come in progressively increasing sizes and require a commitment and maturity on the part of the patient to comply with daily use (20-30 min daily). If done correctly it is possible to achieve a functional vaginal length (6-8 cm), width, and physiologic angle for intercourse in about 6-8 wk of therapy. When the ultimate size that accommodates coitus is reached, then the patient must use the dilator or have coitus with a frequency that maintains adequate length.

Surgical approaches require more expertise and often some postoperative vaginal dilation to ensure a functional result. Controversy exists among surgical subspecialties, because pediatric surgeons and pediatric urologists often recommend creating the neovagina in infancy. Pediatric gynecologists and reproductive endocrinologists believe better outcomes result from creating the neovagina when the young woman is interested in sexual activity and can participate in the decision to have surgery and in her own postoperative recovery. There is no consensus as to the best surgical option; the most-used procedures include 2 surgical approaches followed by dilators or an approach using a loop of bowel out of which to construct a vagina. Patients need to be counseled about the ability to use their own oocytes and a gestational carrier through in vitro fertilization to achieve pregnancy. These therapies can be quite complicated physically and emotionally. They are best approached in a multidisciplinary fashion, often with the assistance of psychologic counseling and surgeons with specialized training.

For transverse vaginal septa, treatment is surgical resection of the obstruction through a vaginal approach. Some surgeons advocate waiting for 1 or more menstrual cycles or using preoperative dilators from below to increase the depth and circumference of the distal vagina and to allow menstrual blood to accumulate and dilate the upper portion of the vagina. Complete resection of the septum, with primary anastomosis of the upper and lower mucosal segments, should be attempted. A vaginal stent is sometimes placed postoperatively in the vagina to maintain patency and allow squamous epithelization of the upper vagina and cervix. Follow-up dilation may be necessary after the stent is removed. Careful preoperative assessment is important because surgeons who begin a case believing they are operating on an imperforate hymen can find themselves in entirely different and more complex surgical planes. Regardless of the approach, vagino-

plasty is often best deferred until the patient is mature and physically and psychologically prepared to participate in the healing process and postoperative dilator treatments.

Longitudinal vaginal septa themselves do not lead to adverse reproductive outcomes but may be symptomatic in a patient, causing dyspareunia, difficulties with tampon insertion, or impedance during vaginal birth. Such complaints can warrant a resection of the vaginal septa. In a small number of patients there may be unilateral obstruction of a hemivagina, which would require incision and resection.

CERVICAL ANOMALIES

Congenital atresia or complete agenesis of the uterine cervix is extremely rare and often manifests at puberty with amenorrhea and pelvic pain. It is associated with significant renal anomalies in 5-10% of patients. A pelvic MRI is often warranted to completely define the abnormality. Usually, pain and obstruction are significant and a hysterectomy is necessary. Attempts to reconnect the uterus to the vagina are rarely successful and associated with significant morbidity and reoperation rates. As with most müllerian anomalies, the ovaries usually remain normal and future reproduction can still occur through the use of in vitro fertilization and a gestational carrier.

VULVAR AND OTHER ANOMALIES
Complete Vulvar Duplication
Duplication of the vulva is a rare congenital anomaly that is seen in infancy and consists of 2 vulvas, 2 vaginas, and 2 bladders, a didelphic uterus, a single rectum and anus, and 2 renal systems.

Labial Asymmetry and Hypertrophy
With the onset of puberty the labia minora enlarge and grow to an adult size. A woman's labia can vary in size and shape. Asymmetry of the labia, where the right and left labia are different in size and appearance, is a normal variant. Some women are uncomfortable with what they perceive to be their asymmetric or enlarged labia minora and complain about self-consciousness and discomfort while wearing tight clothing, exercising, or having sex. The enlarged labia can have a protuberant and abnormal appearance that can be functionally or psychologically bothersome. Local irritation, problems of personal hygiene with bowel movements or menses, interference with sexual intercourse or while sitting or exercising have resulted in requests for labial reduction. Some surgeons are advertising procedures to reduce uneven or enlarged labia minora. The American College of Obstetricians and Gynecologists does not support performing such surgery unless there is significant impairment in function. Medically indicated surgical procedures can include reversal or repair of female genital cutting and treatment for labial hypertrophy or asymmetrical labial growth secondary to congenital conditions, chronic irritation, or excessive androgenic hormones. Complications of labial surgery include loss of sensation, keloid formation, and dyspareunia.

Clitoral Abnormalities
Agenesis of the clitoris is rare. Clitoral duplication has been reported, often associated with pelvic organ abnormalities, including agenesis of other genital tract structures and bladder exstrophy. Exposure to male hormones will result in clitoral enlargement, and is often a sign of a testosterone producing tumor or use of exogenous steroids.

Cloacal Anomalies
Cloacal anomalies are rare lesions representing a common urogenital sinus into which the gastrointestinal, urinary, and vaginal canals all exit. Usually there is an abnormality in all or some of the processes of fusion of the müllerian ducts, development of the sinovaginal bulbs, or development of the vaginal plate. The single opening (cloaca) requires surgical correction, preferably by a multidisciplinary pediatric surgical team.

Ductal Remnants
Even though the opposite duct regresses in both sexes, there can sometimes be a small portion of either the müllerian or wolffian duct that

remains in either the male or female, respectively. Such remnants can form cysts, which is what makes them clinically visible during surgery, examination, or imaging. Most do not cause pain, although torsion of some has been reported, and small asymptomatic ones usually do not require resection. The most commonly reported are hydatid of Morgagni cysts (remnant of a wolffian duct arising from the fallopian tube), cysts of the broad ligament, and Gartner's duct cysts, which can form an ectopic ureter or be found along the cervix or vaginal walls.

Bibliography is available at Expert Consult.

Chapter **555**

Gynecologic Care for Girls with Special Needs

Elisabeth H. Quint

Adolescence presents challenges for all children and their families, but particularly so for teens with special needs and their families. The start of menstrual periods, the mood changes associated with puberty and the concerns about sexual activity with possible unplanned pregnancies, and worries about safety and abuse may present teens with disabilities and their families with additional issues.

SEXUALITY AND SEXUAL EDUCATION
Adolescents with special needs can have physical and/or developmental disabilities. These young women are often seen as asexual by their families, care providers, and society and therefore sexual education might not have been provided or considered necessary. Physically disabled teens are as likely to be sexually active as nondisabled teens. The care provider needs to assess the teen's knowledge of anatomy and sexuality, her social knowledge of relationships, and her ability to consent to sexual activity. Education regarding HIV and other sexually transmitted infections, disease prevention, and contraception, including postcoital contraception, should be offered at a developmentally appropriate level. Teens with disabilities may be more at risk for isolation and depression during adolescence.

ABUSE
The risk for sexual abuse in teens with disabilities is difficult to estimate. Screening for abuse is mandatory. Studies show that teens with physical disabilities are just as sexually active as their nondisabled counterparts but that more of their activity is nonvoluntary. Patients with cognitive impairment are often taught to be cooperative, which may make them more vulnerable. Abuse prevention education can include the No! Go! Tell! model. For teens with limited verbal capacity or developmental delay, abuse may be very hard to detect. The care provider needs to be vigilant in looking for signs on physical exam, such as unexplained bruises or scratches, or changes in behavior, such as regression, which may be indications of sexual abuse in those adolescents (see Chapters 40.1 and 119).

PELVIC EXAMINATION
An internal pelvic exam is rarely indicated in teens that are not sexually active, as Papanicolaou smears are not recommended to start until age 21 yr. An external genital exam can be performed, if there are vulvar issues such as discharge, irregular bleeding, suspicion for abuse, or foreign body. The frogleg position is usually favored over the use of stirrups. If the vagina or cervix needs to be clearly visualized for a medical indication, an exam under anesthesia by a gynecologist should be considered. Testing for sexually transmitted infections can be accomplished by urine testing or vaginal swabs (see Chapter 120).

MENSTRUATION
Irregular menstruation is common in teenagers, especially during the 1st 5 yr after menarche, because of immaturity of the hypothalamic–pituitary–ovarian axis and subsequent anovulation (see Chapter 116). Several conditions in teens with disabilities are associated with an even higher risk of irregular cycles. Teens with Down syndrome have a higher incidence of thyroid disease. There is a higher incidence of reproductive issues, including polycystic ovarian syndrome in teens with epilepsy and on certain antiepileptic drugs (see Chapter 552). Antipsychotic medication can cause hyperprolactinemia, which can affect menstruation.

For teens with disabilities the main issue with menstrual cycles, whether they are regular, irregular, or heavy, is the impact of menstruation on the patient's life, her health, and her ability to perform her normal activities. The history should focus on this aspect, and menstrual calendars may be helpful to document the cycles, behavior, and the impact of treatments. Most adolescents who self-toilet can learn to use menstrual hygiene products appropriately.

The evaluation for abnormal bleeding is the same as for all teens. Areas requiring particular attention for the girl with special needs are the consideration of menstrual suppression for hygiene or cyclical behavioral issues, like crying, tantrums, or withdrawal. A request for birth control, especially coming from a caregiver and not from the teen, requires an evaluation of the teen's ability to consent to sexual activity and evaluate the safety of her environment. Guidelines for abnormal bleeding include menses that are too heavy (in excess of 1 pad/hr for several hours in a row), too long (longer than 10 days), or too frequent (fewer than 20 days apart).

Treatment of Menstruation
If after documenting the impact of the regular or irregular cycles on the patient's well-being (often through menstrual or behavioral charting for several months), the care provider, patient, and family decide on menstrual intervention, several options are available. Menstrual regulation is not different from that in the nondisabled teenager in general, although there are some special considerations. Goals for treatment can be to decrease the heaviness of flow, regulate cycles to predictable bleeding, relieve pain or cyclical behavior symptoms, provide contraception, and/or obtain amenorrhea. Menstrual suppression leading to complete amenorrhea is usually difficult to obtain and infrequent scheduled bleeds may be easier to manage than unpredictable spotting, a common side effect of any suppressive treatment, for certain patients. After treatment has started, continue to monitor cycles, ideally with continued menstrual or behavior calendars.

Nonhormonal Methods
If menorrhagia or dysmenorrhea (occasionally leading to cyclical behavior changes in nonverbal teens) is the main concern, the patient can be started on nonsteroidal antiinflammatory drugs. These can decrease the flow by up to 20% in adequate doses and can be used alone or in combination with other treatments.

Estrogen-Containing Methods
Oral Contraceptives
Cyclical oral contraceptives usually lead to regular, lighter cycles with less cramping. Extended cycling through the use of continuous use of oral contraceptives can suppress cycles, with amenorrhea rates improving with time. Some unpredictable spotting is usually unavoidable, and often teens with special needs prefer to have predictable cycles several times a year. A chewable oral contraceptive is available for those with swallowing issues.

Contraceptive Ring
The contraceptive ring is usually used in a pattern of 3 wk on and 1 wk off, but it can be used (off-label) in a continuous 4-wk pattern, which can lead to less bleeding. However, the contraceptive ring may be difficult to use for a teen with dexterity problems and help with placement has obvious privacy issues.

Contraceptive Patch
The weekly patch can also be used in a continuous fashion. Some teens with developmental disabilities remove their patch erratically, and placement out of reach (e.g., on buttocks or shoulder) is advised.

Estrogen Use, Venous Thromboembolism and Mobility Issues
Immobility per se is not a contraindication to estrogen-containing contraceptives, according to the Centers for Disease Control and Prevention medical eligibility criteria for contraception released in 2010. There are some data to support the concern that higher-dose oral estrogen, the combined estrogen patch, and the newer progestin preparations may have a higher risk for venous thromboembolism. However, there are minimal data on the risk of venous thromboembolism in teens with mobility issues in wheelchairs with or without extraneous estrogen. It is important to obtain a thorough and extended family history for hypercoagulability before initiating estrogen therapy. Careful use of lower-dose (30 or 20 µg) ethinyl estradiol preparations may be advisable and third-generation progestin combinations and the patch should only be used if other methods have failed.

Progestin-Only Methods
Intramuscular Medroxyprogesterone Acetate
Intramuscular medroxyprogesterone acetate (DMPA) has long been used for menstrual suppression. Two issues are particularly relevant to teens with disabilities. Studies documenting a decrease in bone density associated with longer-term use of DMPA and a black box warning by the FDA have raised concerns about use of these products in young women, although research indicates that the bone density improves after the medication is stopped. For teens with mobility issues or those with very low body weight who are already at risk for low bone density, decreased bone density is a real concern, although the risk of fractures is unclear. Adequate calcium and vitamin D is recommended. The second issue for teens with mobility issues is weight gain associated with DMPA, especially among obese teens, which can lead to transfer and mobility issues. If long-term DMPA is considered for a specific patient, calcium and vitamin D supplementation is recommended and bone density could be measured after several years of use, and weight should be monitored closely.

Oral Progestins
Continuous oral progestins can also be very effective to obtain amenorrhea. The progesterone-only minipill causes significant irregular spotting, so if full suppression is the goal, then other progestins can be used daily, such as norethindrone 2.5 or 5 mg or micronized progesterone 200 mg.

Progesterone Intrauterine Device
The 5 yr levonorgestrel-intrauterine device has now been used for many teenagers for contraception as well as heavy menses. Teens with special needs might require anesthesia for insertion if the exam is very difficult because of discomfort, contractures, or a narrow vagina. Checking for strings in a clinic setting may be challenging; however, the intrauterine device location can be confirmed by sonography. There may be a significant amount of irregular bleeding and spotting in the 1st several mo, but there is 20% amenorrhea after insertion and up to 50% amenorrhea after 1 year of use. The bleeding profile of the newer and smaller 3 year progesterone intrauterine device may not be as helpful for menstrual suppression as the amenorrhea rates from the initial studies by the manufacturer are 6% at 1 year, but more studies are needed.

Implants
Progestin subdermal implants have relatively low amenorrhea rates and high rates of unscheduled bleeding and therefore might not be ideal for teens with special needs, as they also require significant patient cooperation for insertion.

Hormones and Antiepileptic Drugs
Certain enzyme-inducing seizure medications can interfere with oral contraceptives, change their effectiveness, and/or lead to intermittent bleeding. Higher estrogen dose or shorter injection intervals for DMPA may be considered. The only antiepileptic medication that is affected by combined oral contraceptives is lamotrigine; consequently, the dose of that medication may need to be adjusted if used in conjunction with hormones.

Surgical Methods
Surgical procedures such as endometrial ablation, a procedure where the lining of the uterus is surgically removed, and hysterectomy are available for treatment of abnormal periods in adults, but they should only rarely be used in extreme situations for teenagers where all other methods have failed and the patient's health is severely compromised by her cycles. Endometrial ablation only leads to amenorrhea approximately 30% of the time and has a higher failure rate in women younger than 40 yr of age. Ethical considerations around these methods leading to infertility and consent issues are complicated, and state law varies on this topic.

CONTRACEPTION
See also Chapter 117.
The menstrual manipulation methods discussed above can also be used for contraception and if a request for birth control is made, an evaluation of the patient's ability to consent to sexual activity and the safety of her environment should be done. The method chosen should be the safest method for her situation with the highest protection rate. If she is dependent on others a long-acting reversible contraceptive method may be advisable. Sexually transmitted infections and condom use should be addressed with the teen and specific guidelines on how to obtain condoms and negotiate its use may be needed. A discussion about postcoital contraception is recommended, as well as ways to help the teen obtain this if indicated.

Bibliography is available at Expert Consult.

555.1 Female Genital Mutilation/Cutting
Robert M. Kliegman

Female genital mutilation/cutting (FGM/C) is a common practice in many parts of the world and is considered a form of child abuse and is illegal in most countries. It is estimated that more than 125 million women in 29 countries have undergone FGM/C (Fig. 555-1). FGM/C breaches international human rights laws and is considered a criminal act.
FGM/C has no health benefit. It threatens the health of girls and women having adverse effects on their psychologic, sexual, and reproductive well-being (Table 555-1). In addition, it increases the risk of HIV infection.

CLASSIFICATIONS
Type I: Partial or complete removal of the clitoris, prepuce, or both
Type II: Mutilation or cutting producing partial or complete removal of the clitoris and labia minora with or without excision of the labia majora
Type III: Infibulation; narrowing and sealing of the vaginal orifice by cutting and apposition of the labia minora or majora with or without excision of the clitoris
Type IV: All other harmful procedures

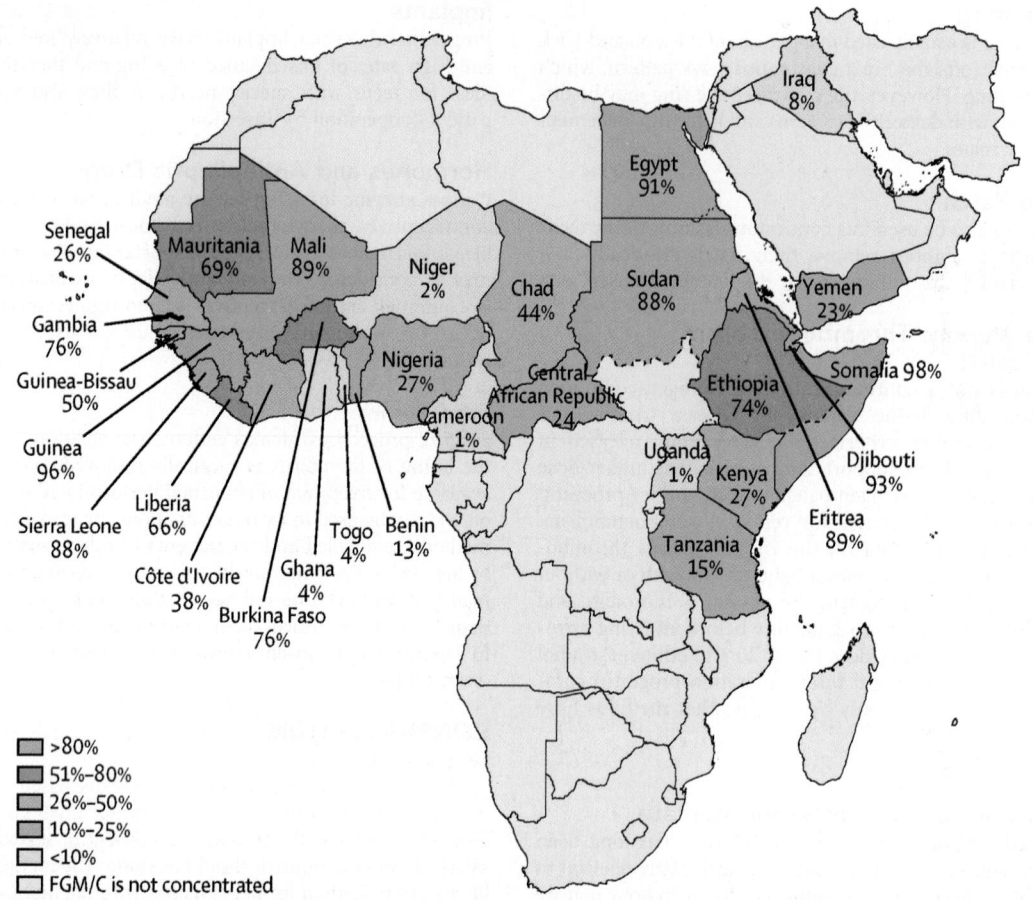

>80%
51%–80%
26%–50%
10%–25%
<10%
FGM/C is not concentrated

Figure 555-1 Proportion of girls and women ages 15-49 yr who have undergone FGM/C, by country. This map is stylized and not to scale; it does not indicate UNICEF's position on the legal status of any country or territory or the delimitation of any frontiers. The final boundary between Sudan and South Sudan has not yet been determined. FGM/C, female genital mutilation/cutting. *(Reproduced from Female genital mutilation/cutting: a statistical overview and exploration of the dynamics of change, by permission of UNICEF. Available at:* http://www.unicef.org/publications/index_69875.html)

Table 555-1	Health Consequences of Female Genital Mutilation

IMMEDIATE RISKS
Pain, shock (caused by pain or hemorrhage, or both), excessive bleeding, difficulty passing urine or feces, infection (including tetanus inoculation and the transmission of bloodborne viruses such as HIV, hepatitis B, and hepatitis C), psychologic consequences (as a result of pain, shock, or physical restraint), unintended labial fusion, death (caused by hemorrhage or infection).

LONG-TERM RISKS
Pain (chronic neuropathic pain), keloid scarring, infections (including chronic pelvic infections, recurrent urinary tract infections, and an increased incidence of certain genital infections), birth complications (cesarean section, postpartum hemorrhage, and episiotomy), danger to the newborn (including death), decreased quality of sexual life, psychologic consequences (including posttraumatic stress disorder, depression, and anxiety)

LONG-TERM RISKS PARTICULAR TO TYPE 3 FEMALE GENITAL MUTILATION
Need for later surgery (deinfibulation), urinary and menstrual problems, painful sexual intercourse, and infertility

From Simpson J, Robinson K, Creighton SM, Hodes D: Female genital mutilation: the role of health professionals in prevention, assessment, and management. BMJ 344:e1361, 2012, Box 3.

West African women are at greater risk of type II FGM/C, while those in northeast and east Africa and the Middle East are subjected to type III FGM/C. Nonetheless because of migration, women and girls in the United States and Western Europe may undergo FGM/C by traditional practitioners or, rarely, ethnic minority obstetricians or other physicians. Many ethnic women at risk for FGM/C living in the United States or Western Europe are more ambivalent about the procedure demonstrating a conflict between 2 cultures.

MANAGEMENT
This is a complex ethnic minority issue that often goes undetected until complications develop, either acutely from the procedure or during pregnancy. Criminalization alone will not eliminate this practice because it is performed in secret, and women are reluctant to discuss this with their healthcare provider, but laws against these procedures are an important step in reducing the number of women subjected to FGM/C.

Surgical repair, such as clitoral reconstruction with removal of scar tissue has been quite beneficial in decreasing pain and enhancing pleasure, including orgasm. Furthermore, women report a positive effect on their self-image and female identity as well as a new sense of "completeness" after reconstructive surgery.

Bibliography is available at Expert Consult.

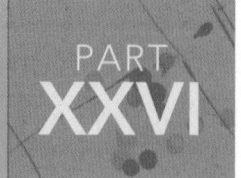

Section 1
Disorders of the Hypothalamus and Pituitary Gland

Chapter 556
Hormones of the Hypothalamus and Pituitary

Eric I. Felner and John S. Parks

The pituitary gland is the major regulator of an elaborate hormonal system. The pituitary gland receives signals from the hypothalamus and responds by sending pituitary hormones to target glands. The target glands produce hormones that provide negative feedback at the level of the hypothalamus and pituitary (Fig. 556-1). This feedback mechanism enables the pituitary to regulate the amount of hormone released into the bloodstream by the target glands. The pituitary's central role in this hormonal system and its ability to interpret and respond to a variety of signals have led to its designation as the "master gland." Table 556-1 lists hypothalamic and pituitary hormones and their functions.

ANATOMY
The pituitary gland is located at the base of the skull in a saddle-shaped cavity of the sphenoid bone called the *sella turcica*. The bony structure protects and surrounds the pituitary bilaterally and inferiorly. The dura, a dense layer of connective tissue, forms the roof of the sella. An external layer of the dura continues into the sella to form its lining. As a result, the pituitary is extradural and is not normally in contact with cerebrospinal fluid. The pituitary gland is connected to the hypothalamus by the pituitary stalk. The pituitary gland is composed of an anterior (adenohypophysis) and a posterior (neurohypophysis) lobe. The anterior lobe constitutes approximately 80% of the gland.

EMBRYOLOGY
The anterior pituitary gland originates from the Rathke pouch as an invagination of the oral ectoderm. It then detaches from the oral epithelium and becomes an individual structure of rapidly proliferating cells. By 6 wk of gestation, the connection between the Rathke pouch and the oropharynx is completely obliterated, and the pouch establishes a direct connection with the downward extension of the hypothalamus, which gives rise to the pituitary stalk. Persistent remnants of the original connection between the Rathke pouch and the oral cavity can develop into **craniopharyngiomas** (see Chapter 497), the most common type of tumor in this area.

VASCULAR SUPPLY
The arterial blood supply of the pituitary gland originates from the internal carotid via the inferior, middle, and superior hypophyseal arteries. This network of vessels forms a unique portal circulation connecting the hypothalamus and pituitary. The branches of the superior hypophyseal arteries penetrate the stalk and form a network of vessels that traverse the pituitary stalk and terminate in a network of capillaries within the anterior lobe. It is through this portal venous system that hypothalamic hormones are delivered to the anterior pituitary gland. Anterior pituitary hormones, in turn, are secreted into a secondary plexus of portal veins that drain into the dural venous sinuses.

ANTERIOR PITUITARY CELL TYPES
A series of sequentially expressed transcriptional activation factors directs the differentiation and proliferation of anterior pituitary cell types. These proteins are members of a large family of DNA-binding proteins resembling homeobox genes. The consequences of mutations in several of these genes are evident in human forms of multiple pituitary hormone deficiency. Five cell types in the anterior pituitary produce 6 peptide hormones. Somatotropes produce growth hormone (GH), lactotropes produce prolactin (PRL), thyrotropes make thyroid-stimulating hormone (TSH), corticotropes express proopiomelanocortin, the precursor of adrenocorticotropic hormone (ACTH), and gonadotropes express luteinizing hormone (LH) and follicle-stimulating hormone (FSH).

Growth Hormone
Human GH is a 191-amino-acid single-chain polypeptide that is synthesized, stored, and secreted by somatotropes in the pituitary. Its gene *(GH1)* is the first in a cluster of 5 closely related genes on the long arm of chromosome 17 (q22-24). The 4 other genes *(CS1, CS2, GH2,* and *CSP)* have >90% sequence identity with the *GH1* gene.

GH is secreted in a pulsatile fashion under the regulation of hypothalamic hormones. The alternating secretion of growth hormone–releasing hormone, which stimulates GH release, and somatostatin, which inhibits GH release, accounts for the rhythmic secretion of GH. Peaks of GH occur when peaks of growth hormone–releasing hormone coincide with troughs of somatostatin. **Ghrelin,** a peptide produced in the arcuate nucleus of the hypothalamus and in much greater quantities by the stomach, also stimulates GH secretion. In addition to the 3 hypothalamic hormones, physiologic factors play a role in stimulating and inhibiting GH. Sleep, exercise, physical stress, trauma, acute illness, puberty, fasting, and hypoglycemia stimulate the release of GH whereas hyperglycemia, hypothyroidism, and glucocorticoids inhibit GH release.

GH binds to receptor molecules on the surface of target cells. The GH receptor is a 620-amino-acid, single-chain molecule with an extracellular domain, a single membrane-spanning domain, and a cytoplasmic domain. Proteolytically cleaved fragments of the extracellular domain circulate in plasma and act as a GH-binding protein. As in other members of the cytokine receptor family, the cytoplasmic domain of the GH receptor lacks intrinsic kinase activity; instead, GH binding induces receptor dimerization and activation of a receptor-associated Janus kinase (Jak2). Phosphorylation of the kinase and other protein substrates initiates a series of events that leads to alterations in nuclear gene transcription. The signal transducer and activator of transcription 5b (STAT5b) plays a critical role in linking receptor activation to changes in gene transcription.

The biologic effects of GH include increases in linear growth, bone thickness, soft tissue growth, protein synthesis, fatty acid release from adipose tissue, insulin resistance, and blood glucose. The mitogenic actions of GH are mediated through increases in the synthesis of **insulin-like growth factor** 1 (IGF-1), formerly named *somatomedin C*, a 70-amino-acid single-chain peptide coded for by a gene on the long arm of chromosome 12. IGF-1 has considerable homology to

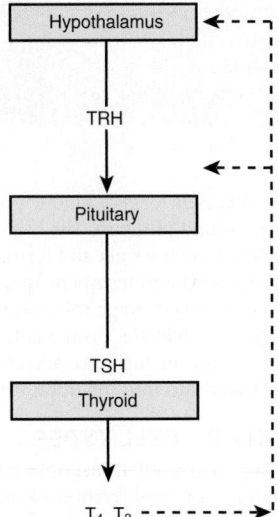

Figure 556-1 Hypothalamic–pituitary–thyroid (HPT) axis. Thyroid-releasing hormone (TRH) from the hypothalamus stimulates the pituitary gland to secrete thyroid-stimulating hormone (TSH). TSH stimulates the thyroid gland to produce and secrete thyroid hormones (T_4 and T_3). High circulating levels of T_3 and T_4 inhibit further TRH and TSH secretion and thyroid hormone production through a negative feedback mechanism (*dashed lines*). T_3, triiodothyronine; T_4, thyroxine; TRH, thyrotropin-releasing hormone; TSH, thyroid-stimulating hormone (thyrotropin); <---, inhibits; ←, stimulates.

insulin. Circulating IGF-1 is synthesized primarily in the liver and formed locally in mesodermal and ectodermal cells, particularly in the growth plates of children, where its effect is exerted by paracrine or autocrine mechanisms. Circulating levels of IGF-1 are related to blood levels of GH and to nutritional status. IGF-1 circulates bound to several different binding proteins. The major one is a 150-kDa complex (IGF-BP3) that is decreased in GH-deficient children. Human recombinant IGF-1 might have therapeutic potential in conditions characterized by end organ resistance to GH such as Laron syndrome and the development of antibodies to administered GH. IGF-2 is a 67-amino-acid single-chain protein that is coded for by a gene on the short arm of chromosome 11. It has homology to IGF-1. Less is known about its physiologic role, but it appears to be an important mitogen in bone cells, where it occurs in a concentration many times higher than that of IGF-1.

Prolactin

PRL is a 199-amino-acid peptide made in pituitary lactotropes. The regulation of PRL is unique because PRL is consistently secreted unless it is actively inhibited by dopamine, a peptide produced by neurons in the hypothalamus. Disruption of the hypothalamus or pituitary stalk can result in elevated PRL levels. Dopamine antagonists, states of primary hypothyroidism, administration of thyrotropin-releasing hormone (TRH), and pituitary tumors result in increased serum levels of PRL. Dopamine agonists and processes causing destruction of the pituitary cause reduced levels of PRL.

The primary physiologic role for PRL is the initiation and maintenance of lactation. PRL prepares the breasts for lactation and stimulates milk production postpartum. During pregnancy, PRL stimulates the development of the milk-secretory apparatus, but lactation does not occur because of the high levels of estrogen and progesterone. After delivery, the estrogen and progesterone levels drop and physiologic stimuli such as suckling and nipple stimulation signal PRL release and initiate lactation.

Thyroid-Stimulating Hormone

TSH consists of 2 glycoprotein chains (α, β) linked by hydrogen bonding; the α-subunit, which is composed of 89 amino acids and is

Table 556-1	Hormones of the Hypothalamus and Pituitary Gland		
HORMONES	**LOCATION**	**S/I**	**FUNCTION**
ACTH	Anterior pituitary	S	Production and secretion of GCs, MCs, and androgens from adrenal gland
ADH	Posterior pituitary	S	Reabsorption of water into the bloodstream via renal collecting ducts
CRH	Hypothalamus	S	Secretion of ACTH
Dopamine	Hypothalamus	S	Secretion of PRL
FSH (females)	Anterior pituitary	I	Secretion of estrogen from ovary
FSH (males)	Anterior pituitary	S	Production of sperm from testis
GH	Anterior pituitary	S	Secretion of IGF-1
GHRH	Hypothalamus	S	Secretion of GH
Ghrelin	Hypothalamus	S	Secretion of GH
GnRH	Hypothalamus	S	Secretion of FSH and LH
LH (females)	Anterior pituitary	S	Ovulation and development of the corpus luteum
LH (males)	Anterior pituitary	S	Production and secretion of testosterone
Oxytocin	Posterior pituitary	S	Contractions of uterus at birth and release of milk from breast
PRL	Anterior pituitary	S	Promotion of milk synthesis
Somatostatin	Hypothalamus	I	Secretion of GH and TSH
TRH	Hypothalamus	S	Secretion of TSH and PRL
TSH	Anterior pituitary	S	Secretion of T_4 and T_3

ACTH, adrenocorticotropic hormone; ADH, antidiuretic hormone; CRH, corticotropin-releasing hormone; FSH, follicle-stimulating hormone; GC, glucocorticoids; GH, growth hormone; GHRH, growth hormone–releasing hormone; GnRH, gonadotropin-releasing hormone; IGF-1, insulin-derived growth factor 1; LH, luteinizing hormone; MC, mineralocorticoids; PRL, prolactin; S/I, stimulate/inhibit; T_3, triiodothyronine; T_4, thyroxine; TRH, thyrotropin-releasing hormone; TSH, thyroid-stimulating hormone (thyrotropin).

identical to other glycoproteins (FSH, LH, and human chorionic gonadotropin), and the β-subunit, composed of 112 amino acids, that is specific for TSH.

TSH is stored in secretory granules and released into circulation primarily in response to TRH, which is produced by the hypothalamus. TRH is released from the hypothalamus into the hypothalamic–pituitary portal system and ultimately stimulates TSH release from pituitary thyrotropes. TSH stimulates release of thyroxine (T_4) and triiodothyronine (T_3) from the thyroid gland through the formation of cyclic adenosine monophosphate and the G protein second messenger system. In addition to the negative feedback inhibition by T_3, the release of TRH and TSH is inhibited by dopamine, somatostatin, and glucocorticoids.

Deficiency of TSH results in inactivity and atrophy of the thyroid gland, whereas excess TSH results in hypertrophy and hyperplasia of the thyroid gland.

Adrenocorticotropic Hormone

ACTH is a 39-amino-acid single-chain peptide that is derived by proteolytic cleavage from proopiomelanocortin, a 240-amino-acid precursor glycoprotein product of the pituitary gland. Proopiomelano-cortin also contains the sequences for the lipotropins, melanocyte-stimulating hormones, and β-endorphin.

Secretion of ACTH is regulated by corticotropin-releasing hormone (CRH), a 41-amino-acid peptide found predominantly in the median eminence but also in other areas in and outside of the brain. ACTH is secreted in a diurnal pattern. It acts on the adrenal cortex to stimulate cortisol synthesis and secretion. ACTH and cortisol levels are highest in the morning at the time of waking, are low in the late afternoon and evening, and reach their nadir 1-2 hr after beginning sleep. ACTH also appears to be the principal pigmentary hormone in humans. Similar to TRH and TSH, CRH and ACTH function through the formation of cyclic adenosine monophosphate and the G protein second-messenger system. Although CRH is the primary regulator of ACTH secretion, other hormones play a role. Arginine vasopressin, oxytocin, angiotensin II, and cholecystokinin stimulate release of CRH and ACTH, whereas atrial natriuretic peptide and opioids inhibit release of CRH and ACTH. Similar to the feedback inhibition T_3 has on TRH and TSH, cortisol also inhibits CRH and ACTH. Physiologic conditions, such as stress, fasting, and hypoglycemia, also stimulate release of CRH and ACTH.

Luteinizing Hormone and Follicle-Stimulating Hormone

Gonadotropic hormones include 2 glycoproteins, LH and FSH. They contain the same α subunit as TSH and human chorionic gonadotropin but distinct β subunits. Receptors for FSH on the ovarian granulosa cells and on testicular Sertoli cells mediate FSH stimulation of follicular development in the ovary and of gametogenesis in the testis. On binding to specific receptors on ovarian theca cells and testicular Leydig cells, LH promotes luteinization of the ovary and Leydig cell function of the testis. The receptors for LH and FSH belong to a class of receptors with 7 membrane-spanning protein domains. Receptor occupancy activates adenylyl cyclase through the mediation of G proteins.

Luteinizing hormone–releasing hormone, a decapeptide, has been isolated, synthesized, and widely used in clinical studies. Because it leads to the release of LH and FSH from the same gonadotropic cells, it appears that it is the only gonadotropin-releasing hormone.

Secretion of LH is inhibited by androgens and estrogens, and secretion of FSH is suppressed by gonadal production of inhibin, a 31-kDa glycoprotein produced by the Sertoli cells. Inhibin consists of α and β subunits joined by disulfide bonds. The β-β dimer (activin) also occurs, but its biologic effect is to stimulate FSH secretion. The biologic features of these more recently identified hormones are being delineated. In addition to its endocrine effect, activin has paracrine effects in the testis. It facilitates LH-induced testosterone production, indicating a direct effect of Sertoli cells on Leydig cells.

POSTERIOR PITUITARY CELL TYPES

The posterior lobe of the pituitary is part of a functional unit, the neurohypophysis, that consists of the neurons of the supraoptic and paraventricular nuclei of the hypothalamus; neuronal axons, which form the pituitary stalk; and neuronal terminals in the median eminence or in the posterior lobe. Arginine vasopressin (antidiuretic hormone [ADH]) and oxytocin are the 2 hormones produced by neurosecretion in the hypothalamic nuclei and released from the posterior pituitary. They are octapeptides and differ by only 2 amino acids.

Antidiuretic Hormone

ADH regulates water conservation at the level of the kidney by increasing the permeability of the renal collecting duct to water. ADH stimulates translocation of water channels through its interaction with vasopressin 2 receptors in the collecting duct, which act through G proteins to increase adenylyl cyclase activity and increase permeability to water. V2 receptors also mediate the von Willebrand factor and tissue plasminogen activator. At higher concentrations, ADH activates V1 receptors in smooth muscle cells and hepatocytes and exerts pressor and glycogenolytic effects through mobilization of intracellular calcium

stores. Separate V3 receptors mediate stimulation of ACTH secretion. These effects involve phosphatidylinositol hydrolysis rather than cyclic adenosine monophosphate production.

ADH and its accompanying protein neurophysin II are encoded by the same gene. A single preprohormone is cleaved and the 2 are transported to neurosecretory vesicles in the posterior pituitary. The 2 are released in equimolar amounts.

ADH has a short half-life and responds quickly to changes in hydration. The stimuli for its release are increased plasma osmolality, perceived by osmoreceptors in the hypothalamus, and decreased blood volume, perceived by baroreceptors in the carotid sinus of the aortic arch.

Oxytocin

Oxytocin stimulates uterine contractions at the time of labor and delivery in response to distention of the reproductive tract and stimulates smooth muscle contraction in the breast during suckling, which results in milk letdown. Studies suggest that oxytocin also plays a role in orgasm, social recognition, pair bonding, anxiety, trust, love, and maternal behavior. Most recently, through the interaction with its G-protein-coupled receptor in pancreatic and adipose tissue, oxytocin appears to play a significant role in appetite regulation and obesity by inducing anorexia.

Bibliography is available at Expert Consult.

Chapter **557**
Hypopituitarism
John S. Parks and Eric I. Felner

Hypopituitarism denotes underproduction of growth hormone (GH) alone or in combination with deficiencies of other pituitary hormones. Affected children have postnatal growth impairment that is specifically corrected by replacement of GH. The incidence of congenital hypopituitarism is thought to be between 1 in 4,000 and 1 in 10,000 live births. With expanding knowledge of the genes that direct pituitary development or hormone production, an increasing proportion of cases can be attributed to specific genetic disorders. Mutations in 7 candidate genes account for 13% of isolated growth hormone deficiency (IGHD) and 20% of multiple pituitary hormone deficiency (MPHD) cases. The likelihood of finding mutations is increased by consanguinity and occurrence in siblings or across generations. The genes, hormonal phenotypes, associated abnormalities, and modes of transmission for such established genetic disorders are shown in Tables 557-1 through 557-4. Acquired hypopituitarism usually has a later onset and different causes (Table 557-5).

MULTIPLE PITUITARY HORMONE DEFICIENCY
Genetic Forms

Sequentially expressed transcriptional activation factors direct the differentiation and proliferation of anterior pituitary cell types. These proteins are members of a large family of DNA-binding proteins resembling homeobox genes. Mutations produce different forms of MPHD. *PROP1* and *POU1F1* genes are expressed fairly late in pituitary development only in cells of the anterior pituitary and result in hypopituitarism without anomalies of other organ systems. The *HESX1*, *LHX3*, *LHX4*, and *PTX2* genes are expressed at earlier stages and are not restricted to the pituitary. Mutations in these genes tend to produce phenotypes that extend beyond hypopituitarism to include abnormalities in other organs.

Table 557-1	Etiologic Classification of Multiple Pituitary Hormone Deficiency	
GENE OR LOCATION	**PHENOTYPE**	**INHERITANCE**
GENETIC FORMS		
POU1F1 (PIT1)	GH, TSH, PRL	R, D
PROP1	GH, TSH, PRL, LH, FSH, ±ACTH, variable AP	R
LHX3	GH, TSH, PRL, LH, FSH, variable AP, ±short neck	R
LHX4	GH, TSH, ACTH, small AP, EPP, ±Arnold-Chiari	D
TPIT	ACTH, severe neonatal form	R
HESX1	GH, variable for others, small AP, EPP	R, D
SOX3	Variable deficiencies, ±MR, EPP, small AP and stalk	XL
PTX2	Rieger syndrome	D
GLI2	Holoprosencephaly, midline defects	D
GLI3	Hall-Pallister syndrome	D
SHH (sonic hedgehog)	GH deficiency with single central incisor	D
ACQUIRED FORMS		
Idiopathic		
Irradiation	GH deficiency precedes other deficiencies	
Inflammation	Histiocytosis, sarcoidosis	
Autoimmune	Hypophysitis	
Postsurgical	Stalk section, vascular compromise	
Tumor	Craniopharyngioma, glioma, pinealoma	
Trauma	Battering, shaken baby, vehicular	
UNCERTAIN ETIOLOGY		
Idiopathic		
Congenital absence of pituitary		
Septooptic dysplasia		
Birth trauma		

ACTH, adrenocorticotropic hormone; AP, anterior pituitary; D, dominant; EPP, ectopic posterior pituitary; FSH, follicle-stimulating hormone; GH, growth hormone; LH, luteinizing hormone; MR, mental retardation; PRL, prolactin; R, recessive; TSH, thyroid-stimulating hormone; XL, X-linked.

PROP1

PROP1 is found in the nuclei of somatotropes, lactotropes, and thyrotropes. Its roles include turning on *POU1F1* expression, hence its name prophet of *PIT1*. Mutations of *PROP1* are the most common explanation for recessive MPHD and are 10 times as common as the combined total of mutations in other pituitary transcription factor genes. Deletions of 1 or 2 base pairs in exon 2 are most common, followed by missense, nonsense, and splice-site mutations. Anterior pituitary hormone deficiencies are seldom evident in the neonatal period. The median age at diagnosis of GH deficiency is around 6 yr. Recognition of thyroid-stimulating hormone (TSH), luteinizing hormone (LH), follicle-stimulating hormone, and adrenocorticotropin (ACTH) deficiencies is delayed relative to recognition of GH deficiency. Anterior pituitary size is small in most patients, but in others there is progressive enlargement of the pituitary.

POU1F1 (PIT1)

POU1F1 (formerly *PIT1*) was identified as a nuclear protein that binds to the GH and prolactin promoters. It is necessary for emergence and mature function of somatotropes, lactotropes, and thyrotropes. Dominant and recessive mutations in *POU1F1* are responsible for

Table 557-2	Established Genetic Defects of the GH-IGF Axis Resulting in IGF Deficiency	
MUTANT GENE	**INHERITANCE**	**PHENOTYPE**
HPA		Developmental abnormalities
HESX1	AR	Septooptic dysplasia; variable involvement of pituitary hormones
PROP1	AR	GH, PRL, TSH, LH, FSH deficiencies; variable ACTH deficiency
POU1F1 (PIT1)	AR, AD	GH, PRL deficiency; variable degree of TSH deficiency
RIEG	AD	Rieger syndrome
LHX3	AR	GH, TSH, LH, FSH, prolactin deficiencies
LHX4	AD	GH, TSH, ACTH deficiencies
SOX3	XL	GH deficiency, mental retardation
GLI2	AD	Holoprosencephaly, hypopituitarism
GLI3	AD	Pallister-Hall syndrome, hypopituitarism
IGHD		
GHRHR	AR	IGHD, type IB form of IGHD
GHS-R	AD	GHD and ISS
GH1	AR	Type IA form of IGHD
	AR	Type IB form of IGHD
	AD	Type II form of IGHD
	XL	Type III form of IGHD; hypogammaglobulinemia
	AD	Bioinactive GH molecule
GHI		
GHR		
Extracellular domain	AR, AD	IGF-I deficiency; decreased or normal GHBP
Transmembrane	AR	IGF-I deficiency; normal or increased GHBP
Intracellular domain	AD	IGF-I deficiency; normal or increased GHBP
IGF		
IGF1	AR	IGF-1 deficiency; IUGR and postnatal growth failure
STAT5b	AR	IGF-1 deficiency, variable immune defect, hyperprolactinemia, chronic pulmonary infections, recurrent eczema
ALS	AR	IGF-1 deficiency; variable postnatal growth failure, delayed puberty

ACTH, adrenocorticotropic hormone (corticotropin); AD, autosomal dominant; ALS, acid labile subunit; AR, autosomal recessive; FSH, follicle-stimulating hormone; GH, growth hormone; GHBP, GH-binding protein; GHD, growth hormone deficiency; GHRHR, GH-releasing hormone receptor; HPA, hypothalamic pituitary; IGF, insulin-like growth factor; IGHD, isolated GHD; ISS, idiopathic short stature; IUGR, intrauterine growth retardation; LH, luteinizing hormone; PRL, prolactin; TSH, thyroid-stimulating hormone; XL, X-linked.

From Sperling MA: Pediatric endocrinology, ed 4, Philadelphia, 2014, Elsevier, Table 10-3, p. 333.

Table 557-3	Clinical and Biochemical Features of Molecular Defects of the GH–IGF-1 Axis

GENE DEFECT/PHENOTYPE	GHR	STAT5B	PTPN11	IGF1	IGFALS	IGFIR	BIOINACTIVE GH	GH1 WITH ANTI-GH ANTIBODIES
Severe growth failure	+/–	+	–	+	–	–	–	+
Mild growth failure	–/+	–	+	–	+	+	+	–
Midface hypoplasia	+/–	+/–	–	–	–	–	–	+
Other facial dysmorphism	–	–	+	+	–	+	–	–
Deafness	–	–	–	+/–	–	–	–	–
Microcephaly	–	–	–	+	–	+	–	–
Intellectual delay	–	–	–/+	+	–	+/–	–	–
Puberty delay	+/–	+/–	+/–	–	+	–	–	–
Immune deficiency	–	+	–	–	–	–	–	–
Hypoglycemia	+	–/+	–	–	–	–	–	–
Hyperinsulinemia	–	–	–	+/–	–	–	–	–
IGF-1 deficiency	+	+	–/+	+/–	+	–	+	+
IGFBP-3 deficiency	+	+	–/+	–	–	–	+	+
ALS deficiency	+	+	–/+	–	+	–	+	+
GH excess	+	+	–	+/–	–	–	–	–
GHBP deficiency	+/–	–	–	–	–	–	–	–
Homozygous or compound heterozygous mutations	+	+	–	+	+	–	–/+	+
Heterozygous mutations	–	–	+	–/+	–	+	+/–	–

+, Positive; –, negative; +/–, predominantly positive; –/+, predominantly negative; ALS, acid labile subunit; GH, growth hormone; GHBP, growth hormone–binding protein; IGF, insulin-like growth factor; IGFBP, insulin-like growth factor–binding protein.
From David A, Hwa V, Metherell L, et al: Evidence for a continuum of genetic, phenotypic, and biochemical abnormalities in children with growth hormone insensitivity. Endocr Rev 32:472–497, 2011, Table 2.

Table 557-4	Proposed Classification of Growth Hormone Insensitivity

Primary GH insensitivity (hereditary defects)
  GH receptor defect (may be positive or negative for GH-binding protein)
  • Extracellular mutation (e.g., Laron syndrome)
  • Cytoplasmic mutation
  • Intracellular mutation
  GH signal transduction defects (distal to cytoplasmic domain of GH receptor)
  • Stat5b mutations
  Insulin-like growth factor-1 defects
  • IGF-1 gene deletion
  • IGF-1 transport defect (ALS mutation)
  • IGF-1 receptor defect
  Bioinactive GH molecule (responds to exogenous GH)
Secondary GH insensitivity (acquired defects)
  • Circulating antibodies to GH that inhibit GH action
  • Antibodies to the GH receptor
  • GH insensitivity caused by malnutrition, liver disease, catabolic states, diabetes mellitus
  • Other conditions that cause GH insensitivity

GH insensitivity: Clinical and biochemical features of IGF-1 deficiency and insensitivity to exogenous GH, associated with GH secretion that would not be considered abnormally low.
GH insensitivity syndrome: GH insensitivity associated with the recognizable dysmorphic features described by Laron.
Partial GH insensitivity: GH insensitivity in the absence of dysmorphic features described by Laron.
ALS, acid labile subunit; GH, growth hormone; IGF, insulin-like growth factor.
From Sperling MA: Pediatric endocrinology, ed 4, Philadelphia, 2014, Elsevier, Box 10-4, p. 347.

complete deficiencies of GH and prolactin and variable TSH deficiency. Affected patients exhibit nearly normal fetal growth but experience severe growth failure in the 1st yr of life. With normal production of LH and follicle-stimulating hormone, puberty develops spontaneously, though at a later than normal age. These patients are not at risk for development of ACTH deficiency. Anterior pituitary size is normal to small.

HESX1

The *HESX1* gene is expressed in precursors of all 5 cell types of the anterior pituitary early in embryologic development. Mutations result in a complex phenotype with defects in development of the optic nerve. Heterozygotes for loss-of-function mutations show the combinations of isolated GH deficiency and optic nerve hypoplasia. Homozygotes can have full expression of septooptic dysplasia. This condition combines incomplete development of the septum pellucidum with optic nerve hypoplasia and other midline abnormalities. Clinical observation of nystagmus and visual impairment in infancy leads to the discovery of optic nerve and brain abnormalities. Septooptic dysplasia is associated with anterior and/or posterior pituitary hormone deficiencies in approximately 25% of the cases. These patients often show the triad of a small anterior pituitary gland, an attenuated pituitary stalk, and an ectopic posterior pituitary bright spot. The great majority of patients with septooptic dysplasia do not have *HESX1* mutations. The etiology might involve mutations in another gene or a nongenetic explanation (see Chapters 591 and 631).

LHX3 and LHX4

The phenotype produced by recessive loss-of-function mutations of the *LHX3* gene resembles that produced by *PROP1* mutations. There are

Table 557-5 | Causes of Acquired Hypopituitarism

BRAIN DAMAGE*
Traumatic brain injury
Subarachnoid hemorrhage
Neurosurgery
Irradiation
Stroke

PITUITARY TUMORS*
Adenomas
Others

NONPITUITARY TUMORS
Craniopharyngiomas
Meningiomas
Gliomas
Chordomas
Ependymomas
Metastases

INFECTION
Abscess
Hypophysitis
Meningitis
Encephalitis

INFARCTION
Apoplexy
Sheehan syndrome

AUTOIMMUNE DISORDER
Lymphocytic hypophysitis

OTHER
Hemochromatosis, granulomatous diseases, histiocytosis
Empty sella
Perinatal insults

*Pituitary tumors are classically the most common cause of hypopituitarism. However, new findings imply that causes related to brain damage might outnumber pituitary adenomas in causing hypopituitarism.
  From Schneider HJ, Aimaretti G, Kreitschmann-Andermahr I, et al: Hypopituitarism, Lancet 369:1461–1470, 2007.

deficiencies of GH, prolactin, TSH, LH, and follicle-stimulating hormone, but not ACTH. Some affected persons show enlargement of the anterior pituitary. The first patients to be described had the unusual findings of a short neck and a rigid cervical spine. They were only able to rotate their necks approximately 90 degrees compared with the normal rotation of 150-180 degrees. Dominantly inherited mutations in the structurally similar *LHX4* gene consistently produce GH deficiency, with the variable presence of TSH and ACTH deficiencies. Additional findings can include a very small V-shaped pituitary fossa, Chiari I malformation, and an ectopic posterior pituitary.

Other Congenital Forms

Pituitary hypoplasia can occur as an isolated phenomenon or in association with more extensive developmental abnormalities such as anencephaly or holoprosencephaly. Midfacial anomalies (cleft lip, palate; see Chapter 310) or the finding of a solitary maxillary central incisor indicates a high likelihood of GH or other anterior or posterior hormone deficiency. At least 12 genes have been implicated in the complex genetic etiology of holoprosencephaly (see Chapter 591.7). The Hall-Pallister syndrome is caused by dominant loss of function mutations in the *GLI3* gene. Absence of the pituitary gland is accompanied by hypothalamic hamartoblastoma, polydactyly, nail dysplasia, bifid epiglottis, imperforate anus, and anomalies of the heart, lungs, and kidneys. The combination of anophthalmia and hypopituitarism has been associated with mutations in the *SIX6, SOX2,* and *OTX2* genes.

Severe, early-onset MPHD including deficiency of ACTH is often associated with the triad of anterior pituitary hypoplasia, absence or attenuation of the pituitary stalk, and an ectopic posterior pituitary

bright spot on MRI. Most cases are sporadic and there is a male predominance. Some are from abnormalities of the *SOX3* gene, located on the X chromosome. As with septooptic dysplasia, the majority of cases have not been explained at the genetic level.

Acquired Forms

Any lesion that damages the hypothalamus, pituitary stalk, or anterior pituitary can cause pituitary hormone deficiency (see Table 557-5). Because such lesions are not selective, multiple hormonal deficiencies are usually observed. Diabetes insipidus is more frequent in acquired than in congenital hypopituitarism. The most common lesion is the craniopharyngioma (see Chapter 497). Central nervous system germinoma, eosinophilic granuloma (histiocytosis), tuberculosis, sarcoidosis, toxoplasmosis, meningitis, and aneurysms can also cause hypothalamic-hypophyseal destruction. Trauma, including abusive head trauma (see Chapter 40), motor vehicle accidents, traction at delivery, anoxia, and hemorrhagic infarction, can also damage the pituitary, its stalk, or the hypothalamus.

ISOLATED GROWTH HORMONE DEFICIENCY AND INSENSITIVITY

Genetic Forms of Growth Hormone Deficiency

IGHD is caused by abnormalities of the GH-releasing hormone receptor, GH genes, and genes located on the X chromosome.

Growth Hormone–Releasing Hormone Receptor

Recessive loss-of-function mutations in the receptor for GH-releasing hormone interfere with proliferation of somatotropes during pituitary development and disrupt the most important signals for release of GH. The anterior pituitary is small, in keeping with the observation that somatotropes normally account for >50% of pituitary volume. There is some compromise of fetal growth followed by severe compromise of postnatal growth.

GH1

The *GH1* gene is one of a cluster of 5 genes on chromosome 17q22-24. This cluster arose through successive duplications of an ancestral GH gene. Unequal crossing over at meiosis has produced a variety of gene deletions. Small deletions (<10 kb) remove only the *GH1* gene, whereas large deletions (45 kb) remove 1 or more of the adjacent genes *(CSL, CS1, GH2,* and *CS2)*. The growth phenotype is identical with deletion of *GH1* alone or *GH1* together with 1 or more of the adjacent genes. Loss of the *CS1, GH2,* and *CS2* genes without loss of *GH1* causes deficiency of chorionic somatomammotropin and placental GH in the maternal circulation, but it does not result in fetal or postnatal growth retardation. Most children with *GH1* gene deletions respond very well to recombinant GH treatment, but some develop antibodies to GH and cease growing.

Recessively transmitted mutations in the *GH1* gene produce a similar phenotype. Missense, nonsense, and frameshift mutations have been described. Autosomal dominant IGHD is also caused by mutations in *GH1*. The mutations usually involve splice-site errors in intron 3 and result in a variant protein that lacks the amino acids normally encoded by exon 3. Accumulation of this protein interferes with the processing, storage, and secretion of the normal GH protein and may result in additional deficiencies of TSH and/or ACTH. There are several reports of mutations in *GH1* that lead to variant proteins with reduced biological activity.

X-Linked Isolated Growth Hormone Deficiency

Two loci on the X chromosome have been associated with hypopituitarism. The first lies at Xq21.3-q22 in the region of the Bruton thymidine kinase *(BTK)* gene. Mutations in this region produce hypogammaglobulinemia as well as IGHD. The second locus maps farther out on the long arm, at Xq24-q27.1, a region containing the *SOX2* transcription factor gene. Abnormalities in this locus have been linked to IGHD with intellectual disability as well as to MPHD with the triad of pituitary hypoplasia, missing pituitary stalk, and ectopic posterior pituitary gland.

Acquired Forms

The GH axis is more susceptible to disruption by acquired conditions than are other hypothalamic-pituitary axes. Recognized causes of acquired GH deficiency include the use of radiotherapy for malignancy, meningitis, histiocytosis, and trauma.

Children who receive radiotherapy for central nervous system tumors or prevention of central nervous system malignancies (e.g., leukemia) are at risk for developing GH deficiency. Spinal irradiation contributes to disproportionately poor growth of the trunk. Growth typically slows during radiation therapy (see Chapter 718) or chemotherapy (see Chapter 494), improves for 1-2 yr, and then declines with the development of GH deficiency. The dose and frequency of radiotherapy are important determinants of hypopituitarism. GH deficiency is almost universal 5 yr after therapy with a total dose ≥35 Gy. More subtle defects are seen with doses around 20 Gy. Deficiency of GH is the most common defect, but deficiencies of TSH and ACTH can also occur. In contrast to other forms of hypopituitarism, puberty tends to be early rather than delayed (see Chapter 562.3). The clinician is likely to encounter children in the 8-10 yr age range who are growing at rates that are normal for chronological age but subnormal for stage of pubertal development.

GROWTH HORMONE INSENSITIVITY
Abnormalities of the Growth Hormone Receptor

GH insensitivity is caused by disruption of pathways distal to production of GH. Laron syndrome involves mutations of the GH receptor. Children with this condition clinically resemble those with severe IGHD. Birth length tends to be about 1 SD below the mean, and severe short stature with lengths >4 SD below the mean is present by 1 yr of age. Resting and stimulated GH levels tend to be high and insulin-like growth factor (IGF) 1 levels are low. The GH receptor has an extracellular GH-binding domain, a transmembrane domain, and an intracellular signaling domain. Mutations in the extracellular domain interfere with binding of GH. Serum GH-binding protein activity, representing the circulating form of the membrane receptor for GH, is generally low. Mutations in the transmembrane domain can interfere with anchoring of the receptor to the plasma membrane. In these cases, circulating GH-binding protein activity is normal or high. Mutations in the intracellular domain interfere with JAK/STAT signaling.

Postreceptor Forms of Growth Hormone Insensitivity

Some children with severe growth failure, high GH and low IGF-1 levels, and normal GH-binding protein levels have abnormalities distal to the GH binding and activation of the GH receptor. Several have been found to have mutations in the gene encoding signal transducer and activator of transcription 5b (STAT5b). Disruption of this key intermediate connecting receptor activation to gene transcription produces growth failure similar to that seen in Laron syndrome. These patients also suffer from chronic pulmonary infections, consistent with important roles for STAT5b in interleukin cytokine signaling.

IGF-1 Gene Abnormalities

Abnormalities of the IGF-1 gene produce severe prenatal and postnatal growth impairment. Microcephaly, intellectual disability, and deafness are present in patients with exon deletion and a missense mutation. These patients can be expected to respond to recombinant IGF-1 treatment.

Insulin-Like Growth Factor–Binding Protein Abnormalities

Mutation of the gene encoding the acid labile subunit of the circulating 165-kDa IGF-1, IGF-BP3, acid labile subunit complex has been associated with short stature. Total IGF-1 levels were very low. The index case, with homozygosity for an acid labile subunit mutation, did not show an increase in IGF-1 levels or an increase in growth rate during GH treatment.

IGF-1 Receptor Gene Abnormalities

Mutations of the IGF-1 receptor also compromise prenatal and postnatal growth. The phenotype does not appear to be as severe as that seen with absence of IGF-1. Adult heights are closer to the normal range, and affected patients do not have intellectual disability or deafness.

CLINICAL MANIFESTATIONS
Congenital Hypopituitarism

The child with hypopituitarism is usually of normal size and weight at birth, although those with MPHD and genetic defects of the GH1 or GHR gene have birth lengths that average 1 SD below the mean. Children with severe defects in GH production or action typically fall more than 4 SD below the mean for length by 1 yr of age. Those with less-severe deficiencies grow at rates below the 25th percentile for age and gradually diverge from normal height percentiles. Delayed closure of the epiphyses permits growth beyond the normal age when growth should be complete. Features of GH insensitivity are noted in Table 557-6.

Infants with congenital defects of the pituitary or hypothalamus may present with neonatal emergencies such as apnea, cyanosis, or severe hypoglycemia with or without seizures. Prolonged neonatal jaundice is common. It involves elevation of conjugated and unconjugated bilirubin and may be mistaken for neonatal hepatitis. Nystagmus can suggest septooptic dysplasia (see Chapter 591). Micropenis in boys provides an additional diagnostic clue. Deficiency of GH may be accompanied by hypoadrenalism (see Chapter 575) and hypothyroidism (see Chapter 565) as well as gonadotropin deficiency (see Chapters 583.2 and 586.2).

On physical examination, the head is round and the face is short and broad. The frontal bone is prominent, and the bridge of the nose is depressed and saddle shaped. The nose is small, and the nasolabial folds are well developed. The eyes are somewhat bulging. The mandible and the chin are underdeveloped, and the teeth, which erupt late, are often crowded. The neck is short and the larynx is small. The voice is high-pitched and remains high after puberty. The extremities are well proportioned, with small hands and feet. Weight for height is usually

Table 557-6	Clinical Features of Growth Hormone Insensitivity

Growth and development
  Birthweight: near-normal
  Birth length: may be slightly decreased
  Postnatal growth: severe growth failure
  Bone age: delayed, but may be advanced relative to height age
  Genitalia: micropenis in childhood; normal for body size in adults
  Puberty: delayed 3-7 yr
  Sexual function and fertility: normal
Craniofacies
  Hair: sparse before the age of 7 yr
  Forehead: prominent; frontal bossing
  Skull: normal head circumference; craniofacial disproportion due to small facies
  Facies: small
  Nasal bridge: hypoplastic
  Orbits: shallow
  Dentition: delayed eruption
  Sclerae: blue
  Voice: high pitched
Musculoskeletal/metabolic/miscellaneous
  Hypoglycemia: in infants and children; fasting symptoms in some adults
  Walking and motor milestones: delayed
  Hips: dysplasia; avascular necrosis of femoral head
  Elbow: limited extensibility
  Skin: thin, prematurely aged
  Osteopenia

From Sperling MA: Pediatric endocrinology, ed 4, Philadelphia, 2014, Elsevier, Table 10-5, p. 355.

normal, but an excess of body fat and a deficiency of muscle mass contribute to a pudgy appearance. The genitals are usually small for age, and sexual maturation may be delayed or absent. Facial, axillary, and pubic hair usually is lacking, and the scalp hair is fine. Intelligence is usually normal for age and the children may seem precocious compared to children of a similar size.

Acquired Hypopituitarism

The child is normal initially, and manifestations similar to those seen in idiopathic pituitary growth failure gradually appear and progress. When complete or almost complete destruction of the pituitary gland occurs, signs of pituitary insufficiency are present. Atrophy of the adrenal cortex, thyroid, and gonads results in loss of weight, asthenia, sensitivity to cold, mental torpor, and absence of sweating. Sexual maturation fails to take place or regresses if already present. There may be atrophy of the gonads and genital tract with amenorrhea and loss of pubic and axillary hair. There is a tendency to hypoglycemia. Growth slows dramatically. Diabetes insipidus (see Chapter 558) may be present but tends to improve spontaneously with development of central adrenal insufficiency.

If the lesion is an expanding tumor, symptoms such as headache, vomiting, visual disturbances, pathologic sleep patterns, decreased school performance, seizures, polyuria, and growth failure can occur (see Chapter 497). Slowing of growth can antedate neurologic signs and symptoms, especially with craniopharyngiomas. Evidence of pituitary insufficiency may first appear after surgical intervention. In children with craniopharyngiomas, visual field defects, optic atrophy, papilledema, and cranial nerve palsy are common.

LABORATORY FINDINGS

GH deficiency should be suspected in children with severe postnatal growth failure (Table 557-7). Criteria for growth failure include height

Table 557-7	Evaluation of Suspected Growth Hormone Deficiency
Growth-related history and patient physical exam	• Infants and children with GHD have growth failure • Short stature and growth failure may be the only clinical features present • GHD affects ~1 in 3,500 children
Imaging and other evaluations	• Diagnosis is based on clinical, auxologic, and biochemical parameters • Radiologic evaluation of bone age • Central nervous system MRI or CT scan to evaluate the hypothalamic-pituitary region and to exclude other conditions • Evaluation and management by a pediatric endocrinologist
Laboratory evaluation	• Measurements of GH, IGF-1, and IGF-1–binding protein levels • Determination of peak GH levels after stimulation test
Special testing (if applicable)	• Family history and genetic analyses (e.g., search for PROP1 and POU1F1 mutations)
Rationale for treatment and treatment modalities	• Replacement therapy with rhGH (GHT) • Predictors of greater benefit with GHT in GHD include early initiation of treatment, higher rhGH dose, and IGF-1–guided dosing • GHT should be started as soon as GHD is diagnosed

GH, growth hormone; GHD, growth hormone deficiency; GHT, growth hormone therapy; IGF, insulin-like growth factor; POU1F1, POU class 1 homeobox 1; PROP1, homeobox protein prophet of Pit1; rhGH, human recombinant growth hormone.

From Rogol AD, Hayden GF: Etiologies and early diagnosis of short stature and growth failure in children and adolescents. J Pediatr 164(5):S1–S14, 2014, Table XIII, p. S10.

below the 1st percentile for age and sex or height >2 SD below sex-adjusted mid-parent height. Acquired GH deficiency can occur at any age, and when it is of acute onset, height may be within the normal range. A strong clinical suspicion is important in establishing the diagnosis because laboratory measures of GH sufficiency lack specificity. Observation of low serum levels of IGF-1 and the GH-dependent IGF-BP3 can be helpful, but IGF-1 and IGF-BP3 levels should be matched to normal values for skeletal age rather than chronological age. Values in the upper part of the normal range for age effectively exclude GH deficiency. IGF-1 values in normally growing children and those with hypopituitarism overlap during infancy and early childhood.

Definitive diagnosis of GH deficiency traditionally requires demonstration of absent or low levels of GH in response to stimulation. A variety of provocative tests have been devised that rapidly increase the level of GH in normal children. These include administration of insulin, arginine, clonidine, or glucagon. In chronic GH deficiency, the demonstration of subnormal linear growth, a delayed skeletal age, and low peak levels of GH (<10 ng/mL) in each of 2 provocative tests are compatible with GH deficiency. In acute GH deficiency, a high clinical suspicion of GH deficiency and low peak levels of GH (<10 ng/mL) in each of 2 provocative tests are compatible with GH deficiency. This rather arbitrary cutoff point is higher than the 3 or 5 ng/mL criteria used for diagnosis of adult GH deficiency. There is no consensus regarding adoption of criteria that take into account age, sex, and GH assay characteristics. Some studies indicate that a majority of normal prepubertal children fail to achieve GH values >10 ng/mL with 2 pharmacologic tests. The researchers suggest that 3 days of estrogen priming should be used before GH testing to achieve greater diagnostic specificity.

In addition to establishing the diagnosis of GH deficiency, it is necessary to examine other pituitary functions. Levels of TSH, free thyroxine, ACTH, cortisol, gonadotropins, and gonadal steroids might provide evidence of other pituitary hormonal deficiencies. Antidiuretic hormone deficiency may be established by appropriate studies.

RADIOLOGIC FINDINGS

Conventional x-ray films of the skull have been replaced by CT and MRI. CT is appropriate for recognizing suprasellar calcification associated with craniopharyngiomas and bony changes accompanying histiocytosis. MRI provides a much more detailed view of hypothalamic and pituitary anatomy. Many cases of severe early-onset MPHD show the triad of a small anterior pituitary gland, a missing or attenuated pituitary stalk, and an ectopic posterior pituitary bright spot at the base of the hypothalamus. Subnormal anterior pituitary height, implying a small anterior pituitary, is common in genetic and idiopathic causes of IGHD. Craniopharyngiomas are common and pituitary adenomas are rare in children with hypopituitarism. Both hypoplastic and markedly enlarged anterior pituitary glands are seen in patients with *PROP1* or *LHX3* mutations.

Skeletal maturation is delayed in patients with IGHD and may be even more delayed when there is combined GH and TSH deficiency. Dual-photon x-ray absorptiometry shows deficient bone mineralization, deficiencies in lean body mass, and a corresponding increase in adiposity.

DIFFERENTIAL DIAGNOSIS

The causes of growth disorders are legion. Systemic conditions, such as inflammatory bowel disease, celiac disease, occult renal disease, and anemia, must be considered. Patients with systemic conditions often have greater loss of weight than length. A few otherwise normal children are short (i.e., >3 SD below the mean for age) and grow 5 cm/yr or less but have normal levels of GH in response to provocative tests and normal spontaneous episodic secretion. Most of these children show increased rates of growth when treated with GH in doses comparable to those used to treat children with hypopituitarism. Plasma levels of IGF-1 in these patients may be normal or low. Several groups of treated children have achieved final or near-final adult heights. Different studies have found changes in adult height that range from −2.5 to +7.5 cm compared with pretreatment predictions. There are no methods that can reliably predict which of these children will become taller in adulthood as a result of GH treatment and which will have compromised adult height.

Diagnostic strategies for distinguishing between permanent GH deficiency and other causes of impaired growth are imperfect. Children with a combination of genetic short stature and constitutional delay of growth have short stature, below-average growth rates, and delayed bone ages. Many of these children exhibit minimal GH secretory responses to provocative stimuli. When children in whom idiopathic or acquired GH deficiency is diagnosed are treated with human GH (hGH) and retested as adults, the majority have peak GH levels within the normal range.

Constitutional Growth Delay

Constitutional growth delay is one of the variants of normal growth commonly encountered by the pediatrician. Length and weight measurements of affected children are normal at birth, and growth is normal for the 1st 4-12 mo of life. Height is sustained at a lower percentile during childhood. The pubertal growth spurt is delayed, so their growth rates continue to decline after their classmates have begun to accelerate. Detailed questioning often reveals other family members (often 1 or both parents) with histories of short stature in childhood, delayed puberty, and eventual normal stature. IGF-1 levels tend to be low for chronological age but within the normal range for bone age. GH responses to provocative testing tend to be lower than in children with a more typical timing of puberty. The prognosis for these children to achieve normal adult height is guarded. Predictions based on height and bone age tend to overestimate eventual height to a greater extent in boys than in girls. Boys with >2 yr of pubertal delay can benefit from a short course of testosterone therapy to hasten puberty after 14 yr of age. The cause of this variant of normal growth is thought to be persistence of the relatively hypogonadotropic state of childhood (see Chapter 15).

Primary Hypothyroidism

Primary hypothyroidism (see Chapter 565) is more common than GH deficiency. Low total or free thyroxine and elevated TSH levels establish the diagnosis. Responses to GH provocative tests may be subnormal and the sella may be enlarged. Pituitary hyperplasia recedes during treatment with thyroid hormone. Because thyroid hormone is a necessary prerequisite for normal GH synthesis, it must always be assessed before GH evaluation.

Psychosocial Causes

Emotional deprivation is an important cause of retardation of growth and mimics hypopituitarism. The condition is known as *psychosocial dwarfism, maternal deprivation dwarfism,* or *hyperphagic short stature.* The mechanisms by which sensory and emotional deprivation interfere with growth are not fully understood. Functional hypopituitarism is indicated by low levels of IGF-1 and by inadequate responses of GH to provocative stimuli. Puberty may be normal or even premature. Appropriate history and careful observations reveal disturbed mother–child or family relations and provide clues to the diagnosis (see Chapter 40). Proof may be difficult to establish because the parents or caregivers often hide the true family situation from professionals, and the children rarely divulge their plight. Emotionally deprived children often have perverted or voracious appetites, enuresis, encopresis, insomnia, crying spasms, and sudden tantrums. The subgroup of children with hyperphagia and a normal body mass index tends to show catch-up growth when placed in a less stressful environment.

TREATMENT

Recombinant hGH has been available by prescription since 1982. There are currently 8 brands marketed in the United States. They are therapeutically equivalent, with the major differences consisting of proprietary devices for subcutaneous injection and availability of solubilized liquid forms or powders needing reconstitution before injection. At present none of the products are available in long-acting repository forms.

The FDA has approved 8 indications for GH treatment to promote growth. They are GH deficiency, Turner syndrome, chronic renal failure before transplantation, idiopathic short stature, small-for-gestational age short stature, Prader-Willi syndrome, *SHOX* gene abnormality, and Noonan syndrome. FDA approval for a given indication does not ensure that a patient's third-party insurance carrier will approve payment for the drug. The Pediatric Endocrine Society, the Academy of Pediatrics, and the GH Research Society have published guidelines for hGH treatment of children with classic GH deficiency. Treatment should be started as soon as possible to narrow the gap in height between patients and their classmates during childhood and to have the greatest effect on mature height. The recommended dose of hGH is 0.18-0.3 mg/kg/wk during childhood. Higher doses have been used during puberty. Recombinant GH is administered subcutaneously in 6 or 7 divided doses. Maximal response to GH occurs in the 1st yr of treatment. Growth velocity during this 1st yr is typically above the 95th percentile for age. With each successive yr of treatment, the growth rate tends to decrease. If growth rate drops below the 25th percentile, compliance should be evaluated before the dose is increased.

Concurrent treatment with GH and a gonadotropin-releasing hormone agonist has been used in the hope that interruption of puberty will delay epiphyseal fusion and prolong growth. This strategy can increase adult height. It can also increase the discrepancy in physical maturity between GH-deficient children and their age peers and can impair bone mineralization. There have also been attempts to forestall epiphyseal fusion in boys by giving drugs that inhibit aromatase, the enzyme responsible for converting androgens to estrogens. Therapy should be continued until near-final height is achieved. Criteria for stopping GH treatment include a decision by the patient that he or she is tall enough, a growth rate <1 inch/yr, and a bone age >14 yr in girls and >16 yr in boys.

Some patients develop either primary or central hypothyroidism while under treatment with GH. Similarly, there is a risk of developing adrenal insufficiency. If unrecognized, this can be fatal. Periodic evaluation of thyroid and adrenal function is indicated for all patients treated with GH.

Recombinant IGF-1 is approved for use in the United States. It is given subcutaneously twice a day. The risk of hypoglycemia is reduced by giving the injections concurrently with a meal or snack. In some situations its use is more efficacious than use of GH. These conditions include abnormalities of the GH receptor and *STAT5b* genes, as well as severe GH deficiency in patients who have developed antibodies to administered GH. Its utility in improving growth rate and adult stature in broader categories of short children is being explored.

The doses of GH used to treat children with classic GH deficiency usually enhance the growth of many non–GH-deficient children as well. Intensive investigation is in progress to determine the full spectrum of short children who may benefit from treatment with GH. The FDA approval for use of GH in idiopathic short stature specifies a height below the 1.2 percentile (−2.25 SD) for age and sex, a predicted height below the 5th percentile, and open epiphyses. Studies of the effect of GH treatment on adult height suggest a median gain of 2-3 inches, depending on dose and duration of treatment.

In children with MPHD, replacement should also be directed at other hormonal deficiencies. In TSH-deficient patients, thyroid hormone is given in full replacement doses. In ACTH-deficient patients, the optimal dose of hydrocortisone should not exceed 10 mg/m²/24 hr. Increases of 2-3–fold are made to provide stress coverage during illness or in anticipation of surgical procedures. In patients with a deficiency of gonadotropins, gonadal steroids are given when bone age reaches the age at which puberty usually takes place. For infants with micropenis, 1 or 2 three-month courses of monthly intramuscular injections of 25 mg of testosterone cypionate or testosterone enanthate can bring the penis to normal size without an inordinate effect on osseous maturation.

COMPLICATIONS AND ADVERSE EFFECTS OF GH TREATMENT

GH treatment influences glucose homeostasis. Fasting and postprandial insulin levels are characteristically low before treatment, and they normalize during GH replacement. Recent studies indicate that GH treatment is associated with a 6-fold increase in the risk for type 2 diabetes and no significant increase in the risk for type 1 diabetes.

Concerns have been raised about the safety of GH treatment in children who become deficient after treatment of brain tumors, leukemia, and other neoplasms. Long-term studies show no increase in risk of recurrence of craniopharyngioma, other brain tumors, or leukemia. At least 3 studies indicate an increased risk of second neoplasms in cancer survivors treated with GH. An unconfirmed study documents a 30% increase in mortality among young adults who received GH in childhood. There appears to be a correlation between risk of mortality and GH doses >0.35 mg/kg/wk.

Other reported side effects include pseudotumor cerebri, slipped capital femoral epiphysis, gynecomastia, and worsening of scoliosis, and in adults treated as a child there is an increased risk of hemorrhagic stroke. The risk of later development of Creutzfeldt-Jakob disease was limited to recipients of contaminated lots of extracted pituitary GH. No comparable risks have been seen with recombinant hGH.

Bibliography is available at Expert Consult.

Chapter 558
Diabetes Insipidus
David T. Breault and Joseph A. Majzoub

Diabetes insipidus (DI) manifests clinically with polyuria and polydipsia and can result from either vasopressin deficiency (central DI) or vasopressin insensitivity at the level of the kidney (nephrogenic DI). Both central DI and nephrogenic DI can arise from inherited defects of congenital or neonatal onset or can be secondary to a variety of causes (Table 558-1).

PHYSIOLOGY OF WATER BALANCE
The control of extracellular tonicity (osmolality) and volume within a narrow range is critical for normal cellular structure and function (see Chapter 55.2). Extracellular fluid tonicity is regulated almost exclusively by water intake and excretion, whereas extracellular volume is regulated by sodium intake and excretion. The control of plasma

Table 558-1	Differential Diagnosis of Polyuria and Polydipsia

Diabetes insipidus (DI)
• Central DI
Genetic (autosomal dominant)
Acquired
Trauma (surgical or accidental)
Congenital malformations (holoprosencephaly, septooptic dysplasia, encephalocele)
Neoplasms (craniopharyngioma, germinoma, metastasis)
Infiltrative (Langerhans cell histiocytosis), autoimmune (lymphocytic infundibuloneurohypophysitis), and infectious diseases
Drugs (chemotherapy)
Idiopathic
• Nephrogenic DI
Genetic (X-linked, autosomal recessive, autosomal dominant)
Acquired
Hypercalcemia, hypokalemia
Drugs (lithium, demeclocycline)
Kidney disease
Primary polydipsia
Sickle cell anemia
• Diabetes mellitus

tonicity and intravascular volume involves a complex integration of endocrine, neural, behavioral, and paracrine systems (Fig. 558-1). Vasopressin, secreted from the posterior pituitary, is the principal regulator of tonicity, with its release largely stimulated by increases in plasma tonicity. Volume homeostasis is largely regulated by the renin–angiotensin–aldosterone system, with contributions from both vasopressin and the natriuretic peptide family.

Vasopressin, a 9-amino-acid peptide, has both antidiuretic and vascular pressor activity and is synthesized in the paraventricular and supraoptic nuclei of the hypothalamus. It is transported to the posterior pituitary via axonal projections, where it is stored awaiting release into the systemic circulation. The half-life of vasopressin in the circulation is 5 min. In addition to responding to osmotic stimuli, vasopressin is secreted in response to significant decreases in intravascular volume and pressure (minimum of 8% decrement) via afferent baroreceptor pathways arising from the aortic arch (carotid sinus) and volume receptor pathways in the cardiac atria and pulmonary veins. Osmotic and hemodynamic stimuli interact synergistically.

The sensation of thirst is regulated by cortical as well as hypothalamic neurons. The thirst threshold is approximately 10 mOsm/kg higher (i.e., 293 mOsm/kg) than the osmotic threshold for vasopressin release. Consequently, under conditions of hyperosmolality, vasopressin is released before thirst is initiated, allowing ingested water to be retained. Chemoreceptors present in the oropharynx rapidly downregulate vasopressin release following water ingestion.

Vasopressin exerts its principal effect on the kidney via V2 receptors located primarily in the collecting tubule, the thick ascending limb of the loop of Henle, and the periglomerular tubules. The human V2 receptor gene is located on the long arm of the X chromosome (Xq28) at the locus associated with **congenital, X-linked, vasopressin-resistant DI.** Activation of the V2 receptor results in increases in intracellular cyclic adenosine monophosphate, which leads to the insertion of the aquaporin-2 water channel into the apical (luminal) membrane. This allows water movement along its osmotic gradient into the hypertonic inner medullary interstitium from the tubule lumen and excretion of concentrated urine. In contrast to aquaporin-2,

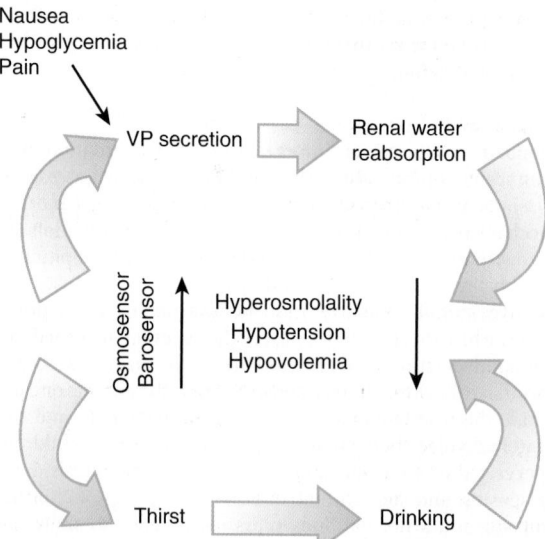

Figure 558-1 Regulation of vasopressin (VP) secretion and serum osmolality. Hyperosmolality, hypovolemia, and hypotension are sensed by osmosensors, volume sensors, and barosensors, respectively. These stimulate both VP secretion and thirst. VP, acting on the kidney, causes increased reabsorption of water (antidiuresis). Thirst causes increased water ingestion. The results of these dual negative feedback loops cause a reduction in hyperosmolality or in hypotension or hypovolemia. Additional stimuli for VP secretion include nausea, hypoglycemia, and pain. *(From Muglia LJ, Majzoub JA: Disorders of the posterior pituitary. In Sperling MA, editor: Pediatric endocrinology, ed 4, Philadelphia, 2014, Elsevier, Fig. 6.)*

aquaporin-3 and aquaporin-4 are expressed on the basolateral membrane of the collecting duct cells and aquaporin-1 is expressed in the proximal tubule. These channels may also contribute to urinary concentrating ability.

Atrial natriuretic peptide, initially isolated from cardiac atrial muscle, has a number of important effects on salt and water balance, including stimulation of natriuresis, inhibition of sodium resorption, and inhibition of vasopressin secretion. Atrial natriuretic peptide is expressed in endothelial cells and vascular smooth muscle, where it appears to regulate relaxation of arterial smooth muscle. Atrial natriuretic peptide is also expressed in the brain, along with other natriuretic family members; the physiologic role of these factors has yet to be defined.

APPROACH TO THE PATIENT WITH POLYURIA, POLYDIPSIA, AND HYPERNATREMIA

The cause of pathologic polyuria or polydipsia (exceeding 2 L/m²/24 hr) may be difficult to establish in children. Infants can present with irritability, failure to thrive, and intermittent fever. Patients with suspected DI should have a careful history taken, which should quantify the child's daily fluid intake and output and establish the voiding pattern, nocturia, and primary or secondary enuresis. A complete physical examination should establish the patient's hydration status, and the physician should search for evidence of visual and central nervous system dysfunction, as well as for other pituitary hormone deficiencies.

If pathologic polyuria or polydipsia is present, the following should be obtained: serum for osmolality, sodium, potassium, blood urea nitrogen, creatinine, glucose, and calcium; urine for osmolality, specific gravity, and glucose determination. The diagnosis of DI is established if the serum osmolality is >300 mOsm/kg and the urine osmolality is <300 mOsm/kg. DI is unlikely if the serum osmolality is <270 mOsm/kg or the urine osmolality is >600 mOsm/kg. If the patient's serum osmolality is <300 mOsm/kg (but >270 mOsm/kg) and pathologic polyuria and polydipsia are present, a water deprivation test is indicated to establish the diagnosis of DI and to differentiate central from nephrogenic causes.

In the inpatient postneurosurgical setting, central DI is likely if hyperosmolality (serum osmolality >300 mOsm/kg) is associated with urine osmolality less than serum osmolality. It is important to distinguish between polyuria resulting from postsurgical central DI and polyuria resulting from the normal diuresis of fluids received intraoperatively. Both cases may be associated with a large volume (>200 mL/m²/hr) of dilute urine, although in patients with DI, the serum osmolality is high in comparison with patients undergoing postoperative diuresis.

CAUSES OF HYPERNATREMIA

Hypernatremia is discussed in Chapter 55.3.

Central Diabetes Insipidus

Central DI can result from multiple etiologies, including genetic mutations in the vasopressin gene; trauma (accidental or surgical) to vasopressin neurons; congenital malformations of the hypothalamus or pituitary; neoplasms; infiltrative, autoimmune, and infectious diseases affecting vasopressin neurons or fiber tracts; and increased metabolism of vasopressin. In approximately 10% of children with central DI, the etiology is idiopathic. Other pituitary hormone deficiencies may be present (see Chapter 557). Over time, up to 35% of those with idiopathic central DI will develop other hormone deficiencies or have an underlying etiology identified.

Autosomal dominant central DI usually occurs within the 1st 5 yr of life and results from mutations in the vasopressin gene. A number of mutations can cause gene-processing defects in a subset of vasopressin-expressing neurons, which have been postulated to result in endoplasmic reticulum stress and cell death. **Wolfram syndrome,** which includes DI, diabetes mellitus, optic atrophy, and deafness, also results in vasopressin deficiency. Mutations in 2 genes, which give rise

to endoplasmic reticulum proteins, are associated with this condition. Congenital brain abnormalities (see Chapter 591) such as **optic nerve hypoplasia syndrome** with agenesis of the corpus callosum, the Niikawa-Kuroki syndrome, holoprosencephaly, and familial pituitary hypoplasia with absent stalk may be associated with central DI and defects in thirst perception. Empty sella syndrome, possibly resulting from unrecognized pituitary infarction (see Chapter 557), can be associated with DI in children.

Trauma to the base of the brain and neurosurgical intervention in the region of the hypothalamus or pituitary are common causes of central DI. The **triphasic response** following surgery refers to an initial phase of transient DI, lasting 12-48 hr, followed by a 2nd phase of syndrome of inappropriate antidiuretic hormone secretion, lasting up to 10 days, which may be followed by permanent DI. The initial phase may be the result of local edema interfering with normal vasopressin secretion; the 2nd phase results from unregulated vasopressin release from dying neurons, whereas in the 3rd phase, permanent DI results if more than 90% of the neurons have been destroyed.

Given the anatomic distribution of vasopressin neurons over a large area within the hypothalamus, tumors that cause DI must either be very large and infiltrative or be strategically located near the base of the hypothalamus, where vasopressin axons converge before their entry into the posterior pituitary. Germinomas and pinealomas typically arise in this region and are among the most common primary brain tumors associated with DI. Germinomas can be very small and undetectable by MRI for several years following the onset of polyuria. Quantitative measurement of α-fetoprotein and β-human chorionic gonadotropin, often secreted by germinomas, should be performed in children with idiopathic or unexplained DI in addition to serial MRI scans. Craniopharyngiomas and optic gliomas can also cause central DI when they are very large, although this is more often a postoperative complication of the treatment for these tumors (see Chapter 497). Hematologic malignancies, such as acute myelocytic leukemia, can cause DI via infiltration of the pituitary stalk and sella.

Langerhans cell histiocytosis (see Chapter 507) and lymphocytic hypophysitis are common types of infiltrative disorders causing central DI, with **hypophysitis** as the cause in 50% of cases of "idiopathic" central DI. Infections involving the base of the brain (see Chapter 603), including meningitis (meningococcal, cryptococcal, listerial, toxoplasmal), congenital cytomegalovirus infection, and nonspecific inflammatory diseases of the brain may give rise to central DI that is often transient. Drugs associated with the inhibition of vasopressin release include ethanol, phenytoin, opiate antagonists, halothane, and α-adrenergic agents.

Nephrogenic Diabetes Insipidus

Nephrogenic (vasopressin-insensitive) DI (NDI) can result from genetic or acquired causes. Genetic causes are less common but more severe than acquired forms of NDI. The polyuria and polydipsia associated with genetic NDI usually occur within the 1st several wk of life, but may only become apparent after weaning or with longer periods of nighttime sleep. Many infants initially present with fever, vomiting, and dehydration. Failure to thrive may be secondary to the ingestion of large amounts of water, resulting in caloric malnutrition. Longstanding ingestion and excretion of large volumes of water can lead to nonobstructive hydronephrosis, hydroureter, and megabladder.

Congenital X-linked NDI results from inactivating mutations of the vasopressin V2 receptor. **Congenital autosomal recessive NDI** results from defects in the aquaporin-2 gene. An **autosomal dominant form of NDI** is associated with processing mutations of the aquaporin-2 gene.

Acquired NDI can result from hypercalcemia or hypokalemia and is associated with lithium, demeclocycline, foscarnet, clozapine, amphotericin, methicillin, and rifampin. Impaired renal concentrating ability can also be seen with ureteral obstruction, chronic renal failure, polycystic kidney disease, medullary cystic disease, Sjögren syndrome, and sickle cell disease. Decreased protein or sodium intake or excessive water intake, as in primary polydipsia, can lead to diminished tonicity of the renal medullary interstitium and NDI.

TREATMENT OF CENTRAL DIABETES INSIPIDUS
Fluid Therapy

With an intact thirst mechanism and free access to oral fluids, a person with complete DI can maintain plasma osmolality and sodium in the high normal range, although at great inconvenience. Neonates and young infants are often best treated solely with fluid therapy, given their requirement for large volumes (3 L/m²/24 hr) of nutritive fluid. The use of vasopressin analogs in patients with obligate high fluid intake is difficult given the risk of life-threatening hyponatremia. Although not FDA approved, the use of diluted parenteral and lyophilized long-acting vasopressin analog DDAVP (desmopressin) has been successfully administered to infants with central DI both subcutaneously and orally without causing severe hyponatremia.

Vasopressin Analogs

Treatment of central DI in older children is best accomplished with the use of DDAVP. DDAVP is available in an intranasal preparation (onset 5-10 min) and as tablets (onset 15-30 min). The intranasal preparation of DDAVP (10 µg/0.1 mL) can be administered by rhinal tube (allowing dose titration) or by nasal spray. Use of DDAVP oral tablets requires at least a 10-fold increase in the dosage compared with the intranasal preparation. Oral dosages of 25-300 µg every 8-12 hr are safe and effective in children. The appropriate dosage and route of administration is determined empirically based on the desired length of antidiuresis and patient preference. The use of DDAVP nasal spray (10 µg/0.1 mL) for the treatment of primary enuresis in older children should be regarded as a temporizing measure, given it does not affect the underlying condition, and should be used with great caution given the risk of hyponatremia if water intake exceeds the capacity for renal clearance. To prevent water intoxication, patients should have at least 1 hr of urinary breakthrough between doses each day and be advised to drink in response to thirst sensation.

Aqueous Vasopressin

Central DI of acute onset following neurosurgery is best managed with continuous administration of synthetic aqueous vasopressin (Pitressin). Under most circumstances, total fluid intake must be limited to 1 L/m²/24 hr during antidiuresis. A typical dosage for intravenous vasopressin therapy is 1.5 mU/kg/hr, which results in a blood vasopressin concentration of approximately 10 pg/mL. On occasion, following hypothalamic (but not transsphenoidal) surgery, higher initial concentrations of vasopressin may be required to treat acute DI, which has been attributed to the release of a vasopressin inhibitory substance. Vasopressin concentrations >1,000 pg/mL should be avoided because they can cause cutaneous necrosis, rhabdomyolysis, cardiac rhythm disturbances, and hypertension. Postneurosurgical patients treated with vasopressin infusion should be switched from intravenous to oral fluids as soon as possible to allow thirst sensation, if intact, to help regulate osmolality.

TREATMENT OF NEPHROGENIC DIABETES INSIPIDUS

The treatment of acquired NDI focuses on eliminating, if possible, the underlying disorder, such as offending drugs, hypercalcemia, hypokalemia, or ureteral obstruction. Congenital nephrogenic DI is often difficult to treat. The main goals are to ensure the intake of adequate calories for growth and to avoid severe dehydration. Foods with the highest ratio of caloric content to osmotic load (Na <1 mmol/kg/24 hr) should be ingested to maximize growth and to minimize the urine volume required to excrete the solute load. Even with the early institution of therapy, however, growth failure and developmental disabilities are common.

Pharmacologic approaches to the treatment of NDI include the use of thiazide diuretics and are intended to decrease the overall urine output. Thiazides appear to induce a state of mild volume depletion by enhancing sodium excretion at the expense of water and by causing a decrease in the glomerular filtration rate, which results in proximal tubular sodium and water reabsorption. Indomethacin and amiloride

may be used in combination with thiazides to further reduce polyuria. High-dose DDAVP therapy, in combination with indomethacin, has been used in some subjects with NDI. This treatment could prove useful in patients with genetic defects in the V2 receptor associated with a reduced binding affinity for vasopressin.

Bibliography is available at Expert Consult.

Chapter 559
Other Abnormalities of Arginine Vasopressin Metabolism and Action
David T. Breault and Joseph A. Majzoub

Hyponatremia (serum sodium <130 mEq/L) in children is usually associated with severe systemic disorders and is most often a result of intravascular volume depletion, excessive salt loss, or hypotonic fluid overload, especially in infants (see Chapter 55).

The initial approach to the patient with hyponatremia begins with determination of the volume status. A careful review of the patient's history, physical examination (including changes in weight), and vital signs helps determine whether the patient is hypovolemic or hypervolemic. Supportive evidence includes laboratory data such as serum electrolytes, blood urea nitrogen, creatinine, uric acid, urine sodium, specific gravity, and osmolality (see Chapter 55; Tables 559-1 and 559-2).

Table 559-1 | Differential Diagnosis of Hyponatremia

DISORDER	INTRAVASCULAR VOLUME STATUS	URINE SODIUM
Systemic dehydration	Low	Low
Decreased effective plasma volume	Low	Low
Primary salt loss (nonrenal)	Low	Low
Primary salt loss (renal)	Low	High
SIADH	High	High
Cerebral salt wasting	Low	Very high
Decreased free water clearance	Normal or high	Normal or high
Primary polydipsia	Normal or high	Normal
Runner's hyponatremia	Low	Low
NSIAD	High	High
Pseudohyponatremia	Normal	Normal
Factitious hyponatremia	Normal	Normal

NSIAD, nephrogenic syndrome of inappropriate antidiuresis; SIADH, syndrome of inappropriate antidiuretic hormone secretion.

| **Table 559-2** | Clinical Parameters to Distinguish Among SIADH, Cerebral Salt Wasting, and Central Diabetes Insipidus |

CLINICAL PARAMETER	SIADH	CEREBRAL SALT WASTING	CENTRAL DI
Serum sodium	Low	Low	High
Urine output	Normal or low	High	High
Urine sodium	High	Very high	Low
Intravascular volume status	Normal or high	Low	Low
Vasopressin level	High	Low	Low

DI, diabetes insipidus; SIADH, syndrome of inappropriate antidiuretic hormone secretion.

CAUSES OF HYPONATREMIA

Syndrome of Inappropriate Antidiuretic Hormone Secretion

Syndrome of inappropriate antidiuretic hormone secretion (SIADH) is characterized by hyponatremia, an inappropriately concentrated urine (>100 mOsm/kg), normal or slightly elevated plasma volume, normal-to-high urine sodium, and low serum uric acid. SIADH is uncommon in children, and most cases result from excessive administration of vasopressin in the treatment of central diabetes insipidus. It can also occur with encephalitis, brain tumors, head trauma, psychiatric disease, prolonged nausea, pneumonia, tuberculous meningitis, and AIDS and in the postictal phase following generalized seizures. SIADH is the cause of the hyponatremic second phase of the triphasic response seen after hypothalamic–pituitary surgery (see Chapter 558). It is found in up to 35% of patients 1 wk after surgery and can result from retrograde neuronal degeneration with cell death and vasopressin release. Common drugs that have been shown to increase vasopressin secretion or mimic vasopressin action, resulting in hyponatremia, include oxcarbazepine, carbamazepine, chlorpropamide, vinblastine, vincristine, and tricyclic antidepressants.

Nephrogenic Syndrome of Inappropriate Antidiuresis

Gain-of-function mutations in the V2 vasopressin receptor gene have been described in male infants presenting with an SIADH-like clinical picture with undetectable vasopressin levels. Activating mutations in the aquaporin-2 gene might also give rise to the same syndrome but have not yet been described.

Systemic Dehydration

The initial manifestation of systemic dehydration is often hypernatremia and hyperosmolality, which subsequently lead to the activation of vasopressin secretion and a decrease in water excretion. As dehydration progresses, hypovolemia and/or hypotension become a major stimulus for vasopressin release, further decreasing free water clearance. Excessive free water intake with ongoing salt loss can also produce hyponatremia. Urinary sodium excretion is low (usually <10 mEq/L) owing to a low glomerular filtration rate and concomitant activation of the renin–angiotensin–aldosterone system, unless primary renal disease or diuretic therapy is present.

Primary Salt Loss

Hyponatremia can result from the primary loss of sodium chloride as seen in specific disorders of the kidney (congenital polycystic kidney disease, acute interstitial nephritis, chronic renal failure), gastrointestinal tract (gastroenteritis), and sweat glands (cystic fibrosis). The hyponatremia is not solely caused by the salt loss, because the latter also causes hypovolemia, leading to an increase in vasopressin. Mineralocorticoid deficiency (hypoaldosteronism), pseudohypoaldosteronism (genetic or sometimes seen in children with urinary tract obstruction or infection), and diuretics can also result in loss of sodium chloride. Hypoaldosterone states are associated with salt wasting, hypovolemia, hyponatremia, hyperkalemia, and failure to thrive (Table 559-3).

Decreased Effective Plasma Volume

Hyponatremia can result from decreased effective plasma volume, as found in congestive heart failure, cirrhosis, nephrotic syndrome, positive pressure mechanical ventilation, severe burns, bronchopulmonary dysplasia in neonates, cystic fibrosis with obstruction, and severe asthma. The resulting decrease in cardiac output leads to reduced water and salt excretion, as with systemic dehydration, and an increase in vasopressin secretion. In patients with impaired cardiac output and elevated atrial volume (congestive heart failure, lung disease), atrial natriuretic peptide concentrations are elevated further, leading to hyponatremia by promoting natriuresis. However, owing to the marked elevation of aldosterone in these patients, their urine sodium remains low (<20 mEq/L) despite this. Unlike dehydrated patients, these patients also have excess total body sodium from activation of the renin–angiotensin–aldosterone system and can demonstrate peripheral edema as well.

Primary Polydipsia (Increased Water Ingestion)

In patients with normal renal function, the kidney can excrete dilute urine with an osmolality as low as 50 mOsm/kg. To excrete a daily solute load of 500 mOsm/m^2, the kidney must produce 10 L/m^2 of urine per day. Therefore, to avoid hyponatremia, the maximum amount of water a person with normal renal function can consume is 10 L/m^2. Neonates, however, cannot dilute their urine to this degree, putting them at risk for water intoxication if water intake exceeds 4 L/m^2/day (approximately 60 mL/hr in a newborn). Many infants develop transient but symptomatic hyponatremic seizures after being fed pure water without electrolytes rather than breast milk or formula.

Decreased Free Water Clearance

Hyponatremia as a consequence of decreased renal free water clearance, even in the absence of an increase in vasopressin secretion, can result from adrenal insufficiency or thyroid deficiency or can be related to a direct effect of drugs on the kidney. Both mineralocorticoids and glucocorticoids are required for normal free water clearance in a vasopressin-independent manner. In patients with unexplained hyponatremia, adrenal and thyroid insufficiency should be considered. In addition, patients with coexisting adrenal failure and diabetes insipidus might have no symptoms of the latter until glucocorticoid therapy unmasks the need for vasopressin replacement. Certain drugs can inhibit renal water excretion through direct effects on the nephron, thus causing hyponatremia; these drugs include high-dose cyclophosphamide, vinblastine, cisplatinum, carbamazepine, and oxcarbazepine.

Cerebral Salt Wasting

Cerebral salt wasting appears to be the result of hypersecretion of atrial natriuretic peptide and is seen primarily with central nervous system disorders including brain tumors, head trauma, hydrocephalus, neurosurgery, cerebrovascular accidents, and brain death. Hyponatremia is accompanied by elevated urinary sodium excretion (often >150 mEq/L), excessive urine output, hypovolemia, normal or high uric acid, suppressed vasopressin, and elevated atrial natriuretic

Table 559-3	Genetic Mutations Associated with Hypoaldosteronism/Pseudohypoaldosteronism (Type IV Renal Tubular Acidosis)

GENE CHROMOSOME OMIM	PATHOPHYSIOLOGY	MUTATION–CLINICAL MANIFESTATIONS–OMIM–INHERITANCE
PRIMARY HYPOALDOSTERONISM		
CYP21A2—cytochrome P450, subfamily XXIA, polypeptide 2 6p21.3 613815	P450c21—steroid 21-hydroxylase that converts 17 α-hydroxyprogesterone to 11-deoxycortisol and progesterone to 11-deoxycorticosterone in the adrenal zona fasciculata	Loss-of-function mutations decrease synthesis of cortisol and aldosterone, the latter resulting in the salt-losing form of classical congenital adrenal hyperplasia, AR–201910
CYP11B2—cytochrome P450, subfamily XIB, polypeptide 2 8q21 124080	P450c11B2—aldosterone synthase/corticosterone methoxidase types I and II expressed only in the zona glomerulosa; hydroxylates deoxycorticosterone at carbon-11 and corticosterone at carbon-18 and oxidizes 18-hydroxycorticosterone to aldosterone	Loss-of-function mutations associated with severe salt loss and volume depletion but not with abnormalities of genital formation or glucocorticoid synthesis AR (CMOI 203400; CMOII 610600)
PSEUDOHYPOALDOSTERONISM TYPE I		
NR3C2—nuclear receptor subfamily 3, group C, member 2 (MR-mineralocorticoid receptor), 4q31.1 600983	Ligand-activated nuclear transcription factor that transmits aldosterone-mediated control of gene expression by binding to the mineralocorticoid response element in the promoter region of the target gene	Loss-of-function mutations lead to mineralocorticoid resistance and pseudohypoaldosteronism type I, AD–177735
SCNN1A—sodium channel, non–voltage-gated, α-subunit 12p13.31 600228	Inactivating mutation of α-subunit of the epithelial sodium channel	Pseudohypoaldosteronism type I, AR–264350
SCNN1B—sodium channel, non–voltage-gated, β-subunit 16p12.2 600760	Inactivating mutation of β-subunit of the epithelial sodium channel	Pseudohypoaldosteronism type I, AR–264350
SCNN1G—sodium channel, non–voltage-gated, γ-subunit 16p12.2 600761	Inactivating mutation of γ-subunit of the epithelial sodium channel	Pseudohypoaldosteronism type I, AR–264350
PSEUDOHYPOALDOSTERONISM TYPE II		
WNK4—protein kinase, lysine-deficient 4 17q21.31 601844	Multifunctional serine-threonine protein kinase whose substrate is SLC12A3, the thiazide-sensitive sodium/chloride cotransporter (NCCT)—OMIM 600968—that also regulates lysosomal degradation of NCCT and endocytosis of the KCNJ1 potassium channel	Pseudohypoaldosteronism type IIB, AD–614491
WNK1—protein kinase, lysine-deficient 1 12p13.33 605232	Serine-threonine protein kinase that inactivates WNK4 by phosphorylating its kinase domain	Pseudohypoaldosteronism type IIC, AD–614492
KLH3—Kelch-like 3 5q31.2 605775	Adaptor protein within the ubiquitination sequence that links WNK1 and WNK4 to CUL3	Pseudohypoaldosteronism type IID, AD/AR–614495
CUL3—Cullin 3 2q36.2 603136	Scaffold protein that links to RING-box E3 ligase facilitating WNK4 ubiquitination and proteasomal destruction of WNK4	Pseudohypoaldosteronism type IIE, AD–614496

AD, autosomal dominant; AR, autosomal recessive; CMO, corticosterone methyloxidase; OMIM, Online Mendelian Inheritance in Man.
From Root AW: Disorders of aldosterone synthesis, secretion, and cellular function. Curr Opin Pediatr 26:480–486, 2014, Table 1, p. 483.

peptide concentrations (>20 pmol/L). Thus, it is distinguished from SIADH, in which normal or decreased urine output, euvolemia, only modestly elevated urine sodium concentration, and an elevated vasopressin level occur. The distinction between cerebral salt wasting and SIADH is important because the treatment of the 2 disorders differs markedly. However, its existence has been questioned, because few patients with the suspected syndrome have documented hypovolemia and thus might truly have SIADH.

Runners' Hyponatremia
Excess fluid ingestion during long-distance running (e.g., marathon running) can result in severe hyponatremia from hypovolemia-induced activation of arginine vasopressin secretion coupled with excessive water ingestion and is correlated with weight gain, long racing time, and extremes of body mass index.

Pseudohyponatremia and Other Causes of Hyponatremia
Pseudohyponatremia can result from hypertriglyceridemia (see Chapter 55). Elevated lipid levels result in a relative decrease in serum water content. As electrolytes are dissolved in the aqueous phase of the serum, they appear low when expressed as a fraction of the total serum volume. As a fraction of serum water, however, electrolyte content is normal. Modern laboratory methods that measure sodium concentration directly, independent of sample volume, do not cause this anomaly. Factitious hyponatremia can result from obtaining a blood sample proximal to the site of intravenous hypotonic fluid infusion.

Hyponatremia is also associated with hyperglycemia, which causes the influx of water into the intravascular space. Serum sodium decreases by 1.6 mEq/L for every 100 mg/dL increment in blood glucose >100 mg/dL. Glucose is not ordinarily an osmotically active agent and does not stimulate vasopressin release, probably because it can equilibrate freely across plasma membranes. In the presence of insulin deficiency and hyperglycemia, however, glucose acts as an osmotic agent, presumably because its normal intracellular access to osmosensor sites is prevented. Under these circumstances, an osmotic gradient exists, stimulating vasopressin release.

TREATMENT
Patients with systemic dehydration and hypovolemia should be rehydrated with salt-containing fluids such as normal saline or lactated Ringer solution. Because of activation of the renin–angiotensin–aldosterone system, the administered sodium is avidly conserved, and water diuresis quickly ensues as volume is restored and vasopressin concentrations decrease. Under these conditions, caution must be taken to prevent a too-rapid correction of hyponatremia, which can

result in central pontine myelinolysis characterized by discrete regions of axonal demyelination and the potential for irreversible brain damage.

Hyponatremia from a decrease in effective plasma volume caused by cardiac, hepatic, renal, or pulmonary dysfunction is more difficult to reverse. The most effective therapy is the least easily achieved: treatment of the underlying systemic disorder. For example, patients weaned from positive pressure ventilation undergo a prompt water diuresis and resolution of hyponatremia as cardiac output is restored and vasopressin concentrations decrease. Vaptans represent a new class of small-molecule arginine vasopressin V2 receptor antagonists (aquaretics) useful for the treatment of hypervolemic hyponatremia associated with severe congestive heart failure and chronic liver failure. Although these agents successfully increase plasma sodium, they also lead to increased thirst and plasma vasopressin levels, which can limit their effectiveness.

Patients with hyponatremia from primary salt loss require supplementation with sodium chloride and fluids. Initially, intravenous replacement of urine volume with fluid containing sodium chloride, 150-450 mEq/L depending on the degree of salt loss, may be necessary; oral salt supplementation may be required subsequently. This treatment contrasts with that of SIADH, in which water restriction without sodium supplementation is the mainstay.

Emergency Treatment of Hyponatremia

The development of acute hyponatremia (onset <12 hr) or a serum sodium concentration <120 mEq/L may be associated with lethargy, psychosis, coma, or generalized seizures, especially in younger children. Acute hyponatremia can cause cell swelling and lead to neuronal dysfunction or to cerebral herniation. The emergency treatment of cerebral dysfunction resulting from acute hyponatremia includes water restriction and can require rapid correction with hypertonic 3% sodium chloride. If hypertonic saline treatment is undertaken, the serum sodium should be raised only high enough to cause an improvement in mental status, and in no case faster than 0.5 mEq/L/hr or 12 mEq/L/24 hr.

Treatment of Syndrome of Inappropriate Antidiuretic Hormone

Chronic SIADH is best treated by oral fluid restriction. With full antidiuresis (urine osmolality of 1,000 mOsm/kg), a normal daily obligate renal solute load of 500 mOsm/m^2 would be excreted in 500 mL/m^2 water. This, plus a daily nonrenal water loss of 500 mL/m^2, would require that oral fluid intake be limited to 1,000 mL/m^2/24 hr to avoid hyponatremia. In young children, this degree of fluid restriction might not provide adequate calories for growth. In this situation, the creation of nephrogenic diabetes insipidus using demeclocycline therapy may be indicated to allow sufficient fluid intake for normal growth. Urea has also been safely used to induce an osmotic diuresis in infants and children.

Treatment of Cerebral Salt Wasting

Treatment of patients with cerebral salt wasting consists of restoring intravascular volume with sodium chloride and water, as for the treatment of other causes of systemic dehydration. The underlying cause of the disorder, which is usually due to acute brain injury, should also be treated if possible. Treatment involves the ongoing replacement of urine sodium losses volume for volume.

Bibliography is available at Expert Consult.

Chapter **560**
Hyperpituitarism, Tall Stature, and Overgrowth Syndromes
Omar Ali

HYPERPITUITARISM

Primary hypersecretion of pituitary hormones rarely occurs in the pediatric population and should be distinguished from **secondary hyperpituitarism,** which occurs in the setting of target hormone deficiencies resulting in decreased hormonal feedback, such as in hypogonadism, hypoadrenalism, or hypothyroidism. In secondary hyperpituitarism, chronic pituitary hypersecretion occurs in response to target hormone deficiencies and leads to pituitary hyperplasia, which can enlarge and erode the sella and, on rare occasions, increase intracranial pressure. Such enlargements should not be confused with primary pituitary tumors; they disappear when the underlying hormone deficiency is treated. The elevated pituitary hormone levels readily suppress to normal following replacement of end-organ hormones. Pituitary hyperplasia can also occur in response to stimulation by ectopic production of releasing hormones such as that seen occasionally in patients with Cushing syndrome secondary to corticotropin-releasing hormone excess or in children with acromegaly secondary to growth hormone–releasing hormone (GHRH) produced by a variety of systemic tumors.

Primary hypersecretion of pituitary hormones by adenoma is uncommon in childhood. The most commonly diagnosed adenoma during childhood is prolactinoma, followed by corticotropinoma, and then somatotropinoma, which secrete prolactin, corticotropin, and growth hormone, respectively. There are a handful of case reports of thyrotropinoma in children and adolescents. There are no pediatric reports of gonadotropinoma, but hypothalamic hamartomas that secrete excess gonadotropin-releasing hormone are responsible for a significant proportion of cases of precocious puberty.

The monoclonal nature of most pituitary adenomas implies that most originate from a clonal event in a single cell. It is suspected that some pituitary tumors result from stimulation with hypothalamic-releasing hormones and in other instances, as in McCune-Albright syndrome (MAS), the tumor is caused by activating mutations of the *GNAS1* gene that codes for the α subunit of $G_s\alpha$, a guanine nucleotide-binding protein. The clinical presentation typically depends on the pituitary hormone that is hypersecreted. Disruptions of growth regulation and/or sexual maturation are common, as a result of either hormone hypersecretion or local compression by the tumor. MAS also features polyostotic fibrous dysplasia of bone and café-au-lait spots in a distinct distribution.

TALL STATURE

The normal distribution of height predicts that 2.3% of the population will be taller than 2 SD (97.7%) above the mean. The social acceptability and even desirability of tallness (heightism) makes tall stature an uncommon complaint in clinical practice. It is exceptionally unusual for boys and men to seek medical attention regarding excessive height. Girls (or their parents) were historically more likely to approach a physician with concern about tall stature, but even in girls this complaint has become less frequent as tallness has become more acceptable and socially desirable in adult women. Concern about side effects of estrogen treatment and reports of dissatisfaction among adult women subjected to this treatment have also led to a decline in estrogen use.

Table 560-1	Differential Diagnosis of Tall Stature and Overgrowth Syndromes

FETAL OVERGROWTH
Maternal diabetes mellitus
Cerebral gigantism (Sotos syndrome)
Weaver syndrome
Beckwith-Wiedemann syndrome
Other IGF-2 excess syndromes

POSTNATAL OVERGROWTH LEADING TO CHILDHOOD TALL STATURE
Nonendocrine Causes
Familial (constitutional) tall stature
Exogenous obesity
Cerebral gigantism (Sotos syndrome)
Weaver syndrome
Marfan syndrome
Fragile X syndrome
Beckwith-Wiedemann syndrome
Klinefelter syndrome (XXY)
SHOX excess syndromes
Homocystinuria
XYY
Endocrine Causes
Excess GH secretion (pituitary gigantism)
McCune-Albright syndrome or MEN associated with excess GH secretion
Precocious puberty
Hyperthyroidism

POSTNATAL OVERGROWTH LEADING TO ADULT TALL STATURE
Familial (constitutional) tall stature
Marfan syndrome
Klinefelter syndrome (XXY)
XYY
Androgen or estrogen deficiency or estrogen resistance
Androgen insensitivity syndrome (testicular feminization)
ACTH or cortisol deficiency or resistance
Excess GH secretion (pituitary gigantism)

ACTH, adrenocorticotropic hormone; GH, growth hormone; IGF, insulin-like growth factor; MEN, multiple endocrine neoplasia.

Differential Diagnosis of Tall Stature

Unusual tall stature can have different causes in each age group. Table 560-1 lists the causes of tall stature in childhood and adolescence. Figure 560-1 shows an approach to diagnosis.

Overgrowth in the Fetus and Neonate

Maternal diabetes is the most common cause of infants large for gestational age. Even in the absence of clinical symptoms or a family history, the birth of a large-for-gestational-age infant should lead to evaluation for maternal (or gestational) diabetes.

A group of disorders associated with excessive somatic growth and growth of specific organs has been described and is collectively referred to as overgrowth syndromes. These disorders appear to be caused in many cases by excess production and availability of insulin-like growth factor 2 (IGF-2) encoded by the gene *Igf2*. The best described of these syndromes is the **Beckwith-Wiedemann syndrome** (BWS), which is an overgrowth malformation syndrome that occurs with an incidence of 1 : 14,000 births, equal in males and females. Approximately 15% of cases are familial, while the rest appear to be sporadic. Most cases of BWS are caused by deregulation of imprinted genes within the chromosome 11p15.5 region. Genetic disruptions affecting this region include gene duplication, loss of heterozygosity, and relaxation or loss of imprinting. The "imprinted" genes involved in BWS and associated childhood tumors include, in addition to *Igf2*, the gene *H19,* which is involved in *Igf2* suppression, as well as *WT-1* (the Wilms tumor gene), cyclin-dependent kinase inhibitor 1C (CDKN1C), potassium channel voltage-gated KQT-like subfamily member 1 (KCNQ1), and KCNQ1-overlapping transcript 1 (KCNQ1OT1, or long QT intronic transcript 1, LIT1).

Affected infants characteristically have macrosomia including macroglossia, hepatosplenomegaly, nephromegaly, and omphalocele. They also have hypoglycemia secondary to hyperinsulinemia as a result of pancreatic β-cell hyperplasia. Children with BWS are predisposed to a specific subset of childhood neoplasms (embryonal tumors), including Wilms tumor, hepatoblastoma, neuroblastoma, and adrenocortical carcinoma. Management focuses on omphalocele, airway issues (a result of macroglossia), and neonatal hypoglycemia. Cancer risk is high until 8 yr of age, and regular surveillance with abdominal ultrasound and measurement of α-fetoprotein is recommended every 3 mo until age 8 yr. Thereafter, renal ultrasound is recommended every 1-2 yr as medullary sponge kidney and nephrocalcinosis may develop later.

Mutations in *GPC3*, a glypican gene (which codes for an IGF-2-neutralizing membrane receptor), cause the related Simpson-Golabi-Behmel overgrowth syndrome. Other syndromic causes of fetal overgrowth include Costello syndrome, Weaver syndrome, Sotos syndrome, and Perlman syndrome.

Overgrowth in Childhood or Adolescence

Normal variant, familial, or constitutional tall stature is by far the most common cause of tall stature. Almost invariably, a family history of tall stature can be obtained, and no organic pathology is present. The child is often taller than the child's peers throughout childhood and enjoys excellent health. The parent of the constitutionally tall adolescent might reflect unhappily upon his or her own adolescence as a tall teenager. There are no abnormalities in the physical examination, and the laboratory studies, if obtained, are negative.

Exogenous obesity is a common condition in adolescence and may be associated with rapid linear growth and early onset of puberty. Bone age is accelerated leading to relative tall stature in childhood but adult height is typically normal.

Klinefelter syndrome (XXY syndrome) is a relatively common (1 in 500-1,000 live male births) abnormality associated with tall stature, learning disabilities (including requirement for speech therapy), gynecomastia, and decreased upper body:lower body segment ratio. Affected boys can have hypotonia, clinodactyly, and hypertelorism. The testes are invariably small, although androgen production by Leydig cells is often in the low-normal range. Spermatogenesis and Sertoli cell function are defective, and infertility results. Other genital abnormalities including relatively small phallus, hypospadias, and cryptorchidism may be present.

XYY syndrome is associated with tall stature, problems in motor and language development, and possible antisocial behavior.

Marfan syndrome is an autosomal dominant connective tissue disorder consisting of tall stature, arachnodactyly, thin extremities, increased arm span, and decreased upper body:lower body segment ratio (see Chapter 702). Additional abnormalities include ocular abnormalities (e.g., lens subluxation), hypotonia, kyphoscoliosis, cardiac valvular deformities, and aortic root dilation.

Homocystinuria is an autosomal recessive inborn error of amino acid metabolism, caused by a deficiency of the enzyme cystathionine synthetase. It is characterized by intellectual disability when untreated, and many of its clinical features resemble Marfan syndrome, particularly ocular manifestations (see Chapter 85).

SOTOS SYNDROME (CEREBRAL GIGANTISM)

Children with cerebral gigantism (also known as Sotos syndrome) are above the 90th percentile for both length and weight at birth; they can also have macrocrania at that time. Most cases of Sotos syndrome are caused by mutations in the *NSD1* (nuclear receptor SET domain-containing protein 1) gene, but in the Japanese population most cases are attributable to microdeletions of the 5q35 region that includes this gene. Inheritance is autosomal dominant, but 95% of cases are a result of new mutations. Incidence is estimated to be approximately 1 in 14,000 live births. The *NSD1* gene is thought to play a role in epigenetic regulation, but the mechanisms by which mutations lead to the features of Sotos syndrome are not clear at this time.

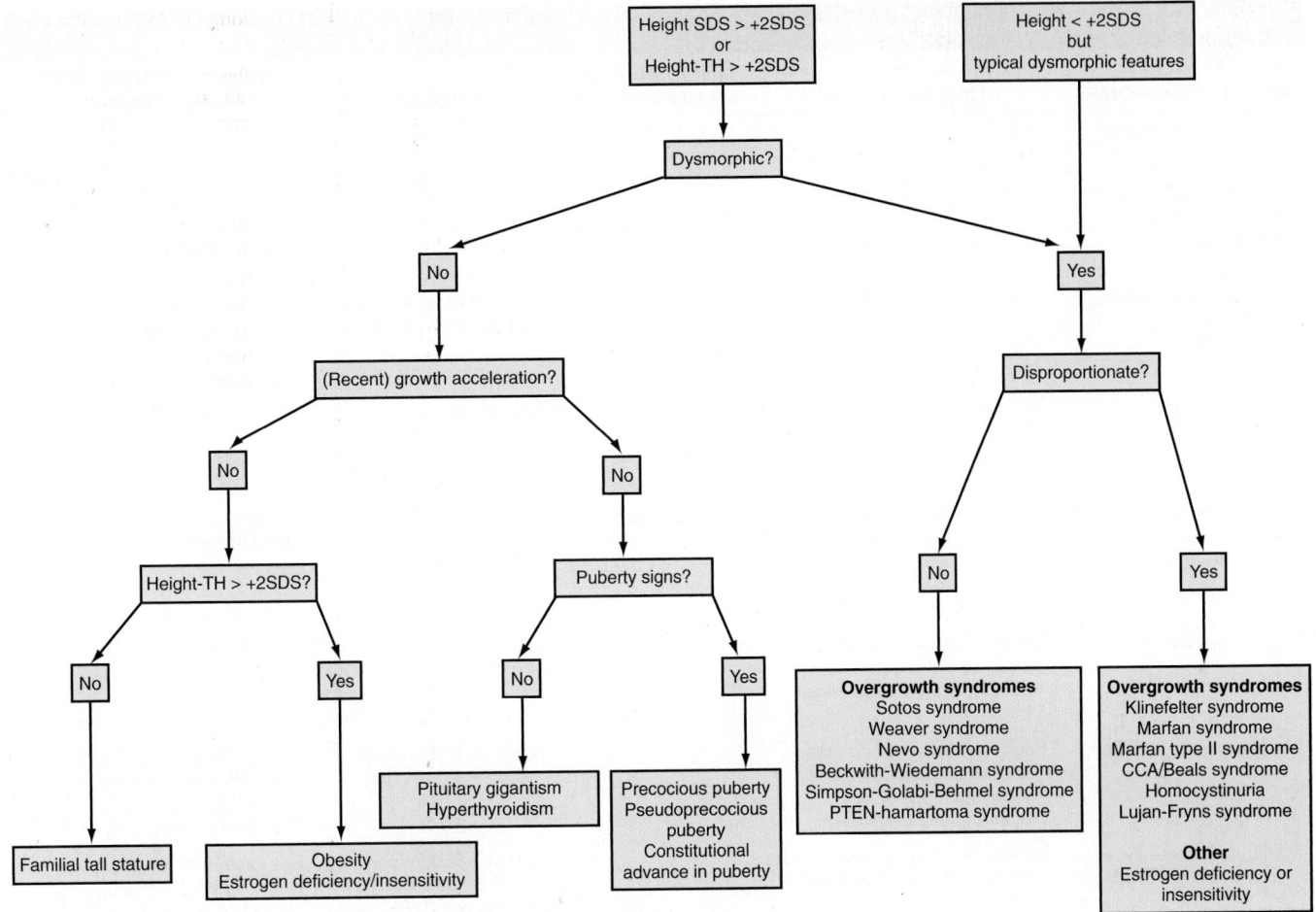

Figure 560-1 Diagnostic flow chart for the differential diagnosis of tall stature and overgrowth syndromes. Height-TH, current height percentile >2 SDS from target height percentile, the latter based on midparental height calculation; SDS, standard deviation score. *(From Neylon OM, Werther GA, Sabin MA: Overgrowth syndromes. Curr Opin Pediatr 24:505–511, 2012, Fig. 1, p. 507.)*

Although it is characterized by rapid growth, there is no evidence that Sotos syndrome is caused by endocrine dysregulation. A hypothalamic defect has been suggested as a cause, but none has been demonstrated functionally or at necropsy. Growth is markedly rapid; by 1 yr of age, affected infants are taller than the 97th percentile in height. Accelerated growth continues for the 1st 4-5 yr and then returns to a normal rate (see Fig. 560-1). Puberty usually occurs at the expected time but may occur slightly early. Adult height is usually in the upper normal range.

Clinically the syndrome is characterized by a large (macrocephaly) dolichocephalic head, prominent forehead and jaw, hypertelorism, antimongoloid slant of the palpebral fissures, high-arched palate, and large hands and feet with thickened subcutaneous tissue. Clumsiness and awkward gait are also noted, and affected children have great difficulty in sports, in learning to ride a bicycle, and in other tasks requiring coordination. Some degree of developmental disability affects most patients; in some affected children perceptual deficiencies may predominate. Many different types of nonfebrile seizures have been reported and up to 25% of patients with Sotos syndrome have seizures at some point in their life. Affected patients may be at somewhat increased risk for neoplasms, including neuroblastoma, hepatoblastoma, and leukemia, with a lifetime risk of between 2% and 4%. Osseous maturation is usually compatible with the patient's height, although advanced bone age has been reported. Scoliosis develops in up to 30% of cases, usually starting in school-age children. Growth hormone (GH), IGF-1, and other endocrine studies are usually normal; there is no distinctive laboratory or radiologic marker for the syndrome. Abnormal electroencephalograms are common; imaging studies often

reveal an enlarged ventricular system, but intracranial pressure is normal. Genetic testing for *NSD1* mutations (or fluorescence in situ hybridization for 5q35 microdeletions in Japanese patients) is available and should be routinely used. Management is symptomatic and includes paying special attention to developmental and behavioral problems (which tend to improve with age), scoliosis, and seizure disorder. No specific treatment is needed for the overgrowth itself. There is no consensus on the need for cancer surveillance at this time. Table 560-2 notes additional features of overgrowth syndromes.

Hyperthyroidism in adolescents is associated with rapid growth but normal final adult height. It is almost always caused by Graves disease and is much more common in girls (see Chapter 568).

Precocious puberty, whether mediated centrally (increased gonadotropin secretion) or peripherally (increased secretion of androgens or estrogens, or both), results in accelerated linear growth during childhood, mimicking the pubertal growth spurt. Because skeletal maturation is also advanced, adult height is often compromised. Chapter 562 discusses the diagnostic evaluation and management of precocious puberty.

Although **delayed puberty** may be associated with short stature in childhood, as with constitutional delay, failure to eventually enter puberty and complete sexual maturation can result in sustained growth during adult life, with ultimate tall stature. The report of tall stature with open epiphyses resulting from a mutation of the estrogen receptor in a man with normal male sexual maturation underscores the fundamental role of estrogen in promoting epiphyseal fusion and termination of normal skeletal growth. Aromatase deficiency leads to tall stature through similar pathways.

| Table 560-2 | Genetic Overgrowth Syndromes |

GENETIC SYNDROMES	CLINICAL FEATURES	INCIDENCE OF MALIGNANCY (%)	ETIOLOGY	INVESTIGATIONS AND MANAGEMENT
Beckwith-Wiedemann syndrome*	Hypoglycemia, large tongue, ear pits, omphalocele or umbilical hernia, hemihyperplasia	~7.5		US heart, kidneys Chromosomes 11p FISH and/or MLPA, methylation studies Tumor surveillance justified
Perlman syndrome*	Macrosomia, unusual facies Nephroblastosis		Rare autosomal recessive	US brain (ACC), heart (coarctation), kidneys
Simpson-Golabi-Behmel syndrome*	Coarse facial features, macroglossia, central groove lower lip, supernumerary nipples	~7.5	X-linked recessive (glypican-3 mutations)	US heart, kidney X-ray spine (vertebral segmentation anomaly) Tumor surveillance justified
Sotos syndrome	Facial gestalt (long, thin face, broad forehead) Feeding difficulties Hypotonia	~4	Usually de novo dominant NSD1 deletion or mutation Rare familial cases	US heart, kidneys Monitor development
PTEN-hamartoma syndrome (Bannayan-Ruvalcaba-Riley)	Macrocephaly (>97th percentile) often progressive from birth, hypotonia, pigmented skin, penile macules, lipomas	Uncertain	Sporadic or autosomal dominant PTEN mutation	US head, heart, and kidney Monitor development
Weaver syndrome	Broad forehead, hypertelorism, small chin, long philtrum, camptodactyly, fetal finger pads	~5-6	Rare, unknown	US heart, brain, kidney
Marfan syndrome type I	Facial gestalt, arachnodactyly, scoliosis, pectus carinatum or excavatum, aortic root dilation, lens dislocation		Autosomal dominant fibrillin-1 (FBN1)	Eye examination and follow-up Heart US and cardiology follow-up Monitor scoliosis
Marfan syndrome type II or Loeys-Dietz syndrome	Marfan-like habitus, aortic root dilation, aortic dissection, vasculopathy		Autosomal dominant, TGF-β pathway anomaly TGFBR1 and TGFBR2 genes	Eye examination usually normal Heart US and follow-up Monitor scoliosis
Beals syndrome	Congenital distal arthrogryposis Crumpled ears		Autosomal dominant fibrillin 2 (FBN2)	Eye examination and heart US usually normal
Homocystinuria	Marfan-like habitus Developmental delay Lens dislocation		Autosomal recessive Cystathionine β-synthase (CBS) mutation	Urine metabolic screen Eye examination Monitor development
Lujan syndrome	Marfanoid habitus plus intellectual disability		X-linked recessive MED12 gene	Eye examination usually normal Heart US usually normal
Sex chromosome aneuploidy Klinefelter 47XXY, 47XYY, 47XXX	Tall stature, small testes, gynecomastia Tall stature, ± learning disability			Androgen replacement from puberty in Klinefelter syndrome Monitor development
Autosomal anomaly Tetrasomy 12p mosaicism,* pat 11pdup, 4pdub, 22q13del, 15q26-qter dup	Congenital overgrowth or childhood tall stature with intellectual disability			Monitor development

*Overgrowth often presenting at birth.
ACC, agenesis of the corpus callosum; FISH, fluorescence in situ hybridization; MLPA, multiple ligation probe amplification; PTEN, phosphatase and tensin homolog; TGF, transforming growth factor; TGFBR, transforming growth factor β receptor; US, ultrasound.
From Verge CF, Mowat D: Overgrowth, Arch Dis Child 95:458–463, 2010.

The purpose of the diagnostic evaluation of tall stature is to distinguish the commonly occurring, normal variant, constitutional variety from the rare pathologic conditions. Often, when the history suggests familial tall stature and the physical examination is entirely normal, no laboratory tests are indicated. It is valuable to obtain a bone age radiograph to be able to predict adult height, which serves as a basis for discussions with the family and for management decisions. If the history suggests any of the aforementioned disorders or the physical examination reveals abnormalities, additional laboratory tests should be obtained. IGF-1 and IGF-binding protein-3 (IGFBP-3) are excellent screening tests for GH excess and can be verified with a glucose suppression test. Laboratory evidence of GH excess mandates MRI evaluation of the pituitary. Chromosome analysis is useful in boys, especially when the ratio of upper to lower body segment is decreased or when developmental disability is present, to rule out Klinefelter syndrome. If Marfan syndrome or homocystinuria is suspected from the physical examination, referral to a cardiologist and an ophthalmologist should be made. Thyroid function tests are useful to diagnose or rule out hyperthyroidism when this disorder is suspected.

Treatment of Normal Variant Tall Stature

Reassurance of the family and the patients is the key to the management of normal variant tall stature. The use of the bone age to predict adult height might provide some comfort for them, as will general supportive discussions on the social acceptability of this condition. Although treatment is possible for girls and boys with excessive growth, its use should be restricted to patients with predicted adult height >3-4 SD above the mean (79 inches or 200 cm in boys, 73 inches or 185 cm in girls) and evidence of significant psychosocial impairment.

Sex steroids have been used in the treatment of tall stature and are designed to accelerate puberty and to promote epiphyseal fusion; these are therefore of little benefit when given in late puberty. The lack of extensive experience with this form of therapy and the risks of estrogen or androgen treatment for tall stature should be carefully weighed and discussed with the family and treatment should be discouraged except in the most extreme cases. Detailed discussion with the child at the child's level is also advisable as up to 40% of those who underwent such treatments are dissatisfied as adults and feel they were not sufficiently consulted about this course of action. Therapy is initiated ideally before puberty or in early puberty. In boys, treatment should begin before the bone age reaches 14 yr. In the extremely rare instances where treatment is desired, testosterone enanthate is used at a dose of 500 mg intramuscularly every 2 wk for 6 mo. In girls, oral estrogens in various doses have been used to reduce the predicted height, but average height reduction may be only 1.1-2.4 cm. Therapy must begin before the bone age has reached 12 yr. In the rare case where treatment is advised, oral ethinyl estradiol at a dose of 0.15-0.5 mg/day until cessation of growth occurs has been used. Short-term side effects have included benign breast disease, cholelithiasis, hypertension, menstrual irregularities, weight gain, nausea, limb pain, galactorrhea, and thrombosis. Reduced fertility later in life may be a potential long-term complication.

EXCESS GROWTH HORMONE SECRETION AND PITUITARY GIGANTISM

In young persons with open epiphyses, overproduction of GH results in **gigantism;** in persons with closed epiphyses, the result is **acromegaly.** Often some acromegalic features are seen with gigantism, even in children and adolescents. After closure of the epiphyses, the acromegalic features become more prominent.

Gigantism is rare, with only several hundred reported cases to date. Most cases are sporadic and are caused by pituitary adenomas or excessive GHRH secretion by the hypothalamus (and, rarely, by tumors in other parts of the body). **Syndromes associated with pituitary GH excess include** MAS, which is caused by mutations resulting in constitutively activated G-proteins, and can include somatotrophic tumors and excess GH secretion. Approximately 20% of patients with gigantism have MAS (commonly consisting of a triad of precocious puberty, café-au-lait spots, and fibrous dysplasia) and 20% of patients with MAS have some degree of GH hypersecretion. GH-secreting tumors are seen in approximately 60% of patients with **multiple endocrine neoplasia type 1,** but almost all these tumors develop in adult life and cause acromegaly rather than pituitary gigantism. Increased GH secretion and GH-secreting adenomas may also be seen in **neurofibromatosis, tuberous sclerosis,** and **Carney complex.**

The cardinal clinical feature of gigantism is longitudinal growth acceleration secondary to GH excess. The usual manifestations consist of coarse facial features and enlarging hands and feet. In young children, rapid growth of the head can precede linear growth. Some patients have behavioral and visual problems. In most recorded cases, the abnormal growth became evident at puberty, but the condition has been established as early as the newborn period in 1 child and at 21 mo of age in another. Giants have rarely been reported to grow to a height of over 8 ft. In some cases the patient may present with local effects of the pituitary tumor (headache, visual field defects, and other pituitary hormone deficiencies) as the main complaint, and there is at least 1 report of a patient presenting with diabetic ketoacidosis induced by

GH excess. The presentation of gigantism is usually dramatic, unlike the insidious onset of acromegaly in adults.

Approximately 50% of the pituitary adenomas that cause gigantism also exhibit hyperprolactinemia because they secrete both GH and prolactin. This is because mammosomatotrophs are the most common type of GH-secreting cells involved in childhood gigantism. GH-secreting tumors of the pituitary are typically eosinophilic or chromophobic adenomas. Adenomas can compromise other anterior pituitary function through growth or cystic degeneration. Secretion of gonadotropins, thyrotropin, or corticotropin may be impaired. Delayed sexual maturation or hypogonadism can occur. When GH hypersecretion is accompanied by gonadotropin deficiency, accelerated linear growth can persist for decades. In some cases, the tumor spreads outside the sella, invading the sphenoid bone, optic nerves, and brain. GH-secreting tumors in pediatric patients are more likely to be locally invasive or aggressive than are those in adults.

Acromegalic features consist chiefly of enlargement of the distal parts of the body, but manifestations of abnormal growth involve all portions. The circumference of the skull increases, the nose becomes broad, and the tongue is often enlarged, with coarsening of the facial features. The mandible grows excessively, and the teeth become separated. Visual field defects and neurologic abnormalities are common; signs of increased intracranial pressure appear later. The fingers and toes grow chiefly in thickness. There may be dorsal kyphosis. Fatigue and lassitude are early symptoms. GH levels are elevated and occasionally exceed 100 ng/mL. There is usually no suppression of GH levels by the hyperglycemia of a glucose tolerance test and IGF-1 and IGFBP-3 levels are consistently elevated in acromegaly and pituitary gigantism.

Diagnosis

Most children with tall stature do not have pituitary gigantism and other etiologies of rapid linear growth such as genetic tall stature, precocious puberty, and hyperthyroidism should be carefully excluded. Coexisting findings (e.g., dysmorphic facial features, neurocognitive problems, hemihypertrophy) may suggest syndromic or chromosomal causes of tall stature, such as Sotos, Weaver, Klinefelter, or XYY syndrome. GH hypersecretion can be screened for by testing IGF-1 and IGFBP-3 levels. An excellent linear dose–response correlation between serum IGF-1 levels and 24 hr mean GH secretion has been demonstrated. An elevated IGF-1 level in a patient with appropriate clinical suspicion usually indicates GH excess. Potential confusion can arise in the evaluation of normal adolescents because significantly higher IGF-1 levels occur during puberty than in adulthood, so the IGF-1 level must be age and gender matched. Serum IGFBP-3 levels are also sensitive markers of GH elevations and will be elevated in almost all cases. If IGF-1 and/or IGFBP-3 levels are elevated, then the next step is to test for GH excess by doing an oral glucose-suppression test. The gold standard for the diagnosis of GH excess in adults is the failure to suppress serum GH levels to <1 ng/dL at any time during a 2 hr oral glucose tolerance test with 1.75 g/kg oral glucose challenge (maximum: 75 g). GH levels may not be suppressed to this level in normal adolescents and a cutoff of 5 ng/mL may be more appropriate in this age group. If laboratory findings suggest GH excess, the presence of a pituitary adenoma should be confirmed by MRI of the brain. In rare cases, a pituitary mass is not identified. This might be from an occult pituitary microadenoma or ectopic production of GHRH or GH. CT is acceptable when MRI is unavailable.

Treatment

The goals of therapy are to remove or shrink the pituitary mass, to restore GH and secretory patterns to normal, to restore IGF-1 and IGFBP-3 levels to normal, to retain the normal pituitary secretion of other hormones, and to prevent recurrence of disease.

For well-circumscribed pituitary adenomas, transsphenoidal surgery is the treatment of choice and may be curative. The tumor should be removed completely. The likelihood of surgical cure depends greatly on the surgeon's expertise as well as on the size and extension of the mass. Intraoperative GH measurements can improve the results of tumor resection. Transsphenoidal surgery to resect the tumors is as safe in children as in adults. At times, a transcranial approach might be necessary. The primary goal of treatment is to normalize GH and IGF-1 levels. GH levels (<1 ng/mL within 2 hr after a glucose load) and serum IGF-1 levels (age-adjusted normal range) are the best tests to define a biochemical cure.

If GH secretion and IGF-1 levels are not normalized by surgery, the options include pituitary irradiation and medical therapy. Further growth of the tumor is prevented by irradiation in >99% of patients. The main disadvantage is the delayed efficacy in decreasing GH levels. GH is reduced by approximately 50% from the initial concentration by 2 yr, by 75% by 5 yr, and approaches 90% by 15 yr. Multiple pituitary hormone deficiency is a predictable outcome, occurring in 40-50% of patients 10 yr after irradiation.

Surgery fails to cure a significant number of patients and radiotherapy may not work fast enough, so medical therapy has an important role in treating patients with GH excess. Treatment is effective and well tolerated with long-acting somatostatin analogs and dopamine agonists, as well as by novel GH antagonists.

The **somatostatin analogs** are highly effective in the treatment of patients with GH excess. Octreotide suppresses GH to <2.5 ng/mL in 65% of patients with acromegaly and normalizes IGF-1 levels in 70%. The effects of octreotide are well sustained over time. Tumor shrinkage also occurs with octreotide but is generally modest. Consistent GH suppression can be obtained with a continuous SC pump infusion of octreotide or with long-acting formulations, including long-acting octreotide and lanreotide. These produce consistent GH and IGF-1 suppression in acromegalic patients with once-monthly or biweekly IM depot injections. These sustained-release preparations have not been formally tested in children. Octreotide injection in the pediatric population has been used at doses of 1-40 μg/kg/24 hr. In adults the long-acting form is used in a dose of 10-40 mg every mo, but no pediatric dose range has been established.

For patients with both GH and prolactin oversecretion, dopamine agonists, such as **bromocriptine and cabergoline,** which bind to pituitary dopamine type 2 receptors and may also suppress GH secretion, should be considered. Prolactin levels are often adequately suppressed, but GH levels and IGF-1 levels are rarely normalized with this treatment modality alone. Tumor shrinkage occurs in a minority of patients. The effectiveness of these agents may be additive to that of octreotide. Cabergoline therapy at doses of 0.25-4.0 mg/wk (given 1-2 times per wk) has been used in adults with acromegaly, and because of its less-frequent dosing and lower incidence of side effects as compared to bromocriptine, this is now considered the dopamine agonist of choice in both adults and children. Side effects can include nausea, vomiting, abdominal pain, arrhythmias, nasal stuffiness, orthostatic hypotension, sleep disturbances, and fatigue.

Pegvisomant is a GH-receptor antagonist that competes with endogenous GH for binding to the GH receptor. It effectively suppresses GH and IGF-1 levels in patients with acromegaly caused by pituitary tumors as well as ectopic GHRH hypersecretion. Normalization of IGF-1 levels occurs in up to 90% of patients treated daily with this drug for 3 mo or longer. The adult dosage is 10-40 mg via subcutaneous injection once daily, although twice-weekly protocols have also been reported as highly successful. IGF-1 levels and hepatic enzymes must be monitored. Combined therapy with somatostatin analogs and weekly pegvisomant injections also is effective. Pediatric experience is limited, but case reports indicate that it can successfully suppress IGF-1 levels when used in doses of 10-30 mg/day.

HYPERSECRETION OF OTHER PITUITARY HORMONES
Prolactinoma

Prolactin-secreting pituitary adenomas are the most common pituitary tumors in adolescents. With the advent of MRI, more of these tumors, particularly microadenomas (<1 cm in diameter), are being detected. The most common presenting manifestations are headache, primary or secondary amenorrhea, and galactorrhea. The disorder affects more than twice as many girls as boys; most patients have undergone normal puberty before becoming symptomatic. Only a few have delayed puberty. In some kindreds with type I multiple endocrine neoplasia, prolactinomas are the presenting feature during adolescence.

Prolactin levels may be elevated mildly (40-50 ng/mL) or markedly (10,000-15,000 ng/mL). Most prolactinomas in children are large (macroadenomas), cause the sella to enlarge, and in some cases cause visual field defects. Approximately 30% of patients with macroadenomas develop other pituitary hormone deficiencies, particularly GH deficiency. Alternatively, prolactin-secreting adenomas might also stain for and secrete excess GH and/or thyroid-stimulating hormone.

Prolactinomas should not be confused with the hyperprolactinemia and pituitary hyperplasia that can occur in patients with **primary hypothyroidism**, which is readily treated with thyroid hormone (see Chapter 565). Moderate elevations (<200 ng/mL) of prolactin are also associated with a variety of **medications** (antipsychotics, metoclopramide, phenothiazines, verapamil), with pituitary stalk dysfunction such as can occur with craniopharyngioma, with chronic stress (rarely >40 ng/mL), and with nipple stimulation.

In some cases, extreme hyperprolactinemia is associated with a "hook effect" that leads to factitiously low values on blood tests. In cases where clinical features are compatible with hyperprolactinemia, serial dilution of the lab specimen should be done to rule out this kind of measurement error. On the other hand, patients may have factitiously elevated prolactin levels on immunoassay as a result of the presence of prolactin polymers and dimers (macroprolactinemia). In cases where an elevated prolactin is detected in an asymptomatic patient, unnecessary diagnostic work-up and treatment can be avoided by performing polyethylene glycol precipitation to exclude the presence of macroprolactinemia, which is clinically benign.

In most patients where the hyperprolactinemia is secondary to an adenoma, it can be effectively treated with dopamine agonists. Treatment leads to lowering of prolactin levels and tumor shrinkage in the vast majority of patients. Because of its greater efficacy and lower incidence of side effects, cabergoline is considered the drug of choice for treatment of hyperprolactinemia in doses ranging from 0.125-1.0 mg twice weekly. Higher doses may be needed in some patients but carry the risk of inducing cardiac valvular abnormalities and should be carefully monitored.

When dopamine agonist treatment has been unsuccessful in lowering the serum prolactin concentration or the size of the adenoma, and when symptoms or signs attributable to hyperprolactinemia or adenoma size persist during treatment, transsphenoidal surgery should be considered.

Corticotropinoma

Corticotropinoma is very rare in children, and its peak occurrence is at age 14 yr. **Cushing disease** refers specifically to an adrenocorticotropic hormone–producing pituitary adenoma that stimulates excess cortisol production and secretion. It is more common than primary adrenal causes of Cushing syndrome, except in younger children (younger than 5 yr of age), in whom adrenal carcinomas and adrenal activating mutations of MAS are rare but dominant causes of the syndrome. Adenomas causing Cushing disease are almost always microadenomas with a diameter of <5 mm and are significantly smaller than all other types of adenomas at presentation. The most sensitive indicator of excess glucocorticoid secretion in children is growth failure, which generally precedes other manifestations. Patients develop weight gain that tends to be centripetal rather than generalized. Pubertal arrest, hypertension, large purplish striae, fatigue, and depression are also common. In prepubertal children, males are more frequently affected than females.

Midnight salivary cortisol measurements can be used as a screening test for cortisol excess, but confirmation requires at least 1 additional test (either 24 hr urinary free cortisol or an overnight dexamethasone suppression test). Location of the microadenoma is usually determined by MRI, and bilateral inferior petrosal sinus sampling may be needed in difficult cases. Transsphenoidal surgery is the treatment of choice for Cushing disease in children. Initial remission rates of 70-98% of patients and long-term success rates of 50-98% are reported. Residual transient hypoadrenalism is often observed after surgery, lasting as long as 30 mo. Pituitary radiotherapy is used if cortisol levels remain elevated and/or adrenocorticotropic hormone levels continue to be detectable. Successful treatment may not correct the height deficit, and GH deficiency may be present after treatment and should be treated as required.

Bibliography is available at Expert Consult.

Chapter 561
Physiology of Puberty
Luigi R. Garibaldi and Wassim Chemaitilly

Between early childhood and approximately 8-9 yr of age (prepubertal stage), the hypothalamic-pituitary-gonadal axis is dormant, as reflected by undetectable serum concentrations of luteinizing hormone (LH) and sex hormones (estradiol in girls, testosterone in boys). One to 3 yr before the onset of clinically evident puberty, low serum levels of LH during sleep become demonstrable. This sleep-entrained LH secretion occurs in a pulsatile fashion and reflects endogenous episodic discharge of hypothalamic gonadotropin-releasing hormone (GnRH). Nocturnal pulses of LH continue to increase in amplitude and, to a lesser extent, in frequency as clinical puberty approaches. This pulsatile secretion of gonadotropins is responsible for enlargement and maturation of the gonads and the secretion of sex hormones. The appearance of the secondary sex characteristics in early puberty is the visible culmination of the sustained, active interaction occurring among hypothalamus, pituitary, and gonads in the peripubertal period. By midpuberty, LH pulses become evident even during the daytime and occur at approximately 90-120 min intervals. A second critical event occurs in middle or late adolescence in girls in whom cyclicity and ovulation occur. A positive feedback mechanism develops whereby increasing levels of estrogen in midcycle cause a distinct increase of LH.

The increasing secretion of hypothalamic GnRH in a pulsatile fashion thus underlies the onset of pubertal development. The resulting "GnRH pulse generator" is regulated by multiple neuropeptides, including glutamic acid, kisspeptin, and neurokinin-B (stimulatory) and γ-aminobutyric acid, preproenkephalin, and dynorphin (inhibitory). GnRH secretion is also regulated by factors produced by the glial cells, such as transforming growth factor α. Loss-of-function mutations of the *KISS1 R*—also known as *GPR54*—gene (the gene encoding a G-protein–coupled receptor whose ligand is kisspeptin) cause an autosomal recessive form of hypogonadotropic hypogonadism, whereas gain-of-function mutations of the gene are associated with precocious puberty. Increased transforming growth factor α signaling is associated with the occurrence of central precocious puberty in patients with hypothalamic hamartoma.

The interpretation of the hormonal changes of puberty is complex. Issues in interpreting LH and follicle-stimulating hormone measurements include the presence of multiple gonadotropin isoforms, immunoassay-related variability, and problems inherent to their pulsatile secretion, which mandates serial sampling in plasma. In addition, important sex differences exist in the maturation of the hypothalamus and pituitary gland, and serum LH concentrations tend to increase earlier in the course of the pubertal process in boys than in girls. Adrenocortical androgens also have a role in sexual maturation. Serum levels of dehydroepiandrosterone (DHEA) and its sulfate (DHEAS) begin to increase at approximately 6-8 yr of age, before any increase in LH or sex hormones and before the earliest physical changes of puberty

are apparent; this process is called *adrenarche*. DHEAS is the most abundant adrenal C-19 steroid in the blood, and its serum concentration remains fairly stable over 24 hr. A single measurement of this hormone is commonly used as a marker of adrenal androgen secretion. Although adrenarche typically antedates the onset of gonadal activity (gonadarche) by a few years, the 2 processes do not seem to be causally related, because adrenarche and gonadarche are dissociated in conditions such as central precocious puberty and adrenocortical failure.

The effects of gonadal steroids (testosterone in boys, estradiol in girls) on bone growth and osseous maturation are critical. Both aromatase deficiency and estrogen receptor defects result in delayed epiphyseal fusion and tall stature in affected males. These observations suggest that estrogens, rather than androgens, are responsible for the process of bone maturation that ultimately leads to epiphyseal fusion and cessation of growth. Estrogens also mediate the increased production of growth hormone, which along with a direct effect of sex steroids on bone growth, is responsible for the pubertal growth spurt.

The age of onset of puberty varies and is more closely correlated with osseous maturation than with chronological age (see Chapter 14). In females, the **breast bud** (thelarche) is usually the first sign of **puberty** (10-11 yr of age), followed by the appearance of pubic hair (pubarche) 6-12 mo later. The interval to the onset of **menstrual activity** (menarche) is usually 2-2.5 yr, but may be as long as 6 yr. In the United States, at least 1 sign of puberty is present in approximately 95% of girls by 12 yr of age and in 99% of females by 13 yr of age. Peak height velocity occurs early (at breast stages II-III, typically between 11 and 12 yr of age) in girls and always precedes menarche. The mean age of menarche is approximately 12.75 yr. There are, however, wide variations in the sequence of changes involving growth spurt, breast bud, pubic hair, and maturation of the internal and external genitalia.

In males, **growth of the testes** (≥4 mL in volume or 2.5 cm in longest diameter) and thinning of the scrotum are the first signs of puberty (11-12 yr). These are followed by pigmentation of the scrotum and growth of the penis (see Chapter 14) and by **pubarche**. Appearance of **axillary hair** usually occurs in midpuberty. In males, unlike in females, acceleration of growth begins after puberty is well under way and is maximal at genital stages IV-V (typically between 13 and 14 yr of age). In males, the growth spurt occurs approximately 2 yr later than in females, and growth may continue beyond 18 yr of age.

Genetic and environmental factors affect the timing for the onset of puberty. Population-based studies in the United States and in Europe suggest secular trends for earlier onset of puberty over the past few decades in females and, to a lesser degree, in males. African-American and, to a lesser extent, Hispanic girls appear to be more advanced in the development of secondary sex characteristics for age than white females. The timing of menarche has, however, remained generally stable with only a marginal advancement (2.5-4 mo) reported in U.S.-based studies and no significant change reported in the Copenhagen Puberty Study. The latter also showed that the earlier onset of breast development observed in girls examined in 2006-2008 when compared to those seen in 1991-1993 (means: 10.88 yr vs 9.86 yr, p < 0.0001) was not associated with different levels of estradiol or gonadotropins when girls of similar chronological ages were compared between the 2 groups. Hence, earlier breast development may not necessarily reflect an earlier activation of the hypothalamic-pituitary-gonadal axis but could be the consequence of other factors such as increased adiposity or increased exposure to certain environmental agents. Positive correlations between the degree of adiposity and earlier pubertal development in girls have, indeed, been reported. Conversely, female athletes in whom leanness and strenuous physical activity have coexisted from early childhood frequently exhibit a marked delay in puberty or menarche, and they frequently have oligomenorrhea or amenorrhea as adults (see Chapter 691). Pubertal delay is also prevalent in males who are physically very active. These observations support the thesis that the energy balance is closely related to the activity of the GnRH pulse generator and the mechanisms initiating and sustaining puberty via hormonal signals such as leptin or other adipokines.

Bibliography is available at Expert Consult.

Chapter **562**
Disorders of Pubertal Development
Luigi R. Garibaldi and Wassim Chemaitilly

Table 562-1	Conditions Causing Precocious Puberty

CENTRAL (GONADOTROPIN-DEPENDENT, TRUE PRECOCIOUS) PUBERTY
Idiopathic
Organic brain lesions
Hypothalamic hamartoma
Brain tumors, hydrocephalus, severe head trauma, myelomeningocele
Hypothyroidism, prolonged and untreated*

COMBINED PERIPHERAL AND CENTRAL
Treated congenital adrenal hyperplasia
McCune-Albright syndrome, late
Familial male precocious puberty, late

PERIPHERAL (GONADOTROPIN-INDEPENDENT, PRECOCIOUS) PSEUDOPUBERTY
GIRLS
Isosexual (feminizing) conditions
McCune-Albright syndrome
Autonomous ovarian cysts
Ovarian tumors
Granulosa–theca cell tumor associated with Ollier disease
Teratoma, chorionepithelioma
SCTAT associated with Peutz-Jeghers syndrome
Feminizing adrenocortical tumor
Exogenous estrogens
Heterosexual (masculinizing) conditions
Congenital adrenal hyperplasia
Adrenal tumors
Ovarian tumors
Glucocorticoid receptor defect
Exogenous androgens
BOYS
Isosexual (masculinizing) conditions
Congenital adrenal hyperplasia
Adrenocortical tumor
Leydig cell tumor
Familial male precocious puberty
Isolated
Associated with pseudohypoparathyroidism
hCG-secreting tumors
   • Central nervous system
   • Hepatoblastoma
Mediastinal tumor associated with Klinefelter syndrome
Teratoma
Glucocorticoid receptor defect
Exogenous androgen
Heterosexual (feminizing) conditions
Feminizing adrenocortical tumor
SCTAT associated with Peutz-Jeghers syndrome
Exogenous estrogens

INCOMPLETE (PARTIAL) PRECOCIOUS PUBERTY
Premature thelarche
Premature adrenarche
Premature menarche

*Central puberty without true gonadotropin dependency (see text).
 hCG, human chorionic gonadotropin; SCTAT, sex-cord tumor with annular tubules.

Precocious puberty is defined by the onset of secondary sexual characteristics before the age of 8 yr in girls and 9 yr in boys. The variation in the age of the onset of puberty in normal children, particularly of different ethnicities, makes this definition somewhat arbitrary. It remains in use by most clinicians.

Depending on the primary source of the hormonal production, precocious puberty may be classified as **central** (also known as **gonadotropin dependent,** or **true**) or **peripheral** (also known as **gonadotropin independent** or **precocious pseudopuberty**) (Table 562-1). **Central** precocious puberty is always isosexual and stems from hypothalamic-pituitary-gonadal activation with ensuing sex hormone secretion and progressive sexual maturation. In **peripheral** precocious puberty, some of the secondary sex characteristics appear, but there is no activation of the normal hypothalamic-pituitary-gonadal interplay. In this latter group, the sex characteristics may be isosexual or heterosexual (contrasexual) (see Chapters 583-588).

Peripheral precocious puberty can induce maturation of the hypothalamic-pituitary-gonadal axis and trigger the onset of central puberty. This mixed type of precocious puberty occurs commonly in conditions such as congenital adrenal hyperplasia, McCune-Albright syndrome, and familial male-limited precocious puberty, when the bone age reaches the pubertal range (10.5-12.5 yr).

562.1 Central Precocious Puberty
Luigi R. Garibaldi and Wassim Chemaitilly

Central precocious puberty is defined by the onset of breast development before the age of 8 yr in girls and by the onset of testicular development (volume ≥4 mL) before the age of 9 yr in boys, as a result of the early activation of the hypothalamic-pituitary-gonadal axis. It occurs 5-10–fold more frequently in girls than in boys and is usually sporadic. A high prevalence of idiopathic central precocious puberty has been reported in girls adopted from developing countries, with the limitation that the exact date of birth may be uncertain.

Although approximately 90% of girls have an idiopathic form, a structural central nervous system (CNS) abnormality can be demonstrated in up to 75% of boys with central precocious puberty. Beyond its etiology, which thus needs to be specifically addressed, central precocious puberty can impact linear growth and affect the child's growth potential.

CLINICAL MANIFESTATIONS
Sexual development may begin at any age and generally follows the sequence observed in normal puberty. In girls, early menstrual cycles may be more irregular than they are with normal puberty. The initial cycles are usually anovulatory, but pregnancy has been reported as early as 5.5 yr of age (Fig. 562-1). In boys, testicular biopsies have shown stimulation of all elements of the testes, and spermatogenesis has been observed as early as 5-6 yr of age. In affected girls and boys, height, weight, and osseous maturation are advanced. The increased rate of bone maturation results in early closure of the epiphyses, and the ultimate stature is less than it would have been otherwise. Without treatment, approximately 30% of girls and an even larger percentage of boys achieve a height less than the 5th percentile as adults. Mental development is usually compatible with chronological age. Emotional behavior and mood swings are common, but serious psychologic problems are rare.

Although the clinical course is variable, 3 main patterns of pubertal progression can be identified. Most girls (particularly those younger than 6 yr of age at the onset) and a large majority of boys have rapidly progressive puberty, characterized by rapid physical and osseous maturation, leading to a loss of height potential. An increasing percentage of girls (older than 6 yr of age at the onset with an idiopathic form) have a slowly progressive variant, characterized by parallel advancement of osseous maturation and linear growth, with preserved height potential. Spontaneously regressive or unsustained central precocious

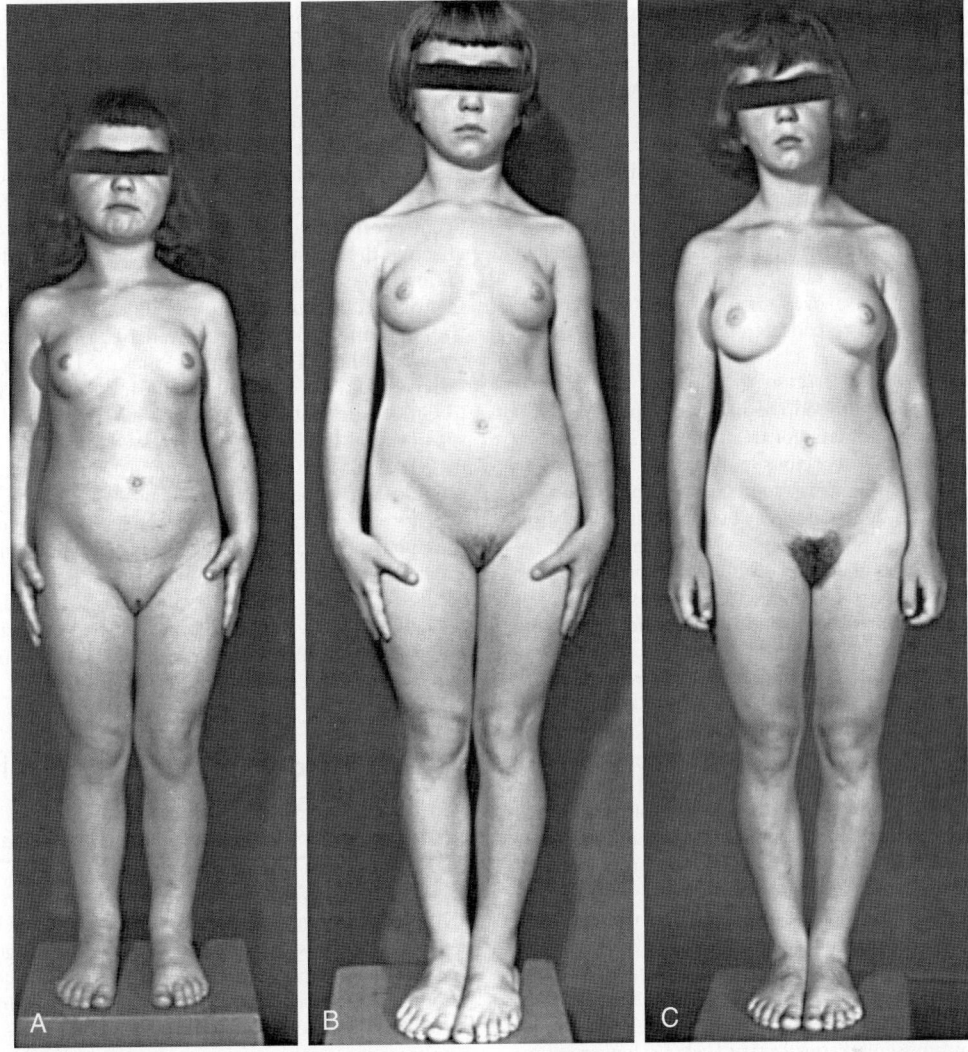

Figure 562-1 Natural course of idiopathic central precocious puberty. Patient **(A)** at $3^{11}/_{12}$, **(B)** at $5^{2}/_{3}$, and **(C)** at 8.5 yr of age. Breast development and vaginal bleeding began at 2.5 yr of age. Bone age was 7.5 yr at $3^{11}/_{12}$ yr of age, and 14 yr at 8 yr of age. Intelligence and dental age were normal for chronological age. Growth was completed at 10 yr; ultimate height was 142 cm (56 in). No effective therapy was available at the time this patient sought medical attention.

puberty is quite rare. This variability in the natural course of sexual precocity underscores the need for longitudinal observation at the onset of sexual development, before treatment is considered.

LABORATORY FINDINGS

Sex hormone concentrations are usually appropriate for the stage of puberty in both sexes. Despite the availability of sensitive and specific (liquid chromatography/tandem mass spectrometry) assays for sex hormones, serum estradiol concentrations are low or undetectable in the early phase of sexual precocity in girls, as they are in normal puberty. In boys, serum testosterone levels are usually detectable or clearly elevated by the time the parents seek medical attention, provided that an early morning blood sample is obtained. With the use of highly sensitive immunofluorometric and chemiluminescent assays, serum luteinizing hormone (LH) concentrations are undetectable in prepubertal children in random blood samples, but become detectable in 50-75% of girls and a higher percentage of boys with central sexual precocity. Unfortunately, a number of hospitals use only moderately sensitive immunoenzymatic assays for LH, and often insensitive assays for estradiol and testosterone, which decrease the diagnostic sensitivity of these measurements. Measurement of LH in serial blood samples obtained during sleep has greater diagnostic power than measurement in a single random sample, and it typically reveals a well-defined pul-

satile secretion of LH. Intravenous administration of gonadotropin-releasing hormone (GnRH stimulation test) or a GnRH agonist (leuprolide stimulation test) is a helpful diagnostic tool, particularly for boys, in whom a "pubertal" LH response (LH peak >5 IU/L) with predominance of LH over follicle-stimulating hormone (FSH) tends to occur early in the course of precocious puberty. In girls with sexual precocity, however, the nocturnal LH secretion and the LH response to GnRH or GnRH agonist may be quite low at breast stages II to early III (immunometric LH peak, <5 IU/L), and the LH:FSH ratio may remain low until mid-advanced puberty. In such girls with "low" LH response, the central nature of sexual precocity can be proven by detecting pubertal levels of estradiol (>50 pg/mL), 20-24 hr after stimulation with leuprolide.

Osseous maturation is variably advanced, often by more than 2-3 SD. Pelvic ultrasonography in girls reveals progressive enlargement of the ovaries, followed by enlargement of the fundus and then of the whole uterus to pubertal size. An MRI scan usually demonstrates physiologic enlargement of the pituitary gland, as seen in normal puberty; it may also reveal CNS pathology (see Chapter 562.2).

DIFFERENTIAL DIAGNOSIS

Organic CNS causes of central sexual precocity are more likely in boys, and those girls who have rapid breast development, have estradiol

>30 pg/mL, or are younger than 6 yr of age. All children in these categories should undergo MRI scans of the brain and pituitary gland. Specific criteria for ordering brain imaging in girls older than age 6 yr are still lacking, although some authorities recommend MRI scans for all children with central precocious puberty.

Gonadotropin-independent causes of isosexual precocious puberty must be considered in the differential diagnosis (see Table 562-1). For girls, these include tumors of the ovaries, autonomously functioning ovarian cysts, feminizing adrenal tumors, McCune-Albright syndrome, and exogenous sources of estrogens. In boys, congenital adrenal hyperplasia, adrenal tumors, Leydig cell tumors, chorionic gonadotropin–producing tumors, exposure to exogenous androgens, and familial male precocious puberty should be considered.

TREATMENT

Virtually all boys and the large subgroup of girls with rapidly progressive precocious puberty are candidates for treatment. Girls with slowly progressive idiopathic central precocious puberty do not seem to benefit in terms of height prognosis from GnRH-agonist therapy. Former small-for-gestational-age infants may be at greater risk of short stature as adults and may require more aggressive treatment of precocious puberty, possibly in conjunction with human growth hormone therapy. Certain patients require treatment solely for psychologic or social reasons, including children with special needs and very young girls at risk of early menarche.

The observation that the pituitary gonadotropic cells require pulsatile, rather than continuous, stimulation by GnRH to maintain the ongoing release of gonadotropins provides the rationale for using GnRH agonists for treatment of central precocious puberty. By virtue of being more potent, and having a longer duration of action, than native GnRH, these GnRH agonists (after a brief period of stimulation) "desensitize" the gonadotropic cells of the pituitary to the stimulatory effect of endogenous GnRH and effectively halt the progression of central sexual precocity.

Long-acting formulations of GnRH agonists, which maintain fairly constant serum concentrations of the drug for weeks or months, constitute the preparations of choice for treatment of central precocious puberty. In the United States, the available preparations include: (1) leuprolide acetate (Lupron Depot-Ped), in a dose of 0.25-0.3 mg/kg (minimum 7.5 mg) intramuscularly once every 4 wk; (2) longer-acting preparations of depot leuprolide, allowing for injections (11.25-30.0 mg intramuscularly) every 90 days; and (3) histrelin (Supprelin LA), a subcutaneous 50 mg implant with effects lasting 12 mo. Other preparations (D-Trp6-GnRH [Decapeptyl], goserelin acetate [Zoladex]) are approved for treatment of precocious puberty in other countries. Recurrent sterile fluid collections at the sites of injections are an uncommon local side effect and occur in less than 1-3% of patients treated with depot leuprolide. Breakage or malfunction of the histrelin implant is very rare. Other available treatment options, usually reserved for children who cannot tolerate the products listed above, include subcutaneous injections of aqueous leuprolide, given once or twice daily (total dose 60 μg/kg/24 hr), or intranasal administration of the GnRH agonist nafarelin (Synarel), 800 μg bid. The potential for irregular compliance with daily administration, as well as the variable absorption of the intranasal route for nafarelin, may limit the long-term benefit of the latter preparations on adult height. GnRH antagonists have not been investigated sufficiently and are not FDA approved. Oral GnRH antagonists are also being investigated.

Treatment results in decrease of the growth rate, generally to age-appropriate values, and an even greater decrease of the rate of osseous maturation. Some children, particularly those with greatly advanced (pubertal) bone age, may show marked deceleration of their growth rate and a complete arrest in the rate of osseous maturation. Treatment results in enhancement of the predicted height, although the actual adult height of patients followed to epiphyseal closure is approximately 1 SD less than their midparental height. In girls, breast development may regress in those with Tanner stages II-III development. Most commonly, the size of the breasts remains unchanged in girls with stages III-V development, or may even increase slightly because of progres-

sive adipose tissue deposition. The amount of glandular tissue decreases. Pubic hair usually remains stable in girls, or may progress slowly during treatment, reflecting the gradual increase in adrenal androgens. Menses, if present, cease. Pelvic sonography demonstrates a decrease of the ovarian and uterine size. In boys, there is decrease of testicular size, variable regression of pubic hair, and decrease in the frequency of erections. Except for a reversible decrease in bone density (of uncertain clinical significance), no serious adverse effects of GnRH analogs have been reported in children treated for sexual precocity. If treatment is effective, the serum sex hormone concentrations decrease to prepubertal levels (testosterone, <10-20 ng/dL in boys; estradiol, <5-10 pg/mL in girls). The serum LH and FSH concentrations, as measured by sensitive immunometric assays, decrease to less than 1 IU/L in most patients, although almost never does the LH return to truly prepubertal levels (<0.1 IU/L). Moreover, the incremental FSH and LH responses to GnRH stimulation decrease to less than 2-3 IU/L. Serum LH and sex hormone levels remain suppressed for as long as therapy is continued, but puberty resumes promptly when therapy is discontinued, typically at a "pubertal" chronological age. In girls, menarche generally appears at an average of 18 mo (range: 6-24 mo) of cessation of intramuscular therapy, and somewhat earlier after removal of the histrelin implant. The addition of human growth hormone to GnRH agonists has been used on an investigational basis in children with precocious puberty, markedly advanced bone age, and prediction of short stature. The available, albeit limited, data indicate that combined therapy may increase the adult height.

562.2 Precocious Puberty Resulting from Organic Brain Lesions

Wassim Chemaitilly and Luigi R. Garibaldi

ETIOLOGY

Hypothalamic hamartomas are the most common brain lesion causing central precocious puberty (Fig. 562-2). This congenital malformation consists of ectopically located neural tissue. Glial cells within the hamartoma have been shown to produce transforming growth factor α, which has the potential to activate the GnRH pulse generator. On MRI, it appears as a small pedunculated mass attached to the tuber cinereum or the floor of the third ventricle or, less often, as a sessile mass (Fig. 562-3) that remains static in size over years. Hypothalamic hamartomas, especially the sessile variant, can be associated with gelastic or psychomotor seizures.

A wide variety of other CNS lesions or insults, usually involving the hypothalamus by scarring, invasion, or pressure, are associated with gonadotropin-dependent sexual precocity. They include postencephalitic scars, tuberculous meningitis, tuberous sclerosis, severe head trauma, and hydrocephalus, either isolated or associated with myelomeningocele. Neoplasms causing precocious puberty include astrocytomas, ependymomas, and optic tract tumors. Tumors of the latter type (typically slowly progressive or indolent optic gliomas) are highly prevalent (15-20%) in children with neurofibromatosis type 1 and constitute the main etiologic factor for the central sexual precocity encountered in a small subset (approximately 3%) of children with neurofibromatosis type 1.

Approximately 50% of the tumors in the pineal region are germ cell tumors or astrocytomas; the remainder consist of a wide variety of histologically distinct tumor types. In boys, pineal or hypothalamic germ cell tumors can cause central precocious puberty by secreting human chorionic gonadotropin (hCG), which stimulates the LH receptors in the Leydig cells of the testes (see Chapter 562.5).

CLINICAL MANIFESTATIONS

Some of these tumors or malformations (hypothalamic hamartomas) remain static in size or grow slowly, producing no signs other than precocious puberty. For lesions causing neurologic symptoms, the neuroendocrine manifestations may be present for 1-2 yr before the tumor can be detected radiologically. Hypothalamic signs or symptoms such

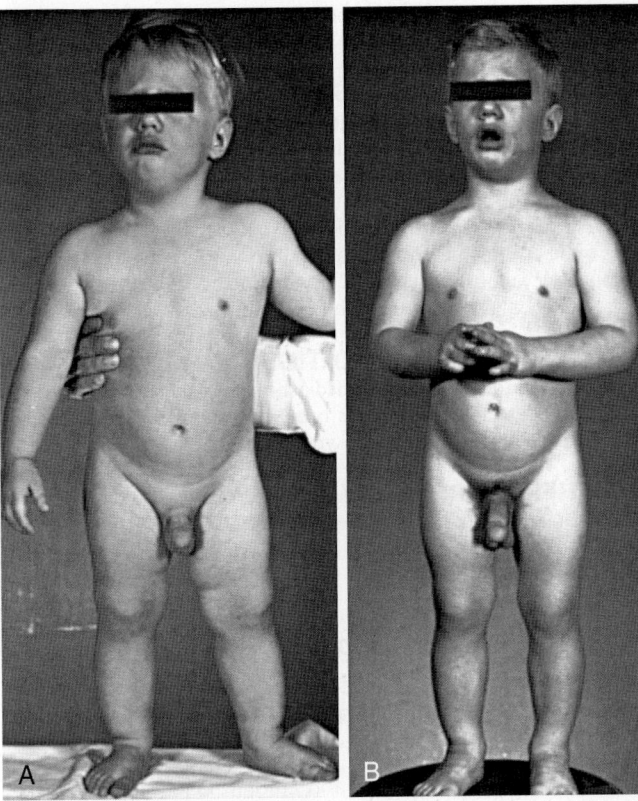

Figure 562-2 Natural course of precocious puberty with central nervous system lesion. Photographs at 1.5 **(A)** and 2.5 **(B)** yr of age. Accelerated growth, muscular development, osseous maturation, and testicular development were consistent with the degree of secondary sexual maturation. In early infancy, the patient began having frequent spells of rapid, purposeless motion; later in life, he had episodes of uncontrollable laughing with ocular movements. At 7 yr, he exhibited emotional lability, aggressive behavior, and destructive tendencies. Although a hypothalamic hamartoma had been suspected, it was not established until CT scanning became available when the patient was 23 yr of age. Epiphyses fused at 9 yr of age; final height was 142 cm (56 in). At 24 yr of age, he developed an embryonal cell carcinoma of the retroperitoneum.

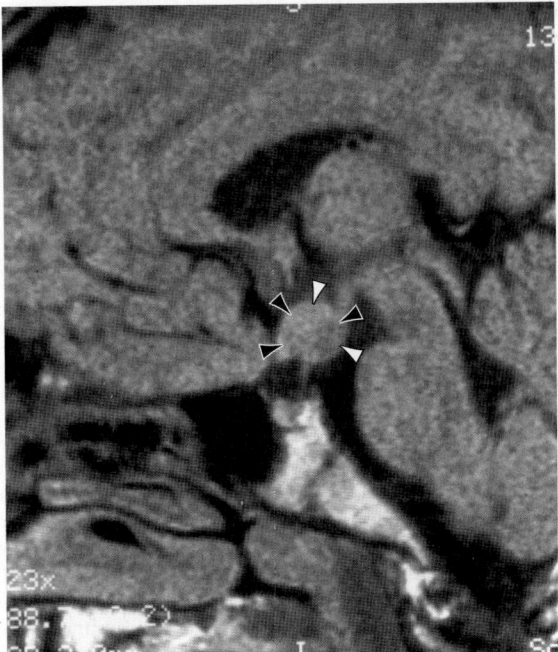

Figure 562-3 MRI of a central nervous system lesion in a child with central precocious puberty. A 6 yr old girl was referred for stage IV breast development and growth acceleration. Serum luteinizing hormone and estradiol concentrations were in the adult range. The midsagittal T1-weighted image shows an isointense hypothalamic mass (*arrowheads*), typical of a hamartoma. (*From Sharafuddin M, Luisiri A, Garibaldi LR, et al: MR imaging diagnosis of central precocious puberty: importance of changes in the shape and size of the pituitary gland, AJR Am J Roentgenol 162:1167–1173, 1994.*)

as diabetes insipidus, adipsia, hyperthermia, unnatural crying or laughing (gelastic seizures), obesity, and cachexia should suggest the possibility of an intracranial lesion. Visual signs (proptosis, decreased visual acuity, visual field defects) may be the first manifestation of an optic glioma.

The sexual precocity is always isosexual, and the endocrine patterns are generally those found in children without demonstrable organic lesions. Rapidly progressive sexual precocity in very young children suggests the likelihood of a hypothalamic hamartoma. In conditions other than hypothalamic hamartoma, growth hormone deficiency can occur and may be masked by the growth-promoting effect of the increased sex hormone levels.

TREATMENT

Regardless of the cause, therapy with GnRH agonists is as effective in children with organic brain lesions causing central precocious puberty, and these analogs are the therapy of choice to halt premature sexual development. This includes patients with a hypothalamic hamartoma, if precocious puberty is its only manifestation. In patients with hypothalamic hamartoma and associated intractable gelastic or psychomotor seizures, however, stereotactic radiation therapy (gamma knife surgery) is effective and less risky than neurosurgical intervention. For other neurologic lesions, therapy depends on the nature and location of the pathologic process. Combined growth hormone therapy

should be considered for patients with associated growth hormone deficiency.

562.3 Precocious Puberty Following Irradiation of the Brain
Wassim Chemaitilly and Luigi R. Garibaldi

Radiation therapy, generally for leukemia or intracranial tumors, increases the risk of precocious puberty considerably, whether the irradiation is directed to the hypothalamic area or to areas of the brain anatomically distant from the hypothalamus. Low-dose radiation (18-24 Gy) hastens the onset of puberty almost exclusively in girls. High-dose radiation (25-47 Gy), conversely, appears to trigger precocious sexual development in both sexes, and the risk of sexual precocity is inversely proportional to the age of the child at the time radiation was given.

This type of sexual precocity is often associated with growth hormone deficiency and may also be combined with other conditions (spinal irradiation, hypothyroidism) adversely affecting the prognosis for a reasonable adult height. Unless careful attention is paid to early signs of pubertal development in these children, the combination of growth hormone deficiency and the growth-promoting effect of sex steroids often results in a "normal" growth rate at the expense of a rapidly advancing bone age and impaired adult height potential.

TREATMENT

GnRH analogs are effective in arresting pubertal progression in this patient population. However, concomitant growth hormone deficiency (and/or thyroid hormone deficiency) should be diagnosed and treated promptly in order for the adult height prognosis to improve.

Paradoxically, hypopituitarism with gonadotropin deficiency may subsequently develop as a late effect of high-dose CNS irradiation in patients with or without a history of precocious puberty, and it may require substitution therapy with sex steroids.

562.4 Syndrome of Precocious Puberty and Hypothyroidism
Luigi R. Garibaldi and Wassim Chemaitilly

In children with untreated hypothyroidism, the onset of puberty is usually delayed until epiphyseal maturation reaches 12-13 yr of age. Precocious puberty in a child with untreated hypothyroidism and a prepubertal bone age presents a strikingly unphysiologic association, yet is common and may occur in as many as 50% of children with severe hypothyroidism of long duration. These children have the usual manifestations of hypothyroidism, including retardation of growth and of osseous maturation (see Chapter 565). The cause of the hypothyroidism is usually Hashimoto thyroiditis, which often goes undiagnosed, especially in children with special needs such as those with trisomy 21, in whom the symptoms of profound hypothyroidism may be more difficult to recognize. Sexual development in girls consists of breast enlargement and menstrual bleeding; the latter may occur even in girls with minimal breast enlargement. Pelvic sonography may reveal large, multicystic ovaries. Boys have testicular enlargement associated with modest or no penile enlargement. No pubic hair development occurs in either girls or boys. Enlargement of the sella, which is typical of long-standing primary hypothyroidism, may be demonstrated by skull film or MRI. Plasma levels of thyroid-stimulating hormone (TSH) are markedly elevated, often greater than 500 µU/mL, and those of pro-lactin and estradiol are mildly elevated. Although serum FSH is low and LH is undetectable, when measured by specific assays, the massively elevated concentrations of TSH appear to interact with the FSH receptor ("specificity spillover"), thus inducing FSH-like effects in the absence of LH effects on the gonads. The FSH-like effect suffices to induce estradiol secretion by the ovaries, while in boys testicular enlargement occurs without substantial testosterone secretion. Thus, the precocious puberty associated with hypothyroidism behaves as an incomplete form of gonadotropin-dependent puberty. Treatment of the hypothyroidism results in rapid return to normal of the biochemical and clinical manifestations. Possible progression to central puberty with rapid bone age advancement could occur in the months following the initiation of thyroid hormone replacement, a complication that would justify delaying puberty with GnRH analogs. Macroorchidism (testicular volume >30 mL) may persist in adult males despite adequate levothyroxine therapy.

562.5 Chorionic Gonadotropin-Secreting Tumors
Luigi R. Garibaldi and Wassim Chemaitilly

These are rare tumors, whose secretion of hCG stimulates the LH receptors in the Leydig cells. The testicles are only minimally enlarged, and the histology reveals interstitial cell hyperplasia with no spermatogenesis. Plasma levels of testosterone are elevated, while those of FSH and LH, as measured by specific immunometric assays, are low. These tumors induce puberty in boys but not in girls, as ovarian production of estrogens cannot take place in the absence of FSH stimulation.

HEPATIC TUMORS
All reported cases of **hepatoblastoma** causing isosexual precocious puberty have been in boys, with the average age of onset of 2 yr (range: 4 mo to 8 yr). An enlarged liver or mass in the right upper quadrant should suggest the diagnosis. Plasma levels of hCG and α-fetoprotein are usually markedly elevated and serve as useful markers for following the effects of therapy. Similarly to other carcinomas of the liver;

the prognosis for survival beyond 1-2 yr from the time of diagnosis is poor.

INTRACRANIAL TUMORS
Nongerminomatous or mixed germ cell tumors, choriocarcinomas, teratomas, teratocarcinomas, and others account for <5% of intracranial tumors. They are usually located in the neurohypophyseal area or the pineal area and may cause precocious puberty in boys if they secrete hCG, and rarely in girls because of mass effect. Marked elevations of hCG and α-fetoprotein often occur in the cerebrospinal fluid, although elevations in the blood may be modest. Treatment includes radiation, chemotherapy, and debulking surgery.

TUMORS IN OTHER LOCATIONS
Very rare locations include the mediastinum, gonads, or even adrenal glands. Mediastinal tumors have been reported to cause precocious puberty in boys with Klinefelter syndrome.

PERIPHERAL PRECOCIOUS PUBERTY
The adrenal causes of pseudopuberty are discussed in Chapter 576, and the gonadal causes are discussed in Chapters 584 and 587.

562.6 McCune-Albright Syndrome (Precocious Puberty with Polyostotic Fibrous Dysplasia and Abnormal Pigmentation)
Wassim Chemaitilly and Luigi R. Garibaldi

This syndrome of endocrine dysfunction is associated with patchy cutaneous pigmentation and fibrous dysplasia of the skeletal system. It is a rare condition with a prevalence between 1 in 100,000 and 1 in 1,000,000 people. A classical cause of peripheral precocious puberty, it can also induce pituitary, thyroid, and adrenal aberrations. It is characterized by autonomous hyperfunction of many glands and is caused by a missense mutation in the gene encoding the α-subunit of G$_s$, the G protein that stimulates cyclic adenosine monophosphate formation, resulting in the formation of the putative gsp oncoprotein. Activation of receptors (corticotropin [adrenocorticotropic hormone (ACTH)], TSH, FSH, and LH receptors) that operate via a cyclic adenosine monophosphate–dependent mechanism, as well as cell proliferation, ensue. Because the mutation is somatic rather than genomic, it is expressed differently in different tissues; hence the variability of clinical expression. Precocious puberty has been described predominantly in girls (Fig. 562-4). The average age at onset in affected girls is about 3 yr, but vaginal bleeding has occurred as early as 4 mo of age and secondary sex characteristics have occurred as early as 6 mo. Young girls have suppressed levels of LH and FSH, and there is no response to GnRH or leuprolide stimulation. Estradiol levels vary from normal to markedly elevated (>900 pg/mL), are often cyclic, and may correlate with the size of the recurrent ovarian cysts. In boys, precocious puberty is less common but has been reported in several instances. Unlike ovarian enlargement in girls, testicular enlargement in boys is fairly symmetric. It is followed by the appearance of phallic enlargement and pubic hair, as in normal puberty. Testicular histology has demonstrated large seminiferous tubules and no or minimal Leydig cell hyperplasia; these findings may simply reflect the fact that biopsy specimens were obtained at an early stage of pubertal development. In girls and boys, when the bone age reaches the usual pubertal age range, gonadotropin secretion begins, and the response to GnRH becomes pubertal. Central precocious puberty overrides the antecedent (gonadotropin-independent) precocious pseudopuberty. In girls, menses become more regular, but often not completely so, and fertility has been documented.

Pubertal progression is variable in these patients. Functioning ovarian cysts often disappear spontaneously; aspiration or surgical excision of cysts is rarely indicated, but ovarian torsion may occur.

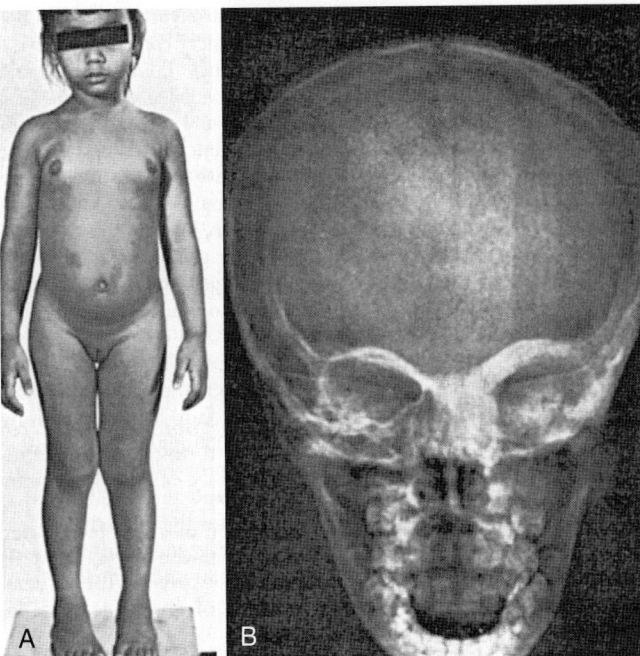

Figure 562-4 Precocious puberty associated with polyostotic fibrous dysplasia (McCune-Albright syndrome) in a girl 4.5 yr of age; at this time, her height age and bone age were normal. Menarche occurred at 4 yr of age. **A,** Note the bilateral breast development, hyperpigmented spots on the abdomen, and prominence of the left side of the face. **B,** Roentgenograms revealed fibrous dysplasia in the distal end of the left ulna and thickening of the bones about the left orbit and the maxillary portion of the frontal bones shown here.

For girls with persistent estradiol secretion, agents that interfere with the final step of estrogen biosynthesis (i.e., aromatase inhibitors such as letrozole [1.25-2.5 mg/day orally]) or antiestrogens (such as tamoxifen 5-20 mg/day orally) may limit, to a variable extent, the estrogen effects on pubertal and osseous maturation. The same compounds have also been used in boys, in combination with anti-androgens (such as spironolactone 50-100 mg bid, flutamide 125-250 mg bid, or bicalutamide 25-50 mg daily). These compounds are not approved by the FDA for this indication; tamoxifen, flutamide, and bicalutamide may be hepatotoxic, and high-dose spironolactone may (rarely) cause hyperkalemia. Associated therapy with long-acting analogs of GnRH is indicated only for patients whose puberty has shifted from a gonadotropin-independent to a predominantly gonadotropin-dependent mechanism.

EXTRAGONADAL MANIFESTATIONS
The hyperthyroidism that occurs in this condition differs from that characteristic of Graves disease. There is an equal distribution between male and female patients; the goiters are multinodular. Clinical hyperthyroidism is uncommon in children, but goiters, mildly elevated triiodothyronine levels, suppressed TSH levels, and abnormalities on ultrasound have been reported. Thyroidectomy is rarely necessary.

In patients with associated Cushing syndrome, bilateral nodular adrenocortical hyperplasia has occurred in early infancy, antedating the sexual precocity. ACTH levels are low, and adrenal function is not suppressed by large doses of dexamethasone. Treatment is bilateral adrenalectomy.

Increased secretion of growth hormone occurs uncommonly and is manifested clinically by gigantism or acromegaly or by increased rates of growth even in the absence of precocious puberty. Girls and boys are equally affected. Serum levels of growth hormone are elevated, increase during sleep, and are poorly inhibited by oral glucose. Serum levels of prolactin are increased in most patients, but fewer than 50% of the patients have a demonstrable pituitary tumor. Depot octreotide

(Sandostatin LAR Depot 10-30 mg IM monthly) or Lanreotide (Somatuline Depot, 60-90 mg SC monthly), long-acting somatostatin analogs, can be used to treat the hypersomatotropism. The prognosis is favorable for longevity, but deformities, repeated fractures, pain, and occasional cranial nerve compression may result from the bony lesions.

Of the extraglandular manifestations, phosphaturia, leading to rickets or osteomalacia, is the most common. Cardiovascular and hepatic involvement is rare but may be life-threatening (severe neonatal cholestasis).

562.7 Familial Male Gonadotropin-Independent Precocious Puberty
Wassim Chemaitilly and Luigi R. Garibaldi

This rare, autosomal dominant form of peripheral precocious puberty is transmitted from affected males and unaffected female carriers of the gene to their male offspring. Signs of puberty appear by 2-3 yr of age. The testes are only slightly enlarged. Testicular biopsies show Leydig cell maturation and, sometimes, marked hyperplasia. Maturation of seminiferous tubules may be present. Testosterone levels are variably and often markedly elevated, even above the adult male range; however, baseline levels of LH are prepubertal, pulsatile secretion of LH is absent, and LH does not respond to stimulation with GnRH or GnRH agonist. The cause for activation of Leydig cells independently of gonadotropin stimulation is a missense mutation of the LH receptor leading to constitutive activation of cyclic adenosine monophosphate production. Osseous maturation may be markedly advanced; when it reaches the pubertal age range, hypothalamic maturation shifts the mechanism of pubertal development to a gonadotropin-dependent one. This sequence of events is similar to that occurring in children with McCune-Albright syndrome (see Chapter 562.6) or in those with congenital adrenal hyperplasia (see Chapter 576.1).

Gonadotropin-independent precocious puberty has been diagnosed in a few unrelated boys with type IA pseudohypoparathyroidism who had a single mutation of the G$_s$α protein. This mutation is inactivating at normal body temperature and causes pseudohypoparathyroidism, but in the cooler temperature of the testes, it is constitutionally activating, resulting in adenyl cyclase stimulation and production of testosterone. Although this mutation differs from the constitutive LH receptor mutation, which usually causes familial male gonadotropin-independent precocious puberty, the end result is the same.

TREATMENT
Young boys have been successfully treated with ketoconazole (600 mg/24 hr in 8 hr divided doses), an antifungal drug that inhibits C-17,20-lyase and testosterone synthesis. Other investigators use a combination of antiandrogens (such as spironolactone 50-100 mg twice a day, flutamide 125–250 mg twice a day, or bicalutamide 25-50 mg daily) and aromatase inhibitors (letrozole 2.5 mg/day, or anastrozole 1 mg/day), because estrogens derived from androgens stimulate bone maturation. These medications are unable to revert the serum testosterone to the normal (prepubertal) concentrations or completely offset the unfavorable effects of the elevated sex hormones. They slow down, but do not halt, the progression of puberty and may not improve the height prognosis. Boys whose GnRH pulse generator has matured require combined therapy with GnRH agonists.

562.8 Incomplete (Partial) Precocious Development
Luigi R. Garibaldi and Wassim Chemaitilly

Isolated manifestations of precocity without development of other signs of puberty are not unusual; development of the breasts in girls and growth of sexual hair in both sexes are the 2 most common forms.

PREMATURE THELARCHE

This term applies to a sporadic, transient condition of isolated breast development that most often appears in the 1st 2 yr of life. In some girls, breast development is present at birth and persists. It may be unilateral or asymmetric and often fluctuates in degree. Growth and osseous maturation are normal or slightly advanced. The genitalia show no evidence of estrogenic stimulation. Breast development may regress after 2 yr, often persists for 3-5 yr, and is rarely progressive. Menarche occurs at the expected age, and reproduction is normal. Basal serum levels of FSH and the FSH response to GnRH stimulation may be greater than that seen in normal controls. Plasma levels of LH and estradiol are consistently less than the limits of detection. Ultrasound examination of the ovaries reveals normal size, but a few small (<9 mm) cysts are not uncommon.

In some girls, breast development may be associated with definite evidence of systemic estrogen effects, such as growth acceleration or bone age advancement. Pelvic sonography may reveal enlarged ovaries or uterus. This condition, referred to as **exaggerated or atypical thelarche,** differs from central precocious puberty because it spontaneously regresses. Leuprolide or GnRH stimulation elicits a robust FSH response, a low LH response, and (after leuprolide only) a moderate estradiol increment at 24 hr (average: 60-90 pg/mL). The pathogenesis of typical and exaggerated forms of thelarche is unclear. Delayed inactivation of the hypothalamic-pituitary-ovarian axis, which is active during the prenatal and early postnatal period, increased peripheral sensitivity to estrogens, and other possibilities have been proposed, yet are unproven hypotheses. Premature thelarche is a benign condition but may be the first sign of true or peripheral precocious puberty, or it may be caused by exogenous exposure to estrogens. In addition to a detailed history, a bone age should be obtained if there are any unusual features. Random serum concentrations of FSH, LH, and estradiol are generally low and not diagnostic. Pelvic ultrasound examination or leuprolide stimulation testing is rarely indicated. Continued observation is important because the condition cannot be readily distinguished from true precocious puberty. Regression and recurrence suggest functioning follicular cysts. Occurrence of thelarche in children older than 3 yr of age most often is caused by a condition other than benign premature thelarche.

PREMATURE PUBARCHE (ADRENARCHE)

Premature adrenarche has traditionally applied to the appearance of sexual hair before the age of 8 yr in girls or 9 yr in boys without other evidence of maturation. It is much more frequent in girls than in boys. The higher prevalence of this condition in African-American and, to a smaller extent, Latino girls in comparison to white girls may suggest that the cutoff age for the definition of "premature" should be adjusted for different ethnic groups on the basis of epidemiologic data. Hair appears on the mons and labia majora in girls and perineal and scrotal area in boys; axillary hair generally appears later. Adult-type axillary odor is common. Affected children are often slightly advanced in height and osseous maturation. Premature adrenarche is an early maturational event of adrenal androgen production. This event coincides with precocious maturation of the zona reticularis, an associated decrease in 3β-hydroxysteroid dehydrogenase activity, and an increase in C-17,20-lyase activity. These enzymatic changes result in increased basal and ACTH-stimulated serum concentrations of the Δ^5-steroids (17-hydroxypregnenolone and dehydroepiandrosterone) and, to a lesser extent, of the Δ^4-steroids (particularly androstenedione) compared with age-matched control subjects. The levels of these steroids and of dehydroepiandrosterone sulfate are usually comparable to those of older children in the early stages of normal puberty. Idiopathic premature adrenarche is a slowly progressive condition that requires no therapy. However, a subset of patients with precocious pubarche has 1 or more features of systemic androgen effect, such as marked growth acceleration, clitoral (girls) or phallic (boys) enlargement, cystic acne, or advanced bone age (>2 SD above the mean for age). In these patients with **atypical premature adrenarche,** an ACTH stimulation test with measurement of steroid intermediates (mainly, serum 17-hydroxyprogesterone concentrations) is indicated to rule out nonclassical congenital adrenal hyperplasia caused by 21-hydroxylase deficiency. Epidemiologic and molecular genetic studies show that the prevalence of nonclassical 21-hydroxylase deficiency is approximately 3-6% of unselected children with precocious pubarche; the prevalence of other enzyme defects (i.e., 3β-hydroxysteroid dehydrogenase or 11β-hydroxylase deficiency) is extremely low. Although idiopathic premature adrenarche has been considered a benign condition, longitudinal observations suggest that approximately 50% of girls with premature adrenarche are at high risk for **hyperandrogenism** and **polycystic ovary syndrome,** alone or more often in combination with other components of the so-called metabolic syndrome (insulin resistance possibly progressing to type 2 diabetes mellitus, dyslipidemia, hypertension, increased abdominal fat) as adults. Whether the unfavorable progression to pubertal hyperandrogenism can be prevented by insulin-sensitizing agents (metformin 850-1,000 mg/day) or lifestyle interventions (diet, exercise) remains to be proven in large studies. An increased risk of premature adrenarche and the metabolic syndrome is documented in children born small for their gestational age. This appears to be associated with insulin resistance and decreased β-cell reserve, perhaps as a consequence of fetal undernutrition.

PREMATURE MENARCHE

This is a rare entity, much less frequent than premature thelarche or premature adrenarche, and is a diagnosis of exclusion. In girls with isolated vaginal bleeding in the absence of other secondary sexual characteristics, more common causes, such as vulvovaginitis, a foreign body (typically associated with malodorous discharge), or sexual abuse, and uncommon causes, such as urethral prolapse and sarcoma botryoides, must be carefully excluded. The majority of girls with idiopathic premature menarche have only 1-3 episodes of bleeding; puberty occurs at the usual time, and menstrual cycles are normal. Plasma levels of gonadotropins are low, but estradiol levels may be occasionally elevated, probably owing to episodic ovarian estrogen secretion associated with ovarian follicular cysts that can be detected on ultrasound.

562.9 Medicational Precocity

Luigi R. Garibaldi and Wassim Chemaitilly

A variety of medicaments can induce the appearance of secondary sexual characteristics that may be confused with precocious puberty. A careful history focused on exploring the possibility of accidental exposure to, or ingestion of, sex hormones is important. Peripheral precocious puberty has occurred in boys and girls from the accidental ingestion of estrogens (including contraceptive pills) and from the administration of anabolic steroids. The most common cause of medicational precocity is currently related to the widespread use of testosterone gels or creams that are applied to the skin for treatment of male hypogonadism. This has resulted in virilization of children and women following skin contact at, and systemic absorption from, the area where the gel/cream was applied by their family member.

Less commonly, estrogens in cosmetics, hair creams, and breast augmentation creams have caused breast development in girls and gynecomastia in boys, via percutaneous absorption. The high prevalence of premature thelarche and peripheral precocious puberty in Puerto Rico has been attributed to contamination of meats, particularly chicken, with estrogens used in animal husbandry, but has not been proved. Exogenous estrogens may produce a darkening of the areola that is not usually seen in endogenous types of precocity. The precocious changes disappear after cessation of exposure to the hormones.

Bibliography is available at Expert Consult.

Section **2**

Disorders of the Thyroid Gland

Chapter **563**

Thyroid Development and Physiology

Stephen H. LaFranchi and
Stephen A. Huang

FETAL DEVELOPMENT

The fetal thyroid arises from an outpouching of the foregut at the base of the tongue (foramen cecum). It migrates to its normal location over the thyroid cartilage by 8-10 wk of gestation. The thyroid bilobed shape is recognized by 7 wk of gestation, and characteristic thyroid follicle cell and colloid formation is seen by 10 wk. Thyroglobulin synthesis occurs from 4 wk, iodine trapping occurs by 8-10 wk, and thyroxine (T_4) and, to a lesser extent, triiodothyronine (T_3) synthesis and secretion occur from 12 wk of gestation. There is evidence that several transcription factors—TTF-1/NKX-2.1, TTF-2 (also termed FOXE1), NKX2.5, and PAX8—are important in thyroid gland morphogenesis and differentiation, and possibly also in its caudal migration to its final location. These factors also bind to the promoters of thyroglobulin and thyroid peroxidase genes and so influence thyroid hormone production. Hypothalamic neurons synthesize thyrotropin-releasing hormone (TRH) by 6-8 wk, the pituitary portal vessel system begins development by 8-10 wk, and thyroid-stimulating hormone (TSH) secretion is evident by 12 wk of gestation. Maturation of the hypothalamic-pituitary-thyroid axis occurs over the second half of gestation, but normal feedback relationships are not mature until approximately 3 mo of postnatal life. Other transcription factors, including PROP-1 and Pit-1, are important for differentiation and growth of thyrotrophs, along with somatotrophs and lactotrophs.

THYROID PHYSIOLOGY

The main function of the thyroid gland is to synthesize T_4 and T_3. The only known physiologic role of iodine (or iodide [I^-] in its ionized form) is in the synthesis of these hormones; the recommended dietary allowance of iodine is 30 μg/kg/24 hr for infants, 90-120 μg/24 hr for children, and 150 μg/24 hr for adolescents and adults.

The median iodine intake in the United States decreased by approximately 50% between the 1970s (320 μg/L) and the 1990s (145 μg/L), but it now appears to have stabilized (2009-2010 = 144 μg/L). Whatever the chemical form ingested, iodine eventually reaches the thyroid gland as iodide. Thyroid tissue has an avidity for iodide and is able to trap (with a gradient of 100 : 1), transport, and concentrate it in the follicular lumen for synthesis of thyroid hormone. Entry of iodide from the circulation into the thyroid is carried out by the sodium–iodide symporter. Iodide diffuses across the cell to the apical membrane where it is transported into the colloid via pendrin.

Before trapped iodide can react with tyrosine, it must be oxidized; this reaction is catalyzed by **thyroidal peroxidase.** Dual oxidase maturation factor 2 (**DUOXA2**) is required to express **DUOX2** enzymatic activity, which is required for H_2O_2 generation, a crucial step in iodide oxidation. The thyroid cells produce **thyroglobulin,** a large globular glycoprotein with a molecular weight of approximately 660,000, containing approximately 120 tyrosine units. Iodination of tyrosine forms

monoiodotyrosine and diiodotyrosine; 2 molecules of diiodotyrosine then couple to form 1 molecule of T_4, or 1 molecule of diiodotyrosine and 1 of monoiodotyrosine to form T_3. Once formed, hormones are stored as thyroglobulin in the lumen of the follicle (colloid) until ready to be delivered to the body cells. T_4 and T_3 are liberated from thyroglobulin by activation of proteases and peptidases.

The metabolic potency of T_3 is 3-4 times that of T_4. In adults, the thyroid produces approximately 100 μg of T_4 and 20 μg of T_3 daily. Only 20% of circulating T_3 is secreted by the thyroid; the remainder is produced by deiodination of T_4 in the liver, kidney, and other extrathyroidal tissues by type I 5′-deiodinase. Selenocysteine is the active center of the iodothyronine deiodinases. Thus, selenium indirectly plays a role in normal growth and development. In the pituitary and brain, approximately 80% of required T_3 is produced locally from T_4 by a different enzyme, type II 5′-deiodinase. The level of T_3 in blood is one fiftieth that of T_4, but T_3 is the physiologically active thyroid hormone.

Thyroid hormones increase oxygen consumption, stimulate protein synthesis, influence growth and differentiation, and affect carbohydrate, lipid, and vitamin metabolism. Specific thyroid hormone transporters, of which the most important is monocarboxylate transporter 8, facilitate entry of T_4 and T_3 into cells. Once into the cell, T_4 is converted to T_3 by type I or II 5′-deiodinase. Intracellular T_3 then enters the nucleus, where it binds to thyroid hormone receptors. Thyroid hormone receptors are members of the steroid hormone receptor superfamily that includes glucocorticoids, estrogen, progesterone, vitamin D, and retinoids. Four different isoforms of the thyroid hormone receptor (α_1, α_2, β_1, and β_2) are expressed in different tissues; the protein product of the formerly designated c-*erb* A protooncogene *(THRA2)* is the α_2 thyroid hormone receptor in the brain and hypothalamus. Thyroid hormone receptors consist of a ligand-binding domain (binds T_3), hinge region, and DNA-binding domain (zinc finger). Binding of T_3 activates the thyroid hormone receptor response element, resulting in production of an encoded messenger RNA and protein synthesis specific for the target cell. In this manner, a single hormone, T_4, acting through tissue-specific thyroid hormone receptor isoforms and gene-specific thyroid response elements, can produce multiple effects in various tissues.

Approximately 70% of the circulating T_4 is firmly bound to T_4-binding globulin (TBG). Less-important carriers are T_4-binding prealbumin, called *transthyretin*, and albumin. Only 0.03% of T_4 in serum is not bound and comprises free T_4. Approximately 50% of circulating T_3 is bound to TBG, and 50% is bound to albumin; 0.30% of T_3 is unbound, or free, T_3. Because the concentration of TBG is altered in many clinical circumstances, its status must be considered when interpreting total T_4 or T_3 levels.

THYROID REGULATION

The thyroid is regulated by TSH, a glycoprotein produced and secreted by the anterior pituitary. This hormone activates adenylate cyclase in the thyroid gland and is important in all steps of thyroid hormone biosynthesis, from trapping of iodine to release of thyroid hormones. TSH is composed of 2 noncovalently bound subunits (chains): α and β. The α subunit is common to luteinizing hormone, follicle-stimulating hormone, and chorionic gonadotropin; the specificity of each hormone is conferred by the β subunit. TSH synthesis and release are stimulated by TRH, which is synthesized in the hypothalamus and secreted into the pituitary. TRH is found in other parts of the brain besides the hypothalamus and in many other organs; aside from its endocrine function, it may be a neurotransmitter. TRH is a simple tripeptide. In states of decreased production of thyroid hormone, TSH and TRH are increased. Exogenous thyroid hormone or increased thyroid hormone synthesis inhibits TSH and TRH production. Except in the neonate, levels of TRH in serum are very low.

Further control of the level of circulating thyroid hormones occurs in the periphery. In many nonthyroidal illnesses, extrathyroidal production of T_3 decreases; factors that inhibit T_4-type I 5′-deiodinase include fasting, chronic malnutrition, acute illness, and certain drugs. Such factors increase type III 5′-deiodinase conversion of T_4 to reverse T_3. Whereas levels of T_3 may be significantly decreased, levels of free

T_4 and TSH may remain normal. The decreased levels of T_3 may be a physiologic adaptation, resulting in decreased rates of oxygen production, of substrate use, and of other catabolic processes.

Bibliography is available at Expert Consult.

563.1 Thyroid Hormone Studies

Stephen H. LaFranchi

SERUM THYROID HORMONES
Methods are available to measure all the thyroid hormones in serum: T_4, free T_4, T_3, and free T_3. A metabolically inert T_3 (3,5′,3′-triiodothyronine), called reverse T_3, is also present in serum. Age must be considered in interpreting results, particularly in the neonate.

Thyroglobulin is a glycoprotein that is secreted through the apical surface of the thyroid follicular cell into the colloid. Small amounts escape into the circulation and are measurable in serum. Levels increase with TSH (also called *thyrotropin*) stimulation and decrease with TSH suppression. Serum thyroglobulin levels are increased in the neonate, in patients with Graves disease and other forms of autoimmune thyroid disease, and in those with endemic goiter. The most marked elevations of thyroglobulin occur in patients with differentiated carcinoma of the thyroid. Athyreotic infants have markedly reduced levels of thyroglobulin in serum.

Serum TSH levels are the most accurate test of thyroid function. Serum TSH levels are elevated in primary hypothyroidism and suppressed in hyperthyroidism. After the neonatal period, normal levels of TSH are <6 mIU/L. With central (secondary) hypothyroidism, serum TSH may be subnormal, though often it is "inappropriately" in the normal range, despite a low serum T_4 or free T_4 level. TSH appears to be less biologically active in central hypothyroidism. These sensitive (third-generation) TSH assays obviate the need for TRH stimulation in the diagnosis of most patients with thyroid disorders.

FETAL AND NEWBORN THYROID
Fetal serum T_4 and free T_4 increase progressively from midgestation to approximately 11.5 μg/dL and 1.5 ng/dL, respectively, at term. Fetal levels of T_3 are low before 20 wk and then gradually increase to approximately 45 ng/dL at term. Reverse T_3 levels (inactive form of T_3), however, are high in the fetus (250 ng/dL at 30 wk) and decrease to 150 ng/dL at term. Serum levels of TSH gradually increase to 10 mU/L at term. Approximately one third of maternal T_4 crosses the placenta to the fetus. Maternal T_4 plays a role in fetal development, especially that of the brain, before the synthesis of fetal thyroid hormone begins. The fetus of a hypothyroid mother may be at risk for neurologic injury, and a hypothyroid fetus may be partially protected by maternal T_4 until delivery. The amount of T_4 that crosses the placenta is not sufficient to interfere with a diagnosis of congenital hypothyroidism in the neonate.

At birth, there is an acute release of TSH; peak serum concentrations reach 60 mU/L 30 min following delivery in full-term infants. A rapid decline occurs in the ensuing 24 hr and a more gradual decline over the next 5 days to <10 mIU/L. The acute increase in TSH produces a dramatic increase in levels of T_4 to approximately 16 μg/dL and of T_3 to approximately 300 ng/dL in about 4 hr. This T_3 seems largely derived from increased peripheral conversion of T_4 to T_3. T_4 levels gradually decrease during the 1st 2 wk of life to 12 μg/dL. T_3 levels decline during the 1st wk of life to levels below 200 ng/mL. Serum free T_4 levels are 0.9-2.3 ng/dL in infancy and decline to 0.7-1.8 ng/dL in childhood. Serum free T_3 concentrations are approximately 180-760 pg/dL in infancy and decline to 230-650 pg/dL in childhood. Reverse T_3 levels are maintained for 2 wk (200 ng/dL) and decrease by 4 wk to around

50 ng/dL. In preterm infants, changes in thyroid function after birth are qualitatively similar to but quantitatively smaller than in full-term infants. Serum T_4 and T_3 levels are decreased in proportion to gestational age and birthweight.

SERUM THYROXINE-BINDING GLOBULIN
The thyroid hormones are transported in plasma bound to TBG, a glycoprotein synthesized in the liver. Estimation of TBG levels is occasionally necessary because TBG is increased or decreased in a variety of clinical situations, with effects on the level of total T_4 and T_3. TBG binds approximately 70% of T_4 and 50% of T_3. TBG levels increase in pregnancy, in the newborn period, with hepatitis, and with administration of estrogens (oral contraceptives), selective estrogen receptor modulators, heroin or methadone, mitotane, 5-fluorouracil, and perphenazine, and they decrease with androgens, anabolic steroids, glucocorticoids, nicotinic acid, and L-asparaginase. These effects are the results of modulation of hepatic synthesis of TBG. TBG levels may be markedly decreased owing to decreased production with hepatocellular disease or loss in the gut with protein-losing enteropathies or in urine, as in the congenital nephrotic syndrome. Decreased or increased levels of TBG also occur as genetic traits (see Chapter 564).

Some drugs, in particular phenytoin, carbamazepine, furosemide, salicylates, nonsteroidal antiinflammatory drugs, and heparin, also inhibit binding of T_4 and T_3 to TBG. In addition, phenytoin and carbamazepine cause abnormalities of thyroid function tests by another mechanism. They stimulate hepatic cytochrome P450 degradation of T_4 and accelerate transport of T_4 into tissues.

IN VIVO RADIONUCLIDE STUDIES
Markedly improved direct tests of thyroid function have made radioiodine uptake studies less necessary. The iodine trapping or concentrating mechanism of the thyroid can be evaluated by measuring the uptake of radioactive isotope [123]I (half-life: 13 hr). The technology allows doses of radioiodine (0.1-0.5 mCi) that are only a fraction of those used with [131]I. Technetium (^{99m}Tc) is a particularly useful radioisotope for children because in contrast to iodine, it is trapped but not organified by the thyroid and has a half-life of only 6 hr. Thyroid scanning may be indicated to assess the presence of thyroid tissue in questions of thyroid dysgenesis and to detect ectopic thyroid tissue, and thyroid uptake may be indicated to evaluate possible "hot" thyroid nodules. Diagnostic studies should be performed with ^{99m}Tc pertechnetate or ^{123}I because they have the advantages of lower radiation exposure and high-quality scintigrams. Radioiodine treatment, which may be used to treat children with Graves hyperthyroidism or differentiated thyroid cancer, employs administration of ^{131}I, which has a longer half-life (8 days) and greater killing effect.

THYROID ULTRASONOGRAPHIC STUDIES
Thyroid ultrasound examinations can determine the location, size, and shape of the thyroid gland, and they are useful for assessing the solid or cystic nature of nodules. Ultrasound is not as reliable as radionuclide studies in evaluating infants with suspected thyroid dysgenesis, particularly ectopic glands. Ultrasound examinations are useful in identifying normal thyroid gland position in children with suspected thyroglossal duct cysts. In children with autoimmune thyroiditis, ultrasound reveals scattered hypoechogenicity. Ultrasound examinations are more accurate than physical examination in estimating goiter size and assessing thyroid nodules. Certain characteristics of thyroid nodules, such as blurred margins, microcalcifications, hypoechogenicity, taller-than-wide shape, capsular extension, and increased vascularity, increase the likelihood of thyroid cancer, although none of these features is 100% sensitive or specific.

Bibliography is available at Expert Consult.

Chapter 564
Defects of Thyroxine-Binding Globulin
Stephen H. LaFranchi and Stephen A. Huang

Abnormalities in levels of thyroxine-binding globulin (TBG) are not associated with clinical disease and do not require treatment. They are usually uncovered by a chance finding of abnormally low or high levels of thyroxine (T_4) and may be a source of confusion in the diagnosis of hypothyroidism or hyperthyroidism.

TBG deficiency occurs as an X-linked dominant disorder. Congenital TBG deficiency is most often discovered through screening programs for neonatal hypothyroidism that measure levels of T_4 as the primary screening test. Affected patients have low levels of total T_4 and elevated resin triiodothyronine uptake, but levels of free T_4 and thyroid-stimulating hormone are normal. The diagnosis is confirmed by the finding of absent or low levels of TBG. TBG deficiency occurs in 1 in 2,400 male newborns, 36% of whom have TBG levels <1 mg/dL. Milder forms of TBG deficiency occur in approximately 1 in 42,000 heterozygous female newborns. Complete TBG deficiency (<5 μg/dL) occurs much less often. To date, more than 25 different mutations have been reported in the TBG gene, resulting in either decreased TBG levels or reduced affinity of TBG for T_4. Table 564-1 lists causes of acquired TBG deficiency.

TBG excess also is a harmless X-linked dominant anomaly, occurring in approximately 1 in 25,000 persons. It has been recognized primarily in adults, but newborn screening programs may uncover the condition in the neonate. The level of T_4 is elevated, triiodothyronine is variably elevated, thyroid-stimulating hormone and free T_4 are normal, and resin triiodothyronine uptake is decreased. The elevated levels of TBG confirm the diagnosis. In affected neonates, levels of T_4 as high as 95 μg/dL have been found, which decrease to 20-30 μg/dL after 2-3 wk. Such high levels of T_4 may be related in part to the normally elevated levels of TBG in neonates, presumably as an effect of maternal estrogens. Affected patients are euthyroid. Family studies may be indicated to alert other affected family members. Table 564-1 lists causes of acquired TBG excess.

Familial dysalbuminemic hyperthyroxinemia is an autosomal dominant disorder that may be confused with hyperthyroidism. Markedly increased binding of T_4 to an abnormal albumin variant leads to increased serum concentrations of T_4. However, the levels of free T_4, free triiodothyronine, and thyroid-stimulating hormone are normal.

Table 564-1	Causes of Acquired Thyroxine-Binding Globulin (TBG) Deficiency and Excess
DECREASED TBG	**INCREASED TBG**
Androgens	Estrogens
Anabolic steroids	Selective estrogen receptor modulators
Glucocorticoids	Pregnancy
Hepatocellular disease	Hepatitis
Severe illness	Porphyria
Protein-losing nephropathies	Heroin, methadone
Protein-losing enteropathies	Mitotane
Nicotinic acid	5-Flurouracil
L-Asparaginase	Perphenazine

Levels of triiodothyronine are normal or only slightly elevated. Affected patients are euthyroid.

Bibliography is available at Expert Consult.

Chapter 565
Hypothyroidism
Stephen H. LaFranchi and Stephen A. Huang

Hypothyroidism results from deficient production of thyroid hormone, either from a defect in the gland itself (primary hypothyroidism) or a result of reduced thyroid-stimulating hormone (TSH) stimulation (central or hypopituitary hypothyroidism; Table 565-1). The disorder may be manifested from birth (congenital) or acquired. When symptoms appear after a period of apparently normal thyroid function, the disorder may be truly acquired or might only appear so as a result of one of a variety of congenital defects in which the manifestation of the deficiency is delayed.

CONGENITAL HYPOTHYROIDISM
Most cases of congenital hypothyroidism are not hereditary and result from thyroid dysgenesis. Some cases are familial; these are usually caused by one of the inborn errors of thyroid hormone synthesis (dyshormonogenesis) and may be associated with a goiter. Most infants with congenital hypothyroidism are detected by newborn screening programs in the 1st few wk after birth, before obvious clinical symptoms and signs develop. In infants born in areas with no screening program, severe cases manifest features in the 1st few wk of life, but in cases of milder deficiency, manifestations may be delayed for months.

Epidemiology
The prevalence of congenital hypothyroidism based on nationwide programs for neonatal screening was initially reported at 1 in 4,000 infants worldwide. Over the last 2 decades, the prevalence has dropped to 1 in 2,000, likely the result of detection of milder cases of hypothyroidism. Studies from the United States report that the prevalence is lower in black Americans and higher in Asian-Americans and Pacific Islanders, Hispanics, and Native Americans as compared to white babies.

Etiology
See Table 565-1.

Primary Hypothyroidism
Thyroid Dysgenesis. Some form of thyroid dysgenesis (aplasia, hypoplasia, or an ectopic gland) is the most common cause of permanent congenital hypothyroidism, accounting for 80-85% of cases. In approximately 33% of cases of dysgenesis, even sensitive radionuclide scans can find no remnants of thyroid tissue (aplasia). In the other 66% of infants, rudiments of thyroid tissue are found in an ectopic location, anywhere from the base of the tongue (lingual thyroid) to the normal position in the neck (hypoplasia). Thyroid dysgenesis has a 2:1 female:male ratio.

The cause of thyroid dysgenesis is unknown in most cases. Thyroid dysgenesis occurs sporadically, but familial cases occasionally have been reported. The finding that thyroid developmental anomalies, such as thyroglossal duct cysts and hemiagenesis, are present in 8-10% of 1st-degree relatives of infants with thyroid dysgenesis supports an underlying genetic component.

Mutations in several transcription factors important for thyroid morphogenesis and differentiation (including TTF-1/NKX2.1, TTF-2 [also termed FOXE1], and PAX8) are monogenic causes of approximately 2% of the cases of thyroid dysgenesis. In addition, genetic

Table 565-1	Etiologic Classification of Congenital Hypothyroidism

PRIMARY HYPOTHYROIDISM
Defect of fetal thyroid development (dysgenesis)
- Aplasia
- Hypoplasia
- Ectopia
Defect in thyroid hormone synthesis (dyshormonogenesis)
- Iodide transport defect from blood into follicular cell: mutation in sodium–iodide symporter gene
- Defective iodide transport from follicular cell into colloid: mutation in Pendrin transport protein
- Thyroid organification, or coupling defect: mutation in thyroid peroxidase gene
- Defects in H_2O_2 generation: mutations in DUOXA2 maturation factor or *DUOX2* gene
- Thyroglobulin synthesis defect: mutation in thyroglobulin gene
- Deiodination defect: mutation in *DEHAL1* gene
TSH unresponsiveness
- Mutation in TSH receptor
- Defective TSH signaling: $G_s\alpha$ mutation (e.g., type IA pseudohypoparathyroidism)
Defect in thyroid hormone transport: mutation in monocarboxylate transporter 8 *(MCT8)* gene
Resistance to thyroid hormone
Maternal antibodies: thyrotropin receptor–blocking antibody (TRBAb, measured as *thyrotropin-binding inhibitor immunoglobulin*)
Iodine deficiency (endemic goiter)
Maternal medications
- Iodides, amiodarone
- Propylthiouracil, methimazole
- Radioiodine

CENTRAL (HYPOPITUITARY) HYPOTHYROIDISM
Isolated TSH deficiency: mutation in TSH β-subunit gene (depending on mutation, TSH may be undetectable, measurable ["normal"], or elevated)
Isolated TRH deficiency: mutation in TRH gene
TRH unresponsiveness: mutation in TRH receptor gene
Multiple congenital pituitary hormone deficiencies (e.g., septooptic dysplasia)
PIT-1 mutations
- Deficiency of TSH
- Deficiency of growth hormone
- Deficiency of prolactin
PROP-1 mutations
- Deficiency of TSH
- Deficiency of growth hormone
- Deficiency of prolactin
- Deficiency of LH
- Deficiency of FSH
- ±Deficiency of ACTH

ACTH, adrenocorticotropic hormone; FSH, follicle-stimulating hormone; LH, luteinizing hormone; TRH, thyroid-releasing hormone; TSH, thyroid-stimulating hormone.

defects leading to absent or ineffective thyrotropin (TSH) receptor binding or signaling have been described.

The transcription factor TTF-1/NKX2.1 is expressed in the thyroid, lung, and central nervous system. Mutations in TTF-1/NKX2.1 are reported to result in congenital hypothyroidism, respiratory distress, and persistent neurologic problems, including chorea and ataxia, despite early thyroid hormone treatment. NKX2.5 is expressed in the thyroid and heart. Mutations in *NKX2.5* are associated with congenital hypothyroidism and cardiac malformations. PAX-8 is expressed in the thyroid and kidney. Mutations in *PAX-8* are associated with congenital hypothyroidism and kidney and ureteral malformations.

The common finding of thyroid dysgenesis confined to only 1 of a pair of monozygotic twins suggests the operation of a deleterious factor during intrauterine life. Maternal antithyroid antibodies might be that factor. Although thyroid peroxidase antibodies have been detected in

some mother–infant pairs, there is little evidence of their pathogenicity. The demonstration of thyroid growth-blocking and cytotoxic antibodies in some infants with thyroid dysgenesis, as well as in their mothers, suggests a more likely pathogenetic mechanism.

Defective Synthesis of Thyroxine (Dyshormonogenesis). A variety of defects in the biosynthesis of thyroid hormone can result in congenital hypothyroidism; these account for 15% of cases detected by neonatal screening programs (1 in 30,000-50,000 live births). These defects are transmitted in an autosomal recessive manner. A **goiter** is almost always present. When the defect is incomplete, compensation occurs, and onset of hypothyroidism may be delayed for years.

Defect of Iodide Transport. Defect of iodide transport is rare and involves mutations in the sodium–iodide symporter. Among the several cases now reported, it has been found in 9 related infants of the Hutterite sect, and approximately 50% of the cases are from Japan. Consanguinity is a factor in approximately 30% of the families.

In the past, clinical hypothyroidism, with or without a goiter, often developed in the 1st few months of life; the condition has been detected in neonatal screening programs. In Japan, however, untreated patients acquire goiter and hypothyroidism after 10 yr of age, perhaps because of the very high iodine content (often 19 mg/24 hr) of the Japanese diet.

The energy-dependent mechanisms for concentrating iodide are defective in the thyroid and salivary glands. In contrast to other defects of thyroid hormone synthesis, uptake of radioiodine and pertechnetate is low; a reduced saliva∶serum ratio of ^{123}I will support the diagnosis, confirmed by finding a mutation in the sodium–iodide symporter gene. This condition responds to treatment with large doses of potassium iodide, but treatment with L-thyroxine is preferable.

Thyroid Peroxidase Defects of Organification and Coupling. Thyroid peroxidase defects of organification and coupling are the most common of the thyroxine (T_4) synthetic defects. After iodide is trapped by the thyroid, it is rapidly oxidized to reactive iodine, which is then incorporated into tyrosine units on thyroglobulin. This process requires generation of H_2O_2, thyroid peroxidase, and hematin (an enzyme cofactor); defects can involve each of these components, and there is considerable clinical and biochemical heterogeneity. In the Dutch neonatal screening program, 23 infants were found with a complete organification defect (1 in 60,000 live births), but its prevalence in other areas is unknown. A characteristic finding in all patients with this defect is a marked "discharge" of thyroid radioactivity when perchlorate or thiocyanate is administered 2 hr after administration of a test dose of radioiodine. In these patients, perchlorate discharges 40-90% of radioiodine compared with <10% in normal persons. Several mutations in the thyroid peroxidase gene have been reported in children with congenital hypothyroidism.

Dual oxidase maturation factor 2 (**DUOXA2**) is required to express **DUOX2** enzymatic activity, which is required for H_2O_2 generation, a crucial step in iodide oxidation. Biallelic *DUOXA2* mutations produce permanent congenital hypothyroidism, whereas monoallelic mutations are associated with transient hypothyroidism. *DUOX2* mutations can also cause permanent or transient congenital hypothyroidism. *DUOX2* mutations are relatively common, present in 30% of cases of apparent dyshormonogenesis, whereas *DUOXA2* mutations are relatively rare, present in 2% of such cases.

Pendred syndrome is an autosomal recessive disorder caused by a mutation in the chloride–iodide transport protein common to the thyroid gland and the cochlea. Pendred syndrome is comprised of sensorineural deafness and goiter; it is the most common cause of syndromic deafness. Pendrin allows transport of iodide from the follicular cell into the colloid where it undergoes organification to iodine and incorporation into the tyrosine residues on thyroglobulin. Patients with a mutation in the pendrin gene have impaired iodide organification and a positive perchlorate discharge.

Defects of Thyroglobulin Synthesis. Defects of thyroglobulin synthesis are a heterogeneous group of disorders characterized by goiter, elevated serum TSH, low T_4 levels, and absent or low levels of thyroglobulin. It has been reported in approximately 100 patients. Molecular defects, primarily point mutations, have been described in several patients.

Defects in Deiodination. Monoiodotyrosine and diiodotyrosine released from thyroglobulin are normally deiodinated within the thyroid or in peripheral tissues by a deiodinase. The liberated iodine is recycled in the synthesis of thyroid hormones. The *DEHAL1* gene encodes iodotyrosine deiodinase in the thyroid. *DEHAL1* mutations are relatively rare; patients with deiodinase deficiency experience severe iodine loss from the constant urinary excretion of nondeiodinated tyrosines, leading to hormonal deficiency and goiter. The deiodination defect may be limited to thyroid tissue only or to peripheral tissue only, or it may be universal.

Thyrotropin Hormone Unresponsiveness. A mutation in the TSH receptor gene is a relatively uncommon autosomal recessive cause of congenital hypothyroidism. Both homozygous and compound heterozygous mutations in the TSH receptor gene have been reported. Infants with a severe defect have elevated TSH levels and will be detected by newborn screening, whereas other patients with a mild defect remain euthyroid without treatment. A study of infants with congenital hypothyroidism detected by newborn screening from Tokyo reported TSH receptor mutations in 4.3% of patients (1 in 118,000 live births), with a founder mutation (p.R450H) accounting for 70% of gene defects.

Mild congenital hypothyroidism has been detected in newborn infants who subsequently proved to have **type Ia pseudohypoparathyroidism.** The molecular cause of resistance to TSH in these patients is the generalized impairment of cyclic adenosine monophosphate activation caused by genetic defect of the α subunit of the guanine nucleotide regulatory protein G$_s$ (see Chapter 572).

Defects in Thyroid Hormone Transport. Passage of thyroid hormone into the cell is facilitated by plasma membrane transporters. A mutation in one such transporter gene, monocarboxylate transporter 8 (*MCT8*), located on the X chromosome (**Allan-Herndon-Dudley syndrome**), has now been reported in multiple patients. The defective transporter impairs passage of T$_4$ and triiodothyronine (T$_3$) into cells; this syndrome is characterized by elevated serum T$_3$ levels, low T$_4$ levels, and normal or mildly elevated TSH levels. Neurologic manifestations include severe developmental delay, reduced muscle mass, initial hypotonia that evolves into spastic paraplegia, dysarthria, and athetoid movements.

Resistance to Thyroid Hormone

This autosomal dominant disorder is caused by mutations in the thyroid hormone receptor. Most patients have a goiter, and levels of T$_4$, T$_3$, free T$_4$, and free T$_3$ are elevated. These findings often have led to the erroneous diagnosis of Graves disease, although most affected patients are clinically euthyroid. The unresponsiveness can vary among tissues. There may be subtle clinical features of hypothyroidism, including developmental delay, growth retardation, and delayed skeletal maturation. On the other hand, there may be clinical features compatible with hyperthyroidism, such as tachycardia and hyperreflexia. It is presumed that these patients have varying tissue resistance to thyroid hormone. One neurologic manifestation is an increased association of attention-deficit/hyperactivity disorder; the converse is not true because patients with attention-deficit/hyperactivity disorder do not have an increased risk of thyroid hormone resistance.

TSH levels are diagnostic in that they are not suppressed as in Graves disease but instead are moderately elevated or normal but inappropriate for the levels of T$_4$ and T$_3$. The failure of TSH suppression indicates that the resistance is generalized and affects the pituitary gland as well as peripheral tissues. More than 40 distinct point mutations in the hormone-binding domain of the β-thyroid receptor are identified. Different phenotypes do not correlate with genotypes. The same mutation has been observed in patients with generalized or isolated pituitary resistance, even in different members of the same family. A child homozygous for the receptor mutation showed unusually severe resistance. These cases support the dominant negative effect of mutant receptors, in which the mutant receptor protein inhibits normal receptor action in heterozygotes. Elevated levels of T$_4$ on neonatal thyroid screening should suggest the possibility of this diagnosis. No treatment is usually required unless growth and skeletal retardation are present.

Two infants of consanguineous matings are known to have an autosomal recessive form of thyroid resistance. These infants had manifestations of hypothyroidism early in life, and genetic studies revealed a major deletion of the β-thyroid receptor in 1 of them. The resistance appears to be more severe in this form of the entity.

Some patients have greater resistance to thyroid hormone in the pituitary gland as compared to peripheral tissues. Because the peripheral tissues are not resistant to thyroid hormones, the patient has a goiter and manifestations of hyperthyroidism. The laboratory findings are the same as those seen with generalized thyroid hormone resistance. This condition must be differentiated from a pituitary TSH-secreting tumor. Different treatments, including D-thyroxine, triiodothyroacetic acid, and tetraiodothyroacetic acid, have been successful in some patients. Bromocriptine administration, which interferes with TSH secretion, was reported to be successful in another patient. Whether isolated pituitary resistance to thyroid hormone exists as a distinct entity is controversial; it may be a variant of generalized resistance to thyroid hormone with varying tissue responsiveness.

Although the majority of patients with resistance have mutations in the thyroid hormone receptor β gene, a child with a mutation in the thyroid hormone receptor α gene has been reported. This patient presented at age 6 yr with growth retardation, delayed development, and constipation. Genetic analysis showed a heterozygous nonsense mutation in the thyroid hormone receptor α gene that, like β gene mutations, inhibited wild-type receptor action in a dominant negative manner.

Thyrotropin Receptor-Blocking Antibody. Maternal TSH receptor-blocking antibody (TRBAb) is an unusual cause of transitory congenital hypothyroidism. Transplacental passage of maternal TRBAb inhibits binding of TSH to its receptor in the neonate. Maternal TRBAb accounts for 2% of cases detected by neonatal screening programs (1 in 50,000-100,000 infants). It should be suspected whenever there is a history of maternal autoimmune thyroid disease, including Hashimoto thyroiditis or Graves disease, maternal hypothyroidism on replacement therapy, or recurrent congenital hypothyroidism of a transient nature in previous siblings. In these situations, maternal levels of TRBAb (measured as thyrotropin-binding inhibitor immunoglobulin) should be determined during pregnancy. Affected infants and their mothers also can have thyrotropin receptor–stimulating antibodies and thyroid peroxidase antibodies. Technetium pertechnetate and ^{123}I scans might fail to detect any thyroid tissue, mimicking thyroid agenesis, but ultrasonography will show a thyroid gland. After the condition remits, a normal thyroid gland is demonstrable by scanning following discontinuation of replacement therapy. The half-life of the antibody is 21 days, and remission of the hypothyroidism occurs in approximately 3-6 mo. Correct diagnosis of this cause of congenital hypothyroidism prevents unnecessary protracted treatment, alerts the clinician to possible recurrences in future pregnancies, and allows a favorable prognosis.

Radioiodine Administration. Hypothyroidism can occur as a result of inadvertent administration of radioiodine during pregnancy for treatment of Graves disease or cancer of the thyroid. The fetal thyroid is capable of trapping iodide by 70-75 days of gestation. Whenever radioiodine is administered to a woman of childbearing age, a pregnancy test must be performed before a therapeutic dose of ^{131}I is given, regardless of the menstrual history or putative history of contraception. Administration of radioactive iodine to lactating women also is contraindicated because it is readily excreted in milk.

Iodine Exposure. Congenital hypothyroidism can result from fetal exposure to excessive iodides. Perinatal exposure can occur with the use of iodine antiseptic to prepare the skin for caesarian section or painting of the cervix before delivery. It has also been reported in infants born to mothers who consumed large amounts of iodine daily (up to 12 mg) in the form of nutritional supplements and in mothers in Japan who consumed large quantities of iodine-rich seaweed. These conditions are transitory and must not be mistaken for the other forms of hypothyroidism. In the neonate, topical iodine-containing antiseptics used in nurseries and by surgeons can also cause transient congenital hypothyroidism, especially in low-birthweight infants, and can lead to abnormal results on neonatal screening tests. In older children, the usual sources of iodides are proprietary preparations used to treat asthma. In a few instances, the cause of hypothyroidism was amiodarone, an antiarrhythmic drug with high iodine content. In most of these instances, goiter is present (see Chapter 567).

Iodine-Deficiency Endemic Goiter. See Chapter 567.3.

Iodine deficiency or endemic goiter is the most common cause of congenital hypothyroidism worldwide. The recommended intake of iodine in adults is 150 μg daily, increasing to 250 μg daily during pregnancy to allow for fetal iodine requirements. Despite efforts at universal iodization of salt in many countries, economic, political, and practical obstacles make achieving this objective difficult. While the U.S. population is iodine-sufficient as a whole, approximately 15% of women of reproductive age fall into the iodine-deficient category. Borderline iodine deficiency is more likely to cause problems in preterm infants who depend on a maternal source of iodine for normal thyroid hormone production.

Central (Hypopituitary) Hypothyroidism
Thyrotropin and Thyrotropin-Releasing Hormone Deficiency.
Deficiency of TSH and central hypothyroidism can occur in any of the conditions associated with developmental defects of the pituitary or hypothalamus (see Chapter 557). More often in these conditions, the deficiency of TSH is secondary to a deficiency of thyrotropin-releasing hormone (TRH). TSH-deficient hypothyroidism is found in 1 in 30,000-50,000 infants; most screening programs are designed to detect primary hypothyroidism, so most of these cases are not detected by neonatal thyroid screening. The majority of affected infants have multiple pituitary deficiencies and present with hypoglycemia, persistent jaundice, and micropenis in association with septooptic dysplasia, midline cleft lip, midface hypoplasia, and other midline facial anomalies.

Mutations in genes coding for transcription factors essential to pituitary development, cell type differentiation, and hormone synthesis are associated with congenital TSH deficiency. *PIT-1* mutations include TSH deficiency associated with growth hormone and prolactin deficiency. Patients with *PROP-1* mutations ("prophet of pit-1") have not only TSH, growth hormone, and prolactin deficiency but also luteinizing hormone and follicle-stimulating hormone deficiency and variable adrenocorticotropic hormone deficiency. *HESX1* mutations are associated with TSH, growth hormone, prolactin, and adrenocorticotropic hormone deficiencies and are found in some patients with optic nerve hypoplasia (septooptic dysplasia syndrome; see Chapter 591).

Isolated deficiency of TSH is a rare autosomal recessive disorder that has been reported in several sibships. DNA studies in affected family members reveal defects in the TSH β-subunit gene, including point mutations, frame shifts causing a stop codon, and splice-site mutations. Depending on the specific mutation, serum TSH levels may be undetectable, measureable, or elevated. The diagnosis is usually delayed because the serum TSH level is not elevated in most cases, and so such patients are not detected by newborn screening programs.

Thyrotropin-Releasing Hormone Receptor Abnormality.
Mutations in the TRH receptor gene, a rare cause of congenital central hypothyroidism, have now been reported in a few families. This condition, which results in isolated TSH deficiency and hypothyroidism, was suspected because of failure of both TSH and prolactin to respond to TRH stimulation.

Thyroid Function in Preterm Babies
Postnatal thyroid function in preterm babies is qualitatively similar but quantitatively reduced compared with that of term infants. The cord serum T_4 is decreased in proportion to gestational age and birthweight. The postnatal TSH surge is reduced, and the more premature, very-low-birthweight infants with complications of prematurity, such as respiratory distress syndrome, actually experience a decrease in serum T_4 in the 1st wk of life. As these complications resolve, the serum T_4 gradually increases so that generally by 6 wk of life it enters the T_4 range seen in term infants. Serum free T_4 concentrations seem less affected, and when measured by equilibrium dialysis, these levels are

often normal. Preterm babies also have a higher incidence of "delayed" TSH elevation and apparent transient primary hypothyroidism. Premature infants of <28 wk of gestation might have problems resulting from a combination of immaturity of the hypothalamic-pituitary-thyroid axis and loss of the maternal contribution of thyroid hormone and so may be candidates for temporary thyroid hormone replacement; further studies are needed.

Clinical Manifestations
Most infants with congenital hypothyroidism are asymptomatic at birth, even if there is complete agenesis of the thyroid gland. This situation is attributed to partial transplacental passage of maternal T_4, which provides fetal levels that are approximately 33% of normal at birth. Despite this maternal contribution of T_4, hypothyroid infants still have a low serum T_4 and elevated TSH level and so will be identified by newborn screening programs.

The clinician depends on neonatal screening tests for the diagnosis of congenital hypothyroidism. Some babies escape newborn screening, and laboratory errors occur, so awareness of early symptoms and signs must be maintained. Congenital hypothyroidism caused by thyroid dysgenesis, the most common etiology, is twice as common in girls as in boys. Before neonatal screening programs, congenital hypothyroidism was rarely recognized in the newborn because the signs and symptoms are usually not sufficiently developed. It can be suspected and the diagnosis established during the early weeks of life if the initial, but less characteristic, manifestations are recognized. Birthweight and length are normal, but head size may be slightly increased because of myxedema of the brain. The anterior and posterior fontanels are open widely; observation of this sign at birth can serve as an initial clue to the early recognition of congenital hypothyroidism. *Only 3% of normal newborn infants have a posterior fontanel larger than 0.5 cm.* Prolongation of physiologic jaundice, caused by delayed maturation of glucuronide conjugation, may be the earliest sign. Feeding difficulties, especially sluggishness, lack of interest, somnolence, and choking spells during nursing, are often present during the 1st mo of life. Respiratory difficulties, partly caused by the large tongue, include apneic episodes, noisy respirations, and nasal obstruction. Some infants may develop respiratory distress syndrome. Affected infants cry little, sleep much, have poor appetites, and are generally sluggish. There may be constipation that does not usually respond to treatment. The abdomen is large, and an umbilical hernia is usually present. The temperature is subnormal, often <35°C (95°F), and the skin, particularly that of the extremities, may be cold and mottled. Edema of the genitals and extremities may be present. The pulse is slow, and heart murmurs, cardiomegaly, and asymptomatic pericardial effusion are common. Macrocytic anemia is often present and is refractory to treatment with hematinics. Because symptoms appear gradually, the clinical diagnosis is often delayed.

Approximately 10% of infants with congenital hypothyroidism have associated congenital anomalies. Cardiac anomalies are most common, but anomalies of the nervous system and eye have also been reported. Infants with congenital hypothyroidism may have associated hearing loss. As noted under "Etiology" above, specific mutations in genes involved in thyroid gland development result in "syndromic" congenital hypothyroidism. Mutations in *NKX2.1 (TTF-1)*, present in the thyroid gland, lungs, and brain, are characterized by congenital hypothyroidism, respiratory distress syndrome, and ataxia, or even choreoathetosis. Mutations in *NKX2.5* result in congenital hypothyroidism and associated congenital heart defects. Mutations in *TTF-2*, present in the thyroid gland, palate, and hair, include congenital hypothyroidism, cleft palate, and spiky hair. Mutations in *PAX-8*, present in the thyroid gland and kidneys, present with congenital hypothyroidism and genitourinary anomalies, including renal agenesis.

If congenital hypothyroidism goes undetected and untreated, these manifestations progress. Retardation of physical and mental development becomes greater during the following months, and by 3-6 mo of age the clinical picture is fully developed (Fig. 565-1). When there is only partial deficiency of thyroid hormone, the symptoms may be milder, the syndrome incomplete, and the onset delayed. Although breast milk contains significant amounts of thyroid hormones,

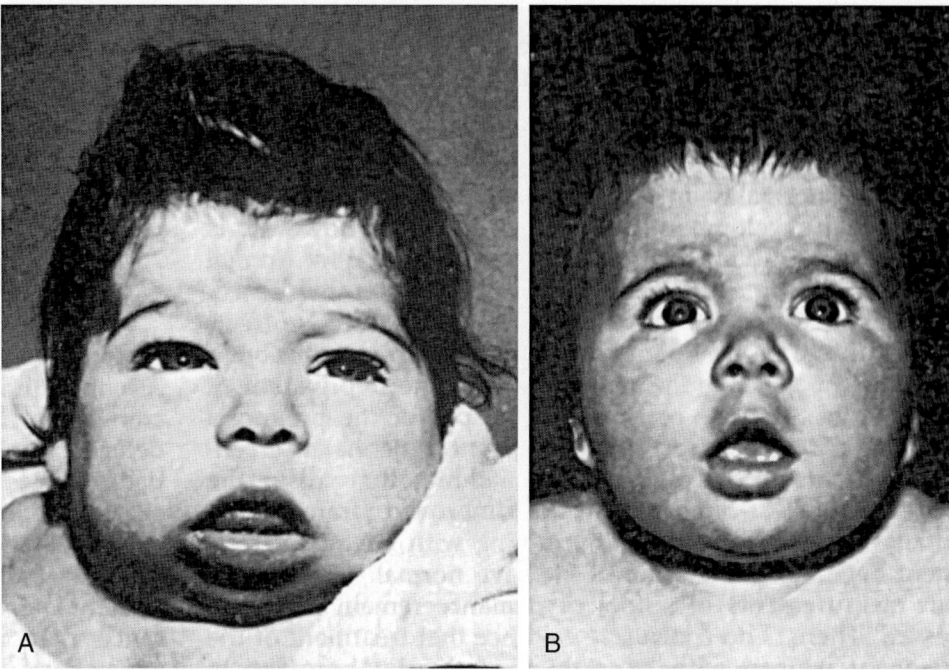

Figure 565-1 Congenital hypothyroidism in an infant 6 mo of age. The infant ate poorly in the neonatal period and was constipated. She had a persistent nasal discharge and a large tongue; she was very lethargic and had no social smile and no head control. **A,** Notice the puffy face, dull expression, and hirsute forehead. Tests revealed a negligible uptake of radioiodine. Osseous development was that of a newborn. **B,** Four mo after treatment, note the decreased puffiness of the face, the decreased hirsutism of the forehead, and the alert appearance.

particularly T_3, it is inadequate to protect the breastfed infant who has congenital hypothyroidism, and it has no effect on neonatal thyroid screening tests.

The child's growth will be stunted, the extremities are short, and the head size is normal or even increased. The anterior fontanel is large and the posterior fontanel may remain open. The eyes appear far apart, and the bridge of the broad nose is depressed. The palpebral fissures are narrow and the eyelids are swollen. The mouth is kept open, and the thick, broad tongue protrudes. Dentition will be delayed. The neck is short and thick, and there may be deposits of fat above the clavicles and between the neck and shoulders. The hands are broad and the fingers are short. The skin is dry and scaly, and there is little perspiration. Myxedema is manifested, particularly in the skin of the eyelids, the back of the hands, and the external genitals. The skin shows general pallor with a sallow complexion. Carotenemia can cause a yellow discoloration of the skin, but the sclerae remain white. The scalp is thickened, and the hair is coarse, brittle, and scanty. The hairline reaches far down on the forehead, which usually appears wrinkled, especially when the infant cries.

Development is usually delayed. Hypothyroid infants appear lethargic and are late in learning to sit and stand. The voice is hoarse, and they do not learn to talk. The degree of physical and intellectual delay increases with age. Sexual maturation may also be delayed or might not take place at all.

The muscles are usually hypotonic, but in rare instances generalized muscular pseudohypertrophy occurs (**Kocher-Debré-Sémélaigne syndrome**). Affected older children can have an athletic appearance because of pseudohypertrophy, particularly in the calf muscles. Its pathogenesis is unknown; nonspecific histochemical and ultrastructural changes seen on muscle biopsy return to normal with treatment. Boys are more prone to development of the syndrome, which has been observed in siblings born from a consanguineous mating. Affected patients have hypothyroidism of longer duration and severity.

Some infants with mild congenital hypothyroidism have normal thyroid function at birth and so are not identified by newborn screening programs. In particular, some children with ectopic thyroid tissue (lingual, sublingual, subhyoid) produce adequate amounts of thyroid hormone for many years, or it eventually fails in early childhood. Affected children come to clinical attention because of a growing mass

at the base of the tongue or in the midline of the neck, usually at the level of the hyoid. Occasionally, ectopia is associated with **thyroglossal duct cysts**. It can occur in siblings. Surgical removal of ectopic thyroid tissue from a euthyroid patient usually results in hypothyroidism, because most such patients have no other thyroid tissue.

Laboratory Findings

In developed countries, infants with congenital hypothyroidism are identified by newborn screening programs. Blood obtained by heelprick between 2 and 5 days of life is placed on a filter paper card and sent to a central screening laboratory. The early approach to newborn screening in North America and Europe began with measure of levels of T_4, followed by measurement of TSH when T_4 is low. This approach identifies infants with primary hypothyroidism, some with central or hypopituitary hypothyroidism, and infants with a delayed elevation in TSH levels. Over time, many neonatal screening programs in North America, Europe, and elsewhere in the world have switched to an initial TSH measurement. This approach will detect infants with primary hypothyroidism and infants with milder, subclinical hypothyroidism (normal T_4, elevated TSH), but it may not detect infants with delayed TSH elevation or with central or hypopituitary hypothyroidism. With any of these tests, special care should be given to the normal range of values for age of the patient, particularly in the 1st weeks of life (Table 565-2). Regardless of the approach used for screening, some infants escape detection because of technical or human errors; clinicians must maintain their vigilance for clinical manifestations of hypothyroidism.

Serum levels of T_4 or free T_4 are low; serum levels of T_3 may be normal and are not helpful in the diagnosis. If the defect is primarily in the thyroid, levels of TSH are elevated, often to >100 mU/L. Serum levels of thyroglobulin are usually low in infants with thyroid agenesis or defects of thyroglobulin synthesis or secretion, whereas they are elevated with ectopic glands and other inborn errors of T_4 synthesis, but there is a wide overlap of ranges.

Special attention should be paid to identical twins; in several reported cases, neonatal screening failed to detect the affected twin with hypothyroidism, and the diagnosis was not made until the infants were 4-5 mo of age. In these cases, transfusion of euthyroid blood from the unaffected twin normalized the serum levels of T_4 and TSH in the

Table 565-2	Thyroid Function Tests		
AGE	**U.S. REFERENCE VALUE**	**CONVERSION FACTOR**	**SI REFERENCE VALUE**
THYROID THYROGLOBULIN, SERUM			
Cord blood	14.7-101.1 ng/mL	×1	14.7-101.1 µg/L
Birth to 35 mo	10.6-92.0 ng/mL	×1	10.6-92.0 µg/L
3-11 yr	5.6-41.9 ng/mL	×1	5.6-41.9 µg/L
12-17 yr	2.7-21.9 ng/mL	×1	2.7-21.9 µg/L
THYROID-STIMULATING HORMONE, SERUM			
Premature Infants (28-36 wk)			
1st wk of life	0.7-27.0 mIU/L	×1	0.7-27.0 mIU/L
Term Infants			
Birth to 4 days	1.0-17.6 mIU/L	×1	1.0-17.6 mIU/L
2-20 wk	0.6-5.6 mIU/L	×1	0.6-5.6 mIU/L
5 mo-20 yr	0.5-5.5 mIU/L	×1	0.5-5.5 mIU/L
THYROXINE-BINDING GLOBULIN, SERUM			
Cord blood	1.4-9.4 mg/dL	×10	14-94 mg/L
1-4 wk	1.0-9.0 mg/dL	×10	10-90 mg/L
1-12 mo	2.0-7.6 mg/dL	×10	20-76 mg/L
1-5 yr	2.9-5.4 mg/dL	×10	29-54 mg/L
5-10 yr	2.5-5.0 mg/dL	×10	25-50 mg/L
10-15 yr	2.1-4.6 mg/dL	×10	21-46 mg/L
Adult	1.5-3.4 mg/dL	×10	15-34 mg/L
THYROXINE, TOTAL, SERUM			
Full-Term Infants			
1-3 days	8.2-19.9 µg/dL	×12.9	106-256 nmol/L
1 wk	6.0-15.9 µg/dL	×12.9	77-205 nmol/L
1-12 mo	6.1-14.9 µg/dL	×12.9	79-192 nmol/L
Prepubertal Children			
1-3 yr	6.8-13.5 µg/dL	×12.9	88-174 nmol/L
3-10 yr	5.5-12.8 µg/dL	×12.9	71-165 nmol/L
Pubertal Children and Adults			
>10 yr	4.2-13.0 µg/dL	×12.9	54-167 nmol/L
THYROXINE, FREE, SERUM			
Full-term (3 days)	2.0-4.9 ng/dL	×12.9	26-63.1 pmol/L
Infants	0.9-2.6 ng/dL	×12.9	12-33 pmol/L
Prepubertal children	0.8-2.2 ng/dL	×12.9	10-28 pmol/L
Pubertal children and adults	0.8-2.3 ng/dL	×12.9	10-30 pmol/L
THYROXINE, TOTAL, WHOLE BLOOD			
Newborn screen (filter paper)	6.2-22 µg/dL	×12.9	80-283 nmol/L
TRIIODOTHYRONINE, FREE, SERUM			
Cord blood	20-240 pg/dL	×0.01536	0.3-0.7 pmol/L
1-3 days	180-760 pg/dL	×0.01536	2.8-11.7 pmol/L
1-5 yr	185-770 pg/dL	×0.01536	2.8-11.8 pmol/L
5-10 yr	215-700 pg/dL	×0.01536	3.3-10.7 pmol/L
10-15 yr	230-650 pg/dL	×0.01536	3.5-10.0 pmol/L
>15 yr	210-440 pg/dL	×0.01536	3.2-6.8 pmol/L
TRIIODOTHYRONINE RESIN UPTAKE TEST (RT$_3$U), SERUM			
Newborn	26-36%	×0.01	0.26-0.36 fractional uptake
Thereafter	26-35%	×0.01	0.26-0.35 fractional uptake
TRIIODOTHYRONINE, TOTAL, SERUM			
Cord blood	30-70 ng/dL	×0.0154	0.46-1.08 nmol/L
1-3 days	75-260 ng/dL	×0.0154	1.16-4.00 nmol/L
1-5 yr	100-260 ng/dL	×0.0154	1.54-4.00 nmol/L
5-10 yr	90-240 ng/dL	×0.0154	1.39-3.70 nmol/L
10-15 yr	80-210 ng/dL	×0.0154	1.23-3.23 nmol/L
>15 yr	115-190 ng/dL	×0.0154	1.77-2.93 nmol/L

Adapted from Nicholson JF, Pesce MA: Reference ranges for laboratory tests and procedures. In Behrman RE, Kliegman RM, Jenson HB, editors: Nelson textbook of pediatrics, ed 17, Philadelphia, 2004, WB Saunders, pp. 2412–2413; TSH from Lem AJ, de Rijke YB, van toor H, et al: Serum thyroid hormone levels in healthy children from birth to adulthood and in short children born small for gestational age. J Clin Endocrinol Metab 97:3170–3178, 2012; free T_3 from Elmlinger MW, Kuhnel W, Lambrecht H-G, Ranke MB: Reference intervals from birth to adulthood for serum thyroxine (T_4), triiodothyronine (T_3), free T_3, free T_4, thyroxine binding globulin (TBG), and thyrotropin (TSH). Clin Chem Lab Med 39:973–979, 2001.

affected twin at the initial screening. Many newborn screening programs perform a routine second test in same-sex twins.

Retardation of osseous development can be shown radiographically at birth in approximately 60% of congenitally hypothyroid infants and indicates some deprivation of thyroid hormone during intrauter-ine life. The distal femoral and proximal tibial epiphyses, normally present at birth, are often absent (Fig. 565-2A). In undetected and untreated patients, the discrepancy between chronologic age and osseous development increases. The epiphyses often have multiple foci of ossification (epiphyseal dysgenesis; Fig. 565-2B); deformity

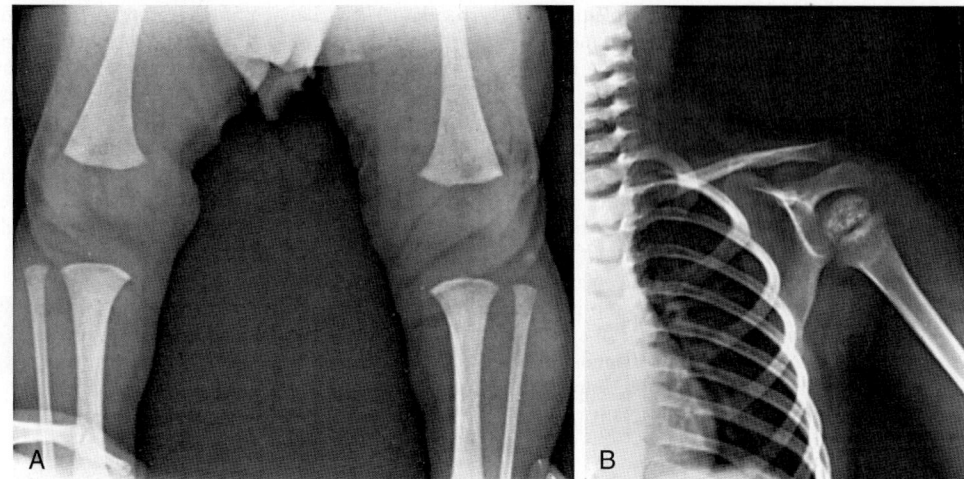

Figure 565-2 Congenital hypothyroidism. **A,** Absence of distal femoral epiphysis in a 3 mo old infant who was born at term. This is evidence for the onset of the hypothyroid state during fetal life. **B,** Epiphyseal dysgenesis in the head of the humerus in a 9 yr old girl who had been inadequately treated with thyroid hormone.

("beaking") of the 12th thoracic or 1st or 2nd lumbar vertebra is common. X-rays of the skull show large fontanels and wide sutures; intersutural (wormian) bones are common. The sella turcica is often enlarged and round; in rare instances, there may be erosion and thinning. Formation and eruption of teeth can be delayed. Cardiac enlargement or pericardial effusion may be present.

Scintigraphy can help to pinpoint the underlying cause in infants with congenital hypothyroidism, but treatment should not be unduly delayed for this study. ^{123}I-sodium iodide is superior to ^{99m}Tc-sodium pertechnetate for this purpose. Ultrasonographic examination of the thyroid is helpful, but studies show it can miss some ectopic glands shown by scintigraphy. Demonstration of ectopic thyroid tissue is diagnostic of thyroid dysgenesis and establishes the need for lifelong treatment with T_4. Failure to demonstrate any thyroid tissue suggests thyroid aplasia, but this also occurs in neonates with hypothyroidism caused by maternal TRBAb and in infants with the iodide-trapping defect. A normally situated thyroid gland with a normal or avid uptake of radionuclide indicates a defect in thyroid hormone biosynthesis. In the past, patients with goitrous hypothyroidism have required extensive evaluation, including radioiodine studies, perchlorate discharge tests, kinetic studies, chromatography, and studies of thyroid tissue, to determine the biochemical nature of the defect. Most can be evaluated by genetic studies looking for a suspected mutation in the steps along the T_4 biosynthetic pathway.

The electrocardiogram may show low-voltage P and T waves with diminished amplitude of QRS complexes and suggest poor left ventricular function and pericardial effusion. Echocardiography can confirm a pericardial effusion. The electroencephalogram often shows low voltage. In children older than 2 yr of age, the serum cholesterol level is usually elevated. Brain MRI before treatment is reportedly normal, although proton magnetic resonance spectroscopy shows high levels of choline-containing compounds, which can reflect blocks in myelin maturation.

Treatment

Levothyroxine (L-T_4) given orally is the treatment of choice. Although T_3 is the biologically active form of thyroid hormone, most of the T_3 in the brain is formed from local deiodination of T_4. Because 80% of circulating T_3 is formed by monodeiodination of T_4, serum levels of T_4 and T_3 return to normal with L-T_4 treatment alone. The recommended initial starting dose is 10-15 µg/kg/day (totaling 37.5-50.0 µg/day for most term infants). The starting dose can be tailored to the severity of hypothyroidism. Rapid normalization of thyroid function has been demonstrated to be important in achieving optimal neurodevelopmental outcome. Newborns with more severe hypothyroidism, as judged by a serum T_4 <5 µg/dL and/or imaging studies

confirming aplasia, should be started at the higher end of the dosage range.

L-T_4 is available only in tablet form in the United States; there is an approved liquid L-T_4 preparation in Europe. The daily tablets should be crushed and mixed with a small volume of liquid. *L-T_4 tablets should not be mixed with soy protein formulas, concentrated iron, or calcium, because these can bind T_4 and inhibit its absorption.* Although it is recommended to administer L-T_4 on an empty stomach and avoid food for 30-60 min, this is not practical in an infant. As long as the method of administration is consistent day to day, dosing can be adjusted based on serum thyroid test results to achieve the desired treatment goals.

Levels of serum T_4 or free T_4 and TSH should be monitored at recommended intervals (every 1-2 mo in the 1st 6 mo of life, and then every 2-4 mo between 6 mo and 3 yr of age). The goals of treatment are to maintain the serum free T_4 or total T_4 in the upper half of the reference range for age (see Table 565-2), with serum TSH in the reference range for age, optimally 0.5-2.0 mU/L. The dose of L-T_4 on a weight basis gradually decreases with age.

Later, confirmation of the diagnosis may be necessary for some infants to rule out the possibility of transient hypothyroidism. This is unnecessary in infants with proven thyroid ectopia or in those who manifest elevated levels of TSH after 6-12 mo of therapy because of poor compliance or an inadequate dose of T_4. Discontinuation of therapy at about 3 yr of age for 3-4 wk results in a marked increase in TSH levels in children with permanent hypothyroidism.

Care should be taken to avoid prolonged undertreatment or overtreatment. The only untoward effects of L-T_4 are related to its dosage. Overtreatment can risk craniosynostosis and temperament problems.

Prognosis

Thyroid hormone is critical for normal cerebral development in the early postnatal months; biochemical diagnosis must be made soon after birth, and effective treatment must be initiated promptly to prevent irreversible brain damage. With the advent of neonatal screening programs for detection of congenital hypothyroidism, the prognosis for affected infants has improved dramatically. Early diagnosis and adequate treatment from the 1st weeks of life result in normal linear growth and development. Most studies report that psychometric testing in infants detected by newborn screening shows verbal, psychomotor, and global IQ scores similar to those of unaffected siblings or classmate controls. Some screening programs report that the most severely affected infants, as judged by the lowest T_4 levels and retarded skeletal maturation, have reduced IQs (by 5-20 points) and other neuropsychologic sequelae, such as incoordination, hypotonia or hypertonia, short attention span, and speech problems, even with early diagnosis and adequate treatment. Psychometric testing can show problems with vocabulary and reading comprehension, arithmetic, and memory. Approximately 20% of children have a neurosensory hearing deficit. Outcome studies in adults, detected and treated as neonates, reveal delayed social development, lower self-esteem, and a lower health-related quality of life. The latter appears to be related to those individuals with lower neurocognitive outcome and associated congenital malformations.

Delay in diagnosis, failure to correct initial hypothyroxinemia rapidly, inadequate treatment, and poor compliance in the 1st 2-3 yr of life result in variable degrees of brain damage. Without treatment, affected infants are profoundly intellectually challenged and growth retarded. When onset of hypothyroidism occurs after 2 yr of age, the outlook for normal development is much better even if diagnosis and treatment have been delayed, indicating how much more important thyroid hormone is to the rapidly growing brain of the infant.

ACQUIRED HYPOTHYROIDISM

Epidemiology

Studies of school-age children report that hypothyroidism occurs in approximately 0.3% (1 in 333). Subclinical hypothyroidism (TSH >4.5 mU/L, normal T_4 or free T_4) is more common, occurring in approximately 2% of adolescents. Acquired hypothyroidism is most commonly a result of chronic lymphocytic thyroiditis; 6% of children age 12-19 yr have evidence of autoimmune thyroid disease, which occurs with a 2:1 female:male preponderance.

Etiology

The most common cause of acquired hypothyroidism (Table 565-3) is chronic lymphocytic (Hashimoto) thyroiditis (see Chapter 566). **Autoimmune thyroid disease** may be part of polyglandular syndromes; children with Down and Turner syndrome, possibly Klinefelter syndrome, and celiac disease or diabetes are at higher risk for associated autoimmune thyroid disease (see Chapter 566) as are those with **autoimmune polyglandular syndromes (APSs)** (Tables 565-4 and 565-5). APS has 4 types, but APS-1 and APS-2 are the most common. APS-1 includes 2 components of the triad of hypoparathyroidism, Addison disease (adrenal insufficiency) and mucocutaneous candidiasis ("HAM" syndrome). Commonly referred to by the acronym APECED (autoimmune polyendocrinopathy-candidiasis-ectodermal dysplasia), it is autosomal recessive, caused by a mutation in the *AIRE* (autoimmune

regulator) gene. Less-common features include thyroiditis (~10%), type 1 diabetes mellitus, primary hypogonadism, pernicious anemia, vitiligo, alopecia, chronic active hepatitis, and malabsorption syndrome. APS-2 (Schmidt syndrome) most commonly consists of autoimmune thyroiditis (~70%), Addison disease, and type 1 diabetes mellitus. Less-common features include primary hypogonadism, pernicious anemia, and vitiligo. APS-2 occurs more commonly than APS-1, generally presents in early adulthood, and has a female preponderance. The underlying immunologic defect remains to be determined.

Table 565-4	Autoimmune Polyglandular Syndromes 1 and 2	
	APS-1	**APS-2**
Incidence	<1 in 100,000 population/yr	1-2 in 10,000 population/yr
Onset	Infancy/early childhood	Late childhood/adulthood
Male:female ratio	3:4	1:3
Inheritance	Monogenic (*AIRE* gene)	Polygenic (HLA-associated)
Mucocutaneous candidiasis	73-100%	None
Hypoparathyroidism	77-89%	None
Addison disease	60-86%	70-100%
Type 1 diabetes	4-18%	41-52%
Autoimmune thyroid disease	8-40%	70%
GONADAL FAILURE		
Male	7-17%	5%
Female	30-60%	3.5-10%
Ectodermal dysplasia	77%	None
Vitiligo	4-13%	4-5%
Pernicious anemia	12-15%	2-25%
Alopecia	27%	2%
Autoimmune hepatitis	10-15%	Rare
Malabsorption	10-18%	Rare

HLA, human leukocyte antigen.
From Nambam B, Winter WE, Schatz DA: IgG₄ antibodies in autoimmune polyglandular disease and IgG₄-related endocrinopathies: pathophysiology and clinical characteristics. Curr Opin Pediatr 26:493–499, 2014, Table 1, p. 494.

Table 565-3	Etiologic Classification of Acquired Hypothyroidism

Autoimmune
- Hashimoto thyroiditis
- Autoimmune polyglandular syndromes types 1 and 2 (APS-1, APS-2)

Drug-induced
- Excess iodide: amiodarone, nutritional supplements, expectorants
- Anticonvulsants: phenytoin, phenobarbital, valproate
- Antithyroid drugs: methimazole, propylthiouracil
- Miscellaneous: lithium, tyrosine kinase inhibitors, interferon alfa, stavudine, thalidomide, aminoglutethimide

Postablative
- Irradiation
- Radioiodine
- Thyroidectomy

Systemic infiltrative disease
- Cystinosis
- Langerhans cell histiocytosis

Hemangiomas (large) of the liver (type 3 iodothyronine deiodinase)

Hypothalamic-pituitary disease with multiple pituitary hormone deficiencies
- Hypothalamic-pituitary tumors (e.g., craniopharyngioma)
- Meningoencephalitis
- Cranial radiation
- Head trauma
- Langerhans cell histiocytosis

Table 565-5	Organ-Specific Autoantigens in Autoimmune Polyglandular Syndromes
DISEASE	**AUTOANTIGENS**
Addison disease	P450c21, P450c17, P450scc
Hashimoto thyroiditis	Thyroid peroxidase, thyroglobulin
Graves disease	TSH receptor
Hypoparathyroidism	Calcium-sensing receptor, NALP 5 (NACHT leucine-rich-repeat protein 5)
Type 1 diabetes	Insulin, glutamic acid decarboxylase-65, IA-2A, ZnT8
Hypogonadism	P450c17, P450scc
Immune gastritis	H+, K+-ATPase
Pernicious anemia	Intrinsic factor
Celiac disease	Transglutaminase, gliadin
Immune hepatitis	P450D6, P4502C9, P4501A2
Alopecia areata	Tyrosine hydroxylase
Vitiligo	Tyrosinase

ATPase, adenosine triphosphatase; TSH, thyroid-stimulating hormone.
From Nambam B, Winter WE, Schatz DA: IgG₄ antibodies in autoimmune polyglandular disease and IgG₄-related endocrinopathies: pathophysiology and clinical characteristics. Curr Opin Pediatr 26:493–499, 2014, Table 2, p. 495.

In children with **Down syndrome**, antithyroid antibodies develop in approximately 30%, and subclinical or overt hypothyroidism occurs in approximately 15-20%. In girls with **Turner syndrome**, antithyroid antibodies develop in approximately 40%, and subclinical or overt hypothyroidism occurs in approximately 15-30%, rising with increasing age. In children with **type 1 diabetes mellitus**, approximately 20% develop antithyroid antibodies and 5% become hypothyroid. Additional autoimmune diseases with an increased risk of hypothyroidism include immune dysregulation–polyendocrinopathy–enteropathy–X-linked syndrome (IPEX) and IPEX-like disorders, immunoglobulin G_4–related diseases, Sjögren syndrome, multiple sclerosis, pernicious anemia, Addison disease, and ovarian failure. Although typically seen in adolescence, it occurs as early as in the 1st yr of life. **Williams syndrome** is associated with subclinical hypothyroidism; this does not appear to be autoimmune, as antithyroid antibodies are negative.

Protracted ingestion of **medications** containing iodides—for example, expectorants or nutritional supplements—can cause hypothyroidism, usually accompanied by goiter (see Chapter 567). Amiodarone, a drug used for cardiac arrhythmias and consisting of 37% iodine by weight, causes hypothyroidism in approximately 20% of treated children. It affects thyroid function directly by its high iodine content as well as by inhibition of 5′-deiodinase, which converts T_4 to T_3. Children treated with this drug should have serial measurements of T_4, T_3, and TSH.

Anticonvulsants, including phenytoin, phenobarbital, and valproate, may cause thyroid dysfunction, usually mild, subclinical hypothyroidism. Certain anticonvulsants stimulate hepatic P450 metabolism and excretion of T_4. Children with Graves disease treated with antithyroid drugs (methimazole or propylthiouracil) can develop hypothyroidism. Additional drugs that can produce hypothyroidism include lithium, tyrosine kinase inhibitors, interferon-α, stavudine, thalidomide, and aminoglutethimide.

Children who receive craniospinal irradiation, as with treatment of Hodgkin disease or other head and neck malignancies or that is administered before bone marrow transplantation, are at risk for thyroid damage. Approximately 30% of such children acquire elevated TSH levels within a year after therapy, and another 15-20% progress to hypothyroidism within 5-7 yr. Central (hypopituitary) hypothyroidism may develop in approximately 10% of children receiving craniospinal irradiation.

Radioactive iodine ablative treatment or **thyroidectomy** for Graves disease or cancer results in hypothyroidism, as can removal of ectopic thyroid tissue. Thyroid tissue in a thyroglossal duct cyst usually constitutes the only source of thyroid hormone, and excision results in hypothyroidism. Ultrasonographic examination or a radionuclide scan before surgery is indicated in these patients.

Children with **nephropathic cystinosis**, a disorder characterized by intralysosomal storage of cystine in body tissues, acquire impaired thyroid function. Hypothyroidism may be overt, but subclinical forms are more common, and periodic assessment of TSH levels is indicated. By 13 yr of age, two thirds of these patients require T_4 replacement.

Histiocytic infiltration of the thyroid in children with **Langerhans cell histiocytosis** (see Chapter 507) can result in hypothyroidism.

Children with chronic **hepatitis C infection** are at risk for subclinical hypothyroidism; this does not appear to be autoimmune, because antithyroid antibodies are negative.

Hypothyroidism can occur in children with large **hemangiomas** of the liver, because of increased type 3 deiodinase activity, which catalyzes conversion of T_4 to reverse T_3 and T_3 to diiodothyronine. Thyroid secretion is increased, but it is not sufficient to compensate for the large increase in degradation of T_4 to reverse T_3.

Some patients with congenital thyroid dysgenesis and residual thyroid function or with incomplete genetic defects in thyroid hormone synthesis do not display clinical manifestations until childhood and appear to have acquired hypothyroidism. Although these conditions are usually now detected by newborn screening programs, very mild defects can escape detection.

Any **hypothalamic** or **pituitary** disease can cause acquired central hypothyroidism (see Chapter 557). TSH deficiency may be the result of a hypothalamic-pituitary tumor (craniopharyngioma is most common in children) or a result of treatment for the tumor. Other causes include cranial radiation, head trauma, or diseases infiltrating the pituitary gland, such as Langerhans cell histiocytosis.

Clinical Manifestations

Deceleration of growth is usually the first clinical manifestation, but this sign often goes unrecognized (Figs. 565-3 and 565-4). Goiter associated with Hashimoto thyroiditis, which may be a presenting feature, typically is nontender and firm, with a rubbery consistency and a pebbly surface. Weight gain is mostly fluid retention (myxedema), not true obesity. Myxedematous changes of the skin, constipation, cold intolerance, decreased energy, and an increased need for sleep develop insidiously. Surprisingly, schoolwork and grades usually do not suffer, even in severely hypothyroid children. Additional features include bradycardia, muscle weakness or cramps, nerve entrapment, and ataxia. Osseous maturation is delayed, often strikingly, which is an indication of the duration of the hypothyroidism. Adolescents typically have delayed puberty; older adolescent girls manifest menometrorrhagia. Younger children might present with galactorrhea or pseudoprecocious puberty. Galactorrhea is a result of increased TRH stimulating prolactin secretion. The precocious puberty, characterized by breast development and vaginal bleeding in girls and macroorchidism in boys, is thought to be the result of abnormally high TSH concentrations binding to the follicle-stimulating hormone receptor with subsequent stimulation.

Some children have headaches and vision problems; they usually have enlargement of the pituitary gland, sometimes with suprasellar extension, after long-standing primary hypothyroidism. This condition, believed to be the result of thyrotroph hyperplasia, may be mistaken for a pituitary tumor (see Chapter 557). Abnormal laboratory studies include hyponatremia, macrocytic anemia, hypercholesterolemia, and elevated creatine phosphokinase. Table 565-6 lists the complications seen in severe hypothyroidism. All these changes return to normal with adequate replacement of T_4.

Diagnostic Studies

Children with suspected hypothyroidism should undergo measurement of serum free T_4 and TSH. Because the normal range for thyroid tests is slightly higher in children than adults, it is important to compare results to age-specific reference ranges. Measurement of antithyroglobulin and antiperoxidase antibodies can pinpoint autoimmune thyroiditis as the cause. In cases with a goiter resulting from autoimmune thyroid disease, an ultrasound examination typically shows diffuse enlargement with scattered hypoechogenicity. However, generally, sonography is not indicated unless there is a suspicion of a thyroid nodule on neck palpation. In such cases, ultrasound examination is the most accurate study to confirm the presence of a nodule and determine if other, smaller nodules are present. In addition, an ultrasound examination can determine the nodule dimensions, texture (solid vs cystic nature), and presence or absence of other features that might influence a decision to undertake fine-needle aspiration, such as microcalcifications, blurred margins, "taller-than-wide" shape, intranodular vascular flow, and pathologic-appearing adjacent lymph nodes (see Chapter 569.1). In children with a nodule and suppressed TSH, a radioactive iodine uptake scan is indicated to determine if this is a "hot" or hyperfunctioning nodule. A bone age x-ray at diagnosis is useful, in that the degree of delay approximates duration and severity of hypothyroidism.

Treatment and Prognosis

L-T_4 is the treatment of choice in children with hypothyroidism. The dose on a weight basis gradually decreases with age. For children age 1-3 yr, the average L-T_4 dosage is 4-6 µg/kg/day; for age 3-10 yr, 3-5 µg/kg/day; and for age 10-16 yr, 2-4 µg/kg/day. Treatment should be monitored by measuring serum free T_4 and TSH every 4-6 mo as well as 6 wk after any change in dosage. In children with central hypothyroidism, where TSH levels are not helpful in monitoring treatment, the goal should be to maintain serum free T_4 in the upper half of the normal reference range for age.

During the 1st yr of treatment, deterioration of schoolwork, poor sleeping habits, restlessness, short attention span, and behavioral

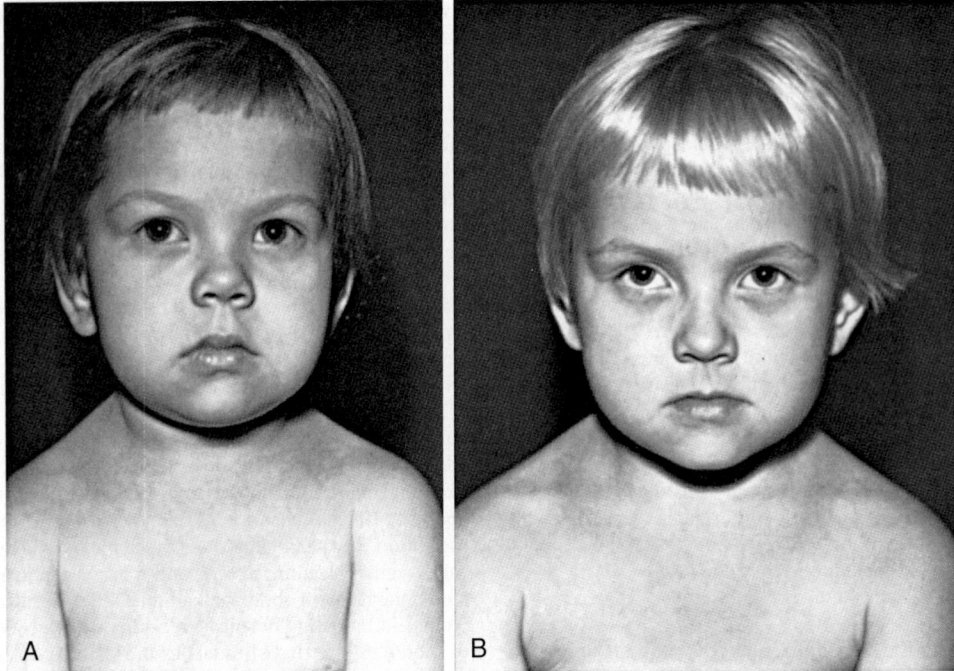

Figure 565-3 A, Acquired hypothyroidism in a girl 6 yr of age. She was treated with a wide variety of hematinics for refractory anemia for 3 yr. She had almost complete cessation of growth, constipation, and sluggishness for 3 yr. The height age was 3 yr; the bone age was 4 yr. She had a sallow complexion and immature facies with a poorly developed nasal bridge. Serum cholesterol, 501 mg/dL; radioiodine uptake, 7% at 24 hr; protein-bound iodine (PBI), 2.8 mg/dL. **B,** After therapy for 18 mo, note the nasal development, increased luster and decreased pigmentation of hair, and maturation of the face. The height age was 5.5 yr; the bone age was 7 yr. There was a decided improvement in her general condition. Menarche occurred at 14 yr. The ultimate height was 155 cm (61 in). She graduated from high school. The disorder was well controlled with sodium–L-thyroxine daily.

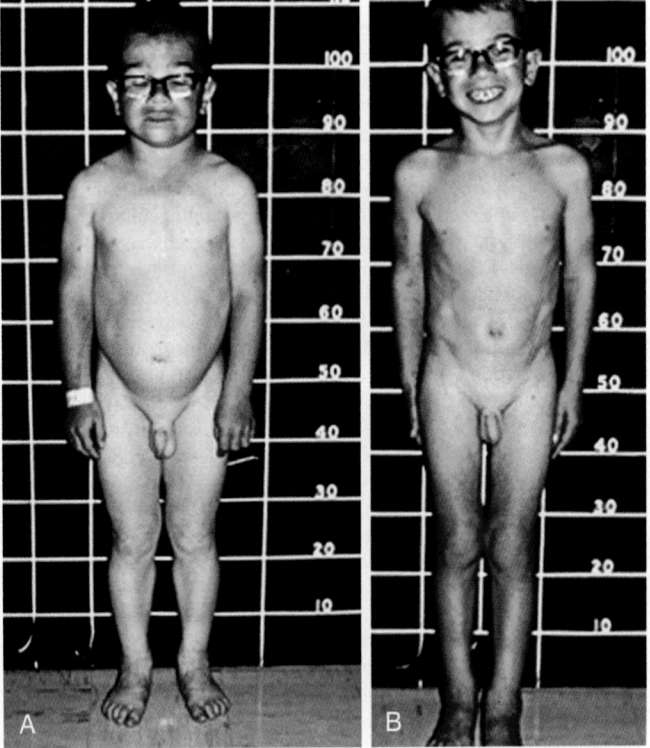

Figure 565-4 A, Short stature (108 cm, <3rd percentile), generalized myxedema, sleepy expression, protuberant abdomen, and coarse hair are signs of hypothyroidism in this 12 yr old boy. Body proportions are immature for his age (1.25:1). **B,** Same boy 4 mo after treatment. His height increased by 4 cm; note the marked change in body habitus owing to loss of generalized myxedema, improved muscle tone, and bright facial expression. *(From LaFranchi SH: Hypothyroidism, Pediatr Clin North Am 26:33–51, 1979.)*

Table 565-6	Pathogenesis of General Complications in Management of Complicated Hypothyroidism
COMPLICATION	**PATHOGENESIS**
Heart failure	Impaired ventricular systolic and diastolic functions and increased peripheral vascular resistance
Ventilatory failure	Blunted hypercapnic and hypoxic ventilatory drives
Hyponatremia	Impaired renal free water excretion and syndrome of inappropriate antidiuretic hormone secretion
Ileus	Bowel hypomotility
Medication sensitivity	Reduced clearance rate and increased sensitivity to sedative, analgesic, and anesthetic agents
Hypothermia and lack of febrile response to sepsis	Decreased calorigenesis
Delirium, dementia, seizure, stupor, and coma	Decreased central nervous system thyroid hormone actions, and encephalopathy from hyponatremia and hypercapnia
Adrenal insufficiency	Associated intrinsic adrenal or pituitary disease, or reversible impairment of hypothalamic-pituitary-adrenal stress response
Coagulopathy	Acquired von Willebrand syndrome (type 1) and decreased factors VIII, VII, V, IX, and X

From Roberts CG, Landenson PW: Hypothyroidism, Lancet 363:793–803, 2004.

problems might ensue, but these are transient; forewarning families about these manifestations enhances appropriate management. These may partially be ameliorated by starting at subreplacement T_4 doses and advancing slowly. The development of persistent headaches or vision changes should prompt an evaluation for papilledema associated with pseudotumor cerebri, a rare complication following initiation of L-T_4 treatment in older children (age 8-13 yr).

In older children, after catch-up growth is complete, the growth rate provides a good index of the adequacy of therapy. Periodic bone age x-rays are useful to monitor treatment and future growth potential. In children with long-standing hypothyroidism, catch-up growth may be incomplete (see Fig. 565-4). During the 1st 18 mo of treatment, skeletal maturation often exceeds expected linear growth, resulting in a loss of approximately 7 cm of predicted adult height.

Bibliography is available at Expert Consult.

Chapter **566**
Thyroiditis
Stephen H. LaFranchi and Stephen A. Huang

CHRONIC LYMPHOCYTIC THYROIDITIS (HASHIMOTO THYROIDITIS, AUTOIMMUNE THYROIDITIS)

Chronic lymphocytic thyroiditis is the most common cause of thyroid disease in children and adolescents and accounts for many of the enlarged thyroids formerly designated "adolescent" or "simple" goiter. It is also the most common cause of acquired hypothyroidism, with or without goiter.

One to 2% of younger school-age children and 6-8% of adolescents have positive antithyroid antibodies as evidence of autoimmune thyroid disease.

Etiology

This typical organ-specific autoimmune disease results from inheritance of susceptible genes involved in immunoregulation and environmental triggers, both as yet poorly characterized. Early in the course of the disease, there may be thyroid hyperplasia only; this is followed by infiltration of lymphocytes and plasma cells between the follicles and by atrophy of the follicles. Lymphoid follicle formation with germinal centers is almost always present; the degree of atrophy and fibrosis of the follicles varies from mild to moderate.

Intrathyroidal lymphocyte subsets differ from those in blood. Approximately 60% of infiltrating lymphoid cells are T cells, and approximately 30% express B-cell markers; the T-cell population is represented by helper (CD4$^+$) and cytotoxic (CD8$^+$) cells. The participation of cellular events in the pathogenesis is clear. Certain human leukocyte antigen (HLA) haplotypes (HLA-DR4, HLA-DR5) are associated with an increased risk of goiter and thyroiditis, and others (HLA-DR3) are associated with the atrophic variant of thyroiditis.

A variety of different thyroid antigen autoantibodies are also involved. Thyroid antiperoxidase antibodies (TPO-Abs) and antithyroglobulin antibodies (anti-Tg Abs) are demonstrable in the sera of 90% of children with chronic lymphocytic thyroiditis and in many patients with Graves disease. TPO-Abs are involved in activation of the complement cascade and in antibody-dependent, cell-mediated cytotoxicity. Anti-Tg Abs do not appear to play a role in the autoimmune destruction of the gland. Thyroid-stimulating hormone (TSH) receptor–blocking antibodies are related to the development of hypothyroidism and thyroid atrophy; they have been demonstrated in 18% of patients with severe hypothyroidism (TSH >20 mU/L) caused by autoimmune thyroiditis. Antibodies to pendrin, an apical protein on thyroid follicular cells, have

been demonstrated in 80% of children with autoimmune thyroiditis. Antibodies also have been found against the sodium–iodide symporter, but their pathogenic role is unclear.

Clinical Manifestations

The disorder is 4-6 times more common in girls than in boys. It can occur during the 1st 3 yr of life, but becomes sharply more common after 6 yr of age and reaches a peak incidence during adolescence. The most common clinical manifestations are goiter and growth retardation. The goiter can appear insidiously and may be small or large. In most patients, the thyroid is diffusely enlarged, firm, and nontender. In approximately 30% of patients, the gland is asymmetric and can seem to be nodular. Most of the affected children are clinically euthyroid and asymptomatic; some may have symptoms of pressure in the neck, including difficulty swallowing and shortness of breath. Some children have clinical signs of hypothyroidism, but others who appear clinically euthyroid have laboratory evidence of hypothyroidism. A few children have manifestations suggesting hyperthyroidism, such as nervousness, irritability, increased sweating, and hyperactivity, but results of laboratory studies are not necessarily those of hyperthyroidism. Occasionally, the disorder coexists with Graves disease ("Hashitoxicosis"). Ophthalmopathy can occur in autoimmune thyroiditis in the absence of Graves disease.

The clinical course is variable. The goiter might become smaller or might disappear spontaneously, or it might persist unchanged for years while the patient remains euthyroid. Most children who are euthyroid at presentation remain euthyroid, although a percentage of patients acquire hypothyroidism gradually within months or years. In children who initially have mild or subclinical hypothyroidism (elevated serum TSH, normal free thyroxine [T_4] level), over several years approximately 40% revert to euthyroidism, 50% continue to have subclinical hypothyroidism, and approximately 10% develop overt hypothyroidism (elevated serum TSH, subnormal free T_4 level). Chronic lymphocytic thyroiditis is the cause of most cases of nongoitrous (atrophic) hypothyroidism.

Familial clusters of chronic lymphocytic thyroiditis are common; the incidence in siblings or parents of affected children may be as high as 25%. TPO-Abs and anti-Tg Abs in these families appear to be inherited in an autosomal dominant fashion, with reduced penetrance in males. The concurrence within families of patients with chronic lymphocytic thyroiditis, hypothyroidism, and Graves disease provides cogent evidence for a basic relationship among these 3 conditions.

The disorder is associated with many other autoimmune disorders. Autoimmune thyroiditis occurs in 10% of patients with type I autoimmune polyglandular syndrome (APS-1), characterized by autoimmune polyendocrinopathy, candidiasis, and ectodermal dysplasia (APECED). APS-1 consists of 2 of the triad of hypoparathyroidism, Addison disease, and mucocutaneous candidiasis (HAM syndrome). This relatively rare autosomal recessive disorder occurs in childhood and is caused by mutations in the autoimmune regulator *(AIRE)* gene on chromosome 21q22.3.

Autoimmune thyroid disease occurs in 70% of patients with APS-2. APS-2 consists of the association of autoimmune thyroiditis and Addison disease (Schmidt syndrome) or autoimmune thyroiditis with type 1 diabetes mellitus (Carpenter syndrome). It typically occurs in later childhood or early adulthood; the etiology is unknown. Autoimmune thyroiditis has been described in children with immunodysregulation polyendocrinopathy enteropathy X-linked (IPEX) syndrome, which includes early-onset diabetes and colitis. Autoimmune thyroid disease also tends to be associated with pernicious anemia, vitiligo, or alopecia. TPO-Abs are found in approximately 20% of white and 4% of black children with type 1 diabetes mellitus. Autoimmune thyroid disease has an increased incidence in children with congenital rubella.

Chronic lymphocytic thyroiditis also is associated with certain chromosomal disorders, particularly Turner syndrome and Down syndrome. In children with Down syndrome, one study reported that 28% had antithyroid antibodies (predominantly anti-TPOs), 7% had subclinical hypothyroidism, 7% had overt hypothyroidism, and 5% had

Table 566-1	Characteristics of Thyroiditis Syndromes					
CHARACTERISTIC	**HASHIMOTO THYROIDITIS**	**PAINLESS POSTPARTUM THYROIDITIS**	**PAINLESS SPORADIC THYROIDITIS**	**PAINFUL SUBACUTE THYROIDITIS**	**ACUTE SUPPURATIVE THYROIDITIS**	**RIEDEL THYROIDITIS**
Sex ratio (F:M)	4-6:1	—	2:1	5:1	1:1	3-4:1
Cause	Autoimmune	Autoimmune	Autoimmune	Unknown (probably viral)	Infectious (bacterial)	Unknown
Pathologic findings	Lymphocytic infiltration, germinal centers, fibrosis	Lymphocytic infiltration	Lymphocytic infiltration	Giant cells, granulomas	Abscess formation	Dense fibrosis
Thyroid function	Usually euthyroidism; some hypothyroidism	Hyperthyroidism, hypothyroidism, or both	Hyperthyroidism, hypothyroidism, or both	Hyperthyroidism, hypothyroidism, or both	Usually euthyroidism	Usually euthyroidism
TPO antibodies	High titer, persistent	High titer, persistent	High titer, persistent	Low titer, or absent, or transient	Absent	Usually present
ESR	Normal	Normal	Normal	High	High	Normal
24 hr ^{123}I uptake	Variable	<5%	<5%	<5%	Normal	Low or normal

ESR, erythrocyte sedimentation rate; ^{123}I, iodine 123; TPO, thyroid peroxidase.
Data from Farwell AP, Braverman LE. Inflammatory thyroid disorders. Otolaryngol Clin North Am 4:541–556, 1996.

hyperthyroidism. In a study of girls with Turner syndrome, 41% had antithyroid antibodies (again, predominantly anti-TPOs), 18% had goiter, and 8% had subclinical or overt hypothyroidism. Another study of 75 girls with Turner syndrome found that autoimmune thyroid disease increased from the 1st (15%) to the 3rd (30%) decade of life. Boys with Klinefelter syndrome appear to be at risk for autoimmune thyroid disease. Table 566-1 compares the characteristics of Hashimoto thyroiditis to other thyroiditis syndromes.

Laboratory Findings
Thyroid function tests (free T_4 and TSH) are often normal, although the level of TSH may be slightly or even moderately elevated in some patients, which is termed *subclinical hypothyroidism*. That many children with chronic lymphocytic thyroiditis do not have elevated levels of TSH indicates that the goiter is caused by the lymphocytic infiltrations or by thyroid growth-stimulating immunoglobulins. Young children with chronic lymphocytic thyroiditis have serum TPO-Abs, but the anti-Tg Abs are positive in <50%. TPO-Abs and anti-Tg Abs are found equally in adolescents with chronic lymphocytic thyroiditis. When both tests are used, approximately 95% of patients with thyroid autoimmunity are detected. Levels in children and adolescents are lower than those in adults with Hashimoto thyroiditis, and repeated measurements are indicated in questionable instances because titers might increase later in the course of the disease. In adolescent females with overt hypothyroidism, measurement of TSH receptor–blocking antibodies may identify patients at future risk of having babies with transient congenital hypothyroidism.

Thyroid scans and ultrasonography usually are not needed. If they are done, thyroid scans reveal irregular and patchy distribution of the radioisotope, and in approximately 60% or more, the administration of perchlorate results in a >10% discharge of iodide from the thyroid gland. Thyroid ultrasonography shows heterogeneous echogenicity in most patients, along with an increased number of benign-appearing hyperplastic lymph nodes in the neck. The definitive diagnosis can be established by biopsy of the thyroid; this procedure is rarely clinically indicated.

Antithyroid antibodies also may be found in almost 50% of the siblings of affected patients and in a significant percentage of the mothers of children with Down syndrome or Turner syndrome without demonstrable thyroid disease.

Treatment
If there is evidence of overt hypothyroidism (elevated TSH, low T_4 or free T_4), replacement treatment with levothyroxine (at doses specific for size and age) is indicated. The goiter usually shows some decrease in size but can persist for years. In a euthyroid patient, treatment with

suppressive doses of levothyroxine is unlikely to lead to a significant decrease in size of the goiter. Antibody levels fluctuate in both treated and untreated patients and persist for years. Because the disease is self-limited in some instances, the need for continued therapy requires periodic reevaluation. Untreated patients should also be checked periodically. Although there is some controversy about treating patients with subclinical hypothyroidism (elevated TSH, normal T_4 or free T_4), many clinicians prefer to treat such children until growth and puberty are complete, and then reevaluate their thyroid function.

Prominent **nodules** (i.e., >1 cm) that persist despite suppressive therapy should be examined histologically using fine-needle aspiration, because thyroid carcinoma or lymphoma has occurred in patients with Hashimoto thyroiditis.

OTHER CAUSES OF THYROIDITIS
Subacute granulomatous thyroiditis (de Quervain disease) is rare in children. It is thought to have a viral cause and remits spontaneously. The disorder becomes manifested by an upper respiratory infection with vague tenderness over the thyroid and low-grade fever, followed by severe pain in the region of the thyroid gland. Inflammation results in leakage of preformed thyroid hormone from the gland into the circulation. Serum levels of T_4 and triiodothyronine are elevated while TSH is suppressed, and mild symptoms of hyperthyroidism may be present, but radioiodine uptake is depressed. The erythrocyte sedimentation rate is increased. The course is variable but usually characterized by 4 phases: hyperthyroidism, usually followed by a euthyroid phase and then a hypothyroid phase, and remission usually occurring in several months, with recovery to euthyroidism.

Acute suppurative thyroiditis is uncommon in children; it is usually preceded by a respiratory infection with pharyngitis. The left lower lobe is affected predominantly. Abscess formation can occur; anaerobic organisms, with or without aerobes, are the typical infectious agents. The most common organism is α-hemolytic streptococci (viridans) followed by *Staphylococcus aureus* and pneumococci. Recurrent episodes or detection of a mixed bacterial flora suggests that the infection arises from a **piriform sinus fistula** or, less commonly, from a **thyroglossal duct** remnant. Exquisite tenderness of the gland, swelling, erythema, dysphagia, and limitation of head motion are characteristic findings. Fever, chills, and sore throat are not uncommon, and leukocytosis is present. Scintigrams of the thyroid often reveal decreased uptake in the affected areas, and ultrasonography might show a complex echogenic mass. Thyroid function is usually normal, but hyperthyroidism caused by escape of thyroid hormone has been encountered in a child with suppurative thyroiditis resulting from *Aspergillus*. When abscesses form, incision and drainage and administration of parenteral antibiotics are indicated. After the infection subsides, a barium esophagram or CT scan with contrast is indicated to search for a fistulous tract; if one is found, surgical excision is indicated.

Specific conditions such as tuberculosis, sarcoidosis, mumps, and cat-scratch disease are rare causes of thyroiditis in children. **Other forms of thyroiditis** seen in adults, such as painless sporadic thyroiditis and Riedel thyroiditis, are rare in children (see Table 566-1).

Bibliography is available at Expert Consult.

Chapter **567**
Goiter
Stephen A. Huang and Stephen H. LaFranchi

A goiter, or thyromegaly, is an enlargement of the thyroid gland. Persons with enlarged thyroids can have normal function of the gland (**euthyroidism**), thyroid deficiency (**hypothyroidism**), or overproduction of the hormones (**hyperthyroidism**). Goiter may be congenital or acquired, endemic or sporadic. Detection of a goiter should prompt an investigation of its cause and the assessment of thyroid function.

Goiter most often results from the increased pituitary secretion of thyroid-stimulating hormone (TSH) in response to decreased circulating levels of thyroid hormones. Activation of the TSH receptor from thyrotropin receptor–stimulating antibodies (in Graves disease), gain-of-function TSH receptor mutations, or inappropriate TSH secretion (from dominant negative thyroid hormone receptor mutations or TSH-secreting adenomas) can also cause thyromegaly. Thyroid enlargement can also result from infiltrative processes that may be inflammatory or neoplastic.

567.1 Congenital Goiter
Stephen A. Huang and Stephen H. LaFranchi

Congenital goiter is usually sporadic and can result from a fetal thyroxine (T_4) synthetic defect or from administration of antithyroid drugs or iodides during pregnancy for the treatment of maternal thyrotoxicosis. Goitrogenic drugs that cross the placenta at high doses can interfere with synthesis of thyroid hormone, resulting in goiter and hypothyroidism in the fetus. These effects are most severe when pharmacologic overtreatment with antithyroid drugs causes concomitant hypothyroidism in the mother and reduces the supply of maternal thyroid hormone available to the fetus. In women with Graves disease receiving antithyroid drugs, fetal effects can occur when the mother takes propylthiouracil at only 100-200 mg/24 hr; consequently, all infants born to women treated with antithyroid drugs in the 3rd trimester should undergo thyroid studies at birth. Even when the infant is clinically euthyroid, there may be retardation of osseous maturation, low levels of T_4, and elevated levels of TSH. Administration of thyroid hormone to affected infants may be indicated to treat clinical hypothyroidism, to hasten the disappearance of the goiter, and to prevent brain damage. Because the condition is rarely permanent, thyroid hormone may be safely discontinued after the antithyroid drug has been excreted by the neonate, usually after 1-2 wk. In addition to antithyroid medications, iodides are included in many proprietary cough preparations used to treat asthma; these preparations should be avoided during pregnancy because they have often been reported to cause congenital goiter. Amiodarone, an antiarrhythmic drug with 37% iodine content, has also caused congenital goiter with hypothyroidism.

Enlargement of the thyroid at birth may occasionally be sufficient to cause respiratory distress that interferes with nursing and can even cause death. The head may be maintained in extreme hyperextension. In pregnant women who are overtreated with antithyroid drugs, the prenatal diagnosis of even massive fetal goiter can often be corrected by withdrawal of the maternal medication, with or without intraamniotic thyroid hormone injection. When postnatal respiratory obstruction is severe, partial thyroidectomy rather than tracheostomy is indicated (Fig. 567-1).

Goiter is almost always present in the infant with neonatal Graves hyperthyroidism. Thyroid enlargement results from transplacental passage of maternal thyroid-stimulating immunoglobulin (see Chapter 568.2). These goiters usually are not large; the infant manifests clinical symptoms of hyperthyroidism. The mother often has a history of Graves disease, or the diagnosis of maternal Graves may be revealed through the evaluation of neonatal hyperthyroidism. TSH receptor–activating mutations are also a recognized cause of congenital goiter and hyperthyroidism.

When no causative factor is identifiable from the maternal or medication history, a **defect in synthesis** of thyroid hormone should be suspected. Neonatal screening programs find congenital hypothyroidism caused by such a defect in 1 in 30,000-50,000 live births. It is advisable to treat immediately with thyroid hormone and to postpone more-detailed studies for later in life. If a specific defect is suspected,

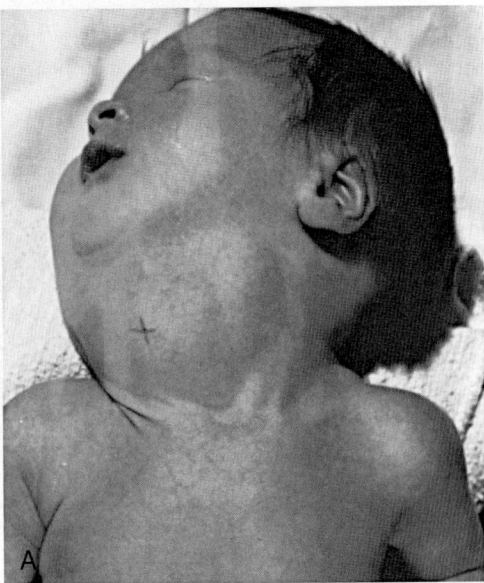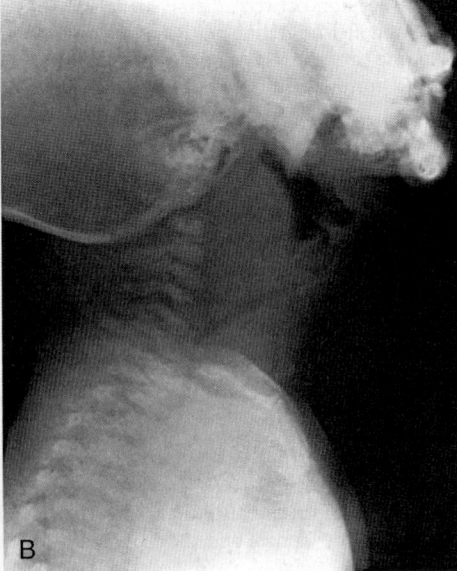

Figure 567-1 Congenital goiter in infancy. **A,** Large congenital goiter in an infant born to a mother with thyrotoxicosis who had been treated with iodides and methimazole during pregnancy. **B,** A different infant, 6 wk old, with increasing respiratory distress and cervical mass since birth. The operation revealed a large goiter that almost completely encircled the trachea. Notice the anterior deviation and posterior compression of the trachea. Partial thyroidectomy completely relieved the symptoms. It is apparent why a tracheostomy is not adequate treatment for these infants. The cause for the goiter was not found.

genetic tests to identify a mutation may be undertaken (see Chapter 565). Because these defects are often caused by recessive mutations, a precise diagnosis is helpful for genetic counseling. Monitoring subsequent pregnancies with ultrasonography can be useful in detecting fetal goiters (see Chapter 96).

Pendred syndrome, characterized by familial goiter and neurosensory deafness, is caused by a mutation in the *SLC26A4* gene, which encodes the pendrin chloride–iodide transport protein expressed in the thyroid gland and cochlea. This defect results in abnormal iodide organification in the thyroid and can cause a goiter at birth. The more common presentation is a euthyroid goiter and sensorineural hearing loss later in life.

Iodine deficiency as a cause of congenital goiter is rare in developed countries but persists in isolated endemic areas (see Chapter 567.3). More important is the recognition that severe iodine deficiency early in pregnancy can cause neurologic damage during fetal development, even in the absence of goiter. The iodine deficiency can result in combined maternal and fetal hypothyroidism, reducing the protective transfer of maternal thyroid hormones.

When the "goiter" is lobulated, asymmetric, firm, or large to an unusual degree, a teratoma within or in the vicinity of the thyroid must be considered in the differential diagnosis (see Chapter 569).

Bibliography is available at Expert Consult.

567.2 Intratracheal Goiter
Stephen A. Huang and Stephen H. LaFranchi

One of the many ectopic locations of thyroid tissue is within the trachea. The intraluminal thyroid lies beneath the tracheal mucosa and is often continuous with the normally situated extratracheal thyroid gland. The thyroid is susceptible to goitrous enlargement, which involves both the eutopic and ectopic thyroid tissue. When there is obstruction of the airway associated with a goiter, it must be ascertained whether the obstruction is extratracheal or endotracheal. If obstructive manifestations are mild, administration of sodium L-thyroxine (levothyroxine) usually causes the goiter to decrease in size. When symptoms are severe, surgical removal of the endotracheal goiter is indicated.

567.3 Endemic Goiter and Cretinism
Stephen A. Huang and Stephen H. LaFranchi

ETIOLOGY
The association between dietary deficiency of iodine and the prevalence of goiter or cretinism is well established. A moderate deficiency of iodine can be overcome by increased efficiency in the synthesis of thyroid hormone. Iodine liberated in the tissues is returned rapidly to the gland, which resynthesizes triiodothyronine (T_3) preferentially at a higher rate than normal. This increased activity is achieved by compensatory hypertrophy and hyperplasia (goiter), which satisfy the demands of the tissues for thyroid hormone. In geographic areas where deficiency of iodine is severe, decompensation and hypothyroidism can result. Recent estimates from the World Health Organization indicate that nearly 2 billion individuals currently have insufficient iodine intake, including one third of the world's school-age children. Thus, despite great progress in the global effort to reduce iodine deficiency, it remains the leading cause of preventable intellectual disability worldwide.

Seawater is rich in iodine; the iodine content of fish and shellfish is also high. As a result, endemic goiter is rare in populations living along the coast. Iodine is deficient in the water and native foods in the Pacific West and the Great Lakes areas of the United States. Deficiency of dietary iodine is even greater in certain Alpine valleys, the Himalayas, the Andes, the Congo, and the highlands of Papua New Guinea. In areas such as the United States, where iodine is provided in foods from other areas and in iodized salt, endemic goiter has disappeared. Iodized salt in the United States contains potassium iodide (100 µg/g), which provides excellent prophylaxis. Further iodine intake in the United States is contributed by iodates used in baking, iodine-containing coloring agents, and iodine-containing disinfectants used in the dairy industry. The recommended daily allowance of iodine is as follows:

◆ Children younger than 2 yr: ≥100 µg/day
◆ School-age children: 100-299 µg/day
◆ Pregnant women: ≥150 µg/day
◆ Lactating women: ≥100 µg/day

While the overall dietary iodine intake in the United States is considered adequate, the most recent NHANES (National Health and Nutrition Examination Survey) from 2007-2010 reports that the median urinary iodine concentration among pregnant U.S. women has dropped to <150 µg/L. This indicates mild iodine deficiency and highlights the risk of iodine deficiency reemergence in industrialized countries as salt intake decreases. These risks can be mitigated by the continued monitoring of iodine status, the adjustment of salt iodization levels, and the targeted supplementation of vulnerable subpopulations (promotion of iodine-containing prenatal vitamins).

CLINICAL MANIFESTATIONS
If the deficiency of iodine is mild, thyroid enlargement does not become noticeable except when there is increased demand for the hormone during periods of rapid growth, as in adolescence and during pregnancy. In regions of moderate iodine deficiency, goiter observed in school children can disappear with maturity and reappear during pregnancy or lactation. Iodine-deficient goiters are more common in girls than in boys. In areas where iodine deficiency is severe, as in the hyperendemic highlands of Papua New Guinea, nearly half the population has large goiters, and endemic cretinism is common (Fig. 567-2).

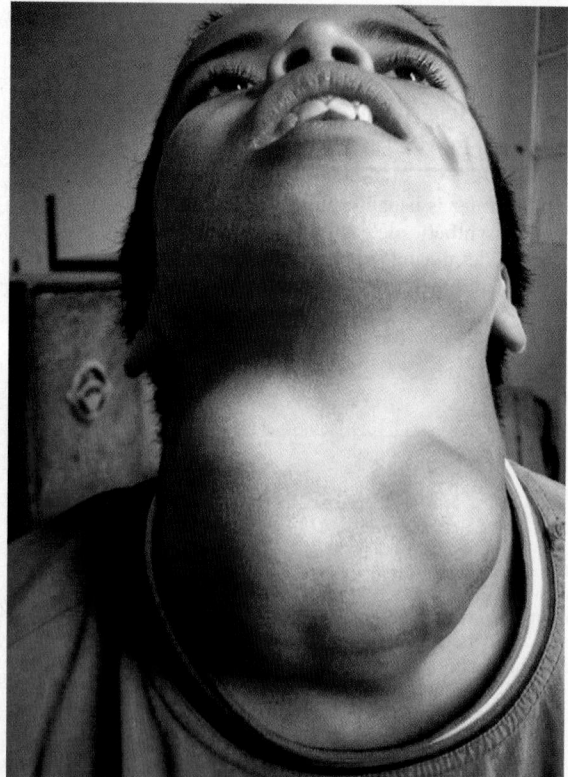

Figure 567-2 A 14 yr old boy with a large nodular goiter was seen in 2004, in an area of severe iodine-deficiency disorders in northern Morocco. He had tracheal and esophageal compression and hoarseness, probably as a result of damage to the recurrent laryngeal nerves. *(From Zimmernamm MB, Jooste PL, Pandav CS: Iodine-deficiency disorders, Lancet 372:1251–1262, 2008, Fig 2.)*

Serum T$_4$ levels are often low in persons with endemic goiter, although clinical hypothyroidism is rare. This is true in New Guinea, the Congo, the Himalayas, and South America. Despite low serum T$_4$ levels, serum TSH concentrations are often normal or only moderately increased. In such patients, circulating levels of T$_3$ are elevated. Moreover, T$_3$ levels are also elevated in patients with normal T$_4$ levels, indicating a preferential secretion of T$_3$ by the thyroid in this disease and an adaptive increase in peripheral T$_4$ to T$_3$ conversion.

Endemic cretinism is the most serious consequence of iodine deficiency; it occurs only in geographic association with endemic goiter. The term *endemic cretinism* includes 2 different but overlapping syndromes: a **neurologic type** and a **myxedematous type.** The incidence of the 2 types varies among different populations. In Papua New Guinea, the neurologic type occurs almost exclusively, whereas in the Congo, the myxedematous type predominates. Both types are found in all endemic areas, and some persons have intermediate or mixed features.

The **neurologic syndrome** is characterized by intellectual disability, deaf-mutism, disturbances in standing and gait, and pyramidal signs such as clonus of the foot, the Babinski sign, and patellar hyperreflexia. Affected persons are goitrous but euthyroid, have normal pubertal development and adult stature, and have little or no impaired thyroid function. Persons with the **myxedematous syndrome** also are intellectually challenged and deaf and have neurologic symptoms, but in contrast to the neurologic type, they have delayed growth and sexual development, myxedema, and absence of goiter. Serum T$_4$ levels are low and TSH levels are markedly elevated. Delayed skeletal maturation may extend into the 3rd decade or later. Ultrasonographic examination shows thyroid atrophy.

PATHOGENESIS

The pathogenesis of the **neurologic syndrome** is attributed to iodine deficiency and hypothyroxinemia during pregnancy, leading to fetal and postnatal hypothyroidism. Although some investigators have attributed brain damage to a direct effect of elemental iodine deficiency in the fetus, most believe the neurologic symptoms are caused by combined fetal and maternal hypothyroxinemia. There is evidence for the presence of thyroid hormone receptors in the fetal brain as early as 7 wk of gestation. Although the normal fetal thyroid gland does not begin to produce significant amounts of thyroid hormone until midgestation, there is measurable T$_4$ in the coelomic fluid as early as 6 wk, almost certainly of maternal origin. These lines of evidence support a role for maternal thyroid hormone in fetal brain development in the 1st trimester. In addition, there is evidence of transplacental passage of maternal thyroid hormone into the fetus, which normally might ameliorate the effects of fetal hypothyroidism on the developing nervous system in the second half of pregnancy. Thus, iodine deficiency in the mother affects fetal brain development both in the 1st trimester and throughout pregnancy. Intake of iodine after birth is often sufficient for normal or only minimally impaired thyroid function.

The pathogenesis of the **myxedematous syndrome** leading to thyroid atrophy is more bewildering. Searches for additional environmental factors that might provoke continuing postnatal hypothyroidism have led to incrimination of selenium deficiency, goitrogenic foods, thiocyanates, and *Yersinia* (Table 567-1). Studies from western China suggest that thyroid autoimmunity might play a role. Children with myxedematous cretinism with thyroid atrophy, but not children with euthyroid cretinism, were found to have thyroid growth-blocking immunoglobulins of the kind found in infants with sporadic congenital hypothyroidism. Others are skeptical about any role of thyroid growth-blocking immunoglobulins to explain these findings.

TREATMENT

In many developing countries, administration of a single intramuscular injection of iodinated poppy seed oil to women prevents iodine deficiency during future pregnancies for approximately 5 yr. This form of therapy given to children younger than 4 yr of age with myxedematous cretinism results in a euthyroid state in 5 mo. Older

Table 567-1	Goitrogens and Their Mechanism
GOITROGEN	**MECHANISM**
FOODS	
Cassava, lima beans, linseed, sorghum, sweet potato	Contain cyanogenic glucosides that are metabolized to thiocyanates that compete with iodine for uptake by the thyroid
Cruciferous vegetables such as cabbage, kale, cauliflower, broccoli, turnips, rapeseed	Contain glucosinolates; metabolites compete with iodine for uptake by the thyroid
Soy, millet	Flavonoids impair thyroid peroxidase activity
INDUSTRIAL POLLUTANTS	
Perchlorate	Competitive inhibitor of the sodium–iodine symporter, decreasing iodine transport into the thyroid
Others (e.g., disulfides from coal processes)	Reduce thyroidal iodine uptake
Smoking	An important goitrogen; smoking during breastfeeding is associated with reduced iodine concentrations in breast milk; high serum concentration of thiocyanate from smoking might compete with iodine for active transport into the secretory epithelium of the lactating breast
NUTRIENTS	
Selenium deficiency	Accumulated peroxides can damage the thyroid, and deiodinase deficiency impairs thyroid hormone activation
Iron deficiency	Reduces heme-dependent thyroperoxidase activity in the thyroid and might blunt the efficacy of iodine prophylaxis
Vitamin A deficiency	Increases TSH stimulation and goiter through decreased vitamin A–mediated suppression of the pituitary TSH-β gene

TSH, thyroid-stimulating hormone.
From Zimmernamm MB, Jooste PL, Pandav CS: Iodine-deficiency disorders, Lancet 372:1251–1262, 2008, Table 1.

children respond poorly and adults not at all to iodized oil injections, indicating an inability of the thyroid gland to synthesize hormone; these patients require treatment with T$_4$. Through the efforts of the World Health Organization and its program of universal salt iodization, the number of households worldwide with access to adequately iodized salt has increased from <10% in 1990 to 70% in 2012. In the Xinjiang province of China, where the usual methods of iodine supplementation had failed, iodination of irrigation water has increased iodine levels in soil, animals, and human beings. In other countries, iodinated salt in school meal programs gives children the dietary iodine they need. Still, political, economic, and practical obstacles have limited penetration of iodized food into regular diets around the world.

Bibliography is available at Expert Consult.

567.4 Acquired Goiter
Stephen A. Huang and Stephen H. LaFranchi

Most acquired goiters are sporadic and develop from a variety of causes; patients are usually euthyroid but may be hypothyroid or hyperthyroid. The most common cause of acquired goiter is lymphocytic thyroiditis (see Chapter 566). Rarer causes in children include painless sporadic thyroiditis and subacute painful thyroiditis (de Quervain disease; see Chapter 566). Other causes include excess iodide ingestion and certain drugs, including amiodarone and lithium. Intrinsic biochemical defects in the synthesis of thyroid hormone are almost always associated with goiter; thyromegaly from milder defects occurs later in childhood. The occurrence of the disorder in siblings, onset in early life, and possible association with hypothyroidism (goitrous hypothyroidism) are important clues to the diagnosis.

IODIDE GOITER

A small percentage of patients treated with iodide preparations for prolonged periods acquire goiters. Iodides are commonly included for their expectorant effect in cough medicines and in proprietary mixtures for asthma. Goiters resulting from iodide administration are firm and diffusely enlarged, and in some instances hypothyroidism develops. In normal persons, acute administration of large doses of iodide inhibits the organification of iodine and the synthesis of thyroid hormone (Wolff-Chaikoff effect). This effect is short-lived and does not lead to permanent hypothyroidism. When iodide administration continues, an autoregulatory mechanism in normal persons limits iodide trapping and permits the level of iodide in the thyroid to decrease and organification to proceed normally. In patients with iodide-induced goiter, this escape does not occur, because of an underlying abnormality of biosynthesis of thyroid hormone. The persons most susceptible to the development of iodide goiter are those with lymphocytic thyroiditis or with a subclinical inborn error in thyroid hormone synthesis and those who have had a partial thyroidectomy.

Lithium carbonate, which is used to treat bipolar disorder, also causes goiters and mild hypothyroidism. Lithium decreases T_4 and T_3 synthesis and release; the mechanism producing the goiter or hypothyroidism is similar to that described for iodide goiter. Lithium and iodide also act synergistically to produce goiter; their combined use should be avoided.

Amiodarone, a drug used to treat cardiac arrhythmias, can cause thyroid dysfunction with goiter because it is rich in iodine. It is also a potent inhibitor of 5′-deiodinase, preventing conversion of T_4 to T_3. It can cause hypothyroidism, particularly in patients with underlying autoimmune disease. In other patients, it can cause thyrotoxicosis through either transient thyroiditis or the Jod-Basedow effect.

SIMPLE GOITER (COLLOID GOITER)

A few children with euthyroid goiters have simple goiters, a condition of unknown cause not associated with hypothyroidism or hyperthyroidism and not caused by inflammation or neoplasia. The condition predominates in girls and has a peak incidence before and during the pubertal years. Histologic examination of the thyroid either is normal or reveals variable follicular size, dense colloid, and flattened epithelium. The goiter may be small or large. It is firm in half the patients and occasionally is asymmetric or nodular. Levels of TSH are normal or low, scintiscans are normal, and thyroid antibodies are absent. Differentiation from lymphocytic thyroiditis might not be possible without a biopsy, but biopsy is usually not indicated. Therapy with thyroid hormone can help prevent progression to a large multinodular goiter, although it is difficult to separate any treatment effects from the natural history, which is for the goiter to decrease in size. Patients should be reevaluated periodically, because some have antibody-negative lymphocytic thyroiditis and therefore are at risk for changes in thyroid function (see Chapter 566).

MULTINODULAR GOITER

Rarely, a firm goiter with a lobulated surface and single or multiple palpable nodules is encountered. Areas of cystic change, hemorrhage, and fibrosis may be present. The incidence of this condition has decreased markedly with the use of iodine-enriched salt. A mild goitrogenic stimulus, acting over a long time, is thought to be the cause. Ultrasonographic examination can reveal multiple nodules that are nonfunctioning on scintiscans. Thyroid studies are usually normal. Some children with chronic lymphocytic thyroiditis develop multinodular goiter; TSH may be elevated, and thyroid antibodies may be present.

Children can develop toxic multinodular goiter, characterized by a suppressed TSH and hyperthyroidism. The condition occurs in children with **McCune-Albright syndrome** (usually resulting in hyperthyroidism), with **TSH receptor–activating mutations,** and it has been described in 3 children (including 2 siblings) with digital anomalies and cystic kidney disease. If hypofunctioning nodules within a multinodular goiter grow to significant size (≥1 cm), fine-needle aspiration should be considered to rule out malignancy (see Chapter 569).

TOXIC GOITER (HYPERTHYROIDISM)

See Chapter 568.

Bibliography is available at Expert Consult.

Chapter 568
Hyperthyroidism
Stephen A. Huang and Stephen H. LaFranchi

Hyperthyroidism results from excessive secretion of thyroid hormone; during childhood, with few exceptions, it is caused by Graves disease (Table 568-1). **Graves disease** is an autoimmune disorder; production of thyroid-stimulating immunoglobulin that binds to and activates the G-protein–coupled **thyroid-stimulating hormone (TSH) receptor** results in diffuse toxic goiter. Other causes of hyperthyroidism include gain-of-function germline mutations in the **TSH receptor,** which are found in both familial (autosomal dominant) and sporadic cases of non–autoimmune hyperthyroidism. These patients, whose disease can appear in the neonatal period or in later childhood, have thyroid hyperplasia with goiter and suppressed levels of TSH. Different activating mutations have been identified in some cases of thyroid adenomas. Hyperthyroidism occurs in some patients with **McCune-Albright syndrome** as a result of an activating mutation of the α subunit of the G-protein; these patients tend to have a multinodular goiter. Other rare causes of thyrotoxicosis that have been observed in children include painless sporadic thyroiditis, subacute painful thyroiditis, acute suppurative thyroiditis, thyrotoxicosis factitia, TSH-secreting adenomas, and hyperfunctioning thyroid carcinoma.

Suppression of plasma TSH indicates that the hyperthyroidism is not pituitary in origin. Hyperthyroidism caused by inappropriate thyrotropin secretion is rare and, in most cases, is caused by dominant negative thyroid hormone receptor mutations and pituitary resistance to thyroid hormone. TSH-secreting pituitary tumors are extremely rare in the pediatric population. In infants born to mothers with Graves disease, hyperthyroidism is almost always a transitory phenomenon; classic Graves disease during the neonatal period is rare. Choriocarcinoma, hydatidiform mole, and struma ovarii have caused hyperthyroidism in adults but have not been recognized as causes in children.

Studies have examined the health and quality of life of individuals with subclinical hyperthyroidism (i.e., with TSH <0.1 mU/L, but normal serum thyroxine [T_4] and triiodothyronine [T_3] concentrations) or who are euthyroid on antithyroid medication. These studies indicate that subclinical hyperthyroidism carries a risk of late-life atrial fibrillation, but no similar risks have been identified in the general pediatric population. There appears to be no difference in long-term quality of life among hyperthyroid patients treated with antithyroid medication, radioiodine ablation, or surgery. Quality of life was diminished relative to control persons in all 3 cases (see Chapter 568.1).

Table 568-1	Causes of Hyperthyroidism		
CAUSES OF HYPERTHYROIDISM	**PATHOPHYSIOLOGIC FEATURES**	**INCIDENCE**	
CIRCULATING THYROID STIMULATORS			
Graves disease	Thyroid-stimulating immunoglobulins	Common	
Neonatal Graves disease	Thyroid-stimulating immunoglobulins	Rare	
Thyrotropin-secreting tumor	Pituitary adenoma	Very rare	
Choriocarcinoma	Human chorionic gonadotropin secretion stimulating the thyroid-stimulating hormone receptor	Rare	
THYROIDAL AUTONOMY			
Toxic multinodular goiter	Activating mutations in thyrotropin receptor or G-protein	Common	
Toxic solitary adenoma	Activating mutations in thyrotropin receptor or G-protein	Common	
Congenital hyperthyroidism	Activating mutations in thyrotropin receptor	Very rare	
Iodine-induced hyperthyroidism (Jod-Basedow phenomenon)	Unknown; excess iodine results in unregulated thyroid hormone production	Uncommon in United States and other iodine-sufficient areas	
DESTRUCTION OF THYROID FOLLICLES (THYROIDITIS)			
Subacute painful thyroiditis	Probable viral infection	Uncommon	
Painless sporadic thyroiditis (or postpartum thyroiditis)	Autoimmune	Common	
Amiodarone-induced thyroiditis	Direct toxic drug effects	Uncommon	
Acute (infectious) thyroiditis	Thyroid infection (e.g., bacterial, fungal) and release of preformed hormone	Uncommon	
EXOGENOUS THYROID HORMONE			
Iatrogenic	Overtreatment with thyroid hormone	Common	
Factitious	Excess ingestion of thyroid hormone	Rare	
Hamburger thyrotoxicosis	Thyroid gland included in ground beef	Probably rare	
ECTOPIC THYROID TISSUE			
Struma ovarii	Ovarian teratoma containing thyroid tissue	Rare	
Metastatic follicular thyroid cancer	Large tumor mass capable of secreting thyroid hormone autonomously	Rare	
Pituitary resistance to thyroid hormone	Mutated thyroid hormone receptor-β	Rare	

Adapted from Cooper DS: Hyperthyroidism, Lancet 362:459–468, 2003.

568.1 Graves Disease

Stephen A. Huang and Stephen H. LaFranchi

EPIDEMIOLOGY

Graves disease occurs in approximately 0.02% of children (1:5,000). It has a peak incidence in the 11-15 yr old age group; there is a 5:1 female:male ratio. Most children with Graves disease have a positive family history of some form of autoimmune thyroid disease. In Japan, familial Graves disease, defined as Graves disease in a 1st-degree relative, occurs in 2-3% of cases.

ETIOLOGY

Enlargement of the thymus, splenomegaly, lymphadenopathy, infiltration of the thyroid gland and retroorbital tissues with lymphocytes and plasma cells, and peripheral lymphocytosis are well-established findings in Graves disease. In the thyroid gland, T-helper cells (CD4$^+$) predominate in dense lymphoid aggregates; in areas of lower cell density, cytotoxic T cells (CD8$^+$) predominate. The percentage of activated B lymphocytes infiltrating the thyroid is higher than in peripheral blood. A postulated failure of T-suppressor cells allows expression of T-helper cells, sensitized to the TSH antigen, which interact with B cells. These cells differentiate into plasma cells, which produce thyrotropin receptor–stimulating antibody (TRSAb). TRSAb binds to the receptor for TSH and stimulates cyclic adenosine monophosphate, resulting in thyroid hyperplasia and unregulated overproduction of thyroid hormone. In addition to TRSAb, thyrotropin receptor–blocking antibody (TRBAb), which binds but does not activate the TSH receptor, may also be produced, and the clinical course of the disease usually correlates with the ratio between the 2 antibodies.

The ophthalmopathy occurring in Graves disease appears to be caused by antibodies against antigens shared by the thyroid and eye muscle. TSH receptors have been identified in retroorbital adipocytes and might represent a target for antibodies. The antibodies that bind to the extraocular muscles and orbital fibroblasts stimulate the synthesis of glycosaminoglycans by orbital fibroblasts and produce cytotoxic effects on muscle cells.

In whites, Graves disease is associated with human leukocyte antigen (HLA)-B8 and HLA-DR3; the latter carries a 7-fold relative risk for Graves disease. Graves disease is also associated with other HLA-D3–related disorders, such as Addison disease, type 1 diabetes mellitus, myasthenia gravis, and celiac disease. Systemic lupus erythematosus, rheumatoid arthritis, vitiligo, idiopathic thrombocytopenic purpura, and pernicious anemia have been described in children with Graves disease. In family clusters, the conditions associated most commonly with Graves disease are autoimmune lymphocytic thyroiditis and hypothyroidism. In Japanese children, Graves disease is associated with different HLA haplotypes: HLA-DRB1*0405 and HLA-DQB1*0401. In the Chinese population, the RNASET2-FGFR1OP-CCR6 region at 6q27 and an intergenic region at 4p14 are important susceptibility loci.

CLINICAL MANIFESTATIONS

Approximately 5% of all patients with hyperthyroidism are younger than 15 yr of age; the peak incidence in these children occurs during adolescence. Although rare, Graves disease has begun between 6 wk and 2 yr of age in children born to mothers without a history of hyperthyroidism. The incidence is approximately 5 times higher in girls than in boys.

The clinical course in children is highly variable but usually is not so fulminant as in many adults (Table 568-2). Symptoms develop gradually; the usual interval between onset and diagnosis is 6-12 mo and may be longer in prepubertal children compared with adolescents. The earliest signs in children may be emotional disturbances accompanied by motor hyperactivity. The children become irritable and excitable, and they cry easily because of emotional lability. They are restless sleepers and tend to kick their covers off. Their schoolwork suffers as a result of a short attention span and poor sleep. Tremor of the fingers can be

Table 568-2	Major Symptoms and Signs of Hyperthyroidism and of Graves Disease and Conditions Associated with Graves Disease

MANIFESTATIONS OF HYPERTHYROIDISM
Symptoms
Hyperactivity, irritability, altered mood, insomnia, anxiety, poor
  concentration
Heat intolerance, increased sweating
Palpitations
Fatigue, weakness
Dyspnea
Weight loss with increased appetite (weight gain in 10% of patients)
Pruritus
Increased stool frequency
Thirst and polyuria
Oligomenorrhea or amenorrhea
Signs
Sinus tachycardia, atrial fibrillation (rare in children), supraventricular
  tachycardia
Fine tremor, hyperkinesis, hyperreflexia
Warm, moist skin
Palmar erythema, onycholysis
Hair loss or thinning
Osteoporosis
Muscle weakness and wasting
High-output heart failure
Chorea
Periodic (hypokalemic) paralysis (primarily in Asian men)
Psychosis (rare)

MANIFESTATIONS OF GRAVES DISEASE
Diffuse goiter
Ophthalmopathy
A feeling of grittiness and discomfort in the eye
Retrobulbar pressure or pain
Eyelid lag or retraction
Periorbital edema, chemosis, scleral or conjunctival injection
Exophthalmos (proptosis)
Extraocular muscle dysfunction
Exposure keratitis
Optic neuropathy
Localized dermopathy (rare in children)
Lymphoid hyperplasia
Thyroid acropachy (rare in children)

CONDITIONS ASSOCIATED WITH GRAVES DISEASE
Type 1 diabetes mellitus
Addison disease
Vitiligo
Pernicious anemia
Alopecia areata
Myasthenia gravis
Celiac disease

Adapted from Weetman AP: Graves disease, N Engl J Med 343:1236–1248, 2000.

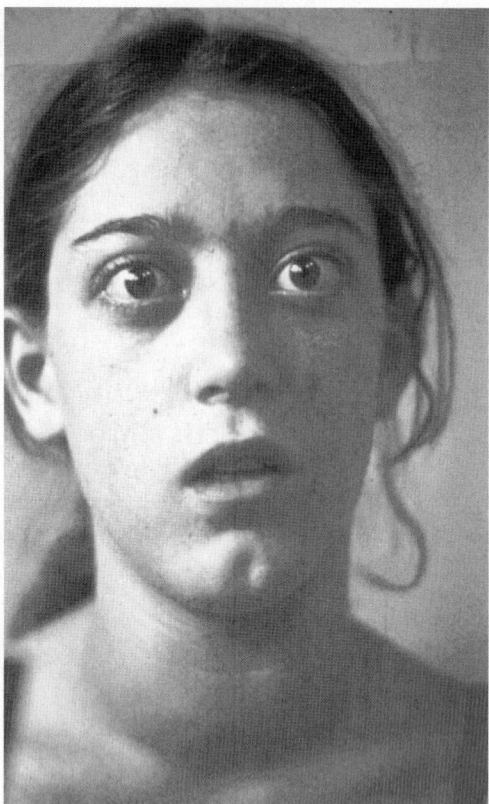

Figure 568-1 A 15 yr old girl with classic Graves disease. Clinical features include a goiter and exophthalmos. She was treated with antithyroid drugs, to which she had a good response.

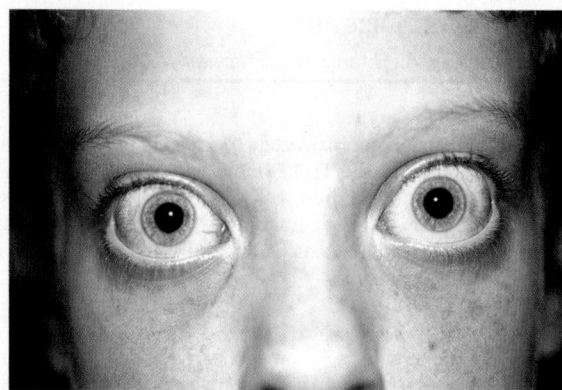

Figure 568-2 Retraction of upper eyelids in the primary gaze (Dalrymple sign). (*From Kanski JJ: Systemic diseases and the eye: signs and differential diagnosis, London, 2001, Mosby.*)

noticed if the arm is extended. There may be a voracious appetite combined with loss of or no increase in weight. Recent height measurements might show acceleration in growth velocity.

The size of the thyroid is variable. It may be so minimally enlarged that it initially escapes detection, but with careful examination, a diffuse goiter, soft with a smooth surface, is found in almost all patients. Exophthalmos is noticeable in most patients but is usually mild. Lagging of the upper eyelid as the eye looks downward, impairment of convergence, and retraction of the upper eyelid and infrequent blinking may be present (Figs. 568-1 and 568-2). Ocular manifestations can produce pain, lid erythema, chemosis, decreased extraocular muscle function, and decreased visual acuity (corneal or optic nerve involvement). The skin is smooth and flushed, with excessive sweating. Muscular weakness is uncommon but may be severe enough to result in

clumsiness. Tachycardia, palpitations, dyspnea, and cardiac enlargement and insufficiency cause discomfort but rarely endanger the patient's life. Atrial fibrillation is a rare complication. Mitral regurgitation, probably resulting from papillary muscle dysfunction, is the cause of the apical systolic murmur present in some patients. The systolic blood pressure and the pulse pressure are increased. Reflexes are brisk, especially the return phase of the Achilles reflex. Many of the findings in Graves disease result from hyperactivity of the sympathetic nervous system.

Thyroid crisis, or thyroid storm, is a form of hyperthyroidism manifested by a severe biochemical derangement, acute onset, hyperthermia, tachycardia, heart failure, and restlessness. There may be rapid progression to delirium, coma, and death. Precipitating events include trauma, infection, radioactive iodine treatment, or surgery. **Apathetic**

(or **masked**) **hyperthyroidism** is another variety of hyperthyroidism characterized by extreme listlessness, apathy, and cachexia. A combination of both forms can occur. These symptom complexes are rare in children.

LABORATORY FINDINGS

Levels of TSH are suppressed to below the lower range of normal. Serum levels of T_4, T_3, free T_4, and free T_3 are typically elevated. In some patients, levels of T_3 may be more elevated than those of T_4. Antithyroid antibodies, including thyroid peroxidase antibodies, are often present. Most patients with newly diagnosed Graves disease have measurable TRSAb; the 2 methods to measure TRSAb are thyroid-stimulating immunoglobulin or thyrotropin-binding inhibitory immunoglobulin. Measurement of thyroid-stimulating immunoglobulin or thyrotropin-binding inhibitory immunoglobulin is useful in confirming the diagnosis of Graves disease. Children who experience an acceleration of growth might also have advanced skeletal maturation. Bone density may be reduced at diagnosis but returns to normal with treatment.

DIFFERENTIAL DIAGNOSIS

Diagnosis is rarely difficult once hyperthyroidism is considered. Elevated levels of T_4 or free T_4 and T_3 in association with suppressed levels of TSH are usually diagnostic (see Table 568-1). The combination of diffuse goiter and prolonged hyperthyroidism is nearly always caused by Graves disease, and the presence of characteristic eye or skin changes is diagnostic. Documentation of elevated TRSAb can confirm the diagnosis.

Other causes of hyperthyroidism are uncommon. In rare cases where clinical assessment cannot distinguish Graves hyperthyroidism from painless sporadic thyroiditis, ^{123}I radioiodine uptake can be measured and used to determine the appropriateness of antithyroid medication. If a discrete thyroid nodule is palpated, a ^{123}I scan should be performed to assess the possibility of a hyperfunctioning nodule(s). Some children with toxic multinodular goiter may have either a TSH receptor–activating mutation or McCune-Albright syndrome. If precocious puberty, polyostotic fibrous dysplasia, or café-au-lait pigmentation is present, the autonomous thyroid disorder of McCune-Albright syndrome is likely. Patients with generalized thyroid hormone resistance have elevated levels of free T_4 and free T_3, but levels of TSH are inappropriately elevated or normal. They must be differentiated from patients with TSH-secreting pituitary tumors who have elevated serum levels of the TSH α subunit. Most other causes of hyperthyroxinemia are uncommon but can result in erroneous diagnosis. Patients with elevated T_4-binding globulin levels or familial dysalbuminemic hyper-

thyroxinemia have normal levels of free T_4 and TSH. Rare patients with mutations in *SLC16A2* (encoding the MCT8 thyroid hormone transporter) or *THRA* (encoding thyroid hormone receptor α) can present with high serum T_3 and inappropriately normal or high TSH but low serum T_4 concentrations.

When hyperthyroxinemia is caused by **exogenous thyroid hormone (thyrotoxicosis factitia),** levels of free T_4 and TSH are the same as those seen in Graves disease but, in contrast to Graves hyperthyroidism, serum thyroglobulin is very low, thyroid size is small, and ^{123}I radioiodine uptake is suppressed.

TREATMENT

Most pediatric endocrinologists recommend initial medical therapy using antithyroid drugs rather than radioiodine or subtotal thyroidectomy, although radioiodine is gaining acceptance as initial treatment in children older than 10 yr of age. All therapeutic options have advantages and disadvantages (Table 568-3). The 2 antithyroid drugs used historically are propylthiouracil and methimazole (Tapazole). Both compounds inhibit incorporation of trapped inorganic iodide into organic compounds. However, there are important differences between the drugs. Methimazole is at least 10 times more potent than propylthiouracil on a weight basis and has a much longer serum half-life (6-8 hr vs 0.5 hr); propylthiouracil generally is administered 3 times daily, but methimazole can be given once daily. Unlike methimazole, propylthiouracil is heavily protein bound and has a lesser ability to cross the placenta and to pass into breast milk; theoretically, therefore, propylthiouracil is the preferred drug during pregnancy and for nursing mothers. Because of reports of **severe liver disease** in patients treated with **propylthiouracil,** with some patients requiring liver transplant or potentially suffering a fatal outcome, the consensus is to **use only methimazole** to treat children with Graves disease.

Adverse reactions occur with antithyroid drugs; most are mild, but some are life-threatening. Minor adverse effects occur in approximately 10-20%, and more-severe adverse effects occur in 2-5% of children. Reactions are unpredictable and can occur after therapy of any duration. Transient granulocytopenia (<2,000/mm^3) is common; it is asymptomatic and is not a harbinger of agranulocytosis, and it usually is not a reason to discontinue treatment. Transient urticarial rashes are common. They may be managed by a short period off therapy, and then restarting the antithyroid drug. The most severe reactions are hypersensitive and include agranulocytosis (0.1-0.5%), hepatitis (0.2-1.0%), a lupus-like polyarthritis syndrome, glomerulonephritis, and an antineutrophilic cytoplasmic antibody–positive vasculitis involving the skin and other organs. **Severe liver disease**, including liver failure requiring transplantation, have been reported **exclusively**

Table 568-3	Treatments for Hyperthyroidism Caused by Graves Disease		
TREATMENT	**ADVANTAGE**	**DISADVANTAGE**	**COMMENT**
Antithyroid drugs	Noninvasive Less initial cost Low risk of permanent hypothyroidism Possible remission	Cure rate 30-80% (average: 40-50%) Adverse drug reactions Drug compliance required	First-line treatment in children and adolescents and in pregnancy Initial treatment in severe cases or preoperative preparation
Radioactive iodine (^{131}I)	Cure of hyperthyroidism Most cost-effective	Permanent hypothyroidism is almost inevitable Might worsen ophthalmopathy Pregnancy must be deferred for 6-12 mo, mother cannot breastfeed; small potential risk of exacerbation of hyperthyroidism	No evidence for infertility, birth defects, cancer when currently recommended doses are applied
Surgery	Rapid, effective treatment especially in patients with large goiter	Most invasive therapy Potential complications (recurrent laryngeal nerve damage, hypoparathyroidism) Most costly therapy Permanent hypothyroidism; pain; scarring	Potential use in pregnancy if major side effect from antithyroid drugs Useful when coexisting suspicious nodule is present or thyromegaly is massive Option for patients who refuse radioiodine

From Cooper DS: Hyperthyroidism, Lancet 362:459–468, 2003.

with propylthiouracil. The most common liver disease associated with methimazole is cholestatic jaundice, reversible when the drug is discontinued. Patients with severe adverse effects should be treated with radioiodine or thyroidectomy. In rare instances where hyperthyroidism is severe and methimazole cannot be used, a short course of propylthiouracil may be offered to restore euthyroidism prior to definitive therapy. Cases of congenital skin defects (aplasia cutis) have been seen in infants exposed in fetal life to methimazole, but this association does not appear to be a strong one.

The initial dosage of methimazole is 0.25-1.0 mg/kg/24 hr given once or twice daily. Smaller initial dosages should be used in early childhood. Careful surveillance is required after treatment is initiated. Rising serum levels of TSH to greater than normal indicates overtreatment and leads to increased size of the goiter. Clinical response becomes apparent in 3-6 wk, and adequate control is evident in 3-4 mo. The dose is decreased to the minimal level required to maintain a euthyroid state.

Most studies report a remission rate of approximately 25% after 2 yr of antithyroid drug treatment in children. Some studies find that longer treatment is associated with higher remission rates, with 1 study reporting a 50% remission rate after 4.5 yr of drug treatment. If a relapse occurs, it usually appears within 3 mo and almost always within 6 mo after therapy has been discontinued. Therapy may be resumed in case of relapse. Patients older than 13 yr of age, boys, those with a higher body mass index, and those with small goiters and modestly elevated T_3 levels appear to have earlier remissions.

A β-adrenergic blocking agent such as propranolol (0.5-2.0 mg/kg/24 hr orally, divided 3 times daily) or atenolol (1-2 mg/kg orally given once daily) is a useful supplement to antithyroid drugs in the management of severely toxic patients. Table 568-4 lists additional therapies for **thyroid storm.** Thyroid hormones potentiate the actions of catecholamines, including tachycardia, tremor, excessive sweating, lid lag, and stare. These symptoms abate with the use of propranolol, which does not, however, alter thyroid function or exophthalmos.

Radioiodine treatment or surgery is indicated when adequate cooperation for medical management is not possible, when an adequate trial of medical management has failed to result in permanent remission, or when severe side effects preclude further use of antithyroid drugs. Either of these treatments may also be preferred by the patient or parent.

Radioiodine is an effective therapy for Graves disease in children. In patients with severe thyrotoxicosis, euthyroidism should be restored with methimazole prior to radioablation in order to deplete the gland of preformed hormone and reduce the risk of thyrotoxic flare from radiation thyroiditis. If a patient is taking thionamides, they must be stopped 3-5 days before radioiodine administration to avoid inhibition of uptake. In children, the goal is to select a dose of radioiodine high enough to ensure complete ablation of thyroid tissue. Most centers obtain a diagnostic radioiodine uptake measurement before treatment and then use this to calculate a ^{131}I dose that delivers an absorbed thyroid dose of >150 μCi/g. Alternatively, an empirical fixed ^{131}I dose (usually 15 mCi) can be offered. The theoretical advantage of calculated doses is that they define for each individual patient the lowest administered dose that achieves the therapeutic target. This benefit is most important in small children, as the absorbed radiation dose to the bone marrow and other normal tissues is inversely proportional to body size. Based upon this concept and theoretical modeling of radiation exposure, current consensus guidelines recommend that ^{131}I therapy be avoided in very small children who are younger than 5 yr of age and that administered doses in children between 5 and 10 yr of age be <10 mCi. As with other Graves therapies, ^{131}I ablation has a low but obligate failure rate (5-20%). Patients with persistent hyperthyroidism more than 6 mo after their first ^{131}I therapy can be offered retreatment.

Thyroidectomy, a safe procedure when performed by an experienced surgeon, is done only after the patient has been brought to a euthyroid state. This may be accomplished with methimazole over 2-3 mo. After a euthyroid state has been attained, a saturated solution of potassium iodide, 3-5 drops 3 times per day, is added to the regimen for 2 wk before surgery to decrease the vascularity of the gland. In expert hands, complications of surgical treatment are rare and include hypoparathyroidism (transient or permanent) and paralysis of the vocal cords. The incidence of residual or recurrent hyperthyroidism or hypothyroidism depends on the extent of the surgery. Most recommend near-total thyroidectomy. The incidence of recurrence is low, and most patients become hypothyroid. Referral to a surgeon with extensive experience in thyroidectomy and a low personal complication rate is paramount.

The **ophthalmopathy** usually remits gradually and independently of the hyperthyroidism. Severe ophthalmopathy can require treatment with high-dose prednisone, orbital radiotherapy (of questionable value), or orbital decompression surgery. Cigarette smoking is a risk factor for thyroid eye disease and should be avoided or discontinued to avoid progression of eye involvement.

Bibliography is available at Expert Consult.

568.2 Congenital Hyperthyroidism

Stephen A. Huang and Stephen H. LaFranchi

ETIOLOGY AND PATHOGENESIS

Neonatal Graves disease is caused by transplacental passage of TRSAb, but the clinical onset, severity, and course may be modified by the concurrent presence of thyrotropin receptor–blocking antibody and by the transplacental passage of antithyroid drugs taken by the mother. Very high levels of TRSAb usually result in classic neonatal hyperthyroidism, but if the infant has been exposed to antithyroid drugs, onset of symptoms is delayed by 3-4 days as the maternally derived antithyroid drug is metabolized. If thyrotropin receptor–blocking antibody is also present, onset of hyperthyroid symptoms may be delayed for several weeks. The mothers of these infants have active Graves disease, Graves disease in remission, a past history of Graves disease managed by radioactive iodine ablation or surgery, or rarely hypothyroidism and a history of lymphocytic thyroiditis.

Neonatal hyperthyroidism occurs in only approximately 2% of infants born to mothers with a history of Graves disease. Fetal tachycardia and goiter can allow prenatal diagnosis and fetal ultrasound

Table 568-4	Management of Thyroid Storm in Adolescents
GOAL	**TREATMENT**
Inhibition of thyroid hormone formation and secretion	Propylthiouracil, 400 mg every 8 hr PO or by nasogastric tube Saturated solution of potassium iodide, 3 drops every 8 hr
Sympathetic blockade	Propranolol, 20-40 mg every 4-6 hr or 1 mg IV slowly (repeat doses until heart rate slows); not indicated in patients with asthma or heart failure that is not rate related
Glucocorticoid therapy	Prednisone 20 mg bid
Supportive therapy	Intravenous fluids (depending on indication: glucose, electrolytes, multivitamins) Temperature control (cooling blankets, acetaminophen; avoid salicylates) O₂ if required Digitalis for heart failure and to slow ventricular response; pentobarbital for sedation Treatment of precipitating event (e.g., infection)

From Goldman L, Ausiello D, editors: Cecil textbook of medicine, ed 22, Philadelphia, 2004, WB Saunders, p. 1401.

surveillance is recommended in mothers with uncontrolled hyperthyroidism, elevated serum titers of TRSAb (thyrotropin-binding inhibitory immunoglobulin more than 3 times the upper limit of normal), or the history of a prior child with neonatal thyroid dysfunction. Unlike Graves disease at all other ages, neonatal hyperthyroidism affects boys as often as girls. One would expect twins to be equally affected, but 1 case reported 1 twin to be hyperthyroid and the other twin to be hypothyroid. Both eventually recovered to euthyroidism.

The disorder usually remits spontaneously within 6-12 wk but can persist longer, depending on the levels of TRSAb. Mild asymptomatic hyperthyroxinemia also occurs. Rarely, classic neonatal Graves disease does not remit but persists for several years or longer. These children have impressive family histories of Graves disease. In these infants, TRSAb transfer from the mother apparently blends with the infantile onset of autonomous Graves disease.

CLINICAL MANIFESTATIONS

Many of the infants are premature and appear to have intrauterine growth restriction. Most have goiters. The infant is extremely restless, irritable, and hyperactive and appears anxious and unusually alert. Microcephaly and ventricular enlargement may be present. The eyes are opened widely and appear exophthalmic (Fig. 568-3). There may be extreme tachycardia and tachypnea, and the temperature is elevated. In severely affected infants, there is a progression of symptoms; weight loss occurs despite a ravenous appetite, hepatosplenomegaly increases, and jaundice can occur. Severe hypertension and cardiac decompensation can occur. The infant can die if therapy is not instituted promptly. The serum levels of T_4 or free T_4 and T_3 are markedly elevated, and TSH is suppressed. Advanced bone age, frontal bossing with triangular facies, and cranial synostosis are common, especially in infants with persistent clinical manifestations of hyperthyroidism.

TREATMENT

Treatment of the neonate consists of oral administration of propranolol (1-2 mg/kg/24 hr, orally in 3 divided doses) and methimazole (0.25-1.0 mg/kg/24 hr given every 12 hr); saturated solution of potassium iodide (1 drop per day) may be added. When propranolol is used during pregnancy to treat thyrotoxicosis, it crosses the placenta and can cause respiratory depression in the newborn infant. If the thyrotoxic state is severe, parenteral fluid therapy and corticosteroids may be indicated. If heart failure occurs, digitalization is indicated. After a euthyroid state is reached, antithyroid medications should be gradually tapered to keep the infant euthyroid. Most cases remit by 3-4 mo of age.

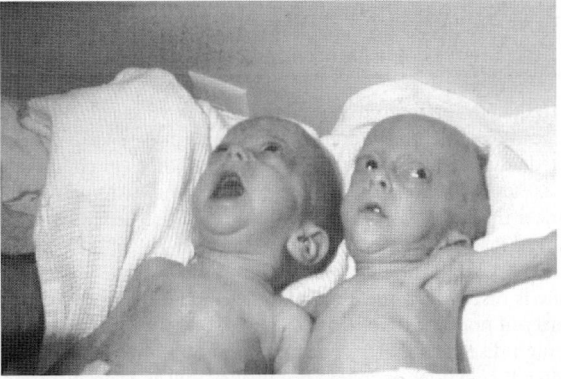

Figure 568-3 Twin boys with neonatal hyperthyroidism confirmed by abnormal thyroid function tests. Clinical features include lack of subcutaneous tissue owing to a hypermetabolic state and a wide-eyed, anxious stare. They were given the diagnosis of neonatal Graves disease, but, in fact, their mother did not have Graves disease; they had persistent, not transient, hyperthyroidism. At age 8 yr, they were treated with radioiodine. They are now believed to have had some other form of neonatal hyperthyroidism, such as a constitutive activation of the thyroid-stimulating hormone receptor.

Occasionally, neonatal hyperthyroidism does not remit but persists into childhood. These patients can have an impressive family history of hyperthyroidism. Neonatal hyperthyroidism, without evidence for autoimmune disease in mother or infant, may be caused by a mutation in the *TSHR* gene that produced constitutive activation of the receptor. Neonatal hyperthyroidism has also been reported in patients with McCune-Albright syndrome, a result of an activating mutation of the α subunit of the G-protein. Under these circumstances, hyperthyroidism recurs when antithyroid drugs are discontinued; these children eventually must be treated with radioiodine or surgery.

PROGNOSIS

Advanced osseous maturation, microcephaly, and cognitive impairment occur when treatment is delayed. Intellectual development is normal in most treated infants with neonatal Graves disease, though some manifest neurocognitive problems from in utero hyperthyroidism. In some infants, in utero hyperthyroidism appears to suppress the hypothalamic-pituitary-thyroid feedback mechanism, and they develop permanent central hypothyroidism, requiring lifelong thyroid hormone treatment.

Bibliography is available at Expert Consult.

Chapter 569
Carcinoma of the Thyroid

Stephen A. Huang and
Stephen H. LaFranchi

EPIDEMIOLOGY

Carcinoma of the thyroid is rare in childhood; the annual incidence in children younger than 15 yr of age is approximately 2 in 100,000 cases, compared with an annual incidence at all ages around the world of 4-10 in 100,000 cases. In the last 2 decades, the incidence in children has increased 2-fold. Compared to adults, childhood thyroid cancers are characterized by dramatically higher rates of metastasis and recurrence. Despite being widespread at discovery, pediatric thyroid cancers usually have an indolent course and, with adequate treatment, most patients have a favorable outcome.

PATHOGENESIS

At all ages, the vast majority of differentiated thyroid cancers are of follicular cell origin and, in North America, **papillary carcinoma** (88%) is the most common subtype. Interestingly, while their histologic features are similar, the thyroid cancers of childhood are genetically distinct from their adult counterparts. Although up to 70% of adults with papillary thyroid cancer exhibit pathogenic somatic mutations in *BRAF* or *RAS,* these mutations are extremely rare in children with papillary cancer. In contrast, *RET-PTC* translocations, which result in chimeric proteins containing the tyrosine kinase domains of RET fused to the regulatory sequences of ubiquitously expressed genes such as *H1* and *ELE1,* are often found in childhood thyroid cancers. After papillary thyroid cancer, follicular cancer (10%) is the next most common type of childhood thyroid cancer. Medullary cancer (2%) and anaplastic thyroid cancers are relatively rare. Of note, only thyroid cancers of follicular cell origin (papillary and follicular carcinomas) respond to the adjunctive therapies of ^{131}I therapy and thyroid-stimulating hormone (TSH) suppression.

Up to 10% of cases of follicular cell–derived thyroid cancers are familial, and these are usually inherited in an autosomal dominant manner. Familial syndromes associated with an increased risk of thyroid neoplasia include Cowden syndrome (characterized by mucocutaneous lesions, breast cancer, macrocephaly, and endometrial tumors) and familial adenomatous polyposis. Germline mutations in the *DICER-1* gene have also been recognized as a cause of thyroid neoplasia. The evaluation of a child with thyroid nodule should include a medical and family history to assess for features of these syndromes.

The thyroid gland of children is unusually sensitive to exposure to external radiation. There probably is no threshold dose; 1 Gy results in a 7.7 relative risk of thyroid cancer. In the past, approximately 80% of children with cancer of the thyroid had received inappropriate therapeutic irradiation of the neck and adjacent areas during infancy for benign conditions such as "enlarged" thymus, hypertrophied tonsils and adenoids, hemangiomas, nevi, eczema, tinea capitis, and "cervical adenitis." With the discontinuation of irradiation for benign conditions, this cause of thyroid cancer has vanished. The long-term survival of children who have received appropriate therapeutic irradiation of areas of the neck for neoplastic disease has made this cause of thyroid cancer and nodules increasingly prevalent; increased dose, younger age at time of treatment, and female sex are factors that increase the risk of thyroid cancer. Long-term risk data for cancer are sparse, but 15-50% of children who have received irradiation and chemotherapy for Hodgkin disease, leukemia, bone marrow transplantation, brain tumors, and other malignancies of the head and neck have elevated levels of TSH within the 1st yr of therapy, and 5-20% progress to hypothyroidism during the next 5-7 yr. Most large groups of treated children have a 10-30% incidence of benign thyroid nodules and an increased incidence of thyroid cancer. The latter begins to appear within 3-5 yr after radiation treatment and reaches a peak in 15-25 yr. It is unknown whether there is a period after which no more tumors develop. Administration of ^{131}I for diagnostic or therapeutic purposes does not appear to increase the risk of thyroid cancer.

Thyroid cancer has been reported in children with congenital goiter or ectopic thyroid tissue. In these patients, and also in children with autoimmune thyroiditis and hypothyroidism, chronic TSH stimulation appears to play a pathogenic role. It is unclear if the course of thyroid cancer differs in these patients compared to the general population. From a practical standpoint, nodules that are detected in the context of these disorders should be fully evaluated for cancer risk as in other children.

CLINICAL MANIFESTATIONS

The incidence of childhood thyroid cancer peaks in adolescence and girls are more commonly affected than boys. A painless nodule in the thyroid or in the neck is the usual presentation of disease. Rapid growth and large nodule size, firmness, fixation to adjacent tissues, hoarseness, dysphagia, and neck lymphadenopathy should heighten the concern for thyroid cancer. Cervical lymph node metastasis is common, so any unexplained cervical lymph node enlargement warrants examination of the thyroid. The lungs are the most common site of distant metastasis. There may be no clinical manifestations referable to them and formal pulmonary function testing may be normal even with widespread macroscopic metastases. Radiologically, they appear as diffuse miliary or nodular infiltrations, typically greatest in the posterior basal portions. They may be mistaken for tuberculosis, histoplasmosis, or sarcoidosis. Other sites of metastasis include the mediastinum, axilla, long bones, skull, and brain. Almost all children are euthyroid, but rarely, the carcinoma is functional and produces symptoms of hyperthyroidism.

DIAGNOSIS

As detailed in the following section, patients usually present with a neck mass and virtually all have a thyroid nodule of significant size upon ultrasound. While several imaging features are significantly associated with thyroid cancer risk, none have sufficient negative predictive value to forgo tissue diagnosis. Papillary thyroid cancer is characterized by nuclear abnormalities that are well identified by cytology and *fine-needle aspiration is the gold standard* in the evaluation of adults with nodules. Growing literature supports its use in the pediatric population. In most cases, operative pathology is required to confirm the diagnosis of thyroid cancer and to stage the extent of disease.

TREATMENT

The primary therapy for thyroid cancer is surgical resection. Because intrathyroidal spread is common in papillary thyroid, near-total thyroidectomy is the favored approach. Prior to this surgery, neck ultrasonography should be performed to screen for sonographically abnormal lymph nodes. Suspicious lymph nodes may be biopsied preoperatively to determine the appropriateness and extent of initial lymph node dissection. With the exception of very-low-risk patients, thyroidectomy is usually followed by adjunctive therapy with both TSH suppression (dosing levothyroxine to lower serum TSH and deprive residual thyroid cancer cells of this growth factor) and ^{131}I therapy (to ablate the normal thyroid remnant and/or to treat residual thyroid cancer).

PROGNOSIS

Although extrathyroidal invasion and distant metastasis are more common in the pediatric population, most children with thyroid cancer have a good outcome. Families should be counseled that the response to ^{131}I therapy is slow and that repeated treatments and years of care may be required to eliminate the disease. They should further be informed that many patients who are unable to achieve complete cure can be maintained in the well state with stable or slowly progressive cancer burden. For rare children with aggressive cancers that progress despite the optimization of conventional therapies, newer options, such as oral tyrosine kinase inhibitors, are available through research trials or on a compassionate basis. As with any cancer, psychosocial supports must be available, including access to social work and other mental health professionals.

Among solid tumors, thyroid cancer is unique in its capacity for late recurrence, sometimes occurring decades after initial presentation. For this reason, all children with thyroid cancer deserve lifelong monitoring for disease progression. For most patients, serum thyroglobulin is a sensitive and specific cancer marker. However, it must be recognized that about one fourth of patients have circulating antithyroglobulin autoantibodies that interfere with standard thyroglobulin assays and produce artifactually low measurements. Because of this, antithyroglobulin autoantibodies must always be measured whenever serum thyroglobulin is assayed to confirm the latter's reliability. As most thyroid cancer recurrences are local, surveillance should include serial neck ultrasounds. Patients with higher recurrence risk or documentation of distant metastases typically benefit from additional anatomic imaging studies and from extended surveillance studies performed during TSH stimulation.

Bibliography is available at Expert Consult.

569.1 Solitary Thyroid Nodule
Stephen A. Huang and Stephen H. LaFranchi

The frequency of thyroid nodules increases with age. While sonographically detectable nodules are present in 19-67% of randomly selected adults, the estimated frequency of nodules in children is only 0.05-2.0%. Although early pediatric series cited extremely high rates of cancer in thyroid nodules (up to 70%), more recent studies of children report lower cancer prevalence (around 20-26%) that is similar to the 5-15% prevalence observed in adults. Thus, when a thyroid nodule is discovered in a child, parents should be counseled that the majority of nodules are benign.

Benign disorders that can occur as a solitary thyroid mass include benign adenomatous or colloid nodules, as well as a variety of congenital cysts (Table 569-1). A suddenly appearing or rapidly enlarging thyroid mass can indicate hemorrhage into a cyst or benign adenoma. When evaluating a child with a thyroid nodule, it is helpful to begin by measuring serum TSH.

In rare patients who present with a suppressed serum TSH, a thyroid scan, preferably using ^{123}I or ^{99m}Tc-pertechnetate, should be performed to assess the possibility of a benign hyperfunctioning thyroid nodule. All other patients should proceed directly to ultrasound and, if a

Table 569-1	Etiologic Classification of Solitary Thyroid Nodules

Lymphoid follicle, as part of chronic lymphocytic thyroiditis
Thyroid developmental anomalies
  Intrathyroidal thyroglossal duct cyst
Thyroid abscess (acute suppurative thyroiditis)
Simple cyst
  Neoplasms
    Benign
      Colloid (adenomatous) nodule
      Follicular adenoma
      Toxic adenoma
      Nonthyroidal (e.g., lymphohemangioma)
    Malignant
      Papillary carcinoma
      Follicular carcinoma
      Mixed papillary-follicular carcinoma
      Undifferentiated (anaplastic)
      Medullary carcinoma
  Nonthyroidal
    Lymphoma
    Teratoma

discrete nodule(s) of significant size is documented by this imaging, it should be biopsied by ultrasound-guided fine-needle aspiration (FNA). FNA cytology may be interpreted as benign, positive for papillary thyroid cancer, indeterminate, or inadequate. When an initial biopsy is nondiagnostic, an adequate sample can usually be obtained by repeating aspiration. Multiple categorization systems exist and most North American centers follow the Bethesda Criteria for interpretation of thyroid cytology. The predictive value of thyroid FNA varies between institutions. In most high-volume centers, the "positive for papillary thyroid cancer" category corresponds to a >98% likelihood of cancer and, in that context, near-total thyroidectomy is appropriate. In children with indeterminate cytology and unilateral nodules, lobectomy is commonly performed. This is followed by completion thyroidectomy if lobectomy pathology shows a significant cancer. Patients with cytologically benign nodules can be offered the option of deferring surgery so long as they are willing to commit to careful surveillance with serial neck imaging.

Bibliography is available at Expert Consult.

569.2 Medullary Thyroid Carcinoma

Stephen H. LaFranchi

Medullary thyroid carcinoma (MTC) arises from the parafollicular cells (C cells) of the thyroid and accounts for approximately 2% of thyroid malignancies in children. The majority of MTC cases are sporadic, but approximately 25% are familial, autosomal dominant disorders. Hereditary MTC is divided into 3 distinct syndromes: multiple endocrine neoplasia type 2A (MEN2A), multiple endocrine neoplasia type 2B (MEN2B), and familial MTC. In contrast to the somatic mutations associated with sporadic MTC, germline mutations in the *RET* protooncogene on chromosome 10q11.2 are inheritable and can cause familial medullary thyroid cancer. Once an index case is diagnosed in a family, it is important to pinpoint the specific *RET* mutation and then genotype all 1st-degree relatives for the mutation. Many *RET* mutations have been well studied and strong genotype–phenotype associations have been established to predict disease aggressiveness. In carriers, thyroidectomy before the MTC has spread outside the gland represents the best chance for a cure and the patient's specific genotype can be used to guide the timing of prophylactic surgery.

The most common presentation of sporadic MTC is an asymptomatic, palpable thyroid nodule. When the tumor occurs sporadically, it is usually unicentric, but in the familial form, it is usually multicentric, and it begins as hyperplasia of parafollicular cells. The diagnosis of

MTC can often be made through routine FNA cytology, but documentation of high calcitonin in an FNA washing or in the patients' serum is helpful as confirmation. The diagnosis of MTC warrants genetic testing for *RET* mutation and screens for MEN2-associated pheochromocytoma and hyperparathyroidism should be obtained prior to anesthesia for thyroidectomy. No clinically recognizable manifestations result from the elevated serum levels of calcitonin or CEA. Nonetheless, these tests are helpful in screening and monitoring therapy.

MULTIPLE ENDOCRINE NEOPLASIA, TYPE 2A

MEN2A is an autosomal dominant disorder characterized by MTC, pheochromocytoma, and parathyroid hyperplasia. At least 19 different specific missense mutations of exon 10 or 11 of the extracellular domain of the *RET* gene have been described for MEN2A and for cases of familial MTC. DNA analysis permits unambiguous identification of carriers of the *RET* protooncogene mutation. Penetrance of MTC is close to 100%, but there is much variability in the other manifestations of MEN2A. C-cell hyperplasia or MTC usually appears earlier than pheochromocytoma. Pheochromocytomas are often bilateral and may be multiple. Adrenal medullary hyperplasia is known to precede pheochromocytoma, but the detectable latent period is short. Hypercalcemia is a late manifestation and indicates hyperparathyroidism. The parathyroid glands might reveal chief-cell hyperplasia or only hypercellularity.

MULTIPLE ENDOCRINE NEOPLASIA, TYPE 2B

MEN2B is an autosomal dominant disorder characterized by MTC and pheochromocytomas but not hyperparathyroidism. The distinguishing feature of MEN2B, also called the **mucosal neuroma syndrome,** is the occurrence of multiple neuromas and a characteristic phenotype that includes Marfan-like facies. A missense mutation of the *RET* protooncogene in exon 16, the tyrosine catalytic domain of *RET,* is found in 93% of families; all patients have had the same point mutation.

The neuromas most often occur on the tongue, buccal mucosa, lips, and conjunctivae. Peripheral neurofibromas and café-au-lait patches may be present, and intestinal ganglioneuromatosis is common. Diffuse proliferation of nerves and ganglion cells is found in mucosal, submucosal, myenteric, and subserosal plexus involving the small and large bowel as well as the esophagus. The patients may be tall, with arachnodactyly and a Marfan-like appearance. Scoliosis, pectus excavatum, pes cavus, and muscular hypotonia are common. The eyelids may be thickened and everted, the lips patulous and blubbery, the jaw prognathic. Feeding difficulties, poor sucking, diarrhea, constipation, and failure to thrive can begin in infancy or early childhood, many years before the appearance of neuromas or endocrine symptoms.

TREATMENT

Total thyroidectomy is indicated for all children who are shown by genetic studies to carry high-risk *RET* mutations. Recognition of familial forms of this tumor is critical to the early diagnosis and intervention in children at risk. MTC develops at an earlier age in patients with MEN2B and is more aggressive than in MEN2A. MTC has been seen in a 6 mo old child with MEN2B and in a 3 yr old child with MEN2A. In MEN2A, there is genotype–phenotype correlation between the specific mutation and the onset of C-cell hyperplasia or MTC. With codon 634 mutations, MTC occurs at an early age, whereas with mutations at codons 618, 620, and 804, MTC tends to occur at a later age. In young children, recommendations for the timing of prophylactic thyroidectomy are available for the common *RET* mutations. All these children should be screened for pheochromocytoma before surgery. Monitoring the serum levels of calcitonin and carcinoembryonic antigen is useful in following the course of the disease after operation and in detecting metastatic lesions. Periodic screening for the development of pheochromocytoma and hyperparathyroidism is indicated. Metastases to the regional lymph nodes and to the liver can occur. Early clinic studies support that prophylactic thyroidectomy is effective in preventing death from MTC.

Bibliography is available at Expert Consult.

Section 3

Disorders of the Parathyroid Gland

Chapter 570

Hormones and Peptides of Calcium Homeostasis and Bone Metabolism

Daniel A. Doyle

Parathyroid hormone (PTH) and vitamin D are the principal regulators of calcium homeostasis (see Chapters 48 and 694). Calcitonin and PTH-related peptide (PTHrP) are important primarily in the fetus.

PARATHYROID HORMONE

PTH is an 84-amino-acid chain (95 kDa), but its biologic activity resides in the first 34 residues. In the parathyroid gland, a pre-pro-PTH (115-amino-acid chain) and a pro-PTH (90 amino acids) are synthesized. Pre-pro-PTH is converted to pro-PTH and pro-PTH to PTH. PTH (consisting of amino acids 1-84) is the major secretory product of the gland, but it is rapidly cleaved in the liver and kidney into smaller COOH-terminal, mid-region, and NH₂-terminal fragments.

The occurrence of these fragments in serum has led to the development of a variety of assays. The 1-34 aminoterminal (N-terminus) fragments possess biologic activity but are present in low amounts in the circulation; assay of these fragments is most useful for detecting acute secretory changes. The carboxyterminal (C-terminus) and midregion fragments, although biologically inert, are cleared more slowly from the circulation and represent 80% of plasma immunoreactive PTH; concentrations of the C-terminal fragment are 50-500 times the level of the active hormone. The C-terminal assays are effective in detecting hyperparathyroidism, but because C-terminal fragments are removed from the circulation by glomerular filtration, these assays are less useful for evaluating the secondary hyperparathyroidism characteristic of renal disease. Only certain sensitive radioimmunoassays for PTH can differentiate the subnormal concentrations that occur in hypoparathyroidism from normal levels.

When serum levels of calcium fall, the signal is transduced through the calcium-sensing receptor, and secretion of PTH increases (Fig. 570-1). PTH stimulates activity of 1α-hydroxylase in the kidney, enhancing production of 1,25-dihydroxycholecalciferol, also written 1,25(OH)₂D₃. The increased level of 1,25(OH)₂D₃ induces synthesis of a calcium-binding protein (calbindin-D) in the intestinal mucosa, with resultant absorption of calcium. PTH also mobilizes calcium by directly enhancing bone resorption, an effect that requires 1,25(OH)₂D₃. The effects of PTH on bone and kidney are mediated through binding to specific receptors on the membranes of target cells and through activation of a transduction pathway involving a G-protein coupled to the adenylate cyclase system (see Chapter 572).

The calcium-sensing receptor regulates the secretion of PTH and the reabsorption of calcium by the renal tubules in response to alterations in serum calcium concentrations. The gene for the receptor is located on chromosome 3q13.3-q21 and encodes a cell surface protein that is expressed in parathyroid glands and kidneys and belongs to the family of G-protein–coupled receptors. In the normally functioning calcium-sensing receptor, hypocalcemia induces increased secretion of PTH and hypercalcemia depresses PTH secretion. Loss-of-function mutations cause an increased set point with respect to serum calcium, resulting in hypercalcemia and in the conditions of **familial hypocalciuric hypercalcemia** and neonatal severe hyperparathyroidism. Acquired hypocalciuric hypercalcemia may be a result of autoantibodies to the calcium-sensing receptor and manifests with hypercalcemia and hyperparathyroidism. Gain-of-function mutations result in depressed secretion of PTH in response to hypocalcemia, leading to the syndrome of familial hypocalcemia with hypercalciuria (see Fig. 570-1).

PARATHYROID HORMONE–RELATED PEPTIDE

PTHrP is homologous to PTH only in the first 13 amino acids of its amino terminus, 8 of which are identical to PTH. Its gene is on the short arm of chromosome 12 and that of PTH is on the short arm of chromosome 11.

PTHrP, like PTH, activates PTH receptors in kidney and bone cells and increases urinary cyclic adenosine monophosphate and renal production of 1,25(OH)₂D₃. It is produced in almost every type of cell of the body, including every tissue of the embryo at some stage of development. PTHrP is critical for normal fetal development. Inactivating mutations of the receptor for PTH/PTHrP result in a lethal bone disorder characterized by short limbs and markedly advanced bone maturation known as *Blomstrand chondrodysplasia* (see Fig. 570-1). PTHrP appears to have a paracrine or autocrine role because serum levels are low except in a few clinical situations. Cord blood contains levels of PTHrP that are 3-fold higher than in serum from adults; it is produced by the fetal parathyroid glands and appears to be the main agent stimulating maternal-fetal calcium transfer. PTHrP appears to be essential for normal skeletal maturation of the fetus, which requires 30 g of calcium during a normal gestation. During pregnancy, maternal absorption of calcium increases from about 150 mg daily to 400 mg during the 2nd trimester.

As in cord blood, PTHrP levels are increased during lactation and in patients with benign breast hypertrophy. Breast milk and pasteurized bovine milk have levels of PTHrP that are 10,000 times higher than those of normal plasma. Most instances of the hormonal hypercalcemia syndrome of malignancy are caused by elevated concentrations of PTHrP.

VITAMIN D

See Chapter 51.

CALCITONIN

Calcitonin is a 32-amino-acid polypeptide. Its gene is on chromosome 11p and is tightly linked to that of PTH. The gene for calcitonin encodes 3 peptides: calcitonin, a 21-amino-acid carboxyterminal flanking peptide (katacalcin), and a calcitonin gene–related peptide. Katacalcin and calcitonin are cosecreted in equimolar amounts by the parafollicular cells (C cells) of the thyroid gland. Calcitonin appears to be of little consequence in children and adults because very high levels in patients with medullary carcinoma of the thyroid (a tumor arising from the C cells) do not cause hypercalcemia. In the fetus, however, circulating levels are high and appear to augment bone metabolism and skeletal growth; these high levels are probably stimulated by the normally high fetal calcium levels. Unlike the high levels in cord blood and circulating concentrations in young children, levels in older children and adults are low. Infants and children with congenital hypothyroidism (and presumed deficiency of C cells) have lower levels of calcitonin than do normal children.

Its action appears to be independent of PTH and vitamin D. Its main biologic effect appears to be the inhibition of bone resorption by decreasing the number and activity of bone-resorbing osteoclasts. This action of calcitonin is the rationale for its use in treatment of Paget disease. Calcitonin is synthesized in other organs, such as the gastrointestinal tract, pancreas, brain, and pituitary. In these organs, calcitonin is thought to behave as a neurotransmitter to impose a local inhibitory effect on cell function.

Bibliography is available at Expert Consult.

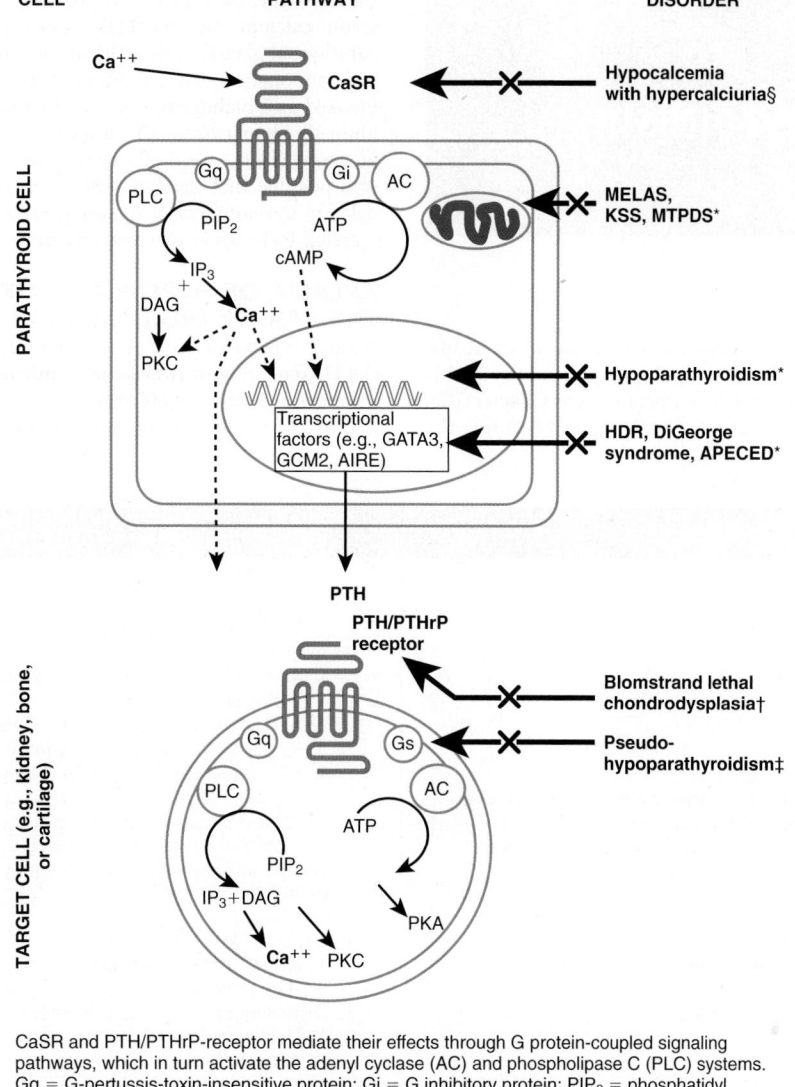

CaSR and PTH/PTHrP-receptor mediate their effects through G protein-coupled signaling pathways, which in turn activate the adenyl cyclase (AC) and phospholipase C (PLC) systems. Gq = G-pertussis-toxin-insensitive protein; Gi = G inhibitory protein; PIP$_2$ = phosphatidyl inositol 4,5-bisphosphate; IP$_3$ = inositol 1,4,5-triphosphate; DAG = diacylglycerol; PKC = protein kinase C.
*Disorders due to PTH deficiency.
†Defect due to defect in the PTH/PTHrP receptor.
‡Defect due to insensitivity to PTH caused by defects downstream of the PTH/PTHrP receptor.
§Defect due to altered set point in the Ca^{++}/PTH axis, associated with a gain-of-function mutation of the CaSR.
MELAS = mitochondrial encephalopathy, stroke-like episodes, and lactic acidosis.
KSS = Kearns Sayre syndrome (progressive external ophthalmoplegia, pigmentary retinopathy, heart block, and cardiomyopathy).
MTPDS = mitochondrial trifunctional protein deficiency syndrome.
HDR = hypoparathyroidism, deafness, and renal anomalies.
APECED = autoimmune polyendocrinopathy-candidosis-ectodermal dystrophy.

Figure 570-1 Some components involved in calcium homeostasis. The calcium-sensing receptor (CaSR) and PTH/PTHrP receptor mediate their effects through G-protein–coupled signaling pathways, which, in turn, activate the adenyl cyclase (AC) and phospholipase C (PLC) systems. *(From Thakker RV: Genetic development in hypoparathyroidism, Lancet 357:974–976, 2001.)*

Chapter **571**

Hypoparathyroidism

Daniel A. Doyle

ETIOLOGY

Hypocalcemia is common in neonates between 12 and 72 hr of life, especially in premature infants, in infants with asphyxia, and in infants of diabetic mothers (early neonatal hypocalcemia; see Chapter 106; Table 571-1 and Fig. 571-1). After the 2nd to 3rd day and during the 1st wk of life, the type of feeding also is a determinant of the level of serum calcium (late neonatal hypocalcemia). The role played by the parathyroid glands in these hypocalcemic infants remains to be clarified, although functional immaturity of the parathyroid glands is invoked as 1 pathogenetic factor. In a group of infants with transient idiopathic hypocalcemia (1-8 wk of age), serum levels of parathyroid hormone (PTH) are significantly lower than those in normal infants. It is possible that the functional immaturity is a manifestation of a delay in development of the enzymes that convert glandular PTH to secreted PTH; other mechanisms are possible.

APLASIA OR HYPOPLASIA OF THE PARATHYROID GLANDS

Aplasia or hypoplasia of the parathyroid glands is often associated with the **DiGeorge/velocardiofacial syndrome** (see Fig. 570-1). This syndrome occurs in 1 in 4,000 newborns. In 90% of patients, the condition is caused by a deletion of chromosome 22q11.2. Approximately 25%

Table 571-1	Causes of Hypocalcemia

I. Neonatal
  A. Maternal Disorders
    Diabetes mellitus
    Toxemia of pregnancy
    Vitamin D deficiency
    High intake of alkali or magnesium sulfate
    Use of anticonvulsants
    Hyperparathyroidism
  B. Neonatal Disorders
    Low birthweight: prematurity, intrauterine growth restriction
    Peripartum asphyxia, sepsis, critical illness
    Hyperbilirubinemia, phototherapy, exchange transfusion
    Hypomagnesemia, hypermagnesemia
    Acute/chronic renal failure
    Nutrients/medications: high phosphate intake, fatty acids, phytates, bicarbonate infusion, citrated blood, anticonvulsants, aminoglycosides
    Hypoparathyroidism
    Vitamin D deficiency or resistance
    Osteopetrosis type II
II. Hypoparathyroidism
  A. Congenital
    1. Transient neonatal
    2. Congenital hypoparathyroidism
      a. Familial isolated hypoparathyroidism
        (1) Autosomal recessive hypoparathyroidism (GCMB, PTH)
        (2) Autosomal dominant hypoparathyroidism (CaSR)
        (3) X-linked hypoparathyroidism (*SOX3*)
      b. DiGeorge syndrome (*TBX1*)
      c. Sanjad-Sakati syndrome (short stature, retardation, dysmorphism; HRD); Kenny-Caffey syndrome 1 (short stature, medullary stenosis) (*TBCE*)
      d. Barakat syndrome (sensorineural deafness, renal dysplasia; HDR) (*GATA3*)
      e. Lymphedema-hypoparathyroidism-nephropathy, nerve deafness
      f. Mitochondrial fatty acid disorders (Kearns-Sayre, Pearson, MELAS)
    3. Insensitivity to PTH
      a. Blomstrand chondrodysplasia (*PTHR1*)
      b. Pseudohypoparathyroidism type IA (*GNAS*)
        Pseudohypoparathyroidism type IB
        Pseudohypoparathyroidism type IC
        Pseudohypoparathyroidism type II
        Pseudopseudohypoparathyroidism
      c. Acrodysostosis with hormone resistance (*PRKAR1A*)
      d. Hypomagnesemia

    4. CaSR-activating mutation
      a. Sporadic
      b. Autosomal dominant (G protein subunit α11 mutation)
  B. Acquired
    1. Autoimmune polyglandular syndrome type I (*AIRE* gene mutation)
    2. Activating antibodies to the CaSR
    3. Postsurgical, radiation destruction
    4. Infiltrate—excessive iron (hemochromatosis, thalassemia) or copper (Wilson disease) deposition; granulomatous inflammation, neoplastic invasion; amyloidosis, sarcoidosis
    5. Maternal hyperparathyroidism
    6. Hypomagnesemia/hypermagnesemia
III. Vitamin D Deficiency
IV. Other Causes of Hypocalcemia
  A. Calcium Deficiency
    1. Nutritional deprivation
    2. Hypercalciuria
  B. Disorders of Magnesium Homeostasis
    1. Congenital hypomagnesemia
    2. Acquired
      a. Acute renal failure
      b. Chronic inflammatory bowel disease, intestinal resection
      c. Diuretics
  C. Hyperphosphatemia
    1. Renal failure
    2. Phosphate administration (intravenous, oral, rectal)
    3. Tumor cell lysis
    4. Muscle injuries (crush, rhabdomyolysis)
  D. Miscellaneous
    1. Hypoproteinemia
    2. Hyperventilation
    3. Drugs: furosemide, aminoglycosides, bisphosphonates, calcitonin, anticonvulsants, ketoconazole, antineoplastic agents (plicamycin, asparaginase, cisplatinum, cytosine arabinoside, doxorubicin), citrated blood products
    4. Hungry bone syndrome
    5. Acute and critical illness: sepsis, acute pancreatitis, toxic shock
      a. Organic acidemia: propionic, methylmalonic, isovaleric

HDR, hypoparathyroidism, sensorineural deafness, and renal anomaly; HRD, hypoparathyroidism, retardation, dysmorphism; MELAS, mitochondrial encephalomyopathy with lactic acidosis and stroke-like episode; PTH, parathyroid hormone.
Modified from Root AW, Diamond JR FB: Disorders of mineral homeostasis in children and adolescents. In Sperling MA, editor: Pediatric endocrinology, ed 4, Philadelphia, 2014, Elsevier, Table 18-2A, p. 739.

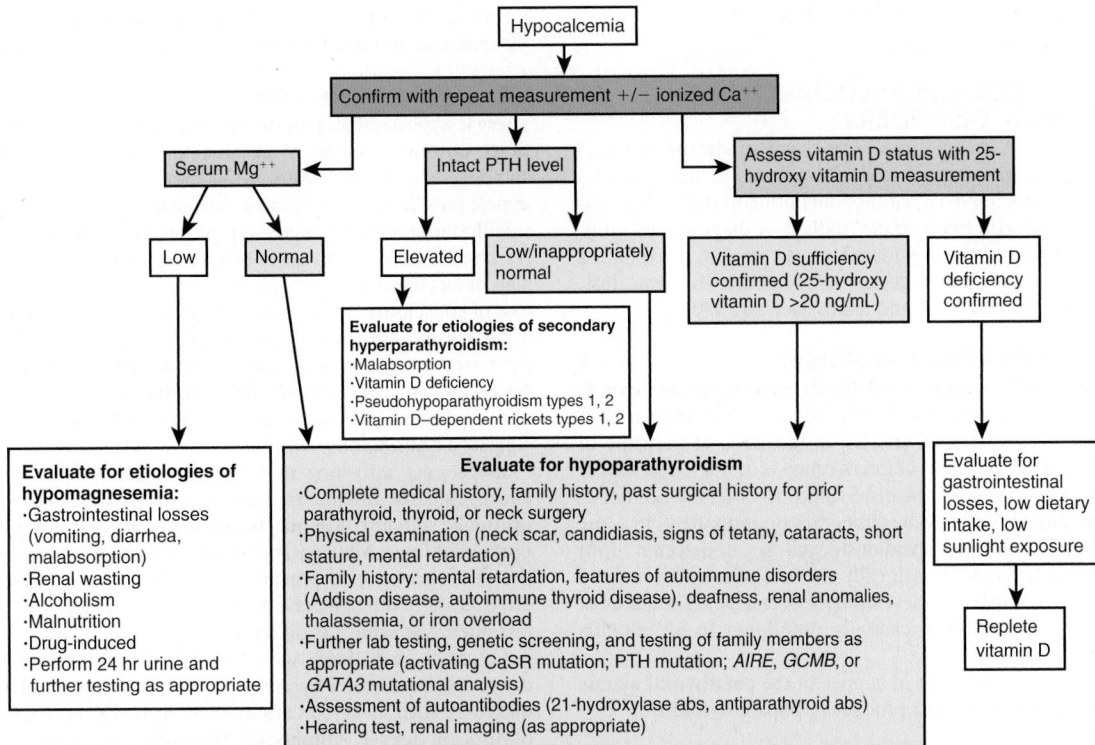

Figure 571-1 Evaluation of hypocalcemia. Abs, autoantibodies; CaSR, calcium-sensing receptor; PTH, parathyroid hormone. *(From Bilezikian JP, Khan A, Potts JT Jr, et al. Hypoparathyroidism in the adult: epidemiology, diagnosis, pathophysiology, target-organ involvement, treatment, and challenges for future research. J Bone Miner Res 26:2317–2337, 2011, Fig. 1.)*

of these patients inherit the chromosomal abnormality from a parent. Neonatal hypocalcemia occurs in 60% of affected patients, but it is transitory in the majority; hypocalcemia can recur or can have its onset later in life. Associated abnormalities of the third and fourth pharyngeal pouches are common; these include conotruncal defects of the heart in 25%, velopharyngeal insufficiency in 32%, cleft palate in 9%, renal anomalies in 35%, and aplasia of the thymus with severe immunodeficiency in 1%. This syndrome has also been reported in a small number of patients with a deletion of chromosome 10p13, in infants of diabetic mothers, and in infants born to mothers treated with retinoic acid for acne early in pregnancy.

X-LINKED RECESSIVE HYPOPARATHYROIDISM

Familial clusters of hypoparathyroidism with various patterns of transmission have been described. In 2 large North American pedigrees, this disorder appears to be transmitted by an X-linked recessive gene located on Xq26-q27. In these families, the onset of afebrile seizures characteristically occurs in infants from 2 wk to 6 mo of age. The absence of parathyroid tissue after detailed examination of a boy with this condition suggests a defect in embryogenesis.

AUTOSOMAL RECESSIVE HYPOPARATHYROIDISM WITH DYSMORPHIC FEATURES

Autosomal recessive hypoparathyroidism with dysmorphic features has been described in Middle Eastern children. Parental consanguinity occurred for almost all of several dozen affected patients. Profound hypocalcemia occurs early in life, and dysmorphic features include microcephaly, deep-set eyes, beaked nose, micrognathia, and large floppy ears. Intrauterine and postnatal growth restriction are severe, and cognitive impairment is common. The putative gene is on chromosome 1q42-43. The autosomal recessive form of hypoparathyroidism that occurs with type I polyglandular autoimmune disease is described subsequently. In a few patients with autosomal recessive inheritance of

isolated hypoparathyroidism, mutations of the *PTH* gene have been found.

HYPOPARATHYROIDISM, SENSORINEURAL DEAFNESS, AND RENAL ANOMALY SYNDROME

Hypoparathyroidism, sensorineural deafness, and renal anomaly occur owing to mutations of the *GATA3* gene. The protein encoded by this gene is essential in the development of the parathyroids, auditory system, and kidneys. The *GATA3* gene is located at chromosome 10p14 and is nonoverlapping with the DiGeorge critical region at 10p13 (see Fig. 570-1).

SUPPRESSION OF NEONATAL PARATHYROID HORMONE SECRETION BECAUSE OF MATERNAL HYPERPARATHYROIDISM

Neonatal PTH secretion can be suppressed by maternal hyperparathyroidism, resulting in transient hypocalcemia in the newborn infant. It appears that neonatal hypocalcemia results from suppression of the fetal parathyroid glands by exposure to elevated levels of calcium in maternal and hence fetal serum. Tetany usually develops within 3 wk but may be delayed by 1 mo or more if the infant is breastfed. Hypocalcemia can persist for weeks or months. When the cause of hypocalcemia in an infant is unknown, measurements of calcium, phosphorus, and PTH should be obtained from the mother. Most affected mothers are asymptomatic, and the cause of their hyperparathyroidism is usually a parathyroid adenoma.

AUTOSOMAL DOMINANT HYPOPARATHYROIDISM

Patients with autosomal dominant hypoparathyroidism have an activating (gain-of-function) mutation of the Ca^{2+}-sensing receptor, forcing the receptor to an "on" state with subsequent depression of PTH secretion even during hypocalcemia. The patients have hypercalciuria. The hypocalcemia is usually mild and might not require treatment beyond childhood (see Fig. 570-1).

HYPOPARATHYROIDISM ASSOCIATED WITH MITOCHONDRIAL DISORDERS

Mitochondrial DNA mutations in Kearns-Sayre syndrome, MELAS (myopathy, encephalopathy, lactic acidosis, and stroke-like episodes) syndrome, and in mitochondrial trifunctional protein–deficiency syndrome are associated with hypoparathyroidism. A diagnosis of mitochondrial cytopathy should be considered in patients with unexplained symptoms, such as ophthalmoplegia, sensorineural hearing loss, cardiac conduction disturbances, and tetany (see Fig. 570-1).

SURGICAL HYPOPARATHYROIDISM

Removal or damage of the parathyroid glands can complicate thyroidectomy. Hypoparathyroidism has developed even when the parathyroid glands have been identified and left undisturbed at the time of operation. This may be the result of interference with the blood supply or of postoperative edema and fibrosis. Symptoms of tetany can occur abruptly postoperatively and may be temporary or permanent. In some instances, symptoms develop insidiously and go undetected until months after thyroidectomy. Occasionally, the first evidence of surgical hypoparathyroidism may be the development of cataract. The status of parathyroid function should be carefully monitored in all patients undergoing thyroidectomy.

Deposition of iron pigment or of copper in the parathyroid glands (thalassemia, Wilson disease) can produce hypoparathyroidism.

AUTOIMMUNE HYPOPARATHYROIDISM

An autoimmune mechanism for hypoparathyroidism is strongly suggested by the finding of parathyroid antibodies and by its frequent association with other autoimmune disorders or organ-specific antibodies. Autoimmune hypoparathyroidism is often associated with Addison disease and chronic mucocutaneous candidiasis. The association of at least 2 of these 3 conditions has been tentatively classified as **autoimmune polyglandular disease type I.** It is also known as autoimmune polyendocrinopathy, candidiasis, and ectodermal dystrophy (APECED). This syndrome is inherited in an autosomal recessive fashion and is not related to any single human leukocyte antigen–associated haplotype. One third of patients with this syndrome have all 3 components; 66% have only 2 of 3 conditions. The candidiasis almost always precedes the other disorders (70% of cases occur in children younger than 5 yr of age); the hypoparathyroidism (90% of cases occur after 3 yr of age) usually occurs before Addison disease (90% of cases occur after 6 yr of age). A variety of other disorders, including alopecia areata or totalis, malabsorption disorder, pernicious anemia, gonadal failure, chronic active hepatitis, vitiligo, and insulin-dependent diabetes, occurs at various times. Some of these associations might not appear until adult life. Autoimmune thyroid disease is a rare concomitant finding.

Affected siblings can have the same or different constellations of disorders (hypoparathyroidism, Addison disease). The disorder is exceptionally prevalent among Finns and Iranian Jews. The gene for this disorder is designated *AIRE* (autoimmune regulator); it is located on chromosome 21q22. It appears to be a transcription factor that plays an essential role in the development of immunologic tolerance. Patients with Addison disease as part of polyendocrinopathy syndrome type I have demonstrated adrenal-specific autoantibody reactivity directed against the side-chain cleavage enzyme.

IDIOPATHIC HYPOPARATHYROIDISM

The term *idiopathic hypoparathyroidism* should be reserved for the small residuum of children with hypoparathyroidism for whom no causative mechanism can be defined. Most children in whom onset of hypoparathyroidism occurs after the 1st few yr of life have an **autoimmune condition.** Autoantibodies to the extracellular domain of the calcium-sensing receptor have been identified in some patients with acquired hypoparathyroidism. One should always consider incomplete forms of DiGeorge syndrome or an activating calcium-sensing receptor mutation in the differential diagnosis.

Clinical Manifestations

There is a spectrum of parathyroid deficiencies with clinical manifestations varying from no symptoms to those of complete and long-standing deficiency. Mild deficiency may be revealed only by appropriate laboratory studies. Muscular pain and cramps are early manifestations; they progress to numbness, stiffness, and tingling of the hands and feet. There may be only a positive Chvostek or Trousseau sign or laryngeal and carpopedal spasms. Convulsions with or without loss of consciousness can occur at intervals of days, weeks, or months. These episodes can begin with abdominal pain, followed by tonic rigidity, retraction of the head, and cyanosis. Hypoparathyroidism is often mistaken for epilepsy. Headache, vomiting, increased intracranial pressure, and papilledema may be associated with convulsions and might suggest a brain tumor.

In patients with long-standing hypocalcemia, the teeth erupt late and irregularly. Enamel formation is irregular, and the teeth may be unusually soft. The skin may be dry and scaly, and the nails might have horizontal lines. Mucocutaneous candidiasis, when present, antedates the development of hypoparathyroidism; the candidal infection most often involves the nails, the oral mucosa, the angles of the mouth, and less often, the skin; it is difficult to treat.

Cataracts in patients with long-standing untreated disease are a direct consequence of hypoparathyroidism; other autoimmune ocular disorders such as keratoconjunctivitis can also occur. Manifestations of Addison disease, lymphocytic thyroiditis, pernicious anemia, alopecia areata or totalis, hepatitis, and primary gonadal insufficiency may also be associated with those of hypoparathyroidism.

Permanent physical and mental deterioration occurs if initiation of treatment is long delayed.

Laboratory Findings

The serum calcium level is low (5-7 mg/dL), and the phosphorus level is elevated (7-12 mg/dL). Blood levels of ionized calcium (usually approximately 45% of the total) more nearly reflect physiologic adequacy but also are low. The serum level of alkaline phosphatase is normal or low, and the level of $1,25(OH)_2D_3$ is usually low, but high levels have been found in some children with severe hypocalcemia. The level of magnesium is normal but should always be checked in hypocalcemic patients. Levels of PTH are low when measured by immunometric assay. Radiographs of the bones occasionally reveal an increased density limited to the metaphyses, suggesting heavy metal poisoning, or an increased density of the lamina dura. Radiographs or CT scans of the skull can reveal calcifications in the basal ganglia. There is a prolongation of the QT interval on the electrocardiogram, which disappears when the hypocalcemia is corrected. The electroencephalogram usually reveals widespread slow activity; the tracing returns to normal after the serum calcium concentration has been within the normal range for a few weeks, unless irreversible brain damage has occurred or unless the parathyroid insufficiency is associated with epilepsy. When hypoparathyroidism occurs concurrently with Addison disease, the serum level of calcium may be normal, but hypocalcemia appears after effective treatment of the adrenal insufficiency.

Treatment

Emergency treatment of neonatal tetany consists of intravenous injections of 5-10 mL or 1-3 mg/kg of a 10% solution of calcium gluconate (elemental calcium 9.3 mg/mL) at the rate of 0.5-1.0 mL/min while the heart rate is monitored and a total dose not to exceed 20 mg of elemental calcium/kg. Additionally, 1,25-dihydroxycholecalciferol (calcitriol) should be given. The initial dosage is 0.25 µg/24 hr; the maintenance dosage ranges from 0.01-0.10 µg/kg/24 hr to a maximum of 1-2 µg/24 hr. Calcitriol has a short half-life and should be given in 2 equal divided doses; it has the advantages of rapid onset of effect (1-4 days) and rapid reversal of hypercalcemia after discontinuation in the event of overdosage (calcium levels begin to fall in 3-4 days). Calcitriol is supplied as an oral solution.

An adequate intake of calcium should be ensured. Supplemental calcium can be given in the form of calcium gluconate or calcium glubionate to provide 800 mg of elemental calcium daily, but it is rarely essential. Foods with high phosphorus content such as milk, eggs, and cheese should be reduced in the diet.

Clinical evaluation of the patient and frequent determinations of the serum calcium levels are indicated in the early stages of treatment to determine the requirement for calcitriol or vitamin D_2. If hypercalcemia occurs, therapy should be discontinued and resumed at a lower dose after the serum calcium level has returned to normal. In long-standing cases of hypercalcemia, repair of cerebral and dental changes is not likely. Pigmentation, lowering of blood pressure, or weight loss can indicate adrenal insufficiency, which requires specific treatment. *Patients with autosomal dominant hypocalcemic hypercalciuria can develop nephrocalcinosis and renal impairment if treated with vitamin D.*

Differential Diagnosis

Magnesium deficiency must be considered in patients with unexplained hypocalcemia. Concentrations of serum magnesium <1.5 mg/dL (1.2 mEq/L) are usually abnormal. Familial hypomagnesemia with secondary hypocalcemia has been reported in approximately 50 patients, most of whom developed tetany and seizures at 2-6 wk of age. Administration of calcium is ineffective, but administration of magnesium promptly corrects both calcium and magnesium levels. Oral supplements of magnesium are necessary to maintain levels of magnesium in the normal range. Two genetic forms have been described. One is caused by an autosomal recessive gene on chromosome 9, resulting in a specific defect in absorption of magnesium. The other is caused by an autosomal dominant gene on chromosome 11q23, resulting in renal loss of magnesium.

Hypomagnesemia also occurs in malabsorption syndromes such as Crohn disease and cystic fibrosis. Patients with autoimmune polyglandular disease type I and hypoparathyroidism can also have concurrent steatorrhea and low magnesium levels. Therapy with aminoglycosides causes hypomagnesemia by increasing urinary losses.

It is not clear how low levels of magnesium lead to hypocalcemia. Evidence suggests that hypomagnesemia impairs release of PTH and induces resistance to the effects of the hormone, but other mechanisms also may be operative.

Poisoning with inorganic phosphate leads to hypocalcemia and tetany. Infants administered large doses of inorganic phosphates, either as laxatives or as sodium phosphate enemas, have had sudden onset of tetany, with serum calcium levels <5 mg/dL and markedly elevated levels of phosphate. Symptoms are quickly relieved by intravenous administration of calcium. The mechanism of the hypocalcemia is not clear (see Chapter 55.6).

Hypocalcemia can occur early in the course of treatment of acute lymphoblastic leukemia. Hypocalcemia is usually associated with hyperphosphatemia resulting from destruction of lymphoblasts.

Episodic symptomatic hypocalcemia occurs in the **Kenny-Caffey syndrome,** which is characterized by medullary stenosis of the long bones, short stature, delayed closure of the fontanel, delayed bone age, and eye abnormalities. Idiopathic hypoparathyroidism and abnormal PTH levels have been found. Autosomal dominant and autosomal recessive modes of inheritance have been reported. Mutations of the TBCE gene (1q 43-44) perturb microtubule organization in diseased cells.

Bibliography is available at Expert Consult.

Chapter 572
Pseudohypoparathyroidism (Albright Hereditary Osteodystrophy)
Daniel A. Doyle

In contrast to the situation in hypoparathyroidism, in pseudohypoparathyroidism (PHP) the parathyroid glands are normal or hyperplastic and they can synthesize and secrete parathyroid hormone (PTH). Serum levels of immunoreactive PTH are elevated even when the patient is hypocalcemic and may be elevated when the patient is normocalcemic. Neither endogenous nor administered PTH raises the serum levels of calcium or lowers the levels of phosphorus. The genetic defects in the **hormone receptor adenylate cyclase system** are classified into various types depending on the phenotypic and biochemical findings.

TYPE IA

Type Ia accounts for the majority of patients with PHP. Affected patients have a genetic defect of the α subunit of the stimulatory guanine nucleotide-binding protein ($G_s\alpha$). This coupling factor is required for PTH bound to cell surface receptors to activate cyclic adenosine monophosphate (cAMP). Heterogeneous mutations of the $G_s\alpha$ gene have been documented; the gene is located on chromosome 20q13.2. Deficiency of the $G_s\alpha$ subunit is a generalized cellular defect and accounts for the association of other endocrine disorders with type Ia PHP. The defect is inherited as an autosomal dominant trait, and the paucity of father-to-son transmissions is thought to be a result of decreased fertility in males.

Tetany is often the presenting sign. Affected children have a short, stocky build and a round face. Brachydactyly with dimpling of the dorsum of the hand is usually present. The 2nd metacarpal is involved least often. As a result, the index finger occasionally is longer than the middle finger. Likewise, the 2nd metatarsal is only rarely affected. There may be other skeletal abnormalities such as short and wide phalanges, bowing, exostoses, and thickening of the calvaria. These patients often have calcium deposits and metaplastic bone formation subcutaneously. Moderate degrees of cognitive impairment, calcification of the basal ganglia, and lenticular cataracts are common in patients whose disease is diagnosed late.

Some members of affected kindreds may have the usual anatomic stigmata of PHP, but serum levels of calcium and phosphorus are normal despite reduced $G_s\alpha$ activity; however, PTH levels may be slightly elevated. Such patients have been labeled as having **pseudopseudohypoparathyroidism.** Transition from normocalcemia to hypocalcemia often occurs with increasing age of the patient. These phenotypically similar but metabolically dissimilar patients may be in the same family and have the same mutations of $G_s\alpha$ protein. It is not known what other factors cause clinically overt hypocalcemia in some affected patients and not in others. There is some evidence to suggest that the $G_s\alpha$ mutation is paternally transmitted in pseudopseudohypoparathyroidism and maternally transmitted in patients with type Ia disease. The gene may be imprinted in a tissue-specific manner.

In addition to resistance to PTH, resistance to other G-protein–coupled receptors for thyroid-stimulating hormone (TSH), gonadotropins, and glucagon can result in various metabolic effects. Clinical hypothyroidism is uncommon, but basal levels of TSH are elevated and thyrotropin-releasing hormone–stimulated TSH responses are exaggerated. Moderately decreased levels of thyroxine and increased levels of TSH have been demonstrated by newborn thyroid-screening programs, leading to the detection of type Ia PHP in infancy. In adults, gonadal dysfunction is common, as manifested by sexual immaturity, amenorrhea, oligomenorrhea, and infertility. Each of these abnormalities can be related to deficient synthesis of cAMP secondary to a deficiency of $G_s\alpha$, but it is not clear why resistance to other G-protein–dependent hormones (corticotropin, vasopressin) is much less affected.

Serum levels of calcium are low, and those of phosphorus and alkaline phosphatase are elevated. Clinical diagnosis can be confirmed by demonstration of a markedly attenuated response in urinary phosphate and cAMP after intravenous infusion of the synthetic 1-34 fragment of human PTH (teriparatide acetate). Definitive diagnosis is established by demonstration of the mutated G protein.

Type Ia with Precocious Puberty

Two boys have been reported with both type Ia PHP and gonadotropin-independent precocious puberty (see Chapter 562.7). They were found to have a temperature-sensitive mutation of the G_s protein. Thus, at normal body temperature (37°C [98.6°F]), the G_s is degraded, resulting in PHP, but in the cooler temperature of the testes (33°C [91.4°F]) the G_s mutation results in constitutive activation of the luteinizing hormone receptor and precocious puberty.

TYPE IB

Affected patients have normal levels of G protein activity and a normal phenotypic appearance. These patients have tissue-specific resistance to PTH but not to other hormones. Serum levels of calcium, phosphorus, and immunoreactive PTH are the same as those in patients with type Ia PHP. These patients also show no rise in cAMP in response to exogenous administration of PTH. Bioactive PTH is not increased. The pathophysiology of the disorder in this group of patients is caused by paternal uniparental isodisomy of chromosome 20q and resulting *GNAS1* methylation. This, along with the loss of the maternal *GNAS1* gene, leads to PTH resistance in the proximal renal tubules, which leads to impaired mineral ion homeostasis.

ACRODYSOSTOSIS WITH HORMONE RESISTANCE

Patients with acrodysostosis resemble those with PHP type Ia, but defects in the $G_s\alpha$ subunit are not present. Instead, in 1 subgroup of patients there is a defect in the gene encoding *PRKAR1A*, the cAMP-dependent regulatory subunit of protein kinase A that confers resistance to multiple hormones, including PTH. Another subgroup has a defect in a phosphodiesterase gene *Pde4d*. This subgroup also carries the phenotype of PHP type Ia but rarely exhibits the hormone resistance.

Bibliography is available at Expert Consult.

Chapter **573**
Hyperparathyroidism
Daniel A. Doyle

Excessive production of parathyroid hormone (PTH) can result from a primary defect of the parathyroid glands such as an adenoma or hyperplasia (**primary hyperparathyroidism**).

More often, the increased production of PTH is compensatory, usually aimed at correcting hypocalcemic states of diverse origins

(**secondary hyperparathyroidism**). In vitamin D–deficient rickets and the malabsorption syndromes, intestinal absorption of calcium is deficient but hypocalcemia and tetany may be averted by increased activity of the parathyroid glands. In **pseudohypoparathyroidism,** PTH levels are elevated because a mutation in the $G_s\alpha$ protein interferes with response to PTH. Early in chronic renal disease, hyperphosphatemia results in a reciprocal fall in the calcium concentration with a consequent increase in PTH, but in advanced stages of renal failure, production of $1,25(OH)_2D_3$ is also decreased, leading to worsening hypocalcemia and further stimulation of PTH. In some instances, if stimulation of the parathyroid glands has been sufficiently intense and protracted, the glands continue to secrete increased levels of PTH for months or years after kidney transplantation, with resulting hypercalcemia.

ETIOLOGY

Childhood hyperparathyroidism is uncommon. Onset during childhood is usually the result of a single benign adenoma. It usually becomes manifested after 10 yr of age. There have been a number of kindreds in which multiple members have hyperparathyroidism transmitted in an autosomal dominant fashion. Most of the affected family members are adults, but children have been involved in approximately 30% of the pedigrees. Some affected patients in these families are asymptomatic, and disease is detected only by careful study. In other kindreds, hyperparathyroidism occurs as part of the constellation known as the **multiple endocrine neoplasia** (MEN) syndromes or of the hyperparathyroidism–jaw tumor syndrome.

Neonatal severe hyperparathyroidism is a rare disorder. Symptoms develop shortly after birth and consist of anorexia, irritability, lethargy, constipation, and failure to thrive. Radiographs reveal subperiosteal bone resorption, osteoporosis, and pathologic fractures. Symptoms may be mild, resolving without treatment, or can have a rapidly fatal course if diagnosis and treatment are delayed. Histologically, the parathyroid glands show diffuse hyperplasia. Affected siblings have been observed in some kindreds, and parental consanguinity has been reported in several kindreds. Most cases have occurred in kindreds with the clinical and biochemical features of **familial hypocalciuric hypercalcemia.** Infants with neonatal severe hyperparathyroidism may be homozygous or heterozygous for the mutation in the Ca^{2+}-sensing receptor gene, whereas most persons with 1 copy of this mutation exhibit autosomal dominant familial hypocalciuric hypercalcemia.

MEN type I is an autosomal dominant disorder characterized by hyperplasia or neoplasia of the endocrine pancreas (which secretes gastrin, insulin, pancreatic polypeptide, and occasionally glucagon), the anterior pituitary (which usually secretes prolactin), and the parathyroid glands. In most kindreds, hyperparathyroidism is usually the presenting manifestation, with a prevalence approaching 100% by 50 yr of age and occurring only rarely in children younger than 18 yr of age. With appropriate DNA probes, it is possible to detect carriers of the gene with 99% accuracy at birth, avoiding unnecessary biochemical screening programs.

The gene for MEN type I is on chromosome 11q13; it appears to function as a tumor-suppressor gene and follows the 2-hit hypothesis of tumor development. The first mutation (germinal) is inherited and is recessive to the dominant allele; this does not result in tumor formation. A second mutation (somatic) is required to eliminate the normal allele, which then leads to tumor formation.

Hyperparathyroidism–jaw tumor syndrome is an autosomal dominant disorder characterized by parathyroid adenomas and fibroosseous jaw tumors. Affected patients can also have polycystic kidney disease, renal hamartomas, and Wilms tumor. Although the condition affects adults primarily, it has been diagnosed as early as age 10 yr.

MEN type II may also be associated with hyperparathyroidism (see Chapter 569.2).

Transient neonatal hyperparathyroidism has occurred in a few infants born to mothers with hypoparathyroidism (idiopathic or surgical) or with pseudohypoparathyroidism. In each case, the maternal disorder had been undiagnosed or inadequately treated during pregnancy. The cause of the condition is chronic intrauterine exposure to hypocalcemia with resultant hyperplasia of the fetal parathyroid glands. In the newborn, manifestations involve the bones primarily, and healing occurs between 4 and 7 mo of age.

CLINICAL MANIFESTATIONS

At all ages, the clinical manifestations of hypercalcemia of any cause include muscle weakness, fatigue, headache, anorexia, abdominal pain, nausea, vomiting, constipation, polydipsia, polyuria, weight loss, and fever. When hypercalcemia is of long duration, calcium may be deposited in the renal parenchyma (nephrocalcinosis), with progressively diminished renal function. Renal calculi can develop and can cause renal colic and hematuria. Osseous changes can produce pain in the back or extremities, disturbances of gait, genu valgum, fractures, and tumors. Height can decrease from compression of vertebrae; the patient can become bedridden. Detection of completely asymptomatic patients is increasing with the advent of automated panel assays that include serum calcium determinations.

Abdominal pain is occasionally prominent and may be associated with **acute pancreatitis.** Parathyroid crisis can occur, manifested by serum calcium levels >15 mg/dL and progressive oliguria, azotemia, stupor, and coma. In infants, failure to thrive, poor feeding, and hypotonia are common.

Cognitive impairment, convulsions, and blindness can occur as sequelae of long-standing hypercalcemia. Psychiatric manifestations include depression, confusion, dementia, stupor, and psychosis.

LABORATORY FINDINGS

The serum calcium level is elevated; 39 of 45 children with adenomas had levels >12 mg/dL. The hypercalcemia is more severe in infants with parathyroid hyperplasia; concentrations ranging from 15-20 mg/dL are common, and values as high as 30 mg/dL have been reported. Even when the total serum calcium level is borderline or only slightly elevated, ionized calcium levels are often increased. The serum phosphorus level is reduced to approximately 3 mg/dL or less, and the level of serum magnesium is low. The urine can have a low and fixed specific gravity, and serum levels of nonprotein nitrogen and uric acid may be elevated. In patients with adenomas who have skeletal involvement, serum phosphatase levels are elevated, but in infants with hyperplasia

the levels of alkaline phosphatase may be normal even when there is extensive involvement of bone.

Serum levels of intact PTH are elevated, especially in relation to the level of calcium. Calcitonin levels are normal. Acute hypercalcemia can stimulate calcitonin release, but with prolonged hypercalcemia, hypercalcitoninemia does not occur.

The most consistent and characteristic radiographic finding is resorption of subperiosteal bone, best seen along the margins of the phalanges of the hands. In the skull, there may be gross trabeculation or a granular appearance resulting from focal rarefaction; the lamina dura may be absent. In more advanced disease, there may be generalized rarefaction, cysts, tumors, fractures, and deformities. Approximately 10% of patients have radiographic signs of rickets. Radiographs of the abdomen can reveal renal calculi or nephrocalcinosis.

DIFFERENTIAL DIAGNOSIS

Other causes of hypercalcemia can result in a similar clinical pattern and must be differentiated from hyperparathyroidism (Table 573-1 and Fig. 573-1). A low serum phosphorus level with hypercalcemia is characteristic of primary hyperparathyroidism; elevated levels of PTH are also diagnostic. With hypercalcemia of any cause except hyperparathyroidism and familial hypocalciuric hypercalcemia, PTH levels are suppressed. Pharmacologic doses of corticosteroids lower the serum calcium level to normal in patients with hypercalcemia from other causes but generally do not affect the calcium level in patients with hyperparathyroidism.

TREATMENT

Surgical exploration is indicated in all instances. All glands should be carefully inspected; if an adenoma is discovered, it should be removed; very few instances of carcinoma are known in children. Most neonates with severe hypercalcemia require total parathyroidectomy; less-severe hypercalcemia remits spontaneously in others. Still others have been treated successfully with bisphosphonates and calcimimetics. The patient should be carefully observed postoperatively for the development of hypocalcemia and tetany; intravenous administration of calcium gluconate may be required for a few days. The serum calcium level then gradually returns to normal, and, under ordinary

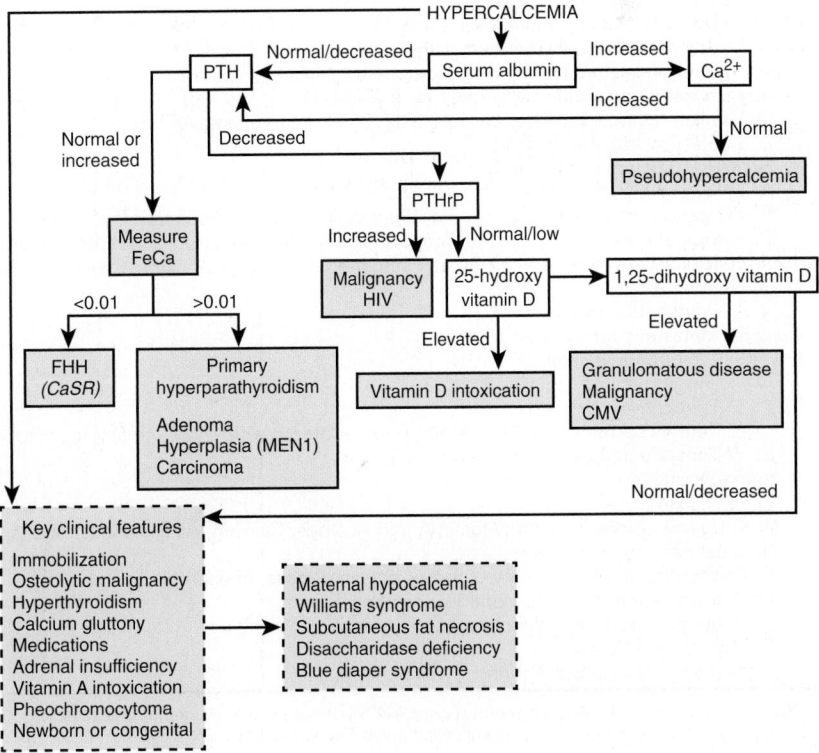

Figure 573-1 Evaluation of hypercalcemia. Ca^{2+}, calcium ions; CaSR, calcium-sensing receptor; CMV, cytomegalovirus; FeCa, fractional excretion of urinary calcium. (*From Lietman SA, Germain-Lee EL, Levine MA. Hypercalcemia in children and adolescents. Curr Opin Pediatr 22:508–515, 2010.*)

Table 573-1	Causes of Hypercalcemia

I. Neonate/Infant
   A. Maternal Disorders
      1. Excessive vitamin D ingestion, hypoparathyroidism, pseudohypoparathyroidism
   B. Neonate/Infant
      1. Iatrogenic: excessive intake of calcium, vitamin D, vitamin A
      2. Phosphate depletion
      3. Subcutaneous fat necrosis
      4. Williams-Beuren syndrome (del7q11.23/*BAZ1B*) (transient receptor potential; 3-channel defect)
      5. Neonatal severe hyperparathyroidism (*CaSR*)
      6. Metaphyseal chondrodysplasia, Murk-Jansen type (*PTH1R*)
      7. Idiopathic infantile hypercalcemia (*CYP24A1*) (25-hydroxyvitamin D 24-hydroxylase)
      8. Persistent parathyroid hormone–related protein
      9. Lactase/disaccharidase deficiency (*LCT*)
      10. Infantile hypophosphatasia (*TNSALP*)
      11. Mucolipidosis type II (*GNPTAB*)
      12. Blue diaper syndrome
      13. Antenatal Bartter syndrome types 1 and 2 (*SLC12A1, KCNJ1*)
      14. Distal renal tubular acidosis
      15. IMAGe syndrome (*CDKN1C*)
      16. Post bone marrow transplantation for osteopetrosis
      17. Endocrinopathies: primary adrenal insufficiency, severe congenital hypothyroidism, hyperthyroidism
II. Hyperparathyroidism
   A. Sporadic
      1. Parathyroid hyperplasia, adenoma, carcinoma
   B. Familial
      1. Neonatal severe hyperparathyroidism (*CaSR*)
      2. Multiple endocrine neoplasia, type I (*MEN1*)
      3. Multiple endocrine neoplasia, type IIA (*RET*)
      4. Multiple endocrine neoplasia, type IIB (*RET*)
      5. Multiple endocrine neoplasia, type IV (*CDKN1B*)
      6. McCune-Albright syndrome (*GNAS*)
      7. Familial isolated hyperparathyroidism 1 (*CDC73*)
      8. Familial isolated hyperparathyroidism 2 (jaw tumor syndrome) (*CDC73*)
      9. Familial isolated hyperparathyroidism 3
      10. Jansen metaphyseal dysplasia (*PTH1R*)
   C. Secondary/Tertiary
      1. Postrenal transplantation
      2. Chronic hyperphosphatemia
   D. Hypercalcemia of Malignancy
      1. Ectopic production of parathyroid hormone–related peptide
      2. Metastatic dissolution of bone
III. Familial Hypocalciuric Hypercalcemia
   A. Familial Hypocalciuric Hypercalcemia I (*CaSR*)
      1. Loss-of-function mutations in *CaSR*
         a. Monoallelic: familial benign hypercalcemia
         b. Biallelic: neonatal severe hyperparathyroidism
   B. Familial Hypocalciuric Hypercalcemia II (*GNA11*)
   C. Familial Hypocalciuric Hypercalcemia III, Oklahoma Variant (*AP2S1*)
   D. *CaSR*-blocking autoantibodies
IV. Excessive Calcium or Vitamin D
   A. Milk-Alkali Syndrome
   B. Exogenous Ingestion of Calcium or Vitamin D or Topical Application of Vitamin D (calcitriol or analog)
   C. Ectopic Production of Calcitriol Associated with Granulomatous Diseases (sarcoidosis, cat-scratch fever; tuberculosis, histoplasmosis, coccidioidomycosis, leprosy; human immunodeficiency virus; cytomegalovirus; chronic inflammatory bowel disease)
   D. Neoplasia
      1. Primary bone tumors
      2. Metastatic tumors with osteolysis
      3. Lymphoma, leukemia
      4. Dysgerminoma
      5. Pheochromocytoma
      6. Tumors secreting parathyroid hormone–related peptide, growth factors, cytokines, prostaglandins, osteoclast-activating factors
   E. Williams-Beuren Syndrome (del7q11.23)
V. Immobilization
VI. Other Causes
   A. Drugs: Thiazides, Lithium, Vitamin A and Analogs, Calcium, Alkali, Antiestrogens, Aminophylline
   B. Total Parenteral Nutrition
   C. Endocrinopathies: Hyperthyroidism, Addison disease, Pheochromocytoma
   D. Vasoactive Intestinal Polypeptide–Secreting Tumor
   E. Acute or Chronic Renal Failure/Administration of Aluminum
   F. Hypophosphatasia
   G. Juvenile Rheumatoid Arthritis: Cytokine Mediated

Adapted from Lietman SA, Germain-Lee EL, Levine MA. Hypercalcemia in children and adolescents. Curr Opin Pediatr 22:508–515, 2010; Benjamin RW, Moats-Staats BM, Calikoglu A, et al. Hypercalcemia in children. Pediatr Endocrinol Rev 5:778–784, 2008; Davies JH. A practical approach to the problems of hypercalcaemia. Endocr Dev 16:93–114, 2009.

circumstances, a diet high in calcium and phosphorus must be maintained for only several months after operation.

CT, real-time ultrasonography, and subtraction scintigraphy using sestamibi/technetium-pertechnetate alone and in combination have proved effective in localizing a single adenoma vs diffuse hyperplasia in 50-90% of adults. Parathyroid surgeons often rely on intraoperative selective venous sampling with intraoperative assay of PTH for localizing and removing the source of increased PTH secretion.

PROGNOSIS

The prognosis is good if the disease is recognized early and there is appropriate surgical treatment. When extensive osseous lesions are present, deformities may be permanent. A search for other affected family members is indicated.

573.1 Other Causes of Hypercalcemia
Daniel A. Doyle

FAMILIAL HYPOCALCIURIC HYPERCALCEMIA (FAMILIAL BENIGN HYPERCALCEMIA)

Patients with familial hypocalciuric hypercalcemia are usually asymptomatic, and the hypercalcemia is identified by chance during routine investigation for other conditions. The parathyroid glands are normal, PTH levels are inappropriately normal, and subtotal parathyroidectomy does not correct the hypercalcemia. Serum levels of magnesium are high normal or mildly elevated. The ratio of calcium-to-creatinine clearance is usually decreased despite hypercalcemia.

The disorder is inherited in an autosomal dominant manner and is caused by a mutant gene on chromosome 3q2. Penetrance is near 100%, and the disorder can be diagnosed early in childhood by serum and urinary calcium concentrations. Detection of other affected family members is important to avoid inappropriate parathyroid surgery. The defect is an inactivating mutation in the Ca^{2+}-sensing receptor gene. This G-protein–coupled receptor senses the level of free Ca^{2+} in the blood and triggers the pathway to increase extracellular Ca^{2+} in the face of hypocalcemia. This receptor functions in the parathyroid and kidney to regulate calcium homeostasis; inactivating mutations lead to an increased set point with respect to serum Ca^{2+}, resulting in mild to moderate hypercalcemia in heterozygotes.

GRANULOMATOUS DISEASES

Hypercalcemia occurs in 30-50% of children with sarcoidosis and less often in patients with other granulomatous diseases such as tuberculosis. Levels of PTH are suppressed, and levels of $1,25(OH)_2D_3$ are elevated. The source of **ectopic $1,25(OH)_2D_3$** is the activated macrophage, through stimulation by interferon-α from T lymphocytes, which are present in abundance in granulomatous lesions. Unlike renal tubular cells, the 1α-hydroxylase in macrophages is unresponsive to homeostatic regulation. Oral administration of prednisone (2 mg/kg/24 hr) lowers serum levels of $1,25(OH)_2D_3$ to normal and corrects the hypercalcemia.

HYPERCALCEMIA OF MALIGNANCY

Hypercalcemia often occurs in adults with a wide variety of solid tumors but is identified much less often in children. It has been reported in infants with malignant rhabdoid tumors of the kidney or congenital mesoblastic nephroma and in children with neuroblastoma, medulloblastoma, leukemia, Burkitt lymphoma, dysgerminoma, and rhabdomyosarcoma. Serum levels of PTH are rarely elevated. In most patients, the hypercalcemia associated with malignancy is caused by elevated levels of parathyroid hormone–related peptide and not PTH. Rarely, tumors produce $1,25(OH)_2D_3$ or PTH ectopically.

MISCELLANEOUS CAUSES OF HYPERCALCEMIA

Hypercalcemia can occur in infants with **subcutaneous fat necrosis.** Levels of PTH are normal. In 1 infant, the level of $1,25(OH)_2D_3$ was elevated and biopsy of the skin lesion revealed granulomatous infiltration, suggesting that the mechanism of the hypercalcemia was akin to that seen in patients with other granulomatous disease. In another infant, although the level of $1,25(OH)_2D_3$ was normal, PTH was suppressed, suggesting the hypercalcemia was not related to PTH. Treatment with prednisone is effective.

Hypophosphatasia, especially the severe infantile form, is usually associated with mild to moderate hypercalcemia (see Chapter 705). Serum levels of phosphorus are normal, and those of alkaline phosphatase are subnormal. The bones exhibit rachitic-like lesions on radiographs. Urinary levels of phosphoethanolamine, inorganic pyrophosphate, and pyridoxal 5′-phosphate are elevated; each is a natural substrate to a tissue-nonspecific (liver, bone, kidney) alkaline phosphatase enzyme. Missense mutations of the tissue-nonspecific alkaline phosphatase enzyme gene result in an inactive enzyme in this autosomal recessive disorder.

Idiopathic hypercalcemia of infancy is manifested by failure to thrive and hypercalcemia during the 1st yr of life, followed by spontaneous remission. Serum levels of phosphorus and PTH are normal. The condition has been defined as resulting from increased absorption of calcium from decreased degradation of $1,25(OH)_2D_3$. Mutations in the *CYP24A1* gene that encodes 25-hydroxyvitamin D 24-hydroxylase, the key enzyme in $1,25(OH)_2D_3$ degradation, cause excessive levels of the active vitamin D metabolite, which, in turn, causes hypercalcemia in a subset of infants who receive supplemental vitamin D. An excessive rise in the level of $1,25(OH)_2D_3$ in response to PTH administration has been reported years after the hypercalcemic phase.

Approximately 10% of patients with **Williams syndrome** also inconsistently exhibit associated infantile hypercalcemia. The phenotype consists of feeding difficulties, slow growth, elfin facies (small mandible, prominent maxilla, upturned nose), renovascular disorders, and a gregarious "cocktail party" personality. Cardiac lesions include supravalvular aortic stenosis, peripheral pulmonic stenosis, aortic hypoplasia, coronary artery stenosis, and atrial or ventricular septal defects. Nephrocalcinosis can develop if hypercalcemia persists. The IQ score of 50-70 is curiously accompanied by enhanced quantity and quality of vocabulary, auditory memory, and social use of language. A contiguous gene deletion syndrome with a submicroscopic deletion at chromosome 7q11.23, which includes deletion of 1 elastin allele, occurs in 90% of patients and seems to account for the vascular problems. Definitive diagnosis can be established by specific fluorescence in situ hybridization. The hypercalcemia and central nervous system symptoms may be caused by deletion of adjacent genes. Hypercalcemia has been successfully controlled with either prednisone or calcitonin.

Hypervitaminosis D resulting in hypercalcemia from drinking milk that has been incorrectly fortified with excessive amounts of vitamin D has been reported. Not all patients with hypervitaminosis D develop hypercalcemia. Affected infants can manifest failure to thrive, nephrolithiasis, poor renal function, and osteosclerosis. Serum levels of 25(OH)D are a better indicator of hypervitaminosis D than levels of $1,25(OH)_2D_3$ because 25(OH)D has a longer half-life.

Prolonged immobilization can lead to hypercalcemia and occasionally to decreased renal function, hypertension, and encephalopathy. Children who have hypophosphatemic rickets and undergo surgery with subsequent long-term immobilization are at risk for hypercalcemia and should therefore have their vitamin D supplementation decreased or discontinued.

Jansen-type metaphyseal chondrodysplasia is a rare genetic disorder characterized by short-limbed dwarfism and severe but asymptomatic hypercalcemia (see Chapter 704). Circulating levels of PTH and parathyroid hormone–related peptide are undetectable. These patients have an activating PTH–parathyroid hormone–related peptide receptor mutation that results in aberrant calcium homeostasis and abnormalities of the growth plate.

Bibliography is available at Expert Consult.

Section **4**
Disorders of the Adrenal Gland

Chapter **574**
Physiology of the Adrenal Gland

574.1 Histology and Embryology

Perrin C. White

The adrenal gland is composed of 2 endocrine tissues: the medulla and the cortex. The chromaffin cells of the adrenal medulla are derived from neuroectoderm, whereas the cells of the adrenal cortex are derived from mesoderm. Mesodermal cells also contribute to the development of the gonads. The adrenal glands and gonads have certain common enzymes involved in steroid synthesis; an inborn error in steroidogenesis in one tissue can also be present in the other.

The adrenal cortex of the older child or adult consists of 3 zones: the zona glomerulosa, the outermost zone located immediately beneath the capsule; the zona fasciculata, the middle zone; and the zona reticularis, the innermost zone, lying next to the adrenal medulla. The zona fasciculata is the largest zone, constituting approximately 75% of the cortex; the zona glomerulosa constitutes approximately 15% and the zona reticularis approximately 10%. Glomerulosa cells are small, with a lower cytoplasmic:nuclear ratio, an intermediate number of lipid inclusions, and smaller nuclei containing more condensed chromatin than the cells of the other 2 zones. The cells of the zona fasciculata are large, with a high cytoplasmic:nuclear ratio and many lipid inclusions that give the cytoplasm a foamy, vacuolated appearance. The cells are arranged in radial cords. The cells of the zona reticularis are arranged in irregular anastomosing cords. The cytoplasmic:nuclear ratio is intermediate, and the compact cytoplasm has relatively little lipid content.

The zona glomerulosa synthesizes aldosterone, the most potent natural mineralocorticoid in humans. The zona fasciculata produces cortisol, the most potent natural glucocorticoid in humans, and the zona fasciculata and zona reticularis synthesize the adrenal androgens.

The adrenal medulla consists mainly of neuroendocrine (chromaffin) cells and glial (sustentacular) cells with some connective tissue and vascular cells. Neuroendocrine cells are polyhedral, with abundant cytoplasm and small, pale-staining nuclei. Under the electron microscope, the cytoplasm contains many large secretory granules that contain catecholamines. Glial cells have less cytoplasm and more basophilic nuclei.

The primordium of the fetal adrenal gland can be recognized at 3-4 wk of gestation just cephalad to the developing mesonephros. At 5-6 wk, the gonadal ridge develops into the steroidogenic cells of the gonads and adrenal cortex; the adrenal and gonadal cells separate, the adrenal cells migrate retroperitoneally, and the gonadal cells migrate caudad. At 6-8 wk of gestation, the gland rapidly enlarges, the cells of the inner cortex differentiate to form the fetal zone, and the outer subcapsular rim remains as the definitive zone. The primordium of the adrenal cortex is invaded at this time by sympathetic neural elements that differentiate into the chromaffin cells capable of synthesizing and storing catecholamines. Catechol O-methyltransferase, which converts norepinephrine to epinephrine, is expressed later in gestation. By the end of the 8th wk of gestation, the encapsulated adrenal gland is associated with the upper pole of the kidney. By 8-10 wk of gestation, the cells of the fetal zone are capable of active steroidogenesis.

In the full-term infant, the combined weight of both adrenal glands is 7-9 g. At birth, the inner fetal cortex makes up approximately 80% of the gland and the outer "true" cortex, 20%. Within a few days the fetal cortex begins to involute, undergoing a 50% reduction by 1 mo of age. Conversely, the adrenal medulla is relatively small at birth and undergoes a proportionate increase in size over the 1st 6 mo after birth. By 1 yr, the adrenal glands each weigh <1 g. Adrenal growth thereafter results in adult adrenal glands reaching a combined weight of 8 g. The zonae fasciculata and glomerulosa are fully differentiated by about 3 yr of age. The zona reticularis is not fully developed until puberty.

Adrenocorticotropic hormone (ACTH) is essential for fetal adrenal growth and maturation; feedback regulation of ACTH by cortisol is apparently established by 8-10 wk of gestation. Additional factors important in fetal growth and steroidogenesis include placental chorionic gonadotropins and a number of peptide growth factors produced by the placenta and fetus.

Several transcription factors are critical for the development of the adrenal glands. The 3 transcription factors associated with adrenal hypoplasia in humans are steroidogenic factor-1 (*SF-1; NR5A1*), *DAX-1* (dosage-sensitive sex reversal, adrenal hypoplasia congenita, X chromosome; NR0B1), and the *GLI3* oncogene. Disruption of *SF-1*, encoded on chromosome 9q33, results in gonadal and often adrenal agenesis, absence of pituitary gonadotropes, and an underdeveloped ventral medial hypothalamus. In-frame deletions and frameshift and missense mutations of this gene are associated with 46,XX ovarian insufficiency and 46,XY gonadal dysgenesis. Mutations in the *DAX1* gene, encoded on Xp21, result in adrenal hypoplasia congenita and hypogonadotropic hypogonadism (see Chapter 575.1). Mutations in *GLI3* on chromosome 7p13 cause Pallister-Hall syndrome, other features of which include hypothalamic hamartoblastoma, hypopituitarism, imperforate anus, and postaxial polydactyly.

The postnatal adrenal cortex is not static but, in fact, is continually regenerated from a population of stem or progenitor cells under the adrenal capsule. These cells move radially inward (i.e., centripetally) and can differentiate into zona glomerulosa or fasciculata cells as needed in response to the appropriate trophic stimuli (see Chapter 574.3). Several signaling pathways, including sonic hedgehog and Wnt, regulate this process. Sonic hedgehog expression is restricted to the peripheral cortical cells that do not express high levels of steroidogenic genes but give rise to the underlying differentiated cells of the cortex. Wnt/β-catenin signaling maintains the undifferentiated state and adrenal fate of adrenocortical stem/progenitor cells, in part through induction of its target genes *DAX1* and inhibin-α, respectively. Adrenal tumors can result from constitutive activation of the Wnt signaling pathway (see Chapter 579), whereas mutations of *DAX1* lead to loss of the ability of the adrenal cortex to regenerate; this condition is termed *adrenal hypoplasia congenita* (see Chapter 575).

Bibliography is available at Expert Consult.

574.2 Adrenal Steroid Biosynthesis

Perrin C. White

Cholesterol is the starting substrate for all steroid biosynthesis (Fig. 574-1). Although adrenal cortex cells can synthesize cholesterol de novo from acetate, circulating plasma lipoproteins provide most of the cholesterol for adrenal cortex hormone formation. Receptors for both low-density lipoprotein and high-density lipoprotein cholesterol are expressed on the surface of adrenocortical cells; the receptor is termed scavenger receptor class B, type I. Patients with familial hypercholesterolemia who lack low-density lipoprotein receptors have unimpaired adrenal steroidogenesis, suggesting that high-density lipoprotein is the more important source of cholesterol. Cholesterol is stored as cholesteryl esters in vesicles and subsequently hydrolyzed by cholesteryl ester hydrolases to liberate free cholesterol for steroid hormone synthesis.

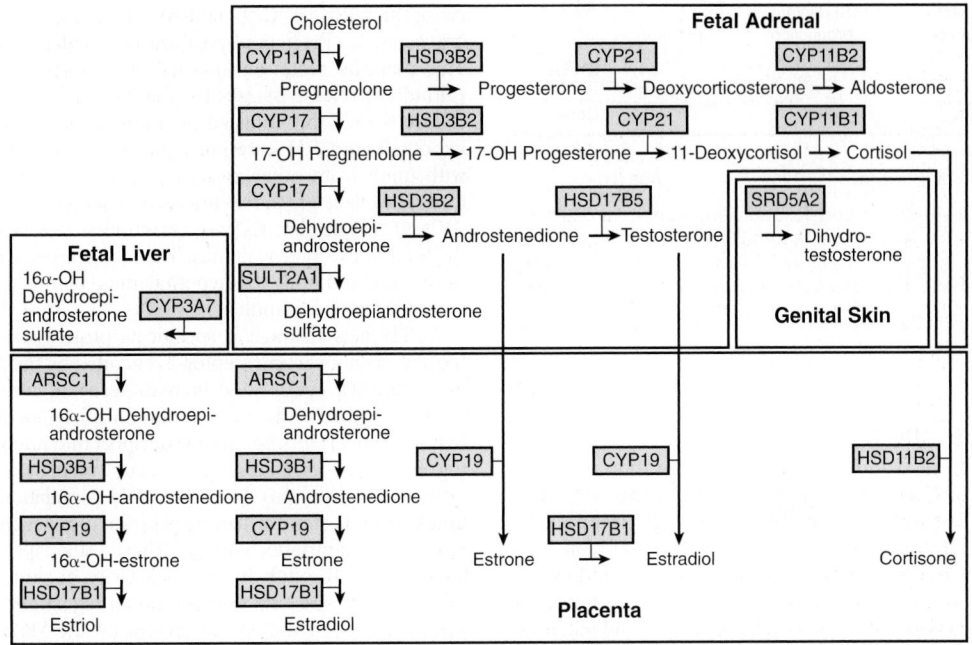

Figure 574-1 Steroid biosynthesis and metabolism during gestation. Conversions within the fetal adrenal cortex, fetal liver, male (i.e., testosterone-exposed) genital skin, and placenta are denoted by *arrows*; the enzyme mediating each conversion is also shown. Enzymatic conversions in the adrenal cortex are the same postnatally as prenatally, but cortisol and aldosterone biosynthesis are more prominent, and normally little testosterone is synthesized. Many of the involved enzymes are cytochromes P450 (CYPs). Adrenal enzymes include CYP 11A, cholesterol side-chain cleavage enzyme (P450scc in older terminology); HSD3B2, 3β-hydroxysteroid dehydrogenase/Δ5,Δ4 isomerase type 2; CYP 17, 17β-hydroxylase/17,20-lyase (P450c17); CYP 21, 21-hydroxylase (P450c21); CYP 11B1, 11β-hydroxylase (P450c11); CYP 11B2, aldosterone synthase (P450aldo; this enzyme mediates successive 11β-hydroxylase, 18-hydroxylase, and 18-oxidase reactions in the zona glomerulosa for the conversion of deoxycorticosterone to aldosterone). Other enzymes important in the fetoplacental unit include ARSC1, arylsulfatase; CYP 19, aromatase (P450arom); HSD3B1, 3β-hydroxysteroid dehydrogenase/Δ5,Δ4 isomerase type 1; HSD11B2, 11β-hydroxysteroid dehydrogenase type 2; HSD17B1 and HSD17B5 are 2 different 17-hydroxysteroid dehydrogenase enzymes; SRD5A2, steroid 5α-reductase type 2; SULT2A1, steroid sulfotransferase.

The rate-limiting step of adrenal steroidogenesis is importation of cholesterol across the mitochondrial outer and inner membrane. This requires several proteins, particularly the steroidogenic acute regulatory (StAR) protein. The steroidogenic acute regulatory protein has a very short half-life, and its synthesis is rapidly induced by trophic factors (corticotropin); thus, it is the main short-term (minutes to hours) regulator of steroid hormone biosynthesis.

At the mitochondrial inner membrane, the side chain of cholesterol is cleaved to yield pregnenolone. This is catalyzed by the cholesterol side-chain cleavage enzyme (cholesterol desmolase, side-chain cleavage enzyme, P450scc, CYP11A1; the last term is the current systematic nomenclature), a cytochrome P450 (CYP) enzyme. Like other P450s, this is a membrane-bound hemoprotein with a molecular mass of approximately 50 kDa. It accepts electrons from a nicotinamide adenine dinucleotide phosphate–dependent mitochondrial electron transport system consisting of 2 accessory proteins, adrenodoxin reductase (a flavoprotein) and adrenodoxin (a small protein containing nonheme iron). P450 enzymes use electrons and O_2 to hydroxylate the substrate and form H_2O. In the case of cholesterol side-chain cleavage, 3 successive oxidative reactions are performed to cleave the C20,22 carbon bond. Pregnenolone then diffuses out of mitochondria and enters the endoplasmic reticulum. The subsequent reactions that occur depend on the zone of the adrenal cortex.

ZONA GLOMERULOSA

In the zona glomerulosa, pregnenolone is converted to progesterone by 3β-hydroxysteroid dehydrogenase type 2, a nicotinamide adenine dinucleotide–positive–dependent enzyme of the short-chain dehydrogenase type. Progesterone is converted to 11-deoxycorticosterone by steroid 21-hydroxylase (P450c21, CYP21), which is another P450. Like other P450s in the endoplasmic reticulum, it uses an electron transport system with only 1 accessory protein, P450 oxidoreductase.

Deoxycorticosterone then reenters mitochondria and is converted to aldosterone by aldosterone synthase (P450aldo, CYP11B2), a P450 enzyme structurally related to cholesterol desmolase. Aldosterone synthase also carries out 3 successive oxidations: 11β-hydroxylation, 18-hydroxylation, and further oxidation of the 18-methyl carbon to an aldehyde.

ZONA FASCICULATA

In the endoplasmic reticulum of the zona fasciculata, pregnenolone and progesterone are converted by 17α-hydroxylase (P450c17, CYP17) to 17-hydroxypregnenolone and 17-hydroxyprogesterone, respectively. This enzyme is not expressed in the zona glomerulosa, which consequently cannot synthesize 17-hydroxylated steroids. 17-Hydroxypregnenolone is converted to 17-hydroxyprogesterone and 11-deoxycortisol by the same 3β-hydroxysteroid and 21-hydroxylase enzymes, respectively, as are active in the zona glomerulosa. Thus, inherited disorders in these enzymes affect both aldosterone and cortisol synthesis (see Chapter 576). Finally, 11-deoxycortisol reenters mitochondria and is converted to cortisol by steroid 11β-hydroxylase (P450c11, CYP11B1). This enzyme is closely related to aldosterone synthase but has low 18-hydroxylase and nonexistent 18-oxidase activity. Thus, under normal circumstances the zona fasciculata cannot synthesize aldosterone.

ZONA RETICULARIS

In the zona reticularis and to some extent in the zona fasciculata, the 17-hydroxylase (CYP17) enzyme has an additional activity, cleavage of the 17,20 carbon–carbon bond. This converts 17-hydroxypregnenolone to dehydroepiandrosterone (DHEA). DHEA is converted to androstenedione by HSD3B. This may be further converted in other tissues to testosterone and estrogens.

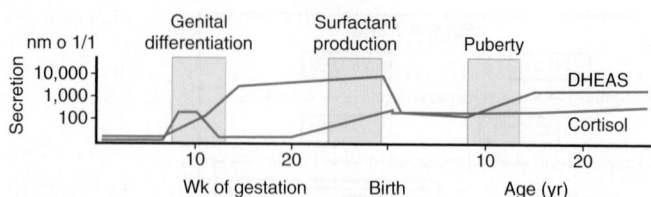

Figure 574-2 Relative levels of cortisol and dehydroepiandrosterone sulfate (DHEAS) secretion by the fetal adrenal cortex during gestation as well as postnatally. Approximate times of several events are shown. Vertical axis is logarithmic, but values are approximate. Horizontal axis is not to scale.

FETOPLACENTAL UNIT

Steroid synthesis in the fetal adrenal varies during gestation (see Figs. 574-1 and 574-2). Shortly after the fetal adrenal gland forms (wk 8-10), it efficiently secretes cortisol, which is able to negatively feedback on the fetal pituitary and hypothalamus to suppress ACTH secretion. This is critical time for differentiation of the external genitalia in both sexes (see Chapter 576.1); to prevent virilization, the female fetus must not be exposed to high levels of androgens of adrenal origin, and placental aromatase activity must remain low during this time to minimize conversion of testosterone to estradiol in male fetuses, which would interfere with masculinization. After wk 12, HSD3B activity in the fetal adrenal gland decreases and steroid sulfokinase activity increases. Thus, the major steroid products of the midgestation fetal adrenal gland are DHEA and DHEA sulfate (DHEAS) and, by 16α-hydroxylation in the liver, 16α-hydroxy DHEAS. Aromatase activity increases in the placenta at the same time, and steroid sulfatase activity is high as well. Thus, the placenta uses DHEA and DHEAS as substrates for estrone and estradiol and 16α-OH DHEAS as a substrate for estriol. Cortisol activity is low during the 2nd trimester, which might serve to prevent premature secretion of surfactant by the developing fetal lungs; surfactant levels can affect the timing of parturition. As term approaches, fetal cortisol concentration increases as a result of increased cortisol secretion and decreased conversion of cortisol to cortisone by 11β-hydroxysteroid dehydrogenase type 2 (HSD11B2). Low levels of aldosterone are produced in mid-gestation, but aldosterone secretory capacity increases near term.

Bibliography is available at Expert Consult.

574.3 Regulation of the Adrenal Cortex
Perrin C. White

REGULATION OF CORTISOL SECRETION

Glucocorticoid secretion is regulated mainly by ACTH (corticotropin), a 39-amino-acid peptide that is produced in the anterior pituitary. It is synthesized as part of a larger-molecular-weight precursor peptide known as proopiomelanocortin. This precursor peptide is also the source of β-lipotropin. ACTH and β-lipotropin are cleaved further to yield α- and β-melanocyte–stimulating hormone, corticotropin-like intermediate lobe peptide, γ-lipotropin, β- and γ-endorphin, and enkephalin (see Chapter 556).

ACTH is released in secretory bursts of varying amplitude throughout the day and night. The normal diurnal rhythm of cortisol secretion is caused by the varying amplitudes of ACTH pulses. Pulses of ACTH and cortisol occur every 30-120 min, are highest at about the time of waking, are low in late afternoon and evening, and reach their lowest point 1 or 2 hr after sleep begins.

Corticotropin-releasing hormone (CRH), synthesized by neurons of the parvicellular division of the hypothalamic paraventricular nucleus, is the most important stimulator of ACTH secretion. Arginine vasopressin (AVP) augments CRH action. Neural stimuli from the brain

cause the release of CRH and AVP (see Chapter 556). AVP and CRH are secreted in the hypophyseal-portal circulation in a pulsatile manner. This pulsatile secretion appears to be responsible for the pulsatile (ultradian) release of ACTH. The circadian rhythm of corticotropin release is probably induced by a corresponding circadian rhythm of hypothalamic CRH secretion, regulated by the suprachiasmatic nucleus with input from other areas of the brain. Cortisol exerts a negative feedback effect on the synthesis and secretion of ACTH, CRH, and AVP. ACTH inhibits its own secretion, a feedback effect mediated at the level of the hypothalamus. Thus the secretion of cortisol is a result of the interaction of the hypothalamus, pituitary, and adrenal glands and other neural stimuli.

ACTH acts through a specific G-protein–coupled receptor (also termed melanocortin receptor-2, encoded by the *MCR2* gene) to activate adenylate cyclase and increase levels of cyclic adenosine monophosphate. Cyclic adenosine monophosphate has short-term (minutes to hours) effects on cholesterol transport into mitochondria by increasing expression of steroidogenic acute regulatory protein. The long-term effects (hours to days) of ACTH stimulation are to increase the uptake of cholesterol and the expression of genes encoding the enzymes required to synthesize cortisol. These transcriptional effects occur at least in part through increased activity of protein kinase A, which phosphorylates several transcriptional regulatory factors. MC2R trafficking and signaling are dependent on the MC2R accessory protein (MRAP). Mutations in either MC2R or MRAP can cause familial glucocorticoid deficiency (see Chapter 575).

REGULATION OF ALDOSTERONE SECRETION

The rate of aldosterone synthesis, which is normally 100- to 1,000-fold less than that of cortisol synthesis, is regulated mainly by the renin–angiotensin system and by potassium levels, with ACTH having only a short-term effect. In response to decreased intravascular volume, renin is secreted by the juxtaglomerular apparatus of the kidney. Renin is a proteolytic enzyme that cleaves angiotensinogen (renin substrate), an α_2-globulin produced by the liver, to yield the inactive decapeptide angiotensin I. Angiotensin-converting enzyme in the lungs and other tissues rapidly cleaves angiotensin I to the biologically active octapeptide angiotensin II. Cleavage of angiotensin II produces the heptapeptide angiotensin III. Angiotensins II and III are potent stimulators of aldosterone secretion; angiotensin II is a more potent vasopressor agent. Angiotensins II and III occupy a G-protein–coupled receptor activating phospholipase C. This protein hydrolyzes phosphatidylinositol bisphosphate to produce inositol triphosphate and diacylglycerol, which raise intracellular calcium levels and activate protein kinase C and calmodulin-activated kinases. Similarly, increased levels of extracellular potassium depolarize the cell membrane and increase calcium influx through voltage-gated L-type calcium channels. Phosphorylation of transcriptional regulatory factors by calmodulin-activated kinases increases transcription of the aldosterone synthase (CYP11B2) enzyme required for aldosterone synthesis.

REGULATION OF ADRENAL ANDROGEN SECRETION

The mechanisms by which the adrenal androgens DHEA and androstenedione are regulated are not completely understood. Adrenarche is a maturational process in the adrenal gland that results in increased adrenal androgen secretion between the ages of 5 and 20 yr. The process begins before the earliest signs of puberty and continues throughout the years when puberty is occurring. Histologically, it is associated with the appearance of the zona reticularis. Whereas ACTH stimulates adrenal androgen production acutely and clearly is the primary stimulus for cortisol release, additional factors have been implicated in the stimulation of the adrenal androgens. These include a relative decrease in expression of HSD3B in the zona reticularis and possibly increases in 17,20-lyase activity owing to phosphorylation of CYP17 or increased cytochrome b5 expression.

Bibliography is available at Expert Consult.

574.4 Adrenal Steroid Hormone Actions

Perrin C. White

Steroid hormones act through several distinct receptors corresponding to the known biologic activities of the steroid hormones: glucocorticoid, mineralocorticoid, progestin, estrogen, and androgen. These receptors belong to a larger superfamily of nuclear transcriptional factors that include, among others, thyroid hormone and retinoic acid receptors. They have a common structure that includes a carboxyterminal ligand-binding domain and a midregion DNA-binding domain. The latter domain contains 2 zinc fingers, each of which consists of a loop of amino acids stabilized by 4 cysteine residues chelating a zinc ion.

Unliganded glucocorticoid and mineralocorticoid receptors are found mainly in the cytosol. Hormone molecules diffuse through the cell membrane and bind receptors, changing their conformation and causing them to be translocated to the nucleus, where they bind DNA at specific hormone-response elements. Bound receptors can recruit other transcriptional coregulatory factors to DNA.

Whereas different steroids can share bioactivities because of their ability to bind to the same receptor, a given steroid can exert diverse biologic effects in different tissues. The diversity of hormonal responses is determined by the different genes that are regulated by each hormone in different tissues. Additionally, different combinations of coregulators are expressed in different tissues, allowing each steroid hormone to have many different effects. Moreover, enzymes can increase or decrease the affinity of steroids for their receptors and thus modulate their activity. 11β-Hydroxysteroid dehydrogenase type 1 (HSD11B1) converts cortisone, which is not a ligand for the glucocorticoid receptor, to cortisol, which is an active glucocorticoid. This increases local glucocorticoid concentrations in several tissues, especially the liver, where glucocorticoids maintain hepatic glucose output (see Chapter 575.4). Overexpression of this enzyme in adipose tissue can predispose to development of obesity. Conversely, HSD11B2 oxidizes cortisol to cortisone, particularly in the kidney, preventing mineralocorticoid receptors from being occupied by high levels of cortisol (see Chapter 575.4).

Although corticosteroid receptors mainly act in the nucleus, some responses to both glucocorticoids and mineralocorticoids begin within minutes, an interval too short to be accounted for by increased gene transcription and protein synthesis. Such "nongenomic" effects can in some cases be mediated by cell membrane–associated isoforms of the classic glucocorticoid and mineralocorticoid receptors, which can couple to a variety of rapid intracellular signaling pathways such as G proteins. Direct interactions with other proteins, such as ion channels, have been documented as well, particularly in the nervous system.

ACTIONS OF GLUCOCORTICOIDS

Glucocorticoids are essential for survival. The term *glucocorticoid* refers to the glucose-regulating properties of these hormones. However, glucocorticoids have multiple effects on carbohydrate, lipid, and protein metabolism. They also regulate immune, circulatory, and renal function. They influence growth, development, bone metabolism, and central nervous system activity.

In stress situations, glucocorticoid secretion can increase up to 10-fold. This increase is believed to enhance survival through increased cardiac contractility, cardiac output, sensitivity to the pressor effects of catecholamines and other pressor hormones, work capacity of the skeletal muscles, and capacity to mobilize energy stores.

Metabolic Effects

The primary action of the glucocorticoids on carbohydrate metabolism is to increase glucose production by increasing hepatic gluconeogenesis. Glucocorticoids also increase cellular resistance to insulin, thereby decreasing entry of glucose into the cell. This inhibition of glucose uptake occurs in adipocytes, muscle cells, and fibroblasts. In addition to opposing insulin action, glucocorticoids can work in parallel with insulin to protect against long-term starvation by stimulating glycogen deposition and production in liver. Both hormones stimulate glycogen synthetase activity and decrease glycogen breakdown. Glucocorticoid excess can cause hyperglycemia, and glucocorticoid deficiency can cause hypoglycemia.

Glucocorticoids increase free fatty acid levels by enhancing lipolysis, decreasing cellular glucose uptake, and decreasing glycerol production, which is necessary for reesterification of fatty acids. This increase in lipolysis is also stimulated through the permissive enhancement of lipolytic action of other factors such as epinephrine. This action affects adipocytes differently according to their anatomic locations. In the patient with glucocorticoid excess, fat is lost in the extremities but it is increased in the trunk (centripetal obesity), neck, and face (moon facies). This may involve effects on adipocyte differentiation.

Glucocorticoids generally exert a catabolic or antianabolic effect on protein metabolism. Proteolysis in fat, skeletal muscle, bone, lymphoid, and connective tissue increases amino acid substrates that can be used in gluconeogenesis. Cardiac muscle and the diaphragm are almost entirely spared from this catabolic effect.

Circulatory and Renal Effects

Glucocorticoids have a positive inotropic influence on the heart, increasing the left ventricular work index. Moreover, they have a permissive effect on the actions of epinephrine and norepinephrine on both the heart and the blood vessels. In the absence of glucocorticoids, decreased cardiac output and shock can develop; in states of glucocorticoid excess, hypertension is often observed. This may be a result of activation of the mineralocorticoid receptor (see Chapter 575.4), which occurs when renal HSD11B is saturated by excessive levels of glucocorticoids.

Growth

In excess, glucocorticoids inhibit linear growth and skeletal maturation in children, apparently through direct effects on the epiphyses. However, glucocorticoids are also necessary for normal growth and development. In the fetus and neonate, they accelerate the differentiation and development of various tissues, including the hepatic and gastrointestinal systems, as well as the production of surfactant in the fetal lung. Glucocorticoids are often given to pregnant women at risk for delivery of premature infants in an effort to accelerate these maturational processes (see Chapters 97.2 and 101.3).

Immunologic Effects

Glucocorticoids play a major role in immune regulation. They inhibit synthesis of glycolipids and prostaglandin precursors and the actions of bradykinin. They also block secretion and actions of histamine and proinflammatory cytokines (tumor necrosis factor-α, interleukin-1, and interleukin-6), thus diminishing inflammation. High doses of glucocorticoids deplete monocytes, eosinophils, and lymphocytes, especially T cells. They do so at least in part by inducing cell-cycle arrest in the G₁ phase and by activating apoptosis through glucocorticoid receptor–mediated effects. The effects on lymphocytes are primarily exerted on T-helper 1 cells and hence on cellular immunity, whereas the T-helper 2 cells are spared, leading to a predominantly humoral immune response. Pharmacologic doses of glucocorticoids can also decrease the size of immunologic tissues (spleen, thymus, and lymph nodes).

Glucocorticoids increase circulating polymorphonuclear cell counts, mostly by preventing their egress from the circulation. Glucocorticoids decrease diapedesis, chemotaxis, and phagocytosis of polymorphonuclear cells. Thus, the mobility of these cells is altered such that they do not arrive at the site of inflammation to mount an appropriate immune response. High levels of glucocorticoids decrease inflammatory and cellular immune responses and increase susceptibility to certain bacterial, viral, fungal, and parasitic infections.

Effects on Skin, Bone, and Calcium

Glucocorticoids inhibit fibroblasts, leading to increased bruising and poor wound healing through cutaneous atrophy. This effect explains the thinning of the skin and striae that are seen in patients with Cushing syndrome.

Glucocorticoids have the overall effect of decreasing serum calcium and have been used in emergency therapy for certain types of hypercalcemia. This hypocalcemic effect probably results from a decrease in the intestinal absorption of calcium and a decrease in the renal reabsorption of calcium and phosphorus. Serum calcium levels, however, generally do not fall below normal because of a secondary increase in parathyroid hormone secretion.

The most significant effect of long-term glucocorticoid excess on calcium and bone metabolism is **osteoporosis.** Glucocorticoids inhibit osteoblastic activity by decreasing the number and activity of osteoblasts. Glucocorticoids also decrease osteoclastic activity but to a lesser extent, leading to low bone turnover with an overall negative balance. The tendency of glucocorticoids to lower serum calcium and phosphate levels causes secondary hyperparathyroidism. These actions decrease bone accretion and cause a net loss of bone mineral. Compliance with oral bisphosphonates, agents that are effective against glucocorticoid-induced osteoporosis, is poor, but evidence suggests that yearly treatment with intravenous zoledronic acid is just as effective.

Central Nervous System Effects

Glucocorticoids readily penetrate the blood–brain barrier and have direct effects on brain metabolism. They decrease certain types of central nervous system edema and are often used to treat increased intracranial pressure. They stimulate appetite and cause insomnia with a reduction in rapid eye movement sleep. There is an increase in irritability and emotional lability, with an impairment of memory and ability to concentrate. Mild to moderate glucocorticoid excess for a limited period often causes a feeling of euphoria or well-being, but glucocorticoid excess and deficiency can both be associated with clinical depression. Glucocorticoid excess produces **psychosis** in some patients.

Glucocorticoid effects in the brain are mediated largely through interactions with both the mineralocorticoid and glucocorticoid receptors (sometimes referred to in this context as type I and type II corticosteroid receptors, respectively). Activation of type II receptors increases sensitivity of hippocampal neurons to the neurotransmitter serotonin, which might help explain the euphoria associated with high doses of glucocorticoids. Glucocorticoids suppress release of CRH in the anterior hypothalamus, but they stimulate it in the central nucleus of the amygdala and lateral bed nucleus of the stria terminalis, where it can mediate fear and anxiety states. Glucocorticoids and other steroids might have nongenomic effects by modulating activities of both γ-aminobutyric acid and N-methyl-D-aspartate receptors.

ACTIONS OF MINERALOCORTICOIDS

The most important mineralocorticoids are aldosterone and, to a lesser degree, 11-deoxycorticosterone; corticosterone and cortisol are normally not important as mineralocorticoids unless secreted in excess. Mineralocorticoids have more limited actions than glucocorticoids. Their major function is to maintain intravascular volume by conserving sodium and eliminating potassium and hydrogen ions. They exert these actions in the kidney, gut, and salivary and sweat glands. Aldosterone can have distinct effects in other tissues. Mineralocorticoid receptors are found in the heart and vascular endothelium, and aldosterone increases myocardial fibrosis in heart failure.

Mineralocorticoids have their most important actions in the distal convoluted tubules and cortical collecting ducts of the kidney, where they induce reabsorption of sodium and secretion of potassium. In the medullary collecting duct, they act in a permissive fashion to allow vasopressin to increase osmotic water flux. Thus, patients with mineralocorticoid deficiency can develop weight loss, hypotension, hyponatremia, and hyperkalemia, whereas patients with mineralocorticoid excess can develop hypertension, hypokalemia, and metabolic alkalosis (see Chapters 575-578).

The mechanisms by which aldosterone affects sodium excretion are incompletely understood. Most effects of aldosterone are presumably due to changes in gene expression mediated by the mineralocorticoid receptor, and indeed levels of subunits of both the Na^+,K^+-adenosine triphosphatase and the epithelial sodium channel increase in response to aldosterone. Additionally, aldosterone increases expression of the serum and glucocorticoid-regulated kinase, which indirectly reduces turnover of epithelial sodium channel subunits and thus increases the number of open sodium channels.

The mineralocorticoid receptor has similar affinities in vitro for cortisol and aldosterone, yet cortisol is a weak mineralocorticoid in vivo. This discrepancy results from the action of HSD11B2, which converts cortisol to cortisone. Cortisone is not a ligand for the receptor, whereas aldosterone is not a substrate for the enzyme. Pharmacologic inhibition (as occurs with excessive consumption of licorice) or genetic deficiency of this enzyme allows cortisol to occupy renal mineralocorticoid receptors and produce sodium retention and hypertension; the genetic condition is termed *apparent mineralocorticoid excess syndrome.*

ACTIONS OF THE ADRENAL ANDROGENS

Many actions of adrenal androgens are exerted through their conversion to active androgens or estrogens such as testosterone, dihydrotestosterone, estrone, and estradiol. In men, <2% of the biologically important androgens are derived from adrenal production, whereas in women approximately 50% of androgens are of adrenal origin. The adrenal contribution to circulating estrogen levels is mainly important in pathologic conditions such as feminizing adrenal tumors. Adrenal androgens contribute to the physiologic development of pubic and axillary hair during normal puberty. They also play an important role in the pathophysiology of congenital adrenal hyperplasia, premature adrenarche, adrenal tumors, and Cushing syndrome (see Chapters 576, 577, and 579).

In humans, circulating levels of DHEA and DHEAS, the chief adrenal androgens, reach a peak in early adulthood and then decline. This has led to speculation that age-related physiologic changes might be reversed by DHEA administration, and beneficial effects have been suggested (but not proved) on insulin sensitivity, bone mineral density, muscle mass, cardiovascular risk, obesity, cancer risk, autoimmunity, and the central nervous system.

Synthetic Corticosteroids

Many synthetic analogs of cortisone and hydrocortisone are available. Prednisone and prednisolone are derivatives with an additional double bond in ring A. Like cortisone, prednisone is not an active steroid but it is converted to prednisolone by HSD11B1 in the liver. Prednisone and prednisolone are 4-5 times as potent in antiinflammatory and carbohydrate activity but have slightly less effect on retention of water and sodium than cortisol. Halogenated derivatives have different effects. Betamethasone and dexamethasone have 25-40 times the glucocorticoid potency of cortisol but have little mineralocorticoid effect. These analogs are usually used in pharmacologic doses for their antiinflammatory or immunosuppressive properties. The antiinflammatory activity of fludrocortisone is about 15 times that of hydrocortisone, but fludrocortisone is more than 125 times as active a mineralocorticoid; it is used to treat aldosterone deficiency.

Bibliography is available at Expert Consult.

574.5 Adrenal Medulla

Perrin C. White

The principal hormones of the adrenal medulla are the physiologically active catecholamines: dopamine, norepinephrine, and epinephrine (Fig. 574-3). Catecholamine synthesis also occurs in the brain, in sympathetic nerve endings, and in chromaffin tissue outside the adrenal medulla. Metabolites of catecholamines are excreted in the urine, principally 3-methoxy-4-hydroxymandelic acid, metanephrine,

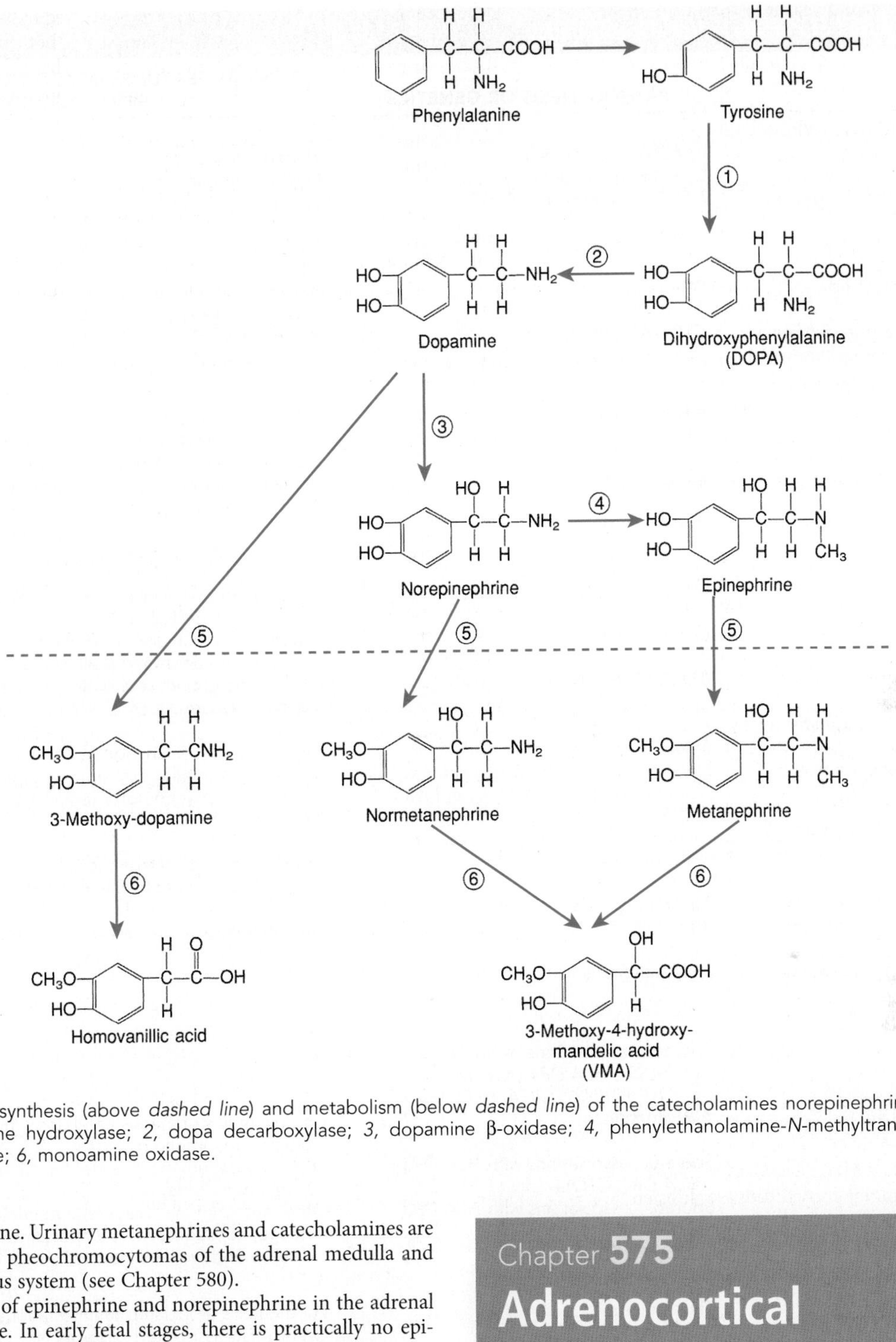

Figure 574-3 Biosynthesis (above *dashed line*) and metabolism (below *dashed line*) of the catecholamines norepinephrine and epinephrine. Enzymes: *1*, tyrosine hydroxylase; *2*, dopa decarboxylase; *3*, dopamine β-oxidase; *4*, phenylethanolamine-*N*-methyltransferase; *5*, catechol *O*-methyltransferase; *6*, monoamine oxidase.

and normetanephrine. Urinary metanephrines and catecholamines are measured to detect pheochromocytomas of the adrenal medulla and sympathetic nervous system (see Chapter 580).

The proportions of epinephrine and norepinephrine in the adrenal gland vary with age. In early fetal stages, there is practically no epinephrine; at birth, norepinephrine remains predominant. However in adults, norepinephrine accounts for only 10-30% of the pressor amines in the medulla.

The effects of catecholamines are mediated through a series of G-protein–coupled adrenergic receptors. Both epinephrine and norepinephrine raise the mean arterial blood pressure, but only epinephrine increases cardiac output. By increasing peripheral vascular resistance, norepinephrine increases systolic and diastolic blood pressures with only a slight reduction in the pulse rate. Epinephrine increases the pulse rate and, by decreasing the peripheral vascular resistance, decreases the diastolic pressure. The hyperglycemic and calorigenic effects of norepinephrine are much less pronounced than are those of epinephrine.

Bibliography is available at Expert Consult.

Chapter 575
Adrenocortical Insufficiency
Perrin C. White

In primary adrenal insufficiency, congenital or acquired lesions of the adrenal cortex prevent production of cortisol and often aldosterone (Table 575-1). Acquired primary adrenal insufficiency is termed *Addison disease.* Dysfunction of the anterior pituitary gland or hypothalamus can cause a deficiency of corticotropin (adrenocorticotropic hormone [ACTH]) and lead to hypofunction of the adrenal cortex, termed *secondary adrenal insufficiency;* the term *tertiary adrenal insufficiency* is sometimes used to denote cases arising from hypothalamic dysfunction (Table 575-2).

| Table 575-1 | Causes of Primary Adrenal Insufficiency |

	PATHOGENESIS OR GENETICS	CLINICAL FEATURES IN ADDITION TO ADRENAL INSUFFICIENCY
CONGENITAL ADRENAL HYPERPLASIA		
21-Hydroxylase deficiency	*CYP21A2* mutations	Hyperandrogenism
11β-Hydroxylase deficiency	*CYP11B1* mutations	Hyperandrogenism, hypertension
3β-Hydroxysteroid dehydrogenase type 2 deficiency	*HSD3B2* mutations	Ambiguous genitalia in boys, postnatal virilization in girls
17α-Hydroxylase deficiency	*CYP17A1* mutations	XY sex reversal, pubertal delay in both sexes, hypertension
P450 oxidoreductase deficiency	*POR* mutations	Skeletal malformation (Antley-Bixler syndrome), abnormal genitalia
P450 side-chain cleavage deficiency	*CYP11A1* mutations	XY sex reversal
Congenital lipoid adrenal hyperplasia	*STAR* mutations	XY sex reversal
OTHER GENETIC DISORDERS		
Adrenoleukodystrophy or adrenomyeloneuropathy	*ABCD1* mutations	Weakness, spasticity, dementia, blindness, quadriparesis. Adrenomyeloneuropathy is a milder variant of adrenoleukodystrophy with slower progression
Triple A syndrome (Allgrove syndrome)	*AAAS* mutations	Achalasia, alacrima, cognitive deficits, neuromuscular deficits, hyperkeratosis
Smith-Lemli-Opitz syndrome	*DHCR7* mutations	Craniofacial malformations, developmental delay growth failure, cholesterol deficiency
Wolman disease	*LIPA* mutations	Bilateral adrenal calcification, hepatosplenomegaly
Kearns-Sayre syndrome	Mitochondrial DNA deletions	External ophthalmoplegia, retinal degeneration, cardiac conduction defects, other endocrine disorders
Pallister-Hall syndrome	*GLI3* mutations	hypothalamic hamartoblastoma, hypopituitarism, imperforate anus, and postaxial polydactyly
IMAGe syndrome	*CDKN1C* mutations	Intrauterine growth retardation, metaphyseal dysplasia, genital abnormalities
Adrenal Hypoplasia Congenita		
X-linked	*NR0B1* mutations	Hypogonadotropic hypogonadism in boys
Xp21 contiguous gene syndrome	Deletion of genes for Duchenne muscular dystrophy, glycerol kinase, and *NR0B1*	Duchenne muscular dystrophy, glycerol kinase deficiency, psychomotor retardation
SF-1 linked	*NR5A1* mutations	XY sex reversal
Familial Glucocorticoid Deficiency or Corticotropin Insensitivity Syndromes		
Type 1	*MC2R* mutations	Tall stature, characteristic facial features, such as hypertelorism and frontal bossing
Type 2	*MRAP* mutations	
Variant of familial glucocorticoid deficiency	*MCM4* mutations	Growth failure, increased chromosomal breakage, natural killer cell deficiency
Variant of familial glucocorticoid deficiency	*NNT* mutations	
AUTOIMMUNE		
Isolated	Sporadic; associations with *HLA-DR3-DQ2, HLA-DR4-DQ8, MICA, CTLA4, PTPN22, CIITA, CLEC16A*	None
APS type 1 (APECED)	*AIRE* mutations	Chronic mucocutaneous candidosis, hypoparathyroidism, other autoimmune diseases
APS type 2	Sporadic; associations with *HLA-DR3, HLA-DR4, CTLA4*	Thyroid autoimmune disease, type 1 diabetes, other autoimmune diseases
APS type 4	Sporadic; associations with *HLA-DR3, CTLA4*	Other autoimmune diseases (autoimmune gastritis, vitiligo, coeliac disease, alopecia), excluding thyroid disease and type 1 diabetes
INFECTIOUS		
Tuberculous adrenalitis	Tuberculosis	Tuberculosis-associated manifestations in other organs
AIDS	HIV-1	Other AIDS-associated diseases
Fungal adrenalitis	Histoplasmosis, cryptococcosis, coccidioidomycosis	Opportunistic infections
Meningococcal sepsis (Waterhouse-Friderichsen syndrome),	*Neisseria meningitidis*	
African trypanosomiasis	*Trypanosoma brucei*	Other trypanosomiasis-associated organ involvement
OTHER ACQUIRED CAUSES		
Bilateral adrenal hemorrhage	Meningococcal sepsis (Waterhouse-Friderichsen syndrome), primary antiphospholipid syndrome, traumatic birth, anticoagulation	Symptoms and signs of underlying disease
Bilateral adrenal metastases	Mainly cancers of the lung, stomach, breast, and colon	Symptoms and signs of underlying disease
Bilateral adrenal infiltration	Primary adrenal lymphoma, amyloidosis, hemochromatosis, sarcoidosis (rare)	Symptoms and signs of underlying disease
Bilateral adrenalectomy		Symptoms and signs of underlying disease

Table 575-1	Causes of Primary Adrenal Insufficiency—cont'd

	PATHOGENESIS OR GENETICS	CLINICAL FEATURES IN ADDITION TO ADRENAL INSUFFICIENCY
DRUG-INDUCED		
Mitotane (o,p-DDD)	Cytotoxicity	None, unless related to drug
Aminoglutethimide	Inhibition of cholesterol side chain cleavage enzyme (CYP11A1)	None, unless related to drug
Trilostane	Inhibition of 3β-hydroxysteroid dehydrogenase type 2	None, unless related to drug
Etomidate	Inhibition of 11β-hydroxylase (CYP11B1)	None, unless related to drug
Ketoconazole, fluconazole	Inhibition of mitochondrial cytochrome P450 enzymes (e.g., CYP11A1, CYP11B1)	None, unless related to drug

AAAS, achalasia, adrenocortical insufficiency, alacrima syndrome; ABCD, ATP-binding cassette, subfamily D; ABCG5, ATP-binding cassette, subfamily G, member 5; ABCG8, ATP-binding cassette, subfamily G, member 8; APECED, autoimmune polyendocrinopathy-candidiasis-ectodermal dystrophy; APS, autoimmune polyendocrinopathy syndrome; CIITA, class II transactivator; CTLA-4, cytotoxic T-lymphocyte antigen 4; DHCR7, 7-dehydrocholesterol reductase; HLA, human leukocyte antigen; IMAGe, intrauterine growth restriction (IUGR), metaphyseal dysplasia, adrenal hypoplasia congenita (AHC), and genitourinary abnormalities; LIPA, lipase A; MC2R, melanocortin 2 receptor; MCM4, minichromosome maintenance complex component 4; MICA, major histocompatibility complex class I chain-related gene A; MRAP, melanocortin 2 receptor accessory protein; PTPN22, protein tyrosine phosphatase, non-receptor type 22; StAR, steroidogenic acute regulatory protein.

Adapted from: Charmandari E, Nicolaides NC, Chrousos GP. Adrenal insufficiency. Lancet 383:2152–2164, 2014, Table 1, pp. 2153–2154.

Table 575-2	Causes of Secondary Adrenal Insufficiency

	ETIOLOGIES	CLINICAL MANIFESTATIONS IN ADDITION TO ADRENAL INSUFFICIENCY
DRUG-INDUCED		
Abrupt cessation of glucocorticoid therapy (systemic or topical)	Suppression of CRH and ACTH secretion leading to atrophy of the adrenal cortex	Primary disease-associated symptoms
OTHER ACQUIRED CAUSES		
Hypothalamic or pituitary tumors	Adenomas, cysts, craniopharyngiomas, ependymomas, meningiomas, rarely carcinomas, metastasis	Panhypopituitarism*; primary disease-associated symptoms
Traumatic brain injury		Panhypopituitarism*; primary disease-associated symptoms
Hypothalamic or pituitary surgery or irradiation		Panhypopituitarism*; primary disease-associated symptoms
Infections or infiltrative processes	Lymphocytic hypophysitis, hemochromatosis, tuberculosis, meningitis, sarcoidosis, actinomycosis, histiocytosis X, Wegener granulomatosis	Panhypopituitarism*; primary disease-associated symptoms
Pituitary apoplexy (when occurring in a peripartum mother, termed Sheehan syndrome)	High blood loss or hypotension	Abrupt onset of severe headache, visual disturbance, nausea, vomiting; panhypopituitarism*; primary disease-associated symptoms
CONGENITAL OR GENETIC CAUSES		
Abnormal Central Nervous System Development		
Anencephaly	Multiple	Primary disease-associated symptoms
Holoprosencephaly	Multiple	Primary disease-associated symptoms
Combined Pituitary Hormone Deficiency (CPHD)†		
CPHD2	Mutations in PROP1 (paired-like homeobox 1)	Panhypopituitarism; corticotropin deficiency occurs in adolescence
CPHD3	Mutations in LHX3 (LIM homeobox 3)	Panhypopituitarism; deafness, short neck
CPHD4	Mutations in LHX4 (LIM homeobox 4)	Panhypopituitarism; small sella, cerebellar defects
Septooptic dysplasia, CPHD5	Mutations in HESX1 (HESX homeobox 1)	Panhypopituitarism; septooptic dysplasia (blindness owing to hypoplasic optic nerves, absence of the septum pellucidum); developmental delay
CPHD6	Mutations in OTX2 (orthodenticle homeobox 2)	Panhypopituitarism; ectopic posterior pituitary gland
X-linked panhypopituitarism	Mutations in SOX3 (SRY(sex-determining region Y) box 3)	Panhypopituitarism; infundibular hypoplasia, developmental delay
Other Genetic Syndromes Affecting Corticotropin Secretion		
Congenital proopiomelanocortin deficiency	Mutations in POMC (proopiomelanocortin)	Early-onset severe obesity, hyperphagia, red hair
Prohormone convertase 1/3 deficiency	Mutations in PC1 (prohormone convertase 1/3)	Obesity, malabsorption or diarrhea, hypogonadotropic hypogonadism
Isolated ACTH (corticotropin) deficiency	Mutations in TBX19 (T-box 19)	
Prader-Willi syndrome	Deletion or silencing of genes on the parental copy of genes within the imprinted chromosome region 15q11-q13 including SNRPN (small nuclear ribonucleoprotein polypeptide N) and NDN (necdin, melanoma antigen (MAGE) family member)	Dysmorphic features, hypotonia, developmental delay, obesity, growth hormone deficiency, hypogonadotropic hypogonadism

*The associated anterior and/or posterior hormone deficiencies may vary.
†CPHD1 (mutations in POUF1) is not associated with corticotropin deficiency.

575.1 Primary Adrenal Insufficiency

Perrin C. White

Primary adrenal insufficiency in children is most frequently caused by genetic conditions that are often but not always manifested in infancy and less often by acquired problems such as autoimmune conditions (Table 575-3). Susceptibility to autoimmune conditions often has a genetic basis, and so these distinctions are not absolute.

INHERITED ETIOLOGIES
Inborn Defects of Steroidogenesis
The most common causes of adrenocortical insufficiency in infancy are the salt-losing forms of congenital adrenal hyperplasia (see Chapter 576). Approximately 75% of infants with 21-hydroxylase deficiency, almost all infants with lipoid adrenal hyperplasia, and most infants with a deficiency of 3β-hydroxysteroid dehydrogenase manifest salt-losing symptoms in the newborn period because they are unable to synthesize either cortisol or aldosterone.

Adrenal Hypoplasia Congenita
Adrenal hypoplasia congenita (AHC) is a relatively frequent cause of adrenal failure in boys along with congenital adrenal hyperplasia, autoimmune disease, and adrenoleukodystrophy. The name of the disorder notwithstanding, AHC is predominantly a failure of development of the definitive zone of the adrenal cortex; the fetal zone may be relatively normal. Consequently, adrenal insufficiency generally becomes evident as the fetal zone involutes postnatally (see Chapter 574), with onset in infancy or in the 1st 2 yr of life, but occasionally in later childhood or even adulthood. In some cases, aldosterone deficiency becomes evident before cortisol deficiency.

The disorder is caused by mutation of the *DAX1 (NR0B1)* gene, a member of the nuclear hormone receptor family, located on Xp21. Boys with AHC often do not undergo puberty owing to hypogonadotropic hypogonadism caused by the same mutated *DAX1* gene. **Cryptorchidism,** sometimes noted in these boys, is probably an early manifestation of hypogonadotropic hypogonadism, but often testicular function in infants is normal, with a typical or even an unusually prolonged testosterone surge in the 1st mo of life.

AHC occasionally occurs as part of a **contiguous gene deletion** syndrome together with Duchenne muscular dystrophy, glycerol

Table 575-3	Frequencies of Etiologies of Primary Adrenal Insufficiency
ETIOLOGY	**AGE AT DIAGNOSIS**
Congenital adrenal hyperplasia	59% Infancy
Autoimmune	16% Childhood-adolescence
APECED (autoimmune polyendocrinopathy–candidiasis–ectodermal dystrophy)	6% Childhood-adolescence
Adrenoleukodystrophy	4% Childhood-adolescence
Isolated glucocorticoid deficiency	4% Infancy
Idiopathic	4% Childhood
Syndromes	3% Infancy
X-linked adrenal hypoplasia congenita	2% Infancy-childhood
Hemorrhage	1% Infancy

Data from Perry R, Kecha O, Paquette J, et al. Primary adrenal insufficiency in children: twenty years' experience at the Sainte-Justine Hospital, Montreal. J Clin Endocrinol Metab 90:3243–3250, 2005; Hsieh S, White PC. Presentation of primary adrenal insufficiency in childhood. J Clin Endocrinol Metab 96:E925–E928, 2011.

kinase deficiency, cognitive impairment, or a combination of these conditions.

Other Genetic Causes of Adrenal Hypoplasia
The transcription factor SF-1 is required for adrenal and gonadal development (see Chapter 574). Males with a heterozygous mutation in SF-1 (*NR5A1*) have impaired development of the testes despite the presence of a normal copy of the gene on the other chromosome and can appear to be female, similar to patients with lipoid adrenal hyperplasia (see Chapter 576). Rarely, such patients have adrenal insufficiency as well.

Adrenal hypoplasia is also occasionally seen in patients with Pallister-Hall syndrome caused by mutations in the GLI3 oncogene (see Chapter 575).

Adrenoleukodystrophy
In adrenoleukodystrophy (ALD), adrenocortical deficiency is associated with demyelination in the central nervous system (see Chapters 86.2 and 599.3). High levels of very-long-chain fatty acids are found in tissues and body fluids, resulting from their impaired β-oxidation in the peroxisomes.

The most common form of ALD is an X-linked disorder with various presentations. The most common clinical picture is of a degenerative neurologic disorder appearing in childhood or adolescence and progressing to severe dementia and deterioration of vision, hearing, speech, and gait, with death occurring within a few years. Neurologic symptoms may be subtle at onset, sometimes consisting only of behavioral changes or deteriorating academic performance. Generalized but incomplete alopecia, resembling that of chemotherapy, is a characteristic but inconsistent finding. A milder form of X-linked ALD is adrenomyeloneuropathy, which begins in later adolescence or early adulthood. Patients may have evidence of adrenal insufficiency before, at the time of, or after neurologic symptoms develop, often with years separating their presentation. X-linked ALD is caused by mutations in the *ABCD1* gene located on Xq28. The gene encodes a transmembrane transporter involved in the importation of very-long-chain fatty acids into peroxisomes. More than 400 mutations have been described in patients with X-linked ALD. Clinical phenotypes can vary even within families, perhaps owing to modifier genes or other unknown factors. There is no correlation between the degree of neurologic impairment and severity of adrenal insufficiency. Prenatal diagnosis by DNA analysis and family screening by very-long-chain fatty acid assays and mutation analysis are available. Women who are heterozygous carriers of the X-linked ALD gene can develop symptoms in midlife or later; adrenal insufficiency is rare.

Neonatal ALD is a rare autosomal recessive disorder. Infants have neurologic deterioration and have or acquire evidence of adrenocortical dysfunction. Most patients have severe, progressive cognitive impairment and die before 5 yr of age. This disorder is a subset of Zellweger (cerebrohepatorenal) syndrome, in which peroxisomes do not develop at all owing to mutations in any of several genes (*PEX5, PEX1, PEX10, PEX13,* and *PEX26*) controlling the development of this organelle.

Familial Glucocorticoid Deficiency
Familial glucocorticoid deficiency is a form of chronic adrenal insufficiency characterized by isolated deficiency of glucocorticoids, elevated levels of ACTH, and generally normal aldosterone production, although salt-losing manifestations as are present in most other forms of adrenal insufficiency occasionally occur. Patients mainly have hypoglycemia, seizures, and increased pigmentation during the 1st decade of life. The disorder affects both sexes equally and is inherited in an autosomal recessive manner. There is marked adrenocortical atrophy with relative sparing of the zona glomerulosa. Mutations in the gene for the ACTH receptor (*MCR2*) have been described in approximately 25% of these patients, most of which affect trafficking of receptor molecules from the endoplasmic reticulum to the cell surface. Another 20% of cases are caused by mutations in *MRAP,* which encodes a melanocyte receptor accessory protein required for this trafficking. Recently, mutations at new genetic loci have been identified, including

the minichromosome maintenance-deficient 4 homolog *(MCM4)* and nicotinamide nucleotide transhydrogenase *(NNT)*. These genes are involved in DNA replication and antioxidant defense, respectively. Patients with *MCM4* mutations also have growth failure, increased chromosomal breakage, and natural killer cell deficiency.

Another syndrome of ACTH resistance occurs in association with **achalasia** of the gastric cardia and **alacrima (triple A or Allgrove syndrome).** These patients often have a progressive neurologic disorder that includes autonomic dysfunction, intellectual disability, motor neuropathy, and occasional deafness. This syndrome is also inherited in an autosomal recessive fashion, and the *AAAS* gene has been mapped to chromosome 12q13. The encoded protein, aladin, might help regulate nucleocytoplasmic transport of other proteins.

Type I Autoimmune Polyendocrinopathy

Although autoimmune Addison disease most often occurs sporadically (see "Autoimmune Addison Disease" in Chapter 575.1), it can occur as a component of 2 syndromes, each consisting of a constellation of autoimmune disorders (see Chapter 566). **Type I autoimmune polyendocrinopathy (APS-1),** also known as *autoimmune polyendocrinopathy–candidiasis–ectodermal dystrophy* (APECED) syndrome, is inherited in a mendelian autosomal recessive manner, whereas APS-2 (see "Autoimmune Addison Disease" in Chapter 575.1) has complex inheritance. **Chronic mucocutaneous candidiasis** is most often the first manifestation of APS-1, followed by hypoparathyroidism and then by Addison disease, which typically develops in early adolescence. Other closely associated autoimmune disorders include gonadal failure, alopecia, vitiligo, keratopathy, enamel hypoplasia, nail dystrophy, intestinal malabsorption, and chronic active hepatitis. Hypothyroidism and type 1 diabetes mellitus occur in less than 10% of affected patients. Some components of the syndrome continue to develop as late as the 5th decade. Patients with APS-1 may have autoantibodies to the adrenal cytochrome P450 enzymes CYP21, CYP17, and CYP11A1. The presence of such antibodies indicates a high likelihood of the development of Addison disease or, in female patients, ovarian failure. Adrenal failure can evolve rapidly in APS-1; death in patients with a previous diagnosis and unexplained deaths in siblings of patients with APS-1 have been reported, indicating the need to closely monitor patients with APS-1 and to thoroughly evaluate apparently unaffected siblings of patients with this disorder.

The gene affected in APS-1 is designated autoimmune regulator-1 *(AIRE1)*; it has been mapped to chromosome 21q22.3. The *AIRE1* gene encodes a transcription factor that controls the expression of many proteins within the thymus, thus playing a critical role in the generation of immune tolerance. Many different mutations in the *AIRE1* gene have been described in patients with APS-1, with 2 mutations (R257X and a 3-bp deletion) being most common. There has been autosomal dominant transmission in 1 kindred owing to a specific missense mutation (G228W).

Disorders of Cholesterol Synthesis and Metabolism

Patients with disorders of cholesterol synthesis or metabolism, including abetalipoproteinemia with deficient lipoprotein B-containing lipoproteins, and familial hypercholesterolemia, with decreased or impaired low-density lipoprotein receptors, have limited adrenocortical function. Adrenal insufficiency has been reported in patients with **Smith-Lemli-Opitz syndrome**, an autosomal recessive disorder manifesting with facial anomalies, microcephaly, limb anomalies, and developmental delay (see Chapter 86.3). Mutations in the gene coding for sterol Δ^7-reductase, mapped to 11q12-q13, resulting in impairment of the final step in cholesterol synthesis with marked elevation of 7-dehydrocholesterol, abnormally low cholesterol, and adrenal insufficiency, have been identified in Smith-Lemli-Opitz syndrome. **Wolman disease** is a rare autosomal recessive disorder caused by mutations in the gene encoding human lysosomal acid lipase on chromosome 10q23.2-23.3. Cholesteryl esters accumulate in lysosomes in most organ systems, leading to organ failure. Infants during the 1st or 2nd mo of life have hepatosplenomegaly, steatorrhea, abdominal

distention, and failure to thrive. Adrenal insufficiency and bilateral adrenal calcification are present, and death usually occurs in the 1st yr of life.

Corticosteroid-Binding Globulin Deficiency and Decreased Cortisol-Binding Affinity

Corticosteroid-binding globulin deficiency and decreased cortisol-binding affinity result in low levels of plasma cortisol but normal urinary free cortisol and normal plasma ACTH levels. A high prevalence of hypotension and fatigue has been reported in some adults with abnormalities of corticosteroid-binding globulin deficiency.

ACQUIRED ETIOLOGIES
Autoimmune Addison Disease

The most common cause of Addison disease is autoimmune destruction of the glands. The glands may be so small that they are not visible at autopsy, and only remnants of tissue are found in microscopic sections. Usually, the medulla is not destroyed, and there is marked lymphocytic infiltration in the area of the former cortex. In advanced disease, all adrenocortical function is lost, but early in the clinical course, isolated cortisol deficiency can occur. Most patients have **antiadrenal cytoplasmic antibodies** in their plasma; 21-hydroxylase (CYP21) is the most commonly occurring biochemically defined autoantigen.

Addison disease can occur as a component of 2 autoimmune polyendocrinopathy syndromes. Type I (APS-1) was discussed previously. **Type II autoimmune polyendocrinopathy (APS-2)** consists of Addison disease associated with autoimmune thyroid disease (Schmidt syndrome) or type 1 diabetes (Carpenter syndrome). Gonadal failure, vitiligo, alopecia, and chronic atrophic gastritis, with or without pernicious anemia, can occur. Frequencies of the human leukocyte antigen (HLA)-D3 and HLA-D4 alleles are increased in these patients and appear to confer an increased risk for development of this disease; particular alleles at the major histocompatibility complex class I chain-related genes A and B *(MICA and MICB)* also are associated with this disorder. Polymorphisms in genes involved in other autoimmune disorders have been inconsistently associated with primary adrenal insufficiency, and their contribution to its pathogenesis must be regarded as uncertain. These include the class II, major histocompatibility complex, transactivator *(CIITA)*, C-type lectin domain family 16, member A *(CLEC16A)*, and protein tyrosine phosphatase, nonreceptor type 22 *(PTPN22)*. The disorder is most common in middle-aged women and can occur in many generations of the same family. Antiadrenal antibodies, specifically antibodies to the CYP21, CYP17, and CYP11A1 enzymes, are also found in these patients. Autoimmune adrenal insufficiency may also be seen in patients with celiac disease (see Chapter 338.2).

Infection

Tuberculosis was a common cause of adrenal destruction in the past but is much less prevalent now. The most common infectious etiology for adrenal insufficiency is meningococcemia (see Chapter 191); adrenal crisis from this cause is referred to as the Waterhouse-Friderichsen syndrome. Patients with AIDS can have a variety of subclinical abnormalities in the hypothalamic-pituitary-adrenal axis, but frank adrenal insufficiency is rare. However, drugs used in the treatment of AIDS can affect adrenal hormone homeostasis.

Drugs

Ketoconazole, an antifungal drug, can cause adrenal insufficiency by inhibiting adrenal enzymes. Mitotane (o,p′-DDD), used in the treatment of adrenocortical carcinoma and refractory Cushing syndrome (see Chapters 577 and 579), is cytotoxic to the adrenal cortex and can also alter extraadrenal cortisol metabolism. Signs of adrenal insufficiency occur in a substantial percentage of patients treated with mitotane. Etomidate, used in the induction and maintenance of general anesthesia, inhibits 11β-hydroxylase (CYP11B1), and a single induction dose can block cortisol synthesis for 4-8 hr or longer. This may be problematic in severely stressed patients, particularly if repeated doses are used in a critical care setting. Atlhough not themselves a cause of adrenal insufficiency, rifampicin and anticonvulsive drugs such as phenytoin and phenobarbital reduce the effectiveness and bioavailability of corticosteroid replacement therapy by inducing steroid metabolizing enzymes in the liver.

Hemorrhage into Adrenal Glands

Hemorrhage into adrenal glands can occur in the neonatal period as a consequence of a difficult labor (especially breech presentation), or its etiology might not be apparent (Fig. 575-1). An incidence rate of 3 in 100,000 live births has been suggested. The hemorrhage may be sufficiently extensive to result in death from exsanguination or hypoadrenalism. An abdominal mass, anemia, unexplained jaundice, or scrotal hematoma may be the presenting sign. Often, the hemorrhage is asymptomatic initially and is identified later by calcification of the adrenal gland. Fetal adrenal hemorrhage has also been reported. Postnatally, adrenal hemorrhage most often occurs in patients being treated with anticoagulants. It can also occur as a result of child abuse.

Clinical Manifestations

Primary adrenal insufficiency leads to cortisol and often aldosterone deficiency. The signs and symptoms of adrenal insufficiency are most easily understood in the context of the normal actions of these hormones (see Chapter 574; Table 575-4).

Hypoglycemia is a prominent feature of adrenal insufficiency. It is often accompanied by ketosis as the body attempts to use fatty acids as an alternative energy source. Ketosis is aggravated by anorexia, nausea, and vomiting, all of which occur frequently.

Cortisol deficiency decreases cardiac output and vascular tone; moreover, catecholamines such as epinephrine have decreased inotropic and pressor effects in the absence of cortisol. These problems are initially manifested as orthostatic hypotension in older children and can progress to frank shock in patients of any age. They are exacerbated by aldosterone deficiency, which results in hypovolemia owing to decreased resorption of sodium in the distal nephron.

Hypotension and decreased cardiac output decrease glomerular filtration and thus decrease the ability of the kidney to excrete free water. Vasopressin (AVP) is secreted by the posterior pituitary in response to hypotension and also as a direct consequence of lack of inhibition by cortisol. These factors decrease plasma osmolality and lead in particular to hyponatremia. Hyponatremia is also caused by aldosterone deficiency and may be much worse when both cortisol and aldosterone are deficient.

In addition to hypovolemia and hyponatremia, aldosterone deficiency causes hyperkalemia by decreasing potassium excretion

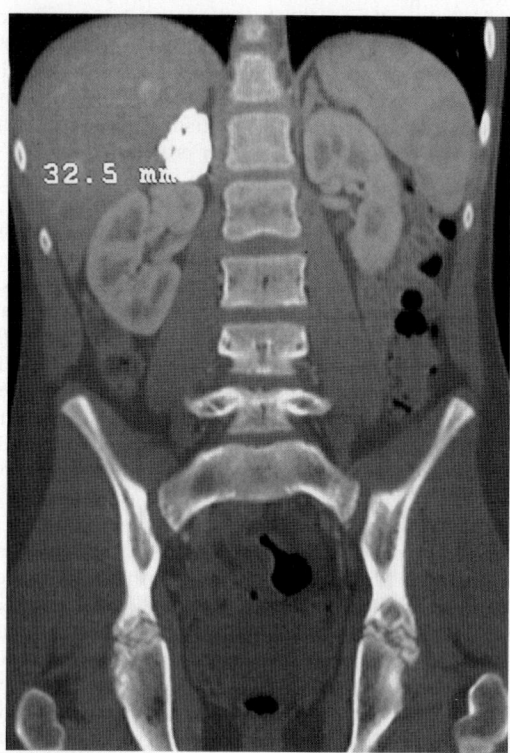

Figure 575-1 Coronal plane of contrast-enhanced computed tomography confirming intraadrenal localization of a round hyperdense lesion compatible with a large calcification. *(From Llano JP, Beaufils E, Nicolino M: Uncommon cause of large paravertebral calcification in a child. J Pediatr 162:881, 2013, Fig. 2.)*

Table 575-4	Clinical Manifestations and Biochemical Findings in Adrenal Insufficiency	
	PATHOPHYSIOLOGIC MECHANISM	**PREVALENCE (%)***
SYMPTOMS		
Fatigue	Glucocorticoid deficiency	90
Anorexia, weight loss	Glucocorticoid deficiency	90
Nausea, vomiting	Glucocorticoid deficiency, mineralocorticoid deficiency	90
Salt craving (primary adrenal insufficiency only)	Mineralocorticoid deficiency	20
Myalgia or joint pain	Glucocorticoid deficiency	
SIGNS		
Low blood pressure, orthostatic hypotension	Mineralocorticoid deficiency, glucocorticoid deficiency	70-100%
Skin or mucosal hyperpigmentation (primary adrenal insufficiency only)	Excess of proopiomelanocortin-derived peptides	70
LABORATORY FINDINGS		
Hyponatremia	Mineralocorticoid deficiency, glucocorticoid deficiency (leading to decreased free water excretion)	90
Hyperkalemia (primary adrenal insufficiency only)	Mineralocorticoid deficiency	50
Hypoglycemia	Glucocorticoid deficiency	30
Ketosis	Glucocorticoid deficiency	30
Low random cortisol level	Glucocorticoid deficiency	80
Eosinophilia, lymphocytosis	Glucocorticoid deficiency	
High ACTH level (primary adrenal insufficiency only)	Glucocorticoid deficiency	100
High plasma renin activity (primary adrenal insufficiency only)	Mineralocorticoid deficiency	100

*Prevalence data are for primary insufficiency only. Blanks indicate that no pediatric prevalence data are available.
Data from Hsieh S, White PC. Presentation of primary adrenal insufficiency in childhood. J Clin Endocrinol Metab 96:E925–E928, 2011

in the distal nephron. Cortisol deficiency alone does not cause hyperkalemia.

Cortisol deficiency decreases negative feedback on the hypothalamus and pituitary, leading to increased secretion of ACTH. Hyperpigmentation is caused by ACTH and other peptide hormones (γ-melanocyte–stimulating hormone) arising from the ACTH precursor proopiomelanocortin. In patients with a fair complexion, the skin can have a bronze cast. Pigmentation may be more prominent in skin creases, mucosa, and scars. In dark-skinned patients, it may be most readily appreciated in the gingival and buccal mucosa.

The clinical presentation of adrenal insufficiency depends on the age of the patient, whether both cortisol and aldosterone secretion are affected, and to some extent on the underlying etiology. The most common causes in early infancy are inborn errors of steroid biosynthesis, sepsis, AHC, and adrenal hemorrhage. Infants have a relatively greater requirement for aldosterone than do older children, possibly owing to immaturity of the kidney and also to the low sodium content of human breast milk and infant formula. Hyperkalemia, hyponatremia, and hypoglycemia are prominent presenting signs of adrenal insufficiency in infants. Ketosis is not consistently present because infants generate ketones less well than do older children. Hyperpigmentation is not usually seen because this takes weeks or months to develop, and orthostatic hypotension is obviously difficult to demonstrate in infants.

Infants can become ill very quickly. There may be only a few days of decreased activity, anorexia, and vomiting before critical electrolyte abnormalities develop.

In older children with Addison disease, symptoms include muscle weakness, malaise, anorexia, vomiting, weight loss, and orthostatic hypotension. These may be of insidious onset. It is not unusual to elicit, in retrospect, an episodic history spanning years with symptoms being noticeable only during intercurrent illnesses. Such patients can present with acute decompensation (**adrenal crisis**) during relatively minor infectious illnesses. *Some of these patients have been initially misdiagnosed with chronic fatigue syndrome, postmononucleosis syndrome, chronic Lyme disease, or psychiatric disorders (depression or anorexia nervosa).*

Hyperpigmentation is often, but not necessarily, present. Hyponatremia is present at diagnosis in almost 90% of patients. Hyperkalemia tends to occur later in the course of the disease in older children than in infants and is present in only half of patients at diagnosis. Normal potassium levels must never be presumed to rule out primary adrenal insufficiency.

Hypoglycemia and ketosis are common. Thus, the clinical presentation can be easily confused with gastroenteritis or other acute infections. Chronicity of symptoms can alert the clinician to the possibility of Addison disease, but this diagnosis should be considered in any child with orthostatic hypotension, hyponatremia, hypoglycemia, and ketosis. Salt craving is seen in primary adrenal insufficiency with mineralocorticoid deficiency. Fatigue, myalgias, fever, eosinophilia, lymphocytosis, hypercalcemia, and anemia may be noted with glucocorticoid deficiency.

LABORATORY FINDINGS

Hypoglycemia, ketosis, hyponatremia, and hyperkalemia have been discussed. An electrocardiogram is useful for quickly detecting hyperkalemia in a critically ill child. Acidosis is often present, and the blood urea nitrogen level is elevated if the patient is dehydrated.

Cortisol levels are sometimes at the low end of the normal range but are invariably low when the patient's degree of illness is considered. ACTH levels are high in primary adrenal insufficiency but can take time to be reported by the laboratory. Similarly, aldosterone levels may be within the normal range but inappropriately low considering the patient's hyponatremia, hyperkalemia, and hypovolemia. Plasma renin activity is elevated. Blood eosinophils may be increased in number, but this is rarely useful diagnostically.

Urinary excretion of sodium and chloride are increased and urinary potassium is decreased, but these are difficult to assess on random urine samples. Accurate interpretation of urinary electrolytes requires more-prolonged (24 hr) urine collections and knowledge of the patient's sodium and potassium intake.

The **most definitive** test for adrenal insufficiency is measurement of serum levels of cortisol before and after administration of ACTH; resting levels are low and do not increase normally after administration of ACTH. Occasionally, normal resting levels that do not increase after administration of ACTH indicate an absence of adrenocortical reserve. A low initial level followed by a significant response to ACTH can indicate secondary adrenal insufficiency. Traditionally, this test has been performed by measuring cortisol levels before and 30 or 60 min after giving 0.250 mg of cosyntropin (ACTH 1-24) by rapid intravenous infusion. Aldosterone will transiently increase in response to this dose of ACTH and may also be measured. A low-dose test (1 μg ACTH 1-24/1.73 m²) is a more sensitive test of pituitary-adrenal reserve, but has somewhat lower specificity (more false-positive tests).

DIFFERENTIAL DIAGNOSIS

Upon presentation, Addison disease often needs to be distinguished from more acute illnesses such as gastroenteritis with dehydration or sepsis. Additional testing is directed at identifying the specific cause for adrenal insufficiency. When congenital adrenal hyperplasia is suspected, serum levels of cortisol precursors (17-hydroxyprogesterone) should be measured along with cortisol in an ACTH stimulation test (see Chapter 576). Elevated levels of very-long-chain fatty acids are diagnostic of ALD (see Chapter 599.3). Many genetic etiologies for primary adrenal insufficiency may be identified by direct genetic testing, but it can take many weeks for results to become available. The presence of antiadrenal antibodies suggests an autoimmune pathogenesis. Patients with autoimmune Addison disease must be closely observed for the development of other autoimmune disorders. In children, hypoparathyroidism is the most commonly associated disorder, and it is suspected if hypocalcemia and elevated phosphate levels are present.

Ultrasonography (which requires an experienced operator), CT, or MRI can help define the size of the adrenal glands.

TREATMENT

Treatment of acute adrenal insufficiency must be immediate and vigorous. If the diagnosis of adrenal insufficiency has not been established, a blood sample should be obtained before therapy to determine electrolytes, glucose, ACTH, cortisol, aldosterone, and plasma renin activity. If the patient's condition permits, an ACTH stimulation test can be performed while initial fluid resuscitation is under way. An intravenous solution of 5% glucose in 0.9% saline should be administered to correct hypoglycemia, hypovolemia, and hyponatremia. Hypotonic fluids (e.g., 5% glucose in water or 0.2% saline) must be avoided because they can precipitate or exacerbate hyponatremia. If hyperkalemia is severe, it can require treatment with intravenous calcium and/or bicarbonate, intrarectal potassium-binding resin (Kayexalate), or intravenous infusion of glucose and insulin. A water-soluble form of hydrocortisone, such as hydrocortisone sodium succinate, should be given intravenously. As much as 10 mg for infants, 25 mg for toddlers, 50 mg for older children, and 100 mg for adolescents should be administered as a bolus and a similar total amount given in divided doses at 6 hr intervals for the 1st 24 hr. These doses may be reduced during the next 24 hr if progress is satisfactory. Adequate fluid and sodium repletion is achieved by intravenous saline administration, aided by the mineralocorticoid effect of high doses of hydrocortisone.

Particular caution should be exercised in the rare patient with concomitant adrenal insufficiency and hypothyroidism, because thyroxine can increase cortisol clearance. Thus, an adrenal crisis may be precipitated if hypothyroidism is treated without first ensuring adequate glucocorticoid replacement.

After the acute manifestations are under control, most patients require chronic replacement therapy for their cortisol and aldosterone deficiencies. *Hydrocortisone (cortisol) may be given orally in daily doses of 10 mg/m²/24 hr in 3 divided doses; some patients require 15 mg/m²/24 hr to minimize fatigue,* especially in the morning.

Timed-release preparations of hydrocortisone are undergoing clinical trials but are not yet generally available. *Equivalent doses (20-25% of the hydrocortisone dose) of prednisone or prednisolone may be divided and given twice daily.* ACTH levels may be used to monitor adequacy of glucocorticoid replacement in primary adrenal insufficiency; in congenital adrenal hyperplasia, levels of precursor hormones are used instead (see Chapter 576). Blood samples for monitoring should be obtained at a consistent time of day and in a consistent relation to (i.e., before or after) the hydrocortisone dose. Normalizing ACTH levels is unnecessary and can require excessive doses of hydrocortisone; generally morning ACTH levels high in the normal range to 3-4 times normal are satisfactory. Because untreated or severely undertreated patients can acutely decompensate during relatively minor illnesses, assessment of symptoms (or lack thereof) must not be used as a substitute for biochemical monitoring. During situations of stress, such as periods of infection or minor operative procedures, the dose of hydrocortisone should be increased 2-3–fold. Major surgery under general anesthesia requires high intravenous doses of hydrocortisone similar to those used for acute adrenal insufficiency.

If aldosterone deficiency is present, *fludrocortisone, a synthetic mineralocorticoid, is given orally in doses of 0.05-0.2 mg daily.* Measurements of plasma renin activity are useful in monitoring the adequacy of mineralocorticoid replacement. Chronic overdosage with glucocorticoids leads to obesity, short stature, and osteoporosis, whereas overdosage with fludrocortisone results in hypertension and occasionally hypokalemia.

Replacement of dehydroepiandrosterone (DHEA) in adults remains controversial; prepubertal children do not normally secrete large amounts of DHEA. Many adults with Addison disease complain of having decreased energy, and replacing DHEA can improve this problem, particularly in women in whom adrenal androgens represent approximately 50% of total androgen secretion.

Additional therapy might need to be directed at the underlying cause of the adrenal insufficiency in regard to infections and certain metabolic defects. Therapeutic approaches to ALD include administration of glycerol trioleate and glycerol trierucate (Lorenzo's oil), bone marrow transplantation, and lovastatin (see Chapter 599.3).

Bibliography is available at Expert Consult.

575.2 Secondary and Tertiary Adrenal Insufficiency

Perrin C. White

ETIOLOGY
Abrupt Cessation of Administration of Corticosteroids

Secondary adrenal insufficiency most commonly occurs when the hypothalamic-pituitary-adrenal axis is suppressed by prolonged administration of high doses of a potent glucocorticoid and that agent is suddenly withdrawn or the dose is tapered too quickly. Patients at risk for this problem include those with leukemia, asthma (particularly when patients are transitioned from oral to inhaled corticosteroids), and collagen vascular disease or other autoimmune conditions and those who have undergone tissue transplants or neurosurgical procedures. The maximal duration and dosage of glucocorticoid that can be administered before encountering this problem is not known, but it is assumed that high-dose glucocorticoids (the equivalent of >10 times physiologic cortisol secretion) can be administered for at least 1 wk without requiring a subsequent taper of dose. On the other hand, when high doses of dexamethasone are given to children with leukemia, it can take up to 2 mo or longer after therapy is stopped before tests of adrenal function return to normal. Signs and symptoms of adrenal insufficiency are most likely in patients who are subsequently subjected to stresses such as severe infections or additional surgical procedures.

Corticotropin (Adrenocorticotropic Hormone) Deficiency

Pituitary or hypothalamic dysfunction can cause corticotropin deficiency (see Chapter 557), usually associated with deficiencies of other pituitary hormones such as growth hormone and thyrotropin. Destructive lesions in the area of the pituitary, such as craniopharyngioma and germinoma, are the most common causes of corticotropin deficiency. In many cases, the pituitary or hypothalamus is further damaged during surgical removal or radiotherapy of tumors in the midline of the brain. Traumatic brain injury (see Chapter 710) frequently causes pituitary dysfunction, especially in the first days after the injury. However, corticotropin deficiency is difficult to detect then owing to frequent use of high doses of dexamethasone to minimize brain swelling, and permanent corticotropin deficiency is unusual after traumatic brain injury. In rare instances, autoimmune hypophysitis is the cause of corticotropin deficiency.

Congenital lesions of the pituitary also occur. The pituitary alone may be affected, or additional midline structures may be involved, such as the optic nerves or septum pellucidum. The latter type of abnormality is termed **septooptic dysplasia,** or de Morsier syndrome (see Chapter 591.9). More-severe developmental anomalies of the brain, such as anencephaly and holoprosencephaly, can also affect the pituitary. These disorders are usually sporadic, although a few cases of autosomal recessive inheritance have occurred. Isolated deficiency of corticotropin has been reported, including in several sets of siblings. Patients with multiple pituitary hormone deficiencies caused by mutations in the *PROP1* gene have been described with progressive ACTH/cortisol deficiency. Isolated deficiency of corticotropin-releasing hormone has been documented in an Arab kindred as an autosomal recessive trait.

It was recently recognized that up to 60% of children with **Prader-Willi syndrome** (see Chapter 81.8) have some degree of secondary adrenal insufficiency as assessed by provocative testing with metyrapone (see "Laboratory Findings" in Chapter 575.2), although diurnal cortisol levels are normal. The clinical significance of this finding is uncertain, but it might contribute to the relatively high incidence of sudden death with infectious illness that occurs in this population. Although it is not yet a standard of care, some endocrinologists advocate treating patients who have Prader-Willi syndrome with hydrocortisone during febrile illness.

CLINICAL PRESENTATION
Aldosterone secretion is unaffected in secondary adrenal insufficiency because the adrenal gland is, by definition, intact and the renin–angiotensin system is not involved. Thus, signs and symptoms are those of cortisol deficiency. Newborns often have hypoglycemia. Older children can have orthostatic hypotension or weakness. Hyponatremia may be present.

When secondary adrenal insufficiency is the consequence of an inborn or acquired anatomic defect involving the pituitary, there may be signs of associated deficiencies of other pituitary hormones. The penis may be small in male infants if gonadotropins are also deficient. Infants with secondary hypothyroidism are often jaundiced. Children with associated growth hormone deficiency grow poorly after the 1st yr of life.

Some children with pituitary abnormalities have hypoplasia of the midface. Children with optic nerve hypoplasia can have obvious visual impairment. They usually have a characteristic wandering nystagmus, but this is often not apparent until several months of age.

LABORATORY FINDINGS
Because the adrenal glands themselves are not directly affected, the diagnosis of secondary adrenal insufficiency is sometimes challenging. Historical gold standard dynamic tests include insulin-induced hypoglycemia, which provides a potent stress to the entire hypothalamic-pituitary-adrenal (HPA) axis. This test requires constant attendance by a physician and is considered by many endocrinologists to be too dangerous for routine use. A second gold standard test uses metyrapone, a specific inhibitor of steroid 11β-hydroxylase (CYP11B1) to

block cortisol synthesis, thus removing the normal negative feedback of cortisol on ACTH secretion. There are several protocols for this test; one version administers 30 mg/kg of metyrapone orally at midnight, with a blood sample obtained for cortisol and 11-deoxycortisol (the substrate for 11β-hydroxylase) at 8 AM. A low cortisol level (<5 μg/dL) demonstrates adequate suppression of cortisol synthesis, and an 11-deoxycortisol level >7 μg/dL indicates that ACTH has responded normally to the cortisol deficiency by stimulating the adrenal cortex. This test should be used with caution outside the research setting because it can precipitate adrenal crises in patients with marginal adrenal function; the drug is not available in all locales.

At present, the most commonly used test to diagnose secondary adrenal insufficiency is low-dose ACTH stimulation testing (1 μg/1.73 m² of cosyntropin given intravenously), the rationale being that there will be some degree of atrophy of the adrenal cortex if normal physiologic ACTH stimulation is lacking. Thus, this test may be falsely negative in cases of acute compromise of the pituitary (e.g., injury or surgery). Such circumstances rarely pose a diagnostic dilemma; in general, this test provides excellent sensitivity and specificity. Although assays vary somewhat, a threshold cortisol level of 18-20 μg/dL 30 min after cosyntropin administration may be used to dichotomize normal and abnormal responses.

At present, there seems to be little reason to use stimulation with corticotropin-releasing hormone instead of ACTH; although the corticotropin-releasing hormone test has the theoretical advantage of testing the ability of the anterior pituitary to respond to this stimulus by secreting ACTH (thus distinguishing secondary and tertiary adrenal insufficiency), in practice it does not provide improved sensitivity and specificity, and the agent is not as widely available.

TREATMENT

Iatrogenic secondary adrenal insufficiency (caused by chronic glucocorticoid administration) is best avoided by use of the smallest effective doses of systemic glucocorticoids for the shortest period of time. When a patient is thought to be at risk, tapering the dose rapidly to a level equivalent to or slightly less than the physiologic replacement (~10 mg/m²/24 hr of hydrocortisone) and further tapering over several weeks can allow the adrenal cortex to recover without development of signs of adrenal insufficiency. Patients with anatomic lesions of the pituitary should be treated indefinitely with glucocorticoids. Mineralocorticoid replacement is not required. In patients with panhypopituitarism, treating cortisol deficiency can increase free water excretion, thus unmasking central diabetes insipidus. Electrolytes must be monitored carefully when initiating cortisol therapy in panhypopituitary patients.

Bibliography is available at Expert Consult.

575.3 Adrenal Insufficiency in the Critical Care Setting
Perrin C. White

ETIOLOGY

Adrenal insufficiency in the context of critical illness is encountered in up to 20-50% of pediatric patients, often as a transient condition. In many cases, it is considered to be "functional" or "relative" in nature, meaning that cortisol levels are within normal limits but cannot increase sufficiently to meet the demands of critical illness. The causes are heterogeneous, and some were discussed in Chapter 575.1. They include adrenal hypoperfusion from shock, particularly septic shock, as is often seen in meningococcemia. Inflammatory mediators during septic shock, particularly interleukin-6, can suppress ACTH secretion, directly suppress cortisol secretion, or both. Etomidate, used as sedation for intubation, inhibits steroid 11β-hydroxylase and thus blocks cortisol biosynthesis. Neurosurgical patients with closed head trauma, or with tumors that involve the hypothalamus or pituitary, might have ACTH deficiency in the context of panhypopituitarism. Some children

have been previously treated with systemic corticosteroids (e.g., children with leukemia) and have suppression of the HPA axis for that reason. In the intensive care nursery, premature infants have not yet developed normal cortisol biosynthetic capacity (see Chapter 574.2) and thus may not be able to secrete adequate amounts of this hormone when ill.

CLINICAL MANIFESTATIONS

Cortisol is required for catecholamines to have their normal pressor effects on the cardiovascular system (see Chapters 574.4 and 574.5). Accordingly, adrenal insufficiency is often suspected in hypotensive patients who do not respond to intravenous pressor agents. Patients may be at increased risk for hypoglycemia or a presentation resembling the syndrome of inappropriate antidiuretic hormone secretion, but these conditions commonly occur in the context of sepsis, and the contribution of adrenal insufficiency may be difficult to distinguish.

LABORATORY FINDINGS

Although low random cortisol levels in severely stressed patients are certainly abnormal, very high levels are also associated with a poor outcome in such patients; the latter situation presumably reflects a maximally stimulated adrenal cortex with diminished reserve. ACTH (cosyntropin) stimulation testing is generally considered the best way to diagnose adrenal insufficiency in this setting (see Chapter 575.1); evidence suggests that the low-dose (1 μg/1.73 m²) test may be superior to the 250 μg standard dose test, although this remains controversial. Generally, a peak cortisol level <18 μg/dL or an increment of <9 μg/dL from baseline is considered suggestive for adrenal insufficiency in this context. In evaluating cortisol levels, it should be remembered that cortisol in the circulation is normally mostly bound to cortisol-binding globulin; in hypoproteinemic states total cortisol levels may be decreased, whereas free cortisol levels might be normal. It may be prudent to measure free cortisol before initiating treatment when total cortisol is low and albumin is <2.5 g/dL, but such measurements are not readily available in all institutions.

TREATMENT

There are limited data regarding treatment efficacy in critically ill children. Based on studies of both children and adults, it is likely that moderate stress doses of hydrocortisone (e.g., 50 mg/m²/day) improve responses to pressor agents in patients with shock and documented adrenal insufficiency. It is uncertain if there is a beneficial effect on overall survival. There seems to be no benefit in using pharmacologic doses of potent synthetic glucocorticoids such as dexamethasone.

Bibliography is available at Expert Consult.

575.4 Altered End-Organ Sensitivity to Corticosteroids
Perrin C. White

Diseases can result from altered actions of hormones at their physiologic targets. These may be caused by abnormal metabolism of hormones, mutations in hormone receptors, or defects in cellular effectors (such as ion channels) that are targets of hormone action.

GENERALIZED GLUCOCORTICOID RESISTANCE
Etiology

Patients with generalized glucocorticoid resistance have target-tissue insensitivity to glucocorticoids. The condition is usually inherited in an autosomal dominant manner but sporadic cases occur. Impairment of normal negative feedback of cortisol at the levels of the hypothalamus and pituitary activates the HPA axis with consequent increases in ACTH and cortisol concentrations. Generalized glucocorticoid resistance is caused by mutations in the glucocorticoid receptor (encoded by the *NR3C1* gene) that impair its action by interfering with ligand binding, DNA binding, transcriptional activation, or some combination of these. Most mutations are heterozygous; glucocorticoid receptors usually bind DNA as dimers, and 3 out of every 4 dimers will contain at least 1 abnormal receptor molecule when a heterozygous mutation is present.

Clinical Manifestations

The excess ACTH secretion causes adrenal hyperplasia with increased production of adrenal steroids with mineralocorticoid activity, including cortisol, deoxycorticosterone, and corticosterone, and also androgens and precursors, including androstenedione, dehydroepiandrosterone, and dehydroepiandrosterone sulfate. The high cortisol concentrations do not cause Cushing syndrome (see Chapter 577) because of the insensitivity to glucocorticoids; conversely, most signs and symptoms of adrenal insufficiency are absent except for the frequent occurrence of chronic fatigue and occasional anxiety (neonatal hypoglycemia was reported in 1 very unusual patient with a homozygous null mutation). On the other hand, the mineralocorticoid and androgen receptors are normally sensitive to their ligands. Signs of mineralocorticoid excess, such as hypertension and hypokalemic alkalosis, are frequently noted. The increased concentrations of adrenal androgens may cause ambiguous genitalia in girls and gonadotropin-independent precocious puberty in children of either gender; acne; hirsutism, and infertility in both sexes; menstrual irregularities in females; and oligospermia in males. Testicular adrenal rest tumors and ACTH-secreting pituitary adenomas occasionally occur.

Laboratory Findings

The diagnosis of generalized glucocorticoid resistance is suggested by elevated serum cortisol concentrations and increased 24 hr urinary free cortisol excretion in the absence of Cushing syndrome. Levels of other adrenal steroids are also increased. Plasma concentrations of ACTH may be normal or high. The circadian pattern of ACTH and cortisol secretion is preserved, although at higher-than-normal concentrations, and there is resistance of the HPA axis to dexamethasone suppression. Sequencing of the *NR3C1* gene can confirm the diagnosis, but is not routinely available.

Differential Diagnosis

Generalized glucocorticoid resistance should be distinguished from relatively mild cases of Cushing syndrome (whether caused by a pituitary adenoma or adrenal tumor, see Chapter 577); the latter is more likely to be associated with excessive weight gain or poor linear growth. Adrenocortical tumors may secrete mineralocorticoids such as deoxycorticosterone and also androgens, but ACTH levels are often suppressed and of course the tumor can usually be visualized with appropriate imaging techniques. Congenital adrenal hyperplasia (see Chapter 576), particularly 11β-hydroxylase deficiency, may present with hypertension and signs of androgen excess, but in that condition cortisol levels are low and levels of cortisol precursors (17-hydroxyprogesterone, 11-deoxycortisol) are elevated. Obese patients may be hypertensive and have hyperandrogenism, but cortisol secretion should be readily suppressed by dexamethasone.

Treatment

The goal of treatment is to suppress the excess secretion of ACTH, thereby suppressing the increased production of adrenal steroids with mineralocorticoid and androgenic activity. This requires administration of high doses of a pure glucocorticoid agonist such as dexamethasone (typically ~20-40 μg/kg/day) with careful titration to suppress endogenous corticosteroid secretion without causing signs of glucocorticoid excess such as excessive weight gain or suppression of linear growth.

CORTISONE REDUCTASE DEFICIENCY
Etiology

Levels of active glucocorticoids in target tissues are modulated by 2 isozymes of 11β-hydroxysteroid dehydrogenase. The 11-HSD2 isozyme converts cortisol to an inactive metabolite, cortisone; the 2 steroids differ in the presence of an 11β-hydroxyl vs an 11-oxo group, respectively. Mutations in this enzyme cause the syndrome of **apparent mineralocorticoid excess**. Conversely, the 11-HSD1 isozyme converts cortisone to cortisol, and so it is sometimes referred to as "cortisone reductase." This isozyme is expressed at high levels in glucocorticoid target tissues, particularly the liver, where it ensures adequate levels of active glucocorticoids (cortisol and corticosterone) to meet metabolic demands without requiring excessive adrenal cortisol secretion.

The 11-HSD1 isozyme is located in the endoplasmic reticulum (i.e., it is a "microsomal" enzyme) and functions as a dimer. It accepts electrons from reduced nicotine–adenine dinucleotide phosphate, which is generated within the endoplasmic reticulum by hexose-6-phosphate dehydrogenase, an enzyme distinct from cytoplasmic glucose-6-phosphate dehydrogenase.

Apparent cortisone reductase deficiency is caused by homozygous mutations in hexose-6-phosphate dehydrogenase that prevent generation of reduced nicotine–adenine dinucleotide phosphate within the endoplasmic reticulum and thus starve 11-HSD1 of its essential cofactor for the reductase reaction. Very rare patients have been reported to have heterozygous mutations in the *HSD11B1* gene encoding 11-HSD1 itself and thus have "true" cortisone reductase deficiency; because the enzyme functions as a homodimer, heterozygous mutations are able to impair three fourths of all dimmers.

Clinical Manifestations

Because circulating cortisone is not converted to cortisol, the circulating half-life of cortisol is decreased and the adrenal cortex must secrete additional cortisol to compensate. This leads to adrenocortical overactivity analogous to, but generally much milder than, that seen in generalized glucocorticoid resistance. This is usually not severe enough to cause hypertension, presenting instead with mild to moderate signs of androgen excess such as hirsutism, oligomenorrhea or amenorrhea, and infertility in females, and precocious pseudopuberty (axillary and pubic hair, and penile enlargement, but not testicular enlargement) in males.

Laboratory Findings

The ratio of cortisol to cortisone in blood is lower than usual. The same is true of urinary metabolites, typically measured as a ratio of the sum of the tetrahydrocortisol and allotetrahydrocortisol excretion to that of tetrahydrocortisone. These determinations are best accomplished by gas chromatography followed by mass spectrometry, and are available in specialized reference laboratories. Absolute levels of cortisol and ACTH are within normal limits.

Differential Diagnosis

Cortisone reductase deficiency has to be distinguished from, and is much less common than, other causes of androgen excess such as polycystic ovarian syndrome and nonclassical congenital adrenal hyperplasia as a result of 21-hydroxylase deficiency.

Treatment

Treatment is aimed at decreasing adrenal overactivity and thus reducing secretion of androgens. This can be accomplished by administration of hydrocortisone.

ALTERED END-ORGAN SENSITIVITY TO MINERALOCORTICOIDS
Pseudohypoaldosteronism
Etiology

Pseudohypoaldosteronism type 1 (PHA1) is a monogenic disease in which aldosterone action is deficient and patients are thus unable to resorb urinary sodium or excrete potassium properly. There are 2 forms. A relatively mild **autosomal dominant** form is caused by mutations in the *NR3C2* gene encoding the human mineralocorticoid receptor. As with generalized glucocorticoid resistance, a heterozygous mutation is sufficient to cause disease because the mineralocorticoid receptor interacts with DNA as a dimer, and three fourths of the dimers are defective in individuals carrying heterozygous mutations (assuming mutant protein is synthesized). A more-severe **autosomal recessive** form is usually the result of homozygous mutations in the α (*SCNN1A*), β (*SCNN1B*), or γ (*SCNN1G*) subunits of the epithelial Na(+) channel, but 1 reported case of severe autosomal recessive disease was caused by homozygous mutations in *NR3C2*.

PHA1 should not be confused with pseudohypoaldosteronism type 2, a rare mendelian syndrome characterized by hyperkalemia and, in contrast to PHA1, by hypertension from excessive renal salt reabsorption. This disorder is caused by mutations in the renal regulatory kinases, WNK1 and WNK4, or components of an E3 ubiquitin ligase complex Kelch-like 3 (KLHL3) and Cullin 3 (CUL3).

Clinical Manifestations

Infants with PHA1 present with hyperkalemia, hyponatremia, hypovolemia, hypotension, and failure to thrive. In more-severe (usually autosomal recessive) cases, salt loss is not confined to the kidney but instead occurs from most epithelia. Mothers may report that the skin of their affected infants tastes salty. Some infants suffer from **cystic fibrosis–like pulmonary symptoms.** It is often difficult to control electrolyte abnormalities in patients with the autosomal recessive form, leading to frequent hospitalizations and a need for close clinical monitoring.

It is noteworthy that signs and symptoms of aldosterone deficiency tend to remit as the patients get older, particularly in the autosomal dominant form. This is similar to what is seen in actual aldosterone deficiency as occurs in the salt-losing forms of congenital adrenal hyperplasia or aldosterone synthase deficiency. The kidney matures after early infancy to become more efficient at excreting potassium, and whereas breast milk and infant formula are low in sodium, the normal adult Western diet is relatively high in sodium, thus compensating for the renal salt wasting.

Laboratory Findings

Infants have marked hyperkalemia and hyponatremia. Both plasma renin and aldosterone are markedly elevated. Levels of cortisol and ACTH are normal. If hypovolemia is severe, patients may develop prerenal azotemia. The electrocardiogram may include tall peaked T waves with severe hyperkalemia or ventricular tachycardia.

Differential Diagnosis

PHA in infants should be distinguished from other causes of hyperkalemia and hyponatremia. These include renal failure of any cause, congenital adrenal hyperplasia, aldosterone synthase deficiency, and other causes of adrenocortical insufficiency such as AHC. Patients with renal failure will have elevated blood urea nitrogen and creatinine, but these may be seen in severely dehydrated patients with PHA. Patients with any form of adrenal insufficiency in this clinical context will have low or low-normal aldosterone levels (with elevated plasma renin), in contrast to the elevated aldosterone levels seen in PHA. Patients with congenital adrenal hyperplasia have elevated levels of steroid precursors such as 17-hydroxyprogesterone (in patients with 21-hydroxylase deficiency), and patients with most forms of adrenal insufficiency have elevated ACTH levels.

Treatment

Infants must be given dietary sodium supplementation (initially intravenous and then oral), typically approximately 8 mEq/kg/day. Potassium levels in the infant formula often need to be reduced, which may be accomplished by mixing the formula with polystyrene resin (Kayexalate) and then decanting the formula prior to feeding. Fludrocortisone, a synthetic mineralocorticoid, may be efficacious in milder autosomal dominant cases if administered in high doses (titrating up to ~0.5 mg daily). Significant electrolyte abnormalities require treatment with intravenous normal saline and rectal polystyrene resin. Severe hyperkalemia may require glucose and insulin infusions to control.

APPARENT MINERALOCORTICOID EXCESS
Etiology

The syndrome of apparent mineralocorticoid excess is an autosomal recessive disorder caused by mutations in the *HSD11B2* gene encoding the 11-HSD2 isozyme of 11β-hydroxysteroid dehydrogenase. The mineralocorticoid receptor actually has nearly identical affinities for aldosterone (the main mineralocorticoid hormone) and cortisol, yet cortisol is normally only a weak mineralocorticoid in vivo. This is because 11-HSD2 is expressed along with the mineralocorticoid receptor in most target tissues such as the renal cortical collecting duct epithelium. It converts cortisol to cortisone, which is not an active steroid, thus preventing it from occupying the mineralocorticoid receptor. In contrast, aldosterone is not a substrate for the enzyme because its 11β-hydroxyl group forms a hemiketal with the 18-aldehyde group of the steroid and is thus not accessible to the enzyme. Thus, in the absence of 11-HSD2, cortisol is able to efficiently occupy the mineralocorticoid receptor, and because cortisol concentrations are normally far higher than those of aldosterone, this results in signs and symptoms of mineralocorticoid excess.

A similar clinical picture occurs with excessive consumption of licorice or licorice-flavored chewing tobacco; licorice contains compounds including glycyrrhetinic and glycyrrhizic acids that inhibit 11-HSD2. Carbenoxolone, an antihypertensive drug that is not marketed in the United States, has similar effects.

Clinical Manifestations

Affected infants often have some degree of intrauterine growth restriction with birth weights of 2 kg typical for term infants. Infants and children often fail to thrive. Severe hypertension (to ~200/120 mm Hg) is almost always present. In some patients, the hypertension tends to be labile or paroxysmal with severe emotional stress as a precipitating factor. Complications of hypertension have included cerebrovascular accidents. Several patients have died during infancy or adolescence, either from electrolyte imbalances leading to cardiac arrhythmias or from vascular sequelae of hypertension. Hypokalemic alkalosis can eventually cause nephrocalcinosis (often visible on renal ultrasound) and nephrogenic diabetes insipidus leading to polyuria and polydipsia. Deleterious effects on muscle range from elevations in serum creatine phosphokinase to frank rhabdomyolysis. Electrocardiograms show left ventricular hypertrophy.

Laboratory Findings

Hypokalemia and alkalosis are common but not persistent. Sodium levels are generally in the upper part of the reference range. Aldosterone and renin levels are very low because the hypertension and hypervolemia are independent of aldosterone concentrations. Serum cortisol and ACTH levels are generally within normal limits. The serum half-life of cortisol is increased, but the test for this requires a radioactive tracer and is not clinically available. Total urinary excretion of cortisol metabolites is markedly decreased. The urinary ratio of free cortisol to free cortisone is elevated, as is the ratio of urinary tetrahydrocortisol plus allotetrahydrocortisol to tetrahydrocortisone.

Differential Diagnosis

The differential diagnosis includes other forms of severe childhood hypertension such as renal artery anomalies, but relatively few conditions present with suppressed renin and aldosterone levels. Liddle syndrome has a similar presentation but no abnormalities in the steroid profile, typically has an autosomal dominant mode of inheritance, and does not respond to treatment with mineralocorticoid receptor antagonists. Hypertensive forms of congenital adrenal hyperplasia (see Chapter 576) also have suppressed renin and aldosterone levels, but they present with signs of androgen excess (11β-hydroxylase deficiency) or androgen deficiency (17α-hydroxylase deficiency); the latter can be difficult to appreciate in young children. The steroid profiles in congenital adrenal hyperplasia differ from those seen in apparent mineralocorticoid excess syndrome.

Patients with severe Cushing syndrome may have high enough cortisol levels to overwhelm renal 11-HSD2, leading to severe hypertension with alterations in urinary cortisol-to-cortisone ratios. This occurs most often in patients with the ectopic ACTH syndrome. This generally does not present a diagnostic dilemma, because of the other signs of Cushing syndrome including high cortisol levels.

Treatment
Treatment includes a low-salt diet, potassium supplementation, and mineralocorticoid receptor blockade with spironolactone or eplerenone; a sodium channel blocker, such as amiloride or triamterene may work at least as well. In principle, suppression of cortisol secretion with dexamethasone (which does not bind the mineralocorticoid receptor) should work, but in practice it is much less effective than mineralocorticoid receptor blockade.

LIDDLE SYNDROME
Etiology
Liddle syndrome is a form of hypertension and hypokalemia that is clinically similar to the syndrome of apparent mineralocorticoid excess, but it is inherited in an autosomal dominant manner. It is caused by activating mutations in the β (*SCNN1B*) or γ (*SCNN1G*) subunits of the epithelial sodium channel. Most of these mutations prevent the channel subunits from being ligated to ubiquitin and targeted to the proteosome for degradation, a process that is normally regulated indirectly by aldosterone. The net effect is to increase the number of open channels at the apical surface of epithelial cells of the renal collecting duct, thus facilitating sodium resorption and potassium excretion. This disorder is thus the exact opposite of the autosomal recessive form of pseudohypoaldosteronism discussed previously.

Clinical Manifestations, Laboratory Findings, and Differential Diagnosis
Liddle syndrome is characterized by severe early-onset hypertension and by hypokalemia, which may not be persistent. Aldosterone and renin levels are suppressed but all steroid hormone levels are normal.

The differential diagnosis is the same as that for apparent mineralocorticoid excess.

Treatment
The mainstays of treatment are a low-salt diet, potassium supplementation, and a sodium channel blocker such as amiloride or triamterene. Mineralocorticoid receptor antagonists such as spironolactone are ineffective.

Bibliography is available at Expert Consult.

Chapter 576
Congenital Adrenal Hyperplasia and Related Disorders
Perrin C. White

Congenital adrenal hyperplasia (CAH) is a family of autosomal recessive disorders of cortisol biosynthesis (normal adrenal steroidogenesis is discussed in Chapter 574). Cortisol deficiency increases secretion of corticotropin (adrenocorticotropic hormone [ACTH]), which, in turn, leads to adrenocortical hyperplasia and overproduction of intermediate metabolites. Depending on the enzymatic step that is deficient, there may be signs, symptoms, and laboratory findings of mineralo-

corticoid deficiency or excess; incomplete virilization or precocious puberty in affected males; and virilization or sexual infantilism in affected females (Figs. 576-1 and 576-2 and Table 576-1).

576.1 Congenital Adrenal Hyperplasia Caused by 21-Hydroxylase Deficiency
Perrin C. White

ETIOLOGY
More than 90% of CAH cases are caused by 21-hydroxylase deficiency. This P450 enzyme (CYP21, P450c21) hydroxylates progesterone and 17-hydroxyprogesterone to yield 11-deoxycorticosterone and 11-deoxycortisol, respectively (see Fig. 574-1 in Chapter 574). These conversions are required for synthesis of aldosterone and cortisol, respectively. Both hormones are deficient in the most-severe, "salt-wasting" form of the disease. Slightly less-severely affected patients are able to synthesize adequate amounts of aldosterone but have elevated levels of androgens of adrenal origin; this is termed "simple virilizing disease". These 2 forms are collectively termed classic 21-hydroxylase deficiency. Patients with nonclassic disease have relatively mildly elevated levels of androgens and may be asymptomatic or have signs of androgen excess at any time after birth. Clinical presentation is dependent, in part, on the genotype (see below, "Genetics,") (Table 576-2).

EPIDEMIOLOGY
Classic 21-hydroxylase deficiency occurs in approximately 1 in 15,000-20,000 births in most populations. Approximately 70% of affected infants have the salt-losing form, whereas 30% have the simple virilizing form of the disorder. In the United States, CAH is less common in African-Americans compared with white children (1:42,000 vs 1:15,500). Nonclassic disease has a prevalence of approximately 1 in 1,000 in the general population, but occurs more frequently in specific ethnic groups such as Ashkenazi Jews and Hispanics.

GENETICS
There are 2 steroid 21-hydroxylase genes—*CYP21P* (*CYP21A1P, CYP21A*) and *CYP21* (*CYP21A2, CYP21B*)—which alternate in tandem with 2 genes for the fourth component of complement (C4A and C4B) in the human leukocyte antigen (HLA) major histocompatibility complex on chromosome 6p21.3 between the HLA-B and HLA-DR loci. Many other genes are located in this cluster. *CYP21* is the active gene; *CYP21P* is 98% identical in DNA sequence to *CYP21* but is a pseudogene because of 9 different mutations. More than 90% of mutations causing 21-hydroxylase deficiency are recombinations between *CYP21* and *CYP21P*. Approximately 20% are deletions generated by unequal meiotic crossing-over between *CYP21* and *CYP21P*, whereas the remainder are nonreciprocal transfers of deleterious mutations from *CYP21P* to *CYP21*, a phenomenon termed gene conversion.

The deleterious mutations in *CYP21P* have different effects on enzymatic activity when transferred to *CYP21*. Several mutations completely prevent synthesis of a functional protein, whereas others are missense mutations (they result in amino acid substitutions) that yield enzymes with 1-50% of normal activity. Disease severity correlates well with the mutations carried by an affected individual; for example, patients with salt-wasting disease usually carry mutations on both alleles that completely destroy enzymatic activity. Patients are frequently compound heterozygotes for different types of mutations (i.e., 1 allele is less-severely affected than the other), in which case the severity of disease expression is largely determined by the activity of the less-severely affected of the 2 alleles.

Closely adjacent to, but on the opposite DNA strand from, *CYP21* is the tenascin-X (*TNX*) gene, which encodes a connective tissue protein. Rarely, deletions of *CYP21* extend into *TNX*. Such patients may have a contiguous gene syndrome (see Chapter 81.1) consisting of CAH and **Ehlers-Danlos syndrome** (see Chapters 484 and 659).

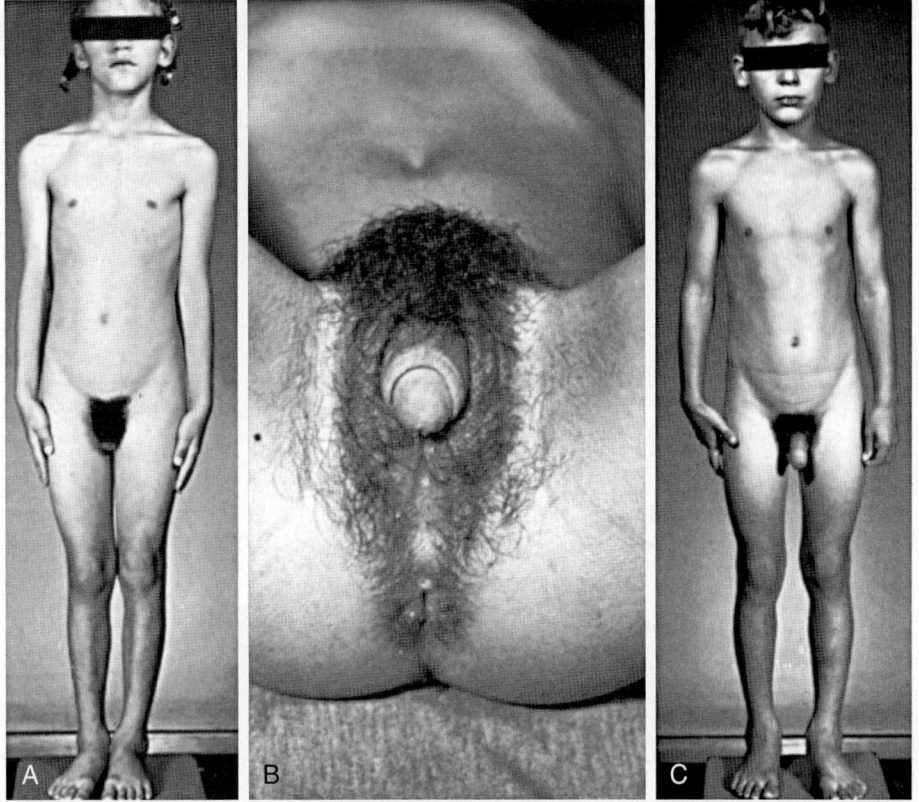

Figure 576-1 A, A 6-yr-old girl with congenital virilizing adrenal hyperplasia. The height age was 8.5 yr, and the bone age was 13 yr. **B,** Notice the clitoral enlargement and labial fusion. **C,** Her 5 yr old brother was not considered to be abnormal by the parents. The height age was 8 yr, and the bone age was 12.5 yr.

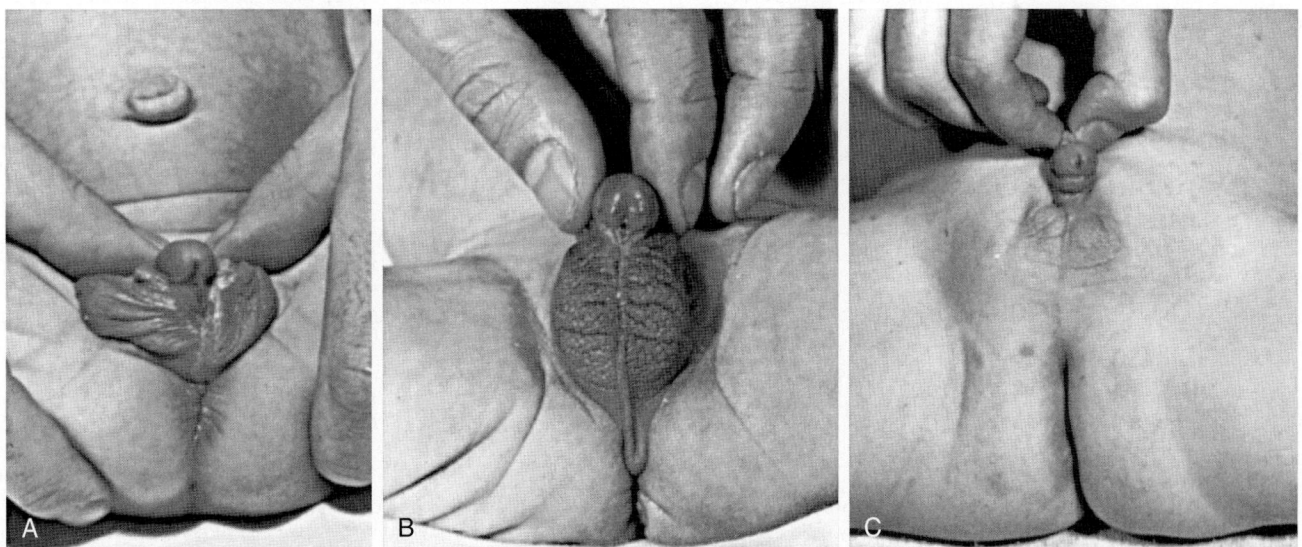

Figure 576-2 Three virilized females with untreated congenital adrenal hyperplasia. All were erroneously assigned male sex at birth, and each had a normal female sex-chromosome complement. Infants **A** and **B** had the salt-wasting form and received the diagnosis early in infancy. Infant **C** was referred at 1 yr of age because of bilateral cryptorchidism. Notice the completely penile urethra; such complete masculinization in females with adrenal hyperplasia is rare; most of these infants have the salt-wasting form.

Table 576-1	Diagnosis and Treatment of Congenital Adrenal Hyperplasia

DISORDER	AFFECTED GENE AND CHROMOSOME	SIGNS AND SYMPTOMS	LABORATORY FINDINGS	THERAPEUTIC MEASURES
21-Hydroxylase deficiency, classic form	*CYP21* 6p21.3	Glucocorticoid deficiency	↓ Cortisol, ↑ACTH ↑↑ Baseline and ACTH-stimulated 17-hydroxy-progesterone	Glucocorticoid (hydrocortisone) replacement
		Mineralocorticoid deficiency (salt-wasting crisis)	Hyponatremia, hyperkalemia ↑ Plasma renin	Mineralocorticoid (fludrocortisone) replacement; sodium chloride supplementation
		Ambiguous genitalia in females	↑ Serum androgens	Vaginoplasty and clitoral recession
		Postnatal virilization in males and females	↑ Serum androgens	Suppression with glucocorticoids
21-Hydroxylase deficiency, nonclassic form	*CYP21* 6p21.3	May be asymptomatic; precocious adrenarche, hirsutism, acne, menstrual irregularity, infertility	↑ Baseline and ACTH-stimulated 17-hydroxyprogesterone ↑ Serum androgens	Suppression with glucocorticoids
11β-Hydroxylase deficiency	*CYP11B1* 8q24.3	Glucocorticoid deficiency	↓ Cortisol, ↑ ACTH ↑↑ Baseline and ACTH-stimulated 11-deoxycortisol and deoxycorticosterone	Glucocorticoid (hydrocortisone) replacement
		Ambiguous genitalia in females	↑ Serum androgens	Vaginoplasty and clitoral recession
		Postnatal virilization in males and females	↑ Serum androgens	Suppression with glucocorticoids
		Hypertension	↓ Plasma renin, hypokalemia	Suppression with glucocorticoids
3β-Hydroxysteroid dehydrogenase deficiency, classic form	*HSD3B2* 1p13.1	Glucocorticoid deficiency	↓ Cortisol, ↑ ACTH ↑↑ Baseline and ACTH-stimulated Δ5 steroids (pregnenolone, 17-hydroxy-pregnenolone, DHEA)	Glucocorticoid (hydrocortisone) replacement
		Mineralocorticoid deficiency (salt-wasting crisis)	Hyponatremia, hyperkalemia ↑ Plasma renin	Mineralocorticoid (fludrocortisone) replacement; sodium chloride supplementation
		Ambiguous genitalia in females and males	↑ DHEA, ↓ androstenedione, testosterone, and estradiol	Surgical correction of genitals and sex hormone replacement as necessary, consonant with sex of rearing
		Precocious adrenarche, disordered puberty	↑ DHEA, ↓ androstenedione, testosterone, and estradiol	Suppression with glucocorticoids
17α-Hydroxylase/ 17,20-lyase deficiency	*CYP17* 10q24.3	Cortisol deficiency (corticosterone is an adequate glucocorticoid)	↓ Cortisol, ↑ ACTH ↑ DOC, corticosterone Low 17α-hydroxylated steroids; poor response to ACTH	Glucocorticoid (hydrocortisone) administration
		Ambiguous genitalia in males	↓ Serum androgens; poor response to hCG	Orchidopexy or removal of intraabdominal testes; sex hormone replacement consonant with sex of rearing
		Sexual infantilism	↓ Serum androgens or estrogens	Sex hormone replacement consonant with sex of rearing
		Hypertension	↓ Plasma renin; hypokalemia	Suppression with glucocorticoids
Congenital lipoid adrenal hyperplasia	*STAR* 8p11.2	Glucocorticoid deficiency	↑ ACTH Low levels of all steroid hormones, with decreased or absent response to ACTH	Glucocorticoid (hydrocortisone) replacement
		Mineralocorticoid deficiency (salt-wasting crisis)	Hyponatremia, hyperkalemia ↓ Aldosterone, ↑ plasma renin	Mineralocorticoid (fludrocortisone) replacement; sodium chloride supplementation
		Ambiguous genitalia in males	Decreased or absent response to hCG in males	Orchidopexy or removal of intraabdominal testes; sex hormone replacement consonant with sex of rearing
		Poor pubertal development or premature ovarian failure in females	↑ FSH, ↑ LH, ↓ estradiol (after puberty)	Estrogen replacement

Table 576-1	Diagnosis and Treatment of Congenital Adrenal Hyperplasia—cont'd			
DISORDER	**AFFECTED GENE AND CHROMOSOME**	**SIGNS AND SYMPTOMS**	**LABORATORY FINDINGS**	**THERAPEUTIC MEASURES**
P450 oxidoreductase deficiency	*POR* 7q11.3	Glucocorticoid deficiency Ambiguous genitalia in males and females Maternal virilization Antley-Bixler syndrome	↓ Cortisol, ↑ ACTH ↑ Pregnenolone, ↑ progesterone ↑ Serum androgens prenatally, ↓ androgens and estrogens at puberty Decreased ratio of estrogens to androgens	Glucocorticoid (hydrocortisone) replacement Surgical correction of genitals and sex hormone replacement as necessary, consonant with sex of rearing

↓, Decreased; ↑, increased; ↑↑, markedly increased; ACTH, adrenocorticotropic hormone; DHEA, dehydroepiandrosterone; DOC, 11-deoxycorticosterone; FSH, follicle-stimulating hormone; hCG, human chorionic gonadotropin; LH, luteinizing hormone.

Table 576-2	Genotype-Phenotype Correlations in Congenital Adrenal Hyperplasia Owing to 21-Hydroxylase Deficiency		
MUTATION GROUP	**A**	**B**	**C**
Enzymatic activity, % normal	Nil	1-2%	20-50%
CYP21 mutations (phenotype generally corresponds to the least affected allele)	Gene deletion Exon 3 del 8 bp Exon 6 cluster Q318X R356W Intron 2 splice	I172N	P30L V281L P453S
Severity	Salt wasting	Simple virilizing	Nonclassic
Aldosterone synthesis	Low	Normal	Normal
Age at diagnosis (without newborn screening)	Infancy	Infancy (females) Childhood (males)	Childhood to adulthood, or asymptomatic
Virilization	Severe	Moderate to severe	None to Mild
Incidence	1/20,000	1/50,000	1/500

PATHOGENESIS AND CLINICAL MANIFESTATIONS

Aldosterone and Cortisol Deficiency

Because both cortisol and aldosterone require 21-hydroxylation for their synthesis, both hormones are deficient in the most-severe, salt-wasting form of the disease. This form constitutes approximately 70% of cases of classic 21-hydroxylase deficiency. The signs and symptoms of cortisol and aldosterone deficiency, and the pathophysiology underlying them, are essentially those described in Chapter 575. These include progressive weight loss, anorexia, vomiting, dehydration, weakness, hypotension, hypoglycemia, hyponatremia, and hyperkalemia. These problems typically first develop in affected infants at approximately 10-14 days of age. Without treatment, shock, cardiac arrhythmias, and death may occur within days or weeks.

CAH differs from other causes of primary adrenal insufficiency in that precursor steroids accumulate proximal to the blocked enzymatic conversion. Because cortisol is not synthesized efficiently, ACTH levels are high, leading to hyperplasia of the adrenal cortex and levels of precursor steroids that may be hundreds of times normal. In the case of 21-hydroxylase deficiency, these precursors include 17-hydroxyprogesterone and progesterone. Progesterone and perhaps other metabolites act as antagonists of the mineralocorticoid receptor and thus may exacerbate the effects of aldosterone deficiency in untreated patients.

Prenatal Androgen Excess

The most important problem caused by accumulation of steroid precursors is that 17-hydroxyprogesterone is shunted into the pathway for androgen biosynthesis, leading to high levels of androstenedione that are converted outside the adrenal gland to testosterone. This problem begins in affected fetuses by 8-10 wk of gestation and leads to abnormal genital development in females (see Figs. 576-1 and 576-2).

The external genitalia of males and females normally appear identical early in gestation (see Chapter 582). Affected females who are exposed in utero to high levels of androgens of adrenal origin have masculinized external genitalia (see Figs. 576-1 and 576-2). This is manifested by enlargement of the clitoris and by partial or complete labial fusion. The vagina usually has a common opening with the urethra (urogenital sinus). The clitoris may be so enlarged that it resembles a penis; because the urethra opens below this organ, some affected females may be mistakenly presumed to be males with hypospadias and cryptorchidism. The severity of virilization is usually greatest in females with the salt-losing form of 21-hydroxylase deficiency (see Table 576-2). The internal genital organs are normal, because affected females have normal ovaries and not testes and thus do not secrete antimüllerian hormone.

Prenatal exposure of the brain to high levels of androgens may influence subsequent sexually dimorphic behaviors in affected females. Girls may demonstrate aggressive play behavior, tend to be interested in masculine toys such as cars and trucks, and often show decreased interest in playing with dolls. Women may have decreased interest in maternal roles. There is an increased frequency of homosexuality in affected females. Nonetheless, most function heterosexually and do not have gender identity confusion or dysphoria. It is unusual for affected females to assign themselves a male role except in some with the severest degree of virilization.

Male infants appear normal at birth. Thus, the diagnosis may not be made in boys until signs of adrenal insufficiency develop. Because patients with this condition can deteriorate quickly, infant boys are more likely to die than infant girls. For this reason, all 50 American states and many countries have instituted newborn screening for this condition (see "Newborn Screening" in Chapter 576.2).

Postnatal Androgen Excess

Untreated or inadequately treated children of both sexes develop additional signs of androgen excess after birth. Boys with the simple virilizing form of 21-hydroxylase deficiency often have a delayed diagnosis because they appear normal and rarely develop adrenal insufficiency.

Signs of androgen excess include rapid somatic growth and accelerated skeletal maturation. Thus, affected patients are tall in childhood but premature closure of the epiphyses causes growth to stop relatively early, and adult stature is stunted (see Fig. 576-1). Muscular development may be excessive. Pubic and axillary hair may appear, and acne and a deep voice may develop. The penis, scrotum, and prostate may become enlarged in affected boys; however, the **testes are usually prepubertal** in size so that they appear relatively small in contrast to the enlarged penis. Occasionally, ectopic adrenocortical cells in the testes of patients become hyperplastic similarly to the adrenal glands, producing testicular adrenal rest tumors (see Chapter 584). The clitoris may become further enlarged in affected females (see Fig. 576-1). Although the internal genital structures are female, breast development and menstruation may not occur unless the excessive production of androgens is suppressed by adequate treatment.

Similar but usually milder signs of androgen excess may occur in **nonclassic 21-hydroxylase deficiency** (see Table 576-2). In this attenuated form, cortisol and aldosterone levels are normal and affected females have normal genitals at birth. Males and females may present with precocious pubarche and early development of pubic and axillary hair. Hirsutism, acne, menstrual disorders, and infertility may develop later in life, but many females and males are completely asymptomatic.

Adrenomedullary Dysfunction

Development of the adrenal medulla requires exposure to the extremely high cortisol levels normally present within the adrenal gland. Thus patients with classic CAH have abnormal adrenomedullary function, as evidenced by blunted epinephrine responses, decreased blood glucose, and lower heart rates with exercise. Ability to exercise is unimpaired and the clinical significance of these findings is uncertain. Adrenomedullary dysfunction may exacerbate the cardiovascular effects of cortisol deficiency in untreated or undertreated patients.

LABORATORY FINDINGS

See Table 576-1.

Patients with salt-losing disease have typical laboratory findings associated with cortisol and aldosterone deficiency, including hyponatremia, hyperkalemia, metabolic acidosis, and, often, hypoglycemia, but these abnormalities can take 10-14 days or longer to develop after birth. Blood levels of **17-hydroxyprogesterone** are markedly elevated. However, levels of this hormone are high during the 1st 2-3 days of life even in unaffected infants and especially if they are sick or premature. After infancy, once the circadian rhythm of cortisol is established, 17-hydroxyprogesterone levels vary in the same circadian pattern, being highest in the morning and lowest at night. Blood levels of cortisol are usually low in patients with the salt-losing type of disease. They are often normal in patients with simple virilizing disease but inappropriately low in relation to the ACTH and 17-hydroxyprogesterone levels. In addition to 17-hydroxyprogesterone, levels of androstenedione and testosterone are elevated in affected females; testosterone is not elevated in affected males, because normal infant males have high testosterone levels compared with those seen later in childhood. Levels of urinary 17-ketosteroids and pregnanetriol are elevated but are now rarely used clinically because blood samples are easier to obtain than 24 hr urine collections. ACTH levels are elevated but have no diagnostic utility over 17-hydroxyprogesterone levels. Plasma levels of renin are elevated, and serum aldosterone is inappropriately low for the renin

level. However, renin levels are high in normal infants in the 1st few wk of life.

Diagnosis of 21-hydroxylase deficiency is most reliably established by measuring 17-hydroxyprogesterone before and 30 or 60 min after an intravenous bolus of 0.125-0.25 mg of cosyntropin (ACTH 1-24). Nomograms exist that readily distinguish normals and patients with nonclassic and classic 21-hydroxylase deficiency. Heterozygous carriers of this autosomal recessive disorder tend to have higher ACTH-stimulated 17-hydroxyprogesterone levels than genetically unaffected individuals, but there is significant overlap between subjects in these 2 categories. However, in infants with frank electrolyte abnormalities or circulatory instability, it may not be possible or necessary to delay treatment to perform this test, as levels of precursors will be sufficiently elevated on a random blood sample to make the diagnosis.

Genotyping is clinically available and may help confirm the diagnosis, but it is expensive and may take weeks. Because the gene conversions that generate most mutant alleles may transfer more than one mutation, at least one parent should be genotyped as well to determine which mutations lie on each allele.

DIFFERENTIAL DIAGNOSIS

Disorders of sexual development are discussed more generally in Chapter 588. The initial step in evaluating an infant with ambiguous genitals is a thorough physical examination to define the anatomy of the genitals, locate the urethral meatus, palpate the scrotum or labia and the inguinal regions for testes (palpable gonads almost always indicate the presence of testicular tissue and thus that the infant is a genetic male), and look for any other anatomic abnormalities. Ultrasonography is helpful in demonstrating the presence or absence of a uterus and can often locate the gonads. A rapid karyotype (such as fluorescence in situ hybridization of interphase nuclei for X and Y chromosomes) can quickly determine the genetic sex of the infant. These results are all likely to be available before the results of hormonal testing and together allow the clinical team to advise the parents as to the genetic sex of the infant and the anatomy of internal reproductive structures. Injection of contrast medium into the urogenital sinus of a virilized female demonstrates a vagina and uterus, and many surgeons utilize this information to formulate a plan for surgical management.

PRENATAL DIAGNOSIS

Prenatal diagnosis of 21-hydroxylase is possible late in the 1st trimester by analysis of DNA obtained by chorionic villus sampling or during the 2nd trimester by amniocentesis. This is usually done because the parents already have an affected child. Most often, the *CYP21* gene is analyzed for frequently occurring mutations; more rare mutations may be detected by DNA sequencing.

NEWBORN SCREENING

Because 21-hydroxylase deficiency is often undiagnosed in affected males until they have severe adrenal insufficiency, all states in the United States and many other countries have instituted newborn screening programs. These programs analyze **17-hydroxyprogesterone** levels in dried blood obtained by heelstick and absorbed on filter paper cards; the same cards are screened in parallel for other congenital conditions, such as hypothyroidism and phenylketonuria. Potentially affected infants are typically quickly recalled for additional testing (electrolytes and repeat 17-hydroxyprogesterone determination) at approximately 2 wk of age. Infants with salt-wasting disease often have abnormal electrolytes by this age but are usually not severely ill. Thus, screening programs are effective in preventing many cases of adrenal crisis in affected males. The nonclassic form of the disease is not reliably detected by newborn screening, but this is of little clinical significance because adrenal insufficiency does not occur in this type of 21-hydroxylase deficiency.

The main difficulty with current newborn screening programs is that to reliably detect all affected infants, the cutoff 17-hydroxyprogesterone levels for recalls are set so low that there is a very high frequency of false-positive results (i.e., the test has a low positive predictive value of approximately 1%). This problem is worst in premature infants. Positive predictive value can be improved by using cutoff levels based on gestational age, and by utilizing more specific second-tier screening methods such as liquid chromatography followed by tandem mass spectrometry.

TREATMENT

Glucocorticoid Replacement

Cortisol deficiency is treated with glucocorticoids. Treatment also suppresses excessive production of androgens by the adrenal cortex and thus minimizes problems such as excessive growth and skeletal maturation and virilization. *This often requires larger glucocorticoid doses than are needed in other forms of adrenal insufficiency, typically 15-20 mg/m²/24 hr of hydrocortisone daily administered orally in 3 divided doses.* Affected infants usually require dosing at the high end of this range. *Double or triple doses are indicated during* **periods of stress,** *such as infection or surgery.* Glucocorticoid treatment must be continued indefinitely in all patients with classic 21-hydroxylase deficiency but may not be necessary in patients with nonclassic disease unless signs of androgen excess are present. Therapy must be individualized. It is desirable to maintain linear growth along percentile lines; crossing to higher height percentiles may suggest undertreatment, whereas loss of height percentiles often indicates overtreatment with glucocorticoids. Overtreatment is also suggested by excessive weight gain. Pubertal development should be monitored by periodic examination, and skeletal maturation is evaluated by serial radiographs of the hand and wrist for bone age. Hormone levels, particularly 17-hydroxyprogesterone and androstenedione, should be measured early in the morning, before taking the morning medications, or at a consistent time in relation to medication dosing. In general, desirable 17- hydroxyprogesterone levels are in the high-normal range or several times normal; low-normal levels can usually be achieved only with excessive glucocorticoid doses.

Menarche occurs at the appropriate age in most girls in whom good control has been achieved; it may be delayed in girls with suboptimal control.

Children with simple virilizing disease, particularly males, are frequently not diagnosed until 3-7 yr of age, at which time skeletal maturation may be 5 yr or more in advance of chronological age. In some children, especially if the bone age is 12 yr or more, **spontaneous central (i.e., gonadotropin-dependent) puberty** may occur when treatment is instituted, because therapy with hydrocortisone suppresses production of adrenal androgens and thus stimulates release of pituitary gonadotropins if the appropriate level of hypothalamic maturation is present. *This form of superimposed true precocious puberty may be treated with a gonadotropin hormone–releasing hormone analog such as leuprolide* (see Chapter 562.1).

Males with 21-hydroxylase deficiency who have had inadequate corticosteroid therapy may develop **testicular adrenal rest tumors,** which usually regress with increased steroid dosage. Testicular MRI, ultrasonography, and color flow Doppler examination help define the character and extent of disease. Testis-sparing surgery for steroid-unresponsive tumors has been reported.

Mineralocorticoid Replacement

Patients with salt-wasting disease (i.e., aldosterone deficiency) require mineralocorticoid replacement with **fludrocortisone.** Infants may have very high mineralocorticoid requirements in the 1st few mo of life, usually 0.1-0.3 mg daily in 2 divided doses but occasionally up to 0.4 mg daily, and often require sodium supplementation (sodium chloride, 8 mmol/kg) in addition to the mineralocorticoid. Older infants and children are usually maintained with 0.05-0.1 mg daily of fludrocortisone. In some patients, simple virilizing disease may be easier to control with a low dose of fludrocortisone in addition to hydrocortisone even when these patients have normal aldosterone levels in the absence of mineralocorticoid replacement. Therapy is evaluated by monitoring of vital signs; tachycardia and hypertension are signs of overtreatment with mineralocorticoids. Serum electro-

lytes should be measured frequently in early infancy as therapy is adjusted. Plasma renin activity is a useful way to determine adequacy of therapy; it should be maintained in or near the normal range but not suppressed.

Additional approaches to improve outcome have been proposed but have not yet become the standard of care. These include an anti-androgen such as flutamide to block the effects of excessive androgen levels, and/or an aromatase inhibitor such as anastrozole, which blocks conversion of androgens to estrogen and thus retards skeletal maturation, a process that is sensitive to estrogens in both boys and girls. Aromatase inhibitors generally should not be used in pubertal girls because they will obviously retard normal puberty and may expose the ovaries to excessive levels of gonadotropins. Growth hormone, with or without luteinizing hormone–releasing hormone agonists to retard skeletal maturation, has been suggested to improve adult height.

Surgical Management of Ambiguous Genitals

Significantly virilized females usually undergo surgery between 2-6 mo of age. If there is severe clitoromegaly, the clitoris is reduced in size, with partial excision of the corporal bodies and preservation of the neurovascular bundle; however, moderate clitoromegaly may become much less noticeable even without surgery as the patient grows. Vaginoplasty and correction of the urogenital sinus usually are performed at the time of clitoral surgery; revision in adolescence is often necessary.

Risks and benefits of surgery should be fully discussed with parents of affected females. There is limited long-term follow-up of functional outcomes in patients who have undergone **modern** surgical procedures. It appears that female sexual dysfunction increases in frequency and severity in those with the most significant degrees of genital virilization and with the degree of enzymatic impairment (prenatal androgen exposure) caused by each patient's mutations (see Table 576-2). Sex assignment of infants with **disorders of sexual differentiation** (including CAH) is usually based on expected sexual functioning and fertility in adulthood with early surgical correction of the external genitals to conform with the sex assignment. Confused gender identity is not common with CAH; it occurs mostly in females with the salt-wasting form of the disease and the greatest degree of virilization.

Lay and medical opponents of genital surgery for other disorders of sexual differentiation state that it ignores any prenatally biased gender role predisposition from androgen exposure and precludes the patient from having any decision as to the patient's own preferred sexual identity and what surgical correction of the genitals should be performed. These individuals and groups say treatment should be aimed primarily at educating the patient, family, and others about the medical condition, its treatment, and how to deal with the intersex condition. They propose that surgery should be delayed until the patient decides on what, if any, correction should be performed. Severely virilized genotypic (XX) females raised as males have generally functioned well in the male gender as adults.

In adolescent and adult females with poorly controlled 21-hydroxylase deficiency (hirsutism, obesity, amenorrhea), bilateral laparoscopic adrenalectomy (with hormone replacement) may be an alternative to standard medical hormone replacement therapy, but patients treated in this way may be more susceptible to acute adrenal insufficiency if treatment is interrupted because the adrenal glands have been removed. Moreover, they may exhibit signs of elevated ACTH levels such as abnormal pigmentation.

Prenatal Treatment

Besides genetic counseling, the main goal of prenatal diagnosis is to facilitate appropriate prenatal treatment of affected females. Mothers with pregnancies at risk are given dexamethasone, a steroid that readily crosses the placenta, in an amount of 20 μg/kg prepregnancy maternal weight daily in 2 or 3 divided doses. This suppresses secretion of steroids by the fetal adrenal, including secretion of adrenal androgens. If started by 6 wk of gestation, it ameliorates virilization of the external genitals in affected females. Chorionic villus biopsy is then performed to determine the sex and genotype of the fetus; therapy is continued only if the fetus is an affected female. DNA analysis of fetal cells isolated from maternal plasma for sex determination and *CYP21* gene analysis may permit earlier identification of the affected female fetus. Children exposed to this therapy have slightly lower birthweights. Effects on personality or cognition, such as increased shyness, have been suggested but not consistently observed. At present there is insufficient information to determine whether the long-term risks are acceptable, particularly in the males and unaffected females who derive no direct benefit from the treatment. Maternal side effects of prenatal treatment have included edema, excessive weight gain, hypertension, glucose intolerance, cushingoid facial features, and severe striae. Prenatal treatment is therefore carried out only under institutional protocols in some locales, but it is offered as an option outside the research setting by high-risk obstetricians in other communities.

Bibliography is available at Expert Consult.

576.2 Congenital Adrenal Hyperplasia Caused by 11β-Hydroxylase Deficiency
Perrin C. White

ETIOLOGY
Deficiency of 11β-hydroxylase is caused by a mutation in the *CYP11B1* gene located on chromosome 8q24. *CYP11B1* mediates 11-hydroxylation of 11-deoxycortisol to cortisol. Because 11-deoxycortisol is not converted to cortisol, levels of corticotropin are high. In consequence, precursors—particularly 11-deoxycortisol and deoxycorticosterone—accumulate and are shunted into androgen biosynthesis in the same manner as occurs in 21-hydroxylase deficiency. The adjacent *CYP11B2* gene encoding aldosterone synthase is generally unaffected in this disorder, so patients are able to synthesize aldosterone normally.

EPIDEMIOLOGY
11β-Hydroxylase deficiency accounts for approximately 5% of cases of adrenal hyperplasia; its incidence in the general population has been estimated as 1 in 250,000 to 1 in 100,000. The disorder occurs relatively frequently in Israeli Jews of North African origin (1 in 15,000-17,000 live births). In this ethnic group almost all alleles carry an Arg448 to His (R448H) mutation in *CYP11B1*, but many other mutations have been identified. This disorder presents in a classic, severe form and very rarely in a nonclassic, milder form.

CLINICAL MANIFESTATIONS
Although cortisol is not synthesized efficiently, aldosterone synthetic capacity is normal, and some corticosterone is synthesized from progesterone by the intact aldosterone synthase enzyme. Thus, it is unusual for patients to manifest signs of adrenal insufficiency such as hypotension, hypoglycemia, hyponatremia, and hyperkalemia. Approximately 65% of patients become **hypertensive,** although this can take several years to develop. Hypertension is probably a consequence of elevated levels of deoxycorticosterone, which has mineralocorticoid activity. Infants may transiently develop signs of mineralocorticoid deficiency after treatment with hydrocortisone is instituted. This is presumably from sudden suppression of deoxycorticosterone secretion in a patient with atrophy of the zona glomerulosa caused by chronic suppression of renin activity.

All signs and symptoms of androgen excess that are found in 21-hydroxylase deficiency may also occur in 11β-hydroxylase deficiency.

LABORATORY FINDINGS
Plasma levels of 11-deoxycortisol and deoxycorticosterone are elevated. Because deoxycorticosterone and metabolites have mineralocor-

ticoid activity, plasma renin activity is suppressed. Consequently, aldosterone levels are low even though the ability to synthesize aldosterone is intact. Hypokalemic alkalosis occasionally occurs.

TREATMENT
Patients are treated with hydrocortisone in doses similar to those used for 21-hydroxylase deficiency. Mineralocorticoid replacement is sometimes transiently required in infancy but is rarely necessary otherwise. Hypertension often resolves with glucocorticoid treatment but may require additional therapy if it is of long standing. Calcium channel blockers may be beneficial under these circumstances.

Bibliography is available at Expert Consult.

576.3 Congenital Adrenal Hyperplasia Caused by 3β-Hydroxysteroid Dehydrogenase Deficiency
Perrin C. White

ETIOLOGY
Deficiency of 3β-hydroxysteroid dehydrogenase (3β-HSD) occurs in fewer than 2% of patients with adrenal hyperplasia. This enzyme is required for conversion of Δ5 steroids (pregnenolone, 17-hydroxypregnenolone, dehydroepiandrosterone [DHEA]) to Δ4 steroids (progesterone, 17-hydroxyprogesterone, and androstenedione). Thus, deficiency of the enzyme results in decreased synthesis of cortisol, aldosterone, and androstenedione but increased secretion of DHEA (see Fig. 574-1 in Chapter 574). The 3β-HSD isozyme expressed in the adrenal cortex and gonad is encoded by the *HSD3B2* gene located on chromosome 1p13.1. Over 30 mutations in the *HSD3B2* gene have been described in patients with 3β-HSD deficiency.

CLINICAL MANIFESTATIONS
Because cortisol and aldosterone are not synthesized in patients with the classic form of the disease, infants are prone to **salt-wasting crises.** Because androstenedione and testosterone are not synthesized, **boys are incompletely virilized.** Varying degrees of hypospadias may occur, with or without bifid scrotum or cryptorchidism. Because DHEA levels are elevated and this hormone is a weak androgen, girls are mildly virilized, with slight to moderate clitoral enlargement. Postnatally, continued excessive DHEA secretion can cause precocious adrenarche. During adolescence and adulthood, hirsutism, irregular menses, and polycystic ovarian disease occur in females. Males manifest variable degrees of hypogonadism, although appropriate male secondary sexual development may occur. A persistent defect of testicular 3β-HSD is demonstrated, however, by the high Δ5:Δ4 steroid ratio in testicular effluent.

LABORATORY FINDINGS
The hallmark of this disorder is the marked elevation of the Δ5 steroids (such as 17-hydroxypregnenolone and DHEA) preceding the enzymatic block. Patients may also have elevated levels of 17-hydroxyprogesterone because of the extraadrenal 3β-HSD activity that occurs in peripheral tissues; these patients may be mistaken for patients with 21-hydroxylase deficiency. The ratio of 17-hydroxypregnenolone:17-hydroxyprogesterone is markedly elevated in 3β-HSD deficiency, in contrast to the decreased ratio in 21-hydroxylase deficiency. Plasma renin activity is elevated in the salt-wasting form.

DIFFERENTIAL DIAGNOSIS
It is not unusual for children with premature adrenarche, or women with signs of androgen excess, to have mild to moderate elevations in DHEA levels. It has been suggested that such individuals have "nonclassic 3β-HSD deficiency." Mutations in the *HSD3B2* gene are usually not found in such individuals, and a nonclassic form of this deficiency must actually be quite rare. The activity of 3β-HSD in the adrenal zonae

fasciculata and reticularis, relative to CYP17 (17-hydroxylase/17,20-lyase) activity, normally decreases during adrenarche to facilitate DHEA synthesis, and so modest elevations in DHEA in preteenage children or women usually represent a normal variant.

TREATMENT

Patients require glucocorticoid and mineralocorticoid replacement with hydrocortisone and fludrocortisone, respectively, as in 21-hydroxylase deficiency. Incompletely virilized genetic males in whom a male sex of rearing is contemplated may benefit from several injections of 25 mg every 4 wk of a depot form of testosterone early in infancy to increase the size of the phallus. They may also require testosterone replacement at puberty.

Bibliography is available at Expert Consult.

576.4 Congenital Adrenal Hyperplasia Caused by 17-Hydroxylase Deficiency
Perrin C. White

ETIOLOGY

Less than 1% of CAH cases are caused by 17-hydroxylase deficiency, but the condition is apparently more common in Brazil and China. A single polypeptide, CYP17, catalyzes 2 distinct reactions: 17-hydroxylation of pregnenolone and progesterone to 17-hydroxypregnenolone and 17-hydroxyprogesterone, respectively, and the 17,20-lyase reaction mediating conversion of 17-hydroxypregnenolone to DHEA and, to a lesser extent, 17-hydroxyprogesterone to Δ4-androstenedione. DHEA and androstenedione are steroid precursors of testosterone and estrogen (see Fig. 574-1 in Chapter 574). The enzyme is expressed in both the adrenal cortex and the gonads and is encoded by a gene on chromosome 10q24.3. Most mutations affect both the hydroxylase and lyase activities, but rare mutations can affect either activity alone.

Mutations in genes other than *CYP17* can have the same phenotype as 17,20-lyase deficiency (i.e., deficient androgen synthesis with normal cortisol synthesis). These include an accessory electron transfer protein, cytochrome b_5, and mutations in 2 aldo-keto reductases, AKR1C2 and AKR1C4. These AKR1C isozymes normally catalyze 3α-hydroxysteroid dehydrogenase activity, which allows synthesis of the potent androgen dihydrotestosterone through an alternative "backdoor" biosynthetic pathway that does not include testosterone as an intermediate.

CLINICAL MANIFESTATIONS AND LABORATORY FINDINGS

Patients with 17-hydroxylase deficiency cannot synthesize cortisol, but their ability to synthesize corticosterone is intact. Because corticosterone is an active glucocorticoid, patients do not develop adrenal insufficiency. Deoxycorticosterone, the immediate precursor of corticosterone, is synthesized in excess. This can cause **hypertension, hypokalemia,** and suppression of renin and aldosterone secretion, as occurs in 11β-hydroxylase deficiency. In contrast to 11β-hydroxylase deficiency, patients with 17-hydroxylase deficiency are unable to synthesize sex hormones. Affected **males are incompletely virilized** and present as phenotypic females (but gonads are usually palpable in the inguinal region or the labia) or with sexual ambiguity. Affected females usually present with **failure of sexual development** at the expected time of **puberty.** 17-Hydroxylase deficiency in females must be considered in the differential diagnosis of primary hypogonadism (see Chapter 586). Levels of deoxycorticosterone are elevated and renin and aldosterone are consequently suppressed. Cortisol and sex steroids are unresponsive to stimulation with ACTH and human chorionic gonadotropin, respectively.

Patients with isolated 17,20-lyase deficiency have deficient androgen synthesis with normal cortisol synthesis, and therefore do not become hypertensive.

TREATMENT

Patients with 17-hydroxylase deficiency require cortisol replacement to suppress secretion of deoxycorticosterone and thus control hypertension. Additional antihypertensive medication may be required. Females require estrogen replacement at puberty. Genetic males may require either estrogen or androgen supplementation depending on the sex of rearing. Because of the possibility of malignant transformation of abdominal testes with androgen insensitivity syndrome (see Chapter 588.2), genetic males with severe 17-hydroxylase deficiency being reared as females require gonadectomy at or before adolescence.

Bibliography is available at Expert Consult.

576.5 Lipoid Adrenal Hyperplasia
Perrin C. White

ETIOLOGY

Lipoid adrenal hyperplasia is a rare disorder, most frequently found in Japanese persons. Patients with this disorder exhibit marked accumulation of cholesterol and lipids in the adrenal cortex and gonads, associated with severe impairment of all steroidogenesis. Lipoid adrenal hyperplasia is usually caused by mutations in the gene for steroidogenic acute regulatory protein (StAR), a mitochondrial protein that promotes the movement of cholesterol from the outer to the inner mitochondrial membrane. However, mutations in the *CYP11A1* gene (which encodes the cholesterol side chain cleavage enzyme) have been reported in several patients.

Some cholesterol is able to enter mitochondria even in the absence of StAR, so it might be supposed that this disorder would not completely impair steroid biosynthesis. However, the accumulation of cholesterol in the cytoplasm is cytotoxic, eventually leading to death of all steroidogenic cells in which StAR is normally expressed. This occurs prenatally in the adrenals and testes. The ovaries do not normally synthesize steroids until puberty, so cholesterol does not accumulate and the ovaries can retain the capacity to synthesize estrogens until adolescence.

Although estrogens synthesized by the placenta are required to maintain pregnancy, the placenta does not require StAR for steroid biosynthesis. Thus, mutations of StAR are not prenatally lethal.

CLINICAL MANIFESTATIONS

Patients with lipoid adrenal hyperplasia are usually unable to synthesize any adrenal steroids. Thus, affected infants are likely to be confused with those with adrenal hypoplasia congenita. Salt-losing manifestations are typical, and many infants die in early infancy. Genetic males are unable to synthesize androgens and thus are **phenotypically female** but with gonads palpable in the labia majora or inguinal areas. Genetic females appear normal at birth and may undergo feminization at puberty with menstrual bleeding. They too, progress to hypergonadotropic hypogonadism when accumulated cholesterol kills granulosa (i.e., steroid synthesizing) cells in the ovary.

LABORATORY FINDINGS

Adrenal and gonadal steroid hormone levels are low in lipoid adrenal hyperplasia, with a decreased or absent response to stimulation (ACTH, human chorionic gonadotropin). Plasma renin levels are increased.

Imaging studies of the adrenal gland demonstrating massive adrenal enlargement in the newborn help establish the diagnosis of lipoid adrenal hyperplasia.

TREATMENT

Patients require glucocorticoid and mineralocorticoid replacement. Genetic males are usually assigned a female sex of rearing; thus both genetic males and females require estrogen replacement at the expected age of puberty.

Bibliography is available at Expert Consult.

576.6 Deficiency of P450 Oxidoreductase (Antley-Bixler Syndrome)

Perrin C. White

ETIOLOGY, PATHOGENESIS, AND CLINICAL MANIFESTATIONS

P450 oxidoreductase (POR, gene located on chromosome 7q11.3) is required for the activity of all microsomal cytochrome P450 enzymes (see Chapter 574) including the adrenal enzymes CYP17 and CYP21. Thus, complete POR deficiency abolishes all microsomal P450 activity. This is embryonically lethal in mice and presumably in humans as well. Patients with mutations that decrease but do not abolish POR activity have partial deficiencies of 17-hydroxylase and 21-hydroxylase activities in the adrenals. A single recurrent mutation, A287P (alanine-287 to proline) is found on approximately 40% of alleles.

Deficiency of 17-hydroxylase leads to incomplete masculinization in males; 21-hydroxylase deficiency may lead to virilization in females. Additionally, aromatase *(CYP19)* activity in the placenta is decreased, leading to unopposed action of androgens produced by the fetal adrenal. This exacerbates virilization of female fetuses and may **virilize the mother** of an affected fetus as well. Although it is puzzling that affected females could be virilized despite a partial deficiency in *CYP17* (which is required for androgen biosynthesis), an alternative ("backdoor") biosynthetic pathway is utilized in which 17-hydroxyprogesterone is converted to 5α-pregnane-3α,17α-diol-20-one, a metabolite that is a much better substrate for the 17,20-lyase activity of *CYP17* than the usual substrate, 17-hydroxypregnenolone (see Chapter 574). The metabolite is then converted in several enzymatic steps to dihydrotestosterone, a potent androgen.

Because many other P450 enzymes are affected, patients often (but not invariably) have other congenital anomalies collectively referred to as **Antley-Bixler syndrome.** These include craniosynostosis; brachycephaly; frontal bossing; severe midface hypoplasia with proptosis and choanal stenosis or atresia; humeroradial synostosis; medial bowing of ulnas; long, slender fingers with camptodactyly; narrow iliac wings; anterior bowing of femurs; and malformations of the heart and kidneys. Studies of mutant mice suggest that the metabolic defects responsible for these anomalies include defective metabolism of retinoic acid, leading to elevated levels of this teratogenic compound, and deficient biosynthesis of cholesterol.

EPIDEMIOLOGY

The prevalence is not known with certainty. It must be rare compared with 21-hydroxylase deficiency but might occur at similar frequencies to the other forms of CAH.

LABORATORY FINDINGS

Serum steroids that are not 17- or 21-hydroxylated are most increased, including pregnenolone and progesterone. 17-Hydroxy, 21-deoxysteroids are also increased, including 17-hydroxypregnenolone, 17-hydroxyprogesterone, and 21-deoxycortisol. Urinary steroid metabolites may be determined by quantitative mass spectrometry. Metabolites excreted at increased levels include pregnanediol, pregnanetriol, pregnanetriolone, and corticosterone metabolites. Urinary cortisol metabolites are decreased. Genetic analysis demonstrates mutations in the *POR* gene.

DIFFERENTIAL DIAGNOSIS

This disorder must be distinguished from other forms of CAH, particularly 21-hydroxylase deficiency in females, which is far more common and has similar laboratory findings. Suspicion for *POR* deficiency may be raised if the mother is virilized or if the associated abnormalities of Antley-Bixler syndrome are present. Conversely, virilization of both the mother and her daughter can result from a luteoma of pregnancy, but in this case postnatal abnormalities of corticosteroid biosynthesis should not be observed. Antley-Bixler syndrome may also occur without abnormalities of steroid hormone biosynthesis, resulting from mutations in the fibroblast growth factor receptor FGFR2.

Bibliography is available at Expert Consult.

576.7 Aldosterone Synthase Deficiency

Perrin C. White

ETIOLOGY

This is a rare autosomal recessive disorder in which conversion of corticosterone to aldosterone is impaired; a group of Iranian Jewish patients has been the most thoroughly studied. The majority of cases result from mutations in the *CYP11B2* gene coding for aldosterone synthase; however, linkage to *CYP11B2* has been excluded in other kindreds. When not caused by *CYP11B2* mutations, the disorder has been termed *familial hyperreninemic hypoaldosteronism type 2;* the causative gene or genes have not yet been identified.

Aldosterone synthase mediates the 3 final steps in the synthesis of aldosterone from deoxycorticosterone (11β-hydroxylation, 18-hydroxylation, and 18-oxidation). Although 11β-hydroxylation is required to convert deoxycorticosterone to corticosterone, this conversion can also be catalyzed by the related enzyme, CYP11B1, located in the fasciculata, which is unaffected in this disorder. For the same reason, these patients have normal cortisol biosynthesis.

The disease has been classified into 2 types, termed *corticosterone methyloxidase deficiency types I and II.* They differ only in levels of the immediate precursor of aldosterone, 18-hydroxycorticosterone; levels are low in type I deficiency and elevated in type II deficiency. These differences do not correspond in a simple way to particular mutations and are of limited clinical importance.

CLINICAL MANIFESTATIONS

Infants with aldosterone synthase deficiency may have severe electrolyte abnormalities with **hyponatremia, hyperkalemia,** and **metabolic acidosis.** Because cortisol synthesis is unaffected, infants rarely become as ill as untreated infants with salt-losing forms of CAH such as 21-hydroxylase deficiency. Thus, some infants escape diagnosis. Later in infancy or in early childhood they may exhibit failure to thrive and poor growth. Adults often are asymptomatic, although they may develop electrolyte abnormalities when depleted of sodium through procedures such as bowel preparation for a barium enema.

LABORATORY FINDINGS

Infants have elevated plasma renin activity. Aldosterone levels are decreased; they may be at the lower end of the normal range but are always inappropriately low for the degree of hyperkalemia or hyperreninemia. Corticosterone levels are often elevated.

Some, but not all, patients have marked elevation of 18-hydroxycorticosterone; however, low levels of this steroid do not exclude the diagnosis. In those kindreds in which 18-hydroxycorticosterone levels are elevated in affected individuals, this biochemical abnormality persists in adults even when they have no electrolyte abnormalities.

DIFFERENTIAL DIAGNOSIS

It is important to distinguish aldosterone synthase deficiency from primary adrenal insufficiency in which both cortisol and aldosterone are affected (including salt-wasting forms of CAH) because the latter condition is usually associated with a much greater risk of shock and hyponatremia. This becomes apparent after the appropriate laboratory studies. Adrenal hypoplasia congenita may initially present with aldosterone deficiency; all male infants with apparently isolated aldosterone deficiency should be carefully monitored for subsequent development of cortisol deficiency. **Pseudohypoaldosteronism** (see Chapter 575.4) may have similar electrolyte abnormalities and hyperreninemia, but aldosterone levels are high, and this condition usually does not respond to fludrocortisone treatment.

TREATMENT

Treatment consists of giving enough fludrocortisone (0.05-0.3 mg daily) or sodium chloride, or both, to return plasma renin levels to normal. With increasing age, salt-losing signs usually improve and drug therapy can often be discontinued.

Bibliography is available at Expert Consult.

576.8 Glucocorticoid-Suppressible Hyperaldosteronism
Perrin C. White

ETIOLOGY

Glucocorticoid-suppressible hyperaldosteronism (glucocorticoid-remediable aldosteronism, familial hyperaldosteronism type I) is an autosomal dominant form of **low-renin hypertension** in which hyperaldosteronism is rapidly suppressed by glucocorticoid administration. This unusual effect of glucocorticoids suggests that aldosterone secretion in this disorder is regulated by ACTH instead of by the renin–angiotensin system. In addition to abnormally regulated secretion of aldosterone, there is marked overproduction of 18-hydroxycortisol and 18-oxocortisol. The synthesis of these steroids requires both 17-hydroxylase (CYP17) activity, which is expressed only in the zona fasciculata, and aldosterone synthase (CYP11B2) activity, which is normally expressed only in the zona glomerulosa. Together, these features imply that aldosterone synthase is being expressed in a manner similar to the closely related enzyme steroid 11-hydroxylase *(CYP11B1)*. The disorder is caused by unequal meiotic crossing-over events between the *CYP11B1* and *CYP11B2* genes, which are closely linked on chromosome 8q24. An additional "hybrid" gene is produced, having regulatory sequences of *CYP11B1* juxtaposed with coding sequences of *CYP11B2*. This results in the inappropriate expression of a *CYP11B2*-like enzyme with aldosterone synthase activity in the adrenal fasciculata.

CLINICAL MANIFESTATIONS

Some affected children have no symptoms, the diagnosis being established after incidental discovery of moderate hypertension, typically approximately 30 mm Hg higher than unaffected family members of the same age. Others have more symptomatic hypertension with headache, dizziness, and visual disturbances. A strong family history of early-onset hypertension or early strokes may alert the clinician to the diagnosis. Some patients have chronic hypokalemia, but this is not a consistent finding and is usually mild.

LABORATORY FINDINGS

Patients have elevated plasma and urine levels of aldosterone and suppressed plasma renin activity. Hypokalemia is not consistently present. Urinary and plasma levels of 18-oxocortisol and 18-hydroxycortisol are markedly increased. The hybrid *CYP11B1/CYP11B2* gene can be readily detected by molecular genetic methods.

DIFFERENTIAL DIAGNOSIS

This condition should be distinguished from primary aldosteronism based on bilateral hyperplasia or an aldosterone-producing adenoma (see Chapter 578). Most cases of primary aldosteronism are sporadic, although several affected kindreds have been reported. Patients with primary aldosteronism may also have elevated levels of 18-hydroxycortisol and 18-oxocortisol, and these biochemical tests should be used cautiously to distinguish primary and glucocorticoid-suppressible aldosteronism. A therapeutic trial of dexamethasone may be helpful if aldosterone secretion is suppressed, and genetic testing should identify the hybrid gene of glucocorticoid-suppressible hyperaldosteronism if it is present.

TREATMENT

Glucocorticoid-suppressible hyperaldosteronism is managed by daily administration of a glucocorticoid, usually dexamethasone, 25 μg/kg/day in divided doses. If necessary, effects of aldosterone can be blocked with a potassium-sparing diuretic such as spironolactone, eplerenone, or amiloride. Hypertension resolves in patients in whom the hypertension is not severe or of long standing. If hypertension is long standing, additional antihypertensive medication may be required, such as a calcium channel blocker.

GENETIC COUNSELING

Because of the autosomal dominant mode of inheritance, at-risk family members should be investigated for this easily treated cause of hypertension.

Bibliography is available at Expert Consult.

Chapter 577
Cushing Syndrome
Perrin C. White

Cushing syndrome is the result of abnormally high blood levels of cortisol or other glucocorticoids. This can be iatrogenic or the result of endogenous cortisol secretion, a result of either an adrenal tumor or of hypersecretion of corticotropin (adrenocorticotropic hormone [ACTH]) by the pituitary (Cushing disease) or by a tumor (Table 577-1).

ETIOLOGY

The most common cause of Cushing syndrome is prolonged exogenous administration of glucocorticoid hormones, especially at the high doses used to treat lymphoproliferative disorders. This rarely represents a diagnostic challenge, but management of hyperglycemia, hypertension, weight gain, linear growth retardation, and osteoporosis often complicates therapy with corticosteroids.

Endogenous Cushing syndrome is most often caused in infants by a functioning adrenocortical tumor (see Chapter 579). Patients with these tumors often exhibit signs of hypercortisolism along with signs of hypersecretion of other steroids such as androgens, estrogens, and aldosterone.

Although extremely rare in infants, the most common etiology of endogenous Cushing syndrome in children older than 7 yr of age is **Cushing disease,** in which excessive ACTH secreted by a pituitary adenoma causes bilateral adrenal hyperplasia. Such adenomas are often too small to detect by imaging techniques and are termed microadenomas. They consist principally of chromophobe cells and frequently show positive immunostaining for ACTH and its precursor, proopiomelanocortin. Whereas the vast majority of such tumors are sporadic, a small number occur in kindreds with familial isolated pituitary adenoma syndrome. This syndrome, which is caused by mutations in the aryl hydrocarbon receptor interacting protein *(AIP)* gene, accounts for perhaps 2% of pituitary adenomas, but more commonly tumors with *AIP* mutations secrete growth hormone or prolactin, and only rarely do they secrete ACTH. Similarly, multiple endocrine neoplasia type 1 (MEN1) patients, who by definition have mutations in the MEN1 (menin) gene, may develop pituitary tumors, but these are typically prolactinomas.

ACTH-dependent Cushing syndrome may also result from ectopic production of ACTH, although this is uncommon in children. Ectopic

Table 577-1	Etiologic Classification of Adrenocortical Hyperfunction

EXCESS ANDROGEN
Congenital adrenal hyperplasia
21-Hydroxylase (P450c21) deficiency
11β-Hydroxylase (P450c11) deficiency
3β-Hydroxysteroid dehydrogenase defect (deficiency or dysregulation)
Tumor

EXCESS CORTISOL (CUSHING SYNDROME)
Bilateral adrenal hyperplasia
Adenoma
Hypersecretion of corticotropin (Cushing disease)
Ectopic secretion of corticotropin
Exogenous corticotropin
Adrenocortical nodular dysplasia
Pigmented nodular adrenocortical disease (Carney complex)
Tumor
McCune-Albright syndrome

EXCESS MINERALOCORTICOID
Primary hyperaldosteronism
Aldosterone-secreting adenoma
Bilateral micronodular adrenocortical hyperplasia
Glucocorticoid-suppressible aldosteronism
Tumor
Deoxycorticosterone excess
Congenital adrenal hyperplasia
11β-Hydroxylase (P450c11)
17α-Hydroxylase (P450c17)
Tumor
Apparent mineralocorticoid excess (deficiency of 11β-hydroxysteroid dehydrogenase type 2)

EXCESS ESTROGEN
Tumor

ACTH secretion in children is associated with islet cell carcinoma of the pancreas, neuroblastoma or ganglioneuroblastoma, hemangiopericytoma, Wilms tumor, and thymic carcinoid. Hypertension is more common in the ectopic ACTH syndrome than in other forms of Cushing syndrome, because very high cortisol levels may overwhelm 11β-hydroxysteroid dehydrogenase in the kidney (see Chapter 575) and thus have an enhanced mineralocorticoid (salt-retaining) effect.

Several syndromes are associated with the development of multiple autonomously hyperfunctioning nodules of adrenocortical tissue, rather than single adenomas or carcinomas (which are discussed in Chapter 579). **Primary pigmented nodular adrenocortical disease** (PPNAD) is a distinctive form of ACTH-independent Cushing syndrome. It may occur as an isolated event or, more commonly, as a familial disorder with other manifestations. The adrenal glands are small and have characteristic multiple, small (<4 mm in diameter), pigmented (black) nodules containing large cells with cytoplasm and lipofuscin; there is cortical atrophy between the nodules. This adrenal disorder occurs as a component of **Carney complex,** an autosomal dominant disorder also consisting of centrofacial lentigines and blue nevi; cardiac and cutaneous myxomas; pituitary, thyroid, and testicular tumors; and pigmented melanotic schwannomas. Carney complex is inherited in an autosomal dominant manner, although sporadic cases occur. Genetic loci for Carney complex have been mapped to the gene for the type 1α regulatory subunit of protein kinase A (PRKAR1A) on chromosome 17q22-24 and less frequently to chromosome 2p16. Patients with Carney complex and PRKAR1A mutations generally develop PPNAD as adults, and those with the disorder mapping to chromosome 2 (and most sporadic cases) develop PPNAD less frequently and later. Conversely, children presenting with PPNAD as an isolated finding rarely have mutations in PRKAR1A, or subsequently

develop other manifestations of Carney complex. Some patients with isolated PPNAD have mutations in the *PDE8B* or *PDE11A* genes encoding different phosphodiesterase isozymes.

ACTH-independent Cushing syndrome with nodular hyperplasia and adenoma formation occurs rarely in cases of **McCune-Albright syndrome,** with symptoms beginning in infancy or childhood. McCune-Albright syndrome is caused by a somatic mutation of the *GNAS* gene encoding the G protein, $G_s\alpha$, through which the ACTH receptor (MCR2) normally signals. This results in inhibition of guanosine triphosphatase activity and constitutive activation of adenylate cyclase, thus increasing levels of cyclic adenosine monophosphate. When the mutation is present in adrenal tissue, cortisol and cell division are stimulated independently of ACTH. Other tissues in which activating mutations may occur are bone (producing fibrous dysplasia), gonads, thyroid, and pituitary. Clinical manifestations depend on which tissues are affected.

Thus the genes causing nodular adrenocortical hyperplasia that have been identified thus far all produce overactivity of the ACTH signaling pathway either by constitutively activating $G_s\alpha$ (McCune-Albright syndrome), by reducing the breakdown of cyclic adenosine monophosphate and thus increasing its intracellular levels (mutations of *PDE8B* or *PDE11A*), or by disrupting the regulation of the cyclic adenosine monophosphate–dependent enzyme, protein kinase A (PRKAR1A mutations).

Additionally, adrenocortical lesions including diffuse hyperplasia, nodular hyperplasia, adenoma, and rarely carcinoma may occur as part of the MEN1 syndrome (see Chapter 573), an autosomal dominant disorder, in which there is homozygous inactivation of the menin (**MEN1**) tumor-suppressor gene on chromosome 11q13.

CLINICAL MANIFESTATIONS

Signs of Cushing syndrome have been recognized in infants younger than 1 yr of age. The disorder appears to be more severe and the clinical findings more flagrant in infants than in older children. The face is rounded, with prominent cheeks and a flushed appearance (moon facies). Generalized obesity is common in younger children. In children with adrenal tumors, signs of abnormal masculinization occur frequently; accordingly, there may be hirsutism on the face and trunk, pubic hair, acne, deepening of the voice, and enlargement of the clitoris in girls. Growth is impaired, with length falling below the 3rd percentile, except when significant virilization produces normal or even accelerated growth. Hypertension is common and may occasionally lead to heart failure. An increased susceptibility to infection may also lead to sepsis.

In older children, in addition to obesity, short stature is a common presenting feature. Gradual onset of obesity and deceleration or cessation of growth may be the only early manifestations. Older children most often have more severe obesity of the face and trunk compared with the extremities. Purplish striae on the hips, abdomen, and thighs are common. Pubertal development may be delayed, or amenorrhea may occur in girls past menarche. Weakness, headache, and emotional lability may be prominent. Hypertension and hyperglycemia usually occur; hyperglycemia may progress to frank diabetes. Osteoporosis is common and may cause pathologic fractures.

LABORATORY FINDINGS

Cortisol levels in blood are normally highest at 8 AM and decrease to less than 50% by midnight except in infants and young children in whom a diurnal rhythm is not always established. In patients with Cushing syndrome this circadian rhythm is lost; midnight cortisol levels >4.4 μg/dL strongly suggest the diagnosis. It is difficult to obtain diurnal blood samples as part of an outpatient evaluation, but cortisol can be measured in saliva samples, which can be obtained at home at the appropriate times of day. Elevated nighttime salivary cortisol levels raise suspicion for Cushing syndrome.

Urinary excretion of free cortisol is increased. This is best measured in a 24 hr urine sample and is expressed as a ratio of micrograms of cortisol excreted per gram of creatinine. This ratio is independent of body size and completeness of the urine collection.

A single-dose dexamethasone suppression test is often helpful; a dose of 25-30 μg/kg (maximum: 2 mg) given at 11 PM results in a plasma cortisol level of less than 5 μg/dL at 8 AM the next morning in normal individuals but not in patients with Cushing syndrome. It is prudent to measure the dexamethasone level in the same blood sample to ensure adequacy of dosing.

A glucose tolerance test is often abnormal but is of no diagnostic utility. Levels of serum electrolytes are usually normal, but potassium may be decreased, especially in patients with tumors that secrete ACTH ectopically.

After the diagnosis of Cushing syndrome has been established, it is necessary to determine whether it is caused by a pituitary adenoma, an ectopic ACTH-secreting tumor, or a cortisol-secreting adrenal tumor. ACTH concentrations are usually suppressed in patients with cortisol-secreting tumors and are very high in patients with ectopic ACTH-secreting tumors but may be normal in patients with ACTH-secreting pituitary adenomas. After an intravenous bolus of corticotropin-releasing hormone, patients with ACTH-dependent Cushing syndrome have an exaggerated ACTH and cortisol response, whereas those with adrenal tumors show no increase in ACTH and cortisol. The 2-step dexamethasone suppression test consists of administration of dexamethasone, 30 and 120 μg/kg/24 hr in 4 divided doses, on consecutive days. In children with pituitary/Cushing syndrome, the larger dose, but not the smaller dose, suppresses serum levels of cortisol. Typically, patients with ACTH-independent Cushing syndrome do not show suppressed cortisol levels with dexamethasone.

CT detects virtually all adrenal tumors larger than 1.5 cm in diameter. MRI may detect ACTH-secreting pituitary adenomas, but many are too small to be seen; the addition of gadolinium contrast increases the sensitivity of detection. Bilateral inferior petrosal blood sampling to measure concentrations of ACTH before and after corticotropin-releasing hormone administration may be required to localize the tumor when a pituitary adenoma is not visualized; this is not routinely available in many centers, and moreover may be of decreased specificity in children.

DIFFERENTIAL DIAGNOSIS

Cushing syndrome is frequently suspected in children with obesity, particularly when striae and hypertension are present. Children with simple obesity are usually tall, whereas those with Cushing syndrome are short or have a decelerating growth rate. Although urinary excretion of cortisol is often elevated in simple obesity, salivary nighttime levels of cortisol are usually normal and cortisol secretion is suppressed by oral administration of low doses of dexamethasone.

Elevated levels of cortisol and ACTH without clinical evidence of Cushing syndrome occur in patients with generalized glucocorticoid resistance (see Chapter 575.4). Affected patients may be asymptomatic or exhibit hypertension, hypokalemia, and precocious pseudopuberty; these manifestations are caused by increased mineralocorticoid and adrenal androgen secretion in response to elevated ACTH levels. Mutations in the glucocorticoid receptor have been identified.

TREATMENT

Transsphenoidal pituitary microsurgery is the treatment of choice in pituitary Cushing disease in children. The overall success rate with follow-up of less than 10 yr is 60-80%. Low postoperative serum or urinary cortisol concentrations predict long-term remission in the majority of cases. Relapses are treated with reoperation or pituitary irradiation.

Cyproheptadine, a centrally acting serotonin antagonist that blocks ACTH release, has been used to treat Cushing disease in adults; remissions are usually not sustained after discontinuation of therapy. This agent is rarely used in children. Inhibitors of adrenal steroidogenesis (metyrapone, ketoconazole, aminoglutethimide, etomidate) have been used preoperatively to normalize circulating cortisol levels and reduce perioperative morbidity and mortality. Mifepristone, a glucocorticoid receptor antagonist, has been used in a limited number of cases.

Pasireotide, a somatostatin analog, can inhibit ACTH secretion, and is approved for use in adults with persistent disease after surgery or in whom surgery is contraindicated.

If a pituitary adenoma does not respond to treatment or if ACTH is secreted by an ectopic metastatic tumor, the adrenal glands may need to be removed. This can often be accomplished laparoscopically. Adrenalectomy may lead to increased ACTH secretion by an unresected pituitary adenoma, evidenced mainly by marked hyperpigmentation; this condition is termed **Nelson syndrome.**

Management of patients undergoing adrenalectomy requires adequate preoperative and postoperative replacement therapy with a corticosteroid. Tumors that produce corticosteroids usually lead to atrophy of the normal adrenal tissue, and replacement with cortisol (10 mg/m^2/24 hr in 3 divided doses after the immediate postoperative period) is required until there is recovery of the hypothalamic-pituitary-adrenal axis. Postoperative complications may include sepsis, pancreatitis, thrombosis, poor wound healing, and sudden collapse, particularly in infants with Cushing syndrome. Substantial catch-up growth, pubertal progress, and increased bone density occur, but bone density remains abnormal and adult height is often compromised. The management of adrenocortical tumors is discussed in Chapter 579.

Bibliography is available at Expert Consult.

Chapter **578**
Primary Aldosteronism
Perrin C. White

Primary aldosteronism encompasses disorders caused by excessive aldosterone secretion independent of the renin–angiotensin system. These disorders are characterized by **hypertension, hypokalemia,** and suppression of the renin–angiotensin system.

ETIOLOGY

Aldosterone-secreting adenomas are unilateral and have been reported in children as young as 3.5 yr of age; they mainly affect girls. Adrenocortical tumors are discussed further in Chapter 579. Bilateral micronodular adrenocortical hyperplasia tends to occur in older children and is more frequent in males. Primary aldosteronism due to unilateral adrenal hyperplasia may also occur. Glucocorticoid-suppressible hyperaldosteronism is discussed in Chapter 576.8.

EPIDEMIOLOGY

These conditions are thought to be rare in children, but they may account for 5-10% of cases of hypertension in adults. Although usually sporadic, kindreds with several affected members have been reported. Genetic linkage to chromosome 7p22 has been identified in some of these kindreds, but the involved gene has not yet been identified. Mutations in the *KCNJ5* gene on chromosome 11q24 have been identified in several kindreds; these mutations (G151R and G151E) altered channel selectivity, producing increased Na$^+$ conductance and membrane depolarization, which increases aldosterone production and proliferation of adrenal glomerulosa cells. Moreover, such mutations have been identified in a subset of sporadic aldosterone-producing adenomas.

CLINICAL MANIFESTATIONS

Some affected children have no symptoms, the diagnosis being established after incidental discovery of moderate hypertension. Others have severe hypertension (up to 240/150 mm Hg), with headache, dizziness, and visual disturbances. Chronic hypokalemia, if present, may lead to polyuria, nocturia, enuresis, and polydipsia. Muscle weakness and discomfort, tetany, intermittent paralysis, fatigue, and growth failure affect children with severe hypokalemia.

LABORATORY FINDINGS

Hypokalemia occurs frequently. Serum pH and the carbon dioxide and sodium concentrations may be elevated and the serum chloride and magnesium levels decreased. Serum levels of calcium are normal, even in children who manifest tetany. The urine is neutral or alkaline, and urinary potassium excretion is high. Plasma levels of aldosterone may be normal or elevated. Aldosterone concentrations in 24 hr urine collections are always increased. Plasma levels of renin are persistently low.

The diagnostic test of choice for primary aldosteronism is controversial. Both renin and aldosterone levels may vary by time of day, posture, and sodium intake, making it difficult to establish consistent reference ranges. It is desirable to establish a consistent sampling protocol, for example, at midmorning after the patient has been sitting for 15 min. If possible, antihypertensive drugs or other medications that can affect aldosterone or renin secretion should be avoided for several weeks prior to testing, including diuretics, β-blockers, angiotensin-converting enzyme inhibitors, angiotensin receptor blockers, clonidine, and nonsteroidal antiinflammatory agents. Patients taking these agents may need to be changed to α-adrenergic blockers or calcium channel blockers that have smaller effects on the biochemical measurements. The ratio of plasma aldosterone concentration to renin activity is always high, and this represents a cost-effective screening test for primary aldosteronism. Aldosterone does not decrease with administration of saline solution or fludrocortisone, and renin does not respond to salt and fluid restriction. Urinary and plasma levels of 18-oxocortisol and 18-hydroxycortisol may be increased but not to the extent seen in glucocorticoid-suppressible hyperaldosteronism.

DIFFERENTIAL DIAGNOSIS

Primary aldosteronism should be distinguished from glucocorticoid-suppressible hyperaldosteronism (see Chapter 576.8), which is specifically treated with glucocorticoids. An autosomal dominant pattern of inheritance should raise suspicion for the latter disorder. Glucocorticoid-suppressible hyperaldosteronism is diagnosed by dexamethasone suppression tests or by specific genetic testing. More generally, primary aldosteronism should be distinguished from other forms of hypertension by means of the testing previously discussed.

TREATMENT

The treatment of an aldosterone-producing adenoma is surgical removal. This is performed primarily by laparotomy and adrenalectomy; successful enucleation of aldosterone-producing adenomas, as well as laparoscopic adrenalectomy, has been reported. *Hyperaldosteronism caused by bilateral adrenal hyperplasia is treated with the mineralocorticoid antagonists spironolactone (1-3 mg/kg/day to a maximum of 100 mg/day) or eplerenone (25-100 mg/day in 2 divided doses),* often normalizing blood pressure and serum potassium levels. There is greater experience with spironolactone, but this agent has antiandrogenic properties that may be unacceptable in pubertal males. Eplerenone is a more specific antimineralocorticoid that is safe in children, but there is little specific experience with primary aldosteronism in the pediatric age group. As an alternative, an epithelial sodium channel blocker, such as amiloride, may be used, with other antihypertensive agents added as necessary. In patients whose condition cannot be controlled medically, unilateral adrenalectomy may be considered.

Bibliography is available at Expert Consult.

Chapter 579
Adrenocortical Tumors
Perrin C. White

EPIDEMIOLOGY

Adrenocortical tumors are rare in childhood, with an incidence of 0.3-0.5 cases per 1 million child-years. They occur in all age groups but most commonly in children younger than 6 yr of age, and are more frequent (1.6-fold) in girls. In 2-10% of cases, the tumors are bilateral. Almost half of childhood adrenocortical tumors are carcinomas.

Symptoms of endocrine hyperfunction are present in 80-90% of children with adrenal tumors (see Table 577-1 in Chapter 577). Tumors that secrete cortisol and aldosterone are also discussed in Chapters 577 and 578, respectively. Tumors may be associated with hemihypertrophy, usually occurring during the 1st few yr of life. They are also associated with other congenital defects, particularly genitourinary tract and central nervous system abnormalities and hamartomatous defects.

ETIOLOGY

The incidence of adrenocortical tumors is increased in several familial cancer syndromes resulting from abnormalities in genes that encode transcription factors implicated in cell proliferation, differentiation, senescence, apoptosis, and genomic instability. These include tumor protein 53 (*TP53*), menin (the *MEN1* gene involved in multiple endocrine neoplasia type 1), the *APC* gene involved in familial adenomatous polyposis coli, and the *PRKAR1A* gene encoding a cyclic adenosine monophosphate–dependent protein kinase regulatory subunit (also see Chapter 577).

Germline mutations in *TP53* (on chromosome 17p13.1) have been found in patients with isolated adrenal carcinoma as well as in patients with familial clustering of unusual malignancies; this latter condition is termed **Li-Fraumeni syndrome**. A 15-fold increased incidence of childhood adrenocortical tumors is found in southern Brazil, associated with a R337H mutation in *TP53*. Overexpression of insulin-like growth factor 2 (encoded by *IGF2*, on chromosome 11p15.5) occurs in 80% of sporadic childhood adrenocortical tumors, as well as in those associated with **Beckwith-Wiedemann syndrome,** in which there is loss of the normal imprinting of genes in this chromosomal region. Further implicating insulin-like growth factors (IGFs) in pathogenesis, many pediatric adrenocortical tumors overexpress the IGF receptor, IGF1R. Overexpression of steroidogenic factor-1 (SF1), a transcription factor required for adrenal development (see Chapter 574) is associated with decreased overall survival and recurrence-free survival when it occurs in adults with adrenocortical carcinomas, but it is seen in most pediatric adrenocortical tumors, where it does not seem to have prognostic significance. Conversely, the messenger RNA encoding the nephroblastoma overexpressed (NOV) protein (also termed cysteine-rich protein 61, or connective tissue growth factor, or nephroblastoma overexpressed gene-3) is significantly downregulated in childhood adrenocortical tumors. NOV is a selective pro-apoptotic factor for human adrenocortical cells, suggesting that abnormal apoptosis may play a role in childhood adrenocortical tumorigenesis.

Aldosterone-producing adenomas constitute a separate category from other adrenocortical tumors. They are very rarely malignant. The majority have mutations that activate the Wnt/β-catenin signaling pathway, either in β-catenin itself, or in the *APC* gene, which regulates this pathway. Additional, somatic mutations are often found in the potassium channel, KCNJ5, which probably first causes cell hypertrophy (see Chapter 576.8).

579.1 Virilizing and Feminizing Adrenal Tumors
Perrin C. White

CLINICAL MANIFESTATIONS
Virilization is the most common presenting symptom in children with adrenocortical tumors, occurring in 50-80%. In males, the clinical picture is similar to that of simple virilizing congenital adrenal hyperplasia: accelerated growth velocity and muscle development, acne, penile enlargement, and the precocious development of pubic and axillary hair. In females, virilizing tumors of the adrenal gland cause masculinization of a previously normal female with clitoral enlargement, growth acceleration, acne, deepening of the voice, and premature pubic and axillary hair development.

Conversely, adrenal tumors can occasionally (less than 10%) secrete high levels of estrogens as a result of overexpression of CYP19 (aromatase). Gynecomastia in males or premature thelarche in girls is often the initial manifestation. Growth and development may be otherwise normal, or concomitant virilization may occur.

In addition to virilization, 15-40% of children with adrenocortical tumors also have Cushing syndrome (see Chapter 577). Whereas isolated virilization occurs relatively frequently, children with adrenal tumors usually do not have Cushing syndrome alone.

In adults, adrenal tumors are frequently detected incident to CT or MRI imaging of the abdomen for other reasons; these are often referred to as **incidentalomas** (see Chapter 581.1). There are no published data on the frequency of the occurrence of such tumors in childhood. They are likely to be infrequent, being found in approximately 7% of autopsies of persons older than age 70 yr but in <1% of those younger than age 30 yr.

LABORATORY FINDINGS
Serum levels of dehydroepiandrosterone, dehydroepiandrosterone sulfate, and androstenedione are usually elevated, often markedly. Serum levels of testosterone are often increased, usually as a result of peripheral conversion of androstenedione, but infants with predominantly testosterone-secreting adenomas have been reported. Levels of estrone and estradiol are elevated in tumors from patients with feminizing signs. Urinary 17-ketosteroids (sex steroid metabolites) are also increased but are no longer routinely measured. Many adrenocortical tumors have a relative deficiency of 11β-hydroxylase activity and secrete increased amounts of deoxycorticosterone; these patients are hypertensive, and their tumors are often malignant.

Tumors can usually be detected by ultrasonography, CT, or MRI. Preoperatively, the presence of metastatic disease should be determined by MRI or CT of the chest, abdomen, and pelvis. Radiochemical imaging of these tumors by positron emission tomography with 11C-metomidate or single photon emission CT with ^{123}I-iodometomidate have been proposed but are not routinely available.

PATHOLOGIC FINDINGS
Differentiation between benign and malignant tumors by histologic criteria (architecture, cytologic atypia, mitotic activity, atypical mitotic figures) is usually not possible; almost all pediatric adrenocortical tumors would be classified as malignant by the criteria used to classify adult tumors. Size is a useful prognostic factor, with tumors weighing less than 200 g, 200-400 g, and >400 g being classified as low, intermediate, and high risk (>10 cm diameter has also been suggested as a high-risk category). Incomplete resection and gross local invasion or metastasis are also associated with a poor prognosis. However, most tumors occurring in children younger than 4 yr of age fall into favorable prognostic categories.

DIFFERENTIAL DIAGNOSIS
For functioning tumors, the differential diagnoses are those of the main presenting signs and symptoms. The differential diagnosis for Cushing syndrome is discussed in Chapter 577. For virilizing signs, the differential includes virilizing forms of adrenal hyperplasia (see Chapter 576) and factitious exposure to androgens, such as topical testosterone preparations. The differential diagnosis for hormonally inactive adrenocortical adenomas includes pheochromocytomas, adrenocortical carcinoma, and metastasis from an extraadrenal primary carcinoma (very rare in children). Careful history, physical examination, and endocrine evaluation must be performed to seek evidence of autonomous cortisol, androgen, mineralocorticoid, or catecholamine secretion. Not infrequently, a low level of autonomous cortisol secretion is detected that does not cause clinically apparent symptoms; this condition is sometimes referred to as "subclinical" Cushing syndrome.

TREATMENT
Functioning adrenocortical tumors should be removed surgically. There are no data on which to base a recommendation regarding nonfunctioning childhood incidentalomas; in adults, such tumors may be closely observed with imaging and repeat biochemical studies if smaller than 4 cm in diameter, but it is not certain that this is prudent in small children. Adrenalectomy may be performed either transperitoneally or laparoscopically. Some adrenocortical neoplasms are highly malignant and metastasize widely, but cure with regression of masculinizing or Cushingoid features may follow removal of less malignant, encapsulated tumors. Postoperatively, patients should be closely monitored biochemically, with frequent determinations of adrenal androgen levels and imaging studies. Recurrent symptoms or biochemical abnormalities should prompt a careful search for metastatic disease. Metastases primarily involve liver, lung, and regional lymph nodes. The majority of metastatic recurrences appear within 1 yr of tumor resection. Repeat surgical resection of metastatic lesions should be performed if possible and adjuvant therapy instituted. Radiation therapy has not been generally helpful. Antineoplastic agents such as cisplatin and etoposide, ifosfamide and carboplatin, and 5-fluorouracil and leucovorin have had limited use in children, and their success is not established. Therapy with o,p′-DDD (mitotane), an adrenolytic agent, may relieve the symptoms of hypercortisolism or virilization in recurrent disease. Treatment with higher doses of mitotane for more than 6 mo is associated with improved survival. Other agents that interfere with adrenal steroid synthesis, such as ketoconazole, aminoglutethimide, and metyrapone, may also relieve symptoms of steroid excess but do not improve survival.

A neoplasm of 1 adrenal gland may produce atrophy of the other because excessive production of cortisol by the tumor suppresses adrenocorticotropic hormone stimulation of the normal gland. Consequently, adrenal insufficiency may follow surgical removal of the tumor. This situation can be avoided by giving 10-25 mg of hydrocortisone every 6 hr, starting on the day of operation and weaned over 3-4 days postoperatively. Adequate quantities of water, sodium chloride, and glucose also must be provided.

Bibliography is available at Expert Consult.

Chapter 580
Pheochromocytoma
Perrin C. White

Pheochromocytomas are catecholamine-secreting tumors arising from chromaffin cells. The most common site of origin (approximately 90%) is the adrenal medulla; however, tumors may develop anywhere along the abdominal sympathetic chain and are likely to be located near the aorta at the level of the inferior mesenteric artery or at its bifurcation.

They also appear in the periadrenal area, urinary bladder or ureteral walls, thoracic cavity, and cervical region. Ten percent occur in children, in whom they present most frequently between 6 and 14 yr of age. Tumors vary from 1-10 cm in diameter; they are found more often on the right side than on the left. In more than 20% of affected children, the adrenal tumors are bilateral; in 30-40% of children, tumors are found in both adrenal and extraadrenal areas or only in an extraadrenal area.

ETIOLOGY
Pheochromocytomas may be associated with genetic syndromes such as **von Hippel-Lindau disease,** as a component of **multiple endocrine neoplasia** (MEN) syndromes MEN2A and MEN2B, and more rarely in association with **neurofibromatosis (type 1) or tuberous sclerosis.** The classic features of von Hippel-Landau syndrome, which occurs in 1 in 36,000 individuals, include retinal and central nervous system hemangioblastomas, renal clear cell carcinomas, and pheochromocytomas, but kindreds differ in their propensity to develop pheochromocytoma; in some kindreds, pheochromocytoma is the only tumor to develop. Germline mutations in the *VHL* tumor-suppressor gene on chromosome 3p25-26 have been identified in patients with this syndrome. Mutations of the *RET* protooncogene on chromosome 10q11.2 have been found in families with MEN2A and MEN2B. Patients with MEN2 are at risk of developing medullary thyroid carcinoma and parathyroid tumors; approximately 50% develop pheochromocytoma, with patients carrying mutations at codon 634 of the *RET* gene being at particularly high risk. Mutations are present in the *NF1* gene on chromosome 17q11.2 in neurofibromatosis type 1 patients.

Pheochromocytomas may occur in kindreds along with paragangliomas, particularly at sites in the head and neck. Such families typically carry mutations in the *SDHB, SDHD,* and, rarely, the *SDHC* genes encoding subunits of the mitochondrial enzyme succinate dehydrogenase.

Pheochromocytomas are also associated with tuberous sclerosis, Sturge-Weber syndrome, and ataxia-telangiectasia. Somatic mutations of the genes mentioned above, particularly *VHL,* have been found in some sporadic cases of pheochromocytoma (see Chapter 596).

CLINICAL MANIFESTATIONS
Pheochromocytomas detected by surveillance of patients who are known carriers of mutations in tumor-suppressor genes may be asymptomatic. Otherwise, patients are detected owing to hypertension, which results from excessive secretion of epinephrine and norepinephrine. All patients have hypertension at some time. Paroxysmal hypertension should particularly suggest pheochromocytoma as a diagnostic possibility, but in contrast to adults, the hypertension in children is more often sustained rather than paroxysmal. When there are paroxysms of hypertension, the attacks are usually infrequent at first, but become more frequent and eventually give way to a continuous hypertensive state. Between attacks of hypertension, the patient may be free of symptoms. During attacks, the patient complains of headache, palpitations, abdominal pain, and dizziness; pallor, vomiting, and sweating also occur. Convulsions and other manifestations of hypertensive encephalopathy may occur. In severe cases, precordial pains radiate into the arms; pulmonary edema and cardiac and hepatic enlargement may develop. Symptoms may be exacerbated by exercise, or with use of nonprescription medications containing stimulants such as pseudoephedrine. Patients have a good appetite but because of the hypermetabolic state may not gain weight, and severe cachexia may develop. Polyuria and polydipsia can be sufficiently severe to suggest diabetes insipidus. Growth failure may be striking. The blood pressure may range from 180-260 mm Hg systolic and from 120-210 mm Hg diastolic, and the heart may be enlarged. Ophthalmoscopic examination may reveal papilledema, hemorrhages, exudate, and arterial constriction.

LABORATORY FINDINGS
The urine may contain protein, a few casts, and occasionally glucose. Gross hematuria suggests that the tumor is in the bladder wall.

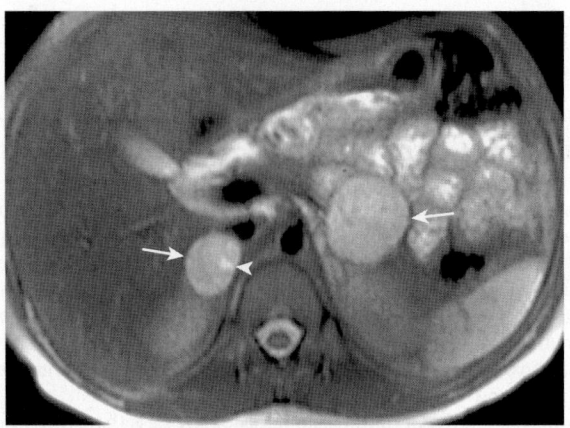

Figure 580-1 Bilateral pheochromocytoma in an 11 yr old boy with von Hippel-Lindau disease and arterial hypertension. An axial fat-suppressed T2-weighted magnetic resonance image shows bilateral adrenal masses *(arrows),* larger on the left. The masses are hyperintense with small cystic change on the right medially. *(From Navarro OM, Daneman A. Acquired conditions. In Coley BD (ed):* Caffey's pediatric diagnostic imaging, ed 12, Philadelphia, 2013, Elsevier, Fig. 123-9, p. 1283.)

Polycythemia is occasionally observed. The diagnosis is established by demonstration of elevated blood or urinary levels of catecholamines and their metabolites.

Pheochromocytomas produce norepinephrine and epinephrine. Normally, norepinephrine in plasma is derived from both the adrenal gland and adrenergic nerve endings, whereas epinephrine is derived primarily from the adrenal gland. In contrast to adults with pheochromocytoma in whom both norepinephrine and epinephrine are elevated, children with pheochromocytoma predominantly excrete norepinephrine in the urine. Total urinary catecholamine excretion usually exceeds 300 µg/24 hr. Urinary excretion of metanephrines (particularly normetanephrine) is also increased (see Fig. 574-3 in Chapter 574). Daily urinary excretion of these compounds by unaffected children increases with age. Although urinary excretion of vanillylmandelic acid (3-methoxy-4-hydroxymandelic acid), the major metabolite of epinephrine and norepinephrine, is increased, vanilla-containing foods and fruits can produce falsely elevated levels of this compound, which therefore is no longer routinely measured.

Elevated levels of free catecholamines and metanephrines can also be detected in plasma. In children, the best sensitivity and specificity are obtained by measuring plasma normetanephrine using gender-specific pediatric reference ranges, with plasma norepinephrine being next best. Plasma metanephrine and epinephrine are not reliably elevated in children. Additionally, the patient should be instructed to abstain from caffeinated drinks, and to avoid acetaminophen, which can interfere with plasma normetanephrine assays. If possible, the blood sample should be obtained from an indwelling intravenous catheter, to avoid acute stress associated with venipuncture.

Most tumors in the area of the adrenal gland are readily localized by CT or MRI (Fig. 580-1), but extraadrenal tumors may be difficult to detect. ^{123}I-metaiodobenzylguanidine is taken up by chromaffin tissue anywhere in the body and is useful for localizing small tumors. Venous catheterization with sampling of blood at different levels for catecholamine determinations is now only rarely necessary for localizing the tumor.

DIFFERENTIAL DIAGNOSIS
Various causes of hypertension in children must be considered, such as renal or renovascular disease; coarctation of the aorta; hyperthyroidism; Cushing syndrome; deficiencies of 11β-hydroxylase, 17α-hydroxylase, or 11β-hydroxysteroid dehydrogenase (type 2 isozyme); primary aldosteronism; adrenocortical tumors; and, rarely, essential hypertension (see Chapter 445). A nonfunctioning kidney may result

from compression of a ureter or of a renal artery by a pheochromocytoma. Paroxysmal hypertension may be associated with porphyria or familial dysautonomia. Cerebral disorders, diabetes insipidus, diabetes mellitus, and hyperthyroidism must also be considered in the differential diagnosis. Hypertension in patients with neurofibromatosis may be caused by renal vascular involvement or by concurrent pheochromocytoma.

Neuroblastoma, ganglioneuroblastoma, and ganglioneuroma frequently produce catecholamines, but urinary levels of most catecholamines are higher in patients with pheochromocytoma, although levels of dopamine and homovanillic acid are usually higher in neuroblastoma. Secreting neurogenic tumors often produce hypertension, excessive sweating, flushing, pallor, rash, polyuria, and polydipsia. Chronic diarrhea may be associated with these tumors, particularly with ganglioneuroma, and at times may be sufficiently persistent to suggest celiac disease.

TREATMENT
These tumors must be removed surgically, but careful preoperative, intraoperative, and postoperative management is essential. Preoperative α- **and** β-**adrenergic blockade** and **fluid loading** are required. Because these tumors are often multiple in children, a thorough transabdominal exploration of all the usual sites offers the best opportunity to find them all. Appropriate choice of anesthesia and expansion of blood volume with appropriate fluids during surgery are critical to avoid a precipitous drop in blood pressure during operation or within 48 hr postoperatively. Manipulation and excision of these tumors result in marked increases in catecholamine secretion that increase blood pressure and heart rate. Surveillance must continue postoperatively.

Although these tumors often appear malignant histologically, the only accurate indicators of malignancy are the presence of metastatic disease or local invasiveness that precludes complete resection, or both. Approximately 10% of all adrenal pheochromocytomas are malignant. Such tumors are rare in childhood; pediatric malignant pheochromocytomas occur more frequently in extraadrenal sites and are often associated with mutations in the *SDHB* gene encoding a subunit of succinate dehydrogenase. Prolonged follow-up is indicated because functioning tumors at other sites may be manifested many years after the initial operation. Examination of relatives of affected patients may reveal other individuals harboring unsuspected tumors that may be asymptomatic.

Bibliography is available at Expert Consult.

Chapter 581
Adrenal Masses

581.1 Adrenal Incidentaloma
Perrin C. White

Adrenal masses are discovered with increasing frequency in patients undergoing abdominal imaging for reasons unrelated to the adrenal gland. The rate of detection of single adrenal masses has ranged from less than 1% to more than 4% of abdominal CT examinations in adults. The unexpected discovery of such a mass presents the clinician with a dilemma in terms of diagnostic steps to undertake and treatment interventions to recommend. The differential diagnosis of adrenal incidentaloma includes benign lesions such as cysts, hemorrhagic cysts, hematomas, and myelolipomas. These lesions can usually be identified on CT or MRI. If the nature of the lesion is not readily apparent, additional evaluation is required. Included in the differential diagnosis of

lesions requiring additional evaluation are benign adenomas, pheochromocytomas, adrenocortical carcinoma, and metastasis from an extraadrenal primary carcinoma. Benign, hormonally inactive adrenocortical adenomas make up the majority of incidentalomas. Careful history, physical examination, and endocrine evaluation must be performed to seek evidence of autonomous cortisol, androgen, mineralocorticoid, or catecholamine secretion. Functional tumors require removal. If the adrenal mass is nonfunctional and larger than 4-6 cm, recommendations are to proceed with surgical resection of the mass. Lesions of 3 cm or less should be followed clinically with periodic reimaging. Treatment must be individualized; nonsecreting adrenal incidentalomas may enlarge and become hyperfunctioning. Nuclear scan, and occasionally fine-needle aspiration, may be helpful in defining the mass.

581.2 Adrenal Calcification
Perrin C. White

Calcification within the adrenal glands may occur in a wide variety of situations, some serious and others of no obvious consequence. Adrenal calcifications are often detected as incidental findings in radiographic studies of the abdomen in infants and children. The physician may elicit a history of anoxia or trauma at birth. Hemorrhage into the adrenal gland at or immediately after birth is probably the most common factor that leads to subsequent calcification (see Fig. 575-1 in Chapter 575). Although it is advisable to assess the adrenocortical reserve of such patients, there is rarely any functional disorder.

Neuroblastomas, ganglioneuromas, cortical carcinomas, pheochromocytomas, and cysts of the adrenal gland may be responsible for calcifications, particularly if hemorrhage has occurred within the tumor. Calcification in such lesions is almost always unilateral.

In the past, tuberculosis was a common cause both of calcification within the adrenals and of Addison disease. Calcifications may also develop in the adrenal glands of children who recover from the Waterhouse-Friderichsen syndrome; such patients are usually asymptomatic. Infants with Wolman disease, a rare lipid disorder caused by a deficiency of lysosomal acid lipase, have extensive bilateral calcifications of the adrenal glands (see Chapter 86.4).

Bibliography is available at Expert Consult.

Section 5
Disorders of the Gonads

Chapter 582
Development and Function of the Gonads
Patricia A. Donohoue

GENETIC CONTROL OF EMBRYONIC GONADAL DIFFERENTIATION
Gonadal differentiation is a complex, multistep process that requires the sequential action and interaction of multiple gene products.

Early in the 1st trimester, the undifferentiated, bipotential fetal gonad begins as a thickening of the urogenital ridge, near the developing kidney and adrenal cortex. At 6 wk of gestation, the gonad contains germ cells, stromal cells that will become Leydig cells in testes, or theca, interstitial, or hilar cells in the ovary; and supporting cells that will develop into Sertoli cells in testes or granulosa cells in ovaries. In males, *SRY* (**s**ex-determining **r**egion on the **Y** chromosome) is transiently expressed, followed by a sequential upregulation of a number of testis-specific genes. SRY may also suppress a putative factor 2 that functions as repressor of male development. In the absence of SRY, the bipotential gonad will be able to develop into an ovary. Ovarian development is also characterized by expression of ovary-specific genes during the same time period. One such gene is *R-spondin1*. During the gestation time period of 6-9 wk, a number of genes are upregulated to the same degree in both the testis and the ovary, including *WNT4* and *CTNNB1*.

A chromosome complement of 46,XX is necessary for the development of **normal ovaries.** Both the long and short arms of the X chromosome contain genes for normal ovarian development. The DSS (**d**osage **s**ensitive/**s**ex reversal) locus associated with the *DAX1* (**D**SS **a**drenal hypoplasia on the **X** chromosome) gene, which is defective in patients with X-linked congenital adrenal hypoplasia and hypogonadotropic hypogonadism, is a member of the nuclear receptor superfamily and acts as a repressor of male gene expression. *DAX1* acts by binding to a related nuclear receptor SF-1 (**s**teroidogenic **f**actor-1). In vitro, the signaling gene *WNT4* stimulates expression of *DAX1*, resulting in the suppression of androgen synthesis in XX females. The WNTs are ligands that activate receptor-mediated signal transduction pathways and are involved in modulating gene expression as well as cell behavior, adhesion, and polarity. A key to its role in humans was elucidated by loss-of-function mutation of the *WNT4* gene that was found in an 18 yr old 46,XX woman. She had absence of müllerian-derived structures (uterus and fallopian tubes), unilateral renal agenesis, and clinical signs of androgen excess.

Mutations of the Wilms tumor 1 *(WT1)* gene, including alternative splicing, may also impact sex differentiation. *WT1* mutations are associated with the **Denys-Drash syndrome** (early-onset renal failure with abnormal external genitalia and Wilms tumor). Haploinsufficiency of a 3-amino-acid (KTS) form of *WT1* has been implicated in the gonadal dysgenesis of patients with **Fraser syndrome** (late-onset progressive glomerulopathy and 46,XY gonadal dysgenesis). Mutations in the *FOXL2* and *SF-1* genes are associated with ovarian failure. Mutation of the *R-spondin1* gene has been described in individuals with 46,XX DSD (**d**isorder of **s**ex **d**evelopment). Other autosomal genes also play a role in normal ovarian organogenesis and testicular development. Several conditions of gonadal dysgenesis are associated with gross abnormalities of both autosomes and sex chromosomes. A deletion affecting the short arm of the X chromosome produces the typical somatic anomalies of Turner syndrome.

Development of the testis requires the short arm of the Y chromosome; this contains the testis-determining factor *SRY* gene. During male meiosis, the Y chromosome must segregate from the X chromosome so that both X and Y chromosomes do not occur in the same spermatozoa. The major portion of the Y chromosome is composed of Y-specific sequences that do not pair with the X chromosome. However, a minor portion of the Y chromosome shares sequences with the X chromosome and pairing does occur in this region. The genes and sequences in this area recombine between the sex chromosomes, behaving like autosomal genes. Therefore, the term *pseudoautosomal region* is used to describe this portion of the chromosome, and the term indicates genetic behavior of these genes relative to pairing and recombinational events. The *SRY* gene is localized to the 35-kb portion proximal to the pseudoautosomal region of the Y chromosome. It contains a high-mobility group (HMG) nonhistone protein (HMG box), supporting SRY's role as a transcriptional regulator of other genes involved in sex differentiation. The gonadal ridge forms at around 33 days of gestation. SRY is detected at 41 days, peaks at 44 days when testis cords are first visible, and persists into adulthood.

Other genes that are found on autosomes are important in this process. *SOX9*, a *SRY*-related gene containing a region homologous with the HMG box 9 of *SRY*, is located on chromosome 17. Mutations of this gene result in XY sex reversal and camptomelic dysplasia. *SF-1* on chromosome 9q33 is important in adrenal and gonadal development, as well as the development of gonadotropin-releasing hormone–secreting neurons in the hypothalamus. *WT1*, especially the KST isoform on chromosome 11p13, is needed for early gonadal, adrenal, and renal development. Fibroblast growth factor-9, GATA-4, XH-2, and SOY9 are also important.

When genetic recombination events on sex chromosomes extend beyond the pseudoautosomal region, X- and Y-specific DNA may be transferred between the chromosomes. Such aberrant recombinations result in X chromosomes carrying *SRY*, resulting in **XX males,** or Y chromosomes that have lost *SRY*, resulting in **XY females.** SRY acts as a transcriptional regulator to increase cellular proliferation, attract interstitial cells from adjacent mesonephros into the genital ridge, and stimulate testicular Sertoli cell differentiation. Sertoli cells act as an organizer of steroidogenic and germ cell lines and produce **antimüllerian hormone** (AMH) that causes the female duct system to regress. Table 582-1 lists additional genes involved in sex development.

Development of the ovary was once thought to be a passive process in the absence of SRY. Although the morphologic changes in the developing ovary are less marked than in the testis, there are a number of sequentially expressed genes and pathways that are required for complete ovarian development as well as maintenance of ovarian integrity postnatally. One of these genes is *R-spondin1*, which if mutated can result in testicular or ovotesticular development in 46,XX individuals. Some peptides in the Wnt-signaling pathway may antagonize testicular development. This effect may be mediated by β-catenin signaling, which is required for suppressing testicular features. Once developed, the ovary requires FAX12 to preserve its differentiation and stability.

FUNCTION OF THE TESTES

Levels of placental chorionic gonadotropin peak at 8-12 wk of gestation and stimulate the fetal Leydig cells to secrete testosterone, the main hormonal product of the testis. In the classical androgen biosynthetic pathway, testosterone is then converted by the enzyme 5α-reductase to its more potent metabolite, dihydrotestosterone. This early period is critical for normal and complete virilization of the XY fetus. Defects in this process lead to different forms of atypical male development (see Chapter 588.2). After virilization occurs, fetal levels of testosterone decrease but are maintained at lower levels in the latter half of pregnancy by luteinizing hormone (LH) secreted by the fetal pituitary; this LH-mediated testosterone secretion is required for continued penile growth, and to some degree also for testicular descent.

As part of the normal transition from intrauterine to extrauterine life, perhaps related to the sudden withdrawal of maternal and placental hormones, newborns and young infants experience a transient surge of gonadotropins and sex steroids. This is the so-called minipuberty.

In males, LH and testosterone peak at 1-2 mo of age and then decline to reach prepubertal levels by 4-6 mo of age. Follicle-stimulating hormone (FSH), along with inhibin B, peak at 3 mo and decline to prepubertal levels by 9 and 15 mo, respectively. The LH rise is more dominant than that of FSH.

The neonatal surge may be important for postnatal maturation of the gonads, stabilization of male external genitalia, and perhaps also for gender identity and sexual behaviors. The postnatal surge in LH and testosterone is absent or blunted in infants with hypopituitarism, cryptorchidism, and complete androgen insensitivity syndrome. The development of nocturnal pulsatile secretion of LH marks the advent of puberty.

Within specific target cells, 6-8% of testosterone is converted by 5α-reductase to dihydrotestosterone, a more potent androgen (Fig. 582-1), and approximately 0.3% is acted on by aromatase to produce estradiol. Approximately half of circulating testosterone is bound to sex hormone–binding globulin and half to albumin; only 2% circulates in the free form. Plasma levels of sex hormone–binding globulin are low at birth, rise rapidly during the 1st 10 days of life, and then remain stable until the onset of puberty. Thyroid hormone may play a role in this

Table 582-1 Genes Known to Be Involved in Disorders of Sex Development (DSd)

GENE	PROTEIN	OMIM DATA BASE NO.	LOCUS	INHERITANCE	GONAD	MÜLLERIAN STRUCTURES	EXTERNAL GENITALS	ASSOCIATED FEATURES/VARIANT PHENOTYPES
46,XY DSD								
Disorders of Gonadal (Testicular) Development: Single-Gene Disorders								
WT1	TF	607102	11p13	AD	Dysgenetic testis	±	Female or ambiguous	Wilms tumor, renal abnormalities, gonadal tumors (WAGR, Denys-Drash, and Frasier syndromes)
SF-1 (NR5A1)	Nuclear receptor TF	184757	9q33	AD/AR	Dysgenetic testis	±	Female or ambiguous	More severe phenotypes include primary adrenal failure; milder phenotypes have isolated partial gonadal dysgenesis; mothers who carry SF-1 mutation have premature ovarian insufficiency
SRY	TF	480000	Yp11.3	Y	Dysgenetic testis or ovotestis	±	Female or ambiguous	
SOX9	TF	608160	17q24-25	AD	Dysgenetic testis or ovotestis	±	Female or ambiguous	Camptomelic dysplasia (17q24 rearrangements milder phenotype than point mutations)
DHH	Signaling molecule	605423	12q13.1	AR	Dysgenetic testis	+	Female	The severe phenotype of 1 patient included monofascicular neuropathy; other patients have isolated gonadal dysgenesis
ATRX	Helicase (?chromatin remodeling)	300032	Xq13.3	X	Dysgenetic testis	−	Female, ambiguous or male	α-Thalassemia, mental retardation
ARX	TF	3003382	Xp22.13	X	Dysgenetic testis	−	Ambiguous	X-linked lissencephaly, epilepsy, temperature instability
Disorders of Gonadal (Testicular) Development: Chromosomal Changes Involving Key Candidate Genes								
DMRT1	TF	602424	9p24.3	Monosomic deletion	Dysgenetic testis	±	Female or ambiguous	Mental retardation
DAX1 (NR0B1)	Nuclear receptor TF	300018	Xp21.3	dupXp21	Dysgenetic testis or ovary	±	Female or ambiguous	
WNT4	Signaling molecule	603490	1p35	dup1p35	Dysgenetic testis	+	Ambiguous	Mental retardation
Disorders in Hormone Synthesis or Action								
LHGCR	G-protein receptor	152790	2p21	AR	Testis	−	Female, ambiguous or micropenis	Leydig cell hypoplasia
DHCR7	Enzyme	602858	11q12-13	AR	Testis	−	Variable	Smith-Lemli-Opitz syndrome: coarse facies, 2nd-3rd toe syndactyly, failure to thrive, developmental delay, cardiac and visceral abnormalities
StAR	Mitochondrial membrane protein	600617	8p11.2	AR	Testis	−	Female	Congenital lipoid adrenal hyperplasia (primary adrenal failure), pubertal failure
CYP11A1	Enzyme	118485	15q23-24	AR	Testis	−	Female or ambiguous	CAH (primary adrenal failure), pubertal failure
HSD3B2	Enzyme	201810	1p13.1	AR	Testis	−	Ambiguous	CAH, primary adrenal failure, partial androgenization caused by ↑DHEA
CYP17A1	Enzyme	202110	10q24.3	AR	Testis	−	Female ambiguous or micropenis	CAH, hypertension caused by ↑corticosterone and 11-deoxycorticosterone (except in isolated 17,20-lyase deficiency)
POR (P450 oxidoreductase)	CYP enzyme electron donor	124015	7q11.2	AR	Testis	−	Male or ambiguous	Mixed features of 21-hydroxylase deficiency, 17α-hydroxylase/17,20-lyase deficiency, and aromatase deficiency; sometimes associated with Antley-Bixler skeletal dysplasia

Continued

Table 582-1 Genes Known to Be Involved in Disorders of Sex Development (DSd)—cont'd

GENE	PROTEIN	OMIM DATA BASE NO.	LOCUS	INHERITANCE	GONAD	MÜLLERIAN STRUCTURES	EXTERNAL GENITALS	ASSOCIATED FEATURES/VARIANT PHENOTYPES
HSD17B3	Enzyme	605573	9q22	AR	Testis	–	Female or ambiguous	Partial androgenization at puberty, ↑androstenedione:testosterone ratio
SRD5A2	Enzyme	607306	2p23	AR	Testis	–	Ambiguous or micropenis	Partial androgenization at puberty, ↑testosterone:DHT ratio
AMH	Signaling molecule	600957	19p13.3-13.2	AR	Testis	+	Normal male	PMDS; male
AMH-receptor	Serine-threonine kinase transmembrane receptor	600956	12q13	AR	Testis	–	Normal male	External genitalia, bilateral cryptorchidism
Androgen receptor	Nuclear receptor TF	3130700	Xq11-12	X	Testis	–	Female, ambiguous, micropenis, or normal male	Phenotypic spectrum from complete androgen insensitivity syndrome (female external genitalia) and partial androgen insensitivity (ambiguous) to normal male genitalia/infertility
AKR1C2	3α-Hydroxysteroid dehydrogenase type III	600450	10p15.1	AR	Testis	–	Ambiguous or female	Originally thought that affected members of this family had isolated 17,20-lyase deficiency (CYP17A1)
46,XX DSD								
Disorders of Gonadal (Ovarian) Development								
SRY	TF	480000	Yp11.3	Translocation	Testis or ovotestis	–	Male or ambiguous	
SOX9	TF	608160	17q24	dup17q24	ND	–	Male or ambiguous	
R-spondin 1	R-spondin	609595	1p34.3		Ovotestis		Ambiguous	Palmoplantar hyperkeratosis
Androgen Excess								
HSD3B2	Enzyme	201810	1p13	AR	Ovary	+	Clitoromegaly	CAH, primary adrenal failure, partial androgenization caused by ↑DHEA
CYP21A2	Enzyme	201910	6p21-23	AR	Ovary	+	Ambiguous	CAH, phenotypic spectrum from severe salt-losing forms associated with adrenal failure to simple virilizing forms with compensated adrenal function, ↑17-hydroxyprogesterone
CYP11B1	Enzyme	20210	8q21-22	AR	Ovary	+	Ambiguous	CAH, hypertension caused by ↑11-deoxycortisol and 11-deoxycorticosterone
POR (P450 oxidoreductase)	CYP enzyme electron donor	124015	7q11.2	AR	Ovary	+	Ambiguous	Mixed features of 21-hydroxylase deficiency, 17α-hydroxylase/17,20-lyase deficiency, and aromatase deficiency; associated with Antley-Bixler skeletal dysplasia
CYP19	Enzyme	107910	15q21	AR	Ovary	+	Ambiguous	Maternal virilization during pregnancy, absent breast development at puberty, except in partial cases
Glucocorticoid receptor	Nuclear receptor TF	138040	5q31	AR	Ovary	+	Ambiguous	↑ACTH, 17-hydroxyprogesterone and cortisol; failure of dexamethasone suppression (patient heterozygous for a mutation in CYP21)

Chromosomal rearrangements likely to include key genes are included.
↑, Increased; ACTH, adrenocorticotropin; AD, autosomal dominant (often de novo mutation); AMH, antimüllerian hormone; AR, autosomal recessive; CAH, congenital adrenal hyperplasia; DAX1, dosage sensitive/sex reversal adrenal hypoplasia on the X chromosome; DHEA, dehydroepiandrosterone; DHT, dihydrotestosterone; DSD, disorder of sex development; ND, not determined; PMDS, persistent müllerian duct syndrome; SF-1, steroidogenic factor-1; SRY, sex-determining region on the Y chromosome; StAR, steroidogenic acute regulatory; TF, transcription factor; WAGR, Wilms, aniridia, genital anomalies, and retardation; WT1, Wilms tumor 1; X, X-chromosomal; Y, Y-chromosomal.
From Lee PA, Houk CP, Ahmed SF, et al: International Consensus Conference on Intersex organized by the Lawson Wilkins Pediatric Endocrine Society and the European Society for Paediatric Endocrinology. Consensus statement on management of intersex disorders. International Consensus Conference on Intersex, Pediatrics 118:e488–e500, 2006.

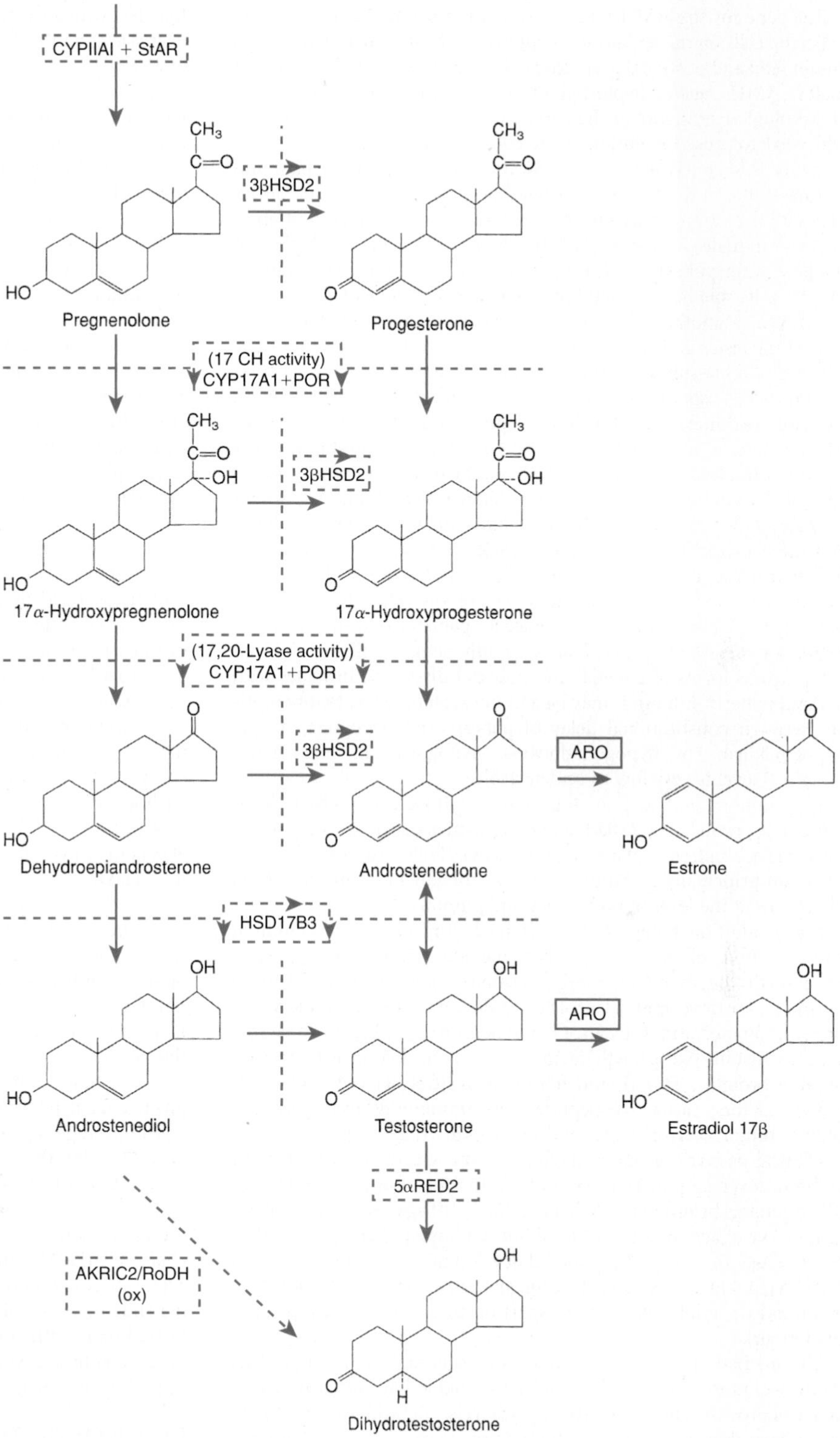

Figure 582-1 Biosynthesis of sex steroids. *Dashed lines* indicate enzymatic defects associated with 46,XY disorder of sex differentiation. *3β-HSD2,* 3β-hydroxysteroid dehydrogenase type 2; *AKR1C2/RoDH (Ox),* one of the enzymes in the recently described alternative androgen biosynthetic pathway; *ARO,* aromatase; *CYP17A1,* the enzyme that catalyzes both 17α-hydroxylase (17-OH) and 17,20-lyase activities; *HSD17B3,* enzyme that catalyzes the 17-ketoreductase reaction; *POR,* P450 oxidoreductase; *StAR,* steroidogenic acute regulatory protein.

physiologic increase because neonates with athyreosis (absence of the thyroid gland) have very low levels of sex hormone–binding globulin.

AMH (antimüllerian hormone; previously referred to as *müllerian inhibitory substance*), **inhibin,** and **activin** are members of the transforming growth factor-β (TGF-β) superfamily of growth factors. This group, which has more than 45 members, also includes bone morphogenetic proteins. Members of the TGF-β superfamily are involved in the regulation of developmental processes and multiple diverse human disease states, including chondrodysplasias and cancer.

AMH, a homodimeric glycoprotein hormone encoded by a gene on chromosome 19, is the earliest secreted product of the Sertoli cells of the fetal testis. Produced as a prohormone, its carboxyterminal fragment is cleaved to make it active. *AMH* transcription is initiated by *SOX9* acting through the HMG box, while its expression is upregulated by SF-1 binding to its promoter and further interacting with *SOX9, WT1,* and *GATA4.* AMH binds to 2 distinct serine/threonine receptors, each having a single transmembrane domain. The activated type 1 receptor signals to the SMAD family of intracellular mediators.

The gene for the AMH receptor (on chromosome 12) is expressed in Sertoli cells. In the female, it is expressed in fetal müllerian duct cells and in fetal and postnatal granulosa cells. During sex differentiation in males, AMH causes involution of the müllerian ducts, which are embryologic precursors of the cervix and uterus. It works in concert with SF-1 to cause involution of the fallopian tubes.

AMH is secreted in males by Sertoli cells during both fetal and postnatal life. In females, it is secreted by granulosa cells from 36 wk of gestation to menopause but at lower levels. The serum concentration of AMH in males is highest at birth, whereas in females it is highest at puberty. After puberty, both sexes have similar serum concentrations of AMH. Its role in postnatal life is not yet fully characterized.

Inhibin is another glycoprotein hormone secreted by the Sertoli cells of the testes and granulosa and theca cells of the ovary. Inhibin A consists of an α-subunit disulfide linked to the β-A subunit, whereas inhibin B consists of the same α subunit linked to the β-B subunit. Activins are dimers of the B subunits, either homodimers (BA/BA, BB/BB) or heterodimers (BA/BB). Inhibins selectively inhibit whereas activins stimulate pituitary FSH secretion. By means of immunoassays specific for inhibin A or B, it has been shown that inhibin A is absent in males and is present mostly in the luteal phase in women. Inhibin B is the principal form of inhibin in males and in females during the follicular phase. Inhibin B may be used as a marker of Sertoli cell function in males. FSH stimulates inhibin B secretion in females and males, but only in males is there also evidence for gonadotropin-independent regulation. Levels of inhibin B are currently being studied in children with various forms of gonadal and pubertal disorders. In males with delayed puberty, inhibin B may be a useful screening test to differentiate between constitutional delay of puberty and hypogonadotropic hypogonadism. In hypogonadotropic hypogonadism, the serum inhibin B level is very low to undetectable.

Like inhibin and activin, follistatin (a single-chain glycosylated protein) is produced by gonads and other tissues such as the hypothalamus, kidney, adrenal gland, and placenta. Follistatin inhibits FSH secretion principally by binding activins, thereby blocking the effects of activins at the level of both ovary and pituitary.

Many additional peptides act as mediators of the development and function of the testis. They include neurohormones such as growth hormone–releasing hormone, gonadotropin-releasing hormone, corticotropin-releasing hormone, oxytocin, arginine vasopressin, somatostatin, substance P, and neuropeptide Y; growth factors such as insulin-like growth factors and insulin-like growth factor–binding proteins, TGF-β, and fibroblast, platelet-derived, and nerve growth factors; vasoactive peptides; and immune-derived cytokines such as tumor necrosis factor and interleukins 1, 2, 4, and 6.

Clinical patterns of pubertal changes vary widely (see Chapters 14 and 561 covering pubertal maturation). In 95% of boys, enlargement of the genitals begins between 9.5 and 13.5 yr of age, reaching maturity at 13-17 yr of age. In a minority of normal boys, puberty begins after 15 yr of age. In some boys, pubertal development is completed in less than 2 yr, but in others it may take longer than 4.5 yr. Pubertal development and the adolescent growth spurt occur at an older age in boys than in girls.

The median age of sperm production (spermarche) is 14 yr. This event occurs in midpuberty as judged by pubic hair, testis size, evidence of growth spurt, and testosterone levels. Nighttime levels of FSH are in the adult male range at the time of spermarche; the first conscious ejaculation occurs at about the same time.

FUNCTION OF THE OVARIES

In the normal female, the undifferentiated gonad can be identified histologically as an ovary by 10-11 wk of gestation, after the upregulation of *R-spondin1*. Oocytes are present from the 4th mo of gestation and reach a peak of 7 million by 5 mo of gestation. For normal maintenance, oocytes need granulosa cells to form primordial follicles. Functional FSH (but not LH) receptors are present in oocytes of primary follicles during follicular development. Normal X chromosomes are needed for maintenance of oocytes. In contrast to somatic cells, in which only 1 X is active, both Xs are active in germ cells. At birth, the ovaries contain approximately 1 million active

follicles, which decrease to 0.5 million by menarche. Thereafter, they decrease at a rate of 1,000/mo, and at an even higher rate after the age of 35 yr.

The hormones of the fetal ovary are provided in most part by the fetoplacental unit. As in males, peak gonadotropin secretion occurs in fetal life and then again at 2-3 mo of life, with the lowest levels at about 6 yr of age. By contrast to males, the FSH surge predominates over LH in females. FSH peaks around 3-6 mo of age, declines by 12 mo, but remains detectable for 24 mo. Under LH influence, estradiol peaks at 2-6 mo of age. The inhibin B response is variable, peaking between 2 and 12 mo and remaining above prepubertal levels until 24 mo. In both infancy and childhood, gonadotropin levels are higher in females than in males.

The most important estrogens produced by the ovary are estradiol-17β (E_2) and estrone (E_1); estriol is a metabolic product of these 2, and all 3 estrogens may be found in the urine of mature females. Estrogens also arise from androgens produced by the adrenal gland and both the female and male gonads (see Fig. 574-1 in Chapter 574). This conversion explains why in certain types of disorders of sex differentiation in males, feminization occurs at puberty. In 17-ketosteroid reductase deficiency, for example, the enzymatic block results in markedly increased secretion of androstenedione, which is converted in the peripheral tissues to estradiol and estrone. These estrogens, in addition to those directly secreted by the testis, result in gynecomastia. Estradiol produced from testosterone in the complete androgen insensitivity syndrome causes complete feminization in XY individuals.

Estrogen regulates a host of functionally different activities in multiple tissues. There are at least 2 distinct estrogen receptors with different expression patterns. The ovary also synthesizes progesterone, the main progestational steroid; the adrenal cortex and testis also synthesize progesterone where it is a precursor for other adrenal and testicular hormones.

A host of other hormones with autocrine, paracrine, and intracrine effects have been identified in the ovary. They include inhibins, activins, relaxin, and growth factors insulin-like growth factor-1, TGF-α and TGF-β, and cytokines.

Plasma levels of estradiol increase slowly but steadily with advancing sexual maturation and correlate well with clinical evaluation of pubertal development, skeletal age, and rising levels of FSH. Levels of LH do not rise until secondary sexual characteristics are well developed. Estrogens, like androgens, inhibit secretion of both LH and FSH (negative feedback). In females, estrogens also provoke the surge of LH secretion that occurs in the mid–menstrual cycle. The capacity for this positive feedback is another maturational milestone of puberty.

The average age at menarche in American girls is approximately 12.5-13 yr, but the range of "normal" is wide, and 1-2% of normal girls have not menstruated by 16 yr of age. The age at onset of pubertal signs varies, with recent studies suggesting earlier ages than previously thought, especially in the U.S. African-American population (see Chapter 561). Menarche generally correlates closely with skeletal age. Maturation and closure of the epiphyses is at least partially estrogen dependent, as demonstrated by a very tall 28 yr old, normally masculinized male with continued growth as a result of incomplete closure of the epiphyses, who proved to have complete estrogen insensitivity caused by an estrogen-receptor defect.

DIAGNOSTIC TESTING

Improved, sensitive, and specific assays for pituitary and gonadal hormones that can be measured in small amounts of blood have contributed to rapid advances in the understanding of normal and abnormal hypothalamic-pituitary-gonadal interactions. In male infants, measurements of LH, FSH, and testosterone can detect pituitary and testicular defects. Leydig cell integrity in childhood can be determined by the testosterone response following human chorionic gonadotropin administration. (One protocol is to use 5,000 IU IM daily for 3 days; other protocols are available.) The integrity, as well as the maturity, of the hypothalamic-pituitary-gonadal axis in males and females can be assessed by measuring serial sex steroid, LH, and FSH levels after the subcutaneous administration of the gonadotropin-releasing hormone analog leuprolide. An ultrasensitive LH assay has been shown to differentiate between boys with delayed puberty and those with complete, but not partial, hypogonadotropic hypogonadism.

The normal range for inhibin B levels has been established in infant boys. Inhibin B may be a marker of spermatogenesis and also of tumors such as granulosa cell tumors. Inhibin may be involved in tumor suppression. Estrogen-receptor assays may be clinically useful in the management of various ovarian cancers. AMH measurements are useful in the evaluation of children with nonpalpable gonads and disorders of sex development.

THERAPEUTIC USE OF SEX STEROIDS

The estrogenic effects of polyhalogenated aromatic hydrocarbons may in part be a result of inhibition of estradiol sulfation by estrogen sulfotransferase, an important pathway of estradiol inactivation. Naturally occurring estrogens administered orally are rapidly destroyed by gastrointestinal and liver enzymes; accordingly, they are usually given as conjugates or esters. The most widely used oral preparations are equine conjugated estrogens (Premarin) and ethinyl estradiol. Estrogen-containing skin patches for transdermal absorption are also used. With improvements in the understanding of estrogen and estrogen-receptor interactions, a new class of compounds called *selective estrogen-receptor modulators* has been synthesized. For example, raloxifene, a nonsteroidal benzothiophene derivative, acts as an estrogen agonist in bone and liver and as an estrogen antagonist in breast and uterus.

Androgens, such as testosterone, are generally injected intramuscularly as long-acting esters (enanthate or cypionate, most commonly) because of their potency and steady response. Transdermal testosterone patches and a cutaneously applied gel have to date been used mostly in adults with hypogonadism because of the difficulty in titrating the doses needed during childhood and adolescence. Oral preparations, such as methyltestosterone or fluoxymesterone, do not produce so potent an androgenic response and may be hepatotoxic. Testosterone undecenoate, another oral preparation, is used in Europe but not in the United States. Sublingual (microspheres or pellets) and buccal (absorption via the buccal mucosa) preparations of testosterone are in development.

Bibliography is available at Expert Consult.

Chapter **583**
Hypofunction of the Testes
Omar Ali and Patricia A. Donohoue

Testicular hypofunction during fetal life can be a component of some types of **disorders of sex development** (see Chapter 588.2) and may lead to varying degrees of ambiguous genitalia. After birth, neonates undergo "minipuberty" with relatively high levels of gonadotropins and sex steroids, but this phenomenon is transient and its absence does not lead to any obvious clinical findings. Because prepubertal children normally do not produce significant amounts of testosterone and are not yet producing sperm, there are no discernible effects of testicular hypofunction in this age group. Testicular hypofunction from the age of puberty onward may lead to testosterone deficiency, infertility, or both. Such hypofunction may be primary in the testes (**primary hypogonadism**) or secondary to deficiency of pituitary gonadotropic hormones (**secondary hypogonadism**). Both types may be caused by inherited genetic defects or acquired causes, and in some cases the etiology may be unclear, but the level of the lesion (primary or secondary) is usually well defined; patients with primary hypogonadism have elevated levels of gonadotropins (hypergonadotropic); those with secondary hypogonadism have inappropriately low or absent levels

Table 583-1	Etiologic Classification of Male Hypogonadism

HYPERGONADOTROPIC HYPOGONADISM (PRIMARY HYPOGONADISM; TESTES)
Congenital
Follicle-stimulating hormone (FSH) and luteinizing hormone (LH) resistance
Mutations in steroid synthetic pathways
Gonadal dysgenesis
Klinefelter syndrome (47,XXY)
Noonan syndrome (*PTPN-11* gene mutation in many cases)
Cystic fibrosis (infertility)
Acquired
Cryptorchidism (some cases)
Vanishing testes
Chemotherapy
Radiation
Infection (e.g., mumps)
Infarction (testicular torsion)
Trauma

HYPOGONADOTROPIC HYPOGONADISM (SECONDARY HYPOGONADISM; HYPOTHALAMIC-PITUITARY)
Congenital
Genetic defects causing Kallmann syndrome and/or normosmic hypogonadotropic hypogonadism (HH)
Other genetic disorders associated with HH: leptin gene, leptin receptor, DAX1 (dosage-sensitive/sex-reversal adrenal hypoplasia on the X chromosome), SF-1 (steroidogenic factor-1)
Inherited syndromes: Prader-Willi, Bardet-Biedl, Laurence-Moon-Biedl, Alström
Isolated HH at pituitary level (gonadotropin-releasing hormone receptor, FSH and LH β-subunit)
Multiple pituitary hormone deficiencies: septooptic dysplasia (*HESX-1* in some cases) and other disorders of pituitary organogenesis (e.g., *PROP1, LHX3, LHX4, SOX-3*)
Idiopathic
Acquired
Anorexia nervosa
Drug use
Malnutrition
Chronic illness, especially Crohn disease
Hyperprolactinemia
Pituitary tumors
Pituitary infarction
Infiltrative disorders (e.g., histiocytosis, sarcoidosis)
Hemosiderosis and hemochromatosis
Radiation

(hypogonadotropic). Table 583-1 details the etiologic classification of male hypogonadism.

583.1 Hypergonadotropic Hypogonadism in the Male (Primary Hypogonadism)
Omar Ali and Patricia A. Donohoue

ETIOLOGY

Some degree of testicular function is essential in the development of phenotypically male newborns. If testicular function is present, sex differentiation is normally complete by the 14th wk of intrauterine life. Hypogonadism may occur after phenotypically male genitalia have developed for a variety of reasons; genetic or chromosomal anomalies may lead to testicular hypofunction that does not become apparent until the time of puberty, when these boys may have delayed or incomplete pubertal development. In other cases, normally developed testes may be damaged by infarction, trauma, radiation, chemotherapy, infections, infiltration, or other causes after sexual differentiation has occurred. In some cases, genetic defects may predispose to atrophy or maldescent; or torsion or infarction or may lead to progressive testicular damage and atrophy after a period of normal development. If testicular compromise is global, both testosterone secretion and fertility (sperm production) are likely to be affected. Even when the primary defect is in testosterone production, low levels of intratesticular testosterone will frequently lead to infertility. The reverse is not necessarily true. Defects in sperm production and in the storage and transit of sperm may not be associated with low testosterone levels; infertility may thus be seen in patients with normal testosterone levels, normal libido, and normal secondary sexual characteristics.

Various degrees of primary hypogonadism also occur in a significant percentage of patients with chromosomal aberrations as in **Klinefelter syndrome, males with more than one X chromosome**, and **XX males.** These chromosomal anomalies are associated with other characteristic findings. Noonan syndrome is associated with cryptorchidism and infertility, but other (nongonadal) features dominate its clinical picture.

Congenital Anorchia or Testicular Regression Syndrome

Boys in whom the external genitalia have developed normally (or nearly normally) and müllerian duct derivatives (uterus, fallopian tubes) are absent have obviously had testicular function for at least some part of gestation. If their testes cannot be palpated at birth, they are said to have **cryptorchidism.** In most such cases, the testes are undescended or retractile, but in some cases no testes are found in any location, even after extensive investigation. This syndrome of absence of testes in a phenotypic male with normal 46,XY karyotype (indicating that there was some period of testicular function in intrauterine life) is known as "vanishing testes," "congenital anorchia," or **"testicular regression syndrome."**

Testicular regression syndrome is not uncommon. Cryptorchidism occurs in 1.5-9% of male births and in 10-20% of these cases, the testes are impalpable. Of children with impalpable testes, up to 50% may have no detectable testes after extensive investigation. Most cases appear to be sporadic and are thought to be a result of torsion or vascular accidents. The incompletely descended testis may be more prone to torsion and this may be one of the causes of "vanishing testes." Most cases are sporadic but in a subset of patients testicular regression syndrome occurs in monozygotic twins or in families with other affected individuals, suggesting a genetic etiology. Some cases are associated with micropenis and in these cases the testicular loss probably occurred after the 14th wk, but well before the time of birth, or this may indicate a preexisting dysfunction of male hormonal development. Low levels of testosterone (<10 ng/dL) and markedly elevated levels of luteinizing hormone (LH) and follicle-stimulating hormone (FSH) are found in the early postnatal months; thereafter, levels of gonadotropins tend to decrease even in agonadal children, rising to very high levels again as the pubertal years approach. Stimulation with human chorionic gonadotropin (hCG) fails to evoke an increase in the level of testosterone. Serum levels of antimüllerian hormone (AMH) are undetectable or low. All patients with undetectable testes should be tested for AMH and should undergo an hCG stimulation test. If the results indicate that no testicular tissue is present (absent AMH and no rise in testosterone after hCG stimulation), then the diagnosis of testicular regression syndrome is confirmed. If testosterone secretion is demonstrated, then imaging with abdominal MRI and/or surgical exploration is indicated. A small fibrotic nodule may be found at the end of the spermatic cord in many cases of testicular regression syndrome. Treatment of male hypogonadism (primary or secondary) is discussed in Chapter 583.2. There is no possibility of normal fertility in these patients.

Chemotherapy and Radiation-Induced Hypogonadism

Testicular damage is a frequent consequence of **chemotherapy** and **radiotherapy** for cancer. The frequency and extent of damage depend on the agent used, total dose, duration of therapy, and posttherapy interval of observation. Another important variable is age at therapy; germ cells are less vulnerable in prepubertal than in pubertal and postpubertal boys. **Chemotherapy** is most damaging if more than 1 agent is used. The use of alkylating agents such as cyclophosphamide in prepubertal children does not impair pubertal development, even

though there may be biopsy evidence of germ cell damage. High doses of cyclophosphamide and ifosfamide are associated with infertility. Cisplatin causes transient azoospermia or oligospermia at lower doses, while higher doses (400-600 mg/m^2) can cause permanent infertility. Interleukin 2 can depress Leydig cell function, whereas interferon-α does not seem to affect gonadal function. Most chemotherapeutic agents produce azoospermia and infertility; Leydig cell damage (leading to low testosterone levels) is less common. In many cases, the damage is transient and sperm counts recover after 12-24 mo. Both chemotherapy and radiotherapy are associated with an increase in the percentage of abnormal gametes, but data concerning the outcomes of pregnancies after such therapy have *not* shown any increase in genetically mediated birth defects, possibly because of selection bias against abnormal sperm.

Radiation damage is dose dependent. Temporary oligospermia can be seen with doses as low as 0.1 Gy, with permanent azoospermia seen with doses greater than 2 Gy. Recovery of spermatogenesis can be seen as long as 5 yr (or more) after irradiation, with higher doses leading to slower recovery. Leydig cells are more resistant to irradiation. Mild damage as determined by elevated LH levels can be seen with up to 6 Gy; doses greater than 30 Gy cause hypogonadism in most patients. Whenever possible, testes should be shielded from irradiation. Testicular function should be carefully evaluated in adolescents after multimodal treatment for cancer in childhood. Replacement therapy with testosterone and counseling concerning fertility may be indicated. The storage of sperm prior to chemotherapy or radiation treatment in postpubertal males is an option. Even in those cases where sperm counts are abnormal, recovery is possible, though the chances of recovery decline with increasing dose of radiation. If sperm counts remain low, fertility is still possible in some cases with testicular sperm extraction and intracytoplasmic sperm injection.

Sertoli Cell–Only Syndrome

Small testes and azoospermia are seen in patients with the extremely rare Sertoli cell–only syndrome (germ cell aplasia, or **Del Castillo syndrome**). These patients have no germ cells in the testes, but usually have normal testosterone production, and present as adults with the complaint of infertility. Most cases are sporadic and idiopathic, but deletions involving the azoospermia factor (AZF) region of the Y chromosome (Yq11) may be found in some cases.

Other Causes of Testicular Hypofunction

Atrophy of the testes may follow damage to the vascular supply as a result of manipulation of the testes during surgical procedures for correction of cryptorchidism or as a result of bilateral torsion of the testes. **Acute orchitis** is common in pubertal or adult males with mumps and may lead to subfertility in 13% of cases, though infertility is rare. Testosterone secretion usually remains normal. The incidence of mumps orchitis in postpubertal males has increased in some areas as a result of decrease in measles, mumps, and rubella vaccination uptake. Autoimmune polyendocrinopathy may be associated with primary hypogonadism (associated with anti-P450scc antibodies) but this appears to be more common in females.

Testicular Dysgenesis Syndrome

The incidence of testicular cancer has increased in many developed societies while the incidence of cryptorchidism, hypospadias, low sperm counts, and sperm abnormalities also appears to have increased in some, but not all, studies. It has been proposed that all these trends are linked by prenatal testicular dysgenesis. The hypothesis is that some degree of testicular dysgenesis develops in intrauterine life from genetic as well as environmental factors, and is associated with increased risk of cryptorchidism, hypospadias, hypofertility, and testicular cancer. The environmental influences that have been implicated in this syndrome include environmental chemicals that act as endocrine disruptors, such as bisphenol A and phthalates (components of many types of plastics), several pesticides, phytoestrogens or mycoestrogens, and other chemicals. The fact that these lesions can be reproduced in some animal models by environmental chemicals has led to efforts to remove these chemicals from products used by infants and pregnant mothers, and from the environment in general. Nonetheless, the evidence is only suggestive and is not conclusive.

CLINICAL MANIFESTATIONS

Primary hypogonadism may be suspected at birth if the testes and penis are abnormally small. Normative data are available for different populations. The condition often is not noticed until puberty, when secondary sex characteristics fail to develop. Facial, pubic, and axillary hair is scant or absent; there is neither acne nor regression of scalp hair; and the voice remains high pitched. The penis and scrotum remain infantile and may be almost obscured by pubic fat; the testes are small or not palpable. Fat accumulates in the region of the hips and buttocks and sometimes in the breasts and on the abdomen. The epiphyses close later than normal; therefore, extremities are long. The span may be several inches longer than the height, and the distance from the symphysis pubis to the soles of the feet (lower segment) is much greater than that from the symphysis to the vertex (upper segment). The proportions of the body are described as **eunuchoid.** The upper to lower segment ratio is considerably less than 0.9. Many individuals with milder degrees of hypogonadism may be detected only by appropriate studies of the pituitary-gonadal axis. Examination of the testes should be performed routinely by pediatricians; testicular volumes as determined by comparison with standard orchidometers or by measurement of linear dimensions should be recorded.

DIAGNOSIS

Levels of serum FSH and, to a lesser extent, of LH are elevated to greater than age-specific normal values in early infancy (when "minipuberty" normally occurs and the gonadotropins are normally disinhibited). This is followed by a period of time when even agonadal children may not exhibit significant elevation in gonadotropins, indicating that the gonadotropins are also suppressed at this stage by some mechanism independent of feedback inhibition by gonadal hormones. In the latter half of childhood and several years prior to the onset of puberty, this inhibition is released and gonadotropin levels again rise above age-matched normals in subjects with primary hypogonadism. These elevated levels indicate that even in the prepubertal child there is an active hypothalamic-gonadal feedback relationship. After the age of 11 yr, FSH and LH levels rise significantly, reaching the castrate range. Measurements of random plasma testosterone levels in prepubertal boys are not helpful because they are ordinarily low in normal prepubertal children, rising during puberty to attain adult levels. During puberty, these levels, when measured in an early-morning blood sample, correlate better with testicular size, stage of sexual maturity, and bone age than with chronological age. In patients with primary hypogonadism, testosterone levels remain low at all ages. There is an attenuated rise or no rise at all after administration of hCG, in contrast to normal males in whom hCG produces a significant rise in plasma testosterone at any stage of development.

AMH is secreted by the Sertoli cells and this secretion is suppressed by testosterone. As a result, AMH levels are elevated in prepubertal boys and suppressed at onset of puberty. Boys with primary hypogonadism continue to have elevated AMH levels in puberty. Detection of AMH may be used in prepubertal years as an indicator of the presence of testicular tissue (e.g., in patients with bilateral cryptorchidism). Inhibin B is also secreted by the Sertoli cells, is present throughout childhood, and rises at onset of puberty (more in boys than in girls). It may be used as another marker of the presence of testicular tissue in bilateral cryptorchidism and as a marker of spermatogenesis (e.g., in delayed puberty, cancer survivors, and patients with Noonan syndrome). Bone age x-rays are useful to document delayed bone age in patients with constitutional growth delay as well as primary hypogonadism.

NOONAN SYNDROME
Etiology

The term *Noonan syndrome* has been applied to males and females with normal karyotypes who have certain phenotypic features that occur also in females with Turner syndrome (although the genetic causes are completely distinct) (see Chapter 81.4). Noonan syndrome occurs in 1 in 1,000-2,500 live births. Approximately 20% of the cases are familial and exhibit autosomal dominant inheritance. Males and females are equally affected. It is now thought that several mutations in the renin-angiotensin system (RAS)–mitogen-activated protein kinase (MAPK) pathway can cause Noonan syndrome and other related disorders and such mutations are currently detected in approximately 70% of the cases of Noonan syndrome. Missense mutations in *PTPN11*—a gene on chromosome 12q24.1 encoding the nonreceptor protein tyrosine phosphatase SHP-2—are seen in about half the cases. Mutations in other genes in this pathway, including *SHOC2, CBL, SOS1, KRAS, NRAS, BRAF,* and *RAF1,* as well as duplications of the 12q24 region, are also seen. Phenotypic features of Noonan syndrome therefore overlap with other syndromes involving the RAS-MAPK pathway, such as Leopard syndrome and cardiofaciocutaneous syndrome.

Clinical Manifestations

The most common abnormalities are short stature, webbing of the neck, pectus carinatum or pectus excavatum, cubitus valgus, right-sided congenital heart disease, and characteristic facies. Hypertelorism, epicanthus, downward-slanting palpebral fissures, ptosis, micrognathia, and ear abnormalities are common. Other abnormalities such as clinodactyly, hernias, and vertebral anomalies occur less frequently. As opposed to Turner syndrome, the mean IQ of school-age children with Noonan syndrome is subnormal at 86, with a range of 53-127. Verbal IQ tends to be better than performance IQ. High-frequency sensorineural hearing loss is common. The cardiac defect is most often pulmonary valvular stenosis, hypertrophic cardiomyopathy, or atrial septal defect. Hepatosplenomegaly and several hematologic diseases, including low clotting factors XI and XII, acute lymphoblastic leukemia, and chronic myelomonocytic leukemia, are noted. Noonan-like features can be part of the phenotypic variation of the *NF1* (neurofibromatosis) gene mutation, possibly as a result of common involvement of the RAS-MAPK pathway in both diseases. Males frequently have cryptorchidism and small testes. Testosterone secretion may be low or normal, but spermatogenesis may be affected even in those with normal testosterone (and normal secondary sexual characteristics). Serum inhibin-B is a useful marker of Sertoli cell function in these patients. Puberty is delayed and adult height is achieved by the end of the 2nd decade and usually reaches the lower limit of the normal population. Prenatal diagnosis should be suspected in fetuses with normal karyotype, edema, or hydrops and short femur length.

Treatment

Human growth hormone results in improvement in growth velocity in many Noonan syndrome patients, comparable to that seen in patients with Turner syndrome, and studies show a mean increase in height standard deviation score ranging from 1.3-1.7, corresponding to 9.5-13 cm for boys and 9.0-9.8 cm for girls. Many patients with Noonan syndrome reach normal height without growth hormone therapy, but treatment is recommended for those who fall below the 3rd percentile for height. The recommended dose is up to 66 µg/kg/day of recombinant growth hormone. Patients with Noonan syndrome and demonstrable *PTNP11* mutations grow less well and are less responsive to growth hormone treatment than those without mutations. They have lower insulin-like growth factor-1 and higher growth hormone levels, suggesting partial growth hormone resistance because of postreceptor-signaling defects. Treatment of male hypogonadism is discussed in Chapter 583.2.

KLINEFELTER SYNDROME
See also Chapter 81.

Etiology

Klinefelter syndrome is the most common sex chromosomal aneuploidy in males, with an incidence of 0.1-0.2% in the general population (1 in 500-1,000) and rising to 4% among infertile males and 10-11% in those with oligospermia or azoospermia. Approximately 80% of them have a 47,XXY chromosome complement, while mosaics and higher degrees of polyX are seen in the remaining 20%. Even with as many as 4 X chromosomes, the Y chromosome determines a male phenotype. The chromosomal aberration most often results from meiotic nondisjunction of an X chromosome during parental gametogenesis; the extra X chromosome is maternal in origin in 54% and paternal in origin in 46% of patients. A national study in Denmark revealed a prenatal prevalence of 213 per 100,000 male fetuses, but in adult men the prevalence was only 40 per 100,000, suggesting that only 1 in 4 of adult males with Klinefelter syndrome was diagnosed.

Clinical Manifestations

In patients who do not have a prenatal diagnosis, the diagnosis is rarely made before puberty because of the paucity or subtleness of clinical manifestations in childhood. Behavioral or psychiatric disorders may be apparent long before defects in sexual development. These children tend to have learning disabilities and deficits in "executive function" (concept formation, problem solving, task switching, and planning), and the condition should be considered in boys with psychosocial, learning, or school adjustment problems. Affected children may be anxious, immature, or excessively shy and tend to have difficulty in social interactions throughout life. In a prospective study, a group of children with 47,XXY karyotypes identified at birth exhibited relatively mild deviations from normal during the 1st 5 yr of life. None had major physical, intellectual, or emotional disabilities; some were inactive, with poorly organized motor function and mild delay in language acquisition. Problems often first become apparent after the child begins school. Full-scale IQ scores may be normal, with verbal IQ being somewhat decreased. Verbal cognitive defects and underachievement in reading, spelling, and mathematics are common. By late adolescence, many boys with Klinefelter syndrome have generalized learning disabilities, most of which are language based. Despite these difficulties, most complete high school.

The patients tend to be tall, slim, and have a specific tendency to have long legs (disproportionate to the arms, and longer than those seen with other causes of hypogonadism), but body habitus can vary markedly. The testes tend to be small for age, but this sign may become apparent only after puberty, when normal testicular growth fails to occur. The phallus tends to be smaller than average, and cryptorchidism is more common than in the general population. Bone mineral density may be low in adults with Klinefelter syndrome and this correlates with lower testosterone levels.

Pubertal development may be delayed, although some children undergo apparently normal or nearly normal virilization. Despite normal testosterone levels, serum LH and FSH concentrations and their responses to gonadotropin-releasing hormone (GnRH) stimulation are elevated starting at around 13 yr of age. Approximately 80% of adults have **gynecomastia;** they have sparser facial hair, most shaving less often than daily. The most common testicular lesions are spermatogenic arrest and Sertoli cell predominance. The sperm have a high incidence of sex chromosomal aneuploidy. Azoospermia and infertility are usual, although rare instances of fertility are known. It is now clear that germ cell numbers and sperm counts are higher in early puberty and decline with age. Testicular sperm extraction followed by intracytoplasmic sperm injection can result in the birth of healthy infants, with success rates declining with increasing age. In nonmosaic Klinefelter patients, most testicular sperm (94%) have a normal pattern of sex chromosome segregation, indicating that meiotic checkpoints can remove most aneuploid cells. Antisperm antibodies have been detected in 25% of tested specimens.

There is an increased incidence in adulthood of central adiposity, metabolic syndrome, pulmonary disease, varicose veins, and cancer of the breast. Among 93 unselected **male breast cancer** patients, 7.5% were found to have Klinefelter syndrome. Mediastinal germ cell tumors have been reported; some of these tumors produce hCG and cause precocious puberty in young boys. They may also be associated with leukemia, lymphoma, and other hematologic neoplasia. The highest cancer risk (relative risk: 2.7) occurs in the 15-30 yr age group. A large cohort study in Britain demonstrated an overall significantly increased standardized mortality ratio (1.5), with particular increases in deaths from diabetes, epilepsy, peripheral and intestinal vascular sufficiency,

pulmonary embolism, and renal disease. Mortality from ischemic heart disease was decreased. In adults, structural brain abnormalities correlate with cognitive deficits.

In adults with XY/XXY mosaicism, the features of Klinefelter syndrome are decreased in severity and frequency. Children with mosaicism have a better prognosis for virilization, fertility, and psychosocial adjustment.

Klinefelter Variants and Other Poly-X Syndromes

When the number of X chromosomes exceeds 2, the clinical manifestations, including mental retardation and impairment of virilization, are more severe. Height decreases with increasing number of X chromosomes. The XXYY variant is the most common variant (1 in 18,000-40,000 male births). In most, mental retardation occurs with IQ scores between 60 and 80, but 10% have IQs greater than 110. The XXYY male phenotype is not distinctively different from that of the XXY patient, except that XXYY adults tend to be taller than the average XXY patient. The 49,XXXXY variant is sufficiently distinctive to be detected in childhood. Its incidence is estimated to be 1 in 80,000-100,000 male births. The disorder arises from sequential nondisjunction in meiosis. Affected patients are severely cognitively impaired and have short necks and typical coarse facies with wide-set eyes with a mild upward slant of the fissures, epicanthus, strabismus, a wide and flat upturned nose, a large open mouth, and large malformed ears. The testes are small and may be undescended, the scrotum is hypoplastic, and the penis is very small. Defects suggestive of Down syndrome (short, incurved terminal 5th phalanges, single palmar creases, and hypotonia) and other skeletal abnormalities (including defects in the carrying angle of the elbows and restricted supination) are common. The most frequent radiographic abnormalities are radioulnar synostosis or dislocation, elongated radius, pseudoepiphyses, scoliosis or kyphosis, coxa valga, and retarded osseous age. Most patients with such extensive changes have a 49,XXXXY chromosome karyotype; several mosaic patterns have also been observed: 48,XXXY/49,XXXXY; 48,XXXY/49,XXXXY/50,XXXXXY; and 48,XXXY/49,XXXXY/50,XXXXYY. Prenatal diagnosis of a 49,XXXXY infant has been reported. The fetus had intrauterine growth retardation, edema, and cystic hygroma colli.

The 48,XXXY variant is relatively rare. The characteristic features are generally less severe than those of patients with 49,XXXXY and more severe than those of 47,XXY patients. Mild intellectual disability, delayed speech and motor development, and immature but passive and pleasant behavior are associated with this condition.

Very few patients have been described with 49,XYYY and 49,XXYYY karyotypes. Dysmorphic features and cognitive impairment are common to both.

Laboratory Findings

Most males with Klinefelter syndrome go through life undiagnosed. The chromosomes should be examined in all patients suspected of having Klinefelter syndrome, particularly those attending child guidance, psychiatric, and cognitive disability clinics. In infancy, inhibin B and AMH levels are normal but testosterone levels are lower than in controls. Before 10 yr of age, boys with 47,XXY Klinefelter syndrome have normal basal plasma levels of FSH and LH. Responses to gonadotropin-stimulating hormone and to hCG are normal. The testes show normal growth early in puberty, but by midpuberty the testicular growth stops, gonadotropins become elevated, and testosterone levels are slightly low. Inhibin B levels are normal in early puberty, decrease in late puberty, and are low in adults with the syndrome. Elevated levels of estradiol, resulting in a high estradiol to testosterone ratio, account for the development of gynecomastia during puberty. Sex hormone–binding globulin levels are elevated, further decreasing free testosterone levels. Long androgen receptor polyglutamine (CAG) repeat length is associated with the more-severe phenotype, including gynecomastia, small testes, and short penile length.

Testicular biopsy before puberty may reveal only deficiency or absence of germinal cells. After puberty, the seminiferous tubular membranes are hyalinized, and there is adenomatous clumping of Leydig cells. Sertoli cells predominate. Azoospermia is characteristic, and infertility is the rule.

Management

Boys known to have Klinefelter syndrome should be monitored closely for speech, learning, and behavioral problems, and referred for early evaluation and treatment as needed. Testosterone, LH, and FSH levels should be checked at 11-12 yr of age and replacement therapy with a testosterone preparation is recommended once FSH and LH begin to rise above normal. Fasting glucose, lipids, and hemoglobin A_{1C} should also be obtained as these children are at risk for central adiposity and metabolic syndrome. A baseline dual-energy x-ray absorptiometry scan to assess bone density is also recommended by some authorities. Although testosterone treatment will normalize testosterone levels, stimulate the development of secondary sexual characteristics, increase bone mass and muscle mass, and improve body composition, it will *not* improve fertility (and will, in fact, suppress spermatogenesis). There is some evidence that it also improves mood and may have a positive effect on cognition and social functioning but the findings are not conclusive at this time. Either long-acting testosterone injections or daily application of testosterone gel may be used (testosterone patches have a high incidence of skin rash and are not frequently used in pediatrics). Testosterone enanthate or cypionate ester may be used in a starting dose of 25-50 mg injected intramuscularly every 3-4 wk, with 50-mg increments every 6-9 mo until a maintenance dose for adults (200-250 mg every 3-4 wk) is achieved. At that time, testosterone patches or testosterone gel may be substituted for the injections. Depending on patient and physician preference, transdermal testosterone may also be used as initial treatment instead of injections. For older boys, larger initial doses and increments can achieve more rapid virilization. The various transdermal preparations differ somewhat from each other and standard references should be consulted for recommendations regarding dosage and mode of application.

Gynecomastia may be treated with aromatase inhibitors (which will also increase endogenous testosterone levels) but medical treatment is not always successful and plastic surgery may be needed. Fertility is usually not an issue in the pediatric age group, but adults can father children using testicular sperm extraction followed by intracytoplasmic sperm injection. Because sperm counts decrease rapidly after onset of puberty in children with Klinefelter syndrome, sperm banking during early puberty is an option that can be discussed with a fertility specialist. Sperm counts can be stimulated using hCG treatment prior to testicular sperm extraction. Therapy, counseling and psychiatric services should be provided as needed for learning difficulties and psychosocial disabilities.

XX MALES

This disorder is thought to occur in 1 in 20,000 newborn males. Affected individuals have a male phenotype, small testes, a small phallus, and no evidence of ovarian or müllerian duct tissue. They appear, therefore, to be distinct from the ovotesticular disorder of sexual development. Undescended testes and hypospadias occur in a minority of patients. Infertility occurs in practically all cases and the histologic features of the testes are essentially the same as in Klinefelter syndrome. Patients with the condition usually come to medical attention in adult life because of hypogonadism, gynecomastia, or infertility. Hypergonadotropic hypogonadism occurs secondary to testicular failure. A few cases have been diagnosed perinatally as a result of discrepancies between prenatal ultrasonography and karyotype findings.

In 90% of XX males with normal male external genitalia, 1 of the X chromosomes carries the *SRY* (sex-determining region on the Y chromosome) gene. The exchange from the Y to the X chromosome occurs during paternal meiosis, when the short arms of the Y and X chromosomes pair. XX males inherit 1 maternal X chromosome and 1 paternal X chromosome containing the translocated male-determining gene. A few cases of 46,XX males with 9P translocations have also been identified. Most XX males who are identified before puberty have hypospadias or micropenis; this group of patients may lack Y-specific sequences, suggesting other mechanisms for virilization. Fluorescent in situ hybridization and primed in situ labeling have been used to identify small *SRY* DNA segments. Yp fragment abnormalities may result in sexually ambiguous phenotypes.

45,X MALES

In a few male patients recognized with a 45,X karyotype, Yp sequences are translocated to an autosomal chromosome. In 1 instance, the terminal short arm of the Y chromosome was translocated onto an X chromosome. In another, *SRY/autosomal* translocation was postulated. A male with 45,X karyotype and Leri-Weill dyschondrosteosis, *SHOX* gene loss, and SRY to Xp translocation also has been described.

47,XXX MALES

A Japanese male with poor pubic hair development, hypoplastic scrotal testes (4 mL), normal penis and normal height, gynecomastia, and severe cognitive impairment had 47,XXX karyotype caused by an abnormal X-Y interchange during paternal meiosis and X-X nondisjunction during maternal meiosis.

Bibliography is available at Expert Consult.

583.2 Hypogonadotropic Hypogonadism in the Male (Secondary Hypogonadism)
Omar Ali and Patricia A. Donohoue

In hypogonadotropic hypogonadism, lack of gonadal function is secondary to deficiency of 1 or both gonadotropins: FSH or LH. The primary defect may lie either in the anterior pituitary or in the hypothalamus. Hypothalamic etiologies result in deficiency of GnRH. The testes are normal but remain in the prepubertal state because stimulation by gonadotropins is lacking. The disorder may be recognized in infancy but is much more commonly recognized because of marked pubertal delay. Rarely, patients with an inherited form of hypogonadotropic hypogonadism (HH) may go through puberty and may present with hypogonadism as adults.

ETIOLOGY

HH may be genetic or acquired. Several different genes can cause inherited forms of HH; the affected genes may be upstream of GnRH, at the level of GnRH receptors, or at the level of gonadotropin production. In addition, various genetic defects in transcription factors such as POUF-1, LHX-3, LHX-4, and HESX-1 lead to defects in pituitary development and multiple pituitary hormone deficiencies, including deficiency of gonadotropins. Acquired pituitary gonadotropin deficiency may develop from various lesions in the hypothalamic-pituitary region (e.g., tumors, infiltrative disease, autoimmune disease, trauma, stroke).

Isolated Gonadotropin Deficiency

Isolated gonadotropin deficiency in which other pituitary hormone levels are normal is more likely to be from defects in the secretion of GnRH from the hypothalamus rather than defects in gonadotropin synthesis in the pituitary. It affects approximately 1 in 10,000 males and 1 in 50,000 females and encompasses a heterogeneous group of entities. Many cases are associated with anosmia and this combination of anosmia and HH defines Kallmann syndrome.

Kallmann syndrome is the most common form of HH and is genetically heterogeneous, with autosomal recessive, X-linked, and autosomal dominant forms of inheritance. Clinically, it is characterized by its association with **anosmia** or **hyposmia;** 85% of the cases are autosomal and 15% are X-linked. The X-linked form (KAL1) is caused by mutations of the *KAL1* gene at Xp22.3. This leads to failure of olfactory axons and GnRH-expressing neurons to migrate from their common origin in the olfactory placode to the brain. The *KAL* gene product anosmin-1, an extracellular 95 kDa matrix glycoprotein, facilitates neuronal growth and migration. The *KAL* gene is also expressed in various parts of the brain, facial mesenchyme, and mesonephros and metanephros, thus explaining some of the associated findings in patients with Kallmann syndrome, such as synkinesia (mirror movements), hearing loss, midfacial defects, and renal agenesis.

Some kindreds contain anosmic individuals with or without hypogonadism; others contain hypogonadal individuals who are anosmic.

Cleft lip and palate, hypotelorism, median facial clefts, sensorineural hearing loss, unilateral renal aplasia, neurologic deficits, and other findings occur in some affected patients. When Kallmann syndrome is caused by terminal or interstitial deletions of the Xp22.3 region, it may be associated with other contiguous gene syndromes, such as steroid sulfatase deficiency, chondrodysplasia punctata, X-linked ichthyosis, or ocular albinism.

The autosomal dominant form of Kallmann syndrome (KAL2) occurs in up to 10% of patients, and is caused by a loss of function mutation in the fibroblast growth factor receptor 1 (*FGFR1*) gene. Cleft lip and palate are associated with KAL2 but not with KAL1. Oligodontia and hearing loss may occur with both KAL1 and KAL2.

A variety of other genes, including *FGF8, PROK2/PROKR2, NELF, CHD7* (responsible for CHARGE [coloboma of the eye, heart anomaly, choanal atresia, retardation, and genital and ear anomalies] syndrome, which includes hypogonadism in its phenotype), *HS6ST1, WDR11,* and *SEMA3A,* are associated with defects in neuronal migration that can result in Kallmann syndrome, but in most patients the affected gene remains undefined.

Hypogonadotropic Hypogonadism Without Anosmia

A specific genetic defect is not found in most cases of normosmic idiopathic hypogonadotropic hypogonadism (IHH) but the list of genes associated with this disorder is growing; mutations in the genes *KISS1/KISS1R, TAC3/TACR3,* and *GNRH1/GNRHR* lead to abnormalities in the secretion and action of GnRH and are seen exclusively in patients with normosmic IHH. Mutations in *FGFR1, FGF8, PROKR2, CHD7,* and *WDR11* more commonly present with anosmia/hyposmia (Kallmann syndrome), but are also associated with normosmic IHH in some cases. It appears that kisspeptin (the gene product of the *KISS1* gene) and its G-protein–coupled receptor (GPCR54) play an important role in triggering puberty in humans and act downstream of the leptin receptor in this pathway. Rare cases of leptin deficiency and leptin receptor defects are also associated with HH. In addition, starvation and anorexia are associated with hypogonadism, most likely acting via the leptin pathway.

There are no known human mutations of the *GnRH* gene, but several families with mutations in the GnRH receptor have been described. These mutations account for 2-14% of idiopathic HH without anosmia. The severity of the defect is variable and many patients will respond to high-dose GnRH with increased gonadotropin secretion, indicating that the receptor defect is partial and not complete.

Mutations in gonadotropin genes are extremely rare. Mutations in the common α-subunit are not known in humans. Mutations in the LH-β subunit have been described in a few individuals and may lead to low, absent, or elevated LH levels, depending on the mutation. Defects in the FSH-β subunit may be the cause of azoospermia in a few rare cases.

Children with **X-linked congenital adrenal hypoplasia** have associated HH as a result of impaired GnRH secretion. In these patients, there is a mutation of the *DAX1* gene at Xp21.2-21.3. Conditions occasionally associated with these patients because of the **contiguous gene syndrome** include glycerol kinase deficiency, Duchenne muscular dystrophy, and ornithine transcarbamoyltransferase deficiency. Most boys with *DAX1* mutations develop HH in adolescence, although a patient with adult-onset adrenal insufficiency and partial HH and 2 females with HH and delayed puberty also have been described, the latter as part of extended families with males with classic HH. The *DAX1* gene defect is, however, rare in patients with delayed puberty or HH without at least a family history of adrenal failure (see Chapter 576).

It should be noted that genotype–phenotype correlations in IHH appear to be complex and pedigrees with digenic or oligogenic inheritance have been described. The same genetic defect may be associated with Kallmann syndrome, normosmic IHH, additional birth defects, delayed normal puberty, or an apparently normal phenotype. This variability has been observed more frequently in kindreds with mutations in *FGF8/FGFR1* and in *PROK2/PROKR2* ligand-receptor pairs, and may be from other interacting genes, epigenetic effects, or environmental factors.

Other Disorders with Hypogonadotropic Hypogonadism

HH has been observed in a few patients with polyglandular autoimmune syndrome, in some with elevated melatonin levels, and in those with a variety of other syndromes such as Bardet-Biedl, Prader-Willi, multiple lentigines, and several ataxia syndromes. In rare cases, HH is associated with complex chromosomal abnormalities.

Hypogonadotropic Hypogonadism Associated with Other Pituitary Hormone Deficiencies

Defects in pituitary transcription factors such as PROP-1, HESX-1, LHX-4, SOX-3, and LHX-3 lead to multiple pituitary deficiencies, including HH. Most of these present with multiple pituitary hormone deficiency in infancy, but some cases (especially with *PROP-1* mutations) may present with hypogonadism or hypoadrenalism in adult life. Growth hormone is almost always affected in multiple pituitary hormone deficiency, but thyroid-stimulating hormone and adrenocorticotropic hormone may be spared in some cases. In patients with organic lesions in or near the pituitary, the gonadotropin deficiency is usually pituitary in origin. Microphallus (<2.5 cm at term) in the newborn male with growth hormone deficiency suggests the possibility of gonadotropin deficiency.

DIAGNOSIS

Levels of gonadotropins and gonadal steroids are elevated for up to 6 mo after birth (minipuberty), and if the diagnosis of HH is suspected in early infancy these levels will be found to be inappropriately low. By the second half of the 1st yr of life these levels normally decline to near zero and remain suppressed until late childhood. Therefore, routine lab tests cannot distinguish HH from normal suppression of gonadotropins in this age group. At the normal age of puberty, these patients fail to show clinical signs of puberty or normal increase in LH and FSH levels. Children with constitutional delay of growth and puberty will have the same clinical picture and similar lab findings (and these cases are far more common than true HH, especially in males), and their differentiation from patients with HH is extremely difficult. Dynamic testing with GnRH or hCG may *not* be able to distinguish these groups in a reliable manner. A testosterone level greater than 50 ng/dL (1.7 nmol/L) generally indicates that normal puberty is likely, but a lower level does not reliably distinguish these groups. At least 1 study shows that an inhibin B level of <35 pg/mL in Tanner stage 1 and <65 pg/mL in Tanner stage 2 may be able to distinguish IHH from constitutional delay in males.

Insulin-like growth factor-1, thyroid-stimulating hormone, free thyroxine, and morning cortisol levels should be checked to assess the status of other anterior pituitary hormones; dynamic testing for growth hormone deficiency and adrenal insufficiency may be necessary if these are abnormal or equivocal. HH is very likely if the patient has evidence of another pituitary deficiency, such as a deficiency of growth hormone, particularly if it is associated with adrenocorticotropic hormone deficiency. **Hyperprolactinemia** is a known cause of delayed puberty and should be excluded by determination of serum prolactin levels in all patients. The presence of **anosmia** usually indicates permanent gonadotropin deficiency, but occasional instances of markedly delayed puberty (18-20 yr of age) have been observed in anosmic individuals. Although anosmia may be present in the family or in the patient from early childhood, its existence is rarely volunteered, and direct questioning is necessary in all patients with delayed puberty. Formal olfactometry, such as the University of Pennsylvania Smell Identification Test, is advisable to determine if partial degrees of hyposmia are present because IHH patients display a broad spectrum of olfactory function.

In the absence of family history, it may not be possible to make the diagnosis of HH with certainty, but the diagnosis will become more and more likely as puberty is delayed further beyond the normal age. If pubertal delay persists beyond age 18 yr with low 8 AM testosterone levels and inappropriately low gonadotropins (normal values are inappropriately low in this setting), then the patient can be presumptively diagnosed with HH. An MRI of the brain is indicated to look for tumors and other anomalies in the hypothalamic-pituitary region. Genetic testing for pituitary transcription factors and several of the genes involved in isolated HH is also available and should be performed when possible. A renal ultrasound is recommended in patients with Kallmann syndrome because of its association with unilateral renal agenesis. Some authorities also recommend obtaining a baseline bone-density evaluation.

Treatment

Constitutional delay of puberty should be ruled out before a diagnosis of HH is established and treatment is initiated. Testicular volume of less than 4 mL by 14 yr of age occurs in approximately 3% of boys, but true HH is a rare condition. Even relatively moderate delays in sexual development and growth may result in significant psychologic distress and require attention. Initially, an explanation of the variations characteristic of puberty and reassurance suffice for the majority of boys. If by 15 yr of age no clinical evidence of puberty is beginning and the testosterone level is <50 ng/dL, a brief course of testosterone may be recommended. Various regimens are used, including testosterone enanthate 100 mg intramuscularly once monthly for 4-6 mo or 150 mg once monthly for 3 mo. Some practitioners use oral oxandrolone, which may have the theoretical advantage that it is not aromatized and may have less effect on bone age advancement (though definitive evidence of advantage is lacking). Oral oxandrolone may cause hepatic dysfunction and liver function tests should be monitored if it is used. Treatment is not necessary in all cases of constitutional delay, but if used, it is usually followed by normal progression through puberty and this may differentiate constitutional delay in puberty from isolated gonadotropin deficiency. The age of initiation of this treatment must be individualized.

Once a diagnosis of HH is made, treatment with testosterone will induce secondary sexual characteristics but will *not* stimulate testicular growth or spermatogenesis. Treatment with gonadotropins (either as a combination of hCG and human menopausal gonadotropins or using GnRH pulse therapy) will lead to testicular development, including spermatogenesis, but is much more complex to manage, so in most cases testosterone treatment is the best option. Either long-acting testosterone injections or daily application of testosterone gel may be used (testosterone patches have a high incidence of skin rash and are infrequently used in pediatrics). Testosterone enanthate or cypionate ester may be used in a starting dose of 25-50 mg injected intramuscularly every 3-4 wk, with 50 mg increments every 6-9 mo until a maintenance dose for adults (200-250 mg every 3-4 wk) is achieved. At that time, testosterone patches or testosterone gel may be substituted for the injections. Depending on patient and physician preference, transdermal testosterone may also be used as initial treatment instead of injections. For older boys, larger initial doses and increments can achieve more rapid virilization.

Treatment with gonadotropins is more physiologic but is expensive and complex, so it is less commonly used in adolescence. This treatment may be attempted in adult life when fertility is desired. The treatment schedule varies from 1,250-5,000 IU hCG in combination with 12.5-150 IU human menopausal gonadotropins 3 times per wk intramuscularly. It may require up to 2 yr of treatment to achieve adequate spermatogenesis in adults. Recombinantly produced gonadotropins (LH and FSH) are also able to stimulate gonadal growth and function but are much more expensive. Treatment with GnRH (when available) is the most physiologically appropriate, but it requires the use of a subcutaneous infusion pump to deliver appropriately pulsed therapy because continuous exposure to GnRH will suppress gonadotropins rather than stimulate them. In some cases, patients with GnRH defects also have pituitary or testicular dysfunction (a "dual defect") and may fail to respond adequately to GnRH or gonadotropin treatment. The rare patient with isolated LH deficiency can be treated effectively using hCG injections.

It has been found that up to 10% of patients diagnosed with HH (with or without anosmia) may exhibit spontaneous reversal of hypogonadism with sustained normal gonadal function when treatment has been discontinued; this may occur in patients with known genetic mutations in various genes, including *FGFR1, PROK2, GNRH, CHD7,* and *TAC/TACR3*. Such recovery is more likely in patients who show an increase in testicular volume during treatment or when treatment has been discontinued. Therefore, a brief trial of interruption of treatment is justified in patients with idiopathic HH. However, the recovery of gonadal function may not be lifelong.

Bibliography is available at Expert Consult.

Chapter **584**
Pseudoprecocity Resulting from Tumors of the Testes

Omar Ali and Patricia A. Donohoue

Leydig cell tumors of the testes are rare causes of precocious pseudopuberty (gonadotropin-independent) and cause asymmetric enlargement of the testes. Leydig cells are sparse before puberty and tumors derived from them are more common in the adult, but rare cases do occur in children and the youngest reported case was in a 1 yr old boy. Although up to 10% of adult tumors may be malignant, metastasizing malignant tumors have not been reported in children, and pediatric Leydig cell tumors are usually unilateral and benign. Some tumors may be due to somatic activating mutations of the luteinizing hormone receptor.

The clinical manifestations are those of puberty in the male; onset usually occurs at 5-9 yr of age. Gynecomastia has been described. The tumor of the testis can usually be readily felt; the contralateral unaffected testis is normal in size for the age of the patient.

Plasma levels of testosterone are markedly elevated, and follicle-stimulating hormone and luteinizing hormone levels are suppressed. Ultrasonography may aid in the detection of small nonpalpable tumors. Fine-needle aspiration biopsy may help define the diagnosis.

Treatment consists of surgical removal of the affected testis. These tumors are generally resistant to chemotherapy. Progression of virilization ceases after removal of the tumor, and partial reversal of the signs of precocity may occur.

Testicular adrenal rests may develop into tumors that mimic Leydig cell tumors. Adrenal rest tumors are usually bilateral and occur in children with inadequately controlled congenital adrenal hyperplasia, usually of the salt-losing variety, during adolescence or young adult life. The stimulus for the growth of the adrenal rests is inadequate corticosteroid suppressive therapy causing excess adrenocorticotropic hormone secretion, and treatment with adequate doses almost always results in their regression. These tumors are histologically similar to primary Leydig cell tumors, but definite evidence of the origin of these may be achieved by demonstrating their 21-hydroxylase activity. Misdiagnosis of these tumors as primary Leydig cell tumors may lead to unnecessary orchidectomy and should be avoided.

Fragile X syndrome (see Chapter 81.5) is caused by the amplification of a polymorphic CGG repeat in the 5′ untranslated region of the *FMRI* gene at Xp17.3. The gene encodes an RNA binding protein that is highly expressed in the brain and the testis. In otherwise normal individuals, 6-50 CGG repeats are present in the gene; the presence of 50-200 repeats (permutation) is associated with mild intellectual disability and other abnormalities, and the presence of more than 200 repeats (fragile X mutation) is associated with the classic fragile X syndrome. Permutations are present in 1 in 1,000 white males, and mutations are found in 1 in 4,000-8,000. A cardinal characteristic of the condition is testicular enlargement (**macroorchidism**), reaching 40-50 mL after puberty. Although the condition has been recognized in a child as young as 5 mo of age, affected boys younger than 6 yr of age rarely have testicular enlargement; by 8-10 yr of age, most have testicular volumes greater than 3 mL. The testes are enlarged bilaterally, are not nodular, and are histologically normal. Results of hormonal studies are normal. Direct DNA analysis searching for CGG repeat sequences permits definitive diagnosis.

Large-cell calcifying Sertoli cell tumors of the testes and **sex cord tumors with annular tubules** are extremely rare Sertoli cell tumors that may be a cause of breast development in young boys. These tumors are usually associated with Peutz-Jeghers syndrome or Carney complex; they often occur bilaterally, are multifocal, and are detectible by ultrasonography. Excessive production of aromatase (P450arom), the enzyme that converts testosterone to estradiol, causes feminization of these boys. Because they are usually benign, they may be left in place if they are not causing pain; the gynecomastia can be treated with aromatase inhibitors.

In boys with **unilateral cryptorchidism,** the contralateral testis is approximately 25% larger than normal for age. Testicular enlargement has also been noted in boys with Henoch-Schönlein purpura and lymphangiectasia. Epidermoid and dermoid cysts of the testes have been reported rarely.

Bibliography is available at Expert Consult.

Chapter **585**
Gynecomastia
Omar Ali and Patricia A. Donohoue

Gynecomastia, the proliferation of mammary glandular tissue in the male, is a common condition. True gynecomastia (the presence of glandular breast tissue) needs to be distinguished from pseudogynecomastia, which is the result of accumulation of adipose tissue in the area of the breast that is commonly seen in overweight boys. True gynecomastia is characterized by the presence of a palpable fibroglandular mass at least 0.5 cm in diameter, located concentrically beneath the nipple and areolar region.

PHYSIOLOGIC FORMS OF GYNECOMASTIA
Gynecomastia occurs in many newborn males as a result of normal stimulation by maternal estrogen; the effect usually disappears in a few weeks. It is then extremely rare in prepubertal boys, in whom it should always be investigated to identify the cause, but again becomes common during normal puberty.

Neonatal Gynecomastia
Transient gynecomastia occurs in 60-90% of male newborns secondary to exposure to estrogens during pregnancy. Breast development may be asymmetrical and galactorrhea is seen in approximately 5%. Most cases resolve within 4-8 wk of birth, but a few can last as long as 12 mo.

Pubertal Gynecomastia
During early puberty to midpuberty, up to 70% of boys develop various degrees of subareolar hyperplasia of the breasts. Incidence peaks at 14 yr of age, at Tanner stage 3-4 and at a testicular volume of 5-10 mL. Physiologic pubertal gynecomastia may involve only 1 breast; it is not unusual for both breasts to enlarge at disproportionate rates or at different times. Tenderness of the breast is common but transitory. Spontaneous regression may occur within a few months; it rarely persists longer than 2 yr. Significant psychosocial distress may be present, especially in obese boys with relatively large breasts.

The cause is thought to be an imbalance between estrogen and androgen action at the level of breast tissue. Testing usually fails to reveal any significant difference in circulating estrogen and androgen levels between affected and unaffected males, but minor degrees of imbalance in free hormone levels may still be present. Other hormones, including leptin and luteinizing hormone, may directly stimulate breast development and may play a role in pubertal gynecomastia. Some cases may be caused by an increased sensitivity to estrogens and/or relative androgen resistance in the affected tissue. As androgen levels continue to rise in later puberty, most cases resolve.

Pathologic Gynecomastia
See Table 585-1.

Monogenic forms of gynecomastia are extremely rare, but do exist. Familial gynecomastia has occurred in several kindreds as an X-linked or autosomal dominant sex-limited trait. Some of these cases were found to be caused by constitutive activation of the P450 aromatase enzyme (*CYP19A1* gene), leading to increased peripheral conversion of C-19 steroids to estrogens (increased aromatization). A report of this syndrome in a father and his son and daughter suggests autosomal dominant inheritance. Excess aromatase activity was shown in skin fibroblasts and transformed lymphocytes in vitro.

Exogenous sources of estrogens are an important cause of gynecomastia in prepubertal children. Very small amounts of estrogens can cause gynecomastia in male children and accidental exposure may occur by inhalation, percutaneous absorption, or ingestion. Common sources of estrogens include oral contraceptive pills and oral and transdermal estrogen preparations. Gynecomastia has been reported in workers involved in the manufacture of estrogens and even in the children of such workers. Gynecomastia can also occur secondary to exposure to medications that decrease the level of androgens (especially free androgens), increase estradiol, or displace androgens from breast androgen receptors. Spironolactone, alkylating agents, anabolic steroids, human chorionic gonadotropin, ketoconazole, cimetidine, and androgen inhibitors such as flutamide are all associated with the occurrence of gynecomastia. Weaker associations are seen with a large number of other medications and drugs of abuse, including opiates, alcohol, and marijuana, although the association with marijuana may not be as strong as previously thought. Lavender, tea oils, and excessive consumption of soy are also implicated as causes of prepubertal gynecomastia.

Klinefelter syndrome and other causes of **male hypogonadism** are strongly associated with gynecomastia. Significant gynecomastia is seen in 50% of adolescents with Klinefelter syndrome; it is also seen in other conditions characterized by male undervirilization, including partial androgen insensitivity syndrome and 17-ketosteroid reductase deficiency. Gynecomastia has also been observed in children with congenital virilizing adrenal hyperplasia (11β-hydroxylase deficiency) and with Leydig cell tumors of the testis or with feminizing tumors of the adrenal gland. Several boys with Peutz-Jeghers syndrome and gynecomastia had sex cord tumors of the testes. The testes may not be enlarged in these cases and the tumor is usually multifocal and bilateral. Excessive aromatase production accounts for the gynecomastia. When gynecomastia is associated with galactorrhea, a prolactinoma should be considered. Hyperthyroidism alters the androgen to estrogen ratio by increasing bound androgen and decreasing the free testosterone and may result in gynecomastia in up to 40% of cases. Gynecomastia is also seen in malnourished patients after restoration of normal nutrition (refeeding syndrome), in whom it may be from hepatic dysfunction or abnormal activation of the gonadotropin axis.

EVALUATION OF GYNECOMASTIA
In pubertal cases a detailed history and physical examination may be all that is needed to exclude rare pathologic causes. Historical evaluation should include family history of male relatives with gynecomastia, history of liver or renal disease, use of medications or drugs of abuse, and exposure to herbal and cosmetic products that may contain phytoestrogens. Physical examination should include special attention to the breasts (looking for overlying skin changes, fixation, local lymphadenopathy, and nipple discharge) as well as a testicular exam. No

Table 585-1	Causes of Gynecomastia
SYMPTOMS	**SIGNS**

FETAL ANDROGEN DEFICIENCY

Ambiguous genitalia	Ambiguous genitalia (47,XY disorders of sex development)
	Normal female genitalia
	Microphallus (resembling clitoromegaly)
	Pseudovaginal perineoscrotal hypospadias
	Bifid scrotum
	Cryptorchidism

PREPUBERTAL ANDROGEN DEFICIENCY

Delayed puberty	Eunuchoidism
Lack of sexual interest or desire (libido)	Infantile genitalia
	Small testes
Reduced nighttime or morning spontaneous erections	Lack of male hair pattern growth, no acne
Breast enlargement and tenderness	Disproportionately long arms and legs relative to height
Reduced motivation and initiative	Pubertal fat distribution
Diminished strength and physical performance	Poorly developed muscle mass
	High-pitched voice
No ejaculate or ejaculation (spermarche)	Reduced peak bone mass, osteopenia, or osteoporosis
	Gynecomastia
Inability to father children (infertility)	Small prostate gland
	Aspermia, severe oligozoospermia, or azoospermia

ADULT ANDROGEN DEFICIENCY

Incomplete sexual development	Eunuchoidism
Lack of sexual interest or desire (libido)	Small or shrinking testes
Reduced nighttime or morning spontaneous erections	Loss of male hair (axillary and pubic hair)
	Gynecomastia
Breast enlargement and tenderness	Aspermia or azoospermia or severe oligozoospermia
Inability to father children (infertility)	Low bone mineral density (osteopenia or osteoporosis)
Height loss, history of minimal-trauma fracture	Height loss, minimal-trauma or vertebral compression fracture
Hot flushes, sweats	
Reduced shaving frequency	Unexplained reduction in prostate size or prostate-specific antigen

Less-Specific Symptoms	**Less-Specific Signs**
Decreased energy, vitality	Mild normocytic, normochromic anemia (normal female range)
Decreased motivation, self-confidence	Depressed mood, mild depression or dysthymia
Feeling sad or blue, irritability	Reduced muscle bulk and strength
Weakness, decreased physical or work performance	Increased body fat or body mass index
Poor concentration and memory	Fine facial skin wrinkling (lateral to orbits and mouth)
Increased sleepiness	

From Matsumoto AM, Bremner WJ: Testicular disorders. In Melmed S, Polonsky KS, Larsen PR, Kronenberg HM, editors: Williams textbook of endocrinology, ed 12, Philadelphia, 2011, WB Saunders, Table 19-3, p. 719.

laboratory evaluation is indicated in routine cases with no other associated abnormality but all prepubertal cases, as well as pubertal cases with suspicious features, should be investigated; initial laboratory evaluation should include thyroid function tests (to rule out hyperthyroidism), testosterone, estradiol, human chorionic gonadotropin, luteinizing hormone, and prolactin levels. Most cases of hyperprolactinemia are associated with galactorrhea, but there are a few reports of hyperprolactinemia causing gynecomastia without associated galactorrhea. Because of circadian variation, these levels should ideally be obtained in the morning. Other tests that may be indicated

in selected cases include a karyotype, dehydroepiandrosterone sulfate, and liver and renal function tests. Gonadotropin levels may be a useful screen for Klinefelter syndrome and will be elevated in pubertal boys with this condition. If elevated, a karyotype should be performed.

TREATMENT

Treatment in case of benign pubertal gynecomastia usually consists of reassuring the boy and his family of the physiologic and transient nature of the phenomenon. When the enlargement is striking and persistent and causes serious emotional disturbance to the patient, specific treatment may be justified. Unfortunately, medical treatment is generally ineffective in long-standing cases. Early cases respond better to medical treatment but it is harder to justify treatment as most cases will resolve spontaneously. Agents that have been used for medical treatment include androgens, aromatase inhibitors, and estrogen antagonists. The effectiveness of synthetic androgens is variable and side effects are a concern, so these are rarely used in pediatrics. Aromatase inhibitors make physiologic sense, but placebo-controlled trials have been disappointing. Estrogen antagonists like tamoxifen and raloxifene are more effective, with raloxifene being the superior agent in at least 1 well-designed trial. If medical treatment is attempted, it should be in early cases (<12 mo standing) using raloxifene (in a dose of 60 mg/day) or tamoxifen (10-20 mg/day) for 3-9 mo, with the understanding that success rates are generally low in severe cases and mild cases will likely resolve on their own without treatment.

In those cases where breast development is excessive (Tanner stages 3-5), causes significant psychologic distress, and fails to regress in 18-24 mo, surgical removal of the enlarged breast tissue may be indicated, particularly in boys who have completed or nearly completed pubertal development. Careful examination and laboratory testing to exclude nonphysiologic causes are advisable before proceeding to surgery.

Bibliography is available at Expert Consult.

Chapter **586**
Hypofunction of the Ovaries
Alvina R. Kansra and Patricia A. Donohoue

Hypofunction of the ovaries can be either primary or central in etiology. It may be caused by congenital failure of development, postnatal destruction (primary or hypergonadotropic hypogonadism), or lack of central stimulation by the pituitary and/or hypothalamus (secondary or tertiary hypogonadotropic hypogonadism). **Primary ovarian insufficiency** (hypergonadotropic hypogonadism), which is also termed *premature ovarian failure*, is characterized by the arrest of normal ovarian function before the age of 40 yr. Certain genetic mutations can result in primary ovarian insufficiency. Hypofunction of the ovaries because of a lack of central stimulation (hypogonadotropic hypogonadism) can be associated with other processes, such as multiple pituitary hormone deficiencies and some chronic diseases. Table 586-1 details the etiologic classification of ovarian hypofunction.

586.1 Hypergonadotropic Hypogonadism in the Female (Primary Hypogonadism)
Alvina R. Kansra and Patricia A. Donohoue

Diagnosis of hypergonadotropic hypogonadism before puberty is difficult. Except in the case of Turner syndrome, most affected patients have no prepubertal clinical manifestations.

Table 586-1	Etiologic Classification of Ovarian Hypofunction

HYPOGONADOTROPIC HYPOGONADISM

Hypothalamic

Genetic defects
- Kallmann syndrome *KAL1, FGFR1, FGF8, PROK2, PROKR2, CHD7, WDR11, NELF, SEMA3A*
- Other gene defects: leptin, leptin receptor, *KISS-1* (deficiency of kisspeptin), *DAX-1, TAC3* (deficiency of neurokinin B), *TACR3, SEMA7A*
- Inherited syndromes: Prader-Willi, Bardet-Biedl, and others
- Marked constitutional growth delay

Acquired defects (reversible)
- Anorexia nervosa
- Drug use
- Malnutrition
- Chronic illness, especially Crohn disease
- Hyperprolactinemia

Pituitary

Genetic defects
- Isolated gonadotropin deficiency (GnRH receptor, FSH, and LH β-subunit)
- Septooptic dysplasia (*HESX-1* in some cases)
- Disorders of pituitary organogenesis (*PROP1, LHX3, LHX4, SOX-3,* etc.)

Acquired defects
- Pituitary tumors
- Pituitary infarction
- Infiltrative disorders (histiocytosis, sarcoidosis)
- Hemosiderosis and hemochromatosis
- Radiation

HYPERGONADOTROPIC HYPOGONADISM

Genetic

Follicle-stimulating hormone and luteinizing hormone resistance
Mutations in steroidogenic pathways
46,XX gonadal dysgenesis
Turner syndrome and its variants
Noonan syndrome (*PTPN-11* gene)
SF-1 gene mutations
Galactosemia
Fragile X–associated disorders
Bloom syndrome
Werner syndrome
Ataxia-telangiectasia
Fanconi anemia

Acquired

Chemotherapy
Radiation
Autoimmune ovarian failure from autoimmune polyendocrine syndromes 1 and 2

TURNER SYNDROME

Turner described a syndrome consisting of sexual infantilism, webbed neck, and cubitus valgus in adult females (see Chapter 81). Ullrich described a girl with short stature and many of the same phenotypic features. The term *Ullrich-Turner syndrome* is frequently used in Europe, but is infrequently used in the United States where the condition is called Turner syndrome. The syndrome is defined as the combination of the characteristic phenotypic features accompanied by complete or partial absence of the second X chromosome with or without mosaicism.

Pathogenesis

Half the patients with Turner syndrome have a 45,X chromosomal complement. Approximately 15% of patients are mosaics for 45,X and a normal cell line (45,X/46,XX). Other mosaics with isochromosomes, 45,X/46,X,i(Xq); with rings, 45,X/46,X,r(X); or with fragments, 45,X/46fra, occur less often. Mosaicism is detected most commonly when more than 1 tissue is examined. The single X is of maternal origin in nearly 80% of 45,X patients. The mechanism of chromosome loss is

unknown, and the risk for the syndrome does not increase with maternal age. The genes involved in the Turner phenotype are X-linked genes that escape inactivation. A major locus involved in the control of linear growth has been mapped within the pseudoautosomal region of the X chromosome (PAR1). *SHOX*, a homeobox-containing gene of 170 kb of DNA within the PAR1, is thought to be important for controlling growth in children with Turner syndrome, Leri-Weill syndrome, and, rarely, in patients having idiopathic short stature. Genes for the control of normal ovarian function are postulated to be on Xp and perhaps 2 "supergenes" on Xq.

Turner syndrome occurs in approximately 1 in 1,500-2,500 liveborn females. The frequency of the 45,X karyotype at *conception* is approximately 3%, but 99% of these are spontaneously aborted, accounting for 5-10% of all abortuses. Mosaicism (45,X/46,XX) occurs in a proportion higher than that seen with any other aneuploid state, but the mosaic Turner constitution is rare among the abortuses; these findings indicate preferential survival for mosaic forms.

The normal fetal ovary contains approximately 7 million oocytes, but these begin to disappear rapidly after the 5th mo of gestation. At birth, there are only 2 million (1 million active follicles); by menarche, there are 400,000-500,000; and at menopause, 10,000 remain. In the absence of 1 X chromosome, this process is accelerated, and nearly all oocytes are gone by 2 yr of age. In aborted 45,X fetuses, the number of primordial germ cells in the gonadal ridge appears to be normal, suggesting that the normal process is accelerated in patients with Turner syndrome. Eventually, the ovaries are described as "streaks" and consist only of connective tissue, with very few germ cells present.

Clinical Manifestations

Many patients with Turner syndrome are recognizable at birth because of a characteristic edema of the dorsa of the hands and feet and loose skinfolds at the nape of the neck. Low birthweight and decreased birth length are common (see Chapter 81). Clinical manifestations in childhood include webbing of the neck, a low posterior hairline, small mandible, prominent ears, epicanthal folds, high arched palate, a broad chest presenting the illusion of widely spaced nipples, cubitus valgus, and hyperconvex fingernails. The diagnosis is often first suspected at puberty when breast development fails to occur.

Short stature, the cardinal finding in virtually all girls with Turner syndrome, may be present with little in the way of other clinical manifestations. The linear growth deceleration begins in infancy and young childhood, gets progressively more pronounced in later childhood and adolescence, and results in significant adult short stature. Sexual maturation (breast development) fails to occur at the expected age; however, signs of adrenarche (pubic hair) are normally present. Among untreated patients with Turner syndrome, the mean adult height is 143-144 cm in the United States and most of northern Europe, but 140 cm in Argentina and 147 cm in Scandinavia (Fig. 586-1). The height is well correlated with the midparental height (average of the parents' heights). Specific growth curves for height have been developed for girls with Turner syndrome.

Associated **cardiac defects** are common. In the girls with Turner syndrome, life-threatening consequences of X-chromosome haploinsufficiency involve the cardiovascular system. There is a 4-5-fold increased rate of premature mortality secondary to congenital heart disease and premature coronary heart disease in adults with Turner syndrome. Clinically silent cardiac defects, mainly bicuspid aortic valve but also ascending aortic dilation, coarctation of the aorta, and partial anomalous pulmonary venous connections, are present in patients with Turner syndrome. Regardless of the age, all patients with Turner syndrome at the time of diagnosis need comprehensive cardiovascular evaluation by a cardiologist specializing in congenital heart disease. Complete cardiologic evaluation, including echocardiography, reveals isolated nonstenotic bicuspid aortic valves in one third to one half of patients. In later life, bicuspid aortic valve disease can progress to dilation of the aortic root. Less-frequent defects include aortic coarctation (20%), aortic stenosis, mitral valve prolapse, and anomalous pulmonary venous drainage. In 1 study, 38% of patients with 45,X chromosomes had cardiovascular malformations compared with 11%

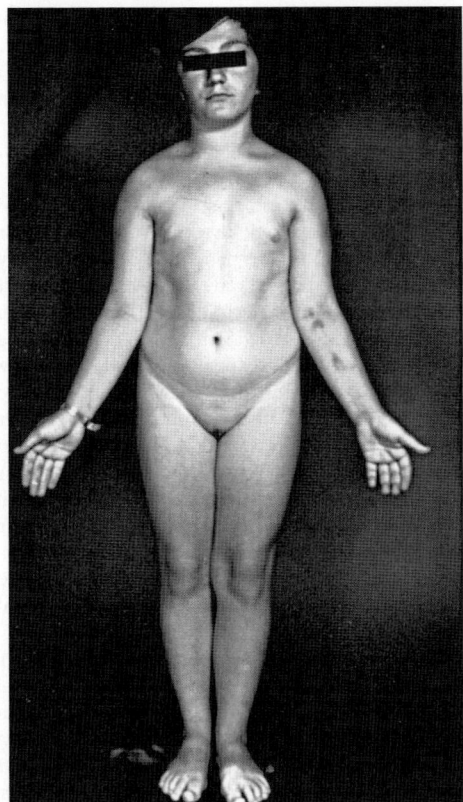

Figure 586-1 Turner syndrome in a 15 yr old girl exhibiting failure of sexual maturation, short stature, cubitus valgus, and a goiter. There is no webbing of the neck. Karyotyping revealed 45,X/46,XX chromosome complement.

of those with mosaic monosomy X; the most common were aortic valve abnormalities and aortic coarctation. *Webbed neck in patients with or without recognized chromosome syndromes is associated with both flow-related and non–flow-related heart defects.* Among patients with Turner syndrome, those with webbed necks have a much greater chance of having coarctation of the aorta than do those without webbed necks. Transthoracic echocardiogram in young girls is adequate if cardiac anatomy is clearly seen; otherwise magnetic resonance angiographic screening studies should be considered in asymptomatic individuals with Turner syndrome. During adolescence, and certainly before pregnancy (when possible) is contemplated, repeat cardiac evaluation should be considered even in those without prior findings of cardiac abnormalities. Blood pressure should be routinely monitored even in the absence of cardiac or renal lesions and especially in those with suggestions of aortic root dilation. Cardiac MRI is a valuable tool to detect and monitor aortic root dilation.

Renal ultrasound should be performed in all girls with Turner syndrome at diagnosis. One fourth to one third of patients have **renal malformations** on ultrasonographic examination (50% of those with 45,X karyotypes). The more serious defects include pelvic kidney, horseshoe kidney, double collecting system, complete absence of 1 kidney, and ureteropelvic junction obstruction. Some of the malformations may increase the risk of hypertension and urinary tract infection. Idiopathic hypertension is also common. Girls with Turner syndrome who had normal baseline renal ultrasound findings did not develop renal disease during a follow-up period averaging 6 yr.

When the ovaries were examined by ultrasonography, older studies found a significant decrease in percentage of detectable ovaries from infancy to later childhood. A subsequent report found no such age-related differences in a cross-sectional and longitudinal study; 27-46% of patients had detectable ovaries at various ages; 76% of those with X mosaicism and 26% of those with 45,X karyotypes had detectable ovaries.

Sexual maturation usually fails to occur, but 10-20% of girls have spontaneous breast development, and a small percentage may have menstrual periods. Primary gonadal failure is associated with early onset of adrenarche (elevation in dehydroepiandrosterone sulfate) but delayed pubarche (pubic hair development). Spontaneous pregnancies have been reported in menstruating patients with Turner syndrome. Premature menopause, increased risk of miscarriage, and offspring with increased risk of trisomy 21 have been reported. A woman with a 45,X/46,X,r(X) karyotype treated with hormone replacement therapy had 3 pregnancies, resulting in a normal 46,XY male infant, a spontaneous abortion, and a healthy term female with Turner syndrome 45,X/46,Xr(X).

Antithyroid antibodies (thyroid peroxidase, and/or thyroglobulin antibodies) occur in 30-50% of patients. The prevalence increases with advancing age. **Autoimmune thyroid disease,** with or without the presence of a goiter, occurs in 10-30% of patients. Age-dependent abnormalities in carbohydrate metabolism characterized by abnormal glucose tolerance and insulin resistance and, only rarely, frank type 2 diabetes occur in older patients with Turner syndrome. Impaired insulin secretion has been described in 45,X women. Cholesterol levels are elevated in adolescence, regardless of body mass index or karyotype.

Inflammatory bowel disease, both Crohn disease and ulcerative colitis, gastrointestinal bleeding because of abnormal mesenteric vasculature, and delayed gastric emptying time have all been reported. Screening for celiac disease is recommended by recent guidelines, as the risk of celiac disease is increased in Turner syndrome, with 4-6% of individuals affected. Although autoimmune diseases have been associated with Turner syndrome, the prevalence of type 1 diabetes with Turner syndrome is not very high.

Sternal malformations can be detected by lateral chest radiography. An increased carrying angle at the elbow is usually not clinically significant. Scoliosis occurs in approximately 10% of adolescent girls. Congenital hip dysplasia occurs more commonly than in the general population. Reported eye findings include anterior segment dysgenesis and keratoconus. Pigmented nevi become more prominent with age; melanocytic nevi are common. Essential hyperhidrosis, torus mandibularis, and alopecia areata occur rarely.

Recurrent bilateral otitis media develops in approximately 75% of patients. Sensorineural hearing deficits are common, and the frequency increases with age. Problems with gross and fine motor-sensory integration, failure to walk before 15 mo of age, and early language dysfunction often raise questions about developmental delay, but intelligence is normal in most patients. However, cognitive impairment does occur in patients with 45,X/46,X,r(X); the ring chromosome is unable to undergo inactivation and leads to 2 functional X chromosomes.

Special attention should be given to psychosocial development in girls with Turner syndrome. In general, the behavior function is normal in girls with Turner syndrome, but they are at an increased risk for social isolation, immaturity, and anxiety. Other conditions, such as dyslexia, nonverbal learning disability, and attention deficit disorder, have been reported in girls with Turner syndrome. In adults, deficits in perceptual spatial skills are more common than they are in the general population. Some unconfirmed data suggest the existence of an imprinted X-linked locus that affects cognitive function such as verbal and higher-order executive function skills. These functions are apparently better when the X is paternal in origin.

The prevalence of mosaicism depends in large part on the techniques used for studying chromosomal patterns. The use of fluorescent in situ hybridization and reverse transcription–polymerase chain reaction (PCR) has increased the reported prevalence of mosaic patterns to as high as 60-74%.

Mosaicism involving the Y chromosome occurs in 5%. A population study using PCR with 5 different primer sets found Y chromosome material in 12.2%. **Gonadoblastoma** among Y-positive patients occurred in 7-10%. Therefore, the recommendation is that prophylactic gonadectomy should be performed even in the absence of MRI or CT evidence of tumors. The recommended timing of this procedure is at the time of diagnosis, but this may need to be reevaluated in the future. The gonadoblastoma locus on the Y chromosome (GBY) maps close to the Y centromere. The presence of only the SRY (sex-determining region on the Y chromosome) locus is not sufficient to confer increased susceptibility for the development of gonadoblastoma. A detailed study of 53 patients with Turner syndrome by nested PCR excluded low-level Y mosaicism in almost all cases. A second round of PCR detected SRY on the distal short arm of the Y chromosome in only 2 subjects. Therefore, routine PCR for Y chromosome detection for the purpose of assigning gonadoblastoma risk is not indicated. High-throughput quantitative genotyping may provide an effective and inexpensive method for the identification of X chromosome abnormalities and Y chromosome material identification.

In patients with 45,X/46,XX mosaicism, the clinical abnormalities are attenuated and fewer; short stature is as frequent as it is in the 45,X patient and may be the only manifestation of the condition other than ovarian failure (see Fig. 586-1).

Laboratory Findings
Chromosomal analysis must be considered routinely in short girls. In a systematic search, using Southern blot analysis of leukocyte DNA, Turner syndrome was detected in 4.8% of girls referred to an endocrinology service because of short stature. Patients with a marker chromosome in some or all cells should be tested for DNA sequences at or near the centromere of the Y chromosome for GBY.

Ultrasonography of the heart, kidneys, and ovaries is indicated after the diagnosis is established. The most common skeletal abnormalities are shortening of the 4th metatarsal and metacarpal bones, epiphyseal dysgenesis in the joints of the knees and elbows, Madelung deformity, scoliosis, and in older patients, inadequate osseous mineralization.

Plasma levels of gonadotropins, particularly follicle-stimulating hormone (FSH), are markedly elevated to greater than those of age-matched controls during infancy; at 2-3 yr of age, a progressive decrease in levels occurs until they reach a nadir at 6-8 yr of age, and by 10-11 yr of age, they rise to adult castrate levels.

Antithyroid peroxidase and antithyroglobulin antibodies should be checked periodically, and if positive, levels of thyroxine and thyroid-stimulating hormone should be obtained. Turner syndrome girls should be screened for **celiac disease** by measuring tissue transglutaminase immunoglobulin A antibodies. Initial testing should be done around age 4 yr and repeated every 2-5 yr. Extensive studies have failed to establish that growth hormone deficiency plays a primary role in the pathogenesis of the growth disorder. Defects in normal secretory patterns of growth hormone are seen in adolescents because of a lack of gonadal steroids, but not in younger girls with Turner syndrome. In vitro, monocytes and lymphocytes show decreased sensitivity to insulin-like growth factor 1.

Treatment
Treatment with recombinant human growth hormone increases height velocity and ultimate stature in most, but not all, children with Turner syndrome. Many girls achieve heights of greater than 150 cm with early initiation of treatment. In a large, multicenter, placebo-controlled clinical trial, 99 patients with Turner syndrome who started receiving growth hormone at a mean age of 10.9 yr at doses between 0.27 and 0.36 mg/kg/wk achieved a mean height of 149 cm, with nearly one third reaching heights greater than 152.4 cm (60 in). In the Netherlands, higher doses of growth hormone (up to 0.63 mg/kg/wk in the 3rd yr of treatment) resulted in 85% of the subjects reaching adult heights in the normal range for the Dutch reference population. Growth hormone treatment should be initiated in early childhood and/or when there is evidence of height velocity attenuation on specific Turner syndrome growth curves. The average starting dose of growth hormone is 0.375 mg/kg/wk. Growth hormone therapy does not significantly aggravate carbohydrate tolerance and does not result in marked adverse events in patients with Turner syndrome. Serum levels of insulin-like growth factor 1 should be monitored if the patient is receiving high doses of growth hormone. If the insulin-like growth factor 1 levels are significantly elevated, the dose of growth hormone may need to be reduced. Treatment with growth hormone can cause

excessive growth of the hands and feet in some girls with Turner syndrome.

Oxandrolone has also been used to treat the short stature associated with Turner syndrome, either alone or in combination with growth hormone. This synthetic anabolic steroid has weak androgenic effects, and patients should be monitored for signs of pubarche, as well as hepatotoxicity. The latter is rare.

Replacement therapy with estrogens is indicated, but there is little consensus about the optimal age at which to initiate treatment. The psychologic preparedness of the patient to accept therapy must be taken into account. The improved growth achieved by girls treated with growth hormone in childhood permits initiation of estrogen replacement at 12-13 yr. Delaying estrogen therapy to optimize height potential until 15 yr of age, as previously recommended, seems unwarranted. This change to starting earlier estrogen therapy was considered because of the psychologic importance of age-appropriate pubertal maturation. Also, delaying estrogen therapy could be deleterious for bone health and other aspects of the child's health. Low-dose estrogen replacement at 12 yr of age permits a normal pace of puberty without interfering with the positive effect of growth hormone on the final adult height. Estrogen therapy improves verbal and nonverbal memory in girls with Turner syndrome. In young women with age-appropriate pubertal development who achieve normal height, health-related quality-of-life questionnaires have yielded normal results.

Although many forms of estrogen are available, oral estrogens have been mostly used. Even though transdermal and injectable depot forms of estradiol may be alternative physiologic options, transdermal patches are increasing in popularity. This is because transdermal patches bypass the first hepatic metabolism, thereby requiring only a small amount of estrogen to attain the adequate levels for its function. For oral preparation a conjugated estrogen (Premarin), 0.15-0.625 mg daily, or micronized estradiol (Estrace), 0.5 mg given daily for 3-6 mo, is usually effective in inducing puberty. The recommendations for transdermal patch are 6.25 µg daily that is gradually increased over 2 yr to the adult dose of 100-200 µg daily. The estrogen then is cycled (taken on days 1-23) and a progestin (Provera) is added (taken on days 10-23) in a dose of 5-10 mg daily. In the remainder of the calendar month, during which no treatment is given, withdrawal bleeding usually occurs.

Prenatal chromosome analysis for advanced maternal age has revealed a frequency of 45,X/46,XX that is 10 times higher than when diagnosed postnatally. Most of these patients have no clinical manifestations of Turner syndrome, and levels of gonadotropins are normal. Awareness of this mild phenotype is important in counseling patients.

Psychosocial support for these girls is an integral component of treatment. A comprehensive psychologic education evaluation is recommended either at the time of Turner syndrome diagnosis, depending on the patient's age, when any of the components of behavior or cognition become obvious, or immediately preceding school entry. The Turner Syndrome Society, which has local chapters in the United States, and similar groups in Canada and other countries provide a valuable support system for these patients and their families in addition to that given by the healthcare team.

Successful pregnancies have been carried to term using ovum donation and in vitro fertilization. Adolescents with few signs of spontaneous puberty may have ovaries with follicles. There remains a future possibility of using cryopreserved ovarian tissue with immature oocytes before the regression of the ovaries for the future pregnancies. In adult women with Turner syndrome, there seems to be a high prevalence of undiagnosed bone mineral density, lipid, and thyroid abnormalities. Glucose intolerance, diminished 1st-phase insulin response, elevated blood pressure, and lowered fat-free mass are common. Glucose tolerance worsens, but fat-free mass and blood pressure and general physical fitness improve with sex hormone replacement. The neurocognitive profile of adult women is unaffected by estrogen status.

XX GONADAL DYSGENESIS
Some phenotypically and genetically normal females have gonadal lesions identical to those in 45,X patients but without somatic features

of Turner syndrome; their condition is termed **pure gonadal dysgenesis** or **pure ovarian dysgenesis**.

The disorder is rarely recognized in prepubertal children because the external genitals are normal, no other abnormalities are visible, and growth is normal. At pubertal age, sexual maturation fails to take place. Plasma gonadotropin levels are elevated. Delay of epiphyseal fusion may result in a **eunuchoid** habitus. Pelvic ultrasonography reveals streak ovaries.

Affected siblings, parental consanguinity, and failure to uncover mosaicism all point to female-limited autosomal recessive inheritance. The disorder appears to be especially frequent in Finland (1 in 8,300 liveborn girls). In this population, several mutations in the FSH receptor gene (on chromosome 2p) were demonstrated as the cause of the condition. FSH receptor gene mutations were not detected in Mexican women with 46,XX gonadal dysgenesis. In some patients, XX gonadal dysgenesis has been associated with sensorineural deafness (**Perrault syndrome**). A patient with this condition and concomitant growth hormone deficiency and virilization has also been reported. There may be distinct genetic forms of this disorder. **Müllerian agenesis**, or the **Mayer-Rokitansky-Küster-Hauser** syndrome, which is second to gonadal dysgenesis as the most common cause of primary amenorrhea, occurring in 1 in 4,000-5,000 females, has been reported in association with 46,XX gonadal dysgenesis in a 17 yr old adolescent with primary amenorrhea and lack of breast development. One case of dysgerminoma with syncytiotrophoblastic giant cells was reported. An 18 yr old woman with primary amenorrhea and an absence of müllerian-derived structures, unilateral renal agenesis, and clinical signs of androgen excess, a phenotype resembling the Mayer-Rokitansky-Küster-Hauser syndrome, was found to have a loss-of-function mutation in the *WNT4* gene. Treatment consists of estrogen replacement therapy.

45,X/46,XY GONADAL DYSGENESIS

45,X/46,XY gonadal dysgenesis, also called **mixed gonadal dysgenesis**, has extreme phenotypic variability postnatally that may extend from a Turner-like syndrome to a male phenotype with a penile urethra; it is possible to delineate 3 major clinical phenotypes. Short stature is a major finding in all affected children. Ninety percent of prenatally diagnosed cases have a normal male phenotype.

Some patients have no evidence of virilization; they have a female phenotype and often have the somatic signs of Turner syndrome. The condition is discovered prepubertally when chromosomal studies are made in short girls, or later when chromosomal studies are made because of failure of sexual maturation. Fallopian tubes and uterus are present. The gonads consist of intraabdominal undifferentiated streaks; chromosomal study of the streak often reveals an XY cell line. The streak gonad differs somewhat from that in girls with Turner syndrome; in addition to wavy connective tissue, there are often tubular or cordlike structures, occasional clumps of granulosa cells, and frequently, mesonephric or hilar cells.

Some children have mild virilization manifested only by prepubertal clitoromegaly. Normal müllerian structures are present, but at puberty virilization occurs. These patients usually have an intraabdominal testis, a contralateral streak gonad, and bilateral fallopian tubes.

Many 45,X/46,XY children present with frank ambiguity of the genitals in infancy. A testis and vas deferens are found on one side in the labioscrotal fold, and a streak gonad is identified on the contralateral side. Despite the presence of a testis, fallopian tubes are often present bilaterally. An infantile or rudimentary uterus is almost always present.

Other genotypes and phenotypes have been described in mixed gonadal dysgenesis. Approximately 25% of 200 analyzed patients have a dicentric Y chromosome (45,X/46,X,dic Y). In some patients, the Y chromosome may be represented by only a fragment (45,X/45,X +fra); application of Y-specific probes can establish the origin of the fragment. It is not clear why the same genotype (45,X/46,XY) can result in such diverse phenotypes. Mutations in the *SRY* gene have been described in some patients.

Children with a female phenotype present no problem in gender of rearing. Patients who are only slightly virilized are usually assigned a female gender of rearing before a diagnosis is established. Patients with ambiguity of the genitals are readily often clinically indistinguishable

from patients with various types of 46,XY disorders of sex development (46,XY DSD). In some instances, there may need to be careful consideration regarding sex of rearing. Factors that may influence this decision include short stature, the need for surgical genital reconstruction, the presence of müllerian structures, and the need for gonadectomy because of predisposition of the gonad to the development of malignancy. In some patients followed to adulthood, the putative normal testis proves to be dysgenetic with eventual loss of Leydig and Sertoli cell function (see Chapter 583). In an analysis of 22 patients with mixed gonadal dysgenesis, no significant associations or correlations were found between internal and external phenotypes or endocrine function and gonadal morphologic features. The sex of rearing was determined by the appearance of the external genitalia. In 11 patients, basal and human chorionic gonadotropin–stimulated testosterone levels were lower than in control subjects.

Gonadal tumors, usually **gonadoblastomas,** occur in approximately 25% of these children. As described above, a gonadoblastoma locus has been localized to a region near the centromere of the Y chromosome (GBY). These germ cell tumors are preceded by the changes of carcinoma in situ. Accordingly, both gonads should be removed in all patients reared as girls, and the undifferentiated gonad should be removed in the patients reared as boys.

There is no correlation among the proportion of 45,X/46,XY cell lines in either blood or fibroblasts with the phenotype. In the past, all patients came to clinical attention because of their abnormal phenotypes. However, 45,X/46,XY mosaicism is found in approximately 7% of fetuses, with true chromosome mosaicism encountered prenatally. Of 76 infants with 45,X/46,XY mosaicism diagnosed prenatally, 72 had a normal male phenotype, 1 had a female phenotype, and only 3 males had hypospadias. Of 12 males whose gonads were examined, only 3 were abnormal. These data must be taken into account when counseling a family in which a 45,X/46,XY infant is discovered prenatally.

XXX, XXXX, AND XXXXX FEMALES
XXX Females
The 47,XXX (trisomy) chromosomal constitution is the most frequent extra–X chromosome abnormality in females, occurring in almost 1 in 1,000 liveborn females. In 68%, this condition is caused by maternal meiotic nondisjunction, but most 45,X and half of 47,XXY constitutions are caused by paternal sex chromosome errors. The phenotype is that of a normal female; affected infants and children are not recognized based on the genital appearance.

Sexual development and menarche are normal. Most pregnancies have resulted in normal infants. By 2 yr of age, delays in speech and language become evident and lack of coordination, poor academic performance, and immature behavior are seen in some. These girls tend to be tall and gangly, manifest behavior disorders, and are placed in special education classes. Using high-resolution MRI, 10 47,XXX subjects had lower amygdala volumes than 20 euploid controls; 10 47,XXY subjects had even lower amygdala volumes. In a review of 155 girls, 62% were physically normal. There is marked variability within the syndrome, and a small proportion of affected girls are well coordinated, socially outgoing, and academically superior.

XXXX and XXXXX Females
The great majority of females with these rare karyotypes have been intellectually challenged. Commonly associated defects are epicanthal folds, hypertelorism, clinodactyly, transverse palmar creases, radioulnar synostosis, and congenital heart disease. Sexual maturation is often incomplete and may not occur at all. Nevertheless, 3 women with the tetra-X syndrome gave birth, but no pregnancies were reported in 49,XXXXX women. Most 48,XXXX women tend to be tall, with an average height of 169 cm, whereas short stature is a common feature of the 49,XXXXX phenotype.

NOONAN SYNDROME
Girls with Noonan syndrome show certain anomalies that also occur in girls with 45,X Turner syndrome, but they have normal 46,XX chromosomes (see Chapter 81.4). The most common abnormalities are

the same as those described for males with Noonan syndrome (see Chapter 583.1). Short stature is one of the cardinal signs of this syndrome. The phenotype differs from Turner syndrome in several respects. Cognitive impairment is often present, the cardiac defect is most often pulmonary valvular stenosis or an atrial septal defect rather than an aortic defect, normal sexual maturation usually occurs but is delayed by 2 yr on average, and premature ovarian failure has been reported. Growth hormone therapy is approved by the FDA for use in Noonan syndrome patients with short stature.

OTHER OVARIAN DEFECTS

Some young women with no chromosomal abnormality are found to have streak gonads that may contain only occasional or no germ cells. Gonadotropins are increased. Cytotoxic drugs, especially alkylating agents such as cyclophosphamide and busulfan, procarbazine, etoposide, and exposure of the ovaries to irradiation for the treatment of malignancy are frequent causes of ovarian failure. Young women with Hodgkin disease demonstrate that combination chemotherapy and pelvic irradiation may be more deleterious than either therapy alone. Teenagers are more likely than older women to retain or recover ovarian function after irradiation or combined chemotherapy; normal pregnancies have occurred after such treatment. Treatment regimens may result in some ovarian damage in most girls treated for cancer. The median lethal dose for the human oocyte is estimated to be approximately 4 Gy; doses as low as 6 Gy have produced primary amenorrhea. Ovarian transposition before abdominal and pelvic irradiation in childhood can preserve ovarian function by decreasing the ovarian exposure to less than 4-7 Gy.

Autoimmune ovarian failure occurs in 60% of children older than 13 yr of age with type I autoimmune polyendocrinopathy (Addison disease, hypoparathyroidism, candidiasis). This condition, also known as *polyglandular autoimmune disease* type 1 is rare worldwide but not in Finland, where, as a result of a founder gene effect, it occurs in 1 in 25,000 people. The gene for this disorder is located on chromosome 21 and is associated with human leukocyte antigen (HLA) DR5. In patients with polyglandular autoimmune disease type 1 and ovarian failure, an association with HLA-A3 has been described. Affected girls may not develop sexually, or secondary amenorrhea may occur in young women. The ovaries may have lymphocytic infiltration or appear simply as streaks. Most affected patients have circulating steroid cell antibodies and autoantibodies to 21-hydroxylase. Among patients with polyglandular autoimmune syndromes, 5% were found to have hypogonadism.

The condition also occurs in young women as an isolated event or in association with other autoimmune disorders, leading to secondary amenorrhea (premature ovarian failure [POF]). It occurs in 0.2-0.9% of women younger than 40 yr of age. Premature ovarian failure is a heterogeneous disorder with many causes: chromosomal, genetic, enzymatic, infectious, and iatrogenic. When associated with autoimmune adrenal disease, steroid cell autoantibodies are always present. These antibodies react with P450scc, 17α-OH, or 21-OH enzymes. When associated with an entire host of endocrine and nonendocrine autoimmune diseases and not adrenal autoimmunity, steroid cell autoantibodies are rarely found. A second autoimmune disorder, often subclinical, is found in 10-39% of adult patients with POF. One 17 yr old with idiopathic thrombocytopenic purpura and 47,XXX chromosomes had autoimmune POF. Patients with POF do not have the neurocognitive defects found in Turner syndrome patients.

Galactosemia, particularly the classical form of the disease, usually results in ovarian damage, beginning during intrauterine life. Levels of FSH and luteinizing hormone (LH) are elevated early in life. Ovarian damage may be caused by deficient uridine diphosphate-galactose (see Chapter 87). The **Denys-Drash syndrome,** caused by a *WT1* mutation, can result in ovarian dysgenesis.

Ataxia-telangiectasia may be associated with ovarian hypoplasia and elevated gonadotropins; the cause is unknown. Gonadoblastomas and dysgerminomas have occurred in a few girls.

Hypergonadotropic hypogonadism has been postulated to also occur because of the resistance of the ovary to both endogenous and

exogenous gonadotropins (Savage syndrome). This condition occurs also in women with POF. Antiovarian antibodies or FSH receptor abnormalities may cause this condition. Mutation of the FSH receptor gene has been reported as an autosomal recessive condition (see Chapter 582). A few females with 46,XX chromosomes presenting in primary amenorrhea with elevated gonadotropin levels were found to have inactivating mutations of the LH receptor gene. This suggests that LH action is needed for normal follicular development and ovulation. Other genetic defects associated with ovarian failure include mutations in *FOXL2, GNAS, CYP17,* and *CYP19.* Some data also suggest that mutations within the gene encoding transcription factor SF-1 are associated with early ovarian failure.

Bibliography is available at Expert Consult.

586.2 Hypogonadotropic Hypogonadism in the Female (Secondary Hypogonadism)

Alvina R. Kansra and Patricia A. Donohoe

Hypofunction of the ovaries can result from failure to secrete normal pulses of the gonadotropins LH (luteinizing hormone) and FSH. Hypogonadotropic hypogonadism may occur if the hypothalamic-pituitary-gonadal axis is interrupted either at the hypothalamic or pituitary level. The mechanisms that result in hypogonadotropic hypogonadism include failure of the hypothalamic luteinizing hormone–releasing hormone (also known as *gonadotropin-releasing hormone*) pulse generator or inability of the pituitary to respond with secretion of LH and FSH. It is often difficult to distinguish between marked constitutional delay and hypogonadotropic hypogonadism.

ETIOLOGY
Hypopituitarism

Hypogonadotropic hypogonadism is most commonly seen with multiple pituitary hormone deficiencies resulting from malformations (e.g., septooptic dysplasia, other midline defects), pituitary transcription factor defects such as in PROP-1, or lesions of the pituitary that are acquired postnatally. Familial isolated gonadotropin deficiency associated with anosmia (Kallmann syndrome) was described in 1944. Many other genetic causes for hypogonadotropic hypogonadism have been identified. A gene important in luteinizing hormone–releasing hormone secretion is named *KISS* (encoding the protein kisspeptin), which is suggested to play a significant role in the development of the luteinizing hormone–releasing hormone–secreting cells. Another set of genes recently implicated in hypogonadotropic hypogonadism are the genes for neurokinin B (*TAC3*) and its receptor (*TAC3R*).

In children with idiopathic hypopituitarism, the defect is usually found in the hypothalamus. In these patients, administration of gonadotropin-releasing hormone results in increased plasma levels of FSH and LH, establishing the integrity of the pituitary gland.

Hypogonadotropic hypogonadism is less common than hypergonadotropic hypogonadism. The latter condition, when associated with LH excess, underlies polycystic ovarian syndrome (Stein-Leventhal syndrome; see Chapter 552).

Isolated Deficiency of Gonadotropins

This heterogeneous group of disorders is characterized more fully with the use of the gonadotropin-releasing hormone analog stimulation test. In most children, the pituitary gland is normal, and the defect causing gonadotropin deficiency resides in the hypothalamus. Patients with hyperprolactinemia, most often caused by a pituitary prolactin-secreting adenoma, often have suppression of gonadotropin secretion. If breast development has occurred, then galactorrhea and amenorrhea are frequently seen.

Several sporadic instances of anosmia with hypogonadotropic hypogonadism have been reported. **Anosmic** hypogonadal females have also been reported in kindreds with Kallmann syndrome, but hypogonadism more frequently affects the males in these families. Mutations in the gene for the β-subunit of FSH and LH have been reported.

Some autosomal recessive disorders, such as the Laurence-Moon-Biedl, multiple lentigines, and Carpenter syndromes, appear in some instances to include gonadotropic hormone deficiency. Patients with Prader-Willi syndrome usually have some degree of hypogonadotropic hypogonadism. Girls with severe thalassemia may have gonadotropin deficiency from pituitary damage caused by chronic iron overload secondary to multiple transfusions. Anorexia nervosa frequently results in hypogonadotropic hypogonadism. The rare patients described with leptin deficiency or leptin receptor defects have failure of pubertal maturation because of gonadotropin deficiency.

DIAGNOSIS

The diagnosis may be apparent in patients with other deficiencies of pituitary tropic hormones, but, as in males, it is difficult to differentiate isolated hypogonadotropic hypogonadism from physiologic delay of puberty. Repeated measurements of FSH and LH, particularly during sleep, may reveal the rising levels that herald the onset of puberty. Stimulation testing with gonadotropin-releasing hormone or one of its analogs may help establish the diagnosis. Morbidity for both men and women with hypogonadism includes infertility and an increased risk of osteoporosis.

Bibliography is available at Expert Consult.

Chapter **587**
Pseudoprecocity Resulting from Lesions of the Ovary
Alvina R. Kansra and Patricia A. Donohoue

Girls with signs of early puberty may, in rare circumstances, have a lesion of the ovary as the etiology. These include tumors or cysts that secrete estrogenic, androgenic, or both types of hormones. In these patients the sex steroid production is not mediated by pituitary gonadotropin secretion, and thus they are said to produce pseudoprecocity.

Ovarian tumors are rare in the pediatric population, occurring at a rate of less than 3 in 100,000. Most ovarian masses are benign, but 10-30% may be malignant. If they occur before 8 yr of age they may cause signs of puberty. Ovarian malignancies, the most common genital neoplasms in adolescence, account for only 1% of childhood cancers. More than 60% are germ cell tumors, most of which are dysgerminomas that can secrete tumor markers as well as sex hormones (see Chapter 503). Five to 10% of germ cell tumors occur in phenotypic females with abnormal gonads associated with the presence of a Y chromosome. Next most common are epithelial cell tumors (20%), and nearly 10% are sex cord/stromal tumors (granulosa, Sertoli cell, and mesenchymal tumors). Multiple tumor markers can be seen in ovarian tumors, including α-fetoprotein, human chorionic gonadotropin, carcinoembryonic antigen, oncoproteins, p105, p53, *KRAS* mutations, cyclin D$_1$, epidermal growth factor–related proteins and receptors, cathepsin B, and others. Variable levels of inhibin–activin subunit gene expression have been detected in ovarian tumors.

Functioning lesions of the ovary consist of benign cysts or malignant tumors. The majority synthesize estrogens; a few synthesize androgens. The most common estrogen-producing ovarian tumor causing precocious puberty is the granulosa cell tumor. Other tumors that can cause precocious puberty are thecomas, luteomas, mixed types, theca-lutein and follicular cysts, and ovarian tumors (i.e., teratoma, choriocarcinoma, and dysgerminoma).

ESTROGENIC LESIONS OF THE OVARY

These lesions cause isosexual precocious sexual development but account for only a small percentage of all cases of precocity. Benign ovarian follicular cysts are the most common tumors associated with isosexual precocious puberty in girls; they may rarely be gonadotropin dependent. Gonadotropin-independent follicular cysts that produce estrogen are often associated with the McCune-Albright syndrome.

Juvenile Granulosa Cell Tumor

In childhood, the most common neoplasm of the ovary with estrogenic manifestations is the granulosa cell tumor, although it makes up only 1-10% of all ovarian tumors. These tumors have distinctive histologic features that differ from those encountered in older women (adult granulosa cell tumor). The cells have high mitotic activity, follicles are often irregular, Call-Exner bodies are rare, and luteinization is frequent. The tumor may be solid or cystic, or both. It usually is benign. In a few instances, this tumor has been associated with multiple enchondromas (**Ollier disease**) and, in fewer still, with multiple subcutaneous hemangiomas (**Maffucci syndrome**).

Clinical Manifestations and Diagnosis

The juvenile granulosa cell tumor has been observed in newborns and may manifest with sexual precocity at 2 yr of age or younger; about half these tumors occurred before 10 yr of age. The mean age at diagnosis is 7.5 yr. The tumors are almost always unilateral. The breasts become enlarged, rounded, and firm, and the nipples prominent. The external genitals resemble those of a normal girl at puberty, and the uterus is enlarged. A white vaginal discharge is followed by irregular or cyclic menstruation. Ovulation, however, does not occur. The presenting manifestation may be abdominal pain or swelling. Pubic hair is usually absent unless there is mild virilization.

A mass is readily palpable in the lower portion of the abdomen in most children by the time sexual precocity is evident. The tumor may be small, however, and escape detection even on careful rectal and abdominal examination; the tumors may be detected by ultrasonography, but multidetector CT scans are most sensitive. Most such tumors (90%) are diagnosed at very early stages of malignancy.

Plasma estradiol levels are markedly elevated. Plasma levels of gonadotropins are suppressed and do not respond to gonadotropin-releasing hormone analog stimulation. Levels of antimüllerian hormone, inhibin B, and α-fetoprotein may be elevated. Activating mutations of G$_S$α are seen in 30%, and GATA-4 expression is retained in the more aggressive tumors while antimüllerian hormone levels are inversely proportional to tumor size. Osseous development is moderately advanced. Several case reports showing the association of 45,X/46,XY karyotype and ambiguous genitalia with ovarian granulosa tumor have been published in literature.

Treatment and Prognosis

The tumor should be removed as soon as the diagnosis is established. Prognosis is excellent because fewer than 5% of these tumors in children are malignant. Advanced-stage tumors, however, behave aggressively and require difficult decisions regarding surgical approaches as well as the use of irradiation and chemotherapy. In adults with granulosa cell tumors, p53 expression is associated with unfavorable prognosis. Vaginal bleeding immediately after removal of the tumor is common. Signs of precocious puberty abate and may disappear within a few months after the operation. The secretion of estrogens returns to normal.

Sex cord tumor with annular tubules is a distinctive tumor, thought to arise from granulosa cells, that occurs primarily in patients with Peutz-Jeghers syndrome. These tumors are multifocal, bilateral, and usually benign. The presence of calcifications aids ultrasonographic detection. Increased aromatase production by these tumors results in gonadotropin-independent precocious puberty. Inhibin A and B levels are elevated and decrease after tumor removal. In 1 study, 9 of 13 sex cord/stromal tumors exhibited follicle-stimulating hormone receptor mutations, suggesting a role for such mutation in the development of these tumors.

Chorioepithelioma has been reported only rarely. This highly malignant tumor is thought to arise from a preexisting teratoma. The usually unilateral tumor produces large amounts of human chorionic gonadotropin, which stimulates the contralateral ovary to secrete estrogen. Elevated levels of human chorionic gonadotropin are diagnostic.

Follicular Cyst

Small ovarian cysts (<0.7 cm in diameter) are common in prepubertal children. At puberty and in girls with true isosexual precocious puberty, larger cysts (1-6 cm) are often seen; these are secondary to stimulation by gonadotropins. However, similar larger cysts occur occasionally in young girls with precocious puberty in the absence of luteinizing hormone and follicle-stimulating hormone. Because surgical removal or spontaneous involution of these cysts results in regression of pubertal changes, there is little doubt that they are its cause. The mechanism of production of these autonomously functioning cysts is unknown. Such cysts may form only once, or they may disappear and recur, resulting in waxing and waning of the signs of precocious puberty. They may be unilateral or bilateral. The sexual precocity that occurs in young girls with **McCune-Albright syndrome** is usually associated with autonomous follicular cysts caused by a somatic-activating mutation of the $G_S\alpha$-protein occurring early in development (see Chapter 562.6). Gonadotropins are suppressed, and estradiol levels are often markedly elevated, but they may fluctuate widely and even temporarily may return to normal. Gonadotropin-releasing hormone analog stimulation fails to evoke an increase in gonadotropins. Ultrasonography is the method of choice for the detection and monitoring of such cysts. Aromatase inhibitors are shown to be the mainstay of the therapy in females with McCune-Albright syndrome and persistent estradiol elevation. A short period of observation to ascertain the lack of spontaneous resolution is advisable before cyst aspiration or cystectomy is considered. Cystic neoplasms must be considered in the differential diagnosis.

ANDROGENIC LESIONS OF THE OVARY

Virilizing ovarian tumors are rare at all ages but particularly so in prepubertal girls. **Arrhenoblastoma** has been reported as early as 14 days of age, but few cases have been reported in girls younger than 16 yr of age.

The **gonadoblastoma** occurs exclusively in dysgenetic gonads, particularly in phenotypic females who have a Y chromosome or a Y fragment in their genotype (46,XY; 45,X/46,XY; 45,X/46,X-fra). As noted above, there is a proposed gonadoblastoma locus on the Y chromosome (GBY). The tumors may be bilateral. Virilization occurs with some but not all tumors. The clinical features are the same as those seen in patients with virilizing adrenal tumors and include accelerated growth, acne, clitoral enlargement, and growth of sexual hair. A palpable, abdominal mass is found in about 50% of patients. Plasma levels of testosterone and androstenedione are elevated, and gonadotropins are suppressed. Ultrasonography, CT, and MRI usually localize the lesion. The dysgenetic gonad of phenotypic females with a Y chromosome or fragment of Y chromosome containing GBY should be removed prophylactically. When a unilateral tumor is removed, the contralateral dysgenetic gonad should also be removed. Association of gonadoblastoma and WAGR (Wilms, aniridia, genitourinary anomalies, mental retardation) syndrome is also reported in the literature. In an immunohistochemical study of 2 gonadoblastomas, expressions of *WT1*, *p53*, and *MIS*, as well as inhibin, were all demonstrated.

Virilizing manifestations occur occasionally in girls with **juvenile granulosa cell tumors.** Adrenal rests and hilum cell tumors rarely lead to virilization. Activating mutations of G-protein genes have been described in ovarian (and testicular) tumors. $G_S\alpha$ mutations, usually seen in gonadal tumors associated with **McCune-Albright syndrome,** were also noted in 4 of 6 Leydig cell tumors (3 ovarian, 1 testicular). Two granulosa cell tumors and 1 thecoma of 10 ovarian tumors studied were found to have *GIP-2* mutations.

Sertoli-Leydig cell tumors, rare sex cord/stromal neoplasms, constitute less than 1% of ovarian tumors. The average age at diagnosis is 25 yr; less than 5% of these tumors occur before puberty. α-Fetoprotein levels may be mildly elevated. In one 12 mo old with Sertoli-Leydig cell tumor presenting with isosexual precocity the only detectable tumor marker was the serum inhibin level, with elevations in both A and B subunits. Five-year survival rates are 70-90%.

Of 102 consecutive patients who underwent surgery because of ovarian masses over a 15 yr period, the presenting symptoms were acute abdominal pain in 56% and abdominal or pelvic mass in 22%. Of 9 children whose cause for surgery was presumed malignancy, 3 had dysgerminomas, 2 had teratomas, 2 had juvenile granulosa cell tumors, 1 had a Sertoli-Leydig cell tumor, and 1 had a yolk sac tumor.

Bibliography is available at Expert Consult.

Chapter **588**
Disorders of Sex Development
Patricia A. Donohoue

SEX DIFFERENTIATION
See also Chapter 582.

In normal differentiation, the final form of all sexual structures is consistent with normal sex chromosomes (either XX or XY). A 46,XX complement of chromosomes as well as genetic factors such as DAX1 (dosage-sensitive/sex-reversal adrenal hypoplasia on the X chromosome), the signaling molecule WNT-4, and R-Spondin1 are among the many needed for the development of normal ovaries. Development of the male phenotype is potentially more complex. It requires a Y chromosome and, specifically, an intact *SRY* (sex-determining region on the Y chromosome) gene, which, in association with other genes such as *SOX9*, *SF-1* (steroidogenic factor-1), *WT1* (Wilms tumor 1), and others (see Chapter 582), directs the undifferentiated gonad to become a testis. Aberrant recombinations may result in X chromosomes carrying *SRY*, resulting in XX males, or Y chromosomes that have lost *SRY*, resulting in XY females. Epigenetic causes of abnormal sex differentiation have been shown in plants, invertebrates, and vertebrates, and will likely contribute to human disorders of sex development (DSDs) as well.

Antimüllerian hormone (AMH) causes the müllerian ducts to regress; in its absence, they persist as the uterus, fallopian tubes, cervix, and upper vagina. AMH activation in the testes may require the *SF-1* gene. By about 8 wk of gestation, the Leydig cells of the testis begin to produce testosterone. During this critical period of male differentiation, testosterone secretion is stimulated by placental human chorionic gonadotropin (hCG), which peaks at 8-12 wk. In the latter half of pregnancy, lower levels of testosterone are maintained by luteinizing hormone (LH) secreted by the fetal pituitary. Testosterone produced locally initiates development of the ipsilateral wolffian duct into the epididymis, vas deferens, and seminal vesicle. Development of the external genitalia also requires dihydrotestosterone (DHT), the more active metabolite of testosterone. DHT is produced largely from circulating testosterone and is necessary to fuse the genital folds to form the penis and scrotum. DHT is also produced via an alternative biosynthetic pathway from androstanediol, and this pathway must be intact for normal and complete prenatal virilization to occur. A functional androgen receptor, produced by an X-linked gene, is required for testosterone and DHT to induce these androgen effects.

In the XX fetus with normal long and short arms of the X chromosome, the bipotential gonad develops into an ovary by about the 10th-11th wk. This occurs only in the absence of SRY, testosterone, and AMH and requires a normal gene in the dosage-sensitive/sex-reversal

Table 588-1	Revised Nomenclature
PREVIOUS	**CURRENTLY ACCEPTED**
Intersex	Disorders of sex development (DSD)
Male pseudohermaphrodite	46,XY DSD
Undervirilization of an XY male	46,XY DSD
Undermasculinization of an XY male	46,XY DSD
46,XY intersex	46,XY DSD
Female pseudohermaphrodite	46,XX DSD
Overvirilization of an XX female	46,XX DSD
Masculinization of an XX female	46,XX DSD
46,XX intersex	46,XX DSD
True hermaphrodite	Ovotesticular DSD
Gonadal intersex	Ovotesticular DSD
XX male or XX sex reversal	46,XX testicular DSD
XY sex reversal	46,XY complete gonadal dysgenesis

From Lee PA, Houk CP, Ahmed SF, et al: Consensus statement on management of intersex disorders, Pediatrics 118:e488–e500, 2006.

Table 588-2	Etiologic Classification of Disorders of Sex Development (DSD)

46,XX DSD
Androgen Exposure
Fetal/Fetoplacental Source
21-Hydroxylase (P450c21 or CYP21) deficiency
11β-Hydroxylase (P450c11 or CYP11B1) deficiency
3β-Hydroxysteroid dehydrogenase II (3β-HSD II) deficiency
Cytochrome P450 oxidoreductase (POR)
Aromatase (P450arom or CYP19) deficiency
Glucocorticoid receptor gene mutation
Maternal Source
Virilizing ovarian tumor
Virilizing adrenal tumor
Androgenic drugs
Disorder of Ovarian Development
XX gonadal dysgenesis
Testicular DSD (SRY+, SOX9 duplication)
Undetermined Origin
Associated with genitourinary and gastrointestinal tract defects

46,XY DSD
Defects in Testicular Development
Denys-Drash syndrome (mutation in *WT1* gene)
WAGR syndrome (Wilms tumor, aniridia, genitourinary malformation, retardation)
Deletion of 11p13
Campomelic syndrome (autosomal gene at 17q24.3-q25.1) and *SOX9* mutation
XY pure gonadal dysgenesis (Swyer syndrome)
Mutation in *SRY* gene
XY gonadal agenesis
Unknown cause
Deficiency of Testicular Hormones
Leydig cell aplasia
Mutation in LH receptor
Lipoid adrenal hyperplasia (P450scc or CYP11A1) deficiency; mutation in StAR (steroidogenic acute regulatory protein)
3β-HSD II deficiency
17-Hydroxylase/17,20-lyase (P450c17 or CYP17) deficiency
Persistent müllerian duct syndrome because of antimüllerian hormone gene mutations or receptor defects for antimüllerian hormone
Defect in Androgen Action
Dihydrotestosterone deficiency because of 5α-reductase II mutations or *AKR1C2/AKR1C4* mutations
Androgen receptor defects:
    Complete androgen insensitivity syndrome
    Partial androgen insensitivity syndrome (Reifenstein and other syndromes)
Smith-Lemli-Opitz syndrome (defect in conversion of 7-dehydrocholesterol to cholesterol, DHCR7)
Ovotesticular DSD
XX
XY
XX/XY chimeras
Sex Chromosome DSD
45,X (Turner syndrome and variants)
47,XXY (Klinefelter syndrome and variants)
45,X/46,XY (mixed gonadal dysgenesis, sometimes a cause of ovotesticular DSD)
46,XX/46,XY (chimeric, sometimes a cause of ovotesticular DSD)

From Lee PA, Houk CP, Ahmed SF, et al: Consensus statement on management of intersex disorders, Pediatrics 118:e488–e500, 2006.

locus DAX1, the WNT-4 molecule, and R-Spondin1. A female external phenotype develops in the absence of fetal gonads. However, the male phenotype development requires androgen production and action. Estrogen is unnecessary for normal prenatal sexual differentiation, as demonstrated by 46,XX patients with aromatase deficiency and by mice without estradiol receptors.

Chromosomal aberrations may result in ambiguity of the external genitalia. Conditions of aberrant sex differentiation may also occur with the XX or XY genotype. The appropriate term for what was previously called *intersex* is **DSD.** This term defines a condition "in which development of chromosomal, gonadal, or anatomical sex is atypical." It is increasingly preferable to use the term "atypical genitalia" rather than "ambiguous genitalia." Tables 588-1 and 588-2 compare previous terms with their revised etiologic classification nomenclature. Table 582-1 in Chapter 582 lists some of the genes that are mutated in various forms of DSD.

The definition of atypical or ambiguous genitalia, in a broad sense, is any case in which the external genitalia do not appear completely male or completely female. Although there are standards for genital size dimensions, variations in size of these structures do not always constitute ambiguity.

Development of the external genitalia begins with the potential to be either male or female (Fig. 588-1). Virilization of a female, the most common form of DSD, results in varying phenotypes (Fig. 588-2), that develop from the basic bipotential genital appearances of the embryo (Fig. 588-1).

DIAGNOSTIC APPROACH TO THE PATIENT WITH ATYPICAL OR AMBIGUOUS GENITALIA

The appearance of the external genitalia is rarely diagnostic of a particular disorder, and thus does not often allow distinction among the various forms of DSD. The most common forms of 46,XX DSD are virilizing forms of congenital adrenal hyperplasia. It is important to note that in 46,XY DSD, the specific diagnosis is not found in up to 50% of cases; partial androgen insensitivity syndrome and pure gonadal dysgenesis are common identifiable etiologies in XY DSD. At 1 center with a large experience, the etiologies of DSD in 250 patients over 25 yr were compiled. The 6 most common diagnoses accounted for 50% of the cases. These included virilizing congenital adrenal hyperplasia (14%), androgen insensitivity syndrome (10%), mixed gonadal dysgenesis (8%), clitoral/labial anomalies (7%), hypogonadotropic hypogonadism (6%), and 46,XY small-for-gestational-age males with hypospadias (6%).

The relative lack of established diagnoses in 46,XY DSD and the resulting lack of specific management emphasizes the need for thorough diagnostic evaluations. These include biochemical characterization of possible steroidogenic enzymatic defects in each patient with genital ambiguity. The parents need counseling about the potentially complex nature of the baby's condition, and guidance as to how to deal with their well-meaning but curious friends and family members. The

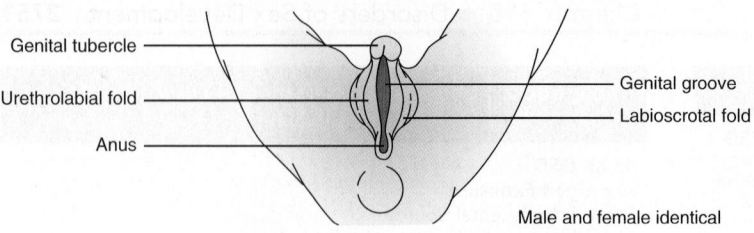

Sexual appearance of fetus at 2nd to 3rd mo of pregnancy

Genital tubercle
Urethrolabial fold
Anus

Genital groove
Labioscrotal fold

Male and female identical

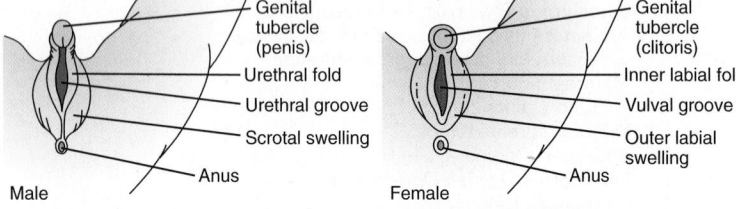

Sexual appearance of fetus at 3rd to 4th mo of pregnancy

Genital
tubercle
(penis)
Urethral fold
Urethral groove
Scrotal swelling
Anus

Male

Genital
tubercle
(clitoris)
Inner labial fold
Vulval groove
Outer labial
swelling
Anus

Female

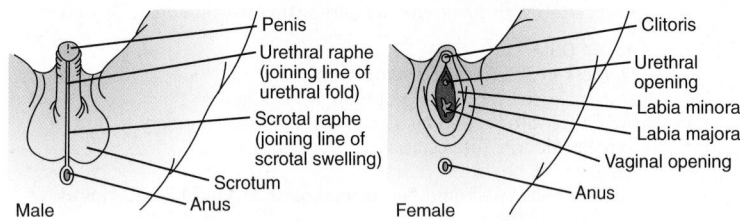

Sexual appearance of fetus at time of birth

Penis
Urethral raphe
(joining line of
urethral fold)
Scrotal raphe
(joining line of
scrotal swelling)
Scrotum
Anus

Male

Clitoris
Urethral
opening
Labia minora
Labia majora
Vaginal opening
Anus

Female

Figure 588-1 Schematic demonstration of differentiation of normal male and female genitalia during embryogenesis. *(From Zitelli BJ, Davis HW: Atlas of pediatric physical diagnosis, ed 4, St. Louis, 2002, Mosby, p. 328.)*

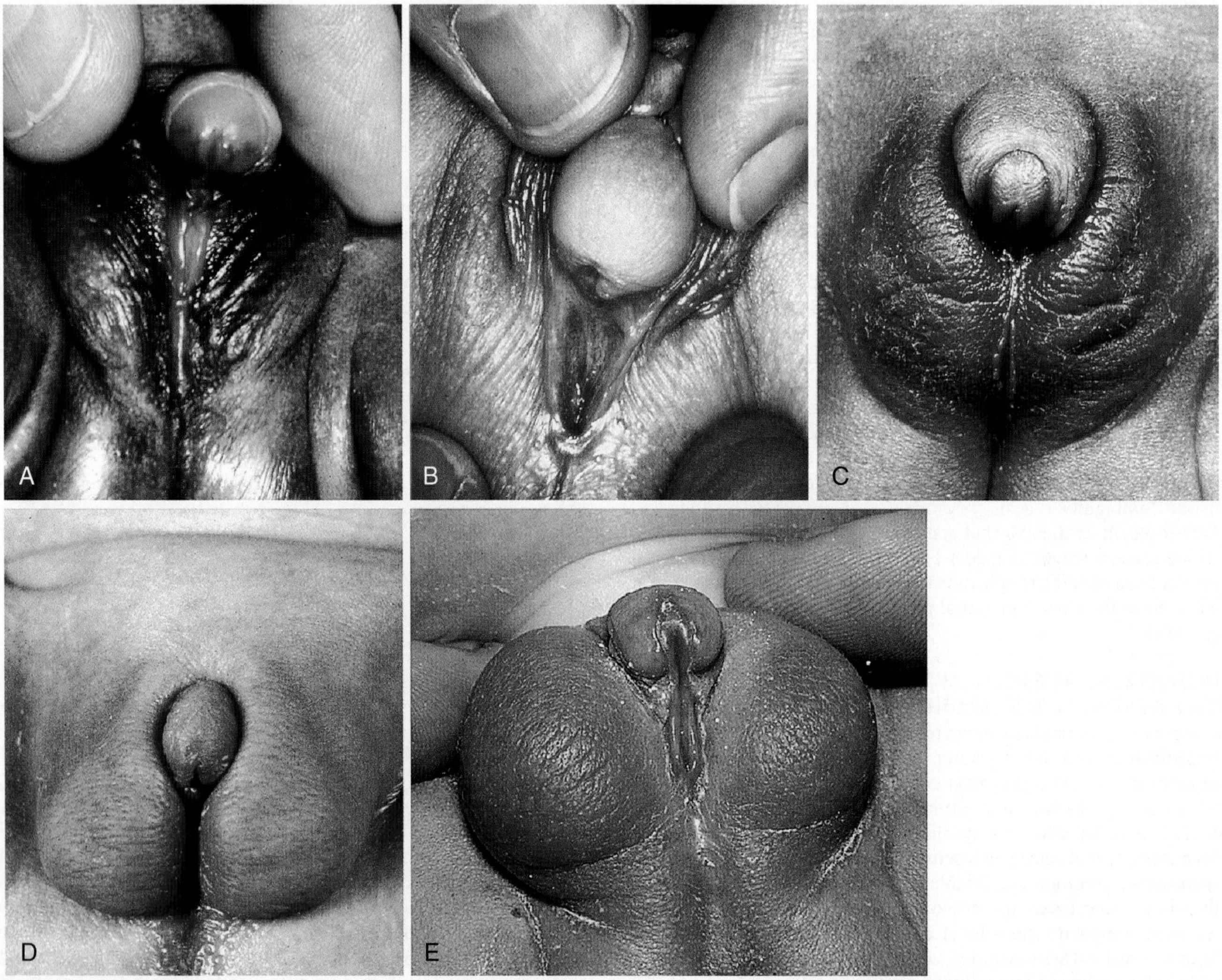

Figure 588-2 Examples of atypical genitalia. These cases include ovotesticular disorder of sexual development **(A)** and congenital virilizing adrenal hyperplasia **(B-E)**. *(B-D courtesy of D. Becker, MD, Pittsburgh. From Zitelli BJ, Davis HW: Atlas of pediatric physical diagnosis, ed 4, St. Louis, 2002, Mosby, p. 329.)*

| Table 588-3 | Ambiguous Genitalia: Steps in Establishing the Diagnosis |

	21-OH DEFICIENCY	GONADAL DYSGENESIS WITH Y CHROMOSOME	OVOTESTICULAR DSD	PARTIAL ANDROGEN INSENSITIVITY	BLOCK IN TESTOSTERONE SYNTHESIS
CLINICAL FEATURE					
Palpable gonad(s)	–	±	±	+	+
Uterus present*	+	+	Usually	–	–
Increased skin pigmentation	±	–	–	–	–
Sick baby	±	–	–	–	±
Dysmorphic features	–	±	–	–	–
DIAGNOSTIC CONSIDERATIONS					
Serum 17-OHP	Elevated	Normal	Normal	Normal	Normal
Electrolytes	Possibly abnormal	Normal	Normal	Normal	Possibly abnormal
Karyotype	46,XX	45,X/46,XY or others	46,XX	46,XY	46,XY
Testosterone response to hCG	NA	Positive	Normal or reduced	Positive response	Reduced or absent
Gonadal biopsy	NA	Dysgenetic gonad	Ovotestis	Normal testis with ± Leydig cell hyperplasia	Normal testis
Other testing				Genital skin fibroblast culture For AR assay Or DNA screening for AR mutations in blood cells	Measure Testosterone Precursors

*As determined by ultrasound or rectal examination.

AR, androgen receptor; DSD, disorders of sex development; hCG, human chorionic gonadotropin; 21-OH, 21-hydroxylase; 17-OHP, 17-hydroxyprogesterone; NA, not applicable.

Adapted from Donohoue PA, Saenger PH: Ambiguous genitalia. In Finberg L, Kleinman RE, editors: Saunders manual of pediatric practice, Philadelphia, 2002, WB Saunders, p. 874.

evaluation and management should be carried out by a multidisciplinary team of experts that includes pediatric endocrinology, pediatric surgery/urology, pediatric radiology, newborn medicine, genetics, and psychology. Once the sex of rearing has been agreed on by the family and team, treatment can be organized. Genetic counseling should be offered when the specific diagnosis is established.

After a complete history and physical exam, the common diagnostic approach includes multiple steps, described in the following outline. These steps are usually performed simultaneously rather than waiting for results of 1 test prior to performing another, because of the sensitive and sometimes urgent nature of the condition. Careful attention to the presence of physical features other than the genitalia is crucial, to determine if a diagnosis of a particular multisystem syndrome is possible. These are described in more detail in Chapters 588.1, 588.2, and 588.3 below. Table 588-3 summarizes many of the features of commonly encountered causes of DSD.

Diagnostic tests include the following:
1. Karyotype, with rapid determination of sex chromosomes (in many centers this is available within 24-48 hr)
2. Other blood tests
   a. Screen for congenital adrenal hyperplasia: cortisol biosynthetic precursors and adrenal androgens (particularly 17-hydroxyprogesterone and androstenedione for 21-hydroxylase deficiency, the most common form)
   b. Screen for androgens and their biosynthetic precursors
   c. Screen for gonadal response to gonadotropin in patients suspected of having testicular gonads: stimulation with injections of hCG; measure testosterone and DHT before and after hCG
   d. Molecular genetic analyses for SRY and other Y-specific loci
   e. Gonadotropin levels
3. The internal anatomy of patients with ambiguous genitalia can be defined with 1 or more of the following studies:
   a. Voiding cystourethrogram
   b. Endoscopic examination of the genitourinary tract
   c. Pelvic ultrasound; renal and adrenal ultrasound
   d. Pelvic CT or MRI
   e. Exploratory laparoscopy

588.1 46,XX DSD
Patricia A. Donohoue

In this condition, the genotype is XX and the gonads are ovaries but the external genitalia are virilized. There is no significant AMH production because the gonads are ovaries. Thus the uterus, fallopian tubes, and cervix develop. The varieties and causes of this condition are relatively few. Most instances result from exposure of the female fetus to excessive exogenous or endogenous androgens during intrauterine life. The changes consist principally of virilization of the external genitalia (clitoral hypertrophy and labioscrotal fusion).

CONGENITAL ADRENAL HYPERPLASIA
See Chapter 576.1.

This is the most common cause of genital ambiguity and of 46,XX DSD. Females with the 21-hydroxylase and 11-hydroxylase defects are the most highly virilized, although minimal virilization also occurs with the type II 3β-hydroxysteroid dehydrogenase defect (see Fig. 588-1). Female patients with salt-losing congenital adrenal hyperplasia tend to have more virilization than do non–salt-losing patients. Masculinization may be so intense that a complete penile urethra results, and the patient may appear to be a male with bilateral cryptorchidism.

AROMATASE DEFICIENCY
In genotypic females, the rare condition of aromatase deficiency during fetal life leads to 46,XX DSD and results in hypergonadotropic hypogonadism at puberty because of ovarian failure to synthesize estrogen.

Two 46,XX infants had enlargement of the clitoris and posterior labial fusion at birth. In 1 instance, maternal serum and urinary levels of estrogen were very low and serum levels of androgens were high. Cord serum levels of estrogen were also extremely low, but those of androgen were elevated. The second patient also had virilization of unknown cause since birth, but the aromatase deficiency was not diagnosed until 14 yr of age, when she had further virilization and failed to go into puberty. At that time, she had elevated levels of gonadotropins and androgens but low estrogen levels, and ultrasonography revealed large ovarian cysts bilaterally. These 2 patients demonstrate the important role of aromatase in the conversion of androgens to estrogens. Additional female and male patients with aromatase deficiency as a consequence of mutations in the *aromatase gene (CYP19)* are known. Two siblings were described. The 28 yr old XX proband was 177.6 cm tall (+2.5 SD) after having received hormonal replacement therapy; her 24 yr old brother was 204 cm tall (+3.7 SD), and had a bone age of 14 yr. Low-dose estradiol replacement, carefully adjusted to maintain normal age-appropriate levels, may be indicated for affected females, even prepubertally.

GLUCOCORTICOID RECEPTOR GENE MUTATION

A 9 yr old girl with 46,XX disorder of sexual development, thought to be caused by 21-hydroxylase deficiency (congenital adrenal hyperplasia) since the age of 5 yr, had elevated cortisol levels both at baseline and after dexamethasone, hypertension, and hypokalemia, suggestive of the diagnosis of generalized glucocorticoid resistance. A novel homozygous mutation in exon 5 of the glucocorticoid receptor was demonstrated. In this Brazilian family, the condition was autosomal recessive.

Cytochrome P450 oxidoreductase, encoded by a gene on 7q11.2, is a cofactor implicated in combined P450C17 and P450C21 steroidogenic defects. Girls are born with ambiguous genitalia, but the virilization does not progress postnatally and androgen levels are normal or low. Boys may be born undervirilized. Both may exhibit bony abnormalities seen in **Antley-Bixler syndrome**. Conversely, in a series of Antley-Bixler syndrome patients, those with ambiguous genitalia and disordered steroidogenesis had cytochrome P450 oxidoreductase deficiency. Those without genital ambiguity with normal steroidogenesis had fibroblast growth factor receptor 2 (*FGFR2*) mutations. The cardinal features of Antley-Bixler syndrome include craniosynostosis, severe midface hypoplasia, proptosis, choanal atresia/stenosis, frontal bossing, dysplastic ears, depressed nasal bridge, radiohumeral synostosis, long bone fractures and femoral bowing, and urogenital abnormalities.

VIRILIZING MATERNAL TUMORS

Rarely, the female fetus has been virilized during fetal life by a maternal androgen-producing tumor. In a few cases, the lesion was a benign adrenal adenoma, but all others were ovarian tumors, particularly androblastomas, luteomas, and Krukenberg tumors (Table 588-4). **Maternal virilization** may be manifested by enlargement of the

Table 588-4	Sources of Maternal-Derived Androgens
ENDOGENOUS	**EXOGENOUS**
BENIGN	SYNTHETIC ANDROGENS
Luteoma of pregnancy	Danazol
Adrenal adenoma	Progestins
	(medroxyprogesterone acetate)
Hyperreactio luteinalis	Potassium-sparing diuretics
Thecoma/fibroma	
Stromal hyperthecosis	
Brenner tumor	
Serous cystadenoma	
Mature cystic teratoma	
(dermoid cyst)	
MALIGNANT	
Metastatic carcinomas	
(Krukenberg tumor)	
Sex-cord stromal tumors—	
granulosa cell and Sertoli-	
Leydig tumors	
Adrenal cortical carcinoma	
Cystadenocarcinoma	
Hilar cell tumor	

From Auchus RJ, Chang AY: 46,XX DSD: the masculinised female. Best Pract Res Clin Endocrinol Metab 24:219–242, 2010, Table 2, p. 237.

clitoris, acne, deepening of the voice, decreased lactation, hirsutism, and elevated levels of androgens. In the infant, there is enlargement of the clitoris of varying degrees, often with labial fusion. Mothers of children with unexplained 46,XX DSD should undergo physical examination and measurements of their own levels of plasma testosterone, dehydroepiandrosterone sulfate, and androstenedione.

ADMINISTRATION OF ANDROGENIC DRUGS TO WOMEN DURING PREGNANCY

Testosterone and 17-methyltestosterone have been reported to cause 46,XX DSD in some instances (see Table 588-4). The greatest number of cases has resulted from the use of certain progestational compounds for the treatment of threatened abortion. These progestins have been replaced by nonvirilizing ones.

Infants with virilization and 46,XX chromosomes and caudal anomalies have been reported for whom no virilizing agent could be identified. In such instances, the disorder is usually associated with other congenital defects, particularly of the urinary and gastrointestinal tracts. Y-specific DNA sequences, including SRY, are absent. In 1 case, a scrotal raphe and elevated testosterone levels were found, but the cause remains unknown.

Bibliography is available at Expert Consult.

588.2 46,XY DSD
Patricia A. Donohoue

In this condition, the genotype is XY but the external genitalia are either not completely virilized, are ambiguous (atypical), or are completely female. When gonads can be found, they invariably contain testicular elements; their development ranges from rudimentary to normal. Because the process of normal virilization in the fetus is so complex, it is not surprising that there are many varieties and causes of 46,XY DSD. As noted earlier, the etiology of 46,XY DSD is not identified in approximately 50% of cases.

DEFECTS IN TESTICULAR DIFFERENTIATION

The first step in male differentiation is conversion of the bipotential gonad into a testis. In the XY fetus, if there is a deletion of the short arm of the Y chromosome or of the *SRY* gene, male differentiation does not occur. The phenotype is female; müllerian ducts are well developed because of the absence of AMH, and gonads consist of undifferentiated streaks. By contrast, even extreme deletions of the long arm of the Y chromosome (Yq−) have been found in normally developed males, most of whom are azoospermic and have short stature. This indicates that the long arm of the Y chromosome normally has genes that prevent these manifestations. In many syndromes in which the testes fail to differentiate, Y chromosomes are morphologically normal.

Denys-Drash Syndrome

The constellation of nephropathy with ambiguous genitalia and **bilateral Wilms tumor** is the major phenotype of this syndrome. Most reported cases have been 46,XY. Müllerian ducts are often present, indicating a global deficiency of fetal testicular function. Patients with a 46,XX karyotype have normal external genitalia. The onset of proteinuria in infancy progresses to **nephrotic syndrome** and end-stage renal failure by 3 yr of age, with focal or diffuse mesangial sclerosis being the most consistent histopathologic finding. Wilms tumor usually develops in children younger than 2 yr of age and is frequently bilateral. Gonadoblastomas have also been reported.

Several mutations of the *WT1* gene, located on chromosome 11p13, have been found. *WT1* functions as a tumor-suppressor gene and a transcriptional factor, and is expressed in the genital ridge and fetal gonads. Nearly all reported mutations have been near or within the zinc finger–coding region. One report found a zinc finger domain mutation in the *WT1* alleles of a patient with no genitourinary abnormalities, suggesting that some cases of sporadic Wilms tumor may carry the *WT1* mutation. Different mutations of the *WT1* gene, constitutional heterozygote mutations at intron 9, have been described in **Fraser syndrome,** a condition of nonspecific focal and segmental glomerulosclerosis, 46,XY gonadal dysgenesis, and frequent gonadoblastoma, but **without** Wilms tumor.

WAGR Syndrome

This acronymic contiguous gene syndrome consists of Wilms tumor, aniridia, genitourinary malformations, and retardation (WAGR). These children have a deletion of 1 copy of chromosome 11p13, which may be visible on karyotype analysis. The deleted region encompasses the aniridia gene *(PAX6)* and the Wilms tumor-suppressor gene *(WT1)*. Only the 46,XY males have genital abnormalities, ranging from cryptorchidism to severe deficiency of virilization. Gonadoblastomas have developed in the dysgenetic gonads. Wilms tumor usually occurs by 2 yr of age. Some cases also had unexplained obesity, raising the question of an obesity-associated gene in this region of chromosome 11 and naming the syndrome **WAGRO.**

Campomelic Syndrome
See Chapter 704.

This form of **short-limbed dysplasia** is characterized by anterior bowing of the femur and tibia, small, bladeless scapulae, small thoracic cavities, and 11 pairs of ribs, along with malformations of other organs. It is usually lethal in early infancy. Approximately 75% of reported 46,XY patients exhibit a completely **female phenotype;** the external and internal genitalia are female. Some 46,XY patients have ambiguous genitals. The gonads appear to be ovaries but histologically may contain elements of both ovaries and testes.

The gene responsible for the condition is *SOX9* (SRY-related HMG [high-mobility group]-box gene) and is on 17q24-q25. This gene is structurally related to *SRY* and also directly regulates development of the type II collagen gene *(COL2A1)*. The same mutations may result in different gonadal phenotypes. Gonadoblastoma was reported in a patient with this condition. The inheritance is autosomal dominant. Adrenal insufficiency and 46,XY gonadal dysgenesis has been described in patients with mutations of the *SF-1* gene. In some of these patients, if the mother shares the *SF-1* mutation, she has premature ovarian insufficiency.

46,XY sex reversal has been described in patients with deletions of parts of autosomal loci on chromosomes 2q, 9p, and 10q.

XY Pure Gonadal Dysgenesis (Swyer Syndrome)

The designation "pure" distinguishes this condition from forms of gonadal dysgenesis that are of chromosomal origin and associated with somatic anomalies. Affected patients have normal stature and a **female phenotype,** including vagina, uterus, and fallopian tubes, but at pubertal age, breast development and menarche fail to occur. None of the other phenotypic features associated with 45,X are present. Patients present at puberty with hypergonadotropic primary amenorrhea. Familial cases suggest an X-linked or a sex-limited dominant autosomal transmission. Most of the patients examined have had mutations of the *SRY* gene. None had a *SOX9* gene mutation. The gonads consist of almost totally undifferentiated streaks despite the presence of a cytogenetically normal Y chromosome. The primitive gonad cannot accomplish any testicular function, including suppression of müllerian ducts. There may be hilar cells in the gonad capable of producing some androgens; accordingly, some virilization, such as clitoral enlargement, may occur at the age of puberty. The streak gonads may undergo neoplastic changes, such as gonadoblastomas and dysgerminomas, and should be removed as soon as the diagnosis is established, regardless of the age of the patient.

Pure gonadal dysgenesis also occurs in XX individuals (see Chapter 586).

XY Gonadal Agenesis Syndrome (Embryonic Testicular Regression Syndrome)

In this rare syndrome, the external genitalia are slightly ambiguous but more nearly **female.** Hypoplasia of the labia; some degree of labioscrotal fusion; a small, clitoris-like phallus; and a perineal urethral opening

are present. No uterus, no gonadal tissue, and usually no vagina can be found. At the age of puberty, no sexual development occurs and gonadotropin levels are elevated. Most children have been reared as females. In several patients with XY gonadal agenesis in whom no gonads could be found on exploration, significant rises in testosterone followed stimulation with hCG, indicating Leydig cell function somewhere. Siblings with the disorder are known.

It is presumed that testicular tissue was active long enough during fetal life for AMH to inhibit development of müllerian ducts but not long enough for testosterone production to result in virilization. In 1 patient, no deletion of the Y chromosome was found by means of Y-specific DNA probes. Testicular degeneration seems to occur between the 8th and the 12th fetal wk. Regression of the testis before the 8th wk of gestation results in Swyer syndrome; between the 14th and the 20th wk of gestation, it results in the rudimentary testis syndrome; and after the 20th wk, it results in anorchia.

In **bilateral anorchia,** sometimes referred to as *vanishing testes syndrome,* testes are absent, but the **male phenotype** is complete; it is presumed that tissue with fetal testicular function was active during the critical period of genital differentiation but that sometime later it was damaged. Bilateral anorchia in identical twins and unilateral anorchia in identical twins and in siblings suggest a genetic predisposition. Coexistence of anorchia and the gonadal agenesis syndrome in a sibship is evidence for a relationship between the disorders. *SRY* defects have not yet been reported for patients with anorchia.

A retrospective review of urologic explorations revealed absent testes in 21% of 691 testes. Of those, 73% had blind-ending cord structures with the suggested site of the vanishing testes being the inguinal canal (59%), abdomen (21%), superficial inguinal ring (18%), and scrotum (2%). It was suggested that the presence of cord structures on laparoscopy should prompt inguinal exploration because viable testicular tissue was found in 4 of these children. No hormonal data (hCG stimulation tests, AMH levels) were reported.

DEFECTS IN TESTICULAR HORMONES

Five genetic defects have been delineated in the enzymatic synthesis of testosterone by the fetal testis, and a defect in Leydig cell differentiation has been described. These defects produce 46,XY males with inadequate masculinization (see Fig. 582-1 in Chapter 582). Because levels of testosterone are normally low before puberty, an hCG stimulation test may be needed in children to assess the ability of the testes to synthesize testosterone.

Leydig Cell Aplasia

Patients with aplasia or hypoplasia of the Leydig cells usually have **female phenotypes,** but there may be mild virilization. Testes, epididymis, and vas deferens are present; the uterus and fallopian tubes are absent because of normal production of AMH. There are no secondary sexual changes at puberty, but pubic hair may be normal. Plasma levels of testosterone are low and do not respond to hCG; LH levels are elevated. The Leydig cells of the testes are absent or markedly deficient. The defect may involve a lack of receptors for LH. In children, hCG stimulation is necessary to differentiate the condition from the androgen insensitivity syndromes (AISs). There is male-limited autosomal recessive inheritance. The human LH receptor is a member of the G-protein–coupled superfamily of receptors that contains 7 transmembrane domains. Several inactivating mutations of the LH receptor have been described in males with hypogonadism suspected of having Leydig cell hypoplasia or aplasia.

High serum LH and low follicle-stimulating hormone were noted in 1 male with hypogonadism owing to a mutation in the gene for the β-subunit of follicle-stimulating hormone (see Table 583-1 in Chapter 583).

Lipoid Adrenal Hyperplasia
See Chapter 576.

The most severe form of congenital adrenal hyperplasia derives its name from the appearance of the enlarged adrenal glands resulting from accumulation of cholesterol and cholesterol esters. The rate-limiting process in steroidogenesis is the transport of free cholesterol through the cytosol to the inner mitochondrial membrane, where the P450 side-chain cleavage enzyme (P450scc; CYP11A1) acts. Cholesterol transport into mitochondria is mediated by the steroidogenetic acute regulatory protein (StAR) whose synthesis occurs via cyclic adenosine monophosphate through a cyclic adenosine monophosphate response element–binding protein. StAR is a 30 kDa protein essential for steroidogenesis and is encoded by a gene on chromosome 8p11.2. The mitochondrial content of StAR increases between 1 and 5 hr after adrenocorticotropic hormone stimulation, long after the acute adrenocorticotropic hormone–induced increase in steroidogenesis. This has led some to suggest that extramitochondrial StAR might also be involved in the acute response to adrenocorticotropic hormone.

All serum steroid levels are low or undetectable, whereas corticotropin and plasma renin levels are quite elevated. The phenotype is female in both genetic females and males. Genetic males have no müllerian structures because the testes can produce normal AMH but no steroid hormones. These children present with acute adrenal crisis and salt wasting in infancy. Most patients are 46,XY. In a few patients, ovarian steroidogenesis is present at puberty.

The regulatory role of StAR-independent steroidogenesis is illustrated by 46,XX 4 mo old twins with lipoid adrenal hyperplasia. One died at 15 mo because of cardiac complications related to coarctation of the aorta. The adrenal glands had characteristic lipid deposits. The surviving twin had spontaneous puberty with feminization at 11.5 yr and menarche at 13.8 yr. When restudied at the age of 15 yr, a homozygous frameshift-inactivating mutation in her *StAR* gene was discovered. This and the fact that she survived as an infant until 4 mo of age without replacement therapy with detectable serum aldosterone levels supports the hypothesis that StAR-independent steroidogenesis was able to proceed until enough intracellular lipid accumulated to destroy steroidogenic activity. Partial defects in only partially virilized males and delayed onset of salt wasting have been described. Complete P450scc defects may be incompatible with life because only this enzyme can convert cholesterol to pregnenolone, which then becomes progesterone, a hormone essential for the maintenance of normal mammalian pregnancy. Heterozygous mutation in *CYP11A1* was described in a 4 yr old with 46,XY sex reversal and late-onset form of lipoid adrenal hyperplasia. At 6-7 wk of gestation, when maternal corpus luteum progesterone synthesis stops, the placenta, which does not express StAR, produces progesterone by StAR-independent steroidogenesis using the CYP11A1 enzyme system.

3β-Hydroxysteroid Dehydrogenase Deficiency

Males with this form of congenital adrenal hyperplasia (see Chapter 576) have various degrees of **hypospadias,** with or without bifid scrotum and cryptorchidism and, rarely, a complete female phenotype. Affected infants usually develop salt-losing manifestations shortly after birth. Incomplete defects, occasionally seen in boys with premature pubarche, as well as late-onset nonclassic forms, have been reported. These children have point mutations of the gene for type II 3β-hydroxysteroid enzyme, resulting in impairment of steroidogenesis in the adrenals and gonads; the impairment may be unequal between adrenals and gonads. Normal pubertal changes in some boys could be explained by the normally present type I 3β-hydroxysteroid dehydrogenase present in many peripheral tissues. Infertility is frequent. There is no correlation between degree of salt wasting and degree of phenotypic abnormality.

Deficiency of 17-Hydroxylase/17,20-Lyase

A single enzyme (CYP17A1) encoded by a single gene on chromosome 10q24.3 has both 17-hydroxylase and 17,20-lyase activities in adrenal and gonadal tissues (see Chapter 576). Many different genetic lesions have been reported. Genetic males usually have a complete female phenotype or, less often, various degrees of undervirilization from labioscrotal fusion to perineal hypospadias and cryptorchidism. Pubertal development fails to occur in both genetic sexes.

In the classical disorder, there is decreased synthesis of cortisol by the adrenals and of sex steroids by the adrenals and gonads. Levels of deoxycorticosterone and corticosterone are markedly increased and

lead to the hypertension and hypokalemia characteristic of this form of male DSD. Although levels of cortisol are low, the elevated corticotropin and corticosterone levels prevent symptomatic cortisol deficiency. The renin–aldosterone axis is suppressed because of the strong mineralocorticoid effect of elevated deoxycorticosterone. Virilization does not occur at puberty; levels of testosterone are low, and those of gonadotropins are increased. Because fetal production of AMH is normal, no müllerian duct remnants are present. In phenotypic XY females, gonadectomy and replacement therapy with hydrocortisone and sex steroids are indicated.

The defect follows autosomal recessive inheritance. Affected XX females are usually not detected until young adult life, when they fail to experience normal pubertal changes and are found to have hypertension and hypokalemia. This condition should be suspected in patients presenting with primary amenorrhea and hypertension whose chromosomal complement is either 46,XX or 46,XY.

Deficiency of 17-Ketosteroid Reductase

This enzyme, also called *17β-hydroxysteroid dehydrogenase*, catalyzes the final step in testosterone biosynthesis. It is necessary to convert androstenedione to testosterone and also dehydroepiandrosterone to androstenediol and estrone to estradiol. Enzymatic defects in the fetal testis give rise to males with complete or near-complete female phenotype in 46,XY males. Müllerian ducts are absent, and a shallow vagina is present. The diagnosis is based on the ratio of androstenedione to testosterone; in prepubertal children, stimulation with hCG may be necessary to make the diagnosis.

The defect is inherited in an autosomal recessive fashion. At least 4 different types of 17β-hydroxysteroid dehydrogenase are recognized, each coded by a different gene or different chromosomes. Type III is the enzyme defect that is especially common in a highly inbred Arab population in Gaza. The gene for the disorder is at 9q22 and is expressed only in the testes, where it converts androstenedione to testosterone. Most patients are diagnosed at puberty because of virilization and the failure to menstruate. Testosterone levels at puberty may approach normal, presumably as a result of peripheral conversion of androstenedione to testosterone; at this time, some patients spontaneously adopt a male gender role.

Type I 17β-hydroxysteroid dehydrogenase, encoded by a gene on chromosome 17q21, converts estrone to estradiol and is found in placenta, ovary, testis, liver, prostate, adipose tissue, and endometrium. Type II, whose gene is on chromosome 16q24, reverses the reactions of types I and III (converting testosterone to androstenedione and estrone to estradiol, respectively). Type IV is similar in action to type II. A late-onset form of 17-ketosteroid reductase deficiency presents as gynecomastia in young adult males.

Persistent Müllerian Duct Syndrome

In this disorder, there is persistence of müllerian duct derivatives in otherwise completely virilized males. Cases have been reported in siblings and identical twins. **Cryptorchidism** is present in 80% of affected males; and during surgery for this or inguinal hernia, the condition is uncovered when a fallopian tube and uterus are found. The degree of müllerian development is variable and may be asymmetric. Testicular function is normal in most, but testicular degeneration has been reported. Some affected males acquire testicular tumors after puberty. In a study of 38 families, 16 families had defects in the AMH gene, located on the short arm of chromosome 19. They had low AMH levels. In 16 families with high AMH levels, the defect was in the AMH type II receptor gene, with 10 of 16 having identical 27-bp deletions on exon 10 in at least 1 allele.

Treatment consists of removal of as many of the müllerian structures as possible without causing damage to the testis, epididymis, or vas deferens.

DEFECTS IN ANDROGEN ACTION

In the following group of disorders, fetal synthesis of testosterone is normal and defective virilization results from inherited abnormalities in androgen action.

Dihydrotestosterone Deficiency

Decreased production of DHT in utero results in marked ambiguity of external genitalia of affected males. Biosynthesis and peripheral action of testosterone are normal.

The phenotype most commonly associated with this condition results in boys who have a small phallus, bifid scrotum, urogenital sinus with perineal hypospadias, and a blind vaginal pouch (Fig. 588-3). Testes are in the inguinal canals or labioscrotal folds and are normal histologically. There are no müllerian structures. Wolffian structures—the vas deferens, epididymis, and seminal vesicles—are present. Most affected patients have been identified as females. At puberty, virilization occurs; the phallus enlarges, the testes descend and grow normally, and spermatogenesis occurs. There is no gynecomastia. Beard growth is scanty, acne is absent, the prostate is small, and recession of the temporal hairline fails to occur. Virilization of the wolffian duct is caused by the action of testosterone itself, although masculinization of the urogenital sinus and external genitals depends on the action of DHT during the critical period of fetal masculinization. Growth of facial hair and of the prostate also appears to be DHT dependent.

The adult height reached is close to that of the father and other male siblings. There is significant phenotypic heterogeneity. This has led to a classification of such patients into 5 types of steroid 5α-reductase deficiency (SRD).

Several different gene defects of SRD5A2 (the 5α-reductase type 2 gene leading to SRD) have been identified, located on the short arm of chromosome 2, in patients from throughout the world. Familial clusters have been reported from the Dominican Republic, Turkey, Papua New Guinea, Brazil, Mexico, and the Middle East. There is no reliable correlation between genotype and phenotype.

The disorder is inherited as an autosomal recessive trait but is limited to males; normal homozygous females with normal fertility indicate that in females DHT has no role in sexual differentiation or in ovarian function later in life. The clinical diagnosis should be made as early as possible in infancy. It is important to distinguish this from partial androgen insensitivity syndrome (PAIS), as patients with PAIS are far less sensitive to androgen than are patients with SRD. The biochemical diagnosis of SRD is based on finding normal serum testosterone levels, normal or low DHT levels with markedly increased basal and especially hCG-stimulated testosterone: DHT ratios (>17), and high ratios of urinary etiocholanolone to androsterone. Children with androgen insensitivity have normal hepatic 5α reduction and, thus, a normal ratio of tetrahydrocortisol to 5α-tetrahydrocortisol, as opposed to those with SRD.

It is important to note that most but not all children with SRD reared as females in childhood have changed to male around the time of puberty. It appears that exposures to testosterone in utero, neonatally, and at puberty have variable contributions to the formation of male gender identity. Much more needs to be learned about the influences of hormones such as androgens as well as the influences of cultural, social, psychologic, genetic, and other biologic factors in gender identity and behavior. Infants with this condition should be reared as boys whenever practical. Treatment of male infants with DHT results in phallic enlargement.

Another cause of DHT deficiency is a block in an alternative pathway of DHT synthesis. Patients previously thought to have 46,XY DSD because of isolated 17,20-lyase deficiency have subsequently been characterized as having mutations in the *AKR1C2* gene (3α-reductase type 3) or both the *AKR1C2* and *AKR1C4* (3α-reductase type 4) genes. These findings showed that both the classical and alternative pathways to DHT must be intact for normal prenatal virilization.

Androgen Insensitivity Syndromes

The AISs are the most common forms of male DSD, occurring with an estimated frequency of 1/20,000 genetic males. This group of heterogeneous X-linked recessive disorders is caused by more than 150 different mutations in the androgen receptor gene, located on Xq11-12: single point mutations resulting in amino acid substitutions or premature stop codons, frameshift and premature terminations, gene deletions, and splice-site mutations.

Clinical Manifestations

The clinical spectrum of patients with AISs, all of whom have a 46,XY chromosomal complement, range from phenotypic females (in complete AIS) to males with various forms of ambiguous genitalia and undervirilization (partial AIS, or clinical syndromes such as **Reifenstein syndrome**) to phenotypically normal-appearing males with infertility. In addition to normal 46,XY chromosomes, the presence of testes and normal or elevated testosterone and LH levels are common to all such children (Figs. 588-4 and 588-5).

In **complete androgen insensitivity syndrome (CAIS),** an extreme form of failure of virilization, genetic males appear female at birth and are invariably reared accordingly. The external genitalia are female. The vagina ends blindly in a pouch, and the uterus is absent as a result of the normal production and effect of AMH by the testes. In about one third of patients, unilateral or bilateral fallopian tube remnants are found. The testes are usually intraabdominal but may descend into the inguinal canal; they consist largely of seminiferous tubules. At puberty, there is normal development of breasts and the habitus is female, but menstruation does not occur and sexual hair is absent. Adult heights of these women are commensurate with those of normal males despite profound congenital deficiency of androgenic effects.

The testes of affected adult patients produce normal male levels of testosterone, which are converted to normal levels of DHT. Failure of normal male differentiation during fetal life reflects a defective response to androgens at that time. The absence of androgenic effects is caused by a striking resistance to the action of endogenous or exogenous testosterone at the cellular level.

Prepubertal girls with this disorder are often detected when inguinal masses prove to be testes or when a testis is unexpectedly found during herniorrhaphy. Approximately 1-2% of girls with an inguinal hernia prove to have this disorder. In infants, elevated LH levels should suggest the diagnosis. In older girls and adults, **amenorrhea** is the usual presenting symptom. In prepubertal children, the condition must

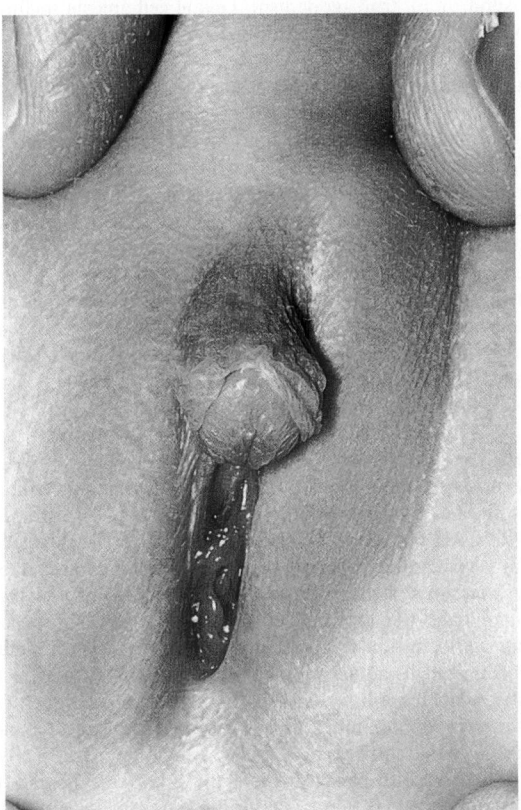

Figure 588-3 5α-Reductase deficiency. *(From Wales JKH, Wit JM, Rogol AD: Pediatric endocrinology and growth, ed 2, Philadelphia, 2003, WB Saunders, p. 165.)*

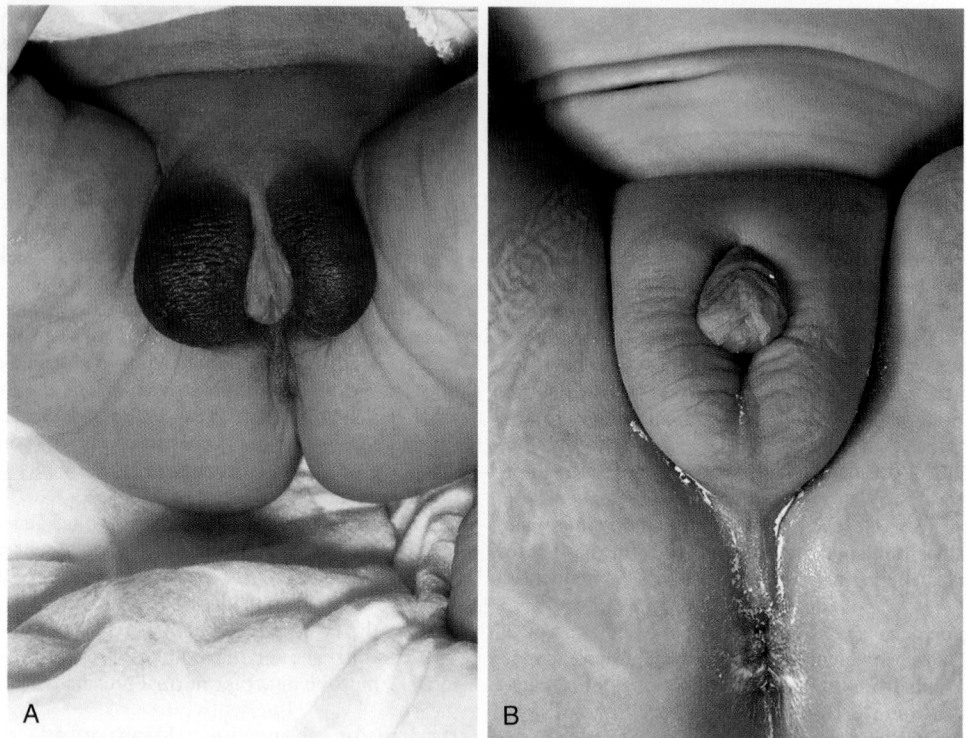

Figure 588-4 A, Partial androgen insensitivity with descended testes in bifid labioscrotal folds. **B,** Less-severe partial androgen insensitivity with severe hypospadias and maldescent of testes. *(From Wales JKH, Wit JM, Rogol AD: Pediatric endocrinology and growth, ed 2, Philadelphia, 2003, WB Saunders, p. 165.)*

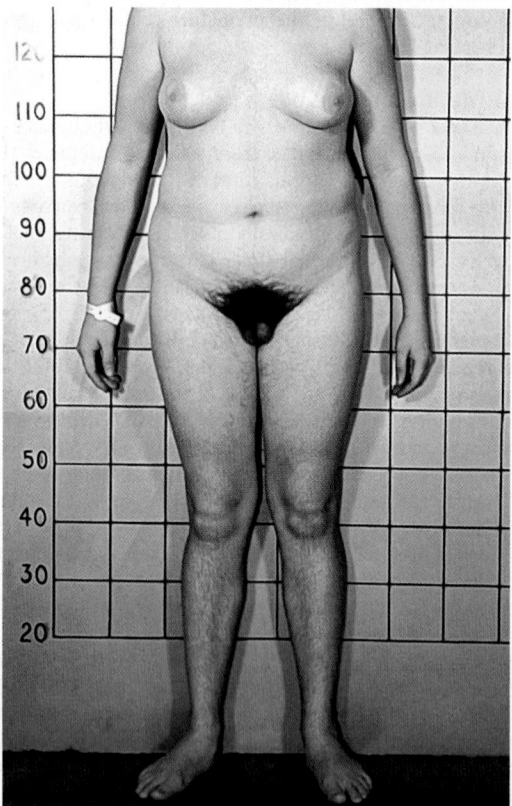

Figure 588-5 Partial androgen insensitivity syndrome at adolescence, male sex of rearing. Note gynecomastia from peripheral aromatase conversion of testosterone to estrogen. Abundant pubic hair implies only partial resistance. *(From Wales JKH, Wit JM, Rogol AD: Pediatric endocrinology and growth, ed 2, Philadelphia, 2003, WB Saunders, p. 165.)*

be differentiated from other types of XY undervirilized males in which there is complete feminization. These include XY gonadal dysgenesis (Swyer syndrome), true agonadism, Leydig cell aplasia including LH receptor defects, and 17-ketosteroid reductase deficiency; all these conditions, unlike CAIS, are characterized by **low levels of testosterone** as neonates and during adult life and by failure to respond to hCG during the prepubertal years.

Although patients with CAIS have unambiguously female external genitals at birth, those with **PAIS** have a wide variety of phenotypic presentations, ranging from **perineoscrotal hypospadias,** bifid scrotum, and cryptorchidism to extreme undervirilization appearing as clitoromegaly and labial fusion. Some forms of PAIS are known as specific syndromes. Patients with **Reifenstein syndrome** have incomplete virilization characterized by hypogonadism, severe hypospadias, and gynecomastia (see Fig. 588-5). **Gilbert-Dreyfus** and **Lubs** syndromes are also classified as PAISs. In all cases, abnormalities in the androgen receptor gene have been identified. Table 588-5 lists other causes of a PAIS-like syndrome.

Diagnosis

The diagnosis of patients with PAIS may be particularly difficult in infancy. The postnatal surge in testosterone and LH is diminished in those with CAIS but not in those with PAIS. In some, especially those sufficiently virilized in infancy, the diagnosis is not suspected until puberty when there is inadequate virilization with lack of facial hair or voice change and the appearance of gynecomastia. Azoospermia and infertility are common. Increasingly, androgen receptor defects are being recognized in adults who have a small phallus and testes and infertility. A single-amino-acid substitution in the androgen receptor was reported in a large Chinese family in whom some affected members were fertile while others had gynecomastia and/or hypospadias. Production of insulin-like growth factor 2 and insulin-like growth factor–binding protein-2, but not insulin-like growth factor–binding protein-3, by genital skin fibroblasts is decreased in CAIS compared with normal genital skin fibroblasts, suggesting a possible role for the insulin-like growth factor system in modulating androgen action.

Table 588-5	Causes of a PAIS-Like Phenotype

DEFECTS IN ANDROGEN PRODUCTION
- Partial gonadal dysgenesis
  - Mutations in *SRY, NR5A1, WT1*
- Mutations of the luteinizing hormone receptor
- Biosynthetic enzyme deficiencies
- 17,20-Lyase deficiency
- P450 oxidoreductase deficiency
- 17β-hydroxysteroid dehydrogenase deficiency type 3
- 5α-Reductase deficiency type 2

GENETIC
- Klinefelter syndrome
- Smith-Lemli-Opitz syndrome
- Denys-Drash syndrome
- Frasier syndrome

PAIS
- Mutations of the androgen receptor gene
- Normal androgen receptor gene with fetal growth restriction

NR5A1, nuclear receptor subfamily 5 A1; PAIS, partial androgen insensitivity syndrome; SRY, sex-determining region Y; WT1, Wilms tumor 1.
From Hughes IA, Davies JD, Bunch TI, et al: Androgen insensitivity syndrome. Lancet 380:1419–1428, 2012, Panel 1, p. 1421.

Treatment and Prognosis

In patients with CAIS whose sexual orientation is unambiguously female, the testes should be removed as soon as they are discovered. Laparoscopic removal of Y chromosome–bearing gonads has been performed in patients with AIS and in those with gonadal dysgenesis. In one third of patients, malignant tumors, usually seminomas, develop by 50 yr of age. Several teenage girls have acquired seminomas. Replacement therapy with estrogens is indicated at the age of puberty.

Normal breasts develop in affected girls who have not had their testes removed by the age of puberty. In these individuals, production of estradiol results from aromatase activity on testicular testosterone. The absence of androgenic activity also contributes to the feminization of these women.

The psychosexual and surgical management of patients with PAIS is extremely complex and depends in large part on the presenting phenotype. Osteopenia is recognized as a late feature of AIS.

Molecular analyses have suggested that phenotype may depend in part on somatic mosaicism of the androgen receptor gene. This was based on the case of a 46,XY patient who had a premature stop codon in exon 1 of the androgen receptor gene, but who also had evidence of virilization (pubic hair and clitoral enlargement) explained by the discovery of the wild-type alleles on careful examination of the sequencing gel. The presence of mosaicism shifts the phenotype to a higher degree of virilization than expected from the genotype of the mutant allele alone.

Genetic counseling is difficult in families with androgen receptor gene mutation. In addition to lack of genotype–phenotype correlations, there is a high rate (27%) of de novo mutations in families.

Sex hormone–binding globulin reduction after exogenous androgen administration (stanozolol) correlates with the severity of the receptor defect and may become a useful clinical tool. Successful therapy with supplemental androgens has been reported in patients with PAIS and various mutations of the androgen receptor in the DNA-binding domain and the ligand-binding domain.

Mutated androgen receptors are also reported in patients with spinal and bulbar muscular atrophy in whom clinical manifestations including testicular atrophy, infertility, gynecomastia, and elevated LH, follicle-stimulating hormone, and estradiol levels usually manifest between the 3rd and 5th decades of life. Androgen receptor mutations have also been described in patients with prostate cancer.

UNDETERMINED CAUSES

Other XY undervirilized males display great variability of the external and internal genitalia and various degrees of phallic and müllerian

development. Testes may be histologically normal or rudimentary, or there may only be 1. No recognized cause is identified in up to 50% of children with 46,XY DSD. Some ambiguity of the genitalia is associated with a wide variety of chromosomal aberrations, which must always be considered in the differential diagnosis, the most common being the 45,X/46,XY syndrome (see Chapter 586.1). It may be necessary to karyotype several tissues to establish mosaicism. Other complex genetic syndromes, many resulting from single gene mutations, are associated with varying degrees of ambiguity of the genitalia, particularly in the male. These entities must be identified on the basis of the associated extragenital malformations.

Smith-Lemli-Opitz syndrome is an autosomal recessive disorder caused by mutations in the sterol Δ7-reductase gene located on chromosome 11q12-q13. It is characterized by prenatal and postnatal growth retardation, microcephaly, ptosis, anteverted nares, broad alveolar ridges, syndactyly of the 2nd-3rd toes, and severe cognitive impairment (see Chapter 86.3). Its incidence is 1 in 20,000 to 30,000 live births in populations of northern and central European origin; 70% are male. Genotypic males usually have genital ambiguity and, occasionally, partial sex reversal with female genital ambiguity or complete sex reversal with female external genitals. Müllerian duct derivatives are usually absent. Affected 46,XX patients have normal genitalia. Two types of Smith-Lemli-Opitz syndrome have been recognized. The **classical form** (type I) described earlier and the acrodysgenital syndrome, which is usually lethal within 1 yr and is associated with severe malformations, postaxial polydactyly, and extremely abnormal external genitalia (type II). Pyloric stenosis is associated with Smith-Lemli-Opitz syndrome type I and Hirschsprung disease with type II. Cleft palate, skeletal abnormalities, and 1 case of a lipoma of the pituitary gland have been seen in **type II** cases. Some authors believe in a spectrum of disease severity rather than in the above classification. Low plasma cholesterol with elevated 7-dehydrocholesterol, its precursor, are found in types I and II, and the levels do not correlate with severity. Maternal apolipoprotein E values do seem to correlate with severity. The most common prenatal expression of Smith-Lemli-Opitz syndrome is intrauterine growth retardation (see Chapter 86.3 for treatment).

46,XY DSD subjects also have been described in siblings with the α-thalassemia/mental retardation syndrome.

Bibliography is available at Expert Consult.

588.3 Ovotesticular DSD

Patricia A. Donohue

In ovotesticular DSD, both ovarian and testicular tissues are present, either in the same or in opposite gonads. Affected patients have ambiguous genitalia, varying from normal female with only slight enlargement of the clitoris to almost normal male external genitalia (see Fig. 588-2A).

Approximately 70% of all patients have a 46,XX karyotype. Ninety-seven percent of affected patients of African descent are 46,XX. Fewer than 10% of persons with ovotesticular DSD are 46,XY. Approximately 20% have 46,XX/46,XY mosaicism. Half of these are derived from more than 1 zygote and are chimeras (chi 46,XX/46,XY). The presence of paternal and both maternal alleles for some blood groups is demonstrated. An ovotesticular DSD chimera, 46,XX/46,XY, was reported as resulting from embryo amalgamation after in vitro fertilization. Each embryo was derived from an independent, separately fertilized ovum.

Examination of 46,XX ovotesticular DSD patients with Y-specific probes has detected fewer than 10% with a portion of the Y chromosome including the *SRY* gene. Ovotesticular DSD is usually sporadic, but a number of siblings have been reported. The cause of most cases of ovotesticular DSD is unknown.

The most frequently encountered gonad in ovotesticular DSD is an ovotestis, which may be bilateral. If unilateral, the contralateral gonad is usually an ovary but may be a testis. The ovarian tissue is normal, but the testicular tissue is dysgenetic. The presence and function of testicular tissue can be determined by measuring basal and hCG-stimulated testosterone levels as well as AMH levels. Patients who are highly virilized and have had adequate testicular function with no uterus are usually reared as males. If a uterus exists, virilization is often mild and testicular function minimal; assignment of female sex may be indicated. Selective removal of gonadal tissue inconsistent with sex of rearing may be indicated. In a few families, 46,XY ovotesticular DSD subjects and 44,XX males have been described in the same sibship.

Defects in R-Spondin1, encoded by the *RSPO1* gene, have been described in 46,XX ovotesticular DSD.

Pregnancies with living offspring have been reported in 46,XX ovotesticular DSD individuals reared as females, but very few males with ovotesticular DSD have fathered children. Approximately 5% of patients will develop gonadoblastomas, dysgerminomas, or seminomas.

DIAGNOSIS AND MANAGEMENT OF DISORDERS OF SEX DEVELOPMENT

In the neonate, ambiguity of the genitals requires immediate attention to decide on the sex of rearing as early in life as possible. The family of the infant needs to be informed of the child's condition as early, completely, compassionately, and honestly as possible. Caution must be used to avoid feelings of guilt, shame, and discomfort. Guidance needs to be provided to alleviate both short-term and long-term concerns and to allow the child to grow up in a completely supportive environment. The initial care is best provided by a team of professionals that include neonatologists and pediatric specialists, endocrinologists, radiologists, urologists, psychologists, and geneticists, all of whom remain focused foremost on the needs of the child. Management of the potential psychologic upheaval that these disorders can generate in the child or the family is of paramount importance and requires physicians and other healthcare professionals with sensitivity, training, and experience in this field.

While awaiting the results of chromosomal analysis, pelvic ultrasonography is indicated to determine the presence of a uterus and ovaries. Presence of a uterus and absence of palpable gonads usually suggests a virilized XX female. A search for the source of virilization should be undertaken; this includes studies of adrenal hormones to rule out varieties of congenital adrenal hyperplasia, and studies of androgens and estrogens occasionally may be necessary to rule out aromatase deficiency. Virilized XX females are generally (but not always) reared as females even when highly virilized.

The absence of a uterus, with or without palpable gonads, often indicates an undervirilized male and an XY karyotype. Measurements of levels of gonadotropins, testosterone, AMH, and DHT are necessary to determine whether testicular production of androgen is present and is normal. Undervirilized males who are totally feminized may be reared as females. Certain significantly feminized infants, such as those with 5α-reductase deficiency, may be reared as males because these children virilize normally at puberty. Sixty percent of individuals with 5α-reductase deficiency assigned as female in infancy live as males as adults. An infant with a comparable degree of feminization resulting from an androgen receptor defect, such as CAIS, is best reared as a female.

When receptor disorders are suspected in the XY male with a small phallus (micropenis), a course of 3 monthly intramuscular injections of testosterone enanthate (25-50 mg) may assist in the differential diagnosis of androgen insensitivity, as well as in treatment.

In some mammals, the female exposed to androgens prenatally or in early postnatal life exhibits nontraditional sexual behavior in adult life. Most, but not all, girls who have undergone fetal masculinization from congenital adrenal hyperplasia or from maternal progestin therapy have female sexual identity, although during childhood they may appear to prefer male playmates and activities over female playmates and feminine play with dolls in mothering roles.

In the past it was thought that surgical treatment of ambiguous genitalia to create a female appearance, particularly when a vagina is present, was more successful than construction of male genitalia. Considerable controversy exists regarding these decisions. Sexual functioning is to a large extent more dependent on neurohormonal and behavioral factors than the physical appearance and functional ability of the genitalia. Similarly, controversy exists regarding the timing of the performance of invasive and definitive procedures, such as surgery. Whenever possible without endangering the physical or psychologic health of the child, an expert multidisciplinary team should consider deferring elective surgical repairs and gonadectomies until the child can participate in the informed consent for the procedure. One study of children (*n* = 59 boys and 18 girls) with gender dysphoria but without documentation of genomic or enzymologic abnormalities indicated that most of these children no longer have gender dysphoria after completion of puberty. Among those who do, homosexuality and bisexuality are the most frequent diagnoses.

For patients with DSD who have Y-chromosome material and intraabdominal gonads, gonadectomy is generally recommended because of the risk of gonadal tumors, many of which are malignant.

The pediatrician, pediatric endocrinologist, and psychologist, along with the appropriate additional specialists, should provide ongoing compassionate, supportive care to the patient and the patient's family throughout childhood, adolescence, and adulthood. Support groups are available for families and patients with many of the conditions discussed.

Bibliography is available at Expert Consult.

Section 6
Diabetes Mellitus in Children

Chapter 589
Diabetes Mellitus

589.1 Classification
Britta M. Svoren and Nicholas Jospe

Diabetes mellitus (DM) is a common, chronic, metabolic disease characterized by hyperglycemia as a cardinal biochemical feature. The major forms of diabetes are differentiated by insulin deficiency vs insulin resistance: type 1 diabetes mellitus (T1DM) results from deficiency of insulin secretion because of pancreatic β-cell damage; type 2 diabetes mellitus (T2DM) is a consequence of insulin resistance occurring at the level of skeletal muscle, liver, and adipose tissue, with various degrees of β-cell impairment. T1DM is the most common endocrine-metabolic disorder of childhood and adolescence, with important consequences for physical and emotional development. Individuals with T1DM confront serious lifestyle alterations, including an absolute daily requirement for exogenous insulin, the need to monitor their own glucose level, and the need to pay attention to dietary intake. Morbidity and mortality stem from a constant potential for acute metabolic derangements and from long-term **complications** (usually in adulthood) that affect small and large blood vessels resulting in retinopathy, nephropathy, neuropathy, ischemic heart disease, and arterial obstruction with gangrene of the extremities. The acute clinical manifestations are caused by hypoinsulinemic hyperglycemic ketoacidosis; the genesis of T1DM owes to autoimmune mechanisms; and the long-term complications are related to metabolic disturbances (hyperglycemia).

Table 589-1	Etiologic Classifications of Diabetes Mellitus

I. Type 1 diabetes (β-cell destruction ultimately leading to complete insulin deficiency)
   A. Immune mediated
   B. Idiopathic
II. Type 2 diabetes (variable combinations of insulin resistance and insulin deficiency)
   A. Typical
   B. Atypical
III. Genetic defects of β-cell function
   A. MODY (maturity-onset diabetes of the young) syndromes
      1. MODY 1 chromosome 20, HNF4α
      2. MODY 2 chromosome 7, glucokinase
      3. MODY 3 chromosome 12, HNF1α, TCF-1
      4. MODY 4 chromosome 13, IPF-1
      5. MODY 5 chromosome 17, HNF1β, TCF-2
      6. MODY 6 chromosome 2q32, neuro-D_1/β_2
   B. Mitochondrial DNA mutations (includes 1 form of Wolfram syndrome, Pearson syndrome, Kearns-Sayre, diabetes mellitus, deafness)
   C. Wolfram syndrome—DIDMOAD (diabetes insipidus, diabetes mellitus, optic atrophy, deafness): WFS1-Wolframin—chromosome 4p
      1. Wolfram locus 2—chromosome 4q22-24
      2. Wolfram mitochondrial
   D. Thiamine responsive megaloblastic anemia and diabetes
IV. Drug or chemical induced
   A. Antirejection—cyclosporine, sirolimus
   B. Glucocorticoids (with impaired insulin secretion; e.g., cystic fibrosis)
   C. L-Asparaginase
   D. β-Adrenergic blockers
   E. Vacor (rodenticide)
   F. Phenytoin (Dilantin)
   G. α-Interferon
   H. Diazoxide
   I. Nicotinic acid
   J. Pentamidine
V. Diseases of exocrine pancreas
   A. Cystic fibrosis–related diabetes
   B. Trauma—pancreatectomy
   C. Pancreatitis—ionizing radiation
   D. Others
VI. Infections
   A. Congenital rubella
   B. Cytomegalovirus
   C. Hemolytic-uremic syndrome
VII. Variants of type 2 diabetes
   A. Genetic defects of insulin action
      1. Rabson-Mendenhall syndrome
      2. Leprechaunism
      3. Lipoatrophic diabetes syndromes
      4. Type A insulin resistance—acanthosis
   B. Acquired defects of insulin action
      1. Endocrine tumors—rare in childhood
   C. Pheochromocytoma
   D. Cushing
   E. Others
      1. Antiinsulin receptor antibodies
VIII. Genetic syndromes with diabetes and insulin resistance/insulin deficiency
   A. Prader-Willi syndrome, chromosome 15
   B. Down syndrome, chromosome 21
   C. Turner syndrome
   D. Klinefelter syndrome
   E. Others
      1. Bardet-Biedel
      2. Alström
      3. Werner
   F. IPEX (immunodysfunction, polyendocrinopathy, enteropathy, X-linked)
   G. Celiac disease
   H. Autoimmune polyendocrinopathy
IX. Gestational diabetes
X. Neonatal diabetes
   A. Transient—chromosome 6q24, KCNJ11, ABCC8, INS, HNF1β, others
   B. Permanent—agenesis of pancreas—glucokinase deficiency, homozygous, KCNJ11, ABCC8, others

Modified from Sperling MA, Tamborlane WV, Battelino T, Weinzimer SA, Phillip M: Diabetes mellitus. In Sperling MA, editor: Pediatric endocrinology, ed 4, Philadelphia, 2014, Elsevier, Box 19-1.

DM is not a single entity but rather a heterogeneous group of disorders in which there are distinct genetic patterns as well as other etiologic and pathophysiologic mechanisms that lead to impairment of glucose tolerance. Table 589-1 presents a classification of diabetes and other categories of glucose intolerance. Three major forms of diabetes and several forms of carbohydrate intolerance are identified.

TYPE 1 DIABETES MELLITUS

Formerly called *insulin-dependent diabetes mellitus* (IDDM) or *juvenile diabetes*, T1DM is characterized by low or absent levels of endogenously produced insulin and by dependence on exogenous insulin to prevent development of ketoacidosis, an acute life-threatening complication of T1DM. The natural history includes 4 distinct stages: (1) preclinical β-cell autoimmunity with progressive defect of insulin secretion, (2) onset of clinical diabetes, (3) transient remission "honeymoon period," and (4) established diabetes during which there may occur acute and/or chronic complications and decreased life expectancy. The onset occurs predominantly in childhood, with a median age of 7-15 yr, but it may present at any age. The incidence of T1DM has steadily increased in nearly all parts of the world (Fig. 589-1). T1DM is characterized by autoimmune destruction of pancreatic islet β cells. Both genetic susceptibility and environmental factors contribute to the pathogenesis. Susceptibility to T1DM is genetically con-

trolled by alleles of the major histocompatibility complex class II genes expressing human leukocyte antigens (HLAs). Autoantibodies to β-cell antigens such as islet cell cytoplasm (ICA), insulin autoantibody (IAA), antibodies to glutamic acid decarboxylase, and ICA512 are detected in serum from affected subjects. These can be detected months to years prior to clinical onset of T1DM. T1DM is associated with other **auto-immune** diseases such as thyroiditis, celiac disease, and Addison disease. In some children and adolescents with apparent T1DM, the β-cell destruction is not immune mediated. This subtype of diabetes occurs in patients of African or Asian origin and is distinct from known causes of β-cell destruction such as drugs or chemicals, viruses, mitochondrial gene defects, pancreatectomy, and ionizing radiation. These individuals may have ketoacidosis, but they have extensive periods of remission with variable insulin deficiency, similar to patients with T2DM.

TYPE 2 DIABETES MELLITUS

Children and adolescents with this type of diabetes are usually obese but are not insulin dependent and infrequently develop ketosis. Some subjects with T2DM may present with or develop ketosis during severe infections or other stresses and may then need insulin for correction of symptomatic hyperglycemia. This category includes the most prevalent form of diabetes in adults, which is characterized by insulin resistance and often a progressive defect in insulin secretion. This type of diabetes was formerly known as *adult-onset diabetes mellitus or non–insulin-dependent diabetes mellitus*.

The presentation of T2DM is typically more insidious than that with T1DM. In contrast to patients with T1DM who are usually ill at the time of diagnosis and whose presentation rarely spans more than a few weeks, children with T2DM often seek medical care because of excessive weight gain and fatigue as a result of insulin resistance and/or the incidental finding of glycosuria during routine physical examination. A history of polyuria and polydipsia is not always a cardinal clinical feature in these patients. The incidence of T2DM in children has increased by more than 10-fold, depending on geography and mostly as a result of the epidemic of childhood obesity (see Chapter 47). Pediatric T2DM may account for as many as 80% of the new cases of diabetes, especially in obese African-American and Mexican-American adolescents. **Acanthosis nigricans** (dark pigmentation of skin creases in the nape of the neck especially), a sign of insulin resistance, is present in the majority of patients with T2DM and is accompanied by a relative hyperinsulinemia at the time of the diagnosis (see Chapter 652). However, the serum insulin elevation is usually disproportionately lower than that of age-, weight-, and sex-matched nondiabetic children and adolescents, suggesting a state of insulin insufficiency. In some individuals, it may represent slowly evolving T1DM.

In some children with a strong family history of diabetes, impaired glucose tolerance (IGT) may occur in a pattern implying dominant inheritance. This pattern of diabetes has been termed **maturity-onset diabetes of the young (MODY)**: it may require insulin treatment, can be treated with sulfonylureas with varying degrees of success, and is often now referred to as monogenic diabetes. MODY may present with hyperglycemia, and consequent polyuria and polydipsia, or may be diagnosed simply by routine screening. In MODY, there is no autoimmune destruction of β cells and no HLA association. MODY results from specific genetic disorders involving mutations in the gene encoding either pancreatic β-cell and liver glucokinase or in the nuclear transcription factors hepatocyte nuclear factor (1α, 4α, or 1β). A defect in the gene regulating glucose transport into the pancreatic β cell, the GLUT2 transporter, may be responsible for other forms of T2DM. The genetic basis of T2DM also includes defects in glycogen synthase,

insulin receptors, Rad (Ras associated with diabetes), and possibly apolipoprotein C-III. A recent metaanalysis suggests that the incidence of T2DM has a complexly inverse relationship with birthweight in some populations, depending on ethnic and genetic factors.

OTHER SPECIFIC TYPES OF SECONDARY DIABETES
Examples include diabetes secondary to exocrine pancreatic diseases (cystic fibrosis), other endocrine diseases (Cushing syndrome), and ingestion of certain drugs or poisons (the rodenticide Vacor). In organ transplantation survivors, there is a linkage between cyclosporine and tacrolimus and posttransplantation DM, ascribed to a number of mechanisms. Certain genetic syndromes, including those with abnormalities of the insulin receptor, also are included in this category. There are no associations with HLA types, autoimmunity, or islet cell antibodies among the entities in this subdivision.

Table 589-2 details the current criteria for the diagnosis of type 1 and type 2 DM. It should be noted that a fasting blood glucose that exceeds 125 mg/dL (6.9 mmol/L) is the accepted criterion for the diagnosis of diabetes.

IMPAIRED GLUCOSE TOLERANCE
The term *impaired glucose tolerance* (IGT) refers to a metabolic stage that is intermediate between normal glucose homeostasis and diabetes. A fasting glucose concentration of 99 mg/dL (5.5 mmol/L) is the upper limit of "normal." This choice is near the level above which acute-phase insulin secretion is lost in response to intravenous administration of glucose and is associated with a progressively greater risk of the development of microvascular and macrovascular complications.

Many individuals with IGT (fasting glucose 100-125 mg/dL) are euglycemic in their daily lives and may have normal or nearly normal glycated hemoglobin levels. Individuals with IGT often manifest hyperglycemia only when challenged with the oral glucose load used in the standardized oral glucose tolerance test.

In the absence of pregnancy, IGT is not a clinical entity but rather a risk factor for future diabetes and cardiovascular disease. This may be observed as an intermediate stage in any of the disease processes listed in Table 589-1. IGT is often associated with the **insulin**

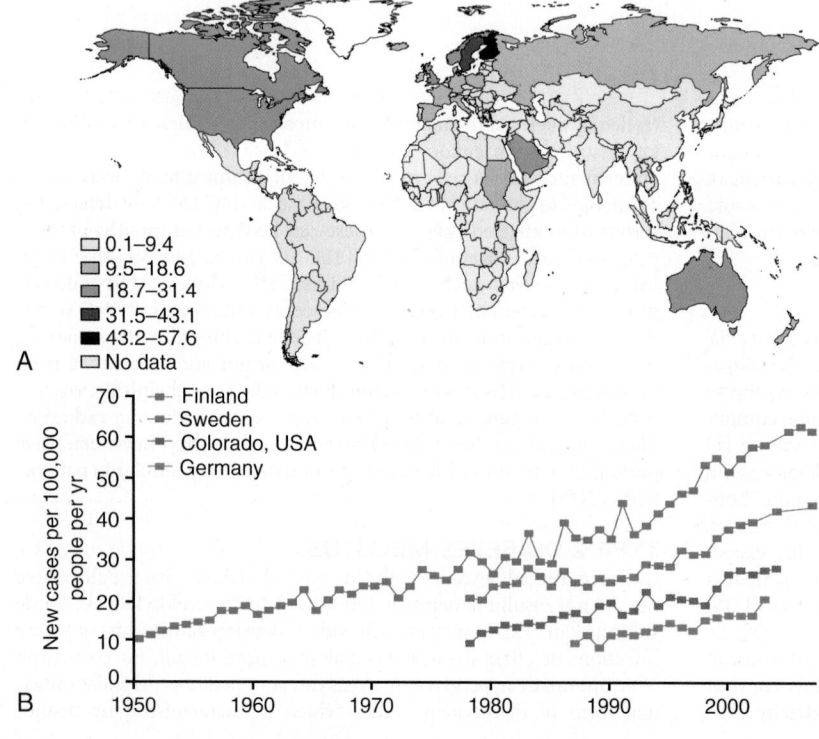

Figure 589-1 Incidence of type 1 diabetes in children ages 0-14 yr, by geographical region and over time. **A,** Estimated global incidence of type 1 diabetes, by region, in 2011. **B,** Time-based trends for the incidence of type 1 diabetes in children ages 0-14 yr in areas with high or high-intermediate rates of disease. (*From Atkinson MA, Eisenbarth GS, Michels AW: Type 1 diabetes. Lancet 383:69–78, 2014, Fig. 1, p. 70.*)

Table 589-2	Diagnostic Criteria for Impaired Glucose Tolerance and Diabetes Mellitus
IMPAIRED GLUCOSE TOLERANCE	**DIABETES MELLITUS**
Fasting glucose 100-125 mg/dL (5.6-7.0 mmol/L)	Symptoms* of diabetes mellitus plus random or casual plasma glucose ≥200 mg/dL (11.1 mmol/L) *or*
2-hr plasma glucose during the OGTT ≥140 mg/dL, but <200 mg/dL (11.1 mmol/L)	Fasting (at least 8 hr) plasma glucose ≥126 mg/dL (7.0 mmol/L) *or* 2 hr plasma glucose during the OGTT ≥200 mg/dL *or* Hemoglobin A$_{1C}$ ≥6.5%[†]

*Symptoms include polyuria, polydipsia, and unexplained weight loss with glucosuria and ketonuria.

[†]Results should be confirmed by repeat testing if in absence of unequivocal hyperglycemia.

OGTT, oral glucose tolerance test.

From Report of the Expert Committee on the Diagnosis and Classification of Diabetes Mellitus, Diabetes Care 20(Suppl 1):S5, 1999; and from Chaing J, Kirkman S, Laffel L, et al: Type 1 diabetes through the life span: A position statement of the American Diabetes Association, Diabetes Care 37:2034–2054, 2014.

resistance syndrome (also known as *syndrome X* or *metabolic syndrome*), which consists of insulin resistance, compensatory hyperinsulinemia to maintain glucose homeostasis, obesity (especially abdominal or visceral obesity), dyslipidemia of the high-triglyceride or low- or high-density lipoprotein type, or both, and hypertension (see Chapter 47). Insulin resistance is directly involved in the pathogenesis of T2DM. IGT appears as a risk marker for this type of diabetes at least in part because of its correlation with insulin resistance. Table 589-2 presents the diagnostic criteria for IGT.

589.2 Type 1 Diabetes Mellitus (Immune Mediated)

Britta M. Svoren and Nicholas Jospe

EPIDEMIOLOGY

T1DM accounts for approximately 10% of all cases of diabetes, affecting up to 3 million people in the United States and more than 15 million people in the world. Using population-based estimates of diabetes incidence and prevalence, a recent study indicates that approximately 15,000 youths are diagnosed with type 1 diabetes each year. While it accounts for most cases of diabetes in childhood, it is not limited to this age group; new cases continue to occur in adult life and approximately 50% of individuals with T1DM present as adults. The incidence of T1DM is highly variable among different ethnic groups (see Fig. 589-1). The overall age-adjusted incidence of T1 DM varies from 0.7 in 100,000 per yr in Karachi (Pakistan) to more than 40 in 100,000 per yr in Finland. The incidence of T1DM is increasing in most (but not all) populations and this increase appears to be most marked in populations where the incidence of autoimmune diseases was historically low. Data from Western European diabetes centers suggest that the annual rate of increase in T1DM incidence is 2-5%, whereas some central and eastern European countries demonstrate an even more rapid increase—up to 9%. The rate of increase is greatest among the youngest children. In the United States, the overall prevalence of diabetes among school-age children is approximately 1.9 in 1,000, increasing from a prevalence of 1 in 1,430 children at 5 yr of age to 1 in 360 children at 16 yr of age. Among African-Americans, the occurrence of T1DM is 30-60% of that seen in American whites. The annual incidence of new cases in the United States is now approximately 19.7

in 100,000 among youth younger than 10 yr and 18.6 in 100,000 of those older than 10 yr, It is estimated that 30,000 new cases occur each year in the United States, affecting 1 in 300 children and as many as 1 in 100 adults during the life span. Rates are similar or higher in most Western European countries and significantly lower in Asia and Africa.

Girls and boys are almost equally affected, but there is a modest female preponderance in some low-risk populations (e.g., the Japanese); there is no apparent correlation with socioeconomic status. Peaks of presentation occur in 2 age groups: at 5-7 yr of age and at the time of puberty. The first peak may correspond to the time of increased exposure to infectious agents coincident with the beginning of school; the second peak may correspond to the pubertal growth spurt induced by gonadal steroids and the increased pubertal growth hormone secretion (which antagonizes insulin). The understanding of the cause of diabetes or of its increased incidence remains elusive. A growing number of cases are presenting between 1 and 2 yr of age, especially in high-risk groups; the average age of presentation is older in low-risk populations. Low-risk groups that migrate to a high-risk country seem to acquire the increased risk of that country. On the other hand, there can be marked differences in incidence rates in various ethnic groups within the same country; for example, incidence rates in the 10-14 yr age group in the United States range from a low of 7.1 in Native Americans, to 17.6 in Hispanics, 19.2 in African-Americans, and 32.9 in whites. These variations also remain unexplained at this time.

GENETICS

There is a clear familial clustering of T1DM, with prevalence in siblings approaching 6%, whereas the prevalence in the general population in the United States is only 0.4%. Risk of diabetes is also increased when a parent has diabetes and this risk differs between the 2 parents; the risk is 3-4% if the mother has diabetes but 5-6% when the father has diabetes. In monozygotic twins, the concordance rate ranges from 30-65%, whereas dizygotic twins have a concordance rate of 6-10%. Because the concordance rate of dizygotic twins is higher than the sibling risk, factors other than the shared genotypes (e.g., the shared intrauterine environment) may play a role in increasing the risk in dizygotic twins. Furthermore, the genetic susceptibility for T1DM in the parents of a child with diabetes is estimated at 3%. It should be kept in mind that although there is a large genetic component in T1DM, 85% of newly diagnosed type 1 diabetic patients do not have a family member with T1DM. Thus, we cannot rely on family history to identify patients who may be at risk for the future development of T1DM as most cases will develop in individuals with no such family history.

Monogenic Type 1 Diabetes Mellitus

Classic single-gene defects are an extremely rare cause of type 1 diabetes, and more than 20 genes have been linked to monogenic diabetes, in children and in adults. In 2 rare syndromes (IPEX and APS-1) the genetic susceptibility that leads to diabetes is caused by a classic single-gene defect. The IPEX (immune dysfunction, polyendocrinopathy, enteropathy, X-linked) syndrome is caused by mutations of the *FOXP3* and other genes. The *FOXP3* (forkhead box P3) is a gene involved in immune system responses. A member of the FOX protein family, *FOXP3* appears to function as the master regulator in the development and function of regulatory T cells. These mutations lead to the lack of a major population of regulatory T lymphocytes with resulting overwhelming autoimmunity and development of diabetes (as early as 2 days of age) in approximately 80% of the children with this disorder.

APS-1 (autoimmune polyendocrinopathy syndrome type 1) is caused by mutations of the *AIRE* (autoimmune regulator) gene, leading to abnormalities in expression of peripheral antigens within the thymus and/or abnormalities of negative selection in the thymus. This results in widespread autoimmunity. Approximately 18% of children with this syndrome develop type 1 diabetes.

Genes Altering the Risk of Autoimmune Type 1 Diabetes Mellitus

For most patients with T1DM, their risk of developing T1DM is modified by the influence of several risk loci. The genomic region with by far the greatest contribution to the risk of T1DM is the major histocompatibility complex on chromosome 6. The region with the next highest odds ratio is the promoter region 5′ of the insulin gene on chromosome 11. Studies have identified more than 50 other risk loci. These loci include insulin *(INS)*, protein tyrosine phosphatase nonreceptor type 22 *(PTPN22)*, protein tyrosine phosphatase nonreceptor type 2 *(PTPN2)*, interleukin (IL)-2 receptor *(CD25)*, a lectin-like gene *(KIAA0350)*, v-erb-b2 erythroblastic leukemia viral oncogene homolog 3e *(ERBB3e)*, cytotoxic T-lymphocyte antigen 4 *(CTLA4)*, and interferon-induced with helicase C domain 1 *(IFIH1)*. However, except for *PTPN22*, their contribution is relatively small, thus making them less useful for predicting the genetic risk of T1DM in a given individual. On balance, the known functions of these genes suggest the primary etiologic pathways of diabetes, namely, HLA class II and class I molecules binding, T and B cell activation, innate pathogen viral responses, chemokine and cytokine signaling, and T regulatory and antigen-presenting cell functions.

Major Histocompatibility Complex/Human Leukocyte Antigen Encoded Susceptibility to Type 1 Diabetes Mellitus

The major histocompatibility complex is a large genomic region that contains a number of genes related to immune system function in humans. These genes are further divided into HLA classes I, II, III, and IV genes. Class II genes are the ones most strongly associated with risk of T1DM, but some of the risk associated with various HLA types is a result of variation in genes in HLA classes other than class II. Overall, genetic variation in the HLA region can explain 40-50% of the genetic risk of T1DM (Fig. 589-2).

Some of the known associations include the HLA DR3/4-DQ2/8 genotype; compared to a population prevalence of T1DM of approximately 1 in 300, DR3/4-DQ2/8 newborns from the general population have a 1 in 20 genetic risk. This risk of development of T1DM is even higher when the high-risk HLA haplotypes are shared with a sibling or parent with T1DM. Thus, if 1 sibling has T1DM and shares the same high-risk DR3/4-DQ2/8 haplotype with another sibling, then the risk of autoimmunity in the other sibling is 50%. And this risk approaches 80% when siblings share both HLA haplotypes identical by descent. This is known as the *relative paradox* and points to the existence of other shared genetic risk factors (most likely in the extended HLA haplotype).

With advances in genotyping, further discrimination is possible and we can identify more specific risk ratios for specific haplotypes. For example, the DRB1*0401-DQA1*0301g-DQB1*0302 haplotype has an odds ratio (OR) of 8.39 whereas the DRB1*0401-DQA1*0301g-DQB1*0301 has an OR of 0.35, implicating the DQB1*0302 allele as a critical susceptibility allele. There are some dramatically protective

DR-DQ haplotypes (e.g., DRB1*1501-DQA1*0102-DQB1*0602 [OR = 0.03], DRB1*1401-DQA1*0101-DQB1*0503 [OR = 0.02], and DRB1*0701-DQA1*0201-DQB1*0303 [OR = 0.02]). The DR2 haplotype (DRB1*1501-DQA1*0102-DQB1*0602) is dominantly protective and is present in 20% of the general population but is seen in only 1% of patients with T1DM.

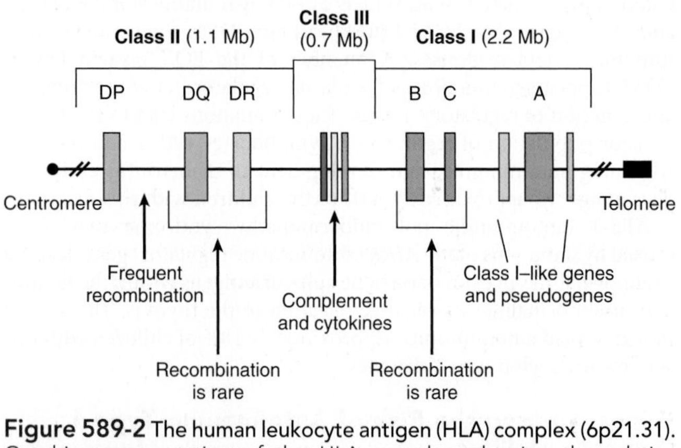

Role of Aspartate at Position 57 in DQB1
DQB1*0302 (high risk for diabetes) differs from DQB1*0301 (protective against diabetes) only at position 57, where it lacks an aspartic acid residue. The DQB1*0201 allele (increased risk for diabetes) also lacks aspartic acid at position 57, and it has been proposed that the presence of aspartate at this position alters the protein recognition and protein binding characteristics of this molecule. Although the absence of aspartate at this position appears to be important in most studies on white individuals, it does not have the same role in Korean and Japanese populations. Moreover, certain low-risk DQB1 genotypes also lack aspartic acid at position 57, including DQB1*0302/DQB1*0201 (DR7) and DQB1*0201 (DR3)/DQB1*0201 (DR7). Thus, the presence of aspartate at this position is usually, but not always, protective in white populations but not necessarily in other populations.

Role of Human Leukocyte Antigen Class I
Although the alleles of class II HLA genes appear to have the strongest associations with diabetes, recent genotyping studies and analyses of pooled data have identified associations with other elements in the HLA complex, especially HLA-A and HLA-B. The most significant association is with HLA-B39, which confers high risk for T1DM in 3 different populations, makes up the majority of the signal from HLA-B, and is associated with a lower age of onset of the disease.

Insulin Gene Locus, *IDDM2*
The second locus found to be associated with risk of T1DM was labeled IDDM2 and has been localized to a region upstream of the insulin gene (i.e., 5′ of the insulin gene). It is estimated that this locus accounts for approximately 10% of the familial risk of T1DM. Susceptibility in this region has been primarily mapped to a variable number of tandem repeats approximately 500 bp upstream of the insulin gene. This highly polymorphic region consists of anywhere from 30 to several hundred repeats of a 14-15 bp unit sequence (ACAGGGGTCTGGGG). A shorter number of repeats is associated with increased risk of T1DM.

PTPN22 (Lymphoid Tyrosine Phosphatase)
A single-nucleotide polymorphism in the *PTPN22* gene on chromosome 1p13 that encodes lymphoid tyrosine phosphatase correlates strongly with the incidence of T1DM in 2 independent populations. This gene has an association with several other autoimmune diseases such as rheumatoid arthritis, systemic lupus erythematosus, vitiligo, and Graves disease.

Cytotoxic T Lymphocyte Antigen 4
The cytotoxic T lymphocyte antigen 4 *(CTLA-4)* gene is located on chromosome 2q33 and is associated with T1DM as well as Graves disease, Hashimoto thyroiditis, celiac disease, and systemic lupus erythematosus. This gene is a negative regulator of T-cell activation.

Interleukin-2 Receptor
Single-nucleotide polymorphisms in or near the gene for the IL-2 receptor have been found to have an association with T1DM risk. Studies with IL-2 in T1DM to date have not been successful in halting progression.

Interleukin-1 Receptor
IL-1 receptor activation and chemokines involved in monocyte/macrophage and neutrophil chemotaxis have been also identified as critical steps in nitric oxide–induced islet necrosis and subsequent apoptosis. Indeed, inhibition of the activation of IL-1β–dependent inflammatory pathways by an IL-1 receptor antagonist in cultured rat islets exposed to nitric oxide prevented necrosis and apoptosis

Figure 589-2 The human leukocyte antigen (HLA) complex (6p21.31). Graphic representation of the HLA complex, showing the relative locations of the 3 classes of HLA genes. *(Courtesy of Dr. George Eisenbarth.)*

supporting evaluation in human islets in vitro and potentially as a posttransplantation therapy. **IL-1 blockade in patients with T1DM has not halted progression.**

Interferon-Induced Helicase
Another gene identified as having a modest effect on the risk of T1DM is the interferon-induced helicase *(IFIH1)* gene. Significant association exists with T1DM as well as Graves disease and multiple sclerosis. This gene is thought to play a role in protecting the host from viral infections and given the specificity of different helicases for different RNA viruses, it is possible that knowledge of this gene locus will help to narrow down the list of viral pathogens that may have a role in T1DM.

CYP27B1
Cytochrome P450, subfamily 27, polypeptide 1 gene encodes vitamin D 1α-hydroxylase. Because of the known role of vitamin D in immune regulation and because of epidemiologic evidence that vitamin D may play a role in T1DM, this gene was examined as a candidate gene and 2 single-nucleotide polymorphisms were found to be associated.

ENVIRONMENTAL FACTORS
That 50% or so of monozygotic twins are discordant for T1DM, the variation seen in urban and rural areas populated by the same ethnic group, the change in incidence that occurs with migration, the increase in incidence that has been seen in almost all populations in the last few decades, and the occurrence of seasonality all provide evidence that environmental factors also play a significant role in the causation of T1DM.

Viral Infections
It is possible that various viruses do play a role in the pathogenesis of T1DM, but no single virus, and no single pathogenic mechanism, stands out in the environmental etiology of T1DM. Instead, a variety of viruses and mechanisms may contribute to the development of diabetes in genetically susceptible hosts. Invoked mechanisms involved direct infection of β cells by viruses resulting in lysis and release of self-antigens, direct viral infection of antigen-presenting cells causing increased expression of cytokines, and "molecular mimicry," the notion that viral antigens exhibit homology to self-epitopes.

Congenital Rubella Syndrome
The clearest evidence of a role for viral infection in human T1DM is seen in congenital rubella syndrome. Prenatal infection with rubella is associated with β-cell autoimmunity in up to 70%, with development of T1DM in up to 40% of infected children. The time lag between infection and development of diabetes may be as high as 20 yr. T1DM after congenital rubella is more likely in patients that carry the higher-risk genotypes. Interestingly, there appears to be no increase in risk of diabetes when rubella infection develops after birth or when live-virus rubella immunization is used.

Enteroviruses
Studies show an increase in evidence of enteroviral infection in patients with T1DM and an increased prevalence of enteroviral RNA in prenatal blood samples from children who subsequently develop T1DM. In addition, there are case reports of association between enteroviral infection and subsequent T1DM. But the true significance of these infections remains unknown at this time.

Mumps Virus
It has been variably observed that mumps infection leads to the development of β-cell autoimmunity with high frequency and to T1DM in some cases. Although mumps may play a role in some cases of diabetes, the fact that T1DM diabetes incidence has increased steadily in several countries after universal mumps vaccination was introduced and that the incidence is extremely low in several populations where mumps is still prevalent indicates that mumps alone is not a major causal factor in diabetes.

The Hygiene Hypothesis: Possible Protective Role of Infections
Although some viral infections may increase the risk of T1DM, infectious agents may also play a protective role against diabetes. The hygiene hypothesis states that T1DM is a disease of industrialized countries, where the observation that there are fewer infections implies that the immune system is less-well trained for its main task, namely host defense. Some call this theory the "microbial deprivation hypothesis." The hygiene hypothesis states that lack of exposure to childhood infections may increase an individual's chances of developing autoimmune diseases, including T1DM. Rates of T1DM and other autoimmune disorders are generally lower in underdeveloped nations with a high prevalence of childhood infections and tend to increase as these countries become more developed. The incidence of T1DM differs almost 6-fold between Russian Karelia and Finland, even though both are populated by a genetically related population and are adjacent to each other and at the same latitude. The incidence of autoimmunity in the 2 populations varies inversely with immunoglobulin (Ig) E antibody levels, and IgE is involved in the response to parasitic infestation. All these observations indicate that decreased exposure to certain parasites and other microbes in early childhood may lead to an increased risk of autoimmunity in later life, including autoimmune diabetes. On the other hand, retrospective case-control studies have been equivocal at best and direct evidence of protection by childhood infections is still lacking.

Diet
Breastfeeding may lower the risk of T1DM, either directly or by delaying exposure to cow's milk protein. Early introduction of cow's milk protein and early exposure to gluten are implicated in the development of autoimmunity and it has been suggested that this is a result of the "leakiness" of the immature gut to protein antigens. Implicated antigens include β-lactoglobulin, a major lipocalin protein in bovine milk, which is homologous to the human protein glycodelin (PP14), a T-cell modulator. Other studies focused on bovine serum albumin as the inciting antigen, but the data are contradictory and not yet conclusive. In addition, milk and milk products are also indicators of the level of contamination of persistent organic pollutants, polychlorinated biphenyls, dioxin, and others. One large study in infants who are at high risk for T1DM did not demonstrate a reduced incidence of diabetes-associated autoantibodies when fed an extensively hydrolyzed vs cow milk–based formula. A smaller study demonstrated a reduced incidence of autoantibody production in infants fed a whey-based formula that was free of bovine insulin. Additional studies are underway and should be available in 2017.

Other dietary factors that have been suggested at various times as playing a role in diabetes risk include omega-3 fatty acids, vitamin D, ascorbic acid, zinc, and vitamin E. Vitamin D is biologically plausible (it has a role in immune regulation), deficiency is more common in northern countries like Finland, and there is some epidemiologic evidence that decreased vitamin D levels in pregnancy or early childhood may be associated with diabetes risk; but the evidence is not yet conclusive and it is hoped that ongoing studies like TEDDY (The Environmental Determinants of Diabetes in the Young) will help to resolve some of the uncertainties in this area.

Psychologic Stress
Several studies show an increased prevalence of stressful psychologic situations among children who subsequently developed T1DM. Whether these stresses only aggravate preexisting autoimmunity or whether they can actually trigger autoimmunity through epigenetic mechanisms remains unknown.

PATHOGENESIS AND NATURAL HISTORY OF TYPE 1 DIABETES MELLITUS
In T1DM, a genetically susceptible host develops autoimmunity against the host's own β cells. What triggers this autoimmune response remains unclear at this time. In some (but not all) patients, this autoimmune process results in progressive destruction of β cells until a critical mass

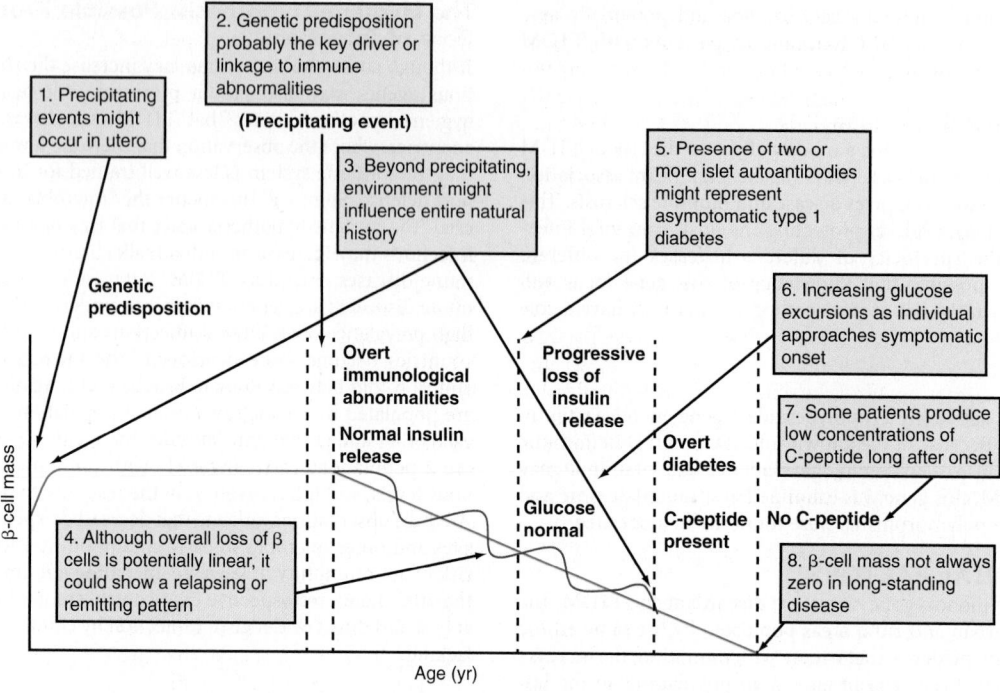

Figure 589-3 The natural history of type 1 diabetes—a 25 yr old concept revisited. A recreation of the model of type 1 diabetes, originally proposed in 1986, is shown in *black*. Additions and conjectures based on recent knowledge gains are shown in *green*. *(From Atkinson MA, Eisenbarth GS, Michels AW: Type 1 diabetes. Lancet 383:69–78, 2014, Fig. 4, p. 73.)*

of β cells is lost and insulin deficiency develops. Insulin deficiency, in turn, leads to the onset of clinical signs and symptoms of T1DM. At the time of diagnosis, some viable β cells are still present and these may produce enough insulin to lead to a partial remission of the disease (honeymoon period) but over time, almost all β cells are destroyed and the patient becomes totally dependent on exogenous insulin for survival (Fig. 589-3). Over time, some of these patients develop secondary complications of diabetes that appear to be related to how well-controlled the diabetes has been. Thus, the natural history of T1DM involves some or all of the following stages:

1. Initiation of autoimmunity
2. Preclinical autoimmunity with progressive loss of β-cell function
3. Onset of clinical disease
4. Transient remission
5. Established disease
6. Development of complications

Initiation of Autoimmunity

Genetic susceptibility to T1DM is determined by several genes (see "Genetics" below), with the largest contribution coming from variants in the HLA system. But it is important to keep in mind that even with the highest-risk haplotypes, most carriers will *not* develop T1DM. Even in monozygotic twins, the concordance is 30-65%. The observed rise in incidence of T1DM within an essentially genetically stable patient population implies that something has accordingly changed in the environment or the way children are raised. A number of factors, including prenatal influences, diet in infancy, viral infections, lack of exposure to certain infections, even psychologic stress, are implicated in the pathogenesis of T1DM, but their exact role and the mechanism by which they trigger or aggravate autoimmunity remains uncertain (Fig. 589-4). What is clear is that markers of autoimmunity are much more prevalent than clinical T1DM, indicating that initiation of autoimmunity is a necessary but not a sufficient condition for T1DM. Whatever the triggering factor, it seems that in most cases of T1DM that are diagnosed in childhood, the onset of autoimmunity occurs very early in life. In a majority of the children diagnosed before age 10 yr, the first signs of autoimmunity appear before age 2 yr. Development of autoimmunity is associated with the appearance of several

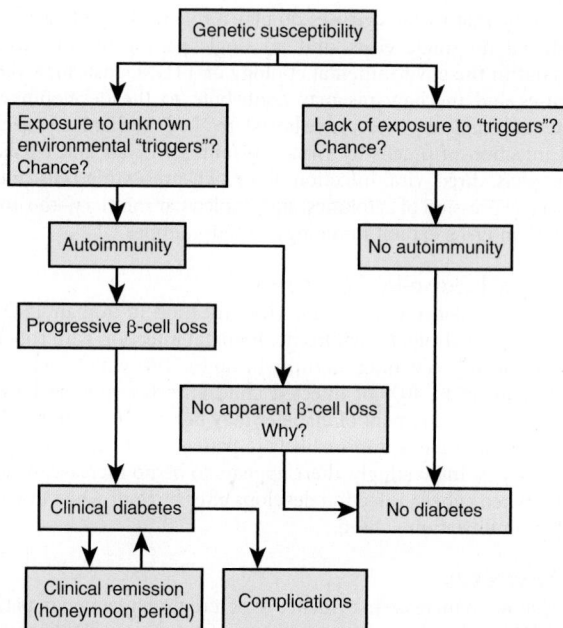

Figure 589-4 Schematic of the natural history of type 1 diabetes mellitus. Unknown triggers act upon a genetically susceptible host to trigger autoimmunity. Some proportion of those with autoimmunity develop progressive β-cell loss that eventually leads to clinical diabetes. This is followed by temporary clinical remission (honeymoon period) in most patients. Over time, insulin secretion is almost completely lost and complications may develop in some patients (in direct proportion to the occurrence of hyperglycemia).

autoantibodies. IAAs are usually the first to appear in young children, followed by glutamic acid decarboxylase 65 kDa, and later by tyrosine phosphatase insulinoma–associated 2 and zinc transporter 8 antibodies. The earliest antibodies are predominantly of the IgG1 subclass. Not only is there "spreading" of autoimmunity to more antigens (IAA, and then glutamic acid decarboxylase 65 and insulinoma-associated 2 and zinc transporter 8) but there is also epitope spreading within 1 antigen. Initial glutamic acid decarboxylase 65 antibodies tend to be against the middle region or the carboxyl-terminal region, whereas aminoterminal antibodies usually appear later and are less common in children.

Preclinical Autoimmunity with Progressive Loss of β-Cell Function

In some, but not all, patients, the appearance of autoimmunity is followed by progressive destruction of β cells. Antibodies are a marker for the presence of autoimmunity, but the actual damage to the β cells is primarily T-cell mediated (Fig. 589-5). Histologic analysis of the pancreas from patients with recent-onset T1DM reveals insulitis, with an infiltration of the islets of Langerhans by mononuclear cells, including T and B lymphocytes, monocytes/macrophages, and natural killer cells. In the nonobese diabetic mouse, a similar cellular infiltrate is followed by linear loss of β cells until they completely disappear. But it appears that the process in human T1DM is not necessarily linear and there may be an undulating downhill course, with remissions and relapses, in the development of T1DM.

Role of Autoantibodies

Even though T1DM does not occur as a direct consequence of autoantibody formation, the risk of developing clinical disease increases dramatically with an increase in the number of antibodies; only 30% of children with 1 antibody will progress to diabetes, but this risk increases to 70% when 2 antibodies are present and 90% when 3 are present. The risk of progression also varies with the intensity of the antibody response and those with higher antibody titers are more likely to progress to clinical disease. Another factor that appears to influence

progression of β-cell damage is the age at which autoimmunity develops; children in whom IAAs appeared within the 1st 2 yr of life rapidly developed anti–islet cell antibodies and progressed to diabetes more frequently than children in whom the first antibodies appeared between ages 5 and 8 yr.

Role of Genetics in Disease Progression

Genetics plays a role in progression to clinical disease. In a large study of healthy children, the appearance of single antibodies is relatively common and usually transient, and does not correlate with the presence of high-risk HLA alleles, but those carrying high-risk HLA alleles are more likely to develop multiple antibodies and progress to disease. Similarly, the appearance of antibodies is more likely to predict diabetes in those with a family history of diabetes vs those with no family history of T1DM. Thus, it may be the case that environmental factors can induce transient autoimmunity in many children, but those with genetic susceptibility are more likely to see progression of autoimmunity and eventual development of diabetes.

Role of Environmental Factors

In addition to genetic factors, environmental factors may also act as accelerators of T1DM after the initial appearance of autoimmunity. This is evident from the fact that the incidence of T1DM can vary several-fold between populations that have the same prevalence of autoimmunity. For instance, the incidence of T1DM in Finland is almost 4-fold higher than in Lithuania, but the incidence of autoimmunity is similar in both countries.

The fact that all children with evidence of autoimmunity and of autoreactive T cells do not progress to diabetes indicates that there are "checkpoints" at which the autoimmune process can be halted or

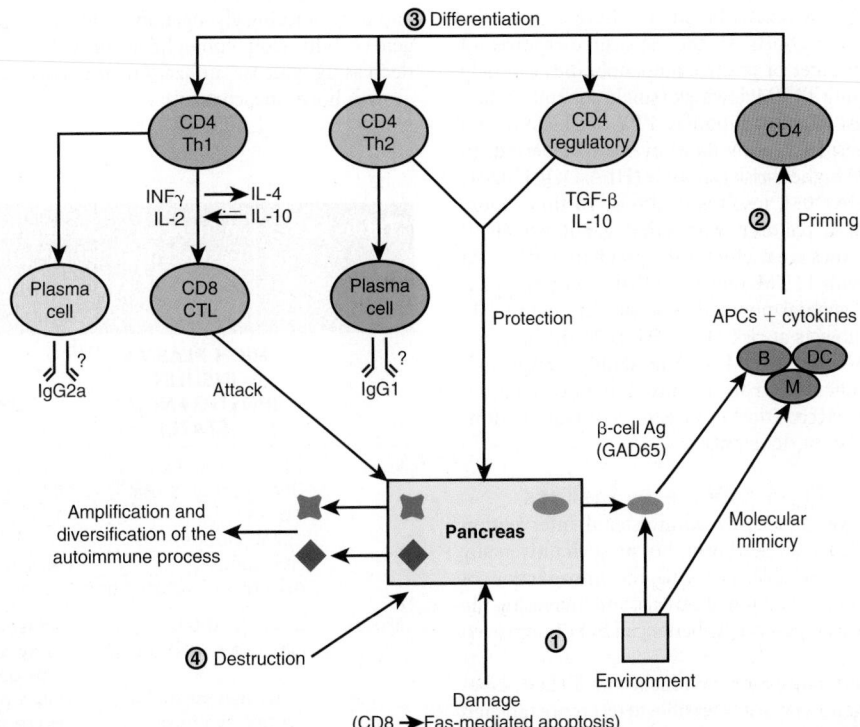

Figure 589-5 Schematic of the autoimmune response against pancreatic β cells. An insult to the pancreas leads to the release of β-cell antigens (GAD65), which are taken up by antigen-presenting cells (APCs) and the epitopes presented to the CD4 T cells. Type and stage of activation of APCs as well as the cytokine environment, in which the CD4 T-cell priming takes place, dictate the differentiation of autoreactive T cells toward diabetogenic T-helper type 1 (Th1) cells, T-helper type 2 (Th2) cells, or antigen-specific regulatory T cells. A predominant Th1 autoimmune response results in the recruitment and differentiation of cytotoxic CD8 cells, which attack the pancreatic β cells, leading to a massive release of β-cell antigens (Ag), epitope spreading, and destruction of the pancreatic islets. B, B lymphocyte; CTL, cytotoxic cell; DC, dendritic cell; IL, interleukin; INFγ, interferon-γ; M, macrophage; TGF-β, tumor growth factor β. (*Adapted from Casares S, Brumeanu TD: Insights into the pathogenesis of T1DM: a hint for novel immunospecific therapies,* Curr Mol Med *1:357–378, 2001.*)

reversed before it progresses to full-blown diabetes. This has raised the possibility of preventing T1DM by intervening in the preclinical stage.

Onset of Clinical Disease

Patients with progressive β-cell destruction will eventually present with clinical T1DM. It was thought that 90% of the total β-cell mass is destroyed by the time clinical disease develops, but later studies have revealed that this is not always the case. It now appears that β-cell destruction is more rapid and more complete in younger children, while in older children and adults the proportion of surviving β cells is greater (10-20% in autopsy specimens) and some β cells (about 1% of the normal mass) survive up to 30 yr after the onset of diabetes. As autopsies are usually done on patients who died of diabetic ketoacidosis, these figures may underestimate the actual β-cell mass present at diagnosis. Functional studies indicate that up to 40% of the insulin secretory capacity may be preserved in adults at the time of presentation of T1DM. Ultrasensitive assays indicate that C-peptide production is measurable decades after onset of T1DM. The fact that newly diagnosed diabetic individuals may still have a significant surviving β-cell mass is important because it raises the possibility of secondary prevention of T1DM. Similarly, the existence of viable β cells years or decades after initial presentation indicates that even patients with long-standing diabetes may be able to exhibit some recovery of β-cell function if the autoimmune destructive process can be halted and islet cell regeneration occurs.

PREDICTION AND PREVENTION

Autoimmunity precedes clinical T1DM, and indicators of maturing autoimmune responses may be useful markers for disease prediction. Individuals at risk for T1DM can be identified by a combination of genetic, immunologic, and metabolic markers. The most informative genetic locus, HLA class II, confers about half of the total genetic risk but has a low positive predictive value (PPV) when used in the general population. Autoantibodies provide a practical readout of β-cell autoimmunity, are easily sampled in venous blood, and have become the mainstay of T1DM prediction efforts. In the 1st-degree relatives of patients with T1DM, the number of positive autoantibodies can help estimate the risk of developing T1DM: low risk (single autoantibodies: PPV of 2-6%), moderate risk (2 autoantibodies: PPV of 21-40%), and high risk (>2 autoantibodies: PPV of 59-80%) over a 5 yr period. In children carrying the T1DM highest-risk genotype (HLA-DQB1*0201-DQA1*05/DQB1*0302-DQA1*03), insulitis is almost 10 times more frequent (PPV 21%) than in children with other genotypes (PPV 2.2%). But while autoantibodies are useful for the prediction of T1DM in the relatives of patients with T1DM, outside of that obvious population, the screening of the general population would be required in order to identify healthy subjects at risk of T1DM. Indeed, close to 9 of 10 individuals with new-onset T1DM have no family background of T1DM. This has been difficult, in part, because the observed autoantibody prevalence greatly exceeds the low disease prevalence in non-relatives, leading to high false-positive rates.

Primary Prevention of Type 1 Diabetes Mellitus

A safe, effective, inexpensive, and easily administered intervention could theoretically be targeted at all newborns, but no such universally effective intervention is yet available. Delaying the introduction of cow's milk protein, delaying introduction of cereals, and increasing the duration of breastfeeding are all potentially beneficial but of unproven value.

In high-risk populations (relatives of individuals with T1DM, especially those with high-risk genotypes), it is feasible to test more targeted interventions. Parenteral insulin and nasal insulin proved similarly ineffective in preventing diabetes, but oral insulin appeared to delay the incidence of diabetes in only some of autoantibody-positive but still prediabetic patients. In the approach to the newly diagnosed patient with T1DM, antigen-specific immunotherapy trials studying the effect of glutamic acid decarboxylase formulated in aluminum hydroxide, IL-1β inhibition, or intranasal insulin have been negative, and anti-CD3 antibodies have been inconclusive.

Secondary Prevention

Immunosuppressants like cyclosporine have been tested after the onset of T1DM, but while they may prolong the honeymoon period, they are associated with significant side effects and are only effective as long as they are being administered, so their use for this purpose has been abandoned.

The possibility of using glucagon-like peptide (GLP)-1 agonists (e.g., exenatide) alone or in combination with immunomodulatory therapies is also being explored as these agents are capable of increasing β-cell mass in animals.

PATHOPHYSIOLOGY

Insulin performs a critical role in the storage and retrieval of cellular fuel. Its secretion in response to feeding is exquisitely modulated by the interplay of neural, hormonal, and substrate-related mechanisms to permit controlled disposition of ingested foodstuff as energy for immediate or future use. Insulin levels must be lowered to then mobilize stored energy during the fasted state. Thus, in normal metabolism, there are regular swings between the postprandial, high-insulin anabolic state and the fasted, low-insulin catabolic state that affect liver, muscle, and adipose tissue (Table 589-3). T1DM is a progressive low-insulin catabolic state in which feeding does not reverse, but rather exaggerates, these catabolic processes. With moderate insulinopenia, glucose utilization by muscle and fat decreases and postprandial hyperglycemia appears. At even lower insulin levels, the liver produces excessive glucose via glycogenolysis and gluconeogenesis, and fasting hyperglycemia begins. Hyperglycemia produces an osmotic diuresis (glycosuria) when the renal threshold is exceeded (180 mg/dL; 10 mmol/L). The resulting loss of calories and electrolytes, as well as the worsening dehydration, produces a physiologic stress with hypersecretion of stress hormones (epinephrine, cortisol, growth hormone, and glucagon). These hormones, in turn, contribute to the metabolic decompensation by further impairing insulin secretion (epinephrine), by antagonizing its action (epinephrine, cortisol, growth hormone), and by promoting glycogenolysis, gluconeogenesis, lipolysis, and ketogenesis (glucagon, epinephrine, growth hormone, and cortisol) while decreasing glucose utilization and glucose clearance (epinephrine, growth hormone, cortisol).

Table 589-3	Influence of Feeding (High Insulin) or of Fasting (Low Insulin) on Some Metabolic Processes in Liver, Muscle, and Adipose Tissue*

	HIGH PLASMA INSULIN (POSTPRANDIAL STATE)	LOW PLASMA INSULIN (FASTED STATE)
Liver	Glucose uptake Glycogen synthesis Absence of gluconeogenesis Lipogenesis Absence of ketogenesis	Glucose production Glycogenolysis Gluconeogenesis Absence of lipogenesis Ketogenesis
Muscle	Glucose uptake Glucose oxidation Glycogen synthesis Protein synthesis	Absence of glucose uptake Fatty acid and ketone oxidation Glycogenolysis Proteolysis and amino acid release
Adipose tissue	Glucose uptake Lipid synthesis Triglyceride uptake	Absence of glucose uptake Lipolysis and fatty acid release Absence of triglyceride uptake

*Insulin is considered to be the major factor governing these metabolic processes. Diabetes mellitus may be viewed as a permanent low-insulin state that, untreated, results in exaggerated fasting.

The combination of insulin deficiency and elevated plasma values of the counterregulatory hormones is also responsible for accelerated lipolysis and impaired lipid synthesis, with resulting increased plasma concentrations of total lipids, cholesterol, triglycerides, and free fatty acids. The hormonal interplay of insulin deficiency and glucagon excess shunts the free fatty acids into ketone body formation; the rate of formation of these ketone bodies, principally β-hydroxybutyrate and acetoacetate, exceeds the capacity for peripheral utilization and renal excretion. Accumulation of these keto acids results in metabolic acidosis (diabetic ketoacidosis [DKA]) and compensatory rapid deep breathing in an attempt to excrete excess CO_2 (Kussmaul respiration). Acetone, formed by nonenzymatic conversion of acetoacetate, is responsible for the characteristic fruity odor of the breath. Ketones are excreted in the urine in association with cations and thus further increase losses of water and electrolyte and bicarbonate regenerating ability. With progressive dehydration, acidosis, hyperosmolality, and diminished cerebral oxygen utilization, consciousness becomes impaired, and the patient ultimately becomes comatose.

CLINICAL MANIFESTATIONS

In diabetes the decreasing β-cell mass with worsening insulinopenia, progressive hyperglycemia, and eventual ketoacidosis all imply that symptoms steadily increase, from early intermittent polyuria to DKA and coma, over weeks usually, rather than months. Initially, when only insulin reserve is limited, occasional postprandial hyperglycemia occurs. When the serum glucose increases above the renal threshold, intermittent polyuria or nocturia begins. With further β-cell loss, chronic hyperglycemia causes a more persistent diuresis, often with nocturnal enuresis, and polydipsia becomes more apparent. Female patients may develop monilial vaginitis from the chronic glycosuria. Calories are lost in the urine (glycosuria), triggering a compensatory hyperphagia. If this hyperphagia does not keep pace with the glycosuria, loss of body fat ensues, with clinical weight loss and diminished subcutaneous fat stores. An average, healthy 10 yr old child consumes approximately 50% of 2,000 daily calories as carbohydrate. As that child becomes diabetic, daily losses of water and glucose may be 5 L and 250 g, respectively, representing 1,000 calories, or 50%, of the average daily caloric intake. Despite the child's compensatory increased intake of food, the body starves because unused calories are lost in the urine.

When extremely low insulin levels are reached, ketoacids accumulate. At this point, the child quickly deteriorates. Ketoacids produce abdominal discomfort or true pain, nausea, and emesis, preventing oral replacement of urinary water losses. Dehydration accelerates, causing weakness or orthostasis—but polyuria persists. As in any hyperosmotic state, the degree of dehydration may be clinically underestimated because intravascular volume is conserved at the expense of intracellular volume. Ketoacidosis exacerbates prior symptoms and leads to Kussmaul respirations (deep, heavy, nonlabored rapid breathing), fruity breath odor (acetone), prolonged corrected Q-T interval, diminished neurocognitive function, and possible coma. Approximately 20-40% of children with new-onset diabetes progress to DKA before diagnosis.

This entire progression happens much more quickly (over a few weeks) in younger children, owing to either more aggressive autoimmune destruction of β cells and/or to lower β-cell mass compared to older subjects. In infants, most of the weight loss is acute water loss because they will not have had prolonged urinary loss of calories from glycosuria, and there will be an increased incidence of DKA at diagnosis. In adolescents, the course is usually more prolonged (over a few months), and most of the weight loss represents fat loss from prolonged starvation. Additional weight loss from acute dehydration may occur just before diagnosis. In any child, the progression of symptoms may be accelerated by the stress of an intercurrent illness or trauma, when counterregulatory (stress) hormones overwhelm the limited insulin secretory capacity.

DIAGNOSIS

The diagnosis of T1DM is usually straightforward (see Table 589-2). Although most symptoms are nonspecific, the most important clue is an inappropriate polyuria in any child with dehydration, poor weight gain, or "the flu." Hyperglycemia, glycosuria, and ketonuria can be determined quickly. Nonfasting blood glucose greater than 200 mg/dL (11.1 mmol/L) with typical symptoms is diagnostic with or without ketonuria. In the obese child, T2DM must be considered (see "Type 2 Diabetes Mellitus" below). Once hyperglycemia is confirmed, it is prudent to determine whether DKA is present (especially if ketonuria is found) and to evaluate electrolyte abnormalities—even if signs of dehydration are minimal. A baseline hemoglobin A_{1c} (HbA_{1c}) will be confirmatory and allows an estimate of the duration of hyperglycemia and provides an initial value by which to compare the effectiveness of subsequent therapy. Falsely low HbA_{1c} levels are noted in hemolytic anemias, pure red cell aplasia, blood transfusions, and anemias associated with hemorrhage, cirrhosis, myelodysplasias, or renal disease treated with erythropoietin.

In the nonobese child, testing for autoimmunity to β cells is not commonly necessary. Other autoimmunities associated with T1DM should be sought, including celiac disease (by tissue transglutaminase IgA and total IgA) and thyroiditis (by antithyroid peroxidase and antithyroglobulin antibodies). Fifteen to 30% of subjects with T1DM have elevated thyroid-stimulating hormone (TSH) and antithyroid antibodies and close to 5-10% have evidence for celiac disease. These diseases share common genes and likely the same interplay between environmental and immunologic factors. Because significant physiologic distress can disrupt the pituitary–thyroid axis, free thyroxine and TSH levels should be checked after the child is stable for a few weeks.

Rarely, a child has transient hyperglycemia with glycosuria while under substantial physical stress. This usually resolves permanently during recovery from the stressors. Stress-produced hyperglycemia can reflect a limited insulin reserve temporarily revealed by counterregulatory hormones. A child with temporary hyperglycemia should therefore be monitored for the development of symptoms of persistent hyperglycemia and tested if such symptoms occur. Formal testing in a child who remains clinically asymptomatic is not necessary; if there is concern for T1DM or T2DM a hemoglobin A_{1c} may be of value.

Routine screening procedures, such as postprandial determinations of blood glucose or screening oral glucose tolerance tests have yielded low detection rates in healthy, asymptomatic children, even among those considered at risk, such as siblings of diabetic children. Accordingly, such screening procedures are not recommended in children.

Diabetic Ketoacidosis

DKA is the end result of the metabolic abnormalities resulting from a severe deficiency of insulin or insulin effectiveness. The latter occurs during stress as counterregulatory hormones block insulin action. DKA occurs in 20-40% of children with new-onset diabetes and in children with known diabetes who omit insulin doses or who do not successfully manage an intercurrent illness. DKA may be arbitrarily classified as mild, moderate, or severe (Table 589-4), and the range of symptoms depends on the depth of ketoacidosis. There is a large amount of ketonuria, an increased ion gap, a decreased serum bicarbonate (or total CO_2) and pH, and an elevated effective serum osmolality, indicating hypertonic dehydration.

TREATMENT

Therapy is tailored to the degree of insulinopenia at presentation. Most children with new diabetes have mild to moderate symptoms, have minimal dehydration with no history of emesis, and have not progressed to ketoacidosis. Once DKA has resolved in the newly diagnosed child, therapy is transitioned to that described for children with nonketotic onset. Children with previously diagnosed diabetes who develop DKA are usually transitioned to their previous insulin regimen.

NEW-ONSET DIABETES WITHOUT KETOACIDOSIS

Excellent diabetes control involves many goals: to maintain a balance between tight glucose control and avoiding hypoglycemia, to eliminate polyuria and nocturia, to prevent ketoacidosis, and to permit normal growth and development with minimal effect on lifestyle. Therapy

Table 589-4	Classification of Diabetic Ketoacidosis			
	NORMAL	**MILD**	**MODERATE**	**SEVERE***
CO_2 (mEq/L, venous)[†]	20-28	16-20	10-15	<10
pH (venous)[†]	7.35-7.45	7.25-7.35	7.15-7.25	<7.15
Clinical	No change	Oriented, alert but fatigued	Kussmaul respirations; oriented but sleepy; arousable	Kussmaul or depressed respirations; sleepy to depressed sensorium to coma

*Severe hypernatremia (corrected Na >150 mEq/L) would also be classified as severe diabetic ketoacidosis.
†CO_2 and pH measurement are method dependent; normal ranges may vary.

Table 589-5	Starting Doses of Insulin (units/kg/day)	
	NO DIABETIC KETOACIDOSIS	**DIABETIC KETOACIDOSIS**
Prepubertal	0.25-0.50	0.75-1.0
Pubertal	0.50-0.75	1.0-1.2
Postpubertal	0.25-0.50	0.8-1.0

Insulin Therapy

Several factors influence the initial daily insulin dose per kilogram of body weight. The dose is usually higher in pubertal children. It is also higher in those who are in DKA at the time of presentation. Table 589-5 shows the recommended starting total daily dose (units/kg/day) of insulin in children.

The optimal insulin dose can only be determined empirically, with frequent self-monitored blood glucose levels and insulin adjustment by the diabetes team. Many children with new-onset diabetes have some residual β-cell function (the honeymoon period), which is associated with reduced exogenous insulin needs shortly after starting on treatment. Residual β-cell function usually fades within a few months and is reflected as a steady increase in insulin requirements and wider glucose excursions.

The initial insulin schedule should be directed toward the optimal degree of glucose control in an attempt to duplicate the activity of the β cell. There are inherent limits to our ability to mimic the β cell. Exogenous insulin does not have a first pass to the liver, whereas 50% of pancreatic portal insulin is taken up by the liver, a key organ for the disposal of glucose; absorption of an exogenous dose continues despite hypoglycemia, whereas endogenous insulin release ceases and serum levels quickly lower with a normally rapid clearance. The absorption rate from an injection varies by injection site and patient activity level, whereas endogenous insulin is secreted directly into the portal circulation. Despite these fundamental physiologic differences, acceptable glucose control can be obtained with insulin analogs used in a basal-bolus regimen, that is, with slow-onset, long-duration background insulin for between-meal glucose control and rapid-onset insulin at each meal.

All preanalog insulins form hexamers, which must dissociate into monomers subcutaneously before being absorbed into the circulation. Thus, a detectable effect for **regular insulin** is delayed by 30-60 min after injection. This, in turn, requires delaying the meal 30-60 min after the injection for optimal effect—a delay rarely attained in a busy child's life. Regular insulin has a wide peak and a long tail for bolus insulin (Figs. 589-6 and 589-7). This profile limits postprandial glucose control, produces prolonged peaks with excessive hypoglycemic effects between meals, and increases the risk of nighttime hypoglycemia. These unwanted between-meal effects often necessitate "feeding the insulin" with snacks and limiting the overall degree of blood glucose control. **Neutral protamine Hagedorn (NPH) and Lente insulins** also have

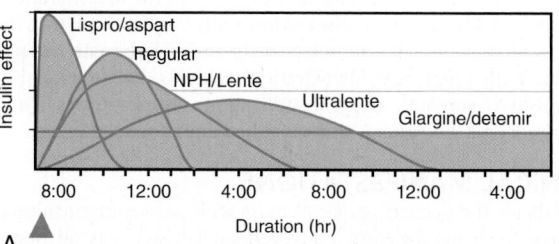

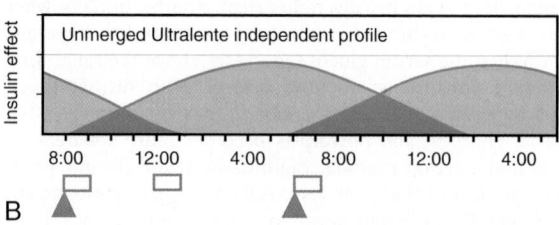

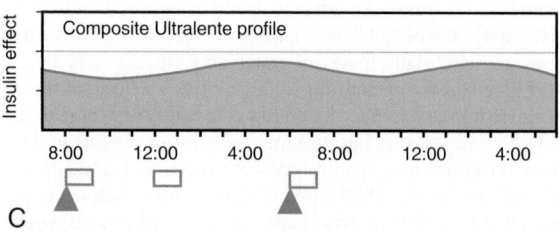

Figure 589-6 Approximate insulin effect profiles. Meals are shown as rectangles below time axis. **A,** The following relative peak effect and duration units are used: lispro/aspart, peak 20 for 4 hr; regular, peak 15 for 7 hr; neutral protamine Hagedorn/Lente, peak 12 for 12 hr; Ultralente, peak 9 for 18 hr; glargine, peak 5 for 24 hr. Although Lente and Ultralente are no longer manufactured, they are shown to give historical comparison to newer insulin analogs. ▲, Injection time. **B,** Two Ultralente injections given at breakfast and supper. Note overlap of profiles. **C,** Composite curve showing approximate cumulative insulin effect for the 2 Ultralente injections. This composite view is much more useful to the patient, parents, and medical personnel because it shows important combined effects of multiple insulin injections with variable absorption characteristics and overlapping durations.

inherent limits because they do not create a peakless background insulin level (see Fig. 589-7C-E). This produces a significant hypoglycemic effect during the midrange of their duration. Thus, it is often difficult to predict their interaction with fast-acting insulins. When regular insulin is combined with NPH or Lente (see Fig. 589-7E), the composite insulin profile poorly mimics normal endogenous insulin secretion. Lente and Ultralente insulins have been discontinued and are no longer available.

Lispro and aspart, insulin analogs, are absorbed much quicker because they do not form hexamers. They provide discrete pulses with little if any overlap and short tail effect. This allows better control of postmeal glucose increase and reduces between-meal or nighttime

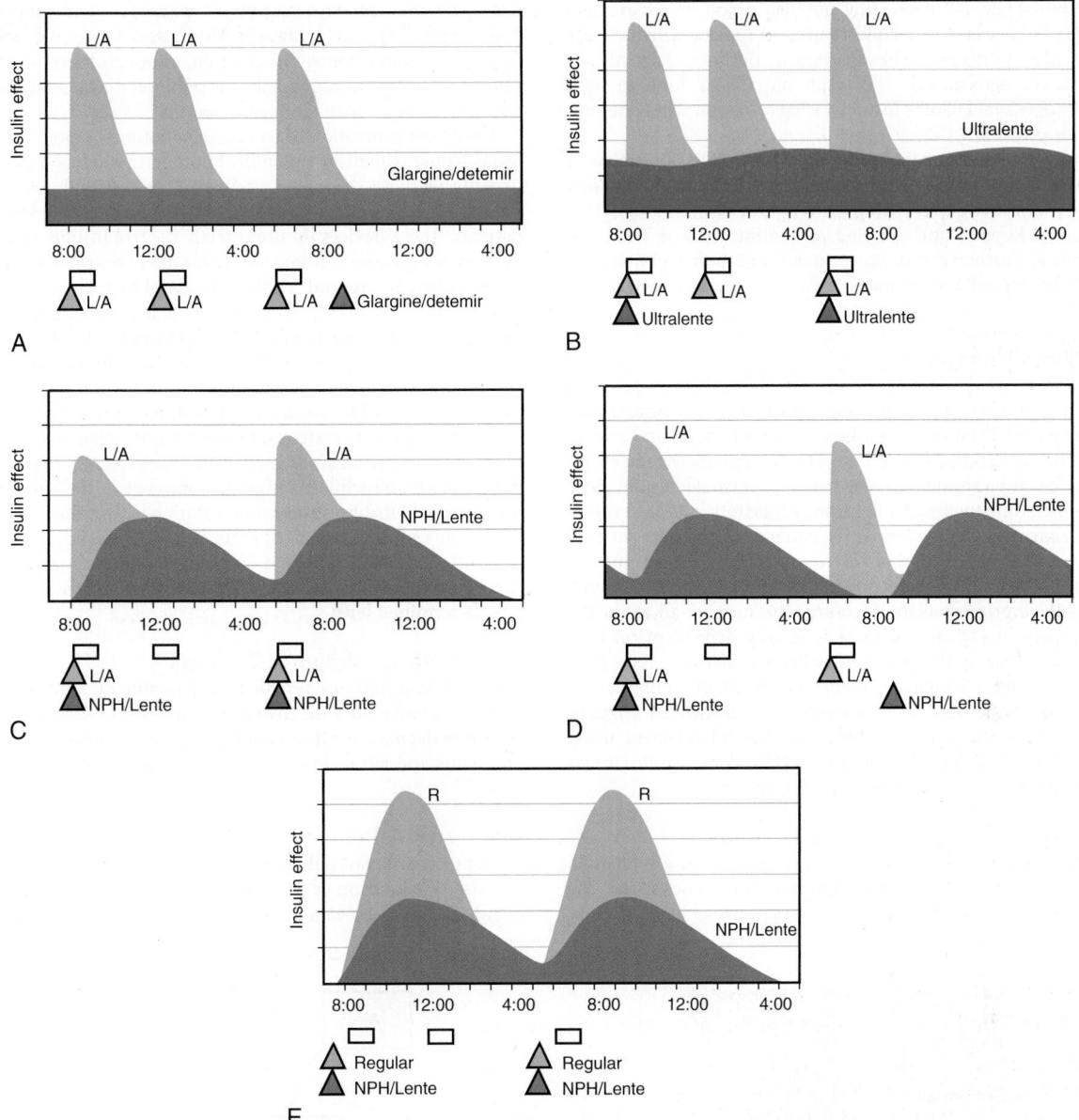

Figure 589-7 Approximate composite insulin effect profiles. Meals are shown as rectangles below time axis. Injections are shown as labeled *triangles*; *L/A*, lispro or aspart. Even though the fast- and long-acting insulins are shaded differently to show the addition of 1 insulin effect to another, the profile is changed to show the combined effect. For example, in the breakfast injection in **C**, the quick decline of L/A effect is blunted by the rising neutral protamine Hagedorn (NPH)/Lente effect, producing a broad tail, which slowly declines to baseline at supper. All profiles are idealized using average absorption and clearance rates. In typical clinical situations, these profiles vary among patients. A given patient has varying rates of absorption depending on the injection site, physical activity, and other variables. **A,** L or A premeal; glargine at bedtime. The rapid onset and short duration of L or A reduce overlap between premeal injections, and there is no extended nighttime action. This reduces the risk of hypoglycemia. Glargine provides a steady basal profile that simplifies prediction of bolus insulin effect. **B,** L or A premeal; Ultralente at breakfast and supper. Ultralente produces a basal profile similar to that seen with glargine. Some excessive insulin effect, however, is seen before supper and at nighttime. **C,** L or A premeal; NPH or Lente at breakfast and supper. The broad peak of NPH or Lente produces substantial risk of hypoglycemia before lunch and during the early hours of the night. The waning insulin effect before supper and breakfast may also allow breakthrough hyperglycemia. **D,** L or A premeal; NPH or Lente at breakfast and bedtime. Moving the evening long-acting insulin helps to cover the prebreakfast hours, but the risk of nighttime lows persists. **E,** Regular and NPH or Lente at breakfast and supper. This produces the least physiologic profile, with large excesses before lunch and during the early night, combined with poor coverage before supper and breakfast. Although Lente and Ultralente are no longer manufactured, they are shown to give historical comparison to newer insulin analogs.

hypoglycemia (see Fig. 589-7*A*). The **long-acting analog glargine** creates a much flatter 24 hr profile, making it easier to predict the combined effect of a rapid bolus (lispro or aspart) on top of the basal insulin, producing a more physiologic pattern of insulin effect (see Fig. 589-7*A*). Postprandial glucose elevations are better controlled, and between-meal and nighttime hypoglycemia are reduced.

Glargine may be given every 12 hr in young children if a single daily dose of glargine does not produce complete 24 hr basal coverage. The basal insulin glargine should be 25-30% of the total dose in toddlers and 40-50% in older children. The remaining portion of the total daily dose is provided as bolus insulin that is dosed by both the carbohydrate content of the meal as well as the preprandial glucose value.

Frequent blood glucose monitoring and insulin adjustment are necessary in the 1st weeks as the child returns to routine activities and adapts to a new nutritional schedule, and as the total daily insulin requirements are determined. The major physiologic limit to tight control is hypoglycemia. Use of insulin analogs moderates but does not eliminate this problem.

Some families may be unable to administer 4 daily injections. In these cases, a compromise may be needed. A 3 injection regimen combining NPH with a rapid analog bolus at breakfast, a rapid-acting analog bolus at supper, and glargine at bedtime may provide fair glucose control. Further compromise to a 2 injection regimen may occasionally be needed and frequently involves use of premix insulin (e.g., 70/30).

Insulin Pump Therapy

Continuous subcutaneous insulin infusion (CSII) via battery-powered pumps provides a closer approximation of normal plasma insulin profiles and increased flexibility regarding timing of meals and snacks compared with conventional insulin injection regimens. Insulin pump models can be programmed with a patient's personal insulin dose algorithms, including the insulin to carbohydrate ratio and the correction scale for premeal glucose levels. The patient can enter the patient's blood glucose level and the carbohydrate content of the meal, and the pump computer will calculate the proper insulin bolus dose. Although CSII frequently improves metabolic control, this may not always be the case. The degree of glycemic control is mainly dependent on how closely patients adhere to the principles of diabetes self-care, regardless of the type of intensive insulin regimen. One benefit of pump therapy may be a reduction in severe hypoglycemia and associated seizures. Randomized trials comparing multiple daily insulin regimens using glargine insulin and CSII in children with T1DM demonstrate similar metabolic control and frequency of hypoglycemic events.

Continuous Glucose Monitoring Systems

Subcutaneous glucose sensors that continuously measure interstitial fluid glucose levels are available and approved for use in children. The 1st generation of continuous glucose monitors provided blood glucose data only after downloading by the physician, and did not provide real-time feedback to the patient. This type of device did not appear to improve glycemic control in children, although there was some educational value in detecting patterns of blood glucose fluctuations and episodes of hypoglycemia during periods of sleep.

The newer generation of continuous monitors report blood glucose levels to the patient in real time. Short-term studies indicate clinical benefits of these devices as compared to conventional methods of blood glucose monitoring, when used by motivated and well-informed patients. These devices do not directly control insulin administration but provide glucose readings to permit finer control of insulin administration by patients and families. To avoid hypoglycemia the glucose sensor sounds an alarm; many episodes of hypoglycemia occur at night and unfortunately the parent may sleep through the alarm. Studies are currently evaluating the efficacy of a fully automated closed-loop system of insulin delivery based on continuous glucose sensing, sometimes mistakenly known as an "artificial pancreas" (Fig. 589-8). Some automated glycemic systems employ a bihormonal approach (insulin, glucagon) or have an automated insulin suspension program to ensure normal glycemia while avoiding hypoglycemia. The latter hypoglycemia threshold insulin suspension feature greatly reduces the incidence of hypoglycemia, especially at night. The FDA has approved an insulin pump in combination with a continuous glucose monitoring system that will stop insulin delivery when interstitial glucose levels fall below a predetermined level.

Amylin-Based Adjunct Therapy

Pramlintide acetate, a synthetic analog of amylin, may be of therapeutic value combined with insulin therapy. In adolescents it has been shown to decrease postprandial hyperglycemia, insulin dosage, gastric emptying, and HbA$_{1c}$ levels. It is given as a subcutaneous dose before meals.

Basic and Advanced Diabetes Education

Therapy consists not only of initiation and adjustment of insulin dose but also of education of the patient and family. Teaching is most efficiently provided by experienced diabetes educators and nutritionists.

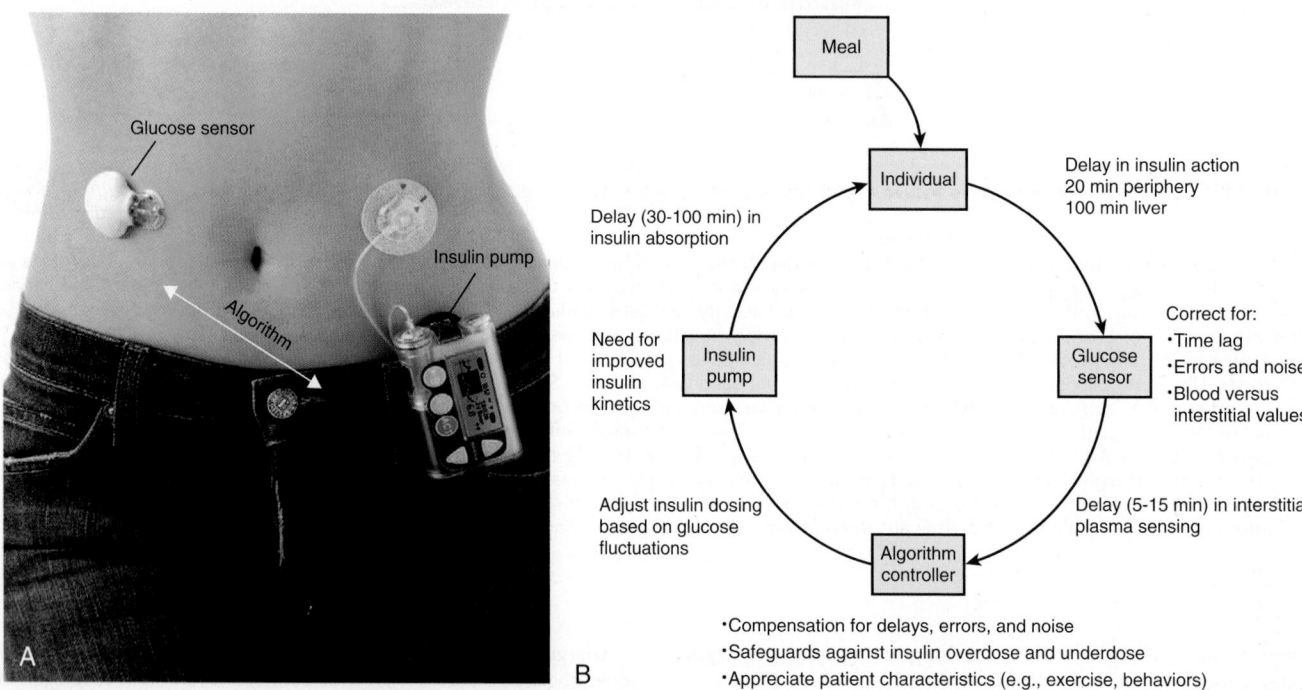

Figure 589-8 Closed-loop system for type 1 diabetes (artificial pancreas). **A,** Prototype of a closed-loop system. **B,** Components of a closed-loop system. Three potential delays in the system include glucose sensing in interstitial fluid, insulin absorption (depends on use of rapid vs regular insulin), and insulin action in peripheral tissues and liver. (*From Atkinson MA, Eisenbarth GS, Michels AW: Type 1 diabetes. Lancet 383:69–78, 2014, Fig. 5, p. 75.*)

In the acute phase, the family must learn the "basics," which includes monitoring the child's blood glucose and urine and/or blood ketones, preparing and injecting the correct insulin dose subcutaneously at the proper time, recognizing and treating low blood glucose reactions, and having a basic meal plan. Most families are trying to adjust psychologically to the new diagnosis of diabetes in their child and thus have a limited ability to retain new information. Written materials covering these basic topics help the family during the 1st few days.

Children and their families are also required to complete advanced self-management classes in order to facilitate implementation of flexible insulin management. These educational classes will help patients and their families acquire skills for managing diabetes during athletic activities and sick days.

Ketoacidosis

Severe insulinopenia (or lack of effective insulin action) results in a physiologic cascade of events in 3 general pathways:
1. Excessive glucose production coupled with reduced glucose utilization raises serum glucose. This produces an osmotic diuresis, with loss of fluid and electrolytes, dehydration, and activation of the renin–angiotensin–aldosterone axis with accelerated potassium loss. If glucose elevation and dehydration are severe and persist for several hours, the risk of cerebral edema increases.
2. Increased catabolic processes result in cellular losses of sodium, potassium, and phosphate.
3. Increased release of free fatty acids from peripheral fat stores supplies substrate for hepatic ketoacid production. When ketoacids accumulate, buffer systems are depleted and a metabolic acidosis ensues. Therapy must address both the initiating event in this cascade (insulinopenia) and the subsequent physiologic disruptions.

Reversal of DKA is associated with inherent risks that include hypoglycemia, hypokalemia, and cerebral edema. Any protocol must be used with caution and close monitoring of the patient. Adjustments based on sound medical judgment may be necessary for any given level of DKA (Table 589-6).

Hyperglycemia and Dehydration

Insulin must be given at the beginning of therapy to accelerate movement of glucose into cells, to subdue hepatic glucose production, and to halt the movement of fatty acids from the periphery to the liver. An initial insulin bolus does not speed recovery and may increase the risk of hypokalemia and hypoglycemia. Therefore, insulin infusion is typically begun **without** a bolus at a rate of 0.1 units/kg/hr. This approximates maximal insulin output in normal subjects during an oral glucose tolerance test. Rehydration also lowers glucose levels by improving renal perfusion and enhancing renal excretion. The combination of these therapies usually causes a rapid initial decline in serum glucose levels. Once glucose goes below 180 mg/dL (10 mmol/L), the osmotic diuresis stops and rehydration accelerates without further increase in the infusion rate.

Repair of hyperglycemia occurs well before correction of acidosis. Therefore, insulin is still needed to control fatty acid release and ketosis after normal glucose levels are reached. To continue the insulin infusion without causing hypoglycemia, glucose must be added to the infusion. We typically recommend that glucose be added as a 5% solution when the serum glucose has decreased <300 mg/dL and as a 10% solution when the serum glucose has decreased <200 mg/dL. The insulin infusion can also be lowered from the initial maximal rate if, despite the above outlined interventions, the serum glucose falls further.

Repair of fluid deficits must be tempered by the potential risk of cerebral edema. It is prudent to approach any child in any hyperosmotic state with cautious rehydration. The effective serum osmolality ($E_{osm} = 2 \times [Na_{uncorrected}] + [glucose]$) is an accurate index of tonicity of the body fluids, reflecting intracellular and extracellular hydration better than measured plasma osmolality. It is calculated with sodium and glucose in mmol/L. This value is usually elevated at the beginning of therapy and should steadily normalize. A rapid decline, or a slow decline to a subnormal range, may indicate an excess of free water entering the vascular space and an increasing risk of cerebral edema. Therefore, patients should not be allowed oral fluids until rehydration is well underway and significant electrolyte shifts are no longer likely. Limited ice chips may be given as a minimal oral intake. All fluid intake and output should be closely monitored.

Calculation of fluid deficits using clinical signs is difficult in children with DKA because intravascular volume is better maintained in the hypertonic state. For any degree of tachycardia, delayed capillary refill, decreased skin temperature, or orthostatic blood pressure change, the child with DKA will be more dehydrated than the child with a normotonic fluid deficit. The protocol in Table 589-6 corrects a deficit of 85 mL/kg (8.5% dehydration) for all patients in the 1st 24 hr. Children with mild DKA rehydrate earlier and can be switched to oral intake,

Table 589-6	Diabetic Ketoacidosis Treatment Protocol		
TIME	**THERAPY**	**COMMENTS**
1st hr	10-20 mL/kg IV bolus 0.9% NaCl or LR Insulin drip at 0.05 to 0.10 units/kg/hr	Quick volume expansion; may be repeated. NPO. Monitor I/O, neurologic status. Use flow sheet. Have mannitol at bedside; 1 g/kg IV push for cerebral edema
2nd hr until DKA resolution	0.45% NaCl: plus continue insulin drip 20 mEq/L KPhos and 20 mEq/L KAc 5% glucose if blood sugar >250 mg/dL (14 mmol/L)	$IV\ rate = \dfrac{85\ mL/kg + maintenance - bolus}{23\ hr}$ If K <3 mEq/L, give 0.5-1.0 mEq/kg as oral K solution *or* increase IV K to 80 mEq/L
Variable	Oral intake with subcutaneous insulin	No emesis; CO_2 ≥16 mEq/L; normal electrolytes

Note that the initial IV bolus is considered part of the total fluid allowed in the 1st 24 hr and is subtracted before calculating the IV rate.

Maintenance (24 hr) = 100 mL/kg (for the first 10 kg) + 50 mL/kg (for the second 10 kg) + 25 mL/kg (for all remaining kg)

Sample calculation for a 30-kg child:
1st hr = 300 mL IV bolus 0.9% NaCl or LR

$$2nd\ and\ subsequent\ hr = \frac{(85\ mL \times 30) + 1750\ mL - 300\ mL}{23\ hr} = \frac{175\ mL}{hr}$$

(0.45% NaCl with 20 mEq/L Kphos and 20 mEq/L KAc)

DKA, diabetic ketoacidosis; I/O, input and output (urine, emesis); K, potassium; KAc, potassium acetate; KPhos, potassium phosphate; LR, lactated Ringer solution; NaCl, sodium chloride; NPO, nothing by mouth.

whereas those with severe DKA and a greater volume deficit require 30-36 hr with this protocol. This more gradual rehydration of the child with severe DKA is an inherent safety feature. The initial intravenous bolus (20 mL/kg of glucose-free isotonic sodium salt solution such as Ringer lactate or 0.9% sodium chloride) for all patients ensures a quick volume expansion and may be repeated if clinical improvement is not quickly seen. This bolus is given as isotonic saline because the patient is inevitably hypertonic, keeping most of the initial infusion in the intravascular space. Subsequent fluid is hypotonic to repair the free water deficit, to allow intracellular rehydration, and to allow a more appropriate replacement of ongoing hypotonic urine losses.

The initial serum sodium is usually normal or low because of the osmolar dilution of hyperglycemia and the effect of an elevated sodium-free lipid fraction. An estimate of the reconstituted, or "true," serum sodium for any given glucose level above 100 mg/dL (5.6 mmol/L) is calculated as follows:

$$[Na^+] + (1.6\ mEq/L\ Na^+\ for\ every\ 100\ mg/dL\ glucose\ in\ excess\ of\ 100)$$

or

$$[Na^+] + (1.6\ mEq/L\ Na^+\ for\ every\ 5.6\ mmol/L\ glucose\ in\ excess\ of\ 5.6)$$

The sodium should increase by approximately 1.6 mmol/L for each 100 mg/dL decline in the glucose. The corrected sodium is usually normal or slightly elevated and indicates moderate hypernatremic dehydration. If the corrected value is greater than 150 mmol/L, severe hypernatremic dehydration may be present and may require slower fluid replacement. The sodium should steadily increase with therapy. *Declining sodium may indicate excessive free water accumulation and increased risk of cerebral edema.*

Catabolic Losses

Both the metabolic shift to a catabolic predominance and the acidosis move potassium and phosphate from the cell to the serum. The osmotic diuresis, the kaliuretic effect of the hyperaldosteronism, and the ketonuria then accelerate renal losses of potassium and phosphate. Sodium is also lost with the diuresis, but free water losses are greater than isotonic losses. With prolonged illness and severe DKA, total body losses can approach 10-13 mEq/kg of sodium, 5-6 mEq/kg of potassium, and 4-5 mEq/kg of phosphate. These losses continue for several hours during therapy until the catabolic state is reversed and the diuresis is controlled. For example, 50% of infused sodium may be lost in the urine during IV therapy. Even though the sodium deficit may be repaired within 24 hr, intracellular potassium and phosphate may not be completely restored for several days.

Although patients with DKA have a total body potassium deficit, the initial serum level is often normal or elevated. This is caused by the movement of potassium from the intracellular space to the serum, both as part of the ketoacid buffering process and as part of the catabolic shift. These effects are reversed with therapy, and potassium returns to the cell. Improved hydration increases renal blood flow, allowing for increased excretion of potassium in the elevated aldosterone state. The net effect is often a dramatic decline in serum potassium levels, especially in severe DKA, and can precipitate changes in cardiac conductivity, flattening of T waves, and prolongation of the QRS complex and can cause skeletal muscle weakness or ileus. The risk of myocardial dysfunction is increased with shock and acidosis. Potassium levels must be closely followed and electrocardiographic monitoring continued until DKA is substantially resolved. If needed, the parenteral potassium can be increased to 80 mEq/L or an oral supplement can be given if there is no emesis. Rarely, the IV insulin must be temporarily stopped.

It is unclear whether phosphate deficits contribute to symptoms of DKA such as generalized muscle weakness. In pediatric patients, a deficit has not been shown to compromise oxygen delivery via a deficiency of 2,3-diphosphoglycerate. Because the patient will receive an excess of chloride, which may aggravate acidosis, it is prudent to use potassium phosphate rather than potassium chloride as a potassium source. Potassium acetate is also used, because it provides an additional buffer.

Pancreatitis is occasionally seen with DKA, especially if prolonged abdominal distress is present; serum amylase may be elevated. If the serum lipase is not elevated, the amylase is likely nonspecific or salivary in origin. Serum creatinine adjusted for age may be falsely elevated owing to interference by ketones in the autoanalyzer methodology. An initial elevated value rarely indicates renal failure and should be rechecked when the child is less ketonemic. Blood urea nitrogen may be elevated with prerenal azotemia and should be rechecked as the child is rehydrated. Mildly elevated creatine or blood urea nitrogen is not a reason to withhold potassium therapy if good urinary output is present.

Keto Acid Accumulation

Low insulin infusion rates (0.02-0.05 units/kg/hr) are usually sufficient to stop peripheral release of fatty acids, thereby eliminating the flow of substrate for ketogenesis. Therefore, the initial infusion rate may be decreased if blood glucose levels go below 150 mg/dL (8 mmol/L) despite the addition of glucose to the infusion. Ketogenesis continues until fatty acid substrates already in the liver are depleted, but this production declines much more quickly without new substrate inflow. Bicarbonate buffers, regenerated by the distal renal tubule and by metabolism of ketone bodies, steadily repair the acidosis once ketoacid production is controlled. *Bicarbonate therapy is rarely necessary and may even increase the risk of hypokalemia and cerebral edema.*

There should be a steady increase in pH and serum bicarbonate as therapy progresses. Kussmaul respirations should abate and abdominal pain resolve. Persistent acidosis may indicate inadequate insulin or fluid therapy, infection, or rarely lactic acidosis. Urine ketones may be positive long after ketoacidosis has resolved because the nitroprusside reaction routinely used to measure urine ketones by dipstick measures only acetoacetate. During DKA, most excess ketones are β-hydroxybutyrate, which increases the normal ratio to acetoacetate from 3:1 to as high as 8:1. With resolution of the acidosis, β-hydroxybutyrate converts to acetoacetate, which is excreted into the urine and detected by the dipstick test. Therefore, persistent ketonuria may not accurately reflect the degree of clinical improvement and should not be relied on as an indicator of therapeutic failure.

All patients with DKA should be checked for initiating events that may have triggered the metabolic decompensation.

Diabetic Ketoacidosis Protocol
See Table 589-6.

Even though DKA can be of variable severity, a common approach to all cases simplifies the therapeutic regimen and can be safely used for most children. Fluids are best calculated based on weight, not body surface area (m²), because heights are rarely available for the acutely critically ill child. A standard water deficit (85 mL/kg) is assumed. This amount, when added to maintenance, yields approximately 4 L/m² for children of all sizes. Children with milder DKA recover in 10-20 hr (and need less total IV fluid before switching to oral intake), whereas those with more severe DKA require 30-36 hr with this protocol. Any child can be easily transitioned to oral intake and subcutaneous insulin when DKA has resolved (total CO_2 >15 mEq/L; pH >7.30; sodium stable between 135 and 145 mEq/L; no emesis). The first dose of short-acting subcutaneous insulin is given with a meal, and the insulin drip is discontinued approximately 30 min later.

A flow sheet is mandatory for accurate monitoring of changes in acidosis, electrolytes, fluid balance, and clinical status, especially if the patient is transferred from the emergency department to an inpatient setting with new caretakers. This flow sheet is best implemented by a central computer system, which allows for rapid update and wide availability of results, as well as rule-driven highlighting of critical values. A paper flow sheet suffices if it stays with the patient, is kept current, and is reviewed frequently by the physician. Any flow sheet should include columns for serial electrolytes, pH, glucose, and fluid balance. Blood testing should occur every 1-2 hr for children with severe DKA and every 3-4 hr for those with mild to moderate DKA.

Cerebral Edema

Cerebral edema complicating DKA remains the major cause of morbidity and mortality in children and adolescents with T1DM. However, its etiology remains unknown. A case-control study of DKA suggested that baseline acidosis and abnormalities of sodium, potassium, and blood urea nitrogen concentrations were important predictors of risk of cerebral edema. Early bolus administration of insulin and high volumes of fluid were also identified as risk factors. The incidence of cerebral edema in children with DKA has not changed over the past 15-20 yr, despite the widespread introduction of gradual rehydration protocols during this interval. Radiographic imaging is frequently unhelpful in making the diagnosis of cerebral edema. Consequently, each patient must be closely monitored. For all but the mildest cases, this includes frequent neurologic checks for any signs of increasing intracranial pressure, such as a change of consciousness, depressed respiration, worsening headache, bradycardia, apnea, pupillary changes, papilledema, posturing, and seizures. Mannitol must be readily available for use at the earliest sign of cerebral edema. The physician must also keep informed of the laboratory changes; hypokalemia or hypoglycemia can occur rapidly. Children with moderate to severe DKA have a higher overall risk and should be treated in an intensive care environment.

Nonketotic Hyperosmolar Coma

This syndrome is characterized by severe hyperglycemia (blood glucose >800 mg/dL), absence of or only slight ketosis, nonketotic acidosis, severe dehydration, depressed sensorium or frank coma, and various neurologic signs that may include grand mal seizures, hyperthermia, hemiparesis, and positive Babinski signs. Respirations are usually shallow, but coexistent metabolic (lactic) acidosis may be manifested by Kussmaul breathing. Serum osmolarity is commonly 350 mOsm/kg or greater. This condition is uncommon in children; among adults, mortality rates are high, possibly in part because of delays in recognition and institution of appropriate therapy. In children, there has been a high incidence of preexisting neurologic damage. Profound hyperglycemia may develop over a period of days and, initially, the obligatory osmotic polyuria and dehydration may be partially compensated for by increasing fluid intake. With progression of disease, thirst becomes impaired, possibly because of alteration of the hypothalamic thirst center by hyperosmolarity and, in some instances, because of a preexisting defect in the hypothalamic osmo-regulating mechanism.

The low production of ketones is attributed mainly to the hyperosmolarity, which in vitro blunts the lipolytic effect of epinephrine and the antilipolytic effect of residual insulin; blunting of lipolysis by the therapeutic use of β-adrenergic blockers may contribute to the syndrome. Depression of consciousness is closely correlated with the degree of hyperosmolarity in this condition as well as in DKA. Hemoconcentration may also predispose to cerebral arterial and venous thromboses.

Treatment of nonketotic hyperosmolar coma is directed at rapid repletion of the vascular volume deficit and very slow correction of the hyperosmolar state. One-half isotonic saline (0.45% NaCl; some use normal saline) is administered at a rate estimated to replace 50% of the volume deficit in the 1st 12 hr, and the remainder is administered during the ensuing 24 hr. The rate of infusion and the saline concentration are titrated to result in a slow decline of serum osmolality. When the blood glucose concentration approaches 300 mg/dL, the hydrating fluid should be changed to 5% dextrose in 0.2 normal saline. Approximately 20 mEq/L of potassium chloride should be added to each of these fluids to prevent hypokalemia. Serum potassium and plasma glucose concentrations should be monitored at 2 hr intervals for the 1st 12 hr and at 4 hr intervals for the next 24 hr to permit appropriate adjustments of administered potassium and insulin.

Insulin can be given by continuous intravenous infusion beginning with the 2nd hr of fluid therapy. Blood glucose may decrease dramatically with fluid therapy alone. The IV insulin dosage should be 0.05 units/kg/hr rather than 0.1 units/kg/hr as advocated for patients with DKA.

Nutritional Management

Nutrition plays an essential role in the management of patients with T1DM. This is of critical importance during childhood and adolescence, when appropriate energy intake is required to meet the needs for energy expenditure, growth, and pubertal development. There are no special nutritional requirements for the diabetic child other than those for optimal growth and development. In outlining nutritional requirements for the child on the basis of age, sex, weight, and activity, food preferences, including cultural and ethnic ones, must be considered.

Total recommended caloric intake is based on size or surface area and can be obtained from standard tables (Tables 589-7 and 589-8). The caloric mixture should comprise approximately 55% carbohydrate, 30% fat, and 15% protein. Approximately 70% of the carbohydrate content should be derived from complex carbohydrates such as starch; intake of sucrose and highly refined sugars should be limited. Complex carbohydrates require prolonged digestion and absorption so that plasma glucose levels increase slowly, whereas glucose from refined sugars, including carbonated beverages, is rapidly absorbed and may cause wide swings in the metabolic pattern; carbonated beverages should be sugar free. Priority should be given to total calories and total carbohydrate consumed rather than its source. Carbohydrate counting has become a mainstay in the nutrition education and management of patients with DM. Patients and their families are provided with information regarding the carbohydrate contents of different foods and food label reading. This allows patients to adjust their insulin dosage to their mealtime carbohydrate intake. The use of carbohydrate counting and insulin to carbohydrate ratios and the use of fast-acting insulin analogs and long-acting basal insulin (detemir and glargine) provide many children with less rigid meal planning. Flexibility in the use of insulin in relation to carbohydrate content of food improves the quality of life.

Although in children there is concern about the potential cumulative effect of saccharin, available data do not support an association of moderate amounts with bladder cancer. Other nonnutritive sweeteners such as aspartame are used in a variety of products.

Diets with high fiber content are useful in improving control of blood glucose. Moderate amounts of sucrose consumed with fiber-rich foods such as whole-grain bread may have no more glycemic effect than their low-fiber, sugar-free equivalents.

The intake of fat is adjusted so that the polyunsaturated:saturated ratio is increased to approximately 1.2:1.0, in contrast to the estimated American average of 0.3:1.0. Dietary fats derived from animal sources are, therefore, reduced and replaced by polyunsaturated fats from vegetable sources. Substituting margarine for butter, vegetable oil for

Table 589-7	Calorie Needs for Children and Young Adults
AGE	**KCAL REQUIRED/KG BODY WEIGHT***
CHILDREN	
0-12 mo	120
1-10 yr	100-75
YOUNG WOMEN	
11-15 yr	35
≥16 yr	30
YOUNG MEN	
11-15 yr	80-55 (65)
16-20 yr	
Average activity	40
Very physically active	50
Sedentary	30

Numbers in parentheses are means.
*Gradual decline in calories per unit weight as age increases.
From Nutrition guide for professionals: diabetes education and meal planning, *Alexandria, VA, and Chicago, IL, 1988, The American Diabetes Association and The American Dietetic Association.*

Table 589-8	Summary of Nutrition Guidelines for Children and/or Adolescents with Type 1 Diabetes Mellitus

NUTRITION CARE PLAN

Promotes optimal compliance.

Incorporates goals of management: normal growth and development, control of blood glucose, maintenance of optimal nutritional status, and prevention of complications. Uses staged approach.

NUTRIENT RECOMMENDATIONS AND DISTRIBUTION

NUTRIENT	(%) OF CALORIES	RECOMMENDED DAILY INTAKE
Carbohydrate	Will vary	High fiber, especially soluble fiber; optimal amount unknown
Fiber	>20 g/day	
Protein	12-20	
Fat	<30	
Saturated	<10	
Polyunsaturated	6-8	
Monounsaturated	Remainder of fat allowance	
Cholesterol		300 mg
Sodium		Avoid excessive; limit to 3,000-4,000 mg if hypertensive

ADDITIONAL RECOMMENDATIONS

Energy: If using measured diet, reevaluate prescribed energy level at least every 3 mo.

Protein: High-protein intakes may contribute to diabetic nephropathy. Low intakes may reverse preclinical nephropathy. Therefore, 12-20% of energy is recommended; lower end of range is preferred. In guiding toward the end of the range, a staged approach is useful.

Alcohol: Safe use of moderate alcohol consumption should be taught as routine anticipatory guidance as early as junior high school.

Snacks: Snacks vary according to individual needs (generally 3 snacks per day for children; midafternoon and bedtime snacks for junior high children or teens).

Alternative sweeteners: Use of a variety of sweeteners is suggested.

Educational techniques: No single technique is superior. Choice of educational method used should be based on patient needs. Knowledge of variety of techniques is important. Follow-up education and support are required.

Eating disorders: Best treatment is prevention. Unexplained poor control or severe hypoglycemia may indicate a potential eating disorder.

Exercise: Education is vital to prevent delayed or immediate hypoglycemia and to prevent worsened hyperglycemia and ketosis.

From Connell JE, Thomas-Doberson D: Nutritional management of children and adolescents with insulin-dependent diabetes mellitus: a review by the Diabetes Care and Education Dietetic Practice Group, J Am Diet Assoc 91:1556, 1991.

animal oils in cooking, and lean cuts of meat, poultry, and fish for fatty meats is advisable. The intake of cholesterol is also reduced by these measures and by limiting the number of egg yolks consumed. These simple measures reduce serum low-density lipoprotein cholesterol, a predisposing factor to atherosclerotic disease. Less than 10% of calories should be derived from saturated fats and up to 10% from polyunsaturated fats; the remaining fat-derived calories should be derived from monounsaturated fats. Table 589-8 summarizes current nutritional guidelines.

Each child/family can and should select a diet based on personal taste with the help of the physician or dietitian (or both). Emphasis should be placed on regularity of food intake and on constancy of carbohydrate intake. Occasional excesses ("treats") for birthdays and other parties are permissible and tolerated to not foster rebellion and stealth in obtaining desired food. Cakes and even candies are permissible on special occasions as long as the food carbohydrate content is adjusted in the meal plan. Adjustments in meal planning must constantly be made to meet the needs as well as the desires of each child. A consistent eating pattern with appropriate supplements for exercise, the pubertal growth spurt, and pregnancy in an adolescent with diabetes is important for metabolic control.

Monitoring

Success in the daily management of the child with diabetes can be measured by the competence acquired by the family, and subsequently by the child, in assuming responsibility for daily self-care. Their initial and ongoing instruction in conjunction with their supervised experience can lead to a sense of confidence in making adjustments in insulin dosage for dietary deviations, for unusual physical activity, and even for some minor intercurrent illnesses. Such acceptance of responsibility should make them relatively independent of the physician for their ordinary care. The physician must maintain ongoing interested supervision and shared responsibility with the family and the child.

Self-monitoring of blood glucose is an essential component of managing diabetes. Monitoring often also needs to include insulin dose, unusual physical activity, dietary changes, hypoglycemia, intercurrent illness, and other items that may influence the blood glucose. These items may be valuable in interpreting the self-monitoring of blood glucose record, prescribing appropriate adjustments in insulin doses, and teaching the family. If there are discrepancies in the self-monitoring of blood glucose and other measures of glycemic control (such as the HbA_{1c}), the clinician should attempt to clarify the situation in a manner that does not undermine their mutual confidence.

Daily blood glucose monitoring has been markedly enhanced by the availability of strips impregnated with glucose oxidase that permit blood glucose measurement from a drop of blood. A portable calibrated reflectance meter can approximate the blood glucose concentration accurately. Many meters contain a memory "chip" enabling recall of each measurement, its average over a given interval, and the ability to display the pattern on a computer screen. Such information is a useful educational tool for verifying degree of control and modifying recommended regimens. A small, spring-loaded device that automates capillary bloodletting (lancing device) in a relatively painless fashion is commercially available. Parents and patients should be taught to use these devices and measure blood glucose at least 4 times daily—before breakfast, lunch, and supper, and at bedtime. When insulin therapy is initiated and when adjustments are made that may affect the overnight glucose levels, self-monitoring of blood glucose should also be performed at 12 midnight and 3 AM to detect nocturnal hypoglycemia. Ideally, the blood glucose concentration should range from approximately 80 mg/dL in the fasting state to 140 mg/dL after meals. In practice, however, a range is acceptable, based on age of the patient (Table 589-9). Blood glucose measurements that are consistently at or outside these limits, in the absence of an identifiable cause such as exercise or dietary indiscretion, are an indication for a change in the insulin dose. If the fasting blood glucose is high, the evening dose of long-acting insulin is increased by 10-15% and/or additional fast-acting insulin (lispro or aspart) coverage for bedtime snack may be considered. If the noon glucose level exceeds set limits, the morning fast-acting insulin (lispro or aspart) is increased by 10-15%. If the presupper glucose is high, the noon dose of fast-acting insulin is increased by 10-15%. If the prebedtime glucose is high, the presupper dose of fast-acting insulin is increased by 10-15%. Similarly, reductions in the insulin type and dose should be made if the corresponding blood glucose measurements are consistently below desirable limits.

A minimum of 4 daily blood glucose measurements should be performed. However, some children and adolescents may need to have more frequent blood glucose monitoring based on their level of physical activity and history of frequent hypoglycemic reactions. Families should be encouraged to become sufficiently knowledgeable about managing diabetes. They can maintain near-normal glycemia for prolonged periods by self-monitoring of blood glucose levels before and

Table 589-9	Target Premeal and 30-Day Average Blood Glucose Ranges and the Corresponding Hemoglobin A₁c for Each Age Group		
AGE GROUP (yr)	TARGET PREMEAL BG RANGE (mg/dL)	30-DAY AVERAGE BG RANGE (mg/dL)	TARGET HbA₁c (%)
<5	100-200	180-250	7.5-9.0
5-11	80-150	150-200	6.5-8.0
12-15	80-130	120-180	6.0-7.5
16-18	70-120	100-150	5.5-7.0

In our laboratory, the nondiabetic reference range for HbA₁c is 4.5-5.7% (95% confidence interval).
BG, blood glucose; HbA₁c, hemoglobin A₁c.

2 hr after meals, and in conjunction with multiple daily injections of insulin, adjusted as necessary.

A continuous glucose monitoring system (CGMS) records data obtained from a subcutaneous sensor every 5 min for up to 72 hr and provides the clinician with a continuous profile of tissue glucose levels. The interstitial glucose levels lag about 13 min behind the blood glucose values at any given level. The CGMS values tend to have a high correlation coefficient for blood glucose values ranging between 40 and 400 mg/dL. CGMS is minimally invasive and entails the placement of a small, subcutaneous catheter that can be easily worn by adults and children. The system provides information that allows the patient and healthcare team to adjust the insulin regimen and the nutrition plan to improve glycemic control. CGMS can be helpful in detecting asymptomatic nocturnal hypoglycemia as well as in lowering HbA₁c values without increasing the risk for severe hypoglycemia. Although there are potential pitfalls in CGMS use, including suboptimal compliance, human error, incorrect technique, and sensor failure, the implementation of CGMS in ambulatory diabetes practice allows the clinician to diagnose abnormal glycemic patterns in a more precise manner.

Real-Time Continuous Glucose Monitoring
Real-time continuous glucose monitoring is a technology with the potential of transforming current concepts of glycemic control and optimal diabetes management. In addition to displaying real-time glucose data, newer generations of continuous glucose monitors also have alarms that can be set at below or above predetermined blood glucose thresholds. This safety feature can help parents of young children to recognize nocturnal hypoglycemia. In addition, continuous glucose monitoring shows the rate and direction of glucose change and alerts patients to trends that could lead to dangerous hypoglycemia or hyperglycemia. However, the use of continuous glucose monitoring without clinical decision-making algorithms and guidelines has not been proven to be very effective in improving glycemic control.

Glycosylated Hemoglobin
A reliable index of long-term glycemic control is provided by measurement of glycosylated hemoglobin. HbA₁c represents the fraction of hemoglobin to which glucose has been nonenzymatically attached in the bloodstream. The formation of HbA₁c is a slow reaction that is dependent on the prevailing concentration of blood glucose; it continues irreversibly throughout the red blood cell's life span of approximately 120 days. The higher the blood glucose concentration and the longer the red blood cell's exposure to it, the higher is the fraction of HbA₁c, which is expressed as a percentage of total hemoglobin. Because a blood sample at any given time contains a mixture of red blood cells of varying ages, exposed for varying times to varying blood glucose concentrations, an HbA₁c measurement reflects the average blood glucose concentration from the preceding 2-3 mo. When measured by standardized methods to remove labile forms, the fraction of HbA₁c is not influenced by an isolated episode of hyperglycemia.

It is recommended that HbA₁c measurements be obtained 3-4 times/yr to obtain a profile of long-term glycemic control. The lower the HbA₁c level, the more likely it is that microvascular complications such as retinopathy and nephropathy will be less severe, delayed in appearance, or even avoided altogether. Depending on the method used for determination, HbA₁c values may be spuriously elevated in thalassemia (or other conditions with elevated hemoglobin F) and spuriously lower in sickle cell disease (or other conditions with high red blood cell turnover). Although values of HbA₁c may vary according to the method used for measurement, in individuals without diabetes, the HbA₁c fraction is usually less than 6%; in individuals with diabetes, values of 6-7.5% represent good metabolic control, values of 7.6-9.9%, fair control, and values of 10% or higher, poor control. The target HbA₁c of <7.5% is the same regardless of the patient's age (see Table 589-9).

Exercise
No form of exercise, including competitive sports, should be forbidden to the child with diabetes. A major complication of exercise in patients with diabetes is the presence of a hypoglycemic reaction during or within hours after exercise. If hypoglycemia does not occur with exercise, adjustments in diet or insulin are not necessary, and glucoregulation is likely to be improved through the increased utilization of glucose by muscles. The major contributing factor to hypoglycemia with exercise is an increased rate of absorption of insulin from its injection site. Higher insulin levels dampen hepatic glucose production so that it is inadequate to meet the increased glucose utilization of exercising muscle. Regular exercise also improves glucoregulation by increasing insulin receptor number. In patients who are in poor metabolic control, vigorous exercise may precipitate ketoacidosis because of the exercise-induced increase in the counterregulatory hormones.

Benefits of Improved Glycemic Control
The Diabetes Control and Complications Trial (DCCT) established conclusively the association between higher glucose levels and long-term microvascular complications. Intensive management produced dramatic reductions of retinopathy, nephropathy, and neuropathy by 47-76%. The data from the adolescent cohort demonstrated the same degree of improvement and the same relationship between the outcome measures of microvascular complications.

The beneficial effect of intensified treatment was determined by the degree of blood glucose normalization, independently of the type of intensified treatment used. Frequent blood glucose monitoring was considered an important factor in achieving better glycemic control for the intensively treated adolescents and adults. Patients who were intensively treated had individualized glucose targets, frequent adjustments based on ongoing capillary blood glucose monitoring, and a team approach that focused on the person with diabetes as the prime initiator of ambulatory care. Care was constantly adjusted toward reaching normal or near-normal glycemic goals while avoiding or minimizing severe episodes of hypoglycemia. Teaching emphasized a preventive approach to blood glucose fluctuations with constant readjustment to counterbalance any high or low blood glucose readings. Target blood glucose goals were adjusted upward if hypoglycemia could not be prevented.

Total duration of diabetes contributes to development and severity of complications. Nonetheless, many professionals have concerns about applying the results of the DCCT to preschool-age children, who often have hypoglycemia unawareness with unique safety issues, and to prepubertal school-age children, who were not included in the DCCT. When the DCCT ended in 1993, researchers continued to study more than 90% of participants. The follow-up study, called Epidemiology of Diabetes Interventions and Complications (EDIC), was assessing the incidence and predictors of cardiovascular disease events such as heart attack, stroke, or needed heart surgery, as well as diabetic complications related to the eye, kidney, and nerves. The EDIC demonstrated that **intensive blood glucose control reduced risk** of any cardiovascular disease event by 42%. In addition, intensive therapy reduced risk of nonfatal heart attack, stroke, or death from cardiovascular causes by 57%.

Current Intensive Insulin Replacement Regimens

The goal of physiologic insulin replacement for T1DM is accomplished with short-acting insulins that more closely mimic the sharp increase and short duration of pancreatic insulin secreted with nutrient intake. The rapid-acting insulin analog lispro has superior pharmacokinetic properties for the control of postprandial glucose. Improved postprandial glucose responses occur with twice-daily injections (conventional insulin), multiple daily insulin injections, or CSII. The use of lispro or aspart insulin reduces the frequency of between-meal hypoglycemic events, especially when it is carefully balanced with the carbohydrate content of meal.

The carbohydrate content of food does not influence glycemic control if premeal rapid-acting insulin (bolus) is adjusted to the carbohydrate content of the meal. Wide variations in carbohydrate intake do not modify long-acting (detemir or glargine) or basal insulin requirements. Insulin replacement strategies stress the importance of administering smaller doses of insulin throughout the day. This approach allows insulin doses to be changed as needed to correct hyperglycemia, supplement for additional anticipated carbohydrate intake, or subtract for exercise. Indeed, bolus-basal treatment with multiple injections is better adapted to the physiologic profiles of insulin and glucose and can therefore provide better glycemic control than the conventional 2-3 dose regimen. Age-adjusted and individualized insulin to carbohydrate ratios and insulin dosage adjustment algorithms have been developed to normalize elevated blood glucose levels and to compensate for alterations in carbohydrate intake. The use of flexible multiple daily injections and CSII in children with T1DM improves glycemic control without an increase in the incidence of severe hypoglycemia.

Hypoglycemic Reactions

Hypoglycemia is the major limitation to tight control of glucose levels. Once injected, insulin absorption and action are independent of the glucose level, thus creating a unique risk of hypoglycemia from an unbalanced insulin effect. Insulin analogs may help reduce but cannot eliminate this risk. Most children with T1DM can expect mild hypoglycemia each week, moderate hypoglycemia a few times each year, and severe hypoglycemia every few years. These episodes are usually not predictable, although exercise, delayed meals or snacks, and wide swings in glucose levels increase the risk. Infants and toddlers are at higher risk for hypoglycemia because they have more variable meals and activity levels, are unable to recognize early signs of hypoglycemia, and are limited in their ability to seek a source of oral glucose to reverse the hypoglycemia. The very young have an increased risk of permanently reduced cognitive function as a long-term sequela of severe hypoglycemia. For this reason, a more relaxed degree of glucose control is necessary until the child matures (see Table 589-9).

Hypoglycemia can occur at any time of day or night. Early symptoms and signs (mild hypoglycemia) may occur with a sudden decrease in blood glucose to levels that do not meet standard criteria for hypoglycemia in children without diabetes. The child may show pallor, sweating, apprehension or fussiness, hunger, tremor, and tachycardia, all as a result of the surge in catecholamines as the body attempts to counter the excessive insulin effect. Behavioral changes such as tearfulness, irritability, and aggression are more prevalent in children. As glucose levels decline further, cerebral glucopenia occurs with drowsiness, personality changes, mental confusion, and impaired judgment (moderate hypoglycemia), progressing to inability to seek help and seizures or coma (severe hypoglycemia). Prolonged severe hypoglycemia can result in a depressed sensorium or stroke-like focal motor deficits that persist after the hypoglycemia has resolved. Although permanent sequelae are rare, severe hypoglycemia is frightening for the child and family and can result in significant reluctance to attempt even moderate glycemic control afterward.

Important counterregulatory hormones in children include growth hormone, cortisol, epinephrine, and glucagon. The latter 2 seem more critical in the older child. Many older patients with long-standing T1DM lose their ability to secrete glucagon in response to hypoglycemia. In the young adult, epinephrine deficiency may also develop as part of a general autonomic neuropathy. This substantially increases the risk of hypoglycemia because the early warning signals of a declining glucose level are as a result of catecholamine release. Recurrent hypoglycemic episodes associated with tight metabolic control may aggravate partial counterregulatory deficiencies, producing a syndrome of hypoglycemia unawareness and reduced ability to restore euglycemia (hypoglycemia-associated autonomic failure). Avoidance of hypoglycemia allows some recovery from this unawareness syndrome.

The most important factors in the management of hypoglycemia are an understanding by the patient and family of the symptoms and signs of the reaction and an anticipation of known precipitating factors such as gym or sports activities. Tighter glucose control increases the risk. Families should be taught to look for typical hypoglycemic scenarios or patterns in the home blood glucose log, so that they may adjust the insulin dose and avert predictable episodes. A source of emergency glucose should be available at all times and places, including at school and during visits to friends. If possible, it is important to document the hypoglycemia before treating, because some symptoms may not always be from hypoglycemia. Any child suspected of having a moderate to severe hypoglycemic episode should be treated before testing. It is important not to give too much glucose; 5-10 g should be given as juice or a sugar-containing carbonated beverage or candy, and the blood glucose checked 15-20 min later. Patients, parents, and teachers should also be instructed in the administration of glucagon when the child cannot take glucose orally. An injection kit should be kept at home and school. The intramuscular dose is 0.5 mg if the child weighs less than 20 kg and 1.0 mg if more than 20 kg. This produces a brief release of glucose from the liver. Glucagon often causes emesis, which precludes giving oral supplementation if the blood glucose declines after the glucagon effects have waned. Caretakers must then be prepared to take the child to the hospital for IV glucose administration, if necessary. Minidose glucagon (10 µg/yr of age up to a maximum of 150 µg subcutaneously) is effective in treating hypoglycemia in children with blood glucose less than 60 mg/dL who fail to respond to oral glucose and remain symptomatic.

Dawn Phenomenon and Somogyi Phenomenon

There are several reasons that blood glucose levels increase in the early morning hours before breakfast. The most common is a simple decline in insulin levels. This usually results in routinely elevated morning glucose. The **dawn phenomenon** is thought to be mainly caused by overnight growth hormone secretion and increased insulin clearance. It is a normal physiologic process seen in most adolescents without diabetes, who compensate with more insulin output. A child with T1DM cannot compensate. The dawn phenomenon is usually recurrent and modestly elevates most morning glucose levels.

Rarely, high morning glucose is caused by the **Somogyi phenomenon,** a theoretical rebound from late-night or early-morning hypoglycemia, thought to be from an exaggerated counterregulatory response. It is unlikely to be a common cause, in that most children remain hypoglycemic (do not rebound) once nighttime glucose levels decline. Continuous glucose monitoring systems may help clarify ambiguously elevated morning glucose levels.

Behavioral/Psychologic Aspects and Eating Disorders

Diabetes in a child affects the lifestyle and interpersonal relationships of the entire family. Feelings of anxiety and guilt are common in parents. Similar feelings, coupled with denial and rejection, are equally common in children, particularly during the rebellious teenage years. Family conflict has been associated with poor treatment adherence and poor metabolic control among youths with T1DM. On the other hand, it has been shown that shared responsibility is consistently associated with better psychologic health, good self-care behavior, and good metabolic control, whereas responsibility assumed by either the child or parent alone does not have outcomes that are equally successful. In some cases, links of shared responsibility to health outcomes were stronger among older adolescents. However, no specific personality disorder or psychopathology is characteristic of diabetes; similar feelings are observed in families with other chronic disorders.

COGNITIVE FUNCTION

There is increasing agreement that children with T1DM are at higher risk of developing small differences in cognitive abilities compared to healthy age-matched peers. Evidence suggests that early-onset diabetes (younger than 7 yr) is associated with cognitive difficulties compared to late-onset diabetes and healthy controls. The cognitive difficulties observed were primarily learning and memory skills (both verbal and visual) and attention/executive function skills. It is likely that the impact of diabetes on pediatric cognition appears shortly after diagnosis. Indeed, it has been observed that early-onset diabetes and longer duration of diabetes in children with diabetes adversely affect their school performance and educational achievements.

COPING STYLES

Children and adolescents with T1DM are faced with a complex set of developmental changes as well as shifting burdens of the disease. Adjustment problems might affect psychologic well-being and the course of the disease by impacting self-management and leading to poor metabolic control. Coping styles refer to typical habitual preferences for ways of approaching problems and might be regarded as strategies that people generally use to cope across a wide range of stressors. Problem-focused coping refers to efforts directed toward rational management of a problem, and it is aimed at changing the situation causing distress. On the other hand, emotion-focused coping implies efforts to reduce emotional distress caused by the stressful event and to manage or regulate emotions that might accompany or result from the stressor. In adolescents with diabetes, avoidance coping and venting emotions have been found to predict poor illness-specific self-care behavior and poor metabolic control. Patients who use more mature defenses and exhibit greater adaptive capacity are more likely to adhere to their regimen. Coping strategies seem to be age dependent, with adolescents using more avoidance coping than younger children with diabetes.

NONADHERENCE

Family conflict, denial, and feelings of anxiety or loss of control find expression in nonadherence to instructions regarding nutritional and insulin therapy and in noncompliance with self-monitoring. When adolescents perceive their parents' involvement as criticism, or when they externalize behavior problems, such behaviors interfere with adherence and may result in deterioration of glycemic control. Such behaviors are very common, whereas episodes of deliberate overdosage with insulin resulting in hypoglycemia, or omission of insulin resulting in ketoacidosis, are far less prevalent. They may, however, be pleas for psychologic help or be manipulative attempts to escape an environment perceived as undesirable or intolerable; occasionally, they may be manifestations of suicidal intent. Frequent admissions to the hospital for ketoacidosis or hypoglycemia should arouse suspicion of an underlying emotional conflict. Overprotection on the part of parents is common and often is not in the best interest of the adolescent patient. Feelings of being different or of being alone, or both, are common and must be acknowledged, but may be addressed by tailoring the insulin administration and timing of meals and blood sugar testings in order to allow for a more individualized lifestyle. Families and patients worry about the risk of complications from diabetes, aggregating what they know about type 1 and type II diabetes, and worry about the decreased life span. Unfortunately, misinformation abounds about the risks of the development of diabetes in siblings or offspring and of pregnancy in young diabetic women. Even appropriate information may cause further anxiety.

All of these issues must be spoken about at the outset, and many of these problems can be averted through continued empathic counseling based on correct information, focusing on normality and on planning to be a productive member of society. Recognizing the potential impact of these problems, peer discussion groups have been organized in many locales; feelings of isolation and frustration tend to be lessened by the sharing of common problems. Summer camps for diabetic children afford an excellent opportunity for learning and sharing under expert supervision. Education about the pathophysiology of diabetes, insulin dose, technique of administration, nutrition, exercise, and hypoglycemic reactions can be reinforced by medical and paramedical personnel. The presence of numerous peers with similar problems offers new insights to the diabetic child. Residential treatment for children and adolescents with difficult to manage T1DM is an option available only in some centers.

ANXIETY AND DEPRESSION

It has been shown that there are significant correlations between poor metabolic control and depressive symptoms, a high level of anxiety, or a previous psychiatric diagnosis. In a similar way, poor metabolic control is related to higher levels of personal, social, school maladjustment, or family environment dissatisfaction. It is estimated that 20-26% of adolescent patients may develop major depressive disorder. The prevalence of depression is 2-fold greater than controls in children with diabetes and 3-fold greater in adolescents. The course characteristics of depression in young diabetic subjects and psychiatric control subjects appear to be similar; however, eventual propensity of diabetic youths for more protracted depressions is greater and there is a higher risk of recurrence among young diabetic females. On balance, anxiety and depression play an important and complex role in T1DM; their relationship to metabolic control does not yet appear clear. Therefore, the healthcare providers managing a child or adolescent with diabetes should be aware of their pivotal role as counselor and advisor and should closely monitor the mental health of patients with diabetes.

FEAR OF SELF-INJECTING AND SELF-TESTING

Extreme fear of self-injecting insulin (injection phobia) is likely to compromise glycemic control as well as emotional well-being. Likewise, fear of finger pricks can be a source of distress and may seriously hamper self-management. Children and adolescents may either omit insulin dosing or refuse to rotate their injection sites because repeated injection in the same site is associated with less pain sensation. Failure to rotate injection sites results in subcutaneous scar formation (lipohypertrophy). Insulin injection into the lipohypertrophic skin is usually associated with poor insulin absorption and/or insulin leakage with resultant suboptimal glycemic control. Children and adolescents with injection phobia and fear of self-testing can be counseled by a trained behavioral therapist and benefit from such techniques as desensitization and biofeedback to attenuate pain sensation and psychologic distress associated with these procedures. Another possibility is to consider using an indwelling subcutaneous soft cannula to minimize the discomfort of repeated injections.

EATING DISORDERS

Treatment of T1DM involves constant monitoring of food intake. In addition, improved glycemic control is sometimes associated with increased weight gain. In adolescent females, these 2 factors, along with individual, familial, and socioeconomic factors, can lead to an increased incidence of both nonspecific and specific eating disorders, which can disrupt glycemic control and increase the risk of long-term complications. Eating disorders and subthreshold eating disorders are almost twice as common in adolescent females with T1DM as in their nondiabetic peers. The reports of the frequencies of specific (anorexia or bulimia nervosa) eating disorders vary from 1.0-6.9% among female patients with T1DM. The prevalence of nonspecific and subthreshold eating disorders is 9% and 14%, respectively. Approximately 11% of T1DM adolescent females take less insulin than prescribed in order to lose weight. Among adolescent females with an eating disorder, approximately 42% of patients misuse insulin, whereas the estimates of insulin misuse prevalence in subthreshold and nondisordered eating groups are 18% and 6%, respectively. Although there is little information regarding the prevalence of eating disorders among male adolescents with T1DM, available data suggest normal eating attitudes in most. Among healthy adolescent males who participate in wrestling, however, the drive to lose weight has led to the seasonal, transient development of abnormal eating attitudes and behaviors, which may lead to insulin dose omission in order to lose weight.

When behavioral/psychologic problems and/or eating disorders are assumed to be responsible for poor adherence with the medical regimen, referral for psychologic evaluation and management is indicated. Behavioral therapists and psychologists usually form part of the pediatric diabetes team in most centers and can help assess and manage emotional and behavioral disorders in diabetic children. Evaluation of nurse-delivered motivational enhancement with and without cognitive behavior therapy in adults revealed the combined therapy resulted in modest improvement in glycemic control. However, motivational enhancement therapy alone did not improve glycemic control. While in some studies the effect of therapist-delivered motivational enhancement therapy on glycemic control in adolescents with T1DM lasted as long as intensive individualized counseling continued, in other studies, motivational interviewing was shown to be an effective method of facilitating changes in a teenager's behavior with T1DM with corresponding improvement in glycemic control.

Management During Infections

Although infections are no more common in diabetic children than in nondiabetic ones, they can often disrupt glucose control and may precipitate DKA. In addition, the diabetic child is at increased risk of dehydration if hyperglycemia causes an osmotic diuresis or if ketosis causes emesis. Counterregulatory hormones associated with stress blunt insulin action and elevate glucose levels. If anorexia occurs from ketosis, lack of caloric intake increases the risk of hypoglycemia. Although children younger than 3 yr of age tend to become hypoglycemic and older children tend toward hyperglycemia, the overall effect is unpredictable. Therefore, frequent blood glucose monitoring and adjustment of insulin doses are essential elements of sick day guidelines (Table 589-10).

The overall goals are to maintain hydration, control glucose levels, and avoid ketoacidosis. This can usually be done at home if proper sick day guidelines are followed and with telephone contact with healthcare providers. The family should seek advice if home treatment does not control ketonuria, hyperglycemia, or hypoglycemia, or if the child shows signs of dehydration. A child with large ketonuria and emesis should be seen in the emergency department for a general examination, to evaluate hydration, and to determine whether ketoacidosis is present by checking serum electrolytes, glucose, pH, and total CO_2. A child whose blood glucose declines to less than 50-60 mg/dL (2.8-3.3 mmol/L) and who cannot maintain oral intake may need IV glucose, especially if further insulin is needed to control ketonemia.

Management During Surgery

Surgery can disrupt glucose control in the same way as can intercurrent infections. Stress hormones associated with the underlying condition as well as with surgery itself cause insulin resistance. This increases glucose levels, exacerbates fluid losses, and may initiate DKA. On the other hand, caloric intake is usually restricted, which decreases glucose levels. The net effect is as difficult to predict as during an infection. Vigilant monitoring and frequent insulin adjustments are required to maintain euglycemia and avoid ketosis.

Maintaining glucose control and avoiding DKA are best accomplished with IV insulin and fluids. A simple insulin adjustment scale based on the patient's weight and blood glucose level can be used in most situations (Table 589-11). The IV insulin is continued after surgery as the child begins to take oral fluids; the IV fluids can be steadily decreased as oral intake increases. When full oral intake is achieved, the IV may be capped and subcutaneous insulin begun. When surgery is elective, it is best performed early in the day, allowing the patient maximal recovery time to restart oral intake and subcutaneous insulin therapy. When elective surgery is brief (less than 1 hr) and full oral intake is expected shortly afterward, one may simply monitor the blood glucose hourly and give a dose of insulin analog according to the child's home glucose correction scale. If glargine or detemir is used as the basal insulin, a full dose is given the evening before planned surgery. If NPH or Lente is used, one half of the morning dose is given before surgery. The child should not be discharged until blood glucose levels are stable and oral intake is tolerated.

Table 589-11	Guidelines for Intravenous Insulin Coverage During Surgery	
BLOOD GLUCOSE LEVEL (mg/dL)	**INSULIN INFUSION (units/kg/hr)**	**BLOOD GLUCOSE MONITORING**
<120	0.00	1 hr
121-200	0.03	2 hr
200-300	0.06	2 hr
300-400	0.08	1 hr*
400	0.10	1 hr*

An infusion of 5% glucose and 0.45% saline solution with 20 mEq/L of potassium acetate is given at 1.5 times maintenance rate.
*Check urine ketones.

Table 589-10	Guidelines for Sick Day Management			
	GLUCOSE TESTING AND EXTRA RAPID-ACTING INSULIN			
URINE KETONE STATUS	**Insulin**	**Correction Doses***		**COMMENT**
Negative or small†	q2hr	q2hr for glucose >250 mg/dL		Check ketones every other void
Moderate to large‡	q1hr	q1hr for glucose >250 mg/dL		Check ketones each void; go to hospital if emesis occurs

Basal insulin: glargine or detemir basal insulin should be given at the usual dose and time. NPH and Lente should be reduced by half if blood glucose <150 mg/dL and the oral intake is limited.
  Oral fluids: sugar-free if blood glucose >250 mg/dL (14 mmol/L); sugar-containing if blood glucose <250 mg/dL.
  Call physician or nurse if blood glucose remains elevated after 3 extra doses; if blood glucose remains less than 70 mg/dL and child cannot take oral supplement; if dehydration occurs.
*Give insulin based on individualized dosing schedule. Also give usual dose for carbohydrate intake if glucose >150 mg/dL.
†For home serum ketones <1.5 mmol/L per commercial kit.
‡For home serum ketones >1.5 mmol/L.

LONG-TERM COMPLICATIONS: RELATION TO GLYCEMIC CONTROL

Complications of DM can be divided into 3 major categories: (1) microvascular complications, specifically, retinopathy and nephropathy; (2) macrovascular complications, particularly accelerated coronary artery disease, cerebrovascular disease, and peripheral vascular disease; and (3) neuropathies, both peripheral and autonomic, affecting a variety of organs and systems (Table 589-12). In addition, cataracts may occur more frequently.

Diabetic retinopathy is the leading cause of blindness in the United States in adults age 20-65 yr. The risk of diabetic retinopathy after 15 yr duration of diabetes is 98% for individuals with T1DM and 78% for those with T2DM. Rates for diabetic retinopathy range from close to 15% to up to 30%. Lens opacities (caused by glycation of tissue proteins and activation of the polyol pathway) are present in at least 5% of those younger than age 19 yr. The metabolic control has an impact on the development of this complication, as prevalence rates are substantially higher with increased duration of diabetes, and higher HbA_{1c}, blood pressure, and cholesterol. Independent of duration, the prevalence of diabetic retinopathy is higher in T1DM. However, genetic factors also have a role, because only 50% of patients develop proliferative retinopathy. The earliest clinically apparent manifestations of diabetic retinopathy are classified as nonproliferative or background diabetic retinopathy—microaneurysms, dot and blot hemorrhages, hard and soft exudates, venous dilation and beading, and intraretinal microvascular abnormalities. These changes do not impair vision. The more severe form is proliferative diabetic retinopathy, which manifests by neovascularization, fibrous proliferation, and preretinal and vitreous hemorrhages. Proliferative retinopathy, if not treated, is relentlessly progressive and impairs vision, leading to blindness. The mainstay of treatment is panretinal laser photocoagulation. In advanced diabetic eye disease—manifested by severe vitreous hemorrhage or fibrosis, often with retinal detachment—vitrectomy is an important therapeutic modality. Eventually, the eye disease becomes quiescent, a stage termed involutional retinopathy. A separate subtype of retinopathy is diabetic maculopathy, which is manifested by severe macular edema impairing central vision, for which focal laser photocoagulation may be effective.

Guidelines suggest that diabetic patients have an initial dilated and comprehensive examination by an ophthalmologist shortly after the diagnosis of diabetes is made in patients with T2DM, and within 3-5 yr after the onset of T1DM (but not before age 10 yr). Any patients with visual symptoms or abnormalities should be referred for ophthalmologic evaluation. Subsequent evaluations for both T1DM and T2DM patients should be repeated annually by an ophthalmologist who is experienced in diagnosing the presence of diabetic retinopathy and is knowledgeable about its management (see Table 589-12).

Diabetic nephropathy is the leading known cause of end-stage renal disease (ESRD) in the United States. Most ESRD from diabetic nephropathy is preventable. Diabetic nephropathy affects 20-30% of patients with T1DM and 15-20% of T2DM patients 20 yr after onset. The mean 5 yr life expectancy for patients with diabetes-related ESRD is less than 20%. The increased mortality risk in long-term T1DM may be due to nephropathy, which may account for approximately 50% of deaths. The risk of nephropathy increases with duration of diabetes (up until 25-30 yr duration, after which this complication rarely begins), degree of metabolic control, and genetic predisposition to essential hypertension. Only 30-40% of patients affected by T1DM eventually experience ESRD. The glycation of tissue proteins results in glomerular basement membrane thickening. The course of diabetic nephropathy is slow. An increased urinary albumin excretion rate of 30-300 mg/24 hr (20-200 µg/min)—microalbuminuria—can be detected and constitutes an early stage of nephropathy from intermittent to persistent (incipient), which is commonly associated with glomerular hyperfiltration and blood pressure elevation. As nephropathy evolves to early overt stage with proteinuria (albumin excretion rate >300 mg/24 hr, or >200 µg/min), it is accompanied by hypertension. Advanced-stage nephropathy is defined by a progressive decline in renal function (declining glomerular filtration rate and elevation of serum blood urea and creatinine), progressive proteinuria, and

Table 589-12	Screening Guidelines				
	WHEN TO COMMENCE SCREENING	FREQUENCY	PREFERRED METHOD OF SCREENING	OTHER SCREENING METHODS	POTENTIAL INTERVENTION
Retinopathy	After 5 yr duration in prepubertal children, after 2 yr in pubertal children	1-2 yearly	Fundal photography	Fluorescein angiography, mydriatic ophthalmoscopy	Improved glycemic control, laser therapy
Nephropathy	After 5 yr duration in prepubertal children, after 2 yr in pubertal children	Annually	Spot urine sample for albumin:creatinine ratio	24 hr excretion of albumin, urinary albumin:creatinine ratio	Improved glycemic control, blood pressure control, ACE inhibitors
Neuropathy	Unclear in children; adults at diagnosis in T2DM and 5 yr after diagnosis in T1DM	Unclear	Physical examination	Nerve conduction, thermal and vibration threshold, pupillometry, cardiovascular reflexes	Improved glycemic control
Macrovascular disease	After age 2 yr	Every 5 yr	Lipids	Blood pressure	Statins for hyperlipidemia Blood pressure control
Thyroid disease	At diagnosis	Every 2-3 yr or more frequently based on symptoms or the presence of antithyroid antibodies	TSH	Thyroid peroxidase, thyroglobulin antibodies	Thyroxine
Celiac disease	At diagnosis	Every 2-3 yr	Tissue transglutaminase, endomysial antibody	Transglutaminase antibodies	Gluten-free diet

ACE, angiotensin-converting enzyme; T1DM, type 1 diabetes mellitus; T2DM, type 2 diabetes mellitus; TSH, thyroid-stimulating hormone.
From Glastras SJ, Mohsin F, Donaghue KC: Complications of diabetes mellitus in childhood, Pediatr Clin North Am 52:1735–1753, 2005.

hypertension. Progression to ESRD is recognized by the appearance of uremia, the nephritic syndrome, and the need for renal replacement (transplantation or dialysis).

Screening for diabetic nephropathy is a routine aspect of diabetes care (see Table 589-12). The American Diabetes Association recommends yearly screening for individuals with T2DM and yearly screening for those with T1DM after 5 yr duration of disease (but not before puberty). A random spot urine sample for albumin to creatinine ratio is obtained. Abnormal results should be confirmed by 2 additional specimens on separate days because of the high variability of albumin excretion in patients with diabetes. Short-term hyperglycemia, strenuous exercise, urinary tract infections, marked hypertension, heart failure, and acute febrile illness can cause transient elevation urinary albumin excretion. There is marked day-to-day variability in albumin excretion, so at least 2 of 3 collections done in a 3-6 mo period should show elevated levels before microalbuminuria is diagnosed and treatment is started. Once albuminuria is diagnosed, a number of factors attenuate the effect of hyperfiltration on kidneys: (1) meticulous control of hyperglycemia, (2) aggressive control of systemic blood pressure, (3) selective control of arteriolar dilation by use of angiotensin-converting enzyme inhibitors (thus decreasing transglomerular capillary pressure), and (4) dietary protein restriction (because high protein intake increases the renal perfusion rate). Tight glycemic control will delay the progression of microalbuminuria and slow the progression of diabetic nephropathy. Previous extensive therapy of diabetes has a persistent benefit for 7-8 yr and may delay or prevent the development of diabetic nephropathy.

DIABETIC NEUROPATHY
Both the peripheral and autonomic nervous systems can be involved, and adolescents with diabetes can show early evidence of neuropathy. This complication can be traced to the metabolic effects of hyperglycemia and/or other effects of insulin deficiency on the various constituents of the peripheral nerve. The polyol pathway, nonenzymatic glycation, and/or disturbances of myoinositol metabolism affecting 1 or more cell types in the multicellular constituents of the peripheral nerve appear likely to have an inciting role. The role of other factors, such as possible direct neurotrophic effects of insulin, insulin-related growth factors, nitric oxide, and stress proteins, seems to be relevant. Peripheral neuropathy may first present in some adolescents with a long-standing history of diabetes. Using quantitative sensory testing, abnormal cutaneous thermal perception is a common finding in both upper and lower limbs in neurologically asymptomatic young diabetic patients. Heat-induced pain threshold in the hand is correlated with the duration of the diabetes. There is no correlation between quantitative sensory testing scores and metabolic control. Subclinical motor nerve impairment as manifested by reduced sensory nerve conduction velocity and sensory nerve action potential amplitude can be detected during late puberty and after puberty in approximately 10% of adolescents. Poor metabolic control during puberty appears to induce deteriorating peripheral neural function in young patients. An early sign of autonomic neuropathy such as decreased heart rate variability may present in adolescents with a history of long-standing disease and poor metabolic control. A number of therapeutic strategies have been attempted with variable results. These treatment modalities include (1) improvement in metabolic control, (2) use of aldose reductase inhibitors to reduce by-products of the polyol pathway, (3) use of α-lipoic acid (an antioxidant) that enhances tissue nitric oxide and its metabolites, (4) use of anticonvulsants (e.g., lorazepam, valproate, gabapentin, carbamazepine, pregabalin, phenytoin, tiagabine, and topiramate) for treatment of neuropathic pain, and (5) antidepressants (amitriptyline, imipramine, and selective serotonin reuptake inhibitors). Additional medications include antiarrhythmics such as lidocaine, topical analgesics, and nonsteroidal antiinflammatory drugs.

Other quite rarely noted complications in diabetic children include dwarfism associated with a glycogen-laden enlarged liver (**Mauriac syndrome**), osteopenia, and a syndrome of limited joint mobility associated with tight, waxy skin; growth impairment; and maturational delay. The Mauriac syndrome is related to chronic underinsulinization;

it is much less common since longer-acting insulins have become available. Clinical features of Mauriac syndrome include moon face, protuberant abdomen, proximal muscle wasting, and enlarged liver from fat and glycogen infiltration. The syndrome of limited joint mobility is frequently associated with the early development of diabetic microvascular complications, such as retinopathy and nephropathy, which may appear before 18 yr of age. In the past decade or two, the prevalence of limited joint mobility has significantly decreased, which is attributed to the improved overall metabolic control of children and adolescents with T1DM.

PROGNOSIS
T1DM is a serious, chronic disease. It has been estimated that the average life span of individuals with diabetes is approximately 10 yr shorter than that of the nondiabetic population. Although diabetic children eventually attain a height within the normal adult range, puberty may be delayed, and the final height may be less than the genetic potential. From studies in identical twins, it is apparent that despite seemingly satisfactory control, the diabetic twin manifests delayed puberty and a substantial reduction in height when onset of disease occurs before puberty. These observations indicate that, in the past, conventional criteria for judging control were inadequate and that adequate control of T1DM was almost never achieved by routine means.

The introduction of portable devices (insulin pumps) that can be programmed to provide CSII with meal-related boluses is 1 approach to the resolution of these long-term problems. In selected individuals, nearly normal patterns of blood glucose and other indices of metabolic control, including HbA$_{1c}$, have been maintained for several years. This approach, however, should be reserved for highly motivated persons committed to rigorous self-monitoring of blood glucose who are alert to the potential complications, such as mechanical failure of the infusion device causing hyperglycemia or hypoglycemia and to infection at the site of catheter insertion.

The changing pattern of metabolic control is having a profound influence on reducing the incidence and the severity of certain complications. For example, after 20 yr of diabetes, there is a decline in the incidence of nephropathy in T1DM in Sweden among children whose disease was diagnosed in 1971-1975 compared with in the preceding decade. In addition, in most patients with microalbuminuria in whom it was possible to obtain good glycemic control, microalbuminuria disappeared. This improved prognosis is directly related to metabolic control.

PANCREAS AND ISLET TRANSPLANTATION AND REGENERATION
In an attempt to cure T1DM, transplantation of a segment of the pancreas or of isolated islets has been performed in adults. These procedures are both technically demanding and associated with the risks of disease recurrence and complications of rejection or its treatment by immunosuppression. Long-term complications of immunosuppression include the development of malignancy. Some antirejection drugs, notably cyclosporine and tacrolimus, are toxic to the islets of Langerhans, impairing insulin secretion and even causing diabetes. Hence, segmental pancreas transplantation is generally only performed in association with transplantation of a kidney for a patient with ESRD due to diabetic nephropathy in which the immunosuppressive regimen is indicated for the renal transplantation. Several thousand such transplants have been performed in adults. With experience and newer immunosuppressive agents, functional survival of the pancreatic graft may be achieved for up to several years, during which time patients may be in metabolic control with no or minimal exogenous insulin and reversal of some of the microvascular complications. However, because children and adolescents with DM are not likely to have ESRD from their diabetes, pancreas transplantation as a primary treatment in children cannot be recommended.

Islet cell transplantation is challenging because of limited survival of the transplanted cells and because of rejection. Research continues to improve techniques for the yield, viability, and reduction of immunogenicity of the islets of Langerhans for transplantation. An islet transplantation strategy (**Edmonton protocol**) infused isolated pancreatic islets into the portal vein of a group of adults with T1DM, along with immunosuppressive medications that had lower side-effect profiles than other drugs. While lasting insulin independence was initially low, engraftment and insulin independence have improved over the last decade, and over a thousand patients having undergone the procedure. There has been improved islet engraftment by the use of improved induction and maintenance immunosuppression. Still, in 5-yr follow-up studies, only 1 in 10 maintain insulin independence, with an average duration of insulin independence in all of only about 15 mo. Long-term challenges remain the toxicity of immunosuppression, the limited procurement of viable tissue, and funding and limitations of engraftment itself.

Alternative means of generating β cells are being sought from islet expansion, encapsulated islet xenografts, human islet cell-lines, and stem cells. Regeneration of islets is an approach that could potentially cure T1DM because β-cell mass is actually dynamically regulated.

589.3 Type 2 Diabetes Mellitus
Britta M. Svoren and Nicholas Jospe

Formerly known as non–insulin dependent diabetes or adult-onset diabetes, T2DM is a heterogeneous disorder, characterized by peripheral insulin resistance and failure of the β cell to keep up with increasing insulin demand. Patients with T2DM have relative rather than absolute insulin deficiency. Generally, they are not ketosis prone, but ketoacidosis may develop in some circumstances. The specific etiology is not known, but these patients do not have autoimmune destruction of β cells, nor do they have any of the known causes of secondary diabetes.

NATURAL HISTORY
T2DM is considered a polygenic disease aggravated by environmental factors, such as low physical activity and excessive caloric intake. Most patients are obese, although the disease can occasionally be seen in normal weight individuals. Asians in particular appear to be at risk for T2DM at lower degrees of total adiposity. Some patients may not necessarily meet overweight or obese criteria for age and gender despite abnormally high percentage of body fat in the abdominal region. Obesity, in particular, central obesity, is associated with the development of insulin resistance. In addition, patients who are at risk for developing T2DM exhibit decreased glucose-induced insulin secretion. Obesity does not lead to the same degree of insulin resistance in all individuals and even those who develop insulin resistance do not necessarily exhibit impaired β-cell function. Thus, many obese individuals have some degree of insulin resistance but compensate for it by increasing insulin secretion. Those individuals who are unable to adequately compensate for insulin resistance by increasing insulin secretion, develop IGT and impaired fasting glucose (usually, although not always, in that order). Hepatic insulin resistance leads to excessive hepatic glucose output (failure of insulin to suppress hepatic glucose output), while skeletal muscle insulin resistance leads to decreased glucose uptake in a major site of glucose disposal. Over time hyperglycemia worsens, a phenomenon that has been attributed to the deleterious effect of chronic hyperglycemia (glucotoxicity) or chronic hyperlipidemia (lipotoxicity) on β-cell function and is often accompanied by increased triglyceride content and decreased insulin gene expression. At some point, blood glucose elevation meets the criteria for diagnosis of T2DM (see Table 589-2), but most patients with T2DM remain asymptomatic for months to years after this point because hyperglycemia is moderate and symptoms are not as dramatic as the polyuria and weight loss accompanying T1DM. Weight gain may even continue. The prolonged hyperglycemia may be accompanied by the development of microvascular and macrovascular complications. In time, β-cell function can decrease to the point that the patient has absolute insulin deficiency and becomes dependent on exogenous insulin. In T2DM, insulin deficiency is rarely absolute, so patients usually do not need insulin to survive. Nevertheless, glycemic control can be improved by exogenous insulin. Although DKA is uncommon in patients with T2DM, it can occur and is usually associated with the stress of another illness such as severe infection. DKA tends to be more common in African-American patients than in other ethnic groups. Although it is generally believed that autoimmune destruction of pancreatic β cells does not occur in T2DM, autoimmune markers of T1DM—namely, glutamic acid decarboxylase antibody, ICA512, and insulin-associated autoantibody—may be positive in up to one third of the cases of adolescent T2DM. The presence of these autoimmune markers does not rule out T2DM in children and adolescents. At the same time, because of the general increase in obesity, the presence of obesity does not preclude the diagnosis of T1DM. Although the majority of newly diagnosed children and adolescents can be confidently assigned a diagnosis of T1DM or T2DM, a few exhibit features of both types and are difficult to classify.

EPIDEMIOLOGY
National Health and Nutritional Examination Surveys data (from 1999-2002) show that the prevalence of T2DM in 12-19 yr olds in the United States is 1.46 in 1,000. The Southeastern Aerosol Research and Characterization (SEARCH) study found that the prevalence of type 2 diabetes in the 10-19 yr old age group in the United States was 15% in 2001 and it is likely that this proportion has increased over time. Certain ethnic groups appear to be at higher risk; for example, Native Americans, Hispanic Americans, and African-Americans (in that order) have higher incidence rates than white Americans. Although a majority of children presenting with diabetes still have T1DM, the percentage of children presenting with T2DM is increasing and represents up to 50% of the newly diagnosed children in some centers.

Prevalence in the rest of the world varies widely and accurate data are not available for many countries, but it is clear that the prevalence is increasing in every part of the world. Asians in general seem to develop T2DM at lower body mass index levels than Europeans. In conjunction with their low incidence of type 1 diabetes, this means that T2DM accounts for a higher proportion of childhood diabetes in many Asian countries.

The epidemic of T2DM in children and adolescents parallels the emergence of the obesity epidemic. Although obesity itself is associated with insulin resistance, diabetes does not develop until there is some degree of failure of insulin secretion. Thus, when measured, insulin secretion in response to glucose or other stimuli is always lower in persons with T2DM than in control subjects matched for age, sex, weight, and equivalent glucose concentration.

GENETICS
T2DM has a strong genetic component; concordance rates among identical twins are in the 60-90% range. It should be kept in mind, however, that twinning itself increases the risk of T2DM (because of intrauterine growth restriction) and this may distort estimates of genetic risk. In at least 1 study from Denmark, both monozygotic and dizygotic twins have a lifetime concordance of T2DM of around 70%, indicating that shared environmental factors (including the prenatal environment) may play a large role in the development of T2DM. The genetic basis for T2DM is complex and incompletely defined; no single identified defect predominates as does the HLA association with T1DM. Genomewide association studies have now identified certain genetic polymorphisms that are associated with increased T2DM risk in most populations studied; the most consistently identified are variants of the TCF7L2 (transcription factor 7–like 2) gene, which may have a role in β-cell function. Other identified risk alleles include variants in *PPARG* and *KCNJ11* as well as many others. But to date, all these identified variants explain only a small portion (probably less than 20%) of the population risk of diabetes and in many cases the mechanism by which these polymorphisms confer risk of T2DM is not clear.

EPIGENETICS AND FETAL PROGRAMMING
Low birthweight and intrauterine growth restriction are associated with increased risk of T2DM. This risk appears to be higher in

low-birthweight infants who gain weight more rapidly in the 1st few years of life. These findings have led to the formulation of the "thrifty phenotype" hypothesis, which postulates that poor fetal nutrition somehow programs these children to maximize storage of nutrients and makes them more prone to future weight gain and development of diabetes. Epigenetic modifications may play a role in this phenomenon, but the detailed molecular mechanisms involved have yet to be determined. Whatever the exact mechanism, prenatal and early childhood environments play an important role in the pathogenesis of T2DM and may do so by epigenetic modification of the DNA (in addition to other factors).

ENVIRONMENTAL AND LIFESTYLE-RELATED RISK FACTORS

Obesity is the most important lifestyle factor associated with development of T2DM. This, in turn, is associated with the intake of high-energy foods, physical inactivity, TV viewing ("screen time"), and low socioeconomic status (in developed countries). Maternal smoking also increases the risk of diabetes and obesity in the offspring. Interestingly, smoking by young adults also increases their own risk of diabetes by as yet unknown mechanisms. In addition, sleep deprivation and psychosocial stress are associated with increased risk of obesity in childhood and with IGT in adults, possibly via overactivation of the hypothalamic-pituitary-adrenal axis. Many antipsychotics (especially the atypical antipsychotics like olanzapine and quetiapine) and antidepressants (both tricyclic antidepressants and newer antidepressants like fluoxetine and paroxetine) induce weight gain. In addition to the risk conferred by increased obesity, some of these medications may also have a direct role in causing insulin resistance, β-cell dysfunction, leptin resistance, and activation of inflammatory pathways. To complicate matters further, there is evidence that schizophrenia and depression themselves increase the risk of T2DM and the metabolic syndrome, independent of the risk conferred by drug treatment. As a result, both obesity and T2DM are more prevalent in this population, and with increasing use of antipsychotics and antidepressants in the pediatric population, this association is likely to become stronger.

CLINICAL FEATURES

In the United States, T2DM in children is more likely to be diagnosed in Native American, Hispanic American, and African-American youth, with the highest incidence being reported in Pima Indian youth. While cases may be seen as young as 6 yr of age, most are diagnosed in adolescence and incidence increases with increasing age. Family history of T2DM is present in practically all cases. Typically, patients are obese and present with mild symptoms of polyuria and polydipsia, or are asymptomatic and detected on screening tests. Presentation with DKA occurs in up to 10% of cases. Physical examination frequently reveals the presence of acanthosis nigricans, most commonly on the neck and in other flexural areas. Other findings may include striae and an increased waist:hip ratio. Laboratory testing reveals elevated HbA_{1c} levels. Hyperlipidemia characterized by elevated triglycerides and low-density lipoprotein cholesterol levels is commonly seen in patients with T2DM at diagnosis. Consequently, lipid screening is indicated in all new cases of T2DM. Because hyperglycemia develops slowly and patients may be asymptomatic for months or years after they develop T2DM, screening for T2DM is recommended in high-risk children (Table 589-13). The American Diabetes Association recommends that all youth who are overweight and have at least 2 other risk factors be tested for T2DM beginning at age 10 yr or at the onset of puberty and every 2 yr after that. Risk factors include family history of T2DM in 1st- or 2nd-degree relatives, history of gestational diabetes in the mother, belonging to certain ethnic groups (i.e., Native American, African-American, Hispanic, or Asian/Pacific Islander groups) and having signs of insulin resistance (e.g., acanthosis nigricans, hypertension, dyslipidemia, or polycystic ovary syndrome). The current recommendation is to use fasting blood glucose as a screening test, but some authorities now recommend that HbA_{1c} be used as a screening tool. In borderline or asymptomatic cases, the diagnosis may be confirmed using a standard oral glucose tolerance test, but this test is not required

Table 589-13	Testing for Type 2 Diabetes in Children

- Criteria*
  Overweight (body mass index >85th percentile for age and sex, weight for height >85th percentile, or weight >120% of ideal for height)
  Plus
  Any 2 of the following risk factors:
    Family history of type 2 diabetes in 1st- or 2nd-degree relative
    Race/ethnicity (Native American, African-American, Hispanic, Asian/Pacific Islander)
    Signs of insulin resistance or conditions associated with insulin resistance (acanthosis nigricans, hypertension, dyslipidemia, polycystic ovary syndrome)
- Age of initiation: age 10 yr or at onset of puberty if puberty occurs at a younger age
- Frequency: every 2 yr
- Test: fasting plasma glucose preferred

*Clinical judgment should be used to test for diabetes in high-risk patients who do not meet these criteria.
From Type 2 diabetes in children and adolescents. American Diabetes Association, Diabetes Care 23:386, 2000. Reproduced by permission.

if typical symptoms are present or fasting plasma glucose or HbA_{1c} is clearly elevated on 2 separate occasions.

TREATMENT

Type 2 diabetes is a progressive syndrome that gradually leads to complete insulin deficiency during the patient's life. A systematic approach for treatment of T2DM should be implemented according to the natural course of the disease, including adding insulin when hypoglycemic oral agent failure occurs. Nevertheless, lifestyle modification (diet and exercise) is an essential part of the treatment regimen, and consultation with a dietitian is usually necessary.

There is no particular dietary or exercise regimen that has been conclusively shown to be superior but most centers recommend a low-calorie, low-fat diet and 30-60 min of physical activity at least 5 times/ wk. Screen time should be limited to 1-2 hr/day. Children with T2DM often come from household environments with a poor understanding of healthy eating habits. Commonly observed behaviors include skipping meals, heavy snacking, and excessive daily television viewing, video game playing, and computer use. Adolescents engage in non–appetite-based eating (i.e., emotional eating, television-cued eating, boredom) and cyclic dieting ("yo-yo" dieting). Treatment in these cases is frequently challenging and may not be successful unless the entire family buys into the need to change their unhealthy lifestyle.

It is recommended that oral hypoglycemic agents be introduced at the time of diagnosis (Table 589-14). Patients who present with DKA or with markedly elevated HbA_{1c} (>9.0%) will require treatment with insulin using protocols similar to those used for treating T1DM. Once blood glucose levels are under control, most cases can be managed with oral hypoglycemic agents and lifestyle interventions, but some patients will continue to require insulin therapy.

The most commonly used and the only FDA-approved oral agent for the treatment of T2DM in children and adolescents is metformin. Renal function must be assessed before starting metformin as impaired renal function has been associated with potentially fatal lactic acidosis. Significant hepatic dysfunction is also a contraindication to metformin use, although mild elevations in liver enzymes may not be an absolute contraindication. The usual starting dose is 500 mg once daily. This may be increased to a maximum dose of 2,000 mg/day. Abdominal symptoms are common early in the course of treatment, but in most cases they will resolve with time.

Other agents such as thiazolidinediones, sulfonylureas, acarbose, pramlintide, and incretin mimetics are being used routinely in adults but are not used as commonly in pediatrics. Sulfonylureas are widely used in adults, but experience in pediatrics is limited. Sulfonylureas cause insulin release by closing the potassium channel (K_{ATP}) on β

Table 589-14 | Oral Hypoglycemic Agents

DRUG	MECHANISM OF ACTION	DURATION OF BIOLOGIC EFFECT (hr)	USUAL DAILY DOSE (mg)	DOSES/DAY	SIDE EFFECTS	CAUTION
Biguanide	Insulin sensitizer				Gastrointestinal disturbance, lactic acidosis	Avoid in hepatic or renal impairment
Metformin			1500-2500	2-3		
Sulfonylureas						
1st generation						
Acetohexamide		12-18	500-750	1 or divided		
Chlorpropamide		27-72	250-500	1		
Tolbutamide		14-16	1000-2000	1 or divided		
2nd generation						
Glipizide		14-16	2.5-10	1 or divided		
			XL: 5-10	1		
Glyburide		20-24+	2.5-10	1 or divided		
Glimepiride		24+	2-4	1		
Glitinides	Promote insulin secretion					Titrate carefully in renal or hepatic dysfunction
Repaglinide		≤24	2-16	3		
Nateglinide		4	360	3		
α-Glucosidase inhibitors	Slow hydrolysis and absorption of complex carbohydrates		150-300	3 (with meals)	Transient gastrointestinal disturbances	
Acarbose			150-300	3 (with meals)		
Miglitol						
Thiazolidinedione	Peripheral insulin sensitizer				Upper respiratory tract infection, headache, edema, weight gain	
Rosiglitazone			4-8	1 or divided		
Pioglitazone			15-45	1		
Sitagliptin	GLP-1 receptor agonist	24	50-100	1	Upper respiratory tract infection, sore throat, diarrhea	No data in children or adolescents

From Jacobson-Dickman E, Levistky L: Oral agents in managing diabetes mellitus in children and adolescents, Pediatr Clin North Am 52:1689–1703, 2005.

cells. They are occasionally used when metformin monotherapy is unsuccessful or contraindicated for some reason (use in certain forms of neonatal diabetes is discussed in the section on neonatal diabetes). Thiazolidinediones are not approved for use in pediatrics. Pramlintide (Symlin) is an analog of IAPP (islet amyloid polypeptide), which is a peptide that is cosecreted with insulin by the β cells and acts to delay gastric emptying, suppress glucagon, and possibly suppress food intake. It is not yet approved for pediatric use. Incretins are gut-derived peptides like GLP-1, GLP-2, and GIP (glucose-dependent insulinotropic peptide, previously known as gastric inhibitory protein) that are secreted in response to meals and act to enhance insulin secretion and action, suppress glucagon production, and delay gastric emptying (among other actions). GLP-1 analogs (e.g., exenatide) and agents that prolong endogenous GLP-1 action (e.g., sitagliptin) are now available for use in adults but are not yet approved for use in children; they may be associated with side effects such as hepatic injury and pancreatitis.

COMPLICATIONS
In the SEARCH study of diabetes in youth, 92% of the patients with T2DM had 2 or more elements of the metabolic syndrome (hypertension, hypertriglyceridemia, decreased high-density lipoprotein, increased waist circumference), including 70% with hypertension. In addition, the incidence of microalbuminuria and diabetic retinopathy appears to be higher in T2DM than it is in T1DM. In the SEARCH study, the incidence of microalbuminuria among patients who had

T2DM of less than 5 yr duration was 7-22%, while retinopathy was present in 18.3%. Thus, all adolescents with T2DM should be screened for hypertension and lipid abnormalities and screening for microalbuminuria and retinopathy may be indicated even earlier than it is in T1DM. Sleep apnea and fatty liver disease are being diagnosed with increasing frequency and may necessitate referral to the appropriate specialists. Complications associated with all forms of diabetes and recommendations for screening are noted in Table 589-12; Table 589-15 lists additional conditions particularly associated with T2DM.

PREVENTION
The difficulties in achieving good glucose control and preventing diabetes complications make prevention a compelling strategy. This is particularly true for T2DM, which is clearly linked to modifiable risk factors (obesity, a sedentary lifestyle). The Diabetes Prevention Program was designed to prevent or delay the development of T2DM in adult individuals at high risk by virtue of IGT. The Diabetes Prevention Program results demonstrated that intensified lifestyle or drug intervention in individuals with IGT prevented or delayed the onset of T2DM. The results were striking. Lifestyle intervention reduced the diabetes incidence by 58%; metformin reduced the incidence by 31% compared with placebo. The effects were similar for men and women and for all racial and ethnic groups. Lifestyle interventions are believed to have similar beneficial effects in obese adolescents with IGT. Screening is indicated for at-risk patients (see Table 589-13).

Table 589-15	Monitoring for Complications and Comorbidities	
CONDITION	**SCREENING TEST**	**COMMENT**
Hypertension	Blood pressure	
Fatty liver	Aspartate aminotransferase, alanine aminotransferase, possibly liver ultrasound	
Polycystic ovary syndrome	Menstrual history, assessment for androgen excess with free/total testosterone, dehydroepiandrosterone	
Microalbuminuria	Urine albumin concentration and albumin:creatinine ratios	
Dyslipidemia	Fasting lipid profile (total, low-density lipoprotein, high-density lipoprotein cholesterol, triglycerides)	Obtain at diagnosis and every 2 yr
Sleep apnea	Sleep study to assess overnight oxygen saturation	

From Liu L, Hironaka K, Pihoker C: Type 2 diabetes in youth, *Curr Probl Pediatr Adolesc Health Care* 34:249–280, 2004.

589.4 Other Specific Types of Diabetes
Britta M. Svoren and Nicholas Jospe

Most cases of diabetes in children as well as adults fall into the 2 broad categories of type 1 and type 2 diabetes, but up to 4% of cases are caused by single-gene disorders. These disorders include hereditary defects of β-cell function and insulin action, as well as rare forms of mitochondrial diabetes.

GENETIC DEFECTS OF β-CELL FUNCTION
Maturity-Onset Diabetes of Youth
Several forms of diabetes are associated with monogenic defects in β-cell function. Before these genetic defects were identified, this subset of diabetics was diagnosed on clinical grounds and described by the term MODY. This subtype of DM consists of a group of heterogeneous clinical entities that are characterized by onset before 25 yr, autosomal dominant inheritance, and a primary defect in insulin secretion. Strict criteria for the diagnosis of MODY include diabetes in at least 3 generations with autosomal dominant transmission and diagnosis before age 25 yr in at least 1 affected subject. Mutations have been found in at least in 10 different genes, accounting for the dominantly inherited monogenic defects of insulin secretion, for which the term MODY is used. The American Diabetes Association groups these disorders together under the broader category of "genetic defects of β-cell function." Eleven of these defects typically meet the clinical criteria for the diagnosis of MODY and are listed in Table 589-16. Just 3 of them (MODY2 and MODY3 and MODY5) account for 90% of the cases in this category in European populations, but the distribution may be different in other ethnic groups. Except for MODY2 (which is caused by mutations in the enzyme glucokinase), all other forms are caused by genetic defects in various transcription factors (Table 589-16).

MODY2
This is the second most common form of MODY and accounts for approximately 15-30% of all patients diagnosed with MODY. Glucokinase plays an essential role in β-cell glucose sensing and heterozygous mutations in this gene lead to mild reductions in pancreatic β-cell response to glucose. Homozygotes with the same mutations are completely unable to secrete insulin in response to glucose and develop a form of permanent neonatal diabetes. Patients with heterozygous mutations have a higher threshold for insulin release but are able to secrete insulin adequately once blood glucose rises above 7 mmol/L. This results in a relatively mild form of diabetes (HbA$_{1c}$ is usually less than 7%), with mild fasting hyperglycemia and IGT in the majority of patients. MODY2 may be misdiagnosed as type 1 diabetes in children, gestational diabetes in pregnant women, or well-controlled type 2 diabetes in adults (Table 589-17). An accurate diagnosis is important because most cases are not progressive, and except for gestational diabetes, may not require treatment. When needed, they can usually be treated with small doses of exogenously administered insulin. Treatment with oral agents (sulfonylureas and related drugs) can be successful and may be more acceptable to many patients.

MODY3
Patients affected with mutations in the transcription factor hepatocyte nuclear factor-1α show abnormalities of carbohydrate metabolism varying from IGT to severe diabetes and often progressing from a mild to a severe form over time. They are also prone to the development of vascular complications. This is the most common MODY subtype and accounts for 50-65% of all cases. These patients are very sensitive to the action of sulfonylureas and can usually be treated with relatively low doses of these oral agents, at least in the early stages of the disease. In children, this form of MODY is sometimes misclassified as T1DM and treated with insulin. Evaluation of autoimmune markers will rule out T1DM, and genetic testing for this form of MODY is now available and is indicated in patients with relatively mild diabetes and a family history suggestive of autosomal dominant inheritance. On the other hand, even patients with relatively mild and gradual onset of diabetes may have T1DM, and in the absence of a family history suggestive of autosomal dominant inheritance, the diagnosis of MODY is not warranted. Accurate diagnosis can lead to avoidance of unnecessary insulin treatment and specific genetic counseling.

Hepatocyte nuclear factor-4α (MODY1), insulin promoter factor (IPF)-1, also known as (PDX-1) (MODY4), hepatocyte nuclear factor 1β/TCF2 (MODY5), and NeuroD1 (MODY6) are all transcription factors that are involved in β-cell development and function and mutations in these lead to various rare forms of MODY. In addition to diabetes they can also have specific findings unrelated to hyperglycemia; for example, MODY1 is associated with low triglyceride and lipoprotein levels and MODY5 is associated with renal cysts and renal dysfunction. In terms of treatment, MODY1 and MODY4 may respond to oral sulfonylureas, but MODY5 does not respond to oral agents and requires treatment with insulin. NeuroD1 defects are extremely rare and not much is known about their natural history.

Primary or secondary defects in the glucose transporter-2, which is an insulin-independent glucose transporter, may also be associated with diabetes. Diabetes may also be a manifestation of a polymorphism in the glycogen synthase gene. This enzyme is crucially important for storage of glucose as glycogen in muscle. Patients with this defect are notable for marked insulin resistance and hypertension, as well as a strong family history of diabetes.

Mitochondrial Gene Defects
Maternally Inherited Diabetes and Deafness. Point mutations in mitochondrial DNA are sometimes associated with maternally inherited DM and deafness. The most common mitochondrial DNA mutation in these cases is the point mutation m.3243A>G in the transfer RNA leucine gene. This mutation is identical to the

Table 589-16	Summary of MODY Types and Special Clinical Characteristics		
	GENE MUTATED	**FUNCTION**	**SPECIAL FEATURE**
MODY1	*HNF4α*	Transcription factor	Decreased levels of triglycerides, apolipoproteins AII and CIII (5-10% of MODY), neonatal hypoglycemia, very sensitive to sulfonylureas
MODY2	Glucokinase (*GCK*)	Enzyme, glucose sensor	Hyperglycemia of early onset but mild and nonprogressive; common (30-70% MODY)
MODY3	*HNF1α*	Transcription factor	Decreased renal absorption of glucose and consequent glycosuria; common (30-70% of cases of MODY); very sensitive to sulfonylureas
MODY4	*IPF-1*	Necessary for pancreatic development	Homozygous mutation causes pancreatic agenesis
MODY5	*HNF1β*	Transcription factor	Renal malformations; associated with uterine abnormalities, hypospadias, joint laxity, and learning difficulties, pancreatic atrophy, pancreatic exocrine insufficiency; 5-10% of MODY
MODY6	*NEUROD1*	Differentiation factor in the development of pancreatic islets	Extremely rare
MODY7	*KFL11*	Zinc finger transcription factor	Early-onset type II diabetes mellitus
MODY8	*CEL*	Bile salt–dependent lipase	Hyperglycemia; fecal elastase deficiency; exocrine pancreatic atrophy
MODY9	*PAX4*	Transcription factor	
MODY10	*INS*	Insulin gene	Usually associated with neonatal diabetes
MODY11	*BLK*	B-lymphocyte tyrosine kinase	Early-onset T1DM without autoantibodies

MODY, maturity-onset diabetes of the young.
From Nakhla M, Polychronakos C: Monogenic and other unusual causes of diabetes mellitus, Pediatr Clin North Am 52:1637–1650, 2005.

Table 589-17	Clinical and Biochemical Features Associated with Type 1 Diabetes, Type 2 Diabetes and the Common Subtypes of Maturity-Onset Diabetes of the Young			
FEATURES	**TYPE 1 DIABETES**	**TYPE 2 DIABETES**	**GCK-MODY**	**HNF1A/4A-MODY**
Typical age of diagnosis (yr)	10-30	>25	Present from birth; presents at any age	15-45
Diabetic ketoacidosis	Common	Rare	Rare	Rare
Insulin dependent	Yes	No	No	No
Parental history of diabetes	<15%	>50% in young onset type 2 diabetes	If tested, 1 parent usually has impaired fasting glycemia (may not be previously known)	60-90%*
Obesity	Uncommon	Common	Uncommon	Uncommon
Insulin resistance	Uncommon	Common	Uncommon	Uncommon
Presence of β-cell antibodies	>90%	Negative	Rare	Rare
C-peptide concentrations	Undetectable/low	Normal/high	Normal	Normal
Optimal first-line treatment	Insulin	Metformin	None	Sulfonylurea

*Family history is often part of the criteria for testing. Some reports cite a parental history of 60-70%.
GCK, glucokinase; HNF1A/4A, hepatocyte nuclear factor 1α/4α; MODY, maturity-onset diabetes of the young.
From Thanabalasingham G, Owen KR: Diagnosis and management of maturity onset diabetes of the young (MODY), BMJ 343:d6044, 2011, Table 2, p. 838.

mutation in MELAS (myopathy, encephalopathy, lactic acidosis, and stroke-like syndrome), but this syndrome is not associated with diabetes; the phenotypic expression of the same defect varies. Diabetes in most of these cases presents insidiously but approximately 20% of patients have an acute presentation resembling T1DM. The mean age of diagnosis of diabetes is 37 yr but cases have been reported as young as 11 yr. This mutation has been estimated to be present in 1.5% of Japanese diabetics, which may be higher than the prevalence in other ethnic groups. Metformin should be avoided in these patients because of the theoretical risk of severe lactic acidosis in the presence of mitochondrial dysfunction.

Another form of IDDM, sometimes associated with mitochondrial mutations, is the **Wolfram syndrome**. **Wolfram syndrome 1** is characterized by diabetes insipidus, DM, optic atrophy, and deafness—thus, the acronym DIDMOAD. Some patients with diabetes appear to have

severe insulinopenia, whereas others have significant insulin secretion as judged by C-peptide. The overall prevalence is 1 in 770,000 live births. The sequence of appearance of the stigmata is as follows: non-autoimmune IDDM in the 1st decade, central diabetes insipidus and sensorineural deafness in two thirds to three fourths of the patients in the 2nd decade, renal tract anomalies in about one half of the patients in the 3rd decade, and neurologic complications such as cerebellar ataxia and myoclonus in one half to two thirds of the patients in the 4th decade. Other features include primary gonadal atrophy in the majority of males and a progressive neurodegenerative course with neurorespiratory death at a median age of 30 yr. Some (but not all) cases are caused by mutations in the *WFS-1* (wolframin) gene on chromosome 4p. **Wolfram syndrome 2** has early-onset optic atrophy, DM, deafness, and a shortened life span but no diabetes insipidus; the associated gene is *CISD2*.

DIABETES MELLITUS OF THE NEWBORN

Neonatal DM is exceedingly rare. Onset of classic autoimmune T1DM before the age of 6 mo is most unusual and most cases of diabetes in this age range are caused by genetic mutations.

Transient Neonatal Diabetes Mellitus

Neonatal diabetes is transient in approximately 50% of cases, but after an interim period of normal glucose tolerance, 50-60% of these patients develop permanent diabetes (at an average age of 14 yr). There are also reports of patients with classic T1DM who formerly had transient diabetes of the newborn. It remains to be determined whether this association of transient diabetes in the newborn followed much later in life by classic T1DM is a chance occurrence or causally related.

The syndrome of transient DM in the newborn infant has its onset in the 1st wk of life and persists several weeks to months before spontaneous resolution. Median duration is 12 wk. It occurs most often in infants who are small for gestational age and is characterized by hyperglycemia and pronounced glycosuria, resulting in severe dehydration and, at times, metabolic acidosis, but with only minimal or no ketonemia or ketonuria. There may also be findings such as umbilical hernia or large tongue. Insulin responses to glucose or tolbutamide are low to absent; basal plasma insulin concentrations are normal. After spontaneous recovery, the insulin responses to these same stimuli are brisk and normal, implying a functional delay in β-cell maturation with spontaneous resolution. Occurrence of the syndrome in consecutive siblings has been reported. About 70% of cases are due to **abnormalities of an imprinted locus on chromosome 6q24**, resulting in overexpression of paternally expressed genes such as pleomorphic adenoma gene–like 1 (PLAGL1/ZAC) and hydatidiform mole associated and imprinted (HYMAI). Most of the remaining cases are caused by mutations in K_{ATP} channels. Mutations in K_{ATP} channels also cause many cases of permanent neonatal diabetes, but there is practically no overlap between the mutations that lead to transient neonatal DM and those causing permanent neonatal DM. This syndrome of transient neonatal DM should be distinguished from the severe hyperglycemia that may occur in hypertonic dehydration; that usually occurs in infants beyond the newborn period and responds promptly to rehydration with minimal or no requirement for insulin.

Administration of insulin is mandatory during the active phase of DM in the newborn. One to 2 units/kg/24 hr of an intermediate-acting insulin in 2 divided doses usually results in dramatic improvement and accelerated growth and gain in weight. Attempts at gradually reducing the dose of insulin may be made as soon as recurrent hypoglycemia becomes manifested or after 2 mo of age. Genetic testing is now available for 6q24 abnormalities as well as potassium channel defects and should be obtained on all patients and recurrence risk assessment by a genetic counselor is recommended.

Permanent Neonatal Diabetes Mellitus

Permanent DM in the newborn period is caused in approximately 50% of the cases by mutations in the *KCNJ11* (potassium inwardly-rectifying channel J, member 11) and *ABCC8* (adenosine triphosphate–binding cassette, subfamily C, member 8) genes. These genes code for the Kir6.2 and SUR1 subunits of the adenosine triphosphate–sensitive potassium channel, which is involved in an essential step in insulin secretion by the β cell. Some cases are caused by pancreatic agenesis as a result of homozygous mutations in the *IPF-1* gene (where heterozygous mutations cause MODY4); homozygous mutations in the glucokinase gene (where heterozygous mutations cause MODY2); and mutations in the insulin gene. Almost all these infants are small at birth because of the role of insulin as an intrauterine growth factor. Instances of affected twins and families with more than 1 affected infant have been reported. Infants with permanent neonatal DM may be initially euglycemic and typically present between birth and 6 mo of life (mean age of presentation is 5 wk). There is a spectrum of severity and up to 20% have neurologic features. The most severely affected patients have the syndrome of *d*evelopmental delay, *e*pilepsy and *n*eonatal *d*iabetes (DEND syndrome). Less-severe forms of DEND are labeled intermediate DEND or i-DEND.

Activating mutations in the *KCNJ11* gene (encoding the adenosine triphosphate–sensitive potassium channel subunit Kir6.2) are associated with both transient neonatal DM and permanent neonatal DM, with particular mutations being associated with each phenotype. More than 90% of these patients respond to sulfonylureas (at higher doses than those used in T2DM), but patients with severe neurologic disease may be less responsive. Mutations in the *ABCC8* gene (encoding the SUR1 subunit of this potassium channel) were thought to be less likely to respond to sulfonylureas (because this is the subunit that binds sulfonylurea drugs), but some of these mutations are reported to respond and patients have been successfully switched from insulin to oral therapy. Several protocols for switching the patient from insulin to glibenclamide are available and patients are usually stabilized on doses ranging from 0.4-1 mg/kg/day. Because approximately 50% of neonatal diabetics have K-channel mutations that can be switched to sulfonylurea therapy, with dramatic improvement in glycemic control and quality of life, *all* patients with diabetes diagnosed before 6 mo of age (and perhaps even those diagnosed before 12 mo of age) should now be screened for these mutations by genetic testing.

IPEX Syndrome

IPEX means immunodysregulation, polyendocrinopathy, and enteropathy, X-linked. In most patients with IPEX, mutations in the *FOXP3* (Forkhead box P3) gene, a specific marker of natural and adaptive regulatory T cells, leads to severe immune dysregulation and rampant autoimmunity. Autoimmune diabetes develops in >90% of cases, usually within the 1st few wk of life and is accompanied by enteropathy, failure to thrive, and other autoimmune disorders (see Chapter 126.5).

Abnormalities of the Insulin Gene

Diabetes of variable degrees may also result from defects in the insulin gene that lead to various amino acid substitutions that impair the effectiveness of insulin at the receptor level. Insulin gene defects are exceedingly rare and may be associated with relatively mild diabetes or even normal glucose tolerance. Diabetes may also develop in patients with faulty processing of proinsulin to insulin (an autosomal dominant defect). These defects are notable for the high concentration of insulin as measured by radioimmunoassay, whereas MODY and glucose transporter-2 defects are characterized by relative or absolute deficiency of insulin secretion for the prevailing glucose concentrations.

GENETIC DEFECTS OF INSULIN ACTION

Various genetic mutations in the insulin receptor can impair the action of insulin at the insulin receptor or impair postreceptor signaling, leading to insulin resistance.

The mildest form of the syndrome with mutations in the insulin receptor was previously known as *type A insulin resistance*. This is associated with hirsutism, hyperandrogenism, and cystic ovaries in females, without obesity. Acanthosis nigricans may be present and life expectancy is not significantly impaired. More-severe forms of insulin resistance are seen in 2 mutations in the insulin receptor gene that cause the pediatric syndromes of Donohue syndrome (formerly called leprechaunism) and Rabson-Mendenhall syndrome.

Donohue Syndrome

This is a syndrome characterized by intrauterine growth restriction, fasting hypoglycemia, and postprandial hyperglycemia in association with profound resistance to insulin; severe hyperinsulinemia is seen compared to age-matched infants during an oral glucose tolerance test. Various defects of the insulin receptor have been described, thereby attesting to the important role of insulin and its receptor in fetal growth and possibly in morphogenesis. Most of these patients die in the 1st yr of life.

Rabson-Mendenhall Syndrome

This entity is defined by clinical manifestations that appear to be intermediate between those of acanthosis nigricans with insulin resistance type A and Donohue syndrome. The features include extreme insulin

Table 589-18	Clinical and Biochemical Features of Inherited Lipodystrophies			
	CONGENITAL GENERALIZED LIPODYSTROPHY		**FAMILIAL PARTIAL LIPODYSTROPHY**	
Subtype	**BSCL1**	**BSCL2**	**FPLD2**	**FPLD3**
Defective gene	*AGPAT2*	*BSCL2*	*LMNA*	*PPARG*
Clinical onset	Soon after birth	Soon after birth	Puberty	Usually puberty, but may present in younger children
Fat distribution	Generalized absence	Generalized absence	Loss of limb and gluteal fat; typically excess facial and nuchal fat; trunk fat often lost	Loss of limb and gluteal fat; preserved facial and trunk fat
Cutaneous features	Acanthosis nigricans and skin tags; hirsutism common in women	Acanthosis nigricans and skin tags; hirsutism common in women	Acanthosis nigricans and skin tags; hirsutism common in women	Acanthosis nigricans and skin tags; hirsutism common in women
Musculoskeletal	Acromegaloid features common	Acromegaloid features common	Frequent muscle hypertrophy; some have overlap features of muscular dystrophy	Nil specific
Nonalcoholic fatty liver disease	Severe	Severe	Yes	Yes
Dyslipidemia	Severe associated with pancreatitis	Severe associated with pancreatitis	Yes, may be severe	Yes, may be severe
Insulin resistance	Severe early onset	Severe early onset	Severe	Severe; early onset in some
Diabetes onset	<20 yr	<20 yr	Variable; generally later in men than women	Variable; generally later in men than women
Hypertension	Common	Common	Common	Very common
Other		Mild mental retardation possible		

From Semple RK, Savage DB, Halsall DJ, O'Rahilly S: Syndromes of severe insulin resistance and/or lipodystrophy. In Weiss RE, Refetoff S, editors: Genetic diagnosis of endocrine disorders, Philadelphia, 2010, Elsevier, Table 4.2.

resistance, acanthosis nigricans, abnormalities of the teeth and nails, and pineal hyperplasia. It is not clear whether this syndrome is entirely distinct from Donohue syndrome; however, by comparison, patients with Rabson-Mendenhall tend to live significantly longer. Therapies with modest benefit have included insulin-like growth factor-1 and leptin.

Lipoatrophic Diabetes
Various forms of lipodystrophy are associated with insulin resistance and diabetes (Table 589-18). Familial partial lipoatrophy is associated with mutations in the *LMNA* gene, encoding nuclear envelope proteins lamin A and C. Severe generalized lipoatrophy is associated with mutations in the seipin and *AGPAT2* genes, but the mechanism by which these mutations lead to insulin resistance and diabetes is not known.

Stiff-Person Syndrome
This is an extremely rare autoimmune central nervous system disorder that is characterized by progressive stiffness and painful spasms of the axial muscles and very high titers of glutamic acid decarboxylase antibodies. About one third of the patients also develop T1DM.

Systemic Lupus Erythematosus
In rare cases, patients with systemic lupus erythematosus may develop autoantibodies to the insulin receptor, leading to insulin resistance and diabetes.

CYSTIC FIBROSIS–RELATED DIABETES
See Chapter 403.

As patients with cystic fibrosis (CF) live longer, an increasing number are being diagnosed with cystic fibrosis–related diabetes (CFRD). Females appear to have a somewhat higher risk of CFRD than males and prevalence increases with increasing age until age 40 yr (there is a decline in prevalence after that, presumably because only the healthiest CF patients survive beyond that age). There is an

association with pancreatic insufficiency and there may be a higher risk in patients with class I and class II CF transmembrane conductance regulator mutations. A large multicenter study in the United States reported prevalence (in all ages) of 17% in females and 12% in males. Cross-sectional studies indicate that the prevalence of IGT may be significantly higher than this and up to 65% of children with CF have diminished 1st phase insulin secretion, even when they have normal glucose tolerance. In Denmark, oral glucose tolerance screening of the entire CF population demonstrated no diabetes in patients younger than 10 yr, diabetes in 12% of patients age 10-19 yr, and diabetes in 48% of adults age 20 yr and older. At a Midwestern center where routine annual oral glucose tolerance screening is performed, only about one half of children and one fourth of adults have normal glucose tolerance.

Patients with CFRD have features of both T1DM and T2DM. In the pancreas, exocrine tissue is replaced by fibrosis and fat and many of the pancreatic islets are destroyed. The remaining islets demonstrate diminished numbers of β-, α-, and pancreatic polypeptide-secreting cells. Secretion of the islet hormones insulin, glucagon, and pancreatic polypeptide is impaired in patients with CF in response to a variety of secretagogs. This pancreatic damage leads to slowly progressive insulin deficiency, of which the earliest manifestation is an impaired 1st phase insulin response. As patients age, this response becomes progressively delayed and less robust than normal. At the same time, these patients develop insulin resistance due to chronic inflammation and the intermittent use of corticosteroids. Insulin deficiency and insulin resistance lead to a very gradual onset of IGT that eventually evolves into diabetes. In some cases, diabetes may wax and wane with disease exacerbations and the use of corticosteroids. The clinical presentation is similar to that of T2DM in that the onset of the disease is insidious and the occurrence of ketoacidosis is rare. Islet antibody titers are negative. Microvascular complications do develop but may do so at a slower rate than in typical T1DM or T2DM. Macrovascular complications do not appear to be of concern in CFRD, perhaps because of the shortened life span of these patients. Several factors unique to CF influence the onset and the course of diabetes. For example: (1) frequent infections are associated with waxing and waning of insulin resistance; (2) energy needs are increased because of infection and pulmonary disease; (3) malabsorption is common, despite enzyme supplementation; (4) nutrient absorption is altered by abnormal intestinal transit time; (5) liver disease is frequently present; (6) anorexia and nausea are common; (7) there is a wide variation in daily food intake based on the patient's acute health status; and (8) both insulin and glucagon secretion are impaired (in contrast to autoimmune diabetes, in which only insulin secretion is affected).

Impaired glucose tolerance and CFRD are associated with poor weight gain and there is evidence that treatment with insulin improves weight gain and slows the rate of pulmonary deterioration. Because of these observations, the CF Foundation recommends routine diabetes screening of all children with CF, starting at age 12 yr. Despite debate over the ideal screening modality, the current recommendation is the 2 hr glucose tolerance test, though it is possible that simply obtaining a single 2 hr postprandial glucose value may be sufficient. When hyperglycemia develops, the accompanying metabolic derangements are usually mild, and relatively low doses of insulin usually suffice for adequate management. Basal insulin may be started initially, but basal-bolus therapy similar to that used in T1DM will eventually be needed. Dietary restrictions are minimal as increased energy needs are present and weight gain is usually desired. Ketoacidosis is very uncommon but may occur with progressive deterioration of islet cell function. Impaired glucose tolerance is not necessarily an indication for treatment, but patients who have poor growth and inadequate weight gain may benefit from the addition of basal insulin even if they do not meet the criteria for diagnosis of diabetes.

AUTOIMMUNE DISEASES

Chronic lymphocytic thyroiditis (Hashimoto thyroiditis) is frequently associated with T1DM in children (see Chapter 566). As many as 1 in 5 insulin-dependent diabetic patients have thyroid antibodies in their serum; the prevalence is 2-20 times greater than in control populations. Only a small proportion of these patients, however, acquire clinical hypothyroidism; the interval between diagnosis of diabetes and thyroid disease averages about 5 yr. Periodic palpation of the thyroid gland is indicated in all diabetic children; if the gland feels firm or enlarged, serum measurements of thyroid antibodies and TSH should be obtained. A confirmed TSH level of greater than 10 μU/mL indicates existing or incipient thyroid dysfunction that warrants replacement with thyroid hormone. Deceleration in the rate of growth may also be caused by thyroid failure and is, in itself, a reason for securing serum measurements of thyroxine and TSH concentrations.

When diabetes and thyroid disease coexist, the possibility of autoimmune adrenal insufficiency should be considered. It may be heralded by decreasing insulin requirements, increasing pigmentation of the skin and buccal mucosa, salt craving, weakness, asthenia and postural hypotension, or even frank Addisonian crisis. This syndrome is most unusual in the 1st decade of life, but it may become apparent in the 2nd decade or later.

Celiac disease, which is caused by hypersensitivity to dietary gluten, is another autoimmune disorder that occurs with significant frequency in children with T1DM (see Chapter 338.2). It is estimated that approximately 7-15% of children with T1DM develop celiac disease within the 1st 6 yr of diagnosis, and the incidence of celiac disease is significantly higher in children younger than 4 yr of age and in girls. Young children with T1DM and celiac disease usually present with gastrointestinal symptoms (abdominal cramping, diarrhea, and gastroesophageal reflux), growth failure as a consequence of suboptimal weight gain, and unexplained hypoglycemic reactions because of nutrient malab-

sorption, including vitamin D; adolescents may remain asymptomatic. The diagnosis of celiac disease is considered if serum tissue transglutaminase antibody titers are elevated in the presence of normal serum total IgA levels. The diagnosis is confirmed on endoscopic evaluation and biopsy of small bowel revealing characteristic atrophy of intestinal villi. Therapy consists of a gluten-free diet, which will alleviate gastrointestinal symptoms and may reduce glycemic excursions.

Circulating antibodies to gastric parietal cells and to intrinsic factor are 2-3 times more common in patients with T1DM than in control subjects. The presence of antibodies to gastric parietal cells is correlated with atrophic gastritis and antibodies to intrinsic factor are associated with malabsorption of vitamin B_{12}. However, megaloblastic anemia is rare in children with T1DM.

A variant of the multiple endocrine deficiency syndrome is characterized by T1DM, idiopathic intestinal mucosal atrophy with associated inflammation and severe malabsorption, IgA deficiency, and circulating antibodies to multiple endocrine organs including the thyroid, adrenal, pancreas, parathyroid, and gonads. In addition, nondiabetic family members have an increased frequency of vitiligo, Graves disease, and multiple sclerosis as well as low complement levels and antibodies to endocrine tissues.

ENDOCRINOPATHIES

The endocrinopathies listed in Table 589-1 are only rarely encountered as a cause of diabetes in childhood. They may accelerate the manifestations of diabetes in those with inherited or acquired defects in insulin secretion or action.

DRUGS

High-dose oral or parenteral steroid therapy usually results in significant insulin resistance leading to glucose intolerance and overt diabetes. The immunosuppressive agents cyclosporin and tacrolimus are toxic to β cells, causing IDDM in a significant proportion of patients treated with these agents. Their toxicity to pancreatic β cells was 1 of the factors that limited their usefulness in arresting ongoing autoimmune destruction of β cells. Streptozotocin and the rodenticide Vacor are also toxic to β cells, causing diabetes.

There are no consensus guidelines regarding treatment of steroid-induced hyperglycemia in children. Many patients on high-dose steroids have elevated blood glucose during the day and evening, but become normoglycemic late at night and early in the morning. In general, significant hyperglycemia in an inpatient setting is treated with short-acting insulin on an as-needed basis. Basal insulin may be added when fasting hyperglycemia is significant. Outpatient treatment can be more difficult, but when treatment is needed, protocols similar to the basal-bolus regimens used in T1DM are used.

GENETIC SYNDROMES ASSOCIATED WITH DIABETES MELLITUS

A number of rare genetic syndromes associated with IDDM or carbohydrate intolerance have been described (see Table 589-1). These syndromes represent a broad spectrum of diseases, ranging from premature cellular aging, as in the Werner and Cockayne syndromes (see Chapter 90) to excessive obesity associated with hyperinsulinism, resistance to insulin action, and carbohydrate intolerance, as in the Prader-Willi syndrome (see Chapters 80 and 81). Some of these syndromes are characterized by primary disturbances in the insulin receptor or in antibodies to the insulin receptor without any impairment in insulin secretion. Although rare, these syndromes provide unique models to understand the multiple causes of disturbed carbohydrate metabolism from defective insulin secretion or from defective insulin action at the cell receptor or postreceptor level.

Bibliography is available at Expert Consult.

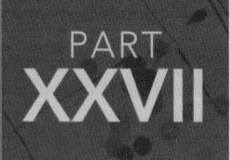
Chapter **590**

Neurologic Evaluation

Rebecca K. Lehman and Nina F. Schor

HISTORY

A detailed history is the cornerstone of any neurologic assessment. Although parents may be the primary informants, most children older than 3-4 yr are capable of contributing to their history and should be questioned directly.

The history should begin with the chief complaint, as well as a determination of the complaint's relative significance within the context of normal development (see Chapters 9-16). The latter step is critical because a 13 mo old who cannot walk may be perfectly normal, whereas a 4 yr old who cannot walk might have a serious neurologic condition.

Next, the history of present illness should provide a chronological outline of the patient's symptoms, with attention paid to location, quality, intensity, duration, associated features, and alleviating or exacerbating factors. It is essential to perform a review of systems, because abnormalities of the central nervous system (CNS) often manifest with vague, nonfocal symptoms that may be misattributed to other organ systems (e.g., vomiting, constipation, urinary incontinence). A detailed history might suggest that vomiting is as a result of increased intracranial pressure (ICP) rather than gastritis or that constipation and urinary incontinence are caused by a spinal cord tumor rather than behavioral stool withholding. In addition, a systemic illness may produce CNS manifestations such as lupus erythematosus (seizures, psychosis, demyelination) or mitochondrial disorders (developmental delay, strokes, hypotonia).

Following the chief complaint and history of present illness, the physician should obtain a complete birth history, particularly if a congenital disorder is suspected. The birth history should begin with a review of the pregnancy, including specific questions about common complications, such as pregnancy-induced hypertension, preeclampsia, gestational diabetes, vaginal bleeding, infections, and falls. It is important to quantify any cigarette, alcohol, or drug (prescription, herbal, illicit) use. Inquiring about fetal movement might provide clues to an underlying diagnosis, because decreased or absent fetal activity can be associated with chromosomal anomalies and CNS or neuromuscular disorders. Finally, any abnormal ultrasound or amniocentesis results should be noted.

A labor history should address the gestational age at delivery and mode of delivery (spontaneous vaginal, vacuum- or forceps-assisted, cesarean section) and should comment on the presence or absence of fetal distress. If delivery was by cesarean section, it is essential to record the indication for surgery.

The birth weight, length, and head circumference provide useful information about the duration of a given problem, as well as insights into the uterine environment. Parents can usually provide a reliable history of their child's postnatal course; however, if the patient was resuscitated or had a complicated hospital stay, it is often helpful to obtain the hospital records. The physician should inquire about the infant's general well-being, feeding and sleeping patterns, activity level, and the nature of the infant's cry. If the infant had jaundice, it is important to determine both the degree of jaundice and how it was managed.

Historical markers of neurologic dysfunction include full-term infants who are unable to breathe spontaneously; have poor, uncoordinated sucks; need an inordinate amount of time to feed; or require gavage feeding. Again, it is important to consider the developmental context, because all of these issues would be expected in premature infants, particularly those with a very-low birthweight. Double-checking the state newborn screening results may provide a clue to abnormal neurologic manifestation in an infant.

The most important component of a neurologic history is the **developmental assessment** (see Chapters 9-14 and 16). Careful evaluation of a child's social, cognitive, language, fine motor, and gross motor skills is required to distinguish normal development from either isolated or global (i.e., in 2 or more domains) developmental delay. An abnormality in development from birth suggests an intrauterine or perinatal cause, but a loss of skills (**regression**) over time strongly suggests an underlying degenerative disease of the CNS, such as an inborn error of metabolism. The ability of parents to recall the precise timing of their child's developmental milestones is extremely variable. It is often helpful to request old photographs of the child or to review the baby book, where the milestones may have been dutifully recorded. In general, parents are aware when their child has a developmental problem, and the physician should show appropriate concern. Table 590-1 outlines the upper limits of normal for attaining specific developmental milestones. Chapter 16 includes a comprehensive review of developmental screening tests and their interpretation.

Family history is extremely important in the neurologic evaluation of a child. Most parents are extremely cooperative in securing medical information about family members, particularly if it might have relevance for their child. The history should document the age and history of neurologic disease, including developmental delay, epilepsy, migraine, stroke, and inherited disorders, for all 1st- and 2nd-degree relatives. It is important to inquire directly about miscarriages or fetal deaths in utero and to document the sex of the embryo or fetus, as well as the gestational age at the time of demise. When available, the results of postmortem examinations should be obtained, as they can have a direct bearing on the patient's condition. The parents should be questioned about their ethnic backgrounds, because some genetic disorders occur more commonly within specific populations (e.g., Tay-Sachs disease in the Ashkenazi Jewish population). They should also be asked if there is any chance that they could be related to each other, because the incidence of metabolic and degenerative disorders of the CNS is increased significantly in children of **consanguineous** marriages.

The social history should detail the child's current living environment, as well as the child's relationship with other family members. It is important to inquire about recent stressors, such as divorce, remarriage, birth of a sibling, or death of a loved one, because they can affect the child's behavior. If the child is in daycare or school, one should document the child's academic and social performance, paying particular attention to any abrupt changes. Academic performance can be assessed by asking about the child's latest report card, and peer relationships can be evaluated by having the child name his or her "best friends." Any child who is unable to name at least 2 or 3 playmates might have abnormal social development. In some cases, discussions with the daycare worker or teacher provide useful ancillary data.

NEUROLOGIC EXAMINATION

The neurologic examination begins at the outset of the interview. Indirect observation of the child's appearance and movements can yield valuable information about the presence of an underlying disorder. For instance, it may be obvious that the child has dysmorphic facies, an

Table 590-1	Screening Scheme for Developmental Delay: Upper Range			
AGE (mo)	**GROSS MOTOR**	**FINE MOTOR**	**SOCIAL SKILLS**	**LANGUAGE**
3	Supports weight on forearms	Opens hands spontaneously	Smiles appropriately	Coos, laughs
6	Sits momentarily	Transfers objects	Shows likes and dislikes	Babbles
9	Pulls to stand	Pincer grasp	Plays pat-a-cake, peek-a-boo	Imitates sounds
12	Walks with 1 hand held	Releases an object on command	Comes when called	1-2 meaningful words
18	Walks upstairs with assistance	Feeds from a spoon	Mimics actions of others	At least 6 words
24	Runs	Builds a tower of 6 blocks	Plays with others	2-3–word sentences

unusual posture, or an abnormality of motor function manifested by a hemiparesis or gait disturbance. The child's behavior while playing and interacting with his or her parents may also be telling. A normal child usually plays independently early in the visit, but then engages in the interview process. A child with attention-deficit/hyperactivity disorder might display impulsive behavior in the examining room, and a child with neurologic impairment might exhibit complete lack of awareness of the environment. Finally, note should be made of any unusual odors about the patient, because some metabolic disorders produce characteristic scents (e.g., the "musty" smell of phenylketonuria or the "sweaty feet" smell of isovaleric acidemia). If such an odor is present, it is important to determine whether it is persistent or transient, occurring only with illnesses.

The examination should be conducted in a nonthreatening, child-friendly setting. The child should be allowed to sit where the child is most comfortable, whether it be on a parent's lap or on the floor of the examination room. The physician should approach the child slowly, reserving any invasive or painful tests (e.g., measurement of head circumference, gag reflex) for the end of the examination. In the end, the more that the examination seems like a game, the more the child will cooperate. Because the neurologic examination of an infant requires a somewhat modified approach from that of an older child, the 2 groups are considered separately (see Chapters 9, 10, and 94 vs Chapters 11-14).

Mental Status

Age aside, the neurologic examination should include an assessment of the patient's mental status in terms of both level of arousal and interaction with the environment. Premature infants born at <28 wk of gestation do not have consistent periods of alertness, whereas slightly older infants arouse from sleep with gentle physical stimulation. Sleep–wake patterns are well developed at term. Because the level of alertness of a neonate depends on many factors, including the time of the last feeding, room temperature, and gestational age, serial examinations are critical when evaluating for changes in neurologic function. Older children's mental status can be assessed by watching them play. Having them tell a story, draw a picture, or complete a puzzle can also be helpful in assessing cognitive function. Memory can be evaluated informally as patients recount their personal information, as well as more formally by asking them to register and recall 3 objects or perform a digit span.

Head

Correct measurement of the **head circumference** is important. It should be performed at every visit for patients younger than 3 yr and should be recorded on a suitable head growth chart. To measure, a nondistensible plastic measuring tape is placed over the mid-forehead and extended circumferentially to include the most prominent portion of the occiput. If the patient's head circumference is abnormal, it is important to document the head circumferences of the parents and siblings. Errors in the measurement of a newborn skull are common owing to scalp edema, overriding sutures, and the presence of cephalohematomas. The average rate of head growth in a healthy

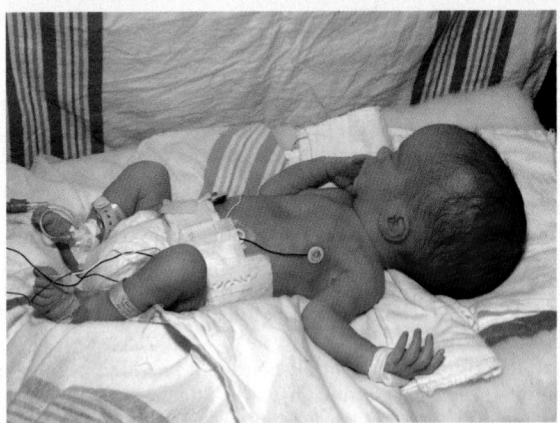

Figure 590-1 Congenital hydrocephalus. Note the enlarged cranium and prominent scalp veins.

premature infant is 0.5 cm in the 1st 2 wk, 0.75 cm in the 3rd wk, and 1.0 cm in the 4th wk and every week thereafter until the 40th wk of development. The head circumference of an average term infant measures 34-35 cm at birth, 44 cm at 6 mo, and 47 cm at 1 yr of age (see Chapters 9 and 10).

If the brain is not growing, the skull will not grow; therefore, a small head frequently reflects a small brain, or **microcephaly**. Conversely, a large head may be associated with a large brain, or **macrocephaly**, which is most commonly familial but may be from a disturbance of growth, neurocutaneous disorder (e.g., neurofibromatosis), chromosomal defect (e.g., Klinefelter syndrome), or storage disorder. Alternatively, the head size may be increased secondary to hydrocephalus (Fig. 590-1) or chronic subdural hemorrhages. In the latter case, the skull tends to assume a square or box-like shape, because the long-standing presence of fluid in the subdural space causes enlargement of the middle fossa.

The shape of the head should be documented carefully. Plagiocephaly, or flattening of the skull, can be seen in normal infants but may be particularly prominent in hypotonic or weak infants, who are less mobile. A variety of abnormal head shapes can be seen when cranial sutures fuse prematurely, as in the various forms of inherited **craniosynostosis** (see Chapter 591.12).

An infant has 2 **fontanels** at birth: a diamond-shaped anterior fontanel at the junction of the frontal and parietal bones that is open at birth, and a triangular posterior fontanel at the junction of the parietal and occipital bones that can admit the tip of a finger or may be closed at birth. If the posterior fontanel is open at birth, it should close over the ensuing 6-8 wk; its persistence suggests underlying hydrocephalus or congenital hypothyroidism. The anterior fontanel varies greatly in size, but it usually measures approximately 2 × 2 cm. The average time of closure is 18 mo, but the fontanel can close normally as early as 9 mo. A very small or absent anterior fontanel at birth might indicate craniosynostosis or microcephaly, whereas a very large fontanel can signify a variety of problems. The fontanel is normally slightly depressed and pulsatile and is best evaluated by holding the infant upright while the infant is asleep or feeding. A bulging fontanel is a potential indicator of increased ICP, but vigorous crying can cause a protuberant fontanel in a normal infant.

Inspection of the head should include observation of the venous pattern, because increased ICP and thrombosis of the superior sagittal sinus can produce marked venous distention. Dysmorphic facial features can indicate a neurodevelopmental aberration. Likewise, cutaneous abnormalities, such as cutis aplasia or abnormal hair whorls, can suggest an underlying brain malformation or genetic disorder.

Palpation of a newborn's skull characteristically reveals **molding** of the skull accompanied by **overriding sutures**—a result of the pressures exerted on the skull during its descent through the pelvis. Marked overriding of the sutures beyond the early neonatal period is cause for alarm, because it suggests an underlying brain abnormality. Palpation additionally might reveal bony bridges between sutures (**craniosynostosis**), cranial defects, or, in premature infants, softening of the parietal bones (**craniotabes**).

Auscultation of the skull is an important adjunct to the neurologic examination. **Cranial bruits** may be noted over the anterior fontanel, temporal region, or orbits, and are best heard using the diaphragm of the stethoscope. Soft symmetric bruits may be discovered in normal children younger than 4 yr of age or in association with a febrile illness. Demonstration of a loud or localized bruit is usually significant and warrants further investigation, because they may be associated with severe anemia, increased ICP, or arteriovenous malformations of the middle cerebral artery or vein of Galen. It is important to exclude murmurs arising from the heart or great vessels, because they may be transmitted to the cranium.

Cranial Nerves
Olfactory Nerve (Cranial Nerve I)
Anosmia, loss of smell, most commonly occurs as a transient abnormality in association with an upper respiratory tract infection or allergies. Permanent causes of anosmia include head trauma with damage to the ethmoid bone or shearing of the olfactory nerve fibers as they cross the cribriform plate, tumors of the frontal lobe, intranasal drug use, and exposure to toxins (acrylates, methacrylates, cadmium). Occasionally, a child who recovers from purulent meningitis or develops hydrocephalus has a diminished sense of smell. Rarely, anosmia is congenital, in which case it can occur as an isolated deficit or as part of Kallmann syndrome, a familial disorder characterized by hypogonadotropic hypogonadism and congenital anosmia. Although not a routine component of the examination, smell can be tested reliably as early as the 32nd wk of gestation by presenting a stimulus and observing for an alerting response, withdrawal, or both. Care should be taken to use appropriate stimuli, such as coffee or peppermint, as opposed to strongly aromatic substances (e.g., ammonia inhalants) that stimulate the trigeminal nerve. Each nostril should be tested individually by pinching shut the opposite side.

Optic Nerve (Cranial Nerve II)
Assessment of the optic disc and retina is a critical component of the neurologic examination. Although the retina is best visualized by dilating the pupil, most physicians do not have ready access to mydriatic agents at the bedside; therefore, it may be necessary to consult an ophthalmologist in some cases. Mydriatics should not be administered to patients whose pupillary responses are being followed as a marker for impending herniation or to patients with cataracts. When mydriatics are used, both eyes should be dilated, because unilateral papillary fixation and dilation can cause confusion and worry in later examiners unaware of the pharmacologic intervention. Examination of an infant's retina may be facilitated by providing a nipple or soother and by turning the head to one side. The physician gently strokes the patient to maintain arousal, while examining the closer eye. An older child should be placed in the parent's lap and should be distracted by bright objects or toys. The color of the optic nerve is salmon-pink in a child but may be gray-white in a newborn, particularly if the newborn has fair coloring. This normal finding can cause confusion and can lead to the improper diagnosis of optic atrophy.

Disc edema refers to swelling of the optic disc, and **papilledema** specifically refers to swelling that is secondary to increased ICP. Papilledema rarely occurs in infancy because the skull sutures can separate to accommodate the expanding brain. In older children, papilledema may be graded according to the Frisen scale (Fig. 590-2). Disc edema must be differentiated from **papillitis**, or inflammation of the optic nerve. Both conditions manifest with enlargement of the blind spot, but visual acuity and color vision tend to be spared in early papilledema in contrast to what occurs in optic neuritis.

Retinal hemorrhages occur in 30-40% of all full-term newborn infants. The hemorrhages are more common after vaginal delivery than after Cesarean section and are not associated with birth injury or with neurologic complications. They disappear spontaneously by 1-2 wk of age. The presence of retinal hemorrhages beyond the early neonatal period should raise a concern for nonaccidental trauma.

Vision
At 28 wk of corrected gestational age, a premature infant blinks in response to a bright light, and at 32 wk, the infant maintains eye closure until the light source is removed. A normal 37 wk infant turns the head and eyes toward a soft light, and a term infant is able to fix on and follow a target, such as the examiner's face. **Optokinetic nystagmus** (OKN), which is conjugate nystagmus that occurs during attempted fixation on a series of rapidly moving objects, can also be used as a crude assessment of the visual system in infants. OKN is elicited by moving an OKN tape—usually a strip of material with alternating 2-inch black and white strips—across the patient's visual field. Although OKN responses can be tested monocularly in neonates, they do not become symmetric until 4-6 mo of age.

Visual fields can be tested in an infant or young child by advancing a brightly colored object from behind the patient's head into the peripheral visual field and noting when the patient first looks at the object. Suspension of the object by a string prevents the patient from focusing on the examiner's hand and arm. The examiner should be certain that the patient is responding to seeing, not hearing, the object.

Visual acuity in term infants approximates 20/150 and reaches the adult level of 20/20 by about 6 mo of age. Children who are too young to read the standard letters on a Snellen eye chart may learn the "E game," which entails pointing to indicate the direction that the E is facing. Children as young as 2.5-3 yr of age can identify the objects on a pediatric eye chart (Allen chart) at a distance of 15-20 ft.

The pupil reacts to light by 29-32 wk of corrected gestational age; however, the pupillary response is often difficult to evaluate, because premature infants resist eye opening and have poorly pigmented irises. Pupillary size, symmetry, and reactivity may be affected by drugs, space-occupying brain lesions, metabolic disorders, and abnormalities of the optic nerves and midbrain. A small pupil may be seen as part of the **Horner syndrome**—characterized by ipsilateral **ptosis** (droopy eyelid), **miosis** (constricted pupil), and **anhidrosis** (lack of sweating) of the face. Horner syndrome may be congenital or may be caused by a lesion of the sympathetic pathway in the hypothalamus, brainstem, cervical spinal cord, or sympathetic plexus. Localization of the lesion within the sympathetic nervous system may be obvious given the other signs present or may be uncertain. In the latter case, serial testing with cocaine drops followed by hydroxyamphetamine drops may be helpful.

During the examination of the pupil, any abnormalities of the iris should also be noted (e.g., heterochromia, Brushfield spots). The physician should also assess the posterior segment of the eye using the **red reflex** test, which is performed in a darkened room using a direct ophthalmoscope held close to the examiner's eye and 12-18 inches from the infant's eyes. If the posterior segment of the eye is normal, the examiner should see symmetric reddish-pink retinal reflections. The absence of any red reflex or the presence of a blunted reflex, white reflex (**leukocoria**), or red reflex with dark spots all signal pathology and should prompt referral to an ophthalmologist.

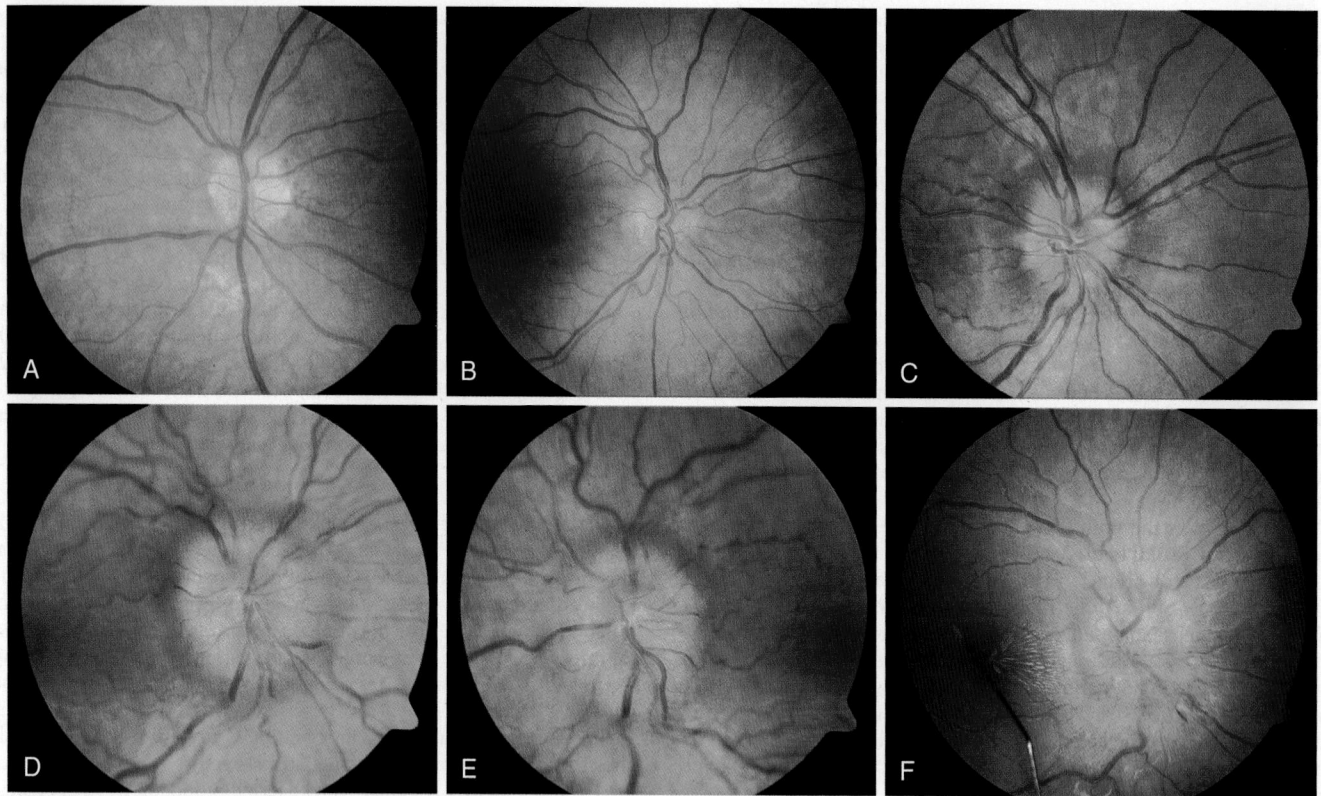

Figure 590-2 Stages of papilledema (Frisen scale). **A,** Stage 0: Normal optic disc. **B,** Stage 1: Very early papilledema with obscuration of the nasal border of the disc only, without elevation of the disc borders. **C,** Stage 2: Early papilledema showing obscuration of all borders, elevation of the nasal border, and a complete peripapillary halo. **D,** Stage 3: Moderate papilledema with elevation of all borders, increased diameter of the optic nerve head, obscuration of vessels at the disc margin, and a peripapillary halo with finger-like extensions. **E,** Stage 4: Marked papilledema characterized by elevation of the entire nerve head and total obscuration a segment of a major blood vessel on the disc. **F,** Stage 5: Severe papilledema with obscuration of all vessels and obliteration of the optic cup. Note also the nerve fiber layer hemorrhages and macular exudate. (**A-C** *courtesy Dr. Deborah Friedman;* **D-F** *courtesy Flaum Eye Institute, University of Rochester.*)

Oculomotor (Cranial Nerve III), Trochlear (Cranial Nerve IV), and Abducens Nerves (Cranial Nerve VI)

The globe is moved by 6 extraocular muscles, which are innervated by the oculomotor, trochlear, and abducens nerves. These muscles and nerves can be assessed by having the patient follow an interesting toy or the examiner's finger in the 6 cardinal directions of gaze. The physician observes the range and nature (conjugate vs dysconjugate, smooth vs choppy or saccadic) of the eye movements, particularly noting the presence and direction of any abnormal eye movements. Premature infants older than 25 wk of gestational age and comatose patients can be evaluated using the oculocephalic (doll's eye) maneuver, in which the patient's head is quickly rotated to evoke reflex eye movements. If the brainstem is intact, rotating the patient's head to the right causes the eyes to move to the left and vice versa. Similarly, rapid flexion and extension of the head elicits vertical eye movement.

Disconjugate gaze can result from extraocular muscle weakness; cranial nerve (CN) III, IV, or VI palsies; or brainstem lesions that disrupt the medial longitudinal fasciculus. Infants who are younger than 2 mo old can have slightly disconjugate gaze at rest, with 1 eye horizontally displaced from the other by 1 or 2 mm (**strabismus**). Vertical displacement of the eyes requires investigation, as it can indicate trochlear nerve (CN IV) palsy or **skew deviation** (supranuclear ocular malalignment that is often associated with lesions of the posterior fossa). Strabismus is discussed further in Chapter 623.

The oculomotor nerve innervates the superior, inferior, and medial recti, as well as the inferior oblique and the levator palpebrae superioris muscles. Complete paralysis of the oculomotor nerve causes ptosis, dilation of the pupil, displacement of the eye outward and downward, and impairment of adduction and elevation. The trochlear nerve supplies the superior oblique muscle, which depresses and intorts the

globe during activities such as reading and walking downstairs. Patients with an isolated paralysis of the trochlear nerve often have a compensatory head tilt away from the affected side, which helps to alleviate their diplopia. The abducens nerve innervates the lateral rectus muscle; its paralysis causes medial deviation of the eye with an inability to abduct beyond the midline. Patients with increased ICP often respond positively when questioned about double vision (**diplopia**) and exhibit incomplete abduction of the eyes on lateral gaze as a result of partial VIth nerve palsies. This false-localizing sign occurs because CN VI has a long intracranial course, making it particularly susceptible to being stretched. **Internuclear ophthalmoplegia,** caused by a lesion in the medial longitudinal fasciculus of the brainstem, that functionally serves conjugate gaze by connecting CN VI on one side to CN III on the other, results in paralysis of medial rectus function in the adducting eye and nystagmus in the abducting eye.

When there is a subtle eye movement abnormality, the **red glass test** may be helpful in localizing the lesion. To perform this test, a red glass is placed over one of the patient's eyes and the patient is instructed to follow a white light in all directions of gaze. The child sees 1 red/white light in the direction of normal muscle function but notes a separation of the red and white images that is greatest in the plane of action of the affected muscle.

In addition to gaze palsies, the examiner might encounter a variety of adventitious movements. **Nystagmus** is an involuntary, rapid movement of the eye that may be subclassified as being **pendular,** in which the 2 phases have equal amplitude and velocity, or **jerk,** in which there is a fast and slow phase. Jerk nystagmus can be further characterized by the direction of its fast phase, which may be left-, right-, up-, or downbeating; rotatory; or mixed. Many patients have a few beats of nystagmus with extreme lateral gaze (**end-gaze nystagmus**), which is of no consequence. Pathologic horizontal nystagmus is most often congenital, drug-induced (e.g., alcohol, anticonvulsants), or a result of vestibular system dysfunction. By contrast, vertical nystagmus is often associated with structural abnormalities of the brainstem and cerebellum. **Ocular bobbing** is characterized by a downward jerk followed by a slow drift back to primary position and is associated with pontine lesions. **Opsoclonus** describes involuntary, chaotic oscillations of the eyes, which are often seen in the setting of neuroblastoma or viral infection.

Trigeminal Nerve (Cranial Nerve V)

The 3 divisions of the trigeminal nerve—ophthalmic, maxillary, and mandibular—convey information about facial protopathic (pain, temperature) and epicritic (vibration, proprioception) sensation. Each modality should be tested and compared to the contralateral side. In patients who are uncooperative or comatose, the integrity of the trigeminal nerve can be assessed by the corneal reflex, elicited by touching the cornea with a small pledget of cotton and observing for symmetric eye closure, and nasal tickle, obtained by stimulating the nasal passage with a cotton swab and observing for symmetric grimace. An absent reflex may be because of a sensory defect (trigeminal nerve) or a motor deficit (facial nerve). The motor division of the trigeminal nerve can be tested by examining the masseter, pterygoid, and temporalis muscles during mastication, as well as by evaluation of the jaw jerk.

Facial Nerve (Cranial Nerve VII)

The facial nerve is a predominantly motor nerve that innervates the muscles of facial expression, buccinator, platysma, stapedius, stylohyoid, and posterior belly of the digastric. It also has a separate division, called the chorda tympani, that contains sensory, special sensory (taste), and parasympathetic fibers. Because the portion of the facial nucleus that innervates the upper face receives bilateral cortical input, lesions of the motor cortex or corticobulbar tract have little effect on upper face strength. Rather, such lesions manifest with flattening of the contralateral nasolabial fold or drooping of the corner of the mouth. Conversely, lower motor neuron or facial nerve lesions tend to involve upper and lower facial muscles equally. Facial strength can be evaluated by observing the patient's spontaneous movements and by asking the patient to mimic a series of facial movements (e.g., smiling, raising the eyebrows, inflating the cheeks). A facial nerve palsy may be congenital; idiopathic (**Bell palsy**); or secondary to trauma, demyelination (Guillain-Barré syndrome), infection (Lyme disease, herpes simplex virus, HIV), granulomatous disease, neoplasm, or meningeal inflammation or infiltration. Facial nerve lesions that are proximal to the junction with the chorda tympani will result in an inability to taste substances with the anterior two-thirds of the tongue. If necessary, taste can be tested by placing a solution of saline or glucose on 1 side of the extended tongue. Normal children can identify the test substance in <10 sec. Other findings that may be associated with facial nerve palsy include hyperacusis, resulting from stapedius muscle involvement, and impaired tearing.

Vestibulocochlear Nerve (Cranial Nerve VIII)

The vestibulocochlear nerve has 2 components within a single trunk: the vestibular nerve, which innervates the semicircular canals of the inner ear and is involved with equilibrium, coordination, and orientation in space, and the cochlear nerve, which innervates the cochlea and subserves hearing.

Dysfunction of the vestibular system results in **vertigo**, the sensation of environmental motion. On examination, patients with vestibular nerve dysfunction typically have nystagmus, in which the fast component is directed away from the affected nerve. With their arms outstretched and eyes closed, their limbs tend to drift toward the injured side. Likewise, if they march in place, they slowly pivot toward the lesion (**Fukuda stepping test**). On Romberg and tandem gait testing, they tend to fall toward the abnormal ear. Vestibular function can be further evaluated with **caloric testing**. Before testing, the tympanic membrane should be visualized to ensure that it is intact and

unobstructed. In an obtunded or comatose patient, 30-50 mL of ice water is then delivered by syringe into the external auditory canal with the patient's head elevated 30 degrees. If the brainstem is intact, the eyes deviate toward the irrigated side. A much smaller quantity of ice water (2 mL) is used in awake, alert patients to avoid inducing nausea. In normal subjects, introduction of ice water produces eye deviation toward the stimulated labyrinth followed by nystagmus with the fast component away from the stimulated labyrinth.

Because hearing is integral to normal language development, the physician should inquire directly about hearing problems. Parents' concern is often a reliable indicator of hearing impairment and warrants a formal audiologic assessment with either audiometry or brainstem auditory evoked potential testing (see Chapter 637). Even in the absence of parents' concern, certain children warrant formal testing within the 1st mo of life, including those with a family history of early life or syndromic deafness or a personal history of prematurity, severe asphyxia, exposure to ototoxic drugs, hyperbilirubinemia, congenital anomalies of the head or neck, bacterial meningitis, and congenital TORCH (*t*oxoplasmosis, *o*ther infections, *r*ubella, *c*ytomegalovirus, *h*erpes simplex virus) infections. For all other infants and children, a simple bedside assessment of hearing is usually sufficient. Newborns might have subtle responses to auditory stimuli, such as changes in breathing, cessation of movement, or opening of the eyes and/or mouth. If the same stimulus is presented repeatedly, normal neonates cease to respond, a phenomenon known as *habituation*. By 3-4 mo of age, infants begin to orient to the source of sound. Hearing-impaired toddlers are visually alert and appropriately responsive to physical stimuli but might have more frequent temper tantrums and abnormal speech and language development.

Glossopharyngeal Nerve (Cranial Nerve IX)

The glossopharyngeal nerve conveys motor fibers to the stylopharyngeus muscle; general sensory fibers from the posterior third of the tongue, pharynx, tonsil, internal surface of the tympanic membrane, and skin of the external ear; special sensory (taste) fibers from the posterior third of the tongue; parasympathetic fibers to the parotid gland; and general visceral sensory fibers from the carotid bodies. The nerve is tested by stimulating 1 side of the lateral oropharynx or soft palate with a tongue blade and observing for symmetric elevation of the palate (**gag reflex**). An isolated lesion of CN IX is rare, because it runs in close proximity to CN X. Potential causes of injury and/or dysfunction include birth trauma, ischemia, mass lesions, motor neuron disease, retropharyngeal abscess, and Guillain-Barré syndrome.

Vagus Nerve (Cranial Nerve X)

The vagus nerve has 10 terminal branches: meningeal, auricular, pharyngeal, carotid body, superior laryngeal, recurrent laryngeal, cardiac, pulmonary, esophageal, and gastrointestinal. The pharyngeal, superior laryngeal, and recurrent laryngeal branches contain motor fibers that innervate all of the muscles of the pharynx and larynx, with the exception of the stylopharyngeus (CN IX) and tensor veli palatini (CN V) muscles. Thus, unilateral injury of the vagus nerve results in weakness of the ipsilateral soft palate and a hoarse voice; bilateral lesions can produce respiratory distress as a result of vocal cord paralysis, as well as nasal regurgitation of fluids, pooling of secretions, and an immobile, low-lying soft palate. Isolated lesions to the vagus nerve may be a complication of thoracotomies or may be seen in neonates with type II Chiari malformations. If such a lesion is suspected, it is important to visualize the vocal cords. In addition to motor information, the vagus nerve carries somatic afferents from the pharynx, larynx, ear canal, external surface of the tympanic membrane, and meninges of the posterior fossa; visceral afferents; taste fibers from the posterior pharynx; and preganglionic parasympathetics.

Accessory Nerve (Cranial Nerve XI)

The accessory nerve innervates the sternocleidomastoid (SCM) and trapezius muscles. The left SCM acts to turn the head to the right side and vice versa; acting together, the SCMs flex the neck. The trapezius acts to elevate the shoulder. Lesions to the accessory nerve result in atrophy and paralysis of the ipsilateral SCM and trapezius muscles, with resultant depression of the shoulder. Because several cervical muscles are involved in head rotation, unilateral SCM paresis might not be evident unless the patient is asked to rotate the head against resistance. Skull base fractures or lesions, motor neuron disease, myotonic dystrophy, and myasthenia gravis commonly produce atrophy and weakness of these muscles; congenital torticollis is associated with SCM hypertrophy.

Hypoglossal Nerve (Cranial Nerve XII)

The hypoglossal nerve innervates the tongue. Examination of the tongue includes assessment of its bulk and strength, as well as observation for adventitious movements. Malfunction of the hypoglossal nucleus or nerve produces atrophy, weakness, and fasciculations of the tongue. If the injury is unilateral, the tongue deviates toward the side of the injury; if it is bilateral, tongue protrusion is not possible and the patient can have difficulty swallowing (**dysphagia**). Werdnig-Hoffmann disease (infantile spinal muscular atrophy, or spinal muscular atrophy type 1) and congenital anomalies in the region of the foramen magnum are the principal causes of hypoglossal nerve dysfunction.

Motor Examination

The motor examination includes assessment of muscle bulk, tone, and strength, as well as observation for involuntary movements that might indicate central or peripheral nervous system pathology.

Bulk

Decreased muscle bulk (**atrophy**) may be secondary to disuse or to diseases of the lower motor neuron, nerve root, peripheral nerve, or muscle. In most cases, neurogenic atrophy is more severe than myogenic atrophy. Increased muscle bulk (**hypertrophy**) is usually physiologic (e.g., body builders). **Pseudohypertrophy** refers to muscle tissue

that has been replaced by fat and connective tissue, giving it a bulky appearance with a paradoxical reduction in strength, as in Duchenne muscular dystrophy.

Tone

Muscle tone, which is generated by an unconscious, continuous, partial contraction of muscle, creates resistance to passive movement of a joint. Tone varies greatly based on a patient's age and state. At 28 wk of gestation, all 4 extremities are extended and there is little resistance to passive movement. Flexor tone is visible in the lower extremities at 32 wk and is palpable in the upper extremities at 36 wk; a normal-term infant's posture is characterized by flexion of all 4 extremities.

There are 3 key tests for assessing postural tone in neonates: the traction response, vertical suspension, and horizontal suspension (Fig. 590-3; see Chapters 94 and 97). To evaluate the **traction response**, the physician grasps the infant's hands and gently pulls the infant to a sitting position. Normally, the infant's head lags slightly behind the infant's body and then falls forward upon reaching the sitting position. To test **vertical suspension**, the physician holds the infant by the axillae without gripping the thorax. The infant should remain suspended with the infant's lower extremities held in flexion; a hypotonic infant will slip through the physician's hands. With **horizontal suspension**, the physician holds the infant prone by placing a hand under the infant's abdomen. The head should rise and the limbs should flex, but a hypotonic infant will drape over the physician's hand, forming a U shape. Assessing tone in the extremities is accomplished by observing the infant's resting position and passively manipulating the infant's limbs. When the upper extremity of a normal-term infant is pulled gently across the chest, the elbow does not quite reach the mid-sternum (**scarf sign**), whereas the elbow of a hypotonic infant extends beyond the midline with ease. Measurement of the **popliteal angle** is a useful method for documenting tone in the lower extremities. The examiner flexes the hip and extends the knee. Normal-term infants allow

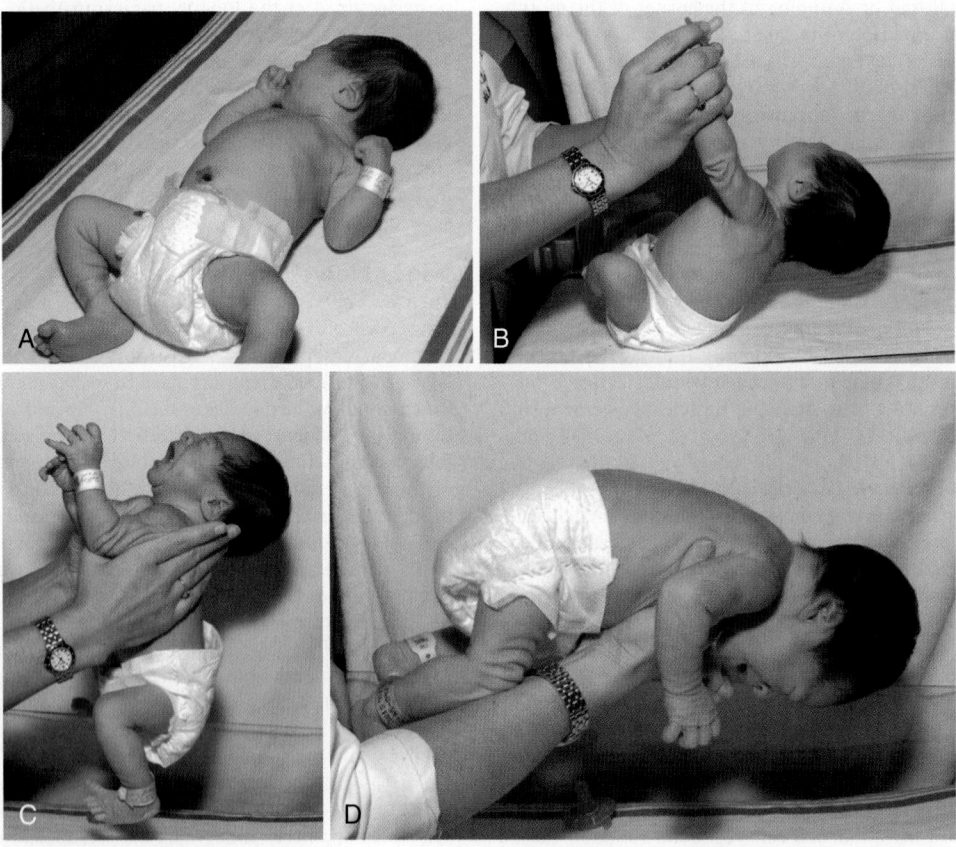

Figure 590-3 Normal tone in a full-term neonate. **A,** Flexed resting posture. **B,** Traction response. **C,** Vertical suspension. **D,** Horizontal suspension.

extension of the knee to approximately 80 degrees. Similarly, tone can be evaluated by flexing the hip and knee to 90 degrees and then internally rotating the leg, in which case the heel should not pass the umbilicus.

Abnormalities of tone include spasticity, rigidity, and hypotonia. (Paratonia, which is rarely seen in the pediatric population, is not discussed here.) **Spasticity** is characterized by an initial resistance to passive movement, followed by a sudden release, referred to as the **clasp-knife** phenomenon. Because spasticity results from upper motor neuron dysfunction, it disproportionately affects the upper-extremity flexors and lower-extremity extensors and tends to occur in conjunction with disuse atrophy, hyperactive deep tendon reflexes, and extensor plantar reflexes **(Babinski sign)**. In infants, spasticity of the lower extremities results in scissoring of the legs upon vertical suspension. Older children can present with prolonged commando crawling or toe-walking. **Rigidity,** seen with lesions of the basal ganglia, is characterized by resistance to passive movement that is equal in the flexors and extensors regardless of the velocity of movement **(lead pipe).** Patients with either spasticity or rigidity might exhibit **opisthotonos**, defined as severe hyperextension of the spine caused by hypertonia of the paraspinal muscles (Fig. 590-4), although similar posturing can be seen in patients with Sandifer syndrome (gastroesophageal reflux or hiatal hernia associated with torsional dystonia). **Hypotonia** refers to abnormally diminished tone and is the most common abnormality of tone in neurologically compromised neonates. A hypotonic infant is

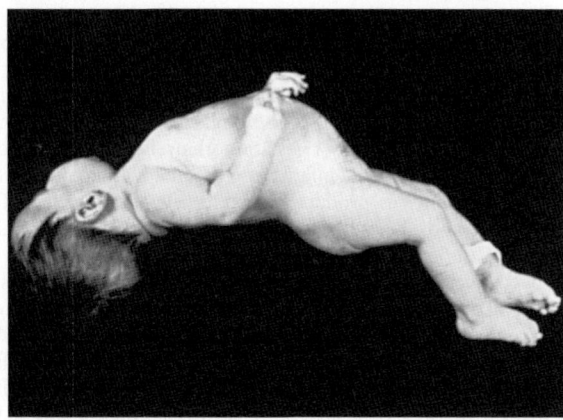

Figure 590-4 Opisthotonus in a brain-injured infant.

floppy and often assumes a frog-leg posture at rest. Hypotonia can reflect pathology of the cerebral hemispheres, cerebellum, spinal cord, anterior horn cell, peripheral nerve, neuromuscular junction, or muscle.

Strength
Older children are usually able to cooperate with formal strength testing, in which case muscle power is graded on a scale of 0-5 as follows: 0 = no contraction; 1 = flicker or trace of contraction; 2 = active movement with gravity eliminated; 3 = active movement against gravity; 4 = active movement against gravity and resistance; 5 = normal power. An examination of muscle power should include all muscle groups, including the neck flexors and extensors and the muscles of respiration. It is important not only to assess individual muscle groups, but also to determine the pattern of weakness (i.e., proximal vs distal; segmental vs regional). Testing for **pronator drift** can be helpful in localizing the lesion in a patient with weakness. This test is accomplished by having the patient extend his or her arms away from the body with the palms facing upward and the eyes closed. *Together, pronation and downward drift of an arm indicate a lesion of the contralateral corticospinal tract.*

Because infants and young children are not able to participate in formal strength testing, they are best assessed with functional measures. Proximal and distal strength of the upper extremities can be tested by having the child reach overhead for a toy and by watching the child manipulate small objects. In infants younger than 2 mo old, the physician can also take advantage of the palmar grasp reflex in assessing distal power and the Moro reflex in assessing proximal power. Infants with decreased strength in the lower extremities tend to have diminished spontaneous activity in their legs and are unable to support their body weight when held upright. Older children may have difficulty climbing or descending steps, jumping, or hopping. They might also use their hands to "climb up" their legs when asked to rise from a prone position, a maneuver called **Gowers sign** (Fig. 590-5).

Involuntary Movements
Patients with lower motor neuron or peripheral nervous system lesions might have **fasciculations**, which are small, involuntary muscle contractions that result from the spontaneous discharge of a single motor unit and create the illusion of a "bag of worms" under the skin. Because most infants have abundant body fat, muscle fasciculations are best observed in the tongue in this age group.

Most other involuntary movements, including tics, dystonia, chorea, and athetosis, stem from disorders of the basal ganglia. Tremor seems

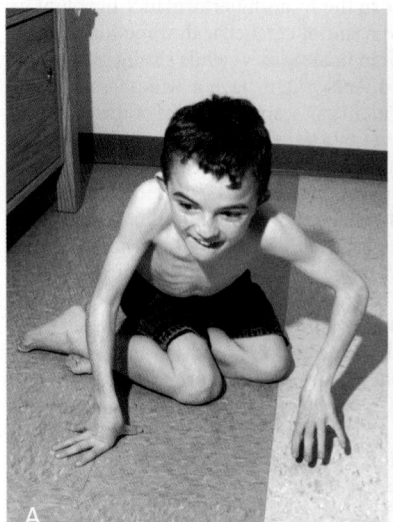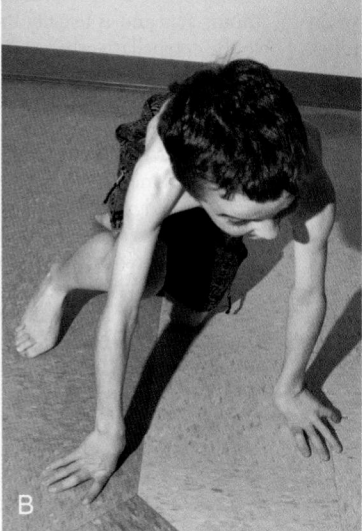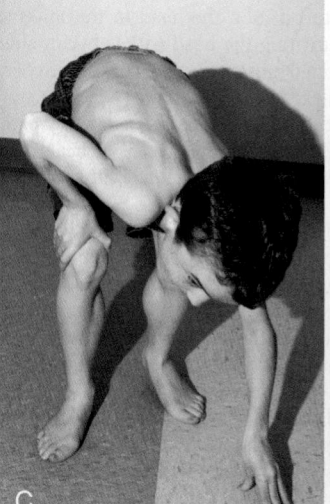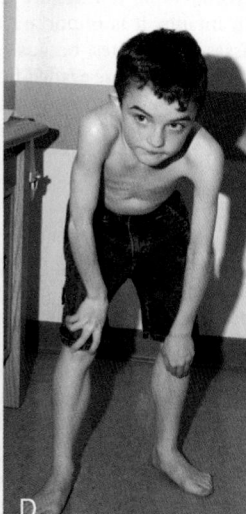

Figure 590-5 A-D, Gowers sign in a boy with hip girdle weakness because of Duchenne muscular dystrophy. When asked to rise from a prone position, the patient uses his hands to walk up his legs to compensate for proximal lower-extremity weakness.

Table 590-2	Timing of Selected Primitive Reflexes		
REFLEX	**ONSET**	**FULLY DEVELOPED**	**DURATION**
Palmar grasp	28 wk gestation	32 wk gestation	2-3 mo postnatal
Rooting	32 wk gestation	36 wk gestation	Less prominent after 1 mo postnatal
Moro	28-32 wk gestation	37 wk gestation	5-6 mo postnatal
Tonic neck	35 wk gestation	1 mo postnatal	6-7 mo postnatal
Parachute	7-8 mo postnatal	10-11 mo postnatal	Remains throughout life

to be an exception, as it is thought to be mediated by cerebellothalamocortical pathways. Further detail on the individual movement disorders is provided in Chapter 597.

Sensory Examination

The sensory examination is difficult to perform on an infant or uncooperative child and has a relatively low yield in terms of the information that it provides. A gross assessment of sensory function can be achieved by distracting the patient with an interesting toy and then touching the patient with a cotton swab in different locations. Normal infants and children indicate an awareness of the stimulus by crying, withdrawing the extremity, or pausing briefly; however, with repeated testing, they lose interest in the stimulus and begin to ignore the examiner. It is critical, therefore, that any areas of concern are tested efficiently and, if necessary, reexamined at an appropriate time.

Fortunately, isolated disorders of the sensory system are less common in the very young pediatric population than in the adult population, so detailed sensory testing is rarely warranted. Furthermore, most patients who are old enough to voice a sensory complaint are also old enough to cooperate with formal testing of light touch, pain, temperature, vibration, proprioception, and corticosensation (e.g., stereognosis, 2-point discrimination, extinction to double simultaneous stimulation). A notable exception is when the physician suspects a spinal cord lesion in an infant or young child and needs to identify a sensory level. In such situations, observation might suggest a difference in color, temperature, or perspiration, with the skin cool and dry below the level of injury. Lightly touching the skin above the level can evoke a squirming movement or physical withdrawal. Other signs of spinal cord injury include decreased anal sphincter tone and strength and absence of the superficial abdominal, anal wink, and cremasteric reflexes.

Reflexes
Deep Tendon Reflexes and the Plantar Response

Deep tendon reflexes are readily elicited in most infants and children. In infants, it is important to position the head in the midline when assessing reflexes, because turning the head to 1 side can alter reflex tone. Reflexes are graded from 0 (absent) to 4+ (markedly hyperactive), with 2+ being normal. Reflexes that are 1+ or 3+ can be normal as long as they are symmetrical. Sustained clonus is always pathologic, but infants younger than 3 mo old can have 5-10 beats of clonus, and older children can have 1-2 beats of clonus, provided that it is symmetrical.

The ankle jerk is hardest to elicit, but it can usually be obtained by passively dorsiflexing the foot and then tapping on either the Achilles tendon or the ball of the foot. The knee jerk is evoked by tapping the patellar tendon. If this reflex is exaggerated, extension of the knee may be accompanied by contraction of the contralateral adductors (**crossed adductor response**). Hypoactive reflexes reflect lower motor neuron or cerebellar dysfunction, whereas hyperactive reflexes are consistent with upper motor neuron disease. The plantar response is obtained by stimulation of the lateral aspect of the sole of the foot, beginning at the heel and extending to the base of the toes. The **Babinski sign,** indicating an upper motor neuron lesion, is characterized by extension of the great toe and fanning of the remaining toes. Too vigorous stimulation may produce withdrawal, which may be misinterpreted as a Babinski sign. Plantar responses have limited diagnostic utility in neonates,

because they are mediated by several competing reflexes and can be either flexor or extensor, depending on how the foot is positioned. Asymmetry of the reflexes or plantar response is a useful lateralizing sign in infants and children.

Primitive Reflexes

Primitive reflexes appear and disappear at specific times during development (Table 590-2), and their absence or persistence beyond those times signifies CNS dysfunction. Although many primitive reflexes have been described, the Moro, grasp, tonic neck, and parachute reflexes are the most clinically relevant. The **Moro reflex** is elicited by supporting the infant in a semierect position and then allowing the infant's head to fall backwards onto the examiner's hand. A normal response consists of symmetric extension and abduction of the fingers and upper extremities, followed by flexion of the upper extremities and an audible cry. An asymmetric response can signify a fractured clavicle, brachial plexus injury, or hemiparesis. Absence of the Moro reflex in a term newborn is ominous, suggesting significant dysfunction of the CNS. The **grasp response** is elicited by placing a finger in the open palm of each hand; by 37 wk of gestation, the reflex is strong enough that the examiner can lift the infant from the bed with gentle traction. The **tonic neck reflex** is produced by manually rotating the infant's head to 1 side and observing for the characteristic fencing posture (extension of the arm on the side to which the face is rotated and flexion of the contralateral arm). An obligatory tonic neck response, in which the infant becomes "stuck" in the fencing posture, is always abnormal and implies a CNS disorder. The **parachute reflex**, which occurs in slightly older infants, can be evoked by holding the infant's trunk and then suddenly lowering the infant as if he or she were falling. The arms will spontaneously extend to break the infant's fall, making this reflex a prerequisite to walking.

Coordination

Ataxia refers to a disturbance in the smooth performance of voluntary motor acts and is usually the result of cerebellar dysfunction. Lesions to the cerebellar vermis result in unsteadiness while sitting or standing (**truncal ataxia**). Affected patients might have a wide-based gait or may be unable to perform tandem gait testing. Lesions of the cerebellar hemispheres cause appendicular ataxia, which may be apparent as the patient reaches for objects and performs finger-to-nose and heel-to-shin movements. Other features of cerebellar dysfunction include errors in judging distance (**dysmetria**), inability to inhibit a muscular action (**rebound**), impaired performance of rapid alternating movements (**dysdiadochokinesia**), intention tremor, nystagmus, scanning dysarthria, hypotonia, and decreased deep tendon reflexes. Acute ataxia suggests an infectious or postinfectious, endocrinologic, toxic, traumatic, vascular, or psychogenic process, and chronic symptoms suggest a metabolic, neoplastic, or degenerative process.

Station and Gait

Observation of a child's station and gait is an important aspect of the neurologic examination. Normal children can stand with their feet close together without swaying; however, children who are unsteady may sway or even fall. On gait testing, the heels should strike either side of an imaginary line, but children with poor balance tend to walk with their legs farther apart to create a more stable base. Tandem gait testing forces patients to have a narrow base, which highlights subtle balance difficulties.

There are a variety of abnormal gaits, many of which are associated with a specific underlying etiology. Patients with a **spastic** gait appear stiff-legged like a soldier. They may walk on tiptoe as a result of tightness or contractures of the Achilles tendons, and their legs may scissor as they walk. A **hemiparetic** gait is associated with spasticity and circumduction of the leg, as well as decreased arm swing on the affected side. **Cerebellar ataxia** results in a wide-based, reeling gait like a drunk person, whereas **sensory ataxia** results in a wide-based **steppage gait,** in which the patient lifts the legs up higher than usual in the swing phase and then slaps the foot down. A **myopathic,** or waddling, gait is associated with hip girdle weakness. Affected children often develop a compensatory lordosis and have other signs of proximal muscle weakness, such as difficulty climbing stairs. During gait testing, the examiner might also note hypotonia or weakness of the lower extremities; extrapyramidal movements, such as dystonia or chorea; or orthopedic deformities, such as pelvic tilt, genu recurvatum, varus or valgus deformities of the knee, pes cavus (high arches) or pes planus (flat feet), and scoliosis.

GENERAL EXAMINATION

Examination of other organ systems is essential because myriad systemic diseases affect the nervous system. Dysmorphic features can indicate a genetic syndrome (see Chapter 108). Heart murmurs may be associated with rheumatic fever (Sydenham chorea), cardiac rhabdomyoma (tuberous sclerosis), cyanotic heart disease (cerebral abscess or thrombosis), and endocarditis (cerebral vascular occlusion). Hepatosplenomegaly can suggest an inborn error of metabolism, storage disease, HIV, or malignancy. Cutaneous lesions may be a feature of a neurocutaneous syndrome (see Chapter 596).

SPECIAL DIAGNOSTIC PROCEDURES
Lumbar Puncture and Cerebrospinal Fluid Examination

Examination of the cerebrospinal fluid (CSF) and measurement of the pressure it creates in the subarachnoid space are essential in confirming the diagnosis of meningitis, encephalitis, and idiopathic intracranial hypertension (previously referred to as pseudotumor cerebri), and it is often helpful in assessing subarachnoid hemorrhage; demyelinating, degenerative, and collagen vascular diseases; and intracranial neoplasms. Having an experienced assistant who can position, restrain, and comfort the patient is critical to the success of the procedure.

The patient should be situated in a lateral decubitus or seated position with the neck and legs flexed to enlarge the intervertebral spaces. As a rule, sick neonates should be maintained in a seated position to prevent problems with ventilation and perfusion. Regardless of the position chosen, it is important to make sure that the patient's shoulders and hips are straight to prevent rotating the spine.

Once the patient is situated, the physician identifies the appropriate interspace by drawing an imaginary line from the iliac crest downward perpendicular to the vertebral column. In adults, lumbar punctures are usually performed in the L3-L4 or L4-L5 interspaces. Next, the physician dons a mask, gown, and sterile gloves. The skin is thoroughly prepared with a cleansing agent, and sterile drapes are applied. The skin and underlying tissues are anesthetized by injecting a local anesthetic (e.g., 1% lidocaine) at the time of the procedure or by applying a eutectic mixture of lidocaine and prilocaine (EMLA) to the skin 30 minutes before the procedure. A 22-gauge, 1.5-3.0 in, sharp, beveled spinal needle with a properly fitting stylet is introduced in the midsagittal plane and directed slightly cephalad. The physician should pause frequently, remove the stylet, and assess for CSF flow. Although a pop can occur as the needle penetrates the dura, it is more common to experience a subtle change in resistance.

Once CSF has been detected, a manometer and 3-way stopcock can be attached to the spinal needle to obtain an opening pressure. If the patient was seated as the spinal needle was introduced, the patient should be moved carefully to a **lateral decubitus position** with the head and legs extended before the manometer is attached. Normal opening pressures are 90-120 mm H_2O in newborns, 60-180 mm H_2O in young children, and 12-120 mm H_2O in older children and adults. The 90th percentile in children has been reported to be 250 mm of H_2O. The most common cause of an elevated opening pressure is an agitated patient. Sedation and high body mass index can also increase the opening pressure.

Contraindications to performing a lumbar puncture include suspected mass lesion of the brain, especially in the posterior fossa or above the tentorium and causing shift of the midline; suspected mass lesion of the spinal cord; symptoms and signs of impending cerebral herniation in a child with probable meningitis; critical illness (on rare occasions); skin infection at the site of the lumbar puncture; and thrombocytopenia with a platelet count $<20 \times 10^9/L$. If disc edema or focal findings suggest a mass lesion, a head CT should be obtained before proceeding with lumbar puncture to prevent uncal or cerebellar herniation as the CSF is removed. In the absence of these findings, routine head imaging is not warranted. The physician should also be alert to clinical signs of impending herniation, including alterations in the respiratory pattern (e.g., hyperventilation; Cheyne-Stokes respirations, ataxic respirations, respiratory arrest), abnormalities of pupil size and reactivity, loss of brainstem reflexes, and decorticate or decerebrate posturing. If any of these signs are present or the child is so ill that the lumbar puncture might induce cardiorespiratory arrest, blood cultures should be drawn and supportive care, including antibiotics, should be initiated. Once the patient has stabilized, it may be possible to perform a lumbar puncture safely.

Normal CSF contains up to 5/mm³ white blood cells, and a newborn can have as many as 15/mm³. Polymorphonuclear cells are always abnormal in a child, but 1-2/mm³ may be present in a normal neonate. An elevated polymorphonuclear count suggests bacterial meningitis or the early phase of aseptic meningitis (see Chapter 603). CSF lymphocytosis can be seen in aseptic, tuberculous, or fungal meningitis; demyelinating diseases; brain or spinal cord tumor; immunologic disorders, including collagen vascular diseases; and chemical irritation (following myelogram, intrathecal methotrexate).

Normal CSF contains no red blood cells; thus, their presence indicates a traumatic tap or a subarachnoid hemorrhage. Progressive clearing of the blood between the first and last samples indicates a traumatic tap. Bloody CSF should be centrifuged immediately. A clear supernatant is consistent with a bloody tap, whereas **xanthochromia** (yellow color that results from the degradation of hemoglobin) suggests a subarachnoid hemorrhage. Xanthochromia may be absent in bleeds <12 hr old, particularly when laboratories rely on visual inspection rather than spectroscopy. Xanthochromia can also occur in the setting of hyperbilirubinemia, carotenemia, and markedly elevated CSF protein.

The normal CSF protein is 10-40 mg/dL in a child and as high as 120 mg/dL in a neonate. The CSF protein falls to the normal childhood range by 3 mo of age. The CSF protein may be elevated in many processes, including infectious, immunologic, vascular, and degenerative diseases, blockage of CSF flow, as well as tumors of the brain (primary CNS tumors, systemic tumors metastatic to the CNS, infiltrative acute lymphoblastic leukemia) and spinal cord. With a traumatic tap, the CSF protein is increased by approximately 1 mg/dL for every 1,000 red blood cells/mm³. Elevation of CSF immunoglobulin G, which normally represents approximately 10% of the total protein, is observed in subacute sclerosing panencephalitis, in postinfectious encephalomyelitis, and in some cases of multiple sclerosis. If the diagnosis of multiple sclerosis is suspected, the CSF should be tested for the presence of oligoclonal bands.

The CSF glucose content is approximately 60% of the blood glucose in a healthy child. To prevent a spuriously elevated blood:CSF glucose ratio in a case of suspected meningitis, it is advisable to collect the blood glucose before the lumbar puncture when the child is relatively calm. Hypoglycorrhachia is found in association with diffuse meningeal disease, particularly bacterial and tubercular meningitis. Widespread neoplastic involvement of the meninges, subarachnoid hemorrhage, disorders involving the glucose transporter protein type 1, fungal meningitis, and, occasionally, aseptic meningitis can produce low CSF glucose as well.

A Gram stain of the CSF is essential if there is a suspicion for bacterial meningitis; an acid-fast stain and India ink preparation can be used to assess for tuberculous and fungal meningitis, respectively. CSF is then plated on different culture media depending on the suspected pathogen. When indicated by the clinical presentation, it can also be helpful to assess for the presence of specific antigens (e.g., latex agglutination for *Neisseria meningitidis*, *Haemophilus influenzae* type b, or *Streptococcus pneumoniae*) or to obtain antibody or polymerase chain reaction studies (e.g., herpes simplex virus-1 and -2, West Nile virus, enteroviruses). In noninfectious cases, levels of CSF metabolites, such as lactate, amino acids, and enolase, can provide clues to the underlying metabolic disease.

Neuroradiologic Procedures

Skull roentgenograms have limited diagnostic utility. They can demonstrate fractures, bony defects, intracranial calcifications, or indirect evidence of increased ICP. Acutely increased ICP causes separation of the sutures, whereas chronically increased ICP is associated with erosion of the posterior clinoid processes, enlargement of the sella turcica, and increased convolutional markings.

Cranial ultrasonography is the imaging method of choice for detecting intracranial hemorrhage, periventricular leukomalacia, and hydrocephalus in infants with patent anterior fontanels. Ultrasound is less sensitive than either CT or MRI for detecting hypoxic–ischemic injury, but the use of color Doppler or power Doppler sonography, both of which show changes in regional cerebral blood flow, improve its sensitivity. In general, ultrasound is not a useful technique in older children, although it can be helpful intraoperatively when placing shunts, locating small tumors, and performing needle biopsies.

CT is a valuable diagnostic tool in the evaluation of many neurologic emergencies, as well as some nonemergent conditions. It is a noninvasive, rapid procedure that can usually be performed without sedation. CT scans use conventional x-ray techniques, meaning that they produce ionizing radiation. Because children younger than 10 yr of age are several times more sensitive to radiation than adults, it is important to consider the whether imaging is actually indicated and, if it is, whether an ultrasound or MRI might be the more appropriate study. In the emergency setting, a noncontrast CT scan can demonstrate skull fractures, pneumocephalus, intracranial hemorrhages, hydrocephalus, and impending herniation. If the noncontrast scan reveals an abnormality and an MRI cannot be performed in a timely fashion, nonionic contrast should be used to highlight areas of breakdown in the blood–brain barrier (e.g., abscesses, tumors) and/or collections of abnormal blood vessels (e.g., arteriovenous malformations). CT is less useful for diagnosing acute infarcts in children, because radiographic changes might not be apparent for up to 24 hr. Some subtle signs of early (<24 hr) infarction include sulcal effacement, blurring of the gray-white junction, and the hyperdense middle cerebral artery sign (increased attenuation in the middle cerebral artery that is often associated with thrombosis). In the routine setting, CT imaging can be used to demonstrate intracranial calcifications or, with the addition of 3-dimensional reformatting, to evaluate patients with craniofacial abnormalities or craniosynostosis. Although other pathologic processes may be visible on CT scan, *MR is generally preferred because it provides a more-detailed view of the anatomy without exposure to ionizing radiation* (Table 590-3).

CT angiography is a useful tool for visualizing vascular structures and is accomplished by administering a tight bolus of iodinated contrast through a large-bore intravenous catheter and then acquiring CT images as the contrast passes through the arteries.

MRI is a noninvasive procedure that is well suited for detecting a variety of abnormalities, including those of the posterior fossa and spinal cord. MR scans are highly susceptible to patient motion artifact; consequently, many children younger than age 8 yr require sedation to ensure an adequate study. (The need for sedation is beginning to change in some centers as MRI technology improves and allows for faster performance of studies.) Because the American Academy of Pediatrics recommends that infants be kept nothing by mouth (NPO) for 4 hr or longer and older children for 6 hr or longer before deep sedation, it is often difficult to obtain an MRI on an infant or young

child in the acute setting. MRI can be used to evaluate for congenital or acquired brain lesions, migrational defects, dysmyelination or demyelination, posttraumatic gliosis, neoplasms, cerebral edema, and acute stroke (see Table 590-3). Paramagnetic MR contrast agents (e.g., gadolinium-diethylenetriaminepentaacetic acid [DTPA]) are efficacious in identifying areas of disruption in the blood–brain barrier, such as those occurring in primary and metastatic brain tumors, meningitis, cerebritis, abscesses, and active demyelination. **MR angiography** and **MR venography** provide detailed images of major intracranial vasculature structures and assist in the diagnosis of conditions such as stroke, vascular malformations, and cerebral venous sinus thrombosis. MR angiography is the procedure of choice for infants and young children owing to the lack of ionizing radiation and contrast; however, CT angiography may be preferable in older children because it is faster and can eliminate the need for sedation; it is particularly useful for looking at blood vessels in the neck, where there is less interference from bone artifact than in the skull-encased brain.

Functional MRI is a noninvasive technique used to map neuronal activity during specific cognitive states and/or sensorimotor functions. Data are usually based on blood oxygenation, although they can also be based on local cerebral blood volume or flow. Functional MRI is useful for presurgical localization of critical brain functions and has several advantages over other functional imaging techniques. Specifically, functional MRI produces high-resolution images without exposure to ionizing radiation or contrast, and it allows coregistration of functional and structural images.

Proton MR spectroscopy (MRS) is a molecular imaging technique in which the unique neurochemical profile of a preselected brain region is displayed in the form of a spectrum. Many metabolites can be detected, the most common of which are *N*-acetylaspartate, creatine and phosphocreatine, choline, myoinositol, and lactate. Changes in the spectral pattern of a given area can yield clues to the underlying pathology, making MRS useful in the diagnosis of inborn errors of metabolism, as well as the preoperative and posttherapeutic assessment of intracranial tumors. MRS can also detect areas of cortical dysplasia in patients with epilepsy, because these patients have low *N*-acetylaspartate:creatine ratios. Finally, MRS may be useful in detecting hypoxic–ischemic injury in newborns in the 1st day of life, because the lactate peak enlarges and the *N*-acetylaspartate peak diminishes before MRI sequences become abnormal.

Catheter angiography is the gold standard for diagnosing vascular disorders of the CNS, such as arteriovenous malformations, aneurysms, arterial occlusions, and vasculitis. A 4-vessel study is accomplished by introducing a catheter into the femoral artery and then injecting contrast media into each of the internal carotid and vertebral arteries. Because catheter angiography is invasive and requires general anesthesia, it is typically reserved for treatment planning of endovascular or open procedures and for cases in which noninvasive imaging results are not diagnostic.

Positron emission tomography provides unique information on brain metabolism and perfusion by measuring blood flow, oxygen uptake, and/or glucose consumption. Positron emission tomography is an expensive technique that is gaining a following in some pediatric centers, particularly those with active epilepsy surgery programs. **Single-photon emission CT** using ^{99m}Tc hexamethylpropyleneamine oxime is a sensitive and inexpensive technique to study regional cerebral blood flow. Single-photon emission CT is particularly useful in assessing for vasculitis, herpes encephalitis, dysplastic cortex, and recurrent brain tumors. Positron emission tomography MRI is only available in a few pediatric centers in the United States; it provides better resolution and tissue definition than single-photon emission CT.

Electroencephalography

An electroencephalogram (EEG) provides a continuous recording of electrical activity between reference electrodes placed on the scalp. Although the genesis of the electrical activity is not certain, it likely originates from postsynaptic potentials in the dendrites of cortical neurons. Even with amplification of the electrical activity, not all potentials are recorded because there is a buffering effect of the scalp, muscles, bone, vessels, and subarachnoid fluid. EEG waves are

Table 590-3	Preferred Imaging Procedures in Neurologic Diseases

ISCHEMIC INFARCTION OR TRANSIENT ISCHEMIC ATTACK
CT/CTA (head and neck) ± CT perfusion for patients who are unstable or are potential candidates for tissue plasminogen activator or other acute interventions
Otherwise, MRI/MRA (head and neck) with and without gadolinium and with diffusion-weighted images
If the examination findings localize to the anterior circulation, carotid ultrasound should be performed rather than neck CTA or MRA
Obtain an MRV if the infarct does not follow an arterial distribution
CT or MRI can detect infarcts more than 24 hr old, although MRI is generally preferred to avoid exposure to ionizing radiation

INTRAPARENCHYMAL HEMORRHAGE
CT if <24 hr; MRI if >24 hr
MRI and MRA to assess for underlying vascular malformation, tumor, etc.
Catheter angiography if MRA is nondiagnostic

ARTERIOVENOUS MALFORMATION
CT for acute hemorrhage; MRI and MRA with and without gadolinium as early as possible
Catheter angiography if noninvasive imaging is nondiagnostic

CEREBRAL ANEURYSM
CT without contrast for acute subarachnoid hemorrhage
MRA or CTA to identify the aneurysm
Catheter angiography may be necessary in some cases
TCD to detect vasospasm

HYPOXIC–ISCHEMIC BRAIN INJURY
Ultrasound in infants
If ultrasound is negative or there is a discrepancy between the clinical course and the sonogram, obtain an MRI
In older children, CT if unstable; otherwise, MRI
MRS can show a lactate peak even in the absence of structural abnormalities and can be useful for prognostication purposes

METABOLIC DISORDERS
MRI, particularly T2-weighted and FLAIR images
Diffusion-weighted images may be useful in distinguishing acute and chronic changes
MRS, SPECT, and PET may be useful in certain disorders

HYDROCEPHALUS
Ultrasound (in infants), CT with and without contrast, or MR with and without gadolinium for diagnosis of communicating hydrocephalus
MR with and without gadolinium for diagnosis of noncommunicating hydrocephalus
Ultrasound (in infants) or CT to follow ventricular size in response to treatment

HEADACHE
CT with and without contrast or MRI with and without gadolinium if a structural disorder is suspected (MRI is preferred in nonemergent situations as it does not involve ionizing radiation and provides a better view of the parenchyma)

HEAD TRAUMA
CT without contrast initially
MRI after initial assessment and treatment if clinically indicated. Diffusion tensor imaging and/or diffusion kurtosis sequences may be useful to detect subtle white matter abnormalities

EPILEPSY
MRI with and without gadolinium. Thin slices through the mesial temporal lobes may be helpful if a temporal focus is suspected
PET
Interictal SPECT

BRAIN TUMOR
MRI with and without gadolinium
MRS
PET

MULTIPLE SCLEROSIS
MRI with and without gadolinium
Obtain sagittal FLAIR images

MENINGITIS OR ENCEPHALITIS
CT without and with contrast before lumbar puncture if there are signs of increased ICP on examination
MRI with and without gadolinium after initial assessment and treatment for patients with complicated meningitis or encephalitis

BRAIN ABSCESS
MRI with and without gadolinium
Diffusion-weighted images and MRS can help to differentiate abscess from necrotic tumor
If the patient is unstable, CT with and without contrast followed by MRI with and without contrast when feasible

MOVEMENT DISORDERS
MRI with and without gadolinium
PET
DaTscan (SPECT scan using ioflupane iodine-123 as the contrast agent for detecting dopamine transporters in suspected parkinsonian syndromes)

CTA, computed tomographic angiography; FLAIR, fluid-attenuated inversion recovery; ICP, intracranial pressure; MRA, magnetic resonance angiography; MRS, magnetic resonance spectroscopy; MRV, magnetic resonance venography; PET, positron emission tomography; SPECT, single-photon emission computed tomography; TCD, transcranial Doppler ultrasonography.

---

classified according to their frequency as delta (1-3/sec), theta (4-7/sec), alpha (8-12/sec), and beta (13-20/sec). These waves are altered by many factors, including age, level of alertness, eye closure, drugs, and disease states.

The normal waking EEG is characterized by the posterior dominant rhythm—a sinusoidal, 8-12 Hz rhythm that is most prominent over the occipital region in a state of relaxed wakefulness with the eyes closed. This rhythm first becomes apparent at 3-4 mo old, and most children have achieved the adult frequency of 8-12 Hz by age 8 yr.

Normal sleep is divided into 3 stages of non–rapid eye movement sleep—designated N1, N2, and N3—and rapid eye movement sleep. N1 corresponds to drowsiness, and N3 represents deep, restorative, slow-wave sleep. Rapid eye movement sleep is rarely captured during a routine EEG but may be seen on an overnight recording. The American Electroencephalography Society Guideline and Technical Standards states that "sleep recordings should be obtained whenever possible"; however, it appears that sleep deprivation—not sleep during the EEG—is what increases the yield of the study, particularly in children with 1 or more clinically diagnosed seizures and in children older than 3 yr of age.

EEG abnormalities can be divided into 2 general categories: epileptiform discharges and slowing. Epileptiform discharges are paroxysmal spikes or sharp waves, often followed by slow waves, which interrupt the background activity. They may be focal, multifocal, or generalized. Focal discharges are often associated with cerebral dysgenesis or irritative lesions, such as cysts, slow-growing tumors, or glial scar tissue; generalized discharges typically occur in children with structurally normal brains. Generalized discharges can occur as an epilepsy trait in children who have never had a seizure and, by themselves, are not an indication for treatment. Epileptiform activity may be enhanced by activation procedures, including hyperventilation and photic stimulation.

As with epileptiform discharges, slowing can be either focal or diffuse. Focal slowing should raise a concern for an underlying functional or structural abnormality, such as an infarct, hematoma, or tumor. Diffuse slowing is the hallmark of encephalopathy and is usually secondary to a widespread disease process or toxic–metabolic insult.

Long-term video EEG monitoring provides precise characterization of seizure types, which allows specific medical or surgical management. It facilitates more accurate differentiation of epileptic seizures from paroxysmal events that mimic epilepsy, including psychogenic nonepileptiform attacks. Long-term EEG monitoring can also be useful during medication adjustments.

Evoked Potentials

An evoked potential is an electrical signal recorded from the CNS following the presentation of a specific visual, auditory, or sensory stimulus. Stimulation of the visual system by a flash or patterned stimulus, such as a black-and-white checkerboard, produces **visual evoked potentials** (VEPs), which are recorded over the occiput and averaged in a computer. Abnormal VEPs can result from lesions to the visual pathway anywhere from the retina to the visual cortex. Many demyelinating disorders and neurodegenerative diseases, such as Tay-Sachs, Krabbe, or Pelizaeus-Merzbacher disease, or neuronal ceroid lipofuscinoses, show characteristic VEP abnormalities. Flash VEPs can also be helpful in evaluating infants who have sustained an anoxic injury; however, detection of an evoked potential does not necessarily mean that the infant will have functional vision.

Brainstem auditory evoked responses (BAERs) provide an objective measure of hearing and are particularly useful in neonates and in children who have failed, or are uncooperative with, audiometric testing. BAERs are abnormal in many neurodegenerative diseases of childhood and are an important tool in evaluating patients with suspected tumors of the cerebellopontine angle. BAERs can be helpful in assessing brainstem function in comatose patients, because the waveforms are unaffected by drugs or by the level of consciousness; however, they are not accurate in predicting neurologic recovery and outcome.

Somatosensory evoked potentials (SSEPs) are obtained by stimulating a peripheral nerve (peroneal, median) and then recording the electrical response over the cervical region and contralateral parietal somatosensory cortex. SSEPs determine the functional integrity of the dorsal column–medial lemniscal system and are useful in monitoring spinal cord function during operative procedures for scoliosis, aortic coarctation, and myelomeningocele repair. SSEPs are abnormal in many neurodegenerative disorders and are the most accurate evoked potential in the assessment of neurologic outcome following a severe CNS insult.

Bibliography is available at Expert Consult.

Chapter **591**
Congenital Anomalies of the Central Nervous System

*Stephen L. Kinsman and
Michael V. Johnston*

Central nervous system (CNS) malformations are grouped into neural tube defects and associated spinal cord malformations; encephaloceles; disorders of structure specification (gray matter structures, neuronal migration disorders, disorders of connectivity, and commissure and tract formation); disorders of the posterior fossa, brainstem, and cerebellum; disorders of brain growth and size; and disorders of skull growth and shape. Classification of these conditions into syndromic, nonsyndromic, and single-gene etiologies is also important. These disorders can also be seen as isolated findings or as being a consequence of environmental exposures. Elucidation of single-gene causes has out-

paced our understanding of the epigenetic and environmental mechanisms causing these malformations.

These disorders are heterogeneous in their presentation. Common presentations and clinical problems include disorders of head size and/or shape; hydrocephalus; fetal ultrasonographic brain abnormalities; neonatal encephalopathy and seizures; developmental delay, cognitive impairment, and intellectual disability; hypotonia, motor impairment, and cerebral palsy; seizures, epilepsy, and drug-resistant epilepsy; cranial nerve dysfunction; and spinal cord dysfunction.

Bibliography is available at Expert Consult.

591.1 Neural Tube Defects
Stephen L. Kinsman and Michael V. Johnston

Neural tube defects (NTDs) account for the largest proportion of congenital anomalies of the CNS and result from failure of the neural tube to close spontaneously between the 3rd and 4th wk of in utero development. Although the precise cause of NTDs remains unknown, evidence suggests that many factors, including hyperthermia, drugs (valproic acid), malnutrition, low red cell folate levels, chemicals, maternal obesity or diabetes, and genetic determinants (mutations in folate-responsive or folate-dependent enzyme pathways) can adversely affect normal development of the CNS from the time of conception. In some cases, an abnormal maternal nutritional state or exposure to radiation before conception increases the likelihood of a congenital CNS malformation. The major NTDs include spina bifida occulta, meningocele, myelomeningocele, encephalocele, anencephaly, caudal regression syndrome, dermal sinus, tethered cord, syringomyelia, diastematomyelia, and lipoma involving the conus medullaris and/or filum terminale and the rare condition iniencephaly.

The human nervous system originates from the primitive ectoderm that also develops into the epidermis. The ectoderm, endoderm, and mesoderm form the three primary germ layers that are developed by the 3rd wk. The endoderm, particularly the notochordal plate and the intraembryonic mesoderm, induces the overlying ectoderm to develop the neural plate in the 3rd wk of development (Fig. 591-1A). Failure of normal induction is responsible for most of the NTDs, as well as disorders of prosencephalic development. Rapid growth of cells within the neural plate causes further invagination of the neural groove and differentiation of a conglomerate of cells, the neural crest, which migrate laterally on the surface of the neural tube (Fig. 591-1B). The notochordal plate becomes the centrally placed notochord, which acts as a foundation around which the vertebral column ultimately develops. With formation of the vertebral column, the notochord undergoes involution and becomes the nucleus pulposus of the intervertebral disks. The neural crest cells differentiate to form the peripheral nervous system, including the spinal and autonomic ganglia and the ganglia of cranial nerves V, VII, VIII, IX, and X. In addition, the neural crest forms the leptomeninges, as well as Schwann cells, which are responsible for myelination of the peripheral nervous system. The dura is thought to arise from the paraxial mesoderm. In the region of the embryo destined to become the head, similar patterns exist. In this region, the notochord is replaced by the prechordal mesoderm.

In the 3rd wk of embryonic development, invagination of the neural groove is completed and the neural tube is formed by separation from the overlying surface ectoderm (see Fig. 591-1C). Initial closure of the neural tube is accomplished in the area corresponding to the future junction of the spinal cord and medulla and moves rapidly both caudally and rostrally. For a brief period, the neural tube is open at both ends, and the neural canal communicates freely with the amniotic cavity (see Fig. 591-1D). Failure of closure of the neural tube allows excretion of fetal substances (α-fetoprotein [AFP], acetylcholinesterase) into the amniotic fluid, serving as biochemical markers for a NTD. Prenatal screening of maternal serum for AFP in the 16th-18th wk of gestation is an effective method for identifying pregnancies at risk for fetuses with NTDs in utero. Normally, the rostral end of the neural tube closes on the 23rd day and the caudal neuropore closes by a process of secondary neurulation by the 27th day of development, before the time that many women realize they are pregnant.

The embryonic neural tube consists of 3 zones: ventricular, mantle, and marginal (see Fig. 591-1*E*). The ependymal layer consists of pluripotential, pseudostratified, columnar neuroepithelial cells. Specific neuroepithelial cells differentiate into primitive neurons or neuroblasts that form the mantle layer. The marginal zone is formed from cells in the outer layer of the neuroepithelium, which ultimately becomes the white matter. Glioblasts, which act as the primitive supportive cells of the CNS, also arise from the neuroepithelial cells in the ependymal zone. They migrate to the mantle and marginal zones and become future astrocytes and oligodendrocytes. The importance of other pathways of progenitor cell generation and migration are also being elucidated. It is likely that microglia originate from mesenchymal cells at a later stage of fetal development when blood vessels begin to penetrate the developing nervous system.

591.2 Spina Bifida Occulta (Occult Spinal Dysraphism)

Stephen L. Kinsman and Michael V. Johnston

Spina bifida occulta is a common anomaly consisting of a midline defect of the vertebral bodies without protrusion of the spinal cord or meninges. Most patients are asymptomatic and lack neurologic signs, and the condition is usually of no consequence. Some consider the term *spina bifida occulta* to denote merely a posterior vertebral body fusion defect. This simple defect does not have an associated spinal cord malformation. Other clinically more significant forms of this closed spinal cord malformation are more correctly termed *occult spinal dysraphism*. In most of these cases, there are cutaneous manifestations such as a hemangioma, discoloration of the skin, pit, lump, dermal sinus, or hairy patch (Fig. 591-2). A spine roentgenogram in simple spina bifida occulta shows a defect in closure of the posterior vertebral arches and laminae, typically involving L5 and S1; there is no abnormality of the meninges, spinal cord, or nerve roots. Occult spinal dysraphism is often associated with more significant developmental abnormalities of the spinal cord, including syringomyelia, diastematomyelia, lipoma, fatty filum, dermal sinus, and/or a tethered cord. A spine x-ray in these cases might show bone defects or may be normal. All cases of occult spinal dysraphism are best investigated with MRI (Fig. 591-3). Initial screening in the neonate may include ultrasonography, but MRI is more accurate at any age.

A dermoid sinus usually forms a small skin opening, which leads into a narrow duct, sometimes indicated by protruding hairs, a hairy patch, or a vascular nevus. Dermoid sinuses occur in the midline at the sites where meningoceles or encephaloceles can occur: the lumbosacral region or occiput, respectively and occasionally in the cervical or thoracic area. Dermoid sinus tracts can pass through the dura, acting as a conduit for the spread of infection. Recurrent meningitis of occult origin should prompt careful examination for a small sinus tract in the posterior midline region, including the back of the head. Lower back sinuses are usually above the gluteal fold and are directed cephalad. Tethered spinal cord syndrome may also be an associated problem. Diastematomyelia commonly has bony abnormalities that require surgical intervention along with untethering of the spinal cord.

An approach to imaging of the spine in patients with cutaneous lesions is noted in Table 591-1.

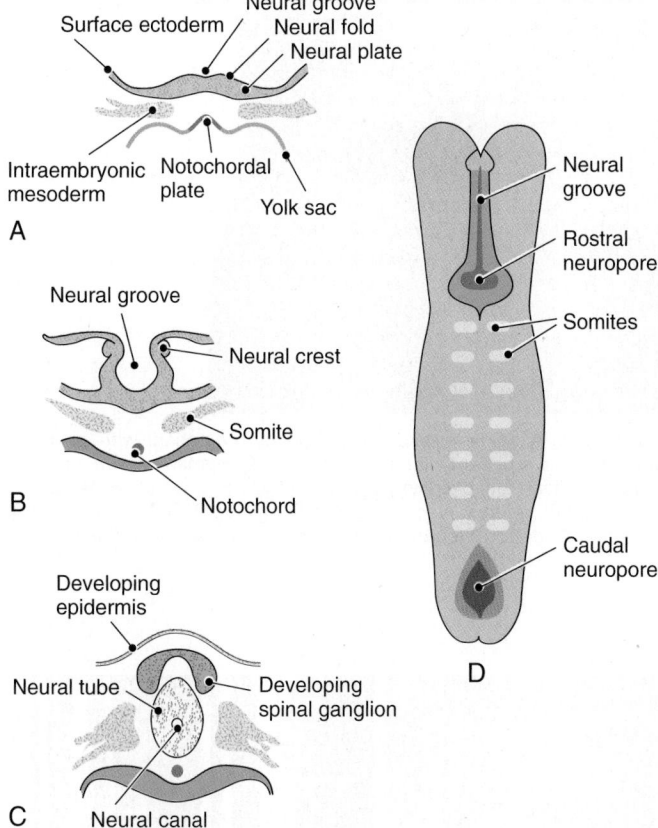

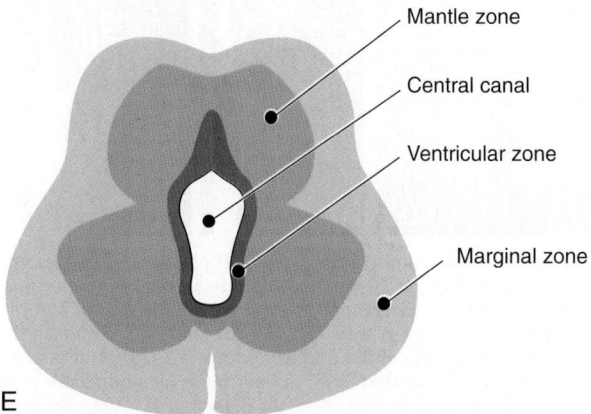

Figure 591-1 Diagrammatic illustration of the developing nervous system. **A,** Transverse sections of the neural plate during the 3rd wk. **B,** Formation of the neural groove and the neural crest. **C,** The neural tube is developed. **D,** Longitudinal drawing showing the initial closure of the neural tube in the central region. **E,** Cross-sectional drawing of the embryonic neural tube (primitive spinal cord).

Table 591-1	Cutaneous Lesions Associated with Occult Spinal Dysraphism

IMAGING INDICATED
Subcutaneous mass or lipoma
Hairy patch
Dermal sinus
Atypical dimples (deep, >5 mm, >25 mm from anal verge)
Vascular lesion, e.g., hemangioma or telangiectasia
Skin appendages or polypoid lesions, e.g., skin tags, tail-like appendages
Scar-like lesions

IMAGING UNCERTAIN
Hyperpigmented patches
Deviation of the gluteal fold

IMAGING NOT REQUIRED
Simple dimples (<5 mm, <25 mm from anal verge)
Coccygeal pits

From Williams H: Spinal sinuses, dimples, pits and patches: what lies beneath? Arch Dis Child Educ Pract Ed 91:ep75–ep80, 2006.

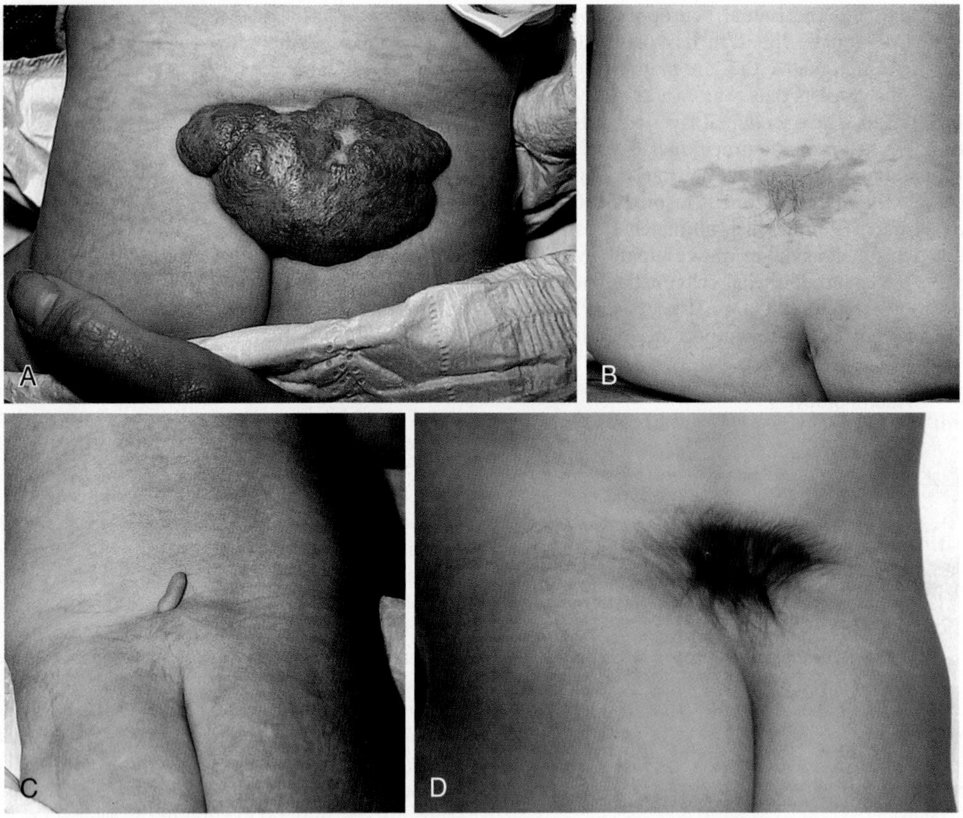

Figure 591-2 Clinical aspects of congenital median lumbosacral cutaneous lesions. **A,** Midline sacral hemangioma in a patient with an occult lipomyelomeningocele. **B,** Capillary malformation with a subtle patch of hypertrichosis in a patient with a dermal sinus. **C,** Human tail with underlying lipoma in an infant with lipomyelomeningocele. **D,** Midline area of hypertrichosis (faun tail) overlying a patch of hyperpigmentation. (**A-C** from Kos L, Drolet BA: Developmental abnormalities. In Eichenfield LF, Frieden IJ, Esterly NB, editors: *Neonatal dermatology*, ed 2, Philadelphia, 2008, WB Saunders. **D** from Spine and spinal cord: developmental disorders. In Schapira A, editor: *Neurology and clinical neuroscience*, Philadelphia, 2007, Mosby.)

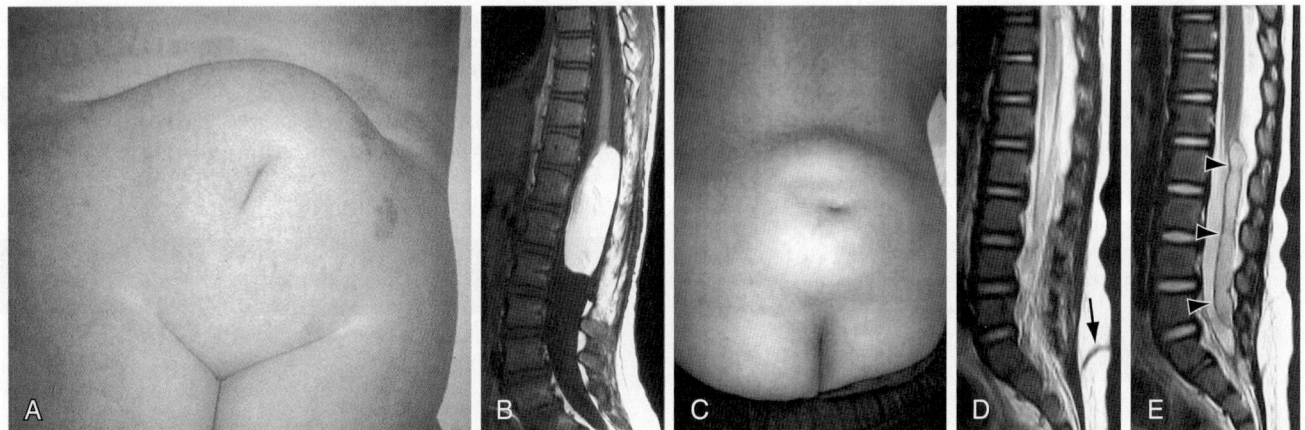

Figure 591-3 Clinical features and imaging findings associated with occult spinal dysraphism. **A,** Lumbosacral lipoma. The subcutaneous lipoma is in continuity with the spinal cord via a defect in the underlying muscles bone and dura. **B,** Sagittal T1-weighted image shows huge intradural lipoma, merging with the conus medullaris superiorly. **C,** Lipoma and central dermal sinus. **D** and **E,** Dermal sinus with dermoid on an 8 yr old girl. Slightly parasagittal T2-weighted image shows sacral dermal sinus coursing obliquely downward in subcutaneous fat *(arrow)* **(D).** Midsagittal T2-weighted image shows huge dermoid in the thecal sac *(arrowheads),* extending upward to the tip of the conus medullaris **(E).** The mass gives a slightly lower signal than cerebrospinal fluid and is outlined by a thin low-signal rim. (**A** from Thompson DNP: Spinal dysraphic anomalies: classification, presentation and management. Paed Child Health 24:431–438, 2014, Fig. 4; **B, D,** and **E** from Rossi A, Biancheri R, Cama A, et al: Imaging in spine and spinal cord malformations, Eur J Radiol 50(2):177–200, 2004, Fig. 9a; and **C,** from Jaiswal AK, Garg A, Mahapatra AK: Spinal ossifying lipoma, J Clin Neurosci 12:714–717, 2005, Fig. 1.)

591.3 Meningocele

Stephen L. Kinsman and Michael V. Johnston

A meningocele is formed when the meninges herniate through a defect in the posterior vertebral arches or the anterior sacrum. The spinal cord is usually normal and assumes a normal position in the spinal canal, although there may be tethering of the cord, syringomyelia, or diastematomyelia. A fluctuant midline mass that might transilluminate occurs along the vertebral column, usually in the lower back. Most meningoceles are well covered with skin and pose no immediate threat to the patient. Careful neurologic examination is mandatory. Orthopedic and urologic examination should also be considered. In asymptomatic children with normal neurologic findings and full-thickness skin covering the meningocele, surgery may be delayed or sometimes not performed.

Before surgical correction of the defect, the patient must be thoroughly examined with the use of plain x-rays, ultrasonography, and MRI to determine the extent of neural tissue involvement, if any, and associated anomalies, including diastematomyelia, lipoma, and possible clinically significant tethered spinal cord. Urologic evaluation usually includes cystometrogram to identify children with neurogenic bladder who are at risk for renal deterioration. Patients with leaking cerebrospinal fluid (CSF) or a thin skin covering should undergo immediate surgical treatment to prevent meningitis. A CT scan or MRI of the head is recommended for children with a meningocele because of the association with hydrocephalus in some cases. An anterior meningocele projects into the pelvis through a defect in the sacrum. Symptoms of constipation and bladder dysfunction develop due to the increasing size of the lesion. Female patients might have associated anomalies of the genital tract, including a rectovaginal fistula and vaginal septa. Plain x-rays demonstrate a defect in the sacrum, and CT scanning or MRI outlines the extent of the meningocele and any associated anomalies.

591.4 Myelomeningocele

Stephen L. Kinsman and Michael V. Johnston

Myelomeningocele represents the most severe form of dysraphism, a so-called aperta or open form, involving the vertebral column and spinal cord, which occurs with an incidence of approximately 1 in 4,000 live births.

ETIOLOGY

The cause of myelomeningocele is unknown, but as with all neural tube closure defects, including anencephaly, a genetic predisposition exists; the risk of recurrence after 1 affected child is 3-4% and increases to 10% with 2 prior affected children. Both epidemiologic evidence and the presence of substantial familial aggregation of anencephaly, myelomeningocele, and craniorachischisis indicate heredity, on a polygenic basis, as a significant contributor to the etiology of NTDs. Nutritional and environmental factors have a role in the etiology of myelomeningocele as well.

Folate is intricately involved in the prevention and etiology of NTDs. Folate functions in single-carbon transfer reactions and exists in many chemical forms. Folic acid (pteroylmonoglutamic acid), which is the most oxidized and stable form of folate, occurs rarely in food but is the form used in vitamin supplements and in fortified food products, particularly flour. Most naturally occurring folates (food folate) are pteroylpolyglutamates, which contain 1-6 additional glutamate molecules joined in a peptide linkage to the γ-carboxyl of glutamate. Folate coenzymes are involved in DNA synthesis, purine synthesis, generation of formate into the formate pool, and amino acid interconversion; the conversion of homocysteine to methionine provides methionine for the synthesis of *S*-adenosylmethionine (SAMe, an agent important for in vivo methylation). Mutations in the genes encoding the enzymes involved in homocysteine metabolism may play

a role in the pathogenesis of meningomyelocele. These enzymes include 5,10-methylenetetrahydrofolate reductase, cystathionine β-synthase, and methionine synthase. An association between a thermolabile variant of 5,10-methylenetetrahydrofolate reductase and mothers of children with NTDs might account for up to 15% of preventable NTDs. Maternal periconceptional use of folic acid supplementation reduces the incidence of NTDs in pregnancies at risk by at least 50%. To be effective, folic acid supplementation should be initiated before conception and continued until at least the 12th wk of gestation, when neurulation is complete. The mechanisms by which folic acid prevents NTDs remain poorly understood.

PREVENTION

The U.S. Public Health Service has recommended that all women of childbearing age and who are capable of becoming pregnant take 0.4 mg of folic acid daily. If, however, a pregnancy is planned in high-risk women (previously affected child), supplementation should be started with 4 mg of folic acid daily, beginning 1 mo before the time of the planned conception. The modern diet provides about half the daily requirement of folic acid. To increase folic acid intake, fortification of flour, pasta, rice, and cornmeal with 0.15 mg folic acid per 100 g was mandated in the United States and Canada in 1998. The added folic acid is insufficient to maximize the prevention of preventable NTDs. Therefore, informative educational programs and folic acid vitamin supplementation remain essential for women planning a pregnancy and possibly for all women of childbearing age. In addition, women should also strive to consume food folate from a varied diet. Certain drugs, including drugs that antagonize folic acid, such as trimethoprim and the anticonvulsants carbamazepine, phenytoin, phenobarbital, and primidone, increase the risk of myelomeningocele. The anticonvulsant valproic acid causes NTDs in approximately 1-2% of pregnancies when administered during pregnancy. Some epilepsy clinicians recommend that all female patients of childbearing potential who take anticonvulsant medications also receive folic acid supplements. There may be a threshold for ideal red blood cell folate levels (900-1,000 nmol/L), which is associated with a markedly reduced risk of NTDs.

CLINICAL MANIFESTATIONS

Myelomeningocele produces dysfunction of many organs and structures, including the skeleton, skin, and gastrointestinal and genitourinary tracts, in addition to the peripheral nervous system and the CNS. A myelomeningocele may be located anywhere along the neuraxis, but the lumbosacral region accounts for at least 75% of the cases. The extent and degree of the neurologic deficit depend on the location of the myelomeningocele and the associated lesions. A lesion in the low sacral region causes bowel and bladder incontinence associated with anesthesia in the perineal area but with no impairment of motor function. Newborns with a defect in the midlumbar or high lumbothoracic region typically have either a sac-like cystic structure covered by a thin layer of partially epithelialized tissue (Fig. 591-4) or an exposed flat

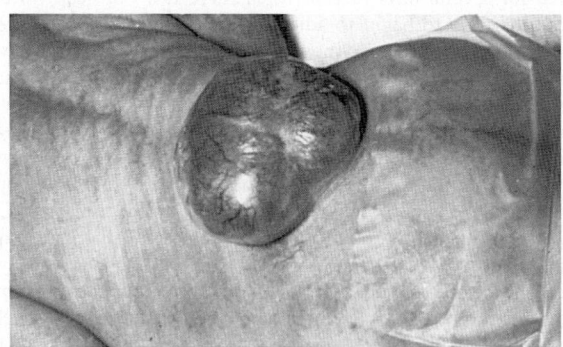

Figure 591-4 A lumbar myelomeningocele is covered by a thin layer of skin.

neural placode without overlying tissues. When a cyst or membrane is present, remnants of neural tissue are visible beneath the membrane, which occasionally ruptures and leaks CSF.

Examination of the infant shows a flaccid paralysis of the lower extremities, an absence of deep tendon reflexes, a lack of response to touch and pain, and a high incidence of lower-extremity deformities (clubfeet, ankle and/or knee contractures, and subluxation of the hips). Some children have constant urinary dribbling and a relaxed anal sphincter. Other children do not leak urine and in fact have a high-pressure bladder and sphincter dyssynergy. Thus, a myelomeningocele above the midlumbar region tends to produce lower motor neuron signs because of abnormalities and disruption of the conus medullaris and above spinal cord structures.

Infants with myelomeningocele typically have increased neurologic deficit as the myelomeningocele extends higher into the thoracic region. These infants sometimes have an associated kyphotic gibbus that requires neonatal orthopedic correction. Patients with a myelomeningocele in the upper thoracic or cervical region usually have a very minimal neurologic deficit and, in most cases, do not have hydrocephalus. They can have neurogenic bladder and bowel.

Hydrocephalus in association with a type II Chiari malformation develops in at least 80% of patients with myelomeningocele. Generally, patients with sacral myelomeningocele have a very low risk of hydrocephalus. The possibility of hydrocephalus developing after the neonatal period should always be considered, no matter what the spinal level. Ventricular enlargement may be indolent and slow growing or may be rapid causing a bulging anterior fontanel, dilated scalp veins, setting-sun appearance of the eyes, irritability, and vomiting in association with an increased head circumference. Approximately 15% of infants with hydrocephalus and Chiari II malformation develop symptoms of hindbrain (brainstem) dysfunction, including difficulty feeding, choking, stridor, apnea, vocal cord paralysis, pooling of secretions, and spasticity of the upper extremities, which, if untreated, can lead to death. This Chiari crisis is caused by downward herniation of the medulla and cerebellar tonsils through the foramen magnum, as well as endogenous malformations in the cerebellum and brainstem, causing dysfunction.

TREATMENT

Management and supervision of a child and family with a myelomeningocele require a multidisciplinary team approach, including surgeons, other physicians, and therapists, with 1 individual (often a pediatrician) acting as the advocate and coordinator of the treatment program. The news that a newborn child has a devastating condition such as myelomeningocele causes parents to feel considerable grief and anger. They need time to learn about the condition and its associated complications and to reflect on the various procedures and treatment plans. A knowledgeable individual in an unhurried and nonthreatening setting must give the parents the facts, along with general prognostic information and management strategies and timelines. If possible, discussions with other parents of children with NTDs are helpful in resolving important questions and issues.

Surgery is often done within a day or so of birth but can be delayed for several days (except when there is a CSF leak) to allow the parents time to begin to adjust to the shock and to prepare for the multiple procedures and inevitable problems that lie ahead. Evaluation of other congenital anomalies and renal function can also be initiated before surgery. Most pediatric centers aggressively treat the majority of infants with myelomeningocele. After repair of a myelomeningocele, most infants require a shunting procedure for hydrocephalus. If symptoms or signs of hindbrain dysfunction appear, early surgical decompression of the posterior fossa is indicated. Clubfeet can require taping or casting, and dislocated hips may require operative procedures.

Careful evaluation and reassessment of the genitourinary system are some of the most important components of the management. Teaching the parents, and, ultimately, the patient, to regularly catheterize a neurogenic bladder is a crucial step in maintaining a low residual volume and bladder pressure that prevents urinary tract infections and reflux leading to pyelonephritis, hydronephrosis, and bladder damage. Latex-free catheters and gloves must be used to prevent development of latex allergy. Periodic urine cultures and assessment of renal function, including serum electrolytes and creatinine as well as renal scans, vesiculourethrograms, renal ultrasonography, and cystometrograms, are obtained according to the risk status and progress of the patient and the results of the physical examination. This approach to urinary tract management has greatly reduced the need for urologic diversionary procedures and significantly decreased the morbidity and mortality associated with progressive renal disease in these patients. Some children can become continent with surgical implantation of an artificial urinary sphincter (these are used less often) or bladder augmentation at a later age.

Although incontinence of fecal matter is common and is socially unacceptable during the school years, it does not pose the same organ-damaging risks as urinary dysfunction, but occasionally fecal impaction and/or megacolon develop. Many children can be bowel-trained with a regimen of timed enemas or suppositories that allows evacuation at a predetermined time once or twice a day. Special attention to low anorectal tone and enema administration and retention is often required. Appendicostomy for antegrade enemas may also be helpful (see Chapter 23.4).

Functional ambulation is the wish of each child and parent and may be possible, depending on the level of the lesion and on intact function of the iliopsoas muscles. Almost every child with a sacral or lumbosacral lesion obtains functional ambulation; approximately half the children with higher defects ambulate with the use of braces, other orthotic devices, and canes. Ambulation is often more difficult as adolescence approaches and body mass increases. Deterioration of ambulatory function, particularly during earlier years, should prompt referral for evaluation of tethered spinal cord and other neurosurgical issues.

In utero surgical closure of a spinal lesion has been successful in a few centers. Preliminary reports suggest a lower incidence of hindbrain abnormalities and hydrocephalus (fewer shunts) as well as improved motor outcomes. This suggests that the defects may be progressive in utero and that prenatal closure might prevent the development of further loss of function. In utero diagnosis is facilitated by maternal serum AFP screening and by fetal ultrasonography (see Chapter 96).

PROGNOSIS

For a child who is born with a myelomeningocele and who is treated aggressively, the mortality rate is 10-15%, and most deaths occur before age 4 yr, although life-threatening complications occur at all ages. At least 70% of survivors have normal intelligence, but learning problems and seizure disorders are more common than in the general population. Previous episodes of meningitis or ventriculitis adversely affect intellectual and cognitive function. Because myelomeningocele is a chronic disabling condition, periodic and consistent multidisciplinary follow-up is required for life. Renal dysfunction is one of the most important determinants of mortality.

Bibliography is available at Expert Consult.

591.5 Encephalocele
Stephen L. Kinsman and Michael V. Johnston

Two major forms of dysraphism affect the skull, resulting in protrusion of tissue through a bony midline defect, called cranium bifidum. A cranial meningocele consists of a CSF-filled meningeal sac only, and a cranial encephalocele contains the sac plus cerebral cortex, cerebellum, or portions of the brainstem. Microscopic examination of the neural tissue within an encephalocele often reveals abnormalities. The cranial defect occurs most commonly in the occipital region at or below the inion, but in certain parts of the world, frontal or nasofrontal encephaloceles (transethmoidal, sphenoethmoidal, sphenomaxillary, sphenoorbital, transsphenoidal) are more common. Some frontal lesions are associated with a cleft lip and palate. These abnormalities are one-tenth as common as neural tube closure defects involving the spine. The etiology is presumed to be similar to that for anencephaly and myelomeningocele; examples of each are reported in the same family.

Infants with a cranial encephalocele are at increased risk for developing hydrocephalus because of **aqueductal stenosis**, **Chiari malformation**, or the **Dandy-Walker syndrome**. Examination might show a small sac with a pedunculated stalk or a large cyst-like structure that can exceed the size of the cranium. The lesion may be completely covered with skin, but areas of denuded lesion can occur and require urgent surgical management. Transillumination of the sac can indicate the presence of neural tissue. A plain x-ray of the skull and cervical spine is indicated to define the anatomy of the cranium and vertebrae. Ultrasonography is most helpful in determining the contents of the sac. MRI or CT further helps define the spectrum of the lesion. Children with a cranial meningocele generally have a good prognosis, whereas patients with an encephalocele are at risk for vision problems, microcephaly, intellectual disability, and seizures. Generally, children with neural tissue within the sac and associated hydrocephalus have the poorest prognosis.

Cranial encephalocele is often part of a syndrome. Meckel-Gruber syndrome is a rare autosomal recessive condition that is characterized by an occipital encephalocele, cleft lip or palate, microcephaly, microphthalmia, abnormal genitalia, polycystic kidneys, and polydactyly. Determination of maternal serum AFP levels and ultrasound measurement of the biparietal diameter, as well as identification of the encephalocele itself, can diagnose encephaloceles in utero. Fetal MRI can help define the extent of associated CNS anomalies and the degree of brain herniated into the encephalocele.

Bibliography is available at Expert Consult.

591.6 Anencephaly
Stephen L. Kinsman and Michael V. Johnston

An anencephalic infant presents a distinctive appearance with a large defect of the calvarium, meninges, and scalp associated with a rudimentary brain, which results from failure of closure of the rostral neuropore, the opening of the anterior neural tube. The primitive brain consists of portions of connective tissue, vessels, and neuroglia. The cerebral hemispheres and cerebellum are usually absent, and only a residue of the brainstem can be identified. The pituitary gland is hypoplastic, and the spinal cord pyramidal tracts are missing owing to the absence of the cerebral cortex. Additional anomalies include folding of the ears, cleft palate, and congenital heart defects in 10-20% of cases. Most anencephalic infants die within several days of birth.

The incidence of anencephaly approximates 1 in 1,000 live births; the greatest incidence is in Ireland, Wales, and Northern China. The recurrence risk is approximately 4% and increases to 10% if a couple has had 2 previously affected pregnancies. Many factors, in addition to genetics, are implicated as a cause of anencephaly, including low socioeconomic status, nutritional and vitamin deficiencies, and a large number of environmental and toxic factors. It is very likely that several noxious stimuli interact on a genetically susceptible host to produce anencephaly. The incidence of anencephaly has been decreasing since the 1990s. Approximately 50% of cases of anencephaly have associated polyhydramnios. Couples who have had an anencephalic infant should have successive pregnancies monitored, including amniocentesis, determination of AFP levels, and ultrasound examination between the 14th and 16th wk of gestation. Prenatal folic acid supplementation decreases the risk of this condition.

591.7 Disorders of Neuronal Migration
Stephen L. Kinsman and Michael V. Johnston

Disorders of neuronal migration can result in minor abnormalities with little or no clinical consequence (small heterotopia of neurons) or devastating abnormalities of CNS structure and/or function (intellectual disability, seizures, lissencephaly, and schizencephaly, particularly the open-lip form) (Fig. 591-5). One of the most important mechanisms in the control of neuronal migration is the radial glial fiber system that guides neurons to their proper site. Migrating neurons attach to the radial glial fiber and then disembark at predetermined sites to form, ultimately, the precisely designed 6-layered cerebral cortex. Another important mechanism is the tangential migration of progenitor neurons destined to become cortical interneurons. The severity and the extent of the disorder are related to numerous factors, including the timing of a particular insult and a host of environmental and genetic contributors. Some cortical malformations may be from somatic mutations, as exemplified by kinesin gene mutations in patients with pachygyria.

LISSENCEPHALY
Lissencephaly, or agyria, is a rare disorder that is characterized by the absence of cerebral convolutions and a poorly formed sylvian fissure, giving the appearance of a 3-4 mo fetal brain. The condition is probably a result of faulty neuroblast migration during early embryonic life and is usually associated with enlarged lateral ventricles and heterotopias in the white matter. In some forms, there is a 4-layered cortex, rather than the usual 6-layered one, with a thin rim of periventricular white matter and numerous gray heterotopias visible by microscopic examination. Milder forms of lissencephaly also exist.

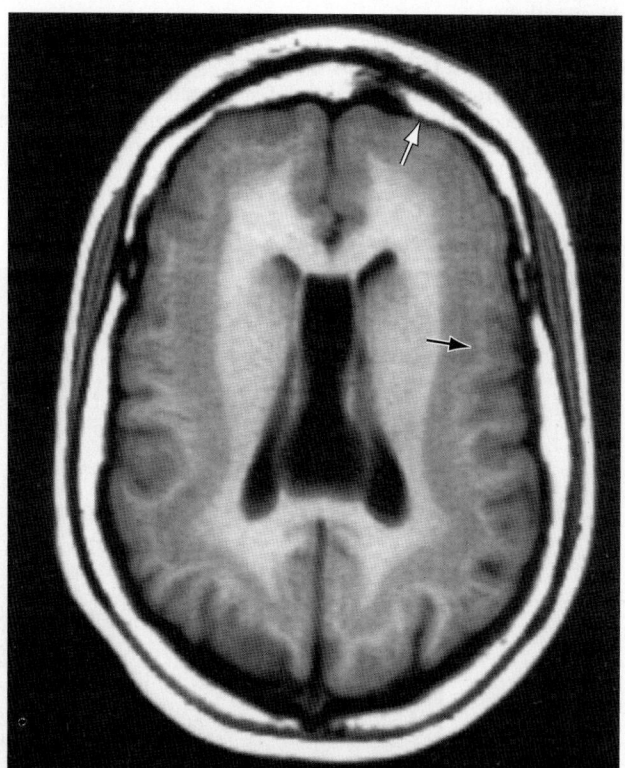

Figure 591-5 T1-weighted MRI scan demonstrating band heterotopia. A thin layer of white matter *(black arrow)* lies between the band of heterotopic gray matter and the cortical surface. Failure of cortical organization with lissencephaly is present in both frontal lobes *(white arrow)*.

These infants present with failure to thrive, microcephaly, marked developmental delay, and a severe seizure disorder. Ocular abnormalities are common, including hypoplasia of the optic nerve and microphthalmia. Lissencephaly can occur as an isolated finding, but it is associated with Miller-Dieker syndrome in approximately 15% of cases. These children have characteristic facies, including a prominent forehead, bitemporal hollowing, anteverted nostrils, a prominent upper lip, and micrognathia. Approximately 70% of children with Miller-Dieker syndrome have visible or submicroscopic chromosomal deletions of 17p13.3.

The gene *LIS-1* (lissencephaly 1) that maps to chromosome region 17p13.3 is deleted in patients with Miller-Dieker syndrome. CT and MRI scans typically show a smooth brain with an absence of sulci (Fig. 591-6). *Doublecortin* is an X chromosome gene that causes lissencephaly when mutated in males and subcortical band heterotopia when mutated in females. Other important forms of lissencephaly include the Walker-Warburg variant and other cobblestone cortical malformations.

SCHIZENCEPHALY

Schizencephaly is the presence of unilateral or bilateral clefts within the cerebral hemispheres owing to an abnormality of morphogenesis (Fig. 591-7). The cleft may be fused or unfused and, if unilateral and large, may be confused with a porencephalic cyst. Not infrequently, the borders of the cleft are surrounded by abnormal brain, particularly microgyria. MRI is the study of choice for elucidating schizencephaly and associated malformations.

When the clefts are bilateral, many patients are severely intellectually challenged, with seizures that are difficult to control, and microcephalic, with spastic quadriparesis. Some cases of bilateral schizencephaly are associated with septooptic dysplasia and endocrinologic disorders. Unilateral schizencephaly is a common cause of congenital hemiparesis. It remains controversial whether genetic causes of schizencephaly exist. Some gene mutations are seen in cases of familial schizencephaly.

NEURONAL HETEROTOPIAS

Subtypes of neuronal heterotopias include periventricular nodular heterotopias, subcortical heterotopia (including band-type), and marginal glioneuronal heterotopias. Intractable seizures are a common feature.

Several genes have been identified that are a cause of these conditions.

POLYMICROGYRIAS

Polymicrogyria is characterized by an augmentation of small convolutions separated by shallow enlarged sulci. Epilepsy, including drug-resistant forms, is a common feature. Truncation of the *KBP* gene has been implicated in a family with multiple members with polymicrogyria.

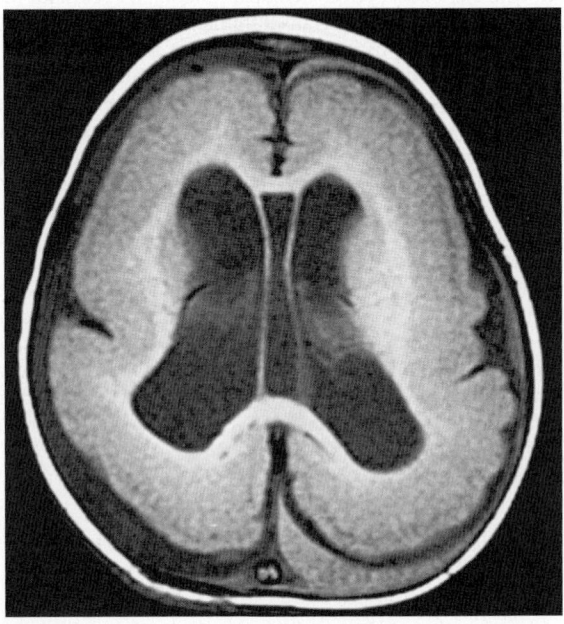

Figure 591-6 MRI of an infant with lissencephaly. Note the absence of cerebral sulci and the maldeveloped sylvian fissures associated with enlarged ventricles.

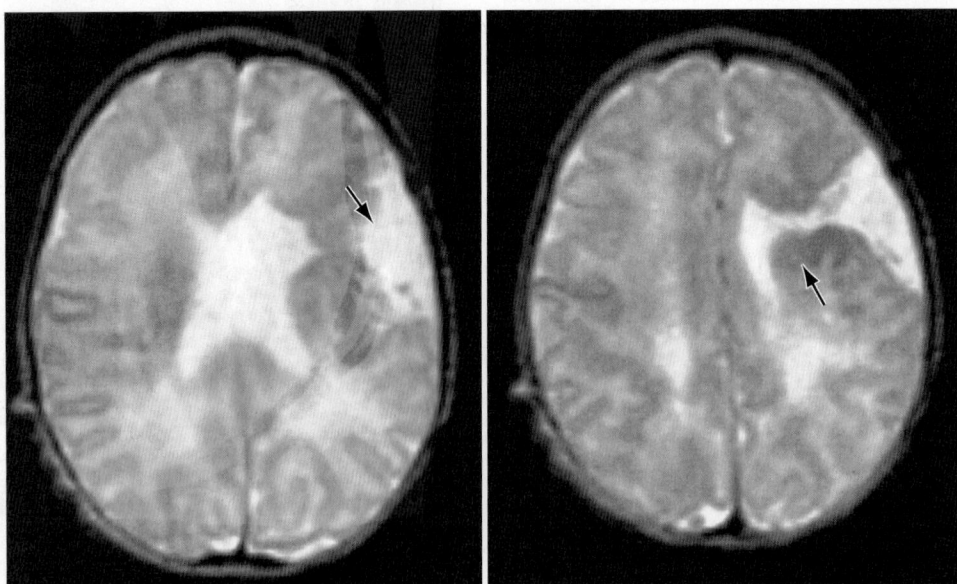

Figure 591-7 Unilateral schizencephaly shown on axial MR images of the brain. Example of an open-lip schizencephaly with a cleft communicating between the ventricle and the extraaxial cranial space *(arrow on left panel)*. Many of these clefts are lined with abnormal gray matter *(arrow on right panel)*.

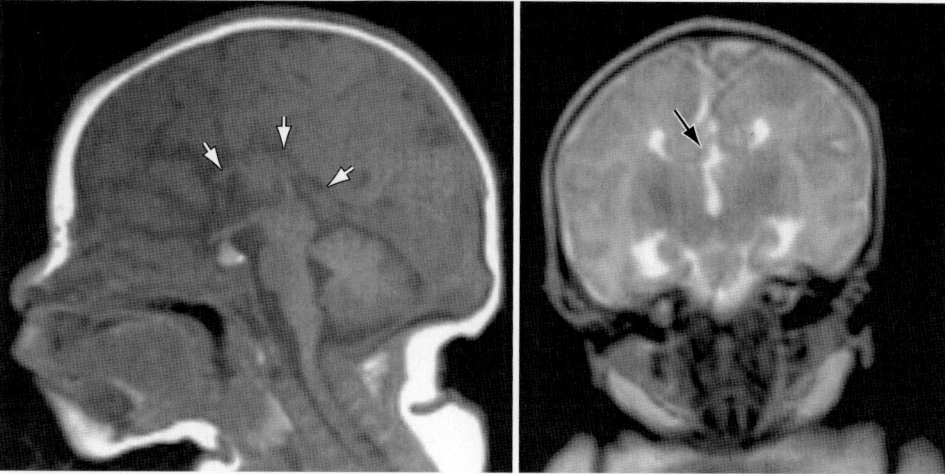

Figure 591-8 Agenesis of the corpus callosum shown on MR images of the brain. Sagittal *(left panel)* and coronal *(right panel)* views of an infant show the total absence of a midsagittal white matter structure *(left panel, arrows)*. The coronal view *(right panel)* demonstrates (despite some motion artifact) the absence of a structure bridging the 2 hemispheres *(area under arrow)*.

FOCAL CORTICAL DYSPLASIAS

Focal cortical dysplasias consist of abnormal cortical lamination in a discrete area of cortex. High-resolution, thin-section MRI can reveal these areas sometimes in the setting of drug-resistant epilepsy.

PORENCEPHALY

Porencephaly is the presence of cysts or cavities within the brain that result from developmental defects or acquired lesions, including infarction of tissue. True porencephalic cysts are most commonly located in the region of the sylvian fissure and typically communicate with the subarachnoid space, the ventricular system, or both. They represent developmental abnormalities of cell migration and are often associated with other malformations of the brain, including microcephaly, abnormal patterns of adjacent gyri, and encephalocele. Affected infants tend to have many problems, including intellectual disability, spastic hemiparesis or quadriparesis, optic atrophy, and seizures.

Several risk factors for porencephalic cyst formation have been identified, including hemorrhagic venous infarctions; various thrombophilias such as protein C deficiency and factor V Leiden mutations; perinatal alloimmune thrombocytopenia; von Willebrand disease; maternal warfarin use; maternal cocaine use; congenital infections; trauma such as amniocentesis; and maternal abdominal trauma. Mutations in the *COL4A1* gene have been described in cases of familial porencephaly.

Pseudoporencephalic cysts characteristically develop during the perinatal or postnatal period and result from abnormalities (infarction, hemorrhage) of arterial or venous circulation. These cysts tend to be unilateral, do not communicate with a fluid-filled cavity, and are not associated with abnormalities of cell migration or CNS malformations. Infants with pseudoporencephalic cysts present with hemiparesis and focal seizures in the 1st yr of life and sometimes present with neonatal encephalopathy or as a floppy newborn or infant.

Bibliography is available at Expert Consult.

591.8 Agenesis of the Corpus Callosum

Stephen L. Kinsman and Michael V. Johnston

Agenesis of the corpus callosum consists of a heterogeneous group of disorders that vary in expression from severe intellectual and neurologic abnormalities to the asymptomatic and normally intelligent patient (Fig. 591-8). The corpus callosum develops from the commissural plate that lies in proximity to the anterior neuropore. Either a direct insult to the commissural plate or disruption of the genetic signaling that specifies and organizes this area during early embryogenesis causes agenesis of the corpus callosum.

It is often said that the outcome of agenesis of the corpus callosum is dictated by *the company it keeps*. When agenesis of the corpus callosum is an isolated phenomenon, the patient may be normal. When it is accompanied by brain anomalies from cell migration defects, such as heterotopias, polymicrogyria, and pachygyria (broad, wide gyri), patients often have significant neurologic abnormalities, including intellectual disability, microcephaly, hemiparesis, diplegia, and seizures.

The anatomic features of agenesis of the corpus callosum are best depicted on MRI or CT scan and include widely separated frontal horns with an abnormally high position of the third ventricle between the lateral ventricles. MRI precisely outlines the extent of the corpus callosum defect.

Absence of the corpus callosum may be inherited as an X-linked recessive trait or as an autosomal dominant trait and on occasion as an autosomal recessive trait. The condition may be associated with specific chromosomal disorders, particularly trisomy 8 and trisomy 18. Single-gene mutations have also been identified, usually in association with other anomalies. Agenesis of the corpus callosum is also seen in some metabolic disorders (Table 591-2).

Aicardi syndrome represents a complex disorder that affects many systems and is typically associated with agenesis of the corpus callosum, distinctive chorioretinal lacunae, and infantile spasms. Patients are almost all female, suggesting a genetic abnormality of the X chromosome (it may be lethal in males during fetal life). Seizures become evident during the 1st few mo and are typically resistant to anticonvulsants. An electroencephalogram shows independent activity recorded from both hemispheres as a result of the absent corpus callosum and shows often hemihypsarrhythmia. All patients have severe intellectual disability and can have abnormal vertebrae that may be fused or only partially developed (hemivertebra). Abnormalities of the retina, including circumscribed pits or lacunae and coloboma of the optic disc, are the most characteristic findings of Aicardi syndrome.

Colpocephaly refers to an abnormal enlargement of the occipital horns of the ventricular system and can be identified as early as the fetal period. It is often associated with agenesis of the corpus callosum, but it can occur in isolation. It is also associated with microcephaly. It can also be seen in anatomic megalencephaly, such as is associated with Sotos syndrome.

HOLOPROSENCEPHALY

Holoprosencephaly is a developmental disorder of the brain that results from defective formation of the prosencephalon and

Table 591-2	Disorders Associated with Agenesis of the Corpus Callosum*

DISORDER	SALIENT FEATURES
WITH IDENTIFIED GENES[†]	
Andermann syndrome (KCC3)	ACC, progressive neuropathy, and dementia
Donnai-Barrow syndrome (LRP2)	Diaphragmatic hernia, exomphalos, ACC, deafness
Frontonasal dysplasia (ALX1)	ACC, bilateral extreme microphthalmia, bilateral oblique facial cleft
XLAG (ARX)	Lissencephaly, ACC, intractable epilepsy
Microcephaly (TBR2)	ACC, polymicrogyria
Microcephaly with simplified gyral pattern and ACC (WDR62)	
Mowat-Wilson syndrome (ZFHX1B)	Hirschsprung disease, ACC
Pyridoxine-dependent epilepsy (ALDH7A1)	ACC, seizures, other brain malformations
Pyruvate dehydrogenase deficiency (PDHA1, PDHB, PDHX)	ACC with other brain changes
ACC with fatal lactic acidosis (MRPS16)	Complexes I and IV deficiency, ACC, brain malformations
HSAS/MASA syndromes (L1CAM)	Hydrocephalus, adducted thumbs, ACC, MR
ACC SEEN CONSISTENTLY (NO GENE YET IDENTIFIED)	
Acrocallosal syndrome	ACC, polydactyly, craniofacial changes, MR
Aicardi syndrome	ACC, chorioretinal lacunae, infantile spasms, MR
Chudley-McCullough syndrome	Hearing loss, hydrocephalus, ACC, colpocephaly
FG syndrome	MR, ACC, craniofacial changes, macrocephaly
Genitopatellar syndrome	Absent patellae, urogenital malformations, ACC
Temtamy syndrome	ACC, optic coloboma, craniofacial changes, MR
Toriello-Carey syndrome	ACC, craniofacial changes, cardiac defects, MR
Vici syndrome	ACC, albinism, recurrent infections, MR
ACC SEEN OCCASIONALLY (PARTIAL LIST)[‡]	
ACC with spastic paraparesis (SPG11; SPG15)	Progressive spasticity and neuropathy, thin corpus callosum
Craniofrontonasal syndrome	Coronal craniosynostosis, facial asymmetry, bifid nose
Fryns syndrome	CDH, pulmonary hypoplasia, craniofacial changes
Marden-Walker syndrome	Blepharophimosis, micrognathia, contractures, ACC
Meckel-Gruber syndrome	Encephalocele, polydactyly, polycystic kidneys
Nonketotic hyperglycinemia (GLDC, GCST, GCSH)	ACC, cerebral and cerebellar atrophy, myoclonus, progressive encephalopathy
Microphthalmia with linear skin defects	Microphthalmia, linear skin markings, seizures
Opitz G syndrome	Pharyngeal cleft, craniofacial changes, ACC, MR
Orofaciodigital syndrome	Tongue hamartoma, microretrognathia, clinodactyly
Pyruvate decarboxylase deficiency	Lactic acidosis, seizures, severe MR and spasticity
Rubinstein-Taybi syndrome	Broad thumbs and great toes, MR, microcephaly
Septooptic dysplasia (de Morsier syndrome)	Hypoplasia of septum pellucidum and optic chiasm
Sotos syndrome	Physical overgrowth, MR, craniofacial changes
Warburg micro syndrome	Microcephaly, microphthalmia, microgenitalia, MR
Wolf-Hirschhorn syndrome	Microcephaly, seizures, cardiac defects, 4p−

*Reliable incidence data are unavailable for these very rare syndromes.

†Gene symbols in parentheses.

‡Many of these also may consistently have a thin of dysplastic corpus callosum, such as Sotos' syndrome or agenesis of the corpus callosum (ACC) with spastic paraparesis (SPG11). The overlap between ACC and these conditions is still under investigation. Other gene symbols are omitted from this section.

4p−, deletion of the terminal region of the short arm of chromosome 4, defines the genotype for Wolf-Hirschhorn patients; ACC, agenesis of the corpus callosum; ARX, Aristaless-related homeobox gene; CDH, congenital diaphragmatic hernia; HSAS/MASA, X-linked hydrocephalus/mental retardation, aphasia, shuffling gait, and adducted thumbs; KCC3, KCl cotransporter 3; L1CAM, L1 cell adhesion molecule; MR, mental retardation; MRPS16, mitochondrial ribosomal protein S16; SPG11, spastic paraplegia 11; XLAG, X-linked lissencephaly with absent corpus callosum and ambiguous genitalia; ZFHX1B, zinc finger homeobox 1b.

From Sherr EH, Hahn JS: Disorders of forebrain development. In Swaiman KF, Ashwal S, Ferriero DM, Schor NF, editors: Swaiman's pediatric neurology, 5th ed. Philadelphia, 2012, WB Saunders, Table 23-2.

inadequate induction of forebrain structures. The abnormality, which represents a spectrum of severity, is classified into 3 groups: alobar, semilobar, and lobar, depending on the degree of the cleavage abnormality (Fig. 591-9). A fourth type, the middle interhemispheric fusion variant or syntelencephaly, involves a segmental area of noncleavage, actually a nonseparation, of the posterior frontal and parietal lobes. Facial abnormalities, including cyclopia, synophthalmia, cebocephaly, single nostril, choanal atresia, solitary central incisor tooth, and premaxillary agenesis are common in severe cases, because the prechordal mesoderm that induces the ventral prosencephalon is also responsible for induction of the median facial structures. Milder facial abnormalities are seen in milder forms. Alobar holoprosencephaly is characterized by a single ventricle, an absent falx, and nonseparated deep cerebral nuclei. Care must be taken not to overdiagnose holoprosencephaly based on ventricular abnormalities alone. Evidence of nonseparated midline deep-brain structures, such as caudate, putamen, globus pallidus, and hypothalamus, is the critical element for diagnosis.

Affected children with the alobar type have high mortality rates, but some live for years. Mortality and morbidity with milder types are more variable, and morbidity is less severe. Care must be taken not to prognosticate severe outcomes in all cases. The incidence of holoprosencephaly ranges from 1 in 5,000-16,000 live births. A prenatal diagnosis can be confirmed by ultrasonography after the 10th wk of gestation for more severe types, but fetal MRI at later gestational ages gives far greater anatomic, and therefore diagnostic, precision.

The cause of holoprosencephaly is often not identified. There appears to be an association with maternal diabetes. Chromosomal abnormalities, including deletions of chromosomes 7q and 3p, 21q, 2p, 18p, and 13q, as well as trisomy 13 and 18, account for upwards of 50% of all cases. Mutations in the *sonic hedgehog* gene at 7q have been shown to cause holoprosencephaly. *Gene Reviews* lists 14 single-gene causes. Clinically, it is important to look for associated anomalies, because many syndromes are associated with holoprosencephaly.

Bibliography is available at Expert Consult.

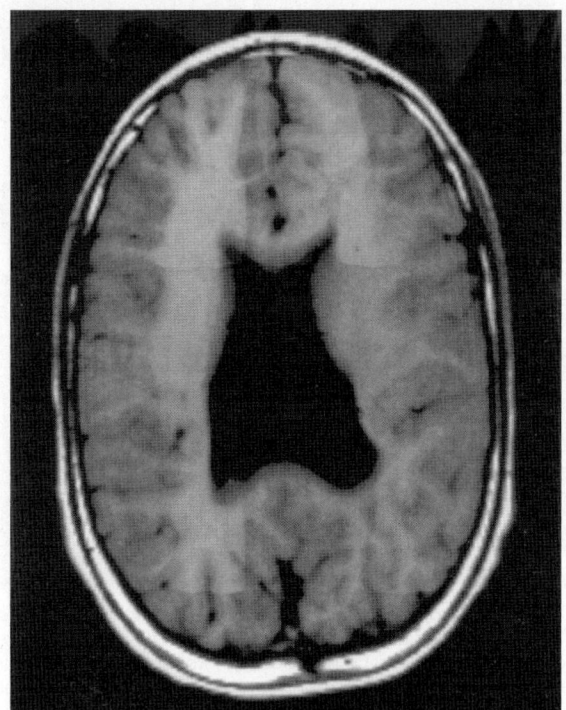

Figure 591-9 Lobar holoprosencephaly. T1-weighted MRI scan demonstrates failure of separation of the hemispheres and a persistent fused ventricle.

591.9 Agenesis of the Cranial Nerves and Dysgenesis of the Posterior Fossa

Stephen L. Kinsman and Michael V. Johnston

Classification of disorders of cranial nerve, brainstem, and cerebellum development remains anatomic, but future classification systems will likely be based on the molecular biology of brain development based on the genes involved and the roles they play in orchestrating brain architecture.

CONGENITAL CRANIAL DYSINNERVATION DISORDERS

Absence of the cranial nerves or the corresponding central nuclei has been described in several conditions and includes the optic nerve defects, congenital ptosis, Marcus Gunn phenomenon (sucking jaw movements causing simultaneous eyelid blinking; this congenital synkinesis results from abnormal innervation of the trigeminal and oculomotor nerves), trigeminal and auditory nerves defects, and cranial nerves IX, X, XI, and XII defects. Increased understanding of these disorders and their genetic causes has led to the term *congenital cranial dysinnervation disorders*.

Optic nerve hypoplasia can occur in isolation or as part of the septooptic dysplasia complex (de Morsier syndrome). Septooptic dysplasia can be caused by a mutation in the *HESX1* gene.

Möbius syndrome is characterized by bilateral facial weakness, which is often associated with paralysis of the abducens nerve. Hypoplasia or agenesis of brainstem nuclei, as well as absent or decreased numbers of muscle fibers, has been reported. Affected infants present in the newborn period with facial weakness, causing feeding difficulties owing to a poor suck. The immobile, dull facies might give the incorrect impression of intellectual impairment; the prognosis for normal development is excellent in most cases. The facial appearance of Möbius syndrome has been improved by facial surgery.

Duane retraction syndrome is characterized by congenital limitation of horizontal globe movement and some globe retraction on attempted adduction and is believed to be the result of abnormal innervation by the oculomotor nerve of the lateral rectus muscle. Abnormalities of cranial nerve development have been demonstrated in this condition.

Less common than Duane retraction syndrome and Möbius syndrome are the group of disorders known as **congenital fibrosis of the extraocular muscles**. Congenital fibrosis of the extraocular muscles is characterized by severe restriction of eye movements and ptosis from abnormal oculomotor and trochlear nerve development and/or from abnormalities of extraocular muscle innervation.

BRAINSTEM AND CEREBELLAR DISORDERS

Disorders of the posterior fossa structures include abnormalities of not only the brainstem and cerebellum, but also the CSF spaces. Commonly encountered malformations include Chiari malformation, Dandy-Walker malformation, arachnoid cysts, mega cisterna magna, persisting Blake pouch, Joubert syndrome, rhombencephalosynapsis, Lhermitte-Duclos disease, and the pontocerebellar hypoplasias.

Chiari malformation is the most common malformation of the posterior fossa and hindbrain. It consists of herniation of the cerebellar tonsils though the foramen magnum. Often, there is also an associated developmental abnormality of the bones of the skull base leading to a small posterior fossa. Cases can be either asymptomatic or symptomatic. When symptoms develop, they often do not do so until late childhood. Symptoms include headaches that are worse with straining and other maneuvers that increase intracranial pressure. Symptoms of brainstem compression such as diplopia, oropharyngeal dysfunction, spasticity, tinnitus, and vertigo can occur. Obstructive hydrocephalus and/or syringomyelia can also occur.

Dandy-Walker malformation is part of a continuum of posterior fossa anomalies that include cystic dilation of the fourth ventricle, hypoplasia of the cerebellar vermis, hydrocephalus, and an enlarged posterior fossa with elevation of the lateral venous sinuses and the tentorium. Extracranial anomalies are also seen. Variable degrees of neurologic impairment are usually present. The etiology of Dandy-Walker malformation includes chromosomal abnormalities, single gene disorders, and exposure to teratogens.

Arachnoid cysts of the posterior fossa can be associated with hydrocephalus. Mega cisterna magna is characterized by an enlarged CSF space inferior and dorsal to the cerebellar vermis and when present in isolation may be considered a normal variant. Persisting Blake pouch is a cyst that obstructs the subarachnoid space and is associated with hydrocephalus.

Joubert syndrome is an autosomal recessive disorder (ciliopathy) with significant genetic heterogeneity that is associated with cerebellar vermis hypoplasia and the pontomesencephalic **molar tooth sign** (a deepening of the interpeduncular fossa with thick and straight superior cerebellar peduncles) (Fig. 591-10). It is associated with hypotonia, ataxia (as toddler), characteristic breathing abnormalities including episodic apnea and hyperpnea (which improves with age), global developmental delay, nystagmus, strabismus, ptosis, and oculomotor apraxia. There can be many associated systemic features (Joubert syndrome and related disorders) including progressive retinal dysplasia (Leber congenital amaurosis), coloboma, congenital heart disease, microcystic kidney disease, liver fibrosis, polydactyly, tongue protrusion, and soft tissue tumors of the tongue (Fig. 591-11).

Rhombencephalosynapsis is an absent or small vermis associated with a nonseparation or fusion of the deep midline cerebellar structures. Ventriculomegaly or hydrocephalus is often seen. There is variable clinical presentation from normal to cognitive and language impairments, epilepsy, and spasticity. **Lhermitte-Duclos** disease is a dysplastic gangliocytoma of the cerebellum leading to focal enlargement of the cerebellum and macrocephaly, cerebellar signs, and seizures.

Pontocerebellar hypoplasias are a group of disorders characterized by impairment of cerebellar and pontine development together with histopathologic features of neuronal death and glial replacement. Clinical features tend to be nonspecific and include hypotonia, feeding difficulties, developmental delay, and breathing difficulties. Classification, associations, and causes include type I (with features of anterior

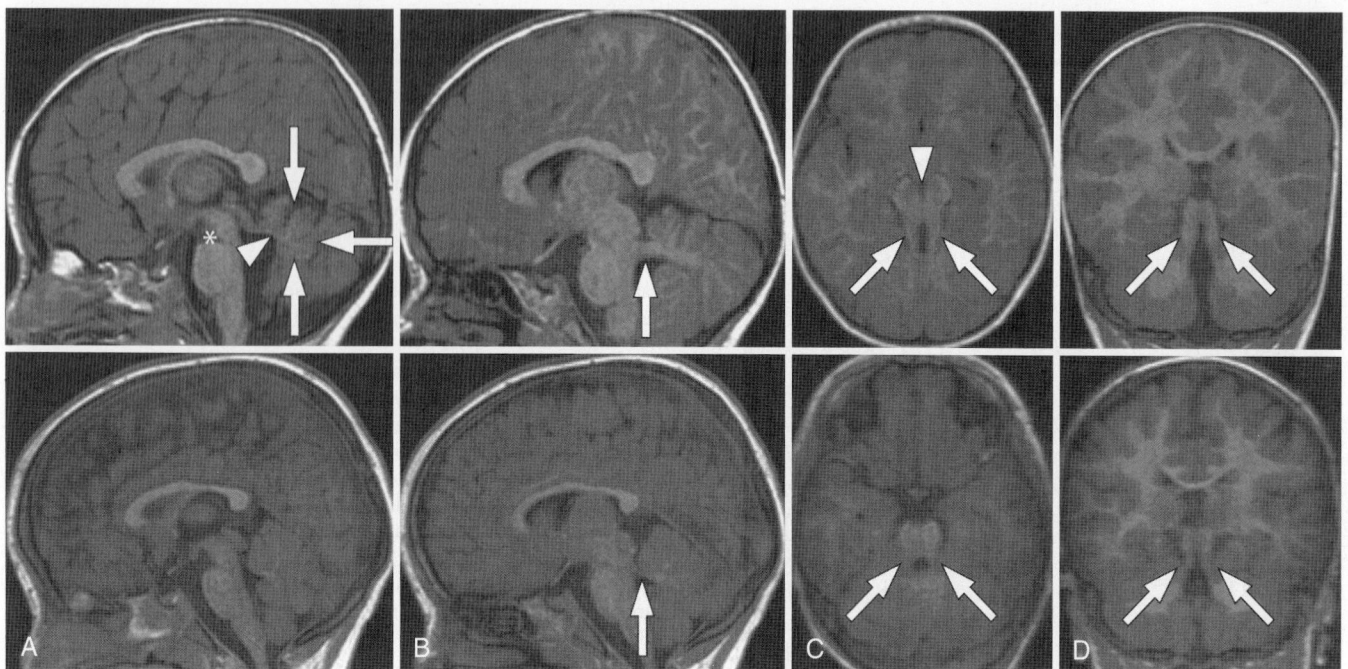

Figure 591-10 Neuroimaging findings in a 2-yr-old child with pure Joubert syndrome *(upper panels)* compared to a healthy control *(lower panels)*. **A,** Parasagittal T1-weighted image shows the thickened, elongated, and horizontally orientated superior cerebellar peduncles *(white arrow)*. **B,** Midsagittal T1-weighted image demonstrates a moderate hypoplasia and dysplasia of the cerebellar vermis *(white arrows)* with secondary distortion and enlargement of the fourth ventricle with rostral shifting of the fastigium *(white arrowhead)*. A deepened interpeduncular fossa is also noted. **C,** Axial T1-weighted image at the level of the pontomesencephalic junction shows the molar tooth sign with a deepened interpeduncular fossa *(white arrowhead)* and elongated, thickened, and horizontally orientated superior cerebellar peduncles *(white arrows)*. Additionally, the cerebellar vermis appears to be hypoplastic and its remnants dysplastic. **D,** Coronal T1-weighted image reveals the thickened superior cerebellar peduncles *(white arrows)*. *(From Romani M, Micalizzi A, Valente EM: Joubert syndrome: congenital cerebellar ataxia with the molar tooth.* Lancet Neurol *12:894–905, 2013, Fig. 1.)*

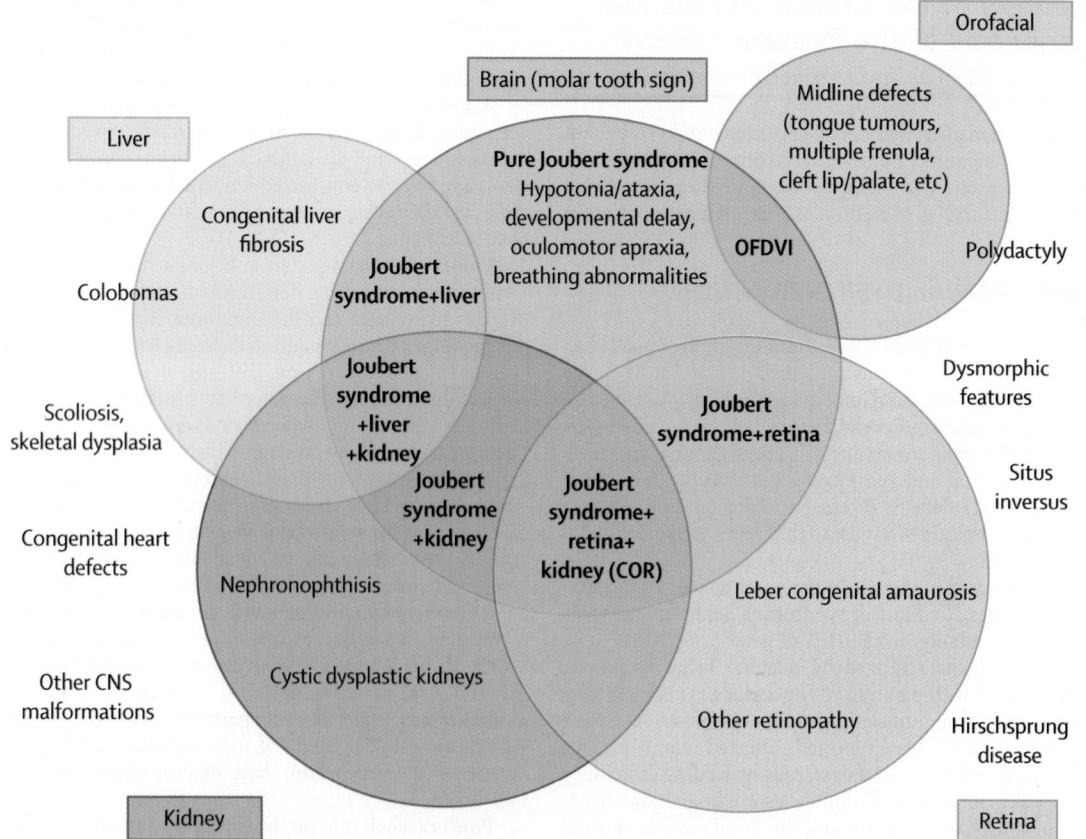

Figure 591-11 Spectrum of organ involvement in Joubert syndrome and classification in clinical subgroups *(in bold)*. Chorioretinal colobomas are more frequently found in the subgroup of Joubert syndrome with liver involvement but can be present also in other subgroups. Similarly, polydactyly (especially if preaxial or mesoaxial) is invariably present in the Orofaciodigital type VI subgroup, but postaxial polydactyly is frequently observed also in association with other Joubert syndrome phenotypes. Other clinical features outside the circles occur more rarely, without a specific association to a clinical subgroup. *CNS,* central nervous system; *COR,* cerebello oculorenal; *K,* kidney involvement; *L,* liver involvement; *MTS,* molar tooth sign; *OFDVI,* orofaciodigital type VI syndrome. *(From Romani M, Micalizzi A, Valente EM: Joubert syndrome: congenital cerebellar ataxia with the molar tooth.* Lancet Neurol *12:894–905, 2013, Fig. 3.)*

horn cell involvement), type II (with extrapyramidal features, seizures, and acquired microcephaly), Walker-Warburg syndrome, muscle-eye-brain disease, congenital disorders of glycosylation type 1A, mitochondrial cytopathies, teratogen exposure, congenital cytomegalovirus infection, 3-methylglutaconic aciduria, PEHO syndrome (progressive encephalopathy with edema, hypsarrhythmia, and optic atrophy), autosomal recessive cerebellar hypoplasia in the Hutterite population, lissencephaly with cerebellar hypoplasia, and other subtypes of ponto-cerebellar hypoplasia.

Bibliography is available at Expert Consult.

591.10 Microcephaly
Stephen L. Kinsman and Michael V. Johnston

Microcephaly is defined as a head circumference that measures more than 3 SD below the mean for age and sex. This condition is relatively common, particularly among developmentally delayed children. Although there are many causes of microcephaly, abnormalities in neuronal migration during fetal development, including heterotopias of neuronal cells and cytoarchitectural derangements, are often found. Microcephaly may be subdivided into 2 main groups: primary (genetic) microcephaly and secondary (nongenetic) microcephaly. A precise diagnosis is important for genetic counseling and for prediction for future pregnancies.

ETIOLOGY
Primary microcephaly refers to a group of conditions that usually have no associated malformations and follow a mendelian pattern of inheritance or are associated with a specific genetic syndrome. Affected infants are usually identified at birth because of a small head circumference. The more common types include familial and autosomal dominant microcephaly and a series of chromosomal syndromes that are summarized in Table 591-3. Primary microcephaly is also associated with at least 7 gene loci, and 7 single etiologic genes have been identified. It is known as autosomal recessive primary microcephaly and has autosomal inheritance. Many X-linked causes of microcephaly are caused by gene mutations that lead to severe structural brain

Table 591-3	Causes of Microcephaly	
CAUSES	**CHARACTERISTIC FINDINGS**	
PRIMARY (GENETIC)		
Familial (autosomal recessive)	Incidence 1 in 40,000 live births	
	Typical appearance with slanted forehead, prominent nose and ears; severe mental retardation and prominent seizures; surface convolutional markings of the brain, poorly differentiated and disorganized cytoarchitecture	
Autosomal dominant	Nondistinctive facies, upslanting palpebral fissures, mild forehead slanting, and prominent ears	
	Normal linear growth, seizures readily controlled, and mild or borderline mental retardation	
Syndromes		
Down (trisomy 21)	Incidence 1 in 800 live births	
	Abnormal rounding of occipital and frontal lobes and a small cerebellum; narrow superior temporal gyrus, propensity for Alzheimer neurofibrillary alterations, ultrastructure abnormalities of cerebral cortex	
Edward (trisomy 18)	Incidence 1 in 6,500 live births	
	Low birthweight, microstomia, micrognathia, low-set malformed ears, prominent occiput, rocker-bottom feet, flexion deformities of fingers, congenital heart disease, increased gyri, heterotopias of neurons	
Cri-du-chat (5 p-)	Incidence 1 in 50,000 live births	
	Round facies, prominent epicanthic folds, low-set ears, hypertelorism, characteristic cry	
	No specific neuropathology	
Cornelia de Lange	Prenatal and postnatal growth delay; synophrys; thin, downturning upper lip	
	Proximally placed thumb	
Rubinstein-Taybi	Beaked nose, downward slanting of palpebral fissures, epicanthic folds, short stature, broad thumbs and toes	
Smith-Lemli-Opitz	Ptosis, scaphocephaly, inner epicanthic folds, anteverted nostrils	
	Low birthweight, marked feeding problems	
SECONDARY (NONGENETIC)		
Congenital Infections		
Cytomegalovirus	Small for dates, petechial rash, hepatosplenomegaly, chorioretinitis, deafness, mental retardation, seizures	
	Central nervous system calcification and microgyria	
Rubella	Growth retardation, purpura, thrombocytopenia, hepatosplenomegaly, congenital heart disease, chorioretinitis, cataracts, deafness	
	Perivascular necrotic areas, polymicrogyria, heterotopias, subependymal cavitations	
Toxoplasmosis	Purpura, hepatosplenomegaly, jaundice, convulsions, hydrocephalus, chorioretinitis, cerebral calcification	
Drugs		
Fetal alcohol	Growth retardation, ptosis, absent philtrum and hypoplastic upper lip, congenital heart disease, feeding problems, neuroglial heterotopia, disorganization of neurons	
Fetal hydantoin	Growth delay, hypoplasia of distal phalanges, inner epicanthic folds, broad nasal ridge, anteverted nostrils	
Other Causes		
Radiation	Microcephaly and mental retardation most severe with exposure before 15th wk of gestation	
Meningitis/encephalitis	Cerebral infarcts, cystic cavitation, diffuse loss of neurons	
Malnutrition	Controversial cause of microcephaly	
Metabolic	Maternal diabetes mellitus and maternal hyperphenylalaninemia	
Hyperthermia	Significant fever during 1st 4-6 wk has been reported to cause microcephaly, seizures, and facial anomalies	
	Pathologic studies show neuronal heterotopias	
	Further studies show no abnormalities with maternal fever	
Hypoxic–ischemic encephalopathy	Initially diffuse cerebral edema; late stages characterized by cerebral atrophy and abnormal signals on MRI	

malformations such as lissencephaly, holoprosencephaly, polymicrogyria, cobblestone dysplasia, neuronal heterotopia, pontocerebellar hypoplasia; these should be sought on MRI. Secondary microcephaly results from a large number of noxious agents that can affect a fetus in utero or an infant during periods of rapid brain growth, particularly the 1st 2 yr of life.

Acquired microcephaly can be seen in conditions such as Rett, Seckel, and Angelman syndromes and in encephalopathy syndromes associated with severe seizure disorders.

CLINICAL MANIFESTATIONS AND DIAGNOSIS

A thorough family history should be taken, seeking additional cases of microcephaly or disorders affecting the nervous system. It is important to measure a patient's head circumference at birth to diagnose microcephaly as early as possible. A very small head circumference implies a process that began early in embryonic or fetal development. An insult to the brain that occurs later in life, particularly beyond the age of 2 yr, is less likely to produce severe microcephaly. Serial head circumference measurements are more meaningful than a single determination, particularly when the abnormality is minimal. The head circumference of each parent and sibling should be recorded.

Laboratory investigation of a microcephalic child is determined by the history and physical examination. If the cause of the microcephaly is unknown, the mother's serum phenylalanine level should be determined. High phenylalanine serum levels in an asymptomatic mother can produce marked brain damage in an otherwise normal nonphenylketonuric infant. A karyotype and/or array comparative genomic hybridization study is obtained if a chromosomal syndrome is suspected or if the child has abnormal facies, short stature, and additional congenital anomalies. MRI is useful in identifying structural abnormalities of the brain such as lissencephaly, pachygyria, and polymicrogyria, and CT scanning is useful to detect intracerebral calcification. Additional studies include a fasting plasma and urine amino acid analysis; serum ammonia determination; *to*xoplasmosis, *r*ubella, *c*ytomegalovirus, and *h*erpes simplex (TORCH) titers as well as HIV testing of the mother and child; and a urine sample for the culture of cytomegalovirus. Single-gene mutations as a cause of both primary microcephaly and syndromic microcephaly are being increasingly identified.

TREATMENT

Once the cause of microcephaly has been established, the physician must provide accurate and supportive genetic and family counseling. Because many children with microcephaly are also intellectually challenged, the physician must assist with placement in an appropriate program that will provide for maximal development of the child (see Chapter 36).

Bibliography is available at Expert Consult.

591.11 Hydrocephalus
Stephen L. Kinsman and Michael V. Johnston

Hydrocephalus is not a specific disease; it represents a diverse group of conditions that result from impaired circulation and/or absorption of CSF or, in rare circumstances, from increased production of CSF by a choroid plexus papilloma (Table 591-4). Because megalencephaly is often discovered as part of an evaluation for hydrocephalus in children with macrocephaly, it is included in this section.

PHYSIOLOGY

The CSF is formed primarily in the ventricular system by the choroid plexus, which is situated in the lateral, third, and fourth ventricles. Although most CSF is produced in the lateral ventricles, approximately 25% originates from extrachoroidal sources, including the capillary endothelium within the brain parenchyma. There is active neurogenic control of CSF formation because adrenergic and cholinergic nerves

Table 591-4	Causes of Hydrocephalus

COMMUNICATING
Achondroplasia
Basilar impression
Benign enlargement of subarachnoid space
Choroid plexus papilloma
Meningeal malignancy
Meningitis
Posthemorrhagic

NONCOMMUNICATING
Aqueductal stenosis
Infectious*
X-linked
Mitochondrial
Autosomal recessive
Autosomal dominant
L1CAM mutations
Chiari malformation
Dandy-Walker malformation
Klippel-Feil syndrome
Mass lesions
Abscess
Hematoma
Tumors and neurocutaneous disorders
Vein of Galen malformation
Walker-Warburg syndrome

HYDRANENCEPHALY
Holoprosencephaly
Massive hydrocephalus
Porencephaly

*Toxoplasmosis, neurocysticercosis mumps.
From Fenichel GM: Clinical pediatric neurology, ed 5, Philadelphia, 2005, Elsevier, p. 354.

innervate the choroid plexus. Stimulation of the adrenergic system diminishes CSF production, whereas excitation of the cholinergic nerves may double the normal CSF production rate. In a normal child, approximately 20 mL/hr of CSF is produced. The total volume of CSF approximates 50 mL in an infant and 150 mL in an adult. Most of the CSF is extraventricular. The choroid plexus forms CSF in several stages; through a series of intricate steps, a plasma ultrafiltrate is ultimately processed into a secretion, the CSF.

CSF flow results from the pressure gradient that exists between the ventricular system and venous channels. Intraventricular pressure may be as high as 180 mm H_2O in the normal state, whereas the pressure in the superior sagittal sinus is in the range of 90 mm H_2O. Normally, CSF flows from the lateral ventricles through the foramina of Monro into the 3rd ventricle. It then traverses the narrow aqueduct of Sylvius, which is approximately 3 mm long and 2 mm in diameter in a child, to enter the fourth ventricle. The CSF exits the fourth ventricle through the paired lateral foramina of Luschka and the midline foramen of Magendie into the cisterns at the base of the brain. Hydrocephalus resulting from obstruction within the ventricular system is called obstructive or noncommunicating hydrocephalus. The CSF then circulates from the basal cisterns posteriorly through the cistern system and over the convexities of the cerebral hemispheres. CSF is absorbed primarily by the arachnoid villi through tight junctions of their endothelium by the pressure forces that were noted earlier. CSF is absorbed to a much lesser extent by the lymphatic channels directed to the paranasal sinuses, along nerve root sleeves, and by the choroid plexus itself. Hydrocephalus resulting from obliteration of the subarachnoid cisterns or malfunction of the arachnoid villi is called nonobstructive or communicating hydrocephalus.

PATHOPHYSIOLOGY AND ETIOLOGY

Obstructive or noncommunicating hydrocephalus develops most commonly in children because of an abnormality of the aqueduct of Sylvius or a lesion in the fourth ventricle. Aqueductal stenosis results from an abnormally narrow aqueduct of Sylvius that is often associated with branching or forking. In a small percentage of cases, aqueductal stenosis is inherited as a sex-linked recessive trait. These patients occasionally have minor neural tube closure defects, including spina bifida occulta. Rarely, aqueductal stenosis is associated with neurofibromatosis. Aqueductal gliosis can also give rise to hydrocephalus. As a result of neonatal meningitis or a subarachnoid hemorrhage in a premature infant, the ependymal lining of the aqueduct is interrupted and a brisk glial response results in complete obstruction. Intrauterine viral infections can also produce aqueductal stenosis followed by hydrocephalus, and mumps meningoencephalitis has been reported as a cause in a child. A vein of Galen malformation can expand to become large and, because of its midline position, obstruct the flow of CSF. Lesions or malformations of the posterior fossa are prominent causes of hydrocephalus, including posterior fossa brain tumors, Chiari malformation, and the Dandy-Walker syndrome.

Nonobstructive or communicating hydrocephalus most commonly follows a subarachnoid hemorrhage, which is usually a result of intraventricular hemorrhage in a premature infant. Blood in the subarachnoid spaces can cause obliteration of the cisterns or arachnoid villi and obstruction of CSF flow. Pneumococcal and tuberculous meningitis have a propensity to produce a thick, tenacious exudate that obstructs the basal cisterns, and intrauterine infections can also destroy the CSF pathways. Leukemic infiltrates can seed the subarachnoid space and produce communicating hydrocephalus.

CLINICAL MANIFESTATIONS

The clinical presentation of hydrocephalus is variable and depends on many factors, including the age at onset, the nature of the lesion causing obstruction, and the duration and rate of increase of the intracranial pressure (ICP). In an infant, an accelerated rate of enlargement of the head is the most prominent sign. In addition, the anterior fontanel is wide open and bulging, and the scalp veins are dilated. The forehead is broad, and the eyes might deviate downward because of impingement of the dilated suprapineal recess on the brainstem tectum, producing the setting-sun eye sign. Long-tract signs, including brisk tendon reflexes, spasticity, clonus (particularly in the lower extremities), and Babinski sign, are common owing to stretching and disruption of the corticospinal fibers originating from the leg region of the motor cortex. In an older child, the cranial sutures are less accommodating so that the signs of hydrocephalus may be subtler. Irritability, lethargy, poor appetite, and vomiting are common to both age groups, and headache is a prominent symptom in older patients. A gradual change in personality and deterioration in academic productivity suggest a slowly progressive form of hydrocephalus. With regard to other clinical signs, serial measurements of the head circumference often indicate an increased velocity of growth. Percussion of the skull might produce a cracked pot sound or Macewen sign, indicating separation of the sutures. A foreshortened occiput suggests Chiari malformation, and a prominent occiput suggests the Dandy-Walker malformation. Papilledema, abducens nerve palsies, and pyramidal tract signs, which are most evident in the lower extremities, are apparent in many cases.

Chiari malformation consists of 2 major subgroups. Type I typically produces symptoms during adolescence or adult life and is usually not associated with hydrocephalus. Patients complain of recurrent headache, neck pain, urinary frequency, and progressive lower-extremity spasticity. The deformity consists of displacement of the cerebellar tonsils into the cervical canal (Fig. 591-12). Syrinx of the spinal cord, especially the cervical region should be looked for on MRI imaging. Although the pathogenesis is unknown, a prevailing theory suggests that obstruction of the caudal portion of the fourth ventricle during fetal development is responsible. Other theories include tethering of the cord or additional anomalies (syrinx).

The type II Chiari malformation is characterized by progressive hydrocephalus with a myelomeningocele. This lesion represents an anomaly of the hindbrain, probably owing to a failure of pontine flexure development during embryogenesis, and results in elongation of the fourth ventricle and kinking of the brainstem, with displacement of the inferior vermis, pons, and medulla into the cervical canal

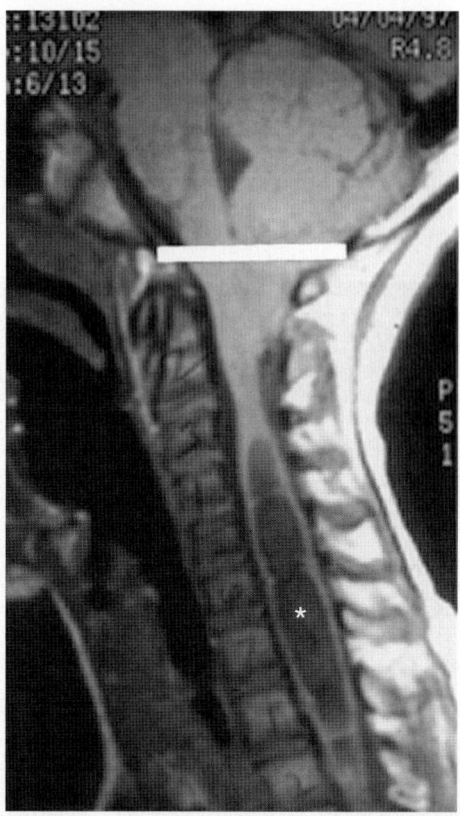

Figure 591-12 Sagittal MR scan of a patient with Chiari malformation type I. Cerebellar tonsils are displaced through the foramen magnum *(white bar)* to the lower aspect of C2 with clear crowding at the foramen. A syrinx *(white asterisk)* is visible extending from C3 to T2. *(From Yassari R, Frim D: Evaluation and management of the Chiari malformation type 1 for the primary care pediatrician, Pediatr Clin North Am 51:477–490, 2004.)*

(Fig. 591-13). Approximately 10% of type II malformations produce symptoms during infancy, consisting of stridor, weak cry, and apnea, which may be relieved by shunting or by decompression of the posterior fossa. A more indolent form consists of abnormalities of gait, spasticity, and increasing incoordination (including the arms and hands) during childhood.

Plain skull radiographs show a small posterior fossa and a widened cervical canal. CT scanning with contrast and MRI display the cerebellar tonsils protruding downward into the cervical canal and the hindbrain abnormalities. The anomaly is treated by surgical decompression, but asymptomatic or mildly symptomatic patients may be managed conservatively.

The Dandy-Walker malformation consists of a cystic expansion of the fourth ventricle in the posterior fossa and midline cerebellar hypoplasia, which results from a developmental failure of the roof of the fourth ventricle during embryogenesis (Fig. 591-14). Approximately 90% of patients have hydrocephalus, and a significant number of children have associated anomalies, including agenesis of the posterior cerebellar vermis and corpus callosum. Infants present with a rapid increase in head size and a prominent occiput. Transillumination of the skull may be positive. Most children have evidence of long-tract signs, cerebellar ataxia, and delayed motor and cognitive milestones, probably due to the associated structural anomalies. The Dandy-Walker malformation is managed by shunting the cystic cavity (and on occasion the ventricles as well) in the presence of hydrocephalus.

DIAGNOSIS AND DIFFERENTIAL DIAGNOSIS

Investigation of a child with hydrocephalus begins with the history. Familial cases suggest X-linked or autosomal hydrocephalus secondary to aqueductal stenosis. A past history of prematurity with intracranial hemorrhage, meningitis, or mumps encephalitis is important to ascertain. Multiple café-au-lait spots and other clinical features of neurofibromatosis point to aqueductal stenosis as the cause of hydrocephalus.

Examination includes careful inspection, palpation, and auscultation of the skull and spine. The occipitofrontal head circumference is recorded and compared with previous measurements. The size and configuration of the anterior fontanel are noted, and the back is

inspected for abnormal midline skin lesions, including tufts of hair, lipoma, or angioma that might suggest spinal dysraphism. The presence of a prominent forehead or abnormalities in the shape of the occiput can suggest the pathogenesis of the hydrocephalus. A cranial bruit is audible in association with many cases of vein of Galen arteriovenous malformation. Transillumination of the skull is positive with massive dilation of the ventricular system or in the Dandy-Walker syndrome. Inspection of the eyegrounds is mandatory because the finding of chorioretinitis suggests an intrauterine infection, such as toxoplasmosis, as a cause of the hydrocephalus. Papilledema is observed in older children but is rarely present in infants because the cranial sutures separate as a result of the increased pressure.

Plain skull films typically show separation of the sutures, erosion of the posterior clinoids in an older child, and an increase in convolutional markings (beaten-silver appearance) on the inside of the skull with long-standing increased ICP. The CT scan and/or MRI along with ultrasonography in an infant are the most important studies to identify the specific cause and severity of hydrocephalus.

The head might appear enlarged (and can be confused with hydrocephalus) secondary to a thickened cranium resulting from chronic anemia, rickets, osteogenesis imperfecta, and epiphyseal dysplasia. Chronic subdural collections can produce bilateral parietal bone prominence. MRI has revealed the common occurrence of benign external hydrocephalus, a growth-limited condition where intervention is rarely required. Various metabolic and degenerative disorders of the CNS produce megalencephaly as a result of abnormal storage of substances within the brain parenchyma. These disorders include lysosomal diseases (Tay-Sachs disease, gangliosidosis, and the mucopolysaccharidoses), the aminoacidurias (maple syrup urine disease), and the leukodystrophies (metachromatic leukodystrophy, Alexander disease, Canavan disease). In addition, cerebral gigantism (Sotos syndrome), other overgrowth syndromes and neurofibromatosis are characterized by increased brain mass. Familial megalencephaly is inherited as an autosomal dominant trait and is characterized by delayed motor milestones and hypotonia but normal or near-normal intelligence. Measurement of parents' head circumferences is necessary to establish the diagnosis.

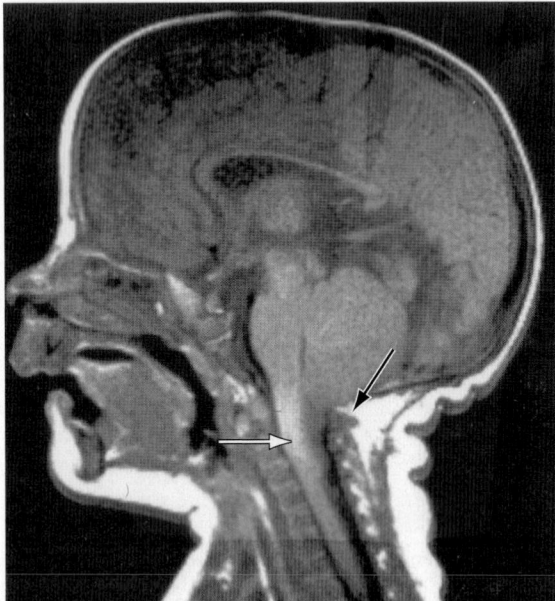

Figure 591-13 A midsagittal T1-weighted MRI of a patient with type II Chiari malformation. The cerebellar tonsils *(white arrow)* have descended below the foramen magnum *(black arrow)*. Note the small, slitlike fourth ventricle, which has been pulled into a vertical position.

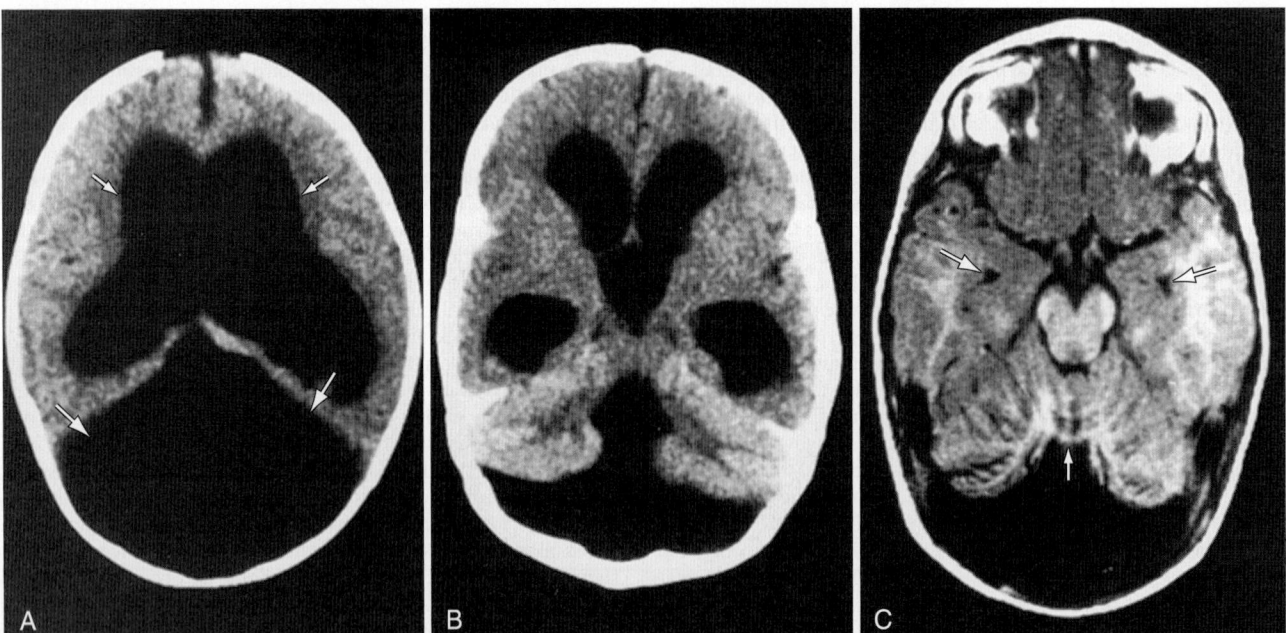

Figure 591-14 Dandy-Walker cyst. **A,** Axial CT scan (preoperative) showing large posterior fossa cyst (Dandy-Walker cyst; *large arrows*) and dilated lateral ventricles *(small arrows),* a complication secondary to cerebrospinal fluid (CSF) pathway obstruction at the fourth ventricular outlet. **B,** Same patient, with a lower axial CT scan showing splaying of the cerebellar hemispheres by the dilated fourth ventricle (Dandy-Walker cyst). The dilated ventricles proximal to the fourth ventricle again show CSF obstruction caused by the Dandy-Walker cyst. **C,** MRI of the same patient showing decreased size of the Dandy-Walker cyst and temporal horns *(arrows)* after shunting. The incomplete vermis *(small arrow)* now becomes recognizable.

MEGALENCEPHALY

Megalencephaly is an anatomic disorder of brain growth defined as a brain weight:volume ratio >98th percentile for age (or ≥2 SD above the mean) that is usually accompanied by macrocephaly (an occipitofrontal circumference >98th percentile). Various storage and degenerative diseases are associated with megalencephaly, but anatomic and genetic causes exist as well. The most common cause of anatomic megalencephaly is benign familial megalencephaly. This condition is easily diagnosed by careful family history and measurement of the parents' head circumferences (occipitofrontal circumferences). On the other hand, macrocephaly is a known feature of more than 100 syndromes.

Anatomic megalencephaly is usually apparent at birth, and head growth continues to run parallel to the upper percentiles. Sometimes, in some syndromes, increased occipitofrontal circumference is the presenting sign. Neuroimaging is critical in identifying the various structural and gyral abnormalities seen in syndromic macrocephaly and determining whether anatomic megalencephaly exists.

Common megalencephaly-associated macrocephaly syndromes include syndromes with prenatal and/or postnatal somatic overgrowth such as Sotos, Simpson-Golabi-Behmel, fragile X, Weaver, macrocephaly-cutis marmorata telangiectatica congenita, and Bannayan-Ruvalcaba-Riley syndromes, and syndromes without somatic overgrowth such as FG, Greig cephalopolysyndactyly, acrocallosal, and Gorlin.

Sotos syndrome (cerebral gigantism) is the most common megalencephalic syndrome, with 50% of patients having prenatal macrocephaly and 100% of patients having macrocephaly by age 1 yr. Early postnatal overgrowth normalizes by adulthood. Facial features include high forehead with frontal bossing, sparse hair in the frontoparietal region, downslanting palpebral fissures, apparent hypertelorism, long narrow face, prominent mandible, and malar flushing. Hypotonia, poor coordination, and speech delay are common. Most children show cognitive impairment, ranging from mild to severe.

HYDRANENCEPHALY

Hydranencephaly may be confused with hydrocephalus. The cerebral hemispheres are absent or represented by membranous sacs with remnants of frontal, temporal, or occipital cortex dispersed over the membrane. The midbrain and brainstem are relatively intact (Fig. 591-15).

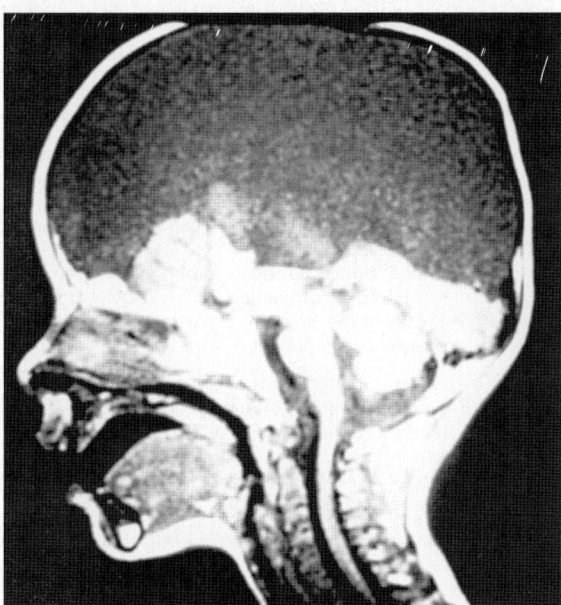

Figure 591-15 Hydranencephaly. MRI scan showing the brainstem and spinal cord with remnants of the cerebellum and the cerebral cortex. The remainder of the cranium is filled with cerebrospinal fluid.

The cause of hydranencephaly is unknown, but bilateral occlusion of the internal carotid arteries during early fetal development would explain most of the pathologic abnormalities. Affected infants can have a normal or enlarged head circumference at birth that grows at an excessive rate postnatally. Transillumination shows an absence of the cerebral hemispheres. The child is irritable, feeds poorly, develops seizures and spastic quadriparesis, and has little or no cognitive development. A ventriculoperitoneal shunt prevents massive enlargement of the cranium.

TREATMENT

Therapy for hydrocephalus depends on the cause. Medical management, including the use of acetazolamide and furosemide, can provide temporary relief by reducing the rate of CSF production, but long-term results have been disappointing. Most cases of hydrocephalus require extracranial shunts, particularly a ventriculoperitoneal shunt. Endoscopic third ventriculostomy has evolved as a viable approach and criteria have been developed for its use, but the procedure might need to be repeated to be effective. Ventricular shunting may be avoided with this approach. The major complications of shunting are occlusion (characterized by headache, papilledema, emesis, mental status changes) and bacterial infection (fever, headache, meningismus), usually caused by *Staphylococcus epidermidis*. With meticulous preparation, the shunt infection rate can be reduced to <5%. The results of intrauterine surgical management of fetal hydrocephalus have been poor (possibly because of the high rate of associated cerebral malformations in addition to the hydrocephalus) except for some promise in cases of hydrocephalus associated with fetal meningomyelocele.

PROGNOSIS

Prognosis depends on the cause of the dilated ventricles and not on the size of the cortical mantle at the time of operative intervention, except in cases in which the cortical mantle has been severely compressed and stretched. Hydrocephalic children are at increased risk for various developmental disabilities. The mean intelligence quotient is reduced compared with the general population, particularly for performance tasks as compared with verbal abilities. Many children have abnormalities in memory function. Vision problems are common, including strabismus, visuospatial abnormalities, visual field defects, and optic atrophy with decreased acuity secondary to increased ICP. The visual evoked potential latencies are delayed and take some time to recover after correction of the hydrocephalus. Although most hydrocephalic children are pleasant and mild mannered, some children show aggressive and delinquent behavior. Accelerated pubertal development in patients with shunted hydrocephalus or myelomeningocele is relatively common, possibly because of increased gonadotropin secretion in response to increased ICP. It is imperative that hydrocephalic children receive long-term follow-up in a multidisciplinary setting.

Bibliography is available at Expert Consult.

591.12 Craniosynostosis
Stephen L. Kinsman and Michael V. Johnston

Craniosynostosis is defined as premature closure of the cranial sutures and is classified as primary or secondary. It is associated with varying types of abnormal skull shape. Primary craniosynostosis refers to closure of 1 or more sutures owing to abnormalities of skull development, whereas secondary craniosynostosis results from failure of brain growth and expansion and is not discussed here. The incidence of primary craniosynostosis approximates 1 in 2,000 live births. The cause is unknown in the majority of children; however, genetic syndromes account for 10-20% of cases. Deformational forces appear important in occipital and frontal plagiocephaly in many cases. Early detection of posterior skull shape is critical and allows successful intervention to be offered in the form of physical therapy for torticollis and other positional asymmetries that lead to plagiocephaly.

DEVELOPMENT AND ETIOLOGY

The bones of the cranium are well developed by the 5th mo of gestation (frontal, parietal, temporal, and occipital) and are separated by sutures and fontanels. The brain grows rapidly in the 1st several yr of life and is normally not impeded because of equivalent growth along the suture lines. The cause of craniosynostosis is unknown, but the prevailing hypothesis suggests that abnormal development of the base of the skull creates exaggerated forces on the dura that act to disrupt normal cranial suture development. Genetic factors have been identified for some isolated and for many syndromic causes of craniosynostosis (Table 591-5).

Table 591-5	Commonly Used Clinical Genetic Classifications of Craniosynostoses
DISORDER	**CAUSE**
ISOLATED CRANIOSYNOSTOSIS	
Morphologically described	Unknown, uterine constraint, or *FGFR3* mutation
SYNDROMIC CRANIOSYNOSTOSIS	
Antler-Bixler syndrome	Unknown
Apert syndrome	Usually 1 of 2 mutations in *FGFR2*
Beare-Stevenson syndrome	Mutation in *GFGR2* or *FGFR3*
Baller-Gerold syndrome	Mutation in *TWIST* heterogenous
Carpenter syndrome	Unknown
Craniofrontonasal dysplasia	Unknown gene at *Xp22*
Crouzon syndrome	Numerous different mutations at *FGFR2*
Crouzonomesodermoskeletal syndrome	Mutation in *FGFR3*
Jackson-Weiss syndrome	Mutation in *FGFR2*
Muenke syndrome	Mutation in *FGFR3*
Pfeiffer syndrome	Mutation in *FGFR1* or numerous mutation in *FGFR2*
Saethre-Chotzen syndrome	Mutation in *TWIST*
Shprintzen-Goldberg syndrome	Mutation in *FBEN1*

From Ridgway EB, Weiner HL: Skull deformities, Pediatr Clin North Am 51:359–387, 2004.

CLINICAL MANIFESTATIONS AND TREATMENT

Most cases of craniosynostosis are evident at birth and are characterized by a skull deformity that is a direct result of premature suture fusion. Palpation of the suture reveals a prominent bony ridge, and fusion of the suture may be confirmed by plain skull roentgenograms, CT scan, or bone scan in ambiguous cases (Table 591-6).

Premature closure of the sagittal suture produces a long and narrow skull, or **scaphocephaly,** the most common form of craniosynostosis. Scaphocephaly is associated with a prominent occiput, a broad forehead, and a small or absent anterior fontanel. The condition is sporadic, is more common in males, and often causes difficulties during labor because of cephalopelvic disproportion. Scaphocephaly does not produce increased ICP or hydrocephalus, and results of neurologic examination of affected patients are normal.

Frontal plagiocephaly is the next most common form of craniosynostosis and is characterized by unilateral flattening of the forehead, elevation of the ipsilateral orbit and eyebrow, and a prominent ear on the corresponding side. The condition is more common in females and is the result of premature fusion of a coronal and sphenofrontal suture. Surgical intervention produces a cosmetically pleasing result. When imaging does not reveal a closed suture, positional factors are of primary importance.

Occipital plagiocephaly is most often a result of positioning during infancy and is more common in an immobile child or a child with a disability, but fusion or sclerosis of the lambdoid suture can cause unilateral occipital flattening and bulging of the ipsilateral frontal bone. **Trigonocephaly** is a rare form of craniosynostosis caused by premature fusion of the metopic suture. These children have a keel-shaped forehead and hypotelorism and are at risk for associated developmental abnormalities of the forebrain. Milder forms of metopic ridging are more common. **Turricephaly** refers to a cone-shaped head from premature fusion of the coronal, and often sphenofrontal and frontoethmoidal, sutures. The **kleeblattschädel deformity** is a peculiarly shaped skull that resembles a cloverleaf. Affected children have very prominent temporal bones, and the remainder of the cranium is constricted. Hydrocephalus is a common complication.

Premature fusion of only 1 suture rarely causes a neurologic deficit. In this situation, the sole indication for surgery is to enhance the child's cosmetic appearance, and the prognosis depends on the suture involved

Table 591-6	Epidemiology and Clinical Characteristics of the Common Craniosynostoses		
TYPE	**EPIDEMIOLOGY**	**SKULL DEFORMITY**	**CLINICAL PRESENTATION**
Sagittal	Most common CSO affecting a single suture, 80% male	Dolicocephaly or scaphocephaly (boat-shaped)	Frontal bossing, prominent occiput, palpable keel ridge. OFC normal and reduced biparietal diameter
Coronal	18% of CSO, more common in girls. Associated with Apert syndrome (with syndactyly) and Crouzon disease, which includes abnormal sphenoid, orbital, and facial bones (hypoplasia of the midface)	Unilateral: plagiocephaly. Bilateral: brachycephaly, acrocephaly	Unilateral: flattened forehead on affected side, flat checks, nose deviation on normal side; higher supraorbital margin leading to harlequin sign on radiograph and outward rotation of orbit can result in amblyopia. Bilateral: broad, flattened forehead. In Apert syndrome accompanied by syndactyly and in Crouzon disease by hypoplasia of the midface and progressive proptosis
Lambdoid	10-20% of CSO, M:F ratio 4:1	Lambdoid/occipital plagiocephaly; right side affected in 70% of cases	Unilateral: flattening of occiput, indentation along synostotic suture, bulging of ipsilateral forehead leading to rhomboid skull, ipsilateral ear is anterior and inferior. Bilateral: brachycephaly with bilateral anteriorly and inferiorly displaced ears
Metopic	Association with 19p chromosome abnormality	Trigonocephaly	Pointed forehead and midline ridge, hypotelorism
Multiple		Oxycephaly	Tower skull with undeveloped sinuses and shallow orbits, and elevated intercranial pressure

CSO, craniosynostosis; OFC, occipital-frontal circumference.
From Ridgway EB, Weiner HL: Skull deformities, Pediatr Clin North Am 51:359–387, 2004.

and on the degree of disfigurement. Neurologic complications, including hydrocephalus and increased ICP, are more likely to occur when 2 or more sutures are prematurely fused, in which case operative intervention is essential. The role of early repositioning efforts and therapy for torticollis and the use of cranial molding devices are beyond the scope of this review.

The most prevalent genetic disorders associated with craniosynostosis include Crouzon, Apert, Carpenter, Chotzen, and Pfeiffer syndromes. Crouzon syndrome is characterized by premature craniosynostosis and is inherited as an autosomal dominant trait. The shape of the head depends on the timing and order of suture fusion but most often is a compressed back-to-front diameter or brachycephaly resulting from bilateral closure of the coronal sutures. The orbits are underdeveloped, and ocular proptosis is prominent. Hypoplasia of the maxilla and orbital hypertelorism are typical facial features.

Apert syndrome has many features in common with Crouzon syndrome. Apert syndrome is usually a sporadic condition, although autosomal dominant inheritance can occur. It is associated with premature fusion of multiple sutures, including the coronal, sagittal, squamosal, and lambdoid sutures. The facies tend to be asymmetric, and the eyes are less proptotic than in Crouzon syndrome. Apert syndrome is characterized by syndactyly of the 2nd, 3rd, and 4th fingers, which may be joined to the thumb and the 5th finger. Similar abnormalities often occur in the feet. All patients have progressive calcification and fusion of the bones of the hands, feet, and cervical spine.

Carpenter syndrome is inherited as an autosomal recessive condition, and the many fusions of sutures tend to produce the kleeblattschädel skull deformity. Soft tissue syndactyly of the hands and feet is always present, and intellectual disability is common. Additional but less common abnormalities include congenital heart disease, corneal opacities, coxa valga, and genu valgum.

Chotzen syndrome is characterized by asymmetric craniosynostosis and plagiocephaly. The condition is the most prevalent of the genetic syndromes and is inherited as an autosomal dominant trait. It is associated with facial asymmetry, ptosis of the eyelids, shortened fingers, and soft tissue syndactyly of the 2nd and 3rd fingers.

Pfeiffer syndrome is most often associated with turricephaly. The eyes are prominent and widely spaced, and the thumbs and great toes are short and broad. Partial soft-tissue syndactyly may be evident. Most cases appear to be sporadic, but autosomal dominant inheritance has been reported.

Mutations of the fibroblast growth factor receptor (FGFR) gene family have been shown to be associated with phenotypically specific types of craniosynostosis. Mutations of the *FGFR1* gene located on chromosome 8 result in Pfeiffer syndrome; a similar mutation of the *FGFR2* gene causes Apert syndrome. Identical mutations of the *FGFR2* gene can result in both Pfeiffer and Crouzon phenotypes.

Each of the genetic syndromes poses a risk of additional anomalies, including hydrocephalus, increased ICP, papilledema, optic atrophy resulting from abnormalities of the optic foramina, respiratory problems secondary to a deviated nasal septum or choanal atresia, and disorders of speech and deafness. Craniectomy is mandatory for management of increased ICP, and a multidisciplinary craniofacial team is essential for the long-term follow-up of affected children. Craniosynostosis may be surgically corrected with good outcomes and relatively low morbidity and mortality, especially for nonsyndromic infants.

Bibliography is available at Expert Consult.

Chapter 592
Deformational Plagiocephaly
René P. Myers, Aubrey N. Duncan, and John A. Girotto

Deformational plagiocephaly (DP), also known as positional plagiocephaly, is the development of cranial flattening and asymmetry in the infant *as a result of extrinsic molding forces placed on the skull, such as consistently sleeping on the same area of the head.* Since the suggestion to place sleeping infants on their backs to sleep for the prevention of the **sudden infant death syndrome**, the incidence of DP has risen dramatically, and this has caused concern for parents and clinicians in the primary care setting.

EPIDEMIOLOGY AND ETIOLOGY
Incidence
The incidence is frequent at 6 wk of age (16%), greatest at 4 mo of age (up to 20%), and then decreases over the next 3 yr (7% at 12 mo and 3.3% at 24 mo). It generally resolves completely by 2-3 yr of age. The American Academy of Pediatrics started a campaign in the 1990s that resulted in the recommendation to place infants on their backs or sides while sleeping, which resulted in a 40% decrease in sudden infant death syndrome cases. Within 4 yr, craniofacial centers and primary care offices reported a 600% increase in referrals for plagiocephaly, which was previously reported to be approximately 1 in 300 infants. This may be a result of increasing awareness or early referral, as point prevalence has not changed in the past 40 yr.

Infants cannot reposition their heads in the 1st few wk of life and are not able to hold their own heads up until about 4 mo of age. It is for this reason that DP is most severe around 4 mo of age. It is also during this time that an infant's head circumference is rapidly increasing: about 2 cm/month in the 1st 3 mo, 1 cm/month from 4-6 mo of age, and 0.5 cm/month after 6 mo of age. Around 6 mo of age, an infant has developed head control, and this ability to actively reposition their own head allows for the gradual improvement of the cranial shape because of pressure offloading and continued brain growth.

Risk Factors
Congenital torticollis, positional preference when sleeping, and lower levels of activity are especially prominent in patients with DP. Table 592-1 delineates other risk factors. Many of these risk factors cannot be prevented, but sleeping supine with the head always turned to the same side has been found to predict DP independent of the other factors, and this *can* be prevented. There may be an association between developmental delay and DP. Although not causal, studies have found significant differences in gross motor development such as sitting up, crawling, and rolling back to side, between babies with and without DP.

Table 592-1	Factors That Increase Risk for Deformational Plagiocephaly

Male
Firstborn child
Limited passive neck rotation at birth (e.g., congenital torticollis)
Developmental delay
Sleep position is supine at birth and at 6 weeks
Bottle feeding only
Tummy time <3 times/day
Lower activity level, slower milestone achievement
Sleeping with head to same side, positional preference

Causes

Prenatal causes of DP include uterine compression and intrauterine constraint, such as occurs with oligohydramnios or multifetus gestation. Postnatal causes of DP include infant sleeping position and congenital muscular torticollis.

Muscular torticollis is a condition that is present in as many as 1 in 6 newborns and causes continuous tightening of muscles in the neck preventing passive rotation. It is thought that this condition typically precedes the development of cranial deformity. However, head position preference may result from cervical asymmetry that leads to torticollis and later flattening of a side of the skull from acquired positional preference (see Chapter 680.1).

Sleeping position plays a major role in the incidence of DP. When an infant continuously sleeps with the same part of the skull resting on a flat surface, a continuous force is placed in this area. During this time of rapid skull development, the growth is inhibited at the area where it rests on a hard surface, causing a "flat spot." Because of this inhibition, growth is increased in opposite directions causing a deformation that can be distinguished from other types of plagiocephaly.

EXAMINATION AND DIFFERENTIATING BETWEEN DEFORMATIONAL PLAGIOCEPHALY AND CRANIOSYNOSTOSIS

Abnormal head shape in an infant is distressing for parents. DP is a clinical diagnosis. Management also requires accurate counseling about its cause and treatment. It is especially important to be able to rule out **craniosynostosis** as a primary cause for cranial asymmetry in infants, as management of this condition is very different from that of DP and requires immediate referral to a craniofacial surgeon for evaluation (see Chapter 591.12). Craniosynostosis occurs in approximately 1 in 2,000 live births and results in plagiocephaly as a consequence of the early closure of skull sutures. Craniosynostosis must be distinguished from DP because the management is different. Lambdoidal craniosynostosis, although extremely rare (1 in 300,000 live births), presents with features most similar to those of DP. It can be distinguished from DP by a variety of historical and physical findings. Bilateral coronal synostosis also presents very similarly to posterior DP.

History and Physical Exam

Tables 592-2 and 592-3 outline the key components of history and physical examination.

Observation of the cranial shape as well as ear displacement are the first steps. It is critical to observe the child anteriorly, laterally, and from a vertex view. When cranial shape is viewed from above, DP typically looks like a **parallelogram**, and the ear on the same side of the flat or bald spot is **displaced anteriorly**. In lambdoidal craniosynostosis, the head has a trapezoid shape and the ear on the same side as the flat spot is posteriorly displaced (Fig. 592-1).

Palpation will help to differentiate these 2 conditions. Craniosynostosis presents with palpable ridges along the suture, whereas DP does not. Additionally, patients with craniosynostosis will not have mobile calvarial bones. This can be tested by applying gentle pressure on 2

Table 592-2	Important Historical and Physical Factors in the Evaluation of a Patient with Plagiocephaly	
	DEFORMATIONAL	**SYNOSTOTIC**
Birth history	• Intrauterine compression • Firstborn child	• Typically no complications
Head shape at birth	• Typically normal	• Can be irregular
Age first noticed shape irregularity	• Usually in 1st few mo of life	• Can be at birth
How patient prefers to sleep	• Same side, same position • Same even during naps	• Variable
Bald spot	• Yes	• No
Motor development for age	• If age atypical for deformational plagiocephaly, typically slow motor development for age • Torticollis present • History of limited activity or mobility	• Varies depending on presence of concomitant syndrome
Tummy time	• Decreased	• Suggested time
Signs/symptoms of increasing intracranial pressure	• No	• Possible

Table 592-3	Key Differences Between Synostotic (Craniosynostosis) and Deformational Plagiocephaly	
	DEFORMATIONAL PLAGIOCEPHALY	**CRANIOSYNOSTOSIS**
Causes	External forces applied to the skull • Prenatal: uterine compression, intrauterine constrained • Postnatal: congenital torticollis, sleeping position	Premature fusion of 1 or more cranial sutures
Common types	• Lateral • Posterior	• Bilateral coronal • Sagittal • Metopic
Common distinguishing features	• Normal round head shape at birth • Parallelogram shape to head • Ipsilateral ear anteriorly displaced • No palpable bony ridges	• Can have abnormal head shape at birth • Trapezoid shape to head • Ipsilateral ear posteriorly displaced • Palpable bony ridges
Management	• Repositioning • Physical therapy • Helmet in some cases	• Surgery • Helmet in some cases

Adapted from Nield LS, Brunner MD, Kamat D: The infant with a misshapen head. Clin Pediatr (Phila) 46:292–298, 2007, Tables 1 and 2.

Figure 592-1 Differentiating physical findings between deformational plagiocephaly and craniosynostosis. Vertex views. **A,** Right-sided deformational plagiocephaly exhibiting a parallelogram head shape. **B,** Right-sided lambdoid craniosynostosis exhibiting a trapezoid-like head shape. *(From Lin AY, Losee JE: Pediatric plastic surgery. In Zitelli BJ, McIntire SC, Norwalk AJ, editors: Zitelli and Davis' atlas of pediatric physical diagnosis, ed 6, Philadelphia, 2012, Elsevier, Fig. 22-5.)*

Positional molding   Unilateral lambdoid synostosis

Contralateral occipital bossing   Flattening   Ipsilateral ear displaced anteriorly

Parietal bossing   Flattening   Ipsilateral ear displaced posteriorly (variable)   Ipsilateral occipitomastoid bossing

A   B

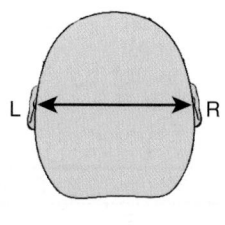
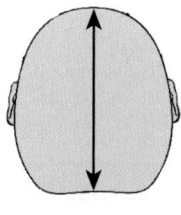
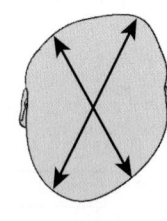

Figure 592-2 Cranial measurements. *(Modified from Looman WS, Flannery AB: Evidence-based care of the child with deformational plagiocephaly, part I: assessment and diagnosis. J Pediatr Health Care 26:242–250, 2012, Table 1.)*

L ⟷ R

Width   Length   Transcranial diagonal difference

adjacent skull bones separated by a suspected synostotic suture. If the plates do not move relative to each other, then the suspicion for craniosynostosis is raised.

Verifying neck muscle tone and range of motion is a key part of the exam because it helps in evaluating motor development and in diagnosing congenital torticollis. Resistance to passive motion raises the concern for torticollis. Decreased tone should prompt further evaluation of motor development. Infants do not gain the muscle control to turn or lift their heads until approximately 4 mo of age, and delays in motor development could increase the infant's risk of DP at later ages than those at which it usually occurs. Decreased range of motion can also be seen in cervical spine abnormalities, although this is rare. Early recognition of these conditions is critical in treatment, management, and outcome.

Accurate and consistent measurements will help to distinguish etiologies and manage infants presenting with an abnormal-shape skull. Along with the usual head circumference measurements, the clinician should also measure cranial width, length, and transcranial diameter (as shown in Figure 592-2), which are best performed with calipers. These measurements allow the clinician to diagnose, determine severity, and monitor the plagiocephaly.

◆ *Cranial length:* Distance from the most prominent point between the eyebrows to the most prominent point of the occiput
◆ *Width:* Maximum transverse diameter, horizontal
◆ *Cephalic index* (cranial index): Ratio of the cranial width to the cranial length
◆ *Occipital-frontal transcranial diameter:* Find the points on either side of the head where the deformation is the worst (2 on the right, 2 on the left), then measure the **diagonal distances** between these points
◆ *Transdiagonal difference* (transcranial diagonal difference): The difference between 2 transcranial diameters

◆ *Cranial vault asymmetry:* Ratio of oblique measurements. This is difficult to implement because different physicians and authors propose varying points to use for these measurements

One technology for the evaluation of the severity and improvement over time of DP is the 3-dimensional photographic system. Advantages of this system include an easy and comfortable ability to image in an unbiased manner. Similarly, the use of laser scanners for the prefabrication scans for helmets is frequently employed by orthotists.

After observations and measurements the clinician can determine the type and severity of the DP (Table 592-4 and Fig. 592-3). For *lateral DP*, bossing of the occiput occurs opposite the flattened deformity and the ear on the same side as the flat area can be anteriorly displaced. This type of DP is typically associated with infants who have torticollis or a head position preference to 1 side. Transdiagonal diameter is typically abnormal in this type of plagiocephaly, and this measurement is the gold standard for determining severity.

In *posterior DP*, the occiput is uniformly flattened, temporal bossing can occur, and the ears are normal. It is usually associated with large head size and a history of limited activity or mobility. Cephalic index is increased with posterior DP.

Time and accurate exam records can help in management. If deformation is worsening when DP typically begins to demonstrate improving head shape, craniosynostosis should be suspected.

TREATMENT
Prevention

Sleep position should be monitored and varied. Alternating the infant's head to face the head and foot of the crib on alternate nights will allow the infant to sleep facing into the room without always lying on the same side of the head. Consistently alternating sleeping position early on allows the infant to have equal time on both sides of the occiput, and this will become a pattern the infant is used to. Infants who have

Table 592-4	Diagnostic Guide for Determining Type and Severity of Lateral and Posterior Deformational Plagiocephaly	

TYPE

CLINICAL FINDINGS	LATERAL DEFORMATIONAL PLAGIOCEPHALY	POSTERIOR DEFORMATIONAL PLAGIOCEPHALY (BRACHYCEPHALY)
Occiput (vertex view)	Ipsilateral occipital flattening; contralateral occipital bossing	Uniform occipital flattening
Ear position (vertex view)	Ipsilateral ear may be anteriorly displaced	Normal
Face, forehead (anterior, lateral, and vertex views)	May be normal; more-severe cases may present with the following: mandibular asymmetry, ipsilateral frontal bossing, contralateral forehead flattening, ipsilateral cheek anteriorly displaced	Temporal bossing, increase in vertical height in severe cases
Other	Torticollis, head position preference	Large size, history of limited activity or limited mobility

SEVERITY

		LATERAL DEFORMATIONAL PLAGIOCEPHALY		POSTERIOR DEFORMATIONAL PLAGIOCEPHALY (BRACHYCEPHALY)	
Mild	TDD 3-10 mm	Type I	Flattening restricted to the back of the skull	CI: 0.82-0.9	Central posterior deformity ("ping-pong ball depression")
Moderate	TDD 10-12 mm	Type II	Malposition of ear	CI: 0.9-1.0	Central posterior deformity and widening of posterior skull
		Type III	Forehead deformity		
Severe	TDD >12 mm	Type IV	Malar deformity	CI: >1.0	Vertical head, head growth, or temporal bossing
		Type V	Vertical or temporal skull growth		

CI, cephalic index (cranial index); TDD, transcranial diameter difference.

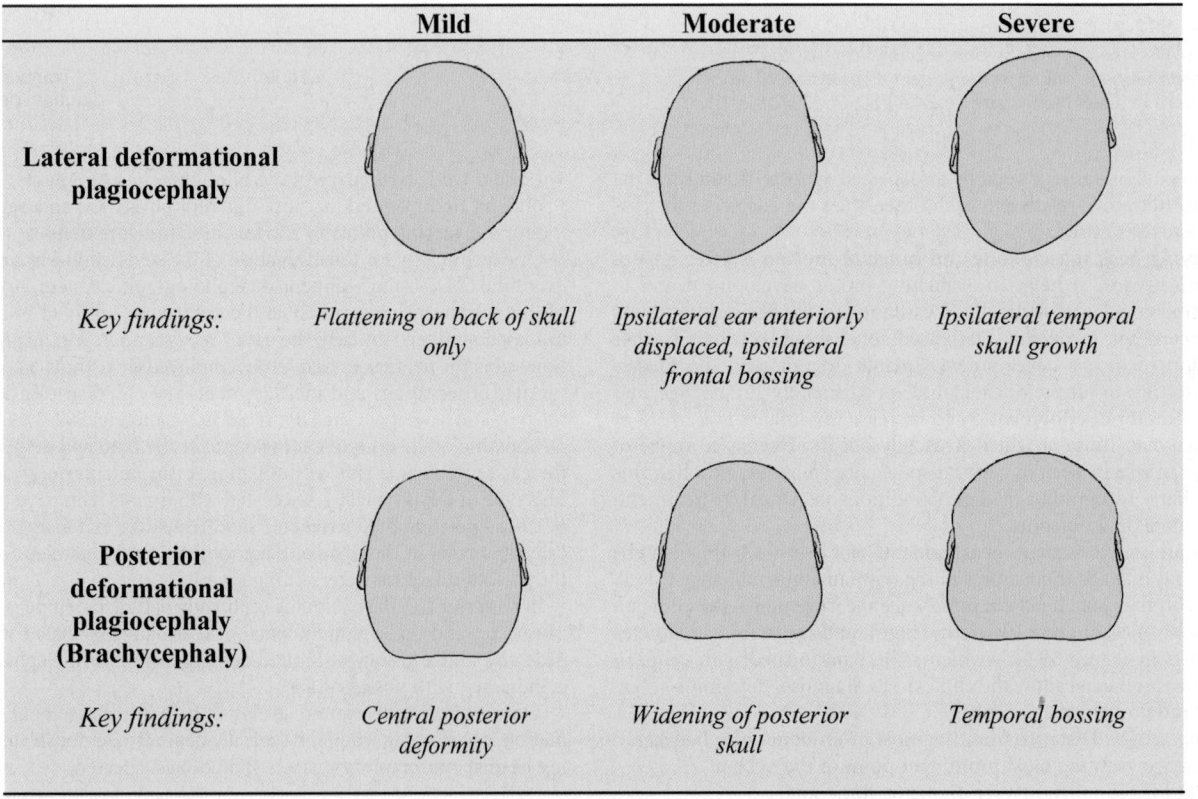

Figure 592-3 Types of deformational plagiocephaly. *(From Looman WS, Flannery AB: Evidence-based care of the child with deformational plagiocephaly, part I: assessment and diagnosis. J Pediatr Health Care 26:242–250, 2012, Fig. 1.)*

an obvious positional preference to a particular side will take more time and effort in purposefully repositioning them counter to their preference. Parents must be counseled in the benefit of this strategy in preventing bald spots or flat spots that can progress to cranial deformity.

"Tummy time" is the term used to describe the infant's awake time spent lying on their stomach. The suggested amount of tummy time is **10-15 minutes at least 3 times a day**. Reassure parents that sleep is the only time during which the prone position should be avoided, and educate the parents as to the benefits for the infant of awake prone positioning to help progression of motor development.

Treatment Options
Cranial asymmetry from DP does not usually spontaneously improve, nor do the more-severe manifestations of facial and ear asymmetry disappear. Once a flat spot develops, it is unlikely that the infant will be able to overcome the pull to lie on the same spot in time to allow for reversal of the asymmetry.

"Watch-and-wait" management is not recommended in infants with DP. Evidence suggests that, at a minimum, repositioning and physiotherapy should be initiated as soon as asymmetry is observed.

Repositioning and physiotherapy (RPPT) include the counseling and teaching for parents as to positional changes and tummy time in their child as well as referral to physical therapy in the case of congenital torticollis. RPPT is the optimal treatment choice for patients younger than 4 mo of age who have mild or moderately severe DP. The earliest types of behavioral modifications can be as simple as increasing tummy time, or repositioning the infant's crib such that everything interesting in the room is on the side opposite the DP.

Molding therapy (helmet therapy) is the use of an orthotic helmet to promote the resolution of cranial asymmetry while the infant's head is still rapidly growing. Orthotic helmets do not actively mold the skull; rather, they protect the areas that are flat and allow the child to "grow into" the flat spot. Studies have shown helmet therapy to achieve correction 3 times faster and better than repositioning alone. This therapy is still debated because of its expense, time requirements, coverage and side effects (irritation, rashes, and pressure sores). The most recent studies suggest that combined treatment with helmet therapy and RPPT is the most beneficial management of infants older than 4 mo with severe DP or with worsening of mild/moderate DP trialed on RPPT. Infants with severe DP should be considered for helmet therapy at any age.

Studies suggest helmet therapy should be started for significant DP between 4 and 8 mo and continued for 7-8 mo. Parents should be counseled on the commitment involved in this treatment as helmets need to be worn more than 20 hr a day.

Patients with craniosynostosis require surgery. Sometimes, a molding helmet can be used as an adjunctive therapy after surgery but never as monotherapy.

OUTCOMES
Outcomes may be better when helmet therapy is started before 6 mo of age, and infants starting therapy later than that do not achieve the same degree of normal head measurements as those whose helmet therapy is started before 6 mo of age do. Significant improvements in asymmetry are usually obvious at 4-11 wk after initiation of helmet therapy.

Studies in patients with a median follow-up age of 9 yr old found that 75% of cases had a what both parents and patients considered to be a normal head appearance. Nine percent of patients and 4% of parents noted residual asymmetry that they considered significant.

Cognitive and academic outcomes may be different depending on the side of deformity. Poorer academic performance and greater speech abnormalities were found in patients with left-sided deformities compared to those with right-sided deformities. This manifested as double the number of patients with expressive speech abnormalities and triple the number of special education needs. It is unclear what the underlying mechanism is; treatment differences were apparently not a factor. In general, children with DP and without comorbid conditions are usually developmentally normal, healthy children. This is in contrast to craniosynostosis, in which increases in intracranial pressure may have deleterious effects on central nervous system function.

Bibliography is available at Expert Consult.

Chapter 593
Seizures in Childhood
Mohamad A. Mikati and Abeer J. Hani

A seizure is a transient occurrence of signs and/or symptoms resulting from abnormal excessive or synchronous neuronal activity in the brain. The International Classification of Epileptic Seizures divides epileptic seizures into 2 large categories: In focal (formerly known as partial) seizures, the first clinical and electroencephalographic (EEG) changes suggest initial activation of a system of neurons limited to part of 1 cerebral hemisphere. The term *simple partial seizures* is an outdated classification that refers to focal seizures with no alteration in consciousness whereas complex partial seizures, currently also referred to as focal dyscognitive, denote focal seizures with altered awareness of the surroundings. In generalized seizures, the first clinical and EEG changes indicate synchronous involvement of all of both hemispheres (Table 593-1). Approximately 30% of patients who have a first afebrile seizure have later epilepsy; the risk is approximately 20% if neurologic exam, EEG, and neuroimaging are normal. Febrile seizures are a separate category. Acute symptomatic seizures occur secondary to an acute problem affecting brain excitability such as electrolyte imbalance. Most children with these types of seizures do well. However, sometimes these seizures signify major structural, inflammatory, or metabolic disorders of the brain, such as meningitis, encephalitis, acute stroke, or brain tumor. Consequently, the prognosis depends on the underlying disorder, including its reversibility or treatability and the likelihood of developing epilepsy from it. An unprovoked seizure is one that is not an acute symptomatic seizure. Remote symptomatic seizure is one that is considered to be secondary to a distant brain injury, such as an old stroke. Reflex seizures are usually precipitated by a sensory stimulus such as flashing lights (see Chapter 593.9).

Epilepsy is a disorder of the brain characterized by an enduring predisposition to generate seizures and by the neurobiologic, cognitive, psychologic, and social consequences of this condition. The clinical diagnosis of epilepsy usually requires the occurrence of at least 1 unprovoked epileptic seizure with either a second such seizure or enough EEG and clinical information to convincingly demonstrate an enduring predisposition to develop recurrences. For epidemiologic and commonly for clinical purposes, epilepsy is considered to be present when 2 or more unprovoked seizures occur in a time frame of longer than 24 hr. Approximately 4-10% of children experience at least 1 seizure (febrile or afebrile) in the 1st 16 yr of life. The cumulative lifetime incidence of epilepsy is 3%, and more than half of the cases start in childhood. The annual prevalence is 0.5-1.0%. Thus, the occurrence of a single seizure or of febrile seizures does not necessarily imply the diagnosis of epilepsy. Seizure disorder is a general term that is usually used to include any 1 of several disorders, including epilepsy, febrile seizures, and possibly single seizures and symptomatic seizures secondary to metabolic, infectious, or other etiologies (e.g., hypocalcemia, meningitis).

An epileptic syndrome is a disorder that manifests 1 or more specific seizure types and has a specific age of onset and a specific prognosis. Several types of epileptic syndromes can be distinguished

Table 593-1	Types of Epileptic Seizures

SELF-LIMITED SEIZURE TYPES
Focal Seizures
Focal sensory seizures
- With elementary sensory symptoms (e.g., occipital and parietal lobe seizures)
- With experiential sensory symptoms (e.g., temporoparietooccipital junction seizures)

Focal motor seizures
- With elementary clonic motor signs
- With asymmetrical tonic motor seizures (e.g., supplementary motor seizures)
- With typical (temporal lobe) automatisms (e.g., mesial temporal lobe seizures)
- With hyperkinetic automatisms
- With focal negative myoclonus
- With inhibitory motor seizures

Gelastic seizures
Hemiclonic seizures
Secondarily generalized seizures
Reflex seizures in focal epilepsy syndromes
Generalized Seizures
Tonic-clonic seizures (includes variations beginning with a clonic or myoclonic phase)
Clonic seizures
- Without tonic features
- With tonic features

Typical absence seizures
Atypical absence seizures
Absence with special features:
- Eyelid myoclonia
- Myoclonic absence

Tonic seizures
Myoclonic seizures
Myoclonic atonic seizures
Negative myoclonus
Atonic seizures
Reflex seizures in generalized epilepsy syndromes
Unknown
Epileptic Spasms

CONTINUOUS SEIZURE TYPES
Generalized Status Epilepticus
Generalized tonic-clonic status epilepticus
Clonic status epilepticus
Absence status epilepticus
Tonic status epilepticus
Myoclonic status epilepticus
Focal Status Epilepticus
Epilepsia partialis continua of Kojevnikov
Aura continua
Limbic status epilepticus (psychomotor status)
Hemiconvulsive status with hemiparesis

PRECIPITATING STIMULI FOR REFLEX SEIZURES
Visual stimuli
- Flickering light—color to be specified when possible
- Patterns
- Other visual stimuli

Thinking
Music
Eating
Praxis
Somatosensory
Proprioceptive
Reading
Hot water
Startle

Modified from Berg AT, Berkovic SF, Brodie MJ et al: Revised terminology and concepts for organization of seizures and epilepsies: report of the ILAE Commission on Classification and Terminology, 2005–2009. Epilepsia 51(4):676–685, 2010.

(Tables 593-2 to 593-5). This classification has to be distinguished from the classification of epileptic seizures that refers to single events rather than to clinical syndromes. In general, seizure type is the primary determinant of the type of medications the patient is likely to respond to, and the epilepsy syndrome determines the type of prognosis one could expect. An **epileptic encephalopathy** is an epilepsy syndrome in which there is a severe EEG abnormality which is thought to result in cognitive and other impairments in the patient. **Idiopathic epilepsy** is an older term that refers to an epilepsy syndrome that is genetic or presumed genetic and in which there is no underlying disorder affecting development or other neurologic function (e.g., petit mal epilepsy). In the International League Against Epilepsy (ILAE) classification of etiology of epilepsy, idiopathic epilepsy was replaced by the term **genetic epilepsy**, which implies that the epilepsy syndrome is the direct result of a known or presumed genetic defect(s) in which the genetic defect is not causative of a brain structural or metabolic disorder other than the epilepsy. **Symptomatic epilepsy** is also an older term referring to an epilepsy syndrome caused by an underlying brain disorder that may or may not be genetic (e.g., epilepsy secondary to tuberous sclerosis or to an old stroke); this is referred to as **structural/metabolic epilepsy**, which would be caused by a distinct structural or metabolic entity that increases the risk for seizures and causes the epilepsy. The older terms of **cryptogenic epilepsy** or of presumed **symptomatic epilepsy** refer to an epilepsy syndrome in which there is a presumed underlying brain disorder causing the epilepsy and affecting neurologic function, but the underlying disorder is not known; this

is referred to as the **unknown epilepsy**, designating that the underlying cause of the epilepsy is as yet unknown.

EVALUATION OF THE FIRST SEIZURE
Initial evaluation of an infant or child during or shortly after a suspected seizure should include an assessment of the adequacy of the airway, ventilation, and cardiac function, as well as measurement of temperature, blood pressure, and glucose concentration. For acute evaluation of the first seizure, the physician should search for potentially life-threatening causes of seizures such as meningitis, systemic sepsis, unintentional or nonaccidental intentional head trauma, and ingestion of drugs of abuse or accidental ingestion of drugs or of other toxins. The history should attempt to define factors that might have promoted the convulsion and to provide a detailed description of the seizure and the child's postictal state (see Chapter 593.9). Most parents vividly recall their child's initial convulsion and can describe it in detail.

The subsequent step in an evaluation is to determine whether the seizure has a focal onset or is generalized. **Focal seizures** may be characterized by motor or sensory symptoms, which could include forceful turning of the head and eyes to 1 side, unilateral clonic movements beginning in the face or extremities, or a sensory disturbance, such as paresthesias or pain localized to a specific area. Focal seizures in an adolescent or adult usually indicate a localized lesion, whereas these seizures during childhood are often, but not always, secondary to a

Text continued on p. 2829

| Table 593-2 | Classification for Epilepsy Syndromes with an Indication of Age of Onset, Duration of Active Epilepsy, Prognosis, and Therapeutic Options |

SPECIFIC SYNDROMES	AGE AT ONSET	AGE AT REMISSION	PROGNOSIS	MONOTHERAPY OR ADD-ON*	POSSIBLE ADD-ON†	SURGERY†
EPILEPSIES OF UNKNOWN CAUSE OF INFANCY AND CHILDHOOD						
Benign infantile seizures (nonfamilial)	Infant	Infant	Good	PB	—	No
Benign childhood epilepsy with centrotemporal spikes	3-13 yr	16 yr	Good	CBZ, LEV, OXC, VPA	—	No
Early and late-onset idiopathic occipital epilepsy	2-8 yr; 6-17 yr	12 yr or younger; 18 yr	Good	CBZ, LEV, OXC, VPA	—	No
FAMILIAL (AUTOSOMAL DOMINANT) EPILEPSIES						
Benign familial neonatal convulsions	Newborn to young infant	Newborn to young infant	Good	PB	—	No
Benign familial infantile convulsions	Infant	Infant	Good	CBZ, PB	—	No
Autosomal dominant nocturnal frontal lobe epilepsy	Childhood		Variable	CBZ, GBP, OXC, PHT, TPM	CLB, LEV, PB, PHT	No
Familial lateral temporal lobe epilepsy	Childhood to adolescence		Variable	CBZ, GBP, OXC, PHT, TPM, VPA	CLB, LEV, PB, PHT	No
Generalized epilepsies with febrile seizures plus	Childhood to adolescence		Variable	ESM, LTG, TPM, VPA	CLB, LEV	No
STRUCTURAL–METABOLIC FOCAL EPILEPSIES						
Limbic Epilepsy						
Mesial temporal lobe epilepsy with hippocampal sclerosis	School-age or earlier	Long lasting	Variable	CBZ, LEV, OXC, TPM, VPA	CLB, GBP, LAC, PB, PHT, ZON	Temporal resection
Mesial temporal lobe epilepsy defined by specific causes	Variable	Long lasting	Variable	CBZ, LEV, OXC, TPM, VPA	CLB, GBP, LAC, PB, PHT, ZON	Temporal resection
Other types defined by location and causes	Variable	Long lasting	Variable	CBZ, LEV, OXC, TPM, VPA	CLB, FBM, GBP, LAC, PB, PHT, ZON	Lesionectomy ± temporal resection
Neocortical Epilepsies						
Rasmussen syndrome	6-12 yr	Progressive	Ominous	Plasmapheresis, immunoglobulins	CBZ, LAC, PB, PHT, TPM	Functional hemispherectomy
Hemiconvulsion-hemiplegia syndrome	1-5 yr	Chronic	Severe	CBZ, LEV, OXC, TPM, VPA	CLB, GBP, LAC, PB, PHT, ZON	Functional hemispherectomy
Other types defined by location and cause	Variable	Long lasting	Variable	CBZ, LEV, OXC, TPM, VPA	PHT, PB, CLB, GBP, LAC, ZON	Lesionectomy ± cortical resection
Migrating partial seizures of early infancy	Infant	No remission	Ominous	Bromides, CBZ, LEV, PB, PHT, TPM, VPA	BDZ, LAC, ZON	No
GENERALIZED EPILEPSIES OF UNKNOWN CAUSE						
Benign myoclonic epilepsy in infancy	3 mo-3 yr	3-5 yr	Variable	LEV, TPM, VPA	BDZ, ZON	No
Epilepsy with myoclonic astatic seizures	3-5 yr	Variable	Variable	ESM, TPM, VPA	BDZ, ketogenic diet, LEV, LTG, steroids, ZON	No
Childhood absence epilepsy	5-6 yr	10-12 yr	Good	ESM, LTG, VPA	Acetazolamide, ketogenic diet, ZON	No
Epilepsy with myoclonic absences	1-12 yr	Variable	Guarded	ESM, VPA	BDZ, ZON	No

*Reflects current trends in practice, which may be off-label and may not be FDA approved for that indication. See Table 593-10 for FDA indications.
†May apply to selected cases only. Vagus nerve stimulation has been used for all types of refractory seizures and epilepsy types.

ACTH, adrenocorticotropic hormone; BDZ, benzodiazepine; CBZ, carbamazepine; CLB, clobazam; DZP: diazepam; ESM, ethosuximide; FBM: felbamate; GBP, gabapentin; IVIG, intravenous immunoglobulin; LAC, lacosamide; LEV, levetiracetam; LTG, lamotrigine; n/a, not applicable; OXC: oxcarbazepine; PB, phenobarbital; PHT, phenytoin; PRM, primidone; RFD, rufinamide; TPM, topiramate; VGB: vigabatrin; VPA, valproic acid; ZON, zonisamide.

Continued

Table 593-2	Classification for Epilepsy Syndromes with an Indication of Age of Onset, Duration of Active Epilepsy, Prognosis, and Therapeutic Options—cont'd					
SPECIFIC SYNDROMES	**AGE AT ONSET**	**AGE AT REMISSION**	**PROGNOSIS**	**MONOTHERAPY OR ADD-ON***	**POSSIBLE ADD-ON†**	**SURGERY†**
GENERALIZED EPILEPSIES OF UNKNOWN CAUSE WITH VARIABLE PHENOTYPES						
Juvenile absence epilepsy	10-12 yr	Usually lifelong	Good	ESM, LTG, VPA	BDZ	No
Juvenile myoclonic epilepsy	12-18 yr	Usually lifelong	Good	LEV, TPM, VPA	BDZ, LTG, PB, PRM, ZON	No
Epilepsy with generalized tonic-clonic seizures only	12-18 yr	Usually lifelong	Good	LEV, LTG, TPM, VPA	BDZ, CBZ, ZON	No
REFLEX EPILEPSIES						
Idiopathic photosensitive occipital lobe epilepsy	10-12 yr	Unclear	Variable	VPA	BDZ, LEV, LTG, ZON	No
Other visual sensitive epilepsies	2-5 yr	Unclear	Variable	VPA	BDZ, LEV, LTG, ZON	No
Startle epilepsy	Variable	Long lasting	Guarded	CBZ, GBP, OXC, PHT, TPM, VPA	CLB, LEV, PB, PHT, ZON	Lesionectomy ± cortical resection in some
EPILEPTIC ENCEPHALOPATHIES						
Early myoclonic encephalopathy and Ohtahara syndrome	Newborn-infant	Poor, Ohtahara syndrome evolves into West syndrome	Ominous	PB, steroids, VGB	BDZ, ZON	No
West syndrome	Infant	Variable	Variable	ACTH, steroids, VGB	BDZ, FBM, IVIG, TPM, ZON	Lesionectomy ± cortical resection
Dravet syndrome (severe myoclonic epilepsy in infancy)	Infant	No remission	Severe	CLB, stiripentol, TPM, VPA	BDZ, ZON	No
Lennox-Gastaut syndrome	3-10 yr	No remission	Severe	CLB, LTG, RFD, TPM, VPA	BDZ, FBM, IVIG, steroids, ZON	Callosotomy
Landau-Kleffner syndrome	3-6 yr	8-12 yr	Guarded	LEV, nocturnal DZP, steroids, VPA	BDZ, ESM, IVIG, LTG	Multiple subpial transections, rarely lesionectomy
Epilepsy with continuous spike waves during slow-wave sleep	4-7 yr	8-12 yr	Guarded	LEV, nocturnal DZP, steroids, VPA	BDZ, ESM, IVIG, LTG	No
PROGRESSIVE MYOCLONUS EPILEPSIES						
Unverricht-Lundborg, Lafora, ceroid lipofuscinoses, etc.	Late infant to adolescent	Progressive	Ominous	TPM, VPA, ZON	BDZ, PB	No
OTHER EPILEPSIES AND SEIZURE DISORDERS OF UNKNOWN OR OTHER CAUSES						
Benign neonatal seizures	Newborn	Newborn	Good	LEV, PB	—	No
Febrile seizures	3-5 yr	3-6 yr	Good	PB or VPA if repeated and prolonged	—	No
Reflex seizures	Variable	n/a		LEV, VPA	LTG, ZON	No
Drug or other chemically induced seizures	Variable	n/a		Withdraw offending agent	—	No
Immediate and early posttraumatic seizures	Variable	n/a		LEV, PHT	—	No

Modified from Guerrini R: Epilepsy in children, Lancet 367:499–524, 2006; and Parisi P, Verrotti A, Paolino MC, et al. "Electro-clinical syndromes" with onset in the pediatric age group: the highlights of the clinical-EEG, genetic and therapeutic advances. Ital J Pediatr 37:58, 2011.

Table 593-3	Identified Genes for Epilepsy Syndromes*†

EPILEPSY TYPE	GENE	PROTEIN
INFANTILE ONSET		
Benign familial neonatal seizures	KCNQ2	Potassium voltage-gated channel
	KCNQ3	Potassium voltage-gated channel
Benign familial neonatal infantile seizures	SCN2A	Sodium channel protein type 2α
Early familial neonatal infantile seizures	SCN2A	Sodium channel protein type 2α
Early infantile epileptic encephalopathy (EIEE)	CDKL5 (EIEE2)	Cyclin-dependent kinase-like 5
	ARX (EIEE1)	Aristaless-related homeobox
	TSC1	Hamartin
	TSC2	Tuberin
	SCN1A (EIEE6)	Sodium channel protein type 1α
	PCDH19(EIEE9)	Protocadherin-19
	KCNQ2 (EIEE7)	Potassium voltage-gated channel
	STXBP1 (EIEE4)	Syntaxin binding protein 1
	SLC2A1	Solute carrier family 2, facilitated glucose transporter member 1
	ALDH7A1	α-Aminoadipic semialdehyde dehydrogenase (antiquitin)
	POLG	DNA polymerase subunit gamma-1
	SCN2A (EIEE11)	Sodium channel protein type 2α
	PLCβ1 (EIEE12)	Phospholipase C β1
	ATP6AP2	Renin receptor
	SPTAN1 (EIEE5)	α₂-Spectrin
	SLC25A22 (EIEE3)	Mitochondrial glutamate carrier 1
	PNPO	Pyridoxine-5′-phosphate oxidase
Generalized epilepsy with febrile seizures plus (early onset)	SCN1A	Sodium channel protein type 1α
	SCN1B	Sodium channel protein type 1β
	GABRG2	γ-Aminobutyric acid receptor subunit γ2
	SCN2A	Sodium channel protein type 1α
CHILDHOOD ONSET		
Childhood onset epileptic encephalopathies	SCN1A	Sodium channel protein type 1α
	PCDH19	Protocadherin-19
	SLC2A1	Solute carrier family 2, facilitated GTM1
	POLG	DNA polymerase subunit γ1
	SCN2A	Sodium channel protein type 2α
Early onset absence seizures, refractory epilepsy of multiple types at times with movement disorder	GLUT-1 deficiency syndrome, SLC2A1gene	Solute carrier family 2, facilitated GTM1
Generalized epilepsy with febrile seizure plus	SCN1A	Sodium channel protein type 1α
	SCN1B	Sodium channel protein type 1β
	GABRG2	γ-Aminobutyric acid receptor subunit γ2
	SCN2A	Sodium channel protein type 1α
Juvenile myoclonic epilepsy (more commonly presents in adolescence)	EFHC1	EF-hand domain-containing protein 1
	CACNB4	Voltage-dependent L-type calcium channel
	GABRA1	γ-Aminobutyric acid receptor subunit α1
Progressive myoclonic epilepsy (different forms present from infancy through adulthood)	EPM2A	Laforin
	NHLRC1	NHL repeat-containing protein 1 (Malin)
	CSTB	Cystatin-B
	PRICKLE1	Prickle-like protein 1
	PPT1, TPP1,CLN3, CLN5, CLN6, CLN8, CTSD, DNAJC5, MFSD8	Multiple proteins causing neuronal ceroid lipofuscinosis
Autosomal dominant nocturnal frontal lobe epilepsies (presents in childhood through adulthood)	CHRNA4	Neuronal acetylcholine receptor α4
	CHRNB2	Neuronal acetylcholine receptor β2
	CHRNA2	Neuronal acetylcholine receptor α2
ADOLESCENT ONSET		
Juvenile myoclonic epilepsy (JME)	See Childhood Onset JME	
Progressive myoclonic epilepsy (PME)	See Childhood Onset PME	
Autosomal dominant nocturnal frontal lobe epilepsies (AD-NFLE)	See Childhood Onset AD-NFLE	
Autosomal dominant lateral temporal lobe epilepsy (AD-LTLE)	See Childhood Onset AD-LTLE	
Autosomal dominant lateral temporal lobe epilepsy (usually presents in adulthood)	LGI1	Leucine-rich glioma-inactivated protein 1

*Note that the same gene (different mutations) often appears as causing different epilepsy syndromes.
†Most of these genes can be tested for through commercially available targeted single-gene sequencing or through commercially available gene panels or though exome sequencing (http://www.ncbi.nlm.nih.gov/sites/GeneTests/review?db=genetests).

Table 593-4	Identified Genes for Syndromic Epilepsy Syndromes*	
SYNDROME	**GENE**	**PROTEIN**
Rett/atypical Rett syndromes	MECP2	Methyl CpG binding protein 2
	CDKL5	Cyclin-dependent kinase-like 5
	FOXG1	Forkhead box protein G1
	MBD5	Methyl-CpG-binding domain protein 5
	MEF2C	Myocyte-specific enhancer factor 2C
Angelman/Angelman-like/Pitt-Hopkins syndromes	UBE3A	Ubiquitin protein ligase E3A
	SLC9A6	Sodium/hydrogen exchanger 6
	MBD5	Methyl-CpG-binding domain protein 5
	TCF4	Transcription factor 4
	NRXN1	Neurexin-1
	CNTNAP2	Contactin-associated protein-like 2
Mowat-Wilson syndrome	ZEB2	Zinc finger E-box-binding homeobox 2
Creatine deficiency syndromes	GAMT	Guanidinoacetate N-methyltransferase
	GATM	Glycine amidinotransferase, mitochondrial
Neuronal ceroid lipofuscinosis (NCL)	PPT1 (CLN1)	Palmitoyl-protein thioesterase 1
	TPP1 (CLN2)	Tripeptidyl-peptidase 1
	CLN3	Battenin
	CLN5	Ceroid-lipofuscinosis neuronal protein 5
	CLN6	Ceroid-lipofuscinosis neuronal protein 6
	MFSD8 (CLN7)	Major facilitator superfamily domain-containing protein 8
	CLN8	Ceroid-lipofuscinosis neuronal protein 8
	CTSD (CLN10)	Cathepsin D
	KCTD7 (CLN14)	BTB/POZ domain-containing protein KCTD7
Adenosuccinate lyase deficiency	ADSL	Adenylosuccinate lyase
Cerebral folate deficiency	FOLR1	Folate receptor alpha
Epilepsy with variable learning and behavioral disorders	GRIN2A	Glutamate receptor ionotropic, N-methyl-D-aspartate (NMDA) 2A
	SYN1	Synapsin-1
17q21.31 microdeletion syndrome	KANSL1	KAT8 regulatory nonspecific lethal (NSL) complex subunit 1
Microcephaly with early-onset intractable seizures and developmental delay (MCSZ)	PNKP	Bifunctional polynucleotide phosphatase/kinase

*Most of these genes can be tested for through commercially available targeted single-gene sequencing or through commercially available gene panels or though exome sequencing.

Table 593-5	Childhood Epileptic Syndromes with Generally Good Prognosis
SYNDROME	**COMMENT**
Benign neonatal familial convulsions	Dominant, may be severe and resistant for a few days Febrile or afebrile seizures (benign) occur later in a minority
Infantile familial convulsions	Dominant; seizures often in clusters
Febrile convulsions plus syndromes (see Table 593-2)	Febrile and afebrile generalized convulsions, absence and myoclonic seizures occur in different members. Seizures usually generalized (GEFS+) but in some families may be focal
Benign myoclonic epilepsy of infancy	Often seizures during sleep; 1 rare variety with reflex myoclonic seizures (touch, noise)
Partial idiopathic epilepsy with rolandic spikes (benign epilepsy with centrotemporal spikes)	Seizures with falling asleep or on awakening; focal sharp waves with centrotemporal location on EEG
Idiopathic occipital partial epilepsy	Early childhood form with seizures during sleep and ictal vomiting; can occur as status epilepticus Later form with occipital spikes that block on eye opening; migrainous symptoms and seizures; not always benign
Petit mal absence epilepsy	Cases with absences only; some have generalized seizures In most cases, absences disappear on therapy but there are resistant cases (unpredictable); 60-80% full remission
Juvenile myoclonic epilepsy	Adolescence onset, with early morning myoclonic seizures and generalized seizures during sleep or upon awakening; often history of absences in childhood

EEG, electroencephalogram; GEFS+, generalized epilepsy with febrile seizures plus.
Modified from Deonna T: Management of epilepsy, Arch Dis Child 90:5–9, 2005; and Seneviratne U: The prognosis of idiopathic generalized epilepsy, Epilepsia 53(12):2079–2090, 2012.

lesion or the result of a genetic, idiopathic, epilepsy. Focal seizures in a neonate may be seen because of focal lesions like perinatal stroke or because of a metabolic abnormality like hypocalcemia caused by immaturity of the brain connections. Focal and generalized motor seizures may be tonic–clonic, tonic, clonic, myoclonic, or atonic. **Tonic seizures** are characterized by increased tone or rigidity, and **atonic seizures** are characterized by flaccidity or lack of movement during a convulsion. **Clonic seizures** consist of rhythmic fast muscle contractions and slightly longer relaxations; **myoclonus** is a "shock-like" contraction of a muscle of <50 msec that is often repeated. The duration of the seizure and state of consciousness (retained or impaired) should be documented. The history should determine whether an **aura** preceded the convulsion and the behavior of the child immediately preceding the seizure. The most common aura experienced by children consists of epigastric discomfort or pain and a feeling of fear. The posture of the patient, presence or absence and distribution of cyanosis, vocalizations, loss of sphincter control (particularly of the urinary bladder), and postictal state (including sleep, headache, and hemiparesis) should be noted.

In addition to the assessment of cardiorespiratory and metabolic status, examination of a child with a seizure disorder should be geared toward the search for an organic cause. The child's head circumference, length, and weight are plotted on a growth chart and compared with previous measurements. A careful general and neurologic examination should be performed. The **eyegrounds** must be examined for the presence of papilledema, optic neuritis, retinal hemorrhages, uveitis, chorioretinitis, coloboma, or macular changes, as well as retinal phakoma. The finding of unusual facial features or of associated physical findings such as hepatosplenomegaly point to an underlying metabolic or storage disease as the cause of the neurologic disorder. The presence of a **neurocutaneous disorder** may be indicated by the presence of vitiliginous ash leaf–type lesions using an ultraviolet light (Wood lamp), of adenoma sebaceum, shagreen patches, or of retinal phakomas (tuberous sclerosis), of multiple café-au-lait spots (neurofibromatosis), or of V1 or V2 distribution nevus flammeus (Sturge-Weber syndrome).

Localizing neurologic signs, such as a subtle **hemiparesis** with hyperreflexia, an equivocal Babinski sign, and a downward-drifting of an extended arm with eyes closed, might suggest a contralateral hemispheric structural lesion, such as a slow-growing glioma, as the cause of the seizure disorder. Unilateral growth arrest of the thumbnail, hand, or extremity in a child with a focal seizure disorder suggests a chronic condition, such as a porencephalic cyst, arteriovenous malformation, or cortical atrophy of the opposite hemisphere.

After the initial acute investigation, which often includes metabolic and CT scanning, depending on the clinical presentation in emergency room, in a child with a first nonfebrile seizure, it is recommended to obtain an EEG to help predict the risk of seizure recurrence. Subsequent imaging studies with MRI should be seriously considered in any child with a significant cognitive or motor impairment of unknown etiology, unexplained abnormalities on neurologic or psychiatric examination, a seizure of focal onset with or without secondary generalization, an EEG that does not represent a benign partial epilepsy of childhood or primary generalized epilepsy, or in children younger than 1 year of age. Other laboratory tests or lumbar punctures may be pursued depending on the specific clinical settings. Further details regarding the approach to a first seizure are included in Chapter 593.2.

593.1 Febrile Seizures
Mohamad A. Mikati and Abeer J. Hani

Febrile seizures are seizures that occur between the age of 6 and 60 mo with a temperature of 38°C (100.4°F) or higher, that are not the result of central nervous system infection or any metabolic imbalance, and that occur in the absence of a history of prior afebrile seizures. A **simple febrile seizure** is a primary generalized, usually tonic–clonic, attack associated with fever, lasting for a maximum of 15 min, and not

recurrent within a 24-hr period. A **complex febrile seizure** is more prolonged (>15 min), is focal, and/or reoccurs within 24 hr. **Febrile status epilepticus** is a febrile seizure lasting longer than 30 min. Some use the term **simple febrile seizure plus** for those with recurrent febrile seizures within 24 hr. Most patients with simple febrile seizures have a very short postictal state and usually return to their baseline normal behavior and consciousness within minutes of the seizure.

Between 2% and 5% of neurologically healthy infants and children experience at least 1, usually simple, febrile seizure. Simple febrile seizures do not have an increased risk of mortality even though they are, understandably, concerning to the parents when they first witness them. Complex febrile seizures may have an approximately 2-fold long-term increase in mortality, as compared to the general population, over the subsequent 2 yr, probably secondary to coexisting pathology. There are no long-term adverse effects of having 1 or more simple febrile seizures. Compared with age-matched controls, patients with febrile seizures do not have any increase in the incidence of abnormalities of behavior, scholastic performance, neurocognitive function, or attention. Children who develop later epilepsy, however, might experience such difficulties. Febrile seizures recur in approximately 30% of those experiencing a first episode, in 50% after 2 or more episodes, and in 50% of infants younger than 1 yr old at febrile seizure onset. Several factors affect recurrence risk (Table 593-6). Although approximately 15% of children with epilepsy have had febrile seizures, only 2-7% of children who experience febrile seizures proceed to develop epilepsy later in life. There are several predictors of epilepsy after febrile seizures (Table 593-7).

GENETIC FACTORS
The genetic contribution to the incidence of febrile seizures is manifested by a positive family history for febrile seizures in many patients. In some families, the disorder is inherited as an autosomal dominant

Table 593-6	Risk Factors for Recurrence of Febrile Seizures

MAJOR
Age <1 yr
Duration of fever <24 hr
Fever 38-39°C (100.4-102.2°F)

MINOR
Family history of febrile seizures
Family history of epilepsy
Complex febrile seizure
Daycare
Male gender
Lower serum sodium at time of presentation

Having no risk factors carries a recurrence risk of approximately 12%; 1 risk factor, 25-50%; 2 risk factors, 50-59%; 3 or more risk factors, 73-100%.

Table 593-7	Risk Factors for Occurrence of Subsequent Epilepsy After a Febrile Seizure

RISK FACTOR	RISK FOR SUBSEQUENT EPILEPSY
Simple febrile seizure	1%
Recurrent febrile seizures	4%
Complex febrile seizures (more than 15 min duration or recurrent within 24 hr)	6%
Fever <1 hr before febrile seizure	11%
Family history of epilepsy	18%
Complex febrile seizures (focal)	29%
Neurodevelopmental abnormalities	33%

trait, and multiple single genes that cause the disorder have been identified in such families. However, in most cases the disorder appears to be polygenic, and the genes predisposing to it remain to be identified. Identified single genes include *FEB 1, 2, 3, 4, 5, 6, 7, 8, 9,* and *10* genes on chromosomes 8q13-q21, 19p13.3, 2q24, 5q14-q15, 6q22-24, 18p11.2, 21q22, 5q34, 3p24.2-p23, and 3q26.2-q26.33. Only the function of *FEB 2* is known: it is a sodium channel gene, *SCN1A*.

Almost any type of epilepsy can be preceded by febrile seizures, and a few epilepsy syndromes typically start with febrile seizures. These are **generalized epilepsy with febrile seizures plus** (GEFS+), **severe myoclonic epilepsy of infancy** (also called **Dravet syndrome**), and, in many patients, temporal lobe epilepsy secondary to mesial temporal sclerosis.

GEFS+ is an autosomal dominant syndrome with a highly variable phenotype. Onset is usually in early childhood and remission is usually in mid-childhood. It is characterized by multiple febrile seizures and by several subsequent types of afebrile generalized seizures, including generalized tonic–clonic, absence, myoclonic, atonic, or myoclonic astatic seizures with variable degrees of severity. A focal febrile seizures plus epilepsy variant, in which the seizures are focal rather than generalized, has also been described.

Dravet syndrome is the most severe of the phenotypic spectrum of febrile seizure-associated epilepsies. It constitutes a distinct entity in the onset of which is in infancy. Its onset is characterized by febrile and afebrile unilateral clonic seizures recurring every 1 or 2 mo. These early seizures are typically induced by fever, but they differ from the usual febrile convulsions in that they are more prolonged, are more frequent, are focal and come in clusters. Seizures subsequently start to occur with lower fevers and then without fever. During the 2nd yr of life, myoclonus, atypical absences, and partial seizures occur frequently and developmental delay usually follows. This syndrome is usually caused by a de novo mutation, although rarely it is inherited in an autosomal dominant manner. The mutated gene is located on 2q24-31 and encodes for *SCN1A*, the same gene mutated in GEFS+ spectrum. However, in Dravet syndrome the mutations lead to loss of function and thus to a more severe phenotype. There are several milder variants of Dravet syndrome that manifest some but not all of the above features and that are referred to as Dravet syndrome spectrum or Borderland. Mutations in other genes may also cause Dravet syndrome or GEFS+ phenotypes.

The majority of patients who had prolonged febrile seizures and encephalopathy after vaccination and who had been presumed to have suffered from **vaccine encephalopathy** (seizures and psychomotor regression occurring after vaccination and presumed to be caused by it) turn out to have Dravet syndrome mutations, indicating that their disease is caused by the mutation and not secondary to the vaccine. This has raised doubts about the very existence of the entity termed vaccine encephalopathy.

EVALUATION

Figure 593-1 delineates the general approach to the patient with febrile seizures. Each child who presents with a febrile seizure requires a detailed history and a thorough general and neurologic examination. Febrile seizures often occur in the context of otitis media, roseola and human herpesvirus (HHV) 6 infection, shigella, or similar infections, making the evaluation more demanding. In patients with febrile status, HHV-6B (more frequently) and HHV-7 infections were found to account for one-third of the cases. Several laboratory studies need to be considered in evaluating the patient with febrile seizures.

Lumbar Puncture

Meningitis should be considered in the differential diagnosis, and lumbar puncture should be performed for all infants younger than 6 mo of age who present with fever and seizure, or if the child is ill-appearing or at any age if there are clinical signs or symptoms of concern. A lumbar puncture is an option in a child 6-12 mo of age who is deficient in *Haemophilus influenzae* type b and *Streptococcus pneumoniae* immunizations or for whom immunization status is unknown. A lumbar puncture is an option in children who have been pretreated

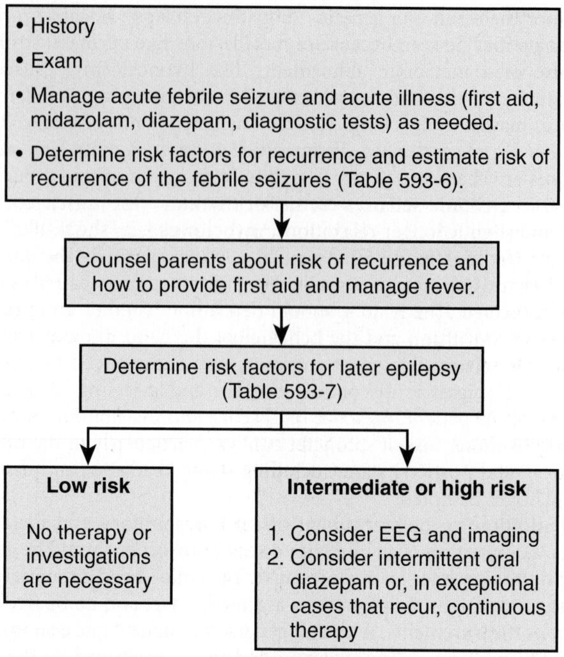

Figure 593-1 Management of febrile seizures. *(Modified from Mikati MA, Rahi A: Febrile seizures: from molecular biology to clinical practice,* Neurosciences (Riyadh) *10:14–22, 2004.)*

with antibiotics. *In patients presenting with febrile status epilepticus in the absence of a central nervous system infection, a nontraumatic lumbar puncture rarely shows cerebrospinal fluid (CSF) pleocytosis (96% have <3 nucleated cells in the CSF) and the CSF protein and glucose are usually normal.*

Electroencephalogram

If the child is presenting with the first simple febrile seizure and is otherwise neurologically healthy, an EEG need not normally be performed as part of the evaluation. An EEG would not predict the future recurrence of febrile seizures or epilepsy even if the result is abnormal. Spikes during drowsiness are often seen in children with febrile seizures, particularly those older than age 4 yr, and these do not predict later epilepsy. EEGs performed within 2 wk of a febrile seizure often have nonspecific slowing, usually posteriorly. Thus, in many cases, if an EEG is indicated, it is delayed until or repeated after more than 2 wk have passed. An EEG should, therefore, generally be restricted to special cases in which epilepsy is highly suspected, and, generally, it should be used to delineate the type of epilepsy rather than to predict its occurrence. If an EEG is done, it should be performed for at least 20 min in wakefulness and in sleep according to international guidelines to avoid misinterpretation and drawing of erroneous conclusions. At times, if the patient does not recover immediately from a seizure, then an EEG can help distinguish between ongoing seizure activity and a prolonged postictal period, sometimes termed a **nonepileptic twilight state.** EEG can also be helpful in patients who present with febrile status epilepticus because the presence of focal slowing present on the EEG obtained within 72 hr of the status has been shown to be highly associated with MRI evidence of acute hippocampal injury.

Blood Studies

Blood studies (serum electrolytes, calcium, phosphorus, magnesium, and complete blood count) are not routinely recommended in the work-up of a child with a first simple febrile seizure. Blood glucose should be determined in children with prolonged postictal obtundation or with poor oral intake (prolonged fasting). Serum electrolyte values may be abnormal in children after a febrile seizure, but this should be suggested by precipitating or predisposing conditions elicited in the history and reflected in abnormalities of the physical examination. If clinically indicated (e.g., in a history or physical examination suggesting dehydration), these tests should be performed. A low sodium level is associated with higher risk of recurrence of the febrile seizure within the following 24 hr.

Neuroimaging

A CT or MRI is not recommended in evaluating the child after a first simple febrile seizure. The work-up of children with complex febrile seizures needs to be individualized. This can include an EEG and neuroimaging, particularly if the child is neurologically abnormal. Approximately 11% of children with febrile status epilepticus are reported to have (usually) unilateral swelling of their hippocampus acutely, which is followed by subsequent long-term hippocampal atrophy. Whether these patients will ultimately develop temporal lobe epilepsy remains to be determined.

TREATMENT

In general, antiepileptic therapy, continuous or intermittent, is not recommended for children with 1 or more simple febrile seizures. Parents should be counseled about the relative risks of recurrence of febrile seizures and recurrence of epilepsy, educated on how to handle a seizure acutely, and given emotional support. If the seizure lasts for longer than 5 min, acute treatment with diazepam, lorazepam, or midazolam is needed (see Chapter 593.8 for acute management of seizures and status epilepticus). Rectal diazepam is often prescribed to be given at the time of reoccurrence of a febrile seizure lasting longer than 5 min (see Table 593-12 for dosing). Alternatively, buccal or intranasal midazolam may be used and is often preferred by parents. Intravenous benzodiazepines, phenobarbital, phenytoin, or valproate may be needed in the case of febrile status epilepticus. If the parents are very anxious concerning their child's seizures, intermittent oral diazepam (0.33 mg/kg every 8 hr during fever) or intermittent rectal diazepam (0.5 mg/kg administered as a rectal suppository every 8 hr), can be given during febrile illnesses. Intermittent oral nitrazepam, clobazam, and clonazepam (0.1 mg/kg/day) have also been used. Such therapies help reduce, but do not eliminate, the risks of recurrence of febrile seizures. Other therapies have included continuous phenobarbital (4-5 mg/kg/day in 1 or 2 divided doses), and continuous valproate (20-30 mg/kg/day in 2 or 3 divided doses). *In the vast majority of cases, it is not justified to use continuous therapy owing to the risk of side effects and lack of demonstrated long-term benefits, even if the recurrence rate of febrile seizures is expected to be decreased by these drugs.*

Antipyretics can decrease the discomfort of the child but do not reduce the risk of having a recurrent febrile seizure, probably because the seizure often occurs as the temperature is rising or falling. Chronic antiepileptic therapy may be considered for children with a high risk for later epilepsy. Currently available data indicate that the possibility of future epilepsy does not change with or without antiepileptic therapy. Iron deficiency is associated with an increased risk of febrile seizures, and thus screening for that problem and treating it appears appropriate.

Bibliography is available at Expert Consult.

593.2 Unprovoked Seizures
Mohamad A. Mikati and Abeer J. Hani

HISTORY AND EXAMINATION

Acute evaluation of a first seizure includes assessment of vital signs and respiratory and cardiac function, and institution of measures to normalize and stabilize them as needed. Signs of head trauma, abuse, drug intoxication, poisoning, meningitis, sepsis, focal abnormalities, increased intracranial pressure, herniation, neurocutaneous stigmata, brainstem dysfunction, and/or focal weakness should all be sought because they could suggest an underlying etiology for the seizure.

The **history** should also include details of the seizure manifestations, particularly those that occurred at its initial onset. These could give clues to the type and brain localization of the seizure. One should also

probe for previous signs or symptoms of other seizures in the preceding weeks, or longer, that the parents may have overlooked and did not report. In some instances, if the events have been going on for a time and there is a question about their nature (e.g., sleep myoclonus vs seizures), then the family could video record the patient and make the video available to the healthcare provider. Having the parents imitate the seizure can also be helpful. Seizure patterns (e.g., clustering), precipitating conditions (e.g., sleep or sleep deprivation, television, visual patterns, mental activity, stress), exacerbating conditions (e.g., menstrual cycle, medications), frequency, duration, time of occurrence, and other characteristics need to be carefully documented (see Chapter 593.9). Parents often overlook, do not report, or underreport absence, complex partial, or myoclonic seizures. A history of personality change or symptoms of increased intracranial pressure can suggest an intracranial tumor. Similarly, a history of cognitive regression can suggest a degenerative or metabolic disease. Certain medications such as stimulants or antihistamines, particularly sedating ones, can precipitate seizures. A history of prenatal or perinatal distress or of developmental delay can suggest etiologic congenital or perinatal brain dysfunction. Details of the spells can suggest nonepileptic paroxysmal disorders that mimic seizures (see Chapter 594).

DIFFERENTIAL DIAGNOSIS

This involves consideration of nonepileptic paroxysmal events (see Chapter 594), determination of the seizure type, as classified by the new ILAE system (see Table 593-1) and consideration of potential underlying etiologies. Some seizures might begin with **auras**, which are sensory experiences reported by the patient and not observed externally. These can take the form of visual (e.g., flashing lights or seeing colors or complex visual hallucinations), somatosensory (tingling), olfactory, auditory, vestibular, or experiential (e.g., déjà vu, déjà vécu feelings) sensations, depending upon the precise localization of the origin of the seizures.

Motor seizures can be **tonic** (sustained contraction), **clonic** (rhythmic contractions), **myoclonic** (rapid shock-like contractions, usually <50 msec in duration, that may be isolated or may repeat but usually are not rhythmic), **atonic**, or **astatic**. **Astatic** seizures often follow myoclonic seizures and cause a very momentary loss of tone with a sudden fall. **Atonic** seizures, on the other hand, are usually longer and the loss of tone often develops more slowly. Sometimes it is difficult to distinguish among tonic, myoclonic, atonic, or astatic seizures based on the history alone when the family reports only that the patient "falls"; in such cases, the seizure may be described as a **drop attack**. Loss of tone or myoclonus in only the neck muscles results in a milder seizure referred to as a **head drop**. Tonic, clonic, myoclonic, and atonic seizures can be focal (including 1 limb or 1 side only), focal with secondary generalization, or primary generalized. Epileptic **spasms** (axial spasms, these terms being preferred over infantile spasms because they can occur beyond infancy) consist of flexion or extension of truncal and extremity musculature that is sustained for 1-2 sec, shorter than what is seen in tonic seizures, which last longer than 2 sec. Focal motor clonic and/or myoclonic seizures that persist for days, months, or even longer are termed **epilepsia partialis continua**.

Absence seizures are generalized seizures consisting of staring, unresponsiveness, and eye flutter lasting usually for few seconds. **Typical absences** are associated with 3 Hz spike–and–slow-wave discharges and with petit mal epilepsy, which has a good prognosis. **Atypical absences** are associated with 1-2 Hz spike–and–slow-wave discharges, and with head atonia and myoclonus during the seizures. They occur in Lennox-Gastaut syndrome, which has a poor prognosis. **Juvenile absences** are similar to typical absences but are associated with 4-5 Hz spike-and-slow waves and occur in juvenile myoclonic epilepsy. Seizure type and other EEG and clinical manifestations determine the type of **epilepsy syndrome** with which a particular patient is afflicted (Table 593-8; see Chapter 593.3 and 593.4).

Family history of certain forms of epilepsy, like benign neonatal seizures, can suggest the specific epilepsy syndrome. More often, however, different members of a family with a positive history of epilepsy have different types of epilepsy. Head circumference can indicate

Table 593-8	Selected Epilepsy Syndromes by Age of Onset

NEONATAL PERIOD
Benign familial neonatal seizures (BFNS)
Early myoclonic encephalopathy (EME)
Ohtahara syndrome

INFANCY
Epilepsy of infancy with migrating focal seizures
West syndrome
Myoclonic epilepsy in infancy (MEI)
Benign infantile seizures
Benign familial infantile epilepsy
Dravet syndrome
Myoclonic encephalopathy in nonprogressive disorders

CHILDHOOD
Febrile seizures plus (FS+) (can start in infancy; this can be with
   generalized [GEFS+] or with focal seizures)
Early-onset benign childhood occipital epilepsy (Panayiotopoulos
   type)
Epilepsy with myoclonic atonic (previously astatic) seizures
Benign epilepsy with centrotemporal spikes (BCECTS)
Late-onset childhood occipital epilepsy (Gastaut type)
Autosomal dominant nocturnal frontal lobe epilepsy (AD-NFLE)
Epilepsy with myoclonic absences
Lennox-Gastaut syndrome
Epileptic encephalopathy with continuous spike-and-wave during
   sleep (CSWS)
Landau-Kleffner syndrome
Childhood absence epilepsy (CAE)

ADOLESCENCE–ADULT
Juvenile absence epilepsy (JAE)
Juvenile myoclonic epilepsy (JME)
Epilepsy with generalized tonic–clonic seizures alone
Progressive myoclonus epilepsies (PME)
Autosomal dominant epilepsy with auditory features (ADEAF)
Other familial temporal lobe epilepsies

AGE-RELATED (AGE OF ONSET LESS SPECIFIC)
Familial focal epilepsy with variable foci (childhood to adult)
Reflex epilepsies

**SEIZURE DISORDERS THAT ARE NOT TRADITIONALLY GIVEN
THE DIAGNOSIS OF EPILEPSY**
Benign neonatal seizures (BNS)
Febrile seizures (FS)

EPILEPTIC ENCEPHALOPATHIES
EME
Ohtahara syndrome
Migrating partial seizures of infancy
West syndrome
Dravet syndrome
Myoclonic encephalopathy in nonprogressive disorders
Epilepsy with myoclonic astatic seizures
Lennox-Gastaut syndrome
Epileptic encephalopathy with CSWS
Landau-Kleffner syndrome

OTHER SECONDARY GENERALIZED EPILEPSIES
Generalized epilepsy secondary to neurodegenerative disease
Progressive myoclonus epilepsies

*Modified from Berg AT, Berkovic SF, Bordie MJ, et al. Revised terminology
and concepts for organization of seizures and epilepsies: report of the
ILAE Commission on Classification and Terminology, 2005-2009. Epilepsia
51:676–685, 2010.*

Table 593-9	Proposed Diagnostic Scheme for People with Epileptic Seizures and with Epilepsy

Epileptic seizures and epilepsy syndromes are to be described
and categorized according to a system that uses standardized
terminology and that is sufficiently flexible to take into account
the practical and dynamic aspects of epilepsy diagnosis:
- Axis 1: Ictal phenomenology, used to describe ictal events with
  any degree of detail needed.
- Axis 2: Seizure type, from the List of types of Epileptic Seizures.
  Localization within the brain and precipitating stimuli for reflex
  seizures should be specified when appropriate.
- Axis 3: Syndrome, from the List of Epilepsy Syndromes, with the
  understanding that a syndromic diagnosis may not always be
  possible.
- Axis 4: Etiology, from a Classification of Diseases Frequently
  Associated with Epileptic Seizures or Epilepsy Syndromes when
  possible, genetic defects, or specific pathologic substrates for
  symptomatic focal epilepsies.
- Axis 5: Impairment; this is often useful to make sure one does not
  overlook the consequences of epilepsy, such as medication side
  effects, and learning and socialization difficulties.

*Modified from Engel J. A proposed diagnostic scheme for people with epileptic
seizures and with epilepsy: report of the ILAE task force on classification and
terminology. Epilepsia. 2001;42:796–803.*

lesions (sometimes associated with tuberous sclerosis and detected
more reliably by viewing the skin under UV light), or other neurocutaneous manifestations such as Shagreen patches and adenoma sebaceum (associated with tuberous sclerosis), or whorl-like hypopigmented
areas (hypomelanosis of Ito, associated with hemimegalencephaly).
Subtle asymmetries on the exam such as drift of 1 of the extended arms,
posturing of an arm on stress gait, slowness in rapid alternating movements, small hand or thumb and thumb nail on 1 side, or difficulty in
hopping on 1 leg relative to the other can signify a subtle hemiparesis
associated with a lesion on the contralateral side of the brain.

Guidelines on the evaluation of a **first unprovoked nonfebrile**
seizure include a careful history and physical examination and brain
imaging by head CT or MRI. Emergency head CT in the child presenting with a first unprovoked nonfebrile seizure is often useful for acute
management of the patient. Laboratory studies are recommended in
specific clinical situations: Spinal tap is considered in patients with
suspected meningitis or encephalitis, in children without brain swelling or papilledema, and in children in whom a history of intracranial
bleeding is suspected without evidence of such on head CT. In the
second of these, examination of the CSF for xanthochromia is essential.
Electrocardiography (ECG) to rule out long QT or other cardiac dysrhythmias and other tests directed at disorders that could mimic seizures may be needed (see Chapter 594). EEG is highly recommended
to assess for focal abnormalities and predict seizure recurrence.

LONG-TERM APPROACH TO THE PATIENT AND ADDITIONAL TESTING

The approach to the patient with epilepsy is based on the diagnostic
scheme proposed by the ILAE Task Force on Classification and Terminology and presented in Table 593-9. This emphasizes the total
approach to the patient, including identification, if possible, of the
underlying etiology of the epilepsy and the impairments that result
from it. The impairments are very often just as important as, if not
more important than, the seizures themselves. Most epilepsy syndromes are potentially caused by any 1 of multiple underlying or still
undetermined etiologies. However, in addition, there are many epilepsy syndromes that are associated with specific gene mutations (see
Table 593-2). Different mutations of the same gene can result in different epilepsy syndromes, and mutations of different genes can cause the
same epilepsy syndrome phenotype. The clinical use of gene testing in
the diagnosis and management of childhood epilepsy has been limited
to patients manifesting specific underlying malformational, metabolic,
or degenerative disorders, patients with severe named epilepsy syndromes (such as West and Dravet syndromes and progressive

the presence of microcephaly or of macrocephaly. Eye exam may show
optic disc edema, retinal hemorrhages, chorioretinitis, colobomata
(associated with brain malformations), a cherry-red spot, optic atrophy,
macular changes (associated with genetic neurodegenerative and
storage diseases), or phakomas (associated with tuberous sclerosis).
Skin exam could show a trigeminal V_1 distribution capillary hemangioma (associated with Sturge-Weber syndrome), hypopigmented

myoclonic epilepsies), and to patients with syndromes of mendelian inheritance (see Table 593-2).

Patients with **recurrent seizures**, specifically with 2 seizures spaced apart by longer than 24 hr, warrant further work-up directed at the underlying etiology. In patients with drug-resistant epilepsy, or in infants with new-onset epilepsy in whom the initial testing did not reveal an underlying etiology, a full metabolic work-up, including amino acids, organic acids, biotinidase, and CSF studies, is needed. Additional testing can include, depending on the case, some or most of the following:

1. Measurement of serum lactate, pyruvate, acyl carnitine profile, creatine, very-long-chain fatty acids, and guanidino-acetic acid.
2. Blood and serum sometimes need to be tested for white blood cell lysosomal enzymes, serum coenzyme Q levels, and serum copper and ceruloplasmin levels (for Menkes syndrome).
3. Serum immune isoelectric focusing is performed for carbohydrate-deficient transferrin.
4. CSF glucose testing looks for glucose transporter deficiency, and CSF can be examined for cells and proteins (for parainfectious and postinfectious syndromes, and for Aicardi-Goutières syndrome, which also shows cerebral calcifications and has a specific gene defect test available).
5. Other laboratory studies include immunoglobulin (Ig) G index, NMDA (N-methyl-D-aspartate) receptor antibodies, and measles titers.
6. CSF tests can also confirm with, the appropriate clinical setup, the diagnosis of cerebral folate deficiency, pyridoxine dependency, pyridoxal dependency, mitochondrial disorders, nonketotic hyperglycinemia, neopterin/biopterin metabolism disorders, adenylosuccinate lyase deficiency, and neurotransmitter deficiencies. In infants who do not respond immediately to antiepileptic therapy, vitamin B$_6$ (100 mg intravenously) is given as a therapeutic trial to help diagnose pyridoxine-responsive seizures, with precautions to guard against possible apnea. The trial is best done with continuous EEG monitoring, including a preadministration baseline recording period. Prior to the vitamin B$_6$ trial, a pipecolic acid level and urine and CSF α-aminoadipic acid semialdehyde levels should be drawn, because they often elevated in this rare syndrome and the therapeutic trial result may not be definitive. Some patients are pyridoxal phosphate, rather than pyridoxine, dependent. Also patients with cerebral folate deficiency can have intractable seizures. Thus trials of pyridoxal phosphate given orally (up to 50 mg/kg) and folinic acid (up to 3 mg/kg) over several weeks can help diagnose these rare disorders while waiting for the definitive diagnosis from CSF or genetic testing for these disorders. Certain EEG changes such as continuous spike–and–slow-wave seizure activity and burst-suppression patterns may also suggest these vitamin-responsive syndromes.
7. Urine may also need to be tested for urinary sulfites indicating molybdenum cofactor deficiency and for oligosaccharides and mucopolysaccharides. MR spectroscopy is performed for lactate and creatine peaks to rule out mitochondrial disease and creatine transporter deficiency.
8. Gene testing looks for specific disorders that can manifest with seizures, including *SCN1A* mutations in Dravet syndrome; *ARX* gene for West syndrome in boys; *MECP2, CDKL5,* and protocadherin 19 for Rett syndrome and similar presentations; syntaxin binding protein for Ohtahara syndrome; and polymerase G for West syndrome and other seizures in infants. Gene testing can also be performed for other dysmorphic or metabolic syndromes.
9. Muscle biopsy can be performed for mitochondrial enzymes and coenzyme Q10 levels, and skin biopsy for inclusion bodies seen in neuronal ceroid lipofuscinosis and Lafora body disease is sometimes needed.
10. Genetic panels are available that include multiple genes that can cause epilepsy at specific ages; whole-exome sequencing is also available. These can be helpful in selected patients.

Most patients do not require a work-up anywhere near the above described extensive testing. The pace and extent of the work-up must depend critically upon the clinical epileptic and nonepileptic features, the family and antecedent personal history of the patient, the medication responsiveness of the seizures, the likelihood of identifying a treatable condition, and the wishes and need of the family to assign a specific diagnosis to the child's illness.

Bibliography is available at Expert Consult.

593.3 Partial Seizures and Related Epilepsy Syndromes
Mohamad A. Mikati and Abeer J. Hani

Partial (now referred to as focal) seizures account for approximately 40% of seizures in children and can be divided into **simple partial seizures** (currently referred to in the most recent ILAE classification as **focal seizures without impairment of consciousness**), in which consciousness is not impaired, and **complex partial seizures** (currently referred to as **focal seizures with impairment of consciousness**, also called **focal dyscognitive seizures**), in which consciousness is affected. Simple and complex partial seizures can each occur in isolation, one can temporally lead to the other (usually simple to complex), and/or each can progress into **secondary generalized seizures** (tonic, clonic, atonic, or most often tonic–clonic).

FOCAL SEIZURES WITHOUT IMPAIRMENT OF CONSCIOUSNESS
These can take the form of sensory seizures (auras) or brief motor seizures, the specific nature of which gives clues as to the location of the seizure focus. Brief motor seizures are the most common and include focal tonic, clonic, or atonic seizures. Often there is a motor (jacksonian) march from face to arm to leg, adversive head and eye movements to the contralateral side, or postictal (Todd) paralysis that can last minutes or hours, and sometimes longer. Unlike tics, motor seizures are not under partial voluntary control; seizures are more often stereotyped and less likely than tics to manifest different types in a given patient.

FOCAL SEIZURES WITH IMPAIRMENT OF CONSCIOUSNESS
These seizures usually last 1-2 min and are often preceded by an **aura**, such as a rising abdominal feeling, déjà vu or déjà vécu, a sense of fear, complex visual hallucinations, micropsia or macropsia (temporal lobe), generalized difficult-to-characterize sensations (frontal lobe), focal sensations (parietal lobe), or simple visual experiences (occipital lobe). Children younger than 7 yr old are less likely than older children to report auras, but parents might observe unusual preictal behaviors that suggest the experiencing of auras. Subsequent manifestations consist of decreased responsiveness, staring, looking around seemingly purposelessly, and automatisms. **Automatisms** are automatic semipurposeful movements of the mouth (oral, alimentary such as chewing) or of the extremities (manual, such as manipulating the sheets; leg automatisms such as shuffling, walking). Often there is salivation, dilation of the pupils, and flushing or color change. The patient might appear to react to some of the stimulation around him or her but does not later recall the epileptic event. At times, walking and/or marked limb flailing and agitation occur, particularly in patients with frontal lobe seizures. Frontal lobe seizures often occur at night and can be very numerous and brief, but other complex partial seizures from other areas in the brain can also occur at night, too. There is often contralateral dystonic posturing of the arm and, in some cases, unilateral or bilateral tonic arm stiffening. Some seizures have these manifestations with minimal or no automatisms. Others consist of altered consciousness with contralateral motor, usually clonic, manifestations. After the seizure, the patient can have postictal automatisms, sleepiness, and/or other transient focal deficits such as weakness (Todd paralysis) or aphasia.

SECONDARY GENERALIZED SEIZURES

Seizures of this type were previously known as focal seizures with impairment of consciousness evolving to bilateral convulsive seizures. Secondary generalized seizures can start with generalized clinical phenomena (from rapid spread of the discharge from the initial focus), or as simple or complex partial seizures with subsequent clinical generalization. There is often adversive eye and head deviation to the side contralateral to the side of the seizure focus followed by generalized tonic, clonic, or tonic–clonic activity. Tongue biting, urinary and stool incontinence, vomiting with risk of aspiration, and cyanosis are common. Fractures of the vertebrae or humerus are rare complications. Most such seizures last 1-2 min. Tonic focal or secondary generalized seizures often manifest adversive head deviation to the contralateral side, or fencing, hemi- or full figure-of-four arm, or Statue of Liberty postures. These postures often suggest frontal origin, particularly when consciousness is preserved during them, indicating that the seizure originated from the medial frontal supplementary motor area.

EEG in patients with focal/partial seizures usually shows focal spikes or sharp waves in the lobe where the seizure originates. A sleep-deprived EEG with recording during sleep increases the diagnostic yield and is advisable in all patients whenever possible (Fig. 593-2). Despite that, approximately 15% of children with epilepsy initially have normal EEGs because the discharges are relatively infrequent or the focus is deep. If repeating the test does not detect paroxysmal findings, then longer recordings in the laboratory or using ambulatory EEG or even inpatient 24-hr video EEG monitoring may be helpful. The latter is particularly helpful if the seizures are frequent enough, because it then can allow visualization of the clinical events and the corresponding EEG tracing.

Brain imaging is critical in patients with focal seizures. In general, MRI is preferable to CT, which misses subtle but occasionally potentially clinically significant lesions. MRI can show pathologies such as changes as a result of previous strokes or hypoxic injury, malforma-

tions, medial temporal sclerosis, arteriovenous malformations, inflammatory pathologies, or tumors (Fig. 593-3).

BENIGN EPILEPSY SYNDROMES WITH FOCAL SEIZURES

The most common such syndrome is **benign childhood epilepsy with centrotemporal spikes** which typically starts during childhood (ages 3-10 yr) and is outgrown in adolescence. The child typically wakes up at night owing to a focal (simple partial) seizure causing buccal and throat tingling and tonic or clonic contractions of 1 side of the face, with drooling and inability to speak but with preserved consciousness and comprehension. Dyscognitive focal (complex partial) and secondary generalized seizures can also occur. EEG shows typical broad-based centrotemporal spikes that are markedly increased in frequency during drowsiness and sleep. MRI is normal. Patients respond very well to antiepileptic drugs (AEDs) such as carbamazepine. In some patients who only have rare and mild seizures treatment might not be needed.

Benign epilepsy with occipital spikes can occur in early childhood (**Panayiotopoulos type**) and manifests with complex partial seizures with ictal vomiting, or they appear in later childhood (**Gastaut type**) with complex partial seizures, visual auras, and migraine headaches. Both are typically outgrown in a few years. Manifestations may include visual hallucinations and postictal headache (epilepsy–migraine sequence).

In infants, several less-common **benign infantile familial convulsion syndromes** have been reported. For some of these, the corresponding gene mutation and its function are known (see Tables 593-2 and 593-5), but for others, the genetic underpinnings are yet to be determined. Specific syndromes include benign infantile familial convulsions with parietooccipital foci linked to chromosomal loci 19q and 2q, benign familial infantile convulsions with associated choreoathetosis linked to chromosomal locus 16p12-q12, and benign

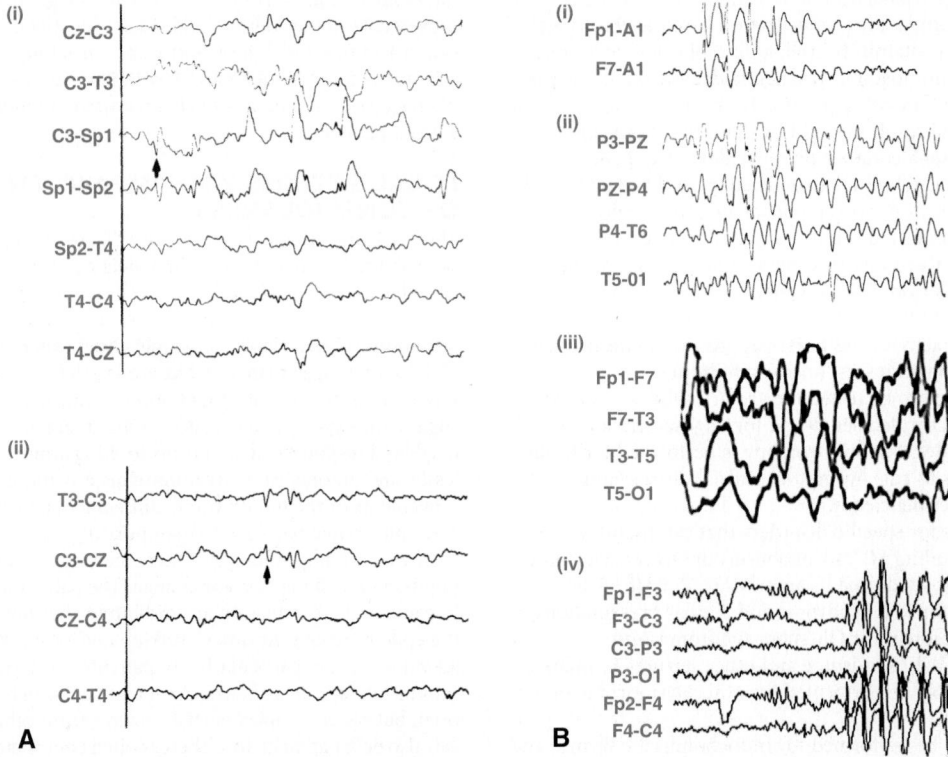

Figure 593-2 A, Representative EEG associated with partial seizures: (i) Spike discharges from the left temporal lobe *(arrow)* in a patient with complex partial seizures caused by mesial temporal sclerosis; (ii) left central-parietal spikes *(arrow)* characteristic of benign partial epilepsy with centrotemporal spikes. **B,** Representative EEGs associated with generalized seizures: (i) 3/sec spike-and-wave discharge of absence seizures with normal background activity; (ii) 1-2/sec interictal slow spike waves in a patient with Lennox-Gastaut syndrome; (iii) hypsarrhythmia with an irregular multifocal high-voltage spike and wave activity with chaotic high-voltage slow background; (iv) juvenile myoclonic epilepsy EEG showing 4-6/sec spike and waves enhanced by photic stimulation.

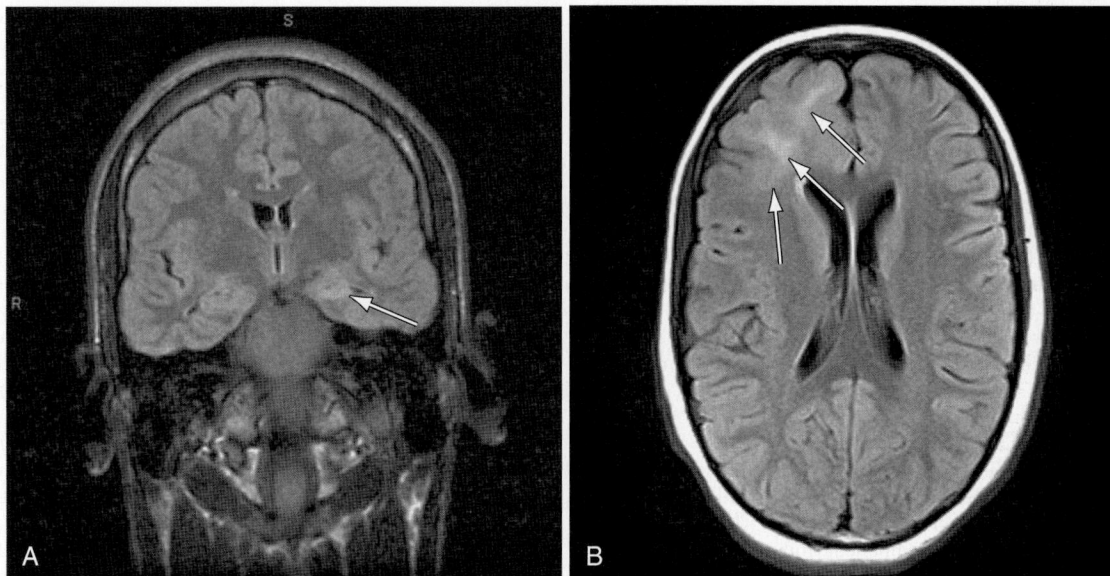

Figure 593-3 A, Coronal fluid-attenuated inversion-recovery (FLAIR) MRI scan of a 13 yr old with intractable seizures and mesial temporal sclerosis (MTS). The *arrow* points at the hippocampus with the high-intensity signal characteristic of MTS. **B,** Axial FLAIR MRI of a 7 yr old with intractable seizures and right frontal cortical dysplasia. The *arrows* point at the high-intensity signal corresponding to the dysplasia. (*A from Lee JYK, Adelson PD: Neurosurgical management of pediatric epilepsy, Pediatr Clin North Am 51:441–456, 2004.*)

infantile familial convulsions with hemiplegic migraine linked to chromosome 1. A number of **benign infantile nonfamilial syndromes** have been reported, including dyscognitive focal (complex partial) seizures with temporal foci, secondary generalized tonic–clonic seizures with variable foci, tonic seizures with midline foci, and partial seizures in association with mild gastroenteritis. All of these have a good prognosis and respond to treatment promptly, often necessitating only short-term (e.g., 6 mo), if any, therapy. **Nocturnal autosomal dominant frontal lobe epilepsy** has been linked to acetylcholine-receptor gene mutations and manifests with nocturnal seizures with dystonic posturing and agitation, screaming, kicking that respond promptly to carbamazepine. Several other less-frequent familial benign epilepsy syndromes with different localizations have also been described, some of which occur exclusively or predominantly in adults (see Table 593-2).

SEVERE EPILEPSY SYNDROMES WITH FOCAL SEIZURES

Symptomatic structural/metabolic epilepsy secondary to focal brain lesions has a higher chance of being severe and refractory to therapy than idiopathic genetic epilepsy. It is important to note that many patients with focal lesions, for example, old strokes or brain tumors, either never have seizures or have well-controlled epilepsy. In infants, drug-resistant epilepsy with focal seizures is often caused by severe metabolic problems, hypoxic–ischemic injury, or congenital malformations. In addition, in this age group, a syndrome of multifocal severe partial seizures with progressive mental regression and cerebral atrophy called **migrating partial seizures of infancy** has been described. In infants and older children, several types of lesions, which can occur in any lobe, can cause intractable epilepsy and seizures and some cases may be secondary to mutations in the calcium sensitive potassium channel KCNT1. Brain malformations causing focal epilepsy include focal cortical dysplasia, hemimegalencephaly, Sturge-Weber hemangioma, tuberous sclerosis, and congenital tumors such as ganglioglioma, and dysembryoplastic neuroepithelial tumors, as well as others. The intractable seizures can be simple partial, complex partial, secondary generalized, or combinations thereof. If secondary generalized seizures predominate and take the form of absence-like seizures and drop attacks, the clinical picture can mimic the generalized epilepsy syndrome of Lennox-Gastaut syndrome and has been termed by some **pseudo–Lennox-Gastaut syndrome.**

Temporal lobe epilepsy can be caused by any temporal lobe lesion. A common cause is **mesial** (also termed **medial**) **temporal sclerosis**, a condition often preceded by febrile seizures and, rarely, genetic in origin. Pathologically, these patients have atrophy and gliosis of the hippocampus and, in some, of the amygdala. It is the most common cause of surgically remediable partial epilepsy in adolescents and adults. Occasionally, in patients with other symptomatic or cryptogenic partial or generalized epilepsies, the focal discharges are so continuous that they cause an epileptic encephalopathy. Activation of temporal discharges in sleep can lead to loss of speech and verbal auditory agnosia (**Landau-Kleffner epileptic aphasia syndrome**). Activation of frontal and secondary generalized discharges in sleep leads to more global delay secondary to the **syndrome of continuous spike waves in slow-wave sleep** (>85% of slow-wave sleep recording dominated by discharges).

The syndrome of **Rasmussen encephalitis** is a form of chronic encephalitis that manifests with unilateral intractable partial seizures, epilepsia partialis continua, and progressive hemiparesis of the affected side, with progressive atrophy of the contralateral hemisphere. The etiology is usually unknown. Some cases have been attributed to cytomegalovirus and others to anti-NMDA receptor autoantibodies.

593.4 Generalized Seizures and Related Epilepsy Syndromes
Mohamad A. Mikati and Abeer J. Hani

ABSENCE SEIZURES

Typical absence seizures usually start at 5-8 yr of age and are often, owing to their brevity, overlooked by parents for many months even though they can occur up to hundreds of times per day. Unlike complex partial seizures they do not have an aura, usually last for only a few seconds, and are accompanied by eye lid flutter or upward rolling of the eyes but typically not by the usually more florid automatisms of complex partial seizures (absence seizures can have simple automatisms like lip-smacking or picking at clothing and the head can minimally fall forward). Absence seizures do not have a postictal period and are characterized by immediate resumption of what the patient was doing before the seizure. Hyperventilation for 3-5 min can precipitate the seizures and the accompanying 3 Hz spike–and–slow-wave discharges. The presence of periorbital, lid, perioral or limb myoclonic jerks with the typical absence seizures usually predicts difficulty in controlling the seizures with medications. Early onset absence seizures (before the age of 4 yr) should trigger evaluation for glucose transporter defect that is often associated with low CSF glucose levels and an abnormal sequencing test of the transporter gene.

Atypical absence seizures have associated myoclonic components and tone changes of the head (head drop) and body and are also usually more difficult to treat. They are precipitated by drowsiness and are usually accompanied by 1-2 Hz spike–and–slow-wave discharges.

Juvenile absence seizures are similar to typical absences but occur at a later age and are accompanied by 4-6 Hz spike–and–slow-wave and polyspike–and–slow-wave discharges. These are usually associated with juvenile myoclonic epilepsy (see "Benign Generalized Epilepsies").

GENERALIZED MOTOR SEIZURE

The most common generalized motor seizures are generalized tonic–clonic seizures that can be either primarily generalized (bilateral) or secondarily generalized (as described in Chapter 593.3) from a unilateral focus. If there is no partial component, then the seizure usually starts with loss of consciousness and, at times, with a sudden cry, upward rolling of the eyes, and a generalized tonic contraction with falling, apnea, and cyanosis. In some, a clonic or myoclonic component precedes the tonic stiffening. The tonic phase is followed by a clonic phase that, as the seizure progresses, shows slowing of the rhythmic contractions until the seizure stops usually 1-2 min later. Incontinence and a postictal period often follow. The latter usually lasts for 30 min to several hours with semicoma or obtundation and postictal sleepiness, weakness, ataxia, hyper- or hyporeflexia, and headaches. There is a risk of aspiration and injury. First aid measures include positioning the patient on his or her side, clearing the mouth if it is open, loosening tight clothes or jewelry, and gently extending the head and, if possible, insertion of an airway by a trained professional. The mouth should not be forced open with a foreign object (this could dislodge teeth, causing aspiration) or with a finger in the mouth (this could result in serious injury to the examiner's finger). Many patients have single **idiopathic generalized tonic–clonic seizures** that may be associated with intercurrent illness or with a cause that cannot be ascertained (see Chapter 593.2). Generalized tonic, atonic, and astatic seizures often occur in severe generalized pediatric epilepsies. Generalized myoclonic seizures can occur in either benign or difficult-to-control generalized epilepsies (see "Benign Generalized Epilepsies" and "Severe Generalized Epilepsies").

BENIGN GENERALIZED EPILEPSIES

Petit mal epilepsy typically starts in mid-childhood, and most patients outgrow it before adulthood. Approximately 25% of patients also develop generalized tonic–clonic seizures, half before and half after the onset of absences. **Benign myoclonic epilepsy of infancy** consists of the onset of myoclonic and other seizures during the 1st yr of life, with generalized 3 Hz spike–and–slow-wave discharges. Often, it is initially difficult to distinguish this type from more-severe syndromes, but follow-up clarifies the diagnosis. **Febrile seizures plus syndrome** manifests febrile seizures and multiple types of generalized seizures in multiple family members, and at times different individuals within the same family manifest different generalized and febrile seizure types (see Chapter 593.1).

Juvenile myoclonic epilepsy (Janz syndrome) is the most common generalized epilepsy in young adults, accounting for 5% of all epilepsies. It has been linked to mutations in many genes including *CACNB4; CLNC2; EJM2, 3, 4, 5, 6, 7, 9; GABRA1; GABRD;* and *Myoclonin1/ EFHC1* (see Table 593-2). Typically, it starts in early adolescence with 1 or more of the following manifestations: myoclonic jerks in the morning, often causing the patient to drop things; generalized tonic–clonic or clonic–tonic–clonic seizures upon awakening; and juvenile absences. Sleep deprivation, alcohol (in older patients), and photic stimulation, or, rarely, certain cognitive activities can act as precipitants. The EEG usually shows generalized 4-5 Hz polyspike–and–slow-

wave discharges. There are other forms of generalized epilepsies such as **photoparoxysmal epilepsy**, in which generalized tonic–clonic, absence or myoclonic generalized seizures are precipitated by photic stimuli such as strobe lights, flipping through TV channels and viewing video games. Other forms of **reflex** (i.e., **stimulus-provoked**) **epilepsy** can occur; associated seizures are usually generalized, although some may be focal (see Table 593-1 and Chapter 593.9).

SEVERE GENERALIZED EPILEPSIES

Severe generalized epilepsies are associated with intractable seizures and developmental delay. **Early myoclonic infantile encephalopathy** starts during the 1st 2 mo of life with severe myoclonic seizures and burst suppression pattern on EEG. It is usually caused by inborn errors of metabolism such as non-ketotic hyperglycinemia. **Early infantile epileptic encephalopathy (Ohtahara syndrome)** has similar age of onset and EEG but manifests tonic seizures and is usually caused by brain malformations or syntaxin binding protein 1 mutations. Severe **myoclonic epilepsy of infancy (Dravet syndrome)** starts as focal febrile status epilepticus or focal febrile seizures and later manifests myoclonic and other seizure types (see Chapter 593.1).

West syndrome starts between the ages of 2 and 12 mo and consists of a triad of infantile epileptic spasms that usually occur in clusters (particularly in drowsiness or upon arousal), developmental regression, and a typical EEG picture called **hypsarrhythmia** (see Fig. 593-2). Hypsarrhythmia is a high-voltage, slow, chaotic background with multifocal spikes. Patients with cryptogenic (sometimes called idiopathic, now referred to as unknown etiology) West syndrome have normal development before onset, while patients with symptomatic West syndrome have preceding developmental delay owing to perinatal encephalopathies, malformations, underlying metabolic disorders, or other etiologies (see Chapter 593.2). In boys, West syndrome can also be caused by *ARX* gene mutations (often associated with ambiguous genitalia and cortical migration abnormalities). West syndrome, especially in cases of unknown etiology (cryptogenic cases, i.e., cases that are not symptomatic of metabolic or structural brain disorder), is a medical emergency because diagnosis delayed for 3 wk or longer can affect long-term prognosis. The spasms are often overlooked by parents and by physicians, being mistaken for startles caused by colic or for other benign paroxysmal syndromes (see Chapter 594).

Lennox-Gastaut syndrome typically starts between the ages of 2 and 10 yr and consists of a triad of developmental delay, multiple seizure types that as a rule include atypical absences, myoclonic, astatic, and tonic seizures. The tonic seizures occur either in wakefulness (causing falls and injuries) or also, typically, in sleep. The third component is the EEG findings (see Fig. 593-2): 1-2 Hz spike–and–slow waves, polyspike bursts in sleep, and a slow background in wakefulness. Patients commonly have myoclonic, atonic, and other seizure types that are difficult to control, and most are left with long-term cognitive impairment and intractable seizures despite multiple therapies. Some, but not all, patients start with Ohtahara syndrome, develop West syndrome, and then progress to Lennox-Gastaut syndrome. **Myoclonic astatic epilepsy** is a syndrome similar to, but milder than, Lennox-Gastaut syndrome that usually does not have tonic seizures or polyspike bursts in sleep. The prognosis is more favorable than that for Lennox-Gastaut syndrome. Another syndrome characterized by atonic seizures causing head nodding as well as tonic, clonic and stimulus sensitive seizures is the **nodding syndrome**, which is a recently described epidemic type of epilepsy seen in some African countries and often associated with encephalopathy, stunted growth, and variable degrees of cognitive deficits. The underlying etiology is unknown.

Progressive myoclonic epilepsies are a group of epilepsies characterized by progressive dementia and worsening myoclonic and other seizures. **Type I** or **Unverricht-Lundborg disease** (secondary to a cystatin B mutation) is more slowly progressive than the other types and usually starts in adolescence. **Type II** or **Lafora body disease** can have an early childhood onset but usually starts in adolescence, is more quickly progressive, and is usually fatal within the 2nd or 3rd decade. It can be associated with photosensitivity, manifests periodic acid–Schiff-positive Lafora inclusions on muscle or skin biopsy (in eccrine sweat gland cells), and has been shown to be caused by laforin (EPM2A) or malin (EPM2B) gene mutations. Other causes of progressive myoclonic epilepsy include myoclonic epilepsy with ragged red fibers, sialidosis type I, neuronal ceroid lipofuscinosis, juvenile neuropathic Gaucher disease, dentatorubral-pallidoluysian atrophy, and juvenile neuroaxonal dystrophy.

Myoclonic encephalopathy in nonprogressive disorders is an epileptic encephalopathy that occurs in some congenital disorders affecting the brain, such as Angelman syndrome, and consists of almost continuous and difficult-to-treat myoclonic and, at times, other seizures.

Landau-Kleffner syndrome is a rare condition of unknown cause characterized by loss of language skills attributed to auditory agnosia in a previously normal child. At least 70% have associated clinical seizures, but some do not. The seizures when they occur are of several types, including focal, generalized tonic–clonic, atypical absence, partial complex, and, occasionally, myoclonic seizures. High-amplitude spike-and-wave discharges predominate and tend to be bitemporal. In the later evolutionary stages of the condition, the EEG findings may be normal. The spike discharges are always more apparent during non–rapid eye movement sleep; thus, a child in whom Landau-Kleffner syndrome is suspected should have an EEG during sleep, particularly if the awake record is normal. CT and MRI studies typically yield normal results. In the related but clinically distinct epilepsy syndrome with **continuous spike waves in slow-wave sleep**, the discharges are more likely to be frontal or generalized and the delays more likely to be global. The approach and therapy to the 2 syndromes are similar. Valproic acid is often the anticonvulsant that is used first to treat the clinical seizures and may help the aphasia. Some children respond to clobazam, to the combination of valproic acid and clobazam, or to levetiracetam. For therapy of the aphasia, nocturnal diazepam therapy (0.2-0.5 mg/kg PO at bedtime for several months) is often used as first- or second-line therapy, as are oral steroids. Oral prednisone is started at 2 mg/kg/24 hr for 1 mo and decreased to 1 mg/kg/24 hr for an additional month. With clinical improvement, the prednisone is reduced further to 0.5 mg/kg/24 hr for up to 6-12 mo. Long-term therapy is often needed irrespective of what the patient responds to. If the seizures and aphasia persist after diazepam and steroids trials, then a course of intravenous immunoglobulins should be considered. It is imperative to initiate speech therapy and maintain it for several years, because improvement in language function occurs over a prolonged period.

Amenably treatable metabolic epilepsies are becoming increasingly recognized. **Pyridoxine-dependent epilepsy** typically presents as neonatal encephalopathy shortly after birth with, at times, report of increased fetal movements (seizure) in utero. There are associated gastrointestinal symptoms with emesis and abdominal distention, neurologic irritability, sleepless and facial grimacing along with recurrent partial motor seizure, generalized tonic seizures, and myoclonus. Seizures are usually refractory and may progress to status epilepticus if no pyridoxine is used. Some cases start in infancy or in childhood. Diagnosis is confirmed by the presence of elevated plasma, urine and CSF α-aminoadipic semialdehyde and elevated plasma and CSF pipecolic acid levels. The presence of either homozygous or compound heterozygous mutations in ALDH7A1 alleles (which encode the protein antiquitin) confirms the diagnosis. The use of pyridoxine 100 mg daily orally (up to 600 mg/day) or intravenously helps stop the seizures. **Pyridoxal phosphate responsive neonatal epileptic encephalopathy** (Pyridox[am]ine 5′-phosphate oxidase [PNPO] deficiency) may present similarly in the absence of gastrointestinal symptoms. Diagnostically, there are reduced pyridoxal phosphate levels in the CSF with increased levels of CSF levodopa and 3-methoxytyrosine along with decreased CSF homovanillic acid and 5-hydroxyindolacetic acid. The EEG may show a burst suppression pattern and treatment is by enteral administration of pyridoxal phosphate (up to 60 mg/kg/day). **Folinic acid–responsive seizures** may also present with neonatal epileptic encephalopathy and intractable seizures. These patients have a similar diagnostic profile as pyridoxine-dependent epilepsy patients and are caused by the same gene mutations but respond to folinic acid

supplementation in addition to pyridoxine use. **Cerebral folate deficiency**, which also responds to high doses of folinic acid (2-3 mg/kg/day), may manifest with epilepsy, intellectual disability, developmental regression, dyskinesias, and autism. CSF 5-methyltetrahydrofolate levels are decreased with normal plasma and red blood cell folate levels. There are usually mutations in the folate receptor (FOLR1) gene or blocking autoantibodies against membrane-associated folate receptors of the choroid plexus. **Tetrahydrobiopterin deficiencies** with or without hyperphenylalaninemia may present with epilepsies, and symptoms resulting from deficiencies of dopamine (parkinsonism, dystonia), noradrenaline (axial hypotonia), serotonin (depression, insomnia, temperature changes) and folate (myelin formation, basal ganglia calcifications, and seizures). Treatment is by substitution therapy with tetrahydrobiopterin and neurotransmitter precursors started as early as possible. **Creatine deficiency syndromes** present typically with developmental delay, seizures, autistic features, and movement disorders and are diagnosed by abnormal levels of urine creatine and guanidinoacetic acid and/or, depending on the type of underlying genetic etiology, with absent creatine peak on MR spectroscopy of the brain. Use of creatine monohydrate and dietary restrictions are helpful. **Biotinidase deficiency** presenting as developmental delay, seizures, ataxia, alopecia, and skin rash and often associated with intermittent metabolic acidosis and organic profile of lactic and propionic acidemia, responds to the use of biotin. Serine biosynthesis defects with low serine levels in plasma or CSF amino acids often present with congenital microcephaly, intractable seizures, and psychomotor retardation and respond to supplemental serine and glycine use. **Developmental delay, epilepsy, and neonatal diabetes** is caused by activating mutations in the adenosine triphosphate-sensitive potassium channels. Sulfonylurea drugs that block the potassium channel treat the neonatal diabetes and probably also favorably affect the central nervous system (CNS) symptoms and affect seizures. Hyperinsulinism-hyperammonemia syndrome is caused by activating mutations of the glutamate dehydrogenase encoded by the GLUD1 gene. Patients present with hypoglycemic seizures after a protein-rich meal with hyperammonemia (ammonia levels 80-150 µmol/L). They are managed with a combination of protein restriction, AEDs, and diazoxide (a potassium channel agonist that inhibits insulin release). **GLUT-1 deficiency syndrome** classically presents with infantile-onset epilepsy, developmental delay, acquired microcephaly, and complex movement disorders. It causes impaired glucose transport to the brain typically diagnosed by genetic testing or finding of low CSF lactate and CSF glucose, or low CSF to serum glucose ratios (less than 0.4). The manifestations of the disease are usually responsive to ketogenic diet.

593.5 Mechanisms of Seizures
Mohamad A. Mikati and Abeer J. Hani

One can distinguish in the pathophysiology of epilepsy 4 distinct, often sequential, mechanistic processes. First is the **underlying etiology**, which is any pathology or pathologic process that can disrupt neuronal function and connectivity and that eventually leads to the second process (epileptogenesis) which makes the brain epileptic. The underlying etiologies of epilepsy are diverse and include, among other entities, brain tumors and malformations, strokes, scarring, or mutations of specific genes. These mutations can involve voltage-gated channels (Na^+, K^+, Ca^{2+}, Cl^-, and HCN [hydrogen cyanide]), ligand-gated channels (nicotinic acetylcholine and γ-aminobutyric acid A receptors [$GABA_A$]) or other proteins. In some but not in all such mutations, the molecular and cellular deficits caused by the mutations have been identified. For example, in Dravet syndrome, the loss of function mutation in the SCN1A gene causes decreased excitability in inhibitory GABAergic interneurons, leading to increased excitability and epilepsy. In human cortical dysplasia, the expression of the NR2B subunit of the NMDA receptor is increased, leading to excessive depolarizing currents. In many other epileptic conditions, a clear etiology is still lacking and in others the etiology may be known, but it is still not known how the identified underlying genetic etiology or brain insult results in epileptogenesis.

Second, **epileptogenesis** is the mechanism through which the brain, or part of it, turns epileptic. The presence of this process explains why some patients with the above pathologies develop epilepsy and some do not. **Kindling** is an animal model for human focal epilepsy in which repeated electrical stimulation of selected areas of the brain with a low-intensity current initially causes no apparent changes but with repeated stimulation results in epilepsy. This repetitive stimulation can lead to temporal lobe epilepsy, for example, through activation of metabotropic and ionotropic glutamate receptors (by glutamate), as well as the tropomyosin-related kinase B receptor (by brain-derived neurotrophic factor and neurotrophin-4). This leads to an increase in the intraneuronal calcium, which, in turn, activates calcium calmodulin–dependent protein kinase and calcineurin, a phosphatase, resulting eventually in calcium-dependent epileptogenic gene expression (e.g., c-fos) and promotion of mossy fiber sprouting. **Mossy fibers** are excitatory fibers that connect the granule cells to the CA3 region within the hippocampus, and their pathologic sprouting underlies increased excitability in medial temporal lobe epilepsy associated with mesial temporal sclerosis in humans and in animal models. The cell loss in the CA3 region that is a characteristic of mesial temporal sclerosis (presumably resulting from an original insult such as a prolonged febrile status epilepticus episode or hypoxia) leads to a pathologic attempt at compensation by sprouting of the excitatory mossy fibers. Consequently, mossy fiber sprouting, which has been demonstrated in humans also, leads to increased excitability and to epilepsy. Complex febrile seizures in rats induce hyperactivation of, paradoxically excitatory, GABA$_A$ receptors leading to granule cell ectopia and to subsequent temporal lobe epilepsy. Possibly similar yet to be fully characterized epileptogenesis mechanisms may underlie other focal epilepsies.

Lately, the role of large-scale molecular cell signaling pathways in epileptogenesis, namely the mammalian target of rapamycin (mTOR), the Ras/ERK, and repressor element 1 (RE1)-silencing transcription factor (REST; also known as neuron-restrictive silencer factor) pathways have been implicated in the mechanisms leading to epilepsy. The mTOR pathway in tuberous sclerosis, hemimegalencephaly and cortical dysplasia-related epilepsies, Ras/ERK in a number of syndromes, and REST in epileptogenesis after acute neuronal injury.

The third process is the resultant **epileptic state of increased excitability** that is present in all patients irrespective of the underlying etiology or mechanism of epileptogenesis. In a seizure focus, each neuron has a stereotypic synchronized response called **paroxysmal depolarization shift** that consists of a sudden depolarization phase, resulting from glutamate and calcium channel activation, with a series of action potentials at its peak followed by an after-hyperpolarization phase, resulting from activation of potassium channels and GABA receptors that open chloride channels. When the after-hyperpolarization is disrupted in a sufficient number of neurons, the inhibitory surround is lost and a population of neurons fire at the same rate and time, resulting in a seizure focus. In childhood absence epilepsy, the discharging neurons also develop a paroxysmal depolarization shift similar to the one found in partial epilepsy. However, the mechanism of paroxysmal depolarization shift generation is different because it involves thalamocortical connections bilaterally. T-type calcium channels on thalamic relay neurons are activated during hyperpolarization by GABAergic interneurons in the reticular thalamic nucleus, which results in enhancement of synchronization in the thalamocortical loop and consequently in the typical generalized spike-wave pattern. In tumor-related epilepsy, particularly in that related to oligodendroglioma, the voltage-gated sodium channels are present on the surface of tumor cells at a higher density than on normal cells, and their inactivation is impaired by the alkaline pH present in this condition. In hypothalamic hamartoma causing gelastic seizures, clusters of GABAergic interneurons spontaneously fire, thus synchronizing the output of the hypothalamic hamartoma neurons projecting to the hippocampus.

The fourth process is **seizure-related neuronal injury** as demonstrated by MRI in patients after prolonged febrile and afebrile status

epilepticus. Many such patients show acute swelling in the hippocampus and long-term hippocampal atrophy with sclerosis on MRI. Nonetheless in most patients with seizure-related MRI abnormalities, the findings are transient. In experimental models, the mechanisms of such injuries have been shown to involve both apoptosis and necrosis of neurons in the involved regions. There is evidence from surgically resected epileptic tissue that apoptotic pathways are activated in foci of intractable epilepsy.

In infantile spasms, recently developed animal models suggest that increases in stress-related corticotropin-releasing hormone, sodium channel blockade, and NMDA receptor stimulation are contributing mechanisms. Prior positron emission tomography data suggest that an interaction between focal cortical lesions and the brainstem raphe nuclei is important at least in some infantile spasms patients.

Bibliography is available at Expert Consult.

593.6 Treatment of Seizures and Epilepsy
Mohamad A. Mikati and Abeer J. Hani

DECIDING ON LONG-TERM THERAPY
After a *first seizure*, if the risk of recurrence is low, such as when the patient has normal neurodevelopmental status, EEG, and MRI (risk approximately 20%), then treatment is usually not started. If the patient has abnormal EEG, MRI, development, and/or neurologic exam, and/or a positive family history of epilepsy, then the risk is higher and often treatment is started. Other considerations are also important, such as motor vehicle driving status and type of employment in older patients or the parents' ability to deal with recurrences or AED drug therapy in children. The decision is therefore always individualized. All aspects of this decision-making process should be discussed with the family. Figure 593-4 presents an overview of the approach to the treatment of seizures and epilepsy.

COUNSELING
An important part of the management of a patient with epilepsy is educating the family and the child about the disease, its management, and the limitations it might impose and how to deal with them. It is important to establish a successful therapeutic alliance. Restrictions on driving (in adolescents) and on swimming are usually necessary (Table 593-10). In most states, the physician is not required to report the epileptic patient to the motor vehicle registry; this is the responsibility of the patient. The physician then is requested to complete a specific form for patients who are being cleared to drive. Also in most states, a seizure-free period of 6 mo, and in some states longer, is required before driving is allowed. Often swimming in rivers, lakes, or sea, and underwater diving are prohibited, but swimming in swimming pools may be allowable. When swimming, even patients with epilepsy that is under excellent control should be under the continuous supervision of an observer who is aware of their condition and capable of lifeguard-level rescue.

The physician, parents, and child should jointly evaluate the risk of involvement in athletic activities. To participate in athletics, proper medical management, good seizure control, and proper supervision are crucial to avoid significant risks. Any activity where a seizure might cause a dangerous fall should be avoided; these activities include rope climbing, use of the parallel bars, and high diving. Participation in collision or contact sports depends on the patient's condition. Epileptic children should not automatically be banned from participating in hockey, baseball, basketball, football, or wrestling. Rather, individual consideration should be based on the child's specific case (see Table 593-10).

Counseling is helpful to support the family and to educate them about the resources available in the community. Educational and, in some cases, psychologic evaluation may be necessary to evaluate for possible learning disabilities or abnormal behavioral patterns that might coexist with the epilepsy. Epilepsy does carry a risk of increased

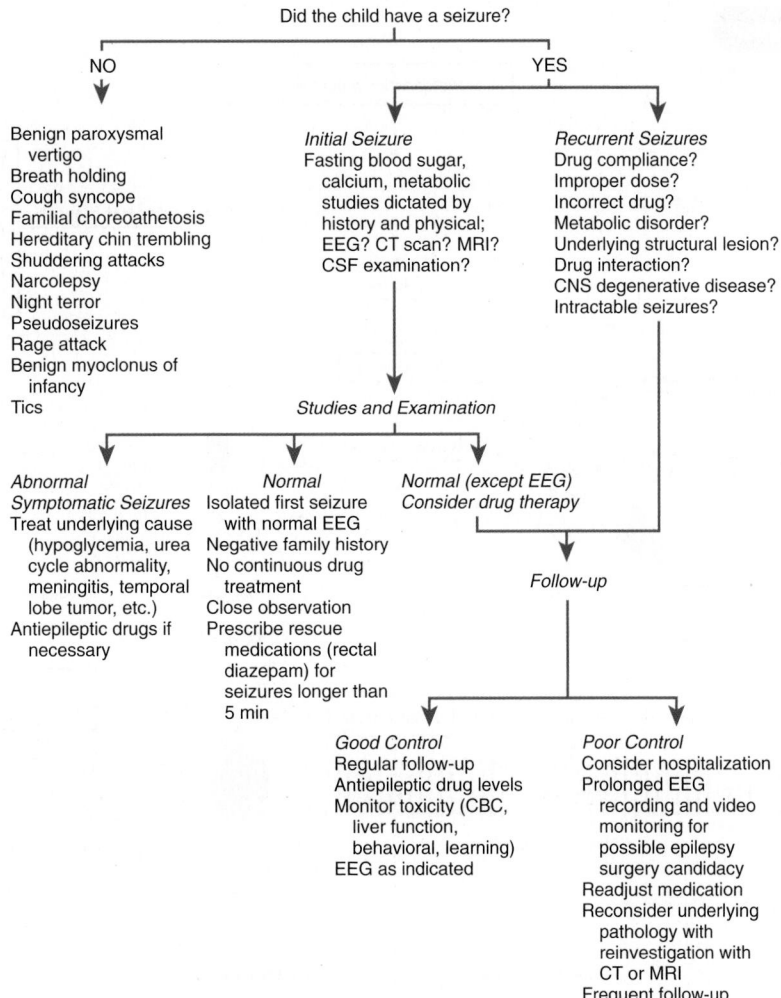

Figure 593-4 Approach to the child with a suspected convulsive disorder.

Table 593-10	Sports and Special Considerations for the Child with Epilepsy*
SPORTS TYPE	**SPECIAL CONSIDERATIONS**
Body contact sports	If there are more than occasional seizures, physician evaluation of benefits and risks of participation should be made based on the child's condition. No contraindications in general except for boxing.
Noncontact sports	Generally recommended. Anxiety and fatigue can cause a problem in some children. Individualization based on clinical history must be the rule.
Gymnastics	A fall can result if the child experiences a sudden seizure, especially with trampolines, parallel bars, and rope climbing, which should be avoided. Individual consideration remains the basic determinant.
Swimming	The child should always be under supervision, and scuba diving should be discouraged in poorly controlled epileptics.

*Specific advice should be individualized depending on the patient's clinical condition. Many patients actually have fewer seizures when they are active than when they are idle.

Modified from Committee on Children with Handicaps: The epileptic child and competitive school athletics, Pediatrics 42:700–702, 1968; and Knowles BD: Athletes with seizure disorders, Curr Sports Med Rep 11(1):16–20, 2012, Table 1.

mortality (2 or more times the standardized mortality rates of the general population) and of sudden unexpected death. This is mostly related to the conditions associated with or underlying the epilepsy (e.g., tumor, metabolic diseases), to poor seizure control (e.g., in patients with severe epileptic encephalopathies, or drug-resistant seizures), and to poor compliance with prescribed therapies. Thus, family members can usually be informed about this increased risk without inappropriately increasing their anxiety. Many family members feel they need to observe the patient continuously in wakefulness and sleep and have the patient sleep in the parents' room to detect seizures. There are currently advertised seizure-detection equipment that use motion sensors placed under the mattress to detect seizures. Some are disappointing and ineffective in detecting seizures, whereas data from other equipment are encouraging in that they were useful in detecting a majority of generalized tonic–clonic seizures during sleep (see bibliography for details). Whether such measures can reduce sudden unexpected death in epilepsy (SUDEP) risk remains to be seen and the parents need to guard against being overprotective to avoid adversely affecting the psychology of the child. Education about what to do in case of seizures, the choices of treatment or no treatment and of medications and their side effects, and potential complications of epilepsy should be provided to the parents and, if the child is old enough, to the child.

MECHANISMS OF ACTION OF ANTIEPILEPTIC DRUGS

AEDs reduce excitability by interfering with the sodium, potassium or calcium ion channels, by reducing excitatory neurotransmitter release

RESPONSE TO ANTIEPILEPTIC DRUGS

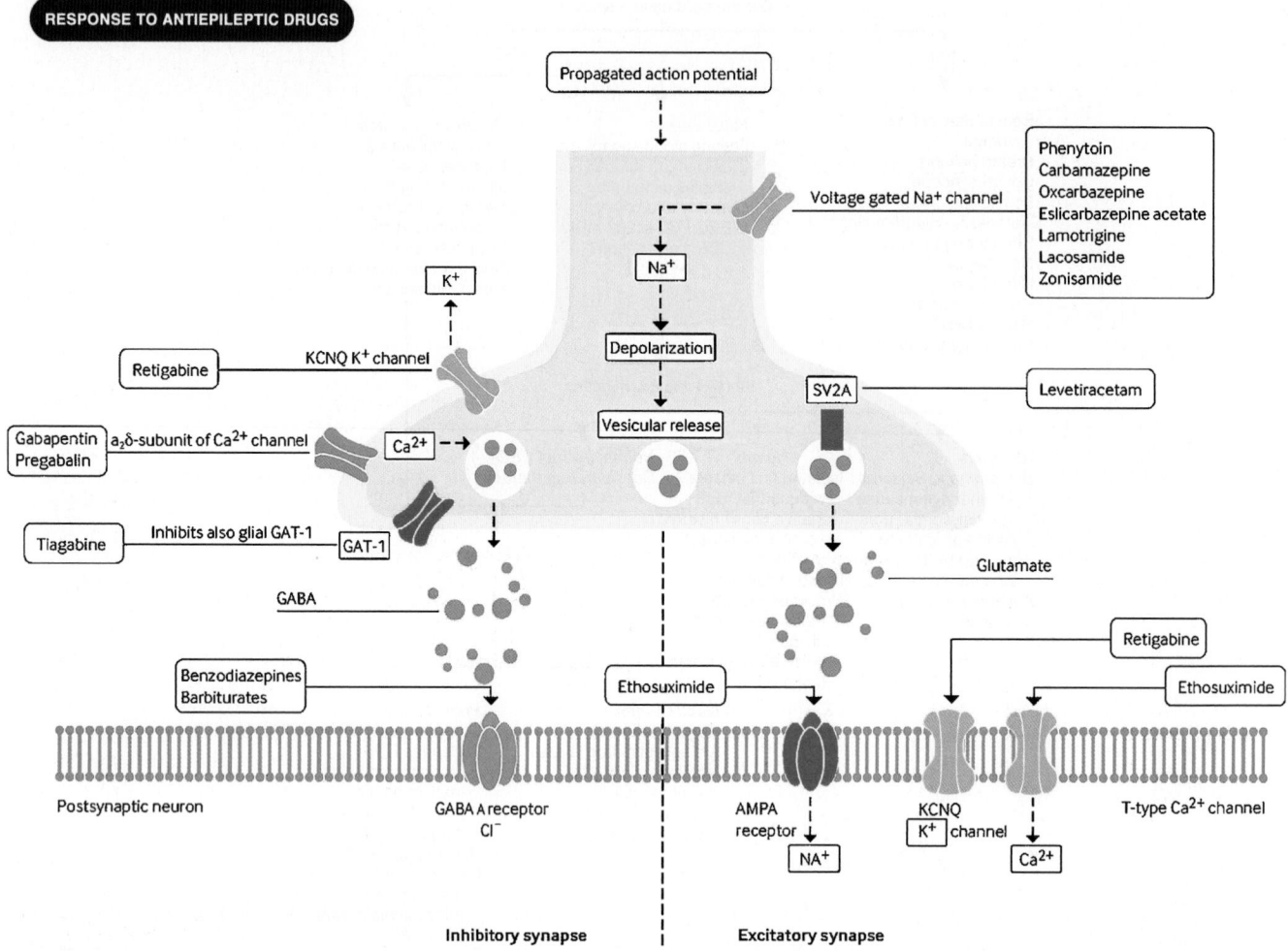

Figure 593-5 Mechanisms of action of antiepileptic drugs, which act by diverse mechanisms, mainly involving modulation of voltage activated ion channels, potentiation of GABA, and inhibition of glutamate. Approved antiepileptic drugs have effects on inhibitory *(left hand side)* and excitatory *(right hand side)* nerve terminals. The antiepileptic efficacy in trials of most of these drugs as initial add-on does not differ greatly, indicating that seemingly similar antiseizure activity can be obtained by mechanisms aimed at diverse targets. However, putative mechanisms of action were determined only after discovering the antiseizure effects; mechanism driven drug discovery has been largely ignored. AMPA, α-amino-3-hydroxy-5-methyl-4-isoxazole propionic acid; GABA, γ-aminobutyric acid; GAT-1, sodium-dependent and chloride-dependent GABA transporter 1; SV2A, synaptic vesicle glycoprotein 2A. *(From Schmidt D, Schachter SC: Drug treatment of epilepsy in adults. BMJ, 348:bmj.g254, 2014.)*

or function, or by enhancing GABAergic inhibition (Fig. 593-5). Most medications have multiple mechanisms of action, and the exact mechanism responsible for their activity in human epilepsy is usually not fully understood. Often, medications acting on sodium channels are effective against partial seizures, and medications acting on T-type calcium channels are effective against absence seizures. Voltage-gated sodium channels are blocked by felbamate, valproate, topiramate, carbamazepine, oxcarbazepine, lamotrigine, phenytoin, rufinamide, lacosamide, and zonisamide. T-type calcium channels, found in the thalamus area, are blocked by valproate, zonisamide, and ethosuximide. Voltage-gated calcium channels are inhibited by gabapentin, pregabalin, lamotrigine, and felbamate. N-type calcium channels are inhibited by levetiracetam. Ezogabine/retigabine opens KCNQ/Kv7 voltage-gated potassium channels.

GABA$_A$ receptors are activated by phenobarbital, benzodiazepines, topiramate, felbamate, and levetiracetam. Tiagabine, by virtue of its binding to GABA transporters 1 (GAT-1) and 3 (GAT-3), is a GABA reuptake inhibitor. GABA levels are increased by vigabatrin via its irreversible inhibition of GABA transaminases. Valproate inhibits GABA transaminases, acts on GABA$_B$ presynaptic receptors (also done by gabapentin), and activates glutamic acid decarboxylase (the enzyme that forms GABA).

Glutaminergic transmission is decreased by felbamate that blocks NMDA and AMPA (α-amino-3-hydroxy-5-methyl-4-isoxazole-

propionic acid)/kainate receptors. Topiramate also blocks AMPA/kainate receptors. Levetiracetam binds to the presynaptic vesicle protein SV2A found in all neurotransmitter vesicles and possibly results in inhibition of presynaptic neurotransmitter release in a use-dependent manner. Perampanel blocks glutamate AMPA receptors.

CHOICE OF DRUG ACCORDING TO SEIZURE TYPE AND EPILEPSY SYNDROME

Drug therapy should be based on the type of seizure and the epilepsy syndrome as well as on other individual factors. In general, the **drugs of first choice** for focal seizures and epilepsies are oxcarbazepine and carbamazepine; for absence seizures, ethosuximide; for juvenile myoclonic epilepsy, valproate and lamotrigine; for Lennox-Gastaut syndrome, clobazam, valproate, topiramate, lamotrigine, and, most recently, as add on, rufinamide; and for infantile spasms, adrenocorticotropic hormone (ACTH). There is significant controversy about these choices, and therapy should always be individualized (see Choice of Drug: Other Considerations below and Table 593-10).

West syndrome is best treated with ACTH. There are several protocols that range in dose from high to intermediate to low. The recommended regimen of ACTH (80 mg/mL) is a daily dose of 150 units/m^2 (divided into twice-daily intramuscular injections of 75 units/m^2, the lot number is recorded) administered over a 2-wk period with a subsequent gradual taper over a 2-wk period (30 units/m^2 in the morning for 3 days; 15 units/m² in the morning for 3 days; 10 units/m² in the morning for 3 days; and 10 units/m² every other morning for 6 days, then stop). The increase in price of ACTH gel in the United States has led many physicians to use the lower-dose regimen because it may be just as effective (initial: 20 units/day for 2 wk, if patient responds, taper and discontinue over a 1-wk period; if patient does not respond, increase dose to 30 units/day for 4 wk then taper and discontinue over a 1-wk period). Response is usually observed within the 1st 7 days; however, if no response is observed within 2 wk, the lot is changed. During the tapering period of any regimen, and especially in symptomatic patients, relapse can occur. Remediation entails increasing the dose to the previously effective dose for 2 wk and then beginning the taper again. Synthetic ACTH has also been used: Synacthen Depot intramuscular 0.25 mg/mL or 1 mg/mL is used; 1 mg is considered to have the potency of 100 IU in stimulating the adrenal gland.

Awake and asleep EEGs are often done 1, 2, and 4 wk after the initiation of ACTH to monitor the patient's response, with the aim of clearing the EEG from hypsarrhythmia and of stopping the seizures. Side effects, more common with the higher doses, include hypertension, electrolyte imbalance, infections, hyperglycemia and/or glycosuria, and gastric ulcers. All should be carefully monitored for and prophylactic therapy for ulcers is desirable. ACTH is generally thought to offer an added advantage, particularly in cryptogenic cases, over vigabatrin and possibly over prednisone and other steroids.

Vigabatrin is considered by some as a drug of second choice for infantile spasms and by some even as an alternative to ACTH as a drug of first choice. Its principal side effect is retinal toxicity that is seen in approximately 30% of the patients, with resultant visual field defects that persist despite withdrawal of the drug. The level of evidence for its efficacy is weaker than that for ACTH but stronger than that of other alternative medications, including valproate, benzodiazepines like nitrazepam and clonazepam, topiramate, lamotrigine, zonisamide, pyridoxine, ketogenic diet, and intravenous gamma globulin (IVIG). None of these alternative drugs offers uniformly satisfactory results. However, they are useful for decreasing the frequency and severity of seizures in patients with symptomatic infantile spasms and as adjunctive therapy in patients with cryptogenic infantile spasms who do not respond completely to ACTH or vigabatrin.

Lennox-Gastaut syndrome is another difficult-to-treat epilepsy syndrome. Treatment of seizures in Lennox-Gastaut syndrome varies according to the preponderant seizure type. For drop attacks (tonic, atonic, or myoclonic astatic seizures), valproate, lamotrigine, topiramate, clobazam, felbamate, and rufinamide are considered to be effective. Felbamate is used as a last resort medication because of its potential toxicity. These drugs might control other types of seizures (partial, generalized tonic–clonic, atypical absence, other tonic, myoclonic) as well. For patients who have a preponderance of atypical absence seizures, lamotrigine or ethosuximide are often suitable drugs to try because they are relatively less toxic than many of the alternative drugs. Valproate is helpful against these seizures, too. Clonazepam is often helpful but produces significant sedation, hyperactivity, and drooling, and often tolerance to its antiepileptic effects develops in a few months. Consequently, clonazepam is often used as a rescue medication for clusters of seizures (disintegrating tablet preparation). In resistant cases of Lennox-Gastaut syndrome and related epilepsies, zonisamide, levetiracetam, acetazolamide, methsuximide, corticosteroids, ketogenic diet, or IVIG can be used.

Dravet syndrome is usually treated with valproate and benzodiazepines such as clobazam or clonazepam. The ketogenic diet can also be useful in patients with this syndrome, including cases with refractory status. Stiripentol, which is available in some countries, is useful, particularly if used in combination with valproate and clobazam, but doses need to be adjusted, since stirpentol can increase clobazam levels and valproate can increase stirpentol levels. Other medications include zonisamide and topiramate. Lamotrigine, carbamazepine, and phenytoin are reported to exacerbate seizures. Barbiturate use during status epilepticus in this syndrome is suspected to be associated with adverse outcomes; consequently, alternative acute therapies in such cases need to be considered.

Very rare cases of patients who have neonatal, infantile, or early childhood seizures who have **pyridoxine-dependent epilepsy** (demonstrated to be caused by antiquitin gene mutation) respond to pyridoxine 10-100 mg/day orally (up to 600 mg/day has been used) within 3-7 days of the initiation of oral therapy and almost immediately if given parenterally. Some patients have seizures that are intractable from onset, but others have seizures that show an initial but transient response to traditional AEDs. Some of these patients also require concurrent folinic acid (5-15 mg/day). Other patients require the active form of vitamin B₆, specifically, pyridoxal phosphate (50 mg/day initial dose that can be increased gradually up to 15 mg/kg every 6 hr) owing to their deficiency of **PNPO**. In both the PNPO-deficient/pyridoxal phosphate–dependent and the pyridoxine-dependent forms, hypotonia and hypopnea can occur after initiation of vitamin therapy. Pyridoxine has also been used by some, specifically in Japan, early in the treatment of West syndrome. Patients with **cerebral folate deficiency** can respond to folinic acid supplementation (usually at doses of 2-3 mg/kg/day). Traditionally these entities have been diagnosed by giving the vitamin B₆ or folinic acid in therapeutic trials, but currently laboratory testing is available to confirm the diagnosis (see Chapter 593.4).

Absence seizures are most often initially treated with ethosuximide, which is, as effective as, but less toxic than, valproate and more effective than lamotrigine. Alternative drugs of first choice are lamotrigine and valproate, especially if generalized tonic–clonic seizures coexist with absence seizures, as these 2 medications are effective against the latter seizures whereas ethosuximide is not. Patients resistant to ethosuximide might still respond to valproate or to lamotrigine. In absence seizures, the EEG is usually helpful in monitoring the response to therapy and is often more sensitive than the parents' observations in detecting these seizures. The EEG often normalizes when complete seizure control is achieved. This is usually not true for partial epilepsies. Other medications that could be used for absence seizures include acetazolamide, zonisamide, or clonazepam.

Benign myoclonic epilepsies are often best treated with valproate, particularly when patients have associated generalized tonic–clonic and absence seizures. Benzodiazepines, clonazepam, lamotrigine, and topiramate are alternatives for the treatment of benign myoclonic epilepsy. **Severe myoclonic epilepsies** are treated with medications effective for Lennox-Gastaut syndrome such topiramate, clobazam, and valproate, as well as zonisamide. Levetiracetam may also have efficacy in myoclonic epilepsies.

Partial and secondary generalized tonic and clonic seizures can be treated with oxcarbazepine, levetiracetam, carbamazepine, phenobarbital, topiramate, valproic acid, lamotrigine, clobazam, or clonazepam (see Table 593-8). Oxcarbazepine, levetiracetam, carbamazepine (United States), or valproate (Europe) are often being used first. One study favored lamotrigine as initial monotherapy for partial seizures and valproate for generalized seizures. Almost any of these medications has been used as first or second choice. depending on the individualization of the therapy.

CHOICE OF DRUG: OTHER CONSIDERATIONS

Because there are many options for each patient, the choice of which drug to use is always an individualized decision based on comparative effectiveness data from randomized controlled trials and on several other considerations delineated below.

Comparative effectiveness (Table 593-11) and **potential for paradoxical seizure aggravation** by some AEDs (e.g., precipitation of myoclonic seizures by lamotrigine in Dravet syndrome and exacerbation of absence seizures by carbamazepine and tiagabine) must be considered.

♦ **Comparative tolerability** (see Table 593-14): Adverse effects can vary according to the profile of the patient. The most prominent example is the increased risk of liver toxicity for valproate therapy in children who are younger than 2 yr of age, on polytherapy, and/or have metabolic disorders. Thus, if metabolic disorders are suspected, other drugs should be considered first and valproate should not be started until the metabolic disorders are ruled out by normal amino acids, organic acids, acylcarnitine profile, lactate,

Table 593-11	Comparison of Recommendations for the Treatment of Pediatric Epilepsy

SEIZURE TYPE OR EPILEPSY SYNDROME	FDA APPROVED	SIGN (2005)	NICE (2012)	AAN (2004)	ILAE (2013)*	PEDIATRIC EXPERT CONSENSUS SURVEY (NORTH AMERICA–2005)	PEDIATRIC EXPERT CONSENSUS SURVEY (EUROPE–2007)
Partial-onset	CBZ, ezogabine, lacosamide, LEV, LTG, OXC, PB, perampanel, PHT, TPM, VGB	CBZ, CLB, LTG, OXC, PHT, TPM, VGB, VPA	CBZ, LEV, LTG, OXC, VPA	CBZ, GBP, LTG, OXC, PB, PHT, TPM	A: OXC B: None C: CBZ, PB, PHT, TPM, VGB, VPA D: CLB, CZP, LTG, ZNS	CBZ, OXC	CBZ, OXC
BCECT	None	Not specifically mentioned	CBZ, LEV, LTG, OXC, VPA	Not surveyed	A, B: None C: CBZ, VPA D: GBP, LEV, OXC, STM	CBZ, OXC	VPA
Childhood absence epilepsy	ESM, VPA	ESM, LTG, VPA	ESM, LTG, VPA	LTG	A: ESM, VPA B: None C: LTG D: None	ESM	VPA
Juvenile myoclonic epilepsy	LEV, LTG, TPM	VPA	LEV, LTG, TPM, VPA	Not surveyed	A, B, C: None D: TPM, VPA	LTG, VPA	VPA
Lennox-Gastaut syndrome	CLB, FLB, LTG, rufinamide (atonic), TPM	CLB, LTG, VPA	VPA	Not surveyed	Not reviewed	LTG, VPA	VPA
Infantile spasms	VGB	Nitrazepam, TPM, VGB, VPA	Corticosteroids, VGB	ACTH, VGB (updated IS guidelines 2012)	Not reviewed	ACTH, VGB	VGB
Primary generalized tonic-clonic seizures	LEV, LTG, TPM	TPM, VPA	LTG, TPM, VPA	No evidence given	A: None B: None C: CBZ, PB, PHT, TPM, VPA D: OXC		

*ILAE recommendations are listed according to levels of evidence supporting the efficacy of the options. Level A: ≥1 class I randomized controlled trial (RCT) or ≥2 class II RCTs; Level B: 1 class II RCT or ≥2 class III RCTs; Level C: ≥2 class III RCTs; Level D: 1 class III double-blind or open-label study or 1 class IV clinical study or data from expert committee reports, opinions from experienced clinicians.

AAN, American Academy of Neurology; ACTH, adrenocorticotropic hormone; BCECT, benign childhood epilepsy with centrotemporal spikes; CBZ, carbamazepine; CLB, clobazam; CZP, clonazepam; ESM, ethosuximide; FDA, Food and Drug Administration; FLB, felbamate; GBP, gabapentin; ILAE, International League against Epilepsy; LEV, levetiracetam; LTG, lamotrigine; NICE, National Institute for Clinical Excellence; OXC, oxcarbazepine; PB, phenobarbital; PHT, phenytoin; SIGN, Scottish Intercollegiate Guidelines Network; STM, sulthiame; TPM, topiramate; VGB, vigabatrin; VPA, valproic acid; ZNS, zonisamide.

Modified and updated from Wheless JW, Clarke DF, Arzimanoglou A, et al: Treatment of pediatric epilepsy: European expert opinion, Epileptic Disord 9:353–412, 2007; and Perucca E, Tomson T; ILAE Subcommission on AED Guidelines. Updated ILAE evidence review of antiepileptic drug efficacy and effectiveness as initial monotherapy for epileptic seizures and syndromes. Epilepsia 54(3):551–563, 2013.

pyruvate, liver function tests, and perhaps other tests. The choice of an AED can also be influenced by the likelihood of occurrence of nuisance side effects such as weight gain (valproate, carbamazepine), gingival hyperplasia (phenytoin), alopecia (valproate), hyperactivity (benzodiazepines, barbiturates, levetiracetam, valproate, gabapentin). Children with behavior problems and/or with attention-deficit disorder can become particularly hyperactive with GABAergic drugs mentioned above. This often affects the choice of medications.

◆ **Cost and availability:** The cost of the newer AEDs often precludes their use, particularly in developing countries where cost is a major issue. Also, many drugs are not available in many countries either because they are too expensive, because, paradoxically, they are too inexpensive (lower profit margin), or because of regulatory restrictions. AEDs have a narrow therapeutic range and thus switching from brand name to generic formulations, or from one generic to another, can result in changes in levels that could result in breakthrough seizures or side effects. Thus, generic substitution is generally best avoided, particularly in fragile patients, if a brand name drug has already proved efficacious.

◆ **Ease of initiation** of the AED: Medications that are started very gradually such as lamotrigine and topiramate should not be chosen in situations when there is a need to achieve a therapeutic level quickly. In such situations, medications that have intravenous preparations or that can be started and titrated more quickly, such as valproate, phenytoin, or levetiracetam, should be considered instead.

◆ **Drug interactions** and presence of background medications: An example is the potential interference of enzyme-inducing drugs with many chemotherapeutic agents. In those cases, medications like gabapentin or levetiracetam are used. Also, valproate inhibits the metabolism and increases the levels of lamotrigine, phenobarbital, and felbamate. It also displaces protein-bound phenytoin from protein-binding sites, increasing the free fraction, and, thus, the free and not the total level needs to be checked when both medications are being used together. Enzyme inducers like phenobarbital, carbamazepine, phenytoin, and primidone reduce levels of lamotrigine, valproate, and, to a lesser extent, topiramate and zonisamide. Medications exclusively excreted by the kidney like levetiracetam and gabapentin are not subject to such interactions.

Table 593-12	Teratogenesis and Perinatal Outcomes of Antiepileptic Drugs	
FINDING	**RECOMMENDATION**	**LEVEL OF RECOMMENDATION**
VPA as part of polytherapy and possibly monotherapy probably contributes to the development of major congenital malformations and adverse cognitive outcome	If possible, avoidance of valproate polytherapy during the 1st trimester of pregnancy should be considered so as to decrease the risk of major congenital malformations and adverse cognitive outcome	B
AED polytherapy, as compared to monotherapy, regimens probably contribute to the development of major congenital malformations and to adverse cognitive outcomes	If possible, avoidance of AED polytherapy during the 1st trimester of pregnancy should be considered to decrease the risk of major congenital malformations and adverse cognitive outcome	B
Monotherapy exposure to phenytoin or phenobarbital possibly increases the likelihood of adverse cognitive outcomes	If possible, avoidance of phenytoin and phenobarbital during pregnancy may be considered to prevent adverse cognitive outcomes	C
Neonates of women with epilepsy taking AEDs probably have an increased risk of being small for gestational age and possibly have an increased risk of a 1 min Apgar score of <7	Pregnancy risk stratification should reflect that the offspring of women with epilepsy taking AEDs are probably at increased risk for being small for gestational age (level B) and possibly at increased risk of 1 min Apgar scores of <7	C

Levels of recommendation: A: strongest recommendation; based on class 1 evidence; B and C: lower levels of recommendations.
    Types of malformations: Prior studies had reported the occurrence of spina bifida with valproate and carbamazepine therapy, and of cardiac malformation and cleft palate after carbamazepine, phenytoin, and phenobarbital exposure. There is variability from study to study. However, in general the relative incidence of major malformations of approximately 10% for valproate monotherapy, higher with valproate polytherapy, and in the range of 5% for monotherapy with the other above 3 AEDs and higher with polytherapy.
    FDA categories: Valproate, phenobarbital, carbamazepine, and phenytoin are classified by the FDA as category D. Ethosuximide, felbamate, gabapentin, lamotrigine, levetiracetam, oxcarbazepine, tiagabine, topiramate, and zonisamide are category C. Category C: Animal studies have shown an adverse effect and there are no adequate and well-controlled studies in pregnant women or no animal studies have been conducted and there are no adequate and well-controlled studies in pregnant women. Category D: Studies, adequate, well-controlled, or observational, in pregnant women have demonstrated a risk to the fetus. However, the benefits of therapy might outweigh the potential risk.
    AED, antiepileptic drug; VPA, valproate.
    Data from Harden CL, Meador KJ, Pennell PB, et al: Practice parameter update: management issues for women with epilepsy—focus on pregnancy (an evidence-based review): teratogenesis and perinatal outcomes. Report of the Quality Standards Subcommittee and Therapeutics and Technology Subcommittee of the American Academy of Neurology and American Epilepsy Society, Neurology 73(2):133–141, 2009.

◆ **The presence of comorbid conditions:** For example, the presence of migraine in a patient with epilepsy can lead to the choice of a medication that is effective against both conditions such as valproate or topiramate. In an obese patient, a medication such as valproate might be avoided, and a medication that decreases appetite such as topiramate might be used instead. In adolescent girls of child-bearing potential, enzyme-inducing AEDs are often avoided because they can interfere with birth control pills; other AEDs, particularly valproate, can increase risks for fetal malformations (Table 593-12). Valproic acid may unmask or exacerbate certain underlying metabolic disorders; these include nonketotic hyperglycinemia, DNA polymerase γ mutations *(POLG)* with mitochondrial DNA depletion (also known as Alpers-Huttenlocher syndrome), other mitochondrial disorders (Leigh syndrome; mitochondrial myopathy, encephalopathy, lactic acidosis, and stroke-like episodes [MELAS]; myoclonic epilepsy with ragged red fibers; myoclonic epilepsy-myopathy-sensory ataxia syndrome), and hyperammonemic encephalopathies. Manifestations may include hepatotoxicity or encephalopathy.

◆ **Coexisting seizures:** In a patient with both absence and generalized tonic–clonic seizures, a drug that has a broad spectrum of antiseizure effects such as lamotrigine or valproate could be used rather than medications that have a narrow spectrum of efficacy, such as phenytoin and ethosuximide.

◆ **History of prior response** to specific AEDs: For example, if a patient or a family member with the same problem had previously responded to carbamazepine, carbamazepine could be a desirable choice.

◆ **Mechanism of drug actions:** At present, the current understanding of the pathophysiology of epilepsy does not allow specific choice of AEDs based on the assumed pathophysiology of the epilepsy. However, in general, it is believed that it is better to avoid combining medications that have similar mechanisms of action, such as phenytoin and carbamazepine (both work on sodium channels). A number of medications, such as lamotrigine and valproate or topiramate and lamotrigine, are reported to have synergistic effects, possibly because they have different mechanisms of action.

◆ **Ease of use:** Medications that are given once or twice a day are easier to use than medications that are given 3 or 4 times a day. Availability of a pediatric liquid preparation, particularly if palatable, also plays a role.

◆ **Ability to monitor the medication** and adjust the dose: Some medications are difficult to adjust and to follow, requiring frequent blood levels. The prototype of such medications is phenytoin, but many of the older medications also require blood level monitoring for optimal titration. However, monitoring in itself can represent a practical or patient satisfaction disadvantage for the older drugs as compared to the newer AEDs, which generally do not require blood-level monitoring except to check for compliance.

◆ **Patient's and family's preferences:** All things being equal, the choice between 2 or more acceptable alternative AEDs might also depend on the patient's or family's preferences. For example, some patients might want to avoid gingival hyperplasia and hirsutism as side effects but might tolerate weight loss, or vice versa.

◆ **Genetics** and genetic testing: A genetic predisposition to developing AED-induced side effects is another factor that may be a consideration. For example, there is a strong association between the human leukocyte antigen HLA-B*1502 allele and severe cutaneous reactions induced by carbamazepine, phenytoin, or lamotrigine in Chinese Han patients and, to a lesser extent, South East Asian populations; hence these AEDs should be avoided in genetically susceptible persons after testing for the allele. The testing for other alleles that predispose to such allergies in other populations is not yet clinically useful. Mutations of the *SCN1A* sodium channel gene indicating Dravet syndrome could also lead to avoiding lamotrigine, carbamazepine, and phenytoin, and to the use of the more appropriate valproate, clobazam, or stiripentol.

2844 Part XXVII ◆ The Nervous System

◆ **Teratogenic profiles:** Some AEDs, including valproate and to a lesser extent carbamazepine, phenobarbital, and phenytoin, are associated with teratogenic effects (see Table 593-12).

Some of these considerations can be addressed by resorting to expert opinion surveys (see Table 593-11) or to guidelines developed by concerned societies such as the ILAE, National Institute for Clinical Excellence (NICE) in England, Scottish Intercollegiate Guidelines Network (SIGN), or the American Academy of Neurology (AAN). Some guidelines are totally evidence based (AAN, ILAE), and others (NICE, SIGN) incorporate other considerations as well. However, no guideline is able to incorporate all the considerations relevant to each patient.

INITIATING AND MONITORING THERAPY

In nonemergency situations, or when loading is not necessary, the **maintenance dose** of the chosen AED is started (Table 593-13). With some medications (e.g., carbamazepine and topiramate), even smaller doses are initially started then **gradually increased** up to the maintenance dose to build tolerance to adverse effects such as sedation. For example, the starting dose of carbamazepine is usually 5-10 mg/kg/day. Increments of 5 mg/kg/day can be added every 3 days until a therapeutic level is achieved and a therapeutic response is established or until unacceptable adverse effects occur. With other medications such as zonisamide, phenobarbital, phenytoin, or valproate, starting at the maintenance dose is usually tolerated. With some, such as levetiracetam and gabapentin, either approach can be used. Patients should be counseled about potential adverse effects, and these should be monitored during follow-up visits (Table 593-14).

Titration

Levels of many AEDs should usually be determined after initiation to ensure compliance and therapeutic concentrations. Monitoring is most helpful for the older AEDs such as phenytoin, carbamazepine, valproate, phenobarbital, and ethosuximide. After starting the maintenance dosage or after any change in the dosage, a steady state is not reached until 5 half-lives have elapsed, which, for most AEDs, is 2-7 days (half-life: 6-24 hr). For phenobarbital, it is 2-4 wk (mean half-life: 69 hr). For zonisamide it is 14 days during monotherapy and less than that during polytherapy with enzyme inducers (half-life: 63 hr in monotherapy and 27-38 hr during combination therapy with enzyme inducers). If a therapeutic level has to be achieved faster, a **loading dose** may be used for some drugs, usually with a single dose that is twice the average maintenance dose per half-life. For valproate it is 25 mg/kg, for phenytoin it is 20 mg/kg, and for phenobarbital it is 10-20 mg/kg. A lower loading dosage of phenobarbital is sometimes given in older children (5 mg/kg, which may be repeated once or more in 24 hr), to avoid excessive sedation.

Only 1 drug should be used initially and the dose increased until complete control is achieved or until side effects prohibit further increases. Then, and only then, may another drug be added and the initial drug subsequently tapered. Control with 1 drug (**monotherapy**) should be the goal, although some patients eventually need to take

Table 593-13	Dosages of Selected Antiepileptic Drugs				
MEDICATION	**FDA APPROVAL (AGE APPROVED)**	**MAINTENANCE ORAL DOSAGE (mg/kg/day) UNLESS OTHERWISE SPECIFIED**	**USUAL DOSING**	**THERAPEUTIC LEVELS**	**PREPARATIONS**
Acetazolamide	Absence seizures (adults)	1-12 mo; 10 <1 yr: 20-30	bid or tid	10-15 mg/L	125, 250, 500 mg tabs
Bromide		50-100	bid or qd	10-15 mEq/L	Supplied as triple bromide soln (240 mg/mL of bromide salt)
Carbamazepine*	Partial and GTC (all ages)	10-20	tid or qid SR usually bid	3-12 mg/L	150, 300 mg ER caps 100, 200, 400 mg ER tabs 100 mg chewable tabs 200 mg tabs 100 mg/5 mL susp
Clobazam†	LGS (all ages above 2 yr)	10-20 mg/day	bid or tid	60-200 µg/L	5 mg, 10 mg, 20 mg tabs 2.5 mg/mL soln
Clonazepam†	Absence sz, LGS, myoclonic sz (all ages)	0.05-0.2	bid or tid	25-85 µg/L	0.5, 1, 2 mg tabs 0.125, 0.25, 0.5 mg orally disintegrating tabs
Diazepam	Partial sz (all ages >6 mo)	0.25-1.5 0.01-0.25 IV 0.2-0.5 mg/kg rectal (according to age; see Table 593-15)	bid or tid	100-700 µg/L	2, 5, 10 mg tabs 5 mg/mL, 5 mg/5 mL soln Rectal gel that can be dialed to dispense 2.5, 5, 7.5, 10, 12.5, 15, 17.5, 20 mg
Ethosuximide	Absence sz (>3 yr)	20-30	bid or tid	40-100 mg/L	250 mg caps 250 mg/5 mL syrup, soln
Ezogabine	Partial sz (adults)	No pediatric dose approved	tid	—	50, 200, 300, 400 mg tabs
Felbamate	LGS (>2 yr) Partial sz (>14 yr)	15-45	bid or tid	50-110 mg/L	400, 600 mg tabs 600 mg/5 mL susp
Gabapentin‡	Partial sz (>3 yr)	30-60	tid	2-20 mg/L	100, 300, 400 mg caps, 600, 800 mg tabs
Lacosamide	Partial sz (>17 yr)	No FDA approved dose. 4-12	bid	<= 15 µg/L	50, 100, 150, 200 mg tabs 10 mg/mL oral soln

Table 593-13 | Dosages of Selected Antiepileptic Drugs—cont'd

MEDICATION	FDA APPROVAL (AGE APPROVED)	MAINTENANCE ORAL DOSAGE (mg/kg/day) UNLESS OTHERWISE SPECIFIED	USUAL DOSING	THERAPEUTIC LEVELS	PREPARATIONS
Lamotrigine	LGS, partial and tonic–clonic sz (age >2 yr)	5-15§ 1-5¶	tid bid	1-15 mg/L	25, 100, 150, 200 mg tabs 5, 25 mg chewable dispersible tabs 25, 50, 100, 200 mg ODTs 25, 50, 100, 200, 250, 300 mg ER tabs
Levetiracetam†	Myoclonic, partial and tonic–clonic sz (age >4-6 yr)	20-40	bid or tid	6-20 mg/L	250, 500, 750 mg tabs 100 mg/mL soln 500, 750 mg SR (ER) tabs
Lorazepam	Status epilepticus (all ages)	0.05-0.1	bid or tid	20-30 µg/L	0.5, 1, 2 mg tabs 2 mg/mL soln
Methsuximide (or methsuximide)	Absence sz (children and older)	10-30	bid or tid	10-50 mg/L	150, 300 mg caps
Nitrazepam	–	0.25-1	bid or tid	<200 µg/L	5 mg tabs
Oxcarbazepine*	Partial sz (>2 yr)	20-40	bid	13-28 mg/L	150, 300, 600 mg tabs 300 mg/5 mL susp
Perampanel	Partial sz (>12 yr)	2-12 mg per day (older than 12 yr)	qhs	-	2 mg, 4 mg, 6 mg, 8 mg, 10 mg, 12 mg tabs
Phenobarbital	Myoclonic, partial, and tonic–clonic sz and status (all ages)	<5 yr, 3-5 >5 yr, 2-3	bid or qd	10-40 mg/L	15, 30, 60, 90, 100 mg tabs 4 mg/mL soln
Phenytoin	Partial, tonic–clonic sz and status (all ages)	<3 yr, 8-10 >3 yr, 4-7	tabs, susp: tid caps: qd	5-20 mg/L	50 mg tabs 30,100 mg caps 125 mg/5 mL susp
Pregabalin	Partial sz (adults)	2-14	bid	Up to 10 µg/mL	25, 50, 75, 100, 150, 200, 225, 300 mg caps 20 mg/mL soln
Primidone	Partial and tonic–clonic sz (all ages)	10-20	bid or tid	4-13 mg/L	50, 250 mg tabs, susp
Rufinamide†	LGS (age >4 yr)	30-45	bid	<60 µg/mL	200, 400 mg tabs
Sulthiame‖		5-15	bid or tid	1.5-20 µg/mL	50, 200 mg caps Not available in all countries
Tiagabine	Partial sz (age >2 yr)	0.5-2	bid, tid, qid	80-450 µg/L	2, 4, 12, 16 mg tabs
Topiramate†	LGS, partial and tonic–clonic sz (all ages)	3-9, slow titration	bid or tid	2-25 mg/L	25, 100, 200 mg tabs 15, 25 mg sprinkle caps
Valproate	Absence, myoclonic, partial and tonic–clonic sz (age >2 yr)	15-40. Higher doses are used if the patient is on enzyme inducers (up to 60 kg/day)	Sprinkle caps: bid Soln: tid	50-100 mg/L	250 mg caps 125 mg sprinkle caps 125, 250, 500 mg tabs 250 mg/5 mL soln
Vigabatrin	Infantile spasms and partial sz (age >1 mo)	50-150	bid	20-160 µg/mL	500 mg tabs 500 mg powder for soln
Zonisamide	Partial sz (age >16 yr)	4-8	bid or qd	10-40 mg/L	100 mg caps

Unless specified otherwise, as above, one would usually target the lower range of therapeutic dose then adjust as needed depending on response and/or levels. Dosing schedule (e.g., bid or tid) can depend on if a sustained release preparation is available and if the patient is on enzyme inducers (e.g., carbamazepine) or inhibitors (e.g., valproic acid) that could affect that drug (as indicated in the dosing in the table and in the text).

*Usually start by one-fourth maintenance dose and increase by one-fourth every 2-3 days to full dose.

†Usually start with one-fourth maintenance dose and increase by one-fourth every 7 days to full dose.

‡Usually start with one-fourth maintenance dose and increase by one-fourth every day to full dose.

§Child on enzyme inducers.

‖Available in some European countries.

¶Child on valproate.

cap, capsule; ER, extended release; GTC, generalized tonic–clonic; LGS, Lennox-Gastaut syndrome; ODT, orally disintegrating tablet; soln, solution; SR, sustained release; susp, suspension; sz, seizure(s); tab, tablet.

Table 593-14	Some Common Adverse Effects of Antiepileptic Drugs*
ANTIEPILEPTIC DRUG	**SIDE EFFECT(S)**
Acetazolamide	Nuisance: dizziness, polyuria, electrolyte imbalance Serious: Stevens-Johnson syndrome
Benzodiazepines	Nuisance: dose-related neurotoxicity (drowsiness, sedation, ataxia), hyperactivity, drooling, increased secretions Serious: apnea
Bromide	Nuisance: irritability, spurious hyperchloremia (falsely high chloride owing to bromide) Serious: psychosis, rash, toxicity developing slowly owing to the very long half-life
Carbamazepine	Nuisance: tics, transient leukopenia; hyponatremia, weight gain, nausea; dizziness Serious: Stevens-Johnson syndrome, agranulocytosis, aplastic anemia, liver toxicity
Ezogabine	Nuisance: dizziness, somnolence tremor, abnormal coordination, disturbance in attention, memory impairment, blurred vision, gait disturbance, and dysarthria Serious: blue discoloration of the skin and retinal pigmentation that requires close ophthalmologic monitoring in follow up, urinary retention
Felbamate	Nuisance: anorexia, vomiting, insomnia, hyperactivity, dizziness Serious: major risks for liver and hematologic toxicity requiring close monitoring (1 in 500 in children >2 yr with complex neurological disorders)
Gabapentin	In children: acute onset of aggression, hyperactivity In adults: euphoria and behavioral disinhibition, weight gain
Lacosamide	Nuisance: diplopia, headache, dizziness, nausea Serious: possibly cardiac arrhythmias (if predisposed)
Lamotrigine	Nuisance: CNS side effects: headache, ataxia, dizziness, tremor, but usually less than other AEDs Serious: Stevens-Johnson syndrome, rarely liver toxicity
Levetiracetam	CNS adverse events: somnolence, asthenia, dizziness, but usually less than other AEDs In children: behavioral symptoms are common In adults: depressive mood
Oxcarbazepine	Somnolence, headache, dizziness, nausea, apathy, rash, hypertrichosis, gingival hypertrophy, hyponatremia
Perampanel	Dizziness, somnolence, fatigue, irritability, falls, nausea, weight gain, vertigo, ataxia, gait disturbance, and balance disorder
Phenobarbital and other barbiturates	Nuisance: neurotoxicity, insomnia, hyperactivity, signs of distractibility, fluctuation of mood, aggressive outbursts Serious: liver toxicity, Stevens-Johnson syndrome
Phenytoin and other hydantoins	Nuisance: gingival hyperplasia, coarsening of the facies, hirsutism, cerebellovestibular symptoms (nystagmus and ataxia) Serious: Stevens-Johnson syndrome, liver toxicity
Pregabalin	Nuisance: dizziness, peripheral edema, blurred vision, weight gain, thrombocytopenia Serious: hypersensitivity reactions, rhabdomyolysis
Primidone	Nuisance: CNS toxicity (dizziness, slurred speech, giddiness, drowsiness, depression) Serious: liver toxicity, Stevens-Johnson syndrome
Rufinamide	Nuisance: somnolence, vomiting Serious: contraindicated in familial short QT interval
Succinimides	Nuisance: nausea, abdominal discomfort, anorexia, hiccups Serious: Stevens-Johnson syndrome, drug-induced lupus
Tiagabine	Nuisance: dizziness, somnolence, asthenia, headache and tremor, precipitation of absence or myoclonic seizures Serious: precipitation of nonconvulsive status epilepticus
Topiramate	Nuisance: cognitive dysfunction, weight loss, renal calculi, hypohidrosis, fever Serious: precipitation of glaucoma
Valproic acid	Nuisance: weight gain; hyperammonemia tremor, alopecia, menstrual irregularities Serious: hepatic and pancreatic toxicity
Vigabatrin	Nuisance: hyperactivity Serious: irreversible visual field deficits, retinopathy that requires frequent ophthalmologic evaluations and follow up
Zonisamide	Fatigue, dizziness, anorexia, psychomotor slowing, ataxia, rarely hallucinations, hypohidrosis and fever

*Essentially all AEDs can cause CNS toxicity and potentially rashes and serious allergic reactions.
  AED, antiepileptic drug; CNS, central nervous system.

multiple drugs. When appropriate, levels should also be checked upon addition (or discontinuation) of a second drug because of potential drug interactions. During follow-up, repeating the EEG every few months may be helpful to evaluate changes in the predisposition to seizures. This is especially true in situations where tapering off of medication is contemplated in any seizure type and during follow-up to assess response for absence seizures, as the EEG mirrors response in such patients.

Monitoring

For the older AEDs, before starting treatment, **baseline laboratory studies,** including complete blood count, platelets, liver enzymes, and possibly kidney function tests and urinalysis, are often obtained and repeated periodically. Laboratory monitoring is more relevant early on, because idiosyncratic adverse effects such as allergic hepatitis and agranulocytosis are more likely to occur in the 1st 3-6 mo of therapy. These laboratory studies are usually initially checked once or twice during the 1st mo, then every 3-4 mo thereafter. Serious concerns have been raised about the real usefulness of routine monitoring (in the absence of clinical signs) because the yield of significant adverse effects is low and the costs may be high. There are currently many advocates of less-frequent routine monitoring.

In approximately 10% of patients, a reversible dose-related leukopenia may occur in patients on carbamazepine or on phenytoin. This adverse effect responds to decreasing the dose or to stopping the medication and should be distinguished from the much-less-common idiosyncratic aplastic anemia or agranulocytosis. One exception requiring frequent (even weekly) monitoring of liver function and of blood counts throughout the therapy is felbamate, owing to the high incidence of liver and hematologic toxicity (1 in 500 children under 2 yr of age with complex neurological disorders who are on the drug). The gum hyperplasia that is seen with phenytoin necessitates good oral hygiene (brushing teeth at least twice per day and rinsing the mouth after taking the phenytoin); in a few cases, it may be severe enough to warrant surgical reduction and/or change of medication. Allergic rash can occur with any medication, but is probably most common with lamotrigine, carbamazepine, and phenytoin.

SIDE EFFECTS

During follow-up the patient should be monitored for **side effects**. Occasionally, a Stevens-Johnson–like syndrome develops, probably most commonly with lamotrigine; it also has been found to be particularly common in Chinese patients who have the allele HLA-B*1502 and are taking carbamazepine and lamotrigine.

Other potential side effects are rickets from phenytoin, phenobarbital, primidone, and carbamazepine (enzyme inducers that reduce 25-hyrdroxy-vitamin D level by inducing its metabolism) and hyperammonemia from valproate. Skeletal monitoring is warranted in patients on chronic AED therapy because it is often associated with vitamin D abnormalities (low bone density, rickets, and hypocalcemia) in children and adults, particularly those on enzyme-inducing medications. Thus, counseling the patient about sun exposure and vitamin D intake, monitoring its levels, and, in most cases, vitamin D supplementation are recommended. There is currently no consensus on the dose to be used for supplementation or prophylaxis, but starting doses of 400-2,000 IU/day with follow-up of the levels are reasonable.

Irreversible hepatic injury and death are particularly feared in young children (<2 yr old) who are on valproate in combination with other AEDs, particularly those who might have inborn errors of metabolism such as acidopathies and mitochondrial disease. Virtually all AEDs can produce sleepiness, ataxia, nystagmus, and slurred speech with toxic levels.

The FDA has determined that the use of AEDs may be associated with an increased risk of suicidal ideation and action and has recommended counseling about this side effect before starting these medications. This is obviously more applicable to adolescents and adults.

When adding a new AED, the doses used are often affected by the background medications. For example, if the patient is on enzyme inducers, the doses needed of valproate and lamotrigine are often double the usual maintenance doses. On the other hand, if the patient is on valproate, the doses of phenobarbital or lamotrigine are approximately half of what is usually needed. Thus, changes in the dosing of the background medication are often done as the interacting medication is being started. Genetic variability in enzymes that metabolize AEDs, and in the presence of inducible multidrug resistance genes, **pharmacogenomics**, might account for some of the variation among individuals in responding to certain AEDs. Although numerous variants of the cytochrome P450 enzymes have been characterized and although several multidrug resistance genes have been identified, the use of this new knowledge is currently largely restricted to research investigations, and it has yet to be applied in routine clinical practice.

Additional Treatments

The principles of monotherapy indicate that a second medication needs to be considered after the first either is pushed as high as tolerated and still does not control the seizures or results in intolerable adverse effects. In those cases, a second drug is started and the first is tapered and then discontinued. The second drug is then again pushed to the dose that controls the seizure or that results in intolerable side effects. If the second drug fails, monotherapy with a third drug or **dual (combination) therapy** is considered.

Patients with **drug-resistant** (previously referred to as intractable or refractory) **epilepsy** (those who have failed at least 2 fair trials of appropriate medications) warrant a careful diagnostic reevaluation to look for degenerative, metabolic, or inflammatory underlying disorders (e.g., mitochondrial disease, Rasmussen encephalitis; see Chapter 593.2) and to investigate them for candidacy for epilepsy surgery. Treatable metabolic disorders that can manifest as intractable epilepsy include pyridoxine-dependent and pyridoxal-responsive epilepsy; folinic acid–responsive seizures (demonstrated to be the same disorder as pyridoxine-dependent epilepsy); cerebral folate deficiency; neurotransmitter disorders; biotinidase deficiency; glucose transporter 1 deficiency (responds to the ketogenic diet); serine synthesis defects; creatine deficiency syndromes; untreated phenylketonuria; developmental delay, epilepsy and neonatal diabetes; and hyperinsulinemia–hyperammonia. Often patients who do not respond to AEDs are candidates for steroids, IVIG, or the ketogenic diet.

Steroids, usually given as ACTH (see the discussion of West syndrome in "Severe Generalized Epilepsies" in Chapter 593.4) or as prednisone 2 mg/kg/day (or equivalent), are often used in epileptic encephalopathies such as West, Lennox-Gastaut, myoclonic astatic, continuous spike-waves in slow-wave sleep, and Landau-Kleffner syndromes. The course usually is for 2-3 mo with a taper over a similar period. Because relapses occur commonly during tapering, and in such syndromes as Landau-Kleffner and continuous spike-waves in slow-wave sleep, therapy for longer than 1 yr is often needed.

IVIG has also been reported to be similarly effective in non–immunodeficient patients with West, Lennox-Gastaut, Landau-Kleffner, and continuous spike-waves in slow-wave sleep syndromes and may also have efficacy in partial seizures. One should check the IgA levels before starting the infusions (to assess the risk for allergic reactions, because these are increased in patients with complete IgA deficiency) and guard against allergic reactions during the infusion. Low IgA, low IgG$_2$, and male sex are reported to possibly predict favorable response. The usual regimen is 2 g/kg divided over 4 consecutive days followed by 1 g/kg once a month for 6 mo. The mechanism of action of steroids and of IVIG are not known but is presumed to be antiinflammatory, because it has been demonstrated that seizures increase cytokines and that these, in turn, increase neuronal excitability by several mechanisms, including activation of glutamate receptors. Steroids and ACTH might also stimulate brain neurosteroid receptors that enhance GABA activity and might reduce corticotrophin-releasing hormone, which is known to be epileptogenic.

The **ketogenic diet** is believed to be effective in glucose transporter protein 1 deficiency, pyruvate dehydrogenase deficiency, myoclonic–astatic epilepsy, tuberous sclerosis complex, Rett syndrome, severe myoclonic epilepsy of infancy (Dravet syndrome), and infantile spasms. There is also suggestion of possible efficacy in selected mitochondrial disorders—glycogenosis type V, Landau-Kleffner syndrome, Lafora body disease, and subacute sclerosing panencephalitis. The diet is absolutely contraindicated in carnitine deficiency (primary); carnitine palmitoyltransferase I or II deficiency; carnitine translocase deficiency; β-oxidation defects; medium-chain acyl dehydrogenase deficiency; long-chain acyl dehydrogenase deficiency; short-chain acyl dehydrogenase deficiency; long-chain 3-hydroxyacyl-coenzyme A deficiency; medium-chain 3-hydroxyacyl-coenzyme A deficiency; pyruvate carboxylase deficiency; and porphyrias. Thus, an appropriate metabolic work-up, depending on the clinical picture, usually needs to be performed before starting the diet (e.g., acyl carnitine profile, total and free carnitine levels). The diet has been used for refractory seizures of various types (partial or generalized) and consists of an initial period of fasting followed by a diet with a 3:1 or 4:1 fat:nonfat ratio, with fats consisting of animal fat, vegetable oils, or medium-chain triglycerides. Many patients do not tolerate it owing to diarrhea, vomiting, hypoglycemia, dehydration, or lack of palatability. Diets such as the low-glycemic-index diet and the Atkins diet are easier to institute, do not require hospitalization, and are also useful, but it is not known yet if they are as effective as the classic diet.

APPROACH TO EPILEPSY SURGERY

If a patient has failed 3 drugs, the chance of achieving seizure freedom using AEDs is generally <10%. Therefore, proper evaluation for surgery is necessary as soon as patients fail 2 or 3 AEDs, usually within 2 yr of the onset of epilepsy and often sooner than 2 yr. Performing epilepsy surgery in children at an earlier stage (e.g., <5 yr of age) allows transfer of function in the developing brain. Candidacy for epilepsy surgery requires proof of resistance to AEDs used at maximum, tolerably nontoxic doses; absence of expected unacceptable adverse consequences of surgery, and a properly defined **epileptogenic zone** (area that needs to be resected to achieve seizure freedom). The epileptogenic zone is identified by careful analysis, by an expert team of epilepsy specialists in an epilepsy center, of the following parameters: seizure semiology, interictal EEG, video-EEG long-term monitoring, neuropsychologic profile, and MRI. Other techniques, such as invasive EEG (depth electrodes, subdurals), single-photon emission CT, magnetoencephalography, and positron emission tomography are also often needed when the epileptogenic zone is difficult to localize or when it is close to eloquent cortex. To avoid resection of eloquent cortex, several techniques can be used, including the **Wada test**. In this test, intracarotid infusion of amobarbital is used to anesthetize 1 hemisphere to lateralize memory and speech by testing them during that unilateral anesthesia. Other tests to localize function include functional MRI, magnetoencephalography, and subdural electrodes with cortical stimulation. Developmental delay or psychiatric diseases must be considered in assessing the potential impact of surgery on the patient. The usual minimal presurgical evaluation includes EEG monitoring, imaging, and age-specific neuropsychologic assessment.

Epilepsy surgery is often used to treat refractory epilepsy of a number of etiologies, including cortical dysplasia, tuberous sclerosis, polymicrogyria, hypothalamic hamartoma, Landau-Kleffner syndrome, and hemispheric syndromes, such as Sturge-Weber syndrome, hemimegalencephaly, and Rasmussen encephalitis. Patients with intractable epilepsy resulting from metabolic or degenerative problems are not candidates for resective epilepsy surgery. **Focal resection** of the epileptogenic zone is the most common procedure. **Hemispherectomy** is used for diffuse hemispheric lesions; **multiple subpial transection**, a surgical technique in which the horizontal connections of the epileptic focus are partially cut without resecting it, is sometimes used for unresectable foci located in eloquent cortex such as in Landau-Kleffner syndrome. In Lennox-Gastaut syndrome, **corpus callosotomy** is used for drop attacks. **Vagal nerve stimulation** is often used for intractable epilepsies of various types and for seizures of diffuse focal or multifocal anatomic origin that do not yield themselves to resective surgery. Focal resection and hemispherectomy result in a high rate (50-80%) of seizure freedom. Corpus callosotomy and vagal nerve stimulation result in lower rates (5-10%) of seizure freedom; however, these procedures do result in significant reductions in the frequency and severity

of seizures, decrease in medication requirements, and meaningful improvements in the patient's quality of life in approximately half or more of eligible patients.

DISCONTINUATION OF THERAPY

Discontinuation of AEDs is usually indicated when children are free of seizures for at least 2 yr. In more-severe syndromes, such as temporal lobe epilepsy secondary to mesial temporal sclerosis, Lennox-Gastaut syndrome, or severe myoclonic epilepsy, a prolonged period of seizure freedom on treatment is often warranted before AEDs are withdrawn, if withdrawal is attempted at all. In self-limited (benign) epilepsy syndromes, the duration of therapy can often be as short as 6 mo.

Many factors should be considered before discontinuing medications, including the likelihood of remaining seizure-free after drug withdrawal based on the type of epilepsy syndrome and etiology; the risk of injury in case of seizure recurrence (e.g., if the patient drives); and the adverse effects of AED therapy. Most children who have not had a seizure for 2 yr or longer and who have a normal EEG when AED withdrawal is initiated, remain free of seizures after discontinuing medication, and most relapses occur within the 1st 6 mo.

Certain risk factors can help the clinician predict the prognosis after AED withdrawal. The most important risk factor for seizure relapse is an abnormal EEG before medication is discontinued. Children who have remote structural (symptomatic) epilepsy are less likely to be able to stop AEDs than are children who have a benign genetic (idiopathic) epilepsy. In patients with absences or in patients treated with valproate for primary generalized epilepsy, the risk of relapse might still be high despite a normal EEG because valproate can normalize EEGs with generalized spike-wave abnormalities. Thus, in these patients, repeating the EEG during drug taper can help identify recurrence of the EEG abnormality and associated seizure risk before clinical seizures recur. Older age of epilepsy onset, longer duration of epilepsy, presence of multiple seizure types, and need to use more than 1 AED are all factors associated with a higher risk of seizure relapse after AED withdrawal.

AED therapy should be discontinued gradually; often over a period of 3-6 mo. Abrupt discontinuation can result in withdrawal seizures or status epilepticus. Withdrawal seizures are especially common with phenobarbital and benzodiazepines; consequently, special attention must be given to a prolonged tapering schedule during the withdrawal of these AEDs. Seizures that occur more than 2-3 mo after AEDs are completely discontinued indicate relapse, and resumption of treatment is usually warranted.

The decision to attempt AED withdrawal must be assessed mutually among the clinician, the parents, and the child depending on the child's age. Risk factors should be identified and precautionary measures should be taken. The patient and family should be counseled fully on what to expect, what precautions to take (including cessation of driving for a period of time), and what to do in case of relapse. A prescription for rectal diazepam or of intranasal midazolam to be given at the time of seizures that might occur during and after tapering is usually warranted (see Table 593-12 for dosing).

Sudden Unexpected Death in Epilepsy

SUDEP is the most common epilepsy related mortality in patients with chronic epilepsy; the incidence is unknown but ranges from 1-5 per 1,000 people with epilepsy. Although the precise etiology is unknown, risk factors include polypharmacology, poorly controlled generalized tonic–clonic seizures, male gender, age younger than 16 yr, long duration of epilepsy, and frequent seizures. Patients are usually found dead in their bed in a prone position with evidence suggesting a recent seizure. Potential mechanisms of SUDEP include respiratory arrest or dysfunction, drug-induced cardiac toxicity, CNS dysfunction (hypoventilation, arrhythmia, suppression of brain electrical activity), or pulmonary edema. Table 593-15 lists possible preventive measures.

Bibliography is available at Expert Consult.

Table 593-15	Measures in Clinical Practice to Reduce the Risk of SUDEP

- **Reduction of tonic–clonic seizures:** optimum treatment, good drug compliance, lifestyle advice (e.g., alcohol intake, sleep deprivation)
- **Treatment changes:** change in a gradual staged manner; when switching drugs, introduce the new drug before withdrawing the old drug; the patients should have access to immediate advice in the event of worsening seizures during periods of change
- **Supervision at night for patients at high risk:** attendance, use of alarms (balancing the benefits of independent living and the penalties of intrusive monitoring)
- **Choice of drugs:** caution with antiepileptic drugs with potential cardiorespiratory adverse effects
- **Act on ictal warning signs:** tonic–clonic seizures that are prolonged, associated with marked cyanosis, severe bradycardia or apnea, and postictal EEG suppression; complex partial seizures with marked atonia (drop attacks); seizure in those with preexisting cardiac or respiratory impairment
- **Supervision after a tonic–clonic seizure:** continuous attendance until full consciousness is restored; call emergency services for high-risk seizures
- **Counseling on the risks:** lifestyle and treatment decisions are the patient's prerogative and the physician's role is to provide a risk-vs-benefit analysis

EEG, electroencephalogram; SUDEP, sudden unexpected death in epilepsy.
From Shorvan S, Tomson T: Sudden unexpected death in epilepsy. Lancet 378:2028–2036, 2011.

593.7 Neonatal Seizures
Mohamad A. Mikati and Abeer J. Hani

Seizures are possibly the most important and common indicator of significant neurologic dysfunction in the neonatal period. Seizure incidence is higher during this period than in any other period in life: 57.5 per 1,000 in infants with birth weights <1,500 g and 2.8 per 1,000 in infants weighing between 2,500 and 3,999 g have seizures.

PATHOPHYSIOLOGY
The immature brain has many differences from the mature brain that render it more excitable and more likely to develop seizures. Based predominantly on animal studies, these are delay in Na^+, K^+-adenosine triphosphatase maturation and increased NMDA and α-amino-3-hydroxy-5-methylisoxazole-4-propionate (AMPA) receptor density. In addition, the specific types of these receptors that are increased are those that are permeable to calcium (GLUR2 AMPA receptors). This contributes to increased excitability and to the long-term consequences associated with seizures, particularly those resulting from perinatal hypoxia. Medications that block AMPA receptors, such as topiramate, may thus prove useful in this clinical setup.

Another difference is delay in the development of inhibitory GABAergic transmission. In fact, GABA in the immature brain has an excitatory function as the chloride gradient is reversed relative to the mature brain, with higher concentrations of chloride being present intracellularly than extracellularly. Thus, opening of the chloride channels in the immature brain results in depolarizing the cell and not in hyperpolarizing it. This phenomenon appears to be more prominent in male neonates, perhaps explaining their greater predisposition to seizures. The reason for this is that the Cl^- transporter, NKCC1, is predominantly expressed in the neonatal period, leading to transport of Cl^- into the cell at rest, and then to cellular depolarization upon activation of $GABA_A$ receptors and opening of Cl^- channels with chloride efflux. This is important for neuronal development but renders the neonatal brain hyperexcitable. With maturation, expression of NCCK1 decreases and KCC2 increases. KCC2 transports Cl^- out of the cell, resulting in reduction of intracellular chloride concentration so that when $GABA_A$ receptors are activated, Cl^- influx and hyperpolarization occur. Bumetanide, a diuretic that blocks NKCC1, can prevent exces-

sive GABA depolarization and avert the neuronal hyperexcitability underlying neonatal seizures. It also prevents, in rats, complex febrile seizure induced hyperactivation of excitatory $GABA_A$ receptors and the resultant granule cell ectopia and temporal lobe epilepsy.

Although it is susceptible to developing seizures, the immature brain appears to be more resistant to the deleterious effects of seizures than the mature brain, as a result of increases in calcium binding proteins that buffer injury-related increases in calcium, increased extracellular space, decreased levels of the second messenger inositol triphosphate, and the immature brain's ability to tolerate hypoxic conditions by resorting to anaerobic energy metabolism.

Many animal studies indicate that seizures are detrimental to the immature brain. Human studies also suggest harmful effects of seizures as shown by MRI and by the association of worse prognosis in neonates with seizures even when correcting for confounding factors. Even electrographic seizures without clinical correlates have been shown to be associated with worse prognosis. However, it is not definite that this association is causal: It is difficult in human studies to distinguish among effects of seizures, of the underlying insult responsible for the seizures (clinical or electrographic), and of the AEDs used to stop the seizures. Most physicians currently believe that it is favorable to control clinical as well as electrographic seizures.

TYPES OF NEONATAL SEIZURES
There are 5 main neonatal seizure types: subtle, clonic, tonic, spasms, and myoclonic. Spasms, focal clonic, focal tonic, and generalized myoclonic seizures are, as a rule, associated with electrographic discharges (epileptic seizures), whereas motor automatisms, the subtle, generalized tonic and multifocal myoclonic episodes are frequently not associated with discharges and thus are thought to often represent release phenomena with abnormal movements secondary to brain injury rather than true epileptic seizures (Table 593-16). To determine clinically whether such manifestations are seizures or release phenomena is often difficult, but precipitation of such manifestations by stimulation and aborting them by restraint or manipulation would suggest that they are not seizures. One needs to keep in mind, however, that epileptic seizures can also be induced by stimulation. Thus, in many cases, specifically in sick neonates with history of neurologic insults, continuous bedside EEG monitoring helps make this distinction. Such monitoring has become the standard of care in most intensive care nurseries.

Subtle Seizures
Subtle seizures include transient eye deviations, nystagmus, blinking, mouthing, abnormal extremity movements (rowing, swimming, bicycling, pedaling, and stepping), fluctuations in heart rate, hypertension episodes, and apnea. Subtle seizures occur more commonly in premature than in full-term infants.

Clonic Seizures
Clonic seizures can be focal or multifocal. Multifocal clonic seizures incorporate several body parts and are migratory in nature. The migration follows a nonjacksonian trend; for example, jerking of the left arm can be associated with jerking of the right leg. Generalized clonic seizures that are bilateral, symmetric, and synchronous are uncommon in the neonatal period presumably due to decreased connectivity associated with incomplete myelination at this age.

Tonic Seizures
Tonic seizures can be focal or generalized (generalized are more common). Focal tonic seizures include persistent posturing of a limb or posturing of trunk or neck in an asymmetric way often with persistent horizontal eye deviation. Generalized tonic seizures are bilateral tonic limb extension or tonic flexion of upper extremities often associated with tonic extension of lower extremities.

Spasms
Spasms are sudden generalized jerks lasting 1-2 sec that are distinguished from generalized tonic spells by their shorter duration and by

Table 593-16	Clinical Characteristics, Classification, and Presumed Pathophysiology of Neonatal Seizures
CLASSIFICATION	**CHARACTERIZATION**
Focal clonic	Repetitive, rhythmic contractions of muscle groups of the limbs, face, or trunk May be unifocal or multifocal May occur synchronously or asynchronously in muscle groups on 1 side of the body May occur simultaneously but asynchronously on both sides Cannot be suppressed by restraint Pathophysiology: epileptic
Focal tonic	Sustained posturing of single limbs Sustained asymmetrical posturing of the trunk Sustained eye deviation Cannot be provoked by stimulation or suppressed by restraint Pathophysiology: epileptic
Generalized tonic	Sustained symmetrical posturing of limbs, trunk, and neck May be flexor, extensor, or mixed extensor/flexor May be provoked or intensified by stimulation May be suppressed by restraint or repositioning Presumed pathophysiology: nonepileptic
Myoclonic	Random, single, rapid contractions of muscle groups of the limbs, face, or trunk Typically not repetitive or may recur at a slow rate May be generalized, focal, or fragmentary May be provoked by stimulation Presumed pathophysiology: may be epileptic or nonepileptic
Spasms	May be flexor, extensor, or mixed extensor/flexor May occur in clusters Cannot be provoked by stimulation or suppressed by restraint Pathophysiology: epileptic
Motor automatisms	
Ocular signs	Random and roving eye movements or nystagmus (distinct from tonic eye deviation) May be provoked or intensified by tactile stimulation Presumed pathophysiology: nonepileptic
Oral-buccal-lingual movements	Sucking, chewing, tongue protrusions May be provoked or intensified by stimulation Presumed pathophysiology: nonepileptic
Progression movements	Rowing or swimming movements Pedaling or bicycling movements of the legs May be provoked or intensified by stimulation May be suppressed by restraint or repositioning Presumed pathophysiology: nonepileptic
Complex purposeless movements	Sudden arousal with transient increased random activity of limbs May be provoked or intensified by stimulation Presumed pathophysiology: nonepileptic

From Mizrahi EM, Kellaway P. Diagnosis and management of neonatal seizures. *Philadelphia, 1998, Lippincott-Raven. Tab 4, p. 21.*

the fact that spasms are usually associated with a single, very brief, generalized discharge.

Myoclonic Seizures

Myoclonic seizures are divided into focal, multifocal, and generalized types. Myoclonic seizures can be distinguished from clonic seizures by the rapidity of the jerks (<50 msec) and by their lack of rhythmicity. Focal myoclonic seizures characteristically affect the flexor muscles of the upper extremities and are sometimes associated with seizure activity on EEG. Multifocal myoclonic movements involve asynchronous twitching of several parts of the body and are not commonly associated with seizure discharges on EEG. Generalized myoclonic seizures involve bilateral jerking associated with flexion of upper and occasionally lower extremities. The latter type of myoclonic jerks is more commonly correlated with EEG abnormalities than the other types.

Seizures vs Jitteriness

Jitteriness can be defined as rapid motor activities, such as a tremor or shake, that can be ended by flexion or holding the limb. Seizures, on the other hand, generally do not end with tactile or motor suppression. Jitteriness, unlike most seizures, is usually induced by a stimulus. Also unlike jitteriness, seizures often involve eye deviation and autonomic changes.

ETIOLOGY

Table 593-17 lists causes of neonatal seizures.

Hypoxic–Ischemic Encephalopathy

This is the most common cause of neonatal seizures, accounting for 50-60% of patients. Seizures secondary to this encephalopathy occur within 12 hr of birth.

Vascular Events

These include intracranial bleeds and ischemic strokes and account for 10-20% of patients. Three types of hemorrhage can be distinguished: primary subarachnoid hemorrhage, germinal matrix–intraventricular hemorrhage, and subdural hemorrhage. Patients with arterial strokes or venous sinus thrombosis can present with seizure and these can be

| Table 593-17 | Causes of Neonatal Seizures According to Common Age of Presentation |

AGES 1-4 DAYS
Hypoxic–ischemic encephalopathy
Drug withdrawal, maternal drug use of narcotic or barbiturates
Drug toxicity: lidocaine, penicillin
Intraventricular hemorrhage
Acute metabolic disorders
- Hypocalcemia
- Sepsis
- Maternal hyperthyroidism, or hypoparathyroidism
- Hypoglycemia
- Perinatal insults, prematurity, small for gestational age
- Maternal diabetes
- Hyperinsulinemic hypoglycemia
- Hypomagnesemia
- Hyponatremia or hypernatremia
- Iatrogenic or inappropriate antidiuretic hormone secretion
Inborn errors of metabolism
- Galactosemia
- Hyperglycinemia
- Urea cycle disorders
Pyridoxine deficiency and pyridoxal-5-phosphate deficiency (must be considered at any age)

AGES 4-14 DAYS
Infection
- Meningitis (bacterial)
- Encephalitis (enteroviral, herpes simplex)
Metabolic disorders
- Hypocalcemia
- Diet, milk formula
- Hypoglycemia, persistent
- Inherited disorders of metabolism
- Galactosemia
- Fructosemia
- Leucine sensitivity
- Hyperinsulinemic hypoglycemia, hyperinsulinism, hyperammonemia syndrome
- Anterior pituitary hypoplasia, pancreatic islet cell tumor
- Beckwith syndrome
Drug withdrawal, maternal drug use of narcotics or barbiturates
Benign neonatal convulsions, familial and nonfamilial
Kernicterus, hyperbilirubinemia
Developmental delay, epilepsy, neonatal diabetes syndrome

AGES 2-8 WK
Infection
- Herpes simplex or enteroviral encephalitis
- Bacterial meningitis
Head injury
- Subdural hematoma
- Child abuse
Inherited disorders of metabolism
- Aminoacidurias
- Urea cycle defects
- Organic acidurias
- Neonatal adrenoleukodystrophy
Malformations of cortical development
- Lissencephaly
- Focal cortical dysplasia
Tuberous sclerosis
Sturge-Weber syndrome

diagnosed by neuroimaging. Venous sinus thrombosis could be missed unless MR or CT venography studies are requested.

Intracranial Infections
Bacterial and nonbacterial infections account for 5-10% of the cases of neonatal seizures and include bacterial meningitis, TORCH (*t*oxoplasmosis, *o*ther infections, *r*ubella, *c*ytomegalovirus, *h*erpes simplex virus) infections, particularly herpes simplex encephalitis.

Brain Malformations
Brain malformations account for 5-10% of neonatal seizure cases. An example is **Aicardi syndrome**, which affects girls only and consists of retinal lacunae, agenesis of the corpus callosum, and severe seizures including subsequent infantile spasms with hypsarrhythmia that is sometimes initially unilateral on EEG.

Metabolic Disturbances
Metabolic disturbances include disturbances in glucose, calcium, magnesium, other electrolytes, amino acids, or organic acids and pyridoxine dependency.

Hypoglycemia can cause neurologic disturbances and is very common in small neonates and neonates whose mothers are diabetic or prediabetic. The duration of hypoglycemia is very critical in determining the incidence of neurologic symptoms.

Hypocalcemia occurs at 2 peaks. The first peak corresponds to low-birthweight infants and is evident in the 1st 2-3 days of life. The second peak occurs later in neonatal life and often involves large, full-term babies who consume milk that has an unfavorable ratio of phosphorus to calcium and phosphorus to magnesium. **Hypomagnesemia** is often associated with hypocalcemia. **Hyponatremia** can cause seizures and is often secondary to inappropriate antidiuretic hormone secretion.

Local anesthetic intoxication seizures can result from neonatal intoxication with local anesthetics administered into the infant's scalp.

Neonatal seizures can also result from disturbances in **amino acid or organic acid** metabolism. These are usually associated with acidosis and/or hyperammonemia. However, even in the absence of these findings, if a cause of the seizures is not immediately evident, then ruling out metabolic causes requires a full metabolic work-up (see Chapter 593.2) including examination of serum amino acids, acyl carnitine profile, lactate, pyruvate, ammonia, very-long-chain fatty acids (for neonatal adrenoleukodystrophy and Zellweger syndrome), examination of urine for organic acids, α-aminoadipic acid semialdehyde and sulfocysteine, as well as examination of CSF for glucose, protein, cells, amino acids, lactate, pyruvate, α-aminoadipic acid semialdehyde, pyridoxal phosphate, 5-MTHF (5-methyltetrahydrofolate), succinyladenosine, and CSF neurotransmitter metabolites. This is because many inborn errors of metabolism, such as nonketotic hyperglycinemia, can manifest with neonatal seizures (often mistaken initially for hiccups that these patients also have) and can be detected only by performing these tests. Definitive diagnosis of **nonketotic hyperglycinemia**, for example, requires measuring the ratio of CSF glycine to plasma glycine.

Pyridoxine and **pyridoxal dependency disorders** can cause severe seizures. These seizures, which are often multifocal clonic, usually start during the 1st few hr of life. Cognitive impairment is often associated if therapy is delayed (see Chapter 593.6).

Drug Withdrawal
Seizures can rarely be caused by the neonate's passive addiction and then drug withdrawal. Such drugs include narcotic analgesics, sedative–hypnotics, and others. The associated seizures appear during the 1st 3 days of life.

Neonatal Seizure Syndromes
Seizure syndromes include **benign idiopathic neonatal seizures (fifth day fits)**, which are usually apneic and focal motor seizures that start around the fifth day of life. Interictal EEG shows a distinctive pattern called *theta pointu alternant* (runs of sharp 4-7 Hz activity), and ictal EEG shows multifocal electrographic seizures. Patients have a good response to medications and a good prognosis. Autosomal dominant **benign familial neonatal seizures** have onset at 2-4 days of age and usually remit at 2-15 wk of age. The seizures consist of ocular deviation, tonic posturing, clonic jerks, and, at times, motor automatisms. Interictal EEG is usually normal. These are caused by mutations in the *KCNQ2* and *KCNQ3* genes. Approximately 16% of patients develop later epilepsy. **Early myoclonic encephalopathy** and **early infantile epileptic encephalopathy (Ohtahara syndrome)** are discussed in Chapter 593.4.

Miscellaneous Conditions

Miscellaneous conditions include benign neonatal sleep myoclonus and hyperekplexia, which are nonepileptic conditions (see Chapter 594).

DIAGNOSIS

Some cases can be correctly diagnosed by simply taking the prenatal and postnatal history and performing an adequate physical examination. Depending on the case, additional tests or procedures can be performed. EEG is considered the main tool for diagnosis. It can show paroxysmal activity (e.g., sharp waves) in between the seizures and electrographic seizure activity if a seizure is captured. However, some neonatal seizures might not be associated with EEG abnormalities as noted above either because they are "release phenomena" or alternatively because the discharge is deep and is not detected by the scalp EEG. Additionally, electrographic seizures can occur without observed clinical signs (**electroclinical dissociation**). This is presumed to be caused by the immaturity of cortical connections, resulting, in many cases, in no or minimal motor manifestations. Continuously monitoring the EEG at the bedside in the neonatal intensive care unit for neonates at risk for neonatal seizures and brain injury is part of routine clinical practice in most centers, providing real-time measurements of the brain's electrical activity and identifying seizure activity. Many centers apply EEG monitoring to at-risk babies even before seizures develop, which is often desirable; others monitor patients who have manifested or are suspected of having seizures. In addition, there are currently attempts to develop methods for continuous monitoring of cerebral activity with automated detection and background analysis of neonatal seizures, similar to the continuous ECG monitoring in intensive care facilities. In infants started on hypothermia protocols following suspected hypoxic–ischemic injuries, it is recommended to continuously monitor the EEG during the cooling and rewarming periods to detect clinical and subclinical events in this high-risk population. The American Clinical Neurophysiology Society recommends continuous EEG monitoring in the neonatal intensive care unit to monitor evolution of EEG background to help with prognostication, to guide titration of anticonvulsant therapy for infants with established seizures, to screen for seizures among infants deemed to be at risk (hypoxic ischemic encephalopathy, stroke, meningitis, intraventricular hemorrhage, metabolic disorders, and congenital cerebral malformations), to screen for seizures among infants who are paralyzed, to characterize clinical events suspected to represent seizures, and to detect impending cerebral ischemia or hemorrhage.

Careful neurologic examination of the infant might uncover the cause of the seizure disorder. Examination of the **retina** might show the presence of chorioretinitis, suggesting a congenital TORCH infection, in which case titers of mother and infant are indicated. The **Aicardi syndrome** is associated with coloboma of the iris and retinal lacunae. Inspection of the **skin** might show hypopigmented lesions characteristic of tuberous sclerosis (seen best on UV light examination) or the typical crusted vesicular lesions of incontinentia pigmenti; both neurocutaneous syndromes are often associated with generalized myoclonic seizures beginning early in life. An unusual body or urine odor suggests an inborn error of metabolism.

Blood should be obtained for determinations of glucose, calcium, magnesium, electrolytes, and blood urea nitrogen. If hypoglycemia is a possibility, serum glucose testing is indicated so that treatment can be initiated immediately. Hypocalcemia can occur in isolation or in association with hypomagnesemia. A lowered serum calcium level is often associated with birth trauma or a CNS insult in the perinatal period. Additional causes include maternal diabetes, prematurity, DiGeorge syndrome, and high-phosphate feedings. Hypomagnesemia (<1.5 mg/dL) is often associated with hypocalcemia and occurs particularly in infants of malnourished mothers. In this situation, the seizures are resistant to calcium therapy but respond to intramuscular magnesium, 0.2 mL/kg of a 50% solution of $MgSO_4$. Serum electrolyte measurement can indicate significant hyponatremia (serum sodium <115 mEq/L) or hypernatremia (serum sodium >160 mEq/L) as a cause of the seizure disorder.

A **lumbar puncture** is indicated in virtually all neonates with seizures, unless the cause is obviously related to a metabolic disorder such as hypoglycemia or hypocalcemia. The latter infants are normally alert interictally and usually respond promptly to appropriate therapy. The CSF findings can indicate a bacterial meningitis or aseptic encephalitis. Prompt diagnosis and appropriate therapy improve the outcome for these infants. Bloody CSF indicates a traumatic tap or a subarachnoid or intraventricular bleed. Immediate centrifugation of the specimen can assist in differentiating the 2 disorders. A clear supernatant suggests a traumatic tap, and a xanthochromic color suggests a subarachnoid bleed. Mildly jaundiced normal infants can have a yellowish discoloration of the CSF that makes inspection of the supernatant less reliable in the newborn period.

Many **inborn errors of metabolism** cause generalized convulsions in the newborn period. Because these conditions are often inherited in an autosomal recessive or X-linked recessive fashion, it is imperative that a careful family history be obtained to determine if there is consanguinity or whether siblings or close relatives developed seizures or died at an early age. Serum ammonia determination is useful for screening for the hypoglycemic hyperammonemia syndrome and for suspected urea cycle abnormalities. In addition to having generalized clonic seizures, these latter infants present during the 1st few days of life with increasing lethargy progressing to coma, anorexia and vomiting, and a bulging fontanel. If the blood gases show an anion gap and a metabolic acidosis with the hyperammonemia, urine organic acids should be immediately determined to investigate the possibility of methylmalonic or propionic acidemia.

Maple syrup urine disease should be suspected when a metabolic acidosis occurs in association with generalized clonic seizures, vomiting, bulging fontanel, and muscle rigidity during the 1st wk of life. The result of a rapid screening test using 2,4-dinitrophenylhydrazine that identifies keto derivatives in the urine is positive in maple syrup urine disease.

Additional metabolic causes of neonatal seizures include nonketotic hyperglycinemia, an intractable condition characterized by markedly elevated plasma and CSF glycine levels, prominent hiccups, persistent generalized seizures, and lethargy rapidly leading to coma; ketotic hyperglycinemia in which seizures are associated with vomiting, fluid and electrolyte disturbances, and a metabolic acidosis; and Leigh disease suggested by elevated levels of serum and CSF lactate or an increased lactate : pyruvate ratio. Biotinidase deficiency should also be considered. A comprehensive description of the diagnosis and management of these metabolic diseases is discussed in Part XI, Metabolic Disorders.

Unintentional **injection of a local anesthetic** into a fetus during labor can produce intense tonic seizures. These infants are often thought to have had a traumatic delivery because they are flaccid at birth, have abnormal brainstem reflexes, and show signs of respiratory depression that sometimes require ventilation. Examination may show a needle puncture of the skin or a perforation or laceration of the scalp. An elevated serum anesthetic level confirms the diagnosis. The treatment consists of supportive measures and promotion of urine output by administering intravenous fluids with appropriate monitoring to prevent fluid overload.

Benign familial neonatal seizures, an autosomal dominant condition, begins on the 2nd-3rd day of life, with a seizure frequency of 10-20/day. Patients are normal between seizures, which stop in 1-6 mo. These are caused by mutations in the voltage-sensitive potassium channel genes Kv7.2, and Kv7.3 (KCNQ2 and KCNQ3). Other mutations in the Kv7.2 gene cause severe neonatal epileptic encephalopathy. **Fifth-day fits** occur on day 5 of life (4-6 days) in normal-appearing neonates. The seizures are multifocal and are often present for <24 hr. The diagnosis requires exclusion of other causes of seizures and sequencing of the above genes. The prognosis is good for the benign form.

Pyridoxine dependency, a rare disorder, must be considered when seizures begin shortly after birth with signs of fetal distress in utero and are resistant to conventional anticonvulsants such as phenobarbital or phenytoin. The history may suggest that similar seizures occurred in utero. When pyridoxine-dependent seizures are suspected, 100-200 mg of pyridoxine or pyridoxal phosphate should be administered intravenously during the EEG, which should be promptly performed once the diagnosis is considered. The seizures abruptly cease, and the EEG often normalizes in the next few hours or longer. Not all cases of pyridoxine dependency respond dramatically to the initial bolus of IV pyridoxine. Therefore, a 6-wk trial of oral pyridoxine (100-200 mg/day) or preferably pyridoxal phosphate (as pyridoxine does not help infants with the related but distinct syndrome of pyridoxal dependency) is recommended for infants in whom a high index of suspicion continues after a negative response to IV pyridoxine. Measurement of serum pipecolic acid and α-aminoadipic acid semialdehyde (elevated) and CSF pyridoxal-5-phosphate (decreased) needs to be performed before initiation of the trials without delay. These children require lifelong supplementation of oral pyridoxine (100 mg/day at times with folinic acid) or pyridoxal phosphate (15-60 mg/kg/day). Cerebral folate deficiency should also be ruled out by medication trial (folinic acid 1-3 mg/kg/day) and by CSF levels of 5-methyltetrahydrofolate assay. Gene sequencing can confirm the diagnosis (see Chapter 593.4). The earlier the therapy is initiated in these vitamin responsive disorders, the more favorable the outcome.

Drug-withdrawal seizures can occur in the newborn nursery but can take several weeks to develop because of prolonged excretion of the drug by the neonate. The incriminated drugs include barbiturates, benzodiazepines, heroin, and methadone. The infant may be jittery, irritable, and lethargic, and can have myoclonus or frank clonic seizures. The mother might deny the use of drugs; a serum or urine drug screen might identify the responsible agent.

Infants with focal seizures, suspected stroke or intracranial hemorrhage, and severe **cytoarchitectural abnormalities** of the brain (including lissencephaly and schizencephaly) who clinically may appear normal or microcephalic should undergo MRI or CT scan. Indeed, it is appropriate to recommend imaging of all neonates with seizures unexplained by serum glucose, calcium, or electrolyte disorders. Infants with chromosome abnormalities and adrenoleukodystrophy are also at risk for seizures and should be evaluated with investigation of a karyotype and serum very-long-chain fatty acids, respectively.

PROGNOSIS
Over the last few decades, prognosis of neonatal seizures has improved owing to advancements in obstetric and intensive neonatal care. Mortality has decreased from 40% to 20%. The correlation between EEG and prognosis is very clear. Although neonatal EEG interpretation is very difficult, EEG was found to be highly associated with the outcome in premature and full-term infants. An abnormal background is a powerful predictor of less-favorable later outcome. In addition, prolonged electrographic seizures (>10 min/hr), multifocal periodic electrographic discharges, and spread of the electrographic seizures to the contralateral hemisphere also correlate with poorer outcome. The underlying etiology of the seizures is the main determinant of outcome. For example, patients with seizures secondary to hypoxic–ischemic encephalopathy have a 50% chance of developing normally, whereas those with seizures caused by primary subarachnoid hemorrhage or hypocalcemia have a much better prognosis.

TREATMENT
A mainstay in the therapy of neonatal seizures is the diagnosis and treatment of the underlying etiology (e.g., hypoglycemia, hypocalcemia, meningitis, drug withdrawal, trauma), whenever one can be identified. There are conflicting approaches regarding the control of neonatal seizures. Most experts advocate complete control of clinical as well electrographic seizures. Others argue for treating clinical seizures only. Most centers favor the first approach. An important consideration before starting anticonvulsants is deciding, based on the severity duration and frequency of the seizures if the patient needs to receive intravenous therapy and loading with an initial bolus or can simply be started on maintenance doses of a long-acting drug. Patients

often require assisted ventilation after receiving intravenous or oral loading doses of AEDs, and thus precautions for observations and for needed interventions are necessary.

Lorazepam
The initial drug used to control acute seizures is usually lorazepam. Lorazepam is distributed to the brain very quickly and exerts its anticonvulsant effect in <5 min. It is not very lipophilic and does not clear out from the brain very rapidly. Its action can last 6-24 hr. Usually, it does not cause hypotension or respiratory depression. The dose is 0.05 mg/kg (range: 0.02-0.10 mg/kg) every 4-8 hr.

Diazepam
Diazepam can be used as an alternative initial drug. It is highly lipophilic, so it distributes very rapidly into the brain and then is cleared very quickly out, carrying the risk of recurrence of seizures. Like other intravenous benzodiazepines, it carries a risk of apnea and hypotension, particularly if the patient is also on a barbiturate, so patients need to be observed for 3-8 hr after administration. The usual dose is 0.1-0.3 mg/kg IV over 3-5 min, given every 15-30 min to a maximum total dose of 2 mg. However, because of the respiratory and blood pressure limitations and because the intravenous preparation contains sodium benzoate and benzoic acid, it is currently not recommended as a first-line agent.

Midazolam
Midazolam can be used as an initial drug as a bolus or as a second- or third-line drug as a continuous drip for patients who did not respond to phenobarbital and/or to phenytoin. The doses used have been in the range of 0.05-0.1 mg/kg IV initial bolus, with a continuous infusion of 0.5-1 μg/kg/min IV that can be gradually titrated upward, if tolerated, every 5 min or longer, to a maximum of approximately 33 μg/kg/min (2 mg/kg/hr).

Phenobarbital
Phenobarbital is considered by many as the first choice long-acting drug in neonatal seizures. Whether to use a benzodiazepine first depends on the clinical situation. The usual loading dose is 20 mg/kg. If this dosage is not effective, then additional doses of 5-10 mg/kg can be given until a dose of 40 mg/kg is reached. Respiratory support may be needed after phenobarbital loading. Twenty-four hours after starting the loading dose, maintenance dosing can be started at 3-6 mg/kg/day usually administered in 2 separate doses. Phenobarbital is metabolized in the liver and is excreted through kidneys. Thus, any abnormality in the function of these organs alters the drug's metabolism and can result in toxicity. In infants with acidosis or critical illness that might alter serum protein content, free (i.e., not protein bound) levels of the drug should be followed carefully.

Phenytoin and Fosphenytoin
For ongoing seizures, if a total loading dose of 40 mg/kg of phenobarbital was not effective, then a loading dose of 15-20 mg/kg of phenytoin can be administered intravenously. The rate at which the dose should be given must not exceed 0.5-1.0 mg/kg/min so as to prevent cardiac problems, and the medication needs to be avoided in patients with significant heart disease. Heart rate should be monitored while administrating the drug. It is not possible to mix phenytoin or fosphenytoin with dextrose solutions. Owing to its reduced solubility, potentially severe local cutaneous reactions, interaction with other drugs, and possible cardiac toxicity, intravenous phenytoin is not widely used.

Fosphenytoin, which is a phosphate ester prodrug, is preferable. It is highly soluble in water, and can be administered very safely intravenously and intramuscularly, without causing injury to tissues. Fosphenytoin is administered in phenytoin equivalents (PE). The usual loading dose of fosphenytoin is 15-20 PE/kg administered over 30 min. Maintenance doses of 4-8 PE/kg/day can be given. As is the case for phenobarbital, free levels of the drug should be monitored in neonates whose serum pH or protein content might not be normal.

Other Medications

Approximately 45% of neonates respond to the first drug used if it is phenobarbital or phenytoin and an additional 15% respond to the second agent. Levetiracetam (which can be given intravenously with later convenient conversion to oral solution) and topiramate (oral) are reported to be the drugs of second and third choice for approximately half of surveyed pediatric neurologists and some have used them even before phenobarbital or phenytoin in selected cases. The dosages used are 10-30 mg/kg/day of levetiracetam, at times higher, and up to 20 mg/kg/day of topiramate. Bumetanide has been used as an adjunct drug, particularly with phenobarbital, because of its effect on the chloride gradient, as discussed above. Lidocaine is another medication used for resistant cases. Primidone, carbamazepine, valproate, and lamotrigine use, although reported in some studies, is rarely warranted. Valproate, for example, is more likely to be toxic in children younger than 2 yr of age than in older children.

Duration of Therapy

Duration of therapy is related to the risk of developing later epilepsy in infants suffering from neonatal seizures, which ranges from 10-30% and depends on the individual neurologic examination, the etiology of the seizures, and the EEG at the time of discharge from the hospital. In general, if the EEG at the time of discharge does not show evidence of epileptiform activity, then medications are usually tapered at that time. If the EEG remains paroxysmal, then the decision is usually delayed for several months after discharge.

Bibliography is available at Expert Consult.

593.8 Status Epilepticus

Mohamad A. Mikati and Abeer J. Hani

Status epilepticus is a medical emergency that should be anticipated in any patient who presents with an acute seizure. It is defined as continuous seizure activity or recurrent seizure activity without regaining of consciousness lasting for more than 5 min as part of an operational definition put forth within the past few years. In the past, the cutoff time was 30 min, but this has been reduced to emphasize the risks involved with the longer durations. The ILAE defines status epilepticus as "a seizure which shows no clinical signs of arresting after a duration encompassing the great majority of seizures of that type in most patients or recurrent seizures without resumption of baseline central nervous system function interictally." The measures used to treat status epilepticus have to be started in any patient with acute seizures that do not stop within a few minutes. The most common type is **convulsive status epilepticus** (generalized tonic, clonic, or tonic–clonic), but other types do occur, including **nonconvulsive status** (complex partial, absence), myoclonic status, epilepsia partialis continua, and neonatal status epilepticus. The incidence of status epilepticus ranges between 10 and 60 per 100,000 population in various studies. Status epilepticus is most common in children younger than 5 yr of age, with an incidence in this age group of >100 per 100,000 children.

Approximately 30% of patients presenting with status epilepticus are having their first seizure, and approximately 40% of these later develop epilepsy. Febrile status epilepticus is the most common type of status epilepticus in children. In the 1950s and 1960s, mortality rates of 6-18% were reported after status epilepticus; currently, with the recognition of status epilepticus as a medical emergency, a lower mortality rate of 4-5% is observed, most of it secondary to the underlying etiology rather than to the seizures. Status epilepticus carries an approximately 14% risk of new neurologic deficits, most of this (12.5%) secondary to the underlying pathology.

Nonconvulsive status epilepticus manifests as a confusional state, dementia, hyperactivity with behavioral problems, fluctuating impairment of consciousness with at times unsteady sitting or walking, fluctuating mental status, confusional state, hallucinations, paranoia,

aggressiveness catatonia, and or psychotic symptoms. It should be considered in any of these situations, especially in an unresponsive or encephalopathic child. Epilepsia partialis continua has been defined previously and can be caused by tumor, vascular etiologies, mitochondrial disease (mitochondrial myopathy, encephalopathy, lactic acidosis, and stroke-like episodes [MELAS]), and Rasmussen encephalitis.

Refractory status epilepticus is status epilepticus that has failed to respond to therapy, usually with at least 2 (such as a benzodiazepine and another medication) medications. Currently, the trend is not to assign a minimum duration, whereas in the past a minimum duration of 30 min, 60 min, or even 2 hr was cited. **New-onset refractory status epilepticus** has been identified as a distinct entity that can be caused by almost any of the causes of status epilepticus in a patient without prior epilepsy. It also is often of unknown etiology, presumed to be encephalitic or postencephalitic, can last several weeks or longer, and often, but not always, has a poor prognosis. Devastating epileptic encephalopathy in school-age children, also called **fever-induced refractory epileptic encephalopathy in school age children (FIRES)** is a syndrome of refractory status epilepticus that is associated with acute febrile infections, appears to be parainfectious in nature, and to be highly drug resistant but responsive to the ketogenic diet.

ETIOLOGY

Etiologies include new-onset epilepsy of any type; drug intoxication (e.g., tricyclic antidepressants) in children and drug and alcohol abuse in adolescents; drug withdrawal or overdose in patients on AEDs; hypoglycemia; hypocalcemia; hyponatremia; hypomagnesemia; acute head trauma; encephalitis; meningitis; autoimmune encephalitis (such as anti-NMDA receptor and anti–voltage-gated potassium channel complex antibody syndromes); ischemic (arterial or venous) stroke; intracranial hemorrhage; folinic acid and pyridoxine and pyridoxal phosphate dependency (these usually present in infancy but childhood onset is also possible); inborn errors of metabolism (see Chapter 593.2) such as nonketotic hyperglycinemia in neonates and mitochondrial encephalopathy with lactic acidosis (MELAS) in infants, children, and adolescents; ion channel–related epilepsies (e.g., sodium and potassium channel mutations reviewed in the sections above); hypoxic–ischemic injury (e.g., after cardiac arrest); systemic conditions (such as hypertensive encephalopathy, posterior reversible encephalopathy, renal or hepatic encephalopathy); brain tumors; and any other disorders that can cause epilepsy (such as brain malformations, neurodegenerative disorders, different types of progressive myoclonic epilepsy, storage diseases).

A rare condition called **hemiconvulsion-hemiplegia-epilepsy syndrome** consists of prolonged febrile status epilepticus presumably caused by focal acute encephalitis with resultant atrophy in the involved hemisphere, contralateral hemiplegia, and chronic epilepsy. It should be suspected early on to attempt to control the seizures as early as possible. This and the somewhat similar condition mentioned above called FIRES are likely to be have a parainfectious-autoimmune etiology. Rasmussen encephalitis often causes epilepsia partialis continua (see Chapter 593.3) and sometimes convulsive status epilepticus. Several types of infections are more likely to cause encephalitis with status epilepticus, such as herpes simplex (complex partial and convulsive status), *Bartonella* (particularly nonconvulsive status), Epstein-Barr virus, and mycoplasma (postinfectious encephalomyelitis with any type of status epilepticus). Postinfectious encephalitis and acute disseminated encephalomyelitis are common causes of status epilepticus, including refractory status epilepticus. HHV6 can cause a distinct epileptic syndrome with limbic status epilepticus in immune-suppressed patients.

MECHANISMS

The mechanisms leading to the establishment of sustained seizure activity seen in status epilepticus appear to involve (1) failure of desensitization of AMPA glutamate receptors, thus persistence of increased excitability, and (2) reduction of GABA-mediated inhibition as a result of intracellular internalization of $GABA_A$ receptors. This explains the clinical observation that status epilepticus is often less likely to stop in the next specific period of time the longer the seizure has lasted and why benzodiazepines appear to be decreasingly effective the longer seizure activity lasts. During status epilepticus there is increased cerebral metabolic rate and a compensatory increase in cerebral blood flow that, after approximately 30 min, is not able to keep up with the increases in cerebral metabolic rate. This leads to a transition from adequate to inadequate cerebral oxygen tensions and, together with other factors, contributes to neuronal injury resulting from status epilepticus. Status epilepticus can cause both neuronal necrosis and apoptosis. The mechanisms of apoptosis are thought to be related to increases in intracellular calcium and proapoptotic factors such as ceramide, Bax, and apoptosis-inducing factor. In addition, inflammation through the cytokines (such as interleukin-1β) released during seizure activity can modify neuronal excitability by modifying neurotransmitter function in a number of ways, such as through phosphorylation of the NR2B subunit rendering the NMDA receptors more permeable to calcium influx, increased expression of highly calcium-permeable AMPA receptors, and induction of endocytosis of $GABA_A$ receptors. Prostaglandins (such as prostaglandin E_2) can increase glutamate release and reduce potassium currents leading to increased excitability.

THERAPY

Status epilepticus is a medical emergency that requires initial and continuous attention to securing airway, breathing, and circulation (with continuous monitoring of vital signs including ECG) and determination and management of the underlying etiology (e.g., hypoglycemia). Laboratory studies, including glucose, sodium, calcium, magnesium, complete blood count, basic metabolic panel, CT scan, and continuous EEG, are needed for all patients. Blood and spinal fluid cultures, toxic screens, and tests for inborn errors of metabolism are often needed. AED levels need to be determined in all patients known already to be taking these drugs. Lumbar puncture, comprehensive toxicologic screens, MRI, and other laboratory tests are performed depending on clinical suspicion and need. EEG is helpful in ruling out **pseudo–status epilepticus** (psychologic conversion reaction mimicking status epilepticus) or other movement disorders (chorea, tics), rigors, clonus with stimulation, and decerebrate/decorticate posturing. The EEG can also be helpful in identifying the type of status epilepticus (generalized vs focal), which can guide further testing for the underlying etiology and further therapy. EEG can also help distinguish between postictal depression and later stages of status epilepticus in which the clinical manifestations are subtle (e.g., minimal myoclonic jerks) or absent (electroclinical dissociation), and can help in monitoring the therapy, particularly in patients who are paralyzed and intubated. Neuroimaging must be considered after the child has been stabilized, especially if it is indicated by the clinical manifestations, by an asymmetric or focal nature of the EEG abnormalities, or by lack of knowledge of the underlying etiology. The EEG manifestations of status epilepticus show several stages that consist of initial distinct electrographic seizures (stage I) followed by waxing and waning electrographic seizures (stage II), continuous electrographic seizures (stage III; many patients start with this directly), continuous ictal discharges punctuated by flat periods (stage IV), and periodic epileptiform discharges on flat background (stage V). The last 2 stages are often associated with subtle clinical manifestations and with a lower chance of response to medications.

The initial **emergent** therapy usually involves intravenous diazepam, lorazepam, or midazolam. Diazepam is at least as effective as intravenous lorazepam but has fewer side effects (Table 593-18). The use of midazolam autoinjector as initial therapy for acute seizures was found to be at least as useful and safe as the use intravenous lorazepam and results in earlier response. If intravenous access is not available, buccal or intranasal midazolam, intranasal lorazepam, or rectal diazepam are effective options. Intramuscular midazolam is equally effective as intravenous lorazepam. With all options, respiratory depression is a potential side effect for which the patient should be monitored and managed as needed. In some infants, a trial of pyridoxine may be warranted. The strongest evidence for initial and emergent therapy is for diazepam or

Table 593-18	Doses of Commonly Used Antiepileptic Drugs in Status Epilepticus	
DRUG*	**ROUTE**	**DOSAGE**
Lorazepam	Intravenous	0.1 mg/kg up to 4 mg total, may repeat in 5-10 min
	Intranasal	0.1 mg/kg
Midazolam	Intravenous	0.2 mg/kg up to 10 mg total dose, may repeat in 5-10 min
		0.08-0.23 mg/kg/hr maintenance
	Intramuscular	0.2 mg/kg
	Intranasal	0.2 mg/kg
	Buccal	0.5 mg/kg
Diazepam	Intravenous	0.15 mg/kg up to a max total dose of 10 mg, may repeat in 5-10 min
	Rectal	2-5 yr: 0.5 mg/kg
		6-11 yr: 0.3 mg/kg
		≥12 yr: 0.2 mg/kg
Fosphenytoin	Intravenous	20 mg/kg PE, then 3-6 mg/kg/24 hr, loading rate up to 50 mg PE per min
Phenobarbital†	Intravenous	5-20 mg/kg
Pentobarbital coma†	Intravenous	13.0 mg/kg, then 1-5 mg/kg/hr
Propofol†	Intravenous	1 mg/kg (bolus), then 1-15 mg/kg/hr (infusion)
Thiopental†	Intravenous	5 mg/kg/1st hr, then 1-2 mg/kg/hr
Valproate†	Intravenous	Loading: 25 mg/kg, then 30-60 mg/kg/24 hr
Lacosamide†	Intravenous	Loading: 4 mg/kg then 4-12 mg/kg/24 hr
Levetiracetam	Intravenous	20-60 mg/kg
Topiramate	Enterally	5-10 mg/kg/24 hr (loading dose) then same or lower for maintenance

*Reflects current trends in use which may not be FDA approved. For FDA indications, see Table 593-13.
†May cause PR prolongation.
PE, phenytoin sodium equivalents.

lorazepam, followed by phenytoin/fosphenytoin and phenobarbital, then valproate and levetiracetam.

After the emergent therapy usually with a benzodiazepine, the subsequent **urgent therapy** medication is usually fosphenytoin, and the loading dose is usually 15-20 PE/kg. A level is usually taken 2 hr later to ensure achievement of a therapeutic concentration. Depending on the level, maintenance dose can be started right away or, more commonly, in 6 hr. With phenytoin and phenobarbital, each 1 mg/kg (1 PE/kg for fosphenytoin) increases the serum concentration by approximately 1 µg/mL; for valproate, each 1 mg/kg increases the serum concentration by approximately 4 µg/mL. Precautions about the rate of infusion of fosphenytoin and phenytoin (not >0.5-1.0 mg/kg/min) and the other medications need to be followed because side effects often depend on infusion rate. The subsequent medication is often phenobarbital. The dose used in neonates is usually 20 mg/kg loading dose, but in infants and children the dose is often 5-10 mg/kg (to avoid respiratory depression), with the dose repeated if there is not an adequate response. Current evidence for the urgent therapy is strongest for valproate, followed by phenytoin/fosphenytoin and midazolam continuous infusion, followed by phenobarbital and levetiracetam, the last of which are currently being increasingly used.

After the second or third medication is given, and sometimes before that, the patient might need to be intubated. All patients with status epilepticus, even the ones who respond, need to be admitted to the ICU for completion of therapy and monitoring. Ideally, emergent and urgent therapies should have been received within less than 30 min so as to initiate the subsequent therapy soon, thus reducing the chances of sequelae. For **refractory status epilepticus treatment**, an intravenous bolus followed by continuous infusion of midazolam, propofol, pentobarbital, or thiopental is used. This is done in the ICU. Subsequent boluses and adjustment of the rate of the infusion are usually made depending on clinical and EEG responses. Because most of these patients need to be intubated and paralyzed, the EEG becomes the method of choice by which to follow them. The goal is to stop electrographic seizure activity before reducing the therapy. Usually this implies achievement of complete flattening of the EEG. Some consider that achieving a burst suppression pattern may be enough, and the periods of flattening in such a case need to be 8-20 sec to ensure interruption of electrographic seizure activity. However, this is an area that is in need of further study. Currently, the level of the evidence for refractory treatment is strongest for midazolam and valproate, followed by propofol and pentobarbital/thiopental, followed by levetiracetam, phenytoin/fosphenytoin, lacosamide, topiramate, and phenobarbital.

Patients on these therapies require careful attention to blood pressure and to systemic complications, and some develop multiorgan failure. It is not unusual for patients put into pentobarbital coma to have to be on multiple pressors to maintain their blood pressure during therapy.

The choice among the above options to treat refractory status epilepticus often depends on the experience of the specific center. Midazolam probably has fewer side effects, but is less effective, and barbiturate coma is more effective, but carries a higher risk of side effects. On propofol, some patients develop a propofol infusion syndrome with lactic acidosis, hemodynamic instability, and rhabdomyolysis with higher infusion rates (>67 µg/kg/min). Thus electrolytes, creatine phosphokinase, and organ function studies need to be monitored. Often, barbiturate coma and similar therapies are maintained for 1 or more days before it is possible to gradually taper the therapy, usually over a few days. However, in some cases, including cases of new-onset refractory status epilepticus (new-onset refractory status epilepticus), such therapies need to be maintained for several weeks or even months. Even though the prognosis in new-onset refractory status epilepticus cases is often poor and many patients do not survive, meaningful recovery despite a prolonged course is still possible. This also appears to apply to the FIRES syndrome. Occasionally, inhalational anesthetics are useful. Probably isoflurane is preferable because halothane can increase intracranial pressure and enflurane can induce seizures. Other therapies have included ketamine, corticosteroids (e.g., for Rasmussen encephalitis, Hashimoto encephalopathy, or other

autoimmune encephalitides), immunoglobulins, and plasma exchange (e.g., in Rasmussen or other autoimmune encephalitides), ketogenic diet (in patients with FIRES and Landau-Kleffner syndrome), vagus nerve stimulation in catastrophic epilepsy in infants, hypothermia, electroconvulsive therapy, magnetic transcranial stimulation, and surgical management with focal resection. Another potential therapy under study for convulsive status epilepticus is induction of acidosis (e.g., by hypercapnia), which could reduce neuronal excitability.

For nonconvulsive status epilepticus and epilepsia partialis continua, therapy needs to be tailored according to the clinical manifestations and often consists of trials of sequential oral or sometimes parenteral AEDs without resorting to barbiturate coma or overmedication that could result in respiratory compromise. The approach to complex partial status epilepticus is sometimes similar to the approach to convulsive status epilepticus and sometimes intermediate between the approach for epilepsia partialis and that for convulsive status, depending on severity. Long-term consequences after complex partial status epilepticus do occur, but the complications are often less severe than those after convulsive status epilepticus of similar duration. Prolonged nonconvulsive complex partial status epilepticus can last for as long as 12 wk, with patients manifesting psychotic symptoms and confusional states. These cases can be resistant to therapy. Despite that, patients still can have a full recovery. Some of these cases appear to improve with the use of steroids or IVIG, which are used if an autoimmune, parainfectious etiology is suspected.

Bibliography is available at Expert Consult.

593.9 Reflex Seizures (Stimulus Precipitated Seizures)
Robert M. Kliegman

Many patients with epilepsy can identify precipitating or provoking events that predispose them to having a seizure. Common events in patients with epilepsy include stress, lack of sleep, fever, or fatigue.

There is another group of patients who have seizures in response to a very specific, identifiable sensory stimulus or activity and are considered to have reflex seizures. Although no known "reflex" may be involved, more appropriate terms may be sensory precipitated or stimulus sensitive seizures (see Table 593-1). Stimuli may be external (light, patterns, music, brushing teeth) or internal (math, reading, thinking, self-induced). Reflex seizures may be generalized, partial, nonconvulsive, absence or myoclonic. One common pattern is photomyoclonic seizures characterized by forehead muscle twitching or repetitive eye opening or closing.

Photosensitive or pattern-induced seizures are a well-recognized disorder stimulated by bright or flashing lights (TV, video games, discotheques, concert light shows) or by patterns (TV, video games, lines on the road while traveling). Visual sensitivity may occur in 0.3-3% of the population, while photosensitive or pattern-induced seizures may occur in 1 in 4,000 people in the at-risk age group of 5-25 yr. When Japanese children were exposed to a Pokémon cartoon that induced seizures, only 24% had a history of spontaneous seizures. Patients tend to outgrow photosensitive or pattern-induced seizures in their 30s. Photoparoxysmal responses, with an abnormal EEG response to photic stimulation may be more common than photic-induced seizures. There are some photo-induced responses that do not demonstrate EEG abnormalities (nonconvulsive).

For patients with isolated photosensitive or pattern-induced seizures, avoidance or modification of stimuli is the initial approach. Such activities may include blue or polarized sunglasses, avoiding high-contrast flashing-light video games, avoiding discotheques, use a TV remote or watch TV in a well-lit room at a distance of >8 feet, and covering 1 eye when in a provocative situation.

Bibliography is available at Expert Consult.

Table 593-19	Consensus Case Definition and Modified Consensus Case Definition for Nodding Syndrome—Uganda, 2012-2013*	
TYPE OF CASE	**CONSENSUS CASE DEFINITION**	**MODIFIED CONSENSUS CASE DEFINITION**
Suspected case	Reported head nodding (repetitive involuntary drops of the head toward the chest on 2 or more occasions) in a previously normal person	Reported head nodding (repetitive involuntary drops of the head toward the chest on 2 or more occasions) in a previously normal person
Probable case	Suspected case of head nodding, with both major criteria: • Age of onset of nodding ranging from 3-18 yr • Frequency of nodding 5-20 per minute Plus at least 1 of the following minor criteria: • Other neurologic abnormalities (cognitive decline, school dropout because of cognitive or behavioral problems, other seizures or neurologic abnormalities) • Clustering in space or time with similar cases • Triggering by food or cold weather • Stunting or wasting • Delayed sexual or physical development • Psychiatric symptoms	Suspected case of head nodding, with 1 major criterion: • Age of onset of nodding ranging from 3-18 yr Plus at least 1 of the following minor criteria: • Other neurologic abnormalities (cognitive decline, school dropout because of cognitive or behavioral problems, other seizures or neurologic abnormalities) • Clustering in space or time with similar cases • Triggering by food or cold weather • Stunting or wasting • Psychiatric symptoms
Confirmed case	Probable case, with documented nodding episode • Observed and recorded by a trained healthcare worker, or • Videotaped nodding episode, or • Video/EEG/EMG documenting head nodding as atonic seizures	Probable case, with documented nodding episode • Observed and recorded by a trained healthcare worker, or • Videotaped nodding episode, or • Video/EEG/EMG documenting head nodding as atonic seizures

*The consensus case definition was drafted at the first International Scientific Meeting on Nodding Syndrome, held July 30–August 1, 2012, in Kampala, Uganda. Meeting report available at http://www.who.int/neglected_diseases/diseases/Nodding_syndrom_Kampala_Report_2012.pdf. The modified consensus case definition was developed during the March 2013 single-stage cluster survey conducted by Centers for Disease Control and Prevention (CDC) and the Ugandan Ministry of Health to assess prevalence of nodding syndrome in Uganda.

EEG, electroencephalographic; EMG, electromyographic.

From Iyengar PJ, Wamala J, Ratto J, et al: Prevalence of nodding syndrome–Uganda, 2012-2013. MMWR Morb Mortal Wkly Rep 63:603–606, 2014, Table 1.

593.10 Nodding Syndrome
Robert M. Kliegman

Nodding syndrome appears to be an epidemic progressive epilepsy encephalopathy syndrome of unknown etiology seen predominantly in Uganda, Liberia, Tanzania, and the southern Sudan, with a prevalence of approximately 6.8 per 1,000 children. Age of onset is 6-13 yr. Nodding episodes are characterized by at least daily, rapid, paroxysmal forward head bobbling spells lasting several minutes; some patients are unresponsive whereas others may respond to commands or continue what they were doing before the episode. Children were previously healthy, although there may be a family history of seizures. In addition to episodes of nodding, there may be associated definable generalized tonic–clonic or absence seizures. Furthermore, patients go on to demonstrate severe and global cognitive impairment (see Table 593-19 for case definitions).

The EEG demonstrates a disorganized slow background and interictal generalized 2.5-3.0 Hz spike and slow waves. During a nodding episode, the EEG demonstrates generalized electrodecrement and paraspinal electromyography dropout suggestive of an atonic seizure. Cerebral spinal fluid analysis is usually negative, while the MRI shows cerebral and cerebellar atrophy.

Nodding episodes may be triggered during meals while eating hot foods or drinking cold liquids; cold environmental temperature may also trigger a nodding episode.

Treatment of seizures are indicated; however, the response to treatment is poor.

Bibliography is available at Expert Consult.

Chapter 594
Conditions That Mimic Seizures
Mohamad A. Mikati and Makram M. Obeid

The misdiagnosis of epilepsy is estimated to be as high as 5-40%, implying that many patients may be subjected to unnecessary therapy and tests. Often all that is needed to differentiate nonepileptic paroxysmal disorders from epilepsy is a careful and detailed history in addition to a thorough exam; but sometimes an electroencephalogram (EEG) or more advanced testing may be necessary. The ready availability of video recording on mobile phones and other devices at home or at school can provide invaluable information. Nonepileptic paroxysmal disorders can be classified according to the age of presentation and the clinical manifestations: (1) syncope and other generalized paroxysms, (2) movement disorders and other abnormal movements and postures, (3) oculomotor abnormalities and visual hallucinations, and (4) sleep-related disorders (Table 594-1).

SYNCOPE AND OTHER GENERALIZED PAROXYSMS
Apnea
Apneic episodes in neonates are usually associated with bradycardia as is usually apnea resulting from brainstem compression. In contrast, apnea associated with seizures is usually accompanied by tachycardia. Of note, exceptions do occur as bradycardia can occur during epileptic seizures, and severe apnea of any cause can be followed by anoxic seizures.

Table 594-1	Conditions That Mimic Seizures According to Age of Presentation			
AGE	**SYNCOPE AND OTHER GENERALIZED PAROXYSMS**	**MOVEMENT DISORDERS AND OTHER ABNORMAL MOVEMENTS**	**OCULOMOTOR ABNORMALITIES**	**SLEEP DISORDERS**
Neonate	Apnea Paroxysmal extreme pain disorder	Jitteriness Hyperekplexia Paroxysmal dystonic choreoathetosis	Paroxysmal tonic up gaze Alternating hemiplegia of childhood	Benign neonatal sleep myoclonus Sleep transition disorders
Infants	Reflex anoxic seizures Breath-holding spells Benign paroxysmal vertigo Paroxysmal extreme pain disorder	Jitteriness Sandifer Paroxysmal dystonic choreoathetosis Benign myoclonus of early infancy Pathologic startle Shuddering attacks Benign paroxysmal torticollis Psychologic disorders Alternating hemiplegia of childhood Jactatio capitis head banging Drug reactions	Paroxysmal tonic upgaze Oculomotor apraxia Spasmus nutans Opsoclonus myoclonus syndrome	Non-REM partial arousal disorders REM sleep disorders Narcolepsy Sleep transition disorders (somnambulism, somniloquy)
Children and adolescents	Benign paroxysmal vertigo Compulsive Valsalva Familial hemiplegic migraine Syncope (long QT, vasovagal, vagovagal, orthostatic, migraine-induced) Psychogenic seizures Transient global amnesia Hyperventilation spells	Tics Tremor Pathologic startle Paroxysmal dyskinesias Alternating hemiplegia of childhood Benign paroxysmal torticollis Episodic ataxia Psychologic disorders including factitious disorder imposed on another, malingering Masturbation Psychogenic seizures Cataplexy Jactatio capitis (head banging) Episodic rage Drug reactions	Daydreaming Drug reactions	Non-REM partial-arousal disorders REM sleep disorders Narcolepsy Sleep transition disorders (somnambulism, somniloquy) Sleep myoclonus Restless legs syndrome

REM, rapid eye movement.

From Obeid M, Mikati MA: Expanding spectrum of paroxysmal events in children: potential mimickers of epilepsy, Pediatr Neurol 37(5):309–316, 2007.

Breath-Holding Spells

The term *breath-holding spells* is actually a misnomer, as these are not self-induced, but result from the immaturity of the autonomic system and occur in 2 different forms. The first type is the **pallid breath-holding spell**, which is caused by reflex vagal–cardiac bradycardia and asystole. The second type is the **cyanotic, or "blue," breath-holding spell**, which does not occur during inspiration, but results from prolonged expiratory apnea and intrapulmonary shunting. Episodes usually start with a cry (often, in the case of the pallid type, a "silent" cry with marked pallor), and progress to apnea and cyanosis. Spells usually begin between 6 and 18 mo of age. Syncope, tonic posturing, and even reflex anoxic seizures may follow the more-severe episodes, particularly in breath-holding spells of the pallid type. Injury, anger, and frustration, particularly with surprise, are common triggers. Education and reassurance of the parents is usually all that is needed, as these episodes are, as a rule, self-limited and are outgrown within a few years. However, treatment of coexisting iron deficiency is needed if it is present as the spells are made worse by iron-deficiency anemia. Anticholinergic drugs (e.g., atropine sulfate 0.01 mg/kg/24 hr in divided doses with a maximum daily dose of 0.4 mg), or antiepileptic drug therapy for coexisting anoxic seizures that are recurrent and not responding to other measures may, rarely, be needed. It is important also to educate parents on how to handle more-severe spells by first-aid measures, or even basic CPR when needed. In severe cases of asystole, a cardiac pacemaker implantation may be needed. All parents should be taught not to provide secondary gain when the episodes occur, because this can reinforce the episodes. Also, preparation for unpleasant experiences (such as receiving a shot) rather than surprising the child with them, can help limit the number of spells (see Chapter 69).

Compulsive Valsalva

In children with intellectual disability, including Rett syndrome, syncopal convulsions may be self-induced by maneuvers like Valsalva. In this case, true breath-holding occurs, and it usually lasts for approximately 10 sec during inspiration. Some clinicians advocate the use of naloxone in such cases.

Neurally Mediated Syncope

Syncope can present with drop attacks and can also lead to generalized convulsions, termed *anoxic seizures*. These convulsions, triggered by a sudden reduction of oxygen to the brain, are clinically similar to and can be misdiagnosed as generalized epileptic seizures. **Vasovagal (neurocardiogenic) syncope** is one of the most common mimickers of generalized tonic–clonic seizures and is usually triggered by dehydration, heat, standing for a long time without movement, hot showers, the sight of blood, pain, swallowing, vomiting, and or sudden stress. History is usually the clue to distinguishing syncope from epileptic seizures: There is initially pallor and sweating followed by blurring of vision, dizziness, nausea, and then gradual collapse with loss of consciousness. These symptoms are present in most, although not necessarily all patients with syncope and can sometimes be manifestations of complex partial seizures. Much more important is the fact that such prodromal features have an insidious onset and build up gradually, often arising from a state of malaise when they precede syncope. However when they precede an epileptic convulsion, such features usually start suddenly are short in duration, paroxysmal and are followed by other manifestations of complex partial seizures such as stereotyped automatisms. Abdominal pain, a common aura in temporal lobe epilepsy, occurs in vasovagal syncope, and can be a trigger or a consequence of that process (intestinal vagal discharge). Urinary incontinence and a brief period of convulsive jerks are not uncommon in vasovagal syncope. These occur with a frequency of 10% and 50%, respectively. Postictal confusion only rarely occurs, and the rule is the occurrence of only brief postictal tiredness with a subsequent remarkable ability to resume planned activities. Most children with vasovagal syncope have an affected 1st-degree relative; reports demonstrate autosomal dominant inheritance at least in some families. The EEG is normal and the tilt test has been used for diagnostic purposes in selected cases. In most cases with typical history, this test is not needed. **Vagovagal syncope** can progress to convulsive seizure if the asystole is sufficiently prolonged. Sudden cold exposure to the face or to the body can also trigger vagal syncope. Syncope has been reported (rarely) to occur in association with cough, tight hair braiding, and hair combing. **Orthostatic hypotension and orthostatic intolerance** manifest symptoms that develop during upright standing and can be relieved by recumbence. **Postural tachycardia syndrome,** the pathophysiology of which presumably involves an excessive sympathetic discharge resulting in increased heart rate and vasoconstriction that can lead to decreased peripheral perfusion, is usually a disease of adolescent females that is characterized by upright syncope/near syncope, and tachycardia with normal or even increased blood pressure during the episode. Primary autonomic failure is rare in children, and familial dysautonomia is the only relatively common form. **Familial dysautonomia** is a disease common in Ashkenazi Jews and is characterized by absence of overflow emotional tears, depressed patellar reflexes, and lack of a flare reaction following intradermal histamine. **Dopamine β-hydroxylase deficiency** is a very rare cause of primary autonomic failure, and is characterized by a complicated perinatal course (hypotension, hypotonia, hypothermia), ptosis, highly arched palate, hyperflexible joints, impaired ejaculation, and nocturia. The tilt test causes a drop in both blood pressure and heart rate in patients with classic vasovagal syncope. It results in a blood pressure drop with minimal change in heart rate in autonomic failure, and in blood pressure drop and an increase in heart rate in postural tachycardia syndrome. Management of syncope centers on avoidance of precipitating factors (maintenance of hydration, avoidance of standing still, rising slowly from sitting, first-aid measures, raising of the legs, positioning) and treatment of any accompanying or underlying medical conditions (anemia, adrenal insufficiency, cardiac, etc.). In addition, **salt supplementation (2-4 g/day),** β-blockers (e.g., metoprolol at a starting dose of 1-2 mg/kg once per day up to a maximum of 6 mg/kg/day), or fluorohydrocortisone (0.05-0.1 mg/day) therapy may be needed in selected cases.

Cardiac Syncope

See Chapter 435.5.

Long QT syndromes (LQT) can cause life-threatening "pallid" or white syncope. Accompanying this are ventricular arrhythmias, usually torsades de pointes or even ventricular fibrillation. There are more than 10 types of prolonged QT syndrome. When accompanied by congenital deafness, it is part of the autosomal recessive Jervell and Lange-Nielson syndrome (type 1, LQT 1, associated with *KvLQT1* potassium channel mutation). The Romano-Ward syndrome is an autosomal dominant syndrome with incomplete penetrance that is characterized by episodes of lying still like a dead body for several seconds before the anoxic convulsive episode (LQT 2 associated with an *HERG* potassium channel mutation). LQT 3 is associated with an *SCN1A* sodium channel mutation, LQT 4 with ankyrin protein mutation, LQT 5 (milder form) with *KCNE1* mutations, LQT 6 with *KCNE2* potassium gene mutations, LQT 9 with caveolin sodium channel–related protein mutations, and LQT 10 with *SCN4B* sodium channel mutations. LQT 7 and LQT 8 are of particular interest because of associated clinical and neurologic manifestations. LQT 7 (Andersen-Tawil) syndrome is associated with periodic paralysis, skeletal developmental abnormalities, clinodactyly, low-set ears, and micrognathia (mutations in *KCNJ2* gene). LQT 8 or the Timothy syndrome (mutations in the calcium channel gene *CACNA1c*) manifests congenital heart disease, autism, syndactyly, and immune deficiency. All family members of an affected LQT syndrome individual should be investigated. Affected individuals need insertion of cardiac defibrillators, and their families should be taught CPR. As a rule, children with new-onset seizure disorder should get an electrocardiogram to rule out LQT syndrome masquerading as seizure disorder. Cardiac syncope is usually sudden without the gradual onset and the symptoms that accompany vagal syncope. Aortic stenosis can cause sudden syncope at the height of the exercise (usually hypertrophic),

or directly at the end (usually valvular) and, if suspected, warrants an echocardiogram.

Other Causes of Syncope

Syncope that is not neurally mediated or cardiac in origin is caused by a decrease in blood volume, or a mechanical disruption of brain perfusion. Systemic diseases that lead to syncope by affecting blood volume (e.g., adrenal insufficiency) are usually first brought to medical attention by other accompanying signs and symptoms. In **stretch syncope,** which occurs mostly in adolescents while stretching the neck and the trunk backward and the arms outward, or during flexion of the neck, the presumed mechanism is mechanical disruption of brain perfusion caused by compression of the vertebral arteries. In some cases, this may be associated with an abnormally prolonged stylomastoid process compressing the carotids. If the latter condition is suspected, then neuroimaging (CT, MRI) is required for proper diagnosis of the stylomastoid anomaly.

Sporadic and Familial Hemiplegic Migraine

This is a rare type of migraine with a motor aura of weakness. Attacks begin as early as 5-7 yr of age. In a genetically susceptible person, attacks may be precipitated by head trauma, exertion, or emotional stress. The 3 genes so far identified are *SCN1A* (neuronal sodium channel subunit), *CACNA1A* (neuronal calcium channel subunit), and *ATP1A2* (sodium potassium adenosine triphosphatase subunit). However at least a quarter of the affected families, and most of the sporadic cases do not carry a mutations in these 3 genes. Headaches occur in all attacks in most patients. The presence of negative phenomena (e.g., numbness, visual scotomas) in addition to positive phenomena (pins and needles, flickering lights), and the progressive and successive occurrence of visual, sensory, motor, aphasic, and basilar signs and symptoms, in that order, help differentiate these attacks from epileptic seizures. Persistent cerebellar deficits (e.g., nystagmus, ataxia) may be present. Verapamil, acetazolamide, and lamotrigine have been successfully used to prevent attacks and verapamil and ketamine have been used for the acute episode, while ergot derivatives, nimodipine, Midrin (isometheptene mucate, dichloralphenazone, and paracetamol), and probably triptans and propranolol are to be avoided because of concerns of exacerbating the attacks. Interestingly, the co-occurrence of epileptic seizures has been reported in a minority of patient with hemiplegic migraine. It is important also to note that recurrent attacks akin to hemiplegic migraine can be symptomatic of Sturge-Weber syndrome or various metabolic diseases (e.g., mitochondrial encephalopathy with lactic acidosis and stroke-like episodes).

Benign Paroxysmal Vertigo of Childhood

This is a common migraine equivalent that consists of brief seconds-to-minutes episodes of vertigo that is often accompanied by postural imbalance and nystagmus. It is important to note that vertigo does not always refer to a spinning motion; it can also refer to a backward or forward motion (vertigo titubant) where children sometimes report that objects are moving toward them. The child appears frightened during the episode. Diaphoresis, nausea, vomiting, and, rarely, tinnitus may be present. Episodes usually remit by 6 yr of age. MRI and EEG are normal, but caloric testing, if done, can show abnormal vestibular function. Diphenhydramine, 5 mg/kg/day (maximum of 300 mg/day) may be used for a cluster of attacks. Preventive therapy with cyproheptadine may be rarely needed for frequent attacks.

Cyclic Vomiting Syndrome

This syndrome is another related periodic migraine variant that can respond to antimigraine or antiepileptic drugs. This and other periodic syndromes have been associated with mutations that also can cause hemiplegic migraine.

The "Alice in Wonderland" Syndrome

This is the episodic experience of transient distortions of body image or visual images that, most often, constitute a migraine equivalent. It also can be an epileptic phenomenon.

Migraine-Induced Syncope

Migraine, usually of the basilar variety, can trigger vasovagal syncope and, less commonly, epileptic seizures. Careful elicitation of the history of a migrainous prelude to the syncope helps in identifying these phenomena.

Psychologic Disorders

Psychogenic nonepileptic seizures are conversion reactions that are usually suspected clinically based on the characteristics of the spells (Table 594-2). The diagnosis can be confirmed by video EEG with capture of an episode to eliminate any residual doubts about their nature, as they can often occur in patients who also have epileptic seizures. They are best managed acutely by reassurance about their relatively benign nature and by a supportive attitude while at the same time avoiding positive reinforcement of the episodes. Psychiatric evaluation and follow-up are needed to uncover underlying psychopathology, and to establish continued support as psychogenic seizures can persist over long periods of time. **Malingering** and **factitious disorder imposed on another (formerly called Munchausen syndrome by proxy)** are often difficult to diagnose but an approach similar to that for psychogenic seizures, including video-EEG monitoring, is often helpful.

Paroxysmal Extreme Pain Disorder

Paroxysmal extreme pain disorder was previously called familial rectal pain syndrome. This syndrome (caused by the *SCN9A* sodium channel gene mutation) usually starts in the neonatal period or infancy and persists throughout life. Autonomic manifestations predominate initially, with skin flushing in all cases and harlequin color change and tonic attacks in most. Dramatic syncope with bradycardia and sometimes asystole are common. Later, the disorder is characterized by attacks of excruciating deep burning pain often in the rectal, ocular, or jaw areas, but also diffusely in some. Attacks are triggered by defecation, cold, wind, eating, and emotion. Carbamazepine is used, but the

response is often incomplete. Gain-of-function Na(v)1.7 mutations are known to cause two neuropathic **pain** syndromes: inherited **erythromelalgia** and **paroxysmal extreme pain syndrome**. These syndromes are inherited in a dominant trait; they usually begin in childhood or infancy, and are characterized by attacks of severe neuropathic **pain** accompanied with autonomic symptoms. In addition, small fiber neuropathy and chronic nonparoxysmal **pain** have been described in patients harboring gain-of-function mutations in Na(v)1.7 channel. Loss-of-function mutations in Na(v)1.7 are extremely rare and invariably cause **congenital inability to perceive pain.**

Autonomic Storms (Diencephalic Seizures)

Spells of hyperhidrosis, changes in blood pressure, temperature and autonomic instability occur in patients with severe diffuse brain injury or localized hypothalamic injury and have been termed autonomic storms. The term *diencephalic seizures* is discouraged as these are not truly seizures. Therapy is difficult and has included, with mixed results, clonidine, anticonvulsants, cyproheptadine, morphine, and sympathectomy. Serotonin syndrome caused by antidepressants, stimulants, opioids, certain herbs like St. John's Wart and some other medications can produce similar symptoms, and if not recognized, can at times be fatal as can be the similar neuroleptic malignant syndrome caused by antipsychotic medications.

MOVEMENT DISORDERS AND OTHER ABNORMAL MOVEMENTS AND POSTURES
Neonatal Jitteriness and Clonus

Jitteriness consists of equal backward and forward movements of limbs, occurring spontaneously, or triggered by touch or loud sounds. Movement suppression by stimulus removal or by relaxing the affected limbs, the lack of autonomic symptoms, and the clear difference from the 2-phased (fast contraction, slow relaxation) clonic activity and the very quick myoclonic jerks, point to a nonepileptic event.

Table 594-2	Comparison of Generalized Seizures and Some Disorders That Can Mimic Them			
CONDITION	**PRECIPITANTS (MAY NOT APPLY TO ALL PATIENTS)**	**PRODROME**	**ICTAL SYMPTOMS**	**POSTICTAL SYMPTOMS**
Generalized seizures	Sleep deprivation, television, video games, visual patterns, and photic stimulation	Rarely irritability or nonspecific behavioral changes	Usually 2-3 min; Consciousness might be preserved if atonic, or in some, tonic seizures; Synchronous bilateral movements; Tongue biting	Delayed recovery with postictal depression, incontinence (may be ictal also)
Syncope: vasovagal	Fatigue, emotional stress, dehydration, vomiting, choking, swallowing	Blurring of vision, tinnitus, dizziness; Crying in breath-holding spells	Loss of consciousness for seconds, pallor and rarely reflex anoxic seizures	Rapid recovery with no postictal depression
Syncope with reflex anoxic seizures	Minor bump to head, upsetting surprises			
Syncope: trigeminal vagal	Cold water on face			
Syncope: orthostatic	Standing up, bathing, awakening			
Hyperekplexia	Auditory and tactile stimuli	None	Tonic stiffening, cyanosis if severe, nonfatigable nose-tap–induced startles	Depending on severity, may have postictal depression
Cardiac	Exercise	None	Loss of consciousness, often only few seconds, pallor	Rarely
Psychogenic	Suggestion, stress	None	Eyes closed; Asynchronous flailing limb movements that vary between attacks; No injury, closed eyelids; May respond to suggestion during "loss of consciousness"; Usually longer than 2-3 min	No postictal depression

Adapted from Obeid M, Mikati MA: Expanding spectrum of paroxysmal events in children: potential mimickers of epilepsy, Pediatr Neurol 37(5):309–316, 2007.

Hypocalcemia, hypoglycemia, drug withdrawal, and hypoxic–ischemic encephalopathy are possible etiologies. **Clonus** as a result of corticospinal tract injury usually occurs in later infancy and childhood and can be stopped by change in position.

Hyperekplexia (Stiff Baby Syndrome) and Pathologic Startles

Hyperekplexia is a rare, sporadic or dominantly inherited disorder with neonatal onset of life-threatening episodes of tonic stiffening that precipitate apnea and convulsive hypoxic seizures.

Stiffness may result in difficulty in swallowing, choking spells, hip dislocations, umbilical or inguinal hernias, and delayed motor development. Stiffness in the neonatal form improves by 1 yr of age and may disappear during sleep.

The genetic cause is a defect in the α or β subunits of the strychnine-sensitive glycine receptors. It is characterized by a triad of generalized stiffness, nocturnal myoclonus, and later a pathologic startle reflex. A specific diagnostic sign can be elicited by tapping the nose, which produces a nonfatigable startle reflex with head retraction. Bathing, sudden awakening, and auditory or tactile stimuli can induce attacks. The differential diagnosis includes congenital stiff person syndrome, startle epilepsy, myoclonic seizures, neonatal tetany, phenothiazine toxicity, and Schwartz-Jampel syndrome. Making a prompt diagnosis is extremely important to initiate treatment with clonazepam as hypoxic brain injury can result from a prolonged episode. Other antiepileptics have also been effective. Repeatedly flexing the baby at the neck and hips (the Vigevano maneuver) can abort the episodes.

In other children after brain injury, and in many patients with cerebral palsy, an exaggerated startle reflex can occur. This is more common than hyperekplexia. In Tay-Sachs disease and similar gangliosidoses, exaggerated startle to sound occurs and has been, inappropriately, interpreted as hyperacusis.

Benign Paroxysmal Torticollis of Infancy

This condition typically presents as morning episodes of painless retrocollis, and later, torticollis, often triggered by changes in posture. Attacks may start with abnormal ocular movements, and progress to stillness in an abnormal posture. This usually lasts for minutes or hours and, at times, days. Neurologic exam between attacks, EEG, and neuroimaging are normal. It affects girls more than boys (3:1), often begins before 3 mo of age, and spontaneously remits before the age of 5 yr. Medical therapy is not needed. It is considered to be a migraine equivalent and cosegregates with migraine in families.

Sandifer Syndrome

Gastroesophageal reflux in infants may cause paroxysmal episodes of generalized stiffening and opisthotonic posturing that may be accompanied by apnea, staring, and minimal jerking of the extremities. Episodes often occur 30 min after a feed. In older children, this syndrome manifests with episodic dystonic or dyskinetic movements consisting of latero-, retro-, or torticollis, the exact pathophysiology of which remains elusive.

Alternating Hemiplegia of Childhood

This is a rare, often severe, disorder that consists of attacks of flaccid hemiplegia affecting 1 or both sides lasting minutes to days, starting in the 1st 18 mo of life. Earlier manifestations include paroxysmal nystagmus, which is often monocular and ipsilateral to the hemiplegia. Dystonic and tonic spells often occur and can be confused with seizures and the hemiplegia with Todd paralysis. Attacks can be triggered by bathing, cold, fatigue, hyperthermia, and emotional stress, and they remit during sleep and for about 15 minutes or so after waking up. Most cases are caused by mutations in the *ATP1A3* gene while, rarely, a similar clinical picture can occur as a result of mutations in *ATP1A2* or in the glucose transporter 1 *(GLUT1/SLC2AI)* gene mutations. Flunarizine 2.5-15 mg/day reduces the frequency of the attacks. Most children ultimately develop ataxia, developmental delay, and persistent choreoathetosis.

Paroxysmal Dyskinesias and Other Movement Disorders

These disorders are characterized by sudden attacks that consist of choreic, dystonic, ballistic, or mixed movements (Table 594-3). A sensation of fatigue or weakness confined to 1 side may herald an attack. Consciousness is preserved and patients may be able perform a motor activity, like walking, despite the attack. The variability in the pattern of severity and localization between different attacks may also help in differentiating them from seizures. The frequency of attacks increases in adolescence, and steadily decreases in the 3rd decade. Neurologic exam between attacks, EEG, laboratory investigations, and imaging studies are normal. These dyskinesias often respond to phenytoin, carbamazepine, clonazepam, or to antidopaminergic drugs such as haloperidol. **Drug reactions** can result in abnormal movements such as **oculogyric crisis** with many antiemetics, choreoathetosis with phenytoin, dystonia and facial dyskinesias with antidopaminergic drugs, and tics with carbamazepine. Strokes, focal brain lesions, connective tissue disorders (e.g., systemic lupus erythematosus), vasculitis, or metabolic and genetic disorders can also cause movement disorders. Mutations of the glucose transporter 1 *(GLUT1/SLC2AI)* gene have been described in patients with **exercise-induced dyskinesia**.

Motor Tics

These are movements that are under partial control, and are associated with an urge to do them and with a subsequent relief. They are usually exacerbated by emotions, and often change in character over time. In patients with tics who have Tourette syndrome, there is often a family history of tics and/or obsessive compulsive disorder or personality traits.

Episodic Ataxias

Episodic ataxia encompasses 7 clinically and genetically heterogeneous syndromes, only 2 of which (types 1 and 2) have been described in a large number of families. Type 1 is caused by mutations in the voltage-gated potassium channel Kv1.1. It consists of brief episodes (seconds to minutes) of cerebellar ataxia, and occasional partial seizures with interictal myokymia as a main diagnostic feature. Type 2 is characterized by longer attacks (minutes to hours) and interictal cerebellar signs. It is caused by mutations in the voltage-gated calcium channel gene *CACNA1A*. This type is more responsive than type 1 to acetazolamide that reduces the frequency and severity of attacks, but not the interictal signs and symptoms.

Benign Myoclonus of Early Infancy, Shuddering Attacks, and Chin Trembling

Benign myoclonus consists of myoclonic jerks of the extremities in wakefulness and sometimes also in sleep. It has been suggested by some that these attacks are in the same spectrum as shuddering attacks. **Shuddering attacks** are characterized by rapid tremor of the head, shoulder, and trunk, lasting a few seconds, often associated with eating, and recurring many times a day. Others have considered shuddering as an early manifestation of essential tremor as family history of essential tremor is often present. The clinical events in either of these can be mistaken for infantile spasms, but ictal and interictal EEG, MRI, and development are normal. Spontaneous remission occurs in both usually within a few months. **Hereditary chin trembling** at a frequency faster than 3 Hz starting shortly after birth and precipitated by stress has been described in several families.

A novel type of nonepileptic attack with infantile onset characterized in 3 patients as clusters of repeated head drops, mimicking epileptic negative myoclonus of the neck, accompanied by crying. The episodes occurred for 5 or 6 mo and disappeared by the end of the 1st yr. Language and cognition were normal This is a different form of myoclonic activity that may complicate the diagnosis of infantile spasms and West syndrome; thorough EEG investigation is needed in such cases.

Brainstem Dysfunction

Decorticate or decerebrate posturing that mimics epileptic tonic seizures may be secondary to decompensated hydrocephalus,

| Table 594-3 | Differential Diagnoses of Various Types of Paroxysmal Dyskinesia |

Features	PKD	PNKD MR1+	PNKD MR1−	PED	PHD
Nomenclature	PKC	PDC, FPC	PDC, FPC	PEDt	ADNFLE
Inheritance	AD–16q	AD–2q35	AD–2q13	AD/AR	AD–20q13, 15q24, 1q21, 8p21
Age at onset (yr)	1-20	<1-12	1-23	Usually childhood	Usually childhood
Triggers	Sudden whole-body movement	Coffee, alcohol, stress	Exercise	After 10-15 minutes of exercise	Sleep
Clinical features	Chorea, athetosis, ballismus, dystonia	Chorea, athetosis, dystonia, ballismus	Chorea, athetosis, dystonia, ballismus	Mainly leg dystonia	Wakes up with dystonic posture
Usual duration	<1-5 min	10 min to 1 hr	10 min to 2-3 hr	10-15 min	<1 min
Frequency	1-20/day	1/week	1/week	Unclear	Several/night
Associations	Infantile seizures, migraine, writer's cramp, essential tremor	Migraine	Epilepsy	RE-PED-WC	
Medication	Carbamazepine Phenytoin Oxcarbazepine	Clonazepam Benzodiazepine	Clonazepam Benzodiazepine	Acetazolamide L-DOPA	Carbamazepine Oxcarbazepine
Prognosis	Excellent	Excellent, worse than PKD	Minimally worse than PNKD MR1+	Poor medication response	Excellent

AD, autosomal-dominant; ADNFLE, autosomal-dominant nocturnal frontal lobe epilepsy; AR, autosomal-recessive; FPC, familial paroxysmal choreoathetosis; MR1+, myofibrillogenesis regulator 1-positive; MR1−, myofibrillogenesis regulator 1-negative; PDC, paroxysmal dystonic choreoathetosis; PED, paroxysmal exercise-induced dyskinesia; PEDt, paroxysmal exercise-induced dystonia; PHD, paroxysmal hypnogenic dyskinesia; PKC, paroxysmal kinesigenic choreoathetosis; PKD, paroxysmal kinesigenic dyskinesia; PNKD, paroxysmal nonkinesigenic dyskinesia; RE-PED-WC, rolandic epilepsy–paroxysmal exercise-induced dystonia–writer's cramp.

From Friedman NR, Ghosh D, Moodley M: Syncope and paroxysmal disorders other than epilepsy. In Swaiman KF, Ashwal S, Ferriero DM, Schor NF, editors: Swaiman's pediatric neurology, ed 5, Philadelphia, 2012, WB Saunders, Table 65-1.

hemorrhage, or other causes of sudden rises in intracranial pressure that lead to brainstem dysfunction. In addition, crowding of the posterior fossa and near herniation, the so-called cerebellar fits can also lead to abnormal extensor posturing, drop attacks, and varying degrees of altered consciousness and respiratory compromise. Historically secondary to undiagnosed posterior fossa tumors in the preneuroimaging era, "cerebellar fits" mostly occur in the context of Chiari I malformations.

Psychologic Disorders

Many psychologic disorders can be mistaken for epileptic seizures. Pleasurable behavior similar to masturbation may occur from infancy onward, and may consist of rhythmical rocking movement in a sitting or lying position, or rhythmic hip flexion and adduction. **Masturbation** may occur in girls 2-3 yr of age and is often associated with perspiration, irregular breathing, and grunting, but no loss of consciousness. Occasionally this is associated with child abuse or with other psychopathology. **Stereotypies,** or repetitive movements that are more complex than tics and do not change and wax and wane like tics (e.g., head banging, head rolling, body rocking, and hand flapping), usually occur in neurologically impaired children. **A mannerism** is a pattern of socially acceptable, situational behavior that is seen in particular situations such as gesturing when talking. Mannerisms should not be confused with stereotypies which are generally pervasive over almost every other activity such as head-shaking or hand-flapping in multiple situations. Stereotypies, unlike mannerisms, increase with stress. Unlike tics and mannerisms, stereotypies usually start before the age of 3 yr, involve more body parts, are more rhythmic and most importantly occur with engrossment with an object or activity of interest and do not have a premonitory urge that increases with attempts to suppress them as children rarely try to suppress stereotypies. **Panic and anxiety attacks** have been described in children; at times, these may be clinically indistinguishable from actual epileptic seizures, and therefore may necessitate video-EEG monitoring. **Rage attacks** usually occur in patients with personality disorder and are usually not seizures although rare cases of partial seizures can manifest as rage attacks.

Hyperventilation spells can be precipitated by anxiety and are associated with dizziness, tingling, and, at times, carpopedal spasm. **Transient global amnesia** consists of isolated short-term memory loss for minutes to hours that occurs mostly in the elderly. The etiology can be epileptic, vascular, or drug related.

OCULOMOTOR ABNORMALITIES AND VISUAL HALLUCINATIONS
Paroxysmal Tonic Upgaze of Childhood
This usually starts before 3 mo of age, and consists of protracted attacks (hours to days) of continuous or episodic upward gaze deviation, during which horizontal eye movements are preserved. A downbeating nystagmus occurs on downward gaze. Symptoms are reduced or relieved by sleep, exacerbated by fatigue and infections, and spontaneously remit after a few years. Up to 50% of patients may have psychomotor and language delay. Imaging, laboratory, and neuropsychologic examinations are usually nonrevealing. Therapy with low-dose levodopa/carbidopa may be helpful.

Oculomotor Apraxia and Saccadic Intrusions
In oculomotor apraxia saccadic eye movements are impaired. Sudden head turns compensating for lateral gaze impairment mimic seizures. This disorder may be idiopathic (Cogan oculomotor apraxia) or may occur in the context of ataxia telangiectasia or lysosomal storage diseases. Genetic defects in DNA repair mechanisms have been implicated in at least 4 spinocerebellar ataxia disorders that are accompanied by oculomotor apraxia. A selective loss of Purkinje cells required to suppress omnipause neurons and initiate saccadic eye movement is believed to occur in those disorders. Saccadic intrusions are involuntary sudden conjugate eye movements away from the desired eye position. These are not necessarily pathologic.

Spasmus Nutans
This disorder presents with a triad of nystagmus, head tilt, and head nodding. If diurnal fluctuation occurs, symptoms may look like epileptic seizures. Brain MRI should be performed, as the triad has been

associated with masses in the optic chiasm and third ventricle. Retinal disease should also be ruled out. In the absence of these associations, remission occurs before 5 yr of age.

Opsoclonus Myoclonus Syndrome

The so-called dancing eyes refers to continuous, random, irregular, and conjugate eye movements that may fluctuate in intensity. They usually accompany myoclonus and ataxia ("dancing feet"). Encephalitis and neuroblastoma are possible causes. Therapy is by treating the underlying etiology, but adrenocorticotropic hormone (ACTH), corticosteroids, and clonazepam may be needed. Rituximab has been studied and preliminary trials suggest it may be effective as well.

Daydreaming and Behavioral Staring

Staring may be a manifestation of absence seizures, which should be differentiated from daydreaming, behavioral staring because of fatigue, and inattention. Episodes of staring only in certain settings (e.g., school) are unlikely to be seizures. In addition, responsiveness to stimulation such as touch and lack of interruption of playing activity characterizes nonepileptic staring.

Visual Hallucinations

Visual perceptions in the absence of external stimuli, or visual hallucinations, are usually accompanied by other neurologic signs and symptoms when they occur in the context of seizures. An exception is occipital seizures, which can manifest with isolated and unformed visual hallucinations and may be accompanied by headache and nausea, making them difficult to differentiate from migraine. However, occipital seizures are characterized by colorful, shapes, circles and spots lasting seconds and confined to 1 hemifield, while migrainous auras usually last minutes, and consist of black-and-white lines, scotomas, and or fortification spectra that start in the center of vision. Hallucinations can also be secondary to drug exposure, midbrain lesions, and psychiatric illnesses. In addition, retinal-associated hallucinations can occur in the form of flashes of light in the context of inflammatory etiologies, trauma, or optic nerve edema.

SLEEP DISORDERS

Paroxysmal nonepileptic sleep events are more common in epileptic patients than in the general population, which makes their diagnosis difficult. Semiology, timing of events, and if needed video-EEG and polysomnography help in distinguishing epileptic from nonepileptic events. Parasomnias typically occur less than once or twice a night; more frequent episodes suggest epileptic seizures. Of note, the EEG pattern of frontal lobe epileptic seizures may be similar to the one seen in a normal arousals, making their diagnosis challenging, especially that they have nonspecific hypermotor manifestations such as thrashing, body rocking, kicking, boxing, pedaling, bending, running, and various vocalizations. The diagnosis of such epileptic seizures is made on the basis of highly stereotyped events arising several times a night from nonrapid eye movement sleep.

Benign Sleep Myoclonus and Neonatal Sleep Myoclonus

Neonatal sleep myoclonus consists of repetitive, usually bilateral rhythmic jerks involving the upper and lower limbs during nonrapid eye movement sleep, sometimes mimicking clonic seizures. A slow (1 Hz) rocking of the infant in a head-to-toe direction is a specific diagnostic test that may reproduce the myoclonus. The lack of autonomic changes, occurrence only in sleep, and suppression by awakenings may help in differentiating these events from epileptic seizures. Remission is spontaneous at 2-3 mo of age. In older children and adults, sleep myoclonus consists of random myoclonic jerks of the limbs.

Nonrapid Eye Movement Partial Arousal Disorders

Brief **nocturnal confusional arousals** occurring 1-2 hr after sleep in stage 4 sleep are normal in children. Such episodes can vary from chewing, sitting up, and mumbling to agitated sleep walking, and

usually last for 10-15 min. **Night terrors** similarly occur a few hours after going to sleep in stage 3 or 4 of sleep, most often at 2-7 yr of age and more so in boys. The child screams; appears terrified; has dilated pupils, tachycardia, tachypnea, unresponsiveness, agitation, and thrashing that increase with attempts to be consoled; is difficult to arouse; and may have little or no vocalization. In older children with persistent night terrors, an underlying psychologic etiology may be present. Diagnosis is based on the history. However, rarely, video EEG monitoring may be needed. At times, the use of bedtime diazepam (0.2-0.3 mg/kg) or clonazepam (0.01 mg/kg) may help control the problem while psychologic factors are being investigated. **Restless leg syndrome** can cause painful leg dysesthesias that cause nocturnal arousals and insomnia. It can be either genetic or associated with iron deficiency, systemic illness, or some drugs. Therapy depends upon treating the underlying cause and, if needed, on dopaminergic drugs such as levodopa/carbidopa, or antiepileptics like gabapentin.

Rapid Eye Movement Sleep Disorders

Nightmares and **sleep paralysis** are common disorders. Unlike night terrors, nightmares tend to occur later during the night and the child has a memory of the event.

Sleep Transition Disorders

Nocturnal head banging (**jactatio capitis nocturna**), rolling, or body rocking often occurs in infants and toddlers as they are trying to fall asleep. These usually remit spontaneously by 5 yr of age. No specific therapy is needed.

Narcolepsy-Cataplexy Syndrome

Narcolepsy is characterized by excessive daytime sleepiness, cataplexy, sleep paralysis, hypnogogic hallucinations, and disturbed nighttime sleep. The persistence of rapid eye movement sleep atonia upon awakening or its intrusion during wakefulness lead to sleep paralysis or cataplexy, respectively. Loss of tone in cataplexy occurs in response to strong emotions, and spreads from the face downwards leading to a fall in a series of stages rather than a sudden one. Consciousness is maintained in cataplexy. A selective loss of hypocretin-secreting neurons in the hypothalamus is at the origin of this disorder. The fact that DQB1*0602 is a predisposing HLA allele identified in 85-95% of patients with narcolepsy-cataplexy suggests an autoimmune-mediated neuronal loss. Diagnosis is based on the **multiple sleep latency test**, and therapy relies on scheduled naps, amphetamines, methylphenidate, tricyclic antidepressants, and counseling about precautions in work and driving.

Bibliography is available at Expert Consult.

Chapter **595**

Headaches

Andrew D. Hershey,
Marielle A. Kabbouche, and
Hope L. O'Brien

Headache is a common complaint in children and adolescents. Headaches can be a primary problem or occur as a symptom of another disorder, representing a secondary problem. Recognizing this difference is essential for choosing the appropriate evaluation and treatment to ensure successful management of the headache. Primary headaches are most often recurrent, episodic headaches and for most children are sporadic in their presentation.

The most common forms of primary headache of childhood are migraine and tension-type headaches (Table 595-1). Other forms of

Table 595-1	Classification of Headaches (ICHD-3 Beta Code Diagnosis)

MIGRAINE
Migraine with or without aura
Migraine with typical aura (with or without headache)
Migraine with brainstem aura
Hemiplegic migraine (sporadic or familial types 1, 2, 3, or other genetic loci)
Retinal migraine
Chronic migraine
Complications of Migraine
Status migrainosus
Persistent aura without infarction
Migrainous infarction
Migraine aura-triggered seizure
Episodic Syndromes That May Be Associated with Migraine
Recurrent gastrointestinal disturbance
Cyclical vomiting syndrome
Abdominal migraine
Benign paroxysmal vertigo
Benign paroxysmal torticollis

TENSION-TYPE HEADACHE (TTH)
Infrequent episodic tension-type headache associated with or without pericranial tenderness
Frequent episodic tension-type headache associated with or without pericranial tenderness
Chronic tension-type headache associated with or without pericranial tenderness
Probable tension-type headaches

TRIGEMINAL AUTONOMIC CEPHALALGIAS (TACS)
Cluster headache (episodic or cluster)
Paroxysmal hemicrania (episodic or cluster)
Short-lasting unilateral neuralgiform headache attacks with or without conjunctival injection and tearing (SUNCT)
Episodic SUNCT
Chronic SUNCT
Short-lasting unilateral neuralgiform headache attacks with or without cranial autonomic symptoms (SUNA)
Episodic SUNA
Chronic SUNA
Hemicrania continua
Probable trigeminal autonomic cephalalgias

OTHER PRIMARY HEADACHE DISORDERS
Primary cough headache
Primary exercise headache
Primary headache associated with sexual activity
Primary thunderclap headache
Cold-stimulus headache (external application, ingestion, or inhalation)
External-pressure headache
External-compression headache
External-traction headache
Primary stabbing headache
Nummular headache
Hypnic headache
New daily persistent headache (NDPH)

HEADACHE ATTRIBUTED TO TRAUMA OR INJURY TO THE HEAD AND/OR NECK
Acute headache attributed to traumatic (mild, moderate, or severe) injury to the head
Persistent headache attributed to traumatic (mild, moderate, or severe) injury to the head
Acute or persistent headache attributed to whiplash
Acute or persistent headache attributed to craniotomy

HEADACHE ATTRIBUTED TO CRANIAL OR CERVICAL VASCULAR DISORDER
Headache attributed to ischemic stroke or transient ischemic attack
Headache attributed to nontraumatic intracerebral hemorrhage
Headache attributed to nontraumatic subarachnoid hemorrhage (SAH)
Headache attributed to nontraumatic acute subdural hemorrhage (ASDH)
Headache attributed to unruptured vascular malformation
Headache attributed to unruptured saccular aneurysm
Headache attributed to arteriovenous malformation (AVM)
Headache attributed to dural arteriovenous fistula (DAVF)
Headache attributed to cavernous angioma
Headache attributed to encephalotrigeminal or leptomeningeal angiomatosis (Sturge-Weber syndrome)
Headache attributed to arteritis
Headache attributed to giant cell arteritis (GCA)
Headache attributed to primary angiitis of the central nervous system (PACNS)
Headache attributed to secondary angiitis of the central nervous system (SACNS)
Headache attributed to cervical carotid or vertebral artery disorder
Headache or facial or neck pain attributed to cervical carotid or vertebral artery dissection
Post-endarterectomy headache
Headache attributed to carotid or vertebral angioplasty
Headache attributed to cerebral venous thrombosis (CVT)
Headache attributed to other acute intracranial arterial disorder
Headache attributed to an intracranial endovascular procedure
Angiography headache
Headache attributed to reversible cerebral vasoconstriction syndrome (RCVS)
Headache attributed to intracranial arterial dissection
Headache attributed to genetic vasculopathy
Cerebral autosomal dominant arteriopathy with subcortical infarcts and leukoencephalopathy (CADASIL)
Mitochondrial encephalopathy, lactic acidosis and stroke-like episodes (MELAS)
Headache attributed to another genetic vasculopathy
Headache attributed to pituitary apoplexy

HEADACHE ATTRIBUTED TO NONVASCULAR INTRACRANIAL DISORDER
Headache attributed to increased cerebrospinal fluid pressure
Headache attributed to idiopathic intracranial hypertension (IIH)
Headache attributed to intracranial hypertension secondary to metabolic, toxic, or hormonal causes
Headache attributed to intracranial hypertension secondary to hydrocephalus
Headache attributed to low cerebrospinal fluid pressure
Postdural puncture headache
Cerebrospinal fluid fistula headache
Headache attributed to spontaneous intracranial hypotension
Headache attributed to noninfectious inflammatory disease
Headache attributed to neurosarcoidosis
Headache attributed to aseptic (noninfectious) meningitis
Headache attributed to other noninfectious inflammatory disease
Headache attributed to lymphocytic hypophysitis
Syndrome of transient headache and neurological deficits with cerebrospinal fluid lymphocytosis (HaNDL)
Headache attributed to intracranial neoplasm
Headache attributed to colloid cyst of the third ventricle
Headache attributed to carcinomatous meningitis
Headache attributed to hypothalamic or pituitary hyper- or hyposecretion
Headache attributed to intrathecal injection
Headache attributed to epileptic seizure
Hemicrania epileptica
Postictal headache
Headache attributed to Chiari malformation type I (CM1)
Headache attributed to other nonvascular intracranial disorder

Table 595-1	Classification of Headaches (ICHD-3 Beta Code Diagnosis)—cont'd

HEADACHE ATTRIBUTED TO A SUBSTANCE OR ITS WITHDRAWAL
Headache attributed to use of or exposure to a substance
Nitric oxide (NO) donor-induced headache
Phosphodiesterase (PDE) inhibitor-induced headache
Carbon monoxide (CO)-induced headache
Alcohol-induced headache
Monosodium glutamate (MSG)-induced headache
Cocaine-induced headache
Histamine-induced headache
Calcitonin gene-related peptide (CGRP)-induced headache
Headache attributed to exogenous acute pressor agent
Headache attributed to occasional or long-term use of nonheadache medication
Headache attributed to exogenous hormone
Medication-Overuse Headache (MOH)
Ergotamine-overuse headache
Triptan-overuse headache
Simple analgesic-overuse headache
Paracetamol (acetaminophen)-overuse headache
Acetylsalicylic acid-overuse headache
Other non-steroidal antiinflammatory drug (NSAID)-overuse headache
Opioid-overuse headache
Combination analgesic-overuse headache
Headache Attributed to Substance Withdrawal
Caffeine-withdrawal headache
Opioid-withdrawal headache
Estrogen-withdrawal headache

HEADACHE ATTRIBUTED TO INFECTION
Acute or chronic headache attributed to bacterial meningitis or meningoencephalitis
Persistent headache attributed to past bacterial meningitis or meningoencephalitis
Acute or chronic headache attributed to intracranial fungal or other parasitic infection
Headache attributed to brain abscess
Headache attributed to subdural empyema
Headache attributed to systemic infection (acute or chronic)

HEADACHE ATTRIBUTED TO DISORDER OF HOMEOSTASIS
Headache attributed to hypoxia and/or hypercapnia
High-altitude headache
Headache attributed to airplane travel
Diving headache
Sleep apnea headache
Dialysis headache
Headache attributed to arterial hypertension
Headache attributed to pheochromocytoma
Headache attributed to hypertensive crisis with or without hypertensive encephalopathy
Headache attributed to preeclampsia or eclampsia
Headache attributed to autonomic dysreflexia
Headache attributed to hypothyroidism
Headache attributed to fasting
Cardiac cephalalgia
Headache attributed to other disorder of homoeostasis

HEADACHE OR FACIAL PAIN ATTRIBUTED TO DISORDER OF THE CRANIUM, NECK, EYES, EARS, NOSE, SINUSES, TEETH, MOUTH, OR OTHER FACIAL OR CERVICAL STRUCTURE
Headache attributed to disorder of cranial bone
Headache attributed to retropharyngeal tendonitis
Headache attributed to craniocervical dystonia
Headache attributed to acute glaucoma
Headache attributed to refractive error
Headache attributed to heterophoria or heterotropia (latent or persistent squint)
Headache attributed to ocular inflammatory disorder
Headache attributed to trachelitis
Headache attributed to disorder of the ears
Headache attributed to acute or chronic or recurring rhinosinusitis
Headache attributed to temporomandibular disorder (TMD)
Head or facial pain attributed to inflammation of the stylohyoid ligament
Headache or facial pain attributed to other disorder of cranium, neck, eyes, ears, nose, sinuses, teeth, mouth, or other facial or cervical structure

HEADACHE ATTRIBUTED TO PSYCHIATRIC DISORDER
Headache attributed to somatization disorder
Headache attributed to psychotic disorder

PAINFUL CRANIAL NEUROPATHIES AND OTHER FACIAL PAINS
Classical trigeminal neuralgia
Classical trigeminal neuralgia, purely paroxysmal or with concomitant persistent facial pain
Painful trigeminal neuropathy
Painful trigeminal neuropathy attributed to acute herpes zoster
Postherpetic trigeminal neuropathy
Painful posttraumatic trigeminal neuropathy
Painful trigeminal neuropathy attributed to multiple sclerosis (MS) plaque
Painful trigeminal neuropathy attributed to space-occupying lesion
Painful trigeminal neuropathy attributed to other disorder
Glossopharyngeal neuralgia
Classical nervus intermedius (facial nerve) neuralgia
Nervus intermedius neuropathy attributed to herpes zoster
Occipital neuralgia
Optic neuritis
Headache attributed to ischemic ocular motor nerve palsy
Tolosa-Hunt syndrome
Paratrigeminal oculosympathetic (Raeder) syndrome
Recurrent painful ophthalmoplegic neuropathy
Burning mouth syndrome (BMS)
Persistent idiopathic facial pain (PIFP)
Central neuropathic pain
Central neuropathic pain attributed to multiple sclerosis (MS)
Central post-stroke pain (CPSP)

From Headache Classification Committee on the International Headache Society (IHS): The International Classification of Headache Disorders, ed 3 (beta version). Cephalalgia 33(9):629–808, 2013.

primary headache, including the trigeminal autonomic cephalalgias, occur much less commonly. Primary headache can progress to very frequent or even daily headaches with chronic migraine and chronic tension-type headaches being increasingly recognized. These more frequent headaches can have an enormous impact on the life of the child and adolescent, as reflected in school absences and decreased school performance, social withdrawal, and changes in family interactions. To reduce this impact, a treatment strategy that incorporates acute treatments, preventive treatments, and biobehavioral therapies must be implemented.

Secondary headache involves headaches that are a symptom of an underlying illness (see Table 595-1). The underlying illness should be clearly present as a direct cause of the headaches. This is often difficult when 2 or more common conditions occur in close temporal association. This frequently leads to the misdiagnosis of a primary headache as a secondary headache. This is, for example, the case when migraine is misdiagnosed as a sinus headache. In general, the key components of a secondary headache are the likely direct cause-and-effect relationship between the headache and the precipitating condition, and the lower likelihood in a specific patient and circumstance of the headaches being the result of a recurrent headache disorder. In addition, once the underlying suspected cause is treated, the secondary headache should resolve. If this does not occur, either the diagnosis must be reevaluated or the effectiveness of the treatment reassessed. *One key clue that additional investigation is warranted is the presence of an abnormal neurologic examination or unusual neurologic symptoms.*

595.1 Migraine

Andrew D. Hershey, Marielle A. Kabbouche,
and Hope L. O'Brien

Migraine is the most frequent type of recurrent headache that is brought to the attention of parents and primary care providers, but it remains underrecognized and undertreated, particularly in children. Migraine is characterized by episodic attacks that may be moderate to severe in intensity, focal in location on the head, have a throbbing quality, and may be associated with nausea, vomiting, light sensitivity, and sound sensitivity. Compared to adults, pediatric migraine is shorter in duration and has a bilateral, often bifrontal, location. Migraine can also be associated with an aura that may be typical (visual, sensory, or dysphasic) or atypical (i.e., hemiplegic, "Alice in Wonderland" syndrome) (Tables 595-2 to 595-6). In addition, a number of migraine variants have been described and, in children, include abdominal related symptoms without headache, and components of the painless periodic syndromes of childhood (see Table 595-1). Treatment of migraine requires the incorporation of an acute treatment plan, a preventive treatment plan if the migraine occurs frequently or is disabling, and a biobehavioral plan to help cope with both the acute attacks and frequent or persistent attacks if present.

EPIDEMIOLOGY

Up to 75% of children report having a significant headache by the time they are 15 yr old. Recurrent headaches are less common, but remain highly frequent. Migraine has been reported to occur in up to 10.6% of children between the ages of 5 and 15 yr, and up to 28% of older

Table 595-2	Migraine Without Aura

A. At least 5 attacks fulfilling criteria B to D
B. Headache attacks lasting 4-72 hr (untreated or unsuccessfully treated)
C. Headache has at least 2 of the following 4 characteristics:
　1. Unilateral location
　2. Pulsating quality
　3. Moderate or severe pain intensity
　4. Aggravation by or causing avoidance of routine physical activity (e.g., walking or climbing stairs)
D. During headache at least 1 of the following:
　1. Nausea and/or vomiting
　2. Photophobia and phonophobia
E. Not better accounted for by another ICHD-3 diagnosis

From Headache Classification Committee on the International Headache Society (IHS): The International Classification of Headache Disorders, ed 3 (beta version). Cephalalgia 33(9):629–808, 2013, Table 4.

Table 595-3	Migraine with Typical Aura

A. At least 2 attacks fulfilling criteria B and C
B. Aura consisting of visual, sensory and/or speech/language symptoms, each fully reversible, but no motor, brainstem or retinal symptoms
C. At least 2 of the following 4 characteristics:
　1. At least 1 aura symptom spreads gradually over 5 or more minutes, and/or 2 or more symptoms occur in succession
　2. Each individual aura symptom lasts 5-60 minutes
　3. At least 1 aura symptom is unilateral
　4. The aura is accompanied, or followed within 60 minutes, by headache
D. Not better accounted for by another ICHD-3 diagnosis, and transient ischemic attack has been excluded

From Headache Classification Committee on the International Headache Society (IHS): The International Classification of Headache Disorders, ed 3 (beta version). Cephalalgia 33(9):629–808, 2013, Table 6.

Table 595-4	Migraine with Brainstem Aura

A. At least 2 attacks fulfilling criteria B to D
B. Aura consisting of visual, sensory and/or speech/language symptoms, each fully reversible, but no motor or retinal symptoms
C. At least 2 of the following brainstem symptoms:
　1. Dysarthria
　2. Vertigo
　3. Tinnitus
　4. Hypacusis
　5. Diplopia
　6. Ataxia
　7. Decreased level of consciousness
D. At least 2 of the following 4 characteristics:
　1. At least 1 aura symptom spreads gradually over 5 or more minutes, and/or 2 or more symptoms occur in succession
　2. Each individual aura symptom lasts 5-60 minutes
　3. At least 1 aura symptom is unilateral
　4. The aura is accompanied, or followed within 60 minutes, by headache
E. Not better accounted for by another ICHD-3 diagnosis, and transient ischemic attack has been excluded.

From Headache Classification Committee on the International Headache Society (IHS): The International Classification of Headache Disorders, ed 3 (beta version). Cephalalgia 33(9):629–808, 2013, Table 7.

Table 595-5	Vestibular Migraine with Vertigo

A. At least 5 episodes fulfilling criteria C and D
B. A current or past history of 1.1 *Migraine without aura* or 1.2 *Migraine with aura*
C. Vestibular symptoms of moderate or severe intensity, lasting between 5 min and 72 hr
D. At least 50% of episodes are associated with at least 1 of the following 3 migrainous features:
　1. Headache with at least 2 of the following 4 characteristics:
　　a. Unilateral location
　　b. Pulsating quality
　　c. Moderate or severe intensity
　　d. Aggravation by routine physical activity
　2. Photophobia and phonophobia
　3. Visual aura
E. Not better accounted for by another ICHD-3 diagnosis or by another vestibular disorder

From Headache Classification Committee on the International Headache Society (IHS): The International Classification of Headache Disorders, ed 3 (beta version). Cephalalgia 33(9):629–808, 2013 (Table 8).

Table 595-6	Chronic Migraine

A. Headache (tension-type-like and/or migraine-like) on 15 or more days per month for more than 3 mo and fulfilling criteria B and C
B. Occurring in a patient who has had at least 5 attacks fulfilling criteria B to D for 1.1 *Migraine without aura* and/or criteria B and C for 1.2 *Migraine with aura*
C. On 8 or more days per month for more than 3 mo, fulfilling any of the following:
　1. Criteria C and D for 1.1 *Migraine without aura*
　2. Criteria B and C for 1.2 *Migraine with aura*
　3. Believed by the patient to be migraine at onset and relieved by a triptan or ergot derivative
D. Not better accounted for by another ICHD-3 diagnosis

From Headache Classification Committee on the International Headache Society (IHS): The International Classification of Headache Disorders, ed 3 (beta version). Cephalalgia 33(9):629–808, 2013, Table 9.

adolescents. When the headaches become frequent, they convert into chronic daily headaches in up to 1% of children. When headaches are occurring more than 15 days a month the risk of conversion to a daily headache becomes more prominent. This explains the necessity to treat the headaches aggressively or prevent the headaches altogether, trying to block transformation to chronic daily headaches.

Migraine can impact a patient's life through school absences, limitation of home activities, and restriction of social activities. As headaches become more frequent, their negative impact increases in magnitude. This can lead to further complications including anxiety and school avoidance, requiring a more extensive treatment plan.

CLASSIFICATION AND CLINICAL MANIFESTATIONS

Criteria have been established to guide the clinical and scientific study of headaches; these are summarized in *The International Classification of Headache Disorders*, 3rd edition (ICHD-3 beta). Table 595-1 contrasts the different clinical types of migraine; Tables 595-2 to 595-6 list the specific criteria for migraine types.

Migraine Without Aura

Migraine without aura is the most common form of migraine in both children and adults. The ICHD-3 beta (see Table 595-2) requires this to be recurrent (at least 5 headaches that meet the criteria, but there is no time limit over which this must occur). The recurrent episodic nature helps differentiate this from a secondary headache, as well as separates migraine from tension-type headache, but may limit the diagnosis in children as they may just be beginning to have headaches.

The duration of the headache is defined as 4-72 hr for adults. It has been recognized that children may have shorter-duration headaches, so an allowance has been made to reduce this duration to 2-72 hr or 1-72 hr with diary confirmation. Note that this duration is for the untreated or unsuccessfully treated headache. Furthermore, if the child falls asleep with the headache, the entire sleep period is considered part of the duration. These duration limits help differentiate migraine from both short-duration headaches, including the trigeminal autonomic cephalalgias, and prolonged headaches, like those caused by idiopathic intracranial hypertension (pseudotumor cerebri). Some prolonged headaches may still be migraine, but a migraine that persists beyond 72 hr is classified as a variant termed **status migrainosus.**

The quality of migraine pain is often, but not always, throbbing or pounding. This may be difficult to elicit in young children and drawings or demonstrations may help confirm the throbbing quality.

The location of the pain has classically been described as **unilateral (hemicrania)**; in young children it is more commonly bilateral. A more appropriate way to think of the location would therefore be focal, to differentiate it from the diffuse pain of tension-type headaches. Of particular concern is the exclusively occipital headache because although these can be migraines, they are more frequently secondary to another more proximate etiology such as posterior fossa abnormalities.

Migraine, when allowed to fully develop, often worsens in the face of and secondarily results in altered activity level. For example, worsening of the pain occurs classically in adults when going up or down stairs. This history is often not elicited in children. A change in the child's activity pattern can be easily observed as a reduction in play or physical activity. Older children may limit or restrict their sports activity or exercise during a headache attack.

Migraine may have a variety of associated symptoms. In younger children, nausea and vomiting may be the most obvious symptoms and often outweigh the headache itself. This often leads to the overlap with several of the gastrointestinal periodic diseases, including recurrent abdominal pain, recurrent vomiting, cyclic vomiting, and abdominal migraine. The common feature among all of these related conditions is an increased propensity among children with them for the later development of migraine. Oftentimes, early childhood recurrent vomiting may in fact be migraine, but the child is not asked about or is unable to describe headache pain. Once this becomes clear, the earlier

diagnosis of a gastrointestinal disorder is no longer appropriate. When headache is present, vomiting raises the concern of a secondary headache, particularly related to increased intracranial pressure. *One of the red flags for this is the daily or near daily early morning vomiting, or headaches waking the child up from sleep.* When the headaches associated with vomiting episodes are sporadic and not worsening, it is more likely that the diagnosis is migraine. Vomiting and headache caused by increased intracranial pressure are frequently present on first awakening and remit with maintenance of upright posture. In contrast, if a migraine is present on first awakening *(a relatively infrequent occurrence in children)*, getting up and going about normal, upright activities usually makes the headache and vomiting worse.

As the child matures, light and sound sensitivity (**photophobia** and **phonophobia**) may become more apparent. This is either by direct report of the patient, or the interpretation by the parents of the child's activity. These symptoms are likely a component of the hypersensitivity that develops during an acute migraine attack and may also include smell sensitivity (**osmophobia**) and touch sensitivity (**cutaneous allodynia with central sensitization**). Although only the photophobia and phonophobia are components of the ICHD-3 beta criteria, these other symptoms are helpful in confirming the diagnosis and may be helpful in understanding the underlying pathophysiology and determining the response to treatment. The final ICHD-3 beta requirement is the exclusion of causes of secondary headaches, and this should be an integral component of the headache history.

Migraine typically runs in families with reports up to 90% of children having a 1st- or 2nd-degree relative with recurrent headaches. Given the underdiagnosis and misdiagnosis in adults, this is often not recognized by the family and a headache family history is required. When a family history is not identified, this may be the result of either a lack of awareness of migraine within the family or an underlying secondary headache in the child. Any child whose family, upon close and both direct and indirect questioning, does not include individuals with migraine or related syndromes (e.g., motion sickness, cyclic vomiting, menstrual headache) should have an imaging procedure performed to look for anatomic etiologies for headache.

In addition to the classifying features, there may additional markers of a migraine disorder. These include such things as triggers (skipping meals, inadequate or irregular sleep, dehydration and weather changes are the most common), pattern recognition (associated with menstrual periods in adolescents or Monday-morning headaches resulting from changes in sleep patterns over the weekend and nonphysiologic early waking on Monday mornings for school), and premonitory symptoms (a feeling of irritability, tiredness, and food cravings prior to the start of the headache). Although these additional features may not be consistent, they do raise the index of suspicion for migraine and provide a potential mechanism of intervention. In the past, food triggers were considered widely common, but the majority have either been discredited with scientific study or represent such a small number of patients that they only need to be addressed when consistently triggering the headache.

Migraine with Aura

The aura associated with migraine is a neurologic warning that a migraine is going to occur. In the common forms this can be the start of a typical migraine or a headache without migraine, or it may even occur in isolation. For a typical aura, the aura needs to be visual, sensory, or dysphasic, lasting longer than 5 min and less than 60 min with the headache starting within 60 min (see Table 595-3). The importance of the aura lasting longer than 5 min is to differentiate the migraine aura from a seizure with a postictal headache, while the 60 min maximal duration is to separate migraine aura from the possibility of a more prolonged neurologic event such as a transient ischemic attack.

The most common type of visual aura in children and adolescents is **photopsia** (flashes of light or light bulbs going off everywhere). These photopsias are often multicolored and when gone, the child may report not being able to see where the flash occurred. Less likely in children are the typical adult auras including *fortification spectra* (brilliant white zigzag lines resembling a starred pattern castle) or *shimmering scotoma* (sometimes described as a shining spot that grows or a sequined curtain closing). In adults, the auras typically involve only half the visual field, whereas in children they may be randomly dispersed. Blurred vision is often confused as an aura but is difficult to separate from photophobia or difficulty concentrating during the pain of the headache.

Sensory auras are less common. They typically occur unilaterally. Many children describe this sensation as insects are worms crawling from their hand, up their arm to their face with a numbness following this sensation. Once the numbness occurs, the child may have difficulty using the arm as they have lost sensory input, and a misdiagnosis of hemiplegic migraine may be made.

Dysphasic auras are the least-common type of typical aura and have been described as an inability or difficulty to respond verbally. The patient afterwards will describe an ability to understand what is being asked, but cannot answer back. This may be the basis of what in the past has been referred to as confusional migraine and special attention needs to be paid to asking the child about this possibility and their degree of understanding during the initial phases of the attack. Most of the time, these episodes are described as a motor aphasia and they are often associated with sensory or motor symptoms.

Much less commonly, *atypical forms of aura can occur,* including hemiplegia (true weakness, not numbness, and may be familial), vertigo or lower cranial nerve symptoms (basilar-type, formerly thought to be caused by basilar artery dysfunction, now thought to be more brainstem based) (see Table 595-4), and distortion ("Alice in Wonderland" syndrome). Whenever these rarer forms of aura are present, further investigation is warranted. Not all motor auras can be classified as hemiplegic migraine spectrum and they should be differentiated from those very specific migrainous events, as the diagnosis of hemiplegic migraine has genetic, pathophysiologic, and therapeutic implications.

Hemiplegic migraine is one of the better known forms of rare auras. This transient unilateral weakness usually lasts only a few hours but may persist for days. Both familial and sporadic forms have been described. The familial hemiplegic migraine is an autosomal dominant disorder with mutations described in 3 separate genes: (1) *CACNA1A*, (2) *ATP1A2*, and (3) *SCN1A*. Some patients with familial hemiplegic migraine have other yet-to-be-identified genetic mutations. Multiple polymorphisms have been described for these genes. Hemiplegic migraines may be triggered by minor head trauma, exertion, or emotional stress. The motor weakness is usually associated with another aura symptom and may progress slowly over 20-30 min first with visual and then followed in sequence by sensory, motor, aphasic, and then basilar auras. Headache is present in more than 95% of patients and usually begins during the aura; headache may be unilateral or bilateral and may have no relationship to the motor weakness. Some patients may develop attacks of coma with encephalopathy, cerebrospinal fluid (CSF) pleocytosis, and cerebral edema. Long-term complications may include seizures, repetitive daily episodes of blindness, cerebellar signs with the development of cerebellar atrophy, and mental retardation.

Basilar-type migraine was formerly considered a disease of the basilar artery as many of the unique symptoms were attributed to dysfunction in this area of the brainstem. Some of the symptoms described include vertigo, tinnitus, diplopia, blurred vision, scotoma, ataxia, and an occipital headache. The pupils may be dilated, and ptosis may be evident.

Syndrome of transient headache and neurological deficits with CSF lymphocytosis (HaNDL) describes transient headaches associated with neurologic deficits, and CSF showing pleocytosis. It is considered a self-limited migraine-like syndrome, and is rarely reported in the pediatric population.

Childhood periodic syndromes are a group of potentially related symptoms that occur with increased frequency in children with migraine. The hallmark of these symptoms is the recurrent episodic nature of the events. Some of these have included gastrointestinal-related symptoms (motion sickness, recurrent abdominal pain, recurrent vomiting including cyclic vomiting, and abdominal migraine),

sleep disorders (sleepwalking, sleeptalking, and night terrors), unexplained recurrent fevers, and even seizures.

The gastrointestinal symptoms span the spectrum from the relatively mild (motion sickness on occasional long car rides) to severe episodes of uncontrollable vomiting that may lead to dehydration and the need for hospital admission to receive fluids. These latter episodes may occur on a predictable time schedule and hence have been called cyclic vomiting. During these attacks, the child may appear pale and frightened but does not lose consciousness. After a period of deep sleep, the child awakens and resumes normal play and eating habits as if the vomiting had not occurred. Many children with cyclic vomiting have a positive family history of migraine, and as they grow older have a higher than average likelihood of developing migraine. Cyclic vomiting may be responsive to migraine-specific therapies with careful attention to fluid replacement if the vomiting is excessive. Cyclic vomiting of migraine must be differentiated from gastrointestinal disorders including intestinal obstruction (malrotation, intermittent volvulus, duodenal web, duplication cysts, superior mesenteric artery compression, and internal hernias), peptic ulcer, gastritis, giardiasis, chronic pancreatitis, and Crohn disease. Abnormal gastrointestinal motility and pelviureteric junction obstruction can also cause cyclic vomiting. Metabolic causes include disorders of amino acid metabolism (heterozygote ornithine transcarbamylase deficiency), organic acidurias (propionic acidemia, methylmalonic acidemia), fatty acid oxidation defects (medium-chain acyl-coenzyme A dehydrogenase deficiency), disorders of carbohydrate metabolism (hereditary fructose intolerance), acute intermittent porphyria, and structural central nervous system lesions (posterior fossa brain tumors, subdural hematomas or effusions). The diagnosis is a diagnosis of exclusion and children will need a full work up prior to be labeled of cyclic vomiting syndrome. Cyclic vomiting syndrome is more frequent in younger children and will gradually transform into a typical migraine attack by puberty.

The diagnosis of **abdominal migraine** can be confusing but can be thought of as a migraine without the headache. Like a migraine, it is an episodic disorder characterized by midabdominal pain with pain-free periods between attacks. At times this pain is associated with nausea and vomiting (thus crossing into the recurrent abdominal pain or cyclic vomiting spectrum). The pain is usually described as "dull" and may be moderate to severe. The pain may persist from 1-72 hr and, although usually midline, may be periumbilical or poorly localized by the child. To meet the criteria of abdominal migraine, the child must complain at the time of the abdominal pain of at least 2 of the following: anorexia, nausea, vomiting, or pallor. As with cyclic vomiting, a thorough history and physical examination with appropriate laboratory studies must be completed to rule out an underlying gastrointestinal disorder as a cause of the abdominal pain. Careful questioning about the presence of headache or head pain needs to be addressed directly with the child, as many times this is truly a migraine, but in the child's mind (as well as the parents' observation) the abdominal symptoms are paramount.

DIAGNOSIS AND DIFFERENTIAL DIAGNOSIS

A thorough history and physical examination including a neurologic examination with special focus on headache has been shown to be the most sensitive indicator of an underlying etiology. The history needs to include a thorough evaluation of the premonitory symptoms, any potential triggering events or timing of the headaches, associated neurologic symptoms, and a detailed characterization of the headache attacks, including frequency, severity, duration, associated symptoms, use of medication, and disability. The disability assessment should include the impact on school, home, and social activities and can easily be assessed with tools such as PedMIDAS. Family history of headaches and any other neurologic, psychiatric, and general health conditions is also important both for identification of migraine within the family as well as the identification of possible secondary headache disorders. The familial penetrance of migraine is so robust that the absence of a family history of migraine or its equivalent phenomena should trigger obtaining of an imaging procedure. When headaches are refractory, a history of potential comorbid conditions, which includes mood disorders and illicit substance use, especially in teenagers, that may influence adherence and acceptability of the treatment plan, may also need to be addressed.

Neuroimaging is warranted when the neurologic examination is abnormal or unusual neurologic features occur during the migraine; when the child has headaches that awaken the child from sleep or that are present on first awakening and remit with upright posture; when the child has brief headaches that only occur with cough or bending over; when the headache is mostly in the occipital area; and when the child has migrainous headache with an absolutely negative family history of migraine or its equivalent (e.g., motion sickness, cyclic vomiting; Table 595-7). In this case, an MRI is the imaging of choice as it provides the highest sensitivity for detecting posterior fossa lesions and does not expose the child to radiation.

In the child with a headache that is instantaneously at its worst at onset, a CT scan looking for blood is the best initial test; and, if it is negative, a lumbar puncture should be done looking especially for xanthochromia of the CSF. There is no evidence that laboratory studies or an electroencephalogram is beneficial in a typical migraine without aura or migraine with aura.

TREATMENT
Table 595-8 outlines the drugs used to manage migraine headaches in children.

The American Academy of Neurology established useful practice guidelines for the management of migraine as follows:
1. Reduction of headache frequency, severity, duration, and disability
2. Reduction of reliance on poorly tolerated, ineffective, or unwanted acute pharmacotherapies
3. Improvement in quality of life
4. Avoidance of acute headache medication escalation
5. Education and enabling of patients to manage their disease to enhance personal control of their migraine
6. Reduction of headache-related distress and psychologic symptoms

Table 595-7	Indications for Neuroimaging in a Child with Headaches

Abnormal neurologic examination
Abnormal or focal neurologic signs or symptoms
- Focal neurologic symptoms or signs developing during a headache (i.e., complicated migraine)
- Focal neurologic symptoms or signs (except classic visual symptoms of migraine) develop during the aura, with fixed laterality; focal signs of the aura persisting or recurring in the headache phase
Seizures or very brief auras (<5 min)
Unusual headaches in children
- Atypical auras including basilar-type, hemiplegic
- Trigeminal autonomic cephalalgia including cluster headaches in child or adolescent
- An acute secondary headache (i.e., headache with known underlying illness or insult)
Headache in children younger than 6 yr old or any child who cannot adequately describe his or her headache
Brief cough headache in a child or adolescent
Headache worst on first awakening or that awakens the child from sleep
Migrainous headache in the child with no family history of migraine or its equivalent

Table 595-8	Drugs Used in the Management of Migraine Headaches in Children			
DRUG	DOSE	MECHANISM	SIDE EFFECTS	COMMENTS
ACUTE MIGRAINE				
Analgesics				
Acetaminophen	15 mg/kg/dose	Analgesic effects	Overdose, fatal hepatic necrosis	Effectiveness limited in migraine
Ibuprofen	7.5-10 mg/kg/dose	Antiinflammatory and analgesic	GI bleeding stomach upset, kidney injury	Avoid overuse (2-3 times per wk)
Triptans				
Almotriptan* (ages 12-17 yr)	12.5 mg	5-HT$_{1b/1d}$ agonist	Vascular constriction, serotonin symptoms such as flushing, paresthesias, somnolence, GI discomfort	Avoid overuse (more than 4-6 times per mo)
Eletriptan	40 mg	Same	Same	Avoid overuse (more than 4-6 times per mo)
Frovatriptan	2.5 mg	Same	Same	May be effective for menstrual migraine prevention Avoid overuse (more than 4-6 times per mo)
Naratriptan	2.5 mg	Same	Same	May be effective for menstrual migraine prevention Avoid overuse (more than 4-6 times per mo)
Rizatriptan* (ages 6-17 yr)	5 mg for child weighing <40 kg, 10 mg	Same	Same	Available in tablets and melts Avoid overuse (more than 4-6 times per mo)
Sumatriptan	Oral: 25 mg, 50 mg, 100 mg Nasal: 10 mg SC: 6 mg	Same	Same	Avoid overuse (more than 4-6 times per mo)
Zolmitriptan	Oral: 2.5 mg, 5 mg Nasal: 5 mg	Same	Same	Available in tablets and melts Avoid overuse (more than 4-6 times per mo)

Continued

Table 595-8	Drugs Used in the Management of Migraine Headaches in Children—cont'd

DRUG	DOSE	MECHANISM	SIDE EFFECTS	COMMENTS
PROPHYLAXIS (NONE APPROVED BY FDA FOR CHILDREN)				
Calcium Channel Blockers				
Flunarizine†	5 mg hs	Calcium channel blocking agent	Headache, lethargy, dizziness	May ↑ to 10 mg hs
Anticonvulsants				
Valproic acid	20 mg/kg/24 hr (begin 5 mg/kg/24 hr)	↑ Brain GABA	Nausea, pancreatitis, fatal hepatotoxicity	↑ 5 mg/kg every 2 wk
Topiramate	100-200 mg divided bid	↑ Activity of GABA	Fatigue, nervousness	Increase slowly over 12-16 wk
Levetiracetam	20-60 mg/kg divided bid	Unknown	Irritability, fatigue	Increase every 2 wk starting at 20 mg/kg divided bid
Gabapentin	900-1800 mg divided bid	Unknown	Somnolence, fatigue aggression, weight gain	Begin 300 mg, ↑ 300 mg/wk
Antidepressants				
Amitriptyline	1 mg/kg/day	↑ CNS serotonin and norepinephrine	Cardiac conduction, abnormalities and dry mouth, constipation, drowsiness, confusion	Increase by 0.25 mg/kg every 2 wk Morning sleepiness reduced by administration at dinnertime
Antihistamines				
Cyproheptadine	0.2-0.4 mg/kg divided bid; max: 0.5 mg/kg/24 hr	H₁-receptor and serotonin agonist	Drowsiness, thick bronchial secretions	Preferred in children who cannot swallow pills; not well tolerated in adolescents
Antihypertensive				
Propranolol	10-20 mg tid	Nonselective β-adrenergic blocking agent	Dizziness, lethargy	Begin 10 mg/24 hr ↑ 10 mg/wk (contraindicated in asthma and depression)
Others				
Coenzyme Q10	1-3 mg/kg/day	Increases fatty acid oxidation in mitochondria	No adverse effects reported	Fat soluble; ensure brand contains small amount of vitamin E to help absorption
Riboflavin	50-400 mg daily	Cofactor in energy metabolism	Bright yellow urine, polyuria and diarrhea	
Magnesium	9 mg/kg divided tid	Cofactor in energy metabolism	Diarrhea or soft stool	
Butterbur	50-150 mg daily	May act similar to a calcium channel blocker	Burping	
OnabotulinumtoxinA	100 units (age 11-17 yr)	Inhibits acetylcholine release from nerve endings	Ptosis, blurred vision, hematoma at injection site	Used off label in children
SEVERE INTRACTABLE				
Prochlorperazine	0.15 mg/kg/IV; max dose 10 mg	Dopamine antagonist	Agitation, drowsiness, muscle stiffness, akinesia and akathisia	May have increased effectiveness when combined with ketorolac and fluid hydration
Metoclopramide	0.2 mg/kg IV; 10 mg max dose	Dopamine antagonist	Drowsiness, urticaria, agitation, akinesia and akathisia	Caution in asthma patients
Ketorolac	0.5 mg/kg IV; 15 mg max dose	Antiinflammatory and analgesic	GI upset, bleeding	
Valproate sodium injection	15 mg/kg IV: 1,000 mg max dose	↑ Brain GABA	Nausea, vomiting, somnolence, thrombocytopenia	Would avoid in hepatic disease
Dihydroergotamine IV	0.5 mg/dose every 8 hr (<40 kg) 1.0 mg/dose every 8 hr (>40 kg)		Nausea, vomiting, vascular constriction, phlebitis	Dose may need to be adjusted for side effects (decrease) or limited effectiveness (increase).
Nasal spray	0.5-1.0 mg/dose 0.5 mg/spray			

*FDA approved in the pediatric population.
†Available in Europe.
↑, Increase; CNS, central nervous system; GABA, γ-aminobutyric acid; GI, gastrointestinal; hs, at night; SC, subcutaneous.

To accomplish these goals, 3 components need to be incorporated into the treatment plan:

1. An acute treatment strategy should be developed for stopping a headache attack on a consistent basis with return to function as soon as possible with the goal being 2 hr maximum.
2. A preventive treatment strategy should be considered when the headaches are frequent (1 or more per week) and disabling.
3. Biobehavioral therapy should be started, including a discussion of adherence, elimination of barriers to treatment, and healthy habit management.

Acute Treatment

Management of an acute attack is to provide headache freedom as quickly as possible with return to normal function. This mainly includes 2 groups of medicines: nonsteroidal antiinflammatory drugs (NSAIDs) and triptans. Most migraine headaches in children will respond to appropriate doses of NSAIDs when administered at the onset of the headache attack. Ibuprofen has been well documented to be effective at a dose of 7.5-10.0 mg/kg and is often preferred; however, acetaminophen (15 mg/kg) can be effective in those with a contraindication to NSAIDs. Special concern for the use of ibuprofen or other NSAIDs includes ensuring that the children can recognize and respond to onset of the headache. This means discussing with the child the importance of telling the teacher when the headache starts at school and ensuring that proper dosing guidelines and permission have been provided to the school. In addition, overuse needs to be avoided, limiting the NSAID (or any combination of nonprescription analgesics) to not more than 2-3 times per week. The limitation of any analgesic to not more than 3 headaches a week is necessary to prevent the transformation of the migraines into medication overuse headaches. If a patient has maximized the weekly allowance of analgesics, the patient's next step is to only use hydrating fluids for the rest of the week as an abortive approach. If ibuprofen is not effective, naproxen sodium also may be tried in similar doses. Aspirin is also a reasonable option but is usually reserved for older children (older than age 15 yr). Use of other NSAIDs have yet to be studied in pediatric migraine. The goal of the primary acute medication should be headache relief within 1 hr with return to function in 10 of 10 headaches.

When a migraine is especially severe, NSAIDs alone may not be sufficient. In this case, a triptan may be considered. Multiple studies have demonstrated their effectiveness and tolerability. There are currently 2 triptans that are approved by the FDA for the treatment of episodic migraine in the pediatric population. Almotriptan is approved for the treatment of acute migraine in adolescents (ages 12-17 yr). Rizatriptan is approved for the treatment of migraine in children as young as age 6 yr. The combination of naproxen sodium and sumatriptan has been studied and may be effective in children. Controlled clinical trials demonstrate that intranasal sumatriptan is safe and effective in children older than age 8 yr with moderate to severe migraine. At present, pediatric studies showing the effectiveness of oral sumatriptan are lacking and there is insufficient evidence to support the use of subcutaneous sumatriptan in children. For most adolescents, dosing is the same as for adults; a reduction in dose is made for children weighing less than 40 kg. The triptans vary by rapidity of onset and biologic half-life. This is related to both their variable lipophilicity and dose. Clinically, 60-70% of patients respond to the first triptan tried, with 60-70% of the patients who did not respond to the first triptan responding to the next triptan. Therefore, in the patient who does not respond to the first triptan in the desired way (rapid reproducible response without relapse or side effects), it is worthwhile to try a different triptan. The most common side effects of the triptans are caused by their mechanism of action—tightness in the jaw, chest, and fingers as a result of vascular constriction and a subsequent feeling of grogginess and fatigue from the central serotonin effect. The vascular constriction symptoms can be alleviated through adequate fluid hydration during an attack.

The most effective way to administer abortive treatment is to use NSAIDs first in mild to severe cases, restricting their use to fewer than 2-3 attacks per week, and adding the triptan for moderate to severe, or attacks that have failed NSAID use, restricting to not more than 4-6 attacks per month. For an acute attack, the NSAIDs can be repeated once in 3-4 hr if needed for that specific attack, and the triptans can be repeated once in 2 hr if needed. It is important to consider the various formulations available and a discussion of these options should be made with pediatric patients and their parents, especially if a child is unable to swallow pills or take an oral dose because of nausea.

As vascular dilation is a common feature of migraine that may be responsible for some of the facial flushing followed by paleness and the lightheaded feeling accompanying the attacks, fluid hydration should be integrated into the acute treatment plan. For oral hydration this can include the sports drinks that combine electrolytes and sugar to provide the intravascular rehydration.

Antiemetics were used for acute treatment of the nausea and vomiting. Further study has identified that their unique mechanism of effectiveness in headache treatment is related to their antagonism of dopaminergic neurotransmission. Therefore, the antiemetics with the most robust dopamine antagonism (i.e., prochlorperazine and metoclopramide) have the best efficacy. These can be very effective for status migrainosus or a migraine that is unresponsive to the NSAIDs and triptans. They require intravenous administration, as other forms of administration of these drugs are less effective than the NSAIDs or triptans. When combined with ketorolac and intravenous fluids in the emergency department or an acute infusion center, intravenous antiemetics can be very effective. When they are not effective, further inpatient treatment may be required using dihydroergotamine (DHE) which will mean an admission to an inpatient unit for more aggressive therapy of an intractable attack.

Emergency Department Treatments for Intractable Headaches

When an acute migraine attack does not respond to an outpatient regimen and is disabling, other therapeutic approaches are available and may be necessary to prevent further increases in the frequency of headaches. These migraines fall into the classification of status migrainosus and need infusion therapy and admission to the emergency room department or to an inpatient unit.

Available specific treatments for migraine headache in an emergency room setting include the following: antidopaminergic medications such as prochlorperazine and metoclopramide; NSAIDs such as ketorolac and DHE; antiepileptic drugs such as sodium valproate; and triptans.

Antidopaminergic Drugs: Prochlorperazine and Metoclopramide. The use of these medications is not limited to controlling the nausea and vomiting often present during a migraine headache. Their potential pharmacologic effect may be a result of their antidopamine property and the underlying pathologic process involving the dopaminergic system during a migraine attack. Prochlorperazine is very effective in aborting an attack in the emergency room when given intravenously with a bolus of IV fluid. Results show a 75% improvement with 50% headache freedom at 1 hr and 95% improvement with 60% headache freedom at 3 hr. Prochlorperazine may be more effective than metoclopramide. The average dose of metoclopramide use is 0.13-0.15 mg/kg with a maximum dose of 10 mg given intravenously over 15 min. The average dose of prochlorperazine is 0.15 mg/kg with a maximum dose of 10 mg. These medications are usually well tolerated, but *extrapyramidal reactions* are more frequent in children compared to the older population. An acute extrapyramidal reaction can be controlled in the emergency room with 25-50 mg of diphenhydramine given IV.

Nonsteroidal Antiinflammatory Drugs: Ketorolac. It is known that an aseptic inflammation occurs in the central nervous system as a result of the effect of multiple reactive peptides in patients with migraines. Ketorolac is often used in the emergency department as monotherapy for a migraine attack or in combination with other drugs. In monotherapy, the response to ketorolac is 55.2% improvement. When combined to prochlorperazine, the response rate jumps to 93%.

Antiepileptic Drugs: Sodium Valproate. Antiepileptic drugs have been used as prophylactic treatment for migraine headache for years with adequate double-blinded, controlled studies on their efficacy in adults. The mechanism in which sodium valproate acutely aborts migraine headaches is not well understood. Sodium valproate is given as a bolus of 15-20 mg/kg push (over 10 min). This intravenous load is followed by an oral dose (15-20 mg/day) in the 4 hr after the injection. Patients may benefit from a short-term preventive treatment with an extended release form after discharge from the emergency room. Sodium valproate is usually well tolerated. Patients should be receiving a fluid load during the procedure to prevent a possible hypotensive episode.

Triptans. Subcutaneous sumatriptan (0.06 mg/kg) has an overall efficacy of 72% at 30 min and 78% at 2 hr, with a recurrence rate of 6%. Because children tend to have a shorter duration of headache, a recurrence rate of 6% would seem appropriate for this population. DHE, if recommended for the recurrences, should not be given in the 24 hr after triptan use. Triptans are contraindicated in patients treated with ergotamine within 24 hr and within 2 wk of treatment with monoamine oxidase inhibitors. Triptans may potentially produce a serotonin syndrome in patients taking a serotonin syndrome reuptake inhibitor. Both triptans and ergotamine are contraindicated in hemiplegic migraines.

Dihydroergotamine. DHE is an old migraine medication used as a vasoconstrictor to abort the vascular phase of migraine headache. The effectiveness is discussed in detail in the section "Inpatient Management of Intractable Migraine and Status Migrainosus" below. One dose of DHE can be effective for abortive treatment in the emergency department. Emergency room treatment of migraine shows a recurrence rate of 29% at 48-72 hr, with 6% who need more aggressive therapy in an inpatient unit.

Inpatient Management of Intractable Migraine and Status Migrainosus

Six percent to 7% of patients fail acute treatment in the emergency department. These patients are usually admitted for a 3-5 day stay and receive extensive parenteral treatment. A child should be admitted to the hospital for a primary headache when the child is in status migrainous, has an exacerbation of a chronic severe headache, or is in an analgesic rebound headache. The goal of inpatient treatment is to control a disabling headache that has been unresponsive to other abortive therapy and is disabling to the child. Treatment protocols include the use of DHE, antiemetics, sodium valproate and other drugs.

Dihydroergotamine. Ergots are one of the oldest treatments for migraine headache. DHE is a parenteral form used for acute exacerbations. Its effect is because of the $5HT_{1A-1B-1D-1F}$ receptor agonist affinity and central vasoconstriction. DHE has a greater α-adrenergic antagonist activity and is less vasoconstrictive peripherally. Before initiation of an IV ergot protocol, a full history and neurologic examination should be obtained. Girls of childbearing age should be evaluated for pregnancy before administering ergots.

The DHE protocol consists of the following: Patients are premedicated with 0.13-0.15 mg/kg of prochlorperazine 30 min prior to the DHE dose (maximum of 3 prochlorperazine doses to prevent extrapyramidal syndrome, then other types of antiemetics should be used, such as ondansetron). A dose of 0.5-1.0 mg of DHE is used (depending on age and tolerability) every 8 hr until headache freedom. When headache ceases, an extra dose is given in an attempt to prevent recurrence after discharge. The response to this protocol is a 97% improvement and 77% headache freedom. Response starts being noticeable by the fifth dose and can reach its maximum effects after the 10th dose. Side effects of DHE include nausea, vomiting, abdominal discomfort, flushed face, increased blood pressure. The maximum dose used in this protocol is 15 mg total of DHE. During the hospital admission the patient is usually started on migraine prophylaxis depending on the patient's history and comorbid problems.

Sodium Valproate. Sodium valproate is used when DHE is contraindicated or has been ineffective. One adult study recommends the use of valproate sodium as follows: Bolus with 15 mg/kg (maximum of 1,000 mg), followed by 5 mg/kg every 8 hr until headache freedom or up to a maximum of 10 doses. Always give an extra dose after headache ceases. This protocol was studied in adults with chronic daily headaches and showed an 80% improvement. It is well tolerated and is useful in children when DHE is ineffective, contraindicated, or not tolerated.

Preventive Therapy

When the headaches are frequent (more than 1 headache/wk) or there are more than 1 disabling headache a month (missing school, home, or social activities, or a PedMIDAS score higher than 20), preventive or **prophylactic therapy** is warranted. The goal of this therapy should to be to reduce frequency (1-2 headaches or fewer per month) and disability (PedMIDAS score <10). Prophylactic agents should be given for at least 4-6 mo at an adequate dose and then weaned over several weeks. Evidence in adult studies has begun to demonstrate that persistent frequent headaches foreshadow an increased risk of progression with decreased responsiveness and increased risk of refractoriness in the future. It is unclear whether this also occurs in children and/or adolescents and whether early treatment of headache in childhood prevents development of refractory headache in adulthood.

Multiple preventive medications have been utilized for migraine prophylaxis in children. When analyzed as part of a practice parameter, only 1 medication, **flunarizine** (a calcium channel blocking agent), demonstrated a level of effectiveness viewed as substantial; it is not available in the United States. Flunarizine is typically dosed at 5 mg orally daily and increased after 1 mo to 10 mg orally daily, with a month off of the drug every 4-6 mo.

The most commonly used preventive therapy for headache and migraine is amitriptyline. Typically, a dose of 1 mg/kg daily at dinner or in the evening is effective. However, this dose needs to be reached slowly (i.e., over weeks: with an increase every 2 wk until goal is reached) to minimize side effects and improve tolerability. The most common side effects are sleepiness and those related to amitriptyline's anticholinergic activity. Weight gain has been observed in adults using amitriptyline but is a less frequent occurrence in children. Amitriptyline does have the potential to exacerbate prolonged QT syndrome, so it should be avoided in patients with this diagnosis and looked for in patients on the drug who complain of rapid or irregular heart rate.

Antiepileptic medications are also used for migraine prophylaxis, with topiramate, valproic acid, and levetiracetam having been demonstrated to be effective in adults. There are limited studies in children for migraine prevention, but all of these medications have been assessed for safety and tolerability in children with epilepsy.

Topiramate has become widely used for migraine prophylaxis in adults. Topiramate was also demonstrated to be effective in an adolescent study. This study demonstrated that a 25 mg dose twice a day was equivalent to placebo, whereas a 50 mg dose twice a day was superior. Thus it appears that the adult dosing schedule is also effective in adolescents with an effective dosage range or 50 mg twice a day to 100 mg twice a day. This dose needs to be reached slowly to minimize the cognitive slowing associated with topiramate use. Additional side effects include weight loss, paresthesias, kidney stones, lowered bicarbonate levels, decreased sweating, and rarely glaucoma and changes in serum transaminases. In addition, in adolescent girls taking birth control pills, the lowering of the effectiveness of the birth control by topiramate needs to be discussed.

Valproic acid has long been used for epilepsy in children and has been demonstrated to be effective in migraine prophylaxis in adults. The effective dose in children appears to be 10 mg/kg orally twice a day. Side effects of weight gain, ovarian cysts, and changes in serum transaminases and platelet counts need to be monitored. Other antiepileptics, including lamotrigine, levetiracetam, zonisamide, gabapentin, and pregabalin, are also used for migraine prevention.

β-Blockers have long been used for migraine prevention. The studies on β-blockers have a mixed response pattern with variability both between β-blockers and between patients with a given β-blocker. Propranolol is the best studied for pediatric migraine prevention with unequivocally positive results. The contraindication for use of propranolol in children with asthma or allergic disorders or diabetes and the increased incidence of depression in adolescents using propranolol limit its use somewhat. It may be very effective for a mixed subtype of migraine (basilar-type migraine with postural orthostatic tachycardia syndrome). This syndrome has been reported to be responsive to propranolol. α-Blockers and calcium channel blockers, aside from flunarizine, also have been used in pediatric migraine; their effectiveness, however, remains unclear.

In very young children, cyproheptadine may be effective in prevention of migraine or the related variants. Young children tend to tolerate the increased appetite induced by the cyproheptadine and tend not to be subject to the lethargy seen in older children and adults; the weight gain is limiting once children start to enter puberty. Typical dosing is 0.1-0.2 mg/kg orally twice a day.

Nutraceuticals have become increasingly popular over the past few years, especially among families who prefer a more "natural" approach to headache treatment. Despite studies showing success of these therapies in adults, few studies have shown effectiveness in pediatric headaches. Riboflavin (vitamin B_2), at doses ranging from 25-400 mg, is the most widely studied with good results. Side effects are minimal and include bright yellow urine, diarrhea, and polyuria. Coenzyme Q10 supplementation may be effective in reducing migraine frequency at doses of 1-2 mg/kg/day. Butterbur is also effective in reducing headaches with minimal side effects, including burping. Use in children has been limited to avoid the potential toxicity of butterbur containing pyrrolizidine alkaloids, which are naturally contained and are a known carcinogen and toxic to the liver.

OnabotulinumtoxinA is the first medication FDA-approved for chronic migraine in adults. There are studies in children indicating its effectiveness; use in children is considered off-label. The limited available studies revealed the following: Average dose used was 188.5 units ± 32 units with a minimum dose of 75 units and maximum of 200 units. The average age of patients receiving the treatment was 16.8 ± 2.0 yr (minimum: 11; maximum: 21 yr old). OnabotulinumtoxinA injections improved disability scores (PedMIDAS) and headache frequency in pediatric chronic daily headache patients and chronic migraine in this age group. OnabotulinumtoxinA not only had a positive effect on the disability scoring for these young patients with headache, but was also able to transform the headaches from chronic daily to intermittent headache in more than 50% of the patients.

Biobehavioral Therapy

Biobehavioral evaluation and therapy is essential for effective migraine management. This includes identification of behavioral barriers to treatment, like a child's shyness or limitation in notifying a teacher of the start of a migraine or a teacher's unwillingness to accept the need for treatment. Additional barriers include a lack of recognition of the significance of their headache problem and reverting to "bad habits" once the headaches have responded to treatment. Adherence is equally important for acute and preventive treatment. The need to have a sustained response for long enough to prevent relapse (i.e., to stay on preventive medication) is often difficult when the child starts to feel better. Establishing a defined treatment goal (1-2 or fewer headaches per month for 4-6 mo) helps with acceptance.

As many of the potential triggers for frequent migraines (skipping meals, dehydration, decreased or altered sleep) are related to a child's daily routine, a discussion of healthy habits is a component of biobehavioral therapy. This should include adequate fluid intake without caffeine, regular exercise, not skipping meals and making healthy food choices, and adequate (8-9 hr) sleep on a regular basis. Sleep is often difficult in adolescents, as middle and high schools often have very early start times, and the adolescent's sleep architecture features a shift to later sleep onset and waking. This has been one of the explanations for worsening headaches during the school year in general and at the beginning of the school year and week.

Biofeedback-assisted relaxation and cognitive behavioral therapy (usually in combination with amitriptyline) are effective for both acute and preventive therapy and may be incorporated into this multiple treatment strategy. This provides the child with a degree of self-control over the headaches and may further help the child cope with frequent headaches.

Bibliography is available at Expert Consult.

595.2 Secondary Headaches

Andrew D. Hershey, Marielle A. Kabbouche, and Hope L. O'Brien

Headaches can be a common symptom of other underlying illnesses. In recognition of this, the ICHD-3 beta has classified the potential secondary headaches (see Table 595-1). The key to the diagnosis of a secondary headache is to recognize the underlying cause and demonstrate a direct cause and effect. Until this has been demonstrated the diagnosis is speculative. This is especially true when the suspected etiology is common.

Common causes or suspected causes of secondary headaches in children include the sequelae of head trauma and sinusitis. **Posttraumatic headaches** sometimes occur in children who have not had a prior history of headaches and are temporally related to the initiating head injury. Frequently, though, these children have a family history of migraine or its equivalent. The head injury may be minor or major and the subsequent headache may be acute (resolves within 3 mo, most typically within 10 days) or chronic (longer than 15 days per month for more than 3 mo). Bed rest appears to be the most effective treatment for acute posttraumatic headache; magnesium supplementation and migraine prophylaxis may also be effective. When a child has a history of episodic headaches, the head trauma or the overuse of daily medications may lead to status migrainosus or chronic migraine and the diagnosis may be difficult to sort out.

Sinus headache is the most overdiagnosed form of recurrent headaches. Although no studies have evaluated the frequency of misdiagnosis of an underlying migraine as a sinus headache in children, in adults, it has been found that up to 90% of adults diagnosed as having a sinus headache by either themselves or their physician appear to have migraine. When headaches are recurrent and respond within hours to analgesics, migraine should be considered first. In the absence of purulent nasal discharge, fever, or chronic cough, the diagnosis of sinus headache should not be made.

Medication overuse headaches frequently complicate primary and secondary headaches. A medication overuse headache is defined as a headache present for more than 15 days/mo for longer than 3 mo and intake of a simple analgesic on more than 15 days/mo and/or prescription medications including triptans or combination medications on more than 10 days/mo. Some of the signs that should raise suspicion of medication overuse are the increasing use of analgesics (nonprescription or prescription) with either decreased effectiveness or frequently wearing off (i.e., analgesic rebound). This can be worsened by using ineffective medications and underdosing or misdiagnosing the headache. Patients should be cautioned against the frequent use of antimigraine medications, including combination analgesics or triptans.

Serious causes of secondary headaches are likely to be related to increased intracranial pressure. This can be caused by a mass (tumor, vascular malformation, cystic structure) or an intrinsic increase in pressure (idiopathic intracranial hypertension also known as pseudotumor cerebri). In the former case, the headache is caused by the mass effect and local pressure on the dura; in the latter case, the headache is caused by diffuse pressure on the dura. The etiology of idiopathic intracranial hypertension may be the intake of excessive amounts of fat-soluble compounds (e.g., vitamin A, retinoic acid, and minocycline), hormonal changes (increased incidence in females) or blockage of venous drainage (as with inflammation of the transverse venous sinus from mastoiditis). When increased pressure is suspected, either by historical suspicion or the presence of papilledema, an MRI with magnetic resonance angiography and magnetic resonance venography should be performed, followed by a lumbar puncture if no mass or vascular anomaly is noted. The lumbar puncture can be diagnostic and therapeutic of idiopathic intracranial hypertension but must be performed with the patient in a relaxed recumbent position with legs extended, as abdominal pressure can artificially raise intracranial pressure. If headache persists or there are visual field changes, pharmaceutical treatment with a carbonic anhydrase inhibitor, optic nerve fenestration, or a shunt needs to be considered.

Additional causes of secondary headaches in children that may not be associated with increased intracranial pressure include arteriovenous malformations, berry aneurysm, collagen vascular diseases affecting the central nervous system, hypertensive encephalopathy, infectious or autoimmune etiologies, acute subarachnoid hemorrhage, and stroke. The management of secondary headache depends on the cause. Helpful laboratory tests and neuroradiologic procedures depend on the clues provided by the history and physical examination. By definition, a secondary headache has a specific cause and should resolve once this cause is treated. If the headache persists, the diagnosis and treatment should be questioned as either the diagnosis, which may include a primary headache, and/or treatment may be incorrect.

Bibliography is available at Expert Consult.

595.3 Tension-Type Headaches
Andrew D. Hershey, Marielle A. Kabbouche, and Hope L. O'Brien

Tension-type headaches (TTHs) may be very common in children and adolescents with prevalence in some studies shown as high as 48%, with those having a combination of migraine and TTH around 20%. Because of their mild to moderate nature, relative lack of associated symptoms and lower degree of associated disability they are often ignored or have a minimal impact. The ICHD-3 beta subclassifies TTHs as infrequent (<12 times/yr) (Table 595-9), frequent (1-15 times/mo), and chronic (>15 headaches/mo). They can further be separated into headaches with or without pericranial muscle tenderness. The classification of TTH can be likened to the opposite of migraine. Whereas migraines are typically moderate to severe, are focal in location, are worsened by physical activity or limit physical activity, and have a throbbing quality, TTH are mild to moderate in severity, are diffuse in location, are not affected by activity (although the patient may not feel like being active), and are nonthrobbing (often described as a constant pressure). TTH is much less frequently associated with nausea, photophobia, or phonophobia and is never associated with more than 1 of these at a time or with vomiting. TTH must be recurrent, but at least 10 headaches are required and the duration can be 30 min to 7 days. Secondary headaches with other underlying etiologies must be ruled out.

Table 595-9	Infrequent Episodic Tension-Type Headache

A. At least 10 episodes of headache occurring on <1 day per month on average (<12 days per year) and fulfilling criteria B to D
B. Lasting from 30 min to 7 days
C. At least 2 of the following 4 characteristics:
  1. Bilateral location
  2. Pressing or tightening (nonpulsating) quality
  3. Mild or moderate intensity
  4. Not aggravated by routine physical activity such as walking or climbing stairs
D. Both of the following:
  1. No nausea or vomiting
  2. No more than 1 of photophobia or phonophobia
E. Not better accounted for by another ICHD-3 beta diagnosis

From Headache Classification Committee on the International Headache Society (IHS): The International Classification of Headache Disorders, ed 3 (beta version). Cephalalgia 33(9):629–808, 2013, Table 10.

Evaluation of patients with suspected TTHs requires a detailed headache history and complete general and neurologic examination. This is to establish the diagnosis and ensure exclusion of secondary etiologies. When secondary headaches are suspected, further, directed evaluation is indicated.

Treatment of TTHs can require acute therapy to stop attacks, preventive therapy when frequent or chronic, and behavioral therapy. It is often suspected that there may be underlying psychologic stressors (hence the misnomer as a "stress" headache), but this is often difficult to identify in children, and although it may be suspected by the parents, it cannot be confirmed in the child. Studies of and conclusive evidence to guide the treatment of TTH in children are lacking, but the same general principles and medications used in migraine can be applied to children with TTHs (see Chapter 595.1). Oftentimes, simple analgesics (ibuprofen or acetaminophen) can be effective for acute treatment. Flupirtine is a nonopioid analgesic that has been approved in Europe for the treatment of TTH in children as young as age 6 yr, but is not available in the United States. Amitriptyline has the most evidence of effective prevention of TTH; biobehavioral intervention, including biofeedback-assisted relaxation training and coping skills, can be useful as well.

Bibliography is available at Expert Consult.

Chapter 596
Neurocutaneous Syndromes
Mustafa Sahin

The neurocutaneous syndromes include a heterogeneous group of disorders characterized by abnormalities of both the integument and central nervous system. Many of the disorders are familial and believed to arise from a defect in differentiation of the primitive ectoderm. Disorders classified as neurocutaneous syndromes include neurofibromatosis, tuberous sclerosis, Sturge-Weber syndrome, von Hippel-Lindau disease, PHACE (posterior fossa malformations, hemangiomas, arterial anomalies, coarctation of aorta, cardiac defects, eye abnormalities) syndrome, ataxia telangiectasia, linear nevus syndrome, hypomelanosis of Ito, and incontinentia pigmenti.

596.1 Neurofibromatosis
Mustafa Sahin

Neurofibromatoses are autosomal dominant disorders that cause tumors to grow on nerves and result in other abnormalities such as skin changes and bone deformities. It was believed that there were 2 types of neurofibromatosis (type 1 and type 2), but it is recognized that they are clinically and genetically distinct diseases and should be considered separate entities: neurofibromatosis type 1 (NF-1) and neurofibromatosis type 2 (NF-2).

CLINICAL MANIFESTATIONS AND DIAGNOSIS
NF-1 is the most prevalent type, with an incidence of 1 in 3,000 live births, and is caused by dominant loss-of-function mutations in the *NF-1* gene. The disease is clinically diagnosed when any 2 of the following 7 features are present: (1) six or more café-au-lait macules larger than 5 mm in greatest diameter in prepubertal individuals and larger than 15 mm in greatest diameter in postpubertal individuals (Fig. 596-1). Café-au-lait spots are the hallmark of neurofibromatosis

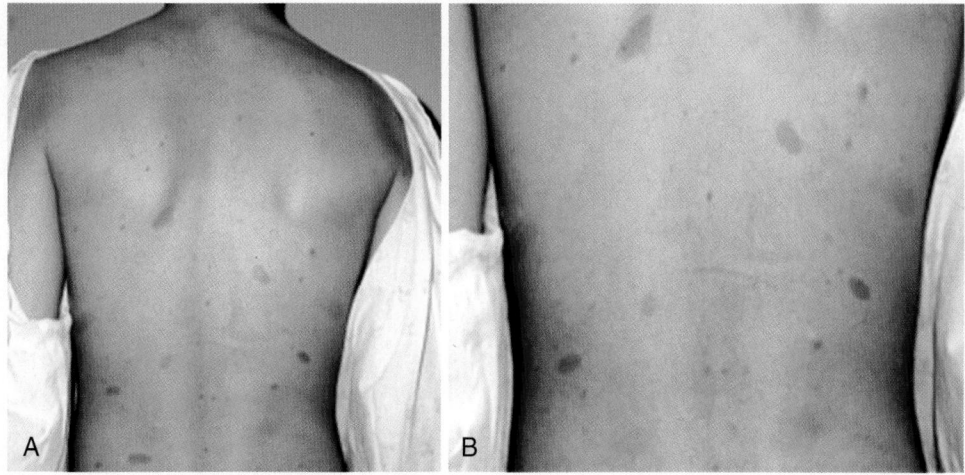

Figure 596-1 A and **B,** Multiple café-au-lait spots over the back. Note the dermal neurofibromas below the right scapula and right side of the lower back. *(From Hersh JH, Committee on Genetics: Health supervision for children with neurofibromatosis, Pediatrics 121:633–642, 2008, Fig. 1.)*

Table 596-1	Diseases Associated with Multiple Café-Au-Lait Spots
DISEASE	**MAJOR FEATURES**
Ataxia telangiectasia	Progressive ataxia, lymphoreticular malignancy
Bannayan-Riley-Ruvalcaba syndrome	Macrosomia, megalencephaly, lipomas, intestinal polyps
Basal cell nevus syndrome	Multiple basal cell epitheliomas, jaw cysts, skeletal anomalies
Bloom syndrome	Short stature, photosensitivity, chromosome breaks, malignancy
Fanconi anemia	Limb anomalies, renal anomalies, pancytopenia
Gaucher disease	Jewish predilection, ataxia, mental retardation
Hunter syndrome	Thickened skin, coarse facies, skin papules, joint contractures
Jaffe-Campanacci syndrome	Fibromas of long bones, hypogonadism, mental retardation, ocular/cardiac anomalies
Maffucci syndrome	Venous malformations, enchondromas
McCune-Albright syndrome	Polyostotic fibrous dysplasia, precocious puberty
Multiple lentigines syndrome	Multiple lentigines, hypertelorism, pulmonic stenosis
Multiple mucosal neuroma syndrome	Mucosal neuromas, thyroid carcinoma, pheochromocytoma, parathyroid adenoma, dysautonomia
Neurofibromatosis	Neurofibromas, central nervous system tumors, iris hamartomas, axillary freckles, skeletal anomalies
Russell-Silver syndrome	Short stature, asymmetry, limb anomalies
Tuberous sclerosis	White macules, multiple hamartomas, central nervous system anomalies
Watson syndrome	Pulmonic stenosis, axillary freckles, low intelligence
Legius syndrome	Axillary freckling macrocephaly, a Noonan-like facial dysmorphism, lipomas

From Marcoux DA, Duran-McKinster C, Baselga E, et al: Pigmentary abnormalities. In: Schachner LA, Hansen RC, editors: Pediatric dermatology, ed 4, Philadelphia, 2011, Mosby, Table 10-2.

and are present in almost 100% of patients. They are present at birth but increase in size, number, and pigmentation, especially during the 1st few yr of life. The spots are scattered over the body surface, with predilection for the trunk and extremities but sparing the face. (2) Axillary or inguinal freckling consisting of multiple hyperpigmented areas 2-3 mm in diameter. Skinfold freckling usually appears between 3 and 5 yr of age. The frequency of axillary and inguinal freckling is reported to be >80% by 6 yr of age. Café-au-lait macules are not specific for NF-1; they may be seen in Noonan syndrome, constitutional mismatch repair deficiency syndrome, Legius syndrome, Peutz-Jeghers syndrome, Carney complex, and those diseases listed in Table 596-1. (3) Two or more iris Lisch nodules. Lisch nodules are hamartomas located within the iris and are best identified by a slit-lamp examination (Fig. 596-2). They are present in more than 74% of patients with

NF-1 but are not a characteristic of NF-2. The prevalence of Lisch nodules increases with age, from only 5% of children younger than 3 yr of age, to 42% among children 3-4 yr of age, and virtually 100% of adults older than 21 yr of age. (4) Two or more neurofibromas or 1 plexiform neurofibroma. Neurofibromas typically involve the skin, but they may be situated along peripheral nerves and blood vessels and within viscera including the gastrointestinal tract. These lesions appear characteristically during adolescence or pregnancy, suggesting a hormonal influence. They are usually small, rubbery lesions with a slight purplish discoloration of the overlying skin. Plexiform neurofibromas are usually evident at birth and result from diffuse thickening of nerve trunks that are frequently located in the orbital or temporal region of the face. The skin overlying a plexiform neurofibroma may be hyperpigmented to a greater degree than a café-au-lait macule. Plexiform

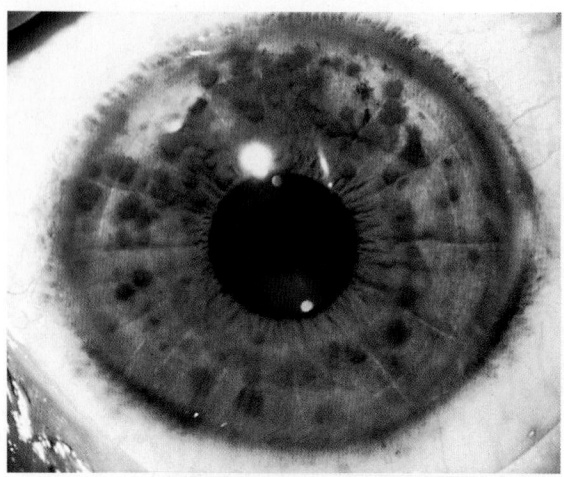

Figure 596-2 Neurofibromatosis type 1 (NF-1). Pigmented hamartomas of the iris (Lisch nodules). *(From Zitelli BJ, McIntire S, Nowalk AJ, editors:* Zitelli and Davis' atlas of pediatric physical diagnosis, *ed 6, Philadelphia, 2012, Mosby, Fig. 15-9.)*

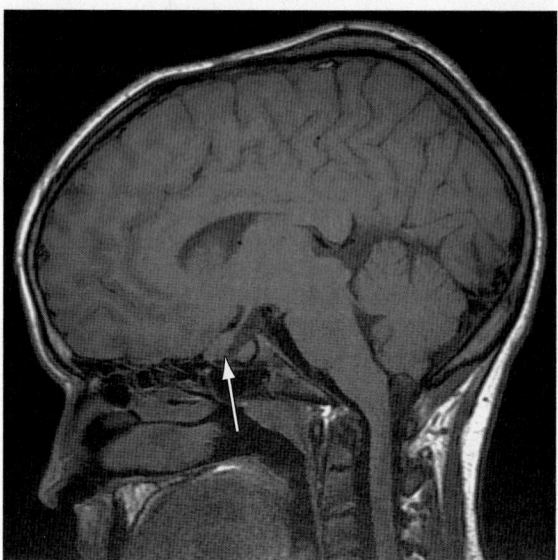

Figure 596-3 Optic glioma. Sagittal T1-weighted MRI scan of a patient with NF-1 shows thickening of the optic nerve *(arrow).*

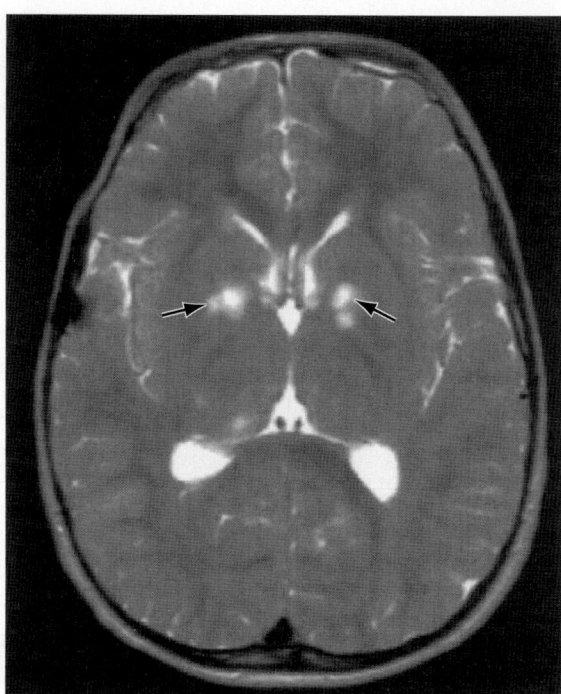

Figure 596-4 T2-weighted MRI scan of a patient with NF-1. Note the high-signal areas (unidentified bright objects) in the basal ganglia *(black arrows).*

neurofibromas may produce overgrowth of an extremity and a deformity of the corresponding bone. (5) A distinctive osseous lesion such as sphenoid dysplasia (which may cause pulsating exophthalmos) or cortical thinning of long bones with or without pseudoarthrosis (e.g., tibia). (6) Optic gliomas are present in approximately 15% of patients with NF-1 and represent mostly low-grade astrocytomas. They are the main central nervous system tumor with a marked increased frequency in NF-1. Because of their growth, it is recommended that all children age 10 yr or younger with NF-1 undergo annual ophthalmologic examinations. When they progress, visual symptoms occur because the tumors enlarge and put pressure on the optic nerves and chiasm resulting in impaired visual acuity and visual fields. Extension into the hypothalamus can lead to endocrine deficiencies or failure to thrive. The MRI findings of an optic glioma include diffuse thickening, localized enlargement, or a distinct focal mass originating from the optic nerve or chiasm (Fig. 596-3). (7) A 1st-degree relative with NF-1 whose diagnosis was based on the aforementioned criteria.

Children with NF-1 are susceptible to **neurologic complications.** MRI studies of selected children have shown abnormal hyperintense T2-weighted signals in the optic tracts, brainstem, globus pallidus, thalamus, internal capsule, and cerebellum (Fig. 596-4). These signals, **"unidentified bright objects,"** tend to disappear with age; most have disappeared by 30 yr of age. It is unclear what the unidentified bright objects represent pathologically, and there is disagreement as to the relationship between the presence and number of unidentified bright objects and the occurrence of learning disabilities, attention-deficit disorders, behavioral and psychosocial problems, and abnormalities of speech among affected children. Therefore, imaging studies such as brain MRIs should be reserved for patients with clinical symptoms only.

One of the most common complications is learning disability affecting approximately 30% of children with NF-1. Seizures are observed in approximately 8% of NF-1 patients. The cerebral vessels may develop aneurysms or stenosis resulting in moyamoya syndrome (see Chapter 601). Neurologic sequelae of these vascular abnormalities include transient cerebrovascular ischemic attacks, hemiparesis, and cognitive defects. Precocious puberty may become evident in the presence or absence of lesions of the optic pathway tumors. Malignant neoplasms are also a significant problem in patients with NF-1, affecting approximately 3% of patients. A neurofibroma occasionally differentiates into a malignant peripheral nerve sheath tumor. The incidence of pheochromocytoma, rhabdomyosarcoma, leukemia, and Wilms tumor is higher than in the general population. Scoliosis is a common complication found in approximately 10% of the patients. Patients with NF-1 are at risk for hypertension, which may result from renal vascular stenosis or a pheochromocytoma.

MANAGEMENT

Because of the diverse and unpredictable complications associated with NF-1, close multidisciplinary follow-up is necessary. Patients with NF-1 should have regular clinical assessments at least yearly, focusing the history and examination on the potential problems for which they are at increased risk. These assessments include yearly ophthalmologic examination, neurologic assessment, blood pressure monitoring, and scoliosis evaluation. Neuropsychologic and educational testing should be considered as needed. The National Institutes of Health (NIH) Consensus Development Conference has advised against routine imaging studies of the brain and optic tracts because treatment in these

Table 596-2	Frequency of Lesions Associated with Neurofibromatosis Type 2	
		FREQUENCY OF ASSOCIATION WITH NF-2
NEUROLOGIC LESIONS		
Bilateral vestibular schwannomas		90-95%
Other cranial nerve schwannomas		24-51%
Intracranial meningiomas		45-58%
Spinal tumors		63-90%
Extramedullary		55-90%
Intramedullary		18-53%
Peripheral neuropathy		Up to 66%
OPHTHALMOLOGIC LESIONS		
Cataracts		60-81%
Epiretinal membranes		12-40%
Retinal hamartomas		6-22%
CUTANEOUS LESIONS		
Skin tumors		59-68%
Skin plaques		41-48%
Subcutaneous tumors		43-48%
Intradermal tumors		Rare

From Asthagiri AR, Parry DM, Butman JA, et al: Neurofibromatosis type 2, Lancet 373:1974–1984, 2009, Table 1.

asymptomatic NF-1 children is rarely required. However, all symptomatic cases (i.e., those with visual disturbance, proptosis, increased intracranial pressure) must be studied without delay.

GENETIC COUNSELING

Although NF-1 is an autosomal dominant disorder, more than half the cases are sporadic, representing de novo mutations. The *NF-1* gene on chromosome region 17q11.2 encodes for a protein also known as neurofibromin. Neurofibromin acts as an inhibitor of the oncogene Ras. The diagnosis of NF-1 is based on the clinical features. However, molecular testing for the *NF-1* gene mutations is available and can be useful in a number of cases. Some scenarios in which genetic testing is helpful include for patients who meet only 1 of the criteria for clinical diagnosis, those with unusually severe disease, and those seeking prenatal/preimplantation diagnosis.

NF-2 is a rarer condition, with an incidence of 1 in 25,000 births, and may be diagnosed when 1 of the following 4 features is present: (1) bilateral vestibular schwannomas; (2) a parent, sibling, or child with NF-2 and either unilateral vestibular schwannoma or any 2 of the following: meningioma, schwannoma, glioma, neurofibroma, posterior subcapsular lenticular opacities; (3) unilateral vestibular schwannoma and any 2 of the following: meningioma, schwannoma, glioma, neurofibroma, posterior subcapsular lenticular opacities; or (4) multiple meningiomas (2 or more) and unilateral vestibular schwannoma or any 2 of the following: schwannoma, glioma, neurofibroma, cataract. Symptoms of tinnitus, hearing loss, facial weakness, headache, or unsteadiness may appear during childhood, although signs of a cerebellopontine angle mass are more commonly present in the 2nd and 3rd decades of life. Although café-au-lait macules and skin neurofibromas are classic findings in NF-1, they are much less common in NF-2. Posterior subcapsular lens opacities are identified in approximately 50% of patients with NF-2. The NF-2 gene (which codes for a protein known as merlin or schwannomin) is located on chromosome 22q1.11. Table 596-2 notes the frequency of lesions in NF-2.

Legius syndrome (caused by *SPRED1* mutations) resembles a mild form of NF-1. Patients with Legius syndrome present with multiple café-au-lait macules and macrocephaly, with and without skinfold freckling. However, other typical features of NF-1, such as Lisch nodules, neurofibromas, optic nerve gliomas, and malignant peripheral nerve sheath tumors, are not seen with *SPRED1* mutations.

Bibliography is available at Expert Consult.

596.2 Tuberous Sclerosis
Mustafa Sahin

Tuberous sclerosis complex (TSC) is inherited in an autosomal dominant manner with variable expression and a prevalence of 1 in 6,000 newborns. Spontaneous genetic mutations occur in 65% of the cases. Molecular genetic studies have identified 2 foci for TSC: the *TSC1* gene is located on chromosome 9q34, and the *TSC2* gene is on chromosome 16p13. The *TSC1* gene encodes a protein called *hamartin,* while the *TSC2* gene encodes the protein *tuberin.* Within a cell, these 2 proteins bind to one another and work together. Consequently, a mutation in either the *TSC1* gene or the *TSC2* gene results in a similar disease in patients. The *TSC1* and *TSC2* genes are tumor-suppressor genes. The loss of either tuberin or hamartin protein results in the formation of numerous benign tumors (hamartomas). Tuberin and hamartin are involved in a key pathway in the cell that regulates protein synthesis and cell size. One of the ways cells regulate their growth is by controlling the rate of protein synthesis. A protein called mTOR (mammalian target of rapamycin) was identified as one of the master regulators of cell growth. mTOR, in turn, is controlled by rheb, a small cytoplasmic guanosine triphosphatase. When rheb is activated, the protein synthesis machinery is turned on, most likely via mTOR, and the cell grows in size. Of interest in TSC, rheb is activated by the protein complex formed by hamartin and tuberin.

TSC is an extremely heterogeneous disease with a wide clinical spectrum varying from severe intellectual disability and intractable epilepsy to normal intelligence and a lack of seizures; this variation is often seen within the same family, thus with individuals carrying the same mutation. The disease affects many organ systems other than the skin and brain, including the heart, kidney, eyes, lungs, and bone (Fig. 596-5).

CLINICAL MANIFESTATIONS AND DIAGNOSIS
Definite TSC is diagnosed when at least 2 major or one major plus 2 minor features are present (Tables 596-3 and 596-4 list the major and minor features).

The hallmark of TSC is the involvement of the central nervous system. Retinal lesions consist of two types: hamartomas (elevated mulberry lesions or plaque-like lesions; Fig. 596-6) and white depigmented patches (similar to the hypopigmented skin lesions). The characteristic brain lesion is a cortical tuber (Fig. 596-7). Brain MRI is the best way of identifying cortical tubers, which can form before birth.

Subependymal nodules are lesions found along the wall of the lateral ventricles where they undergo calcification and project into the ventricular cavity, producing a candle-dripping appearance. These lesions do not cause any problems; however, in 5-10% of cases, these benign lesions can grow into subependymal giant cell astrocytomas (SEGAs). These tumors can grow and block the circulation of cerebrospinal fluid around the brain and cause hydrocephalus, which requires immediate neurosurgical intervention. Thus, it is recommended that all asymptomatic TSC patients undergo brain MRI every 1-3 yr to monitor for new occurrence of SEGA. Patients with large or growing SEGA, or with SEGA causing ventricular enlargement but yet are still asymptomatic, should undergo MRI scans more frequently and the patients and their families should be educated regarding the potential of new symptoms due to increased intracranial pressure. Surgical resection should be performed for acutely symptomatic SEGA. For growing but otherwise asymptomatic SEGA, either surgical resection or medical treatment with an mTOR inhibitor may be used. Presymptomatic treatment with everolimus is effective in slowing the growth or even reducing the size of SEGAs. Everolimus is also effective in treating refractory seizures and reducing the volume of renal angiomyolipomas and lymphangioleiomyomatosis as well as facial angiofibromas.

The most common neurologic manifestations of TSC consist of epilepsy, cognitive impairment, and autism spectrum disorders. TSC may present during infancy with infantile spasms and a hypsarrhythmic electroencephalogram pattern. However, it is important to remember

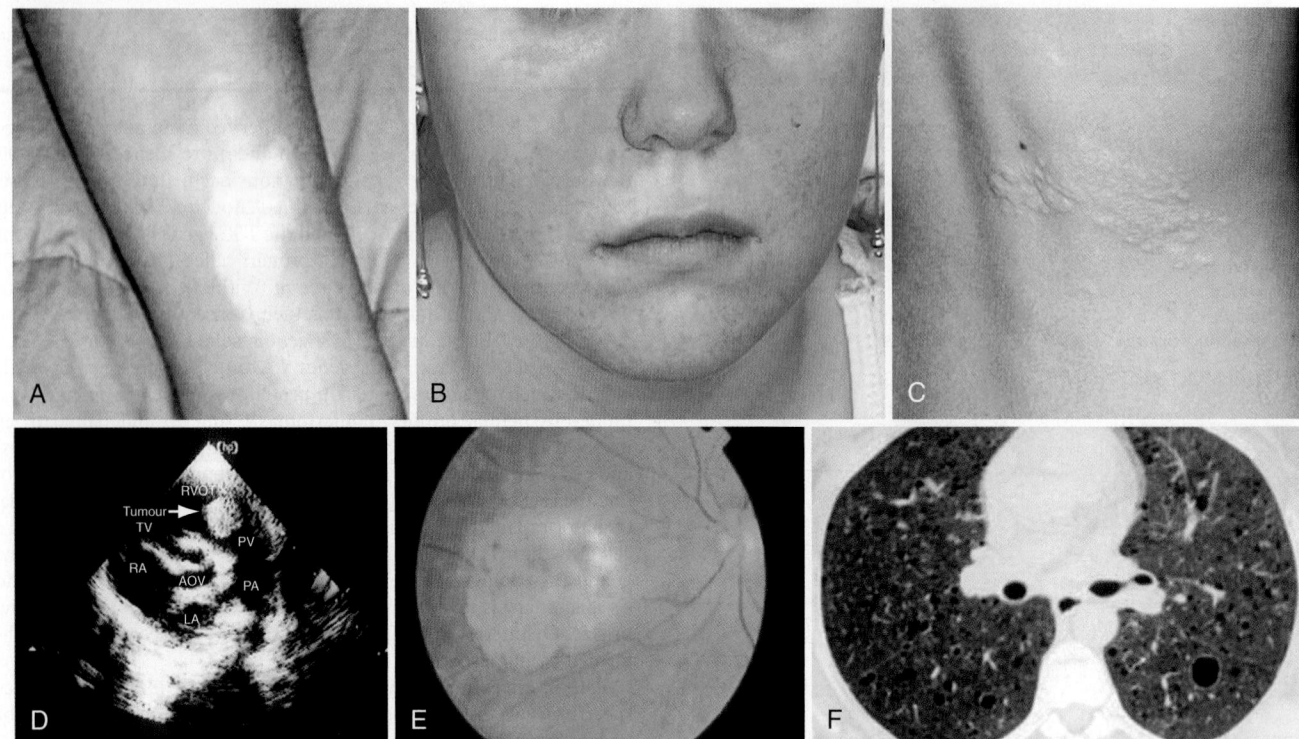

Figure 596-5 Dermatologic, cardiac, and pulmonary manifestations of tuberous sclerosis. **A,** Hypomelanotic macules. **B,** Facial angiofibromas. **C,** Shagreen patch. **D,** Hyperechoic rhabdomyoma detected by echocardiography. **E,** Retinal hamartoma. **F,** Lymphangioleiomyomatosis. *(From Curatolo P, Bombardieri R, Jozwiak S: Tuberous sclerosis, Lancet 372:657–668, 2008, Fig. 7.)*

Table 596-3	Major Features of TSC

Cortical tuber
Subependymal nodule
Subependymal giant cell astrocytoma
Facial angiofibroma or forehead plaque
Ungual or periungual fibroma (non-traumatic)
Hypomelanotic macules (>3)
Shagreen patch
Multiple retinal hamartomas
Cardiac rhabdomyoma
Renal angiomyolipoma
Pulmonary lymphangioleiomyomatosis

Table 596-4	Minor Features of TSC

Cerebral white matter migration lines
Multiple dental pits
Gingival fibromas
Bone cysts
Retinal achromatic patch
Confetti skin lesions
Nonrenal hamartomas
Multiple renal cysts
Hamartomatous rectal polyps

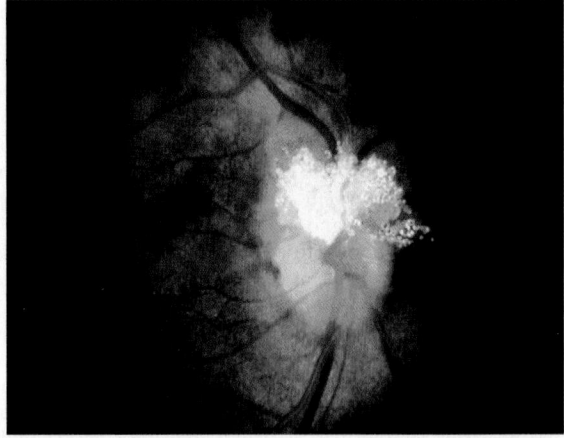

Figure 596-6 A mulberry lesion involving the superior part of the optic nerve in a patient with tuberous sclerosis. *(From Yanoff M, Sassani JW: Ocular pathology, ed 7, Philadelphia, 2015, WB Saunders, Fig. 2-7.)*

SKIN LESIONS

More than 90% of patients show the typical hypomelanotic macules that have been likened to an ash leaf on the trunk and extremities. Visualization of the hypomelanotic macule is enhanced by the use of a Wood ultraviolet lamp (see Chapter 653). To count as a major feature, at least three hypomelanotic macules must be present (see Fig. 596-5). Facial angiofibromas develop between 4 and 6 yr of age; they appear as tiny red nodules over the nose and cheeks and are sometimes confused with acne (see Fig. 596-5). Later, they enlarge, coalesce, and assume a fleshy appearance. A shagreen patch is also characteristic of TSC and consists of a roughened, raised lesion with an orange-peel consistency located primarily in the lumbosacral region (see Fig. 596-5). During adolescence or later, small fibromas or nodules

that you can have infantile spasms without hypsarrhythmia in TSC patients. The seizures may be difficult to control and, at a later age, they may develop into myoclonic epilepsy (see Chapter 593). Vigabatrin is the first-line therapy for infantile spasms. ACTH can be used if treatment with vigabatrin fails. Anticonvulsant therapy of other seizure types in TSC should generally follow that of other epilepsies, and epilepsy surgery should be considered for medically refractory TSC patients.

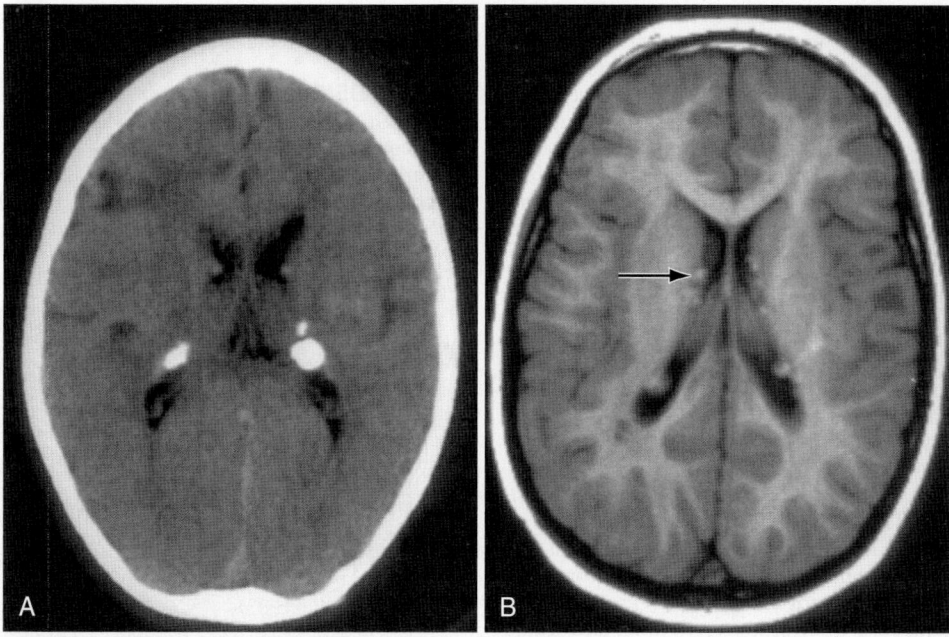

Figure 596-7 Tuberous sclerosis. **A,** CT scan with subependymal calcifications characteristic of tuberous sclerosis. **B,** The MRI demonstrates multiple subependymal nodules in the same patient *(black arrow)*. Parenchymal tubers are also visible on both the CT and the MRI scan as low-density areas in the brain parenchyma.

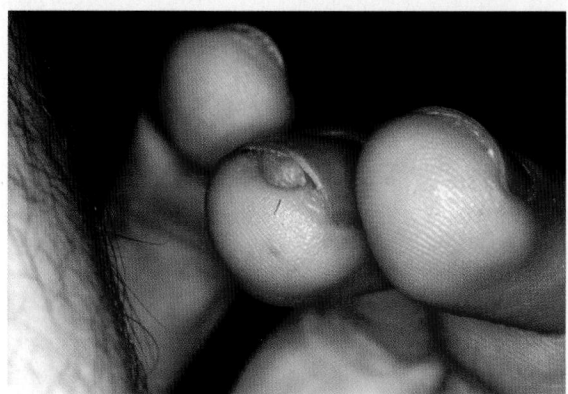

Figure 596-8 Periungual fibroma in a patient tuberous sclerosis complex (TSC).

of skin may form around fingernails or toenails in 15-20% of the TSC patients (Fig. 596-8).

OTHER ORGAN INVOLVEMENT

Approximately 50% of children with TSC have cardiac rhabdomyomas, which may be detected in the fetus at by an echocardiogram. The rhabdomyomas may be numerous or located at the apex of the left ventricle, and although they can cause congestive heart failure and arrhythmias in a minority of patients, they tend to slowly resolve spontaneously. In 75-80% of patients older than 10 yr of age, the kidneys display angiomyolipomas that are usually benign tumors. Angiomyolipomas begin in childhood in many individuals with TSC, but they may not be problematic until young adulthood. By the third decade of life, they may cause lumbar pain and hematuria from slow bleeding, and rarely they may result in sudden retroperitoneal bleeding. Embolization followed by corticosteroids is first-line therapy for angiomyolipoma presenting with acute hemorrhage. Nephrectomy should be avoided. For asymptomatic, growing angiomyolipomas measuring larger than 3 cm in diameter, an mTOR inhibitor, everolimus, is FDA-approved for treatment. Selective embolization or kidney-sparing resection is alternative therapies for asymptomatic angiomyolipoma.

The current recommendation is to follow the angiomyolipoma by yearly imaging, and when the size of the lesion reaches more than 4 cm, to use transcatheter tumor embolization for treatment. Single or multiple renal cysts are also commonly present in TSC. Lymphangioleiomyomatosis is the classical pulmonary lesion in TSC and only affects women after the age of 20 yr.

Diagnosis of TSC relies on a high index of suspicion when assessing a child with infantile spasms. A careful evaluation for the typical skin and retinal lesions should be completed in all patients with a seizure disorder or autism spectrum disorder. Brain MRI confirms the diagnosis in most cases. Genetic testing for *TSC1* and *TSC2* mutations is available and may be considered when the individual patient does not meet all the clinical criteria. Prenatal testing may be offered when a known TSC mutation exists in that family.

MANAGEMENT

As for routine follow-up of individuals with TSC, the following are recommended in addition to physical examination: brain MRI every 1-3 yr, renal imaging (US, CT or MRI) every 1-3 yr and neurodevelopmental testing at the time of beginning 1st grade. Based on the complications of the disease, additional follow-up testing may be required for each individual. Symptoms and signs of increased intracranial pressure suggest obstruction of the foramen of Monro by a SEGA and warrant immediate investigation and surgical intervention.

Bibliography is available at Expert Consult.

596.3 Sturge-Weber Syndrome
Mustafa Sahin

Sturge-Weber syndrome (SWS) is a sporadic vascular disorder and consists of a constellation of symptoms and signs including a facial capillary malformation (port-wine stain), abnormal blood vessels of the brain (leptomeningeal angioma) and abnormal blood vessels of the eye leading to glaucoma. Patients present with seizures, hemiparesis, stroke-like episodes, headaches, and developmental delay. Approximately 1 in 50,000 live births are affected with SWS.

ETIOLOGY

The sporadic incidence and focal nature of SWS suggests the presence of somatic mutations. Whole-genome sequencing from affected and unaffected skin of 3 patients with SWS identified a single-nucleotide variant (c.548G→A, p.Arg183Gln) in the *GNAQ* gene. This mutation has been confirmed in samples of affected tissue from 88% of a larger cohort of SWS patients as well as 92% of the participants with apparently nonsyndromic port-wine stains. Brain tissue from SWS patients also demonstrated the same change in the *GNAQ* gene. These results strongly suggest that SWS occurs as a result of mosaic mutations in *GNAQ*.

The condition is thought to result from anomalous development of the embryonic vascular bed in the early stages of facial and cerebral development. There are hypotheses about aberrant sympathetic innervation, increased vascular growth factors and defects in extracellular matrix, but these remain to be tested. Low flow angiomatosis of the leptomeninges appears to result in a chronic hypoxic state leading to cortical atrophy and calcifications.

CLINICAL MANIFESTATIONS

The facial port-wine stain is present at birth, tends to be unilateral, and always involves the upper face and eyelid, in a distribution consistent with the ophthalmic division of the trigeminal nerve (Fig. 596-9). The capillary malformation may also be evident over the lower face, trunk, and in the mucosa of the mouth and pharynx. It is important to note that not all children with facial port-wine stain have SWS even though the genetic defect appears to be the same. In fact, the overall incidence of SWS has been reported to be 8-33% in those with a port-wine stain. Buphthalmos and glaucoma of the ipsilateral eye are common complications. The incidence of epilepsy in patients with SWS is 75-90%, and seizures develop in most patients in the 1st yr of life. They are typically focal tonic–clonic and contralateral to the side of the facial capillary malformation. The seizures may become refractory to anticonvulsants and are associated with a slowly progressive hemiparesis in many cases. Transient stroke-like episodes or visual defects persisting for several days and unrelated to seizure activity are common and probably result from thrombosis of cortical veins in the affected region. Although neurodevelopment appears to be normal in the 1st yr of life, intellectual disability or severe learning disabilities are present in at least 50% in later childhood, probably the result of intractable epilepsy and increasing cerebral atrophy.

DIAGNOSIS

MRI with contrast is the imaging modality of choice for demonstrating the leptomeningeal angioma in SWS (Fig. 596-10). White matter abnormalities are common and are thought to be a result of chronic hypoxia. Often, atrophy is noted ipsilateral to the leptomeningeal angiomatosis. Calcifications can be seen best with a head CT (Fig. 596-11).

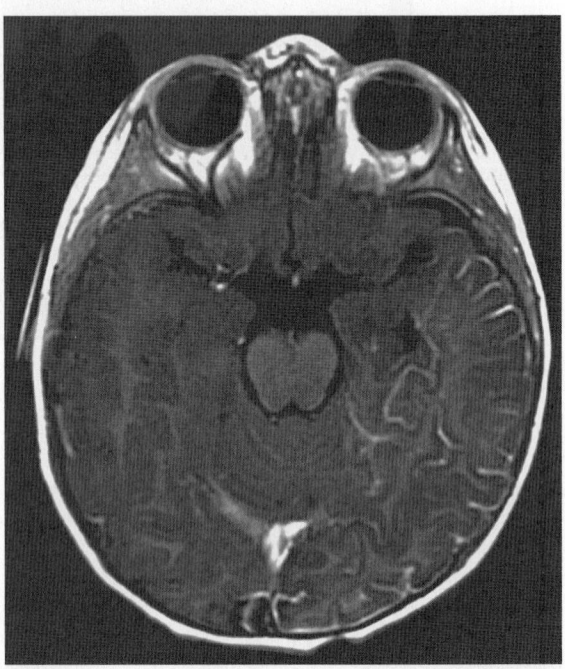

Figure 596-10 Gadolinium-enhanced axial T1 fluid-attenuated inversion recovery (FLAIR) images of a 15 mo old with Sturge-Weber syndrome shows leptomeningeal enhancement in left hemisphere.

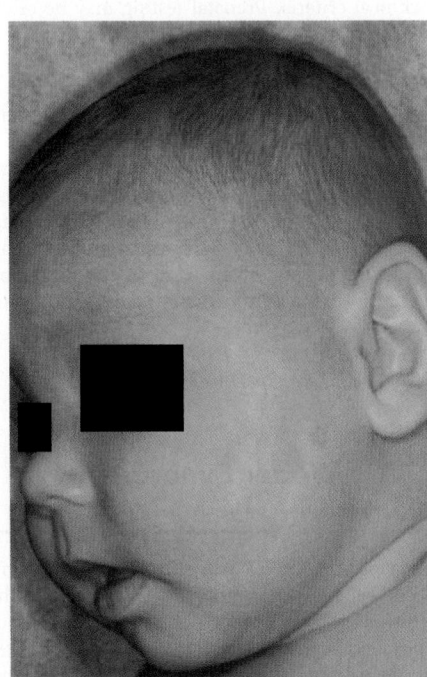

Figure 596-9 Port-wine stain involving both V1 and V2 dermatomes. *(Courtesy of Dr. Anne W. Lucky, Cincinnati Children's Hospital.)*

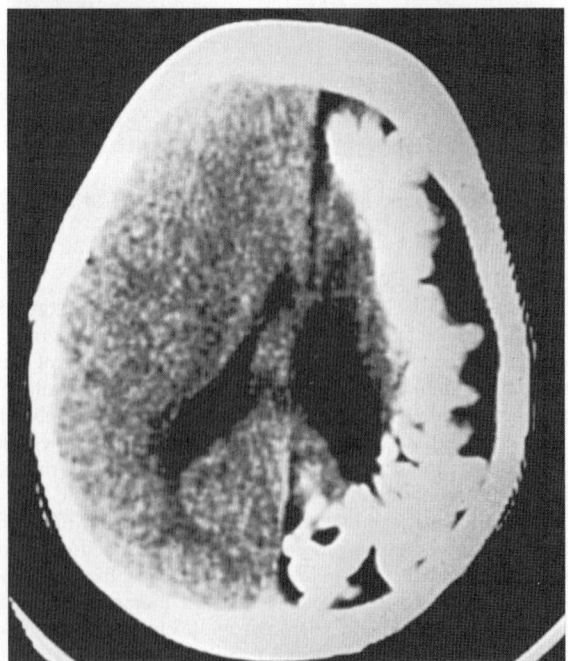

Figure 596-11 CT scan of a patient with Sturge-Weber syndrome showing unilateral calcification and underlying atrophy of a cerebral hemisphere.

Ophthalmologic evaluation examining for glaucoma is also necessary. Based on the involvement of the brain and the face, there are 3 types of SWS according to the Roach Scale:
1. Type I—Both facial and leptomeningeal angiomas; may have glaucoma
2. Type II—Facial angioma alone (no central nervous system involvement); may have glaucoma
3. Type III—Isolated leptomeningeal angiomas; usually no glaucoma

MANAGEMENT

Management of SWS is symptomatic and multidisciplinary but not well studied by prospective studies. It is aimed at seizure control, treatment of headaches, and prevention of stroke-like episodes, as well as monitoring of glaucoma and laser therapy for the cutaneous capillary malformations. Seizures beginning in infancy are not always associated with a poor neurodevelopmental outcome. For patients with well-controlled seizures and normal or near-normal development, management consists of anticonvulsants and surveillance for complications including glaucoma, buphthalmos, and behavioral abnormalities. If the seizures are refractory to anticonvulsant therapy, especially in infancy and the 1st 1-2 yr, and arise from primarily 1 hemisphere, most medical centers advise a hemispherectomy. Because of the risk of glaucoma, regular measurement of intraocular pressure is indicated. The facial port-wine stain is often a target of ridicule by classmates, leading to psychologic trauma. Pulsed-dye laser therapy often provides excellent clearing of the port-wine stain, particularly if it is located on the forehead.

Bibliography is available at Expert Consult.

596.4 Von Hippel-Lindau Disease
Mustafa Sahin

von Hippel-Lindau disease affects many organs, including the cerebellum, spinal cord, retina, kidney, pancreas, and epididymis. Its incidence is around 1 in 36,000 newborns. It results from an autosomal-dominant mutation affecting a tumor suppressor gene, *VHL*. Approximately 80% of individuals with von Hippel-Lindau syndrome have an affected parent, and approximately 20% have a de novo gene mutation. Molecular testing is available and detects mutations in almost 100% of probands.

The major neurologic features of the condition include cerebellar hemangioblastomas and retinal angiomas. Patients with cerebellar hemangioblastoma present in early adult life with symptoms and signs of increased intracranial pressure. A smaller number of patients have hemangioblastoma of the spinal cord, producing abnormalities of proprioception and disturbances of gait and bladder dysfunction. A CT or MRI scan typically shows a cystic cerebellar lesion with a vascular mural nodule. Total surgical removal of the tumor is curative.

Approximately 25% of patients with cerebellar hemangioblastoma have retinal angiomas. Retinal angiomas are characterized by small masses of thin-walled capillaries that are fed by large and tortuous arterioles and venules. They are usually located in the peripheral retina so that vision is unaffected. Exudation in the region of the angiomas may lead to retinal detachment and visual loss. Retinal angiomas are treated with photocoagulation and cryocoagulation, and both have produced good results.

Cystic lesions of the kidneys, pancreas, liver, and epididymis as well as pheochromocytoma are frequently associated with von Hippel-Lindau disease. Renal carcinoma is the most common cause of death. Regular follow-up and appropriate imaging studies are necessary to identify lesions that may be treated at an early stage.

Bibliography is available at Expert Consult.

596.5 Linear Nevus Syndrome
Mustafa Sahin

This sporadic condition is characterized by a facial nevus and neurodevelopmental abnormalities. The nevus is located on the forehead and nose and tends to be midline in its distribution. It may be quite faint during infancy but later becomes hyperkeratotic, with a yellow-brown appearance. Two thirds of the patients with linear nevus syndrome demonstrate associated neurologic findings, including cortical dysplasia, glial hamartomas, and low-grade gliomas. Cerebral and cranial anomalies, predominantly hemimegalencephaly and enlargement of the lateral ventricles, were reported in 72% of cases. The incidence of epilepsy has been reported as high as 75% and intellectual disability as high as 60%. Focal neurologic signs including hemiparesis and homonymous hemianopia may also be seen.

Bibliography is available at Expert Consult.

596.6 PHACE Syndrome
Mustafa Sahin

See also Chapter 650.

The syndrome denotes *p*osterior fossa malformations, *h*emangiomas, *a*rterial anomalies, *c*oarctation of the aorta and other cardiac defects, and *e*ye abnormalities. It is also referred to as *PHACES syndrome* when ventral developmental defects, including *s*ternal clefting and/or a supraumbilical raphe, are present. Large facial hemangiomas may be associated with a Dandy-Walker malformation, vascular anomalies (coarctation of aorta, aplasia or hypoplastic carotid arteries, aneurysmal carotid dilation, aberrant left subclavian artery), glaucoma, cataracts, microphthalmia, optic nerve hypoplasia, and ventral defects (sternal clefts). The facial hemangioma is typically ipsilateral to the aortic arch. The Dandy-Walker malformation is the most common developmental abnormality of the brain. Other anomalies include hypoplasia or agenesis of the cerebellum, cerebellar vermis, corpus callosum, cerebrum, and septum pellucidum. Cerebrovascular anomalies can result in acquired, progressive vessel stenosis and acute ischemic stroke. According to a case series of 29 children with PHACE syndrome, 44% had language delay, 36% gross motor delay, and 8% fine motor delay; 52% had an abnormal neurologic exam, with speech abnormalities as the most common finding. Overall, there is a female predominance. The underlying pathogenesis of PHACE syndrome remains unknown. Propranolol is starting to be used for treatment of the infantile hemangiomas associated with PHACE syndrome.

Bibliography is available at Expert Consult.

596.7 Incontinentia Pigmenti
Mustafa Sahin

This rare, heritable, multisystem ectodermal disorder features dermatologic, dental, and ocular abnormalities. The phenotype is produced by functional mosaicism caused by random X-inactivation of an X-linked dominant gene that is lethal in males (*IKBKG [inhibitor of kappa B kinase gamma,* previously *NEMO]* gene). The paucity of affected males, the occurrence of female-to-female transmission, and an increased frequency of spontaneous abortions in carrier females support this supposition.

CLINICAL MANIFESTATIONS AND DIAGNOSIS

This disease has 4 phases, not all of which may occur in a given patient. The **1st phase** is evident at birth or in the 1st few wk of life and consists of erythematous linear streaks and plaques of vesicles (Fig. 596-12) that are most pronounced on the limbs and circumferentially

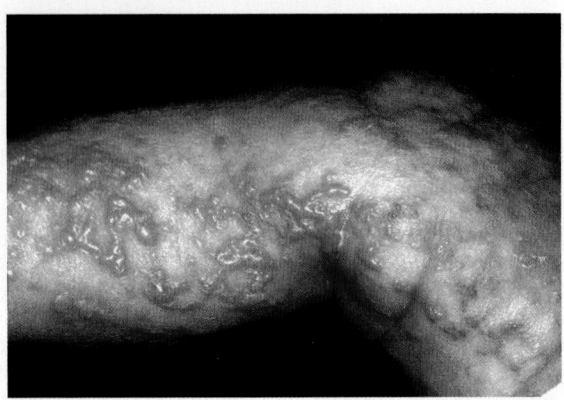

Figure 596-12 Whorled vesicular phase of incontinentia pigmenti.

on the trunk. The lesions may be confused with those of herpes simplex, bullous impetigo, or mastocytosis, but the linear configuration is unique. Histopathologically, epidermal edema and eosinophil-filled intraepidermal vesicles are present. Eosinophils also infiltrate the adjacent epidermis and dermis. Blood eosinophilia as high as 65% of the white blood cell count is common. The **1st stage** generally resolves by 4 mo of age, but mild, short-lived recurrences of blisters may develop during febrile illnesses. In the **2nd phase**, as blisters on the distal limbs resolve, they become dry and hyperkeratotic, forming verrucous plaques. The verrucous plaques rarely affect the trunk or face and generally involute within 6 mo. Epidermal hyperplasia, hyperkeratosis, and papillomatosis are characteristic. The **3rd or pigmentary stage** is the hallmark of incontinentia pigmenti. It generally develops over weeks to months and may overlap the earlier phases, be evident at birth, or, more commonly, begin to appear in the 1st few wk of life. Hyperpigmentation is more often apparent on the trunk than the limbs and is distributed in macular whorls, reticulated patches, flecks, and linear streaks that follow Blaschko lines. The axillae and groin are invariably affected. The sites of involvement are not necessarily those of the preceding vesicular and warty lesions. The pigmented lesions, once present, persist throughout childhood. They generally begin to fade by early adolescence and often disappear by age 16 yr. Occasionally, the pigmentation remains permanently, particularly in the groin. The lesion, histopathologically, shows vacuolar degeneration of the epidermal basal cells and melanin in melanophages of the upper dermis as a result of incontinence of pigment. In the **4th stage**, hairless, anhidrotic, hypopigmented patches or streaks occur as a late manifestation of incontinentia pigmenti; they may develop, however, before the hyperpigmentation of stage 3 has resolved. The lesions develop mainly on the flexor aspect of the lower legs and less often on the arms and trunk.

Approximately 80% of affected children have other defects. Alopecia, which may be scarring and patchy or diffuse, is most common on the vertex and occurs in up to 40% of patients. Hair may be lusterless, wiry, and coarse. Dental anomalies, which are present in up to 80% of patients and are persistent throughout life, consist of late dentition, hypodontia, conical teeth, and impaction. Central nervous system manifestations, including seizures, intellectual disability, hemiplegia, hemiparesis, spasticity, microcephaly, and cerebellar ataxia, are found in up to 30% of affected children. Ocular anomalies, such as neovascularization, microphthalmos, strabismus, optic nerve atrophy, cataracts, and retrolenticular masses, occur in >30% of children. Nonetheless, >90% of patients have normal vision. Less common abnormalities include dystrophy of nails (ridging, pitting) and skeletal defects.

Diagnosis of incontinentia pigmenti is made on clinical grounds, although major and minor criteria have been established to aid in diagnosis. Wood's lamp examination may be useful in older children and adolescents to highlight pigmentary abnormalities. Clinical molecular testing is available, and in 80% of the affected patients a deletion that removes exons 4 through 10 of *IKBKG* gene can be detected. Differential diagnosis includes hypomelanosis of Ito, which presents with similar skin manifestations and is often associated with chromosomal mosaicism.

MANAGEMENT

The choice of investigative studies and the plan of management depend on the occurrence of particular noncutaneous abnormalities since the skin lesions are benign. The high incidence of associated major anomalies warrants genetic counseling.

Bibliography is available at Expert Consult.

Chapter **597**
Movement Disorders
Jonathan W. Mink

Movement disorders are characterized by abnormal or excessive involuntary movements that may result in abnormalities in posture, tone, balance, or fine motor control. Most movement disorders in children are characterized by involuntary movements. These involuntary movements can represent the sole disease manifestation, or they may be one of many signs and symptoms.

Evaluation of movement disorders begins with a comprehensive history and careful neurologic examination. It is often difficult for children and caregivers to describe abnormal movements, which makes observation of the movements by the clinician an essential component of the evaluation. If the movements are not apparent at the time of the examination, video examples from home or school can be invaluable. With the increasing availability of high quality video capability on cellular phones, obtaining a short video is feasible for most families. Resources are available to guide families in gathering useful video data.

There is no specific diagnostic test to differentiate among movement disorders. The category of movement assists in localizing the pathologic process, whereas the onset, age, and degree of abnormal motor activity and associated neurologic findings help organize the investigation.

When considering the type of movement disorder, the following questions concerning the history and examination of the movement are helpful.

- What is the distribution of the movements across body parts?
- Are the movements symmetric?
- What is the speed of the involuntary movements? Are they rapid and fast or slow and sustained?
- When do the movements occur? Are they present at rest? Are they present with maintained posture or with voluntary actions?
- Are the movements seen in relation to certain postures or boy positions?
- Do the abnormal movements occur only with specific tasks?
- Can the child voluntarily suppress the movements, even for a short time?
- Are the movements stereotyped?
- Are the movements rhythmic?
- What is the temporal pattern of the movements? Are they continuous or intermittent? Do they occur in discrete episodes?
- Are the involuntary movements preceded by an urge to make the movement?
- Do the movements persist during sleep?
- Are the movements associated with impairment of motor function?
- What factors aggravated or alleviate the movements?

Table 597-1	Selected Types of Involuntary Movement in Childhood
TYPE	**CHARACTERISTICS**
Stereotypies (see Chapter 24)	Involuntary, patterned, coordinated, repetitive, rhythmic movements that occur in the same fashion with each repetition
Tics (see Chapter 24)	Involuntary, sudden, rapid, abrupt, repetitive, nonrhythmic, simple or complex motor movements or vocalizations (phonic productions). Tics are usually preceded by an urge that is relieved by carrying out the movement
Tremor	Oscillating, rhythmic movements about a fixed point, axis, or plane
Dystonia (see Chapter 597.3)	Intermittent and sustained involuntary muscles contractions that produce abnormal postures and movements of different parts of the body, often with a twisting quality
Chorea (see Chapter 597.2)	Involuntary, continual, irregular movements or movement fragments with variable rate and direction that occur unpredictably and randomly
Ballism	Involuntary, high amplitude, flinging movements typically occurring proximally. Ballism is essentially a large amplitude chorea
Athetosis	Slow, writhing, continuous, involuntary movements
Myoclonus	Sudden, quick, involuntary muscle jerks

The first decision to be made is whether the movement disorder is "hyperkinetic"(characterized by excessive and involuntary movements) or "hypokinetic" (characterized by slow voluntary movements and a general paucity of movement). Hyperkinetic movement disorders are much more common than hypokinetic disorders in children. Once the category of movement disorder is recognized, etiology can be considered. Clinical history, including birth history, medication/toxin exposure, trauma, infections, family history, progression of the involuntary movements, developmental progress, and behavior should be explored as the underlying cause is established. Table 597-1 lists types and clinical characteristics of selected hyperkinetic movement disorders.

597.1 Ataxias
Denia Ramirez-Montealegre and Jonathan W. Mink

Ataxia is the inability to make smooth, accurate, and coordinated movements, usually because of a dysfunction of the cerebellum, its inputs or outputs, sensory pathways in the posterior columns of the spinal cord, or a combination of these. Ataxias may be generalized or primarily affect gait or the hands and arms or trunk; they may be acute or chronic; acquired or genetic (Tables 597-2 to 597-5).

Signs and symptoms of ataxia include clumsiness, difficulty walking or sitting, falling to 1 side, slurred speech, hypotonia, intention tremor, dizziness, and delayed motor development. Genetic or chronic causes of cerebellar ataxia are often characterized by a long duration of symptoms, a positive family history, muscle weakness and abnormal gait, abnormal tone and strength, abnormal deep tendon reflexes, pes cavus, and sensory defects. Distinguishing ataxia from vestibular dysfunction may be difficult; however, labyrinth disorders are often characterized by severe vertigo, nausea and vomiting, position-induced vertigo, and a severe sense of unsteadiness.

Congenital anomalies of the posterior fossa, including the Dandy-Walker malformation, Chiari malformation, and encephalocele, are prominently associated with ataxia because of their destruction or replacement of the cerebellum (see Chapter 591.9). *MRI is the method of choice for investigating congenital abnormalities of the cerebellum, vermis, and related structures.* **Agenesis of the cerebellar vermis** presents in infancy with generalized hypotonia and decreased deep-tendon reflexes. Delayed motor milestones and truncal ataxia are typical. **Joubert syndrome and related disorders** are autosomal recessive disorders marked by developmental delay, hypotonia, abnormal eye movements, abnormal respirations, and a distinctive malformation of the cerebellum and brainstem that manifests as the "molar tooth sign" on MRI. Mutations in more than 21 different genes are associated with

Joubert syndrome, but only approximately 50% of cases have a demonstrated causal mutation (see Chapter 591).

The major **infectious causes of ataxia** include cerebellar abscess, acute labyrinthitis, and acute cerebellar ataxia. **Acute cerebellar ataxia** occurs primarily in children 1-3 yr of age and is a diagnosis of exclusion. The condition often follows a viral illness, such as varicella virus, coxsackievirus, or echovirus infection by 2-3 wk and is thought to represent an autoimmune response to the viral agent affecting the cerebellum (see Chapters 250, 253, and 603). The onset is sudden, and the truncal ataxia can be so severe that the child is unable to stand or sit. Vomiting may occur initially, but fever and nuchal rigidity are absent. Horizontal nystagmus is evident in approximately 50% of cases and, if the child is able to speak, dysarthria may be impressive. Examination of the cerebrospinal fluid is typically normal at the onset of ataxia but a mild lymphocytic pleocytosis (10-30/mm³) is not unusual. Later in the course, the cerebrospinal fluid protein undergoes a moderate elevation. The ataxia begins to improve in a few weeks but may persist for as long as 3 mo and rarely longer than that. The incidence of acute cerebellar ataxia appears to have declined with increased rates of vaccination against varicella. The prognosis for complete recovery is excellent; a small number have long-term sequelae, including behavioral and speech disorders as well as ataxia and incoordination. **Acute cerebellitis** in contrast is a more severe form of cerebellar ataxia demonstrating abnormal MRI scans, more severe symptoms, and a poorer long-term prognosis. Infectious agents include Epstein-Barr virus, mycoplasma, mumps, and influenza virus, although in many the etiology is unknown; autoimmune cerebellitis may represent some of these unknown cases. Patients may present with ataxia, increased intracranial pressure from obstructive hydrocephalus, headache and fever. **Acute labyrinthitis** may be difficult to differentiate from acute cerebellar ataxia in a toddler. The condition is associated with middle-ear infections and presents with intense vertigo, vomiting, and abnormalities in labyrinthine function.

Toxic causes of ataxia include alcohol, thallium (which is used occasionally in homes as a pesticide), and the anticonvulsants, particularly phenytoin and carbamazepine when serum levels exceed the usual therapeutic range.

Brain tumors (see Chapter 497), including tumors of the cerebellum and frontal lobe, as well as peripheral nervous system neuroblastoma, may present with ataxia. Cerebellar tumors cause ataxia because of direct disruption of cerebellar function or indirectly because of increased intracranial pressure from compression of the fourth ventricle. Frontal lobe tumors may cause ataxia as a consequence of destruction of the association fibers connecting the frontal lobe with the cerebellum or because of increased intracranial pressure. Neuroblastoma (see Chapter 498) may be associated with a paraneoplastic encephalopathy characterized by progressive ataxia, myoclonic jerks,

Table 597-2	Selected Causes of Ataxia in Childhood

CONGENITAL
- Agenesis of vermis of the cerebellum
- Aplasia or dysplasia of the cerebellum
- Basilar impression
- Cerebellar dysplasia with microgyria, macrogyria, or agyria
- Cervical spinal bifida with herniation of the cerebellum (Chiari malformation type 3)
- Chiari malformation
- Dandy-Walker syndrome
- Encephalocele
- Hydrocephalus (progressive)
- Hypoplasia of the cerebellum

DEGENERATIVE AND/OR GENETIC
- Acute intermittent cerebellar ataxia
- Ataxia, retinitis pigmentosa, deafness, vestibular abnormality, and intellectual deterioration
- Ataxia-telangiectasia
- Biemond posterior column ataxia
- Cerebellar ataxia with deafness, anosmia, absent caloric responses, nonreactive pupils, and hyporeflexia
- Cockayne syndrome
- Dentate cerebellar ataxia (dyssynergia cerebellaris progressiva)
- Familial ataxia with macular degeneration
- Friedreich ataxia
- Hereditary cerebellar ataxia, intellectual retardation, choreoathetosis, and eunuchoidism
- Hereditary cerebellar ataxia with myotonia and cataracts
- Hypertrophic interstitial neuritis
- Marie ataxia
- Marinesco-Sjögren syndrome
- Multiple-system atrophy
- Pelizaeus-Merzbacher disease
- Periodic attacks of vertigo, diplopia, and ataxia–autosomal-dominant inheritance
- Posterior and lateral column difficulties, nystagmus, and muscle atrophy
- Progressive cerebellar ataxia and epilepsy
- Ramsay Hunt syndrome (myoclonic seizures and ataxia)
- Roussy-Lévy disease
- Spinocerebellar ataxia (SCA); olivopontocerebellar ataxias
- Vanishing white matter syndrome

ENDOCRINOLOGIC
- Acquired hypothyroidism
- Cretinism

INFECTIOUS, POSTINFECTIOUS, INFLAMMATORY
- Acute cerebellar ataxia
- Acute disseminated encephalomyelitis
- Autoimmune (anti-glutamic acid decarboxylase, anti–γ-aminobutyric acid_B receptor antibodies)
- Cerebellar abscess
- Cerebellitis
- Coxsackievirus
- Diphtheria
- Echovirus
- Fisher syndrome
- Infectious mononucleosis (Epstein-Barr virus infection)
- Infectious polyneuropathy
- Japanese B encephalitis
- Mumps encephalitis
- *Mycoplasma* pneumonia
- Paraneoplastic (opsoclonus-myoclonus-ataxia syndrome)
- Pertussis
- Polio
- Postbacterial meningitis
- Rubeola
- Tuberculosis
- Typhoid
- Varicella

METABOLIC
- Abetalipoproteinemia
- Argininosuccinic aciduria
- Ataxia with vitamin E deficiency (AVED)
- Congenital disorders of glycosylation
- GM$_2$ gangliosidosis (late)
- Hartnup disease
- Hyperalaninemia
- Hyperammonemia I and II (urea cycle defects)
- Hypoglycemia
- Kearns-Sayre syndrome
- Leigh disease
- Maple syrup urine disease (intermittent)
- Myoclonic epilepsy with ragged red fibers (MERRF)
- Metachromatic leukodystrophy
- Mitochondrial complex defects (I, III, IV)
- Multiple carboxylase deficiency (biotinidase deficiency)
- Neuronal ceroid-lipofuscinosis
- Neuropathy, ataxia, retinitis pigmentosa (NARP)
- Niemann-Pick disease (late infantile)
- 5-Oxoprolinuria
- Pyruvate decarboxylase deficiency
- Refsum disease
- Sialidosis
- Triose-phosphate isomerase deficiency
- Tryptophanuria
- Wernicke encephalopathy

NEOPLASTIC
- Frontal lobe tumors
- Hemispheric cerebellar tumors
- Midline cerebellar tumors
- Neuroblastoma
- Pontine tumors (primarily gliomas)
- Spinal cord tumors

PRIMARY PSYCHOGENIC
- Conversion reaction

TOXIC
- Alcohol
- Benzodiazepines
- Carbamazepine
- Clonazepam
- Lead encephalopathy
- Neuroblastoma
- Phenobarbital
- Phenytoin
- Primidone
- Tic paralysis poisoning

TRAUMATIC
- Acute cerebellar edema
- Acute frontal lobe edema

VASCULAR
- Angioblastoma of cerebellum
- Basilar migraine
- Cerebellar embolism
- Cerebellar hemorrhage
- Cerebellar thrombosis
- Posterior cerebellar artery disease
- Vasculitis
- von Hippel-Lindau disease

Modified from Jafar-Nejad P, Maricich SM, Zoghbi HY: The cerebellum and the hereditary ataxias. In Swaiman KF, Ashwal S, Ferriero DM, Schor NF, editors: Swaiman's pediatric neurology, ed 5, Philadelphia, 2012, WB Saunders, Box 67-1.

Table 597-3	Treatable Causes of Inherited Ataxia

DISORDER	METABOLIC ABNORMALITY	DISTINGUISHING CLINICAL FEATURES	TREATMENT
Acute disseminated encephalomyelitis	Demyelination	Positive MRI findings	Steroids, IVIG, rituximab
Ataxia with vitamin E deficiency	Mutation in α-tocopherol transfer protein	Ataxia, areflexia, retinopathy	Vitamin E
Bassen-Kornzweig syndrome	Abetalipoproteinemia	Acanthocytosis, retinitis pigmentosa, fat malabsorption	Vitamin E
Hartnup disease	Tryptophan malabsorption	Pellagra rash, intermittent ataxia	Niacin
Familial episodic ataxia type 1 and type 2	Mutations in potassium channel (KCNA1) and α$_{1A}$ voltage-gated calcium channel, respectively	Episodic attacks, worse with pregnancy or birth control pills	Acetazolamide
Multiple carboxylase deficiency	Biotinidase deficiency	Alopecia, recurrent infections, variable organic aciduria	Biotin
Mitochondrial complex defects	Complexes I, III, IV	Encephalomyelopathy	Possibly riboflavin, CoQ10, dichloroacetate
Opsoclonus-myoclonus-ataxia syndrome	Paraneoplastic or spontaneous autoimmune	Underlying neuroblastoma or autoantibodies	Steroids, IVIG, rituximab
Pyruvate dehydrogenase deficiency	Block in E-M and Krebs cycle interface	Lactic acidosis, ataxia	Ketogenic diet, possibly dichloroacetate
Refsum disease	Phytanic acid, α-hydroxylase	Retinitis pigmentosa, cardiomyopathy, hypertrophic neuropathy, ichthyosis	Dietary restriction of phytanic acid
Urea cycle defects	Urea cycle enzymes	Hyperammonemia	Protein restriction, arginine, benzoate, α-ketoacids

CoQ10, Coenzyme Q10; E-M, mitochondrial electron transport; IVIG, intravenous immunoglobulin.
Modified from Stumpf DA: The inherited ataxias. Pediatr Neurol 1:129-133, 1985, Table 1; and from Jafar-Nejad P, Maricich SM, Zoghbi HY: The cerebellum and the hereditary ataxias. In Swaiman KF, Ashwal S, Ferriero DM, Schor NF, editors: Swaiman's pediatric neurology, ed 5, Philadelphia, 2012, WB Saunders, Table 67-1.

Table 597-4	Autosomal-Recessive Cerebellar Ataxias

ATAXIA	CHROMOSOME	GENE	GENE PRODUCT	MECHANISM	AGE OF ONSET (yr)
Friedreich ataxia	9q13	*X25*	Frataxin	GAA repeat	2-51
Friedreich ataxia 2	9p23–p11	Unknown	Unknown	Unknown	5-20
AVED	8q13	*TTP1*	TTPA	Missense mutation, deletion, insertion	2-52
Ataxia-telangiectasia	11q22.3	*ATM*	ATM	Missense and deletion mutations	Infancy
ATLD	11q21	*hMRE11*	MRE11A	Missense and deletion mutations	9-48 mo
Ataxia-ocular apraxia 1	9p13.3	*APTX*	Aprataxin	Frameshift, missense, nonsense mutations	2-18
SCAR1	9q34	*SETX*	Senataxin	Frameshift, missense, nonsense mutations	9-22
SCAR2	9q34–qter	Unknown	Unknown	Unknown	Congenital
SCAR3	6p23–p21	Unknown	Unknown	Unknown	3-52
SCAR4	1p36	Unknown	Unknown	Unknown	23-39
SCAR5	15q24–q26	Unknown	Unknown	Unknown	1-10
SCAR6	20q11–q13	Unknown	Unknown	Unknown	Infancy
SCAR7	11p15	Unknown	Unknown	Unknown	Childhood
SCAR8	11p15	*SYNE1*	SYNE1	Splice site mutation, nonsense mutations	17-46

Continued

Table 597-4	Autosomal-Recessive Cerebellar Ataxias—cont'd				
ATAXIA	**CHROMOSOME**	**GENE**	**GENE PRODUCT**	**MECHANISM**	**AGE OF ONSET (yr)**
SCAR9	1q41	*ADCK3*	ADCK3	Splice site mutation, missense, nonsense mutations	3-11
Ataxia, Cayman type	19q13.3	*ATCAY*	Caytaxin	Missense mutation	Birth
IOSCA	10q24	*C10orf2*	Twinkle	Missense, silent mutations	9-24 mo
Progressive myoclonic epilepsy	21q22.3	*CST6*	Cystatin B	5' dodecamer repeat	6–13
ARSACS	13q12	*SACS*	Sacsin	Frameshift and nonsense mutations	1–20
Congenital disorders of glycosylation	Multiple	Multiple	Multiple		Birth

ARSACS, autosomal-recessive spastic ataxia of Charlevoix-Saguenay; ATLD, ataxia-telangiectasia-like disorder; AVED, ataxia with vitamin E deficiency; IOSCA, infantile-onset spinocerebellar ataxia; SCAR, spinocerebellar ataxia, autosomal-recessive.

From Jafar-Nejad P, Maricich SM, Zoghbi HY: The cerebellum and the hereditary ataxias. In Swaiman KF, Ashwal S, Ferriero DM, Schor NF, editors: Swaiman's pediatric neurology, ed 5, Philadelphia, 2012, WB Saunders, Table 67-2.

Table 597-5	Autosomal-Dominant Cerebellar Ataxias							
ATAXIA	**CHROMOSOME**	**GENE**	**GENE PRODUCT**	**MECHANISM**	**AGE OF ONSET (yr)**	**NORMAL REPEAT**	**EXPANDED REPEAT**	**DURATION OF EPISODES**
POLYGLUTAMINE EXPANSION								
SCA1	6p23	*SCA1*	Ataxin-1	CAG repeat	6-60	6-44*	39-82*	
SCA2	12q24	*SCA2*	Ataxin-2	CAG repeat	2-65	15-24	35-59	
SCA3/MJD	14q24.3-q31	*MJD1*	Ataxin-3	CAG repeat	11-70	13-47*	45-84*	
SCA6	19q13	*CACNA1A*	CACNA1A	CAG repeat	16-v73	4-20	21-33	
SCA7	3p21.1-p12	*SCA7*	Ataxin-7	CAG repeat	Birth-53	4-35	37-460	
SCA17	6q27	*SCA17*	TBP	CAG repeat	3-48	25-42	45-66	
DRPLA	12p13.31	*DRPLA*	Atrophin-1	CAG repeat	4-55 mo	7-34	53-93	
NONCODING EXPANSION								
SCA8	13q21	*SCA8*	SCA8 RNA	CTG repeat in 3' UTR	18-72	2-91*	110-155*	
SCA10	22q13	*SCA10*	Ataxin-10	ATTCT repeat in intron 9	14-45	10-29	750-4500	
SCA12	5q31-q33	*SCA12*	P2R2B	CAG repeat in 5' UTR	8-55	7-32	55-78	
SCA31	16q22.1	*BEAN/TK2*	BEAN/TK2	TGGAA repeat insertion in intron of BEAN and TK	45-72	Rarely (0.23%) 1.5-2.0 kb	2.5-3.8 kb	
OTHER MUTATIONS								
SCA14	19q13.4	*PKC-γ*	PKC-γ	Missense mutation	10-69			
SCA27	13q34	*FGF14*	FGF14	Fibroblast growth factor deficiency	15-20			
SCA5	11p11-q11	*SPTBN2*	β-3 spectrin	Deletion, missense mutations	10-68			
SCA11	15q14-q21.3	*TTBK2*	TTBK2	Truncation mutation	15-43			
SCA13	19q13.3-q13.4	*KCNC3*	KCNC3	Missense mutations	<1-60			
SCA15	3p24.2-3pter	*ITPR1*	ITPR1	Deletion, missense mutation	Child–adult			
SCA28	18p11.22-q11.2.	*AFG3L2*	AFG3L2	Missense mutations	12-36			

| Table 597-5 | Autosomal-Dominant Cerebellar Ataxias—cont'd |

ATAXIA	CHROMOSOME	GENE	GENE PRODUCT	MECHANISM	AGE OF ONSET (yr)	NORMAL REPEAT	EXPANDED REPEAT	DURATION OF EPISODES
MUTATION UNKNOWN								
SCA4	16q22	Unknown	Unknown	Unknown	19-59			
SCA18/SMNA	7q31-q32	Unknown	Unknown	Unknown	12-25			
SCA19	1p21-q21	Unknown	Unknown	Unknown	10-45			
SCA20	11	Unknown	Unknown	Unknown	19-64			
SCA21	7p21.3–p15.1	Unknown	Unknown	Unknown	6-30			
SCA22	1p21-q23	Unknown	Unknown	Unknown	10-46			
SCA23	20p13-p12.2	Unknown	Unknown	Unknown	43-56			
SCA25	2p	Unknown	Unknown	Unknown	1.5-39			
SCA26	19p13.3	Unknown	Unknown	Unknown	26-60			
SCA30	4q34.3-q35.1	Unknown	Unknown	Unknown	45-76			
SAX1	12p13	Unknown	Unknown	Unknown	Early childhood to early 20s			
SPAR	Unknown	Unknown	Unknown	Unknown	15-35			
EPISODIC ATAXIA								
EA1	12p13	*EA1*	KCNA1	Channelopathy	Early childhood			Secs to mins
EA2/FHM	19p13	*CACNA1A*	CACNA1A	Channelopathy: missense and nonsense mutations	4-30			Hours
EA3	1q42	Unknown	Unknown	Unknown	1-42			1 min to 6 h
EA4	Unknown	Unknown	Unknown	Unknown	23-42			Short to constant
EA5	2q22-q23	*CACNB4*	CACNB4	Channelopathy: missense and nonsense mutations	Juvenile			Hours
EA6	5p13	*SLC1A3*	EAAT1	Missense mutation	5			Hours to days
EA7	19q13	Unknown	Unknown	Unknown	<20			Hours to days

*Some overlap of pathogenic and nonpathogenic repeat length.

DRPLA, dentatorubral-pallidoluysian atrophy; EA, episodic ataxia; FHM, familial hemiplegic migraine; MJD, Machado-Joseph disease; SAX, spastic ataxia; SCA, spinocerebellar ataxia; SMNA, sensorimotor neuropathy with ataxia; SPAR, spastic paraplegia, ataxia, and mental retardation; TBP, TATA-binding protein; UTR, untranslated region.

From Jafar-Nejad P, Maricich SM, Zoghbi HY: The cerebellum and the hereditary ataxias. In Swaiman KF, Ashwal S, Ferriero DM, Schor NF, editors: Swaiman's pediatric neurology, ed 5, Philadelphia, 2012, WB Saunders, Table 67-3.

and opsoclonus (nonrhythmic, conjugate horizontal and vertical oscillations of the eyes).

Several **metabolic disorders** are characterized by ataxia, including abetalipoproteinemia, arginosuccinic aciduria, and Hartnup disease. **Abetalipoproteinemia** (Bassen-Kornzweig disease) begins in childhood with steatorrhea and failure to thrive (see Chapters 86.3 and 600). A blood smear shows acanthocytosis. Serum chemistries reveal decreased levels of cholesterol and triglycerides; serum β-lipoproteins are absent. Neurologic signs become evident by late childhood and consist of ataxia, retinitis pigmentosa, peripheral neuritis, abnormalities of position and vibration sense, muscle weakness, and intellectual disability. Vitamin E is undetectable in the serum of patients with neurologic symptoms.

Degenerative diseases of the central nervous system represent an important group of ataxic disorders of childhood because of the genetic consequences and poor prognosis. **Ataxia-telangiectasia,** an autosomal recessive condition, is the most common of the degenerative ataxias and is heralded by ataxia beginning at approximately age 2 yr and progressing to loss of ambulation by adolescence. Ataxia-telangiectasia is caused by mutations in the *ATM* gene located at 11q22-q23. ATM is a phosphytidylinositol-3 kinase that phosphorylates proteins involved in DNA repair and cell-cycle control. Oculomotor apraxia of horizontal gaze, defined as difficulty shifting gaze from one object to another and overshooting the target with lateral movement of the head, followed by refixating the eyes, is a frequent finding, as is strabismus, hypometric saccade pursuit abnormalities, and

nystagmus. Ataxia-telangiectasia may present with chorea (see Chapter 597.2) rather than ataxia. The telangiectasia becomes evident by midchildhood and is found on the bulbar conjunctiva, over the bridge of the nose, and on the ears and exposed surfaces of the extremities. Examination of the skin shows a loss of elasticity. Abnormalities of immunologic function that lead to frequent sinopulmonary infections include decreased serum and secretory immunoglobulin (Ig) A as well as diminished IgG$_2$, IgG$_4$, and IgE levels in more than 50% of patients. Children with ataxia-telangiectasia have a 50-100–fold increased risk of developing lymphoreticular tumors (lymphoma, leukemia, and Hodgkin disease) as well as brain tumors. Additional laboratory abnormalities include an increased incidence of chromosome breaks, particularly of chromosome 14, and elevated levels of α-fetoprotein. Death results from infection or tumor dissemination.

Friedreich ataxia is inherited as an autosomal-recessive disorder involving the spinocerebellar tracts, dorsal columns in the spinal cord, the pyramidal tracts, and the cerebellum and medulla. The majority of patients are homozygous for a GAA repeat expansion in the noncoding region of the gene coding for the mitochondrial protein frataxin. Mutations cause oxidative injury associated with excessive iron deposits in mitochondria. The onset of ataxia is somewhat later than in ataxia-telangiectasia, but usually occurs before age 10 yr. The ataxia is slowly progressive and involves the lower extremities to a greater degree than the upper extremities. The Romberg test result is positive; the deep-tendon reflexes are absent (particularly at the ankle), and the plantar response is typically extensor (Babinski sign). Patients develop a characteristic explosive, dysarthric speech, and nystagmus is present in most children. Although patients may appear apathetic, their intelligence is preserved. They may have significant weakness of the distal musculature of the hands and feet. Marked loss of vibration and joint position sense is common and is caused by degeneration of the posterior columns. Friedreich ataxia is also characterized by skeletal abnormalities, including high-arched feet (pes cavus) and hammertoes, as well as progressive kyphoscoliosis. Results of electrophysiologic studies, including visual, auditory brainstem, and somatosensory-evoked potentials, are often abnormal. Hypertrophic cardiomyopathy with progression to intractable congestive heart failure is the cause of death for most patients.

Several forms of **spinocerebellar ataxia** are similar to Friedreich ataxia but are less common. **Roussy-Levy disease** has, in addition to ataxia, atrophy of the muscles of the lower extremity with a pattern of wasting similar to that observed in Charcot-Marie-Tooth disease; **Ramsay Hunt syndrome** has an associated myoclonic epilepsy.

There are more than 20 dominantly inherited spinocerebellar ataxias, some of which present in childhood. These include those associated with CAG (polyglutamine) repeats and noncoding microsatellite expansions. Dominantly inherited episodic ataxias caused by potassium or calcium channel dysfunction present as episodes of ataxia and muscle weakness. Some of these disorders may respond to acetazolamide. The dominantly inherited **olivopontocerebellar atrophies** include ataxia, cranial nerve palsies, and abnormal sensory findings in the 2nd or 3rd decade, but can present in children with rapidly progressive ataxia, nystagmus, dysarthria, and seizures.

Additional degenerative ataxias include **Pelizaeus-Merzbacher disease, neuronal ceroid lipofuscinoses,** and late-onset **GM₂ gangliosidosis** (see Chapters 86.4 and 600). Rare forms of progressive cerebellar ataxia have been described in association with **vitamin E deficiency.** A number of autosomal-dominant progressive spinocerebellar ataxias have been defined at the molecular level, including those caused by unstable trinucleotide repeat expansions.

597.2 Chorea, Athetosis, Tremor
Rebecca K. Lehman and Jonathan W. Mink

Chorea, meaning "dance-like" in Greek, refers to rapid, chaotic movements that seem to flow from 1 body part to another. Affected individuals exhibit motor impersistence, with difficulty keeping the tongue protruded ("darting tongue") or maintaining grip ("milkmaid grip"). Chorea tends to occur both at rest and with action. Patients often attempt to incorporate the involuntary movements into more purposeful movements, making them appear fidgety. *Chorea increases with stress and disappears in sleep.* Chorea can be divided into primary (i.e., disorders in which chorea is the dominant symptom and the etiology is presumed to be genetic) and secondary forms, with the vast majority of pediatric cases falling into the latter category (Tables 597-6 and 597-7).

Sydenham chorea (St. Vitus dance) is the most common acquired chorea of childhood. It occurs in 10-20% of patients with **acute rheumatic fever,** typically weeks to months after a group A β-hemolytic streptococcal infection (see Chapter 183.1). Peak incidence is at age 8-9 yr, with a female predominance of 2:1. There is evidence that group A β-hemolytic streptococci promote the generation of cross-reactive or polyreactive antibodies through molecular mimicry between streptococcal and host antigens. Specifically, antibodies against the *N*-acetyl-β-D-glucosamine epitope (GlcNAc) of streptococcal group A carbohydrate target intracellular β-tubulin and extracellular lysoganglioside GM₁ in human caudate-putamen preparations. These antibodies are also capable of directing calcium/calmodulin–dependent protein kinase II activation, which may cause the neurologic manifestations of Sydenham chorea by increasing dopamine release into the synapse.

The clinical hallmarks of Sydenham chorea are chorea, hypotonia, and emotional lability. Onset of the chorea is usually insidious but may

Table 597-6	Etiologic Classification of Choreic Syndromes

GENETIC CHOREAS
Huntington disease (rarely presents with chorea in childhood)
Huntington disease–like 2 and other Huntington disease –like syndromes
Dentatorubropallidoluysian atrophy
Neuroacanthocytosis
Leigh syndrome and other mitochondrial disorders
Ataxia telangiectasia
Benign hereditary chorea
Wilson disease
Spinocerebellar ataxia (types 2, 3, or 17)
Pantothene kinase–associated neurodegeneration (PKAN)
Paroxysmal kinesigenic choreoathetosis
Paroxysmal nonkinesigenic choreoathetosis
Fahr syndrome
Rett syndrome

STRUCTURAL BASAL-GANGLIA LESIONS
Vascular chorea in stroke, vasculitis, Moyamoya disease
Mass lesions (e.g., central nervous system lymphoma, metastatic brain tumors)
Joubert syndrome and related disorders
Multiple sclerosis plaques
Extrapontine myelinolysis
Trauma

PARAINFECTIOUS AND AUTOIMMUNE DISORDERS
Sydenham chorea
Systemic lupus erythematosus
Chorea gravidarum
Antiphospholipid antibody syndrome
Postinfectious or postvaccinal encephalitis
Anti-N-methyl-D-aspartate (NMDA)–receptor antibody syndrome (Limbic encephalitis)
Paraneoplastic choreas

INFECTIOUS CHOREA
HIV encephalopathy
Toxoplasmosis
Cysticercosis
Diphtheria
Bacterial endocarditis
Neurosyphilis
Scarlet fever
Viral encephalitis (mumps, measles, varicella)

METABOLIC DRUG OR TOXIC ENCEPHALOPATHIES
Acute intermittent porphyria
Hypo-/hypernatremia
Hypocalcemia
Hyperthyroidism
Hypoparathyroidism
Hepatic/renal failure
Carbon monoxide poisoning
Manganese poisoning
Mercury poisoning
Organophosphate poisoning
Pheochromocytoma

DRUG-INDUCED CHOREA (see Table 597-8)

Modified from Cardoso F, Seppi K, Mair KJ, et al: Seminar on choreas, Lancet Neurol 5:589–602, 2006.

be abrupt. Most patients have generalized chorea but the majority have asymmetric manifestations and up to 20% have hemichorea. Hypotonia manifests with the "pronator sign" (arms and palms turn outward when held overhead) and the "choreic hand" (spooning of the extended hand by flexion of the wrist and extension of the fingers). When chorea and hypotonia are severe, the child may be incapable of feeding, dressing, or walking without assistance. Speech is often involved, sometimes to the point of being unintelligible. Periods of uncontrollable crying and extreme mood swings are characteristic and may precede the onset of the movement disorder.

Table 597-7	Genetic Choreas				
	MODE OF INHERITANCE	**GENE, LOCATION**	**PROTEIN PRODUCT**	**USUAL AGE AT ONSET (yr)**	**CLINICAL SIGNS**
HDL2*	AD†	*JPH3*, 16q	Junctophilin-3	20-40	Huntington disease phenotype, sometimes acanthocytosis; almost exclusively African ethnicity
SCA17	AD†	*TBP*, 6q	TBP	10-30	Cerebellar ataxia, chorea, dystonia, hyperreflexia, cognitive decline
DRPLA	AD†	*DRPLA*, 12p	Atrophin-1	About 20	Variable phenotypic picture including chorea, ataxia, seizures, psychiatric disturbances, dementia; more common in Japan than in Europe or United States
SCA3/MJD	AD†	*MJD*, 14q	Ataxin-3	35-40	Wide phenotypic variability with cerebellar ataxia, protruded eyes, chorea, dystonia, parkinsonian features, neuropathy, pyramidal tract features
SCA2	AD†	*Ataxin-2*, 12q	Ataxin-2	30-35	Cerebellar ataxia, chorea, markedly reduced velocity of saccadic eye movements, hyporeflexia
Chorea-acanthocytosis	AR	*VPS13A* (formerly *CHAC*), 9q	Chorein	20-50	Orofacial self-mutilation, dystonia, neuropathy, myopathy, seizures, acanthocytosis
McLeod syndrome	X-linked, recessive	*XK*, Xp	XK-protein	40-70	Dystonia, neuropathy, myopathy, cardiomyopathy, seizures, acanthocytosis, raised creatine kinase, weak expression of Kell antigen
Neuroferritinopathy	AD	*FTL*, 19q	FTL	20-55	Chorea, dystonia, parkinsonian features; usually reduced serum ferritin; MR abnormalities with cyst formation and increased T2 signal in globus pallidus and putamen
AT and ATLD	AR	*ATM*, 11q (AT) *MRE11*, 11q (ATLD)	ATM (AT) MRE11 (ATLD)	Childhood	Ataxia, neuropathy, oculomotor apraxia, other extrapyramidal manifestations including chorea, dystonia, and myoclonus In AT: oculocutaneous telangiectasias; predisposition to malignancies, IgA and IgG deficiency, high α-fetoprotein in serum and high concentrations of carcinoembryonic antigen
AOA 1 and 2	AR	*APTX*, 9p (AOA 1) *SETX*, 9q (AOA 2)	Aprataxin (AOA 1) Senataxin (AOA 2)	Childhood or adolescence (later onset in AOA 2)	Ataxia, neuropathy, oculomotor apraxia, other extrapyramidal manifestations including chorea and dystonia; ataxia with oculomotor apraxia type 1: hypoalbuminemia and hypercholesterolemia; ataxia with oculomotor apraxia type 2: raised α-fetoprotein in serum
Pantothenate kinase associated neurodegeneration (formerly Hallervorden-Spatz syndrome)	AR	*PANK2*, 20p	Pantothenate kinase 2	Childhood, but also adult-onset subtype	Chorea, dystonia, parkinsonian features, pyramidal tract features; MR abnormalities with decreased T2 signal in the globus pallidus and substantia nigra, "eye of the tiger" sign (hyperintense area within the hypointense area); sometimes acanthocytosis, abnormal cytosomes in lymphocytes

Continued

Table 597-7	Genetic Choreas—cont'd				
	MODE OF INHERITANCE	**GENE, LOCATION**	**PROTEIN PRODUCT**	**USUAL AGE AT ONSET (yr)**	**CLINICAL SIGNS**
Lesch-Nyhan syndrome	X-linked, recessive	*HPRT*, Xq	Hypoxanthine-guanine phosphoribosyl-transferase	Childhood	Chorea, dystonia, hypotonia, self-injurious behavior with biting of fingers and lips, mental retardation; short stature, renal calculi, hyperuricemia
Wilson disease	AR	*ATP7B*, 13q	Copper transporting P-type adenosine triphosphatase (ATPase)	<40	Parkinsonian features, dystonia, tremor, rarely chorea, behavioral and cognitive change, corneal Kayser-Fleischer rings, liver disease
PKC syndrome and ICCA syndrome	AD	Unknown, 16p	Unknown	<1-40	Paroxysmal movement disorders presenting with recurrent brief episodes of abnormal involuntary movements with dramatic response to low-dose carbamazepine (PKC); recurrent brief episodes of abnormal involuntary movements in association with infantile convulsions (ICCA)
Benign hereditary chorea	AD	*TITF-1*, 14q; other	Thyroid transcription factor 1	Childhood	Chorea, mild ataxia; genetically heterogeneous

*HDL1, HDL3, and HDL4 are very rare conditions (only 1 family known) and therefore not included in the table.
†Disorders based on expanded CAG repeats (HDL2 based on CAG/CTG repeats; SCA 17 based on CAG/CAA repeats); age of symptom onset inversely related to repeat size.
AD, autosomal dominant; AOA, ataxia with oculomotor apraxia (types 1 or 2); AR, autosomal recessive; AT, ataxia telangiectasia; ATLD, ataxia telangiectasia–like disorder; DRPLA, dentatorubropallidoluysian atrophy; ICCA, infantile convulsions and paroxysmal choreoathetosis syndrome; MJD, Machado-Joseph disease; PKC, paroxysmal kinesigenic choreoathetosis; SCA, spinocerebellar ataxia (types 2, 3, or 17).
Modified from Cardoso F, Seppi K, Mair KJ, et al: Seminar on choreas, Lancet Neurol 5:589–602, 2006.

Sydenham chorea is a clinical diagnosis; a combination of acute *and* convalescent serum antistreptolysin O titers may help to confirm an acute streptococcal infection. Negative titers do not exclude the diagnosis. All patients with Sydenham chorea should be evaluated for carditis and started on long-term antibiotic prophylaxis (e.g., penicillin G benzathine 1.2 million units IM every 4 wk or penicillin V 250 mg PO twice daily) to decrease the risk of rheumatic heart disease with recurrence. For patients with chorea that is impairing, treatment options include valproate, carbamazepine, and dopamine receptor antagonists. Historically, there have been conflicting data regarding the efficacy of prednisone, intravenous immunoglobulin, and other immunomodulatory agents in Sydenham chorea, making it difficult to recommend their routine use. A more recent randomized, double-blinded study of 37 children with Sydenham chorea compared high-dose prednisone (2 mg/kg/day, max: 60 mg) for 4 wk vs a placebo and found that steroids significantly reduced time to remission (54.3 days vs 119.9 days in controls). There is no evidence that treatment with prednisone alters recurrence rate or long-term outcome.

Sydenham chorea usually resolves spontaneously within 6-9 mo, although it can persist for up to 2 yr and, in rare cases, can remain a lifelong condition. Relapse in the 1st few yr is relatively common, occurring in 37.9% of patients in 1 series. Remote recurrence of chorea is rare, but may be provoked by streptococcal infections, pregnancy **(chorea gravidarum),** or oral contraceptive use.

Although much rarer than Sydenham chorea, **systemic lupus erythematosus** (see Chapter 158) is a well-known cause of chorea in children. In some cases, chorea may be the presenting sign of systemic lupus erythematosus. A recent retrospective study of a large pediatric lupus cohort examined the prevalence of antiphospholipid antibodies and evaluated their association with neuropsychiatric symptoms. There was a significant association between a persistently positive lupus anticoagulant and chorea (p = 0.02); however, only 2 of the 137 patients in the cohort had chorea. Regardless, a child with chorea of unknown cause should be investigated for the presence of antiphospholipid antibodies.

Table 597-8	Drugs That Can Induce Chorea
DOPAMINE RECEPTOR BLOCKING AGENTS (UPON WITHDRAWAL OR AS A TARDIVE SYNDROME) Phenothiazines Butyrophenones Benzamides **ANTIPARKINSONIAN DRUGS** L-DOPA Dopamine agonists Anticholinergics **ANTIEPILEPTIC DRUGS** Phenytoin Carbamazepine Valproic acid **PSYCHOSTIMULANTS** Amphetamines Methylphenidate Cocaine	**CALCIUM CHANNEL BLOCKERS** Cinnarizine Flunarizine Verapamil **OTHERS** Lithium Baclofen Digoxin Tricyclic antidepressants Cyclosporine Steroids/oral contraceptives Theophylline Propofol

Modified from Cardoso F, Seppi K, Mair KJ, et al: Seminar on choreas, Lancet Neurol 5:589–602, 2006.

Additional causes of secondary chorea include metabolic (hyperthyroidism, hypoparathyroidism), infectious (Lyme disease), immune-mediated (systemic lupus erythematosus; anti–*N*-methyl-D-aspartate receptor antibody syndrome), vascular (stroke, moyamoya disease), heredodegenerative disorders (Wilson disease), and drugs (Table 597-8). Although chorea is a hallmark of Huntington disease in adults, children who develop Huntington disease tend to present with rigidity and bradykinesia **(Westphal variant)** or dystonia rather than chorea.

Athetosis is characterized by slow, continuous, writhing movements that repeatedly involve the same body part(s), usually the distal extremities, face, neck, or trunk. Like chorea, athetosis may occur at rest and is often worsened by voluntary movement. Because athetosis tends to co-occur with other movement disorders, such as chorea (**choreoathetosis**) and dystonia, it is often difficult to distinguish as a discrete entity. Choreoathetosis is associated with cerebral palsy, kernicterus, and other forms of basal ganglia injury; therefore, it is often seen in conjunction with **rigidity**—increased muscle tone that is equal in the flexors and extensors in all directions of passive movement regardless of the velocity of the movement. This is to be differentiated from **spasticity,** a velocity-dependent ("clasp-knife") form of hypertonia that is seen with upper motor neuron dysfunction. As with chorea, athetosis/choreoathetosis can also be seen with hypoxic-ischemic injury and dopamine-blocking drugs.

Tremor is a rhythmic, oscillatory movement around a central point or plane that results from the action of antagonist muscles. Tremor can affect the extremities, head, trunk, or voice and can be classified by both its frequency (slow [4 Hz], intermediate [4-7 Hz], and fast [>7 Hz]) and by the context in which it is most pronounced. **Rest tremor** is maximal when the affected body part is inactive and supported against gravity, whereas **postural tremor** is most notable when the patient sustains a position against gravity. **Action tremor** occurs with performance of a voluntary activity and can be subclassified into **simple kinetic tremor**, which occurs with limb movement, and **intention tremor**, which occurs as the patient's limb approaches a target and is a feature of cerebellar disease.

Essential tremor (ET) is the most common movement disorder in adults, and 50% of persons diagnosed with ET report an onset in childhood; thus ET may be the most common tremor disorder in children as well. Clinical experience in pediatric movement disorders clinic suggests that ET is more common in the pediatric population than the literature would suggest. ET is an autosomal-dominant condition with variable expressivity but complete penetrance by the age of 60 yr. Although the genetics of ET are not fully understood, at least 3 different genes—*EMT1* on chromosome 3q13, *EMT2* on chromosome 2p22-25, and *LINGO1* on chromosome 15q24—are linked to the condition. Based on functional imaging studies, the defect is thought to localize to cerebellar circuits.

ET is characterized by a slowly progressive, bilateral, 4-9 Hz postural tremor that involves the upper extremities and occurs in the absence of other known causes of tremor. Mild asymmetry is common, but ET is rarely unilateral. ET may be worsened by actions, such as trying to pour water from cup to cup. Affected adults may report a history of ethanol responsiveness. Most young children present for evaluation because a parent, teacher, or therapist has noticed the tremor, rather than because the tremor causes impairment. Most children with ET do not require pharmacologic intervention. If they are having difficulty with their handwriting or self-feeding, an occupational therapy evaluation and/or assistive devices, such as wrist weights and weighted silverware, may be helpful. Teenagers tend to report more impairment from ET. Teenagers who do require pharmacotherapy usually respond to the same medications that are used in adults—propranolol and primidone. Propranolol, which is generally considered the first-line treatment, can be started at 20–40 mg daily and titrated to effect, with most patients responding to doses of 60-80 mg/day. Propranolol should not be used in patients with reactive airway disease. Primidone can be started at 12.5-25 mg at bedtime and increased gradually in a twice daily schedule. Most patients respond to doses of 50-200 mg/day. Other treatments options for ET reported in the adult literature include atenolol, gabapentin, topiramate, and alprazolam. Surgical treatments, which include deep brain stimulation of the thalamus and unilateral thalamotomy, are generally reserved for adults with medically refractory disabling tremor.

In addition to ET, there are numerous secondary etiologies of tremor in children (Table 597-9). **Holmes tremor,** previously referred to as midbrain or rubral tremor, is characterized by a slow frequency, high-amplitude tremor that is present at rest and with intention. It is a symptomatic tremor, which usually results from lesions of the brainstem, cerebellum, or thalamus. **Psychogenic tremor** is distinguished by its variable appearance, abrupt onset and remission, nonprogressive

Table 597-9	Selected Causes of Tremor in Children

BENIGN
Enhanced physiologic tremor
Shuddering attacks
Jitteriness
Spasmus nutans

STATIC INJURY/STRUCTURAL
Cerebellar malformation
Stroke (particularly in the midbrain or cerebellum)
Multiple sclerosis

HEREDITARY/DEGENERATIVE
Familial essential tremor
Fragile X premutation
Wilson disease
Huntington disease
Juvenile parkinsonism (tremor is rare)
Pallidonigral degeneration

METABOLIC
Hyperthyroidism
Hyperadrenergic state (including pheochromocytoma and
   neuroblastoma)
Hypomagnesemia
Hypocalcemia
Hypoglycemia
Hepatic encephalopathy
Vitamin B_{12} deficiency
Inborn errors of metabolism
Mitochondrial disorders

DRUGS/TOXINS
Valproate, phenytoin, carbamazepine, lamotrigine, gabapentin,
   lithium, tricyclic antidepressants, stimulants (cocaine,
   amphetamine, caffeine, thyroxine, bronchodilators), neuroleptics,
   cyclosporine, toluene, mercury, thallium, amiodarone, nicotine,
   lead, manganese, arsenic, cyanide, naphthalene, ethanol, lindane,
   serotonin reuptake inhibitors

PERIPHERAL NEUROPATHIES

PSYCHOGENIC

course, and association with selective but not task-specific disabilities. In some cases, tremor may even occur as a manifestation of another movement disorder, as is seen with position- or task-specific tremor (e.g., writing tremor), dystonic tremor, and myoclonic tremor.

When evaluating a child with tremor, it is important to screen for common metabolic disturbances, including electrolyte abnormalities and thyroid disease, assess the child's caffeine intake, and review the child's medication list for known tremor-inducing agents. It is also critical to exclude Wilson disease in teenagers with characteristic "wing-beating" tremor, as this is a treatable condition.

597.3 Dystonia
Erika F. Augustine and Jonathan W. Mink

Dystonia is a disorder of movement characterized by sustained muscle contraction, frequently causing twisting and repetitive movements or abnormal postures. Major causes of dystonia include primary generalized dystonia, medications, metabolic disorders, and perinatal asphyxia (Tables 597-10 and 597-11).

INHERITED PRIMARY DYSTONIAS
Primary generalized dystonia, also referred to as primary torsion dystonia or *dystonia musculorum deformans*, is caused by a group of genetic disorders with onset in childhood. One form, which occurs more commonly in the Ashkenazi Jewish population, is caused by a dominant mutation in the ***DYT1*** gene coding for the adenosine

Table 597-10	Causes of Dystonia in Childhood

STATIC INJURY/STRUCTURAL DISORDERS
Cerebral palsy
Hypoxic–ischemic injury
Kernicterus
Head trauma
Encephalitis
Tumors
Stroke in the basal ganglia (which may be a result of vascular abnormalities or varicella)
Congenital malformations

HEREDITARY/DEGENERATIVE DISORDERS
DYT1 (9q34, encodes torsinA)
DYT2 (autosomal-recessive)
DYT3 (X-linked dystonia-parkinsonism syndrome of Lubag–Xq13)
DYT4
DYT5 (14q22.1-2, encodes GTP cyclohydrolase I, leading to dopa-responsive dystonia or Segawa disease)
DYT6 (8p21-q22)
DYT7 (18p)
DYT8 (2q33-q35, causing paroxysmal nonkinesigenic choreoathetosis [PNKC])
DYT9 (1p, causing paroxysmal nonkinesigenic dyskinesia [PNKD] and spasticity)
DYT10 (16p11.2-q12.1, causing paroxysmal kinesigenic choreoathetosis [PKC])
DYT11 (heterogeneous, causing familial myoclonus-dystonia)
Rapid-onset dystonia-parkinsonism (DYT12)
Fahr disease (often caused by hypoparathyroid disease)
Pantothenate kinase-associated neurodegeneration (PKAN; neuronal brain iron accumulation type 1, formerly Hallervorden-Spatz disease, caused by mutations in PANK2)
Huntington disease (particularly the Westphal variant, IT15-4p16.3)
Spinocerebellar ataxias (SCAs, including SCA3/Machado-Joseph disease)
Neuronal ceroid-lipofuscinoses (NCL)
Rett syndrome
Striatal necrosis
Leigh disease
Neuroacanthocytosis
HARP syndrome (hypoprebetalipoproteinemia, acanthocytosis, retinitis pigmentosa, and pallidal degeneration)
Ataxia-telangiectasia
Tay-Sachs disease
Sandhoff's disease
Niemann-Pick type C
GM$_1$ gangliosidosis
Metachromatic leukodystrophy (MLD)
Lesch-Nyhan disease

METABOLIC DISEASE
Glutaric aciduria types 1 and 2
Acyl-coenzyme A (CoA) dehydrogenase deficiencies
Dopa-responsive dystonia (tyrosine hydroxylase deficiency, guanosine triphosphate [GTP] cyclohydrolase 1 deficiency, DYT5)
Dopamine agonist-responsive dystonia (aromatic l-amino acid decarboxylase deficiency, aminolevulinic acid dehydrase [ALAD])
Biotin responsive basal ganglia disease
Mitochondrial disorders
Wilson disease
Vitamin E deficiency
Homocystinuria
Methylmalonic aciduria
Tyrosinemia

DRUGS/TOXINS
Neuroleptic and antiemetic medications (haloperidol, chlorpromazine, olanzapine, risperidone, prochlorperazine)
Calcium channel blockers
Stimulants (amphetamine, cocaine, ergot alkaloids)
Anticonvulsants (carbamazepine, phenytoin)
Thallium
Manganese
Carbon monoxide
Ethylene glycol
Cyanide
Methanol
Wasp sting

PAROXYSMAL DISORDERS
Paroxysmal kinesigenic choreoathetosis (PKC)
Paroxysmal nonkinesigenic choreoathetosis (PNKC)
Exercise-induced dystonia
Complex migraine
Alternating hemiplegia of childhood (AHC)
Paroxysmal torticollis of infancy

DISORDERS THAT MIMIC DYSTONIA
Tonic seizures (including paroxysmal nocturnal dystonia caused by nocturnal frontal lobe seizures)
Arnold-Chiari malformation type II
Atlantoaxial subluxation
Syringomyelia
Posterior fossa mass
Cervical spine malformation (including Klippel-Feil syndrome)
Skew deviation with vertical diplopia causing neck twisting
Juvenile rheumatoid arthritis
Sandifer syndrome (associated with hiatal hernia in infants)
Spasmus nutans
Tics
Infant masturbation
Spasticity
Myotonia
Rigidity
Stiff-person syndrome
Isaac syndrome (neuromyotonia)
Startle disease (hyperekplexia)
Neuroleptic malignant syndrome
Central herniation with posturing
Psychogenic dystonia

From Sanger TD, Mink JW: Movement disorders. In Swaiman KF, Ashwal S, Ferriero DM, Schor NF, editors: Swaiman's pediatric neurology: principles and practice, ed 5, Philadelphia, 2012, WB Saunders, Box 68-2.

Table 597-11	Examples of Primary and Secondary Dystonia in Childhood		
DIAGNOSIS	**ADDITIONAL CLINICAL FEATURES**	**DIAGNOSIS**	**ADDITIONAL CLINICAL FEATURES**
Aicardi-Goutières syndrome	Encephalopathy, developmental regression Acquired microcephaly Sterile pyrexias Lesions on the digits, ears (chilblain) Epilepsy CT: calcification of the basal ganglia	Leigh syndrome	Motor delays, weakness, hypotonia Ataxia, tremor Elevated lactate MRI: bilateral symmetric hyperintense lesions in the basal ganglia or thalamus
Alternating hemiplegia of childhood	Episodic hemiplegia/quadriplegia Abnormal ocular movements Autonomic symptoms Epilepsy Global developmental impairment Environmental triggers for spells	Lesch-Nyhan syndrome (X-linked)	Male Self-injurious behavior Hypotonia Oromandibular dystonia, inspiratory stridor Oculomotor apraxia Cognitive impairment Elevated uric acid
Aromatic amino acid decarboxylase deficiency (AADC)	Developmental delay Oculogyric crises Autonomic dysfunction Hypotonia	Myoclonus dystonia	Myoclonus Head, upper limb involvement
ARX gene mutation (X-linked)	Male Cognitive impairment Infantile spasms, epilepsy Brain malformation	Niemann-Pick type C	Hepatosplenomegaly Hypotonia Supranuclear gaze palsy Ataxia, dysarthria Epilepsy Psychiatric symptoms
Benign paroxysmal torticollis of infancy	Episodic Cervical dystonia only Family history of migraine	Neuroacanthocytosis	Oromandibular and lingual dystonia
Complex regional pain syndrome	Lower limb involvement Prominent pain	Neurodegeneration with brain iron accumulation	Cognitive impairment Retinal pigmentary degeneration, optic atrophy
Dopa-responsive dystonia (DRD)	Diurnal variation	Rapid onset dystonia parkinsonism (DYT12)	Acute onset Distribution face > arm > leg Prominent bulbar signs
Drug-induced dystonia			
Dystonia-deafness optic neuropathy syndrome	Sensorineural hearing loss in early childhood Psychosis Optic atrophy in adolescence	Rett syndrome	Female Developmental regression following a period of normal development Stereotypic hand movements Acquired microcephaly Epilepsy
DYT1 dystonia	Lower limb onset followed by generalization	Spinocerebellar ataxia 17 (SCA17)	Ataxia Dementia, psychiatric symptoms Parkinsonism
Glutaric aciduria type 1	Macrocephaly Encephalopathic crises MRI: striatal necrosis	Tics	Stereotyped movements Premonitory urge, suppressible
GM$_1$ gangliosidosis type 3	Short stature, skeletal dysplasia Orofacial dystonia Speech/swallowing disturbance Parkinsonism MRI: putaminal hyperintensity	Tyrosine hydroxylase deficiency	Infantile encephalopathy, hypotonia Oculogyric crises, ptosis Autonomic symptoms Less diurnal fluctuation than DRD
Huntington disease	Parkinsonism Epilepsy Family history of Huntington disease		
Kernicterus	Jaundice in infancy Hearing loss Impaired upgaze Enamel dysplasia MRI: hyperintense lesions in the globus pallidus		

triphosphate (ATP) binding protein torsinA. The initial manifestation of *DYT1* dystonia is often intermittent unilateral posturing of a lower extremity, which assumes an extended and rotated position. Ultimately, all 4 extremities and the axial musculature can be affected, but the dystonia may also remain localized to one limb. Cranial involvement can occur in *DYT1* dystonia, but it is uncommon compared to non-*DYT1* dystonias. There is a wide clinical spectrum, varying even within families. If a family history of dystonia is absent, the diagnosis

should still be considered, given the intrafamilial variability in clinical expression.

More than a dozen loci for genes for torsion dystonia have been identified (*DYT1-DYT24*). One is the autosomal dominant disorder **dopa-responsive dystonia (DRD, DYT5a)**, also called Segawa syndrome. The gene for DRD codes for guanosine triphosphate cyclohydrolase 1, the rate-limiting enzyme for tetrahydrobiopterin synthesis, which is a cofactor for synthesis of the neurotransmitters dopamine and serotonin. Thus, the genetic mutation results in dopamine deficiency. The hallmark of the disorder, particularly in adolescents and adults, is diurnal variation: symptoms worsen as the day progresses and may transiently improve with sleep. Early-onset patients, who tend to present with delayed or abnormal gait from dystonia of a lower extremity, can easily be confused with patients with dystonic cerebral palsy. It should be noted that in the presence of a progressive dystonia, diurnal fluctuation, or if loss of previously achieved motor skills occurs, a prior diagnosis of cerebral palsy should be reexamined. DRD responds dramatically to small daily doses of levodopa. The responsiveness to levodopa is a sustained benefit, even if the diagnosis is delayed several years, as long as contractures have not developed.

Myoclonus dystonia (DYT11), caused by mutations in the epsilon-sarcoglycan *(SCGE)* gene, is characterized by dystonia involving the upper extremities, head, and/or neck, as well as myoclonic movements in these regions. Although a combination of myoclonus and dystonia typically occurs, each manifestation can present in isolation. When repetitive, the myoclonus may take on a tremor-like appearance, termed *dystonic tremor.* Improvement in symptoms following alcohol ingestion, reported by affected adult family members, may be a helpful clue to this diagnosis.

Common to the inherited dystonias, there is considerable intrafamilial variability in clinical manifestations, distribution, and severity of dystonia. In primary dystonias, although the main clinical features are motor, there may be an increased risk for major depression. Anxiety, obsessive-compulsive disorder, and depression have all been reported in the myoclonus–dystonia syndrome. Screening for psychiatric comorbidities cannot be overlooked in this population.

DRUG-INDUCED DYSTONIAS
A number of medications are capable of inducing involuntary movements, drug-induced movement disorders, in children and adults. Dopamine-blocking agents, including antipsychotics (e.g., haloperidol) and antiemetics (e.g., metoclopramide, prochlorperazine), as well as atypical antipsychotics (e.g., risperidone) can produce acute dystonic reactions or delayed (tardive) drug-induced movement disorders. **Acute dystonic reactions,** occurring in the 1st days of exposure, typically involve the face and neck, manifesting as torticollis, retrocollis, oculogyric crisis, or tongue protrusion. Life-threatening presentations with laryngospasm and airway compromise can also occur, requiring prompt recognition and treatment of this entity. Intravenous diphenhydramine, 1-2 mg/kg/dose, may rapidly reverse the drug-related dystonia. The high potency of the dopamine blocker, young age, and prior dystonic reactions may be predisposing factors. Acute dystonic reactions have also been described with cetirizine.

Severe rigidity combined with high fever, autonomic symptoms (tachycardia, diaphoresis), delirium, and dystonia are signs of **neuroleptic malignant syndrome**, which typically occurs a few days after starting or increasing the dose of a neuroleptic drug, or in the setting of withdrawal from a dopaminergic agent. In contrast to acute dystonic reactions, which take place within days, neuroleptic malignant syndrome occurs within a month of medication initiation or dose increase.

Delayed onset involuntary movements, **tardive dyskinesias,** develop in the setting of chronic (>3 mo duration) neuroleptic use. Involvement of the face, particularly the mouth, lips, and/or jaw with chewing or tongue thrusting is characteristic. The risk of tardive dyskinesia, which is much less frequent in children compared to adults, increases as medication dose and duration of treatment increase. There are data to suggest that children with autism spectrum disorders may also be at increased risk for this drug-induced movement disorders. Unlike acute dystonic reactions and neuroleptic malignant syndrome, discontinuation of the offending agent may not result in clinical improvement. In these patients, use of dopamine-depletors, such as reserpine or tetrabenazine, may prove helpful.

Therapeutic doses of phenytoin or carbamazepine rarely cause progressive dystonia in children with epilepsy, particularly in those who have an underlying structural abnormality of the brain.

During evaluation of new onset dystonia, a careful history of prescriptions and potential medication exposures is critical.

CEREBRAL PALSY
See Chapter 598.

METABOLIC DISORDERS
Disorders of monamine neurotransmitter metabolism, of which DRD is one, present in infancy and early childhood with dystonia, hypotonia, oculogyric crises, and/or autonomic symptoms. The more common disorders among this group of rare diseases include DRD, tyrosine hydroxylase deficiency, and aromatic amino acid decarboxylase deficiency. Abnormalities of the dopamine transporter (DAT) can also present in infancy with dystonia. Detailed discussion is beyond the scope of this chapter; reviews, however, are available for reference.

Wilson disease is an autosomal recessive inborn error of copper transport characterized by cirrhosis of the liver and degenerative changes in the central nervous system, particularly the basal ganglia (see Chapter 357.2). It has been determined that there are multiple mutations in the Wilson disease gene *(WND)*, accounting for the variability in presentation of the condition. The neurologic manifestations of Wilson disease rarely appear before age 10 yr, and the initial sign is often progressive dystonia. Tremors of the extremities develop, unilaterally at first, but they eventually become coarse, generalized, and incapacitating. Other neurologic signs of Wilson disease relate to progressive basal ganglia disease, such as parkinsonism, dysarthria, dysphonia, and choreoathetosis. Less frequent are ataxia and pyramidal signs. The MRI or CT scan shows ventricular dilation in advanced cases with atrophy of the cerebrum, cerebellum, and/or brainstem, along with signal intensity change in the basal ganglia, thalamus, and/or brainstem, particularly the midbrain.

Pantothenate kinase–associated neurodegeneration (formerly known as *Hallervorden-Spatz disease*) is a rare autosomal recessive neurodegenerative disorder. Many patients have mutations in pantothenate kinase 2 *(PANK2)* localized to mitochondria in neurons. The condition usually begins before 6 yr of age and is characterized by rapidly progressive dystonia, rigidity, and choreoathetosis. Spasticity, extensor plantar responses, dysarthria, and intellectual deterioration become evident during adolescence, and death usually occurs by early adulthood. MRI shows lesions of the globus pallidus, including low signal intensity in T2-weighted images (corresponding to iron pigments) and an anteromedial area of high signal intensity (tissue necrosis and edema), or "eye-of-the-tiger" sign (Fig. 597-1). Neuropathologic examination indicates excessive accumulation of iron-containing pigments in the globus pallidus and substantia nigra. More recently, similar disorders of high brain iron content without *PANK2* mutations, including infantile neuroaxonal dystrophy, neuroferritinopathy, and aceruloplasminemia, have been grouped as disorders of neurodegeneration with brain iron accumulation. Patterns of iron deposition visualized by brain MRI have shown utility in differentiating these disorders.

Biotin-responsive basal ganglia disease manifests with episodes of acute dystonia, external ophthalmoplegia and encephalopathy. *SLC19A3* is the responsible mutated gene. MRI demonstrates involvement of the basal ganglia, with vasogenic edema and the "bat-wing" sign (Fig. 597-2). Treatment with biotin and thiamine results in improvement in 2-4 days.

Although dystonia may present in isolation as the first sign of a metabolic or neurodegenerative disorder, this group of diseases should be considered mainly in those who demonstrate signs of systemic disease, (e.g., organomegaly, short stature, hearing loss, vision impairment, epilepsy), those with episodes of severe illness, evidence of regression, or cognitive impairment. Table 597-11 outlines additional features suggestive of specific disorders.

OTHER DISORDERS
Although uncommon, movement disorders, including dystonia, may be part of the presenting symptoms of **complex regional pain syndrome**. Onset of involuntary movements within 1 yr of the traumatic event, affected lower limb, pain disproportionate to inciting event, and changes in the overlying skin and blood flow to the affected area suggest complex regional pain syndrome. Although sustained dystonia

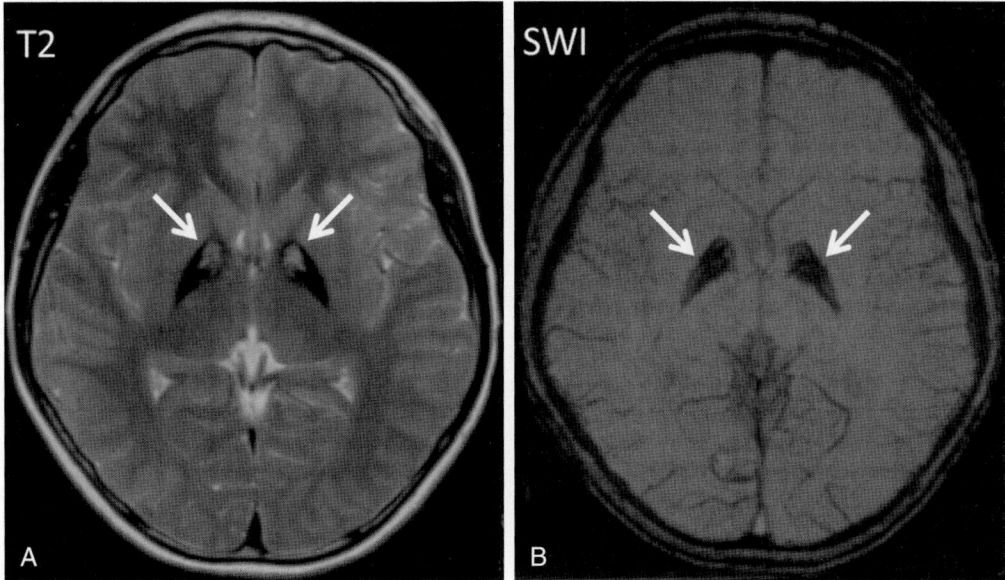

Figure 597-1 Pantothenate kinase–associated neurodegeneration (PKAN). **A,** Axial T2-weighted image showing symmetric hypointensity in the bilateral globi pallidi with central hyperintensity ("eye-of-the-tiger sign," *arrows*). **B,** Axial susceptibility-weighted image (SWI) image showing hypointensity in the globi pallidi representing increased iron accumulation *(arrows). (From From Bosemani T, Meoded A, Poretti A: Susceptibility-weighted imaging in pantothenate kinase-associated neurodegeneration. J Pediatr 164:212, 2014.)*

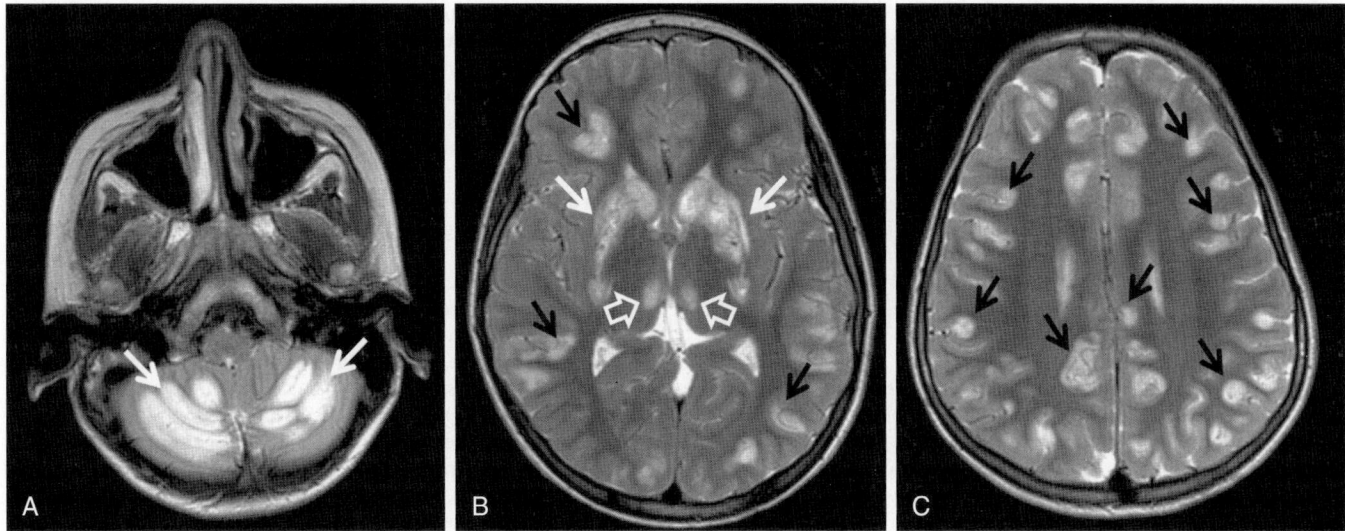

Figure 597-2 Biotin-responsive basal ganglia disease. An initial brain MRI showed high-signal intensity alterations on T2-weighted images bilaterally involving the **(A)** cerebellum *(arrows)*, **(B)** basal ganglia *(white arrows)*, and medial nucleus of the thalamus *(open arrows)*, and **(B, C)** cerebral cortex *(black arrows). (Modified from Tabarki B, Al-Sheikh F, Al-Shahwan S, Zuccoli G: Bilateral external ophthalmoplegia in biotin-responsive basal ganglia disease. J Pediatr 162:1291–1292, 2013.)*

can produce pain or discomfort, complex regional pain syndrome should be considered in those who have a prominent component of pain and recent history of trauma to the affected limb.

There are disorders unique to childhood that warrant exploration in this section. **Benign paroxysmal torticollis of infancy** is characterized by recurrent episodes of cervical dystonia beginning in the 1st few mo of life. The torticollis may alternate sides from 1 episode to the next and may also persist during sleep. Associated signs and symptoms include irritability, pallor, vomiting, vertigo, ataxia, and occasionally limb dystonia. Family history is often notable for migraine and/or motion sickness in 1st-degree relatives. Despite the high frequency of spells, imaging studies are normal, and the outcome is uniformly benign with resolution by 3 yr of age.

In **alternating hemiplegia of childhood**, episodic hemiplegia affecting either side of the body is the hallmark of the disorder. However,

patients are also affected by episodes of dystonia, ranging from minutes to days in duration. On average, both features of the disorder commence at approximately 6 mo of age. Episodic abnormal eye movements are observed in a large proportion of patients (93%) with onset as early as the 1st wk of life. Alternating hemiplegia of childhood is associated with mutations in the *ATP1A2* and *ATP1A3* genes. Alternating hemiplegia of childhood can similarly be triggered by fluctuations in temperature, certain foods, or water exposure. Over time, epilepsy and cognitive impairment emerge, and the involuntary movements change from episodic to constant. Infantile onset and the paroxysmal nature of symptoms early in the disease course are key features to this diagnosis.

Finally, although a diagnosis of exclusion, the presence of odd movements or selective disability may indicate a psychogenic dystonia in older children. There is considerable overlap in features of organic and

psychogenic movement disorders, making the diagnosis difficult to establish. For instance, both organic and psychogenic movement disorders have the potential to worsen in the setting of stress and may dissipate with relaxation or sleep. History should include review of recent stressors, psychiatric symptoms, and exposure to others with similar disorders. On examination, a changing movement disorder, inconsistent motor or sensory exam, or response to suggestion, are supportive of a possible psychogenic movement disorder. Early recognition of this disorder may lessen morbidity caused by unnecessary diagnostic and interventional procedures.

TREATMENT

Children with generalized dystonia, including those with involvement of the muscles of swallowing, may respond to the anticholinergic agent trihexyphenidyl (Artane). Titration occurs slowly over the course of months in an effort to limit untoward side effects, such as urinary retention, mental confusion, or blurred vision. Additional drugs that have been effective include levodopa and diazepam. Segmental dystonia, such as torticollis, often responds well to botulinum toxin injections. Intrathecal baclofen delivered through implantable constant infusion pump may be helpful in some patients. Deep brain stimulation with leads implanted in the globus pallidus is most helpful for children with severe primary generalized dystonia. Recent data suggest, however, that deep brain stimulation may also be of benefit in children with secondary dystonias, such as cerebral palsy.

In the case of drug-induced dystonias, removal of the offending agent and treatment with intravenous diphenhydramine typically suffices. For neuroleptic malignant syndrome, dantrolene may be indicated.

Bibliography is available at Expert Consult.

Chapter 598

Encephalopathies

Michael V. Johnston

Encephalopathy is a generalized disorder of cerebral function that may be acute or chronic, progressive, or static. The etiologies of the encephalopathies in children include infectious, toxic (carbon monoxide, drugs, lead), metabolic, genetic, and ischemic causes. Hypoxic–ischemic encephalopathy is discussed in Chapter 99.5.

598.1 Cerebral Palsy

Michael V. Johnston

See Chapters 36, 97.2, and 597.3.

Cerebral palsy (CP) is a diagnostic term used to describe a group of permanent disorders of movement and posture causing activity limitation, that are attributed to nonprogressive disturbances in the in the developing fetal or infant brain. The motor disorders are often accompanied by disturbances of sensation, perception, cognition, communication, and behavior as well as by epilepsy and secondary musculoskeletal problems. CP is caused by a broad group of developmental, genetic, metabolic, ischemic, infectious, and other acquired etiologies that produce a common group of neurologic phenotypes. CP has historically been considered a static encephalopathy, but some of the neurologic features of CP, such as movement disorders and orthopedic complications, including scoliosis and hip dislocation, can change or progress over time. Many children and adults with CP function at a high educational and vocational level, without any sign of cognitive dysfunction.

EPIDEMIOLOGY AND ETIOLOGY

CP is the most common and costly form of chronic motor disability that begins in childhood; data from the Centers for Disease Control and Prevention indicate that the incidence is 3.6 per 1,000 children with a male:female ratio of 1.4:1. The Collaborative Perinatal Project, in which approximately 45,000 children were regularly monitored from in utero to the age of 7 yr, found that most children with CP had been born at term with uncomplicated labors and deliveries. In 80% of cases, features were identified pointing to antenatal factors causing abnormal brain development. A substantial number of children with CP had congenital anomalies external to the central nervous system (CNS). Fewer than 10% of children with CP had evidence of intrapartum asphyxia. Intrauterine exposure to maternal infection (chorioamnionitis, inflammation of placental membranes, umbilical cord inflammation, foul-smelling amniotic fluid, maternal sepsis, temperature >38°C [100.4°F] during labor, urinary tract infection) was associated with a significant increase in the risk of CP in normal birthweight infants. Elevated levels of inflammatory cytokines have been reported in heelstick blood collected at birth from children who later were identified with CP. Genetic factors may contribute to the inflammatory cytokine response, and a functional polymorphism in the interleukin-6 gene is associated with a higher rate of CP in term infants.

The prevalence of CP has increased somewhat as a result of the enhanced survival of very premature infants weighing <1,000 g, who go on to develop CP at a rate of approximately 15 per 100. However, the gestational age at birth-adjusted prevalence of CP among 2 yr old former premature infants born at 20-27 wk of gestation has decreased over the past decade. The major lesions that contribute to CP in preterm infants are **intracerebral hemorrhage** and **periventricular leukomalacia** (PVL). Although the incidence of intracerebral hemorrhage has declined significantly, PVL remains a major problem. PVL reflects the enhanced vulnerability of immature oligodendroglia in premature infants to oxidative stress caused by ischemia or infectious/inflammatory insults. White matter abnormalities (loss of volume of periventricular white matter, extent of cystic changes, ventricular dilation, thinning of the corpus callosum) present on MRI at 40 wk of gestational age among former preterm infants are a predictor of later CP.

In 2006, the European Cerebral Palsy Study examined prenatal and perinatal factors as well as clinical findings and results of MRI in a contemporary cohort of more than 400 children with CP. In agreement with the Collaborative Perinatal Project study, more than half the children with CP in this study were born at term, and less than 20% had clinical or brain imaging indicators of possible intrapartum factors such as asphyxia. The contribution of intrapartum factors to CP is higher in some underdeveloped regions of the world. Also in agreement with earlier data, antenatal infection was strongly associated with CP and 39.5% of mothers of children with CP reported having an infection during the pregnancy, with 19% having evidence of a urinary tract infection and 11.5% reporting taking antibiotics. Multiple pregnancy was also associated with a higher incidence of CP and 12% of the cases in the European CP study resulted from a multiple pregnancy, in contrast to a 1.5% incidence of multiple pregnancy in the study. Other studies have also documented a relationship between multiple births and CP, with a rate in twins that is 5-8 times greater than in singleton pregnancies and a rate in triplets that is 20-47 times greater. Death of a twin in utero carries an even greater risk of CP that is 8 times that of a pregnancy in which both twins survive and approximately 60 times the risk in a singleton pregnancy. Infertility treatments are also associated with a higher rate of CP, probably because these treatments are often associated with multiple pregnancies. Among children from multiple pregnancies, 24% were from pregnancies after infertility treatment compared with 3.4% of the singleton pregnancies in the study. CP is more common and more severe in boys compared to girls and this effect is enhanced at the extremes of body weight. Male infants with intrauterine growth retardation and a birthweight less than the 3rd percentile are 16 times more likely to have CP than males with optimal growth, and infants with weights above the 97th percentile are 4 times more likely to have CP.

| Table 598-1 | Classification of Cerebral Palsy and Major Causes |

MOTOR SYNDROME (APPROX. % OF CP)	NEUROPATHOLOGY/MRI	MAJOR CAUSES
Spastic diplegia (35%)	Periventricular leukomalacia Periventricular cysts or scars in white matter, enlargement of ventricles, squared off posterior ventricles	Prematurity Ischemia Infection Endocrine/metabolic (e.g., thyroid)
Spastic quadriplegia (20%)	Periventricular leukomalacia Multicystic encephalomalacia Cortical malformations	Ischemia, infection Endocrine/metabolic, genetic/developmental
Hemiplegia (25%)	Stroke: in utero or neonatal Focal infarct or cortical, subcortical damage Cortical malformations	Thrombophilic disorders Infection Genetic/developmental Periventricular hemorrhagic infarction
Extrapyramidal (athetoid, dyskinetic) (15%)	Asphyxia: symmetric scars in putamen and thalamus Kernicterus: scars in globus pallidus, hippocampus Mitochondrial: scaring globus pallidus, caudate, putamen, brainstem No lesions: ? dopa-responsive dystonia	Asphyxia Kernicterus Mitochondrial Genetic/metabolic

CLINICAL MANIFESTATIONS

CP is generally divided into several major motor syndromes that differ according to the pattern of neurologic involvement, neuropathology, and etiology (Table 598-1). The physiologic classification identifies the major motor abnormality, whereas the topographic taxonomy indicates the involved extremities. CP is also commonly associated with a spectrum of developmental disabilities, including intellectual impairment, epilepsy, and visual, hearing, speech, cognitive, and behavioral abnormalities. The motor handicap may be the least of the child's problems.

Infants with **spastic hemiplegia** have decreased spontaneous movements on the affected side and show hand preference at a very early age. The arm is often more involved than the leg and difficulty in hand manipulation is obvious by 1 yr of age. Walking is usually delayed until 18-24 mo, and a circumductive gait is apparent. Examination of the extremities may show growth arrest, particularly in the hand and thumbnail, especially if the contralateral parietal lobe is abnormal, because extremity growth is influenced by this area of the brain. Spasticity refers to the quality of increased muscle tone, which increases with the speed of passive muscle stretching and is greatest in antigravity muscles. It is apparent in the affected extremities, particularly at the ankle, causing an equinovarus deformity of the foot. An affected child often walks on tiptoe because of the increased tone in the antigravity gastrocnemius muscles, and the affected upper extremity assumes a flexed posture when the child runs. Ankle clonus and a Babinski sign may be present, the deep tendon reflexes are increased, and weakness of the hand and foot dorsiflexors is evident. About one-third of patients with spastic hemiplegia have a seizure disorder that usually develops in the 1st yr or 2; approximately 25% have cognitive abnormalities including mental retardation. MRI is far more sensitive than CT for most lesions seen with CP, although a CT scan may be useful for detecting calcifications associated with congenital infections. In the European CP study, 34% of children with hemiplegia had injury to the white matter that probably dated to the in utero period and 27% had a focal lesion that may have resulted from a stroke. Other children with hemiplegic CP had had malformations from multiple causes including infections (e.g., cytomegalovirus), lissencephaly, polymicrogyria, schizencephaly, or cortical dysplasia. Focal cerebral infarction (stroke) secondary to intrauterine or perinatal thromboembolism related to thrombophilic disorders, like the presence of anticardiolipin antibodies, is an important cause of hemiplegic CP (see Chapter 601). Family histories suggestive of thrombosis and inherited clotting disorders, such as factor V Leiden mutation, may be present and evaluation of the mother may provide information valuable for future pregnancies and other family members.

Spastic diplegia is bilateral spasticity of the legs that is greater than in the arms. Spastic diplegia is strongly associated with damage to the immature white matter during the vulnerable period of immature oligodendroglia between 20-34 wk of gestation. However, approximately 15% of cases of spastic diplegia result from in utero lesions in infants who go on to delivery at term. The first clinical indication of spastic diplegia is often noted when an affected infant begins to crawl. The child uses the arms in a normal reciprocal fashion but tends to drag the legs behind more as a rudder (commando crawl) rather than using the normal 4-limbed crawling movement. If the spasticity is severe, application of a diaper is difficult because of the excessive adduction of the hips. If there is paraspinal muscle involvement, the child may be unable to sit. Examination of the child reveals spasticity in the legs with brisk reflexes, ankle clonus, and a bilateral Babinski sign. When the child is suspended by the axillae, a scissoring posture of the lower extremities is maintained. Walking is significantly delayed, the feet are held in a position of equinovarus, and the child walks on tiptoe. Severe spastic diplegia is characterized by disuse atrophy and impaired growth of the lower extremities and by disproportionate growth with normal development of the upper torso. The prognosis for normal intellectual development for these patients is good, and the likelihood of seizures is minimal. Such children often have learning disabilities and deficits in other abilities, such as vision, because of disruption of multiple white matter pathways that carry sensory as well as motor information.

The most common neuropathologic finding in children with spastic diplegia is PVL, which is visualized on MRI in more than 70% of cases. MRI typically shows scarring and shrinkage in the periventricular white matter with compensatory enlargement of the cerebral ventricles. However, neuropathology has also demonstrated a reduction in oligodendroglia in more widespread subcortical regions beyond the periventricular zones, and these subcortical lesions may contribute to the learning problems these patients can have. MRI with diffusion tensor imaging is being used to map white matter tracks more precisely in patients with spastic diplegia, and this technique has shown that thalamocortical sensory pathways are often injured as severely as motor corticospinal pathways (Fig. 598-1). These observations have led to greater interest in the importance of sensory deficits in these patients, which may be important for designing rehabilitative techniques.

Spastic quadriplegia is the most severe form of CP because of marked motor impairment of all extremities and the high association with intellectual disability and seizures. Swallowing difficulties are common as a result of supranuclear bulbar palsies, often leading to aspiration pneumonia. The most common lesions seen on pathologic examination or on MRI scanning are severe PVL and multicystic cortical encephalomalacia. Neurologic examination shows increased tone and spasticity in all extremities, decreased spontaneous movements, brisk reflexes, and plantar extensor responses. Flexion contractures of the knees and elbows are often present by late childhood. Associated

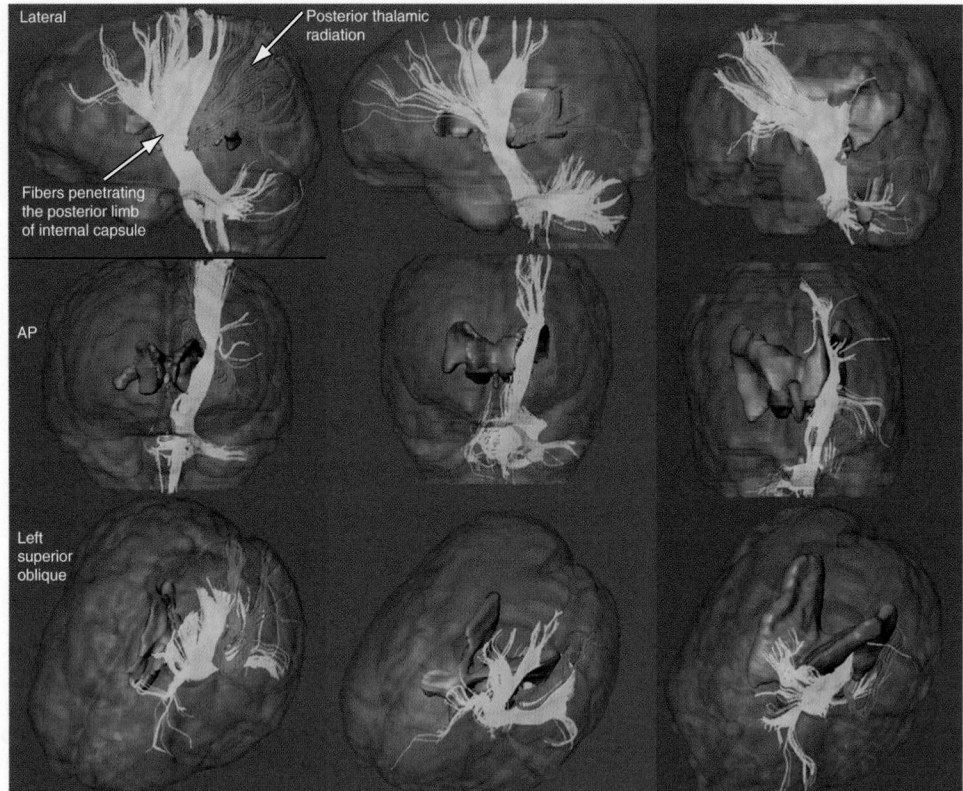

Figure 598-1 Diffusion tensor image of white matter pathways in the brains of 2 patients with spastic diplegia on the right compared to a normal child on the far left. Yellow fibers are corticospinal pathways projected from the motor cerebral cortex at the top downward into the brainstem, whereas the red fibers are thalamocortical sensory fibers projected from the thalamus upward to the cortex. In the children with spastic diplegia, both the corticospinal and thalamocortical pathways are reduced in size, but the ascending thalamocortical pathways are more affected. *(From Nagae LM, Hoon AH Jr, Stashinko E, et al: Diffusion tensor imaging in children with periventricular leukomalacia: variability of injuries to white matter tracts, AJNR Am J Neuroradiol 28:1213–1222, 2007.)*

developmental disabilities, including speech and visual abnormalities, are particularly prevalent in this group of children. Children with spastic quadriparesis often have evidence of athetosis and may be classified as having mixed CP.

Athetoid CP, also called **choreoathetoid, extrapyramidal,** or **dyskinetic** CP, is less common than spastic CP and makes up approximately 15-20% of patients with CP. Affected infants are characteristically hypotonic with poor head control and marked head lag and develop variably increased tone with rigidity and dystonia over several years. The term *dystonia* refers to the abnormality in tone in which muscles are rigid throughout their range of motion and involuntary contractions can occur in both flexors and extensors leading to limb positioning in fixed postures. Unlike spastic diplegia, the upper extremities are generally more affected than the lower extremities in extrapyramidal CP. Feeding may be difficult, and tongue thrust and drooling may be prominent. Speech is typically affected because the oropharyngeal muscles are involved. Speech may be absent or sentences are slurred, and voice modulation is impaired. Generally, upper motor neuron signs are not present, seizures are uncommon, and intellect is preserved in many patients. This form of CP is also referred to in Europe as dyskinetic CP and is the type most likely to be associated with **birth asphyxia.** In the European CP study, 76% of patients with this form of CP had lesions in the basal ganglia and thalamus. Extrapyramidal CP secondary to acute intrapartum near-total asphyxia is associated with bilaterally symmetric lesions in the posterior putamen and ventrolateral thalamus. These lesions appear to be the correlate of the neuropathologic lesion called *status marmoratus* in the basal ganglia. Athetoid CP can also be caused by **kernicterus** secondary to high levels of bilirubin, and in this case the MRI scan shows lesions in the globus pallidus bilaterally. Extrapyramidal CP can also be associated with lesions in the basal ganglia and thalamus caused by metabolic genetic

disorders such as mitochondrial disorders and glutaric aciduria. MRI scanning and possibly metabolic testing are important in the evaluation of children with extrapyramidal CP to make a correct etiologic diagnosis. In patients with dystonia who have a normal MRI, it is important to have a high level of suspicion for dihydroxyphenylalanine (DOPA)-responsive dystonia (Segawa disease), which causes prominent dystonia that can resemble CP. These patients typically have diurnal variation in their signs with worsening dystonia in the legs during the day; however, this may not be prominent. These patients can be tested for a response to small doses of L-dopa and/or cerebrospinal fluid can be sent for neurotransmitter analysis.

Associated comorbidities are common and include pain (in 75%), cognitive disability (50%), hip displacement (30%), seizures (25%), behavioral disorders (25%), sleep disturbances (20%), visual impairment (19%), and hearing impairment (4%).

DIAGNOSIS

A thorough history and physical examination should preclude a **progressive disorder** of the CNS, including degenerative diseases, metabolic disorders, spinal cord tumor, or muscular dystrophy. The possibility of anomalies at the base of the skull or other disorders affecting the cervical spinal cord needs to be considered in patients with little involvement of the arms or cranial nerves. An MRI scan of the brain is indicated to determine the location and extent of structural lesions or associated congenital malformations; an MRI scan of the spinal cord is indicated if there is any question about spinal cord pathology. Additional studies may include tests of hearing and visual function. Genetic evaluation should be considered in patients with congenital malformations (chromosomes) or evidence of metabolic disorders (e.g., amino acids, organic acids, MR spectroscopy). In addition to the genetic disorders mentioned earlier that can present as CP, the urea cycle disorder arginase deficiency is a rare cause of spastic diplegia and a deficiency of sulfite oxidase or molybdenum cofactor can present as CP caused by perinatal asphyxia. Tests to detect inherited thrombophilic disorders may be indicated in patients in whom an in utero or neonatal stroke is suspected as the cause of CP.

Because CP is usually associated with a wide spectrum of developmental disorders, a multidisciplinary approach is most helpful in the assessment and treatment of such children.

TREATMENT

Some progress has been made in both prevention of CP before it occurs and treatment of children with the disorder. Preliminary results from controlled trials of magnesium sulfate given intravenously to mothers in premature labor with birth imminent before 32 wk gestation showed significant reduction in the risk of CP at 2 yr of age. Nonetheless, one study that followed preterm infants whose mothers received magnesium sulfate demonstrated no benefit in terms of the incidence of CP and abnormal motor, cognitive, or behavioral function at school age. Furthermore, several large trials have shown that cooling term infants with hypoxic–ischemic encephalopathy to 33.3°C (91.9°F) for 3 days, starting within 6 hr of birth, reduces the risk of dyskinetic or spastic quadriplegia form of CP.

For children who have a diagnosis of CP, a team of physicians, including neurodevelopmental pediatricians, pediatric neurologists, and physical medicine and rehabilitation specialists, as well as occupational and physical therapists, speech pathologists, social workers, educators, and developmental psychologists, is important to reduce abnormalities of movement and tone and to optimize normal psychomotor development. Parents should be taught how to work with their child in daily activities such as feeding, carrying, dressing, bathing, and playing in ways that limit the effects of abnormal muscle tone. They also need to be instructed in the supervision of a series of exercises designed to prevent the development of contractures, especially a tight Achilles tendon. Physical and occupational therapies are useful for promoting mobility and the use of the upper extremities for activities of daily living. Speech language pathologists promote acquisition of a functional means of communications. These therapists help children to achieve their potential and often recommend further evaluations and adaptive equipment.

Children with spastic diplegia are treated initially with the assistance of adaptive equipment, such as walkers, poles, and standing frames. If a patient has marked spasticity of the lower extremities or evidence of hip dislocation, consideration should be given to performing surgical soft-tissue procedures that reduce muscle spasm around the hip girdle, including an adductor tenotomy or psoas transfer and release. A rhizotomy procedure in which the roots of the spinal nerves are divided produces considerable improvement in selected patients with severe spastic diplegia (Fig. 598-2). A tight heel cord in a child with spastic hemiplegia may be treated surgically by tenotomy of the Achilles tendon. Quadriplegia is managed with motorized wheelchairs, special feeding devices, modified typewriters, and customized seating arrange-

ments. The function of the affected extremities in children with **hemiplegic CP** can often be improved by therapy in which movement of the good side is constrained with casts while the impaired extremities perform exercises which induce improved hand and arm functioning. This constraint-induced movement therapy is effective in patients of all ages.

Several drugs have been used to **treat spasticity,** including the benzodiazepines and baclofen. These medications have beneficial effects in some patients but can also cause side effects such as sedation for benzodiazepines and lowered seizure threshold for baclofen. Several drugs can be used to **treat spasticity,** including oral diazepam (0.01-0.3 mg/kg/day, divided bid or qid), baclofen (0.2-2 mg/kg/day, divided bid or tid) or dantrolene (0.5-10 mg/kg/day, bid). Small doses of levodopa (0.5-2 mg/kg/day) can be used to treat dystonia or DOPA-responsive dystonia. Artane (trihexyphenidyl, 0.25 mg/day, divided bid or tid and titrated upward) is sometimes useful for treating dystonia and can increase use of the upper extremities and vocalizations. Reserpine (0.01-0.02 mg/kg/day, divided bid to a maximum of 0.25 mg daily) or tetrabenazine (12.5-25.0 mg, divided bid or tid) can be useful for hyperkinetic movement disorders including athetosis or chorea.

Intrathecal baclofen delivered with an implanted pump has been used successfully in many children with severe spasticity, and can be useful because it delivers the drug directly around the spinal cord where it reduces neurotransmission of afferent nerve fibers. Direct delivery to the spinal cord overcomes the problem of CNS side effects caused by the large oral doses needed to penetrate the blood–brain barrier. This therapy requires a team approach and constant follow-up for complications of the infusion pumping mechanism and infection. **Botulinum toxin** injected into specific muscle groups for the management of spasticity shows a very positive response in many patients. Botulinum toxin injected into salivary glands may also help reduce the severity of drooling, which is seen in 10-30% of patients with CP and has been traditionally treated with anticholinergic agents. Patients with rigidity, dystonia, and spastic quadriparesis sometimes respond to levodopa, and children with dystonia may benefit from carbamazepine or trihexyphenidyl. Hyperbaric oxygen has not been shown to improve the condition of children with CP.

Communication skills may be enhanced by the use of Bliss symbols, talking typewriters, electronic speech generating devices, and specially adapted computers including artificial intelligence computers to augment motor and language function. Significant behavior problems may substantially interfere with the development of a child with CP; their early identification and management are important, and the assistance of a psychologist or psychiatrist may be necessary. Learning and attention deficit disorders and mental retardation are assessed and managed by a psychologist and educator. Strabismus, nystagmus, and optic atrophy are common in children with CP; an ophthalmologist should be included in the initial assessment. Lower urinary tract dysfunction should receive prompt assessment and treatment.

Bibliography is available at Expert Consult.

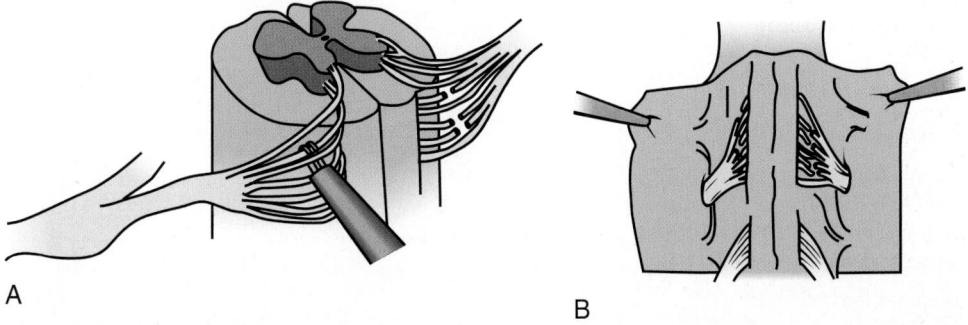

Figure 598-2 Schematic of the technique of selected dorsal rhizotomy. **A,** After laminectomy, the dura is opened and the dorsal spinal rootlets are exposed. The rootlets are stimulated so that abnormal rootlet activity can be identified. **B,** A proportion of rootlets are transected. *(From Koman LA, Smith BP, Shilt JS: Cerebral palsy, Lancet 363:1619–1631, 2004. Reproduced with permission from Wake Forest University Orthopaedic Press.)*

598.2 Mitochondrial Encephalomyopathies

Michael V. Johnston

See Chapters 87.4 and 611.4.

Mitochondrial encephalomyopathies are a heterogeneous group of clinical syndromes caused by genetic lesions that impair energy production through oxidative phosphorylation. The signs and symptoms of these disorders reflect the vulnerability of the nervous system, muscles, and other organs to energy deficiency. Signs of brain and muscle dysfunction (seizures, weakness, ptosis, external ophthalmoplegia, psychomotor regression, hearing loss, movement disorders, and ataxia) in association with lactic acidosis are prominent features of mitochondrial disorders. Cardiomyopathy and diabetes mellitus can also result from mitochondrial disorders.

Children with mitochondrial disorders often have multifocal signs that are intermittent or relapsing–remitting, often in association with intercurrent illness. Many of these disorders were described as clinical syndromes before their genetics were understood. Children with mitochondrial encephalomyopathy with lactic acidosis and stroke-like episodes (MELAS) present with developmental delay, weakness, and headaches, as well as focal signs that suggest a stroke. Brain imaging indicates that injury does not fit within the usual vascular territories. Children with myoclonic epilepsy with ragged red fibers (MERRF) present with myoclonus and myoclonic seizures as well as intermittent muscle weakness. The ragged red fibers referred to in the name of this disorder are clumps of abnormal mitochondria seen within muscle fibers in sections from a muscle biopsy stained with Gomori trichrome stain. NARP syndrome (neuropathy, ataxia, and retinitis pigmentosa), Kearns-Sayre syndrome (KSS; ptosis, ophthalmoplegia, heart block), Leigh disease (subacute necrotizing encephalomyelopathy), and Leber hereditary optic neuropathy (LHON) are also defined as relatively homogeneous clinical subgroups (Table 598-2). It is important to keep in mind that mitochondrial disorders can be difficult to diagnose. They often present with novel combinations of signs and symptoms as a consequence of high mutation rates for mitochondrial DNA (mtDNA), and the severity of disease varies from person to person.

Mitochondrial diseases can be caused by mutations of nuclear DNA (nDNA) or mtDNA (see Chapters 80, 86, and 87). Oxidative phosphorylation in the respiratory chain is mediated by 4 intramitochondrial enzyme complexes (complexes I-IV) and 2 mobile electron carriers (coenzyme Q and cytochrome c) that create an electrochemical proton gradient utilized by complex V (adenosine triphosphate [ATP] synthase) to create the ATP required for normal cellular function. The maintenance of oxidative phosphorylation requires coordinated regulation of nuclear DNA and mtDNA genes. Human mtDNA is a small (16.6 kb), circular, double-stranded molecule that has been completely sequenced and encodes 37 genes including 13 structural proteins, all of which are subunits of the respiratory chain complexes, as well as 2 ribosomal RNAs and 22 transfer RNAs (tRNAs) needed for translation. The nuclear DNA is responsible for synthesizing approximately 70 subunits, transporting them to the mitochondria via chaperone proteins, ensuring their passage across the inner mitochondrial membrane, and coordinating their correct processing and assembly. Diseases of mitochondrial oxidative phosphorylation can be divided into 3 groups: (1) defects of mtDNA, (2) defects of nDNA, and (3) defects of communication between the nuclear and mitochondrial genome. mtDNA is distinct from nDNA for the following 4 reasons: (1) its genetic code differs from nDNA, (2) it is tightly packed with information because it contains no introns, (3) it is subject to spontaneous mutations at a higher rate than nDNA, (4) it has less efficient repair mechanisms.

Inheritance of mutations present on mtDNA is nonmendelian and can be complex. At fertilization, mtDNA is present in hundreds or thousands of copies per cell and is transmitted by maternal inheritance from her oocyte to all her children, but only her daughters can pass it on to their children. Through the process called heteroplasmy or threshold effect, mtDNA containing mutations can be distributed unequally between cells in specific tissues. Some cells receive few or no mutant genomes (**normal** or **wild-type homoplasmy**), whereas

Table 598-2	Clinical Manifestations of Mitochondrial Encephalomyopathies						
TISSUE	**SYMPTOMS/SIGNS**	**MELAS**	**MERRF**	**NARP**	**KSS**	**LEIGH**	**LHON**
CNS	Regression	+	+		+	+	
	Seizures	+	+				
	Ataxia	+	+	+	+		
	Cortical blindness	+					
	Deafness	+		+			
	Migraine	+					
	Hemiparesis	+					
	Myoclonus	+	+				
	Movement disorder	+					+
Nerve	Peripheral neuropathy	+	+	+	+		
Muscle	Ophthalmoplegia				+		
	Weakness	+	+	+	+	+	
	RRF on muscle biopsy	+	+		+		
	Ptosis				+		
Eye	Pigmentary retinopathy			+	+		
	Optic atrophy				+	+	+
	Cataracts						
Heart	Conduction block				+		+
	Cardiomyopathy				+		
Blood	Anemia	+					
	Lactic acidosis		+		+	+	
Endocrine	Diabetes mellitus				+		
	Short stature	+	+		+		
Kidney	Fanconi syndrome	+	+		+		

KSS, Kearns-Sayre syndrome; LHON, Leber hereditary optic neuropathy; MELAS, mitochondrial myopathy, encephalopathy, lactic acidosis, and stroke-like episodes; MERRF, myoclonic epilepsy with ragged red fibers; NARP, neuropathy, ataxia and retinitis pigmentosa; RRF, ragged red fibers.

others receive a mixed population of **mutant** and **wild-type** mtDNAs (**heteroplasmy**), and still others receive primarily or exclusively **mutant** genomes (**mutant homoplasmy**). The important implications of maternal inheritance and heteroplasmy are as follows: (1) inheritance of the disease is maternal, but both sexes are equally affected; (2) phenotypic expression of an mtDNA mutation depends on the relative proportions of mutant and wild-type genomes, with a minimum critical number of mutant genomes being necessary for expression (**threshold effect**); (3) at cell division, the proportional distribution may shift between daughter cells (mitotic segregation), leading to a corresponding phenotypic change; and (4) subsequent generations are affected at a higher rate than in autosomal dominant diseases. The critical number of mutant mtDNAs required for the threshold effect may vary, depending on the vulnerability of the tissue to impairments of oxidative metabolism as well as on the vulnerability of the same tissue over time that may increase with aging. In contrast to maternally inherited disorders caused by mutations in mtDNA, diseases resulting from defects in nDNA follow mendelian inheritance. Mitochondrial diseases caused by defects in nDNA include defects in substrate transport (plasmalemmal carnitine transporter, carnitine palmitoyltransferases I and II, carnitine acylcarnitine translocase defects), defects in substrate oxidation (pyruvate dehydrogenase complex, pyruvate carboxylase, intramitochondrial fatty acid oxidation defects), defects in the Krebs cycle (α-ketoglutarate dehydrogenase, fumarase, aconitase defects), and defects in the respiratory chain (complexes I-V), including defects of oxidation/phosphorylation coupling (Luft syndrome), and defects in mitochondrial protein transport.

Diseases caused by defects in mtDNA can be divided into those associated with point mutations that are maternally inherited (e.g., LHON, MELAS, MERRF, and NARP syndromes) and those caused by deletions or duplications of mtDNA that reflect altered communication between the nucleus and the mitochondria (KSS; Pearson syndrome, a rare severe encephalopathy with anemia and pancreatic dysfunction; and progressive external ophthalmoplegia). These disorders can be inherited by sporadic, autosomal dominant or recessive mechanisms and mutations in multiple genes, including mitochondrial mtDNA polymerase γ catalytic subunit (POLG), have been identified. **POLG mutations** have also been identified in patients with Alpers-Huttenlocher syndrome, which causes a refractory seizure disorder and hepatic failure as well as autosomal dominant and recessive progressive external ophthalmoplegia, childhood myocerebrohepatopathy spectrum disorders, myoclonic epilepsy myopathy sensory ataxia syndrome, and *POLG*-related ataxia neuropathy spectrum disorders. Other genes that regulate the supply of nucleotides for mtDNA synthesis are associated with severe encephalopathy and liver disease, and new disorders are being identified that result from defects in the interactions between mitochondria and their milieu in the cell.

MITOCHONDRIAL MYOPATHY, ENCEPHALOPATHY, LACTIC ACIDOSIS, AND STROKELIKE EPISODES

Children with MELAS may be normal for the 1st several yr, but they gradually display delayed motor and cognitive development and short stature. The clinical syndrome is characterized by (1) recurrent stroke-like episodes of hemiparesis or other focal neurologic signs with lesions most commonly seen in the posterior temporal, parietal, and occipital lobes (CT or MRI evidence of focal brain abnormalities); (2) lactic acidosis, ragged red fibers (RRF), or both; and (3) at least 2 of the following: focal or generalized seizures, dementia, recurrent migraine headaches, and vomiting. In 1 series, onset was before age 15 yr in 62% of patients, and hemianopia or cortical blindness was the most common manifestation. Cerebrospinal fluid protein is often increased. The MELAS 3243 mutation on mtDNA is the most common mutation to produce MELAS and can also be associated with different combinations of exercise intolerance, myopathy, ophthalmoplegia, pigmentary retinopathy, hypertrophic or dilated cardiomyopathy, cardiac conduction defects, deafness, endocrinopathy (diabetes mellitus), and proximal renal tubular dysfunction. A number of other mutations have been reported, and 2 patients have been described with bilateral

rolandic lesions and epilepsia partialis continua associated with mtDNA mutations at 10158T>C and 10191T>C. MELAS is a progressive disorder that has been reported in siblings. However, most maternal relatives of MELAS patients are mildly affected or unaffected. MELAS is punctuated with episodes of stroke leading to dementia (see Chapter 611.4).

Regional cerebral hypoperfusion can be detected by single-photon emission CT studies and MR spectroscopy can detect focal areas of lactic acidosis in the brain. Neuropathology may show cortical atrophy with infarct-like lesions in both cortical and subcortical structures, basal ganglia calcifications, and ventricular dilation. Muscle biopsy specimens usually show RRF. Mitochondrial accumulations and abnormalities have been shown in smooth muscle cells of intramuscular vessels and of brain arterioles and in the epithelial cells and blood vessels of the choroid plexus, producing a mitochondrial angiopathy. Muscle biochemistry shows complex I deficiency in many cases; however, multiple defects have also been documented involving complexes I, III, and IV. Targeted molecular testing for specific mutations or sequence analysis and mutation scanning are generally used to make a diagnosis of MELAS when clinical evaluation suggests the diagnosis. Because the number of mutant genomes is lower in blood than in muscle, muscle is the preferable tissue for examination. Inheritance is maternal, and there is a highly specific, although not exclusive, point mutation at nt 3243 in the tRNA$^{Leu(UUR)}$ gene of mtDNA in approximately 80% of patients. An additional 7.5% have a point mutation at nt 3271 in the tRNA$^{Leu(UUR)}$ gene. A third mutation has been identified at nt 3252 in the tRNA$^{Leu(UUR)}$ gene. The prognosis in patients with the full syndrome is poor. Therapeutic trials reporting some benefit have included corticosteroids, coenzyme Q10, nicotinamide, carnitine, creatine, riboflavin and various combinations of these; L-arginine and preclinical studies reported some success with resveratrol.

MYOCLONUS EPILEPSY AND RAGGED RED FIBERS

MERRF syndrome is characterized by progressive myoclonic epilepsy, mitochondrial myopathy, and cerebellar ataxia with dysarthria and nystagmus. Onset may be in childhood or in adult life, and the course may be slowly progressive or rapidly downhill. Other features include dementia, sensorineural hearing loss, optic atrophy, peripheral neuropathy, and spasticity. Because some patients have abnormalities of deep sensation and pes cavus, the condition may be confused with Friedreich ataxia. A significant number of patients have a positive family history and short stature. This condition is maternally inherited.

Pathologic findings include elevated serum lactate concentrations, RRF on muscle biopsy, and marked neuronal loss and gliosis affecting, in particular, the dentate nucleus and inferior olivary complex with some dropout of Purkinje cells and neurons of the red nucleus. Pallor of the posterior columns of the spinal cord and degeneration of the gracile and cuneate nuclei occur. Muscle biochemistry has shown variable defects of complex III, complexes II and IV, complexes I and IV, or complex IV alone. More than 80% of cases are caused by a heteroplasmic G to A point mutation at nt 8344 of the tRNA^{Lys} gene of mtDNA. Additional patients have been reported with a T to C mutation at nt 8356 in the tRNA^{Lys} gene. Targeted mutation analysis or mutation analysis after sequencing of the mitochondrial genome is used to diagnosis MERRF.

There is no specific therapy, although coenzyme Q10 appeared to be beneficial in a mother and daughter with the MERRF mutation. The anticonvulsant levetiracetam is reported to help reduce myoclonus and myoclonic seizures in this disorder.

NEUROPATHY, ATAXIA, AND RETINITIS PIGMENTOSA SYNDROME

This maternally inherited disorder presents with either Leigh syndrome or with neurogenic weakness and NARP syndrome, as well as seizures. It is caused by a point mutation at nt 8993 within the ATPase subunit 6 gene. The severity of the disease presentation appears to have close correlation with the percentage of mutant mtDNA in leukocytes.

Two clinical patterns are seen in patients with NARP syndrome: (1) neuropathy, ataxia, retinitis pigmentosa, dementia, and ataxia, and (2) severe infantile encephalopathy resembling Leigh syndrome with lesions in the basal ganglia on MRI.

LEBER HEREDITARY OPTIC NEUROPATHY

LHON is characterized by onset usually between the ages of 18 and 30 yr of acute or subacute visual loss caused by severe bilateral optic atrophy, although children as young as 5 yr have been reported to have LHON. Three mtDNA mutations account for most cases of LHON and at least 85% of patients are young men. An X-linked factor may modulate the expression of the mtDNA point mutation. The classic ophthalmologic features include circumpapillary telangiectatic microangiopathy and pseudoedema of the optic disc. Variable features may include cerebellar ataxia, hyperreflexia, Babinski sign, psychiatric symptoms, peripheral neuropathy, or cardiac conduction abnormalities (preexcitation syndrome). Some cases are associated with widespread white matter lesions as seen with multiple sclerosis. Lactic acidosis and RRF tend to be conspicuously absent in LHON. More than 11 mtDNA point mutations have been described, including a usually homoplasmic G to A transition at nt 11,778 of the ND4 subunit gene of complex I. The latter leads to replacement of a highly conserved arginine residue by histidine at the 340th amino acid and accounts for 50-70% of cases in Europe and more than 90% of cases in Japan. Certain LHON pedigrees with other point mutations are associated with complex neurologic disorders and may have features in common with MELAS syndrome and with infantile bilateral striatal necrosis. One family has been reported with pediatric onset of progressive generalized dystonia with bilateral striatal necrosis associated with a homoplasmic G14459A mutation in the mtDNA *ND6* gene, which is also associated with LHON alone and LHON with dystonia.

KEARNS-SAYRE SYNDROME

KSS is a characteristic multiorgan disorder involving external ophthalmoplegia, heart block, and retinitis pigmentosa with onset before age 20 yr caused by single deletions in mtDNA. There must also be at least 1 of the following: heart block, cerebellar syndrome, or cerebrospinal fluid protein >100 mg/dL. Other nonspecific but common features include dementia, sensorineural hearing loss, and multiple endocrine abnormalities, including short stature, diabetes mellitus, and hypoparathyroidism. The prognosis is guarded, despite placement of a pacemaker, and progressively downhill, with death resulting by the 3rd or 4th decade. Unusual clinical presentations can include renal tubular acidosis and Lowe syndrome. There are also a few overlap cases of children with KSS and stroke-like episodes. Muscle biopsy shows RRF and variable cytochrome c oxidase (COX)-negative fibers. Most patients have mtDNA deletions, and some have duplications. These may be new mutations accounting for the generally sporadic nature of KSS. A few pedigrees have shown autosomal dominant transmission. Patients should be monitored closely for endocrine abnormalities, which can be treated. Coenzyme Q is reported anecdotally to have some beneficial effect; a positive effect of folinic acid for low folate levels also is reported. A report of positive effects of a cochlear implant for deafness is also reported.

Sporadic progressive external ophthalmoplegia with ragged red fibers is a clinically benign condition characterized by adolescent or young adult–onset ophthalmoplegia, ptosis, and proximal limb girdle weakness. It is slowly progressive and compatible with a relatively normal life. The muscle biopsy material demonstrates RRF and COX-negative fibers. Approximately 50% of patients with progressive external ophthalmoplegia have mtDNA deletions, and there is no family history.

REVERSIBLE INFANTILE CYTOCHROME C OXIDASE DEFICIENCY MYOPATHY

Mutations in mtDNA are also responsible for a reversible form of severe neuromuscular weakness and hypotonia in infants that is the result of a maternally inherited homoplasmic m.14674T>C mt-tRNA^{Glu} mutation associated with a deficiency of COX. Affected children present within the 1st few wk of life with hypotonia, severe muscle weakness, and very elevated serum lactate levels, and they often require mechanical ventilation. However, feeding and psychomotor development are not affected. Muscle biopsies taken from these children in the neonatal period show RRF and deficient COX activity, but these findings disappeared within 5-20 mo when the infants recovered spontaneously. It is difficult to distinguish these infants from those with lethal mitochondrial disorders without waiting for them to improve. The mechanism for this recovery is not established, but it may reflect a developmental switch in mitochondrial RNAs later in infancy. This reversible disorder is observed only in COX deficiency associated with the 14674T>C mt-tRNA^{Glu} mutation, so it is suggested that infants with this type of severe weakness in the neonatal period be tested for this mutation to help with prognosis.

LEIGH DISEASE (SUBACUTE NECROTIZING ENCEPHALOMYOPATHY)

Leigh disease is a progressive degenerative disorder presenting in infancy with feeding and swallowing problems, vomiting, and failure to thrive associated with lactic acidosis and lesions seen in the brainstem and/or basal ganglia on MRI (Table 598-3). There are several genetically determined causes of Leigh disease that result from nuclear DNA mutations in genes that code for components of the respiratory chain: pyruvate dehydrogenase complex deficiency, complex I or II deficiency, complex IV (COX) deficiency, complex V (ATPase) deficiency, and deficiency of coenzyme Q10. These defects may occur sporadically or be inherited by autosomal recessive transmission, as in the case of COX deficiency; by X-linked transmission, as in the case of pyruvate dehydrogenase E₁α deficiency; or by maternal transmission, as in complex V (ATPase 6 nt 8993 mutation) deficiency. Approximately 30% of cases are caused by mutations in mtDNA. Delayed motor and language milestones may be evident, and generalized seizures, weakness, hypotonia, ataxia, tremor, pyramidal signs, and nystagmus are prominent findings. Intermittent respirations with associated sighing or sobbing are characteristic and suggest brainstem dysfunction. Some patients have external ophthalmoplegia, ptosis, retinitis pigmentosa, optic atrophy, and decreased visual acuity. Abnormal results on CT or MRI scan consist of bilaterally symmetric areas of low attenuation in the basal ganglia and brainstem as well as elevated lactic acid on MR spectroscopy (Fig. 598-3). Pathologic changes consist of focal symmetric areas of necrosis in the thalamus, basal ganglia, tegmental gray matter, periventricular and periaqueductal regions of the brainstem, and posterior columns of the spinal cord. Microscopically, these spongiform lesions show cystic cavitation with neuronal loss, demyelination, and vascular proliferation. Elevations in serum lactate levels are characteristic and hypertrophic cardiomyopathy, hepatic failure and rental tubular dysfunction can occur. The overall outlook is poor, but a few patients experience prolonged periods of remission. There is no definitive treatment for the underlying disorder, but a range of vitamins including riboflavin, thiamine, and coenzyme Q are often given to try to improve mitochondrial function. Biotin, creatine, succinate, and idebenone, as well as a high-fat diet have also been used, but phenobarbital and valproic acid should be avoided because of their inhibitory effect on the mitochondrial respiratory chain.

REYE SYNDROME

This encephalopathy, which has become uncommon, is associated with pathologic features characterized by fatty degeneration of the viscera (microvesicular steatosis) and mitochondrial abnormalities and biochemical features consistent with a disturbance of mitochondrial metabolism (see Chapter 361).

Recurrent Reye-like syndrome is encountered in children with genetic defects of fatty acid oxidation, such as deficiencies of the plasmalemmal carnitine transporter, carnitine palmitoyltransferases I and II, carnitine acylcarnitine translocase, medium- and long-chain acyl-coenzyme A dehydrogenase, multiple acyl-coenzyme A dehydrogenase, and long-chain L-3 hydroxyacyl-coenzyme A dehydrogenase or trifunctional protein. These disorders are manifested by recurrent hypoglycemic and hypoketotic encephalopathy, and they are inherited

| Table 598-3 | Clinical Features of Congenital Leigh Syndrome or Leigh-Like Syndrome |

NEUROLOGIC MANIFESTATIONS

Brainstem
Bradypnea, hypopnea, episodes of apnea
Bradycardia
Tetraparesis
Hypotonia (floppy infant)
Failure to thrive, poor sucking
Swallowing difficulties, dysphagia, poor feeding, poor sucking
Vomiting
Spasticity, brisk tendon reflexes
Dysphasia, dysarthria
Squint
Absence of optic or acoustic blink

Other Cerebral Manifestations
Stroke-like episodes
Delay of developmental milestones
Paralysis of vertical gaze
Myoclonic jerks of limbs or eyelids
Hypothermia
Drowsiness, dizziness
Psychomotor (mental) retardation
Ataxia, tremor
Seizures, convulsions
Growth retardation
Dystonia
Clumsiness, dullness
Nystagmus, uncoordinated eye movement, slow saccades
Optic atrophy
Visual loss
Facial dyskinesia
Ocular apraxia
Drooling
Gaze fixation difficulty

Peripheral Nervous System Manifestations
Cranial nerve palsies
Generalized wasting
Bilateral ptoses
Chronic progressive external ophthalmoplegia, strabismus
Reduced tendon reflexes
Polyneuropathy
Muscle weakness
Myopathy

NONNEUROLOGIC MANIFESTATIONS

Dysmorphic Features
Lip cleft
Short distal phalanges
Single palmar crease
Rostral vertebrae
Round face
Frontal bossing
Flat nasal root
Microcephaly
Thin lips
Small chin
Long, featureless philtrum
Hypospadia

Others
Inguinal hernia
Stiff neck
Retinal dystrophy, retinopathy
Deafness, hypoacusis
Hypertrophic, dilated cardiomyopathy
Pancreatitis
Diarrhea
Urinary excretion of Krebs-cycle intermediates
Intrauterine growth retardation
Hypertrichosis
Villous atrophy
Nephrotic syndrome
Nephropathy
Hyperhidrosis
Scoliosis

From Finsterer J: Leigh and Leigh-like syndrome in children and adults. Pediatr Neurol 39:223–235, 2008, Table 1.

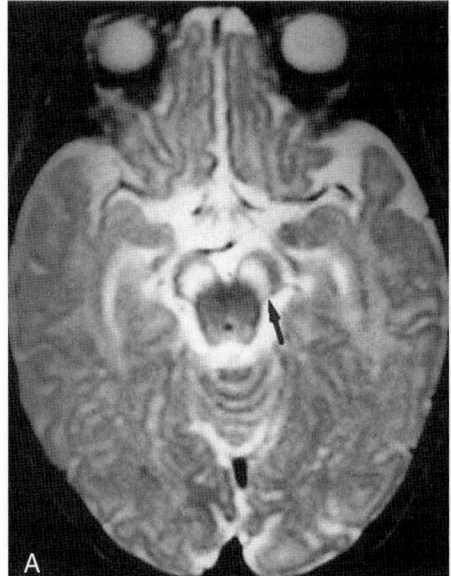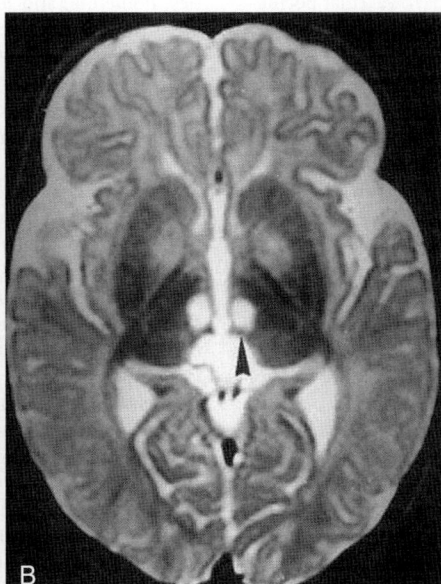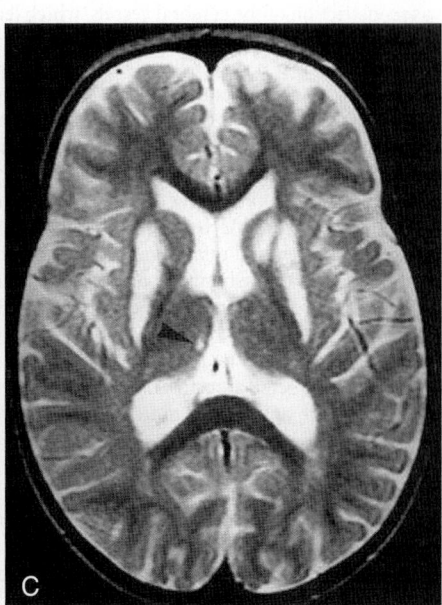

Figure 598-3 Leigh syndrome. Axial T2-weighted magnetic resonance images (TR/TE/NEX = 3,000/120/1 msec) of 8 mo old girl with Leigh syndrome because of a *SURF1* mutation indicate hyperintense lesions in substantia nigra and medial thalamic nuclei **(A, B).** Follow-up images (TR/TE/NEX = 2,028/120/2 msec) at age 26 mo **(C)** indicate hyperintense putamina and hyperintense left caudate nucleus. *(From Farina L, Chiapparini L, Uziel G, et al: MR findings in Leigh syndrome with COX deficiency and SURF-1 mutations, AJNR Am J Neuroradiol 23:1095–1100, 2002, Fig. 2.)*

in an autosomal recessive pattern. Other potential inborn errors of metabolism presenting with Reye syndrome include urea cycle defects (ornithine transcarbamylase, carbamyl phosphate synthetase) and certain of the organic acidurias (glutaric aciduria type I), respiratory chain defects, and defects of carbohydrate metabolism (fructose intolerance).

Bibliography is available at Expert Consult.

598.3 Other Encephalopathies

Michael V. Johnston

HIV ENCEPHALOPATHY
Encephalopathy is an unfortunate and common manifestation in infants and children with HIV infection (see Chapter 276).

LEAD ENCEPHALOPATHY
See Chapter 721.

BURN ENCEPHALOPATHY
An encephalopathy develops in approximately 5% of children with significant burns in the 1st several wk of hospitalization (see Chapter 75). There is no single cause of burn encephalopathy but rather a combination of factors that include anoxia (smoke inhalation, carbon monoxide poisoning, laryngospasm), electrolyte abnormalities, bacteremia and sepsis, cortical vein thrombosis, a concomitant head injury, cerebral edema, drug reactions, and emotional distress. Seizures are the most common clinical manifestation of burn encephalopathy, but altered states of consciousness, hallucinations, and coma may also occur. Management of burn encephalopathy is directed to a search for the underlying cause and treatment of hypoxemia, seizures, specific electrolyte abnormalities, or cerebral edema. The prognosis for complete neurologic recovery is generally excellent, particularly if seizures are the primary abnormality.

HYPERTENSIVE ENCEPHALOPATHY
Hypertensive encephalopathy is most commonly associated with renal disease in children, including acute glomerulonephritis, chronic pyelonephritis, and end-stage renal disease (see Chapters 445 and 535). In some cases, hypertensive encephalopathy is the initial manifestation of underlying renal disease. Marked systemic hypertension produces vasoconstriction of the cerebral vessels, which leads to vascular permeability, causing areas of focal cerebral edema and hemorrhage. The onset may be acute, with seizures and coma, or more indolent, with headache, drowsiness and lethargy, nausea and vomiting, blurred vision, transient cortical blindness, and hemiparesis. Examination of the eyegrounds may be nondiagnostic in children, but papilledema and retinal hemorrhages may occur. MRI often shows increased signal intensity in the occipital lobes on T2-weighted images, which is known as **posterior reversible leukoencephalopathy (PRES)** and may be confused with cerebral infarctions. These high signal areas may appear in other regions of the brain as well. PRES may also be seen in children without hypertension. In all circumstances, PRES manifests with generalized motor seizures, headache, mental status changes, and visual disturbances. CT may be normal in PRES; MRI is the study of choice. Treatment is directed at restoration of a normotensive state and control of seizures with appropriate anticonvulsants.

RADIATION ENCEPHALOPATHY
Acute radiation encephalopathy is most likely to develop in young patients who have received large daily doses of radiation. Excessive radiation injures vessel endothelium, resulting in enhanced vascular permeability, cerebral edema, and numerous hemorrhages. The child may suddenly become irritable and lethargic, complain of headache, or present with focal neurologic signs and seizures. Patients occasionally develop hemiparesis as the result of an infarct secondary to vascular occlusion of the cerebral vessels. Steroids are often beneficial in

Table 598-4	Diagnostic Criteria for Acute Necrotizing Encephalopathy of Childhood

1. Acute encephalopathy following (1-3 days) a febrile disease. Rapid deterioration in the level of consciousness. Seizures.
2. No cerebrospinal fluid pleocytosis. Increase in cerebrospinal fluid protein.
3. CT or MRI evidence of symmetric, multifocal brain lesions. Involvement of the bilateral thalami. Lesions also common in the cerebral periventricular white matter, internal capsule, putamen, upper brainstem tegmentum and cerebellar medulla. No involvement of other central nervous system regions.
4. Elevation of serum aminotransferases of variable degrees. No increase in blood ammonia.
5. Exclusion of resembling diseases.
   A. Differential diagnosis from clinical viewpoints. Overwhelming bacterial and viral infections, and fulminant hepatitis; toxic shock, hemolytic uremic syndrome, and other toxin-induced diseases; Reye syndrome, hemorrhagic shock and encephalopathy syndrome, and heat stroke.
   B. Differential diagnosis from radiologic viewpoints. Leigh encephalopathy and related mitochondrial cytopathies; glutaric acidemia, methylmalonic acidemia, and infantile bilateral striatal necrosis; Wernicke encephalopathy and carbon monoxide poisoning; acute disseminated encephalomyelitis, acute hemorrhagic leukoencephalitis, other types of encephalitis, and vasculitis; arterial or venous infection, and the effects of severe hypoxia or head trauma

Modified from Hoshino A, Saitoh M, Oka, et al: Epidemiology of acute encephalopathy in Japan, with emphasis on the association of viruses and syndromes. Brain Dev 34:337–343, 2012, Table 1.

reducing the cerebral edema and reversing the neurologic signs. Late-radiation encephalopathy is characterized by headaches and slowly progressive focal neurologic signs, including hemiparesis and seizures. Exposure of the brain to radiation for treatment of childhood cancer increases the risk of later cerebrovascular disease, including stroke, moyamoya disease, aneurysm, vascular malformations, mineralizing microangiopathy, and stroke-like migraines. Some children with acute lymphocytic leukemia treated with a combination of intrathecal methotrexate and cranial irradiation develop neurologic signs months or years later; signs consist of increasing lethargy, loss of cognitive abilities, dementia, and focal neurologic signs and seizures (see Chapter 494). The CT scan shows calcifications in the white matter, and the postmortem examination demonstrates a necrotizing encephalopathy. This devastating complication of the treatment of leukemia has prompted re-evaluation and reduction in the use of cranial radiation in the treatment of these children.

ACUTE NECROTIZING ENCEPHALOPATHY
Acute necrotizing encephalopathy is a rare, severe encephalopathy seen more commonly in Asian countries. It is thought to be triggered by a viral infection (influenza, HHV-6) in a genetically susceptible host. Table 598-4 lists the diagnostic criteria. The elevation of hepatic enzymes without hyperammonemia is a unique feature. A familial or recurrent form is associated with mutations in the *RANBP2* gene and is designated ANE1. MRI finding are characterized by symmetric lesions that must be present in the thalami (Fig. 598-4). The prognosis is usually poor, however some patients have responded to steroids and intravenous immunoglobulin (IVIG).

CYSTIC LEUKOENCEPHALOPATHY
An autosomal recessive disorder caused by mutations of RNASET2 proteins produces a brain MRI study that closely resembles congenital cytomegalovirus infection. Cystic leukoencephalopathy is manifest as a static encephalopathy without megalencephaly.

Bibliography is available at Expert Consult.

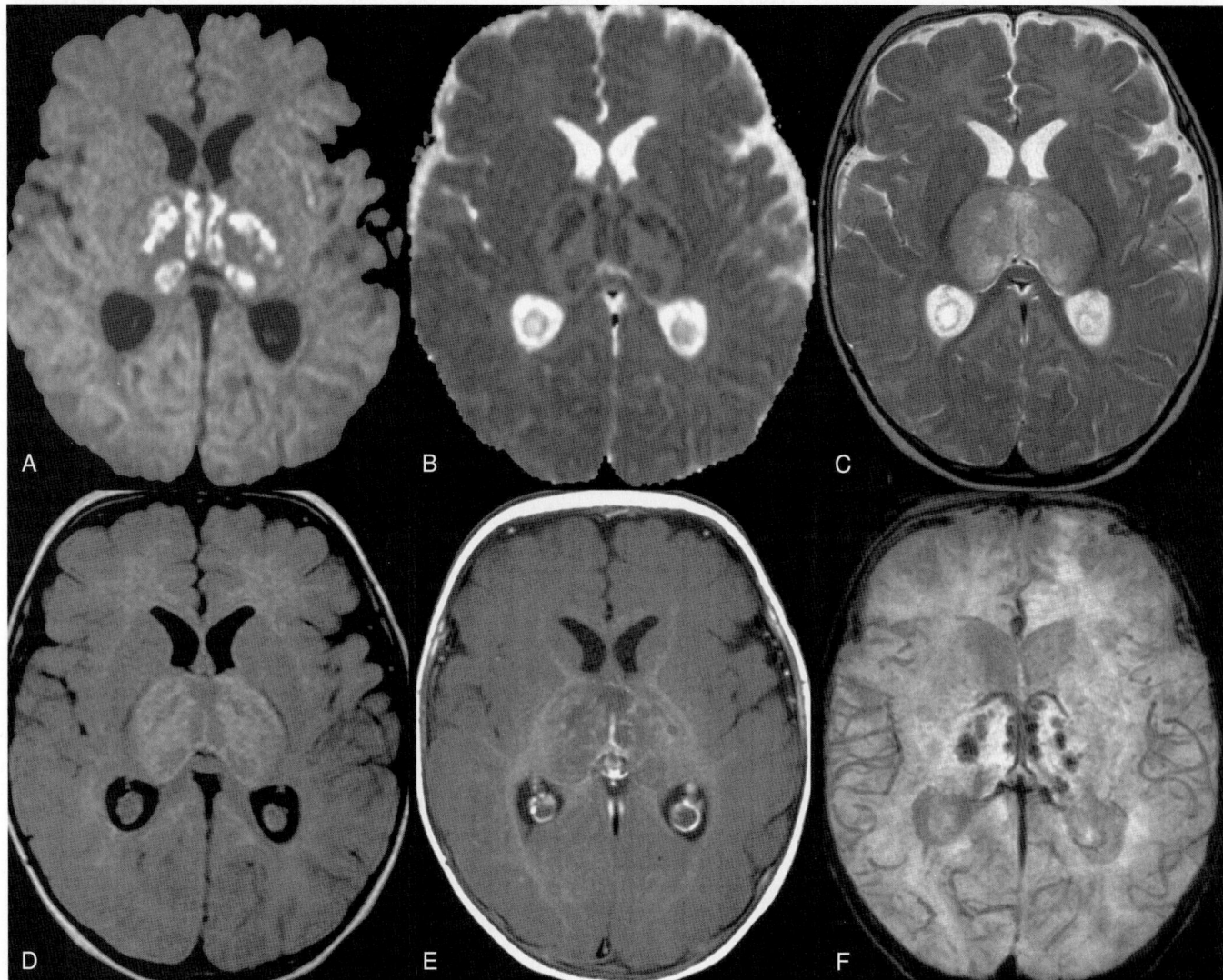

Figure 598-4 Acute necrotizing encephalopathy. MRI at presentation. **A,** Axial diffusion-weighted image; **B,** axial apparent diffusion coefficient (ADC) map; **C,** axial T2-weighted image; **D,** axial fluid-attenuated inversion recovery (FLAIR) image; **E,** contrast-enhanced axial T1-weighted image; **F,** axial susceptibility weighted image. Diffusion-weighted images **(A)** and corresponding ADC map **(B)** clearly show multiple areas of restricted diffusion against a background of increased diffusion involving both thalami, which are swollen. On T2-weighted **(C)** and FLAIR **(D)** images, the thalami are markedly swollen and hyperintense. On T1-weighted images obtained after intravenous gadolinium chelate injection **(E),** multiple necrotic portions are well delineated by peripheral faint, linear enhancement. Incidental choroid plexus cysts are detected. Susceptibility weighted image **(F)** shows multiple hypointense spots, consistent with petechial hemorrhage. *(From Bergamino L, Capra V, Biancheri R, et al: Immunomodulatory therapy in recurrent acute necrotizing encephalopathy ANE1: is it useful? Brain Dev 34:384–391, 2012, Fig. 1.)*

598.4 Autoimmune Encephalitis

Thaís Armangué and Josep O. Dalmau

Autoimmune encephalitis comprises an expanding group of clinical syndromes that can occur at all ages (<1 yr to adult) but preferentially affect younger adults and children (Table 598-5). These disorders associate with antibodies against neuronal cell surface proteins and synaptic receptors involved in synaptic transmission, plasticity, or neuronal excitability. The syndromes vary according to the associated antibody with phenotypes that resemble those in which the function of the target antigen is pharmacologically or genetically modified.

Most of these disorders are severe and potentially fatal but patients frequently respond to immunotherapy with good outcomes. Moreover, because of the broad spectrum of symptoms—including alterations of behavior, psychosis, catatonia, memory deficits, seizures, abnormal movements, and autonomic dysregulation—patients usually require a multidisciplinary treatment approach often in an intensive care unit.

The identification of these disorders provides a definitive diagnosis to many cases of encephalitis previously considered idiopathic, infectious, or postinfectious, although no causative agents were found. Because the etiology and pathogenic mechanisms were unknown, some of these disorders were previously defined with descriptive terms. More than half of cases under the ill-defined term "encephalitis lethargica" and some cases of "choreoathetosis post–herpes simplex encephalitis" are known to be anti–N-methyl-D-aspartate receptor (NMDAR) encephalitis.

The mechanisms that trigger the production of the antibodies are unknown. In a small subgroup of adolescent or young adult patients, the presence of a tumor that expresses the target neuronal antigen likely contributes in triggering the immune response. In addition, the high prevalence of prodromal viral-like symptoms has suggested that nonspecific viral infections may contribute to breaking immune tolerance and increase the permeability of the blood–brain barrier to antibodies. Nonetheless in many of these disorders the blood–brain barrier appears intact and there is evidence that the autoantibodies are

| Table 598-5 | Autoimmune Encephalitis in Children | | | | |

	MECHANISMS	TUMOR ASSOCIATION	SYNDROME	ANCILLARY TEST	TREATMENT/ PROGNOSIS
DEMONSTRATED IMMUNE MECHANISMS					
Anti-NMDAR encephalitis	Antibodies against NR1 subunit of NMDAR, disrupt function by crosslinking and internalization of receptors	Age and gender related: 41% in females older than 12 yr; <6% in girls younger than 12 yr. No tumors identified in young boys	Psychiatric symptoms, seizures, orofacial dyskinesias and other abnormal movements, autonomic dysfunction	EEG: almost always abnormal; it may show "extreme delta brush" pattern Brain MRI: nonspecific findings in ~35% CSF: pleocytosis and/or increased protein in >80%	80% complete recovery after immunotherapy and tumor removal (if appropriate). Frequently second-line drug* immunotherapy is required. Relapses in ~15% of patients
Limbic encephalitis	**Antibodies against intraneuronal antigens:** Hu, Ma2, amphiphysin, GAD **Antibodies against synaptic antigens:** GABA$_B$R, mGluR5	Extremely rare in children (see text)	Severe short-term memory loss, seizures	EEG: temporal lobe epileptic activity; focal or generalized slowing MRI: increased T2 and FLAIR signal in limbic region CSF: pleocytosis and increased proteins	If autoantigens are intracellular, poor response to immunotherapy If autoantigens are on the cell surface, ~80% are responsive to immunotherapy
STRONGLY SUSPECTED IMMUNE MECHANISMS					
Opsoclonus-myoclonus and other cerebellar-brainstem encephalitis	Most patients do not have detectable antibodies (a few patients have Hu antibodies)	Neuroblastoma occurs in 50% of children <2 year old; teratoma in teenagers and young adults	Opsoclonus often accompanied by irritability, ataxia, falling, myoclonus, tremor, and drooling	CSF abnormalities suggesting B-cell activation MRI: in some cases cerebellar atrophy	Partial response to immunotherapy in neuroblastoma-related opsoclonus High response to immunotherapy in teratoma-associated opsoclonus
Bickerstaff encephalitis	GQ1b antibodies	No tumor association	Ophthalmoplegia, ataxia, hyperreflexia. May overlap with Miller-Fisher syndrome	MRI: abnormal in ~30% (T2-signal abnormalities in the brainstem, thalamus, and cerebellum) Nerve conduction studies: abnormal in ~44% (predominant axonal degeneration, less frequent demyelination)	Often good outcome with steroids, IVIG and/or plasma exchange
Hashimoto encephalitis	TPO antibodies	No tumor association	Stroke-like symptoms, tremor, myoclonus, aphasia, sleep and behavioral problems seizures, ataxia	48% hypothyroidism, MRI often normal EEG: slow activity CSF: elevated protein	Steroid-responsive. Partial responses are frequent
Rasmussen encephalitis	Most likely immune mediated (unclear mechanism)	No tumor association	Progressive refractory partial seizures, cognitive decline, focal deficits, and brain hemiatrophy	MRI: progressive unilateral hemispheric atrophy	Limited response to immunotherapy. Patients may need functional hemispherectomy
Basal ganglia encephalitis	Antibodies to D2R in some cases	No tumor association	Abnormal movement and behavior disorder	Variable basal ganglia T2/FLAIR abnormalities	Mostly monophasic, can relapse
POSSIBLE IMMUNE MECHANISMS					
CLIPPERS	No antibodies	No tumor association	Episodic diplopia or facial paresthesias with subsequent development of symptoms of brainstem and occasionally spinal cord dysfunction	MRI: symmetric curvilinear gadolinium enhancement peppering the pons and extending variably into the medulla, brachium pontis, cerebellum, midbrain, and, occasionally, spinal cord	Steroid-responsive but may require chronic steroid or other immunosuppressive therapy
ROHHAD	Unknown. Autoimmune and genetic origin postulated.	Neural crest tumor in ~50% of cases†	Rapid onset obesity, hyperphagia, abnormal behavior, autonomic dysfunction, and central hypoventilation	Brain MRI, usually normal	Symptomatic; in some patients limited response to immunotherapy

*Includes rituximab and cyclophosphamide.
†Exact frequency is unknown.
CLIPPERS, Chronic lymphocytic inflammation with pontine perivascular enhancement responsive to steroids; CSF, cerebrospinal fluid; D2R, dopamine 2 receptor; EEG, electroencephalography; FLAIR, fluid-attenuated inversion recovery; GABA$_B$R, γ-aminobutyric acid-B receptor, GAD, glutamic acid decarboxylase; IVIG, intravenous immunoglobulin; mGluR5, metabotropic glutamate receptor 5; MRI, magnetic resonance imaging; NMDAR, N-methyl-D-aspartate receptor; ROHHAD, rapid onset obesity with hypothalamic dysfunction, hypoventilation, and autonomic dysregulation; TPO, thyroid peroxidase.

synthesized within the CNS by plasma cells that form part of local brain and meningeal inflammatory infiltrates.

ANTI-N-METHYL-D-ASPARTATE RECEPTOR ENCEPHALITIS

In this disorder, the antibodies target the NR1 subunit of the NMDA receptor. The exact frequency of this syndrome is unknown but it is considered the second most common cause of autoimmune encephalitis after acute disseminated encephalomyelitis in children and adolescents. Overall, the disorder predominates in females (80%), although in patients younger than 12 yr the frequency of males is higher (40%). The resulting syndrome is highly predictable and usually evolves in stages. In teenagers and young adults, the disorder usually presents with prominent psychiatric manifestations that may include rapidly progressive anxiety, agitation, delusional thoughts, bizarre behavior, labile affect, mood disturbances (mania), catatonic features, memory deficit, language disintegration, aggression, and insomnia or other sleep disturbances. In many cases, these symptoms had been preceded by a few days of prodromal headache, fever or viral-like symptoms. As a result of this symptom presentation, patients are often misdiagnosed with new-onset psychosis or a primary psychiatric disorder. However, in a few days or weeks, additional symptoms occur, including a decreased level of consciousness, seizures (including status epilepticus), limb or oral dyskinesias, choreoathetoid movements, and autonomic instability which usually includes tachycardia, bradycardia, fluctuations of blood pressure, hypoventilation, hyperthermia and sialorrhea. In rare instances, bradycardia and cardiac pauses occur, at times requiring the transient use of a pacemaker. The disorder also occurs in toddlers and infants (the youngest patient identified to date was 6 mo old), and although the evolution of the syndrome is similar to that of adults, young patients more frequently present with motor or complex seizures and movement disorders. Because of their age, the psychiatric–behavioral features may be missed. In this young age group, behavior changes include irritability, new-onset temper tantrums, agitation, aggression, reduced speech, mutism, and autistic-like regression. Moreover, compared with adults some children also develop cerebellar ataxia and hemiparesis; in contrast, autonomic dysfunction is usually milder and less severe in children. There is often an abrupt on–off phenomenon in alterations of responsiveness or level of consciousness.

Brain MRI is abnormal in approximately 35% of cases, usually showing nonspecific cortical and subcortical T2–fluid-attenuated inversion recovery (FLAIR) signal abnormalities, sometimes with transient cortical or meningeal enhancement; nonspecific white matter abnormalities are common. Lesions may also involve the spinal cord producing symptoms of myelitis. The cerebrospinal fluid (CSF) is initially abnormal in approximately 80% of cases, showing moderate lymphocytic pleocytosis and less frequently increased protein synthesis and oligoclonal bands. The electroencephalogram (EEG) is abnormal in virtually all patients, and usually shows focal or diffuse slow activity in the delta and theta range, which does not correlate with abnormal movements. In addition, many patients develop epileptic activity, requiring video-monitoring for adequate clinical management. A characteristic EEG pattern called "extreme delta brush" characterized by beta-delta complexes occurs in 30% of adults and has been described in children (Fig. 598-5).

The diagnosis of the disorder is established by demonstrating NMDAR antibodies in CSF or serum. The sensitivity is higher in CSF compared with serum (100% vs 85%), and the levels of antibodies in CSF appear to correlate better with outcome. Antibodies may remain detectable, albeit at lower titers, after patients recover.

The presence of an underlying tumor, mostly teratomas, is age and sex dependent. Whereas 40% of females older than 12 yr have an underlying teratoma of the ovary, less than 6% of females younger than 12 yr have a tumor. In young boys with anti-NMDAR encephalitis, the presence of an underlying tumor is exceptional; in young adults, the presence of a testicular teratoma is also rare (<15% of cases). In children, MRI of abdomen and pelvis and abdominal and testicular ultrasound are the preferred tumor screening tests.

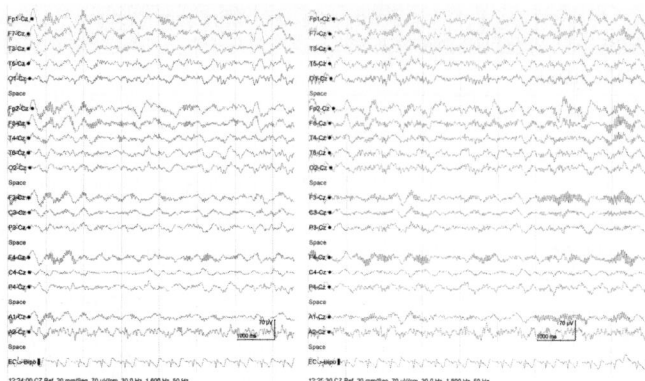

Figure 598-5 Electroencephalogram showing a pattern named "extreme delta brush" in a 14 yr old girl with anti-N-methyl-D-aspartate receptor (NMDAR) encephalitis. This pattern has been found to be characteristic of anti-NMDAR encephalitis. It consists of a nearly continuous combination of delta activity with superimposed fast activity, usually in the beta range, symmetrically involving all head regions, with a frontal preference in patients who are not under effects of sedation or anesthetics. *(From Armangue T, Titulaer MJ, Málaga I, et al: Pediatric anti-N-methyl-D-aspartate receptor encephalitis—clinical analysis and novel findings in a series of 20 patients. J Pediatr 162:850–856, 2012, Fig. 2.)*

In a small number of patients, anti-NMDAR encephalitis occurs simultaneously or after infections with a variety of pathogens, including *Mycoplasma pneumoniae*, human herpes simplex viruses 1 and 6 (HSV), enterovirus, and influenza. A pathogenic link with most of these infections has not established; there is evidence that some patients with HSV encephalitis develop antibodies against the NR1 subunit of the NMDAR. These patients may progress to develop relapsing neurologic symptoms post-HSV encephalitis. In a subgroup of patients with noninfectious relapsing neurologic symptoms post-HSV encephalitis, or "choreoathetosis post-HSV encephalitis," the disorder is in fact anti-NMDAR encephalitis (see Videos 598-1, 598-2, and 598-3).

Although no prospective clinical trials have been done, there is evidence that tumor removal, when appropriate, and prompt immunotherapy improve outcome. Most children receive first-line immunotherapies, including corticosteroids, IVIG, or plasma exchange. However, because these treatments fail in almost 50% of patients, and with an increasing number of reports showing that rituximab can be effective, this treatment is increasingly being used in combination with IVIG and steroids, or after first-line immunotherapies. Cyclophosphamide can be effective when there has been no response to these treatments.

Although anti-NMDAR encephalitis has a mortality rate of 7%, approximately 80% of patients have substantial or full recovery. Recovery is usually slow and can take as long as 2 yr after symptom onset. The last symptoms to improve are social interactions, and language and executive functions. Relapses occur in approximately 15% of patients; they can develop as partial syndromes, are usually milder than the initial episode and respond equally to immunotherapy. Initial comprehensive immunotherapy appears to prevent or reduce the number of relapses. The efficacy of chronic immunosuppression with drugs such as azathioprine or mycophenolate mofetil in preventing relapses is unknown.

The differential diagnosis of anti-NMDAR encephalitis is extensive and varies according to the stage of the disease (Table 598-6). The most frequently considered disorders are viral encephalitis, neuroleptic malignant syndrome, acute psychosis, and drug abuse.

LIMBIC ENCEPHALITIS

This disorder refers to an inflammatory process of the limbic system including, the medial temporal lobes, amygdala, and cingulate gyri. In adults, the most frequent immune-mediated limbic encephalitis occurs

Table 598-6	Differential Diagnosis of Anti-NMDAR Encephalitis in Children
DISORDER	**COMMENTS**
Viral encephalitis	Viral encephalitis is often suggested by the acute onset of symptoms, CSF pleocytosis, and hyperthermia. Most viral encephalitides (except rabies) occur with higher levels of CSF pleocytosis and protein concentration. Psychosis and dyskinesias are significantly less frequent in viral encephalitis than in anti-NMDAR encephalitis.
Relapsing post–herpes simplex virus encephalitis	Occurs ~4-6 wk after successful treatment of herpes simplex encephalitis. This may represent a true viral relapse of encephalitis (CSF PCR-positive, progression of necrotic MRI changes, response to acyclovir), or an autoimmune disorder (CSF PCR-negative, no new necrotic lesions on MRI, lack of response to acyclovir). In a proportion of the latter patients, the disorder is anti-NMDAR encephalitis.
New-onset psychosis	Because most patients with anti-NMDAR encephalitis present with psychosis, a primarily psychiatric disorder is frequently considered. As the disease evolves, the development of neurological symptoms usually reveals the diagnosis.
Drugs/toxins	The acute development of personality and behavioral changes, and symptoms suggesting involvement of dopaminergic pathways (rigidity, dystonia, orofacial movements) usually leads to a suspicion of drug abuse (e.g., ketamine, phencyclidine, among others). Carbon monoxide.
Neuroleptic malignant syndrome	The occurrence of altered level of consciousness, episodes of rigidity, hyperthermia, and autonomic instability often suggest NMS. In addition, some patients with anti-NMDAR encephalitis have elevated serum creatine kinase and rhabdomyolysis (in the absence of antipsychotic medication). The frequent use of neuroleptics to control the abnormal behavior adds further confusion between both syndromes. The presence of dyskinesias and catatonia suggest anti-NMDAR encephalitis.
Limbic encephalitis	Criteria of LE are well defined. Patients with LE do not have dyskinesias or central hypoventilation; the MRI usually shows abnormalities restricted to the medial temporal lobes, and the EEG findings (epileptic or slow activity) are largely restricted to the temporal lobes.
Encephalitis lethargica	This is an ill-defined entity, likely representing multiple disorders. Criteria include: acute or subacute encephalitis with at least 3 of the following: signs of basal ganglia involvement; oculogyric crises; ophthalmoplegia; obsessive-compulsive behavior; akinetic mutism; central respiratory irregularities; and somnolence and/or sleep inversion. Approximately, 50% of patients categorized as encephalitis lethargica hyperkinetica have anti-NMDAR encephalitis.
Childhood disintegrative disorder/late-onset autism	Children with anti-NMDAR encephalitis often show cognitive regression, rapid loss of language function, autistic features, and seizures, suggesting a childhood disintegrative disorder. While the prognosis of CDD is poor, most patients with anti-NMDAR encephalitis respond to immunotherapy and have substantial clinical recovery.
Kleine-Levin syndrome	Symptoms of hypersomnia, compulsive hyperphagia, hypersexuality, apathy, and child-like behavior, which are typical components of Kleine-Levin syndrome, may occur transiently during the process of recovery of anti-NMDAR encephalitis, or as permanent sequelae.
Inborn errors of metabolism	Glutaric aciduria type I can present in previously asymptomatic patients as episodes of encephalopathy with dystonia, coinciding with an infection or febrile process. Several inborn errors of metabolism can also occur with acute or subacute encephalopathy with extrapyramidal signs, including 3-methylglutaconic aciduria, creatine transport deficiency, mitochondrial disorders (Leigh syndrome), Wilson, and Lesch-Nyhan syndromes. Pantothenate kinase associated neurodegeneration, porphyria, and urea cycle defects should also be considered.
Monoamine neurotransmitter disorders	Deficiency of dopamine, serotonin or both can result in encephalopathy, epilepsy, and pyramidal and extrapyramidal symptoms. The diagnosis is established by examining the CSF for levels of these neurotransmitters.
Demyelinating disorders	Acute disseminated encephalomyelitis and neuromyelitis optica are immune-mediated inflammatory and demyelinating disorders of the central nervous system. These disorders should be considered in the differential diagnosis of multifocal neurologic abnormalities and encephalopathy in children. As with anti-NMDAR encephalitis these disorders may be preceded by an infection and can show pleocytosis. The diagnosis is suggested by the MRI findings. In NMO the presence of aquaporin 4 antibodies in serum or CSF is associated with relapses and poor prognosis.
CNS vasculitis	CNS vasculitis results in neurologic deficits and psychiatric manifestations. The diagnosis is established by angiography in large vessel angiitis, and brain biopsy in small vessel angiitis. In the latter, serum inflammatory markers (erythrocyte sedimentation rate, C-reactive protein, Complement 3, von Willebrand factor antigen) are usually elevated, and the MRI shows FLAIR/T2 abnormalities in the white and/or gray matter, not restricted to vascular territories with frequent leptomeningeal and/or local enhancement.
Systemic rheumatic disorders	Systemic lupus erythematosus and other rheumatic disorders can result in encephalopathy and multifocal neurologic and psychiatric manifestations. These disorders are usually suggested by the presence of signs and symptoms of involvement of systemic organs: skin, joints, kidneys, blood-forming cells, and blood vessels.

CDD, childhood disintegrative disorder; CNS, central nervous system; CSF, cerebrospinal fluid; EEG, electroencephalography; FLAIR, fluid-attenuated inversion recovery; LE, limbic encephalitis; MRI, magnetic resonance imaging; NMDAR, N-methyl-D-aspartate receptor; NMO, neuromyelitis optica; NMS, neuroleptic malignant syndrome; PCR, polymerase chain reaction.

in association with antibodies against proteins that were once thought to be voltage-gated potassium channels (VGKC), but which, in fact, target a secreted neuronal protein called leucine-rich glioma-inactivated 1 (LGI1), and a protein called Caspr2 expressed in brain and juxtaparanodal regions of myelinated nerves. Patients with LGI1 antibody associated limbic encephalitis often develop *hyponatremia*; in some patients the disorder is preceded by short-lasting episodes of distinctive dystonic or myoclonic-like movements, described as *faciobrachial dystonic seizures*, but with EEG features of tonic seizures. Patients with antibodies to Caspr2 usually develop Morvan syndrome, which includes encephalopathy, seizures, autonomic dysfunction, and neuromyotonia. How the clinical significance of antibodies called "VGKC-complex proteins" differs from LGI1 and Caspr2 is unknown.

Other less frequent types of autoimmune limbic encephalitis in adults are paraneoplastic and may occur with antibodies against intracellular antigens (e.g., Hu, CRMP5, Ma2) or neuronal cell surface and synaptic proteins (e.g., AMPA, GABA$_B$ receptor, mGluR5). While the disorders associated with antibodies against intracellular antigens appear to be mediated by cytotoxic T-cell responses and are poorly responsive to treatment, those associated with antibodies to cell surface and synaptic antigens are likely mediated by the antibodies and treatment responsive.

In children, autoimmune or paraneoplastic limbic encephalitis is exceptional. Unfortunately, any type of encephalopathy resulting in seizures and alteration of memory and behavior is frequently labeled as "limbic encephalitis," making data based on literature searches using the term "limbic encephalitis" unreliable. Fewer than 30 children with limbic encephalitis have been described in the English literature, some of them with antibodies against intracellular or cell surface antigens (Hu, Ma2, GAD, amphiphysin, GABA$_B$, and VGKC-complex proteins different from LGI1 and Caspr2). In some cases an underlying tumor was identified and included, leukemia, ganglioneuroblastoma, neuroblastoma, and small-cell carcinoma of the ovary.

The **Ophelia syndrome** is a form of limbic encephalitis that occurs in association with Hodgkin's lymphoma and predominantly affects young adults, teenagers or children. Some patients develop antibodies against mGluR5, a receptor involved in learning and memory; symptoms are usually responsive to chemotherapy.

HASHIMOTO ENCEPHALOPATHY

Hashimoto encephalopathy is defined by the detection of thyroid peroxidase (TPO) antibodies in patients with acute or subacute encephalitis that responds to corticosteroids. Since almost 50% of patients have normal thyroid function and not all patients respond to steroids, the term "encephalopathy associated with autoimmune thyroid disease" is considered more accurate than the previous term "steroid-responsive encephalopathy associated with autoimmune thyroiditis." Clinical features are not specific and may include stroke-like symptoms, tremor, myoclonus, transient aphasia, sleep and behavior abnormalities, hallucinations, seizures, and ataxia. The CSF usually shows elevated protein level with less-frequent pleocytosis. EEG studies almost always are abnormal frequently showing generalized slowing. Brain MRI is usually normal, although it may show diffuse white matter abnormalities and meningeal enhancement that can resolve with steroid therapy. As TPO antibodies occur in approximately 10% of asymptomatic children (nonencephalopathic and most cases euthyroid), as well as in patients who have more relevant antibody-associated disorders, such as GABA$_B$, LGI1, or NMDAR antibodies, TPO antibodies should be viewed as a marker of autoimmunity rather than a neurologic disease-specific or pathogenic antibody. Importantly the presence of TPO antibodies should not prevent testing for more relevant antibodies.

OPSOCLONUS–MYOCLONUS AND OTHER BRAINSTEM–CEREBELLAR ENCEPHALITIDES

Opsoclonus-myoclonus occurs in infants, teenagers and adults, although it probably represents different diseases and pathogenic mechanisms. In infants, the syndrome usually develops in the 1st 2 yr of life (mean: 20 mo), and at least 50% of patients have an underlying neuroblastoma. The child often presents with irritability, ataxia, falling, myoclonus, tremor, and drooling. Additional symptoms may include refusal to walk or sit, speech problems, hypotonia, and the typical features of opsoclonus characterized by rapid, chaotic, multidirectional eye movements without saccadic intervals. Because opsoclonus may be absent at symptom presentation, patients may initially be diagnosed with acute cerebellitis or labyrinthitis. Typically CSF abnormalities suggest B-cell activation, and the presence of antibodies against neuronal proteins has been demonstrated in several studies, although the identification of a specific autoantigen has been elusive.

Immunosuppressive treatment, including corticosteroids, IVIG, rituximab, and cyclophosphamide often improves the abnormal eye movements, but residual behavioral, language, and cognitive problems persist in the majority of patients, often requiring special education. In addition, insomnia and abnormal response to pain are common. Relapses occur in 50% of the patients, usually as a result of an intercurrent infection or drug tapering. Delay in treatment appears to associate with a poorer neurologic outcome; therefore, in cases with neuroblastoma, removal of the tumor should not delay the start of immunotherapy.

In teenagers and young adults, opsoclonus–myoclonus and brainstem–cerebellar encephalitis without opsoclonus are often considered "idiopathic" or "postinfectious"; however, there is evidence that some of these patients have an underlying teratoma, usually in the ovaries. These patients do not harbor NMDAR antibodies, and compared with those with anti-NMDAR encephalitis are less likely to initially present with psychosis and behavioral changes, and rarely develop dyskinesias. Although these patients do not appear to have neuronal antibodies, the CSF often shows pleocytosis and elevated protein concentration. Identification of this subphenotype of opsoclonus–myoclonus is important because patients usually have full recovery after treatment with immunotherapy (corticosteroids, IVIG, and/or plasma exchange) and if present, removal of the ovarian teratoma. The prognosis of this disorder seems better than that of neuroblastoma-associated opsoclonus, or the paraneoplastic opsoclonus of older patients, usually related to breast, ovarian, or lung cancer.

BICKERSTAFF ENCEPHALITIS

This term is used to describe patients with subacute progressive ophthalmoplegia and ataxia in addition to drowsiness or hyperreflexia. Although this entity has been described more frequently in adults, children as young as 3 yr old have been identified. Most patients are treated with steroids, IVIG, and/or plasma exchange, and often have good outcome. Serum GQ1b immunoglobulin G antibodies are found in 66% of patients. Brain MRI abnormalities occur in 30% of the patients and usually include increased T2-signal abnormalities in the brainstem, thalamus, cerebellum, and sometimes cerebral white matter. Some patients develop hyporeflexia and limb weakness, with predominant axonal involvement, overlapping with symptoms of the Miller-Fisher syndrome and the axonal subtype of the Guillain-Barré syndrome.

CHRONIC LYMPHOCYTIC INFLAMMATION WITH PONTINE PERIVASCULAR ENHANCEMENT RESPONSIVE TO STEROIDS

This is a clinically and radiologically distinct pontine-predominant encephalomyelitis. To date fewer than 30 patients have been reported and two of them were children (13 and 16 yr). Patients usually present with episodic diplopia or facial paresthesias with subsequent development of symptoms of brainstem and occasionally spinal cord dysfunction. Brain MRI shows symmetric curvilinear gadolinium enhancement peppering the pons and extending variably into the medulla, brachium pontis, cerebellum, midbrain and occasionally spinal cord. The clinical and radiological findings usually respond to high dose steroids but may worsen after the steroid taper, requiring chronic steroid or other immunosuppressive therapy. The differential diagnosis is extensive and includes infections, granulomatous disease, lymphoma or vasculitis. Biopsy studies may be needed to exclude these and other conditions.

AUTOIMMUNE ENCEPHALOPATHIES ASSOCIATED WITH EPILEPSY AND STATUS EPILEPTICUS

Rasmussen encephalitis is an inflammatory encephalopathy characterized by progressive refractory partial seizures, cognitive deterioration, and focal deficits that occur with gradual atrophy of 1 brain hemisphere. The disorder frequently presents in 6-8 yr old children, although adolescents and adults can be affected. The etiology is unknown and, therefore, multiple theories are proposed, including the presence of antibodies against the GluR3 subunit of the AMPA receptor and T-cell mediated mechanisms triggered by a viral infection. None of these mechanisms satisfactorily explains the unilateral brain involvement characteristic of the disorder. Treatment with high-dose steroids, plasma exchange, or IVIG can ameliorate symptoms in early stages of the disease. Rituximab and intraventricular γ-interferon have been effective in a few isolated cases. In a small series, patients treated with tacrolimus showed better outcomes of neurologic function and slower progression of cerebral hemiatrophy, but not improved seizure control. The only definitive treatment is functional hemispherectomy that consists in surgical disconnection of the affected hemisphere.

The discovery of treatment-responsive encephalitis associated with antibodies against cell surface or synaptic proteins has resumed the interest for a potential autoimmune basis of several devastating encephalopathies with refractory seizures. Some well-defined autoimmune encephalitis such as **anti-NMDAR encephalitis** can present in children with refractory seizures or status epilepticus. In these patients, the development over a short period of time of the characteristic spectrum of symptoms (altered behavior, orofacial dyskinesias, and autonomic dysfunction) and demonstration of NMDAR antibodies leads to the correct diagnosis and initiation of immunotherapy.

A devastating epileptic encephalopathy associated with fever named **fever-induced refractory epileptic encephalopathy syndrome,** among other terms, is suspected to be an infection-triggered autoimmune process because of its biphasic clinical course and the occasional finding of neuronal antibodies in a few patients. However, the lack of response to most treatments including immunotherapy, and the rare and inconsistent association to different types of antibodies cast doubts on an autoimmune pathogenesis. Other investigators suggest a genetic error in metabolism.

Antibodies to VGKC-complex proteins different from LGI1 and Caspr2 have been described in a few children with encephalitis with or without status epilepticus. Given that the target antigens are unknown and the response to immunotherapy is unpredictable, the significance of these antibodies is unclear.

OTHER SUSPECTED AUTOIMMUNE ENCEPHALITIDES

Demyelinating disorders, vasculitis of the CNS, and rheumatic diseases associate with autoimmune mechanisms can result in encephalitis.

Rapid onset obesity with hypothalamic dysfunction, hypoventilation, and autonomic dysregulation (**ROHHAD**) usually affects children who had normal development until 2-4 yr of age and then develop rapid onset of hyperphagia, weight gain, and abnormal behavior (social disinhibition, irascibility, impulsivity, lethargy, outburst of euphoria and laughing, impaired concentration), followed by autonomic dysfunction (abnormal pupillary responses, thermal dysregulation, gastrointestinal dysmotility), and central hypoventilation. An autoimmune or paraneoplastic etiology of ROHHAD syndrome is supported by the frequent association to neural crest tumors, the identification in some patients of genetic factors predisposing to autoimmunity, and the finding of intrathecal oligoclonal bands and infiltrates of lymphocytes and histiocytes in the hypothalamus of some patients. Furthermore, responses to immunotherapy have been described in a few patients. A possible genetic origin is suggested because of the similarities of this syndrome with the congenital central hypoventilation syndrome (Ondine curse) related to a *PHOX2B* mutation, which presents in the neonatal period and also associates with autonomic problems (Hirschsprung disease) and neural crest tumors (see Chapter 418.2).

However, no mutations in *PHOX2B* and other candidate genes have been found in patients with ROHHAD.

The term **basal ganglia encephalitis** is used to describe patients with predominant or isolated involvement of the basal ganglia. These patients typically have abnormal movements and neuropsychiatric disease. Although these disorders probably have multiple etiologies, including metabolic, toxic, genetic, and infectious processes, an immune-mediated etiology has been postulated in some patients. There have been no clinical trials, but case reports and small noncontrolled case series describe the potential benefit of immunotherapy. Antibodies against the dopamine-2 receptor have been identified in some of these patients as well as in patients with Sydenham chorea and Tourette syndrome.

Pseudomigraine syndrome with CSF pleocytosis (PMP) or **headache with neurologic deficits and CSF lymphocytosis (HaNDL)** is an ill-defined entity that predominantly affects young male adults with a family history of migraine, although adolescents can be affected. This syndrome is characterized by repeated episodes of severe headache with transient neurologic deficits, accompanied by aseptic CSF lymphocytosis and normal brain MRI. Patients frequently show high CSF opening pressure, elevated CSF protein concentration, and focal EEG slowing, which normalize after the episodes of headache. Because of the inflammatory characteristics of the CSF and the high prevalence of prodromal viral-like symptoms, an infectious-autoimmune mediated mechanism has been proposed. Other theories include spreading cortical depression and trigeminal-vascular activation.

An immune-mediated mechanism and trigeminal-vascular activation are also considered as possible mechanisms of **ophthalmoplegic migraine,** also named **recurrent cranial neuralgia.** This disorder predominantly affects young children and is characterized by recurrent bouts of head pain in addition to cranial nerves III, IV, and/or VI involvement. In contrast to PMP/HaNDL, CSF studies do not show pleocytosis, and in approximately 75% of cases, the MRI shows focal nerve thickening and contrast enhancement. Observational data suggest that treatment with steroids may be beneficial. In this syndrome, as well as in PMP/HaNDL, the differential diagnosis includes structural, neoplastic, traumatic, metabolic, and infectious disorders.

Bibliography is available at Expert Consult.

Chapter **599**
Neurodegenerative Disorders of Childhood
Jennifer M. Kwon

Neurodegenerative disorders of childhood encompass a large, heterogeneous group of diseases that result from specific genetic and biochemical defects, chronic viral infections, and varied unknown causes. Children with suspected neurodegenerative disorders were once subjected to brain and rectal (neural) biopsies, but with modern neuroimaging techniques and specific biochemical and molecular diagnostic tests, these invasive procedures are rarely necessary. The most important component of the diagnostic investigation continues to be a thorough history and physical examination. The hallmark of a neurodegenerative disease is **regression and progressive deterioration** of neurologic function with loss of speech, vision, hearing, or locomotion, often associated with seizures, feeding difficulties, and impairment of intellect. The age of onset, rate of progression, and principal

Table 599-1	Neurometabolic Conditions Associated with Developmental Regression	
AGE AT ONSET (yr)	**CONDITIONS**	**COMMENTS**
<2 with hepatomegaly	Fructose intolerance	Vomiting, hypoglycemia, poor feeding, failure to thrive (when given fructose)
	Galactosemia	Lethargy, hypotonia, icterus, cataract, hypoglycemia (when given lactose)
	Glycogenosis (glycogen storage disease) types I-IV	Hypoglycemia, cardiomegaly (type II)
	Mucopolysaccharidosis types I and II	Coarse facies, stiff joints
	Niemann-Pick disease, infantile type	Gray matter disease, failure to thrive
	Tay-Sachs disease	Seizures, cherry-red macula, edema, coarse facies
	Zellweger syndrome	Hypotonia, high forehead, flat facies
	Gaucher disease (neuronopathic form)	Extensor posturing, irritability
	Carbohydrate-deficient glycoprotein syndromes	Dysmyelination, cerebellar hypoplasia
<2, without hepatomegaly	Krabbe disease	Irritability, extensor posturing, optic atrophy, and blindness
	Rett syndrome	Girls with deceleration of head growth, loss of hand skills, hand wringing, impaired language skills, gait apraxia
	Maple syrup urine disease	Poor feeding, tremors, myoclonus, opisthotonos
	Phenylketonuria	Light pigmentation, eczema, seizures
	Menkes kinky hair disease	Hypertonia, irritability, seizures, abnormal hair
	Subacute necrotizing encephalopathy of Leigh disease	White matter disease
	Canavan disease	White matter disease, macrocephaly
	Neurodegeneration with brain iron accumulation disease	White matter disease, movement disorder
2-5	Niemann-Pick disease types III and IV	Hepatosplenomegaly, gait difficulty
	Wilson disease	Liver disease, Kayser-Fleischer ring; deterioration of cognition is late
	Gangliosidosis type II	Gray matter disease
	Neuronal ceroid lipofuscinosis	Gray matter disease
	Mitochondrial encephalopathies (e.g., myoclonic epilepsy with ragged red fibers [MERRF])	Gray matter disease
	Ataxia-telangiectasia	Basal ganglia disease
	Huntington disease (chorea)	Basal ganglia disease
	Neurodegeneration with brain iron accumulation syndrome	Basal ganglia disease
	Metachromatic leukodystrophy	White matter disease
	Adrenoleukodystrophy	White matter disease, behavior problems, deteriorating school performance, quadriparesis
5-15	Adrenoleukodystrophy	Same as for adrenoleukodystrophy in 2-5 yr olds
	Multiple sclerosis	White matter disease
	Neuronal ceroid lipofuscinosis, juvenile and adult (Spielmeyer-Vogt and Kufs disease)	Gray matter disease
	Schilder disease	White matter disease, focal neurologic symptoms
	Refsum disease	Peripheral neuropathy, ataxia, retinitis pigmentosa
	Sialidosis II, juvenile form	Cherry-red macula, myoclonus, ataxia, coarse facies
	Subacute sclerosing panencephalitis	Diffuse encephalopathy, myoclonus; may occur years after measles

From Kliegman RM, Greenbaum LA, Lye PS: *Practical strategies in pediatric diagnosis and therapy,* ed 2, Philadelphia, 2004, WB Saunders, p. 542.

neurologic findings determine whether the disease affects primarily the white or the gray matter. Upper motor neuron signs and progressive spasticity are the hallmarks of white matter disorders; convulsions and intellectual and visual impairments that occur early in the disease course are the hallmarks of gray matter disorders. A precise history confirms regression of developmental milestones, and the neurologic examination localizes the process within the nervous system. Although the outcome of a neurodegenerative condition is usually fatal and available therapies are often limited in effect, it is important to make the correct diagnosis so that genetic counseling may be offered and prevention strategies can be implemented. Bone marrow transplantation and other novel therapies may prevent the progression of disease in certain individuals who are either presymptomatic or very early in their disease course. For all conditions in which the specific enzyme defect is known, prevention by prenatal diagnosis (chorionic villus sampling or amniocentesis) is possible. Carrier detection is also often possible by enzyme assay. Table 599-1 summarizes selected inherited neurodegenerative and metabolic disorders by their usual age of onset.

599.1 Sphingolipidoses
Jennifer M. Kwon

The sphingolipidoses are characterized by intracellular storage of lipid substrates resulting from defective catabolism of the sphingolipids comprising cellular membranes (Fig. 599-1). The sphingolipidoses are subclassified into 6 categories: Niemann-Pick disease, Gaucher disease, GM_1 gangliosidosis, GM_2 gangliosidosis, Krabbe disease, and metachromatic leukodystrophy. Niemann-Pick disease and Gaucher disease are discussed in Chapter 86.4.

GANGLIOSIDOSES
See also Chapter 86.4.

Gangliosides are glycosphingolipids, normal constituents of the neuronal and synaptic membranes. The basic structure of GM_1 ganglioside consists of an oligosaccharide chain attached to a hydroxyl group of ceramide and sialic acid bound to galactose. The gangliosides are catabolized by sequential cleavage of the sugar molecules

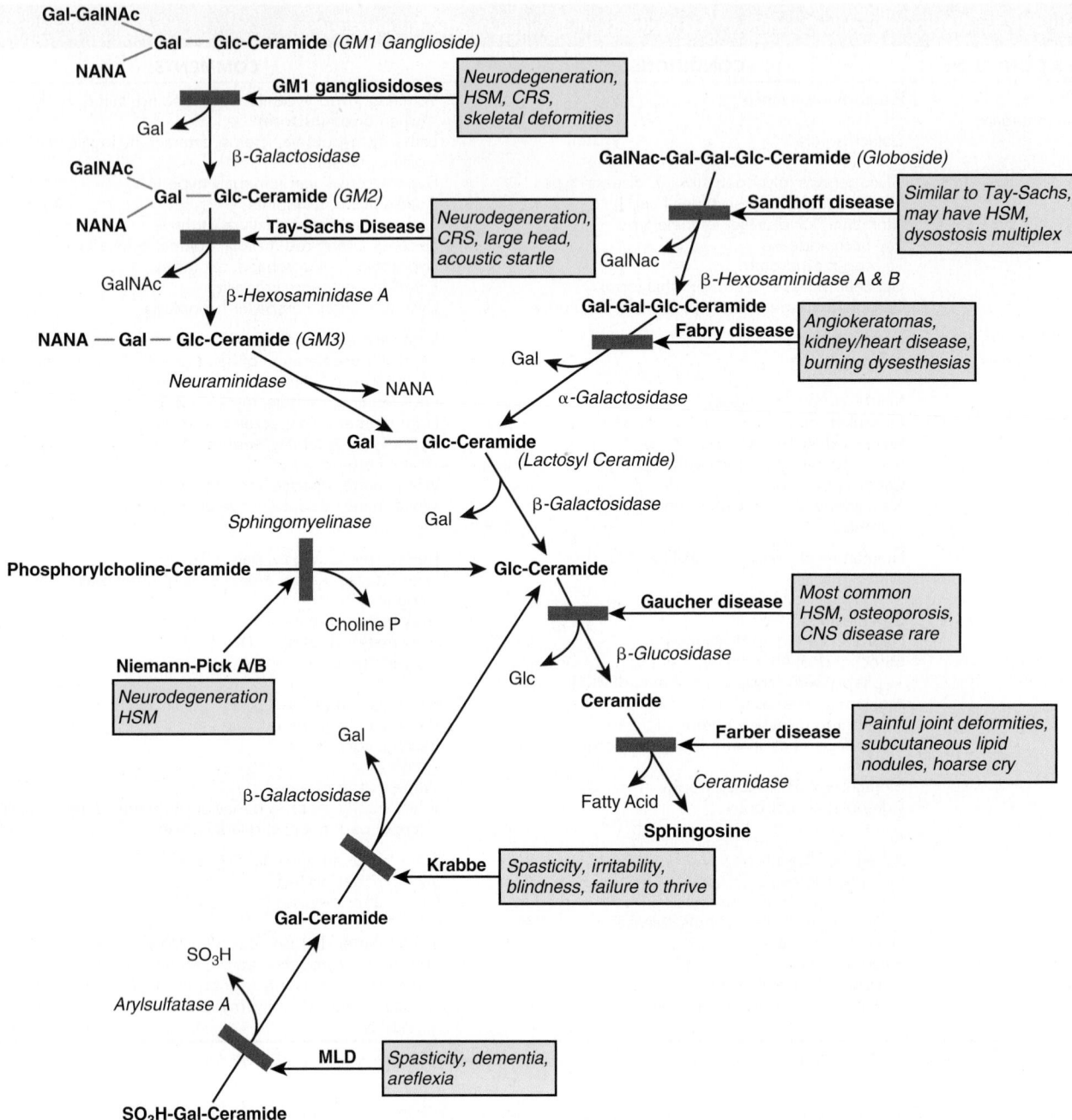

Figure 599-1 Sphingolipid degradation pathway showing the sites of enzyme deficiencies and their associated disorders. Sphingolipids are composed of a ceramide backbone with oligosaccharide side chains. CRS, cherry-red spot (retinal); Gal-, galactosyl-; GalNAc, N-acetyl-galactose; Glc-, glucosyl-; HSM, hepatosplenomegaly; MLD, metachromatic leukodystrophy; NANA, N-acetyl-neuraminic acid.

by specific exoglycosidases. Abnormalities in catabolism result in an accumulation of the ganglioside within the cell. Defects in ganglioside degradation can be classified into 2 groups: the GM$_1$ gangliosidoses and the GM$_2$ gangliosidoses.

GM$_1$ Gangliosidoses

The 3 subtypes of GM$_1$ gangliosidoses are classified according to age at presentation: infantile (type 1), juvenile (type 2), and adult (type 3). The condition is inherited as an autosomal recessive trait and results from a marked deficiency of acid β-galactosidase. This enzyme may be assayed in leukocytes and cultured fibroblasts. The acid β-galactosidase gene has been mapped to chromosome 3p14.2. Prenatal diagnosis is possible by measurement of acid β-galactosidase in cultured amniotic cells.

Infantile GM$_1$ gangliosidosis presents at birth or during the neonatal period with anorexia, poor sucking, and inadequate weight gain.

Development is globally delayed, and generalized seizures are prominent. The phenotype is striking and shares many characteristics with Hurler syndrome. The facial features are coarse, the forehead is prominent, the nasal bridge is depressed, the tongue is large (macroglossia), and the gums are hypertrophied. Hepatosplenomegaly is present early in the course as a result of accumulation of foamy histiocytes, and kyphoscoliosis is evident because of anterior beaking of the vertebral bodies. The neurologic examination is dominated by apathy, progressive blindness, deafness, spastic quadriplegia, and decerebrate rigidity. A cherry-red spot in the macular region is visualized in approximately 50% of cases. The **cherry-red spot** is characterized by an opaque ring (sphingolipid-laden retinal ganglion cells) encircling the normal red fovea (Fig. 599-2). Children rarely survive beyond age 2-3 yr, and death may be from aspiration pneumonia.

Juvenile GM$_1$ gangliosidosis has a delayed onset beginning about 1 yr of age. The initial symptoms consist of incoordination, weakness,

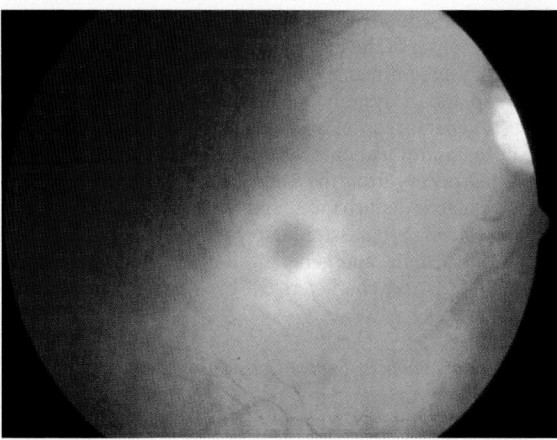

Figure 599-2 A cherry-red spot in a patient with GM₁ gangliosidosis. Note the whitish ring of sphingolipid-laden ganglion cells surrounding the fovea. *(From Leavitt JA, Kotagal S: The "cherry red" spot. Pediatr Neurol 37(1):74–75, 2007, Fig. 1.)*

ataxia, and regression of language. Thereafter, convulsions, spasticity, decerebrate rigidity, and blindness are the major findings. Unlike the infantile type, this type is not usually marked by coarse facial features and hepatosplenomegaly. Radiographic examination of the lumbar vertebrae may show minor beaking. Children rarely survive beyond 10 yr of age. **Adult GM₁ gangliosidosis** is a slowly progressive disease consisting of spasticity, ataxia, dysarthria, and a gradual loss of cognitive function.

GM₂ Gangliosidoses

The GM₂ gangliosidoses are a heterogeneous group of autosomal recessive inherited disorders that consist of several subtypes, including Tay-Sachs disease (TSD), Sandhoff disease, juvenile GM₂ gangliosidosis, and adult GM₂ gangliosidosis. **TSD** is most prevalent in the Ashkenazi Jewish population and has an approximate carrier rate of 1 in 30 Jews in the United States. TSD is caused by mutations in the *HEXA* gene located on chromosome 15q23-q24. Affected infants appear normal until approximately 6 mo of age, except for a marked startle reaction to noise that is evident soon after birth. Affected children then begin to lag in developmental milestones and, by 1 yr of age, they lose the ability to stand, sit, and vocalize. Early hypotonia develops into progressive spasticity, and relentless deterioration follows, with convulsions, blindness, deafness, and cherry-red spots in almost all patients (see Fig. 599-2). Macrocephaly becomes apparent by 1 yr of age and results from the 200-300–fold normal content of GM₂ ganglioside deposited in the brain. Few children live beyond 3-4 yr of age, and death is usually associated with aspiration or bronchopneumonia. A deficiency of the isoenzyme hexosaminidase A is found in tissues of patients with TSD. Mass screening for prenatal diagnosis of TSD is a reliable and cost-effective method of prevention because the condition occurs most frequently in a defined population (Ashkenazi Jews). Targeted screening is responsible for the fact that currently, the rare children with TSD born in the United States are most commonly born to non-Jewish parents who are not routinely screened. An accurate and inexpensive carrier detection test is available (serum or leukocyte hexosaminidase A), and the disease can be reliably diagnosed by chorionic villus sampling in the 1st trimester of pregnancy in couples at risk (heterozygote parents).

Sandhoff disease is very similar to TSD in the mode of presentation, including progressive loss of motor and language milestones beginning at 6 mo of age. Seizures, cherry-red spots, macrocephaly, and doll-like facies are present in most patients; however, children with Sandhoff disease may also have splenomegaly. The visual evoked potentials (VEPs) are normal early in the course of Sandhoff disease and TSD, but become abnormal or absent as the disease progresses. The auditory brainstem responses show prolonged latencies. The diagnosis of Sandhoff disease is established by finding deficient levels of hexosamini-

dases A and B in serum and leukocytes. Children usually die by 3 yr of age. Sandhoff disease is caused by mutations in the *HEXB* gene located on chromosome 5q13.

Juvenile GM₂ gangliosidosis develops in mid-childhood, initially with clumsiness followed by ataxia. Signs of spasticity, athetosis, loss of language, and seizures gradually develop. Progressive visual loss is associated with optic atrophy, but cherry-red spots rarely occur in juvenile GM₂ gangliosidosis. A deficiency of hexosaminidase is variable (total deficiency to near normal) in these patients. Death occurs around 15 yr of age.

Adult GM₂ gangliosidosis is characterized by a myriad neurologic signs, including slowly progressive gait ataxia, spasticity, dystonia, proximal muscle atrophy, and dysarthria. Generally, visual acuity and intellectual function are unimpaired. Hexosaminidase A activity alone or hexosaminidases A and B activity is reduced significantly in the serum and leukocytes.

Krabbe Disease (Globoid Cell Leukodystrophy)

Krabbe disease (KD) is a rare autosomal recessive neurodegenerative disorder characterized by severe myelin loss and the presence of globoid bodies in the white matter. The gene for KD *(GALC)* is located on chromosome 14q24.3-q32.1. The disease results from a marked deficiency of the lysosomal enzyme galactocerebroside β-galactosidase. KD is a disorder of myelin destruction rather than abnormal myelin formation. Normally, myelination begins in the 3rd trimester, corresponding with a rapid increase of galactocerebroside β-galactosidase activity in the brain. In patients with KD, galactocerebroside cannot be metabolized during the normal turnover of myelin because of deficiency of galactocerebroside β-galactosidase. When galactocerebroside is injected into the brains of experimental animals, a globoid cell reaction ensues. It is postulated that a similar phenomenon occurs in humans; nonmetabolized galactocerebroside stimulates the formation of globoid cells that reflect the destruction of oligodendroglial cells. Because oligodendroglial cells are responsible for the elaboration of myelin, their loss results in myelin breakdown, thus producing additional galactocerebroside and causing a vicious circle of myelin destruction.

The symptoms of KD become evident in the 1st few mo of life and include excessive irritability and crying, unexplained episodes of hyperpyrexia, vomiting, and difficulty feeding. In the initial stage of KD, children are often treated for colic or milk allergy with frequent formula changes. Generalized seizures may appear early in the course of the disease. Alterations in body tone with rigidity and opisthotonos and visual inattentiveness as a result of optic atrophy become apparent as the disease progresses. In the later stages of the illness, blindness, deafness, absent deep-tendon reflexes, and decerebrate rigidity constitute the major physical findings. Most patients die by 2 yr of age. MRI and magnetic resonance spectroscopy are useful for evaluating the extent of demyelination in KD. Umbilical cord blood (stem cell) transplantation from unrelated donors in asymptomatic babies may favorably alter the natural history but will not help patients who already have neurologic symptoms.

Late-onset KD has been described beginning in childhood or adolescence. Patients present with optic atrophy and cortical blindness, and their condition may be confused with adrenoleukodystrophy. Slowly progressive gait disturbances, including spasticity and ataxia, are prominent. As with classic KD, globoid cells are abundant in the white matter, and leukocytes are deficient in galactocerebroside β-galactosidase. An examination of the cerebrospinal fluid shows an elevated protein content, and the nerve conduction velocities are markedly delayed as a result of segmental demyelination of the peripheral nerves. The VEPs decrease gradually in amplitude with no response in the late stages of the disease, and the auditory brainstem responses are characterized by the presence of only waves I and II. CT scans and MRI studies highlight the marked decrease in white matter, especially of the cerebellum and centrum semiovale, with sparing of the subcortical U fibers. Prenatal diagnosis is possible by the assay of galactocerebroside β-galactosidase activity in chorionic villi or in cultured amniotic fluid cells. Newborn screening may identify patients at risk for late onset disease.

Metachromatic Leukodystrophy

This disorder of myelin metabolism is inherited as an autosomal recessive trait and is characterized by a deficiency of arylsulfatase A activity. The *ARSA* gene is located on chromosome 22q13-13qter. The absence or deficiency of arylsulfatase A leads to accumulation of cerebroside sulfate within the myelin sheath of the central nervous system (CNS) and peripheral nervous system because of the inability to cleave sulfate from galactosyl-3-sulfate ceramide. The excessive cerebroside sulfate is thought to cause myelin breakdown and destruction of oligodendroglia. Prenatal diagnosis of metachromatic leukodystrophy (MLD) is made by assaying of arylsulfatase A activity in chorionic villi or cultured amniotic fluid cells. Cresyl violet applied to tissue specimens produces metachromatic staining of the sulfatide granules, giving the disease its name. Some individuals with low arylsulfatase A enzyme activity are clinically normal and have a pseudodeficiency state that can only be confirmed by additional genetic or biochemical tests. Those affected with MLD are generally classified according to age of onset: late infantile, juvenile, and adult.

Late infantile MLD begins with insidious onset of gait disturbances between 1 and 2 yr of age. The child initially appears awkward and frequently falls, but locomotion is gradually impaired significantly and support is required to walk. The extremities are hypotonic, and the deep-tendon reflexes are absent or diminished. Within the next several months, the child can no longer stand, and deterioration in intellectual function becomes apparent. The speech is slurred and dysarthric, and the child appears dull and apathetic. Visual fixation is diminished, nystagmus is present, and examination of the retina shows optic atrophy. Within 1 yr from the onset of the disease, the child is unable to sit unsupported, and progressive decorticate postures develop. Feeding and swallowing are impaired because of pseudobulbar palsies, and a feeding gastrostomy is required. Patients ultimately become stuporous and die of aspiration or bronchopneumonia by age 5-6 yr. Neurophysiologic evaluation shows slowing of peripheral nerve conduction velocities and progressive changes in the VEPs, auditory brainstem responses, and somatosensory evoked potentials. CT and MRI images of the brain indicate diffuse symmetric attenuation of the cerebellar and cerebral white matter, and examination of the cerebrospinal fluid shows an elevated protein content. Bone marrow transplantation is a promising experimental therapy for the management of late infantile MLD, and early trials of enzyme replacement are being conducted. As with KD, favorable outcomes have been reported only in patients treated with less-severe disease or those identified very early in the course of the disease.

Juvenile MLD has many features in common with late infantile MLD, but the onset of symptoms is delayed to 5-10 yr of age.

Deterioration in school performance and alterations in personality may herald the onset of the disease. This is followed by incoordination of gait, urinary incontinence, and dysarthria. Muscle tone becomes increased, and ataxia, dystonia, or tremor may be present. In the terminal stages, generalized tonic–clonic convulsions are prominent and are difficult to control. Patients rarely live beyond mid-adolescence.

Adult MLD occurs from the 2nd to 6th decade. Abnormalities in memory, psychiatric disturbances, and personality changes are prominent features. Slowly progressive neurologic signs, including spasticity, dystonia, optic atrophy, and generalized convulsions, lead eventually to a bedridden state characterized by decorticate postures and unresponsiveness.

Bibliography is available at Expert Consult.

599.2 Neuronal Ceroid Lipofuscinoses
Jennifer M. Kwon

The neuronal ceroid lipofuscinoses (NCLs) are a group of inherited, neurodegenerative, lysosomal storage disorders characterized by visual loss, progressive dementia, seizures, motor deterioration, and early death. The NCLs are so named because of the intracellular accumulation of fluorescent lipopigments, ceroid and lipofuscin. They comprise a genetically and phenotypically heterogeneous group of disorders (currently there are at least 9 NCL types) that have traditionally been subclassified by age of onset, among other clinical features. They differ from one another in the associated ultrastructural patterns of the inclusions as seen by electron microscopy. Evaluation of neuronal biopsies (either brain, rectal, conjunctival, or skin) was once required for diagnosis. With the advent of enzymatic and molecular testing methods, clinicians can make specific NCL diagnoses using less-invasive methods (Table 599-2).

Infantile-type neuronal ceroid lipofuscinose (INCL, Haltia-Santavuori) begins in the 1st yr of life with myoclonic seizures, intellectual deterioration, and blindness. Optic atrophy and brownish discoloration of the macula are evident on examination of the retina, and cerebellar ataxia is prominent. The electroretinogram typically shows small-amplitude or absent waveforms. Death occurs during childhood. The infantile form is caused by recessive mutations of the gene for the lysosomal enzyme palmitoyl-protein thioesterase-1 (PPT1) on chromosome 1p32. A number of cell types in INCL patients show characteristic intracellular fine granular osmiophilic deposits discernible by electron microscopy.

Table 599-2	Clinical and Genetic Characteristics of the Neuronal Ceroid Lipofuscinoses (NCL)			
NCL TYPE	**GENE***	**PROTEIN**	**AGE OF ONSET**	**CLINICAL PRESENTATION**
Congenital	CLN10	Cathepsin‡	Birth (but can present later)	Severe seizures, blindness, rigidity, early death Can also present similar to late infantile forms
Infantile	CLN1	Palmitoyl-protein thioesterase-1 (PPT1)‡	6-24 months	Early onset, often rapid progression of seizures; cognitive and motor decline with visual loss
Variant infantile	CLN1		3 yr to adulthood	Chronic course Initial visual loss followed then by slow mental and motor decline and seizures
Late infantile	CLN2 CLN5 CLN6 CLN7	Tripeptidyl peptidase-1 (TPP1)‡ Partially soluble protein Membrane protein Membrane protein	2-8 yr	Seizures, often severe and intractable; cognitive and motor decline; and visual loss
	CLN8	Membrane protein	5-10 yr	Severe epilepsy, progressive with mental retardation
Juvenile	CLN3	Membrane protein	4-10 yr	Visual loss is usually the initial presenting complaint Also have mental, motor disorder and seizures

*Note that all the NCL genes have the prefix CLN. The adult form (also called Kufs disease, with locus CLN4, caused by mutations in DNAJC5) is not well characterized and is not included in the table.
†Direct genetic testing is available for all.
‡Enzyme testing available.

A subset of children with PPT1 enzyme deficiency has a much less-severe course with clinical features resembling those of the juvenile-onset NCL patients. Clinically, these variant INCL patients have a course that is often quite distinct from the typical, classic rapidly degenerating infantile form. Yet they have PPT1 deficiency and granular osmiophilic deposits on pathology. There is no clear *CLN1* genotype that predicts severity of phenotype.

Late infantile-type neuronal ceroid lipofuscinose (LINCL, Jansky-Bielschowsky) generally presents with myoclonic seizures beginning between 2 and 4 yr of age in a previously normal child. Dementia and ataxia are combined with a progressive loss of visual acuity and microcephaly. Examination of the retina shows marked attenuation of vessels, peripheral black bone spicule pigmentary abnormalities, optic atrophy, and a subtle brown pigment in the macular region. The electroretinogram and VEP are abnormal early in the course of disease. The autofluorescent material is deposited in neurons, fibroblasts, and secretory cells. Electron microscopic examination of the storage material in skin or conjunctival biopsy material typically shows curvilinear profiles. LINCL can be caused by autosomal recessive mutations of several different genes: *CLN2* gene, which codes for a tripeptidyl peptidase-1 (TPP1) that is essential for the degradation of cholecystokinin-8, as well as the *CLN5, CLN6,* and *CLN8* genes that code for membrane proteins that have not been completely characterized. *CLN8* is also known as the locus of Northern epilepsy syndrome, which is often called progressive epilepsy with mental retardation.

Juvenile type neuronal ceroid lipofuscinose (JNCL, Spielmeyer-Vogt or Batten disease) is the most common form of NCL disease and is generally caused by autosomal-recessive mutations in *CLN3*. (Patients who present clinically with JNCL but have PPT1 or TPP1 deficiency are said to have variant INCL or LINCL, respectively.) Children affected with JNCL tend to develop normally for the 1st 5 yr of life. Their initial symptom is usually progressive visual loss and their retinal pigmentary changes often results in an initial diagnosis of retinitis pigmentosa. The funduscopic changes are similar to those for the late infantile type. After disease onset, there may be rapid decline with changes in cognition and personality, motor incoordination, and seizures. Myoclonic seizures are not as prominent as in LINCL, but parkinsonism can develop and impair ambulation. Patients die in their late twenties to early thirties. In JNCL caused by *CLN3*, the electron microscopy of tissues show deposits called fingerprint profiles, and routine light microscopy of a peripheral blood smear may show lymphocyte vacuoles.

Bibliography is available at Expert Consult.

599.3 Adrenoleukodystrophy
Jennifer M. Kwon

See Chapter 86.2.

599.4 Sialidosis
Jennifer M. Kwon

Sialidosis is the result of lysosomal sialidase deficiency, secondary to autosomal recessive mutations in the sialidase (α-neuraminidase, *NEU1*) gene on chromosome 6p21.3. The accumulation of sialic acid–oligosaccharides with markedly increased urinary excretion of sialic acid–containing oligosaccharides is associated with clinical presentations that range from the milder sialidosis type I to the more severe sialidosis type II associated with both neurologic and somatic features.

Sialidosis type I, the **cherry-red spot myoclonus syndrome,** usually presents in the 2nd decade of life, when a patient complains of visual deterioration. Inspection of the retina shows a cherry-red spot, but, unlike patients with TSD, visual acuity declines slowly in individuals with cherry-red spot myoclonus syndrome. Myoclonus of the extremities is gradually progressive and often debilitating and eventually renders patients nonambulatory. The myoclonus is triggered by voluntary movement, touch, and sound and is not controlled with anticonvulsants. Generalized convulsions responsive to antiepileptic drugs occur in most patients.

Sialidosis type II patients present at a younger age and have cherry-red spots and myoclonus, as well as somatic involvement, including coarse facial features, corneal clouding (rarely), and dysostosis multiplex, producing anterior beaking of the lumbar vertebrae. Type II patients may be further subclassified into congenital and infantile (childhood) forms, depending on the age at presentation. Examination of lymphocytes shows vacuoles in the cytoplasm, biopsy of the liver demonstrates cytoplasmic vacuoles in Kupffer cells, and membrane-bound vacuoles are found in Schwann cell cytoplasm, all attesting to the multiorgan nature of sialidosis type II. No distinctive neuroimaging findings or abnormalities in electrophysiologic studies are noted in this group of disorders. Patients with sialidosis have been reported to live beyond the 5th decade.

Some cases of what appears to be sialidosis type II are the result of combined deficiencies of β-galactosidase and α-neuraminidase resulting from deficiency of protective protein/cathepsin A that prevents premature intracellular degradation of these 2 enzymes. These patients have galactosialidosis and they are clinically indistinguishable from those with sialidosis type II. Consequently, patients who have features of sialidosis type II with marked urinary excretion of oligosaccharides should be tested for protective protein/cathepsin A deficiency as well as sialidase deficiency.

Bibliography is available at Expert Consult.

599.5 Miscellaneous Disorders
Jennifer M. Kwon

PELIZAEUS-MERZBACHER DISEASE
Pelizaeus-Merzbacher disease (PMD) is an X-linked recessive disorder characterized by nystagmus and abnormalities of myelin. PMD is caused by mutations in the proteolipid protein *(PLP1)* gene, on chromosome Xq22, which is essential for CNS myelin formation and oligodendrocyte differentiation. Mutations in the same gene can cause familial spastic paraparesis (progressive spastic paraparesis type 2, SPG2). *PLP1* mutations causing disease include point mutations, deletions, gene duplications, and other gene dosage changes.

Clinically, classic PMD is recognized by nystagmus and roving eye movements with head nodding during infancy. Developmental milestones are delayed; ataxia, choreoathetosis, and spasticity ultimately develop. Optic atrophy and dysarthria are associated findings, and death occurs in the 2nd or 3rd decade. The major pathologic finding is a loss of myelin with intact axons, suggesting a defect in the function of oligodendroglia. An MRI scan shows a symmetric pattern of delayed myelination. Multimodal-evoked potential studies demonstrate early in the course a pattern consisting of loss of waves III-V on the auditory brainstem response. This finding is useful in the investigation of nystagmus in infant boys. VEPs show prolonged latencies, and somatosensory evoked potentials show absent cortical responses or delayed latencies. It is now recognized that a broad spectrum of phenotypes, including SPG2 and peripheral nerve abnormalities, can also result from mutations in the *PLP1* gene.

There is a PMD-like syndrome caused by autosomal recessive mutations in the gap junction protein alpha 12 (*GJA12*, or connexin 47). Individuals with *GJA12* mutations have a clinical and radiologic phenotype like PMD including hypomyelinating leukodystrophy.

ALEXANDER DISEASE
This is a rare disorder that causes progressive macrocephaly and leukodystrophy. Alexander disease is caused by dominant mutations in the glial fibrillary acidic protein *(GFAP)* gene, on chromosome 17q21

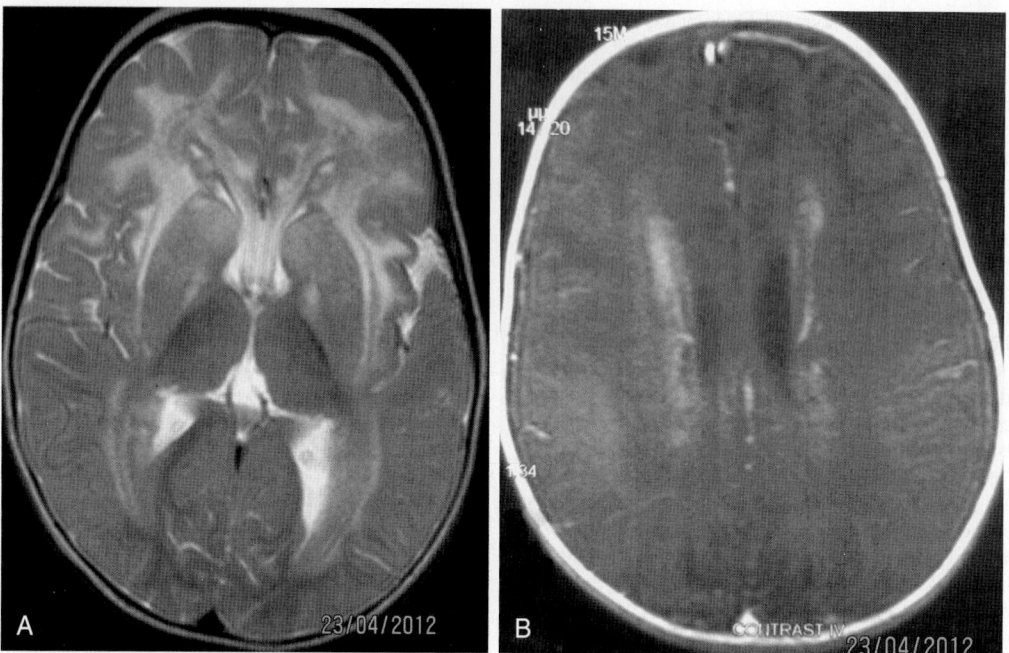

Figure 599-3 Alexander disease. MRI of the index patient at the age of 15 mo. **A,** Axial T2-weighted sequences (TR/TE: 4000/99) at the basal ganglia and thalamus level demonstrating diffuse bilateral, symmetric increased signal predominantly of the frontal periventricular, but also of the subcortical white matter and of the basal ganglia. **B,** Significant periventricular rim after intravenous gadolinium infusion (T1-weighted sequences; TR/TE: 400/88). *(From Zafeiriou DI, Dragoumi P, Vargiami E: Alexander disease. J Pediatr 162:648, 2013.)*

and cases are usually sporadic in their families. Pathologic examination of the brain discloses deposition of eosinophilic hyaline bodies called Rosenthal fibers in astrocyte processes. These accumulate in a perivascular distribution throughout the brain. In the classic infantile form of Alexander disease, degeneration of white matter is most prominent frontally. Diagnosis may be suggested by MRI (Fig. 599-3) and MR spectroscopy demonstrating abnormal metabolic substrates. Affected children develop progressive loss of intellect, spasticity, and unresponsive seizures causing death by 5 yr of age. However, there are milder forms that present later in life and that may not have the characteristic frontal predominance or megalencephaly.

CANAVAN SPONGY DEGENERATION
See Chapter 85.15.

OTHER LEUKODYSTROPHIES
Metabolic and degenerative disorders can present with significant cerebral white matter changes, such as some mitochondrial disorders (see Chapters 86.1 and 598.2) and glutaric aciduria type 1 (see Chapter 85.14). In addition, the broader use of MRI has brought to light new leukodystrophies. One example is vanishing white matter disease or childhood ataxia with CNS hypomyelination characterized by ataxia and spasticity. Some patients also have optic atrophy, seizures, and cognitive deterioration. The age of presentation and the rapidity of decline can be quite variable. In the early-onset forms, decline is usually rapid and followed quickly by death; in the later-onset forms, mental decline is usually slower and milder. Interestingly, acute demyelination in these disorders can be triggered by fever or fright. The diagnosis of vanishing white matter disease or childhood ataxia with CNS hypomyelination is based on clinical findings, characteristic abnormalities on cranial MRI, and autosomal recessive mutations in 1 of 5 causative genes (*EIF2B1, EIF2B2, EIF2B3, EIF2B4,* and *EIF2B5*) encoding the 5 subunits of the eucaryotic translation initiation factor, eIF2B.

MENKES DISEASE
Menkes disease (kinky hair disease) is a progressive neurodegenerative condition inherited as a X-linked recessive trait. The Menkes gene codes for a copper-transporting, P-type adenosine triphosphatase, and

mutations in the protein are associated with low serum copper and ceruloplasmin levels, as well as a defect in intestinal copper absorption and transport. Symptoms begin in the 1st few mo of life and include hypothermia, hypotonia, and generalized myoclonic seizures. The facies are distinctive, with chubby, rosy cheeks and kinky, colorless, friable hair. Microscopic examination of the hair shows several abnormalities, including trichorrhexis nodosa (fractures along the hair shaft) and pili torti (twisted hair). Feeding difficulties are prominent and lead to failure to thrive. Severe mental retardation and optic atrophy are constant features of the disease. Neuropathologic changes include tortuous degeneration of the gray matter and marked changes in the cerebellum with loss of the internal granule cell layer and necrosis of the Purkinje cells. Death occurs by 3 yr of age in untreated patients.

Copper-histidine therapy may be effective in preventing neurologic deterioration in some patients with Menkes disease, particularly when treatment is begun in the neonatal period or, preferably, with the fetus. These presymptomatic children are currently identified because of a family history of an affected brother. Copper is essential in the early stages of CNS development, and its absence probably accounts for the neuropathologic changes. Infants diagnosed presymptomatically in the 1st 10 days of life can be started on an experimental protocol of daily copper-histidine subcutaneous injections (as of 2015, only available at NIH under a program supervised by Dr. Stephen Kaler). Optimal response to copper-histidine injection treatment appears to occur only in patients who are identified in the newborn period and whose mutations permit residual copper-transport activity.

The **occipital horn syndrome,** a skeletal dysplasia caused by different mutations in the same gene as that involved in Menkes disease, is a relatively mild disease. The 2 diseases are often confused, because the biochemical abnormalities are identical. Resolution of the uncertainty about treatment of patients with Menkes disease will require careful genotype-phenotype correlation, along with further clinical trials of copper therapy.

RETT SYNDROME
This syndrome is not strictly speaking a degenerative disease, but a disorder of early brain development marked by a period of developmental regression and deceleration of brain growth after a relatively

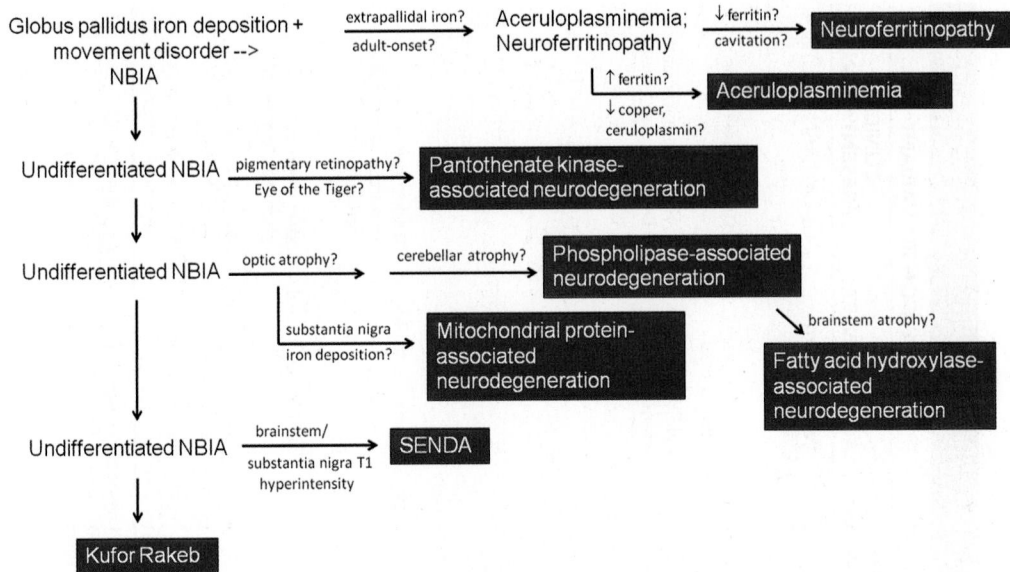

Figure 599-4 Clinical and radiographic approach to neurodegeneration with brain iron accumulation. NBIA, neurodegeneration with brain iron accumulation; SENDA, static encephalopathy of childhood with neurodegeneration in adulthood. *(From Kruer MC, Boddaert N: Neurodegeneration with brain iron accumulation: a diagnostic algorithm. Semin Pediatr Neurol 19:67–74, 2012, Fig. 1.)*

normal neonatal course. It occurs predominantly in girls. The frequency is approximately 1 in 15,000-22,000 children. Rett syndrome is caused by mutations in *MeCP2*, a transcription factor that binds to methylated CpG islands and silences transcription. Development may proceed normally until 1 yr of age, when regression of language and motor milestones and acquired microcephaly become apparent. An ataxic gait or fine tremor of hand movements is an early neurologic finding. Most children develop peculiar sighing respirations with intermittent periods of apnea that may be associated with cyanosis. The hallmark of Rett syndrome is repetitive hand-wringing movements and a loss of purposeful and spontaneous use of the hands; these features may not appear until 2-3 yr of age. Autistic behavior is a typical finding in all patients. Generalized tonic-clonic convulsions occur in the majority and are usually well controlled by anticonvulsants. Feeding disorders and poor weight gain are common. After the initial period of neurologic regression, the disease process appears to plateau, with persistence of the autistic behavior. Cardiac arrhythmias may result in sudden, unexpected death at a rate that is higher than the general population. Generally girls survive into adulthood.

Postmortem studies show significantly reduced brain weight (60-80% of normal) with a decrease in the number of synapses, associated with a decrease in dendritic length and branching. The phenotype may be related to failure to suppress expression of genes that are normally silent in the early phases of postnatal development. Although very few males survive with the classic Rett syndrome phenotype, genotyping of boys without the classic Rett syndrome phenotype but with intellectual disability and other atypical neurologic features has detected a significant number with mutations in *MeCP2*. Mutations in *MeCP2* have been demonstrated in normal female carriers, females with Angelman syndrome, and in males with fatal encephalopathy, Klinefelter (47 XXY) syndrome, and familial X-linked mental retardation.

Some girls have an atypical Rett phenotype associated with severe myoclonic seizures in infancy, slowing of head growth, and developmental arrest and have mutations in another X-linked gene encoding for cyclin-dependent kinase–like 5 (CDKL5), which may interact with MeCP2 and other proteins regulating gene expression.

SUBACUTE SCLEROSING PANENCEPHALITIS

This is a rare, progressive neurologic disorder caused by persistent measles virus infection of the CNS (see Chapter 246). The number of

reported cases has decreased dramatically to 0.06 cases/million population, paralleling the decline in reported measles cases. The initial clinical manifestations include personality changes, aggressive behavior, and impaired cognitive function in individuals who have been exposed to natural measles virus in early childhood. Myoclonic seizures soon dominate the clinical picture. Later, generalized tonic-clonic convulsions, hypertonia, and choreoathetosis become evident, followed by progressive bulbar palsy, hyperthermia, and decerebrate postures. Funduscopic examination early in the course of the disease reveals papilledema in approximately 20% of the cases. Optic atrophy, chorioretinitis, and macular pigmentation are observed in most patients. The diagnosis is established by the typical clinical course and 1 of the following: (1) measles antibody detected in the cerebrospinal fluid, (2) a characteristic electroencephalogram consisting of bursts of high-voltage slow waves interspersed with a normal background that occur with a constant periodicity in the early stages of the disease, and (3) typical histologic findings in the brain biopsy or postmortem specimen. Treatment with a series of antiviral agents has been attempted without success. Death occurs usually within 1-2 yr from the onset of symptoms.

NEURODEGENERATION WITH BRAIN IRON ACCUMULATION

Neurodegeneration with brain iron accumulation represents multiple, age-of-onset-dependent disorders characterized by extrapyramidal symptoms, intellectual deterioration and regression, with iron deposition in the basal ganglia. There is significant phenotype variability of these disorders; however, a characteristic finding on MRI demonstrates symmetric T2 signal homogeneous *hypointensity*. Common neurodegeneration with brain iron accumulation disorders are distinguished in Table 599-3 and an approach to their diagnosis is noted in Figure 599-4. Clinical features, which are highly variable, may include dystonia, parkinsonism, ataxia, spasticity, psychiatric symptoms, and intellectual impairment. Treatment should focus on the specific disorder and is usually symptomatic relief rather than curative. Iron chelation has been attempted without major long-term benefit.

Bibliography is available at Expert Consult.

Table 599-3 | Overview of Neurodegeneration with Brain Iron Accumulation Conditions and Genes (if Known)

CONDITION (ACRONYM)	SYNONYM	GENE	CHROMOSOMAL POSITION	LB PATHOLOGY	CHILDHOOD-ONSET VARIANT		LATE-ONSET VARIANT	
					AGE OF ONSET	CLINICAL PRESENTATION	AGE OF ONSET	CLINICAL PRESENTATION
PKAN	NBIA1	PANK2	20p13	No	Early childhood, around age 3	Typical PKAN	Teens or early adulthood	Atypical PKAN
PLAN	NBIA2, PARK14	PLA2G6	22q12	√	Infancy	Infantile neuroaxonal dystrophy	Teens or early adulthood	Dystonia parkinsonism
FAHN	SPG35	FA2H	16q23	Not known	Childhood	Leukodystrophy, hereditary spastic paraplegia	Adulthood (age range up to 30 yr)	May resemble idiopathic PD
MPAN	—	C19orf12	19q12	√	—	Pyramidal extrapyramidal syndrome		
Kufor-Rakeb disease	PARK9	ATP13A2	1p36	√	Childhood-teens	Parkinsonism, pyramidal tract signs, eye movement disorder		
BPAN	SENDA syndrome	WDR45	Xp11.23	Not known	Childhood	Encephalopathy with psychomotor regression, then static	Then: 20s to 30s	Sudden onset progressive dystonia parkinsonism
Aceruloplasminemia	—	CP	3q23	No	—	—	50s (range: 16-70)	Extrapyramidal, diabetes, dementia
Neuroferritinopathy	—	FTL	19q13	No	—	—	40s	Chorea, dystonia, dementia
Idiopathic late-onset cases	—	Probably heterogeneous	Probably heterogeneous	Heterogeneous	—	—	Heterogeneous	Parkinsonism, in may resemble idiopathic PD

√, Present; BPAN, beta-propeller associated neurodegeneration; CP, ceruloplasmin; FA2H, fatty acid 2-hydroxylase; FAHN, fatty acid 2-hydroxylase-associated neurodegeneration; FTL, ferritin light chain; MPAN, mitochondrial membrane-associated neurodegeneration; NBIA, neurodegeneration with brain iron accumulation; PANK2, pantothenate kinase 2; PD, Parkinson disease; PKAN, pantothenate kinase-associated neurodegeneration; PLA2G6, phospholipase A2; PLAN, PLA2G6-associated neurodegeneration; SENDA, static encephalopathy of childhood with neurodegeneration in adulthood; SPG, spastic paraplegia.
From Schneider SA, Zorzi G, Nardocci N: Pathophysiology and treatment of neurodegeneration with brain iron accumulation in the pediatric population, Curr Treat Option Neurol 15:652-667, 2013, Table 1.

Chapter **600**
Demyelinating Disorders of the Central Nervous System

Jayne M. Ness

Acquired demyelinating disorders of the central nervous system (CNS) result in neurologic dysfunction caused by immune-mediated attacks on white matter insulating the brain, optic nerves and spinal cord. The white matter insulation is formed by myelin contained within oligodendrocytes wrapping around nerve axons. In contrast to genetically determined leukodystrophies (sometimes called dysmyelinating disorders) that produce disrupted white matter, acquired demyelinating disorders generally target normally formed white matter. Pediatric demyelinating syndromes are characterized clinically by (1) localization of neurologic deficits (i.e., single site, such as spinal cord [transverse myelitis], optic nerves [optic neuritis] or brainstem, vs polyregional demyelination); (2) the presence vs absence of encephalopathy; and (3) disease course (i.e., monophasic vs repeated attacks involving either the same or new CNS regions). Major demyelinating disorders in childhood include acute disseminated encephalomyelitis (ADEM), typically a self-limited disorder, and relapsing–remitting multiple sclerosis (MS). MRI of brain and spine is useful to initially characterize symptomatic and clinically silent demyelinating lesions, but serial MRI is often required to distinguish self-limited vs chronic demyelinating syndromes, especially in the younger child. Additional studies, such as cerebrospinal fluid (CSF) analysis, autoimmune and genetic testing, and sometimes even brain biopsy, may be required to evaluate for mimickers of demyelination, such as neoplasm, infection, systemic rheumatologic disorders, isolated CNS angiitis, mitochondrial disease, and leukodystrophies (Tables 600-1 and 600-2).

600.1 Multiple Sclerosis
Jayne M. Ness

Pediatric MS is a chronic demyelinating disorder of the brain, spinal cord, and optic nerves characterized by a relapsing–remitting course of neurologic events without encephalopathy separated in time and space.

EPIDEMIOLOGY
Pediatric MS is rare, with an estimated 2-5% of MS patients experiencing their first symptoms before age 18 yr. Pediatric MS has a slight male predominance when disease onset is before age 6 yr, but by age 12 yr, females outnumber males 2:1.

PATHOGENESIS
A complex interplay of environmental, infectious, and genetic factors influence MS susceptibility. Immune system dysregulation involving T and B lymphocytes triggers inflammation, axonal demyelination, axonal loss, and regeneration within both white and gray matter. Inflammatory infiltrates within actively demyelinating lesions of relapsing-remitting MS are targets for disease modifying agents (DMAs). Neurodegenerative changes predominate in progressive forms of MS.

Table 600-1	Differential Diagnosis of Demyelinating Disorders

Acute disseminated encephalomyelitis (ADEM)
Multiple sclerosis (including tumefactive MS)
Acute hemorrhagic leukoencephalopathy
Clinically isolated syndrome (CIS)
Neuromyelitis optica spectrum disorder
N-methyl-D-aspartate receptor (NMDAR) antibody and other autoimmune encephalitis
Vasculitis/angiopathies
Hashimoto encephalitis (anti–thyroid peroxidase [TPO] antibody)
Familial hemophagocytic lymphohistiocytosis
Langerhans cell histiocytosis
Lymphoma
Gliomatosis cerebri
Glioma
Sarcoidosis
Mitochondrial disorders (Leigh syndrome)
Vitamin E deficiency
Vitamin B_{12} deficiency
Celiac disease
Herpes simplex virus (HSV), enterovirus, arbovirus, Powassan and other viral encephalitides
Rabies
Subacute sclerosing pan-encephalitis (SSPE) (chronic measles)
Charcot-Marie-Tooth syndrome
Leukoencephalopathies (Aicardi-Goutières syndrome)
Vanishing white matter disease
Schilder disease (possibly an adrenoleukodystrophy)
X-linked adrenoleukodystrophy
Griscelli syndrome type 2

CLINICAL MANIFESTATIONS
Presenting symptoms in pediatric MS include hemiparesis or paraparesis; unilateral or, less often, bilateral optic neuritis; focal sensory loss; ataxia; diplopia; dysarthria; or bowel/bladder dysfunction (Table 600-3). Polyregional symptoms are reported in 30% of patients. Encephalopathy is less common and suggests consideration of ADEM or possibly neuromyelitis optica (NMO).

LABORATORY FINDINGS
Cranial MRI exhibits discrete T2 lesions in cerebral white matter, particularly periventricular regions as well as brainstem, cerebellum, and juxtacortical and deep gray matter. Alternatively, large tumefactive T2 lesions may be seen. Spine MRI typically shows partial-width cord lesions restricted to 1-2 spine segments. CSF may be normal or exhibit mild pleocytosis, particularly in younger children. Abnormal MS profiles (increased immunoglobulin [Ig] G index, and/or CSF oligoclonal bands) increase likelihood of MS but may be negative in 10-60% of pediatric MS patients, particularly prepubertal children; they also may be occasionally positive in ADEM or autoimmune encephalitis (Fig. 600-1). Abnormal evoked potential studies can localize disruptions in visual, auditory, or somatosensory pathways.

DIAGNOSIS AND DIFFERENTIAL DIAGNOSIS
Pediatric MS can usually be diagnosed following 2 demyelinating episodes without encephalopathy localizing to distinct CNS regions, lasting longer than 24 hr and separated by more than 30 days, provided no other plausible explanation exists. Current MS diagnostic criteria use MRI to serve as a surrogate for recurrent demyelination, enabling MS diagnosis after the first event. For adults and children >12 yr, the initial MRI may be sufficient to diagnose MS if it demonstrates dissemination in space (≥2 T2 lesions involving juxtacortical, periventricular, infratentorial, or spine regions) and time (presence of asymptomatic gadolinium-enhancing lesion and nonenhancing T2 lesion in same scan). Alternatively, MS can be diagnosed with a follow-up MRI at any time interval exhibiting accumulation of T2 or gadolinium-enhancing lesions in the brain or spine. Challenges arise in distinguishing pediatric MS from other acquired demyelinating

Table 600-2	IPMSSG 2012 Definitions for Pediatric Acute Demyelinating Disorders of the Central Nervous System

DISORDER	IPMSSG 2012
CIS	• A first monofocal or multifocal CNS demyelinating event; encephalopathy is absent, **unless caused by fever**
Monophasic ADEM	• A first polyfocal clinical CNS event with presumed inflammatory cause • Encephalopathy that **cannot be explained by fever** is present MRI typically shows **diffuse, poorly demarcated, large, >1-2 cm lesions** involving predominantly the cerebral white matter; **T1 hypointense white matter lesions are rare**; deep gray-matter lesions (e.g., thalamus or basal ganglia) can be present • No new symptoms, signs or MRI findings after 3 mo of the incident ADEM
Recurrent ADEM	• **See multiphasic ADEM**
Multiphasic ADEM	• New event of ADEM 3 mo or more after the initial event that can be associated with **new or reemergence of prior clinical and MRI findings. Timing in relation to steroids is no longer pertinent**
MS	Any of the following: • Two or more nonencephalopathic CNS clinical events separated by more than 30 days, involving more than 1 area of the CNS • Single clinical event and MRI features rely on 2010 Revised McDonald criteria for DIS and DIT (but criteria relative for DIT for a single attack and single MRI only apply to children ages 2-12 yr and only apply to cases without an ADEM onset)
NMO	All are required: • Optic neuritis • Acute myelitis At least 2 of 3 supportive criteria • Contiguous spinal cord MRI lesion S3 vertebral segments • **Brain MRI not meeting diagnostic criteria for MS** • Anti–aquaporin-4 immunoglobulin G–seropositive status • ADEM followed 3 mo later by a nonencephalopathic clinical event with new lesions on brain MRI consistent with MS

The 2001 McDonald MRI criteria for DIS require 3 of the following 4 MRI features: 29 T2 lesions or 1 gadolinium-enhancing lesion; 23 periventricular lesions; 21 infratentorial lesion(s); 21 juxtacortical lesion(s). The DIT criteria require subsequent white-matter lesions whose timing depends on the temporal relation of the initial MRI with the onset of the clinical symptoms.

The 2010 Revised McDonald MRI criteria for DIS require the presence of at least 2 of the following 4 criteria: 21 lesions in each of the 4 locations; periventricular, juxtacortical, infratentorial, and spinal cord. The 2010 Revised McDonald MRI criteria for DIT can be satisfied either by the emergence of newT2 lesions (with or without enhancement) on serial scan(s) or can be met on a single baseline scan if there exists simultaneous presence of a clinically silent gadolinium-enhancing lesion and a nonenhancing lesion.

ADEM, acute disseminated encephalomyelitis; CIS, clinically isolated syndrome; CNS, central nervous system; DIS, dissemination in space; DIT, dissemination in time; IPMSSG, International Pediatric Multiple Sclerosis Study Group; MS, multiple sclerosis; NMO, neuromyelitis optica.

Modified from Krupp LB, Tardieu M, Amato MP, et al: International Pediatric Multiple Sclerosis Study Group criteria for pediatric multiple sclerosis and immune-mediated central nervous system demyelinating disorders: revision to the 2007 definitions. Mult Scler 19(10):1261–1267, 2013, Appendix 1, p. 1266.

Table 600-3	Symptoms and Signs of Multiple Sclerosis by Site

	SYMPTOMS	SIGNS
Cerebrum	Cognitive impairment	Deficits in attention, reasoning, and executive function (early); dementia (late)
	Hemisensory and motor	Upper motor neuron signs
	Affective (mainly depression)	
	Epilepsy (rare)	
	Focal cortical deficits (rare)	
Optic nerve	Unilateral painful loss of vision	Scotoma, reduced visual acuity, color vision, and relative afferent papillary defect
Cerebellum and cerebellar pathways	Tremor	Postural and action tremor, dysarthria
	Clumsiness and poor balance	Limb incoordination and gait ataxia
Brainstem	Diplopia, oscillopsia	Nystagmus, internuclear and other complex ophthalmoplegias
	Vertigo	
	Impaired swallowing	Dysarthria
	Impaired speech and emotional lability	Pseudobulbar palsy
	Paroxysmal symptoms	
Spinal cord	Weakness	Upper motor neuron signs
	Stiffness and painful spasms	Spasticity
	Bladder dysfunction	
	Erectile impotence	
	Constipation	
Other	Pain	
	Fatigue	
	Temperature sensitivity and exercise intolerance	

Modified from Compston A, Coles A: Multiple sclerosis, Lancet 372:1502–1517, 2008, p. 1503.

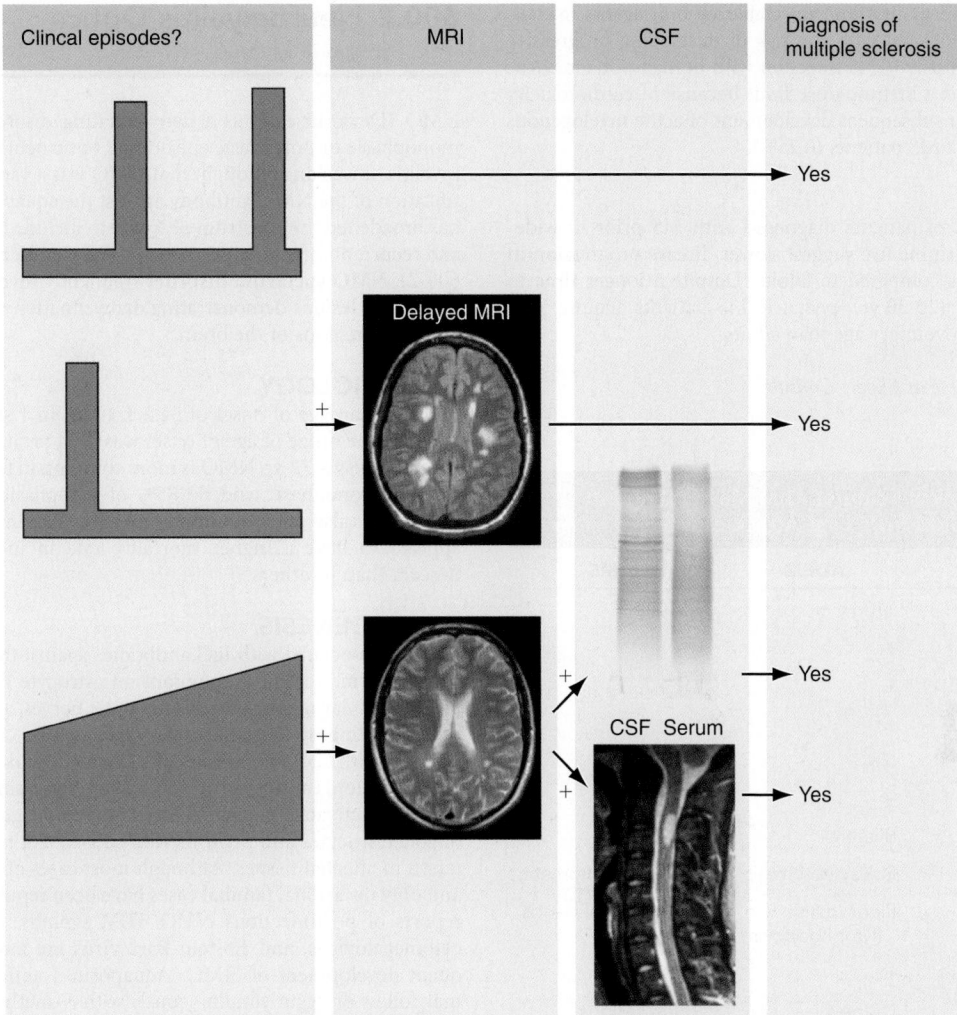

Clinical episodes?	MRI	CSF	Diagnosis of multiple sclerosis
			Yes
	Delayed MRI		Yes
			Yes
		CSF Serum	Yes

Figure 600-1 Criteria for the diagnosis of multiple sclerosis. The principle is to establish dissemination in time and place of lesions, meaning that episodes affecting separate sites within the central nervous system have occurred at least 30 days apart. MRI can substitute for 1 of these clinical episodes. Dissemination in time of magnetic resonance lesions requires simultaneous presence of asymptomatic gadolinium-enhancing and asymptomatic lesions or followup MRI showing accumulation of a new gadolinium-enhancing lesion or T2 lesion. Criteria for MRI definition of dissemination in space require 2 or more lesions in periventricular, juxtacortical, or infratentorial regions or spine. Primary progressive MS is very rare in childhood but can be diagnosed after 1 yr of a progressive deficit and 2 of the following: (1) a positive brain MRI; (2) a positive spinal cord MRI; and (3) positive oligoclonal bands. Patients having an appropriate clinical presentation but who do not meet all of the diagnostic criteria can be classified as having possible MS. CSF, cerebrospinal fluid. (From Compston A, Coles A: Multiple sclerosis, Lancet 372:1502–1517, 2008, Fig. 1.)

syndromes such as ADEM or NMO, especially in the prepubertal child. ADEM is a self-limited syndrome characterized by encephalopathy, polyregional neurologic deficits, and diffuse multifocal MRI T2 abnormalities followed by subsequent clinical improvement and resolution of MRI T2 lesions (see Tables 600-1, 600-2, 600-4, and 600-5). However, a subset of pediatric MS patients (10-25%) presents with an ADEM phenotype and then experiences multiple relapses with accumulation of MRI T2 lesions. NMO, traditionally thought of as a combined myelitis and optic neuritis with normal brain MRI, now has a broader phenotype with the identification of the NMO antibody against the CNS water channel aquaporin-4 and MRI lesions in the brain. The NMO spectrum includes isolated bilateral optic neuritis or longitudinally extensive transverse myelitis even in the presence of brain MRI abnormalities or encephalopathy.

COMPLICATIONS
Similar to adults with MS, pediatric MS patients can acquire fixed neurologic deficits affecting vision and other cranial nerves, motor and sensory function, balance, and bowel/bladder function. Cognitive impairment can impede academic achievement.

TREATMENT
Relapses causing functional disability may be treated with methylprednisolone, 20-30 mg/kg/day (max: 1,000 mg/day) for 3-5 days, with or without prednisone taper. DMAs reduce relapse frequency and T2 lesion load, mainly by targeting the inflammatory response that predominates during the relapsing-remitting phase of MS (Table 600-6). There are 4 injectable DMAs, 3 oral DMAs, and 2 infused DMAs approved by the FDA for adult MS, but to date, none of these agents has a pediatric MS indication. Injectable agents, first approved in the mid-1990s (interferon-beta1α SC or IM or interferon-beta1β SC; glatiramer acetate SC) have some side effects such as flu-like side effects and risk of transaminase elevation with interferon-beta or requirement for daily injections with glatiramer acetate but otherwise have an excellent safety record so are still recommended as first-line therapy in pediatric MS. Three oral DMAs (fingolimod, teriflunomide, dimethyl fumarate) have been FDA-approved since 2010, but despite ease of oral administration, enthusiasm is tempered by reports of severe side effects or even death from reactivation of latent viruses (fingolimod, dimethyl fumarate) and potential of severe birth defects (teriflunomide). Intravenous DMAs (natalizumab, mitoxantrone) are second-line agents

used only after failure of first-line injectable or oral agents. Natalizumab therapy is associated with the risk of developing progressive multifocal encephalopathy (CNS infection with human polyomavirus JC). Mitoxantrone has a lifetime dose limit because of cardiotoxicity and is associated with subsequent development of acute myelogenous lymphoma in 2 of 802 MS patients (0.25%).

PROGNOSIS

Retrospective studies of patients diagnosed with MS prior to widespread dimethyltryptamine use suggest slower disease progression in pediatric MS patients compared to adults. Despite a longer time to irreversible disability (20-30 yr), pediatric MS patients acquire irreversible disability at a younger age than adults.

Bibliography is available at Expert Consult.

Table 600-4	Clinical Features That May Distinguish ADEM from First Attack of MS	
	ADEM	**MS**
Age	<10 yr	>10 yr
Stupor/coma	+	−
Encephalopathy	+	−
Fever/vomiting	+	−
Family history	No	20%
Sensory complaints	+	+
Optic neuritis	Bilateral	Unilateral
Manifestations	Polysymptomatic	Monosymptomatic
CSF	Pleocytosis (lymphocytosis)	Oligoclonal bands
Response to steroids	+	+
Follow-up	No new lesions	New lesions

Some features that may help distinguish an initial acute episode of demyelination from a first attack of MS in children. Final diagnosis of MS is based on follow-up evaluation and possibly MRI.

+, More likely to be present; −, less likely to be present; ADEM, acute disseminated encephalomyelitis; CSF, cerebrospinal fluid; MS, multiple sclerosis.

600.2 Neuromyelitis Optica
Jayne M. Ness

NMO (Devic disease) is a demyelinating disorder characterized by monophasic or polyphasic episodes of optic neuritis and/or transverse myelitis. It was once thought that NMO was a variant of MS; but identification of the NMO antibody against the aquaporin-4 water channel has broadened the spectrum of NMO to include brainstem syndromes and recurrent forms of optic neuritis and transverse myelitis (see Table 600-2). **NMO spectrum disorder** frequently involves symptomatic or silent MRI lesions demonstrating demyelination of the cerebral cortex and other regions of the brain.

EPIDEMIOLOGY
NMO has an age of onset of 31.2 ± 11 yr. In 1 study, in monophasic patients, the range of age of onset was 1-54 yr; in polyphasic patients, the range was 6-72 yr. NMO is more common in females than in males; 65% of monophasic and 80-85% of polyphasic NMO patients are female. It is also more common in Asians than in blacks or whites and appears to have a higher mortality rate in individuals of African descent than in others.

PATHOGENESIS
NMO is associated with IgG antibodies against the aquaporin-4 water channel, which is most abundant on astrocyte foot processes within periventricular regions, brainstem, optic nerves, and spinal cord. Antibody binding to aquaporin-4 activates the classical complement pathway with C5b-C9 components leading to leukocytes attraction and degranulation, causing astrocyte death. Chemokines from dying astrocytes and activated leukocytes attract macrophages, leading to death of oligodendrocytes and neurons with subsequent necrosis or even cavitation in affected tissues. Although most cases of NMO are idiopathic and only occasional familial cases have been reported, there have been reports of postinfectious NMO. HIV, syphilis, chlamydia, varicella, cytomegalovirus, and Epstein-Barr virus are associated with subsequent development of NMO. Aquaporin-4 antibody–positive NMO may follow or occur simultaneously with *N*-methyl-D-aspartate receptor antibody autoimmune encephalitis.

CLINICAL MANIFESTATIONS
NMO presents with optic neuritis or transverse myelitis or brainstem symptoms such as intractable vomiting or hiccups, diplopia, facial

Table 600-5	MRI Characteristics for Dissemination in Space That Increase the Likelihood of a Pediatric Multiple Sclerosis Diagnosis				
BARKHOF*	**MIKAELOFF (KIDMUS)†**	**CALLEN (MS VS ADEM)‡**	**CALLEN (DIAGNOSTIC MS)§**	**VERHEY (DIFFERENTIAL)‖**	**POLMAN (2010 REVISED MCDONALD CRITERIA)¶**
3 of 4: ≥9 T2 lesions or 1 gadolinium enhancing ≥3 Periventricular ≥1 Infratentorial ≥1 Juxtacortical	1 of 2: Lesions perpendicular to long axis of the corpus callosum Sole presence of well-defined lesions	2 of 3: Absence of a diffuse bilateral lesion pattern Presence of black holes ≥2 Periventricular lesions	2 of 3: ≥5 Lesions on T2-weighted images 2 Periventricular lesions ≥1 Brainstem lesions	2 of 2: ≥1 Periventricular lesions ≥1 Hypointense lesions on T1 images	2 of 4: ≥1 Periventricular ≥1 Juxtacortical ≥1 Infratentorial ≥1 Spinal cord

*Barkhof F, Filippi M, Miller DH, et al: Comparison of MRI criteria at first presentation to predict conversion to clinically definite multiple sclerosis. *Brain* 120:2059–2069, 1997.
†Mikaeloff Y, Adamsbaum C, Husson HM, et al: MRI prognostic factors for relapse after acute CNS inflammatory demyelination in childhood. Brain 127:1942–1947, 2004.
‡Callen DJ, Shroff MM, Branson HM, et al: Role of MRI in the differentiation of ADEM from MS in children. *Neurology* 72:968–973, 2009.
§Callen DJ, Shroff MM, Branson HM, et al: MRI in the diagnosis of pediatric multiple sclerosis. *Neurology* 72:961–967, 2009.
‖Verhay LH, Branson HM, Shroff MM, et al: MRI parameters for prediction of multiple sclerosis diagnosis in children with acute CNS demyelination: a prospective national cohort study. *Lancet Neurol* 10:1065–1073, 2011.
¶Polman CH, Reingold SC, Banwell B, et al. Diagnostic criteria for multiple sclerosis: 2010 revisions to the McDonald criteria. *Ann Neurol* 69:292–302, 2011.
ADEM, acute disseminated encephalomyelitis; MS, multiple sclerosis.
From Krupp LB, Tardieu M, Amato MP, et al: International Pediatric Multiple Sclerosis Study Group criteria for pediatric multiple sclerosis and immune-mediated central nervous system demyelinating disorders: revision to the 2007 definitions. Mult Scler 19(10):1261–1267, 2013, Appendix 3, p. 1267.

Table 600-6	Overview of Available and Emerging Therapies in Pediatric Multiple Sclerosis			
MEDICATION	**MEDICATION CLASS**	**MECHANISM IN MS**	**SIDE EFFECTS**	**STUDIES DESCRIBING DRUG EFFICACY IN PEDIATRIC MS**
FIRST-LINE THERAPIES				
Interferon-α or β	Immunomodulator	Modulates T cells and cytokine production	Flu-like symptoms; transaminitis; leukopenia; tissue necrosis at injection site (rare)	Retrospective Prospective multicenter
Glatiramer acetate*	Immunomodulator	Modulates T cells and reduces antigen presentation	Flushing, lipodystrophy at injection sites	Prospective single center Prospective multicenter
SECOND-LINE THERAPIES				
Natalizumab*	Monoclonal antibody	Targets α₄-integrin; prevents T-cell migration into CNS and other tissues	Overall PML rate ~1 in 500 patients, but lower in subgroups; immune reconstitution syndrome after discontinuation; melanoma; infusion reaction; transaminitis (rare)	Retrospective Prospective multicenter
Cyclophosphamide	Chemotherapeutic	DNA alkylation; effects include cytotoxic immune cell depletion	Hemorrhagic cystitis; bladder cancer; late-onset malignancy; infection; infertility	Retrospective multicenter
Mitoxantrone*	Chemotherapeutic	Disrupts DNA synthesis; effects include cytotoxic immune cell depletion	Significant long-term safety risks, including cardiotoxicity (1 in 200 patients) and secondary leukemia (1 in 125 patients); opportunistic infections	Retrospective single center
Daclizumab	Monoclonal antibody	Targets/inactivates interleukin-2 receptor; inhibits activated T cells	Glucose intolerance; pulmonary edema; infusion reaction; gastrointestinal upset; skin reactions	Retrospective multicenter
Rituximab	Monoclonal antibody	Targets CD20, a marker of immature B cells; depletes B-cell populations	PML (rate undefined); infusion-related side effects	No efficacy assessments available in pediatric MS
Azathioprine	Chemotherapeutic	Disrupts purine metabolism; effects include cytotoxic immune cell depletion	Transaminitis; leukopenia; lymphoma	No efficacy assessments available in pediatric MS
Fingolimod*†	Immunomodulator	Sphingosine-1-phosphate agonist; causes T-cell sequestration in lymphoid compartments	Systemic viral infection; cardiac arrhythmia; macular edema; transaminitis	FDA approved for adult MS in September 2010; no reports of use in pediatric MS to date
Teriflunomide*†	Immunomodulator	Impairs immune cell proliferation via pyrimidine synthesis inhibition	Infections; headaches; diarrhea; transaminitis; alopecia; teratogenicity	FDA approved for adult MS in September 2012; no reports of use in pediatric MS to date
EMERGING THERAPIES				
Vitamin D†	Vitamin/hormone	Modulates immune cell expression	Hypercalcemia and kidney stones at a serum 25(OH) vitamin D level >100 ng/mL	Prospective trials in pediatric and adult MS are currently underway
Ocrelizumab	Monoclonal antibody	Targets CD20, a marker of immature B cells; depletes B-cell populations	Headache; infusion-related side effects; theoretical risk of PML (undefined)	Recently completed phase III trial in adult MS; no use in pediatric MS to date
Dimethyl fumarate†	Immunomodulator	Neuroprotectant; antioxidant	Flushing reaction; gastrointestinal upset; headache	FDA approved for adult MS in March 2013; no use in pediatric MS to date
Alemtuzumab	Monoclonal antibody	Anti-CD52 antibody target; depletes mature T cells	Opportunistic infection, autoimmune thyroiditis (20-30% risk), immune thrombocytopenia (1%)	Recently completed phase III trial in adult MS; no use in pediatric MS to date
Laquinimod†	Immunomodulator	Modulates T cell and cytokine production	Transaminitis	Recently completed phase III trial in adult MS; no use in pediatric MS to date

*FDA approved for the treatment of adult MS.
†Orally administered therapy.
CNS, central nervous system; MS, multiple sclerosis; PML, progressive multifocal leukoencephalopathy.

weakness or numbness or dysphagia. Optic neuritis or transverse myelitis may occur simultaneously or may be separated in time by weeks or even years. Some present with an encephalopathy mimicking ADEM. Others exhibit endocrinopathies such as the syndrome of inappropriate antidiuretic hormone secretion, diabetes insipidus, or disrupted puberty. The symptoms and signs of transverse myelitis depend on the spinal level and completeness of the inflammatory changes. NMO differs from MS in that recovery of visual and spinal cord function is generally not as complete after each episode; optic neuritis is more frequently bilateral in NMO than in MS.

LABORATORY FINDINGS

CSF in patients with NMO often has 50 or more white blood cells per microliter. Unlike MS, it is devoid of oligoclonal bands. Serum positivity for anti–aquaporin-4 antibodies (so-called NMO antibodies) has a sensitivity of 73% and a specificity of 91% for NMO. Neuroimaging studies should include the entire spine, optic nerves as well as the cortex that may reveal lesions in the brainstem or thalami or hazy ill-defined lesions in the hemispheres in contrast to the discrete, well-defined oval lesions in the periventricular white matter seen in MS.

DIAGNOSIS AND DIFFERENTIAL DIAGNOSIS

Clinical diagnosis of NMO currently requires optic neuritis and transverse myelitis plus at least 2 of 3 supporting criteria: (1) brain MRI not diagnostic of MS, (2) seropositivity for anti–aquaporin-4 antibody, or (3) spine MRI with longitudinally extensive transverse myelitis involving at least 3 spinal segments (see Table 600-2). NMO spectrum disorder may be diagnosed in relapsing forms of transverse myelitis or optic neuritis with aquaporin-4 seropositivity. The differential diagnosis includes MS; ADEM (see Chapter 600.3); rheumatologic etiologies producing transverse myelitis, and/or optic neuritis, including systemic lupus erythematosus, Behçet disease, and neurosarcoidosis (usually accompanied by other nonneurologic manifestations); idiopathic transverse myelitis, tropical spastic paraparesis, and viral encephalomyelitis (none of which have NMO antibodies in the serum or CSF); and metabolic and idiopathic causes of isolated optic neuritis or other acute monocular or binocular visual loss (see Chapter 631). Additional considerations depending on the location of the lesions include lymphoma, Langerhans cell histiocytosis, tuberculosis, and vitamin B_{12} or E deficiencies.

COMPLICATIONS

Similar to adults with NMO, pediatric NMO patients often are left with fixed neurologic deficits affecting visual acuity, visual fields, color vision, motor and sensory function, balance, and bowel/bladder function.

TREATMENT

Initial episodes and relapses may be treated acutely with methylprednisolone, 20-30 mg/kg/day (max: 1,000 mg/day) for 3-5 days, followed by a slow prednisone taper. Rituximab is effective in preventing relapses of NMO and NMO spectrum disorder. Preliminary evidence suggests that eculizumab also reduced recurrences and may improve disability in patients with severe NMO spectrum disorder.

PROGNOSIS

The prognosis is generally poor for patients with NMO. In 1 study, approximately 20% remained functionally blind (i.e., 20/200 vision or worse) in at least 1 eye and 31% had permanent monoplegia or paraplegia. Five-year survival of the patients with paraplegia is approximately 90%.

Bibliography is available at Expert Consult.

600.3 Acute Disseminated Encephalomyelitis

Jayne M. Ness

ADEM is an initial inflammatory, demyelinating event with multifocal neurologic deficits, typically accompanied by encephalopathy (see Table 600-2).

EPIDEMIOLOGY

ADEM can occur at any age but most series report a mean age between 5 and 8 yr with a slight male predominance. Reported incidence ranges from 0.07-0.4 per 100,000 per year in the pediatric population.

PATHOGENESIS

Molecular mimicry induced by infectious exposure or vaccine may trigger production of CNS autoantigens. Many patients experience a transient febrile illness in the month prior to ADEM onset. Preceding infections associated with ADEM include influenza, Epstein-Barr virus, cytomegalovirus, varicella, enterovirus, measles, mumps, rubella, herpes simplex, and *Mycoplasma pneumoniae*. Postvaccination ADEM has been reported following immunizations for rabies, smallpox, measles, mumps, rubella, Japanese encephalitis B, pertussis, diphtheria-polio-tetanus, and influenza.

CLINICAL MANIFESTATIONS

Initial symptoms of ADEM may include lethargy, fever, headache, vomiting, meningeal signs, and seizures, including status epilepticus. **Encephalopathy** is a hallmark of ADEM, ranging from ongoing confusion to persistent irritability to coma. Focal neurologic deficits can be difficult to ascertain in the obtunded or very young child but common neurologic signs in ADEM include visual loss, cranial neuropathies, ataxia, motor and sensory deficits, plus bladder/bowel dysfunction with concurrent spinal cord demyelination.

NEUROIMAGING

Head CT may be normal or show hypodense regions. Cranial MRI, the imaging study of choice, typically exhibits large, multifocal and sometimes confluent or large edematous mass-like tumefactive T2 lesions with variable enhancement within white and often gray matter of the cerebral hemispheres, cerebellum, and brainstem (Fig. 600-2). Deep gray-matter structures (thalami, basal ganglia) are often involved, although this may not be specific to ADEM. Spinal cord may have abnormal T2 signal or enhancement, with or without clinical signs of myelitis. MRI lesions of ADEM typically appear to be of similar age but their evolution may lag behind the clinical presentation. Serial MRI imaging 3-12 mo following ADEM shows improvement and often complete resolution of T2 abnormalities, although residual gliosis may remain.

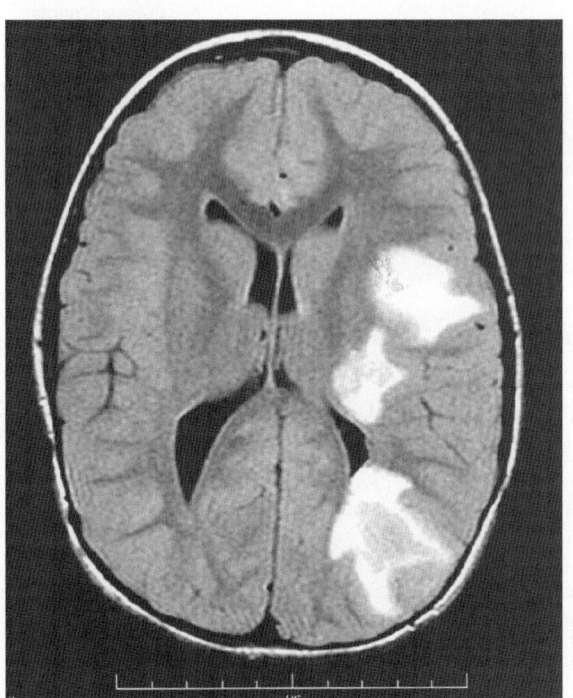

Figure 600-2 Axial T2-weighted fluid-attenuated inversion recovery MRI of the brain in a child with acute disseminated encephalomyelitis. High signal (white) lesions in the T2-weighted image reflect areas of demyelination and edema in deep subcortical and periventricular white matter as well as the basal ganglia and thalamus on the left side.

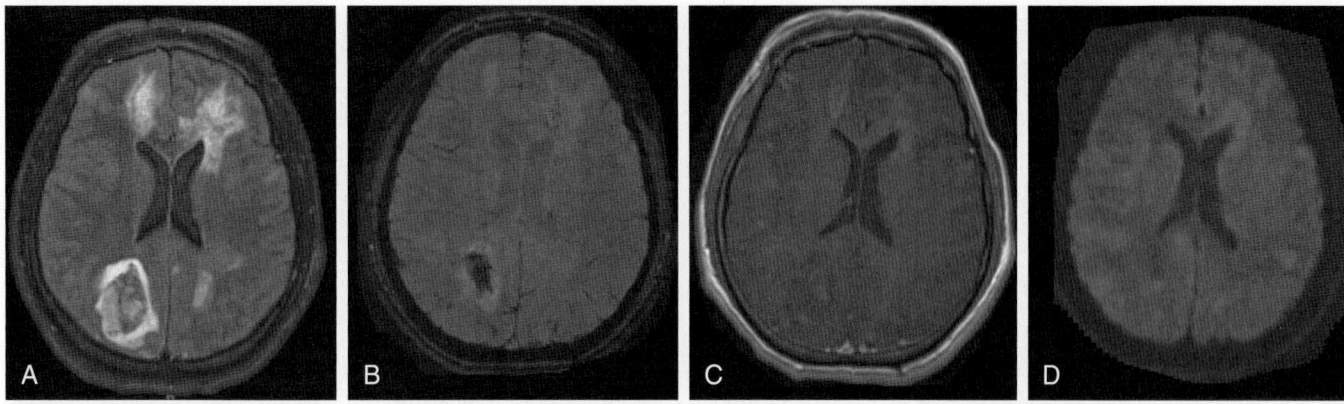

Figure 600-3 MRI findings in acute disseminated encephalomyelitis. Multiple scattered T2 hyperintensities are appreciated on fluid-attenuated inversion recovery images **(A)** with evidence of hemorrhage on susceptibility-weighted images **(B)**, contrast enhancement on T1 postgadolinium images **(C)**, and without diffusion restriction on diffusion-weighted imaging **(D)**. *(From Virmani T, Agarwal A, Klawiter EC: Clinical reasoning: a young adult presents with focal weakness and hemorrhagic brain lesions. Neurology 76:e105–e109, 2011, Fig. 2.)*

Severe involvement may progress to an **acute hemorrhagic leukoencephalopathy (Hurst disease)** with large lesions, edema, mass affect, and a polymorphonucleated cell pleocytosis (in contrast to lymphocytic pleocytosis in the CSF noted in typical ADEM) (Fig. 600-3).

LABORATORY FINDINGS
There is no biologic marker for ADEM and laboratory findings can vary widely. CSF studies often exhibit pleocytosis with lymphocytic or monocytic predominance. CSF protein can be elevated, especially on repeat studies. Up to 10% of patients with ADEM have oligoclonal bands in the CSF and/or elevated CSF immune globulin production. Patients with ADEM may occasionally demonstrate antibodies against myelin oligodendrocyte glycoprotein, or anti–N-methyl-D-aspartate receptor antibodies. Electroencephalograms often show generalized slowing, consistent with encephalopathy, although polyregional demyelination of ADEM can also cause focal slowing or epileptiform discharges.

DIFFERENTIAL DIAGNOSIS
The differential diagnosis for ADEM is broad but can be narrowed by careful history, appropriate laboratory evaluations, and MRI (see Table 600-1). Empirical antibiotic and antiviral treatment should be considered while infectious evaluations are pending. Follow-up MRI examinations 3-12 mo after ADEM should show improvement; new or enlarging T2 lesions should prompt reevaluation for other etiologies such as MS, leukodystrophies, tumor, vasculitis, or mitochondrial, metabolic, or rheumatologic disorders (see Table 600-1 and Table 600-5).

TREATMENT
Although there are no randomized controlled trials to compare acute treatments for ADEM or other demyelinating disorders of childhood, high-dose intravenous steroids are commonly employed (typically methylprednisolone 20-30 mg/kg per day for 5 days with a maximum dose of 1,000 mg per day). An oral prednisone taper over 1 mo may prevent relapse. Other treatment options include intravenous immune globulin (usually 2 g/kg administered over 2-5 days) or plasmapheresis (typically 5-7 exchanges administered every other day). In severe cases of suspected ADEM, rituximab or cyclophosphamide have been used. There is no consensus about timing of these treatments for ADEM.

PROGNOSIS
Many children experience full recovery after ADEM but some are left with residual motor and/or cognitive deficits. ADEM is usually a monophasic illness but demyelinating symptoms can fluctuate for several months. Repeated bouts of demyelination more than 3 mo after ADEM later raise the question of MS vs repeated ADEM.

Bibliography is available at Expert Consult.

Chapter 601
Pediatric Stroke
Adam Kirton and Gabrielle A. deVeber

Stroke is an important cause of acquired brain injury in newborns and children. The ischemic varieties of arterial ischemic stroke (AIS) and cerebral sinovenous thrombosis (CSVT) are more common than brain malignancy (incidence approximately 5 in 100,000 children per year). Perinatal stroke is even more common and is the leading cause of hemiparetic cerebral palsy. A similar number of children suffer from hemorrhagic stroke (HS) and other forms of cerebrovascular disease. Acute stroke is a neurologic emergency; however, delays in recognition are common and delayed treatment worsens outcomes. In contrast to stroke in adults, there are a diverse group of disorders producing stroke in neonates and children.

601.1 Arterial Ischemic Stroke
Adam Kirton and Gabrielle A. deVeber

Arterial blood reaches the brain via the anterior (internal carotid) and posterior (vertebrobasilar) circulations, converging at the circle of Willis. Strokes most often involve the middle cerebral artery territory but can occur in any cerebral artery of any size. AIS is the focal brain infarction that results from occlusion of these arteries and is a leading cause of acquired brain injury in children with the perinatal period carrying the highest risk.

The diagnosis of stroke in children is frequently delayed. This is a consequence of subtle and nonspecific clinical presentations, poor awareness by primary care pediatric physicians, a complicated differential diagnosis (see Chapter 601.4), and a high frequency (>50%) of negative initial CT scan. **The acute onset of a focal neurologic deficit in a child is stroke until proven otherwise.** The most common focal presentation is hemiparesis, but acute visual, speech, sensory, or balance deficits also occur. Children with these presentations require urgent neuroimaging and consultation with a child neurologist, as emergency interventions may be indicated. AIS is a clinical and radiographic diagnosis. Although CT imaging can demonstrate mature AIS and exclude hemorrhage, MRI is required to identify early and small infarcts. **Diffusion-weighted MRI** demonstrates AIS within minutes of onset and up to 7 days postonset; MR angiography can confirm vascular occlusion and suggest possible arteriopathy (Fig. 601-1). Diffusion-weighted MRI can also demonstrate wallerian degeneration

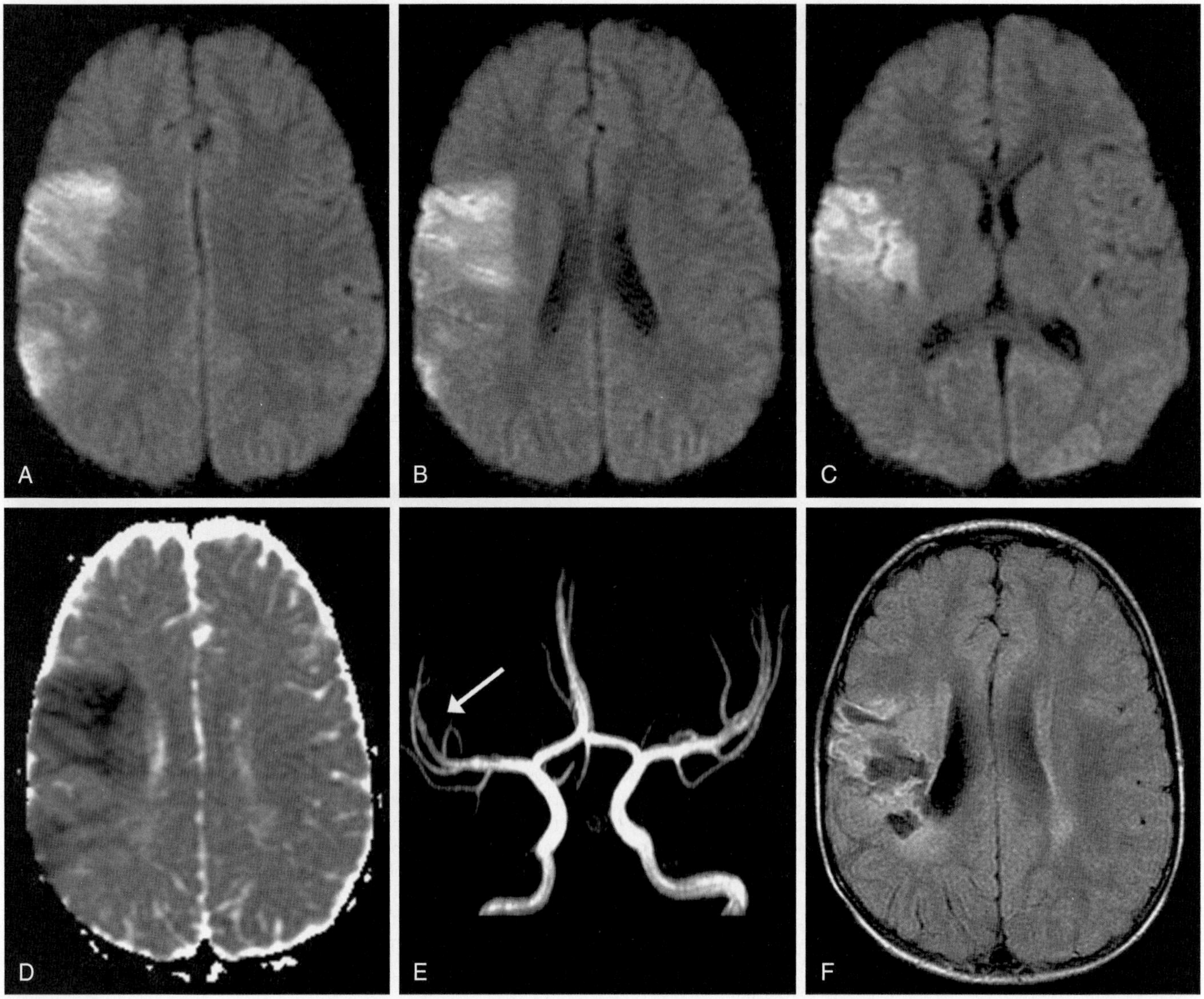

Figure 601-1 Arterial ischemic stroke. A healthy 3 yr old boy had sudden onset of left-sided weakness. Examination also demonstrated left-sided hemisensory loss and neglect. **A** to **C,** Diffusion-weighted MRI shows focal increased signal in the right temporal–parietal region in the territory of the middle cerebral artery (MCA). **D,** Apparent diffusion coefficient map confirms restricted diffusion consistent with infarction (ischemic stroke). **E,** MR angiogram shows decreased flow in the corresponding branch of the MCA. **F,** Follow-up MRI at 3 mo shows atrophy and gliosis in the same region.

in the descending corticospinal tract, which correlates with chronic hemiparesis.

Many possible risk factors for AIS are recognized (Table 601-1), although the specific pathophysiologic mechanisms are often poorly understood. Three main categories of etiology should be considered: **arteriopathy, cardiac,** and **hematologic;** full investigation, however, often reveals multiple risk factors per individual.

Arteriopathy refers to disorders of the cerebral arteries and is a leading cause of childhood AIS, present in more than 50% of children. A common syndrome affecting healthy school-age children features unilateral irregular stenosis of the proximal middle cerebral artery and neighboring arteries presenting with basal ganglia infarction. The description of this entity has been published under multiple names—**transient cerebral arteriopathy,** postvaricella angiopathy, nonprogressive childhood primary angiitis of the central nervous system, and focal cerebral arteriopathy—reflecting uncertainty regarding the pathogenesis.

This entity may represent focal inflammation or intracranial dissection or early moyamoya disease, although it is nearly always self-limited. Diffuse, bilateral, progressive **vasculitis** is rare and can represent progressive childhood primary angiitis of the central nervous system or be associated with systemic vasculitides (Table 601-2). Cranial infections (e.g., bacterial meningitis) also produce arteritis and thrombophlebitis

of surface vessels. A**rterial dissection** can be spontaneous or posttraumatic and can affect extra- or intracranial arteries. **Moyamoya syndrome** may be idiopathic or associated with other conditions (neurofibromatosis type 1, trisomy 21, Alagille syndrome, sickle cell anemia, chromosomal microdeletions/microduplications, postirradiation) and demonstrates progressive occlusion of the distal internal carotid arteries. Congenital malformations of the craniocervical arteries, including PHACES (posterior fossa abnormalities, hemangioma, and arterial, cardiac, eye, and sternal abnormalities) syndrome, or fibromuscular dysplasia may predispose to AIS. Vasospasm as occurs in migraine, subarachnoid hemorrhage or reversible cerebral vasoconstriction syndrome (sometimes called Call-Fleming syndrome) can cause AIS.

Cardioembolic stroke makes up approximately 25% of childhood AIS with maximal embolic risk concurrent with catheterization, surgical repair, or ventricular assistive device use. AIS complicates approximately 0.5% of pediatric cardiac surgeries and reoperation increases the risk. Although **complex congenital heart diseases** are most frequently associated with AIS, acquired conditions, including arrhythmia, cardiomyopathy, and infective endocarditis, also should be considered. A patent foramen ovale provides the possibility of paradoxical venous thromboembolism but is not likely an independent risk factor. All children with suspected AIS require thorough cardiovascular examination, electrocardiogram, and echocardiogram.

Table 601-1	Risk Factors for Arterial Ischemic Stroke in Children
MAJOR CATEGORY	**EXAMPLES**
Arteriopathy	Transient cerebral arteriopathy (TCA) (synonyms: childhood primary angiitis of the central nervous system [cPACNS]; focal cerebral arteriopathy [FCA]) Postvaricella and other viruses angiopathy (PVA) Systemic/secondary vasculitis (e.g., Takayasu arteritis) Moyamoya disease/syndrome Arterial infection (e.g., bacterial meningitis, tuberculosis) Fibromuscular dysplasia Traumatic or spontaneous carotid or vertebral artery dissection Vasospasm (e.g., Call-Fleming syndrome) Migraine (migrainous infarction?) Congenital arterial hypoplasia (e.g., PHACES syndrome)
Cardiac	Complex congenital heart diseases (cyanotic ≫ acyanotic) Cardiac catheterization/procedure (e.g., balloon atrial septostomy) Ventricular assistive device use Cardiac surgery Arrhythmia Valvular heart disease Endocarditis Cardiomyopathy, severe ventricular dysfunction Intracardiac lesions (e.g., atrial myxoma) Septal defects (atrial septal defect, ventricular septal defect, patent foramen ovale [possible paradoxical emboli])
Hematologic	Sickle cell anemia Iron-deficiency anemia Inherited prothrombotic (e.g., factor V Leiden, prothrombin gene mutation 20210A) Acquired prothrombotic (e.g., protein C/S deficiency, antithrombin III deficiency, lipoprotein a, antiphospholipid antibodies, oral contraceptives, pregnancy)

Other including metabolic/genetic etiologies	Acute systemic illness (e.g., dehydration, sepsis, diabetic ketoacidosis)
	Chronic systemic illness (e.g., systemic lupus erythematosus, leukemia)
	Illicit drugs and toxins (e.g., cocaine)
	Extracorporeal membrane oxygenation (ECMO)
	Hereditary dyslipoproteinemia
	  Familial hypoalphalipoproteinemia
	  Familial hypercholesterolemia
	  Type IV, type III hyperlipoproteinemia
	  Tangier disease
	  Progeria
	Fabry disease (α-galactosidase A deficiency)
	Subacute necrotizing encephalomyelopathy (Leigh disease)
	Sulfite oxidase deficiency
	11β-Ketoreductase deficiency
	17α-Hydroxylase deficiency
	Purine nucleoside phosphorylase deficiency
	Ornithine transcarbamylase deficiency
	Neurofibromatosis type 1
	HERNS
	Heritable disorders of connective tissue
	  Ehlers-Danlos syndrome (type IV)
	  Marfan syndrome
	  Pseudoxanthoma elasticum
	  Homocystinuria (cystathionine β-synthase deficiency, or 5,20-methylenetetrahydrofolate reductase)
	  Menkes syndrome
	Organic acidemias
	  Methylmalonic academia
	  Propionic academia
	  Isovaleric academia
	  Glutaric aciduria type II
	Mitochondrial encephalomyopathies
	  MELAS
	  MERRF
	  MERRF/MELAS overlap syndrome
	  Kearns-Sayre syndrome
	See also: stroke mimics (see Chapter 601.4)

HERNS, hereditary endotheliopathy with retinopathy, nephropathy, and stroke; MELAS, mitochondrial myopathy, encephalopathy, lactic acidosis, and stroke-like episodes; MERRF, myoclonic epilepsy with ragged red fibers; PHACES, posterior fossa abnormalities, hemangioma, and arterial, cardiac, eye, and sternal abnormalities.

Modified from Roach ES, Golomb MR, Adams R, et al: Management of stroke in infants and children. Stroke 39:2644–2691, 2008, Table 2, p. 6.

Table 601-2	Classification of Cerebral Vasculitis

Infectious vasculitis
  Bacterial, fungal, parasitic
  Spirochetal (syphilis, Lyme disease, leptospirosis)
  Viral, rickettsial, mycobacterial, free-living amebae, cysticercosis,
    other helminths
Necrotizing vasculitides
  Classic polyarteritis nodosa
  Wegener granulomatosis
  Allergic angiitis and granulomatosis (Churg-Strauss syndrome)
  Necrotizing systemic vasculitis overlap syndrome
  Lymphomatoid granulomatosis
Vasculitis associated with collagen vascular disease
  Systemic lupus erythematosus
  Rheumatoid arthritis
  Scleroderma
  Sjögren syndrome
Vasculitis associated with other systemic diseases
  Behçet disease
  Ulcerative colitis
  Sarcoidosis
  Relapsing polychondritis
  Kohlmeier-Degos disease
Takayasu arteritis
Hypersensitivity vasculitides
  Henoch-Schönlein purpura
  Drug-induced vasculitides
  Chemical vasculitides
  Essential mixed cryoglobulinemia
Miscellaneous
  Vasculitis associated with neoplasia
  Vasculitis associated with radiation
  Cogan syndrome
  Dermatomyositis-polymyositis
  X-linked lymphoproliferative syndrome
  Kawasaki disease

Primary central nervous system vasculitis
From Roach ES, Golomb MR, Adams R, et al: Management of stroke in infants and children, Stroke 39:2644–2691, 2008, Table 5, p. 8.

Prothrombotic coagulation disorders and infection at index stroke increase stroke recurrence risk.

Hematologic disorders associated with AIS include **sickle cell anemia,** in which stroke risk is increased 400-fold, although effective screening (transcranial Doppler) and treatments (transfusions) have reduced the incidence. Iron-deficiency anemia also increases the risk and is easily treatable. Coagulation disorders are associated with childhood AIS. They include hereditary (e.g., factor V Leiden) and acquired (e.g., antiphospholipid antibodies, lipoprotein-a elevation) **prothrombotic states** and **prothrombotic medications,** including oral contraceptives and asparaginase chemotherapy. Additional AIS risk factors include migraine, acute childhood illnesses, chronic systemic illnesses, illicit drugs and toxins, and rare inborn errors of metabolism.

Treatment of childhood AIS is multifaceted and multiple consensus-based guidelines are available. Given the inadequate safety data, emergency thrombolysis is not recommended for children, but safety studies are underway. Early initiation of **antithrombotic strategies** is paramount to prevent early reinfarction. Depending on the suspected cause, this includes anticoagulation with heparins or antiplatelet strategies, usually aspirin. Hyperacute **neuroprotective strategies** are essential to initiate with suspected stroke as they prevent progressive ischemic brain injury. These include control of blood glucose, temperature and seizures and maintenance of cerebral perfusion pressure. Early malignant cerebral edema is life-threatening, more common in children and predictable, and emergency surgical decompression can be life-saving. Disease-specific treatments include transfusion therapy in sickle cell disease, immunosuppression in vasculitis, and revascularization surgery in moyamoya. Long-term treatment goals include **secondary stroke prevention**, including antiplatelet therapy in arteriopathy and anticoagulation in cardiogenic causes. Multimodal, family-centered **rehabilitation** programs are required for most survivors, targeting motor deficits, language and intellectual impairments, behavioral and social disabilities, and epilepsy. Long-term attention to arterial health lifestyle factors may also be important. Outcomes after childhood stroke include recurrent stroke ranging from 10-50% depending on cause and preventative treatment, death in 6-10%, neurologic deficits in 60-70%, and seizure disorders in up to 30%.

PERINATAL ARTERIAL ISCHEMIC STROKE
Perinatal stroke is very common, differs from childhood stroke, and has 2 distinct clinical presentations. Acute symptomatic neonatal AIS presents with focal seizures at 24-28 hr of life (Fig. 601-2). MRI diffusion

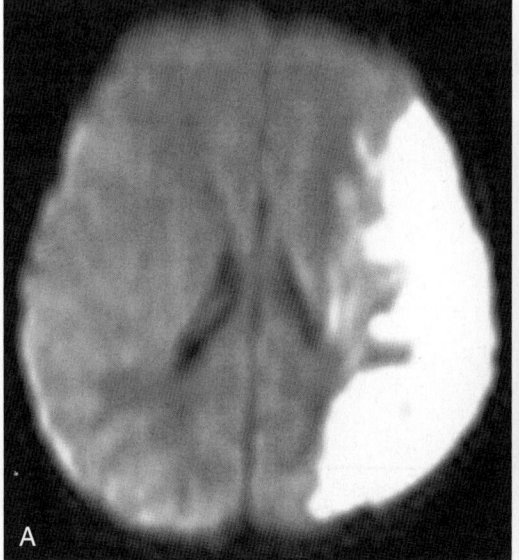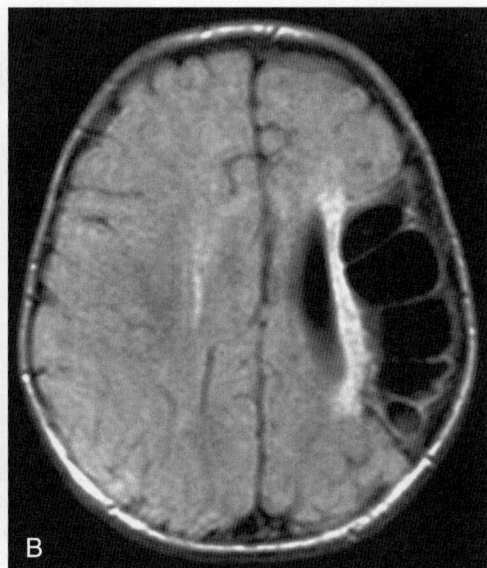

Figure 601-2 Perinatal arterial ischemic stroke. A term newborn developed focal right-sided seizures at 16 hr of life. **A,** Diffusion-weighted MRI on day 2 diagnoses neonatal arterial ischemic stroke by demonstrating restricted diffusion in the left middle cerebral artery territory. **B,** Repeat MRI at 12 mo shows cystic encephalomalacia and scarring in the same territory, a similar appearance to children diagnosed with presumed perinatal arterial ischemic stroke later in infancy.

abnormalities in an arterial territory confirm recent infarction. Alternatively, infants are asymptomatic at birth and present in later infancy with signs of early hand preference and congenital hemiparesis. Hand dominance within the 1st yr of life is abnormal and may be the result of perinatal stroke. Imaging reveals focal encephalomalacia in an arterial territory, typically large middle cerebral artery lesions.

In acute neonatal AIS, seizure control is important, but antithrombotic agents are rarely required (exception: cardiac embolism). Pathophysiology is complex and poorly understood. Most are idiopathic, although established causes include congenital heart disease, thrombotic placentopathy, and other prothrombotic disorders and meningitis. Many other maternal, prenatal, perinatal, obstetrical, and neonatal factors have been investigated with several strong associations found (e.g., infertility, primiparity, multiple gestation). Outcomes are poor, with most children having lifelong disability. Perinatal stroke accounts for most cases of hemiparetic cerebral palsy (congenital hemiplegia, see Chapter 598.1). Additional morbidity, seen in approximately 25%, includes disorders of language, learning, cognition, and behavior and longer-term epilepsy. Stroke recurrence rates for both the child and subsequent pregnancies are extremely low.

Bibliography is available at Expert Consult.

601.2 Cerebral Sinovenous Thrombosis
Adam Kirton and Gabrielle A. deVeber

Cerebral venous drainage occurs via the cerebral sinovenous system. This includes superficial (cortical veins, superior sagittal sinus) and deep (internal cerebral veins, straight sinus) systems that converge at the torcula to exit via the paired transverse and sigmoid sinuses and jugular veins. In CSVT, thrombotic occlusion of these venous structures can create increased intracranial pressure, cerebral edema, and, in 50% of cases, venous infarction or hemorrhage (stroke). CSVT may be more common in children than in adults, and risk is greatest risk in the neonatal period.

Clinical presentations are typically gradual, variable, and nonspecific compared to AIS. Neonates often present with encephalopathy and seizures. Children may present with symptoms mimicking idiopathic intracranial hypertension, including progressive headache, papilledema, diplopia secondary to 6th nerve palsy, or with acute focal deficits. Seizures, lethargy, and confusion are common. Diagnosis requires a high clinical suspicion and purposeful imaging of the cerebral venous system. Nonenhanced CT is very insensitive for CSVT, and contrast **CT venography** or MR venography is necessary to demonstrate filling defects in the cerebral venous system (Fig. 601-3). MRI offers superior parenchymal imaging compared to CT.

Table 601-3 lists the risk factors for CSVT. **Prothrombotic states** associated with childhood CSVT include inherited (e.g., prothrombin gene 20210A mutation) and acquired (e.g., antiphospholipid antibodies) conditions, prothrombotic medications (asparaginase, oral contraceptives) and common childhood illnesses including otitis media, iron-deficiency anemia, and **dehydration. Systemic diseases** associated with increased CSVT risk include leukemia, inflammatory bowel disease, and nephrotic syndrome.

Head and neck disorders can directly involve cerebral veins and sinuses causing CSVT. Common **infections,** including meningitis, otitis media, and mastoiditis, can cause **septic thrombophlebitis** of venous channels. CSVT can complicate head **trauma** especially adjacent to skull fractures. Neurosurgical procedures in proximity to cerebral venous structures may lead to injury and CSVT. Finally, obstruction of the jugular veins and proximal stasis may result in CSVT. In neonates, the unfused status of cranial sutures enables mechanical distortion of underlying venous sinuses during delivery, or postnatally occipital bone compression of the posterior sagittal sinus during supine lying predisposing to CSVT.

Anticoagulation therapy plays an important role in childhood CSVT treatment. Substantial indirect evidence has led to consensus to recommend anticoagulation with unfractionated or low-molecular-weight heparins in most children. Hemorrhagic transformation of venous infarcts is not an absolute contraindication. Treatment is usually planned for 6 mo, although if reimaging at 3 mo confirms recanalization, treatment is usually discontinued. However anticoagulation of neonates is more controversial and guidelines differ. Evidence suggests that 30% of untreated neonates and children will extend their thrombosis in the 1st wk postdiagnosis and additional venous infarction can result. Therefore, if anticoagulation is withheld, early (e.g., 5-7

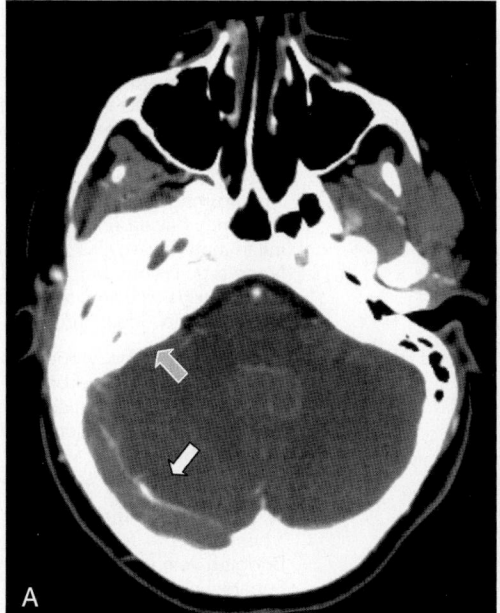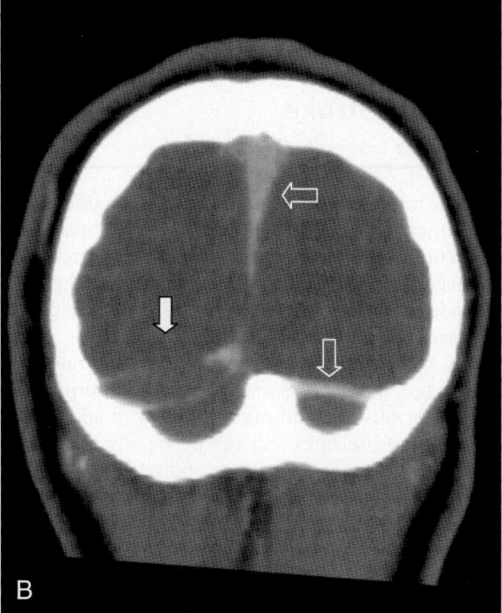

Figure 601-3 Cerebral sinovenous thrombosis. A 9 yr old girl presented with fever and progressive right-sided headache. She complained of double vision and had papilledema on examination. Axial **(A)** and coronal **(B)** CT venography demonstrates a large thrombus in the right transverse sinus that fails to opacify with contrast *(full arrows)*. Note normal filling in superior sagittal and in smaller left transverse sinuses *(empty arrows, right)* and opacification of the mastoid air cells *(hatched arrow, left)*. Cause was otitis media/mastoiditis with septic thrombophlebitis of transverse sinus.

Table 601-3	Common Risk Factors for Cerebral Sinovenous Thrombosis in Children
MAJOR CATEGORIES	**EXAMPLES**
Blood coagulation	Prothrombotic conditions Factor V Leiden, prothrombin gene mutation 20210A, protein C deficiency, protein S deficiency, antithrombin III deficiency, lipoprotein a, antiphospholipid antibodies (lupus anticoagulant, anticardiolipin antibodies), pregnancy/puerperium Dehydration (e.g., gastroenteritis, neonatal failure to thrive) Iron-deficiency anemia Drugs and toxins (e.g., L-asparaginase, oral contraceptives) Acute systemic illness (e.g., sepsis, disseminated intravascular coagulation) Chronic systemic illness (e.g., inflammatory bowel disease, systemic lupus erythematosus, leukemia) Nephrotic syndrome Inborn errors of metabolism (e.g., homocystinuria)

Blood vessel	Infection/thrombophlebitis
	    Otitis media, mastoiditis, bacterial meningitis, sinusitis, dental abscess, pharyngitis
	    Lemierre syndrome
	    Sepsis
	Trauma: skull fractures, closed hear trauma
	Compression: birth, occipital bone compression in neonates in supine lying
	Iatrogenic: neurosurgery, jugular lines, extracorporeal membrane oxygenation
	Venous malformations (e.g., dural arteriovenous fistulas)

days) repeat venous imaging is paramount. Protocols supporting initial anticoagulation recommend shorter treatment durations (i.e., 6 wk to 3 mo) in neonates. Children with persistent risk factors may require prophylactic long-term anticoagulation. At initial diagnosis, supportive interventions include management of infection, detection and treatment of seizures, and neuroprotective measures (normothermia, normotension, normovolemia, normoglycemia). **Optic neuropathy** secondary to increased intracranial pressure is an important and easily missed complication of CSVT. Regular funduscopic examination by an ophthalmologist and measures to reduce intracranial pressure (e.g., acetazolamide, serial lumbar puncture) may be required to avoid visual loss. Most neurologic morbidity is suffered by those incurring venous infarction and children with bilateral venous infarction can be devastated. Consistent with other forms of childhood stroke, a comprehensive neurorehabilitation program is required.

Bibliography is available at Expert Consult.

601.3 Hemorrhagic Stroke
Adam Kirton and Gabrielle A. deVeber

HS includes nontraumatic intracranial hemorrhage and is classified by the intracranial compartment containing the hemorrhage. Intraparenchymal bleeds may occur in any location, whereas intraventricular hemorrhage may be isolated or an extension of intraparenchymal hemorrhage. Bleeding outside the brain may occur in the subarachnoid, subdural, or epidural spaces.

Clinical presentations vary according to location, cause, and rate of bleeding. Acute hemorrhages may feature instantaneous or **thunderclap headache,** loss of consciousness, and nuchal rigidity in addition to focal neurologic deficits and seizures. HS can be rapidly fatal. In bleeds associated with vascular malformations, pulsatile tinnitus, cranial bruit, macrocephaly, and high-output heart failure may be present. Diagnosis relies on imaging and CT is highly sensitive to acute HS. However, lumbar puncture may be required to exclude subarachnoid hemorrhage. MRI is highly sensitive to even small amounts of both acute and chronic hemorrhage and offers improved diagnostic accuracy (Fig. 601-4). Angiography by CT, MR, or conventional catheter means is often required to exclude underlying vascular abnormalities (e.g., vascular malformations, aneurysms).

Abusive head trauma with intracranial bleeding in children may present as primary subdural or parenchymal hemorrhage with no apparent history of trauma. Subtle scalp, suborbital, or ear bruising; retinal hemorrhages in multiple layers; and chronic failure to thrive should always be sought, and in infants with subdural bleeds, x-rays performed to rule out fractures. Epidural hematoma is nearly always caused by trauma, including middle meningeal artery injury typically associated with skull fracture. Subdural hematoma can occur spontaneously in children with brain atrophy because of stretching of bridging veins.

Causes of and risk factors for HS (Table 601-4) include vascular malformations and systemic disorders. **Arteriovenous malformations**

Table 601-4	Potential Risk Factors for Hemorrhagic Stroke in Children
MAJOR CATEGORIES	**EXAMPLES**
Vascular disorder	Arteriovenous malformations Cavernous malformations ("cavernomas") Venous angiomas and other venous anomalies Hereditary hemorrhagic telangiectasia Intracranial aneurysm Choroid plexus angiomas (pure intraventricular hemorrhage) Moyamoya disease/syndrome Inflammatory vasculitis (see Chapter 601.1) Neoplastic lesions with unstable vasculature Drugs/toxins (cocaine, amphetamine) Cerebral sinovenous thrombosis
Blood disorder	Idiopathic thrombocytopenic purpura Hemolytic uremic syndrome Hepatic disease/failure coagulopathy Vitamin K deficiency (hemorrhagic disease of the newborn) Disseminated intravascular coagulopathy
Trauma	Middle meningeal artery injury (epidural hematoma) Bridging vein injury (subdural hematoma) Subarachnoid hemorrhage Hemorrhagic contusions (coup and contrecoup) Nonaccidental trauma (subdural hematomas of different ages) Iatrogenic (neurosurgical procedures, angiography) Rupture of arachnoid cyst

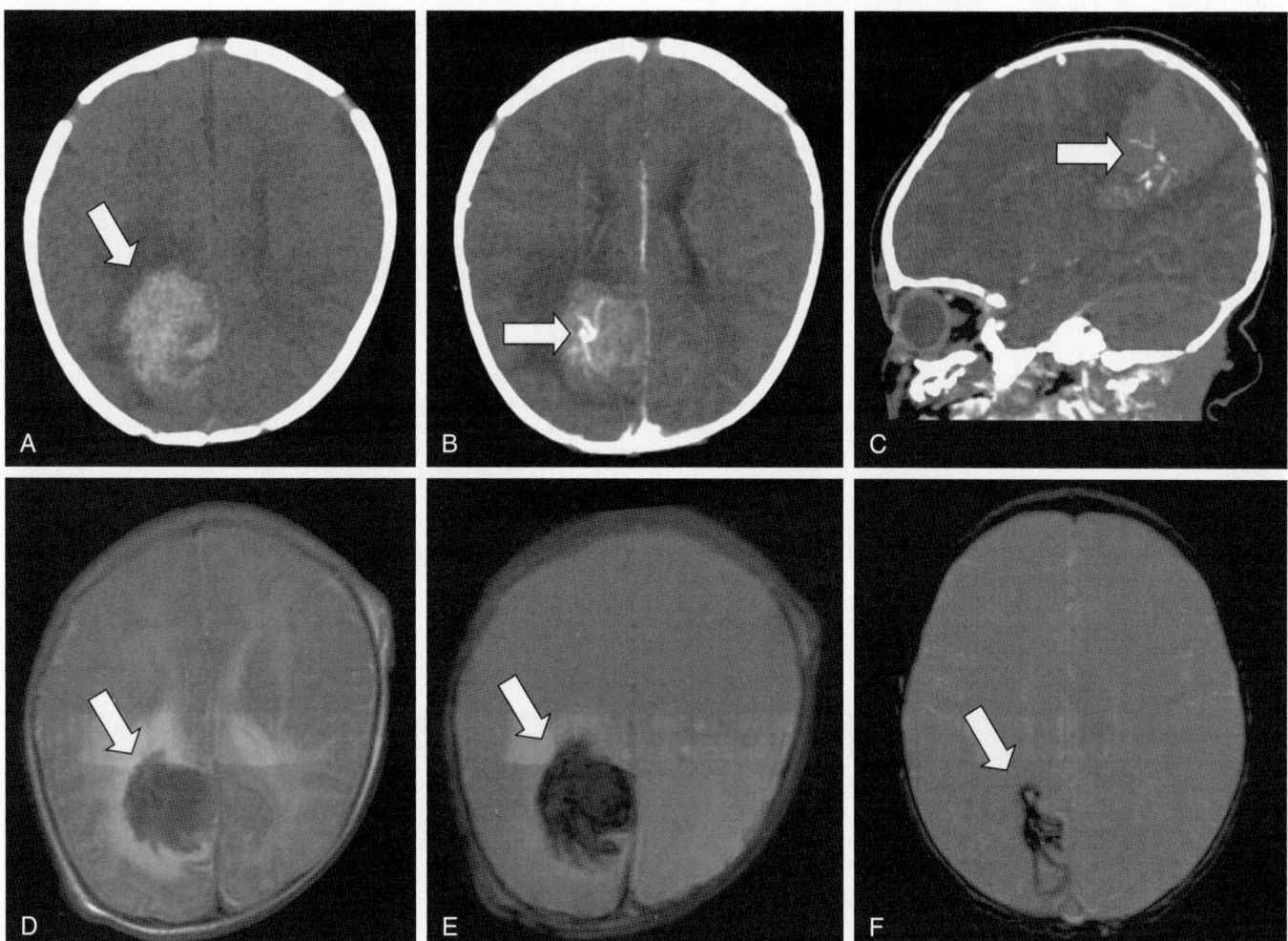

Figure 601-4 Hemorrhagic stroke. A healthy 1 mo old presented with sudden-onset irritability followed by focal left body seizures. Plain CT head demonstrates a large hyperdense lesion in the right parietal region with surrounding edema consistent with acute hemorrhage **(A)**. Axial **(B)** and sagittal **(C)** contrast CT scans suggest an abnormal cluster of vessels in the center of the hemorrhage consistent with an AVM. T2-weighted MRI differentiates the acute hemorrhage from surrounding edema **(D)**. Gradient echo MRI, both acutely **(E)** and at 3 mo **(F)**, demonstrates the presence of blood product.

are the most common cause of childhood subarachnoid and intraparenchymal HS and may occur anywhere. Neonates with vein of Galen malformations may present with heart failure, progressive macrocephaly, or, rarely, hemorrhage. In older children with arteriovenous malformations, the risk of bleeding is approximately 2-4% per year throughout life. Other vascular malformations leading to HS include cavernous angiomas (**"cavernomas"**), dural arteriovenous fistulas, and vein of Galen malformations. Cerebral aneurysms are an uncommon cause of subarachnoid hemorrhage in children and may suggest an underlying disorder (e.g., polycystic kidney disease, infective endocarditis). A common cause for HS is bleeding from a preexisting brain tumor. Arterial diseases that usually cause ischemic stroke, including fibromuscular dysplasia, vasculitis, and moyamoya, can also predispose to HS. Additional causes of parenchymal HS include hypertensive hemorrhage and hematologic disorders such as thrombocytopenic purpura, hemophilia, acquired coagulopathies (e.g., disseminated intravascular coagulopathy, liver failure), anticoagulant therapy (e.g., warfarin), or illicit drug use. Ischemic infarcts may undergo hemorrhagic transformation, particularly in CSVT, and may be difficult to differentiate from primary HS.

Management of acute childhood HS may require emergent neurosurgical intervention for large or rapidly expanding hemorrhage. The same principles of neuroprotection for vulnerable brain suggested in the ischemic stroke sections also apply to HS. Reversal of anticoagulant therapy (with, for example, vitamin K, fresh-frozen plasma) may be required, but the role of other medical interventions, such as factor VII, are unstudied in children. Recurrence risk for those with structural lesions is significant and serial imaging may be required. Definitive repair or removal of the vascular malformation may require a combined approach with interventional endovascular methods or neurosurgery. Outcomes from childhood HS are not well studied but likely depend on lesion size, location, and etiology. Compared with ischemic stroke, HS mortality is higher while long-term deficits are less common.

Neonatal HSs have unique features. Cranial ultrasound can detect many neonatal parenchymal bleeds, especially In the preterm infant where bleeds are located centrally within the cranium and include germinal matrix bleeding and intraventricular hemorrhage (see Chapter 99.3). Germinal matrix injury or bleeding may also occur in utero, resulting in periventricular venous infarction that becomes symptomatic in later infancy as congenital hemiparesis. Subarachnoid and subdural blood may be imaged in up to 25% of normal term newborns. Term HS is poorly studied and includes the etiologies listed above, although HS may be idiopathic in more than 50% of cases. Term intraventricular bleeding is often secondary to deep CSVT with specific management implications.

Bibliography is available at Expert Consult.

601.4 Differential Diagnosis of Stroke-Like Events

Adam Kirton and Gabrielle A. deVeber

The diagnosis of stroke in childhood requires a high index of suspicion balanced with awareness of the differential diagnosis for stroke-like events (Table 601-5). Acute onset of a focal neurologic deficit should be considered stroke until proven otherwise and assessed with neuroimaging. However, pediatric stroke must be differentiated from other stroke-like disorders that may require their own urgent specific treatment.

MIGRAINE

Careful history and examination can often suggest migraine as the cause of acute focal deficits. Migraine auras should last between 5 and 60 min and resolve completely. Neurologic deficits associated with migraine typically evolve slowly compared with stroke, with sensory disturbance or weakness "marching" across body areas over minutes. Although evolution into a migrainous headache is expected, headache may also accompany acute infarction. Furthermore, a group of uncommon migraine subtypes can occur without headache and can more closely mimic stroke in children. These include familial hemiplegic migraine, basilar migraine, and migraine aura without headache.

Migraine can also (rarely) cause a stroke, referred to as migrainous infarction.

SEIZURE

Prolonged focal seizure activity is frequently followed by a period of focal neurologic deficit ("Todd's paresis") which typically resolves within an hour. Very rarely, focal seizures can manifest with only "negative" symptoms producing acute onset, focal neurologic deficits. A history of clonic jerks or tonic posturing at onset, a known past history of seizures, and electroencephalogram findings may be helpful. Imaging is required in all new cases of seizure with persisting Todd's paresis because stroke in children is often associated with seizures at onset.

INFECTION

Life-threatening and treatable brain infections, including bacterial meningitis and herpes encephalitis, can be mistaken for stroke. However, symptom onset in primary central nervous system infection is typically more gradual and less focal with fever as a consistent feature. Children with bacterial meningitis are at risk for both venous and arterial stroke.

DEMYELINATION

Acute disseminated encephalomyelitis, clinically isolated syndrome, multiple sclerosis, and other demyelinating conditions can present

Table 601-5	Differential Diagnosis of Stroke-Like Episodes in Children	
DISORDER	**CLINICAL DISTINCTION FROM STROKE**	**IMAGING DISTINCTION FROM STROKE**
Migraine	Evolving or "marching" symptoms, short duration, complete resolution, headache, personal or family history of migraine	Typically normal Migrainous infarction is rare
Seizure	Positive symptoms, Todd paralysis is postseizure and limited	Normal or may identify source of seizures (e.g., malformation, old injury, etc.)
Infection	Fever, encephalopathy, gradual onset, meningismus	Normal or signs of encephalitis/cerebritis, which are typically diffuse and bilateral. Arterial ischemic stroke and cerebral sinovenous thrombosis can occur in bacterial meningitis
Demyelination	Gradual onset, multifocal symptoms, encephalopathy Accompanying optic neuritis or transverse myelitis	Multifocal lesions, characteristic appearance (e.g., patchy in acute disseminated encephalomyelitis, ovoid in multiple sclerosis), typical locations (e.g., pericallosal in multiple sclerosis), less likely to show restricted diffusion
Hypoglycemia	Risk factor (e.g., insulin therapy), related to meals, additional systemic symptoms	Bilateral, symmetrical May see restricted diffusion Posterior dominant pattern
Watershed infarction caused by global hypoxic–ischemic encephalopathy	Risk factor (e.g., hypotension, sepsis, heart disease), bilateral deficits	Bilateral, symmetric restricted diffusion in border zones between major arteries (watershed zones)
Hypertensive encephalopathy (posterior reversible leukoencephalopathy)	Documented hypertension, bilateral visual symptoms, encephalopathy	Posterior dominant, bilateral, patchy lesions involving gray and white matter, usually no restricted diffusion
Inborn errors of metabolism	Preexisting delays/regression, multisystem disease, abnormal biochemical profiles	May have restricted diffusion lesions but bilateral, symmetrical, not within vascular territories. MR spectroscopy changes (e.g., high lactate in mitochondrial myopathy, encephalopathy, lactic acidosis, and stroke-like episodes)
Vestibulopathy	Symptoms limited to vertigo, imbalance (i.e., no weakness). Gradual onset	Normal
Acute cerebellar ataxia	Sudden-onset bilaterally symmetric ataxia; postviral	Normal
Channelopathy	Syndromic cluster of symptoms not localizing to single lesion. Gradual onset, progressive evolution	Normal
Alternating hemiplegia	History contralateral events Choreoathetosis/dystonia	Normal

with acute focal neurologic deficits. Symptom onset and initial progression is more gradual (typically hours or days) compared with stroke onset (minutes). Multifocal deficits, or concurrent encephalopathy in the case of acute disseminated encephalomyelitis, would decrease the probability of stroke.

HYPOGLYCEMIA

Acute lowering of blood glucose levels can produce focal deficits mimicking stroke. New-onset hypoglycemia in otherwise healthy children is rare, but predisposing conditions include insulin-dependent diabetes, adrenal insufficiency, steroid withdrawal, and ketogenic diet.

GLOBAL HYPOXIC–ISCHEMIC ENCEPHALOPATHY

Generalized decreases in cerebral perfusion can produce focal areas of watershed brain infarction which can be asymmetric and mimic stroke. Watershed ischemic injury should be accompanied by recognized hypotension or conditions predisposing to low cerebral perfusion such as sepsis, dehydration, or cardiac dysfunction. Clinical presentations would involve more generalized and bilateral cerebral dysfunction compared to stroke and the anatomic location of the infarct is in typical bilateral watershed zones rather than a single arterial territory.

HYPERTENSIVE ENCEPHALOPATHY

The posterior reversible leukoencephalopathy syndrome is seen in children with hypertension, often in the context of an acute rise in blood pressure. Posterior regions are selectively involved, possibly resulting in symptoms of bilateral cortical visual dysfunction in addition to encephalopathy and seizures.

INBORN ERRORS OF METABOLISM

Mitochondrial myopathy, encephalopathy, lactic acidosis, and stroke-like episodes (MELAS; see Chapter 598.2) are the classic examples, though other mitochondrial disease can mimic stroke. Features favoring MELAS would include a history of developmental regression, posterior (and often bilateral) lesions not respecting vascular territories on MRI, and elevated serum or cerebrospinal fluid lactate (MR spectroscopy). In contrast to these types of "metabolic infarction," children with Fabry disease (see Chapter 613.6) and homocystinuria (see Chapter 85.4) are at risk of true ischemic stroke.

VESTIBULOPATHY/ATAXIA

Acute onset vertigo and/or ataxia can be confused with brainstem or cerebellar stroke. Simple bedside tests of vestibular function with otherwise intact brainstem functions are reassuring. This differential diagnosis includes acute vestibular neuronopathy, viral labyrinthitis, and the benign paroxysmal vertigos as well as acute cerebellar ataxia and episodic ataxias.

CHANNELOPATHIES

An increasing number of nervous system ion channel mutations are described that feature sudden focal neurological deficits thereby mimicking stroke. These include the migraine syndromes mentioned above as well as a growing list of episodic ataxias. A strong family history raises suspicion but most require additional investigation.

ALTERNATING HEMIPLEGIA OF CHILDHOOD

Alternating hemiplegia of childhood typically presents in infancy with acute intermittent episodes of hemiplegia that alternate from 1 side of the body to the other. The hemiplegia persists for minutes to weeks and then resolves spontaneously. Choreoathetosis and dystonic movements are commonly observed in the hemiparetic extremity. Signs spontaneously regress with sleep but recur with awakening. Neuroimaging including MRA should be completed to exclude moyamoya disease. Alternating hemiplegia of childhood is linked to mutations in the *ATP1A3* gene.

Chapter 602
Central Nervous System Vasculitis

Heather A. Van Mater, William B. Gallentine, and Susanne M. Benseler

Autoimmune-mediated inflammatory brain diseases are recognized as an etiology for neurologic and neuropsychiatric symptoms in children and adults and include primary central nervous system (CNS) vasculitis, secondary CNS vasculitis, and autoimmune encephalitis (Fig. 602-1; see Chapter 598.4).

Primary angiitis of the CNS (PACNS) is recognized as the underlying etiology of a broad spectrum of neurologic and psychiatric symptoms in children. Criteria characteristic of childhood CNS vasculitis (cPACNS) include (1) newly acquired focal and/or diffuse neurologic deficits and/or psychiatric symptoms in a child 18 yr of age or younger, **plus** (2) angiographic and/or histologic evidence of vasculitis **in the absence of** (3) a systemic underlying condition known to cause or mimic the findings. Two broad categories of cPACNS are recognized based on the predominant vessel size affected: large/medium-vessel cPACNS and small-vessel cPACNS. Large/medium-vessel cPACNS is diagnosed on angiography demonstrating features of vessel wall inflammation, wall swelling and edema, and resulting luminal stenosis. Based on the clinical course and the corresponding distribution of vessel stenosis within the vascular tree of the CNS, children with large/medium-vessel cPACNS are classified as a monophasic, nonprogressive (NPcPACNS) or a progressive subtype (PcPACNS). The latter is characterized by chronic, progressive vessel wall inflammation affecting both proximal and distal vessel segments in 1 or both hemispheres. In contrast, NPcPACNS is a monophasic illness; vessel inflammation occurs in a characteristic distribution and is limited to the proximal vessel segments of the anterior and/or middle cerebral artery and/or distal internal carotid artery of 1 hemisphere. Small vessel cPACNS (SVcPACNS) is considered a progressive illness; the diagnosis is confirmed on brain biopsies because angiography is normal.

Secondary childhood CNS vasculitis can affect all cerebral vessel segments and can occur in the context of infections, rheumatic or other inflammatory conditions or as a result of systemic or local vascular irritation (Table 602-1). The neuropsychiatric manifestations of secondary CNS vasculitis are the same as those of primary CNS vasculitis. Secondary CNS vasculitis is distinguished from primary CNS vasculitis largely by the non-CNS manifestations of the underlying systemic vasculitic disease.

EPIDEMIOLOGY

The incidence and prevalence of primary CNS vasculitis is undetermined. In the past, the majority of children have been diagnosed at autopsy. Increased physician awareness, improved diagnostic markers, sensitive neuroimaging techniques, and brain biopsies have led to dramatically increased recognition and decreased mortality. Exploring the epidemiology of primary CNS vasculitis remains a challenge: the disease has many names including isolated angiitis of the CNS, transient cerebral angiitis, postvaricella angiopathy, and focal cerebral arteriopathy. Furthermore, children are frequently diagnosed with their presenting clinical phenotype, such as stroke, movement disorder, hallucination, or cognitive decline. Within clinical phenotypes, such as arterial ischemic stroke or status epilepticus in children without preexisting epilepsy, cPACNS should be considered an important etiology.

CLINICAL MANIFESTATIONS

Recognition of childhood CNS vasculitis requires a very high level of suspicion; any neurologic or psychiatric presentation can be the result

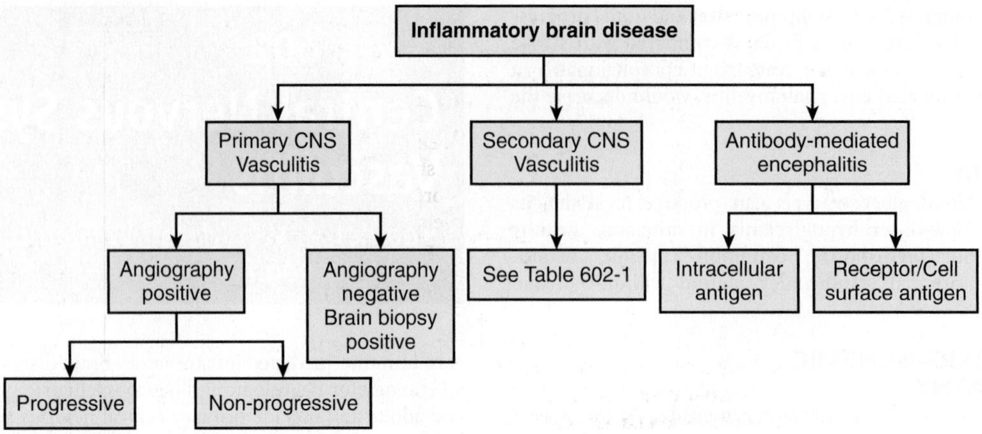

Figure 602-1 CNS vasculitis within the spectrum of immune-mediated inflammatory brain diseases.

Table 602-1	Causes of Secondary CNS Vasculitis

VIRAL INFECTIONS
Varicella zoster virus, HIV, hepatitis C virus, cytomegalovirus, parvovirus B19

BACTERIAL INFECTIONS
Treponema pallidum, Borrelia burgdorferi, Mycobacterium tuberculosis, Mycoplasma pneumoniae, Bartonella henselae, Rickettsia spp.

FUNGAL INFECTIONS
Aspergillosis, mucormycosis, coccidioidomycosis, candidosis

PARASITIC INFECTIONS
Cysticercosis

SYSTEMIC VASCULITIDES
Wegener granulomatosis, Churg-Strauss syndrome, Behçet disease, polyarteritis nodosa, Henoch-Schönlein purpura, Kawasaki disease, giant-cell arteritis, Takayasu arteritis

CONNECTIVE TISSUE DISEASES
Systemic lupus erythematosus, rheumatoid arthritis, Sjögren syndrome, dermatomyositis, mixed connective tissue disease

MISCELLANEOUS
Antiphospholipid antibodies syndrome, Hodgkin and non-Hodgkin lymphomas, neurosarcoidosis, inflammatory bowel disease, graft-versus-host disease, bacterial endocarditis, acute bacterial meningitis, drug-induced CNS vasculitis (cocaine, amphetamine, ephedrine, phenylpropanolamine)

From Salvarani C, Brown Jr. RD, Hunder GG: Adult primary central nervous system vasculitis. Lancet 380:767–776, 2012, Panel, p. 768.

of an underlying CNS vasculitis. The clinical phenotype may provide clues to the size of the primarily affected vessel segments and resulting cPACNS subtype: the majority of children with large/medium cPACNS present with arterial ischemic stroke features. Focal neurologic deficits, such as hemiparesis, facial droop, aphasia or any other distinct gross or fine motor deficits, may be the result of large vessel inflammation causing stenosis and decreased blood supply to the specific functional areas of the brain. Initially, these focal deficits wax and wane; they may even briefly resolve without therapeutic intervention and can therefore be easily overlooked. Headaches are a symptom of vascular disease in general and are commonly reported in cPACNS. New onset of vascular-type (e.g., migraine) headaches in children without any family history of migraine can serve as a diagnostic clue. Cognitive dysfunction in cPACNS often includes loss of higher executive function, concentration difficulties, learning and memory problems, atypical behavior or personality changes, and loss of social and emotional control. Seizures are a hallmark of SVcPACNS, as more than 80% of children with SVcPACNS present with seizures; all seizure types are seen. Often there

is a disconnection between the clinical presentation and the child's electroencephalogram findings. In many centers, refractory status epilepticus is increasingly recognized as the presenting phenotype of SVcPACNS. Optic neuritis and spinal cord disease are also recognized in SVcPACNS.

Constitutional features of fever or fatigue may point toward an underlying systemic illness causing a secondary CNS vasculitis. All children with suspected or confirmed CNS vasculitis require a careful assessment for a systemic illness.

DIAGNOSIS

The first step is considering vasculitis as a possible underlying etiology of newly acquired neurologic deficits and/or psychiatric symptoms (Table 602-2). The likelihood of CNS vasculitis in general and a specific subtype of CNS vasculitis in particular depends on the demographic characteristics of the patient, the CNS and non-CNS features of the clinical presentation, the preceding symptoms, and the mode of onset of the disease. SVcPACNS is more commonly seen in girls of all ages, whereas large/medium cPACNS has a clear male preponderance. Seizures are a hallmark of SVcPACNS, whereas strokes often reflect large/medium-vessel inflammation. Laboratory markers of vasculitis typically include C-reactive protein, erythrocyte sedimentation rate, and complete blood counts. But inflammatory markers lack sensitivity and specificity in cPACNS, particularly when the CNS is involved in isolation. More than 50% of children with large/medium-vessel cPACNS have normal inflammatory markers at diagnosis. In contrast, the majority of children with SVcPACNS present with mild-moderately raised markers. Von Willebrand factor antigen, an endothelial cell–derived protein, is a proposed biomarker of vasculitis correlating closely with disease activity in cPACNS. It may be of particular importance for distinguishing SVcPACNS from demyelinating diseases. Cerebrospinal fluid (CSF) analysis is abnormal in up to 90% of SVcPACNS patients and less than half of large/medium-vessel cPACNS. Within the latter group, children with the progressive subtype have a higher likelihood of presenting with abnormal CSF findings, including high opening pressure, raised CSF cell count, typically with lymphocyte predominance, and raised CSF protein. Oligoclonal bands are seen in 20% of children with SVcPACNS. They are rarely seen in other subtypes. Autoimmune encephalitis (see Chapter 598.4) is one of the key differential diagnoses of SVcPACNS.

Neuroimaging is a valuable diagnostic modality for cPACNS. Parenchymal lesions may be inflammatory or ischemic in nature and are best viewed on MRI including T2/fluid attenuated inversion recovery (FLAIR) sequences and diffusion-weighted images (DWI) (Fig. 602-2). CNS lesions in children with large/medium-vessel cPACNS are predominantly ischemic in nature and restricted to large vascular territories. In contrast, MRI lesions in children with SVcPACNS are not restricted to major vascular territories; lesions are primarily inflammatory and may enhance with contrast. In this subtype, focal or

Table 602-2	Proposed Diagnostic Evaluation of Suspected Childhood Primary CNS Vasculitis

1. Clinical evaluation: Newly acquired symptom or deficit in a previously healthy child
   • Focal neurologic deficit: hemiparesis, hemisensory loss, aphasia, ataxia, movement abnormality, paresthesia, facial droop, ataxia, vision loss, spinal cord symptoms, others
   • Seizures or (refractory) seizure status
   • Diffuse neurologic deficit including cognitive decline with loss of higher executive function, concentration difficulties, learning or memory problems, behavior or personality changes, loss of social skills or emotional/impulse control, others
   • Headaches
   • Meningitis symptoms, abnormal level of consciousness
   • Psychiatric symptoms including hallucinations, pseudoseizures
   Differential diagnosis approach:
   • Underlying illness known to cause, be associated or mimic CNS vasculitis: check all potential clinical features
2. Laboratory tests
   • Blood inflammatory markers: C-reactive protein, erythrocyte sedimentation rate and complete blood counts
   • Endothelial markers: von Willebrand factor (vWF) antigen
   • Cerebrospinal fluid (CSF) inflammatory markers: opening pressure, cell count, protein, oligoclonal bands
   Differential diagnosis approach:
   • Infections/postinfectious inflammation: cultures, serologies, Gram stains
   • Autoimmune encephalitis: check neuronal antibodies in CSF and blood
   • Systemic inflammation/rheumatic disease: characteristic laboratory markers such as complement, autoantibodies
   • Thromboembolic conditions: procoagulatory profile
3. Neuroimaging
   • Parenchymal imaging on MRI:
      • Inflammatory lesions: T2/fluid attenuated inversion recovery sequences plus gadolinium contrast (lesion enhancement)
      • Ischemic lesions: diffusion-weighted images/apparent diffusion coefficient mapping
   • Vessel imaging
4. Brain biopsy

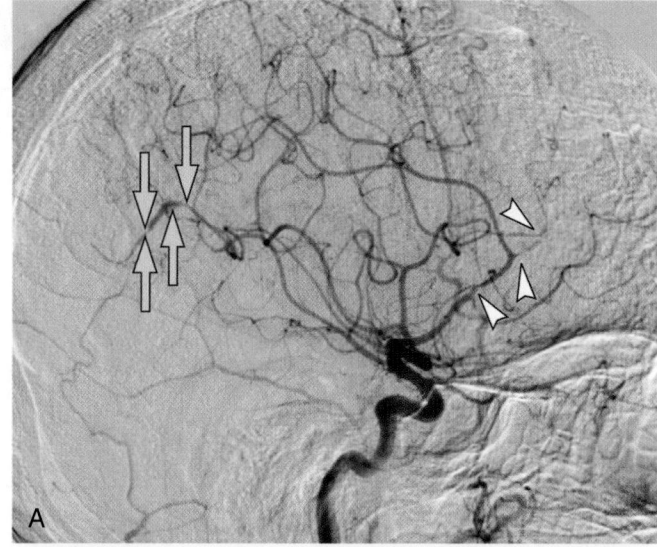

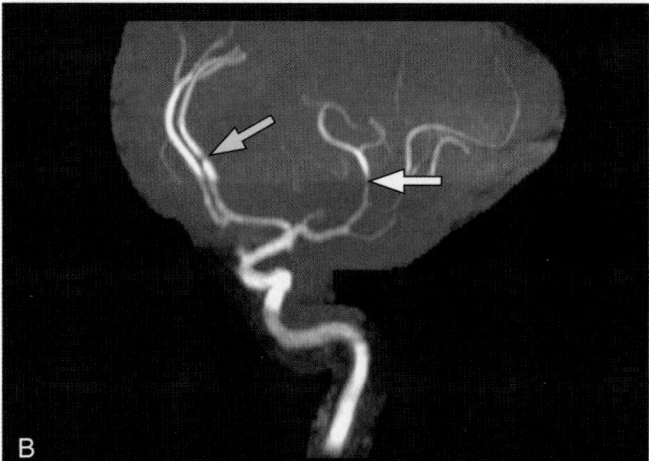

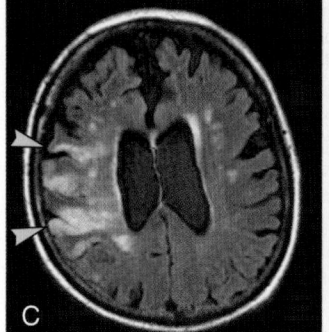 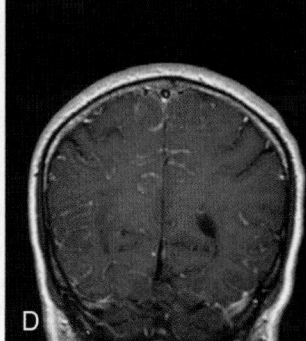

generalized meningeal enhancement is commonly seen if children are imaged prior to immunosuppressive therapy. Spinal cord parenchymal imaging is challenging; defining the nature of lesions is often difficult.

Evidence of vessel stenosis confirms the diagnosis in large/medium-vessel cPACNS subtypes; brain biopsies are not required. Important information about the disease activity can be obtained from post–gadolinium contrast studies of the vascular wall. The vessel wall of an inflamed cerebral vessel in active large/medium-vessel cPACNS subtypes is thickened and enhances contrast. Conventional angiography when compared to MR angiography has a higher sensitivity in detecting vessel stenosis in the distal vessel segments, the posterior circulation, and in very young children. Vessel wall imaging is often normal in children with SVcPACNS, sometimes mandating an elective brain biopsy to definitively make the diagnosis. Studies of regional blood flow or therapeutic trials of antiinflammatory or immunosuppressive agents are nonsurgical alternatives that do not afford specific diagnostic information. Biopsies should target low-risk, nonfunctional areas identified on MRI. In the appropriate clinical context, nonlesional biopsies have a high yield for confirming the diagnosis of SVcPACNS. Characteristic findings in SVcPACNS include an intramural and/or perivascular mononuclear infiltrate, evidence of endothelial activation, and reactive astrocyte activation. Gliosis and perivascular demyelination are hallmarks of long-standing disease. Findings typically seen in adult PACNS, including granulomas or vessel wall necrosis, are rarely seen in children with SVcPACNS. In children, the diagnostic yield of brain biopsies is 70%. Biopsy-related complications are rarely seen.

Figure 602-2 Imaging of patients with primary CNS vasculitis. **A,** Cerebral angiogram shows alternating stenosis and dilation of the distal middle cerebral artery (*arrows*) and the anterior cerebral artery (*arrowheads*). **B,** Magnetic resonance angiography of the brain shows a short-segment stenosis of the anterior cerebral artery (*green arrow*) and stenosis of the distal middle cerebral artery (*white arrow*). **C,** Fluid attenuation inversion recovery–weighted MRI shows a large abnormality within the right cerebral hemisphere consistent with ischemia (*arrowheads*). **D,** MRI shows diffuse, asymmetric, nodular, and linear leptomeningeal enhancement, with dura only slightly affected. (*From Salvarani C, Brown Jr. RD, Hunder GG: Adult primary central nervous system vasculitis. Lancet 380:767–776, 2012, Fig. 2.*)

Table 602-3	Characteristics of Primary CNS Vasculitis and Reversible Cerebral Vasoconstriction Syndrome	
	PCNSV	**RCVS**
Precipitating factor	None	Postpartum onset or onset after exposure to vasoactive substances
Onset	More insidious, progressive course	Acute onset followed by a monophasic course
Headaches	Chronic and progressive	Acute, thunderclap type
CSF findings	Abnormal (leucocytosis and high total protein concentration)	Normal to near normal
MRI	Abnormal in almost all patients	Normal in 70% of patients
Angiography	Possibly normal; otherwise, diffuse abnormalities are often indistinguishable from RCVS; irregular and asymmetrical arterial stenoses or multiple occlusions are more suggestive of PCNSV; abnormalities might be irreversible	Always abnormal, strings of beads appearance of cerebral arteries; abnormalities reversible within 6-12 wk
Cerebral biopsy	Vasculitis	No vasculitic changes
Drug treatment	Prednisone with or without cytotoxic agents	Nimodipine

CSF, cerebrospinal fluid; PCNSV, primary CNS vasculitis; RCVS, reversible cerebral vasoconstriction syndrome.
From Salvarani C, Brown Jr. RD, Hunder GG: Adult primary central nervous system vasculitis. Lancet 380:767–776, 2012, Table 2.

Disorders that may be seen in adolescents and young adults that produce the reversible vasoconstriction syndrome must also be considered. These include migraine, drug-induced vasospasm, and postpartum angiopathy. Differentiating vasculitis is important for therapy and prognosis (Table 602-3).

TREATMENT
Corticosteroids are the mainstay of acute immunosuppressive management of cPACNS. Usually IV pulse therapy is initially given. Antithrombotic therapy is equally important, particularly in large/medium-vessel cPACNS subtypes, because children are at high risk for recurrent ischemic events. For the distinct cPACNS subtypes, different treatment regimens should be considered. Nonprogressive cPACNS is a monophasic inflammatory attack with the highest risk of poor neurologic outcome. Vessel wall inflammation causes severe proximal stenosis and a high restroke risk. High-dose corticosteroid pulses are commonly given followed by a 6-12 wk course of oral steroids at tapering doses. Second-line immunosuppressive agents are uncommonly used. All children require antithrombotic therapy. No unifying regimen exists. Many centers initially use low-molecular-weight heparin followed by long-term antiplatelet therapy. When reimaged at 3 mo follow-up, children should have stable or improved vessel disease, no newly affected vessel segments, and no evidence of contrast wall enhancement. At this point the immunosuppressive therapy is commonly discontinued and children are only kept on antiplatelet agents.

Progressive cPACNS and SVcPACNS are considered chronic progressive vasculitis subtypes requiring a prolonged course of combination immunosuppression. High-dose corticosteroids are initially used followed by long-term oral corticosteroids with slow taper. Many centers use an induction-maintenance protocol adding IV cyclophosphamide to the corticosteroids as the induction medication, followed by mycophenolate mofetil or other oral second-line agents during maintenance therapy. Symptomatic therapy is essential including anticonvulsants or psychotropic medication if required. Supportive therapy includes bone protection with calcium and vitamin D, prophylaxis against pneumocystis pneumonia, and gastric mucosal protection as required.

PROGNOSIS
The mortality rate of cPACNS has significantly improved. Some treatment protocols for SVcPACNS report a good outcome, defined as no functional neurologic deficits in two-thirds of children. Children presenting with status epilepticus and SVcPACNS have the poorest cognitive outcome.

Bibliography is available at Expert Consult.

Chapter 603
Central Nervous System Infections
Charles G. Prober, Nivedita S. Srinivas, and Roshni Mathew

Infection of the central nervous system (CNS) is the most common cause of fever associated with signs and symptoms of CNS disease in children. Many microorganisms can cause infection. Nonetheless, specific pathogens are identifiable and are influenced by the age and immune status of the host and the epidemiology of the pathogen. In general, viral infections of the CNS are much more common than bacterial infections, which, in turn, are more common than fungal and parasitic infections. Infections caused by rickettsiae (Rocky Mountain spotted fever, *Ehrlichia*) are relatively uncommon but assume important roles under certain epidemiologic circumstances. *Mycoplasma* spp. can also cause infections of the CNS, although their precise contribution is often difficult to determine.

Regardless of etiology, most patients with CNS infection have similar clinical manifestations. **Common symptoms** include headache, nausea, vomiting, anorexia, restlessness, altered state of consciousness, and irritability; most of these symptoms are nonspecific. **Common signs** of CNS infection, in addition to fever, include photophobia, neck pain and rigidity, obtundation, stupor, coma, seizures, and focal neurologic deficits. The severity and constellation of signs are determined by the specific pathogen, the host, and the area of the CNS affected.

Infection of the CNS may be diffuse or focal. Meningitis and encephalitis are examples of diffuse infection. Meningitis implies primary involvement of the meninges, whereas encephalitis indicates brain parenchymal involvement. Because these anatomic boundaries are often not distinct, many patients have evidence of both meningeal and parenchymal involvement and should be considered to have meningoencephalitis. Brain abscess is the best example of a focal infection of the CNS. The neurologic expression of this infection is determined by the site and extent of the abscess(es) (see Chapter 604).

The diagnosis of diffuse CNS infections depends on examination of cerebrospinal fluid (CSF) obtained by lumbar puncture (LP). Table 603-1 provides an overview of the expected CSF abnormalities with various CNS disorders.

| Table 603-1 | Cerebrospinal Fluid Findings in Central Nervous System Disorders | | | | |

CONDITION	PRESSURE (mm H$_2$O)	LEUKOCYTES (mm^3)	PROTEIN (mg/dL)	GLUCOSE (mg/dL)	COMMENTS
Normal	50-80	<5, ≥75% Lymphocytes	20-45	>50 (or 75% serum glucose)	
COMMON FORMS OF MENINGITIS					
Acute bacterial meningitis	Usually elevated (100-300)	100-10,000 or more; usually 300-2,000; PMNs predominate	Usually 100-500	Decreased, usually <40 (or <50% serum glucose)	Organisms usually seen on Gram stain and recovered by culture
Partially treated bacterial meningitis	Normal or elevated	5-10,000; PMNs usual but mononuclear cells may predominate if pretreated for extended period of time	Usually 100-500	Normal or decreased	Organisms may be seen on Gram stain. Pretreatment may render CSF sterile. Antigen may be detected by agglutination test
Viral meningitis or meningoencephalitis	Normal or slightly elevated (80-150)	Rarely >1,000 cells. Eastern equine encephalitis and lymphocytic choriomeningitis may have cell counts of several thousand. PMNs early but mononuclear cells predominate through most of the course	Usually 50-200	Generally normal; may be decreased to <40 in some viral diseases, particularly mumps (15-20% of cases)	HSV encephalitis is suggested by focal seizures or by focal findings on CT or MRI scans or EEG. Enteroviruses and HSV infrequently recovered from CSF. HSV and enteroviruses may be detected by PCR of CSF
UNCOMMON FORMS OF MENINGITIS					
Tuberculous meningitis	Usually elevated	10-500; PMNs early, but lymphocytes predominate through most of the course	100-3,000; may be higher in presence of block	<50 in most cases; decreases with time if treatment is not provided	Acid-fast organisms almost never seen on smear. Organisms may be recovered in culture of large volumes of CSF. *Mycobacterium tuberculosis* may be detected by PCR of CSF
Fungal meningitis	Usually elevated	5-500; PMNs early but mononuclear cells predominate through most of the course. Cryptococcal meningitis may have no cellular inflammatory response	25-500	<50; decreases with time if treatment is not provided	Budding yeast may be seen. Organisms may be recovered in culture. Cryptococcal antigen (CSF and serum) may be positive in cryptococcal infection
Syphilis (acute) and leptospirosis	Usually elevated	50-500; lymphocytes predominate	50-200	Usually normal	Positive CSF serology. Spirochetes not demonstrable by usual techniques of smear or culture; dark-field examination may be positive
Amebic (*Naegleria*) meningoencephalitis	Elevated	1,000-10,000 or more; PMNs predominate	50-500	Normal or slightly decreased	Mobile amebas may be seen by hanging-drop examination of CSF at room temperature
BRAIN ABSCESSES AND PARAMENINGEAL FOCUS					
Brain abscess	Usually elevated (100-300)	5-200; CSF rarely acellular; lymphocytes predominate; if abscess ruptures into ventricle, PMNs predominate and cell count may reach >100,000	75-500	Normal unless abscess ruptures into ventricular system	No organisms on smear or culture unless abscess ruptures into ventricular system
Subdural empyema	Usually elevated (100-300)	100-5,000; PMNs predominate	100-500	Normal	No organisms on smear or culture of CSF unless meningitis also present; organisms found on tap of subdural fluid
Cerebral epidural abscess	Normal to slightly elevated	10-500; lymphocytes predominate	50-200	Normal	No organisms on smear or culture of CSF
Spinal epidural abscess	Usually low, with spinal block	10-100; lymphocytes predominate	50-400	Normal	No organisms on smear or culture of CSF
Chemical (drugs, dermoid cysts, myelography dye)	Usually elevated	100-1,000 or more; PMNs predominate	50-100	Normal or slightly decreased	Epithelial cells may be seen within CSF by use of polarized light in some children with dermoids

Continued

Table 603-1	Cerebrospinal Fluid Findings in Central Nervous System Disorders—cont'd				
CONDITION	PRESSURE (mm H$_2$O)	LEUKOCYTES (mm^3)	PROTEIN (mg/dL)	GLUCOSE (mg/dL)	COMMENTS
NONINFECTIOUS CAUSES					
Sarcoidosis	Normal or elevated slightly	0-100; mononuclear	40-100	Normal	No specific findings
Systemic lupus erythematosus with CNS involvement	Slightly elevated	0-500; PMNs usually predominate; lymphocytes may be present	100	Normal or slightly decreased	No organisms on smear or culture. Positive neuronal and ribosomal P protein antibodies in CSF
Tumor, leukemia	Slightly elevated to very high	0-100 or more; mononuclear or blast cells	50-1,000	Normal to decreased (20-40)	Cytology may be positive
Acute disseminated encephalomyelitis	Normal or elevated	~100 lymphocytes	Normal to elevated	Normal	MRI adds to diagnosis
Autoimmune encephalitis	Normal	~100 lymphocytes	Normal to elevated	Normal	Anti-NMDAR antibody–positive

CSF, cerebrospinal fluid; EEG, electroencephalogram; HSV, herpes simplex virus; NMDAR, N-methyl-D-aspartate receptor; PCR, polymerase chain reaction; PMN, polymorphonuclear neutrophils.

603.1 Acute Bacterial Meningitis Beyond the Neonatal Period

Charles G. Prober and Roshni Mathew

Bacterial meningitis is one of the most potentially serious infections occurring in infants and older children. This infection is associated with a high rate of acute complications and risk of long-term morbidity. The incidence of bacterial meningitis is sufficiently high in febrile infants that it should be included in the differential diagnosis of those with altered mental status and other evidence of neurologic dysfunction.

ETIOLOGY

The most common causes of bacterial meningitis in children older than 1 mo of age in the United States are *Streptococcus pneumoniae and Neisseria meningitidis*. Bacterial meningitis caused by *S. pneumoniae* and *Haemophilus influenzae* type b has become much less common in developed countries since the introduction of universal immunization against these pathogens beginning at 2 mo of age. Demonstrating the importance of vaccination, invasive *H. influenzae* disease was reported in Minnesota in 2008 in 5 children with no relationship to one another and who were partially or not immunized. It is the largest number of children with invasive *H. influenzae* in Minnesota since 1992. Infection caused by *S. pneumoniae* or *H. influenzae* type b must be considered in incompletely vaccinated individuals or those in developing countries. Those with certain underlying immunologic (HIV infection, immunoglobulin [Ig] G subclass deficiency) or anatomic (splenic dysfunction, cochlear defects or implants) disorders also may be at increased risk of infection caused by these bacteria.

Alterations of host defense resulting from anatomic defects or immune deficits also increase the risk of meningitis from less-common pathogens such as *Pseudomonas aeruginosa, Staphylococcus aureus*, coagulase-negative staphylococci, *Salmonella* spp., anaerobes, and *Listeria monocytogenes*.

EPIDEMIOLOGY

A major risk factor for meningitis is the lack of immunity to specific pathogens associated with young age. Additional risks include recent colonization with pathogenic bacteria, close contact (household, daycare centers, college dormitories, military barracks) with individuals having invasive disease caused by *N. meningitidis* or *H. influenzae* type b, crowding, poverty, black or Native American race, and male gender. The mode of transmission is probably person-to-person contact through respiratory tract secretions or droplets. The risk of meningitis is increased among infants and young children with occult

bacteremia; the odds ratio is greater for meningococcus (85 times) and *H. influenzae* type b (12 times) relative to that for pneumococcus.

Specific host defense defects as a result of altered immunoglobulin production in response to encapsulated pathogens may be responsible for the increased risk of bacterial meningitis in Native Americans and Eskimos. Defects of the complement system (C5-C8) are associated with recurrent meningococcal infection, and defects of the properdin system are associated with a significant risk of lethal meningococcal disease. Splenic dysfunction (sickle cell anemia) or asplenia (caused by trauma or congenital defect) is associated with an increased risk of pneumococcal, *H. influenzae* type b (to some extent), and, rarely, meningococcal sepsis and meningitis. T-lymphocyte defects (congenital or acquired by chemotherapy, AIDS, or malignancy) are associated with an increased risk of *L. monocytogenes* infections of the CNS.

A congenital or acquired CSF leak across a mucocutaneous barrier, such as a lumbar dural sinus, cranial or midline facial defects (cribriform plate), and middle ear (stapedial foot plate) or inner ear fistulas (oval window, internal auditory canal, cochlear aqueduct), or CSF leakage through a rupture of the meninges as a result of a basal skull fracture into the cribriform plate or paranasal sinus, is associated with an increased risk of pneumococcal meningitis. The risk of bacterial meningitis, caused by *S. pneumoniae*, in children with cochlear implants, used for the treatment of hearing loss, is more than 30 times the risk in the general U.S. population. Lumbosacral dermal sinus and meningomyelocele are associated with staphylococcal, anaerobic, and Gram-negative enteric bacterial meningitis. CSF shunt infections increase the risk of meningitis caused by staphylococci (especially coagulase-negative species) and other low-virulence bacteria that typically colonize the skin.

Streptococcus pneumoniae
See Chapter 182.

The 7-valent pneumococcal protein polysaccharide conjugate vaccine (PCV7) was introduced into the routine vaccination schedule in 2000 and contained the serotypes 4, 6B, 9V, 14, 18C, 19F, and 23F. These serotypes caused most of the invasive pneumococcal infections in the United States at that time. The vaccine led to a dramatic decrease in rates of invasive pneumococcal disease. However, an increase in invasive disease caused by serotypes not contained in the original vaccine, such as serotype 19A, was observed. As a result, a 13-valent pneumococcal polysaccharide-protein conjugate vaccine (PCV13) was licensed in the United States in February 2010. PCV13 contains the serotypes in PCV7 plus serotypes 1, 3, 5, 6A, 7F, and 19A. This vaccine is recommended for routine administration to all children 2-59 mo of age. The PCV13 vaccine is given as a 4-dose series at 2, 4, 6, and 12-15 mo of age. The incidence of invasive pneumococcal infections peaks in the 1st 2 yr of life, reaching rates of 228 per 100,000 in children 6-12 mo of age. Children with anatomic or functional asplenia secondary to sickle cell disease and those infected with HIV have infection rates that are 20-100–fold higher than in those of healthy children in the 1st 5 yr of life. Additional risk factors for contracting pneumococcal meningitis include otitis media, sinusitis, pneumonia, CSF otorrhea or rhinorrhea, the presence of a cochlear implant, and chronic graft-versus-host disease following bone marrow transplantation.

Neisseria meningitidis
See Chapter 191.

Five serogroups of meningococcus—A, B, C, Y, and W-135—are responsible for disease. Meningococcal meningitis may be sporadic or may occur in epidemics. In the United States, serogroups B, C, and Y each account for approximately 30% of cases, although serogroup distribution varies by location and time. Epidemic disease, especially in developing countries, is usually caused by serogroup A. Cases occur throughout the year but may be more common in the winter and spring and following influenza virus infections. Nasopharyngeal carriage of *N. meningitidis* occurs in 1-15% of adults. Colonization may last weeks to months; recent colonization places nonimmune younger children at greatest risk for meningitis. The incidence of disease occurring in association with an index case in the family is 1%, a rate that is 1,000-fold the risk in the general population. The risk of secondary cases occurring in contacts at daycare centers is approximately 1 in 1,000. Most infections of children are acquired from a contact in a daycare facility, a colonized adult family member, or an ill patient with meningococcal disease. Children younger than 5 yr have the highest rates of meningococcal infection. A second peak in incidence occurs in persons between 15 and 24 yr of age. College freshmen living in dormitories have an increased incidence of infection compared to non–college-attending, age-matched controls.

The Centers for Disease Control and Prevention (CDC) recommends vaccination against meningococcus (types A, C, W, and Y) with 1 dose of a quadrivalent conjugate meningococcal vaccine between the ages of 11 and 12 yr and for persons 2 mo to 18 yr who are at increased risk for meningococcal disease. The CDC also has specific recommendations for meningococcal vaccination of infants at high risk of meningococcal infection as a consequence of complement pathway deficiencies. College freshmen living in dormitories who have not been previously vaccinated should also be vaccinated.

Haemophilus influenzae Type B
See Chapter 194.

Before universal *H. influenzae* type b vaccination in the United States, approximately 70% of cases of bacterial meningitis occurring in the 1st 5 yr of life were caused by this pathogen. Invasive infections occurred primarily in infants 2 mo to 2 yr of age; peak incidence was at 6-9 mo of age, and 50% of cases occurred in the 1st yr of life. The risk to children was markedly increased among family or daycare center contacts of patients with *H. influenzae* type b disease. Incompletely vaccinated individuals, those in underdeveloped countries who are not vaccinated, and those with blunted immunologic responses to vaccine (such as children with HIV infection) remain at risk for *H. influenzae* type b meningitis.

PATHOLOGY AND PATHOPHYSIOLOGY

A meningeal purulent exudate of varying thickness may be distributed around the cerebral veins, venous sinuses, convexity of the brain, and cerebellum, and in the sulci, sylvian fissures, basal cisterns, and spinal cord. Ventriculitis with bacteria and inflammatory cells in ventricular fluid may be present (more often in neonates), as may subdural effusions and, rarely, empyema. Perivascular inflammatory infiltrates also may be present, and the ependymal membrane may be disrupted. Vascular and parenchymal cerebral changes characterized by polymorphonuclear infiltrates extending to the subintimal region of the small arteries and veins, vasculitis, thrombosis of small cortical veins, occlusion of major venous sinuses, necrotizing arteritis producing subarachnoid hemorrhage, and, rarely, cerebral cortical necrosis in the absence

of identifiable thrombosis have been described at autopsy. **Cerebral infarction,** resulting from vascular occlusion because of inflammation, vasospasm, and thrombosis, is a frequent sequela. Infarct size ranges from microscopic to involvement of an entire hemisphere.

Inflammation of spinal nerves and roots produces meningeal signs, and inflammation of the cranial nerves produces cranial neuropathies of optic, oculomotor, facial, and auditory nerves. Increased intracranial pressure (ICP) also produces oculomotor nerve palsy because of the presence of temporal lobe compression of the nerve during tentorial herniation. Abducens nerve palsy may be a nonlocalizing sign of elevated ICP.

Increased ICP is a result of cell death (cytotoxic cerebral edema), cytokine-induced increased capillary vascular permeability (vasogenic cerebral edema), and, possibly, increased hydrostatic pressure (interstitial cerebral edema) after obstructed reabsorption of CSF in the arachnoid villus or obstruction of the flow of fluid from the ventricles. ICP may exceed 300 mm H_2O; cerebral perfusion may be further compromised if the cerebral perfusion pressure (mean arterial pressure minus ICP) is <50 cm H_2O as a result of systemic hypotension with reduced cerebral blood flow. The syndrome of inappropriate antidiuretic hormone secretion (SIADH) may produce excessive water retention and potentially increase the risk of elevated ICP (see Chapter 559). Hypotonicity of brain extracellular spaces may cause cytotoxic edema after cell swelling and lysis. Tentorial, falx, or cerebellar herniation does not usually occur because the increased ICP is transmitted to the entire subarachnoid space and there is little structural displacement. Furthermore, if the fontanels are still patent, increased ICP is not always dissipated.

Hydrocephalus can occur as an acute complication of bacterial meningitis. It most often takes the form of a communicating hydrocephalus caused by adhesive thickening of the arachnoid villi around the cisterns at the base of the brain. Thus, there is interference with the normal resorption of CSF. Less often, obstructive hydrocephalus develops after fibrosis and gliosis of the aqueduct of Sylvius or the foramina of Magendie and Luschka.

Raised CSF protein levels are partly a result of increased vascular permeability of the blood–brain barrier and the loss of albumin-rich fluid from the capillaries and veins traversing the subdural space. Continued transudation may result in subdural effusions, usually found in the later phase of acute bacterial meningitis. **Hypoglycorrhachia** (reduced CSF glucose levels) is attributable to decreased glucose transport by the cerebral tissue.

Damage to the cerebral cortex may be a result of the focal or diffuse effects of vascular occlusion (infarction, necrosis, lactic acidosis), hypoxia, bacterial invasion (cerebritis), toxic encephalopathy (bacterial toxins), elevated ICP, ventriculitis, and transudation (subdural effusions). These pathologic factors result in the clinical manifestations of impaired consciousness, seizures, cranial nerve deficits, motor and sensory deficits, and later psychomotor retardation.

PATHOGENESIS
Bacterial meningitis most commonly results from hematogenous dissemination of microorganisms from a distant site of infection; **bacteremia** usually precedes meningitis or occurs concomitantly. Bacterial colonization of the nasopharynx with a potentially pathogenic microorganism is the usual source of the bacteremia. There may be prolonged carriage of the colonizing organisms without disease or, more likely, rapid invasion after recent colonization. Prior or concurrent viral upper respiratory tract infection may enhance the pathogenicity of bacteria producing meningitis.

N. meningitidis and *H. influenzae* type b attach to mucosal epithelial cell receptors by pili. After attachment to epithelial cells, bacteria breach the mucosa and enter the circulation. *N. meningitidis* may be transported across the mucosal surface within a phagocytic vacuole after ingestion by the epithelial cell. Bacterial survival in the bloodstream is enhanced by large bacterial capsules that interfere with opsonic phagocytosis and are associated with increased virulence. Host-related developmental defects in bacterial opsonic phagocytosis also contribute to the bacteremia. In young, nonimmune hosts, the defect may be from an absence of preformed IgM or IgG anticapsular antibodies, whereas in immunodeficient patients, various deficiencies of components of the complement or properdin system may interfere with effective opsonic phagocytosis. Splenic dysfunction may also reduce opsonic phagocytosis by the reticuloendothelial system.

Bacteria gain entry to the CSF through the choroid plexus of the lateral ventricles and the meninges and then circulate to the extracerebral CSF and subarachnoid space. Bacteria rapidly multiply because the CSF concentrations of complement and antibody are inadequate to contain bacterial proliferation. Chemotactic factors then incite a local inflammatory response characterized by polymorphonuclear cell infiltration. The presence of bacterial cell wall lipopolysaccharide (endotoxin) of Gram-negative bacteria (*H. influenzae* type b, *N. meningitidis*) and of pneumococcal cell wall components (teichoic acid, peptidoglycan) stimulates a marked inflammatory response, with local production of tumor necrosis factor, interleukin 1, prostaglandin E, and other inflammatory mediators. The subsequent inflammatory response is characterized by neutrophilic infiltration, increased vascular permeability, alterations of the blood–brain barrier, and vascular thrombosis. Meningitis-associated brain injury is not simply caused by viable bacteria but occurs as a consequence of the host reaction to the inflammatory cascade initiated by bacterial components.

Rarely, meningitis may follow bacterial invasion from a contiguous focus of infection such as paranasal sinusitis, otitis media, mastoiditis, orbital cellulitis, or cranial or vertebral osteomyelitis or may occur after introduction of bacteria via penetrating cranial trauma, dermal sinus tracts, or meningomyeloceles.

CLINICAL MANIFESTATIONS

The onset of acute meningitis has 2 predominant patterns. The more dramatic and, fortunately, less common presentation is sudden onset with rapidly progressive manifestations of shock, purpura, disseminated intravascular coagulation, and reduced levels of consciousness often resulting in progression to coma or death within 24 hr. More often, meningitis is preceded by several days of fever accompanied by upper respiratory tract or gastrointestinal symptoms, followed by nonspecific signs of CNS infection, such as increasing lethargy and irritability.

The signs and symptoms of meningitis are related to the nonspecific findings associated with a systemic infection and to manifestations of meningeal irritation. Nonspecific findings include fever, anorexia and poor feeding, headache, symptoms of upper respiratory tract infection, myalgias, arthralgias, tachycardia, hypotension, and various cutaneous signs, such as petechiae, purpura, or an erythematous macular rash. Meningeal irritation is manifested as nuchal rigidity, back pain, **Kernig sign** (flexion of the hip 90 degrees with subsequent pain with extension of the leg), and **Brudzinski sign** (involuntary flexion of the knees and hips after passive flexion of the neck while supine). In children, particularly in those younger than 12-18 mo, Kernig and Brudzinski signs are not consistently present. Indeed fever, headache, and nuchal rigidity are present in only 40% of adults with bacterial meningitis. Increased ICP is suggested by headache, emesis, bulging fontanel or diastasis (widening) of the sutures, oculomotor (anisocoria, ptosis) or abducens nerve paralysis, hypertension with bradycardia, apnea or hyperventilation, decorticate or decerebrate posturing, stupor, coma, or signs of herniation. Papilledema is uncommon in uncomplicated meningitis and should suggest a more chronic process, such as the presence of an intracranial abscess, subdural empyema, or occlusion of a dural venous sinus. Focal neurologic signs usually are a result of vascular occlusion. Cranial neuropathies of the ocular, oculomotor, abducens, facial, and auditory nerves may also be the result of focal inflammation. Overall, approximately 10-20% of children with bacterial meningitis have focal neurologic signs.

Seizures (focal or generalized) caused by cerebritis, infarction, or electrolyte disturbances occur in 20-30% of patients with meningitis. Seizures that occur on presentation or within the 1st 4 days of onset are usually of no prognostic significance. Seizures that persist after the 4th day of illness and those that are difficult to treat may be associated with a poor prognosis.

Alterations of mental status are common among patients with meningitis and may be the consequence of increased ICP, cerebritis, or hypotension; manifestations include irritability, lethargy, stupor, obtundation, and coma. Comatose patients have a poor prognosis. Additional manifestations of meningitis include photophobia and tache cérébrale, which is elicited by stroking the skin with a blunt object and observing a raised red streak within 30-60 sec.

DIAGNOSIS

The diagnosis of acute pyogenic meningitis is confirmed by analysis of the CSF, which typically reveals microorganisms on Gram stain and culture, a neutrophilic pleocytosis, elevated protein, and reduced glucose concentrations (see Table 603-1). LP should be performed when bacterial meningitis is suspected. **Contraindications** for an immediate LP include (1) evidence of increased ICP (other than a bulging fontanel), such as 3rd or 6th cranial nerve palsy with a depressed level of consciousness, or hypertension and bradycardia with respiratory abnormalities (see Chapter 590); (2) severe cardiopulmonary compromise requiring prompt resuscitative measures for shock or in patients in whom positioning for the LP would further compromise cardiopulmonary function; and (3) infection of the skin overlying the site of the LP. Thrombocytopenia is a relative contraindication for LP. If an LP is delayed, empirical antibiotic therapy should be initiated. CT scanning for evidence of a brain abscess or increased ICP should not delay therapy. LP may be performed after increased ICP has been treated or a brain abscess has been excluded.

Blood cultures should be performed in all patients with suspected meningitis. Blood cultures reveal the responsible bacteria in up to 80-90% of cases of meningitis. Elevations of the C-reactive protein, erythrocyte sedimentation rate, and procalcitonin have been used to differentiate bacterial (usually elevated) from viral causes of meningitis.

Lumbar Puncture
See Chapter 590.

The CSF leukocyte count in bacterial meningitis usually is elevated to >1,000/mm³ and, typically, there is a neutrophilic predominance (75-95%). Turbid CSF is present when the CSF leukocyte count exceeds 200-400/mm³. Normal healthy neonates may have as many as 30 leukocytes/mm³ (usually <10), but older children without viral or bacterial meningitis have <5 leukocytes/mm³ in the CSF; in both age groups there is a predominance of lymphocytes or monocytes.

A CSF leukocyte count <250/mm³ may be present in as many as 20% of patients with acute bacterial meningitis; pleocytosis may be absent in patients with severe overwhelming sepsis and meningitis and is a poor prognostic sign. Pleocytosis with a lymphocyte predominance may be present during the early stage of acute bacterial meningitis; conversely, neutrophilic pleocytosis may be present in patients in the early stages of acute viral meningitis. The shift to lymphocytic-monocytic predominance in viral meningitis invariably occurs within 8-24 hr of the initial LP. The Gram stain is positive in 70-90% of patients with untreated bacterial meningitis.

A diagnostic conundrum in the evaluation of children with suspected bacterial meningitis is the analysis of CSF obtained from children already receiving antibiotic (usually oral) therapy. This is an important issue, because 25-50% of children being evaluated for bacterial meningitis are receiving oral antibiotics when their CSF is obtained. CSF obtained from children with bacterial meningitis, after the initiation of antibiotics, may be negative on Gram stain and culture. Pleocytosis with a predominance of neutrophils, elevated protein level, and a reduced concentration of CSF glucose usually persist for several days after the administration of appropriate intravenous antibiotics. Therefore, despite negative cultures, the presumptive diagnosis of bacterial meningitis can be made. Some clinicians test CSF for the presence of bacterial antigens if the child has been pretreated with antibiotics and the diagnosis of bacterial meningitis is in doubt. These tests have technical limitations. Polymerase chain reactions using broad-based bacterial 16S ribosomal RNA gene patterns may be useful in diagnosing the cause of culture-negative meningitis because of prior antibiotic therapy or the presence of a nonculturable fastidious pathogen.

A traumatic LP may complicate the diagnosis of meningitis. Repeat LP at a higher interspace may produce less hemorrhagic fluid, but this fluid usually also contains red blood cells. Interpretation of CSF leukocytes and protein concentration are affected by LPs that are traumatic, although the Gram stain, culture, and glucose level may not be influenced. Although methods for correcting for the presence of red blood cells have been proposed, it is prudent to rely on the bacteriologic results rather than attempt to interpret the CSF leukocyte and protein results of a traumatic LP. Children with seizure, particularly those with fever associated status epilepticus *do not* have a CSF pleocytosis in the absence of CNS infection or inflammatory disease.

Differential Diagnosis

In addition to *S. pneumoniae*, *N. meningitidis*, and *H. influenzae* type b, many other microorganisms can cause generalized infection of the CNS with similar clinical manifestations. These organisms include less-typical bacteria, such as *Mycobacterium tuberculosis*, *Nocardia* spp., *Treponema pallidum* (syphilis), and *Borrelia burgdorferi* (Lyme disease); fungi, such as those endemic to specific geographic areas (*Coccidioides*, *Histoplasma*, and *Blastomyces*) and those responsible for infections in compromised hosts (*Candida*, *Cryptococcus*, and *Aspergillus*); parasites, such as *Toxoplasma gondii* and those that cause cysticercosis and, most frequently, viruses (see Chapter 603.2; Table 603-2). Focal infections of the CNS including brain abscess and parameningeal abscess (subdural empyema, cranial and spinal epidural abscess) may also be confused with meningitis. In addition, noninfectious illnesses can cause generalized inflammation of the CNS. Relative to infections, these disorders are uncommon and include malignancy, collagen vascular syndromes, and exposure to toxins (Table 603-2).

Determining the specific cause of CNS infection is facilitated by careful examination of the CSF with specific stains (Kinyoun carbol fuchsin for mycobacteria, India ink for fungi), cytology, antigen detection *(Cryptococcus),* serology (syphilis, West Nile virus, arboviruses), viral culture (enterovirus), and polymerase chain reaction (herpes simplex, enterovirus, and others). Other potentially valuable diagnostic tests include blood cultures, CT or MRI of the brain, serologic tests, and, rarely, meningeal or brain biopsy. A unique MRI finding in patients suspected of CNS infection is pachymeningitis (Fig. 603-1). In addition to bacterial, tuberculous, or fungal infection (Fig. 603-1), the differential diagnosis also includes immune or inflammatory diseases such as Sweet syndrome, CNS vasculitis, sarcoidosis, lymphoma, and neonatal-onset multisystem inflammatory disease.

Acute viral meningoencephalitis is the most likely infection to be confused with bacterial meningitis (see Tables 603-2 and 603-3). Although, in general, children with viral meningoencephalitis appear less ill than those with bacterial meningitis, both types of infection have a spectrum of severity. Some children with bacterial meningitis may have relatively mild signs and symptoms, whereas some with viral meningoencephalitis may be critically ill. Although classic CSF profiles associated with bacterial vs viral infection tend to be distinct (see Table 603-1), specific test results may have considerable overlap.

TREATMENT

The therapeutic approach to patients with presumed bacterial meningitis depends on the nature of the initial manifestations of the illness. A child with rapidly progressing disease of less than 24 hr duration, in the absence of increased ICP, should receive antibiotics as soon as possible after an LP is performed. If there are signs of increased ICP or focal neurologic findings, antibiotics should be given without performing an LP and before obtaining a CT scan. Increased ICP should be treated simultaneously (see Chapter 68). Immediate treatment of associated multiple organ system failure, shock (see Chapter 70), and acute respiratory distress syndrome (see Chapter 71) is also indicated.

Patients who have a more protracted subacute course and become ill over a 4-7 day period should also be evaluated for signs of increased ICP and focal neurologic deficits. Unilateral headache, papilledema, and other signs of increased ICP suggest a focal lesion, such as a brain or epidural abscess, or subdural empyema. Under these circumstances, antibiotic therapy should be initiated before LP and CT scanning. If signs of increased ICP and/or focal neurologic signs are present, CT scanning should be performed first to determine the safety of performing an LP.

Initial Antibiotic Therapy

The initial (empirical) choice of therapy for meningitis in immunocompetent infants and children is primarily influenced by the antibiotic susceptibilities (Table 603-4) of *S. pneumoniae*. Selected antibiotics should achieve bactericidal levels in the CSF. Although there are substantial geographic differences in the frequency of resistance of *S. pneumoniae* to antibiotics, rates are increasing throughout the world. In the United States, 25-50% of strains of *S. pneumoniae* are currently resistant to penicillin; relative resistance (minimal inhibitory concentration = 0.1-1.0 μg/mL) is more common than high-level resistance (minimal inhibitory concentration = 2.0 μg/mL). Resistance to cefotaxime and ceftriaxone is also evident in up to 25% of isolates. In contrast, most strains of *N. meningitidis* are sensitive to penicillin and cephalosporins, although rare resistant isolates have been reported. Approximately 30-40% of isolates of *H. influenzae* type b produce β-lactamases and, therefore, are resistant to ampicillin. These β-lactamase–producing strains are sensitive to the extended-spectrum cephalosporins.

Based on the substantial rate of resistance of *S. pneumoniae* to β-lactam drugs, vancomycin (60 mg/kg/24 hr, given every 6 hr) is recommended as part of initial empirical therapy. Because of the efficacy of third-generation cephalosporins in the therapy of meningitis caused by sensitive *S. pneumoniae*, *N. meningitidis*, and *H. influenzae* type b, cefotaxime (300 mg/kg/24 hr, given every 6 hr) or ceftriaxone (100 mg/kg/24 hr administered once per day or 50 mg/kg/dose, given every 12 hr) should also be used in initial empirical therapy. Patients allergic to β-lactam antibiotics and >1 mo of age can be treated with chloramphenicol, 100 mg/kg/24 hr, given every 6 hr. Another option for patients with allergy to β-lactam antibiotics is a combination of vancomycin and rifampin. Alternatively, patients can be desensitized to the antibiotic (see Chapter 152).

If *L. monocytogenes* infection is suspected, as in young infants or those with a T-lymphocyte deficiency, ampicillin (200 mg/kg/24 hr, given every 6 hr) also should also be given because cephalosporins are inactive against *L. monocytogenes*. Intravenous trimethoprim-sulfamethoxazole is an alternative treatment for *L. monocytogenes*.

If a patient is immunocompromised and Gram-negative bacterial meningitis is suspected, initial therapy might include ceftazidime and an aminoglycoside or meropenem.

DURATION OF ANTIBIOTIC THERAPY

Therapy for uncomplicated penicillin-sensitive *S. pneumoniae* meningitis should be for 10-14 days with a third-generation cephalosporin or intravenous penicillin (400,000 units/kg/24 hr, given every 4-6 hr). If the isolate is resistant to penicillin and the third-generation cephalosporin, therapy should be completed with vancomycin. Intravenous penicillin (300,000 units/kg/24 hr) for 5-7 days is the treatment of choice for uncomplicated *N. meningitidis* meningitis. Uncomplicated *H. influenzae* type b meningitis should be treated for 7-10 days. Patients who receive intravenous or oral antibiotics before LP and who do not have an identifiable pathogen, but do have evidence of an acute bacterial infection on the basis of their CSF profile, should continue to receive therapy with ceftriaxone or cefotaxime for 7-10 days. If focal signs are present or the child does not respond to treatment, a parameningeal focus may be present and a CT or MRI scan should be performed.

A routine repeat LP is not indicated in all patients with uncomplicated meningitis caused by antibiotic-sensitive *S. pneumoniae*, *N. meningitidis*, or *H. influenzae* type b. Repeat examination of CSF is indicated in some neonates, in all patients with Gram-negative bacillary meningitis, or in infection caused by a β-lactam–resistant *S. pneumoniae*. The CSF should be sterile within 24-48 hr of initiation of appropriate antibiotic therapy.

Table 603-2 | Clinical Conditions and Infectious Agents Associated with Aseptic Meningitis

VIRUSES
Enteroviruses (coxsackievirus, echovirus, poliovirus, enterovirus)
Arboviruses: Eastern equine, Western equine, Venezuelan equine,
  St. Louis encephalitis, Powassan and California encephalitis, West
  Nile virus, Colorado tick fever
Parechovirus
Herpes simplex (types 1, 2)
Human herpesvirus type 6
Varicella-zoster virus
Epstein-Barr virus
Parvovirus B19
Cytomegalovirus
Adenovirus
Variola (smallpox)
Measles
Mumps
Rubella
Influenza A and B
Parainfluenza
Rhinovirus
Rabies
Lymphocytic choriomeningitis
Rotaviruses
Coronaviruses
Human immunodeficiency virus type 1

BACTERIA
Mycobacterium tuberculosis (early and late)
Leptospira species (leptospirosis)
Treponema pallidum (syphilis)
Borrelia species (relapsing fever)
Borrelia burgdorferi (Lyme disease)
Nocardia species (nocardiosis)
Brucella species
Bartonella species (cat-scratch disease)
Rickettsia rickettsii (Rocky Mountain spotted fever)
Rickettsia prowazekii (typhus)
Ehrlichia canis
Coxiella burnetii
Mycoplasma pneumoniae
Mycoplasma hominis
Chlamydia trachomatis
Chlamydia psittaci
Chlamydia pneumoniae
Partially treated bacterial meningitis

BACTERIAL PARAMENINGEAL FOCUS
Sinusitis
Mastoiditis
Brain abscess
Subdural-epidural empyema
Cranial osteomyelitis

FUNGI
Coccidioides immitis (coccidioidomycosis)
Blastomyces dermatitidis (blastomycosis)
Cryptococcus neoformans (cryptococcosis)
Histoplasma capsulatum (histoplasmosis)
Candida species
Other fungi (*Alternaria, Aspergillus, Cephalosporium, Cladosporium,
  Drechslera hawaiiensis, Paracoccidioides brasiliensis, Petriellidium
  boydii, Sporotrichum schenckii, Ustilago* spp., *Zygomycetes*)

PARASITES (EOSINOPHILIC)
Angiostrongylus cantonensis
Gnathostoma spinigerum
Baylisascaris procyonis
Strongyloides stercoralis
Trichinella spiralis
Toxocara canis
Taenia solium (cysticercosis)
Paragonimus westermani
Schistosoma spp.
Fasciola spp.

PARASITES (NONEOSINOPHILIC)
Toxoplasma gondii (toxoplasmosis)
Acanthamoeba spp.
Naegleria fowleri
Malaria

POSTINFECTIOUS
Vaccines: rabies, influenza, measles, poliovirus
Demyelinating or allergic encephalitis

SYSTEMIC OR IMMUNOLOGICALLY MEDIATED
Acute Disseminated Encephalomyelitis (ADEM)
Autoimmune Encephalitis
Bacterial endocarditis
Kawasaki disease
Systemic lupus erythematosus
Vasculitis, including polyarteritis nodosa
Sjögren syndrome
Mixed connective tissue disease
Rheumatoid arthritis
Behçet syndrome
Wegener granulomatosis
Lymphomatoid granulomatosis
Granulomatous arteritis
Sarcoidosis
Familial Mediterranean fever
Vogt-Koyanagi-Harada syndrome

MALIGNANCY
Leukemia
Lymphoma
Metastatic carcinoma
Central nervous system tumor (e.g., craniopharyngioma, glioma,
  ependymoma, astrocytoma, medulloblastoma, teratoma)

DRUGS
Intrathecal infections (contrast media, serum, antibiotics,
  antineoplastic agents)
Nonsteroidal antiinflammatory agents
OKT3 monoclonal antibodies
Carbamazepine
Azathioprine
Intravenous immune globulins
Antibiotics (trimethoprim-sulfamethoxazole, sulfasalazine,
  ciprofloxacin, isoniazid)

MISCELLANEOUS
Heavy metal poisoning (lead, arsenic)
Foreign bodies (shunt, reservoir)
Subarachnoid hemorrhage
Postictal state
Postmigraine state
Mollaret syndrome (recurrent)
Intraventricular hemorrhage (neonate)
Familial hemophagocytic syndrome
Postneurosurgery
Dermoid–epidermoid cyst
Headache, neurologic deficits
CSF lymphocytosis (syndrome of transient headache and neurologic
  deficits with cerebrospinal fluid lymphocytosis [HaNDL])

Compiled from Cherry JD: Aseptic meningitis and viral meningitis. In Feigin RD, Cherry JD, editors: *Textbook of pediatric infectious diseases*, ed 4, Philadelphia,
1998, WB Saunders, p. 450; Davis LE: Aseptic and viral meningitis. In Long SS, Pickering LK, Prober CG, editors: *Principles and practice of pediatric infectious disease*,
New York, 1997, Churchill Livingstone, p. 329; and Kliegman RM, Greenbaum LA, Lye PS: *Practical strategies in pediatric diagnosis therapy*, ed 2, Philadelphia, 2004,
Elsevier, p. 961.

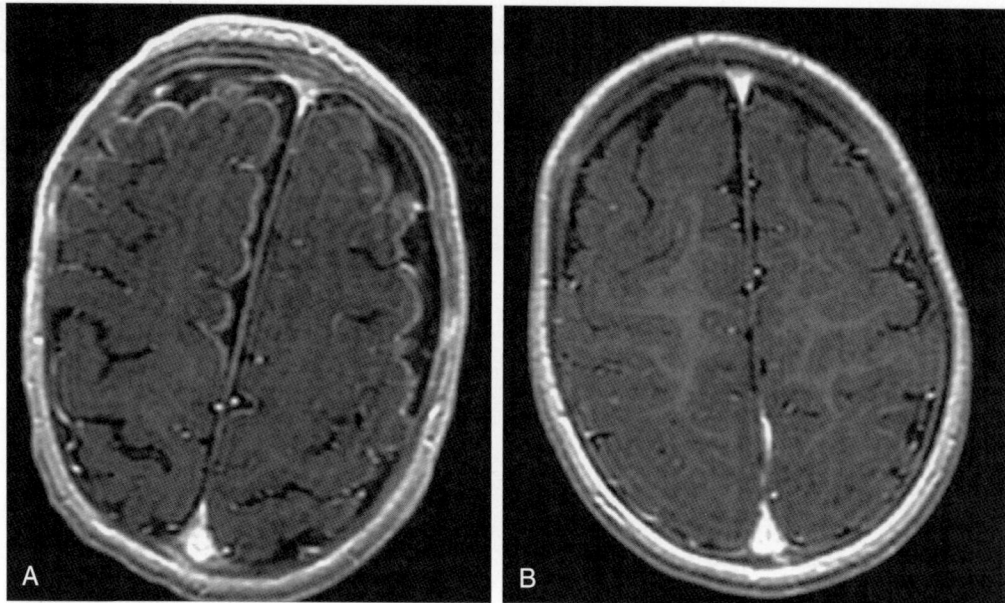

Figure 603-1 Cerebral MRI. Three-dimensional T1 sequence with fast-spoiled gradient-echo gadolinium injection. **A,** Day 11 following meningococcal infection. **B,** Day 9 following meningococcal infection. *(From Toubiana J, Heilbronner C, Gitiaux C, et al: Pachymeningitis after meningococcal infection. Lancet 381:1596–1597, 2013.)*

Meningitis caused by *Escherichia coli* or *P. aeruginosa* requires therapy with a third-generation cephalosporin active against the isolate in vitro. Most isolates of *E. coli* are sensitive to cefotaxime or ceftriaxone, and most isolates of *P. aeruginosa* are sensitive to ceftazidime. Gram-negative bacillary meningitis should be treated for 3 wk or for at least 2 wk after CSF sterilization, which may occur after 2-10 days of treatment.

Side effects of antibiotic therapy of meningitis include phlebitis, drug fever, rash, emesis, oral candidiasis, and diarrhea. Ceftriaxone may cause reversible gallbladder pseudolithiasis, detectable by abdominal ultrasonography. This is usually asymptomatic but may be associated with emesis and upper right quadrant pain.

Corticosteroids

Rapid killing of bacteria in the CSF effectively sterilizes the meningeal infection but releases toxic cell products after cell lysis (cell wall endotoxin) that precipitate the cytokine-mediated inflammatory cascade. The resultant edema formation and neutrophilic infiltration may produce additional neurologic injury with worsening of CNS signs and symptoms. Therefore, agents that limit production of inflammatory mediators may be of benefit to patients with bacterial meningitis.

Data support the use of intravenous dexamethasone, 0.15 mg/kg/dose given every 6 hr for 2 days, in the treatment of children older than 6 wk with acute bacterial meningitis caused by *H. influenzae* type b. Among children with meningitis caused by *H. influenzae* type b, corticosteroid recipients have a shorter duration of fever, lower CSF protein and lactate levels, and a reduction in sensorineural hearing loss. Data in children regarding benefits, if any, of corticosteroids in the treatment of meningitis caused by other bacteria are inconclusive. Early steroid treatment of adults with bacterial meningitis, especially those with pneumococcal meningitis, results in improved outcome.

Corticosteroids appear to have maximum benefit if given 1-2 hr before antibiotics are initiated. They also may be effective if given concurrently with or soon after the first dose of antibiotics. Complications of corticosteroids include gastrointestinal bleeding, hypertension, hyperglycemia, leukocytosis, and rebound fever after the last dose.

Supportive Care

Repeated medical and neurologic assessments of patients with bacterial meningitis are essential to identify early signs of cardiovascular, CNS, and metabolic complications. Pulse rate, blood pressure, and respiratory rate should be monitored frequently. Neurologic assessment, including pupillary reflexes, level of consciousness, motor strength, cranial nerve signs, and evaluation for seizures, should be made frequently in the 1st 72 hr, when the risk of neurologic complications is greatest. Important laboratory studies include an assessment of blood urea nitrogen; serum sodium, chloride, potassium, and bicarbonate levels; urine output and specific gravity; complete blood and platelet counts; and, in the presence of petechiae, purpura, or abnormal bleeding, measures of coagulation function (fibrinogen, prothrombin, and partial thromboplastin times).

Patients should initially receive nothing by mouth. If a patient is judged to be normovolemic, with normal blood pressure, intravenous fluid administration should be restricted to one-half to two-thirds of maintenance, or 800-1,000 mL/m²/24 hr, until it can be established that increased ICP or SIADH is not present. Fluid administration may be returned to normal (1,500-1,700 mL/m²/24 hr) when serum sodium levels are normal. Fluid restriction is not appropriate in the presence of systemic hypotension because reduced blood pressure may result in reduced cerebral perfusion pressure and CNS ischemia. Therefore, shock must be treated aggressively to prevent brain and other organ dysfunction (acute tubular necrosis, acute respiratory distress syndrome). Patients with shock, a markedly elevated ICP, coma, and refractory seizures require intensive monitoring with central arterial and venous access and frequent vital signs, necessitating admission to a pediatric intensive care unit. Patients with septic shock may require fluid resuscitation and therapy with vasoactive agents such as dopamine and epinephrine. The goal of such therapy in patients with meningitis is to avoid excessive increases in ICP without compromising blood flow and oxygen delivery to vital organs.

Neurologic complications include increased ICP with subsequent herniation, seizures, and an enlarging head circumference because of a subdural effusion or hydrocephalus. Signs of increased ICP should be treated emergently with endotracheal intubation and hyperventilation (to maintain the pCO₂ at approximately 25 mm Hg). In addition, intravenous furosemide (Lasix, 1 mg/kg) and mannitol (0.5-1.0 g/kg) osmotherapy may reduce ICP (see Chapter 68). Furosemide reduces brain swelling by venodilation and diuresis without increasing intracranial blood volume, whereas mannitol produces an osmolar gradient between the brain and plasma, thus shifting fluid from the CNS to the plasma, with subsequent excretion during an osmotic diuresis. Another approach to treating reductions of cerebral perfusion pressure caused by elevations of intracranial pressure is to increase systemic blood

Table 603-3	Classification of Encephalitis by Cause and Source

I. INFECTIONS: VIRAL
  A. Spread: person to person only
    1. Mumps: frequent in an unimmunized population; often mild
    2. Measles: may have serious sequelae
    3. Enteroviruses: frequent at all ages; more serious in newborns
    4. Parechovirus
    5. Rubella: uncommon; sequelae rare except in congenital rubella
    6. Herpesvirus group
      a. Herpes simplex (types 1 and 2, possibly 6): relatively common; sequelae frequent; devastating in newborns
      b. Varicella-zoster virus: uncommon; serious sequelae not rare
      c. Cytomegalovirus, congenital or acquired: may have delayed sequelae in congenital type
      d. Epstein-Barr virus (infectious mononucleosis): not common
    7. Pox group
      a. Vaccinia and variola: uncommon, but serious CNS damage occurs
    8. Parvovirus (erythema infectiosum): not common
    9. Influenzas A and B
    10. Adenovirus
    11. Other: reoviruses, respiratory syncytial, parainfluenza, hepatitis B
  B. Arthropod-borne agents
  C. Arboviruses: spread to humans by mosquitoes or ticks; seasonal epidemics depend on ecology of the insect vector; the following occur in the United States:

Eastern equine	California
Western equine	Powassan
Venezuelan equine	Dengue
St. Louis	Colorado tick fever
West Nile	

  D. Spread by warm-blooded mammals
    1. Rabies: saliva of many domestic and wild mammalian species
    2. Herpesvirus simiae ("B" virus): monkeys' saliva
    3. Lymphocytic choriomeningitis: rodents' excreta
II. INFECTIONS: NONVIRAL
  A. Rickettsial: in Rocky Mountain spotted fever and typhus; encephalitic component from cerebral vasculitis
  B. Mycoplasma pneumoniae: interval of some days between respiratory and CNS symptoms
  C. Bacterial: tuberculous and other bacterial meningitis; often has encephalitic component
  D. Spirochetal: syphilis, congenital or acquired; leptospirosis; Lyme disease
  E. Cat-scratch disease
  F. Fungal: immunologically compromised patients at special risk: cryptococcosis; histoplasmosis; aspergillosis; mucormycosis; candidosis; coccidioidomycosis
  G. Protozoal: Plasmodium, Trypanosoma, Naegleria, and Acanthamoeba spp.; Toxoplasma gondii
  H. Metazoal: trichinosis; echinococcosis; cysticercosis; schistosomiasis

III. PARAINFECTIOUS: POSTINFECTIOUS, ALLERGIC, AUTOIMMUNE
Patients in whom an infectious agent or 1 of its components plays a contributory role in etiology, but the intact infectious agent is not isolated in vitro from the nervous system; it is postulated that in this group, the influence of cell-mediated antigen–antibody complexes plus complement is especially important in producing the observed tissue damage
  A. Associated with specific diseases (these agents may also cause direct CNS damage; see I and II)
    Measles
    Rickettsial infections
    Rubella
    Influenzas A and B
    Mumps
    Varicella-zoster
    M. pneumoniae
  B. Associated with vaccines
    Rabies
    Measles
    Vaccinia
    Yellow fever
  C. Autoimmune encephalitis
  D. Acute disseminated encephalomyelitis (ADEM)
    Paraneoplastic
    Idiopathic
IV. HUMAN SLOW-VIRUS DISEASES
Accumulating evidence that viruses frequently acquired earlier in life, not necessarily with detectable acute illness, participate in later chronic neurologic disease (similar events also known to occur in animals)
  A. Subacute sclerosing panencephalitis; measles; rubella?
  B. Creutzfeldt-Jakob disease (spongiform encephalopathy)
  C. Progressive multifocal leukoencephalopathy
  D. Kuru (Fore tribe in New Guinea only)
  E. Human immunodeficiency virus
V. UNKNOWN: COMPLEX GROUP
This group constitutes more than two-thirds of the cases of encephalitis reported to the Centers for Disease Control and Prevention, Atlanta, Georgia; the yearly epidemic curve of these undiagnosed cases suggests that the majority are probably caused by enteroviruses and/or arboviruses.
There is also a miscellaneous group that is based on clinical criteria: Reye syndrome is 1 current example; others include the extinct von Economo encephalitis (epidemic during 1918-1928); myoclonic encephalopathy of infancy; retinomeningoencephalitis with papilledema and retinal hemorrhage; recurrent encephalomyelitis (? allergic or autoimmune); pseudotumor cerebri; and epidemic neuromyasthenia (Iceland disease).
An encephalitic clinical pattern may follow ingestion or absorption of a number of known and unknown toxic substances; these include ingestion of lead and mercury, and percutaneous absorption of hexachlorophene as a skin disinfectant and gamma benzene hexachloride as a scabicide.

CNS, central nervous system.
Modified from Behrman RE, editor: Nelson textbook of pediatrics, ed 14, Philadelphia, 1992, WB Saunders, p. 667. From Kliegman RM, Greenbaum LA, Lye PS: Practical strategies in pediatric diagnosis and therapy, ed 2, Philadelphia, 2004, Elsevier, p. 967.

pressure using fluids (normal saline) and vasopressor agents (dopamine, norepinephrine). This method reduces the risk of systemic hypotension and may improve survival and reduce disability.

Seizures are common during the course of bacterial meningitis. Immediate therapy for seizures includes intravenous diazepam (0.1-0.2 mg/kg/dose) or lorazepam (0.05-0.10 mg/kg/dose), and careful attention paid to the risk of respiratory suppression. Serum glucose, calcium, and sodium levels should be monitored. After immediate management of seizures, patients should receive phenytoin (15-20 mg/ kg loading dose, 5 mg/kg/24 hr maintenance) to reduce the likelihood of recurrence. Phenytoin is preferred to phenobarbital because it produces less CNS depression and permits assessment of a patient's level of consciousness. Serum phenytoin levels should be monitored to maintain them in the therapeutic range (10-20 µg/mL).

COMPLICATIONS

During the treatment of meningitis, acute CNS complications can include seizures, increased ICP, cranial nerve palsies, stroke,

Table 603-4	Antibiotics Used for the Treatment of Bacterial Meningitis*		
	Neonates		
DRUGS	**0-7 DAYS**	**8-28 DAYS**	**INFANTS AND CHILDREN**
Amikacin†‡	15-20 divided q12h	30 divided q8h	20-30 divided q8h
Ampicillin	150 divided q8h	200 divided q6h or q8h	300 divided q6h
Cefotaxime	100-150 divided q8h or q12h	150-200 divided q6h or q8h	225-300 divided q6h or q8h
Ceftriaxone§	—	—	100 divided q12h or q24h
Ceftazidime	100-150 divided q8h or q12h	150 divided q8h	150 divided q8h
Gentamicin†‡	5 divided q12h	7.5 divided q8h	7.5 divided q8h
Meropenem	—	—	120 divided q8h
Nafcillin	75 divided q8h or q12h	100-150 divided q6h or q8h	200 divided q6h
Penicillin G	150,000 divided q8h or q12h	200,000 divided q6h or q8h	300,000 divided q4h or q6h
Rifampin	—	10-20 divided q12h	10-20 divided q12h or q24h
Tobramycin†‡	5 divided q12h	7.5 divided q8h	7.5 divided q8h
Vancomycin†‡	20-30 divided q8h or q12h	30-45 divided q6h or q8h	60 divided q6h

*Dosages in mg/kg (units/kg for penicillin G) per day.
†Smaller doses and longer dosing intervals, especially for aminoglycosides and vancomycin for very-low-birthweight neonates, may be advisable.
‡Monitoring of serum levels is recommended to ensure safe and therapeutic values.
§Use in neonates is not recommended because of inadequate experience in neonatal meningitis.
Adapted from Tunkel AR, Hartman BJ, Kaplan SL, et al: Practice guidelines for the management of bacterial meningitis. *Clin Infect Dis* 39(9):1267–1284, 2004, Table 6.

cerebral or cerebellar herniation, and thrombosis of the dural venous sinuses.

Collections of fluid in the subdural space develop in 10-30% of patients with meningitis and are asymptomatic in 85-90% of patients. **Subdural effusions** are especially common in infants. Symptomatic subdural effusions may result in a bulging fontanel, diastasis of sutures, enlarging head circumference, emesis, seizures, fever, and abnormal results of cranial transillumination. CT or MRI scanning confirms the presence of a subdural effusion. In the presence of increased ICP or a depressed level of consciousness, symptomatic subdural effusion should be treated by aspiration through the open fontanel (see Chapters 68 and 590). Fever alone is not an indication for aspiration.

SIADH occurs in some patients with meningitis, resulting in hyponatremia and reduced serum osmolality. This may exacerbate cerebral edema or result in hyponatremic seizures (see Chapter 55).

Fever associated with bacterial meningitis usually resolves within 5-7 days of the onset of therapy. **Prolonged fever** (>10 days) is noted in approximately 10% of patients. Prolonged fever is usually caused by intercurrent viral infection, nosocomial or secondary bacterial infection, thrombophlebitis, or drug reaction. Secondary fever refers to the recrudescence of elevated temperature after an afebrile interval. Nosocomial infections are especially important to consider in the evaluation of these patients. Pericarditis or arthritis may occur in patients being treated for meningitis, especially that caused by *N. meningitidis*. Involvement of these sites may result either from bacterial dissemination or from immune complex deposition. In general, infectious pericarditis or arthritis occurs earlier in the course of treatment than does immune-mediated disease.

Thrombocytosis, eosinophilia, and anemia may develop during therapy for meningitis. Anemia may be a result of hemolysis or bone marrow suppression. Disseminated intravascular coagulation is most often associated with the rapidly progressive pattern of presentation and is noted most commonly in patients with shock and purpura. The combination of endotoxemia and severe hypotension initiates the coagulation cascade; the coexistence of ongoing thrombosis may produce symmetric peripheral gangrene.

PROGNOSIS

Appropriate antibiotic therapy and supportive care have reduced the mortality of bacterial meningitis after the neonatal period to <10%.

The highest mortality rates are observed with pneumococcal meningitis. Severe neurodevelopmental sequelae may occur in 10-20% of patients recovering from bacterial meningitis, and as many as 50% have some, albeit subtle, neurobehavioral morbidity. The prognosis is poorest among infants younger than 6 mo and in those with high concentrations of bacteria/bacterial products in their CSF. Those with seizures occurring more than 4 days into therapy or with coma or focal neurologic signs on presentation have an increased risk of long-term sequelae. There does not appear to be a correlation between duration of symptoms before diagnosis of meningitis and outcome.

The most common neurologic sequelae include hearing loss, cognitive impairment, recurrent seizures, delay in acquisition of language, visual impairment, and behavioral problems. **Sensorineural hearing** loss is the most common sequela of bacterial meningitis and, usually, is already present at the time of initial presentation. It is a result of cochlear infection and occurs in as many as 30% of patients with pneumococcal meningitis, 10% with meningococcal, and 5-20% of those with *H. influenzae* type b meningitis. Hearing loss may also be caused by direct inflammation of the auditory nerve. All patients with bacterial meningitis should undergo careful audiologic assessment before or soon after discharge from the hospital. Frequent reassessment on an outpatient basis is indicated for patients who have a hearing deficit.

PREVENTION

Vaccination and antibiotic prophylaxis of susceptible at-risk contacts represent the 2 available means of reducing the likelihood of bacterial meningitis. The availability and application of each of these approaches depend on the specific infecting bacteria.

Neisseria meningitidis

Chemoprophylaxis is recommended for all close contacts of patients with meningococcal meningitis regardless of age or immunization status. Close contacts should be treated with rifampin 10 mg/kg/dose every 12 hr (maximum dose of 600 mg) for 2 days as soon as possible after identification of a case of suspected meningococcal meningitis or sepsis. Close contacts include household, daycare center, and nursery school contacts, and healthcare workers who have direct exposure to oral secretions (mouth-to-mouth resuscitation, suctioning, intubation). Exposed contacts should be treated immediately on suspicion of infection in the index patient; bacteriologic confirmation of infection should not be awaited. In addition, all contacts should be educated about the early signs of meningococcal disease and the need to seek prompt medical attention if these signs develop.

Two quadrivalent (A, C, Y, W-135), conjugated vaccines (MCV-4; Menactra and Menveo) are licensed by the FDA. The Advisory Committee on Immunization Practices (ACIP) to the CDC recommends routine administration of this vaccine to 11-12 yr old adolescents. Menactra is licensed for use in infants older than 9 mo of age, and Menveo for use in children older than 2 yr of age. There is also a bivalent meningococcal polysaccharide protein conjugate vaccine that provides protection against serogroups C and Y along with *H. influenzae* type b. This vaccine is licensed for use in children ages 6 wk through 18 mo. High-risk patients include those with anatomic or functional asplenia or deficiencies of terminal complement proteins. Use of meningococcal vaccine should be considered for college freshmen, especially those who live in dormitories, because of an observed increased risk of invasive meningococcal infections compared to the risk in non–college-attending, age-matched controls.

Haemophilus influenzae Type B

Rifampin prophylaxis should be given to all household contacts of patients with invasive disease caused by *H. influenzae* type b, if any close family member younger than 48 mo has not been fully immunized or if an immunocompromised person, of any age, resides in the household. A household contact is one who lives in the residence of the index case or who has spent a minimum of 4 hr with the index case for at least 5 of the 7 days preceding the patient's hospitalization. Family members should receive rifampin prophylaxis immediately after the diagnosis is suspected in the index case because >50% of secondary family cases occur in the 1st wk after the index patient has been hospitalized.

The dose of rifampin is 20 mg/kg/24 hr (maximum dose of 600 mg) given once each day for 4 days. Rifampin colors the urine and perspiration red-orange, stains contact lenses, and reduces the serum concentrations of some drugs, including oral contraceptives. Rifampin is contraindicated during pregnancy.

The most striking advance in the prevention of childhood bacterial meningitis followed the development and licensure of conjugated vaccines against *H. influenzae* type b. Three conjugate vaccines are licensed in the United States. Although each vaccine elicits different profiles of antibody response in infants immunized at 2-6 mo of age, all result in protective levels of antibody with an efficacy rate against invasive infections after primary series at 93%. Efficacy is not as consistent in Native American populations, a group recognized as having an especially high incidence of disease. All children should be immunized with *H. influenzae* type b conjugate vaccine beginning at 2 mo of age (see Chapter 172).

Streptococcus pneumoniae

Routine administration of conjugate vaccine against *S. pneumoniae* is recommended for children younger than 5 yr of age. The initial dose is given at about 2 mo of age. Children who are at high risk of invasive pneumococcal infections, including those with functional or anatomic asplenia and those with underlying immunodeficiency (such as infection with HIV, primary immunodeficiency, and those receiving immunosuppressive therapy) should also receive the vaccine.

Bibliography is available at Expert Consult.

603.2 Viral Meningoencephalitis

Charles G. Prober and Nivedita S. Srinivas

Viral meningoencephalitis is an acute inflammatory process involving the meninges and, to a variable degree, brain tissue. These infections are relatively common and may be caused by a number of different agents. The CSF is characterized by pleocytosis and the absence of microorganisms on Gram stain and routine bacterial culture. In most instances, the infections are self-limited. In some cases, substantial morbidity and mortality occur.

ETIOLOGY

Enteroviruses are the most common cause of viral meningoencephalitis. As of 2014, more than 70 serotypes of these small RNA viruses have been identified. The severity of infection caused by enteroviruses ranges from mild, self-limited illness with primarily meningeal involvement to severe encephalitis resulting in death or significant sequelae. Human enterovirus 68 has been associated with neurologic symptoms including flaccid paralysis. **Parechoviruses** may be an important cause of aseptic meningitis or encephalitis in infants. The clinical manifestations are similar to that of the enteroviruses with the exception of more severe MRI lesions of the cerebral cortex and at times an absence of a CSF pleocytosis.

Arboviruses are arthropod-borne agents, responsible for some cases of meningoencephalitis during summer months. Mosquitoes and ticks are the most common vectors, spreading disease to humans and other vertebrates, such as horses, after biting infected birds or small animals. Encephalitis in horses ("blind staggers") may be the first indication of an incipient epidemic. Although rural exposure is most common, urban and suburban outbreaks also are frequent. The most common arboviruses responsible for CNS infection in the United States are West Nile virus (WNV), La Crosse, Powassan, and St. Louis encephalitis viruses (see Chapter 267). WNV made its appearance in the Western hemisphere in 1999. It has gradually made its way from the east to the west coast over successive summers. Cumulatively, from 1999 through 2008, a total of 47 states reported roughly 30,000 human infections caused by WNV. WNV may also be transmitted by blood transfusion, organ transplantation, or vertically across the placenta. Most children with WNV are either asymptomatic or have a nonspecific viral-like illness. Approximately 1% develop CNS disease; adults are more severely affected than children.

Several members of the **herpes family** of viruses can cause meningoencephalitis. Herpes simplex virus (HSV) type 1 is an important cause of severe, sporadic encephalitis in children and adults. Brain involvement usually is focal; progression to coma and death occurs in 70% of cases without antiviral therapy. Severe encephalitis with diffuse brain involvement is caused by HSV type 2 in neonates who usually contract the virus from their mothers at delivery. A mild transient form of meningoencephalitis may accompany genital herpes infection in sexually active adolescents; most of these infections are caused by HSV type 2. Varicella-zoster virus may cause CNS infection in close temporal relationship with chickenpox. The most common manifestation of CNS involvement is cerebellar ataxia, and the most severe is acute encephalitis. After primary infection, varicella-zoster virus becomes latent in spinal and cranial nerve roots and ganglia, expressing itself later as herpes zoster, sometimes with accompanying mild meningoencephalitis. Cytomegalovirus infection of the CNS may be part of congenital infection or disseminated disease in immunocompromised hosts, but it does not cause meningoencephalitis in normal infants and children. Epstein-Barr virus is associated with myriad CNS syndromes (see Chapter 254). Human herpes virus 6 can cause encephalitis, especially among immunocompromised hosts.

Mumps is a common pathogen in regions where mumps vaccine is not widely used. Mumps meningoencephalitis is mild, but deafness from damage of the 8th cranial nerve may be a sequela. Meningoencephalitis is caused occasionally by respiratory viruses (adenovirus, influenza virus, parainfluenza virus), rubeola, rubella, or rabies; it may follow live virus vaccinations against polio, measles, mumps, or rubella.

EPIDEMIOLOGY

The epidemiologic pattern of viral meningoencephalitis is primarily determined by the prevalence of enteroviruses, the most common etiology. Infection with enteroviruses is spread directly from person to person, with a usual incubation period of 4-6 days. Most cases in temperate climates occur in the summer and fall. Epidemiologic considerations in aseptic meningitis due to agents other than enteroviruses also include season, geography (travel), climatic conditions, animal exposures, mosquito or tick bites, and factors related to the specific pathogen.

PATHOGENESIS AND PATHOLOGY

Neurologic damage is caused by direct invasion and destruction of neural tissues by actively multiplying viruses or by a host reaction to viral antigens. Tissue sections of the brain generally are characterized by meningeal congestion and mononuclear infiltration, perivascular cuffs of lymphocytes and plasma cells, some perivascular tissue necrosis with myelin breakdown, and neuronal disruption in various stages, including, ultimately, neuronophagia and endothelial proliferation or necrosis. A marked degree of demyelination with preservation of neurons and their axons is considered to represent predominantly "postinfectious" or an autoimmune encephalitis.

The cerebral cortex, especially the temporal lobe, is often severely affected by HSV; the arboviruses tend to affect the entire brain; rabies has a predilection for the basal structures. Involvement of the spinal cord, nerve roots, and peripheral nerves is variable.

CLINICAL MANIFESTATIONS

The progression and severity of disease are determined by the relative degree of meningeal and parenchymal involvement, which, in part, is determined by the specific etiology. The clinical course resulting from infection with the same pathogen varies widely. Some children may appear to be mildly affected initially, only to lapse into coma and die suddenly. In others, the illness may be ushered in by high fever, violent convulsions interspersed with bizarre movements, and hallucinations alternating with brief periods of clarity, followed by complete recovery.

The onset of illness is generally acute, although CNS signs and symptoms are often preceded by a nonspecific febrile illness of a few days' duration. The presenting manifestations in older children are headache and hyperesthesia, and in infants, irritability and lethargy. Headache is most often frontal or generalized; adolescents frequently complain of retrobulbar pain. Fever, nausea and vomiting, photophobia, and pain in the neck, back, and legs are common. As body temperature increases, there may be mental dullness, progressing to stupor in combination with bizarre movements and convulsions. Focal neurologic signs may be stationary, progressive, or fluctuating. WNV and nonpolio enteroviruses may cause anterior horn cell injury and a flaccid paralysis. For those reported with WNV, encephalitis is more common than aseptic meningitis; acute flaccid paralysis may be noted in approximately 5% of patients. Nonetheless, many patients have a nonspecific febrile illness "West Nile fever" and may never seek medical attention. Loss of bowel and bladder control and unprovoked emotional outbursts may occur.

Exanthems often precede or accompany the CNS signs, especially with echoviruses, coxsackieviruses, varicella-zoster virus, measles, rubella, and, occasionally, WNV. Examination often reveals nuchal rigidity without significant localizing neurologic changes, at least at the onset.

Specific forms or complicating manifestations of CNS viral infection include Guillain-Barré syndrome, transverse myelitis, hemiplegia, and cerebellar ataxia.

DIAGNOSIS

The diagnosis of viral encephalitis is usually made on the basis of the clinical presentation of nonspecific prodrome followed by progressive CNS symptoms. The diagnosis is supported by examination of the CSF, which usually shows a mild mononuclear predominance (see Table 603-1). Other tests of potential value in the evaluation of patients with suspected viral meningoencephalitis include an electroencephalogram (EEG) and neuroimaging studies. The EEG typically shows diffuse slow-wave activity, usually without focal changes. Neuroimaging

studies (CT or MRI) may show swelling of the brain parenchyma. Focal seizures or focal findings on EEG, CT, or MRI, especially involving the temporal lobes, suggest HSV encephalitis.

Differential Diagnosis

A number of clinical conditions that cause CNS inflammation mimic viral meningoencephalitis (see Table 603-2). The most important group of alternative infectious agents to consider is bacteria. Most children with acute bacterial meningitis appear more critically ill than those with CNS viral infection. Parameningeal bacterial infections, such as brain abscess or subdural or epidural empyema, may have features similar to viral CNS infections. Infections caused by *M. tuberculosis*, *T. pallidum* (syphilis), *B. burgdorferi* (Lyme disease), and *Bartonella henselae*, the bacillus associated with cat scratch disease, tend to result in indolent courses. Analysis of CSF and appropriate serologic tests are necessary to differentiate these various pathogens.

Infections caused by fungi, rickettsiae, mycoplasma, protozoa, and other parasites may also need to be included in the differential diagnosis. Consideration of these agents usually arises as a result of accompanying symptoms, geographic locality of infection, or host immune factors.

Various noninfectious disorders may be associated with CNS inflammation and have manifestations overlapping with those associated with viral meningoencephalitis. Some of these disorders include malignancy, autoimmune diseases, intracranial hemorrhage, and exposure to certain drugs or toxins. Attention to history and other organ involvement usually allow elimination of these diagnostic possibilities. Autoimmune encephalitis owing to anti–N-methyl-D-aspartate receptor antibodies is an important cause of noninfectious encephalitis in children. Detection of these antibodies in the serum or CSF confirms this diagnosis. Acute disseminated encephalomyelitis may also initially be confused with encephalitis.

Laboratory Findings

The CSF contains from a few to several thousand cells per cubic millimeter. Early in the disease, the cells are often polymorphonuclear; later, mononuclear cells predominate. This change in cellular type is often demonstrated in CSF samples obtained as little as 8-12 hr apart. The protein concentration in CSF tends to be normal or slightly elevated, but concentrations may be very high if brain destruction is extensive, such as that accompanying HSV encephalitis. The glucose level is usually normal, although with certain viruses, for example, mumps, a substantial depression of CSF glucose concentrations may be observed. The CSF may be normal with parechovirus and in those who have encephalitis in the absence of meningeal involvement.

The success of isolating viruses from the CSF of children with viral meningoencephalitis is determined by the time in the clinical course that the specimen is obtained, the specific etiologic agent, whether the infection is a meningitic as opposed to a localized encephalitic process, and the skill of the diagnostic laboratory staff. Isolating a virus is most likely early in the illness, and the enteroviruses tend to be the easiest to isolate, although recovery of these agents from the CSF rarely exceeds 70%. To increase the likelihood of identifying the putative viral pathogen, specimens for culture should also be obtained from nasopharyngeal swabs, feces, and urine. Although isolating a virus from 1 or more of these sites does not prove causality, it is highly suggestive. *Detection of viral DNA or RNA by polymerase chain reaction is the test of choice in the diagnosis of CNS infection caused by HSV, parechovirus and enteroviruses, respectively.* CSF serology is the diagnostic test of choice for WNV.

A serum specimen should be obtained early in the course of illness and, if viral cultures are not diagnostic, again 2-3 wk later for serologic studies. Serologic methods are not practical for diagnosing CNS infections caused by the enteroviruses because there are too many serotypes. This approach may be useful, however, in confirming that a case is caused by a known circulating serotype. Serologic tests may also be of value in determining the etiology of nonenteroviral CNS infection, such as arboviral infection.

TREATMENT

With the exception of the use of acyclovir for HSV encephalitis (see Chapter 252), treatment of viral meningoencephalitis is supportive. Treatment of mild disease may require only symptomatic relief. Headache and hyperesthesia are treated with rest, non–aspirin-containing analgesics, and a reduction in room light, noise, and visitors. Acetaminophen is recommended for fever. Opioid agents and medications to reduce nausea may be useful, but if possible, their use in children should be minimized because they may induce misleading signs and symptoms. Intravenous fluids are occasionally necessary because of poor oral intake. More-severe disease may require hospitalization and intensive care.

It is important to monitor patients with severe encephalitis closely for convulsions, cerebral edema, inadequate respiratory exchange, disturbed fluid and electrolyte balance, aspiration and asphyxia, and cardiac or respiratory arrest of central origin. In patients with evidence of increased ICP, placement of a pressure transducer in the epidural space may be indicated. The risks of cardiac and respiratory failure or arrest are high with severe disease. All fluids, electrolytes, and medications are initially given parenterally. In prolonged states of coma, parenteral alimentation is indicated. SIADH is common in acute CNS disorders; monitoring of serum sodium concentrations is required for early detection (see Chapter 559). Normal blood levels of glucose, magnesium, and calcium must be maintained to minimize the likelihood of convulsions. If cerebral edema or seizures become evident, vigorous treatment should be instituted.

PROGNOSIS

Supportive and rehabilitative efforts are very important after patients recover from the acute phase of illness. Motor incoordination, convulsive disorders, total or partial deafness, and behavioral disturbances may follow viral CNS infections. Visual disturbances from chorioretinopathy and perceptual amblyopia may also occur. Special facilities and, at times, institutional placement may become necessary. Some sequelae of infection may be very subtle. Therefore, neurodevelopmental and audiologic evaluations should be part of the routine follow-up of children who have recovered from viral meningoencephalitis.

Most children completely recover from viral infections of the CNS, although the prognosis depends on the severity of the clinical illness, the specific causative organism, and the age of the child. If the clinical illness is severe and substantial parenchymal involvement is evident, the prognosis is poor, with potential deficits being intellectual, motor, psychiatric, epileptic, visual, or auditory in nature. Severe sequelae should also be anticipated in those with infection caused by HSV. Although some literature suggests that infants who contract viral meningoencephalitis have a poorer long-term outcome than older children, most other data refute this observation. Approximately 10% of children younger than 2 yr of age with enteroviral CNS infections suffer an acute complication such as seizures, increased ICP, or coma. Almost all have favorable long-term neurologic outcomes.

PREVENTION

Widespread use of effective viral vaccines for polio, measles, mumps, rubella, and varicella has almost eliminated CNS complications from these diseases in the United States. The availability of domestic animal vaccine programs against rabies has reduced the frequency of rabies encephalitis. Control of encephalitis caused by arboviruses has been less successful because specific vaccines for the arboviral diseases that occur in North America are not available. Control of insect vectors by suitable spraying methods and eradication of insect breeding sites, however, reduces the incidence of these infections. Furthermore, minimizing mosquito bites through the application of N,N-diethyl-3-methylbenzamide (DEET)-containing insect repellents on exposed skin and wearing long-sleeved shirts, long pants, and socks when outdoors, especially at dawn and dusk, reduces the risk of arboviral infection.

Bibliography is available at Expert Consult.

603.3 Eosinophilic Meningitis

Charles G. Prober and Nivedita S. Srinivas

Eosinophilic meningitis is defined as 10 or more eosinophils/mm^3 of CSF. The most common cause worldwide of eosinophilic pleocytosis is CNS infection with helminthic parasites. In countries such as the United States, where helminthic infestation is uncommon, however, the differential diagnosis of CSF eosinophilic pleocytosis is broad.

ETIOLOGY

Although any tissue-migrating helminth may cause eosinophilic meningitis, the most common cause is human infection with the rat lungworm, *Angiostrongylus cantonensis* (see Chapter 297). Other parasites that can cause eosinophilic meningitis include *Gnathostoma spinigerum* (dog and cat roundworm) (see Chapter 297), *Baylisascaris procyonis* (raccoon roundworm), *Ascaris lumbricoides* (human roundworm), *Trichinella spiralis, Toxocara canis, T. gondii, Paragonimus westermani, Echinococcus granulosus, Schistosoma japonicum, Onchocerca volvulus,* and *Taenia solium.* Eosinophilic meningitis may also occur as an unusual manifestation of more common viral, bacterial, or fungal infections of the CNS. Noninfectious causes of eosinophilic meningitis include multiple sclerosis, malignancy, hypereosinophilic syndrome, or a reaction to medications or a ventriculoperitoneal shunt.

EPIDEMIOLOGY

A. cantonensis is found in Southeast Asia, the South Pacific, Japan, Taiwan, Egypt, Ivory Coast, and Cuba. Infection is acquired by eating raw or undercooked freshwater snails, slugs, prawns, or crabs containing infectious 3rd-stage larvae. *Gnathostoma* infections are found in Japan, China, India, Bangladesh, and Southeast Asia. Gnathostomiasis is acquired by eating undercooked or raw fish, frog, bird, or snake meat.

CLINICAL MANIFESTATIONS

When eosinophilic meningitis results from helminthic infestation, patients become ill 1-3 wk after exposure. This reflects the transit time for parasites to migrate from the gastrointestinal tract to the CNS. Common concomitant findings include fever, peripheral eosinophilia, vomiting, abdominal pain, creeping skin eruptions, or pleurisy. Neurologic symptoms may include headache, meningismus, ataxia, cranial nerve palsies, and paresthesias. Paraparesis or incontinence can result from radiculitis or myelitis.

DIAGNOSIS

The presumptive diagnosis of helminth-induced eosinophilic meningitis is most often based on travel and exposure history in the presence of typical clinical and laboratory findings. Direct visualization of helminths in CSF is affected by the relatively low organism burden, resulting in limited diagnostic sensitivity. Serologic assays for helminthic infections are also of limited utility because they are not readily available commercially and there is substantial cross-reactivity between different helminth species.

TREATMENT

Treatment is supportive, because infection is self-limited and anthelmintic drugs do not appear to influence the outcome of infection. Analgesics should be given for headache and radiculitis, and CSF removal or shunting should be performed to relieve hydrocephalus, if present. Steroids may decrease the duration of headaches in adults with eosinophilic meningitis.

PROGNOSIS

The prognosis is good; 70% of patients improve sufficiently to leave the hospital in 1-2 wk. Mortality associated with eosinophilic meningitis is <1%.

Bibliography is available at Expert Consult.

Chapter 604
Brain Abscess
Charles G. Prober and Roshni Mathew

Brain abscesses can occur in children of any age but are most common in children between 4 and 8 yr old and in neonates. The causes of brain abscess include embolization as a result of congenital heart disease with right-to-left shunts (especially tetralogy of Fallot), endocarditis, meningitis, chronic otitis media and mastoiditis, sinusitis, soft-tissue infection of the face or scalp, orbital cellulitis, dental infections, severe complicated pneumonia, penetrating head injuries, immunodeficiency states, and infection of ventriculoperitoneal shunts.

PATHOLOGY
Cerebral abscesses are evenly distributed between the 2 hemispheres, and 80% of cases are divided equally between the frontal, parietal, and temporal lobes. Brain abscesses in the occipital lobe, cerebellum, and brainstem account for approximately 20% of the cases. Most brain abscesses are single, but 30% are multiple and may involve more than 1 lobe. The pathogenesis is undetermined in 10-15% of cases. An abscess in the frontal lobe is often caused by extension from sinusitis or orbital cellulitis, whereas abscesses located in the temporal lobe or cerebellum are frequently associated with chronic otitis media and mastoiditis. Abscesses resulting from penetrating injuries tend to be singular and caused by *Staphylococcus aureus,* whereas those resulting from septic emboli, congenital heart disease, or meningitis often have several causal organisms.

ETIOLOGY
The predominant organisms causing brain abscesses in children are aerobic and anaerobic streptococci (60-70% of the cases) with *Streptococcus milleri* gp (*Streptococcus anginosus, Streptococcus constellatus,* and *Streptococcus intermedius*) being increasingly isolated from surgically drained brain abscesses. Other important streptococci include group A and *B streptococci, Streptococcus pneumoniae,* and *Enterococcus faecalis.* Other bacteria isolated from brain abscesses include anaerobic organisms (Gram-positive cocci, *Bacteroides* spp., *Fusobacterium* spp., *Prevotella* spp., *Actinomyces* spp.) and Gram-negative aerobic bacilli (*Haemophilus aphrophilus, Haemophilus parainfluenzae, Haemophilus influenzae, Enterobacter, Escherichia coli, Proteus* spp.). *Citrobacter* is most common in neonates. One organism is cultured in 70% of abscesses, 2 in 20%, and 3 or more in 10% of cases. Abscesses associated with mucosal infections (sinusitis) frequently have anaerobic bacteria. Fungi (*Aspergillus, Candida*), *Nocardia, Mycobacterium,* and *Listeria* spp. are more common in children with impaired host defenses.

CLINICAL MANIFESTATIONS
The early stages of cerebritis and abscess formation are associated with nonspecific symptoms, including low-grade fever, headache, and lethargy. The significance of these symptoms is generally not recognized, and an oral antibiotic is often prescribed with resultant transient relief. As the inflammatory process proceeds, vomiting, severe headache, seizures, papilledema, focal neurologic signs (hemiparesis), and coma may develop. A cerebellar abscess is characterized by nystagmus, ipsilateral ataxia and dysmetria, vomiting, and headache. If the abscess ruptures into the ventricular cavity, overwhelming shock and death usually ensue.

DIAGNOSIS
The peripheral white blood cell count can be normal or elevated, and the blood culture is positive in 10% of cases. Examination of the cerebrospinal fluid shows variable results; the white blood cells and protein

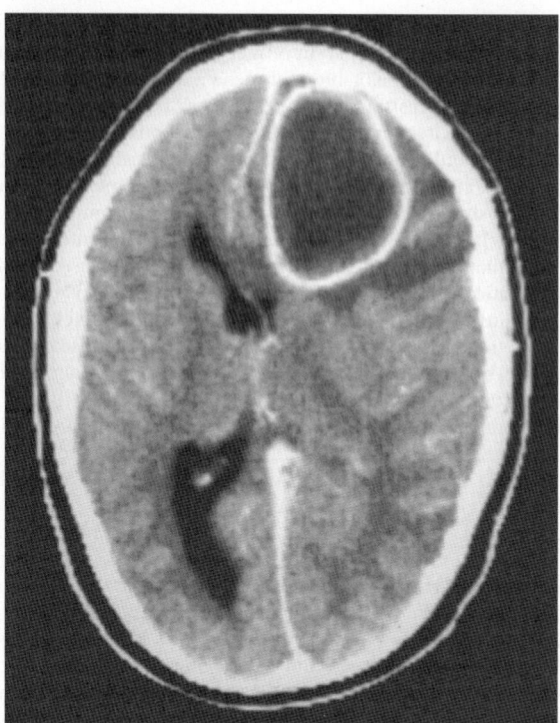

Figure 604-1 CT with contrast. Note the large, wall-enhancing abscess in the left frontal lobe causing a shift of the brain to the right. The patient had no neurologic signs until just before the CT scan because the abscess is located in the frontal lobe, a "silent" area of the brain.

may be minimally elevated or normal, and the glucose level may be low. Cerebrospinal fluid cultures are rarely positive; culture of pus from the neurosurgical drainage is the key to establishing a bacteriologic diagnosis. However, the culture can be sterile in a substantial number of cases and 16S bacterial ribosomal RNA polymerase chain reaction amplification and sequencing may be used to identify unculturable bacteria in brain abscesses. Because examination of the cerebrospinal fluid is seldom useful and a lumbar puncture may cause herniation of the cerebellar tonsils, the procedure should not be undertaken in a child suspected of having a brain abscess. The electroencephalogram shows corresponding focal slowing, and the radionuclide brain scan indicates an area of enhancement caused by disruption of the blood–brain barrier in more than 80% of cases. CT with contrast and MRI are the most reliable methods of demonstrating cerebritis and abscess formation (Fig. 604-1). MRI is the diagnostic test of choice. The CT findings of cerebritis are characterized by a parenchymal low-density lesion, and MRI T2-weighted images indicate increased signal intensity. An abscess cavity shows a ring-enhancing lesion by contrast CT, and the MRI also demonstrates an abscess capsule with gadolinium administration.

TREATMENT
The initial management of a brain abscess includes prompt diagnosis and institution of an antibiotic regimen that is based on the probable pathogenesis and the most likely organism. When the cause is unknown, the combination of vancomycin, a third-generation cephalosporin, and metronidazole is commonly used. The same regimen is initiated when otitis media, sinusitis, or mastoiditis is the likely cause. If there is a history of penetrating head injury, head trauma, or neurosurgery, vancomycin plus a third-generation cephalosporin is appropriate. When cyanotic congenital heart disease is the predisposing factor, ampicillin-sulbactam alone or a third-generation cephalosporin plus metronidazole may be used. Meropenem has good activity against Gram-negative bacilli, anaerobes, staphylococci, and streptococci,

including most antibiotic-resistant pneumococci, and may be used alone to replace the combination of metronidazole and a β-lactam in the previous regimens. Notably, meropenem does not provide activity against methicillin-resistant *S. aureus* and may have decreased activity against penicillin-resistant strains of *S. pneumoniae*, indicating that vancomycin should remain a part of the initial regimen when these organisms are suspected. Abscesses secondary to an infected ventriculoperitoneal shunt may be initially treated with vancomycin and ceftazidime. When *Citrobacter* meningitis (often in neonates) leads to abscess formation, a third-generation cephalosporin is used, typically in combination with an aminoglycoside. *Listeria monocytogenes* may cause a brain abscess in the neonate and if suspected, ampicillin should be added to the cephalosporin. In immunocompromised patients, broad-spectrum antibiotic coverage is used, and amphotericin B therapy should be considered.

A brain abscess can be treated with antibiotics without surgery if the abscess is <2 cm in diameter, the illness is of short duration (<2 wk), there are no signs of increased intracranial pressure, and the child is neurologically intact. If the decision is made to treat with antibiotics alone, the child should have follow-up neuroimaging studies to ensure the abscess is decreasing in size. An encapsulated abscess, particularly if the lesion is causing a mass effect or increased intracranial pressure, should be treated with a combination of antibiotics and aspiration. Surgical excision of an abscess is rarely required, because the procedure may be associated with greater morbidity compared with aspiration of a cavity. Surgery is indicated when the abscess is >2.5 cm in diameter, gas is present in the abscess, the lesion is multiloculated, the lesion is located in the posterior fossa, or a fungus is identified. Associated infectious processes, such as mastoiditis, sinusitis, or a periorbital abscess, may require surgical drainage. The duration of antibiotic therapy depends on the organism and response to treatment but is usually 4-6 wk.

PROGNOSIS

Mortality rates prior to 1980s ranged from 11-53%. More recent mortality rates accompanying wider use of CT and MRI, improved microbiologic techniques and prompt antibiotic and surgical management, range from 5-10%. Factors associated with high mortality rate at the time of admission include age younger than 1 yr, multiple abscesses and coma. Long-term sequelae occur in about one-third of the survivors and include hemiparesis, seizures, hydrocephalus, cranial nerve abnormalities, and behavior and learning problems.

Bibliography is available at Expert Consult.

Chapter **605**

Idiopathic Intracranial Hypertension/ Pseudotumor Cerebri

Misha L. Pless

Idiopathic intracranial hypertension, also known as pseudotumor cerebri, is a clinical syndrome that mimics brain tumors and is characterized by increased intracranial pressure ≥280 mm Hg in sedated or obese children; ≥250 mm Hg in nonobese, nonsedated children with a normal cerebrospinal fluid (CSF) cell count and protein content and normal to slightly decreased ventricular size, and normal ventricular anatomy and position documented by MRI. Papilledema is universally present in children old enough to have a closed fontanel (Fig. 605-1).

ETIOLOGY

Table 605-1 lists the many causes of pseudotumor cerebri. There are many explanations for the development of pseudotumor cerebri, including alterations in CSF absorption and production, subtle cerebral edema, abnormalities in vasomotor control and cerebral blood flow, and venous obstruction. The causes of pseudotumor are numerous and include metabolic disorders (galactosemia, hypoparathyroidism, pseudohypoparathyroidism, hypophosphatasia, prolonged corticosteroid therapy or rapid corticosteroid withdrawal, possibly growth hormone treatment, refeeding of a significantly malnourished child, hypervitaminosis A, severe vitamin A deficiency, Addison disease, obesity, menarche, oral contraceptives, and pregnancy), infections (roseola infantum, sinusitis, chronic otitis media and mastoiditis, Guillain-Barré syndrome), drugs (nalidixic acid, doxycycline, minocycline, tetracycline, nitrofurantoin, isotretinoin used for acne therapy especially when combined with tetracycline), hematologic disorders (polycythemia, hemolytic and iron-deficiency anemias [see Fig. 605-1],

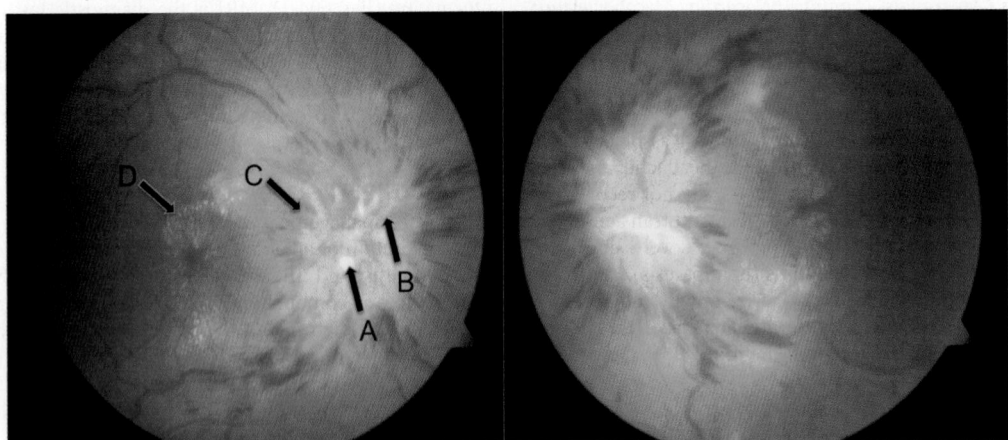

Figure 605-1 Optic nerve photos of the right and left eyes, respectively, demonstrating grade 5 optic nerve head edema with characteristics, including **(A)** total obscuration of the optic cup; **(B)** total obscuration of a segment of a major blood vessel; **(C)** total obscuration of disc margin; and **(D)** macular star. *(From Vickers AL, El-Dairi MA: Subacute vision loss in young, obese female. J Pediatr 163:1518–1519, 2013, Fig. 1.)*

Table 605-1	Etiology of Childhood Pseudotumor Cerebri

HEMATOLOGIC
Wiskott-Aldrich syndrome
Iron-deficiency anemia
Aplastic anemia
Sickle cell disease
Polycythemia?
Bone marrow transplantation and associated treatments?
Prothrombotic states
Fanconi anemia

INFECTIONS
Acute sinusitis
Otitis media (lateral sinus thrombosis)
Mastoiditis
Tonsillitis
Measles
Roseola
Varicella, recurrent varicella-zoster virus infection
Lyme disease?
HIV or associated treatment complications?

DRUGS
Tetracyclines
Sulfonamides
Nalidixic acid
Fluoroquinolones
Corticosteroid therapy and withdrawal
Nitrofurantoin
Cytarabine
Cyclosporine
Phenytoin
Mesalamine
Isotretinoin
Amiodarone?
1-Deamino-8-D-arginine vasopressin (DDAVP)?
Lithium?
Levonorgestrel implants?
Oral contraceptive pills

RENAL
Nephrotic syndrome
Chronic renal insufficiency?
Post–renal transplantation?
Peritoneal dialysis?

NUTRITIONAL
Hypovitaminosis A
Vitamin A intoxication
Hyperalimentation in malnourished patient
Vitamin D–dependent rickets

CONNECTIVE TISSUE DISORDERS
Antiphospholipid antibody syndrome
Systemic lupus erythematosus?
Behçet disease

ENDOCRINE
Menarche
Polycystic ovarian syndrome
Hypothyroidism
Hypoparathyroidism/hyperparathyroidism
Congenital adrenal hyperplasia
Addison disease
Recombinant growth hormone

OTHER
Dural sinus thrombosis
Obesity (in pubertal patients)
Bariatric surgery
Head trauma
Superior vena cava syndrome
Arteriovenous malformation
Sleep apnea
Guillain-Barré syndrome
Crohn disease
Ulcerative colitis?
Turner syndrome

POSSIBLE ASSOCIATIONS
Cystic fibrosis
Cystinosis
Down syndrome
Hypomagnesemia–hypercalciuria
Galactokinase deficiency
Galactosemia
Atrial septal defect repair
Moebius syndrome
Sarcoidosis?

Wiskott-Aldrich syndrome), obstruction of intracranial drainage by venous thrombosis (lateral sinus or posterior sagittal sinus thrombosis), head injury, and obstruction of the superior vena cava. When a cause is not identified, the condition is classified as idiopathic intracranial hypertension.

CLINICAL MANIFESTATIONS

The most frequent symptom is chronic (weeks to months), progressive, frontal headache that may worsen with postural changes or a Valsalva maneuver, and although vomiting also occurs, the vomiting is rarely as persistent and insidious as that associated with a posterior fossa tumor. Transient visual obscuration lasting seconds and diplopia (secondary to dysfunction of the abducens nerve) may also occur as may pulsatile tinnitus. Most patients are alert and lack constitutional symptoms. Examination of the infant with pseudotumor cerebri characteristically reveals a bulging fontanel and a "cracked pot sound" or Macewen sign (percussion of the skull produces a resonant sound) resulting from separation of the cranial sutures. **Papilledema** with an enlarged blind spot is the most consistent sign in a child beyond infancy. Papilledema may be absent or mild in infants with pseudotumor cerebri because high CSF pressure may be transmitted to the soft fontanels earlier than the optic nerves. Early optic nerve edema may be noted with orbit ultrasonography. Inferior nasal or peripheral visual field defects may be detected on formal tangent screen testing. The presence of focal neurologic signs should prompt an investigation to uncover a process other than pseudotumor cerebri. Any patient suspected of pseudotumor cerebri should undergo an MRI. MR angiography/MR venography should be considered in patients suspected of having dural sinus thrombosis.

TREATMENT

The key objective in management is recognition and treatment of the underlying cause. There are no randomized clinical trials to guide the treatment of pseudotumor cerebri. Pseudotumor cerebri can be a self-limited condition, but optic atrophy and blindness are the most significant complications of untreated pseudotumor cerebri (Fig. 605-2). The obese patient should be treated with a weight-loss regimen, and if a drug is thought to be responsible, it should be discontinued. For most patients old enough to participate in such testing, serial monitoring of visual function is required. Serial determination of visual acuity, color vision, and visual fields is critical in this disease. Serial optic nerve examination is essential as well. Optical coherence tomography is useful to serially follow changes in papilledema. Serial visual-evoked potentials are useful if the visual acuity cannot be reliably documented. The initial lumbar tap that follows a CT or MRI scan is diagnostic and may be therapeutic. The spinal needle produces a small rent in the dura that allows CSF to escape the subarachnoid space, thus reducing the intracranial pressure. Several additional lumbar taps and the removal

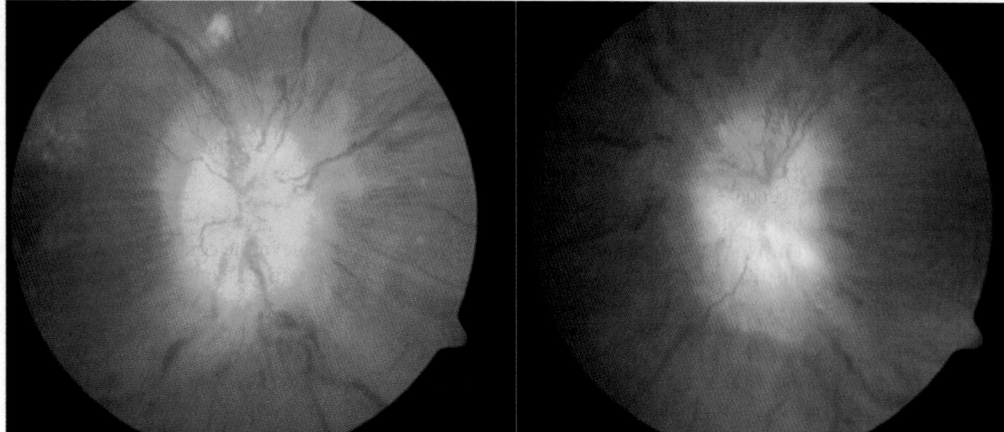

Figure 605-2 Bilateral optic atrophy is evident upon resolution of the papilledema, 1 mo after bilateral optic nerve sheath fenestrations. *(From Vickers AL, El-Dairi MA: Subacute vision loss in young, obese female. J Pediatr 163:1518–1519, 2013, Fig. 2.)*

of sufficient CSF to reduce the opening pressure by 50% occasionally lead to resolution of the process. Acetazolamide, 10-30 mg/kg/24 hr, is an effective regimen. Corticosteroids are not routinely administered, although they may be used in a patient with severe intracranial pressure elevation who is at risk of losing visual function and is awaiting a surgical decompression. Sinus thrombosis is typically addressed by anticoagulation therapy. Rarely, a ventriculoperitoneal shunt or subtemporal decompression is necessary, if the aforementioned approaches are unsuccessful and optic nerve atrophy supervenes. Some centers perform optic nerve sheath fenestration to prevent visual loss. Any patient whose intracranial pressure proves to be refractory to treatment warrants consideration for repeat neuroradiologic studies. A **slow-growing tumor** or **obstruction of a venous sinus** may become evident by the time of reinvestigation.

Bibliography is available at Expert Consult.

Chapter **606**
Spinal Cord Disorders
Harold L. Rekate

606.1 Tethered Cord
Harold L. Rekate

Beyond infancy the spinal cord in humans ends in the conus medullaris at about the level of L1. The position of the conus below L2 is consistent with a congenital tethered spinal cord. For normal humans as the spine flexes and extends, the spinal cord is free to move up and down within the spinal canal. If the spinal cord is fixed at any point, this movement is restricted and the spinal cord and nerve roots become stretched. This fixing of the spinal cord, regardless of the underlying cause of the fixation, is called a tethered cord. When severe pain or neurologic deterioration occurs in response to the fixation, it is called the **tethered cord syndrome.**

In its simplest form the tethered cord syndrome results from a thickened filum terminale, which normally extends as a thin, very mobile structure from the tip of the conus to the sacrococcygeal region where it attaches. When this structure is thickened and shortened, the conus is found to end at levels below L2. This stretching between 2 points is likely to cause symptoms later in life. Fatty infiltration is often seen in the thickened filum (Fig. 606-1).

Any condition that fixes the spinal cord can be the cause of the tethered cord syndrome. Conditions that are well established to cause symptomatic tethering include various forms of occult dysraphism such as lipomyelomeningocele, myelocystocele, and diastematomyelia. These conditions are associated with cutaneous manifestations such as midline lipomas often with asymmetry of the gluteal fold (Fig. 606-2), and hairy patches called hypertrichosis (Fig. 606-3). Probably the most common type of symptomatic tethered cord involves patients who had previously undergone closure of an open myelomeningocele and later become symptomatic with pain or neurologic deterioration. Tethered cord syndrome can also be associated with attachment of the spinal cord in patients who undergo surgical procedures that disrupt the pial surface of the spinal cord.

It is possible that a patient can be suffering from a tethered cord with the conus medullaris in a completely normal position. Although this concept remains controversial, recent reports suggest that half of children with new onset of incontinence found to be neurologic in nature by urodynamic measurements can be successfully treated by sectioning

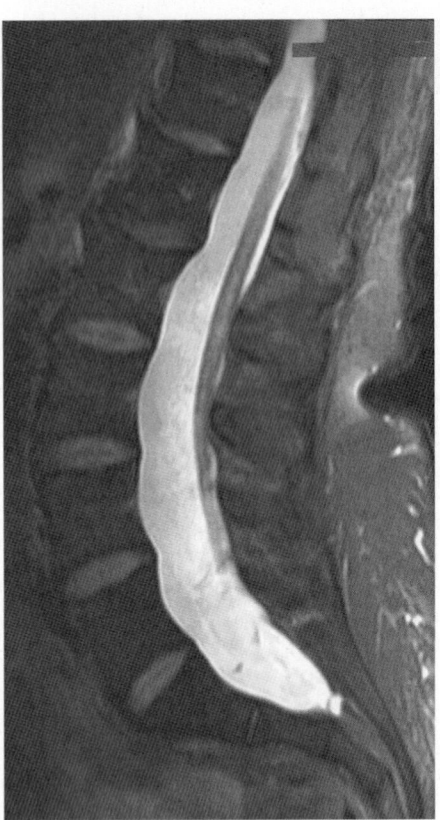

Figure 606-1 Sagittal MRI showing thickening of the filum terminale in a patient with a symptomatic tethered spinal cord. *(Used with permission from Barrow Neurological Institute.)*

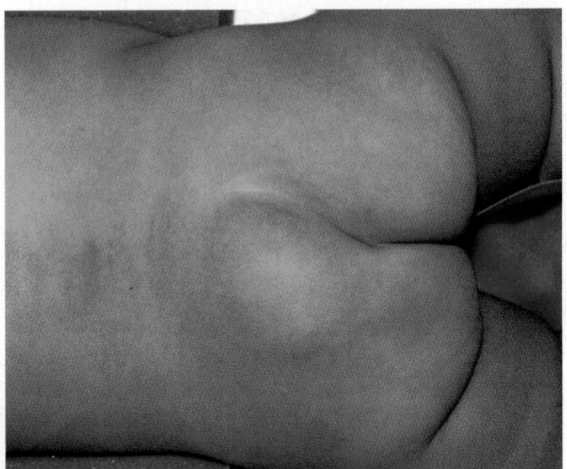

Figure 606-2 Child with a lipomyelomeningocele demonstrating an extraspinal mass and an asymmetry of the gluteal fold indicative of underlying occult dysraphism. *(Used with permission from Barrow Neurological Institute.)*

of the filum terminale in the context of normal radiology. This concept will require a randomized controlled trial to evaluate the efficacy of this approach.

CLINICAL MANIFESTATIONS
Patients at risk for the subsequent development of the tethered cord syndrome can often be identified at birth by the presence of an open myelomeningocele or by cutaneous manifestations of dysraphism. It is important to examine the back of the newborn for cutaneous midline lesions (lipoma, dermal sinus, tail, or hairy patch) that may signal an

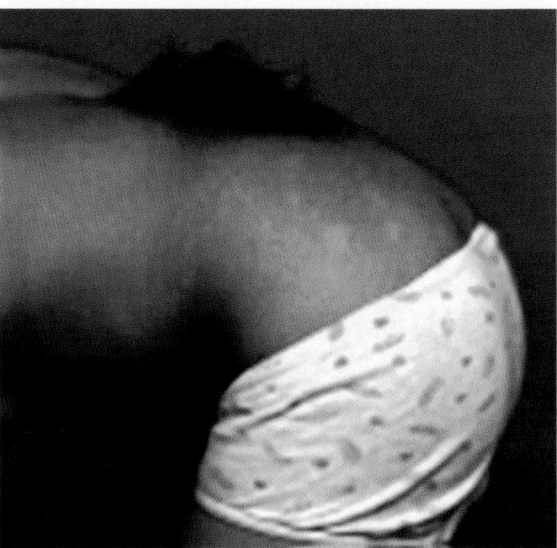

Figure 606-3 Hairy patch or hypertrichosis usually associated with diastematomyelia. *(Used with permission from Barrow Neurological Institute.)*

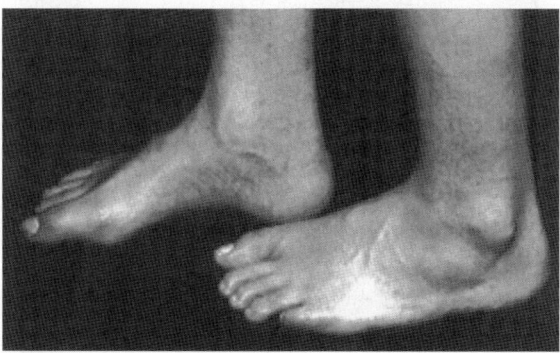

Figure 606-4 Example of the neuroorthopedic syndrome involving a larger left foot than right foot, a high arch, and absent ankle jerk frequently associated with tethered cord regardless of the etiology. *(Used with permission from Barrow Neurological Institute.)*

underlying form of occult dysraphism. Dermal sinuses are usually located above the gluteal fold. Cutaneous abnormalities are not found in patients with an isolated thickened filum terminale. Patients who become symptomatic later in life often exhibit an asymmetry of the feet (i.e., 1 is smaller than the other). The smaller foot will show a high arch and clawing of the toes (Fig. 606-4). Characteristically, there is no ankle jerk on the involved side and the calf is atrophied. This condition is termed the **neuroorthopedic syndrome**.

Three clinical syndromes can occur at the time of deterioration. The most likely clinical presentation is increasing urinary urgency and, finally, incontinence. Deterioration of motor and sensory function in the lower extremities is a compelling reason for intervention. Finally, severe generalized back pain, often radiating into the lower extremities, can occur, particularly in older adolescents and adults.

DIAGNOSTIC EVALUATION

When patients present with symptoms related to the tethered cord syndrome, a thorough motor and sensory examination of the patient must be documented. Assessment of bladder function with an ultrasound of the bladder and urodynamic studies is useful in analyzing bladder innervation. MRI is the diagnostic study of choice to reflect the anatomy of the tethering lesion and to provide information about the risks of surgical intervention.

TREATMENT

There are no nonsurgical options for the management of tethered cord syndrome. Because the presence of tethering is most likely to be at least suspected in the newborn, prophylactic surgery to prevent late deterioration has been advocated by some neurosurgeons. This strategy remains controversial and depends to some extent on a careful assessment of the risks compared to the benefits. If surgical intervention is chosen, microsurgical dissection with release of the spinal cord attachment to the overlying dura is the goal of treatment.

OUTCOME

The outcome of releasing a thickened filum terminale or detethering of patients with diastematomyelia is routinely good, and the chance of recurrent symptoms is very low. Patients with symptomatic tethered cord who undergo repair of a myelomeningocele or a lipomyelomeningocele have a significant possibility of recurrent tethering and recurrent symptoms.

Bibliography is available at Expert Consult.

606.2 Diastematomyelia
Harold L. Rekate

DIASTEMATOMYELIA: SPLIT-CORD MALFORMATION

Diastematomyelia is a relatively rare form of occult dysraphism in which the spinal cord is divided into 2 halves. In type 1 split-cord malformation, there are 2 spinal cords, each in its own dural tube and separated by a spicule of bone and cartilage (Fig. 606-5A). In a type 2 split-cord malformation, the 2 spinal cords are enclosed in a single dural sac with a fibrous septum between the 2 spinal segments (Fig. 606-5B). In both cases the anatomy of the outer half of the spinal cord is essentially normal while the medial half is extremely underdeveloped. Undeveloped nerve roots and dentate ligaments terminate medially into the medial dural tube in type 1 cases and terminate in the membranous septum in type 2 cases. Both types have an associated defect in the bony spinal segment. In the case of type 2 lesions, this defect can be quite subtle.

CLINICAL MANIFESTATIONS

Patients with both type 1 and type 2 split-cord malformations may have subtle signs of neurologic involvement such as unilateral calf atrophy and a high arch to 1 or both feet early in life, but they are more likely to be neurologically normal. These patients are tethered by the adherence of the spinal cord to the median membrane or dural sac. Later they may develop progressive loss of bowel and bladder function and sensory and motor difficulties in the lower extremities. Back pain is a common symptom in adolescents and adults with split-cord malformation but is uncommon in small children.

Cutaneous manifestations of dysraphism are present in 90% of patients with split-cord malformations. Large, hairy, midline patches called hypertrichosis, the most common cutaneous manifestations, are present in approximately 60% of the cases.

DIAGNOSTIC EVALUATION

MRI, the study of choice, shows the 2 spinal cords. The frequent association of bony abnormalities in this condition may require further evaluation with radiography or computed tomography.

TREATMENT

The treatment of split-cord malformations is surgical. This abnormality is a form of tethered cord syndrome, and its treatment is to release the spinal cord to move freely with movement of the spine. In type 1 split-cord malformations, the 2 half cords are in separate dural sacs with medial attachment to the dura and bony septum. In this case the dura needs to be opened, the bony septum removed, the medial attachments to the dura lysed, and a single dural tube created. For type 2 lesions,

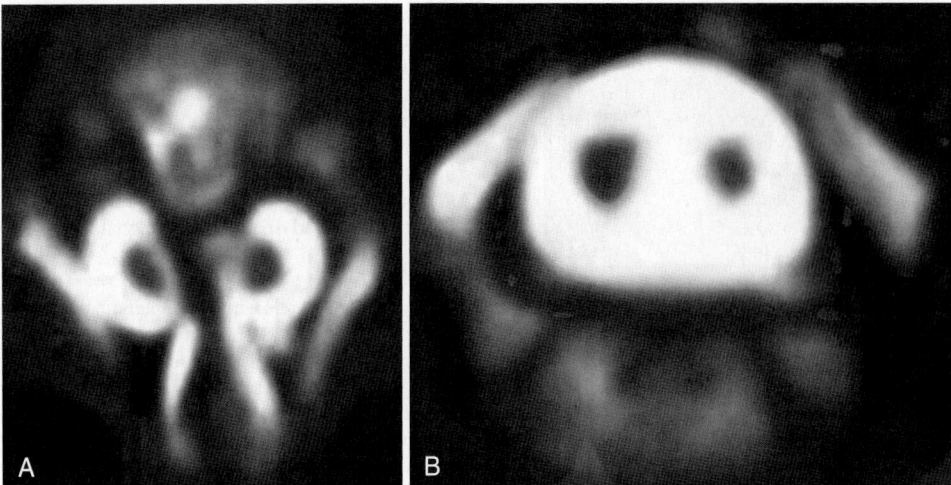

Figure 606-5 A, T2-weighted axial MRI of a type 1 split cord malformation showing the 2 spinal cords within 2 separate dural compartments. **B,** Type 2 split cord malformation with 2 spinal cords sharing a single dural compartment. (*A and B used with permission from Barrow Neurological Institute.*)

the membranous septum should be lysed. An attachment of this membrane to the anterior dura should be explored and lysed as well. Retethering of this type is rare as there is no reason to disrupt the pial layer of the spinal cord.

Bibliography is available at Expert Consult.

606.3 Syringomyelia
Harold L. Rekate

Syringomyelia is a cystic distention of the spinal cord caused by obstruction of the flow of spinal fluid from within the spinal cord to its point of absorption. There are 3 recognized forms of syringomyelia depending on the underlying cause. Communicating syringomyelia implies that cerebrospinal fluid (CSF) from within the ventricles communicates with the fluid within the spinal cord and is assumed to be the source of the CSF that distends the spinal cord. Noncommunicating syringomyelia implies that ventricular CSF does not communicate with the fluid within the spinal cord. It primarily occurs in the context of intramedullary tumors and obstructive lesions. In the final form of syringomyelia, that is, posttraumatic syringomyelia, spinal cord injury results in damage and subsequent softening of the spinal cord. This softening, combined with the scarring of the surrounding spinal cord tissue, results in progressive distention of the cyst. Syringomyelia has been associated with Chiari anomalies and in patients with Ehlers-Danlos syndrome; most are isolated findings unassociated with syndromes.

CLINICAL MANIFESTATIONS
Signs and symptoms of syringomyelia develop insidiously over years or decades. The classic presentation is the **central cord syndrome.** In this situation the patient develops numbness beginning in the shoulder in a cape-like distribution followed by the development of atrophy and weakness in the upper extremities. Trophic ulcers of the hands are characteristic of advanced cases. The central cord syndrome results from damage to the central spinal cord and the orientation of spinal tracts from proximal to distal leading to selective involvement of the upper rather than the lower extremities.

Other forms of presentation include scoliosis that may be rapidly progressive and often can be presumed from the absence of superficial abdominal reflexes. Urgency and bladder dysfunction as well as lower extremity spasticity also may be part of the presentation.

In patients with syringomyelia related to spinal cord injury, the presentation is usually severe pain in the area of the spinal cord

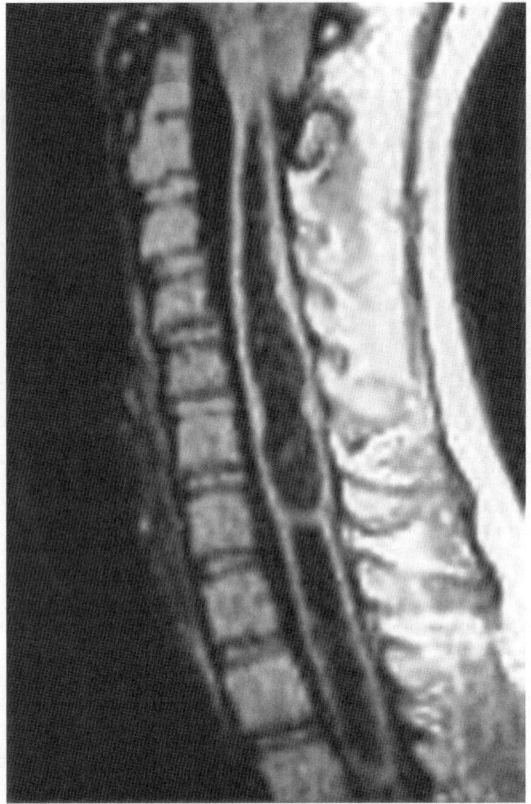

Figure 606-6 Sagittal MRI of patient with a Chiari I malformation and a holocord syrinx. (*Used with permission from Barrow Neurological Institute.*)

distention above the level of the initial injury. There is also an ascending level of motor and sensory dysfunction.

DIAGNOSTIC EVALUATION
MRI is the radiologic study of choice (Figs. 606-6 and 606-7). The study should include the entire spine and should include gadolinium-enhanced sequences. Specific attention should be paid to the craniovertebral junction because of the frequent association of syringomyelia with Chiari I and II malformations. Obstruction to the flow of CSF from the fourth ventricle can cause syringomyelia; therefore, most patients also should undergo imaging of the brain.

TREATMENT

The treatment of syringomyelia should be tailored to the underlying cause. If that cause can be removed or ameliorated, the syrinx should improve. Traumatic syrinxes result from hematomyelia in the substance of the spinal cord coupled with severe arachnoidal scarring around the circumference of the spinal cord. When progressive this form of syringomyelia is treated by exploration and lysis of the adhesions that fix the spinal cord to the overlying dura. In cases of complete spinal cord injury, as is usually found in the thoracic spinal cord, the most effective treatment is the transection of the spinal cord, which would both drain the syrinx and detether the spinal cord. Doing so drains the fluid from the spinal cord. In cases of incomplete spinal cord injury, functioning neurologic elements must be protected. Microscopic lysis of the scar surrounding the spinal cord at the point of injury allows the spinal cord to collapse and prevents it from being distorted by a hydrostatic column.

Communicating syringomyelia is most frequently seen in the context of abnormalities at the craniovertebral junction caused by inflammatory conditions such as chronic meningitis as seen in tuberculosis or meningeal carcinomatosis. There is frequently a causative association with hindbrain herniation as in Chiari malformations (see Fig. 606-6). In such cases decompression of the craniovertebral junction is usually effective in the management of the syringomyelia. In the context of the Chiari II malformation associated with spina bifida, syringomyelia usually results from an insidious failure of the shunt used to treat the hydrocephalus. This distention of the spinal cord results in a rapid development of scoliosis and occasionally spasticity in the lower extremities. Repair of the shunt is effective treatment.

Noncommunicating syringomyelia results from blocking the flow of spinal cord extracellular fluid or CSF within the central canal by an intramedullary spinal cord tumor or severe external compression of the spinal cord. In such cases, management should be directed to tumor resection or to decompression of constricting elements.

Drainage procedures can result in symptomatic and radiographic improvement. Syrinx-to-subarachnoid shunting with a small piece of shunt tubing is 1 form of treatment. Syrinx-to-pleural or syrinx-to-peritoneal shunting is more likely to result in improvement in the radiographic appearance of the syrinx. In patients with syringomyelia that extends to the conus medullaris, remnants of the central canal can be found in the filum terminale. Lysis of this structure near the conus can provide effective drainage.

Some children who show no testable neurologic findings are being referred to pediatric neurosurgeons with the diagnosis of syringomyelia. Many of these children were scanned because of back pain or as part of a screening for scoliosis. They are found on MRI to have a **persistent central canal** and the diagnosis of syringomyelia is made. Some have been scanned sequentially for follow up and banned from athletic activities. These syrinxes are 1-3 mm in diameter and extend over 2 segments (see Fig. 606-7). There is no distortion of the spinal cord in the region and no change in signal of the surrounding spinal cord. These syrinxes have been called "idiopathic" syrinxes. Follow-up of significant numbers of such children has shown them to be benign in nature and probably represent a normal variant. There does not seem to be a need for routine follow-up imaging without new symptoms. They need no treatment and do not require limitations of activity.

Bibliography is available at Expert Consult.

606.4 Spinal Cord Tumors
Harold L. Rekate

Tumors of the spine and spinal cord are rare in children. Different types of tumors have different relationships with the spinal cord, meninges, and bony elements of the spine (Fig. 606-8). Intramedullary spinal cord tumors arise within the substance of the spinal cord itself (Fig. 606-9). They represent between 5% and 15% of primary central nervous system tumors. This percentage may well reflect the total volume of spinal cord as opposed to brain. Approximately 10% of intramedullary spinal cord tumors are malignant astrocytic tumors, but most are World Health Organization grade I or II tumors of glial or ependymal origin. In children, low-grade astrocytomas and gangliogliomas represent the most common tumor types with ependymomas being less common than in adults. Ependymomas in children are frequently associated with neurofibromatosis (NF-2).

Except in the context of NF-1 and NF-2, intradural extramedullary tumors are extremely rare in children. Most are nerve sheath tumors,

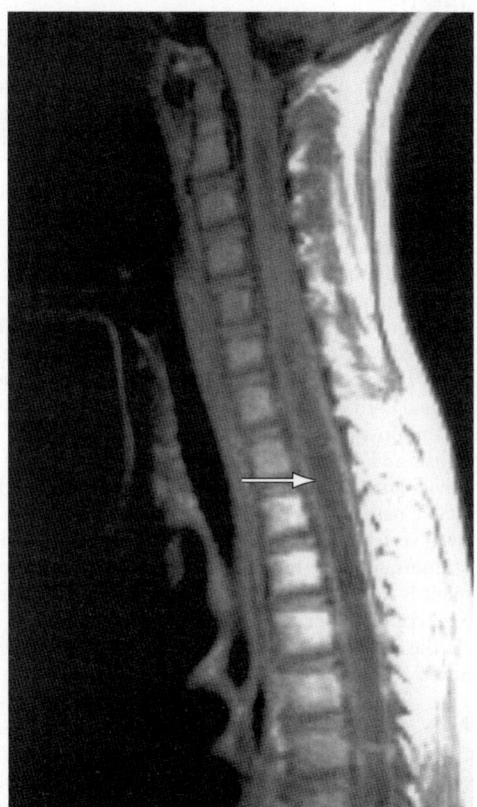

Figure 606-7 T1-weighted MRI scan of upper spinal cord showing an extensive syringomyelia *(arrow)*.

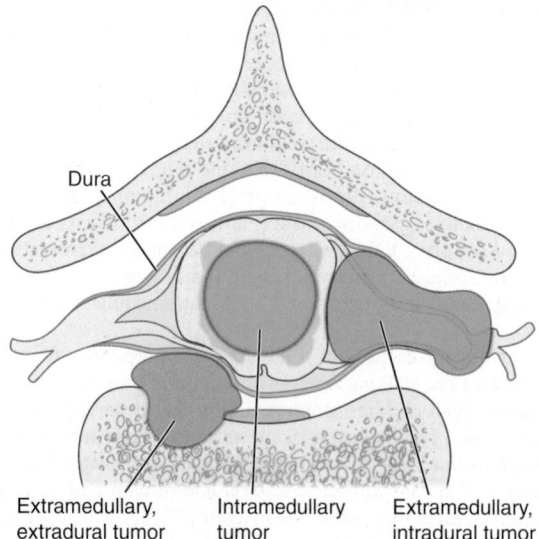

Figure 606-8 Diagram of the relationship of various tumors to the spine, nerve roots, and spinal cord. *(Used with permission from Barrow Neurological Institute.)*

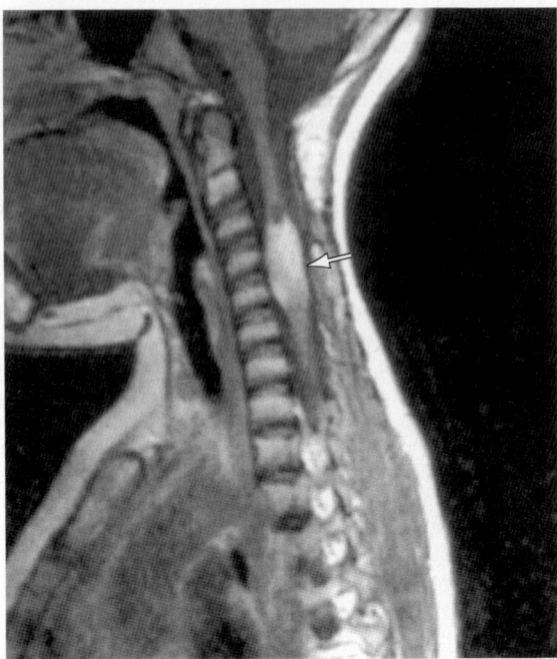

Figure 606-9 T1-weighted MRI scan of a spinal cord tumor *(arrow)*. The fusiform expansion of the cervical cord enhances after intravenous gadolinium injection.

either schwannomas or, in the case of NF-2, neurofibromas. Intraspinal meningiomas in children are essentially found only in patients with NF-2. The intradural extramedullary compartment is also a site for metastatic tumors from primary cancers such as leukemia or primitive neuroectodermal tumors.

Extradural spinal tumors characteristically begin in the bones of the spine. Primary tumors in this location include aneurysmal bone cysts, Langerhans cell histiocytosis (formerly called eosinophilic granuloma), and giant cell tumors. In infants, the extradural space is often the site of neuroblastomas or ganglioneuroblastomas, which tend to be present in the epidural space and in the paraspinous tissue through the intervertebral foramen. In older patients, the bones of the spine may be the site of multiple myeloma and metastases from common malignant tumors.

CLINICAL MANIFESTATIONS
With the exception of the uncommon malignant glial tumors of the spinal cord, which tend to present precipitously, intramedullary spinal cord tumors present in a very insidious manner. Back pain related to the level of the tumor is a common presenting complaint. It is likely that this pain will awaken the child from sleep and improve as the day progresses. Before the use of MRI became routine, the time from the first onset of symptoms to diagnosis of the tumor could be as long as 9 yr. Weakness, gait disturbance, and sensory deficits are usually minor and are often found when formal neurologic examinations are performed. Scoliosis, urinary urgency, and incontinence may be the presenting complaints associated with intramedullary spinal cord tumors.

Extramedullary extradural tumors have a propensity to cause an acute block of the CSF pathways owing to rapid growth within a confined space. Such children present with a flaccid paraplegia, urinary retention, and a patulous anus. Some extramedullary tumors produce the *Brown-Séquard syndrome,* which consists of ipsilateral weakness, spasticity, and ataxia, with contralateral loss of pain and temperature sensation. Papilledema is observed in a few patients, usually in association with markedly elevated CSF protein levels that presumably interfere with normal CSF flow dynamics.

Nerve sheath tumors primarily arise from the sensory rootlet of the exiting spinal nerve. They are very slow-growing tumors and

present with symptoms and signs relative to the nerve root involved. Pain in a band-like distribution around the chest or into an extremity is the most common presenting complaint. Tumor growth eventually leads to spinal cord compression and involvement of adjacent nerve roots.

Tumors rarely arise in the fat of the epidural space; most epidural tumors arise in the bony compartment of the spine. They can present abruptly with severe pain and neurologic deficit at the time of pathologic fracture of the vertebral body. Benign tumors such as giant cell tumors and aneurysmal bone cysts present more insidiously as the tumor slowly grows and begins to compress neural structures.

DIAGNOSTIC EVALUATION
MRI with and without gadolinium enhancement of the spinal cord is the diagnostic study of choice and is essential in the diagnosis of spinal cord tumors, especially intramedullary spinal cord tumors. Most astrocytic tumors of the spinal cord and most ependymomas show diffuse enhancement and will distend the spinal cord focally. These tumors may involve the entire length of the spinal cord (holocord astrocytomas). MRI also shows the relationship between the normal spinal cord and tumor embedded within spinal cord tissue. These tumors are frequently associated with a syrinx, which is usually distal to the tumor. Nerve sheath tumors characteristically enhance and are focal. They may exit through the neural foramen and distend the canal as can be seen on MRI. They also may be visualized on plain radiographs of the affected area of the spine.

Plain radiographs of the spine are helpful in defining the relationship of extradural tumors to the bony spine and in documenting evidence of instability in the case of pathologic compression fractures. When a pathologic fracture occurs, CT is essential to determine the effect of the tumor on the bone. Because many of these tumors occur as metastatic lesions, a general staging of the extent of disease is essential. In the case of Langerhans cell histiocytosis, a thorough bone survey should be conducted to look for other lesions. Radionucleotide bone scanning is also useful in determining the extent of the disease.

TREATMENT
The primary treatment of both intramedullary and extramedullary intradural tumors is surgical removal. For both low-grade astrocytomas and ependymomas, microsurgical removal with the intent of total removal is the treatment of choice. This goal should be attainable in all patients with ependymomas and in most patients with low-grade astrocytomas and gangliogliomas. Adjunctive treatment of these tumors is unwarranted in patients treated with adequate surgical resection. Likewise, schwannomas should be resectable. Occasionally, however, the nerve root must be resected. Doing so may be of no consequence in the thoracic spinal cord, but an attempt to remove the tumor while salvaging the motor root in the cervical and lumbosacral region is critical to preserve movement. Malignant astrocytic tumors cannot be resected without major morbidity and, in any case, carry an extremely poor prognosis. In the case of grades III and IV astrocytomas of the spinal cord, decompression and biopsy followed by radiation therapy and possibly chemotherapy are utilized.

The diagnosis and treatment of extramedullary spinal cord tumors must be individualized. Patients with distention of the vertebral body or with unstable pathologic fractures benefit from extensive resection of the involved vertebral bodies and will likely need fusion. For extramedullary tumors with soft-tissue components such as neuroblastomas, treatment is determined by the nature of the tumor and degree of spinal cord compression, and directed following needle biopsy of the lesion. In the absence of significant neurologic compression, surgical intervention is rarely indicated.

OUTCOME
The prognosis for patients with benign intramedullary spinal cord tumors depends, to some extent, on the patient's condition at the time of surgical intervention. It is very unlikely that nonambulatory patients will improve after surgery. If, however, patients are ambulatory at the time of surgery, they may experience increased weakness after surgery.

They are likely to recover at least their preoperative level of function. Malignant spinal cord tumors are usually lethal with death resulting from diffuse metastases via the CSF pathways. Successful resection of nerve sheath tumors should be curative. In the context of neurofibromatosis, however, many more tumors can be found at other levels or can be expected to develop later in life. Surgical intervention in the context of neurofibromatoses should be performed only on clearly symptomatic lesions.

The outcome of treatment of extramedullary tumors depends on the cell type and, in most cases, on the efficacy of nonsurgical, adjunctive therapies. For aneurysmal bone cysts and giant cell tumors, resection of the tumor and fusion of the spine are the treatments of choice.

The significant majority of spinal cord tumors in children are benign (World Health Organization grades 2 and 3). The intramedullary low-grade glial tumors for the most part act the same as the same histology in the brain. The evidence would point to the fact that intramedullary ependymomas act in a more benign fashion than they do in the fourth ventricle. Gross total removal without adjuvant treatment is the preferred method of treatment and carries not only much longer progression free survival but improved quality of life as well.

Bibliography is available at Expert Consult.

606.5 Spinal Cord Injuries in Children
Harold L. Rekate

Spine and spinal cord injuries are very rare in children, particularly in young children. The spine of a small child is very mobile, and fractures of the spine are exceedingly rare. This increased mobility is not always a positive feature. Transfer of energy leading to spinal distortion can maintain the structural integrity of the spine but lead to significant injuries of the spinal cord. Spinal cord injury without radiographic bone (vertebral) abnormalities, called **SCIWORA,** is more common in children than adults. There seem to be 2 distinct forms. The infantile form involves severe injury of the cervical or thoracic spine. These patients have a poor likelihood of complete recovery. In older children and adolescents, SCIWORA is more likely to cause a less-severe injury and the likelihood of complete recovery over time is high. The adolescent form is assumed to be a spinal cord concussion or mild contusion as opposed to the severe spinal cord injury related to the mobility of the spine in small children.

Although the mechanisms of spinal cord injury in children include birth trauma, falls, and child abuse, the major cause of morbidity and mortality remains motor vehicle injuries. Although the mechanisms of injury and diagnosis are distinct in very small children, adolescents incur spinal cord injuries with epidemiology similar to that of adults, including significant male predominance and a high likelihood of fracture dislocations of the lower cervical spine or thoracolumbar region. In infants and children younger than age 5 yr, fractures and mechanical disruption of spinal elements are limited to the upper cervical spine between the occiput and C3.

CLINICAL MANIFESTATIONS
One in 3 patients with significant trauma to the spine and spinal cord will have a concomitant severe head injury, which makes early diagnosis challenging. For these patients clinical evaluation may be difficult. They need to be maintained in a protective environment such as a collar until the appropriate radiographs can be obtained. A careful neurologic examination is necessary for infants with suspected spinal cord injuries. Complete spinal cord injury will lead to **spinal shock** with early areflexia. Severe cervical spinal cord injuries will usually lead to paradoxical respiration in patients who are breathing spontaneously. Paradoxical respiration occurs when the diaphragm functions because the phrenic nerves from C3, C4, and C5 are functioning normally but the intercostal musculature innervated by the thoracic spinal cord is paralyzed. In this situation, inspiration fails to expand of the chest wall but distends the abdomen.

The *mildest injury* to the spinal cord is transient quadriparesis evident for seconds or minutes with complete recovery in 24 hr. This injury follows a concussion of the cord.

A transverse injury in the high cervical cord level (C1-C2) causes respiratory arrest and death in the absence of ventilatory support. *Fracture dislocations at the C5-C6 level* resulting in spinal cord injuries are characterized by flaccid quadriparesis, loss of sphincter function, and a sensory level corresponding to the upper sternum. Fractures or dislocations in the low thoracic (T12-L1) region may produce the **conus medullaris syndrome,** which includes a loss of urinary and rectal sphincter control, flaccid weakness, and sensory disturbances of the legs. A **central cord lesion** may result from contusion and hemorrhage and typically involves the upper extremities to a greater degree than the legs. There are lower motor neuron signs in the upper extremities and upper motor neuron signs in the legs, bladder dysfunction, and loss of sensation caudal to the lesion. There may be considerable recovery, particularly in the lower extremities.

Thoracolumbar injuries are usually fracture–dislocations such as occur in severe motor vehicle accidents when children are wearing lap belts but not shoulder harnesses. These injuries lead to a conus medullaris syndrome. These patients exhibit a loss of bowel and bladder function and lower motor neuron injuries involving the innervation of the lower extremities.

CLEARING THE CERVICAL SPINE IN CHILDREN
The management of children following major trauma is challenging. Clearing the cervical spine in children carries some of the same issues as it does in comatose adults in that with small children you cannot count on their cooperation with positioning for radiographs and complaints of pain are difficult to assess. There has been an increasing emphasis on the use of MRI for the evaluation of potential cervical spine instability but in small children this study requires sedation and, in most centers, the presence of an anesthesiologist. Despite the radiation dose, it is clear that the CT scan is the most important study with 100% sensitivity and 95% specificity. A multiply injured child is likely to be in the scanner having other anatomic studies done in any case and no other study has been shown to be better for detection of unstable cervical spine injury. This test detects all significant injuries to the cervical spine and has very few false-positives as opposed to MRI scanning, which overcalls the injury 1 in 4 times.

TREATMENT
The initial management of spine and spinal cord injuries in children is similar to that in adults. The cervical spine should be immobilized in the field by the emergency medical technicians. In cases of acute spinal cord injury, some data support the acute infusion of a bolus of high-dose (30 mg/kg) methylprednisolone followed by a 23 hr infusion (5.4 mg/kg/hr). The data for this treatment in children are controversial.

Surgical management of unstable spinal injuries must be tailored to the patient's age. For occipitocervical dislocations, early surgery with fusion from the occiput to C2 or C3 should be performed, even in babies older than 6 mo. Fixation of the subaxial spine must be tailored to the size of the pedicles and other osseus structures of the developing axial skeleton.

PREVENTION
The most important aspect of the care of spinal cord injuries in children relates to injury prevention. In this regard, the use of appropriate child restraints in automobiles is the most important precaution. In older children and adolescents, rules against spear tackling in football and the "Feet First, First Time Program" from the Think First Foundation aimed at adolescents diving into swimming pools and natural water areas are important ways to help prevent severe cervical spinal cord injuries.

Bibliography is available at Expert Consult.

606.6 Transverse Myelitis

Harold L. Rekate

Transverse myelitis (TM) is a condition characterized by rapid development of both motor and sensory deficits at any level of the spinal cord. TM presents acutely as either partial or complete cord involvement and is defined as evidence of spinal cord inflammation by an MRI-documented enhancing lesion, or CSF pleocytosis (>10 cells), or increased immunoglobulin G index. The progression is rapid and the time to maximal disability is more than 4 hr and fewer than 21 days. It has multiple causes and tends to occur in 2 distinct contexts. Small children, 3 yr of age and younger, develop spinal cord dysfunction over hours to a few days. They have a history of an infectious disease, usually of viral origin, or of an immunization within the few weeks preceding the development of their neurologic difficulties. The clinical loss of function is often severe and may seem complete. Although a slow recovery (weeks to months) is common in these cases, it is likely to be incomplete. The likelihood of independent ambulation in these small children is approximately 40%. The pathologic findings of perivascular infiltration with mononuclear cells imply an infectious or inflammatory basis. Overt necrosis of spinal cord may rarely be seen.

In older children, the syndrome is somewhat different. Although the onset is also rapid with a nadir in neurologic function occurring between 2 days and 2 wk, recovery is more rapid and more likely to be complete. Pathologic or imaging examination shows acute demyelination.

CLINICAL MANIFESTATIONS

TM is often preceded within the previous 1-3 wk by a mild nonspecific illness, minimal trauma, or perhaps an immunization. In both forms the patient shows or complains of discomfort or overt pain in the neck or back, depending on the level of the lesion. The most common involved segments are in the thoracic region. Depending on its severity, the condition progresses to numbness, anesthesia, ataxia, areflexia, and motor weakness in the truncal and appendicular musculature at or distal to the lesion. Paralysis begins as flaccidity (paraparesis, tetraparesis), but over a few weeks spasticity develops and is evident by hyper-

reflexia and clonus. Rarely is the weakness unilateral. Urinary retention is an early finding; incontinence occurs later in the course. Most have sensory loss manifest as anesthesia, paresthesia, or allodynia. Other findings may include priapism and vision loss (neuromyelitis optica), as well as spinal shock and subsequent autonomic dysreflexia.

The differential diagnosis includes demyelinating disorders, overt meningitis, spinal cord infarction, or mass lesions such as bony distortion, abscess, and spine and spinal cord tumors (Table 606-1).

DIAGNOSTIC EVALUATION

MRI with and without contrast enhancement is essential to rule out a mass lesion requiring neurosurgical intervention. In both conditions, T1-weighted images of the spine at the anatomic level of involvement may be normal or may show distention of the spinal cord. In the infantile form, T2-weighted images show high signal intensity that extends over multiple segments. In the adolescent form, the high signal intensity may be limited to 1 or 2 segments. A limited degree of contrast enhancement after the administration of gadolinium is expected, especially in the infantile form, and denotes an inflammatory condition (Fig. 606-10). MRI of the brain is also indicated and shows evidence of other foci of demyelination in at least 30% of patients; in these patients and those with encephalopathy, acute disseminated encephalomyelitis must be considered (Fig. 606-11).

After a mass lesion associated with spinal cord compression or complete subarachnoid column block from spinal cord swelling have been ruled out, a lumbar puncture is indicated. In both forms of disease, the number of mononuclear cells is usually elevated. The level of CSF protein maybe elevated or normal. CSF should be analyzed for myelin basic protein and immunoglobulin levels, which are usually elevated in TM. The presence of inflammatory cells is essential for the diagnosis of TM.

Because one of the most important possibilities for this condition is neuromyelitis optica (NMO; Devic syndrome) the serum of all patients should be analyzed for the NMO antibody. This test is positive in most patients with NMO (see Chapter 600.2). NMO is associated with bilateral optic neuritis and recurrent or long segment TM (≥3 segments). NMO may involve any spinal segment in addition to the brainstem or conus medullaris and cauda equina (myeloradiculitis). As in adults with

Table 606-1	Clinical and Radiologic Mimics of Transverse Myelitis

EXTRAAXIAL COMPRESSION DISEASE	SPINAL CORD DISORDERS
1. Vertebral spine disorders	1. Congenital malformation
a. Trauma	a. Neurenteric cysts
i. Blunt	b. Spinal cord tethering
ii. Penetrating	2. Infection
iii. Surfing	a. Nonpolio enteroviruses
b. Atlantoaxial subluxation	b. West Nile virus
i. Trisomy 21	c. Human T-lymphocyte virus 1
ii. Mucopolysaccharidosis type IV	d. Neurocysticercosis
iii. Grisel syndrome	3. Vascular disorders
c. Destructive lesions	a. Arteriovenous malformation
i. Tuberculosis	b. Cavernomas
ii. Lymphoma	c. Cobb syndrome
iii. Langerhans cell histiocytosis	d. Fibrocartilaginous embolization
d. Scheuermann disease	e. Spinal cord infarction
2. Epidural disease	4. Vasculitis
a. Tumor	a. Systemic lupus erythematosus
i. Neuroblastoma	b. Behçet disease
ii. Wilms tumor	5. Nutritional disorders
iii. Ewing sarcoma	a. Vitamin B_{12} deficiency (Subacute combined degeneration)
b. Abscess	6. Toxic injury
i. Associated dermal sinus, vertebral body infection	a. Chemotherapy (e.g., methotrexate)
c. Hematoma	b. Radiation
3. Arachnoiditis	7. Immune mediated
a. Tuberculosis	a. Acute disseminated encephalomyelitis
b. Cryptococcosis	b. Neuromyelitis optica
c. Carcinomatous infiltration	c. Multiple sclerosis
4. Spinal nerve root inflammation	
a. Guillain-Barré syndrome	

Modified from Thomas T, Branson HM: Childhood transverse myelitis and its mimics. Neuroimaging Clin N Am 23:267–278, 2013, Box 11.

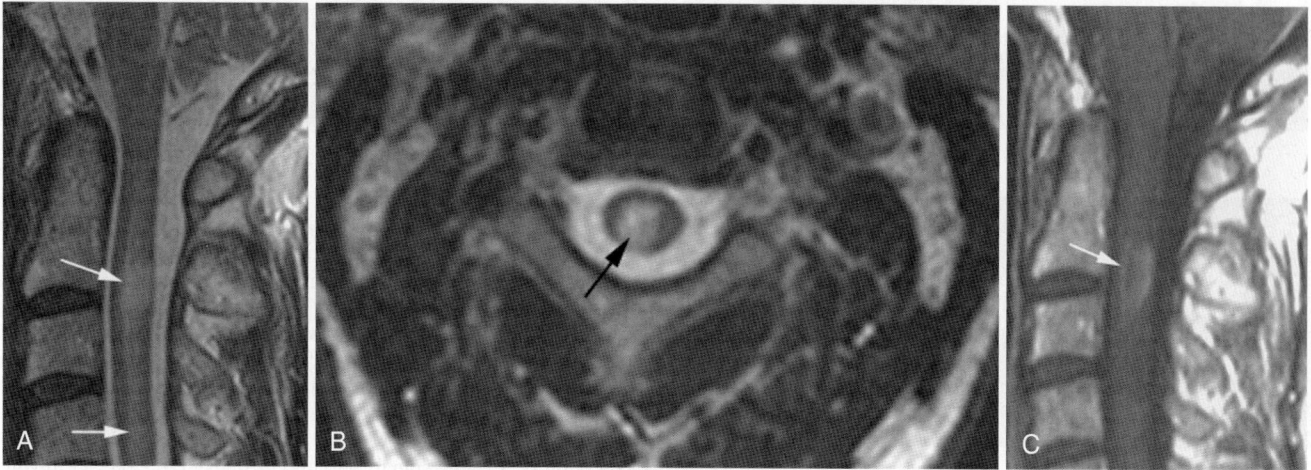

Figure 606-10 Transverse myelitis. **A,** Sagittal T2-weighted image demonstrates a longitudinal hyperintense spinal cord lesion spanning three vertebral segments *(arrows)*. **B,** On an axial T2-weighted image, the lesion involves more than two-thirds of the cord's cross-sectional area *(arrow)*. **C,** Sagittal T1-weighted postcontrast image shows an enhancing area within the lesion *(arrow)*. *(From Ajtai B, Lindzen E, Masdeu JC: Structural imaging: magnetic resonance imaging and computed tomography. In Daroff RB, Fenichel GM, Jankovic J, Mazziotta JC, editors: Bradley's neurology in clinical practice, ed 6. Philadelphia, 2012, WB Saunders, Fig. 33A.96.)*

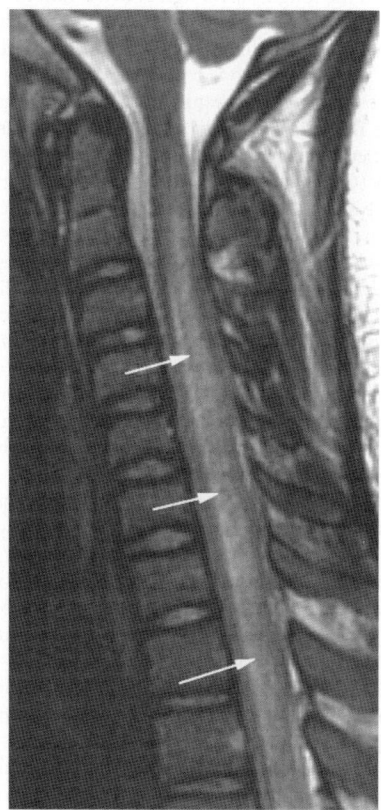

Figure 606-11 Acute disseminated encephalomyelitis. Sagittal T2-weighted image shows a diffuse hyperintense lesion spanning the length of the cervical cord *(arrows)*. Note the enlarged caliber of the cord, which is a result of swelling. *(From Ajtai B, Lindzen E, Masdeu JC: Structural imaging: magnetic resonance imaging and computed tomography. In Daroff RB, Fenichel GM, Jankovic J, Mazziotta JC, editors: Bradley's neurology in clinical practice, ed 6. Philadelphia, 2012, WB Saunders, Fig. 33A.95.)*

TM, older children with the condition should have serum studies sent for autoimmune disorders, especially systemic lupus erythematosus.

TREATMENT
There are no standards for the treatment of TM. Available evidence suggests that modulation of the immune response may be effective in decreasing the severity and duration of the condition. The use of high-dose steroids, particularly methylprednisolone, is the initial approach to treatment of childhood forms of TM. If there is a poor response to high-dose steroids, other therapeutic approaches include intravenous immunoglobulin, plasma exchanges, rituximab, and cyclophosphamide.

Follow-up of children with TM often reveals poor ambulation, continued bowel or bladder symptoms and dysesthesias.

Bibliography is available at Expert Consult.

606.7 Spinal Arteriovenous Malformations
Harold L. Rekate

Arteriovenous malformations of the spinal cord are rare lesions in children. Only about 60 patients younger than age 18 yr are treated in the United States each year. These lesions are complex. Despite their rarity there are multiple subtypes, which require different treatment strategies. Patients commonly present with back or neck pain, depending on the segments of the spinal cord involved, and they may experience the insidious onset of motor and sensory disturbances. Sudden onset of paraplegia secondary to hemorrhage has been reported. Occasionally, patients present with subarachnoid hemorrhage without overt neurologic deficits, similar to the presentation associated with cerebral aneurysms. In some cases, bruits are audible upon auscultation over the bony spine.

DIAGNOSTIC EVALUATION
When a spinal arteriovenous malformation is suspected, MRI of the spinal cord is first needed to make the diagnosis and to obtain a general idea of the location of the lesion. MR angiography or CT angiography may provide further information, but formal catheter angiography of the spinal cord is needed to obtain an adequate understanding of the complex anatomy of the lesion and to plan the intervention.

TREATMENT
Open microsurgery had been the mainstay of treatment for spinal cord arteriovenous fistulas and arteriovenous malformations. With the rapid development of interventional techniques, the percentage of patients undergoing microsurgery has decreased from 70% to approximately 30%. Stereotactic radiosurgery may be used adjunctively. Treatment of these complex lesions requires the commitment of an organized neurovascular treatment program.

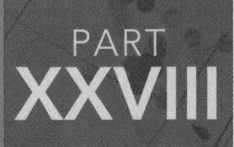
Chapter 607

Evaluation and Investigation

Harvey B. Sarnat

The term **neuromuscular disease** defines disorders of the motor unit and excludes influences on muscular function from the brain, such as spasticity. The motor unit has 4 components: a motor neuron in the brainstem or ventral horn of the spinal cord; its axon, which together with other axons forms the peripheral nerve; the neuromuscular junction; and all muscle fibers innervated by a single motor neuron. The size of the motor unit varies among different muscles and with the precision of muscular function required. In large muscles, such as the glutei and quadriceps femoris, hundreds of muscle fibers are innervated by a single motor neuron; in small, finely tuned muscles, such as the stapedius or the extraocular muscles, a 1:1 ratio can prevail. The motor unit is influenced by suprasegmental or upper motor neuron control that alters properties of muscle tone, precision of movement, reciprocal inhibition of antagonistic muscles during movement, and sequencing of muscle contractions to achieve smooth, coordinated movements. Suprasegmental impulses also augment or inhibit the monosynaptic stretch reflex; the corticospinal tract is inhibitory upon this reflex.

Diseases of the motor unit are common in children. These neuromuscular diseases may be genetically determined, congenital or acquired, acute or chronic, and progressive or static. Because specific therapy is available for many diseases and because of genetic and prognostic implications, precise diagnosis is important; laboratory confirmation is required for most diseases because of overlapping clinical manifestations.

Many chromosomal loci are identified with specific neuromuscular diseases as a result of genetic linkage studies and the isolation and cloning of a few specific genes. In some cases, such as Duchenne muscular dystrophy, the genetic defect is a deletion of nucleotide sequences and is associated with a defective protein product, dystrophin. In other cases, such as myotonic muscular dystrophy, the genetic defect is an expansion or repetition, rather than a deletion, in a codon (a set of 3 consecutive nucleotide repeats that encodes for a single amino acid), with many copies of a particular codon (in this example they are also associated with abnormal messenger RNA). Some diseases manifest as autosomal dominant and autosomal recessive traits in different pedigrees; these distinct mendelian genotypes can result from different genetic mutations on different chromosomes (nemaline myopathy) or from small differences in the same gene at the same chromosomal locus (myotonia congenita), despite many common phenotypic features and shared histopathologic findings in a muscle biopsy specimen. Among the several clinically defined mitochondrial myopathies, specific mitochondrial DNA deletions and transfer RNA point mutations are recognized. The inheritance patterns and chromosomal and mitochondrial loci of common neuromuscular diseases affecting infants and children are summarized in Table 608-1 in Chapter 608.

CLINICAL MANIFESTATIONS

Examination of the neuromuscular system includes an assessment of muscle bulk, tone, and strength. Tone and strength should not be confused: **Passive tone** is range of motion around a joint; **active tone** is physiologic resistance to movement. Head lag when an infant is pulled to a sitting position from supine is a sign of weakness, not of low tone. Hypotonia may be associated with normal strength or with weakness; enlarged muscles may be weak or strong; thin, wasted muscles may be weak or have unexpectedly normal strength. The distribution of these components is of diagnostic importance. In general, myopathies follow a proximal distribution of weakness and muscle wasting (with the notable exception of myotonic muscular dystrophy); neuropathies are generally distal in distribution (with the notable exception of juvenile spinal muscular atrophy; Table 607-1). Involvement of the face, tongue, palate, and extraocular muscles provides an important distinction in the differential diagnosis. **Tendon stretch reflexes** are generally lost in neuropathies and in motor neuron diseases and are diminished but preserved in myopathies (Table 607-1). A few specific clinical features are important in the diagnosis of some neuromuscular diseases. **Fasciculations** of muscle, which are often best seen in the tongue, are a sign of denervation. Sensory abnormalities indicate neuropathy. Fatigable weakness is characteristic of neuromuscular junctional disorders. Myotonia is specific for a few myopathies.

Some features do not distinguish myopathy from neuropathy. Muscle pain or **myalgias** are associated with acute disease of either myopathic or neurogenic origin. Acute dermatomyositis and acute polyneuropathy (Guillain-Barré syndrome) are characterized by myalgias. Muscular dystrophies and spinal muscular atrophies are not associated with muscle pain. Myalgias also occur in several metabolic diseases of muscle and in ischemic myopathy, including vascular diseases such as dermatomyositis. Myalgias denote the acuity, rather than the nature, of the process, so that progressive but chronic diseases, such as muscular dystrophy and spinal muscular atrophy, are not painful but acute stages of inflammatory myopathies and acute denervation of muscle often do present with muscular pain and tenderness to palpation. **Contractures** of muscles, whether present at birth or developing later in the course of an illness, occur in both myopathic and neurogenic diseases.

Infant boys who are weak in late fetal life and in the neonatal period often have **undescended testes**. The testes are actively pulled into the scrotum from the anterior abdominal wall by a pair of cords that consist of smooth and striated muscle called the gubernacula. The gubernacula are weakened in many congenital neuromuscular diseases, including spinal muscular atrophy, myotonic muscular dystrophy, and many congenital myopathies.

The thorax of infants with congenital neuromuscular disease often has a funnel shape, and the ribs are thin and radiolucent as a result of intercostal muscle weakness during intrauterine growth. This phenomenon is characteristically found in infantile spinal muscular atrophy but also occurs in myotubular myopathy, neonatal myotonic dystrophy, and other disorders (Fig. 607-1). Because of the small muscle mass, birthweight may be low for gestational age.

Generalized hypotonia and motor developmental delay are the most common presenting manifestations of neuromuscular disease in infants and young children (Table 607-2). These features can also be expressions of neurologic disease, endocrine and systemic metabolic diseases, and Down syndrome, or they may be nonspecific neuromuscular expressions of malnutrition or chronic systemic illness (Table 607-3). A prenatal history of decreased fetal movements and intrauterine growth retardation is often found in patients who are symptomatic at birth. Developmental disorders tend to be of slow onset and are progressive. Acute flaccid paralysis in older infants and children has a different differential diagnosis (Table 607-4).

LABORATORY FINDINGS
Serum Enzymes

Several lysosomal enzymes are released by damaged or degenerating muscle fibers and may be measured in serum. The most useful of these enzymes is **creatine kinase (CK)**, which is found in only 3 organs and may be separated into corresponding isozymes: MM for skeletal muscle, MB for cardiac muscle, and BB for brain. Serum CK determination is not a universal screening test for neuromuscular disease because many diseases of the motor unit are not associated with elevated enzymes. The CK level is characteristically elevated in certain diseases, such as Duchenne muscular dystrophy, and the magnitude of increase is characteristic for particular diseases.

Table 607-1	Distinguishing Features of Disorders of the Motor System							
LOCUS OF LESION	**WEAKNESS**				**DEEP TENDON REFLEXES**	**ELECTRO-MYOGRAPHY**	**MUSCLE BIOPSY**	**OTHER**
	Face	Arms	Legs	Proximal–Distal				
Central	0	+	+	≥	Normal or ↑	Normal	Normal	Seizures, hemiparesis, and delayed development
Ventral horn cell	Late	++++	++++	≥	0	Fasciculations and fibrillations	Denervation pattern	Fasciculations (tongue)
Peripheral nerve	0	+++	+++	<	↓	Fibrillations	Denervation pattern	Sensory deficit, elevated cerebrospinal fluid protein, depressed nerve biopsy
Neuromuscular junction	+++	+++	+++	=	Normal	Decremental response (myasthenia); incremental response and BSAP (botulism)	Normal	Response to neostigmine or edrophonium (myasthenia); constipation and fixed pupils (botulism)
Muscle	Variable (+ to ++++)	++	+	>	↓	Short duration, small-amplitude motor unit potentials and myopathic polyphasic potentials	Myopathic pattern*	Elevated muscle enzyme levels (variable)

*Can also show unique features, such as in central core disease, nemaline myopathy, myotubular myopathy, and congenital fiber type disproportion.
 + to ++++, varying degrees of severity; BSAP, brief duration, small amplitude, overly abundant motor unit potentials.
 From Volpe J: Neurology of the newborn, ed 4, Philadelphia, 2001, WB Saunders, p. 706.

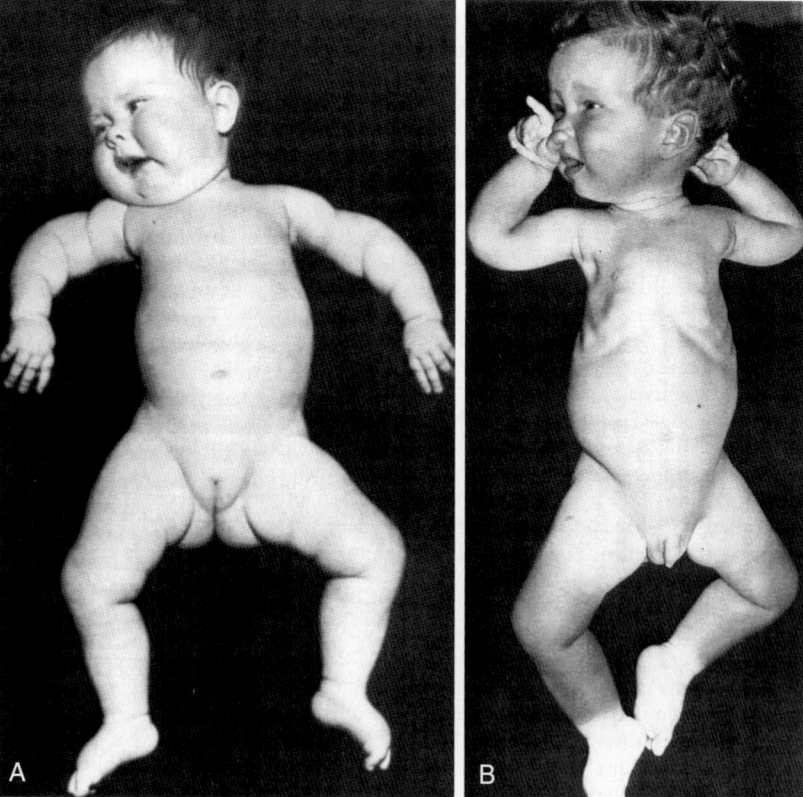

Figure 607-1 Type 1 spinal muscular atrophy (Werdnig-Hoffmann disease). Characteristic postures in 6 wk old **(A)** and 1 yr old **(B)** infants with severe weakness and hypotonia from birth. Note the frogleg posture of the lower limbs and internal rotation ("jug handle") **(A)** or external rotation **(B)** at the shoulders. Note also intercostal recession, especially evident in **B**, and normal facial expressions. *(From Volpe J: Neurology of the newborn, ed 4, Philadelphia, 2001, WB Saunders, p. 645.)*

Table 607-2	Pattern of Weakness and Localization in the Floppy Infant	
ANATOMIC REGION OF HYPOTONIA	**CORRESPONDING DISORDERS**	**PATTERN OF WEAKNESS AND INVOLVEMENT**
Central nervous system	Chromosomal disorders Inborn errors of metabolism Cerebral dysgenesis Cerebral, spinal cord trauma	Central hypotonia Axial hypotonia more prominent Hyperactive reflexes
Motor neuron	Spinal muscular atrophy	Generalized weakness; often spares the diaphragm, facial muscles, pelvis, and sphincters
Nerve	Peripheral neuropathies	Distal muscle groups involved Weakness with wasting
Neuromuscular junction	Myasthenia syndromes Infantile botulism	Bulbar, oculomotor muscles exhibit greater degree of involvement
Muscle	Congenital myopathies Metabolic myopathies Congenital muscular dystrophy Congenital myotonic dystrophy	Weakness is prominent Proximal musculature Hypoactive reflexes Joint contractures

From Prasad AN, Prasad C: The floppy infant: contribution of genetic and metabolic disorders, Brain Dev 27:457–476, 2003.

Molecular Genetic Markers

Many DNA markers of hereditary myopathies, including the muscular dystrophies, and neuropathies are available from leukocytes in blood samples. If the clinical manifestations suggest a particular disease, these tests can provide a definitive diagnosis and not subject the child to more-invasive procedures, such as muscle biopsy. Other molecular markers are available only in muscle biopsy tissue.

Nerve Conduction Velocity

Motor and sensory nerve conduction velocity may be measured electrophysiologically by using surface electrodes. Neuropathies of various types are detected by decreased conduction. The site of a traumatic nerve injury may also be localized. The nerve conduction value at birth is about half of the mature value achieved by age 2 yr. Tables are available for normal values at various ages in infancy, including for preterm infants. Because the nerve conduction velocity study measures only the fastest conducting fibers in a nerve, 80% of the total nerve fibers must be involved before slowing in conduction is detected.

Electromyography

Electromyography (EMG) requires insertion of a needle into the belly of a muscle and recording of the electric potentials in various states of contraction. It is less useful in pediatrics than in adult medicine, in part because of technical difficulties in recording these potentials in young children and in part because the best results require the patient's cooperation for full relaxation and maximal voluntary contraction of a muscle. Many children are too frightened to provide such cooperation. Characteristic EMG patterns distinguish denervation from myopathic involvement. The specific type of myopathy is not usually definitively diagnosed, but certain specialized myopathic conditions, such as myotonia, may be demonstrated. An EMG can transiently raise the serum CK level.

EMG combined with repetitive electrical stimulation of a motor nerve supplying a muscle to produce tetany is useful in demonstrating myasthenic decremental responses. Small muscles, such as the abductor digiti quinti of the hypothenar eminence, are used for such studies. Additional specialized tests, such as single myofiber EMG, may provide supplementary evidence in selected cases, but are performed only in large neuromuscular centers.

Imaging of Muscle and Central Nervous System

Ultrasonography, CT scans, and, more often, MRI are used to image muscle in many neuromuscular diseases. Although these methods are not always definitively diagnostic, in experienced hands, they provide a supplementary means of following the progression of disease over time. MRI is quite useful in identifying inflammatory myopathies of immune (dermatomyositis) or infectious (viral, bacterial, parasitic) origin. MRI is the study of choice to image the spinal cord, if a tumor or other structural lesion of the spinal cord is suspected as the cause of muscular dysfunction, and nerve roots and plexus (e.g., brachial plexus). Brain MRI is indicated in some myopathies, such as the congenital muscular dystrophies, in which cerebral malformations often accompany the myopathy because the mutated gene responsible is expressed in both muscle and the developing brain.

Muscle Biopsy

The muscle biopsy is traditionally the most important and specific diagnostic study of most neuromuscular disorders, if the definitive diagnosis of a hereditary disease is not provided by molecular genetic testing in blood. Not only are neurogenic and myopathic processes distinguished, but also the type of myopathy and specific enzymatic deficiencies may be determined. The vastus lateralis (quadriceps femoris) is the muscle that is most commonly sampled. The deltoid muscle should be avoided in most cases because it normally has a 60-80% predominance of type I fibers so that the distribution patterns of fiber types are difficult to recognize. Muscle biopsy is a simple outpatient procedure that may be performed under local anesthesia with or without femoral nerve block. Needle biopsies are preferred in some centers but are not percutaneous and require an incision in the skin similar to open biopsy; numerous samples must be taken to conduct an adequate examination of the tissue, and they provide inferior specimens. The volume of tissue from a needle biopsy is usually not adequate for all required studies, including supplementary biochemical studies, such as mitochondrial respiratory chain enzymes; a small, clean, open biopsy is therefore advantageous.

Histochemical studies of frozen sections of the muscle are obligatory in all pediatric muscle biopsies because many congenital and metabolic myopathies cannot be diagnosed from paraffin sections using conventional histologic stains. Immunohistochemistry is a useful supplement in some cases, such as for demonstrating dystrophin in suspected Duchenne muscular dystrophy or merosin in congenital muscular dystrophy. A portion of the biopsy specimen should be fixed for potential electron microscopy, but ultrastructure has additional diagnostic value only in selected cases. Interpretation of muscle biopsy samples is complex and should be performed by an experienced pathologist. A portion of frozen muscle tissue should also be routinely saved for possible biochemical analysis (mitochondrial cytopathies, carnitine palmitoyltransferase, acid maltase).

Immunocytochemical reactivities can be applied to formalin-fixed, paraffin-embedded sections and do not require frozen sections. Some reactivities, such as slow and fast myosin, can distinguish fiber types and hence substitute for myofibrillar adenosine triphosphatase histochemical stains in frozen sections. An increasing number of sarcolemmal regional proteins can be demonstrated that are specific for

Table 607-3	Differential Diagnosis of Infantile Hypotonia

Cerebral hypotonia
- Benign congenital hypotonia
- Chromosome disorders
- Prader-Willi syndrome
- Trisomy
- Chronic nonprogressive encephalopathy
- Cerebral malformation
- Perinatal distress
- Postnatal disorders
- Peroxisomal disorders
- Cerebrohepatorenal syndrome (Zellweger syndrome)
- Neonatal adrenoleukodystrophy
- Other genetic defects
- Familial dysautonomia
- Oculocerebrorenal syndrome (Lowe syndrome)
- Other metabolic defects
- Acid maltase deficiency (see "Metabolic Myopathies")
- Infantile G_M gangliosidosis

Spinal cord disorders
Spinal muscular atrophies
- Acute infantile
  - Autosomal dominant
  - Autosomal recessive
- Cytochrome-c oxidase deficiency
- X-linked
- Chronic infantile
  - Autosomal dominant
  - Autosomal recessive
- Congenital cervical spinal muscular atrophy
- Infantile neuronal degeneration
- Neurogenic arthrogryposis

Polyneuropathies
- Congenital hypomyelinating neuropathy
- Giant axonal neuropathy
- Hereditary motor-sensory neuropathies

Disorders of neuromuscular transmission
- Familial infantile myasthenia
- Infantile botulism
- Transitory myasthenia gravis

Fiber-type disproportion myopathies
- Central core disease
- Congenital fiber-type disproportion myopathy
- Myotubular (centronuclear) myopathy
- Acute
- Chronic
- Nemaline (nemaline rod) myopathy
- Autosomal dominant
- Autosomal recessive

Metabolic myopathies
- Acid maltase deficiency (Pompe disease)
- Cytochrome-c oxidase deficiency
- Other mitochondrial disorders
- Muscular dystrophies
- Bethlem myopathy
- Congenital dystrophinopathy
- Congenital muscular dystrophy
- Merosin deficiency primary
- Merosin deficiency secondary
- Merosin positive
- Congenital myotonic dystrophy

From Fenichel GM: The hypotonic infant. In Fenichel GM, editor: Clinical pediatric neurology: a signs and symptoms approach, ed 5, Philadelphia, 2005, Saunders, p. 150.

Table 607-4	Differential Diagnosis of Acute Flaccid Paralysis

Brainstem stroke
Brainstem encephalitis
Acute anterior poliomyelitis
- Caused by poliovirus
- Caused by other neurotropic viruses

Acute myelopathy
- Space-occupying lesions
- Acute transverse myelitis

Peripheral neuropathy
- Guillain-Barré syndrome
- Post–rabies vaccine neuropathy
- Diphtheritic neuropathy
- Heavy metals, biologic toxins, or drug intoxication
- Acute intermittent porphyria
- Vasculitic neuropathy
- Critical illness neuropathy
- Lymphomatous neuropathy

Disorders of neuromuscular transmission
- Myasthenia gravis
- Biologic or industrial toxins
- Tic paralysis

Disorders of muscle
- Hypokalemia
- Hypophosphatemia
- Inflammatory myopathy
- Acute rhabdomyolysis
- Trichinosis
- Familial periodic paralyses (normokalemic, hypokalemic, hyperkalemic)

From Hughes RAC, Camblath DR: Guillain-Barré syndrome, Lancet 366:1653–1666, 2005.

Nerve Biopsy

The most commonly sampled nerve is the sural nerve, a pure sensory nerve that supplies a small area of skin on the lateral surface of the foot. Whole or fascicular biopsy specimens of this nerve may be taken. When the sural nerve is severed behind the lateral malleolus of the ankle, regeneration of the nerve occurs in more than 90% of cases, so that permanent sensory loss is not experienced. The sural nerve is often involved in many neuropathies whose clinical manifestations are predominantly motor.

Electron microscopy is performed on most nerve biopsy specimens because many morphologic alterations cannot be appreciated at the resolution of a light microscope. Teased fiber preparations are sometimes useful in demonstrating segmental demyelination, axonal swellings, and other specific abnormalities, but these time-consuming procedures are not done routinely. Special stains may be applied to ordinary frozen or paraffin sections of nerve biopsy material to demonstrate myelin, axoplasm, and metabolic products.

The molecular genetic identification of the specific mutation in many of the hereditary motor and sensory neuropathies, determined from blood samples, has rendered the nerve biopsy much less often performed than in the past, but it retains a great value in selected cases for which the etiology remains elusive despite genetic and electrophysiological testing.

Cardiac Assessment

Cardiac evaluation is important if myopathy is suspected because of involvement of the heart in muscular dystrophies and in inflammatory and metabolic myopathies. Electrocardiography often detects early cardiomyopathy or conduction defects that are clinically asymptomatic. At times, a more complete cardiac work-up, including echocardiography and consultation with a pediatric cardiologist, is indicated. Serial pulmonary function tests also should be performed in muscular dystrophies and in other chronic or progressive diseases of the motor unit.

Bibliography is available at Expert Consult.

each of the various muscular dystrophies and include the dystrophins, merosin, sarcoglycans, and dystroglycans. Ryanodine receptors, important in myasthenia gravis and in malignant hyperthermia, also now can be demonstrated. In addition, immunocytochemical reactivities can distinguish the various types of inflammatory cells in autoimmune myopathies, including T and B lymphocytes and macrophages.

Chapter **608**

Developmental Disorders of Muscle

Harvey B. Sarnat

A heterogeneous group of congenital neuromuscular disorders is known as the **congenital myopathies** (Tables 608-1 and 608-2). Most of these disorders have subcellular abnormalities that can be demonstrated only by muscle biopsy, by means of histochemistry and electron microscopy. In others, the muscle biopsy abnormality is not a subcellular anatomic defect but an aberration in the ratio and sizes of specific myofiber types. A genetic basis is demonstrated in many of the congenital myopathies, and molecular genetic testing from blood samples may confirm the diagnosis without muscle biopsy.

Most congenital myopathies are nonprogressive conditions, but some patients show slow clinical deterioration accompanied by additional changes in their muscle histology. In some congenital myopathies, such as severe neonatal nemaline myopathy, the clinical expression can be life-threatening because of dysphagia and respiratory and/or cardiac insufficiency. *Cardiomyopathy develops in some patients with congenital myopathies* (Table 608-3). Most of the diseases in the category of congenital myopathies are hereditary; others are

sporadic. Although clinical features, including phenotype, can raise a strong suspicion of a congenital myopathy, the definitive diagnosis is determined by the histopathologic findings in the muscle biopsy specimen. In conditions for which the defective gene has been identified, the diagnosis may be established by the specific molecular analysis of the suspected gene expressed in lymphocytes. The morphologic and histochemical abnormalities differ considerably from those of the muscular dystrophies, spinal muscular atrophies, and neuropathies. Many are reminiscent of the embryologic development of muscle, thus suggesting possible defects in the genetic regulation of muscle development.

Congenital myopathies often show closer genetic relationships than previously appreciated between entities that have quite distinct pathologic phenotypes in the muscle biopsy and also distinctiveness in clinical expression with a degree of overlap. For example, mutation of the *tropomyosin-3* (*TPM3*) gene is one of the well-documented etiologies of nemaline myopathy, but identical genetic mutations of this gene are more recently also shown to be capable of causing isolated congenital fiber-type disproportion without nemaline rods, cap myopathy, centronuclear ("myotubular") myopathy, and central core/minicore disease.

MYOGENIC REGULATORY GENES AND GENETIC LOCI OF INHERITED DISEASES OF MUSCLE

A family of 4 myogenic regulatory genes shares encoding transcription factors of "basic helix-loop-helix" proteins associated with common DNA nucleotide sequences. These genes direct the differentiation of striated muscle from any undifferentiated mesodermal cell. The earliest basic helix-loop-helix gene to program the differentiation of myoblasts is myogenic factor 5 (*MYF5*). The second gene, *myogenin*, promotes

Text continued on p. 2970

Table 608-1	Classification of Muscular Dystrophies					
	INHERITANCE	**OMIM NUMBER**	**LOCUS**	**GENE SYMBOL**	**PROTEIN**	**MAIN LOCALIZATION**
Duchenne or Becker muscular dystrophy	X-R	310200 (Duchenne); 300376 (Becker)	Xq21·2	*DMD*	Dystrophin	Sarcolemma-associated protein
LIMB-GIRDLE MUSCULAR DYSTROPHY						
Type 1A	AD	159000	5q31	*MYOT*	Myotilin	Sarcomere-associated protein (Z disc)
Type 1B	AD	159001	1q21·2	*LMNA*	Lamin A/C	Nuclear lamina-associated protein
Type 1C	AD	607780	3p25	*CAV3*	Caveolin-3	Sarcolemma-associated protein
Type 1D	AD	603511	7q	*DNAJB6*	Co-chaperone DNAJB6	Sarcomere-associated protein (Z disc)
Type 1E	AD	602067	6q23	*DES*	Desmin	Intermediate filament protein
Type 1F	AD	608423	7q32	Unknown	Unknown	Unknown
Type 1G	AD	609115	4p21	Unknown	Unknown	Unknown
Type 1H	AD	613530	3p23–p25	Unknown	Unknown	Unknown
Type 2A	AR	253600	15q15·1	*CAPN3*	Calpain-3	Myofibril-associated proteins
Type 2B	AR	253601	2p13	*DYSF*	Dysferlin	Sarcolemma-associated protein
Type 2C	AR	253700	13q12	*SGCG*	γ-Sarcoglycan	Sarcolemma-associated protein
Type 2D	AR	608099	17q12–q21·33	*SGCA*	α-Sarcoglycan	Sarcolemma-associated protein
Type 2E	AR	604286	4q12	*SGCB*	β-Sarcoglycan	Sarcolemma-associated protein
Type 2F	AR	601287	5q33	*SGCD*	δ-Sarcoglycan	Sarcolemma-associated protein

Table 608-1 | Classification of Muscular Dystrophies—cont'd

	INHERITANCE	OMIM NUMBER	LOCUS	GENE SYMBOL	PROTEIN	MAIN LOCALIZATION
Type 2G	AR	601954	17q12	TCAP	Titin cap (telethonin)	Sarcomere-associated protein (Z disc)
Type 2H	AR	254110	9q31–q34	TRIM32	Tripartite motif-containing 32 (ubiquitin ligase)	Sarcomeric-associated protein (Z disc)
Type 2I	AR	607155	19q13·3	FKRP	Fukutin-related protein	Putative glycosyltransferase enzymes
Type 2J	AR	608807	2q31	TTN	Titin	Sarcomeric protein
Type 2K	AR	609308	9q34	POMT1	Protein-1-O-mannosyltransferase 1	Glycosyltransferase enzymes
Type 2L	AR	611307	11p14·3	ANO5	Anoctamin 5	Transmembrane protein, possible sarcoplasmic reticulum
Type 2M	AR	611588	9q31	FKTN	Fukutin	Putative glycosyltransferase enzymes
Type 2N	AR	613158	14q24	POMT2	Protein-O-mannosyltransferase 2	Glycosyltransferase enzymes
Type 2O	AR	613157	1p34	POMGNT1	Protein-O-linked mannose β 1,2-N-aminyltransferase 1	Glycosyltransferase enzymes
Type 2P	AR	613818	3p21	DAG1	Dystrophin-associated glycoprotein 1	Sarcomeric-associated protein
Type 2Q	AR	613723	8q24	PLEC1	Plectin 1	Sarcolemma-associated protein (Z disc)
FACIOSCAPULOHUMERAL MUSCULAR DYSTROPHY						
Type 1	AD	158900	4q35	Unknown	DUX4 and chromatin rearrangement	Nuclear
Type 2	AD	158901	18	Unknown	SMCHD1	Structural maintenance of chromosome's flexible hinge domain containing 1
EMERY-DREIFUSS MUSCULAR DYSTROPHY						
X-linked type 1	X-R	310300	Xq28	EMD	Emerin	Nuclear membrane protein
X-linked type 2	X-R	300696	Xq27·2	FHL1	Four and a half LIM domain 1	Sarcomere and sarcolemma
Autosomal dominant	AD	2181350	1q21·2	LMNA	Lamin A/C	Nuclear membrane protein
Autosomal recessive	AR	604929	1q21·2	LMNA	Lamin A/C	Nuclear membrane protein
With nesprin-1 defect	AD	612998	6q25	SYNE1	Spectrin repeat containing, nuclear envelope 1 (nesprin-1)	Nuclear membrane protein
With nesprin-2 defect	AD	5612999	4q23	SYNE2	Spectrin repeat containing, nuclear envelope 2 (nesprin-2)	Nuclear membrane protein
Congenital muscular dystrophy with merosin deficiency (MDC1A)	AR	607855	6q2	LAMA2	Laminin α₂ chain of merosin	Extracellular matrix proteins
Congenital muscular dystrophy	AR	604801	1q42	Unknown	Unknown	Unknown
Congenital muscular dystrophy and abnormal glycosylation of dystroglycan (MDC1C)	AR	606612	19q13	FKRP	Fukutin-related protein	Putative glycosyltransferase enzymes
Congenital muscular dystrophy and abnormal glycosylation of dystroglycan (MDC1D)	AR	608840	22q12	LARGE	Like-glycosyl transferase	Putative glycosyltransferase enzymes
Fukuyama congenital muscular dystrophy	AR	253800	9q31–q33	FCMD	Fukutin	Putative glycosyltransferase enzymes

Continued

Table 608-1 | Classification of Muscular Dystrophies—cont'd

	INHERITANCE	OMIM NUMBER	LOCUS	GENE SYMBOL	PROTEIN	MAIN LOCALIZATION
WALKER–WARBURG SYNDROME						
With fukutin defect	AR	236670	9q31–q33	FCMD	Fukutin	Putative glycosyltransferase enzymes
With protein-O-mannosyltransferase 1 defect	AR	236670	9q34	POMT1	Protein-1-O-mannosyltransferase 1	Glycosyltransferase enzymes
With protein-O-mannosyltransferase 2 defect	AR	236670	14q24	POMT2	Protein-O-mannosyltransferase 2	Glycosyltransferase enzymes
With protein-O-linked mannose β 1,2-N-aminyltransferase 1 defect	AR	236670	1p34	POMGNT1	Protein-O-linked mannose β 1,2-N-aminyltransferase 1	Glycosyltransferase enzymes
With fukutin-related protein defect	AR	236670	19q13	FKRP	Fukutin-related protein	Putative glycosyltransferase enzymes
MUSCLE-EYE-BRAIN DISEASE						
With protein-O-linked mannose β 1,2-N-aminyltransferase 1 defect	AR	253280	1p34	POMGNT1	Protein-O-linked mannose β 1,2-N-aminyltransferase 1	Glycosyltransferase enzymes
With fukutin-related protein defect	AR	253280	19q13	FKRP	Fukutin-related protein	Putative glycosyltransferase enzymes
With protein-O-mannosyltransferase 2 defect	AR	253280	14q24	POMT2	Protein-O-mannosyltransferase 2	Glycosyltransferase enzymes
Congenital muscular dystrophy caused by glycosylation disorder	AR	NA	9q34.1	DPM2	Dolichyl-phosphate mannosyltransferase polypeptide 2	Glycosyltransferase enzymes
Congenital muscular dystrophy caused by glycosylation disorder	AR	NA	1q21.3	DPM3	Dolichyl-phosphate mannosyltransferase polypeptide 3	Glycosyltransferase enzymes
Congenital muscular dystrophy with mitochondrial structural abnormalities	mtDNA	602541	22q13	CHKB	Choline kinase	Sarcolemmal and mitochondrial membrane
Congenital muscular dystrophy with rigid spine syndrome	AR	602771	1p36	SEPN1	Selenoprotein N1	Endoplasmic reticulum protein
ULLRICH SYNDROME						
With collagen type VI subunit α_1 defect	AR	254090	21q22.3	COL6A1	Collagen type VI, subunit α_1	Extracellular matrix proteins
With collagen type VI subunit α_2 defect	AR	254090	21q22.3	COL6A2	Collagen type VI, subunit α_2	Extracellular matrix proteins
With collagen type VI subunit α_3 defect	AR	254090	2q37	COL6A3	Collagen type VI, subunit α_3	Extracellular matrix proteins
Congenital muscular dystrophy with integrin α_7 defect	AR	613204	12q13	ITGA7	Integrin α_7	External sarcolemmal protein
Congenital muscular dystrophy with integrin α_9 defect	AR	NA	3p21.3	ITGA9	Integrin α_9	External sarcolemmal protein
Muscular dystrophy with generalized lipodystrophy	AR	NA	17q21–q23	PTRF	Polymerase I and transcript release factor (cavin-1)	T tubules and sarcolemma
Oculopharyngeal muscular dystrophy	AD or AR	164300	14q11.2	PABPN1	Polyadenylate-binding protein nuclear 1	Unknown

AD, autosomal dominant; AR, autosomal recessive; NA, not assigned; OMIM, Online Mendelian Inheritance in Man; X-R, X-linked recessive.
From Mercuri E, Muntoni F: Muscular dystrophies. Lancet 381:845–858, 2013, Table 1.

Table 608-2 | Clinical Signs of Muscular Dystrophy

	MOTOR FUNCTION	DISTRIBUTION OF WEAKNESS	RIGID SPINE	CARDIOMYOPATHY	RESPIRATORY IMPAIRMENT	DISEASE COURSE	INCREASED CK	OTHER SIGNS
CONGENITAL-ONSET MUSCULAR DYSTROPHY								
Congenital muscular dystrophy with merosin deficiency	Independent ambulation generally not achieved in patients with absent merosin	Upper limbs > lower limbs	−	Not frequent	++	Slowly progressive	++	White matter changes on brain MRI
Congenital muscular dystrophy and abnormal glycosylation of dystroglycan (Walker-Warburg syndrome, muscle-eye-brain disease, congenital muscular dystrophy type 1C, etc.)	Independent ambulation generally not achieved	Upper limbs > lower limbs	−	Not frequent	+	Slowly progressive	++	Frequent structural brain changes
Congenital muscular dystrophy with rigid spine syndrome type 1 (SEPN1)	Ambulation achieved	Axial muscles > limbs	++	−	Early respiratory failure	Progression of respiratory signs > motor signs	N or +	Scoliosis
Ullrich syndrome	Ambulation achieved in ~50% but lost by middle teens	Proximal and axial	++	−	Early respiratory failure	Progression of respiratory and motor signs	N or +	Distal laxity
FROM EARLY-ONSET TO CHILDHOOD-ONSET MUSCULAR DYSTROPHY								
Duchenne muscular dystrophy	Independent ambulation achieved, but lost before age of 13 yr	Proximal > distal (pattern A)	−	++	++	Progression of motor, cardiac, and respiratory signs	++	Mental retardation in 30%
Emery-Dreifuss muscular dystrophy AC deficiency (type 2)	Ambulation achieved in all cases except for rare cases with congenital onset	Scapuloperoneal (pattern B)	++	++	In adulthood in the typical form, but also in childhood (congenital variants)	Slowly progressive	+ (+)	Frequent association with Dunningham-type lipodystrophy
Limb-girdle muscular dystrophy with lamin AC deficiency (type 1B)	Independent ambulation achieved, variable progression	Proximal > distal (pattern A)	+	++	In adulthood	Progression of cardiac signs > motor signs	+ (+)	None
Limb-girdle muscular dystrophy with calpain deficiency (type 2A)	Ambulation achieved	Proximal > distal (pattern A)	+	−	Not frequent	Slow progression	++	None

Continued

Table 608-2 Clinical Signs of Muscular Dystrophy—cont'd

	MOTOR FUNCTION	DISTRIBUTION OF WEAKNESS	RIGID SPINE	CARDIOMYOPATHY	RESPIRATORY IMPAIRMENT	DISEASE COURSE	INCREASED CK	OTHER SIGNS
CHILDHOOD-ONSET AND ADULTHOOD-ONSET MUSCULAR DYSTROPHY								
Becker muscular dystrophy	Independent ambulation achieved, variable progression	Proximal > distal (pattern A)	−	++	Not frequent	Progressive with substantial variability	++	None
Limb-girdle muscular dystrophy with sarcoglycan deficiency (types 2C, 2D, 2E, 2F)	Independent ambulation achieved, generally lost in the 2nd decade	Proximal > distal (pattern A)	−	++	++	Progression of motor, cardiac, and respiratory signs	++	None
Limb-girdle muscular dystrophy with abnormal glycosylation of dystroglycan (types 2I, 2K, 2L, 2M, 2N, 2O)	Independent ambulation achieved, variable progression	Proximal > distal (pattern A)	−	++	+(+)	Progressive	++	Mental retardation reported in some cases
Limb-girdle muscular dystrophy with dysferlin deficiency (type 2B)	Independent ambulation always achieved	Both pattern A and pattern E	−	−	−	Progressive in adulthood	++	None
Limb-girdle muscular dystrophy with telethonin deficiency (type 2G)	Independent ambulation achieved, generally lost in the 4th decade	Proximal > distal (pattern A); in some pattern B	−	+	+	Progressive in adulthood	+ (+)	None
Limb-girdle muscular dystrophy with titin deficiency (type 2J)	Independent ambulation achieved	Proximal > distal (pattern A) but also pattern E	−	−	−	Roughly half lose ambulation in adulthood	++	None
Facioscapulohumeral dystrophy	Independent ambulation achieved, variable progression	Pattern D	−	−	Uncommon and mild	Slowly progressive	N or +	Neurosensory hearing loss and retinal degeneration
Emery-Dreifuss muscular dystrophy with merin deficiency (type 1)	Independent ambulation achieved, variable progression	Scapuloperoneal (pattern B)	+	++	Not frequent	Progression of cardiac signs > motor signs	+ (+)	None
ADULT-ONSET MUSCULAR DYSTROPHY								
Limb-girdle muscular dystrophy with anoctamin deficiency (type 2L)	Onset in adulthood, 8:1 ratio of men to women	Mainly lower limbs pattern A, rarely pattern E	−	−	−	Slowly progressive in adulthood	++	None
Limb-girdle muscular dystrophy type 1A (myotilin)	Independent ambulation achieved	Proximal > distal (pattern A)	−	−	−	Generally slowly progressive in adulthood	+	Dysarthria in some cases
Limb-girdle muscular dystrophy with caveolin deficiency (type 1C)	Independent ambulation achieved; rippling might be seen before weakness	Proximal and distal	−	+	−	Slowly progressive, variable	++	Cramps, rippling, percussion-induced repetitive contractions

−, Absent; +, mild; ++, severe; +(+), variable; CK, creatine kinase; N, normal.
From Mercuri E, Muntoni F: Muscular dystrophies. Lancet 381:845–858, 2013, Table 2.

Table 608-3	Cardiac Involvement in Muscular Dystrophies			
	ONSET AND FIRST SIGNS	**PROGRESSION**	**CARDIAC DEATH**	**SURVEILLANCE**
Duchenne muscular dystrophy	Dilated cardiomyopathy with reduced left-ventricular ejection fraction after 10 yr of age	Dilated cardiomyopathy in almost all patients by 18 yr of age. Ventricular dysrhythmias occur in older patients	Congestive heart failure or sudden death in 20% of patients, although the contribution of heart to death of ventilated patients is now well established	Echocardiography every 2 yr in the 1st decade of life and annually after 10 yr of age (or more frequently if abnormalities are identified)
Becker muscular dystrophy	Dilated cardiomyopathy, generally after 10 yr of age	Present in 40% of patients older than 18 yr and more than 80% of those older than 40 yr. Most patients develop dilated cardiomyopathy followed by ventricular arrhythmias	Death from congestive heart failure and arrhythmias is estimated to occur in up to 50% of cases. Cardiac transplants reported	Echocardiography at least every 5 yr
Myotonic dystrophy	Cardiac abnormalities can occur as early as the 2nd decade of life	Conduction deficits occur in about 65% of adult patients	20-30% of patients; mean 54 yr of age. Sudden death is mainly caused by conduction blocks, but ventricular tachyarrhythmias are also a possible cause of death	ECG yearly. Holter monitoring is recommended in patients with ECG abnormalities to detect asymptomatic conduction blocks and arrhythmias
EMERY-DREIFUSS MUSCULAR DYSTROPHY				
X-linked recessive Emery-Dreifuss muscular dystrophy (type 1)	Conduction disturbances generally in the 2nd decade	Ventricular myocardium might become involved, leading to mild ventricular dilation and low-to-normal systolic function	Sudden death is by far the most common cause of death and can be very unpredictable	ECG and yearly Holter monitoring are indicated. Pacemaker implantation should be considered if sinus node or atrioventricular node disease develops. Defibrillator might be needed in some patients
Emery-Dreifuss muscular dystrophy 2 and limb-girdle muscular dystrophy 1B	Conduction disease and cardiac failure	Dysrhythmias (sinus bradycardia, atrioventricular conduction block, or atrial arrhythmias) present in 92% of patients older than 30 yr	Sudden death reported also in patients with pacemaker. Rare death with defibrillator also reported. Cardiac failure. Cardiac transplants reported	ECG and yearly Holter monitoring are indicated. Defibrillator implantation should be considered as pacemaker does not have a substantial effect on mortality
LIMB-GIRDLE MUSCULAR DYSTROPHY				
Sarcoglycanopathies	ECG and/or echocardiographic abnormalities reported in 20-30% of patients (especially β and δ variants; less common in α variant)	Severe dilated cardiomyopathy and lethal ventricular arrhythmias might occur in patients with Duchenne muscular dystrophy–like dystrophy	Typically by cardiac failure. Cardiac transplants reported	No evidence-based standards of care exist, but experts have made recommendations
Limb-girdle muscular dystrophy 2I	Cardiac involvement reported in 29-62% of limb-girdle muscular dystrophy 2I. Dilated cardiomyopathy may start in teenage yr	Symptomatic cardiac failure over time, at a mean age of 38 yr (range: 18-58 yr)	Cardiac failure. Cardiac transplants reported	No evidence-based standards of care exist, but experts have made recommendations
Limb-girdle muscular dystrophy 1E	Dilated, restrictive, hypertrophic cardiomyopathies and arrhythmias. Cardiac involvement can precede muscle weakness in some patients	Major cardiac signs, such as atrioventricular block, can be the presenting symptom or occur within a decade of onset of muscle weakness	Life-threatening cardiac complications in roughly 50% of patients, at a mean age of 40 yr, including sudden death, end-stage heart failure, atrioventricular block, and syncope	No evidence-based standards of care exist, but experts have made recommendations

Continued

Table 608-3	Cardiac Involvement in Muscular Dystrophies—cont'd			
	ONSET AND FIRST SIGNS	**PROGRESSION**	**CARDIAC DEATH**	**SURVEILLANCE**
CONGENITAL MUSCULAR DYSTROPHY				
Congenital muscular dystrophy merosin muscular dystrophy type C1A	Occasional reports of reduced left ventricular systolic function	Not well characterized	Rare by cardiac failure	No evidence-based standards of care exist, but experts have made recommendations
Fukuyama congenital muscular dystrophy	Systolic left-ventricular dysfunction may develop in the 2nd decade	Symptomatic cardiac failure over time	Death from congestive heart failure might occur by the age of 20 yr	No evidence-based standards of care exist, but experts have made recommendations
Muscular dystrophy type C1C	Dilated cardiomyopathy reported in young children	Not well characterized	Not reported	No evidence-based standards of care exist, but experts have made recommendations
Facioscapulohumeral muscular dystrophy	Uncommon	Not well characterized	Not reported	No evidence-based standards of care exist, but experts have made recommendations

ECG, electrocardiogram.

From Mercuri E, Muntoni F: Muscular dystrophies. Lancet 381:845–858, 2013, Table 3.

fusion of myoblasts to form myotubes. *Herculin* (also known as *MYF6*) and *MYOD1* are the other 2 myogenic genes. *Myf5* cannot support myogenic differentiation without myogenin, *MyoD,* and *MYF6.* Each of these 4 genes can activate the expression of at least 1 other and, under certain circumstances, can autoactivate as well. Another recently discovered gene known as **myomaker** also facilitates myoblast fusion. The expression of *MYF5* and of *herculin* is transient in early ontogenesis but returns later in fetal life and persists into adult life.

The human locus of the *MYOD1* gene is on chromosome 11, very near to the domain associated with embryonal rhabdomyosarcoma. The genes *Myf5* and *herculin* are on chromosome 12, and *myogenin* is on chromosome 1.

The myogenic genes are activated during muscle regeneration, recapitulating the developmental process; *MyoD* in particular is required for myogenic stem cell (satellite cell) activation in adult muscle. *PAX3, PAX7,* and *WNT3a* genes also play important roles in myogenesis and interact with each of the 4 basic genes mentioned above. Another gene, *myostatin,* is a negative regulator of muscle development by preventing myocytes from differentiating. The precise integrative roles of the myogenic genes in developmental myopathies are not yet fully defined.

The myogenic genes are important not only for fetal myogenesis but also for regeneration of muscle at any age, particularly in degenerative diseases such as muscular dystrophies and autoimmune inflammatory myopathies and in injuries of muscle secondary to trauma or to toxins. Satellite cells in mature muscle that mediate regeneration have the same somitic origin as embryonic muscle progenitor cells, but the genes that regulate them differ. *Pax3* and *Pax7* mediate the migration of primitive myoblast progenitors from the myotomes of the somites to their peripheral muscle sites in the embryo, but only 1 of 2 *Pax7* genes continues to act postnatally for satellite cell survival. Then it, too, no longer is required after the juvenile period for muscle satellite (i.e., stem) cells to become activated for muscle regeneration.

Bibliography is available at Expert Consult.

608.1 Myotubular Myopathy (Centronuclear Myopathy)

Harvey B. Sarnat

The term **myotubular myopathy** is a misnomer because it implies maturational arrest of fetal muscle during the myotubular stage of

development at 8-15 wk of gestation. It was based on the morphologic appearance of myofibers as a row of central nuclei and mitochondria within a core of cytoplasm, with contractile myofibrils forming a cylinder around this core (Fig. 608-1). These morphologically abnormal myofibers are not true fetal myotubes, however; hence the more neutral and descriptive term **centronuclear myopathy** is preferred.

PATHOGENESIS
The common pathogenesis involves loss of myotubularin protein, leading to structural and functional abnormalities in the organization of T-tubules and sarcoplasmic reticulum and defective excitation-contraction coupling.

CLINICAL MANIFESTATIONS
Fetal movements can decrease in late gestation. Polyhydramnios is a common complication because of pharyngeal weakness of the fetus and inability to swallow amniotic fluid.

At birth, affected infants have a thin muscle mass involving axial, limb girdle, and distal muscles; severe generalized hypotonia; and diffuse weakness. Respiratory efforts may be ineffective, requiring ventilatory support. Gavage feeding may be required because of weakness of the muscles of sucking and deglutition. The testes are often undescended. Facial muscles may be weak, but infants do not have the characteristic facies of myotonic dystrophy. Ptosis may be a prominent feature. Ophthalmoplegia is observed in a few cases. The palate may be high. The tongue is thin, but fasciculations are not seen. Tendon stretch reflexes are weak or absent.

Myotubular myopathy is not associated with cardiomyopathy (mature cardiac muscle fibers normally have central nuclei), but one report describes complete atrioventricular block without cardiomyopathy in a patient with confirmed X-linked myotubular myopathy. Congenital anomalies of the central nervous system or of other systems are not associated. A single patient with progressive dementia was reported, who had a mutation removing the start signal of exon 2. Patients with much milder symptoms or a much later age of onset with mutations in the same gene are now known. Some of these are manifesting carriers.

LABORATORY FINDINGS
Serum levels of creatine kinase (CK) are normal. Electromyography does not show evidence of denervation; results are usually normal or show minimal nonspecific myopathic features in early infancy. Nerve conduction velocity may be slow but is usually normal. The

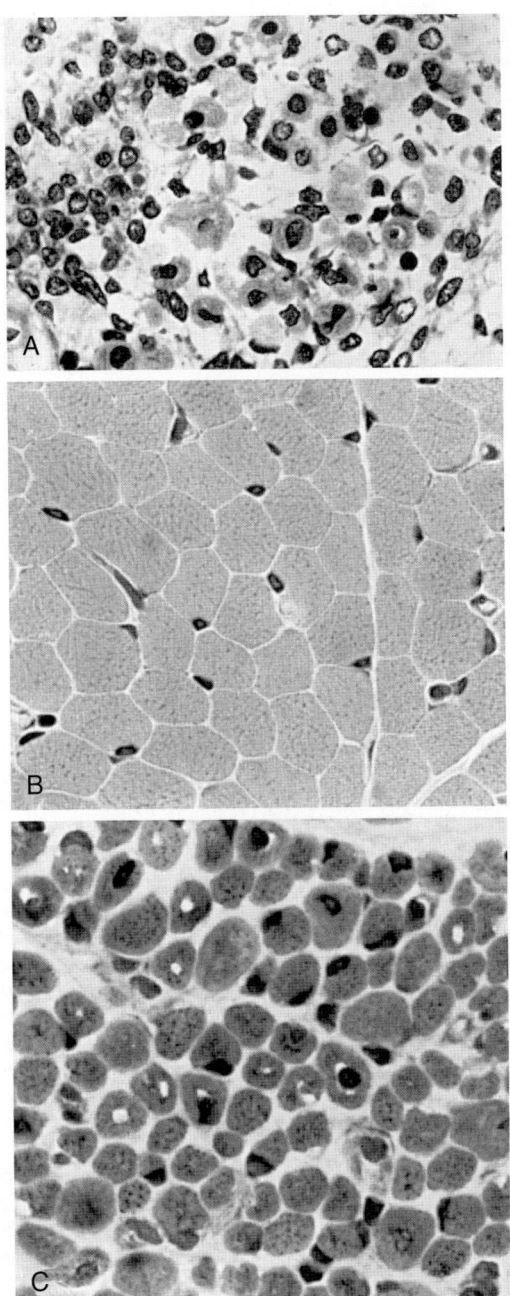

Figure 608-1 Cross section of muscle from a 14 wk old human fetus **(A)**, a normal full-term neonate **(B)**, and a term neonate with X-linked recessive myotubular myopathy **(C)**. Myofibers have large central nuclei in the fetus and in myotubular myopathy patient, and nuclei are at the periphery of the muscle fiber in the term neonate as in the adult (hematoxylin and eosin, ×500).

electrocardiogram appears normal. Chest radiographs show no cardiomegaly; the ribs may be thin.

DIAGNOSIS

If the diagnosis is strongly suspected from the clinical presentation, especially if this diagnosis was confirmed in a sibling, genetic tests can be performed in the neonatal period. In most cases the diagnosis is not so evident, but the muscle biopsy findings are diagnostic at birth, even in premature infants. More than 90% of muscle fibers are small and have centrally placed, large vesicular nuclei in a single row. Spaces between nuclei are filled with sarcoplasm containing mitochondria.

Histochemical stains for oxidative enzymatic activity and glycogen reveal a central distribution as in fetal myotubes. The cylinder of myofibrils shows mature histochemical differentiation with adenosine triphosphatase stains. The connective tissue of muscle spindles, blood vessels, intramuscular nerves, and motor end plates is mature. Ultrastructural features other than those that define the disease are also mature. Electron microscopy shows disorganized triads and focal loss of myofilaments. Vimentin and desmin show strong immunoreactivity in muscle fibers in congenital centronuclear myopathy and no demonstrable activity in normal term neonatal muscle. The molecular genetic marker in blood is available also for early prenatal diagnosis if suspicion is strong because of family history. Table 608-4 distinguishes centronuclear myopathy from other congenital myopathies.

GENETICS

At least 5 genes are involved in this disorder and account for approximately 80% of patients. These include mutations in myotubularin (*MTM1* gene) with X-linked severe manifestations; dynamin 2 (*DNM2*) with autosomal dominant or sporadic occurrence; amphiphysin 2 (*BIN1*) and titin (*TTN*) mutations with autosomal recessive inheritance and ryanodine receptor 1 (*RYR1*), with autosomal recessive or sporadic occurrence.

X-linked recessive inheritance is the most common trait in this disease affecting boys. The mothers of affected infants are clinically asymptomatic, but their muscle biopsy specimens show minor alterations. Genetic linkage on the X chromosome has been localized to the Xq28 site, a locus different from the Xp21 gene of Duchenne and Becker muscular dystrophies. A deletion in the responsible *MTM1* gene has been identified. It encodes a protein called myotubularin. This gene belongs to a family of similar genes encoding enzymatically active and inactive forms of phosphatidylinositol-3-phosphatases that form dimers. *MTM1*, dynamin-2, and amphiphysin all are localized to the T-tubule wall in triads. This crucial region is where the action potential releases a signal to the ryanodine receptor to release calcium. The pathogenesis is in the regulation of enzymatic activity and binding to other proteins induced by dimer interactions. Although only a single *MTM1* gene is involved, 5 distinct point mutations and many different alleles, as well as large duplications, can produce the same clinical disease. Mutations in the dynamin-2 protein result in an autosomal dominant form of centronuclear myopathy and may account for up to half of all patients with centronuclear myopathy, but these cases usually are mild and might not manifest clinically until adult life as diffuse, slowly progressive weakness and generalized muscular pseudohypertrophy.

Other **rarer centronuclear myopathies** also are known; some are autosomal recessive and affect both sexes and others are sporadic and of unknown genetic origin. The recessive forms are sometimes divided into an early-onset form with or without ophthalmoplegia and a late-onset form without ophthalmoplegia.

TREATMENT

Only supportive and palliative treatment is presently available. Progressive scoliosis may be treated by long posterior fusion. Genetic and neuropathologic studies of X-linked centronuclear ("myotubular") myopathy have led to effective gene therapy in mice and in dogs, so that even after a single dose the animals are more ambulatory and have much improved weakness. Gene replacement therapy in this disease is now being studied in humans.

PROGNOSIS

Approximately 75% of severely affected neonates with the X-linked disease die within the 1st few wk or mo of life. Survivors do not experience a progressive course but have major physical handicaps, rarely walk, and remain severely hypotonic. Late-onset and especially autosomal dominant forms have a much better prognosis, often with mild static weakness.

Bibliography is available at Expert Consult.

Table 608-4	Specific Congenital Myopathies: Distinguishing Clinical Features				
MYOPATHY	**NEONATAL HYPOTONIA AND WEAKNESS**	**SEVERE FORM WITH NEONATAL DEATH**	**FACIAL WEAKNESS**	**PTOSIS**	**EXTRAOCULAR MUSCULAR WEAKNESS**
Central core disease	+	0	±	0	0
Nemaline myopathy	+	+	+	0	0
Myotubular myopathy (centronuclear myopathy)	+	+	+	+	+
Congenital fiber-type disproportion	+	±	±	0	+

+, Often a prominent feature; ±, variably a prominent feature; 0, not a prominent feature.
    From Volpe JJ: Neurology of the newborn, ed 5, Philadelphia, 2008, Elsevier Saunders, p. 820.

608.2 Congenital Muscle Fiber-Type Disproportion

Harvey B. Sarnat

Congenital muscle fiber-type disproportion (CMFTD) occurs as an isolated congenital myopathy but also develops in association with various unrelated disorders that include nemaline rod disease, Krabbe disease (globoid cell leukodystrophy) early in the course before expression of the neuropathy, cerebellar hypoplasia and certain other brain malformations, fetal alcohol syndrome, some glycogenoses, multiple sulfatase deficiency, Lowe syndrome, rigid spine myopathy, and some infantile cases of myotonic muscular dystrophy. CMFTD should, therefore, be regarded as a syndrome, unless a specific genetic mutation is confirmed.

PATHOGENESIS
The association of CMFTD with cerebellar hypoplasia suggests that the pathogenesis may be an abnormal suprasegmental influence on the developing motor unit during the stage of histochemical differentiation of muscle between 20 and 28 wk of gestation. Muscle fiber types and growth are determined by innervation and are mutable even in adults. Although CMFTD does not actually correspond with any normal stage of development, it appears to be an embryologic disturbance of fiber type differentiation and growth.

CLINICAL MANIFESTATIONS
As an isolated condition not associated with other diseases, CMFTD is a nonprogressive disorder present at birth. Patients have generalized hypotonia and weakness, but the weakness is usually not severe and respiratory distress and dysphagia are rare. Contractures are present at birth in 25% of patients. Poor head control and developmental delay for gross motor skills are common in infancy. Walking is usually delayed until 18-24 mo but is eventually achieved. Because of the hypotonia, subluxation of the hips can occur. Muscle bulk is reduced. The muscle wasting and hypotonia are proportionately greater than the weakness, and the child may be stronger than expected during examination. Cardiomyopathy is a rare complication.

The facies of children with CMFTD often raise suspicion, especially if the child is referred for assessment of developmental delay and hypotonia. The head is dolichocephalic, and facial weakness is present. The palate is usually high arched. Thin muscles of the trunk and extremities give a thin, wasted appearance. The phenotype is very similar to that of nemaline myopathy that also includes CMFTD as part of the pathologic picture. Patients do not complain of myalgias. The clinical course is nonprogressive.

LABORATORY FINDINGS
Serum CK, electrocardiogram, electromyography, and nerve conduction velocity results are normal in simple CMFTD. If other diseases are associated, laboratory investigation of those conditions discloses the specific features.

DIAGNOSIS
CMFTD is diagnosed by muscle biopsy that shows disproportion in size and relative ratios of histochemical fiber types: Type I fibers are uniformly small, and type II fibers are hypertrophic; type I fibers are more numerous than type II fibers. Degeneration of myofibers and other primary myopathic features are absent. The biopsy is diagnostic at birth. Table 608-2 lists the features that distinguish CMFTD from other congenital myopathies.

GENETICS
Many cases of simple CMFTD are sporadic, although autosomal recessive inheritance is well documented in some families and an autosomal dominant trait is suspected in others. The genetic basis is heterogeneous in hereditary forms; a mutation in the insulin receptor gene at 19p13.2 is reported. Translocation t(10;17) was seen in 1 family. X-linked transmission with linkage to Xp23.12-p11.4 and Xq13.1-q22.1 also is described. In 3 unrelated families with CMFTD, a heterozygous missense mutation of the skeletal muscle α-actin gene (*ACTA1*) was demonstrated, but this genetic defect represents a minority; mutations in *TPM3* are a more common genetic finding. As with X-linked myotubular myopathy, large duplications in the *TPM3* gene can cause CMFTD. In CMFTD associated with cerebellar hypoplasia, the genetic effect is on cerebellar development and the muscular expression is secondary.

TREATMENT
No drug therapy is available. Physiotherapy may be helpful for some patients in strengthening muscles that do not receive sufficient exercise in daily activities. Mild congenital contractures often respond well to gentle range-of-motion exercises and rarely require plaster casting or surgery.

Bibliography is available at Expert Consult.

608.3 Nemaline Rod Myopathy

Harvey B. Sarnat

Nemaline rods (derived from the Greek *nema*, meaning "thread") are rod-shaped, inclusion-like abnormal structures within muscle fibers. They are difficult to demonstrate histologically with conventional hematoxylin-and-eosin stain, but are easily seen with special stains. They are not foreign inclusion bodies but rather consist of excessive Z-band material with a similar ultrastructure (Fig. 608-2). Chemically, the rods are composed of actin, α-actinin, tropomyosin-3, and the protein nebulin. Nemaline rod formation may be an unusual reaction of muscle fibers to injury because these rod structures have rarely been found in other diseases. They are most abundant in the congenital myopathy known as *nemaline rod disease*. Most rods are within the myofibrils, but intranuclear rods are occasionally demonstrated by electron microscopy. Intranuclear rods occur mainly in neonates with

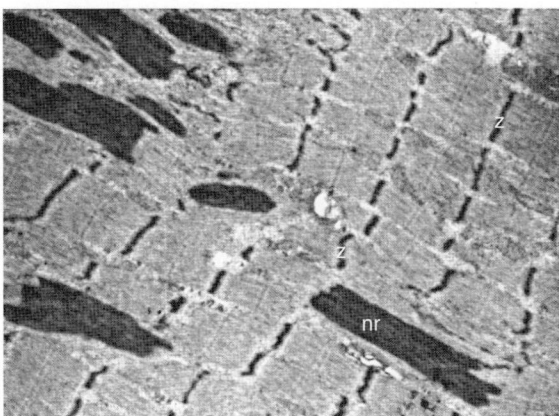

Figure 608-2 Electron micrograph of the muscle from a patient shown in Figure 608-4. Nemaline rods *(nr)* are seen within many myofibrils. They are identical in composition to the normal Z bands *(z)* (×6,000).

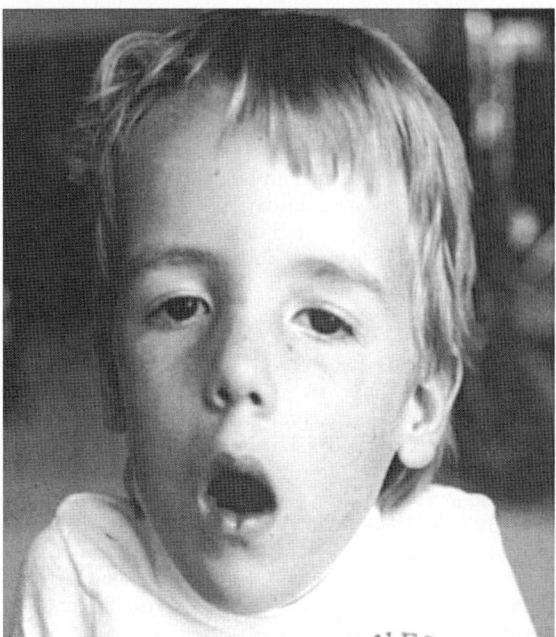

Figure 608-4 Infantile form of nemaline rod disease in a 6 yr old boy. Facial weakness and generalized muscle wasting are severe. The head is dolichocephalic. The mouth is usually open because the masseters are too weak to lift the mandible against gravity for more than a few seconds.

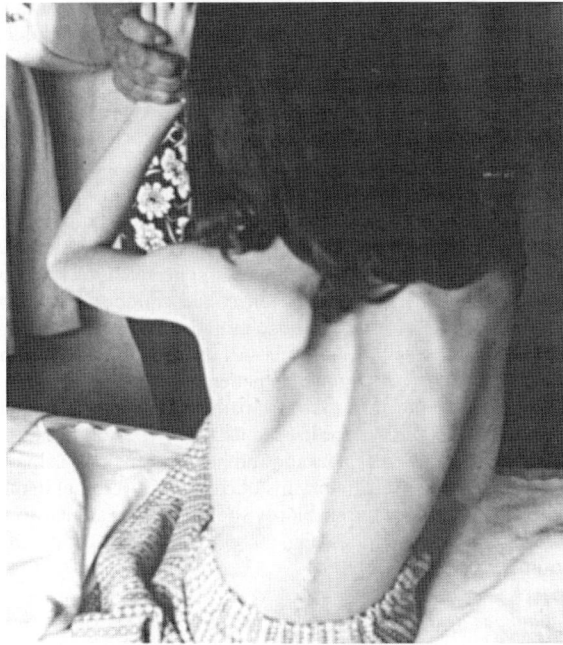

Figure 608-3 Back of a 13 yr old girl with the juvenile form of nemaline rod disease. The paraspinal muscles are very thin, and winging of the scapulas is evident. The muscle mass of the extremities is also greatly reduced proximally and distally.

The head is dolichocephalic, and the palate high arched or even cleft. Muscles of the jaw may be too weak to hold it closed (Fig. 608-4). Decreased fetal movements are reported by the mother, and neonates suffer from hypoxia and dysphagia; arthrogryposis may be present. Infants with severe neonatal and infantile nemaline myopathy have facies and phenotype that are nearly indistinguishable from those of neonatal myotonic dystrophy, but their mothers have normal facies. The juvenile form is the mildest and is not associated with respiratory failure, but the phenotype, including facial involvement, is similar.

LABORATORY FINDINGS
Serum CK level is normal or mildly elevated. The muscle biopsy is diagnostic. In addition to the characteristic nemaline rods, it also shows CMFTD or at least fiber type I predominance. In some patients, uniform type I fibers are seen with few or no type II fibers. Focal myofibrillar degeneration and an increase in lysosomal enzymes have been found in a few severe cases associated with progressive symptoms. Intranuclear nemaline rods, demonstrated by electron microscopy, correlate with the most severe neonatal manifestations. Because nemaline bodies can occur in other myopathies, their presence in the muscle biopsy is not pathognomonic in the absence of the supportive clinical manifestations. Adult-onset cases may be associated with monoclonal gammopathy.

GENETICS
Autosomal dominant and autosomal recessive forms of nemaline rod disease occur, and an X-linked dominant form in girls also can occur. Nemaline myopathy can be caused by mutation in at least 7 genes, including α-actin, α-tropomyosin, β-tropomyosin, troponin-T, nebulin, cofilin-2, and Kelch-like family member *(KLML40)*. The latter causes severe neonatal autosomal recessive nemaline myopathy. The proteins encoded for by all these genes are related to the thin filaments of myofibrils. Dominant nemaline myopathy is most often caused by mutations in *ACTA-1* or α-tropomyosin *(TPM3* at the 1q21-q23 locus); recessive mutations most frequently result from nebulin mutations (2q21.2-q22 locus), which account for about half the cases of nemaline myopathy and are particularly prevalent in Ashkenazi Jews. Some

severe weakness; they usually indicate *ACTA1* mutations and may coexist with the more usual cytoplasmic rods. Nemaline myopathy caused by *ACTA1* mutation is one of a spectrum of "actinopathies."

Mutations in tropomyosin-2 *(TPM2)* can cause a congenital myopathy related to nemaline rod myopathy, designated **cap myopathy**, in which accumulations of distorted myofilaments are focally present on the periphery of fibers. They may coexist with myofibrillar nemaline rods. Somatic mosaicism is demonstrated in *TPM2*-related nemaline myopathy with cap structures.

CLINICAL MANIFESTATIONS
Neonatal, infantile, and juvenile forms of the disease are known. The neonatal form is severe and usually fatal because of respiratory failure since birth. In the infantile form, generalized hypotonia and weakness, which can include bulbar-innervated and respiratory muscles, and a very thin muscle mass are characteristic (Fig. 608-3).

mutations in the α-actin gene give rise to a severe neonatal myopathy with masses of exclusively thin filaments, with or without rods. Mutations in tropomyosin-2 can cause a congenital myopathy with nonspecific findings. In α-actin defects both autosomal dominant and recessive varieties occur at the same 1q42.1 locus. The autosomal dominantly inherited defect of β-tropomyosin at 9q13 and the α-tropomyosin defects are rare and account for only 3% of patients with nemaline myopathy. An autosomal recessive troponin-T defect is at locus 19q13 and has been found only in the Amish population, in whom the incidence of nemaline myopathy is as high as 1 in 500, whereas in Australia in non-Amish ethnic groups it is estimated at 1 in 500,000.

TREATMENT AND PROGNOSIS

Therapy is supportive. Survivors are confined to an electric wheelchair and are usually unable to overcome gravity. Both proximal and distal muscles are involved. Congenital arthrogryposis can occur and predicts a poor prognosis. Gastrostomy may be needed for chronic dysphagia. In the juvenile form, patients are ambulatory and are able to perform most tasks of daily living. Weakness is not usually progressive, but some patients have more difficulty over time or enter a phase of progressive weakness. Cardiomyopathy is an uncommon complication. Death usually results from respiratory insufficiency, with or without superimposed pneumonia.

Bibliography is available at Expert Consult.

608.4 Central Core, Minicore, and Multicore Myopathies

Harvey B. Sarnat

Central core disease most often manifests itself in children with slow motor development who are hypotonic and have mild weakness especially in the hip girdle; congenital dislocation or dysplasia of the hips may be diagnosed in the neonatal period. In older children, central core disease is an important differential diagnosis of progressive thoracolumbar scoliosis. Central core myopathies are transmitted as either an autosomal dominant or recessive trait and are caused by the same abnormal gene at the 19q13.1 locus. This gene programs the ryanodine receptor *(RYR1)*, a tetrameric receptor that contains a non–voltage-gated calcium channel; it is prevalent in the sarcoplasmic reticulum and especially at the junction of the T-tubule with the cisternae of the sarcoplasmic reticulum. It contains the channel by which calcium is released among the myofilaments. Mutations in the *RYR1* gene are also the cause of **malignant hyperthermia**.

Infantile hypotonia, proximal weakness, muscle wasting, and involvement of facial muscles and neck flexors are the typical features in both the dominant and recessive forms. Contractures of the knees, hips, and other joints are common, and kyphoscoliosis and pes cavus often develop, even without much axial or distal muscle weakness. There is a high incidence of cardiac abnormalities. The course is not progressive, except for the contractures. In one variant, external ophthalmoplegia also is present. Rare cases of minicore myopathy also show hypertrophic cardiomyopathy associated with short-chain acyl-coenzyme A dehydrogenase deficiency.

The disease is characterized pathologically by central cores within muscle fibers in which only amorphous, granular cytoplasm is found with an absence of myofibrils and organelles. Histochemical stains show a lack of enzymatic activities of all types within these cores, as well as absence of contractile proteins (actin and myosin) that form the thin and thick myofilaments. Variants of central cores, called *minicores* and *multicores*, are described in some families.

Minicores or multicores are small areas, usually multiple within muscle fibers, that lack mitochondria and show Z-disc streaming. They can be caused by mutations in the gene *(SEPN1)* for the selenoprotein N, localized to triads, but *RYR1* mutations also are reported. The distinction previously made between single and multiple cores in

myofibers is now believed to be of little importance and they represent the same basic disease process.

The serum CK value is normal in central core disease except during crises of malignant hyperthermia, which can result in rhabdomyolysis or extensive acute myofiber necrosis (see Chapter 611.2). Central core disease is consistently associated with malignant hyperthermia, which can precede the diagnosis of central core disease. All patients should have special precautions with pretreatment with dantrolene before an anesthetic agent is administered.

Bibliography is available at Expert Consult.

608.5 Myofibrillar Myopathies

Harvey B. Sarnat

Most myofibrillar myopathies are not symptomatic in childhood, but occasionally older children and adolescents show early symptoms of nonspecific proximal and distal weakness. An infantile form also occurs and can cause mild neonatal hypotonia and weakness with disproportionately severe dysphagia and respiratory insufficiency, at times leading to early death. It is not progressive, however, and some patients show improvement in later infancy and early childhood, acquiring the ability to swallow by 3 yr of age. Cardiomyopathy is a complication in a minority.

The diagnosis is by muscle biopsy: some sarcomeres of myofibers have disorganization or dissolution of myofibrils adjacent to other areas of normal sarcomeres within the same fiber. These zones are associated with streaming of the Z bands and focally increased desmin intermediate filaments, myotilin, and αB-crystallin. Immunocytochemical and ultrastructural study of the muscle biopsy tissue is required. Mutation in the desmin gene is implicated as a contributory factor in the etiology of both adult-onset and childhood myofibrillar myopathies, but the primary defect is a mutation in, not just an upregulation of, the αB-crystallin molecule. An associated secondary mitochondrial defect is detected in some patients.

A unique autosomal recessive myopathy in Cree native infants is characterized by severe generalized muscular hypertonia that is not relieved by neuromuscular blockade and hence is myopathic in origin. Most die in infancy of respiratory insufficiency as a result of diaphragmatic involvement. The muscle biopsy shows findings similar to many other myofibrillar myopathies (Fig. 608-5); a novel αB-crystallin gene mutation is the cause.

Bibliography is available at Expert Consult.

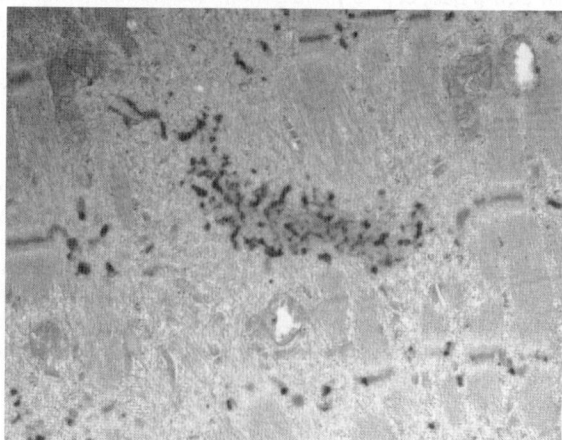

Figure 608-5 Electron micrograph of quadriceps femoris muscle biopsy of a 1 mo old native girl with Cree myofibrillar myopathy. Within the same myofiber, some sarcomeres are well formed and others exhibit disarray of the thick and thin myofilaments and fragmentation of Z bands. Mitochondria appear normal (×21,400).

608.6 Brain Malformations and Muscle Development
Harvey B. Sarnat

Infants with **cerebellar hypoplasia** are hypotonic and developmentally delayed, especially in gross motor skills. Muscle biopsy is sometimes performed to exclude a congenital myopathy. A biopsy specimen can show delayed maturation of muscle, fiber-type predominance, or CMFTD. Other malformations of the brain may also be associated with abnormal histochemical patterns, but supratentorial lesions are less likely than brainstem or cerebellar lesions to alter muscle development. Abnormal descending impulses along bulbospinal pathways probably alter discharge patterns of lower motor neurons that determine the histochemical differentiation of muscle at 20-28 wk of gestation. The corticospinal tract does not participate because it is not yet functional during this period of fetal life.

In several congenital muscular dystrophies (see Chapter 609.6), including the Walker-Warburg syndrome, Fukuyama disease, and muscle-eye-brain disease of Santavuori, major cerebral malformations, such as pachygyria and lissencephaly, are present. It is clear that in at least some of these cases, the abnormal protein implicated in pathogenesis of the syndrome is expressed in both muscle and brain and is important for both stabilization of muscle and migration of central neurons.

Bibliography is available at Expert Consult.

608.7 Amyoplasia
Harvey B. Sarnat

Congenital absence of individual muscles is common and is often asymmetric. A common aplasia is the *palmaris longus muscle* of the ventral forearm, which is absent in 30% of normal subjects and is fully compensated for by other flexors of the wrist. Unilateral absence of a *sternocleidomastoid muscle* is one cause of congenital torticollis. Absence of 1 *pectoralis major muscle* is part of the **Poland anomalad**.

When innervation does not develop, as in the lower limbs in severe cases of *myelomeningocele*, muscles can fail to develop. In *sacral agenesis*, the abnormal somites that fail to form bony vertebrae can also fail to form muscles from the same defective mesodermal plate, a disorder of induction resulting in segmental amyoplasia. Skeletal muscles of the extremities fail to differentiate from embryonic myomeres if the long bones do not form. Absence of 1 long bone, such as the radius, is associated with variable aplasia or hypoplasia of associated muscles, such as the flexor carpi radialis. End-stage neurogenic atrophy of muscle is sometimes called **amyoplasia**, but this use is semantically incorrect.

Generalized amyoplasia usually results in fetal death, and liveborn neonates rarely survive. A mutation in 1 of the myogenic genes is the suspected etiology because of genetic knockout studies in mice, but it has not been proven in humans.

608.8 Muscular Dysgenesis (Proteus Syndrome Myopathy)
Harvey B. Sarnat

Proteus syndrome is a disturbance of cellular growth involving ectodermal and mesodermal tissues, representing a cellular mosaicism. The genetic defect is a mutation in the *AKT1* gene, of the same genetic family as *AKT3*, which causes hemimegalencephaly; indeed many cases of Proteus syndrome also have hemimegalencephaly. These genes participate in the mammalian target of rapamycin pathway. Proteus syndrome also manifests as asymmetric overgrowth of the extremities, verrucous cutaneous lesions, angiomas of various types, thickening of

bones, and excessive growth of muscles without weakness. Severe seizures, beginning in neonates, are uncommon. Histologically, the muscle demonstrates a unique *muscular dysgenesis*. Abnormal zones are adjacent to zones of normal muscle formation and do not follow anatomic boundaries.

Bibliography is available at Expert Consult.

608.9 Benign Congenital Hypotonia
Harvey B. Sarnat

Benign congenital hypotonia is not a disease, but it is a descriptive term for infants or children with nonprogressive hypotonia of unknown origin. The hypotonia is not usually associated with weakness or developmental delay, although some children acquire gross motor skills more slowly than normal. Tendon stretch reflexes are normal or hypoactive. There are no cranial nerve abnormalities, and intelligence is normal.

The **diagnosis** is one of exclusion (see Table 607-2 in Chapter 607) after results of laboratory studies, including muscle biopsy and imaging of the brain with special attention to the cerebellum, are normal. Muscle biopsy is deferred in some mild cases to follow the clinical evolution over time, but the diagnosis in these infants is more provisional. No known molecular genetic basis for this syndrome has been identified. Table 607-3 in Chapter 607 lists the differential diagnosis.

The **prognosis** is generally good; no specific therapy is required. Contractures do not develop. Physical therapy might help achieve motor milestones (walking) sooner than expected. Hypotonia persists into adult life. The disorder is not always as "benign" as its name implies because a common complication is recurrent dislocation of joints, especially the shoulders. Excessive motility of the spine can result in stretch injury, compression, or vascular compromise of nerve roots or of the spinal cord. These are particular hazards for patients who perform gymnastics or who become circus performers because of agility of joints without weakness or pain.

Bibliography is available at Expert Consult.

608.10 Arthrogryposis
Harvey B. Sarnat

Arthrogryposis multiplex congenita is not a disease but is a descriptive term that signifies multiple congenital contractures and is heterogeneous in etiology (see Chapter 682).

Bibliography is available at Expert Consult.

Chapter 609
Muscular Dystrophies
Harvey B. Sarnat

The term *dystrophy* means abnormal growth, derived from the Greek *trophe*, meaning "nourishment." A muscular dystrophy is distinguished from all other neuromuscular diseases by 4 obligatory criteria: It is a primary myopathy, it has a genetic basis, the course is progressive, and degeneration and death of muscle fibers occur at some stage in the disease. This definition excludes neurogenic diseases such as spinal muscular atrophy, nonhereditary myopathies such as dermatomyositis, nonprogressive, and nonnecrotizing congenital myopathies such as congenital muscle fiber-type disproportion, and nonprogressive inherited metabolic myopathies. Some metabolic myopathies can fulfill the definition of a progressive muscular dystrophy but are not traditionally classified as dystrophies (muscle carnitine deficiency).

All muscular dystrophies might eventually be reclassified as metabolic myopathies once the biochemical defects are better defined. Muscular dystrophies are a group of unrelated diseases, each transmitted by a different genetic trait and each differing in its clinical course and expression. Some are severe diseases at birth that lead to early death; others follow very slow progressive courses over many decades, may be compatible with normal longevity, and might not even become symptomatic until late adult life. Some categories of dystrophies, such as limb-girdle muscular dystrophy (LGMD), are not homogeneous diseases but rather syndromes encompassing several distinct myopathies. Relationships among the various muscular dystrophies are resolved by molecular genetics rather than by similarities or differences in clinical and histopathologic features.

609.1 Duchenne and Becker Muscular Dystrophies

Harvey B. Sarnat

Duchenne muscular dystrophy (DMD) is the most common hereditary neuromuscular disease affecting all races and ethnic groups. Its characteristic clinical features are progressive weakness, intellectual impairment, hypertrophy of the calves, and proliferation of connective tissue in muscle. The incidence is 1 in 3,600 liveborn infant boys. This disease is inherited as an X-linked recessive trait. The abnormal gene is at the Xp21 locus and is one of the largest genes. **Becker muscular dystrophy** (BMD) is a disease that is fundamentally similar to DMD, with a genetic defect at the same locus, but clinically it follows a milder and more protracted course.

CLINICAL MANIFESTATIONS

Infant boys are rarely symptomatic at birth or in early infancy, although some are mildly hypotonic. Early gross motor skills, such as rolling over, sitting, and standing, are usually achieved at the appropriate ages or may be mildly delayed. Poor head control in infancy may be the first sign of weakness. Distinctive facies are not an early feature because facial muscle weakness is a late event; in later childhood, a "transverse" or horizontal smile may be seen. Walking is often accomplished at the normal age of approximately 12 mo, but hip girdle weakness may be seen in subtle form as early as the 2nd yr. Toddlers might assume a lordotic posture when standing to compensate for gluteal weakness. An early Gowers sign is often evident by age 3 yr and is fully expressed by age 5 or 6 yr (see Fig. 590-5 in Chapter 590). A Trendelenburg gait, or hip waddle, appears at this time. Common presentations in toddlers include delayed walking, falling, toe walking, and trouble running or walking upstairs, developmental delay, and, less often, malignant hyperthermia after anesthesia.

The length of time a patient remains ambulatory varies greatly. Some patients are confined to a wheelchair by 7 yr of age; most patients continue to walk with increasing difficulty until age 10 yr without orthopedic intervention. With orthotic bracing, physiotherapy, and sometimes minor surgery (Achilles tendon lengthening), most are able to walk until age 12 yr. Ambulation is important not only for postponing the psychologic depression that accompanies the loss of an aspect of personal independence but also because scoliosis usually does not become a major complication as long as a patient remains ambulatory, even for as little as 1 hr per day; scoliosis often becomes rapidly progressive after confinement to a wheelchair.

The relentless progression of **weakness** continues into the 2nd decade. The function of distal muscles is usually relatively well enough preserved, allowing the child to continue to use eating utensils, a pencil, and a computer keyboard. Respiratory muscle involvement is expressed as a weak and ineffective cough, frequent pulmonary infections, and decreasing respiratory reserve. Pharyngeal weakness can lead to episodes of aspiration, nasal regurgitation of liquids, and an airy or nasal voice quality. The function of the extraocular muscles remains well preserved. Incontinence due to anal and urethral sphincter weakness is an uncommon and very late event.

Contractures most often involve the ankles, knees, hips, and elbows. **Scoliosis** is common. The thoracic deformity further compromises pulmonary capacity and compresses the heart. Scoliosis usually progresses more rapidly after the child becomes nonambulatory and may be uncomfortable or painful. Enlargement of the calves (pseudohypertrophy) and wasting of thigh muscles are classic features. The enlargement is caused by hypertrophy of some muscle fibers, infiltration of muscle by fat, and proliferation of collagen. After the calves, the next most common site of muscular hypertrophy is the tongue, followed by muscles of the forearm. Fasciculations of the tongue do not occur. The voluntary sphincter muscles rarely become involved.

Unless ankle contractures are severe, ankle deep tendon reflexes remain well preserved until terminal stages. The knee deep tendon reflexes may be present until about 6 yr of age but are less brisk than the ankle jerks and are eventually lost. In the upper extremities, the brachioradialis reflex is usually stronger than the biceps or triceps brachii reflexes.

Cardiomyopathy, including persistent tachycardia and myocardial failure, is seen in 50-80% of patients with this disease. The severity of cardiac involvement does not necessarily correlate with the degree of skeletal muscle weakness. Some patients die early of severe cardiomyopathy while still ambulatory; others in terminal stages of the disease have well-compensated cardiac function. Smooth muscle dysfunction, particularly of the gastrointestinal tract, is a minor, but often overlooked, feature.

Intellectual impairment occurs in all patients, although only 20-30% have an IQ <70. The majority have learning disabilities that still allow them to function in a regular classroom, particularly with remedial help. A few patients are profoundly intellectually impaired, but there is no correlation with the severity of the myopathy. Epilepsy is slightly more common than in the general pediatric population. Autism-like behavior may develop but is uncommon. Dystrophin is expressed in brain and retina, as well as in striated and cardiac muscle, though the level is lower in brain than in muscle. This distribution might explain some of the central nervous system manifestations. Abnormalities in cortical architecture and of dendritic arborization may be detected neuropathologically; cerebral atrophy is demonstrated by MRI late in the clinical course. The degenerative changes and fibrosis of muscle constitute a painless process. Myalgias and muscle spasms do not occur. Calcinosis of muscle is rare.

Death occurs usually at about 18-20 yr of age. The causes of death are respiratory failure during sleep, intractable heart failure, pneumonia, or, occasionally, aspiration and airway obstruction.

In **BMD,** boys remain ambulatory until late adolescence or early adult life. Calf pseudohypertrophy, cardiomyopathy, and elevated serum levels of creatine kinase (CK) are similar to those of patients with DMD. Learning disabilities are less common. The onset of weakness is later in BMD than in DMD. Death often occurs in the mid to late 20s; fewer than half of patients are still alive by age 40 yr; these survivors are severely disabled.

LABORATORY FINDINGS

The serum CK level is consistently greatly elevated in DMD, even in presymptomatic stages, including at birth. The usual serum concentration is 15,000-35,000 IU/L (normal <160 IU/L). A normal serum CK level is incompatible with the diagnosis of DMD, although in terminal stages of the disease, the serum CK value may be considerably lower than it was a few years earlier because there is less muscle to degenerate. Other lysosomal enzymes present in muscle, such as aldolase and aspartate aminotransferase, are also increased but are less specific.

Cardiac assessment by echocardiography, electrocardiography (ECG), and radiography of the chest is essential and should be repeated periodically. After the diagnosis is established, patients should be referred to a pediatric cardiologist for long-term cardiac care.

Electromyography (EMG) shows characteristic myopathic features but is not specific for DMD. No evidence of denervation is found. Motor and sensory nerve conduction velocities are normal.

DIAGNOSIS

Polymerase chain reaction (PCR) for the dystrophin gene mutation is the primary test, if the clinical features and serum CK are consistent with the diagnosis. If the blood PCR is diagnostic, muscle biopsy may be deferred, but if it is normal and clinical suspicion is high, the more specific dystrophin immunocytochemistry performed on muscle biopsy sections detects the 30% of cases that do not show a PCR abnormality. Immunohistochemical staining of frozen sections of muscle biopsy tissue detects differences in the rod domain, the carboxyl-terminus (that attaches to the sarcolemma), and the aminoterminus (that attaches to the actin myofilaments) of the large dystrophin molecule, and may be prognostic of the clinical course as Duchenne or Becker disease. More-severe weakness occurs with truncation of the dystrophin molecule at the carboxyl-terminus than at the aminoterminus. The diagnosis should be confirmed by blood PCR or muscle biopsy in every case. Dystroglycans and other sarcolemmal regional proteins, such as merosin and sarcoglycans, also can be measured because they may be secondarily decreased.

The **muscle biopsy** is diagnostic and shows characteristic changes (Figs. 609-1 and 609-2). Myopathic changes include endomysial connective tissue proliferation, scattered degenerating and regenerating myofibers, foci of mononuclear inflammatory cell infiltrates as a reaction to muscle fiber necrosis, mild architectural changes in still-functional muscle fibers, and many dense fibers. These hypercontracted fibers probably result from segmental necrosis at another level,

allowing calcium to enter the site of breakdown of the sarcolemmal membrane and trigger a contraction of the whole length of the muscle fiber. Calcifications within myofibers are correlated with secondary β-dystroglycan deficiency.

The decision about whether muscle biopsy should be performed to establish the diagnosis sometimes presents problems. If there is a family history of the disease, particularly in the case of an involved brother whose diagnosis has been confirmed, a patient with typical

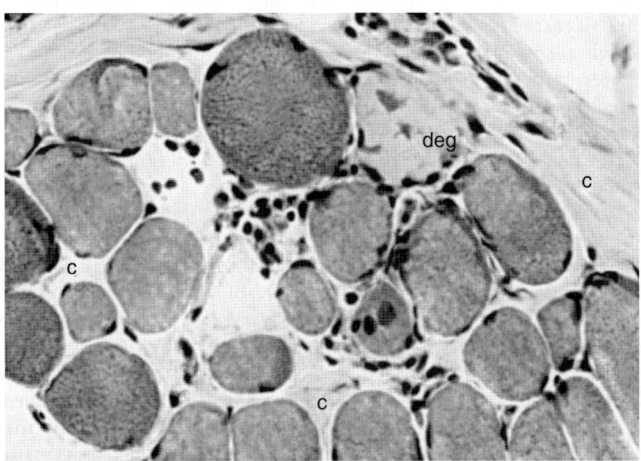

Figure 609-1 Muscle biopsy of a 4 yr old boy with Duchenne muscular dystrophy. Both atrophic and hypertrophic muscle fibers are seen, and some fibers are degenerating (*deg*). Connective tissue (*c*) between muscle fibers is increased (hematoxylin and eosin, ×400).

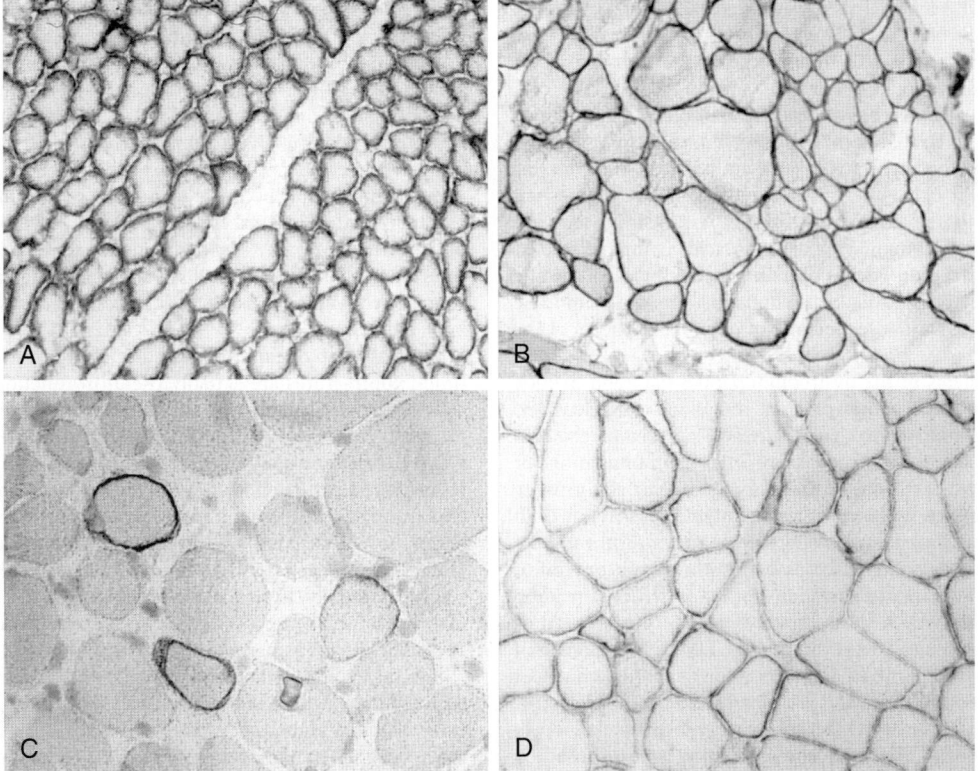

Figure 609-2 Dystrophin is demonstrated by immunohistochemical reactivity in the muscle biopsies of a normal term male neonate **(A)**, a 10 yr old boy with limb-girdle muscular dystrophy **(B)**, a 6 yr old boy with Duchenne muscular dystrophy **(C)**, and a 10 yr old boy with Becker muscular dystrophy **(D)**. In the normal condition, and also in non–X-linked muscular dystrophies in which dystrophin is not affected, the sarcolemmal membrane of every fiber is strongly stained, including atrophic and hypertrophic fibers. In Duchenne dystrophy, most myofibers express no detectable dystrophin, but a few scattered fibers known as revertant fibers show near-normal immunoreactivity. In Becker muscular dystrophy, the abnormal dystrophin molecule is thin, with pale staining of the sarcolemma, in which reactivity varies not only between myofibers but also along the circumference of individual fibers (×250).

clinical features of DMD and high concentrations of serum CK probably does not need to undergo biopsy. The result of the PCR might also influence whether to perform a muscle biopsy. A first case in a family, even if the clinical features are typical, should have the diagnosis confirmed to ensure that another myopathy is not masquerading as DMD. The most common muscles sampled are the vastus lateralis (quadriceps femoris) and the gastrocnemius.

GENETIC ETIOLOGY AND PATHOGENESIS

Despite the X-linked recessive inheritance in DMD, approximately 30% of cases are new mutations, and the mother is not a carrier. The female carrier state usually shows no muscle weakness or any clinical expression of the disease, but affected girls are occasionally encountered, usually having much milder weakness than boys. These symptomatic girls are explained by the Lyon hypothesis in which the normal X chromosome becomes inactivated and the one with the gene deletion is active (see Chapter 80). The full clinical picture of DMD has occurred in several girls with Turner syndrome in whom the single X chromosome must have had the Xp21 gene deletion.

The asymptomatic carrier state of DMD is associated with elevated serum CK values in 80% of cases. The level of increase is usually in the magnitude of hundreds or a few thousand but does not have the extreme values noted in affected males. Prepubertal girls who are carriers of the dystrophy also have increased serum CK values, with highest levels at 8-12 yr of age. Approximately 20% of carriers have normal serum CK values. If the mother of an affected boy has normal CK levels, it is unlikely that her daughter can be identified as a carrier by measuring CK. Muscle biopsy of suspected female carriers can detect an additional 10% in whom serum CK is not elevated; a specific genetic diagnosis using PCR on peripheral blood is definitive. Some female carriers suffer cardiomyopathy without weakness of striated muscles.

A 427-kDa cytoskeletal protein known as *dystrophin* is encoded by the gene at the Xp21.2 locus. This gene contains 79 exons of coding sequence and 2.5 Mb of DNA, 10 times larger than the next largest gene yet identified. This subsarcolemmal protein attaches to the sarcolemmal membrane overlying the A and M bands of the myofibrils and consists of 4 distinct regions or domains: the aminoterminus contains 250 amino acids and is related to the *N*-actin binding site of α-actinin; the second domain is the largest, with 2,800 amino acids, and contains many repeats, giving it a characteristic rod shape; a third, cysteine-rich domain is related to the carboxyl-terminus of α-actinin; and the final carboxyl-terminal domain of 400 amino acids is unique to dystrophin and to a dystrophin-related protein encoded by chromosome 6. "Dystrophin deficiency" at the sarcolemma disrupts the membrane cytoskeleton and leads to loss secondarily of other components of the cytoskeleton.

The molecular defects in the dystrophinopathies vary and include intragenic deletions, duplications, or point mutations of nucleotides. Approximately 65% of patients have deletions; approximately 10% exhibit duplications while approximately 10% have point mutations or smaller rearrangements. The site or size of the intragenic abnormality does not always correlate well with the phenotypic severity; in both Duchenne and Becker forms the mutations are mainly near the middle of the gene, involving deletions of exons 46-51. Phenotypic or clinical variations are explained by the alteration of the translational reading frame of messenger RNA (mRNA), which results in unstable, truncated dystrophin molecules and severe, classic DMD; mutations that preserve the reading frame still permit translation of coding sequences further downstream on the gene and produce a semifunctional dystrophin, expressed clinically as BMD. An even milder form of adult-onset disease, formerly known as **quadriceps myopathy,** is also caused by an abnormal dystrophin molecule. The clinical spectrum of the dystrophinopathies not only includes the classic Duchenne and Becker forms but also ranges from a severe neonatal muscular dystrophy to asymptomatic children with persistent elevation of serum CK levels >1,000 IU/L.

Analysis of the dystrophin protein requires a muscle biopsy and is demonstrated by Western blot analysis or in tissue sections by immunohistochemical methods using either fluorescence or light microscopy of antidystrophin antisera (see Fig. 609-2). In classic DMD, levels of <3% of normal are found; in BMD, the molecular weight of dystrophin is reduced to 20-90% of normal in 80% of patients, but in 15% of patients the dystrophin is of normal size but reduced in quantity, and 5% of patients have an abnormally large protein caused by excessive duplications or repeats of codons. Selective immunoreactivity of different parts of the dystrophin molecule in sections of muscle biopsy material distinguishes the Duchenne and Becker forms (Fig. 609-3). The demonstration of deletions and duplications also can be made from blood samples by the more rapid PCR, which identifies as many as 98% of deletions by amplifying 18 exons but cannot detect duplications. The diagnosis can thus be confirmed at the molecular genetic level from either the muscle biopsy material or from peripheral blood, although as many as 30% of boys with DMD or BMD have a false-normal blood PCR; all cases of dystrophinopathy are detected by muscle biopsy.

The same methods of DNA analysis from blood samples may be applied for carrier detection in female relatives at risk, such as sisters and cousins, and to determine whether the mother is a carrier or whether a new mutation occurred in the embryo. Prenatal diagnosis is possible as early as the 12th wk of gestation by sampling chorionic villi for DNA analysis by Southern blot or PCR and is confirmed in aborted fetuses with DMD by immunohistochemistry for dystrophin in muscle.

TREATMENT

There is no medical cure for this disease. Much can be done to treat complications and to improve the quality of life of affected children. **Cardiac decompensation** often responds initially well to digoxin. **Pulmonary infections** should be promptly treated. Patients should avoid contact with children who have obvious respiratory or other contagious illnesses. Immunizations for influenza virus and other routine vaccinations are indicated.

Preservation of a good **nutritional state** is important. DMD is not a vitamin-deficiency disease, and excessive doses of vitamins should be avoided. Adequate calcium intake is important to minimize osteoporosis in boys confined to a wheelchair, and fluoride supplements may also be given, particularly if the local drinking water is not fluoridated. Because sedentary children burn fewer calories than active children and because depression is an additional factor, these children tend to eat excessively and gain weight. Obesity makes a patient with myopathy even less functional because part of the limited reserve muscle strength is dissipated in lifting the weight of excess subcutaneous adipose tissue. Dietary restrictions with supervision may be needed.

Physiotherapy delays but does not always prevent contractures. At times, contractures are actually useful in functional rehabilitation. If contractures prevent extension of the elbow beyond 90 degrees and the muscles of the upper limb no longer are strong enough to overcome gravity, the elbow contractures are functionally beneficial in fixing an otherwise flail arm and in allowing the patient to eat and write. Surgical correction of the elbow contracture may be technically feasible, but the result may be deleterious. Physiotherapy contributes little to muscle strengthening because patients usually are already using their entire reserve for daily function, and exercise cannot further strengthen involved muscles. Excessive exercise can actually accelerate the process of muscle fiber degeneration.

Special vigilance should be maintained in watching for progressive scoliosis, which should be treated early by orthopedists using external braces or corsets and occasionally by surgeons. Scoliosis often becomes rapidly progressive once the patient is confined to a wheelchair.

Another recommended treatment of patients with DMD involves the use of prednisone, prednisolone, deflazacort, or other steroids. Glucocorticoids decrease the rate of apoptosis or programmed cell death of myotubes during ontogenesis and can decelerate the myofiber necrosis in muscular dystrophy. Strength usually improves initially, but the long-term complications of chronic steroid therapy, including

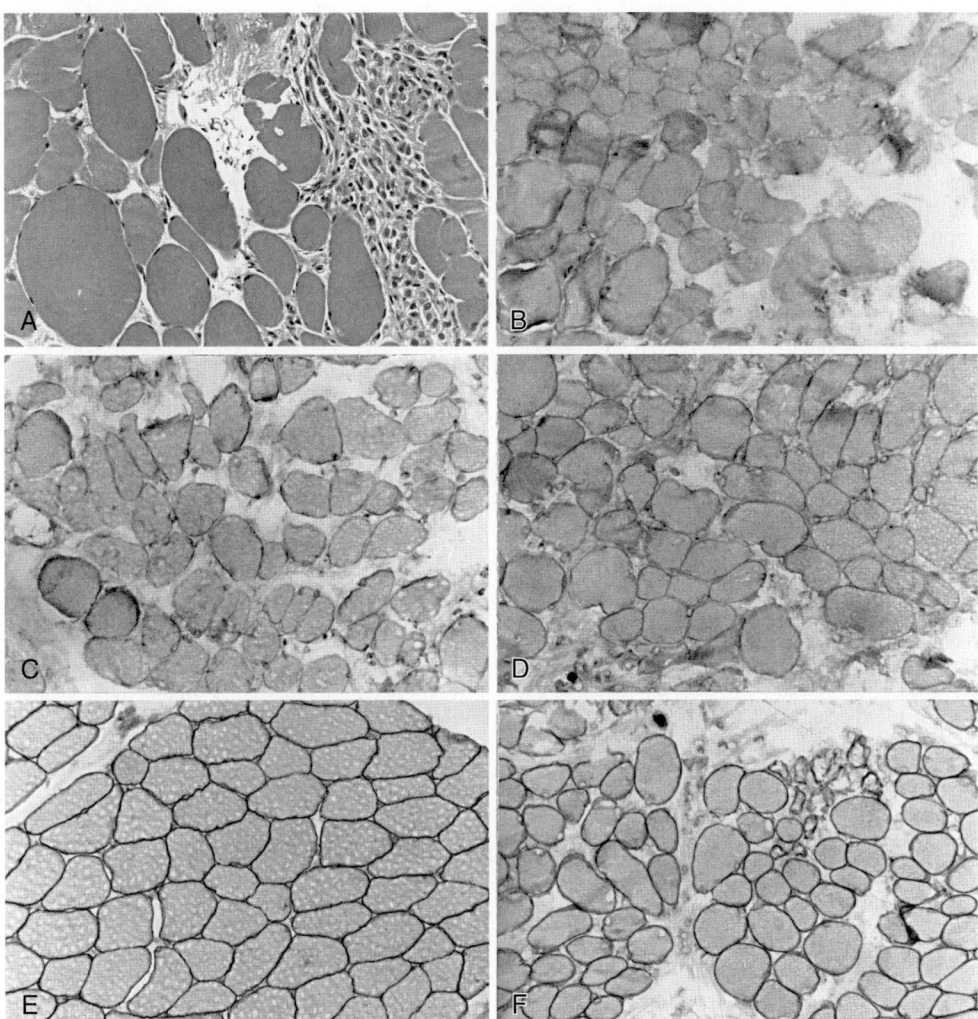

Figure 609-3 Quadriceps femoris muscle biopsy specimens from a 4 yr old boy with Becker muscular dystrophy. **A,** Myofibers vary greatly in size, with both atrophic and hypertrophic forms; at the right is a zone of degeneration and necrosis infiltrated by macrophages, similar to Duchenne muscular dystrophy (hematoxylin and eosin, ×250). Immunoreactivity using antibodies against the dystrophin molecule in the rod domain **(B),** carboxyl-terminus **(C),** and aminoterminus **(D)** all show deficient but not totally absent dystrophin expression; most fibers of all sizes retain some dystrophin in parts of the sarcolemma but not around the entire circumference in cross section. Alternatively, the prominence of dystrophin is less, appearing weak, when compared with the simultaneously incubated normal control from another child of similar age **(E). F,** Merosin expression is normal in this patient with Becker dystrophy, in both large and small myofibers, and is lacking only in frankly necrotic fibers. Compare with classic Duchenne muscular dystrophy illustrated in Figure 609-2C and with Figure 609-6.

considerable weight gain and osteoporosis, can offset this advantage or even result in greater weakness than might have occurred in the natural course of the disease. Nevertheless, some patients with DMD treated early with steroids appear to have an improved long-term prognosis in muscle and myocardial outcome, as well as short-term improvement in muscle strength, and steroids can help keep patients ambulatory for more years than expected without treatment. One protocol gives prednisone (0.75 mg/kg/day) for the 1st 10 days of each month to avoid chronic complications. Deflazacort, administered as 0.9 mg/kg/day, may be more effective than prednisone. Fluorinated steroids, such as dexamethasone or triamcinolone, should be avoided because they induce myopathy by altering the myotube abundance of ceramide. The American Academy of Neurology and the Child Neurology Society recommend administering corticosteroids during the ambulatory stage of the disease.

Another potential treatment still under investigation is intravenous or subcutaneous injection of antisense oligonucleotide drugs that induce exon skipping during mRNA splicing in patients with susceptible mutations (~15% of patients) to restore the open reading frame in the DMD gene. Drisapersen and eteplirsen are exon 51 skipping antisense oligonucleotides that bind RNA and skip (bridge) over the defective exon, thus producing a shorter but potentially functional dystrophin protein. The shortened protein has been demonstrated to appear in muscle biopsies after treatment with these agents.

Bibliography is available at Expert Consult.

609.2 Emery-Dreifuss Muscular Dystrophy
Harvey B. Sarnat

Emery-Dreifuss muscular dystrophy, also known as **scapuloperoneal or scapulohumeral muscular dystrophy,** is a rare X-linked recessive dystrophy. The usual locus of its associated genetic abnormality is on the long arm within the large Xq28 region that includes other mutations that cause myotubular myopathy, neonatal adrenoleukodystrophy, and the Bloch-Sulzberger type of incontinentia pigmenti; it is far from the gene for DMD on the short arm of the X chromosome. Another, rarer form of Emery-Dreifuss dystrophy is transmitted as an autosomal dominant trait and is localized at 1q. This form can manifest quite late, in adolescence or early adult life, although the muscular and cardiac symptoms and signs are similar, and sudden death from ventricular fibrillation is a risk.

Clinical manifestations begin at between 5 and 15 yr of age, but many patients survive to late adult life because of the slow progression of the disease's course. A rarer severe infantile presentation also is documented. Muscles do not exhibit pseudohypertrophy. Contractures of elbows and ankles develop early, and muscle becomes wasted in a scapulohumeroperoneal distribution. Facial weakness does not occur; this disease is thus distinguished clinically from autosomal dominant scapulohumeral and scapuloperoneal syndromes of neurogenic origin. Myotonia is absent. Intellectual function is normal. Dilated cardiomyopathy is severe and is often the cause of death, more commonly from conduction defects such as atrial fibrillation/flutter and sudden ventricular fibrillation than from intractable myocardial failure. Stroke is another complication, secondary to the cardiac arrhythmia. The serum CK value is only mildly to moderately elevated, further distinguishing this disease from other X-linked recessive muscular dystrophies.

Nonspecific myofiber necrosis and endomysial fibrosis are seen in the muscle biopsy. Many centronuclear fibers and selective histochemical type I muscle fiber atrophy can cause confusion with myotonic dystrophy.

GENETICS

The defective gene in the X-linked form is called *EMD* or *EDMD* and encodes a protein, emerin. Unlike other dystrophies in which the defective gene is expressed at the sarcolemmal membrane, emerin is expressed at the inner nuclear membrane; this protein stabilizes the nuclear membrane against the mechanical stresses that occur during muscular contraction. It interacts with *Nesprin-1* and *Nesprin-2* genes, also critical for nuclear membrane integrity. Complete deletion of *EDMD* occurs in approximately 25% of cases and results from an inversion in the Xq28 region; total absence of emerin is demonstrated by both Western blotting and immunoreactivity in tissue sections. Another gene, *LMNA*, at the 1q21 locus, is linked to the nuclear envelope and encodes lamins A and C, sometimes termed *laminopathy*. This genetic mutation causes an identical clinical phenotype to EMD defects, except that both sexes are affected and it is transmitted as either an autosomal dominant or recessive trait. Most *EDMD* deletions are null mutations, whereas most *LMNA* alterations are mainly missense mutations with a minority being nonsense or out-of-frame mutations. Desmin protein also may be mutated and seen to be abnormally expressed in the muscle biopsy. Homozygous nonsense mutations in these *lamin A/C* genes are lethal owing to cardiomyopathy and conduction disturbances.

DIAGNOSIS AND INVESTIGATIONS

In suspected cases, emerin deficiency may be demonstrated not only in the muscle biopsy by immunoreactivity and Western blotting techniques but also in a variety of other tissues, including circulating lymphocytes in peripheral blood, exfoliative buccal mucosal cells, and skin fibroblasts. Emerin is absent in varying proportions in female carriers. Genetic testing of the specific genes also is available. Patients should all have careful cardiac evaluation, including electrocardiogram and echocardiogram. Serum CK should be measured because it may be moderately elevated; though nonspecific, it provides a baseline for comparison with future measurements. Muscle MRI of the glutei and lower extremities may be helpful, particularly in *LMNA* mutations. EMG is not definitively diagnostic, but it provides a serial means of following the progression of the myopathy. Muscle biopsy is diagnostic from the onset of symptoms. In the differential diagnosis, an Emery-Dreifuss–like syndrome with joint contractures, mild weakness, and later-onset cardiac symptoms is caused by *FHL1* mutations of myofibrillar myopathy, but reducing bodies are absent.

Treatment should be supportive, with special attention to cardiac conduction defects, and can require medications or a pacemaker. Implantable cardioverter-defibrillators are now available and have prevented sudden death in some patients with Emery-Dreifuss muscular dystrophy.

Bibliography is available at Expert Consult.

609.3 Myotonic Muscular Dystrophy

Harvey B. Sarnat

Myotonic dystrophy (Steinert disease) is the second most common muscular dystrophy in North America, Europe, and Australia, having an incidence varying from 1 in 100,000 to 1 in 300,000 in the general population. It is inherited as an autosomal dominant trait. Classic myotonic dystrophy (type 1) (DM1) is caused by a CTG trinucleotide expansion on chromosome 19q13.3 in the 3′ untranslated region of *DMPK*, the gene that encodes a serine-threonine protein kinase. Type 2 (DM2) is associated with unstable CCTG tetranucleotide repeat expansion on chromosome 3q21 of an intron of the zinc finger 9 protein gene. A third, late form (DM3) is identified, at locus 15q21-q24.

Myotonic dystrophy is an example of a genetic defect causing dysfunction in multiple organ systems. Not only is striated muscle severely affected, but smooth muscle of the alimentary tract and uterus is also involved, cardiac function is altered, and patients have multiple and variable endocrinopathies, immunologic deficiencies, cataracts, dysmorphic facies, increased risk for malignancies, intellectual impairment, and other neurologic abnormalities.

CLINICAL MANIFESTATIONS

DM1 becomes symptomatic at any age, but DM2 is rarely expressed in infancy or early childhood. In the usual clinical course, **excluding the severe neonatal** form, DM1 infants can appear almost normal at birth, or facial wasting and hypotonia can already be early expressions of the disease. The facial appearance is characteristic, consisting of an inverted V-shaped upper lip, thin cheeks, and scalloped, concave temporalis muscles (Fig. 609-4). The head may be narrow, and the palate is high and arched because the weak temporal and pterygoid muscles in late fetal life do not exert sufficient lateral forces on the developing head and face.

Weakness is mild in the 1st few yr. Progressive wasting of distal muscles becomes increasingly evident, particularly involving intrinsic muscles of the hands. The thenar and hypothenar eminences are flattened, and the atrophic dorsal interossei leave deep grooves between the fingers. The dorsal forearm muscles and anterior compartment muscles of the lower legs also become wasted. The tongue is thin and atrophic. Wasting of the sternocleidomastoids gives the neck a long, thin, cylindrical contour. Proximal muscles also eventually undergo atrophy, and scapular winging appears. Difficulty with climbing stairs

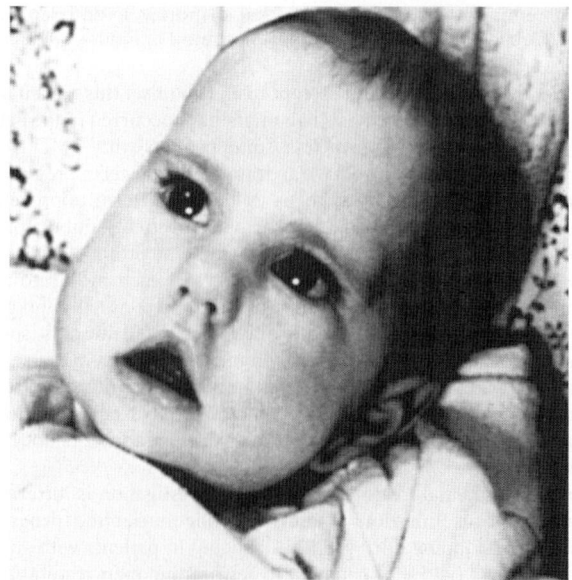

Figure 609-4 Facial weakness, inverted V–shaped upper lip, and loss of muscle mass in the temporal fossae are characteristic of myotonic muscular dystrophy, even in infancy, as seen in this 8 mo old girl.

and Gowers sign are progressive. Tendon stretch reflexes are usually preserved.

The distal distribution of muscle wasting in myotonic dystrophy is an *exception* to the general rule of myopathies having proximal and neuropathies having distal distribution patterns. The muscular atrophy and weakness in myotonic dystrophy are slowly progressive throughout childhood and adolescence and continue into adulthood. It is rare for patients with myotonic dystrophy to lose the ability to walk even in late adult life, although splints or bracing may be required to stabilize the ankles.

Myotonia, a characteristic feature shared by few other myopathies, does not occur in infancy and is usually not clinically or even electromyographically evident until about age 5 yr. Exceptional patients develop it as early as age 3 yr. Myotonia is a very slow relaxation of muscle after contraction, regardless of whether that contraction was voluntary or was induced by a stretch reflex or electrical stimulation. During physical examination, myotonia may be demonstrated by asking the patient to make tight fists and then to quickly open the hands (grip myotonia; Fig. 609-5). It may be induced by striking the thenar eminence with a rubber percussion hammer (percussion myotonia), and it may be detected by watching the involuntary drawing of the thumb across the palm. Myotonia can also be demonstrated in the tongue by pressing the edge of a wooden tongue blade against its dorsal surface and by observing a deep furrow that disappears slowly. The severity of myotonia does not necessarily parallel the degree of weakness, and the weakest muscles often have only minimal myotonia. *Myotonia is not a painful muscle spasm.* Myalgias do not occur in myotonic dystrophy.

The **speech** of patients with myotonic dystrophy is often articulated poorly and is slurred because of the involvement of the muscles of the face, tongue, and pharynx. Difficulties with swallowing sometimes occur. Aspiration pneumonia is a risk in severely involved children. Incomplete external ophthalmoplegia sometimes results from extraocular muscle weakness.

Smooth muscle involvement of the **gastrointestinal tract** results in slow gastric emptying, poor peristalsis, and constipation. Some patients have encopresis associated with anal sphincter weakness. Women with myotonic dystrophy can have ineffective or abnormal uterine contractions during labor and delivery.

Cardiac involvement is usually manifested as heart block in the Purkinje conduction system and arrhythmias (and sudden death) rather than as cardiomyopathy, unlike most other muscular dystrophies. Atrial or ventricular tachyarrhythmias have also resulted in sudden death in adults and older children.

Endocrine abnormalities involve many glands and appear at any time during the course of the disease so that endocrine status must be

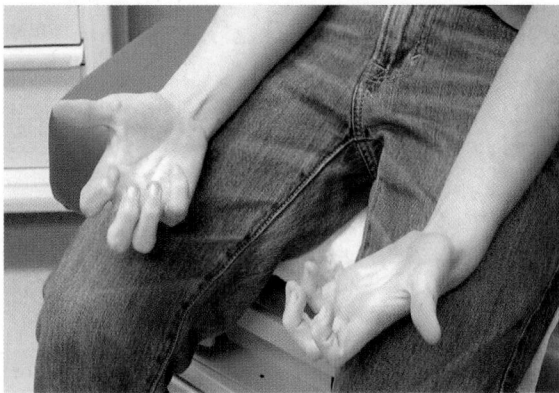

Figure 609-5 The patient was asked to squeeze with both of his hands for several seconds and then suddenly release his grasp, and several seconds passed before full relaxation was achieved, an exam finding known as grip myotonia. *(From Hughes BN, Hogue JS, Hsieh DT: Grip and percussion myotonia in myotonic dystrophy type 1, J Pediatr 164:1234, 2014.)*

reevaluated annually. Hypothyroidism is common; hyperthyroidism occurs rarely. Adrenocortical insufficiency can lead to an addisonian crisis even in infancy. Diabetes mellitus is common in patients with myotonic dystrophy; some children have a disorder of insulin release rather than defective insulin production. Onset of puberty may be precocious or, more often, delayed. Testicular atrophy and testosterone deficiency are common in adults and are responsible for a high incidence of male infertility. Ovarian atrophy is rare. Frontal baldness is also characteristic in male patients and often begins in adolescence.

Immunologic deficiencies are common in myotonic dystrophy. The plasma immunoglobulin G level is often low.

Cataracts often occur in myotonic dystrophy. They may be congenital, or they can begin at any time during childhood or adult life. Early cataracts are detected only by slit-lamp examination; periodic examination by an ophthalmologist is recommended. Visual evoked potentials are often abnormal in children with myotonic dystrophy and are unrelated to cataracts. They are not usually accompanied by visual impairment.

About half of the patients with myotonic dystrophy are **intellectually impaired,** but severe intellectual impairment is unusual. The remainder are of average or occasionally above-average intelligence. Epilepsy is not common. Cognitive impairment might result from accumulations of mutant *DMPK* mRNA and aberrant alternative splicing in cerebral cortical neurons. A higher than expected incidence of autism occurs in children with DM1.

A severe **congenital form** of myotonic dystrophy appears in a minority of involved infants born to mothers with symptomatic myotonic dystrophy. All patients with this severe congenital disease to date have had the DM1 form. Clubfoot deformities alone or more extensive congenital contractures of many joints can involve all extremities (arthrogryposis multiplex congenita) and even include the cervical spine. Generalized hypotonia and weakness are present at birth. Facial wasting is prominent. Infants can require gavage feeding or ventilator support for respiratory muscle weakness or apnea. Those requiring ventilation for <30 days often survive, and those with prolonged ventilation have an infant mortality of 25%. Children ventilated for <30 days have better motor, language, and daily activity skills than those requiring prolonged ventilation. One or both leaves of the diaphragm may be nonfunctional. The abdomen becomes distended with gas in the stomach and intestine because of poor peristalsis from smooth muscle weakness. The distention further compromises respiration. Inability to empty the rectum can compound the problem.

LABORATORY FINDINGS

The classic myotonic electromyogram is not found in infants but can appear in toddlers or children in the early school years. The levels of serum CK and other serum enzymes from muscle may be normal or only mildly elevated in the hundreds (never the thousands).

ECG should be performed annually in early childhood. Ultrasound imaging of the abdomen may be indicated in affected infants to determine diaphragmatic function. Radiographs of the chest and abdomen and contrast studies of gastrointestinal motility may be needed.

Endocrine assessment should be undertaken to determine thyroid and adrenal cortical function and to verify carbohydrate metabolism (glucose tolerance test). Immunoglobulins should be examined, and, if needed, more extensive immunologic studies should be performed.

DIAGNOSIS

The primary diagnostic test is a DNA analysis of blood to demonstrate the abnormal expansion of the CTG or CCTG repeat. Prenatal diagnosis also is feasible. The muscle biopsy specimen in older children shows many muscle fibers with central nuclei and selective atrophy of histochemical type I fibers, but degenerating fibers are usually few and widely scattered, and there is little or no fibrosis of muscle. Intrafusal fibers of muscle spindles are also abnormal. In young children with the common form of the disease, the biopsy specimen can even appear normal or at least not show myofiber necroses, which is a striking contrast with DMD. In the severe neonatal form of myotonic dystrophy, the muscle biopsy reveals maturational arrest in various stages of development in some and congenital muscle fiber-type disproportion in others. It is likely that the sarcolemmal membrane of muscle fibers not only has abnormal properties of electrical polarization but is also incapable of responding to trophic influences of the motor neuron. Muscle biopsy is not usually required for diagnosis, which in typical cases can be based on the clinical manifestations, including family history. **Neonatal myotonic dystrophy** must be distinguished from amyoplasia, congenital muscular dystrophy with or without merosin expression, congenital myasthenia gravis, spinal muscular atrophy, and arthrogryposis secondary to oligohydramnios.

GENETICS
The genetic defect in myotonic muscular dystrophy is on chromosome 19 at the 19q13 locus. It consists of an expansion of the *DM* gene that encodes a serine-threonine kinase *(DMPK)*, with numerous repeats of the CTG codon. Expansions range from 50 to >2,000, with the normal alleles of this gene ranging in size from 5-37; the larger the expansion, the more severe the clinical expression, with the largest expansions seen in the severe neonatal form. Rarely, the disease is associated with no detectable repeats, perhaps a spontaneous correction of a previous expansion but a phenomenon still incompletely understood. Another myotonic dystrophy (proximal myotonic myopathy) is a clinical entity linked to at least 2 different chromosomal loci than classic myotonic dystrophy but to 1 locus that shares a common unique pathogenesis in being mediated by a mutant mRNA. Defects in RNA splicing explain the insulin resistance in myotonic dystrophies as well as the myotonia.

Clinical and genetic expression can vary between siblings or between an affected parent and child. In the severe neonatal form of the disease, the mother is the transmitting parent in 94% of cases, a fact not explained by increased male infertility alone. Several cases of paternal transmission have been reported. Genetic analysis reveals that symptomatic neonates usually have many more repeats of the CTG codon than do patients with the more classic form of the disease, regardless of which parent is affected. Myotonic dystrophy often exhibits a pattern of **anticipation** in which each successive generation has a tendency to be more severely involved than the previous generation. Prenatal genetic diagnosis of myotonic dystrophy is available.

Treatment
There is no specific medical treatment, but the cardiac, endocrine, gastrointestinal, and ocular complications can often be treated. Physiotherapy and orthopedic treatment of contractures in the neonatal form of the disease may be beneficial. Myotonia may improve with exercise (warm-up phenomenon). Cardiac pacemaker implantation might be considered for heart block and antiarrhythmic drugs might be indicated but are needed only rarely in children.

Myotonia may be diminished, and function may be restored by drugs that raise the depolarization threshold of muscle membranes, such as mexiletine, phenytoin, carbamazepine, procainamide, and quinidine sulfate. These drugs also have cardiotropic effects; thus, cardiac evaluation is important before prescribing them. Phenytoin and carbamazepine are used in doses similar to their use as antiepileptics (see Chapter 593.6); serum concentrations of 10-20 μg/mL for phenytoin and 5-12 μg/mL for carbamazepine should be maintained. If a patient's disability is caused mainly by weakness rather than by myotonia, these drugs will be of no value.

OTHER MYOTONIC SYNDROMES
Most patients with myotonia have myotonic dystrophy. However, myotonia is not specific for this disease and occurs in several rarer conditions.

Myotonic chondrodystrophy (Schwartz-Jampel disease) is a rare congenital disease characterized by generalized muscle hypertrophy and weakness. Dysmorphic phenotypical features and the radiographic appearance of long bones are reminiscent of Morquio disease (see Chapter 88), but abnormal mucopolysaccharides are not found. Dwarfism, joint abnormalities, and blepharophimosis are present. Several patients have been the products of consanguinity, suggesting autosomal recessive inheritance. The muscle protein perlecan, encoded by the *SJS1* gene, a large heparan sulfate proteoglycan of basement membranes and cartilage, is defective in some cases of Schwartz-Jampel disease and explains both the muscular hyperexcitability and the chondrodysplasia.

EMG reveals continuous electrical activity in muscle fibers closely resembling or identical to myotonia. Muscle biopsy reveals nonspecific

Table 609-1	Channelopathies and Related Disorders			
DISORDER	**PATTERN OF CLINICAL FEATURES**	**INHERITANCE**	**CHROMOSOME**	**GENE**
CHLORIDE CHANNELOPATHIES				
Myotonia Congenita				
Thomsen disease	Myotonia	Autosomal dominant	7q35	*CLC1*
Becker disease	Myotonia and weakness	Autosomal recessive	7q35	*CLC1*
SODIUM CHANNELOPATHIES				
Paramyotonia congenita	Paramyotonia	Autosomal dominant	17q13.1-13.3	*SCNA4A*
Hyperkalemic periodic paralysis	Periodic paralysis with myotonia and paramyotonia	Autosomal dominant	17q13.1-13.3	*CNA4A*
Hypokalemic periodic paralysis	Periodic paralysis	Autosomal dominant	17q13.1-13.3	*SCNA4A*
POTASSIUM-AGGRAVATED MYOTONIAS				
Myotonia fluctuans	Myotonia	Autosomal dominant	17q13.1-13.3	*SCNA4A*
Myotonia permanens	Myotonia	Autosomal dominant	17q13.1-13.3	*SCNA4A*
Acetazolamide-responsive myotonia	Myotonia	Autosomal dominant	17q13.1-13.3	*SCNA4A*
CALCIUM CHANNELOPATHIES				
Hypokalemic periodic paralysis	Periodic paralysis	Autosomal dominant	1q31-32	Dihydropyridine receptor
Schwartz-Jampel syndrome (chondrodystrophic myotonia)	Myotonia; dysmorphic	Autosomal recessive	1q34.1-36.1	*Perlecan*
Rippling muscle disease	Muscle mounding, stiffness	Autosomal dominant	1q41	*Caveolin-3*
Anderson syndrome	Periodic paralysis, cardiac arrhythmia, distinctive facies	Autosomal dominant	17q23	*KCNJ2-Kir2.1*
Brody disease	Delayed relaxation, no electromyogram myotonia	Autosomal recessive	16p12	Calcium adenosine triphosphatase
Malignant hyperthermia	Anesthetic-induced delayed relaxation	Autosomal dominant	19q13.1	Ryanodine receptor

From Goldman L, Ausiello D: Cecil textbook of medicine, ed 22, Philadelphia, 2004, WB Saunders.

myopathic features, which are minimal in some cases and pronounced in others. The sarcotubular system is dilated.

Myotonia congenita (Thomsen disease) is a channelopathy (Table 609-1) and is characterized by weakness and generalized muscular hypertrophy so that affected children resemble bodybuilders. Myotonia is prominent and can develop at age 2-3 yr, earlier than in myotonic dystrophy. The disease is clinically stable and is apparently not progressive for many years. Muscle biopsy specimens show minimal pathologic changes, and the EMG demonstrates myotonia. Various families are described as showing either autosomal dominant (Thomsen disease) or recessive (Becker disease, not to be confused with BMD or DMD) inheritance. Rarely, myotonic dystrophy and myotonia congenita coexist in the same family. The autosomal dominant and autosomal recessive forms of myotonia congenita have been mapped to the same 7q35 locus. This gene is important for the integrity of chloride channels of the sarcolemmal and T-tubular membranes.

Paramyotonia is a temperature-related myotonia that is aggravated by cold and alleviated by warm external temperatures. Patients have difficulty when swimming in cold water or if they are dressed inadequately in cold weather. *Paramyotonia congenita* (Eulenburg disease) is a defect in a gene at the 17q13.1-13.3 locus, the identical locus identified in hyperkalemic periodic paralysis. By contrast with myotonia congenita, paramyotonia is a disorder of the voltage-gated sodium channel caused by a mutation in the α subunit. Myotonic dystrophy also is a sodium channelopathy (see Table 609-1).

In sodium channelopathies, exercise produces increasing myotonia, whereas in chloride channelopathies, exercise reduces the myotonia. This is easily tested during examination by asking patients to close the eyes forcefully and open them repeatedly; it becomes progressively more difficult in sodium channel disorders and progressively easier in chloride channel disorders.

Bibliography is available at Expert Consult.

609.4 Limb-Girdle Muscular Dystrophies

Harvey B. Sarnat

Limb-girdle muscular dystrophies (LGMDs) encompass a heterogeneous group of progressive hereditary muscular dystrophies that mainly affect muscles of the hip and shoulder girdles (Table 609-2). Distal muscles also eventually become atrophic and weak. Hypertrophy of the calves and ankle contractures develop in some forms, causing potential confusion with BMD. Sixteen genetic forms of LGMD are now described, each at a different chromosomal locus and expressing different protein defects. Some include diseases classified with other traditional groups, such as the lamin-A/C defects of the nuclear membrane (see Emery-Dreifuss muscular dystrophy, above), and some forms of congenital muscular dystrophy. LGMD1 denotes autosomal dominant inheritance and LGMD2 implies an autosomal recessive trait, but neither term defines the genetic etiology. LGMD2 is mainly a group of several sarcoglycanopathies, calpainopathy resulting from a mutation in the *calpain-3* gene (*CAPN3*), or dysferlinopathies that include Miyoshi myopathy, which usually does not become symptomatic until adult life.

The initial **clinical manifestations** rarely appear before middle or late childhood or may be delayed until early adult life. Low back pain may be a presenting complaint because of the lordotic posture resulting from gluteal muscle weakness. Confinement to a wheelchair usually becomes obligatory at about 30 yr of age. The rate of progression varies from one pedigree to another but is uniform within a kindred. Although weakness of neck flexors and extensors is universal, facial, lingual, and other bulbar-innervated muscles are rarely involved. As weakness and muscle wasting progress, tendon stretch reflexes become diminished. Cardiac involvement is unusual. Intellectual function is generally normal. The clinical **differential diagnosis** of LGMD includes juvenile spinal muscular atrophy (Kugelberg-Welander disease), myasthenia gravis, and metabolic myopathies.

The EMG and muscle biopsy show confirmatory evidence of muscular dystrophy, but none of the findings is specific enough to make the definitive **diagnosis** without additional clinical criteria. In some cases, α-sarcoglycan (formerly known as *adhalin*), a dystrophin-related glycoprotein of the sarcolemma, is deficient; this specific defect may be demonstrated in the muscle biopsy by immunocytochemistry, as may deficiency of 3 other forms of sarcoglycan as well. Increased serum CK level is usual, but the magnitude of elevation varies among families. The ECG is usually unaltered.

In one autosomal dominant form of LGMD, a genetic defect has been localized to the long arm of chromosome 5. In the autosomal recessive disease, it is on the long arm of chromosome 15. A mutated dystrophin-associated protein in the sarcoglycan complex (sarcoglycanopathy; LGMD types 2C, 2E, and 2F) is responsible for some cases of autosomal recessive LGMD. Most sarcoglycanopathies result from a mutation in α-sarcoglycan; other LGMDs resulting from deficiencies in β-, γ-, and δ-sarcoglycan also occur. In normal smooth muscle, α-sarcoglycan is replaced by ε-sarcoglycan, and the others are the same. A dystroglycan mutation also is implicated in some cases.

Another group of LGMDs (type 2B) are caused by allelic mutations of the dysferlin (*DYSF*) gene, another gene expressing a protein essential to structural integrity of the sarcolemma, though not associated with the dystrophin-glycoprotein complex. *DYSF* interacts with caveolin-3 or calpain-3, and *DYSF* deficiency may be secondary to defects in these other gene products. Primary calpain-3 defect (type 2A) is reported in Amish families and in families from French Reunion Island and from Brazil. Autosomal recessive (Miyoshi myopathy) and autosomal dominant traits are documented. Both are slowly progressive myopathies with onset in adolescence or young adult life and can affect distal as well as proximal muscles. Cardiomyopathy is rare. Chronically elevated serum CK in the thousands is found in dysferlinopathies. Ultrastructure shows a thickened basal lamina over defects in the sarcolemma and replacement of the sarcolemma by multiple

Table 609-2	Autosomal Recessive Limb-Girdle Muscular Dystrophies		
TYPE	**LOCATION**	**GENE PRODUCT**	**CLINICAL FEATURES**
LGMD2A	15q	Calpain 3	Onset at 8-15 yr, progression variable
LGMD2B	2p13-16	Dysferlin	Onset at adolescence, mild weakness; gene site is the same as for Miyoshi myopathy
LGMD2C	13q12	Sarcoglycan	Duchenne-like, severe childhood autosomal recessive muscular dystrophy (SCARMD1)
LGMD2D	17q12	α-Sarcoglycan (adhalin)	Duchenne-like, severe childhood autosomal recessive muscular dystrophy (SCARMD2)
LGMD2E	4q12	β-Sarcoglycan	Phenotype between Duchenne and Becker muscular dystrophies
LGMD2F	5q33-34	Sarcoglycan	Slowly progressive, growth retardation

LGMD, limb-girdle muscular dystrophy.
From Fenichel GM: Clinical pediatric neurology: a signs and symptoms approach, ed 5, Philadelphia, 2005, Elsevier Saunders, p. 176, Table 7-5.

layers of small vesicles. Regenerating myofibers outnumber degenerating myofibers. These disorders were formerly called *hyperCKemia* and *rippling muscle disease,* the latter sometimes confused with myotonia. An autosomal recessive mutation in the calcium-activated chloride channel anoctamin-5 can cause proximal LGMD2.

There is overlap of the group of LGMDs with the congenital muscular dystrophies, such as Walker-Warburg syndrome with *POMT,* Fukuyama muscular dystrophy with *FKRP* genetic defects, and Ullrich muscular dystrophy of collagen VI subunits.

Bibliography is available at Expert Consult.

609.5 Facioscapulohumeral Muscular Dystrophy
Harvey B. Sarnat

Facioscapulohumeral muscular dystrophy, also known as **Landouzy-Dejerine disease,** is probably not a single disease entity but a group of diseases with similar clinical manifestations. Autosomal dominant inheritance is the rule; genetic anticipation is often found within several generations of a family, the succeeding more severely involved at an earlier age than the preceding. The frequency is 1 : 20,000 population. Though the clinical onset is generally in later childhood or adult life, early molecular defects arising during myogenesis are demonstrated in the human fetus. The genetic mechanism in autosomal dominant facioscapulohumeral dystrophy involves integral deletions of a 3.3-kb tandem repeat (D4Z4) in the subtelomeric region at the 4q35 locus. Several other genes clustered at the 4q35 locus are upregulated in fetuses with facioscapulohumeral dystrophy. D4Z4 acts as a lamins-dependent insulator exhibiting both enhancer-blocking and barrier activities and displaces the telomere toward the nuclear periphery. A 3.3-kb repeat array at the subtelomeric locus 10q26 is closely homologous, with chromosomal translocation or sequence conversion between these 2 regions, possibly predisposing to the DNA rearrangement causing facioscapulohumeral dystrophy. Approximately 10% of families with this phenotype do not map to the 4q35 locus.

CLINICAL MANIFESTATIONS
Facioscapulohumeral dystrophy shows the earliest and most severe weakness in facial and shoulder girdle muscles. The facial weakness differs from that of myotonic dystrophy; rather than an inverted V–shaped upper lip, the mouth in facioscapulohumeral dystrophy is rounded and appears puckered because the lips protrude. Inability to close the eyes completely in sleep is a common expression of upper facial weakness; some patients have extraocular muscle weakness, although ophthalmoplegia is rarely complete. Facioscapulohumeral dystrophy has been associated with Möbius syndrome on rare occasions. Pharyngeal and tongue weakness may be absent and is never as severe as the facial involvement. Hearing loss, which may be subclinical, and retinal vasculopathy (indistinguishable from Coats disease) are associated features, particularly in severe cases of facioscapulohumeral dystrophy with early-childhood onset.

Scapular winging is prominent, often even in infants. Flattening or even concavity of the deltoid contour is seen, and the biceps and triceps brachii muscles are wasted and weak. Muscles of the hip girdle and thighs also eventually lose strength and undergo atrophy, and Gowers sign and a Trendelenburg gait appear. Contractures of the extremities are rare. Finger and wrist weakness occasionally is the first symptom. Weakness of the anterior tibial and peroneal muscles can lead to footdrop; this complication usually occurs only in advanced cases with severe weakness. Lumbar lordosis and kyphoscoliosis are common complications of axial muscle involvement. Calf pseudohypertrophy is not a usual feature but is described rarely.

Facioscapulohumeral muscular dystrophy can also be a mild disease causing minimal disability. Clinical manifestations might not be expressed in childhood and are delayed into middle adult life. Unlike most other muscular dystrophies, asymmetry of weakness is common.

About 30% of affected patients are asymptomatic or show only mild scapular winging and decreased tendon stretch reflexes, of which they were unaware until formal neurologic examination was performed.

LABORATORY FINDINGS
Serum levels of CK and other enzymes vary greatly, ranging from normal or near-normal to elevations of several thousand. An ECG should be performed, although the anticipated findings are usually normal. EMG reveals nonspecific myopathic muscle potentials. Diagnostic molecular testing in individual cases and within families is indicated for prediction.

DIAGNOSIS AND DIFFERENTIAL DIAGNOSIS
Molecular genetic diagnosis is the most specific confirmation if clinical suspicion is high, with or without a family history of the disease. Muscle biopsy distinguishes more than one form of facioscapulohumeral dystrophy, consistent with clinical evidence that several distinct diseases are embraced by the term *facioscapulohumeral dystrophy.* Muscle biopsy and EMG also distinguish the primary myopathy from a neurogenic disease with a similar distribution of muscular involvement. The general histopathologic findings in the muscle biopsy material are extensive proliferation of connective tissue between muscle fibers, extreme variation in fiber size with many hypertrophic as well as atrophic myofibers, and scattered degenerating and regenerating fibers. An "inflammatory" type of facioscapulohumeral muscular dystrophy is also distinguished, characterized by extensive lymphocytic infiltrates within muscle fascicles. Despite the resemblance of this form to inflammatory myopathies, such as polymyositis, there is no evidence of autoimmune disease, and steroids and immunosuppressive drugs do not alter the clinical course. A precise histopathologic diagnosis has important therapeutic implications. Mononuclear cell "inflammation" in a muscle biopsy sample of infants younger than 2 yr old is usually facioscapulohumeral dystrophy or, less often, a congenital muscular dystrophy.

TREATMENT
Physiotherapy is of no value in regaining strength or in retarding progressive weakness or muscle wasting. Footdrop and scoliosis may be treated by orthopedic measures. In selected cases, surgical wiring of the scapulas to the thoracic wall provides improved shoulder stability and abduction of the arm, but brachial plexopathy, frozen shoulder, and scapular fractures are reported complications. Cosmetic improvement of the facial muscles of expression may be achieved by reconstructive surgery, which grafts a fascia lata to the zygomatic muscle and to the zygomatic head of the quadratus labii superioris muscle. Exercise of facial muscles can help minimize secondary disuse atrophy. No effective pharmacologic or genetic treatment is presently available.

Bibliography is available at Expert Consult.

609.6 Congenital Muscular Dystrophies
Harvey B. Sarnat

The term *congenital muscular dystrophy* is misleading because all muscular dystrophies are genetically determined. It is used to encompass several distinct diseases that have a common characteristic of severe involvement at birth but that, ironically, often follow a more benign clinical course than the early onset and the histopathological changes in the muscle biopsy would suggest. A distinguishing feature of the congenital dystrophies, by contrast with other muscular dystrophies, is a high association with brain malformations, particularly disorders of cortical development such as lissencephaly/pachygyria and polymicrogyria, often complicated by severe epilepsy. Autosomal recessive inheritance is the rule.

CLINICAL MANIFESTATIONS
In several distinct clinical and genetic diseases grouped under the umbrella term *congenital muscular dystrophies,* infants often have

contractures or arthrogryposis at birth and are diffusely hypotonic. The muscle mass is thin in the trunk and extremities. Head control is poor. Facial muscles may be mildly involved, but ophthalmoplegia, pharyngeal weakness, and weak sucking are not common. A minority has severe dysphagia and requires gavage or gastrostomy. Tendon stretch reflexes may be hypoactive or absent. Arthrogryposis is common in all forms of congenital muscular dystrophy (see Chapter 608.10). Congenital contractures of the elbows have a high association with the **Ullrich type of congenital muscular dystrophy** owing to a defect in 1 or more of the 3 collagen VI genes, each at a different locus.

The congenital muscular dystrophies can be classified according to the type of protein altered by the specific genetic mutations. Diseases of extracellular matrix proteins include merosin deficiency (*LAMA2* mutation at locus 6q22-q23) and Ullrich disease (*COL6A1, -A2* and *-A3* mutations at 21q22 and 2q37 loci). A protein of the endoplasmic reticulum (*SEPN1* mutation at 1p35) is the basis of rigid spine syndrome. Abnormal glycosylation of α-dystroglycan causes Walker-Warburg syndrome (*POMT1* mutation at 9q34), muscle-eye-brain disease of Santavuori (*POMGnT1* mutation at 1p32), Fukuyama muscular dystrophy (*FCMD* mutation at 8q31-q33 and 9q31), and congenital muscular dystrophy with secondary merosin deficiency (*FKRP* mutation at 19q13). Glycosylation defects (dystroglycanopathies) result in defective neuroblast migration in the fetal brain and also can cause dilated cardiomyopathy. The dystroglycan molecule interacts with both proteins of the plasma (sarcolemmal) membrane and those of the extracellular matrix and basal lamina not only in muscle but also in brain, where defective dystroglycan and poor glycosylation result in gaps in the pial limiting membrane, a discontinuous glia limitans, causing cobblestone lissencephaly and glioneuronal heterotopia of overmigrated neural cells during formation of the cerebral cortex.

The **Fukuyama type** of congenital muscular dystrophy is the second most common muscular dystrophy in Japan (after DMD); it has also been reported in children of Dutch, German, Scandinavian, and Turkish ethnic backgrounds. In the Fukuyama variety, severe cardiomyopathy and malformations of the brain usually accompany the skeletal muscle involvement. Signs and symptoms related to these organs are prominent: cardiomegaly and heart failure, intellectual disability, seizures, microcephaly, and failure to thrive.

Central neurologic disease can accompany forms of congenital muscular dystrophy other than Fukuyama disease. Mental and neurologic status is the most variable feature; an apparently normal brain and normal intelligence do not preclude the diagnosis if other manifestations indicate this myopathy. The cerebral malformations that occur are not consistently of one type and vary from severe dysplasias (holoprosencephaly, lissencephaly) to milder conditions (agenesis of the corpus callosum, focal heterotopia of the cerebral cortex and subcortical white matter, cerebellar hypoplasia). Seizures are a frequent complication, as early as the neonatal period, and may include infantile spasms and other severe infantile epilepsies.

Congenital muscular dystrophy is a constant association with cerebral dysgenesis in the **Walker-Warburg syndrome** and in **muscle-eye-brain disease of Santavuori.** The neuropathologic findings are those of neuroblast migratory abnormalities in the cerebral cortex, cerebellum, and brainstem. Studies indicate considerably more genetic overlap between Walker-Warburg, Fukuyama, and muscle-eye-brain forms of congenital muscular dystrophy that explain mixed and transitional phenotypes, so that, for example, a *Fukutin*-related (*FKRP*) gene can cause a Walker-Warburg or muscle-eye-brain presentation, or *POMGnT1* also can produce phenotypes other than classic Walker-Warburg disease.

LABORATORY FINDINGS

Serum CK level is usually moderately elevated from several hundred to many thousand IU/L; only marginal increases are sometimes found. EMG shows nonspecific myopathic features. Investigation of all forms of congenital muscular dystrophy should include cardiac assessment and an imaging study of the brain. Muscle biopsy is essential for the diagnosis, but if there is a high degree of suspicion (e.g., a confirmed

genetic defect in a sibling), specific genetic testing might avoid the muscle biopsy.

DIAGNOSIS

Muscle biopsy is diagnostic in the neonatal period or thereafter. An extensive proliferation of endomysial collagen envelops individual muscle fibers even at birth, also causing them to be rounded in cross-sectional contour by acting as a rigid sleeve, especially during contraction. The perimysial connective tissue and fat are also increased, and the fascicular organization of the muscle may be disrupted by the fibrosis. Tissue cultures of intramuscular fibroblasts exhibit increased collagen synthesis, but the structure of the collagen is normal. Muscle fibers vary in diameter, and many show central nuclei, myofibrillar splitting, and other cytoarchitectural alterations. Scattered degenerating and regenerating fibers are seen. No inflammation or abnormal inclusions are found.

Immunocytochemical reactivity for merosin (α₂ chain of laminin) at the sarcolemmal region is absent in approximately 40% of cases and normally expressed in the others (Figs. 609-6 and 609-7).

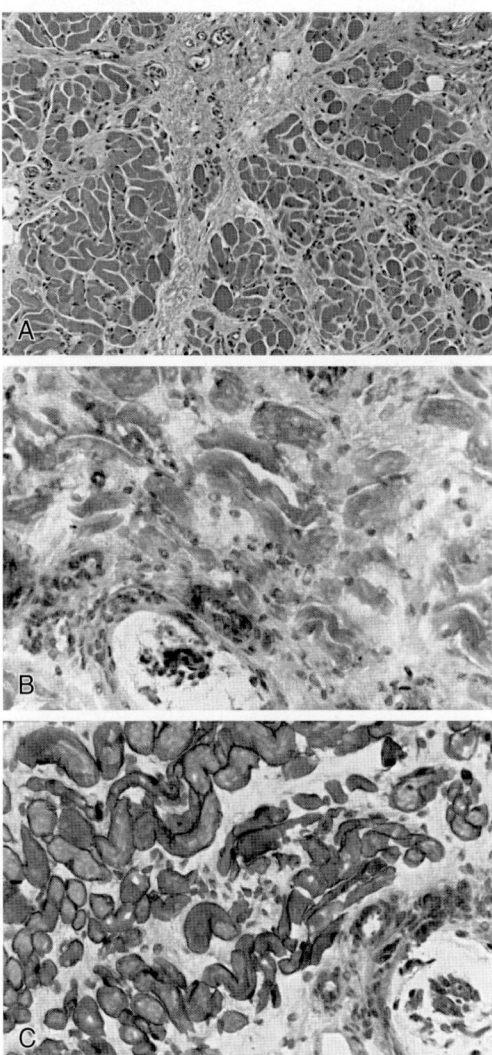

Figure 609-6 Quadriceps femoris muscle biopsy of a 6 mo old girl with congenital muscular dystrophy associated with merosin (α₂-laminin) deficiency. **A,** Histologically, the muscle is infiltrated by a great proliferation of collagenous connective tissue; myofibers vary in diameter, but necrotic fibers are rare. **B,** Immunocytochemical reactivity for merosin (α₂-laminin) is absent in all fibers, including the intrafusal myofibers of a muscle spindle seen at bottom. **C,** Dystrophin expression (rod domain) is normal. Compare with Figures 609-2, 609-3, and 609-7.

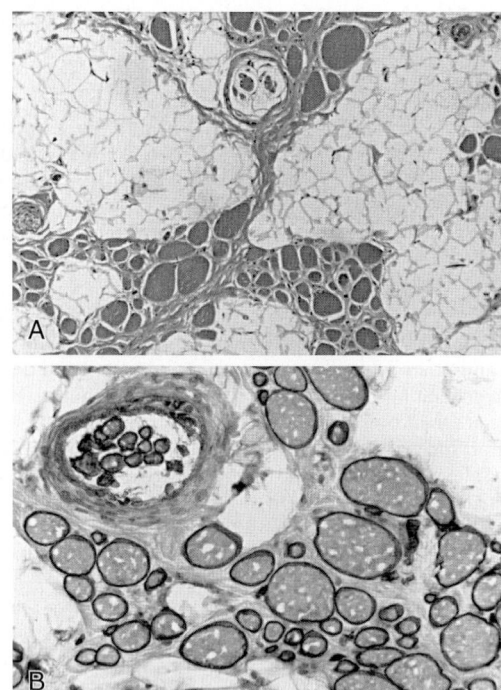

Figure 609-7 Quadriceps femoris muscle biopsy specimen of a 2 yr old girl with congenital muscular dystrophy. **A,** The fascicular architecture of the muscle is severely disrupted, and muscle is replaced by fat and connective tissue; the remaining small groups of myofibers of variable size are seen, including a muscle spindle at top. **B,** Merosin expression is normal in both extrafusal fibers of all sizes and in intrafusal spindle fibers. The severity of the myopathy does not relate to the presence or absence of merosin in congenital muscular dystrophy. Compare with Figure 609-6.

Merosin is a protein that binds the sarcolemmal membrane of the myofiber to the basal lamina or basement membrane. Merosin also is expressed in brain and in Schwann cells. The presence or absence of merosin does not always correlate with the severity of the myopathy or predict its course, but cases with merosin deficiency tend to have more severe cerebral involvement. Adhalin (α-dystroglycan) may be secondarily reduced in some cases. Collagen VI is selectively reduced or absent in Ullrich disease because of a mutation in the *COL6A* gene. Mitochondrial dysfunction may be another secondary defect.

TREATMENT

Only supportive therapy is available in general. Cyclosporine might correct the mitochondrial dysfunction and muscular apoptosis in collagen VI myopathy. Though no curative treatment is presently available for the congenital muscular dystrophies, a consensus statement on the standard of supportive care was issued at a special workshop in 2009 and published the following year. It covers aspects of various organ systems that could be involved, including neurologic, pulmonary, gastroenterologic, cardiac, orthopedic/rehabilitation, and palliative care.

Bibliography is available at Expert Consult.

Chapter **610**
Endocrine and Toxic Myopathies
Harvey B. Sarnat

THYROID MYOPATHIES

See also Chapters 563-568.

Thyrotoxicosis causes proximal weakness and wasting accompanied by myopathic electromyographic changes. Thyroxine binds to myofibrils and, if in excess, impairs contractile function. **Hyperthyroidism** can also induce myasthenia gravis and hypokalemic periodic paralysis, the latter mainly affecting East Asian males who have a genetic predisposition. Mutation in the gene *KCNJ18* may be responsible for altering the potassium channel Kir2.6 in up to one third of cases. Potassium supplementation and propranolol are useful in treating thyrotoxic periodic paralysis.

Hypothyroidism, whether congenital or acquired, consistently produces hypotonia and a proximal distribution of weakness. Although muscle wasting is most characteristic, one form of cretinism, the Kocher-Debré-Sémélaigne syndrome, is characterized by generalized pseudohypertrophy of weak muscles. Infants can have a Herculean appearance reminiscent of myotonia congenita. The serum creatine kinase (CK) level is elevated in hypothyroid myopathy and returns to normal after thyroid replacement therapy.

Results of muscle biopsy in hypothyroidism reveal acute myopathic changes, including myofiber necrosis and sometimes central cores. In hyperthyroidism, the muscle biopsy specimen shows only mild, nonspecific myopathic changes without necrosis of myofibers.

The clinical and pathologic features of hyperthyroid myopathy and hypothyroid myopathy resolve after appropriate treatment of the thyroid disorder. Many of the systemic symptoms of hyperthyroidism, including myopathic weakness and ophthalmoparesis, improve with the administration of β-blockers.

Most patients with primary **hyperparathyroidism** (see Chapter 573) develop weakness, fatigability, fasciculations, and muscle wasting that is reversible after removal of the parathyroid adenoma. The serum creatine kinase and muscle biopsy remain normal, but the electromyography can show nonspecific myopathic features. A minority of patients develop myotonia that could be confused with myotonic dystrophy.

STEROID-INDUCED MYOPATHY

Natural Cushing disease and iatrogenic Cushing syndrome from exogenous corticosteroid administration can cause painless, symmetric, progressive proximal weakness, increased serum creatine kinase levels, and a myopathic electromyogram and muscle biopsy specimen (see Chapter 577). Myosin filaments may be selectively lost. The 9α-fluorinated steroids, such as dexamethasone, betamethasone, and triamcinolone, are the most likely to produce *steroid myopathy.* Dexamethasone alters the abundance of ceramides in myotubes in developing muscle. In patients with dermatomyositis or other myopathies treated with steroids, it is sometimes difficult to distinguish refractoriness of the disease from steroid-induced weakness, especially after long-term steroid administration. Vitamin D is another factor altering muscle metabolism and particularly its sensitivity to insulin; vitamin D deficiency may be accentuated and contribute to steroid myopathy, especially in type 2 diabetic patients and insulin resistance.

All patients who have been taking steroids for long periods develop reversible type II myofiber atrophy; this is a *steroid effect* but is not steroid myopathy unless it progresses to become a necrotizing myopathy. At greatest risk in the pediatric age group are children requiring long-term steroid therapy for asthma, rheumatoid arthritis, dermatomyositis, lupus, and other autoimmune or inflammatory diseases or who are being treated for leukemia or other hematologic diseases.

Table 610-1	Toxic Myopathies

INFLAMMATORY	MALIGNANT HYPERTHERMIA
Cimetidine	Halothane
D-Penicillamine	Ethylene
Procainamide	Diethyl ether
L-Tryptophan	Methoxyflurane
L-DOPA	Ethyl chloride
	Trichloroethylene
NONINFLAMMATORY	Gallamine
NECROTIZING OR VACUOLAR	Succinylcholine
Cholesterol-lowering agents	
Chloroquine	**MITOCHONDRIAL**
Colchicine	Zidovudine
Emetine	
ε-Aminocaproic acid	**MYOTONIA**
Labetalol	2,4-d-Chlorophenoxyacetic acid
Cyclosporine and tacrolimus	Anthracene-9-carboxycyclic acid
Isoretinoic acid (vitamin A	Cholesterol-lowering drugs
analog)	Chloroquine
Vincristine	Cyclosporine
Alcohol	
	MYOSIN LOSS
RHABDOMYOLYSIS AND	Nondepolarizing neuromuscular
MYOGLOBINURIA	blocking agents
Cholesterol-lowering drugs	Intravenous glucocorticoids
(especially statins)	
Alcohol	
Heroin	
Amphetamine	
Toluene	
Cocaine	
ε-Aminocaproic acid	
Pentazocine	
Phencyclidine	

From Goldman L, Ausiello D: Cecil textbook of medicine, ed 22, Philadelphia, 2004, WB Saunders, p. 2399.

In addition to steroids, the drugs listed in Table 610-1 can cause acute or chronic toxic myopathies. An incompletely understood entity known as critical illness myopathy is a progressive weakness of patients with extended illnesses who remain in the intensive care unit; it is associated pathologically with selective loss of thick (myosin) myofilaments; immobility and excessive steroid treatment are believed to be important factors. Various steroids are sometimes used chronically in the treatment of Duchenne muscular dystrophy; they may actually exaggerate the weakness because of steroid myopathy superimposed on the dystrophic process (see Chapter 609).

Hyperaldosteronism (Conn syndrome) is accompanied by episodic and reversible weakness similar to that of periodic paralysis. The proximal myopathy can become irreversible in chronic cases. Elevated creatine kinase levels and even myoglobinuria sometimes occur during acute attacks. Arterial hypertension is a frequent manifestation and, in children, aldosterone-secreting adenomas should be considered in the differential diagnosis of idiopathic hypertension. Hereditary primary aldosteronism is due to a mutation in one of the potassium channel genes *KCNJ5* and *GIRK4*.

Chronic growth hormone excess (sometimes illicitly acquired by adolescent athletes or seen in acromegaly) produces atrophy of some myofibers and hypertrophy of others, and scattered myofiber degeneration. Despite the augmented protein synthesis induced by growth hormone, it impairs myofibrillar adenosine triphosphatase activity and reduces sarcolemmal excitability, with resultant diminished, rather than increased, strength corresponding to the larger muscle mass. It has been used therapeutically in muscular dystrophy with both a positive effect and complications. *Ghrelin* is an intestinal hormone that activates a growth hormone secretagog receptor and stimulates growth hormone release. In addition to its effect as a "hunger hormone" that involves food intake and fat deposition, it also prevents muscular atrophy by inducing myodifferentiation and myoblast fusion.

Bibliography is available at Expert Consult.

Chapter 611
Metabolic Myopathies
Harvey B. Sarnat

Table 611-1 describes the differential diagnosis of metabolic myopathies.

611.1 Periodic Paralyses (Potassium-Related) and Other Muscle Channelopathies
Harvey B. Sarnat

Episodic, reversible weakness or paralysis, known as **periodic paralysis,** is associated with transient alterations in serum potassium levels, usually hypokalemia but occasionally hyperkalemia. All familial forms of periodic paralysis are caused by mutations in genes encoding voltage-gated ion channels in muscle: sodium, calcium, and potassium. Mutations in the *CACNA1S* voltage-gated calcium (not potassium) channel are the etiology of hypokalemic periodic paralysis. Nonhereditary causes of periodic paralysis are caused by a diverse group of disorders that affect potassium balance (Table 611-2). During

Table 611-1	Metabolic and Mitochondrial Myopathies

GLYCOGEN METABOLISM DEFICIENCIES
Type II: α-1,4-Glucosidase (acid maltase)
Type III: Debranching
Type IV: Branching
Type V: Phosphorylase (McArdle disease)*
Type VII: Phosphofructokinase (Tarui disease)*
Type VIII: Phosphorylase B kinase*
Type IX: Phosphoglycerate kinase*
Type X: Phosphoglycerate mutase*
Type XI: Lactate dehydrogenase*

LIPID METABOLISM DEFICIENCIES
Carnitine palmitoyltransferase*
Primary systemic/muscle carnitine deficiency
Secondary carnitine deficiency
β-Oxidation defects
Medications (valproic acid)

PURINE METABOLISM DEFICIENCIES
Myoadenylate deaminase deficiency

MITOCHONDRIAL MYOPATHIES
Alpers-Huttenlocher syndrome
Chronic progressive external ophthalmoplegia
Kearns-Sayre syndrome
Pearson syndrome
Mitochondrial encephalomyopathy with lactic acidosis and
stroke-like episodes (MELAS)
Mitochondrial neurogastrointestinal encephalomyopathy (MNGIE)
Myoclonic epilepsy with ragged red fibers (MERRF)
Leber hereditary optic neuropathy
Leigh syndrome
Infantile myopathy and lactic acidosis

*Deficiency can produce exercise intolerance and myoglobinuria.
*From Chinnery PF: Muscle diseases. In Goldman L, Schafer AI, editors: Goldman's Cecil medicine, ed 24, Philadelphia, 2012, Elsevier, Table 429-7, p. 2413.

Table 611-2	Secondary Causes of Periodic Paralysis

HYPOKALEMIC
Thyrotoxic
Primary hyperaldosteronism (Conn syndrome)
Renal tubular acidosis (e.g., Fanconi syndrome)
Juxtaglomerular apparatus hyperplasia (Bartter syndrome)
Gastrointestinal potassium wastage
Villous adenoma
Laxative abuse
Pancreatic non–insulin-secreting tumors with diarrhea
Nontropical sprue
Barium intoxication
Potassium-depleting diuretics
Amphotericin B
Licorice
Corticosteroids
Toluene toxicity
p-Aminosalicylic acid
Carbenoxolone

HYPERKALEMIC
Addison disease
Hypoaldosteronism
Excessive potassium supplementation
Potassium-sparing diuretics
Chronic renal failure

From Chinnery PF: Muscle diseases. In Goldman L, Schafer AI, editors: Goldman's Cecil medicine, ed 24, Philadelphia, 2012, Elsevier, Table 429-8, p. 2415.

attacks, myofibers are electrically unexcitable, although the contractile apparatus can respond normally to calcium. The genetic disorder is inherited as an autosomal dominant trait. It is precipitated in some patients by a heavy carbohydrate meal, insulin, epinephrine including that induced by emotional stress, hyperaldosteronism or hyperthyroidism, administration of amphotericin B, or ingestion of licorice. The defective genes are at the 17q13.1-13.3 locus in **hyperkalemic periodic paralysis,** the same as in paramyotonia congenita, and at the 1q31-32 locus in **hypokalemic periodic paralysis.**

Attacks often begin in infancy, particularly in the hyperkalemic form, and the disease is nearly always symptomatic by 10 yr of age, affecting both sexes equally. Late childhood or adolescence is the more typical age of onset of the hypokalemic form, Andersen-Tawil syndrome, and paramyotonia congenita. Periodic paralysis is an episodic event; patients are unable to move after awakening and gradually recover muscle strength during the next few minutes or hours. All 4 extremities are involved. Muscles that remain active in sleep, such as the diaphragm, extraocular muscles (rapid eye movements), and cardiac muscle, are not affected. Patients are normal between attacks, but in adult life the attacks become more frequent, and the disorder causes progressive myopathy with permanent weakness even between attacks. The usual frequency of attacks in childhood is once a week. The differential diagnosis includes thyrotoxic periodic paralysis, myotonia congenita, and paramyotonia congenita. A triad of periodic paralysis, potentially fatal cardiac ventricular ectopy (caused by a defect in Kir2.1 channels for terminal repolarization), and characteristic physical features is known as **Andersen-Tawil syndrome.**

Alterations in serum potassium levels occur only during acute episodes and are accompanied by T-wave changes in the electrocardiogram. Hypokalemia may be caused by alterations in calcium gradients. The creatine kinase (CK) level may be mildly elevated at those times. Plasma phosphate levels often decrease during symptomatic periods. Muscle biopsy findings are often normal between attacks, but during an attack a vacuolar myopathy is demonstrated. Pathologic changes in the periodic paralyses are similar, whether the disease is the result of a sodium or a potassium channel defect, suggesting that the changes might result from the recurrent paralytic state rather than the specific channelopathy. The vacuoles are dilated sarcoplasmic reticulum and invaginations of the extracellular space into the cytoplasm, and they

may be filled with glycogen. Muscle biopsy is not essential to diagnose periodic paralysis, however. Hypoglycemia does not occur. Loci for the majority of periodic paralyses have been demonstrated and the genes at least partially characterized, but many patients with the same clinical phenotype exhibit no mutations in the identified genes.

TREATMENT
Paralytic attacks of hypokalemic periodic paralysis are best treated by the oral administration of potassium or even fruit juices that contain potassium. A low sodium intake and the administration of acetazolamide, 125-250 mg bid or tid in school-age children, often is effective in abolishing attacks or at least reducing their frequency and severity. Spironolactone, in a dose of 100-200 mg/day PO in school-age children, may be beneficial as well.

OTHER MUSCLE CHANNELOPATHIES
Disorders of ion channels other than the well-documented potassium channelopathies also are recognized. A rare, severe **neonatal myotonia** is secondary to a mutation of the voltage-gated sodium-channel *SCN4A* gene; it is unrelated to neonatal myotonic dystrophy, myotonia congenita, or infantile myofibrillar myopathies. This same gene also is responsible for severe neonatal episodic laryngospasm. Mexiletine is effective treatment of the myotonia, but the long-term prognosis remains poor, with death by 2 yr of age. Sodium channel blockers, such as carbamazepine, phenytoin, and procainamide, are alternatives.

Neuromyotonia, a continuous muscle activity of neurogenic origin, may be caused by mutations in genes encoding or antibodies against potassium channels, but is rare in childhood. **Schwartz-Jampel disease,** resulting from, an autosomal recessive trait, involves severe muscle stiffness, myotonia, blepharospasm, and chondroplasia. It becomes symptomatic in the 1st yr of life and is slowly progressive until midadolescence, after which it is stable. It is no longer considered a variant of myotonic dystrophy and is caused by mutation in the *HSPG2* gene that encodes perlecan, the major heparin sulphate proteoglycan of basement membranes. Sodium channel blockers may be useful.

Bibliography is available at Expert Consult.

611.2 Malignant Hyperthermia
Harvey B. Sarnat

See also Chapters 61 and 608.4.

This syndrome is usually inherited as an autosomal dominant trait. It occurs in all patients with central core disease but is not limited to that particular myopathy. The gene is at the 19q13.1 locus in both central core disease and malignant hyperthermia without this specific myopathy. At least 15 separate mutations in this gene are associated with malignant hyperthermia. The gene programs the ryanodine receptor, a tetrameric calcium release channel in the sarcoplasmic reticulum, in apposition to the voltage-gated calcium channel of the transverse tubule. It occurs rarely in Duchenne and other muscular dystrophies, in various other myopathies, in some children with scoliosis, and in an isolated syndrome not associated with other muscle disease. Affected children sometimes have peculiar facies. All ages are affected, including premature infants whose mothers underwent general anesthesia for cesarean section.

Acute episodes are precipitated by exposure to general anesthetics and occasionally to local anesthetic drugs. Patients suddenly develop extreme fever, rigidity of muscles, and metabolic and respiratory acidosis; the serum CK level rises to as high as 35,000 IU/L. Myoglobinuria can result in tubular necrosis and acute renal failure.

The muscle biopsy specimen obtained during an episode of malignant hyperthermia or shortly afterward is not indicated but shows widely scattered necrosis of muscle fibers known as **rhabdomyolysis**. Between attacks, the muscle biopsy specimen is normal unless there is an underlying chronic myopathy.

It is important to recognize patients at risk of malignant hyperthermia because the attacks may be prevented by administering dantrolene sodium before an anesthetic is given. Patients at risk, such as siblings, are identified by the caffeine contracture test: a portion of fresh muscle biopsy tissue in a saline bath is attached to a strain gauge and exposed to caffeine and other drugs; an abnormal spasm is diagnostic. The syndrome-associated receptor also may be demonstrated by immunochemistry in frozen sections of the muscle biopsy. The gene defect of the ryanodine receptor is present in 50% of patients; gene testing is available only for this genetic group. This receptor also may be seen in the muscle biopsy by immunoreactivity. Another candidate gene is at the 1q31 locus.

Apart from the genetic disorder of malignant hyperthermia, some drugs can induce acute rhabdomyolysis with myoglobinuria and potential renal failure, but this usually occurs in patients who are predisposed by some other metabolic disease (mitochondrial myopathies). Valproic acid can induce this process in children with mitochondrial cytopathies or with carnitine palmitoyltransferase deficiency.

611.3 Glycogenoses
Harvey B. Sarnat

See also Chapter 87.1.

Glycogenosis I (von Gierke disease) is not a true myopathy because the deficient liver enzyme glucose-6-phosphatase is not normally present in muscle. Nevertheless, children with this disease are hypotonic and mildly weak for unknown reasons.

Glycogenosis II (Pompe disease) is an autosomal recessively inherited deficiency of the glycolytic lysosomal enzyme α-glucosidase (formerly known as acid maltase) that cleaves the α-1,4 and α-1,6 glycosidic linkages. Of the 12 known glycogenoses, type II is the only one with a defective lysosomal enzyme. The defective gene is at locus 17q23, with more than 200 distinct mutations identified. Two clinical forms are described. The **infantile** form is a severe generalized myopathy and cardiomyopathy. Patients have cardiomegaly and hepatomegaly and are diffusely hypotonic and weak. The serum CK level is greatly elevated. A muscle biopsy specimen reveals a vacuolar myopathy with abnormal lysosomal enzymatic activities such as acid and alkaline phosphatases. Evidence of a secondary mitochondrial cytopathy is often demonstrated; it includes electron microscopic demonstration of paracrystallin structures within muscle mitochondria and low concentrations of respiratory chain enzymes. Death in infancy or early childhood is usual; however, enzyme replacement therapy has improved the outcome.

The **late childhood** or **adult** form is a much milder myopathy without cardiac or hepatic enlargement. It might not become clinically expressed until later childhood or early adult life but may be symptomatic as myopathic weakness and hypotonia even in early infancy. Even in late adult-onset acid maltase deficiency, >50% of the patients report difficulties with muscle strength dating from childhood. Ultrastructural evidence of secondary mitochondrial cytopathy also occurs, as with infantile Pompe disease. MRI of muscle may show distinctive changes that differ from other myopathies.

The serum CK level is greatly elevated, and the muscle biopsy findings are diagnostic even in the presymptomatic stage. The diagnosis of glycogenosis II is confirmed by quantitative assay of acid maltase activity in muscle or liver biopsy specimens. A rare variant of the milder form of acid maltase deficiency can show muscle acid maltase activity in the low normal range with only intermittent decreases to subnormal values; the muscle biopsy findings are similar although milder. In another form, **Danon disease,** transmitted as an X-linked recessive trait at the Xq24 locus, the primary deficiency is lysosomal membrane protein-2 (LAMP2) and results in hypertrophic cardiomyopathy, proximal myopathy, and intellectual disability.

Glycogenosis III (Cori-Forbes disease), a deficiency of debrancher enzyme (amylo-1,6-glucosidase), is more common than is usually diagnosed, and it is generally the least severe. Hypotonia, weakness, hepatomegaly, and fasting hypoglycemia in infancy are common, but these features often resolve spontaneously, and patients become asymptomatic in childhood and adult life. Others experience slowly progressive distal muscle wasting, hepatic cirrhosis, recurrent hypoglycemia, and heart failure. This more serious chronic course is particularly seen in the Inuit population. Minor myopathic findings including vacuolation of muscle fibers are found in the muscle biopsy specimen.

Glycogenosis IV (Andersen disease) is a deficiency of brancher enzyme, resulting in the formation of an abnormal glycogen molecule, amylopectin, in the liver, reticuloendothelial cells, and skeletal and cardiac muscle. Hypotonia, generalized weakness, muscle wasting, and contractures are the usual signs of myopathic involvement. Most patients die before age 4 yr because of hepatic or cardiac failure. A few children without neuromuscular manifestations have been described.

Glycogenosis V (McArdle disease) is caused by muscle glycogen phosphorylase deficiency inherited as an autosomal recessive trait at locus 11q13, encoded by the *PMGM* gene. Exercise intolerance is the cardinal clinical feature. Physical exertion results in cramps, weakness, and myoglobinuria, but strength is normal between attacks. The serum CK level is elevated only during exercise. A characteristic clinical feature is lack of the normal rise in serum lactate levels during ischemic exercise because of inability to convert pyruvate to lactate under anaerobic conditions in vivo. Myophosphorylase deficiency may be demonstrated histochemically and biochemically in the muscle biopsy tissue. Some patients have a defect in adenosine monophosphate–dependent muscle phosphorylase β-kinase, a phosphorylase enzyme activator. Muscle phosphorylase deficiency was the first neuromuscular disease to be diagnosed by MR spectroscopy, which shows that the intramuscular pH does not decrease with exercise and there is no depletion of adenosine triphosphatase but that the phosphocreatine concentration falls excessively. This noninvasive technique may be useful in some patients if the radiologist is experienced with the disease.

A rare **neonatal form of myophosphorylase deficiency** causes feeding difficulties in early infancy, may be severe enough to result in neonatal death, or can follow a course of slowly progressive weakness resembling a muscular dystrophy. The long-term prognosis is good. Patients must learn to moderate their physical activities, but they do not develop severe chronic myopathic handicaps or cardiac involvement.

Glycogenosis VII (Tarui disease) is muscle phosphofructokinase deficiency. Although this disease is rarer than glycogenosis V, the symptoms of exercise intolerance, clinical course, and inability to convert pyruvate to lactate are identical. The distinction is made by biochemical study of the muscle biopsy specimen. It is transmitted as an autosomal recessive trait at the 1cenq32 locus and some mutations are particularly prevalent in the Ashkenazi Jewish population.

Bibliography is available at Expert Consult.

611.4 Mitochondrial Myopathies
Harvey B. Sarnat

See also Chapters 87.4 and 598.2.

Several diseases involving muscle, brain, and other organs are associated with structural and functional abnormalities of mitochondria, producing defects in aerobic cellular metabolism, the electron transport chain, and the Krebs cycle. Because mitochondria are found in all cells, except mature erythrocytes, the term **mitochondrial cytopathy** is used preferentially to emphasize the multisystemic nature of these diseases. The structural aberrations are best demonstrated by electron microscopy of the muscle biopsy sample, revealing a proliferation of abnormally shaped cristae, including stacked or whorled cristae and paracrystallin structures that occupy the space between cristae and are formed from CK. Muscle biopsies of neonates, infants, and toddlers show more severe involvement of endothelial cells of intramuscular capillaries than of myofibers, unlike the reverse in adults, but endothelial paracrystallin structures are globular rather than brick shaped as in myofibers. The endoplasmic reticulum becomes abnormally adherent to mitochondria. Similar endothelial mitochondrial alterations are seen in brain in Leigh and other infantile mitochondrial encephalopathies. Histochemical study of the muscle biopsy specimen reveals abnormal clumping of oxidative enzymatic activity and scattered myofibers, with loss of cytochrome-c oxidase activity and with increased neutral lipids within myofibers. Ragged red muscle fibers occur in some mitochondrial myopathies, particularly those with a combination of respiratory chain complexes I and IV deficiencies. Accumulations of this membranous material beneath the muscle fiber membrane are best demonstrated by special stains, such as modified Gomori trichrome.

These characteristic histochemical and ultrastructural changes are most consistently seen with point mutations in mitochondrial transfer RNA. The large mitochondrial DNA (mtDNA) deletions of 5 or 7.4 kb (the single mitochondrial chromosome has 16.5 kb) are associated with defects in mitochondrial respiratory oxidative enzyme complexes, if as few as 2% of the mitochondria are affected, but minimal or no morphologic or histochemical changes may be noted in the muscle biopsy specimen, even by electron microscopy; hence, quantitative biochemical studies of the muscle tissue are needed to confirm the diagnosis. Because most of the subunits of the respiratory chain complexes are encoded by nuclear DNA (nDNA) rather than mtDNA, mendelian autosomal inheritance is possible, rather than maternal transmission as with pure mtDNA point mutations. Complex II (succinate dehydrogenase) is the only enzyme complex in which all of its subunits are encoded by nDNA; hence it is histochemically reactive in all mitochondrial diseases with mtDNA point mutations. Serum lactate is elevated in some diseases, and cerebrospinal fluid lactate is more consistently elevated, even if serum concentrations are normal.

Several distinct mitochondrial diseases that primarily affect striated muscle or muscle and brain are identified. These can be divided into the ragged red fiber diseases and non–ragged fiber diseases. The ragged red fiber diseases include Kearns-Sayre, MELAS (*mitochondrial encephalopathy, lactic acidosis, and stroke-like episodes*) syndrome, MERRF (*myoclonic epilepsy with ragged red fibers*) syndrome, and progressive external ophthalmoplegia syndromes, which are associated with a combined defect in respiratory chain complexes I and IV. The non–ragged fiber diseases include Leigh encephalopathy and Leber hereditary optic atrophy; they involve complex I or IV alone or, in children, the common combination of defective complexes III and V. **Kearns-Sayre syndrome** is characterized by the triad of progressive external ophthalmoplegia, pigmentary degeneration of the retina, and onset before age 20 yr. Heart block, cerebellar deficits, and high cerebrospinal fluid protein content are often associated. Visual evoked potentials are abnormal. Patients usually do not experience weakness of the trunk or extremities or dysphagia. Most cases are sporadic.

Chronic progressive external ophthalmoplegia may be isolated or accompanied by limb muscle weakness, dysphagia, and dysarthria. A few patients described as having *ophthalmoplegia plus* have additional central nervous system involvement. Autosomal dominant inheritance is found in some pedigrees, but most cases are sporadic.

MERRF and **MELAS syndromes** are other mitochondrial disorders affecting children. The latter is characterized by stunted growth, episodic vomiting, seizures, and recurring cerebral insults causing hemiparesis, hemianopia, or even cortical blindness, and dementia. The disease behaves as a degenerative disorder, and children die within a few years.

Other "degenerative" diseases of the central nervous system that also involve myopathy with mitochondrial abnormalities include **Leigh subacute necrotizing encephalopathy** (see Chapter 87.4) and **cerebrohepatorenal (Zellweger) disease, primarily a peroxisomal disease with secondary mitochondrial alterations** (see Chapter 86.2). Another recognized mitochondrial myopathy is **cytochrome-c oxidase deficiency. Oculopharyngeal muscular dystrophy** is also fundamentally a mitochondrial myopathy.

Mitochondrial depletion syndrome of early infancy is characterized by severely decreased oxidative enzymatic activities in most or all 5 of the complexes; in addition to diffuse muscle weakness, neonates and young infants can show multisystemic involvement and the syndrome occurs in several forms: myopathic; encephalomyopathic; hepatoencephalopathic; and intestinal encephalopathic. Cardiomyopathy and sometimes bullous skin lesions or generalized edema also can occur. **Alpers syndrome** is genetically homogeneous and is caused by mtDNA depletion and mutations in the *POLG1* gene. Several other

genes are identified, mostly in later-onset forms; hence mitochondrial depletion is a syndrome and not a single disease. **Barth syndrome** is an X-linked recessive mitochondrial disorder characterized by cardiomyopathy, myopathy of striated muscle, growth retardation, neutropenia, and high serum and urinary concentrations of 3-methylglutaconic acid.

Many rare diseases with only a few case reports are suspected of being mitochondrial disorders. It is also now recognized that secondary mitochondrial defects occur in a wide range of nonmitochondrial diseases, including inflammatory autoimmune myopathies, Pompe disease, and some cerebral malformations, and also may be induced by certain drugs and toxins, so that interpretation of mitochondrial abnormalities as primary defects must be approached with caution.

mtDNA is distinct from the DNA of the cell nucleus and is inherited exclusively from the mother; mitochondria are present in the cytoplasm of the ovum but not in the head of the sperm, the only part that enters the ovum at fertilization. The rate of mutation of mtDNA is 10 times higher than that of nDNA. The mitochondrial respiratory enzyme complexes each have subunits encoded either in mtDNA or nDNA. Complex II (succinate dehydrogenase, a Krebs cycle enzyme) has 4 subunits, all encoded in nDNA; complex III (ubiquinol or cytochrome-b oxidase) has 9 subunits, only 1 of which is encoded by mtDNA and 8 of which are programmed by nDNA; complex IV (cytochrome-c oxidase) has 13 subunits, only 3 of which are encoded by mtDNA. For this reason, mitochondrial diseases of muscle may be transmitted as autosomal recessive traits rather than by strict maternal transmission, even though all mitochondria are inherited from the mother.

In Kearns-Sayre syndrome, a single large mtDNA deletion has been identified, but other genetic variants are known; in MERRF and MELAS syndromes of mitochondrial myopathy, point mutations occur in transfer RNA.

INVESTIGATIONS
Investigation for mitochondrial cytopathies begins with serum lactate. Lactic acid is not increased in all mitochondrial cytopathies, so that a normal result is not necessarily reassuring; cerebrospinal fluid lactate is increased in some cases in which serum lactate is normal, particularly if there are clinical signs of encephalopathy. Serum 3-methylglutaconic acid often is increased in mitochondrial cytopathies in general, demonstrated in more than 50 different genetic mutations, and hence is a good screening measurement; it rarely is increased in other metabolic diseases. This product also may be increased in urine. Hepatic enzymes (transaminases) should be measured in blood. Cardiac evaluation often is warranted. Molecular markers in blood for the common diseases with known mtDNA point mutations identify many of the mitochondrial cytopathies presenting in adult life or adolescence, but less frequently in children and least in young infants. MRI of the brain may reveal hyperintense lesions of the basal ganglia and MR spectroscopy can demonstrate an increased lactate peak. The muscle biopsy provides the best evidence of all mitochondrial myopathies and should include histochemistry for oxidative enzymes, electron microscopy, and quantitative biochemical assay of respiratory chain enzyme complexes and coenzyme-Q10; muscle tissue also can be analyzed for mtDNA. Many mitochondrial disorders also can affect the Schwann cells and axons of peripheral nerves and present clinically with neuropathy; hence motor and sensory nerve conduction velocities can be measured in selected patients; sural nerve biopsy is required only rarely if neuropathy is the predominant finding and the diagnosis is not evident from other studies.

TREATMENT
There is no effective treatment of mitochondrial cytopathies, but various "cocktails" are often used empirically to try to overcome the metabolic deficits. These include oral carnitine supplements, riboflavin, coenzyme-Q10, ascorbic acid (vitamin C), vitamin E, and other antioxidants. Although some anecdotal reports are encouraging, no controlled studies that prove efficacy have been published.

Bibliography is available at Expert Consult.

611.5 Lipid Myopathies
Harvey B. Sarnat

See Chapter 86.4.

Considered as metabolic organs, skeletal muscles are the most important sites in the body for long-chain fatty acid metabolism because of their large mass and their rich density of mitochondria where fatty acids are metabolized. They are the major source of energy for skeletal muscle during sustained exercise or fasting. Hereditary disorders of lipid metabolism that cause progressive myopathy are an important, relatively common, and often treatable group of muscle diseases. Increased lipid within myofibers is seen in the muscle biopsy of some mitochondrial myopathies and is a constant, rather than an unpredictable, feature of specific diseases. Among the ragged red fiber diseases, Kearns-Sayre syndrome always shows increased neutral lipid, whereas MERRF and MELAS syndromes do not, a useful diagnostic marker for the pathologist. Free fatty acids are converted to acyl-coenzyme A by fatty acyl-coenzyme A synthetases; the resulting long-chain fatty acids bind to carnitine and are transported into mitochondria where β-oxidation is carried out. Disorders of lipid fuel utilization and lipid storage disorders can be divided into defects of transport and oxidation of exogenous fatty acids within mitochondria and defects of endogenous triglyceride catabolism.

Muscle carnitine deficiency is an autosomal recessive disease caused by mutations in the *SLC22A5* gene, involving deficient transport of dietary carnitine across the intestinal mucosa. Carnitine is acquired from dietary sources but is also synthesized in the liver and kidneys from lysine and methionine; it is the obligatory carrier of long- and medium-chain fatty acids into muscle mitochondria.

The clinical course may be one of sudden exacerbations of weakness or can resemble a progressive muscular dystrophy with generalized proximal myopathy and sometimes facial, pharyngeal, and cardiac involvement. Symptoms usually begin in late childhood or adolescence or may be delayed until adult life. Progression is slow but can end in death.

Serum CK level is mildly elevated. Muscle biopsy material shows vacuoles filled with lipid within muscle fibers in addition to nonspecific changes suggestive of a muscular dystrophy. Mitochondria can appear normal or abnormal. Carnitine measured in muscle biopsy tissue is reduced, but the serum carnitine level is normal.

Treatment stops the progression of the disease and can even restore lost strength if the disease is not too advanced. It consists of special diets low in long-chain fatty acids. Steroids can enhance fatty acid transport. Specific therapy with L-carnitine taken orally in large doses overcomes the intestinal barrier in some patients. Some patients also improve when given supplementary riboflavin, and other patients seem to improve with propranolol.

Systemic carnitine deficiency is a disease of impaired renal and hepatic synthesis of carnitine rather than a primary myopathy. Patients with this autosomal recessive disease experience progressive proximal myopathy and show muscle biopsy changes similar to those of muscle carnitine deficiency; however, the onset of weakness is earlier and may be evident at birth. Endocardial fibroelastosis also can occur. Episodes of acute hepatic encephalopathy resembling Reye syndrome can occur. Hypoglycemia and metabolic acidosis complicate acute episodes. Cardiomyopathy may be the predominating feature in some cases and result in death.

Cerebral infarctions and myopathy occur in children, particularly when accompanied by hypoglycemia. Mean age at presentation is approximately 9 yr. Brain MRI shows distinctive changes related to multiple infarcts of various sizes.

The concentration of carnitine is reduced in serum as well as in muscle and liver. L-Carnitine deficiency can be corrected by oral administration of carnitine on a daily basis.

A similar clinical syndrome may be a complication of renal Fanconi syndrome because of excessive urinary loss of carnitine or loss during chronic hemodialysis.

Treatment with L-carnitine improves the maintenance of blood glucose and serum carnitine levels but does not reverse the ketosis or acidosis or improve exercise capacity.

Muscle carnitine palmitoyltransferase (CPT) deficiency manifests as episodes of rhabdomyolysis, coma, and elevated serum CK levels that may be indistinguishable from Reye syndrome. It is the most common identified cause of recurrent myoglobinuria in adults, but myoglobinuria is not a constant feature in all. CPT transfers long-chain fatty acid acyl-coenzyme A residues to carnitine on the outer mitochondrial membrane for transport into the mitochondria. Exercise intolerance and myoglobinuria resemble glycogenoses V and VII. The degree of exercise that triggers an attack varies among individuals, ranging from casual walking to strenuous exercise. Fasting hypoglycemia can occur. Some patients present only in late adolescence or adult life with myalgias. Genetic transmission is autosomal recessive and is caused by a defect on chromosome 1 at the 1p32 locus. Administration of valproic acid can precipitate acute rhabdomyolysis with myoglobinuria in patients with CPT deficiency; it should be avoided in the treatment of seizures or migraine if they occur. *Very long-chain acyl-coenzyme A dehydrogenase deficiency* has a similar clinical presentation but mainly with adult onset.

Bibliography is available at Expert Consult.

611.6 Vitamin E Deficiency Myopathy
Harvey B. Sarnat

In experimental animals, deficiency of vitamin E (α-tocopherol, an antioxidant also important in mitochondrial superoxide generation) produces a progressive myopathy closely resembling a muscular dystrophy. Myopathy and neuropathy are recognized in humans who lack adequate intake of this antioxidant. Patients with chronic malabsorption, those undergoing long-term dialysis, and premature infants who do not receive vitamin E supplements are particularly vulnerable. Treatment with high doses of vitamin E can reverse the deficiency. Myopathy caused by chronic hypervitaminosis E also occurs.

Bibliography is available at Expert Consult.

Chapter **612**
Disorders of Neuromuscular Transmission and of Motor Neurons
Harvey B. Sarnat

612.1 Myasthenia Gravis
Harvey B. Sarnat

AUTOIMMUNE MYASTHENIA GRAVIS
Myasthenia gravis is a chronic autoimmune disease of neuromuscular blockade, characterized clinically by rapid fatigability of striated muscle, particularly extraocular and palpebral muscles and those of swallowing. It must be distinguished from congenital myasthenic

syndrome, a genetic disorder of receptors on the postsynaptic membrane of the neuromuscular junction and toxin-induced myasthenia, such as botulism (see below). The release of acetylcholine (ACh) into the synaptic cleft by the axonal terminal is normal, but the postsynaptic muscle membrane (i.e., *sarcolemma*) or *motor end plate* is less responsive than normal. A decreased number of available ACh receptors is as a result of circulating receptor-binding antibodies in most cases of autoimmune myasthenia.

A rare **familial** myasthenia gravis is an autosomal recessive trait not associated with increased plasma anti-ACh antibodies. One familial form is a deficiency of motor end plate acetylcholinesterase (AChE). Most congenital (familial) forms are postsynaptic defects. Infants born to myasthenic mothers can have a **transient neonatal myasthenic syndrome** secondary to placentally transferred anti-ACh receptor antibodies, distinct from congenital myasthenic syndromes (Tables 612-1 and 612-2).

Clinical Manifestations

In juvenile autoimmune myasthenia gravis, unilateral or bilateral but usually asymmetrical ptosis and some degree of extraocular muscle weakness are the earliest and most constant signs. Extraocular weakness is not confined to muscles innervated by just 1 or 2 of the 3 corresponding brainstem nuclei and is progressive. Older children might complain of diplopia, and young children might hold open their eyes with their fingers or thumbs if the ptosis is severe

Table 612-1	Classification of the Congenital Myasthenic Syndromes

PRESYNAPTIC DEFECTS
- Paucity of synaptic vesicles and decreased quantal release
- Congenital myasthenic syndromes with episodic apnea (choline acetyltransferase deficiency)
- Lambert-Eaton syndrome–like form

SYNAPTIC DEFECTS
- End plate acetylcholinesterase deficiency

POSTSYNAPTIC DEFECTS
- Primary acetylcholine receptor deficiency
- Reduced receptor expression as a result of acetylcholine receptor mutations
- Reduced receptor expression because of rapsyn mutations
- Reduced receptor expression with plectin deficiency
- Primary acetylcholine receptor kinetic abnormality with or without acetylcholine receptor deficiency
- Slow-channel syndrome
- Fast-channel syndrome
- Sodium-channel mutations
- *Dok7* mutations

From Muppidi S, Wolfe GI, Barhon RJ: Diseases of the neuromuscular junction. In Swaiman KF, Ashwal S, Ferriero DM, Schor NF, editors: Swaiman's pediatric neurology, ed 5, Philadelphia, 2012, Elsevier, Box 91-3.

Table 612-2	Distinctive Clinical and Electrodiagnostic Features of Congenital Myasthenic Syndromes

	Presynaptic		Synaptic	Postsynaptic			
	CHOLINE ACETYLTRANSFERASE DEFICIENCY	**LEMS-LIKE FORM**	**AChE DEFICIENCY**	**PRIMARY AChR DEFICIENCY**	**SLOW-CHANNEL CMS**	**FAST-CHANNEL CMS**	***DOK7* MUTATIONS**
Autosomal dominant inheritance					X (most mutations)		
Episodic apnea triggered by stressors	X						
Neonatal hypotonia and respiratory insufficiency	X	X	X (in severe cases)	X (in severe cases)			
Skeletal deformities			X	X		X (in severe cases)	
Delayed pupillary light responses			X				
Prominent neck, wrist, and finger extensor weakness					X		
Repetitive CMAPs after single stimulus			X		X		
Progressive decrement with prolonged exercise or repetitive stimulation	X			X			
Marked increment (>200%) with high-frequency repetitive stimulation		X					
Decrement repairs with AChE inhibitors				X		X	
Clinical improvement with AChE inhibitors						X	
Clinical worsening with AChE inhibitors			X		X		X

AChE, acetylcholinesterase; AChR, acetylcholine receptor; CMAPs, compound muscle action potentials; CMS, congenital myasthenic syndrome; LEMS, Lambert-Eaton myasthenic syndrome.
From Muppidi S, Wolfe GI, Barhon RJ: Diseases of the neuromuscular junction. In Swaiman KF, Ashwal S, Ferriero DM, Schor NF, editors: Swaiman's pediatric neurology, ed 5, Philadelphia, 2012, Elsevier, Table 91-3.

enough to obstruct vision. Pupillary responses to light are preserved. Dysphagia and facial weakness also are common and, in early infancy, feeding difficulties are frequent as the cardinal sign of myasthenia; in severe cases, aspiration and airway obstruction may occur. Poor head control because of weakness of the neck flexors may be prominent. Involvement initially may appear to be limited to bulbar-innervated muscles, but the disease is systemic and progressive weakness eventually involves limb-girdle muscles and distal muscles of the hands in most cases. Fasciculations of muscle, myalgias, and sensory symptoms do not occur. Tendon stretch reflexes may be diminished but rarely are lost. Ocular myasthenia gravis may prove to be transitory over time, but in some patients weakness never progresses to involve axial or appendicular muscles. This group accounts for approximately 25% of all juvenile myasthenia gravis patients and is most frequent in children of Chinese and southeastern Asian descent, suggesting an ethnic genetic predisposition.

Rapid fatigue of muscles is a characteristic feature of myasthenia gravis that distinguishes it from most other neuromuscular diseases. Ptosis increases progressively as patients are asked to sustain an upward gaze for 30-90 sec. Holding the head up from the surface of the examining table while lying supine is very difficult, and gravity cannot be overcome for more than a few seconds. Repetitive opening and closing of the fists produces rapid fatigue of hand muscles, and patients cannot elevate their arms for more than 1-2 min because of fatigue of the deltoids. Patients are more symptomatic late in the day or when tired. Dysphagia can interfere with eating, and the muscles of the jaw soon tire when an affected child chews. Reviewing activities of daily living helps determine the severity of symptoms (Table 612-3).

Left untreated, myasthenia gravis is usually progressive and can become life-threatening because of respiratory muscle involvement and the risk of aspiration, particularly at times when the child is otherwise unwell, such as with an upper respiratory tract infection. Familial myasthenia gravis usually is not progressive.

Myasthenic crisis is an acute or subacute severe increase in weakness in patients with myasthenia gravis, usually precipitated by an intercurrent infection, surgery, or even emotional stress. It may require intravenous cholinesterase inhibitors, immunoglobulin, plasma exchange, gavage feeding, and even transitory ventilator support. It must be distinguished from **cholinergic crisis** secondary to overdosing with anticholinesterase medications. The muscarinic effects include abdominal cramps, diarrhea, profuse sweating, salivation, bradycardia, increased weakness, and miosis. Cholinergic crisis requires only supportive care and withholding of further doses of cholinergic drugs, and it passes within a few hours; the dose of medication to be restarted

should be reconsidered, unless the patient had taken an overdose that was not prescribed.

Approximately 30% of affected adolescents show elevations, but anti-AChR antibodies are only occasionally demonstrated in the plasma of prepubertal children. Some with negative titers of AChE exhibit anti–muscle-specific tyrosine kinase (MuSK) circulating antibodies. MuSK is localized at the neuromuscular junction and appears essential to fetal development of this junction. MuSK myasthenia usually occurs in female infants and toddlers and severe bulbar involvement with dysphagia is frequent, but clinical features alone cannot distinguish between these 2 different antibody forms of the disease.

Infants born to myasthenic mothers can have respiratory insufficiency, inability to suck or swallow, and generalized hypotonia and weakness. They might show little spontaneous motor activity for several days to weeks. Some require ventilatory support and feeding by gavage during this period. After the abnormal antibodies disappear from the blood and muscle tissue, these infants regain normal strength and are not at increased risk of developing myasthenia gravis in later childhood. A small minority develop *fetal akinesia sequence* with multiple joint contractures (*arthrogryposis*) that develop in utero from lack of fetal movement. AChR antibodies can usually be demonstrated in maternal blood, but at times maternal antibodies may not be detected.

CONGENITAL MYASTHENIC SYNDROMES

A heterogeneous group of genetic diseases of neuromuscular transmission is collectively called **congenital myasthenic syndromes.** The etiology and pathogenesis of these syndromes are unrelated to either transitory neonatal myasthenia caused by placental transfer of maternal antibodies or to autoimmune myasthenia gravis, despite overlap of clinical symptoms. Congenital myasthenic syndromes are nearly always permanent static disorders without spontaneous remission (see Tables 612-1 and 612-2). Several distinct genetic forms are recognized, all with onset at birth or in early infancy with hypotonia, external ophthalmoplegia, ptosis, dysphagia, weak cry, facial weakness, easy muscle fatigue generally, and sometimes respiratory insufficiency or failure, the last often precipitated by a minor respiratory infection. Cholinesterase inhibitors have a favorable effect in most, but in some forms the symptoms and signs are actually worsened. Most congenital myasthenic syndromes are transmitted as autosomal recessive traits, but the slow channel syndrome is autosomal dominant.

Mutations responsible for congenital myasthenic syndromes have been identified in 18 different genes. The genetic mutations are known in less than half of children with congenital myasthenic syndromes. Of

Table 612-3	Myasthenia Gravis Activities of Daily Living Scale (MG-ADL)			
GRADE	**0**	**1**	**2**	**3**
Talking	Normal	Intermittent slurring or nasal speech	Constant slurring or nasal, but can be understood	Difficult to understand speech
Chewing	Normal	Fatigue with solid food	Fatigue with soft food	Gastric tube
Swallowing	Normal	Rare episode of choking	Frequent choking, necessitating changes in diet	Gastric tube
Breathing	Normal	Shortness of breath with exertion	Shortness of breath at rest	Ventilator dependence
Impairment of ability to brush teeth or comb hair	None	Extra effort, but no rest periods needed	Rest periods needed	Cannot do 1 of these functions
Impairment of ability to arise from a chair	None	Mild, sometimes uses arms	Moderate, always uses arms	Severe, requires assistance
Double vision	None	Occurs, but not daily	Daily, but not constant	Constant
Eyelid droop	None	Occurs, but not daily	Daily, but not constant	Constant
TOTAL MG-ADL SCORE				

From Wolfe GI, Herbelin L, Nations SP, et al: Myasthenia gravis activities of daily living profile. Neurology 52:1487–1489, 1999.

known genetic defects, *rapsyn* and *downstream-of-kinase-7* (*DOK7*) are demonstrated in 85% of cases. Acetylcholine receptor deficiencies have more than 60 identified genetic mutations. Basal lamina–associated synaptic defects from mutations of the *COLQ* gene that encodes the collagen tail of AChR account for another 10% of cases. Another 5% of cases are presynaptic, attributed to mutations in *ChAT*, encoding choline acetyltransferase. Anti-AChR and anti-MuSK antibodies are usually, but not always, absent in serum, unlike in autoimmune forms of myasthenia gravis affecting older children and adults.

Three **presynaptic congenital myasthenic syndromes** are recognized, all as autosomal recessive traits; some of these have anti-MuSK antibodies. These children exhibit weakness of extraocular, pharyngeal, and respiratory muscles and later show shoulder girdle weakness as well. **Episodic apnea** is a problem in congenital myasthenia gravis. Another synaptic form is caused by congenital absence or marked deficiency of motor end plate AChE in the synaptic basal lamina; this was the first form recognized as caused by an enzymatic deficiency at the neuromuscular junction. Postsynaptic forms of congenital myasthenia are caused by mutations in ACh receptor subunit genes that alter the synaptic response to ACh. An abnormality of the ACh receptor channels appearing as high conductance and excessively fast closure may be the result of a point mutation in a subunit of the receptor affecting a single amino acid residue. Children with congenital myasthenia gravis do not experience myasthenic crises and rarely exhibit elevations of anti-ACh antibodies in plasma.

RARE OTHER CAUSES OF MYASTHENIA

Myasthenia gravis is occasionally associated with hypothyroidism, usually as caused by **Hashimoto thyroiditis.** Other collagen vascular diseases may also be associated with myasthenia gravis. Thymomas, noted in some adults, rarely coexist with myasthenia gravis in children, nor do carcinomas of the lung occur, which produce a unique form of myasthenia in adults called **Eaton-Lambert syndrome.** The Eaton-Lambert syndrome in children is rare but is reported with lymphoproliferative disorders and with neuroblastoma. Postinfectious myasthenia gravis in children is transitory and usually follows a varicella-zoster infection by 2-5 wk as an immune response.

Laboratory Findings and Diagnosis

Myasthenia gravis is one of the few neuromuscular diseases in which electromyography (EMG) is more specifically diagnostic than a muscle biopsy. A *decremental response* is seen to repetitive nerve stimulation; the muscle potentials diminish rapidly in amplitude until the muscle becomes refractory to further stimulation. Motor nerve conduction velocity remains normal. This unique EMG pattern is the electrophysiologic correlate of the fatigable weakness observed clinically and is reversed after a cholinesterase inhibitor is administered. A myasthenic decrement may be absent or difficult to demonstrate in muscles that are not involved clinically. This feature may be confusing in early cases or in patients showing only weakness of extraocular muscles. Microelectrode studies of end plate potentials and currents reveal whether the transmission defect is presynaptic or postsynaptic. Special electrophysiologic studies are required in the classification of congenital myasthenic syndromes and involve estimating the number of ACh receptors per end plate and in vitro study of end plate function. These special studies and patch-clamp recordings of kinetic properties of channels are performed on special biopsy samples of intercostal muscle strips that include both origin and insertion of the muscle but are only performed in specialized centers. If myasthenia is limited to the extraocular, levator palpebrae, and pharyngeal muscles, evoked-potential EMG of the muscles of the extremities and spine, diagnostic in the generalized disease, usually is normal.

Anti-AChR antibodies should be assayed in the plasma but are inconsistently demonstrated. Antibodies against the MuSK receptor should be sought in children without circulating AChR antibodies, a diagnostic finding when elevated, which further delineates the etiology. Many cases of congenital myasthenia gravis result from failure to synthesize or release ACh at the presynaptic membrane. In some cases, the gene that mediates the enzyme choline acetyltransferase for the

synthesis of ACh is mutated. In others, there is a defect in the quantal release of vesicles containing ACh. The treatment of such patients with cholinesterase inhibitors is futile. Assays of anti-rapsyn, anti-*Dok7*, *COLQ*, and *ChAT* antibodies are available in a few specialized laboratories.

Other serologic tests of autoimmune disease, such as antinuclear antibodies and abnormal immune complexes, should also be sought. If these are positive, more extensive autoimmune disease involving vasculitis or tissues other than muscle is likely. A thyroid profile should always be examined. The serum creatine kinase level is normal in myasthenia gravis.

The heart is not involved, and electrocardiographic findings remain normal. Radiographs of the chest often reveal an enlarged thymus, but the hypertrophy is not a thymoma. It may be further defined by tomography or by CT or MRI of the anterior mediastinum if the radiographic findings are uncertain, but these imaging modalities are not recommended routinely because of radiation exposure and anesthetic risk, which is higher in myasthenic patients than in normal children.

The role of conventional muscle biopsy in myasthenia gravis is limited. It is not required in most cases, but approximately 17% of patients show inflammatory changes, sometimes called *lymphorrhages,* that are interpreted by some physicians as a mixed myasthenia-polymyositis immune disorder. Muscle biopsy tissue in myasthenia gravis shows nonspecific type II muscle fiber atrophy, similar to that seen with disuse atrophy, steroid effects on muscle, polymyalgia rheumatica, and many other conditions. The ultrastructure of motor end plates shows simplification of the membrane folds; the ACh receptors are located in these postsynaptic folds, as shown by bungarotoxin (snake venom), which binds specifically to the ACh receptors.

A **clinical test for myasthenia gravis** is administration of a short-acting cholinesterase inhibitor, usually edrophonium chloride. Ptosis and ophthalmoplegia improve within a few seconds, and fatigability of other muscles decreases.

Recommendations on the Use of Cholinesterase Inhibitors as a Diagnostic Test for Myasthenia Gravis in Infants and Children
Children 2 Yr and Older

◆ The child should have a specific fatigable weakness that can be measured, such as ptosis of the eyelids, dysphagia, or inability of the cervical muscles to support the head. Nonspecific generalized weakness without cranial nerve motor deficits is not a criterion.

◆ An IV infusion should be started to enable the administration of medications in the event of an adverse reaction.

◆ Electrocardiographic monitoring is recommended during the test.

◆ A dose of atropine sulfate (0.01 mg/kg) should be available in a syringe, ready for IV administration at the bedside during the edrophonium test, to block acute muscarinic effects of the cholinesterase inhibitor, mainly abdominal cramps and/or sudden diarrhea from increased peristalsis, profuse bronchotracheal secretions that can obstruct the airway, or, rarely, cardiac arrhythmias. Some physicians pretreat all patients with atropine before administering edrophonium, but this is not recommended unless there is a history of reaction to tests. Atropine can cause the pupils to be dilated and fixed for as long as 14 days after a single dose, and the pupillary effects of homatropine can last 4-7 days.

◆ Edrophonium chloride (Tensilon) is administered IV. Initially, a test dose of 0.01 mg/kg is given to ensure that the patient does not have an allergic reaction or is otherwise very sensitive to muscarinic side effects. In children weighing <30 kg, 0.1 mg/kg is the maximum total delivered dose; in children weighing >30 kg, the total delivered dose is 0.2 mg/kg. After the test dose, intravenous injection of 0.01-0.02 mg is administered every 30-45 sec, as long as dosing does not exceed the recommended maximum dose. In adults, the average edrophonium dose to show positive responses is approximately 3.3 mg for ptosis and approximately 2.6 mg for oculomotor symptoms. Side effects include nausea and emesis; light-headedness from bradycardia (atropine is the antidote) and bronchospasm are less common side effects. These doses may be given IM or subcutaneously, but these routes are not recommended because the results are much more variable owing to unpredictable absorption, and the test may be ambiguous or falsely negative.

◆ Effects should be seen within 10 sec and disappear within 120 sec. Weakness is measured as, for example, distance between upper and lower eyelids before and after administration, degree of external ophthalmoplegia, or ability to swallow a sip of water.

◆ Long-acting cholinesterase inhibitors, such as pyridostigmine (Mestinon), are generally not as useful for the acute assessment of myasthenic weakness. The Prostigmin test may be used (as outlined later) but might not be as definitively diagnostic as the edrophonium test.

For Children Younger Than 2 Yr

◆ Infants ideally should have a specific fatigable weakness that can be measured, such as ptosis of the eyelids, dysphagia, and inability of cervical muscles to support the head. Nonspecific generalized weakness without cranial nerve motor deficits makes it less easy to assess results but may be a criterion at times.

◆ An IV infusion should be started as a rapid route for medications in the event of an adverse effect of the test medication.

◆ Electrocardiographic monitoring is recommended during the test.

◆ Pretreatment with atropine sulfate to block the muscarinic effects of the test medication is not recommended, but atropine sulfate should be available at the bedside in a prepared syringe. If needed, it should be administered IV in a dose of 0.01 mg/kg.

◆ Edrophonium is not recommended for use in infants; its effect is too brief for objective assessment and an increased incidence of acute cardiac arrhythmias is reported in infants, especially neonates, with this drug.

◆ Prostigmin methylsulfate (neostigmine) is administered IM at a dose of 0.04 mg/kg. If the result is negative or equivocal, another dose of 0.04 mg/kg may be administered 4 hr after the first dose (a typical dose is 0.5-1.5 mg). The peak effect is seen in 20-40 min. IV Prostigmin is contraindicated because of the risk of cardiac arrhythmias, including fatal ventricular fibrillation, especially in young infants.

◆ Long-acting cholinesterase inhibitors administered orally, such as pyridostigmine (Mestinon), are generally not as useful for the acute assessment of myasthenic weakness because onset and duration are less predictable.

The test should be performed in the emergency department, hospital ward, or intensive care unit; the important issue is preparation for potential complications such as cardiac arrhythmia or cholinergic crisis, as outlined.

Treatment

Some patients with mild myasthenia gravis require no treatment. **Cholinesterase-inhibiting drugs** are the primary therapeutic agents. Neostigmine methylsulfate (0.04 mg/kg) may be given IM every 4-6 hr, but most patients tolerate oral neostigmine bromide, 0.4 mg/kg every 4-6 hr. If dysphagia is a major problem, the drug should be given approximately 30 min before meals to improve swallowing. Pyridostigmine is an alternative; the dose required is approximately 4 times greater than that of neostigmine, but it may be slightly longer acting. Overdoses of cholinesterase inhibitors produce cholinergic crises; atropine blocks the muscarinic effects but does not block the nicotinic effects that produce additional skeletal muscle weakness. In the rare familial myasthenia gravis caused by absence of end plate AChE, cholinesterase inhibitors are not helpful and often cause increased weakness; these patients can be treated with ephedrine or diaminopyridine, both of which increase ACh release from terminal axons.

Because of the autoimmune basis of the disease, long-term **steroid treatment** with prednisone may be effective. **Thymectomy** should be considered and might provide a cure. Thymectomy is most effective in patients who have high titers of anti-ACh receptor antibodies in the plasma and who have been symptomatic for <2 yr. Thymectomy is ineffective in congenital and familial forms of myasthenia gravis. Treatment of hypothyroidism usually abolishes an associated myasthenia without the use of cholinesterase inhibitors or steroids.

If the specific genetic mutation can be identified in a patient with one of the congenital myasthenic syndromes, specific therapeutic approaches are available for some that differ from the treatments listed above; these are well outlined by Eyemard et al (2013).

Plasmapheresis is effective treatment in some children, particularly those who do not respond to steroids, but plasma exchange therapy provides only temporary remission. **IV immunoglobulin** is beneficial and should be tried before plasmapheresis because it is less invasive. Plasmapheresis and IV immunoglobulin appear to be most effective in patients with high circulating levels of anti-ACh receptor antibodies. Refractory patients might respond to rituximab, a monoclonal antibody to the B-cell CD20 antigen.

Neonates with transient maternally transmitted myasthenia gravis require cholinesterase inhibitors for only a few days or occasionally for a few weeks, especially to allow feeding. No other treatment is usually necessary. In non–maternally transmitted congenital myasthenia gravis, identification of the specific molecular defect is important for treatment; Table 612-4 summarizes specific therapies for each type.

Complications

Children with myasthenia gravis do not tolerate neuromuscular-blocking drugs, such as succinylcholine and pancuronium, and may be paralyzed for weeks after a single dose. An anesthesiologist should carefully review myasthenic patients who require a surgical anesthetic and such anesthetics should be administered only by an experienced physician/anesthesiologist. Also, certain antibiotics can potentiate myasthenia and should be avoided; these include the aminoglycosides (gentamicin and others).

Prognosis

Some patients with autoimmune myasthenia gravis experience spontaneous remission after a period of months or years; others have a permanent disease extending into adult life. Immunosuppression, thymectomy, and treatment of associated hypothyroidism might provide a cure. Genetically determined congenital myasthenic syndromes may show initial worsening in infancy but then remain static throughout childhood and into adult life.

Other Causes of Neuromuscular Blockade

Organophosphate chemicals, commonly used as insecticides, can cause a myasthenia-like syndrome in children exposed to these toxins (see Chapter 63).

Botulism results from ingestion of food containing the toxin of *Clostridium botulinum*, a Gram-positive, spore-bearing, anaerobic bacillus (see Chapter 210). The mechanism is cleavage by the botulinum toxin of several of the structural glycoproteins of the wall (i.e., membrane) of synaptic vesicles within axonal terminals. These glycoproteins include synaptobrevin and synaptotagmin, but synaptophysin is resistant. Honey is a common source of contamination. The incubation period is short, only a few hours, and symptoms begin with nausea, vomiting, and diarrhea. Cranial nerve involvement soon follows, with diplopia, dysphagia, weak suck, facial weakness, and absent gag reflex. Generalized hypotonia and weakness then develop and can progress to respiratory failure. Neuromuscular blockade is documented by EMG with repetitive nerve stimulation. Respiratory support may be required for days or weeks until the toxin is cleared from the body. No specific antitoxin is available. Guanidine, 35 mg/kg/24 hr, may be effective for extraocular and limb muscle weakness but not for respiratory muscle involvement.

Tick paralysis is a disorder of ACh release from axonal terminals due to a neurotoxin that blocks depolarization. It also affects large

Table 612-4	Potential Therapies in Congenital Myasthenic Syndromes
AChE	Ephedrine 3 mg/kg/day in 3 divided doses; begin with 1 mg/kg; not obtainable in several countries If ephedrine is not obtainable, 3,4-diaminopyridine 1 mg/kg/day in 4 divided doses, up to 60 mg/day in adults Avoid AChE inhibitors
AChR deficiency	AChE inhibitors: pyridostigmine bromide (Mestinon) 4-5 mg/kg/day in 4-6 divided doses If necessary add 3,4-diaminopyridine 1 mg/kg/day in 4 divided doses, up to 60 mg/day in adults
AChR fast channel	AChE inhibitors: pyridostigmine bromide (Mestinon) 4-5 mg/kg/day in 4-6 divided doses If necessary add 3,4-diaminopyridine 1 mg/kg/day in 4 divided doses, up to 60 mg/day in adults
AChR slow channel	Quinidine sulfate • Adults: Begin for 1 wk with 200 mg tid; gradual increase to maintain a serum level of 1-25 µg/mL • Children: 15-60 mg/kg/day in 4-6 divided doses; not available in several countries If quinidine sulfate is not available, fluoxetine 80-100 mg/day in adults Avoid AChE inhibitors
ChAT	AChE inhibitors: pyridostigmine bromide (Mestinon) 4-5 mg/kg/day in 4-6 divided doses If necessary add 3,4-diaminopyridine 1 mg/kg/day in 4 divided doses, up to 60 mg/day in adults
Dok7	Ephedrine 3 mg/kg/day in 3 divided doses; begin with 1 mg/kg; not obtainable in several countries If ephedrine is not obtainable, 3,4-diaminopyridine 1 mg/kg/day in 4 divided doses, up to 60 mg/day in adults Avoid AChE inhibitors
Laminin β_2	Ephedrine 3 mg/kg/day in 3 divided doses; begin with 1 mg/kg; not obtainable in several countries Avoid AChE inhibitors
MuSK	AChE inhibitors: pyridostigmine bromide (Mestinon) 4-5 mg/kg/day in 4-6 divided doses 3,4-Diaminopyridine 1 mg/kg/day in 4 divided doses, up to 60 mg/day in adults
Rapsyn	AChE inhibitors: pyridostigmine bromide (Mestinon) 4-5 mg/kg/day in 4-6 divided doses If necessary add 3,4-diaminopyridine 1 mg/kg/day in 4 divided doses, up to 60 mg/day in adults

Modified from Eyemard B, Hantaï D, Estounet B: Congenital myasthenic syndromes, Handb Clin Neurol 113:1469-1480, 2013.

myelinated motor and sensory nerve fibers. This toxin is produced by the wood tick or dog tick, insects common in the Appalachian and Rocky Mountains of North America. The tick embeds its head into the skin, usually the scalp, and neurotoxin production is maximal about 5-6 days later. Motor symptoms include weakness, loss of coordination, and sometimes an ascending paralysis resembling Guillain-Barré syndrome. Tendon reflexes are lost. Sensory symptoms of tingling paresthesias can occur in the face and extremities. The diagnosis is confirmed by EMG and nerve conduction studies and by identifying the tick. The tick must be removed completely and the buried head not left beneath the skin. Patients then recover completely within hours or days.

Bibliography is available at Expert Consult.

612.2 Spinal Muscular Atrophies
Harvey B. Sarnat

Spinal muscular atrophies (SMAs) are degenerative diseases of motor neurons that begin in fetal life and continue to be progressive in infancy and childhood. The progressive denervation of muscle is compensated for in part by reinnervation from an adjacent motor unit, but giant motor units are thus created with subsequent atrophy of muscle fibers when the reinnervating motor neuron eventually becomes involved. Motor neurons of cranial nerves III, IV, and VI to extraocular muscles, as well as those of the sacral spinal cord innervating striated muscle of the urethral and anal sphincters, are selectively spared. Upper motor neurons (layer 5 pyramidal neurons in the cerebral cortex) also remain normal.

SMA is classified clinically into a severe infantile form, also known as **Werdnig-Hoffmann disease** or SMA type 1; a late infantile and more slowly progressive form, SMA type 2; and a more chronic or juvenile form, also called **Kugelberg-Welander disease,** or SMA type 3. A severe fetal form that is usually fatal in the perinatal period has been described as SMA type 0, with motor neuron degeneration demonstrated in the spinal cord as early as midgestation. These distinctions of types are based upon age at onset, severity of weakness, and clinical course; muscle biopsy does not distinguish types 1 and 2, though type 3 shows a more adult than perinatal pattern of denervation and reinnervation. Type 0 can show biopsy features more similar to myotubular myopathy because of maturational arrest; scattered myotubes and other immature fetal fibers also are demonstrated in the muscle biopsies of patients with types 1 and 2, but they do not predominate. Approximately 25% of patients have type 1, 50% type 2, and 25% type 3; type 0 is rare and accounts for <1%. Some patients are transitional between types 1 and 2 or between types 2 and 3 in terms of clinical function. A variant of SMA, **Fazio-Londe disease,** is a progressive bulbar palsy resulting from motor neuron degeneration more in the brainstem than the spinal cord, but cranial nerves of extraocular muscles also are spared in this form. Table 612-5 lists other variants.

Autonomic motor neurons of both the sympathetic and parasympathetic systems are not spared, but usually do not show clinical manifestations until late stages. Autonomic deficits may involve the detrusor muscle of the urinary bladder or the smooth muscle urethral and anal sphincters, in all 3 forms of SMA. In some patients with type 1 SMA and respiratory distress there may be severe autonomic dysregulation with dysautonomia and cardiovascular collapse leading to death or to severe ischemic brain damage.

ETIOLOGY
The cause of SMA is genetic as an autosomal recessive mendelian trait. Neuropathologically it appears to be a pathologic continuation of a process of programmed cell death (apoptosis) that is normal in embryonic life. A surplus of motor neuroblasts and other neurons is generated from primitive neuroectoderm, but only about half survive and mature to become neurons; the excess cells have a limited life cycle and degenerate. If the process that arrests physiologic cell death fails to intervene by a certain stage, neuronal death can continue in late fetal life and postnatally. The survivor motor neuron gene *(SMN)* arrests apoptosis of motor neuroblasts. Unlike most genes that are highly conserved in evolution, *SMN* is a uniquely mammalian gene. An additional function of *SMN*, both centrally and peripherally, is to transport RNA-binding proteins to the axonal growth cone to ensure an adequate

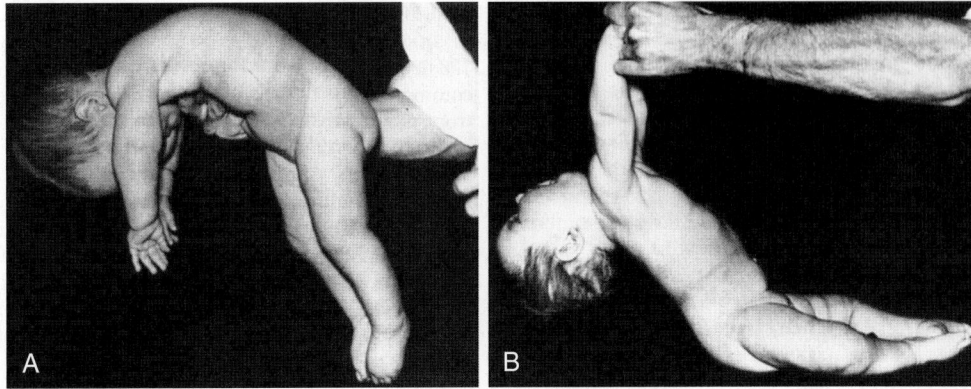

Figure 612-1 Type 1 spinal muscular atrophy (Werdnig-Hoffmann disease). Clinical manifestations of weakness of limb and axial musculature in a 6 wk old infant with severe weakness and hypotonia from birth. Note the marked weakness of the limbs and trunk on ventral suspension **(A)** and of neck on pull to sit **(B)**. *(From Volpe JJ: Neurology of the newborn, ed 4, Philadelphia, 2001, WB Saunders, p. 644.)*

Table 612-5	Spinal Muscular Atrophy Variants: Progressive or Severe Neonatal Anterior Horn Cell Disease Not Linked to *SMN*
VARIANT	**MAJOR FEATURES**
SMA with respiratory distress type 1 (SMARD1)	Mild hypotonia, weak cry, distal contractures initially Respiratory distress from diaphragmatic paralysis 1-6 mo, progressive distal weakness Autosomal recessive, locus 11q13.2, gene: immunoglobulin mu-binding protein 2 (IGHMBP2)
Pontocerebellar hypoplasia type 1	Arthrogryposis, hypotonia, weakness, bulbar deficits early; later, microcephaly, extraocular defects, cognitive deficits: pontocerebellar hypoplasia Molecular defect unknown Likely autosomal recessive
X-linked infantile SMA with bone fractures	Arthrogryposis, hypotonia, weakness, congenital bone fractures, respiratory failure Lethal course as in severe type 1 SMA Most cases X-linked (X9/11.3-q11.2), a few cases likely autosomal recessive
Congenital SMA with predominant lower limb involvement	Arthrogryposis, hypotonia, weakness, especially distal lower limbs early Nonprogressive but severe disability Autosomal dominant or sporadic; locus 12q23-24

SMA, spinal muscular atrophy; *SMN*, survivor motor neuron gene.
From Volpe JJ: Neurology of the newborn, ed 5, Philadelphia, 2008, Saunders Elsevier, Table 18-7, p. 775.

amount of protein-encoding transcripts essential for growth cone mobility both during fetal development and in postnatal synaptic remodeling.

CLINICAL MANIFESTATIONS
The cardinal features of **SMA type 1** are severe hypotonia (Fig. 612-1); generalized weakness; thin muscle mass; absent tendon stretch reflexes; involvement of the tongue, face, and jaw muscles; and sparing of extraocular muscles and sphincters. Diaphragmatic involvement is late. Infants who are symptomatic at birth can have respiratory distress and are unable to feed. Congenital contractures, ranging from simple clubfoot to generalized arthrogryposis, occur in approximately 10% of severely involved neonates. Infants lie flaccid with little movement, unable to overcome gravity (see Fig. 607-1 in Chapter 607). They lack head control. More than 65% of children die by 2 yr of age, and many die early in infancy.

In **type 2 SMA,** affected infants are usually able to suck and swallow, and respiration is adequate in early infancy. These children show progressive weakness, but many survive into the school years or beyond, although confined to an electric wheelchair and severely handicapped. Nasal speech and problems with deglutition develop later. Scoliosis becomes a major complication in many patients with long survival. Gastroesophageal reflux may lead to malnutrition or to aspiration with acute airway obstruction or pneumonia.

Kugelberg-Welander disease is the mildest **SMA (type 3),** and patients can appear normal in infancy. The progressive weakness is proximal in distribution, particularly involving shoulder girdle muscles. Patients are ambulatory. Symptoms of bulbar muscle weakness are rare. Approximately 25% of patients with this form of SMA have muscular hypertrophy rather than atrophy, and it may easily be confused with a muscular dystrophy. Longevity can extend well into middle adult life. Fasciculations are a specific clinical sign of denervation of muscle. In thin children, they may be seen in the deltoid and biceps brachii muscles and occasionally the quadriceps femoris muscles, but the continuous, involuntary, worm-like movements may be masked by a thick pad of subcutaneous fat. Fasciculations are best observed in the tongue, where almost no subcutaneous connective tissue separates the muscular layer from the epithelium. If the intrinsic lingual muscles are contracted, such as in crying or when the tongue protrudes, fasciculations are more difficult to see than when the tongue is relaxed. Cramps and myalgias of appendicular and axial muscles are common, especially in later stages, and problems of micturition may present, though adolescent patients may be too embarrassed to state them unless the physician directly inquires.

The outstretched fingers of children with SMA often show a characteristic tremor owing to fasciculations and weakness. It should not be confused with a cerebellar tremor.

The heart is not involved in SMA. Intelligence is normal, and children often appear brighter than their normal peers because the effort they cannot put into physical activities is redirected to intellectual development, and they are often exposed to adult speech more than to juvenile language because of the social repercussions of the disease. Progressive deterioration of ambulation and the high risk of falling and fracturing long bones or the pelvis eventually require use of a

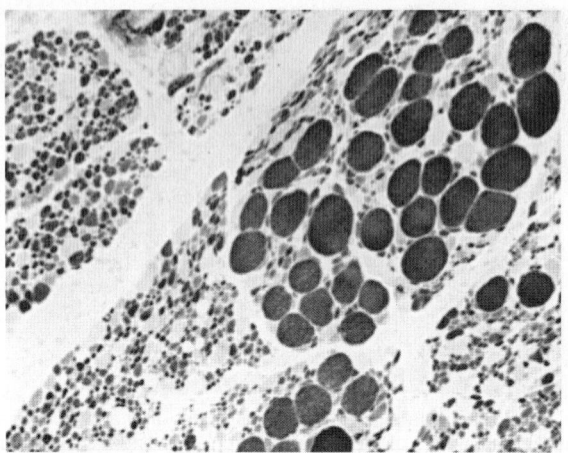

Figure 612-2 Muscle biopsy of neonate with infantile spinal muscular atrophy. Groups of giant type I (darkly stained) fibers are seen within muscle fascicles of severely atrophic fibers of both histochemical types. This is the characteristic pattern of perinatal denervation of muscle. Myofibrillar adenosine triphosphatase, preincubated at pH 4.6 (×400).

wheelchair; an electric wheelchair often is needed because weakness of the upper extremities does not allow the patient to manually push the wheels. Progressive scoliosis is another serious complication and may have a further adverse effect on respiration.

LABORATORY FINDINGS
The serum creatine kinase level may be normal but more commonly is mildly elevated in the hundreds. A creatine kinase level of several thousand is rare. The chest x-ray in early-onset disease demonstrates thin ribs. Results of motor nerve conduction studies are normal, except for mild slowing in terminal stages of the disease, an important feature distinguishing SMA from peripheral neuropathy. EMG shows fibrillation potentials and other signs of denervation of muscle. A secondary mitochondrial DNA depletion is sometimes demonstrated in the muscle biopsy of infants with SMA. The molecular genetic test of the *SMN* gene provides definite confirmation of the diagnosis.

DIAGNOSIS
The simplest, most definitive diagnostic test is a molecular genetic marker in blood for the *SMN* gene. Muscle biopsy used to be the diagnostic test before the genetic marker from blood samples became available, and muscle biopsy now is used more selectively in patients showing equivocal or negative genetic findings. The muscle biopsy in infancy reveals a characteristic pattern of perinatal denervation that is unlike that of mature muscle. Groups of giant type I fibers are mixed with fascicles of severely atrophic fibers of both histochemical types (Fig. 612-2). Scattered immature myofibers resembling myotubes also are demonstrated. In juvenile SMA, the pattern may be more similar to adult muscle that has undergone many cycles of denervation and reinnervation. Neurogenic changes in muscle also may be demonstrated by EMG, but the results are less definitive than by muscle biopsy in infancy. Sural nerve biopsy is now performed only occasionally, but shows mild sensory neuropathic changes, and sensory nerve conduction velocity may be slowed; hypertrophy of unmyelinated axons also is seen. At autopsy, mild degenerative changes are seen in sensory neurons of dorsal root ganglia and in somatosensory nuclei of the thalamus, but these alterations are not perceived clinically as sensory loss or paresthesias. The most pronounced neuropathologic lesions are the extensive neuronal degeneration and gliosis in the ventral horns of the spinal cord and brainstem motor nuclei, especially the hypoglossal nucleus.

GENETICS
Molecular genetic diagnosis by DNA probes in blood samples or in muscle biopsy or chorionic villi tissues is available for diagnosis of

suspected cases and for prenatal diagnosis. Most cases are inherited as an autosomal recessive trait. The incidence of SMA is 10-15 in 100,000 live births, affecting all ethnic groups; it is the second most common neuromuscular disease, following Duchenne muscular dystrophy. The incidence of heterozygosity for autosomal recessive SMA is 1 in 50.

The genetic locus for all 3 of the common forms of SMA is on chromosome 5, a deletion at the 5q11-q13 locus, indicating that they are variants of the same disease rather than different diseases. The affected *SMN1* gene has a molecular weight of 38 kDa and contains 8 exons that span 20 kb and telomeric and centromeric exons that differ only by 5bp and produce a transcript encoding 294 amino acids. *SMN1* is duplicated in a highly homologous gene called *SMN2* and both genes are transcribed. *SMN2* remains present in all patients with SMA, but cannot fully compensate the *SMN1* defect. However, a molecular basis for correlation between the SMN2 copy number and clinical severity of the SMA is the capability of *SMN2* to encode a small amount of an identical *SMN* protein. The critical difference between *SMN1* and *SMN2* genes is a cytosine (C) to thymine (T) transition in exon 7 of *SMN2*. Another gene, the *neuronal apoptosis inhibitory gene (NAIP),* is located next to the *SMN* gene and in many cases there is an inverted duplication with 2 copies, telomeric and centromeric, of both genes; isolated mutations or deletions of *NAIP* do not produce clinical SMA and generate a mostly nonfunctional isoform lacking the carboxy-terminus amino acids encoded by exon 7. Milder forms of SMA have more than 2 copies of *SMN2*, and in late-onset patients with homozygous deletion of the *SMN1* gene, there are 4 copies of *SMN2*. An additional gene mapped to 11q13-q21 in SMA may help explain early respiratory failure in some patients. Nucleotide expansions account for only 5-10% of cases of SMA, and deletions or splicing out of exons 7 and 8 are the genetic mechanism in the great majority of cases. Another pair of genes adjacent to the *SMN1* and *SMN2* genes, *SERF1* and *SERF2*, also may play a secondary role. The *SMN* gene product modulates axonal growth and localization of β-actin messenger RNA in growth cones of motor neurons.

Infrequent families with autosomal dominant inheritance are described, and a rare X-linked recessive form also occurs. Carrier testing by dose analysis is available.

TREATMENT
No medical treatment is able to delay the progression. Supportive therapy includes orthopedic care with particular attention to scoliosis and joint contractures, mild physiotherapy, and mechanical aids for assisting the child to eat and to be as functionally independent as possible. Most children learn to use a computer keyboard with great skill but cannot use a pencil easily. Valproic acid is sometimes administered because it increases SMN2 protein, and gabapentin and oral phenylbutyrate also may slow the progression, but these treatments do not alter the course in all patients. A benefit of antioxidants is unproved. Gene replacement and protein replacement therapies remain theoretical and experimental. Potential therapeutic genetic strategies in SMA include upregulation of *SMN2* gene expression, preventing exon 7 skipping of SMN2 transcripts and improving the stability of the protein lacking the amino acid sequence encoded by exon 7.

Bibliography is available at Expert Consult.

612.3 Other Motor Neuron Diseases
Harvey B. Sarnat

Motor neuron diseases other than SMA are rare in children. *Poliomyelitis* used to be a major cause of chronic disability, but with the routine use of polio vaccine, this viral infection is now rare (see Chapter 249). Other enteroviruses, such as coxsackievirus and echovirus, or the live polio vaccine virus can also cause an acute infection of motor neurons with symptoms and signs similar to poliomyelitis, although usually milder. Specific polymerase chain reaction tests and viral cultures of cerebrospinal fluid are diagnostic. Motor neuron infection with the West Nile virus also occurs.

A **juvenile form of amyotrophic lateral sclerosis** is rare. Upper and lower motor neuron loss is evident clinically, unlike in SMA. The course is progressive and ultimately fatal.

Pena-Shokeir and **Marden-Walker syndromes** are progressive motor neuron degenerations associated with severe arthrogryposis and congenital anomalies of many organ systems. **Pontocerebellar hypoplasias** are progressive degenerative diseases of the central nervous system that begin in fetal life; type 1 also involves motor neuron degeneration resembling an SMA, but the *SMN* gene on chromosome 5 is normal.

Motor neurons become involved in several metabolic diseases of the nervous system, such as gangliosidosis (Tay-Sachs disease), ceroid lipofuscinosis (Batten disease), and glycogenosis II (Pompe disease), but the signs of denervation may be minor or obscured by the more prominent involvement of other parts of the central nervous system or of muscle.

Chapter 613

Hereditary Motor-Sensory Neuropathies

Harvey B. Sarnat

The hereditary motor-sensory neuropathies (HMSNs) are a group of progressive diseases of peripheral nerves (Table 613-1). Motor components generally dominate the clinical picture, but sensory and autonomic involvement is expressed later. Sural nerve biopsy used to be the most definitive means of diagnosis, but with the expanded knowledge *Text continued on p. 3003*

Table 613-1	Hereditary Peripheral Neuropathies		
DISORDER (OMIM NO.)	**CLINICAL FEATURES**	**NERVE CONDUCTION STUDIES**	**GENE OR LOCUS**
CMT1 (DEMYELINATING)			
CMT1 A-F (HMSN type I)	Autosomal dominant. Onset 1st-4th decade. Predominant distal weakness, decreased DTRs, mild distal sensory loss, hypertrophy of nerves common	Delayed motor and sensory conduction studies. Motor studies typically <38 m/s	
1A (118220)	Commonest form recognized, seen in all ages (but more adults)		*PMP22* duplication or point mutation
1B (118200)	Approximately 5% of CMT1 group		*MPZ*
1C (601098)	Childhood onset, starts with abnormal gait, then distal weakness and wasting, occasional nerve hypertrophy. Rarely, early-onset hearing loss		*LITAF*
1D (607678)	Possible cranial nerve involvement. Late onset in childhood or early adulthood		*EGR2*
1E (118300)	Associated with deafness (29-45%)		*PMP22*
1F (607734)			*NEFL*
Hereditary neuropathy with liability to pressure palsies (tomaculous neuropathy) (162500)	Autosomal dominant. Recurrent mononeuropathy simplex or multiplex frequently related to trauma	Significant slowing of motor and sensory conduction velocities in clinically affected nerves but also in unaffected nerves	*PMP 22* deletion
Slowed NCVs Asymptomatic	Often a miscellaneous group. Incidentally detected with no clinical symptoms. Autosomal dominant	Moderately slowed conduction velocities	*ARHGEF10*
CMT2 (AXONAL)			
CMT2 A-L (HMSN type II)	Autosomal dominant (A, B, D, E, F, G, I) Autosomal recessive (BI, B2, H, K) Clinically similar to CMT type 1, except for later onset, absence of peripheral nerve enlargement, and less marked weakness	Nerve conduction velocities greater than HMSN type I (>38 m/s) but below normal range occasionally	
2A1 (118210)	CMT2A: prominent distal weakness, proximal weakness also present in 60%. Optic atrophy and central involvement reported. Main form related to *MFN2* mutations		2A1: *KIF1B* (one family)
2A2 (609260)			2A2: *MFN2*
2B (600882)	CMT2B: severe sensory loss: often complications with infections, arthropathy, amputations, foot ulcers, distal weakness		2B: *RAB7*
2B1 (605588)			2B1: *LMNA*
2B2 (605589)	Average onset 34 yr (Costa Rican family)		?*MED25*
2C (606071)	Vocal cord, diaphragm, and respiratory involvement, decreased longevity. Allelic with congenital dSMA (600175) and scapuloperoneal muscular atrophy (181405)		*TRP4* 12q23–q24 *TRP4*
2D (601472) (allelic to dSMA)	Upper limb predominance		*GARS*
2E (607684) (1F dominant is allelic to CMT2E)	30% associated with deafness, early childhood onset with gait abnormalities, occasional hyperkeratosis, increased sensory involvement	Intermediate/slow nerve conduction studies	*NEFL*

Continued

Table 613-1 Hereditary Peripheral Neuropathies—cont'd

DISORDER (OMIM NO.)	CLINICAL FEATURES	NERVE CONDUCTION STUDIES	GENE OR LOCUS
2F (606595)	Trophic changes feet and knees		*HSPB1* (*HSP27*)
2G (608591)	Onset age 9-76 yr, average age 20 yr, large Spanish family. Also severe form with early onset		12q12–q13
2H (607731) 2H (allelic to CMT4A–CMT4C2 in original publication)	Pyramidal involvement, vocal cord involvement	Intermediate/slow nerve conduction studies	*GDAP1*
2I (607677)	CMT I and J: possible late onset, pupillary anomalies, pain, hearing loss, dysphagia		*MPZ*
2J (607736)	Vocal cord paralysis, more severe early-onset form		*MPZ*
2K (607831)	Occasional proximal leg weakness (like dHMN II), large Chinese family, with onset at age 15-33 yr. Scoliosis		*GDAP1*
2L (608673)			*HSPB8* 12q24
HMSN II with onset in early childhood (EOHMSN) Severe early-onset axonal neuropathy (SEOAN)	Autosomal dominant or recessive. Weakness within 1st 5 yr, rapid progression of weakness, usually complete paralysis below elbows and knees by teens, absent DTRs, moderate sensory changes in most cases. Normal CSF protein. Occasional optic atrophy or spasticity	Axonal pattern with axonal-degenerative polyneuropathy. Absent SNAPs, no response to stimulation in cerebral palsy nerve, upper limb nerves normal or mildly slowed. EMG: denervation	*MFN2*; *GDAP1* Heterogeneous
Spinal muscular atrophy with respiratory distress type 1 (SMARD1)/severe infantile axonal neuropathy with respiratory failure (SIANR) Allelic to dHMN6 dSMA1 (604320)	Autosomal recessive. Onset in infancy (3-6 mo), respiratory failure, progressive distal weakness, eventual plateau. No recovery	Absent conduction in most cases	*IGHMBP2*
Hereditary motor and sensory neuropathy (HMSN-P) (Okinawa type)	Adult onset (after 30 yr). Autosomal dominant. Slowly progressive proximal dominant area of weakness. Fasciculations of extremities and trunk. Raised creatine kinase, hyperlipidemia, diabetes mellitus, eventual loss of ambulation, absent DTRs, sensory disturbances. Most patients described from Japan	Motor and sensory axonal neuropathy. SNAPs, CMAPs, MNCVs, and SNCVs reduced or absent EMG: fasciculations, fibrillations, and neuromyotonic picture early on	3q13
CMT3* AND 4			
CMT3 (Dejerine-Sottas syndrome) (145900)	Onset 1st 2 yr, overall disability ?less severe than CMT4. Hypotonia, motor delay by 1st yr, poor coordination, ataxia, distal weakness (max. lower limbs), short stature. By 2nd decade, proximal weakness, hand and foot deformities. Nerve hypertrophy. Moderate to severe sensory loss. Scoliosis. Common cranial nerve involvement, nystagmus, deafness, and mild bifacial weakness. Raised CSF protein	Motor conduction velocities usually <10 m/s. SAPs absent. EMG: chronic denervation	*PMP22*, *MPZ*, *PRX*, *EGR2*, *FIG4*
CMT4 (A-J) Autosomal recessive	Clinical picture similar to or slightly more severe than in CMT1 form, increased ataxia, areflexia, scoliosis. Nerve hypertrophy rare	Moderate slowing of nerve conduction studies	
4A (214400)	Onset <2 yr, Tunisian and Moroccan families. Severe progressive. Less-severe European phenotypes	25-35 m/s	*GDAP1*
4B1 (601382)	Ophthalmoplegia, vocal cord paralysis, facial, bulbar weakness (all infrequent). Weakness below 5 yr, proximal and distal weakness, absent DTRs	9-20 m/s	*MTMR2*, (*MPZ*)
4B2 (604563)	Early onset: 1st decade; glaucoma and deafness sometimes. Recorded in Tunisia, Japan, and Turkey	15-30 m/s	*SBF2*, *MTMR13*
4C (601596)	Early-onset scoliosis, commoner in Algerians, glaucoma and neutropenia. 1st and 2nd decades	4-37 m/s	*SH3TC2* (*KIAA1985*)
4D (601455) (HMSN-Lom)	Closed gypsy pedigree; onset <10 yr. Deafness (by 2nd-3rd decade). Tongue atrophy	10-20 m/s	*NDRG1*
4E (605253)	Congenital hypomyelinating neuropathy	5-20 m/s	*ERG2/KROX 20*, *MPZ*

Table 613-1	Hereditary Peripheral Neuropathies—cont'd		
DISORDER (OMIM NO.)	**CLINICAL FEATURES**	**NERVE CONDUCTION STUDIES**	**GENE OR LOCUS**
4F (145900)	Severely affected at birth or by 7 yr; arthrogryposis multiplex congenita common; respiratory and feeding difficulties; often die young	<5 m/s	PRX
4G (605285)	Type Russe. Onset 8-16 yr. Origin Bulgaria	30-35 m/s	10q22
4H (609311)	Increased in Lebanese/Turkish. Onset infancy to childhood (1-2 yr). Delayed motor milestones. Occasional scoliosis, increased distal weakness, usually absent DTRs	<10 m/s or absent	FDG4
4J (611228)	Onset by 5 yr. Severe disorder. Similarities to motor neuron disease	2-7 m/s; some cases higher	FIG4
CCFDN (604168)	Congenital cataract, microcornea, facial dysmorphism, mental retardation, distal motor peripheral neuropathy	19-33 m/s	CTDP1
MIXED PATHOLOGY (AXONAL AND DEMYELINATING)			
CMT X X-linked CMT X1 (302800)	X-linked dominant. Onset 1st-2nd decade. Progressive wasting and weakness of distal limb musculature, especially hands, more marked in affected males than carrier females	Median nerve motor conduction studies <40 m/s (but faster than CMT1A). Intermediate slowing less uniform along nerves with dispersion more pronounced	GJB1
X2 (302801)	X-linked recessive. Rare infantile onset, intellectual disability, females very mildly affected	Mixed demyelinating/axonal	Xp22.2
X3 (302802)	X-linked recessive. ± Spasticity. Females unaffected	Mixed demyelinating/axonal	Xq26
X4 (310490)	X-linked (Cowchock syndrome). Severe neuropathy, females very mildly affected. Isolated case reports. Onset birth to early childhood. Slowly progressive. Many develop deafness by 5 yr. Mental retardation commonly seen. Occasional optic atrophy	Axonal neuropathy. Motor conduction velocities: mild delay (33-56 m/s). Sensory very abnormal. EMG: denervation, large motor unit potential, and fasciculation	Xq24–26.1
X5 (311070)	X-linked. Mild to moderate neuropathy, deafness, optic atrophy. Allelic with Rosenberg-Chutorian (opticoacoustic neuropathy) and Arts syndromes	Axonal neuropathy–mild demyelinating changes	Xq21.32–q24 PRPS1
Intermediate forms of CMT	Patients have neurophysiologic results that fall between axonal and demyelinating ranges	"Intermediate values" 30-40 m/s–most accurate from median motor nerves. Some forms have normal nerve conduction studies (DI-CMTB)	
DI-CMTA DI-CMTB (606482) DI-CMTC (608323) DI-CMTD (607791) A–autosomal recessive form (608340)	Italian family American family Myelin protein zero Overlap conditions: Recessive CMT with GADP1 mutations: (CMT2K and 4A) Spanish and Tunisian family–severe childhood forms reported. Also called DI-CMTA autosomal recessive form CMT with NF-L: (CMT1F and 2E)		10q24.1–q25.1 DNM2 YARS MPZ Overlap: GJB1 NF-L GDAP1
OTHER HMSN AND HMN SYNDROMES			
HMSN V/spastic paraplegia with HMSN type V/CMT5 (CMT with pyramidal signs) (600631)	Variable inheritance. Spasticity in lower limbs causing difficulty walking and toe walking. Autosomal recessive form associated with mental retardation. Lower limb marked spasticity with little weakness, increased DTRs, extensor plantars, pes cavus, often distal amyotrophy. Expanding field with multiple subforms, n = 37. Not all associated with peripheral neuropathy CMT with pyramidal signs: part of HMSN V but described without spasticity	Small/absent SNAPs. Motor studies axonal in type	SPG3A, SPAST, NIPA1, BSCL2, SPG4, SPG7, SPG20, SPG21, SPG30, PLP1 CMT with pyramidal signs: MFN2
HMSN VI (allelic CMT2A)	Visual impairment due to optic atrophy. Dominant and recessive forms. Onset in 1st decade. Distal weakness, often proximal involvement too. Less sensory involvement. Scoliosis	No response or motor conduction around 45 m/s. Sensory nerves often cannot be stimulated	MFN2
HMSN VII	HMSN with retinitis pigmentosa. CSF protein raised. Usually adult onset. Rare entity described in a few families, mainly of adult onset		

Continued

Table 613-1 | Hereditary Peripheral Neuropathies—cont'd

DISORDER (OMIM NO.)	CLINICAL FEATURES	NERVE CONDUCTION STUDIES	GENE OR LOCUS
DISTAL HEREDITARY MOTOR NEURONOPATHIES (DHMN)			
dHMNI (182960)	Autosomal dominant. Juvenile onset. Distal weakness and wasting	Normal nerve conduction studies, occasional mild slowing. EMG neurogenic	HSPB1 7q34–q36
dHMNII (608634)	Autosomal dominant. Adult onset, distal weakness and wasting		HSPB8, HSPB3
dHMNIIjuv (158590)	(Allelic CMT2F, CMT2L)		HSPB1
dHMNIII	Autosomal recessive. Infantile to adult onset. Slow, progressive muscle wasting and weakness, variable diaphragmatic paralysis		11q13.3
dHMNIV (607088) Distal SMA type 3	Autosomal recessive. Juvenile onset. Severe muscle wasting and weakness and diaphragmatic paralysis		11q13
dHMNV (600794)	(Allelic CMT2D) Autosomal dominant. Upper limb predominance, occasional pyramidal features		GARS
dHMN type V (Silver syndrome) (270685)	Autosomal dominant. Prominent hand muscle weakness and wasting, mild to severe spasticity of lower limbs		BSCL2
dHMNVI (604320)	(Allelic SMARD1) Autosomal recessive. Severe infantile form with respiratory distress		IGHMBP2
dHMNVIIA (158580)	Autosomal dominant. Onset with vocal cord paralysis		DCTN1
dHMNVIIB (607641)	Autosomal dominant. Onset with vocal cord paralysis and facial weakness		2q14 Xq13–q21
X-linked dHMN			
dHMN/ALS4 (602433)	X-linked recessive. Juvenile onset with distal wasting and weakness		SETX
dHMN-J (Jerash)	Autosomal dominant. Early onset symptomatic in 2nd decade with pyramidal tract signs		9p21.1–p12
Congenital distal SMA (600175)	Autosomal recessive. Onset from 6-10 yr with pyramidal features in 1 Jordanian family Autosomal dominant congenital nonprogressive distal HMN with contractures		12q23–q24
Peripheral neuropathy with agenesis of corpus callosum (Charlevoix disease or Andermann syndrome) (218000)	Autosomal recessive. Increased in French Canadian populations. Progressive axonal neuropathy. CNS malformations—absence/hypoplasia of corpus callosum in most, early onset, developmental delay, areflexia, dysmorphology. Later, increased motor disability, hallucinatory psychosis. Death by 3rd decade	EMG: denervation. Axonal neuropathy	SLC12A6 (KCC3)
Hereditary neuralgic amyotrophy (brachial plexus neuropathy) (162100)	Autosomal dominant. Episodes of paralysis and muscle weakness initiated by severe pain. Onset can be from birth or later childhood but usually adult onset. Outcome usually good but some left with residual dysfunction. Episodes often triggered by infections, immunizations, and stress. Some pedigrees dysmorphic with hypotelorism	Normal or mildly prolonged MNCVs distal to affected brachial plexus	SEPT9
HEREDITARY SENSORY AND AUTONOMIC NEUROPATHIES			
HSN (HSAN) 1 (162400)	Type 1: Autosomal dominant. Onset 2nd–5th decade. Predominant loss of pain and temperature sensation, preservation of vibration sense, lancinating pain, variable distal motor involvement	Normal to low-normal MNCVs, disturbance of sensory conduction of variable severity Type 1B: Autosomal dominant. Predominantly sensory neuropathy with cough and gastroesophageal reflux, rarely foot ulcers. More often adult onset. Hearing often abnormal	SPTLC1 RAB7 3p24–p22
HSN (HSAN) 2(A) (201300)	Autosomal recessive. Onset in infancy/early childhood–1st 2 decades. Mutilating acropathy. Often unrecognized fractures. Marked sensory loss affecting all cutaneous modalities, most marked distally in all limbs. Autonomic dysfunction less marked. Absent or decreased DTRs	Normal MNCVs; SNAPs are absent	WNK1
HSN (HSAN) 2B (223900)	Autosomal recessive. Impaired sensation, ulcers, and arthropathy develop in childhood		FAM134B

Table 613-1	Hereditary Peripheral Neuropathies—cont'd		
DISORDER (OMIM NO.)	**CLINICAL FEATURES**	**NERVE CONDUCTION STUDIES**	**GENE OR LOCUS**
HSN (HSAN) 3 (Riley-Day syndrome, familial dysautonomia) (223900)	Autosomal recessive. History of neurologic abnormality and of difficult feeding from birth. Failure to produce tears regularly. Absent or reduced DTRs. Absent corneal reflexes, postural hypotension, emotional lability. Relative indifference to pain, absence of fungiform papillae on tongue, absence of flare with intradermal histamine. Normal intelligence	Motor conduction velocities usually slightly below control values. Sensory conduction normal or decreased	*IKBAP*
HSN (HSAN) 4 (congenital insensitivity to pain with anhidrosis, CIPA) (256800)	Autosomal recessive. Onset from infancy, often high fevers due to truncal anhidrosis during hot weather. Painless injuries of extremities and oral structures, often self-mutilation. Lack of pain sensation, both peripheral and visceral, inability to distinguish hot and cold. Preservation of DTRs. Mild mental retardation. Hyperactivity and emotional lability common	Nerve conduction studies normal. Sympathetic skin responses are absent (histamine test)	*NTRK1*
HSN (HSAN) 5 (608654)	Autosomal recessive. Onset in early life. Rare disorder. Painless injuries of the extremities. Lack of pain and thermal sensitivity in the limbs but preservation of response to tactile and mechanical stimuli. Preservation of muscle strength and DTRs. Distal anhidrosis. Bone and joint fractures; arthropathy. Normal intelligence	Normal motor and sensory nerve conduction studies	*NGFβ*

*The term CMT3 should be reserved for hereditary neuropathies in which hypomyelination is the dominant feature. This would include congenital hypomyelinating neuropathy, Dejerine-Sottas disease, and congenital amyelinating neuropathy.

CCFDN, congenital cataract, microcornea, facial dysmorphism, mental retardation, distal motor peripheral neuropathy; CIPA, congenital insensitivity to pain with anhidrosis; CMAP, compound motor unit action potential; CMT, Charcot-Marie-Tooth disease; CP, common peroneal; CSF, cerebrospinal fluid; dHMN, distal hereditary motor neuronopathy; DI, dominant intermediate; dSMA, distal spinal muscular atrophy; DTR, deep tendon reflex; EMG, electromyography; EOHMSN, early-onset HMSN; HMN, hereditary motor neuropathy; HMSN, hereditary motor and sensory neuropathy; HSAN, hereditary sensory and autonomic neuropathy; HSN, hereditary sensory neuropathy; MNCV, motor nerve conduction velocity; OMIM, Online Mendelian Inheritance in Man; SAP, sensory action potential; SEOAN, severe early-onset axonal neuropathy; SMA, spinal muscular atrophy; SNAP, sensory nerve action potential.

From Wilmshurst JM, Ouvrier R: Hereditary peripheral neuropathies of childhood: an overview for clinicians, Neuromuscul Disord 21(11):763–775, 2011.

of the molecular genetics of this group of diseases, the diagnosis of most can be confirmed by less invasive genetic testing. Electromyography (EMG) remains a useful adjunct to clinical diagnosis and helps distinguish between **demyelinating** or **hypomyelinating** and **axonal** forms.

Classification of HMSNs is difficult because no simple unifying scheme is capable of incorporating all the clinical presentations and overlapping genetics (see Table 613-1). In some neuropathies, a diverse genotype of mutations of different genes at different chromosomal loci may produce a similar phenotype. One classification identifies: I. Hereditary neuropathies secondary to general diseases; II. Primary neuropathies as: IIa. Hereditary motor sensory neuropathies; IIb. Distal hereditary motor neuropathies; IIc. Hereditary sensory ± autonomic neuropathies; III. Syndromic neuropathies including congenital hypomyelinating neuropathies; and IV. Hereditary sensory neuropathy (Refsum disease).

613.1 Peroneal Muscular Atrophy (Charcot-Marie-Tooth Disease, Hereditary Motor-Sensory Neuropathy Type IIa)

Harvey B. Sarnat

Charcot-Marie-Tooth disease is the most common genetically determined neuropathy and has an overall prevalence of 3.8/100,000 population. It is transmitted as an autosomal dominant trait with 83% expressivity; the 17p11.2 locus is the site of the abnormal gene. Autosomal recessive transmission also is described but is rarer. The gene product is peripheral myelin protein 22 (PMP22). A much rarer X-linked HMSN type I results from a defect at the Xq13.l locus, causing mutations in the gap junction protein connexin-32. Other forms have been reported (see Table 613-1).

CLINICAL MANIFESTATIONS

Most patients are asymptomatic until late childhood or early adolescence, but young children sometimes manifest gait disturbance as early as the 2nd yr of life. The peroneal and tibial nerves are the earliest and most severely affected. Children with the disorder are often described as being clumsy, falling easily, or tripping over their own feet. Application of the Cumberland Ankle Instability Tool for Youth is a means of objectively documenting and following this manifestation. The onset of symptoms may be delayed until after the 5th decade.

Muscles of the anterior compartment of the lower legs become wasted, and the legs have a characteristic stork-like contour. The muscular atrophy is accompanied by progressive weakness of dorsiflexion of the ankle and eventual footdrop. The process is bilateral but may be slightly asymmetric. Pes cavus deformities invariably develop as a result of denervation of intrinsic foot muscles, further destabilizing the gait. Atrophy of muscles of the forearms and hands is usually not as severe as that of the lower extremities, but in advanced cases contractures of the wrists and fingers produce a claw hand. Proximal muscle weakness is a late manifestation and is usually mild. Axial muscles are not involved.

The disease is slowly progressive throughout life, but patients occasionally show accelerated deterioration of function over a few years. Most patients remain ambulatory and have normal longevity, although orthotic appliances are required to stabilize the ankles.

Sensory involvement mainly affects large myelinated nerve fibers that convey proprioceptive information and vibratory sense, but the threshold for pain and temperature can also increase. Some children complain of tingling or burning sensations of the feet, but pain is rare. Because the muscle mass is reduced, the nerves are more vulnerable to trauma or compression. Autonomic manifestations may be expressed as poor vasomotor control with blotching or pallor of the skin of the feet and inappropriately cold feet.

Nerves often become palpably enlarged. Tendon stretch reflexes are lost distally. Cranial nerves are not affected. Sphincter control remains well preserved. Autonomic neuropathy does not affect the heart, gastrointestinal tract, or bladder. Intelligence is normal. A unique point mutation in *PMP22* causes progressive auditory nerve deafness in addition, but this is usually later in onset than the peripheral neuropathy.

Davidenkow syndrome is a variant of HMSN type I with a scapuloperoneal distribution.

LABORATORY FINDINGS AND DIAGNOSIS

Motor and sensory nerve conduction velocities are greatly reduced, sometimes as slow as 20% of normal conduction time. In new cases without a family history, both parents should be examined, and nerve conduction studies should be performed.

EMG and muscle biopsy are not usually required for diagnosis, but they show evidence of many cycles of denervation and reinnervation. Serum creatine kinase level is normal. Cerebrospinal fluid (CSF) protein may be elevated, but no cells appear in the CSF.

Sural nerve biopsy is diagnostic. Large- and medium-size myelinated fibers are reduced in number, collagen is increased, and characteristic **onion bulb formations** of proliferated Schwann cell cytoplasm surround axons. This pathologic finding is called **interstitial hypertrophic neuropathy.** Extensive segmental demyelination and remyelination also occur.

The definitive molecular genetic diagnosis may be made in blood.

TREATMENT

Stabilization of the ankles is a primary concern. In early stages, stiff boots that extend to the midcalf often suffice, particularly when patients walk on uneven surfaces such as ice and snow or stones. As the dorsiflexors of the ankles weaken further, lightweight plastic splints may be custom made to extend beneath the foot and around the back of the ankle. They are worn inside the socks and are not visible, reducing self-consciousness. External short-leg braces may be required when footdrop becomes complete. Surgical fusion of the ankle may be considered in some cases.

The leg should be protected from traumatic injury. In advanced cases, compression neuropathy during sleep may be prevented by placing soft pillows beneath or between the lower legs. Burning paresthesias of the feet are not common but are often abolished by phenytoin, carbamazepine, or gabapentin. No medical treatment is available to arrest or slow the progression.

613.2 Peroneal Muscular Atrophy (Axonal Type)
Harvey B. Sarnat

Peroneal muscular atrophy is clinically similar to HMSN type I, but the rate of progression is slower and the disability is less. EMG shows denervation of muscle. Sural nerve biopsy reveals axonal degeneration rather than the demyelination and whorls of Schwann cell processes typical in type I. The locus is on chromosome 1 at 1p35-p36; this is a different disease than HMSN type I, although both diseases are transmitted as autosomal dominant traits. An autosomal recessive infantile motor axonal neuropathy can closely mimic infantile spinal muscular atrophy.

613.3 Congenital Hypomyelinating Neuropathy and Dejerine-Sottas Disease (Hereditary Motor-Sensory Neuropathy Type III)
Harvey B. Sarnat

Congenital hypomyelinating neuropathy is an interstitial hypertrophic neuropathy of autosomal dominant transmission, clinically similar to

HMSN type I but more severe. Symptoms develop in early infancy and are rapidly progressive, with hypotonia and breathing and feeding difficulties. Pupillary abnormalities, such as lack of reaction to light and *Argyll Robertson pupil,* are common. Kyphoscoliosis and pes cavus deformities complicate approximately 35% of cases. Nerves become palpably enlarged at an early age. Dejerine-Sottas disease is a more slowly progressive variant with onset usually before age 5 yr.

An autosomal recessive form of congenital hypomyelinating neuropathy also is known and may be caused by various genetic mutations, including *MTMR2, PMP22, EGR2,* and *MPZ.* Neonatal hypotonia and developmental delay in infancy are hallmark clinical features. Many patients exhibit congenital insensitivity to pain. Cranial nerves are inconsistently involved, and respiratory distress and dysphagia are rare complications. Tendon reflexes are absent. **Arthrogryposis** is present at birth in at least half the cases.

The onion bulb formations seen in the sural nerve biopsy specimen are pronounced. Hypomyelination also occurs. In the recessive form, hypomyelination may not be accompanied by interstitial hypertrophy in all cases.

The genetic locus of 17p11.2 is identical to that of HMSN type I or Charcot-Marie-Tooth disease. Monoallelic mutations in *MPZ* (myelin protein zero), *PMP22,* or *EGR2* (early grow response 2) are the most frequent genetic causes. The clinical and pathologic differences may be phenotypical variants of the same disease, analogous to the situation in Duchenne and Becker muscular dystrophies. An autosomal recessive form of Dejerine-Sottas disease is incompletely documented.

613.4 Roussy-Lévy Syndrome
Harvey B. Sarnat

Roussy-Lévy syndrome is defined as a combination of HMSN type II and cerebellar deficit resembling Friedreich ataxia, but it does not have cardiomyopathy.

613.5 Refsum Disease (Hereditary Sensory Neuropathy Type IV) and Infantile Refsum Disease
Harvey B. Sarnat

See Chapter 86.2.

Refsum disease is a rare autosomal recessive disease caused by an enzymatic block in β-oxidation of phytanic acid to pristanic acid. Phytanic acid is a branched-chain fatty acid that is derived mainly from dietary sources: spinach, nuts, and coffee. Levels of phytanic acid are greatly elevated in plasma, CSF, and brain tissue. The CSF shows an albuminocytologic dissociation, with a protein concentration of 100-600 mg/dL. Genetic linkage studies identify 2 distinct loci at 10p13 and 6q22-q24 with *PHYH* and *PEX7* genetic mutations, respectively. The infantile form also can be caused by *PEX1, PEX2,* or *PEX26* genes, which produce both clinical and biochemical differences from the classical form, and include minor facial dysmorphism, retinitis pigmentosa, sensorineural hearing loss, hypercholesterolemia, hepatomegaly, and failure to thrive. Phytanic acid accumulation in infantile Refsum disease is secondary to a primary peroxisomal disorder; hence autosomal recessive Refsum disease is really a different disease.

Clinical onset of classical Refsum disease is usually between 4 and 7 yr of age, with intermittent motor and sensory neuropathy. Ataxia, progressive neurosensory hearing loss, retinitis pigmentosa with loss of night vision, ichthyosis, and liver dysfunction also develop in various degrees. Skeletal malformations from birth and cardiac findings of conduction disturbances and cardiomyopathy appear in the majority. Motor and sensory nerve conduction velocities are delayed. Sural nerve biopsy shows loss of myelinated axons. Treatment is by dietary management and periodic plasma exchange. With careful management, life expectancy can be normal.

613.6 Fabry Disease
Harvey B. Sarnat

See Chapter 86.4.

Fabry disease, a rare X-linked recessive trait, results in storage of ceramide trihexose because of deficiency of the enzyme ceramide trihexosidase, which cleaves the terminal galactose from ceramide trihexose (ceramide-glucose-galactose-galactose), resulting in tissue accumulation of this trihexose lipid in central nervous system neurons, Schwann cells and perineurial cells, ganglion cells of the myenteric plexus, skin, kidneys, blood vessel endothelial and smooth muscle cells, heart, sweat glands, cornea, and bone marrow. It results from a missense mutation disrupting the crystallographic structure of α-galactosidase A.

CLINICAL MANIFESTATIONS
The presentation is in late childhood or adolescence, with recurrent episodes of burning pain and paresthesias of the feet and lower legs so severe that patients are unable to walk. These episodes are often precipitated by fever or by physical activity. Objective sensory and motor deficits are not demonstrated on neurologic examination, and reflexes are preserved. Characteristic skin lesions are seen in the perineal region, scrotum, buttocks, and periumbilical zone as flat or raised red-black telangiectases known as **angiokeratoma corporis diffusum.** Hypohidrosis may be present. Corneal opacities, cataracts, and necrosis of the femoral heads are inconstant features. Tortuosity of retinal vessels and of the vertebral and basilar arteries can occur. The disease is progressive. Hypertension and renal failure are usually delayed until early adult life. Recurrent strokes result from vascular wall involvement. Death often occurs in the 5th decade owing to cerebral infarction or renal insufficiency, but a significant morbidity already occurs in childhood despite the absence of major organ failure. Heterozygous female carriers may be asymptomatic or, rarely, are as affected as males; corneal opacities involve 70-80%, though cataracts are rare.

LABORATORY FINDINGS
Motor and sensory nerve conduction velocities are normal to only mildly slow, showing preservation of large myelinated nerve fibers. CSF protein is normal. Proteinuria is present early in the course.

Calcifications often are seen in pulvinar of the thalamus, as demonstrated by CT or MRI and are specific imaging findings, believed caused by cerebral hyperperfusion. Positron tomography, by contrast, shows reduced cerebral blood flow velocity and impaired autoregulation because of the glycosphingolipid storage in vascular endothelial cells.

Pathologic features are usually first detected in skin or sural nerve biopsy specimens. Electron microscopy demonstrates crystalline glycosphingolipids, appearing as *zebra bodies*, in lysosomes of endothelial cells, in smooth myocytes of arterioles, and in Schwann cells. Nerves show a selective loss of small myelinated fibers and relative preservation of large and medium-sized axons, contrasting to most axonal neuropathies in which large myelinated fibers are most involved.

Assay for the deficient enzyme, α-galactosidase-A, may be performed from skin fibroblasts, leukocytes, and other tissues. This test permits detection of the female carrier state and provides a reliable means of prenatal diagnosis.

TREATMENT
See Chapter 86.4 for specific therapy of Fabry disease, including enzyme replacement.

Medical therapy of painful neuropathies includes management of the initiating disease and therapy directed to the neuropathic pain independent of etiology. Pain may be burning or associated with paresthesia, hyperalgesia (abnormal response to noxious stimuli), or allodynia (induced by non–noxious stimuli; see Chapter 62). Neuropathic pain is often successfully managed by tricyclic antidepressants; selective serotonin reuptake inhibitors are less effective. Anticonvulsants (carbamazepine, phenytoin, gabapentin, lamotrigine) are effective, as are narcotic and nonnarcotic analgesics. Enzyme replacement therapy has improved the short- and long-term prognosis of the clinical neuropathy and also reverses the increased blood flow velocity in the brain.

613.7 Giant Axonal Neuropathy
Harvey B. Sarnat

Giant axonal neuropathy is a rare autosomal recessive disease with onset in early childhood. It is a progressive mixed peripheral neuropathy and degeneration of central white matter, similar to the leukodystrophies. Ataxia and nystagmus are accompanied by signs of progressive peripheral neuropathy. A large majority of affected children have frizzy hair, which microscopically shows variation in diameter of the shaft and twisting, similar to that in Menkes disease; hence, microscopic examination of a few scalp hairs provides a simple screening tool in suspected cases. Focal axonal enlargements are seen in both the peripheral nervous system and the central nervous system, but the myelin sheath is intact. The disease is a general proliferation of intermediate filaments, including neurofilaments in axons, glial filaments (i.e., Rosenthal fibers) in brain, cytokeratin in hair, and vimentin in Schwann cells and fibroblasts.

Nonsense and missense mutations or deletions occur in the *GAN* gene, with allelic heterogeneity, at 16q24. These mutations are responsible for defective synthesis of the protein gigaxonin, a member of the cytoskeletal BTB/kelch superfamily, crucial to linkage between intermediate proteins and the cell membrane. MRI shows white matter lesions of the brain similar to leukodystrophies, and MR spectroscopy demonstrates increased ratios of choline : creatine and myoinositol : creatine, with a normally preserved ratio of *N*-acetyl aspartate : creatine, indicating demyelination and glial proliferation without axonal loss. Gigaxonin is expressed in a wide variety of neuronal cell types and is localized to the Golgi apparatus and endoplasmic reticulum.

The diagnosis is established by microscopy of scalp hair and by MRI and MR spectroscopy of the brain; it is confirmed by sural nerve biopsy and/or by genetic studies, if available, of the *GAN* gene. A mutation of *BAG3*, one of several genes associated with myofibrillar myopathy (see Chapter 608.5), also can cause giant axonal neuropathy as another genetic etiology not associated with the more frequent *GAN* gene.

613.8 Tomaculous (Hypermyelinating) Neuropathy; Hereditary Neuropathy with Liability to Pressure Palsies
Harvey B. Sarnat

This hereditary neuropathy is characterized by redundant overproduction of myelin around each axon in an irregular segmental fashion so that tomaculous (sausage-shaped) bulges occur in the individual myelinated nerve fibers. Other sections of the same nerve can show loss of myelin. Such nerves are particularly prone to pressure palsies, and patients, usually beginning in adolescence, present with recurrent or intermittent mononeuropathies secondary to minor trauma or entrapment neuropathies, such as carpal tunnel syndrome, peroneal palsies, and even "writer's cramp." It is transmitted as an autosomal dominant trait, with loci identified at 17p11.2 and 17p12, deletion of exons in the *PMP22* gene, in some patients only microdeletions. Duplication of the same 17p12 locus leads to Charcot-Marie-Tooth disease type 1A, myelin protein zero *(MPZ)* gene mutation. Sural nerve biopsy is diagnostic, but special teased fiber preparations should be made to demonstrate the myelin abnormalities most clearly. Skin or conjunctival biopsies also may be diagnostic. Electrophysiologic nerve conduction studies are abnormal but nonspecific. Genetic studies are definitive.

Treatment is supportive and includes avoiding trauma and prolonged nerve compression, including postures when sitting or lying.

Surgical release of entrapped nerves is indicated at times, particularly of the ulnar nerve.

613.9 Leukodystrophies
Harvey B. Sarnat

Several hereditary degenerative diseases of white matter of the central nervous system also cause peripheral neuropathy. The most important are Krabbe disease (globoid cell leukodystrophy), metachromatic leukodystrophy, and adrenoleukodystrophy (see Chapters 86 and 599).

Bibliography is available at Expert Consult.

Chapter 614
Toxic Neuropathies
Harvey B. Sarnat

Many chemicals (organophosphates), toxins, and drugs can cause peripheral neuropathy (Table 614-1). Heavy metals are well-known neurotoxins. Lead poisoning, especially if chronic, causes mainly a motor neuropathy selectively involving large nerves, such as the common peroneal, radial, and median nerves, a condition known as **mononeuritis multiplex** (see Chapter 721). Arsenic produces painful burning paresthesias and motor polyneuropathy. Exposure to industrial and agricultural chemicals is a less-common cause of toxic neuropathy in children than in adults, but insecticides are neurotoxins for both insects and humans, and if they are used as sprays in closed spaces, they may be inhaled and induce lethargy, vomiting, seizures, and neuropathy, particularly with recurrent or long-term exposure. Working adolescents and children in developing countries are also at risk. Puffer fish poisoning, which can be acquired even when fish contaminated with the venom has been cooked, produces a Guillain-Barré–like syndrome. Ethanol abuse can be neurotoxic and particularly affects the optic nerves, but optic neuritis is not a true peripheral neuropathy.

The most frequent cause of toxic neuropathies in children is prescribed medications, though street drugs also can be neurotoxic. Antimetabolic and immunosuppressive drugs, such as vincristine, cisplatin, and paclitaxel, produce polyneuropathies as complications of chemotherapy for neoplasms and immunologic disorders, such as juvenile idiopathic arthritis. This "iatrogenic" cause is usually an axonal degeneration rather than primary demyelination, unlike primary autoimmune neuropathies. Excessive vitamin intake ("megavitamins") can be neurotoxic.

Chronic uremia is associated with toxic neuropathy and myopathy. The neuropathy is caused by excessive levels of circulating parathyroid hormone. Reduction in serum parathyroid hormone levels is accompanied by clinical improvement and a return to normal of nerve conduction velocity. Peripheral nerve axonal damage, particularly of small fibers, can be secondary to mitochondrial loss or dysfunction in toxic neuropathies. Abnormal toxic complex lipids, generated in Schwann cells by deficient mitochondrial respiration, are capable of damaging or destroying neighboring axons, a secondary mitochondrial toxic neuropathy. Small heat-shock proteins can be provoked that also may contribute to toxic neuropathy.

Biologic neurotoxins associated with diphtheria, Lyme disease, West Nile virus disease, leprosy, herpesviruses (Bell palsy), and rabies also produce peripheral nerve– or ventral horn cell–induced weakness or paralysis. HIV infections also produce neuropathy and this infection

Table 614-1	Toxic and Metabolic Neuropathies
METALS Arsenic (insecticide, herbicide) Lead (paint, batteries, pottery) Mercury (metallic, vapor) Thallium (rodenticides) Gold **OCCUPATIONAL OR INDUSTRIAL CHEMICALS** Acrylamide (grouting, flocculation) Carbon disulfide (solvent) Cyanide Dichlorophenoxyacetate Dimethylaminopropionitrite Ethylene oxide (gas sterilization) Hexacarbons (glue, solvents) Organophosphates (insecticides, petroleum additive) Polychlorinated biphenyls Tetrachlorbiphenyl Trichloroethylene **DRUGS** Amiodarone Chloramphenicol Chloroquine Cisplatin Colchicine Dapsone Ethambutol Ethanol Fluoroquinolones Gold Hydralazine Isoniazid Metronidazole	Nitrofurantoin Nitrous oxide Nucleosides (antiretroviral agents dideoxycytidine [ddC], didanosine [ddI], d4T, others) Penicillamine Pentamidine Phenytoin Pyridoxine (excessive) Statins Stilbamidine Suramin Tacrolimus Taxanes (paclitaxel, docetaxel) Thalidomide Tryptophan (eosinophilia-myalgia syndrome) Vincristine **METABOLIC DISORDERS** Fabry disease Krabbe disease Leukodystrophies Porphyria Tangier disease Tyrosinemia Uremia **BIOLOGIC AND INFECTIOUS NEUROPATHIES** Diphtheria Herpesviruses HIV Leprosy Lyme disease Rabies West Nile virus

is particularly prevalent in children in several African countries, including those who immigrate to western countries as refugees. Tick paralysis, botulism, and paralytic shellfish poisoning cause neuromuscular junction blockade rather than true neuropathy. Various inborn errors of metabolism are also associated with peripheral neuropathy from metabolite toxicity or deficiencies (see Part XI and Table 614-1).

Bibliography is available at Expert Consult.

Chapter 615
Autonomic Neuropathies
Harvey B. Sarnat

Involvement of small, lightly or unmyelinated autonomic nerve fibers may be seen in many peripheral neuropathies; the autonomic manifestations are usually mild or subclinical. Certain autonomic neuropathies are more symptomatic and demonstrate varying degrees of involvement of the autonomic nervous system regulation of the cardiovascular, gastrointestinal, genitourinary, thermoregulatory, sudomotor, and pupillomotor systems. Figure 615-1 shows the classification of autonomic disorders (dysautonomias).

The differential diagnosis is noted in Tables 613-1 (in Chapter 613) and 615-1; Table 615-2 compares the neonatal-infantile onset

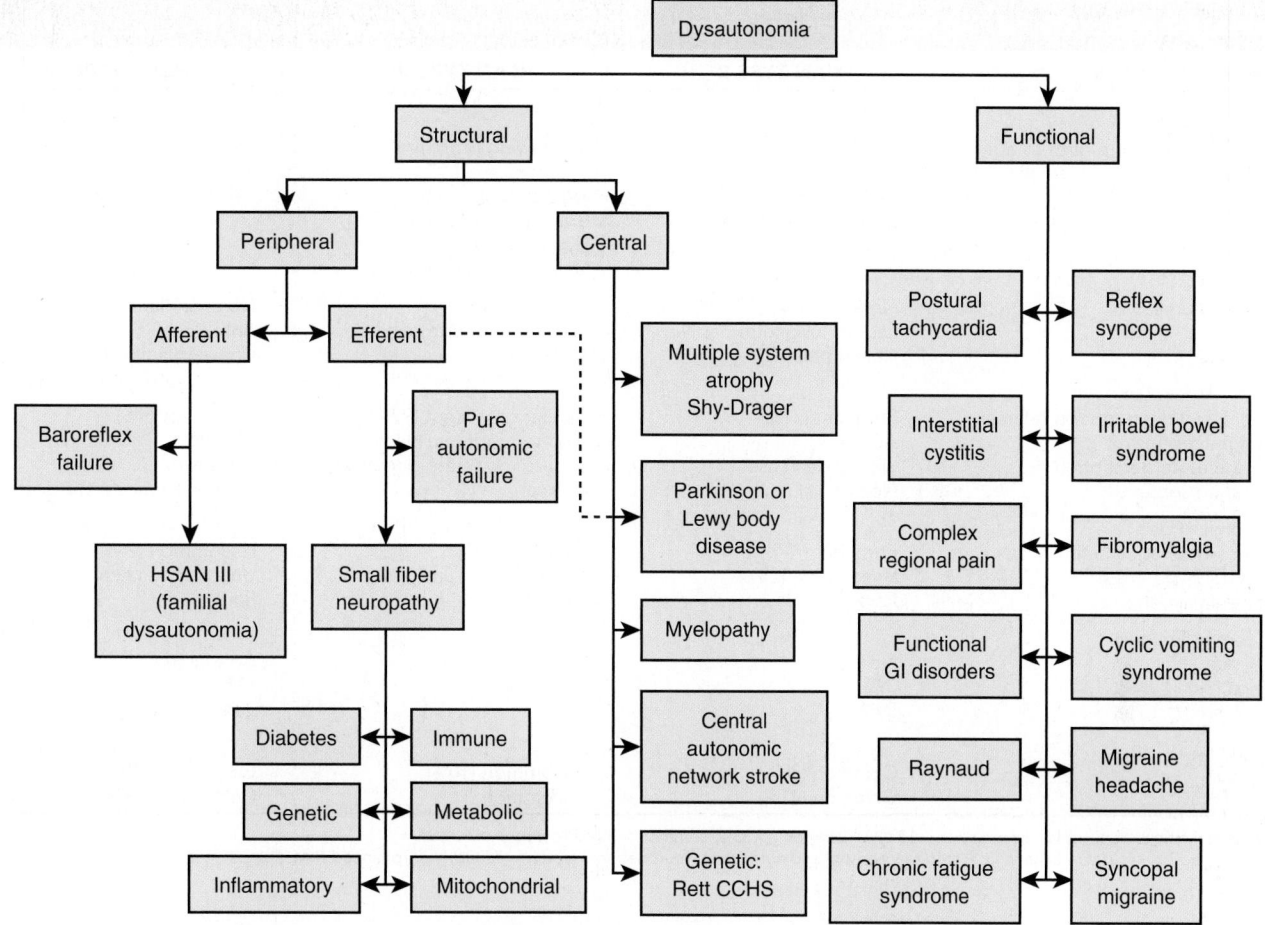

Figure 615-1 Classification of autonomic disorders or dysautonomias. The first conceptual division is between a structural and functional disorder. The word "functional" is being used in its true meaning of a disturbance in autonomic function, without clear evidence of structural damage to the autonomic nervous system, akin to the use of the word "functional" in functional gastrointestinal disorders, and without implication of a psychiatric etiology. In the absence of any evidence of consistent structural abnormalities functional disorders clearly cannot be localized in the nervous system. In contrast, structural disorders can be further divided into those localized in the central and peripheral nervous systems, with the division point usually taken at the sympathetic ganglion. Finally, peripheral nervous system disorders can be further classified based on whether they primarily involve afferent or efferent nerves. It should be emphasized that there is overlap between these groups, for example, diabetes will often involve afferent nerve fibers, but this classification emphasizes the predominant fiber involvement. A *dotted line* links Parkinson disease to a peripheral efferent group as Lewy bodies are present in the both parasympathetic and sympathetic ganglia, impairing peripheral autonomic function. See below for discussion of specific disorders. *CCHS,* Congenital central hypoventilation syndrome; *HSAN,* hereditary sensory autonomic neuropathy. *(From Chelimsky T, Robertson D, Chelimsky G: Disorders of the autonomic nervous system. In Daroff RB, Fenichel GM, Jankovic J, Mazziotta JC, editors: Bradley's neurology in clinical practice, ed 6, Philadelphia, 2012, WB Saunders, Fig. 77-1, p. 2018.)*

Table 615-1	Autonomic Neuropathies

Guillain-Barré syndrome (see Chapter 608) Non–Guillain-Barré syndrome autoimmunity • Paraneoplastic (type I antineuronal nuclear antibody) • Lambert-Eaton syndrome • Antibodies to neuronal nicotinic acetylcholine receptors • Antibodies to P/Q-type calcium channels • Other autoantibodies • Systemic lupus erythematosus Hereditary sensory and autonomic neuropathies • Type I autosomal dominant • Type II autosomal recessive (Morvan disease) • Type III autosomal recessive (Riley-Day) • Type IV autosomal recessive (congenital insensitivity to pain with anhidrosis) • Type V absence of pain	Metabolic • Fabry disease • Diabetes mellitus • Tangier disease • Porphyria Infectious • HIV • Chagas disease • Botulism • Leprosy • Diphtheria Other • Triple A (Allgrove) syndrome • Navajo Indian neuropathy • Multiple endocrine neoplasia type 2b Toxins (see Table 614-1 in Chapter 614)

Table 615-2 | Major Clinical Features of Hereditary Sensory-Autonomic Neuropathy Types II, III, and IV

CLINICAL FEATURES	HSAN TYPE II	HSAN TYPE III	HSAN TYPE IV
Onset	Birth	Birth	Birth
Initial symptoms (from birth to age 3 yr)	Swallowing problems	Swallowing problems	Fevers
	Self-mutilation (65%) Delayed development	Aspiration pneumonia Breech presentation (37%) Hypothermia Delayed development	Self-mutilation (88%)
Unique features	No axon flare Lack of fungiform papilla Hearing loss (30%)	No axon flare Lack of fungiform papilla Alacrima	No axon flare Anhidrosis Consanguinity 50%
Sensory dysfunction			
Depressed deep tendon reflexes	Frequent (71%)	Almost consistent (99%)	Infrequent (9%)
Pain perception	Absent	Mild to moderate decrease	Absent
Temperature perception	Severe decrease	Mild to moderate decrease	Absent
Vibration sense	Normal	Normal	Normal to moderate decrease
Autonomic			
Gastroesophageal reflux	Frequent (71%)	Frequent (67%)	Uncommon (24%)
Postural hypotension	Uncommon (25%)	Almost consistent (99%)	Uncommon (29%)
Episodic hypertension	Rare	Frequent	Rare
Ectodermal features			
Dry skin	No	No	Consistent
Fractures	29%	40%	71%
Scoliosis	59%	85%	23%
Intelligence			
IQ <65	Common (38%)	Uncommon (10%)	Common (33%)
Hyperactivity	Common (41%)	Uncommon	Common (54%)

Frequency definitions: rare = <1%; infrequent = <10%; uncommon = <30%; common = 30-65%; frequent = >65%.
From Axelrod FB, Gold-von Simson G: Hereditary sensory and autonomic neuropathies: types II, III, and IV, Orphanet J Rare Dis 2:39, 2007, Table 2.

Table 615-3 | Autonomic Function Testing

Sympathetic and parasympathetic divisions of the autonomic nervous system are involved in all tests of autonomic function

CARDIAC PARASYMPATHETIC NERVOUS SYSTEM FUNCTION
Heart rate variability with deep respiration (respiratory sinus arrhythmia); time-domain and frequency-domain assessments
Heart rate response to Valsalva maneuver
Heart rate response to standing

SYMPATHETIC ADRENERGIC FUNCTION
Blood pressure response to upright posture (standing or tilt table)
Blood pressure response to Valsalva maneuver
Microneurography

SYMPATHETIC CHOLINERGIC FUNCTION
Thermoregulatory sweat testing
Quantitative sudomotor-axon reflex test
Sweat imprint methods
Sympathetic skin response

From Freeman R: Autonomic peripheral neuropathy, Lancet 365:1259–1270, 2005.

Table 615-4 | Management of Autonomic Neuropathies

PROBLEM	TREATMENT
Orthostatic hypotension	Volume and salt supplements Fluorohydrocortisone (mineralocorticoid) Midodrine (α agonist)
Gastroparesis	Prokinetic agents (metoclopramide, domperidone, erythromycin)
Hypomotility	Fiber, laxatives
Urinary dysfunction	Timed voiding; bladder catheterization
Hyperhidrosis	Anticholinergic agents (glycopyrrolate, propantheline) Intracutaneous botulism toxin

---

hereditary sensory-autonomic neuropathies (HSANs). Table 615-3 lists autonomic nervous system functional tests. The general treatment of acquired autonomic dysfunction includes treating the primary disorder (systemic lupus erythematosus, diabetes) and long-term management of specific organ system manifestations (Table 615-4). Acute fluctuations of autonomic symptoms may be seen in Guillain-Barré syndrome. Rapid fluctuations of hypertension or tachycardia changing to hypotension or bradycardia should be managed carefully and with very short-acting medications.

615.1 Familial Dysautonomia
Harvey B. Sarnat

Familial dysautonomia (Riley-Day syndrome) is an autosomal recessive disorder that is common in Eastern European Jews, among whom the incidence is 1 in 10,000-20,000, and the carrier state is estimated to be 1%. It is rare in other ethnic groups but is the most common HSAN. The defective gene is at the 9q31-q33 locus. The familial dysautonomia gene is identified as *IKBKAP* (IκB kinase–associated protein), with aberrant splicing and a truncated protein (see Table 615-2). This and other autonomic neuropathies are often regarded as **neurocristopathies** because the abnormal target tissues are largely derived from neural crest.

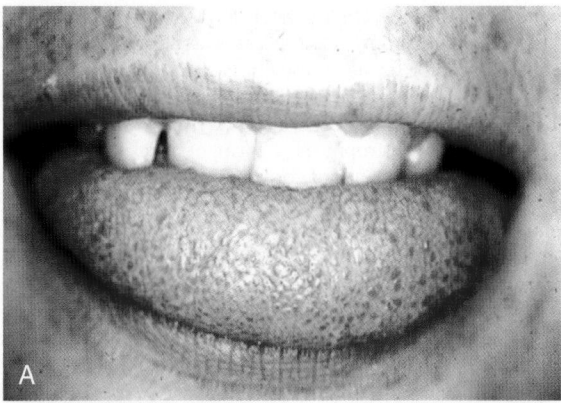

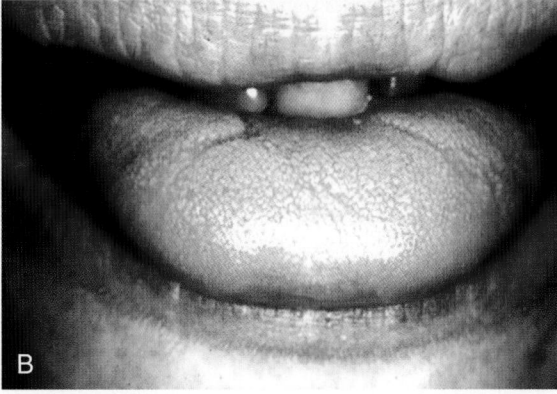

Figure 615-2 A, Normal tongue with fungiform papillae present on the tip. **B,** Dysautonomic tongue. Note the absence of the highly vascularized fungiform papillae from the tongue tip, which gives the appearance of a smooth tongue. *(From Axelrod FB, Gold-von Simson G: Hereditary sensory and autonomic neuropathies: types II, III, and IV, Orphanet J Rare Dis 2:39, 2007, Fig. 4.)*

PATHOLOGY

This disease of the peripheral nervous system is characterized pathologically by a reduced number of small unmyelinated nerve fibers that carry pain, temperature, and taste sensations and that mediate autonomic functions including baroreceptors. Large myelinated afferent nerve fibers that relay impulses from muscle spindles and Golgi tendon organs also are deficient. The degree of demonstrable anatomic change in peripheral and especially autonomic nerves is variable. Optic neuropathy with predominant loss of papillomacular nerve fibers may impair visual acuity. Fungiform papillae of the tongue (taste buds) are absent or reduced in number (Fig. 615-2). The number of parasympathetic ganglion cells in the myenteric plexuses is reduced. There is terminal vessel hyperperfusion in tissues, despite an overall hypoperfusion of organs and extremities.

CLINICAL MANIFESTATIONS

Clinical manifestations are highly variable between individuals. The disease is expressed in infancy by poor sucking and swallowing. Aspiration pneumonia can occur. Feeding difficulties with oral incoordination is a major symptom throughout childhood. Vomiting crises can occur, and indeed nausea, retching, and hyperemesis (dysautonomic crisis) are the most disabling symptoms in some children. Apart from dysphagia, esophageal dysmotility can contribute to these symptoms. Episodic somnolence can occur in infants, as does hypotonia. Excessive sweating and blotchy erythema of the skin are common, especially at mealtime or when the child is excited. Infants are vulnerable to heatstroke. Episodic hyperhidrosis is caused by chemical hypersensitivity of the remaining sudomotor axons rather than of the sweat gland secretory cells. Breathholding spells followed by syncope are common

in the 1st 5 yr of life. Episodic arterial hypertension and hypotension may be related to loss of baroreceptor modulation of muscle vasoconstrictor drive, and an acute fall in blood pressure manifests as orthostatic hypotension. Chronic and progressive renal disease may result from renal hypoperfusion. Responses to hypoxia are reduced.

As affected children become older, insensitivity to pain becomes evident and traumatic injuries are frequent. Pain and temperature sensation is reduced but is not as severe as in other HSANs (see Table 615-2). Corneal ulcerations are common partly as a result of decreased corneal reflexes and perhaps because of alacrima (absence of tears with emotional crying), which is a universal finding. Newly erupting teeth cause tongue ulcerations and, in older children, dental trauma and oral soft tissue mutilation may be prominent. Walking is delayed or clumsy or appears ataxic because of poor sensory feedback from muscle spindles. The ataxia is probably related more to deficient muscle spindle feedback and to vestibular nerve dysfunction than to cerebellar involvement, but defective ocular saccades also may indicate cerebellar dysfunction and cerebellar atrophy. Tendon stretch reflexes are absent. Scoliosis or kyphosis is a serious complication in the majority of patients and usually is progressive. Overflow tearing with crying does not normally develop until 2-3 mo of age but fails to develop after that time or is severely reduced or absent in children with familial dysautonomia. There is an increased incidence of urinary incontinence. Bradycardia and other cardiac arrhythmias can occur, and some patients require a cardiac pacemaker.

Approximately 40% of patients have generalized major motor seizures; some of these are associated with acute hypoxia during breathholding and some with extreme fevers, but most do not have an apparent precipitating event. Body temperature is poorly controlled; both hypothermia and extreme fevers occur. Impaired intellectual function is not secondary to epilepsy. Emotional lability and learning disabilities are common in school-age children with the disorder. Puberty is often delayed, especially in girls. Short stature can occur, but growth velocity can be accelerated by treatment with growth hormone. Speech is often slurred or nasal.

After 3 yr of age, autonomic crises begin, usually with attacks of cyclic vomiting lasting 24-72 hr or even several days. Retching and vomiting occur every 15-20 min and are associated with hypertension, profuse sweating, blotching of the skin, apprehension, and irritability. Prominent gastric distention can occur, causing abdominal pain and even respiratory distress. Hematemesis can complicate pernicious vomiting. Activation of dopamine receptors may explain the cyclic vomiting and retching.

Allgrove syndrome (triple A syndrome) is a clinical variant, involving early-onset alacrima, feeding difficulties and achalasia, autonomic dysfunction with orthostatic hypotension, altered heart rate variability, hyperreflexia, ataxia, muscle weakness, sensorimotor polyneuropathy, and adrenocorticotropic hormone–resistant adrenal insufficiency (develops in 1st decade). The gene *AAAS* (alacrima-achalasia-adrenal insufficiency neurologic disorder) is located on chromosome 12q13.

LABORATORY FINDINGS

Electrocardiography discloses prolonged corrected QT intervals with lack of appropriate shortening with exercise, a reflection of the aberration in autonomic regulation of cardiac conduction. Chest radiographs show atelectasis and pulmonary changes resembling cystic fibrosis. Urinary vanillylmandelic acid level is decreased, and the homovanillic acid level is increased. Plasma level of dopamine β-hydroxylase (the enzyme that converts dopamine to epinephrine) is diminished. Sural nerve biopsy shows a decreased number of unmyelinated fibers. Electroencephalography is useful for evaluating seizures.

DIAGNOSIS

Slow IV infusion of norepinephrine produces an exaggerated pressor response. The hypotensive response to infusion of methacholine is increased. Intradermal injection of 1:1,000 histamine phosphate fails to produce a normal axon flare, and local pain is absent or diminished.

Because the skin of a normal infant reacts more intensely to histamine, a 1 : 10,000 dilution should be used. Instillation of 2.5% methacholine into the conjunctival sac produces miosis in patients with familial dysautonomia and no detectable effect on a normal pupil; this is a nonspecific sign of parasympathetic denervation from any cause. Methacholine is applied to only 1 eye in this test, with the other eye serving as a control; the pupils are compared at 5 min intervals for 20 min. The combination of alacrima, absent fungiform papillae, decreased patellar reflexes, and an abnormal histamine test with Ashkenazi Jewish lineage is diagnostic. Because of variable expression and potential overlap with other HSANs, genetic testing should be used to confirm the diagnosis.

TREATMENT

Symptomatic treatment includes special attention to the respiratory and gastrointestinal systems to prevent aspiration and malnutrition, methylcellulose eyedrops or topical ocular lubricants to replace tears and prevent corneal ulceration, orthopedic management of scoliosis and joint problems, and appropriate anticonvulsants for epilepsy. Chlorpromazine is an effective antiemetic and may be given as rectal suppositories during autonomic crises; however, clonidine may be more effective. It also reduces apprehension and lowers the blood pressure. Diazepam has also been effective in some cases. Dehydration and electrolyte disturbances should be anticipated. A more specific and promising approach is the administration of carbidopa, an inhibitor of dopa-decarboxylase, particularly for the hyperemesis that is so prominent and disabling in many patients. Blockers of dopamine receptors are alternative drugs for cyclic vomiting. It is also useful for enuresis, another common complication, and augments tear production. Protection from injuries is important because of the lack of pain as a protective mechanism. Scoliosis often requires surgical treatment. Antiepileptic drugs may be required. A cardiac pacemaker may be required by some children. Blood pressure monitoring may be important in some cases. A promising genetic approach to treatment, which corrects the splicing defect, is the use of oral kinetin to regulate the expression of *IKBKAP* transcripts. Specific compounds identified from stem cells obtained from dysautonomia patients provide a potential therapy to rescue IKBKAP expression.

PROGNOSIS

Sixty percent of patients die in childhood before the age of 20 yr, usually of chronic pulmonary failure or aspiration. Treatment in a center familiar with the diverse complications greatly extends the life expectancy; some have survived to age 40 yr. Prevention of aspiration with fundoplication, gastrostomy, and tube feeding reduces the risk of aspiration. Newer measures to better control vasomotor stability and vomiting improve the quality of life, but whether they change longevity is not yet known.

Bibliography is available at Expert Consult.

615.2 Other Autonomic Neuropathies
Harvey B. Sarnat

CONGENITAL INSENSITIVITY TO PAIN AND ANHIDROSIS

Congenital insensitivity to pain and anhidrosis is an autosomal recessive disorder HSAN type IV (see Table 615-2). Onset is in infancy. Patients have episodes of extreme fevers related to warm environmental temperatures because they have absent or reduced sweating. Frequent burns and traumatic injuries result from apparent lack of pain perception. Poor healing of fractures occurs, as does osteomyelitis. Neonatal hypotonia improves with growth but learning problems may develop. Intelligence is normal. Nerve biopsy reveals an almost total absence of unmyelinated nerve fibers that convey impulses of pain, temperature, and autonomic functions. Some cases of hypomyelinating neuropathy manifest clinically as congenital insensitivity to pain (see

Chapter 613.3). The sympathetic skin response as an electrophysiologic study is a reliable diagnostic test in cases associated with a mutation in the TrKA receptor for nerve growth factor.

REFLEX SYMPATHETIC DYSTROPHY

Reflex sympathetic dystrophy is a form of local causalgia, usually involving a hand or foot but not corresponding to the anatomic distribution of a peripheral nerve (see Chapter 168.2). A continuous burning pain and hyperesthesia are associated with vasomotor instability in the affected zone, resulting in increased skin temperature, erythema, and edema caused by vasodilation and hyperhidrosis. In the chronic state, atrophy of skin appendages, cool and clammy skin, and disuse atrophy of underlying muscle and bone occur. More than 1 extremity is occasionally involved. The pain is disabling and is exacerbated by the movement of an associated joint, although no objective signs of arthritis are seen; immobilization provides some relief. The most common preceding event is local trauma in the form of a contusion, laceration, sprain, or fracture that occurred days or weeks earlier.

Several theories of pathogenesis have been proposed to explain this phenomenon. The most widely accepted is reflexive overactivity of autonomic nerves in response to injury, and regional sympathetic blockade often affords temporary relief. Physiotherapy also is helpful. Some cases resolve spontaneously after weeks or months, but others continue to be symptomatic and require sympathectomy. A psychogenic component is suspected in some cases but is difficult to prove.

Bibliography is available at Expert Consult.

Chapter 616
Guillain-Barré Syndrome
Harvey B. Sarnat

Guillain-Barré syndrome is an autoimmune disorder often considered a postinfectious polyneuropathy involving mainly motor but also sensory and sometimes autonomic nerves. This syndrome affects people of all ages and is not hereditary. Most patients in the United States and Europe have a demyelinating neuropathy, but primarily axonal degeneration is documented in some cases, mainly in China, Mexico, Bangladesh, and Japan.

CLINICAL MANIFESTATIONS

The paralysis usually follows a nonspecific gastrointestinal or respiratory infection by approximately 10 days. The original infection might have caused only gastrointestinal (especially *Campylobacter jejuni,* but also *Helicobacter pylori*) or respiratory tract (especially *Mycoplasma pneumoniae*) symptoms. Consumption of undercooked poultry, unpasteurized milk, and contaminated water are the main sources of gastrointestinal infections. West Nile virus also can mimic Guillain-Barré–like syndrome, but more often it causes motor neuron disease similar to poliomyelitis. Guillain-Barré syndrome is reported following administration of vaccines against rabies, influenza, and poliomyelitis (oral) and following administration of conjugated meningococcal vaccine, particularly serogroup C. Additional infectious precursors of Guillain-Barré syndrome include mononucleosis, Lyme disease, cytomegalovirus, and *Haemophilus influenzae* (for the Miller-Fisher syndrome).

Initial symptoms include numbness and paresthesia, followed by weakness. There may be associated neck, back, buttock, and leg pain. Weakness usually begins in the lower extremities and progressively involves the trunk, the upper limbs, and, finally, the bulbar muscles, a pattern known as **Landry ascending paralysis.** Proximal and distal muscles are involved relatively symmetrically, but asymmetry is found in 9% of patients. The onset is gradual and progresses over days or weeks; the process plateaus in 1-28 days. Particularly in cases with an abrupt onset, tenderness on palpation and pain in muscles are common in the initial stages. Affected children are irritable. Weakness can progress to inability or refusal to walk and later to flaccid tetraplegia. Maximal severity of weakness is usually reached by 4 wk after onset. The differential diagnosis of acute weakness is noted in Table 607-3 (in Chapter 607) and of Guillain-Barré syndrome in Table 616-1.

Bulbar involvement occurs in about half of cases. Respiratory insufficiency can result. Dysphagia and facial weakness are often impending signs of respiratory failure. They interfere with eating and increase the risk of aspiration. The facial nerves may be involved. Some young patients exhibit symptoms of viral meningitis or meningoencephalitis. Extraocular muscle involvement is rare, but in an uncommon variant, oculomotor and other cranial neuropathies are severe early in the course.

Miller-Fisher syndrome (MFS) consists of acute external and occasionally internal ophthalmoplegia, ataxia, and areflexia. The 6th cranial nerve is most often involved in MFS. Papilledema may precede or follow MFS and suggests a diagnosis of pseudotumor; optic neuritis may also be noted. Although areflexia is seen in MFS, patients do not have significant lower extremity weakness compared with Guillain-Barré syndrome. Distal paresthesias are noted in MFS. Urinary incontinence or retention of urine is a complication in approximately 20% of cases but is usually transient. MFS overlaps with Bickerstaff brainstem encephalitis, which also shares many features with Guillain-Barré syndrome with lower motor neuron involvement.

Tendon reflexes in Guillain-Barré syndrome are lost, usually early in the course, but are sometimes preserved until later; areflexia is common but hyporeflexia may be seen; 10% may have normal reflexes. This variability can cause confusion when attempting early diagnosis. The **autonomic nervous system** is also involved in some cases. Lability of blood pressure and cardiac rate, postural hypotension, episodes of profound bradycardia, or tachycardia and occasional asystole occur. Cardiovascular monitoring is important. A few patients require insertion of a temporary venous cardiac pacemaker.

Subtypes of Guillain-Barré syndrome include an acute inflammatory demyelinating polyneuropathy and an acute motor axonal neuropathy; these are distinguished by nerve conduction studies, geography, and the pattern of antiganglioside antibodies (Table 616-2). Localized forms also occur and include a pattern of facial diplegia with paresthesias and a pattern of pharyngeal-cervical-brachial weakness.

Chronic inflammatory demyelinating polyradiculoneuropathies (CIDPs, sometimes called *chronic inflammatory relapsing polyneuritis* or *chronic unremitting polyradiculoneuropathy*) are chronic varieties of Guillain-Barré syndrome that recur intermittently, or do not improve, or progress slowly and relentlessly for periods of months to years. Approximately 7% of children with Guillain-Barré syndrome suffer an acute relapse. Patients are usually severely weak and can have a flaccid tetraplegia with or without bulbar and respiratory muscle involvement. Hyporeflexia or areflexia is almost universal. Motor deficits occur in 94% of cases, sensory paresthesias in 64%, and cranial nerve involvement in less than a third of patients. Autonomic and micturitional involvement is variable. Cerebrospinal fluid (CSF) shows no pleocytosis and protein is variably normal or mildly elevated. Nerve conduction

Table 616-1	Differential Diagnosis of Childhood Guillain-Barré Syndrome

SPINAL CORD LESIONS
Acute transverse myelitis
Epidural abscess
Tumors
Poliomyelitis (natural or live virus)
Enteroviruses
Hopkins syndrome
Vascular malformations
Cord infarction
Fibrocartilaginous embolism
Cord compression from vertebral subluxation related to congenital abnormalities or trauma
Acute disseminated encephalomyelitis
Bickerstaff brainstem encephalitis for Miller-Fisher syndrome

PERIPHERAL NEUROPATHIES
Toxic
• Vincristine
• Glue sniffing
• Heavy metal: gold, arsenic, lead, thallium
• Organophosphate pesticides
• Fluoroquinolones
Infections
• HIV
• Diphtheria
• Lyme disease
Inborn errors of metabolism
• Leigh disease
• Tangier disease
• Porphyria
Critical illness: polyneuropathy/myopathy
Vasculitis syndromes
Porphyria
Mitochondrial neurogastrointestinal encephalomyopathy
CD59 deficiency

NEUROMUSCULAR JUNCTION DISORDERS
Tick paralysis
Myasthenia gravis
Botulism
Hypercalcemia
Myopathies
Periodic paralyses
Dermatomyositis
Critical illness myopathy/polyneuropathy

From Agrawal S, Peake D, Whitehouse WP: Management of children with Guillain Barré syndrome, Arch Dis Child Educ Pract Ed 92:161–168, 2007.

Table 616-2	Classification of Guillain-Barré Syndrome and Related Disorders and Typical Antiganglioside Antibodies By Pathology

DISORDER	ANTIBODIES
Acute inflammatory demyelinating polyradiculoneuropathy	Unknown
Acute motor and sensory axonal neuropathy	GM_1, GM_{1b}, GD_{1a}
Acute motor axonal neuropathy	GM_1, GM_{1b}, GD_{1a}, GalNac-GD_{1a}
Acute sensory neuronopathy	GD_{1b}
ACUTE PANDYSAUTONOMIA	
Regional Variants	
Fisher syndrome	GQ_{1b}, GT_{1a}
Oropharyngeal	GT_{1a}
Overlap	
Fisher/Guillain-Barré overlap syndrome	GQ_{1b}, GM_1, GM_{1b}, GD_{1a}, GalNac-GD_{1a}

From Hughes RAC: Treatment of Guillain-Barré syndrome with corticosteroids: lack of benefit? Lancet 363:181–182, 2004.

velocity studies and sural nerve biopsy are abnormal. Polymorphic nucleotide repeats in the *SH2D2A* gene are associated with a predisposition to CIDP.

Congenital Guillain-Barré syndrome is described rarely, manifesting as generalized hypotonia, weakness, and areflexia in an affected neonate, fulfilling all electrophysiologic and CSF criteria and in the absence of maternal neuromuscular disease. Treatment might not be required, and there is gradual improvement over the 1st few mo and no evidence of residual disease by 1 yr of age. In 1 case, the mother had ulcerative colitis treated with prednisone and mesalamine from the 7th mo of gestation until delivery at term.

LABORATORY FINDINGS AND DIAGNOSIS

CSF studies are essential for diagnosis. The CSF protein is elevated to more than twice the upper limit of normal, the glucose level is normal, and there is no pleocytosis. Fewer than 10 white blood cells/mm³ may be found. The results of bacterial cultures are negative, and viral cultures rarely isolate specific viruses. The dissociation between high CSF protein and a lack of cellular response in a patient with an acute or subacute polyneuropathy is diagnostic of Guillain-Barré syndrome. MRI of the spinal cord may be indicated to rule out disorders listed in

Table 616-1. MRI findings include thickening of the cauda equina and intrathecal nerve roots with gadolinium enhancement. These finds are fairly sensitive and are present in >90% of patients (Fig. 616-1). Imaging in CIDP is similar but demonstrates greater enhancement of spinal nerve roots (Fig. 616-2).

Motor nerve conduction velocities are greatly reduced, and sensory nerve conduction time is often slow. Electromyography shows evidence of acute denervation of muscle. *Serum creatine kinase level may be mildly elevated or normal.* Antiganglioside antibodies, mainly against GM_1 and GD_1, are sometimes elevated in the serum in Guillain-Barré syndrome, particularly in cases with primarily axonal rather than demyelinating neuropathy, and suggest that they might play a role in disease propagation and/or recovery in some cases (see Table 616-1). Muscle biopsy is not usually required for diagnosis; specimens appear normal in early stages and show evidence of denervation atrophy in chronic stages. Sural nerve biopsy tissue shows segmental demyelination, focal inflammation, and wallerian degeneration but also is usually not required for diagnosis.

Serologic testing for *Campylobacter* and *Helicobacter* infections helps establish the cause if results are positive but does not alter the course of treatment. Results of stool cultures are rarely positive because

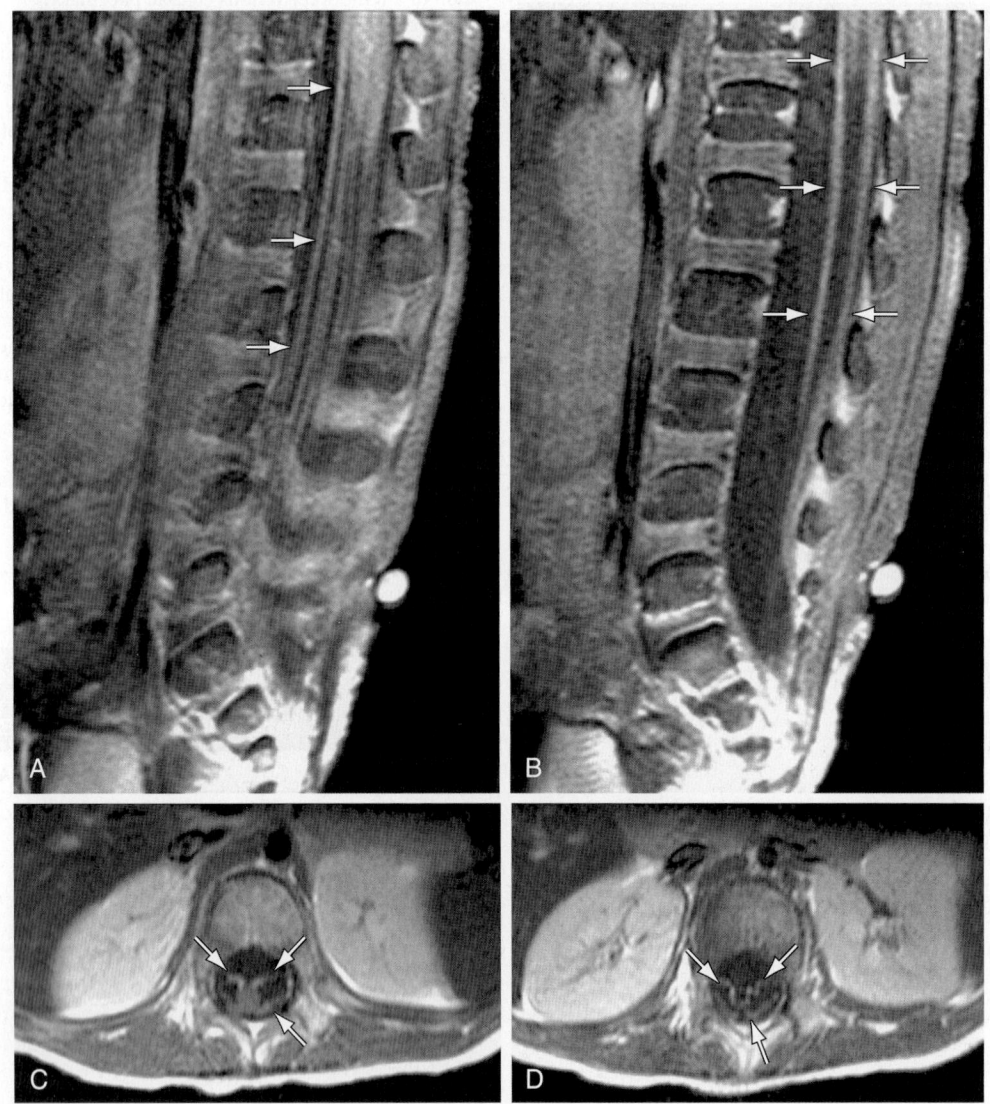

Figure 616-1 Guillain-Barré syndrome. Sagittal off-midline **(A)** and midline **(B)** postgadolinium T1-weighted fat-saturated images through the lumbar spine of a patient who could not ambulate. **C** and **D,** Axial postcontrast T1-weighted images through the conus medullaris and proximal lumbar nerve roots, respectively. The images show extensive contrast enhancement of nerve roots (*arrows* in **A-D**), in keeping with changes of Guillain-Barré. (*From Slovis TL, editor:* Caffey's pediatric diagnostic imaging, *ed 11, Philadelphia, 2008, Mosby, Fig. 65-6.*)

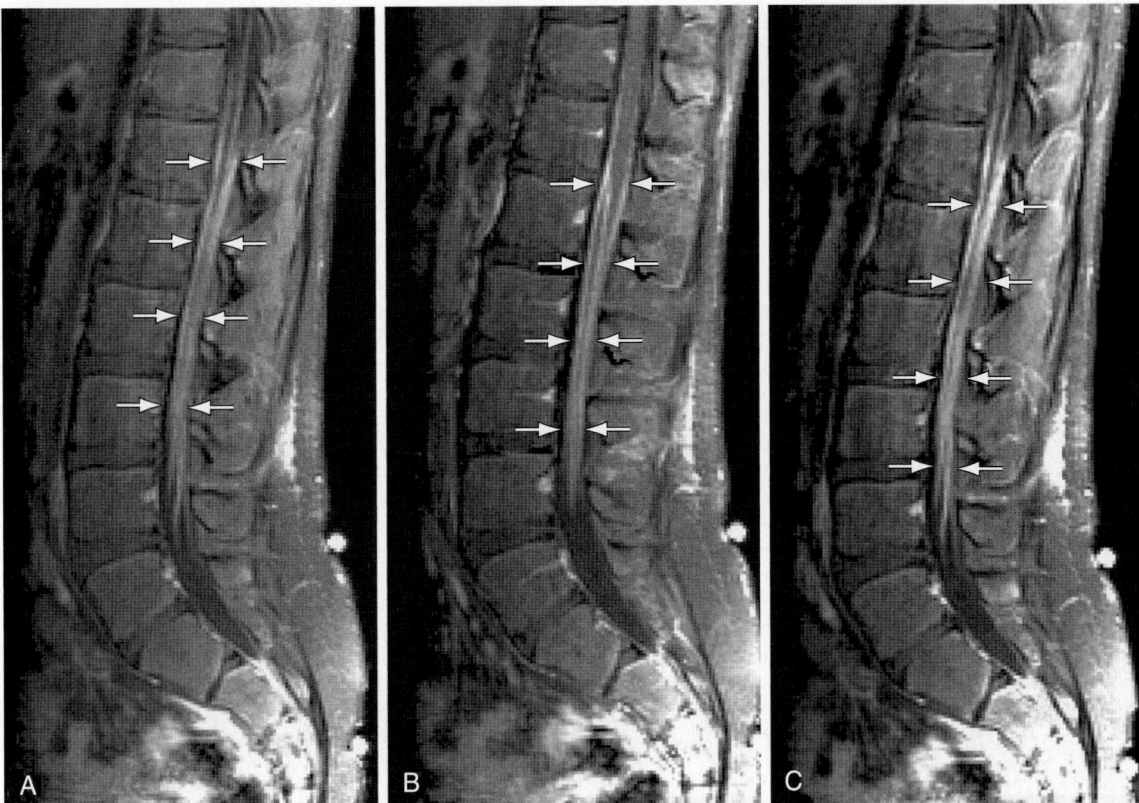

Figure 616-2 Chronic inflammatory demyelinating polyneuropathy (CIDP) in a 13 yr old boy with peripheral neuropathy and gait disturbance. Sagittal fat-saturated T1-weighted images off the midline to the right **(A)**, at the midline **(B)**, and off the midline to the left **(C)**. *(From Slovis TL, editor: Caffey's pediatric diagnostic imaging, ed 11, Philadelphia, 2008, Mosby, Fig. 65-7.)*

the infection is self-limited and only occurs for about 3 days, and the neuropathy follows the acute gastroenteritis.

TREATMENT

Patients in early stages of this acute disease should be admitted to the hospital for observation because the ascending paralysis can rapidly involve respiratory muscles during the next 24 hr. Respiratory effort (negative inspiratory force, spirometry) **must** be monitored to prevent respiratory failure and respiratory arrest. Patients with slow progression might simply be observed for stabilization and spontaneous remission without treatment. Rapidly progressive ascending paralysis is treated with intravenous immunoglobulin (IVIG), administered for 2, 3, or 5 days. A commonly recommended protocol is IVIG 0.4 g/kg/day for 5 consecutive days, but some studies suggest that larger doses are more effective (1 g/kg/day for 2 consecutive days) and related to improved outcome. Plasmapheresis and/or immunosuppressive drugs are alternatives if IVIG is ineffective. Steroids are not effective. Supportive care, such as respiratory support, prevention of decubiti in children with flaccid tetraplegia, nutritional support, pain management, prevention of deep vein thrombosis, and treatment of secondary bacterial infections, is important.

CIDPs, whether relapsing-remitting or unremitting, also are treated with oral or pulsed steroids and IVIG. Subcutaneous immunoglobulin infusion may be an alternative to the intravenous route. Plasma exchange, sometimes requiring as many as 10 exchanges daily, is an alternative. Remission in these cases may be sustained, but relapses can occur within days, weeks, or even after many months; relapses usually respond to another course of plasmapheresis. Steroid and immunosuppressive drugs are another alternative, but their effectiveness is less predictable. High-dose pulsed methylprednisolone given intravenously is successful in some cases. The prognosis in chronic forms of the Guillain-Barré syndrome is more guarded than in the acute form, and many patients are left with major residual handicaps.

Even if *C. jejuni* infection is documented by stool culture or serologic tests, treatment of the infection is not necessary because it is self-limited, and the use of antibiotics does not alter the course of the polyneuropathy.

For the treatment of chronic neuropathic pain following Guillain-Barré syndrome, gabapentin is more effective than carbamazepine, and the requirement for fentanyl is reduced. But no pharmacologic treatments for neuropathic pain in this disease are wholly effective.

PROGNOSIS

The clinical course is usually benign, and spontaneous recovery begins within 2-3 wk. Most patients regain full muscular strength, although some are left with residual weakness. The tendon reflexes are usually the last function to recover. Improvement usually follows a gradient opposite the direction of involvement: bulbar function recovering first, and lower extremity weakness resolving last. Bulbar and respiratory muscle involvement can lead to death if the syndrome is not recognized and treated. Although prognosis is generally good and the majority of children recover completely, 3 clinical features are predictive of poor outcome with sequelae: cranial nerve involvement, intubation, and maximum disability at the time of presentation. The electrophysiologic features of conduction block are predictive of good outcome. Long-term follow-up studies of patients who recover from an attack of Guillain-Barré syndrome reveal that many do have some permanent axonal loss, with or without residual clinical signs of chronic neuropathy. Easy fatigue is one of the most common chronic symptoms, but it is not the rapid fatigability of muscles seen in myasthenia gravis. Most patients with the axonal form of Guillain-Barré syndrome had a slow recovery over the 1st 6 mo and could eventually walk, although some required years to recover. Electromyography and nerve conduction velocity electrophysiologic studies do not necessarily predict the long-term outcome.

Bibliography is available at Expert Consult.

Chapter 617
Bell Palsy
Harvey B. Sarnat

Bell palsy is an acute unilateral peripheral facial nerve palsy that is not associated with other cranial neuropathies or brainstem dysfunction. It is a common disorder at all ages from infancy through adolescence and usually develops abruptly about 2 wk after a systemic viral infection. The preceding infection is caused by the herpes simplex virus, varicella-zoster virus, Epstein-Barr virus, Lyme disease, mumps virus, *Toxocara, Rickettsia, Mycoplasma,* or HIV infection (Table 617-1). Ramsay Hunt syndrome (herpes zoster oticus) is associated with vesicles in the external auditory canal or auricle and an ipsilateral facial palsy. Active or reactivation of herpes simplex or varicella-zoster virus may be the most common cause of Bell palsy (Fig. 617-1). The disease is occasionally a postinfectious allergic or immune demyelinating facial neuritis. It also may be a focal toxic or inflammatory neuropathy and has been associated with ribavirin and interferon-α therapy for hepatitis C. Hereditary forms are rare, but it may be associated with other genetic polyneuropathies. Rarely, Bell palsy occurs in the context of hypertension or juvenile type 1 diabetes mellitus, most often associated with concomitant viral infections.

Table 617-1	**Etiologies of Acute Peripheral Facial Palsy**

COMMON
Idiopathic
Herpes simplex virus type 1*
Varicella-zoster virus*
 	
LESS-COMMON INFECTIONS
Otitis media ± cholesteatoma
Lyme disease
Epstein-Barr virus
Cytomegalovirus
Mumps
Human herpesvirus 6
Intranasal influenza vaccine
Mycoplasma
Toxocara
Rickettsia
AIDS/HIV
	OTHER LESS-COMMON CONDITIONS
	Trauma
	Schwannoma of facial nerve
	Infiltrative tumor
	Aneurysm or vascular
	  malformation
	Anomalous narrowing of facial
	  canal
	Hypertension
	Sjögren syndrome
	Diabetes mellitus, type 1
	Guillain-Barré syndrome
	Sarcoidosis
	Melkersson-Rosenthal syndrome†
	Ribavirin
	Interferon

*Implicated in idiopathic Bell palsy.
†Noncaseating granulomas with facial (lips, eyelids) edema, recurrent alternating facial paralysis, family history, migraines, or headaches.

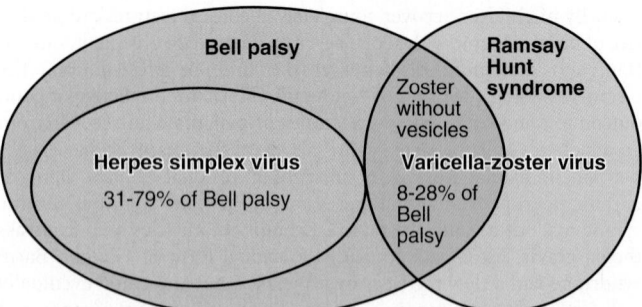

Figure 617-1 Involvement of herpes simplex and varicella-zoster viruses in acute facial palsy. *(Modified from Hato N, Murakami S, Gyo K: Steroid and antiviral treatment for Bell's palsy, Lancet 371:1818–1820, 2008.)*

CLINICAL MANIFESTATIONS
The upper and lower portions of the face are paretic, and the corner of the mouth droops. Patients are unable to close the eye on the involved side and can develop an exposure keratitis at night. Taste on the anterior two thirds of the tongue is lost on the involved side in approximately 50% of cases; this finding helps to establish the anatomic limits of the lesion as being proximal or distal to the chorda tympani branch of the facial nerve. Numbness and paresthesias do not usually occur, but ipsilateral numbness of the face is reported in a few cases and probably is caused by viral (especially herpes) or postviral immunologic impairment of the trigeminal and the facial nerves. Pain behind the ear may precede weakness. Acute hearing loss may occur in Bell palsy associated with *Rickettsia* infection. Several grading systems have been devised for Bell palsy, including the Sunnybrook, House-Brackmann, and Yanagihara systems.

IMAGING THE FACIAL NERVE AND ITS BONY CANAL
Modern high-resolution MRI, particularly with multiplanar reconstruction, is able to visualize the facial nerve within its canal and determine whether there are bony anomalies, compressive aneurysms, vascular malformations, or nerve sheath or infiltrative tumors that might explain a palsy anatomically. The two sides can be compared and, in particular, the labyrinthine segment within the petrous bone, which is the narrowest site in the facial nerve canal, can be examined. Ultrasound of the facial nerve also has been used, in part as a predictor of functional outcome in Bell palsy. More recently, diffusion tensor tractography enables a tridimensional display of facial nerve axons.

TREATMENT
Oral prednisone (1 mg/kg/day for 1 wk, followed by a 1 wk taper) started within the 1st 3-5 days results in improved outcome and is a traditional treatment, its efficacy confirmed in a recent long-term prospective study in the United Kingdom. Because of the recovery of herpes simplex virus in the neural fluid of the 7th nerve, some also recommend adding oral acyclovir or valacyclovir to the prednisone therapy. Alone, antiviral agents are not effective in reducing adverse sequelae (synkinesis, autonomic dysfunction), but added to prednisone may be associated with an additional small benefit. If a specific infection can be identified as a predisposing cause, specific antiviral or antibacterial treatment is more justified. Surgical decompression of the facial canal, theoretically to provide more space for the swollen facial nerve, is not of value unless imaging provides evidence of nerve compression or an anatomic lesion. Both high- and low-level laser therapy has been used with good results in some cases as a form of physiotherapy. Traditional physiotherapy to the facial muscles is recommended in some chronic cases with poor recovery, but the efficacy of this treatment is uncertain. Protection of the cornea with methylcellulose eyedrops or an ocular lubricant is especially important at night. Botulinum toxin has been applied in adults to the contralateral normal facial muscles for cosmetic purposes to minimize the apparent asymmetry or to treat chronic unilateral ptosis, but this has little application in pediatric patients.

PROGNOSIS
The prognosis for functional recovery is excellent. More than 85% of patients recover spontaneously with no residual facial weakness. Another 10% have mild facial weakness as a sequela, often perceived only as a mild facial asymmetry, and only 5% are left with permanent severe facial weakness. In patients who do not recover within a few weeks (chronic), electrophysiologic examination of the facial nerve helps to determine the degree of neuropathy and regeneration. In chronic cases, other causes of facial neuropathy should be considered, including facial nerve tumors such as schwannomas and neurofibromas, infiltration of the facial nerve by leukemic cells or by a rhabdomyosarcoma of the middle ear, brainstem infarcts or tumors, and traumatic injury of the facial nerve.

Nerve regrowth may be misdirected and result in **synkinesis**, where activation of one muscle group may produce activation of another inappropriate muscle group; blinking may result in mouth twitching, smiling may cause eye blinking, and lacrimation (crocodile tears) may occur while eating.

FACIAL PALSY AT BIRTH
Facial palsy at birth is usually a compression neuropathy from forceps application during delivery and recovers spontaneously in a few days or weeks in most cases. **Congenital absence of the depressor angularis oris muscle** causes facial asymmetry, especially when an affected infant cries, and is often associated with other congenital anomalies, especially of the heart. It is not a facial nerve lesion but is a cosmetic defect that does not interfere with feeding. Infants with **Möbius syndrome** can have bilateral or, less commonly, unilateral facial palsy; this syndrome is usually caused by symmetric calcified infarcts in the tegmentum of the pons and medulla oblongata during midgestation or late fetal life, although it rarely is a developmental anomaly of the brainstem.

Bibliography is available at Expert Consult.

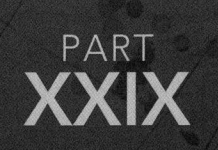

Chapter 618

Growth and Development

*Scott E. Olitsky, Denise Hug,
Laura S. Plummer, Erin D. Stahl,
Michelle M. Ariss, and
Timothy P. Lindquist*

The eye of a normal full-term infant at birth is approximately 65% of adult size. Postnatal growth is maximal during the 1st yr, proceeds at a rapid, but decelerating rate until the 3rd yr, and continues at a slower rate thereafter until puberty, after which little change occurs. The anterior structures of the eye are relatively large at birth but thereafter grow proportionately less than the posterior structures. This results in a progressive change in the shape of the globe such that it becomes more spherical.

In an infant, the sclera is thin and translucent, with a bluish tinge. The cornea is relatively large in newborns (averaging 10 mm) and attains adult size (nearly 12 mm) by the age of 2 yr or earlier. Its curvature tends to flatten with age, resulting in a progressive change in the refractive properties of the eye. A normal cornea is perfectly clear. In infants born prematurely, however, the cornea may have a transient opalescent haze. The anterior chamber in a newborn appears shallow, and the angle structures, important in the maintenance of normal intraocular pressure, must undergo further differentiation after birth. The iris, typically light blue or gray at birth in white individuals, undergoes progressive change of color as the pigmentation of the stroma increases in the 1st 6 mo of life. The pupils of a newborn infant tend to be small and are often difficult to dilate. This is the result of an immature iris dilator muscle. Remnants of the **pupillary membrane** (anterior vascular capsule) are often evident on ophthalmoscopic examination, appearing as cobweb-like lines crossing the pupillary aperture, especially in preterm infants.

The lens of a newborn infant is more spherical than that of an adult; its greater refractive power helps to compensate for the relative shortness of the young eye. The lens continues to grow throughout life; new fibers added to the periphery continually push older fibers toward the center of the lens. With age, the lens becomes progressively denser and more resistant to change of shape during accommodation.

The fundus of a newborn's eye is less pigmented than that of an adult; the choroidal vascular pattern is highly visible, and the retinal pigment pattern often has a fine peppery or mottled appearance. In some darkly pigmented infants, the fundus has a gray or opalescent sheen. In a newborn, the macular landmarks, particularly the foveal light reflex, are less-well defined and may not be readily apparent. The peripheral retina appears pale or grayish, and the peripheral retinal vasculature is immature, especially in premature infants. The optic nerve head color varies from pink to slightly pale, sometimes grayish. Within 4-6 mo, the appearance of the fundus approximates that of the mature eye.

Superficial retinal hemorrhages may be observed in many newborn infants. These are usually absorbed promptly and rarely leave any permanent effect. The majority of birth-related **retinal hemorrhages** resolve within 2 wk, with complete resolution of all such hemorrhages within 4-6 wk of birth. Conjunctival hemorrhages also may occur at birth and are resorbed spontaneously without consequence.

Remnants of the **primitive hyaloid vascular** system may also be seen as small tufts or wormlike structures projecting from the disc (Bergmeister papilla) or as a fine strand traversing the vitreous; in some cases, only a small dot (Mittendorf dot) remains on the posterior aspect of the lens capsule.

An infant's eye is somewhat hyperopic **(farsighted)**. The general trend is for hyperopia to increase from birth until age 7 yr. Thereafter, the level of hyperopia tends to decrease rapidly until age 14 yr. Elimination of the hyperopic state may occur during this time. If the process continues, myopia (nearsightedness) develops. A slower continuation of the decrease in hyperopia, or increase in myopia, continues into the 3rd decade of life. The refractive state at any time in life depends on the net effect of many factors: the size of the eye, the state of the lens, and the curvature of the cornea.

Newborn infants tend to keep their eyes closed much of the time, but normal newborns can see, respond to changes in illumination, and fixate points of contrast. The visual acuity in newborns is estimated to be approximately 20/400. This poor vision is a result of the immature, multilayered foveal anatomy. Retinal development continues postnatally, maturing completely during the 1st few yr of life. One of the earliest responses to a formed visual stimulus is an infant's regard for the mother's face, evident especially during feeding. By 2 wk of age, an infant shows more sustained interest in large objects, and by 8-10 wk of age, a normal infant can follow an object through an arc of 180 degrees. The acuity improves rapidly and may reach 20/30-20/20 by the age of 2-3 yr.

Many normal infants may have imperfect coordination of the eye movements and alignment during the early days and weeks, but proper coordination should be achieved by 3-6 mo, usually sooner. Persistent deviation of an eye in an infant at 6 mo of age requires evaluation.

Tears often are not present with crying until after 1-3 mo. Preterm infants have reduced reflex and basal tear secretion, which may allow topically applied medications to become concentrated and lead to rapid drying of their corneas.

Bibliography is available at Expert Consult.

Chapter 619

Examination of the Eye

*Scott E. Olitsky, Denise Hug,
Laura S. Plummer, Erin D. Stahl,
Michelle M. Ariss, and
Timothy P. Lindquist*

The eye exam is a routine part of the pediatric wellness evaluation, which begins in the newborn period. The primary care physician plays a critical role in the detection of both obvious and insidious, asymptomatic eye diseases. School and community screening programs can also be effective in identifying problems at an early age. The American Academy of Ophthalmology recommends preschool vision screening as a means of reducing preventable visual loss (Table 619-1). The screening process begins with the pediatrician during well child visits. Referrals to an ophthalmologist should be made when a significant ocular abnormality or visual acuity deficit is suspected. An

Table 619-1	Vision Screening Guidelines		
FUNCTION	**RECOMMENDED TESTS**	**REFERRAL CRITERIA**	**COMMENTS**
AGES 3-5 YR			
Distance visual acuity	Snellen letters Snellen numbers Tumbling E test HOTV test	<4 of 6 correct on 20-ft line with either eye tested at 10 ft monocularly (i.e., <10/20 or 20/40), or Two-line difference between eyes, even within the passing range (i.e., 10/12.5 and 10/20 or 20/25 and 20/40)	Tests are listed in decreasing order of cognitive difficulty; the highest test that the child is capable of performing should be used; in general, the tumbling E or the HOTV test should be used for ages 3-5 yr and Snellen letters or numbers for ages 6 yr and older.
	Picture tests		Testing distance of 3 m (10 ft) is recommended for all visual acuity tests.
	-Allen figures -Lea symbols		A line of figures is preferred over a single figure. The nontested eye should be covered by an occluder held by the examiner or by an adhesive occluder patch applied to eye; the examiner must ensure that it is not possible to peek with the nontested eye.
Ocular alignment	Cross cover test at 3 m (10 ft) or Random dot E stereo test at 40 cm (630 sec of arc)	Any eye movement <4 of 6 correct	
	Simultaneous red reflex test (Bruckner test)	Any asymmetry of pupil color, size, brightness	Direct ophthalmoscope used to view both red reflexes simultaneously in a darkened room from 2-3 ft away; detects asymmetric refractive errors as well.
Ocular media clarity (cataracts, tumors, etc.)	Red reflex	White pupil, dark spots, absent reflex	Direct ophthalmoscope, darkened room. View eyes separately at 12-18 inches; white reflex indicates possible retinoblastoma.
AGES 6 YR AND OLDER			
Distance visual acuity	Snellen letters Snellen numbers Tumbling E test HOTV test	<4 of 6 correct on 4.5 m (15 ft) line with either eye tested at 3 m (10 ft) monocularly (i.e., <10/15 or 20/30)	Tests are listed in decreasing order of cognitive difficulty; the highest test that the child is capable of performing should be used; in general, the tumbling E or the HOTV test should be used for ages 3-5 yr and Snellen letters or numbers for ages 6 yr and older.
	Picture tests	Two-line difference between eyes, even within the passing range (i.e., 10/10 and 10/15 or 20/20 and 20/30)	Testing distance of 3 m (10 ft) is recommended for all visual acuity tests.
	-Allen figures -Lea symbols		A line of figures is preferred over a single figure. The nontested eye should be covered by an occluder held by the examiner or by an adhesive occluder patch applied to the eye; the examiner must ensure that it is not possible to peek with the nontested eye.
Ocular alignment	Cross cover test at 3 m (10 ft) or Random dot E stereo test at 40 cm (630 sec of arc)	Any eye movement <4 of 6 correct	

ophthalmologist should also examine high-risk children, such as those with a family history of eye disease, or various systemic or genetic disorders, such as Down syndrome.

The basic eye exam, whether performed by a pediatrician or an ophthalmologist, must include: visual acuity and visual field testing, assessment of pupils, ocular motility and alignment, a general external/facial examination, and finally, examination of the media and fundus via ophthalmoscopy. When indicated, biomicroscopy (slit-lamp examination), cycloplegic refraction, and tonometry are performed by an ophthalmologist. Special diagnostic procedures, such as ultrasound, fluorescein angiography, electroretinography, or visual evoked response testing, are also indicated for specific conditions.

VISUAL ACUITY

There are various means of assessing visual acuity in the pediatric population. A child's age and ability to cooperate, as well as clinician preference, all factor in deciding which test to use. The most common visual acuity test in infants is an assessment of their ability to fixate and follow a target. If appropriate targets are used, this response can be demonstrated by approximately 6 wk of age.

The test begins by seating the child comfortably in the caretaker's lap. The object of visual interest, usually a bright-colored toy, or target with lights, is slowly moved to the right and to the left. The examiner observes whether the infant's eyes turn toward the object and follow its movements. The examiner can use a thumb or palm of the hand to occlude one of the infant's eyes, in order to test each eye separately. Although a sound-producing object might compromise the purity of the visual stimulus, in practice, toys that squeak or rattle heighten an infant's awareness and interest in the test.

The human face is a better target than test objects. The examiner can exploit this by moving his or her face slowly in front of the infant's face. If the appropriate following movements are not elicited, the test should be repeated with the caretaker's face as the test stimulus. It should be remembered that even children with poor vision can follow a large object without apparent difficulty, especially if only 1 eye is affected.

An objective measurement of visual acuity is usually possible when children reach the age of 2.5-3 yr. Children this age are tested using a schematic picture or other illiterate eye chart. Examples include Allen or Lea symbols and tumbling E. Each eye should be tested separately. It is essential to prevent peeking. The examiner should hold the occluder in place and observe the child throughout the test. The child should be reassured and encouraged throughout the test as many children are intimidated by the process and fear a "bad grade" or punishment for errors.

The tumbling **E test,** in which the child indicates which direction the E is facing, is the most widely used visual acuity test for preschool children. Right–left presentations are more confusing than up–down presentations. With pretest practice, the test can be performed by most children ages 3-4 yr.

An adult-type **Snellen acuity chart** can be used at 5-6 yr of age if the child knows letters. A visual acuity of 20/40 is generally accepted as normal for 3 yr old children. At 4 yr of age, 20/30 is acceptable. By 5 or 6 yr of age, most children attain 20/20 vision.

Optokinetic nystagmus (the response to a sequence of moving targets; "railroad" nystagmus) can also be used to assess vision; this can be calibrated by targets of various sizes (stripes or dots) or by a rotating drum (known as an OKN drum) at specified distances.

The visual evoked response, an electrophysiologic method of evaluating the response to light and special visual stimuli, such as calibrated stripes or a checkerboard pattern, can also be used to study visual function in selected cases.

Preferential looking tests are used for evaluating vision in infants and children who cannot respond verbally to standard acuity tests. This is a behavioral technique based on the observation that, given a choice, an infant prefers to look at patterned rather than unpatterned stimuli. Because these tests require the presence of a skilled examiner, their use is often limited to research protocols involving preverbal children.

VISUAL FIELD ASSESSMENT

Like visual acuity testing, visual field assessment must be geared to a child's age and abilities. Formal visual field examination (perimetry and scotometry) can often be accomplished in school-age children. In younger children and in the pediatrician's office, the examiner must often rely on confrontation techniques and finger counting in quadrants of the visual field. In many such children, only testing by attraction can be accomplished; the examiner observes a child's response to familiar objects brought into each of the 4 quadrants of the visual field of each eye in turn. The child's bottle, a favorite toy, and lollipops are particularly effective attention-getting items. These gross methods can often detect diagnostically significant field changes such as the bitemporal hemianopia of a chiasmal lesion or the homonymous hemianopia of a cerebral lesion.

COLOR VISION TESTING

Color vision testing can be accomplished when a child is able to name or trace the test symbols, which include numbers, shapes, or other symbols. The common color vision testing tools include Ishihara color plates or Hardy Rand Littler. Color vision testing is not frequently necessary in young children; however, parents may request testing, particularly if their child seems to be slow in learning colors or if there is a family history of color vision deficiency. It is important to keep in mind, and reassure parents that "color-deficient" children do not misname colors, and that true "color blindness" is very rare and not compatible with normal vision. Defective color vision is common in

male patients but rare in females, as the gene is transmitted in an X-linked manner. Achromatopsia, which may be encountered occasionally, is a condition of complete color blindness associated with subnormal visual acuity, nystagmus, and photophobia.

Color discrimination is a means of assessing the intensity of a hue, typically red. Patients describe the intensity of red depicted from the test object. A change in color discrimination (often referred to as color "desaturation") can be a sign of optic nerve or retinal disease.

PUPILLARY EXAMINATION

The pupil exam includes evaluations of both the direct and consensual responses to light, accommodation (a near target), and reduced illumination, noting the size and symmetry of the pupils under each testing condition. Special care must be taken to differentiate the reaction to light from the reaction to near gaze. A child's natural tendency is to look directly at the approaching light, inducing the near gaze reflex when one is attempting to test only the reaction to light; accordingly, every effort must be made to control fixation on a distance target. The swinging flashlight test is especially useful for detecting unilateral or asymmetric prechiasmatic afferent defects in children (see "Marcus Gunn Pupil" section in Chapter 622).

OCULAR MOTILITY

Ocular motility testing assesses alignment and extraocular muscle function. This is tested by having a child follow an object in various positions of gaze, known as the cardinal positions. The cardinal positions are those in which one extraocular muscle predominantly functions and a deficit can be identified if present. Movements of each eye individually (ductions) and of the 2 eyes together (versions, conjugate movements, and convergence) are assessed.

Alignment can be assessed in 2 ways. The first is symmetry of the corneal light reflexes. The second method is to occlude each eye in an alternating fashion and observe for a change in fixation of the viewing eye (see discussion on cover testing for strabismus in Chapter 623).

BINOCULAR VISION

Attaining binocular visual function is one of the primary goals of amblyopia therapy and ocular realignment surgery. Just as there are multiple methods for assessing visual acuity, there are various means of testing the level of binocular vision. The Titmus test is probably the most frequently used test; a series of three-dimensional images are shown to the child while he or she wears a set of polarized glasses. The level of difficulty with which these images can be detected correlates with the degree of binocular vision present.

EXTERNAL EXAMINATION

The external examination begins with general inspection, in good illumination of the face, paying close attention to the orbits and lids, noting the size, shape, and symmetry of the orbits; position and movement of the lids; and position and symmetry of the globes. Viewing the eyes and lids in such a manner aids in detecting orbital asymmetry, lid masses, proptosis **(exophthalmos),** and abnormal pulsations. Palpation is also important in detecting orbital and lid masses. Orbital dermoids and capillary hemangiomas are frequently evaluated during the external examination.

The lacrimal system is assessed by looking for evidence of tear deficiency, overflow of tears **(epiphora),** erythema, and swelling in the region of the tear sac or gland. The lacrimal gland is located in the superotemporal orbit, beneath the eyebrow. The tear drain system, which includes the lacrimal sac, is located within the medial wall of the orbit, where the eyelids meet the bridge of the nose. The sac is massaged to check for reflux when obstruction is suspected. The presence and position of the puncta are also checked.

The lids and conjunctivae are specifically examined for focal lesions, foreign bodies, and inflammatory signs; loss and misdirection of lashes should also be noted. When necessary, the lids can be everted in the following manner: (1) instruct the patient to look down; (2) grasp the lashes of the patient's upper lid between the thumb and index finger of 1 hand; (3) place a probe, a cotton-tipped applicator, or the thumb of the other hand at the upper margin of the tarsal plate; and (4) pull the lid down and outward and evert it over the probe, using the instrument as a fulcrum. Foreign bodies commonly lodge in the concavity just above the lid margin and are exposed only by fully everting the lid.

The anterior segment of the eye is then evaluated with oblique focal illumination, noting the luster and clarity of the cornea, the depth and clarity of the anterior chamber, and the features of the iris. Transillumination of the anterior segment aids in detecting opacities and in demonstrating atrophy or hypopigmentation of the iris; these latter signs are important when ocular albinism is suspected. When necessary, fluorescein dye can be used to aid in diagnosing abrasions, ulcerations, and foreign bodies.

BIOMICROSCOPY (SLIT-LAMP EXAMINATION)
The slit-lamp exam provides a highly magnified view of the various structures of the eye and an optical section through the media of the eye—the cornea, aqueous humor, lens, and vitreous. Lesions can be identified and localized according to their depth within the eye; the resolution is sufficient to detect individual inflammatory cells in the aqueous and anterior vitreous. With the addition of special lenses and prisms, the angle of the anterior chamber and components of the fundus also can be examined with a slit lamp. Biomicroscopy is often crucial in trauma and in examining for iritis. It is also helpful in diagnosing many metabolic and genetic diseases of childhood.

FUNDUS EXAMINATION (OPHTHALMOSCOPY)
The ideal setting for ophthalmoscopy is with a well-dilated pupil, unless there are neurologic or other contraindications. Tropicamide (Mydriacyl) 0.5-1% and phenylephrine (Neo-Synephrine) 2.5% are recommended as mydriatics of short duration. These are safe for most children, but the possibility of adverse systemic effects must be recognized. For very small infants, especially 6 mo or younger, more dilute preparations may be advisable. Beginning with posterior landmarks, the disc and the macula, the 4 quadrants are systematically examined by following each of the major vessel groups to the periphery. Retinal hemorrhages, vascular anomalies, and posterior uveitis are often appreciated during this segment of the examination. Color, cup, and contour of the optic nerve should be noted as well. Abnormalities are frequently followed with further imaging studies such as a CT or MRI or diagnostic testing such as automated perimetry (see "Visual Field Assessment" above). The midperipheral retina can be seen if a child is directed to look up and down and to the right and left. Even with care, only a limited fraction of the fundus can be seen with a direct or handheld ophthalmoscope. For examination of the far periphery, an indirect ophthalmoscope is used, and full dilation of the pupil is essential.

REFRACTION
Refraction determines the focusing power of the eye: the degree of nearsightedness (hypermetropia), farsightedness (myopia), or astigmatism. Retinoscopy provides an objective determination of the amount of correction needed and can be performed at any age, including the newborn period. In young children, it is best done with cycloplegia using cyclopentolate 1% eyedrops in an ophthalmologist's office. Subjective refinement of refraction involves asking patients for preferences in the strength and axis of corrective lenses; it can be accomplished in many school-age children. Refraction and determination of visual acuity with appropriate corrective lenses in place are essential steps in deciding whether a patient has a visual defect or amblyopia. Photoscreening cameras aid ancillary medical personnel in screening for refractive errors in preverbal children. The accuracy and practical usefulness of these devices are still being investigated.

TONOMETRY
Tonometry is the method of assessing intraocular pressure. It may be performed with a portable, stand-alone instrument or by the applanation method during slit-lamp examination. Alternative methods are pneumatic, electronic, or rebound tonometry. When accurate measurement of the pressure is necessary in a child who cannot cooperate, it may be performed with sedation or general anesthesia. A gross estimate of pressure can be made by palpating the globe with the index fingers placed side by side on the upper lid above the tarsal plate.

Bibliography is available at Expert Consult.

Chapter **620**
Abnormalities of Refraction and Accommodation

Scott E. Olitsky, Denise Hug, Laura S. Plummer, Erin D. Stahl, Michelle M. Ariss, and Timothy P. Lindquist

Emmetropia is the state in which parallel rays of light come to focus on the retina with the eye at rest (nonaccommodating). Even though such an ideal optical state is common, the opposite condition, ametropia, often occurs. Three principal types of **ametropia** exist: **hyperopia** (farsightedness), **myopia** (nearsightedness), and **astigmatism** (Fig. 620-1). The majority of children are physiologically hyperopic at birth. Yet a significant number, especially those born prematurely, are myopic and often have some degree of astigmatism. With growth the refractive state tends to change and should be evaluated periodically.

Measurement of the refractive state of the eye (refraction) can be accomplished both objectively and subjectively. The objective method involves directing a beam of light from a retinoscope onto a patient's retina. Using loose lenses of various strengths held in front of the eye, the retinal light reflex (viewed through the pupil) can be neutralized, yielding a precise refraction. An objective refraction is obtainable at any age because it requires no response from the patient. In infants and children, it is generally more accurate to perform a refraction after instillation of eyedrops that produce mydriasis (dilation of the pupil) and cycloplegia (paralysis of accommodation); those used most commonly are tropicamide (Mydriacyl), cyclopentolate (Cyclogyl), and atropine sulfate. A subjective refraction involves placing lenses in front of the eye and having the patient report which lenses provide the clearest image of the letters on a chart. This method is dependent on a patient's ability to discriminate and communicate, but can be used for some children and can be helpful in determining the best refractive correction for children who are developmentally capable.

HYPEROPIA
If parallel rays of light come to focus posterior to the retina with the eye in a neutral state, hyperopia or farsightedness exists. This may result from a shorter anteroposterior diameter of the eye or a lower refractive power of the cornea or lens.

In hyperopia, the additional refracting power needed to bring objects into focus at distance and near is generated through the accommodative mechanism. If the accommodative effort required for focus is within that child's accommodative amplitude, the vision is clear. In high degrees of hyperopia requiring greater accommodative effort, vision may be blurred, and the child may complain of eyestrain, headaches, or fatigue. Squinting, eye rubbing, and lack of interest in reading are frequent manifestations. If the induced discomfort is great enough, a child may not make an effort to focus and may develop bilateral amblyopia (ametropic amblyopia). Esotropia may also be associated (see discussion on convergent strabismus, accommodative esotropia in Chapter 623). Convex lenses (spectacles or contact lenses) of sufficient

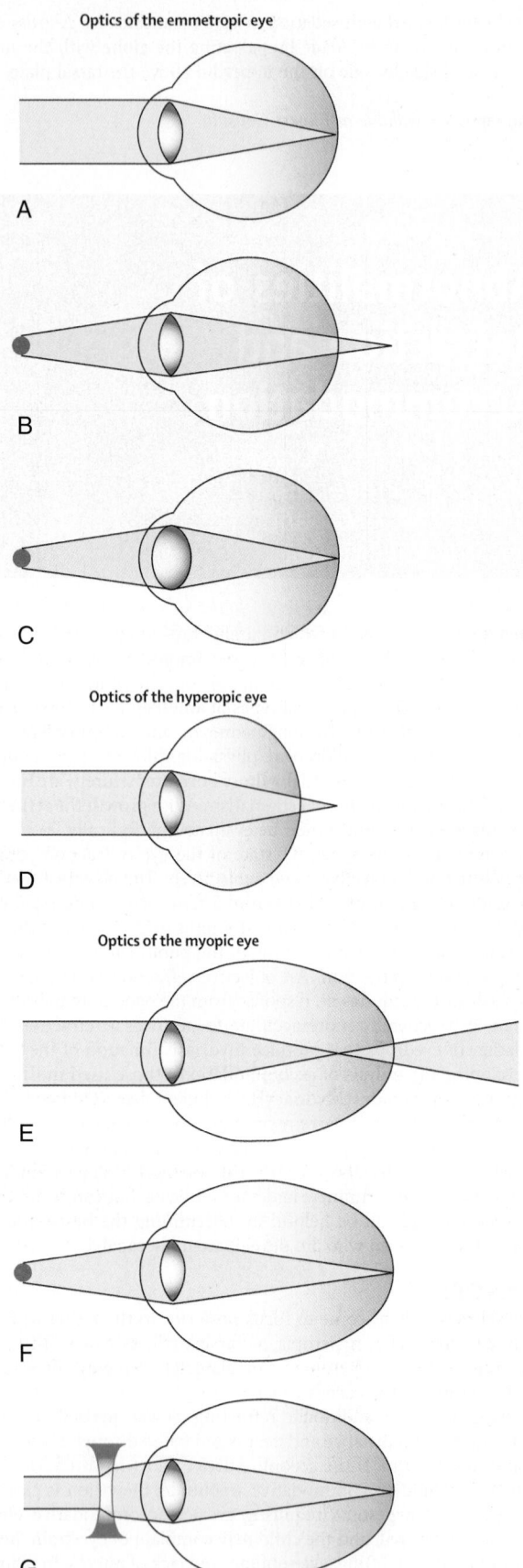

Figure 620-1 Schematic optics of the eye. **A, B,** and **C,** Emmetropic eyes. **D,** Hyperopic eyes. **E, F,** and **G,** Myopic eyes. **A,** In emmetropic eyes, the parallel rays of a distant object are focused on the photoreceptors. **B,** When a closer object is viewed, the image is in focus behind the photoreceptors. The image can be brought forward into focus on the photoreceptors by the process of accommodation—increasing the optical power of the lens **(C).** In hyperopic eyes **(D),** the eye is too short, and the image of a distant object is focused behind the photoreceptors, and can be brought into focus by accommodation. Myopic eyes are eyes that have grown too long **(E),** and the image of a distant object falls in front of the photoreceptors, and cannot be brought into focus by accommodation. When closer objects are viewed, the image moves back toward the photoreceptors, and at a certain distance (the far point), which is related inverse to the severity of the myopia, it comes into focus **(F).** Closer objects can then be brought into focus using accommodation. Optical correction for myopia is achieved with concave (diverging) lenses, which move the image into focus on the photoreceptors **(G).** Contact lenses work in a similar way, whereas refractive surgery reduces the power of the cornea to bring the image of distant objects into focus. For equal corneal power, myopic eyes have longer axial lengths than emmetropic eyes, with deeper anterior and vitreal chambers. Their lenses tend to be thinner and of lower power than those of emmetropic eyes. *(From Morgan IG, Ohno-Matusi K, Saw SM: Myopia. Lancet 379:1739–1746, 2012, Fig. 1, p. 1740.)*

strength to provide clear vision and comfort are prescribed when indicated. Even children who have high degrees of hyperopia but who have good vision will happily wear glasses because they provide comfort by eliminating the excessive accommodation required to see well. Preverbal children should also be given glasses for high levels of hyperopia to prevent the development of esotropia or amblyopia. Children with normal levels of hyperopia do not require correction in the majority of cases.

MYOPIA

In myopia, parallel rays of light come to focus anterior to the retina. This is a result of either a long anteroposterior diameter of the eye or a higher refractive power of the cornea or lens. The principal symptom is blurred vision for distant objects. The far point of clear vision varies inversely with the degree of myopia; as the myopia increases, the far point of clear vision moves closer to the eye. With myopia of 1 diopter, for example, the far point of clear focus is 1 m from the eye; with myopia of 3 diopters, the far point of clear vision is only ⅓ m from the eye. Thus, myopic children tend to hold objects and reading material closer, prefer to be close to the blackboard, and may be uninterested in distant activities. Squinting is common because the visual acuity is improved when the lid aperture is reduced, also known as the pinhole effect.

Myopia is infrequent in infants and preschool-age children. It is more common in infants with a history of **retinopathy of prematurity.** A hereditary tendency to myopia is also observed, and children of myopic parents should be examined at an early age. The incidence of myopia increases during the school years, especially during the preteen and teen years. The degree of myopia also increases with age during the growing years.

Concave lenses (spectacles or contact lenses) of appropriate strength to provide clear vision and comfort are prescribed. Changes are usually needed periodically, from every few months to every 1-2 yr. Excessive accommodation during near work has been considered by some to lead to progression of myopia. Based on this philosophy, some practitioners advocate the use of cycloplegic agents, bifocals, intentional undercorrection of myopic refractive errors, or mandatory removal of myopic glasses for near work in an effort to retard the progression of myopia. The value of such treatment has not been scientifically proven.

Excimer laser correction for myopia has been approved for adults since 1995. The laser is applied to the corneal stroma to reshape the cornea, changing its refractive power. LASIK (laser-assisted in situ keratomileusis) uses either a microkeratome or a femtosecond laser to produce an epithelial-stromal flap permitting the underlying corneal tissue to be ablated. The flap is then reseated and assumes the altered corneal shape. Photorefractive keratectomy (PRK) uses manual removal of the epithelium following treatment with alcohol to expose the Bowman layer and stroma, which is then treated by the excimer laser. The epithelium regenerates to cover the defect over a period of 4-10 days. Visual improvement is usually significant and remains stable over time. Risks are greatest with high degrees of myopia (>10 diopters) and include starbursts, halos, and distorted images or multiple images (usually at night). Refractive surgery is not approved for pediatric patients but is being used off-label to treat of some forms of amblyopia and certain circumstances of myopia and astigmatism, usually by PRK.

In most cases, myopia is not a result of pathologic alteration of the eye and is referred to as simple or physiologic myopia. Some children may have pathologic myopia, a rare condition caused by a pathologically abnormal axial length of the eye; this is usually associated with thinning of the sclera, choroid, and retina and often with some degree of uncorrectable visual impairment. Tears or breaks in the retina may occur as it becomes increasingly thin, leading to the development of retinal detachments. Myopia may also occur as a result of other ocular abnormalities, such as keratoconus, ectopia lentis, congenital stationary night blindness, and glaucoma. Myopia is also a major feature of Stickler syndrome, a genetic disorder of connective tissue involving problems with vision, hearing, and facial and skeletal development.

ASTIGMATISM

In astigmatism, the refractive powers of the various meridians of the eye differ. Most cases are caused by irregularity in the curvature of the cornea, although some astigmatism results from changes in the lens. Mild degrees of astigmatism are common and may produce no symptoms. With greater degrees, distortion of vision can occur. To achieve a clearer image, a person with astigmatism uses accommodation or squints to obtain a pinhole effect. Symptoms include eyestrain, headache, and fatigue. Cylindrical or spherocylindrical lenses are used to provide optical correction when indicated. Glasses may be needed constantly or only part time, depending on the degree of astigmatism and the severity of the attendant symptoms. In some cases, contact lenses are used.

Infants and children with corneal irregularity resulting from injury, ptosis, or hemangiomas of the periorbita or eyelid are at increased risk of astigmatism and associated amblyopia.

ANISOMETROPIA

When the refractive state of one eye is significantly different from the refractive state of the other eye, anisometropia exists. If uncorrected, 1 eye may always be out of focus, leading to the development of amblyopia. Early detection and correction are essential if normal visual development in both eyes is to be achieved.

ACCOMMODATION

During accommodation, the ciliary muscle contracts, the suspensory fibers of the lens relax, and the lens assumes a more rounded shape, adding power to the lens. The amplitude of accommodation is greatest during childhood and gradually diminishes with age. The physiologic decrease in accommodative ability that occurs with age is called presbyopia.

Disorders of accommodation in children are relatively rare. Premature presbyopia is occasionally encountered in young children. The most common cause of paralysis of accommodation in children is intentional or inadvertent use of cycloplegic substances, topically or systemically; included are all the anticholinergic drugs and poisons, as well as plants and plant substances having these effects. Neurogenic causes of accommodative paralysis include lesions affecting the oculomotor nerve (3rd cranial nerve) in any part of its course. Differential diagnoses include tumors, degenerative diseases, vascular lesions, trauma, and infectious etiologies. Systemic disorders that may cause impairment of accommodation include botulism, diphtheria, Wilson disease, diabetes mellitus, and syphilis. Adie tonic pupil may also lead to a deficiency of accommodation after some viral illnesses (see

Chapter 622). An apparent defect in accommodation may be psychogenic in origin; it is common for a child to feign inability to read when it can be demonstrated that visual acuity and ability to focus are normal.

Bibliography is available at Expert Consult.

Chapter **621**
Disorders of Vision

Scott E. Olitsky, Denise Hug, Laura S. Plummer, Erin D. Stahl, Michelle M. Ariss, and Timothy P. Lindquist

Severe visual impairment (corrected vision poorer than **6/60**) and blindness in children have many etiologies and may be caused by multiple defects affecting any structure or function along the visual pathways (Table 621-1). The overall incidence is approximately 2.5 per 100,000 children; the incidence is higher in developing countries, in low birthweight infants, and in the 1st yr of life. The most common causes occur during the prenatal and perinatal time periods; the cerebral-visual pathways, optic nerve, and retinal sites are most often affected. Important prenatal causes include autosomal recessive (most common), autosomal dominant, and X-linked genetic disorders as well as hypoxia and chromosomal syndromes. Perinatal/neonatal causes include retinopathy of prematurity, hypoxia–ischemia, and infection. Severe visual impairment starting in older children may be due to central nervous system or retinal tumors, infections, hypoxia–ischemia, injuries, neurodegenerative disorders, or juvenile idiopathic arthritis.

AMBLYOPIA

This is a decrease in visual acuity, unilateral or bilateral, that occurs in visually immature children as a result of a lack of a clear image projecting onto the retina. The unformed retinal image may occur secondary to a deviated eye **(strabismic amblyopia),** an unequal need for vision correction between the eyes **(anisometropic amblyopia),** a high refractive error in both eyes **(ametropic amblyopia),** or a media opacity within the visual axis **(deprivation amblyopia).**

The development of visual acuity normally proceeds rapidly in infancy and early childhood. Anything that interferes with the formation of a clear retinal image during this early developmental period can produce amblyopia. Amblyopia occurs only during the critical period of development before the cortex has become visually mature, within the 1st decade of life. The younger the child, the more susceptible he or she is to the development of amblyopia.

The **diagnosis** of amblyopia is confirmed when a complete ophthalmologic examination reveals reduced acuity that is unexplained by an organic abnormality. If the history and ophthalmologic examination do not support the diagnosis of amblyopia in a child with poor vision, consideration must be given to other causes (neurologic, psychologic). Amblyopia is usually asymptomatic and can avoid detection until vision screening, which may delay diagnosis as screening programs often target school-age children. This is problematic as amblyopia is more resistant to treatment at an older age, being reversed more rapidly in younger children whose visual system is less mature. Thus, one key to the successful treatment of amblyopia is early detection and prompt intervention.

Most often **treatment** first consists of removing any media opacity or prescribing appropriate glasses, if needed, so that a well-focused retinal image can be produced in each eye. The sound eye is then

Table 621-1	Causes of Childhood Severe Visual Impairment or Blindness

CONGENITAL
Optic nerve hypoplasia or aplasia
Septooptic dysplasia
Optic coloboma
Congenital hydrocephalus
Hydranencephaly
Porencephaly
Micrencephaly
Encephalocele, particularly occipital
Morning glory disc
Aniridia
Microphthalmia/anophthalmia
Peters anomaly
Rieger anomaly
Persistent pupillary membrane
Glaucoma
Cataracts
Persistent hyperplastic primary vitreous

PHAKOMATOSES
Tuberous sclerosis
Neurofibromatosis (special association with optic glioma)
Sturge-Weber syndrome
von Hippel-Lindau disease

TUMORS
Retinoblastoma
Optic glioma
Perioptic meningioma
Craniopharyngioma
Cerebral glioma
Astrocytoma
Posterior and intraventricular tumors when complicated by
  hydrocephalus
Pseudotumor cerebri

NEURODEGENERATIVE DISEASES
Cerebral storage disease
Gangliosidoses, particularly Tay-Sachs disease, Sandhoff variant,
  generalized gangliosidosis
Other lipidoses and ceroid lipofuscinoses, particularly the late-onset
  disorders such as those of Jansky-Bielschowsky and of Batten-
  Mayou-Spielmeyer-Vogt
Mucopolysaccharidoses, particularly Hurler syndrome and Hunter
  syndrome
Leukodystrophies (dysmyelination disorders), particularly
  metachromatic leukodystrophy and Canavan disease
Demyelinating sclerosis (myelinoclastic diseases), especially Schilder
  disease and Devic neuromyelitis optica

Special types: Dawson disease, Leigh disease, the Bassen-Kornzweig
  syndrome, Refsum disease
Retinal degenerations: retinitis pigmentosa and its variants and Leber
  congenital type
Optic atrophies: congenital autosomal recessive type, infantile and
  congenital autosomal dominant types, Leber disease, and atrophies
  associated with hereditary ataxias—the types of Behr, of Marie, and
  of Sanger-Brown

INFECTIOUS/INFLAMMATORY PROCESSES
Encephalitis, especially in the prenatal infection syndromes caused by
  Toxoplasma gondii, cytomegalovirus, rubella virus, *Treponema
  pallidum*, herpes simplex virus
Meningitis; arachnoiditis
Chorioretinitis
Endophthalmitis
Trachoma
Keratitis
Uveitis

HEMATOLOGIC DISORDERS
Leukemia with central nervous system involvement

VASCULAR AND CIRCULATORY DISORDERS
Collagen vascular diseases
Arteriovenous malformations—intracerebral hemorrhage,
  subarachnoid hemorrhage
Central retinal occlusion

TRAUMA
Contusion or avulsion of optic nerves, chiasm, globe, cornea
Cerebral contusion or laceration
Intracerebral, subarachnoid, or subdural hemorrhage
Retinal detachment
Laser injury

DRUGS AND TOXINS
Quinine
Ethambutol
Methanol
Many others

OTHER
Retinopathy of prematurity
Sclerocornea
Conversion reaction
Optic neuritis
Osteopetrosis

Modified from Kliegman R: Practical strategies in pediatric diagnosis and therapy. Philadelphia, 1996, WB Saunders.

covered (occlusion therapy) or blurred with glasses (fogging) or drops (penalization therapy) to stimulate proper visual development of the more severely affected eye. Occlusion therapy may provide a more rapid improvement in vision, but some children may better tolerate atropine penalization. The best treatment for any one patient should be selected on an individual basis. The goals of treatment should be thoroughly understood, and the treatment carefully supervised. Close monitoring of amblyopia therapy by an ophthalmologist is essential, especially in the very young, to avoid deprivation amblyopia in the good eye. Many families need reassurance and support throughout the trying course of treatment. Although full-time occlusion has historically been considered the best way to treat children with amblyopia, a series of prospective studies has shown that some children can achieve similar results with part-time patching or through the use of atropine drops. Historical thought was that older children would not respond to amblyopia therapy. Recent studies now suggest children deemed visually mature who demonstrate amblyopia, particularly refractive or anisometropic in etiology, can demonstrate improvement in vision with appropriate therapy.

DIPLOPIA

Diplopia, or double vision, is generally a result of a misalignment of the visual axes. Occluding either eye relieves the diplopia if it is binocular in origin. Affected children commonly squint, cover 1 eye with a hand, or assume an abnormal head posture (a face turn or head tilt) to alleviate the bothersome sensation. These behaviors, especially in preverbal children, are important clues to diplopia. *The onset of diplopia in any child warrants prompt evaluation; it may signal the onset of a serious problem such as increased intracranial pressure, a brain tumor, infection (Lyme disease), migraine, Guillain-Barré syndrome, or an orbital mass.*

Monocular diplopia results from dislocation of the lens, cataract, dry eyes, or some defect in the media or macula. With this type of diplopia, occluding the nondiplopic eye will not relieve the symptoms. *Monocular diplopia may often have psychological causes.*

SUPPRESSION

In the presence of strabismus, diplopia occurs secondary to the same image falling on different regions of the retina in each eye. In a visually immature child, a process may occur in the cortex that eliminates the disability of seeing double. This is an active process and is termed *suppression*. It develops only in children. Although suppression eliminates the annoying symptom of diplopia, it is the potential awareness of a second image that tends to keep our eyes properly aligned. Once suppression develops, it may allow an intermittent strabismus to become constant or strabismus to redevelop later in life, even after successful treatment during childhood.

AMAUROSIS

Amaurosis is partial or total loss of vision; the term is usually reserved for profound impairment, blindness, or near blindness. When amaurosis exists from birth, primary consideration in the differential diagnosis must be given to developmental malformations, damage consequent to gestational or perinatal infection, anoxia or hypoxia, perinatal trauma, and the genetically determined diseases that can affect the eye itself or the visual pathways. Often, the reason for amaurosis can be readily determined by objective ophthalmic examination; examples are severe microphthalmia, corneal opacification, dense cataracts, chorioretinal scars, macular defects, retinal dysplasia, and severe optic nerve hypoplasia. In other cases, an intrinsic retinal disease may not be apparent on initial ophthalmoscopic examination or the defect may involve the brain and not the eye. Neuroradiologic (MRI or CT) and electrophysiologic (electroretinography) evaluation may be especially helpful in these cases.

Amaurosis that develops in a child who once had useful vision has different implications. In the absence of obvious ocular disease (cataract, chorioretinitis, retinoblastoma, retinitis pigmentosa), consideration must be given to many neurologic and systemic disorders that can affect the visual pathways. Amaurosis of rather rapid onset may indicate an encephalopathy (hypertension), infectious or parainfectious processes, vasculitis, migraine, leukemia, toxins, or trauma. It may be caused by acute demyelinating disease affecting the optic nerves, chiasm, or cerebrum. In some cases, precipitous loss of vision is a result of increased intracranial pressure, rapidly progressive hydrocephalus, or dysfunction of a shunt. More slowly progressive visual loss suggests tumor or neurodegenerative disease. Gliomas of the optic nerve and chiasm and craniopharyngiomas are primary diagnostic considerations in children who show progressive loss of vision.

Clinical manifestations of impairment of vision vary with the age and abilities of a child, the mode of onset, and the laterality and severity of the deficit. The first clue to amaurosis in an infant may be **nystagmus** or **strabismus,** with the vision deficit itself passing undetected for some time. Timidity, clumsiness, or behavioral change may be the initial clues in the very young. Deterioration in school progress and indifference to school activities are common signs in an older child. School-age children often try to hide their disability and, in the case of very slowly progressive disorders, may not themselves realize the severity of the problem; some detect and promptly report small changes in their vision.

Any evidence of loss of vision requires prompt and thorough ophthalmic evaluation. Complete delineation of childhood amaurosis and its cause may require extensive investigation involving neurologic evaluation, electrophysiologic tests, neuroradiologic procedures, and sometimes metabolic and genetic studies. Furthermore, attendant special educational, social, and emotional needs must be met.

NYCTALOPIA

Nyctalopia, or night blindness, is vision that is defective in reduced illumination. It generally implies impairment in function of the rods, particularly in dark adaptation time and perceptual threshold. Stationary congenital night blindness may occur as an autosomal dominant, autosomal recessive, or X-linked recessive condition. It may be associated with myopia and nystagmus. Children may have excessive problems going to sleep in a dark room, which may be mistaken for a behavioral problem. Progressive night blindness usually indicates primary or secondary retinal, choroidal, or vitreoretinal degeneration (see Chapter 630); it occurs also in vitamin A deficiency or as a result of retinotoxic drugs such as quinine.

PSYCHOGENIC DISTURBANCES

Vision problems of psychogenic origin are common in school-age children. Both conversion reactions and willful feigning are encountered. The usual manifestation is a report of reduced visual acuity in 1 or both eyes. Another common manifestation is constriction of the visual field. In some cases, the symptom is diplopia or polyopia (see Chapters 22 and 25).

Important clues to the diagnosis are inappropriate affect, excessive grimacing, inconsistency in performance, and suggestibility. A thorough ophthalmologic examination is essential to differentiate organic from functional visual disorders.

Affected children usually fare well with reassurance and positive suggestions. In some cases, psychiatric care is indicated. In all cases, the approach must be supportive and nonpunitive.

DYSLEXIA

This is the inability to develop the capability to read at an expected level despite an otherwise normal intellect. The terms *reading disability* and *dyslexia* are often used interchangeably. Most dyslexic individuals also display poor writing ability. Dyslexia is a primary reading disorder and should be differentiated from secondary reading difficulties caused by intellectual disability, environmental or educational deprivation, and systemic physical or other organic brain or eye diseases. Because there is no one standard test for dyslexia, the diagnosis is usually made by comparing reading ability with intelligence and standard reading expectations. Dyslexia is a language-based disorder and is not caused by any defect in the eye or visual acuity per se, nor is it attributable to a defect in ocular motility or binocular alignment. Although ophthalmologic evaluation of children with a reading problem is recommended to diagnose and correct any concurrent ocular problems such as a refractive error, amblyopia, or strabismus, treatment directed to the eyes themselves cannot be expected to correct developmental dyslexia (see Chapter 34).

Bibliography is available at Expert Consult.

Chapter **622**

Abnormalities of Pupil and Iris

Scott E. Olitsky, Denise Hug, Laura S. Plummer, Erin D. Stahl, Michelle M. Ariss, and Timothy P. Lindquist

ANIRIDIA

The term *aniridia* is a misnomer because iris tissue is usually present, although it is hypoplastic (Fig. 622-1). Two thirds of the cases are dominantly transmitted with a high degree of penetrance. The other third of cases are sporadic and are considered to be new mutations. The condition is bilateral in 98% of all patients, regardless of the means of transmission, and is found in approximately 1/50,000 persons. *PAX6* is the mutated gene at the chromosome 11p3 region.

Aniridia is a panocular disorder and should not be thought of as an isolated iris defect. Macular and optic nerve hypoplasias are commonly present and lead to decreased vision and sensory nystagmus. The visual acuity is measured as 20/200 in most patients, although the vision may occasionally be better. Other ocular deformities are common and may involve the lens and cornea. The cornea may be small, and a cellular infiltrate (pannus) occasionally develops in the superficial layers of

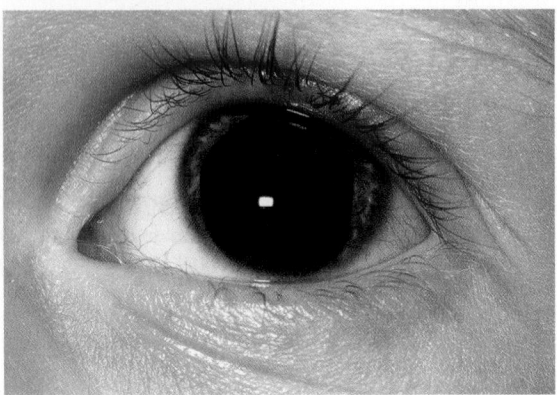

Figure 622-1 Partial aniridia in a member of an autosomal dominant pedigree. *(From Hoyt CS, Taylor D, editors: Pediatric ophthalmology and strabismus, ed 4, Philadelphia, 2013, Elsevier Saunders, Fig. 32.22, p. 304.)*

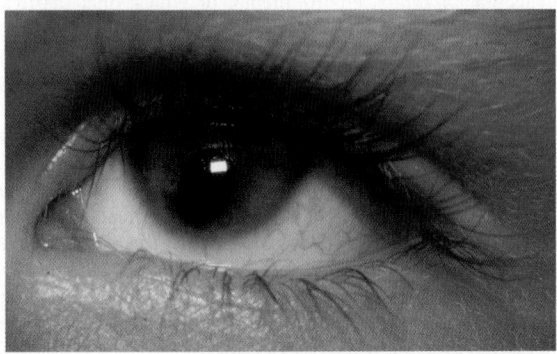

Figure 622-2 Coloboma ("keyhole pupil"). *(From Hoyt CS, Taylor D, editors: Pediatric ophthalmology and strabismus, ed 4, Philadelphia, 2013, Elsevier Saunders, Fig. 38.11, p. 372.)*

the peripheral cornea. Clinically, this appears as a gray opacification. Lens abnormalities include cataract formation and partial or total lens dislocation. **Glaucoma** develops in as many as 75% of individuals with aniridia.

One fifth of **sporadic** aniridic patients may develop **Wilms tumor** (see Chapter 499.1).

The gene for aniridia is very close to the Wilms tumor gene; deletions in this area cause the association. Of particular interest is the association of aniridia, genitourinary anomalies, mental retardation, and a partial deletion of the short arm of chromosome 11. Among individuals thus affected, the appearance of Wilms tumor is more common. It is thought that only patients with sporadic aniridia are at risk for developing Wilms tumor, although Wilms tumor has occurred in a patient with familial aniridia. Wilms tumor usually presents before the 5th yr. Therefore, these children should be screened using renal ultrasonography every 3-6 mo until approximately 5 yr of age if there is an 11p13 region deletion placing the child at risk for Wilms tumor.

COLOBOMA OF THE IRIS

This developmental defect may present as a defect in a sector of the iris, a hole in the substance of the iris, or a notch in the pupillary margin (Fig. 622-2). Simple colobomas are frequently transmitted as an autosomal dominant trait and may occur alone or in association with other anomalies. A coloboma is formed when the embryonic fissure fails to close completely. Because of the anatomic location of the embryonic fissure, an iris coloboma is always located inferiorly, giving the iris a keyhole appearance. An iris coloboma may be the only

externally visible part of an extensive malclosure of the embryonic fissure that also involves the fundus and optic nerve. When this occurs, vision is likely to be severely affected. Therefore, all children with an iris coloboma should undergo a full ophthalmologic examination.

MICROCORIA

Microcoria (congenital miosis) appears as a small pupil that does not react to light or accommodation and that dilates poorly, if at all, with medication. The condition may be unilateral or bilateral. In bilateral cases, the degree of miosis may be different in each eye. The eye may be otherwise normal or may demonstrate other abnormalities of the anterior segment. Congenital microcoria is usually transmitted as an autosomal dominant trait, although it may occur sporadically.

CONGENITAL MYDRIASIS

In this disorder, the pupils appear dilated, do not constrict significantly to light or near gaze, and respond minimally to miotic agents. The iris is otherwise normal, and affected children are usually healthy. Trauma, pharmacologic mydriasis, and neurologic disorders should be considered. Many apparent cases of congenital mydriasis show abnormalities of the central iris structures and may be considered a form of aniridia.

DYSCORIA AND CORECTOPIA

Dyscoria is abnormal shape of the pupil, and corectopia is abnormal pupillary position. They may occur together or independently as congenital or acquired anomalies.

Congenital corectopia is usually bilateral and symmetric and rarely occurs as an isolated anomaly; it is usually accompanied by dislocation of the lens (ectopia lentis et pupillae), and the lens and pupil are commonly dislocated in opposite directions. Ectopia lentis et pupillae is transmitted as an autosomal recessive disorder; consanguinity is common. It is associated with mutations in ADAMTSL4, a secreted glycoprotein widely distributed in the eye, which binds fibrillin-1 microfibrils and accelerates microfibril biogenesis.

When acquired, distortion and displacement of the pupil are frequently a result of trauma or intraocular inflammation. Prolapse of the iris after perforating injuries of the eye leads to peaking of the pupil in the direction of the perforation. Posterior synechiae (adhesions of the iris to the lens) are commonly seen when inflammation due to any cause occurs in the anterior segment.

ANISOCORIA

This is inequality of the pupils. The difference in size may be a result of local or neurologic disorders. As a rule, if the inequality is more pronounced in the presence of bright focal illumination or on near gaze, there is a defect in pupillary constriction and the larger pupil is abnormal. If the anisocoria is worse in reduced illumination, a defect in dilation exists and the smaller pupil is abnormal. Neurologic causes of anisocoria (parasympathetic or sympathetic lesions) must be differentiated from local causes such as synechiae (adhesions), congenital iris defects (colobomas, aniridia), and pharmacologic effects. **Horner syndrome** is an important cause of anisocoria (see below). Simple central anisocoria may occur in otherwise healthy individuals.

DILATED FIXED PUPIL

Differential diagnosis of a dilated unreactive pupil includes internal ophthalmoplegia caused by a central or peripheral lesion, Hutchinson pupil of transtentorial herniation, tonic pupil, pharmacologic blockade, and iridoplegia secondary to ocular trauma.

The most common cause of a dilated unreactive pupil is purposeful or accidental instillation of a cycloplegic agent, particularly atropine and related substances. Central nervous system lesions, such as a pinealoma, may cause internal ophthalmoplegia in children. Because the external surface of the oculomotor nerve carries the fibers responsible for pupillary constriction, compression of the nerve along its intracranial course may be associated with internal ophthalmoplegia, even before the development of ptosis or an ocular motility deficit. Although ophthalmoplegic migraine is a common cause of a 3rd nerve palsy with pupillary involvement in children, an intracranial aneurysm must also be considered in the differential diagnosis. The **blown pupil** of transtentorial herniation, occurring with increasing intracranial pressure, is generally unilateral, and patients usually are obviously ill. The pilocarpine test can help differentiate neurologic iridoplegia from pharmacologic blockade. In the case of neurologic iridoplegia, the dilated pupil constricts within minutes after instillation of 1 or 2 drops of 0.5–1% pilocarpine; if the pupil has been dilated with atropine, pilocarpine has no effect. Because pilocarpine is a long-acting drug, this test is not to be used in acute situations in which pupillary signs must be carefully monitored. Because of the consensual pupil response to light, even complete uniocular blindness does not cause a unilaterally dilated pupil.

TONIC PUPIL
This is typically a large pupil that reacts poorly to light (the reaction may be very slow or essentially nil), reacts poorly and slowly to accommodation, and redilates in a slow, tonic manner. The features of tonic pupil are explained by cholinergic supersensitivity of the sphincter after peripheral (postganglionic) denervation and imperfect reinnervation. A distinctive feature of a tonic pupil is its sensitivity to dilute cholinergic agents. Instillation of 0.125% pilocarpine causes significant constriction of the involved pupil and has little or no effect on the unaffected side. The condition is usually unilateral.

Tonic pupil may develop after the acute stage of a partial or complete iridoplegia. It can be seen after trauma to the eye or orbit and may occur in association with toxic or infectious conditions. For those in the pediatric age group, tonic pupil is uncommon. Infectious processes (primarily viral syndromes) and trauma are the primary causes. Features of tonic pupil may also be seen in infants and children with familial dysautonomia (Riley-Day syndrome), although the significance of these findings has been questioned. Tonic pupil has also been reported in young children with Charcot-Marie-Tooth disease. The occurrence of tonic pupil in association with decreased deep tendon reflexes in young women is referred to as **Adie syndrome.**

MARCUS GUNN PUPIL
This relative afferent pupillary defect indicates an asymmetric, prechiasmatic, afferent conduction defect. It is best demonstrated by the swinging flashlight test, which allows comparison of the direct and consensual pupillary responses in both eyes. With patients fixing on a distant target (to control accommodation), a bright focal light is directed alternately into each eye in turn. In the presence of an afferent lesion, both the direct response to light in the affected eye and the consensual response in the other eye are subnormal. Swinging the light to the better or normal eye causes both pupils to react (constrict) normally. Swinging the light back to the affected eye causes both pupils to redilate to some degree, reflecting the defective conduction. This is a very sensitive and useful test for detecting and confirming optic nerve and retinal disease. This test is only abnormal if there is a "relative" difference in the conduction properties of the optic nerves. Therefore, patients with bilateral and symmetrical optic nerve disease will not demonstrate an afferent pupillary defect. A subtle relative afferent defect may be found in some children with amblyopia.

HORNER SYNDROME
The principal signs of oculosympathetic paresis (Horner syndrome) are homolateral miosis, mild ptosis, and apparent enophthalmos with slight elevation of the lower lid as a result of the slight ptosis. Patients may also have decreased facial sweating, increased amplitude of accommodation, and transient decrease in intraocular pressure. If paralysis of the ocular sympathetic fibers occurs before the age of 2 yr, heterochromia iridis with hypopigmentation of the iris may occur on the affected side (Fig. 622-3).

Oculosympathetic paralysis may be caused by a lesion (tumor, trauma, infarction) in the midbrain, brainstem, upper spinal cord, neck, middle fossa, or orbit. Congenital oculosympathetic paresis, often as part of Klumpke brachial palsy, is common, although the

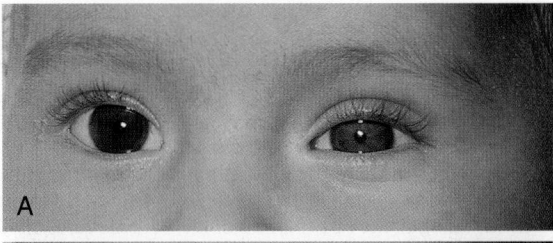
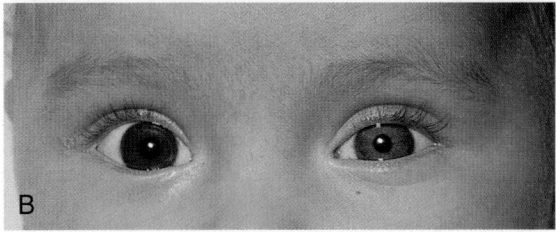

Figure 622-3 Left congenital Horner syndrome showing upper- and lower-lid ptosis and an iris heterochromia, with the lighter eye being the affected eye. **A,** In bright light and **(B)** in the dark. *(From Hoyt CS, Taylor D, editors: Pediatric ophthalmology and strabismus, ed 4, Philadelphia, 2013, Elsevier Saunders, Fig. 63.9, p. 661.)*

ocular signs, particularly the anisocoria, may pass undetected for years. Horner syndrome is also seen in some children after thoracic surgery. Congenital Horner syndrome may occur in association with vertebral anomalies and with enterogenous cysts. In some infants and children, Horner syndrome is the presenting sign of tumor in the mediastinal or cervical region, particularly neuroblastoma. Rare causes of Horner syndrome, such as vascular lesions, also occur in the pediatric age group. In many cases, no cause of congenital Horner syndrome can be identified. Occasionally, the condition is familial.

When the cause of Horner syndrome is in question, investigative procedures should be implemented and may include imaging of the head, neck, and chest as well as 24-hr urinary catecholamine assay. Examining old photographs and old records can sometimes be helpful in establishing the age at onset of Horner syndrome.

The cocaine test is useful in diagnosing oculosympathetic paralysis; a normal pupil dilates within 20–45 min after instillation of 1 or 2 drops of 4% cocaine, whereas the miotic pupil of an oculosympathetic paresis dilates poorly, if at all, with cocaine. In some cases, there is denervation supersensitivity to dilute phenylephrine; 1 or 2 drops of a 1% solution dilates the affected pupil but not the normal one. Furthermore, instillation of 1% hydroxyamphetamine hydrobromide dilates the pupil only if the postganglionic sympathetic neuron is intact.

PARADOXICAL PUPIL REACTION
Some children exhibit paradoxical constriction of the pupils to darkness. An initial brisk constriction of the pupils occurs when the light is turned off, followed by slow redilation of the pupils. The response to direct light stimulation and the near response are normal. The mechanism is not clear, but paradoxical constriction of the pupils in reduced light can be a sign of retinal or optic nerve abnormalities. The phenomenon has been observed in children with congenital stationary night blindness, albinism, retinitis pigmentosa, Leber congenital retinal amaurosis, and Best disease. It has also been observed in those with optic nerve anomalies, optic neuritis, optic atrophy, and possibly amblyopia. Thus, children with paradoxical pupillary constriction to darkness should have a thorough ophthalmologic examination.

PERSISTENT PUPILLARY MEMBRANE
Involution of the pupillary membrane and anterior vascular capsule of the lens is usually completed during the 5th–6th mo of fetal development. It is common to see some remnants of the pupillary membrane in newborns, particularly in premature infants. These membranes are

nonpigmented strands of obliterated vessels that cross the pupil and may secondarily attach to the lens or cornea. The remnants tend to atrophy in time and usually present no problem. In some cases, however, significant remnants that remain obscure the pupil and interfere with vision. Rarely, there is patency of the vascular elements; hyphema may result from rupture of persistent vessels.

Intervention must be considered to minimize amblyopia in infants with extensive persistent pupillary membrane of sufficient degree to interfere with vision in the early months of life. In some cases, mydriatics and occlusion therapy may be effective, but in others, surgery may be needed to provide an adequate pupillary aperture.

HETEROCHROMIA

In heterochromia, the 2 irides are of different color (heterochromia iridium) or a portion of an iris differs in color from the remainder (heterochromia iridis). Simple heterochromia may occur as an autosomal dominant characteristic. Congenital heterochromia is also a feature of Waardenburg syndrome, an autosomal dominant condition characterized principally by lateral displacement of the inner canthi and puncta, pigmentary disturbances (usually a median white forelock and patches of hypopigmentation of the skin), and defective hearing. Change in the color of the iris may occur as a result of trauma, hemorrhage, intraocular inflammation (iridocyclitis, uveitis), intraocular tumor (especially retinoblastoma), intraocular foreign body, glaucoma, iris atrophy, oculosympathetic palsy (Horner syndrome), melanosis oculi, previous intraocular surgery, and some glaucoma medications.

OTHER IRIS LESIONS

Discrete nodules of the iris, referred to as **Lisch nodules,** are commonly seen in patients with neurofibromatosis (see Chapter 596.1). Lisch nodules represent melanocytic hamartomas of the iris and vary from slightly elevated pigmented areas to distinct ball-like excrescences. The nodules cause no visual disturbance. Lisch nodules are found in 92-100% of individuals older than 5 yr of age who have neurofibromatosis. Slit-lamp identification of these nodules may help to fulfill the criteria required to confirm the diagnosis of neurofibromatosis.

In leukemia (see Chapter 495), there may be infiltration of the iris, sometimes with **hypopyon,** an accumulation of white blood cells in the anterior chamber, which may herald relapse or involvement of the central nervous system.

The lesion of **juvenile xanthogranuloma** (nevoxanthoendothelioma; see Chapter 670) may occur in the eye as a yellowish fleshy mass or plaque of the iris. Spontaneous hyphema (blood in the anterior chamber), glaucoma, or a red eye with signs of uveitis may be associated. A search for the skin lesions of xanthogranuloma should be made in any infant or young child with spontaneous hyphema. In many cases, the ocular lesion responds to topical corticosteroid therapy.

LEUKOCORIA

This includes any white pupillary reflex, or so-called cat's-eye reflex. Primary diagnostic considerations in any child with leukocoria are cataract, persistent hyperplastic primary vitreous, cicatricial retinopathy of prematurity, retinal detachment and retinoschisis, larval granulomatosis, and retinoblastoma (Fig. 622-4). Also to be considered are endophthalmitis, organized vitreous hemorrhage, leukemic ophthalmopathy, exudative retinopathy (as in Coats disease), and less-common conditions such as medulloepithelioma, massive retinal gliosis, the

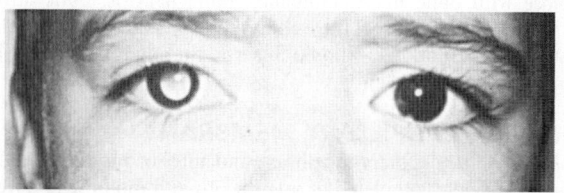

Figure 622-4 Leukocoria. White pupillary reflex in a child with retinoblastoma.

retinal pseudotumor of Norrie disease, the so-called pseudoglioma of the Bloch-Sulzberger syndrome, retinal dysplasia, and the retinal lesions of the phakomatoses. A white reflex may also be seen with fundus coloboma, large atrophic chorioretinal scars, and ectopic medullation of retinal nerve fibers. Leukocoria is an indication for prompt and thorough evaluation.

The diagnosis can often be made by direct examination of the eye by ophthalmoscopy and biomicroscopy. Ultrasonographic and radiologic examinations are often helpful. In some cases, the final diagnosis rests with a pathologist.

Bibliography is available at Expert Consult.

Chapter **623**
Disorders of Eye Movement and Alignment
Scott E. Olitsky, Denise Hug, Laura S. Plummer, Erin D. Stahl, Michelle M. Ariss, and Timothy P. Lindquist

STRABISMUS

Strabismus, or misalignment of the eyes, is one of the most common eye problems encountered in children, affecting approximately 4% of children younger than 6 yr of age. Strabismus can result in vision loss (amblyopia) and can have significant psychological effects. Early detection and treatment of strabismus are essential to prevent permanent visual impairment. Of children with strabismus, 30-50% develop amblyopia. Restoration of proper alignment of the visual axis must occur at an early stage of visual development to allow these children a chance to develop normal binocular vision. The word strabismus means "to squint or to look obliquely." Many terms are used in discussing and characterizing strabismus.

Orthophoria is the ideal condition of exact ocular balance. It implies that the oculomotor apparatus is in perfect equilibrium so that the eyes remain coordinated and aligned in all positions of gaze and at all distances. Even when binocular vision is interrupted, as by occlusion of one eye, truly orthophoric individuals maintain perfect alignment. Orthophoria is seldom encountered because the majority of individuals have a small latent deviation (heterophoria).

Heterophoria is a latent tendency for the eyes to deviate. This latent deviation is normally controlled by fusional mechanisms that provide binocular vision or avoid diplopia (double vision). The eye deviates only under certain conditions, such as fatigue, illness, or stress, or during tests that interfere with maintenance of these normal fusional abilities (such as covering one eye). If the amount of heterophoria is large, it may give rise to bothersome symptoms, such as transient diplopia (double vision), headaches, or asthenopia (eyestrain). Some degree of heterophoria is found in normal individuals; it is usually asymptomatic.

Heterotropia is a misalignment of the eyes that is constant. It occurs because of an inability of the fusional mechanism to control the deviation. Tropias can be alternating, involving both eyes, or unilateral. In an alternating tropia, there is no preference for fixation of either eye, and both eyes drift with equal frequency. Because each eye is used periodically, vision usually develops normally. A unilateral tropia is a more serious situation because only 1 eye is constantly misaligned. The undeviated eye becomes the preferred eye, resulting in loss of vision or amblyopia of the deviated eye.

It is common in ocular misalignments to describe the type of deviation. This helps to make decisions on the cause and treatment of the strabismus. The prefixes *eso-, exo-, hyper-,* and *hypo-* are added to the terms *phoria* and *tropia* to further delineate the type of strabismus. Esophorias and esotropias are inward or convergent deviations of the eyes, commonly known as crossed eyes. Exophorias and exotropias are divergent or outward-facing eye deviations, walleyed being the lay term. Hyperdeviations and hypodeviations designate upward or downward, respectively, deviations of an eye. In cases of unilateral strabismus, the deviating eye is often part of the description of the misalignment (left esotropia).

Diagnosis

Many techniques are used to assess ocular alignment and movement of the eyes to aid in diagnosing strabismic disorders. In a child with strabismus or any other ocular disorder, assessment of visual acuity is mandatory. Decreased vision in 1 eye requires evaluation for a strabismus or other ocular abnormalities, which may be difficult to discern on a brief screening evaluation. Even strabismic deviations of only a few degrees in magnitude, too small to be evident by gross inspection, may lead to amblyopia and significant vision loss.

Corneal light reflex tests are perhaps the most rapid and easily performed diagnostic tests for strabismus. They are particularly useful in children who are uncooperative and in those who have poor ocular fixation. To perform the **Hirschberg corneal reflex test,** the examiner projects a light source onto the cornea of both eyes simultaneously as a child looks directly at the light. Comparison should then be made of the placement of the corneal light reflex in each eye. In straight eyes, the light reflection appears symmetric and, because of the relationship between the cornea and the macula, slightly nasal to the center of each pupil. If strabismus is present, the reflected light is asymmetric and appears displaced in one eye. The Krimsky method of the corneal reflex test uses prisms placed over one or both eyes to align the light reflections. The amount of prism needed to align the reflections is used to measure the degree of deviation. Although it is a useful screening test, corneal light reflex testing may not detect a small angle or an intermittent strabismus.

Cover tests for strabismus require a child's attention and cooperation, good eye movement capability, and reasonably good vision in each eye. If any of these are lacking, the results of these tests may not be valid. These tests consist of the cover–uncover test and the alternate cover test. In the cover–uncover test, a child looks at an object in the distance, preferably 6 m away. An eye chart is commonly used for fixation in children older than 3 yr of age. For younger children, a noise-making toy or movie helps hold their attention for the test. As the child looks at the distant object, the examiner covers 1 eye and watches for movement of the uncovered eye. If no movement occurs, there is no apparent misalignment of that eye. After 1 eye is tested, the same procedure is repeated on the other eye. When performing the alternate cover test, the examiner rapidly covers and uncovers each eye, shifting back and forth from one eye to the other. If the child has an ocular deviation, the eye rapidly moves as the cover is shifted to the other eye. Both the cover–uncover test and the alternate cover test should be performed at both distance and near fixation. The cover–uncover test differentiates tropias, or manifest deviations, from latent deviations, called phorias.

Clinical Manifestations and Treatment

The etiologic classification of strabismus is complex, and the causative types must be distinguished; there are comitant and noncomitant forms of strabismus.

Comitant Strabismus

Comitant strabismus is the most common type of strabismus. The individual extraocular muscles usually have no defect. The amount of deviation is constant, or relatively constant, in the various directions of gaze.

Pseudostrabismus (pseudoesotropia) is one of the most common reasons a pediatric ophthalmologist is asked to evaluate an infant. This condition is characterized by the false appearance of strabismus when the visual axes are aligned accurately. This appearance may be caused by a flat, broad nasal bridge, prominent epicanthal folds, or a narrow interpupillary distance. The observer may see less white sclera nasally than would be expected, and the impression is that the eye is turned in toward the nose, especially when the child gazes to either side. Parents frequently comment that when their child looks to the side, the eye almost disappears from view. Pseudoesotropia can be differentiated from a true misalignment of the eyes when the corneal light reflex is centered in both eyes and when the cover–uncover test shows no refixation movement. Once pseudoesotropia has been confirmed, parents can be reassured that the child will outgrow the appearance of esotropia. As the child grows, the bridge of the nose becomes more prominent and displaces the epicanthal folds, and the medial sclera becomes proportional to the amount visible on the lateral aspect. It is the appearance of crossing that the child will outgrow. Some parents of children with pseudoesotropia erroneously believe that their child has an actual esotropia that will resolve on its own. Because true esotropia can develop later in children with pseudoesotropia, parents and pediatricians should be cautioned that reassessment is required if the apparent deviation does not improve.

Esodeviations are the most common type of ocular misalignment in children and represent >50% of all ocular deviations. *Congenital esotropia* is a confusing term. Few children who are diagnosed with this disorder are actually born with an esotropia. Most reports in the literature have, therefore, considered infants with confirmed onset earlier than 6 mo as having the same condition, which some observers have designated **infantile esotropia**.

Between 2 and 4 mo of age, many infants have infantile esotropia (neonatal misalignments), which in most resolve spontaneously. Those that resolve without treatment do so before 10-12 wk of age and had intermittent or variable deviations, while those who may benefit from active treatment have persistent esotropia (10 weeks–6 mo of age), a constant esotropia (40 PD), a refractive error ≤ +3.00 D, and the absence of prematurity, developmental delay, meningitis, nystagmus, eye anomalies, and incomitant or paralytic strabismus. The evaluation is noted in Figure 623-1.

The characteristic angle of congenital esodeviations is large and constant (Fig. 623-2). Because of the large deviation, cross-fixation is frequently encountered. This is a condition in which the child looks to the right with the left eye and to the left with the right eye. With cross-fixation, there is no need for the eye to turn away from the nose (abduction) as the adducting eye is used in side gaze; this condition simulates a 6th nerve palsy. Abduction can be demonstrated by the doll's-head maneuver or by patching 1 eye for a short time. Children with congenital esotropia tend to have refractive errors similar to those of normal children of the same age. This contrasts with the characteristic high level of farsightedness associated with accommodative esotropia. **Amblyopia** is common in children with congenital esotropia.

The primary goal of treatment in congenital esotropia is to eliminate or reduce the deviation as much as possible. Ideally, this results in normal sight in each eye, in straight-looking eyes, and in the development of binocular vision. Early treatment is more likely to lead to the development of binocular vision, which helps to maintain long-term ocular alignment. Once any associated amblyopia is treated, surgery is performed to align the eyes. Even with successful surgical alignment, it is common for vertical deviations to develop in children with a history of congenital esotropia. The 2 most common forms of vertical deviations to develop are inferior oblique muscle overaction and dissociated vertical deviation. In inferior oblique muscle overaction, the overactive inferior oblique muscle produces an upshoot of the eye closest to the nose when the patient looks to the side (Fig. 623-3). In dissociated vertical deviation, 1 eye drifts up slowly with no movement of the other eye. Surgery may be necessary to treat either or both of these conditions.

It is important that parents realize that early successful surgical alignment is only the beginning of the treatment process. Because many children may redevelop strabismus or amblyopia, they need to be monitored closely during the visually immature period of life.

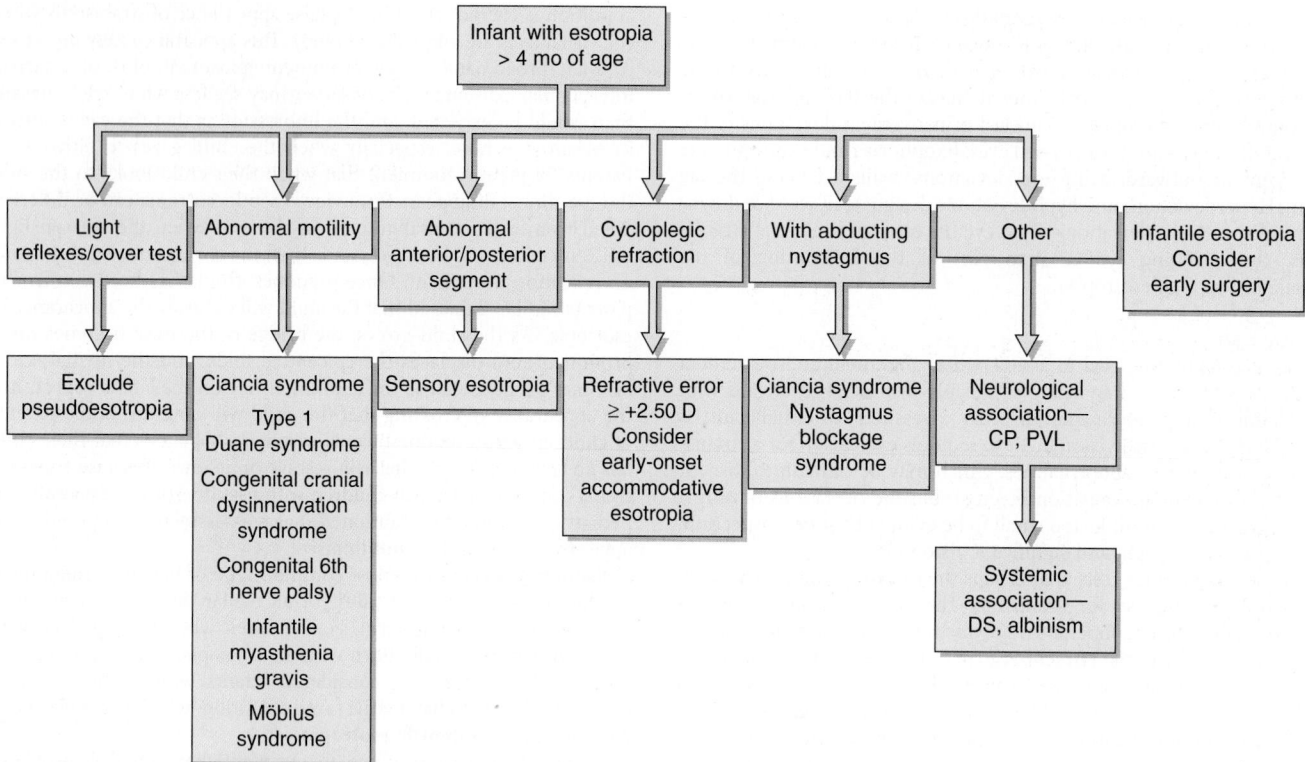

Figure 623-1 Work-up of infant ≥4 mo of age with esotropia. *CP,* cerebral palsy; *DS,* Down syndrome; *PVL,* periventricular leukomalacia. *(From Hoyt CS, Taylor D, editors:* Pediatric ophthalmology and strabismus, *ed 4, Philadelphia, 2013, Elsevier Saunders, Fig. 74.4, p. 767.)*

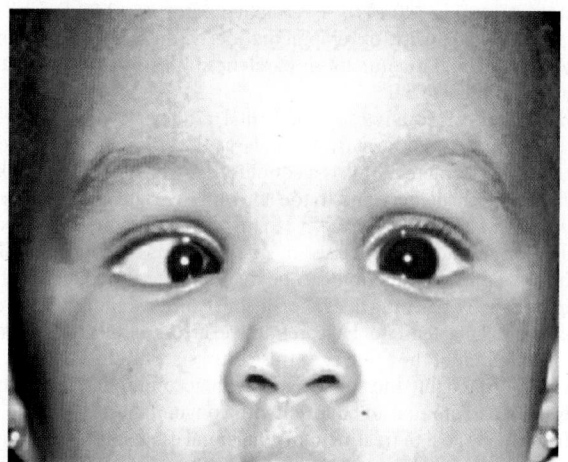

Figure 623-2 Congenital esotropia. Note the large angle of crossing.

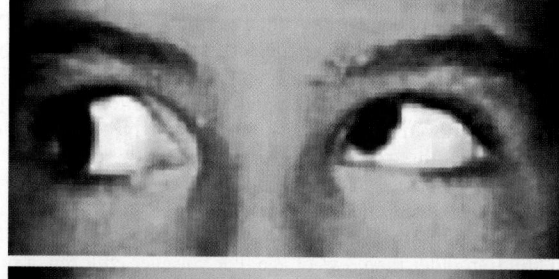
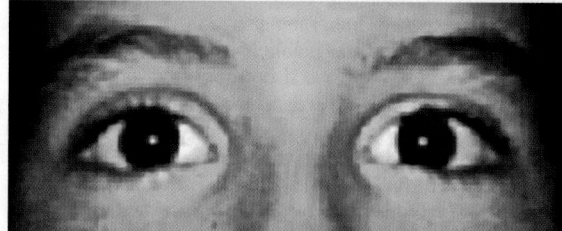
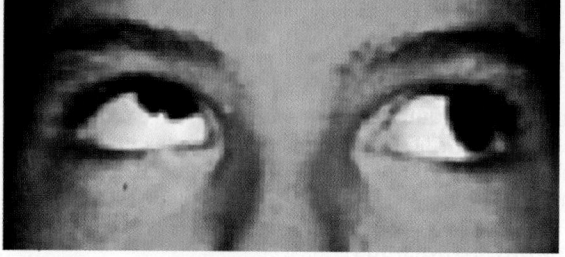

Figure 623-3 Inferior oblique muscle overaction.

Accommodative esotropia is defined as a "convergent deviation of the eyes associated with activation of the accommodative (focusing) reflex." It usually occurs in a child who is between 2 and 3 yr of age and who has a history of acquired intermittent or constant crossing. Amblyopia occurs in the majority of cases.

The mechanism of accommodative esotropia involves uncorrected hyperopia, accommodation, and accommodative convergence. The image entering a hyperopic (farsighted) eye is blurred. If the amount of hyperopia is not significant, the blurred image can be sharpened by accommodating (focusing of the lens of the eye). Accommodation is closely linked with convergence (eyes turning inward). If a child's hyperopic refractive error is large or if the amount of convergence that occurs in response to each unit of accommodative effort is great, esotropia may develop.

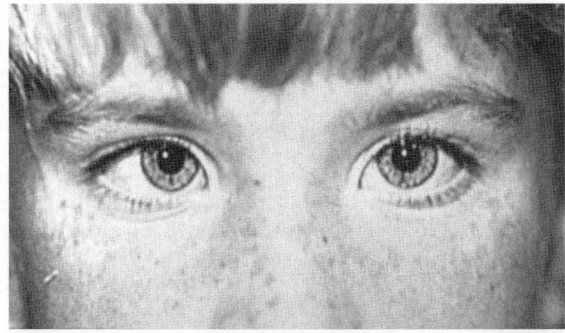
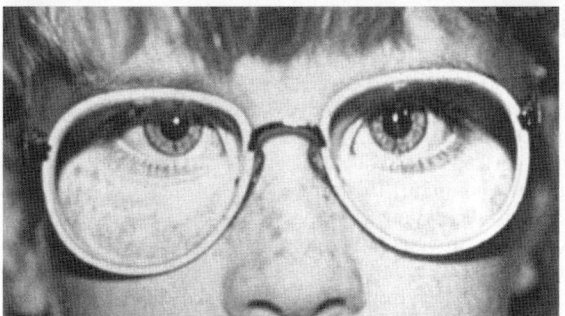

Figure 623-4 Accommodative esotropia. Control of deviation with corrective lenses.

To treat accommodative esotropia, the full hyperopic (farsighted) correction is initially prescribed. These glasses eliminate a child's need to accommodate and therefore correct the esotropia (Fig. 623-4). Although many parents are initially concerned that their child will not want to wear glasses, the benefits of binocular vision and the decrease in the focusing effort required to see clearly provide a strong stimulus to wear glasses, and they are generally accepted well. The full hyperopic correction sometimes straightens the eye position at distance fixation but leaves a residual deviation at near fixation; this may be observed or treated with bifocal lenses or surgery.

It is important to warn parents of children with accommodative esotropia that the esodeviation may appear to increase without glasses after the initial correction is worn. Parents frequently state that before wearing glasses, their child had a small esodeviation, whereas after removal of the glasses, the esodeviation becomes quite large. Parents often blame the increased esodeviation on the glasses. This apparent increase is a result of a child's using the appropriate amount of accommodative effort after the glasses have been worn. When these children remove their glasses, they continue to use an accommodative effort to bring objects into proper focus and increase the esodeviation.

Most children maintain straight eyes once initially treated. Because hyperopia generally decreases with age, patients may outgrow the need to wear glasses to maintain alignment. In some patients, a residual esodeviation persists even when wearing their glasses. This condition commonly occurs when there is a delay between the onset of accommodative esotropia and treatment. In others, the esotropia may initially be eliminated with glasses but crossing redevelops and is not correctable with glasses. The crossing that is no longer correctable with glasses is the deteriorated or nonaccommodative portion. Surgery for this portion of the crossing may be indicated to restore binocular vision.

Exodeviations are the second most common type of misalignment. The divergent deviation may be intermittent or constant. Intermittent exotropia is the most common exodeviation in childhood. It is characterized by outward drifting of 1 eye, which usually occurs when a child is fixating at distance. The deviation is generally more frequent with fatigue or illness. Exposure to bright light may cause reflex closure of the exotropic eye. Because the eyes initially can be kept straight most of the time, visual acuity tends to be good in both eyes and binocular vision is initially normal.

The age at onset of intermittent exotropia varies but is often between age 6 mo and 4 yr. The decision to perform eye muscle surgery is based on the amount and frequency of the deviation. If the deviation is small and infrequent, it is reasonable to observe the child. If the exotropia is large or increasing in frequency, surgery is indicated to maintain normal binocular vision.

Constant exotropia may rarely be congenital. Congenital exotropia may be associated with neurologic disease or abnormalities of the bony orbit, as in Crouzon syndrome. Exotropia that occurs later in life may represent a deterioration of an intermittent exotropia that was present in childhood. Surgery can restore binocular vision even in long-standing cases.

Noncomitant Strabismus

When an eye muscle is paretic, palsied, or restricted, a muscle imbalance occurs in which the deviation of the eye varies according to the direction of gaze. Recent onset of a paretic muscle can be suggested by the symptom of double vision that increases in one direction, the findings of an ocular deviation that increases in the field of action of the paretic muscle, and an increase in the deviation when the child fixates with the paretic eye. It is important to differentiate a noncomitant strabismus from a comitant deviation because noncomitant forms of strabismus are often associated with trauma, systemic disorders, or neurologic abnormalities.

3rd Nerve Palsy

In the pediatric population, 3rd nerve palsies are usually congenital. The congenital form is often associated with a developmental anomaly or birth trauma. Acquired 3rd nerve palsies in children can be an ominous sign and may indicate a neurologic abnormality such as an intracranial neoplasm or an aneurysm. Other less-serious causes include an inflammatory or infectious lesion, head trauma, postviral syndromes, and migraines.

A 3rd nerve palsy, whether congenital or acquired, usually results in an exotropia and a hypotropia, or downward deviation of the affected eye, as well as complete or partial ptosis of the upper lid. This characteristic strabismus results from the action of the normal, unopposed muscles, the lateral rectus muscle, and the superior oblique muscle. If the internal branch of the 3rd nerve is involved, pupillary dilation may be noted as well. Eye movements are usually limited nasally in elevation and in depression. In addition, clinical findings and treatment may be complicated in congenital and traumatic cases of 3rd nerve palsy owing to misdirection of regenerating nerve fibers, referred to as aberrant regeneration. This results in anomalous and paradoxical eyelid, eye, and pupil movement such as elevation of the eyelid, constriction of the pupil, or depression of the globe on attempted medial gaze.

4th Nerve Palsy

These palsies can be congenital or acquired. Because the 4th nerve has a long intracranial course, it is susceptible to damage resulting from head trauma. In children, however, 4th nerve palsies are more frequently congenital than traumatic. A palsied 4th nerve results in weakness in the superior oblique muscle, which causes an upward deviation of the eye, a hypertropia. Because the antagonist muscle, the inferior oblique, is relatively unopposed, the affected eye demonstrates an upshoot when looking toward the nose. Children typically present with a head tilt to the shoulder opposite the affected eye, their chin down, and their face turned away from the affected side. This head position places the eye away from the area of greatest action of the affected muscle and therefore minimizes the deviation and the associated double vision. Long-standing head tilts may lead to facial asymmetry. Because the abnormal head posture maintains the child's ocular alignment, amblyopia is uncommon. Because no abnormality exists in the neck muscles, attempts to correct the head tilt by exercises and neck muscle surgery are ineffective. Recognition of a superior oblique paresis can be difficult because deviation of the head and the eye may be minimal. Eye muscle surgery can be performed to improve the ocular alignment and eliminate the abnormal head posture.

6th Nerve Palsy

These palsies produce markedly crossed eyes with limited ability to move the afflicted eye laterally. Children frequently present with their head turned toward the palsied muscle, a position that helps preserve binocular vision. The esotropia is largest when the eye is moved toward the affected muscle.

Congenital 6th nerve palsies are rare. Decreased lateral gaze in infants is often associated with other disorders, such as congenital esotropia or Duane retraction syndrome. In neonates, a transient 6th nerve paresis can occur; it usually clears spontaneously by 6 wk. It is believed that increased intracranial pressure associated with labor and delivery is the contributing factor.

Acquired 6th nerve palsies in childhood are often an ominous sign because the 6th nerve is susceptible to increased intracranial pressure associated with hydrocephalous and intracranial tumors. Other causes of 6th nerve defects in children include trauma, vascular malformations, meningitis, and Gradenigo syndrome. A benign 6th nerve palsy, which is painless and acquired, can be noted in infants and older children. This is frequently preceded by a febrile illness or upper respiratory tract infection and may be recurrent. Complete resolution of the palsy is usual. Although not uncommon, other causes of an acute 6th nerve palsy should be eliminated before this diagnosis is made.

Strabismus Syndromes

Special types of strabismus have unusual clinical features. Most of these disorders are caused by structural anomalies of the extraocular muscles or adjacent tissues. Most strabismus syndromes produce noncomitant misalignments.

Monocular Elevation Deficiency

A monocular elevation deficit in both abduction and adduction is referred to as monocular elevation deficiency (previously called double-elevator palsy). It may represent a paresis of both elevators, the superior rectus and inferior oblique muscles, or a possible restriction to elevation from a fibrotic inferior rectus muscle. When an affected child fixates with the nonparetic eye, the paretic eye is hypotropic and the ipsilateral upper eyelid may appear ptotic. Fixation with the paretic eye causes a hypertropia of the nonparetic eye and a disappearance of the ptosis (Fig. 623-5). Because the apparent ptosis is actually secondary to the strabismus, correction of the hypotropia treats the pseudoptosis.

Duane Syndrome

This congenital disorder of ocular motility is characterized by retraction of the globe on adduction. This is attributed to the absence of the 6th nerve nucleus and anomalous innervation of the lateral rectus muscle, which results in cocontraction of the medial and lateral rectus muscles on attempted adduction of the affected eye. Within the spectrum of Duane syndrome, patients may exhibit impairment of abduction, impairment of adduction, or upshoot or downshoot of the involved eye on adduction. They may have esotropia, exotropia, or relatively straight eyes. Many exhibit a compensatory head posture to maintain single vision. Some develop amblyopia. Surgery to improve alignment or to reduce a noticeable face turn can be helpful in selected cases. Duane syndrome usually occurs sporadically. It is sometimes inherited as an autosomal dominant trait. It usually occurs as an isolated condition but may occur in association with various other ocular and systemic anomalies.

Möbius Syndrome

The distinctive features of Möbius syndrome are congenital facial paresis and abduction weakness. The facial palsy is commonly bilateral, frequently asymmetric, and often incomplete, tending to spare the lower face and platysma. Ectropion, epiphora, and exposure keratopathy may develop. The abduction defect may be unilateral or bilateral. Esotropia is common. The cause is unknown. Whether the primary defect is maldevelopment of cranial nerve nuclei, hypoplasia of the muscles, or a combination of central and peripheral factors is unclear. Some familial cases have been reported. Associated developmental defects may include ptosis, palatal and lingual palsy, hearing loss, pectoral and lingual muscle defects, micrognathia, syndactyly, supernumerary digits, and the absence of hands, feet, fingers, or toes. Surgical correction of the esotropia is indicated and any attendant amblyopia should be treated.

Brown Syndrome

In this syndrome, elevation of the eye in the adducted position is restricted (Fig. 623-6). An associated downward deviation of the affected eye in adduction may also occur. A compensatory head posture may be evident. Brown syndrome occurs as a result of restriction of the superior oblique tendon as it moves through the trochlea. Cases may be congenital or acquired. Acquired Brown syndrome may follow trauma to the orbit involving the region of the trochlea or sinus surgery. It may also occur with inflammatory processes, particularly sinusitis and juvenile idiopathic arthritis.

Acquired inflammatory Brown syndrome may respond to treatment with either nonsteroidal medications or corticosteroids. Surgery may be helpful for selected cases of Brown syndrome.

Parinaud Syndrome

This eponym designates a palsy of vertical gaze, isolated or associated with pupillary or nuclear oculomotor (3rd cranial nerve) paresis. It indicates a lesion affecting the mesencephalic tegmentum. The ophthalmic signs of midbrain disease include vertical gaze palsy, dissociation of the pupillary responses to light and to near focus, general pupillomotor paralysis, corectopia, dyscoria, accommodative disturbances, pathologic lid retraction, ptosis, extraocular muscle paresis, and convergence paralysis. Some cases have associated spasms of convergence, convergent retraction nystagmus, and vertical nystagmus, particularly on attempted vertical gaze. Combinations of these signs are referred to as the sylvian aqueduct syndrome.

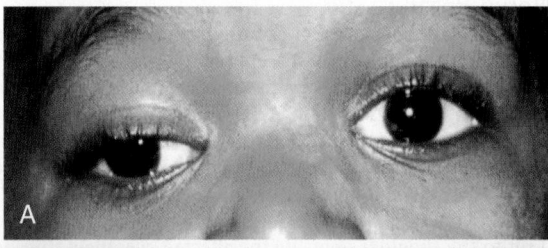
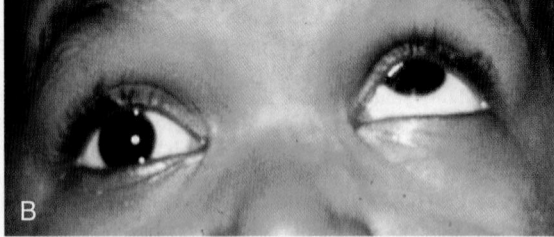

Figure 623-5 Double-elevator palsy of the right eye. Note the disappearance of the apparent ptosis when fixating with the involved eye.

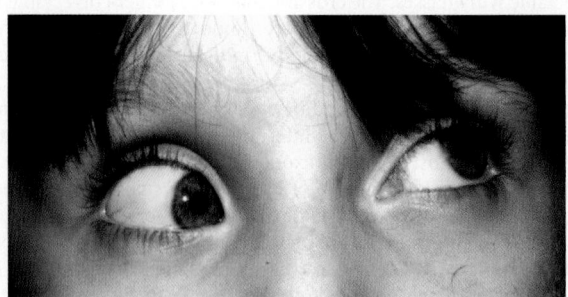

Figure 623-6 Brown syndrome of the right eye.

A principal cause of vertical gaze palsy and associated mesencephalic signs in children is tumor of the pineal gland or third ventricle. Differential diagnosis includes trauma and demyelinating disease. In children with hydrocephalus, impairment of vertical gaze and pathologic lid retraction are referred to as the setting-sun sign. A transient supranuclear disorder of gaze is sometimes seen in healthy neonates.

CONGENITAL OCULAR MOTOR APRAXIA

This congenital disorder of conjugate gaze is characterized by a defect in voluntary horizontal gaze, compensatory jerking movement of the head, and retention of slow pursuit and reflexive eye movements. Additional features are absence of the fast (refixation) phase of optokinetic nystagmus and obligate contraversive deviation of the eyes on rotation of the body. Affected children typically are unable to look quickly to either side voluntarily in response to a command or in response to an eccentrically presented object but may be able to follow a slowly moving target to either side. To compensate for the defect in purposive lateral eye movements, children jerk their head to bring the eyes into the desired position and may also blink repetitively in an attempt to change fixation. The signs tend to become less conspicuous with age.

The pathogenesis of congenital ocular motor apraxia is unknown. It may be a result of delayed myelination of the ocular motor pathways. Structural abnormalities of the central nervous system have been found in a few patients, including agenesis of the corpus callosum and cerebellar vermis, porencephaly, hamartoma of the foramen of Monro, and macrocephaly. Many children with congenital ocular motor apraxia show delayed motor and cognitive development.

NYSTAGMUS

Nystagmus (rhythmic oscillations of 1 or both eyes) may be caused by an abnormality in any one of the 3 basic mechanisms that regulate position and movement of the eyes: the fixation, conjugate gaze, or vestibular mechanism. In addition, physiologic nystagmus may be elicited by appropriate stimuli (Table 623-1).

Congenital sensory nystagmus is generally associated with ocular abnormalities that lead to decreased visual acuity; common disorders that lead to early-onset nystagmus include albinism, aniridia, achromatopsia, congenital cataracts, congenital macular lesions, and congenital optic atrophy. In some instances, nystagmus occurs as a dominant or X-linked characteristic without obvious ocular abnormalities.

Congenital idiopathic motor nystagmus is characterized by horizontal jerky oscillations with gaze preponderance; the nystagmus is coarser in one direction of gaze than in the other, with the jerk toward the direction of gaze. There are no ocular anatomic defects that cause the nystagmus, and the visual acuity is generally near normal. There may be a null point in which the nystagmus lessens and the vision improves; a compensatory head posture will develop that places the eyes into the position of least nystagmus. The cause of congenital idiopathic motor nystagmus is unknown; in some instances, it is familial. Eye muscle surgery may be performed to eliminate an abnormal head posture by bringing the point of best vision into straight-ahead gaze.

Acquired nystagmus requires prompt and thorough evaluation. Worrisome pathologic types are the gaze-paretic or gaze-evoked oscillations of cerebellar, brainstem, or cerebral disease.

Nystagmus retractorius or **convergent nystagmus** is repetitive jerking of the eyes into the orbit or toward each other. It is usually seen with vertical gaze palsy as a feature of Parinaud (sylvian aqueduct) syndrome. The causal condition may be neoplastic, vascular, or inflammatory. In children, nystagmus retractorius suggests particularly the presence of pinealoma or hydrocephalus.

A diagnostic approach to nystagmus is noted in Figures 623-7 and 623-8.

Spasmus nutans is a special type of acquired nystagmus in childhood (see also Chapter 597). In its complete form, it is characterized by the **triad** of pendular nystagmus, head nodding, and torticollis. The nystagmus is characteristically very fine, very rapid, horizontal, and pendular; it is often asymmetric, sometimes unilateral. Signs usually develop within the 1st yr or 2 of life. Components of the triad may develop at various times. In many cases, the condition is benign and self-limited, usually lasting a few months, sometimes years. The cause of this classic type of spasmus nutans, which usually resolves spontaneously, is unknown. Some children exhibiting signs resembling those of spasmus nutans have underlying brain tumors, particularly hypothalamic and chiasmal optic gliomas. Appropriate neurologic and neuroradiologic evaluation and careful monitoring of infants and children with nystagmus are therefore recommended.

Table 623-1	Specific Patterns of Nystagmus	
PATTERN	**DESCRIPTION**	**ASSOCIATED CONDITIONS**
Latent nystagmus	Conjugate jerk nystagmus toward viewing eye	Congenital vision defects, occurs with occlusion of eye
Manifest latent nystagmus	Fast jerk to viewing eye	Strabismus, congenital idiopathic nystagmus
Periodic alternating	Cycles of horizontal or horizontal-rotary that change direction	Caused by both visual and neurologic conditions
Seesaw nystagmus	One eye rises and intorts as other eye falls and extorts	Usually associated with optic chiasm defects
Nystagmus retractorius	Eyes jerk back into orbit or toward each other	Caused by pressure on mesencephalic tegmentum (Parinaud syndrome)
Gaze-evoked nystagmus	Jerk nystagmus in direction of gaze	Caused by medications, brainstem lesion, or labyrinthine dysfunction
Gaze-paretic nystagmus	Eyes jerk back to maintain eccentric gaze	Cerebellar disease
Downbeat nystagmus	Fast phase beating downward	Posterior fossa disease, drugs
Upbeat nystagmus	Fast phase beating upward	Brainstem and cerebellar disease; some visual conditions
Vestibular nystagmus	Horizontal-torsional or horizontal jerks	Vestibular system dysfunction
Asymmetric or monocular nystagmus	Pendular vertical nystagmus	Disease of retina and visual pathways
Spasmus nutans	Fine, rapid, pendular nystagmus	Torticollis, head nodding; idiopathic or gliomas of visual pathways

From Kliegman R: Practical strategies in pediatric diagnosis and therapy. Philadelphia, 1996, WB Saunders.

Work-up and treatment as per ocular malformation, tumor, dysgenesis
Yes
? Obvious ocular malformation, tumor
No
Aniridia
Iridocorneal dysgenesis
Congenital cataracts
Congenital glaucoma
Retinoblastoma
Toxoplasmosis
Ocular coloboma
Cicatricial ROP
Bilateral PHPV
Bilateral retinal dysplasia
Macular coloboma
Juvenile retinoschisis
? Asymmetric, rapid, pendular
Yes
⊕ MRI scan
Yes
Neurologic disorder
No
Spasmus nutans
No
? Searching nystagmus
Yes
? ERG flat
Yes
Leber
No
No
Congenital motor efferent or idiopathic nystagmus
Yes
? Vision normal
Yes
? Pendular nystagmus
? Optic nerve pale/small
Yes
⊕ MRI scan
Yes
Neurologic disorder
No
Idiopathic optic nerve disorder
No
Albinism
Yes
? Foveal hypoplasia ± iris transillumination
No
X-linked retinoschisis
Yes
? Macular NFL schisis ⊕ ERG abnormality
No
No
No
Achromatopsia
Yes
? ⊕ Photophobia
? ⊕ Sloan test/⊖ Flicker ERG
No
CSNB
Yes
? Myopia
? ⊖ Rod dark adaptation
⊕ ERG abnormality
No
? Associated with strabismus
Yes
Nystagmus blockage syndrome
Manifest latent nystagmus
No
Congenital motor efferent or idiopathic nystagmus

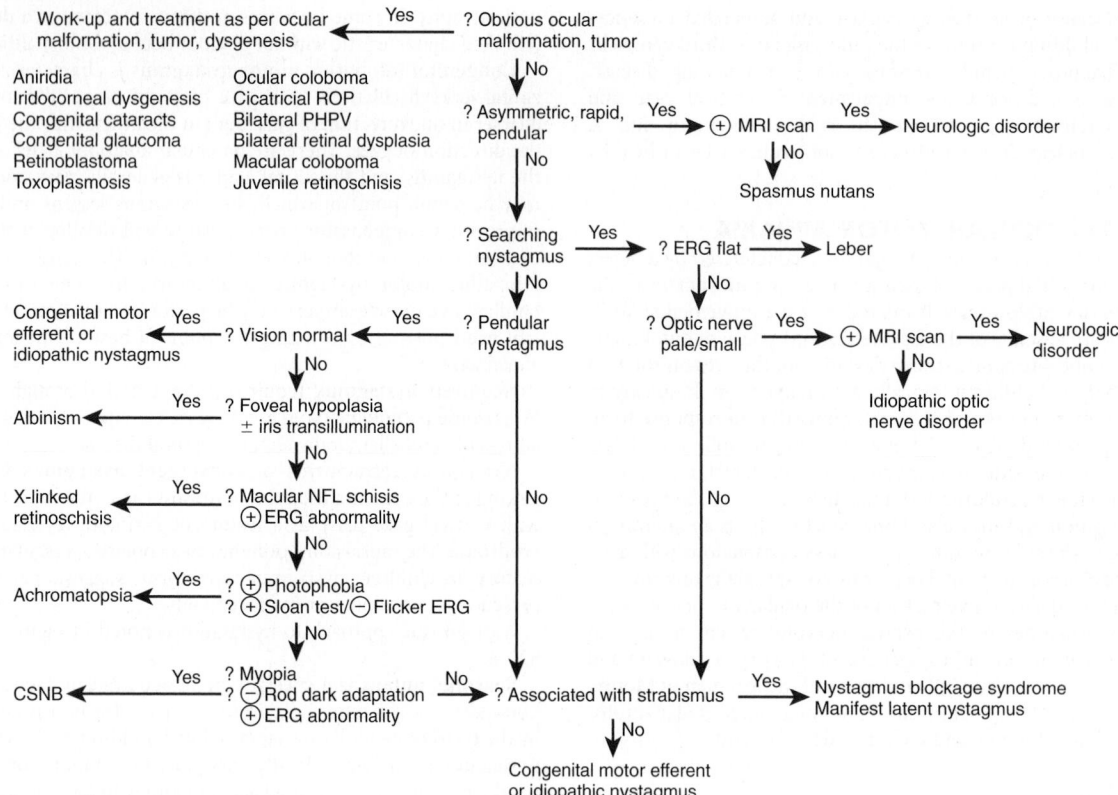

Figure 623-7 Algorithm for the work-up of an infant with nystagmus. ⊕, positive; ⊖, negative; CSNB, congenital stationary night blindness; ERG, electroretinogram; NFL, nerve fiber layer; PHPV, persistent hyperplastic primary vitreous; ROP, retinopathy of prematurity. *(From Nelson LB: Harley's pediatric ophthalmology, ed 4, Philadelphia, 1998, WB Saunders, p. 470.)*

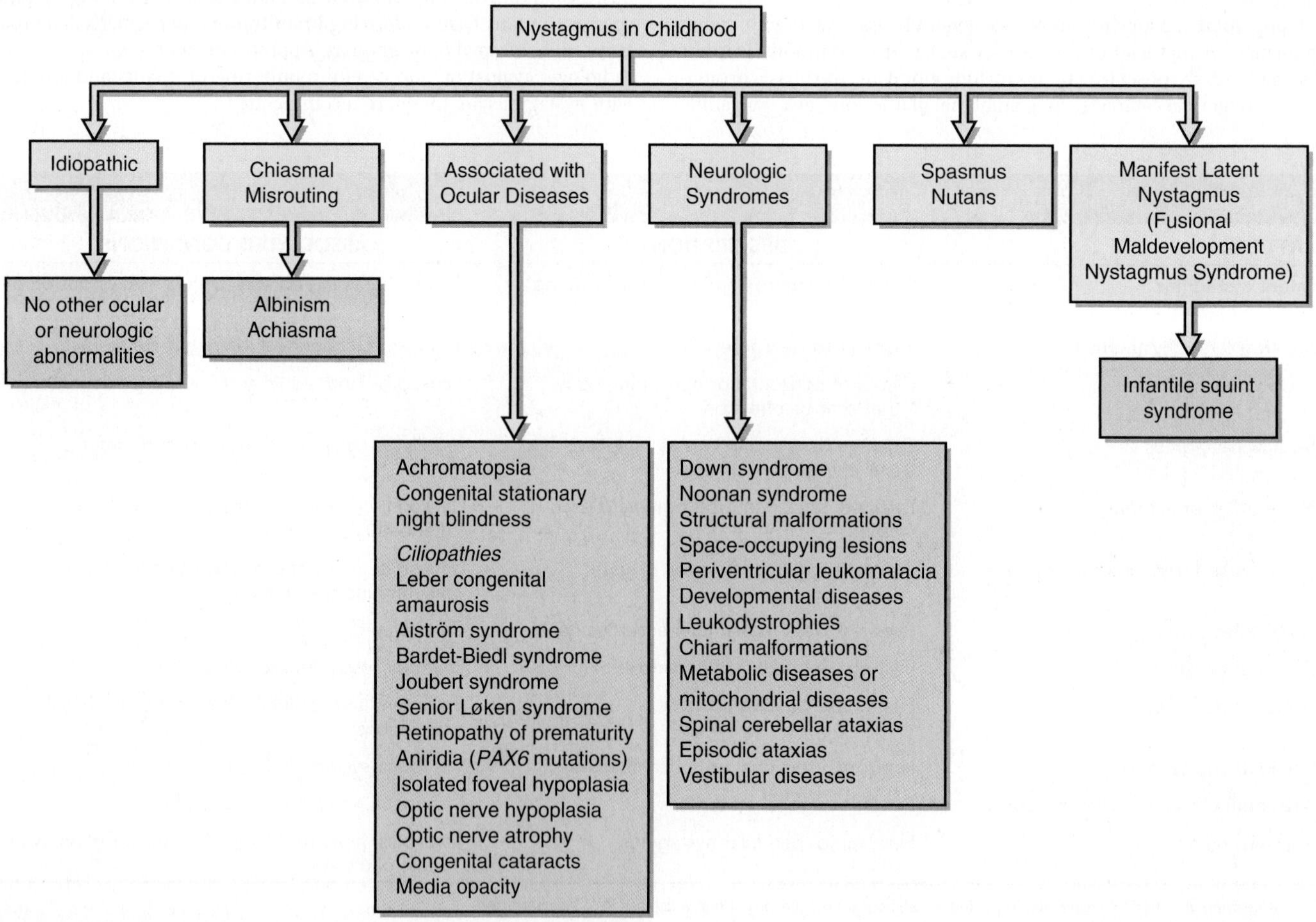

Nystagmus in Childhood
Idiopathic
Chiasmal Misrouting
Associated with Ocular Diseases
Neurologic Syndromes
Spasmus Nutans
Manifest Latent Nystagmus (Fusional Maldevelopment Nystagmus Syndrome)
No other ocular or neurologic abnormalities
Albinism Achiasma
Infantile squint syndrome
Achromatopsia
Congenital stationary night blindness
Ciliopathies
Leber congenital amaurosis
Aiström syndrome
Bardet-Biedl syndrome
Joubert syndrome
Senior Løken syndrome
Retinopathy of prematurity
Aniridia (PAX6 mutations)
Isolated foveal hypoplasia
Optic nerve hypoplasia
Optic nerve atrophy
Congenital cataracts
Media opacity
Down syndrome
Noonan syndrome
Structural malformations
Space-occupying lesions
Periventricular leukomalacia
Developmental diseases
Leukodystrophies
Chiari malformations
Metabolic diseases or mitochondrial diseases
Spinal cerebellar ataxias
Episodic ataxias
Vestibular diseases

Figure 623-8 Classification of nystagmus based on associated diseases. *(From Hoyt CS, Taylor D, editors:* Pediatric ophthalmology and strabismus, *ed 4, Philadelphia, 2013, Elsevier Saunders, Fig. 89.2, p. 910.)*

Table 623-2	Specific Patterns of Nonnystagmus Eye Movements	
PATTERN	**DESCRIPTION**	**ASSOCIATED CONDITIONS**
Opsoclonus	Multidirectional conjugate movements of varying rate and amplitude	Hydrocephalus, diseases of brainstem and cerebellum, neuroblastoma, paraneoplasia syndrome
Ocular dysmetria	Overshoot of eyes on rapid fixation	Cerebellar dysfunction
Ocular flutter	Horizontal oscillations with forward gaze and sometimes with blinking	Cerebellar disease, hydrocephalus, or central nervous system neoplasm
Ocular bobbing	Downward jerk from primary gaze, remains for a few sec, then drifts back	Pontine disease
Ocular myoclonus	Rhythmic to-and-fro pendular oscillations of the eyes, with synchronous nonocular muscle movement	Damage to red nucleus, inferior olivary nucleus, and ipsilateral dentate nucleus

From Kliegman R: Practical strategies in pediatric diagnosis and therapy. Philadelphia, 1996, WB Saunders.

OTHER ABNORMAL EYE MOVEMENTS

To be differentiated from true nystagmus are certain special types of abnormal eye movements, particularly opsoclonus, ocular dysmetria, and flutter (Table 623-2).

Opsoclonus

Opsoclonus and ataxic conjugate movements are spontaneous, non-rhythmic, multidirectional, chaotic movements of the eyes. The eyes appear to be in agitation, with bursts of conjugate movement of varying amplitude in varying directions. Opsoclonus is most often associated with infectious or autoimmune encephalitis. It may be the first sign of neuroblastoma or other tumors producing a paraneoplastic syndrome.

Ocular Motor Dysmetria

This is analogous to dysmetria of the limbs. Affected individuals show a lack of precision in performing movements of refixation, characterized by an overshoot (or undershoot) of the eyes with several corrective to-and-fro oscillations on looking from one point to another. Ocular motor dysmetria is a sign of cerebellar or cerebellar pathway disease.

Flutter-Like Oscillations

These intermittent to-and-fro horizontal oscillations of the eyes may occur spontaneously or on change of fixation. They are characteristic of cerebellar disease.

Bibliography is available at Expert Consult.

Chapter 624

Abnormalities of the Lids

Scott E. Olitsky, Denise Hug,
Laura S. Plummer, Erin D. Stahl,
Michelle M. Ariss, and
Timothy P. Lindquist

PTOSIS

In blepharoptosis, the upper eyelid droops below its normal level. Congenital ptosis is usually a result of a localized dystrophy of the levator muscle in which the striated muscle fibers are replaced with fibrous tissue. The condition may be unilateral or bilateral and can be familial, transmitted as a dominant trait.

Parents often comment that the eye looks smaller because of the drooping eyelid. The lid crease is decreased or absent where the levator muscle would normally insert below the skin surface. Because the levator is replaced by fibrous tissue, the lid does not move downward fully in downgaze (lid lag). If the ptosis is severe, affected children often attempt to raise the lid by lifting their brow or adapting a chin-up head posture to maintain binocular vision. **Marcus Gunn jaw-winking ptosis** accounts for 5% of ptoses in children. In this syndrome, an abnormal synkinesis exists between the 5th and 3rd cranial nerves; this causes the eyelid to elevate with movement of the jaw. The wink is produced by chewing or sucking and may be more noticeable than the ptosis itself.

Although ptosis in children is often an isolated finding, it may occur in association with other ocular or systemic disorders. Systemic disorders include myasthenia gravis, muscular dystrophy, and botulism. Ocular disorders include mechanical ptosis secondary to lid tumors, blepharophimosis syndrome, congenital fibrosis syndrome, combined levator/superior rectus maldevelopment, and congenital or acquired 3rd nerve palsy. A small degree of ptosis is seen in Horner syndrome (see Chapter 622). A complete ophthalmic and systemic examination is therefore important in the evaluation of a child with ptosis.

Amblyopia may occur in children with ptosis. The amblyopia may be secondary to the lid's covering the visual axis (deprivation) or induced astigmatism (anisometropia). When amblyopia occurs, it should generally be treated before treating the ptosis.

Treatment of ptosis in a child is indicated for elimination of an abnormal head posture, improvement in the visual field, prevention of amblyopia, and restoration of a normal eyelid appearance. The timing of surgery depends on the degree of ptosis, its cosmetic and functional severity, the presence or absence of compensatory posturing, the wishes of the parents, and the discretion of the surgeon. Surgical treatment is determined by the amount of levator function that is present. A levator resection may be used in children with moderate to good function. In patients with poor or absent function, a frontalis suspension procedure may be necessary. This technique requires that a suspension material be placed between the frontalis muscle and the tarsus of the eyelid. It allows patients to use their brow and frontalis muscle more effectively to raise their eyelid. Amblyopia remains a concern even after surgical correction and should be monitored closely.

EPICANTHAL FOLDS

These vertical or oblique folds of skin extend on either side of the bridge of the nose from the brow or lid area, covering the inner canthal region. They are present to some degree in most young children and become less apparent with age. The folds may be sufficiently broad to cover the medial aspect of the eye, making the eyes appear crossed (pseudoesotropia). Epicanthal folds are a common feature of many syndromes, including chromosomal aberrations (trisomies) and disorders of single genes.

LAGOPHTHALMOS

This is a condition in which complete closure of the lids over the globe is difficult or impossible. It may be paralytic because of a facial palsy involving the orbicularis muscle, or spastic, as in thyrotoxicosis. It may be structural when retraction or shortening of the lids results from scarring or atrophy consequent to injury (burns) or disease. For example, children with various craniosynostosis syndromes can have problematic lagophthalmos. Infants with collodion membrane may have temporary lagophthalmos caused by the restrictive effect of the membrane on the lids. Lagophthalmos may accompany proptosis or buphthalmos (enlarged cornea because of elevated intraocular pressure) when the lids, although normal, cannot effectively cover the enlarged or protuberant eye. A degree of physiologic lagophthalmos may occur normally during sleep, but functional lagophthalmos in an unconscious or debilitated patient can be a problem.

In patients with lagophthalmos, exposure of the eye may lead to drying, infection, corneal ulceration, or perforation of the cornea; the result may be loss of vision, even loss of the eye. In lagophthalmos, protection of the eye by artificial tear preparations, ophthalmic ointment, or moisture chambers is essential. Gauze pads are to be avoided because the gauze may abrade the cornea. In some cases, surgical closure of the lids (tarsorrhaphy) may be necessary for long-term protection of the eye.

LID RETRACTIONS
Pathologic retraction of the lid may be myogenic or neurogenic. Myogenic retraction of the upper lid occurs in thyrotoxicosis, in which it is associated with 3 classic signs: a staring appearance (Dalrymple sign), infrequent blinking (Stellwag sign), and lag of the upper lid on downward gaze (von Graefe sign).

Neurogenic retraction of the lids may occur in conditions affecting the anterior mesencephalon. Lid retraction is a feature of the syndrome of the sylvian aqueduct. In children, it is commonly a sign of hydrocephalus. It may occur with meningitis. Paradoxical retraction of the lid is seen in the Marcus Gunn jaw-winking syndrome. It may also be seen with attempted eye movement after recovery from a 3rd nerve palsy, if aberrant regeneration of the oculomotor nerve fibers has occurred.

Simple staring and the physiologic or reflexive lid retraction ("eye popping"), in contrast to pathologic lid retractions, occur in infants in response to a sudden reduction in illumination or as a startle reaction.

ECTROPION, ENTROPION, AND EPIBLEPHARON
Ectropion is eversion of the lid margin; it may lead to overflow of tears (epiphora) and subsequent maceration of the skin of the lid, inflammation of exposed conjunctiva, or superficial exposure keratopathy. Common causes are scarring consequent to inflammation, burns, or trauma and weakness of the orbicularis muscle as a result of facial palsy; these forms may be corrected surgically. Protection of the cornea is essential. Ectropion is also seen in certain children who have faulty development of the lateral canthal ligament; this may occur in Down syndrome.

Entropion is inversion of the lid margin, which may cause discomfort and corneal damage because of the inward turning of the lashes (trichiasis). A principal cause is scarring secondary to inflammation such as occurs in trachoma or as a sequela of Stevens-Johnson syndrome. There is also a rare congenital form. Surgical correction is effective in many cases.

Epiblepharon is commonly seen in childhood and may be confused with entropion. In epiblepharon, a roll of skin beneath the lower eyelid lashes causes the lashes to be directed vertically and to touch the cornea (Fig. 624-1). Unlike entropion, the eyelid margin itself is not rotated toward the cornea. Epiblepharon usually resolves spontaneously. If corneal scarring begins to occur, surgical correction may be necessary.

BLEPHAROSPASM
This spastic or repetitive closure of the lids may be caused by irritative disease of the cornea, conjunctiva, or facial nerve; fatigue or uncorrected refractive error; or common tic. Thorough ophthalmic examina-

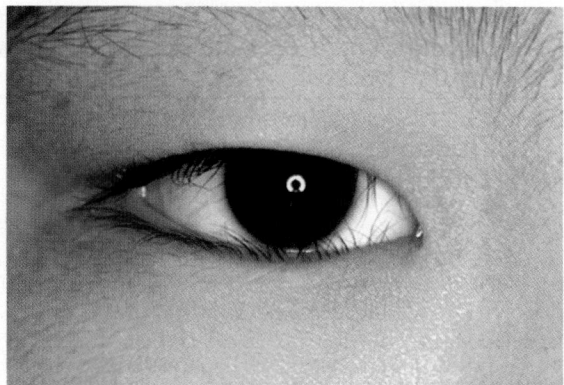

Figure 624-1 Epiblepharon.

tion for pathologic causes, such as trichiasis, keratitis, conjunctivitis, or foreign body, is indicated. Local injection of botulinum toxin may give relief, but frequently must be repeated.

BLEPHARITIS
This inflammation of the lid margins is characterized by erythema and crusting or scaling; the usual symptoms are irritation, burning, and itching. The condition is commonly bilateral and chronic or recurrent. The 2 main types are **staphylococcal** and **seborrheic.** In staphylococcal blepharitis, ulceration of the lid margin is common, the lashes tend to fall out, and conjunctivitis and superficial keratitis are often associated. In seborrheic blepharitis, the scales tend to be greasy, the lid margins are less red, and ulceration usually does not occur. The blepharitis is often of mixed type.

Thorough daily cleansing of the lid margins with a cloth or moistened cotton applicator to remove scales and crusts is important in the **treatment** of both forms. Staphylococcal blepharitis is treated with an antistaphylococcal antibiotic applied directly to the lid margins. When a child also has seborrhea, concurrent treatment of the scalp is important.

Pediculosis of the eyelashes may produce a clinical picture of blepharitis. The lice can be smothered with ophthalmic-grade petrolatum ointment applied to the lid margin and lashes. Nits should be mechanically removed from the lashes. It should be remembered that pediculosis can represent a sexually transmitted disease. Molluscum virus involvement of the lids can also cause blepharitis.

HORDEOLUM (STYE)
Infection of the glands of the lid may be acute or subacute; tender focal swelling and redness are noted. The usual agent is *Staphylococcus aureus*. When the meibomian glands are involved, the lesion is referred to as an internal hordeolum; the abscess tends to be large and may point through either the skin or the conjunctival surface. When the infection involves the glands of Zeis or Moll, the abscess tends to be smaller and more superficial and points at the lid margin; it is then referred to as an external hordeolum or stye.

Treatment is frequent warm compresses and, if necessary, surgical incision and drainage. In addition, topical antibiotic preparations are often used. Untreated, the infection may progress to cellulitis of the lid or orbit, requiring the use of systemic antibiotics.

CHALAZION
A chalazion is a granulomatous inflammation of a meibomian gland characterized by a firm, nontender nodule in the upper or lower lid. This lesion tends to be chronic and differs from internal hordeolum in the absence of acute inflammatory signs. Although many chalazia subside spontaneously, excision may be necessary if they become large enough to distort vision (by inducing astigmatism by exerting pressure on the globe) or to be a cosmetic blemish. Patients who experience frequent chalazia formation, or those who have significant corneal changes secondary to the underlying blepharitis,

may benefit from systemic, low-dose erythromycin or azithromycin treatment.

COLOBOMA OF THE EYELID

This cleft-like deformity may vary from a small indentation or notch of the free margin of the lid to a large defect involving almost the entire lid. If the gap is extensive, ulceration and corneal opacities may result from exposure. Early surgical correction of the lid defect is recommended. Other deformities frequently associated with lid colobomas include dermoid cysts or dermolipomas on the globe; they often occur in a position corresponding to the site of the lid defect. Lid colobomas may also be associated with extensive facial malformation, as in mandibulofacial dysostosis (Franceschetti or Treacher Collins syndrome).

TUMORS OF THE LID

A number of lid tumors arise from surface structures (the epithelium and sebaceous glands). Nevi may appear in early childhood; most are junctional. Compound nevi tend to develop in the prepubertal years and dermal nevi at puberty. Malignant epithelial tumors (basal cell carcinoma, squamous cell carcinoma) are rare in children, but the basal cell nevus syndrome and the malignant lesions of xeroderma pigmentosum and of Rothmund-Thomson syndrome may develop in childhood.

Other lid tumors arise from deeper structures (the neural, vascular, and connective tissues). Capillary hemangiomas are especially common in children (Fig. 624-2). Many tend to regress spontaneously, although they may show alarmingly rapid growth in infancy. In many cases, the best management of such hemangiomas is patient observation, allowing spontaneous regression to occur (see Chapter 650). In the case of a rapidly expanding lesion, which may cause amblyopia by obstructing the visual axis or inducing astigmatism, corticosteroid, interferon, or surgical treatment should be considered. Systemic propranolol has been shown to be an effective treatment without the risks associated with corticosteroid use. Other treatment options include corticosteroids, systemically or by direct injection, and surgical excision. Nevus flammeus (port-wine stain), a noninvoluting hemangioma, occurs as an isolated lesion or in association with other signs of Sturge-Weber syndrome. Affected patients should be monitored for the development of glaucoma. Lymphangiomas of the lid appear as firm masses at or soon after birth and tend to enlarge slowly during the growing years. Associated conjunctival involvement, appearing as a clear, cystic, sinuous conjunctival mass, may provide a clue to the diagnosis. In some cases, there is also orbital involvement. The **treatment** is surgical excision.

Plexiform neuromas of the lids occur in children with neurofibromatosis, often with ptosis as the first sign. The lid may take on an S-shaped configuration. The lids may also be involved by other tumors, such as retinoblastoma, neuroblastoma, and rhabdomyosarcoma of the orbit; these conditions are discussed elsewhere.

Bibliography is available at Expert Consult.

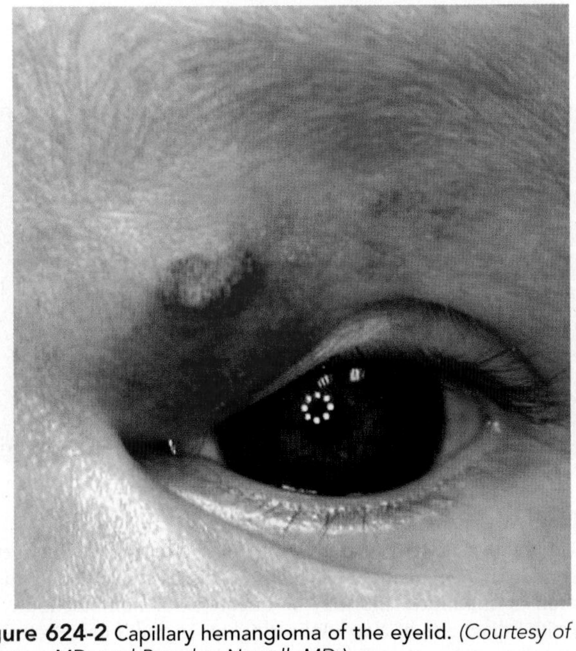

Chapter **625**
Disorders of the Lacrimal System

Scott E. Olitsky, Denise Hug, Laura S. Plummer, Erin D. Stahl, Michelle M. Ariss, and Timothy P. Lindquist

THE TEAR FILM

This film, which bathes the eye, is actually a complex structure composed of 3 layers. The innermost mucin layer is secreted by the goblet and epithelial cells of the conjunctiva and the acinar cells of the lacrimal gland. It adds stability and provides an attachment for the tear film to the conjunctiva and cornea. The middle aqueous layer constitutes 98% of the tear film and is produced by the main lacrimal gland and accessory lacrimal glands. It contains various electrolytes and proteins as well as antibodies. The outermost lipid layer is produced largely from the sebaceous meibomian glands of the eyelid and retards evaporation of the tear film. Tears drain medially into the punctal openings of the lid margin and flow through the canaliculi into the lacrimal sac and then through the nasolacrimal duct into the nose (Fig. 625-1). Preterm infants have reduced tear secretion. This may mask the diagnosis of a nasolacrimal duct obstruction and concentrate topically applied medications. Tear production reaches adult levels near term.

Figure 624-2 Capillary hemangioma of the eyelid. *(Courtesy of Amy Nopper, MD, and Brandon Newell, MD.)*

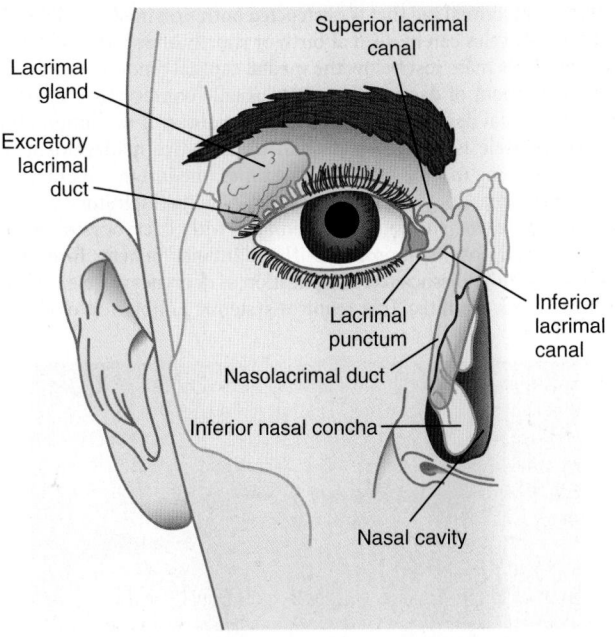

Figure 625-1 The lacrimal apparatus.

DACRYOSTENOSIS

Congenital nasolacrimal duct obstruction (CNLDO), or dacryostenosis, is the most common disorder of the lacrimal system, occurring in up to 20% of newborn infants. It is usually caused by a failure of canalization of the epithelial cells that form the nasolacrimal duct as it enters the nose (valve of Hasner). Signs of CNLDO may be present at the time of birth, although the condition may not become evident until normal tear production develops. Signs of CNLDO include an excessive tear lake, overflow of tears onto the lid and cheek, and reflux of mucoid material that is produced in the lacrimal sac. Erythema or maceration of the skin may result from irritation and rubbing produced by dripping of tears and discharge. If the blockage is complete, these signs may be severe and continuous. If obstruction is only partial, the nasolacrimal duct may be capable of draining the basal tear film that is produced. However, under periods of increased tear production (exposure to cold, wind, sunlight) or increased closure of the distal end of the nasolacrimal duct (nasal mucosal edema), tear overflow may become evident or may increase.

Infants at increased risk for CNLDO include those with trisomy 21, EEC (ectrodactyly, ectodermal dysplasia, clefting) syndrome, branchiooculofacial syndrome, craniometaphyseal or craniodiaphyseal dysplasias, LADD (lacrimo-auriculo-dento-digital) syndrome, CHARGE (coloboma, heart anomaly, choanal atresia, retardation, genital and ear anomalies) syndrome, and Goldenhar syndrome.

Infants with CNLDO may develop acute infection and inflammation of the nasolacrimal sac (**dacryocystitis**), inflammation of the surrounding tissues (**pericystitis**), or, rarely, periorbital cellulitis. With dacryocystitis, the sac area is swollen, red, and tender, and patients may have systemic signs of infection such as fever and irritability.

The primary **treatment** of uncomplicated nasolacrimal duct obstruction is a regimen of nasolacrimal massage, usually 2-3 times daily, accompanied by cleansing of the lids with warm water. Topical antibiotics are used for control of mucopurulent drainage. A bland ophthalmic ointment may be used on eyelids if the skin is macerated. Most cases of CNLDO resolve spontaneously; 96% before 1 yr of age. For cases that do not resolve by 1 yr, the nasolacrimal duct may be probed in the office with topical anesthesia, with a cure rate of approximately 80%. Some ophthalmologists intubate the nasolacrimal system at the same time as this has been shown to improve the outcome of the procedure.

Acute dacryocystitis or cellulitis requires prompt treatment with systemic antibiotics. In such cases, some form of definitive surgical intervention is usually indicated.

A **dacryocystocele** (mucocele) is an unusual presentation of a non-patent nasolacrimal sac that is obstructed both proximally and distally. Dacryocystoceles can be seen at birth or shortly after birth as a bluish subcutaneous mass just below the medial canthal tendon (Fig. 625-2). Initial treatment of dacryocystocele is usually conservative, involving massage/digital decompression of the lacrimal sac. If resolution of the dacryocystocele is not achieved with conservative management, the surgical probing may be beneficial. At times, the intranasal portion of the nasolacrimal duct becomes distended, causing respiratory compromise. In a recent study, 9.5% of infants with dacryocystocele had related respiratory compromise. These infants benefit from early probing. Another associated complication of dacryocystocele is that of dacryocystitis/cellulitis. This requires systemic antibiotics, often with

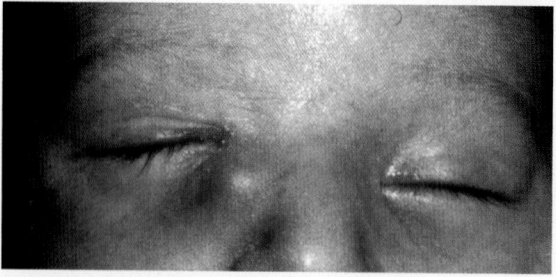

Figure 625-2 Dacryocystocele below inner canthus of the right eye.

hospitalization. In the aforementioned study, 65% of infants with dacryocystocele developed dacryocystitis/cellulitis. Once the cellulitis has improved, the nasolacrimal system should be probed if spontaneous resolution has not occurred.

Not all tearing in infants and children is caused by nasolacrimal obstruction. Tearing may also be a sign of glaucoma, intraocular inflammation, or external irritation, such as that from a corneal abrasion or foreign body.

ALACRIMA AND "DRY EYE"

Alacrima refers to a wide spectrum of disorders with reduced or absent tear secretion. Occasionally, normal basal tearing occurs with an absence of emotional tearing. Etiologies can be divided into syndromes that have a pathologic association or are inherited. Associated syndromes include familial dysautonomia (Riley-Day syndrome), anhidrotic ectodermal dysplasia, and triple-A syndrome (Allgrove syndrome). Examples of pathologic association include aplasia of cranial nerve nuclei and lacrimal gland aplasia/hypoplasia. Both autosomal recessive and autosomal dominant inheritance has been reported in isolated congenital alacrima. In addition, medications with anticholinergic side effects can decrease tear production. The patients with alacrima have variable presentation including no symptoms, photophobia, foreign body sensation, eye pain, and decreased vision. The symptoms, if present, often occur early in life. Because the dryness can be severe, damage to the cornea and subsequent loss of vision may occur. The goal of treatment is to minimize corneal irritation, corneal scarring, and loss of vision. Aggressive ocular lubrication is used to prevent these sequelae.

An acquired abnormality of any layer of the tear film may produce a dry eye. Commonly acquired disorders that may lead to a decreased or unstable tear film include Sjögren syndrome, Stevens-Johnson syndrome, toxic epidermal necrolysis, vitamin A deficiency, viral infections of the lacrimal gland, ocular pemphigoid, trachoma, chemical burns, irradiation, isotretinoin treatment of acne, graft-versus-host disease, and meibomian gland dysfunction. Exposure as a consequence of poor lid closure or other pathologic states can quickly lead to pathologically dry eyes. Examples of conditions leading to such exposure include ichthyosis, xeroderma pigmentosum, and certain craniosynostoses syndromes such as Crouzon, Apert, or Pfeiffer. Any tear deficiency can lead to corneal ulceration, scarring, or infection. **Treatment** includes correction of the underlying disorder when possible and frequent instillation of an ocular lubricant. In some cases, occlusion of the lacrimal puncta is helpful. In severe cases, tarsorrhaphy may be necessary to protect the cornea.

Bibliography is available at Expert Consult.

Chapter **626**
Disorders of the Conjunctiva

*Scott E. Olitsky, Denise Hug,
Laura S. Plummer, Erin D. Stahl,
Michelle M. Ariss, and
Timothy P. Lindquist*

CONJUNCTIVITIS

The conjunctiva reacts to a wide range of bacterial and viral agents, allergens, irritants, toxins, and systemic diseases. Conjunctivitis is common in childhood and may be infectious or noninfectious. The differential diagnosis of a red-appearing eye includes conjunctival as well as other ocular sites (Table 626-1).

Table 626-1	The Red Eye		
CONDITION	**ETIOLOGY**	**SIGNS AND SYMPTOMS**	**TREATMENT**
Bacterial conjunctivitis	*Haemophilus influenzae, Haemophilus aegyptius, Streptococcus pneumoniae, Staphylococcus aureus, Moraxella catarrhalis*	Mucopurulent unilateral or bilateral discharge, normal vision, photophobia	Topical antibiotics, parenteral ceftriaxone for gonococcus, *H. influenzae*
Hyperacute bacterial conjunctivitis	*Neisseria gonorrhoeae, Neisseria meningitides*	Conjunctival injection and edema (chemosis); gritty sensation	
Viral conjunctivitis	Adenovirus, ECHO virus, coxsackievirus, herpes simplex virus	As above; may be hemorrhagic, unilateral	Self-limited
Neonatal conjunctivitis	*Chlamydia trachomatis,* gonococcus, chemical (silver nitrate), *S. aureus*	Palpebral conjunctival follicle or papillae; as above	Ceftriaxone for gonococcus and erythromycin for *C. trachomatis*
Allergic conjunctivitis	Seasonal pollens or allergen exposure	Itching, incidence of bilateral chemosis (edema) greater than that of erythema, tarsal papillae	Antihistamines, topical mast cell stabilizers or prostaglandin inhibitors, steroids
Keratitis	Herpes simplex virus, adenovirus, *S. pneumoniae, S. aureus, Pseudomonas, Acanthamoeba,* chemicals	Severe pain, corneal swelling, clouding, limbus erythema, hypopyon, cataracts; contact lens history with amebic infection	Specific antibiotics for bacterial/ fungal infections; keratoplasty, acyclovir for herpes
Endophthalmitis	*S. aureus, S. pneumoniae, Candida albicans,* associated surgery or trauma	Acute onset, pain, loss of vision, swelling, chemosis, redness; hypopyon and vitreous haze	Antibiotics
Anterior uveitis (iridocyclitis)	JIA, postinfectious with arthritis and rash, sarcoidosis, Behçet disease, Kawasaki disease, inflammatory bowel disease	Unilateral/bilateral; erythema, ciliary flush, irregular pupil, iris adhesions; pain, photophobia, small pupil, poor vision	Topical steroids, plus therapy for primary disease
Posterior uveitis (choroiditis)	Toxoplasmosis, histoplasmosis, *Toxocara canis*	No signs of erythema, decreased vision	Specific therapy for pathogen
Episcleritis/scleritis	Idiopathic autoimmune disease (e.g., SLE, Henoch-Schönlein purpura)	Localized pain, intense erythema, unilateral; blood vessels bigger than in conjunctivitis; scleritis may cause globe perforation	Episcleritis is self-limiting; topical steroids for fast relief
Foreign body	Occupational exposure	Unilateral, red, gritty feeling; visible or microscopic size	Irrigation, removal; check for ulceration
Blepharitis	*S. aureus, Staphylococcus epidermidis,* seborrheic, blocked lacrimal duct; rarely molluscum contagiosum, *Phthirus pubis, Pediculus capitis*	Bilateral, irritation, itching, hyperemia, crusting, affecting lid margins	Topical antibiotics, warm compresses, lid hygiene
Dacryocystitis	Obstructed lacrimal sac: *S. aureus, H. influenzae,* pneumococcus	Pain, tenderness, erythema, and exudates in area of lacrimal sac (inferomedial to inner canthus); tearing (epiphora); possible orbital cellulitis	Systemic, topical antibiotics; surgical drainage
Dacryoadenitis	*S. aureus, Streptococcus,* CMV, measles, EBV, enteroviruses; trauma, sarcoidosis, leukemia	Pain, tenderness, edema, erythema over gland area (upper temporal lid); fever, leukocytosis	Systemic antibiotics; drainage of orbital abscesses
Orbital cellulitis (postseptal cellulitis)	Paranasal sinusitis: *H. influenzae, S. aureus, S. pneumoniae,* streptococci Trauma: *S. aureus* Fungi: *Aspergillus, Mucor* spp. if immunodeficient	Rhinorrhea, chemosis, vision loss, painful extraocular motion, proptosis, ophthalmoplegia, fever, lid edema, leukocytosis	Systemic antibiotics, drainage of orbital abscesses
Periorbital cellulitis (preseptal cellulitis)	Trauma: *S. aureus,* streptococci Bacteremia: pneumococcus, streptococci, *H. influenzae, S. aureus*	Cutaneous erythema, warmth, normal vision, minimal involvement of orbit; fever, leukocytosis, toxic appearance	Systemic antibiotics

CMV, cytomegalovirus; EBV, Epstein-Barr virus; JIA, juvenile idiopathic arthritis; SLE, systemic lupus erythematosus.
From Behrman R, Kliegman R: Nelson's essentials of pediatrics, *ed 3, Philadelphia, 1998, WB Saunders.*

Ophthalmia Neonatorum

This form of conjunctivitis, occurring in infants younger than 4 wk of age, is the most common eye disease of newborns. Its many different causal agents vary greatly in their virulence and outcome. Silver nitrate instillation may result in a mild self-limited chemical conjunctivitis, whereas *Neisseria gonorrhoeae* and *Pseudomonas* are capable of causing corneal perforation, blindness, and death. The risk of conjunctivitis in newborns depends on frequencies of maternal infections, prophylactic measures, circumstances during labor and delivery, and postdelivery exposure to microorganisms.

Epidemiology

Conjunctivitis during the neonatal period is usually acquired during vaginal delivery and reflects the sexually transmitted infections prevalent in the community. In 1880, 10% of European children developed gonococcal conjunctivitis at birth. Ophthalmia neonatorum was the leading cause of blindness during that period. The epidemiology of this condition changed dramatically in 1881, when Crede reported that 2% silver nitrate solution instilled in the eyes of newborns reduced the incidence of gonococcal ophthalmia from 10% to 0.3%.

During the 20th century, the incidence of gonococcal ophthalmia neonatorum decreased in industrialized countries secondary to widespread use of silver nitrate prophylaxis and prenatal screening and treatment of maternal gonorrhea. Gonococcal ophthalmia neonatorum has an incidence of 0.3/1,000 live births in the United States. In comparison, *Chlamydia trachomatis* is the most common organism causing ophthalmia neonatorum in the United States, with an incidence of 8.2/1,000 births.

Clinical Manifestations

The clinical manifestations of the various forms of ophthalmia neonatorum are not specific enough to allow an accurate diagnosis. Although the timing and character of the signs are somewhat typical for each cause of this condition, there is considerable overlap and physicians should not rely solely on clinical findings. Regardless of its cause, ophthalmia neonatorum is characterized by redness and chemosis (swelling) of the conjunctiva, edema of the eyelids, and discharge, which may be purulent.

Neonatal conjunctivitis is a potentially blinding condition. The infection may also have associated systemic manifestations that require treatment. Therefore, any newborn infant who develops signs of conjunctivitis needs a prompt and comprehensive systemic and ocular evaluation to determine the agent causing the infection and the appropriate treatment.

The onset of inflammation caused by silver nitrate drops usually occurs within 6-12 hr after birth, with clearing by 24-48 hr. The usual incubation period for conjunctivitis caused by *N. gonorrhoeae* is 2-5 days, and for that caused by *C. trachomatis,* 5-14 days. Gonococcal infection may be present at birth or be delayed beyond 5 days of life owing to partial suppression by ocular prophylaxis. Gonococcal conjunctivitis may also begin in infancy after inoculation by the contaminated fingers of adults. The time of onset of disease with other bacteria is highly variable.

Gonococcal conjunctivitis begins with mild inflammation and a serosanguineous discharge. Within 24 hr, the discharge becomes thick and purulent, and tense edema of the eyelids with marked chemosis occurs. If proper treatment is delayed, the infection may spread to involve the deeper layers of the conjunctivae and the cornea. Complications include corneal ulceration and perforation, iridocyclitis, anterior synechiae, and rarely panophthalmitis. Conjunctivitis caused by *C. trachomatis* (inclusion blennorrhea) may vary from mild inflammation to severe swelling of the eyelids with copious purulent discharge. The process involves mainly the tarsal conjunctivae; the corneas are rarely affected. Conjunctivitis caused by *Staphylococcus aureus* or other organisms is similar to that produced by *C. trachomatis*. Conjunctivitis caused by *Pseudomonas aeruginosa* is uncommon, acquired in the nursery, and a potentially serious process. It is characterized by the appearance on days 5-18 of edema, erythema of the lids, purulent discharge, pannus formation, endophthalmitis, sepsis, shock, and death.

Diagnosis

Conjunctivitis appearing after 48 hr should be evaluated for a possibly infectious cause. Gram stain of the purulent discharge should be performed and the material cultured. If a viral cause is suspected, a swab should be submitted in tissue culture media for virus isolation. In chlamydial conjunctivitis, the diagnosis is made by examining Giemsa-stained epithelial cells scraped from the tarsal conjunctivae for the characteristic intracytoplasmic inclusions, by isolating the organisms from a conjunctival swab using special tissue culture techniques, by immunofluorescent staining of conjunctival scrapings for chlamydial inclusions, or by tests for chlamydial antigen or DNA. The differential diagnosis of ophthalmia neonatorum includes dacryocystitis caused by congenital nasolacrimal duct obstruction with lacrimal sac distention (dacryocystocele; see Chapter 625).

Treatment

Treatment of infants in whom gonococcal ophthalmia is suspected and the Gram stain shows the characteristic intracellular Gram-negative diplococci should be initiated immediately with ceftriaxone, 50 mg/kg/24 hr for 1 dose, not to exceed 125 mg. The eye should also be irrigated initially with saline every 10-30 min, gradually increasing to 2-hr intervals until the purulent discharge has cleared. An alternative regimen includes cefotaxime (100 mg/kg/24 hr given IV or IM every 12 hr for 7 days or 100 mg/kg as a single dose). Treatment is extended if sepsis or other extraocular sites are involved (meningitis, arthritis). Neonatal conjunctivitis secondary to chlamydial infections is treated with oral erythromycin (50 mg/kg/24 hr in 4 divided doses) for 2 wk. This cures conjunctivitis and may prevent subsequent chlamydial pneumonia. *Pseudomonas* neonatal conjunctivitis is treated with systemic antibiotics, including an aminoglycoside, plus local saline irrigation and gentamicin ophthalmic ointment. Staphylococcal conjunctivitis is treated with parenteral methicillin and local saline irrigation.

Prognosis and Prevention

Before the institution of topical ophthalmic prophylaxis at birth, gonococcal ophthalmia was a common cause of blindness or permanent eye damage. If properly applied, this form of prophylaxis is highly effective unless infection is present at birth. Drops of 0.5% erythromycin or 1% silver nitrate are instilled directly into the open eyes at birth using wax or plastic single-dose containers. Saline irrigation after silver nitrate application is unnecessary. Silver nitrate is ineffective against active infection and may have limited use against *Chlamydia*. Povidone-iodine (2% solution) may also be an effective prophylactic agent, especially in developing countries.

Identification of maternal gonococcal infection and appropriate treatment has become a standard element of routine prenatal care. An infant born to a woman who has untreated gonococcal infection should receive a single dose of ceftriaxone, 50 mg/kg (maximum 125 mg) IV or IM, in addition to topical prophylaxis. The dose should be reduced for premature infants. Penicillin (50,000 units) should be used if the mother's gonococcal isolate is known to be penicillin sensitive.

Neither topical prophylaxis nor topical treatment prevents the afebrile pneumonia that occurs in 10-20% of infants exposed to *C. trachomatis*. Although chlamydial conjunctivitis is often a self-limiting disease, chlamydial pneumonia may have serious consequences. It is important that infants with chlamydial disease receive systemic treatment. Treatment of colonized pregnant women with erythromycin may prevent neonatal disease.

Acute Purulent Conjunctivitis

This is characterized by more or less generalized (bilateral in 50-75%) conjunctival hyperemia, edema, mucopurulent exudate, glued eyes (lids stuck together after sleeping), and various degrees of ocular pain and discomfort. It is usually a result of bacterial infection. In addition, there is usually little or no pruritus or periauricular lymph node enlargement; the peak season is between December and April. Bacterial conjunctivitis is more common in young children (<5 yr), whereas viral conjunctivitis is more common among adults. The most frequent causes are nontypeable *Haemophilus influenzae* (60-80%) (associated

Table 626-2	Topical Antibiotics Used to Treat Bacterial Conjunctivitis: Adult Dosages
DRUG	**DOSAGE**
Bacitracin (AK-Tracin, Bacticin) ointment	Apply 0.5 inch in eye q3-4h
Ciprofloxacin (Ciloxan) 0.3% ophthalmic solution	1-2 gtt in eye q15min × 6h, then q30min × 18h, then q1h × 1 day, then q4h × 12 days*
Gatifloxacin (Zymar) 0.3% ophthalmic solution	1 gt in eye q2h up to 8 × per day × 2 days, then 1 gt qid × 5 days
Gentamicin (Gentak, Gentasol) 0.3% ophthalmic solution or ointment	Ointment: 0.5 inch applied to eye 2-3 × per day Solution: 1-2 gtt in eye q4h
Levofloxacin (Quixin) 0.5% ophthalmic solution	1-2 gtt in eye q2h × 2 days while awake, then q4h × 5 days while awake
Moxifloxacin (Vigamox) 0.5% ophthalmic solution	1 gt in eye tid × 7 days
Neomycin/polymyxin B/gramicidin (Neosporin) ophthalmic solution	1-2 gtt in eye q4h × 7-10 days
Ofloxacin (Ocuflox) 0.3% ophthalmic solution	1-2 gtt in eye q2-4h × 2 days, then 1-2 gtt in eye qid × 5 days
Polymyxin B and trimethoprim (Polytrim) ophthalmic solution	1 gt in eye q3h × 7-10 days
Sulfacetamide (Isopto Cetamide, Ocusulf-10, Sodium Sulamyd, Sulf-10, AK-Sulf) 10% ophthalmic solution, ointment	Ointment: 0.5-inch ribbon in eye q3-4h and qhs × 7 days Solution: 1-2 gtt in eye q2-3h × 7-10 days
Tobramycin (AK-Tob, Tobrex) 0.3% ophthalmic solution	1-2 gtt in eye q4h

*Exceeds dosage recommended by the manufacturer.
From: Bope ET, Kellerman RD, editors: Conn's current therapy, Philadelphia, 2014, Elsevier/Saunders, Table 2, p. 321.

with ipsilateral otitis media), pneumococci (20%), and staphylococci (5-10%). Bacterial purulent conjunctivitis, especially that caused by pneumococcus or *H. influenzae,* may occur in epidemics. Conjunctival smear and culture are helpful in differentiating specific types. These common forms of acute purulent conjunctivitis usually respond well to warm compresses and topical instillation of antibiotic drops, which shortens the duration of illness and hastens return to school. Topical antibiotics include aminoglycosides (gentamicin, tobramycin), quinolones (ciprofloxacin, ofloxacin, moxifloxacin), and combinations of antibiotics and chloramphenicol (Table 626-2). Brazilian purpuric fever caused by *Haemophilus aegyptius* manifests as conjunctivitis and sepsis. **Hyperacute bacterial conjunctivitis** is caused by gonococcal or meningococcal infection and requires systemic, not topical, antimicrobial therapies. Concerning symptoms that should require an ophthalmology referral include vision loss, severe purulent discharge, corneal involvement, conjunctival scarring, cutaneous-conjunctival involvement (Stevens-Johnson syndrome), recurrent symptoms, severe pain, herpes simplex virus infection, severe photophobia, and involvement with a contact (cosmetic or prescription) lens.

Viral Conjunctivitis

This is generally characterized by a watery discharge. Follicular changes (small aggregates of lymphocytes) are often found in the palpebral conjunctiva. Involvement is often unilateral and associated with periauricular nodes. Viral conjunctivitis occurs more often in the summer and in older children (>5 yr). Conjunctivitis resulting from adenovirus infection is relatively common, sometimes with corneal involvement as well as pharyngitis or pneumonia. Outbreaks of conjunctivitis caused by enterovirus are also encountered; this type may be hemorrhagic (Fig. 626-1). Acute hemorrhagic conjunctivitis may be epidemic because of enterovirus CA24 or 70 and is characterized by red, swollen, and painful eyes with a hemorrhagic watery discharge. Conjunctivitis is commonly associated with such systemic viral infections as the childhood exanthems, particularly measles. Viral conjunctivitis is usually self-limited.

Epidemic Keratoconjunctivitis

This is caused by adenovirus type 8 and is transmitted by direct contact. It initially presents as a sensation of a foreign body beneath the lids, with itching and burning. Edema (chemosis) and photophobia develop rapidly, and large oval follicles appear within the conjunctiva. Preauricular adenopathy and a pseudomembrane on the conjunctival surface occur frequently. Subepithelial corneal infiltrates may develop and may cause blurring of vision; these usually disappear but may permanently

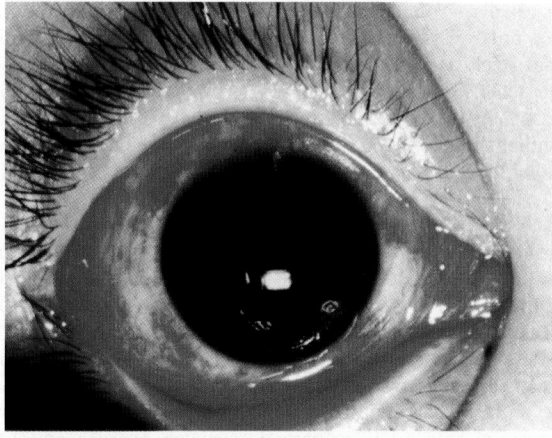

Figure 626-1 Hemorrhagic conjunctivitis caused by enterovirus 70. *(From Kono R, Uchida Y. Acute haemorrhagic conjunctivitis. Ophthalmol Dig 39:14, 1977.)*

reduce visual acuity. Corneal complications are less common in children than in adults. Children may have associated upper respiratory tract infection and pharyngitis. No specific medical therapy is available to decrease the symptoms or shorten the course of the disease. Emphasis must be placed on prevention of spread of the disease. Replicating virus is present in 95% of patients 10 days after the appearance of symptoms.

Pharyngoconjunctival fever presents with high fever, pharyngitis, bilateral conjunctivitis, and periauricular lymphadenopathy. It is highly contagious.

Membranous and Pseudomembranous Conjunctivitis

These types of conjunctivitis can be encountered in a number of diseases. The classic membranous conjunctivitis is that of diphtheria, accompanied by a fibrin-rich exudate that forms on the conjunctival surface and permeates the epithelium; the membrane is removed with difficulty and leaves raw bleeding areas. In pseudomembranous conjunctivitis, the layer of fibrin-rich exudate is superficial and can often be stripped easily, leaving the surface smooth. This type occurs with many bacterial and viral infections, including staphylococcal, pneumococcal, streptococcal, or chlamydial conjunctivitis, and in epidemic keratoconjunctivitis. It is also found in vernal conjunctivitis and in Stevens-Johnson disease.

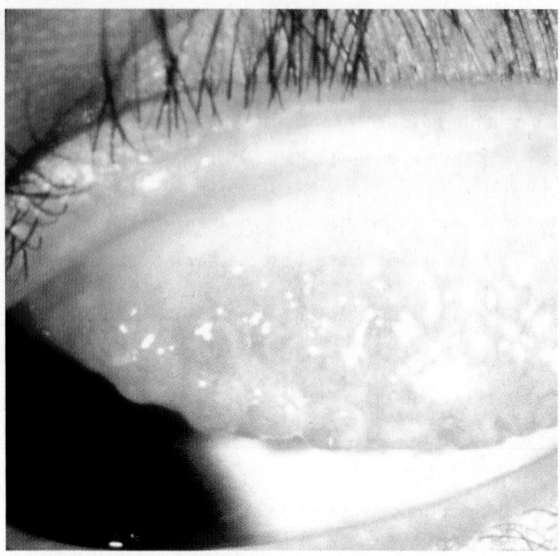

Figure 626-2 Vernal conjunctivitis.

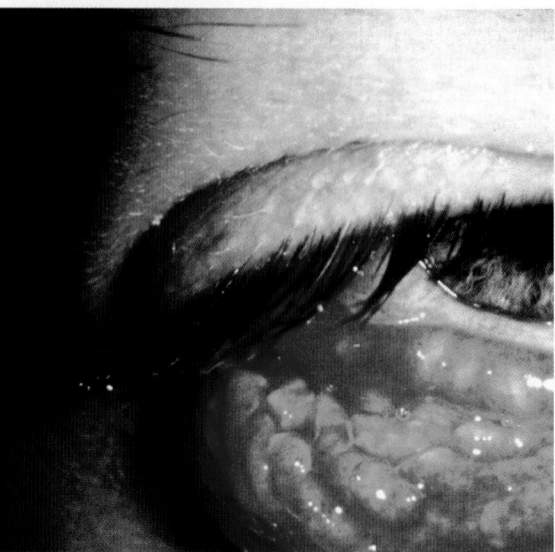

Figure 626-3 Conjunctival granulomas in Parinaud oculoglandular syndrome.

Allergic Conjunctivitis

This is usually accompanied by intense itching, clear watery discharge, and conjunctival edema (chemosis). It is commonly seasonal (spring-summer). Cold compresses and topical antihistamine drops give symptomatic relief. Topical mast cell stabilizers or prostaglandin inhibitors may also help. In selected cases, topical corticosteroids are used under an ophthalmologist's supervision but should not be used routinely or for a long time.

Vernal Conjunctivitis

This usually begins in the prepubertal years and may recur for many years. Atopy appears to have a role in its origin, but the pathogenesis is uncertain. Extreme itching and tearing are the usual complaints. Large, flattened, cobblestone-like papillary lesions of the palpebral conjunctivae are characteristic (Fig. 626-2). A stringy exudate and a milky conjunctival pseudomembrane are frequently present. Small elevated lesions of the bulbar conjunctiva adjacent to the limbus (limbal form) may be found. Smear of the conjunctival exudate reveals many eosinophils. Topical corticosteroid therapy and cold compresses afford some relief. Topical mast cell stabilizers or prostaglandin inhibitors are useful when long-term control is needed. The long-term use of corticosteroids should be avoided.

Parinaud Oculoglandular Syndrome

This represents a form of cat-scratch disease and is caused by *Bartonella henselae,* which is transmitted from cat to cat by fleas (see Chapter 209). Kittens are more likely than adult cats to be infected. Humans can become infected when they are scratched by a cat. In addition, bacteria may pass from a cat's saliva to its fur during grooming. The bacteria can then be deposited on the conjunctiva after rubbing one's eyes after handling the cat. Lymphadenopathy and conjunctivitis are hallmarks of the disease. Conjunctival granulomas may develop (Fig. 626-3). The course is generally self-limited, but antibiotics may be used in some cases.

Chemical Conjunctivitis

This can result when an irritating substance enters the conjunctival sac (as in the acute but benign conjunctivitis caused by silver nitrate in newborns). Other common offenders are household cleaning substances, sprays, smoke, smog, and industrial pollutants. Alkalis tend to linger in the conjunctival tissues and continue to inflict damage for hours or days. Acids precipitate the proteins in tissues and so produce their effect immediately. In either case, prompt, thorough, and copious irrigation is crucial. Extensive tissue damage, even loss of the eye, can result, especially if the offending agent is an alkali.

Other Conjunctival Disorders

Subconjunctival hemorrhage is manifested by bright or dark red patches in the bulbar conjunctiva and may result from injury or inflammation. It commonly occurs spontaneously. It may occasionally result from severe sneezing or coughing. Rarely, it may be a manifestation of a blood dyscrasia. Subconjunctival hemorrhages are self-limiting and require no treatment.

Pinguecula is a yellowish-white, slightly elevated mass on the bulbar conjunctiva, usually in the interpalpebral region. It represents elastic and hyaline degenerative changes of the conjunctiva. No treatment is required except for cosmetic reasons, in which case simple excision suffices.

Pterygium is a fleshy triangular conjunctival lesion that may encroach on the cornea. It typically occurs in the nasal interpalpebral region. The pathologic findings are similar to those of a pinguecula. The development of pterygia is related to exposure to ultraviolet light, and it therefore is more commonly found among people who live near the equator. Removal is suggested when the lesion encroaches far onto the cornea. Recurrence after removal is common.

Dermoid cyst and **dermolipoma** are benign lesions, clinically similar in appearance. They are smooth, elevated, round to oval lesions of various sizes. The color varies from yellowish white to fleshy pink. The most frequent site is the upper outer quadrant of the globe; they also commonly occur near or straddling the limbus. Dermolipoma is composed of adipose and connective tissue. Dermoid cysts may also contain glandular tissue, hair follicles, and hair shafts. Excision for cosmetic reasons is feasible. Dermolipomas are often connected to the extraocular muscles, making their complete removal impossible without sacrificing ocular motility.

Conjunctival nevus is a small, slightly elevated lesion that may vary in pigmentation from pale salmon to dark brown. It is usually benign, but careful observation for progressive growth or changes suggestive of malignancy is advised.

Symblepharon is a cicatricial adhesion between the conjunctiva of the lid and the globe; the lower lid is usually affected. It follows operation or injuries, especially burns from lye, acids, or molten metals. It is a serious complication of Stevens-Johnson syndrome. It may interfere with motion of the eyeball and may cause diplopia. The adhesions should be separated and the raw surfaces kept from uniting during healing. Grafts of oral mucous membrane may be necessary.

Bibliography is available at Expert Consult.

Chapter 627

Abnormalities of the Cornea

Scott E. Olitsky, Denise Hug,
Laura S. Plummer, Erin D. Stahl,
Michelle M. Ariss, and
Timothy P. Lindquist

MEGALOCORNEA

This is a nonprogressive symmetric condition characterized by an enlarged cornea (>12 mm in diameter) and an anterior segment in which there is no evidence of previous or concurrent ocular hypertension. High myopia is frequently present and may lead to reduced vision. A frequent complication is the development of lens opacities in adult life. All modes of inheritance have been described, although X-linked recessive is the most common; therefore, this disorder more commonly affects males. Systemic abnormalities that may be associated with megalocornea include Marfan syndrome, craniosynostosis, and Alport syndrome. The cause of the enlargement of the cornea and the anterior segment is unknown, but possible explanations include a defect in the growth of the optic cup and an arrest of congenital glaucoma. The region on the X chromosome responsible for this disorder has been identified.

Pathologic corneal enlargement caused by glaucoma is to be differentiated from this anomaly. Any progressive increase in the size of the cornea, especially when accompanied by photophobia, lacrimation, or haziness of the cornea, requires prompt ophthalmologic evaluation.

MICROCORNEA

Microcornea, or anterior microphthalmia, is an abnormally small cornea in an otherwise relatively normal eye. It may be familial, with transmission being dominant more often than recessive. More commonly, a small cornea is just one feature of an otherwise developmentally abnormal or microphthalmic eye; associated defects include colobomas, microphakia, congenital cataract, glaucoma, and aniridia.

KERATOCONUS

This is a disease of unclear pathogenesis characterized by progressive thinning and bulging of the central cornea, which becomes cone shaped. Although familial cases are known, most cases are sporadic. It is a common ocular condition with an incidence of 1 in 2,000 adults. Eye rubbing and contact lens wear have been implicated as pathogenic, but the evidence to support this is equivocal. The incidence is increased in individuals with atopy, Down syndrome, Marfan syndrome, and retinitis pigmentosa.

Most cases are bilateral, but involvement may be asymmetric. The disorder usually presents and progresses rapidly during adolescence; progression slows and stabilizes when patients reach full growth. Descemet membrane may occasionally be stretched beyond its elastic breaking point, causing an acute rupture in the membrane with resultant sudden and marked corneal edema (acute hydrops, Fig. 627-1) and decrease in vision. The corneal edema resolves as endothelial cells cover the defective area. Some degree of corneal scarring occurs, but the visual acuity is often better than before the initial incident. Signs of keratoconus include Munson sign (bulging of the lower eyelid on looking downward) and the presence of a Fleischer ring (a deposit of iron in the epithelium at the base of the cone). Glasses and contact lenses are the first step in treating the visual distortion caused by keratoconus. Emerging research now suggests that a corneal cross-linking procedure using riboflavin and UV light may arrest the progression of

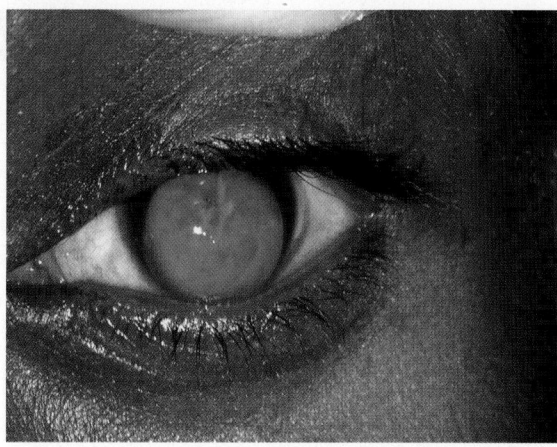

Figure 627-1 Acute hydrops from keratoconus with significant corneal edema.

keratoconus. If the cornea vaults too severely for the vision to be corrected with contact lenses then a corneal transplant must be performed to restore vision.

NEONATAL CORNEAL OPACITIES

Loss of the normal transparency of the cornea in neonates may occur secondary to either intrinsic hereditary or extrinsic environmental causes (Table 627-1).

SCLEROCORNEA

In sclerocornea, the normally translucent cornea is replaced by sclera-like tissue. Instead of a clearly demarcated cornea, white, feathery, often ill-defined and vascularized tissue develops in the peripheral cornea, appearing to blend with and extend from the sclera. The central cornea is usually clearer, but total replacement of the cornea with sclera may occur. The curvature of the cornea is often flatter, similar to the sclera. Potentially coexisting abnormalities include a shallow anterior chamber, iris abnormalities, and microphthalmos. This condition is usually bilateral. In approximately 50% of cases, a dominant or recessive inheritance has been described. Sclerocornea has been reported in association with numerous systemic abnormalities including limb deformities, craniofacial defects, and genitourinary disorders. In generalized sclerocornea, especially if bilateral, early corneal transplantation should be considered in an effort to provide vision.

Sclerocornea is classified into one of the congenital corneal opacity disorders with cornea plana if it involves peripheral scleralization or total sclerocornea disorders such as Peters anomaly.

PETERS ANOMALY

Peters anomaly is a central corneal opacity (leukoma) that is present at birth (Fig. 627-2). It is often associated with iridocorneal adhesions that extend from the iris collarette to the border of the corneal opacity. Approximately 50% of patients have other ocular abnormalities, which may include cataracts, glaucoma, and microcornea. As many as 80% of cases may be bilateral and 60% are associated with systemic malformations (Peters plus syndrome) that may include short stature, developmental delay, dysmorphic facial features, and cardiac, genitourinary, and central nervous system malformations. Some investigators have divided Peters anomaly into 2 types: a mesodermal or neuroectodermal form (type I), which does not show associated lens changes, and a surface ectodermal form (type II), which does. Histologic findings include a focal absence of Descemet membrane and corneal endothelium in the region of the opacity. Peters anomaly may be caused by incomplete migration and differentiation of the precursor cells of the central corneal endothelium and Descemet membrane or a defective separation between the primitive lens and cornea during embryogenesis.

Table 627-1	STUMPED: Differential Diagnosis of Neonatal Corneal Opacities

DIAGNOSIS	LATERALITY	OPACITY	OCULAR PRESSURE	OTHER OCULAR ABNORMALITIES	NATURAL HISTORY	INHERITANCE
S—Sclerocornea	Unilateral or bilateral	Vascularized, blends with sclera, clearer centrally	Normal (or elevated)	Cornea plana	Nonprogressive	Sporadic
T—Tears in endothelium and Descemet membrane						
Birth trauma	Unilateral	Diffuse edema	Normal	Possible hyphema, periorbital ecchymoses	Spontaneous improvement in 1 mo	Sporadic
Infantile glaucoma	Bilateral	Diffuse edema	Elevated	Megalocornea, photophobia and tearing, abnormal angle	Progressive unless treated	Autosomal recessive
U—Ulcers						
Herpes simplex keratitis	Unilateral	Diffuse with geographic epithelial defect	Normal	None	Progressive	Sporadic
Congenital rubella	Bilateral	Disciform or diffuse edema, no frank ulceration	Normal or elevated	Microphthalmos, cataract, pigment epithelial mottling	Stable, may clear	Sporadic
Neurotrophic exposure	Unilateral or bilateral	Central ulcer	Normal	Lid anomalies, congenital sensory neuropathy	Progressive	Sporadic
M—Metabolic (rarely present at birth) (mucopolysaccharidoses IH, IS; mucolipidosis type IV)*	Bilateral	Diffuse haze, denser peripherally	Normal	Few	Progressive	Autosomal dominant
P—Posterior corneal defect	Unilateral or bilateral	Central, diffuse haze or vascularized leukoma	Normal or elevated	Anterior chamber cleavage syndrome	Stable, sometimes early clearing or vascularization	Sporadic, autosomal recessive
E—Endothelial dystrophy						
Congenital hereditary endothelial dystrophy	Bilateral	Diffuse corneal edema, marked corneal thickening	Normal	None	Stable	Autosomal dominant or recessive
Posterior polymorphous dystrophy	Bilateral	Diffuse haze, normal corneal thickness	Normal	Occasional peripheral anterior synechiae	Slowly progressive	Autosomal dominant
Congenital hereditary stromal dystrophy	Bilateral	Flaky, feathery stromal opacities; normal corneal thickness	Normal	None	Stable	Autosomal dominant
D—Dermoid	Unilateral or bilateral	White vascularized mass, hair, lipid arc	Normal	None	Stable	Sporadic

*Mucopolysaccharidosis IH (Hurler syndrome); mucopolysaccharidosis IS (Scheie syndrome).
From Nelson LB, Calhoun JH, Harley RD: Pediatric ophthalmology, ed 3, Philadelphia, 1991, WB Saunders, p. 210.

CORNEAL DYSTROPHIES

These are rare inherited disorders that may present during childhood or early adulthood with bilateral involvement (although severity may be asymmetric) that progresses with time. In most, inheritance is autosomal dominant with variable expression; the most common mutation is in *TGFB1*, which is associated with the granular corneal dystrophy types 1 and 2, as well as lattice corneal dystrophy. Congenital hereditary endothelial dystrophy is both an autosomal recessive (*SLC4A11*) and dominant (unknown gene) disorder; the recessive form presents at birth and is more severe.

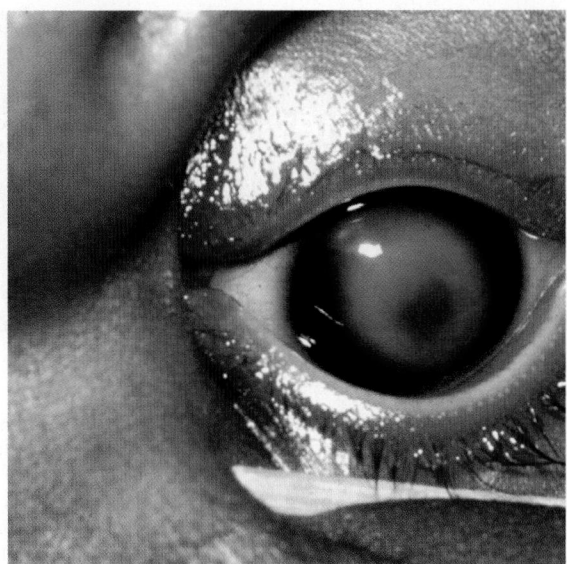

Figure 627-2 Peters anomaly. Central opacity in a patient with Peters anomaly.

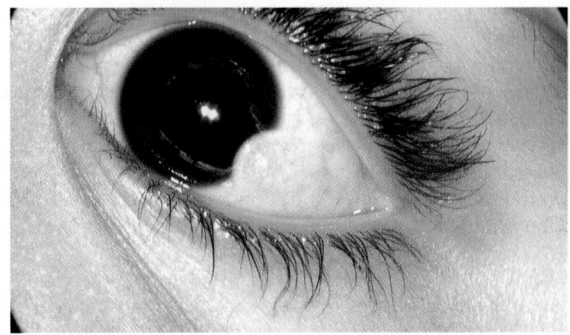

Figure 627-3 Limbal dermoid. Inferotemporal lesion in a patient with Goldenhar syndrome.

DERMOIDS

Epibulbar dermoids are choristomas. They are often present at birth and may increase in size with age. They occur most frequently in the lower temporal quadrant. They most commonly straddle the limbus and extend into the peripheral cornea (Fig. 627-3). Rarely, they may be confined entirely to the cornea or conjunctiva. Epibulbar (or limbal) dermoids may cause visual disturbance by encroaching on the visual axis or by contributing to the development of astigmatism, which may lead to amblyopia.

A dermoid usually appears as a well-circumscribed rounded or oval, gray or pinkish-yellow mass with a dry surface from which short hairs may protrude. It may affect only the superficial layers of the cornea, although full-thickness involvement is common. Associated ocular anomalies include eyelid and iris colobomas, microphthalmos, and retinal and choroidal defects. A total of 30% of dermoids are associated with systemic abnormalities. Many of the associated anomalies involve developmental defects of the first branchial arch (vertebral anomalies, dysostosis of the facial bones, ear anomalies and dental anomalies, and Goldenhar syndrome). Epibulbar dermoids are found in 75% of cases of Goldenhar syndrome.

DENDRITIC KERATITIS

Infection of the cornea with the herpes simplex virus produces a characteristic lesion of the corneal epithelium, referred to as a dendrite; it has a branching tree-like pattern that can be demonstrated by fluorescein staining. The acute episode is accompanied by pain, photophobia, tearing, blepharospasm, and conjunctival injection. Specific treatment may include mechanical debridement of the involved corneal epithelium to remove the source of infection and eliminate an antigenic stimulus to inflammation in the adjacent stroma. Medical treatment involves the use of trifluridine, topical ganciclovir, or systemic acyclovir. In addition, a cycloplegic agent is useful to relieve pain from spasm of the ciliary muscle. Overly aggressive topical antiviral treatment itself can be toxic to the cornea and should be avoided. Recurrent infection and deep stromal involvement can lead to corneal scarring and loss of vision.

Topical use of corticosteroids causes exacerbation of superficial herpetic disease of the eye and may lead to corneal perforation; eyedrops combining steroids and antibiotics are therefore to be avoided in treatment of red eye unless there are clear-cut indications for their use and close supervision during therapy.

Infants born to mothers infected with herpes simplex virus should be examined carefully for signs of ocular involvement. Intravenous acyclovir is required for treatment of ocular herpes in newborns.

CORNEAL ULCERS

The usual signs and symptoms are focal or diffuse corneal haze, hyperemia, lid edema, pain, photophobia, tearing, and blepharospasm. Hypopyon (pus in the anterior chamber) is common. Corneal ulcers require prompt treatment. They result most frequently from contact lens wear and traumatic lesions that become secondarily infected. Many organisms are capable of infecting the cornea. One of the most serious is *Pseudomonas aeruginosa;* it can rapidly destroy stromal tissue and lead to corneal perforation. *Neisseria gonorrhoeae* also is particularly damaging to the cornea. Indolent ulcers may be caused by fungi, often in association with the use of contact lenses. In each case, scrapings of the cornea must be studied in an effort to identify the infectious agent and to determine the best therapy. Although aggressive local treatment is generally needed to save the eye, systemic treatment may be necessary in some cases as well. Perforation or scarring resulting from corneal ulceration is an important cause of blindness throughout the world and is estimated to be responsible for 10% of blindness in the United States.

Unexplained corneal ulcers in infants and young children should raise the question of a sensory defect, as in Riley-Day or Goldenhar-Gorlin syndrome, or of a metabolic disorder such as tyrosinemia (Fig. 627-4). Corneal ulceration can also occur as a consequence of severe vitamin deficiencies, such as those seen with cystic fibrosis.

PHLYCTENULES

These are small, yellowish, slightly elevated lesions usually located at the corneal limbus; they may encroach on the cornea and extend centrally. A small corneal ulcer is often found at the head of the advancing lesion, with a fascicle of blood vessels behind the head of the lesion. Although once thought to represent a sign of systemic tuberculin infection, phlyctenular keratoconjunctivitis is now accepted as a morphologic expression of delayed hypersensitivity to diverse antigens. In children, it commonly occurs as a result of a hypersensitivity reaction to nonpathogenic staphylococcal strains at the eyelid margin. Treatment usually consists of eliminating the underlying disorder, usually staphylococcal blepharitis or meibomianitis, and suppressing the immune response with the use of topical corticosteroid therapy. A superficial stromal pannus and scarring sometimes remain after treatment.

INTERSTITIAL KERATITIS

This denotes nonulcerative inflammation of the corneal stroma. There is a diverse list of causes of interstitial keratitis (IK), including bacterial, viral, parasitic, and inflammatory etiologies. In the United States, herpesvirus infections and congenital syphilis account for the majority of cases of IK. Although the corneal findings may regress with time, "ghost vessels," which represent the previous vascular changes, and patchy corneal scarring remain and serve as permanent stigmata of the disease.

Cogan syndrome is IK associated with hearing loss and vestibular symptoms. Although its cause is unknown, a systemic vasculitis is

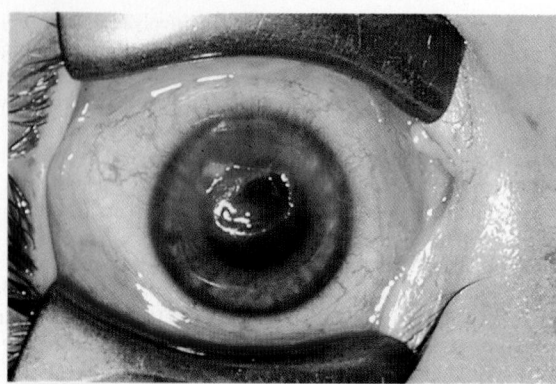
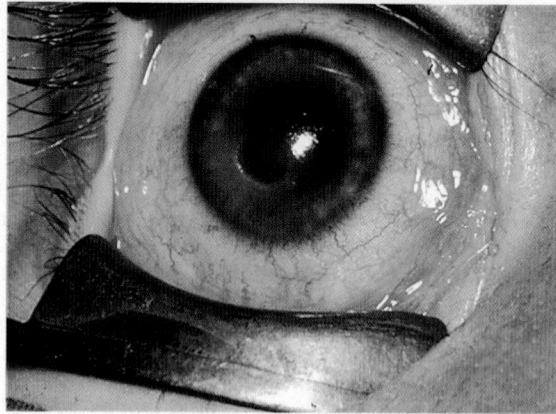

Figure 627-4 Riley-Day syndrome. This child had a combination of anesthetic corneas and dry eyes that had been treated for several months by topical wetting agents without success. He responded well to a bilateral tarsorrhaphy and lubricant ointment. Later, punctal occlusion allowed enough wetting of his eyes to allow the tarsorrhaphies to be undone. *(From Hoyt CS, Taylor D, editors: Pediatric ophthalmology and strabismus, ed 4, Philadelphia, 2013, Elsevier Saunders, Fig. 33-9, p. 315.)*

suspected. Prompt treatment is required to avoid permanent hearing loss. Both the corneal changes and the auditory involvement may respond to the use of immunosuppressive agents.

CORNEAL MANIFESTATIONS OF SYSTEMIC DISEASE

Several metabolic diseases produce distinctive corneal changes in childhood. Refractile polychromatic crystals are deposited throughout the cornea in cystinosis (see Chapter 85.4). Corneal deposits producing various degrees of corneal haze also occur in certain types of mucopolysaccharidosis (MPS; see Chapter 88), particularly MPS IH (Hurler), MPS IS (Scheie), MPS I H/S (Hurler-Scheie compound), MPS IV (Morquio), MPS VI (Maroteaux-Lamy), and sometimes MPS VII (Sly). Corneal deposits may develop in patients with GM_1 (generalized) gangliosidosis (see Chapter 86.4). In Fabry disease, fine opacities radiating in a whorl or fan-like pattern occur, and corneal changes can be important in identifying the carrier state (see Chapter 86.4). A spray-like pattern of corneal opacities may also be seen in the Bloch-Sulzberger syndrome (incontinentia pigmenti; see Chapter 596.7). In Wilson disease (see Chapter 357.2), the distinctive corneal sign is the Kayser-Fleischer ring, a golden brown ring in the peripheral cornea resulting from changes in Descemet's membrane. Pigmented corneal rings may develop in neonates with cholestatic liver disease. Corneal changes may occur in autoimmune hypoparathyroidism and band keratopathy in patients with hypercalcemia (see Chapter 570). Transient keratitis may occur with rubeola and sometimes with rubella (see Chapter 247).

Bibliography is available at Expert Consult.

Chapter 628
Abnormalities of the Lens
Scott E. Olitsky, Denise Hug, Laura S. Plummer, Erin D. Stahl, Michelle M. Ariss, and Timothy P. Lindquist

CATARACTS

A cataract is any opacity of the lens (Fig. 628-1). Some are clinically unimportant; others significantly affect visual function. The incidence of infantile cataracts is approximately 2-13/10,000 live births. An epidemiologic study of infantile cataracts published in 2003 suggests that approximately 60% of cataracts are an isolated defect; 22% are part of a syndrome; and the remainder are associated with other unrelated major birth defects. Cataracts are more common in low birthweight infants. Infants who weigh at or below 2,500 g have 3-4–fold increased odds of developing infantile cataracts. Some cataracts are associated with other ocular or systemic diseases.

Differential Diagnosis

The differential diagnosis of cataracts in infants and children includes a wide range of developmental disorders, infectious and inflammatory processes, metabolic diseases, and toxic and traumatic insults (Table 628-1). Cataracts may also develop secondary to intraocular processes, such as retinopathy of prematurity, persistent hyperplastic primary vitreous, retinal detachment, retinitis pigmentosa, and uveitis. Finally, a fraction of cataracts in children are inherited (Fig. 628-2).

Developmental Variants

Early developmental processes may lead to various congenital lens opacities. Discrete dots or white plaque-like opacities of the lens capsule are common and sometimes involve the contiguous subcapsular region. Small opacities of the posterior capsule may be associated with persistent remnants of the primitive hyaloid vascular system (the common Mittendorf dot), whereas those of the anterior capsule may be associated with persistent strands of the pupillary membrane or vascular sheath of the lens. Congenital cataracts of this type are usually stationary and rarely interfere with vision, but in some cases, progression occurs.

Prematurity

A special type of lens change seen in some preterm newborn infants is the so-called cataract of prematurity. The appearance is of a cluster of tiny vacuoles in the distribution of the Y sutures of the lens. They

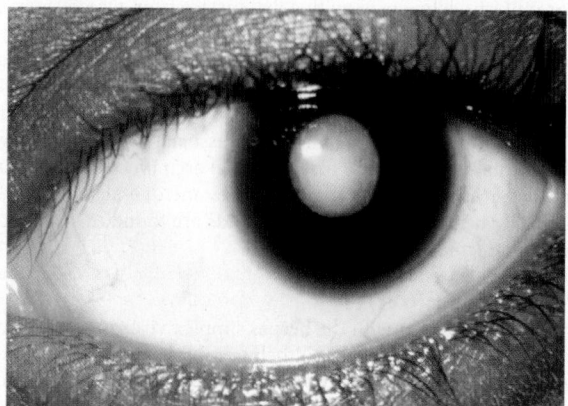

Figure 628-1 Leukocoria secondary to cataract.

Table 628-1	Differential Diagnosis of Cataracts

DEVELOPMENTAL VARIANTS
Prematurity (Y-suture vacuoles) with or without retinopathy of prematurity
Mittendorf dot (remnant of hyaloid artery)
Persistent pupillary membrane (remnant of embryonic lens vasculature)

GENETIC DISORDERS
Simple Mendelian Inheritance
Autosomal dominant (most common)
Autosomal recessive
X-linked
Major Chromosomal Defects
Trisomy disorders (13, 18, 21)
Turner syndrome (45X)
Deletion syndromes (11p13, 18p, 18q)
Duplication syndromes (3q, 20p, 10q)
Multisystem Genetic Disorders
Alport syndrome (hearing loss, renal disease)
Alström syndrome (nerve deafness, diabetes mellitus)
Apert disease (craniosynostosis, syndactyly)
Cerebrooculofacial syndrome
Cockayne syndrome (premature senility, skin photosensitivity)
Conradi disease (chondrodysplasia punctata)
Crouzon disease (dysostosis craniofacialis)
Ectodermal dysplasia
Hallermann-Streiff syndrome (microphthalmia, small pinched nose, skin atrophy, and hypotrichosis)
Hypohidrotic ectodermal dysplasia (anomalous dentition, hypohidrosis, hypotrichosis)
Ichthyosis (keratinizing disorder with thick, scaly skin)
Incontinentia pigmenti (dental anomalies, mental retardation, cutaneous lesions)
Lowe syndrome (oculocerebrorenal syndrome: hypotonia, renal disease)
Marfan syndrome
Meckel-Gruber syndrome (renal dysplasia, encephalocele)
Myotonic dystrophy
Nail–patella syndrome (renal dysfunction, dysplastic nails, hypoplastic patella)
Marinesco-Sjögren syndrome (cerebellar ataxia, hypotonia)
Nevoid basal cell carcinoma syndrome (autosomal dominant, basal cell carcinoma erupts in childhood)
Peters anomaly (corneal opacifications with iris-corneal dysgenesis)
Progeria
Rieger syndrome (iris dysplasia, myotonic dystrophy)
Rothmund-Thomson syndrome (poikiloderma: skin atrophy)
Rubinstein-Taybi syndrome (broad great toe, mental retardation)
Smith-Lemli-Opitz syndrome (toe syndactyly, hypospadias, mental retardation)
Sotos syndrome (cerebral gigantism)
Spondyloepiphyseal dysplasia (dwarfism, short trunk)
Werner syndrome (premature aging in 2nd decade of life)

Inborn Errors of Metabolism
Abetalipoproteinemia (absent chylomicrons, retinal degeneration)
Fabry disease (α-galactosidase A deficiency)
Galactokinase deficiency
Galactosemia (galactose-1-phosphate uridyltransferase deficiency)
Homocystinemia (subluxation of lens, mental retardation)
Infantile neuronal ceroid lipofuscinosis
Mannosidosis (acid α-mannosidase deficiency)
Niemann-Pick disease (sphingomyelinase deficiency)
Refsum disease (phytanic acid α-hydrolase deficiency)
Wilson disease (accumulation of copper leads to cirrhosis and neurologic symptoms)
Zellweger syndrome

ENDOCRINOPATHIES
Hypocalcemia (hypoparathyroidism)
Hypoglycemia
Diabetes mellitus

CONGENITAL INFECTIONS
Toxoplasmosis
Cytomegalovirus infection
Syphilis
Rubella
Perinatal herpes simplex infection
Measles (rubeola)
Poliomyelitis
Influenza
Varicella-zoster

OCULAR ANOMALIES
Microphthalmia
Coloboma
Aniridia
Mesodermal dysgenesis
Persistent pupillary membrane
Posterior lenticonus
Persistent fetal vasculature
Primitive hyaloid vascular system
Retinitis pigmentosa

MISCELLANEOUS DISORDERS
Atopic dermatitis
Drugs (corticosteroids)
Radiation
Trauma
Juvenile idiopathic arthritis
Retinopathy of prematurity

IDIOPATHIC

can be visualized with an ophthalmoscope and are best seen with the pupil well dilated. The pathogenesis is unclear. In most cases, the opacities disappear spontaneously, often within a few weeks.

Mendelian Inheritance

Many cataracts unassociated with other diseases are hereditary. The most common mode of inheritance is autosomal dominant. Penetrance and expressivity vary. Autosomal recessive inheritance occurs less frequently; it is sometimes found in populations with high rates of consanguinity. X-linked inheritance of cataracts unassociated with disease is relatively rare.

Congenital Infection Syndrome

Cataracts in infants and children can be a result of prenatal infection. Lens opacity may occur in any of the major congenital infection syndromes (e.g., toxoplasmosis, cytomegalovirus, syphilis, rubella, herpes simplex virus). Cataracts may also occur secondary to other perinatal infections, including measles, poliomyelitis, influenza, varicella-zoster, and vaccinia.

Metabolic Disorders

Cataracts are a prominent manifestation of many metabolic diseases, particularly certain disorders of carbohydrate, amino acid, calcium, and copper metabolism. A primary consideration in any infant with cataracts is the possibility of **galactosemia** (see Chapter 87.2). In classic infantile galactosemia, galactose-1-phosphate uridyl transferase deficiency, the cataract is typically of the zonular type, with haziness or opacification of 1 or more of the perinuclear layers of the lens. Haziness or clouding of the nucleus also often occurs. In its early stages, the cataract generally has a distinctive oil droplet appearance and is best

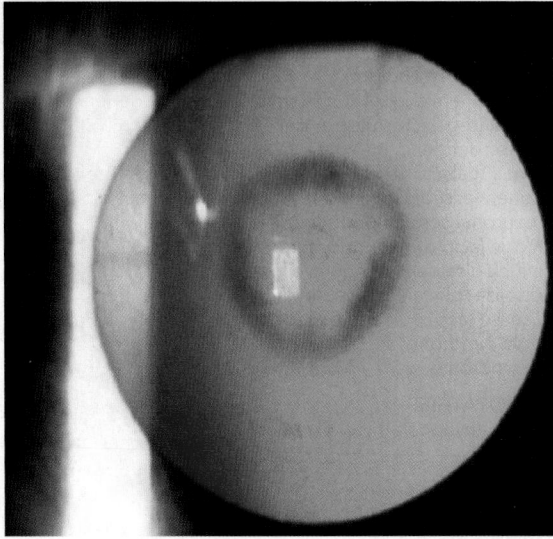

Figure 628-2 Central lamellar cataract.

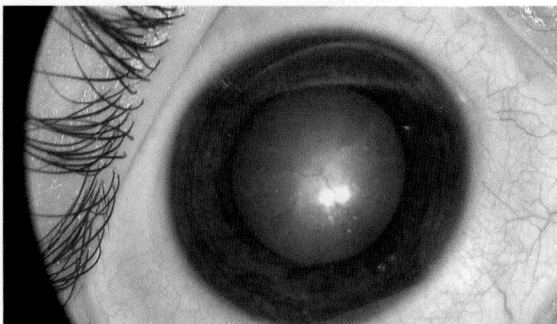

Figure 628-3 Diffuse cataract related to blunt trauma.

detected with the pupil fully dilated. Progression to complete opacification of the lens may occur within weeks. With early treatment (galactose-free diet), the lens changes may be reversible.

In **galactokinase deficiency,** cataracts are the sole clinical manifestation. The cataracts are usually zonular and may appear in the 1st few mo of life, 1st few yr of life, or later in childhood.

In children with juvenile-onset diabetes mellitus, lens changes are uncommon. Some develop snowflake-like white opacities and vacuoles of the lens. Others develop cataracts that may progress and mature rapidly, sometimes in a matter of days, especially during adolescence. An antecedent event may be the sudden development of myopia caused by changes in the optical density of the lens. Congenital lens opacities may be seen in children of diabetic and prediabetic mothers (see Chapter 107.1).

Hypoglycemia in neonates can also be associated with early development of cataracts. Ketotic hypoglycemia is also associated with cataracts.

An association between cataracts and hypocalcemia is well established. Various lens opacities may be seen in patients with hypoparathyroidism (see Chapter 570).

The **oculocerebral renal syndrome of Lowe** is associated with cataracts in infants. Affected male children frequently have dense bilateral cataracts at birth, often in association with glaucoma and miotic pupils. Punctate lens opacities are frequently present in heterozygous females.

The distinctive sunflower cataract of **Wilson disease** is not commonly seen in children. Various lens opacities may be seen in children with certain of the sphingolipidoses, mucopolysaccharidoses, and mucolipidoses, particularly Niemann-Pick disease, mucosulfatidosis, Fabry disease, and aspartylglycosaminuria (see Chapter 86).

Chromosomal Defects

Lens opacities of various types may occur in association with chromosomal defects, including trisomies 13, 18, and 21; Turner syndrome; and a number of deletion (11p13, 18p, 18q) and duplication (3q, 20p, 10q) syndromes.

Drugs, Toxic Agents, and Trauma

Of the various drugs and toxic agents that may produce cataracts, corticosteroids are of major importance in the pediatric age group. Steroid-related cataracts characteristically are posterior subcapsular lens opacities. The incidence and severity vary. The relative significance of dose, mode of administration, duration of treatment, and individual susceptibility is controversial, and the pathogenesis of steroid-induced cataracts is unclear. The effect on vision depends on the extent and density of the opacity. In many cases, the acuity is only minimally or moderately impaired. Reversibility of steroid-induced cataracts may

occur in some cases. All children receiving long-term steroid treatment should have periodic eye examinations.

Trauma to the eye is a major cause of cataracts in children (Fig. 628-3). Opacification of the lens may result from blunt or penetrating injury. Cataracts can be an important manifestation of child abuse.

Cataract formation after exposure to radiation is dose and duration dependent. Adult research shows 50% occurrence in lens dose of 15 Gy. Delayed onset is the rule.

Miscellaneous Disorders

The list of multisystem syndromes and diseases associated with lens opacities and other eye anomalies is extensive (see Table 628-1).

Treatment

The treatment of cataracts that significantly interfere with vision includes the following: (1) surgical removal of lens material to provide an optically clear visual axis; (2) correction of the resultant aphakic refractive error with spectacles, contact lenses, or intraocular lens implantation; and (3) correction of any associated sensory deprivation amblyopia. Because the use of spectacles may not be possible in children after cataract removal, the use of contact lenses for visual rehabilitation is sometimes a medical necessity. Intraocular lens implantation has become a mainstay for visual rehabilitation in children 2 yr or older. A multicenter trial is underway to try to determine visual outcomes in very young children treated with a contact lens versus an intraocular lens implant. One yr after treatment, the children randomized into the intraocular lens implant group had more statistically significant intraoperative complications, adverse events, and need for additional intraocular surgery. Grating visual acuity at 1 yr was measured and 86% of patients in the contact lens group and 77% in the intraocular lens group had 20/200 vision or better. The median visual acuity between the groups was analyzed and although the median acuity was better in the contact lens group, the difference did not reach statistical significance. Final outcome will be the comparison of visual acuity at 4.5 yr of age. Treatment of the amblyopia may be the most demanding and difficult step in the visual rehabilitation of infants or children with cataracts. Not all cataracts require surgical intervention. Cataracts that are not visually significant should be monitored for change and the child should be monitored for development of amblyopia.

Prognosis

Prognosis depends on many factors, including the nature of the cataract, the underlying disease, age at onset, age at intervention, duration and severity of any attendant amblyopia, and presence of any associated ocular abnormalities (e.g., microphthalmia, retinal lesions, optic atrophy, glaucoma, nystagmus, and strabismus). Persistent amblyopia is the most common cause of poor visual recovery after cataract surgery in children. Secondary conditions and complications may develop in children who have had cataract surgery, including inflammatory sequelae, secondary membranes, glaucoma, retinal detachment, and changes in the axial length of the eye. All of these should be considered in planning treatment.

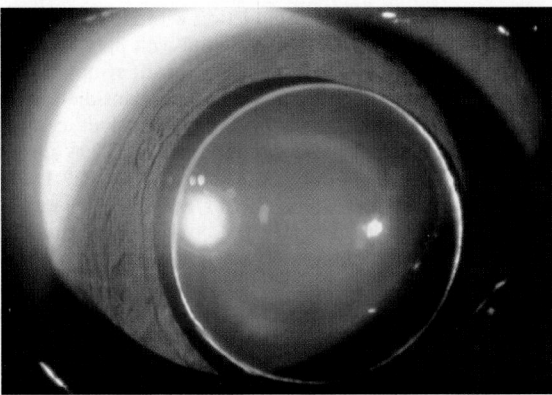

Figure 628-4 Complete dislocation of lens into the anterior chamber seen in Weill-Marchesani syndrome.

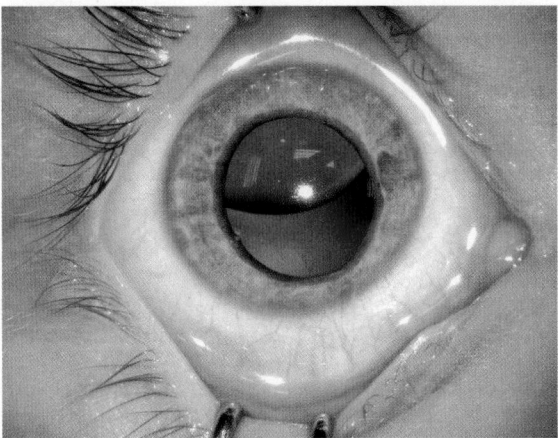

Figure 628-5 Marfan syndrome. Upward lens subluxation. *(From Hoyt CS, Taylor D: Pediatric ophthalmology and strabismus, ed 4, Philadelphia, 2013, Elsevier Saunders, Fig. 35.9A, p. 333.)*

Ectopia Lentis

Normally, the lens is suspended in place behind the iris diaphragm by the zonular fibers of the ciliary body. Abnormalities of the suspensory system resulting from a developmental defect, disease, or trauma may result in instability or displacement of the lens. Displacement of the lens is classified as luxation, which is complete displacement of the lens (also known as dislocation) (Fig. 628-4), or as subluxation, which is a partial displacement (Fig. 628-5). Symptoms include blurring of vision, which is often the result of refractive changes such as myopia, astigmatism, or aphakic hyperopia. Some patients experience diplopia (double vision). An important sign of displacement is iridodonesis, a tremulousness of the iris caused by the loss of its usual support. Also, the anterior chamber may appear deeper than normal. Sometimes the equatorial region ("edge") of the displaced lens may be visible in the pupillary aperture. On ophthalmoscopy, this may appear as a black crescent. Also, the difference between the phakic and aphakic portions can be appreciated when focusing on the fundus.

Differential Diagnosis

A major cause of lens displacement is trauma. Displacement may also occur as a result of ocular disease such as uveitis, intraocular tumor, congenital glaucoma, high myopia, megalocornea, or aniridia or in association with cataract. Ectopia lentis may also be inherited or associated with systemic disease.

Displacement of the lens occurring as a heritable ocular condition unassociated with systemic abnormalities is referred to as simple ectopia lentis. Simple ectopia lentis is usually transmitted as an autosomal dominant condition. The lens is generally displaced upward and temporally. The ectopia may be present at birth or may appear later in life. Another form of heritable dislocation is ectopia lentis et pupillae

(see Chapter 622). In this condition, both the lens and pupil are displaced, usually in opposite directions. This condition is generally bilateral, with 1 eye being almost a mirror image of the other. Ectopia lentis et pupillae is an autosomal recessive condition, although variable expression with some intermingling with simple ectopia lentis has been reported.

Systemic disorders associated with displacement of the lens include Marfan syndrome, homocystinuria, Weill-Marchesani syndrome, and sulfite oxidase deficiency. Ectopia lentis occurs in approximately 80% of patients with Marfan syndrome. In approximately 50% of patients with Marfan syndrome, the ectopia is evident by 5 yr of age. In most cases, the lens is displaced superiorly and temporally; it is almost always bilateral and relatively symmetric. In homocystinuria, the lens is usually displaced inferiorly and somewhat nasally. The subluxation of the lens occurs early in life and is often evident by 5 yr of age. In Weill-Marchesani syndrome, the displacement of the lens is often downward and forward, and the lens tends to be small and round.

Ectopia lentis is also associated occasionally with other conditions, including Ehlers-Danlos, Sturge-Weber, Crouzon, and Klippel-Feil syndromes; oxycephaly; and mandibulofacial dysostosis. A syndrome of dominantly inherited blepharoptosis, high myopia, and ectopia lentis has also been described.

Treatment and Prognosis

Displacement of the lens often results only in optical problems. In some cases, however, more serious complications may develop, such as glaucoma, uveitis, retinal detachment, or cataract. Management must be individualized according to the type of displacement, its cause, and the presence of any complicating ocular or systemic conditions. For many patients, optical correction by spectacles or contact lenses can be provided. Manipulation of the iris diaphragm with mydriatic or miotic drops may sometimes help improve vision. In selected cases, the best treatment is surgical removal of the lens. In many children, treatment of any associated amblyopia must be instituted early. In addition, for children with ectopia lentis, safety precautions should be taken to prevent injury to the eye.

Microspherophakia

The term microspherophakia refers to a small, round lens that may occur as an isolated anomaly (probably autosomal recessive) or in association with other ocular abnormalities, such as ectopia lentis, myopia, or retinal detachment (possibly autosomal dominant). Microspherophakia may also occur in association with various systemic disorders, including Marfan syndrome, Weill-Marchesani syndrome, Alport syndrome, mandibulofacial dysostosis, and Klinefelter syndrome.

Anterior Lenticonus

Anterior lenticonus is a rare bilateral condition in which the anterior capsule of the lens thins, allowing the lens to bulge forward centrally. It may be accompanied by lens opacities or other eye anomalies and is a prominent feature of Alport syndrome. The increased curvature of the central area may cause high myopia. Spontaneous rupture of the anterior capsule may occur, requiring prompt surgical intervention.

Posterior Lenticonus

Posterior lenticonus, which occurs more commonly than anterior lenticonus, is characterized by a circumscribed round or oval bulge of the posterior lens capsule and cortex, involving the central region of the lens. In the early stages, by the red reflex test, this may look like an oil droplet. It occurs in infants and young children and tends to increase with age. Usually the lens material within and surrounding the capsular bulge eventually becomes opacified. Posterior lenticonus usually occurs as an isolated ocular anomaly. It is generally unilateral but may be bilateral. It is believed to be sporadic, although autosomal dominant and X-linked inheritance has been suggested in some cases. Infants or children with posterior lenticonus may require optical correction, amblyopia treatment, and surgery for progressive cataract.

Bibliography is available at Expert Consult.

Chapter 629

Disorders of the Uveal Tract

Scott E. Olitsky, Denise Hug, Laura S. Plummer, Erin D. Stahl, Michelle M. Ariss, and Timothy P. Lindquist

UVEITIS (IRITIS, CYCLITIS, CHORIORETINITIS)

The uveal tract (the inner vascular coat of the eye, consisting of the iris, ciliary body, and choroid) is subject to inflammatory involvement in a number of systemic diseases, both infectious and noninfectious, and in response to exogenous factors, including trauma and toxic agents (Table 629-1). Inflammation may affect any one portion of the uveal tract preferentially or all parts together.

Table 629-1	Uveitis in Childhood

ANTERIOR UVEITIS
Juvenile idiopathic arthritis (pauciarticular)
Sarcoidosis
Trauma
Tuberculosis
Kawasaki disease
Ulcerative colitis
Crohn syndrome
Postinfectious (enteric or genital) with arthritis and rash
Spirochetal (syphilis, leptospiral)
Brucellosis
Heterochromic iridocyclitis (Fuchs)
Viral (herpes simplex, herpes zoster)
Ankylosing spondylitis
Stevens-Johnson syndrome
Chronic infantile neurologic cutaneous arthritis syndrome (CINCA)
Familial Mediterranean fever
Hyperimmunoglobulin D syndrome
Tumor necrosis factor receptor–associated periodic syndrome
Muckle-Wells syndrome
Blau syndrome
Psoriasis
Multiple sclerosis
Cyclic neutropenia
Chronic granulomatous disease
X-linked lymphoproliferative disease
Hypocomplementemic vasculitis
Idiopathic
Drugs

POSTERIOR UVEITIS (CHOROIDITIS—MAY INVOLVE RETINA)
Toxoplasmosis
Toxocariasis
Parasites (toxocariasis)
Sarcoidosis
Cat-scratch disease
Tuberculosis
Viral (rubella, herpes simplex, HIV, cytomegalovirus, West Nile)
Subacute sclerosing panencephalitis
Tubulointestinal nephritis and uveitis syndrome
Idiopathic

ANTERIOR AND/OR POSTERIOR UVEITIS
Sympathetic ophthalmia (trauma to other eye)
Vogt-Koyanagi-Harada syndrome (uveootocutaneous syndrome: poliosis, vitiligo, deafness, tinnitus, uveitis, aseptic meningitis, retinitis)
Behçet syndrome
Lyme disease

Iritis may occur alone or in conjunction with inflammation of the ciliary body as iridocyclitis or in association with pars planitis. Pain, photophobia, and lacrimation are the characteristic symptoms of acute anterior uveitis, but the inflammation may develop insidiously without disturbing symptoms. Signs of anterior uveitis include conjunctival hyperemia, particularly in the perilimbal region (ciliary flush), and cells and protein ("flare") in the aqueous humor (Fig. 629-1). Inflammatory deposits on the posterior surface of the cornea (keratic precipitates) and congestion of the iris may also be seen. More chronic cases may show degenerative changes of the cornea (band keratopathy), lenticular opacities (cataract), development of glaucoma, and impairment of vision. The cause of anterior uveitis is often obscure; primary considerations in children are rheumatoid disease, particularly pauciarticular arthritis, Kawasaki disease, Reiter syndrome, and sarcoidosis. Iritis may be secondary to corneal disease, such as herpetic keratitis or a bacterial or fungal corneal ulcer, or to a corneal abrasion or foreign body. Traumatic iritis and iridocyclitis are especially common in children.

Iridocyclitis that occurs in children with arthritis deserves special mention. Unlike most forms of anterior uveitis, it rarely creates pain, photophobia, or conjunctival hyperemia. Loss of vision may not be noticed until severe and irreversible damage has occurred. Because of the lack of symptoms and the high incidence of uveitis in these children, routine periodic screening is necessary. Ophthalmic screening guidelines are based on 3 factors that predispose children with arthritis to uveitis:
1. Type of arthritis
2. Age of onset of arthritis
3. Antinuclear antibody (ANA) status
Table 629-2 has been developed by the American Academy of Pediatrics for children with juvenile idiopathic arthritis without known iridocyclitis.

Choroiditis, inflammation of the posterior portion of the uveal tract, invariably also involves the retina; when both are obviously affected, the condition is termed chorioretinitis. The causes of posterior uveitis are numerous; the more common are toxoplasmosis, histoplasmosis, cytomegalic inclusion disease, sarcoidosis, syphilis, tuberculosis, and toxocariasis (Fig. 629-2). Depending on the etiology, the inflammatory signs may be diffuse or focal. Vitreous reaction often occurs as well. With many types, the result is atrophic chorioretinal scarring demarcated by pigmentation, often with visual impairment. Secondary complications include retinal detachment, glaucoma, and phthisis.

Panophthalmitis is inflammation involving all parts of the eye. It is frequently suppurative, most often as a result of a perforating injury or of septicemia. It produces severe pain, marked congestion of the eye, inflammation of the adjacent orbital tissues and eyelids, and loss of vision. In many cases, the eye is lost despite intensive treatment of the infection and inflammation. Enucleation of the eye or evisceration of the orbit may be necessary.

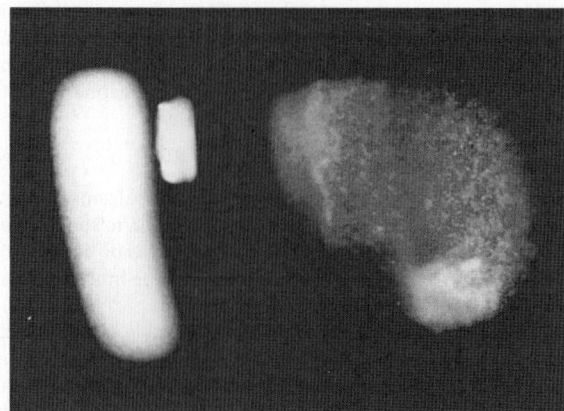

Figure 629-1 Cell and flare in the anterior chamber. The flare represents protein leakage. *(Courtesy of Peter Buch, CRA.)*

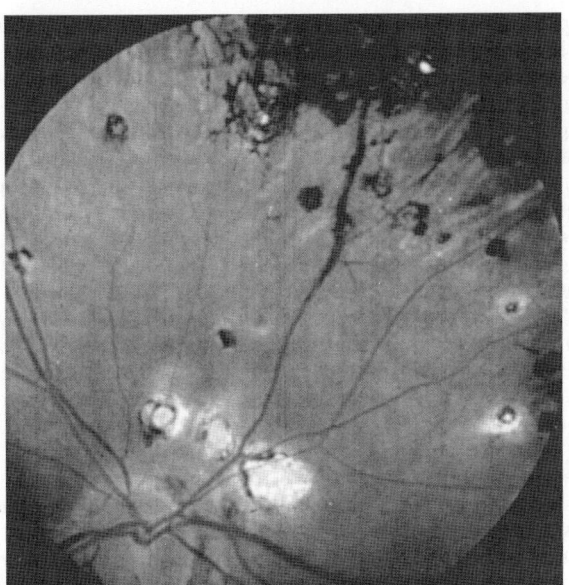

Figure 629-2 Focal atrophic and pigmented scars of chorioretinitis.

Table 629-2	Examination Schedule for Children with JIA Without Known Iridocyclitis

	AGE OF ONSET	
JIA SUBTYPE	**≤6 yr**	**>6 yr**
OLIGOARTHRITIS OR POLYARTHRITIS		
Positive ANA		
Less than 4 yr duration	Every 3 mo	Every 6 mo
4-7 yr duration	Every 6 mo	Annually
More than 7 yr duration	Annually	Annually
Negative ANA		
Less than 4 yr duration	Every 6 mo	Annually
4-7 yr duration	Annually	Annually
More than 7 yr duration	Annually	Annually
Systemic	Annually regardless of duration	Annually regardless of duration

ANA, antinuclear antibody; JIA, juvenile idiopathic arthritis; JRA, juvenile rheumatoid arthritis.

Sympathetic ophthalmia is a rare type of inflammatory response that affects the uninjured eye after a perforating injury. It may occur weeks, months, or even years after the injury. A hypersensitivity phenomenon is the most probable cause. Loss of vision in the uninjured (sympathizing) eye may result. Removal of the injured eye prevents the development of sympathetic ophthalmia but does not stop the progression of the disease once it has occurred. Therefore, early enucleation should be considered if there is no hope of visual recovery after a severe injury.

Treatment

The various forms of intraocular inflammation are treated according to their underlying systemic causal factors. When infection is proved or suspected, appropriate systemic antimicrobial or antiviral therapy is used. In some cases, intravitreal injection is indicated.

Elimination of the intraocular inflammation is important to reduce the risk of severe, and often permanent, vision loss. Untreated, the inflammatory process may lead to the development of band keratopathy (calcium deposition in the cornea), cataracts, glaucoma, and irreversible retinal damage. Anterior inflammation may respond well to topical corticosteroid treatment. Posterior cases often require systemic therapy. The use of topical and systemic corticosteroids can lead to the development of glaucoma and cataracts. To reduce the need for topical and systemic corticosteroids, systemic immunosuppression is often used in patients requiring long-term treatment. Commonly used immunosuppressive agents include methotrexate, cyclosporine, and tumor necrosis factor inhibitors. Multiple agents may be needed in recalcitrant cases. Cycloplegic agents, particularly atropine, are also used to reduce inflammation and to prevent adhesion of the iris to the lens (posterior synechiae), especially in anterior uveitis. Extensive posterior synechiae formation can lead to acute angle closure glaucoma.

Surgery may be required for patients who develop glaucoma because of the underlying disease process or the need for corticosteroid treatment. Cataract surgery should be delayed until the inflammation has been under control for a period of time. Cataract surgery in children with a history of prolonged uveitis can carry significant risk. There is no universal agreement concerning the use of intraocular lenses in these patients.

Pars planitis is an uncommon idiopathic form of intermediate uveitis characterized by anterior chamber involvement, anterior vitreous cells and condensations, and peripheral retinal vasculitis. The average age of onset is 9 yr. It is predominantly bilateral and seen more frequently in males. Painless decreased vision is the usual presenting sign. The prognosis is good when adequate medical treatment is sought early in the course of the disease.

Masquerade syndromes can sometimes mimic intraocular inflammation. Retinoblastoma, leukemia, retained intraocular foreign body, juvenile xanthogranuloma, and peripheral retinal detachments may produce signs similar to those seen in uveitis. These syndromes should be kept in mind when evaluating a patient with suspected uveitis or if a patient does not respond as anticipated to antiinflammatory treatment.

Bibliography is available at Expert Consult.

Chapter 630
Disorders of the Retina and Vitreous

Scott E. Olitsky, Denise Hug, Laura S. Plummer, Erin D. Stahl, Michelle M. Ariss, and Timothy P. Lindquist

RETINOPATHY OF PREMATURITY

Retinopathy of prematurity (ROP) is a complex disease of the developing retinal vasculature in premature infants. It may be acute (early stages) or chronic (late stages). Clinical manifestations range from mild, usually transient changes of the peripheral retina to severe progressive vasoproliferation, scarring, and potentially blinding retinal detachment. ROP includes all stages of the disease and its sequelae. Retrolental fibroplasia, the previous name for this disease, described only the cicatricial stages.

Pathogenesis

Beginning at 16 wk of gestation, retinal angiogenesis normally proceeds from the optic disc to the periphery, reaching the outer rim of the retina (ora serrata) nasally at about 36 wk and extending temporally by approximately 40 wk. Injury to this process results in various pathologic and clinical changes. The first observation in the acute phase is cessation of vasculogenesis. Rather than a gradual transition from vascularized to avascular retina, there is an abrupt termination of the vessels, marked by a line in the retina. The line may then grow into a ridge composed of mesenchymal and endothelial cells. Cell division and differentiation may later resume, and vascularization of the retina may proceed. Alternatively, there may be progression to an abnormal proliferation of vessels out of the plane of the retina, into the vitreous, and over the surface of the retina. Cicatrization and traction on the retina may follow, leading to retinal detachment.

The risk factors associated with ROP are not fully known, but prematurity and the associated retinal immaturity at birth represent the major factors. Oxygenation, respiratory distress, apnea, bradycardia, heart disease, infection, hypercarbia, acidosis, anemia, and the need for transfusion are thought by some to be contributory factors. Generally, the lower the gestational age, the lower the birthweight, and the sicker the infant are, the greater the risk is for ROP.

The basic pathogenesis of ROP is still unknown. Exposure to the extrauterine environment, including the necessarily high inspired oxygen concentrations, produces cellular damage, perhaps mediated by free radicals. Later in the course of the disease, peripheral hypoxia develops and vascular endothelial growth factors (VEGFs) are produced in the nonvascularized retina. These growth factors stimulate abnormal vasculogenesis, and neovascularization may occur. Because of poor pulmonary function, a state of relative retinal hypoxia occurs. This causes upregulation of VEGF, which, in susceptible infants, can cause abnormal fibrovascular growth. This neovascularization may then lead to scarring and vision loss.

Classification

The currently used international classification of ROP describes the location, extent, and severity of the disease. To delineate location, the retina is divided into 3 concentric zones, centered on the optic disc (Fig. 630-1). Zone I, the posterior or inner zone, extends twice the disc-macular distance, or 30 degrees in all directions from the optic disc. Zone II, the middle zone, extends from the outer edge of zone I to the ora serrata nasally and to the anatomic equator temporally. Zone III, the outer zone, is the residual crescent that extends from the outer border of zone II to the ora serrata temporally. The extent of involvement is described by the number of circumferential clock hours involved.

The phases and severity of the disease process are classified into 5 stages. Stage 1 is characterized by a demarcation line that separates vascularized from avascular retina. This line lies within the plane of

the retina and appears relatively flat and white. Often noted is abnormal branching or arcading of the retinal vessels that lead into the line. Stage 2 is characterized by a ridge; the demarcation line has grown, acquiring height, width, and volume and extending up and out of the plane of the retina. Stage 3 is characterized by the presence of a ridge and by the development of extraretinal fibrovascular tissue (Fig. 630-2A). Stage 4 is characterized by subtotal retinal detachment caused by traction from the proliferating tissue in the vitreous or on the retina. Stage 4 is subdivided into 2 phases: (a) subtotal retinal detachment not involving the macula and (b) subtotal retinal detachment involving the macula. Stage 5 is total retinal detachment.

When signs of posterior retinal vascular changes accompany the active stages of ROP, the term *plus disease* is used (see Fig. 630-2B and C). Patients reaching the point of dilation and tortuosity of the retinal vessels also frequently demonstrate the associated findings of engorgement of the iris, pupillary rigidity, and vitreous haze.

Clinical Manifestations and Prognosis

In more than 90% of at-risk infants, the course is one of spontaneous arrest and regression, with little or no residual effects or visual disability. Fewer than 10% of infants have progression toward severe disease, with significant extraretinal vasoproliferation, cicatrization, detachment of the retina, and impairment of vision.

Some children with arrested or regressed ROP are left with demarcation lines, undervascularization of the peripheral retina, or abnormal branching, tortuosity, or straightening of the retinal vessels. Some are left with retinal pigmentary changes, dragging of the retina (so-called dragged disc), ectopia of the macula, retinal folds, or retinal breaks. Others proceed to total retinal detachment, which commonly assumes a funnel-like configuration. The clinical picture is often that of a retrolental membrane, producing leukokoria (a white reflex in the pupil). Some patients develop cataract, glaucoma, and signs of inflammation. The end stage is often a painful blind eye or a degenerated phthisical eye. The spectrum of ROP also includes myopia, which is often progressive and of significant degree in infancy. The incidence of anisometropia, strabismus, amblyopia, and nystagmus may also be increased.

Diagnosis

Systematic serial screening ophthalmologic examinations of infants at risk are recommended. Infants with a birthweight of less than 1,500 g or gestational age of 32 wk or less, and selected infants with a birthweight between 1,500 and 2,000 g or gestational age of more than

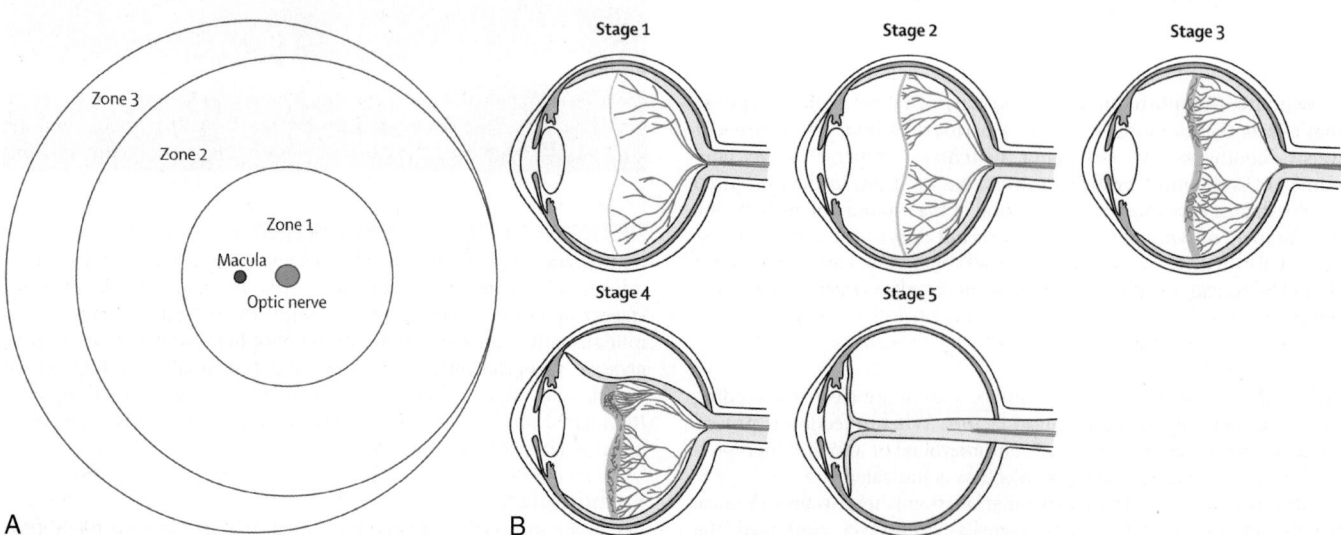

Figure 630-1 The retina is divided into 3 zones (**A,** diagram shows right eye) and the extent or severity of retinopathy in these zones is classified as stages (**B**). Stage 1 is characterized by a thin demarcation line between vascularized and nonvascularized retina, stage 2 by a ridge, stage 3 by extraretinal fibrovascular proliferation, stage 4 by partial retinal detachment, and stage 5 by total retinal detachment. In stage 3, extraretinal neovascularization can become severe enough to cause retinal detachment (stages 4-5), which usually leads to blindness. (*B courtesy Lisa Hård. From Hellström A, Smith LEH, Dammann O: Retinopathy of prematurity. Lancet 382:1445-1454, 2013, Fig. 3, p. 1450.*)

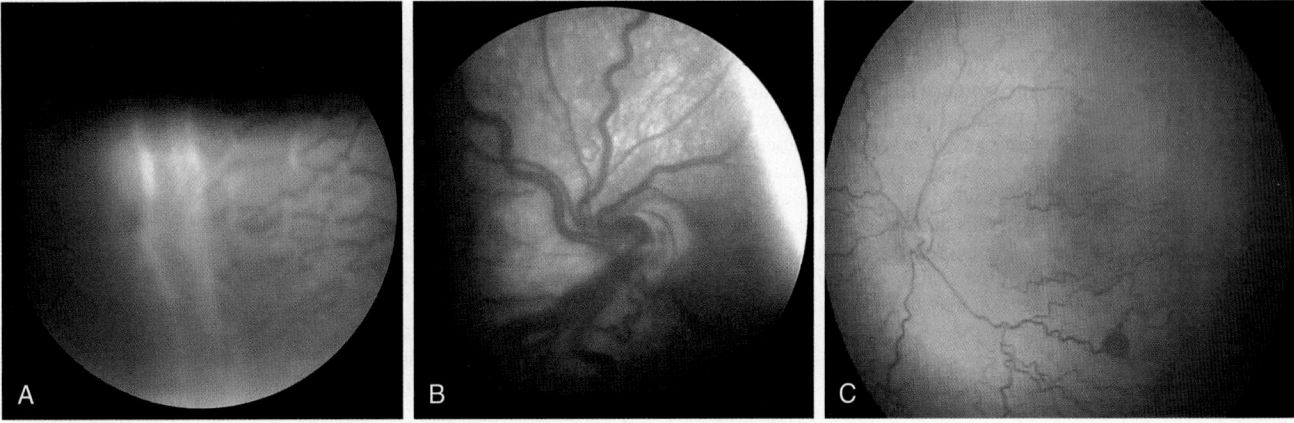

Figure 630-2 Retinopathy of prematurity (ROP). **A,** In stage 3, there is a ridge and extraretinal vascular tissue. **B,** Retinal vessels are dilated and tortuous in active zone 1 ROP with plus disease. **C,** Zone 1 ROP with plus disease.

Table 630-1	Timing of First Eye Examination Based on Gestational Age at Birth	
GESTATIONAL AGE AT BIRTH	**AGE AT INITIAL EXAMINATION IN WEEKS**	
	POSTMENSTRUAL	**CHRONOLOGIC**
22	31	9
23	31	8
24	31	7
25	31	6
26	31	5
27	31	4
28	32	4
29	33	4
30	34	4
31	35	4
32	36	4

32 wk with an unstable clinical course, including those requiring cardiorespiratory support and who are believed by their attending pediatrician or neonatologist to be at high risk, should have retinal screening examinations. The timing of the initial screening exam is based on the infant's age. Table 630-1 was developed from an evidence-based analysis of the Multicenter Trial of Cryotherapy for ROP. The examination can be stressful to fragile preterm infants, and the dilating drops can have untoward side effects. Infants must be carefully monitored during and after the examination. Some neonatologists and ophthalmologists advocate the use of topical tetracaine and/or oral sucrose to reduce the discomfort and stress to the infant. Follow-up is based on the initial findings and risk factors but is usually 2 wk or less.

Treatment
In selected cases, cryotherapy or laser photocoagulation of the avascular retina reduces the more severe complications of progressive ROP. Advances in vitreoretinal surgical techniques have led to limited success in reattaching the retina in infants with total retinal detachment (stage 5 ROP), but the visual results are often disappointing. The Early Treatment for Retinopathy of Prematurity Cooperative study did find improved structural and visual outcomes with the redefined threshold for treatment. It demonstrated the importance of plus disease and the presence of posterior retinal involvement in the determination of when to treat ROP. This study also supported the fact that laser is

the **treatment modality of choice.** Peripheral retinal ablation should be considered for any eye with type 1 ROP. Serial examinations are indicated for any eye with type 2 ROP; treatment is considered if type 2 progresses to type 1 or if threshold ROP develops.

Clinical trials using systemic propranolol or intravitreal VEGF antagonists are ongoing and being evaluated for efficacy and risk.

Prevention
Prevention of ROP ultimately depends on prevention of premature birth and its attendant problems (see Chapters 95 and 97.2). However, a number of other potential factors have been studied in order to decrease the occurrence of ROP in these premature infants. Ambient light had been considered by some to be a potential agent that could hopefully be manipulated. The LIGHT-ROP study definitively found that ambient light reduction had no impact on ROP. The association between ROP and oxygen saturation has been studied for decades. Recent research has focused on maintaining oxygen saturation levels for severely premature infants at levels sufficiently low to minimize the risk of ROP and sufficiently high to optimize survival.

PERSISTENT FETAL VASCULATURE
Persistent fetal vasculature (PFV; formerly called persistent hyperplastic primary vitreous) includes a spectrum of manifestations caused by the persistence of various portions of the fetal hyaloid vascular system and associated fibrovascular tissue.

Pathogenesis
During development of the eye, the hyaloid artery extends from the optic disc to the posterior aspect of the lens; it sends branches into the vitreous and ramifies to form the posterior portion of the vascular capsule of the lens. The posterior portion of the hyaloid system normally regresses by the 7th fetal mo and the anterior portion by the 8th fetal mo. Small remnants of the system, such as a tuft of tissue at the disc (Bergmeister papilla) or a tag of tissue on the posterior capsule of the lens (Mittendorf dot), are common findings in healthy persons. More extensive remnants and associated complications constitute PFV. Two major forms are described, anterior PFV and posterior PFV. Variability is great, and mixed or intermediate forms occur.

Clinical Manifestations
The usual clinical feature of anterior PFV is the presence of a vascularized plaque of tissue on the back surface of the lens in an eye that is microphthalmic or slightly smaller than normal. The condition is usually unilateral and may occur in infants with no other abnormalities and no history of prematurity. The fibrovascular tissue tends to undergo gradual contracture. The ciliary processes become elongated, and the anterior chamber may become shallow. The lens usually is smaller than normal and may be clear but often becomes cataractous and may swell or absorb fluid. Large or anomalous vessels of the iris may be present.

The anterior chamber angle may have abnormalities. In time, the cornea may become cloudy.

Anterior PFV is usually noted in the 1st wk or mo of life. The most frequent presenting signs are leukocoria (white pupillary reflex), strabismus, and nystagmus. The course is usually progressive and the outcome poor. Major complications are spontaneous intraocular hemorrhage, swelling of the lens caused by rupture of the posterior capsule, and glaucoma. The eye may eventually deteriorate. The spectrum of posterior PFV includes fibroglial veils around the disc and macula, vitreous membranes and stalks containing hyaloid artery remnants projecting from the disc, and meridional retinal folds. Traction detachment of the retina may occur. Vision may be impaired, but the eye is usually retained.

Treatment

Surgery is performed in an effort to prevent complications, to preserve the eye and a reasonably good cosmetic appearance, and, in some cases, to salvage vision. Surgical treatment usually involves aspirating the lens and excising the abnormal tissue. If useful vision is to be attained, refractive correction and aggressive amblyopia therapy are required. In some cases, the affected eye is enucleated because distinguishing between this white mass and retinoblastoma can be difficult. Ultrasonography and CT are valuable diagnostic aids.

RETINOBLASTOMA

Also see Chapter 502.

Retinoblastoma (Fig. 630-3) is the most common primary malignant intraocular tumor of childhood. It occurs in approximately 1/15,000 live births; 250-300 new cases are diagnosed in the United States annually. Hereditary and nonhereditary patterns of transmission occur; there is no gender or race predilection. The hereditary form occurs earlier and is usually bilateral and multifocal, whereas the nonhereditary form is generally unilateral and unifocal. Fifteen percent of unilateral cases are hereditary. Bilateral cases often present earlier than unilateral cases. Unilateral tumors are often large by the time they are discovered. The average age at diagnosis is 15 mo for bilateral cases, compared with 27 mo for unilateral cases. It is unusual for a child to present with a retinoblastoma after 3 yr of age. Rarely, the tumor is discovered at birth, during adolescence, or even in early adulthood.

Clinical Manifestations

The clinical manifestations of retinoblastoma vary, depending on the stage at which the tumor is detected. The initial sign in the majority of patients is a white pupillary reflex (leukocoria). Leukocoria results because of the reflection of light off the white tumor. The second most frequent initial sign of retinoblastoma is strabismus. Less-frequent presenting signs include pseudohypopyon (tumor cells layered inferiorly in front of the iris) caused by tumor seeding in the anterior chamber of the eye, hyphema (blood layered in front of the iris) secondary to iris neovascularization, vitreous hemorrhage, and signs of orbital cellulitis. On examination, the tumor appears as a white mass, sometimes small and relatively flat, sometimes large and protuberant. It may appear nodular. Vitreous haze or tumor seeding may be evident.

The retinoblastoma gene is a recessive suppressor gene located on chromosome 13 at the 13q14 region. Because of the hereditary nature of retinoblastoma, family members of affected children should undergo

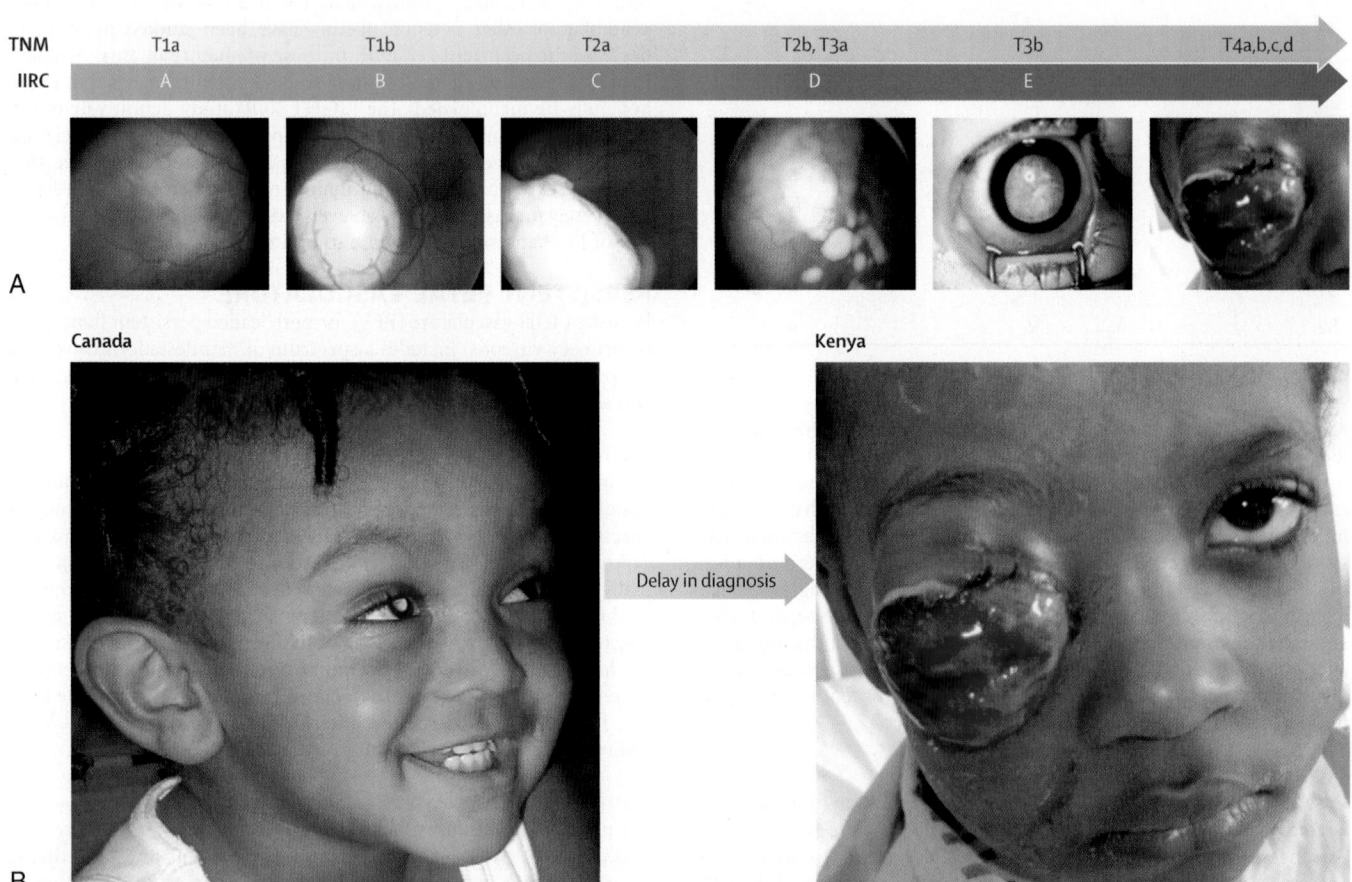

Figure 630-3 Progression of retinoblastoma from small intraretinal tumors to massive orbital retinoblastoma probably extending into the brain. Progression of retinoblastoma **(A)** from small intraretinal tumors that can be cured by laser treatment and cryotherapy (TNM T1a, IIRC A) to massive orbital retinoblastoma probably extending into the brain (TNM T4a-b). A difference in age at diagnosis recorded between Canada and Kenya could be the difference between possible cure and certain death **(B).** The Canadian child with leukocoria was diagnosed because of the left-hand image, which was taken by his sister with his mother's mobile phone. *IIRC,* International Intraocular Retinoblastoma Classification; *TNM,* Tumor Node Metastasis Cancer Staging. *(From Dimaras H, Kimani K, Dimba EAO, et al: Retinoblastoma. Lancet 379:1436-1444, 2012, Fig. 1, p. 1438.)*

a complete ophthalmologic examination and genetic counseling. Newborn siblings and children of affected patients should be referred to an ophthalmologist shortly after birth, when the peripheral retina can be evaluated without the need for an examination under anesthesia.

Diagnosis

This is made by direct observation by an experienced ophthalmologist. Ancillary testing such as CT or ultrasonography may help to confirm the diagnosis and demonstrate calcification within the mass. MRI may better detect the presence of an associated pineoblastoma (trilateral retinoblastoma). A definitive diagnosis occasionally cannot be made, and removal of the eye must be considered to avoid the possibility of lethal metastasis of the tumor. Because a biopsy can lead to spread of the tumor, histologic confirmation before enucleation is not possible in most cases. Therefore, removal of a blind eye in which the diagnosis of retinoblastoma is likely may be appropriate.

Treatment

Therapy varies, depending on the size and location of the tumor as well as whether it is unilateral or bilateral. Advanced tumors may be treated by enucleation. Other treatment modalities include the use of external beam irradiation, radiation plaque therapy, laser or cryotherapy, and chemotherapy. During the last decade there has been a dramatic shift in the treatment of retinoblastomas. Chemoreduction (systemic chemotherapy) followed by local therapies (i.e., laser therapy, cryotherapy, and brachytherapy) has markedly reduced the use of external beam radiation and is a more vision-sparing technique. Those children who are irradiated during their 1st yr of life are 2-8 times more likely to develop second cancers as those irradiated after 1 yr of age. Patients treated with radiation tend to develop brain tumors and sarcomas of the head and neck. Secondary cataracts can also develop from radiation.

Nonocular secondary tumors are common in patients with germinal mutations estimated to occur with an incidence of 1% per yr of life. The most common secondary tumor is osteogenic sarcoma of the skull and long bones; the risk is higher in patients treated with radiation. Other malignancies include lung, brain, soft tissue, and skin.

The prognosis for children with retinoblastoma depends on the size and extension of the tumor. When confined to the eye, most tumors can be cured. The prognosis for long-term survival is poor when the tumor has extended into the orbit or along the optic nerve.

RETINITIS PIGMENTOSA

This progressive retinal degeneration is characterized by pigmentary changes, arteriolar attenuation, usually some degree of optic atrophy, and progressive impairment of visual function. Dispersion and aggregation of the retinal pigment produce various ophthalmoscopically visible changes, ranging from granularity or mottling of the retinal pigment pattern to distinctive focal pigment aggregates with the configuration of bone spicules (Fig. 630-4). Other ocular findings include subcapsular cataract, glaucoma, and keratoconus.

Impairment of night vision or dark adaptation is often the first clinical manifestation. Progressive loss of peripheral vision, often in the form of an expanding ring scotoma or concentric contraction of the field, is usual. There may be loss of central vision. Retinal function, as measured by electroretinography (ERG), is characteristically reduced. The disorder may be autosomal recessive, autosomal dominant, or X linked. Children with autosomal recessive retinitis pigmentosa are more likely to become symptomatic at an earlier age (median age 10.7 yr). Those with autosomal dominant retinitis pigmentosa are more likely to present in their 20s. Only supportive treatment is available.

A special form of retinitis pigmentosa is **Leber congenital retinal amaurosis,** in which the retinal changes tend to be pleomorphic, with various degrees of pigment disorder, arteriolar attenuation, and optic atrophy. The retina may appear normal during infancy. Vision impairment, nystagmus, and poor pupillary reaction are usually evident soon after birth, and the ERG findings are abnormal early and confirm the diagnosis. Retinal pigment epithelium–specific 65-kDa deficiency is the cause of autosomal recessive disease. Gene replacement therapy

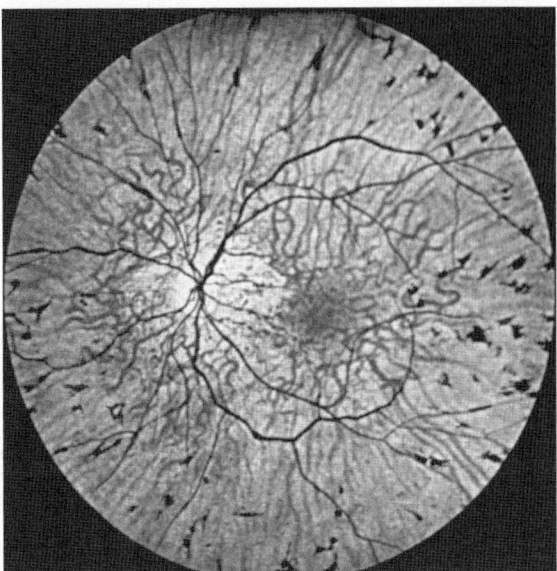

Figure 630-4 Retinitis pigmentosa.

(subretinal injection) presently shows early promise for people affected with Leber congenital retinal amaurosis.

Usher syndrome, an autosomal recessive disorder, is the most common cause of retinitis pigmentosa and sensorineural deafness (incidence 1 : 25,000). Type 1 Usher syndrome presents at birth with profound hearing loss and poor balance; visional loss progresses more slowly and begins during adolescence. Patients with type 3 disease have normal hearing at birth but develop hearing loss and night blindness around puberty. To date, 11 genetic loci have been located (5 for type 1; 3 for type 2; 1 for type 3).

Clinically similar, secondary pigmentary retinal degenerations that need to be differentiated from retinitis pigmentosa occur in a wide variety of metabolic diseases, neurodegenerative processes, and multifaceted syndromes. Examples include the progressive retinal changes of the mucopolysaccharidoses (particularly Hurler, Hunter, Scheie, and Sanfilippo syndromes; see Chapter 88) and certain of the late-onset gangliosidoses (Batten-Mayou, Spielmeyer-Vogt, and Jansky-Bielschowsky diseases; see Chapters 86.4 and 599.2), the progressive retinal degeneration that is associated with progressive external ophthalmoplegia (Kearns-Sayre syndrome; see Chapter 598.2), and the retinitis pigmentosa–like changes in the Laurence-Moon and Bardet-Biedl syndromes. The retinal manifestations of abetalipoproteinemia (Bassen-Kornzweig syndrome; see Chapter 86) and Refsum disease (see Chapter 86.2) are also similar to those found in retinitis pigmentosa. The diagnosis of these latter two disorders in a patient with presumed retinitis pigmentosa is important because treatment is possible. There is also an association of retinitis pigmentosa and congenital hearing loss, as in Usher syndrome.

STARGARDT DISEASE (FUNDUS FLAVIMACULATUS)

This autosomal recessive retinal disorder is characterized by slowly progressive bilateral macular degeneration and vision impairment. It usually appears at 8-14 yr of age, and affected children are often initially misdiagnosed as having functional visual loss. The foveal reflex becomes obtunded or appears grayish, pigment spots develop in the macular area, and macular depigmentation and chorioretinal atrophy eventually occur. Macular hemorrhages also may develop. Some patients also have white or yellow spots beyond the macula or pigmentary changes in the periphery; the term *fundus flavimaculatus* is commonly used for this condition. It is now recognized that Stargardt disease and fundus flavimaculatus represent different entities on the spectrum of the same disease. Central visual acuity is reduced, often to 20/200, but total loss of vision does not occur. ERG findings vary. The condition is not associated with central nervous system abnormalities and is to be

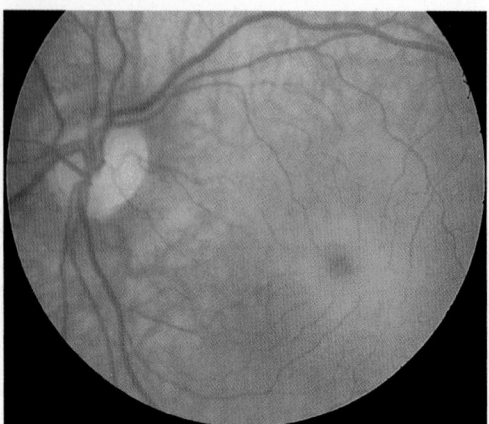

Figure 630-5 Cherry-red spot seen in a case of Tay-Sachs disease. Because the parafoveal area has many retinal ganglion cells and the fovea has none, the fovea retains its orange-red color but is surrounded by retina that is whitish. This produces the cherry-red spot in the macula. *(From Cheng KP, Biglan AW: Ophthalmology. In Zitelli BJ, McIntire S, Nowalk AJ (eds): Zitelli and Davis' atlas of pediatric physical diagnosis, ed 6, Philadelphia: Saunders, 2012. Fig. 19-102.)*

differentiated from the macular changes of many progressive metabolic neurodegenerative diseases. The genetic mutation responsible for Stargardt macular dystrophy has been identified.

BEST VITELLIFORM DEGENERATION

This macular dystrophy is characterized by a distinctive yellow or orange discoid subretinal lesion in the macula, resembling the intact yolk of a fried egg. Diagnosis is usually made at 3-15 yr of age with a mean age of presentation of 6 yr. Vision is usually normal at this stage. The condition may be progressive; the yolk-like lesion may eventually degenerate ("scramble") and result in pigmentation, chorioretinal atrophy, and vision impairment. The condition is usually bilateral. There is no association with systemic abnormalities. Inheritance is usually autosomal dominant. The vitelliform macular dystrophy gene *(VMD2)* has been identified and DNA testing is available. In vitelliform macular degeneration, the ERG response is normal. Electrooculographic findings are abnormal in affected patients and carriers, and this test is useful in diagnosis and in genetic counseling.

CHERRY-RED SPOT

Because of the special histologic features of the macula, certain pathologic processes affecting the retina produce an ophthalmoscopically visible sign referred to as a cherry-red spot, a bright to dull red spot at the center of the macula surrounded and accentuated by a grayish-white or yellowish halo (Fig. 630-5). The halo is a result of a loss of transparency of the retinal ganglion cell layer secondary to edema or lipid accumulation, or both. Because ganglion cells are not present in the fovea, the retina surrounding the fovea is opacified but the fovea transmits the normal underlying choroidal color (red), accounting for the presence of the cherry-red spot. A cherry-red spot typically occurs in certain sphingolipidoses, principally in Tay-Sachs disease (GM_2 type 1), in the Sandhoff variant (GM_2 type 2), and in generalized gangliosidosis (GM_1 type 1). Similar but less distinctive macular changes occur in some cases of metachromatic leukodystrophy (sulfatide lipidosis), in some forms of neuronopathic Niemann-Pick disease, galactosialidosis, and in certain mucolipidoses. The cherry-red spot that characteristically occurs as a result of retinal ischemia secondary to vasospasm, ocular contusion, or occlusion of the central retinal artery must be differentiated from the cherry-red spot of neurodegenerative disease (see Chapters 86.4 and 599).

PHAKOMAS

See also Chapter 596.

These are the herald lesions of the hamartomatous disorders. In Bourneville disease (tuberous sclerosis), the distinctive ocular lesion is

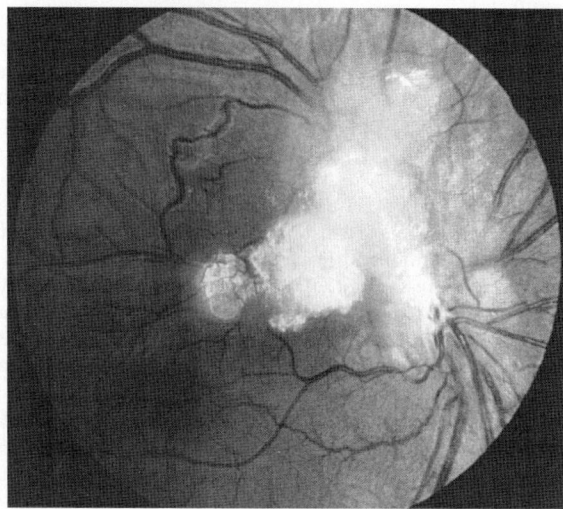

Figure 630-6 Retinal phakoma of tuberous sclerosis.

a refractile, yellowish, multinodular cystic lesion arising from the disc or retina; the appearance of this typical lesion is often compared with that of an unripe mulberry (Fig. 630-6). Equally characteristic and more common in tuberous sclerosis are flatter, yellow to whitish retinal lesions, varying in size from minute dots to large lesions approaching the size of the disc. These lesions are benign astrocytic proliferations. Rarely, similar retinal phakomas occur in von Recklinghausen disease (neurofibromatosis). In von Hippel-Lindau disease (angiomatosis of the retina and cerebellum), the distinctive fundus lesion is a hemangioblastoma; this vascular lesion usually appears as a reddish globular mass with large paired arteries and veins passing to and from the lesion. In Sturge-Weber syndrome (encephalofacial angiomatosis), the fundus abnormality is a choroidal hemangioma; the hemangioma may impart a dark color to the affected area of the fundus, but the lesion is best seen with fluorescein angiography.

RETINOSCHISIS

Congenital hereditary retinoschisis, also referred to as juvenile X-linked retinoschisis, is a bilateral vitreoretinal dystrophy that has a bimodal age of presentation. The first group presents with strabismus and nystagmus at a mean age of 1.5-2 yr and is the most severely affected group. The second group presents at 6-7 yr with poor vision. It is characterized by splitting of the retina into inner and outer layers. The usual ophthalmoscopic finding in affected males is an elevation of the inner layer of the retina, most commonly in the inferotemporal quadrant of the fundus, often with round or oval holes visible in the inner layer. Schisis of the fovea is virtually pathognomonic and is found in almost 100% of patients. Ophthalmoscopically, this appears in early stages as small, fine striae in the internal limiting membrane. These striae radiate outward in a petaloid or spoke wheel configuration. In some cases, frank retinal detachment or vitreous hemorrhage occurs.

Vision impairment varies from mild to severe; visual acuity may worsen with age, but good vision is often retained. Carrier females are asymptomatic, but linkage studies may be useful to help detect carriers.

RETINAL DETACHMENT

A retinal detachment is a separation of the outer layers of the retina from the underlying retinal pigment epithelium (RPE). During embryogenesis, the retina and RPE are initially separated. During ocular development, they join together and are held in apposition to each other by various physiologic mechanisms. Pathologic events leading to a retinal detachment return the retina–RPE to its former separated state. The detachment can occur as a congenital anomaly but more commonly arises secondary to other ocular abnormalities or trauma. Three types of detachment are described; each may occur in children. Rhegmatogenous detachments result from a break in the

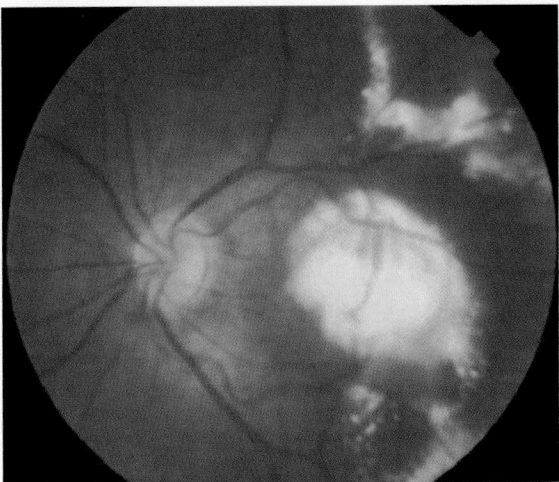

Figure 630-7 Coats disease with massive retinal exudation.

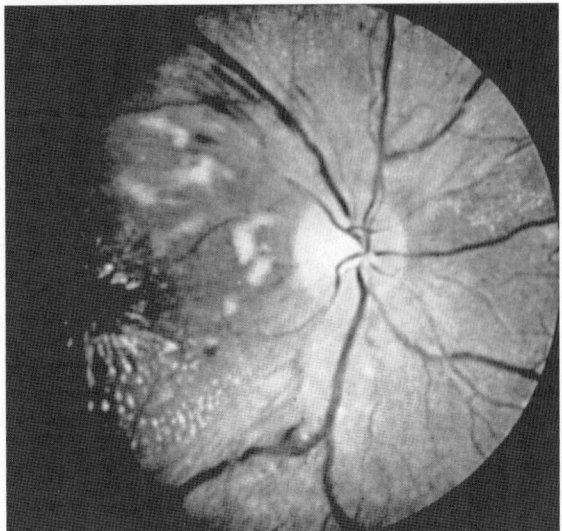

Figure 630-8 Hypertensive retinopathy.

retina that allows fluid to enter the subretinal space. In children, these are usually a result of trauma (such as child abuse) but may occur secondary to myopia or ROP or after congenital cataract surgery. Tractional retinal detachments result when vitreoretinal membranes pull on the retina. They can occur in diabetes, sickle cell disease, and ROP. Exudative retinal detachments result when exudation exceeds absorption. This can be seen in Coats disease, retinoblastoma, and ocular inflammation.

The presenting sign of retinal detachment in an infant or child may be loss of vision, secondary strabismus or nystagmus, or leukocoria (white pupillary reflex). In addition to direct examination of the eye, special diagnostic studies such as ultrasonography and neuroimaging (CT, MRI) may be necessary to establish the cause of the detachment and the appropriate treatment. Prompt treatment is essential if vision is to be salvaged.

COATS DISEASE

This exudative retinopathy of unknown cause is characterized by telangiectasia of retinal vessels with leakage of plasma to form intraretinal and subretinal exudates and by retinal hemorrhages and detachment (Fig. 630-7). The condition is usually unilateral. It predominantly affects boys, usually appearing in the 1st decade. The condition is nonfamilial and for the most part occurs in otherwise healthy children. The most frequent presenting signs are blurring of vision, leukocoria, and strabismus. Rubeosis of the iris, glaucoma, and cataract may develop. **Treatment** with photocoagulation or cryotherapy may be helpful.

FAMILIAL EXUDATIVE VITREORETINOPATHY

This progressive retinal vascular disorder is of unknown cause, but clinical and angiographic findings suggest an aberration of vascular development. Avascularity of the peripheral temporal retina is a significant finding in most cases, with abrupt cessation of the retinal capillary network in the region of the equator. The avascular zone often has a wedge- or V-shaped pattern in the temporal meridian. Glial proliferation or well-marked retinochoroidal atrophy may be found in the avascular zone. Excessive branching of retinal arteries and veins, dilation of the capillaries, arteriovenous shunt formation, neovascularization, and leakage from retinal vessels of the farthest vascularized retina occur. Vitreoretinal adhesions are usually present at the peripheral margin of the vascularized retina. Traction, retinal dragging and temporal displacement of the macula, falciform retinal folds, and retinal detachment are common. Intraretinal or subretinal exudation, retinal hemorrhage, and recurrent vitreous hemorrhages may develop. Patients may also develop cataracts and glaucoma. Vision impairment of varying severity occurs. The condition is usually bilateral. Familial exudative vitreoretinopathy (FEVR) is usually an autosomal dominant

condition with incomplete penetrance. Asymptomatic family members often display a zone of avascular peripheral retina.

The findings in FEVR may resemble those of ROP in the cicatricial stages, but unlike ROP, the neovascularization of FEVR seems to develop years after birth and most patients with FEVR have no history of prematurity, oxygen therapy, prenatal or postnatal injury or infection, or developmental abnormalities. FEVR is also to be differentiated from Coats disease, angiomatosis of the retina, peripheral uveitis, and other disorders of the posterior segment.

HYPERTENSIVE RETINOPATHY

In the early stages of hypertension, no retinal changes may be observable. Generalized constriction and irregular narrowing of the arterioles are usually the first signs in the fundus. Other alterations include retinal edema, flame-shaped hemorrhages, cotton-wool spots (retinal nerve fiber layer infarcts), and papilledema (Fig. 630-8). These changes are reversible if the hypertension can be controlled in the early stages, but in long-standing hypertension, irreversible changes may occur. Thickening of the vessel wall may produce a silver- or copper-wire appearance. Hypertensive retinal changes in a child should alert the physician to renal disease, pheochromocytoma, collagen disease, and cardiovascular disorders, particularly coarctation of the aorta.

DIABETIC RETINOPATHY

The retinal changes of diabetes mellitus are classified as nonproliferative or proliferative. Nonproliferative diabetic retinopathy is characterized by retinal microaneurysms, venous dilation, retinal hemorrhages, and exudates. The microaneurysms appear as tiny red dots. The hemorrhages may be of both the dot and blot type, representing deep intraretinal bleeding, and the splinter or flame-shaped type, involving the superficial nerve fiber layer. The exudates tend to be deep and to appear waxy. There may also be superficial nerve fiber infarcts called cytoid bodies or cotton-wool spots, as well as retinal edema. These signs may wax and wane. They are seen primarily in the posterior pole, around the disc and macula, well within the range of direct ophthalmoscopy. Involvement of the macula may lead to decreased vision.

Proliferative retinopathy, the more serious form, is characterized by neovascularization and proliferation of fibrovascular tissue on the retina, extending into the vitreous. Neovascularization may occur on the optic disc, elsewhere on the retina, or on the iris and in the anterior chamber angle (or rubeosis irides) (Fig. 630-9). Traction on these new vessels leads to hemorrhage and, eventually, scarring. The vision-threatening complications of proliferative diabetic retinopathy are retinal and vitreous hemorrhages, cicatrization, traction, and retinal detachment. Neovascularization of the iris may lead to secondary glaucoma if not treated promptly.

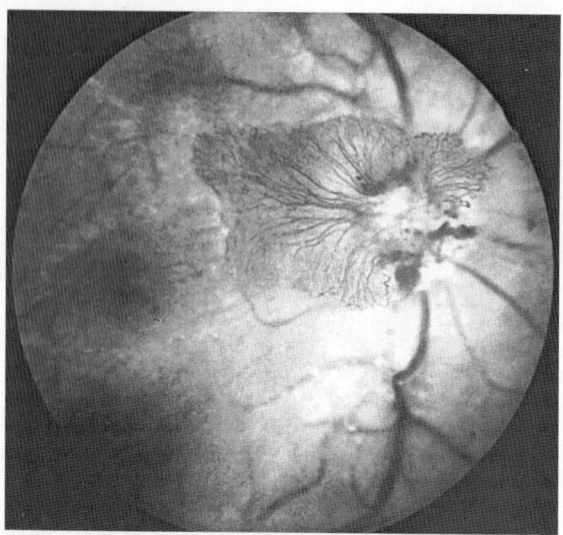

Figure 630-9 Proliferative diabetic retinopathy with neovascularization of the disc.

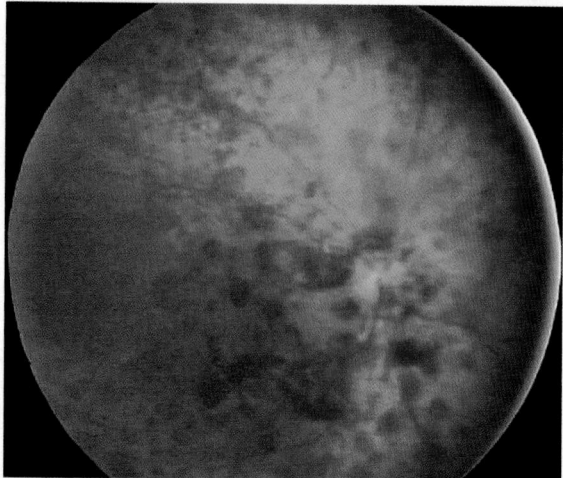

Figure 630-10 Shaken baby syndrome (inflicted neurotrauma). Retinal hemorrhages in multiple layers too numerous to count into far periphery.

Diabetic retinopathy involves the alteration and nonperfusion of retinal capillaries, retinal ischemia, and neovascularization, but its pathogenesis is not yet completely understood, either in terms of location of the primary pathogenetic mechanism (retinal vessels vs surrounding neuronal or glial tissue) or the specific biochemical factors involved. The better the degree of long-term metabolic control, the lower the risk of diabetic retinopathy.

Clinically, the prevalence and course of retinopathy relate to a patient's age and to disease duration. Detectable microvascular changes are rare in prepubertal children, with the prevalence of retinopathy increasing significantly after puberty, especially after the age of 15 yr. The incidence of retinopathy is low during the 1st 5 yr of disease and increases progressively thereafter, with the incidence of proliferative retinopathy becoming substantial after 10 yr and with increased risk of visual impairment after 15 yr or more.

Ophthalmic examination guidelines have been proposed by the American Academy of Pediatrics. An initial exam is recommended at age 9 yr if the diabetes is poorly controlled. If the diabetes is well controlled, an initial exam 3 yr after puberty with annual follow-up is recommended.

In addition to retinopathy, patients with juvenile-onset diabetes may develop optic neuropathy, characterized by swelling of the disc and blurring of vision. Patients with diabetes may also develop cataracts, even at an early age, sometimes with rapid progression.

Treatment
Macular edema is the leading cause of visual loss in diabetic persons. Photocoagulation may be used to decrease the risk of continued vision loss in patients with macular edema.

Proliferative retinopathy causes the most severe vision loss and can lead to total loss of vision and even loss of the eye. Patients who have proliferative disease and who display certain high-risk characteristics should undergo panretinal photocoagulation to preserve their central vision. Neovascularization of the iris is also treated with panretinal photocoagulation to stop the development of neovascular glaucoma.

Vitrectomy and other intraocular surgery may be necessary in patients with nonresolving vitreous hemorrhage or traction retinal detachment. The value of technologic advances, such as insulin infusion pumps and pancreatic transplants, in preventing ocular complications is under investigation (see Chapter 589).

SUBACUTE BACTERIAL ENDOCARDITIS
At some time during the course of the disease, retinopathy is present in approximately 40% of cases of subacute bacterial endocarditis. The lesions include hemorrhages, hemorrhages with white centers (Roth spots), papilledema, and, rarely, embolic occlusion of the central retinal artery.

BLOOD DISORDERS
In primary and secondary anemias, retinopathy in the form of hemorrhages and cotton-wool patches may occur. Vision can be affected if hemorrhage occurs in the macular area. The hemorrhages may be light and feathery or dense and preretinal. In polycythemia vera, the retinal veins are dark, dilated, and tortuous. Retinal hemorrhages, retinal edema, and papilledema may be observed. In leukemia, the veins are characteristically dilated, with sausage-shaped constrictions; hemorrhages, particularly white-centered hemorrhages and exudates, are common during the acute stage. In the sickling disorders, fundus changes include vascular tortuosity, arterial and venous occlusions, "salmon patches," refractile deposits, pigmented lesions, arteriolar-venous anastomoses, and neovascularization (with "sea-fan" formations), sometimes leading to vitreous hemorrhage and retinal detachment. Individuals with sickle cell hemoglobin C and sickle cell hemoglobin β-thalassemia hemoglobinopathies are at a higher risk of the development of retinopathy than are those with homozygous hemoglobin S disease. It is thought that the more anemic state of those patients with homozygous hemoglobin S disease offers protection from vascular occlusions in the retina.

TRAUMA-RELATED RETINOPATHY
Retinal changes may occur in patients who suffer trauma to other parts of the body. The occurrence of retinal hemorrhages in infants who have been physically abused is well documented (Fig. 630-10; see Chapter 40). Retinal, subretinal, subhyaloid, and vitreous hemorrhages have been described in infants and young children with inflicted neurotrauma. Often there are no signs of direct trauma to the eye, periocular region, or head. Such cases may result from violent shaking of an infant, and permanent retinal damage may result.

In patients with severe head or chest compressive trauma, a traumatic retinal angiopathy known as **Purtscher retinopathy** may occur. This is characterized by retinal hemorrhage, cotton-wool spots, possible disc swelling, and decreased vision. The pathogenesis is unclear, but there is evidence of arteriolar obstruction in this condition. A Purtscher-like fundus picture may also occur in several nontraumatic settings, such as acute pancreatitis, lupus erythematosus, and childbirth.

MYELINATED NERVE FIBERS
Myelination of the optic nerve fibers normally terminates at the level of the disc, but in some individuals, ectopic myelination extends to nerve fibers of the retina. The condition is most commonly seen adjacent to the disc, although more peripheral areas of the retina may be

involved. The characteristic ophthalmoscopic picture is a focal white patch with a feathered edge or brushstroke appearance. Because the macula is generally unaffected, the visual prognosis is good. A relative or absolute visual field defect corresponding to areas of ectopic myelination is usually the only associated ocular abnormality. Extensive unilateral involvement, however, is associated with ipsilateral myopia, amblyopia, and strabismus. If unilateral high myopia and amblyopia are present, appropriate optical correction and occlusion therapy should be instituted. For unknown reasons, the disorder is more commonly encountered in patients with craniofacial dysostosis, oxycephaly, neurofibromatosis, and Down syndrome.

COLOBOMA OF THE FUNDUS

The term *coloboma* describes a defect such as a gap, notch, fissure, or hole. The typical fundus coloboma is a result of malclosure of the embryonic fissure, which leaves a gap in the retina, RPE, and choroid, thus baring the underlying sclera. The defect may be extensive, involving the optic nerve, ciliary body, and iris and even the lens, or it may be localized to 1 or more portions of the fissure. The usual appearance is of a well-circumscribed, wedge-shaped white area extending inferonasally below the disc, sometimes involving or engulfing the disc. In some cases, there is ectasia or cyst formation in the area of the defect. Less-extensive colobomatous defects may appear as only single or multiple focal punched-out chorioretinal defects or anomalous pigmentation of the fundus in the line of the embryonic fissure. Colobomas may occur in 1 or both eyes. A visual field defect usually corresponds to the chorioretinal defect. Visual acuity may be impaired, particularly if the defect involves the disc or macula.

Fundus colobomas may occur in isolation as sporadic defects or as an inherited condition. Isolated colobomatous anomalies are commonly inherited in an autosomal dominant manner with highly variable penetrance and expressivity. Family members of affected patients should receive appropriate genetic counseling. Colobomas may also be associated with such abnormalities as microphthalmia, glioneuroma of the eye, cyclopia, or encephalocele. They occur in children with various chromosomal disorders, including trisomies 13 and 18, triploidy, cat's-eye syndrome, and 4p–. Ocular colobomas also occur in many multisystem disorders, including the CHARGE (*C,* coloboma; *H,* heart disease; *A,* atresia choanae; *R,* retarded growth and development and/or central nervous system anomalies; *G,* genetic anomalies and/or hypogonadism; *E,* ear anomalies and/or deafness) association; Joubert, Aicardi, Meckel, Warburg, and Rubinstein-Taybi syndromes; linear sebaceous nevus; Goldenhar and Lenz microphthalmia syndromes; and Goltz focal dermal hypoplasia.

Bibliography is available at Expert Consult.

Chapter **631**
Abnormalities of the Optic Nerve

Scott E. Olitsky, Denise Hug, Laura S. Plummer, Erin D. Stahl, Michelle M. Ariss, and Timothy P. Lindquist

OPTIC NERVE APLASIA

This rare congenital anomaly is typically unilateral. The optic nerve, retinal ganglion cells, and retinal blood vessels are absent. A vestigial dural sheath usually connects with the sclera in a normal position, but no neural tissue is present within this sheath. Optic nerve aplasia typically occurs sporadically in an otherwise healthy person.

OPTIC NERVE HYPOPLASIA

Hypoplasia of the optic nerve is a nonprogressive condition characterized by a subnormal number of optic nerve axons with normal mesodermal elements and glial supporting tissue. In typical cases, the nerve head is small and pale, with a pale or pigmented peripapillary halo or double-ring sign.

This anomaly is associated with defects of vision and of visual fields of varying severity, ranging from blindness to normal or near-normal vision. It may be associated with systemic anomalies that most commonly involve the central nervous system (CNS). Protean CNS defects such as hydranencephaly or anencephaly or more focal lesions compatible with continued development of a patient may accompany optic nerve hypoplasia, but unilateral or bilateral optic nerve hypoplasia may be found without any concomitant defects.

Optic nerve hypoplasia is a principal feature of **septooptic dysplasia of de Morsier,** a developmental disorder characterized by the association of anomalies of the midline structures of the brain with hypoplasia of the optic nerves, optic chiasm, and optic tracts; typically noted are agenesis of the septum pellucidum, partial or complete agenesis of the corpus callosum, and malformation of the fornix, with a large chiasmatic cistern. Patients may have hypothalamic abnormalities and endocrine defects, ranging from panhypopituitarism to isolated deficiency of growth hormone, hypothyroidism, or diabetes insipidus. Neonatal hypoglycemia and seizures are important presenting signs in affected infants.

MRI is preferred for evaluating CNS abnormalities in patients with optic nerve hypoplasia. During MRI, special attention should be directed to the pituitary infundibulum, where ectopia of the posterior pituitary may be found. Posterior pituitary ectopia appears on MRI as an absence of the pituitary infundibulum with an abnormal bright spot at the upper infundibulum area. This abnormality is present in approximately 15% of patients and suggests posterior pituitary hormone deficiency, requiring further endocrinologic work-up. Endocrine function should be watched closely in patients with optic nerve hypoplasia. The cause of optic nerve hypoplasia remains unclear.

Children with **periventricular leukomalacia** display an unusual form of optic nerve hypoplasia. The optic nerves demonstrate a large cup within a normal-size optic disc. This form of optic nerve hypoplasia occurs secondary to transsynaptic degeneration of optic axons caused by the primary bilateral lesion in the optic radiation (periventricular leukomalacia).

OPTIC NERVE COLOBOMA

Optic nerve colobomas can be unilateral or bilateral. The visual acuity can range from normal to complete blindness. The coloboma develops secondary to incomplete closure of the embryonic fissure. The defect may produce a partial or total excavation of the optic disc (Fig. 631-1).

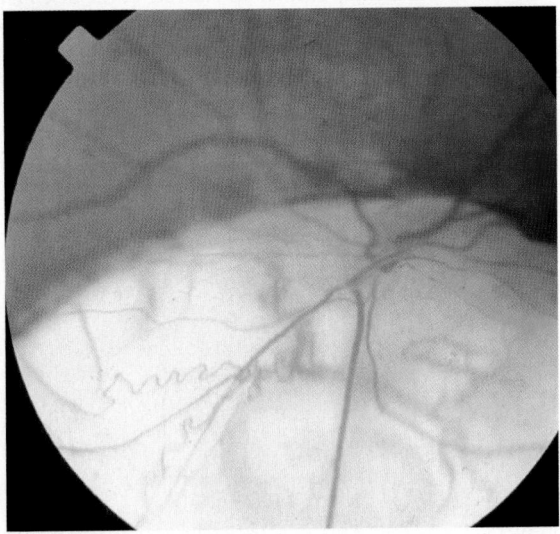

Figure 631-1 Optic nerve coloboma.

Chorioretinal and iris colobomas may also occur. Optic nerve colobomas may be seen in a multitude of ocular and systemic abnormalities including the CHARGE (*C*, coloboma; *H*, heart disease; *A*, atresia choanae; *R*, retarded growth and development and/or CNS anomalies; *G*, genetic anomalies and/or hypogonadism; *E*, ear anomalies and/or deafness) association.

MORNING GLORY DISC ANOMALY

This term describes a congenital malformation of the optic nerve characterized by an enlarged, excavated, funnel-shaped disc with an elevated rim, resembling a morning glory flower. White glial tissue is present in the central part of the disc. The retinal vessels are abnormal and appear at the peripheral disc and course over the elevated pink rim in a radial fashion. Pigmentary mottling of the peripapillary region is usually seen. Most cases are unilateral. Females are affected twice as often as males. Visual acuity is usually severely reduced. Morning glory disc anomaly has been associated with basal encephalocele in patients with midfacial anomalies. Abnormalities of the carotid circulation can also be seen in patients with morning glory anomaly. Moyamoya disease is a well-described associated finding.

TILTED DISC

In this congenital anomaly, the vertical axis of the optic disc is directed obliquely, so that the upper temporal portion of the nerve head is more prominent and anterior to the lower nasal portion of the disc. The retinal vessels emerge from the upper temporal portion of the disc rather than from the nasal side. Often noted is a peripapillary crescent or conus. Associated visual field defects and myopic astigmatism may be found. Clinical recognition of the tilted disc syndrome is important to avoid confusion of its disc and visual field signs with those of papilledema and intracranial tumor.

DRUSEN OF THE OPTIC NERVE

These globular, acellular bodies are thought to arise from axoplasmic derivatives of disintegrating nerve fibers. Drusen may be buried within the optic nerve, producing elevation of the optic nerve head (which can be confused with papilledema), or they may be partially or completely exposed, appearing as refractile bodies at the surface of the disc. Visual field defects and spontaneous peripapillary nerve fiber layer hemorrhages may occur in association with drusen. Drusen may occur as an autosomal dominant condition. B scan ultrasonography can help positively identify drusen suspected on clinical ophthalmic exam (Fig. 631-2).

PAPILLEDEMA

The term *papilledema* is reserved to describe swelling of the nerve head secondary to increased intracranial pressure (ICP). Clinical manifestations of papilledema include edematous blurring of the disc margins, fullness or elevation of the nerve head, partial or complete obliteration of the disc cup, capillary congestion and hyperemia of the nerve head, generalized engorgement of the veins, loss of spontaneous venous

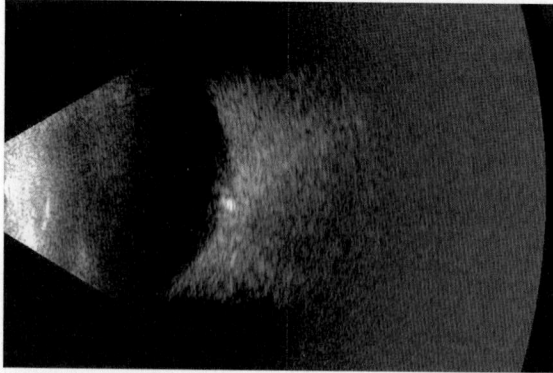

Figure 631-2 Optic nerve drusen seen on B scan ultrasonography.

pulsation, nerve fiber layer hemorrhages around the disc, and peripapillary exudates (see Fig. 590-1 in Chapter 590). In some cases, edema extending into the macula may produce a fan- or star-shaped figure. In addition, concentric peripapillary retinal wrinkling (Paton lines) may be noted. Transient obscuration of vision may occur, lasting seconds and associated with postural changes. Vision, however, is usually normal in acute papilledema. Normally, when the ICP is relieved, the papilledema resolves and the disc returns to a normal or nearly normal appearance within 6-8 wk. Sustained chronic papilledema or long-standing unrelieved increased ICP may, however, lead to permanent nerve fiber damage, atrophic changes of the disc, macular scarring, and impairment of vision.

The *pathophysiology* of papilledema is probably as follows: elevation of intracranial subarachnoid cerebrospinal fluid (CSF) pressure, elevation of CSF pressure in the sheath of the optic nerve, elevation of tissue pressure in the optic nerve, stasis of axoplasmic flow and swelling of the nerve fibers in the optic nerve head, and secondary vascular changes and the characteristic ophthalmoscopic signs of venous stasis. Associated neuroophthalmic signs of increased ICP in infants and children include 6th cranial nerve palsy and attendant esotropia, lid retraction, paresis of upward gaze, tonic downward deviation of the eyes, and convergent nystagmus.

The common **etiologies** of papilledema in childhood are intracranial tumors and obstructive hydrocephalus, intracranial hemorrhage, the cerebral edema of trauma, meningoencephalitis, toxic encephalopathy, and certain metabolic diseases. Whatever the cause, the optic disc signs of increased ICP in early childhood may occasionally be modified by the distensibility of the young skull. In the absence of conditions associated with early closure of sutures and early obliteration of the fontanel (craniosynostosis, Crouzon disease, and Apert syndrome), infants with increased ICP may not develop papilledema.

The **differential diagnosis** of papilledema includes structural changes of the disc (pseudopapilledema, pseudoneuritis, drusen, and myelinated nerve fibers), with which it may be confused, and the disc swelling of papillitis associated with optic neuritis in addition to the disc changes of hypertension and diabetes mellitus. Unless retinal hemorrhage or edema involves the macular area, the preservation of good central vision and the absence of an afferent pupillary defect (Marcus Gunn pupil) help to differentiate acute papilledema from the edema of the optic nerve head found in acute optic neuritis.

Papilledema is a neurologic emergency. It can be accompanied by other signs of increased ICP, including headaches, nausea, and vomiting. Neuroimaging should be performed; if no intracranial masses are detected, a lumbar puncture and determination of CSF pressure should follow.

OPTIC NEURITIS

This is any inflammation or demyelinization of the optic nerve with attendant impairment of function. The process is usually acute, with rapidly progressive loss of vision. It may be unilateral or bilateral. Pain on movement of the globe or pain on palpation of the globe may precede or accompany the onset of visual symptoms. There is decreased visual activity, decreased color vision and contrast sensitivity, a relative afferent pupillary defect, and a normal macula and peripheral retina.

When the retrobulbar portion of the nerve is affected without ophthalmoscopically visible signs of inflammation at the disc, the term *retrobulbar optic neuritis* is applied. When there is ophthalmoscopically visible evidence of inflammation of the nerve head, the term *papillitis* or *intraocular optic neuritis* is used. When there is involvement of both the retina and the papilla, the term optic *neuroretinitis* is used.

In childhood, optic neuritis may occur as an isolated condition or as a manifestation of a neurologic or systemic disease. Optic neuritis may be secondary to inflammatory diseases (systemic lupus erythematosus, sarcoidosis, Behçet disease, autoimmune optic neuritis); infections (tuberculosis, syphilis, Lyme disease, meningitis, viral encephalitis, HIV, or postinfectious disease); and toxic or nutritional disorders (methanol, ethambutol, vitamin B_{12} deficiency). It may signify one of the many demyelinating diseases of childhood (see Chapter 600). Although a significant percentage of adults who experience an episode of optic neuritis eventually develop other symptoms associated with multiple sclerosis (MS), young children with optic neuritis are seemingly at less risk (risk of MS is 19% within 20 yr). High-risk features suggestive of MS include visual acuity better than no light perception, periocular pain, acutely normal-appearing optic nerve, no retinal abnormalities, and abnormal MRI suggesting a demyelinating disease. Bilateral optic neuritis in children may be associated with acute disseminated encephalomyelitis or **neuromyelitis optica (NMO or Devic disease)**. NMO is characterized by rapid and severe bilateral visual loss accompanied by transverse myelitis and paraplegia. Brainstem and occasionally involvement of the cortex may be seen on MRI. NMO-specific immunoglobulin G (directed to the aquaporin 4 water channel) is the diagnostic test of choice for Devic syndrome. Optic neuritis may also be secondary to an exogenous toxin or drug, such as with lead poisoning or as a complication of long-term high-dose treatment with chloramphenicol or vincristine. Extensive pediatric neurologic and ophthalmic investigation, including MRI and lumbar puncture, is usually required. Idiopathic NMO is associated with antiaquaporin 4 antibodies, otherwise known as NMO antibodies.

In most cases of acute optic neuritis, some improvement in vision begins within 1-4 wk after onset, and vision may improve to normal or near normal within weeks or months. The course varies with cause. Although central vision may fully recover, it is common to find permanent defects in other areas of visual function (contrast sensitivity, color, brightness sense, and motion perception). Recurrences may occur especially, but not universally, in patients who go on to develop MS.

A **treatment** trial demonstrated that high-dose intravenous methylprednisolone may help to speed the visual recovery in young adults, and it may prevent the development of MS in those at risk. Orally administered corticosteroids should not be used because they are associated with a significant increase in the recurrence rate of optic neuritis. It is unknown to what degree the results of the aforementioned trial may be extrapolated to optic neuritis in childhood. Eculizumab, an inhibitor of complement C5, has had some success in reducing relapses in patients with NMO.

LEBER OPTIC NEUROPATHY

This entity is characterized by sudden loss of central vision occurring in the 2nd and 3rd decades of life, and primarily affects young males. A characteristic peripapillary telangiectatic microangiopathy occurs not only in the presymptomatic phase of involved eyes but also in a high number of asymptomatic offspring in the female line. Disc hyperemia and edema mark the acute phase of visual loss. One eye is usually affected before the other. Visual field loss and impaired color vision are also present. In time, progressive optic atrophy and vision loss usually ensue. The tortuous angiopathy becomes less obvious. Although visual function after the initial loss generally remains stable, a significant and sometimes complete recovery may occur in as many as 30% of affected individuals. This recovery may take place years or decades after the initial episode of acute vision loss. The peripapillary angiopathy, the lack of short-term remission, and the degree of symmetry serve to distinguish most cases of Leber disease from the optic neuritis of MS.

Leber optic neuropathy is maternally inherited and is caused by defective cytoplasmic mitochondrial DNA. Multiple point mutations in the mitochondrial DNA that lead to the development of the disorder have been found. Because of the mitochondrial nature of the disorder, skeletal and cardiac muscle disorders, including electrocardiographic abnormalities, may also be encountered in affected individuals.

OPTIC ATROPHY

This term denotes degeneration of optic nerve axons, with attendant loss of function. The ophthalmoscopic signs of optic atrophy are pallor of the disc and loss of substance of the nerve head, sometimes with enlargement of the disc cup. The associated vision defect varies with the nature and site of the primary disease or lesion.

Optic atrophy is the common expression of a wide variety of congenital or acquired pathologic processes. The cause may be traumatic, inflammatory, degenerative, neoplastic, or vascular; intracranial tumors and hydrocephalus are principal causes of optic atrophy in children. In some cases, progressive optic atrophy is hereditary. **Dominantly inherited infantile optic atrophy** is a relatively mild heredodegenerative type that tends to progress through childhood and adolescence. **Autosomal recessively inherited congenital optic atrophy** is a rare condition that is evident at birth or develops at a very early age; the visual defect is usually profound. **Behr optic atrophy** is a hereditary type associated with hypertonia of the extremities, increased deep tendon reflexes, mild cerebellar ataxia, some degree of mental deficiency, and possibly external ophthalmoplegia. This disorder afflicts principally boys age 3-11 yr. Some forms of heredodegenerative optic atrophy are associated with sensorineural hearing loss, as may occur in some children with juvenile-onset (insulin-dependent) diabetes mellitus. In the absence of an obvious cause, optic atrophy in an infant or child warrants extensive etiologic investigation.

OPTIC NERVE GLIOMA

Optic nerve glioma, more properly referred to as **juvenile pilocytic astrocytoma,** is the most frequent tumor of the optic nerve in childhood. This neuroglial tumor may develop in the intraorbital, intracanalicular, or intracranial portion of the nerve; the chiasm is often involved.

The tumor is a cytologic benign hamartoma that is generally stationary or only slowly progressive. The principal *clinical manifestations* when the tumor occurs in the intraorbital portion of the nerve are unilateral loss of vision, proptosis, and deviation of the eye; optic atrophy or congestion of the optic nerve head may occur. Chiasmal involvement may be attended by defects of vision and visual fields (often bitemporal hemianopia), increased ICP, papilledema or optic atrophy, hypothalamic dysfunction, pituitary dysfunction, and sometimes nystagmus or strabismus. Juvenile pilocytic astrocytomas occur with increased frequency in patients with neurofibromatosis.

Treatment of optic pathway gliomas is controversial. The best management is usually periodic observation with serial radiography (preferably MRI). Only symptomatic and radiographically progressing optic nerve gliomas require strong consideration for treatment. Surgical removal may be appropriate when the tumor is confined to the intraorbital, intracanalicular, or prechiasmal portion of the nerve if a patient has unsightly proptosis with complete or nearly complete loss of vision of the affected eye. When the chiasm is involved, resection is not usually indicated and radiation and chemotherapy may be necessary.

TRAUMATIC OPTIC NEUROPATHIES

Injury to the optic nerve may result from both direct and indirect trauma. Direct trauma to the optic nerve is a result of a penetrating injury to the orbit with transection or contusion of the nerve. Blunt trauma to the orbit may also lead to severe visual loss if the traumatic force is transmitted to the optic canal and causes disruption of the blood supply to the intracanalicular portion of the nerve. Treatment with high-dose corticosteroids has not been proven to be effective, and similar regimens have shown there is an increased relative risk of death when such regimens are given to patients after significant head injury.

Bibliography is available at Expert Consult.

Chapter 632

Childhood Glaucoma

Scott E. Olitsky, Denise Hug,
Laura S. Plummer, Erin D. Stahl,
Michelle M. Ariss, and
Timothy P. Lindquist

Glaucoma is a general term used to indicate damage to the optic nerve with visual field loss that is caused by or related to elevated pressure within the eye. It is classified according to the age of the affected individual at presentation and the association of other ocular or systemic conditions. Glaucoma that begins within the 1st 3 yr of life is called infantile (congenital); that which begins between the ages of 3 and 30 yr is called juvenile.

Primary glaucoma indicates that the cause is an isolated anomaly of the drainage apparatus of the eye (trabecular meshwork). More than 50% of infantile cases are primary glaucoma. In secondary glaucoma, other ocular or systemic abnormalities are associated, even if a similar developmental defect of the trabecular meshwork is also present. Primary infantile glaucoma occurs with an incidence of 0.03% (Table 632-1).

CLINICAL MANIFESTATIONS

The symptoms of infantile glaucoma include the classic triad of epiphora (tearing), photophobia (sensitivity to light), and blepharospasm (eyelid squeezing; Fig. 632-1). Each can be attributed to corneal irritation. Only approximately 30% of affected infants demonstrate the classic symptom complex. Signs of glaucoma include corneal edema, corneal and ocular enlargement, and conjunctival injection (Fig. 632-2).

Table 632-1	Primary and Secondary Childhood Glaucomas

I. PRIMARY GLAUCOMAS
A. Congenital open-angle glaucoma
   1. Congenital
   2. Infantile
   3. Late recognized
B. Autosomal dominant juvenile glaucoma
C. Primary angle-closure glaucoma
D. Associated with systemic abnormalities
   1. Sturge-Weber syndrome
   2. Neurofibromatosis type 1 (NF-1)
   3. Stickler syndrome
   4. Oculocerebrorenal (Lowe) syndrome
   5. Rieger syndrome
   6. Hepatocerebrorenal syndrome
   7. Marfan syndrome
   8. Rubinstein-Taybi syndrome
   9. Infantile glaucoma associated with mental retardation and paralysis
   10. Oculodentodigital dysplasia
   11. Open-angle glaucoma associated with microcornea and absence of frontal sinuses
   12. Mucopolysaccharidosis
   13. Trisomy 13
   14. Cutis marmorata telangiectasia congenita
   15. Warburg syndrome
   16. Kniest syndrome (skeletal dysplasia)
   17. Michel syndrome
   18. Nonprogressive hemiatrophy
E. Associated with ocular abnormalities
   1. Congenital glaucoma with iris and pupillary abnormalities
   2. Aniridia
      a. Congenital glaucoma
      b. Acquired glaucoma
   3. Congenital ocular melanosis
   4. Sclerocornea
   5. Iridotrabecular dysgenesis
   6. Peters syndrome
   7. Iridotrabecular dysgenesis and ectropion uveae
   8. Posterior polymorphous dystrophy
   9. Idiopathic or familial elevated episcleral venous pressure
   10. Anterior corneal staphyloma
   11. Congenital microcornea with myopia
   12. Congenital hereditary endothelial dystrophy
   13. Congenital hereditary iris stromal hypoplasia

II. SECONDARY GLAUCOMAS
A. Traumatic glaucoma
   1. Acute glaucoma
      a. Angle concussion
      b. Hyphema
      c. Ghost cell glaucoma
   2. Late-onset glaucoma with angle recession
   3. Arteriovenous fistula
B. Secondary to intraocular neoplasm
   1. Retinoblastoma
   2. Juvenile xanthogranuloma
   3. Leukemia
   4. Melanoma
   5. Melanocytoma
   6. Iris rhabdomyosarcoma
   7. Aggressive nevi of the iris
C. Secondary to uveitis
   1. Open-angle glaucoma
   2. Angle-blockage glaucoma
      a. Synechial angle closure
      b. Iris bombé with pupillary block
D. Lens-induced glaucoma
   1. Subluxation–dislocation and pupillary block
      a. Marfan syndrome
      b. Homocystinuria
   2. Spherophakia and pupillary block
   3. Phacolytic glaucoma
E. Secondary to surgery for congenital cataract
   1. Lens material blockage of the trabecular meshwork (acute or subacute)
   2. Pupillary block
   3. Chronic open-angle glaucoma associated with angle defects
F. Steroid-induced glaucoma
G. Secondary to rubeosis
   1. Retinoblastoma
   2. Coats disease
   3. Medulloepithelioma
   4. Familial exudative vitreoretinopathy
H. Secondary angle-closure glaucoma
   1. Retinopathy of prematurity
   2. Microphthalmos
   3. Nanophthalmos
   4. Retinoblastoma
   5. Persistent hyperplastic primary vitreous
   6. Congenital pupillary iris–lens membrane
I. Glaucoma associated with increased venous pressure
   1. Carotid or dural-venous fistula
   2. Orbital disease
J. Secondary to maternal rubella
K. Secondary to intraocular infection
   1. Acute recurrent toxoplasmosis
   2. Acute herpetic iritis

From Nelson LB: Harley's pediatric ophthalmology, ed 4, Philadelphia, 1998, WB Saunders, p. 294.

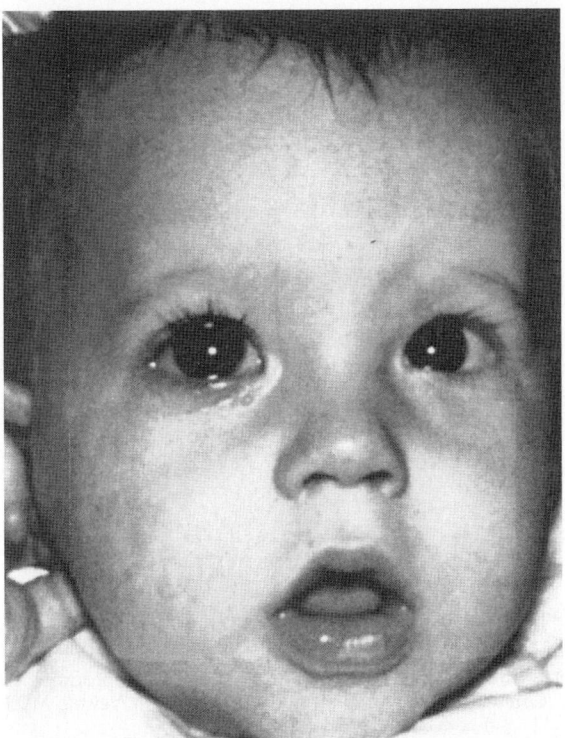

Figure 632-1 Tearing of the right eye caused by glaucoma. Note the increased corneal diameter of the right eye. *(From Nelson LB: Harley's pediatric ophthalmology, ed 4, Philadelphia, 1998, WB Saunders, p. 285.)*

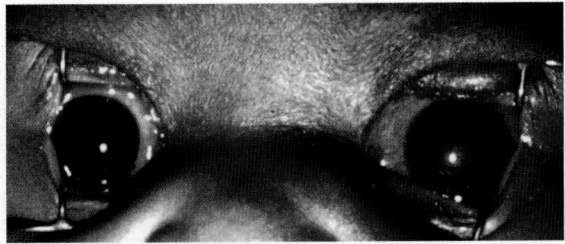

Figure 632-2 Infantile glaucoma. The left cornea is enlarged and edematous.

The sclera and cornea are more elastic in early childhood than later in life. An increase in intraocular pressure (IOP), therefore, leads to an expansion of the globe, including the cornea, and the development of buphthalmos ("ox eye"). If the cornea continues to enlarge, breaks occur in the endothelial basement membrane (Descemet membrane) and may lead to permanent corneal scarring. These breaks in Descemet membrane (Haab striae) are visible as horizontal edematous lines that cross or curve around the central cornea. They rarely occur beyond 3 yr of age or in corneas <12 mm in diameter. The cornea also becomes edematous and cloudy, with increased IOP. The corneal edema leads to tearing and photophobia. Glaucoma should be considered in a child suspected of having a nasolacrimal duct obstruction if any of these other signs or symptoms are present.

Children with unilateral glaucoma generally present early because the difference in the corneal size between the eyes can be noticed. When the disease is bilateral, parents may not recognize the increased corneal size. Many parents view the large eyes as attractive and do not seek help until other symptoms develop.

Cupping of the optic nerve head is detected by ocular examination. The optic nerve of an infant is easily distended by excessive pressure. Deep, central cupping readily occurs and may regress with normalization of pressure.

Some infants and children with early-onset glaucoma have more extensive maldevelopment of the anterior segment of the eye. The neurocristopathies comprise a spectrum of conditions relating to abnormal embryologic development of the anterior segment. They are usually bilateral and may include abnormalities of the iris, cornea, and lens. Other ocular anomalies that may be associated with glaucoma in infants and children are aniridia, cataract, spherophakia, and ectopia lentis. Glaucoma may also develop secondary to persistent hyperplastic primary vitreous or retinopathy of prematurity.

Trauma, intraocular hemorrhage, ocular inflammatory disease, and intraocular tumor are also important causes of glaucoma in the pediatric population. Systemic disorders associated with glaucoma in infants and children are Sturge-Weber syndrome (see Chapter 596.3), neurofibromatosis (see Chapter 596.1), Lowe syndrome, Marfan syndrome (see Chapter 702), congenital rubella (see Chapters 109.6 and 247), and a number of chromosomal syndromes (see Chapter 81).

Glaucoma occurs frequently in children with a history of congenital cataracts. Glaucoma may develop in up to 25% of children who have undergone cataract surgery early in life. The cause of aphakic glaucoma is not known but is thought to be the result of a coexistent anterior chamber deformity. Children treated for cataracts need to be monitored closely for this complication that may threaten vision.

DIAGNOSIS AND TREATMENT

The diagnosis of infantile glaucoma is made on recognition of the signs and symptoms. Once the diagnosis is established, treatment is started promptly. Unlike adult glaucoma, in which medication is often the first line of therapy, for infantile glaucoma, the treatment is primarily surgical. Procedures used to treat glaucoma in children include surgery to establish a more normal anterior chamber angle (goniotomy and trabeculotomy), to create a site for aqueous fluid to exit the eye (trabeculectomy and seton surgery), or to reduce aqueous fluid production (cyclocryotherapy and cyclophotocoagulation). Many children frequently require several operations to lower and maintain their IOP adequately, and long-term medical therapy may be necessary as well. Patients with multiple ocular abnormalities and those with aphakic glaucoma generally require more surgeries to achieve and maintain adequate IOP control. Although vision may be reduced secondary to glaucomatous optic nerve damage or corneal scarring, amblyopia is the most common cause of loss of vision in these children.

Bibliography is available at Expert Consult.

Chapter **633**
Orbital Abnormalities
Scott E. Olitsky, Denise Hug, Laura S. Plummer, Erin D. Stahl, Michelle M. Ariss, and Timothy P. Lindquist

HYPERTELORISM AND HYPOTELORISM

Hypertelorism is wide separation of the eyes or an increased interorbital distance, which may occur as a morphogenetic variant, a primary deformity, or a secondary phenomenon in association with developmental abnormalities, such as frontal meningocele or encephalocele or the persistence of a facial cleft. Often associated are strabismus, generally exotropia, and sometimes optic atrophy.

Hypotelorism refers to narrowness of the interorbital distance, which may occur as a morphogenetic variant alone or in association with other anomalies, such as epicanthus or holoprosencephaly, or secondary to a cranial dystrophy, such as scaphocephaly.

EXOPHTHALMOS AND ENOPHTHALMOS

Protrusion of the eye is referred to as exophthalmos or proptosis and is a common indicator of orbital disease. It may be caused by shallowness of the orbits, as in many craniofacial malformations, or by increased tissue mass within the orbit, as with neoplastic, vascular, and inflammatory disorders. Ocular complications include exposure keratopathy, ocular motor disturbances, and optic atrophy with loss of vision.

Posterior displacement or sinking of the eye back into the orbit is referred to as enophthalmos. This may occur with orbital fracture or with atrophy of orbital tissue.

ORBITAL INFLAMMATION

Inflammatory disease involving the orbit may be primary or secondary to systemic disease. Idiopathic orbital inflammation (**orbital pseudotumor**) represents a wide spectrum of clinical entities. Symptoms at the time of presentation may include pain, eyelid swelling, proptosis, a red eye, and fever. The inflammation may involve a single extraocular muscle (myositis) or the entire orbit. Orbital apex syndrome is a serious condition that may also involve the cavernous sinus and may compress or displace the optic nerve. Confusion with orbital cellulitis is common but can be differentiated by the lack of associated sinus disease, its appearance on CT scan, and lack of improvement with systemic antibiotics. Orbital pseudotumor is associated with systemic lupus erythematosus, Crohn disease, myasthenia gravis, and lymphoma. **Treatment** includes the use of high-dose systemic corticosteroids. Often, the symptoms improve dramatically shortly after treatment is initiated. Bilateral involvement, associated uveitis, disc edema, and recurrence of inflammation are not uncommon in the pediatric population. Immunotherapy or radiation treatment may be necessary for resistant or recurrent cases.

Thyroid-related ophthalmopathy (see also Chapter 563) is believed to be secondary to an immune mechanism, leading to inflammation and deposition of mucopolysaccharides and collagen in the extraocular muscles and orbital fat. Involvement of the extraocular muscles may lead to a restrictive strabismus. Lid retraction and exophthalmos may cause corneal exposure and infection or perforation. Involvement of the posterior orbit can compress the optic nerve. Treatment of thyroid-related ophthalmopathy may include the use of systemic corticosteroids, radiation of the orbit, eyelid surgery, strabismus surgery, or orbital decompression to eliminate symptoms and protect vision. The degree of orbital involvement is often independent of the status of the systemic disease.

Other systemic disorders that may cause inflammatory disease within the orbit include lymphoma (see Chapter 496), sarcoidosis (see Chapter 165), amyloidosis (see Chapter 164), polyarteritis nodosa (see Chapter 167.3), systemic lupus erythematosus (see Chapter 158), dermatomyositis (see Chapter 159), Wegener granulomatosis (see Chapter 167), and juvenile xanthogranuloma (see Chapter 507).

TUMORS OF THE ORBIT

Various tumors occur in and about the orbit in childhood. Among benign tumors, the most common are vascular lesions (principally hemangiomas) (Fig. 633-1) and dermoids. Among malignant neoplasms, rhabdomyosarcoma, lymphosarcoma, and metastatic neuroblastoma are the most frequent. Optic nerve gliomas (see Chapter 631) are most commonly seen in patients with neurofibromatosis and may present with poor vision or proptosis. Retinoblastoma (see Chapter 502) may extend into the orbit if it is discovered late or goes untreated. Teratomas are rare tumors that typically grow rapidly after birth and exhibit explosive proptosis.

The effects of orbital tumors vary with their locations and growth patterns. The principal signs are proptosis, resistance to retroplacement of the eye, and impairment of eye movement. A palpable mass may be found. Other significant signs are ptosis, optic nerve head congestion, optic atrophy, and loss of vision. Bruit and visible pulsation of the globe are important clues to vascular lesions.

Evaluation of orbital tumors includes ultrasonography, MRI, and CT. Pseudotumor of the orbit also must be considered in children with

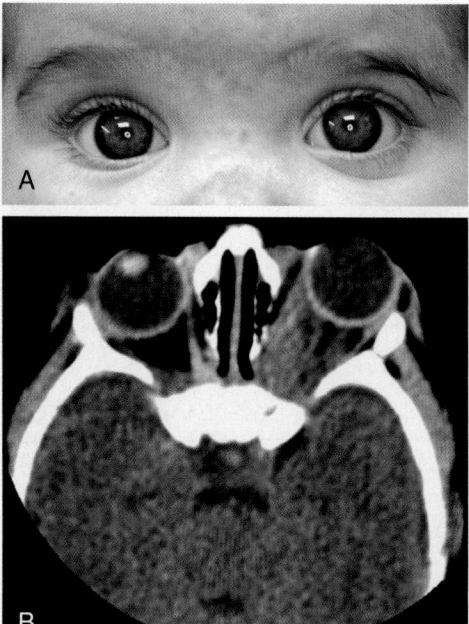

Figure 633-1 Orbital hemangioma. **A,** Note the proptosis. **B,** CT scan. *(Courtesy of Amy Nopper, MD, and Brandon Newell, MD.)*

signs of a mass lesion. In selected cases, an incisional or excisional biopsy of the lesion may be warranted.

Bibliography is available at Expert Consult.

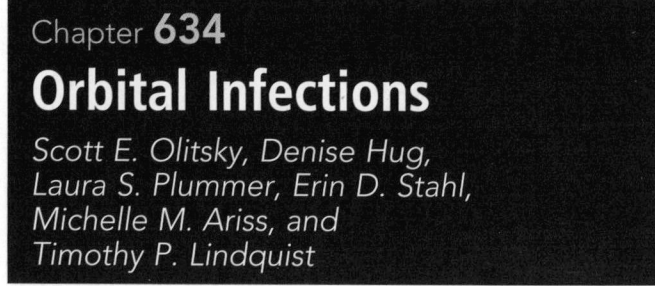

Chapter 634

Orbital Infections

Scott E. Olitsky, Denise Hug, Laura S. Plummer, Erin D. Stahl, Michelle M. Ariss, and Timothy P. Lindquist

Orbital infections are common in children. It is important to be able to distinguish the different forms of infection that occur in the orbital region to allow rapid diagnosis and treatment to prevent loss of vision or spread of the infection to the nearby intracranial structures (Table 634-1).

DACRYOADENITIS

Dacryoadenitis, or inflammation of the lacrimal gland, is uncommon in childhood. It may occur with mumps (in which case it is usually acute and bilateral, subsiding in a few days or weeks) or with infectious mononucleosis. *Staphylococcus aureus* may produce a suppurative dacryoadenitis. Chronic dacryoadenitis is associated with certain systemic diseases, particularly sarcoidosis, tuberculosis, and syphilis. Some systemic diseases may produce enlargement of the lacrimal and salivary glands (Mikulicz syndrome).

DACRYOCYSTITIS

Dacryocystitis is an infection of the lacrimal sac. Dacryocystitis generally requires obstruction of the nasolacrimal system to allow its development. Acute dacryocystitis presents with redness and swelling over the region of the lacrimal sac (Fig. 634-1). It is treated with warm compresses and systemic antibiotics. This helps to control the

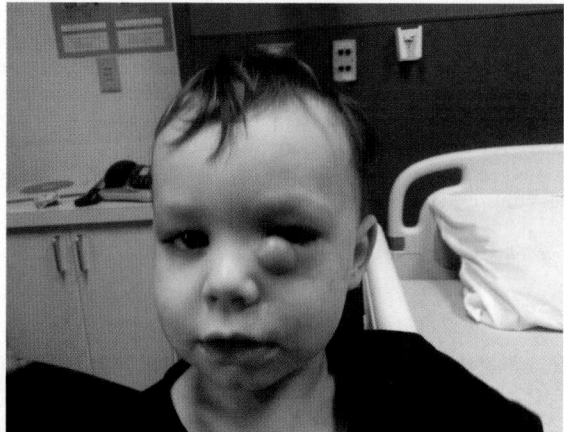

Figure 634-1 Dacrycystitis in a child previously treated for nasolacrimal duct obstruction.

Table 634-1	Chandler Classification of Orbital Complications of Sinusitis, a Clinical Description	
CHANDLER CLASS	**STAGE**	**CLINICAL DESCRIPTION AND DEFINITION**
I	Inflammatory edema	Eyelid edema and erythema Normal extraocular movement Normal visual acuity
II	Orbital cellulitis	Diffuse edema of orbital contents without discrete abscess formation
III	Subperiosteal abscess	Collection of purulent exudate* beneath periosteum of lamina papyracea Displacement of globe downward/laterally
IV	Orbital abscess	Purulent collection within orbit* Proptosis Chemosis Ophthalmoplegia Decreased vision
V	Cavernous sinus thrombosis	Bilateral eye findings Prostration Meningismus

*The radiographic correlation of a subperiosteal or orbital abscess seen with CT is a contrast-enhancing mass in the extraconal or intraconal space, possibly with areas of cavitation, because purulence cannot be determined with CT scanning.
From Rudloe TF, Harper M, Prabhu SP, et al: Acute periorbital infections: who needs emergent imaging? Pediatrics 125:e719–e726, 2010.

infection, but the obstruction usually requires definitive treatment to reduce the risk of recurrence.

Dacryocystitis may occur in newborns as a complication of a congenital dacryocystocele (see Chapter 625). If present, systemic antibiotics and digital pressure for decompression are recommended. The obstruction of the nasolacrimal system may resolve once the infection clears. If spontaneous resolution does not occur, probing should be considered within a short time frame. An intranasal cyst may be present in conjunction with the dacryocystocele. If this occurs, marsupialization of the cyst may be needed at the time of the probing.

PRESEPTAL CELLULITIS
Inflammation of the lids and periorbital tissues without signs of true orbital involvement (such as proptosis or limitation of eye movement) is generally referred to as periorbital or preseptal cellulitis and is a form of facial cellulitis. This is common in young children and may be

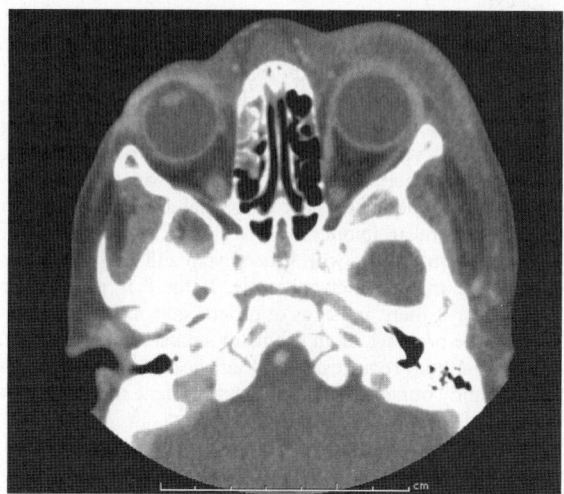

Figure 634-2 CT scan of a patient with preseptal cellulitis.

caused by bacteremia, sinusitis, trauma, an infected wound, or an abscess of the lid or periorbital region (pyoderma, hordeolum, conjunctivitis, dacryocystitis, insect bite). Patients present with eyelid swelling; the edema may be so intense as to make it difficult to evaluate the globe. Prior to the *Haemophilus influenzae* type B vaccine, the most common cause of pediatric preseptal (facial) cellulitis was bacteremia caused by *H. influenzae* type B. Group A streptococcus, *S. aureus*, and pneumococcus are common etiologic agents. Clinical examination will show lack of proptosis, normal ocular movement, and normal pupil function. CT examination will demonstrate edema of the lids and subcutaneous tissues anterior to the orbital septum (Fig. 634-2). Antibiotic therapy and careful monitoring for signs of sepsis and local progression are essential.

ORBITAL CELLULITIS
This is a condition involving inflammation of the tissues of the orbit, with proptosis, limitation of movement of the eye, edema of the conjunctiva (chemosis), and inflammation and swelling of the eyelids with potentially decreased visual acuity (see Table 634-1). The mean age is approximately 7 yr but the range is 10 mo–18 yr. Patients often feel ill with general symptoms of toxicity, fever, and leukocytosis (also see Chapter 194).

Orbital cellulitis may follow direct infection of the orbit from a wound, metastatic deposition of organisms during bacteremia, or **more often** direct extension or venous spread of infection from contiguous sites such as the lids, conjunctiva, globe, lacrimal gland, or nasolacrimal sac or, **more commonly**, from the paranasal (ethmoid) sinuses. In some cases, primary or metastatic tumor in the orbit can produce the clinical picture of orbital cellulitis. The most common cause of orbital cellulitis in children is paranasal sinusitis. The spread of infection to the orbit from the sinuses is more prevalent in children because of their thinner bony septa and sinus wall, greater porosity of bones, open suture lines, and larger vascular foramina. The spread of infection is also facilitated by the venous and lymphatic communication between the sinuses and surrounding structures, which allow flow in either direction, facilitating retrograde thrombophlebitis. Frequent pathogenic organisms include *S. aureus*, including methicillin-resistant *S. aureus*, streptococcus species (*Streptococcus anginosus*), and *Haemophilus* species.

The potential for complications is great. Visual loss can occur secondary to an increase in orbital pressure that causes retinal artery occlusion or optic neuritis. This is more likely to occur in the presence of an orbital abscess. Extension of infection from the orbit into the cranial cavity may lead to cavernous sinus thrombosis or meningitis, epidural or subdural empyema, or brain abscesses. Additional complications include optic atrophy, exposure keratitis, and retinal or choroidal ischemia. The **differential diagnosis** includes idiopathic orbital inflammation, myositis, sarcoidosis, granulomatous vasculitis, leukemia, lymphoma, histiocytic disorders, rhabdomyosarcoma, ruptured dermoid cyst, orbital trauma, and orbital foreign body.

Orbital cellulitis must be recognized promptly and treated aggressively. Hospitalization and systemic antibiotic therapy are usually indicated. All patients require CT imaging of the orbit, including the surrounding central nervous system, preferably with intravenous contrast to detect a subperiosteal abscess, orbital abscess, or intracranial extension. Parenteral antibiotics must be started immediately. Antimicrobial agents should begin with vancomycin and cefotaxime (or ceftriaxone); some include metronidazole. If there is no evidence of improvement or if there are signs of progression, sinus drainage may be required. The presence of an orbital or subperiosteal abscess (Figs. 634-3 and 634-4) may require urgent drainage of the orbit. The clinical presentation and course of each individual patient should dictate the need and timing of abscess drainage.

Children <9 yr of age with a medial **subperiosteal abscess** can initially be managed with a trial of intravenous antibiotics, which usually is sufficient for resolution of the abscess. They must be examined frequently (every 6 hr until improvement) for signs of visual deterioration or pupillary abnormalities. Most will become afebrile within 48 hr and have exam improvement by 72 hr. If there are

pupillary abnormalities, decreased vision, or failure to improve, the subperiosteal abscess should be drained. Many recommend routine drainage for a subperiosteal abscess in children >9 yr of age. If there is an **orbital abscess** with an abnormal physical exam, the recommendation is that drainage be performed and antibiotics given at the time of diagnosis. The use of adjunctive corticosteroids and anticoagulation for cavernous venous thrombosis and or superior ophthalmic vein thrombosis is controversial.

Bibliography is available at Expert Consult.

Chapter **635**
Injuries to the Eye

Scott E. Olitsky, Denise Hug, Laura S. Plummer, Erin D. Stahl, Michelle M. Ariss, and Timothy P. Lindquist

Approximately 30% of all blindness in children results from trauma. Children and adolescents account for a disproportionate number of episodes of ocular trauma. Boys ages 11-15 yr are the most vulnerable; their injuries outnumber those in girls by a ratio of about 4:1. The majority of injuries are related to sports, sticks, stones, fireworks, paint balls, air-powered BB guns, and other projectiles. High-velocity projectiles and fireworks cause particularly devastating ocular and orbital injuries. Much of the trauma is avoidable (see Chapter 5.1). Any part of the orbit or globe may be affected (Fig. 635-1).

ECCHYMOSIS AND SWELLING OF THE EYELIDS
Ecchymosis and edema of the eyelids are common after blunt trauma (Fig. 635-2). These disorders are self-limiting, absorb spontaneously, and can be treated with iced compresses and analgesics. Periorbital ecchymosis should prompt careful examination of the eye and surrounding structures for more serious injuries such as orbital bone fracture, intraocular hemorrhage, or rupture of the globe.

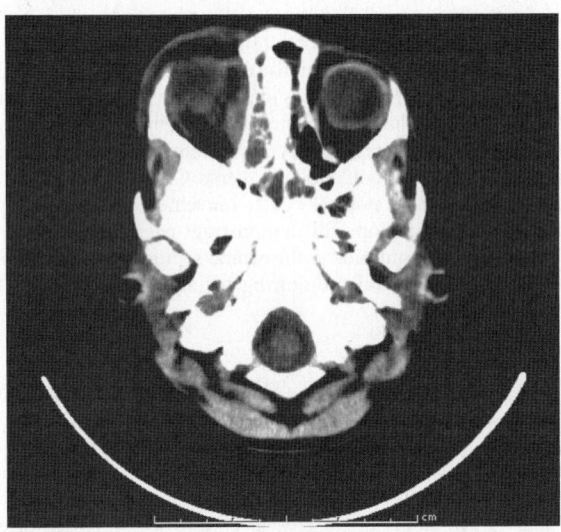

Figure 634-3 CT scan demonstrating a subperiosteal abscess along the medial wall of the orbit.

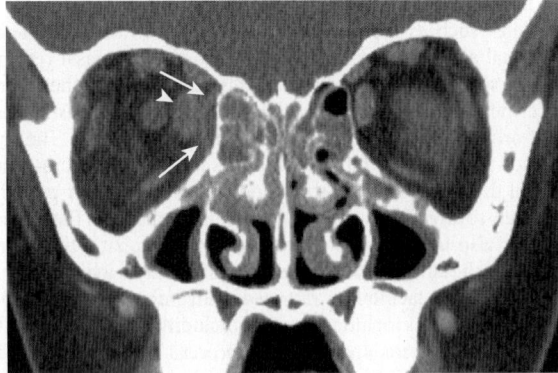

Figure 634-4 An orbital subperiosteal abscess in a 9 yr old girl. A coronal contrast-enhanced computed tomography image shows a small, low-attenuation, rim-enhancing fluid collection consistent with an abscess (arrows) in the medial aspect of the orbit with mass effect on the medial rectus muscle (arrowhead), which is thickened. Bilateral ethmoid sinus disease with infiltration of the right retroorbital fat is demonstrated. (From Coley BD, editor: Caffey's Pediatric diagnostic imaging, ed 12, Vol 1, Philadelphia, 2013, Elsevier Saunders, Fig. 8-17, p. 80.)

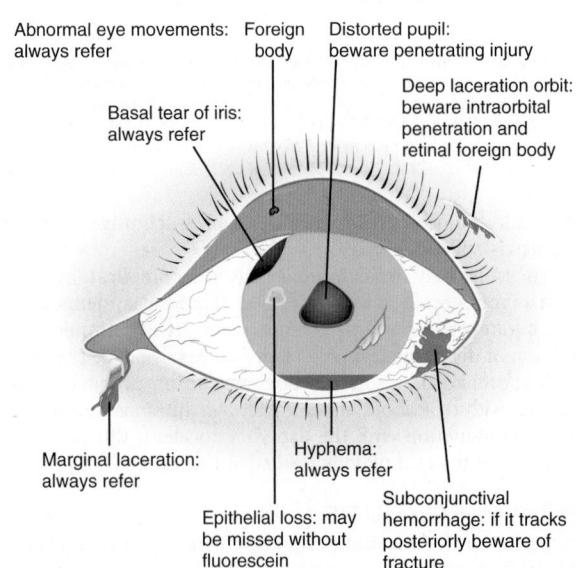

Figure 635-1 The injured eye. (From Khaw PT, Shah P, Elkington AR: Injury to the eye. BMJ 2004;328:36–38.)

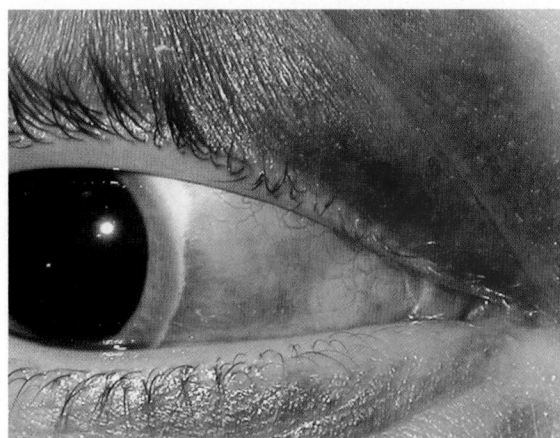

Figure 635-2 Eyelid ecchymosis and subconjunctival hemorrhage.

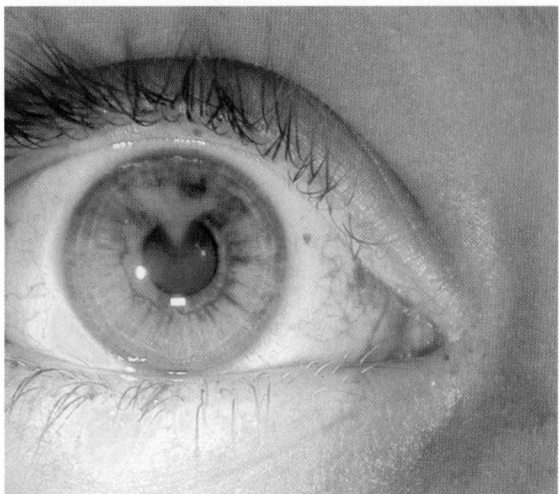

Figure 635-4 Corneal abrasion with fluorescein staining.

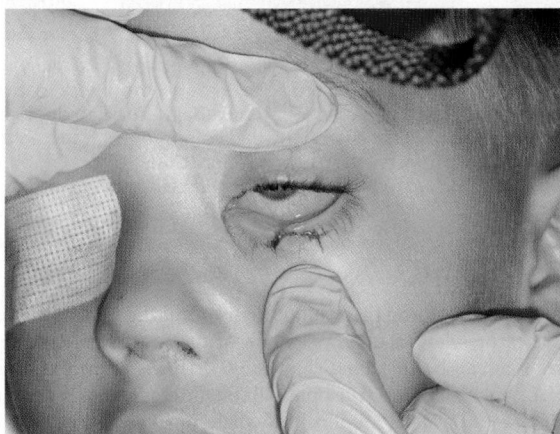

Figure 635-3 Eyelid margin laceration.

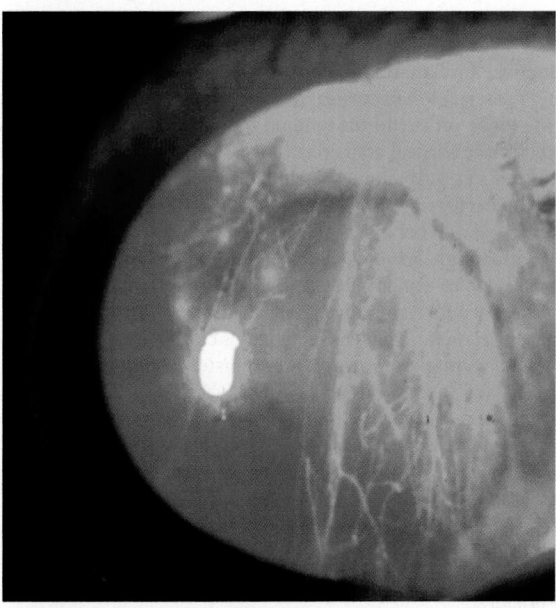

Figure 635-5 Vertically oriented linear corneal abrasions secondary to a foreign body underneath the upper eyelid.

LACERATIONS OF THE EYELIDS

Eyelid lacerations may vary from simple to complex. When evaluating an eyelid laceration, key findings include depth of the laceration, its location, and whether there is involvement of the canaliculus. Most superficial eyelid lacerations may be closed by the primary caregiver, but if a laceration is deep, involves the lid margin, or involves the canaliculus, it should be evaluated by an ophthalmologist. The levator muscle is responsible for elevation of the upper eyelid and runs deep to the skin and orbicularis oculi muscle. If the levator muscle is compromised and not recognized at initial repair, ptosis will occur. Therefore, if orbital fat is visible in the laceration, the laceration has compromised the skin, orbicularis oculi and levator muscles, and orbital septum and must be meticulously repaired to avoid ptosis. Eyelid margin involvement (Fig. 635-3) also requires careful repair to avoid lid malposition and notch formation. These can lead to ocular surface problems in the future, resulting in corneal scarring and loss of vision. Lacerations involving the canaliculus require intubation of the nasolacrimal system in addition to repair of the laceration of the eyelid to avoid future tearing problems. Proper primary repair of eyelid lacerations often achieves a superior outcome to secondary repair at a later date. As with any eyelid injury, careful examination of the eye and surrounding tissue is required.

SUPERFICIAL ABRASIONS OF THE CORNEA

When the corneal epithelium is scratched, abraded, or denuded, it exposes the underlying epithelial basement layer and superficial corneal nerves. This is accompanied by pain, tearing, photophobia, and decreased vision. Corneal abrasions are detected by instilling fluorescein dye and inspecting the cornea using a blue-filtered light

(Fig. 635-4). A slit lamp is ideal for this examination, but a direct ophthalmoscope with blue filter or a handheld Wood lamp is adequate for young children.

Treatment of a corneal abrasion is directed at promoting healing and relieving pain. Abrasions are treated with frequent applications of a topical antibiotic ointment until the epithelium is completely healed. The use of a semipressure patch does not improve healing time or decrease pain. An improperly applied patch may itself abrade the cornea. A topical cycloplegic agent (cyclopentolate hydrochloride 1%) can relieve the pain from ciliary spasm in patients with large abrasions. Topical anesthetics should not be given at home because they retard epithelial healing and inhibit the natural blinking reflex.

FOREIGN BODY INVOLVING THE OCULAR SURFACE

This usually produces acute discomfort, tearing, and inflammation. Most foreign bodies can be detected by examination in good light with the aid of magnification (Fig. 635-5) or a direct ophthalmoscope set on a high plus lens (+10 or +12). In many cases, slit-lamp examination is necessary, especially if the particle is deep or metallic. Some

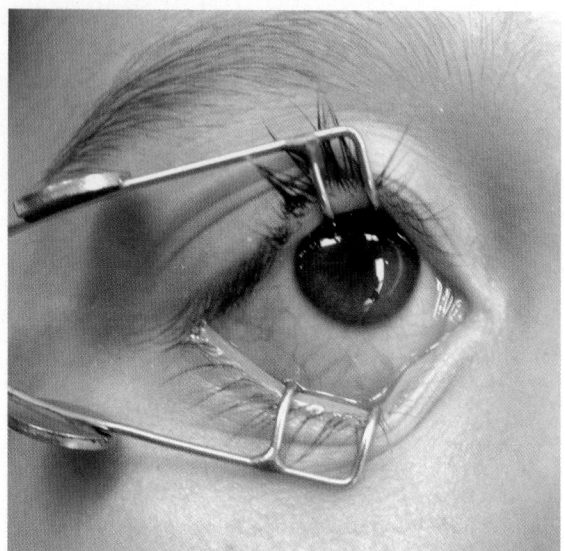

Figure 635-6 Superficial corneal foreign body.

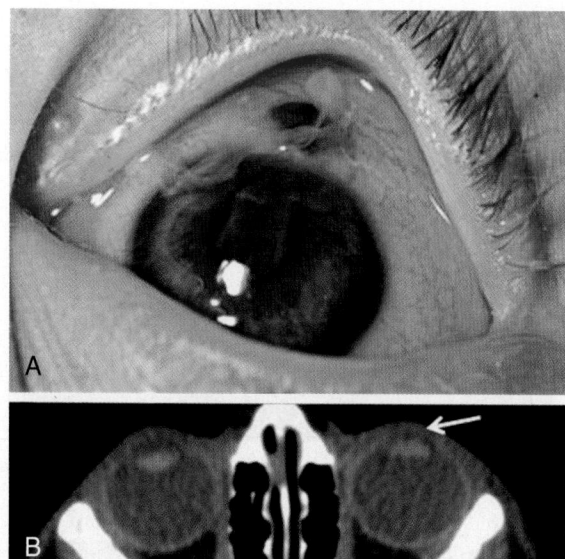

Figure 635-7 A, External photograph of an open globe injury with a peaked pupil because of iris prolapse through the sclera, a shallow anterior chamber, and a traumatic cataract. **B,** CT imaging demonstrating a shallow left anterior chamber when compared with the right, but without evidence of an intraocular foreign body. *(From Hwang RY, Schoenberger SD: Imaging a peaked pupil in a traumatic open globe injury. J Pediatr 163:1517, 2013, Figs. A and B, p. 1517.)*

conjunctival foreign bodies tend to lodge under the upper eyelid, causing the sensation of corneal foreign body as they come into contact with the globe on eyelid movement; they may also produce vertically oriented linear corneal abrasions (Fig. 635-6). Finding these abrasions should lead to a suspicion of such a foreign body, and eversion of the lid may be necessary (see Chapter 619). If a foreign body is suspected but not found, further examination is indicated. If the history suggests injury with a high-velocity particle, radiologic examination of the eye may be needed to explore the possibility of an intraocular foreign body.

Removal of a foreign body can be facilitated by instillation of a drop of topical anesthetic. Many foreign bodies can be removed by irrigation or by gently wiping them away with a moistened cotton-tipped applicator. Embedded foreign bodies or foreign bodies in the central cornea should be treated by an ophthalmologist. Removal of corneal foreign bodies may leave epithelial defects, which are treated as corneal abrasions. Metallic foreign bodies may cause rust to form in the corneal tissues; examination by an ophthalmologist 1 or 2 days after removal of a foreign body is recommended because a rust ring might require further treatment.

HYPHEMA
This is the presence of blood in the anterior chamber of the eye. It may occur with either a blunt or perforating injury and represents a situation that may threaten vision. Hyphema appears as a bright or dark red fluid level between the cornea and iris or as a diffuse murkiness of the aqueous humor. Children with hyphema present with acute loss of vision, with or without pain. The treatment of hyphema involves efforts to minimize the vision-threatening sequelae such as rebleeding, glaucoma, and corneal blood staining. Bedrest is necessary, with elevation of the head of the bed to 30 degrees. A shield (without underlying patch) is placed on the affected eye, and a cycloplegic agent is used to immobilize the iris. Additionally, topical or systemic steroids are used to minimize intraocular inflammation. Antiemetics should be considered if the patient is experiencing nausea. All nonsteroidal anti-inflammatories and aspirin must be avoided. Rarely, hospitalization and sedation may be necessary to ensure compliance in some children. If the intraocular pressure is elevated, topical and systemic pressure-lowering medications are used. If the pressure is not controllable by such measures, then surgical evacuation of the clot may be required to minimize the risk of permanent vision loss. Patients with sickle cell disease or trait are at higher risk of acute loss of vision secondary to elevated intraocular pressure or optic nerve infarction and may require more aggressive intervention. Individuals with a history of traumatic hyphema have an increased incidence of glaucoma later in life and should be monitored on a regular basis throughout their lives.

OPEN GLOBE
A penetrating, perforating, or blunt injury resulting in compromise of the cornea or sclera of the eye is one of the most sight-threatening injuries that can be sustained (Fig. 635-7). This is known as an open globe. An open globe is a true ophthalmologic emergency that requires prompt, careful evaluation and immediate repair to minimize vision loss. Permanent vision loss can result from corneal scarring, loss of intraocular contents, or infection. Evaluation involves careful history including time and mechanism of the injury, as well as visual acuity and inspection of the eye. A full-thickness corneal wound will often present with prolapsed iris tissue through the wound. If this is not immediately evident, a peaked or irregular pupil may be a sign of full-thickness laceration. Scleral compromise may be more difficult to identify because of overlying structures. The thinnest part of the sclera is at the corneoscleral junction (the limbus) and just posterior to the insertion of the rectus muscles. When an open globe is caused by blunt force injury, these are the 2 areas most likely involved. The overlying conjunctiva may not be compromised but a subconjunctival hemorrhage may be present, obscuring the view. In these cases, look for a shallow anterior chamber, low intraocular pressure, or pigment within the involved area. If the patient has been diagnosed with an open globe, the examination should be stopped, an eye shield placed immediately, and the ophthalmologist contacted to minimize further ocular compromise.

OPTIC NERVE TRAUMA
The optic nerve may be injured in both penetrating and blunt trauma. The injury may occur at any point between the globe and the chiasm. Traumatic injury to the optic nerve, regardless of cause or location, results in reduced vision and a pupillary defect. Direct trauma to the intraorbital optic nerve may cause transection, partial transection, or optic sheath hemorrhage. Fractures involving the skull base may cause injury to the intracranial portions of the optic nerve. Treatment decisions are difficult because there are no universally accepted guidelines, and the prognosis for good visual outcome is often poor. Medical management involves observation and the use of high-dose corticosteroids, although the use of corticosteroids has not been proven to improve visual outcomes and has been shown to increase the risk of death in patients with significant head injury. Surgical intervention

involves optic nerve sheath decompression for nerve sheath hemorrhages. If compression of the optic nerve is secondary to orbital hemorrhage, prompt lateral canthotomy and cantholysis should be performed to relieve intraorbital pressure. Decompression of the optic canal may be performed if there is compression of the optic nerve by a bone fragment. Optic canal decompression is controversial in the absence of direct bone compression.

CHEMICAL INJURIES
Chemical burns of the cornea and adnexal tissue are among the most urgent of ocular emergencies. Alkali burns are usually more destructive than acid burns because they react with fats to form soaps, which damage cell membranes, allowing further penetration of the alkali into the eye. Acids generally cause less severe, more localized tissue damage. The corneal epithelium offers moderate protection against weak acids, and little damage occurs unless the pH is 2.5 or less. Most stronger acids precipitate tissue proteins, creating a physical barrier against their further penetration.

Mild acid or alkali burns are characterized by conjunctival injection and swelling and mild corneal epithelial erosions. The corneal stroma may be mildly edematous, and the anterior chamber may have mild to moderate cell and flare reactions. With strong acids, the cornea and conjunctiva rapidly become white and opaque. The corneal epithelium may slough, leaving a relatively clear stroma; this appearance may initially mask the severity of the burn. Severe alkali burns are characterized by corneal opacification.

Emergency treatment of a chemical burn begins with immediate, copious irrigation with water or saline. Local debridement and removal of foreign particles should be performed as irrigation continues. If the nature of the chemical injury is unknown, the use of pH test paper is helpful in determining whether the agent was basic or acidic. Irrigation should continue for at least 30 min or until 2 L of irrigant has been instilled in mild cases and for 2-4 hr or until 10 L of irrigant has been instilled in severe cases. At the end of irrigation, the pH should be within a normal range (7.3-7.7). The pH should be checked again approximately 30 min after irrigation to ensure that it has not changed. The goal of treatment is to minimize sequelae that may threaten vision, such as conjunctival scarring, corneal scarring/opacification, glaucoma, cataract, and phthisis.

ORBITAL FRACTURES
The orbit is the bony structure surrounding the eye. Any of these bones may fracture in a traumatic incident. Superior and lateral wall fractures are the least common of the fracture sites, but superior orbital fracture is the most significant because of the potential of intracranial injury. The medial wall of the orbit is very susceptible to fracture because of the thin nature of the lamina papyracea. Perhaps the most common site of fracture from blunt trauma is the orbital floor. This is often referred to as blowout fracture. At times, the fracture may act as a trapdoor, entrapping orbital contents within the fracture site.

The patient often presents with a recent history of periorbital trauma and pain. Diplopia, eyelid swelling, eye movement restriction, or hypesthesia may or may not be present. Eye symptoms may be associated with nausea and bradycardia if the inferior rectus is entrapped in the fracture site. A complete ophthalmic examination, including visual acuity, examination of the pupil for ocular alignment, ocular motility, anterior segment and fundus status, as well as the history of the injury, is required because there are often accompanying ocular injuries. The diagnosis of fracture is suspected if eye misalignment, eye movement restriction, or enophthalmos (sunken eye) is present. The diagnosis is verified by orbital CT scan.

Medical management includes iced compresses to the orbit and elevation for the head of the bed for the 1st 24-48 hr. Broad-spectrum antibiotics are sometimes recommended for 14 days because of the exposure of the orbital contents to the sinus cavity. In medial wall fractures, instructions not to blow one's nose should be given to the patient to avoid orbital emphysema and subsequent optic nerve compression. Consider neurosurgical consultation in orbital roof fractures. Indications for surgical repair of orbital fractures are diplopia in primary gaze or downgaze that persists for 2 wk, enophthalmos, or fracture of the orbital floor involving more than half of the floor. Extraocular muscle entrapment often requires prompt surgical repair because affected patients have significant pain, nausea, and vomiting that are difficult to control. Rarely, extraocular muscle entrapment can cause activation of the oculocardiac reflex, requiring urgent fracture repair.

PENETRATING WOUNDS OF THE ORBIT
These demand careful evaluation for possible damage to the eye, optic nerve, orbital contents, or brain. Examination should include investigation for a retained foreign body. Orbital hemorrhage and infection are common with penetrating wounds of the orbit; such injuries must be treated as emergencies.

CHILD ABUSE
See Chapter 40.

This is a major cause of injuries to the eye and orbital region. The possibility of nonaccidental trauma must be considered in any child with ecchymosis or laceration of the lids, hemorrhage in or about the eye, cataract or dislocated lens, retinal detachment, or fracture of the orbit. Inflicted childhood neurotrauma (shaken baby syndrome) occurs secondary to violent, nonaccidental, repetitive, unrestrained acceleration-deceleration head and neck movements, with or without blunt head trauma in children typically younger than 3 yr of age. Inflicted childhood neurotrauma accounts for approximately 10% of all cases of child abuse and carries a mortality rate of up to 25%. Detection of abuse is not only important in order to treat the pathology that is discovered but also to prevent further abuse or even death. The ocular manifestations are numerous and may have a prominent role in recognition of this syndrome. Retinal hemorrhage is the most common ophthalmic finding and occurs at all levels of the retina. The pattern of hemorrhage helps to distinguish this disorder from other causes of retinal hemorrhage or from accidental injuries (Fig. 635-8). Retinal hemorrhages can occur without associated intracranial pathology.

FIREWORKS-RELATED INJURIES
Injuries related to the use of fireworks can be the most devastating of all ocular traumas that occur in children. At least 20% of emergency department visits for fireworks-related injuries are for ocular trauma. In the United States, a majority of these injuries take place around Independence Day, and most occur despite adult supervision.

SPORTS-RELATED OCULAR INJURIES AND THEIR PREVENTION
Although sports injuries occur in all age groups, far more children and adolescents participate in high-risk sports than do adults. The

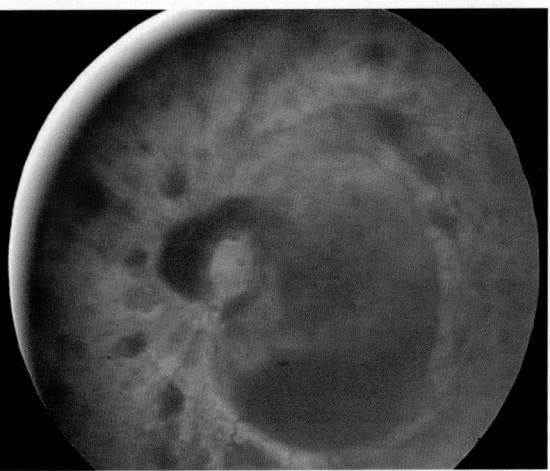

Figure 635-8 Retinal hemorrhages in an abused child.

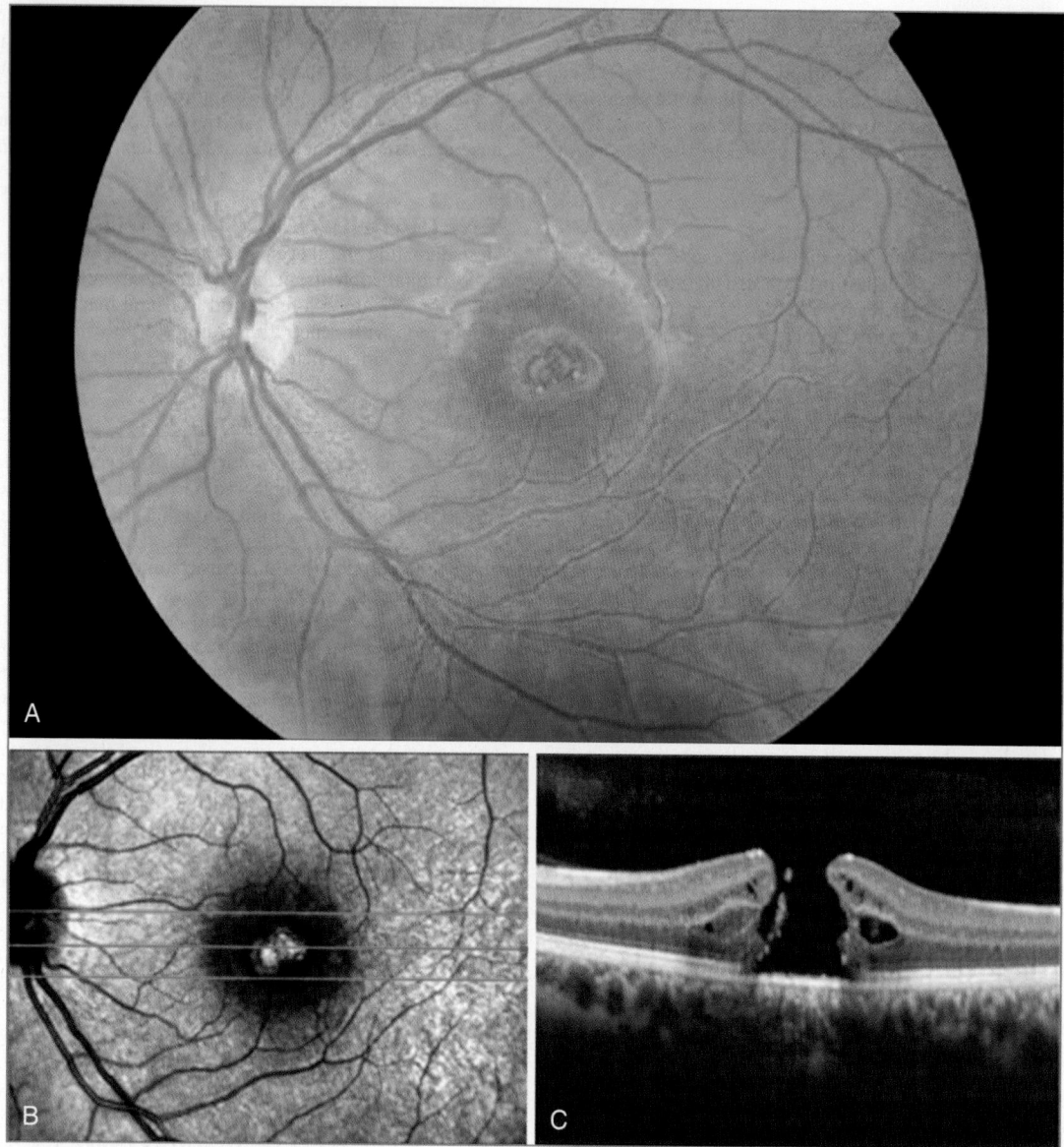

Figure 635-9 Laser damage to the left eye. **A,** Color photo of the fundus of the left eye showing a macular hole. Note the changes at the retinal pigment epithelium. **B,** Infrared photo of the left fundus. **C,** Optical coherence tomography (OCT) of the left eye showing the macular hole. *(From Petrou P, Patwary S, Banerjee PJ, et al: Bilateral macular hole from a handheld laser pointer, Lancet 383:1780, 2014.)*

greater number of participating children, their athletic immaturity, and the increased likelihood of their using inadequate or improper eye protection account for their disproportionate share of sports-related eye injuries (see Chapters 688 and 693).

The sports with the highest risk of eye injury are those in which no eye protection can be worn, including boxing, wrestling, and martial arts. Other high-risk sports include those that use a rapidly moving ball or puck, bat, stick, racquet, or arrow (baseball, hockey, lacrosse, racquet sports, and archery) or involve aggressive body contact (football and basketball). Related to both risk and frequency of participation, the highest percentage of eye injuries are in basketball and baseball.

Protective eyewear, designed for a specific activity, is available for most sports. For basketball, racquet sports, and other recreational activities that do not require a helmet or face mask, molded polycarbonate sports goggles that are secured to the head by an elastic strap

are suggested. For hockey, football, lacrosse, and baseball (batter), specific helmets with polycarbonate face shields and guards are available. Children should also wear sports goggles under the helmets. For baseball, goggles and helmets should be worn for batting, catching, and base running; goggles alone are usually sufficient for other positions.

HANDHELD LASER RETINAL INJURY

Handheld laser pointers, often purchased to light cigarettes or for other purposes, may produce significant retinal damage if the power output is ≥150 mW. If a person looks directly at the light, direct foveal injury may occur before he or she has time to blink. Central (foveal) blurring and decreased visual activity are the chief complaints. Retinal injuries include retinal disruption, subretinal edema, and macular holes (Fig. 635-9), which usually require surgical repair.

Bibliography is available at Expert Consult.

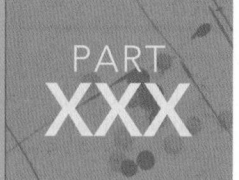

Chapter **636**
General Considerations and Evaluation

Joseph Haddad Jr. and Sarah Keesecker

CLINICAL MANIFESTATIONS

Diseases of the ear and temporal bone typically manifest with 1 or more of 8 clinical signs and symptoms.

Otalgia usually is associated with inflammation of the external or middle ear, but it can represent pain referred from involvement of the teeth, temporomandibular joint, or pharynx. In young infants, pulling or rubbing the ear along with general irritability or poor sleep, especially when associated with fever, may be the only signs of ear pain. Ear pulling alone is not diagnostic of ear pathology.

Purulent otorrhea is a sign of otitis externa, otitis media with perforation of the tympanic membrane (TM), drainage from the middle ear through a patent tympanostomy tube, or, rarely, drainage from a first branchial cleft sinus. Bloody drainage may be associated with acute or chronic inflammation (often with granulation tissue and/or an ear tube), trauma, neoplasm, foreign body, or blood dyscrasia. Clear drainage suggests a perforation of the TM with a serous middle-ear effusion or, rarely, a cerebrospinal fluid leak draining through defects (congenital or traumatic) in the external auditory canal or from the middle ear.

Hearing loss results either from disease of the external or middle ear (conductive hearing loss) or from pathology in the inner ear, retrocochlear structures, or central auditory pathways (sensorineural hearing loss). The most common cause of hearing loss in children is otitis media (OM).

Swelling around the ear most commonly is a result of inflammation (e.g., external otitis, perichondritis, mastoiditis), trauma (e.g., hematoma), benign cystic masses, or neoplasm.

Vertigo is a specific type of dizziness that is defined as any illusion or sensation of motion. **Dizziness** is less specific than vertigo and refers to a sensation of altered orientation in space. Vertigo is an uncommon complaint in children; the child or parent might not volunteer information about balance unless asked specifically. The most common cause of dizziness in young children is eustachian tube–middle-ear disease, but true vertigo also may be caused by labyrinthitis, perilymphatic fistula between the inner and middle ear as a result of trauma or a congenital inner ear defect, cholesteatoma in the mastoid or middle ear, vestibular neuronitis, benign paroxysmal vertigo, Ménière disease, or disease of the central nervous system. Older children might describe a feeling of the room spinning or turning; younger children might express the dysequilibrium only by falling, stumbling, or clumsiness.

Nystagmus may be unidirectional, horizontal, or jerk nystagmus. It is vestibular in origin and usually is associated with vertigo.

Tinnitus rarely is described spontaneously by children, but it is common, especially in patients with eustachian tube–middle-ear disease or sensorineural hearing loss (SNHL). Children can describe tinnitus if asked directly about it, including laterality and the quality of the sound.

FACIAL PARALYSIS

The facial nerve may be dehiscent in its course through the middle ear in as many as 50% of patients. Infection with local inflammation, most commonly in acute OM, can lead to a temporary paralysis of the facial nerve. It also can result from Lyme disease, cholesteatoma, Bell palsy, Ramsay Hunt syndrome (herpes zoster oticus), fracture, neoplasm, or infection of the temporal bone. Congenital facial paralysis can result from birth trauma or congenital abnormality of the 7th nerve or from a syndrome such as Möbius or CHARGE (coloboma, heart defects, atresia choanae, retarded growth, genital hypoplasia, and ear anomalies), or it may be associated with other cranial nerve abnormalities and craniofacial anomalies.

PHYSICAL EXAMINATION

Complete examination with special attention to the head and neck can reveal a condition that can predispose to or be associated with ear disease in children. The facial appearance and the character of speech can give clues to an abnormality of the ear or hearing. Many craniofacial anomalies, such as cleft palate, mandibulofacial dysostosis (Treacher Collins syndrome), and trisomy 21 (Down syndrome), are associated with disorders of the ear and eustachian tube. Mouth breathing and hyponasality can indicate intranasal or postnasal obstruction. **Hypernasality** is a sign of velopharyngeal insufficiency. Examining the oropharyngeal cavity might uncover an overt cleft palate or a submucous cleft (usually associated with a bifid uvula), both of which predispose to OM with effusion. A nasopharyngeal tumor with nasal and eustachian tube blockage may be associated with OM.

The position of the patient for examination of the ear, nose, and throat depends on the patient's age and ability to cooperate, the clinical setting, and the examiner's preference. The child can be examined on an examination table or in the parent's lap. The presence of a parent or assistant usually is necessary to minimize movement and provide better examination results (Fig. 636-1). An examining table may be desirable for uncooperative older infants or when a procedure, such as microscopic evaluation or tympanocentesis, is performed. Wrapping the child in a sheet or using a papoose board can help to minimize movement. Lap examination is adequate and preferable in most infants and young children; the parent may assist in restraining the child by folding the child's wrists and arms over the child's own abdomen with one hand and holding the child's head against the parent's chest with the other hand. If necessary, the child's legs can be held between the parent's knees. To avoid ear trauma with movement, the examiner should hold the otoscope with the hand placed firmly against the child's head or face, so that the otoscope moves with the head. Pulling up and out on the pinna straightens the ear canal and allows better exposure of the TM.

When examining the ear, inspecting the auricle and external auditory meatus for infection can aid in evaluating complications of OM. External otitis can result from acute OM with discharge, or inflammation of the posterior auricular area can indicate a periostitis or subperiosteal abscess extending from the mastoid air cells. The presence of preauricular pits or skin tags also should be noted because affected children have a slightly higher incidence of sensorineural hearing loss; ear pits can develop chronic infection.

Cerumen is a protective, waxy, water-repellent coating in the ear canal that can interfere with examination. Cerumen usually is removed using the surgical head of the otoscope, which allows passage of a wire loop or a blunt curette under direct visualization. Other methods include gentle irrigation of the ear canal with warm water, which should be performed only if the TM is intact, or instillation of a solution such as diluted hydrogen peroxide in the ear canal (with intact TM only) for a few minutes to soften the wax for suction removal or irrigation. Some commercial preparations such as trolamine polypeptide oleate–condensate (Cerumenex) can cause dermatitis of the external canal with chronic use and should be used only under a physician's supervision.

Inflammation of the ear canal with associated pain often indicates external otitis. Abnormalities of the external auditory canal include stenosis (common in children with trisomy 21), bony exostoses, otorrhea, and the presence of foreign bodies. Cholesteatoma of the middle ear can manifest in the canal as intermittent foul-smelling drainage, sometimes associated with white debris; cholesteatoma of the external canal can appear as a white, pearl-like mass in the canal skin. White or gray debris of the canal suggests fungal external otitis. Newborn ear canals are filled with vernix caseosa, which is soft and pale yellow and should disappear shortly after birth.

The TM and its mobility are best assessed with a pneumatic otoscope. The normal TM is in a neutral position; a bulging TM may be caused by increased middle-ear air pressure, with or without pus or effusion in the middle ear; a bulging drum can obscure visualization of the malleus and annulus. Retraction of the TM usually indicates negative middle-ear pressure, but it also can result from previous

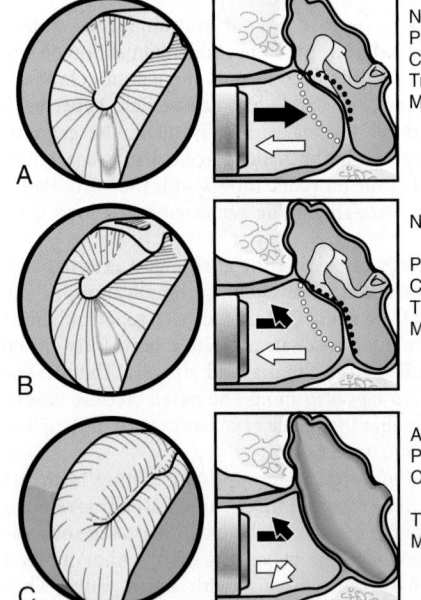

Figure 636-1 Methods of restraining an infant for examination and for procedures such as tympanocentesis or myringotomy. *(From Bluestone CD, Klein JO: Otitis media in infants and children, ed 2, Philadelphia, 1995, WB Saunders, p. 91.)*

middle-ear disease with fixation of the ossicles, ossicular ligaments, or TM. When retraction is present, the bony malleus appears more prominent, and the incus may be more visible posterior to the malleus.

The normal TM has a silvery-gray, "waxed paper" appearance (Fig. 636-2). A white or yellow TM can indicate a middle-ear effusion. A red TM alone might not indicate pathology, because the blood vessels of the membrane may be engorged as a result of crying, sneezing, or nose blowing. A normal TM is translucent, allowing the observer to visualize the middle-ear landmarks: incus, promontory, round window niche, and, often, the chorda tympani nerve. If a middle-ear effusion is present, an air–fluid level or bubbles may be visible (Fig. 636-2). Inability to visualize the middle-ear structures indicates opacification of the drum, usually caused by thickening of the TM or a middle-ear effusion, or both. Assessment of the light reflex often is not helpful, because a middle ear with effusion reflects light as well as a normal ear.

TM mobility is helpful in assessing middle-ear pressures and the presence or absence of fluid (see Fig. 636-2). To best perform pneumatic otoscopy, a speculum of adequate size is used to obtain a good seal and allow air movement in the canal. A rubber ring around the tip of the speculum can help to obtain a better canal seal. Normal middle-ear pressure is characterized by a neutral TM position and brisk TM movement to both positive and negative pressures.

Eardrum retraction is most common when negative middle-ear pressure is present; with even moderate negative middle-ear pressure there is no visible inward movement with applied positive pressure in the ear canal (see Fig. 636-1). However, negative canal pressure, which is produced by releasing the rubber bulb of the pneumatic otoscope, can cause the TM to bounce out toward the neutral position. The TM can retract in both the presence and absence of middle-ear fluid, and if the middle-ear fluid is mixed with air, the TM might still have some mobility. Outward eardrum movement is less likely in the presence of severe negative middle-ear pressure or middle-ear effusion.

The TM that exhibits fullness (bulging) moves to applied positive pressure but not to applied negative pressure if the pressure within the middle ear is positive. A full TM and positive middle-ear pressure without an effusion may be seen in young infants who are crying during the otoscopic examination, in older infants and children with nasal obstruction, and in the early stage of acute OM. When the middle-ear–mastoid air cell system is filled with an effusion and little or no air is present, the mobility of the TM is severely decreased or absent in response to both applied positive and negative pressures.

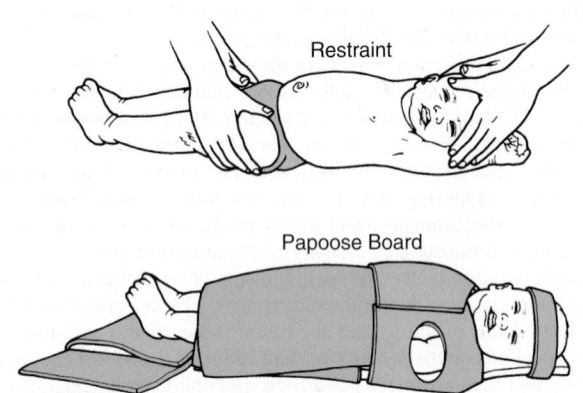
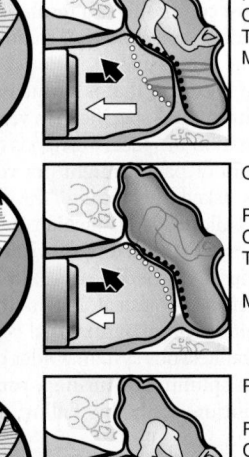

A NORMAL
Position—neutral
Color—normal
Translucency—translucent
Mobility—moves briskly with slight positive and negative pressure

B NEGATIVE MIDDLE-EAR PRESSURE
Position—retracted
Color—normal
Translucency—translucent
Mobility—moves only with applied negative pressure

C ACUTE OTITIS MEDIA
Position—full to bulging
Color—red (can be pink, white, or yellow)
Translucency—opaque
Mobility—poor when both positive and negative pressures are applied

D FLUID LEVEL
Position—retracted
Color—yellow or amber
Translucency—translucent
Mobility—same as with high negative pressure, but fluid level and bubbles change with applied pressure

E OTITIS MEDIA WITH EFFUSION
Position—usually retracted
Color—white (or yellow or blue)
Translucency—opaque (may be translucent)
Mobility—poor when both positive and negative pressures are applied

F PERFORATION (OR PATENT TYMPANOSTOMY TUBE)
Position—neutral or retracted
Color—white, pink, red, or normal
Translucency—translucent or opaque
Mobility—none

Figure 636-2 A-F, Common conditions of the middle ear, as assessed with the otoscope. *(From Bluestone CD, Klein JO: Otitis media in infants and children, ed 3, Philadelphia, 2001, WB Saunders, p. 131.)*

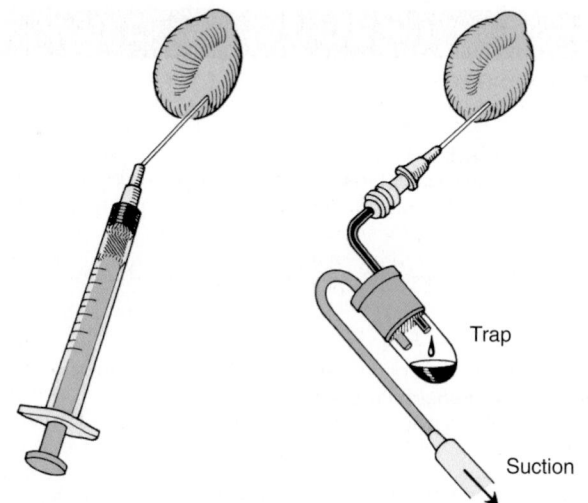

Figure 636-3 Tympanocentesis can be performed with a needle attached to a tuberculin syringe *(left)* or by using an Alden-Senturia collection trap (Storz Instrument Co, St. Louis). *(From Bluestone CD, Klein JO:* Otitis media in infants and children, *ed 2, Philadelphia, 1995, WB Saunders, p. 127.)*

Tympanocentesis, or aspiration of the middle ear, is the definitive method of verifying the presence and type of a middle-ear effusion and is performed by inserting, through the inferior portion of the TM, an 18-gauge spinal needle attached to a syringe or a collection trap (Fig. 636-3). Culturing of the ear canal and alcohol cleansing should precede tympanocentesis and culture of the middle-ear aspirate; a canal culture is taken first to help determine whether organisms cultured from the middle ear are contaminants from the external canal or true middle-ear pathogens.

Further diagnostic studies of the ear and hearing include audiometric evaluation, impedance audiometry (tympanometry), acoustic reflectometry, and specialized eustachian tube function studies. Diagnostic imaging studies, including CT and MRI, often provide further information about anatomic abnormalities and the extent of inflammatory processes or neoplasms. Specialized assessment of labyrinthine function should be considered in the evaluation of a child with a suspected vestibular disorder (see Chapter 641).

Bibliography is available at Expert Consult.

Chapter **637**
Hearing Loss
Joseph Haddad Jr. and Sarah Keesecker

INCIDENCE AND PREVALENCE

Bilateral neural hearing loss is categorized as mild (20-30 dB), moderate (30-50 dB), severe (50-70 dB), or profound (>70 dB). The World Health Organization estimates that approximately 360 million people (5% of the world's population, including 32 million children) have disabling hearing loss. An additional 364 million people have mild hearing loss. Half of these cases could have been prevented. In the United States, the average incidence of neonatal hearing loss is 1.1 in 1,000 infants; the rate by state varies from 0.22-3.61 in 1,000. Among children and adolescents, the rate of mild or greater hearing loss is 3.1% and is higher among Latin Americans, African-Americans, and persons from lower-income families.

The onset of hearing loss among children can occur at any time in childhood. When less-severe hearing loss or the transient hearing loss that commonly accompanies middle-ear disease in young children is considered, the number of affected children increases substantially.

TYPES OF HEARING LOSS

Hearing loss can be peripheral or central in origin. Peripheral hearing loss can be conductive, sensorineural, or mixed. **Conductive hearing loss (CHL)** commonly is caused by dysfunction in the transmission of sound through the external or middle ear or by abnormal transduction of sound energy into neural activity in the inner ear and the 8th nerve. CHL is the most common type of hearing loss in children and occurs when sound transmission is physically impeded in the external and/or middle ear. Common causes of CHL in the *ear canal* include atresia or stenosis, impacted cerumen, or foreign bodies. In the *middle ear*, perforation of the tympanic membrane (TM), discontinuity or fixation of the ossicular chain, otitis media (OM) with effusion, otosclerosis, and cholesteatoma can cause CHL.

Damage to or maldevelopment of structures in the inner ear can cause **sensorineural hearing loss (SNHL).** Causes include hair cell destruction from noise, disease, or ototoxic agents; cochlear malformation; perilymphatic fistula of the round or oval window membrane; and lesions of the acoustic division of the 8th nerve. A combination of CHL and SNHL is considered a **mixed hearing loss.**

An auditory deficit originating along the central auditory nervous system pathways from the proximal 8th nerve to the cerebral cortex usually is considered **central (or retrocochlear) hearing loss.** Tumors or demyelinating disease of the 8th nerve and cerebellopontine angle can cause hearing deficits but spare the outer, middle, and inner ear. These causes of hearing loss are rare in children. Other forms of central auditory deficits, known as **central auditory processing disorders,** include those that make it difficult even for children with normal hearing to listen selectively in the presence of noise, to combine information from the 2 ears properly, to process speech when it is slightly degraded, and to integrate auditory information when it is delivered faster although they can process it when delivered at a slow rate. These deficits can manifest as poor attention or as academic or behavior problems in school. Strategies for coping with such disorders are available for older children, and identification and documentation of the central auditory processing disorder often is valuable so that parents and teachers can make appropriate accommodations to enhance learning.

ETIOLOGY

Most CHL is acquired, with middle-ear fluid the most common cause. Congenital causes include anomalies of the pinna, external ear canal, TM, and ossicles. Rarely, congenital cholesteatoma or other masses in the middle ear manifest as CHL. TM perforation (e.g., trauma, OM), ossicular discontinuity (e.g., infection, cholesteatoma, trauma), tympanosclerosis, acquired cholesteatoma, or masses in the ear canal or middle ear (Langerhans cell histiocytosis, salivary gland tumors, glomus tumors, rhabdomyosarcoma) also can manifest as CHL. Uncommon diseases that affect the middle ear and temporal bone and can manifest with CHL include otosclerosis, osteopetrosis, fibrous dysplasia, and osteogenesis imperfecta.

SNHL may be congenital or acquired. Acquired SNHL may be caused by genetic, infectious, autoimmune, anatomic, traumatic, ototoxic, and idiopathic factors (Tables 637-1, 637-2, 637-3, and 637-4). The recognized risk factors account for approximately 50% of cases of moderate to profound SNHL.

Sudden SNHL in a previously healthy child is uncommon but may be from OM or other middle-ear pathologies such as autoimmunity. Usually these causes are obvious from the history and physical examination. Sudden loss of hearing in the absence of obvious causes often is the result of a vascular event affecting the cochlear apparatus or nerve, such as embolism or thrombosis (secondary to prothrombotic conditions), or an autoimmune process. Additional causes include perilymph fistula, drugs, trauma, and the first episode of Ménière syndrome. In adults, sudden SNHL is often idiopathic and unilateral;

Table 637-1	Indicators Associated with Hearing Loss

INDICATORS ASSOCIATED WITH SENSORINEURAL AND/OR CONDUCTIVE HEARING LOSS
Neonates (Birth-28 Days) When Universal Screening Is Not Available
Family history of hereditary childhood sensorineural hearing loss
In utero infection, such as cytomegalovirus, rubella, syphilis, herpes simplex, or toxoplasmosis
Craniofacial anomalies, including those with morphologic abnormalities of the pinna, ear canal, ear tags, ear pits, and temporal bone anomalies
Birthweight <1500 g (3.3 lb)
Hyperbilirubinemia at a serum level requiring exchange transfusion
Ototoxic medications, including but not limited to the aminoglycosides, used in multiple courses or in combination with loop diuretics
Bacterial meningitis
Apgar scores of 0-4 at 1 min or 0-6 at 5 min
Mechanical ventilation lasting ≥5 days; extracorporeal membrane oxygenation
Stigmata or other findings associated with a syndrome known to include a sensorineural and/or conductive hearing loss; white forelock
Infants and Toddlers (Age 29 Days-2 Yr) When Certain Health Conditions Develop That Require Rescreening
Parent or caregiver concern regarding hearing, speech, language, and/or developmental delay
Bacterial meningitis and other infections associated with sensorineural hearing loss
Head trauma associated with loss of consciousness or skull fracture
Stigmata or other findings associated with a syndrome known to include a sensorineural and/or conductive hearing loss; neurofibromatosis, osteopetrosis, and Usher Hunter, Waardenburg, Alport, Pendred, or Jervell and Lange-Nielsen syndrome
Ototoxic medications, including but not limited to chemotherapeutic agents or aminoglycosides used in multiple courses or in combination with loop diuretics
Recurrent or persistent otitis media with effusion for 3 mo or longer
Skeletal dysplasia
Infants and Toddlers (Age 29 Days-3 Yr) Who Require Periodic Monitoring of Hearing
Some newborns and infants pass initial hearing screening but require periodic monitoring of hearing to detect delayed-onset sensorineural and/or conductive hearing loss. Infants with these indicators require hearing evaluation at least every 6 mo until age 3 yr, and at appropriate intervals thereafter

INDICATORS ASSOCIATED WITH DELAYED-ONSET SENSORINEURAL HEARING LOSS
Family history of hereditary childhood hearing loss
In utero infection, such as cytomegalovirus, rubella, syphilis, herpes simplex, or toxoplasmosis
Neurofibromatosis type 2 and neurodegenerative disorders
Cogan syndrome (vasculitis: keratitis, uveitis, vertigo, arthritis, dermatitis)

INDICATORS ASSOCIATED WITH CONDUCTIVE HEARING LOSS
Recurrent or persistent otitis media with effusion
Anatomic deformities and other disorders that affect eustachian tube function
Neurodegenerative disorders

Note: At all ages, parents' concern about hearing loss must be taken seriously even in the absence of risk factors.
Adapted from American Academy of Pediatrics, Joint Committee on Infant Hearing: Joint Committee on Infant Hearing 1994 position statement, Pediatrics 95:152, 1995.

Table 637-2	Common Types of Early-Onset Hereditary Nonsyndromic Sensorineural Hearing Loss

LOCUS	GENE	AUDIO PHENOTYPE
DFN3	*POU3F4*	Conductive hearing loss as a result of stapes fixation mimicking otosclerosis; superimposed progressive SNHL
DFNA1	*DIAPH1*	Low-frequency loss beginning in the 1st decade and progressing to all frequencies to produce a flat audio profile with profound losses throughout the auditory range
DFNA2	*KCNQ4*	Symmetric high-frequency sensorineural loss beginning in the 1st decade and progressing over all frequencies
	GJB3	Symmetric high-frequency sensorineural loss beginning in the 3rd decade
DFNA3	*GJB2*	Childhood-onset, progressive, moderate-to-severe high-frequency sensorineural hearing impairment
	GJB6	Childhood-onset, progressive, moderate-to-severe high-frequency sensorineural hearing impairment
DFNA6, 14, and 38	*WFS1*	Early-onset low-frequency sensorineural loss; approximately 75% of families dominantly segregating this audio profile carry missense mutations in the C-terminal domain of wolframin
DFNA8, and 12	*TECTA*	Early-onset stable bilateral hearing loss, affecting mainly mid to high frequencies
DFNA10	*EYA4*	Progressive loss beginning in the 2nd decade as a flat to gently sloping audio profile that becomes steeply sloping with age
DFNA11	*MYO7A*	Ascending audiogram affecting low and middle frequencies at young ages and then affecting all frequencies with increasing age
DFNA13	*COL11A2*	Congenital midfrequency sensorineural loss that shows age-related progression across the auditory range
DFNA15	*POU4F3*	Bilateral progressive sensorineural loss beginning in the 2nd decade

LOCUS	GENE	AUDIO PHENOTYPE
Table 637-2		Common Types of Early-Onset Hereditary Nonsyndromic Sensorineural Hearing Loss—cont'd
DFNA20, and 26	ACTG1	Bilateral progressive sensorineural loss beginning in the 2nd decade; with age, the loss increases with threshold shifts in all frequencies, although a sloping configuration is maintained in most cases
DFNA22	MYO6	Postlingual, slowly progressive, moderate to severe hearing loss
DFNB1	GJB2, GJB6	Hearing loss varies from mild to profound. The most common genotype, 35delG/35delG, is associated with severe to profound SNHL in about 90% of affected children; severe to profound deafness is observed in only 60% of children who are compound heterozygotes carrying 1 35delG allele and any other GJB2 SNHL-causing allele variant; in children carrying 2 GJB2 SNHL-causing missense mutations, severe to profound deafness is not observed
DFNB3	MYO7A	Severe to profound sensorineural hearing loss
DFNB4	SLC26A4	DFNB4 and Pendred syndrome (see Table 637-3) are allelic. DFNB4 hearing loss is associated with dilation of the vestibular aqueduct and can be unilateral or bilateral. In the high frequencies, the loss is severe to profound; in the low frequencies, the degree of loss varies widely. Onset can be congenital (prelingual), but progressive postlingual loss also is common
DFNB7, and 11	TMC1	Severe-to-profound prelingual hearing impairment
DFNB9	OTOF	OTOF-related deafness is characterized by 2 phenotypes: prelingual nonsyndromic hearing loss and, less frequently, temperature-sensitive nonsyndromic auditory neuropathy. The nonsyndromic hearing loss is bilateral severe-to-profound congenital deafness
DFNB12	CDH23	Depending on the type of mutation, recessive mutations of CDH23 can cause nonsyndromic deafness or type 1 Usher syndrome (USH1), which is characterized by deafness, vestibular areflexia, and vision loss as a result of retinitis pigmentosa
DFNB16	STRC	Early-onset nonsyndromic autosomal recessive sensorineural hearing loss
mtDNA 1555A > G	12S rRNA	Degree of hearing loss varies from mild to profound but usually is symmetric; high frequencies are preferentially affected; precipitous loss in hearing can occur after aminoglycoside therapy

SNHL, sensorineural hearing loss.
Adapted from Smith RJH, Bale JF Jr, White KR: Sensorineural hearing loss in children, Lancet 365:879–890, 2005.

SYNDROME	GENE	PHENOTYPE
Table 637-3		Common Types of Syndromic Sensorineural Hearing Loss
DOMINANT		
Waardenburg (WS1)	PAX3	Major diagnostic criteria include dystopia canthorum, congenital hearing loss, heterochromic irises, white forelock, and an affected 1st-degree relative. Approximately 60% of affected children have congenital hearing loss; in 90%, the loss is bilateral.
Waardenburg (WS2)	MITF, others	Major diagnostic criteria are as for WS1 but without dystopia canthorum. Approximately 80% of affected children have congenital hearing loss; in 90%, the loss is bilateral.
Branchiootorenal	EYA1	Diagnostic criteria include hearing loss (98%), preauricular pits (85%), and branchial (70%), renal (40%), and external-ear (30%) abnormalities. The hearing loss can be conductive, sensorineural, or mixed, and mild to profound in degree.
CHARGE syndrome	CHD7	Choanal atresia, colobomas, heart defect, retardation, genital hypoplasia, ear anomalies, deafness. Can lead to sensorineural or mixed hearing loss. Can be autosomal dominant or isolated cases.
Goldenhar syndrome	Unknown	Part of the hemifacial microsomia spectrum. Facial hypoplasia, ear anomalies, hemivertebrae, parotid gland dysfunction. Can cause conductive or mixed hearing loss. Can be autosomal dominant or sporadic.
RECESSIVE		
Pendred syndrome	SLC26A4	Diagnostic criteria include sensorineural hearing loss that is congenital, nonprogressive, and severe to profound in many cases, but can be late-onset and progressive; bilateral dilation of the vestibular aqueduct with or without cochlear hypoplasia; and an abnormal perchlorate discharge test or goiter.
Alport syndrome	COL4A3, COL4A4, and COL4A5	Nephritis, deafness, lens defects, retinitis. Can lead to bilateral sensorineural hearing loss in the 2,000-8,000 Hz range. The hearing loss develops gradually and is not generally present in early infancy.
Usher syndrome type 1 (USH1)	USH1A, MYO7A, USH1C, CDH23, USH1E, PCDH15, USH1G	Diagnostic criteria include congenital, bilateral, and profound hearing loss, vestibular areflexia, and retinitis pigmentosa (commonly not diagnosed until tunnel vision and nyctalopia become severe enough to be noticeable).
Usher syndrome type 2 (USH2)	USH2A, USH2B, USH2C, others	Diagnostic criteria include mild to severe, congenital, bilateral hearing loss and retinitis pigmentosa; hearing loss may be perceived as progressing over time because speech perception decreases as diminishing vision interferes with subconscious lip reading.
Usher syndrome type 3 (USH3)	USH3	Diagnostic criteria include postlingual, progressive sensorineural hearing loss, late-onset retinitis pigmentosa, and variable impairment of vestibular function.

Adapted from Smith RJH, Bale JF Jr, White KR: Sensorineural hearing loss in children, Lancet 365:879–890, 2005.

Table 637-4	Infectious Pathogens Implicated in Sensorineural Hearing Loss in Children

CONGENITAL INFECTIONS
Cytomegalovirus
Lymphocytic choriomeningitis virus
Rubella virus
Toxoplasma gondii
Treponema pallidum

ACQUIRED INFECTIONS
Borrelia burgdorferi
Epstein-Barr virus
Haemophilus influenzae
Lassa virus
Measles virus
Mumps virus
Neisseria meningitidis
Nonpolio enteroviruses
Plasmodium falciparum
Streptococcus pneumoniae
Varicella-zoster virus

From Smith RJH, Bale JF Jr, White KR: Sensorineural hearing loss in children, Lancet 365:879–890, 2005.

it may be associated with tinnitus and vertigo. Identifiable causes of sudden SNHL include infections (Epstein-Barr virus, varicella-zoster virus, herpes simplex virus), vascular injury to the cochlea, endolymphatic hydrops, and autoimmune inflammatory diseases. In most patients with sudden SNHL, no etiology is discovered, and it is termed **idiopathic sudden SNHL.**

Infectious Causes

The most common infectious cause of congenital SNHL is **cytomegalovirus (CMV),** which infects 1 in 100 newborns in the United States (see Chapters 255 and 638). Of these, 6,000-8,000 infants each yr have clinical manifestations, including approximately 75% with SNHL. Congenital CMV warrants special attention because it is associated with hearing loss in its symptomatic and asymptomatic forms, and the hearing loss may be progressive. Some children with congenital CMV have suddenly lost residual hearing at 4-5 yr of age. Much less common congenital infectious causes of SNHL include toxoplasmosis and syphilis. Congenital CMV, toxoplasmosis, and syphilis also can manifest with delayed onset of SNHL months to years after birth. Rubella, once the most common viral cause of congenital SNHL, is very uncommon because of effective vaccination programs. In utero infection with herpes simplex virus is rare, and hearing loss is not an isolated manifestation.

Other postnatal infectious causes of SNHL include neonatal group B streptococcal sepsis and bacterial meningitis at any age. *Streptococcus pneumoniae* is the most common cause of bacterial meningitis that results in SNHL after the neonatal period and has become less common with the routine administration of pneumococcal conjugate vaccine. *Haemophilus influenzae* type b, once the most common cause of meningitis resulting in SNHL, is rare owing to the *H. influenzae* type b conjugate vaccine. Uncommon infectious causes of SNHL include Lyme disease, parvovirus B19, and varicella. Mumps, rubella, and rubeola, all once common causes of SNHL in children, are rare owing to vaccination programs.

Genetic Causes

Genetic causes of SNHL probably are responsible for as many as 50% of SNHL cases (see Tables 637-2 and 637-3). These disorders may be associated with other abnormalities, may be part of a named syndrome, or can exist in isolation. SNHL often occurs with abnormalities of the ear and eye and with disorders of the metabolic, musculoskeletal, integumentary, renal, and nervous systems.

Autosomal dominant hearing losses account for approximately 10% of all cases of childhood SNHL. Waardenburg (types I and II) and

branchiootorenal syndromes represent 2 of the most common autosomal dominant syndromic types of SNHL. Types of SNHL are coded with a 4 letter code and a number, as follows: **DFN** = deafness, A = dominant, B = recessive, and number = order of discovery, for example, DFNA 13. Autosomal dominant conditions in addition to those just discussed include DFNA 1-18, 20-25, 30, 36, 38, and mutations in the crystallin gene *(CRYM).*

Autosomal recessive genetic SNHL, both syndromic and nonsyndromic, accounts for approximately 80% of all childhood cases of SNHL. Usher syndrome (types 1, 2, and 3: all associated with blindness, retinitis pigmentosa), Pendred syndrome, and the Jervell and Lange-Nielsen syndrome (one form of the long Q-T syndrome) are 3 of the most common syndromic recessive types of SNHL. Other autosomal recessive conditions include Alström syndrome, type 4 Bartter syndrome, biotinidase deficiency, and DFNB 1-18, 20-23, 26-27, 29-33, 35-40, 42, 44, 46, 48, 49, 53, and 55.

Unlike children with an easily identified syndrome or with anomalies of the outer ear, who may be identified as being at risk for hearing loss and consequently monitored adequately, children with nonsyndromic hearing loss present greater diagnostic difficulty. Mutations of the connexin-26 and -30 genes have been identified in autosomal recessive (DNFB 1) and autosomal dominant (DNFA 3) SNHL and in sporadic patients with nonsyndromic SNHL; up to 50% of nonsyndromic SNHLs may be related to a mutation of connexin-26. Mutations of the *GJB2* gene colocalize with DFNA 3 and DFNB 1 loci on chromosome 13, are associated with autosomal nonsyndromic susceptibility to deafness, and are associated with as many as 30% of cases of sporadic severe to profound congenital deafness and 50% of cases of autosomal recessive nonsyndromic deafness. In addition, mutations in *GJB6* are associated with approximately 5% of recessive nonsyndromic deafness. Sex-linked disorders associated with SNHL, thought to account for 1-2% of SNHLs, include Norrie disease, the otopalatal digital syndrome, Nance deafness, and Alport syndrome. Chromosomal abnormalities such as trisomy 13-15, trisomy 18, and trisomy 21 also can be accompanied by hearing impairment. Patients with Turner syndrome have monosomy for all or part of 1 X chromosome and can have CHL, SNHL, or mixed hearing loss. The hearing loss may be progressive. Mitochondrial genetic abnormalities also can result in SNHL (see Table 637-2).

Many genetically determined causes of hearing impairment, both syndromic and nonsyndromic, do not express themselves until sometime after birth. Alport, Alström, Down, and Hunter-Hurler syndromes and von Recklinghausen disease are genetic diseases that can have SNHL as a late manifestation.

Physical Causes

Agenesis or malformation of cochlear structures, including the Scheibe, Mondini (Fig. 637-1), Alexander, and Michel anomalies, enlarged vestibular aqueducts (which may be associated with Pendred syndrome), and semicircular canal anomalies, may be genetic. These anomalies probably occur before the 8th wk of gestation and result from arrest in normal development or aberrant development, or both. Many of these anomalies also have been described in association with other congenital conditions such as intrauterine CMV and rubella infections. These abnormalities are quite common; in as many as 20% of children with SNHL, obvious or subtle temporal bone abnormalities are seen on high-resolution CT scanning or MRI.

Conditions, diseases, or syndromes that include craniofacial abnormalities may be associated with CHL and possibly with SNHL. Pierre Robin, Treacher Collins, Klippel-Feil, Crouzon, and branchiootorenal syndromes and osteogenesis imperfecta often are associated with hearing loss. Congenital anomalies causing CHL include malformations of the ossicles and middle-ear structures and atresia of the external auditory canal.

SNHL also can occur secondary to exposure to toxins, chemicals, and antimicrobials. Early in pregnancy, the embryo is particularly vulnerable to the effects of toxic substances. Ototoxic drugs, including aminoglycosides, loop diuretics, and chemotherapeutic agents (cisplatin) also can cause SNHL. Congenital SNHL can occur secondary to

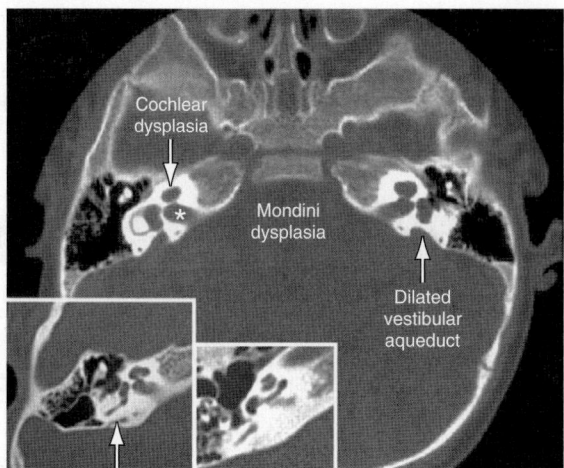

Figure 637-1 Mondini dysplasia shown by CT of the temporal bone in a child with Pendred syndrome. Both dilation of the vestibular aqueduct and cochlear dysplasia are present in this section. In the larger of the 2 inset images of a normal temporal bone, the vestibular aqueduct is visible but much smaller *(arrow)*. The cochlea appears normal, and in the smaller inset image of a more inferior axial section, the expected number of cochlear turns can be clearly counted. *Internal auditory canal. *(From Smith RJH, Bale JF Jr, White KR: Sensorineural hearing loss in children, Lancet 365:879–890, 2005.)*

exposure to these drugs as well as to thalidomide and retinoids. Certain chemicals, such as quinine, lead, and arsenic, can cause hearing loss both prenatally and postnatally.

Trauma, including temporal bone fractures, inner ear concussion, head trauma, iatrogenic trauma (e.g., surgery, extracorporeal membrane oxygenation), radiation exposure, and noise, also can cause SNHL. Other uncommon causes of SNHL in children include immune disease (systemic or limited to the inner ear), metabolic abnormalities, and neoplasms of the temporal bone.

EFFECTS OF HEARING IMPAIRMENT

The effects of hearing impairment depend on the nature and degree of the hearing loss and on the individual characteristics of the child. Hearing loss may be unilateral or bilateral, conductive, sensorineural, or mixed; mild, moderate, severe, or profound; of sudden or gradual onset; stable, progressive, or fluctuating; and affecting a part or all of the audible spectrum. Other factors, such as intelligence, medical or physical condition (including accompanying syndromes), family support, age at onset, age at time of identification, and promptness of intervention, also affect the impact of hearing loss on a child.

Most hearing-impaired children have some usable hearing. Only 6% of those in the hearing-impaired population have bilateral profound hearing loss. Hearing loss very early in life can affect the development of speech and language, social and emotional development, behavior, attention, and academic achievement. Some cases of hearing impairment are misdiagnosed because affected children have sufficient hearing to respond to environmental sounds and can learn some speech and language but when challenged in the classroom cannot perform to full potential.

Even mild or unilateral hearing loss can have a detrimental effect on the development of a young child and on school performance. Children with such hearing impairments have greater difficulty when listening conditions are unfavorable (e.g., background noise and poor acoustics), as can occur in a classroom. The fact that schools are auditory-verbal environments is unappreciated by those who minimize the impact of hearing impairment on learning. Hearing loss should be considered in any child with speech and language difficulties or below-par performance, poor behavior, or inattention in school (Table 637-5).

Children with moderate, severe, or profound hearing impairment and those with other handicapping conditions often are educated in classes or schools for children with special needs. The auditory management and choices regarding modes of communication and education for children with hearing handicaps must be individualized, because these children are not a homogeneous group. A team approach to individual case management is essential, because each child and family unit has unique needs and abilities.

HEARING SCREENING

Hearing impairment can have a major impact on a child's development, and because early identification improves prognosis, screening programs have been widely and strongly advocated. The National Center for Hearing Assessment and Management estimates that the detection and treatment at birth of hearing loss saves $400,000 per child in special education costs; screening costs approximately $8-50/child. Data from the Colorado newborn screening program suggest that if hearing-impaired infants are identified and treated by age 6 mo, these children (with the exception of those with bilateral profound impairment) should develop the same level of language as their age-matched peers who are not hearing impaired. This is compelling support for the establishment of mandated newborn hearing screening programs for all children. The American Academy of Pediatrics endorses the goal of universal detection of hearing loss in infants before 3 mo of age, with appropriate intervention no later than 6 mo of age. Newborn screening rates in the United States have increased significantly; the Centers for Disease Control and Prevention estimates that of the approximately 4 million infants born in the United States in 2009, 97% were screened for hearing loss.

Until mandated screening programs are established universally, many hospitals will continue to use other criteria to screen for hearing loss. Some use the high-risk criteria (see Table 637-1) to decide which infants to screen; some screen all infants who require intensive care; and some do both. The problem with using high-risk criteria to screen is that 50% of cases of hearing impairment will be missed, either because the infants are hearing impaired but do not meet any of the high-risk criteria or because they develop hearing loss after the neonatal period.

The recommended hearing screening techniques are either otoacoustic emissions (OAE) testing or auditory brainstem evoked responses (ABRs). The ABR test, an auditory evoked electrophysiologic response that correlates highly with hearing, has been used successfully and cost-effectively to screen newborns and to identify further the degree and type of hearing loss. OAE tests, used successfully in most universal newborn screening programs, are quick, easy to administer, and inexpensive, and they provide a sensitive indication of the presence of hearing loss. Results are relatively easy to interpret. OAE tests elicit no response if hearing is worse than 30-40 dB, no matter what the cause; children who fail OAE tests undergo an ABR for a more definitive evaluation. Screening methods such as observing behavioral responses to uncalibrated noisemakers or using automated systems such as the Crib-o-gram (Canon) or the auditory response cradle (in which movement of the infant in response to sound is recorded by motion sensors) are not recommended.

Many children become hearing impaired after the neonatal period and therefore are not identified by newborn screening programs. Often it is not until children are in preschool or kindergarten that further hearing screening takes place. Primary care physicians and pediatricians should be alert to the signs and symptoms of childhood hearing impairment, so that children with hearing impairment who have not been screened formally can be identified as early as possible. Figure 637-2 identifies recommendations for postneonatal screening.

IDENTIFICATION OF HEARING IMPAIRMENT

The impact of hearing impairment is greatest on an infant who has yet to develop language; consequently, identification, diagnosis, description, and treatment should begin as soon as possible. In general, infants with a prenatal or perinatal history that puts them at risk (see Table 637-2) or those who have failed a formal hearing screening should be monitored closely by an experienced clinical audiologist until a reliable assessment of auditory function has been obtained. Pediatricians should encourage families to cooperate with the follow-up plan. Infants who are born at risk but who were not screened as neonates (often because of transfer from one hospital to another) should have a hearing screening by age 3 mo.

Hearing-impaired infants, who are born at risk or are screened for hearing loss in a neonatal hearing screening program, account for only a portion of hearing-impaired children. Children who are congenitally deaf because of autosomal recessive inheritance or subclinical congenital infection often are not identified until 1-3 yr of age. Usually, those

Table 637-5	Hearing Handicap as a Function of Average Hearing Threshold Level of the Better Ear				
AVERAGE THRESHOLD LEVEL (dB) AT 500-2,000 Hz (ANSI)	**DESCRIPTION**	**COMMON CAUSES**	**WHAT CAN BE HEARD WITHOUT AMPLIFICATION**	**DEGREE OF HANDICAP (IF NOT TREATED IN 1ST YR OF LIFE)**	**PROBABLE NEEDS**
0-15	Normal range	Conductive hearing loss	All speech sounds	None	None
16-25	Slight hearing loss	Otitis media, TM perforation, tympanosclerosis; eustachian tube dysfunction; some SNHL	Vowel sounds heard clearly, may miss unvoiced consonant sounds	Mild auditory dysfunction in language learning Difficulty in perceiving some speech sounds	Consideration of need for hearing aid, speech reading, auditory training, speech therapy, appropriate surgery, preferential seating
26-30	Mild	Otitis media, TM perforation, tympanosclerosis, severe eustachian dysfunction, SNHL	Hears only some speech sounds, the louder voiced sounds	Auditory learning dysfunction Mild language retardation Mild speech problems Inattention	Hearing aid Lip reading Auditory training Speech therapy Appropriate surgery
31-50	Moderate hearing loss	Chronic otitis, ear canal/middle ear anomaly, SNHL	Misses most speech sounds at normal conversational level	Speech problems Language retardation Learning dysfunction Inattention	All of the above, plus consideration of special classroom situation
51-70	Severe hearing loss	SNHL or mixed loss due to a combination of middle-ear disease and sensorineural involvement	Hears no speech sound of normal conversations	Severe speech problems Language retardation Learning dysfunction Inattention	All of the above; probable assignment to special classes
71+	Profound hearing loss	SNHL or mixed	Hears no speech or other sounds	Severe speech problems Language retardation Learning dysfunction Inattention	All of the above; probable assignment to special classes or schools

ANSI, American National Standards Institute; SNHL, sensorineural hearing loss; TM, tympanic membrane.
Modified from Northern JL, Downs MP: Hearing in children, ed 4, Baltimore, 1991, Williams & Wilkins.

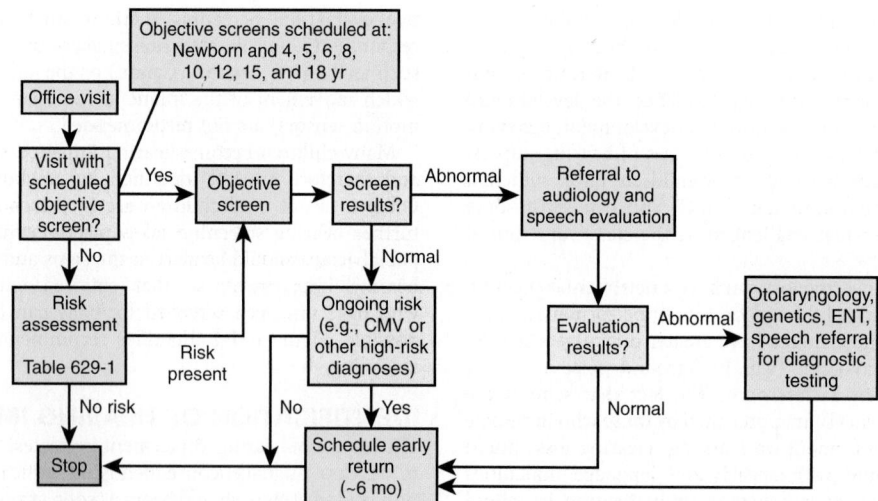

Figure 637-2 Hearing-assessment algorithm within an office visit. CMV, cytomegalovirus; ENT, ear, nose, and throat. (*From Harlor AD Jr, Bower C: Clinical report—hearing assessment in infants and children: recommendations beyond neonatal screening, Pediatrics 124:1252–1263, 2009, Fig. 1, p. 1254.*)

Table 637-6	Criteria for Referral for Audiologic Assessment

AGE (mo)	REFERRAL GUIDELINES FOR CHILDREN WITH "SPEECH" DELAY
12	No differentiated babbling or vocal imitation
18	No use of single words
24	Single-word vocabulary of ≤10 words
30	<100 words; no evidence of 2 word combinations; unintelligible
36	<200 words; no use of telegraphic sentences; clarity <50%
48	<600 words; no use of simple sentences; clarity ≤80%

From Matkin ND: Early recognition and referral of hearing-impaired children, Pediatr Rev 6:151–156, 1984. Reproduced by permission of Pediatrics.

Table 637-7	Guidelines for Referral of Children with Suspected Hearing Loss

AGE (mo)	NORMAL DEVELOPMENT
0-4	Should startle to loud sounds, quiet to mother's voice, momentarily cease activity when sound is presented at a conversational level
5-6	Should correctly localize to sound presented in a horizontal plane, begin to imitate sounds in own speech repertoire or at least reciprocally vocalize with an adult
7-12	Should correctly localize to sound presented in any plane. Should respond to name, even when spoken quietly
13-15	Should point toward an unexpected sound or to familiar objects or persons when asked
16-18	Should follow simple directions without gestural or other visual cues; can be trained to reach toward an interesting toy at midline when a sound is presented
19-24	Should point to body parts when asked; by 21-24 mo, can be trained to perform play audiometry

From Matkin ND: Early recognition and referral of hearing-impaired children, Pediatr Rev 6:151–156, 1984.

with more-severe hearing loss are identified at an earlier age, but identification often occurs later than the age at which intervention can provide an optimal outcome. Children who hear normally develop an extensive language by 3-4 yr of age (Table 637-6) and exhibit behavior reflecting normal auditory function (Table 637-7). Failure to fulfill these criteria should be the reason for an audiologic evaluation. Parents' concern about hearing and any delayed development of speech and language should alert the pediatrician, because parents' concern usually precedes formal identification and diagnosis of hearing impairment by 6 mo to 1 yr of age.

CLINICAL AUDIOLOGIC EVALUATION
Even the youngest infants can be evaluated for auditory function. When hearing impairment is suspected in a young child, reliable and valid estimates of auditory function can be obtained. Successful treatment strategies for hearing-impaired children rely on prompt identification and ongoing assessment to define the dimensions of auditory function. Cooperation among the pediatrician and specialists in areas such as audiology, speech and language pathology, education, and child development is necessary to optimize auditory-verbal development.

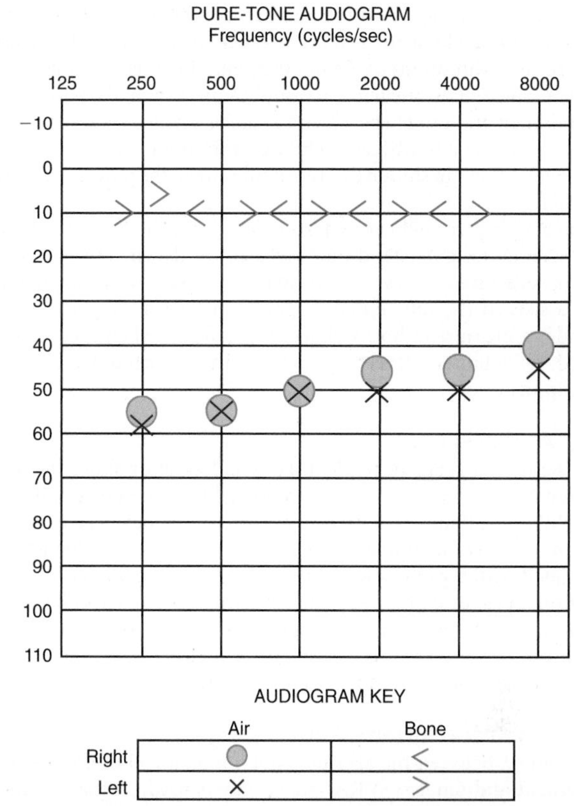

Figure 637-3 Audiogram showing bilateral conductive hearing loss.

Therapy for hearing-impaired children includes considering and often fitting an amplification device, using a **frequency modulation** system in the classroom, monitoring hearing and auditory skills, counseling parents and families, advising teachers, and dealing with public agencies.

Audiometry
The technique of the audiologic evaluation varies as a function of the age or developmental level of the child, the reason for the evaluation, and the child's otologic condition or history. An audiogram provides the fundamental description of hearing sensitivity (Fig. 637-3). Hearing thresholds are assessed as a function of frequency using pure tones (sine waves) at octave intervals from 250-8,000 Hz. Earphones typically are used when age-appropriate, and hearing is assessed independently for each ear. **Air-conducted signals** are presented through earphones (or loudspeakers) and are used to provide information about the sensitivity of the auditory system. These same test sounds can be delivered to the ear through an oscillator that is placed on the head, usually on the mastoid. Such signals are considered bone-conducted because the bones of the skull transmit vibrations as sound energy directly to the inner ear, essentially bypassing the outer and middle ears. In a normal ear, and also in children with SNHL, the air- and bone-conduction thresholds are the same. In those with CHL, the air- and bone-conduction thresholds differ. This is called the **air–bone gap,** which indicates the amount of hearing loss attributable to dysfunction in the outer and/or middle ear. With mixed hearing loss, both the bone- and air-conduction thresholds are abnormal, and there is an air–bone gap.

Speech-Recognition Threshold
Another measure useful for describing auditory function is the **speech-recognition threshold (SRT)**, which is the lowest intensity level at which a score of approximately 50% correct is obtained on a task of recognizing spondee words. Spondee words are 2 syllable words or phrases that have equal stress on each syllable, such as baseball, hotdog,

and pancake. Listeners must be familiar with all the words for a valid test result to be obtained. The SRT should correspond to the average of pure-tone thresholds at 500, 1,000, and 2,000 Hz, the pure-tone average. The SRT is relevant as an indicator of a child's potential for development and use of speech and language; it also serves as a check of the validity of a test because children with nonorganic hearing loss (malingerers) might show a discrepancy between the pure-tone average and SRT.

The basic battery of hearing tests concludes with an assessment of a child's ability to understand monosyllabic words when presented at a comfortable listening level. Performance on such word intelligibility tests assists in the differential diagnosis of hearing impairment and provides a measure of how well a child performs when speech is presented at loudness levels similar to those encountered in the environment.

Play Audiometry

Hearing testing is age dependent. For children at or above the developmental level of a 5-6 yr old, conventional test methods can be used. For children 30 mo to 5 yr of age, play audiometry can be used. Responses in play audiometry usually are conditioned motor activities associated with a game, such as dropping blocks in a bucket, placing rings on a peg, or completing a puzzle. The technique can be used to obtain a reliable audiogram for a preschool child. For those who will not or cannot repeat words clearly for the SRT and word intelligibility tasks, pictures can be used with a pointing response.

Visual Reinforcement Audiometry

For children between the ages of about 6 mo and 30 mo, **visual reinforcement audiometry (VRA)** commonly is used. In this technique, the child is observed for a head-turning response on activation of an animated (mechanical) toy reinforcer. If infants are properly conditioned, by giving sounds associated with the visual toy cue, VRA can provide reliable estimates of hearing sensitivity for tones and speech sounds. In most applications of VRA, sounds are presented by loudspeakers in a sound field, so no *ear-specific* information is obtained. Assessment of an infant often is designed to rule out hearing loss that would affect the development of speech and language. Normal sound-field response levels of infants indicate sufficient hearing for this purpose despite the possibility of different hearing levels in the 2 ears.

Behavioral Observation Audiometry

Used as a screening device for infants <5 mo of age, **behavioral observation audiometry** is limited to unconditioned, reflexive responses to complex (not frequency-specific) test sounds such as noise, speech, or music presented using calibrated signals from a loudspeaker or uncalibrated noisemakers. Response levels can vary widely within and among infants and usually do not provide a reliable estimate of sensitivity.

Assessment of a child with suspected hearing loss is not complete until pure-tone hearing thresholds and SRTs (a reliable audiogram) have been obtained in each ear. Behavioral observation audiometry and VRA in sound-field testing give estimates of hearing responsivity in the *better-hearing ear*.

Acoustic Immittance Testing

Acoustic immittance testing is a standard part of the clinical audiologic test battery and includes tympanometry. It is a useful objective assessment technique that provides information about the status of the middle ear. Tympanometry can be performed in a physician's office and is helpful in the diagnosis and management of OM with effusion, a common cause of mild to moderate hearing loss in young children.

Tympanometry

Tympanometry provides a graph of the middle ear's ability to transmit sound energy (admittance, or compliance) or impede sound energy (impedance) as a function of air pressure in the external ear canal. Because most immittance test instruments measure acoustic admittance, the term *admittance* is used here. The principles apply to whatever units of measurement are used.

A probe is inserted into the entrance of the external ear canal so that an airtight seal is obtained. The probe varies air pressure, presents a tone, and measures sound pressure level in the ear canal through the probe assembly. The sound pressure measured in the ear canal relative to the known intensity of the probe signal is used to estimate the acoustic admittance of the ear canal and middle-ear system. Admittance can be expressed in a unit called a millimho (mmho) or as a volume of air (mL) with equivalent acoustic admittance. The test is performed so that an estimate can be made of the volume of air enclosed between the probe tip and TM. The acoustic admittance of this volume of air is deducted from the overall admittance measure to obtain a measure of the admittance of the middle-ear system alone. Estimating ear canal volume also has a diagnostic benefit, because an abnormally large value is consistent with the presence of an opening in the TM (perforation or tube).

Once the admittance of the air mass in the external auditory canal has been eliminated, it is assumed that the remaining admittance measure accurately reflects the admittance of the entire middle-ear system. Its value is controlled largely by the dynamics of the TM. Abnormalities of the TM can dictate the shape of tympanograms, thus obscuring abnormalities medial to the TM. In addition, the frequency of the probe tone, the speed and direction of the air pressure change, and the air pressure at which the tympanogram is initiated can all influence the outcome.

When air pressure in the ear canal is equal to that in the middle ear, the middle-ear system is functioning optimally. Therefore, the ear canal pressure at which there is the greatest flow of energy (admittance) should be a reasonable estimate of the air pressure in the middle-ear space. This pressure is determined by finding the maximum or **peak admittance** on the tympanogram and obtaining its value on the x-axis. The value on the y-axis at the tympanogram peak is an estimate of peak admittance based on admittance tympanometry (Table 637-8). This peak measure sometimes is referred to as **static acoustic admittance,** even though it is estimated from a dynamic measure.

Tympanometry in Otitis Media with Effusion

Children who have OM with effusion often have reduced peak admittance or high negative tympanometric peak pressures (see Fig. 640-5C in Chapter 640). However, in the diagnosis of effusion, the tympanometric measure with the greatest sensitivity and specificity is the shape of the tympanogram rather than its peak pressure or admittance. This shape sometimes is referred to as the tympanometric gradient or width; it measures the degree of roundness or **peakedness** of the tympanogram. The more rounded the peak (or, in an absent peak, a flat

Table 637-8	Norms for Peak (Static) Admittance Using a 226-Hz Probe Tone for Children and Adults		
AGE GROUP	**ADMITTANCE (mL)**	**Speed of Air Pressure Sweep**	
		≤50 daPa/sec*	200 daPa/sec†
Children (3-5 yr)	Lower limit	0.30	0.36
	Median	0.55	0.61
	Upper limit	0.90	1.06
Adults	Lower limit	0.56	0.27
	Median	0.85	0.72
	Upper limit	1.36	1.38

*Ear canal volume measurement based on admittance at lowest tail of tympanogram.
†Ear canal measurement based on admittance at lowest tail of tympanogram for children and at +200 daPa for adults.
daPa, decaPascals.
Adapted from Margolis RH, Shanks JE: Tympanometry: basic principles of clinical application. In Rintelman WS, editor: Hearing assessment, ed 2, Austin, 1991, PRODED, pp. 179–245.

tympanogram), the higher is the probability that an effusion is present (see Fig. 640-5*B* in Chapter 640). It is important to know which instrument is used, because some compute gradient automatically but others do not.

Acoustic Reflex Test

The **acoustic reflex test** also is part of the immittance test battery. With a properly functioning middle-ear system, admittance at the TM changes on activation of the stapedius and tensor tympani muscles. In healthy ears, the stapedial reflex occurs after exposure to loud sounds. Admittance instruments are designed to present reflex activating signals (pure tones of various frequencies or noise), either to the same ear or the contralateral ear, while monitoring admittance. Very small admittance changes that are time locked to presentations of the signal are considered to be a result of middle-ear muscle reflexes. Admittance changes may be absent when the hearing loss is sufficient to prevent the signal from reaching the loudness level necessary to elicit the reflex or when a middle-ear condition affects the ear's ability to monitor a small admittance change. Reflexes usually are absent in patients with CHL because of the presence of an abnormal transfer system; thus, the acoustic reflex test is useful in the differential diagnosis of hearing impairment. The acoustic reflex test also is used in the assessment of SNHL and the integrity of the neurologic components of the reflex arc, including cranial nerves VII and VIII.

Auditory Brainstem Response

The auditory brainstem response (ABR) test is used to screen newborn hearing, confirm hearing loss in young children, obtain ear-specific information in young children, and test children who cannot, for whatever reason, cooperate with behavioral test methods. It also is important in the diagnosis of auditory dysfunction and of disorders of the auditory nervous system. The ABR test is a far-field recording of minute electrical discharges from numerous neurons. The stimulus, therefore, must be able to cause simultaneous discharge of the large numbers of neurons involved. Stimuli with very rapid onset, such as clicks or tone bursts, must be used. Unfortunately, the rapid onset required to create a measurable ABR also causes energy to be spread in the frequency domain, reducing the frequency-specificity of the response.

The ABR result is not affected by sedation or general anesthesia. Infants and children from about 4 mo to 4 yr of age routinely are sedated to minimize electrical interference caused by muscle activity during testing. The ABR also can be performed in the operating room when a child is anesthetized for another procedure. Children younger than 4 mo of age might sleep for a long enough period of time after feeding to allow an ABR to be done.

The ABR is recorded as 5-7 waves. Waves I, III, and V can be obtained consistently in all age groups; waves II and IV appear less consistently. The latency of each wave (time of occurrence of the wave peak after stimulus onset) increases, and the amplitude decreases with reductions in stimulus intensity or loudness; latency also decreases with increasing age, with the earliest waves reaching mature latency values earlier in life than the later waves.

The ABR test has 2 major uses in a pediatric setting. As an audiometric test, it provides information on the ability of the peripheral auditory system to transmit information to the auditory nerve and beyond. It also is used in the differential diagnosis or monitoring of central nervous system pathology. For audiometry, the goal is to find the minimum stimulus intensity that yields an observable ABR. Plotting latency vs intensity for various waves also aids in the differential diagnosis of hearing impairment. A major advantage of auditory assessment using the ABR test is that ear-specific threshold estimates can be obtained on infants or patients who are difficult to test. ABR thresholds using click stimuli correlate best with behavioral hearing thresholds in the higher frequencies (1,000-4,000 Hz); responsivity in the low frequencies requires different stimuli (tone bursts or filtered clicks) or the use of masking, neither of which isolates the low-frequency region of the cochlea in all cases, and this can affect interpretation.

The ABR test does not assess "hearing." It reflects auditory neuronal electrical responses that can be correlated to behavioral hearing thresholds, but a normal ABR result only suggests that the auditory system, up to the level of the midbrain, is responsive to the stimulus used. Conversely, a failure to elicit an ABR indicates an impairment of the system's synchronous response but does not necessarily mean that there is no "hearing." The behavioral response to sound sometimes is normal when no ABR can be elicited, such as in neurologic demyelinating disease. The ABR test may be used to infer whether and at what level of the auditory system impairment exists.

Hearing losses that are sudden, progressive, or unilateral are indications for ABR testing. Although it is believed that the different waves of the ABR reflect activity in increasingly rostral levels of the auditory system, the neural generators of the response have not been precisely determined. Each ABR wave beyond the earliest waves probably is the result of neural firing at many levels of the system, and each level of the system probably contributes to several ABR waves. High-intensity click stimuli are used for the neurologic application. The morphology of the response and wave and interwave latencies are examined in respect to age-appropriate forms. Delayed or missing waves in the ABR result often have diagnostic significance.

The ABR and other electrical responses are extremely complex and difficult to interpret. A number of factors, including instrumentation design and settings, environment, degree and configuration of hearing loss, and patients' characteristics, can influence the quality of the recording. Therefore, testing and interpretation of electrophysiologic activity as it possibly relates to hearing should be carried out by trained audiologists to avoid the risk that unreliable or erroneous conclusions will affect a patient's care.

Otoacoustic Emissions

During normal hearing, OAEs originate from the hair cells in the cochlea and are detected by sensitive amplifying processes. They travel from the cochlea through the middle ear to the external auditory canal, where they can be detected using miniature microphones. Transient evoked OAEs (TEOAEs) may be used to check the integrity of the cochlea. In the neonatal period, detection of OAEs can be accomplished during natural sleep, and TEOAEs can be used as screening tests in infants and children for hearing at the 30 dB level of hearing loss. They are less time consuming and elaborate than ABRs and are more sensitive than behavioral tests in young children. TEOAEs are reduced or absent owing to various dysfunctions in the middle and inner ears. They are absent in patients with >30 dB of hearing loss and are not used to determine the hearing threshold; rather, they provide a screen for whether hearing is present at >30-40 dB. Diseases such as OM or congenitally abnormal middle-ear structures reduce the transfer of TEOAEs and may incorrectly indicate a cochlear hearing disorder. If a hearing loss is suspected based on the absence of OAEs, the ears should be examined for evidence of pathology, and then ABR testing should be used for confirmation and identification of the type, degree, and laterality of hearing loss.

Acoustic Reflectometry

In acoustic reflectometry, a handheld instrument is placed next to the opening of a child's ear canal and an 80 dB sound is delivered that varies in frequency from 2,000-4,500 Hz in a 100 msec period. The instrument measures the total level of reflected and transmitted sound. Some physicians have found this device useful to help gauge the presence or absence of middle-ear fluid, and a commercial version is marketed to parents as a way to monitor ear fluid. The instrument does not provide any information about hearing; if the presence of chronic fluid is suggested, audiometric evaluation should be obtained.

TREATMENT

With the use of universal hearing screening in the majority of states within the United States, the early diagnosis and treatment of children with hearing loss is common. Testing for hearing loss is possible even in very young children, and it should be done if parents suspect a

Table 637-9	Recommended Pneumococcal Vaccination Schedule for Persons with Cochlear Implants			
AGE AT FIRST PCV13 DOSE (mo)*	PCV12 PRIMARY SERIES	PCV13 ADDITIONAL DOSE	PPV23 DOSE
2-6	3 doses, 2 mo apart†	1 dose at 12-15 mo of age‡	Indicated at ≥24 mo of age§
7-11	2 doses, 2 mo apart†	1 dose at 12-15 mo of age‡	Indicated at ≥24 mo of age§
12-23	2 doses, 2 mo apart¶	Not indicated	Indicated at ≥24 mo of age§
24-59	2 doses, 2 mo apart¶	Not indicated	Indicated§
≥60	Not indicatedǀ	Not indicatedǀ	Indicated

*A schedule with a reduced number of total 13-valent pneumococcal conjugate vaccine (PCV13) doses is indicated if children start late or are incompletely vaccinated. Children with a lapse in vaccination should be vaccinated according to the catch-up schedule (see Chapter 182).
†For children vaccinated at younger than age 1 yr, minimum interval between doses is 4 wk.
‡The additional dose should be administered 8 wk or more after the primary series has been completed.
§Children younger than age 5 yr should complete the PCV13 series first; 23-valent pneumococcal polysaccharide vaccine (PPV23) should be administered to children 24 mo of age or older 8 wk or more after the last dose of PCV13 (see Chapter 182). (Centers for Disease Control and Prevention Advisory Committee on Immunization Practices: Preventing pneumococcal disease among infants and young children: recommendations of the Advisory Committee on Immunization Practices [ACIP], *MMWR Recomm Rep* 49[RR-9]:1–35, 2000, and Licensure of a 13-valent pneumococcal conjugate vaccine [PCV13] and recommendations for use among children—Advisory Committee on Immunization Practices [ACIP], 2010, *MMWR Morb Mortal Wkly Rep* 59(9);258–261, 2010.)
¶Minimum interval between doses is 8 wk.
ǀPCV13 is not recommended generally for children age 5 yr or older.
PCV, pneumococcal conjugate vaccine; PPV, pneumococcal polysaccharide vaccine.
From Centers for Disease Control and Prevention Advisory Committee on Immunization Practices: Pneumococcal vaccination for cochlear implant candidates and recipients: Updated recommendations of the Advisory Committee on Immunization Practices, MMWR Morb Mortal Wkly Rep 52(31):739–740, 2003.

problem. Any child with a known risk factor for hearing loss should be evaluated in the 1st 6 mo of life.

Once a hearing loss is identified, a full developmental and speech and language evaluation is needed. Counseling and involvement of parents are required in all stages of the evaluation and treatment or rehabilitation. A CHL often can be corrected through treatment of a middle-ear effusion (i.e., ear tube placement) or surgical correction of the abnormal sound-conducting mechanism. Children with SNHL should be evaluated for possible hearing aid use by a pediatric audiologist. Hearing aids may be fitted for children as young as 2 mo of age. Compelling evidence from the hearing screening program in Colorado shows that identification and amplification before age 6 mo makes a very significant difference in the speech and language abilities of affected children, compared with cases identified and amplified after the age of 6 mo. In these children, repeat audiologic testing is needed to reliably identify the degree of hearing loss and to fine-tune the use of hearing aids.

Infants and young children with profound congenital or prelingual onset of deafness have benefited from **multichannel cochlear implants** (Fig. 637-4). These implants bypass injury to the organ of Corti and provide neural stimulation by way of an external microphone and a signal processor that digitizes auditory stimuli into digital radiofrequency impulses. Cochlear implantation before age 2 yr (and even 1 yr) improves hearing and speech, enabling more than 90% of children to be in mainstream education. Most develop age-appropriate auditory perception and oral language skills.

A serious complication of cochlear implants is an excessively high incidence of pneumococcal meningitis. All children receiving a cochlear implant must be vaccinated with the pneumococcal polyvalent vaccine PCV13 (Table 637-9).

The best approach to the education of children with significant hearing loss is a subject of ongoing controversy. Because we live in a predominantly speaking world, some have advocated a pure auditory and oral approach to hearing therapy. However, because affected children often are slow to develop communication skills, many advocate a total communication approach; depending on the individual child's needs, this technique uses a mixture of sign language, lip reading, hearing aids, and speech. The appropriate program for each child depends on the patient, family, and available resources.

Management of **idiopathic sudden SNHL** is controversial and has included oral prednisone, intratympanic (also called transtympanic) dexamethasone perfusion, or a combination of both; the latter combination may be the most useful, although the data are not conclusive.

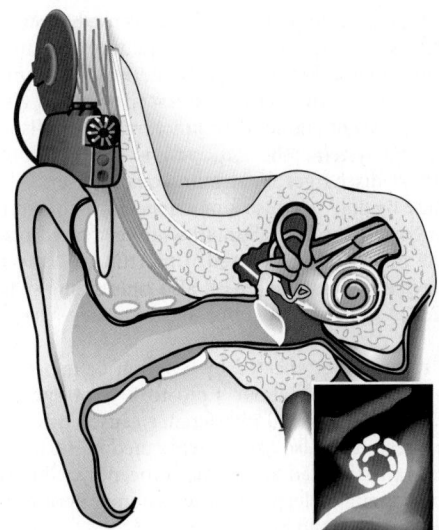

Figure 637-4 All cochlear implants share key components, including a microphone, speech processor, and transmitter coil, shown in a behind-the-ear position in this diagram. The microphone and speech processor pick up environmental sounds and digitize them into coded signals. The signals are sent to the transmitter coil and relayed through the skin to the internal device imbedded in the skull. The internal device converts the code to electronic signals, which are transmitted to the electrode array wrapping around the cochlea. The inset shows the radiographic appearance of the stimulating electrode array. *(Reproduced with permission from MED-EL Corporation, Innsbruck, Austria. From Smith RJH, Bale JF Jr, White KR: Sensorineural hearing loss in children, Lancet 365:879–890, 2005.)*

GENETIC COUNSELING

Families of children with the diagnosis of SNHL or a syndrome associated with SNHL and/or CHL should consider genetic counseling, which will allow a discussion of the likelihood of similar diagnoses in future pregnancies. The geneticist also can help in the evaluation and further testing of the patient with hearing loss to establish a diagnosis.

Bibliography is available at Expert Consult.

Chapter **638**
Congenital Malformations
Joseph Haddad Jr. and Sarah Keesecker

The external and middle ears, derived from the first and second branchial arches and grooves, grow throughout puberty, but the inner ear, which develops from the otocyst, reaches adult size and shape by midfetal development. The ossicles are derived from the first and second arches (malleus and incus), and the stapes arises from the second arch and the otic capsule. The malleus and incus achieve adult size and shape by the 15th wk of gestation, and the stapes achieves adult size and shape by the 18th wk of gestation. Although the pinna, ear canal, and tympanic membrane (TM) continue to grow after birth, congenital abnormalities of these structures develop during the first half of gestation. Malformed external and middle ears may be associated with serious renal anomalies, mandibulofacial dysostosis, hemifacial microsomia, and other craniofacial malformations. Facial nerve abnormalities may be associated with any of the congenital abnormalities of the ear and temporal bone. Malformations of the external and middle ears also may be associated with abnormalities of the inner ear and both conductive (CHL) and sensorineural hearing loss (SNHL).

Congenital ear problems may be minor and mainly cosmetic, or major, affecting both appearance and function. Any child born with an abnormality of the pinna, external auditory canal, or TM should have a complete audiologic evaluation in the neonatal period. Imaging studies are necessary for evaluation and treatment; in the patient with other craniofacial abnormalities a team approach with other specialists can assist in guiding therapy.

PINNA MALFORMATIONS
Severe malformations of the external ear are rare, but minor deformities are common. Isolated abnormalities of the external ear occur in approximately 1% of children. A pit-like depression just in front of the helix and above the tragus may represent a cyst or an epidermis-lined fistulous tract. These are common, with an incidence of approximately 8 in 1,000 children, and may be unilateral or bilateral and familial. The pits require surgical removal only if there is recurrent infection. Accessory skin tags, with an incidence of 1-2/1,000 live births, can be removed for cosmetic reasons by simple ligation if they are attached by a narrow pedicle. If the pedicle is broad based or contains cartilage, the defect should be corrected surgically. An unusually prominent or "lop" ear results from lack of bending of the cartilage that creates the antihelix. It may be improved cosmetically in the neonatal period by applying a firm framework (sometimes soldering wire is used) attached by Steri-Strips to the pinna and worn continuously for weeks to months. Otoplasty for cosmetic correction can be considered in children older than 5 yr of age, when the pinna has reached approximately 80% of its adult size.

The term **microtia** may indicate subtle abnormalities of the size, shape, and location of the pinna and ear canal, or major abnormalities with only small nubbins of skin and cartilage and the absence of the ear canal opening; **anotia** indicates complete absence of the pinna and ear canal. Microtia can have a genetic or environmental predisposition. Several hereditary forms of microtia have been identified that exhibit either autosomal dominant or recessive mendelian inheritance. In addition, some forms due to chromosomal aberrations have been reported. Most of the responsible genes that have been identified are homeobox genes. Microtic ears often are more anterior and inferior in placement than normal auricles, and the location and function of the facial nerve may be abnormal. Surgery to correct microtia is

considered for both cosmetic and functional reasons; children who have some pinna can wear regular glasses, a hearing aid, and earrings and feel more normal in appearance. If the microtia is severe, some patients may opt for creation and attachment of a prosthetic ear, which cosmetically closely resembles a real ear. Surgery to correct severe microtia may involve a multistage procedure, including carving and transplantation of autogenous cartilage rib grafts and local soft tissue flaps. Cosmetic reconstruction of the auricle usually is performed between 5-7 yr of age and is performed before canal atresia repair in children deemed appropriate for this surgery.

CONGENITAL STENOSIS OR ATRESIA OF THE EXTERNAL AUDITORY CANAL
Stenosis or atresia of the ear canal often occurs in association with malformation of the auricle and middle ear. Malformations can occur in isolation or as part of a genetic syndrome. For example, the ear canal is narrow in trisomy 21 and external canal stenosis or atresia is common in branchiooculofacial syndrome, leading to CHL. Audiometric evaluation of these children should be undertaken as early in life as possible. Most children with significant CHL secondary to bilateral atresia wear bone conduction hearing aids for the 1st several yr of life. Diagnosis, evaluation, and surgical planning often are aided by CT, and sometimes MRI, of the temporal bone. Mild cases of ear canal stenosis do not require surgical enlargement unless the patient develops chronic external otitis or severe cerumen impaction that affects hearing.

Reconstructive ear canal and middle-ear surgery for atresia usually is considered for children older than 5 yr of age who have bilateral deformities resulting in a significant CHL. The aim of reconstructive surgery is to improve hearing to a point where the child may not need a hearing aid or to provide an ear canal and pinna so that the child can derive improved benefit from an air-conduction hearing aid. Hearing results for atresiaplasty range from fair to excellent. CT evidence of an adequate middle-ear cleft, ossicles, and mastoid is required to perform the surgery; the position of the facial nerve, which often is in an abnormal location in these children, also must be considered (Fig. 638-1). The use of bone-anchored hearing aids is a safe, reliable, and low-risk alternative to atresiaplasty and hearing results are generally excellent. Bone-anchored hearing aids may also be useful for rehabilitation of nonoptimal atresiaplasty hearing results. These devices are approved by the U.S. Food and Drug Administration for surgical placement in children age 5 yr and older; prior to age 5 yr, they can be worn with a soft band around the head. Disadvantages include the fact that cosmesis is not very good (a bone-anchored hearing aid has a visible titanium abutment and snap-on hearing aid) and frequent wound care is required.

CONGENITAL MIDDLE-EAR MALFORMATIONS
Children may have congenital abnormalities of the middle ear as an isolated defect or in association with other abnormalities of the temporal bone, especially the ear canal and pinna, or as part of a syndrome. Affected children usually have CHL but may have mixed CHL and SNHL. Most malformations involve the ossicles, with the incus most commonly affected. Other less-common abnormalities of the middle ear include persistent stapedial artery, high-riding jugular bulb, and abnormalities of the shape and volume of the aerated portion of the middle ear and mastoid; all present problems for a surgeon. Depending on the type of abnormality and the presence of other anomalies, surgery may be considered to improve hearing.

CONGENITAL INNER EAR MALFORMATIONS
Congenital inner ear malformations have been identified and classified as a result of improvements in imaging modalities, especially CT and MRI. As many as 20% of children with SNHL may have anatomic abnormalities identified on CT or MRI. Congenital malformations of the inner ear usually are associated with SNHL of various degrees, from mild to profound. These malformations may occur as isolated anomalies or in association with other syndromes, genetic abnormalities, or structural abnormalities of the head and neck. Enlarged vestibular

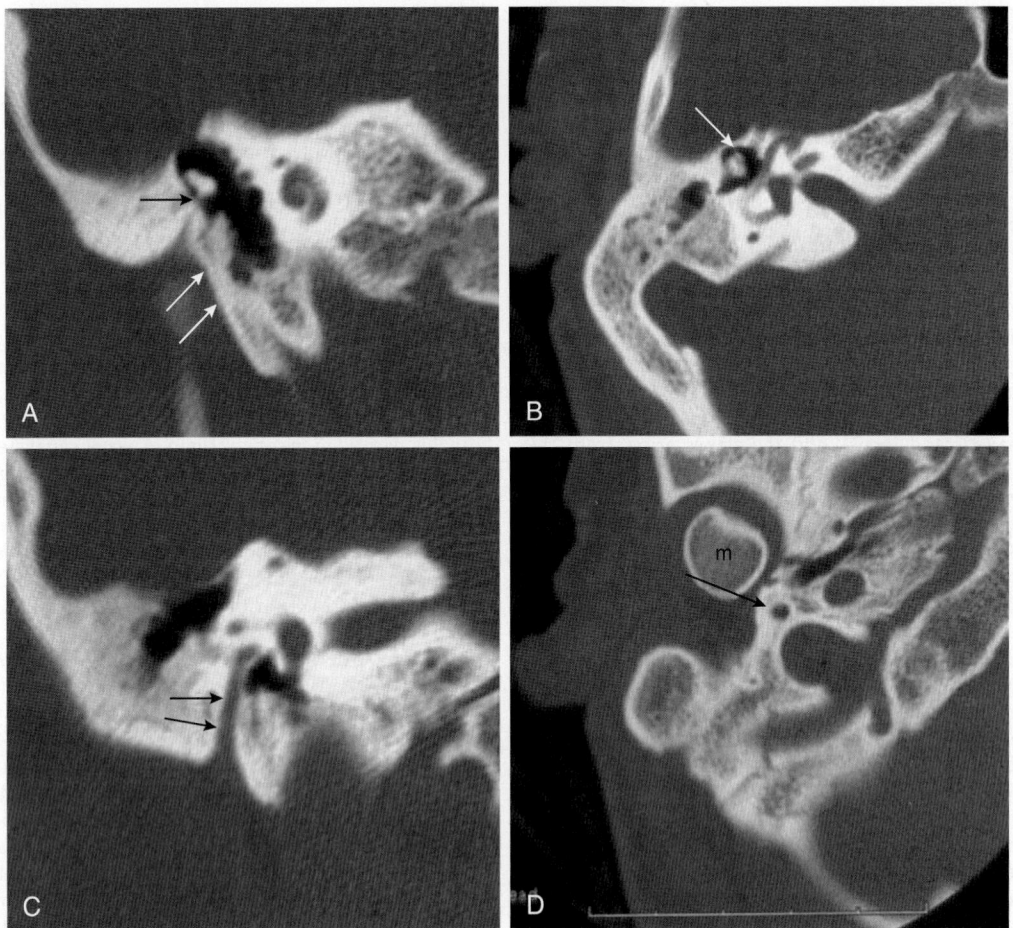

Figure 638-1 External auditory canal atresia on CT scans. **A,** Coronal scan of right ear shows absent external auditory canal with thick bony atresia plate *(white arrows)*. Malleus neck is rotated and fused to superior portion of atresia plate *(black arrow)*. **B,** Axial scan through attic shows fused ossicular mass *(arrow)*. **C,** Coronal scan more posterior to **A** shows mastoid segment of facial nerve canal positioned more anteriorly than normal *(arrows)*. **D,** Axial scan more inferior to **B** shows anterior-posterior mastoid segment of the facial nerve en face *(arrow)*. Note abnormally close relationship to mandibular condoyle. *(From Faerber EN, Booth TN, Swartz JD. Temporal bone and ear. In Slovis TL, editor: Caffey's pediatric diagnostic imaging, ed 11, Philadelphia, 2008, Mosby, Fig. 44-7, p. 584.)*

aqueducts have been identified on imaging studies in association with SNHL; although no therapy exists for this condition, it may be associated with progressive SNHL in some children, and, therefore, diagnosis may have some prognostic value.

Congenital perilymphatic fistula of the oval or round window membrane may present as a rapid-onset, fluctuating, or progressive SNHL with or without vertigo and often is associated with congenital inner ear abnormalities. Middle-ear exploration may be required to confirm this diagnosis, because no reliable nonoperative diagnostic test exists. It may be necessary to repair a perilymphatic fistula to prevent possible spread of infection from the middle ear to the labyrinth, to stabilize hearing loss, and to improve vertigo when present.

CONGENITAL CHOLESTEATOMA

A congenital cholesteatoma (approximately 2% of all cholesteatomas) is a nonneoplastic, destructive, cystic lesion that usually appears as a white, round, cyst-like structure medial to an intact TM. Cysts are seen most commonly in the anterior-superior portion of the middle ear, although they can present in other locations and within the TM or in the skin of the ear canal. Affected children often have no prior history of otitis media. One theory for the pathogenesis is that the cyst derives from a congenital rest of epithelial tissue that persists beyond 33 wk of gestation, when it ordinarily would disappear. Other theories include squamous metaplasia of the middle ear, entrance of squamous epithelium through a nonintact eardrum into the middle ear, ectoder-

mal implants between the first and second branchial arch remnants, and residual amniotic fluid squamous debris. Congenital or acquired cholesteatoma should be suspected when deep retraction pockets, keratin debris, chronic drainage, aural granulation tissue, or a mass behind or involving the TM is present. Besides acting as a benign tumor causing local bone destruction, the keratinaceous debris of a cholesteatoma is a good culture medium and may become a focus of infection for chronic otitis media. Complications include ossicular erosion with hearing loss, bone erosion into the inner ear with dizziness, or exposure of the dura, with consequent meningitis or a brain abscess. Cholesteatoma should be removed surgically after CT scan (Fig. 638-2) and hearing evaluation, and appropriate antibiotic therapy. A second-look procedure 6-9 mo after primary surgery is often recommended to prevent further recurrence. Higher initial stage of disease, erosion of ossicles, cholesteatoma abutting or enveloping the incus or stapes, and need for removal of the ossicles are associated with increased likelihood of residual cholesteatoma. In addition, more extensive disease at initial surgery is associated with poorer hearing outcomes. Recurrence rates vary and are related to the extent of involvement at the time of surgery. In a large case series, recurrence rates were found to be as follows: 14% when disease was confined to 1 quadrant, 33% when more than 1 quadrant was involved but the ossicles and mastoids were not, 41% with ossicular involvement, and 67% with mastoid involvement. Overall recurrence may be as high as 57%. Congenital cholesteatoma is an aggressive disease, and early surgical

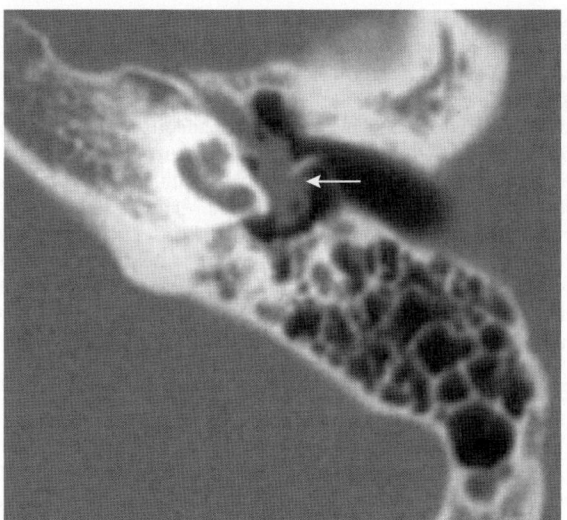

Figure 638-2 Congenital cholesteatoma. Axial CT of left ear shows soft tissue mass *(arrow)* in the middle ear. This mass was noted otoscopically behind an intact membrane. *(From Faerber EN, Booth TN, Swartz JD. Temporal bone and ear. In Slovis TL, editor: Caffey's pediatric diagnostic imaging, ed 11, Philadelphia, 2008, Mosby, Fig. 44-31, p. 598.)*

removal and close monitoring will help prevent permanent damage to the middle and inner ear.

Bibliography is available at Expert Consult.

Chapter **639**
External Otitis (Otitis Externa)
Joseph Haddad Jr. and Sarah Keesecker

In an infant, the outer two thirds of the ear canal is cartilaginous and the inner one third is bony. In an older child and adult the outer one third is cartilaginous and the inner two thirds is bony. The epithelium is thinner in the bony portion than in the cartilaginous portion, there is no subcutaneous tissue, and epithelium is tightly applied to the underlying periosteum; hair follicles, sebaceous glands, and apocrine glands are scarce or absent. The skin in the cartilaginous area has well-developed dermis and subcutaneous tissue and contains hair follicles, sebaceous glands, and apocrine glands. The highly viscid secretions of the sebaceous glands and the watery, pigmented secretions of the apocrine glands in the outer portion of the canal combine with exfoliated surface cells of the skin to form **cerumen,** a protective, waxy, water-repellent coating.

The normal flora of the external canal consists mainly of aerobic bacteria and includes coagulase-negative staphylococci (see Chapter 181.3), *Corynebacterium* (diphtheroids) (see Chapter 187), *Micrococcus,* and, occasionally, *Staphylococcus aureus* (see Chapter 181.1), viridans streptococci (see Chapter 185), and *Pseudomonas aeruginosa* (see Chapter 205.1). **Excessive wetness** (swimming, bathing, increased environmental humidity), **dryness** (dry canal skin and lack of cerumen), the presence of other skin pathologic conditions (previous infection, eczema, or other forms of dermatitis), and trauma (due to digital or foreign body, use of cotton-tip applicators [Q-tips]) make the skin of the canal vulnerable to infection by the normal flora or exogenous bacteria.

ETIOLOGY
External otitis (**swimmer's ear,** although it can occur without swimming) is caused most commonly by *P. aeruginosa,* but *S. aureus, Enterobacter aerogenes, Proteus mirabilis, Klebsiella pneumoniae,* streptococci, coagulase-negative staphylococci, diphtheroids, and fungi such as *Candida* and *Aspergillus* also may be isolated. External otitis results from chronic irritation and maceration from excessive moisture in the canal. The loss of protective cerumen may play a role, as may trauma, but cerumen impaction with trapping of water also can cause infection. Inflammation of the ear canal due to herpesvirus, varicella-zoster virus, other skin exanthems, and eczema also may predispose to external otitis.

CLINICAL MANIFESTATIONS
The predominant symptom is acute rapid onset of ear pain (otalgia), often severe, accentuated by manipulation of the pinna or by pressure on the tragus and by jaw motion. The severity of the pain and tenderness (tragus or pinna, or both) may be disproportionate to the degree of inflammation, because the skin of the external ear canal is tightly adhered to the underlying perichondrium and periosteum. Itching often is a precursor of pain and usually is characteristic of chronic inflammation of the canal or resolving acute otitis externa. Conductive hearing loss (CHL) may result from edema of the skin and tympanic membrane (TM), serous or purulent secretions, or the canal skin thickening associated with chronic external otitis.

Edema of the ear canal, erythema, and thick, clumpy otorrhea are prominent signs of the acute disease. The cerumen usually is white and soft in consistency, as opposed to its usual yellow color and firmer consistency. The canal often is so tender and swollen that the entire ear canal and TM cannot be adequately visualized, and complete otoscopic examination may be delayed until the acute swelling subsides. If the TM can be visualized, it may appear either normal or opaque. TM mobility may be normal or, if the TM is thickened, mobility may be reduced in response to positive and negative pressure.

Other physical findings may include palpable and tender lymph nodes in the periauricular region, and erythema and swelling of the pinna and periauricular skin. Rarely, facial paralysis, other cranial nerve abnormalities, vertigo, and/or sensorineural hearing loss are present. If these occur, **necrotizing (malignant) otitis externa** is probable. This invasive infection of the temporal bone and skull base requires immediate culture, intravenous antibiotics, and imaging studies to evaluate the extent of the disease. Surgical intervention to obtain cultures or debride devitalized tissue may be necessary. *P. aeruginosa* (see Chapter 205.1) is the most common causative organism of necrotizing otitis externa. Fortunately, this disease is rare in children and is seen only in association with immunocompromise or severe malnourishment. In adults, it is associated with diabetes mellitus.

DIAGNOSIS
Diffuse external otitis may be confused with **furunculosis, otitis media (OM),** and **mastoiditis.** Furuncles occur in the lateral hair-bearing part of the ear canal; furunculosis usually causes a localized swelling of the canal limited to 1 quadrant, whereas external otitis is associated with concentric swelling and involves the entire ear canal. In OM, the TM may be perforated, severely retracted, or bulging and immobile; hearing usually is impaired. If the middle ear is draining through a perforated TM or tympanostomy tube, secondary external otitis may occur; if the TM is not visible owing to drainage or ear canal swelling, it may be difficult to distinguish acute OM with drainage from an acute external otitis. Pain on manipulation of the auricle and significant lymphadenitis are not common features of OM, and these findings assist in the differential diagnosis. In some patients with external otitis, the periauricular edema is so extensive that the auricle is pushed forward, creating a condition that may be confused with acute mastoiditis and a subperiosteal abscess. In mastoiditis, the postauricular fold is obliterated, whereas in external otitis, the fold is usually

better preserved. In acute mastoiditis, a history of OM and hearing loss is usual; tenderness is noted over the mastoid and not on movement of the auricle; and otoscopic examination may show sagging of the posterior canal wall.

Referred otalgia may come from disease in the paranasal sinuses, teeth, pharynx, parotid gland, neck and thyroid, and cranial nerves (trigeminal neuralgia) (herpes simplex virus, varicella-zoster virus).

TREATMENT

Topical otic preparations containing acetic acid with or without hydrocortisone, or neomycin (active against Gram-positive organisms and some Gram-negative organisms, notably *Proteus* spp.), polymyxin (active against Gram-negative bacilli, notably *Pseudomonas* spp.), and hydrocortisone are highly effective in treating most forms of acute external otitis. *Other preparations of eardrops (e.g., ofloxacin, ciprofloxacin with hydrocortisone or dexamethasone) are preferable and do not contain potentially ototoxic antibiotics.* If canal edema is marked, the patient may need referral to a specialist for cleaning and possible wick placement. An otic antibiotic and corticosteroid eardrop is often recommended. A wick can be inserted into the ear canal and topical antibiotics applied to the wick 3 times a day for 24-48 hr. The wick can be removed after 2-3 days, at which time the edema of the ear canal usually is markedly improved, and the ear canal and TM are better seen. Topical antibiotics are then continued by direct instillation. When the pain is severe, oral analgesics (e.g., ibuprofen, codeine) may be necessary for a few days. Careful evaluation for underlying conditions should be undertaken in patients with severe or recurrent otitis externa. Figure 639-1 outlines an approach to managing acute external otitis.

As the inflammatory process subsides, cleaning the canal with a suction or cotton-tipped applicator to remove the debris enhances the effectiveness of the topical medications. In subacute and chronic infections, periodic cleansing of the canal is essential. In severe, acute external otitis associated with fever and lymphadenitis, oral or parenteral antibiotics may be indicated; an ear canal culture should be done, and empirical antibiotic treatment can then be modified if necessary, based on susceptibility of the organism cultured. A fungal infection of the external auditory canal, or **otomycosis,** is characterized by fluffy white debris, sometimes with black spores seen; treatment includes cleaning and application of antifungal solutions such as clotrimazole or nystatin; other antifungal agents include m-cresyl acetate 25%, gentian violet 2%, and thimerosal 1:1,000.

PREVENTION

Preventing external otitis may be necessary for individuals susceptible to recurrences, especially children who swim. The most effective prophylaxis is instillation of dilute alcohol or acetic acid (2%) immediately after swimming or bathing. During an acute episode of otitis externa, patients should not swim and the ears should be protected from excessive water during bathing. A hair dryer may be used to clear moisture from the ear after swimming as a method of prevention.

OTHER DISEASES OF THE EXTERNAL EAR
Furunculosis

Furunculosis is caused by *S. aureus* and affects only the hair-containing outer third of the ear canal. Mild forms are treated with oral antibiotics active against *S. aureus*. If an abscess develops, incision and drainage may be necessary.

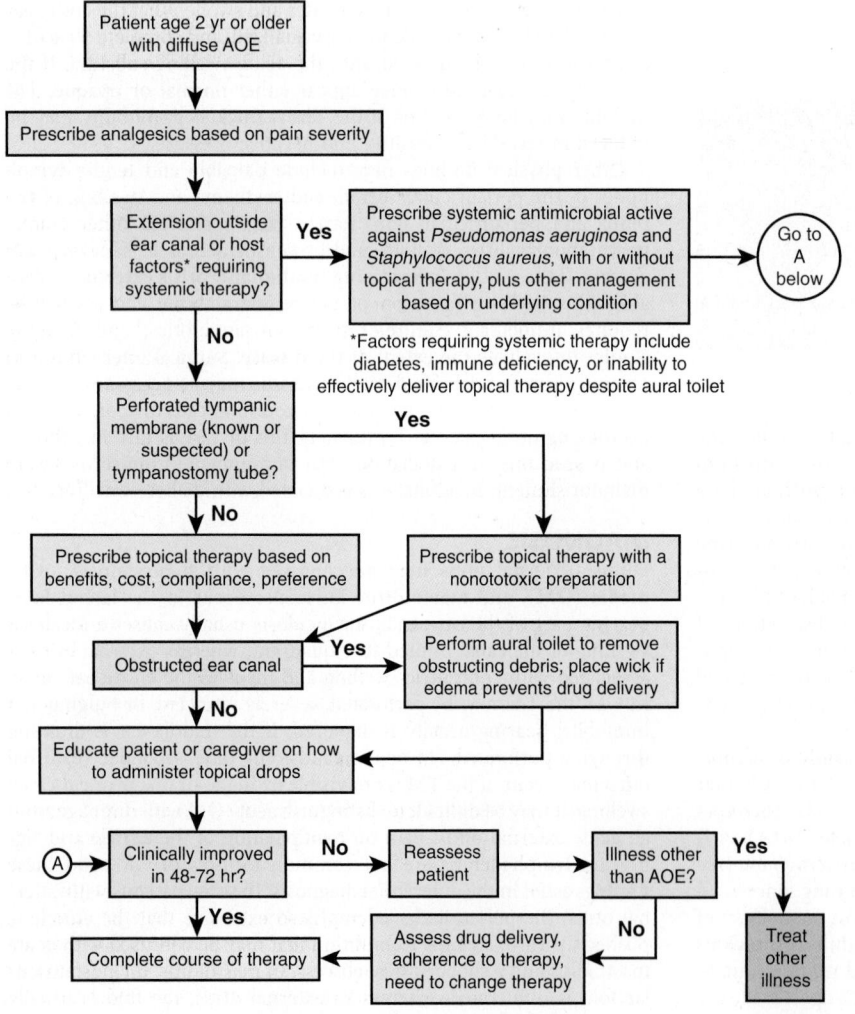

Figure 639-1 Flow chart for managing acute otitis externa (AOE). *(From Rosenfeld RM, Brown L, Cannon CR, et al: Clinical practice guideline: acute otitis externa, Otolaryngol Head Neck Surg 134:S4–S23, 2006. Copyright 2006 American Academy of Otolaryngology-Head and Neck Surgery Foundation, Inc.)*

Acute Cellulitis

Acute cellulitis of the auricle and external auditory canal usually is caused by group A streptococcus and occasionally by *S. aureus*. The skin is red, hot, and indurated, without a sharply defined border. Fever may be present with little or no exudate in the canal. Parenteral administration of penicillin G or a penicillinase-resistant penicillin is the therapy of choice.

Perichondritis and Chondritis

Perichondritis is an infection involving the skin and perichondrium of the auricular cartilage; extension of infection to the cartilage is termed **chondritis.** The ear canal, especially the lateral aspect, also may be involved. Early perichondritis may be difficult to differentiate from cellulitis because both are characterized by skin that is red, edematous, and tender. The main cause of perichondritis/chondritis and cellulitis is trauma (accidental or iatrogenic, laceration or contusion), including ear piercing, especially when done through the cartilage. The most commonly isolated organism in perichondritis and chondritis is *P. aeruginosa,* although other Gram-negative and, occasionally, Gram-positive organisms may be found. Treatment involves systemic, often parenteral, antibiotics; surgery to drain an abscess or remove nonviable skin or cartilage may also be needed. Removal of all ear jewelry is mandatory in the presence of infection.

Dermatoses

Various dermatoses (seborrheic, contact, infectious eczematoid, or neurodermatoid) are common causes of inflammation of the external canal; scratching and the introduction of infecting organisms cause acute external otitis in these conditions.

Seborrheic dermatitis is characterized by greasy scales that flake and crumble as they are detached from the epidermis; associated changes in the scalp, forehead, cheeks, brow, postauricular areas, and concha are usual.

Contact dermatitis of the auricle or canal may be caused by earrings or by topical otic medications such as neomycin, which may produce erythema, vesiculation, edema, and weeping. Poison ivy, oak, and sumac also may produce contact dermatitis. Hair care products have been implicated in sensitive individuals.

Infectious eczematoid dermatitis is caused by a purulent infection of the external canal, middle ear, or mastoid; the purulent drainage infects the skin of the canal or auricle, or both. The lesion is weeping, erythematous, or crusted.

Atopic dermatitis occurs in children with a familial or personal history of allergy; the auricle, particularly the postauricular fold, becomes thickened, scaly, and excoriated.

Neurodermatitis is recognized by intense itching and erythematous, thickened epidermis localized to the concha and orifice of the meatus.

Treatment of these dermatoses depends on the type but should include application of an appropriate topical medication, elimination of the source of infection or contact when identified, and management of any underlying dermatologic problem. In addition to topical antibiotics (or antifungals), topical steroids are helpful if contact dermatitis, atopic dermatitis, or eczematoid dermatitis is suspected.

Herpes Simplex Virus
See Chapter 252.

Herpes simplex virus may appear as vesicles on the auricle and lips. The lesions eventually become encrusted and dry and may be confused with impetigo. Topical application of a 10% solution of carbamide peroxide in anhydrous glycerol is symptomatically helpful. The **Ramsay Hunt syndrome** (herpes zoster oticus with facial paralysis) may present with herpes vesicles in the ear canal and on the pinna and with facial paralysis and pain. Other cranial nerves may be affected as well, especially the 8th nerve. The current recommended treatment of herpes zoster oticus includes systemic antiviral agents, such as acyclovir, and corticosteroids. As many as 50% of patients with Ramsay Hunt syndrome do not completely recover their facial nerve function.

Bullous Myringitis

Commonly associated with an acute upper respiratory tract infection, bullous myringitis presents as an ear infection with more severe pain than usual. On examination, hemorrhagic or serous blisters (bullae) may be seen on the TM. The disease sometimes is difficult to differentiate from acute OM, because a large bulla may be confused with a bulging TM. The organisms involved are the same as those that cause acute OM, including both bacteria and viruses. Treatment consists of empiric antibiotic therapy and pain medications. In addition to ibuprofen or codeine for severe pain, a topical anesthetic eardrop may also provide some relief. Incision of the bullae, although not necessary, promptly relieves the pain.

Exostoses and Osteomas

Exostoses represent benign hyperplasia of the perichondrium and underlying bone. Those involving the auditory canal tend to be found in people who swim often in cold water. Exostoses are broad based, often multiple, and bilateral. Osteomas are benign bony growths in the ear canal of uncertain cause (see Chapter 501.2). They usually are solitary and attached by a narrow pedicle to the tympanosquamous or tympanomastoid suture line. Both are more common in males; exostoses are more common than osteomas. Surgical treatment is recommended when large masses cause cerumen impaction, ear canal obstruction, or hearing loss.

Bibliography is available at Expert Consult.

Chapter **640**
Otitis Media
Joseph E. Kerschner and Diego Preciado

The term **otitis media (OM)** has 2 main categories: acute infection, which is termed suppurative or **acute otitis media (AOM),** and inflammation accompanied by **middle-ear effusion (MEE),** termed nonsuppurative or **secretory OM,** or **otitis media with effusion (OME).** These 2 main types of OM are interrelated: acute infection usually is succeeded by residual inflammation and effusion that, in turn, predispose children to recurrent infection. MEE is a feature of both AOM and of OME and is an expression of the underlying middle-ear mucosal inflammation. MEE results in the conductive hearing loss (CHL) associated with OM, ranging from none to as much as 50 dB of hearing loss.

The peak incidence and prevalence of OM is during the 1st 2 yr of life. More than 80% of children will have experienced at least 1 episode of OM by the age of 3 yr. OM is a leading reason for physician visits and for use of antibiotics and figures importantly in the differential diagnosis of fever. OM often serves as the sole or the main basis for undertaking the most frequently performed operations in infants and young children: myringotomy with insertion of tympanostomy tubes and adenoidectomy. OM is also the most common cause of hearing loss in children. OM has a propensity to become chronic and recur. The earlier in life a child experiences the first episode, the greater the degree of subsequent difficulty the child is likely to experience in terms of frequency of recurrence, severity, and persistence of middle-ear effusion.

Accurate diagnosis of AOM in infants and young children may be difficult (Table 640-1). Symptoms may not be apparent, especially in early infancy and in chronic stages of the disease. Accurate visualization of the tympanic membrane and middle-ear space may be difficult because of anatomy, patient cooperation, or blockage by cerumen, removal of which may be arduous and time consuming. Abnormalities of the eardrum may be subtle and difficult to appreciate. In the face of these difficulties, both underdiagnosis and overdiagnosis occur.

Table 640-1	Treatments for Otalgia in Acute Otitis Media
TREATMENT MODALITY	**COMMENTS**
Acetaminophen, ibuprofen	Effective analgesia for mild to moderate pain. Readily available. Mainstay of pain management for AOM
Home remedies (no controlled studies that directly address effectiveness) Distraction External application of heat or cold Oil drops in external auditory canal	May have limited effectiveness
Benzocaine, procaine, lidocaine (topical)	Additional, but brief, benefit over acetaminophen in patients older than 5 yr
Naturopathic agents	Comparable to amethocaine/phenazone drops in patients older than 6 yr
Homeopathic agents	No controlled studies that directly address pain
Narcotic analgesia with codeine or analogs	Effective for moderate or severe pain. Requires prescription; risk of respiratory depression, altered mental status, gastrointestinal tract upset, and constipation
Tympanostomy/myringotomy	Requires skill and entails potential risk

From Lieberthal AS, Carroll AE, Chonmaitree T, et al. The diagnosis and management of acute otitis media. Pediatrics 131:e964-e999, 2013, Table 3.

EPIDEMIOLOGY

Several factors have been demonstrated to affect the occurrence of OM, including age, gender, race, genetic background, socioeconomic status, breast milk feeding, degree of exposure to tobacco smoke, degree of exposure to other children, presence or absence of respiratory allergy, season of the yr, and vaccination status. Children with certain types of congenital craniofacial anomalies are particularly prone to OM.

Age

The age of onset of OM is an important predictor of the development of recurrent and chronic OM, with earlier age of onset having an increased risk for exhibiting these difficulties later in life. The development of at least 1 episode of OM has been reported as 63-85% by 12 mo and 66-99% by 24 mo of age. The percentage of days with MEE has been reported as 5-27% during the 1st yr of life and 6-18% during the 2nd yr of life. Across groups, rates were highest at 6-20 mo of age. After the age of 2 yr, the incidence and prevalence of OM decline progressively, although the disease remains relatively common into the early school-age years. The most likely reasons for the higher rates in infants and younger children include less-well–developed immunologic defenses and less-favorable eustachian tubal factors involving both the structure and function of the tube.

Gender

Epidemiologic data suggest an incidence of OM greater in boys than in girls, although some studies have found no gender-related differences in the occurrence of OM.

Race

OM is especially prevalent and severe among Native American, Inuit, and indigenous Australian children. Studies comparing the occurrence of OM in white children and black children have given conflicting results.

Genetic Background

That middle-ear disease tends to run in families is a commonplace observation, suggesting that OM has a heritable component. The degree of concordance for the occurrence of OM is much greater among monozygotic than among dizygotic twins.

Socioeconomic Status

Poverty has long been considered an important contributing factor to both the development and the severity of OM. Elements contributing to this relationship include crowding, limited hygienic facilities, suboptimal nutritional status, limited access to medical care, and limited resources for complying with prescribed medical regimens.

Breast Milk Compared to Formula Feeding

Most studies have found a protective effect of breast milk feeding against OM. This protective effect may be greater in socioeconomically disadvantaged than in more advantaged children. The protective effect is attributable to the milk itself rather than to the mechanics of breastfeeding.

Exposure to Tobacco Smoke

Exposure to tobacco smoke is thought to be an important preventable risk factor in the development of OM. Studies that have used objective measures to determine infant exposure to second-hand tobacco smoke, such as cotinine levels, have more consistently identified a significant linkage between tobacco smoke and OM.

Exposure to Other Children

Many studies have established that a strong, positive relationship exists between the occurrence of OM and the extent of repeated exposure to other children—measured mainly by the number of other children involved—whether at home or in out-of-home group daycare. Together, but independently, family socioeconomic status and the extent of exposure to other children appear to constitute 2 of the most important identifiable risk factors for developing OM.

Season

In keeping with the pattern of occurrence of upper respiratory tract infections in general, highest rates of occurrence of OM are observed during cold weather months and lowest rates during warm weather months. In OM, it is likely that these findings strongly depend on the significant association of OM with viral respiratory illnesses.

Congenital Anomalies

OM is universal among infants with unrepaired palatal clefts, and is also highly prevalent among children with submucous cleft palate, other craniofacial anomalies, and Down syndrome (see Chapter 81.2). The common feature in these congenital anomalies is a deficiency in the functioning of the eustachian tubes, which predisposes these children to middle-ear disease.

Vaccination Status

See "Immunoprophylaxis" below.

Other Factors

Pacifier use is linked with an increased incidence of OM and recurrence of OM, although the effect is small. Neither maternal age nor birthweight nor season of birth appears to influence the occurrence of OM once other demographic factors are taken into account. Very limited data are available regarding the association of OM with bottle feeding in the recumbent position.

ETIOLOGY
Acute Otitis Media

Pathogenic bacteria can be isolated by standard culture techniques from middle-ear fluid in a majority of well-documented AOM cases. Three pathogens predominate in AOM: *Streptococcus pneumoniae* (see Chapter 182), nontypeable *Haemophilus influenzae* (see Chapter 194), and *Moraxella catarrhalis* (see Chapter 196). The overall incidence of these organisms has changed with the use of the conjugate pneumococcal vaccine. In countries where this vaccine is employed, nontypeable *H. influenzae* initially overtook *S. pneumoniae* as the most common pathogen, being found in 40-50% of cases. However, over time, *S. pneumoniae* serotypes not covered in the conjugate vaccine have emerged, with *S. pneumoniae* again overtaking nontypeable *H. influenzae* as the most common pathogen in many studies. *M. catarrhalis* represents the majority of the remaining cases. Other pathogens include group A streptococcus (see Chapter 183), *Staphylococcus aureus* (see Chapter 181), and Gram-negative organisms. *S. aureus* and Gram-negative organisms are found most commonly in neonates and very young infants who are hospitalized; in outpatient settings, the distribution of pathogens in these young infants is similar to that in older infants. Molecular techniques to identify nonculturable bacterial pathogens have suggested the importance of other bacterial species such as *Alloiococcus otitidis*.

Evidence of respiratory viruses also may be found in middle-ear exudates of children with AOM, either alone or, more commonly, in association with pathogenic bacteria. Of these viruses, rhinovirus and respiratory syncytial virus are found most often. AOM is a known complication of bronchiolitis; middle-ear aspirates in children with bronchiolitis regularly contain bacterial pathogens, suggesting that respiratory syncytial virus is rarely, if ever, the sole cause of their AOM. Using more precise measures of viable bacteria than standard culture techniques, such as polymerase chain reaction assays, a much higher rate of bacterial pathogens can be demonstrated. It remains uncertain whether viruses alone can cause AOM, or whether their role is limited to setting the stage for bacterial invasion, and perhaps also to amplifying the inflammatory process and interfering with resolution of the bacterial infection. Viral pathogens have a negative impact on eustachian tube function, can impair local immune function, and increase bacterial adherence, and can change the pharmacokinetic dynamics, reducing the efficacy of antimicrobial medications.

Otitis Media with Effusion

Using standard culture techniques, the pathogens typically found in AOM are recoverable in only 30% of children with OME. However, in studies of children with OME using polymerase chain reaction assays, middle-ear effusions have been found to contain evidence of bacterial DNA and viral RNA in much larger proportions of these children. These studies suggest that patients do not have sterile effusions as previously thought. Biofilms of pathogenic bacteria have been demonstrated to be present on the middle-ear mucosa and adenoid pad in a majority of children with chronic OM. Biofilms consist of aggregated and adherent bacteria, embedded in an extracellular matrix, allowing for protection against antimicrobials, and their presence may contribute to the persistence of pathogens and the recalcitrance of chronic OM to antibiotic treatment (see Chapter 171).

PATHOGENESIS

A multifactorial disease process, risk profile, and host–pathogen interactions have become recognized as playing important roles in the pathogenesis of OM. Such events as alterations in mucociliary clearance through repeated viral exposure experienced in daycare settings or through exposure to tobacco smoke may tip the balance of pathogenesis in less-virulent OM pathogens in their favor, especially in children with a unique host predisposition.

Anatomic Factors

Patients with significant craniofacial abnormalities affecting the eustachian tube function have an increased incidence of OM. During the pathogenesis of OM the eustachian tube demonstrates decreased effectiveness in ventilating the middle-ear space.

Under usual circumstances the eustachian tube is passively closed and is opened by contraction of the tensor veli palatini muscle. In relation to the middle ear, the tube has 3 main functions: ventilation, protection, and clearance. The middle-ear mucosa depends on a continuing supply of air from the nasopharynx delivered by way of the eustachian tube. Interruption of this ventilatory process by tubal obstruction initiates an inflammatory response that includes secretory metaplasia, compromise of the mucociliary transport system, and effusion of liquid into the tympanic cavity. Measurements of eustachian tube function have demonstrated that the tubal function is suboptimal during the events of OM with increased opening pressures.

Eustachian tube obstruction may result from extraluminal blockage via hypertrophied nasopharyngeal adenoid tissue or tumor, or may result from intraluminal obstruction via inflammatory edema of the tubal mucosa, most commonly as a consequence of a viral upper respiratory tract infection. Progressive reduction in tubal wall compliance with increasing age may explain the progressive decline in the occurrence of OM as children grow older. The protection and clearance functions of the eustachian tube may also be involved in the pathogenesis of OM. Thus, if the eustachian tube is patulous or excessively compliant, it may fail to protect the middle ear from reflux of infective nasopharyngeal secretions, whereas impairment of the mucociliary clearance function of the tube might contribute to both the establishment and persistence of infection. The shorter and more horizontal orientation of the tube in infants and young children may increase the likelihood of reflux from the nasopharynx and impair passive gravitational drainage through the eustachian tube.

In special patient populations with craniofacial abnormalities there exists an increased incidence of OM that has been associated with the abnormal eustachian tube function. In children with cleft palate, where OM is a universal finding, a main factor underlying the chronic middle-ear inflammation appears to be impairment of the opening mechanism of the eustachian tube. Possible factors include muscular changes, tubal compliance factors, and defective velopharyngeal valving, which may result in disturbed aerodynamic and hydrodynamic relationships in the nasopharynx and proximal portions of the eustachian tubes. In children with other craniofacial anomalies and with Down syndrome, the high prevalence of OM has also been attributed to structural and/or functional eustachian tubal abnormalities.

Host Factors

The effectiveness of a child's immune system in response to the bacterial and viral insults of the upper airway and middle ear during early childhood probably is the most important factor in determining which children are otitis prone. The maturation of this immune system during early childhood is most likely the primary event leading to the decrease in incidence of OM as children move through childhood. Immunoglobulin (Ig) A deficiency is found in some children with recurrent AOM, but the significance is questionable, inasmuch as IgA deficiency is also found not infrequently in children without recurrent AOM. Selective IgG subclass deficiencies (despite normal total serum IgG) may be found in children with recurrent AOM in association with recurrent sinopulmonary infection, and these deficiencies probably underlie the susceptibility to infection. Children with HIV infection have recurrent and difficult to treat episodes of AOM in the 1st and 2nd yr of life. Children with recurrent OM that is not associated with recurrent infection at other sites rarely have a readily identifiable immunologic deficiency. Evidence that subtle immune deficits play a role in the pathogenesis of recurrent AOM is provided by studies involving antibody responses to various types of infection and immunization; by the observation that breast milk feeding, as opposed to formula feeding, confers some protection against the occurrence of OM in infants with cleft palate; and by studies in which young children with recurrent AOM achieved a measure of protection from intramuscularly administered bacterial polysaccharide immune globulin or intravenously administered polyclonal immunoglobulin. This evidence, along with the documented decrease in incidence of upper respiratory tract infections and OM as children's immune systems develop and mature, is indicative of the importance of a child's innate immune system in the pathogenesis of OM (see Chapter 124).

Viral Pathogens

Although OM may develop and certainly may persist in the absence of apparent respiratory tract infection, many, if not most, episodes are initiated by viral or bacterial upper respiratory tract infection. In children in group daycare, AOM was observed in approximately 30-40% of children with respiratory illness caused by respiratory syncytial virus (see Chapter 260), influenzaviruses (see Chapter 258), or adenoviruses (see Chapter 262), and in approximately 10-15% of children with respiratory illness caused by parainfluenza viruses (see Chapter 259), rhinoviruses (see Chapter 263), or enteroviruses (see Chapter 250). Viral infection of the upper respiratory tract results in release of cytokines and inflammatory mediators, some of which may cause eustachian tube dysfunction.

Respiratory viruses also may enhance nasopharyngeal bacterial colonization and adherence and impair host immune defenses against bacterial infection.

Allergy

Evidence that respiratory allergy is a primary etiologic agent in OM is not convincing; however, in children with both conditions it is possible that the otitis is aggravated by the allergy.

CLINICAL MANIFESTATIONS

Symptoms of AOM are variable, especially in infants and young children. In young children, evidence of ear pain may be manifested by irritability or a change in sleeping or eating habits and occasionally, holding or tugging at the ear. *Pulling at the ear alone has a low sensitivity and specificity.* Fever may also be present and may occasionally be the only sign. Rupture of the tympanic membrane with purulent otorrhea is uncommon. Systemic symptoms and symptoms associated with upper respiratory tract infections also occur; occasionally there may be no symptoms, the disease having been discovered at a routine health examination. OME often is not accompanied by overt complaints of the child but can be accompanied by hearing loss. This hearing loss may manifest as changes in speech patterns but often goes undetected if unilateral or mild in nature, especially in younger children. Balance

difficulties or disequilibrium can also be associated with OME and older children may complain of mild discomfort or a sense of fullness in the ear (see Chapter 636).

EXAMINATION OF THE TYMPANIC MEMBRANE
Otoscopy

Two types of otoscope heads are available: **surgical** or **operating**, and **diagnostic** or **pneumatic**. The surgical head embodies a lens that can swivel over a wide arc and an unenclosed light source, thus providing ready access of the examiner's instruments to the external auditory canal and tympanic membrane. Use of the surgical head is optimal for removing cerumen or debris from the canal under direct observation, and is necessary for satisfactorily performing tympanocentesis or myringotomy. The diagnostic head incorporates a larger lens, an enclosed light source, and a nipple for the attachment of a rubber bulb and tubing. When an attached speculum is fitted snugly into the external auditory canal, an airtight chamber is created comprising the vault of the otoscope head, the bulb and tubing, the speculum, and the proximal portion of the external canal. Although examination of the ear in young children is a relatively invasive procedure that is often met with lack of cooperation by the patient, this task can be enhanced if done with as little pain as possible. The outer portion of the ear canal contains hair-bearing skin and subcutaneous fat and cartilage that allow a speculum to be placed with relatively little discomfort. Closer to the tympanic membrane the ear canal is made of bone and is lined only with skin and no adnexal structures or subcutaneous fat; a speculum pushed too far forward and placed in this area often causes skin abrasion and pain. Using a rubber-tipped speculum or adding a small sleeve of rubber tubing to the tip of the plastic speculum may serve to minimize patient discomfort and enhance the ability to achieve a proper fit and an airtight seal, facilitating pneumatic otoscopy.

Learning to perform pneumatic otoscopy is a critical skill in being able to assess a child's ear and in making an accurate diagnosis of AOM. By observing as the bulb is alternately squeezed gently and released, the degree of tympanic membrane mobility in response to both positive and negative pressure can be estimated, providing a critical assessment of middle-ear fluid, which is a hallmark sign of both AOM and OME (Fig. 640-1). With both types of otoscope heads, bright illumination is also critical for adequate visualization of the tympanic membrane.

Clearing the External Auditory Canal

Many children's ears are "self-cleaning" because of squamous migration of ear canal skin. Parental cleaning of cerumen with cotton swabs often complicates cerumen impaction by pushing cerumen deeper into the canal compacting it. If the tympanic membrane is obscured by cerumen, the cerumen should be removed. This can be accomplished through

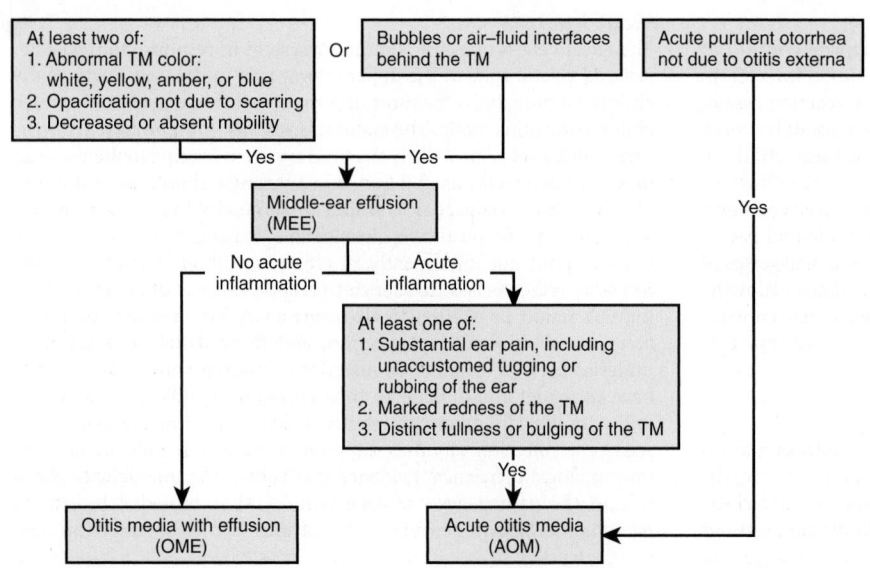

Figure 640-1 Algorithm for distinguishing between acute otitis media and otitis media with effusion. TM, tympanic membrane.

direct visualization using a headlight or through the surgical head of the otoscope by using an ear curette or gentle suction with a No. 5 or 7 French ear suction tube. During this procedure it may be most advantageous to restrain the infant or young child in the prone position, turning the child's head to the left or right as each ear is cleared. In children old enough to cooperate, usually beginning at about 5 yr of age, clearing of the external canal may be achieved more easily and less traumatically by lavage than by mechanical removal, provided one can be certain that a tympanic membrane perforation is not present.

Tympanic Membrane Findings

Important characteristics of the tympanic membrane (TM) consist of contour, color, translucence, structural changes if any, and mobility. The TM is anatomically divided into the pars tensa and pars flaccida. The pars tensa comprises the lower two thirds of the drum inferior to the lateral process of the malleus. Its contour is normally **slightly concave;** abnormalities consist of fullness or bulging or, conversely, extreme retraction. The normal color of the pars tensa is **pearly gray**, with the pars flaccida being slightly more vascular in nature. Erythema may be a sign of inflammation or infection, but unless intense, erythema alone may result from crying or vascular flushing. Abnormal whiteness of the membrane may result from either scarring or the presence of effusion in the middle-ear cavity; this effusion also may impart an amber, pale yellow, or, rarely, bluish color. Rarely a persistent focal white area may be indicative of a congenital cholesteatoma in the middle-ear space. Normally, the membrane is translucent, although some degree of opacity may be normal in the 1st few mo of life; later, opacification denotes either scarring or, more commonly, underlying effusion. Structural changes include scars, perforations, and retraction pockets. Retractions or perforations, especially in the posterior-superior quadrant, or pars flaccida, of the TM may be a sign of cholesteatoma formation. Of all the visible characteristics of the TM, mobility is the most sensitive and specific in determining the presence or absence of MEE. Mobility is generally not an all-or-none phenomenon. A total absence of mobility does exist with a TM perforation that can develop following a substantial increase in middle-ear pressure associated with effusion. When a perforation is not present, substantial impairment of mobility is the more common finding with MEE. Bulging of the TM is the most specific finding of AOM (97%) but has lower specificity (51%) (Fig. 640-2).

Diagnosis

The 2013 guidelines from the American Academy of Pediatrics for diagnosis of AOM are more restrictive than were the earlier (2004) guidelines. The 2004 guidelines employed a 3-part definition: (1) acute onset of symptoms; (2) presence of an MEE; and (3) signs of acute middle-ear inflammation. This definition was thought by the 2013 American Academy of Pediatrics to lack sufficient precision and thereby liable to include cases of OME and/or enable the diagnosis of AOM to be made without visualizing the TM.

A diagnosis of AOM according to the 2013 guideline should be made in children who present with:
- moderate to severe bulging of the TM or new-onset otorrhea not caused by otitis externa
- mild bulging of the TM and recent (<48 hr) onset of ear pain or intense TM erythema

A **diagnosis of AOM should *not*** be made in children without MEE.

AOM and OME may evolve into the other without any clearly differentiating physical findings; any schema for distinguishing between them is to some extent arbitrary. In an era of increasing bacterial resistance, distinguishing between AOM and OME is important in determining treatment, because OME in the absence of acute infection does not require antimicrobial therapy. Purulent otorrhea of recent onset is indicative of AOM; thus, difficulty in distinguishing clinically between AOM and OME is limited to circumstances in which purulent otorrhea is not present. Both AOM without otorrhea and OME are accompanied by physical signs of MEE, namely, the presence of at least 2 of 3 TM abnormalities: white, yellow, amber, or (rarely) blue discoloration; opacification other than that caused by scarring; and decreased or absent mobility. Alternatively in OME, either air–fluid levels or air

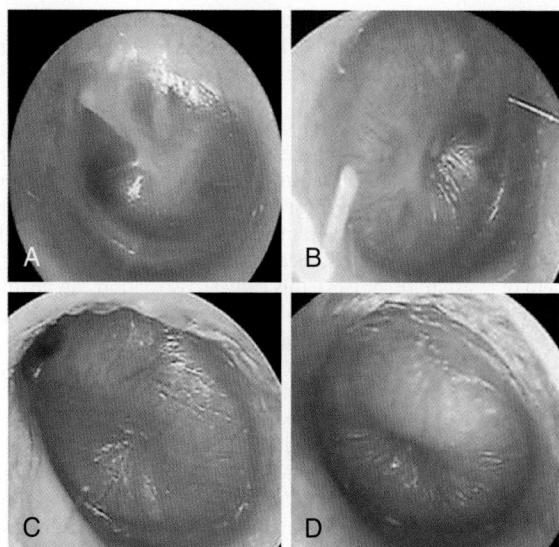

Figure 640-2 Examples of normal tympanic membrane **(A)** and of mild bulging **(B)**, moderate bulging **(C)**, and severe bulging **(D)** of the tympanic membrane from middle-ear effusion. *(Courtesy of Alejandro Hoberman, MD.)*

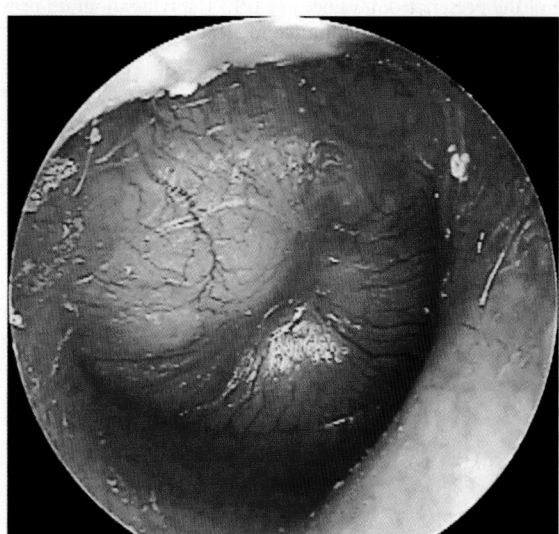

Figure 640-3 Tympanic membrane in acute otitis media.

bubbles outlined by small amounts of fluid may be visible behind the TM, a condition often indicative of impending resolution (Fig. 640-3).

To support a diagnosis of AOM instead of OME in a child with MEE, distinct fullness or bulging of the TM may be present, with or without accompanying erythema, or, at a minimum, MEE should be accompanied by ear pain that appears clinically important. Unless intense, erythema alone is insufficient because erythema, without other abnormalities, may result from crying or vascular flushing. In AOM, the malleus may be obscured and the TM may resemble a bagel without a hole but with a central depression (see Fig. 640-3). Rarely, the TM may be obscured by surface bullae or may have a cobblestone appearance. Bullous myringitis is a physical manifestation of AOM and not an etiologically discrete entity. Within days after onset, fullness of the membrane may diminish, even though infection may still be present.

In OME, bulging of the TM is absent or slight or the membrane may be retracted (Fig. 640-4); erythema also is absent or slight, but may increase with crying or with superficial trauma to the external auditory canal incurred in clearing the canal of cerumen.

Both before and after episodes of OM and also in the absence of OM, the TM may be retracted as a consequence of negative middle-ear air pressure. The presumed cause is diffusion of air from the middle-ear cavity more rapidly than it is replaced via the eustachian tube. Mild retraction is generally self-limited, although in some children it is accompanied by mild conductive hearing loss. More extreme retraction is of concern, as discussed later in the section on sequelae of OM.

Conjunctivitis-Associated Otitis Media

Simultaneous appearance of purulent and erythematous conjunctivitis with an ipsilateral OM is a well-recognized presentation, caused by nontypeable *H. influenzae* in most children.

The disease often is present in multiple family members and affects young children and infants. Topical ocular antibiotics are ineffective. In an era of resistant organisms, this clinical association can be important in antibiotic selection, with oral antibiotics (see later) effective against resistant forms of nontypeable *H. influenzae.*

Asymptomatic Purulent Otitis Media

Rarely, a child will present during a routine exam without fever, irritability, or other overt signs of infection, but on exam, the patient will demonstrate an obvious purulent MEE and bulging TM. Although an uncommon presentation of "acute" OM, the bulging nature of the TM and the obvious purulence of the effusion do warrant antimicrobial therapy.

Tympanometry

Tympanometry, or **acoustic immittance testing,** is a simple, rapid, atraumatic test that, when performed correctly, offers objective evidence of the presence or absence of MEE. The tympanogram provides information about **TM compliance** in electroacoustic terms that can

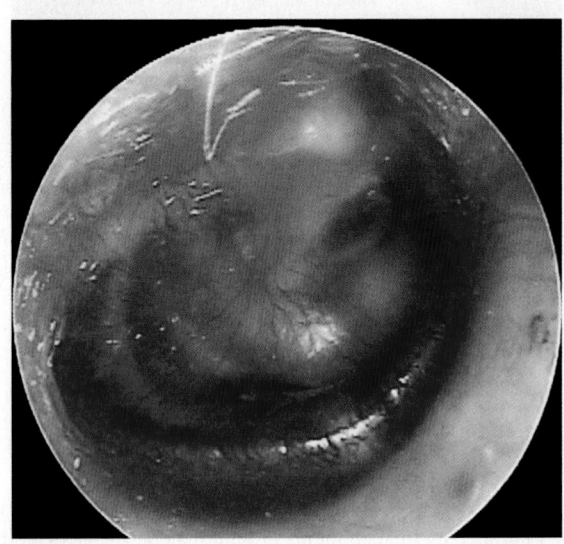

Figure 640-4 Tympanic membrane in otitis media with effusion.

be thought of as roughly equivalent to TM mobility as perceived visually during pneumatic otoscopy. The absorption of sound by the TM varies inversely with its stiffness. The stiffness of the membrane is least, and accordingly its compliance is greatest, when the air pressures impinging on each of its surfaces—middle-ear air pressure and external canal air pressure—are equal. In simple terms, anything tending to stiffen the TM, such as TM scarring or middle-ear fluid, reduces the TM compliance, which is recorded as a flattening of the curve of the tympanogram. An ear filled with middle-ear fluid generally has a very noncompliant TM and, therefore, a flattened tympanogram tracing.

Tympanograms may be grouped into 1 of 3 categories (Fig. 640-5). Tracings characterized by a relatively steep gradient, sharp-angled peak, and middle-ear air pressure (location of the peak in terms of air pressure) that approximates atmospheric pressure (Fig. 640-5A) (type A curve) are assumed to indicate normal middle-ear status. Tracings characterized by a shallow peak or no peak are often termed "flat" or type B (Fig. 640-5B), and usually are assumed to indicate the presence of a middle-ear abnormality that is causing decreased TM compliance. The most common such abnormality in infants and children is MEE. Tracings characterized by intermediate findings—somewhat shallow peak, often in association with a gradual gradient (obtuse-angled peak) or negative middle-ear air pressure peak (often termed type "C"), or combinations of these features (Fig. 640-5C)—may or may not be associated with MEE, and must be considered nondiagnostic or equivocal with respect to OM. However, type C tympanograms do suggest eustachian tube dysfunction and some ongoing pathology in the middle ear and warrant follow-up.

When reading a tympanogram it is important to look at the volume measurement. The type B tympanometric response has to be analyzed within the context of the recorded volume. A flat, "low"-volume (≤1 mL) tracing typically reflects the volume of the ear canal only, representing MEE, which impedes the movement of an intact ear drum. A flat, high-volume (>1 mL) tracing typically reflects the volume of the ear canal and middle-ear space, representing a perforation (or patent tympanostomy tube) in the TM. In a child with a tympanostomy tube present, a flat tympanogram with a volume <1 mL would suggest a plugged or nonfunctioning tube and middle-ear fluid, whereas a flat tympanogram with a volume >1 mL would suggest a patent tympanostomy tube.

Although tympanometry is quite sensitive in detecting MEE, it can be limited by patient cooperation, the skill of the individual administering the test, and the age of the child, with less-reliable results in very young children. Use of tympanometry may be helpful in office screening, may supplement the examination of difficult to examine patients, and may help identify patients who require further attention because their tympanograms are abnormal. Tympanometry also may be used to help confirm, refine, or clarify questionable otoscopic findings; to objectify the follow-up evaluation of patients with known middle-ear disease; and to validate otoscopic diagnoses of MEE. Even

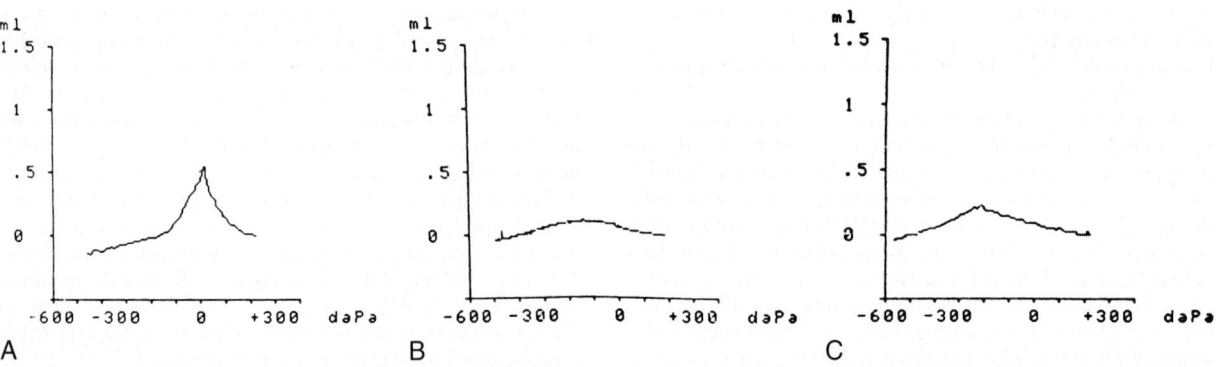

Figure 640-5 Tympanograms obtained with a Grason-Stadler GSI 33 Middle Ear Analyzer, exhibiting **(A)** high admittance, steep gradient (i.e., sharp-angled peak), and middle-ear air pressure approximating atmospheric pressure (0 decaPascals [daPa]); **(B)** low admittance and indeterminate middle-ear air pressure; and **(C)** somewhat low admittance, gradual gradient, and markedly negative middle-ear air pressure.

though tympanometry can predict the probability of MEE, it cannot distinguish the effusion of OME from that of AOM.

PREVENTION

General measures to prevent OM that have been supported by a number of investigations include avoiding exposure to individuals with respiratory infection; appropriate vaccination strategies against pneumococci and influenzae; avoiding environmental tobacco smoke; and breast milk feeding.

IMMUNOPROPHYLAXIS

Heptavalent pneumococcal conjugate vaccine (PCV7) reduced the overall number of episodes of AOM by only 6-8% but with a 57% reduction in serotype-specific episodes. Reductions of 9-23% are seen in children with histories of frequent episodes, and a 20% reduction is seen in the number of children undergoing tympanostomy tube insertion. A 13-valent pneumococcal polysaccharide-protein conjugate vaccine (PCV13) was licensed by the FDA in 2010. PCV13 contains the 7 serotypes included in PCV7 (serotypes 4, 6B, 9V, 14, 18C, 19F, and 23F) and 6 additional serotypes (serotypes 1, 3, 5, 6A, 7F, and 19A). The effects of PCV13 on AOM incidence reduce pneumococcal nasopharyngeal carriage, including serotypes 19A, 7F, and 6C, in young children (younger than age 2 yr) with AOM. Given that 19A is a particularly invasive pneumococcal serotype, the effect of PCV13 on reducing complicated AOM will hopefully be of significance. Early data indicate a significant reduction in the number of invasive pneumococcal mastoiditis cases since the introduction of PCV13. With the widespread use of PCV13, continued surveillance will be necessary to detect other emerging serotypes, which are also demonstrating increasing resistance. Although the influenza vaccine also provides a measure of protection against OM, the relatively limited time during which individuals and even communities are exposed to influenzaviruses limits the vaccine's effectiveness in broadly reducing the incidence of OM. Limitation of OM disease is only a portion of the benefit realized from the vaccinations for pneumococci and influenza viruses. Support for these vaccination programs requires an understanding of the preventive benefit for OM in concert with the other benefits.

TREATMENT
Management of Acute Otitis Media

AOM can be very painful. Whether or not antibiotics are employed for treatment, pain should be assessed and if present, treated (see Table 640-1).

Individual episodes of AOM have traditionally been treated with antimicrobial drugs. Concern about increasing bacterial resistance has prompted some clinicians to recommend withholding antimicrobial treatment in some or most cases unless symptoms persist for 2 or 3 days, or worsen (Table 640-2). Three factors argue in favor of routinely prescribing antimicrobial therapy for children who have documented AOM using the diagnostic criteria outlined previously (see "Diagnosis" above). First, pathogenic bacteria cause a large majority of cases.

Second, symptomatic improvement and resolution of infection occur more promptly and more consistently with antimicrobial treatment than without, even though most untreated cases eventually resolve. Third, prompt and adequate antimicrobial treatment may prevent the development of suppurative complications. The sharp decline in such complications during the last half-century seems likely attributable, at least in part, to the widespread routine use of antimicrobials for AOM. In the Netherlands, where initial antibiotic treatment is routinely withheld from most children older than 6 mo of age, and where only approximately 30% of children with AOM receive antibiotics at all, the incidence of acute mastoiditis, although low (in children younger than age 14 yr, 3.8 per 100,000 person-years), appears slightly higher than rates in other countries with higher antibiotic prescription rates by about 1-2 episodes per 100,000 person-years. Groups in other countries where initial conservative management of AOM is the standard in children older than 6 mo, such as Denmark, report acute mastoiditis rates similar to those of the Netherlands (4.8 per 100,000 person-years).

Given that most episodes of OM will spontaneously resolve, consensus guidelines have been published by the American Academy of Pediatrics to assist clinicians who wish to consider a period of "watchful waiting" or observation prior to treating AOM with antibiotics (see Tables 640-2 and 640-3; Fig. 640-6). The most important aspect of these guidelines is that close follow-up of the patient must be ensured to assess for lack of spontaneous resolution or worsening of symptoms and that patients should be provided with adequate analgesic medications (acetaminophen, ibuprofen) during the period of observation. When pursuing the practice of watchful waiting in patients with AOM, the certainty of the diagnosis, the patient's age, and the severity of the disease should be considered. For younger patients, <2 yr of age, it is recommended to treat all confirmed diagnoses of AOM. In very young patients, <6 mo of age, even presumed episodes of AOM should be treated because of the increased potential of significant morbidity from infectious complications. In children between 6 and 24 mo of age who have a questionable diagnosis of OM but severe disease, defined as temperature of >39°C (102°F), significant otalgia, or toxic appearance, antibiotic therapy is also recommended. Children in this age group with a questionable diagnosis and nonsevere disease can be observed for a period of 2-3 days with close follow-up. In children older than 2 yr of age, observation might be considered in all episodes of nonsevere OM or episodes of questionable diagnosis, while antibiotic therapy is reserved for confirmed, severe episodes of AOM. Information from Finland suggests that the "watchful waiting" or delayed treatment approach does not worsen the recovery from AOM, or increase the complication rates. However, watchful waiting may be associated with transient worsening of the child's condition and longer overall duration of symptoms.

Accurate diagnosis is the most crucial aspect of the treatment of OM. In studies utilizing stringent criteria for diagnosis of AOM the benefit of antimicrobial treatment is enhanced. Additionally, subpopulations of patients clearly receive more benefit from oral antimicrobial

Table 640-2	Recommendations for Initial Management for Uncomplicated Acute Otitis Media*			
AGE	**OTORRHEA WITH AOM***	**UNILATERAL OR BILATERAL AOM* WITH SEVERE SYMPTOMS†**	**BILATERAL AOM* WITHOUT OTORRHEA**	**UNILATERAL AOM* WITHOUT OTORRHEA**
6 mo to 2 yr	Antibiotic therapy	Antibiotic therapy	Antibiotic therapy	Antibiotic therapy or additional observation
≥2 yr	Antibiotic therapy	Antibiotic therapy	Antibiotic therapy or additional observation	Antibiotic therapy or additional observation‡

*Applies only to children with well-documented AOM with high certainty of diagnosis.
†A toxic-appearing child, persistent otalgia more than 48 hr, temperature ≥39°C (102.2°F) in the past 48 hr, or if there is uncertain access to follow-up after the visit.
‡This plan of initial management provides an opportunity for shared decision making with the child's family for those categories appropriate for additional observation. If observation is offered, a mechanism must be in place to ensure follow-up and begin antibiotics if the child worsens or fails to improve within 48-72 hr of AOM onset.
NOTE: For infants younger than age 6 mo, a suspicion of AOM should result in antibiotic therapy.
From Lieberthal AS, Carroll AE, Chonmaitree T, et al. The diagnosis and management of acute otitis media. Pediatrics 131:e964–e999, 2013, Table 4.

| **Table 640-3** | Recommended Antibiotics for (Initial or Delayed) Treatment and for Patients Who Have Failed Initial Antibiotic Treatment |

Initial Immediate or Delayed Antibiotic Treatment		Antibiotic Treatment After 48-72 hr of Failure of Initial Antibiotic Treatment	
RECOMMENDED FIRST-LINE TREATMENT	**ALTERNATIVE TREATMENT (IF PENICILLIN ALLERGY)**	**RECOMMENDED FIRST-LINE TREATMENT**	**ALTERNATIVE TREATMENT**
Amoxicillin (80-90 mg/kg/day in 2 divided doses)	Cefdinir‡ (14 mg/kg/day in 1 or 2 doses)	Amoxicillin-clavulanate* (90 mg/kg/day of amoxicillin, with 6.4 mg/kg/day of clavulanate in 2 divided doses)	Ceftriaxone (50 mg IM or IV for 3 days, every other day until clinical improvement; max 3 doses) Clindamycin (30-40 mg/kg/day in 3 divided doses), with or without third-generation cephalosporin
or	Cefuroxime‡ (30 mg/kg/day in 2 divided doses)	or	Failure of second antibiotic
Amoxicillin-clavulanate* (90 mg/kg/day of amoxicillin, with 6.4 mg/kg/day of clavulanate [amoxicillin:clavulanate ratio, 14:1] in 2 divided doses) or Ceftriaxone (50 mg IM or IV for 3 days, every other day until improvement; max 3 doses)	Cefpodoxime‡ (10 mg/kg/day in 2 divided doses) Ceftriaxone‡ (50 mg IM or IV per day for 1 or 3 days)	Ceftriaxone (50 mg IM or IV for 3 days, every other day until clinical improvement or for a maximum of 3 doses)	Clindamycin (30-40 mg/kg/day in 3 divided doses) with or without third-generation cephalosporin Tympanocentesis† Consult specialist†

IM, intramuscular; IV, intravenous.

*May be considered in patients who have received amoxicillin in the previous 30 days or who have the otitis–conjunctivitis syndrome.

†Perform tympanocentesis/drainage if skilled in the procedure, or seek a consultation from an otolaryngologist for tympanocentesis/drainage. If the tympanocentesis reveals multidrug-resistant bacteria, seek an infectious disease specialist consultation.

‡Cefdinir, cefuroxime, cefpodoxime, and ceftriaxone are highly unlikely to be associated with cross reactivity with penicillin allergy on the basis of their distinct chemical structures.

From Lieberthal AS, Carroll AE, Chonmaitree T, et al. The diagnosis and management of acute otitis media. Pediatrics 131:e964–e999, 2013, Table 5.

therapy than others. *Younger children, children with otorrhea, and children with bilateral AOM have a significantly enhanced benefit from antimicrobial therapy in comparison to older children, children without otorrhea, or children with unilateral AOM.*

Bacterial Resistance

Persons at greatest risk of harboring resistant bacteria are those who are younger than 2 yr of age, who are in regular contact with large groups of other children, especially in daycare settings, or who recently have received antimicrobial treatment. Bacterial resistance is a particular problem in relation to OM. The development of resistant bacterial strains and their rapid spread have been fostered and facilitated by selective pressure resulting from extensive use of antimicrobial drugs, the most common target of which, in children, is OM. Many strains of each of the pathogenic bacteria that commonly cause AOM are resistant to commonly used antimicrobial drugs.

Although antimicrobial resistance rates vary between countries, in the United States approximately 40% of strains of nontypeable *H. influenzae* and almost all strains of *M. catarrhalis* are resistant to aminopenicillins (e.g., ampicillin and amoxicillin). In most cases, the resistance is attributable to production of β-lactamase and can be overcome by combining amoxicillin with a β-lactamase inhibitor (clavulanate) or by using a β-lactamase–stable antibiotic. Occasional strains of nontypeable *H. influenzae* that do not produce β-lactamase are resistant to aminopenicillins and other β-lactam antibiotics by virtue of alterations in their penicillin-binding proteins. It is worth noting that bacterial resistance rates in northern European countries where antibiotic usage is less are comparatively exceedingly lower (β-lactamase resistance in 6-10% of isolates) than in the United States.

In the United States, approximately 50% of strains of *S. pneumoniae* are penicillin-nonsusceptible, divided approximately equally between penicillin-intermediate and, even more difficult to treat, penicillin-resistant strains. A much higher incidence of resistance is seen in children attending daycare. Resistance by *S. pneumoniae* to the penicillins and other β-lactam antibiotics is mediated not by β-lactamase production but by alterations in penicillin-binding proteins. This mechanism of resistance can be overcome if higher concentrations of

β-lactam antibiotics at the site of infection can be achieved for a sufficient time interval. Many penicillin-resistant strains of *S. pneumoniae* are also resistant to other antimicrobial drugs, including sulfonamides, macrolides, and cephalosporins. In general, as penicillin resistance increases, so also does resistance to other antimicrobial classes. Resistance to macrolides, including azithromycin and clarithromycin, by *S. pneumoniae* has increased rapidly, rendering these antimicrobials far less effective in treating AOM. One mechanism of resistance to macrolides also results in resistance to clindamycin, which otherwise is generally effective against resistant strains of *S. pneumoniae*. Unlike resistance to β-lactam antibiotics, macrolide resistance cannot be overcome by increasing the dose.

First-Line Antimicrobial Treatment

Amoxicillin remains the drug of first choice for uncomplicated AOM under many circumstances because of its excellent record of safety, relative efficacy, palatability, and low cost. In particular, amoxicillin is the most efficacious of available oral antimicrobial drugs against both penicillin-susceptible and penicillin-nonsusceptible strains of *S. pneumoniae*. Increasing the dose from the traditional 40-45 mg/kg/24 hr to 80-90 mg/kg/24 hr will generally provide efficacy against penicillin-intermediate and some penicillin-resistant strains. This higher dose should be used particularly in children younger than 2 yr of age, in children who have recently received treatment with β-lactam drugs, and in children who are exposed to large numbers of other children because of their increased likelihood of an infection with a nonsusceptible strain of *S. pneumoniae*. A limitation of amoxicillin is that it may be inactivated by the β-lactamases produced by many strains of nontypeable *H. influenzae* and most strains of *M. catarrhalis*. Episodes of AOM caused by these pathogens often resolve spontaneously. Allergies to penicillin antibiotics should be categorized into type I hypersensitivity, consisting of urticaria or anaphylaxis, and those that fall short of type I reactions, such as rash formation. For children with a non–type I reaction in which cross reactivity with cephalosporins is less of a concern, first-line therapy with cefdinir would be an appropriate choice. In children with a type I reaction or known sensitivity to cephalosporin antibiotics there are far fewer choices. Resistance to

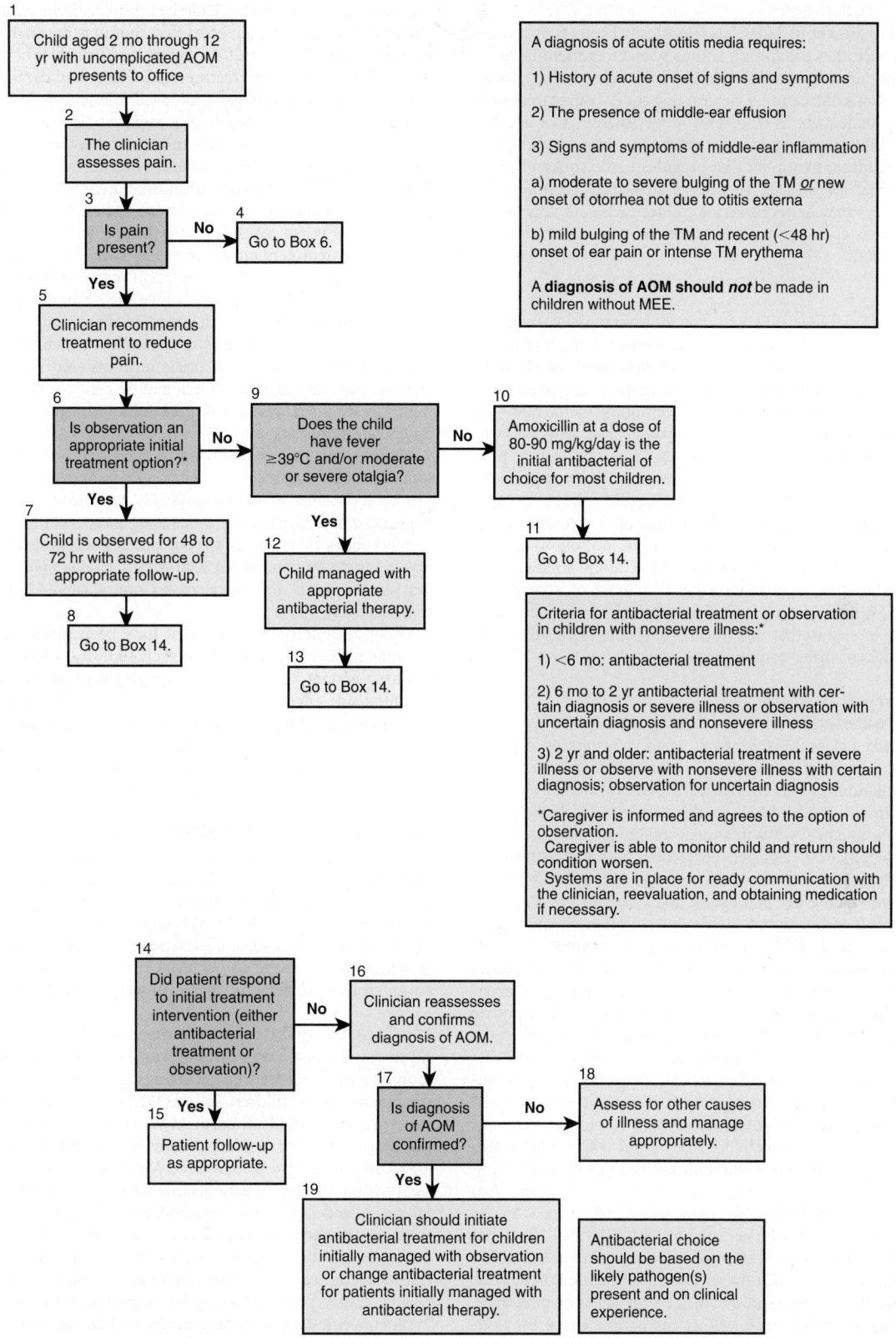

Figure 640-6 Management of acute otitis media. *(From Subcommittee on Management of Acute Otitis Media: Diagnosis and management of acute otitis media, Pediatrics 113:1451–1465, 2004.)*

trimethoprim-sulfamethoxazole by many strains of both nontypeable *H. influenzae* and *S. pneumoniae* and a reported high clinical failure rate in children with AOM treated initially with this antimicrobial argue against its use. Similarly, increasing rates of macrolide resistance argue against the efficacy of azithromycin. Although not approved by the FDA for use in children, many clinicians have employed quinolones in this patient population. Early alternative management in these allergic patients with tympanostomy tubes can allow for lessening of the severity of their disease and the utilization of topical antimicrobials.

Duration of Treatment

The duration of treatment of AOM has historically been set at 10 days and most efficacy studies examining antimicrobial treatment in AOM have utilized this duration as a benchmark. Studies comparing shorter with longer durations of treatment suggest that short-course treatment will often prove inadequate in children younger than 6 yr of age and particularly in children younger than 2 yr of age. Thus, for most episodes in most children, treatment that provides tissue concentrations of an antimicrobial for at least 10 days is advisable. Treatment for longer than 10 days may be required for children who are very young or are having severe episodes or whose previous experience with OM has been problematic.

Follow-Up

The principal goals of follow-up are to assess the outcome of treatment and to differentiate between inadequate response to treatment and early recurrence. The appropriate interval for follow-up should be individualized. Follow-up within days is advisable in the young infant with a severe episode or in a child of any age with continuing pain. Follow-up within 2 wk is appropriate for the infant or young child who has been having frequent recurrences. At that point, the TM is not likely to have returned to normal, but substantial improvement in its appearance should be evident. In the child with only a sporadic episode of AOM and prompt symptomatic improvement, follow-up 1 mo after initial examination is early enough, or in older children, no follow-up may be necessary. The continuing presence of MEE alone following an episode of AOM is not an indication for additional or second-line antimicrobial treatment. However, persisting MEE does warrant additional follow-up to ensure that this resolves and does not lead to persisting hearing loss or other complications.

Unsatisfactory Response to First-Line Treatment

AOM is essentially a closed-space infection and its resolution depends both on eradication of the offending organism and restoration of middle-ear ventilation. Factors contributing to unsatisfactory response to first-line treatment, in addition to inadequate antimicrobial efficacy, include poor compliance with treatment regimens; concurrent or intercurrent viral infection; persistent eustachian tube dysfunction and middle-ear underaeration; reinfection from other sites or from incompletely eradicated middle-ear pathogens; and immature or impaired host defenses. The identification of biofilm formation in the middle ear of children with chronic OM also indicates that, in some children, eradication with standard antimicrobial therapy is likely to be unsuccessful. Despite these many potential factors, switching to an alternative or second-line drug is reasonable when there has been inadequate improvement in symptoms or in middle-ear status as reflected in the appearance of the TM, or when the persistence of purulent nasal discharge suggests that the antimicrobial drug being used has less-than-optimal efficacy. Second-line drugs may also appropriately be used when AOM develops in a child already receiving antimicrobial therapy, or in an immunocompromised child, or in a child with severe symptoms whose previous experience with OM has been problematic.

Second-Line Treatment

When treatment of AOM with a first-line antimicrobial drug has proven inadequate, a number of second-line alternatives are available (see Table 640-3). Drugs chosen for second-line treatment should be effective against β-lactamase–producing strains of nontypeable *H. influenzae* and *M. catarrhalis* and against susceptible and most non-susceptible strains of *S. pneumoniae*. Only 4 antimicrobial agents meet these requirements: amoxicillin-clavulanate, cefdinir, cefuroxime axetil, and intramuscular ceftriaxone. Because high-dose amoxicillin (80-90 mg/kg/24 hr) is effective against most strains of *S. pneumoniae* and because the addition of clavulanate extends the effective antibacterial spectrum of amoxicillin to include β-lactamase–producing bacteria, high-dose amoxicillin-clavulanate is particularly well-suited as a second-line drug for treating AOM. The 14 : 1 amoxicillin-clavulanate formulation contains twice as much amoxicillin as the previously available 7 : 1 formulation. Diarrhea, especially in infants and young children, is a common adverse effect, but may be ameliorated in some cases by feeding active culture yogurt, and usually is not severe enough to require cessation of treatment. Cefdinir has demonstrated broad efficacy in treatment, is generally well tolerated with respect to taste, and can be given as a once-daily regimen. The ability to also utilize cefdinir in most children with mild type 1 hypersensitivity reactions has further added to its favorable selection as a second-line agent. Both cefuroxime axetil and intramuscular ceftriaxone have important limitations for use in young children. The currently available suspension of cefuroxime axetil is not palatable and its acceptance is low. Ceftriaxone treatment entails both the pain of intramuscular injection and substantial cost, and the injection may need to be repeated once or twice at 2 day intervals to achieve the desired degree of effectiveness. Nonetheless, use of ceftriaxone is appropriate in severe cases of AOM when oral treatment is not feasible, or in highly selected cases after treatment failure using orally administered second-line antimicrobials (i.e., amoxicillin-clavulanate or cefuroxime axetil), or when highly resistant *S. pneumoniae* is found in aspirates obtained from diagnostic tympanocentesis.

Clarithromycin and azithromycin have only limited activity against nonsusceptible strains of *S. pneumoniae* and against β-lactamase–producing strains of nontypeable *H. influenzae*. Macrolide use also appears to be a major factor in causing increases in rates of resistance to macrolides by group A streptococcus and *S. pneumoniae*. Clindamycin is active against most strains of *S. pneumoniae*, including resistant strains, but is not active against nontypeable *H. influenzae* or *M. catarrhalis*.

Other antimicrobial agents that have been traditionally utilized in the management of AOM have such significant lack of effectiveness against resistant organisms that employment seldom outweighs the potential side effects or complications possible from the medications. This includes cefprozil, cefaclor, loracarbef, cefixime, trimethoprim-sulfamethoxazole, and erythromycin-sulfisoxazole. Cefpodoxime has demonstrated reasonable effectiveness in some investigations but is generally poorly tolerated because of its taste.

ANTIMICROBIAL PROPHYLAXIS

In children who have developed frequent episodes of AOM, antimicrobial prophylaxis with subtherapeutic doses of an aminopenicillin or a sulfonamide has been utilized in the past to provide protection against recurrences of AOM (although not of OME). However, because of the increased incidence of resistant organisms and the contribution of antimicrobial usage to bacterial resistance, the risks of sustained antimicrobial prophylaxis clearly outweigh potential benefits.

Myringotomy and Tympanocentesis

Myringotomy is a long-standing treatment for AOM but is not commonly needed in children receiving antimicrobials. **Indications for myringotomy** in children with AOM include severe, refractory pain; hyperpyrexia; complications of AOM such as facial paralysis, mastoiditis, labyrinthitis, or central nervous system infection; and immunologic compromise from any source. Myringotomy should be considered as third-line therapy in patients that have failed 2 courses of antibiotics for an episode of AOM. In children with AOM in whom clinical response to vigorous, second-line treatment has been unsatisfactory, either diagnostic tympanocentesis or myringotomy is indicated to enable identification of the offending organism and its sensitivity profile. Either procedure may be helpful in effecting relief of pain. Tympanocentesis with culture of the middle-ear aspirate may also be indicated as part of the sepsis work-up in very young infants with AOM who show systemic signs of illness such as fever, vomiting, or lethargy, and whose illness accordingly cannot be presumed to be limited to infection of the middle ear. Performing tympanocentesis can be facilitated by use of a specially designed tympanocentesis aspirator. Studies reporting the usage of strict, individualized criteria for the diagnosis of AOM that include office tympanocentesis with bacterial culture followed by culture-guided antimicrobial therapy demonstrate significant reduction in the frequency of recurrent AOM episodes and tympanostomy tube surgery. However, many primary care physicians do not feel comfortable performing this procedure, there is the potential for complications, and parents may view this procedure as traumatic. Often children requiring this intervention have a strong enough history of recurrent OM to warrant the consideration of tympanostomy tube placement, so that the procedure can be performed under general anesthesia.

Early Recurrence After Treatment

Recurrence of AOM after apparent resolution may be caused by either incomplete eradication of infection in the middle ear or upper respiratory tract reinfection by the same or a different bacteria or bacterial strain. Recent antibiotic therapy predisposes patients to an increased incidence of resistant organisms, which should also be considered in choosing therapy, and, generally, initiating therapy with a second-line agent is advisable (see Table 640-3).

Myringotomy and Insertion of Tympanostomy Tubes

When AOM is recurrent, despite appropriate medical therapy, consideration of surgical management of AOM with tympanostomy tube insertion is warranted. This procedure is effective in reducing the rate of AOM in patients with recurrent OM and in significantly improving the quality of life in patients with recurrent AOM. Individual patient factors, including the risk profile, severity of AOM episodes, child's development and age, presence of a history of adverse drug reactions, concurrent medical problems, and parental wishes, will affect the timing of a decision to consider referral for this procedure. When a patient experiences 3 episodes of AOM in a 6 mo period or 4 episodes in a 12 mo period with 1 episode in the preceding 6 mo, potential surgical management of the child's AOM should be discussed with the parents. Additionally, often patients with recurrent AOM may have persisting MEE between episodes with accompanying hearing loss, which may add to the indication for tympanostomy tube placement.

Tube Otorrhea

Although tympanostomy tubes often reduce the incidence of AOM in most children, patients with tympanostomy tubes may still develop AOM. One advantage of tympanostomy tubes in children with recurrent AOM is that if patients do develop an episode of AOM with a functioning tube in place, these patients will manifest purulent drainage from the tube. By definition, children with functioning tympanostomy tubes without otorrhea do not have bacterial AOM as a cause for a presentation of fever or behavioral changes and should not be treated with oral antibiotics. If tympanostomy tube otorrhea develops, ototopical treatment should be considered as first-line therapy. With a functioning tube in place, the infection is able to drain, there is usually negligible pain associated with the infection, and the possibility of developing a serious complication from an episode of AOM is extremely remote. The current quinolone otic drops approved by the U.S. Food and Drug Administration for use in the middle-ear space in children are formulated with ciprofloxacin/dexamethasone (Ciprodex) and ofloxacin (Floxin). The topical delivery of these otic drops allows them to utilize a higher antibiotic concentration than can be tolerated by administering oral antibiotics and they have excellent coverage of even the most resistant strains of common middle-ear pathogens as well as coverage of *S. aureus* and *Pseudomonas aeruginosa*. The high rate of success of these topical preparations, their broad coverage, the lower likelihood of their contributing to the development of resistant organisms, the relative ease of administration, the lack of significant side effects, and the lack of ototoxicity makes them the first choice for tube otorrhea. Oral antibiotic therapy should generally be reserved for cases of tube otorrhea that have other associated systemic symptoms, patients who have difficulty in tolerating the use of topical preparations, or, possibly, patients who have failed an attempt at topical otic drops. Despite these advantages of ototopical therapy, survey data have indicated that, compared to otolaryngologists, primary care practitioners are less likely to prescribe ototopicals as first-line therapy in tympanostomy tube otorrhea. As a result of the relative ease in obtaining fluid

for culture and the possibility of the development of fungal otitis, which has shown an increase with the utilization of broad-spectrum quinolone ototopicals, patients that fail topical therapy should also have culture performed to rule out the development of fungal otitis. Other otic preparations are available; although these either have some risk of ototoxicity or have not received approval for use in the middle ear, many of these preparations were widely used prior to the development of the current quinolone drops and were generally considered reasonably safe and effective. In all cases of tube otorrhea, attention to aural toilet (e.g., cleansing the external auditory canal of secretions, and avoidance of external ear water contamination) is important. In some cases with very thick, tenacious discharge, topical therapy may be inhibited due to lack of delivery of the medication to the site of infection. Suctioning and removal of the secretions, often done through referral to an otolaryngologist, may be quite helpful. When children with tube otorrhea fail to improve satisfactorily with conventional outpatient management, they may require tube removal, or hospitalization to receive parenteral antibiotic treatment, or both.

MANAGEMENT OF OTITIS MEDIA WITH EFFUSION

Management of OME depends on an understanding of its natural history and its possible complications and sequelae. Most cases of OME resolve without treatment within 3 mo. To distinguish between persistence and recurrence, examination should be conducted monthly until resolution; hearing should be assessed if effusion has been present for longer than 3 mo. When MEE persists for longer than 3 mo, consideration of referral to an otolaryngologist may be appropriate. For young children, this referral is warranted for the assessment of hearing levels. In older children (generally older than age 4 yr), and depending upon the expertise in the primary care physician's office, hearing screening may be achieved by the primary care physician. For any child who fails a hearing screening in the primary care physician's office, referral to an otolaryngologist is warranted. In considering the decision to refer the patient for consultation, the clinician should attempt to determine the impact of the OME on the child. Although hearing loss may be of primary concern, OME causes a number of other difficulties in children that should also be considered. These include predisposition to recurring AOM, pain, disturbance of balance, and tinnitus. In addition, long-term sequelae that have been demonstrated to be associated with OME include pathologic middle-ear changes; atelectasis of the TM and retraction pocket formation; adhesive OM; cholesteatoma formation and ossicular discontinuity; and conductive and sensorineural hearing loss. Long-term adverse effects on speech, language, cognitive, and psychosocial development have also been demonstrated. This impact is related to the duration of effusion present, whether the effusion is unilateral or bilateral, the degree of underlying hearing loss, and other developmental and social factors affecting the child. In considering the impact of OME on development, it is especially important to take into consideration the overall presentation of the child. Although it is unlikely that OME causing unilateral hearing loss in the mild range will have long-term negative effects on an otherwise healthy and developmentally normal child, even a mild hearing loss in a child with other developmental or speech delays certainly has the potential to compound this child's difficulties (Table 640-4). At a minimum, children with OME persisting longer than 3 mo deserve close monitoring of their hearing levels with skilled audiologic evaluation; frequent assessment of developmental milestones, including speech and language assessment; and attention paid to their rate of recurrent AOM.

Variables Influencing Otitis Media with Effusion Management Decisions

Patient-related variables that affect decisions on how to manage OME include the child's age; the frequency and severity of previous episodes of AOM and the interval since the last episode; the child's current speech and language development; the presence of a history of adverse drug reactions, concurrent medical problems, or risk factors such as daycare attendance; and the parental wishes. In considering surgical management of OME with tympanostomy tubes, particular benefit is

Table 640-4	Sensory, Physical, Cognitive, or Behavioral Factors That Place Children Who Have Otitis Media with Effusion at an Increased Risk for Developmental Difficulties (Delay or Disorder)

Permanent hearing loss independent of otitis media with effusion
Suspected or diagnosed speech and language delay or disorder
Autism-spectrum disorder and other pervasive developmental disorders
Syndromes (e.g., Down) or craniofacial disorders that include cognitive, speech, and language delays
Blindness or uncorrectable visual impairment
Cleft palate with or without associated syndrome
Developmental delay

From American Academy of Family Physicians; American Academy of Otolaryngology-Head and Neck Surgery; American Academy of Pediatrics Subcommittee on Otitis Media with Effusion: Otitis media with effusion, Pediatrics 113(5):1412–1429, 2004, Table 3, p. 1416.

seen in patients with persisting OME punctuated by episodes of AOM, as the tubes generally provide resolution of both conditions. Disease-related variables that most otolaryngologists consider in the treatment of OME include whether the effusion is unilateral or bilateral; the apparent quantity of effusion; the duration, if known; the degree of hearing impairment; the presence or absence of other possibly related symptoms, such as tinnitus, vertigo, or disturbance of balance; and the presence or absence of mucopurulent or purulent rhinorrhea, which, if sustained for longer than 2 wk, would suggest that concurrent naso-pharyngeal or paranasal sinus infection is contributing to continuing compromise of middle-ear ventilation.

Medical Treatment

In some studies, antimicrobials have demonstrated some efficacy in resolving OME, presumably because they help eradicate nasopharyn-geal infection or unapparent middle-ear infection, or both. The most significant effects of antibiotics for OME have been shown with treat-ment durations of 4 wk and 3 mo. However, in the current era of bacte-rial antimicrobial resistance, the small potential benefit of antimicrobial therapy is outweighed by the negative potential of treatment and is not recommended. Instead, treatment should be limited to cases in which there is evidence of associated bacterial upper respiratory tract infec-tion or untreated middle-ear infection. For this purpose, the most broadly effective drug available should be used as recommended for AOM.

The efficacy of corticosteroids in the treatment of OME is probably short term. The risk: benefit ratio for steroids would argue against their use. Antihistamine-decongestant combinations are not effective in treating children with OME. Antihistamines alone, decongestants alone, and mucolytic agents are unlikely to be effective. The risk profile for decongestants and antihistamines in children suggests that they are not indicated in the treatment of OME. Allergic management, includ-ing antihistamine therapy, might prove helpful in children with prob-lematic OME who also have evidence of environmental allergies, although supporting data specifically analyzing this patient population are not conclusive. Recent randomized controlled trials do not support the usage of topical intranasal steroid sprays to treat the manifestations of eustachian tube dysfunction. Inflation of the eustachian tube by the Valsalva maneuver or other means has not demonstrated long-term efficacy but is unlikely to lead to significant harm. Other "alternative" therapies, including spinal manipulation, currently have no demon-strated efficacy or role in children with OME.

Myringotomy and Insertion of Tympanostomy Tubes

When OME persists despite an ample period of watchful waiting, generally 3-6 mo or perhaps longer in children with unilateral effusion, consideration of surgical intervention with tympanostomy tubes is appropriate. Myringotomy alone, without tympanostomy tube inser-tion, permits evacuation of middle-ear effusion and may sometimes be effective, but often the incision heals before the middle-ear mucosa returns to normal and the effusion soon reaccumulates. Inserting a tympanostomy tube offers the likelihood that middle-ear ventilation will be sustained for at least as long as the tube remains in place and functional. Tympanostomy tubes have a variable duration of efficacy based on design. Tubes that are designed for a shorter duration, 6-12 mo, have a lesser impact on disease-free middle-ear spaces in children. Some studies comparing the efficacy of tympanostomy tube types, including shorter-acting tubes, with watchful waiting provide a less helpful assessment of the differences between these approaches. Tubes that are somewhat longer acting, effective for 12-18 mo, are generally more appropriate for most children undergoing tube place-ment. Regardless of type, tympanostomy tube placement nearly uni-formly reverses the conductive hearing loss associated with OME. Occasional episodes of obstruction of the tube lumen and premature tube extrusion may limit the effectiveness of tympanostomy tubes, and tubes can also be associated with otorrhea. However, placement of tympanostomy tubes is generally quite effective in providing resolution of OME in children. Tympanostomy tubes generally extrude on their own but rarely require surgical removal after several years in place. Sequelae following tube extrusion include residual perforation of the eardrum, tympanosclerosis, localized or diffuse atrophic scarring of the eardrum that may predispose to the development of atelectasis or a retraction pocket, or both, residual conductive hearing loss, and cholesteatoma. The more serious of these sequelae are quite infrequent. Recurrence of middle-ear effusion following the extrusion of tubes does develop, especially in younger children; most children without underlying craniofacial abnormalities only require 1 set of tympanos-tomy tubes, with developmental changes providing improved middle-ear health and resolution of chronic OME by the time of tube extrusion. Because even previously persistent OME often clears spontaneously during the summer mo, watchful waiting through the summer season is also advisable in most children with OME who are otherwise well. In considering surgical management of OME in children, primarily in those with bilateral disease and hearing loss, it has been demonstrated that placement of tympanostomy tubes results in a significant improve-ment in their quality of life.

Adenoidectomy

Adenoidectomy is efficacious to some extent in reducing the risk of subsequent recurrences of both AOM and OME in children who have undergone tube insertion and in whom, after extrusion of tubes, OM continues to be a problem. Efficacy appears to be independent of adenoid size and probably derives from removal of the focus of infec-tion in the nasopharynx as a site of biofilm formation, chronic inflam-mation impacting eustachian tube function, and recurrent seeding of the middle ear via the eustachian tube. In younger children with recur-rent AOM who have not previously undergone tube insertion, ade-noidectomy is usually not recommended along with tube insertion, unless significant nasal airway obstruction or recurrent rhinosinusitis is associated, in which case, performing adenoidectomy might be considered.

Complications of Acute Otitis Media

Most complications of AOM consist of the spread of infection to adjoining or nearby structures or the development of chronicity, or both. Suppurative complications are relatively uncommon in children in developed countries but occur not infrequently in disadvantaged children whose medical care is limited. The complications of AOM may be classified as either intratemporal or intracranial.

Intratemporal Complications

Direct but limited extension of AOM leads to complications within the local region of the ear and temporal bone. These complications include dermatitis, TM perforation, chronic suppurative OM (CSOM), mas-toiditis, hearing loss, facial nerve paralysis, cholesteatoma formation, and labyrinthitis.

Infectious Dermatitis

This is an infection of the skin of the external auditory canal resulting from contamination by purulent discharge from the middle ear. The skin is often erythematous, edematous, and tender. Management consists of proper hygiene combined with systemic antimicrobials and ototopical drops as appropriate for treating AOM and tube otorrhea.

Tympanic Membrane Perforation

Rupture of the TM can occur with episodes of either AOM or OME. Although damage to the TM from these episodes generally heals spontaneously, chronic perforations can develop in a small number of cases and require further surgical intervention in the future.

Chronic Suppurative Otitis Media

CSOM consists of persistent middle-ear infection with discharge through a TM perforation. The disease is initiated by an episode of AOM with rupture of the membrane. The mastoid air cells are invariably involved. The most common etiologic organisms are *P. aeruginosa* and *S. aureus;* however, the typical AOM bacterial pathogens may also be the cause, especially in younger children or in the winter months. Treatment is guided by the results of microbiologic investigation. If an associated cholesteatoma is not present, parenteral antimicrobial treatment combined with assiduous aural cleansing is likely to be successful in clearing the infection, but in refractory cases, tympanomastoidectomy can be required.

Acute Mastoiditis

Technically, all cases of AOM are accompanied by mastoiditis by virtue of the associated contiguous inflammation of the mastoid air cells. However, early in the course of the disease, no signs or symptoms of mastoid infection are present, and the inflammatory process usually is readily reversible, along with the AOM, in response to antimicrobial treatment. Spread of the infection to the overlying periosteum, but without involvement of bone, constitutes **acute mastoiditis with periosteitis.** In such cases, signs of mastoiditis are usually present, including redness and swelling in the postauricular area, often with protrusion and displacement of the pinna inferiorly and anteriorly (Fig. 640-7 and Table 640-5). Treatment with myringotomy and parenteral antibiotics, if instituted promptly, usually provides satisfactory resolution.

In acute mastoid osteitis, or **coalescent mastoiditis,** infection has progressed further to cause destruction of the bony trabeculae of the mastoid. Frank signs and symptoms of mastoiditis are usually, but not always, present. In acute **petrositis,** infection has extended further to involve the petrous portion of the temporal bone. Eye pain, a result of irritation of the ophthalmic branch of cranial nerve V, is a prominent symptom. Cranial nerve VI palsy is a later finding, suggesting further extension of the infectious process along the cranial base. **Gradenigo syndrome** is the triad of suppurative OM, paralysis of the external rectus muscle, and pain in the ipsilateral orbit. Rarely, mastoid infection spreads external to the temporal bone into the neck musculature that attaches to the mastoid tip, resulting in an abscess in the neck, termed a **Bezold abscess.**

When mastoiditis is suspected or diagnosed clinically, CT scanning of the temporal bones can be considered to further clarify the nature and extent of the disease. Bony destruction of the mastoid must be differentiated from the simple clouding of mastoid air cells that is found often in uncomplicated cases of OM. The most common causative organisms in all variants of acute mastoiditis are *S. pneumoniae,* group A streptococcus, and nontypeable *H. influenzae. P. aeruginosa* is also a causative agent, primarily in patients with CSOM. Children with acute mastoid osteitis generally require intravenous antimicrobial treatment and mastoidectomy, with the extent of the surgery dependent on the extent of the disease process. Early cases of mastoid osteitis may respond to myringotomy and parenteral antibiotics. Insofar as possible, choice of the antimicrobial regimen should be guided by the findings of microbiologic examination from cultures.

Each of the variants of mastoiditis may also occur in subacute or chronic form. Symptoms are correspondingly less prominent. Chronic mastoiditis is always accompanied by CSOM, and occasionally will

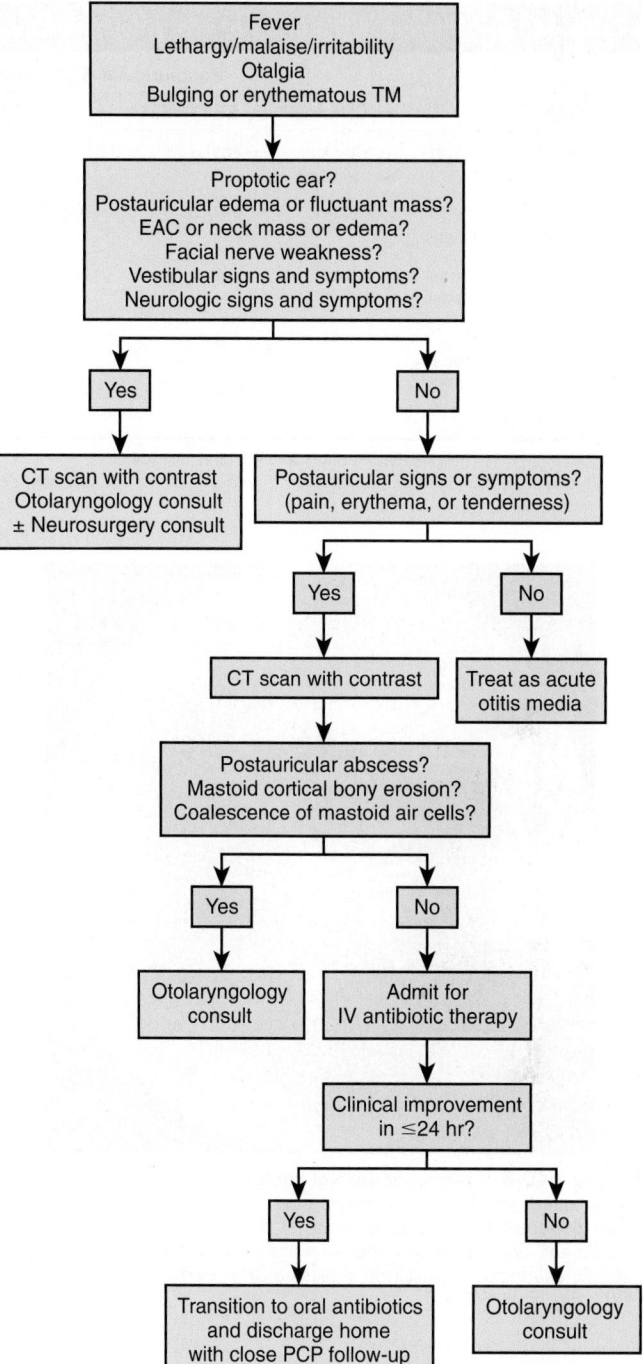

Figure 640-7 Diagnosis and treatment algorithm for cases of suspected acute mastoiditis. (*From Lin HW, Shargorodsky J, Gopen Q. Clinical strategies for the management of acute mastoiditis in the pediatric population. Clin Pediatr (Phila) 49(2):110–115, 2010, Fig. 5.*)

respond to the conservative regimen recommended for that condition. In most cases, mastoidectomy also is required.

Facial Paralysis

The facial nerve, as it traverses the middle ear and mastoid bone, may be affected by adjacent infection. Facial paralysis occurring as a complication of AOM is uncommon, and often resolves after myringotomy and parenteral antibiotic treatment. Facial paralysis in the presence of AOM requires urgent attention as prolonged infection can result in the development of permanent facial paralysis, which can have a devastating effect on a child. Facial paralysis in an infant or child requires complete and unequivocal examination of the TM and middle-ear

Table 640-5	Differential Diagnosis of Postauricular Involvement of Acute Mastoiditis with Periosteitis/Abscess					
	Postauricular Signs and Symptoms				**EXTERNAL CANAL INFECTION**	**MIDDLE-EAR EFFUSION**
DISEASE	**CREASE***	**ERYTHEMA**	**MASS**	**TENDERNESS**		
Acute mastoiditis with periosteitis	May be absent	Yes	No	Usually	No	Usually
Acute mastoiditis with subperiosteal abscess	Absent	Maybe	Yes	Yes	No	Usually
Periosteitis of pinna with postauricular extension	Intact	Yes	No	Usually	No	No
External otitis with postauricular extension	Intact	Yes	No	Usually	Yes	No
Postauricular lymphadenitis	Intact	No	Yes (circumscribed)	Maybe	No	No

*Postauricular crease (fold) between pinna and postauricular area.
From Bluestone CD, Klein JO, editors: Otitis media in infants and children, ed 3, Philadelphia, 2001, WB Saunders, p. 333.

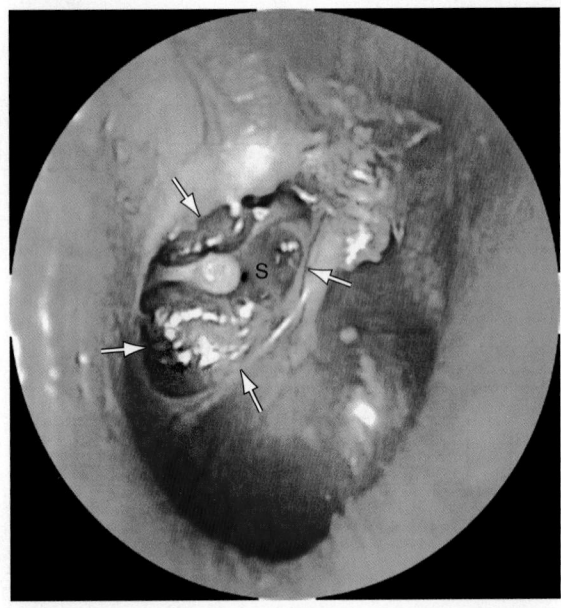

Figure 640-8 A retraction pocket cholesteatoma of the posterosuperior quadrant. The incus long process is eroded, which leaves the drum adherent to the stapes head (S). An effusion is present in the middle ear, and squamous debris emanates from the attic. (From Isaacson G: Diagnosis of pediatric cholesteatoma, Pediatrics 120:603–608, 2007, Fig. 9, p. 607.)

space. Any difficulty in examination requires urgent consultation with an otolaryngologist. Any examination that demonstrates an ear abnormality also requires urgent referral to an otolaryngologist. If facial paralysis develops in a child with mastoid osteitis or with chronic suppurative OM, mastoidectomy should be undertaken urgently.

Cholesteatoma

Cholesteatoma is a cyst-like growth originating in the middle ear, lined by keratinized, stratified squamous epithelium and containing desquamated epithelium and/or keratin (see Chapter 638; Fig. 640-8).

Acquired cholesteatoma develops most often as a complication of long-standing chronic OM. The condition also may develop from a deep retraction pocket of the TM or as a consequence of epithelial implantation in the middle-ear cavity from traumatic perforation of the TM or insertion of a tympanostomy tube. Cholesteatomas tend to expand progressively, causing bony resorption, often extend into the mastoid cavity, and may extend intracranially with potentially life-threatening consequences. Acquired cholesteatoma commonly presents as a chronically draining ear in a patient with a history of previous ear disease. Cholesteatoma should be suspected if otoscopy demonstrates an area of TM retraction or perforation with white, caseous debris persistently overlying this area. Along with otorrhea from this area, granulation tissue or polyp formation identified in conjunction with this history and presentation should prompt suspicion of cholesteatoma. The most common location for cholesteatoma development is in the superior portion of the TM (pars flaccida). Most patients also present with conductive hearing loss on audiologic evaluation. When cholesteatoma is suspected, otolaryngology consultation should be sought immediately. Delay in recognition and treatment can have significant long-term consequences, including the need for more extensive surgical treatment, permanent hearing loss, facial nerve injury, labyrinthine damage with loss of balance function, and intracranial extension. The required treatment for cholesteatoma is tympanomastoid surgery.

Congenital cholesteatoma is an uncommon condition generally identified in younger patients (Fig. 640-9). The etiology of congenital cholesteatoma is thought to be a result of epithelial implantation in the middle-ear space during otologic development in utero. Congenital cholesteatoma most commonly presents in the anterior-superior quadrant of the TM but can be found elsewhere. Congenital cholesteatoma appears as a discrete, white opacity in the middle-ear space on otoscopy. Unlike patients with acquired cholesteatoma, there is generally not a strong history of OM or chronic ear disease, history of otorrhea, or changes in the TM anatomy such as perforation or retraction. Similar to acquired cholesteatoma many patients do have some degree of abnormal findings on audiologic evaluation, unless identified very early. Congenital cholesteatoma also requires surgical resection.

Labyrinthitis

This occurs uncommonly as a result of the spread of infection from the middle ear and/or mastoid to the inner ear (see Chapter 641). Cholesteatoma or CSOM is the usual source. Symptoms and signs include vertigo, tinnitus, nausea, vomiting, hearing loss, nystagmus, and clumsiness. Treatment is directed at the underlying condition and must be undertaken promptly to preserve inner-ear function and prevent the spread of infection.

INTRACRANIAL COMPLICATIONS

Meningitis, epidural abscess, subdural abscess, focal encephalitis, brain abscess (see Chapters 603 and 604), sigmoid sinus thrombosis (also called lateral sinus thrombosis), and otitic hydrocephalus each may develop as a complication of acute or chronic middle-ear or mastoid infection, through direct extension, hematogenous spread, or thrombophlebitis. Bony destruction adjacent to the dura is often involved, and a cholesteatoma may be present. In a child with middle-ear or mastoid infection, the presence of any systemic symptom, such as high

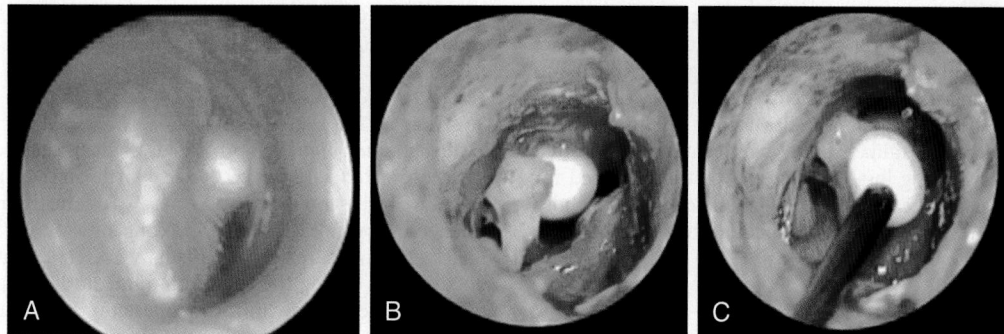

Figure 640-9 A, Congenital cholesteatoma of the anterosuperior quadrant. **B,** The eardrum is reflected downward to reveal a white spherical lesion. **C,** Removal of the lesion. *(From Isaacson G: Diagnosis of pediatric cholesteatoma, Pediatrics 120:603–608, 2007, Fig. 3, p. 605.)*

spiking fevers, headache, or lethargy of extreme degree, or a finding of meningismus or of any central nervous system sign on physical examination should prompt suspicion of an intracranial complication.

When an intracranial complication is suspected, lumbar puncture should be performed only after imaging studies establish that there is no evidence of mass effect or hydrocephalus. In addition to examination of the cerebrospinal fluid, culture of middle-ear exudate obtained via tympanocentesis may identify the causative organism, thereby helping guide the choice of antimicrobial medications. Myringotomy should be performed to permit middle-ear drainage. Concurrent tympanostomy tube placement is preferable to allow for continued decompression of the "infection under pressure" that is the causative event leading to intracranial spread of the infection.

Treatment of intracranial complications of OM requires urgent, otolaryngologic, and, often, neurosurgical consultation, intravenous antibiotic therapy, drainage of any abscess formation, and tympanomastoidectomy in patients with coalescent mastoiditis.

Sigmoid sinus thrombosis may be complicated by dissemination of infected thrombi with resultant development of septic infarcts in various organs. With prompt recognition and wide availability of MRI, which facilitates diagnosis, this complication is exceedingly rare. Mastoidectomy may be required even in the absence of osteitis or coalescent mastoiditis, especially in the case of propagation or embolization of infected thrombi. In the absence of coalescent mastoiditis, sinus thrombosis can often be treated with tympanostomy tube placement and intravenous antibiotics. Anticoagulation therapy may also be considered in the treatment of sigmoid sinus thrombosis; however, otolaryngology consultation should be obtained before initiating this therapy to coordinate the possible need for surgical intervention prior to anticoagulation.

Otitic hydrocephalus, a form of **pseudotumor cerebri** (see Chapter 605), is an uncommon condition that consists of increased intracranial pressure without dilation of the cerebral ventricles, occurring in association with acute or chronic OM or mastoiditis. The condition is commonly also associated with lateral sinus thrombosis, and the pathophysiology is thought to involve obstruction by thrombus of intracranial venous drainage into the neck, producing a rise in cerebral venous pressure and a consequent increase in cerebrospinal fluid pressure. Symptoms are those of increased intracranial pressure. Signs may include, in addition to evidence of OM, paralysis of 1 or both lateral rectus muscles and papilledema with or without visual acuity loss. MRI can confirm the diagnosis. Treatment measures include the use of antimicrobials and medications such as acetazolamide or furosemide to reduce intracranial pressure, mastoidectomy, repeated lumbar puncture, lumboperitoneal shunt, and ventriculoperitoneal shunt. If left untreated, otitic hydrocephalus may result in loss of vision secondary to optic atrophy.

PHYSICAL SEQUELAE

The physical sequelae of OM consist of structural middle-ear abnormalities resulting from long-standing middle-ear inflammation. In most instances, these sequelae are consequences of severe and/or

chronic infection, but some may also result from the noninfective inflammation of long-standing OME. The various sequelae may occur singly, or interrelatedly in various combinations.

Tympanosclerosis consists of whitish plaques in the TM and nodular deposits in the submucosal layers of the middle ear. The changes involve hyalinization with deposition of calcium and phosphate crystals. Uncommonly, there may be associated conductive hearing loss. In developed countries, probably the most common cause of tympanosclerosis is tympanostomy tube insertion.

Atelectasis of the TM is a descriptive term applied to either severe retraction of the TM caused by high negative middle-ear pressure or loss of stiffness and medial prolapse of the membrane as a consequence of long-standing retraction or severe or chronic inflammation. A **retraction pocket** is a localized area of atelectasis. Atelectasis is often transient and usually unaccompanied by symptoms, but a deep retraction pocket may lead to erosion of the ossicles and adhesive otitis, and may serve as the nidus of a cholesteatoma. For a deep retraction pocket, and for the unusual instance in which atelectasis is accompanied by symptoms such as otalgia, tinnitus, or conductive hearing loss, the required treatment is tympanostomy tube insertion and, at times, tympanoplasty. Patients with persisting atelectasis and retraction pockets should have referral to an otolaryngologist.

Adhesive OM consists of proliferation of fibrous tissue in the middle-ear mucosa, which may, in turn, result in severe TM retraction, conductive hearing loss, impaired movement of the ossicles, ossicular discontinuity, and cholesteatoma. The hearing loss may be amenable to surgical correction.

Cholesterol granuloma is an uncommon condition in which the TM may appear to be dark blue secondary to middle-ear fluid of this color. Cholesterol granulomas are rare, benign cysts that occur in the temporal bone. They are expanding masses that contain fluids, lipids, and cholesterol crystals surrounded by a fibrous lining and generally require surgical removal. Tympanostomy tube placement will not provide satisfactory relief. This lesion requires differentiation from bluish middle-ear fluid, which can also rarely develop in patients with the more common OME.

Chronic perforation may rarely develop after spontaneous rupture of the TM during an episode of AOM or from acute trauma, but more commonly results as a sequelae of CSOM or as a result of failure of closure of the TM following extrusion of a tympanostomy tube. Chronic perforations are generally accompanied by conductive hearing loss. Surgical repair of a TM perforation is recommended to restore hearing, prevent infection from water contamination in the middle-ear space, and prevent cholesteatoma formation. Chronic perforations are almost always amenable to surgical repair, usually after the child has been free of OM for an extended period.

Permanent **conductive hearing loss** (see Chapter 637) may result from any of the conditions just described. Rarely, permanent sensorineural hearing loss may occur in association with acute or chronic OM, secondary to spread of infection or products of inflammation through the round window membrane, or as a consequence of suppurative labyrinthitis.

POSSIBLE DEVELOPMENTAL SEQUELAE

Permanent hearing loss in children has a significant negative impact on development, particularly in speech and language. The degree to which OM impacts long-term development in children is difficult to assess and there have been conflicting studies examining this question. Developmental impact is most likely to be significant in children that have greater levels of hearing loss, hearing loss that is sustained for longer periods of time, or hearing loss that is bilateral and in those children that have other developmental difficulties or risk factors for developmental delay (see Table 640-4).

Bibliography is available at Expert Consult.

Chapter 641

The Inner Ear and Diseases of the Bony Labyrinth

Joseph Haddad Jr. and Sarah Keesecker

Genetic factors can impact the anatomy and function of the inner ear. Infectious agents, including viruses, bacteria, and protozoa, also can cause abnormal function, most commonly as sequelae of congenital infection or bacterial meningitis. Other acquired diseases of the labyrinthine capsule include otosclerosis, osteopetrosis, Langerhans cell histiocytosis, fibrous dysplasia, and other types of bony dysplasia. All of these can cause both conductive hearing loss (CHL) and sensorineural hearing loss (SNHL) as well as vestibular dysfunction. Use of currently available vaccines reduces the risk for bacterial meningitis and the associated sensorineural hearing loss.

VIRUSES

The most common cause of childhood sensorineural hearing loss (SNHL) is congenital cytomegalovirus (CMV) infection (see Chapter 255). Although the pathogenesis of hearing loss has not been elucidated, there is histologic evidence of infection in the cells of both the cochlear and vestibular endolabyrinth. The strongest predictor of delayed hearing loss appears to be the presence of symptoms at birth; prolonged viral shedding may also be a risk factor. In one large study, children who passed initial audiologic examinations but who had CMV-related symptoms at birth were approximately 6 times more likely to develop hearing loss than those who were asymptomatic. Stabilization (or even reversal) of the hearing loss may be possible by using ganciclovir in very young infants with congenital CMV infection. Administering ganciclovir for 6 wk improved hearing outcomes in neonates with symptomatic congenital CMV infections involving the central nervous system.

Other viral causes of SNHL include congenital rubella as well as acquired mumps (see Chapter 248), rubella (see Chapter 247), rubeola (measles; see Chapter 246), and fifth disease, caused by parvovirus B19 (see Chapter 251). Many other viruses also occasionally are associated with SNHL. In as many as 50% of cases, hearing loss, which usually is bilateral and often is asymmetric, progresses and worsens over weeks to years.

Before an effective vaccine was introduced, rubella was responsible for as many as 60% of cases of childhood SNHL. Vaccination in developed countries has reduced the rate of rubella by >97%. Similarly, measles and mumps are now uncommon causes of SNHL in the United States because of successful vaccination programs.

Herpes simplex encephalitis can also be associated with SNHL, which is more common in children with congenital herpesvirus infection. Acyclovir and other antiviral agents can help the hearing loss and other central nervous system manifestations (see Chapter 245).

TOXOPLASMOSIS

See Chapter 290.

Toxoplasma gondii is a protozoan that can cause congenital SNHL. In an estimated 1-10 per 10,000 live births in the United States, 1 per 3,000 live births in France, and 1 per 770 live births in southeast Brazil, infants are born each year with congenital toxoplasmosis; approximately 25% of untreated patients have SNHL. If maternal infection is documented during the fetal period, medical therapy may be able to prevent some of the clinical manifestations, including SNHL of the offspring.

BACTERIAL MENINGITIS

Since the *Haemophilus influenzae* type b vaccine was introduced, *Streptococcus pneumoniae* (see Chapter 182) and *Neisseria meningitidis* (see Chapter 191) have become the leading causes of bacterial meningitis in children in the United States. Hearing loss occurs more commonly with *S. pneumoniae*, with an estimated incidence of 15-20%. Approximately 60% of the associated hearing loss is bilateral, although it often is asymmetric. If hearing loss is present at the time of presentation with meningitis, and especially if it is severe to profound, the likelihood of significant improvement is low. However, if the hearing loss develops after admission for treatment and is not severe, stabilization or improvement is possible. Late progression of SNHL also has been noted in some children years after meningitis. In the United States and many other developed countries, bacterial meningitis is one of the major causes of profound deafness leading to cochlear implantation in children. Gadolinium-enhanced MRI could be utilized to detect meningitic labyrinthitis and therefore to predict which patients are at high risk for postmeningitic hearing loss. Gadolinium-enhanced MRI was found to be 87% sensitive and 100% specific for predicting which ears would develop permanent SNHL. The introduction of pneumococcal conjugate vaccine is expected to lead to a reduction in SNHL caused by pneumococcal meningitis, although pneumococcal strains not sensitive to the vaccine appear to be associated with rates of deafness equivalent to those that are sensitive.

Studies have shown favorable trends in the course and outcome after administration of dexamethasone for hearing loss and other neurologic deficits associated with bacterial meningitis (see Chapter 603.1), although its effectiveness, especially for *S. pneumoniae* and *N. meningitidis* meningitis, generally has not reached statistical significance because of the small number of cases in the trials. A metaanalysis of 2,029 patients from randomized, double-blinded, placebo-controlled trials of dexamethasone for bacterial meningitis found that adjunctive dexamethasone does not seem to significantly reduce death or neurologic disability but does reduce hearing loss among survivors. Dexamethasone has been shown to reduce severe hearing loss associated with *H. influenzae* type b meningitis regardless of the timing of administration of dexamethasone (before or with antibiotics vs later) or of the antibiotic used. For pneumococcal meningitis, dexamethasone might confer benefit only when given early and only for protection against severe hearing loss.

SYPHILIS

See Chapter 218.

Congenital syphilis, caused by *Treponema pallidum*, causes SNHL in 3-38% of affected children. The exact incidence is difficult to ascertain, because the hearing loss might not develop until adolescence or even adulthood. When the condition is identified, treatment with antibiotics and corticosteroids can improve the hearing loss.

OTHER DISEASES OF THE INNER EAR

Labyrinthitis (also called **vestibular neuritis**) may be a complication of direct spread of infection from acute or chronic otitis media or mastoiditis and also can complicate bacterial meningitis as a result of organisms entering the labyrinth through the internal auditory meatus, endolymphatic duct, perilymphatic duct, vascular channels, or hematogenous spread. Clinical manifestations of vestibular neuritis can include a sudden onset of rotatory vertigo, dysequilibrium, postural imbalance (furniture walking) with falls to the affected side, deep-seated ear pain, nausea, vomiting, and spontaneous horizontal (occasionally rotary) nystagmus.

The dizziness may last a few days, but balance issues, particularly following rapid head movements toward the affected ear, may last for mo. Vestibular neuritis is usually unilateral and is not associated with other neurologic defects; subjective hearing loss is unusual in vestibular neuritis. If hearing loss is present, idiopathic SNHL should be considered, as well as classical labyrinthitis (vestibular and cochlear nerves). Treatment of vestibular neuritis may include prednisone and vestibular rehabilitative exercises. Recurrent episodes should suggest another diagnosis such as vestibular migraine or benign paroxysmal positional vertigo.

In children, viral labyrinthitis is often associated with hearing loss. Acute suppurative labyrinthitis, characterized by abrupt, severe onset of these symptoms, requires intensive antimicrobial therapy. Vestibular suppressants (dimenhydrinate 1-2 mg/kg) can also be used in the acute stage but should not be given for more than 3 days. If it is secondary to otitis media, otologic surgery may be required to remove underlying cholesteatoma or drain the middle ear and mastoid, in addition to antibiotics. Acute serous labyrinthitis, with milder symptoms of vertigo and hearing loss, can develop secondary to middle-ear infection as well. It usually responds well to antibiotics and corticosteroids, with improvement in both vertigo and hearing. Chronic labyrinthitis, most commonly associated with cholesteatoma, manifests with SNHL and vestibular dysfunction that develops over time; surgery is required to remove the cholesteatoma. Chronic labyrinthitis also occurs uncommonly secondary to long-standing otitis media, with the slow development of SNHL, usually starting in the higher frequencies, and possibly with vestibular dysfunction. Additionally, and more commonly, children with chronic middle-ear fluid often are unsteady or off balance, a situation that improves immediately when the fluid resolves.

Vertigo and dizziness are common among older children and adolescents. Benign **paroxysmal vertigo** is common and is characterized by short periods of vertigo or dizziness lasting seconds to a few min and is associated with imbalance and nystagmus; tinnitus or hearing loss is unusual. **Basilar/vestibular migraine** is a common cause of episodic vertigo or dizziness and is associated with headache (50-70% of patients), rotary or to and fro nystagmus, and sensitivity to noise and bright light (see Chapter 595.1). **Benign paroxysmal positional vertigo** is less common in young children and more common with increasing age into adulthood. Particles form in the semicircular canals (canalolithiasis), most often the posterior canal; symptoms occur with position changes of the head and may last sec to min. Vertigo and nystagmus may be demonstrated by changing position (sitting to lying down on the right or left). Treatment involves canalith repositioning maneuvers to shift the debris from the canals into the utricle.

Otosclerosis, an autosomal dominant disease that affects only the temporal bones, causes abnormal bone growth that can result in fixation of the stapes in the oval window, leading to progressive hearing loss. In one series in North America, otosclerosis was found in 0.6% of temporal bones of children younger than 5 yr of age and 4% of those ages 5-18 yr. The hearing loss is usually conductive at first, but SNHL can develop. White girls and women are affected most commonly, with onset of otosclerosis in teenagers or young adults, often associated with pregnancy. Corrective surgery to replace the stapes with a mobile prosthesis often is successful.

Osteogenesis imperfecta is a systemic disease that can involve both the middle and inner ears (see Chapter 701). Hearing loss occurs in approximately 20% of young children and as many as 90% of adults with this disease. The hearing loss most commonly is conductive because of abnormalities of the ossicles, but SNHL can occur if other areas of the otic capsule become affected. Hearing loss may be the result of clinical or cochlear otosclerosis, fracture or atrophy of the ossicles, and/or cochlear degeneration due to an unidentified mechanism. An association between bone mineral density and hearing loss in osteogenesis imperfecta has been demonstrated, suggesting that patients with lower bone mineral density are more susceptible to microfractures, which may lead to the conductive hearing loss component. If the hearing loss is severe enough, a hearing aid may be a preferable alternative to surgical correction of the fixed stapes, because stapedectomy in children with osteogenesis imperfecta can be technically very difficult, and the disease and the hearing loss may be progressive.

Osteopetrosis, a very uncommon skeletal dysplasia, can involve the temporal bone, including the middle ear and ossicles, resulting in a moderate to severe, usually conductive hearing loss. Recurrent facial nerve paralysis also can occur as a result of excess bone deposition; with each recurrence, less facial function might return (see Chapter 699).

Bibliography is available at Expert Consult.

Chapter **642**
Traumatic Injuries of the Ear and Temporal Bone
Joseph Haddad Jr. and Sarah Keesecker

AURICLE AND EXTERNAL AUDITORY CANAL

Auricle trauma is common in certain sports. Hematoma, with accumulation of blood between the perichondrium and the cartilage, can follow trauma to the pinna and is especially common in teenagers related to wrestling or boxing. Prompt drainage of a hematoma can prevent irreversible damage. Immediate needle aspiration or, when the hematoma is extensive or recurrent, incision and drainage and a pressure dressing are necessary to prevent perichondritis, which can result in cartilage loss and a "cauliflower ear deformity." Sports helmets should be worn when appropriate during activities when head trauma is possible.

Frostbite of the auricle should be managed by rapidly rewarming the exposed pinna with warm irrigation or warm compresses.

Foreign bodies in the external canal are common in childhood. Often these can be removed in the office setting without general anesthesia if the child is mature enough to understand and cooperate and is properly restrained; if an adequate headlight, surgical head otoscope, or otomicroscope is used for visualizing the object; and if appropriate instruments such as alligator forceps, wire loops or a blunt cerumen curette, or suction are used, depending on the shape of the object. Gentle irrigation of the ear canal with body temperature water or saline may be used to remove very small objects, but only if the tympanic membrane (TM) is intact. Attempts to remove an object from a struggling child or with poor visualization and inadequate tools result in a terrified child with a swollen and bleeding ear canal and can then mandate general anesthesia to remove the object. Difficult foreign bodies, especially those that are large, deeply embedded, or associated with canal swelling, are best removed by an otolaryngologist and/or under general anesthesia. Disk batteries are removed emergently because they leach a basic fluid that can cause severe tissue destruction. Insects in the canal are first killed with mineral oil or lidocaine and are then removed under otomicroscopic examination.

After a foreign body is removed from the external canal, the TM should be inspected carefully for possible traumatic perforation or for a preexisting middle-ear effusion. If a foreign body has resulted in acute inflammation of the canal, ear drop treatment as described for acute external otitis should be instituted (see Chapter 639).

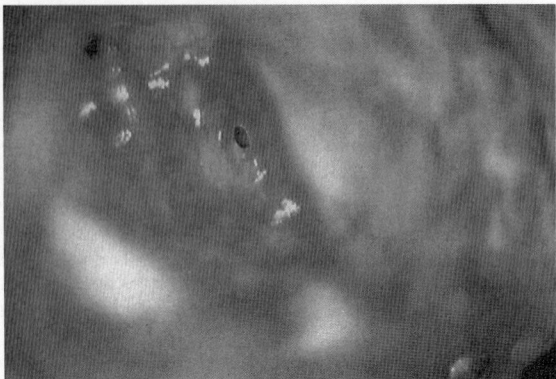

Figure 642-1 Intraoperative view of traumatic oval window perilymphatic fistula. *(From Kim SH, Kazahaya K, Handler SD. Traumatic perilymphatic fistulas in children: etiology, diagnosis and management. Int J Pediatr Otorhinolaryngol 60(2):147–153, 2001, Fig. 2.)*

TYMPANIC MEMBRANE AND MIDDLE EAR

Traumatic perforation of the TM usually occurs as a result of a sudden external compression, such as a slap, or penetration by a foreign object such as a stick or cotton-tipped applicator. The perforation may be linear or stellate. It is most commonly in the anterior portion of the pars tensa when it is caused by compression, and it may be in any quadrant of the TM when caused by a foreign object. Systemic antibiotics and topical otic medications are not required unless suppurative otorrhea is present. Traumatic TM perforations often heal spontaneously, but it is important to evaluate and monitor the patient's hearing to ensure that spontaneous healing occurs. If the TM does not heal within several mo, surgical graft repair should be considered. As long as the perforation is present, otorrhea can occur from water entering the middle ear from the ear canal, which can occur during swimming or bathing; appropriate precautions should be taken. Perforations resulting from penetrating foreign bodies are less likely to heal than those caused by compression. Audiometric examination reveals a conductive hearing loss, with larger air–bone gaps seen in larger perforations. Immediate surgical exploration may be indicated if the injury is accompanied by 1 or more of the following: vertigo, nystagmus, severe tinnitus, moderate to severe hearing loss, or cerebrospinal fluid (CSF) otorrhea. At the time of exploration, it is necessary to inspect the ossicles, especially the stapes, for possible dislocation or fracture and to clear sharp objects that might have penetrated the oval or round windows. SNHL results if the stapes subluxates or dislocates into the oval window or if either the oval or round window is penetrated. Children should not be given access to cotton-tipped applicators, because the applicators commonly cause ear trauma. Contact with small objects should be limited to times of parental supervision.

   Perilymphatic fistula can occur after barotrauma or an increase in CSF pressure. It should be suspected in a child who develops a sudden SNHL or vertigo after physical exertion, deep water diving, air travel, playing a wind instrument, or significant head trauma. The leak characteristically is at the oval (Fig. 642-1) or the round window and may be associated with congenital abnormalities of these structures or an anatomic abnormality of the cochlea or semicircular canals. Perilymphatic fistulas occasionally close spontaneously, but immediate surgical repair of the fistula is recommended to control vertigo and to stop any progression of the SNHL; even timely surgery does not usually restore the SNHL. No reliable test is known for perilymphatic fistula, so middle-ear exploration is required for diagnosis and treatment.

TEMPORAL BONE FRACTURES

Children are particularly prone to basilar skull fractures, which usually involve the temporal bone. Temporal bone trauma should be considered in head injuries, and the status of the ear and hearing should be evaluated. Temporal bone fractures are divided into longitudinal (70-80%), transverse, and mixed. Longitudinal fractures (Fig. 642-2) are

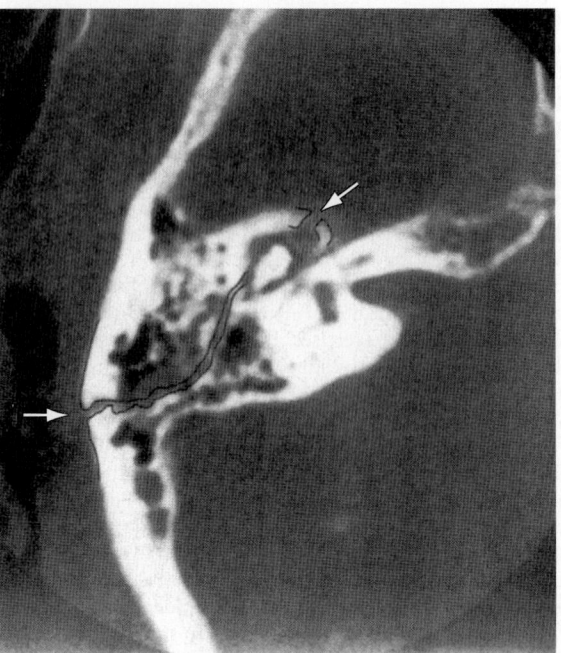

Figure 642-2 High-resolution axial CT of uncomplicated longitudinal fracture *(arrows)*. A hematoma is present. The course of the fracture has been touched. *(From Schubiger O, Valavanis A, Stuckman G, et al: Temporal bone fractures and their complications: examination with high resolution CT. Neuroradiology 28:93–99, 1986.)*

commonly manifested by bleeding from a laceration of the external canal or TM; postauricular ecchymosis **(Battle sign); hemotympanum** (blood behind an intact TM); conductive hearing loss resulting from TM perforation, hemotympanum, or ossicular injury; delayed onset of facial paralysis (which usually improves spontaneously); and temporary CSF otorrhea or rhinorrhea (from CSF running down the eustachian tube). Transverse fractures of the temporal bone have a graver prognosis than longitudinal fractures and are often associated with immediate facial paralysis. Facial paralysis might improve if caused by edema, but surgical decompression of the nerve is often recommended if there is no evidence of clinical recovery and facial nerve studies are unfavorable. If the facial nerve has been transected, surgical decompression and anastomosis offer the possibility of some functional recovery. Transverse fractures are also associated with severe SNHL, vertigo, nystagmus, tinnitus, nausea, and vomiting associated with loss of cochlear and vestibular function; hemotympanum; rarely, external canal bleeding; and CSF otorrhea, either in the external auditory canal or behind the TM, which can exit the nose via the eustachian tube.

   If temporal bone fracture is suspected or seen on radiographs, gentle examination of the pinna and ear canal is indicated; lacerations or avulsion of soft tissue is common with temporal bone fractures. Vigorous removal of external auditory canal blood clots or tympanocentesis is not indicated, because removing the clot can further dislodge the ossicles or reopen CSF leaks. The effectiveness of prophylactic antibiotics to prevent meningitis in patients with basilar skull fractures and CSF otorrhea or rhinorrhea cannot be determined because studies to date are flawed by biases. If a patient is afebrile and the drainage is not cloudy, watchful waiting without antibiotics is indicated. Surgical intervention is reserved for children who require repair of a nonhealing TM perforation, who have suffered dislocation of the ossicular chain, or who need decompression of the facial nerve. SNHL can also follow a blow to the head without an obvious fracture of the temporal bone (labyrinthine concussion).

ACOUSTIC TRAUMA

Acoustic trauma results from exposure to high-intensity sound (fireworks, gunfire, loud music, heavy machinery) and is initially manifested by a temporary decrease in the hearing threshold, most commonly at 4,000 Hz on an audiometric examination, and tinnitus. If the sound is between 85 and 140 dB, the loss is usually temporary (after a rock concert), but both the hearing loss and the tinnitus can become permanent with chronic noise exposure; the frequencies from 3,000-6,000 Hz are most often involved. Sudden, extremely loud (>140 dB), short-duration noises with loud peak components (gunfire, bombs) can cause permanent hearing loss after a single exposure. Noise-induced hearing loss results from interactions between genes and the environment. Ear protection and avoidance of chronic exposure to loud noise are preventive measures. Hearing loss from chronic noise exposure should be entirely preventable. Parents should be made aware of the dangers of acoustic trauma, from the environment and from the use of headphones, and should take measures to minimize exposure. Treatment with high-dose steroids for 1-2 wk should be considered to treat acute hearing loss related to noise trauma.

Bibliography is available at Expert Consult.

Chapter 643
Tumors of the Ear and Temporal Bone
Joseph Haddad Jr. and Sarah Keesecker

Benign tumors of the external canal include osteomas and monostotic and polyostotic fibrous dysplasia. Osteomas manifest as bony masses in the canal and require removal only if hearing is impaired or external otitis results; osteomas may be confused clinically with exostoses (see Chapter 501.2). Masses occurring over the mastoid bone, such as first branchial cysts, dermoid cysts, and lipomas, may be confused with primary mastoid tumors; imaging can help with the diagnosis and treatment plan.

Eosinophilic granuloma, which can occur in isolation or as part of the systemic Langerhans cell histiocytosis (see Chapter 507), should be suspected in patients with otalgia, otorrhea (sometimes bloody), hearing loss, abnormal tissue within the middle ear or ear canal, and roentgenographic findings of a sharply delineated destructive lesion of the temporal bone. Definitive diagnosis is made by biopsy. Treatment depends on the site of the lesion and histology. Depending on the site, it may be treated by surgical excision, curettage, or local radiation. If the lesion is part of a systemic presentation of Langerhans cell histiocytosis, chemotherapy in addition to local therapy (surgery with or without radiation) is indicated. Long-term follow-up is necessary whether the temporal bone lesion is a single isolated lesion or part of a multisystem disease.

Symptoms and signs of rhabdomyosarcoma (see Chapter 500) originating in the middle ear or ear canal include a mass or polyp in the middle ear or ear canal, bleeding from the ear, otorrhea, otalgia, facial paralysis, and hearing loss. Other cranial nerves also may be involved. Diagnosis is based on biopsy, but the extent of disease is determined by both CT and MRI of the temporal and facial bones, skull base, and brain (Fig. 643-1). Management usually involves a combination of chemotherapy, radiation, and surgery.

Non-Hodgkin lymphoma (see Chapter 496.2) and leukemia (see Chapter 495) also occur rarely in the temporal bone. Although primary neoplasms of the middle ear are very uncommon in children, they include adenoid cystic carcinoma, adenocarcinoma, and squamous cell carcinoma. Benign tumors of the temporal bone include glomus tumors. The initial signs and symptoms of the more common nasopharyngeal neoplasms (angiofibroma, rhabdomyosarcoma, epidermoid carcinoma) may be associated with insidious onset of chronic otitis media with effusion (often unilateral). A high index of suspicion is needed for diagnosing these tumors early.

Bibliography is available at Expert Consult.

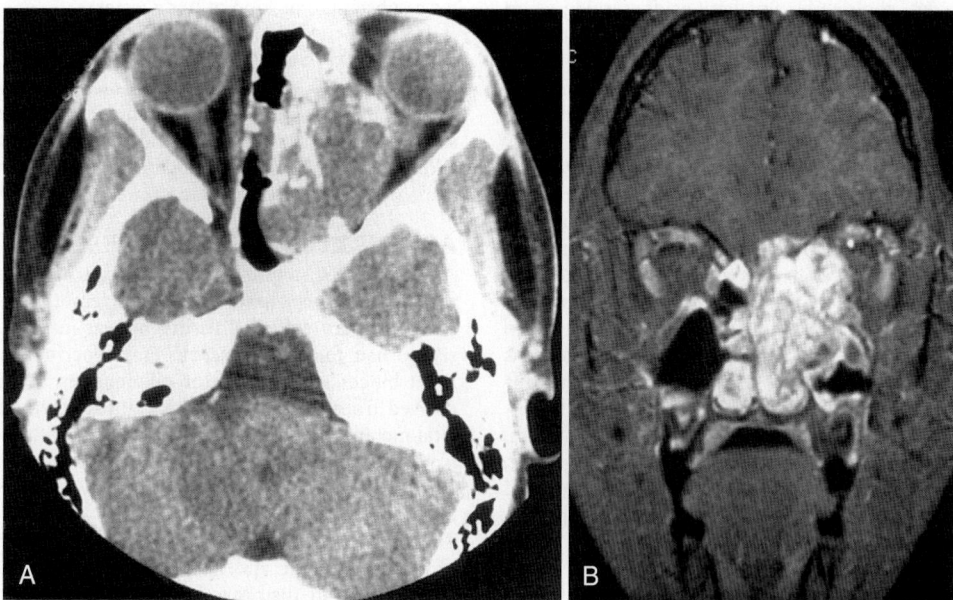

Figure 643-1 Rhabdomyosarcoma in a 2 yr old child presenting with a large mass in the nose. **A,** CT scan of the head shows destruction of the nose and lamina papyracea; a large soft tissue mass is present. **B,** MRI shows enhancement of the mass. *(From Slovis T, editor:* Caffey's pediatric diagnostic imaging, *ed 11, Philadelphia, 2008, Mosby, p. 560.)*

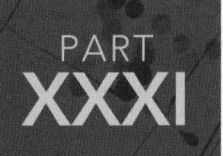

The Skin

Chapter **644**

Morphology of the Skin

Brianne Z. Dickey and Yvonne E. Chiu

EPIDERMIS

The mature epidermis is a stratified epithelial tissue composed predominantly of keratinocytes. The function of the epidermis is protection of the organism from the external environment, through physical, chemical, and immunologic barrier functions, and the prevention of water loss. The process of epidermal differentiation results in the formation of a functional barrier to the external world. The epidermis comprises four histologically recognizable layers, described here from deepest to most superficial. The first or basal layer consists of columnar cells that rest on the dermal–epidermal junction. Basal keratinocytes are connected to the dermal–epidermal junction by hemidesmosomes. Basal keratinocytes are attached to themselves and to the cells in the spinous layer by desmosomal, tight, gap, and adherens junctions. The role of the basal keratinocyte is to serve as a continuing supply of keratinocytes for the normally differentiating epidermis as well as a reservoir of cells to repair epidermal damage. The second layer is the spinous layer, composed of 3-4 layers of spinous cells. Their role is to synthesize keratin, which makes up the keratin intermediate filament network. The third layer is the granular layer, which consists of 2-3 layers of granular cells. Granular cells contain keratohyalin and lamellar granules, containing the protein and lipid components that make up the cornified layer. The fourth layer, or cornified layer, is composed of multiple layers of dead, highly compacted cells. The dead cells are composed mainly of disulfide-bonded keratins crosslinked by filaggrins. The intercellular spaces are composed of hydrophobic lipids, predominantly ceramides, cholesterol, and fatty acids, serving as an effective barrier against water and salt loss as well as permeation of water-soluble substances. As the cornified layer is replenished, the oldest or most superficial layer is shed in a highly regulated process. The normal process of epidermal differentiation from basal cell to shedding of cornified layer takes 28 days.

The epidermis also contains 3 other cell types. The **melanocytes** are pigment-forming cells, which are responsible for skin color and protection from ultraviolet radiation. Epidermal melanocytes are derived from the neural crest and migrate to the skin during embryonic life. They reside in the interfollicular epidermis and in the hair follicles. Melanocytes produce intracellular organelles (melanosomes) containing melanin, which they transfer via dendrites to the keratinocytes to protect the keratinocyte nucleus from ultraviolet damage. **Merkel** cells are type I slow-adapting mechanosensory receptors for touch that differentiate within the epidermis from epidermal progenitor cells. **Langerhans** cells are dendritic cells of the mononuclear phagocyte system. They are recognized electron microscopically by a specific organelle, the Birbeck granule. These cells are derived from bone marrow and participate in immune reactions in the skin, playing an active part in antigen presentation and processing.

The junction of the epidermis and dermis is the basement membrane zone. This complex structure is a result of contributions from both epidermal and mesenchymal cells. The dermal-epidermal junction extends from the basal cell plasma membrane to the uppermost region of the dermis. Ultrastructurally, the basement membrane appears as a trilaminar structure, consisting of a lamina lucida immediately adjacent to the basal cell plasma membrane, a central lamina densa, and the subbasal lamina on the dermal side of the lamina densa. Several structures within this zone act to anchor the epidermis to the dermis. The plasma membrane of basal cells contains electron-dense plates known as hemidesmosomes; tonofilaments course within basal cells to insert at these sites. The **hemidesmosomes** are composed of 180- and 230-kDa bullous pemphigoid antigens (BP180 [type XVII collagen] and BP230, respectively), $\alpha_6\beta_4$ and $\alpha_3\beta_1$ integrins, and plectin. Anchoring filaments originate in the plasma membrane, primarily near the hemidesmosomes, and insert into the lamina densa. Anchoring fibrils, composed predominantly of type VII collagen, extend from the lamina densa into the uppermost dermis, where they loop through collagen fibrils before reinserting into the lamina densa.

DERMIS

The dermis provides the skin with most of its mechanical properties. The dermis forms a tough, pliable, fibrous supporting structure between the epidermis and the subcutaneous fat. The predominant dermal cell is a spindle-shaped fibroblast that is responsible for the synthesis of collagen, elastic fibers, and mucopolysaccharides. Phagocytic histiocytes, mast cells, and motile leukocytes are also present. Within the dermis are blood vessels, lymphatics, neural structures, eccrine and apocrine sweat glands, hair follicles, sebaceous glands, and smooth muscle. Morphologically, the dermis can be divided into 2 layers: the superficial papillary layer that interdigitates with the rete ridges of the epidermis and the deeper reticular layer that lies beneath the papillary dermis. The papillary layer is less dense and more cellular, whereas the reticular layer appears more compact because of the coarse network of interlaced collagen and elastic fibers.

The extracellular matrix of the dermis consists of collagen and elastic fibers embedded in an amorphous ground substance. Collagen provides strength and stability to the dermis, while elastic fibers allow for elasticity. The gelatinous ground substance serves as a supporting medium for the fibrillar and cellular components and as a storage place for a substantial portion of body water.

SUBCUTANEOUS TISSUE

The **panniculus,** or subcutaneous tissue, consists of fat cells and fibrous septa that divide it into lobules and anchor it to the underlying fascia and periosteum. Blood vessels and nerves are also present in this layer, which serves as a storage depot for lipid, an insulator to conserve body heat, and a protective cushion against trauma.

APPENDAGEAL STRUCTURES

Appendageal structures are derived from aggregates of epidermal cells that become specialized during early embryonic development. Small buds (primary epithelial germs) appear in the 3rd fetal mo and give rise to hair follicles, sebaceous and apocrine glands, and the attachment bulges for the arrector pili muscles. Eccrine sweat glands are derived from separate epidermal downgrowths that arise in the 2nd fetal mo and are completely formed by the 5th mo. Formation of nails is initiated in the 3rd intrauterine mo.

Hair Follicles

The pilosebaceous unit includes the hair follicle, sebaceous gland, arrector pili muscle, and, in areas such as the axillae, an apocrine gland. Hair follicles are distributed throughout the skin, except in the palms, soles, lips, and glans penis. Individual follicles extend from the surface of the epidermis to the deep dermis. The hair follicle is divided into 4 segments: the infundibulum, which extends from the skin surface to the opening of the sebaceous duct; the isthmus, extending from the sebaceous duct opening to the bulge; the lower follicle between the bulge and the hair bulb; and the hair bulb. The bulge is at the insertion of the arrector pili muscle and is a focus of epidermal stem cells. The bulb is where the matrix cells and the dermal papilla are involved in formation and maintenance of the hair. The growing hair consists of the hair shaft, made of dead keratinocytes, and its supporting inner and outer root sheaths.

Human hair growth is cyclic, with alternate periods of growth (anagen), transition (catagen), and rest (telogen). The length of the anagen phase varies from months to years. At birth, all hairs are in the anagen phase. Subsequent generative activity lacks synchrony, so an overall random pattern of growth and shedding prevails. At any time, approximately 85% of hairs are in the anagen phase. Scalp hair usually grows about 1 cm per month.

The types of hair are lanugo, terminal, and vellus hairs. Lanugo hair is thin and short; this hair is shed in utero and is replaced by vellus hair by 36-40 wk of gestation. Vellus hair is short, soft, and frequently unpigmented and is distributed over the rest of the body. Terminal hair is long and coarse and is found on the scalp, beard, eyebrows, eyelashes, and axillary and pubic areas. During puberty, androgenic hormone stimulation causes pubic, axillary, and beard hair to change from vellus hair to terminal hair.

Sebaceous Glands
Sebaceous glands occur in all areas except the palms, soles, and dorsal feet and are most numerous on the face, upper chest, and back. Their ducts open into the hair follicles except on the lips, prepuce, and labia minora, where they emerge directly onto the mucosal surface. These holocrine glands are saccular structures that are often branched and lobulated and consist of a proliferative basal layer of small flat cells peripheral to the central mass of lipidized cells. The latter cells disintegrate as they move toward the duct and form the lipid secretion known as sebum, which consists of triglycerides, wax esters, squalene, and cholesterol esters. The purpose of sebum production likely relates to hydrophobic skin barrier function. Sebaceous glands depend on hormonal stimulation and are activated by androgens at puberty. Fetal sebaceous glands are stimulated by maternal androgens, and their lipid secretion, together with desquamated stratum corneum cells, constitutes the vernix caseosa.

Apocrine Glands
The apocrine glands are located in the axillae, areolae, perianal and genital areas, and the periumbilical region. These large, coiled, tubular structures continuously secrete an odorless milky fluid that is discharged in response to adrenergic stimuli, usually as a result of emotional stress. Bacterial biotransformation of apocrine sweat components (fatty acids, thioalcohols, and steroids) accounts for the unpleasant odor associated with perspiration. Apocrine glands remain dormant until puberty, when they enlarge and secretion begins in response to androgenic activity. The secretory coil of the gland consists of a single layer of cells enclosed by a layer of contractile myoepithelial cells. The duct is lined with a double layer of cuboidal cells and opens into the pilosebaceous complex. Although apocrine glands do not function in thermoregulation, they are involved in certain disease processes.

Eccrine Sweat Glands
Eccrine sweat glands are distributed over the entire body surface and are most abundant on the palms and soles. Those on the hairy skin respond to thermal stimuli and serve to regulate body temperature by delivering water to the skin surface for evaporation; in contrast, sweat glands on the palms and soles respond mainly to psychophysiologic stimuli.

Each eccrine gland consists of a secretory coil located in the reticular dermis or subcutaneous fat and a secretory duct that opens onto the skin surface. Sweat pores can be identified on the epidermal ridges of the palm and fingers with a magnifying lens but are not readily visualized elsewhere. Two types of cells constitute the single-layered secretory coil: small dark cells and large clear cells. These rest on a layer of contractile myoepithelial cells and a basement membrane. The glands are supplied by sympathetic nerve fibers, but the pharmacologic mediator of sweating is acetylcholine rather than epinephrine. Sweat from these glands consists of water, sodium, potassium, calcium, chloride, phosphorus, lactate, and small quantities of iron, glucose, and protein. The composition varies with the rate of sweating but is always hypotonic in normal children.

Nails
Nails are specialized protective epidermal structures that form convex, translucent, tight-fitting plates on the distal dorsal surfaces of the fingers and toes. The nail plate, which is derived from a metabolically active matrix of multiplying cells situated beneath the posterior nail fold, is composed of anucleate keratinocytes. Nail growth is relatively slow; complete fingernail regrowth takes 6 mo, while complete toenail regrowth requires 12-18 mo. The nail plate is bounded by the lateral and posterior nail folds; a thin eponychium (the cuticle) protrudes from the posterior fold over a crescent-shaped white area called the lunula. The eponychium serves as a sealant barrier to protect the germinal matrix of the nail plate. The pink color beneath the nail reflects the underlying vascular bed. Nail health relies on several factors, including nutrition, hydration, local infection/irritation, and systemic disease.

Bibliography is available at Expert Consult.

Chapter 645
Evaluation of the Patient
Brianne Z. Dickey and Yvonne E. Chiu

HISTORY AND PHYSICAL EXAMINATION
Although many skin disorders are easily recognized by simple inspection, the history and physical examination are often necessary for accurate assessment. The skin examination should be performed under adequate illumination. In addition to the skin covering the entire body surface, mucous membranes (conjunctiva, oropharynx, nasal mucosa, anogenital mucosa), hair, and nails should be examined when appropriate. The color, turgor, texture, temperature, and moisture of the skin and the growth, texture, caliber, and luster of the hair and nails should be noted. Skin lesions should be palpated, inspected, and classified on the bases of morphology, size, color, texture, firmness, configuration, location, and distribution. One must also decide whether the changes are those of the *primary* lesion itself or whether the clinical pattern has been altered by a *secondary* factor such as infection, trauma, or therapy.

Primary lesions are classified as macules, papules, patches, plaques, nodules, tumors, vesicles, bullae, pustules, wheals, and cysts. A **macule** represents an alteration in skin color but cannot be felt. When the lesion is >1 cm, the term **patch** is used. **Papules** are palpable solid lesions <1 cm. **Plaques** are palpable lesions >1 cm in size and have a flat surface. **Nodules** are palpable lesions >1 cm with a rounded surface. The word **tumor** may be used for a large nodule that is suspected to be neoplastic in origin. Vesicles are raised, fluid-filled lesions <1 cm in diameter; when larger, they are called **bullae. Pustules** contain purulent material. **Wheals** are flat-topped, palpable lesions of variable size, duration, and configuration that represent dermal collections of edema fluid. **Cysts** are circumscribed, thick-walled lesions; they are covered by a normal epidermis and contain fluid or semisolid material.

Primary lesions may change into secondary lesions, or secondary lesions may develop over time where no primary lesion existed.

Primary lesions are usually more helpful for diagnostic purposes than secondary lesions. Secondary lesions include scales, purpura, petechiae, ulcers, erosions, excoriations, fissures, crusts, and scars. **Scales** consist of compressed layers of stratum corneum cells that are retained on the skin surface. **Purpura** are the result of bleeding into the skin and have a red-purple color; they may be flat or palpable. **Petechiae** are small purpura <2-3 mm. **Erosions** involve focal loss of the epidermis, and they heal without scarring. **Ulcers** extend into the dermis and tend to heal with scarring. Ulcerated lesions inflicted by scratching are often linear or angular in configuration and are called **excoriations.** **Fissures** are caused by splitting or cracking. **Crusts** consist of matted, retained accumulations of blood, serum, pus, and epithelial debris on the surface of a weeping lesion. **Scars** are end-stage lesions that can be thin, depressed, and atrophic; raised and hypertrophic; or flat and pliable. **Lichenification** is a thickening of skin with accentuation of normal skin lines that is caused by chronic irritation (rubbing, scratching) or inflammation.

If the diagnosis is not clear after a thorough examination, 1 or more diagnostic procedures may be indicated.

BIOPSY OF SKIN

Biopsy of skin is occasionally required for diagnosis. Punch biopsy is a simple, relatively painless procedure and usually provides adequate tissue for examination if the appropriate lesion is sampled. The selection of a fresh, well-developed primary lesion is extremely important to obtain an accurate diagnosis. The site of the biopsy should have relatively low risk for damage to underlying dermal structures. After cleansing of the site, the skin is anesthetized by intradermal injection of 1-2% lidocaine, with or without epinephrine, with a 27- or 30-gauge needle. A punch, 3 or 4 mm in diameter, is pressed firmly against the skin and rotated until it sinks to the proper depth. All 3 layers (epidermis, dermis, subcutis) should be contained in the plug. The plug should be lifted gently with forceps or extracted with a needle and separated from the underlying tissue with iris scissors. Bleeding abates with firm pressure and with suturing. The biopsy specimen should be placed in 10% formaldehyde solution (Formalin) for appropriate processing.

WOOD LAMP

A Wood lamp emits ultraviolet light mainly at a wavelength of 365 nm. The examination, which is performed in a darkened room, is useful in accentuating changes in pigmentation and detecting fluorescence in certain infectious disorders. Discrete areas of altered pigment can often be visualized more clearly by using a Wood lamp, particularly if the pigmentary change is epidermal. Hyperpigmented lesions appear darker, and hypopigmented lesions (e.g., those seen in **tuberous sclerosis**), lighter than the surrounding skin. Blue-green fluorescence is detectable at the base of each infected hair shaft in ectothrix infections, such as tinea capitis caused by *Microsporum* species. Scales and crusts may appear pale yellow, but this color is not evidence of a fungal infection. Dermatophyte lesions of the skin (tinea corporis) do not fluoresce; macules of tinea versicolor have a golden fluorescence under a Wood lamp. **Erythrasma**, an intertriginous infection caused by *Corynebacterium minutissimum*, may fluoresce pink-orange, whereas *Pseudomonas aeruginosa* is yellow-green under a Wood lamp.

POTASSIUM HYDROXIDE PREPARATION

Potassium hydroxide (KOH) preparation is a rapid and reliable method for detecting fungal elements of both yeasts and dermatophytes. Scaly lesions should be scraped at the active border for optimal recovery of mycelia and spores. Vesicles should be unroofed, and the blister roof should be clipped and placed on a slide for examination. In tinea capitis, infected hairs must be plucked from the follicle; scales from the scalp do not usually contain mycelia. A few drops of 20% KOH are added to the specimen. Dimethyl sulfoxide is usually in solution with the KOH, negating the need to heat the specimen. If using KOH without dimethyl sulfoxide, the specimen is gently heated over an alcohol lamp or on a hot plate until the KOH begins to bubble. Alternatively, sufficient time (10-20 min) can be allowed for dissolution of the keratin at room temperature. The preparation is examined under low-intensity light microscopy for fungal elements.

TZANCK SMEAR

Tzanck smear is useful in the diagnosis of infections caused by herpes simplex virus or varicella zoster virus and for the detection of acantholytic cells in pemphigus. An intact, fresh vesicle is ruptured and drained of fluid. The roof and base of the blister are then carefully scraped with a no. 15 scalpel blade, with care taken to avoid drawing a significant amount of blood; the material is smeared on a clear glass slide and air dried. Staining with Giemsa stain is preferable, but Wright stain is acceptable. Balloon cells and multinucleated giant cells are diagnostic of herpesvirus infection; acantholytic epidermal cells are characteristic of pemphigus.

Direct fluorescent assay and polymerase chain reaction tests have largely replaced Tzanck smears in the diagnosis of herpes simplex and varicella zoster infections. Both of these are rapid, sensitive, and specific, with the polymerase chain reaction even more so. When obtaining specimens for these tests, the vesicles should be ruptured prior to sample collection with the swab.

IMMUNOFLUORESCENCE STUDIES

Immunofluorescence studies of skin can be used to detect tissue-fixed antibodies to skin components and complement; characteristic staining patterns are specific for certain skin disorders (Table 645-1). Direct immunofluorescence detects autoantibodies bound to cutaneous antigens in the skin, while indirect immunofluorescence detects circulating autoantibodies present in the serum.

Skin biopsy specimens for direct immunofluorescence should be obtained from involved sites except in those diseases for which perilesional skin or uninvolved skin is required. A punch biopsy sample is obtained, and the tissue is placed in a special transport medium or immediately frozen in liquid nitrogen for transport or storage. Thin cryostat sections of the specimen are incubated with fluorescein-conjugated antibodies to the specific antigens.

Serum of patients can be examined by indirect immunofluorescence techniques using sections of normal human skin, guinea pig lip, or monkey esophagus as substrate. The substrate is incubated with fresh or thawed frozen serum and then with fluorescein-conjugated antihuman globulin. If the serum contains antibody to epithelial components, its specific staining pattern can be seen on fluorescence microscopy. By serial dilution, the titer of circulating antibody can be estimated.

645.1 Cutaneous Manifestations of Systemic Diseases

Brianne Z. Dickey and Yvonne E. Chiu

Selected diseases have signature skin findings, often as the presenting signs of illness, that can facilitate the assessment of patients with complex medical states (Table 645-2).

CONNECTIVE TISSUE DISEASES

Lupus Erythematosus

Lupus erythematosus (LE; see Chapter 158) is an idiopathic autoimmune inflammatory disease that may be multisystemic (i.e., systemic LE or SLE) or confined to the skin. Distinct cutaneous lupus subtypes seen in children include acute cutaneous LE, subacute cutaneous LE, chronic cutaneous LE (including discoid LE, discussed under "Discoid Lupus Erythematosus"), and neonatal LE (discussed under "Neonatal Lupus Erythematosus").

Systemic Lupus Erythematosus

SLE is a chronic inflammatory multisystem disease. It is diagnosed when 4 of 11 well-defined criteria are present (see Chapter 158). Three of the criteria are skin findings. Criterion 1 is the classic malar or "butterfly" rash (Fig. 645-1). It must be distinguished from other causes of a "red face," most notably seborrheic dermatitis, atopic dermatitis, and

Table 645-1	Immunofluorescence Findings in Immune-Mediated Cutaneous Diseases				
DISEASE	**INVOLVED SKIN**	**UNINVOLVED SKIN**	**DIRECT IF FINDINGS**	**INDIRECT IF FINDINGS**	**CIRCULATING ANTIBODIES**
Dermatitis herpetiformis	Negative	Positive	Granular IgA ± C in papillary dermis	None	IgA antiendomysial and transglutaminase antibodies
Bullous pemphigoid	Positive	Positive	Linear IgG and C band in BMZ, occasionally IgM, IgA, IgE	IgG to BMZ	IgG anti-BP180 and anti-BP230
Pemphigus (all variants)	Positive	Positive	IgG in intercellular spaces of epidermis between keratinocytes	IgG to intercellular spaces of epidermis between keratinocytes	IgG antidesmoglein 1 and 3 (pemphigus vulgaris and foliaceus). IgA antidesmocollin 1 (IgA pemphigus).
Linear IgA bullous dermatosis (chronic bullous dermatosis of childhood)	Positive	Positive	Linear IgA at BMZ, occasionally C	Low titer, rare IgA, anti-BP180	None
Discoid lupus erythematosus	Positive	Negative	Linear IgG, IgM, IgA, and C3 at BMZ (lupus band)	None	Usually ANA-negative
Systemic lupus erythematosus	Positive	Variable; exposed to sun, 30-50%; nonexposed, 10-30%	Linear IgG, IgM, IgA, and C3 at BMZ (lupus band)	None	ANA Anti-Ro (SSA), anti-La (SSB) Anti-RNP Anti-dsDNA Anti-Sm
Henoch-Schönlein purpura	Positive	Positive	IgA around vessel walls	None	None

ANA, antinuclear antibody; BMZ, basement membrane zone at the dermal–epidermal junction; BP, bullous pemphigoid; C, complement; dsDNA, double-stranded deoxyribonucleic acid; IF, immunofluorescence; Ig, immunoglobulin; Sm, Smith; SSA/SSB, Sjögren syndrome A/B; RNP, ribonucleoprotein.

rosacea. Criterion 2 is discoid lupus lesions. Criterion 3 is a photosensitive erythematous macular or papular eruption (Fig. 645-2). Other associated but not diagnostic cutaneous findings include purpuric lesions, livedo reticularis, mucosal ulcerations, Raynaud phenomenon, urticaria, and nonscarring alopecia.

On histology, cutaneous LE demonstrates varying degrees of epidermal atrophy, plugging of hair follicles, and a vacuolar alteration at an inflamed dermal-epidermal junction. Deposition of immunoglobulins (IgM, IgG) and complement in lesional skin may help confirm the diagnosis. Immune deposits in nonlesional sun-exposed skin are found in the majority of patients with SLE (lupus band test), although clinical use of this test has been mostly abandoned in favor of serologic testing.

The skin lesions often respond to treatment of the SLE with systemic agents. Oral hydroxychloroquine is used most commonly, but many other systemic therapies are effective, including both classic and biologic immunosuppressants. Low- to mid-potency topical corticosteroids, topical calcineurin inhibitors, and intralesional corticosteroid injection may be considered for adjunctive therapy.

Neonatal Lupus Erythematosus
Neonatal LE (see Chapter 158.1) manifests at birth or during the 1st few wk of life as annular, erythematous, scaly plaques, typically on the head, neck, and upper trunk (Fig. 645-3). Telangiectasias are also common. Ultraviolet light may exacerbate or initiate cutaneous lesions. Passive transplacental transfer of maternal anti-Ro/SSA and anti-La/SSB antibodies causes the transient skin lesions, though most infants are born to mothers without a known rheumatologic diagnosis. Antibody levels wane by 6 mo, generally resulting in clearance of the rash. Congenital heart block occurs in 30% of affected infants, but only 10% of affected infants have both skin and cardiac abnormalities. Noncardiac extracutaneous manifestations, such as anemia, thrombocytopenia, and cholestatic liver disease are less common. Neonatal LE is often misdiagnosed as infantile eczema, seborrheic dermatitis, or tinea corporis. Skin lesions are typically managed conservatively given the transient nature of neonatal LE, and strict sun avoidance and protection

are important. If necessary, low- to mid-potency topical corticosteroids may be used. Systemic agents should be avoided. Maternal antinuclear antibody testing is indicated.

Discoid Lupus Erythematosus
Discoid LE (DLE) is uncommon in early childhood and manifests in late adolescence. The signature skin findings in DLE are chronic, erythematous, scaly, atrophic plaques (Fig. 645-4) on sun-exposed skin that frequently heal with scarring and dyspigmentation. Extracutaneous features may include involvement of the nasal and oral mucosa, eyes, and nails. The differential diagnosis includes other photodermatoses, such as polymorphous light eruption, juvenile springtime eruption, and juvenile dermatomyositis. There is a distinct overlap between SLE and DLE, with common histopathologic features and photoexacerbation; most patients with DLE have normal laboratory results and do not progress to systemic disease.

First-line treatment of DLE consists of low- to mid-potency topical corticosteroids. Other topical options include calcineurin inhibitors, retinoids, and topically-applied R-salbutamol. Intralesional corticosteroid injection is also effective for severe localized lesions. Oral hydroxychloroquine is used first-line for severe skin disease or as a second-line agent when lesions are not controlled with topical or local agents. Strict ultraviolet light avoidance is important.

Juvenile Dermatomyositis
Characteristic skin findings are often the presenting sign of juvenile dermatomyositis (JDM; see Chapter 159). An ill-defined, erythematous to violaceous, scaly, minimally pruritic eruption occurs in photodistributed areas such as the face, upper trunk, and extensor extremities. Circumscribed periocular involvement of this **heliotrope** rash involving the eyelids may take the appearance of "raccoon eyes," particularly in young children. Distinctive erythematous, scaly papules overlying the knuckles and other joints (**Gottron papules**) are helpful in suggesting the diagnosis in the absence of associated muscle weakness (Fig. 645-5). Other cutaneous features include nail fold and gingival margin telangiectasia, palmar hyperkeratosis ("mechanic's hands"),

Table 645-2 Characteristics of Cutaneous Signs of Systemic Diseases

DISEASE	AGE OF ONSET	SKIN LESIONS	DISTRIBUTION	DIAGNOSTIC EVALUATION(S) AND FINDINGS	ASSOCIATED SYMPTOMS/SIGNS	DIFFERENTIAL DIAGNOSIS
Systemic lupus erythematosus	Any	Erythematous patches; palpable purpura; livedo reticularis; Raynaud phenomenon; thrombocytopenic and nonthrombocytopenic purpura	Photodistribution; "malar" face	ANA panel Anti-dsDNA Leukopenia/lymphopenia Thrombocytopenia Complement levels Urinalysis	Arthritis Nephritis Cerebritis Serositis	Seborrheic dermatitis Atopic dermatitis Juvenile dermatomyositis
Discoid lupus erythematosus	Any	Annular, scaly plaques; atrophy; dyspigmentation	Photodistribution	ANA	Scarring	Subacute cutaneous lupus Polymorphous light eruption Juvenile dermatomyositis
Neonatal lupus erythematosus	Newborn	Annular, erythematous, scaly plaques	Head/neck	ANA Anti-Ro (SSA), anti-La (SSB)	Heart block Thrombocytopenia	Tinea capitis Atopic dermatitis Seborrheic dermatitis
Juvenile dermatomyositis	Any	Erythematous to violaceous scaly, macules; discrete papules overlying knuckles	Periocular face; shoulder girdle; extensor extremities; knuckles; palms	ANA AST ALT Aldolase Creatine kinase Lactate dehydrogenase	Proximal muscle weakness Calcifications Vasculopathy	Atopic dermatitis Allergic contact dermatitis Lupus erythematosus
Henoch-Schönlein purpura	Childhood and adolescence	Purpuric papules and plaques	Buttocks; lower extremities	Urinalysis Blood urea nitrogen/creatinine ratio Skin biopsy	Abdominal pain Arthritis	Vasculitis Drug eruption Infantile hemorrhagic edema Viral exanthem
Kawasaki disease	Infancy, childhood	Erythematous maculopapular to urticarial plaques; acral and groin erythema, edema, desquamation	Diffuse	Leukocytosis ESR C-reactive protein Thrombocytosis	Strawberry tongue Conjunctivitis Lymphadenopathy Cardiovascular complications	Viral syndrome Drug eruption Staphylococcal/streptococcal illness
Inflammatory bowel disease	Childhood and adolescence	Aphthae; erythema nodosum; pyoderma gangrenosum; thrombophlebitis	Oral ulcers; perianal fissures	Skin biopsy	Abdominal pain Diarrhea Cramping Arthritis Conjunctivitis	Behçet syndrome Vasculitis Yersinia colitis
Sweet syndrome	Any	Infiltrated erythematous, edematous plaques	Diffuse	Skin biopsy Leukocytosis ESR	Fever Flu-like illness Conjunctivitis	Infection Urticaria Erythema multiforme Urticarial vasculitis
Graft-versus-host disease	Any	Acute: erythema, papules, vesicles, bulla	Head and neck; palms/soles; diffuse	Skin biopsy Liver function	Fever Mucositis Hepatitis	Drug eruption Infectious exanthem
Drug rash with eosinophilia and systemic symptoms (DRESS syndrome)	Any	Erythema; urticarial macules and plaques	Diffuse	Liver function Eosinophilia Atypical lymphocytosis	Perioral edema Lymphadenopathy Fever Hepatitis	Stevens-Johnson syndrome Infectious exanthem
Serum sickness–like reaction (SSLR)	Any	Edematous, urticarial plaques	Acral; diffuse	None	Fever Lymphadenopathy Arthritis, nephritis	Kawasaki disease Urticaria

ANA, antinuclear antibodies; ALT, alanine aminotransferase; AST, aspartate aminotransferase; dsDNA, double-stranded deoxyribonucleic acid; ESR, erythrocyte sedimentation rate; SSA/SSB, Sjögren's syndrome A/B.

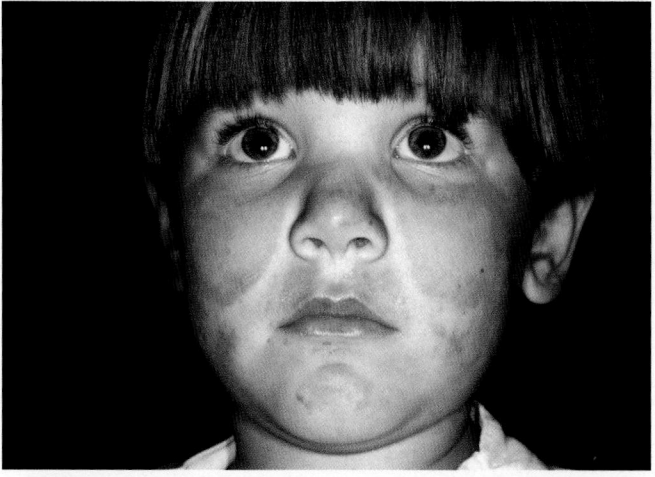

Figure 645-1 Malar rash of systemic lupus erythematosus.

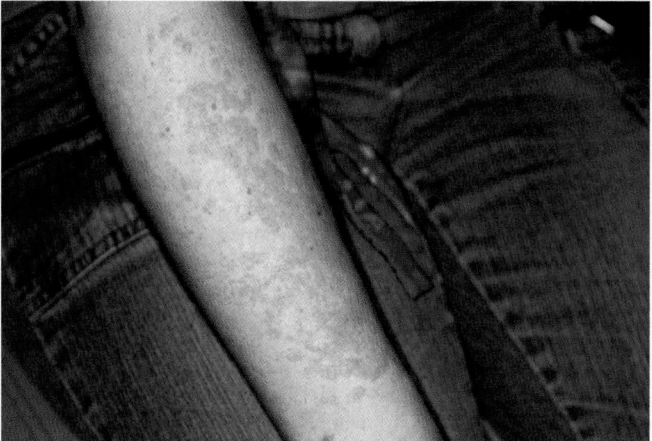

Figure 645-2 Photosensitive rash of systemic lupus erythematosus.

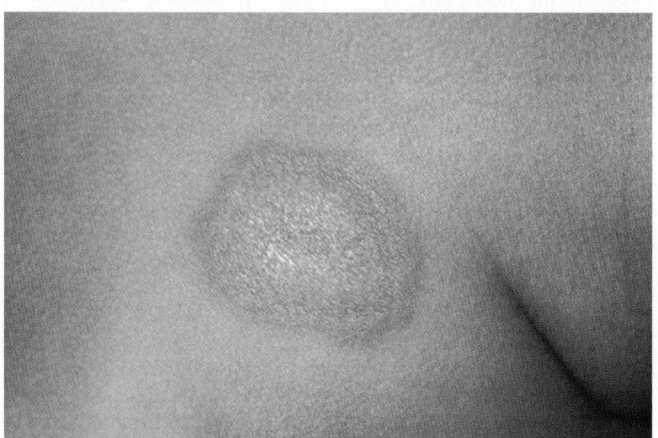

Figure 645-3 Annular plaque in neonatal lupus erythematosus.

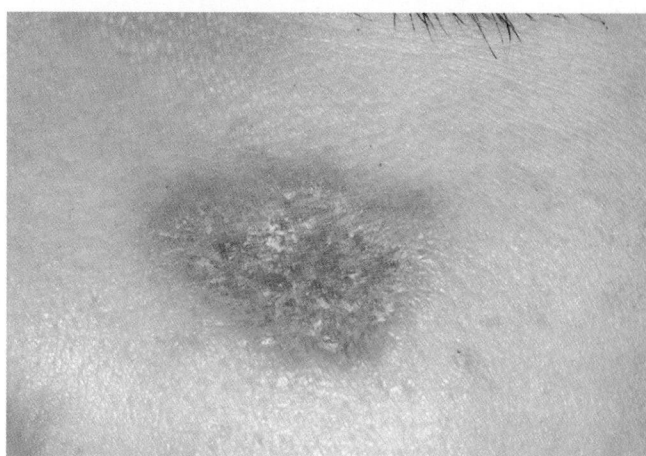

Figure 645-4 Erythematous scaly plaque of discoid lupus erythematosus.

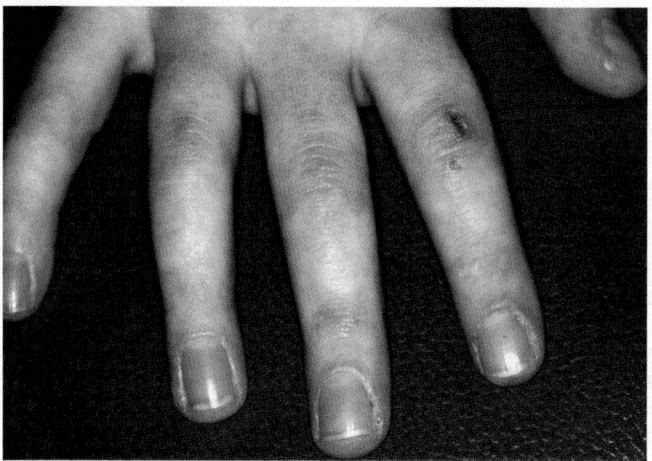

Figure 645-5 Gottron papules in juvenile dermatomyositis.

ulceration resulting from vasculopathy or underlying calcinosis, lipodystrophy, and a poikilodermatous (dyspigmentation and telangiectasia) eruption over the shoulder girdle ("shawl sign"). Cutaneous features may precede the systemic illness, which is primarily characterized by muscle weakness and pain. The differential diagnosis includes atopic dermatitis, other connective tissue diseases, lichen planus, medication reactions, and infectious exanthems. Lesional skin demonstrates epidermal atrophy and vacuolar degeneration at the dermal-epidermal junction, often similar to LE. JDM is distinct from adult dermatomyositis in both presentation and prognosis. Pediatric patients have more difficulty with gastrointestinal vasculopathy and cutaneous calcifications, and JDM is not a paraneoplastic phenomenon as in adults. A rare clinical variant known as **amyopathic dermatomyositis** occurs when only skin, and not muscle, is involved.

Skin lesions benefit from systemic immunosuppressive therapy as discussed in detail in Chapter 159. Additional treatment options for localized skin disease include topical corticosteroids and calcineurin inhibitors. In case reports, the cutaneous calcinosis of JDM has been difficult to manage with a variety of agents, and no treatment consensus exists. Strict photoprotection and sunlight avoidance are vital to prevent cutaneous exacerbations.

Systemic Sclerosis

Systemic sclerosis frequently manifests as acral (sclerodactyly, ulceration, nail fold telangiectasia, or Raynaud phenomenon) and facial changes (pinched nose, furrowed perioral skin, or "scleroderma facies") (see Chapter 160). Overlap syndromes such as **mixed connective tissue disease** may include some physical and laboratory features of scleroderma.

VASCULITIDES

The vasculitides (see Chapter 167) encompass a broad group of disorders having considerable overlap with connective tissue diseases. Immune-mediated inflammation of blood vessels of varying size may be caused by an underlying inflammatory state, infection, medication, or malignancy. Common clinical features include **palpable**

Part XXXI ◆ The Skin

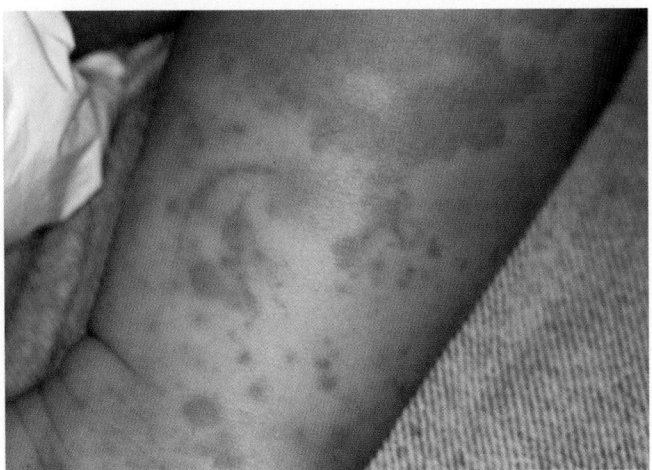

Figure 645-6 Purpura of the lower leg in Henoch-Schönlein purpura.

nonthrombocytopenic purpuric skin lesions, arthritis, fever, myalgia, fatigue, and weight loss as well as an elevated erythrocyte sedimentation rate. Extracutaneous organs that may be involved include the joints, lungs, kidneys, and central nervous system.

Henoch-Schönlein Purpura (Immunoglobulin A Vasculitis)

Henoch-Schönlein purpura (see Chapter 167.1) is a vasculitis that manifests in school-age children as palpable purpuric lesions in gravity dependent areas, predominantly the buttocks and lower extremities (Fig. 645-6). **Infantile hemorrhagic edema (IHE;** also called acute hemorrhagic edema of infancy) shares some clinical features with Henoch-Schönlein purpura but appears in infants and toddlers. Infantile hemorrhagic edema is characterized by the sudden onset of circumscribed edema with purpuric papules and plaques on the trunk and extremities but, unlike Henoch-Schönlein purpura, commonly affects the face and lacks other organ involvement. Henoch-Schönlein purpura must also be differentiated from infectious causes of purpuric skin lesions, such as meningococcemia, Rocky Mountain spotted fever, and purpuric viral exanthems such as those caused by enteroviruses, as well as from juvenile rheumatoid arthritis and other vasculitides. Diagnosis is confirmed by histologic confirmation of a small vessel vasculitis with the immunofluorescence finding of IgA in blood vessel walls. Skin lesions are generally managed conservatively and self-resolve in 3-4 wk. Systemic treatment is discussed in detail in Chapter 167.1.

Kawasaki Disease

Kawasaki disease (see Chapter 166) is a clinical diagnosis based on both cutaneous and extracutaneous features in children younger than age 5 yr. The skin eruption of Kawasaki disease may be polymorphic, manifesting variously as maculopapular or morbilliform patches and plaques or rarely urticarial on the trunk and extremities. Early involvement with erythema and peeling in the perineum/inguinal region may be an initial clue to the diagnosis. Acral edema and desquamation are also prominent features but typically occur later. Classic mucocutaneous features include erythematous cracked lips, nonpurulent conjunctivitis with sparing of the limbus, and lingual plaques ("white strawberry tongue") that shed to produce denuded, erythematous patches with prominent papilla ("strawberry tongue"). Extracutaneous features include high fever, cervical lymphadenopathy, arthritis, and occasionally cardiac or gastrointestinal disease. First-line treatment is with aspirin and intravenous immunoglobulin, as discussed in Chapter 166.

Behçet Disease

Behçet disease (see Chapter 161) is a multisystem disease that includes oral and genital ulceration and ocular disease (uveitis, relapsing iridocyclitis) in older children and adults. Recurrent aphthous stomatitis is present in almost all patients and is commonly the presenting symptom. Genital ulcerations may resemble aphthae; can occur on the penis, scrotum, or vulva; and may be particularly painful in females. Perianal ulceration is more common in children than adults. Additional skin findings may include folliculitis, purpuric lesions, erythema nodosum, and pustule formation after venipuncture or skin trauma (**pathergy**). Differential diagnosis of oral lesions includes recurrent aphthous stomatitis, herpes simplex, and rare oculocutaneous syndromes (e.g., MAGIC [mouth and genital ulcers with inflamed cartilage] syndrome). Skin biopsy demonstrates nongranulomatous vasculitis in all vessel sizes. Oral lesions may respond to swish and spit/swallow preparations variably including corticosteroids, antihistamines, antibiotics, and analgesics. Skin lesions are managed with topical corticosteroids, topical anesthetics such as sucralfate, and systemic agents as outlined in Chapter 161.

GASTROINTESTINAL DISEASES
Inflammatory Bowel Disease

Inflammatory bowel disease includes ulcerative colitis (see Chapter 336.1) and Crohn disease (see Chapter 336.2). Skin lesions of inflammatory bowel disease are classified as specific or reactive. Specific cutaneous manifestations have the same histologic features and pathologic mechanism as the underlying inflammatory bowel disease lesions and include aphthous ulcers, perianal fistulas and fissures, and metastatic Crohn disease (discussed below). Reactive cutaneous manifestations occur secondary to immune-mediated antigen cross-reactivity between gut and skin components; examples include erythema nodosum and pyoderma gangrenosum.

Up to 30% of patients with **ulcerative colitis** present with cutaneous manifestations. Aphthous ulcers are common and may worsen with gastrointestinal exacerbations. Erythema nodosum, occurring in up to 10% of patients, manifests as warm, erythematous nodules, often on the distal lower extremities. Pyoderma gangrenosum is a focal, ulcerative process that has distinctive, inflamed, undermined borders and a purulent, boggy center. Thrombophlebitis also occurs at an increased rate in patients with ulcerative colitis.

Crohn disease classically manifests as perianal fissures and skin tags, abscesses, sinuses, and fistulas; these may be presenting signs. A cobblestone appearance of oral mucosa may also be present. As in ulcerative colitis, aphthae, erythema nodosum, and pyoderma gangrenosum occur at increased frequency and may improve with treatment of the underlying disease. Noncaseating granulomatous inflammation is seen on routine histopathology, and when found in skin not contiguous with the intestinal tract, is labeled **metastatic Crohn disease.** Metastatic lesions may appear as solitary or multiple, localized plaques or nodules and may be located on perianal, perioral, or other cutaneous surfaces, including scars and ileostomy sites. In most cases of inflammatory bowel disease–associated skin disease, treatment of the underlying condition improves the cutaneous sequelae. Azathioprine, a common treatment, causes increased risk for nonmelanoma skin cancers.

CUTANEOUS MANIFESTATIONS OF MALIGNANCY

Skin disease associated with malignancy has a wide variety of presentations, including both metastatic lesions and nonmalignant paraneoplastic conditions. Cutaneous metastases manifest as firm nodules and occur at any cutaneous site. Paraneoplastic reaction patterns are often distinctive and can aid in the diagnosis of the underlying malignancy. Some genetic syndromes have an increased malignancy risk that may be suggested initially by cutaneous signs. Other cutaneous findings that may signal an underlying malignancy include pruritus, ichthyosis, acanthosis nigricans, urticaria, pemphigus, and erythroderma.

Sweet Syndrome

Also known as **acute febrile neutrophilic dermatosis,** Sweet syndrome (see Chapter 169) occurs in several forms, including classical (usually idiopathic or infection-related, Fig. 645-7), malignancy-associated, immunodeficiency-related, and drug-induced; pathogenesis

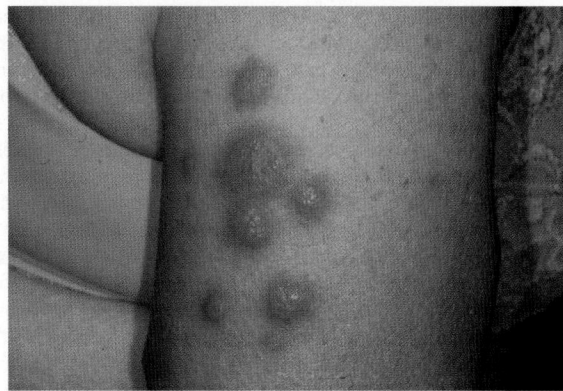

Figure 645-7 Clinical picture of idiopathic Sweet syndrome. *(From Prat L, Bouaziz JD, Wallach D, et al: Neutrophilic dermatoses as systemic diseases. Clin Dermatol 32:376–388, 2014, Fig. 1.)*

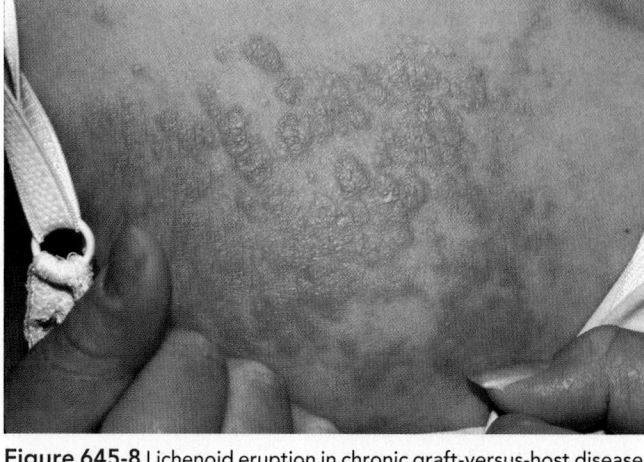

Figure 645-8 Lichenoid eruption in chronic graft-versus-host disease.

for all 3 forms remains unclear. Malignancy-associated Sweet syndrome is most commonly associated with hematologic malignancies, especially **acute myelogenous leukemia**. It manifests abruptly before, during, or after the malignancy course and is characterized by tender, erythematous, edematous plaques or nodules that may be pustular or targetoid, often accompanied by fever, anemia, and leukocytosis. Oral ulcers are more common in malignancy-associated Sweet syndrome than in other forms of the disease, and extracutaneous manifestations involving various organ systems may also occur. Diagnosis is confirmed by the presence of a dense neutrophilic infiltrate without evidence of vasculitis. The differential diagnosis includes other neutrophilic dermatoses-like pyoderma gangrenosum as well as cellulitis, erythema multiforme, Behçet disease, and erythema nodosum. First-line treatment for both malignancy-associated and nonmalignancy-associated Sweet syndrome is oral glucocorticoids (prednisone 1-2 mg/kg/day for 2-4 wk) in combination with high-potency topical or intralesional corticosteroids. Systemic steroid-sparing agents include colchicine and dapsone.

Necrolytic Migratory Erythema (Glucagonoma Syndrome)

Necrolytic migratory erythema is a distinctive migratory erythema that often signals an underlying neoplasm, usually an α-cell pancreatic tumor. Polycyclic, weeping, erythematous patches and plaques on the face, extremities, and groin occur in association with glossitis and cheilitis. The lesions are painful or pruritic, enlarge and coalesce over time and may develop central clearing with vesicles, crusts, and scales peripherally. Skin biopsy reveals superficial necrolysis with perivascular infiltrate. Elevated glucagon levels, hyperglycemia, and hypoaminoacidemia confirm the diagnosis, and tumor resection leads to resolution of the rash. Other treatments for necrolytic migratory erythema include somatostatin analogs (octreotide) and nutritional support; however, these measures do not affect the underlying tumor burden.

CUTANEOUS REACTIONS IN THE SETTING OF IMMUNOSUPPRESSION

Medication reactions, infectious etiologies, and graft-versus-host disease (GVHD) are included in the differential diagnosis in immunosuppressed patients; cutaneous and histologic similarities can be confounding.

Medication Reactions

The majority of medication reactions are mild morbilliform or exanthematous eruptions of little clinical consequence. Identifying the suspect medication may be difficult owing to the many medications used in immunosuppressed patients. Features that may help identify suspect medications include rash onset relative to exposure, character

of distribution and spread, associated symptoms, and laboratory data. Medication eruptions begin on the trunk 7-10 days after exposure; they spread peripherally and are associated with pruritus and, less commonly, with fever, arthralgia, and lymphadenopathy. Eosinophilia may support a diagnosis of drug eruption but may be absent in the setting of bone marrow suppression. Penicillins, sulfa drugs, cephalosporins, nonsteroidal antiinflammatory drugs, anticonvulsants, and aminoglycosides are common offenders. Medication eruptions may resolve despite continued use of the offending agent, or they may progress to more severe involvement. A careful drug history, elimination of all nonessential, suspect medications or change to medications of dissimilar class, and treatment of pruritus with emollients, topical steroids, antihistamines, and antipruritics are indicated. Skin biopsies are rarely useful in distinguishing medication eruptions from infectious exanthems, although GVHD, if sufficiently advanced, may have signature histopathologic findings.

Graft-Versus-Host Disease

GVHD (see Chapter 137) may have florid cutaneous expression in addition to characteristic extracutaneous features such as fever, mucositis, diarrhea, and hepatitis. It may be either acute or chronic. **Acute GVHD** occurs in 20-70% of hematopoietic stem cell transplants, depending on histocompatibility differences. It may be mistaken for a medication reaction or infectious exanthem because of the nonspecific erythematous maculopapular (morbilliform) eruption that often starts focally and then generalizes. Features that suggest acute GVHD include timing of eruption (typically 1-3 wk after transplantation, at the time of hematopoietic reconstitution), initial involvement of the head and neck including the ears, and subsequent spread to the trunk, extremities, palms, and soles. In severe cases of acute GVHD, blistering, necrolysis, and erythroderma occur. **Chronic GVHD** occurs in approximately 65% of long-term transplant survivors who may or may not have experienced prior acute GVHD. Cutaneous manifestations of chronic GVHD are distinctive, with sclerotic, poikilodermic scaly plaques and lichen planus-like papules predominating on the trunk and distal extremities (Fig. 645-8). Sclerotic areas are prone to contracture and chronic wound development. Involvement of the hair, nails, and oral mucosa is also common in chronic GVHD. First-line treatment for GVHD includes systemic glucocorticoids and other immunosuppressants supplemented by mid- to high-potency topical corticosteroids. In mild disease, topical corticosteroids or topical calcineurin inhibitors alone may be effective. Second-line treatment approaches include phototherapy (narrow band UVB or UVA1) and extracorporeal photopheresis. All patients with GVHD benefit from sunlight protection, emollient use, and topical or oral antipruritics.

Bibliography is available at Expert Consult.

645.2 Multisystem Medication Reactions

Brianne Z. Dickey and Yvonne E. Chiu

See also Chapter 152.

Most cutaneous reactions that result from the use of systemic medications are confined to the skin and resolve without sequelae after discontinuation of the offending agent (Table 645-3). More severe drug eruptions may be life-threatening, making rapid recognition vital (see Chapter 654). Genetics and, particularly, ethnicity appear to play a major role in determination of the occurrence of multisystem medication reactions, particularly to anticonvulsants.

DRUG RASH WITH EOSINOPHILIA AND SYSTEMIC SYMPTOMS (DRESS SYNDROME)

DRESS syndrome, or drug rash with eosinophilia and systemic symptoms, is also called drug hypersensitivity syndrome or anticonvulsant hypersensitivity syndrome. It is classically seen 2-6 wk after initial exposure to an anticonvulsant (carbamazepine, phenobarbital, phenytoin, lamotrigine) or other drugs (allopurinol, minocycline, sulfonamides [dapsone, sulfasalazine], other antibiotics) and often manifests as the triad of **fever, rash,** and **hepatitis.** The skin rash is initially located on the head, upper trunk, and arms. A diffuse exanthem of pruritic, morbilliform papules is most common, though any morphology may be present (Fig. 645-9). Exfoliation early in the course, as seen in toxic epidermal necrolysis, is uncommon. If mucous membrane involvement occurs, it is usually mild. Prominent periocular or facial edema, cervical lymphadenopathy, pharyngitis, and malaise accompany this dramatic cutaneous eruption. *Eosinophilia (≥500/μL) and atypical lymphocytosis are common but not always present.* Hepatitis ranging from mild elevation of liver transaminase values to frank hepatic failure may also be accompanied by interstitial nephritis, pneumonitis, myocarditis, shock, and encephalitis; mortality rate from these complications approaches 10%. Late-onset thyroiditis and hypothyroidism may occur months later as a result of antimicrosomal antibodies directed against thyroid peroxidases involved in drug metabolism.

The proposed pathogenesis of anticonvulsant-induced DRESS syndrome relates to a heritable defect in the epoxide hydrolase pathway leading to accumulation of toxic metabolites and subsequent

Table 645-3	Drug Eruptions in Pediatric Patients		
ERUPTION	**KEY DRUGS**	**LESIONAL PATTERN**	**MUCOSAL CHANGES**
Urticaria	Penicillins, cephalosporins, sulfonamides, aspirin/NSAIDs, radiocontrast media, TNF inhibitors	Pruritic erythematous wheals	None
Angioedema	Aspirin/NSAIDs, angiotensin-converting enzyme inhibitors	Swelling of subcutaneous and deep dermal tissues	May be present
Serum sickness–like reaction	Cephalosporins, penicillins, minocycline, bupropion, sulfonamides	Annular urticarial plaques	None
Exanthematous	Any drug	Erythematous macules and/or papules	None
Drug rash with eosinophilia and systemic symptoms (DRESS syndrome)	Phenytoin, phenobarbital, carbamazepine, lamotrigine, allopurinol, sulfonamides, dapsone, minocycline	Edema; erythematous macules and/or papules; sometimes vesicles or bullae	May be present
Lichenoid	Captopril, enalapril, β-blockers, gold salts, hydrochlorothiazide, hydroxychloroquine, penicillamine, griseofulvin, tetracycline, carbamazepine, phenytoin, NSAIDs	Discrete flat-topped, reddish purple papules and plaques	May be present
Fixed drug	Sulfonamides, ibuprofen, acetaminophen, tetracyclines, pseudoephedrine, barbiturates, lamotrigine, metronidazole, penicillin	Solitary to few erythematous, hyperpigmented plaques	Unusual
Pustular (acute generalized exanthematous pustulosis)	β-Lactam antibiotics, macrolides, clindamycin, terbinafine, calcium channel blockers, antimalarials	Generalized small pustules and papules	Unusual
Acneiform	Corticosteroids, androgens, lithium, iodides, phenytoin, isoniazid, tetracycline, B vitamins, azathioprine	Follicle-based inflammatory papules and pustules predominate	None
Pseudoporphyria	NSAIDs, cyclooxygenase-2 inhibitors, tetracyclines, furosemide	Photodistributed blistering and skin fragility	None
Vasculitis	Penicillins, NSAIDs, sulfonamides, cephalosporins	Purpuric papules, especially on the lower extremities; urticaria, hemorrhagic bullae, digital necrosis, pustules, ulcers	Rarely
Stevens-Johnson/toxic epidermal necrolysis	Sulfonamides, anticonvulsants, NSAIDs, allopurinol, dapsone	Target lesions, bullae, epidermal necrosis with detachment	Present
Drug-induced lupus	Minocycline, procainamide, hydralazine, isoniazid, penicillamine, carbamazepine, chlorpromazine, infliximab	Rarely has skin manifestations but may be urticarial, vasculitic, erythematous	Rare

NSAIDs, nonsteroidal antiinflammatory drugs; TNF, tumor necrosis factor.
Adapted from Paller AS, Mancini AJ, editors: Hurwitz clinical pediatric dermatology, *ed 3, Philadelphia, 2006, Elsevier/Saunders, p. 526.*

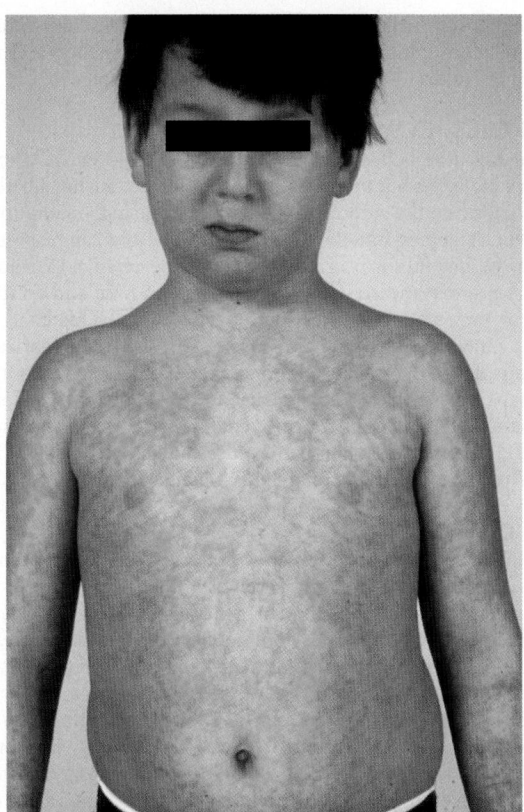

Figure 645-9 A 9 yr old boy with cerebral palsy and seizures treated with carbamazepine. Seventeen days after start of therapy he demonstrated fever, rash (exanthematous), lymphadenopathy, and nephritis, all part of a drug-induced hypersensitivity syndrome. *(From Schachner LA, Hansen RC, editors:* Pediatric dermatology, *ed 3, Philadelphia, 2003, Mosby, p. 1269.)*

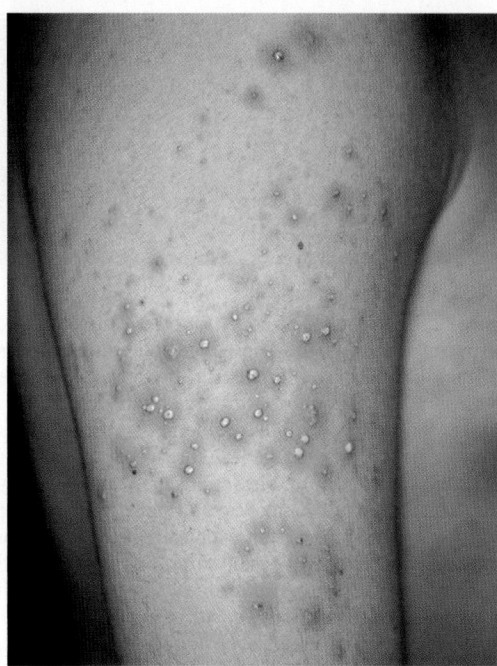

Figure 645-10 Acute generalized exanthematous pustulosis is characterized by the acute onset of fever and generalized erythema with numerous, small, discrete, sterile, nonfollicular pustules. Pustules may appear in a few days after the drug therapy is started. Pustules resolve in less than 15 days, followed by desquamation. *(From Habif TP, editor:* Clinical dermatology, *ed 4, Philadelphia, 2004, Mosby, p. 490.)*

lymphocyte activation. Reactivation of herpesviruses, especially human herpesvirus 6, is also commonly associated with DRESS syndrome via an unknown pathogenic mechanism. The differential diagnosis includes Stevens-Johnson syndrome, viral exanthem, macrophage activation, and hemophagocytic syndromes, and GVHD in the appropriate clinical setting. DRESS syndrome is often distinguished from other medication reactions by its later onset following drug exposure and more persistent course. In addition to anticonvulsants, sulfonamides may cause similar symptoms on first exposure because of abnormalities in glutathione *S*-transferase pathways.

Withdrawal of the medication is the primary therapeutic intervention. Lymphocyte transformation tests and patch testing are helpful for identifying the offending drug when multiple suspect agents are present, but drug discontinuation should not be delayed while awaiting results. Symptomatic treatment of pruritus and pain can be accomplished with emollients and mid- to high-potency topical corticosteroids (twice daily for 1 wk). Oral corticosteroid therapy is necessary in the setting of rapidly evolving or severe hepatic or renal involvement. Counseling about increased risk with similar medications and in siblings is important. DRESS syndrome can have a relapsing course, both in the skin and other organ systems, well after the medication has been withdrawn and initial improvement achieved, necessitating close follow-up for several months.

SERUM SICKNESS–LIKE REACTION

Serum sickness–like reaction (SSLR) manifests as annular, urticarial, sharply marginated, coalescing plaques; these often have a lavender hue to the center. In addition, acral erythema/edema, arthritis/ arthralgia, lymphadenopathy, and fever are often present. Unlike with true serum sickness (see Chapter 150), laboratory evidence of circulating immune complexes and multisystem involvement of vasculitis are typically absent. The differential diagnosis includes Kawasaki disease, connective tissue diseases, acute annular urticaria, and DRESS syndrome. SSLR is most commonly seen after exposure to various drugs (especially cefaclor and other antibiotics), as well as after certain infections and vaccinations. The cause of drug-related SSLR is unknown, but a toxic metabolite is suspected. In contrast to DRESS syndrome, SSLR typically occurs after repeated drug exposures. Medication withdrawal and symptomatic treatment with oral antihistamines and analgesics are recommended. Systemic glucocorticoids are indicated for severe joint involvement or extensive rashes.

ACUTE GENERALIZED EXANTHEMATOUS PUSTULOSIS

Acute generalized exanthematous pustulosis is often drug-related (most commonly aminopenicillins, macrolides, sulfonamides), occurring within hours to days after drug exposure. It is characterized by many nonfollicular sterile pustules with underlying edema and erythema, typically beginning on the face and intertriginous regions (Fig. 645-10). Neutrophilia and fever are common, whereas eosinophilia is less common than in DRESS syndrome. The rash may burn or itch; mucous membrane involvement is rare and often mild. Internal organ involvement is not common and often is asymptomatic. A pustular smear is always indicated to rule out infection in the setting of leukocytosis, fever, and a pustular rash. Therapy consists of stopping the causative drug and offering symptomatic relief with moist dressings, emollients, and mid-potency topical corticosteroids (applied twice daily for 1 wk).

Bibliography is available at Expert Consult.

Chapter **646**
Principles of Therapy
Stephen R. Humphrey and Beth A. Drolet

Competent skin care requires an appreciation of primary vs secondary lesions, a specific diagnosis, and knowledge of the natural course of the disease. If the diagnosis is uncertain, it is better to err on the side of less-aggressive rather than more-aggressive treatment.

In the use of topical medication, consideration of vehicle is as important as the specific therapeutic agent. Acute **weeping lesions** respond best to wet compresses, followed by lotions or creams. For **dry, thickened,** scaly skin, or for treatment of a contact allergic reaction possibly the consequence of a component of a topical medication, an ointment base is preferable, as it helps to occlude and moisten the affected area. Gels and solutions are most useful for the scalp and other hairy areas because of their faster absorption. The site of involvement is of considerable importance because the most desirable vehicle may not be cosmetically or functionally appropriate, such as an ointment on the face or hands. A patient's preference should also play a part in the choice of vehicle because compliance is poor if a medication is not acceptable to a patient. Ointments tend to sting less and are the least irritating. Cosmetically acceptable foam delivery systems have been developed, and the number of products and formulations available is increasing.

Most **lotions** are mixtures of water and oil that can be poured. After the water evaporates, the small amount of remaining oil covers the skin. Some shake lotions are a suspension of water and insoluble powder; as the water evaporates, cooling the skin, a thin film of powder covers the skin. **Creams** are emulsions of oil and water that are viscous and do not pour (more oil than in lotions). **Ointments** have oils and a small amount of water or no water at all; they feel greasy, lubricate dry skin, trap water, and aid in occlusion. Ointments without water usually require no preservatives because microorganisms require water to survive. Because of this, ointments often have the lowest number and concentration of ingredients, decreasing the risk of sensitizing the skin.

Therapy should be kept as simple as possible, and specific written instructions about the frequency and duration of application should be provided. Physicians should become familiar with one or two preparations in each category and should learn to use them appropriately. Prescribing nonspecific proprietary medications that may contain sensitizing agents should be avoided. Certain preparations, such as topical antihistamines and sensitizing anesthetics, are never indicated.

WET DRESSINGS
Wet dressings cool and dry the skin by evaporation and cleanse it by removing crusts and exudate, which would cause further irritation if permitted to remain. The dressings decrease pruritus, burning, and stinging sensations and are indicated for acutely inflamed moist or oozing dermatitis. Although various astringent and antiseptic substances may be added to the solution, cool or tepid tap water compresses are just as effective. Dressings of multiple layers of Kerlix, gauze, or soft cotton material may be saturated with water and remoistened as often as necessary. Compresses should be applied for 10-20 min at least every 4 hr and should usually be continued for 24-48 hr.

Alternatively, cotton long johns can be soaked in water and then wrung as dry as possible. These are placed on the child and covered with dry pajamas, preferably sleeper pajamas with feet. The child should sleep in these overnight. This type of dressing can be used nightly for up to 1 wk.

Wet dressings or wet wraps in conjunction with topical steroids may also be used in more severe cases of dermatitis (e.g., atopic dermatitis). In this method, a thin layer of the topical steroid is applied to the affected areas, which are then covered with warm, wet wraps for approximately 30 min to 1 hr 2-3 times daily. This method is especially effective in children with extensive and severe dermatitis.

BATH OILS, COLLOIDS, SOAPS
Bath oil has little benefit in the treatment of children. It offers little moisturizing effect but increases the risk of injury during a bath. Bath oil may lubricate the surface of the bathtub, causing an adult or child to fall when stepping into the tub. Tar bath solutions can be prescribed and may be helpful for psoriasis and atopic dermatitis. Colloids such as starch powder and colloidal oatmeal are soothing and antipruritic for some patients when added to the bathwater. Oilated colloidal oatmeal contains mineral oil and lanolin derivatives for lubrication if the skin is dry. These can also lubricate the bathtub surface. Ordinary bath soaps may be irritating and drying if patients have dry skin or dermatitis. Synthetic soaps are much less irritating. Fragrance-free soaps and cleansers are often better tolerated and less likely to irritate skin. When skin is acutely inflamed, avoidance of soap is advised.

LUBRICANTS
Lubricants, such as lotions, creams, and ointments, can be used as moisturizers for dry skin and as vehicles for topical agents such as corticosteroids and keratolytics. In general, ointments are the most effective emollients. Numerous commercial preparations are available. Some patients do not tolerate ointments, and some may be sensitized to a component of the lubricant; some preservatives in creams are also sensitizers. These preparations can be applied several times a day if necessary and tolerated. Maximal effect is achieved when they are applied to dry skin 2 or 3 times daily. Lotions containing menthol and camphor in an emollient vehicle can help control pruritus and dryness, but the use of moisturizers in addition to these products is best to decrease skin dryness.

SHAMPOOS
Special shampoos containing sulfur, salicylic acid, zinc, and selenium sulfide are useful for conditions in which there is scaling of the scalp, such as seborrheic dermatitis or psoriasis. Tar-containing shampoos are useful in these conditions. Most shampoos also contain surfactants and detergents. They should be used as frequently as necessary to control scaling. Patients should be instructed to leave the lathered shampoo in contact with the scalp for 5-10 minutes before thorough rinsing.

SHAKE LOTIONS
Shake lotions are useful antipruritic agents; they consist of a suspension of powder in a liquid vehicle. Water-dispersible oil may be added for lubrication. These preparations can be used effectively in combination with wet dressings for exudative dermatitis. Cooling occurs as the lotion evaporates and the powder deposited on the skin absorbs moisture.

POWDERS
Powders are hygroscopic and serve as absorptive agents in areas of excessive moisture. When dry, powders decrease friction between 2 surfaces. They are most useful in the intertriginous areas and between the toes, where maceration and abrasion may result from friction on movement. Coarse powders may cake; therefore, they should be of fine particle size and inert, unless medication has been incorporated in the formulation. The use of cornstarch-based powders in inflamed or broken skin may serve as a good growth environment for microorganisms and should be avoided.

PASTES
Pastes contain fine powder in ointment vehicles and are not often prescribed in current dermatologic therapy; in certain situations, however, they can be used effectively to protect vulnerable or damaged skin. A stiff zinc oxide paste is bland and inert and can be applied to the diaper area to prevent further irritation due to diaper dermatitis. Zinc oxide paste should be applied in a thick layer completely

obscuring the skin and is removed more easily with mineral oil than with soap and water.

KERATOLYTIC AGENTS

Urea-containing agents are hydrophilic; they hydrate the stratum corneum and make the skin more pliable. In addition, because urea dissolves hydrogen bonds and epidermal keratin, it is effective in treating scaling disorders. Concentrations of 10-40% are available in several commercial lotions and creams, which can be applied once or twice daily as tolerated. Salicylic acid is an effective keratolytic agent and can be incorporated into various vehicles in concentrations up to 6% to be applied 2 or 3 times daily. Salicylic acid preparations should not be used in treating small infants or on large surface areas or denuded skin; percutaneous absorption may result in salicylism. The α-hydroxy acids, particularly lactic acid and glycolic acid, are available in commercial preparations or can be incorporated in an ointment vehicle in concentrations up to 12%. Some creams contain both urea and lactic acid. The α-hydroxy acid preparations are useful for the treatment of keratinizing disorders and may be applied once or twice daily. Some patients complain of burning with the use of these agents; in such cases, the frequency of application should be decreased.

TAR COMPOUNDS

Tars are obtained from bituminous coal, shale, petrolatum (coal tars), and wood. They are antipruritic and astringent and appear to promote normal keratinization. They may be useful for chronic eczema and psoriasis, and their efficacy may be increased if the affected area is exposed to UV light after the tar has been removed. Tars should not be used for acute inflammatory lesions. Tars are often messy and unacceptable because they may stain and they have an odor. They may be incorporated into shampoos, bath oils, lotions, and ointments. A useful preparation for pediatric patients is liquor carbonis detergens 2-5% in a cream or ointment vehicle. Tar gel and tar in light body oil are relatively pleasant cosmetic preparations that cause minimal staining of skin and fabrics. Tars can also be incorporated into a vehicle with a topical corticosteroid. The frequency of application varies from 1-3 times daily, according to tolerance. Many children refuse to use tar preparations because of their odor and staining characteristics.

ANTIFUNGAL AGENTS

Antifungal agents are available as powders, lotions, creams, and ointments for the treatment of dermatophyte and yeast infections. Nystatin, naftifine, and amphotericin B are specific for *Candida albicans* and are ineffective in other fungal disorders. Tolnaftate is effective against dermatophytes but not against yeast. The spectrum for ciclopirox olamine includes the dermatophytes, *Malassezia furfur*, and *C. albicans*. The azoles clotrimazole, econazole, ketoconazole, miconazole, oxiconazole, and sulconazole have a similar broad spectrum. Butenafine has a similar broad spectrum and also has antiinflammatory properties. Terbinafine has greater activity against dermatophytes but poorer activity against yeasts than the azoles. The topical antifungal agents should be applied 1-2 times a day for most fungal infections. All have low sensitizing potential; additives such as preservatives and stabilizers in the vehicles may cause allergic contact dermatitis. Ointments containing 6% benzoic acid and 3% salicylic acid are potent keratolytic agents that have also been used for the treatment of dermatophyte infections. Irritant reactions are common.

TOPICAL ANTIBIOTICS

Topical antibiotics have been used for many years to treat local cutaneous infections, although their efficacy, with the exception of mupirocin, fusidic acid and retapamulin, has been questioned. Ointments are the preferred vehicles (except in the treatment of acne vulgaris; see Chapter 669) and combinations with other topical agents such as corticosteroids are, in general, inadvisable. Whenever possible, the etiologic agent should be identified and treated specifically. Antibiotics in wide use as systemic preparations should be avoided because of the risk of bacterial resistance. The sensitizing potential of certain topical antibiotics, such as neomycin and nitrofurazone, should be kept in mind and

avoided when possible. Mupirocin, fusidic acid, and retapamulin are the most effective topical agents currently available and are as effective as oral erythromycin in treatment of mild to moderate impetigo. Polysporin and bacitracin are not as effective.

TOPICAL CORTICOSTEROIDS

Topical corticosteroids are potent antiinflammatory agents and effective antipruritic agents. Successful therapeutic results are achieved in a wide variety of skin conditions. Corticosteroids can be divided into 7 different categories on the basis of strength (Table 646-1), but for practical purposes, 4 categories can be used: low, moderate, high, and super. Low-potency preparations include hydrocortisone, desonide, and hydrocortisone butyrate. Medium-potency compounds include amcinonide, betamethasone, flurandrenolide, fluocinolone, mometasone furoate, and triamcinolone. High-potency topical steroids include fluocinonide and halcinonide. Betamethasone dipropionate and clobetasol propionate are superpotent preparations and should be prescribed with care. Some of these compounds are formulated in several strengths according to clinical efficacy and degree of vasoconstriction. Physicians using topical steroids should become familiar with preparations within each class.

All corticosteroids can be obtained in various vehicles, including creams, ointments, solutions, gels, and aerosols. Some are available in a foam vehicle. Absorption is enhanced by an ointment or gel vehicle, but the vehicle should be selected on the basis of the type of disorder and the site of involvement. Frequency of application should be determined by the potency of the preparation, the location on the body, and the severity of the eruption. Applying a thin film 2 times daily usually suffices. Adverse local effects include cutaneous atrophy, striae, telangiectasia, acneiform eruptions, purpura, hypopigmentation, and increased hair growth. Systemic adverse effects of high-potency and superpotent topical steroids occur with long-term use and include poor growth, cataracts, and suppression of adrenal function.

Table 646-1	Potency of Topical Glucocorticosteroids

CLASS 1—SUPERPOTENT
Betamethasone dipropionate, 0.05% gel, ointment
Clobetasol propionate cream, ointment, 0.05%
Halobetasol propionate cream, ointment, 0.05%

CLASS 2—POTENT
Betamethasone dipropionate cream 0.05%
Desoximetasone cream, ointment, gel 0.05% and 0.25%
Fluocinonide cream, ointment, gel, 0.05%

CLASS 3—UPPER MID-STRENGTH
Betamethasone dipropionate cream, 0.05%
Betamethasone valerate ointment, 0.1%
Fluticasone propionate ointment, 0.005%
Mometasone furoate ointment, 0.1%
Triamcinolone acetonide cream, 0.5%

CLASS 4—MID-STRENGTH
Desoximetasone cream, 0.05%
Fluocinolone acetonide ointment, 0.025%
Triamcinolone acetonide ointment, 0.1%

CLASS 5—LOWER MID-STRENGTH
Betamethasone valerate cream/lotion, 0.1%
Fluocinolone acetonide cream, 0.025%
Fluticasone propionate cream, 0.05%
Triamcinolone acetonide cream/lotion, 0.1%

CLASS 6—MILD STRENGTH
Desonide cream, 0.05%

CLASS 7—LEAST POTENT
Topicals with hydrocortisone, dexamethasone, flumethasone, methylprednisolone, and prednisolone

From Weston WL, Lane AT, Morelli JG: Color textbook of pediatric dermatology, ed 4, St. Louis, 2007, Mosby, p. 418.

The relative skin thickness should be considered in regard to the selection of class of steroid (see Table 646-1). Thin skin such as the eyelids, face, groin, and genitalia will absorb a substantial amount of medication compared to the thickest skin on the palms and soles. One adult fingertip's worth of medication is enough to cover an area the size of an adult palm and is approximately half a gram of medication. Knowing the area being treated and which medication class to prescribe can decrease potential for side effects.

In selected circumstances, corticosteroids may be administered by intralesional injection (acne cysts, keloids, psoriatic plaques, alopecia areata, persistent insect bite reactions). Only experienced physicians should use this method of administration.

TOPICAL NONSTEROIDAL ANTIINFLAMMATORY AGENTS

Calcineurin-inhibiting antiinflammatory agents that inhibit T-cell activation may be used instead of topical steroids for the treatment of atopic dermatitis and other inflammatory conditions. These agents are pimecrolimus and tacrolimus. They do not have the adverse local effects seen with topical steroid. Stinging with application is the most common complaint and may be lessened by mixing the medication with an ointment such as petrolatum jelly for the initial applications. These agents are only as strong as medium-potency topical steroids. They should be used with caution owing to evidence from animal experiments and case reports of an increased risk of lymphoma.

SUNSCREENS

Sunscreens are of 2 general types: (1) those, such as zinc oxide and titanium dioxide, that absorb all wavelengths of the UV and visible spectrums; and (2) a heterogeneous group of chemicals that selectively absorb energy of various wavelengths within the UV spectrum. In addition to the spectrum of light that is blocked, other factors to be considered include cosmetic acceptance, sensitizing potential, retention on skin while swimming or sweating, required frequency of application, and cost. Sunscreen ingredients include para-aminobenzoic acid (PABA) with ethanol, PABA esters, cinnamates, and benzophenone. These block transmission of the majority of solar UVB and some UVA wavelengths. Avobenzone and ecamsule are more effective in blocking UVA. Antioxidants may also be found in some sunscreens. Lip protectants that absorb in the UVB range are also available. Sunscreens are designated by sun protection factor (SPF). The SPF is defined as the amount of time to develop a mild sunburn with the sunscreen compared with the amount of time without the sunscreen. A minimum SPF factor of 15 is required for most fair-skinned individuals to prevent sunburn; however, an SPF of 30 should be recommended most often. The higher the SPF, the better the protection is against UVB rays. Sunscreens do not include any measurement of the efficacy in blocking UVA. The efficacy of these agents depends on careful attention to instructions for use. Chemical sunscreens should be applied at least 30 min before sun exposure to permit penetration into the epidermis, again on arrival at the destination, and every subsequent hour when exposed to direct sunlight. Most patients with photosensitivity eruptions require protection by agents that absorb both UVB and UVA wavelengths (see Chapter 656).

Although sunscreens do confer photoprotection and may decrease the development of nevi, protection is incomplete against all harmful UV light. Midday (10 AM to 4 PM) sun avoidance is the primary method of photoprotection. Clothing, hats, and staying in the shade offer additional sun protection.

LASER THERAPY

The vascular-specific pulsed dye laser therapy is used mainly for the treatment of capillary malformations (port-wine stains). Spider telangiectasia, small facial pyogenic granulomas, superficial and ulcerated hemangioma, and warts may also be treated. Vascular-specific pulsed dye lasers produce light that is readily absorbed by oxyhemoglobin, producing selective photothermolysis of vascular lesions.

Bibliography is available at Expert Consult.

Chapter **647**
Diseases of the Neonate
Kari L. Martin

Minor evanescent lesions of newborn infants, particularly when florid, may cause undue concern. Most of the entities are relatively common, benign, and transient and do not require therapy.

SEBACEOUS HYPERPLASIA

Minute, profuse, yellow-white papules are frequently found on the forehead, nose, upper lip, and cheeks of a term infant; they represent hyperplastic sebaceous glands (Fig. 647-1). These tiny papules diminish gradually in size and disappear entirely within the 1st few wk of life.

MILIA

Milia are superficial epidermal inclusion cysts that contain laminated keratinized material. The lesion is a firm cyst, 1-2 mm in diameter, and pearly, opalescent white. Milia may occur at any age but in neonates are most frequently scattered over the face and gingivae and on the midline of the palate, where they are called **Epstein pearls**. Milia exfoliate spontaneously in most infants and may be ignored; those that appear in scars or sites of trauma in older children may be gently unroofed and the contents extracted with a fine-gauge needle.

SUCKING BLISTERS

Solitary or scattered superficial bullae present at birth on the upper limbs of infants at birth are presumably induced by vigorous sucking on the affected part in utero. Common sites are the radial aspect of the forearm, thumb, and index finger. These bullae resolve rapidly without sequelae and should be distinguished from sucking pads (calluses), which are found on the lips in the 1st few mo and are a result of combined intracellular edema and hyperkeratosis. The diagnosis can be confirmed by observing the neonate sucking the affected area.

CUTIS MARMORATA

When a newborn infant is exposed to low environmental temperatures, an evanescent, lacy, reticulated red and/or blue cutaneous vascular

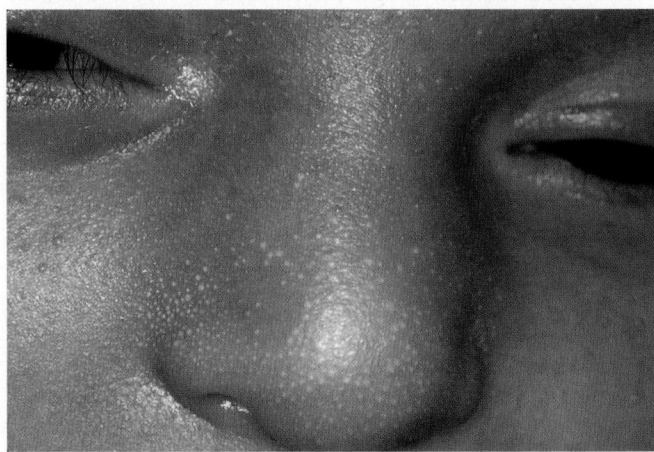

Figure 647-1 Sebaceous hyperplasia. Minute white-yellow papules on the nose of a newborn.

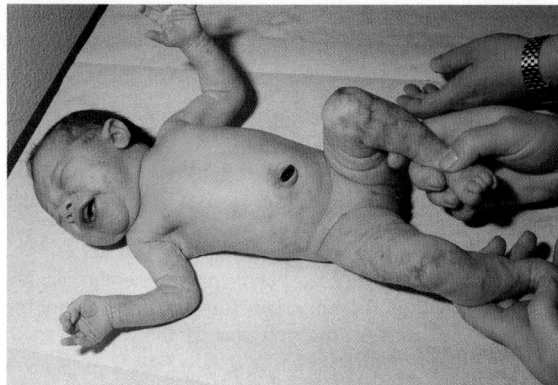

Figure 647-2 Newborn girl with reticulate erythema/livedo on legs, right arm, and cheeks. *(From Pleimes M, Gottler S, Weibel L: Characteristic congenital reticular erythema: cutis marmorata telangiectatica congenital. J Pediatr 163:604, 2013, Fig. 1.)*

pattern appears over most of the body surface. This vascular change represents an accentuated physiologic vasomotor response that disappears with increasing age, although it is sometimes discernible even in older children. **Cutis marmorata telangiectatica congenita** is clinically similar, but the lesions are more intense, may be segmental, are persistent, and may be associated with loss of dermal tissue, epidermal atrophy, and ulceration (Fig. 647-2). The lower extremities are usually affected with limb atrophy noted on the affected side. Gradual fading of the livid erythema occurs over 3-5 yr, but limb asymmetry is permanent.

HARLEQUIN COLOR CHANGE
A rare but dramatic vascular event, harlequin color change occurs in the immediate newborn period and is most common in low-birthweight infants. It probably reflects an imbalance in the autonomic vascular regulatory mechanism. When the infant is placed on 1 side, the body is bisected longitudinally into a pale upper half and a deep red dependent half. The color change lasts only for a few minutes and occasionally affects only a portion of the trunk or face. Changing the infant's position may reverse the pattern. Muscular activity causes generalized flushing and obliterates the color differential. Repeated episodes may occur but do not indicate permanent autonomic imbalance.

NEVUS SIMPLEX (SALMON PATCH)
Nevus simplex is a small, pale pink, ill-defined, vascular macule that occurs most commonly on the glabella, eyelids, upper lip, and nuchal area of 30-40% of normal newborn infants. These lesions, which represent localized **vascular ectasia,** persist for several months and may become more visible during crying or changes in environmental temperature. Most lesions on the face eventually fade and disappear completely, although lesions occupying the entire central forehead often do not. Those on the posterior neck and occipital areas usually persist. The facial lesion should not be confused with a port-wine stain, which is a permanent lesion and may be associated with Sturge-Weber syndrome. Nevus simplex is usually symmetric, with lesions on both eyelids or on both sides of midline. Port-wine stains are often larger and unilateral, and they usually end along the midline (see Chapter 650).

DERMAL MELANOCYTOSIS (MONGOLIAN SPOTS)
Dermal melanocytosis, which appears as blue or slate-gray macular lesions, has variably defined margins. It occurs most commonly in the presacral area but may be found over the posterior thighs, legs, back, and shoulders (Fig. 647-3). The spots may be solitary or numerous and

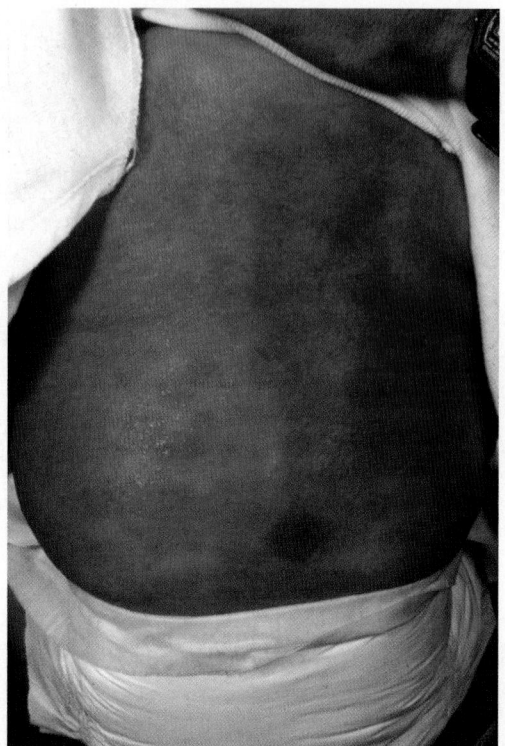

Figure 647-3 Extensive Mongolian spot on the back of a newborn. *(Courtesy of Fitzsimons Army Medical Center teaching file.)*

often involve large areas. The incidence of these lesions varies widely across ethnicities, being most common in African-American, Asian, and Hispanic infants (25-80% depending on the study) and less common in white infants (around 6%). The peculiar hue of these macules is a result of the dermal location of melanin-containing melanocytes (mid-dermal melanocytosis) that are presumably arrested in their migration from neural crest to epidermis. They usually fade during the 1st few yr of life as a result of darkening of the overlying skin. Malignant degeneration does not occur. The characteristic appearance and congenital onset distinguish these spots from the bruises of child abuse. Rarely Mongolian spots are associated with Hurler syndrome or GM_1 gangliosidosis type 1.

ERYTHEMA TOXICUM
A benign, self-limited, evanescent eruption, erythema toxicum occurs in approximately 50% of full-term infants; preterm infants are affected less commonly. The lesions are firm, yellow-white, 1-2 mm papules or pustules with a surrounding erythematous flare (Fig. 647-4). At times, splotchy erythema is the only manifestation. Lesions may be sparse or numerous and either clustered in several sites or widely dispersed over much of the body surface. The palms and soles are usually spared. Peak incidence occurs on the 2nd day of life, but new lesions may erupt during the 1st few days as the rash waxes and wanes. Onset may occasionally be delayed for a few days to weeks in premature infants. The pustules form below the stratum corneum or deeper in the epidermis and represent collections of eosinophils that also accumulate around the upper portion of the pilosebaceous follicle. The **eosinophils** can be demonstrated in Wright-stained smears of the intralesional contents. Cultures are sterile.

The cause of erythema toxicum is unknown. The lesions can mimic pyoderma, candidiasis, herpes simplex, transient neonatal pustular melanosis, and miliaria but can be differentiated by the characteristic infiltrate of eosinophils and the absence of organisms on a stained smear. The course is brief, and no therapy is required. Incontinentia pigmenti and eosinophilic pustular folliculitis also have eosinophilic

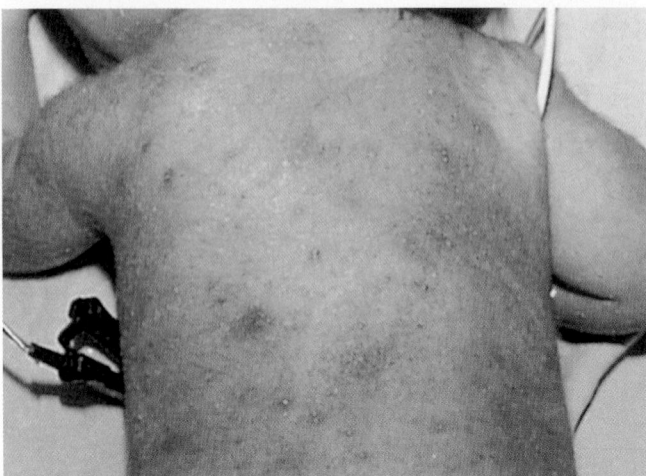

Figure 647-4 Erythema toxicum on the trunk of a newborn infant.

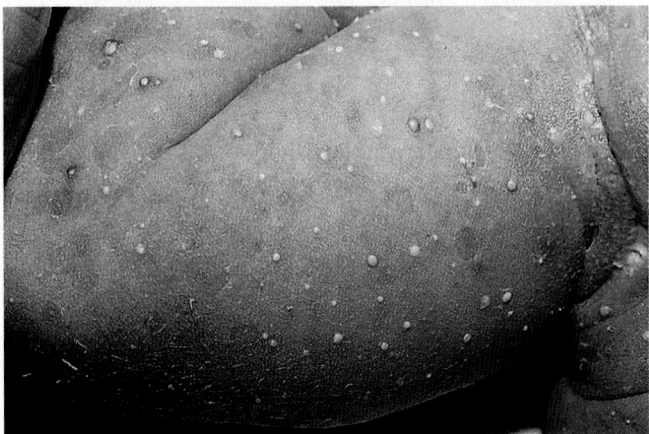

Figure 647-5 Transient neonatal pustular melanosis. Multiple papules present at birth on the arm of an infant. *(From Weston WL, Lane AT, Morelli JG, editors: Color textbook of pediatric dermatology, ed 3, Philadelphia, 2002, Mosby, p. 331.)*

infiltration but can be distinguished by their distribution, histologic type, and chronicity.

TRANSIENT NEONATAL PUSTULAR MELANOSIS

Pustular melanosis, which is more common among African-American than among white infants, is a transient, benign, self-limited dermatosis of unknown etiology that is characterized by 3 types of lesions: (1) evanescent superficial pustules, (2) ruptured pustules with a collarette of fine scale, at times with a central hyperpigmented macule, and (3) hyperpigmented macules (Fig. 647-5). Lesions are present at birth, and 1 or all types of lesions may be found in a profuse or sparse distribution. Pustules represent the early phase of the disorder, and macules, the late phase. The pustular phase rarely lasts more than 2-3 days; hyperpigmented macules may persist for as long as 3 mo. Sites of predilection are the anterior neck, forehead, and lower back, although the scalp, trunk, limbs, palms, and soles may be affected.

The active phase shows an intracorneal or subcorneal pustule filled with **polymorphonuclear leukocytes,** debris, and an occasional eosinophil. The macules are characterized only by increased melanization

of epidermal cells. Cultures and smears can be used to distinguish these pustules from those of pyoderma and erythema toxicum, because the lesions of pustular melanosis do not contain bacteria or dense aggregates of eosinophils. No therapy is required.

INFANTILE ACROPUSTULOSIS

Onset of infantile acropustulosis generally occurs at 2-10 mo of age; lesions are occasionally noted at birth. Darkly pigmented males have a predisposition, but infants of both sexes and all races may be affected. The cause is unknown.

The lesions are initially discrete erythematous papules that become vesiculopustular within 24 hr and subsequently crust before healing. They are intensely pruritic. Preferred sites are the palms of the hands and the soles and sides of the feet, where the lesions may be extensive. A less dense eruption may be found on the dorsum of the hands and feet, ankles, and wrists. Pustules occasionally occur elsewhere on the body. Each episode lasts 7-14 days, during which time pustules continue to appear in crops. After a 2-4 wk remission, a new outbreak follows. This cyclic pattern continues for approximately 2 yr; permanent resolution is often preceded by longer intervals of remission between periods of activity. Infants with acropustulosis are otherwise well.

Wright-stained smears of intralesional contents show abundant neutrophils or, occasionally, a predominance of eosinophils. Histologically, well-circumscribed, subcorneal, neutrophilic pustules, with or without eosinophils, are noted.

The **differential diagnosis** in neonates includes transient neonatal pustular melanosis, erythema toxicum, milia, cutaneous candidiasis, and staphylococcal pustulosis. In older infants and toddlers, additional diagnostic considerations include scabies, dyshidrotic eczema, pustular psoriasis, subcorneal pustular dermatosis, and hand-foot-and-mouth disease. A therapeutic trial of a scabicide is warranted in equivocal cases.

Therapy is directed at minimizing discomfort for infants. Topical corticosteroid preparations and/or oral antihistamines decrease the severity of the pruritus and an infant's irritability. Dapsone (2 mg/kg/day taken orally twice daily) is effective but has potentially serious side effects—notably, hemolytic anemia and methemoglobinemia—and should be used with caution.

EOSINOPHILIC PUSTULAR FOLLICULITIS

Eosinophilic pustular folliculitis is defined as recurrent crops of pruritic, coalescing, follicular papulopustules on the face, trunk, and extremities. Fifty percent of patients have peripheral eosinophilia with eosinophil counts exceeding 5%, and approximately 30% have leukocytosis (>10,000 leukocytes/mm^3).

Infants account for <10% of all cases of eosinophilic pustular folliculitis. The clinical and histologic appearances of this disorder in infants closely resemble those in immunocompetent adults, with minor exceptions. In infants, the lesions are most prominent on the scalp, although they also occur on the trunk and extremities and occasionally are found on the palms and soles. The classic annular and polycyclic appearance with centrifugal enlargement is not seen in infants. Adults have an eosinophilic infiltrate that invades sebaceous glands and the outer root sheath of hair follicles, often leading to spongiosis in the outer root sheath. The eosinophilic infiltrate in most infants, however, is perifollicular, without spongiosis in the outer root sheath. Because of the slight differences between clinical findings and course in immunocompetent adults, immunocompromised adults and those in infants, it has been proposed that eosinophilic pustular folliculitis be **subclassified** into classic, HIV-related, and infantile forms. The **differential diagnosis** includes erythema toxicum neonatorum, infantile acropustulosis, localized pustular psoriasis, pustular folliculitis, and transient neonatal pustular melanosis.

High-potency or superpotent topical corticosteroids are the most effective treatment (see Table 646-1 in Chapter 646).

Bibliography is available at Expert Consult.

Chapter **648**
Cutaneous Defects
Kari L. Martin

SKIN DIMPLES

Cutaneous depressions over bony prominences and in the acral area, at times associated with pits and creases, may occur in normal children and in association with dysmorphologic syndromes. Skin dimples may develop in utero as a result of interposition of tissue between a sharp bony point and the uterine wall, which leads to decreased subcutaneous tissue formation.

Dimples may also be present overlying an area of **bone hypoplasia**. Bilateral acromial skin dimples are usually an isolated finding, but they are also seen in association with deletion of the long arm of chromosome 18. Dimples tend to occur over the patella in congenital rubella, over the lateral aspects of the knees and elbows in prune-belly syndrome, on the pretibial surface in campomelic dwarfs, and in the shape of an H on the chin in whistling-face syndrome.

Sacral dimples are common and usually are isolated findings. They may be seen in multiple syndromes or in association with spina bifida occulta and diastomyelia. Association with a mass or other cutaneous stigma (hair, aplasia cutis, lipoma, hemangioma) should increase concern for underlying **spinal dysraphism** (see Chapter 591). Ultrasonography during the 1st 3 mo of life, before ossification of the posterior elements of the lower spine, may provide a cost-effective, noninvasive method of assessing any associated lumbosacral spine abnormalities in infants with an isolated sacral dimple. *Nonetheless, MRI of the spine is indicated if there is a strong suspicion of a spinal dysraphism.*

REDUNDANT SKIN

Loose folds of skin must be differentiated from a congenital defect of elastic tissue or collagen such as cutis laxa, Ehlers-Danlos syndrome, or pseudoxanthoma elasticum. Redundant skin over the posterior part of the neck is common in the Turner, Noonan, Down, and Klippel-Feil syndromes and monosomy 1p36; more generalized folds of skin occur in infants with trisomy 18 and short-limbed dwarfism.

AMNIOTIC CONSTRICTION BANDS

Partial or complete constriction bands that produce defects in extremities and digits are found in 1 in 10,000-45,000 otherwise normal infants. Constrictive tissue bands are caused by primary amniotic rupture, with subsequent entanglement of fetal parts, particularly limbs, in shriveled fibrotic amniotic strands. This event is probably sporadic, with negligible risk of recurrence. Formation of constrictive tissue bands is associated with abdominal trauma, amniocentesis, and hereditary defects of collagen such as Ehlers-Danlos syndrome and osteogenesis imperfecta.

Adhesive bands involve the craniofacial area and are associated with severe defects such as encephalocele and facial clefts. Adhesive bands result from broad fusion between disrupted fetal tissue and an intact amniotic membrane. The craniofacial defects appear not to be caused by constrictive amniotic bands but to result from a vascular disruption sequence with or without cephaloamniotic adhesion (see Chapter 108).

The **limb–body wall complex** involves vascular disruption early in development, affecting several embryonic structures; it includes at least 2 of the following 3 characteristics: exencephaly or encephalocele with facial clefts, thoracoschisis and/or abdominoschisis, and limb defects.

PREAURICULAR SINUSES AND PITS

Pits and sinus tracts anterior to the pinna may be a result of imperfect fusion of the tubercles of the 1st and 2nd branchial arches. These anomalies may be unilateral or bilateral, may be familial, are more

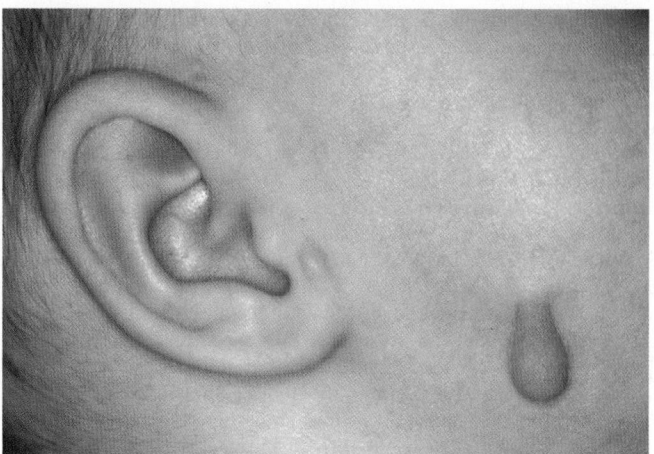

Figure 648-1 Accessory tragus on cheek along jaw line.

common among females and African-Americans, and at times are associated with other anomalies of the ears and face. Preauricular pits are present in **branchiootorenal dysplasia 1 syndrome** (*EYA-1* gene), an autosomal dominant disorder that consists of external ear malformations, branchial fistulas, hearing loss, and renal anomalies. When the tracts become chronically infected, retention cysts may form and drain intermittently; such lesions may require excision.

ACCESSORY TRAGI

An accessory tragus typically appears as a single pedunculated, flesh-colored papule in the preauricular region anterior to the tragus. Less commonly, accessory tragi are multiple or bilateral, and may be located in the preauricular area, on the cheek along the line of the mandible (Fig. 648-1), or on the lateral aspect of the neck anterior to the sternocleidomastoid muscle. In contrast to the rest of the pinna, which develops from the 2nd branchial arch, the tragus and accessory tragi derive from the 1st branchial arch. Accessory tragi may occur as isolated defects or in chromosomal 1st branchial arch syndromes that include anomalies of the ears and face, such as cleft lip, cleft palate, and mandibular hypoplasia. An accessory tragus is consistently found in **oculoauriculovertebral syndrome** (**Goldenhar syndrome**). Surgical excision is appropriate.

BRANCHIAL CLEFT AND THYROGLOSSAL CYSTS AND SINUSES

Cysts and sinuses in the neck may be formed along the course of the 1st, 2nd, 3rd, or 4th branchial clefts as a result of improper closure during embryonic life. Second branchial cleft cysts are the most common. The lesions may be unilateral or bilateral (2-3%) and may open onto the cutaneous surface or drain into the pharynx. Secondary infection is an indication for systemic antibiotic therapy. These anomalies may be inherited as autosomal dominant traits.

Thyroglossal cysts and fistulas are similar defects located in or near the midline of the neck; they may extend to the base of the tongue. A pathognomonic sign is vertical motion of the mass with swallowing and tongue protrusion. In nearly 50% of affected children, the cyst or fistula manifests as an infected midline upper neck mass. Cysts in the tongue base may be differentiated from an undescended lingual thyroid by radionuclide scanning. Unlike branchial cysts, a thyroglossal duct cyst often appears after an upper respiratory infection (see Chapter 563).

SUPERNUMERARY NIPPLES

Solitary or multiple accessory nipples may occur in a unilateral or bilateral distribution along a line from the anterior axillary fold to the inguinal area. They are more common among African-American (3.5%) than white (0.6%) children. Accessory nipples may or may not have areolae and may be mistaken for congenital nevi. They may be excised for cosmetic reasons. Renal or urinary tract anomalies and hematologic abnormalities may rarely occur in children with this finding (see Chapter 551).

APLASIA CUTIS CONGENITA (CONGENITAL ABSENCE OF SKIN)

Developmental absence of skin is usually noted on the scalp as multiple or solitary (70%), noninflammatory, well-demarcated, oval or circular 1-2 cm ulcers (Table 648-1). The appearance of lesions varies, depending on when they occurred during intrauterine development. Those that form early in gestation may heal before delivery and appear as atrophic, fibrotic scars with associated alopecia, whereas more recent defects may manifest as ulcerations. Most occur at the vertex of the scalp just lateral to the midline, but similar defects may also occur on the face, trunk, and limbs, where they are often symmetric and usually associated with an intrauterine fetal demise of a twin (**fetus papyraceus**). The depth and size of the ulcer varies. Only the epidermis and upper dermis may be involved, resulting in minimal scarring or hair loss, or less often the defect may extend to the deep dermis, to the subcutaneous tissue, and, rarely, to the periosteum, skull, and dura. Lesions may be surrounded by a collar of hair (Fig. 648-2).

Diagnosis is made on the basis of physical findings indicative of in utero disruption of skin development. Lesions are sometimes mistakenly attributed to scalp electrodes or obstetric trauma. Most are sporadic, but autosomal dominant and recessive cases occur as well; some are due to mutations in *BMS1*, a ribosomal guanosine triphosphatase.

Although most individuals with aplasia cutis congenita have no other abnormalities, these lesions may be associated with isolated physical anomalies or with malformation syndromes, including Opitz, Adams-Oliver, oculocerebrocutaneous, Johanson-Blizzard, and 4p(−), X-p22 microdeletion syndromes, trisomy 13-15, and chromosome 16-18 defects (see Table 648-1). Aplasia cutis congenita may also be found in association with an overt or underlying embryologic malformation, such as meningomyelocele, gastroschisis, omphalocele, or spinal dysraphism. Aplasia cutis congenita in association with fetus papyraceus is apparently caused by ischemic or thrombotic events in the placenta and fetus. Blistering or skin fragility and/or absence or deformity of nails in association with aplasia cutis congenita is a well-recognized manifestation of **epidermolysis bullosa.**

Major complications are rare and more often associated with large, stellate lesions of the midline parietal scalp. Hemorrhage, secondary local infection, and meningitis have been reported. If the defect is small, recovery is uneventful, with gradual epithelialization and formation of a hairless atrophic scar over a period of several weeks. Small bony defects usually close spontaneously in the 1st yr of life. Large or numerous scalp defects may require repair, but care must be taken as abnormal underlying venous structures have complicated surgical repair. Truncal and limb defects, despite being large, usually epithelialize and form atrophic scars, which can later be revised.

FOCAL FACIAL DERMAL DYSPLASIAS

The focal facial dermal dysplasias (FFDDs) are a rare group of conditions sharing bitemporal or preauricular lesions resembling scars or aplasia cutis congenita. FFDD1 (Brauer syndrome) is inherited in an autosomal dominant fashion and typically mild associated facial features. FFDD2 (Brauer-Setleis syndrome) and FFDD3 (Setleis syndrome) are associated with thin, puckered periorbital skin, distichiasis and/or absent eyelashes, upslating palpebral fissures, flat nasal bridge, large lips and redundant facial skin. FFDD2 is inherited in an autosomal dominant fashion whereas FFDD3 is autosomal recessive and caused by mutations in *TWIST2*. FFDD4 has no other related skin findings; it is inherited both in autosomal dominant and recessive manners and is caused by mutations in *CYP26C1*.

FOCAL DERMAL HYPOPLASIA (GOLTZ SYNDROME)

A rare congenital mesoectodermal and ectodermal disorder, focal dermal hypoplasia is characterized by dysplasia of connective tissue in the skin and skeleton. This disorder is an X-linked dominant disorder caused by mutations in the *PORCN* gene. It manifests as numerous soft tan papillomas. Other cutaneous findings include linear atrophic

Table 648-1	Freiden's Classification of Aplasia Cutis Congenita	
GROUP	**DEFINITION**	**INHERITANCE**
1	Isolated scalp involvement; may be associated with single defects	AD
2	Scalp ACC with limb reduction defects (Adams-Oliver syndrome); may be associated with encephalocele	AD
3	Scalp ACC with epidermal nevus	Sporadic
4	ACC overlying occult spinal dysraphism, spina bifida, or meningoencephalocele	Sporadic
5	ACC with placental infarcts, and/ or fetus papyraceus	Sporadic
6	ACC with epidermolysis bullosa	AD or AR
7	ACC localized to extremities without blistering; usually affecting pretibial areas and dorsum of hands and feet	AD or AR
8	ACC caused by teratogens (e.g., varicella, herpes, methimazole)	Sporadic
9	ACC associated with malformation syndromes (e.g., trisomy 13, deletion 4p−, deletion Xp22.1, ectodermal dysplasia, Johanson-Blizzard syndrome, Adams-Oliver syndrome)	Variable

ACC, Aplasia cutis congenital; AD, autosomal dominant; AR, autosomal recessive.

Modified from Frieden IJ: Aplasia cutis congenital: a clinical review and proposal for classification. J Am Acad Dermatol 14:646–660, 1986.

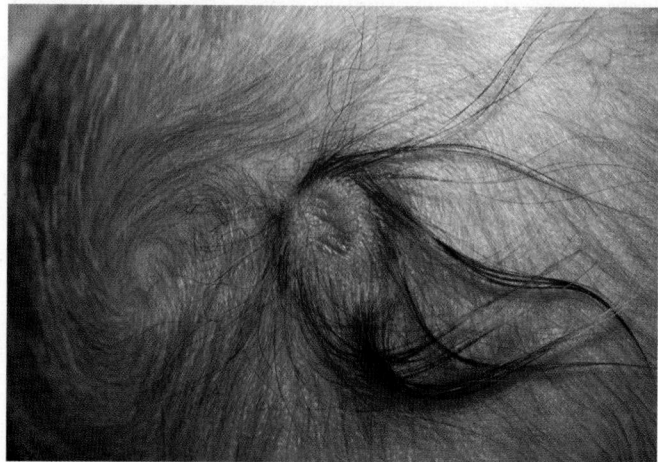

Figure 648-2 Solitary scalp vertex lesion of aplasia cutis congenita with hair collar.

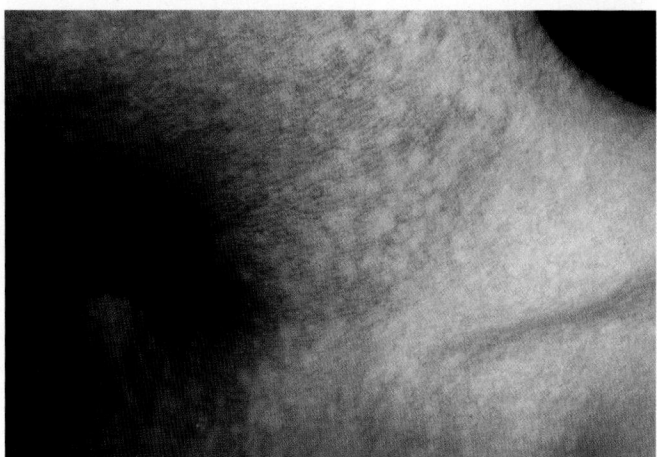

Figure 648-3 Reticulated dyspigmentation on neck of patient with dyskeratosis congenita.

lesions; reticulated hypopigmentation and hyperpigmentation; telangiectasias; congenital absence of skin; angiofibromas presenting as verrucous excrescences; and papillomas of the lips, tongue, circumoral region, vulva, anus, and the inguinal, axillary, and periumbilical areas. Partial alopecia, sweating disorders, and dystrophic nails are additional, less common ectodermal anomalies. The most frequent skeletal defects are syndactyly, clinodactyly, polydactyly, and scoliosis. **Osteopathia striata** are fine parallel vertical stripes noted on radiographs in the metaphyses of long bones of patients with this disorder; these are highly characteristic of focal dermal hypoplasia but are not pathognomonic. Many ocular abnormalities, the most common of which are colobomas, strabismus, nystagmus, and microphthalmia, are also characteristic. Small stature, dental defects, soft tissue anomalies, and peculiar dermatoglyphic patterns are also common. Cognitive impairment occurs occasionally.

DYSKERATOSIS CONGENITA (ZINSSER-ENGMAN-COLE SYNDROME)
Dyskeratosis congenita, a rare familial syndrome, consists classically of the triad of reticulated hyperpigmentation of the skin (Fig. 648-3), dystrophic nails, and mucous membrane leukoplakia in association with immunologic and hematologic abnormalities. Patients with dyskeratosis congenita also show signs of premature aging and increased occurrence of cancer, especially squamous cell carcinoma. Dyskeratosis congenita may be X-linked recessive (*DKC-1* gene), autosomal dominant (*hTERC* and *TINF2* genes), or autosomal recessive (*NOLA3* gene). Onset occurs in childhood, most commonly as **nail dystrophy.** The nails become atrophic and ridged longitudinally with progression to pterygia and complete nail loss. Skin changes usually appear after onset of nail changes and consist of reticulated gray-brown pigmentation, atrophy, and telangiectasia, especially on the neck, face, and chest. Hyperhidrosis and hyperkeratosis of the palms and soles, sparse scalp hair, and easy blistering of the hands and feet are also characteristic. Blepharitis, ectropion, and excessive tearing because of atresia of the lacrimal ducts are occasional manifestations. Oral leukokeratosis may give rise to squamous cell carcinoma. Other mucous membranes, including conjunctival, urethral, and genital, may be involved. Infection, malignancy, pulmonary fibrosis and bone marrow failure are common, and death before age 40 yr is typical.

CUTIS VERTICIS GYRATA
Cutis verticis gyrata, an unusual alteration of the scalp that is more common in males, may be present from birth or may develop during adolescence. The scalp is characterized by convoluted elevated folds, 1-2 cm in thickness, usually in the fronto-occipital axis. Unlike the lax skin of other disorders, the convolutions cannot generally be flattened

by traction. Primary cutis gyrata may be associated with intellectual disability, retinitis pigmentosa, sensorineural deafness, and thyroid aplasia. Secondary cutis gyrata may be due to chronic inflammatory diseases, tumors, nevi, and acromegaly.

Bibliography is available at Expert Consult.

Chapter **649**
Ectodermal Dysplasias
Kari L. Martin

Ectodermal dysplasia (ED) is a heterogeneous group of disorders characterized by a constellation of findings involving defects of 2 or more of the following: teeth, skin, and appendageal structures including hair, nails, and eccrine and sebaceous glands. Although more than 150 EDs have been described, the majority are rare.

HYPOHIDROTIC ECTODERMAL DYSPLASIA
The syndrome known as hypohidrotic ectodermal dysplasia (HED) manifests as a triad of defects: partial or complete absence of sweat glands, anomalous dentition, and hypotrichosis. There are 4 recognized types of HED (Table 649-1); HED-1 (X-linked recessive) is most common.

In HED, affected patients are unable to sweat and may experience episodes of high fever in warm environments, which may be mistakenly considered to be fevers of **unknown origin.** This error is particularly common in infancy, when the facial changes are not easily appreciated. Diagnosis at this time may be made using the starch-iodine test or palmar or scalp biopsy. Scalp biopsy is the most sensitive and is 100% specific. The typical facies are characterized by frontal bossing; malar hypoplasia; a flattened nasal bridge; recessed columella; thick, everted lips; wrinkled, hyperpigmented periorbital skin; and prominent, low-set ears (Fig. 649-1). The skin over the entire body is dry, finely wrinkled, and hypopigmented, often with a prominent venous pattern. Extensive peeling of the skin is a clinical clue to diagnosis in the newborn period. The paucity of sebaceous glands may account for the dry skin. The scalp hair is sparse, fine, and lightly pigmented, and eyebrows and lashes are sparse or absent. Other body hair is also sparse or absent. Sexual hair growth is normal. Anodontia or hypodontia with widely spaced, conical teeth is a consistent feature (Fig. 649-1). Otolaryngic and ophthalmologic abnormalities secondary to decreased saliva and tear production are seen. The incidence of atopic diseases in children with HED is high. Gastroesophageal reflux is common and may play a role in failure to thrive, which is seen in 20% of cases. Sexual development is usually normal. Historically, the infant mortality rate has been 30%. Carrier females of X-linked HED have no or variable clinical manifestations.

Hypohidrotic ED with immune deficiencies causes similar findings in sweating and hair and nail development, in association with a **dysgammaglobulinemia.** Significant mortality is seen from recurrent infections.

Treatment of children with HED includes protecting them from exposure to high ambient temperatures. Early dental evaluation is necessary so that prostheses can be provided for cosmetic reasons and for adequate nutrition. The use of artificial tears prevents damage to the cornea in patients with defective lacrimation. Alopecia may necessitate the wearing of a wig to improve appearance.

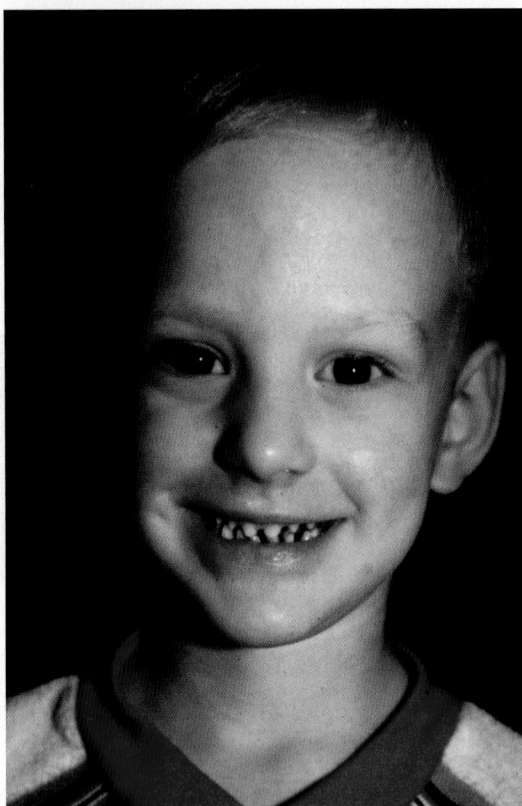

Figure 649-1 Hypohidrotic ectodermal dysplasia is characterized by pointed ears, fine hair, periorbital hyperpigmentation, midfacial hypoplasia, and pegged teeth. *(Courtesy of the Fitzsimons Army Medical Center teaching file.)*

Table 649-1	Four Recognized Types of Anhidrotic Ectodermal Dysplasia	
TYPE	**INHERITANCE**	**GENE DEFECT**
ED-1	X-linked recessive	Ectodysplasin A (*EDA*)
ED-2	Autosomal recessive	Ectodysplasin A anhidrotic receptor (*EDAR*) EDAR-associated death gene (*EDARADD*)
ED-3	Autosomal dominant	*EDAR* *EDARADD*
ED-anhidrotic with immune deficiency	X-linked recessive Autosomal dominant	IκK-γ (*NEMO*) *NFκB-IA*

HIDROTIC ECTODERMAL DYSPLASIA (CLOUSTON SYNDROME)

The salient features of the autosomal dominant disorder hidrotic ED are dystrophic, hypoplastic, or absent nails; sparse hair; and hyperkeratosis of the palms and soles. Conjunctivitis and blepharitis are common. The dentition and sweating are always normal. Absence of eyebrows and eyelashes and hyperpigmentation over the knees, elbows, and knuckles have been noted in some affected individuals. Mutations in the *GJB6* gene encoding the gap junction protein connexin 30 are responsible for this disorder. A similar disorder associated with deafness has been described with mutations in the *GJB2* gene encoding the connexin 26 protein.

Bibliography is available at Expert Consult.

Chapter 650
Vascular Disorders
Kari L. Martin

Nearly all vascular lesions of childhood may be divided into vascular malformations and vascular tumors (Table 650-1). Vascular malformations are developmental errors in blood vessel formation. Malformations do not regress but slowly enlarge. They should be named after the predominant vessel(s) forming the lesion. Genetic disorders may involve arterial, capillary, lymph, or venous malformations. Vascular tumors exhibit endothelial cell hyperplasia and proliferation.

VASCULAR MALFORMATIONS
Capillary Malformation (Port-Wine Stain)
Capillary malformations (CMs) are present at birth. These vascular malformations consist of mature dilated dermal capillaries. The lesions are macular, sharply circumscribed, pink to purple, and tremendously varied in size (Fig. 650-1). The head and neck region is the most common site of predilection; most lesions are unilateral. The mucous

Table 650-1	International Society for the Study of Vascular Anomalies (ISSVA) Classification System
VASCULAR MALFORMATION	**VASCULAR TUMOR**
Slow-flow malformations	Infantile hemangioma
Capillary malformation	Congenital hemangioma
Venous malformation	Rapidly involuting congenital hemangioma
Lymphatic malformation	
Fast-flow malformations	Noninvoluting congenital hemangioma
Arterial malformation	
Arteriovenous malformation	Kaposiform hemangioendothelioma
Arteriovenous fistula	Tufted angioma
Combined vascular malformations	Spindle cell hemangioendothelioma
	Epithelioid hemangioendothelioma
	Other rare hemangioendotheliomas
	Angiosarcoma
	Acquired vascular tumors: pyogenic granuloma

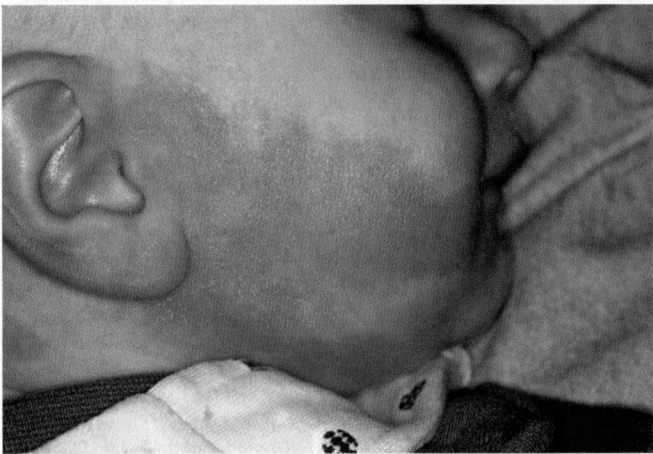

Figure 650-1 Capillary malformation. Pink macule on the cheek of an infant.

membranes can be involved. As a child matures into adulthood, the CM may become darker in color and pebbly in consistency; it may occasionally develop elevated areas that bleed spontaneously.

True CM should be distinguished from **nevus simplex**, which, in contrast, is a relatively transient lesion often located in the midline (see Chapter 647). When a CM is lateral and localized to the forehead, and upper eyelid the diagnosis of **Sturge-Weber syndrome** (glaucoma, leptomeningeal venous angioma, seizures, hemiparesis contralateral to the facial lesion, intracranial calcification) must be considered (see Chapter 596.3). Early screening for glaucoma is important to prevent additional damage to the eye. CMs also occur as a component of Klippel-Trenaunay syndrome and with moderate frequency in other syndromes, including Cobb (spinal arteriovenous malformation, port-wine stain), Proteus, Beckwith-Wiedemann, and Bonnet-Dechaume-Blanc syndromes. In the absence of associated anomalies, morbidity from these lesions may include a poor self-image, hypertrophy of underlying structures, and traumatic bleeding. In contrast to unilateral lesions associated with Sturge-Weber syndrome, medial *frontofacial CMs* are bilateral and involve the forehead, glabella, upper eyelids, nose, philtrum, and upper lip. These lesions may be familial, complete (involving all 7 areas), or incomplete, and are associated with other CMs on the occiput, neck or lumbosacral areas. Atypical cases are associated with Beckwith-Wiedemann and Rubinstein-Taybi syndromes.

The most effective **treatment** for CM is with the pulsed-dye laser. This therapy is targeted to hemoglobin within the lesion and avoids thermal injury to the surrounding normal tissue. After such treatment, the texture and pigmentation of the skin are generally normal without scarring. Therapy can begin in infancy, when the surface area of involvement is smaller. There may be advantages to treating within the 1st yr of life. Although this approach is quite effective, redarkening of the stain may occur 10 yr after therapy. Masking cosmetics may also be used.

Angiokeratoma Circumscriptum

Several forms of angiokeratoma have been described. Angiokeratomas are characterized by ectasia of superficial lymphatic vessels and capillaries with hyperkeratosis of the overlying epidermis. Angiokeratoma circumscriptum is a rare disorder consisting of a solitary lesion or multiple lesions that manifest as a plaque or plaques of blue-red crusted papules or nodules. The limbs are the sites of predilection. If therapy is desired, surgical excision is the treatment of choice.

Venous Malformation

Venous malformations include vein-only malformations and combination malformations. Malformations consisting of veins only run the gamut from nodules containing a mass of venules (Fig. 650-2) to diffuse large vein abnormalities that may consist of either a superficial component resembling varicose veins, deeper venous malformations, or both. Most venous malformations are sporadic, although inherited forms exist as well. Inherited forms and up to 40% of sporadic venous malformations are caused by *TIE2* mutations. Treatment is reserved for painful or symptomatic lesions. Surgical excision is best for small or superficial nodular lesions and sclerotherapy or laser ablation is used for larger, diffuse lesions. Localized intravascular coagulopathy can be problematic in these lesions because of the chronic slow flow. This leads to both painful thrombotic episodes and the risk of progression to systemic disseminated intravascular coagulopathy.

Cutis Marmorata Telangiectatica Congenita

Cutis marmorata telangiectatica congenital is a benign vascular anomaly that represents dilation of superficial capillaries and veins and is apparent at birth. Involved areas of skin have a reticulated red or purple hue that resembles physiologic cutis marmorata but is more pronounced and relatively unvarying (Fig. 650-3). The lesions may be restricted to a single limb and a portion of the trunk or may be more widespread. The lesions become more pronounced during changes in environmental temperature, physical activity, or crying. In some cases, the underlying subcutaneous tissue is atrophic, and ulceration may occur within the reticulated bands. Rarely, defective growth of bone and other congenital abnormalities may be present. No specific therapy is indicated. Mild vascular-only cases may show gradual improvement. Cutis marmorata telangiectatica congenita may be associated with CM, Adams-Oliver syndrome, patent ductus arteriosus, and a variety of other anomalies. It must be differentiated from reticulate CM and physiologic cutis marmorata.

Blue Rubber Bleb Nevus Syndrome

Blue rubber bleb nevus is a rare syndrome consisting of numerous venous malformations of the skin, mucous membranes, and gastrointestinal tract. Typical lesions are blue-purple and rubbery in consistency; they vary in size from a few millimeters to a few centimeters in diameter. They are sometimes painful or tender. The nodules occasionally are present at birth but usually are progressive during childhood. New lesions may continue to develop throughout life. Large disfiguring and irregular blue marks may also occur. The lesions, which can rarely be located in the liver, spleen, and central nervous system in addition to the skin and gastrointestinal tract, do not involute spontaneously. Recurrent gastrointestinal hemorrhage due to lesions in the gastrointestinal tract may lead to severe anemia. Palliation can be achieved by excision of involved bowel.

KLIPPEL-TRENAUNAY AND PARKES-WEBER SYNDROMES

Klippel-Trenaunay syndrome is a term historically used to describe complex, mixed vascular malformation with overgrowth of bone and

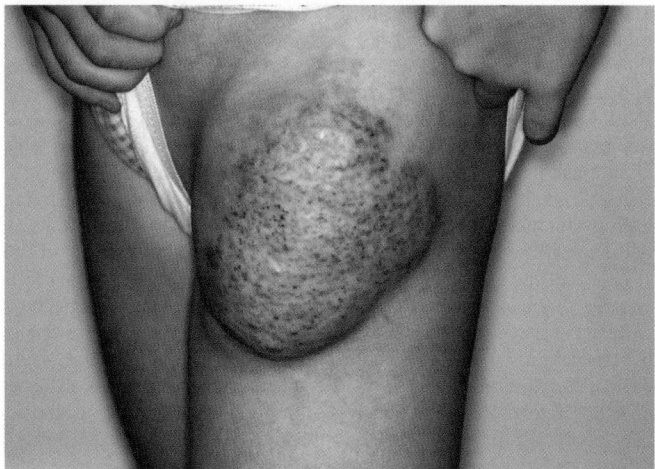

Figure 650-2 Nodular venous malformation on the leg of an adolescent.

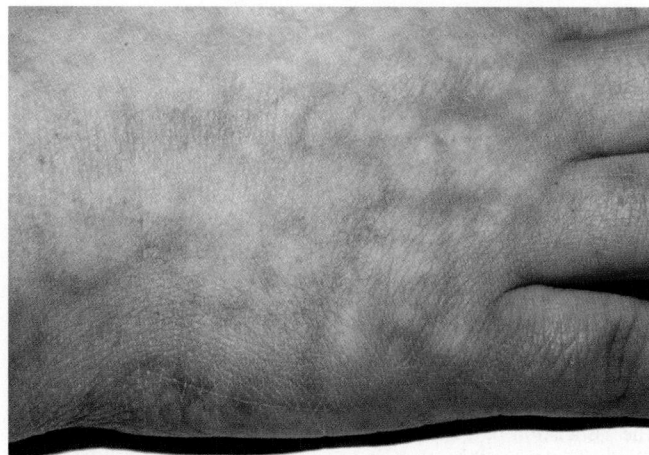

Figure 650-3 Mottled pattern of cutis marmorata telangiectatica congenita on the right hand.

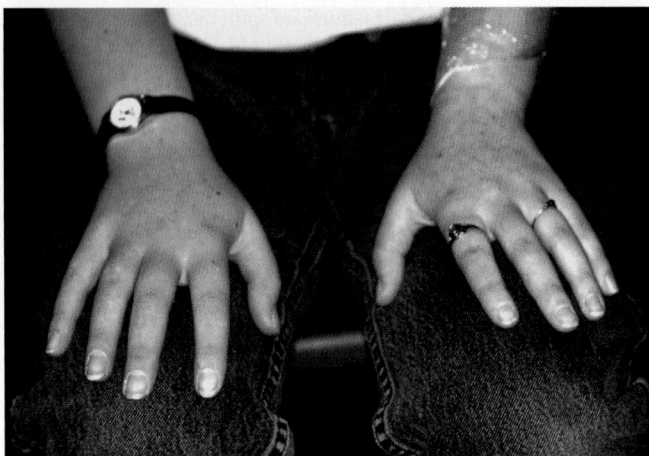

Figure 650-4 Overgrowth of the right arm and hand in and adolescent with Klippel-Trenaunay syndrome.

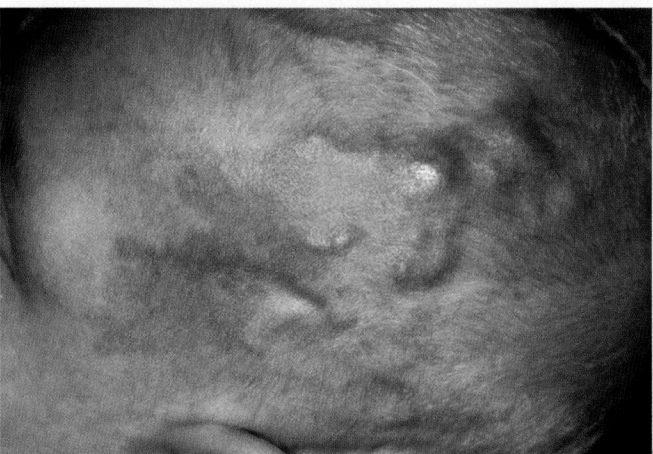

Figure 650-5 Arteriovenous malformation in conjunction with a portwine stain of the scalp of a newborn.

soft tissue (Fig. 650-4). The anomaly is present at birth and usually involves a lower limb but may involve more than 1 limb, as well as portions of the trunk or face. Enlargement of the soft tissues may be gradual and may involve the entire extremity, a portion of it, or selected digits. The vascular lesion most often is a capillary malformation, generally localized to the hypertrophied area. The deep venous system may be absent or hypoplastic. Venous blebs and/or vesicular lymphatic lesions may be present on the malformation's surface. Thick-walled venous varicosities typically become apparent ipsilateral to the vascular malformation after the child begins to ambulate. If there is an associated arteriovenous malformation (AVM), the disorder is called Parkes-Weber syndrome.

These disorders can be confused with **Maffucci syndrome** or, if the surface vascular lesion is minimal, with **Milroy disease**. Pain, limb swelling, and cellulitis may occur. Thrombophlebitis, dislocations of joints, hematuria secondary to angiomatous involvement of the urinary tract, rectal bleeding from lesions of the gastrointestinal tract, pulmonary lesions, and malformations of the lymphatic vessels are infrequent complications. MRI may delineate the extent of the anomaly, but surgical correction or palliation is often difficult. Sclerotherapy or endovenous laser ablation may be of benefit when a venous component is the dominant vessel in the malformation. The indications for radiologic studies of viscera and bones are best determined by clinical evaluation. Supportive care includes compression bandages for varicosities; surgical treatment may help carefully selected patients. Leg-length differences should be treated with orthotic devices to prevent the development of spinal deformities. Corrective bone surgery may eventually be needed to treat significant leg-length discrepancy.

ARTERIOVENOUS MALFORMATION
AVMs are direct connections of artery to vein that bypass the capillary bed (Fig. 650-5). AVMs of the skin are very rare. Skin changes are often noted at birth, but they tend to be very subtle presenting as a red-pink patch. Over time the lesions deepen in color and often result in thickening of the skin and surrounding tissue. They are diagnosed from their obvious arterial palpation. Some AVMs are progressive and can lead to significant morbidity and even mortality, so early diagnosis and evaluation by an experienced multidisciplinary team is essential.

LYMPHATIC MALFORMATIONS
See Chapter 489.

PHAKOMATOSIS PIGMENTOVASCULARIS
Phakomatosis pigmentovascularis is a rare disorder characterized by the association of a capillary malformation and melanocytic lesions. Typically, the capillary malformation is extensive, and associated pigmentary lesions may include dermal melanocytosis (mongolian spots), café-au-lait macules, or a nevus spilus (speckled nevus). Nonpig-

mented skin lesions that may occur in this setting include nevus anemicus and epidermal nevi. Systemic anomalies are seen in rare cases.

NEVUS ANEMICUS
Although present at birth, nevus anemicus may not be detectable until early childhood. The nevus consists of solitary or numerous, sharply delineated pale macules or patches that are most often on the trunk but may also occur on the neck or limbs. These nevi may simulate plaques of vitiligo, leukoderma, or nevoid pigmentary defects, but they can be readily distinguished because of their response to firm stroking. Stroking evokes an erythematous line and flare in normal surrounding skin, but the skin of a nevus anemicus does not redden. They can also be diagnosed by diascopy, in which pressure of the skin with a glass slide will obscure the borders of a nevus anemicus. Although the cutaneous vasculature appears normal histologically, the blood vessels within the nevus do not respond to injection of vasodilators. It has been postulated that the persistent pallor may represent a sustained localized adrenergic vasoconstriction.

VASCULAR TUMORS
Vascular tumors include infantile hemangiomas, tufted angiomas, kaposiform hemangioendotheliomas, rapidly involuting congenital hemangiomas, and noninvoluting congenital hemangiomas.

Infantile Hemangioma
Infantile hemangiomas (IHs) are proliferative, benign vascular tumors of vascular endothelium that may be present at birth or, more commonly, may become apparent in the 1st 2 wk of life, predictably enlarge, and then spontaneously involute. IHs are the most common tumor of infancy, occurring in 5% of newborns. Risk factors include prematurity, low birthweight, female sex, and white race. IHs should be classified as superficial, deep, or mixed. The terms *strawberry* and *cavernous* should not be used to describe hemangiomas. The immunohistochemical marker GLUT-1 is specifically expressed in an IH, which helps distinguish it histologically from other vascular anomalies. Superficial IHs are bright red, protuberant, compressible, sharply demarcated lesions that may occur on any area of the body (Figs. 650-6 and 650-7). Although sometimes present at birth, they more often appear in the 1st 2 mo of life and are heralded by an erythematous or blue mark or an area of pallor, which subsequently develops a fine telangiectatic pattern before the growth phase. The presenting sign may occasionally be an ulceration of the perineum or lip. Favored sites are the face, scalp, back, and anterior chest; lesions may be solitary or multiple. Patterns of facial involvement include frontotemporal, maxillary, mandibular, and frontonasal regions. IHs that are more deeply situated are more diffuse and are less defined than superficial IHs. The lesions are cystic, firm, or compressible, and the overlying skin may appear normal in color or may have a bluish hue (Fig. 650-8).

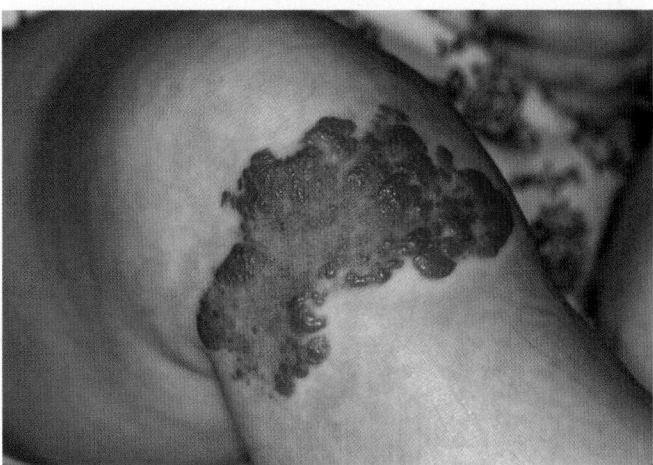

Figure 650-6 Superficial hemangioma on the right knee.

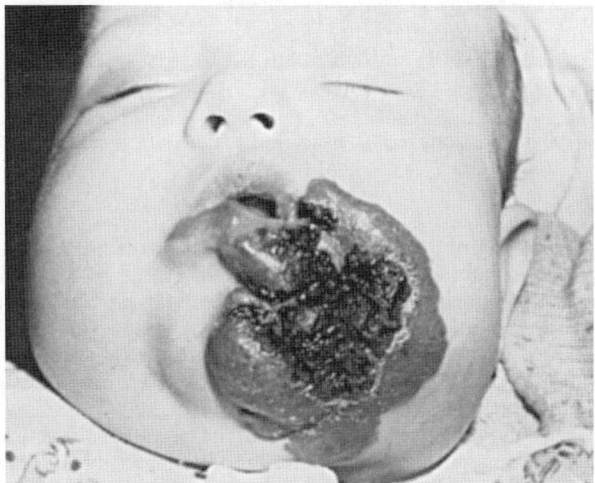

Figure 650-7 Large hemangioma with central crusted ulcer.

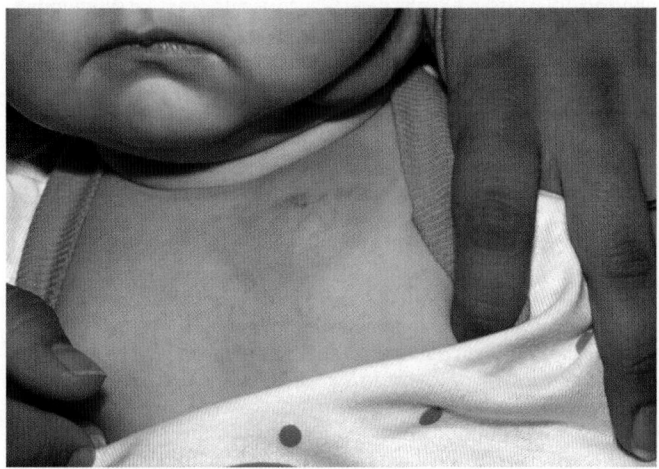

Figure 650-8 Deep hemangioma of the chest.

Table 650-2	Complications of Hemangioma and Their Treatment
CLINICAL FINDING	**RECOMMENDED TREATMENT**
Severe ulceration/ maceration	Encourage twice-daily cleansing regimen Dilute sodium bicarbonate soaks ± Flashlamp pulsed-dye laser ± Oral corticosteroids or propranolol ± Culture-directed systemic antibiotics for infection
Bleeding (not KMP)	Gelfoam or Surgifoam or propranolol Compression therapy ± embolization
Hemangioma with ophthalmologic sequelae	Patching therapy as directed by ophthalmologist Intralesional vs oral corticosteroids vs propranolol
Subglottic hemangioma	Oral corticosteroids, propranolol, ± potassium titanyl phosphate (KtP) laser Tracheotomy if required
KMP	Corticosteroids, aminocaproic acid, vincristine, interferon-α ± embolization
High-flow hepatic hemangioma	Corticosteroids or interferon ± embolization

KMP, Kasabach-Merritt phenomenon.
From Blei F: Vascular anomalies: From bedside to bench and back again.
Curr Probl Pediatr Adolesc Health *32:72–93, 2002.*

involvement, but lip lesions seem to persist most often. Complications include impairment of a vital function, ulceration, secondary infection, and permanent disfigurement (Table 650-2). The location of a lesion may interfere with a vital function (e.g., on eyelid interfering with vision, on urethra with urination, on airway with respiration). IHs in a "beard" distribution may be associated with upper airway or subglottic involvement. Stridor should suggest a tracheobronchial lesion. Large visceral IHs may be complicated by coexistent hypothyroidism because of type 3 iodothyronine deiodinase, and symptoms may be difficult to detect in this age group. Table 650-3 lists other concerning features.

In the usual patient with an IH who has no serious complications or extensive growth resulting in tissue destruction and severe disfigurement, treatment consists of expectant observation. Because almost all lesions regress spontaneously, therapy is rarely indicated. Parents require repeated reassurance and support. After spontaneous involution, many patients are left with small cosmetic defects, such as telangiectasia, hypopigmentation, fibrofatty deposits, and scars if the lesion has ulcerated. Residual telangiectasias may be treated with pulsed-dye laser therapy. Other defects can be treated or minimized by judicious surgical repair if desired.

In the rare case in which intervention is required, topical timolol solution (0.5% gel; maximum dose 0.5 mg/day) is effective, especially in small, superficial, nonulcerating and nonmucosal IH. At this time, topical timolol treatment appears a very safe alternative to observation alone for a superficial IH. Timolol solution may also be used with caution in the treatment of an ulcerated IH, with or without occlusion.

In a disfiguring, life- or vision-threatening, or ulcerated IH that is not responding to other treatment, oral propranolol is the first-line treatment in most cases. IHs typically respond with growth arrest and often early signs of involution within a couple weeks of treatment initiation. Dosing varies ranging from 1-3 mg/kg/day. Some recommend inpatient initiation of propranolol for infants younger than 8 wk gestational age or those with comorbid conditions. The dose is initiated at 1 mg/kg/day divided into 3 doses with heart rate and blood pressure monitoring at 1 and 2 hr after each dose. If that dose is tolerated, the dose is increased to 2 mg/kg/day tid. The outpatient initiation assumes

Most IHs are mixed, having both superficial and deep components. IHs undergo a phase of rapid expansion, followed by a stationary period and finally by spontaneous involution. Regression may be anticipated when the lesion develops pale gray areas centrally. The course of a particular lesion is unpredictable, but approximately 60% of these lesions reach maximal involution by 5 yr of age, and 90-95% by 9 yr. Spontaneous involution cannot be correlated with size or site of

Table 650-3	Clinical "Red Flags" Associated with Hemangiomas
CLINICAL FINDING	**RECOMMENDED EVALUATION**
Facial hemangioma involving significant area of face	Evaluate for PHACES (posterior fossa abnormalities, hemangioma, and arterial, cardiac, eye, and sternal abnormalities): MRI for orbital hemangioma ± posterior fossa malformation Cardiac, ophthalmologic evaluation Evaluate for midline abnormality: supraumbilical raphe, sternal atresia, cleft palate, thyroid abnormality
Cutaneous hemangiomas in beard distribution	Evaluate for airway hemangioma, especially if manifesting with stridor
Periocular hemangioma	MRI of orbit Ophthalmologic evaluation
Paraspinal midline vascular lesion	Ultrasonography or MRI to evaluate for occult spinal dysraphism
Hemangiomatosis (multiple small cutaneous hemangiomas)	Evaluate for parenchymal hemangiomas, especially hepatic/central nervous system Guaiac stool test
Large hemangioma, especially hepatic	Ultrasonography with Doppler flow study MRI Thyroid function studies
Thrill and/or bruit associated with hemangioma	Consider cardiac evaluation and echocardiography to rule out diastolic reversal of flow in aorta MRI to evaluate extent and flow characteristics
Head tilting	Evaluate appropriately for specific site of lesion, and consider physical therapy evaluation
Delayed milestones	Consider side effect of corticosteroids (myopathy, weight-related) Consider side effect of interferon (especially spastic diplegia)
LUMBAR syndrome	MRI of spine, kidneys

LUMBAR, lower body infantile hemangiomas and other skin defects, urogenital anomalies and ulceration, myelopathy, boney deformities, anorectal malformations and arterial anomalies, renal anomalies.
From Blei F: Vascular anomalies: from bedside to bench and back again. Curr Probl Pediatr Adolesc Health 32:67–102, 2002.

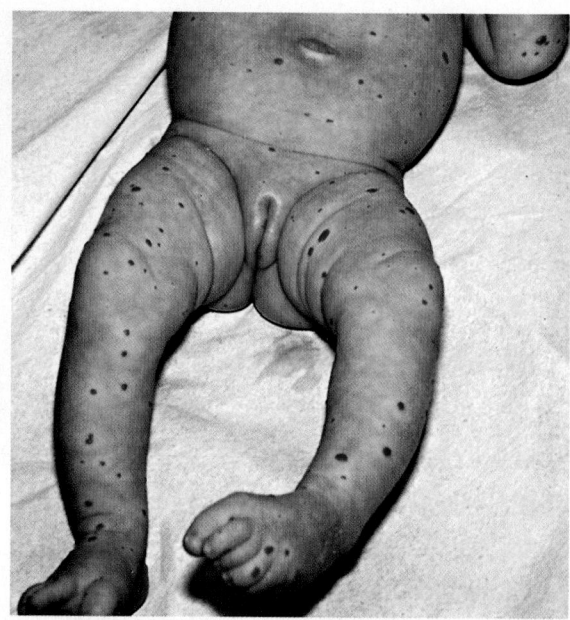

Figure 650-9 Disseminated cutaneous (and liver) neonatal hemangiomatosis. *(From Eichenfield LF, Frieden IJ, Esterly NB: Textbook of neonatal dermatology, ed 2, Philadelphia, 2008, WB Saunders, p. 359.)*

good social support and access to the hospital. The initial dose and monitoring is similar to the inpatient plan; if the dose is tolerated for 3-7 days, the dose is increased to 1.5 mg/kg/day tid. If the latter dose is tolerated after 3-7 days, the dose is increased to 2 mg/kg/day tid. *In all situations, propranolol must be given a minimum of 6 hr after the last dose.* Risks of propranolol treatment include hypoglycemia, bradycardia, hypotension, gastroesophageal reflux disease or worsening of existing disease, hyperkalemia, and bronchospasm/wheezing. Nonetheless, reports of side effects of propranolol used for IH treatment are rare. Increased propranolol levels occur with inhibitors of CYP2D6 (cimetidine, amiodarone, fluoxetine, quinidine, ritonavir) and CPY1A2 (cimetidine, ciprofloxacin, isoniazid, ritonavir, theophylline); decreased blood levels occur with inducers of hepatic drug metabolism (rifampin, phenytoin, phenobarbital).

In patients unable to tolerate propranolol, or if the IH has not responded after a couple of weeks of treatment, systemic oral corticosteroids may be used. Termination of growth and sometimes regression may be evident after 2-4 wk of therapy. When a response is obtained, the dose should be decreased gradually, though most patients will require treatment until about 1 year of age.

Intralesional corticosteroid injection in the hands of an experienced physician can also induce rapid involution of a localized IH, but has risks of ulceration, tissue atrophy, and blindness if used near the orbit. Vincristine is used by some oncologists to treat significant IH. Interferon-α therapy may also be effective, but spastic diplegia is seen in 10% of cases. Use of these therapies has become less necessary since the introduction of propranolol.

In patients with large segmental IH of the face, PHACE syndrome should be considered. **PHACE stands for p**osterior fossa brain defects such as Dandy-Walker malformation or cerebellar hypoplasia, large segmental facial infantile **h**emangioma, **a**rterial cerebrovascular abnormalities such as aneurysms and stroke, **c**oarctation of the aorta, **e**ye abnormalities. **S**ternal raphe defects such as pits, scars, or **s**upraumbilical raphe are infrequently observed. Evaluation of children at risk for PHACE is important both to detect any underlying abnormalities and also before starting systemic therapy, which may be indicated given the size and location of the IH typically associated with this syndrome. PHACE children with cervical and intracranial arterial abnormalities are at increased risk of cerebrovascular accidents and specialized care by an experienced multidisciplinary team is essential.

Multifocal Infantile Hemangioma

Diffuse neonatal hemangiomatosis (or benign neonatal hemangiomatosis) is a historical term to describe a condition in which numerous or multifocal vascular lesions are widely distributed (Fig. 650-9). In the past, several distinct diagnoses have been lumped together under this clinical phenotype with mortality cited as high as 60-80%. Upon further analysis, this group of disorders has been found to comprise several distinct entities which are important to distinguish from one another given their varying prognoses and management strategies. Multifocal IHs may occur in the skin as well as visceral organs, but remain GLUT-1–positive when biopsied, have a relatively good prognosis with low morbidity, and respond to systemic propranolol just as solitary cutaneous IH. **Multifocal lymphangioendotheliomatosis** (also known as cutaneovisceral angiomatosis) also presents with many vascular tumors in the skin and visceral organs, but is GLUT-1–negative and complicated by severe thrombocytopenia and gastrointestinal bleeding with high mortality. Therefore accurate diagnosis in patients who present with multifocal vascular tumors is critical so early, appropriate management may be initiated.

Kaposiform Hemangioendothelioma

Kaposiform hemangioendothelioma (KHE) is a rare and potentially life-threatening vascular tumor. Initial cases described IHs with purpura and coagulopathy, but these are now known to have been KHE. KHE classically present as a red to purple firm plaque on the lateral neck, axilla, trunk or extremities. Visceral tumors occur as well. Lesions may occasionally get smaller over time but rarely resolve completely. **Tufted angioma,** once thought to be a separate tumor on the same clinical spectrum as KHE, is considered under the umbrella term of KHE (Fig. 650-10). The main complication of these tumors is the development of Kasabach-Merritt phenomenon (KMP), which may be fatal; therefore, early diagnosis and treatment is important. Retroperitoneal or intrathoracic lesions in the absence of cutaneous lesions are uncommon but are often associated with KMP.

Kasabach-Merritt Phenomenon

KMP is a life-threatening combination of a rapidly enlarging KHE, thrombocytopenia, microangiopathic hemolytic anemia, and an acute or chronic consumption coagulopathy. The clinical manifestations are usually evident during early infancy. The vascular lesion is usually cutaneous and is only rarely located in viscera. The associated thrombocytopenia may lead to precipitous hemorrhage accompanied by ecchymoses, petechiae, and a rapid increase in the size of the vascular lesion. Severe anemia from hemorrhage or microangiopathic hemolysis may ensue. The platelet count is depressed, but the bone marrow contains increased numbers of normal or immature megakaryocytes. The thrombocytopenia has been attributed to sequestration or increased destruction of platelets within the lesion. Hypofibrinogenemia and decreased levels of consumable clotting factors are relatively common (see Chapter 484.6).

Treatment includes surgical excision of small lesions, although this is often difficult because of coagulopathy. Additional pharmacologic treatments include systemic steroids with or without vincristine as first-line therapy in most cases. Antiplatelet, antifibrinolytic, and other chemotherapeutic agents have been used with mixed results. Ongoing studies of sirolimus use in KHE patients are underway; initial case reports have been promising. The mortality rate overall once patients have KMP is significant.

Pyogenic Granuloma (Lobular Capillary Hemangioma)

A pyogenic granuloma (PG) is a small red, glistening, sessile, or pedunculated papule that often has a discernible epithelial collarette (Fig. 650-11). The surface may be weeping and crusted or completely epithelialized. PGs initially grow rapidly, may ulcerate, and bleed easily when traumatized because they consist of exuberant granulation tissue. They are relatively common in children, particularly on the face, arms, and hands. Such a lesion located on a finger or hand may appear as a subcutaneous nodule. PGs may arise at sites of injury, but a history of trauma often cannot be elicited.

PGs are benign but a nuisance because they bleed easily with trauma and may recur if incompletely removed. Numerous satellite papules have developed after surgical excision of PGs from the back, particularly in the interscapular region. Small lesions may regress after cauterization with silver nitrate; larger lesions require excision and electrodesiccation of the base of the granuloma. Small (<5 mm) lesions may be treated successfully with pulsed-dye laser therapy.

Angiokeratoma of Mibelli

Angiokeratoma of Mibelli is characterized by 1-8 mm red, purple, or black scaly, verrucous, occasionally crusted papules and nodules that appear on the dorsum of the fingers and toes and on the knees and the elbows. Less commonly, palms, soles, and ears may be affected. In many patients, onset has followed frostbite or chilblains. These nodules bleed freely after injury and may involute in response to trauma. They may be effectively eradicated by cryotherapy, electrofulguration, excision, or laser ablation.

Spider Angioma

A vascular spider (nevus araneus) consists of a central feeder artery with many dilated radiating vessels and a surrounding erythematous flush, varying from a few millimeters to several centimeters in diameter (Fig. 650-12). Pressure over the central vessel causes blanching; pulsations visible in larger nevi are evidence for the arterial source of the lesion. Spider angiomas are associated with conditions in which there are increased levels of circulating estrogens, such as cirrhosis and pregnancy, but they also occur in up to 15% of normal preschool-age children and 45% of school-age children. Sites of predilection in children are the dorsum of the hand, forearm, nose, infraocular region,

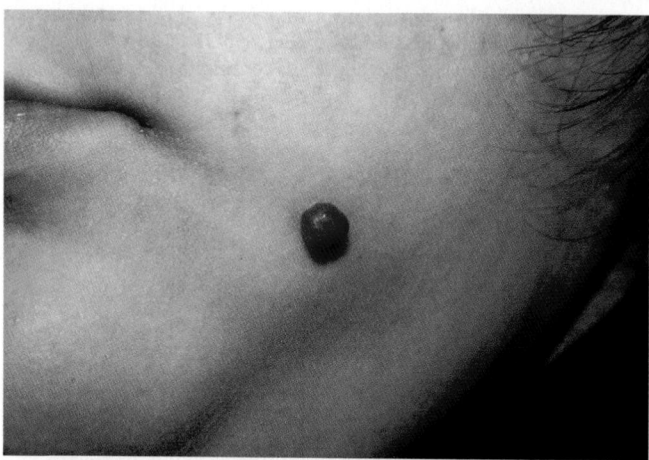

Figure 650-11 Pyogenic granuloma on the left cheek.

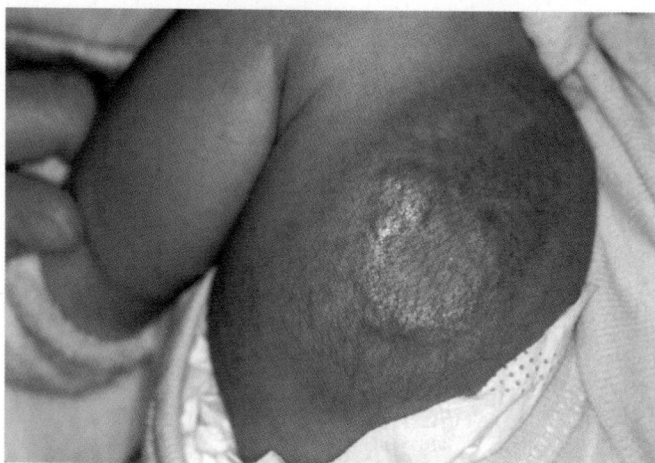

Figure 650-10 Nodular tufted angioma on the left thigh.

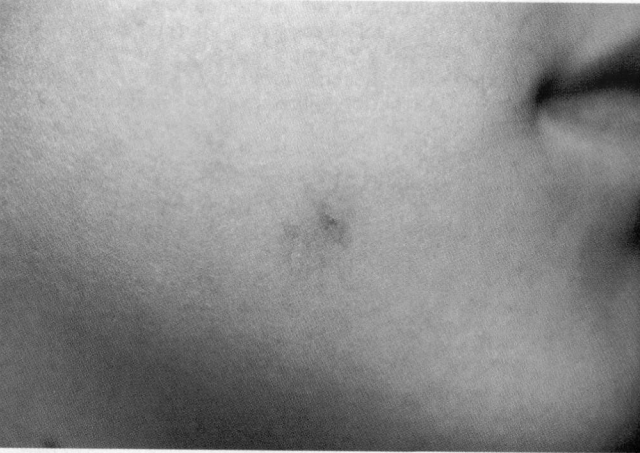

Figure 650-12 Spider telangiectasia with visible central arteriole component.

lips, and ears. Lesions often regress spontaneously after puberty. If removal is desired, pulsed dye laser therapy is the mode of choice; resolution is achieved in 90% of cases with a single treatment.

Maffucci Syndrome

The association of spindle cell hemangiomas with **nodular enchon-dromas** in the metaphyseal or diaphyseal cartilaginous portion of long bones is known as Maffucci syndrome. Maffucci syndrome is caused by somatic mosaic mutations in the *IDH1* and *IDH2* genes. Vascular lesions are typically soft, compressible, asymptomatic blue to purple subcutaneous masses that grow in proportion to a child's growth and stabilize by adulthood. Mucous membranes or viscera may also be involved. Onset occurs during childhood. Bone lesions may produce limb deformities and pathologic fractures. Malignant transformation of enchondromas (chondrosarcoma, angiosarcoma) or primary malignancies (ovarian, fibrosarcoma, glioma, pancreatic) may be a complication (see Chapter 501).

Hereditary Hemorrhagic Telangiectasia (Osler-Weber-Rendu Disease)

Hereditary hemorrhagic telangiectasia (HHT), which is inherited as an autosomal dominant trait, occurs in 2 types. The gene in HHT-1 encodes endoglin (*ENG*), a membrane glycoprotein on endothelial cells that binds transforming growth factor-β. HHT-2 is caused by mutations in the *ACVRL1* gene (activin A receptor type 2-like kinase 1) and is associated with increased risk for hepatic involvement and pulmonary hypertension. Affected children may experience recurrent epistaxis before detection of the characteristic skin and mucous membrane lesions. The mucocutaneous lesions, which usually develop at puberty, are 1-4 mm, sharply demarcated red to purple macules, papules, or spider-like projections, each composed of a tightly woven mat of tortuous telangiectatic vessels (Fig. 650-13). The nasal mucosa, lips, and tongue are usually involved; less commonly, cutaneous lesions occur on the face, ears, palms, and nail beds. Vascular ectasias may

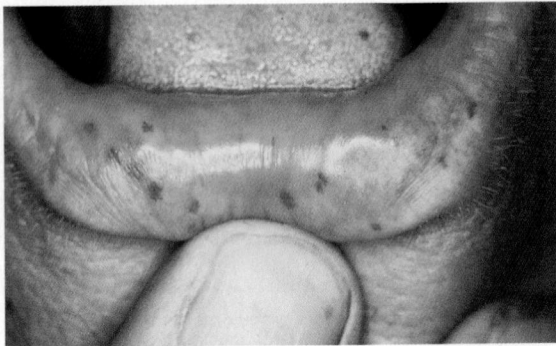

Figure 650-13 Hereditary hemorrhagic telangiectasia. Telangiectases are found on the lips, oral mucosa, nasal mucosa, skin, and conjunctiva. Epistaxis is the most common manifestation of the disease. Blood transfusions may be required. *(From Habif TP: Clinical dermatology: a color guide to diagnosis and therapy, ed 4, Philadelphia, 2004, Mosby, Fig. 23-22, p. 831.)*

also arise in the conjunctivae, larynx, pharynx, gastrointestinal tract, bladder, vagina, bronchi, brain, and liver.

Massive hemorrhage is the most serious complication of HHT and may result in severe anemia. Bleeding may occur from the nose, mouth, gastrointestinal tract, genitourinary tract, or lungs; epistaxis is often the only complaint occurring in 80% of patients. Approximately 15-20% of patients with AVMs in the lungs present with stroke due to embolic abscesses (Fig. 650-14). Persons with HHT have normal levels of clotting factors and an intact clotting mechanism. In the absence of serious complications, the life span of a person with HHT is normal. Local lesions may be ablated temporarily with chemical cautery or electrocoagulation. More drastic surgical measures may be required for lesions in critical sites, such as the lung or gastrointestinal tract. Bevacizumab, an antivascular endothelial growth factor agent, has been effective in treating affected patients with HHT, who have high cardiac output secondary to hepatic AVMs.

Ataxia-Telangiectasia
See Chapter 597.1.

Ataxia-telangiectasia is transmitted as an autosomal recessive trait because of a mutation in the *ATM* gene. The characteristic telangiectasias develop at approximately 3 yr of age, first on the bulbar conjunctivae and later on the nasal bridge, malar areas, external ears, hard palate, upper anterior chest, and antecubital and popliteal fossae. Additional cutaneous stigmata include café-au-lait spots, premature graying of the hair, and sclerodermatous changes. Progressive cerebellar ataxia, neurologic deterioration, sinopulmonary infections, and malignancies are also seen.

Angiokeratoma Corporis Diffusum (Fabry Disease)
See Chapter 86.4.

An inborn error of glycolipid metabolism (α-galactosidase), angiokeratoma corporis diffusum is an X-linked recessive disorder that is fully penetrant in males and is of variable penetrance in carrier females. Angiokeratomas appear before puberty and occur in profusion over the genitalia, hips, buttocks, and thighs and in the umbilical and inguinal regions. They consist of 0.1-3.0 mm red to blue-black papules that may have a hyperkeratotic surface. Telangiectasias are seen in the mucosa and conjunctiva. On light microscopy, these angiokeratomas appear as blood-filled, dilated, endothelium-lined vascular spaces. Granular lipid deposits are demonstrable in dermal macrophages, fibrocytes, and endothelial cells.

Additional clinical manifestations include recurrent episodes of fever and agonizing pain, cyanosis and flushing of the acral limb areas, paresthesias of the hands and feet, corneal opacities detectable on slit-lamp examination, and hypohidrosis. Renal involvement and cardiac involvement are the usual causes of death. The biochemical defect is a deficiency of the lysosomal enzyme α-galactosidase, with accumulation of ceramide trihexoside in tissues, particularly vascular endothelium, and excretion in urine (see Chapter 86.4 for therapy). Similar cutaneous lesions have also been described in another lysosomal enzyme disorder, α-L-fucosidase deficiency, and in sialidosis, a storage disease with neuraminidase deficiency.

Bibliography is available at Expert Consult.

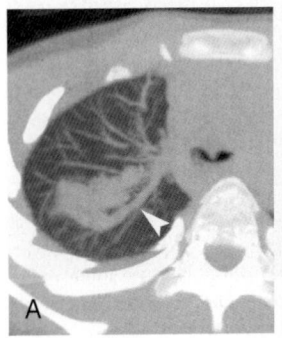
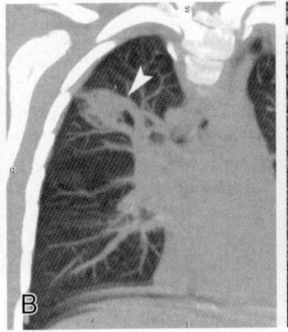
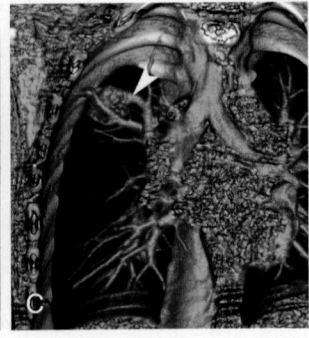

Figure 650-14 Chest multislice spiral CT in patient 2 showing a large pulmonary arteriovenous malformation in the posterior segment of right upper lobe *(arrowhead)*. **A,** Axial maximum intensity projection image. **B,** Coronal maximum intensity projection image. **C,** Three-dimensional volume rendering. *(From Giordano P, Lenato GM, Suppressa P, et al: Hereditary hemorrhagic telangiectasia: arteriovenous malformations in children. J Pediatr 163:179–186, 2013, Fig. 1, p. 182.)*

Chapter **651**
Cutaneous Nevi
Kari L. Martin

Nevus skin lesions are characterized histopathologically by collections of well-differentiated cell types normally found in the skin. Vascular nevi are described in Chapter 650. Melanocytic nevi are subdivided into 2 broad categories: those that appear after birth (acquired nevi) and those that are present at birth (congenital nevi).

ACQUIRED MELANOCYTIC NEVUS
Melanocytic nevus is a benign cluster of melanocytic nevus cells that arises as a result of alteration and proliferation of melanocytes at the epidermal–dermal junction.

Epidemiology
The number of acquired melanocytic nevi increases gradually during childhood and more slowly in early adulthood. The number reaches a plateau in the 3rd or 4th decade and then slowly decreases thereafter. The mean number of melanocytic nevi in an adult varies depending on genetics, skin color, and sun exposure. The greater the number of nevi present, the greater is the risk for development of **melanoma,** though the majority of melanomas arise de novo. Sun exposure during childhood, particularly intermittent, intense exposure of an individual with light skin, and a propensity to burn and freckle rather than tan are important determinants of the number of melanocytic nevi that develop. Red-haired children, despite their light skin and propensity to freckle and sunburn, have fewer nevi than other children. Increased numbers of nevi are also associated with immunosuppression and administration of chemotherapy.

Clinical Manifestations
Nevocellular nevi have a well-defined life history and are classified as **junctional, compound,** or **dermal** in accordance with the location of the nevus cells in the skin. In childhood, >90% of nevi are junctional; melanocyte proliferation occurs at the junction of the epidermis and dermis to form nests of cells. Junctional nevi appear anywhere on the body in various shades of brown; they are relatively small, discrete, flat, and variable in shape. The melanized nevus cells are cuboidal or epithelioid in configuration and occur in nests on the epidermal side of the basement membrane. Although some nevi, particularly those on the palms, soles, and genitalia, remain junctional throughout life, most become compound as melanocytes migrate into the papillary dermis to form nests at both the epidermal–dermal junction and within the dermis. If the junctional melanocytes stop proliferating, nests of melanocytes remain only within the dermis, forming an intradermal nevus. With maturation, compound and intradermal nevi may become raised, dome-shaped, verrucous, or pedunculated. Slightly elevated lesions are usually compound. Distinctly elevated lesions are usually intradermal. With age, the dermal melanocytic nests regress and the nevi gradually disappear.

Prognosis and Treatment
Acquired pigmented nevi are benign, but a very small percentage undergo malignant transformation. Suspicious changes are indications for excision and histopathologic evaluation; they include rapid increase in size; development of satellite lesions; variegation of color, particularly with shades of red, brown, gray, black, and blue; pigmentary incontinence; notching or irregularity of the borders; changes in texture such as scaling, erosion, ulceration, and induration; and regional lymphadenopathy. Most of these changes are from irritation, infection, or maturation; darkening and gradual increase in size and elevation normally occur during adolescence and should not be cause for concern. Two common benign changes are clonal nevi (fried-egg

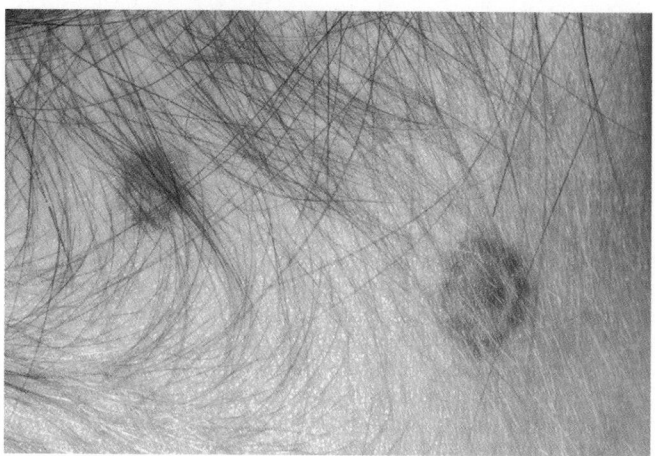

Figure 651-1 Eclipse nevi (rim moles) in the scalp.

moles) and eclipse nevi. A clonal nevus is light brown with a dark raised center representing a clonal change of a subset of nevus cells within the lesion. Eclipse nevi are flat and light brown with dark brown rims. They are seen primarily in the scalp (Fig. 651-1). Consideration should be given to the presence of risk factors for development of melanoma and the patient's parents' wishes about removal of the nevus. If doubt remains about the benign nature of a nevus, excision is a safe and simple outpatient procedure that may be justified to allay anxiety.

ATYPICAL MELANOCYTIC NEVUS
Atypical melanocytic nevi occur both in an **autosomal dominant familial melanoma-prone** setting (familial mole–melanoma syndrome, dysplastic nevus syndrome, BK mole syndrome) and as a sporadic event. Only 2% of all pediatric melanomas occur in individuals with this familial syndrome; melanoma develops before age 20 yr in 10% of individuals with the syndrome. Malignant melanoma has been reported in children with the dysplastic nevus syndrome as young as 10 yr. Risk for development of melanoma is essentially 100% in individuals with dysplastic nevus syndrome who have 2 family members who have had melanomas. The term *atypical mole syndrome* describes lesions in those individuals without an autosomal dominant familial history of melanoma but with more than 50 nevi, some of which are atypical. The lifetime risk of melanoma associated with dysplastic nevi in this context is estimated to be 5-10%.

Atypical nevi tend to be large (5-15 mm) and round to oval. They have irregular margins and variegated color, and portions of them are elevated. These nevi are most common on the posterior trunk, suggesting that intermittent, intense sun exposure has a role in their genesis. They may also occur in sun-protected areas such as the breasts, buttocks, and scalp. Atypical nevi do not usually develop until puberty, although scalp lesions may be present earlier. Atypical nevi demonstrate disordered proliferation of atypical intraepidermal melanocytes, lymphocytic infiltration, fibroplasia, and angiogenesis. It may be helpful to obtain histopathologic documentation of dysplastic change by biopsy to identify these individuals. It is prudent to excise borderline atypical nevi in immunocompromised children or in those treated with irradiation or chemotherapeutic agents. Although chemotherapy is associated with the development of a greater number of melanocytic nevi, it has not been directly linked to increased risk for development of melanoma. The threshold for removal of clinically atypical nevi is also lower at sites that are difficult to observe, such as the scalp. Children with atypical nevi should undergo a complete skin examination every 6-12 mo. In these children, photographic mole mapping serves as a useful adjunct in following nevus change. Parents must be counseled about the importance of sun protection and avoidance and should be instructed to look for early signs of melanoma on a regular basis, approximately every 3-4 mo.

CONGENITAL MELANOCYTIC NEVUS

Congenital melanocytic nevi are present in ≈1% of newborn infants. These nevi have been categorized by size: giant congenital nevi are >20 cm in diameter (adult size) or >5% of the body surface; small congenital nevi are <1.5 cm in diameter, and intermediate nevi are in between these dimensions. Congenital nevi are characterized by the presence of nevus cells in the lower reticular dermis; between collagen bundles; surrounding cutaneous appendages, nerves, and vessels in the lower dermis; and occasionally extending to the subcuticular fat. They often harbor *NRAS* mutations, but not *BRAF* mutations typically seen in regular melanocytic nevi. Identification is often uncertain, however, because they may have the histologic features of ordinary junctional, compound, or intradermal nevi. Some nevi that were not present at birth display histopathologic features of congenital nevi; these should not be considered congenital. Furthermore, congenital nevi may be difficult to distinguish clinically from other types of pigmented lesions, adding to the difficulty that parents may have in identifying nevi that were present at birth. The clinical differential diagnosis includes dermal melanocytosis, café-au-lait macules, and smooth muscle hamartoma.

Sites of predilection for small congenital nevi are the lower trunk, upper back, shoulders, chest, and proximal limbs. The lesions may be flat, elevated, verrucous, or nodular and may be various shades of brown, blue, or black. Given the difficulty in identifying small congenital nevi with certainty, data regarding their malignant potential are controversial and likely overstated. The true incidence of melanoma in congenital nevi, especially small and medium-sized lesions, is unknown. Removal of all small congenital nevi is not warranted because the development of melanoma in a small congenital nevus is an exceedingly rare event before puberty. A number of factors must be weighed in the decision about whether or not to remove a nevus, including its location, the ability to monitor it clinically, the potential for scarring, the presence of other risk factors for melanoma, and the presence of atypical clinical features.

Giant congenital pigmented nevi (<1 in 20,000 births) occur most commonly on the posterior trunk (Fig. 651-2) but may also appear on the head or extremities. These nevi are of special significance because of their association with leptomeningeal melanocytosis (neurocutaneous melanocytosis) and their predisposition for development of malignant melanoma. Leptomeningeal involvement occurs most often when the nevus is located on the head or midline on the trunk, particularly when associated with multiple "satellite" melanocytic nevi (>20 lesions). Nevus cells within the leptomeninges and brain parenchyma may cause increased intracranial pressure, hydrocephalus, seizures, intellectual disability, and motor deficits and may result in melanoma. Malignancy can be identified by careful cytologic examination of the cerebrospinal fluid for melanin-containing cells. MRI

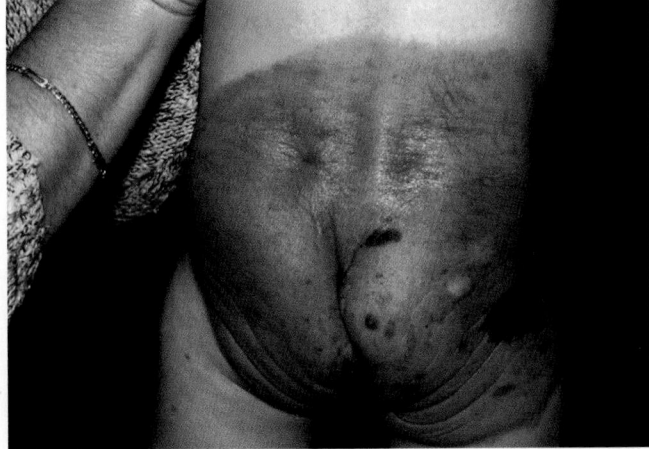

Figure 651-2 "Bathing suit" large congenital melanocytic nevus.

demonstrates asymptomatic leptomeningeal melanosis in ≈30% of individuals with giant congenital nevus of the type described above. The overall incidence of malignant melanoma arising in a giant congenital nevus has been estimated to be ≈5-10% but is more likely to be approximately 1-2%. The median age at diagnosis of the melanomas that arise within a giant congenital nevus is 7 yr. The mortality rate approaches 100%. The risk of melanoma is greater in patients in whom the predicted adult size of the nevus is >40 cm, lesions on trunk, and presence of satellite lesions. Management of giant congenital nevi remains controversial and should involve the parents, pediatrician, dermatologist, and plastic surgeon. If the nevus lies over the head or spine, MRI may allow detection of **neural melanosis,** the presence of which makes gross removal of a nevus from the skin a futile effort. In the absence of neural melanosis, early excision and repair aided by tissue expanders or grafting may reduce the burden of nevus cells and thus the potential for development of melanoma, but at the cost of many potentially disfiguring operations. Nevus cells deep within subcutaneous tissues may evade excision. Random biopsies of the nevus are not helpful, but biopsy of newly expanding nodules is indicated. Follow-up every 6 mo for 5 yr and every 12 mo thereafter is recommended. Serial photographs of the nevus may aid in detecting changes.

MELANOMA

Malignant melanoma accounts for 1-3% of all pediatric malignancies, and approximately 2% of all melanomas occur before age 20 yr. The incidence of melanoma continues to increase. Melanoma is 7 times more frequent in the 2nd decade of life than in the 1st decade of life. Melanoma develops primarily in white individuals, on the head and trunk in males, and on the extremities in females. Risk factors for development of melanoma include the presence of the familial atypical mole–melanoma syndrome or xeroderma pigmentosum; an increased number of acquired melanocytic nevi, or atypical nevi; fair complexion; excessive sun exposure, especially intermittent exposure to intense sunlight; a personal or family (1st-degree relative) history of a previous melanoma, giant congenital nevus, and immunosuppression. In previously well children, UV radiation is responsible for most melanomas. Fewer than 5% of childhood melanomas develop within giant congenital nevi or in individuals with the familial atypical mole–melanoma syndrome. Approximately 40-50% of the time, melanoma develops at a site where there was no apparent nevus. The mortality rate from melanoma is related primarily to tumor thickness and the level of invasion into the skin. The overall mortality rate reaches ≈40%, regardless of whether the tumor arises in a child or adult.

Given the lack of effective therapy for melanoma, prevention and early detection are the most effective measures. Emphasis should be given to avoidance of intense midday sun exposure between 10 AM and 3 PM; wearing of protective clothing such as a hat, long sleeves, and pants; and use of sunscreen. Early detection includes frequent clinical and photographic examinations of patients at risk (dysplastic nevus syndrome) and prompt response to rapid changes in nevi (size, shape, color, inflammation, bleeding or crusting, and sensation). The **ABCD rule** (asymmetry, border irregularities, color variability, diameter >6 mm), which is a useful screening tool for adults, may not be as effective for children.

HALO NEVUS

Halo nevi occur primarily in children and young adults, most commonly on the back (Fig. 651-3). Development of the lesion may coincide with puberty or pregnancy. Several pigmented nevi frequently develop halos simultaneously. Subsequent disappearance of the central nevus over several months is the usual outcome, and the depigmented area usually repigments. Excision and histopathologic examination of the lesion is indicated only when the nature of the central lesion is in question. An acquired melanocytic nevus occasionally develops a peripheral zone of depigmentation over a period of days to weeks. There is a dense inflammatory infiltrate of lymphocytes and histiocytes in addition to the nevus cells. The pale halo reflects disappearance of the melanocytes. This phenomenon is associated with congenital nevi,

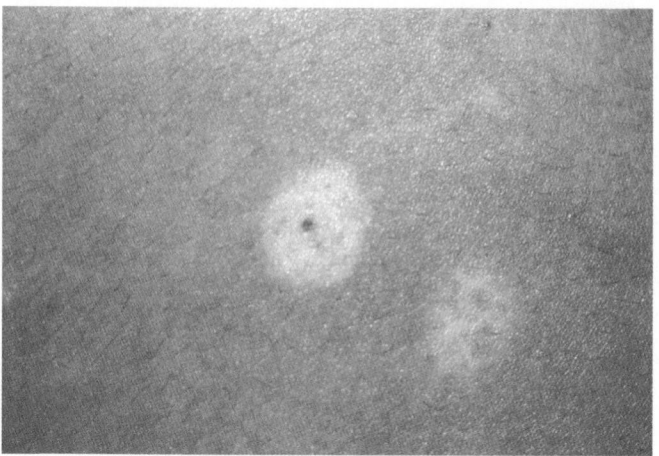

Figure 651-3 Well-developed halo nevus.

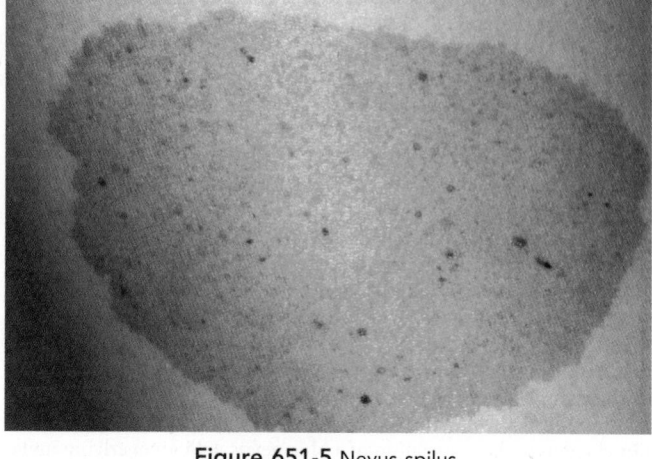

Figure 651-5 Nevus spilus.

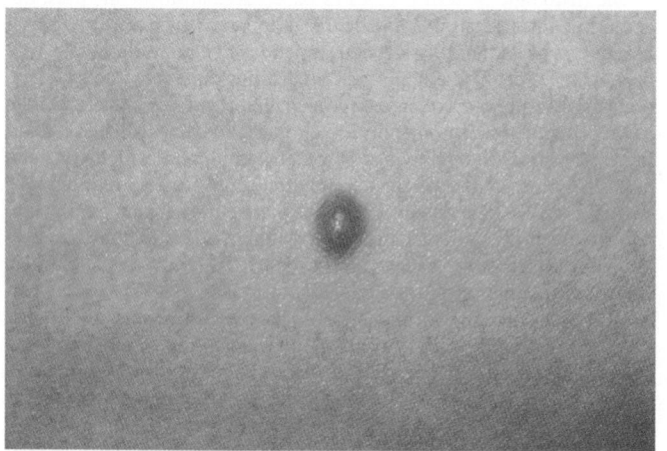

Figure 651-4 Dome-shaped red Spitz nevus.

blue nevi, Spitz nevi, dysplastic nevi, neurofibromas, and primary and secondary malignant melanoma, and occasionally with poliosis, Vogt-Koyanagi-Harada syndrome, and pernicious anemia. Patients with vitiligo have an increased incidence of halo nevi. Individuals with halo nevi have circulating antibodies against the cytoplasm of melanocytes and nevus cells.

SPITZ NEVUS (SPINDLE AND EPITHELIOID CELL NEVUS)
Spitz nevus manifests most commonly in the 1st 2 decades of life as a pink to red, smooth, dome-shaped, firm, hairless papule on the face, shoulder, or upper limb (Fig. 651-4). Most are <1 cm in diameter, but they can achieve a size of 3 cm. Rarely, they occur as numerous grouped lesions. Visually similar lesions include pyogenic granuloma, hemangioma, nevocellular nevus, juvenile xanthogranuloma, and basal cell carcinoma, but these entities are histologically distinguishable. Spitz nevus may be difficult to distinguish histopathologically from malignant melanoma because nuclear atypia is a common feature, particularly after local recurrence of the nevus. Difficulty arises in the fact that many other clinical types of melanocytic nevi have a similar histologic appearance. Local recurrence after excision may occur up to 5% of the time. If a nevus arouses clinical suspicion that it may be a melanoma, an excisional biopsy of the entire lesion is recommended. If the margins of excision of a Spitz nevus are positive, reexcision of the site is prudent to avoid difficulties in histopathologic interpretation of the lesion in the future.

ZOSTERIFORM LENTIGINOUS NEVUS (AGMINATED LENTIGINES)
Zosteriform lentiginous nevus is a unilateral, linear, band-like collection of numerous 2-10 mm brown or black macules on the face, trunk, or limbs. The nevus may be present at birth or may develop during childhood. There are higher numbers of melanocytes in elongated rete ridges of the epidermis.

NEVUS SPILUS (SPECKLED LENTIGINOUS NEVUS)
Nevus spilus is a flat brown patch within which are darker flat or raised brown melanocytic elements (Fig. 651-5). It varies considerably in size and can occur anywhere on the body. The color of the macular component may vary from light to dark brown, and the number of darker lesions may be low or high. Nevus spilus is rare at birth and is commonly acquired in late infancy or early childhood. Dark elements within the nevus are usually present initially and tend to increase in number gradually over time. The darker macules represent nevus cells in a junctional or dermal location; the patch has increased numbers of melanocytes in a lentiginous epidermal pattern. The malignant potential of these nevi is uncertain; nevus spilus is found more commonly in individuals with melanoma than in matched control subjects. The nevi need not be excised, unless atypical features or recent clinical changes are noted.

NEVUS OF OTA AND NEVUS OF ITO
Nevus of Ota is more common among females and Asian, and African-American patients. This nevus consists of a permanent patch composed of partially confluent blue, black, and brown macules. Enlargement and darkening may occur with time. Occasionally, some areas of the nevus are raised. The macular nevi resemble the more common dermal melanocytosis of the lower back and buttocks in color and occur unilaterally in the areas supplied by the 1st and 2nd divisions of the trigeminal nerve. Nevus of Ota differs from a more common dermal melanocytosis patch, not only by its distribution but also by having a speckled rather than a uniform appearance. Both are forms of mid-dermal melanocytosis. Nevus of Ota also has a greater concentration of elongated, dendritic dermal melanocytes located in the upper rather than the lower portion of the dermis. This nevus is sometimes present at birth; in other cases, it may arise during the 1st or 2nd decade of life. Patchy involvement of the conjunctiva, hard palate, pharynx, nasal mucosa, buccal mucosa, or tympanic membrane occurs in some patients. Malignant change is exceedingly rare. Laser therapy may effectively decrease the pigmentation but can be unpredictable.

Nevus of Ito is localized to the supraclavicular, scapular, and deltoid regions. This nevus tends to be more diffuse in its distribution and less mottled than nevus of Ota. It is also a form of mid-dermal melanocytosis. The only available treatments are masking with cosmetics and laser therapy.

BLUE NEVI

The common blue nevus is a solitary, asymptomatic, smooth, dome-shaped, blue to blue-gray papule <10 mm in diameter on the dorsal aspect of the hands and feet. Rarely, common blue nevi form large plaques. Blue nevus is nearly always acquired, often during childhood and more commonly in females. Microscopically, it is characterized by groups of intensely pigmented spindle-shaped melanocytes in the dermis. This nevus is benign.

The cellular blue nevus is typically 1-3 cm in diameter and occurs most frequently on the buttocks and in the sacrococcygeal area. In addition to collections of deeply pigmented dermal dendritic melanocytes, cellular islands composed of large spindle-shaped cells are noted in the dermis and may extend into the subcutaneous fat. A histologic continuum may be seen from blue nevi to cellular blue nevi. A combined nevus is the association of a blue nevus with an overlying melanocytic nevus.

The blue-gray that is characteristic of these nevi is an optical effect caused by dermal melanin. Longer wavelengths of visible light penetrate to the deep dermis and are absorbed there by melanin; shorter-wavelength blue light cannot penetrate deeply but instead is reflected back to the observer.

NEVUS DEPIGMENTOSUS (ACHROMIC NEVUS)

Nevi depigmentosi are usually present at birth; they are localized macular hypopigmented patches or streaks, often with bizarre, irregular borders (Fig. 651-6). They can resemble hypomelanosis of Ito clinically, except that they are more localized and often unilateral. Small lesions may also resemble the ash leaf macules of tuberous sclerosis. Nevi depigmentosi appear to represent a focal defect in transfer of melanosomes to keratinocytes.

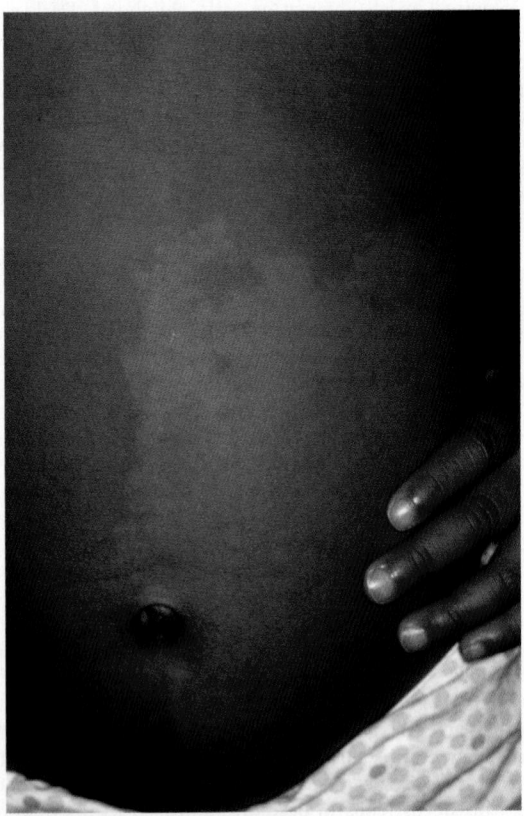

Figure 651-6 Large nevus depigmentosus of the abdomen.

EPIDERMAL NEVI

Epidermal nevi may be visible at birth or may develop in the 1st few mo or yr of life. They affect both sexes equally and usually occur sporadically. Epidermal nevi are hamartomatous lesions characterized by hyperplasia of the epidermis and/or adnexal structures in a focal area of the skin.

Epidermal nevi are classified into a number of variants, depending on the morphology and extent of the individual nevus and the predominant epidermal structure. An epidermal nevus may appear initially as a discolored, slightly scaly patch that, with maturation, becomes more linear, thickened, verrucous, and hyperpigmented. *Systematized* refers to a diffuse or extensive distribution of lesions, and *ichthyosis hystrix* indicates that the distribution is extensive and bilateral (Fig. 651-7). Morphologic types include pigmented papillomas, often in a linear distribution; unilateral hyperkeratotic streaks involving a limb and perhaps a portion of the trunk; velvety hyperpigmented plaques; and whorled or marbled hyperkeratotic lesions in localized plaques or over extensive areas of the body along Blaschko lines. An inflammatory linear verrucous variant is markedly pruritic and tends to become erythematous, scaling, and crusted. Many harbor *RAS* mutations.

The histologic pattern evolves as an epidermal nevus matures, but epidermal hyperplasia of some degree is apparent in all stages of development. One or another dermal appendage may predominate in a particular lesion. These nevi must be distinguished from lichen striatus, lymphangioma circumscriptum, shagreen patch of tuberous sclerosis, congenital hairy nevi, linear porokeratosis, linear lichen planus, linear psoriasis, the verrucous stage of incontinentia pigmenti, and nevus sebaceus (Jadassohn). Keratolytic agents such as retinoic acid and salicylic acid may be moderately effective in reducing scaling and controlling pruritus, but definitive treatment requires full-thickness excision; recurrence is usual if more superficial removal is attempted. Alternatively, the nevus may be left intact. Epidermal nevi are occasionally associated with other abnormalities of the skin and soft tissues, eyes, and nervous, cardiovascular, musculoskeletal, and urogenital systems. In these instances, the disorder is referred to as epidermal nevus syndrome. This syndrome, however, is not a distinct clinical entity. The well-established syndromes that involve a type of epidermal nevus and distinct birth defects include the **proteus** and **CHILD** (congenital hemidysplasia with ichthyosiform erythroderma and limb defects) syndromes.

Nevus Sebaceus (Jadassohn)

A relatively small, sharply demarcated, oval or linear, elevated yellow-orange plaque that is usually devoid of hair, nevus sebaceus occurs on the head and neck of infants (Fig. 651-8). Although the lesion is characterized histopathologically by an abundance of sebaceous glands, all

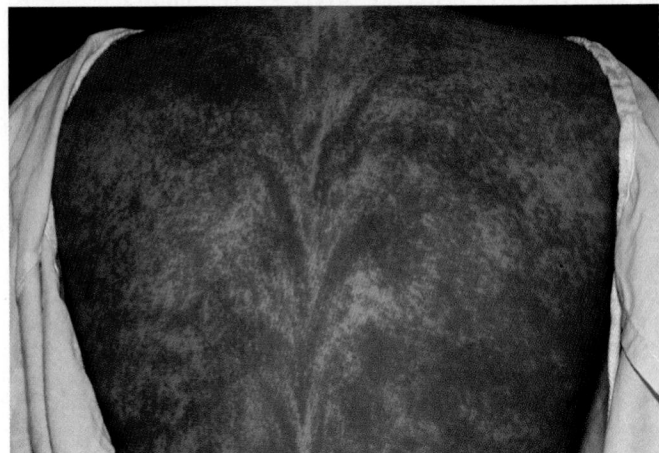

Figure 651-7 Epidermal nevus (ichthyosis hystrix type).

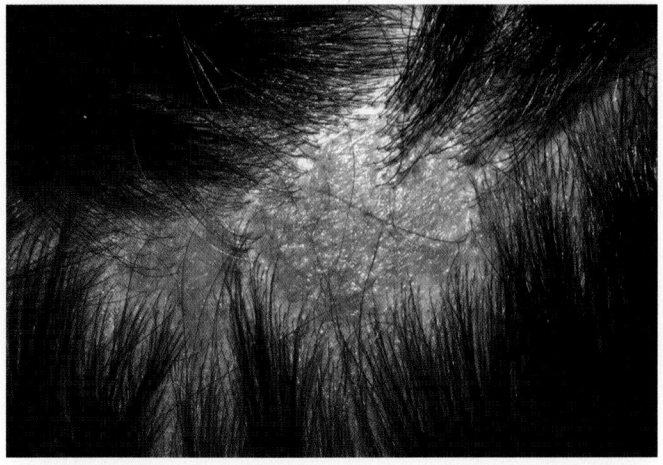

Figure 651-8 Orange-yellow nevus sebaceus of the scalp.

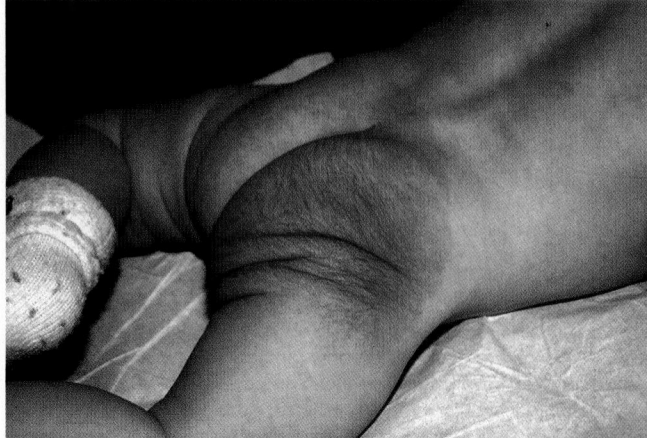

Figure 651-10 Large smooth muscle hamartoma of the buttock.

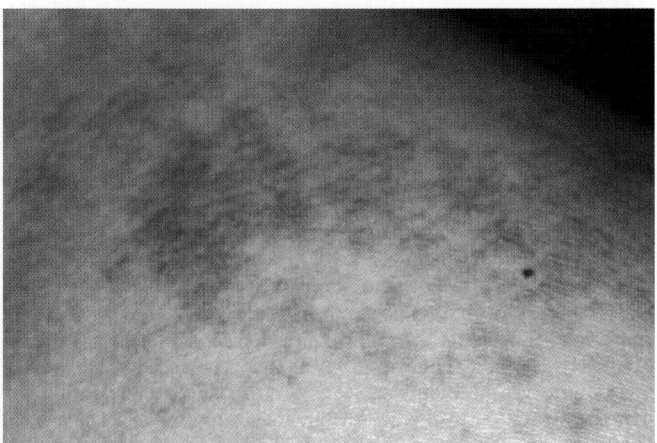

Figure 651-9 Becker nevus on the shoulder of an adolescent male.

elements of the skin are represented. It is frequently flat and inconspicuous in early childhood. With maturity, usually during adolescence, the lesions become verrucous and studded with large rubbery nodules. The changing clinical appearance reflects the histologic pattern, which is characterized by a variable degree of hyperkeratosis, hyperplasia of the epidermis, malformed hair follicles, and often a profusion of sebaceous glands and the presence of ectopic apocrine glands. Sebaceous nevi are caused by somatic mosaic mutations in *HRAS* and *KRAS*. The disruption of these oncogenes helps explain the 14% incidence of these lesions developing tumors throughout a patient's lifetime. Most tumors are benign (trichoblastomas, syringocystadenoma papilliferum, trichilemmomas), but basal cell carcinoma can occur as well. The *treatment of choice* is total excision before adolescence. Sebaceous nevi associated with central nervous system, skeletal, and ocular defects represent a variant of the epidermal nevus syndrome.

Becker Nevus (Becker Melanosis)
Becker nevus develops predominantly in males, during childhood or adolescence, initially as a hyperpigmented patch. The lesion commonly develops hypertrichosis, limited to the area of hyperpigmentation, and evolves into a unilateral, slightly thickened, irregular, hyperpigmented plaque. The most common sites are the upper torso and upper arm (Fig. 651-9). The nevus shows an increased number of basal melanocytes and variable epidermal hyperplasia. Becker melanosis is commonly associated with a smooth muscle hamartoma, which may appear as slight perifollicular papular elevations or slight induration. Stroking of such a lesion may induce smooth muscle contraction and make the hairs stand up (pseudo-Darier sign). The nevus is benign,

has no risk for malignant change, and is rarely associated with other anomalies.

NEVUS COMEDONICUS
An uncommon organoid nevus of epithelial origin, nevus comedonicus consists of linear plaques of plugged follicles that simulate comedones; they may be present at birth or may appear during childhood. The horny plugs represent keratinous debris within dilated, malformed pilosebaceous follicles. The lesions are most often unilateral and may develop at any site. Rarely, they are associated with other congenital malformations, including skeletal defects, cerebral anomalies, and cataracts. Although these lesions are often asymptomatic, some affected individuals experience recurrent inflammation, resulting in cyst formation, fistulas, and scarring. There is no effective treatment except full-thickness excision; palliation of larger lesions may be achieved by regular applications of a retinoic acid preparation.

CONNECTIVE TISSUE NEVUS
Connective tissue nevus is a hamartoma of collagen, elastin, and/or glycosaminoglycans of the dermal extracellular matrix. It may occur as a solitary defect or as a manifestation of an associated disorder. These nevi may occur at any site but are most common on the back, buttocks, arms, and thighs. They are skin-colored, ivory, or yellow plaques, 2-15 cm in diameter, composed of many tiny papules or grouped nodules that are frequently difficult to appreciate visually because of the subtle color changes. The plaques have a rubbery or cobblestone consistency on palpation. Biopsy findings are variable and include increased amounts and/or degeneration or fragmentation of dermal collagen, elastic tissue, or ground substance. Similar lesions occurring with tuberous sclerosis are called shagreen patches; however, shagreen patches consist only of excessive amounts of collagen. The association of many small papular connective tissue nevi with osteopoikilosis is called dermatofibrosis lenticularis disseminata (**Buschke-Ollendorf syndrome**).

SMOOTH MUSCLE HAMARTOMA
Smooth muscle hamartoma is a developmental anomaly resulting from hyperplasia of the smooth muscle (arrector pili) associated with hair follicles. It is usually evident at birth or shortly thereafter as a flesh-colored or lightly pigmented plaque with overlying hypertrichosis on the trunk or limbs (Fig. 651-10). Transient elevation or a rippling movement of the lesion, caused by contraction of the muscle bundles, can sometimes be elicited by stroking of the surface (pseudo-Darier sign). Smooth muscle hamartoma can be mistaken for congenital pigmented nevus, but the distinction is important because the former has no risk for malignant melanoma and need not be removed.

Bibliography is available at Expert Consult.

Chapter **652**
Hyperpigmented Lesions
Anna M. Juern and Beth A. Drolet

DISORDERS OF PIGMENT

Normal pigmentation requires migration of melanoblasts from the neural crest to the dermal–epidermal junction, enzymatic processes to form pigment, structural components to contain the pigment (melanosomes), and transfer of pigment to the surrounding keratinocytes. Increased skin color may be generalized or localized and may result from various defects in any of these requirements. Some of these aberrations are a manifestation of systemic disease, others represent generalized or focal developmental or genetic defects, and still others may be nonspecific and the result of cutaneous inflammation.

EPHELIDES (FRECKLES)

Ephelides are light or dark brown, round, oval or irregularly shaped, well-demarcated, macules usually <3 mm in diameter that occur in sun-exposed areas such as the face, upper back, arms, and hands. They are induced by exposure to sun, particularly during the summer, and may fade or disappear during the winter. They are a result of increased sun-induced melanogenesis and melanosome transport from melanocytes to keratinocytes, and not increased number of melanocytes. They are more common in redheads and fair-haired individuals and first appear in the preschool years. Histologically, they are marked by increased melanin pigment in epidermal basal cells, which have more numerous and larger dendritic processes than the melanocytes of the surrounding paler skin. The lack of melanocytic proliferation or elongation of epidermal rete ridges distinguishes them from lentigines. Freckles have been identified as a marker for increased risk for UV-induced neoplasia and hence melanoma, independent of melanocytic nevi.

LENTIGINES

Lentigines, often mistaken for freckles or junctional nevi, are small (<3 cm), round, dark brown macules that can appear anywhere on the body with an early age of onset. They are more common in darkly pigmented than in lightly pigmented individuals. They are unrelated to sun exposure and remain permanently. Histologically, they have elongated, club-shaped, epidermal rete ridges with increased numbers of melanocytes and dense epidermal deposits of melanin. No nests of melanocytes are found. The lesions are benign and, when few, may be viewed as a normal occurrence and are seen most commonly on the lower lip.

Eruptive/generalized lentiginosis (lentiginosis profusa) involves innumerable small, pigmented macules that are present at birth or appear during childhood. There are no associated abnormalities, and mucous membranes are spared. **Carney complex** is an autosomal dominant syndrome characterized by multiple lentigines and multiple neoplasias, including: myxomas of the skin, heart (atrial) and breast; psammomatous melanotic schwannomas; epithelioid blue nevi of skin and mucosae; growth hormone-producing pituitary adenomas; and testicular Sertoli cell tumors. Components of the Carney complex have been described previously as the NAME (nevi, atrial myxoma, myxoid neurofibroma, ephelides) and LAMB (lentigines, atrial myxoma, mucocutaneous myxoma, blue nevi) syndromes. It is inherited in an autosomal dominant pattern and caused by an inactivating mutation of the *PRKAR1* gene.

The **multiple lentigines syndrome** (formerly LEOPARD) is an autosomal dominant entity consisting of a generalized, symmetric distribution of *l*entigines (Fig. 652-1) in association with *e*lectrocardiogram *a*bnormalities, *o*cular hypertelorism, *p*ulmonary stenosis, *a*bnormal

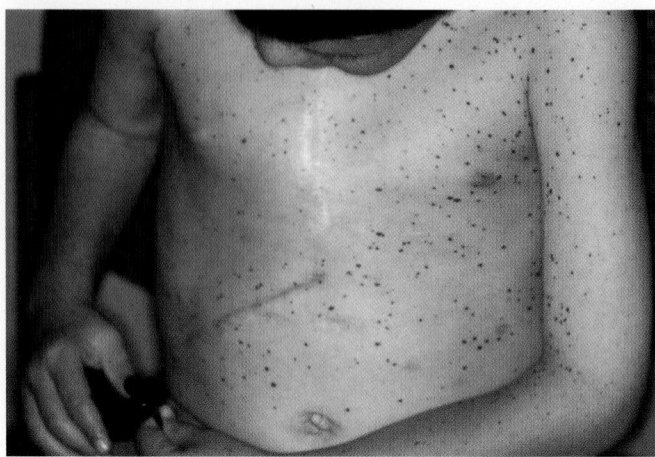

Figure 652-1 Multiple lentigines in LEOPARD (*l*entigines in association with *e*lectrocardiogram abnormalities, *o*cular hypertelorism, *p*ulmonary stenosis, *a*bnormal genitals [cryptorchidism, hypogonadism, hypospadias], growth *r*etardation, and sensorineural *d*eafness) syndrome.

genitals (cryptorchidism, hypogonadism, hypospadias), growth *r*etardation, and sensorineural *d*eafness (type 1, *PTPN11* gene; type 2, *RAF1* gene). Other features include hypertrophic obstructive cardiomyopathy and pectus excavatum or carinatum.

The **Peutz-Jeghers syndrome** is characterized by melanotic macules on the lips and mucous membranes and by gastrointestinal (GI) polyposis. It is inherited as an autosomal dominant trait (*STK11* gene). Onset is noted in infancy and early childhood when pigmented macules appear on the lips and buccal mucosa. The macules are usually a few millimeters in size but may be as large as 1-2 cm. Macules also appear occasionally on the palate, gums, tongue, and vaginal mucosa. Cutaneous lesions may develop on the nose, hands, and feet; around the mouth, eyes, and umbilicus; and as longitudinal bands or diffuse hyperpigmentation of the nails. Pigmented macules often fade from the lips and skin during puberty and adulthood but generally do not disappear from mucosal surfaces. Buccal mucosal macules are the most constant feature of the disorder; in some families, occasional members may be affected only with the pigmentary changes. Indistinguishable pigmentary changes beginning in adult life, without intestinal involvement, also occur sporadically in individuals.

Polyposis usually involves the jejunum and ileum but may also occur in the stomach, duodenum, colon, and rectum (see Chapter 345). Episodic abdominal pain, diarrhea, melena, and intussusception are frequent complications. Patients have a significantly increased risk of GI tract and non–GI tract tumors at a young age. GI cancer has been reported in ≈2-3% of patients; the lifetime relative risk for GI malignancy is 13. The relative risk of non–GI tract malignancies, including ovarian, cervical, and testicular tumors, is 9. Peutz-Jeghers syndrome must be differentiated from other syndromes associated with multiple lentigines (Laugier-Hunziker syndrome), from ordinary freckling, from Gardner syndrome, and from Cronkhite-Canada syndrome, a disorder characterized by GI polyposis, alopecia, onychodystrophy, and diffuse pigmentation of the palms, volar aspects of the fingers, and dorsal hands. Treatment of Peutz-Jeghers melanotic macules is not required or indicated, but multiple different lasers have been successful for cosmesis, in some cases.

CAFÉ-AU-LAIT SPOTS

Café-au-lait spots are uniformly hyperpigmented, sharply demarcated macular lesions, the hues of which vary with the normal degree of pigmentation of the individual: They are tan or light brown in white individuals and may be dark brown in black children (Figs. 652-2 and 652-3). Café-au-lait spots vary tremendously in size and may be large, covering a significant portion of the trunk or limb. Generally the borders are smooth, but some have exceedingly irregular borders. The lesions are characterized by increased numbers of melanocytes and

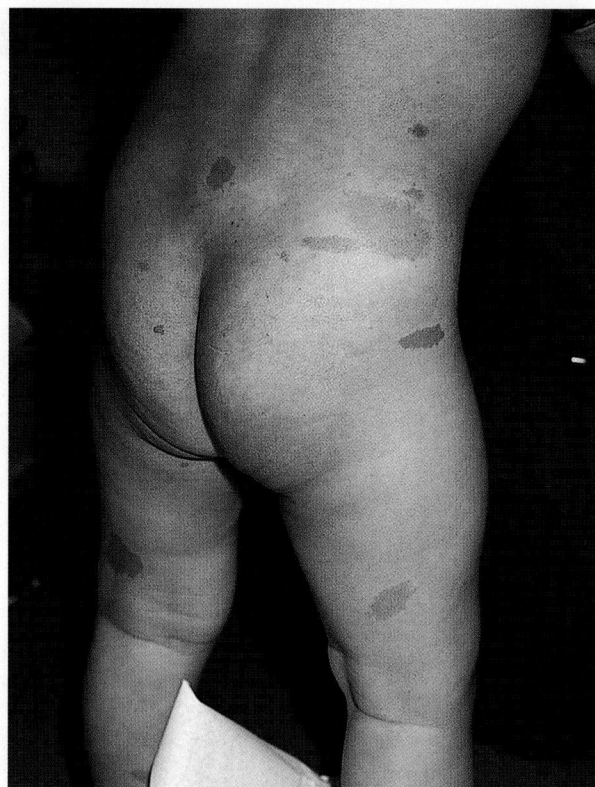

Figure 652-2 Multiple café-au-lait macules on a child with neurofibromatosis type 1. *(From Eichenfield LF, Frieden IJ, Esterly NB: Textbook of neonatal dermatology, Philadelphia, 2001, WB Saunders, p. 372.)*

melanin in the epidermis but lack the clubbed rete ridges that typify lentigines. One to 3 café-au-lait spots are common in normal children; ≈10% of normal children have café-au-lait macules. The spots may be present at birth or may develop during childhood.

Large, often asymmetric café-au-lait spots with irregular borders are characteristic of patients with Albright (**McCune-Albright**) syndrome (*GNAS1* gene; see Chapter 562.6). This disorder includes polyostotic fibrous dysplasia of bone, leading to pathologic fractures; precocious puberty; and numerous hyperfunctional endocrinopathies. The macular hyperpigmentation may be present at birth or may develop late in childhood (see Fig. 652-3). Cutaneous pigmentation is typically most extensive on the side showing the most severe bone involvement.

Neurofibromatosis Type 1 (von Recklinghausen Disease)

The café-au-lait spot (macule) is the most familiar cutaneous hallmark of the autosomal dominant neurocutaneous syndrome known as neurofibromatosis type 1 (*NF-1*, neurofibromin gene; see Fig. 652-2 and Chapter 596.1). Included in the criteria for this diagnosis is the presence of 5 or more café-au-lait spots >5 mm in diameter in prepubertal patients or 6 or more café-au-lait spots >15 mm in diameter in postpubertal patients. Multiple café-au-lait macules commonly produce a freckled appearance of non–sun-exposed areas such as the axillae (Crowe sign), the inguinal and inframammary regions, and under the chin. Café-au-lait macules can also be seen in segmental NF-1 which results from somatic mosaicism arising from postzygotic mutations in the *NF-1* gene such that the clinical manifestations of NF-1 are present only in a localized body segment. Another variant of NF-1 is hereditary spinal neurofibromatosis, which is a rare disorder that generally presents with multiple café-au-lait macules and multiple, symmetric spinal root neurofibromas but other stigmata of NF-1 are typically absent. The lesions also occur with certain other disorders, including other types of neurofibromatosis, but in these disorders the café-au-lait spots are not a major feature of the disorder (Table 652-1).

Table 652-1	**Other Syndromes Associated with Café-Au-Lait Macules**		
STRENGTH OF ASSOCIATION	**SYNDROME**	**CLINICAL FEATURES**	**GENE OR LOCUS**
Strong	Neurofibromatosis type 2	Acoustic neuromas, schwannomas, neurofibromas, meningiomas, juvenile posterior subcapsular lenticular opacity; café-au-lait seen but not a criterion for diagnosis	*NF-2*
	Multiple familial café-au-lait	Multiple café-au-lait without other stigmata of NF-1	?
	Legius (NF-1–like) syndrome	Multiple café-au-lait and skinfold freckling without other stigmata of NF-1	*SPRED1*
	McCune-Albright syndrome	Segmental café-au-lait, precocious puberty, other endocrinopathies, polyostotic fibrous dysplasia	*GNAS1*
	Constitutional mismatch repair deficiency syndrome	Multiple café-au-lait, adenomatous colonic polyps, multiple malignancies, including colonic adenocarcinoma, glioblastoma, medulloblastoma, and lymphoma	*MLH1, MSH2, MSH6, PMS2*
	Ring chromosome syndromes	Multiple café-au-lait, microcephaly, mental retardation, short stature, skeletal anomalies	Chromosomes 7, 11, 12, 15, 17
	LEOPARD/multiple lentigines syndrome	Café-au-lait, café-noir, lentigines, cardiac conduction defects, ocular hypertelorism, pulmonary stenosis, genitourinary anomalies, growth retardation, hearing loss	*PTPN11*
	Cowden syndrome (multiple hamartoma syndrome)	Facial trichilemmomas, cobblestoning of the oral mucosa, predisposition to soft tissue tumors (lipomas, neuromas), gastrointestinal polyps, fibrocystic breast disease and breast carcinoma, thyroid adenoma, and thyroid cancer	*PTEN*

Continued

Table 652-1	Syndromes Associated with Café-Au-Lait Macules—cont'd		
STRENGTH OF ASSOCIATION	**SYNDROME**	**CLINICAL FEATURES**	**GENE OR LOCUS**
	Bannayan-Riley-Ruvalcaba syndrome	Facial trichilemmomas, oral papillomas, pigmented genital macules, gastrointestinal polyps, macrocephaly, vascular anomalies, mental retardation	*PTEN*
Weak	Ataxia-telangiectasia	Cerebellar ataxia, cutaneous and ocular telangiectasias, immunodeficiency, hypogonadism, predisposition to lymphoreticular malignancy	*ATM*
	Bloom syndrome	Photosensitivity, immunodeficiency, chronic lung disease, cryptorchidism, syndactyly, short stature, susceptibility to malignancy	*RECQL3*
	Fanconi anemia	Bone marrow failure, multiple congenital anomalies, predisposition to malignancy, mental retardation, microcephaly	*FANCA, FANCB* (putative), *FANCC, FANCD* locus on chromosome 3, *FANCE* locus on chromosome 6, *FANCF, FANCG, FANCH* (putative)
	Russell-Silver syndrome	Short stature, craniofacial and body asymmetry, low birthweight, microcephaly, triangular facies, fifth finger clinodactyly, congenital cardiac defects	?
	Tuberous sclerosis	Facial angiofibromas, cutaneous collagenomas, seizures, mental retardation, hypomelanotic macules, periungual fibromas, subependymal nodules, subependymal giant cell astrocytoma, cardiac rhabdomyoma, pulmonary lymphangiomyomatosis renal angiomyolipoma, retinal hamartomas	*TSC1, TSC2*
	Turner syndrome	Short stature, lymphedema, congenital heart disease, valgus deformity	X-chromosomal anomalies (XO karyotype or Xp deletion)
	Noonan syndrome	Facial dysmorphism, pulmonary valve stenosis, webbed neck, pectus excavatum, mental retardation, short stature, cryptorchidism, hematologic malignancies	*PTPN11, SOS1, RAF1, KRAS*
	Multiple mucosal neuroma (MEN) syndrome 1	Parathyroid adenoma, pituitary adenoma, pancreatic islet adenoma, lipoma, gingival papules, facial angiofibromas, collagenomas	*MENIN*
	MEN syndrome 2B	Mucosal neuromas, pheochromocytoma, medullary thyroid carcinoma, parathyroid adenoma, marfanoid habitus	*RET*
	Johanson-Blizzard syndrome	Short stature, failure to thrive, microcephaly, sensorineural hearing loss, dental anomalies, congenital heart disease, exocrine pancreatic insufficiency, imperforate anus, genitourinary anomalies, mental retardation, hypothyroidism	*UBR1*
	Microcephalic osteodysplastic primordial dwarfism, type II	Short stature, microcephaly, intrauterine growth retardation, dysmorphic facies, skeletal anomalies, developmental delay, premature puberty	*PCNT2*
	Nijmegen breakage syndrome	Short stature, growth retardation, microcephaly, cleft lip/palate, dysmorphic facies, bronchiectasis, sinusitis, dysgammaglobulinemia with recurrent urinary tract and gastrointestinal infections, mental retardation, spontaneous chromosomal instability, predisposition to malignancy	*NBS1*
	Rubinstein-Taybi syndrome	Short stature, microcephaly, dysmorphic facies, congenital cardiac disease, sternal anomalies, skeletal anomalies, mental retardation	*CREBBP, EP300*
	Kabuki syndrome	Postnatal growth retardation, microcephaly, dysmorphic facies, congenital cardiac defects, malabsorption, anal stenosis, genitourinary anomalies, congenital hip dysplasia, hirsutism, mental retardation	?

From Shah KN: The diagnostic and clinical significance of café-au-lait macules. Pediatr Clin North Am 57(5):1131–1153, 2010, Table 2.

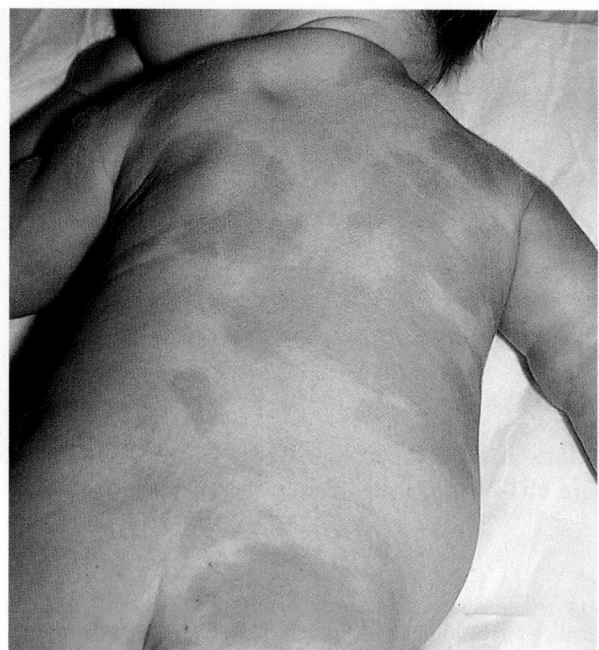

Figure 652-3 Multiple patterned café-au-lait spots in a child with McCune-Albright syndrome. *(From Eichenfield LF, Frieden IJ, Esterly NB: Textbook of neonatal dermatology, Philadelphia, 2001, WB Saunders, p. 373.)*

INCONTINENTIA PIGMENTI (BLOCH-SULZBERGER DISEASE)

See Chapter 596.7.

POSTINFLAMMATORY PIGMENTARY CHANGES

Either hyperpigmentation or hypopigmentation can occur as a result of cutaneous inflammation. Alteration in pigmentation usually follows a severe inflammatory reaction but may result from mild dermatitis. Dark-skinned children are more likely to show these changes than fair-skinned ones. Although altered pigmentation may persist for weeks to months, patients can be reassured that these lesions are usually temporary.

Bibliography is available at Expert Consult.

Chapter **653**
Hypopigmented Lesions
Sheila S. Galbraith

ALBINISM

Several types of congenital oculocutaneous albinism (OCA) consist of partial or complete failure of melanin production in the skin, hair, and eyes despite the presence of normal number, structure, and distribution of melanocytes. They may be divided into 2 major classes: those with abnormal protein function involved in the formation and transfer of melanin, and those with defects in melanosomes (Table 653-1).

Table 653-1	Genes Associated with Hypopigmentation
DISORDER	**GENE DEFECT**
OCULOCUTANEOUS ALBINISM	
OCA1	Tyrosinase
OCA2	P protein
OCA3	*TRP-1*
OCA4	*MATP*
HERMANSKY-PUDLAK	
Type 1	HPS-1 Mouse (pale ear)
Type 2	HPS-2 b3A subunit of AP3
Type 3	HPS-3 Mouse (cocoa)
Type 4	HPS-4 Mouse (light ear)
Type 5	HPS-5 KIAA107
Type 6	HPS-6 Mouse (ruby eye)
Type 7	HPS-7 DTNBP1
Type 8	HPS-8 Bloc153
CHÉDIAK-HIGASHI	*CHS1/LYST*
PIEBALDISM	C-KIT receptor
	Heterozygous SLUG
WAARDENBURG	
Type 1	Heterozygous PAX-3
Type 2a	*MITF*
Type 2b	Chromosome 1p
Type 2c	Chromosome 8p23
Type 2d	*SNAIL*
Type 2e	*SOX10*
Type 3	Homozygous PAX-3
Type 4	*SOX10*
	Endothelin 3
	Endothelin B receptor

Tyrosinase is the copper-containing enzyme that catalyzes at multiple steps in melanin biosynthesis (see Chapter 85.2). Tyrosinase-positive variants are characterized by darkening of the hair bulb on incubation with tyrosine.

Oculocutaneous albinism type 1 (OCA1) is characterized by great reduction in or absence of tyrosinase activity. OCA1A, the most severe form, is characterized by a lack of visible pigment in hair, skin, and eyes (Fig. 653-1). This manifests as photophobia, nystagmus, defective visual acuity, white hair, and white skin. The irises are blue-gray in oblique light and prominent pink in reflected light. OCA1B, or yellow mutant albinism, manifests at birth as white hair, pink skin, and gray eyes. This type is particularly prevalent in Amish communities. Progressively the hair becomes yellow-red, the skin tans lightly on exposure to the sun, and the irises may accumulate some brown pigment, with a resultant improvement in visual acuity. Photophobia and nystagmus are present but mild. OCATS is a temperature-sensitive type of albinism. The abnormal tyrosinase has decreased activity at 35-37°C (95-98.6°F). Therefore, cooler regions of the body such as the limbs and head pigment to some degree, whereas other areas remain depigmented.

OCA2 ranges from nearly normal to closely resembling type 1 albinism. This is the most common form of albinism seen worldwide. Little or no melanin is present at birth, but pigment, particularly red-yellow pigment, may accumulate during childhood to produce straw-colored or light brown skin in white individuals. Pigmented nevi may develop. Progressive improvement in visual acuity and nystagmus occurs with aging. Black individuals may have yellow-brown skin, dark-brown freckles in sun-exposed areas, and brown coloration of the irises. **Brown OCA** is an allelic variant of OCA2. Prader-Willi and Angelman syndromes, which include hypopigmentation, have deletions that include the gene involved in OCA2.

OCA3 (rufous albinism) is seen predominantly in patients of African descent. It is characterized by red hair, reddish brown skin, pigmented nevi, freckles, reddish brown to brown eyes, nystagmus, photophobia, and decreased visual acuity.

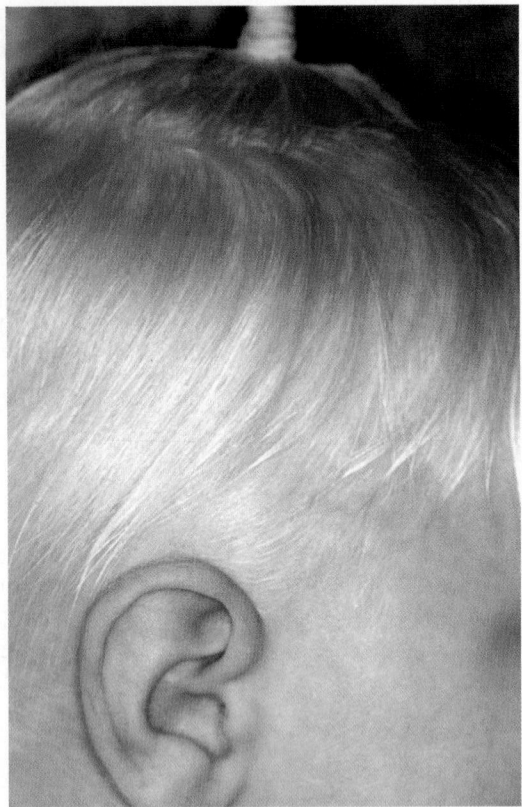

Figure 653-1 White hair and skin in oculocutaneous albinism type 1 (OCA1).

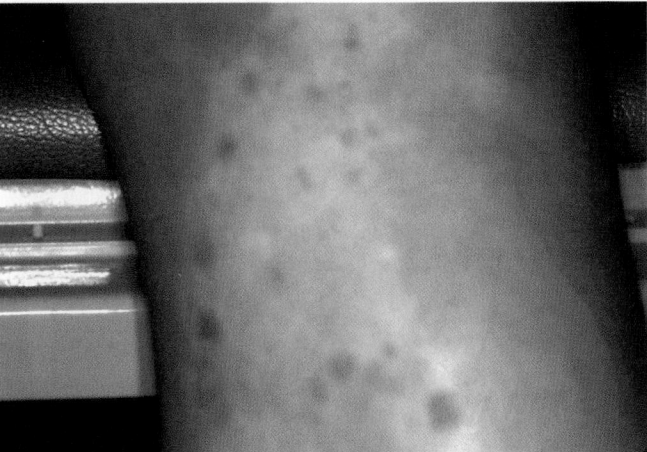

Figure 653-2 Depigmented macule with islands of hyperpigmentation in piebaldism.

OCA4 is a rare OCA with clinical findings similar to those in OCA2.

The **Cross-McKusick-Breen syndrome** consists of tyrosinase-positive albinism with ocular abnormalities, cognitive impairment, spasticity, and athetosis. The genetic defect is unidentified.

Because of the absence of normal protection by adequate amounts of epidermal melanin, persons with albinism are predisposed to development of actinic keratoses and cutaneous carcinoma secondary to skin damage by ultraviolet light. Protective clothing and a broad-spectrum sunscreen (see Chapter 656) should be worn during exposure to sunlight.

Oculocutaneous Albinism with Melanosomal Abnormalities
See Table 653-1.

Hermansky-Pudlak syndrome is a collection of autosomal recessive genetic disorders characterized by OCA, ceroid accumulation in lysosomes, and prolonged bleeding time. In mice, 16 distinct genetic loci that produce coat color mutant phenotypes associated with platelet deficiencies are recognized; eight have been identified in humans.

Chédiak-Higashi syndrome (see Chapter 130) is another genetic abnormality associated with dysfunction of lysosome-related organelles. Patients with Chédiak-Higashi syndrome have hypopigmentation of the skin, eyes, and hair; prolonged bleeding times and easy bruising; recurrent infections; abnormal natural killer cell function; and peripheral neuropathy. Chédiak-Higashi syndrome is caused by mutations in the *CHS1/LYST* gene, which is a lysosomal trafficking regulatory gene.

MELANOBLAST MIGRATION ABNORMALITIES
See Table 653-1.

Piebaldism
A congenital autosomal dominant disorder, piebaldism is characterized by sharply demarcated amelanotic patches that occur most frequently on the forehead, anterior scalp (producing a white forelock),

ventral trunk, elbows, and knees. Islands of normal or darker-than-normal pigmentation may be present within the amelanotic areas (Fig. 653-2). The plaques are a result of a permanent localized absence of melanocytes as a result of a defect in the *KIT* protooncogene, which encodes the cell surface receptor transmembrane tyrosine kinase. The pattern of depigmentation arises from defective melanoblast migration from the neural crest during development. The reason that piebaldism is a localized and not a generalized process remains unknown. Piebaldism must be differentiated from vitiligo, which may be progressive and is not usually congenital, nevus depigmentosus, and Waardenburg syndrome.

Waardenburg Syndrome
Waardenburg syndrome also manifests at birth as localized areas of depigmented skin and hair. There are 4 types of Waardenburg syndrome. The hallmark of Waardenburg type 1 is the white forelock, which is seen in 20-60% of patients. Only 15% of patients have areas of depigmented skin. Deafness occurs in 9-37%, heterochromia irides in 20%, and unibrow (synophrys) in 17-69% of those affected. Dystopia canthorum (i.e., telecanthus) is seen in all patients with Waardenburg type 1. Waardenburg type 2 is similar to type 1, except that patients with type 2 lack dystopia canthorum, but they also have a higher incidence of deafness. Waardenburg type 3 is similar to Waardenburg type 1, except that patients also have limb abnormalities. It is also called the Klein-Waardenburg syndrome. Waardenburg type 4 is also called the Shah-Waardenburg syndrome. Patients with this type all have Hirschsprung disease. Dystopia canthorum is seldom seen in these patients.

Tuberous Sclerosis Complex (*TSC1*, *TSC2* Genes)
See Chapter 596.2 for a discussion of this complex.

Hypomelanosis of Ito
Hypomelanosis of Ito is a rare congenital skin disorder affecting children of both sexes that can have associated defects in several organ systems. There is no evidence for genetic transmission; chromosomal mosaicism and chromosomal translocations have been reported. Hypomelanosis of Ito is currently a descriptive rather than definitive diagnosis. Blaschkoid or mosaic hypomelanosis is a better descriptive term.

The skin lesions of hypomelanosis of Ito are generally present at birth but may be acquired in the 1st 2 yr of life. The lesions are similar to a negative image of those present in incontinentia pigmenti, consisting of bizarre, patterned, hypopigmented macules arranged over the body surface in sharply demarcated whorls, streaks, and patches that follow the lines of Blaschko (Fig. 653-3). The palms, soles, and mucous

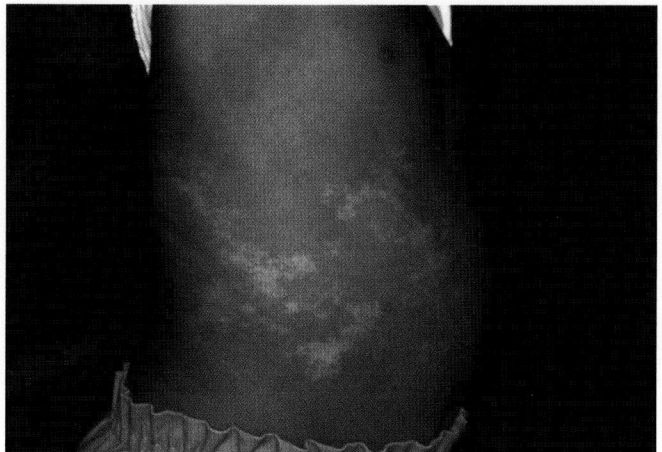

Figure 653-3 Marbled hypopigmented streaks on the abdomen in hypomelanosis of Ito.

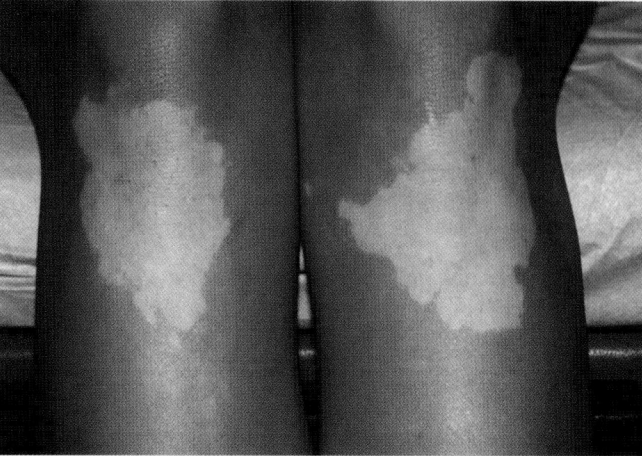

Figure 653-4 Sharply demarcated, symmetric, depigmented areas of vitiligo.

membranes are spared. The hypopigmentation remains unchanged throughout childhood but fades during adulthood. The degree of depigmentation varies from hypopigmented to achromic. Neither inflammatory nor vesicular lesions precede the development of the pigmentary changes as in incontinentia pigmenti. The hypopigmented areas demonstrate fewer and smaller melanocytes and a decreased number of melanin granules in the basal cell layer than normal. Inflammatory cells and pigment incontinence are lacking.

The majority of patients with mosaic hypomelanosis have no associated abnormalities, but involvement of other organs systems can rarely occur. The most commonly associated abnormalities involve the nervous system, including intellectual disability (70%), seizures (40%), microcephaly (25%), and muscular hypotonia (15%). The musculoskeletal system is the second most frequently involved system, affected by scoliosis and thoracic and limb deformities. Minor ophthalmologic defects (strabismus, nystagmus) are present in 25% of patients, and 10% have cardiac defects. These frequencies are likely to be overestimated because patients with isolated skin disease often do not seek further evaluation. The differential diagnosis includes systematized nevus depigmentosus, which is a stable leukoderma not associated with systemic manifestations. Differentiation from incontinentia pigmenti, particularly the hypopigmented fourth stage, is critical for genetic counseling because incontinentia pigmenti, unlike hypomelanosis of Ito, is inherited.

Vitiligo
Epidemiology and Etiology
Vitiligo is macular depigmentation associated with the destruction of melanocytes. The disorder represents a clinical end-point resulting from a complex interaction of environmental, genetic, and immunologic factors. Autoimmune, genetic, autocytotoxic, and neural theories have been postulated. The prevalence is 0.5% of most populations.

There is definitely an **autoimmune** component to vitiligo. Eighty percent of patients with active disease have an antibody to a surface antigen on pigmented melanocytes. These antibodies appear to be cytotoxic for melanocytes. There is also a correlation between disease activity and the titer of serum antimelanocyte antibody. Melanocyte-specific CD8+ T lymphocytes are also involved in the pathogenesis of vitiligo. These antibodies and T cells recognize a variety of melanocyte enzymatic and structural proteins.

The genetic epidemiology of vitiligo is part of a broader genetically determined autoimmune and autoinflammatory diathesis. Fifteen to 20% of patients with generalized vitiligo have 1 or more affected 1st-degree relatives. In these families the genetic pattern is suggestive of polygenic, multifactorial inheritance. In the other patients, the disease occurs sporadically.

Many authorities believe that the cause of melanocyte destruction in vitiligo is an endogenous cellular abnormality. It has been suggested

Table 653-2	Typical Features of Segmental and Nonsegmental Vitiligo
SEGMENTAL VITILIGO	**NONSEGMENTAL VITILIGO**
Often begins in childhood	Can begin in childhood, but later onset is more common
Has rapid onset and stabilizes	Is progressive, with flare-ups
Involves hair compartment soon after onset	Involves hair compartment in later stages
Is usually not accompanied by other autoimmune diseases	Is often associated with personal or family history of autoimmunity
Often occurs in the face	Commonly occurs at sites sensitive to pressure and friction and prone to trauma
Is usually responsive to autologous grafting, with stable repigmentation	Frequently relapses in situ after autologous grafting
Can be difficult to distinguish from nevus depigmentosus, especially in cases with early onset	

From Taïeb A, Picardo M: Vitiligo, N Engl J Med 360:160–168, 2009.

that melanocytes are destroyed because of the accumulation of a toxic melanin synthesis intermediate and/or lack of protection from hydrogen peroxide and other oxygen radicals. There is in vitro evidence that some of these metabolites may be lethal to melanocytes. Others believe that neurochemical factors damage melanocytes and cause depigmentation. This possibility would explain the pattern of involvement in segmental vitiligo that runs roughly along the course of a dermatome.

Clinical Manifestations
There are 2 subtypes of vitiligo, generalized (nonsegmental) and segmental, which probably are distinctly different diseases (Table 653-2). Generalized vitiligo (85-90% of cases) may be divided into widespread (type A) and localized (type B). Approximately 50% of all patients with vitiligo have onset before 18 yr of age, and 25% demonstrate depigmentation before age 8 yr. Most children have the generalized form, but the segmental type is more common among children than among adults. Patients with the generalized form usually present with a remarkably symmetric pattern of white macules and patches (Fig. 653-4); the margins may be somewhat hyperpigmented. The

patches tend to be acral and/or periorificial. Occasionally, almost the entire skin surface becomes depigmented.

There are several varieties of localized vitiligo. A form of localized vitiligo is the halo nevus phenomenon, whereby benign moles develop depigmented rings at the periphery. Premature graying of scalp hair (canities) has also been considered a form of localized vitiligo. In segmental vitiligo, depigmented areas are limited to a quasidermatomal distribution. This type of vitiligo has a rapid onset and progression in a localized area without the development of depigmentation in other areas.

A number of **autoimmune diseases** occur in patients with vitiligo, including Addison disease, Hashimoto thyroiditis, pernicious anemia, diabetes mellitus, hypoparathyroidism, and polyglandular autoimmune syndrome with selective immunoglobulin A deficiency. In addition, other diseases with possible immune defects, such as alopecia areata and morphea, have been seen in patients with vitiligo.

Vogt-Koyanagi-Harada syndrome is vitiligo associated with uveitis, dysacusia, meningoencephalitis, and depigmentation of the skin, scalp hair, eyebrows, and eyelashes. In the **Alezzandrini syndrome**, vitiligo is associated with tapetoretinal degeneration and deafness.

Light microscopic examination of early lesions shows mild inflammatory change. Over time, degenerative changes occur in melanocytes, leading to their complete disappearance.

The differential diagnosis of vitiligo includes other causes of widespread acquired leukoderma. The two most common problem diagnoses are tinea versicolor and postinflammatory hypopigmentation.

Treatment

Localized areas of vitiligo may respond to potent topical steroid, topical tacrolimus, or topical pimecrolimus. In patients with more extensive involvement, narrow-band ultraviolet light B (UVB) [UVB311] is the treatment of choice. In all forms of vitiligo, response to therapy is slow, taking many months to years. For those not interested in treatment, cover-up cosmetics may be used. All areas of vitiligo are susceptible to sun damage, and care should be taken to minimize sun exposure of affected areas. Spontaneous remission may be seen in a small percentage of cases.

Bibliography is available at Expert Consult.

Chapter 654
Vesiculobullous Disorders
Joel C. Joyce

Many diseases are characterized by vesiculobullous lesions; they vary considerably in cause, age of onset, and pattern. The morphology and distribution of the blister often provides a visual clue to the location of the lesion within the skin. Blisters localized to the **epidermal layers** are thin-walled, relatively flaccid, and easily ruptured. **Subepidermal blisters** are tense, thick-walled, and more durable. Biopsies of blisters can be diagnostic because the level of cleavage within the skin and associated findings, such as the nature of the inflammatory infiltrate, are characteristic for a particular disorder. Other diagnostic procedures, such as immunofluorescence and electron microscopy, can often help distinguish vesiculobullous disorders that have nearly identical histopathologic findings (Table 654-1).

Table 654-1	Sites of Blister Formation and Diagnostic Studies for the Vesiculobullous Disorders

DISORDER	BLISTER CLEAVAGE SITE	DIAGNOSTIC STUDIES
Acrodermatitis enteropathica	IE	Zn level
Bullous impetigo	GL	Smear, culture
Bullous pemphigoid	SE (junctional)	Direct and indirect immunofluorescence studies
Candidosis	SC	KOH preparation, culture
Dermatitis herpetiformis	SE	Direct immunofluorescence studies
Dermatophytosis	IE	KOH preparation, culture
Dyshidrotic eczema	IE	Routine histopathology
EB—simplex	IE	Electron microscopy; immunofluorescence mapping
EB of the hands and feet	IE	Electron microscopy; immunofluorescence mapping
Junctional EB (lethalis)	SE (junctional)	Electron microscopy; immunofluorescence mapping
Recessive dystrophic EB	SE	Electron microscopy; immunofluorescence mapping
Dominant dystrophic EB	SE	Electron microscopy; immunofluorescence mapping
Epidermolytic hyperkeratosis	IE	Routine histopathology
Erythema multiforme	SE	Routine histopathology
Erythema toxicum	SC, IE	Smear for eosinophils
Incontinentia pigmenti	IE	Smear for eosinophils Routine histopathology
Insect bites	IE	Routine histopathology
Kindler syndrome	IE, SE	Electron microscopy; immunostaining
Linear immunoglobulin A dermatosis	SE	Direct immunofluorescence studies

Table 654-1	Sites of Blister Formation and Diagnostic Studies for the Vesiculobullous Disorders—cont'd	
DISORDER	**BLISTER CLEAVAGE SITE**	**DIAGNOSTIC STUDIES**
Mastocytosis	SE	Routine histopathology
Miliaria crystallina	IC	Routine histopathology
Neonatal pustular melanosis	SC, IE	Smear for cells
Pemphigus foliaceus	GL	Direct and indirect immunofluorescence studies Tzanck smear
Pemphigus vulgaris	Suprabasal	Direct and indirect immunofluorescence studies Tzanck smear
Scabies	IE	Scraping
Staphylococcal scalded skin syndrome	GL	Routine histopathology
Toxic epidermal necrolysis	SE	Routine histopathology
Viral blisters	IE	Tzanck smear for herpesvirus infections Direct immunofluorescence for herpes simplex virus and varicella-zoster virus Culture Routine histopathology

EB, epidermolysis bullosa; GL, granular layer; IC, intracorneal; IE, intraepidermal; KOH, potassium hydroxide; SC, subcorneal; SE, subepidermal.

654.1 Erythema Multiforme
Joel C. Joyce

ETIOLOGY
Among the numerous factors implicated in the etiology of erythema multiforme (EM), infection with herpes simplex virus (HSV) is the most common. Infection with *Mycoplasma pneumoniae* is implicated, particularly in children and young adults, but differentiation from Stevens-Johnson syndrome and the so-called *M. pneumoniae*-associated mucositis (see below) can be confusing. HSV labialis and, less commonly, HSV genitalis are implicated in 60-70% of episodes of EM and are believed to trigger nearly all episodes of recurrent EM, frequently in association with sun exposure. HSV antigens and DNA are present in skin lesions of EM but are absent in nonlesional skin. The presence of the human leukocyte antigens A33, B62, B35, DQw3 (DQB1*0301 split), and DR53 is associated with an increased risk of HSV-induced EM, particularly the recurrent form. Most patients experience a single self-limited episode of EM. Lesions of HSV-induced recurrent EM typically develop 10-14 days after onset of recurrent HSV eruptions, have a similar appearance from episode to episode, but may vary in frequency and duration in a given patient. Not all episodes of recurrent HSV evolve into EM in susceptible patients.

Drug-related EM is less common (<10% of patients) and may be associated with nonsteroidal antiinflammatory agents, including acetaminophen, sulfonamides, and other antibiotics. The differential diagnosis in drug-related EM should include toxic epidermal necrolysis and drug hypersensitivity syndrome.

CLINICAL MANIFESTATIONS
EM has numerous morphologic manifestations on the skin, varying from erythematous macules, papules, vesicles, bullae, or urticaria-appearing plaques to patches of confluent erythema. The eruption appears most commonly in patients between the ages of 10 and 40 yr (with highest incidence in males in the 2nd decade) and usually is asymptomatic, although a burning sensation or pruritus may be present. The diagnosis of EM is established by finding the classic lesion: doughnut-shaped, target-like (iris or bull's-eye) papules with an erythematous outer border, an inner pale ring, and a dusky purple to necrotic center (which sometimes blisters and erodes; Figs. 654-1 and 654-2).

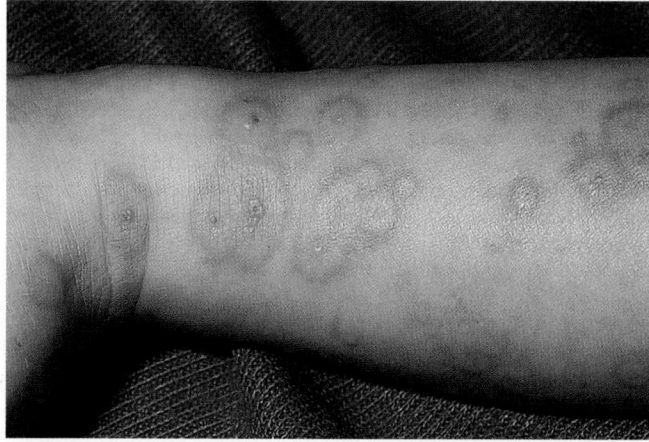

Figure 654-1 Early fixed papules with a central dusky zone on the dorsum of the hand of a child with erythema multiforme caused by herpes simplex virus. *(From Weston WL, Lane AT, Morelli J: Color textbook of pediatric dermatology, ed 3, St. Louis, 2002, Mosby, p. 156.)*

EM is characterized by an abrupt, symmetric cutaneous eruption, most commonly on the extensor upper extremities; lesions are relatively sparse on the face, trunk, and legs. Lesions can be seen on the palms and soles. The eruption often appears initially as red macules or urticarial plaques that expand centrifugally to form lesions up to 2 cm in diameter with a dusky to necrotic center. Lesions of a particular episode typically appear within 72 hr and remain fixed in place (average duration: 7 days). Oral lesions may occur with a predilection for the vermilion border of the lips and the buccal mucosa, but other mucosal surfaces are spared. EM may manifest initially as urticarial-like lesions, but in distinction to urticaria, a given lesion of EM does not fade within 24 hr. Prodromal symptoms are generally absent. Prognosis is favorable with limited long-term morbidity. Lesions typically resolve without sequelae in approximately 2 wk, but in darker pigmented individuals, pigmentary alterations at the site of lesions can be long-standing. Progression to Stevens-Johnson syndrome does not occur. Many authors distinguish between EM minor (mainly cutaneous typical or atypical targetoid lesions affecting less than 10% body surface area plus no or limited mucosal involvement, often limited to 1 site,

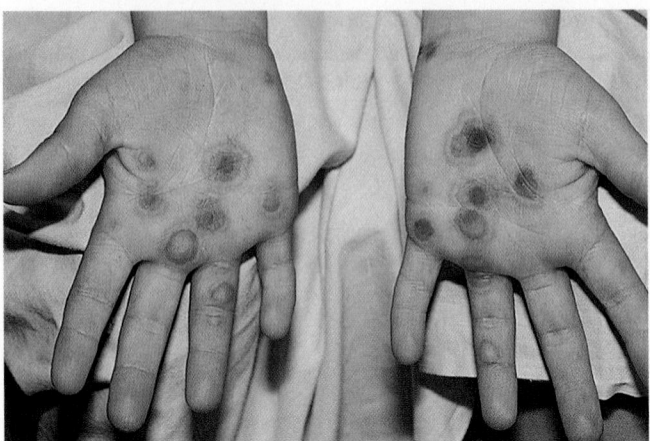

Figure 654-2 "Target" or "iris" lesions with characteristic central dusky zone on palms of a child with erythema multiforme caused by herpes simplex virus. *(From Weston WL, Lane AT, Morelli J: Color textbook of pediatric dermatology, ed 3, St. Louis, 2002, Mosby, p. 156.)*

such as the mouth) from EM major (same cutaneous involvement pattern as EM minor plus 2 or more mucosal sites with more-severe oral involvement). EM major and Stevens-Johnson syndrome are accepted to be separate entities.

Pathogenesis

The pathogenesis of EM is unclear, but it may be a host-specific, cell-mediated immune response to an antigenic stimulus, resulting in damage to keratinocytes. HSV *Pol1* gene expressed in HSV-induced recurrent EM lesions upregulates/activates the transcription factor SP1 and inflammatory cytokines. These cytokines, released by activated mononuclear cells and keratinocytes, may contribute to epidermal cell death and constitutional symptoms.

Pathology

Microscopic findings in EM are variable but may aid in diagnosis. Early lesions typically show slight intercellular edema, rare dyskeratotic keratinocytes, and basal vacuolation in the epidermis and a perivascular lymphohistiocytic infiltrate with edema in the upper dermis. More mature lesions show an accentuation of these characteristics and the development of lymphocytic exocytosis and an intense, perivascular, and interstitial mononuclear infiltrate in the upper third of the dermis. In severe cases, the entire epidermis becomes necrotic.

Differential Diagnosis

The **differential diagnosis** of EM also includes bullous pemphigoid, pemphigus, linear immunoglobulin (Ig) A dermatosis, graft-versus-host disease, fixed-drug eruption, bullous-drug eruption, urticaria, viral infections such as HSV, reactive arthritis syndromes, Kawasaki disease, Sweet syndrome, Behçet disease, allergic vasculitis, erythema annulare centrifugum, polymorphous-drug eruption, and periarteritis nodosa. EM that primarily involves the oral mucosa may be confused with Stevens-Johnson syndrome, bullous pemphigoid, pemphigus vulgaris, vesiculobullous or erosive lichen planus, Behçet syndrome, recurrent aphthous stomatitis, and primary herpetic gingivostomatitis. Serum sickness–like reaction to cefaclor (or other antibiotics) may also manifest as EM-like lesions; the lesions may develop a dusky to purple center, but in most cases, the eruption of cefaclor-induced serum sickness–like reaction is pruritic, transient, and migratory and is probably urticarial rather than true EM.

Treatment

Treatment of EM is supportive. Topical emollients, systemic antihistamines, and nonsteroidal antiinflammatory agents do not alter the course of the disease but may provide symptomatic relief. For individuals with severe mucosal disease, opioids can be used to control pain and diligent oral hygiene is essential. No controlled, prospective studies support the use of corticosteroids in the management of EM. Prophylactic oral acyclovir given for 6 mo may be effective in controlling *recurrent episodes of HSV-associated EM*. On discontinuation of acyclovir, both HSV and EM may recur, although episodes may be less frequent and milder. For recurrent cases not responsive to antiviral therapy, steroid-sparing agents used to decrease frequency of recurrence include azathioprine, mycophenolate mofetil, and dapsone. Appropriate laboratory monitoring is recommended.

Bibliography is available at Expert Consult.

654.2 Stevens-Johnson Syndrome

Joel C. Joyce

ETIOLOGY

Drugs, particularly sulfonamides, nonsteroidal antiinflammatory agents, antibiotics, and anticonvulsants, are the most common precipitants of Stevens-Johnson syndrome and toxic epidermal necrolysis. Stevens-Johnson syndrome (SJS) and toxic epidermal necrolysis (TEN; see below) exist along a spectrum: SJS is defined as affected body surface area <10%, SJS-TEN overlap syndrome is affected body surface area between 10% and 30%, and TEN is affected body surface area >30%. **TEN** is the most-severe disorder in the clinical spectrum of the disease, involving considerable constitutional toxicity and extensive necrolysis of the mucous membranes and >30% of the body surface area. Human leukocyte antigen (HLA)-B*1502 and HLA-B*5801 are implicated in the development of these 2 disorders in Han Chinese patients receiving carbamazepine and in Japanese patients receiving allopurinol, respectively.

Infections, particularly in children, also are associated with SJS, although current thinking defines most cases of classic SJS as secondary to medications. Terms such as "***M. pneumoniae*-associated mucositis**" or "**atypical SJS**" have caused difficulty with diagnosis and classification. Individuals, typically children or young adults, often with upper respiratory symptoms from *M. pneumoniae* infection, suffer from variable degrees of mucosal ulceration and erosion (typically mouth but including other mucosae) but lack other cutaneous involvement (unlike traditional SJS-TEN) and are found to have evidence of infection with *M. pneumoniae*, typically by polymerase chain reaction evaluation. In addition to supportive treatment below, affected individuals benefit from antimicrobial treatment for *M. pneumoniae*. Morbidity is typically less severe than for SJS-TEN spectrum disease.

Clinical Manifestations

Cutaneous lesions in SJS generally consist initially of erythematous macules that rapidly and variably develop central necrosis to form vesicles, bullae, and areas of denudation on the face, trunk, and extremities. The skin lesions are typically more widespread than in EM and are accompanied by involvement of **2 or more mucosal surfaces,** namely the eyes, oral cavity, upper airway or esophagus, gastrointestinal tract, or anogenital mucosa (Fig. 654-3). A burning sensation, edema, and erythema of the lips and buccal mucosa are often the presenting signs, followed by development of bullae, ulceration, and hemorrhagic crusting. Lesions may be preceded by a flu-like upper respiratory illness. Pain from mucosal ulceration is often severe, but skin tenderness is minimal to absent in SJS, in contrast to pain in TEN. Corneal ulceration, anterior uveitis, panophthalmitis, bronchitis, pneumonitis, myocarditis, hepatitis, enterocolitis, polyarthritis, hematuria, and acute tubular necrosis leading to renal failure may occur. Disseminated cutaneous bullae and erosions may result in increased insensible fluid loss and a high risk of bacterial superinfection and sepsis. New lesions occur in crops, and complete healing may take 4-6 wk; ocular scarring, visual impairment, and strictures of the

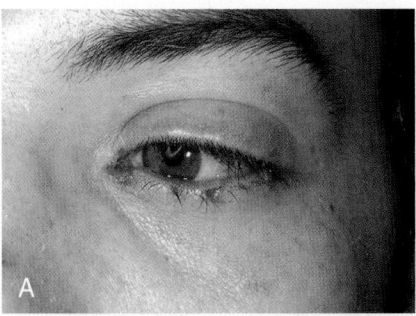
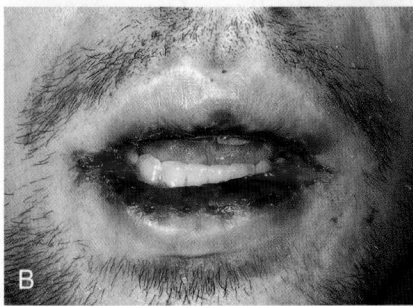
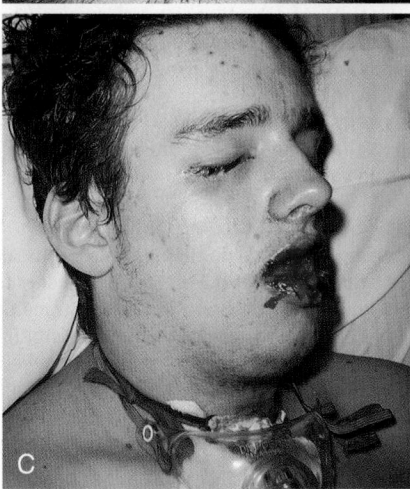

Figure 654-3 Bullae are present on the conjunctivae **(A)** and in the mouth **(B)** with Stevens-Johnson syndrome. **C,** Sloughing, ulceration, and necrosis in the oral cavity interfere with eating. Genital lesions cause dysuria and interfere with voiding. *(From Habif TP, editor: Clinical dermatology, ed 4, Philadelphia, 2004, Mosby, p. 631.)*

esophagus, bronchi, vagina, urethra, or anus may remain. Nonspecific laboratory abnormalities in SJS include leukocytosis, elevated erythrocyte sedimentation rate, and, occasionally, increased liver transaminase levels and decreased serum albumin values.

Pathogenesis
Pathogenesis is related to drug-specific CD8+ cytotoxic T cells, with perforin/granzyme B and granulysin triggering keratinocyte apoptosis. This process is followed by expanded enactment of apoptosis involving the interaction of soluble Fas ligand with Fas receptor. Recently, consideration has been given to the role that macrophages/monocytes play in development of SJS/TEN via tumor necrosis factor-α, tumor necrosis factor–related apoptosis-inducing ligand (TRAIL), and tumor necrosis factor–inducer of apoptosis weak (TWEAK) signaling pathways. It is likely that many affected individuals have yet unrecognized underlying genetic predispositions.

Differential Diagnosis
The differential diagnosis of SJS includes TEN, urticaria, *M. pneumoniae*–associated mucositis, DRESS (drug rash [or reaction]

with eosinophilia and systemic symptoms) syndrome (see Chapter 645.2) and other drug eruptions and viral exanthems, including Kawasaki disease. SJS has rarely been reported in patients with systemic lupus erythematosus.

Treatment
Management of SJS is supportive and symptomatic. Potentially offending drugs must be discontinued as soon as possible. Ophthalmologic consultation is mandatory because ocular sequelae such as corneal scarring can lead to vision loss. Application of cryopreserved amniotic membrane to the ocular surface during the acute phase of the disease limits the destructive and long-term sequelae. Early topical steroid treatment may also reduce ocular sequelae. Oral lesions should be managed with mouthwashes and glycerin swabs. Vaginal lesions should be observed closely and treated to prevent vaginal stricture or fusion. Topical anesthetics (diphenhydramine, dyclonine, viscous lidocaine) may provide relief from pain, particularly when applied before eating. Denuded skin lesions can be cleansed with saline or Burrow solution compresses. Antibiotic therapy is appropriate for documented secondary bacterial infection. Treatment may require admission to an intensive care unit; IV fluids; nutritional support; sheepskin or air-fluid bedding; daily saline or Burrow solution compresses; paraffin gauze or colloidal gel (Hydrogel) dressing of denuded areas; saline compresses on the eyelids, lips, or nose; analgesics; and urinary catheterization (when needed). A daily examination for infection and ocular lesions, which constitute the major cause of long-term morbidity, is essential. Systemic antibiotics are indicated for documented urinary or cutaneous infections and for suspected bacteremia (*Staphylococcus aureus* or *Pseudomonas aeruginosa*) because infection is the leading cause of death. Prophylactic systemic antibiotics are not necessary. Although corticosteroids are sometimes advocated in early, severe cases of SJS, no prospective double-blind studies evaluating their efficacy have been reported. Most authorities discourage their use because of reports of increased morbidity and mortality (sepsis) with their administration, although definitive trials in children are lacking. IV immunoglobulin (IVIG; 1.5-2.0 g/kg/day × 3 days) should be considered in early disease. Total dose greater than 2 g/kg has shown improved but not statistically significant outcomes in children compared to adults. Other immunosuppressive treatment regimens have not demonstrated clear benefit or repeated success in multiple controlled studies.

Bibliography is available at Expert Consult.

654.3 Toxic Epidermal Necrolysis
Joel C. Joyce

EPIDEMIOLOGY AND ETIOLOGY
The pathogenesis of TEN is not proved but may involve a hypersensitivity phenomenon that results in damage primarily to the basal cell layer of the epidermis. Epidermal damage appears to result from keratinocyte apoptosis (see Chapter 654.2). This condition is triggered by many of the same factors that are thought to be responsible for SJS, principally drugs such as the sulfonamides, amoxicillin, phenobarbital, hydantoin, and allopurinol. TEN is defined by (1) widespread blister formation and morbilliform or confluent erythema, associated with skin tenderness; (2) absence of target lesions; (3) sudden onset and generalization within 24-48 hr; (4) histologic findings of full-thickness epidermal necrosis and a minimal-to-absent dermal infiltrate. These criteria categorize TEN as a separate entity from EM.

CLINICAL MANIFESTATIONS
The prodrome consists of fever, malaise, localized skin tenderness, and diffuse erythema. Inflammation of the eyelids, conjunctivae, mouth, and genitals may precede skin lesions. Flaccid bullae may develop,

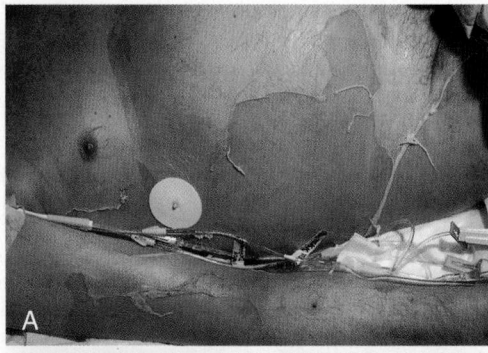
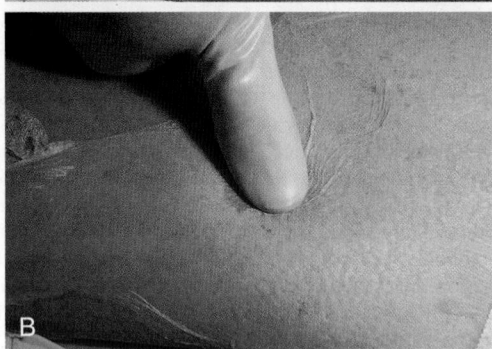

Figure 654-4 A, Large sheets of full-thickness epidermis are shed. **B,** Toxic epidermal necrolysis begins with diffuse, hot erythema. In hours the skin becomes painful, and with slight thumb pressure, the skin wrinkles, slides laterally, and separates from the dermis (Nikolsky sign). *(From Habif TP, editor: Clinical dermatology, ed 4, Philadelphia, 2004, Mosby, p. 633.)*

although this is not a prominent feature. Characteristically, full-thickness epidermis is lost in large sheets (Fig. 654-4). The **Nikolsky sign** (denudation of the skin with gentle tangential pressure) is present but only in the areas of erythema (Fig. 654-4). Healing takes place over 14 or more days. Scarring, particularly of the eyes, may result in corneal opacity. The course may be relentlessly progressive, complicated by severe dehydration, electrolyte imbalance, shock, and secondary localized infection and septicemia. Loss of nails and hair may also occur. Long-term morbidity includes alterations in skin pigmentation, eye problems (lack of tears, conjunctival scarring, loss of lashes), and strictures of mucosal surfaces. The **differential diagnosis** includes staphylococcal scalded skin syndrome, in which the blister cleavage plane is intraepidermal; graft-versus-host disease; chemical burns; drug eruptions; toxic shock syndrome; and pemphigus. The use of skin histopathology to differentiate SJS-TEN from other similar blistering disorders can be difficult, but early full-thickness epidermal necrosis tends to portend a worse clinical prognosis.

Anticonvulsant hypersensitivity syndrome (DRESS syndrome; see Chapter 645.2) is a multisystem reaction that appears approximately 3 wk to 3 mo after the start of therapy with the offending agent. The skin eruption is red-pink morbilliform eruption often associated with facial swelling, lymphadenopathy, fever, hepatic, renal and pulmonary disease, eosinophilia, atypical lymphocytosis, and leukocytosis.

TREATMENT
Appreciation of the specific etiologic factor is crucial. As most cases are drug-induced, cessation of the offending agent is critical as soon as possible. Management is similar to that for severe burns and may be best accomplished in a burn unit (see Chapter 75). It may include strict reverse isolation, meticulous fluid and electrolyte therapy, use of an air–fluid bed, and daily cultures. Systemic antibiotic therapy is indicated when secondary infection is evident or suspected. Skin care consists of cleansing with isotonic saline or Burrow solution. Biologic or colloid gel (Hydrogel) dressings alleviate pain and reduce fluid loss.

Narcotics are often required for pain relief. Mouth and eye care, as for EM major and SJS, may be necessary. Because of an immune mechanism, systemic glucocorticosteroids and IVIG have been used with apparent success. Nonetheless, this treatment remains controversial although trends toward decreased morbidity and mortality in children receiving high-dose IVIG have been demonstrated (see Chapter 654.2).

Bibliography is available at Expert Consult.

654.4 Mechanobullous Disorders
Joel C. Joyce

EPIDERMOLYSIS BULLOSA
Diseases categorized under the general term epidermolysis bullosa (EB) are a heterogeneous group of congenital, genetic blistering disorders. They differ in severity and prognosis, clinical and histologic features, and inheritance patterns but are all characterized by induction of blisters by trauma and exacerbation of blistering in warm weather. The disorders can be categorized under 3 major headings with multiple subgroupings: epidermolysis bullosa simplex (EBS), junctional epidermolysis bullosa (JEB), and dystrophic epidermolysis bullosa (DEB) (Table 654-2). **Kindler syndrome**, which includes poikiloderma and photosensitivity as well as easy blistering, is also considered a separate form of EB. Epidermolysis bullosa acquisita is an autoimmune disorder producing antibodies to the α chain of type VII collagen. Affected mothers may pass the autoantibody to the fetus resulting in similar but transient lesions in the newborn.

EPIDERMOLYSIS BULLOSA SIMPLEX
EBS is a nonscarring, autosomal dominant disorder. The defect in most common types of EBS is in keratin 5 or 14, which makes up intermediate filaments of the basal keratinocytes. The intraepidermal bullae result from cytolysis of the basal cells. There are multiple other rare variants with defects that also result in intraepidermal blistering.

In **EBS–generalized other (formerly Koebner)**, blisters are usually present at birth or during the neonatal period. Sites of predilection are the hands, feet, elbows, knees, legs, and scalp. Intraoral lesions are minimal, nails rarely become dystrophic and usually regrow even when they are shed, and dentition is normal. Bullae heal with minimal to no scar or milia formation. Secondary infection is the primary complication. The propensity to blister decreases with age, and the long-term prognosis is good. Blisters should be drained by puncturing, but the blister top should be left intact to protect the underlying skin. Erosions may be covered with a semipermeable dressing.

EBS–localized (formerly Weber-Cockayne) predominantly affects the hands and feet and often manifests when a child begins to walk; onset may be delayed until puberty or early adulthood, when heavy shoes are worn or the feet are subjected to increased trauma. Bullae are usually restricted to the hands and feet (Fig. 654-5); rarely, they occur elsewhere, such as the dorsal aspect of the arms and the shins. The disorder ranges from mildly incapacitating to crippling at times of severe exacerbations.

EBS–Dowling-Meara (herpetiformis) is characterized by grouped blisters resembling those of herpes simplex (Fig. 654-6). During infancy, blistering may be severe and extensive, may involve mucous membranes, and may result in shedding of nails, formation of milia, and mild pigmentary changes, without scarring. After the 1st few mo of life, warm temperatures do not appear to exacerbate blistering. Hyperkeratosis and hyperhidrosis of the palms and soles may develop, but generally, the condition improves with age.

JUNCTIONAL EPIDERMOLYSIS BULLOSA
JEB–Herlitz is an autosomal recessive condition that is life-threatening. Blisters appear at birth or develop during the neonatal period, particularly on the perioral area, scalp, legs, diaper area, and thorax. Nails eventually become dystrophic and then often permanently lost.

| Table 654-2 | Clinical Presentation and Diagnosis of Selected Epidermolysis Bullosa Subtypes in the Neonatal Period |

| EB SUBTYPE (USUAL INHERITANCE) | CLINICAL FEATURES | | DIAGNOSIS |
	Cutaneous	Extracutaneous	
EB simplex–generalized (AD)	Mild to moderate blistering, often generalized Rare scarring, milia	Occasional mucosal blistering	EM: Intrabasal layer split IF: BPAG1 (BP230), BP-180 (BPAG2, collagen XVII), $\alpha_6\beta_4$ integrin, laminin 1, laminin 332, type IV collagen, type VII collagen (EBA antigen) at base of blister
EB simplex–localized (AD)	Mild blistering, often localized, sometimes in 1st 24 mo, but often not until later infancy or childhood Rare scarring, milia	Rare mucosal involvement	EM: Intrastratum basale split IF: Same as for EB simplex—generalized
EB simplex–Dowling-Meara (AD)	Moderate to severe blistering, which starts generalized, then is grouped (herpetiform); milia; nail dystrophy, shedding	Mild mucosal blistering	EM: Intrastratum basale split; clumped keratin filaments IF: Same as for EB simplex—generalized
Junctional EB–non-Herlitz (AR)	Moderate blistering; atrophic scars; nail dystrophy	Mild mucosal blistering; enamel hypoplasia	EM: Intralamina lucida cleavage; variable reduction in hemidesmosomes IF: Absence of staining with 19-DEJ-1 (uncein); variable staining with GB3 and other laminin 332 antibodies, including 46 and K140; BPAG1 (BP230) BP180 (BPAG2, type XVII collagen), $\alpha_6\beta_4$ integrin in blister roof; laminin 1, type IV collagen, type VII collagen (EBA antigen) at base of blister
Junctional EB–Herlitz (AR)	Severe generalized blistering that heals poorly; granulation tissue; scarring; nail dystrophy	Severe mucosal blistering; GI involvement common; laryngeal involvement with airway obstruction; urologic involvement	EM: Cleavage intralamina lucida; markedly reduced or no hemidesmosomes; absence of sub-basal dense plates IF: Absence of staining with 19-DEJ-1 (uncein) and GB3 (laminin 332) and of staining with other laminin 332 antibodies, including 46 and K140; BPAG1 (BP230) and BP180 (BPAG2, type XVII collagen) in blister roof; laminin-1, type IV collagen, and type VII collagen at base of blister
Junctional EB–pyloric atresia (AR)	Severe blistering	Polyhydramnios; pyloric atresia; urologic involvement: uretovesicular obstruction, hydronephrosis	EM: Cleavage intralamina lucida and intraplasma membrane; small hemidesmosomes IF: BPAG1 (BP230) and BP180 (BPAG2, type XVII collagen) in blister roof; laminin-1, type IV collagen, and type VII collagen at base of blister; Absence of 19-DEJ-1(uncein), $\alpha_6\beta_4$ integrin absent or reduced
Dominant dystrophic EB (AD)	Mild to moderate blistering (but may be more severe in newborn period) Milia, scarring Nail dystrophy	Mild mucosal blistering	EM: Cleavage sublamina densa; variable reduction in anchoring fibrils IF: BPAG1 (BP230), BPAG2 (BP180, type XVII collagen), $\alpha_6\beta_4$ integrin, laminin 1, type IV collagen at top of blister Staining for type VII collagen (EBA antigen) is normal, variable, or absent
Recessive dystrophic EB–Hallopeau-Siemens (AR)	Severe blistering Milia, scarring	Severe mucosal blistering; GI involvement common; urologic involvement	EM: Cleavage sublamina densa; absence of anchoring fibrils IF: BPAG1 (BP230), BP-180 (BPAG2, type XVII collagen), $\alpha_6\beta_4$ integrin, laminin 1, type IV collagen at top of blister Variability or absence of staining for type VII collagen (EBA antigen)

AD, autosomal dominant; AR, autosomal recessive; EB, epidermolysis bullosa; EBA, epidermolysis bullosa acquisita; EM, electron microscopy; GI, gastrointestinal; IF, immunohistochemical and immunofluorescence antigen mapping findings.
Modified from Eichenfield LF, Frieden IJ, Esterly NB: Textbook of neonatal dermatology, Philadelphia, 2001, WB Saunders, p. 159.

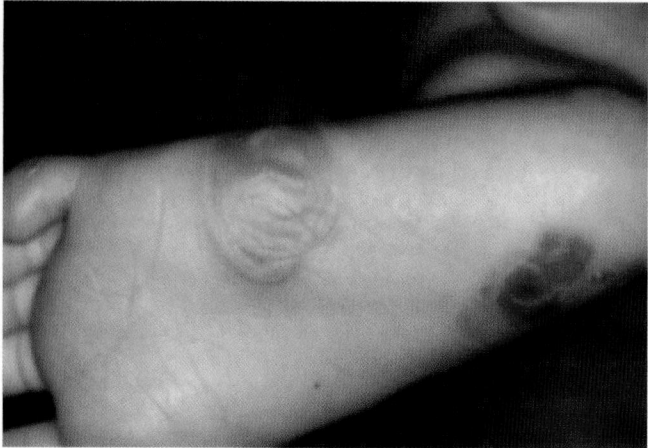

Figure 654-5 Bullae of the feet in epidermolysis bullosa simplex–localized (Weber-Cockayne).

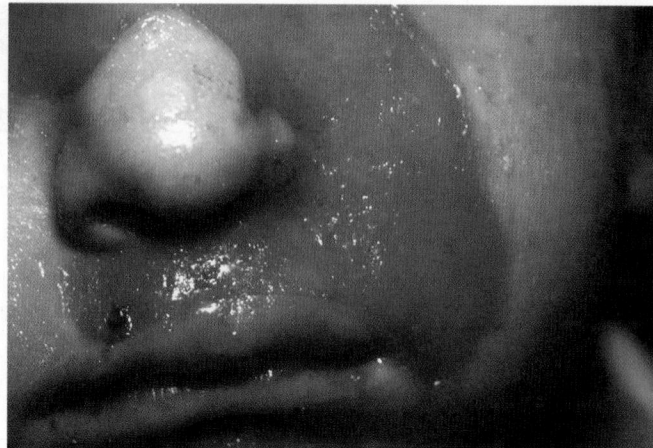

Figure 654-7 Nonhealing granulation tissue in junctional epidermolysis bullosa.

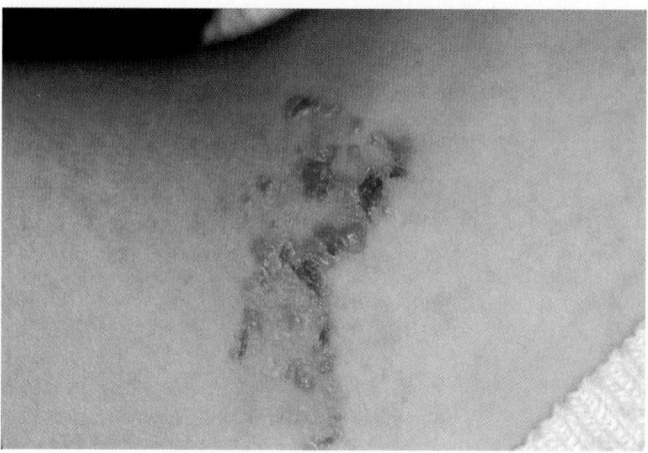

Figure 654-6 Grouped vesicle on an erythematous base in epidermolysis bullosa simplex–Dowling-Meara.

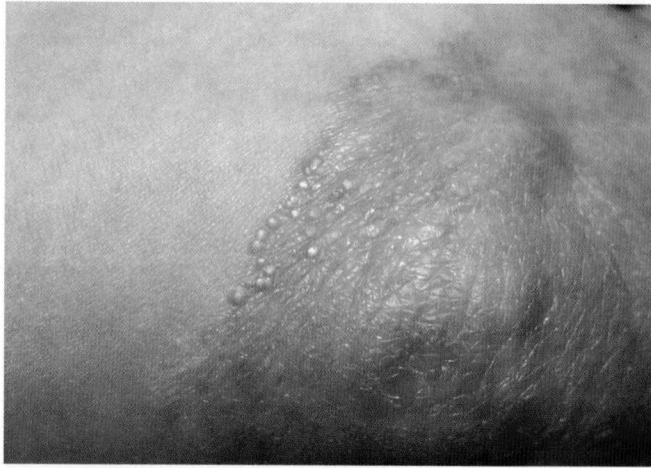

Figure 654-8 Scarring with milia formation over the knee in dominant dystrophic epidermolysis bullosa.

Mucous membrane involvement may be severe, and ulceration of the respiratory, gastrointestinal, and genitourinary epithelium has been documented in many affected children, although less frequently than in severe recessive dystrophic epidermolysis bullosa. Healing is delayed, and vegetating granulomas may persist for a long time. Large, moist, erosive plaques (Fig. 654-7) may provide a portal of entry for bacteria, and septicemia is a frequent cause of death. Mild atrophy may be seen in areas of recurrent blistering. Defective dentition with early loss of teeth as a result of rampant caries is characteristic. Growth retardation and recalcitrant anemia are almost invariable. In addition to infection, cachexia and circulatory failure are common causes of death. Most patients die within the 1st 3 yr of life.

JEB–non-Herlitz is a heterogeneous group of disorders. Blistering may be severe in the neonatal period, making differentiation from the Herlitz type difficult. All conditions associated with the Herlitz type may be seen but are usually milder. **JEB–non-Herlitz generalized (formerly generalized atrophic benign EB)** is included as a variant of non-Herlitz JEB. Another variant of non-Herlitz JEB is associated with **pyloric atresia**.

In all types of JEB, a subepidermal blister is found on light microscopic examination, and electron microscopy demonstrates a cleavage plane in the lamina lucida, between the plasma membranes of the basal cells and the basal lamina. Absence or a great reduction of hemidesmosomes is seen on electron micrographs in **JEB–Herlitz** and some cases of **JEB–non-Herlitz**. The defect is in laminin 332 (formerly laminin 5 or epiligrin), a glycoprotein associated with anchoring filaments beneath the hemidesmosomes. In JEB–non-Herlitz, defects have also been described in other hemidesmosomal components, such as type XVII collagen (BP180). In **JEB–pyloric atresia**, the defect is in the $\alpha_6\beta_4$ integrin.

Treatment for JEB is supportive. The diet should provide adequate calories and supplemental iron. Infections should be treated promptly. Transfusions of packed red blood cells may be required if the patient shows no response to iron and erythropoietin therapy. Strict adherence to wound care regimens is essential. Tissue-engineered skin grafts (artificial skin derived from human keratinocytes and fibroblasts) may be beneficial.

DYSTROPHIC EPIDERMOLYSIS BULLOSA

All forms of DEB result from mutations in collagen VII, a major component of anchoring fibrils that tether the basement membrane and overlying epidermis to its dermal foundation. The blister is subepidermal in all types of DEB. The type and location of the mutation dictate the severity of the phenotype.

Dominant DEB is the most common type of DEB. The spectrum of dominant DEB is varied. Blisters may be manifest at birth and are often limited and characteristically form over acral bony prominences. The lesions heal promptly, with the formation of soft, wrinkled scars, milia, and alterations in pigmentation (Fig. 654-8). Abnormal nails and nail loss are common. In many cases, the blistering process is mild, causing little restriction of activity and not impairing growth and development. Mucous membrane involvement tends to be minimal.

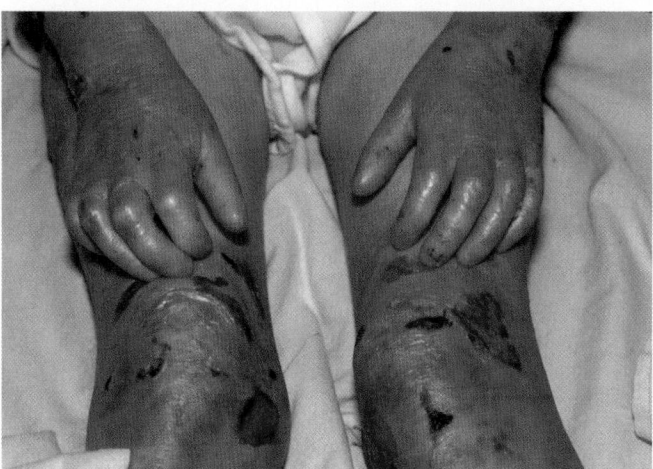

Figure 654-9 Severe scarring of the hands and knees in recessive dystrophic epidermolysis bullosa.

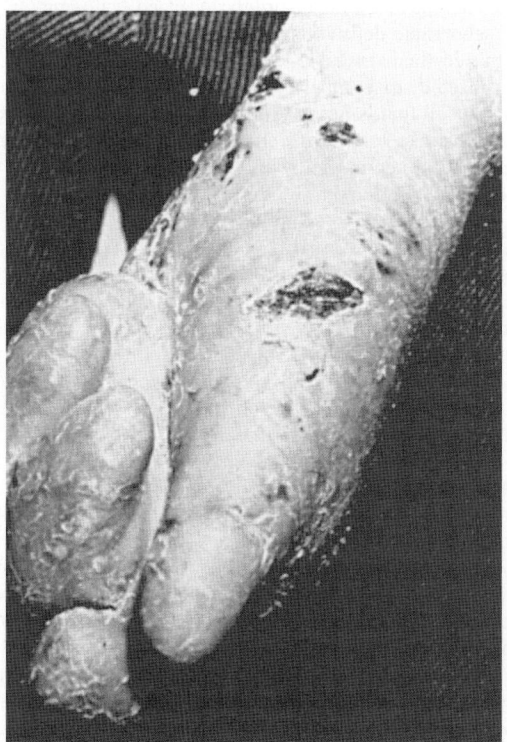

Figure 654-10 Mitten-hand deformity of recessive dystrophic epidermolysis bullosa.

Recessive DEB–severe generalized (formerly recessive DEB–Hallopeau-Siemens) is the most incapacitating form of EB, although the clinical spectrum is wide. Some patients have blisters, scarring, and milia formation primarily on the hands, feet, elbows, and knees (Fig. 654-9). Others have extensive erosions and blister formation at birth that seriously impede their care and feeding. Mucous membrane lesions are common and may cause severe nutritional deprivation, even in older children, whose growth may be retarded. During childhood, esophageal erosions and strictures, scarring of the buccal mucosa, flexion contractures of joints secondary to scarring of the integument, development of cutaneous squamous cell carcinomas, and the development of digital fusion may significantly limit the quality of life (Fig. 654-10). Squamous cell carcinomas and infection are major causes of morbidity and mortality.

Although the skin becomes less sensitive to trauma with aging in patients with recessive DEB, the progressive and permanent deformities complicate management, and the overall prognosis is poor. Foods that traumatize the buccal or esophageal mucosa should be avoided. If esophageal scarring develops, a semiliquid diet and esophageal dilatations may be required. Stricture excision or colonic interposition may be needed to relieve esophageal obstruction. In infants, severe oropharyngeal involvement may necessitate the use of special feeding devices such as a gastrostomy tube. Iron therapy for anemia, intermittent antibiotic therapy for secondary infections, and periodic surgery for release of digits may reduce morbidity. Newer generation wound care dressings, including non-stick dressings made from silicone, are a mainstay of treatment and the daily maintenance of the skin barrier to reduce new skin trauma and promote healing. Tissue-engineered skin grafts containing keratinocytes and fibroblasts are of some benefit. Transdermal gene therapy with allogeneic fibroblasts and the delivery of functional collagens is being pursued. Allogeneic bone marrow transplantation may also be beneficial as may the induction of pluripotent stem cells.

KINDLER SYNDROME
Kindler syndrome, often considered a distant subtype of EB, contains features of both EB such as congenital blistering, and features of the congenital poikilodermas, such as Rothmund-Thomson syndrome and Bloom syndrome (see Chapter 656), which include photosensitivity, congenital poikiloderma, and progressive cutaneous atrophy. Blisters tend to appear on acral sites in infancy or early childhood and are provoked by trauma. Photosensitivity can appear as increased susceptibility to sunburn. Both blistering and photosensitivity can improve greatly with advancing age, but poikilodermatous changes can be progressive. Sclerodermoid-like changes and nail abnormalities of the hands and feet as well as dental abnormalities have been reported.

Kindler syndrome is an autosomal recessive disorder caused by mutations in *KIND1* (also known as *FERMT1*), which encodes kindlin-1, a protein thought to regulate interactions between the extracellular matrix and actin filaments. Blister formation has been shown to occur within the epidermis, within the basement membrane zone, and below the basement membrane. As Kindler syndrome is often confused with EB, at least initially, it can be confirmed by electron microscopy, immunostaining for anti-kindlin-1 antibodies within the skin, or by mutation analysis of the *KIND1* gene.

Treatment is similar to that for EB above, with efforts to reduce trauma to the skin, meticulous wound care, and treatment of skin infections. In addition, sun avoidance measures are beneficial as they can slow the rate of the development of poikiloderma.

Bibliography is available at Expert Consult.

654.5 Pemphigus
Joel C. Joyce

PEMPHIGUS VULGARIS
Etiology/Pathogenesis
Pemphigus vulgaris (PV) is a rare autoimmune blistering disorder caused by circulating antibodies to desmoglein III that result in suprabasal cleaving with consequent blister formation. Desmoglein III is a 30-kDa glycoprotein that is complexed with plakoglobin, a plaque protein of desmosomes. The desmogleins are a subfamily of the cadherin family of cell adhesion molecules.

Clinical Manifestations
PV usually first appears as painful oral ulcers, which may be the only evidence of the disease for weeks or months. Subsequently, large, flaccid bullae emerge on nonerythematous skin, most commonly on the face, trunk, pressure points, groin, and axillae. The **Nikolsky sign**

is present. The lesions rupture and enlarge peripherally, producing painful, raw, denuded areas that have little tendency to heal. When healing occurs, it is without scarring, but hyperpigmentation is common. Malodorous, verrucous, and granulomatous lesions may develop at sites of ruptured bullae, particularly in the skinfolds; as this pattern becomes more pronounced, the condition may be more properly referred to as *pemphigus vegetans*. Because the course may rapidly lead to debility, malnutrition, and death, prompt diagnosis is essential. **Neonatal PV** develops in utero as a result of placental transfer of maternal antidesmoglein antibodies from women who have active PV, although it may occur when the mother is in remission. High antepartum maternal titers of PV antibodies and increased maternal disease activity correlate with a poor fetal outcome, including demise.

Pathology
Biopsy of a fresh small blister reveals a suprabasal (intraepidermal) blister containing loose, acantholytic epidermal cells that have lost their intercellular bridges and thus their contact with one another. Immunofluorescence staining with an IgG antibody produces a characteristic pattern ("chicken wire") on direct immunofluorescence preparations of both involved and uninvolved skin of essentially all patients. Serum IgG antibody titers to desmoglein correlate with the clinical course in many patients; thus, serial determinations may have predictive value.

Differential Diagnosis
PV must be differentiated from EM, bullous pemphigoid, SJS, and TEN.

Treatment
The disease is best treated initially with systemic methylprednisolone 1-2 mg/kg/day. Azathioprine, cyclophosphamide, and methotrexate therapy all have been useful in maintenance regimens. IVIG given in cycles may be beneficial to patients whose disease does not respond to steroids. Rituximab with IVIG replacement has been effective in the management of severe pemphigus. Excellent control of the disease may be obtained, but relapse is common. It has been successfully used in children.

PEMPHIGUS FOLIACEUS
Etiology/Pathogenesis
Pemphigus foliaceus is caused by circulating antibodies to a 50-kDa portion of the 160-kDa desmosomal glycoprotein desmoglein I, which result in subcorneal cleavage leading to superficial erosions. This extremely rare disorder is characterized by subcorneal blistering; the site of cleavage is high in the epidermis rather than suprabasal as in PV.

Clinical Manifestations
The superficial blisters rupture quickly, leaving erosions surrounded by erythema that heal with crusting and scaling (Fig. 654-11). The **Nikolsky sign** is present. Focal lesions are usually localized to the scalp, face, neck, and upper trunk. Mucous membrane lesions are minimal or absent. Pruritus, pain, and a burning sensation are frequent complaints. The clinical course varies but is generally more benign than that of PV. **Fogo selvagem (endemic pemphigus foliaceus),** which is endemic in certain areas of Brazil, is identical clinically, histopathologically, and immunologically to pemphigus foliaceus. Recently, it was shown that anti–desmoglein-1 antibodies in individuals with fogo selvagem crossreact with sand fly (*Lutzomyia* sp.) salivary proteins, suggesting an environmental trigger for this autoimmune disease.

Pathology
An intraepidermal acantholytic bulla high in the epidermis is diagnostic. It is imperative to select an early lesion for biopsy. Immunofluorescent staining with an IgG antibody reveals a characteristic intercellular staining pattern similar to that of PV but higher in the epidermis.

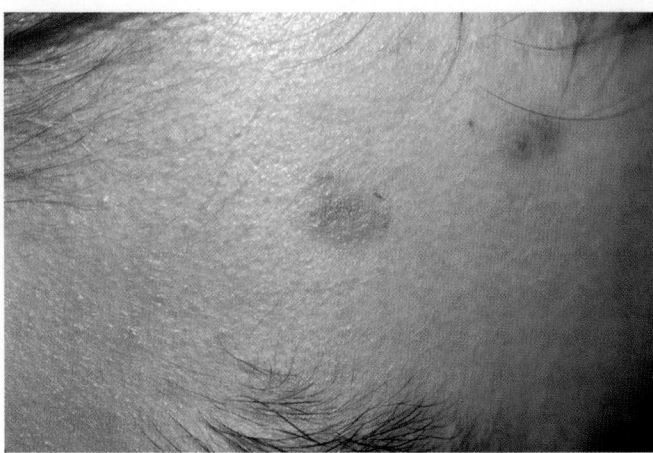

Figure 654-11 Superficial erosions in pemphigus foliaceus.

Differential Diagnosis
When generalized, the eruption may resemble exfoliative dermatitis or any of the chronic blistering disorders; localized erythematous plaques simulate seborrheic dermatitis, psoriasis, impetigo, eczema, and systemic lupus erythematosus.

For localized disease, superpotent topical corticosteroids used twice a day may be all that is needed for control until remission. For more generalized disease, long-term remission is usual after suppression of the disease by systemic methylprednisolone (1 mg/kg/day) therapy. Dapsone (25-100 mg/day) also may be used.

BULLOUS PEMPHIGOID
Etiology/Pathogenesis
Bullous pemphigoid (BP) is caused by circulating antigens to either the 180-kDa or 230-kDa BP antigen that result in a subepidermal blister. The 230-kDa protein (BP230) is part of the hemidesmosome, whereas the 180-kDa protein (BP180, now known as type XVII collagen) localizes to both the hemidesmosome and the upper lamina lucida and is a transmembrane collagenous protein.

Clinical Manifestations
The blisters of BP typically arise in crops on a normal, erythematous, eczematous, or urticarial base. Bullae appear predominantly on the flexural aspects of the extremities, in the axillae, and on the groin and central abdomen. Infants have involvement of the palms, soles, and face more frequently than older children. Individual lesions vary greatly in size, are tense, and are filled with serous fluid that may become hemorrhagic or turbid. Oral lesions occur less frequently and are less severe than in PV. Pruritus, a burning sensation, and subcutaneous edema may accompany the eruption, but constitutional symptoms are not prominent.

Pathology
Biopsy material should be taken from an early bulla arising on an erythematous base. A subepidermal bulla and a dermal inflammatory infiltrate, predominantly of eosinophils, can be identified histopathologically. In sections of a blister or perilesional skin, a band of Ig (usually IgG) and C3 can be demonstrated in the basement membrane zone by direct immunofluorescence. Indirect immunofluorescence studies of serum have positive results in ≈70% of cases for IgG antibodies to the basement membrane zone; the titers, however, do not correlate well with the clinical course.

Diagnosis and Differential Diagnoses
BP rarely occurs in children but must be considered in the differential diagnosis of any chronic blistering disorder. The **differential diagnosis** includes bullous EM, pemphigus, linear IgA dermatosis, bullous drug eruption, dermatitis herpetiformis, herpes simplex infection,

and bullous impetigo, which can be differentiated by histologic examination, immunofluorescence studies, and cultures. The large, tense bullae of BP can generally be distinguished from the smaller, flaccid bullae of PV.

Treatment

Localized bullous pemphigoid can be successfully suppressed with superpotent topical corticosteroids twice a day. Generalized disease usually requires systemic methylprednisolone (1 mg/kg/day) therapy. Rarely are other immunosuppressive treatments necessary, such as azathioprine or mycophenolate mofetil. Refractory cases have been treated with rituximab, but the condition usually remits within a year in most children.

Bibliography is available at Expert Consult.

654.6 Dermatitis Herpetiformis
Joel C. Joyce

ETIOLOGY/PATHOGENESIS

In dermatitis herpetiformis (DH), IgA antibodies are directed at epidermal transglutaminase (transglutaminase 3). **Gluten-sensitive enteropathy (celiac disease)** is found in all patients with DH, although the majority are asymptomatic or have minimal gastrointestinal symptoms (see Chapter 338.2). The severity of the skin disease and the responsiveness to gluten restriction do not correlate with the severity of the intestinal inflammation. An antibody to smooth muscle endomysium is found in 70-90% of patients with DH. Ninety percent of patients with the disease express HLA-DQ2. HLA-DQ2–negative patients with DH usually express HLA-DQ8.

CLINICAL MANIFESTATIONS

DH is characterized by symmetric, grouped, small, tense, erythematous, stinging, intensely pruritic papules and vesicles. The eruption is pleomorphic, including erythematous, urticarial, papular, vesicular, and bullous lesions. Sites of predilection are the knees, elbows, shoulders, buttocks, forehead, and scalp; mucous membranes are usually spared. Hemorrhagic lesions may develop on the palms and soles. When pruritus is severe, excoriations may be the only visible sign (Fig. 654-12).

PATHOLOGY

Subepidermal blisters composed predominantly of neutrophils are found in dermal papillae. The presence of granular IgA on direct immunofluorescence in the dermal papillary tips is diagnostic.

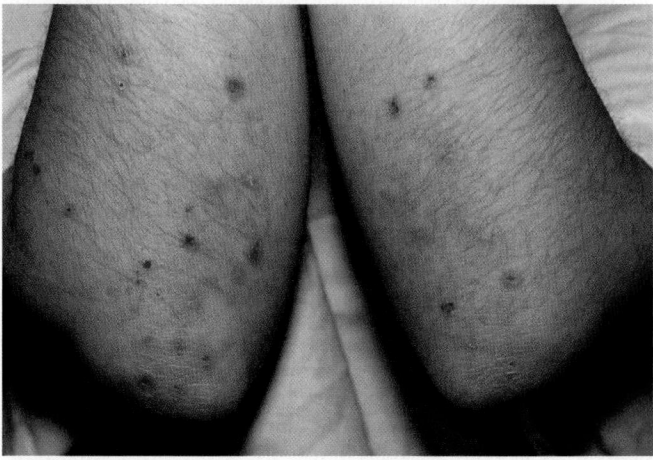

Figure 654-12 Multiple excoriations around the elbows in dermatitis herpetiformis.

DIFFERENTIAL DIAGNOSIS

DH may mimic other chronic blistering diseases and may also resemble scabies, papular urticaria, insect bites, contact dermatitis, and papular eczema.

TREATMENT

Patients with DH show response within weeks to months to a gluten-free diet. Oral administration of dapsone (0.5-2.0 mg/kg/day divided qd or bid) provides immediate relief from the intense pruritus but must be used with caution because of possible serious side effects (methemoglobinemia, hemolysis, and hypersensitivity syndrome [sulfone syndrome]). Dapsone alone may not relieve the intestinal inflammation of celiac disease. Local antipruritic measures may also be useful. Jejunal biopsy is indicated to diagnose gluten-sensitive enteropathy, because cutaneous manifestations may precede malabsorption. The disease is chronic and either a gluten-free diet or dapsone must be continued indefinitely to prevent relapse.

Bibliography is available at Expert Consult.

654.7 Linear Immunoglobulin A Dermatosis (Chronic Bullous Dermatosis of Childhood)
Joel C. Joyce

ETIOLOGY/PATHOGENESIS

Linear IgA dermatosis is a heterogeneous autoimmune disorder with antibodies targeting multiple antigens. It is caused by circulating IgA antibodies, most commonly to LABD97 and LAD-1, which are degradation proteins of BP180 (type XVII collagen). Linear IgA dermatosis may also be seen as a drug eruption. Most cases of drug-induced linear IgA dermatosis are related to vancomycin, although anticonvulsants, ampicillin, cyclosporine, and captopril are implicated.

CLINICAL MANIFESTATIONS

This rare dermatosis is most common in the 1st decade of life, with a peak incidence during the preschool years. The eruption consists of many large symmetrically located, tense bullae filled with clear or hemorrhagic fluid. The bullae are often clustered together and develop on a normal or erythematous, urticarial base. Areas of predilection are the genitals and buttocks (Fig. 654-13), the perioral region, and the scalp. Sausage-shaped bullae may be arranged in an annular or rosette-like fashion around a central crust (Fig. 654-14). Erythematous plaques with gyrate margins bordered by intact bullae may develop over larger areas. Pruritus may be absent or very intense, and systemic signs or symptoms are absent.

PATHOLOGY

The subepidermal bullae are infiltrated with a mixture of inflammatory cells. Neutrophilic abscesses may be noted in the dermal papillary tips, indistinguishable from those of DH. The infiltrate may also be largely eosinophilic, resembling that in BP. Therefore, direct immunofluorescence studies are required for a definitive diagnosis of linear IgA dermatosis; perilesional skin demonstrates linear deposition of IgA and sometimes IgG and C3 at the dermal–epidermal junction. Immuno-electron microscopy has localized the immunoreactants to the sublamina densa, although a combined sublamina densa and lamina lucida pattern has also been seen.

DIFFERENTIAL DIAGNOSIS

The eruption can be distinguished by histopathologic and immunofluorescence studies from pemphigus, BP, DH, and EM. Gram stain and culture preclude the diagnosis of bullous impetigo.

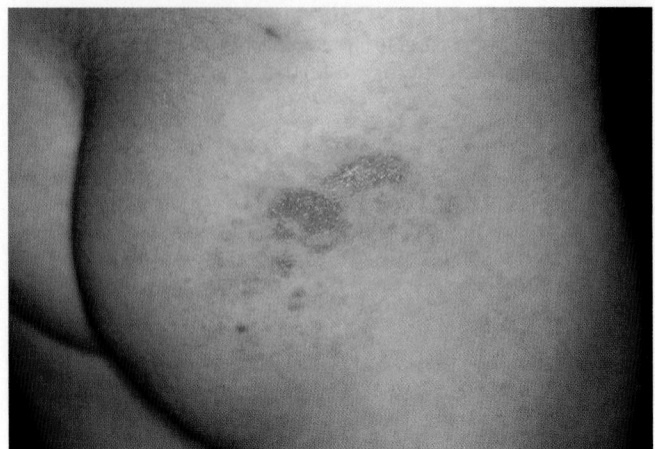

Figure 654-13 Erosion on an erythematous base after loss of blister roof in linear IgA dermatosis.

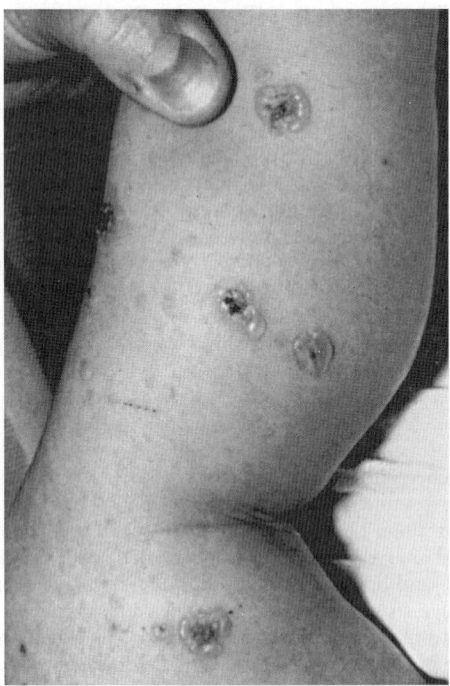

Figure 654-14 Rosette-like blisters around a central crust typical of linear IgA dermatosis (chronic bullous dermatosis of childhood).

TREATMENT

Many cases of linear IgA dermatosis respond favorably to oral dapsone (see treatment of DH) or sulfapyridine. Other antibiotics, including erythromycin and dicloxacillin have been used, but the response is often transient. Children who show no response to dapsone may benefit from oral therapy with methylprednisolone (1 mg/kg/day) or a combination of these drugs. The usual course is 2-4 yr, although some children have persistent or recurrent disease; there are typically no long-term sequelae. IgA nephropathy is a rare complication.

Bibliography is available at Expert Consult.

Chapter 655
Eczematous Disorders
Brianne Z. Dickey and Yvonne E. Chiu

Eczematous skin disorders are a broad group of cutaneous eruptions characterized by erythema, edema, and pruritus. Acute eczematous lesions demonstrate erythema, weeping, oozing, and the formation of microvesicles within the epidermis. Chronic lesions are generally thickened, dry, and scaly, with coarse skin markings (lichenification) and altered pigmentation. Many types of eczema occur in children; the most common is **atopic dermatitis** (see Chapter 145), although seborrheic dermatitis, allergic and irritant contact dermatitis, nummular eczema, and acute palmoplantar eczema (dyshidrosis) are also relatively common in childhood.

Once the diagnosis of eczema has been established, it is important to classify the eruption more specifically for proper management. Pertinent historical data often provide the clue. In some instances, the subsequent course and character of the eruption permit classification. Histologic changes are relatively nonspecific, but all types of eczematous dermatitis are characterized by intraepidermal edema known as spongiosis.

655.1 Contact Dermatitis
Brianne Z. Dickey and Yvonne E. Chiu

The form of eczema known as contact dermatitis can be subdivided into irritant dermatitis, in which nonspecific injury to the skin causes immediate inflammation, and allergic contact dermatitis, resulting from a delayed hypersensitivity reaction. Irritant dermatitis is more frequent in children, particularly during the early years of life. Allergic reactions increase in frequency upon maturation of the immune system.

IRRITANT CONTACT DERMATITIS

Irritant contact dermatitis can result from prolonged or repetitive contact with physical, chemical, or mechanical irritants, including saliva, urine, feces, fragrance, detergents, dyes, henna, plants, caterpillars, abrasive materials, and chafing.

Irritant contact dermatitis may be difficult to distinguish from atopic dermatitis or allergic contact dermatitis. A detailed history and consideration of the sites of involvement, the age of the child, and contactants usually provide clues to the etiologic agent. The propensity for development of irritant dermatitis varies considerably among children; some may respond to minimal injury, making it difficult to identify the offending agent through history. Children with atopic dermatitis are more prone to irritant contact dermatitis as an exacerbating factor. Irritant contact dermatitis usually clears after removal of the stimulus and temporary treatment with a topical corticosteroid preparation (see Chapter 646). Education of patients and parents about the causes of contact dermatitis is crucial to successful therapy.

Dry skin dermatitis results from repetitive wet-to-dry behaviors such as lip-licking (Fig. 655-1), thumb-sucking, frequent hand washing, or excessive sweating. Involved skin is erythematous and fissured, localized to the area of exposure. Treatment of dry skin dermatitis begins with eliminating the offending wet-to-dry behavior. Moisturizer cream applied twice daily decreases transepidermal water loss and replenishes skin lipids to improve hydration. A topical steroid is usually necessary to treat the inflammation.

Juvenile plantar dermatosis occurs mainly in prepubertal children with hyperhidrosis who wear occlusive synthetic footwear. Weight-bearing surfaces of the foot may be pruritic or painful and

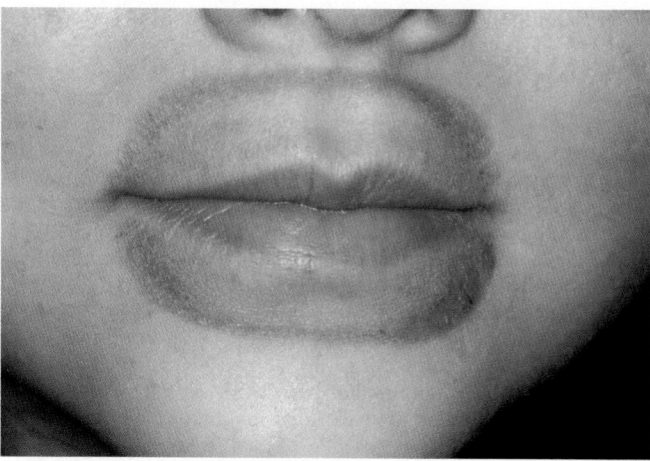

Figure 655-1 Perioral irritant contact dermatitis from lip licking.

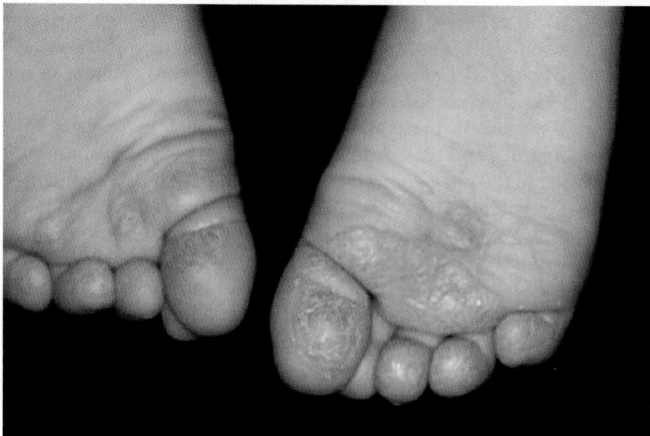

Figure 655-2 Red, scaly juvenile plantar dermatosis.

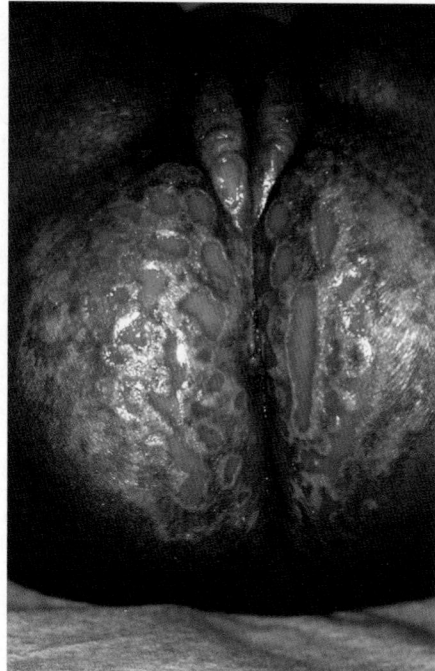

Figure 655-3 Severe, erosive diaper dermatitis.

develop a fissured or glazed appearance (Fig. 655-2). Immediate application of a thick emollient when socks and shoes are removed or immediately after swimming usually minimizes juvenile plantar dermatosis. Severe inflammatory cases may require short-term (1-2 wk) application of a medium- to high-potency topical steroid.

DIAPER DERMATITIS

Diaper dermatitis refers to any rash in the diaper region; the most common of these is irritant diaper dermatitis. Elevated pH in the diaper area and synergistic activity of urinary and fecal enzymes lead to inflammation, which disrupts the normal skin barrier and increases susceptibility to other irritants and organisms. Additional factors are occlusion, friction, and use of diaper wipes and topical preparations. Loose or frequent stooling predisposes an infant to diaper dermatitis. Diaper dermatitis presents with erythema and scaling, often with papulovesicular or bullous lesions, fissures, and erosions in a patchy or confluent pattern (Fig. 655-3). The genitocrural folds are often spared because concave areas are relatively protected. Chronic hypertrophic, flat-topped papules and infiltrative nodules may occur. **Candidal infection** typically represents a secondary process. It is characterized by "beefy" red-pink, tender skin that has numerous 1-2 mm pustules and satellite papules and involves both concave and convex areas. Discomfort may be marked because of intense inflammation. Allergic contact dermatitis, seborrheic dermatitis, psoriasis, candidiasis, atopic dermatitis, child abuse, and rare disorders such as Langerhans cell histiocytosis, nutritional deficiencies, and acrodermatitis enteropathica should be considered when the eruption is persistent or is recalcitrant to simple therapeutic measures.

Diaper dermatitis often responds to simple measures; some infants are predisposed to diaper dermatitis, and management may be difficult. The damaging effects of overhydration of the skin and prolonged contact with feces and urine can be obviated by frequent changing of the diapers and periods of "rest" free of diaper use. Cleansing of affected skin is best accomplished with a soft cloth and lukewarm water, patted dry. Overwashing should be avoided because it leads to chapping and a worsening of the dermatitis. Disposable diapers containing a superabsorbent material may help maintain a relatively dry environment. First-line therapy for diaper dermatitis is application of a protective barrier agent (ointment or paste) containing petroleum or zinc oxide at every diaper change. Topical sucralfate is an effective barrier with some antibacterial activity, useful for recalcitrant cases. Low-potency nonhalogenated topical corticosteroids, such as 2.5% hydrocortisone, may be used for short time periods (3-5 days). Treatment with a topical anticandidal agent is indicated for secondary candidal infection. Topical preparations containing triamcinolone-nystatin and betamethasone dipropionate–clotrimazole are generally inappropriate for diaper dermatitis in infants because of the higher potency of the corticosteroid component. If using multiple topical agents, the protective barrier should be applied last. When diaper dermatitis does not respond to typical prevention and treatment strategies, non–diaper-associated causes must be considered.

ALLERGIC CONTACT DERMATITIS

Allergic contact dermatitis is common in childhood and should be considered in any child with recalcitrant eczema. This is a T-cell–mediated hypersensitivity reaction that is provoked by application of an antigen to the skin surface. The antigen penetrates the skin, where it is conjugated with a cutaneous protein, and the hapten–protein complex is transported to the regional lymph nodes by antigen-presenting Langerhans cells. A primary immunologic response occurs locally in the nodes and becomes generalized, presumably because of dissemination of sensitized T cells. Sensitization requires several days and, when followed by a fresh antigenic challenge, manifests as allergic contact dermatitis. Generalized distribution may also occur if enough antigen finds its way into the circulation, such as by consumption. Once sensitization has occurred, each new antigenic challenge may provoke an inflammatory reaction within 8-12 hr; sensitization to a particular antigen usually persists for many years.

Acute allergic contact dermatitis is an erythematous, intensely pruritic, eczematous dermatitis. Acute cases may be edematous and vesiculobullous. The chronic condition has the features of long-standing eczema: lichenification, scaling, fissuring, and pigmentary change. The distribution of the eruption often provides a clue to the diagnosis. Airborne sensitizers usually affect exposed areas, such as the face and arms. Jewelry, topical agents, shoes, clothing, henna tattoo dyes, plants, and even toilet seats cause dermatitis at points of contact.

Rhus dermatitis (poison ivy, poison sumac, poison oak), a response to the plant allergen urushiol, is the most common allergic contact dermatitis. It is often vesiculobullous and may be distinguished by linear streaks of vesicles where the plant leaves have brushed against the skin (Fig. 655-4). Fluid from ruptured cutaneous vesicles does not spread the eruption; antigen retained on skin, clothing, or under fingernails initiates new plaques of dermatitis if not removed by washing with soap and water. Antigen may also be carried by animals on their fur. "Black spot" poison ivy dermatitis is a rare variant that results from oxidation of concentrated urushiol left on the skin and manifests as small discrete black lacquer–like glossy papules with surrounding erythema and edema. Sensitization to 1 plant produces crossreactions with the others. Spontaneous resolution occurs in 1-3 wk, with the most common complication being secondary bacterial infection with normal skin flora. Exposure avoidance and thorough washing after exposure are the mainstays for prevention. Barrier creams or organoclay compounds such as bentoquatam may be effective if applied prior to expected exposure.

Nickel dermatitis develops from contact with jewelry, metal closures on clothing, or even cell phones. Metal closures on pants frequently cause periumbilical dermatitis (Fig. 655-5). Some children are exquisitely sensitive to nickel, with even the trace amounts found in gold jewelry provoking eruptions. The most frequently involved sites from jewelry are the earlobes from nickel-containing earrings. Early ear piercing increases risk of sensitization, and it is recommended to delay piercing until after 10 yr of age. Patch testing for nickel sensitivity

is unreliable in infants and toddlers and should only be performed if there is high clinical suspicion.

Shoe dermatitis typically affects the dorsum or soles of the feet and toes, sparing the interdigital spaces; it is usually symmetric. Other forms of allergic contact dermatitis, in contrast to irritant dermatitis, rarely involve the palms and soles. Common allergens are the antioxidants and accelerators in shoe rubber, adhesives, and the chromium salts in tanned leather or shoe dyes. Excessive sweating often leaches these substances from their source.

Apparel contains a number of sensitizers, including dyes, dye fixative, fabric finishes, fibers, resins, and cleaning solutions. Dye may be poorly fixed to clothing and so may be leached out with sweating, as can partially cured formaldehyde resins. The elastic in garments is a frequent cause of clothing dermatitis, and contact allergy to the ink "tag" of tagless baby clothing has been reported. Exposure to other items with fabric, such as infant car seats, may induce reactions similar to clothing.

Topical medications and cosmetics may be unsuspected as allergens, particularly if a medication is being used for a preexisting dermatitis. The most common offenders are neomycin, topical antihistamines, topical anesthetics, fragrances, topical corticosteroids, oxybenzone and octocrylene in chemical sunscreens, preservatives, dye in temporary tattoos, and ethylenediamine, a stabilizer present in many medications. All types of cosmetics can cause facial dermatitis; involvement of the eyelids is characteristic for nail polish sensitivity.

Neomycin sulfate is present in many nonprescription topical antibiotic preparations, and thus children are frequently exposed at an early age. It is one of the most common causes of allergic contact dermatitis, and use of combination products of neomycin with other antibiotics, antifungals, or corticosteroids may induce co-reactivity with these chemically-unrelated substances.

Diagnosis of allergic contact dermatitis is usually based on history; however, patch testing may be helpful, especially in older children. Identification and avoidance of the offending agent is the mainstay of

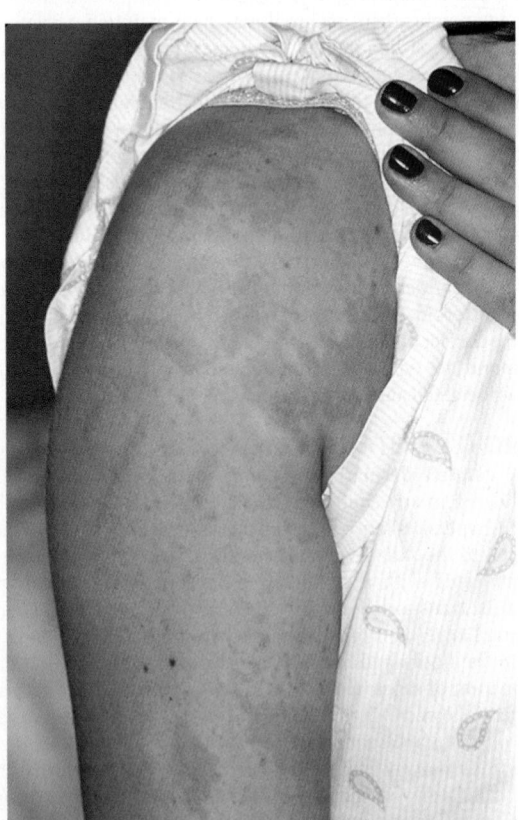

Figure 655-4 Linear lesions in poison ivy.

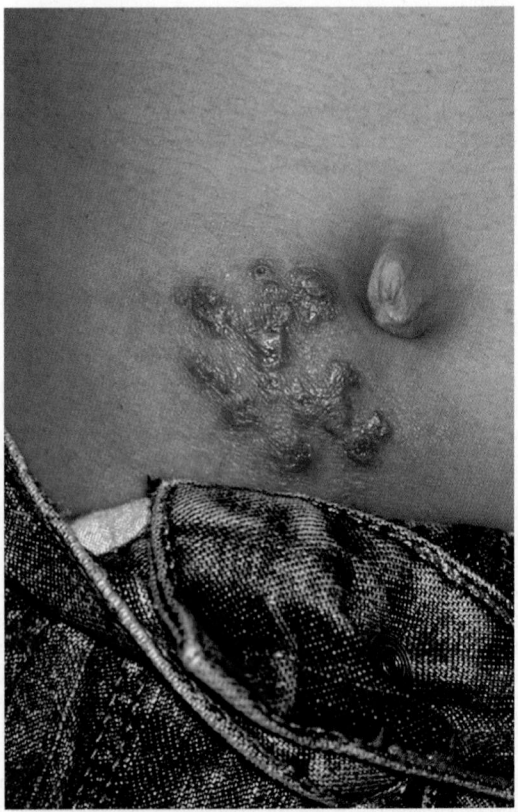

Figure 655-5 Chronic periumbilical nickel dermatitis.

managing allergic contact dermatitis. First-line treatment for acute eruption is with midpotency topical corticosteroid ointment for 2-3 wk, as well as symptom management with wet dressings and sedating antihistamines to allow for sleep. Systemic corticosteroids are used when >10% of skin is involved (0.5-1.0 mg/kg prednisone for 7-10 days, followed by a 7-10 day taper). More chronic allergic contact dermatitis is treated with low- to midpotency topical corticosteroids. Desensitization therapy is rarely indicated. Differential diagnosis of allergic contact dermatitis includes herpes simplex virus, impetigo, cellulitis, atopic dermatitis, irritant contact dermatitis, and dermatophytoses.

Bibliography is available at Expert Consult.

655.2 Nummular Eczema
Brianne Z. Dickey and Yvonne E. Chiu

Nummular eczema is characterized by coin-shaped, severely pruritic, eczematous plaques, commonly involving the extensor surfaces of the extremities (Fig. 655-6), buttocks, and shoulders with facial sparing. The plaques are relatively discrete, boggy, vesicular, slightly scaly, and exudative; when chronic, they often become thickened and lichenified, and may develop central clearing. The etiology remains unclear, although nummular eczema possibly represents an atypical morphology of atopic dermatitis. Flares are generally sporadic but may be precipitated by xerosis, irritants, allergens, or occult staphylococcal infection. Most frequently, these lesions are mistaken for tinea corporis, but plaques of nummular eczema are distinguished by the lack of a raised, sharply circumscribed border, the lack of fungal organisms on a potassium hydroxide (KOH) preparation, and frequent weeping or bleeding when scraped. First-line treatment is with emollients, wet dressings, and potent topical corticosteroids. Steroid-impregnated tapes may simultaneously treat and provide barrier protection to these circumscribed eczematous plaques. An oral antihistamine may be helpful, particularly a sedating antihistamine at night. Antibiotics are indicated for secondary infection.

Bibliography is available at Expert Consult.

655.3 Pityriasis Alba
Brianne Z. Dickey and Yvonne E. Chiu

Pityriasis alba occurs mainly in children and causes lesions that are hypopigmented, ill-defined, round or oval patches (Fig. 655-7). They may be mildly erythematous and finely scaly. Lesions occur on the face, neck, upper trunk, and proximal portions of the arms, and are most pronounced on darker skin tones or after tanning of surrounding skin. Itching is minimal or absent. The cause is unknown, but the eruption appears to be exacerbated by dryness and is often regarded as a mild form of eczema. Pityriasis alba is frequently misdiagnosed as vitiligo, tinea versicolor, or tinea corporis. The lesions wax and wane but eventually disappear, and normal pigmentation often takes months to return. Application of a lubricant or emollient may ameliorate the condition. If pruritus is troublesome, a low-potency topical steroid or calcineurin inhibitor may be used.

Bibliography is available at Expert Consult.

655.4 Lichen Simplex Chronicus
Brianne Z. Dickey and Yvonne E. Chiu

Lichen simplex chronicus is a secondary skin disorder resulting from excessive scratching. It is characterized by a chronic pruritic, eczematous, circumscribed plaque that is usually lichenified and hyperpigmented (Fig. 655-8). All affected areas must be accessible to scratching, with the most common sites being the posterior neck, genitalia, wrists, ankles, and dorsal feet. Although the initiating event may be a transient lesion such as an insect bite, trauma from rubbing and scratching accounts for persistence of the plaque. Pruritus must be controlled to

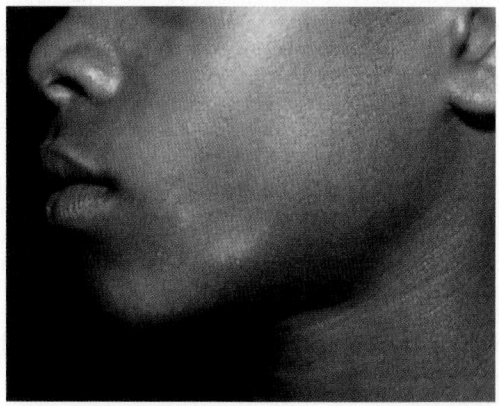

Figure 655-7 Patchy hypopigmented lesions with diffuse borders characteristic of pityriasis alba.

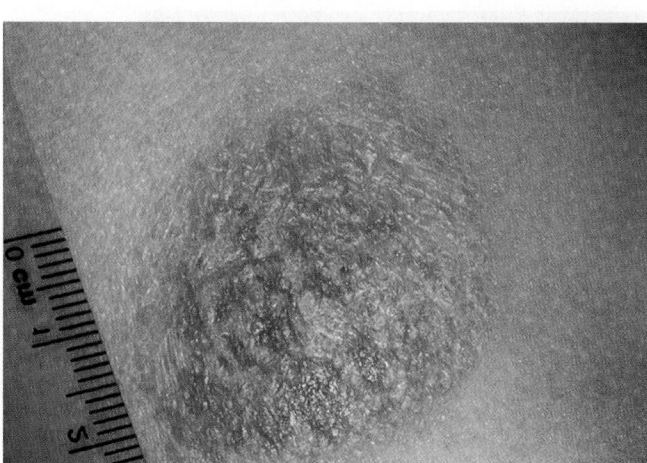

Figure 655-6 Discrete, boggy plaque of nummular dermatitis.

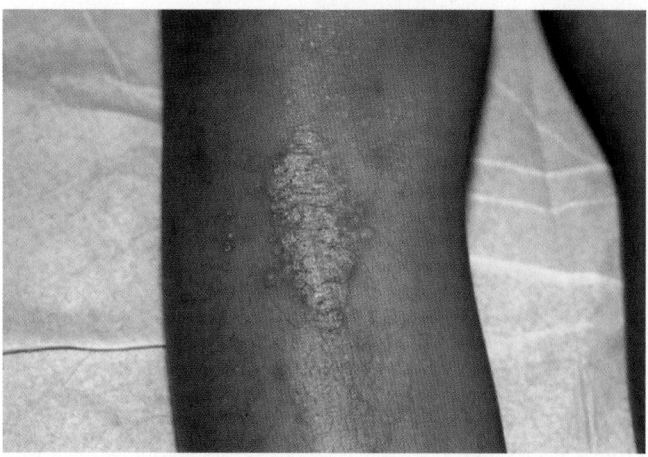

Figure 655-8 Thickened plaque of lichen simplex chronicus.

permit healing, thus a covering to prevent scratching may be necessary. A high potency topical corticosteroid under occlusion is often helpful. Second-line therapy includes adding 6% salicylic acid gel to the topical corticosteroid preparation.

655.5 Acute Palmoplantar Eczema (Dyshidrotic Eczema, Dyshidrosis, Pompholyx)

Brianne Z. Dickey and Yvonne E. Chiu

A recurrent, sometimes seasonal, blistering disorder of the hands and feet, acute palmoplantar eczema occurs in all age groups but is uncommon in infancy. The pathogenesis is unknown, although possible predisposing factors include a history of atopy, exposure to contact allergens or irritants, or IV immunoglobulin therapy. The disease is characterized by recurrent crops of small, deep-seated "tapioca-like" vesicles, which are intensely pruritic and may coalesce into tense bullae (Fig. 655-9). Sites of predilection are the palms, soles, and lateral aspects of the fingers and toes. Primary lesions are noninflammatory and are filled with clear fluid, which, unlike sweat, has a physiologic pH and contains protein. Maceration and secondary infection are frequent because of scratching. The chronic phase is characterized by thickened, fissured plaques that may cause considerable discomfort, as well as dystrophic nails. Hyperhidrosis is common in many patients, but the association may be fortuitous. The diagnosis is made clinically. The disorder may be confused with allergic contact dermatitis, which usually affects the dorsal rather than the volar surfaces, and with dermatophytosis, which can be distinguished by a KOH preparation of the roof of a vesicle and by appropriate cultures.

Acute palmoplantar eczema responds to wet dressings, liberal emollient use, and potent topical corticosteroid ointment applied twice daily for 2-4 wk. Weeping skin benefits from twice daily soaking in an astringent solution, such as aluminum subacetate. Second-line treatment is topical tacrolimus 0.1% ointment. Severe disease may require oral corticosteroids with 2 wk taper, or even psoralen UVA therapy. Control of the chronic stage is difficult; lubricants containing mild keratolytic agents in conjunction with a potent topical fluorinated corticosteroid preparation may be indicated. Secondary bacterial infection should be treated systemically with an appropriate antibiotic. Patients should be told to expect recurrence and should protect their hands and feet from the damaging effects of excessive sweating, chemicals, harsh soaps, and adverse weather. Unfortunately, it is impossible to prevent recurrence or to predict its frequency.

655.6 Seborrheic Dermatitis

Brianne Z. Dickey and Yvonne E. Chiu

ETIOLOGY
Seborrheic dermatitis is a chronic inflammatory disease most common in infancy and adolescence that parallels the distribution, size, and activity of the sebaceous glands. The cause is unknown, as is the role of the sebaceous glands in the disease. *Malassezia furfur* is implicated as a causative agent, although it remains unclear whether dermatitis results from the action of the fungus, its byproducts, or an exaggerated response of the host. In adolescence, seborrheic dermatitis typically occurs after puberty, indicating a possible role for sex hormones.

It is also unknown whether infantile seborrheic dermatitis and adolescent seborrheic dermatitis are the same or different entities. There is no evidence that children with infantile seborrheic dermatitis will experience seborrheic dermatitis as adolescents.

CLINICAL MANIFESTATIONS
The disorder may begin in the 1st mo of life and typically self-resolves by 1 yr. Diffuse or focal scaling and crusting of the scalp, sometimes called cradle cap (Fig. 655-10), may be the initial and at times the only manifestation. A greasy, scaly, erythematous papular dermatitis, which is usually nonpruritic in infants, may involve the face, neck, retroauricular areas, axillae, umbilicus, and diaper area. The dermatitis may be patchy and focal or may spread to involve almost the entire body (Fig. 655-11). Postinflammatory pigmentary changes are common, particularly in black infants. When the scaling becomes pronounced, the condition may resemble psoriasis and, at times, can be distinguished only with difficulty. The possibility of coexistent atopic dermatitis must be considered when there is an acute weeping dermatitis with pruritus, and the two are often clinically inseparable at an early age. An intractable seborrhea-like dermatitis with chronic diarrhea and failure to thrive may reflect systemic dysfunction of the immune system. A chronic seborrhea-like pattern, which responds poorly to treatment, may also result from cutaneous histiocytic infiltrates in infants with Langerhans cell histiocytosis. Seborrheic dermatitis is a common cutaneous manifestation of AIDS in young adults and is characterized by thick, greasy scales on the scalp and large hyperkeratotic erythematous plaques on the face, chest, and genitals.

During adolescence, seborrheic dermatitis is more localized and may be confined to the scalp and intertriginous areas. Also noted may be marginal blepharitis and involvement of the external auditory canal. Scalp changes vary from diffuse, brawny scaling to focal areas of

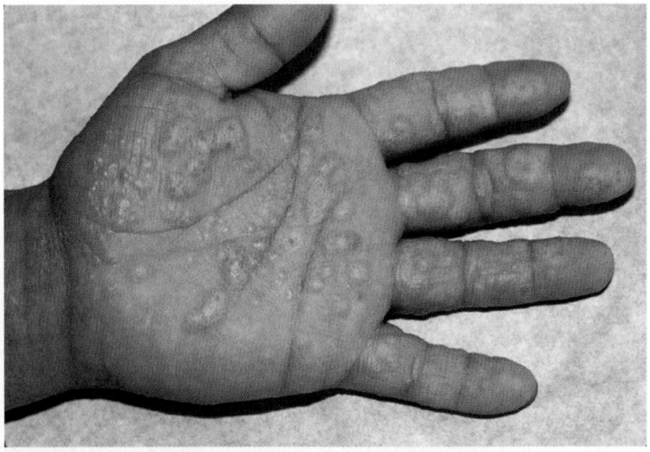

Figure 655-9 Vesicular palmar lesions of dyshidrotic eczema with large bullae.

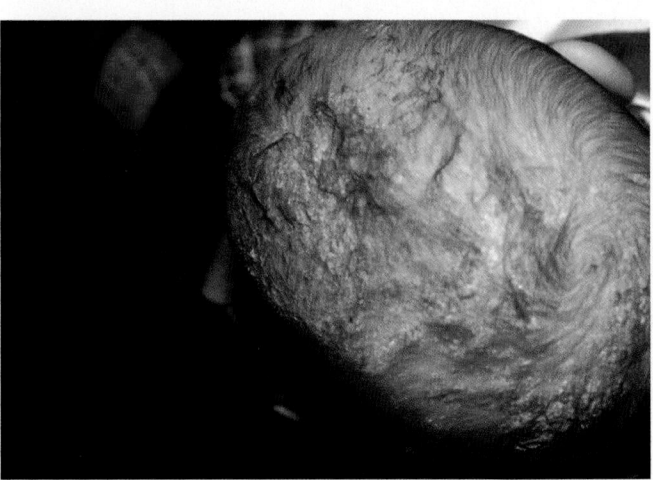

Figure 655-10 Cradle cap in an infant.

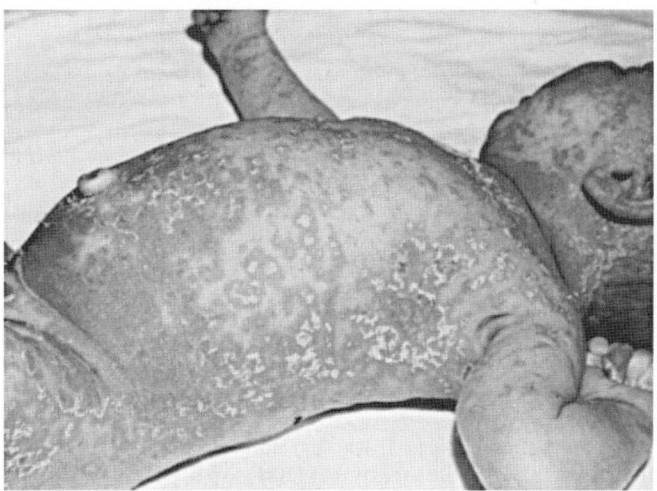

Figure 655-11 Widespread seborrheic dermatitis.

thick, oily, yellow crusts with underlying erythema. Loss of hair is common, and pruritus may be absent to marked. When the dermatitis is severe, erythema and scaling occur at the frontal hairline, the medial aspects of the eyebrows, and in the nasolabial and retroauricular folds. Red, scaly plaques may appear in the axillae, inguinal region, gluteal cleft, and umbilicus. On the extremities, seborrheic plaques may be more eczematous and less erythematous and demarcated. Unlike infantile seborrheic dermatitis, adolescent seborrheic dermatitis generally does not self-resolve and has a chronic relapsing course.

DIFFERENTIAL DIAGNOSIS

The differential diagnosis of seborrheic dermatitis includes psoriasis, atopic dermatitis, dermatophytosis, histiocytic disorders, and candidiasis. Secondary bacterial infections and superimposed candidiasis are common.

TREATMENT

Initial management for infantile seborrheic dermatitis is generally conservative given the self-limited nature of this condition. Emollients, baby oil, gentle shampooing with nonmedicated baby shampoo, and gentle use of a soft brush to remove scales are usually effective measures. Persistent lesions may be treated with low-potency topical corticosteroids if inflamed (applied once daily for 1 wk) and a topical antifungal (e.g., ketoconazole 2% cream twice daily). Antifungal shampoos such as ketoconazole 2% shampoo should be used cautiously as they are not tear-free.

First-line therapy for children and adolescents with scalp seborrheic dermatitis is antifungal shampoo used several times weekly to daily (selenium sulfide, ketoconazole, ciclopirox, zinc pyrithione, salicylic acid, or tar). Midpotency topical corticosteroids such as fluocinolone 0.01% shampoo may also be used for inflamed lesions, applied once daily for 2-4 wk. Nonscalp lesions are treated with topical corticosteroid cream (low-potency for facial lesions, midpotency elsewhere), as well as topical antifungals such as ketoconazole 2% cream or ketoconazole 2% shampoo used as a body wash. Second-line therapy for seborrheic dermatitis includes topical calcineurin inhibitors and keratolytic agents such as urea. Severe adult cases improve with oral antifungal agents; however, pediatric studies are lacking. Once acute disease is controlled, antifungal shampoo used on a weekly basis is effective maintenance to reduce risk of relapse.

Bibliography is available at Expert Consult.

Chapter **656**
Photosensitivity
Brianne Z. Dickey and Yvonne E. Chiu

Photosensitivity denotes a qualitatively or quantitatively abnormal cutaneous reaction to sunlight or artificial light because of UV radiation. The UV light spectrum contains UVA (320-400 nm wavelength), UVB (290-320 nm wavelength), and UVC (100-290 nm wavelength) subtypes. Transmitted radiation <300 nm is largely absorbed in the epidermis, whereas that >300 nm is mostly transmitted to the dermis after variable epidermal melanin absorption. Children vary in susceptibility to UV radiation, depending on their skin type (i.e., its amount of pigment; Table 656-1).

ACUTE SUNBURN REACTION

The most common photosensitive reaction seen in children is acute sunburn. Sunburn is caused mainly by UVB radiation. Sunlight contains many times more UVA than UVB radiation, but UVA must be encountered in much larger quantities than UVB radiation to produce sunburn. Immediate pigment darkening is caused by UVA radiation–induced photooxidative darkening of existing melanin and its transfer from melanocytes to keratinocytes. This effect generally lasts for a few hours and is not photoprotective. UVB-induced effects appear 6-12 hr after initial exposure and reach a peak in 24 hr. Effects include redness, tenderness, edema, and blistering (Fig. 656-1). Severe sunburn induces systemic symptoms of fever, nausea, and headache. Reactive oxidation species generated by UVB induce keratinocyte

Table 656-1	Sun-Reactive Skin Types
FITZPATRICK SKIN TYPE	**SUNBURN, TANNING HISTORY**
I	Always burns easily, no tanning
II	Usually burns, minimal tanning
III	Sometimes burns, gradual light brown tan
IV	Minimal to no burning, always tans
V	Rarely burns, tans profusely dark brown
VI	Never burns, pigmented black

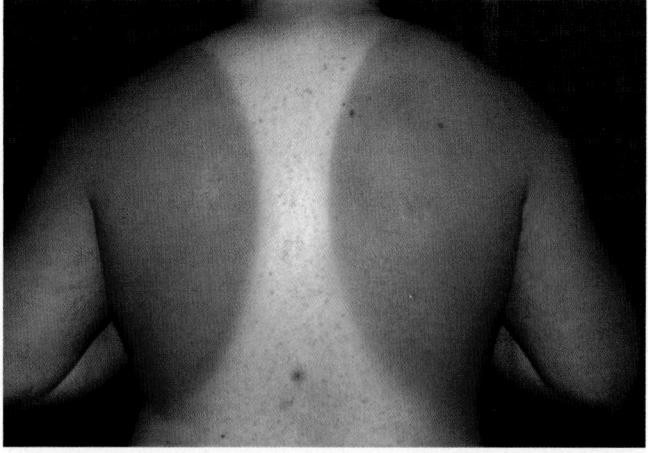

Figure 656-1 Sunburn. Well-demarcated, severe erythema.

membrane damage and are involved in the pathogenesis of sunburn. A portion of the vasodilation seen in UVB-induced erythema is mediated by prostaglandins E_2, E_3, and F_{2A}. Other inflammatory cytokines induced by UVB include interleukins 1, 6, and 8, and tumor necrosis factor-α. Acute sunburn is a self-limited condition that resolves within 1 wk with desquamation and without scarring. Delayed melanogenesis as a result of UVB radiation begins in 2-3 days and lasts several days to a few weeks. Manufacture of new melanin in melanocytes, transfer of melanin from melanocytes to keratinocytes, increase in size and arborization of melanocytes, and activation of quiescent melanocytes produce delayed melanogenesis. This effect reduces skin sensitivity to development of UV-induced erythema. The amount of protection afforded depends on the skin type of the patient. Additional effects and possible complications of sun exposure include increased thickness of the stratum corneum, recurrence or exacerbation of herpes simplex labialis, lupus erythematosus, and many other conditions (Table 656-2).

Acute sunburn should be managed conservatively with cool compresses, aloe vera products, and calamine lotion. Oral analgesics such as ibuprofen and acetaminophen may decrease pain. Topical corticosteroids are only helpful in the acute phase and generally should not be used to treat sunburn once peak erythema has been reached. Topical anesthetics are relatively ineffective and potentially hazardous because of their propensity to cause contact dermatitis. A bland emollient is effective in the desquamative phase.

The long-term sequelae of chronic and intense sun exposure are not often seen in children, but most individuals receive >50% of their lifetime UV dose by age 20 yr; therefore, pediatricians have a pivotal role in educating patients and their parents about the harmful effects, potential malignancy risks, and irreversible skin damage that result from prolonged exposure to the sun and tanning lights. Premature aging, senile elastosis, actinic keratoses, squamous and basal cell carcinomas, and melanomas all occur with greater frequency in sun-damaged skin. In particular, blistering sunburns in childhood and adolescence significantly increase the risk for development of malignant melanoma.

Sun protection is best achieved by sun avoidance, which includes minimizing time in the midday sun (10 AM to 3 PM), staying in the shade, and wearing protective clothing including wide-brimmed hats. Protection is enhanced by a wide variety of sunscreen agents. Physical sunscreens (zinc oxide, titanium dioxide) block UV light, whereas chemical sunscreens (para-aminobenzoic acid [PABA], PABA esters, salicylates, benzophenones, avobenzone, cinnamates, ecamsule) absorb damaging radiation. Most chemical sunscreens are effective for only UVB wavelengths but benzophenones and avobenzone provide protection in both the UVA and UVB ranges; ecamsule is a UVA sunscreen. Stabilizers such as octocrylene and diethyl 2,6-naphthalate increase the time of function of the chemical sunscreens. "Broad-spectrum" sunscreens are combination products that absorb both UVA and UVB, and families should be advised to use products labeled as "broad spectrum" with a sun protective factor (SPF) of at least 30, reapply liberally at least every 2 hr while outdoors, and reapply after swimming. Infants younger than 6 mo of age should not be exposed to direct sunlight but may have SPF 15 physical sunscreens applied to small areas of skin if sunlight avoidance is not possible. SPF is defined as the minimal dose of sunlight required to produce cutaneous erythema after application of a sunscreen, divided by the dose required with no use of sunscreen. SPF applies only to UVB protection; there is no associated rating for UVA protection in the United States aside from the "broad spectrum" designation.

PHOTOSENSITIVE REACTIONS

Photosensitizers in combination with a particular wavelength of light (typically UVA) cause dermatitis that can be classified as phototoxic or photoallergic reactions. Contact of the skin with the photosensitizer may occur externally, internally by enteral or parenteral administration, or through host synthesis of photosensitizers in response to an administered drug.

Photoallergic reactions occur in only a small percentage of persons exposed to photosensitizers and light and require a time interval for sensitization to take place. Thereafter, dermatitis appears within 24 hr of reexposure to the photosensitizer and light. Photoallergic dermatitis is a T-cell–mediated delayed hypersensitivity reaction in which the drug, acting as a hapten, may combine with a skin protein to form the antigenic substance. Photoallergic reactions vary in morphology and may occur on partially covered and on light-exposed skin. Table 656-2 lists some of the important classes of drugs and chemicals responsible for photosensitivity reactions. The most common photoallergens are chemicals present in sunscreens.

Phototoxic reactions occur in all individuals who accumulate adequate amounts of a photosensitizing drug or chemical within the skin. UV radiation excites the agent to a state capable of causing cell or tissue damage through reactive oxygen species formation. Prior sensitization is not required. Dermatitis develops within hours after exposure to radiation in the range of 285-450 nm. The eruption is confined to light-exposed areas and often resembles exaggerated sunburn, but it may be urticarial or bullous. It results in postinflammatory hyperpigmentation. All the drugs that cause photoallergic reactions may also cause a phototoxic dermatitis if given in sufficiently high doses. Several

Table 656-2	Cutaneous Reactions to Sunlight

SUNBURN
Photoallergic drug eruptions:
- Systemic drugs include tetracyclines, psoralens, chlorothiazides, sulfonamides, barbiturates, griseofulvin, thiazides, quinidine, phenothiazines
- Topical agents include coal tar derivatives, psoralens, halogenated salicylanilides (soaps), perfume oils (e.g., oil of bergamot), sunscreens (e.g., para-aminobenzoic acid [PABA], cinnamates, benzophenones)

Phototoxic drug eruptions:
- Systemic agents include nalidixic acid, furosemide, nonsteroidal antiinflammatory agents (naproxen, piroxicam), and high doses of agents causing photoallergic eruptions
- Topical agents include 5-fluorouracial, furocoumarins (e.g., lime, lemon, carrot, celery, dill, parsnip, parsley), and high doses of agents causing photoallergic eruptions

Genetic disorders with photosensitivity:
- Xeroderma pigmentosum
- Bloom syndrome
- Cockayne syndrome
- Rothmund-Thomson syndrome
- Trichothiodystrophy
- Smith-Lemli-Opitz syndrome
- Kindler syndrome

Inborn errors of metabolism:
- Porphyrias, protoporphyria
- Hartnup disease and pellagra

Infectious diseases associated with photosensitivity:
- Recurrent herpes simplex infection
- Viral exanthems (accentuated photodistribution; e.g., varicella)

Skin disease exacerbated or precipitated by light:
- Lichen planus
- Darier disease
- Lupus erythematosus including neonatal
- Dermatomyositis
- Psoriasis
- Erythema multiforme
- Atopic dermatitis
- Hailey-Hailey disease

Deficient protection because of a lack of pigment:
- Vitiligo
- Oculocutaneous albinism
- Phenylketonuria
- Chédiak-Higashi syndrome
- Hermansky-Pudlak syndrome
- Waardenburg syndrome
- Piebaldism

additional drugs and contactants cause phototoxic reactions (see Table 656-2). Differentiating contact phototoxicity from contact dermatitis caused by poison ivy or poison oak may be difficult, but itching is prominent in contact dermatitis while burning is more prominent in photodermatitis. Postinflammatory hyperpigmentation develops rapidly and can be the presenting sign. Contact with furoucoumarin-containing plants causes a disorder called **phytophotodermatitis.** The most common phytophotodermatitis seen in children is caused by lime juice, which presents as hyperpigmentation in streaky patterns on sun-exposed skin consistent with dripping juice or handprints.

Diagnosis of photosensitive reactions caused by drugs or chemicals relies on a high index of suspicion, an appreciation of the distribution pattern of the eruption, and a history of application or ingestion of a known photosensitizing agent. Phototesting and photopatch testing are also helpful when available. First-line treatment for both photoallergy and phototoxicity consists of discontinuation of the offending agent and good sun protection practices, including avoidance of sun exposure. Photoallergic reactions are treated similarly to contact dermatitis, with a topical corticosteroid to alleviate pruritus when necessary. Severe reactions may necessitate a 2-3 wk course of systemic corticosteroid therapy. Phototoxic reactions are treated similarly to sunburn, with comfort measures such as cool compresses, emollients, and oral analgesics.

PORPHYRIAS
See Chapter 91.

Porphyrias are acquired or inborn disorders due to abnormalities of specific enzyme mutations in the heme biosynthetic pathway. Some have childhood photosensitivity as a consistent feature. The pathogenesis of photosensitivity in porphyria relates to deposition of excess porphyrins in the skin; UV radiation excites these molecules, causing cell and tissue damage via generation of reactive oxygen species. Signs and symptoms may be negligible during the winter, when sun exposure is minimal.

Congenital erythropoietic porphyria (Günther disease) is a rare autosomal recessive disorder affecting the enzyme uroporphyrinogen III synthase. It may cause hydrops fetalis, but more typically manifests in the 1st few mo of life as hemolytic anemia and exquisite sensitivity to light, which may induce repeated severe bullous eruptions that result in mutilating scars (Fig. 656-2). **Hyperpigmentation,** hyperkeratosis, vesiculation, and fragility of skin as well as various nail changes develop in light-exposed areas. Light therapy for an affected neonate presenting with jaundice may inadvertently induce skin manifestations. **Hirsutism** in areas of mild involvement, scarring **alopecia** in severely affected areas, pink to red urine, brown teeth (erythrodontia), splenomegaly, and corneal ulceration are additional characteristic manifestations.

Laboratory findings include uroporphyrin I and coproporphyrin I in urine, plasma, and erythrocytes, and coproporphyrin I in feces. Teeth and urine from affected patients fluoresce reddish pink under a Wood lamp as a result of the presence of porphyrins. Skin findings for **hepatoerythropoietic porphyria** closely resemble those seen in congenital erythropoietic porphyria; this extremely rare disorder presents in early childhood and is discussed in greater depth in Chapter 91.

Erythropoietic protoporphyria may be autosomal dominant, autosomal recessive, or X-linked and most commonly involves the enzyme ferrochelatase (FECH). Symptoms develop in early childhood and manifest as intense pain, tingling, or pruritus within 30 minutes of sun exposure, followed by erythema, edema, urticaria, or mild systemic symptoms; these acute manifestations resolve completely within days. The absence of blistering distinguishes erythropoietic protoporphyria from the other cutaneous porphyrias. Nail changes consist of opacification of the nail plate, onycholysis, pain, and tenderness. Recurrent sun exposure produces a subtle chronic eczematous dermatitis with thickened, lichenified skin, especially over the finger joints (Fig. 656-3A), as well as mild facial scarring (Fig. 656-3B). Pigmentation, hypertrichosis, skin fragility, and mutilation are not seen. Gallstones develop frequently; however, severe liver disease occurs in <5% of patients. Protoporphyrin is detected in plasma, erythrocytes, and feces.

The wavelengths of light mainly responsible for eliciting cutaneous reactions in porphyria are in the region of 400 nm (UVA light). Window glass, including that in automobiles, transmits wavelengths >320 nm and is not protective, and fluorescent indoor lights may be pathogenic. Patients must avoid direct sunlight, wear protective clothing, and use a sunscreen agent that effectively blocks UVA light. Oral beta-carotene also provides some photoprotective benefit. Cutaneous porphyria symptoms are typically constant throughout life, and secondary bacterial infections commonly complicate disease course. Cutaneous porphyrias do not appear to increase risk for skin malignancies. Diagnostic and treatment recommendations for **congenital erythropoietic porphyria** and **erythropoietic protoporphyria** are outlined in Chapter 91.

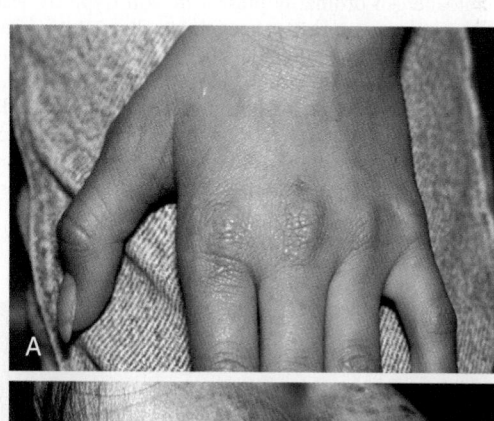
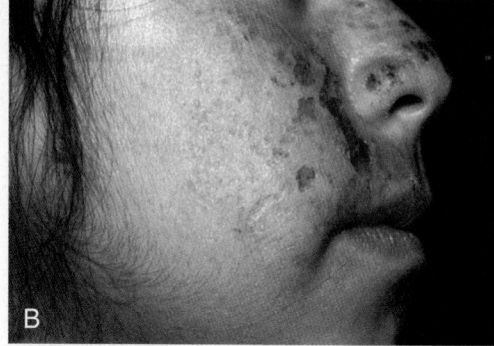

Figure 656-3 Erythropoietic protoporphyria. **A,** Erythematous thickening over the metacarpal phalangeal joints. **B,** Linear crusts and scarring.

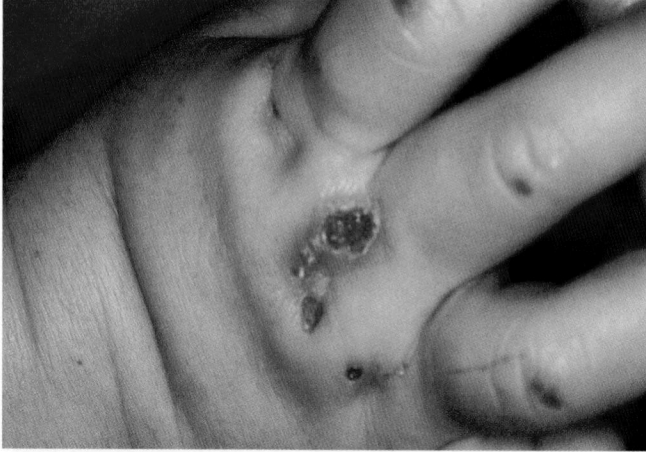

Figure 656-2 Crusted ulcerations in an infant with congenital erythropoietic porphyria.

COLLOID MILIUM

Colloid milium is a rare, asymptomatic disorder that occurs on the face (nose, upper lip, upper cheeks) and may extend to the dorsum of the hands and the neck as a profuse eruption of tiny, ivory to yellow, firm, grouped papules. Lesions appear before puberty on otherwise normal skin, unlike the adult variant that develops on sun-damaged skin. Onset may follow an acute sunburn or long-term sun exposure. Most cases reach maximal severity within 3 yr and remain unchanged thereafter, although the condition may remit spontaneously after puberty. Treatment is usually not necessary.

HYDROA VACCINIFORME

Hydroa vacciniforme is a vesiculobullous disorder with unclear etiology, although chronic or latent Epstein-Barr virus infections or lymphoproliferative disorders have been implicated. It begins in early childhood and may remit at puberty, with peak incidence in the spring and summer. Erythematous, pruritic macules develop symmetrically within hours of sun exposure over the ears, nose, lips, cheeks, and dorsal surfaces of the hands and forearms. Lesions progress to stinging tender papules and hemorrhagic vesicles and bullae, resembling chickenpox. They become umbilicated, ulcerated, and crusted, eventually healing with pitted scars and telangiectasias. Associated features are rare but include fever, malaise, hypersensitivity to mosquito bites, conjunctivitis, and other ocular symptoms. This eruption should be distinguished from erythropoietic protoporphyria, which rarely shows vesicles. Typical lesions have been reproduced with repeated doses of UVA or UVB light. First-line treatment includes sun avoidance, broad-spectrum sunscreens, and other sun-protective habits. Other potential therapies include mid-potency topical corticosteroids for inflamed lesions, low-dose courses of narrow-band UVB (NB-UVB) therapy, beta-carotene, hydroxychloroquine, or antiviral agents such as acyclovir.

SOLAR URTICARIA

Solar urticaria is a rare disorder induced by UV or visible irradiation. The disorder is mediated by immunoglobulin E antibodies to either an abnormal photoallergen present only in affected patients (type I) or a normal photoallergen ordinarily present in skin (type II), leading to mast cell degranulation and histamine release. Classic urticarial lesions consisting of erythematous pruritic wheals develop on sun-exposed skin (Fig. 656-4) within 5-10 minutes of sun exposure and fade within 24 hr. Severe reactions involving large areas of skin may lead to systemic symptoms or anaphylaxis. Diagnosis is achieved by history alone or with phototesting. First-line treatment is an oral H_1 antihistamine, plus sun avoidance and protection. Second-line therapy possibilities include oral or topical corticosteroids, photodesensitization using NB-UVB, omalizumab, or intravenous immunoglobulin.

POLYMORPHOUS LIGHT ERUPTION

Polymorphous light eruption (PMLE) is a common photosensitivity reaction that develops most commonly in females. The first eruption typically appears in the spring after the first episode of prolonged sun exposure of the season. Onset of the eruption is delayed by hours to days after sun exposure and lasts for days to sometimes weeks. PMLE usually resolves with increased sun exposure throughout the spring and summer. Areas of involvement tend to be symmetric and are characteristic for a given patient, including some but not all of the exposed or lightly covered skin on the face, neck, upper chest, and distal extremities. Lesions have various morphologies but most commonly are pruritic, 2-5 mm, grouped, erythematous papules or papulovesicles or >5 cm, edematous plaques; lesions are nonscarring. A PMLE variant known as **juvenile spring eruption** characteristically occurs on affected boys' ears each spring, while **pinpoint papular PMLE** is a variant characterized by pinpoint-sized lesions occurring in darker-skinned individuals. Most PMLE cases involve sensitivity to UVA radiation, although some are UVB induced. PMLE most likely results from a delayed-type hypersensitivity reaction to a photo-induced antigen within the skin, with individuals having a genetic predisposition. Provocative phototesting, as well as skin biopsy (showing epidermal spongiosis and superficial and deep lymphocytic infiltrate), aid in diagnosis. Treatment is aimed at prevention with sun avoidance, protective clothing, and broad-spectrum sunscreens. Topical corticosteroids (low-potency for facial lesions, high-potency for lesions elsewhere) can be used for mild eruptions. Second-line approaches include prophylactic NB-UVB phototherapy or hydroxychloroqine in early spring and short course systemic glucocorticoids for severe flares.

ACTINIC PRURIGO

Actinic prurigo, often classified as a variant of PMLE, is a chronic familial photodermatitis inherited as an autosomal dominant trait seen most commonly in Native Americans of North and South America. Human leukocyte antigen (HLA) DRB1*0407 (60-70%) and HLA DRB1*0401 (20%) are strongly associated with actinic prurigo. Most patients are female and are sensitive to UVA radiation. The first episode generally occurs in early childhood, several hr to 2 days after intense sun exposure. The papulonodular lesions are intensely pruritic, erythematous, and crusted. Areas of predilection include the face (Fig. 656-5), lower lip, distal extremities, and, in severe cases, buttocks. Facial lesions may heal with minute pitted or linear scarring. Lesions often become chronic, without periods of total clearing, merging into

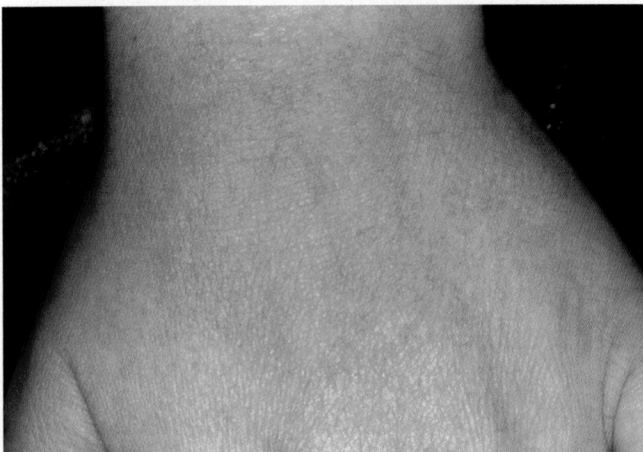

Figure 656-4 Urticaria after 5 minutes of exposure to artificial ultraviolet A radiation.

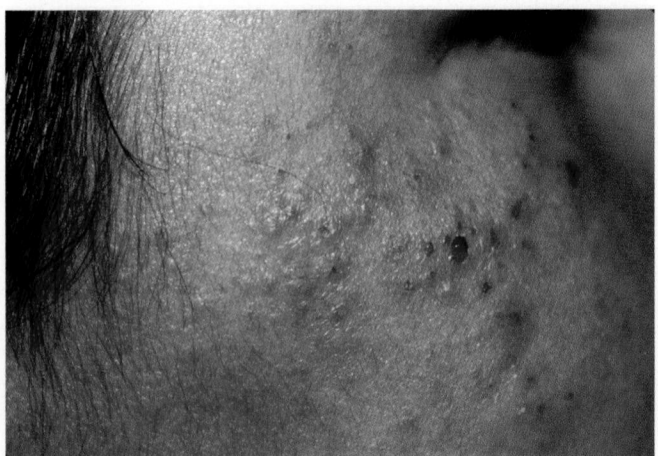

Figure 656-5 Erythematous, excoriated papules in actinic prurigo.

eczematous plaques that become lichenified and occasionally secondarily infected. Associated features that distinguish this disorder from other photoeruptions and atopic dermatitis include cheilitis, conjunctivitis, and traumatic alopecia of the outer half of the eyebrows. Actinic prurigo is a chronic condition that generally persists into adult life, although it may improve spontaneously in the late teenage years. Sun avoidance, protective clothing, and broad-spectrum sunscreens may be helpful in preventing the eruption. Mid- to high-potency topical corticosteroids and antihistamines palliate the pruritus and inflammation. Severe acute eruptions may require oral glucocorticoids. Treatment with NB-UVB beginning in springtime has shown improved tolerance of sunlight during summer months; however, it may induce symptoms in some patients. Thalidomide 50-100 mg/day is very effective, but its use is limited by toxicity, especially severe birth defects when taken by pregnant females.

COCKAYNE SYNDROME

Cockayne syndrome is a rare autosomal recessive disorder. Onset occurs at 1 year of age and is characterized by facial erythema in a butterfly distribution after sun exposure. Later characteristics include loss of adipose tissue and development of thin, atrophic, hyperpigmented skin, particularly over the face. Associated features include dwarfism; microcephaly; mental retardation; progressive dementia; distinct facies (aged look, pinched nose, sunken eyes, large protuberant ears); long limbs; disproportionately large hands and feet; cool and cyanotic extremities; carious teeth; unsteady gait with tremor; limitation of joint mobility; progressive deafness; cataracts; retinal degeneration; optic atrophy; decreased sweating and tearing; and premature graying of the hair. Complications include diabetes and hepatic or renal impairment. Diffuse extensive demyelination of the peripheral and central nervous systems ensues, and patients generally die of atheromatous vascular disease or infections (especially pneumonia) before the 3rd decade. There are 2 types of Cockayne syndrome. Type I (*CSA* gene) is less severe than type II (*CSB* gene). Patients may have xeroderma pigmentosum–Cockayne syndrome overlap, which is phenotypically more like Cockayne syndrome. Photosensitivity in Cockayne syndrome is a result of deficient nucleotide excision repair of UV-induced damage, specifically within actively transcribing regions of DNA (transcription-coupled DNA repair). The etiology of neurologic and other associated features remains unclear; however, evidence points toward a mitochondriopathy. The syndrome is distinguished from progeria (see Chapter 90) by the presence of photosensitivity and ocular abnormalities and from xeroderma pigmentosum by the fact that patients with Cockayne syndrome do not develop skin cancers. Diagnosis is accomplished by genetic testing and performing various tests on cultured fibroblasts. The mainstay of treatment for the photosensitivity of Cockayne syndrome is strict sunlight avoidance and protective measures.

XERODERMA PIGMENTOSUM

Xeroderma pigmentosum is a rare autosomal recessive disorder that results from a defect in nucleotide excision repair. Eight genetic groups have been recognized on the basis of each group's separate defect in ability to repair (xeroderma pigmentosum A through G) or replicate (xeroderma pigmentosum V [variant]) damaged DNA. The wavelength of light that induces the DNA damage ranges from 280-340 nm. Skin changes are first noted during infancy or early childhood in sun-exposed areas though lesions may occur at other sites, including the scalp. The skin lesions consist of erythema, scaling, bullae, crusting, ephelides (freckles), telangiectasia, keratoses (Fig. 656-6), basal and squamous cell carcinomas, and malignant melanomas. Interestingly, although most patients experience exaggerated acute sunburn reactions following minimal UV exposure, up to half of affected patients do not and instead develop progressive freckling. This difference in presentation depends on genetic subtype. Ocular manifestations include photophobia, lacrimation, blepharitis, symblepharon, keratitis, corneal opacities, tumors of the lids, and possible

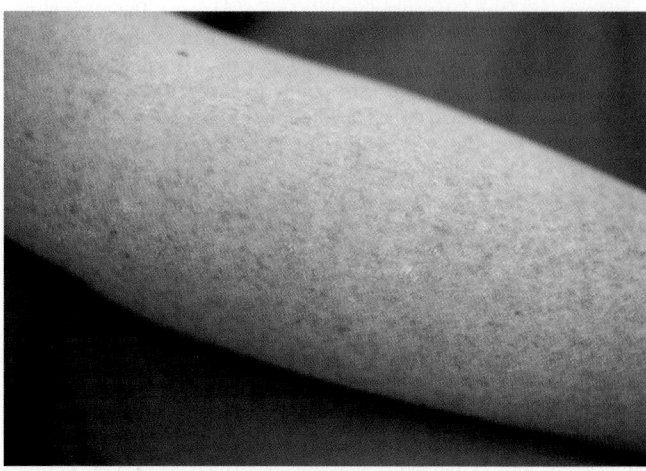

Figure 656-6 Dyspigmentation and actinic keratoses in child with xeroderma pigmentosum.

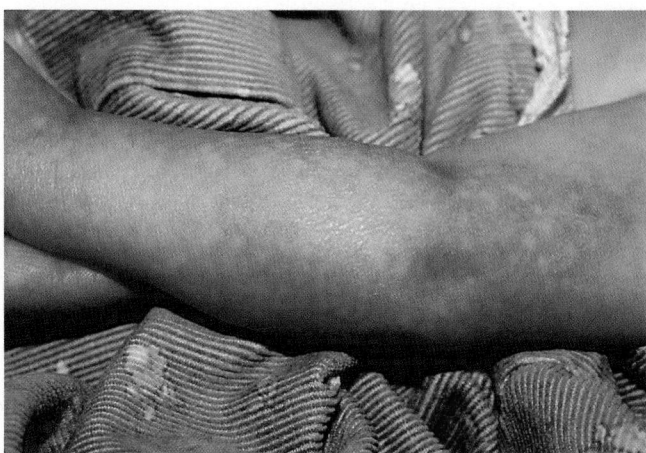

Figure 656-7 Poikiloderma on the arm of an infant with Rothmund-Thomson syndrome.

eventual blindness. Neurologic abnormalities such as cognitive deterioration and sensorineural deafness develop in approximately 20% of patients.

This disease is a serious mutilating disorder, and the life span of an affected patient is often brief. Affected families should have genetic counseling. Xeroderma pigmentosum is detectable in cells cultured from amniotic fluid or DNA analysis of chorionic villous samples. Cultured skin fibroblast tests and genetic testing after birth also confirm diagnosis. Affected children should be totally protected from sun exposure; protective clothing, sunglasses, and opaque broad-spectrum sunscreens should be used even for mildly affected children. Light from unshielded fluorescent bulbs and sunlight passing through glass windows (including vehicle windows) are also harmful, thus applied window films are recommended. Early detection and removal of malignancies is mandatory, and oral isotretinoin may be used to prevent nonmelanoma skin cancers. There is crossover between several subtypes of xeroderma pigmentosum and both Cockayne syndrome and trichothiodystrophy.

ROTHMUND-THOMSON SYNDROME

Rothmund-Thomson syndrome is also known as poikiloderma congenitale because of the striking skin changes (Fig. 656-7). It is inherited as an autosomal recessive trait. Mutations in the *RECQL4* gene, which encodes a DNA helicase involved in repair and replication of DNA and telomeres, are found in approximately 65% of patients. The other mutations causing Rothmund-Thomson syndrome are unknown. Skin changes are noted as early as 3 mo of age and begin on the face. Plaques of erythema and edema appear in a butterfly distribution, as well as on the forehead, ears, neck, dorsal portions of the hands, extensor surfaces of the arms, and buttocks. These are replaced gradually by poikiloderma (reticulated, atrophic, hyperpigmented and hypopigmented telangiectatic patches or plaques). Palmoplantar hyperkeratosis develops in one-third of patients. Light sensitivity is present in many cases, and exposure to the sun may provoke formation of bullae. Areas of involvement, however, are not strictly photodistributed. Short stature; small hands and feet; sparse eyebrows, eyelashes, and pubic and axillary hair, and sparse, fine, prematurely gray scalp hair or alopecia; dystrophic nails; various tooth and skeletal abnormalities; and hypogenitalism are common. Cataracts may also occur at an early age. Most patients have normal mental development. Keratoses and later squamous cell carcinomas may develop on exposed skin. The most worrisome association is that with osteosarcoma, which occurs only in those patients with Rothmund-Thomson syndrome and *RECQL4* mutations. Genetic testing aids diagnosis. Management of dermatologic findings begins with sun avoidance and protection behaviors, and telangiectatic lesions have been shown to respond to pulsed dye laser therapy. In the absence of malignancy, life expectancy is normal.

BLOOM SYNDROME

Bloom syndrome is inherited in an autosomal recessive manner, most commonly in the Ashkenazi Jewish population. It is caused by a mutation in the *BLM/RECQL3* gene, encoding a DNA helicase. Patients are sensitive to UV radiation, with increased rates of chromosomal breaks and sister chromatid exchanges. Erythema and telangiectasia develop during infancy in a butterfly distribution on the face after exposure to sunlight. A bullous eruption on the lips and telangiectatic erythema on the hands and forearms may develop. Café-au-lait spots and hypopigmented macules may be present. Intrauterine growth deficiency developing into short stature and a distinctive facies consisting of a prominent nose and ears and a small, narrow face are generally found. Intellect is average to low average. Immunodeficiency is seen in all patients, manifesting as recurrent ear and pulmonary infections. Gastrointestinal malabsorption, gastroesophageal reflux, and hypogonadism are common. Affected children have an unusual tendency to develop both solid tumors (especially of the skin) and lymphoreticular malignancies, which often result in death during childhood or early adulthood. Sister chromatid exchange analysis is generally performed to confirm diagnosis. The only effective measures to reduce skin disease are sun protection and avoidance.

HARTNUP DISEASE

See Chapter 85.5.

Hartnup disease is a rare inborn error of metabolism with autosomal recessive inheritance. Neutral amino acids, including tryptophan, are not transported across the brush border epithelium of the intestine and kidneys due to mutation of the SLC6A19 gene encoding the transporter. This results in deficiency of nicotinamide synthesis and causes a photo-induced **pellagra-like syndrome.** The urine contains increased amounts of monoamine monocarboxylic amino acids, distinguishing Hartnup disease from dietary pellagra. Cutaneous signs, which precede neurologic manifestations, initially develop during the early months of life. An eczematous, occasionally vesiculobullous, eruption occurs on the face and extremities in a glove-and-stocking photodistribution. Hyperpigmentation and hyperkeratosis may supervene and are intensified by further exposure to sunlight. Episodic flares may be precipitated by febrile illness, sun exposure, emotional stress, and poor nutrition. In most cases, mental development is normal, but some patients display emotional instability and episodic cerebellar ataxia. Neurologic symptoms are fully reversible. Administration of nicotinamide and protection from sunlight results in improvement of both cutaneous and neurologic manifestations.

Bibliography is available at Expert Consult.

Chapter 657
Diseases of the Epidermis

657.1 Psoriasis
Brianne Z. Dickey and Yvonne E. Chiu

ETIOLOGY/PATHOGENESIS
Psoriasis is an inflammatory autoimmune-related disease characterized by inflammation and keratinocyte proliferation. Within the dermis, dendritic cells are activated by self-antigens and release cytokines such as interferon-γ, tumor necrosis factor, and interleukin (IL)-12, IL-17, IL-22, and IL-23, which recruit T cells. Once activated, the T cells release cytokines that induce proliferation and abnormal differentiation of epidermal keratinocytes; in turn, more cytokines are produced to perpetuate the cycle. Psoriasis has a complex multifactorial genetic basis. The major psoriasis-susceptibility gene *(PSORS1)* is human leukocyte antigen (HLA)-CW*0602, encoding a class I major histocompatibility complex protein involved in recognition of self-antigens. Numerous other psoriasis susceptibility genes have been identified.

Factors contributing to disease onset/flares in some patients include bacterial and viral infections, trauma, physical or emotional stress, tobacco use/secondhand exposure, and certain medications. There is an association between psoriasis and childhood obesity worldwide.

CLINICAL MANIFESTATIONS
This common, chronic skin disorder is first evident within the 1st 2 decades of life for approximately 30% of affected individuals. **Plaque psoriasis**, the most common (>80%) subtype, is characterized by erythematous papules that coalesce to form plaques with sharply demarcated, irregular borders. If they are unaltered by treatment, a thick silvery or yellow-white scale (resembling mica) develops (Fig. 657-1*A*). Removal of the scale may result in pinpoint bleeding (**Auspitz sign**). The **Koebner phenomenon,** in which new lesions appear at sites of trauma, is a valuable diagnostic feature. Lesions may occur anywhere, but preferred sites are the scalp, knees, elbows, umbilicus, superior intergluteal fold, genitals, and ear canal. Nail involvement, a valuable diagnostic sign, is characterized by pitting of the nail plate, detachment of the plate (onycholysis), yellowish-brown subungual discoloration, and accumulation of subungual debris (Fig. 657-1*B*). Plaques are generally asymptomatic; however, pruritus is more common in children than adults.

Guttate psoriasis, a variant that occurs predominantly in children, is characterized by an acute eruption of many oval or round papules smaller than 1.5 cm that are morphologically identical to the larger plaques of psoriasis (see Fig. 657-1*C*). Sites of predilection are the trunk, face, and proximal portions of the limbs. The onset usually follows a **streptococcal** infection such as pharyngitis; thus, throat culture and serologic titers should be obtained. Guttate psoriasis has also been observed after perianal streptococcal infection, viral infections, sunburn, and withdrawal of systemic corticosteroid therapy or tumor necrosis factor (TNF)-α inhibitors. Clinical course ranges from spontaneous resolution to chronic disease.

Pustular psoriasis is a multisystem autoinflammatory disease characterized by recurrent episodes with the sudden onset of fever, malaise, extracutaneous organ involvement, and a diffuse erythematous-pustular exanthema. It may be associated with plaque psoriasis in some patients; unregulated cytokine production as a result of mutations in the IL-36Ra gene is implicated.

Psoriasis is rare in infants but may be severe and recalcitrant and may pose a diagnostic problem. Psoriatic diaper rash is a common presentation in children younger than 2 yr old. Other rare forms

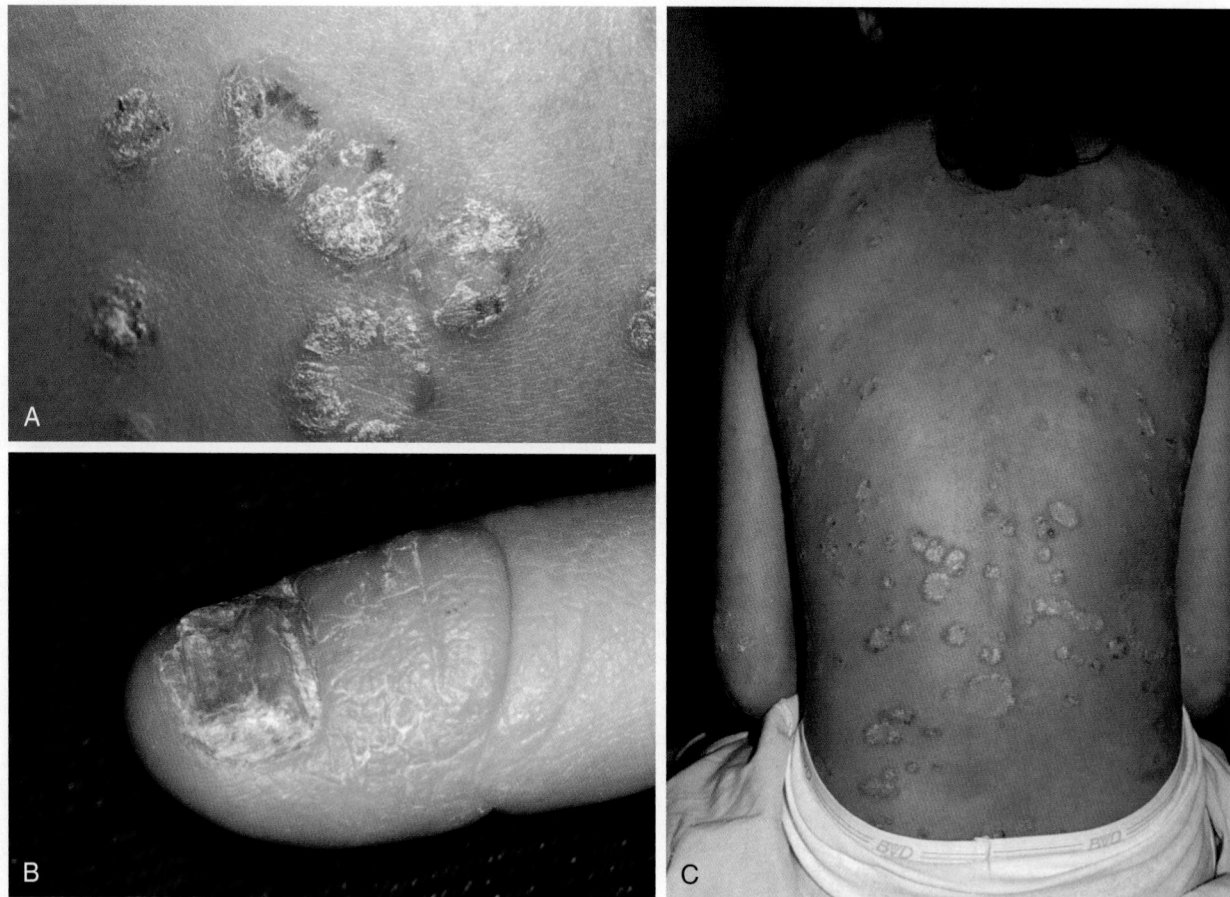

Figure 657-1 A, Chronic psoriatic plaques. **B,** Psoriatic nail dystrophy. **C,** Guttate psoriasis in widespread distribution over the trunk.

include psoriatic erythroderma, localized or generalized pustular psoriasis, linear psoriasis, palmoplantar psoriasis, and inverse psoriasis (occurring in intertriginous areas).

DIFFERENTIAL DIAGNOSIS

Psoriasis is a clinical diagnosis. The differential diagnosis of plaque-type psoriasis includes nummular dermatitis, tinea corporis, seborrheic dermatitis, postinfectious arthritis syndromes, and pityriasis rubra pilaris. Scalp lesions may be confused with seborrheic dermatitis, atopic dermatitis, or tinea capitis. Diaper area psoriasis may mimic seborrheic dermatitis, eczematous diaper dermatitis, perianal streptococcal disease, or candidiasis. Guttate psoriasis can be confused with viral exanthems, secondary syphilis, pityriasis rosea, and pityriasis lichenoides chronica (PLC). Nail psoriasis must be differentiated from onychomycosis, lichen planus, and other causes of onychodystrophy.

PATHOLOGY

When the diagnosis is in doubt, histopathologic examination of an untreated lesion can be helpful. Characteristic changes of psoriasis include parakeratosis, acanthosis, elongated rete ridges, neutrophilic infiltrate in the epidermis sometimes forming microabscesses, dilated dermal blood vessels, and lymphocytic infiltrate in the dermis.

TREATMENT

The therapeutic approach varies with the age of the child, type of psoriasis, sites of involvement, and extent of the disease. Physical and chemical trauma to the skin should be avoided as much as possible to prevent Koebner response lesions. The treatment of psoriasis should be viewed as a 4-tier process.

The **first tier** is **topical therapy.** The first-line topical agents for lesions on the body are emollients, vitamin D analogs (calcipotriene or calcitriol, although calcitriol is less irritating for children), and mid- to high-potency corticosteroids (see Chapter 646). A proprietary formulation containing both calcipotriene and betamethasone dipropionate (a high-potency topical corticosteroid) exists in ointment and solution forms. The preparation that is least potent but effective should be applied twice a day. Second-line topical options for lesions on the body include retinoids (tazarotene), tar preparations, anthralin, and keratolytics (salicylic acid or urea). Facial or intertriginous lesions may be treated with low-potency topical corticosteroids, and/or topical vitamin D analogs or calcineurin inhibitors as corticosteroid-sparing agents. For scalp lesions, applications of a phenol and saline solution (e.g., Baker Cummins P & S liquid) followed by a tar shampoo are effective in the removal of scales. A high- to superpotency corticosteroid in a foam, solution, or lotion base may be applied when the scaling is diminished. Nail lesions are difficult to treat topically; the first-line approach is a high-potency topical corticosteroid to the proximal nail fold.

The **second tier** of therapy is **phototherapy.** Narrow-band UVB (311 nm; NB-UVB) irradiation is the primary form of UVB therapy used in childhood. If available, phototherapy should be used alone or with tar ("Goeckerman treatment") for older children with extensive disease in whom topical therapy alone has failed. Excimer (308 nm) laser UVB irradiation may be used for localized treatment-resistant plaques. Exposure to natural sunlight is often effective for less-severe psoriasis.

The **third tier** is **systemic therapy, required rarely for** children with severe and generalized psoriasis. Methotrexate (0.2-0.7 mg/kg/wk) is the first-line systemic agent for children; other options include oral retinoids (0.5-1.0 mg/kg/day) and cyclosporine (3-5 mg/kg/day). Oral retinoids may be cautiously combined with phototherapy, although doses may need to be decreased because of the photosensitizing effects of the medication.

The **fourth tier** of therapy is the **biologic response modifiers**, including the TNF-α inhibitors etanercept, infliximab, and adalimumab, and the T-cell function inhibitor alefacept. Ustekinumab is a human monoclonal antibody that prevents interactions between IL-12 and IL-23 and their cell-surface receptors. Anti–IL-17 and anti–IL-17 receptor agents also demonstrate some efficacy. Adult studies with all of these agents show efficacy in treating moderate to severe chronic psoriasis and psoriatic arthritis, although experience in children is limited. Novel small molecules that inhibit the inflammatory response are being tested; these include A3 adenosine receptor agonists, Janus kinase inhibitors, and phosphodiesterase 4 inhibitors.

PROGNOSIS

Prognosis is best for children with limited disease. Psoriasis is a lifelong disease characterized by remissions and exacerbations. Arthritis or various eye diseases may be extracutaneous complications. Metabolic and cardiovascular disorders also occur with increased frequency in patients with psoriasis. For example, increasing degree of obesity and the associated metabolic syndrome (hyperglycemia, hyperlipidemia, hypertension) correlates with psoriasis severity. Patients with psoriasis also have increased rates of stroke, myocardial infarction, and other vascular diseases later in adult life. A proposed mechanism involves the systemic proinflammatory state induced by both psoriasis and these associated conditions, although the direction of causality remains unclear.

Bibliography is available at Expert Consult.

657.2 Pityriasis Lichenoides
Brianne Z. Dickey and Yvonne E. Chiu

Pityriasis lichenoides encompasses a disease spectrum ranging from pityriasis lichenoides chronica (PLC) to pityriasis lichenoides et varioliformis acuta (PLEVA; Mucha-Habermann disease). The designation of pityriasis lichenoides as acute or chronic refers to the morphologic appearance of the lesions rather than to the duration of the disease. No correlation is found between the type of lesion at the onset of the eruption and the duration of the disease. Many patients have both acute and chronic lesions simultaneously, and transition of lesions from 1 form into another occurs occasionally. Febrile ulceronecrotic Mucha-Habermann disease (FUMHD) is a rare subtype of PLEVA that is more severe and potentially life-threatening.

ETIOLOGY/PATHOGENESIS

Two main theories exist for the etiology of pityriasis lichenoides. The first is that it arises in a genetically susceptible individual as a hypersensitivity reaction to an infection. The second is that it represents a monoclonal T-cell lymphocytic proliferation on the pathway to cutaneous T-cell dyscrasia.

CLINICAL MANIFESTATIONS

Pityriasis lichenoides most commonly manifests in the 2nd and 3rd decades of life; 30% of cases manifest before age 20 yr. The overall eruption persists for months to years with a tendency to eventually remit.

PLC manifests gradually as generalized, multiple, 3-5 mm, brown-red papules that are covered by a fine grayish scale (Fig. 657-2). Lesions may be asymptomatic or may cause minimal pruritus and occasionally become vesicular, hemorrhagic, crusted, or superinfected. Individual papules become flat and brownish in 2-6 wk, ultimately leaving a hyperpigmented or hypopigmented macule. Scarring is unusual. Various stages of lesions are present most commonly on the trunk and

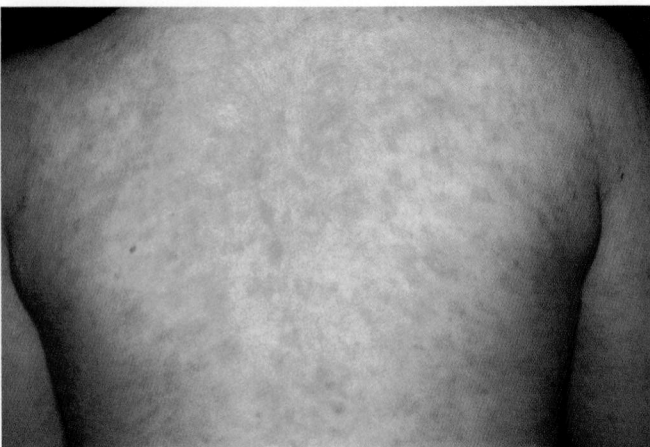

Figure 657-2 Widespread plaques with fine scale in pityriasis lichenoides chronica.

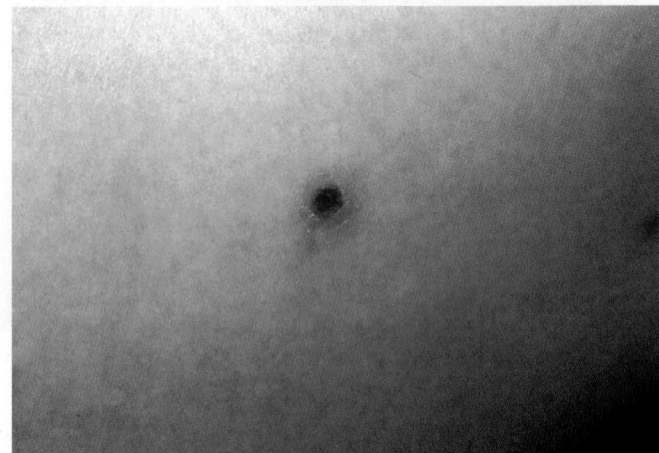

Figure 657-3 Necrotic lesion with erythematous halo in pityriasis lichenoides et varioliformis acuta.

extremities and generally spare the face, palmoplantar surfaces, scalp, and mucous membranes.

PLEVA manifests as an abrupt eruption of numerous papules that have a vesiculopustular and then a purpuric center, are covered by a dark adherent hemorrhagic or necrotic crust, and are surrounded by an erythematous halo (Fig. 657-3). Constitutional symptoms, such as fever, malaise, headache, and arthralgias, may be present for 2-3 days after the initial outbreak. Lesions are distributed diffusely on the trunk and extremities, as in PLC. Individual lesions heal within a few weeks, sometimes leaving a varioliform scar, and successive crops of papules produce the characteristic polymorphous appearance of the eruption, with lesions in various stages of evolution.

FUMHD manifests as fever and ulceronecrotic nodules up to a few centimeters in diameter, which are most common on the anterior trunk and flexor surfaces of the proximal upper extremities. Hemorrhagic bullae, mucosal ulcers, arthritis, cardiomyopathy, vasculitis, abdominal complaints, and superinfection of cutaneous lesions with *Staphylococcus aureus* may also develop. The ulceronecrotic lesions heal with hypopigmented scarring in a few weeks.

PATHOLOGY

PLC histologically shows a parakeratotic, thickened corneal layer; epidermal spongiosis; a superficial perivascular infiltrate of macrophages and predominantly CD8 lymphocytes that may extend into the epidermis; and small numbers of extravasated erythrocytes in the papillary dermis.

The histopathologic changes of PLEVA and FUMHD reflect their more-severe nature. Intercellular and intracellular edema in the epidermis may lead to degeneration of keratinocytes. A dense perivascular mononuclear cell infiltrate, endothelial cell swelling, and extravasation of erythrocytes into the epidermis and dermis are additional characteristic features.

DIFFERENTIAL DIAGNOSIS

The differential diagnosis of pityriasis lichenoides includes guttate psoriasis, pityriasis rosea, drug eruptions, secondary syphilis, viral exanthems, lymphomatoid papulosis, and lichen planus. The chronicity of pityriasis lichenoides helps preclude pityriasis rosea, viral exanthems, and some drug eruptions. A skin biopsy helps distinguish pityriasis lichenoides from other entities in the differential diagnosis.

TREATMENT

In general, pityriasis lichenoides should be considered a benign condition that does not alter the health of the child. A lubricant to remove excessive scaling may be all that is necessary if the patient is asymptomatic. If treatment is required, first-line agents are oral anti-inflammatory antibiotics such as erythromycin (30-50 mg/kg/day for 2-3 mo). Topical corticosteroids (mid-potency, applied twice daily) and topical calcineurin inhibitors may help the pruritus and inflammation, but do not alter the course of the disease. Phototherapy (NB-UVB) is the second-line treatment option. Methotrexate should be reserved for severely symptomatic cases. The rare FUMHD usually requires inpatient treatment; initially, systemic corticosteroids, methotrexate, intravenous immunoglobulin, or cyclosporine may be necessary, with eventual transition to another form of treatment, as mentioned above, once the disease improves and stabilizes.

Bibliography is available at Expert Consult.

657.3 Keratosis Pilaris
Brianne Z. Dickey and Yvonne E. Chiu

Keratosis pilaris is a common papular eruption resulting from keratin plugging of hair follicles. It displays an autosomal dominant transmission with variable penetrance. Typical areas of involvement include the upper extensor surfaces of the arms and thighs, cheeks, and buttocks. The lesions may resemble gooseflesh; they are noninflammatory, scaly, follicular papules that do not coalesce. They are generally asymptomatic but may be pruritic. Irritation of the follicular plugs occasionally causes erythema surrounding the keratotic papules (Fig. 657-4). A

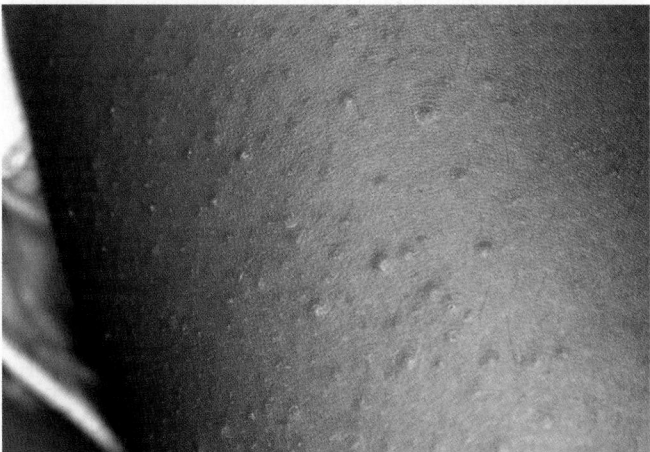

Figure 657-4 Keratotic follicular plugs with surrounding erythema in keratosis pilaris.

subset of patients have keratosis pilaris associated with facial telangiectasia and ulerythema ophryogenes, a rare cutaneous disorder characterized by inflammatory keratotic facial papules that may result in scars, atrophy, and alopecia. Because the lesions of keratosis pilaris are associated with and accentuated by dry skin, they are often more prominent during the winter. Keratosis pilaris is more frequent in patients with atopic dermatitis and is most common during childhood and early adulthood, tending to subside in the 3rd decade of life. Treatment of keratosis pilaris is optional. Measures to decrease pruritus include moisturization with a bland emollient. Regular applications of a 10-40% urea cream or an α-hydroxy acid preparation such as 12% lactic acid cream or lotion can improve the appearance of keratosis pilaris but may further contribute to pruritus and irritation. Therapy may improve the condition but does not cure it.

657.4 Lichen Spinulosus
Brianne Z. Dickey and Yvonne E. Chiu

Lichen spinulosus is an uncommon disorder that occurs principally in children and more frequently in boys. The cause is unknown. The lesions consist of sharply circumscribed irregular plaques of spiny, keratotic, follicular plugs. Plaques may occur anywhere on the body and are often distributed symmetrically on the trunk, elbows, knees, and extensor surfaces of the limbs. Although sometimes erythematous or pruritic, the lesions are usually skin colored and asymptomatic.

Treatment is usually unnecessary. For patients who regard the eruption as a cosmetic defect, urea-containing lubricants (10-40%) are often effective in flattening the projections. The plaques usually disappear spontaneously after several months or years.

657.5 Pityriasis Rosea
Brianne Z. Dickey and Yvonne E. Chiu

ETIOLOGY/PATHOGENESIS

The cause of pityriasis rosea is unknown; a viral agent is suspected, and there is debate over the role of human herpesviruses 6, 7, and 8 in this condition. Supporting evidence for an infectious etiology is the tendency for it to occur in case clusters, although the rash itself is not contagious.

CLINICAL MANIFESTATIONS

This benign, common eruption occurs most frequently in children and young adults. Although a prodrome of fever, malaise, arthralgia, and pharyngitis may precede the eruption, children rarely complain of such symptoms. A **herald patch** classically precedes the generalized eruption and may occur anywhere on the body. Herald patches are generally larger than other lesions and vary from 1-10 cm in diameter; they are annular in configuration and have a raised border with fine, adherent scales. Approximately 5-10 days after the appearance of the herald patch, a widespread, symmetric eruption involving mainly the trunk and proximal limbs becomes evident (Fig. 657-5). In the inverse form of pityriasis rosea, the face, scalp, and distal limbs may be preferentially involved. Lesions may appear in crops for several days. Typical lesions are oval or round, <1 cm in diameter, slightly raised, and pink to brown. The developed lesion is covered by a fine scale, which gives the skin a crinkly appearance. Some lesions clear centrally and produce a collarette of scale that is attached only at the periphery. Papular (more common in black children), vesicular, urticarial, hemorrhagic, large annular, and mucosal lesions are unusual variants. The long axis of each lesion is usually aligned with the cutaneous cleavage lines, a feature that creates the so-called **Christmas tree pattern** on the back. Conformation to skin lines is often more discernible in the anterior and posterior axillary folds and supraclavicular areas. The lesions most commonly are asymptomatic but may be mildly to severely pruritic.

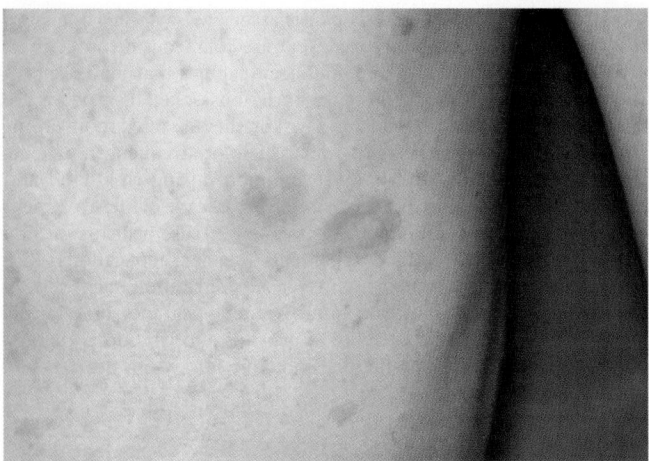

Figure 657-5 Herald patch and surrounding pityriasis rosea.

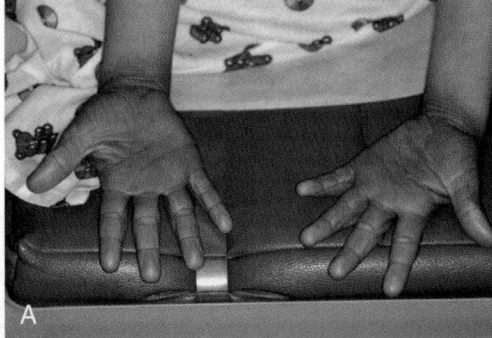

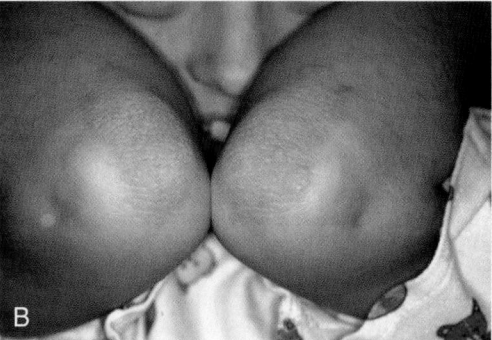

Figure 657-6 Pityriasis rubra pilaris. **A,** Orange palmar hyperkeratosis. **B,** Elbow lesions.

Duration of the eruption varies from 2-12 wk, with self-resolution. After the eruption has resolved, postinflammatory hypopigmentation or hyperpigmentation may be pronounced, particularly in dark-skinned patients. These changes disappear in subsequent weeks to months.

DIFFERENTIAL DIAGNOSIS
The herald patch may be mistaken for tinea corporis, a pitfall that can be avoided if microscopic evaluation of a potassium hydroxide preparation of scrapings of the lesion is performed. The generalized eruption resembles a number of other diseases; secondary syphilis is the most important. Drug eruptions, viral exanthems, guttate psoriasis, PLC, and nummular dermatitis can also be confused with pityriasis rosea.

TREATMENT
Therapy is unnecessary for asymptomatic patients with pityriasis rosea. If scaling is prominent, a bland emollient may suffice. Pruritus may be suppressed by a lubricating lotion containing menthol and camphor or by an oral antihistamine for sedation, particularly at night, when itching may be troublesome. Occasionally, a mid-potency topical corticosteroid preparation may be necessary to alleviate pruritus. Exposure to natural sunlight and NB-UVB phototherapy may reduce disease duration and severity.

Bibliography is available at Expert Consult.

657.6 Pityriasis Rubra Pilaris
Brianne Z. Dickey and Yvonne E. Chiu

ETIOLOGY/PATHOGENESIS
The cause of pityriasis rubra pilaris is unknown. Although genetic forms with autosomal dominant or recessive transmission may account for some cases in childhood, most cases are sporadic. Some studies have indicated a role for TNF-α in disease development, while other hypotheses for causal factors include abnormal vitamin A metabolism, trauma, infections, immunosuppression, and UV light exposure.

CLINICAL MANIFESTATIONS
This rare inflammatory dermatosis is known for its variability in clinical presentation and course of disease. It often has an insidious onset with diffuse scaling and erythema of the scalp, which is indistinguishable from the findings in seborrheic dermatitis, and with thick hyperkeratosis of the palms and soles (Fig. 657-6A). Lesions over the elbows and knees are also common (Fig. 657-6B), and generalized erythroderma develops in some patients. The characteristic primary lesion is a firm, dome-shaped, tiny, acuminate, pink to red papule, which has a central keratotic plug pierced by a vellus hair. Masses of these papules coalesce to form large, erythematous, sharply demarcated orange-pink plaques with overlying scale, within which islands of normal skin can be distinguished. Typical papules on the dorsum of the proximal phalanges are readily palpated. Gray plaques or papules resembling lichen planus may be found in the oral cavity. Dystrophic changes in the nails may occur and mimic those of psoriasis. Lesions are commonly pruritic. In childhood, the prognosis for eventual resolution is relatively good.

DIFFERENTIAL DIAGNOSIS
Differential diagnosis includes ichthyosis, seborrheic dermatitis, keratoderma of the palms and soles, and psoriasis.

HISTOLOGY
Skin biopsy revealing follicular plugging, epidermal acanthosis, perivascular infiltrate, checkerboard pattern of orthokeratosis and parakeratosis, and an intact granular layer may differentiate this condition from psoriasis and seborrheic dermatitis.

TREATMENT
The numerous therapeutic regimens recommended are difficult to evaluate because pityriasis rubra pilaris has a capricious course with exacerbations and remissions. Moisturization alone is useful in mild cases. Topical agents, such as mid- to high-potency corticosteroids, keratolytics (urea, salicylic acid), vitamin D analogs (calcipotriene), retinoids (tazarotene, tretinoin), and tar, are used in combination with systemic agents for widespread disease and as monotherapy for localized disease. When further treatment is necessary, oral retinoids (isotretinoin 1 mg/kg/day or acitretin 0.5 mg/kg/day) are used as first-line agents, while methotrexate is used as a second-line agent. Third-line treatment options include biologic TNF-α inhibitors, cyclosporine, azathioprine, and NB-UVB phototherapy.

Bibliography is available at Expert Consult.

657.7 Darier Disease (Keratosis Follicularis)
Brianne Z. Dickey and Yvonne E. Chiu

ETIOLOGY/PATHOGENESIS
A rare genetic disorder, Darier disease is inherited as an autosomal dominant trait and is caused by mutations in the *ATP2A2* gene. This gene encodes a cellular calcium pump, and dysfunction results in loss of adhesion between epidermal cells and abnormal keratinization.

CLINICAL MANIFESTATIONS
Onset usually occurs in late childhood. Typical lesions are small, firm, skin-colored, warty papules that are not always follicular in location. The lesions eventually acquire yellow, malodorous, greasy crusts and coalesce to form large, gray-brown, vegetative plaques (Fig. 657-7). The scalp, face, neck, shoulders, chest, back, axillae, limb flexures, and groin are symmetrically involved. Papules, fissures, crusts, and ulcers may appear on the mucous membranes of the lips, tongue, buccal mucosa, pharynx, larynx, and vulva. Hyperkeratosis of the palms and soles and nail dystrophy with subungual hyperkeratosis and longitudinal red and white banding are variable features. Severe pruritus, secondary infection, offensive odor, and pain may occur. Several exacerbating triggers have been identified: sweating, UV light exposure, heat, friction, and infections. Thus, Darier disease has a chronic relapsing course that usually worsens in summertime.

HISTOLOGY
Histologic changes seen in Darier disease are diagnostic. Hyperkeratosis with keratin plugging, intraepidermal separation (acantholysis) with formation of suprabasal clefts, and dyskeratotic epidermal cells are characteristic features.

DIFFERENTIAL DIAGNOSIS
Darier disease is most likely to be confused with seborrheic dermatitis, flat warts, or Hailey-Hailey disease.

TREATMENT
Treatment is nonspecific and begins with emollients and avoidance of triggers. First-line treatment for mild/localized disease is low- to mid-potency corticosteroids; second-line is topical retinoids. Further treatment options include topical keratolytic agents (urea, lactic acid), antiseptic washes (triclosan, chlorhexidine gluconate, or bleach), or calcineurin inhibitors. More severe/generalized disease is treated with oral isotretinoin or acitretin (0.5-1.0 mg/kg/day for 3-4 mo). Secondary infections must be treated appropriately.

Bibliography is available at Expert Consult.

657.8 Lichen Nitidus
Brianne Z. Dickey and Yvonne E. Chiu

ETIOLOGY/PATHOGENESIS
The etiology of lichen nitidus is unknown.

CLINICAL MANIFESTATIONS
This chronic, benign, papular eruption is characterized by minute (1-2 mm), flat-topped, shiny, firm papules of uniform size. The papules are most often skin-colored but may be pink or red. In black individuals, they are usually hypopigmented (Fig. 657-8). Sites of predilection are the genitals, abdomen, chest, forearms, wrists, and inner aspects of the thighs. The lesions may be sparse or numerous and may form large plaques; careful examination usually discloses linear papules in a line of scratch (Koebner phenomenon), a valuable clue to the diagnosis because it occurs in only a few diseases. Lichen nitidus occurs in all age groups. The cause is unknown. Patients with lichen nitidus are usually asymptomatic and constitutionally well, although pruritus may be severe. The lesions may be confused with those of lichen planus, and lichen nitidus can rarely occur concurrently with lichen planus.

DIFFERENTIAL DIAGNOSIS
Widespread keratosis pilaris can also be confused with lichen nitidus, but the follicular localization of the papules and the absence of Koebner phenomenon in the former distinguish them. Verruca plana (flat warts), if small and uniform in size, may occasionally resemble lichen nitidus.

HISTOLOGY
Although the diagnosis can be made clinically, a biopsy is occasionally indicated. The lichen nitidus papule consists of sharply circumscribed nests of lymphocytes and histiocytes in the upper dermis enclosed by claw-like epidermal rete ridges.

TREATMENT
The course of lichen nitidus spans months to years, but the lesions eventually involute completely. No treatment is necessary, but mid- to high-potency topical steroids may be used for pruritus.

Bibliography is available at Expert Consult.

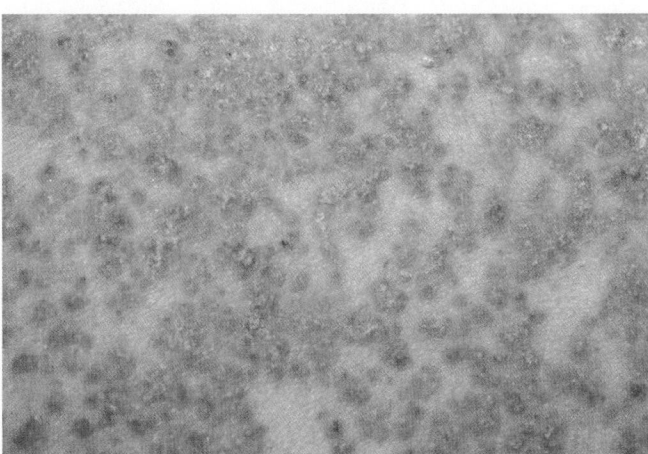

Figure 657-7 Papules coalescing into large plaque on the back of a patient with Darier disease.

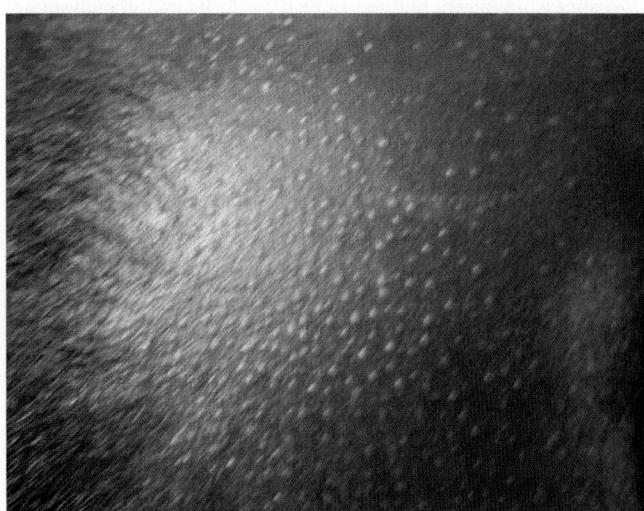

Figure 657-8 Slightly hypopigmented, uniform papules of lichen nitidus.

657.9 Lichen Striatus

Brianne Z. Dickey and Yvonne E. Chiu

ETIOLOGY/PATHOGENESIS

Lichen striatus is hypothesized to be caused by a combination of genetic predisposition present in a mosaic manner (following the lines of Blaschko) and an infectious trigger.

CLINICAL MANIFESTATIONS

A benign, self-limited eruption, lichen striatus consists of a continuous or discontinuous linear band of papules in a Blaschkoid distribution. The primary lesion is a flat-topped, hypopigmented or pink papule covered with fine scale. Aggregates of these papules form multiple bands or plaques. The papules are gradually replaced by hypopigmented macules, which may be the presenting lesion in some cases. The eruption evolves over a period of days or weeks in an otherwise healthy child, remains stationary for weeks to months, and finally remits without sequelae usually within 2 yr. Symptoms are usually absent, although some children complain of itching. Nail dystrophy may occur when the eruption involves the proximal nail fold and matrix (Fig. 657-9).

DIFFERENTIAL DIAGNOSIS

Lichen striatus is occasionally confused with other disorders. The initial plaque may resemble papular eczema or lichen nitidus until the linear configuration becomes apparent. Linear lichen planus and linear psoriasis are usually associated with typical individual lesions elsewhere on the body. Linear epidermal nevi are permanent lesions that often become more hyperkeratotic and hyperpigmented than those of lichen striatus.

TREATMENT

Treatment is not necessary and generally not very effective. A low-potency topical corticosteroid preparation can be used when pruritus is a problem in a patient with lichen striatus.

Bibliography is available at Expert Consult.

657.10 Lichen Planus

Brianne Z. Dickey and Yvonne E. Chiu

ETIOLOGY/PATHOGENESIS

Lichen planus is the result of an attack on the skin by cytotoxic T cells. The cause is unknown, but granzyme B, perforin, and granulysin are markedly increased in skin involved with lichen planus. A genetic predisposition may exist, and other proposed triggers include metal exposure, certain medications, liver disease, vaccinations (especially hepatitis B vaccination), and infections (especially hepatitis C virus).

CLINICAL MANIFESTATIONS

This is a rare disorder in young children and uncommon in older ones. It is more often seen in children from the Indian subcontinent and of African-American background. The classic form of lichen planus is the most common subtype in children, often exhibiting an acute eruptive onset. The lesions erupt in an explosive fashion, much like a viral exanthem, and spread to involve most of the body surface. The primary lesion is a violaceous, sharply demarcated, polygonal papule with fine white lines (Wickham's striae) or scale on the surface. Papules may coalesce to form large plaques (Fig. 657-10). The papules are intensely pruritic, and additional papules are often induced by scratching (Koebner phenomenon) so that lines of them are detected. Sites of predilection are the flexor surfaces of the wrists, the forearms, the inner aspects of the thighs, and the ankles.

Hypertrophic, linear, bullous, atrophic, annular, follicular, erosive, ulcerative, and actinic forms of lichen planus may also occur in children. Characteristic lesions of mucous membranes consist of pinhead-size white papules that coalesce to form reticulated and lacy patterns on the buccal mucosa. Erosive ulcers are also common in the oral mucosa, and may also involve the gastrointestinal tract. Nail involvement causes nail dystrophy. The disorder may persist for months to years, but the acute eruptive form is most likely to involute permanently. Self-resolution eventually occurs. Intense hyperpigmentation frequently persists for a long time after the resolution of lesions.

HISTOLOGY

The histopathologic findings in lichen planus are specific, consisting of hyperkeratosis, irregular acanthosis, wedge-shaped hypergranulosis, apoptotic keratinocytes in the lower epidermis and upper dermis, and basal cell degeneration with a bandlike lymphocytic infiltrate at the epidermal-dermal junction. Pigment incontinence is frequently seen. Biopsy is indicated if the diagnosis is unclear.

TREATMENT

Treatment is directed at alleviation of the intense pruritus and amelioration of the skin lesions. First-line treatment with a high-potency topical corticosteroid applied twice daily is effective for localized disease on the trunk or extremities; lesions on the face and genitals may be treated with low- to mid-potency corticosteroids. Alternatives to topical steroids include topical calcineurin inhibitors or vitamin D analogs. Thick lesions may require intralesional corticosteroid injection. Oral antihistamines (hydroxyzine) are often added for the

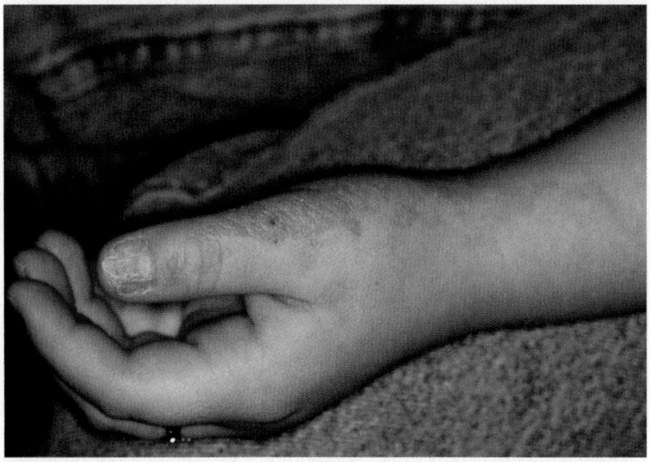

Figure 657-9 Lichen striatus with nail dystrophy.

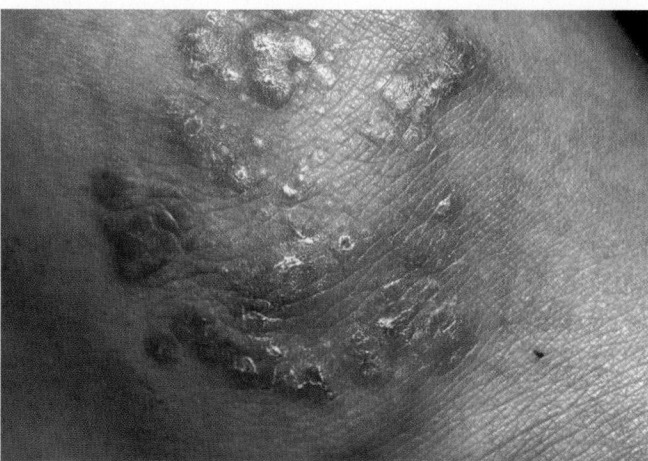

Figure 657-10 Flat-topped, purple polygonal papules of lichen planus.

pruritus. A short course of systemic glucocorticoids or phototherapy (NB-UVB) are used as second-line approaches for rare cases of widespread, intractable lesions. Other medications with efficacy include oral retinoids (acitretin), dapsone, metronidazole, griseofulvin, and methotrexate.

Bibliography is available at Expert Consult.

657.11 Porokeratosis
Brianne Z. Dickey and Yvonne E. Chiu

ETIOLOGY/PATHOGENESIS
Porokeratosis is a disorder of epidermal keratinization. The etiology is unknown except for the disseminated actinic form, which is secondary to chronic sun exposure. Genetic susceptibility, with autosomal dominant transmission, and immunosuppression may also be involved.

CLINICAL MANIFESTATIONS
Porokeratosis is a rare, chronic, progressive disease of keratinization. The prototypical lesion is an atrophic papule or plaque with a surrounding ridge of hyperkeratosis, called cornoid lamella. Several forms have been delineated: solitary plaques, linear porokeratosis, hyperkeratotic lesions of the palms and soles, disseminated eruptive lesions, and superficial actinic porokeratosis. **Classic porokeratosis of Mibelli** begins in childhood and is more common in males. Sites of predilection are the limbs, face, genitals, mucous membranes, palms, and soles. The primary lesion is a small, keratotic papule that slowly enlarges peripherally so that the center becomes depressed, with the edge forming an elevated wall or collar (Fig. 657-11). The configuration of the plaque may be round, oval, or gyrate. The elevated border is split by a thin groove from which minute cornified projections protrude. The central atrophic area is yellow, gray, or tan, and sclerotic, smooth, and dry, whereas the hyperkeratotic border is a darker gray, brown, or black. **Linear porokeratosis** is also more common in childhood and typically follows the lines of Blaschko. The disease is slowly progressive but relatively asymptomatic; some patients experience pruritus or pain. Malignant degeneration to **squamous cell carcinoma** has been reported in long-standing cases.

HISTOLOGY
A skin biopsy is usually unnecessary, but will disclose the characteristic cornoid lamella (plug of stratum corneum cells with retained nuclei), which is responsible for the invariable linear ridge of the lesion. The granular layer is absent beneath the cornoid lamella.

DIFFERENTIAL DIAGNOSIS
The differential diagnosis of porokeratosis includes warts, epidermal nevi, lichen planus, granuloma annulare, tinea corporis, nummular eczema, pityriasis rosea, and elastosis perforans serpiginosa.

TREATMENT
No treatment is uniformly successful, thus therapeutic decisions depend largely on lesion size, location, symptoms, and patient preference. Most lesions are asymptomatic and do not require any intervention; however, when treatment is necessary options include pharmacologic management (topical retinoids, topical 5-fluorouracil, topical imiquimod, or oral retinoids [severe cases only]), destructive therapy (liquid nitrogen cryotherapy, electrodessication and curettage, or various lasers), and surgical removal. In general, the less-invasive topical agents should be attempted first. Good sunlight protection should also be encouraged to decrease risk of malignant transformation.

Bibliography is available at Expert Consult.

657.12 Gianotti-Crosti Syndrome (Papular Acrodermatitis)
Brianne Z. Dickey and Yvonne E. Chiu

ETIOLOGY/PATHOGENESIS
The pathogenesis of Gianotti-Crosti syndrome, also known as papular acrodermatitis, is unclear, but an immunologic reaction to viral infections and immunizations has been postulated. Historically, the most common associations are with Epstein-Barr virus, hepatitis B virus (primarily in countries without routine childhood vaccination programs), coxsackievirus A16, and parainfluenza virus, as well as with many childhood immunizations.

CLINICAL MANIFESTATIONS
This distinctive eruption is benign and predominantly occurs in children younger than 5 yr old about 1 wk after a viral illness. Cases are usually sporadic, but epidemics have been recorded. Skin lesions are monomorphic, firm, dusky or coppery red papules ranging in size from 1-10 mm (Fig. 657-12), although there is considerable variation in lesion appearance between patients. The papules often have the appearance of vesicles; when opened, however, no fluid is obtained. The papules sometimes become hemorrhagic. Lines of papules (**Koebner phenomenon**) may be noted on the extremities following minor local

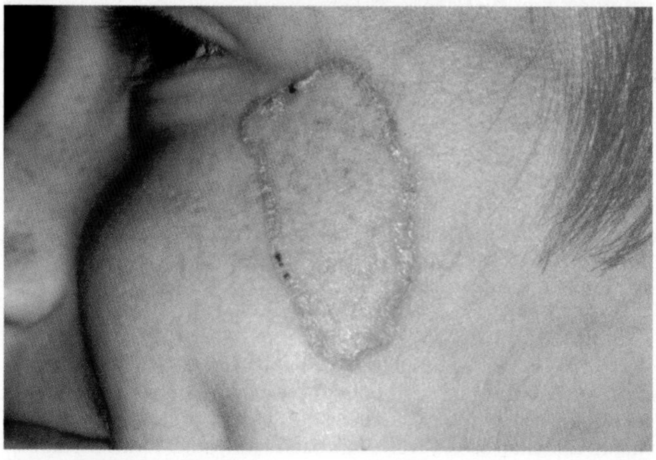

Figure 657-11 Large plaque of porokeratosis of Mibelli with raised border and depressed center.

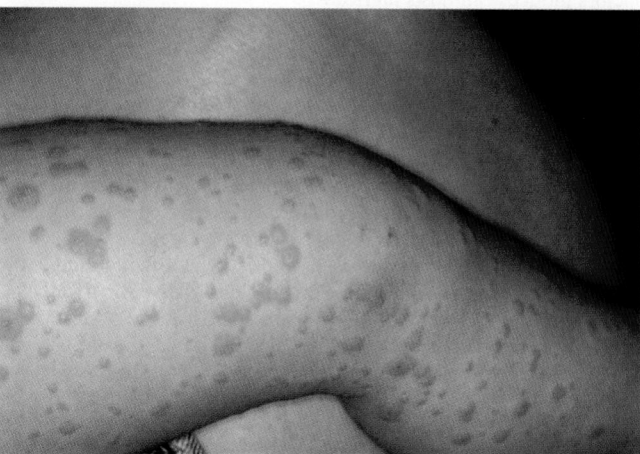

Figure 657-12 Numerous, flat-topped, red papules in Gianotti-Crosti syndrome.

trauma. The papules occur in crops and may become profuse and coalesce into plaques, forming a symmetric eruption on the face, ears, buttocks, and limbs, including the palms and soles. The trunk is relatively spared, as are the scalp and mucous membranes. The eruption is occasionally associated with malaise and low-grade fever but few other constitutional symptoms. Generalized lymphadenopathy and hepatomegaly (in patients with hepatitis B viremia) constitute the only other abnormal physical findings; jaundice is classically absent despite hepatic enzyme elevation. The eruption resolves spontaneously but may take up to 2 mo. Some residual pigment change may occur but not scarring.

HISTOLOGY

Skin biopsy in Gianotti-Crosti syndrome is not specific, being characterized by a dermal perivascular mononuclear cell infiltrate, capillary endothelial swelling, and epidermal spongiosis and parakeratosis.

DIFFERENTIAL DIAGNOSIS

Gianotti-Crosti syndrome can be confused with other viral exanthems, erythema infectiosum, lichen planus, erythema multiforme, and Henoch-Schönlein purpura.

TREATMENT

The lesions are typically asymptomatic and resolve spontaneously, thus requiring no treatment. If present, pruritus may be relieved by emollients or calamine lotion. Mid-potency topical steroids may relieve pruritus but do not alter disease course. Sedating antihistamines at bedtime are also helpful.

Bibliography is available at Expert Consult.

657.13 Acanthosis Nigricans

Brianne Z. Dickey and Yvonne E. Chiu

See also Chapter 47.

ETIOLOGY/PATHOGENESIS

The skin lesions of acanthosis nigricans may be genetic due to mutations in the fibroblast growth factor receptor gene, or acquired as a manifestation of insulin resistance. In familial cases, acanthosis nigricans is inherited as an autosomal dominant trait and develops in infancy. Insulin resistance with compensatory hyperinsulinism may lead to insulin binding to and activation of insulin-like growth factor receptors, promoting epidermal growth. Common causes of insulin resistance in children are obesity and diabetes mellitus, with acanthosis nigricans seen in >60% of children with a body mass index >98%. In the paraneoplastic form (rare in children), tumor-secreted growth factors induce acanthosis nigricans.

CLINICAL MANIFESTATIONS

Acanthosis nigricans is characterized by symmetric, hyperpigmented, velvety, hyperkeratotic plaques with exaggerated skin lines in intertriginous areas. The most common locations are the posterior neck and axillae (Fig. 657-13), but it is also seen in the inframammary areas, groin, inner thighs, and anogenital region. Prior to plaque development, patients notice a "dirty" appearance of affected skin that does not wash clean. Skin lesions remain asymptomatic unless maceration or secondary infection occurs. Acanthosis nigricans is found more commonly in African-American, Hispanic, and Native American children. The clinical severity and histopathologic features of acanthosis nigricans correlate positively with the degree of hyperinsulinism and with the degree of obesity.

HISTOLOGY

The histologic changes are those of papillomatosis and hyperkeratosis rather than acanthosis or excessive pigment formation. A mild dermal inflammatory infiltrate may be present.

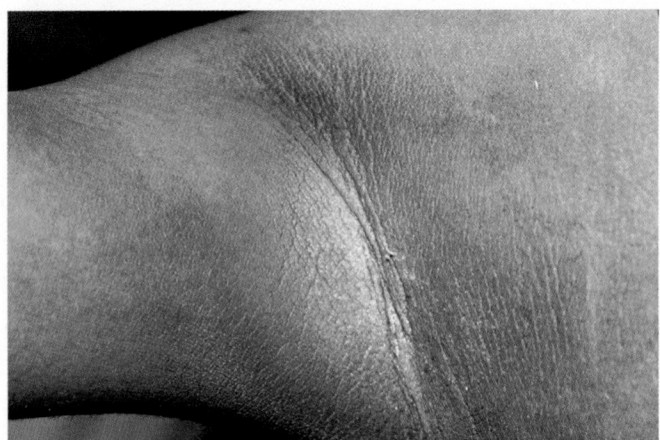

Figure 657-13 Velvety hyperpigmentation of the axilla in acanthosis nigricans.

TREATMENT

Treatment is aimed at palliation of the underlying disorder. Acanthosis nigricans in the obese child is associated with risk factors for glucose homeostasis abnormalities, and counseling families on its causes and consequences may motivate them to make healthy lifestyle changes that can decrease the risk for development of cardiac disease and diabetes mellitus. In children with obesity-related acanthosis nigricans, weight loss should be the primary goal. Appearance of skin lesions responds poorly to local medical management; some patients benefit from topical keratolytic agents (40% urea cream or 12% ammonium lactate cream) and agents that inhibit keratinocyte proliferation (topical vitamin D analogs).

Bibliography is available at Expert Consult.

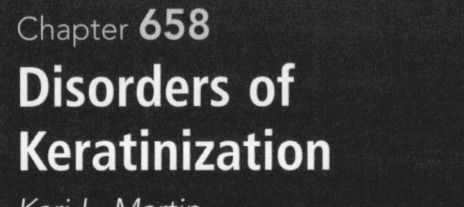

Chapter **658**
Disorders of Keratinization
Kari L. Martin

DISORDERS OF CORNIFICATION

Mendelian disorders of cornification (**ichthyoses**) are a primary group of inherited conditions characterized clinically by patterns of scaling and histopathologically by hyperkeratosis. They are usually distinguishable on the basis of inheritance patterns, clinical features, associated defects, and histopathologic changes (Table 658-1). Much work is currently underway to better categorize the genotype-phenotype correlation of these diseases.

COLLODION BABY

Collodion baby is not a single entity but a newborn phenotype that is most often seen in babies who will eventually demonstrate **lamellar ichthyosis** or congenital **ichthyosiform erythroderma**. Less commonly, collodion babies evolve into babies with other forms of ichthyosis or Gaucher disease. A small subset become otherwise healthy babies without chronic skin disease.

Table 658-1 | Disorders of Cornification That Usually Manifest in the First Weeks of Life

DISORDER	INHERITANCE	CLINICAL FEATURES	MUTATION	VISUAL METHOD OF DIAGNOSIS
Harlequin ichthyosis	AR	Thick, armor-like scale with fissuring	*ABCA12*	Clinical
Collodion baby	Usually AR	Shiny collodion membrane	Various	Clinical
Recessive X-linked ichthyosis	Recessive X-linked	Collodion membrane May have genital anomalies	Steroid sulfatase	Plasma cholesterol sulfate
Lamellar ichthyosis	Usually AR	Collodion membrane	Transglutaminase I *ABCA12* *CYP4F22*	Clinical
Congenital ichthyosiform erythroderma	AR	Collodion membrane	Transglutaminase 1 *ALOX12B* *ALOXE3*	Clinical
Epidermolytic ichthyosis	AD	Scaling and blistering	Keratins 1, 10, 2e	Clinical and histologic
Ichthyosis hystrix	AD	Plaques of hyperkeratosis	Keratin 1, *GJB2*	Clinical
Familial peeling skin	AR	Superficial peeling	Unknown	Clinical and histologic
Sjögren-Larsson syndrome	AR	Variable skin thickening Mental, developmental retardation Spastic diplegia Seizures "Glistening dots"	*FAD*	Clinical and fibroblast cultures for FAD
Neutral lipid storage disease	AR	Collodion membrane or ichthyosiform erythroderma	CGI58	Blood smear for vacuolated polymorphonuclear leukocytes
Netherton syndrome	AR	Ichthyosiform erythroderma	SPINK 5	Clinical; hair exam later in infancy
		Scant hair, often failure to thrive	Unknown	Clinical and hair microscopy; hair sulfur content
Trichothiodystrophy	AR	Collodion membrane Broken hair	XPB XPD	
KID (keratitis with ichthyosis and deafness) syndrome	May be AD, AR	Erythrokeratodermatous or thick, leathery skin with stippled papules	GJB2	Clinical; auditory evoked potentials
CHILD (congenital hemidysplasia with ichthyosiform erythroderma and limb defects) syndrome	X-linked dominant	Alopecia Unilateral waxy yellow, scaling Hemidysplasia Limb defects	NSDHL	Clinical
Conradi-Hünermann syndrome	X-linked dominant	Thick, psoriasiform scale over erythroderma, patterned along Blaschko lines Proximal limb shortening	ARSE	Clinical
Ichthyosis follicularis	Usually X-linked recessive	Prominent follicular hyperkeratoses Alopecia Photophobia	MBTPS2	Clinical
CHIME (colobomas of the eyes, heart defects, ichthyosiform dermatosis, mental retardation, and ear abnormalities) syndrome	AR	Ichthyotic erythematous plaques Cardiac defects; typical facies Retinal colobomas	Unknown	Clinical
Gaucher disease	AR	Collodion membrane Hepatosplenomegaly	β-Glucocerebrosidase	Clinical; fibroblast cultures

AD, autosomal dominant; AR, autosomal recessive.; FAD, fatty aldehyde.
From Eichenfield LF, Frieden IJ, Esterly NB: Textbook of neonatal dermatology, Philadelphia, 2001, WB Saunders, p. 277.

Collodion babies are covered at birth by a thick, taut membrane resembling oiled parchment or collodion (Fig. 658-1), which is subsequently shed. Affected neonates have ectropion, flattening of the ears and nose, and fixation of the lips in an O-shaped configuration. Hair may be absent or may perforate the abnormal covering. The membrane cracks with initial respiratory efforts and, shortly after birth, begins to desquamate in large sheets. A high-humidity environment and application of nonocclusive lubricants facilitates shedding of the membrane. Complete shedding may take several weeks, and a new membrane may occasionally form in localized areas.

Neonatal morbidity and mortality may be due to cutaneous infection, aspiration pneumonia (squamous material), hypothermia, or hypernatremic dehydration from excessive transcutaneous fluid losses as a result of increased skin permeability. The outcome is uncertain,

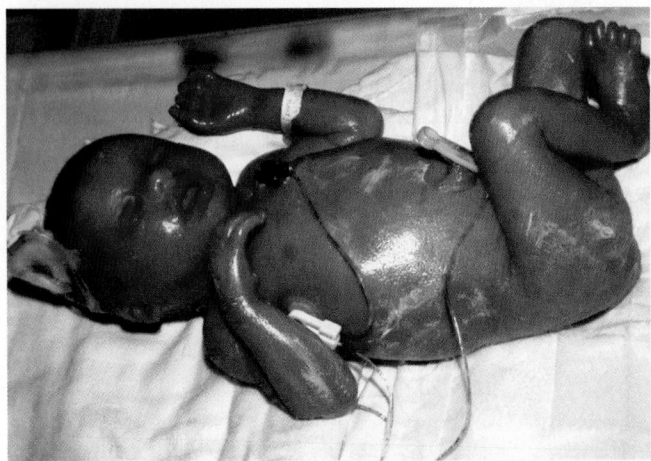

Figure 658-1 Typical appearance of a collodion baby.

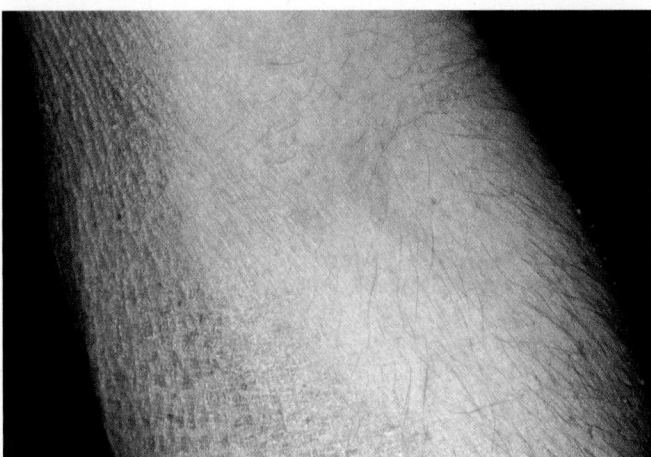

Figure 658-3 Sparing of the antecubital fossa in X-linked ichthyosis.

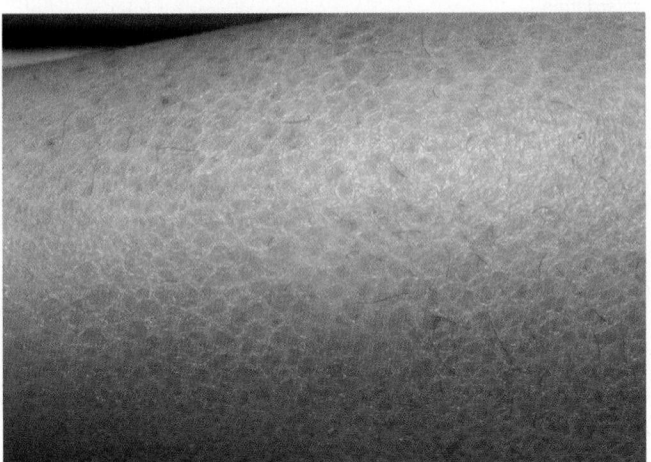

Figure 658-2 Scale over the shin in ichthyosis vulgaris.

and accurate prognosis depends on identification of the underlying ichthyosis.

COMMON ICHTHYOSES
Ichthyosis Vulgaris
Etiology/Pathogenesis
Autosomal dominant or recessive mutations in the filaggrin gene cause ichthyosis vulgaris (IV). Filaggrin is a filament-aggregating protein that assembles the keratin filament cytoskeleton, causing collapse of the granular cells into classic flattened squamous cell shape. Mutations in filaggrin lead to absence or marked reductions in keratohyalin granules.

Clinical Manifestations
IV is the **most common** of the disorders of keratinization, with an incidence of 1/250 live births. Onset generally occurs in the 1st yr of life. In most cases, it is trivial, consisting only of slight roughening of the skin surface. Scaling is most prominent on the extensor aspects of the extremities, particularly the legs (Fig. 658-2). Flexural surfaces are spared, and the abdomen, neck, and face are relatively uninvolved. **Keratosis pilaris**, particularly on the upper arms and thighs, accentuated markings, and hyperkeratosis on the palms and soles, and atopy are relatively common. Scaling is most pronounced during the winter mo and may abate completely during warm weather. There is no accompanying disorder of hair, teeth, mucosal surfaces, or other organ systems.

Treatment
Scaling may be diminished by daily applications of an emollient or a lubricant containing urea (10-40%), salicylic acid, or an α-hydroxy acid such as lactic acid (5-12%).

X-Linked Ichthyosis
Etiology/Pathogenesis
X-linked ichthyosis (XLI) involves a deficiency of steroid sulfatase, which hydrolyzes cholesterol sulfate and other sulfated steroids to cholesterol. Cholesterol sulfate accumulates in the stratum corneum and plasma. In the epidermis this accumulation causes malformation of intercellular lipid layers, leading to barrier defects and delay of corneodesmosome degradation, resulting in corneocyte retention.

Clinical Manifestations
Skin peeling may be present at birth but typically begins at 3-6 mo of life. Scaling is most pronounced on the sides of the neck, lower face, preauricular areas, anterior trunk, and the limbs, particularly the legs. The elbow (Fig. 658-3) and knee flexures are generally spared but may be mildly involved. The palms and soles may be slightly thickened but are also usually spared. The condition gradually worsens in severity and extent. Keratosis pilaris is not present, and there is no increased incidence of atopy. Deep corneal opacities that do not interfere with vision develop in late childhood or adolescence and are a useful marker for the disease because they may also be present in carrier females. Some patients have larger deletions on the X chromosome that encompass neighboring genes, generating *contiguous gene deletion syndromes*. These include **Kallmann syndrome** (*KAL1* gene), which consists of hypogonadotrophic hypogonadism and anosmia, **X-linked chondroplasia punctata** (*ARSE* gene), **short stature,** and **ocular albinism.** The rate of testicular cancer may be increased in patients with coexistent Kallmann syndrome. There is also an increased risk of attention deficit hyperactivity disorder and autism owing to a contiguous gene defect in neuroligin 4.

Reduced steroid sulfatase enzyme activity can be detected in fibroblasts, keratinocytes, and leukocytes and, prenatally, in amniocytes or chorionic villus cells. In affected families, an affected male can be detected by restriction enzyme analysis of cultured chorionic villus cell DNA or amniocytes or by in situ hybridization, which identifies steroid sulfatase gene deletions prenatally in chorionic villus cells. A placental steroid sulfatase deficiency in carrier mothers may result in low urinary and serum estriol values, prolonged labor, and insensitivity of the uterus to oxytocin and prostaglandins.

Treatment
Daily application of emollients and a urea-containing lubricant (10-40%) is usually effective. Glycolic or lactic acid (5-12%) in an

emollient base and propylene glycol (40-60%) in water with occlusion overnight are alternative forms of therapy.

AUTOSOMAL RECESSIVE CONGENITAL ICHTHYOSES (ARCI)
Harlequin Ichthyosis
Etiology/Pathogenesis
Harlequin ichthyosis (HI) is caused by mutations in the *ABCA12* gene. Mutation in the gene leads to defective lipid transport and *ABCA12* activity is required for the generation of long-chain ceramides that are essential for the development of the normal skin barrier.

Clinical Manifestations
At birth, markedly thickened, ridged, and cracked skin forms horny plates over the entire body, disfiguring the facial features and constricting the digits. Severe ectropion and chemosis obscure the orbits, the nose and ears are flattened, and the lips are everted and gaping. Nails and hair may be absent. Joint mobility is restricted, and the hands and feet appear fixed and ischemic. Affected neonates have respiratory difficulty, suck poorly, and are subject to severe cutaneous infection. HI used to be uniformly fatal in the neonatal period, but with the use of oral retinoids, more patients survive (~80%) beyond infancy and have severe ichthyosis usually resembling lamellar ichthyosis or nonbullous congenital ichthyosiform erythroderma as adolescents and adults. Those with a compound heterozygous genotype have a better prognosis.

Treatment
Initial treatment includes high fluid intake to avoid dehydration from transepidermal water loss and use of a humidified heated incubator, emulsifying ointments, careful attention to hygiene, and oral retinoids (1 mg/kg/day). Prenatal diagnosis has been accomplished by fetoscopy, fetal skin biopsy, and microscopic examination of cells from amniotic fluid.

Lamellar Ichthyosis and Congenital Ichthyosiform Erythroderma (Nonbullous Congenital Ichthyosiform Erythroderma)
Lamellar ichthyosis (LI) and congenital ichthyosiform erythroderma (CIE; nonbullous congenital ichthyosiform erythroderma; non-HI ARCI) are the most common types of autosomal recessively inherited ichthyosis. Both forms are present at or shortly after birth. Most infants with these forms of ichthyosis present with erythroderma and scaling; but among collodion babies, most turn out to have one of these ichthyosis variants.

Etiology/Pathogenesis
Six genes have been identified that cause non-HI ARCI: *TGM* (the gene encoding transglutaminase), *ABCA12*, *NIPAL4* (also known as *ICHTHYIN*), *CYP4F22*, and the lipoxygenase genes *ALOX12B* and *ALOX3*. Transglutaminase mutations lead to abnormalities in the cornified envelope, whereas defects in *ABCA12* cause abnormal lipid transport and those in *CYP4F22* produce abnormal lamellar granules. The lipoxygenases are likely to play a role in epidermal barrier formation by affecting lipid metabolism.

Clinical Manifestations
After shedding of the collodion membrane, if present, lamellar ichthyosis evolves into large, quadrilateral, dark scales that are free at the edges and adherent at the center. Scaling is often pronounced and involves the entire body surface, including flexural surfaces (Fig. 658-4). The face is often markedly involved, including ectropion and small, crumpled ears. The palms and soles are generally hyperkeratotic. The hair may be sparse and fine, but the teeth and mucosal surfaces are normal. Unlike in congenital ichthyosiform erythroderma, there is little erythema.

In congenital ichthyosiform erythroderma, erythroderma tends to be persistent, and scales, although they are generalized, are finer and whiter than in lamellar ichthyosis (Fig. 658-5). Hyperkeratosis is

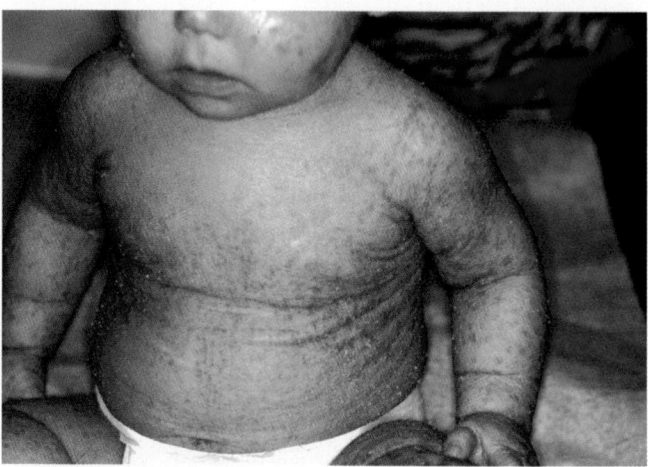

Figure 658-4 Generalized scaling of lamellar ichthyosis.

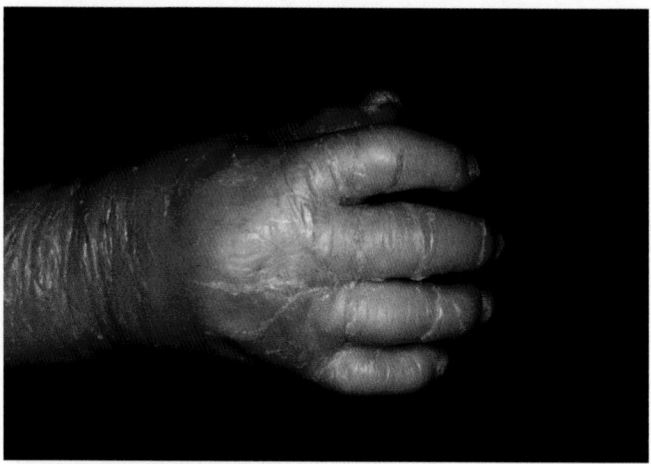

Figure 658-5 Prominent erythema and scale in congenital ichthyosiform erythroderma.

particularly noticeable around the knees, elbows, and ankles. Palms and soles are uniformly hyperkeratotic. Patients have sparse hair, cicatricial alopecia, and nail dystrophy. Neither form includes blistering.

Treatment
Pruritus may be severe and responds minimally to antipruritic therapy. The unattractive appearance of the child and the bad odor from bacterial colonization of macerated scales may create serious psychologic problems. A high-humidity environment in winter and air conditioning in summer reduce discomfort. Generous and frequent applications of emollients and keratolytic agents such as lactic or glycolic acid (5-12%), urea (10-40%), tazarotene (0.1% gel), and retinoic acid (0.1% cream) may lessen the scaling to some extent, although these agents produce stinging if applied to fissured skin. Oral retinoids (1 mg/kg/day) have a beneficial effect in these conditions but do not alter the underlying defect and, therefore, must be administered indefinitely. The long-term risks of these compounds (teratogenic effects and toxicity to bone) may limit their usefulness. Ectropion requires ophthalmologic care and, at times, plastic surgical procedures.

KERATINOPATHIC ICHTHYOSES
Epidermolytic Ichthyosis (Bullous Congenital Ichthyosiform Erythroderma; Epidermolytic Hyperkeratosis)
Etiology/Pathogenesis
Epidermolytic ichthyosis (EI) is an autosomal dominant trait that has been shown to be due to defects in either keratin 1 or keratin 10. These

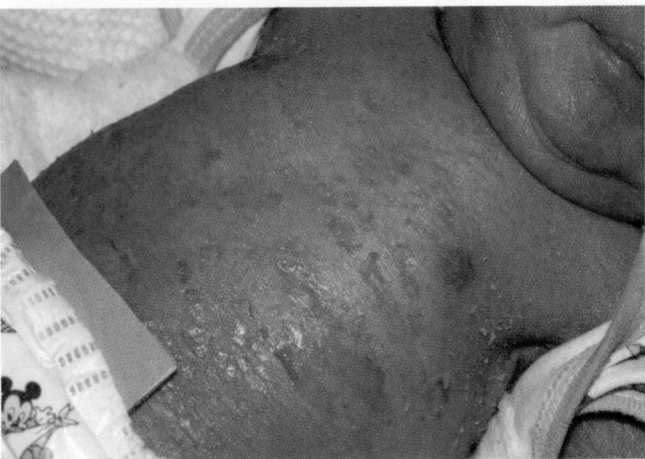

Figure 658-6 Superficial erosions and hyperkeratosis in epidermolytic hyperkeratosis.

keratins are required to form the keratin-intermediate filaments in cells of the suprabasilar layers of the epidermis.

Clinical Manifestations

The clinical manifestations are initially characterized by the onset at birth of widespread blisters and erosions on a background of generalized erythroderma (Fig. 658-6). Recurrent blistering may be widespread in neonates and may cause diagnostic confusion with other blistering disorders. With time, the blister formation ceases, erythema decreases, and generalized hyperkeratosis develops. The scales are small, hard, and verrucous. Distinctive, parallel hyperkeratotic ridges develop over the joint flexures, including the axillary, popliteal, and antecubital fossae, and on the neck and hips. **Palmoplantar keratoderma** is associated with keratin 1 defects. The hair, nails, mucosa, and sweat glands are normal. Malodorous secondary bacterial infection is common and requires appropriate antibiotic therapy.

Histopathology

The histopathology is diagnostic of EI, consisting of hyperkeratosis, degeneration of the epidermal granular layer with an increased number of keratohyalin granules, clear spaces around nuclei, and indistinct cellular boundaries of cells in the upper epidermis. On electron microscopic examination, keratin-intermediate filaments are clumped, and many desmosomes are attached to only one keratinocyte instead of connecting neighboring keratinocytes. Localized forms of the disease may resemble epidermal nevi or keratoderma of the palms and soles but share the distinctive histopathologic changes of EI.

Treatment

Treatment of EI is difficult. Morbidity is increased in the neonatal period as a result of prematurity, sepsis, and fluid and electrolyte imbalance. Bacterial colonization of macerated scales produces a distinctive bad odor that can be controlled somewhat by use of an antibacterial cleanser. Intermittent oral antibiotics are generally necessary. Keratolytic agents are often poorly tolerated. Oral retinoids (1 mg/kg/day) may produce significant improvement. Prenatal diagnosis for affected families is possible by examination of DNA extracts from chorionic villus cells or amniocytes, provided that the specific mutation in the affected parent is known.

OTHER NONSYNDROMIC ICHTHYOSES
Erythrokeratoderma Variabilis
Etiology/Pathogenesis

An autosomal dominant disorder, erythrokeratoderma variabilis (EKV) is caused by mutations in connexins 31 and 30.3. Connexins are proteins that form gap junctions between cells that allow for transport and signaling between neighboring epidermal cells.

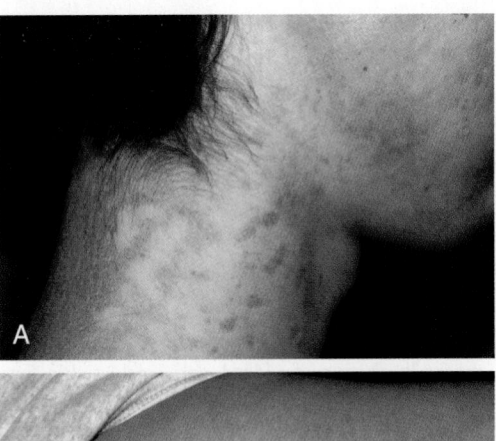

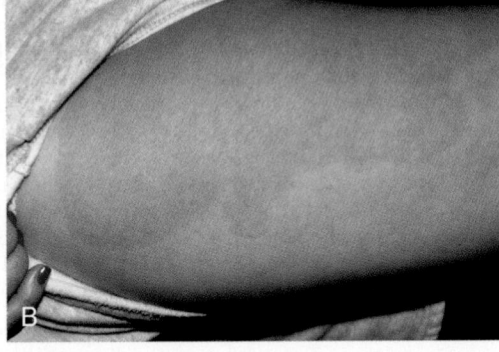

Figure 658-7 Erythrokeratoderma variabilis. **A,** Fixed, hyperkeratotic plaques, **B,** Migratory, erythematous lesion.

Clinical Manifestations

EKV usually manifests in the early mo of life, progresses in childhood, and stabilizes in adolescence. It is characterized by two distinctive manifestations: sharply demarcated, hyperkeratotic plaques (Fig. 658-7A) and transient figurate erythema (Fig. 658-7B). The distribution is generalized but sparse; sites of predilection are the face, buttocks, axillae, and extensor surfaces of the limbs. The palms and soles may be thickened, but hair, teeth, and nails are normal.

Treatment

There are case reports that topical tazarotene gel 0.1% and oral retinoids (1 mg/kg/day) are effective for treatment of EKV.

Symmetric Progressive Erythrokeratoderma
Etiology/Pathogenesis

Symmetric progressive erythrokeratoderma is an autosomal dominant disorder caused by mutations in the gene encoding loricrin. Loricrin is a major component of the epidermal cornified cell envelope.

Clinical Manifestations

The disorder manifests in childhood as large, fixed, geographic and symmetric, fine, scaling, hyperkeratotic, erythematous plaques primarily on the extremities, buttocks, face, ankles, and wrists. The primary feature distinguishing this disorder from EKV is the lack of variable erythema seen in the latter condition.

Treatment

Symmetric progressive erythrokeratoderma is a very rare disorder, but reports of response to topical and oral retinoids (1 mg/kg/day) exist.

SYNDROMIC ICHTHYOSES
Sjögren-Larsson Syndrome
Etiology/Pathogenesis

The autosomal recessive inborn error of metabolism known as Sjögren-Larsson syndrome is an abnormality of fatty alcohol oxidation that results from a deficiency of fatty aldehyde dehydrogenase (*FALDH3A2*), a component of the fatty alcohol–nicotinamide adenine dinucleotide oxidoreductase enzyme complex.

hands and feet, elbows, and knees later in childhood. The PPK may be either diffuse, striate, or punctuate. This syndrome is characterized by periodontal inflammation, leading to loss of teeth by age 4-5 yr if untreated.

Other Syndromes

Keratoderma of palms and soles also occurs as a feature of some forms of ichthyosis and ectodermal dysplasia. **Richner-Hanhart syndrome** is an autosomal recessive focal palmoplantar keratoderma with corneal ulcers, progressive mental impairment, and a deficiency of tyrosine aminotransferase, which leads to tyrosinemia. **Pachyonychia congenita** is transmitted as an autosomal dominant trait with variable expressivity. The classic type I form (**Jadassohn-Lewandowski syndrome**) is due to mutations in the gene for keratin 16. Major features of the syndrome are onychogryposis; palmoplantar keratoderma; follicular hyperkeratosis, especially of the elbows and knees; and oral leukokeratosis. The nail dystrophy is the most striking feature and may be present at birth or develop early in life. The nails are thickened and tubular, projecting upward at the free edge to form a conical roof over a mass of subungual keratotic debris. Repeated paronychial inflammation may result in shedding of the nails. The feature seen most consistently among patients with this condition is keratoderma of the palms and soles. Additional associated features include hyperhidrosis of the palms and soles, and bullae and erosions on the palms and soles. Some patients have shown a selective cell-mediated defect in recognition and processing of *Candida*. Surgical removal of the nails and excision of the nail matrix have been helpful in some patients.

Treatment

Treatment for PPK is the same no matter what its cause. In mild cases, emollient therapy may suffice. Keratolytic agents such as salicylic acid, lactic acid, and urea creams may be required. Oral retinoids are the treatment of choice for severe cases unresponsive to topical therapy.

Bibliography is available at Expert Consult.

Chapter 659
Diseases of the Dermis
Sheila S. Galbraith

KELOID
Etiology and Pathogenesis

Keloids are usually induced by trauma and commonly follow ear piercing, burns, scalds, and surgical procedures. The resulting keloid is larger than the initial area of trauma to the skin. Certain individuals are predisposed to keloid formation; a familial tendency (recessive or dominant inheritance) or the presence of foreign material in the wound may have a pathogenic role. *Keloids are a rare feature of Ehlers-Danlos syndrome, Rubinstein-Taybi syndrome*, and pachydermoperiostosis. Keloids result from an abnormal fibrous wound healing response in which tissue repair and regeneration–regulation control mechanisms are lost. Collagen production is 20 times that seen in normal scars and the type I : type III collagen ratio is abnormally high. In keloids, tissue values of tumor growth factor-β and platelet-derived growth factor are elevated; fibroblasts are more sensitive to their effects, and their degradation rate is decreased.

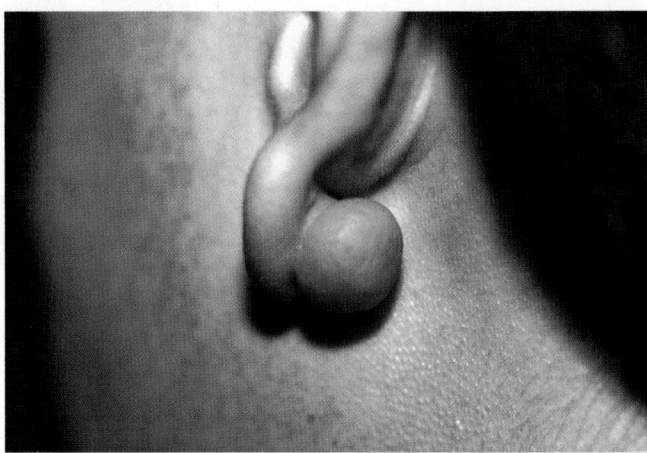

Figure 659-1 Keloid of earlobe after piercing.

Clinical Manifestations

A *keloid* is a sharply demarcated, benign, dense growth of connective tissue that forms in the dermis after trauma. The lesions are firm, raised, pink to hyperpigmented, and rubbery; they may be tender or pruritic. Sites of predilection are the face, earlobes (Fig. 659-1), neck, shoulders, upper trunk, sternum, and lower legs. In both keloids and hypertrophic scars, new collagen forms over a much longer period than in wounds that heal normally.

Histology

A keloid consists of whorled and interlaced hyalinized collagen fibers.

Differential Diagnosis

Keloids should be differentiated from *hypertrophic scars*, which remain confined to the site of injury and gradually involute over time.

Treatment

Young keloids may diminish in size if injected intralesionally at 4 wk intervals with triamcinolone suspension (10-40 mg/mL). At times, a more concentrated suspension is required. Large or old keloids may require surgical excision followed by intralesional injections of corticosteroid. The risk of recurrence at the same site argues against surgical excision alone, although earlobe keloids respond well to surgical excision, pressure dressings, and intralesional steroids. Placement of topical silicone gel sheeting over the keloid for several hours per day for several weeks may help in some patients.

STRIAE CUTIS DISTENSAE (STRETCH MARKS)
Etiology and Pathogenesis

Striae formation is common in adolescence. The most frequent causes are rapid growth, pregnancy, obesity, Cushing disease, and prolonged corticosteroid therapy. The pathogenesis is unknown, but the occurrence of alterations in elastic fibers is thought to be the primary process.

Clinical Manifestations

These thinned, depressed, erythematous bands of atrophic skin eventually become silvery, opalescent, and smooth. They occur most frequently in areas that have been subject to distention, such as the lower back (Fig. 659-2), buttocks, thighs, breasts, abdomen, and shoulders.

Differential Diagnosis

Striae distensae resemble atrophic scars.

Treatment

Controlled trials of treatments for striae are lacking; however, striae tend to spontaneously become less conspicuous as the color fades with time.

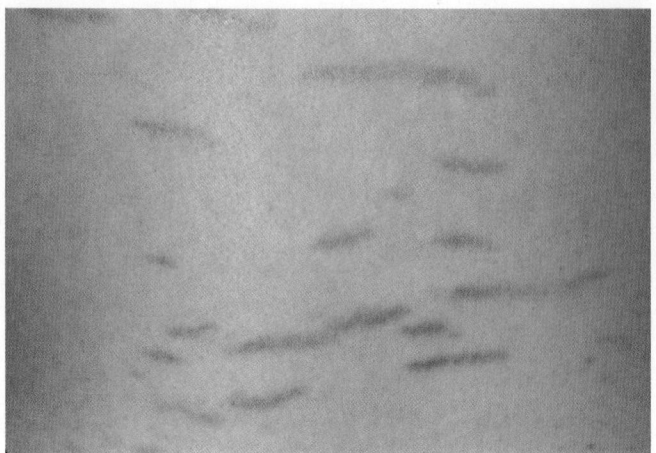

Figure 659-2 Striae on the back of an adolescent.

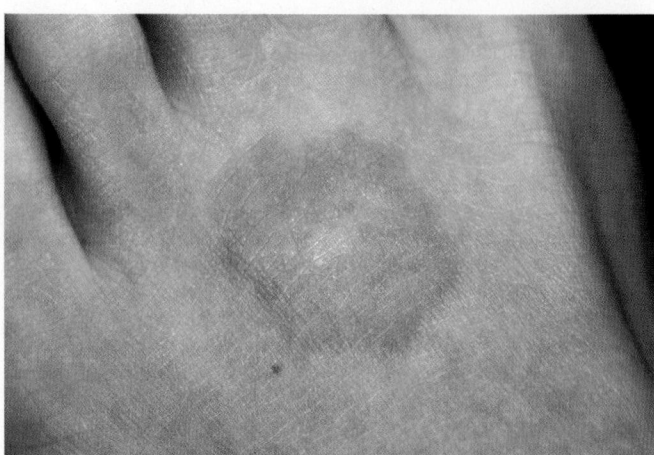

Figure 659-3 Annular lesion with a raised papular border and depressed center, characteristic of granuloma annulare.

CORTICOSTEROID-INDUCED ATROPHY
Etiology and Pathogenesis
Both topical and systemic corticosteroid treatment can result in cutaneous atrophy. This is particularly common when a potent or superpotent topical corticosteroid is applied under occlusion or to an intertriginous area for a prolonged period. Keratinocyte growth is decreased, but epidermal maturation is accelerated, resulting in a thinning of the epidermis and stratum corneum. Fibroblast growth and function are also decreased, leading to the dermal changes. The mechanism involves inhibition of synthesis of collagen type I, noncollagenous proteins, and total protein content of the skin, along with progressive reduction of dermal proteoglycans and glycosaminoglycans.

Clinical Manifestations
Affected skin is thin, fragile, smooth, and semitransparent, with telangiectasias, prominent veins, and loss of normal skin markings.

Histology
Histopathologically, one sees thinning of the epidermis. Spaces between dermal collagen and elastic fibers are small, producing a more compact but thin dermis.

Treatment
Optimal treatment is prevention by proper use of topical steroids to avoid side effects.

GRANULOMA ANNULARE
Etiology and Pathogenesis
The cause of granuloma annulare is unknown. Some cases of granuloma annulare, particularly the generalized form, may be associated with diabetes mellitus or with anterior uveitis. However, most cases are seen in healthy children.

Clinical Manifestations
This common dermatosis occurs predominantly in children and young adults. Affected children are usually healthy. Typical lesions begin as firm, smooth, erythematous papules. They gradually enlarge to form annular plaques with a papular border and a normal, slightly atrophic or discolored central area up to several centimeters in size. Lesions may occur anywhere on the body, but mucous membranes are spared. Favored sites include the dorsum of the hands (Fig. 659-3) and feet. The disseminated papular form is rare in children. Subcutaneous granuloma annulare tends to develop on the scalp and limbs, particularly in the pretibial area. These lesions are firm, usually nontender, skin-colored nodules. Perforating granuloma annulare is characterized by the development of a yellowish center in some of the superficial papular lesions as a result of transepidermal elimination of altered collagen.

Differential Diagnosis
Annular lesions are often mistaken for tinea corporis because of the elevated advancing border. They differ in that they are not scaly. Papular lesions, another variant, may simulate rheumatoid nodules, particularly when grouped on the fingers and elbows.

Histology
The lesion of granuloma annulare consists of a granuloma with a central area of necrotic collagen; mucin deposition; and a peripheral palisading infiltrate of lymphocytes, histiocytes, and foreign body giant cells. The pattern resembles that of necrobiosis lipoidica and rheumatoid nodule, but subtle histologic differences usually permit differentiation.

Treatment
The eruption persists for months to years, but spontaneous resolution without residual change is usual; 50% of lesions clear within 2 yr. Application of a potent or superpotent topical corticosteroid preparation or intralesional injections (5-10 mg/mL) of corticosteroid may hasten involution, but nonintervention is usual.

NECROBIOSIS LIPOIDICA
Etiology and Pathogenesis
The cause of necrobiosis lipoidica is unknown, but 50-75% of patients have **diabetes mellitus**; necrobiosis lipoidica occurs in 0.3% of all diabetic patients.

Clinical Manifestations
This disorder manifests as erythematous papules that evolve into irregularly shaped, sharply demarcated, yellow, sclerotic plaques with central telangiectasia and a violaceous border. Scaling, crusting, and ulceration are frequent. Lesions develop most commonly on the shins (Fig. 659-4). Slow extension of a given lesion over the years is usual, but long periods of quiescence or complete healing with scarring may occur.

Histology
Poorly defined areas of necrobiotic collagen are seen throughout, but primarily low in the dermis, associated with mucin deposition. Surrounding the necrobiotic, disordered areas of collagen is a palisading lymphohistiocytic granulomatous infiltrate. Some lesions are more characteristically granulomatous, with limited necrobiosis of collagen.

Differential Diagnosis
Necrobiosis lipoidica must be differentiated clinically from xanthomas, morphea, granuloma annulare, erythema nodosum, and pretibial myxedema.

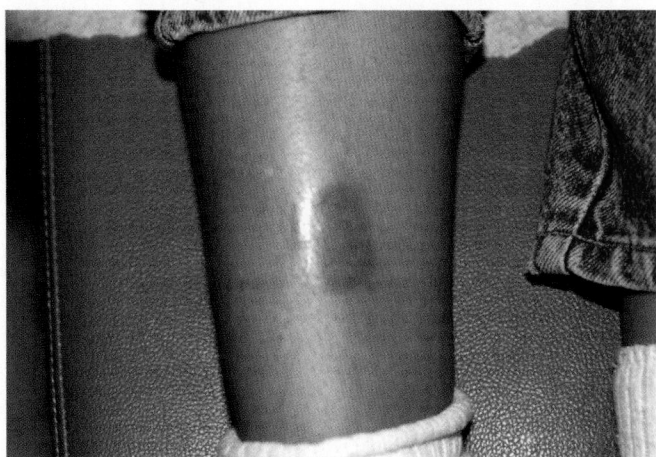

Figure 659-4 Yellow sclerotic plaque of necrobiosis lipoidica on the shin.

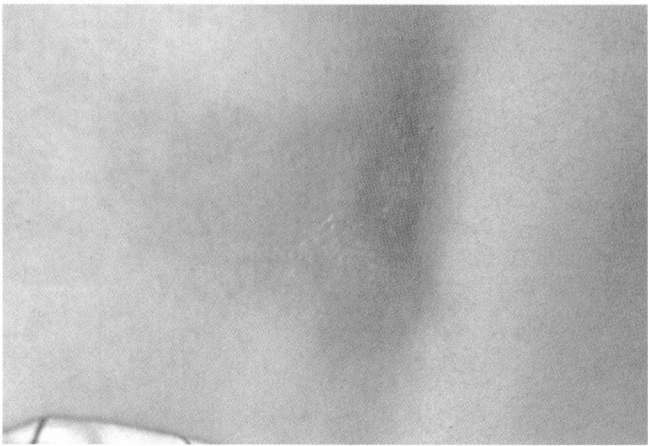

Figure 659-6 Erythematous, hyperpigmented plaque of early morphea.

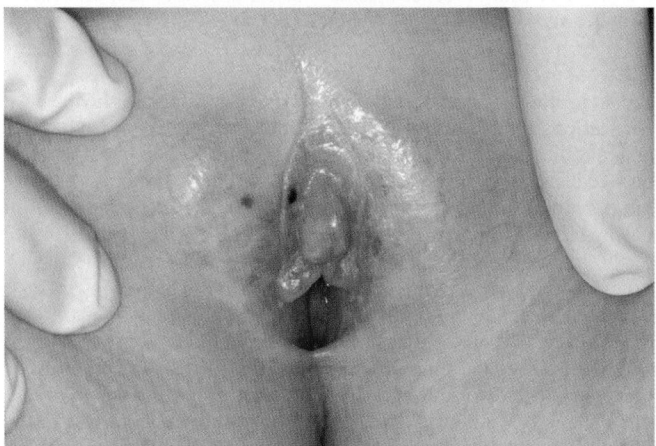

Figure 659-5 Ivory-colored perivaginal plaque with hemorrhage.

the neck, the axillae, the flexor surfaces of wrists, and the areas around the umbilicus and the eyes. Pruritus may be severe.

Differential Diagnosis
In children, lichen sclerosus is most frequently confused with focal morphea (see Chapter 160), with which it may coexist. In the genital area, it may be mistakenly attributed to sexual abuse.

Histology
Biopsy is diagnostic, revealing hyperkeratosis with follicular plugging, hydropic degeneration of basal cells, a bandlike dermal lymphocytic infiltrate, homogenized collagen, and thinned elastic fibers in the upper dermis.

Treatment
Vulvar lichen sclerosus in childhood usually improves with puberty but does not always resolve completely, and symptoms can recur throughout life. Long-term observation for the development of squamous cell carcinoma is necessary. Superpotent topical corticosteroids provide relief from pruritus and produce clearing of lesions, including those in the genital area. Topical tacrolimus and pimecrolimus have also been used. It is not known how response to treatment affects long-term cancer risk.

MORPHEA
Etiology and Pathogenesis
Morphea is a sclerosing condition of the dermis and subcutaneous tissue of unknown etiology.

Clinical Manifestations
Morphea is characterized by solitary, multiple, or linear circumscribed areas of erythema that evolve into indurated, sclerotic, atrophic plaques (Fig. 659-6), later healing, or "burning out" with pigment change. It is seen more commonly in females. The most common types of morphea are plaque and linear. Morphea can affect any area of skin. When confined to the frontal scalp, forehead, and midface in a linear band, it is referred to as **en coup de sabre**. When located on one side of the face, it is called **progressive hemifacial atrophy**. These forms of morphea carry a poorer prognosis because of the associated underlying central nervous system involvement or musculoskeletal atrophy that can be cosmetically disfiguring. Linear morphea over a joint may lead to restriction of mobility (Fig. 659-7). Pansclerotic morphea is a rare, severe, disabling variant.

Differential Diagnosis
The differential diagnosis of morphea includes granuloma annulare, necrobiosis lipoidica, lichen sclerosis, and late-stage Lyme disease (acrodermatitis chronica atrophicans).

Treatment
The lesions persist despite good control of the diabetes but may improve minimally after applications of high-potency topical steroids or local injection of a corticosteroid. Pentoxifylline has also been used.

LICHEN SCLEROSUS
Etiology and Pathogenesis
The cause of lichen sclerosis is unknown. Several studies have identified the presence of autoantibodies to the glycoprotein extracellular matrix protein 1 (ECM-1). The exact role of these antibodies are currently under investigation, however.

Clinical Manifestations
Lichen sclerosus manifests initially as shiny, indurated, ivory-colored papules, often with a violaceous halo. The surface shows prominent dilated pilosebaceous or sweat duct orifices that often contain yellow or brown plugs. The papules coalesce to form irregular plaques of variable size, which may develop hemorrhagic bullae in their margins. In the later stages, atrophy results in a depressed plaque with a wrinkled surface. This disorder occurs more commonly in girls than in boys. Sites of predilection in girls are the vulvar (Fig. 659-5), perianal, and perineal skin. Extensive involvement may produce a sclerotic, atrophic plaque of hourglass configuration; shrinkage of the labia and stenosis of the introitus may result. Vaginal discharge precedes vulvar lesions in approximately 20% of patients. In boys, the prepuce and glans penis are often involved, usually in association with phimosis; most boys with the disorder were not circumcised early in life. Sites elsewhere on the body that are most commonly involved include the upper trunk,

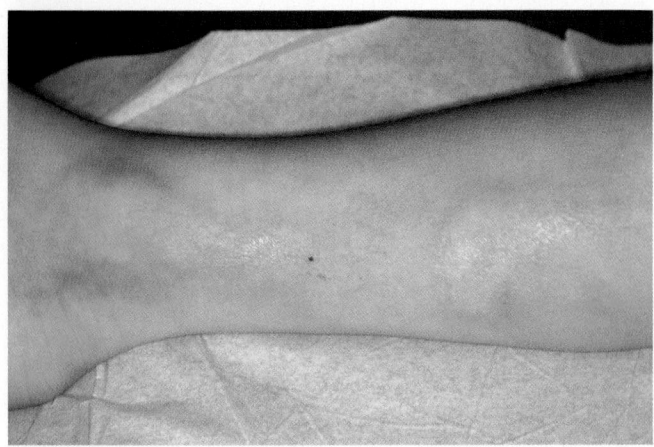

Figure 659-7 Linear morphea with involvement over the ankle.

Histology
Thickening or sclerosis of the dermis with collagen degeneration is seen in morphea.

Treatment
Morphea tends to persist, with gradual outward expansion on the skin for 3-5 yr until spontaneous cessation of the inflammatory phase occurs. Topical calcipotriene alone or in combination with high- to superpotency topical steroids or topical tacrolimus have been used for less-severe disease. For the various forms of linear morphea and for severe plaque morphea, ultraviolet A-1 (UVA-1) phototherapy, or methotrexate with or without pulsed intravenous or oral glucocorticosteroids may halt progression and help shorten the disease course. There are no good comparison studies to suggest which therapy is optimal. Physical therapy is needed in linear morphea over a joint to maintain mobility. Significant postinflammatory pigment alteration may persist for years.

SCLEREDEMA (SCLEREDEMA ADULTORUM, SCLEREDEMA OF BUSCHKE)
Etiology and Pathogenesis
The cause of scleredema is unknown. There are 3 types. Type 1 (55% of cases) is preceded by a febrile illness, often related to an upper or lower respiratory infection (streptococcal most commonly). Type 2 (25%) is associated with paraproteinemias, including multiple myeloma. Type 3 (20%) is seen in diabetes mellitus.

Clinical Manifestations
Fifty percent of patients with scleredema are younger than 20 yr old and almost always have type 1. Onset of type 1 is sudden, with brawny edema of the face and neck that spreads rapidly to involve the thorax and arms in a sweater distribution; the abdomen and legs are usually spared. The face acquires a waxy, mask-like appearance. The involved areas feel indurated and woody, are nonpitting, and are not sharply demarcated from normal skin. The overlying skin is normal in color and is not atrophic.

Onset in patients with type 2 and type 3 scleredema may occur insidiously. Systemic involvement, which is uncommon and usually associated with types 2 and 3, is marked by thickening of the tongue; dysarthria; dysphagia; restriction of eye and joint movements; and pleural, pericardial, and peritoneal effusions. Electrocardiographic changes may also be observed. Laboratory data are not helpful.

Differential Diagnosis
Scleredema must be differentiated from scleroderma (see Chapter 160), morphea, myxedema, trichinosis, dermatomyositis, sclerema neonatorum, and subcutaneous fat necrosis.

Histology
Skin biopsy demonstrates an increase in dermal thickness as a result of swelling and homogenization of the collagen bundles, which are separated by large interfibrous spaces. Special stains can identify increased amounts of mucopolysaccharides in the dermis of patients with scleredema.

Treatment
In type 1 scleredema, the active phase of the disease persists for 2-8 wk; spontaneous and complete resolution usually occurs in 6 mo to 2 yr. Recurrent attacks are unusual. In type 2 and 3, disease is slowly progressive. There is no specific therapy.

LIPOID PROTEINOSIS (URBACH-WIETHE DISEASE, HYALINOSIS CUTIS ET MUCOSAE)
Etiology and Pathogenesis
Lipoid proteinosis, an autosomal recessive disorder, is caused by mutations in the *ECM-1* gene, which encodes the ECM-1 protein. ECM-1 has a functional role in the structural organization of the dermis by binding to perlecan, matrix metalloproteinase 9, and fibulin. Pathogenesis involves infiltration of hyaline material into the skin, oral cavity, larynx, and internal organs.

Clinical Manifestations
Lipoid proteinosis may be noted initially in early infancy as hoarseness. Skin lesions appear during childhood and consist of yellowish papules and nodules that may coalesce to form plaques. The classic sign is beaded papules on the eyelids. Lesions also occur on the face, forearms, neck, genitals, dorsum of the fingers, and scalp, where they result in patchy alopecia. Similar deposits are found on the lips, undersurface of the tongue, fauces, uvula, epiglottis, and vocal cords. The tongue becomes enlarged and feels firm on palpation. The patient may be unable to protrude the tongue. Pock-like atrophic scars may develop on the face. Hypertrophic, hyperkeratotic nodules occur at sites of friction, such as the elbows and knees; the palms may be diffusely thickened. The disease progresses until early adult life, but the prognosis is good. Symmetric ossification lateral to the sella turcica in the medial temporal region, identifiable roentgenographically, is pathognomonic but is not always present. Involvement of the larynx can lead to respiratory compromise, particularly in infancy, necessitating tracheostomy. Associated anomalies include dental abnormalities, epilepsy, and recurrent parotitis as a result of infiltrates in the Stensen duct. Virtually any organ can be involved.

Histology
The distinctive histologic pattern in lipoid proteinosis includes dilation of dermal blood vessels and infiltration of homogeneous eosinophilic extracellular hyaline material along capillary walls and around sweat glands. Hyaline material in homogeneous bundles, diffusely arranged in the upper dermis, produces a thickened dermis. The infiltrates appear to contain both lipid and mucopolysaccharide substances.

Treatment
There is no specific treatment for lipoid proteinosis.

MACULAR ATROPHY (ANETODERMA)
Etiology and Pathogenesis
Anetoderma is characterized by circumscribed areas of slack skin associated with loss of dermal substance. This disorder may have no associated underlying disease (primary macular atrophy) or may develop after an inflammatory skin condition. Secondary macular atrophy may be a result of direct destruction of dermal elastin or elastolysis on an immunologic basis, especially the presence of antiphospholipid antibodies, which are related to autoimmune disorders. The elastolysis may then be a result of release of elastase from inflammatory cells.

Clinical Manifestations
Lesions vary from 0.5-1.0 cm in diameter and, if inflammatory, may initially be erythematous. They subsequently become thin, wrinkled,

and blue-white or hypopigmented. The lesions often protrude as small outpouchings that, on palpation, may be readily indented into the subcutaneous tissue because of the dermal atrophy. Sites of predilection include the trunk, thighs, upper arms, and, less commonly, the neck and face. Lesions remain unchanged for life; new lesions often continue to develop for years.

Histology
All types of macular atrophy show focal loss of elastic tissue on histopathologic examination, a change that may not be recognized unless special stains are used.

Differential Diagnosis
Lesions of anetoderma occasionally resemble morphea, lichen sclerosus, focal dermal hypoplasia, atrophic scars, or end-stage lesions of chronic bullous dermatoses.

Treatment
There is no effective therapy for macular atrophy.

CUTIS LAXA (DERMATOMEGALY, GENERALIZED ELASTOLYSIS)
Etiology and Pathogenesis
Cutis laxa is a heterogenous group of disorders related to abnormalities in elastic tissue. It may be autosomal recessive (type I: *fibulin* 5 and *fibulin* 4 genes; type II: *ATP6V0A2* gene), autosomal dominant (*elastin* and *fibulin* 5 genes), X-linked (*Cu²⁺-transporting adenosine triphosphatase, α-polypeptide*), or acquired. Acquired cutis laxa has developed after a febrile illness, inflammatory skin diseases such as lupus erythematosus or erythema multiforme, amyloidosis, urticaria, angioedema, and hypersensitivity reactions to penicillin, and in infants born to women who were taking penicillamine.

Clinical Manifestations
There may be widespread folds of lax skin, or changes may be mild and limited in extent, resembling anetoderma. Patients with severe cutis laxa have characteristic facial features, including an aged appearance with sagging jowls (bloodhound appearance; Fig. 659-8), a hooked nose with everted nostrils, a short columella, a long upper lip, and everted lower eyelids. The skin is also lax elsewhere on the body and may resemble an ill-fitting suit. Hyperelasticity and hypermobility of the joints are not present as they are in the Ehlers-Danlos syndrome. Many infants have a hoarse cry, probably as a result of laxity of the vocal cords. Tensile strength of the skin is normal.

The dominant form of cutis laxa may develop at any age and is generally benign. When it manifests in infancy, it may be associated with intrauterine growth restriction, ligamentous laxity, and delayed closure of the fontanels. Pulmonary emphysema and mild cardiovascular manifestations may also occur. Patients with the more *common recessive* form of the disease are susceptible to severe complications, such as multiple hernias, rectal prolapse, diaphragmatic atony, diverticula of the gastrointestinal and genitourinary tracts, cor pulmonale, emphysema, pneumothoraces, peripheral pulmonary artery stenosis, and aortic dilation. Characteristic facial features include downward-slanting palpebral fissures, a broad, flat nose, and large ears. Skeletal anomalies, dental caries, growth retardation, and developmental delay also occur. Such patients often have a shortened life span.

Cutis laxa–like skin changes may also be seen in association with multiple other syndromes, including De Barsy syndrome, Lenz-Majewski syndrome, hyperostotic dwarfism, SCARF (**s**keletal abnormalities, **c**utis laxa craniostenosis, **a**mbiguous genitalia, **r**etardation, **f**acial abnormalities) syndrome, wrinkling skin syndrome, and Costello syndrome.

Histology
Histologically, elastic tissue is reduced throughout the dermis, with fragmentation, distention, and clumping of the elastic fibers.

Treatment
Treatment for cutis laxa is supportive.

EHLERS-DANLOS SYNDROME
Ehlers-Danlos syndrome (EDS) is a group of genetically heterogeneous connective tissue disorders. Affected children appear normal at birth, but skin hyperelasticity, fragility of the skin and blood vessels, delayed wound healing, and joint hypermobility (Fig. 659-9) develop. The essential defect is a quantitative deficiency of fibrillar collagen. Additional features include autonomic dysfunction (hypermobility types) characterized by recurrent or chronic musculoskeletal pain, orthostatic intolerance, sudomotor dysfunction, and gastrointestinal disturbances (gastroparesis, diarrhea, constipation). Dysautonomic features may be exacerbated by vasoactive medications. In addition, patients with EDS have an increased incidence of Chiari type 1 malformations, perhaps due to hypermobility of the occipitoatlantal and atlantoaxial joints or poor connective tissue support. Basilar impression symptoms from herniation may contribute to the morbidity of EDS. In patients with a Chiari type 1 malformation there may also be a spinal cord syrinx distal to the malformation. Pulmonary complications may include pneumothorax, hemoptysis, bullous lung disease, and tracheomegaly.

Classification
EDS has been reclassified into 6 clinical recognized forms and 1 unclassified group (Table 659-1).

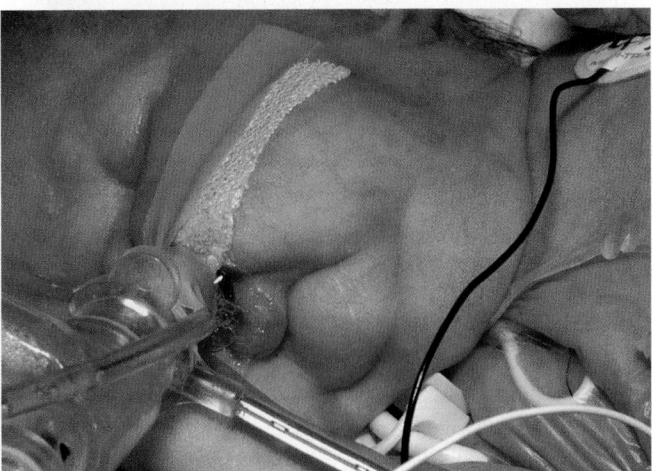

Figure 659-8 Pendulous folds of skin of an infant with cutis laxa.

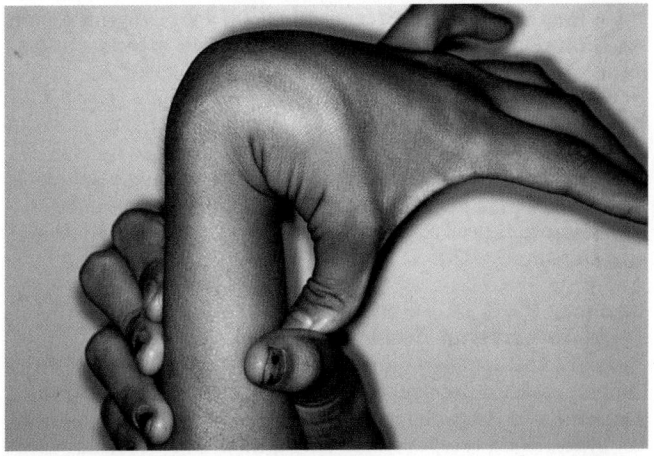

Figure 659-9 Joint hyperextensibility in classic Ehlers-Danlos syndrome.

TYPE	FORMER NAME	CLINICAL FEATURES*	INHERITANCE	OMIM†	MOLECULAR DEFECT
Classic	EDS I and II	Joint hypermobility; skin hyperextensibility; atrophic scars; smooth, velvety skin; subcutaneous spheroids	AD	130000 130010	Structure of type V collagen because of mutations in COL5A1, COL5A2
Hypermobility	EDS III	Joint hypermobility; some skin hyperextensibility, with or without smooth, velvety texture	AD AR	130020 225320	? Tenascin-X (TNX)
Vascular	EDS IV	Thin skin; easy bruising; pinched nose; acrogeria; rupture of large-caliber and medium-caliber arteries, uterus, and large bowel	AD	130050 (225350) (225360)	Deficient type III collagen (COL3A1)
Kyphoscoliotic	EDS VI	Joint hypermobility; congenital, progressive rupture; scoliosis; scleral fragility with globe rupture; tissue fragility, aortic dilation, MVP	AR	225400	Deficiency of lysyl hydroxylase
Arthrochalasis	EDS VII A	Joint hypermobility, severe, with subluxations, congenital hip dislocation; skin hyperextensibility; tissue fragility	AD	130060	No cleavage of amino terminus of type I procollagen because of mutations in COL1A1 or COL1A2
Dermatosparaxis	EDS VII C	Severe skin fragility; decreased skin elasticity, easy bruising; hernias; premature rupture of fetal membranes	AR	225410	No cleavage of amino terminus of type I procollagen because of deficiency of peptidase
Unclassified types	EDS V	Classic features	XL	305200	?
	EDS VIII	Classic features and periodontal disease	AD	130080	?
	EDS X	Mild classic features, MVP	?	225310	?
	EDS XI	Joint instability	AD	147900	?
	EDS IX	Classic features; occipital horns	XL	309400	Allelic to Menkes syndrome
	EDS, progeroid form	Classic features and premature aging	AR	130700	Deficiency of galactosyltransferase I

Table 659-1 | Ehlers-Danlos Syndrome

*Listed in order of diagnostic importance.
†Entries in Online Mendelian Inheritance in Man, OMIM. McKusick-Nathans Institute of Genetic Medicine, Johns Hopkins University (Baltimore, MD). Available at: http://omim.org/
AD, autosomal dominant; AR, autosomal recessive; EDS, Ehlers-Danlos syndrome; MVP, mitral valve prolapse; XL, X-linked.
  From Pyeritz RD: Inherited diseases of connective tissue. In Goldman L, Schafer AI, editors: Goldman's Cecil medicine, ed 24, Philadelphia, 2012, Elsevier, Table 268-2.

Classic (COL5A1, COL5A2, COL1A1 Genes; Previously EDS Type I—Gravis, EDS Type II—MITIS)

This autosomal dominant disorder is characterized by premature birth caused by rupture of membranes, skin hyperelasticity and fragility, easy bruising, generalized and severe joint hypermobility, scoliosis, and mitral valve prolapse. Insignificant lacerations may form gaping wounds that leave broad, atrophic, papyraceous scars. Additional cutaneous manifestations include molluscoid pseudotumors over pressure points from accumulations of connective tissue and piezogenic papules (fat herniation into the dermis) (Fig. 659-10). Life expectancy is not reduced.

Hypermobile (COL3A1 Gene; Previously EDS Type III)

This disorder has autosomal dominant inheritance and manifests as generalized severe joint hypermobility and minimal skin manifestations. Musculoskeletal pain is common, and osteoarthritis may develop prematurely.

Vascular (COL3A1 Gene; Previously EDS Type IV—Arterial Ecchymotic)

This autosomal dominant disorder shows the most pronounced dermal thinning of all. Consequently, the underlying venous network is prominent. The skin has minimal hyperextensibility, and the joints are not hypermobile, except perhaps during childhood. Premature birth, extensive ecchymoses from trauma, a high incidence of keloids, rupture of the bowel (especially the colon), uterine rupture during pregnancy,

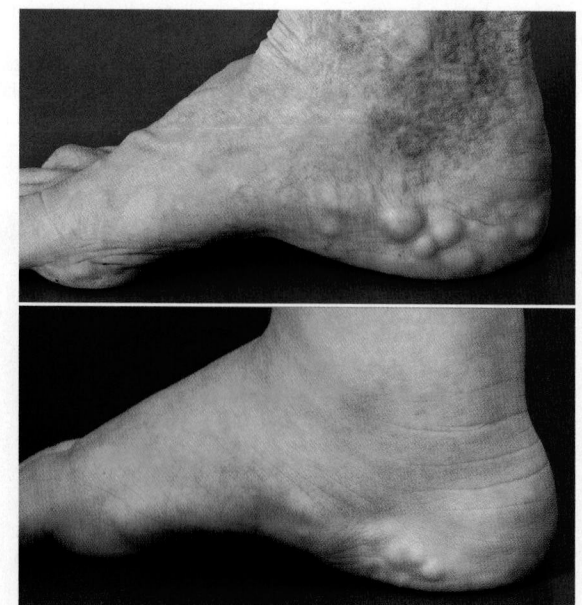

Figure 659-10 Piezogenic papules on the medial aspects of the heels in a 41-year-old patient with Ehlers-Danlos syndrome (top) and his 2-year-old daughter (bottom). (From Poppe H, Hamm H: Piezogenic papules in Ehlers-Danlos syndrome. J Pediatr 163:1788, 2013.)

rupture of the great vessels, dissecting aortic aneurysm, and stroke all contribute to the increased morbidity and shortened life span. Patients should be advised to avoid becoming pregnant, avoid activities that raise intracranial pressure as a result of a Valsalva maneuver, such as trumpet playing, and minimize trauma to the skin. Celiprolol, a β_1 antagonist and a β_2 agonist (vasodilates), may reduce vascular events.

Kyphoscoliosis (Lysyl Hydroxylase [*PLOD* Gene] Deficiency; Previously EDS Type VI)

Patients with this autosomal recessive type have joint hyperextensibility, hypotonia, kyphoscoliosis, fragile cornea, keratoconus, skin hyperelasticity, and fragile bones. Prenatal diagnosis is available through measurement of lysyl hydroxylase activity in amniocytes. The diagnosis can also be confirmed by detection of decreased lysyl hydroxylase activity in cultured dermal fibroblasts.

Arthrochalasia (*COLA1A* Gene, Type A; *COL1A2* Gene, Type B; Previously EDS Types VIIA and B—Arthrochalasis Multiplex Congenita)

The A type is an autosomal dominant disorder characterized by short stature, marked joint hyperextensibility and dislocation, and moderate hyperelasticity and bruisability of skin. The B type is autosomal dominant and is characterized by skin hyperelasticity and marked joint hypermobility.

Dermatosparaxis (Type 1 Collagen *N*-Peptidase; Previously EDS Type VIIC)

This autosomal recessive condition that includes premature rupture of membranes; delayed closure of fontanels; skin fragility and laxity; easy bruisability; growth retardation; short limbs; umbilical hernia; and characteristic facies with micrognathia, jowls, and prominent, puffy eyelids.

Differential Diagnosis

EDS has been confused with cutis laxa, but the features of the 2 disorders differ considerably. The skin of patients with cutis laxa hangs in redundant folds, whereas the skin of those with EDS is hyperextensible and snaps back into place when stretched. Because of the marked skin fragility in EDS, minor trauma results in ecchymoses, bleeding, and poor healing with atrophic cigarette-paper scars, which are most prominent on the forehead and lower legs and over pressure points. Surgical procedures are fraught with risk; dehiscence of wounds is common.

Joint hypermobility is seen in other connective tissue disorders (Fig. 659-11). Joint hypermobility is scored with the 9 point Beighton score (Table 659-2) and can be assessed by history (Table 659-3).

Figure 659-12 provides an initial approach to the diagnosis of EDS.

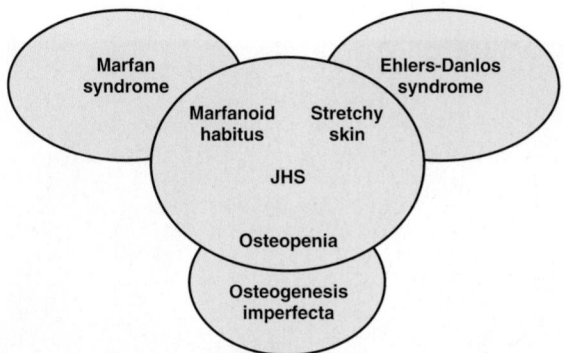

Figure 659-11 A Venn diagram illustrating the overlap features between the 4 major heritable disorders of connective tissue. Joint hypermobility syndrome (JHS) maintains a central position sharing key features with Marfan syndrome, osteogenesis imperfecta, and Ehlers-Danlos syndrome, and is seen as a benign forme fruste of all 3 heritable disorders of connective tissue "rolled into one." (*From Hakim A, Grahame R: Joint hypermobility. Best Pract Res Clin Rheumatol 17:989–1004, 2003, Fig. 1.*)

Table 659-2	The Nine-Point Beighton Hypermobility Score		
The ability to:		**RIGHT**	**LEFT**
1. Passively dorsiflex the fifth metacarpophalangeal joint to ≥90°		1	1
2. Oppose the thumb to the volar aspect of the ipsilateral forearm		1	1
3. Hyperextend the elbow to ≥10°		1	1
4. Hyperextend the knee to ≥10°		1	1
5. Place hands flat on the floor without bending the knees		1	
		Total 9	

One point may be gained for each side for maneuvers 1-4 so the hypermobility score will have a maximum of 9 points if all are positive.
From Hakim A, Grahame R: Joint hypermobility. Best Pract Res Clin Rheumatol 17:989–1004, 2003, Table 1.

Table 659-3	A Five-Part Questionnaire for Identifying Hypermobility
1. Can you now (or could you ever) place your hands flat on the floor without bending your knees?	
2. Can you now (or could you ever) bend your thumb to touch your forearm?	
3. As a child did you amuse your friends by contorting your body into strange shapes *or* could you do the splits?	
4. As a child or teenager did your shoulder or kneecap dislocate on more than one occasion?	
5. Do you consider yourself double-jointed?	

Answer in the affirmative to 2 or more questions suggests hypermobility with sensitivity 80-85% and specificity 80-90%
From Hakim A, Grahame R: Joint hypermobility. Best Pract Res Clin Rheumatol 17:989–1004, 2003, Table 3.

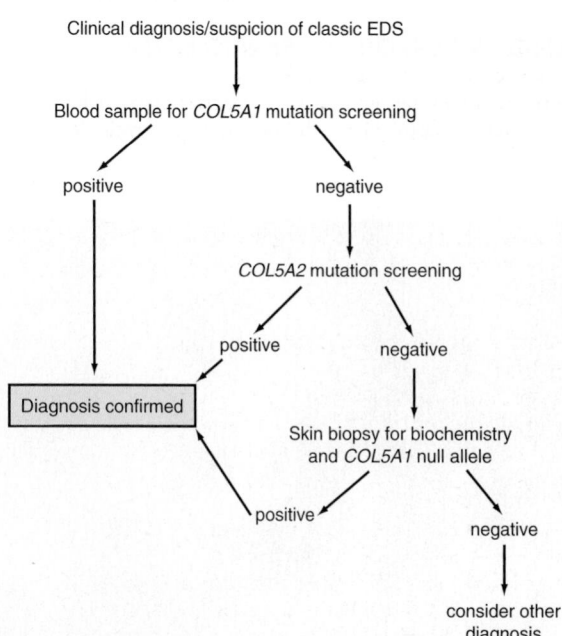

Figure 659-12 Diagnostic flow chart for Ehlers-Danlos syndrome, classic type. (*From De Paepe A, Malfait F: The Ehlers-Danlos syndrome, a disorder with many faces. Clin Genet 82:1–11, 2012, Fig. 3.*)

PSEUDOXANTHOMA ELASTICUM
Etiology and Pathogenesis
Pseudoxanthoma elasticum (PXE) is a primary disorder of elastic tissue. The overwhelming majority of cases are caused by mutations in the *ABCC6* gene. The primary abnormality seen in PXE is an accumulation of mineralized tissue in the skin, Bruch membrane in the retina, and vessel walls. Although other forms of PXE have been postulated, their existence is now debated.

Clinical Manifestations
Onset of skin manifestations often occurs during childhood, but the changes produced by early lesions are subtle and may not be recognized. The characteristic **pebbly, "plucked chicken skin" cutaneous lesions** are 1-2 mm, asymptomatic, yellow papules that are arranged in a linear or reticulated pattern or in confluent plaques. Preferred sites are the flexural neck (Fig. 659-13), axillary and inguinal folds, umbilicus, thighs, and antecubital and popliteal fossae. As the lesions become more pronounced, the skin acquires a velvety texture and droops in lax, inelastic folds. The face is usually spared. Mucous membrane lesions may involve the lips, buccal cavity, rectum, and vagina. There is involvement of the connective tissue of the media, and intima of blood vessels, Bruch membrane of the eye, and endocardium or pericardium may result in visual disturbances, angioid streaks in Bruch membrane, intermittent claudication, cerebral and coronary occlusion, hypertension, and hemorrhage from the gastrointestinal tract, uterus, or mucosal surfaces. Women with PXE have an increased risk of miscarriage in the 1st trimester. Arterial involvement generally manifests in adulthood, but claudication and angina have occurred in early childhood.

Pathology
Histopathologic examination shows fragmented, swollen, and clumped elastic fibers in the middle and lower third of the dermis. The fibers stain positively for calcium. Collagen in the vicinity of the altered elastic fibers is reduced in amount and is split into small fibers. Aberrant calcification of the elastic fibers of the internal elastic lamina of arteries in PXE leads to narrowing of vessel lumina.

Treatment
There is no effective treatment for PXE, although laser therapy may help prevent retinal hemorrhage. The use of oral phosphate binders has shown promise in decreasing calcification of elastic fibers.

ELASTOSIS PERFORANS SERPIGINOSA
Etiology and Pathogenesis
Elastosis perforans serpiginosa (EPS) is characterized by the extrusion of altered elastic fibers through the epidermis. The primary abnormality is probably in the dermal elastin, which provokes a cellular response that ultimately leads to extrusion of the abnormal elastic tissue.

Clinical Manifestations
This is an unusual skin disorder in which 1-3 mm, firm, skin-colored, keratotic papules tend to cluster in arcuate and annular patterns on the posterolateral neck and limbs (Fig. 659-14) and occasionally on the face and trunk. Onset usually occurs in childhood or adolescence. A papule consists of a circumscribed area of epidermal hyperplasia that communicates with the underlying dermis by a narrow channel. There is a great increase in the amount and size of elastic fibers in the upper dermis, particularly in the dermal papillae. Approximately 30% occur in association with osteogenesis imperfecta, Marfan syndrome, PXE, EDS, Rothmund-Thomson syndrome, scleroderma, acrogeria, and Down syndrome. EPS has also occurred in association with penicillamine therapy.

Histology
Histopathology reveals a hyperplastic epidermis with extrusion of abnormal elastic fibers and a lymphocytic superficial infiltrate.

Differential Diagnosis
Differential diagnosis of EPS includes tinea corporis, perforating granuloma annulare, reactive perforating collagenosis, lichen planus, creeping eruption, and porokeratosis of Mibelli.

Treatment
Treatment of EPS is ineffective; however, the lesions are asymptomatic and may disappear spontaneously.

REACTIVE PERFORATING COLLAGENOSIS
Etiology and Pathogenesis
The primary process in reactive perforating collagenosis represents transepidermal elimination of altered collagen. A familial autosomal recessive form has been described.

Clinical Manifestations
Reactive perforating collagenosis usually manifests in early childhood as small papules on the dorsal areas of the hands and forearms, elbows, knees, and, sometimes, face and trunk. Over a period of several weeks, the papules enlarge to 5-10 mm, become umbilicated, and develop keratotic plugs in their centers (Fig. 659-15). Individual lesions resolve spontaneously in 2-4 mo, leaving hypopigmented macules or scars. Lesions may recur in crops; may undergo a linear Koebner phenomenon; and may form in response to cold temperatures or superficial trauma such as abrasions, insect bites, and acne lesions.

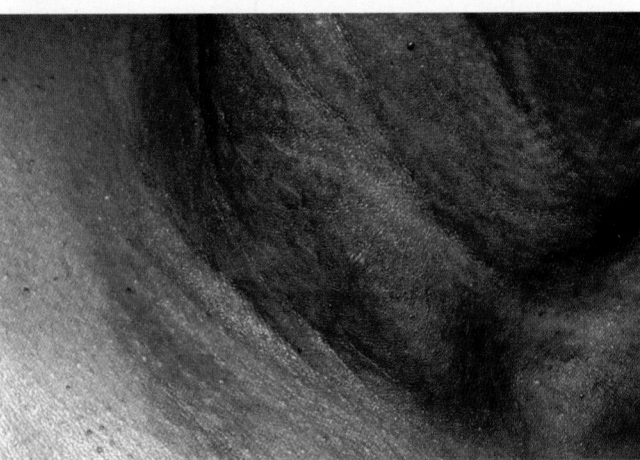

Figure 659-13 Confluent plaque of pebbly skin in pseudoxanthoma elasticum.

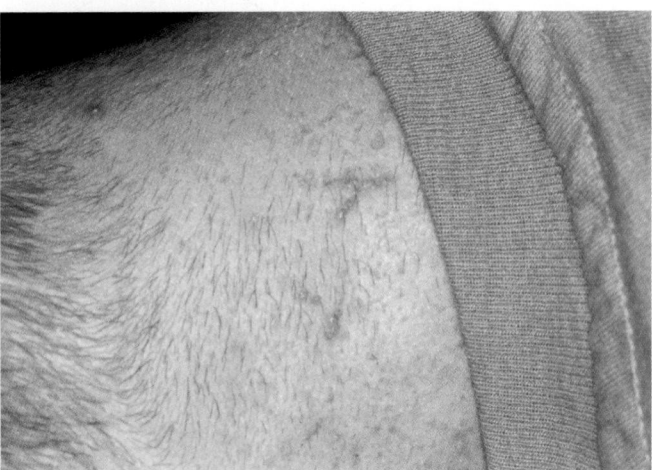

Figure 659-14 Arcuate keratotic papule of elastosis perforans serpiginosa.

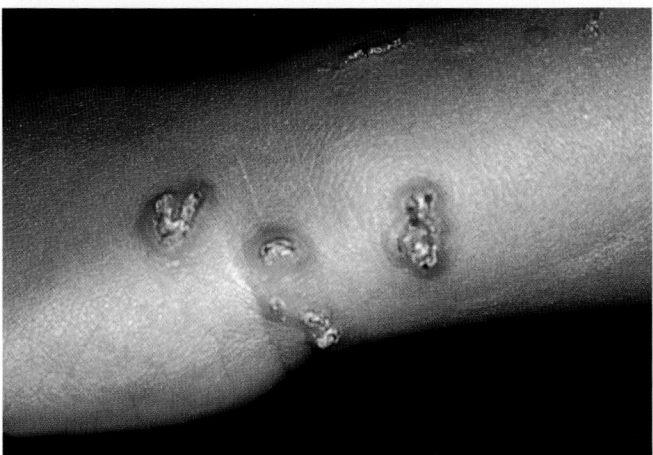

Figure 659-15 Hyperkeratotic papules in reactive perforating collagenosis.

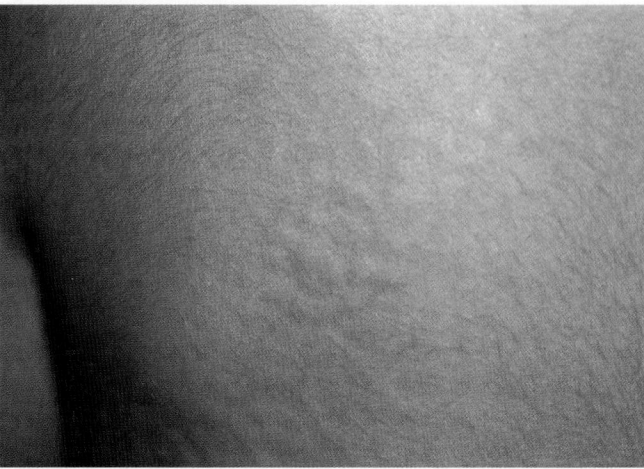

Figure 659-16 Ivory-colored papules on the upper back in Hunter syndrome.

Histology

Collagen in the papillary dermis is engulfed within a cup-shaped perforation in the epidermis. The central crater contains pyknotic inflammatory cells and keratinous debris.

Differential Diagnosis

EPS and Kyrle disease may mimic reactive perforating collagenosis.

Treatment

Reactive perforating collagenosis resolves spontaneously in 6-8 wk. Topical retinoic acid enhances the resolution.

XANTHOMAS

See Chapter 86.

FABRY DISEASE

See Chapter 86.

MUCOPOLYSACCHARIDOSES

See Chapter 88.

In several of the mucopolysaccharidoses, thick, rough, inelastic skin, particularly on the extremities, and generalized hirsutism are characteristic but nonspecific features. Telangiectasias on the face, forearms, trunk, and legs have been observed in Scheie and Morquio syndromes. In some patients with Hunter syndrome, ivory-colored, distinctive firm papulonodules with a corrugated surface texture are grouped into symmetric plaques on the upper trunk (Fig. 659-16), arms, and thighs. Onset of these unusual lesions occurs in the 1st decade of life, and spontaneous disappearance has been noted.

MASTOCYTOSIS
Etiology and Pathogenesis

Mastocytosis encompasses a spectrum of disorders that range from solitary cutaneous nodules to diffuse infiltration of skin associated with involvement of other organs (Table 659-4). All of the disorders are characterized by aggregates of mast cells in the dermis. There are 4 types of mastocytoses: solitary mastocytoma, urticaria pigmentosa (2 forms), diffuse cutaneous mastocytosis, and telangiectasia macularis eruptiva perstans. The 2 forms of urticaria pigmentosa are the childhood variant, which resolves without sequelae, and the form that may start in either childhood or adult life and is associated with a mutation (most commonly the *D816V* mutation) in the stem cell factor gene. Stem cell factor (mast cell growth factor), which can be secreted by keratinocytes, stimulates the proliferation of mast cells and increases the production of melanin by melanocytes. The local and systemic

Table 659-4 | Mastocytosis Classification

Cutaneous mastocytosis:
1. Urticaria pigmentosa:
   (a) Classic infantile type; (b) Chronic with stem cell factor mutations
2. Diffuse cutaneous mastocytosis
3. Mastocytoma of the skin
4. Telangiectasia macularis eruptive perstans
Systemic mastocytosis (without an associated hematologic non–mast cell disorder or leukemic mast cell disease):
1. Systemic indolent mastocytosis
2. Systemic smoldering mastocytosis
Systemic mastocytosis with an associated hematologic non–mast cell disorder:
1. Myeloproliferative syndrome
2. Myelodysplastic syndrome
3. Acute myeloid leukemia
4. Non-Hodgkin lymphoma
Systemic aggressive mastocytosis
Mast cell leukemia
Mast cell sarcoma
Extracutaneous mastocytoma

Adapted from Valent PHH, Li CY, Longley BJ, et al. World Health Organization classification of tumours, pathology and genetics of tumours of the haematopoietic and lymphoid tissues, Lyon, France, 2001, IARC Press; and Carter MC, Metcalfe DD: Paediatric mastocytosis, Arch Dis Child 86:315–319, 2002, Table 3.

manifestations of the disease are at least partly a result of the release of histamine and heparin from mast cell granules; although heparin is present in significant amounts in mast cells, coagulation disturbances occur only rarely. The vasodilator prostaglandin D$_2$ or its metabolite appears to exacerbate the flushing response. Serum tryptase values can be elevated.

Clinical Manifestations

Solitary mastocytomas are usually 1-5 cm in diameter. Lesions may be present at birth or may arise in early infancy at any site. The lesions may manifest as recurrent, evanescent wheals or bullae; in time, an infiltrated, pink, yellow, or tan, rubbery plaque develops at the site of whealing or blistering (Fig. 659-17). The surface acquires a pebbly, orange peel–like texture, and hyperpigmentation may become prominent. Stroking or trauma to the nodule may lead to urtication (Darier sign) as a result of local histamine release; rarely, systemic signs of histamine release become apparent.

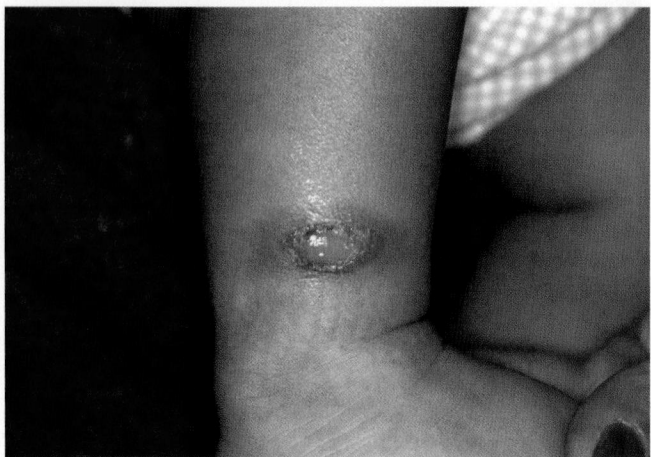

Figure 659-17 Solitary mastocytoma that is partially blistered.

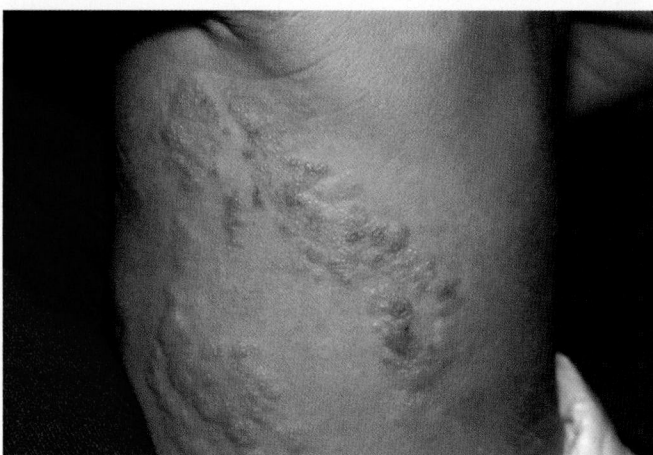

Figure 659-19 Severe blistering in diffuse cutaneous mastocytosis.

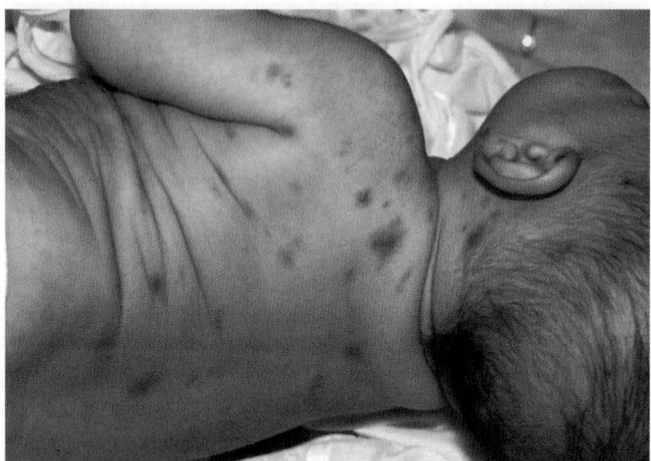

Figure 659-18 Hyperpigmented papular lesions of urticaria pigmentosa.

Urticaria pigmentosa is the most common form of mastocytosis. In the first type of urticaria pigmentosa, the classic infantile type, lesions may be present at birth but more often erupt in crops in the 1st several mo to 2 yr of age. New lesions seldom arise after age 3-4 yr. In some cases, early bullous or urticarial lesions fade, only to recur at the same site, ultimately becoming fixed and hyperpigmented. In others, the initial lesions are hyperpigmented. Vesiculation usually abates by 2 yr of age. Individual lesions range in size from a few millimeters to several centimeters and may be macular, papular, or nodular. They range in color from yellow-tan to chocolate brown and often have ill-defined borders (Fig. 659-18). Larger nodular lesions, like solitary mastocytomas, may have a characteristic orange peel texture. Lesions of urticaria pigmentosa may be sparse or numerous and are often symmetrically distributed. Palms, soles, and face are sometimes spared, as are the mucous membranes. The rapid appearance of erythema and whealing in response to vigorous stroking of a lesion can usually be elicited; dermographism of intervening normal skin is also common. Affected children can have intense pruritus. Systemic signs of histamine release, such as hypotension, syncope, headache, episodic flushing, tachycardia, wheezing, colic, and diarrhea, are uncommon and occur most frequently in the more severe types of mastocytosis. Flushing is by far the most common symptom seen.

The second type of urticaria pigmentosa may begin in infancy but typically develops in adulthood. This type does not resolve, and new lesions continue to develop throughout life. It is associated with mutations in the stem cell factor gene. Patients with this type of mastocytosis are the population in whom systemic involvement may develop.

Systemic mastocytosis is marked by an abnormal increase in the number of mast cells in other than cutaneous tissues. It occurs in approximately 5-10% of patients with mutant stem cell factor–related mastocytosis and is uncommon in children. Bone lesions may be silent but are detectable radiologically as osteoporotic or osteosclerotic areas, principally in the axial skeleton. Gastrointestinal tract involvement may produce complaints of abdominal pain, nausea, vomiting, diarrhea, steatorrhea, and bloating. Mucosal infiltrates may be detectable by barium studies or by small bowel biopsy. Peptic ulcers also occur. Hepatosplenomegaly as a result of mast cell infiltrates and fibrosis has been described, as has mast cell proliferation in lymph nodes, kidneys, periadrenal fat, and bone marrow. Abnormalities in the peripheral blood, such as anemia, leukocytosis, and eosinophilia, are noted in approximately 30% of patients. Mast cell leukemia may occur.

Diffuse cutaneous mastocytosis is characterized by diffuse involvement of the skin rather than discrete hyperpigmented lesions. Affected patients are usually normal at birth and demonstrate features of the disorder after the 1st few mo of life. Rarely, the condition may present with intense generalized pruritus in the absence of visible skin changes. The skin usually appears thickened and pink to yellow and may have a doughy feel and a texture resembling an orange peel. Surface changes are accentuated in flexural areas. Recurrent bullae (Fig. 659-19), intractable pruritus, and flushing attacks are common, as is systemic involvement.

Telangiectasia macularis eruptiva perstans is another variant that consists of telangiectatic hyperpigmented macules that are usually localized to the trunk. These lesions do not urticate when stroked. This form of the disease is seen primarily in adolescents and adults.

Differential Diagnosis
The differential diagnosis of solitary mastocytomas includes recurrent bullous impetigo, herpes simplex, congenital melanocytic nevi, and juvenile xanthogranuloma.

Urticaria pigmentosa can be confused with drug eruptions, postinflammatory pigmentary change, juvenile xanthogranuloma, pigmented nevi, ephelides, xanthomas, chronic urticaria, insect bites, and bullous impetigo. Diffuse cutaneous mastocytoma may be confused with epidermolytic hyperkeratosis.

Telangiectasia macularis eruptiva perstans must be differentiated from other causes of telangiectasia.

Table 659-5	Pharmacologic Agents and Physical Stimuli That May Exacerbate Mast Cell Mediator Release in Patients with Mastocytosis

IMMUNOLOGIC STIMULI
Venoms (immunoglobulin E–mediated bee venom)
Complement-derived anaphylatoxins
Biologic peptides (substance P, somatostatin)
Polymers (dextran)

NONIMMUNOLOGIC STIMULI
Physical stimuli (heat, cold, rubbing, trauma, sunlight)
Drugs
Acetylsalicylic acid and related nonsteroidal analgesics*
Thiamine
Ketorolac tromethamine
Alcohol
Vancomycin
Dextromethorphan
Narcotics (codeine, morphine)*
Radiographic dyes (iodine containing)

EMOTIONAL ISSUES
Anxiety
Sleep deprivation
Stress

*Appears to be a problem in <10% of patients.
From Carter MC, Metcalfe DD: Paediatric mastocytosis, Arch Dis Child 86:315–319, 2002, Table 4.

Prognosis

Spontaneous involution occurs in all patients with solitary mastocytomas and classic infantile urticaria pigmentosa. The incidence of systemic manifestations in these patients is very low. The continued development of lesions past the age of 4 yr implies likely chronic disease with stem cell factor gene mutation and a higher risk for systemic involvement.

Treatment

Solitary mastocytomas usually do not require treatment. Lesions that blister may be treated with topical steroids following each blistering episode.

In urticaria pigmentosa, flushing can be precipitated by excessively hot baths, vigorous rubbing of the skin, and certain drugs, such as codeine, aspirin, morphine, atropine, ketorolac, alcohol, tubocurarine, iodine-containing radiographic dyes, and polymyxin B (Table 659-5). Avoidance of these triggering factors is advisable; it is notable that general anesthesia may be safely performed with appropriate precautions.

For patients who are symptomatic, oral antihistamines may be palliative. H_1 receptor antagonists (hydroxyzine) are the initial drugs of choice for systemic signs of histamine release. If H_1 antagonists are unsuccessful, H_2 receptor antagonists may be helpful in controlling pruritus or gastric hypersecretion. Topical steroids are of benefit in controlling skin urtication and blistering. Oral mast cell–stabilizing agents, such as cromolyn sodium or ketotifen, may also be effective for diarrhea or abdominal cramping and some systemic symptoms such as headache or muscle pain.

For patients with diffuse cutaneous mastocytosis, the treatment is the same as for urticaria pigmentosa, although in early life. Phototherapy with narrow-band UV (UVB or UVA-1) or psoralen with UVA treatment may be required to control symptoms.

Lesions of telangiectasia macularis eruptiva perstans may be cautiously treated with vascular pulsed-dye lasers.

Bibliography is available at Expert Consult.

Chapter 660
Diseases of Subcutaneous Tissue
JiaDe Yu and Beth A. Drolet

Diseases involving the subcutis are usually characterized by necrosis and/or inflammation; they may occur either as a primary event or as a secondary response to various stimuli or disease processes. The principal diagnostic criteria relate to the appearance and distribution of the lesions, associated symptoms, results of laboratory studies, histopathology, and natural history and exogenous provocative factors of these conditions.

CORTICOSTEROID-INDUCED ATROPHY

Intradermal or subcutaneous injection of a corticosteroid can produce deep atrophy accompanied by surface pigmentary changes and telangiectasia (Fig. 660-1). These changes occur approximately 2-8 wks after injection and may last for months.

660.1 Panniculitis and Erythema Nodosum
JiaDe Yu

Inflammation of fibrofatty subcutaneous tissue may primarily involve the fat lobule or, alternatively, the fibrous septum that compartmentalizes the fatty lobules. Lobular panniculitis that spares the subcutaneous vasculature includes poststeroid panniculitis, lupus erythematosus profundus, pancreatic panniculitis, α_1-antitrypsin deficiency, subcutaneous fat necrosis of the newborn, sclerema neonatorum, cold panniculitis, subcutaneous sarcoidosis, and factitial panniculitis. Lobar panniculitis with vasculitis occurs in erythema induratum and, occasionally, as a feature of Crohn disease (see Chapter 336.2). Inflammation predominantly within the septum, sparing the vasculature, may be seen in erythema nodosum (Table 660-1 and Fig. 660-2), necrobiosis lipoidica, progressive systemic sclerosis (see Chapter 160), and subcutaneous granuloma annulare (see Chapter 659). Septal panniculitis that includes inflammation of the vessels is found primarily in leukocytoclastic vasculitis and polyarteritis nodosa (see Chapter 167).

Figure 660-1 Localized fat atrophy with overlying erythema after steroid injection.

ERYTHEMA NODOSUM
Etiology and Pathogenesis
The etiology is unknown in 30-50% of pediatric cases of erythema nodosum; Table 660-1 lists other etiologies. Most common etiologies in children include: group A streptococcal infection, *Yersinia enterocolitica* gastroenteritis, medications (cephalosporins, penicillins, macrolides), and inflammatory disorders (inflammatory bowel disease); sarcoidosis should be considered in young adults.

Clinical Manifestations
Erythema nodosum is a nodular, erythematous hypersensitivity reaction that typically appears with multiple lesions on the anterior surfaces of the arms and legs in the pretibial area (more common) and less often in other cutaneous areas containing subcutaneous fat. The lesions vary in size from 1-6 cm, are symmetric, and are oval with the longer axis

Table 660-1	Etiology of Erythema Nodosum

VIRUSES
Epstein-Barr, hepatitis B, mumps

FUNGI
Coccidioidomycosis, histoplasmosis, blastomycosis, sporotrichosis

BACTERIA AND OTHER INFECTIOUS AGENTS
Group A streptococcus,* tuberculosis,* *Yersinia*, cat-scratch disease, leprosy, leptospirosis, tularemia, mycoplasma, Whipple disease, lymphogranuloma venereum, psittacosis, brucellosis

OTHER
Sarcoidosis, inflammatory bowel disease,* estrogen-containing oral contraceptives,* systemic lupus erythematosus, Behçet syndrome, severe acne, Hodgkin disease, lymphoma, sulfonamides, bromides, Sweet syndrome, pregnancy, idiopathic*

*Common.

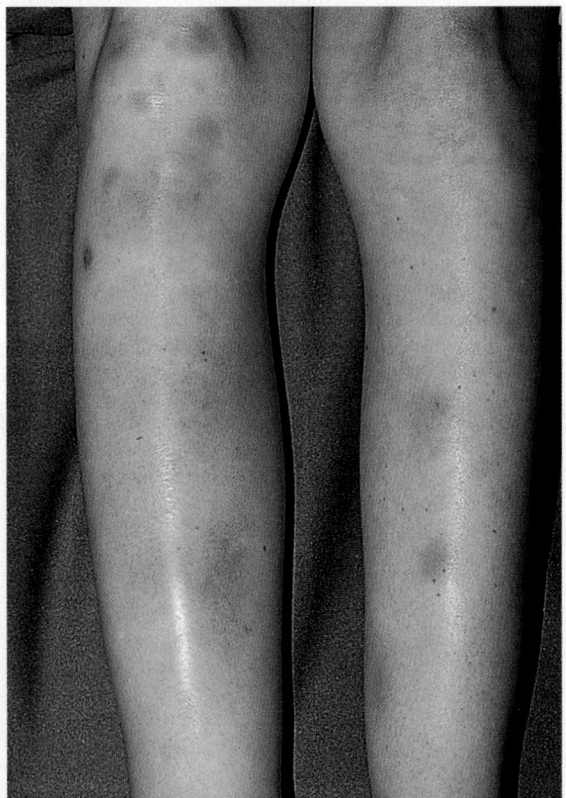

Figure 660-2 Tender red nodules with indistinct borders in a teenage girl with erythema nodosum. *(From Weston AL, Lane AT, Morelli JG: Color textbook of pediatric dermatology, ed 3, St. Louis, 2002, Mosby, p. 212.)*

parallel to the extremity. They initially appear bright or dull red but progress to a brown or purple; they are painful and usually do not ulcerate (see Fig. 660-2). Initial lesions may resolve in 1-2 wk, but new lesions may continue to appear for 2-6 wk. Repeat episodes may occur weeks to months later. Prior to or immediately at the onset of lesions, there may be systemic manifestations that include fever, malaise, arthralgias (50-90%) and rheumatoid factor negative arthritis.

Histology
A septal panniculitis with thickening of the septa with inflammatory cells infiltrate comprised of neutrophils acutely. Monocytes and histiocytes predominate in chronic erythema nodosum.

Treatment
Treatment includes that of the underlying disease as well as symptomatic relief with nonsteroidal antiinflammatory agents. Salicylates, supersaturated solution of potassium iodide (oral), colchicine, intralesional injections of steroids and, in severe, persistent, or recurrent lesions, oral steroids have been employed. The idiopathic form is a self-limited disorder. Protracted or recurrent cases may warrant further workup including antistreptolysin O/deoxyribonuclease B, complete blood count, throat culture, purified protein derivative, QuantiFERON-TB gold assay, chest radiograph, erythrocyte sedimentation rate, and C-reactive protein.

POST-STEROID PANNICULITIS
Etiology and Pathogenesis
The mechanism of the inflammatory reaction in the fat in poststeroid panniculitis is unknown.

Clinical Manifestations
Majority of the cases of post-steroid panniculitis have been reported in children. The disorder occurs in children who have received high-dose corticosteroids. In 1-2 wk after discontinuation of the drug, multiple subcutaneous nodules usually appear on the cheeks, although other areas may be involved. Nodules range in size from 0.5-4.0 cm, are erythematous or skin colored, and may be pruritic or painful.

Histology
A lobular panniculitis with a mixed infiltrate of lymphocytes, histiocytes, and neutrophils is seen. Scattered swollen adipocytes with eosinophilic, needle-shaped crystals are also seen. The epidermis, dermis, and fibrous septa of the fat are normal. Vasculitis is not seen.

Treatment
Treatment of poststeroid panniculitis is unnecessary because the lesions remit spontaneously over a period of months without scarring.

LUPUS ERYTHEMATOSUS PROFUNDUS (LUPUS ERYTHEMATOSUS PANNICULITIS)
Etiology and Pathogenesis
It is unknown what separates those patients in whom lupus erythematosus profundus develops from other patients with systemic lupus erythematosus. This variant of chronic cutaneous lupus erythematosus is rare in childhood. Recent studies show only 2-5% of patients with lupus erythematosus profundus have associated systemic lupus erythematosus. Mean age of onset in reported pediatric cases is 9.8 yr.

Clinical Manifestations
Lupus erythematosus profundus manifests as 1 to several firm, tender, well-defined, purple plaques or nodules 1-3 cm in diameter. Majority of pediatric cases involve the face and proximal upper extremities. This condition may occur in patients with systemic or discoid lupus erythematosus and may precede or follow the development of other cutaneous lesions. The overlying skin is usually normal but may be erythematous, atrophic, poikilodermatous, or hyperkeratotic (Fig. 660-3). On healing, a shallow depression generally remains or, rarely, soft pink areas of anetoderma result.

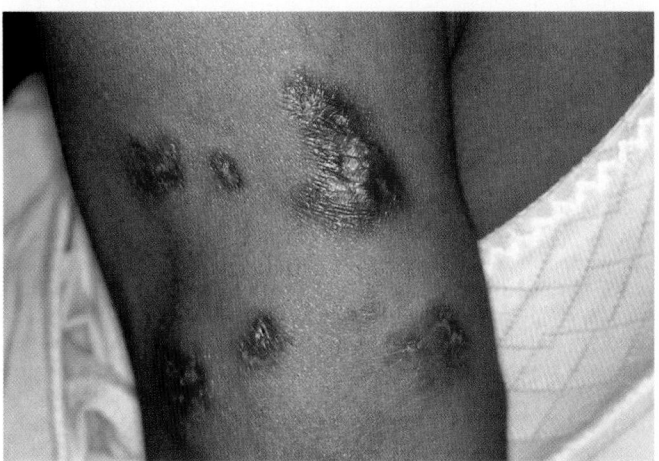

Figure 660-3 Deep nodule of lupus profundus with overlying hyperkeratotic lesion of discoid lupus erythematosus.

Histology

The histopathologic changes in lupus erythematosus profundus are distinctive and may allow the clinician to make the diagnosis in the absence of other cutaneous lesions of lupus erythematosus. The panniculitis is characterized by a mostly nodular dense infiltrate of lymphocytes and plasma cells. Necrosis of the fat lobule is characteristic. A dense perivascular and periappendiceal lymphocytic infiltrate is seen in the dermis. Lichenoid changes may be identified at the epidermal–dermal junction. Histopathologic differentiation from subcutaneous panniculitis–like T-cell lymphoma may be difficult. Results of lupus band and antinuclear antibody tests are usually positive.

Treatment

Nodules tend to be persistent and frequently ulcerate. Long-term follow-up for possible systemic involvement is warranted. There is no consensus on the utility of laboratory testing. antinuclear antibody is positive in only a small subset of patients. Few case reports show slight neutropenia, leukopenia, and mildly elevated liver function tests. Hydroxychloroquine (2-5 mg/kg/day) is the **treatment of choice** for lupus erythematosus profundus. Intralesional corticosteroids may worsen the residual lipoatrophy. Immunosuppressive agents are indicated only for treatment of other severe manifestations of systemic lupus erythematosus. Avoidance of sun exposure and trauma is also important.

α₁-ANTITRYPSIN DEFICIENCY
Etiology and Pathogenesis

Individuals with α_1-antitrypsin deficiency have severe homozygous deficiency or, rarely, a partial deficiency of the protease inhibitor α_1-antitrypsin, which inhibits trypsin activity and the activity of elastase, serine proteases, collagenase, factor VIII, and kallikrein (see Chapter 393). Panniculitis occurs with severe α_1-antitrypsin deficiency or the Z subtype.

Clinical Manifestations

Cellulitis-like areas or tender, red nodules occur on the trunk or proximal extremities (see Chapter 393). Nodules tend to ulcerate spontaneously and discharge an oily yellow fluid. Panniculitis may be associated with other manifestations of the disease, such as panacinar emphysema, noninfectious hepatitis, cirrhosis, persistent cutaneous vasculitis, cold contact urticaria, and acquired angioedema. Diagnosis can be substantiated by a decreased level of serum α_1-antitrypsin activity.

Histology

Extensive septal and lobular neutrophilic infiltrate with necrosis of the fat is observed.

Treatment

Treatment of the panniculitis in with α_1-antitrypsin deficiency is part of the overall treatment of the disease (see Chapter 393).

PANCREATIC PANNICULITIS
Etiology and Pathogenesis

Pathogenesis of pancreatic panniculitis appears to be multifactorial, involving liberation of the lipolytic enzymes lipase, trypsin, and amylase into the circulation, causing adipocyte membrane damage and intracellular lipolysis. There is no correlation, however, between the occurrence of panniculitis and the serum concentration of pancreatic enzymes.

Clinical Manifestations

Pancreatic panniculitis manifests most commonly on the pretibial regions, thighs, or buttocks as tender, erythematous nodules that may be fluctuant and occasionally discharge an oily yellowish substance. It appears most often in males with alcoholism but may also occur in patients with pancreatitis as a result of cholelithiasis or abdominal trauma, with rupture of a pancreatic pseudocyst, with pancreatic ductal adenocarcinoma, or with pancreatic acinar cell carcinoma. Associated features may include polyarthritis (pancreatitis-panniculitis-polyarthritis syndrome). In almost 65% of patients, abdominal signs are absent or mild, making the diagnosis difficult.

Histology

Microscopic changes consist of multiple foci of fat necrosis that contain ghost cells with thick, shadowy walls and no nuclei. A polymorphous inflammatory infiltrate surrounds the areas of fat necrosis.

Treatment

The primary pancreatic disorder must be treated. The arthritis may be chronic and responds poorly to treatment with nonsteroidal antiinflammatory drugs and oral corticosteroids.

SUBCUTANEOUS FAT NECROSIS
Etiology and Pathogenesis

The cause of subcutaneous fat necrosis (SCFN) is unknown. The disease in infants may be a result of ischemic injury from various perinatal complications, such as maternal preeclampsia, birth trauma, asphyxia, and prolonged hypothermia. Whole-body cooling for neonatal encephalopathy is increasingly associated with SCFN. Susceptibility is attributed to differences in composition between the subcutaneous tissue of young infants and that of older infants, children, and adults. Neonatal fat solidifies at a relatively high temperature because of its relatively greater concentration of high-melting-point saturated fatty acids, such as palmitic and stearic acids.

Clinical Manifestations

This inflammatory disorder of adipose tissue occurs primarily in the 1st 4 wk of life in full-term or postterm infants. Typical lesions are asymptomatic, indurated, erythematous to violaceous, sharply demarcated plaques or nodules on the cheeks, buttocks, back, thighs, or upper arms (Fig. 660-4). Lesions may be focal or extensive and are generally asymptomatic, although they may be tender during the acute phase. Uncomplicated lesions involute spontaneously within weeks to months, usually without scarring or atrophy. Calcium deposition may occasionally occur within areas of fat necrosis, which may sometimes result in rupture and drainage of liquid material. These areas may heal with atrophy. A rare but potentially life-threatening complication is **hypercalcemia**. It manifests at 1-6 mo of age (in a review of 20 cases, average age at onset was 6.7 wk) as lethargy, poor feeding, vomiting, failure to thrive, irritability, seizures, shortening of the QT interval on electrocardiography, or renal failure. The origin of the hypercalcemia is unknown, but an accepted hypothesis is that the macrophages present produce 1,25-dihydroxyvitamin D₃ which, in turn, increases calcium uptake. Infants with SCFN should be followed for several months to monitor for delayed hypercalcemia.

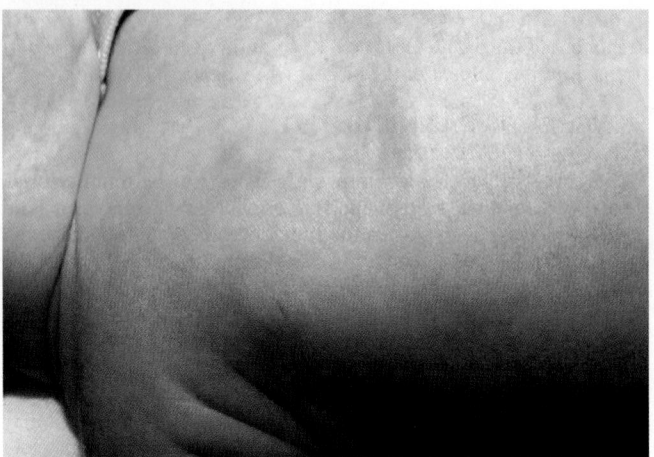

Figure 660-4 Red-purple nodular infiltration of the skin of the chest caused by subcutaneous fat necrosis.

Histology
Histopathologic changes in SCFN are diagnostic, consisting of: necrosis of fat; a granulomatous cellular infiltrate composed of lymphocytes, histiocytes, multinucleated giant cells, and fibroblasts; and radially arranged clefts of crystalline triglyceride within fat cells and multinucleated giant cells. Calcium deposits are commonly found in areas of fat necrosis.

Differential Diagnosis
SCFN can be confused with sclerema neonatorum, panniculitis, cellulitis, and hematoma.

Treatment
Because the lesions are self-limited, therapy is not required for uncomplicated cases of SCFN. Needle aspiration of fluctuant lesions may prevent rupture and subsequent scarring but is rarely needed. Treatment of hypercalcemia is aimed at enhancing renal calcium excretion with hydration and furosemide (1-2 mg/kg/dose) and at limiting dietary calcium and vitamin D intake. Reduction of intestinal calcium absorption and alteration of vitamin D metabolism may be accomplished by administration of corticosteroids (0.5-1.0 mg/kg/day). Pamidronate (0.25-0.5 mg/kg/day) has been used in severe cases.

SCLEREMA NEONATORUM
Etiology and Pathogenesis
Although the cause remains unknown, 4 theories of pathogenesis for sclerema neonatorum have been proposed. It is theorized that sclerema neonatorum results from hardening of the subcutaneous fat because of a decrease in body temperature as a consequence of circulatory shock; a defect in lipolytic enzymes or in lipid transport; association with an underlying severe disease; or a special form of edema affecting the connective tissue that supports the adipocytes.

Clinical Manifestations
This uncommon disorder of adipose tissue manifests abruptly in preterm, gravely ill infants as diffuse, yellowish white woody induration of the skin. It begins on the legs and buttocks then quickly progresses to other areas, sparing palms and soles. Affected skin becomes stony in consistency, cold, and nonpitting. The face assumes a masklike expression, and joint mobility may be compromised because of inflexibility of the skin.

Histology
Histopathologic changes in sclerema neonatorum consist of increases in the size of fat cells and in the width of the fibrous connective tissue septa. In contrast to SCFN, with which this disorder is most apt to be confused, fat necrosis, inflammation, giant cells, and calcium crystals are generally absent.

Treatment
Sclerema neonatorum is almost always associated with serious illness, such as sepsis, congenital heart disease, multiple congenital anomalies, or hypothermia. The appearance of sclerema in a sick infant should be regarded as an ominous prognostic sign. The outcome depends on the response of the underlying disorder to treatment.

COLD PANNICULITIS
Etiology and Pathogenesis
The pathogenic mechanism of cold panniculitis may be similar to that of SCFN, involving a greater propensity of fat to solidify in infants than in older children and adults as a result of the higher percentage of saturated fatty acids in the subcutaneous fat of infants. Lesions occur in infants after prolonged cold exposure, especially on the cheeks, or after prolonged application of a cold object such as an ice cube, ice bag, or fruit ice pop to any area of the skin.

Clinical Manifestations
Ill-defined, erythematous to bluish, indurated plaques or nodules arise within hours to a couple days of exposure on exposed surfaces (face, arms, legs), persist for 2-3 wk, and heal without residua.

Histology
Histopathologic examination reveals an infiltrate of lymphoid and histiocytic cells around blood vessels at the dermal–subdermal junction and in the fat lobules; by the 3rd day, some of the fat cells in the subcutis may have ruptured and coalesced into cystic structures.

Differential Diagnosis
Cold panniculitis may be confused with facial cellulitis caused by *Haemophilus influenzae* type b. Unlike in buccal cellulitis, the area may be cold to the touch, and the patient is afebrile and appears well.

Treatment
Treatment is unnecessary because cold panniculitis spontaneously resolves. Recurrence of the lesions is common, emphasizing the importance of parental education in treating affected patients.

CHILBLAINS (PERNIO)
Etiology and Pathogenesis
Vasospasm of arterioles from damp cold exposure with resultant hypoxemia and localized perivascular mononuclear inflammation appears to be responsible for chilblains. The disease is associated with cryoglobulins, lupus erythematosus with antiphospholipid antibodies, anorexia nervosa, and thin body habitus.

Clinical Manifestations
The condition is characterized by localized symmetric erythematous to purplish edematous plaques and nodules in areas exposed to cold, typically acral areas (distal hands and feet, ears, face; see Chapter 76). Lesions develop 12-24 hr after cold exposure and may be associated with itching, burning, or pain. Blister formation and ulceration are rare.

Histology
Histopathologic examination reveals marked dermal edema and a perivascular and periappendiceal, predominantly T-cell lymphocytic infiltrate in the papillary and reticular dermis.

Differential Diagnosis
Raynaud phenomenon is more acute in nature than chilblains, with characteristic color changes and no chronic lesions. Frostbite due to extreme cold exposure is painful and involves freezing of the tissue with resultant tissue necrosis.

Treatment
Most cases of chilblains resolve spontaneously but can last 2-3 wk. Prevention is the treatment of choice. Nifedipine (0.25-0.5 mg/kg tid,

maximum 10 mg/dose) may be used in severe cases. Unusual or persistent cases of perniosis in children may warrant further work-up including antinuclear antibody titer, cryoglobulins, complete blood count, and cold agglutinins.

FACTITIAL PANNICULITIS
Etiology and Pathogenesis
Factitial panniculitis results from subcutaneous injection by the patient or a proxy of a foreign substance, the most common types of which are organic materials, such as milk and feces; drugs, such as the opiates and pentazocine; oily materials, such as mineral oil and paraffin; and the synthetic polymer povidone.

Clinical Manifestations
Indurated plaques, ulcers, or nodules that liquefy and drain may be noted clinically in factitial panniculitis.

Histology
The histopathology is variable, depending on the injected substance, but may include the presence of birefringent crystals, oil cysts surrounded by fibrosis and inflammation, and an acute inflammatory reaction with fat necrosis. Vessels are characteristically spared.

Treatment
Treatment of factitial panniculitis must address the primary reason the patient is performing the self-destructive act. Munchausen syndrome by proxy should be considered in young children.

Bibliography is available at Expert Consult.

660.2 Lipodystrophy
JiaDe Yu

Several rare conditions are associated with loss of fatty tissue in a partial or generalized distribution and can be familial or acquired. Loss of adipose at certain sites is often accompanied by fat redistribution and consequent hypertrophy of adipose at other sites. Extent of fatty tissue loss or expansion correlates with the degree of clinical and metabolic abnormalities.

PARTIAL LIPODYSTROPHY
Partial lipodystrophy may be familial or acquired. Loss of adipose tissue is not preceded by an inflammatory phase, and histopathologic examination reveals only absence of subcutaneous fat.

There are 5 forms of familial partial lipodystrophy (FPLD):
◆ **Type I (FPLD1–Kobberling)** is characterized by loss of adipose tissue confined to the extremities and gluteal region. Fat distribution of the face, neck, and trunk may be normal or increased. Hyperlipidemia, insulin-resistant diabetes mellitus, and eruptive xanthomas may be seen. The gene is unknown, but only females are affected.
◆ **Type 2 (FPLD2–Dunnigan)** is the most common form of FPLD and caused by mutations in the *laminin A/C* gene leading to premature death of adipocytes. Fat distribution is normal in childhood, but atrophy commences with puberty. Lipodystrophy is seen in the trunk, gluteal region, and extremities. Adipose tissue accumulates in the face and neck and may also be seen in the axillae, back, labia majora, and infraabdominal region. Insulin-resistant diabetes mellitus and hypertriglyceridemia develop, but high-density lipoprotein and cholesterol levels are low. Both males and females are affected, but the diagnosis may be more difficult in males owing to body habitus.
◆ **Type 3 (FPLD3)** is caused by mutations in the peroxisome proliferation–activated receptor γ *(PPARG)* gene inhibiting adipocyte differentiation. Lipodystrophy is seen in the distal limbs and gluteal region. Insulin-resistant diabetes mellitus, primary

amenorrhea, acanthosis nigricans, hypertension, and fatty infiltration of the liver are present.
◆ **Type 4 (FPLD4)** and **Type 5 (FPLD5)** are caused by mutations in *AKT2* and *Perilipin-1 (PLIN1)*, respectively. Both types are also characterized by loss of subcutaneous fat primarily from the extremities.

Acquired partial lipodystrophy (Barraquer-Simons syndrome) is caused by mutations in the *LMNB2* gene. Females are more commonly affected. Fat loss begins in childhood or adolescence and progresses in a cephalotruncal direction, beginning on the face and sparing the lower extremities. Excess fat deposition is seen in the hips and legs, especially in females. Low levels of complement C3 are almost universally seen because of the presence of C3 nephritic factor that stabilizes C3 convertase, allowing for unopposed activation of the alternate complement pathway leading to decreased level of C3. Membranous proliferative glomerulonephritis and other autoimmune diseases may develop. Insulin-resistant diabetes mellitus is rare.

GENERALIZED LIPODYSTROPHY
Generalized lipodystrophy may also be congenital or acquired.

Congenital generalized lipodystrophy is seen in 4 forms:
◆ **Type 1 (Berardinelli-Seip congenital lipodystrophy type 1 [BSCL1])** is an autosomal recessive disorder caused by mutations in the 1-acylglycerol-3-phosphate-*O*-acyltransferase *(AGPAT2)* gene.
◆ **Type 2 (Berardinelli-Seip congenital lipodystrophy type 2 [BSCL2])** is also autosomal recessive and caused by mutations in the seipin gene.
◆ **Type 3 *(CAV1)*** is autosomal recessive and caused by mutations in the caveolin 1 gene.
◆ **Type 4 *(PTRF)*** is autosomal recessive and caused by mutations in the polymerase I and transcript release factor gene. In addition to the classic phenotype of congenital generalized lipodystrophy, these patients also have muscular dystrophy and cardiac conduction abnormalities (QT prolongation).

Marked lipodystrophy occurs at birth or in early infancy with prominent muscularity. Diabetes mellitus, hypertriglyceridemia, hepatic steatosis, acanthosis nigricans, and muscular hypertrophy occur. Congenital generalized lipodystrophy type 1 and type 2 are the most common, with the latter having a more severe phenotype characterized by extensive fat loss, cardiomyopathy, intellectual impairment, and premature death in ≈15% of cases.

Acquired generalized lipodystrophy is more common in females. The most common associated disorder is juvenile dermatomyositis (78%). Panniculitis preceding the loss of fat is seen in 17% of affected individuals. More than half of the children may have other complications, including acanthosis nigricans, hyperpigmentation, hepatomegaly, hypertension, protuberant abdomen, and hyperlipidemia.

Localized lipoatrophy can be idiopathic or secondary to subcutaneous medication injections, pressure, and panniculitis. Unlike generalized or partial lipodystrophy, localized lipoatrophy involve a small part of the body and have no accompanying metabolic derangements. Idiopathic localized lipoatrophy manifests as annular atrophy at the ankles; a bandlike semicircular depression 2-4 cm in diameter on the thighs, abdomen, and/or upper groin or as a centrifugally spreading, depressed, bluish plaque with an erythematous margin. **Insulin lipoatrophy** usually occur approximately 6 mo to 2 yr after initiation of relatively high doses of insulin. A dimple or well-circumscribed depression at or surrounding the site of injection is typically seen. Biopsy reveals a marked decrease or absence of subcutaneous tissue, without inflammation or fibrosis. In some patients, hypertrophy occurs clinically. In these cases, the mid-dermal collagen is replaced by hypertrophic fat cells on histopathologic sections. A recent study shows that adipocytes chronically exposed to high insulin concentrations become insulin-resistant, leading to lipolysis and atrophy. Lesions may also be prevented by frequent alteration of injection sites.

Bibliography is available at Expert Consult.

Chapter **661**
Disorders of the Sweat Glands
Kari L. Martin

Eccrine glands are found over nearly the entire skin surface and provide the primary means, through evaporation of the water in sweat, of cooling the body. These glands have no anatomic relationship to hair follicles and secrete a relatively large amount of odorless aqueous sweat. In contrast, apocrine sweat glands are limited in distribution to the axillae, anogenital skin, mammary glands, ceruminous glands of the ear, Moll glands in the eyelid, and selected areas of the face and scalp. Each apocrine gland duct enters the pilosebaceous follicle at the level of the infundibulum and secretes a small amount of a complex, viscous fluid that, on alteration by microorganisms, produces a distinctive body odor. Some disorders of these 2 types of sweat glands are similar pathogenetically, whereas others are unique to a given gland.

ANHIDROSIS

Neuropathic anhidrosis results from a disturbance in the neural pathway from the control center in the brain to the peripheral efferent nerve fibers that activate sweating. Disorders in this category, which are characterized by generalized anhidrosis, include tumors of the hypothalamus and damage to the floor of the third ventricle. Pontine or medullary lesions may produce anhidrosis of the ipsilateral face or neck and ipsilateral or contralateral anhidrosis of the rest of the body. Peripheral or segmental neuropathies, caused by leprosy, amyloidosis, diabetes mellitus, alcoholic neuritis, or syringomyelia, may be associated with anhidrosis of the innervated skin. Various autonomic disorders are also associated with altered eccrine sweat gland function.

At the level of the sweat gland, anticholinergics (drugs such as atropine and scopolamine) may paralyze the sweat glands. Acute intoxication with barbiturates or diazepam has produced necrosis of sweat glands, resulting in anhidrosis with or without erythema and bullae. Eccrine glands are largely absent throughout the skin or are present in a localized area among patients with **hypohidrotic ectodermal dysplasia** or **localized congenital absence of sweat glands,** respectively. Infiltrative or destructive disorders that may produce atrophy of sweat glands by pressure or scarring include scleroderma, acrodermatitis chronica atrophicans, radiodermatitis, burns, Sjögren syndrome, multiple myeloma, and lymphoma. Obstruction of sweat glands may occur in miliaria and in a number of inflammatory and hyperkeratotic disorders, such as the ichthyoses, psoriasis, lichen planus, pemphigus, porokeratosis, atopic dermatitis, and seborrheic dermatitis. Occlusion of the sweat pore may also occur with the topical agents aluminum and zirconium salts, formaldehyde, or glutaraldehyde.

Diverse disorders that are associated with anhidrosis by unknown mechanisms include dehydration; toxic overdose with lead, arsenic, thallium, fluorine, or morphine; uremia; cirrhosis; endocrine disorders such as Addison disease, diabetes mellitus, diabetes insipidus, and hyperthyroidism; and inherited conditions such as autonomic neuropathies, Fabry disease, Franceschetti-Jadassohn syndrome, which combines features of incontinentia pigmenti and hypohidrotic ectodermal dysplasia, congenital insensitivity to pain with anhidrosis syndrome, and familial anhidrosis with neurolabyrinthitis.

Anhidrosis may be complete, but in many cases, what appears clinically to be anhidrosis is actually **hypohidrosis** caused by anhidrosis of many, but not all, eccrine glands. Compensatory, localized hyperhidrosis of the remaining functional sweat glands may occur, particularly in diabetes mellitus and miliaria. The primary complication of anhidrosis is **hyperthermia,** seen primarily in anhidrotic ectodermal dysplasia or

in otherwise normal preterm or full-term neonates who have immature eccrine glands.

HYPERHIDROSIS
Etiology and Pathogenesis
Hyperhidrosis is excessive sweating beyond what is physiologically necessary for temperature control and occurs in 3% of the population with about half having axillary hyperhidrosis. The numerous disorders that may be associated with increased production of eccrine sweat may also be classified into those with neural mechanisms involving an abnormality in the pathway from the neural regulatory centers to the sweat gland and those that are nonneurally mediated and occur by direct effects on the sweat glands (Table 661-1).

Clinical Manifestations
The average age at onset of hyperhidrosis is 14-25 yr. The excess sweating may be continuous or may occur in response to emotional stimuli. In severe cases, sweat may be seen to drip constantly from the hands.

Treatment
Excessive sweating of the palms and soles (volar hyperhidrosis) and axillary sweating may respond to 20% aluminum chloride in anhydrous ethanol applied under occlusion for several hours, iontophoresis, injection with botulinum toxin, therapy with oral anticholinergics, or in severe, refractory cases, cervicothoracic or lumbar sympathectomy. Reports of successful treatment of hyperhidrosis with microwave technology are available, but studies are faulted with small sample size and lack of controls.

Table 661-1	Causes of Hyperhidrosis

CORTICAL Emotional Familial dysautonomia Congenital ichthyosiform 　erythroderma Epidermolysis bullosa Nail-patella syndrome Jadassohn-Lewandowsky 　syndrome Pachyonychia congenita Palmoplantar keratoderma Stroke **HYPOTHALAMIC** Drugs: 　Alcohol 　Antipyretics 　Cocaine 　Emetics 　Insulin 　Opiates (including withdrawal) 　Ciprofloxacin Exercise Infection: 　Defervescence 　Chronic illness Metabolic: 　Carcinoid syndrome 　Debility 　Diabetes mellitus 　Hyperpituitarism 　Hyperthyroidism 　Hypoglycemia 　Obesity 　Pheochromocytoma 　Porphyria 　Pregnancy 　Rickets 　Infantile scurvy	Cardiovascular: 　Heart failure 　Shock 　Vasomotor 　Cold injury 　Raynaud phenomenon 　Rheumatoid arthritis Neurologic: 　Abscess 　Familial dysautonomia 　Postencephalitic 　Tumor Miscellaneous: 　Chédiak-Higashi syndrome 　Compensatory 　Lymphoma 　Phenylketonuria 　Vitiligo **MEDULLARY** Physiologic gustatory sweating Encephalitis Granulosis rubra nasi Syringomyelia Thoracic sympathetic trunk injury **SPINAL** Cord transection Syringomyelia **CHANGES IN BLOOD FLOW** Maffucci syndrome Arteriovenous fistula Klippel-Trenaunay syndrome Glomus tumor Blue rubber-bleb nevus 　syndrome

MILIARIA

Etiology and Pathogenesis

Miliaria results from retention of sweat in occluded eccrine sweat ducts. The keratinous plug does not form until the later stages of the disease and therefore does not appear to be the primary cause of the sweat duct obstruction. The initial obstruction is postulated to be caused by swelling of the ductal epidermal cells, perhaps from imbibition of water. Retrograde pressure may result in rupture of the duct and leakage of sweat into the epidermis and/or the dermis. The eruption is most often induced by hot, humid weather, but it may also be caused by high fever. Infants who are dressed too warmly may demonstrate this eruption indoors, even during the winter.

Clinical Manifestations

In **miliaria crystallina,** asymptomatic, noninflammatory, pinpoint, clear vesicles may suddenly erupt in profusion over large areas of the body surface, leaving brawny desquamation on healing (Fig. 661-1). This type of miliaria occurs most frequently in newborn infants because of the relative immaturity and delayed patency of the sweat duct and the tendency for infants to be nursed in relatively warm, humid conditions. It may also occur in older patients with hyperpyrexia.

Miliaria rubra is a less superficial eruption characterized by erythematous, minute papulovesicles that may impart a prickling sensation. The lesions are usually localized to sites of occlusion or to flexural areas, such as the neck, groin, and axillae, where friction may have a role in their pathogenesis. Involved skin may become macerated and eroded. Lesions of miliaria rubra, however, are extrafollicular.

Repeated attacks of miliaria rubra may lead to **miliaria profunda,** which is caused by rupture of the sweat duct deeper in the skin, at the level of the dermal–epidermal junction. Severe, extensive miliaria rubra or miliaria profunda may result in disturbance of heat regulation. Lesions of miliaria rubra may become infected, particularly in malnourished or debilitated infants, leading to development of **periporitis staphylogenes,** which involves extension of the process from the sweat duct into the sweat gland.

Histology

Histologically, miliaria crystallina reveals an intracorneal or subcorneal vesicle in communication with the sweat duct, whereas in miliaria rubra, one sees focal areas of spongiosis and spongiotic vesicle formation in close proximity to sweat ducts that generally contain a keratinous plug.

Differential Diagnosis

The clarity of the fluid, superficiality of the vesicles, and absence of inflammation permit differentiation of miliaria crystalline from other blistering disorders. Miliaria rubra may be confused with or superimposed on other diaper area eruptions, including candidosis and folliculitis.

Figure 661-1 Superficial clear vesicles of miliaria crystallina.

Treatment

All forms of miliaria respond dramatically to cooling of the patient by regulation of environmental temperatures and by removal of excessive clothing; administration of antipyretics is also beneficial to patients with fever. Topical agents are usually ineffective and may exacerbate the eruption.

BROMHIDROSIS

The excessive odor that characterizes bromhidrosis may result from alteration of either apocrine or eccrine sweat. Apocrine bromhidrosis develops after puberty as a result of the formation of short-chain fatty acids and ammonia by the action of anaerobic diphtheroids on axillary apocrine sweat. Eccrine bromhidrosis is caused by microbiologic degradation of stratum corneum that has become softened by excessive eccrine sweat. The soles of the feet and the intertriginous areas are the primary affected sites. Hyperhidrosis, warm weather, obesity, intertrigo, and diabetes mellitus are predisposing factors. **Treatments** that may be helpful include cleansing with germicidal soaps, topical clindamycin or erythromycin, or topical application of aluminum or zirconium. Treatment of any associated hyperhidrosis is mandatory.

HIDRADENITIS SUPPURATIVA

Etiology and Pathogenesis

Hidradenitis suppurativa is a disease of the apocrine gland–bearing areas of the skin. Pathogenesis of hidradenitis suppurativa is controversial. It is believed that it is a primary inflammatory disorder of the hair follicle and not solely an alteration of apocrine glands. It is considered a part of the follicular occlusion tetrad, along with acne conglobata, dissecting cellulites of the scalp, and pilonidal sinus. The natural history of the disease involves progressive dilation below the follicular obstruction, leading to rupture of the duct, inflammation, sinus tract formation, and destructive scarring.

Clinical Manifestations

Hidradenitis suppurativa is a chronic, inflammatory, suppurative disorder of the follicular units in the axillae, the anogenital area, and, occasionally, the scalp, posterior aspect of the ears, female breasts, and periumbilical area. Onset of clinical manifestations is sometimes preceded by pruritus or discomfort and usually occurs during puberty or early adulthood. Solitary or multiple painful erythematous nodules, deep abscesses, and contracted scars are sharply confined to areas of skin containing apocrine glands. When the disease is severe and chronic, sinus tracts, ulcers, and thick, linear fibrotic bands develop. Hidradenitis suppurativa tends to persist for many years, punctuated by relapses and partial remissions. Complications include cellulitis, ulceration, and burrowing abscesses that may perforate adjacent structures, forming fistulas to the urethra, bladder, rectum, or peritoneum. Episodic inflammatory arthritis develops in some patients.

Histology

Early lesions are characterized by a keratinous plug in the apocrine duct or hair follicle orifice and by cystic distention of the follicle. The process generally but not necessarily extends into the apocrine gland. Later changes include inflammation within and around apocrine glands. Scarring may obliterate skin appendages.

Differential Diagnosis

Early lesions of hidradenitis suppurativa are often mistaken for infected epidermal cysts, furuncles, scrofuloderma, actinomycosis, cat-scratch disease, granuloma inguinale, or lymphogranuloma venereum. Sharp localization to areas of the body that bear apocrine glands, however, should suggest hidradenitis. When involvement is limited to the anogenital region, the condition may be difficult to distinguish from Crohn disease.

Treatment

Conservative management includes cessation of smoking, weight loss, and avoidance of irritation of the affected area. Warm compresses and topical antiseptic or antibacterial soaps may also be helpful. For mild, early disease, topical clindamycin 1% may be helpful. For more-severe disease, therapy may be initiated with doxycycline (100 mg bid) or minocycline (100 mg bid). Some patients require intermittent or long-term antibiotic treatment. Combination therapy with clindamycin and rifampin is helpful in some patients. Oral retinoids (1 mg/kg/day) for 5-6 mo may also be effective. Oral contraceptive agents, which contain a high estrogen:progesterone ratio and low androgenicity of the progesterone, are another alternative. Laser hair ablation has proven helpful in some studies as well. Systemic immunosuppressants (infliximab, adalimumab, cyclosporine) and medications targeted at glucose metabolism and the metabolic syndrome (metformin) have been helpful. Surgical measures may be required for control or cure, especially in localized, recalcitrant cases.

FOX-FORDYCE DISEASE
Etiology and Pathogenesis
The cause of Fox-Fordyce disease is unknown.

Clinical Manifestations
This disease is most common in females and manifests during puberty to the 3rd decade of life as pruritus in the axillae. Pruritus is exacerbated by emotional stress and stimuli that induce apocrine sweating. Dome-shaped, skin-colored to slightly hyperpigmented, follicular papules develop in the pruritic areas.

Histology
Histopathologically, one sees keratinous plugging of the distal apocrine duct, rupture of the intraepidermal portion of the apocrine duct, periductal microvesicle formation, and periductal acanthosis.

Treatment
Fox-Fordyce disease is difficult to treat. Oral contraceptive pills and topical corticosteroids or retinoic acid may help some patients.

Bibliography is available at Expert Consult.

Chapter 662
Disorders of Hair
Kari L. Martin

Disorders of hair in infants and children may be a result of intrinsic disturbances of hair growth, underlying biochemical or metabolic defects, inflammatory dermatoses, or structural anomalies of the hair shaft. Excessive and abnormal hair growth is referred to as hypertrichosis or hirsutism. **Hypertrichosis** is excessive hair growth at inappropriate locations; hirsutism is an androgen-dependent male pattern of hair growth in women. **Hypotrichosis** is deficient hair growth. Hair loss, partial or complete, is called *alopecia*. Alopecia may be classified as nonscarring or scarring; the latter type is rare in children and, if present, is most often caused by prolonged or untreated inflammatory conditions, such as pyoderma and tinea capitis.

HYPERTRICHOSIS
Hypertrichosis is rare in children and may be localized or generalized and permanent or transient. Table 662-1 lists some of the many causes of hypertrichosis.

HYPOTRICHOSIS AND ALOPECIA
Table 662-2 lists some of the disorders associated with hypotrichosis and alopecia. True alopecia is rarely congenital; it is more often related

Table 662-1	Causes of and Conditions Associated with Hypertrichosis

INTRINSIC FACTORS
Racial and familial forms such as hairy ears, hairy elbows, intraphalangeal hair, or generalized hirsutism

EXTRINSIC FACTORS
Local trauma
Malnutrition
Anorexia nervosa
Long-standing inflammatory dermatoses
Drugs: Diazoxide, phenytoin, corticosteroids, Cortisporin, cyclosporine, androgens, anabolic agents, hexachlorobenzene, minoxidil, psoralens, penicillamine, streptomycin

HAMARTOMAS OR NEVI
Congenital pigmented nevocytic nevus, hair follicle nevus, Becker nevus, congenital smooth muscle hamartoma, fawn-tail nevus associated with diastematomyelia

ENDOCRINE DISORDERS
Virilizing ovarian tumors, Cushing syndrome, acromegaly, hyperthyroidism, hypothyroidism, congenital adrenal hyperplasia, adrenal tumors, gonadal dysgenesis, male pseudohermaphroditism, non–endocrine hormone–secreting tumors, polycystic ovary syndrome

CONGENITAL AND GENETIC DISORDERS
Hypertrichosis lanuginosa, mucopolysaccharidosis, leprechaunism, congenital generalized lipodystrophy, de Lange syndrome, trisomy 18, Rubinstein-Taybi syndrome, Bloom syndrome, congenital hemihypertrophy, gingival fibromatosis with hypertrichosis, Winchester syndrome, lipoatrophic diabetes (Lawrence-Seip syndrome), fetal hydantoin syndrome, fetal alcohol syndrome, congenital erythropoietic or variegate porphyria (sun-exposed areas), porphyria cutanea tarda (sun-exposed areas), Cowden syndrome, Seckel syndrome, Gorlin syndrome, partial trisomy 3q, Ambras syndrome

Table 662-2	Disorders Associated with Alopecia and Hypotrichosis

Congenital total alopecia: Atrichia with papules, Moynahan alopecia syndrome
Congenital localized alopecia: Aplasia cutis, triangular alopecia, sebaceous nevus
Hereditary hypotrichosis: Marie-Unna syndrome, hypotrichosis with juvenile macular dystrophy, hypotrichosis–Mari type, ichthyosis with hypotrichosis, cartilage-hair hypoplasia, Hallermann-Streiff syndrome, trichorhinophalangeal syndrome, ectodermal dysplasia "pure" hair and nail and other ectodermal dysplasias
Diffuse alopecia of endocrine origin: Hypopituitarism, hypothyroidism, hypoparathyroidism, hyperthyroidism
Alopecia of nutritional origin: Marasmus, kwashiorkor, iron deficiency, zinc deficiency (acrodermatitis enteropathica), gluten-sensitive enteropathy, essential fatty acid deficiency, biotinidase deficiency
Disturbances of the hair cycle: Telogen effluvium
Toxic alopecia: Anagen effluvium
Autoimmune alopecia: Alopecia areata
Traumatic alopecia: Traction alopecia, trichotillomania
Cicatricial alopecia: Lupus erythematosus, lichen planopilaris, pseudopelade, morphea (en coup de saber) dermatomyositis, infection (kerion, favus, tuberculosis, syphilis, folliculitis, leishmaniasis, herpes zoster, varicella), acne keloidalis, follicular mucinosis, sarcoidosis
Hair shaft abnormalities: Monilethrix, pili annulati, pili torti, trichorrhexis invaginata, trichorrhexis nodosa, woolly hair syndrome, Menkes disease, trichothiodystrophy, trichodentoosseous syndrome, uncombable hair syndrome (spun-glass hair, pili trianguli et canaliculi)

Table 662-3	Helpful Historical Clues in Diagnosis of Hair Disorders			
HISTORICAL CONSIDERATIONS	**TELOGEN EFFLUVIUM**	**TRICHOTILLOMANIA**	**TINEA CAPITIS**	**ALOPECIA AREATA**
Are the spots itchy?	Negative	Negative	Positive	Usually negative
Do the spots come and go?	Negative	Sometimes positive	Negative	Sometimes positive
Is the hair falling out in clumps?	Positive	Negative	Negative	Usually negative
Are there any anxiety disorders or obsessive–compulsive tendencies?	Negative	Positive	Negative	Negative

From Lio PA: What's missing from this picture? An approach to alopecia in children, Arch Dis Child Educ Pract Ed 92:193–198, 2007.

Table 662-4	Helpful Physical Examination Clues in Diagnosis of Hair Disorders			
PHYSICAL FINDINGS	**TELOGEN EFFLUVIUM**	**TRICHOTILLOMANIA**	**TINEA CAPITIS**	**ALOPECIA AREATA**
Scarring?	Negative	Negative	Usually negative	Negative
Exclamation-point hairs?	Negative	Negative	Negative	Positive
Irregular pattern with mixed length and stubbly hairs?	Negative	Positive	Negative	Negative
Scaling, pustules or kerion?	Negative	Negative	Positive	Negative
Positive hair-pull test result?	Positive	Negative	Negative	Usually negative
Nail pitting or grooves?	Negative	Negative	Negative	Positive

From Lio PA: What's missing from this picture? An approach to alopecia in children, Arch Dis Child Educ Pract Ed 92:193–198, 2007.

to an inflammatory dermatosis, mechanical factors, drug ingestion, infection, endocrinopathy, nutritional disturbance, or disturbance of the hair cycle. Any inflammatory condition of the scalp, such as atopic dermatitis or seborrheic dermatitis, if severe enough, may result in partial alopecia; hair growth returns to normal if the underlying condition is treated successfully, unless the hair follicle has been permanently damaged.

Hair loss in childhood should be divided into the following 4 categories: congenital diffuse, congenital localized, acquired diffuse, and acquired localized.

Acquired localized hair loss is the most common type of hair loss seen in childhood. Three conditions—traumatic alopecia, alopecia areata, tinea capitis—are predominantly seen (Tables 662-3 and 662-4).

TRAUMATIC ALOPECIA (TRACTION ALOPECIA, HAIR PULLING, TRICHOTILLOMANIA)

Traction Alopecia

Traction alopecia is common and is seen in almost 20% of African-American schoolgirls. It is caused by trauma to hair follicles from tight braids or ponytails, headbands, rubber bands, curlers, or rollers (Fig. 662-1). There is a greater risk of traction alopecia if hair trauma is combined with chemically relaxed hair. Broken hairs and inflammatory follicular papules in circumscribed patches at the scalp margins are characteristic and may be subtended by regional lymphadenopathy. Children and parents must be encouraged to avoid devices that cause trauma to the hair and, if necessary, to alter the hairstyle. Otherwise, scarring of hair follicles may occur.

Hair Pulling

Hair pulling in childhood is usually an acute reactional process related to emotional stress or a habit (especially in young children). It may also be seen in trichotillomania (obsessive–compulsive disorder) and as part of more severe psychiatric disorders usually in adolescents.

Trichotillomania

Etiology and Pathogenesis. The diagnostic criteria for trichotillomania include visible hair loss attributable to pulling; mounting tension preceding hair pulling; gratification or release of tension

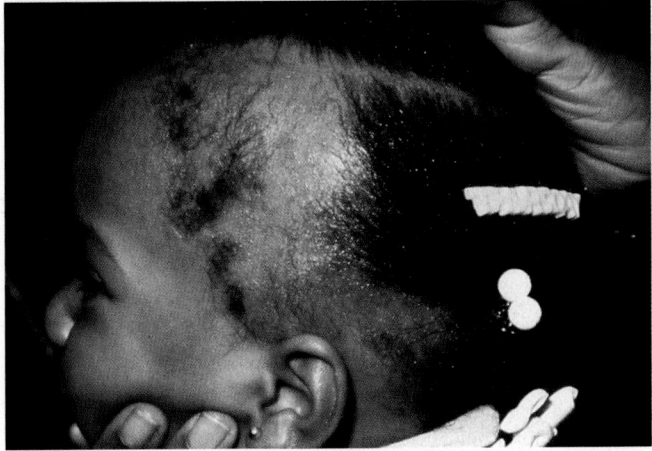

Figure 662-1 Traction alopecia.

after hair pulling; and absence of hair pulling attributable to hallucinations, delusions, or an inflammatory skin condition.

Clinical Manifestations. Compulsive pulling, twisting, and breaking of hair produces irregular areas of incomplete hair loss, most often on the crown and in the occipital and parietal areas of the scalp. Occasionally, eyebrows, eyelashes, and body hair are traumatized. Some plaques of alopecia may have a linear outline. The hairs remaining within the areas of loss are of various lengths (Fig. 662-2) and are typically blunt-tipped because of breakage. The scalp usually appears normal, although hemorrhage, crusting (Fig. 662-3), and chronic folliculitis may also occur. Trichophagy, resulting in **trichobezoars,** may complicate this disorder.

Differential Diagnosis. Acute reactional hair pulling, tinea capitis, and alopecia areata must be considered in the differential diagnosis of trichotillomania (see Tables 662-3 and 662-4).

Histology. Histologic changes include coexistent normal and damaged follicles, perifollicular hemorrhage, atrophy of some follicles, and catagen transformation of hair. In late stages, perifollicular fibrosis may occur. Long-term repeated trauma may result in irreversible damage and permanent alopecia.

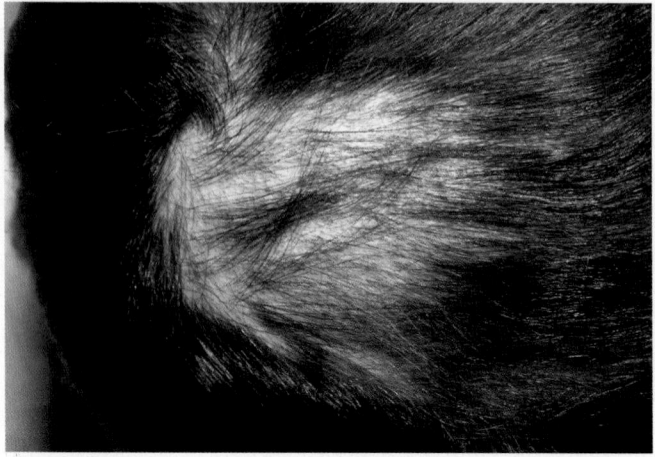

Figure 662-2 Hair pulling. Hairs are broken off at various lengths.

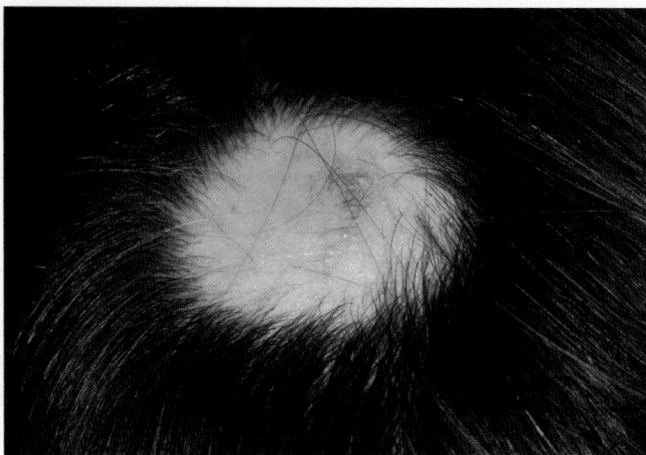

Figure 662-4 Circular patch of alopecia areata with normal-appearing scalp.

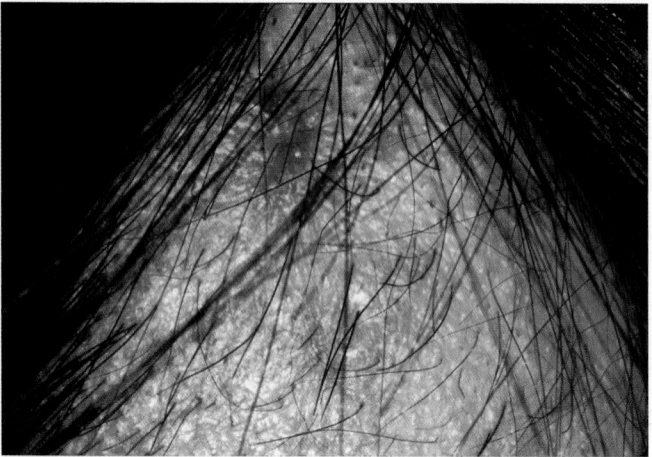

Figure 662-3 Hemorrhage and crusting secondary to hair pulling.

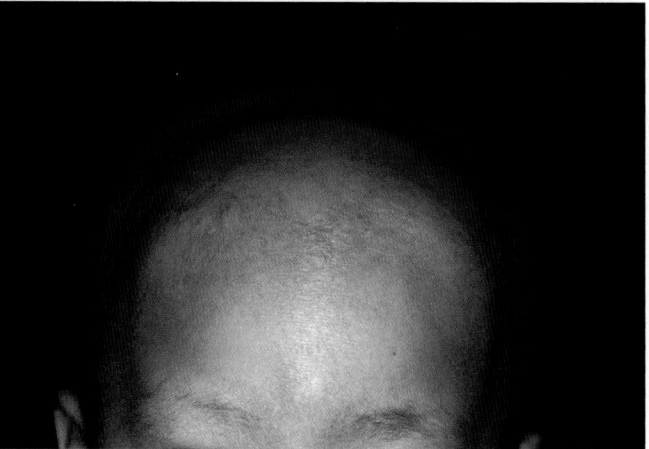

Figure 662-5 Alopecia totalis: total loss of scalp hair.

Treatment. Trichotillomania is closely related to obsessive-compulsive disorder and may be an expression of it for some children. When trichotillomania occur secondary to **obsessive–compulsive disorder**, clomipramine 50-150 mg/day or fluoxetine 40-80 mg/day may be helpful, particularly when combined with behavioral interventions (see Chapter 24). *N*-Acetylcysteine may also be helpful.

ALOPECIA AREATA
Etiology and Pathogenesis
Alopecia areata is a T-cell driven autoimmune disorder producing nonscarring alopecia. The cause is unknown. It is hypothesized that in genetically susceptible individuals, loss of immune privilege of the hair follicle allows for T-cell inflammation against anagen hairs, follicles, leading to stoppage of hair growth.

Clinical Manifestations
Alopecia areata is characterized by rapid and complete loss of hair in round or oval patches on the scalp (Fig. 662-4) and on other body sites. In alopecia totalis, all the scalp hair is lost (Fig. 662-5); alopecia universalis involves all body and scalp hair. The lifetime incidence of alopecia areata is 0.1-0.2% of the population. More than half of affected patients are younger than 20 yr.

The skin within the plaques of hair loss appears normal. Alopecia areata is associated with atopy and with nail changes such as pits (Fig. 662-6), longitudinal striations, and leukonychia. **Autoimmune diseases** such as Hashimoto thyroiditis, Addison disease, pernicious anemia, ulcerative colitis, myasthenia gravis, collagen vascular diseases,

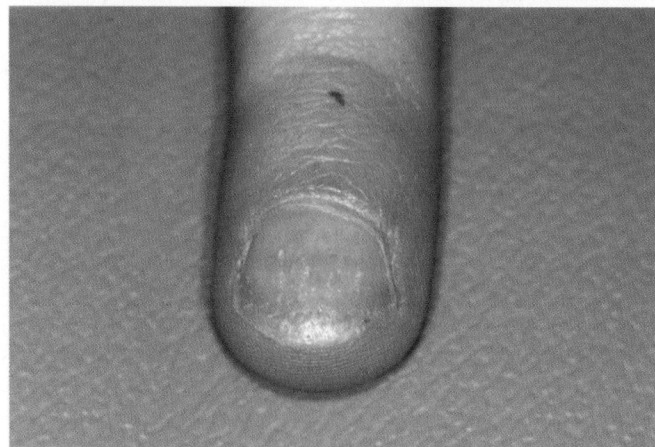

Figure 662-6 Multiple nail pits in alopecia areata.

and vitiligo may also be seen. An increased incidence of alopecia areata has been reported in patients with Down syndrome (5-10%).

Differential Diagnosis
Tinea capitis, seborrheic dermatitis, trichotillomania, traumatic alopecia, and lupus erythematosus should be considered in the differential diagnosis of alopecia areata (see Tables 662-3 and 662-4).

Histology

A perifollicular infiltrate of inflammatory round cells is found in biopsy specimens from active areas of alopecia areata.

Treatment

The course is unpredictable, but spontaneous resolution in 6-12 mo is usual, particularly when relatively small, stable patches of alopecia are present. Recurrences are common. Onset at a young age, extensive or prolonged hair loss, and numerous episodes are usually poor prognostic signs. Alopecia universalis, alopecia totalis, and alopecia ophiasis (Fig. 662-7)—a type of alopecia areata in which hair loss is circumferential—are also less likely to resolve. Therapy is difficult to evaluate because the course is erratic and unpredictable. The use of high- or superpotency topical corticosteroids is effective in some patients. Intradermal injections of steroid (triamcinolone 5 mg/mL) every 4-6 wk may also stimulate hair growth locally, but this mode of treatment is impractical in young children or in patients with extensive hair loss. Systemic corticosteroid therapy (prednisone 1 mg/kg/day) is associated with good results; the permanence of cure is questionable, however, and the side effects of chronic oral corticosteroids are a serious deterrent. Some patients may maintain hair growth by switching to a more appropriate long-term immunosuppressant such as methotrexate. Additional therapies that are sometimes effective include short-contact anthralin, topical minoxidil, and contact sensitization with squaric acid dibutylester or diphencyprone. In general, parents and patients can be reassured that spontaneous remission of alopecia areata usually occurs. New hair growth may initially be of finer caliber and lighter color, but replacement by normal terminal hair can be expected.

ACQUIRED DIFFUSE HAIR LOSS
Telogen Effluvium

Telogen effluvium manifests as sudden loss of large amounts of hair, often with brushing, combing, and washing of hair. Diffuse loss of scalp hair occurs from premature conversion of growing, or anagen, hairs, which normally constitute 80-90% of hairs, to resting, or telogen, hairs. Hair loss is noted 6 wk to 3 mo after the precipitating cause, which may include childbirth; a febrile episode; surgery; acute blood loss, including blood donation; sudden severe weight loss; discontinuation of high-dose corticosteroids or oral contraceptives; and psychiatric stress. Telogen effluvium also accounts for the loss of hair by infants in the 1st few mo of life; friction from bed sheets, particularly in infants with pruritic, atopic skin, may exacerbate the problem. There is no inflammatory reaction; the hair follicles remain intact, and telogen bulbs can be demonstrated microscopically on shed hairs. Because >50% of the scalp hair is rarely involved, alopecia is usually not severe. Parents should be reassured that normal hair growth will return within approximately 3-6 mo.

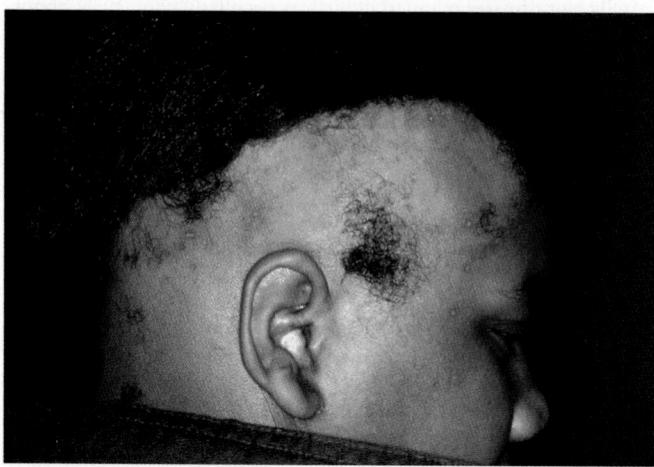

Figure 662-7 Ophiasis pattern of alopecia areata.

Toxic Alopecia (Anagen Effluvium)

Anagen effluvium is an acute, severe, diffuse inhibition of growth of anagen follicles, resulting in loss of >80-90% of scalp hair. Hairs become dystrophic, and the hair shaft breaks at the narrowed segment. Loss is diffuse, rapid (1-3 wk after treatment), and temporary, as regrowth occurs after the offending agent is discontinued. Causes of anagen effluvium include radiation; cancer chemotherapeutic agents such as antimetabolites, alkylating agents, and mitotic inhibitors; thallium; thiouracil; heparin; the coumarins; boric acid; and hypervitaminosis A.

CONGENITAL DIFFUSE HAIR LOSS

Congenital diffuse hair loss is defined as congenitally thin hair diffusely related to either hypoplasia of hair follicles or to structural defects in hair shafts.

Structural Defects of Hair

Structural defects of the hair shaft may be congenital, reflect known biochemical aberrations, or relate to damaging grooming practices. All the defects can be demonstrated by microscopic examination of affected hairs, particularly with scanning and transmission electron microscopy, though many can even be seen by simple trichogram done in the office.

Trichorrhexis Nodosa

Congenital trichorrhexis nodosa is an autosomal dominant condition. The hair is dry, brittle, and lusterless, with irregularly spaced grayish white nodes on the hair shaft. Microscopically, the nodes have the appearance of two interlocking brushes (Fig. 662-8A). The defect results from a fracture of the hair shaft at the nodal points caused by disruption of the cells in the hair cortex. Trichorrhexis nodosa has also been observed in some infants with Menkes syndrome, trichothiodystrophy, citrullinemia, and argininosuccinic aciduria.

Acquired Trichorrhexis Nodosa

Acquired trichorrhexis nodosa, the most common cause of hair breakage, occurs in 2 forms. Proximal defects are found most frequently in African-American children, whose complaint is not of alopecia but of failure of the hair to grow. The hair is short, and longitudinal splits, knots, and whitish nodules can be demonstrated in hair mounts. Easy breakage is demonstrated by gentle traction on the hair shafts. A history of other affected family members may be obtained. The problem may be caused by a combination of genetic predisposition and the cumulative mechanical trauma of rough combing and brushing, hair-straightening procedures, and "permanents." Patients must be cautioned to avoid damaging grooming techniques. A soft, natural-bristle brush and a wide-toothed comb should be used. The condition is self-limited, with resolution in 2-4 yr, if patients avoid damaging practices. Distal trichorrhexis nodosa is seen more frequently in white and Asian children. The distal portion of the hair shaft is thinned, ragged, and faded; white specks, sometimes mistaken for nits, may be noted along the shaft. Hair mounts reveal the paintbrush defect and the sites of excessive fragility and breakage. Localized areas of the moustache or beard may also be affected. Avoidance of traumatic grooming, regular trimming of affected ends, and the use of cream rinses to lessen tangling ameliorate this condition.

Pili Torti

Patients with pili torti present with spangled, brittle, coarse hair of different lengths over the entire scalp. There is a structural defect in which the hair shaft is grooved and flattened at irregular intervals and is twisted on its axis to various degrees. Minor twists that occur in normal hair should not be misconstrued as pili torti. Curvature of the hair follicle apparently leads to the flattening and rotation of the hair shaft. The genetic defect in isolated pili torti is unknown, and both autosomal dominant and recessive forms have been described. **Syndromes** in which the hair shaft abnormalities of pili torti are seen in association with other cutaneous and systemic abnormalities include Menkes kinky hair syndrome, Björnstad syndrome (pili torti with deafness; *BCS1L* gene), and multiple ectodermal dysplasia syndromes.

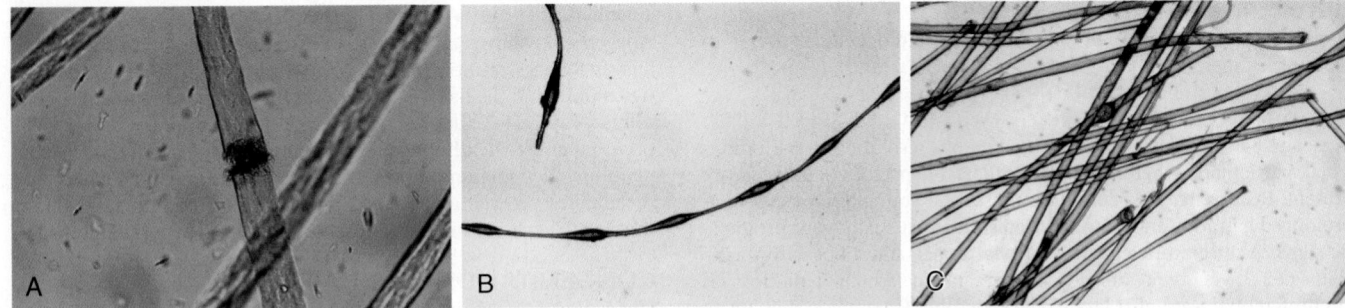

Figure 662-8 A, Microscopic hair fracture in trichorrhexis nodosa. **B,** Beading of hair in monilethrix. **C,** Cup-like abnormality of hair in Netherton syndrome.

Menkes Kinky Hair Syndrome (Trichopoliodystrophy)

Males with Menkes kinky hair syndrome, an X-linked recessive trait, are born to an unaffected mother after a normal pregnancy. Neonatal problems include hypothermia, hypotonia, poor feeding, seizures, and failure to thrive. Hair is normal to sparse at birth but is replaced by short, fine, brittle, light-colored hair that may have features of trichorrhexis nodosa, pili torti, or monilethrix. The skin is hypopigmented and thin, cheeks typically appear plump, and the nasal bridge is depressed. Progressive psychomotor retardation is noted in early infancy. Mutations in the *ATP7A* gene, encoding a copper-transporting adenosine triphosphatase protein, cause Menkes kinky hair syndrome. It is a result of maldistribution of the copper in the body. Copper uptake across the brush-border of the small intestine is increased, but copper transport from these cells into the plasma is defective, resulting in low total body copper stores. Parenteral administration of copper-histidine is helpful if begun in the 1st 2 mo of life.

Monilethrix

The hair shaft defect known as monilethrix is inherited as an autosomal dominant trait with variable age of onset, severity, and course. Mutations in the hair keratins HB1, HB3, and HB6 have been identified in autosomal dominant cases, and mutations in desmoglein 4 are found in autosomal recessive cases. The hair appears dry, lusterless, and brittle, and it fractures spontaneously or with mild trauma. Eyebrows, lashes, body and pubic hair, and scalp hair may be affected. Monilethrix may be present at birth, but the hair is usually normal at birth and is replaced in the 1st few mo of life by abnormal hairs; the condition is sometimes first apparent in childhood. Follicular papules may appear on the nape of the neck and the occiput and, occasionally, over the entire scalp. Short, fragile beaded hairs that emerge from the horny follicular plugs give a distinctive appearance. Keratosis pilaris and koilonychia of fingernails and toenails may also be present. Microscopically, a distinctive, regular beading pattern of the hair shaft is evident, characterized by elliptic nodes that are separated by narrower internodes (see Fig. 662-8B). Not all hairs have nodes, and both normal and beaded hairs may break. Patients should be advised to handle the hair gently to minimize breakage. Treatment is generally ineffective.

Trichothiodystrophy

Hair in trichothiodystrophy is sparse, short, brittle, and uneven; the scalp hair, eyebrows, or eyelashes may be affected. Microscopically, the hair is flattened, folded, and variable in diameter; has longitudinal grooving; and has nodal swellings that resemble those seen in trichorrhexis nodosa. Under a polarizing microscope, distinctive alternating dark and light bands are seen. The abnormal hair has a cystine content that is <50% of normal because of a major reduction in and altered composition of constituent high-sulfur matrix proteins. Trichothiodystrophy may occur as an isolated finding or in association with various syndrome complexes that include intellectual impairment, short stature, ichthyosis, nail dystrophy, dental caries, cataracts,

decreased fertility, neurologic abnormalities, bony abnormalities, and immunodeficiency (*TTDN1* gene). Some patients are photosensitive and have impairment of DNA repair mechanisms, similar to that seen in groups B and D xeroderma pigmentosum; the incidence of skin cancers, however, is not increased. Patients with trichothiodystrophy tend to resemble one another, with a receding chin, protruding ears, raspy voice, and sociable, outgoing personality. Trichoschisis, a fracture perpendicular to the hair shaft, is characteristic of the many syndromes that are associated with trichothiodystrophy. Perpendicular breakage of the hair shaft has also been described in association with other hair abnormalities, particularly monilethrix.

Trichorrhexis Invaginata (Bamboo Hair)

Short, sparse, fragile hair without apparent growth is characteristic of trichorrhexis invaginata, which is found primarily in association with Netherton syndrome (see Chapter 658). It has also been reported in other ichthyosiform dermatoses. The distal portion of the hair is invaginated into the cup-like proximal portion, forming a fragile nodal swelling (see Fig. 662-8C).

Pili Annulati

Alternate light and dark bands of the hair shaft characterize pili annulati. When viewed under the light microscope, the region of the hair shaft that appeared bright in reflected light instead appears dark in the transmitted light as a result of focal aggregates of abnormal air-filled cavities within the shaft. The hair is not fragile. The defect may be autosomal dominant or sporadic in inheritance. Pseudopili annulati is a variant of normal blond hair; an optical effect caused by the refraction and reflection of light from the partially twisted and flattened shaft creates the impression of banding.

Woolly Hair Disease

Woolly hair diseases manifest at birth as peculiarly tight, curly, abnormal hair in a non-black person. Autosomal dominant and recessive (*PKRY5* gene) types have been described. Woolly hair nevus, a sporadic form, involves only a circumscribed portion of the scalp hair. The affected hair is fine, tightly curled, and light colored, and it grows poorly. Microscopically, an affected hair is oval and shows twisting of 180 degrees on its axis.

Uncombable Hair Syndrome (Spun-Glass Hair)

The hair of patients with uncombable hair syndrome appears disorderly, is often silvery blond (Fig. 662-9), and may break because of repeated, futile efforts to control it. The condition is probably autosomal dominant in inheritance. Eyebrows and eyelashes are normal. A longitudinal depression along the hair shaft is a constant feature, and most hair follicles and shafts are triangular (pili trianguli et canaliculi). The shape of the hair varies along its length, however, preventing the hairs from lying flat.

Bibliography is available at Expert Consult.

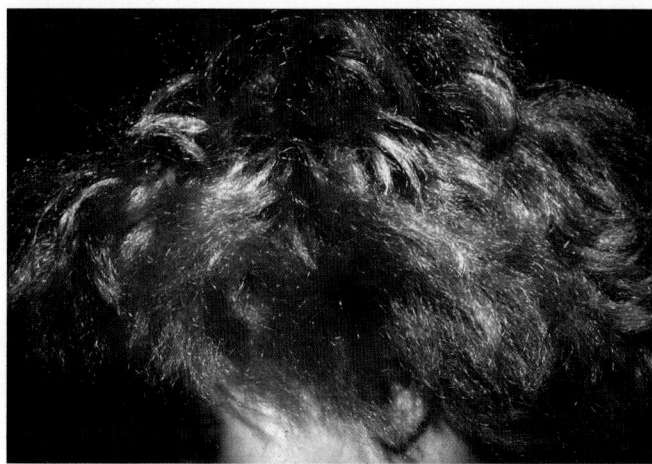

Figure 662-9 Disorderly, silvery blond hair in uncombable hair syndrome.

Chapter 663
Disorders of the Nails
Kari L. Martin

Nail abnormalities in children may be manifestations of generalized skin disease, skin disease localized to the periungual region, systemic disease, drugs, trauma, or localized bacterial and fungal infections (Table 663-1). Nail anomalies are also common in certain congenital disorders (Table 663-2).

ABNORMALITIES IN NAIL SHAPE OR SIZE
Anonychia is absence of the nail plate, usually a result of a congenital disorder or trauma. It may be an isolated finding or may be associated with malformations of the digits. **Koilonychia** is flattening and concavity of the nail plate with loss of normal contour, producing a spoon-shaped nail (Fig. 663-1). Koilonychia occurs as an autosomal dominant trait or in association with iron-deficiency anemia, Plummer-Vinson syndrome, or hemochromatosis. The nail plate is relatively thin for the 1st yr or 2 of life and, consequently, may be spoon-shaped in otherwise normal children.

Congenital nail dysplasia, an autosomal dominant disorder, manifests at birth as longitudinal streaks and thinning of the nail plate. There is platyonychia and koilonychia, which may overgrow the lateral folds and involve all nails of the toes and fingers.

Nail–patella syndrome is an autosomal dominant disorder in which the nails are 30-50% of their normal size and often have triangular or pyramidal lunulae. The thumbnails are always involved, although in some cases only the ulnar half of the nail may be affected or may be missing. The nails from the index finger to the little finger are progressively less damaged. The patella is also smaller than usual, and this anomaly may lead to knee instability. Bony spines arising from the posterior aspect of the iliac bones, overextension of joints, skin laxity, and renal anomalies may also be present. Nail–patella syndrome is caused by mutations in the transcription factor *LMX1B* gene.

For a discussion of **pachyonychia congenita,** see Chapter 658.

Habit tic deformity consists of a depression down the center of the nail with numerous horizontal ridges extending across the nail from it. One or both thumbs are usually involved as a result of chronic rubbing and picking at the nail with an adjacent finger.

Table 663-1	White Nail or Nail Bed Changes
DISEASE	**CLINICAL APPEARANCE**
Anemia	Diffuse white
Arsenic	Mees lines: transverse white lines
Cirrhosis	Terry nails: most of nail, zone of pink at distal end (see Fig. 663-3)
Congenital leukonychia (autosomal dominant; variety of patterns)	Syndrome of leukonychia, knuckle pads, deafness; isolated finding; partial white
Darier disease	Longitudinal white streaks
Half-and-half nail	Proximal white, distal pink azotemia
High fevers (some diseases)	Transverse white lines
Hypoalbuminemia	Muehrcke lines: stationary paired transverse bands
Hypocalcemia	Variable white
Malnutrition	Diffuse white
Pellagra	Diffuse milky white
Punctate leukonychia	Common white spots
Tinea and yeast	Variable patterns
Thallium toxicity (rat poison)	Variable white
Trauma	Repeated manicure: transverse striations
Zinc deficiency	Diffuse white

From Habif TP, editor: Clinical dermatology, ed 4, Philadelphia, 2004, Mosby, p. 887.

Table 663-2	Congenital Diseases with Nail Defects
Large nails	Pachyonychia congenita, Rubinstein-Taybi syndrome, hemihypertrophy
Smallness or absence of nails	Ectodermal dysplasias, nail-patella, dyskeratosis congenita, focal dermal hypoplasia, cartilage-hair hypoplasia, Ellis–van Creveld, Larsen, epidermolysis bullosa, incontinentia pigmenti, Rothmund-Thomson, Turner, popliteal web, trisomy 13, trisomy 18, Apert, Gorlin-Pindborg, long arm 21 deletion, otopalatodigital, fetal alcohol, fetal hydantoin, elfin facies, anonychia, acrodermatitis enteropathica
Other	Congenital malalignment of the great toenails, familial dystrophic shedding of the nails

Clubbing of the nails (hippocratic nails) is characterized by swelling of each distal digit, an increase in the angle between the nail plate and the proximal nail fold (Lovibond angle) to >180 degrees, and a spongy feeling when one pushes down and away from the interphalangeal joint, because of an increase in fibrovascular tissue between the matrix and the phalanx (Fig. 663-2). The pathogenesis is not known. Nail clubbing is seen in association with diseases of numerous organ systems, including pulmonary, cardiovascular (cyanotic heart disease), gastrointestinal (celiac disease, inflammatory bowel disease), and hepatic (chronic hepatitis) systems, as well as in healthy individuals as an idiopathic or familial finding.

CHANGES IN NAIL COLOR
Leukonychia is a white opacity of the nail plate that may involve the entire plate or may be punctate or striate (see Table 663-1). The nail

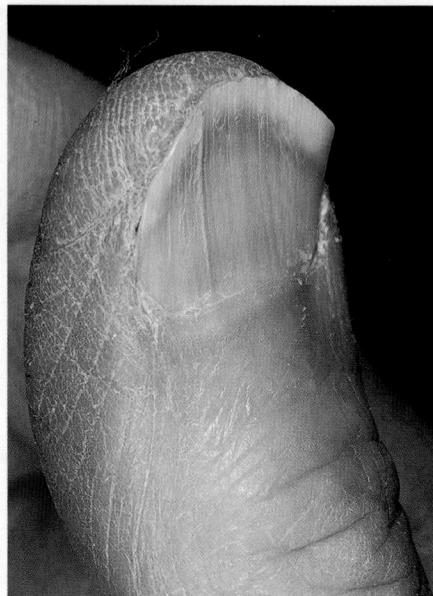

Figure 663-1 Spoon nails (koilonychia). Most cases are a variant of normal. *(From Habif TP, editor: Clinical dermatology, ed 4, Philadelphia, 2004, Mosby, p. 885.)*

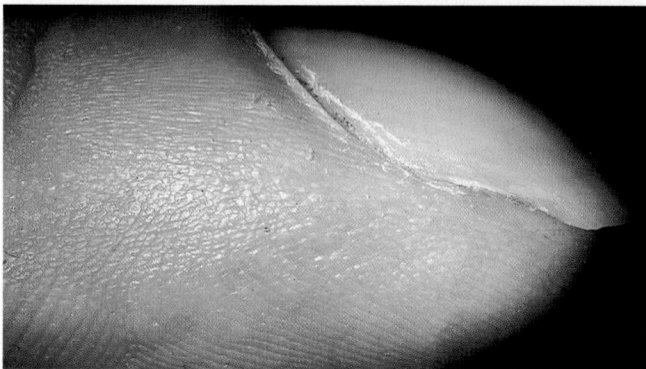

Figure 663-2 Finger clubbing. The distal phalanges are enlarged to a rounded bulbous shape. The nail enlarges and becomes curved, hard, and thickened. *(From Habif TP, editor: Clinical dermatology, ed 4, Philadelphia, 2004, Mosby, p. 885.)*

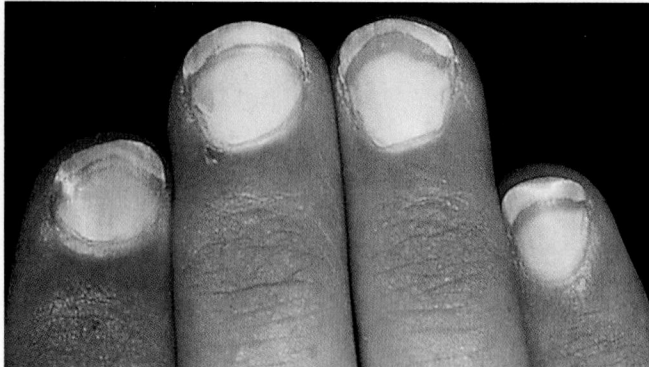

Figure 663-3 Terry nails. The nail bed is white with only a narrow zone of pink at the distal end. *(From Habif TP, editor: Clinical dermatology, ed 4, Philadelphia, 2004, Mosby, p. 885.)*

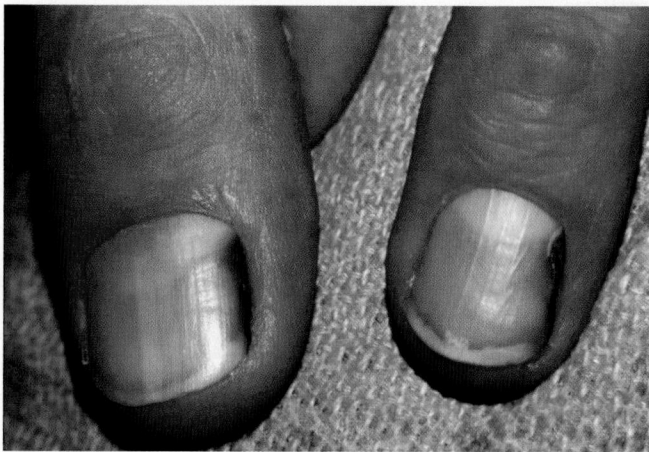

Figure 663-4 Green/black discoloration at the edge of the nails secondary to *Pseudomonas* infection.

plate itself remains smooth and undamaged. Leukonychia can be traumatic or associated with infections such as leprosy and tuberculosis, dermatoses such as lichen planus and Darier disease, malignancies such as Hodgkin disease, anemia, and arsenic poisoning (Mees lines). Leukonychia of all nail surfaces is an uncommon hereditary autosomal dominant trait that may be associated with congenital epidermal cysts and renal calculi. Paired parallel white bands that do not change position with growth of the nail and thus reflect a change in the nail bed are associated with hypoalbuminemia and are called Muehrcke lines. When the proximal portion of the nail is white and the distal 20-50% of the nail is red, pink, or brown, the condition is called half-and-half nails or Lindsay nails; this is seen most commonly in patients with renal disease but may occur as a normal variant. White nails of **cirrhosis,** or Terry nails (Fig. 663-3), are characterized by a white ground-glass appearance of the entire or the proximal end of the nail and a normal pink distal 1-2 mm of the nail; this finding is associated with hypoalbuminemia.

Black pigmentation of an entire nail plate or linear bands of pigmentation (melanonychia striata) is common in African-American (90%) and Asian (10-20%) individuals, but is unusual in white individuals (<1%). Most often, the pigment is melanin, which is produced by melanocytes of a junctional nevus in the nail matrix and nail bed

and is of no consequence. Extension or alteration in the pigment should be evaluated by biopsy because of the possibility of malignant change.

Bluish black to greenish nails may be caused by *Pseudomonas* infection (Fig. 663-4), particularly in association with onycholysis or chronic paronychia. The coloration is caused by subungual debris and pyocyanin pigment from the bacterial organisms.

Yellow nail syndrome manifests as thickened, excessively curved, slow-growing yellow nails without lunulae. All nails are affected in most cases. Associated systemic diseases include bronchiectasis, recurrent bronchitis, chylothorax, and focal edema of the limbs and face. Deficient lymphatic drainage, caused by hypoplastic lymphatic vessels, is believed to lead to the manifestations of this syndrome.

Splinter hemorrhages most often result from minor trauma but may also be associated with subacute bacterial endocarditis, vasculitis, Langerhans cell histiocytosis, severe rheumatoid arthritis, peptic ulcer disease, hypertension, chronic glomerulonephritis, cirrhosis, scurvy, trichinosis, malignant neoplasms, and psoriasis.

NAIL SEPARATION

Onycholysis indicates separation of the nail plate from the distal nail bed. Common causes are trauma, long-term exposure to moisture, hyperhidrosis, cosmetics, psoriasis, fungal infection (distal onycholysis), atopic or contact dermatitis, porphyria, drugs (bleomycin, vincristine, retinoid agents, indomethacin, chlorpromazine [Thorazine]), and drug-induced phototoxicity from tetracyclines (Fig. 663-5) or chloramphenicol.

Beau lines are transverse grooves in the nail plate (Fig. 663-6) that represent a temporary disruption of formation of the nail plate. The

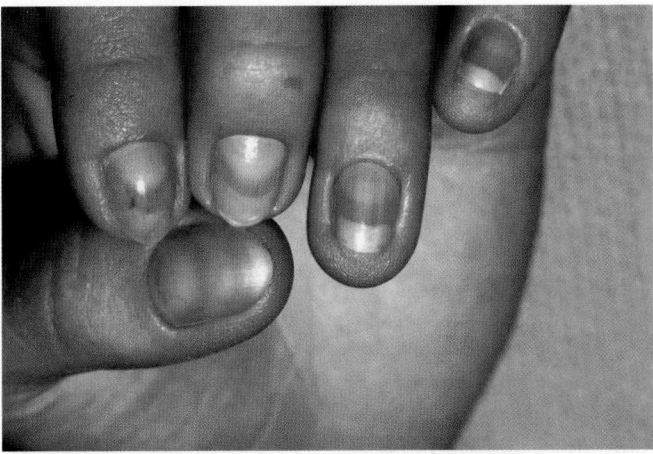

Figure 663-5 Distal onycholysis secondary to oral tetracycline usage and ultraviolet light exposure.

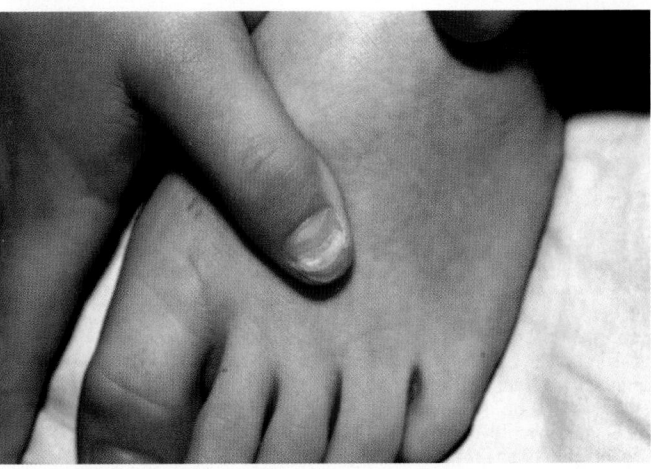

Figure 663-6 Beau lines. Longitudinal disruption of nail.

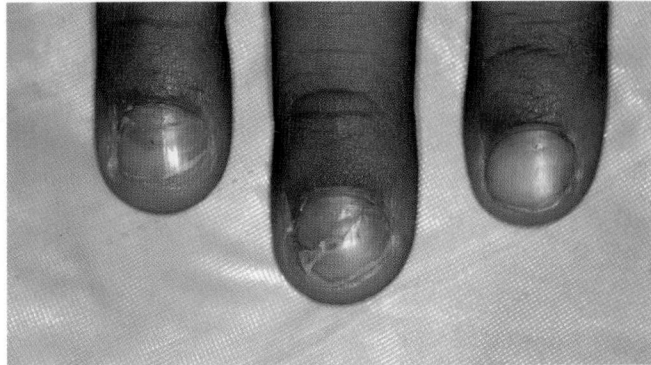

Figure 663-7 Onychomadesis. Proximal nail bed separation.

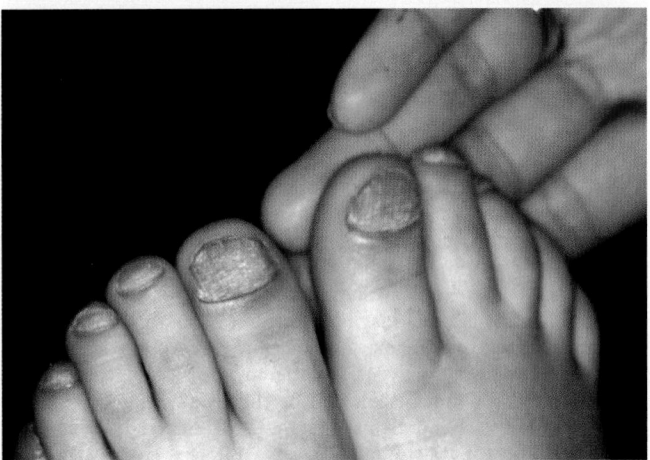

Figure 663-8 Dystrophy of all nails in trachyonychia.

lines first appear a few weeks after the event that caused the disruption in nail growth. A single transverse ridge appears at the proximal nail fold in most 4-6 wk old infants and works its way distally as the nail grows; this line may reflect metabolic changes after delivery. At other ages, Beau lines are usually indicative of periodic trauma or episodic shutdown of the nail matrix secondary to a systemic disease such as hand-foot-and-mouth disease, measles, mumps, pneumonia, or zinc deficiency. **Onychomadesis** is an exaggeration of Beau lines leading to proximal separation of the nail bed (Fig. 663-7).

NAIL CHANGES ASSOCIATED WITH SKIN DISEASE

Nail changes may be particularly associated with various other diseases. Nail changes of **psoriasis** most characteristically include pitting, onycholysis, yellow-brown discoloration, and thickening. Nail changes in lichen planus include violaceous papules in the proximal nail fold and nail bed, leukonychia, longitudinal ridging, thinning of the entire nail plate, and pterygium formation, which is abnormal adherence of the cuticle to the nail plate or, if the plate is destroyed focally, to the nail bed. Postinfectious reactive arthritis syndromes may include painless erythematous induration of the base of the nail fold; subungual parakeratotic scaling; and thickening, opacification, or ridging of the nail plate. Dermatitis that involves the nail folds may produce dystrophy, roughening, and coarse pitting of the nails. Nail changes are more common in atopic dermatitis than in other forms of dermatitis that affect the hands. Darier disease is characterized by red or white streaks that extend longitudinally and cross the lunula. Where the streak meets the distal end of the nail, a V-shaped notch may be present. Total

leukonychia may also occur. Transverse rows of fine pits are characteristic of alopecia areata. In severe cases, the entire nail surface may be rough. Patients with acrodermatitis enteropathica may have transverse grooves (Beau lines) and nail dystrophy as a result of periungual dermatitis.

TRACHYONYCHIA (20-NAIL DYSTROPHY)

Trachyonychia is characterized by longitudinal ridging, pitting, fragility, thinning, distal notching, and opalescent discoloration of all the nails (Fig. 663-8). Patients have no associated skin or systemic diseases and no other ectodermal defects. Its occasional association with alopecia areata has led some authorities to suggest that trachyonychia may reflect an abnormal immunologic response to the nail matrix, whereas histopathologic studies have suggested that it may be a manifestation of lichen planus, psoriasis, or spongiotic (eczematous) inflammation of the nail matrix. The disorder must be differentiated from fungal infections, psoriasis, nail changes of alopecia areata, and nail dystrophy secondary to eczema. Eczema and fungal infections rarely produce changes in all the nails simultaneously. The disorder is self-limited and eventually remits by adulthood.

NAIL INFECTION

Fungal infection (onychomycosis) of the nails has been classified into 4 types. *White superficial onychomycosis* manifests as diffuse or speckled white discoloration of the surface of the toenails. It is caused primarily by *Trichophyton mentagrophytes,* which invades the nail plate. The organism may be scraped off the nail plate with a blade, but **treatment** is best accomplished by the addition of a topical azole antifungal agent. *Distal subungual onychomycosis* involves foci of onycholysis under the distal nail plate or along the lateral nail groove, followed by development of hyperkeratosis and yellow-brown discoloration. The process extends proximally, resulting in nail plate thickening,

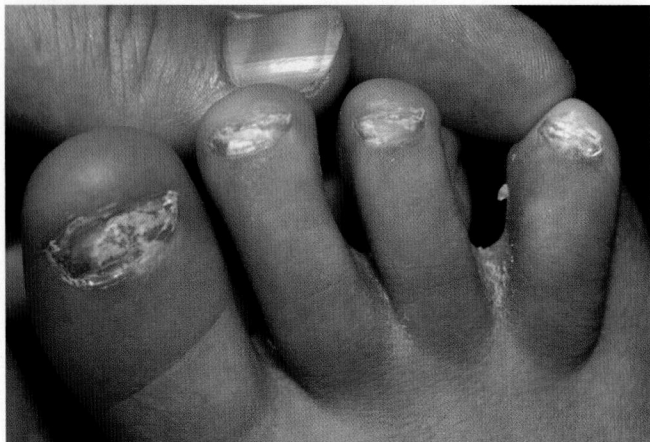

Figure 663-9 Discoloration, hyperkeratosis, and crumbling of nail secondary to dermatophyte infection.

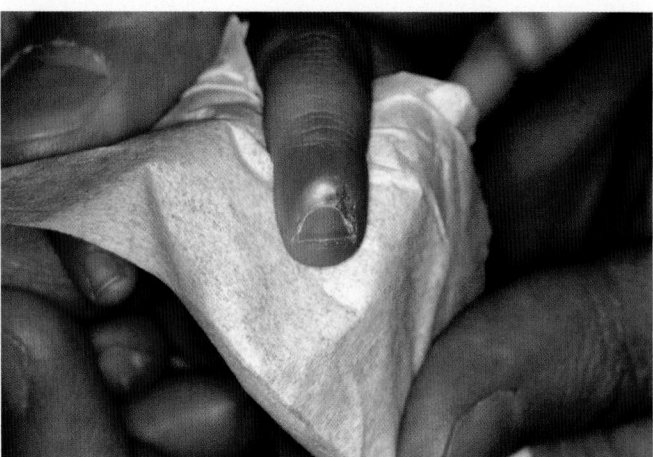

Figure 663-10 Acute paronychia secondary to *Staphylococcus aureus.*

crumbling (Fig. 663-9), and separation from the nail bed. *Trichophyton rubrum* and, occasionally, *T. mentagrophytes* infect the toenails; fingernail disease is almost exclusively caused by *T. rubrum,* which may be associated with superficial scaling of the plantar surface of the feet and often of one hand. The dermatophytes are found most readily at the most proximal area of the nail bed or adjacent ventral portion of the involved nail plates. **Topical therapies** such as ciclopirox 8% lacquer or amorolfine 5% lacquer, may be effective for solitary nail infection. Topical efinaconazole 10% may also be effective; laser treatment is an expensive but safe alternative to oral therapy. Because of its long half-life in the nail, oral itraconazole may be effective when given as pulse therapy (1 wk of each month for 3-4 mo). Dosage is weight dependent. Oral daily terbinafine is also quite effective. Either agent is superior to griseofulvin, fluconazole, or ketoconazole. The risks, the most concerning of which is hepatic toxicity, and costs of oral therapy are minimized with the use of pulsed dosing.

Proximal white subungual onychomycosis occurs when the organism, generally *T. rubrum,* enters the nail through the proximal nail fold, producing yellow-white portions of the undersurface of the nail plate. The surface of the nail is unaffected. This occurs almost exclusively in immunocompromised patients and is a well-recognized manifestation of AIDS. Treatment includes oral terbinafine or itraconazole.

Candidal onychomycosis involves the entire nail plate in patients with chronic mucocutaneous candidiasis. It is also commonly seen in patients with AIDS. The organism, generally *Candida albicans,* enters distally or along the lateral nail folds, rapidly involves the entire thickness of the nail plate, and produces thickening, crumbling, and deformity of the plate. Topical azole antifungal agents may be sufficient for treatment of candidal onychomycosis in an immunocompetent host, but oral antifungal agents are necessary for treatment of patients with immune deficiencies. Table 663-3 outlines the differential diagnosis of onychomycosis.

PARONYCHIAL INFLAMMATION

Paronychial inflammation may be acute or chronic and generally involves 1 or 2 nail folds on the fingers. **Acute paronychia** manifests as erythema, warmth, edema, and tenderness of the proximal nail fold, most commonly as a result of pathogenic staphylococci, streptococci, or candidal (Fig. 663-10). Warm soaks and oral agents are generally effective; incision and drainage may be occasionally necessary. Development of chronic paronychia follows prolonged immersion in water (Fig. 663-11), such as occurs in finger or thumb sucking, exposure to irritating solutions, nail fold trauma, or diseases, including Raynaud phenomenon, collagen vascular diseases, and diabetes. Swelling of the proximal nail fold is followed by separation of the nail fold from the underlying nail plate and suppuration. Foreign material, embedded in the dermis of the nail fold, becomes a nidus for inflammation and infection with *Candida* species and mixed bacterial flora. A

Table 663-3	Differential Diagnosis of Onychomycosis

Psoriasis
- As in onychomycosis: onycholysis, subungual hyperkeratosis, splinter hemorrhages, leuconychia, dystrophy
- Pitting
- Oil drop sign (a translucent yellow-red discoloration seen in the nail bed)
- Other cutaneous features of psoriasis, family history of psoriasis

Lichen planus
- Cutaneous disease at other sites
- Thin nail plate and ridging
- Dorsal pterygium—scarring at proximal aspect of nail

Trauma
- Nail plate can appear abnormal
- Nail bed should be normal
- Distal onycholysis with repeated trauma
- Single nail affected, shape of nail changed, homogenous alteration of nail color

Eczema
- Irregular buckled nails with ridging
- Cutaneous signs of eczema

Yellow nail syndrome
- Nail plate is discolored green-yellow
- Nails are hard with elevated longitudinal curvature
- Nails may be shed, painful
- Associations with bronchiectasis, lymphoedema, and chronic sinusitis

Lamellar onychoschizia (lamellar splitting)
- History of repeated soaking in water
- Usually distal portion of nail

Periungual squamous cell carcinoma/Bowens disease
- Single nail, warty changes of nail fold, ooze from edge of nail

Malignant melanoma
- Black discoloration of nail plate or nail bed
- Pigment can extend onto nail fold
- Can get associated bleeding

Myxoid (mucous) cyst
- Cyst at base of nail, groove in nail extending length of nail

Alopecia areata
- Pits, longitudinal ridging, brittleness
- Hair loss

From Eisman S, Sinclair R: Fungal nail infection: diagnosis and management. BMJ 348:g1800, 2014.

combination of attention to predisposing factors, meticulous drying of the hands, and long-term topical antifungal agents and topical potent corticosteroids may be required for successful treatment of chronic paronychia.

Ingrown nail occurs when the lateral edge of the nail, including spicules that have separated from the nail plate, penetrates the soft

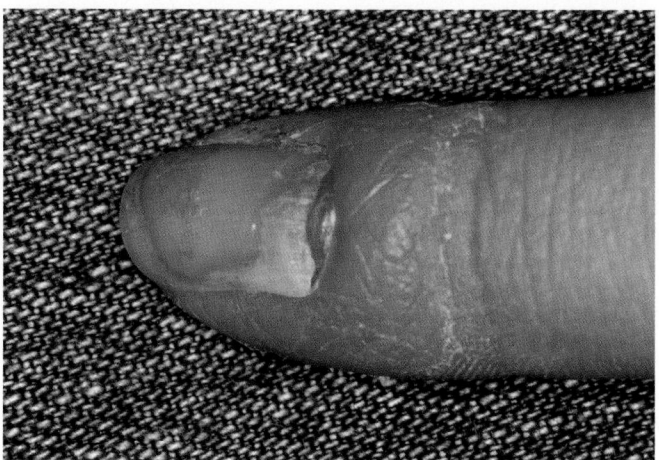

Figure 663-11 Chronic paronychia with erythema and lateral nail fold separation.

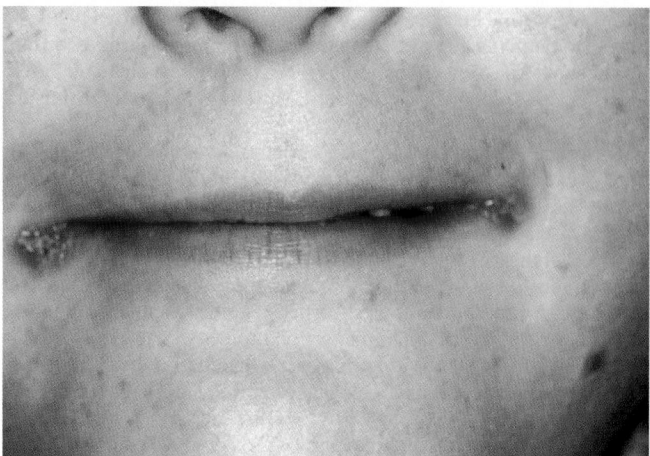

Figure 664-1 Angular cheilitis.

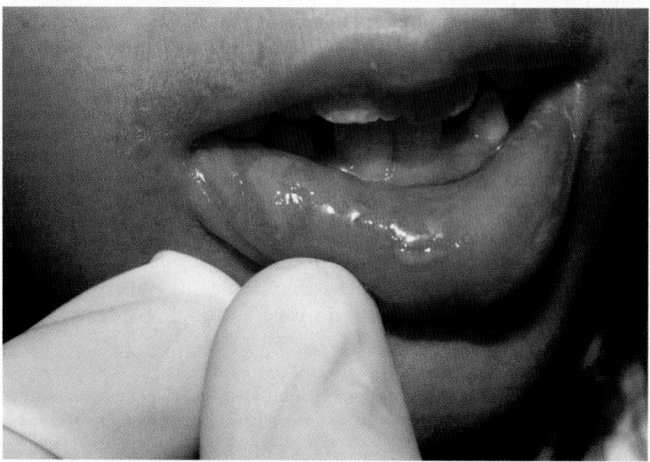

Figure 664-2 Aphthous ulceration on lower lip.

tissue of the lateral nail fold. Erythema, edema, and pain, most often involving the lateral great toes, are noted acutely; recurrent episodes may lead to formation of granulation tissue. Predisposing factors include (1) congenital malalignment (especially of the great toes); (2) compression of the side of the toe from poorly fitting shoes, particularly if the great toes are abnormally long and the lateral nail folds are prominent; and (3) improper cutting of the nail in a curvilinear manner rather than straight across. **Management** includes proper fitting of shoes; allowing the nail to grow out beyond the free edge before cutting it straight across; warm water soaks; oral antibiotics if cellulitis affects the lateral nail fold; and, in severe, recurrent cases, application of silver nitrate to granulation tissue, nail avulsion, or excision of the lateral aspect of the nail followed by matricectomy.

PARONYCHIAL TUMORS
Tumors in the paronychial area include pyogenic granulomas, mucous cysts, subungual exostoses, and junctional nevi. Periungual fibromas that appear in late childhood should suggest a diagnosis of tuberous sclerosis.

Bibliography is available at Expert Consult.

Chapter **664**
Disorders of the Mucous Membranes
Michelle L. Bayer and Beth A. Drolet

The mucous membranes may be involved in developmental disorders, genodermatoses, infections, acute and chronic skin diseases, or benign and malignant tumors.

ANGULAR CHEILITIS
Angular cheilitis (perlèche) is characterized by inflammation and fissuring at the corners of the mouth, often with associated erosion, maceration, and crusting (Fig. 664-1). Chapping or moisture collection at the angles of the mouth predispose children to developing angular cheilitis. Children who are chronic lip lickers or who have excessive salivation or drooling related to neurologic deficits, orthodontic

appliances, or mouth breathing are at increased risk. Atopic dermatitis or contact dermatitis related to toothpaste, chewing gum, mouthwash, or cosmetics are also common causes. Nutritional deficiencies are a less-frequent etiology. Protection can be provided by frequent application of a bland ointment such as petrolatum. Candidosis should be treated with an appropriate antifungal agent, and contact dermatitis of the perioral skin should be treated with a low-potency topical corticosteroid ointment preparation and frequent use of petrolatum or a similar emollient. Correction of the underlying predisposing factors (if possible) will prevent recurrence.

APHTHOUS STOMATITIS (CANKER SORES)
Aphthous stomatitis consists of solitary or multiple painful ulcerations occur on the labial (Fig. 664-2), buccal, lingual, sublingual, palatal, or gingival mucosa (see Chapter 315). Lesions may manifest initially as erythematous, indurated papules that erode rapidly to form sharply circumscribed, necrotic ulcers with a gray fibrinous exudate and an erythematous halo. Minor aphthous ulcers are 2-10 mm in diameter and heal spontaneously in 7-10 days. Major aphthous ulcers are >10 mm in diameter, take from 10-30 days to heal, and may heal with scarring. A third type of aphthous ulceration is herpetiform in appearance, manifesting as a few to numerous grouped 1-2 mm lesions which tend to coalesce into plaques and heal over 7-10 days. Approximately 30% of patients with recurrent lesions have a family history of the disorder (see Chapter 315 for the differential diagnosis).

The etiology of aphthous stomatitis is multifactorial; the condition probably represents an oral manifestation of a number of conditions. Altered local regulation of the cell-mediated immune system, after activation and accumulation of cytotoxic T cells, may contribute to the localized mucosal breakdown. It is a common misconception that aphthous stomatitis is a manifestation of herpes simplex virus infection. Recurrent herpes infections remain localized to the lips and rarely cross the mucocutaneous junction; involvement of the oral mucosa occurs only in primary infections.

Treatment of aphthous stomatitis is palliative. The majority of mild cases do not require therapy. Relief of pain, particularly before eating, may be achieved with the use of a topical anesthetic such as viscous lidocaine or an oral rinse with a combined solution of elixir of diphenhydramine, viscous lidocaine, and an oral antacid. Caution must be taken to avoid hot food and drink after topical anesthetic use. A superpotent topical corticosteroid in a mucosa-adhering agent may help reduce inflammation, and topical tetracycline mouthwash may also hasten healing. In severe, debilitating cases, systemic therapy with corticosteroids, colchicine, dapsone, or thalidomide may be helpful.

FORDYCE SPOTS

Fordyce spots (Fordyce granules) are asymptomatic, 1-3 mm, yellow-white macules and papules on the vermilion lips and buccal mucosa. They are a common clinical finding and represent a normal anatomic variant of sebaceous glands. They can present in either sex from infancy to adulthood and may become more prominent during puberty due to the influence of androgens. No therapy is required.

EPSTEIN PEARLS (GINGIVAL CYSTS OF THE NEWBORN)

Epstein pearls are white, keratin-containing cysts on the palatal or alveolar mucosa of approximately 80% of neonates. They are epidermal inclusion cysts that form when the soft and hard palates fuse and are analogous to facial milia. They cause no symptoms and are generally shed within a few weeks; no therapy is necessary.

MUCOCELE

Mucus retention cysts are painless, fluctuant, tense, 2-10 mm, bluish papules on the lips (Fig. 664-3), tongue, palate, or buccal mucosa. Traumatic severance of the duct of a minor salivary gland leads to submucosal retention of mucus secretion. Lesions on the floor of the mouth are known as ranulas when the sublingual or submandibular salivary gland ducts are involved. Fluctuations in size are typical, and the lesions may disappear temporarily after traumatic rupture. Recurrence is prevented by surgical excision of the mucus deposit and associated salivary gland(s).

FISSURED TONGUE

Fissured tongue (scrotal tongue, or lingua plicata) is a common benign developmental anomaly of the tongue. The dorsal tongue has many folds with deep grooves and a pebbled appearance. Fissured tongue can be seen in individuals with Melkersson-Rosenthal syndrome and Down syndrome, and it is often seen in association with geographic tongue. Food particles and debris may become trapped in the fissures, resulting in irritation, inflammation, and halitosis. Careful cleansing with a mouth rinse and soft-bristled toothbrush is recommended.

GEOGRAPHIC TONGUE (BENIGN MIGRATORY GLOSSITIS)

Geographic tongue consists of single or multiple sharply demarcated, irregular, smooth red patches surrounded by an elevated yellowish-white serpiginous border on the dorsum of the tongue. Onset is rapid, and the pattern may change over hours to days. The smooth patches correspond to atrophic filiform papillae, and the elevated margins represent hypertrophic papillae (Fig. 664-4). The etiology of this condition remains unclear. Lesions are typically asymptomatic, but some patients may experience a burning sensation or sensitivity to spicy, hot, or cold foods. No therapy other than reassurance is necessary.

BLACK HAIRY TONGUE

Black hairy tongue is a dark coating on the dorsum of the tongue caused by hyperplasia and elongation of the filiform papillae; overgrowth of chromogenic bacteria and fungi and entrapped pigmented residues that adsorb to microbial plaque and desquamating keratin may contribute to the dark coloration. Changes often begin posteriorly and extend anteriorly on the dorsum of the tongue. The condition is most common in adults but may also manifest during adolescence. Poor oral hygiene, lack of oral feeding, treatment with systemic antibiotics such as tetracycline (which promote the growth of *Candida* spp.), and smoking are predisposing factors. Improved oral hygiene and brushing with a soft-bristled toothbrush may be all that is necessary for treatment.

ORAL HAIRY LEUKOPLAKIA

Oral hair leukoplakia occurs in approximately 25% of patients with AIDS but is rare in the pediatric population. It manifests as corrugated and shaggy white plaques on the lateral margins of the tongue which cannot be removed by rubbing. The lesions occasionally may spread to the ventral tongue surface, floor of the mouth, tonsillar pillars, and pharynx. The condition is caused by Epstein-Barr virus, which is present in the upper layer of the affected epithelium. The plaques have no malignant potential. The disorder occurs predominantly in HIV-infected patients but may also be found in individuals who are immunosuppressed for other reasons, such as organ transplantation, leukemia, chemotherapy, and long-term use of inhaled steroids. The condition is generally asymptomatic and does not require therapy.

ACUTE NECROTIZING ULCERATIVE GINGIVITIS (VINCENT STOMATITIS, FUSOSPIROCHETAL GINGIVITIS, TRENCH MOUTH)

Acute necrotizing ulcerative gingivitis manifests as painful punched-out ulceration, necrosis, and bleeding of the interdental papillae. A

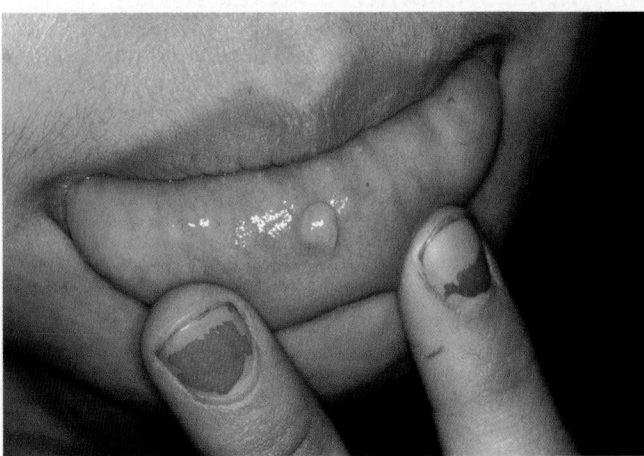

Figure 664-3 Mucocele on lower lip.

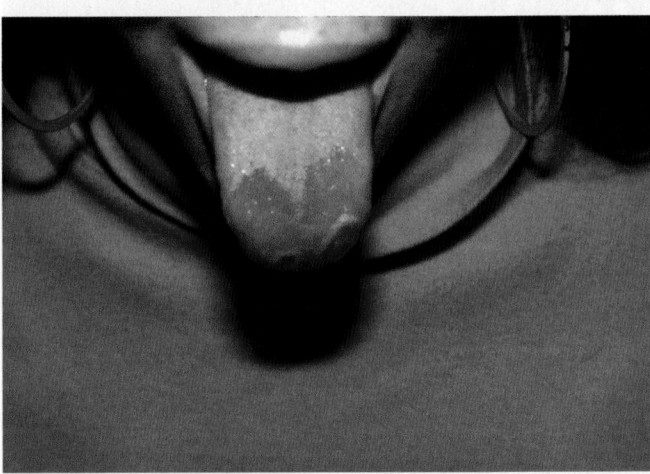

Figure 664-4 Geographic tongue.

grayish white pseudomembrane may cover the ulcerations. Lesions may spread to involve the buccal mucosa, lips, tongue, tonsils, and pharynx and may be associated with dental pain, a bad taste, low-grade fever, and lymphadenopathy. It occurs most commonly in the 2nd or 3rd decade, particularly in the context of poor dental hygiene, poor nutrition, smoking, and stress.

NOMA
Noma is a severe form of fusospirillary gangrenous stomatitis that occurs primarily in malnourished, impoverished children 2-5 yr of age who have had a preceding illness such as measles, scarlet fever, tuberculosis, malignancy, or immunodeficiency. The disease is most prevalent in Africa, but also occurs in Asia and Latin America. Sporadic cases associated with immunodeficiency have been reported in developed countries. It manifests as a painful, red, indurated papule on the alveolar margin, followed by ulceration and mutilating gangrenous destruction of tissue in the oronasal region. The process may also involve the scalp, neck, shoulders, perineum, and vulva. Noma neonatorum manifests in the 1st mo of life as gangrenous lesions of the lips, nose, mouth, and anal regions. Affected infants are usually small for gestational age, malnourished, premature, and frequently ill (particularly with *Pseudomonas aeruginosa* sepsis). Care consists of nutritional support, conservative debridement of necrotic soft tissues, empirical broad-spectrum antibiotics such as penicillin and metronidazole, and, in the case of noma neonatorum, antipseudomonal antibiotics (see Chapter 46).

COWDEN SYNDROME (MULTIPLE HAMARTOMA SYNDROME)
Cowden syndrome is an autosomal dominant condition caused by loss-of-function mutations in the *PTEN* tumor-suppressor gene. Mucocutaneous lesions typically appear in the 2nd or 3rd decade. Oral papillomas are 1-3 mm smooth, pink or whitish papules on the palatal, gingival, buccal, and labial mucosae and may coalesce into a cobblestone appearance. Numerous flesh-colored papules also develop on the face, particularly around the mouth, nose, and ears. These papules are most commonly trichilemmomas, a benign neoplasm of the hair follicle. Associated findings may include acral keratoses, thyroid adenoma, goiter, gastrointestinal polyps, fibrocystic breast nodules, and carcinoma of the breast or thyroid.

Bibliography is available at Expert Consult.

Cutaneous Bacterial Infections

665.1 Impetigo
Anna M. Juern and Beth A. Drolet

ETIOLOGY/PATHOGENESIS
Impetigo is the most common skin infection in children throughout the world. There are 2 classic forms of impetigo: nonbullous and bullous.

Staphylococcus aureus is the predominant organism of nonbullous impetigo in the United States; group A β-hemolytic streptococci

(GABHS) are implicated in the development of some lesions. The staphylococcal types that cause nonbullous impetigo are variable but are not generally from phage group 2, the group that is associated with scalded skin and toxic shock syndromes. Staphylococci generally spread from the nose to normal skin and then infect the skin. In contrast, the skin becomes colonized with GABHS an average of 10 days before development of impetigo. The skin serves as the source for acquisition of GABHS and the probable primary source for spread of impetigo. Lesions of nonbullous impetigo that grow staphylococci in culture cannot be distinguished clinically from those that grow pure cultures of GABHS.

Bullous impetigo is always caused by *S. aureus* strains that produce exfoliative toxins. The staphylococcal exfoliative toxins (ETA, ETB, ETD) blister the superficial epidermis by hydrolyzing human desmoglein 1, resulting in a subcorneal vesicle. This is also the target antigen of the autoantibodies in pemphigus foliaceus (see Chapters 181 and 183).

CLINICAL MANIFESTATIONS
Nonbullous Impetigo
Nonbullous impetigo accounts for more than 70% of cases. Lesions typically begin on the skin of the face or on extremities that have been traumatized. The most common lesions that precede nonbullous impetigo are insect bites, abrasions, lacerations, chickenpox, scabies pediculosis, and burns. A tiny vesicle or pustule forms initially and rapidly develops into a honey-colored crusted plaque that is generally <2 cm in diameter (Fig. 665-1). The infection may be spread to other parts of the body by the fingers, clothing, and towels. Lesions are associated with little to no pain or surrounding erythema, and constitutional symptoms are generally absent. Pruritus occurs occasionally, regional adenopathy is found in up to 90% of cases, and leukocytosis is present in approximately 50%.

Bullous Impetigo
Bullous impetigo is mainly an infection of infants and young children. Flaccid, transparent bullae develop most commonly on skin of the face, buttocks, trunk, perineum, and extremities. **Neonatal bullous impetigo** can begin in the diaper area. Rupture of a bulla occurs easily, leaving a narrow rim of scale at the edge of shallow, moist erosion. Surrounding erythema and regional adenopathy are generally absent. Unlike those of nonbullous impetigo, lesions of bullous impetigo are a manifestation of localized staphylococcal scalded skin syndrome and develop on intact skin.

Differential Diagnosis
The differential diagnosis of **nonbullous impetigo** includes viruses (herpes simplex, varicella-zoster), fungi (tinea corporis, kerion),

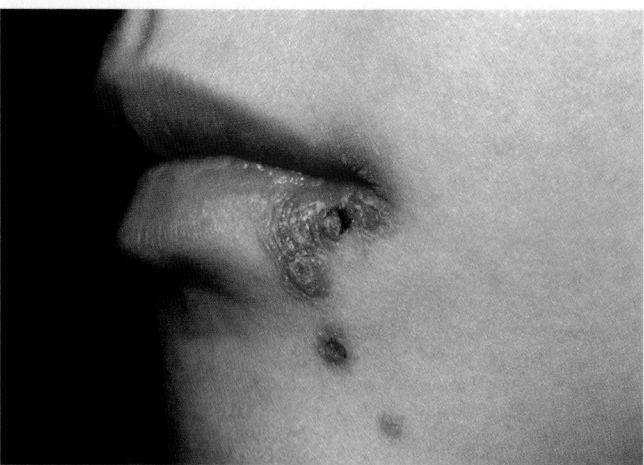
Figure 665-1 Multiple crusted and oozing lesions of impetigo.

arthropod bites, and parasitic infestations (scabies, pediculosis capitis), all of which may become impetiginized.

The differential diagnosis of **bullous impetigo** in neonates includes epidermolysis bullosa, bullous mastocytosis, herpetic infection, and early scalded skin syndrome. In older children, allergic contact dermatitis, burns, erythema multiforme, linear immunoglobulin A dermatosis, pemphigus, and bullous pemphigoid must be considered, particularly if the lesions do not respond to therapy.

COMPLICATIONS

Potential but very rare complications of either nonbullous or bullous impetigo include osteomyelitis, septic arthritis, pneumonia, and septicemia. Positive blood culture results are very rare in otherwise healthy children with localized lesions. Cellulitis has been reported in up to 10% of patients with nonbullous impetigo and rarely follows the bullous form. Lymphangitis, suppurative lymphadenitis, guttate psoriasis, and scarlet fever occasionally follow streptococcal disease. There is no correlation between number of lesions and clinical involvement of the lymphatics or development of cellulitis in association with streptococcal impetigo.

Infection with nephritogenic strains of GABHS may result in **acute poststreptococcal glomerulonephritis** (see Chapter 511.1). The clinical character of impetigo lesions is not predictive of the development of poststreptococcal glomerulonephritis. The most commonly affected age group is children 3-7 yr of age. The latent period from onset of impetigo to development of poststreptococcal glomerulonephritis averages 18-21 days, which is longer than the 10-day latency period after pharyngitis. Poststreptococcal glomerulonephritis occurs epidemically after either pharyngeal or skin infection. Impetigo-associated epidemics have been caused by M groups 2, 49, 53, 55, 56, 57, and 60. Strains of GABHS that are associated with endemic impetigo in the United States have little or no nephritogenic potential. Acute rheumatic fever does not occur as a result of impetigo.

TREATMENT

The decision on how to treat impetigo depends on the number of lesions and their locations. Topical therapy with mupirocin 2%, and retapamulin 1% 2-3 times a day for 10-14 days is acceptable for localized disease caused by S. aureus.

Systemic therapy with oral antibiotics should be prescribed for patients with streptococcal or widespread involvement of staphylococcal infections; when lesions are near the mouth, where topical medication may be licked off; or in cases with evidence of deep involvement, including cellulitis, furunculosis, abscess formation, or suppurative lymphadenitis. Cephalexin, 25-50 mg/kg/day in 3-4 divided doses for 7-10 days, is an excellent choice for initial therapy. No evidence suggests that a 10-day course of therapy is superior to a 7-day course. The emergence of methicillin-resistant S. aureus (MRSA) dictates that if a satisfactory clinical response is not achieved within 7 days, a culture should be performed and an appropriate antibiotic based on drug sensitivity should be given for an additional 7 days. If MRSA is suspected, clindamycin, doxycycline or sulfamethoxazole-trimethoprim is indicated.

Bibliography is available at Expert Consult.

665.2 Subcutaneous Tissue Infections
Anna M. Juern and Beth A. Drolet

The principal determinations for soft-tissue infections is whether it is *nonnecrotizing* or *necrotizing*, as well as *purulent* or *nonpurulent* (see Fig. 665-1). The former responds to antibiotic therapy alone, whereas the latter requires prompt surgical removal of all devitalized tissue in addition to antimicrobial therapy. Necrotizing soft-tissue infections are life-threatening conditions that are characterized by rapidly advancing local tissue destruction and systemic toxicity. Tissue necrosis distinguishes them from cellulitis. In cellulitis, an inflammatory infectious process involves subcutaneous tissue but does not destroy it. Necrotizing soft-tissue infections characteristically manifest with a paucity of early cutaneous signs relative to the rapidity and degree of destruction of the subcutaneous tissues.

CELLULITIS
Etiology

Cellulitis is characterized by infection and inflammation of loose connective tissue, with limited involvement of the dermis and relative sparing of the epidermis. A break in the skin from previous trauma, surgery, or an underlying skin lesion predisposes to cellulitis. Cellulitis is also more common in individuals with lymphatic stasis, diabetes mellitus, or immunosuppression.

Streptococcus pyogenes (group A streptococcus) and *S. aureus* are the most common etiologic agents. In patients who are immunocompromised or have diabetes mellitus, a number of other bacterial or fungal agents may be involved, notably *Pseudomonas aeruginosa; Aeromonas hydrophila* and, occasionally, other Enterobacteriaceae; *Legionella* spp.; the Mucorales, particularly *Rhizopus* spp., *Mucor* spp., and *Absidia* spp.; and *Cryptococcus neoformans*. Children with relapsed nephrotic syndrome may experience cellulitis caused by *Escherichia coli*. In children age 3 mo to 5 yr, *Haemophilus influenzae* type b was once an important cause of facial cellulitis, but its incidence has declined significantly since the institution of immunization against this organism.

Clinical Manifestations

Cellulitis manifests clinically as an area of edema, warmth, erythema, and tenderness. The lateral margins tend to be indistinct because the process is deep in the skin, primarily involving the subcutaneous tissues in addition to the dermis. Application of pressure may produce pitting. Although distinction cannot be made with certainty in any particular patient, cellulitis due to *S. aureus* tends to be more localized and may suppurate, whereas infections caused by *S. pyogenes* (group A streptococci) tend to spread more rapidly and may be associated with lymphangitis. Regional adenopathy and constitutional signs and symptoms such as fever, chills, and malaise are common. Complications of cellulitis are uncommon but include subcutaneous abscess, bacteremia, osteomyelitis, septic arthritis, thrombophlebitis, endocarditis, and necrotizing fasciitis. Lymphangitis or glomerulonephritis can also follow infection with *S. pyogenes*.

Diagnosis

Aspirates from the site of inflammation, skin biopsy, and blood cultures allow identification of the causal organism in approximately 25% of cases of cellulitis. Blood cultures are usually negative in immunocompetent patients with mild to moderate infection. Yield of the causative organism is approximately 30% when the site of origin of the cellulitis is apparent, such as an abrasion or ulcer. An aspirate taken from the point of maximum inflammation yields the causal organism more often than a leading-edge aspirate. Lack of success in isolating an organism stems primarily from the low number of organisms present within the lesion. *Ultrasonography is used if an associated subcutaneous abscess is suspected.*

The differential diagnosis should include an exuberant immune-allergic reaction to insect bites particularly mosquito bites (Skeeter syndromes) (see Chapter 146). The skeeter syndrome is characterized by swelling disproportionate to erythremia; there is pruritus but usually no tenderness. In addition, cold panniculitis may appear as an erythematous but usually nontender swelling after exposure to cold, such as sledding or eating a cold Popsicle (see Chapter 660.1).

Treatment

Empirical therapy for cellulitis should be directed by the history of the illness, the location and severity of the cellulitis, and the age and immune status of the patient (Fig. 665-2). Cellulitis in a neonate should prompt a full sepsis evaluation, followed by initiation of empirical intravenous therapy with a β-lactamase–stable antistaphylococcal antibiotic such as methicillin or vancomycin and an aminoglycoside such as gentamicin or a cephalosporin such as cefotaxime. Treatment of

MANAGEMENT OF SSTIs

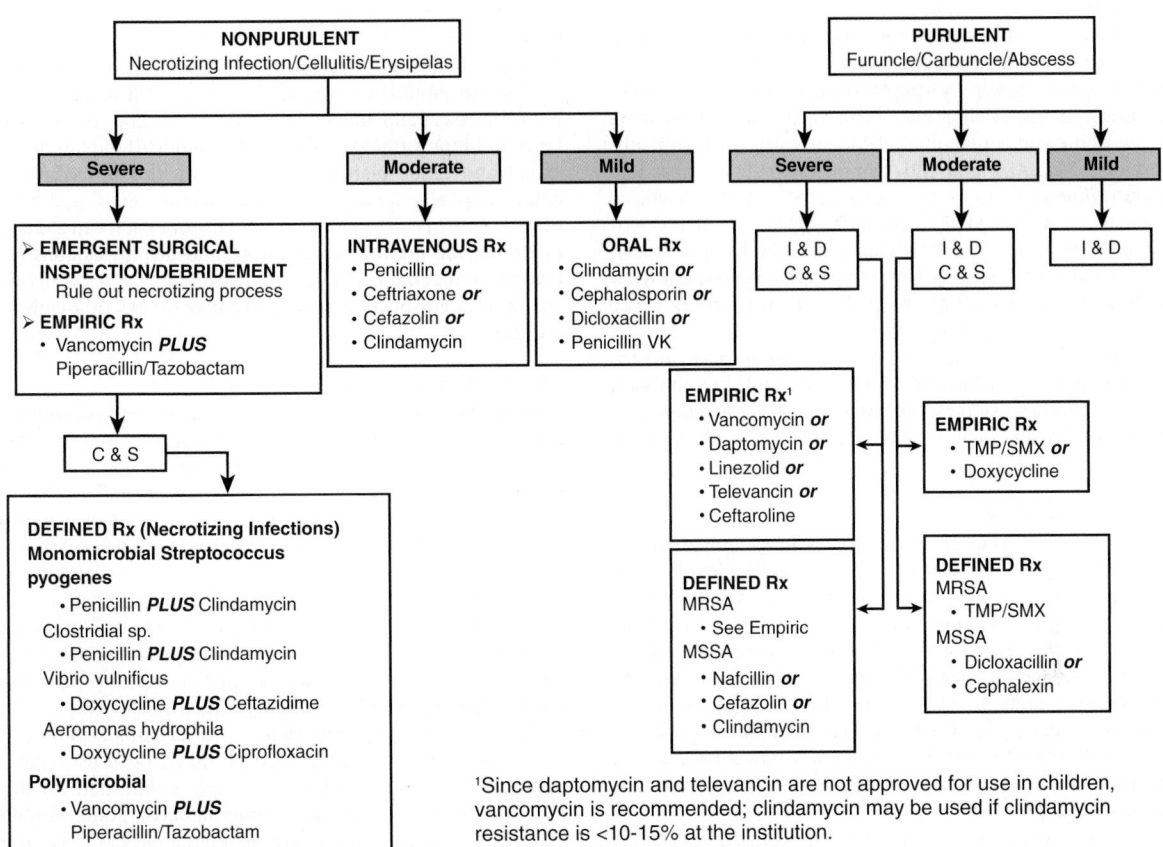

Figure 665-2 Purulent skin and soft-tissue infections (SSTIs)—*Mild infection:* For purulent SSTI, incision and drainage is indicated. *Moderate infection:* Patients with purulent infection with systemic signs of infection. *Severe infection:* Patients who have failed incision and drainage plus oral antibiotics or those with systemic signs of infection such as temperature >38°C (100.4°F), tachycardia (heart rate >90 beats/min), tachypnea (respiratory rate >24 breaths/min) or abnormal white blood cell count (<12,000 or <400 cells/μL), or immunocompromised patients. **Nonpurulent SSTIs**—*Mild infection:* Typical cellulitis/erysipelas with no focus of purulence. *Moderate infection:* Typical cellulitis/erysipelas with systemic signs of infection. *Severe infection:* Patients who have failed oral antibiotic treatment or those with systemic signs of infection (as defined above under purulent infection), or those who are immunocompromised, or those with clinical signs of deeper infection such as bullae, skin sloughing, hypotension, or evidence of organ dysfunction. Three newer agents, oritavancin, tedizolid, and dalbavancin, are also effective agents in SSTIs, including those caused by methicillin-resistant *Staphylococcus aureus*. *C & S,* culture and sensitivity; *I & D,* incision and drainage; *MRSA,* methicillin-resistant *Staphylococcus aureus; MSSA,* methicillin-susceptible *Staphylococcus aureus; Rx,* treatment; *TMP/SMX,* trimethoprim-sulfamethoxazole. *(Modified from Stevens DL, Bisno AL, Chambers HF, et al: Practice guidelines for the diagnosis and management of skin and soft tissue infections: 2014 update by the Infectious Diseases Society of America. Clin Infect Dis 59:147–159, 2014, Fig. 1.)*

cellulitis in an infant or child younger than about 5 yr of age should provide coverage for *S. pyogenes* and *S. aureus* as well as *H. influenzae* type b and *Streptococcus pneumoniae.* The evaluation should include a blood culture, and if the infant is younger than 1 yr of age, if signs of systemic toxicity are present, or if an adequate examination cannot be carried out, a lumbar puncture should also be performed. In most cases of cellulitis on an extremity, regardless of age, *S. aureus* and *S. pyogenes* are the cause and bacteremia is highly unlikely in an otherwise well-appearing child. Blood cultures should be performed if sepsis is suspected.

If fever, lymphadenopathy, and other constitutional signs are absent (white blood cell count <15,000), treatment of cellulitis on an extremity may be initiated orally on an outpatient basis with a penicillinase-resistant penicillin such as dicloxacillin or cloxacillin or a first-generation cephalosporin such as cephalexin or, if MRSA is suspected, with clindamycin. If improvement is not noted or the disease progresses significantly in the 1st 24-48 hr of therapy, parenteral therapy is necessary. If fever, lymphadenopathy, or constitutional signs are present, parenteral therapy should be initiated. Oxacillin or nafcillin is effective in most cases, although if systemic toxicity is significant, consideration should be given to the addition of clindamycin or

vancomycin. Three new agents for skin and skin structure infections have been approved by the FDA in adults. Dalbavancin (intravenous given once weekly; active against MRSA; *S. pyogenes,* and vancomycin-resistant enterococcus and *S. aureus*), tedizolid (oral or IV given bid, active against MRSA, *S. pyogenes,* coagulase-negative *Staphylococcus*), and oritavancin (IV; active against MRSA, *S. pyogenes*). Once the erythema, warmth, edema, and fever have decreased significantly, a 10-day course of treatment may be completed on an outpatient basis. Immobilization and elevation of an affected limb, particularly early in the course of therapy, may help reduce swelling and pain. *If present, a subcutaneous abscess should be drained.*

NECROTIZING FASCIITIS
Etiology
Necrotizing fasciitis is a subcutaneous tissue infection that involves the deep layer of superficial fascia but may spare adjacent epidermis, deep fascia, and muscle.

Relatively few organisms possess sufficient virulence to cause necrotizing fasciitis when acting alone. The majority (55-75%) of cases of necrotizing fasciitis are polymicrobial in nature (synergistic necrotizing fasciitis), with an average of 4 different organisms isolated. The organisms most commonly isolated in polymicrobial necrotizing fasciitis are *S. aureus*, streptococcal species, *Klebsiella* species, *E. coli,* and anaerobic bacteria.

The rest of the cases and the most fulminant infections, associated with toxic shock syndrome and a high case fatality rate, are usually caused by *S. pyogenes* (group A streptococcus) (see Chapter 183). Streptococcal necrotizing fasciitis may occur in the absence of toxic shock–like syndrome and is potentially fatal and associated with substantial morbidity. Necrotizing fasciitis can occasionally be caused by *S. aureus; Clostridium perfringens; Clostridium septicum; P. aeruginosa; Vibrio* spp., particularly *Vibrio vulnificus;* and fungi of the order Mucorales, particularly *Rhizopus* spp., *Mucor* spp., and *Absidia* spp. Necrotizing fasciitis has also been reported, on rare occasions, to result from non–group A streptococci such as group B, C, F, or G streptococci, *S. pneumoniae,* or *H. influenzae* type b.

Infections caused by any 1 organism or combination of organisms cannot be distinguished clinically from one another, although development of **crepitans** signals the presence of *Clostridium* spp. or Gram-negative bacilli such as *E. coli, Klebsiella, Proteus,* or *Aeromonas.*

Clinical Manifestations

Necrotizing fasciitis may occur anywhere on the body. Polymicrobial infections tend to occur on perineal and trunk areas. The incidence of necrotizing fasciitis is highest in hosts with systemic or local tissue immunocompromise, such as those with diabetes mellitus, neoplasia, or peripheral vascular disease as well as those who have recently undergone surgery, who abuse intravenous drugs, or who are undergoing immunosuppressive treatment, particularly with corticosteroids. The infection can also occur in healthy individuals after minor puncture wounds, abrasions, or lacerations; blunt trauma; surgical procedures, particularly of the abdomen, gastrointestinal or genitourinary tracts, or the perineum; or hypodermic needle injection.

There has been a resurgence of fulminant necrotizing soft-tissue infections caused by *S. pyogenes,* which may occur in previously healthy individuals. Streptococcal necrotizing fasciitis is classically located on an extremity. There may be a history of recent trauma to or operation in the area. Necrotizing fasciitis due to *S. pyogenes* may also occur after superinfection of varicella lesions. Children with this disease have tended to display onset, recrudescence, or persistence of high fever and signs of toxicity after the 3rd or 4th day of varicella. Common predisposing conditions in neonates are omphalitis and balanitis after circumcision.

Necrotizing fasciitis begins with acute onset of local, and at times tense, edema, erythema, tenderness, and heat. Fever is usually present, and pain, tenderness, and constitutional signs are disproportionate to cutaneous signs, especially with involvement of fascia and muscle. Lymphangitis and lymphadenitis may or may not be present. The infection advances along the superficial fascial plane, and initially there are few cutaneous signs to herald the serious nature and extent of the subcutaneous tissue necrosis that is occurring. Skin changes may appear over 24-48 hr as nutrient vessels are thrombosed and cutaneous ischemia develops. Early clinical findings include ill-defined cutaneous erythema and edema that extends beyond the area of erythema. Additional signs include formation of bullae filled initially with straw-colored and later bluish to hemorrhagic fluid, and darkening of affected tissues from red to purple to blue. Skin anesthesia and, finally, frank tissue gangrene and slough develop owing to the ischemia and necrosis. Vesiculation or bulla formation, ecchymoses, crepitus, anesthesia, and necrosis are ominous signs indicative of advanced disease. Children with varicella lesions may initially show no cutaneous signs of superinfection with invasive *S. pyogenes,* such as erythema or swelling. Significant systemic toxicity may accompany necrotizing fasciitis, including shock, organ failure, and death. Advance of the infection in this setting can be rapid, progressing to death within hours. Patients with involvement of the superficial or deep fascia and muscle tend to be more acutely and systemically ill and have more rapidly advancing disease than those with infection confined solely to subcutaneous tissues above the fascia. In an extremity, a **compartment syndrome** may develop, manifesting as tight edema, pain on motion, and loss of distal sensation and pulses; this is a surgical emergency.

Diagnosis

Definitive diagnosis of necrotizing fasciitis is made by surgical exploration, which should be undertaken as soon as the diagnosis is suspected. Necrotic fascia and subcutaneous tissue are gray and offer little resistance to blunt probing. Although CT and MRI aids in delineating the extent and tissue planes of involvement, this procedure should not delay surgical intervention. Frozen-section incisional biopsy specimens obtained early in the course of the infection can aid management by decreasing the time to diagnosis and helping establish margins of involvement. Gram staining of tissue can be particularly useful if chains of Gram-positive cocci, indicative of infection with *S. pyogenes,* are seen.

Treatment

Early supportive care, surgical debridement, and parenteral antibiotic administration are mandatory for necrotizing fasciitis. All devitalized tissue should be removed to freely bleeding edges, and repeat exploration is generally indicated within 24-36 hr to confirm that no necrotic tissue remains. This procedure may need to be repeated on several occasions until devitalized tissue has ceased to form. Meticulous daily wound care is also paramount.

Parenteral antibiotic therapy should be initiated as soon as possible with broad-spectrum agents against all potential pathogens. Initial empirical therapy should be instituted with vancomycin, linezolid, daptomycin, or quinupristin to cover Gram-positive and piperacillin-tazobactam to cover Gram-negative organisms. An alternative is to add ceftriaxone with metronidazole to cover mixed aerobic–anaerobic organisms. Therapy should then be based on sensitivity of isolated organisms. Penicillin with clindamycin is indicated for documented group A streptococcal necrotizing fasciitis. Some centers employ hyperbaric oxygen therapy, although it should not delay resuscitation or surgical debridement.

Prognosis

The combined case fatality rate among children and adults with necrotizing fasciitis and syndrome due to polymicrobial infection or *S. pyogenes* has been as high as 60%. Death is less common in children, however, and in cases not complicated by toxic shock–like syndrome.

Bibliography is available at Expert Consult.

665.3 Staphylococcal Scalded Skin Syndrome (Ritter Disease)

Anna M. Juern and Beth A. Drolet

ETIOLOGY AND PATHOGENESIS

Staphylococcal scalded skin syndrome is caused predominantly by phage group 2 staphylococci, particularly strains 71 and 55, which are present at localized sites of infection. Foci of infection include the nasopharynx and, less commonly, the umbilicus, urinary tract, a superficial abrasion, conjunctivae, and blood. The clinical manifestations of staphylococcal scalded skin syndrome are mediated by hematogenous spread, in the absence of specific antitoxin antibody of staphylococcal epidermolytic or exfoliative toxins A or B. The toxins have reproduced the disease in both animal models and human volunteers. Decreased renal clearance of the toxins may account for the fact that the disease is most common in infants and young children, as well as lack of protection from antitoxin antibodies. Epidermolytic toxin A is heat stable and is encoded by bacterial chromosomal genes. Epidermolytic toxin B is heat labile and is encoded on a 37.5-kb plasmid. The site of blister cleavage is subcorneal. The epidermolytic toxins produce the split by binding to and cleaving desmoglein 1. Intact bullae are consistently

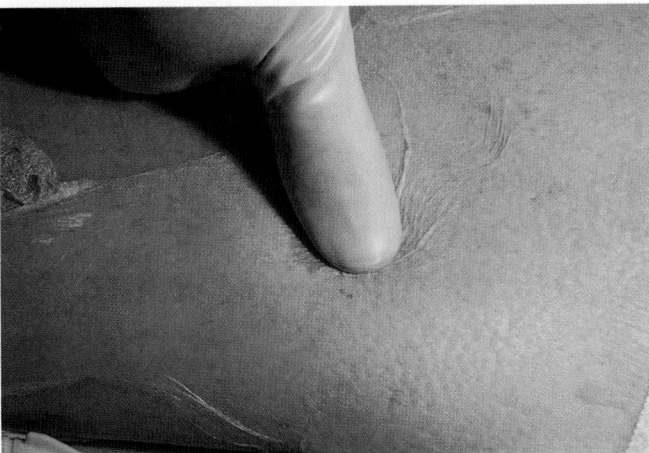

Figure 665-3 Nikolsky sign. With slight thumb pressure the skin wrinkles, slides laterally, and separates from the dermis. (*From Habif TP, editor: Clinical dermatology, ed 4, Philadelphia, 2004, Mosby.*)

sterile, unlike those of bullous impetigo, but culture specimens should be obtained from all suspected sites of localized infection and from the blood to identify the source for elaboration of the epidermolytic toxins.

CLINICAL MANIFESTATIONS

Staphylococcal scalded skin syndrome, which occurs predominantly in infants and children younger than 5 yr of age, includes a range of disease from localized bullous impetigo to generalized cutaneous involvement with systemic illness. Onset of the rash may be preceded by malaise, fever, irritability, and exquisite tenderness of the skin. **Scarlatiniform erythema** develops diffusely and is accentuated in flexural and periorificial areas. The conjunctivae are inflamed and occasionally become purulent. The brightly erythematous skin may rapidly acquire a wrinkled appearance, and in severe cases, sterile, flaccid blisters and erosions develop diffusely. Circumoral erythema is characteristically prominent, as is radial crusting and fissuring around the eyes, mouth, and nose. At this stage, areas of epidermis may separate in response to gentle shear force (Nikolsky sign; Fig. 665-3). As large sheets of epidermis peel away, moist, glistening, denuded areas become apparent, initially in the flexures and subsequently over much of the body surface (Fig. 665-4). This development may lead to secondary cutaneous infection, sepsis, and fluid and electrolyte disturbances. The desquamative phase begins after 2-5 days of cutaneous erythema; healing occurs without scarring in 10-14 days. Patients may have pharyngitis, conjunctivitis, and superficial erosions of the lips, but intraoral mucosal surfaces are spared. Although some patients appear ill, many are reasonably comfortable except for the marked skin tenderness.

DIFFERENTIAL DIAGNOSIS

A presumed **abortive** form of the disease manifests as diffuse, scarlatiniform, tender erythroderma that is accentuated in the flexural areas but does not progress to blister formation. In patients with this form, Nikolsky sign may be absent. Although the exanthem is similar to that of streptococcal scarlet fever, strawberry tongue and palatal petechiae are absent. Staphylococcal scalded skin syndrome may be mistaken for a number of other blistering and exfoliating disorders, including bullous impetigo, epidermolysis bullosa, epidermolytic hyperkeratosis, pemphigus, drug eruption, erythema multiforme, and drug-induced toxic epidermal necrolysis. Toxic epidermal necrolysis can often be distinguished by a history of drug ingestion, the presence of Nikolsky sign only at sites of erythema, absence of perioral crusting, full-thickness epidermal necrosis, and a blister cleavage plane in the lowermost epidermis.

HISTOLOGY

A subcorneal, granular layer split can be identified on skin biopsy. Absence of an inflammatory infiltrate is characteristic. Histology is

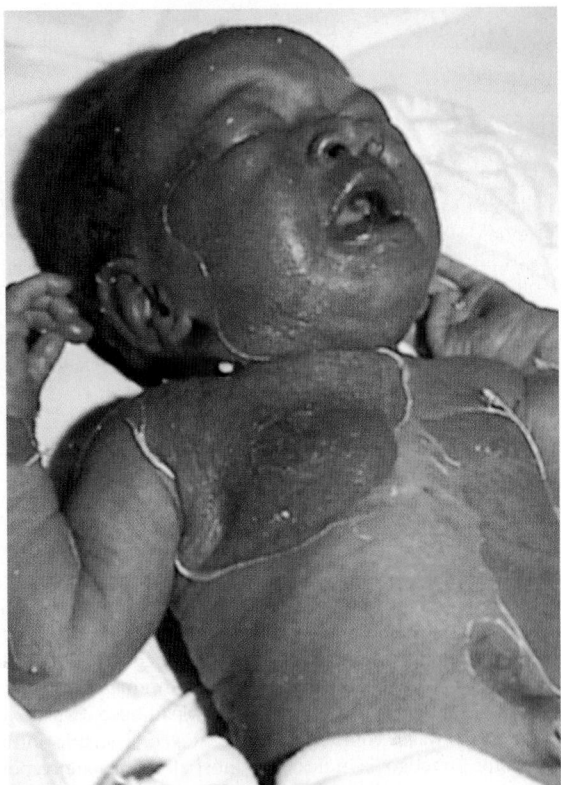

Figure 665-4 Infant with staphylococcal scalded skin syndrome.

identical to that seen in pemphigus foliaceus and subcorneal pustular dermatosis.

TREATMENT

Systemic therapy, given either orally in cases of localized involvement or parenterally with a semisynthetic penicillinase-resistant penicillin or vancomycin if MRSA is considered, should be prescribed. Clindamycin should be added to inhibit bacterial protein (toxin) synthesis. The skin should be gently moistened and cleansed. Application of an emollient provides lubrication and decreases discomfort. Topical antibiotics are unnecessary. In neonates, or in infants or children with severe infection, hospitalization is mandatory, with attention to fluid and electrolyte management, infection control measures, pain management, and meticulous wound care with contact isolation. In particularly severe disease, care in an intensive care or burn unit is required. Recovery is usually rapid, but complications such as excessive fluid loss, electrolyte imbalance, faulty temperature regulation, pneumonia, septicemia, and cellulitis may cause increased morbidity.

Bibliography is available at Expert Consult.

665.4 Ecthyma
Anna M. Juern and Beth A. Drolet

See also Chapters 181, 183, 205.

Ecthyma resembles nonbullous impetigo in onset and appearance but gradually evolves into a deeper, more chronic infection. The initial lesion is a vesicle or vesicular pustule with an erythematous base that erodes through the epidermis into the dermis to form an ulcer with elevated margins. The ulcer becomes obscured by a dry, heaped-up, tightly adherent crust (Fig. 665-5) that contributes to the persistence of the infection and scar formation. Lesions may be spread by autoinoculation, may be as large as 4 cm, and occur most frequently on the

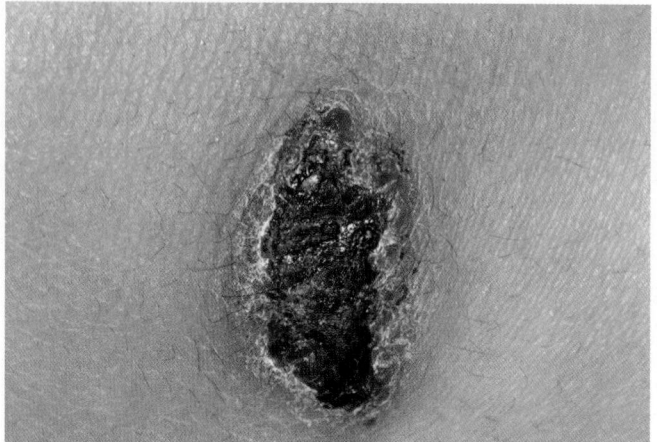

Figure 665-5 Dry, tightly adherent crust in ecthyma.

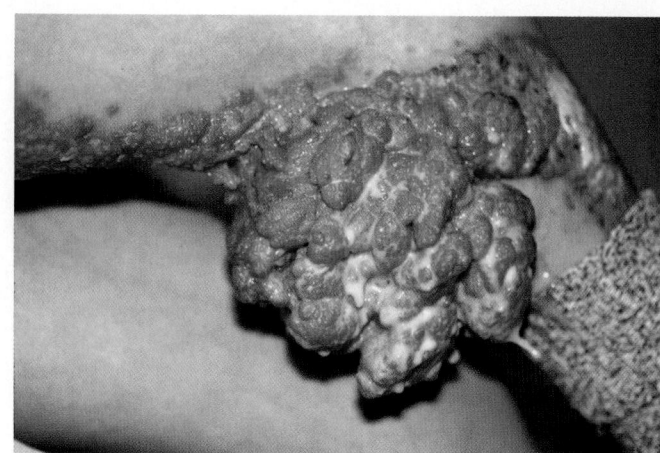

Figure 665-6 Large vegetating lesion of pyoderma vegetans.

legs. Predisposing factors include the presence of pruritic lesions, such as insect bites, scabies, or pediculosis, that are subject to frequent scratching; poor hygiene; and malnutrition. Complications include lymphangitis, cellulitis, and, rarely, poststreptococcal glomerulonephritis. The causative agent is usually GABHS; *S. aureus* is also cultured from most lesions but is probably a secondary pathogen. Crusts should be softened with warm compresses and removed. Systemic antibiotic therapy, as for impetigo, is indicated; almost all lesions are responsive to treatment with penicillin.

Ecthyma gangrenosa is a necrotic ulcer covered with a gray-black eschar. It is usually a sign of *P. aeruginosa* sepsis and usually occurs in immunosuppressed patients. Neutropenia is a risk factor for ecthyma gangrenosum. Ecthyma gangrenosum occurs in up to 6% of patients with systemic *P. aeruginosa* infection but can also occur as a primary cutaneous infection by inoculation. The lesion begins as a red or purpuric macule that vesiculates and then ulcerates. There is a surrounding rim of pink to violaceous skin. The punched-out ulcer develops raised edges with a dense, black, depressed, crusted center. Lesions may be single or multiple. Patients with bacteremia commonly have lesions in apocrine areas. Clinically similar lesions may also develop as a result of infection with other agents, such as *S. aureus, A. hydrophila, Enterobacter* spp., *Proteus* spp., *Burkholderia cepacia, Serratia marcescens, Aspergillus* spp., Mucorales, *E. coli,* and *Candida* spp. There is bacterial invasion of the adventitia and media of dermal veins but not arteries. The intima and lumina are spared. Blood and skin biopsy specimens for culture should be obtained, and empirical broad-spectrum, systemic therapy that includes coverage for *Pseudomonas* (i.e., aminoglycoside and an antipseudomonal penicillin) should be initiated as soon as possible.

Bibliography is available at Expert Consult.

665.5 Other Cutaneous Bacterial Infections
Anna M. Juern and Beth A. Drolet

BLASTOMYCOSIS-LIKE PYODERMA (PYODERMA VEGETANS)
Blastomycosis-like pyoderma is an exuberant cutaneous reaction to bacterial infection that occurs primarily in children who are malnourished and immunosuppressed. The organisms most commonly isolated from lesions are *S. aureus* and group A streptococcus, but several other organisms have been associated with these lesions, including *P. aeruginosa, Proteus mirabilis,* diphtheroids, *Bacillus* spp., and *C. perfringens.* Crusted, hyperplastic plaques on the extremities are characteristic, sometimes forming from the coalescence of many pinpoint, purulent, crusted abscesses (Fig. 665-6). Ulceration and sinus tract formation

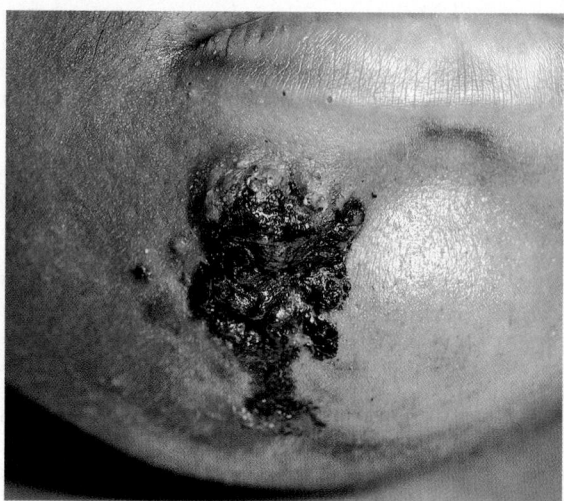

Figure 665-7 Cutaneous blastomycosis. Verrucous, crusted, erythematous plaque on the chin in a 15 yr old boy with respiratory symptoms and bone pain. *(From Paller AS, Mancini AJ, editors: Hurwitz clinical pediatric dermatology, ed 3, Philadelphia, 2006, Elsevier, Fig. 14-13.)*

may develop, and additional lesions may appear at sites distant from the site of inoculation. Regional lymphadenopathy is common, but fever is not. Histopathologic examination reveals pseudoepitheliomatous hyperplasia and abscesses composed of neutrophils and/or eosinophils. Giant cells are usually lacking. The **differential diagnosis** includes deep fungal infection, particularly blastomycosis (Fig. 665-7) and tuberculous and atypical mycobacterial infection. Underlying immunodeficiency should be ruled out, and the selection of antibiotics should be guided by susceptibility testing because the response to antibiotics is often poor.

BLISTERING DISTAL DACTYLITIS
Blistering distal dactylitis is a superficial blistering infection of the volar fat pad on the distal portion of the finger or thumb (Fig. 665-8). More than 1 finger may be involved, as may the volar surfaces of the proximal phalanges, palms, and toes. Blisters are filled with a watery purulent fluid that contains polymorphonuclear leukocytes and, usually, chains of Gram-positive cocci. Patients commonly have no preceding history of trauma, and systemic symptoms are generally absent. Poststreptococcal glomerulonephritis has not occurred after blistering distal dactylitis. The infection is caused most commonly by group A streptococcus but has also occurred as a result of infection with *S. aureus.* If left untreated, blisters may continue to enlarge and

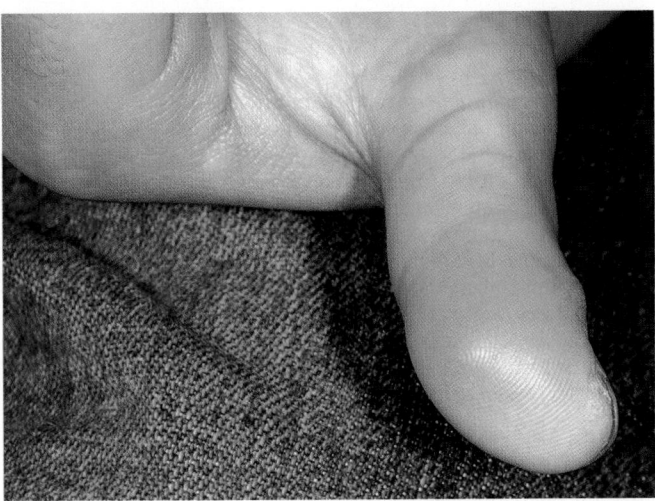

Figure 665-8 Blistering dactylitis. Edema and a tense bulla on the thumb of this 7 yr old girl. Culture of the blister fluid yielded *Staphylococcus aureus* rather than the more commonly seen group A β-hemolytic streptococcus (GABHS). *(From Paller AS, Mancini AJ, editors: Hurwitz clinical pediatric dermatology, ed 3, Philadelphia, 2006, Elsevier, Fig. 14-14.)*

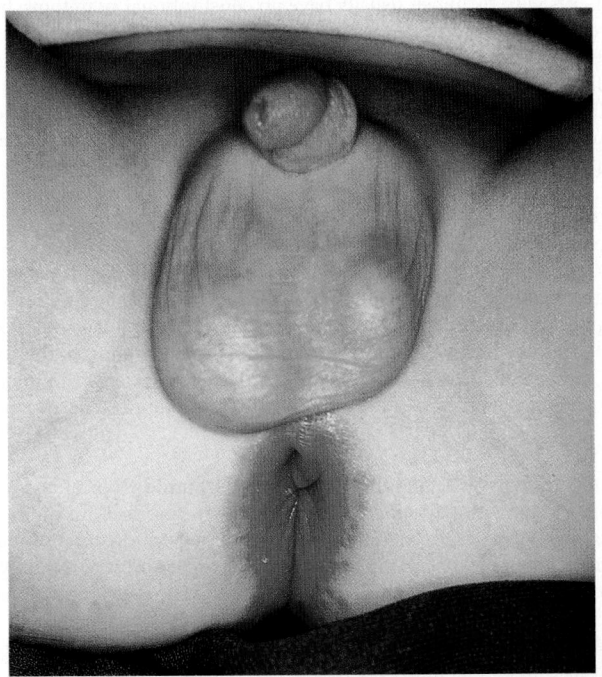

Figure 665-9 Perianal streptococcal dermatitis. Bright red erythema with a moist, tender surface. *(From Paller AS, Mancini AJ, editors: Hurwitz clinical pediatric dermatology, ed 3, Philadelphia, 2006, Elsevier, Fig. 17-38.)*

extend to the paronychial area. The infection responds to incision and drainage and a 10-day course of systemic cephalosporin therapy.

PERIANAL INFECTIOUS DERMATITIS

Perianal infectious dermatitis presents most commonly in boys (70% of cases) between the ages of 6 mo and 10 yr as perianal dermatitis (90% of cases) and pruritus (80% of cases; Fig. 665-9). The incidence of perianal infectious dermatitis is not known precisely but ranges from 1 in 2,000 to 1 in 218 patient visits. The rash is superficial, erythematous, well marginated, nonindurated, and confluent from the anus outward. Acutely (<6 wk), the rash tends to be bright red, moist,

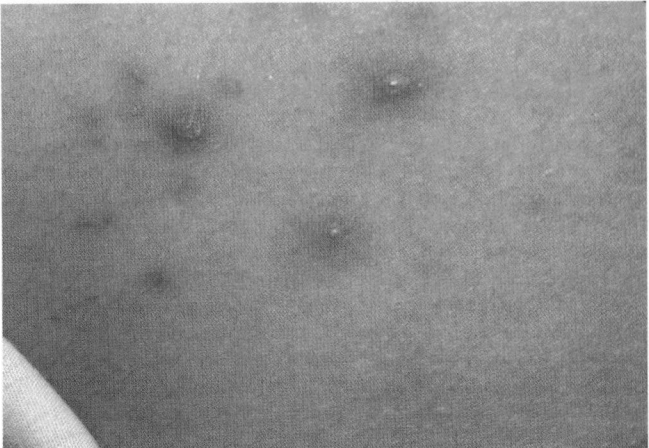

Figure 665-10 Folliculitis. Multiple follicular pustules.

and tender to touch. At this stage, a white pseudomembrane may be present. As the rash becomes more chronic, the perianal eruption may consist of painful fissures, a dried mucoid discharge, or psoriasiform plaques with yellow peripheral crust. In girls, the perianal rash may be associated with vulvovaginitis. In boys, the penis may be involved. Approximately 50% of patients have rectal pain, most commonly described as burning inside the anus during defecation, and 33% have blood-streaked stools. Fecal retention is a frequent behavioral response to the infection. Patients also have presented with guttate psoriasis. Although local induration or edema may occur, constitutional symptoms such as fever, headache, and malaise are absent, suggesting that subcutaneous involvement, as in cellulitis, is absent. Familial spread of perianal infectious dermatitis is common, particularly when family members bathe together or use the same water.

Perianal infectious dermatitis is usually caused by GABHS, but it may also be caused by *S. aureus*. The index case and family members should undergo culture; follow-up cultures to document bacteriologic cure after a course of treatment are recommended.

The **differential diagnosis** of perianal infectious dermatitis includes psoriasis, seborrheic dermatitis, candidiasis, pinworm infestation, sexual abuse, and inflammatory bowel disease.

For GABHS perianal infectious dermatitis, treatment with a 7-day course of cefuroxime (20 mg/kg/day in 2 divided doses) is superior to treatment with penicillin. Concomitant topical mupirocin ointment 2-3 times a day also may be used. If *S. aureus* is cultured, treatment should be based on sensitivities.

ERYSIPELAS

See Chapter 183.

FOLLICULITIS

Folliculitis, or superficial infection of the hair follicle, is most often caused by *S. aureus* (Bockhart impetigo). The lesions are typically small, discrete, dome-shaped pustules with an erythematous base, located at the ostium of the pilosebaceous canals (Fig. 665-10). Hair growth is unimpaired, and the lesions heal without scarring. Favored sites include the scalp, buttocks, and extremities. Poor hygiene, maceration, drainage from wounds and abscesses, and shaving of the legs can be provocative factors. Folliculitis can also occur as a result of tar therapy or occlusive wraps. The moist environment encourages bacterial proliferation. In HIV-infected patients, *S. aureus* may produce confluent erythematous patches with satellite pustules in intertriginous areas and violaceous plaques composed of superficial follicular pustules in the scalp, axillae, or groin. The **differential diagnosis** include *Candida*, which may cause satellite follicular papules and pustules surrounding erythematous patches of intertrigo, and *Malassezia furfur,* which produces 2-3 mm, pruritic, erythematous, perifollicular papules and pustules on the back, chest, and extremities, particularly in patients who have diabetes mellitus or are taking corticosteroids or antibiotics.

Diagnosis is made by examining potassium hydroxide–treated scrapings from lesions. Detection of *Malassezia* may require a skin biopsy, demonstrating clusters of yeast and short, branching hyphae ("macaroni and meatballs") in widened follicular ostia mixed with keratinous debris.

Topical antibiotic therapy (e.g., clindamycin 1% lotion or solution twice a day) is usually all that is needed for mild cases, but more severe cases may require use of a systemic antibiotic such as dicloxacillin or cephalexin. Bacterial culture should be performed in treatment-resistant cases. In chronic recurrent folliculitis, daily application of a benzoyl peroxide 5% gel or wash may facilitate resolution.

Folliculitis barbae (sycosis barbae) is a deeper, more severe recurrent inflammatory form of folliculitis caused by *S. aureus* that involves the entire depth of the follicle. Erythematous follicular papules and pustules develop on the chin, upper lip, and angle of the jaw, primarily in young black males. Papules may coalesce into plaques, and healing may occur with scarring. Affected individuals are frequently found to be *S. aureus* carriers. **Treatment** with warm saline compresses and topical antibiotics such as mupirocin generally clears the infection. More extensive, recalcitrant cases may require therapy with β-lactamase–resistant systemic antibiotics for several weeks, and elimination of *S. aureus* from sites of carriage.

Pseudomonal folliculitis (hot tub folliculitis) is attributable to *P. aeruginosa,* predominantly serotype O-11. It occurs after exposure to poorly chlorinated hot tubs/whirlpools and swimming pools, as well as to a contaminated water slide, or loofah sponge. The lesions are pruritic papules and pustules or deeply erythematous to violaceous nodules that develop 8-48 hr after exposure and are most dense in areas covered by a bathing suit (Fig. 665-11). Patients occasionally experience fever, malaise, and lymphadenopathy. The organism is readily cultured from pus. The eruption usually resolves spontaneously in 1-2 wk, often leaving postinflammatory hyperpigmentation. Consideration should be given to use of systemic antibiotics (ciprofloxacin) in adolescent patients with constitutional symptoms. Immunocompromised children are susceptible to complications of *Pseudomonas* folliculitis (cellulitis) and should avoid hot tubs.

FURUNCLES AND ABSCESSES
Etiology
The causative agent in furuncles ("boils") and carbuncles is usually *S. aureus,* which penetrates abraded perifollicular skin. Conditions predisposing to furuncle formation include obesity, hyperhidrosis, maceration, friction, and preexisting dermatitis. Furunculosis is also more common in individuals with low serum iron levels, diabetes, malnutrition, HIV infection, or other immunodeficiency states. Recurrent furunculosis is frequently associated with carriage of *S. aureus* in the nares, axillae, or perineum or close contact with someone such as a family member who is a carrier. Other bacteria or fungi may occasionally cause furuncles or carbuncles.

Community-acquired MRSA abscesses can also complicate folliculitis. Community-acquired MRSA infections commonly affect children and young adults, especially athletes where spread of the infection is enhanced by skin-to-skin contact. Infection can also be spread by crowding conditions, shared personal hygiene items, and a compromised skin barrier. They may occur in any location, however, they are most common on the lower abdomen, buttocks, and legs. Abscesses which are a common manifestation of community-acquired MRSA should be incised and drained. If oral antibiotics are needed, those with coverage against MRSA are recommended and commonly include oral trimethoprim-sulfamethoxazole (8-12 mg trimethoprim/kg/day in divided doses every 12 hr) or clindamycin (10-20 mg/kg/day in divided doses 3 times daily). To reduce colonization and hence reinfection, bleach baths for patients, and mupirocin intranasally in patients and in family members has been recommended.

Clinical Manifestations
This follicular lesion may originate from a preceding folliculitis or may arise initially as a deep-seated, tender, erythematous, perifollicular nodule. Although lesions are initially indurated, central necrosis and suppuration follow, leading to rupture and discharge of a central core of necrotic tissue and destruction of the follicle (Fig. 665-12). Healing occurs with scar formation. Sites of predilection are the hair-bearing areas on the face, neck, axillae, buttocks, and groin. Pain may be intense if the lesion is situated in an area where the skin is relatively fixed, such as in the external auditory canal or over the nasal cartilages. Patients with furuncles usually have no constitutional symptoms; bacteremia may occasionally ensue. Rarely, lesions on the upper lip or cheek may lead to cavernous sinus thrombosis. Infection of a group of contiguous follicles, with multiple drainage points, accompanied by inflammatory changes in surrounding connective tissue is a **carbuncle**. Carbuncles may be accompanied by fever, leukocytosis, and bacteremia.

Treatment
Treatment for furuncle and carbuncle includes regular bathing with antimicrobial soaps (chlorhexidine) and wearing of loose-fitting clothing to minimize predisposing factors for furuncle formation. Frequent application of a hot, moist compress may facilitate drainage of lesions. Large lesions may be drained by a small incision. Carbuncles and large or numerous furuncles should be treated with systemic antibiotics chosen on the basis of culture and sensitivity testing results.

PITTED KERATOLYSIS
Pitted keratolysis occurs most frequently in humid tropical and subtropical climates, particularly in individuals whose feet are moist for prolonged periods, for example, as a result of hyperhidrosis, prolonged wearing of boots, or immersion in water. It occurs most commonly in young males from early adolescence to the late 20s. The lesions consist

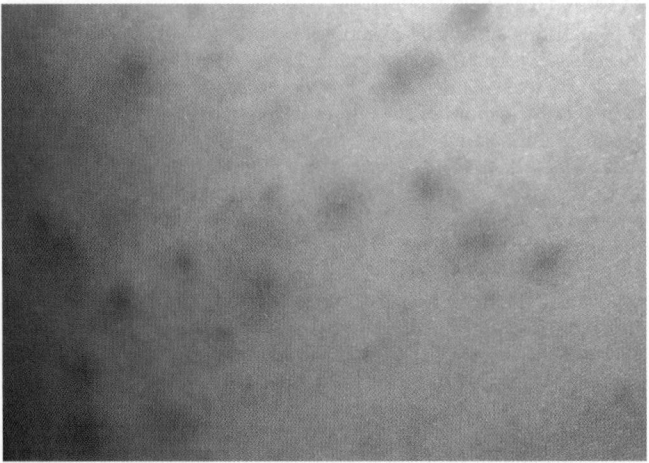

Figure 665-11 Papules and pustules in hot tub folliculitis.

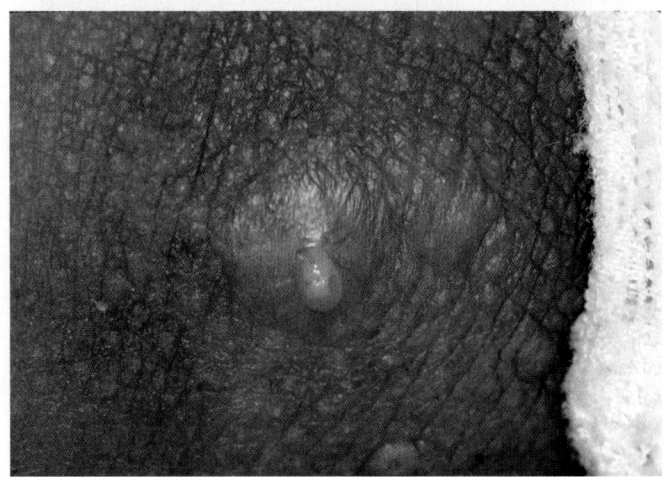

Figure 665-12 Rupture and discharge of pus in a furuncle.

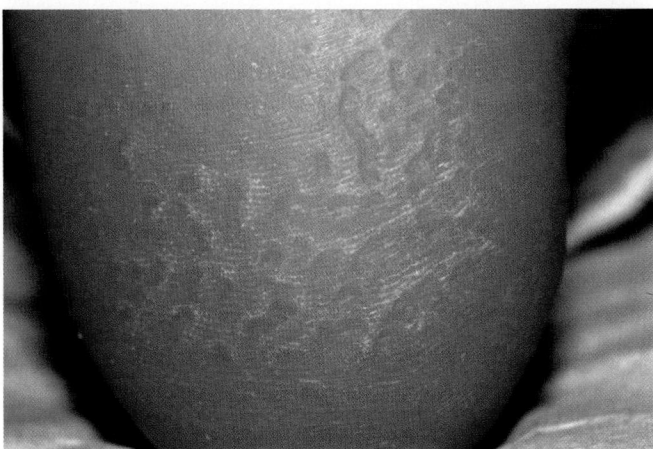

Figure 665-13 Superficial erosions of the horny layer in pitted keratolysis.

of 1-7 mm, irregularly shaped, superficial erosions of the horny layer on the soles, particularly at weight-bearing sites (Fig. 665-13). Brownish discoloration of involved areas may be apparent. A rare variant manifests as thinned, erythematous to violaceous plaques in addition to the typical pitted lesions. The condition is frequently malodorous, and is painful in approximately 50% of cases. The most likely etiologic agent is *Corynebacterium (Kytococcus) sedentarius*. Treatment of hyperhidrosis is mandatory with prescription-strength aluminum chloride products or 40% formaldehyde in petrolatum ointment. Avoidance of moisture and maceration produces slow, spontaneous resolution of the infection. Topical or systemic erythromycin and topical imidazole creams are standard therapy.

ERYTHRASMA

Erythrasma is a benign chronic superficial infection caused by *Corynebacterium minutissimum*. Predisposing factors include heat, humidity, obesity, skin maceration, diabetes mellitus, and poor hygiene. Approximately 20% of affected patients have involvement of the toe webs. Other frequently affected sites are moist, intertriginous areas such as the groin and axillae. The inframammary and perianal regions are occasionally involved. Sharply demarcated, irregularly bordered, slightly scaly, brownish red patches are characteristic of the disease. Mild pruritus is the only constant symptom. *C. minutissimum* is a complex of related organisms that produce porphyrins that fluoresce brilliant coral red under ultraviolet light. The diagnosis is readily made, and erythrasma is differentiated from dermatophyte infection and from tinea versicolor on Wood lamp examination. Bathing within 20 hr of Wood lamp examination, however, may remove the water-soluble porphyrins. Staining of skin scrapings with methylene blue or Gram stain reveals the pleomorphic, filamentous coccobacillary forms.

Effective **treatment** can be achieved with topical erythromycin, clindamycin, miconazole, or a 10-14 day course of oral erythromycin or an oral tetracycline.

ERYSIPELOID

A rare cutaneous infection, erysipeloid is caused by inoculation of *Erysipelothrix rhusiopathiae* from handling contaminated animals, birds, fish, or their products. The localized cutaneous form is most common, characterized by well-demarcated diamond-shaped erythematous to violaceous patches at sites of inoculation. Local symptoms are generally not severe, constitutional symptoms are rare, and the lesions resolve spontaneously after weeks but can recur at the same site or develop elsewhere weeks to months later. The diffuse cutaneous form manifests as lesions at several areas of the body in addition to the site of inoculation. It is also self-limited. The systemic form, caused by hematogenous spread, is accompanied by constitutional symptoms and may include endocarditis, septic arthritis, cerebral infarct and abscess, meningitis, and pulmonary effusion. Diagnosis is confirmed by skin biopsy, which reveals the Gram-positive organisms, and culture. The **treatment** of choice is parenteral penicillin or erythromycin.

TUBERCULOSIS OF THE SKIN

See Chapters 215 and 217.

Cutaneous tuberculosis infection occurs worldwide, particularly in association with HIV infection, malnutrition, and poor sanitary conditions. Primary cutaneous tuberculosis is rare in the United States. All forms of cutaneous disease are caused by *Mycobacterium tuberculosis, Mycobacterium bovis*, and occasionally by the bacillus Calmette-Guérin (BCG), an attenuated vaccine form of *M. bovis*. The manifestations caused by a given organism are indistinguishable from one another. After invasion of the skin, mycobacteria either multiply intracellularly within macrophages, leading to progressive disease, or are controlled by the host immune reaction.

Primary cutaneous tuberculosis (tuberculous chancre) results when *M. tuberculosis* or *M. bovis* gains access to the skin or mucous membranes through trauma in a previously uninfected individual without immunity to the organism. Sites of predilection are the face, lower extremities, and genitals. The initial lesion develops 2-4 wk after introduction of the organism into the damaged tissue. A red-brown papule gradually enlarges to form a shallow, firm, sharply demarcated ulcer. Satellite abscesses may be present. Some lesions acquire a crust resembling impetigo, and others become heaped up and verrucous at the margins. The primary lesion can also manifest as a painless ulcer on the conjunctiva, gingiva, or palate and occasionally as a painless acute paronychia. Painless regional adenopathy may appear several weeks after the development of the primary lesion and may be accompanied by lymphangitis, lymphadenitis, or perforation of the skin surface, forming **scrofuloderma**. Untreated lesions heal with scarring within 12 mo but may reactivate, may form lupus vulgaris, or, rarely, may progress to the acute miliary form. Therefore, antituberculous therapy is indicated (see Chapter 215).

M. tuberculosis or *M. bovis* can be cultured from the skin lesion and local lymph nodes, but acid-fast staining of histologic sections, particularly of a well-controlled infection, often does not reveal the organism. The **differential diagnosis** is broad, including a syphilitic chancre; deep fungal or atypical mycobacterial infection; leprosy; tularemia; cat-scratch disease; sporotrichosis; nocardiosis; leishmaniasis; reaction to foreign substances such as zirconium, beryllium, silk or nylon sutures, talc, and starch; papular acne rosacea; and lupus miliaris disseminatus faciei.

Scrofuloderma results from enlargement, cold abscess formation, and breakdown of a lymph node, most frequently in a cervical chain, with extension to the overlying skin from underlying foci of tuberculous infection. Linear or serpiginous ulcers and dissecting fistulas and subcutaneous tracts studded with soft nodules may develop. Spontaneous healing may take years, eventuating in cordlike keloid scars. Lupus vulgaris may also develop. Lesions may also originate from an underlying infected joint, tendon, bone, or epididymis. The **differential diagnosis** includes syphilitic gumma, deep fungal infections, actinomycosis, and hidradenitis suppurativa. The course is indolent, and constitutional symptoms are typically absent. Antituberculous therapy is indicated (see Chapter 215).

Direct cutaneous inoculation of the tubercle bacillus into a previously infected individual with a moderate to high degree of immunity initially produces a small papule with surrounding inflammation. **Tuberculosis verrucosa cutis** (warty tuberculosis) forms when the papule becomes hyperkeratotic and warty, and several adjacent papules coalesce or a single papule expands peripherally to form a brownish red to violaceous, exudative, crusted verrucous plaque. Irregular extension of the margins of the plaque produces a serpiginous border. Children have the lesions most commonly on the lower extremities after trauma and contact with infected material such as sputum or soil. Regional lymph nodes are involved only rarely. Spontaneous healing with atrophic scarring takes place over months to years. Healing is also gradual with antituberculous therapy.

Lupus vulgaris is a rare, chronic, progressive form of cutaneous tuberculosis that develops in individuals with a moderate to high degree of tuberculin sensitivity induced by previous infection. The incidence is greater in cool, moist climates, particularly in females. Lupus vulgaris develops as a result of direct extension from underlying joints or lymph nodes; through lymphatic or hematogenous spread; or, rarely, by cutaneous inoculation with BCG vaccine. It most commonly follows cervical adenitis or pulmonary tuberculosis. Approximately 33% of cases are preceded by scrofuloderma, and 90% of cases manifest on the head and neck, most commonly on the nose or cheek. Involvement of the trunk is uncommon. A typical solitary lesion consists of a soft, brownish red papule that has an apple-jelly color when examined by diascopy. Peripheral expansion of the papule or, occasionally, the coalescence of several papules forms an irregular lesion of variable size and form. One or several lesions may develop, including nodules or plaques that are flat and serpiginous, hypertrophic and verrucous, or edematous in appearance. Spontaneous healing occurs centrally, and lesions characteristically reappear within the area of atrophy. Chronicity is characteristic, and persistence and progression of plaques over many years is common. Lymphadenitis is present in 40% of those with lupus vulgaris, and 10-20% has infection of the lungs, bones, or joints. Extensive deformities may be caused by vegetative masses and ulceration involving the nasal, buccal, or conjunctival mucosa; the palate; the gingiva; or the oropharynx. Squamous cell carcinoma, with a relatively high metastatic potential, may develop, usually after several years of the disease. After a temporary impairment in immunity, particularly after measles infection (lupus exanthematicus), multiple lesions may form at distant sites as a result of hematogenous spread from a latent focus of infection. The histopathology reveals a tuberculoid granuloma without caseation; organisms are extremely difficult to demonstrate. The **differential diagnosis** includes sarcoidosis, atypical mycobacterial infection, blastomycosis, chromoblastomycosis, actinomycosis, leishmaniasis, tertiary syphilis, leprosy, hypertrophic lichen planus, psoriasis, lupus erythematosus, lymphocytoma, and Bowen disease. Small lesions can be excised. Antituberculous drug therapy usually halts further spread and induces involution.

Orificial tuberculosis (tuberculosis cutis orificialis) appears on the mucous membranes and periorificial skin after autoinoculation of mycobacteria from sites of progressive infection. It is a sign of advanced internal disease and carries a poor prognosis and occurs in s sensitized host with impaired cellular immunity. Lesions appear as painful, yellowish or red nodules that form punched-out ulcers with inflammation and edema of the surrounding mucosa. **Treatment** consists of identification of the source of infection and initiation of antituberculous therapy.

Miliary tuberculosis (hematogenous primary tuberculosis) rarely manifests cutaneously and occurs most commonly in infants and in individuals who are immunosuppressed after chemotherapy or infection with measles or HIV. The eruption consists of crops of symmetrically distributed, minute, erythematous to purpuric macules, papules, or vesicles. The lesions may ulcerate, drain, crust, and form sinus tracts or may form subcutaneous gummas, especially in malnourished children with impaired immunity. Constitutional signs and symptoms are common, and a leukemoid reaction or aplastic anemia may develop. Tubercle bacilli are readily identified in an active lesion. A fulminant course should be anticipated, and aggressive antituberculous therapy is indicated.

Single or multiple metastatic tuberculous abscesses (**tuberculous gummas**) may develop on the extremities and trunk by hematogenous spread from a primary focus of infection during a period of decreased immunity, particularly in malnourished and immunosuppressed children. The fluctuant, nontender, erythematous subcutaneous nodules may ulcerate and form fistulas.

Vaccination with BCG characteristically produces a papule approximately 2 wk after vaccination. The papule expands in size, typically ulcerates within 2-4 mo, and heals slowly with scarring. In 1-2 per million vaccinations, a complication caused specifically by the BCG organism occurs, including regional lymphadenitis, lupus vulgaris, scrofuloderma, and subcutaneous abscess formation.

Tuberculids are skin reactions that exhibit tuberculoid features histologically but do not contain detectable mycobacteria. The lesions appear in a host who usually has moderate to strong tuberculin reactivity, has a history of previous tuberculosis of other organs, and usually shows a therapeutic response to antituberculous therapy. The cause of tuberculids is poorly understood. Most affected patients are in good health with no clear focus of disease at the time of the eruption. The most commonly observed tuberculid is the papulonecrotic tuberculid. Recurrent crops of symmetrically distributed, asymptomatic, firm, sterile, dusky-red papules appear on the extensor aspects of the limbs, the dorsum of the hands and feet, and the buttocks. The papules may undergo central ulceration and eventually heal, leaving sharply delineated, circular, depressed scars. The duration of the eruption is variable, but it usually disappears promptly after treatment of the primary infection. Lichen scrofulosorum, another form of tuberculid, is characterized by asymptomatic, grouped, pinhead-sized, often follicular pink or red papules that form discoid plaques, mainly on the trunk. Healing occurs without scarring.

Atypical mycobacterial infection may cause cutaneous lesions in children. *Mycobacterium marinum* is found in saltwater, freshwater, and diseased fish. In the United States, it is most commonly acquired from tropical fish tanks and swimming pools. Traumatic abrasion of the skin serves as a portal of entry for the organism. Approximately 3 wk after inoculation, a single reddish papule develops and enlarges slowly to form a violaceous nodule or, occasionally, a warty plaque (Fig. 665-14). The lesion occasionally breaks down to form a crusted ulcer or a suppurating abscess. Sporotrichoid erythematous nodules along lymphatics may also suppurate and drain. Lesions are most common on the elbows, knees, and feet of swimmers, and on the hands and fingers in persons with aquarium-acquired infection. Systemic signs and symptoms are absent. Regional lymph nodes occasionally become slightly enlarged but do not break down. Rarely, the infection becomes disseminated, particularly in an immunosuppressed host. A biopsy specimen of a fully developed lesion demonstrates a granulomatous infiltrate with tuberculoid architecture. Treatment options include tetracycline, doxycycline, minocycline, clarithromycin, and rifampin plus ethambutol. Application of heat to the affected site may be a useful adjunctive therapy (see Chapter 217).

Mycobacterium kansasii primarily causes pulmonary disease; skin disease is rare, often occurring in an immunocompromised host. Most commonly, sporotrichoid nodules develop after inoculation of traumatized skin. Lesions may develop into ulcerated, crusted, or verrucous plaques. The organism is relatively sensitive to antituberculous medications, which should be chosen on the basis of susceptibility testing.

Mycobacterium scrofulaceum causes cervical lymphadenitis (scrofuloderma) in young children, typically in the submandibular region. Nodes enlarge over several weeks, ulcerate, and drain. The local reaction is nontender and circumscribed, constitutional symptoms are absent, and there generally is no evidence of lung or other organ involvement. Other atypical mycobacteria may cause a similar

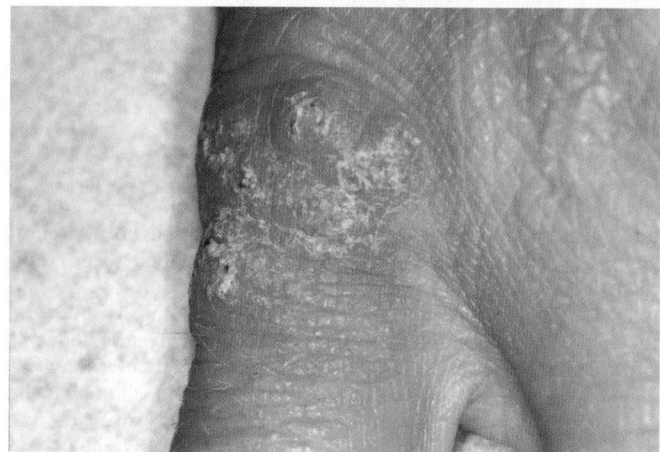

Figure 665-14 Violaceous, warty plaque of *Mycobacterium marinum* infection.

presentation, including *Mycobacterium avium* complex, *Mycobacterium kansasii,* and *Mycobacterium fortuitum.* **Treatment** is accomplished by excision and administration of antituberculous drugs (see Chapter 217).

Mycobacterium ulcerans (Buruli ulcer) causes a painless subcutaneous nodule after inoculation of abraded skin. Most infections occur in children in tropical rain forests. The nodule usually ulcerates, develops undermined edges, and may spread over large areas, most commonly on an extremity. Local necrosis of subcutaneous fat, producing a septal panniculitis, is characteristic. Ulcers persist for months to years before healing spontaneously with scarring and sometimes with lymphedema. Constitutional symptoms and lymphadenopathy are absent. Diagnosis is made by culturing the organism at 32-33°C (89.6-91.4°F). **Treatment of choice** is early excision of the lesion. Local heat therapy and oral chemotherapy may benefit some patients.

M. avium complex, composed of more than 20 subtypes, most commonly causes chronic pulmonary infection. Cervical lymphadenitis and osteomyelitis occur occasionally, and papules or purulent leg ulcers occur rarely by primary inoculation. Skin lesions may be an early sign of disseminated infection. The lesions may take various forms, including erythematous papules, pustules, nodules, abscesses, ulcers, panniculitis, and sporotrichoid spread along lymphatics. For treatment, see Chapter 217.

M. fortuitum complex causes disease in an immunocompetent host principally by primary cutaneous inoculation after traumatic injury, injection, or surgery. A nodule, abscess, or cellulitis develops 4-6 wk after inoculation. In an immunocompromised host, numerous subcutaneous nodules may form, break down, and drain. **Treatment** is based on identification and susceptibility testing of the organism.

Bibliography is available at Expert Consult.

Chapter 666
Cutaneous Fungal Infections
Anna M. Juern and Beth A. Drolet

TINEA VERSICOLOR

A common, innocuous, chronic fungal infection of the stratum corneum, tinea versicolor is caused by the dimorphic yeast *Malassezia globosa.* The synonyms *Pityrosporum ovale* and *Pityrosporum orbiculare* were used previously to identify the causal organism.

Etiology

M. globosa is part of the indigenous flora, predominantly in the yeast form, and is found particularly in areas of skin that are rich in sebum production, and is part of normal skin flora. Proliferation of filamentous forms occurs in the disease state. Predisposing factors include a warm, humid environment, excessive sweating, occlusion, high plasma cortisol levels, immunosuppression, malnourishment, and genetically determined susceptibility. The disease is most prevalent in adolescents and young adults.

Clinical Manifestations

The lesions of tinea versicolor vary widely in color. In white individuals, they are typically reddish brown, whereas in black individuals they may be either hypopigmented or hyperpigmented. The characteristic macules are covered with a fine scale. They often begin in a perifollicular location, enlarge, and merge to form confluent patches, most

Figure 666-1 Hyperpigmented, sharply demarcated macules of varying sizes on the upper trunk characteristic of tinea versicolor.

commonly on the neck, upper chest, back, and upper arms (Fig. 666-1). Facial lesions are common in adolescents; lesions occasionally appear on the forearms, dorsum of the hands, and pubis. There may be little or no pruritus. Involved areas do not tan after sun exposure. A papulopustular perifollicular variant of the disorder may occur on the back, chest, and sometimes the extremities.

Differential Diagnosis

Examination with a Wood lamp discloses a yellowish gold fluorescence. A potassium hydroxide (KOH) preparation of scrapings is diagnostic, demonstrating groups of thick-walled spores and myriad short, thick, angular hyphae resembling macaroni/spaghetti and meatballs. Skin biopsy, including culture and special stains for fungi (periodic acid–Schiff), are often necessary to make the diagnosis in cases of primarily follicular involvement. Microscopically, organisms and keratinous debris can be seen within dilated follicular ostia.

Tinea versicolor must be distinguished from dermatophyte infections, seborrheic dermatitis, pityriasis alba, and secondary syphilis. Tinea versicolor may mimic nonscaling pigmentary disorders, such as postinflammatory pigmentary change, if a patient has removed the scales by scrubbing. *M. globosa* folliculitis must be distinguished from the other forms of folliculitis.

Treatment

Many therapeutic agents can be used to treat this disease successfully. The causative agent, a normal human saprophyte, is not eradicated from the skin, however, and the disorder recurs in predisposed individuals. Appropriate topical therapy may include 1 of the following: selenium 2% shampoo applied for 10 minutes before rinsing for 2 wk; ketoconazole 2% shampoo 3 times a wk for a month or a single application daily for 3 days; and terbinafine spray once to twice daily for 1-2 wk. Antifungal creams are available and can be used; however, these can be impractical to apply given the large surface of skin involved. Oral therapy may be more convenient and may be achieved successfully with ketoconazole or fluconazole, 400 mg, repeated in 1 wk, or itraconazole, 200 mg/24 hr for 5-7 days. Recurrent episodes continue to respond promptly to these agents. Oral therapy is particularly helpful in those with severe disease or recurrent disease, or in those where topical therapies have failed. Maintenance therapy with selenium sulfide shampoo or ketoconazole 2% shampoo once a week may be used.

DERMATOPHYTOSES

Dermatophytoses are caused by a group of closely related filamentous fungi with a propensity for invading the stratum corneum, hair, and nails. The 3 principal genera responsible for infections are *Trichophyton, Microsporum,* and *Epidermophyton.*

Etiology

Trichophyton spp. cause lesions of all keratinized tissue, including skin, nails, and hair. *Trichophyton rubrum* is the most common dermatophyte pathogen. *Microsporum* spp. principally invade the hair, and the *Epidermophyton* spp. invade the intertriginous skin. Dermatophyte infections are designated by the word **tinea** followed by the Latin word for the anatomic site of involvement. The dermatophytes are also classified according to source and natural habitat. Fungi acquired from the soil are called *geophilic*. They infect humans sporadically, inciting an inflammatory reaction. Dermatophytes that are acquired from animals are *zoophilic*. Transmission may be through direct contact or indirectly by infected animal hair or clothing. Infected animals are frequently asymptomatic. Dermatophytes acquired from humans are referred to as *anthropophilic*. These infestations range from chronic low-grade to acute inflammatory disease. *Epidermophyton* infections are transmitted only by humans, but various species of *Trichophyton* and *Microsporum* can be acquired from both human and nonhuman sources.

Epidemiology

Host defense has an important influence on the severity of the infection. Disease tends to be more severe in individuals with diabetes mellitus, lymphoid malignancies, immunosuppression, and states with high plasma cortisol levels, such as Cushing syndrome. Some dermatophytes, most notably the zoophilic species, tend to elicit more severe, suppurative inflammation in humans. Some degree of resistance to reinfection is acquired by most infected persons and may be associated with a delayed hypersensitivity response. No relationship has been demonstrated, however, between antibody levels and resistance to infection. The frequency and severity of infection are also affected by the geographic locale, the genetic susceptibility of the host, and the virulence of the strain of dermatophyte. Additional local factors that predispose to infection include trauma to the skin, hydration of the skin with maceration, occlusion, and elevated temperature.

Occasionally, a secondary skin eruption, referred to as a dermatophytid or "id" reaction, appears in sensitized individuals and has been attributed to circulating fungal antigens derived from the primary infection. The eruption is characterized by grouped papules (Fig. 666-2) and vesicles and, occasionally, by sterile pustules. Symmetric urticarial lesions and a more generalized maculopapular eruption also can occur. Id reactions are most often associated with tinea pedis but also occur with tinea capitis.

Tinea Capitis
Clinical Manifestations

Tinea capitis is a dermatophyte infection of the scalp most often caused by *Trichophyton tonsurans*, occasionally by *Microsporum canis*, and, much less commonly, by other *Microsporum* and *Trichophyton* spp. It is particularly common in black children age 4-14 yr. In *Microsporum*

and some *Trichophyton* infections, the spores are distributed in a sheath-like fashion around the hair shaft (**ectothrix** infection), whereas *T. tonsurans* produces an infection within the hair shaft (endothrix). **Endothrix** infections may continue past the anagen phase of hair growth into telogen and are more chronic than infections with ectothrix organisms that persist only during the anagen phase. *T. tonsurans* is an anthropophilic species acquired most often by contact with infected hairs and epithelial cells that are on such surfaces as theater seats, hats, and combs. Dermatophyte spores may also be airborne within the immediate environment, and high carriage rates have been demonstrated in noninfected schoolmates and household members. *M. canis* is a zoophilic species that is acquired from cats and dogs.

The clinical presentation of tinea capitis varies with the infecting organism. Endothrix infections such as those caused by *T. tonsurans* create a pattern known as "black-dot ringworm," characterized initially by many small circular patches of alopecia in which hairs are broken off close to the hair follicle (Fig. 666-3). Another clinical variant manifests as diffuse scaling, with minimal hair loss secondary. It strongly resembles seborrheic dermatitis, psoriasis, or atopic dermatitis (Fig. 666-4). *T. tonsurans* may also produce a chronic and more diffuse alopecia. Lymphadenopathy is common (Fig. 666-5). A severe inflammatory response produces elevated, boggy granulomatous masses (**kerions**), which are often studded with pustules (Fig. 666-6*A*). Fever, pain, and regional adenopathy are common, and permanent scarring and alopecia may result (Fig. 666-6*B*). The zoophilic organism *M. canis* or the geophilic organism *Microsporum gypseum* also may cause kerion formation. The pattern produced by *Microsporum audouinii*, the most

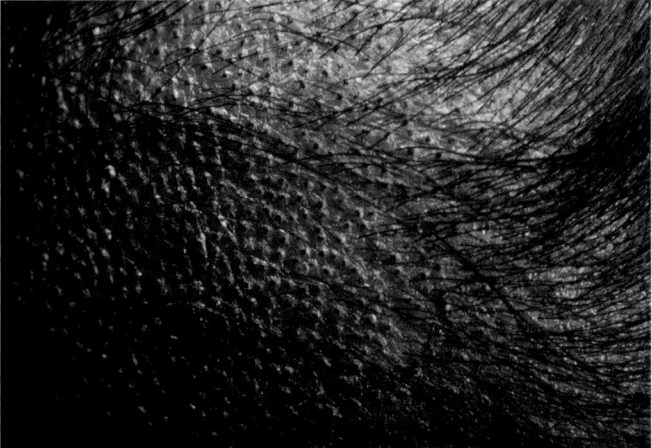

Figure 666-3 Black-dot ringworm with hairs broken off at the scalp.

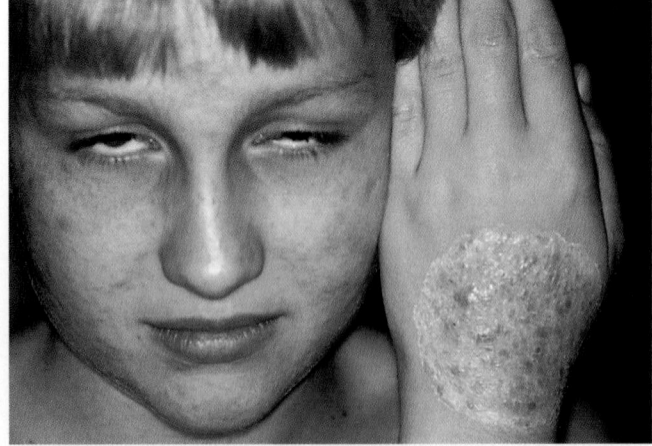

Figure 666-2 Id reaction. Papular eruption of the face associated with severe tinea infection of the hand.

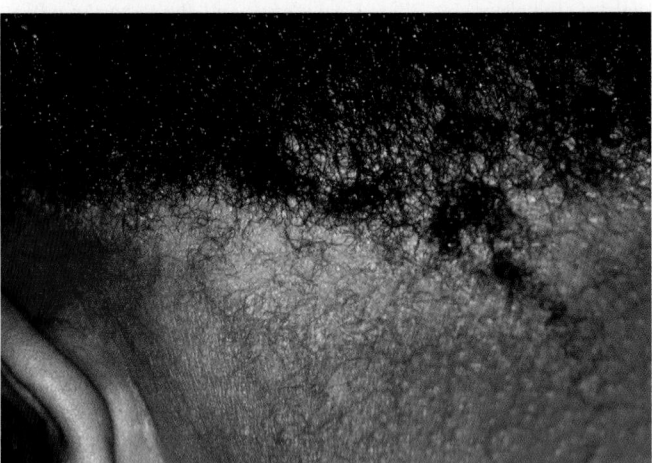

Figure 666-4 Tinea capitis mimicking seborrheic dermatitis.

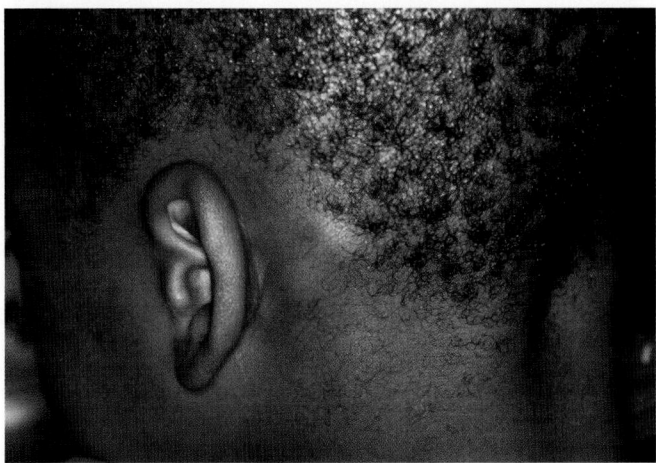

Figure 666-5 Lymphadenopathy associated with tinea capitis.

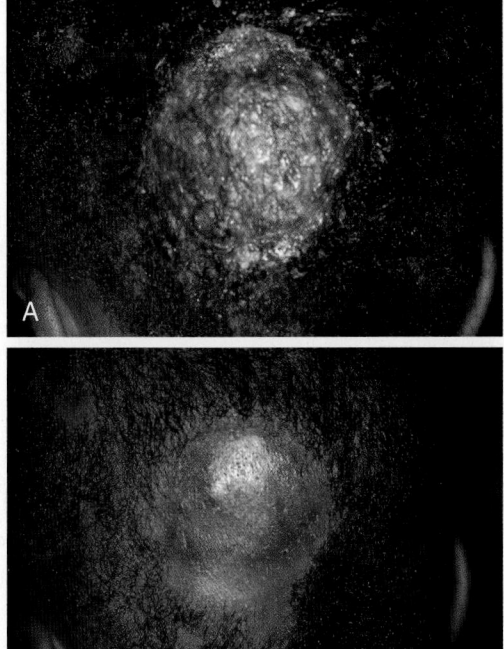

Figure 666-6 A, Kerion. Boggy granulomatous mass of the scalp. B, Scarring after kerion.

common cause of tinea capitis in the 1940s and 1950s, is characterized initially by a small papule at the base of a hair follicle. The infection spreads peripherally, forming an erythematous and scaly circular plaque (**ringworm**) within which the infected hairs become brittle and broken. Numerous confluent patches of alopecia develop, and patients may complain of severe pruritus. *M. audouinii* infection is no longer common in the United States. **Favus** is a chronic form of tinea capitis that is rare in the United States and is caused by the fungus *Trichophyton schoenleinii*. Favus starts as yellowish red papules at the opening of hair follicles. The papules expand and coalesce to form cup-shaped, yellowish, crusted patches that fluoresce dull green under a Wood lamp.

Differential Diagnosis

Tinea capitis can be confused with seborrheic dermatitis, psoriasis, alopecia areata, trichotillomania, and certain dystrophic hair disorders. When inflammation is pronounced, as in kerion, primary or secondary bacterial infection must also be considered. In adolescents, the patchy, moth-eaten type of alopecia associated with secondary syphilis may

resemble tinea capitis. If scarring occurs, discoid lupus erythematosus and lichen planopilaris must also be considered in the differential diagnosis.

The important diagnostic procedures for the various dermatophyte diseases include examination of infected hairs with a Wood lamp, microscopic examination of KOH preparations of infected material, and identification of the etiologic agent by culture. Hairs infected with common *Microsporum* spp. fluoresce a bright blue-green. Most *Trichophyton*-infected hairs do not fluoresce.

Microscopic examination of a KOH preparation of infected hair from the active border of a lesion discloses tiny spores surrounding the hair shaft in *Microsporum* infections and chains of spores within the hair shaft in *T. tonsurans* infections. Fungal elements are not usually seen in scales. A specific etiologic diagnosis of tinea capitis may be obtained by planting broken off infected hairs on Sabouraud medium with reagents to inhibit growth of other organisms. Such identification may require 2 wk or more.

Treatment

Oral administration of griseofulvin microcrystalline (20-25 mg/kg/24 hr, or 10-15 mg/kg per day if the ultramicrosize form is used) is the recommended treatment for all forms of tinea capitis. Absorption of griseofulvin is enhanced by ingestion of a fatty meal and should be recommended for the patient. It may be necessary for 8-12 wk and should be terminated only after fungal culture results are negative. Treatment for 1 mo after a negative culture result minimizes the risk of recurrence. Adverse reactions to griseofulvin are rare but include nausea, vomiting, headache, blood dyscrasias, phototoxicity, and hepatotoxicity. Terbinafine is also effective at a dosage of 3-6 mg/kg/24 hr for 4-6 wk or possibly in pulse therapy, although it has limited activity against *M. canis*. The oral granules formulation of terbinafine is approved by the FDA for tinea capitis in children 4 yr of age and older. Oral itraconazole is useful in instances of griseofulvin resistance, intolerance, or allergy. Itraconazole is given for 4-6 wk at a dosage of 3-5 mg/kg/24 hr with food. Capsules are preferable to the syrup, which may cause diarrhea. Itraconazole is not approved by the FDA for treatment of dermatophyte infections in the pediatric population. Topical therapy alone is ineffective, but it may be an important adjunct because it may decrease the shedding of spores, and should be recommended in all patients. Asymptomatic dermatophyte carriage in family members is common. Because 1 in 3 families have at least 1 member who is a carrier, treatment of both patient and potential carriers with a sporicidal shampoo may hasten clinical resolution. Vigorous shampooing with a 2.5% selenium sulfide, zinc pyrithione, or ketoconazole shampoo is helpful. It is not necessary to shave the scalp.

Tinea Corporis
Clinical Manifestations

Tinea corporis, defined as infection of the glabrous skin, excluding the palms, soles, and groin, can be caused by most of the dermatophyte species, although *T. rubrum* and *Trichophyton mentagrophytes* are the most prevalent etiologic organisms. In children, infections with *M. canis* are also common. Tinea corporis can be acquired by direct contact with infected persons or by contact with infected scales or hairs deposited on environmental surfaces. *M. canis* infections are usually acquired from infected pets.

The most typical clinical lesion begins as a dry, mildly erythematous, elevated, scaly papule or plaque that spreads centrifugally and clears centrally to form the characteristic annular lesion responsible for the designation ringworm (Fig. 666-7). At times, plaques with advancing borders may spread over large areas. Grouped pustules are another variant. Most lesions clear spontaneously within several months, but some may become chronic. Central clearing does not always occur (Fig. 666-8), and differences in host response may result in wide variability in the clinical appearance—for example, granulomatous lesions called **Majocchi granuloma,** which are caused by penetration of organisms along the hair follicle to the level of the dermis, produce a fungal folliculitis and perifolliculitis (Fig. 666-9), and the kerion-like lesions referred to as tinea profunda. Majocchi granuloma is more

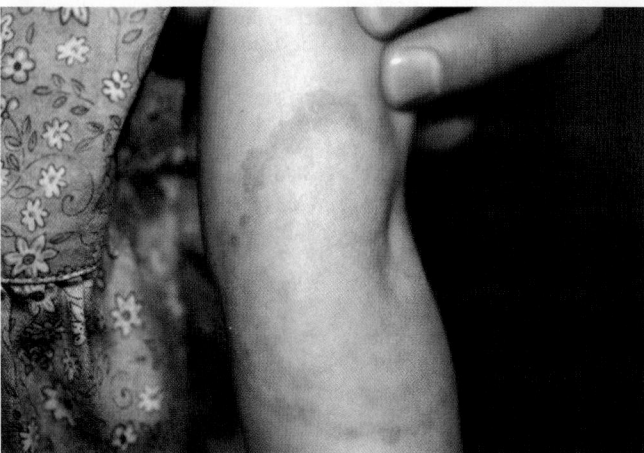

Figure 666-7 Annular plaque of tinea corporis with central clearing.

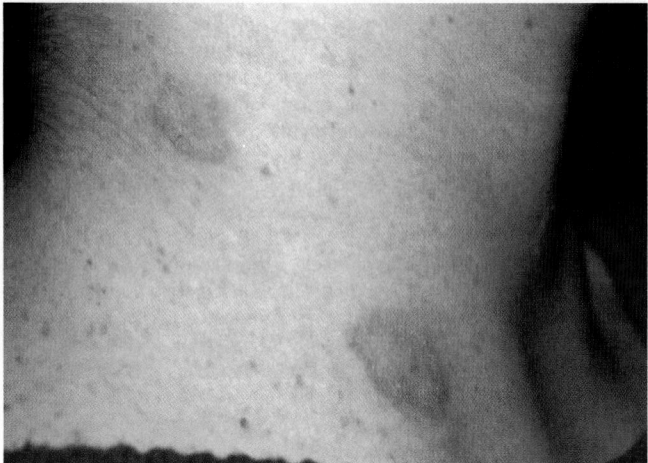

Figure 666-8 Minimal central clearing with tinea corporis.

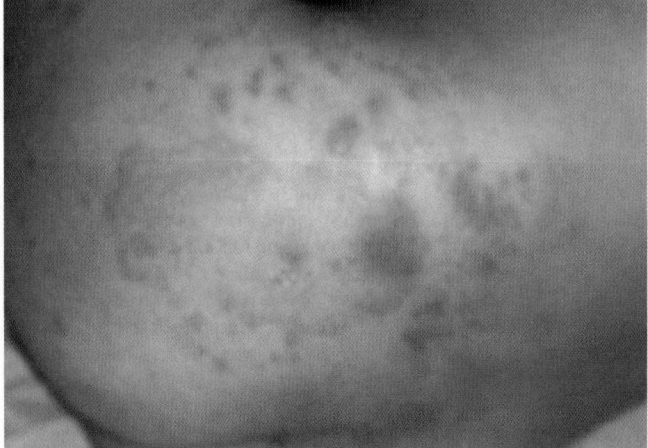

Figure 666-9 Follicular papule and pustule in Majocchi granuloma after use of a superpotent topical steroid.

common after inappropriate treatment with topical corticosteroids, especially the superpotent class.

Differential Diagnosis

Many skin lesions, both infectious and noninfectious, must be differentiated from the lesions of tinea corporis. Those most frequently confused are granuloma annulare, nummular eczema, pityriasis rosea, psoriasis, seborrheic dermatitis, erythema chronicum migrans, and tinea versicolor. Microscopic examination of KOH wet mount preparations and cultures should always be performed when fungal infection is considered. Tinea corporis usually does not fluoresce with a Wood lamp.

Treatment

Tinea corporis usually responds to treatment with one of the topical antifungal agents (e.g., imidazoles, terbinafine, naftifine) twice daily for 2-4 wk. In unusually severe or extensive disease, a course of therapy with oral griseofulvin microcrystalline may be required for 4 wk. Itraconazole has produced excellent results in many cases with a 1-2 wk course of oral therapy. Combination topical corticosteroid/antifungal preparations should not be used as it may result in worsening or persistent infection.

Tinea Cruris
Clinical Manifestations

Tinea cruris, or infection of the groin, occurs most often in adolescent males and is usually caused by the anthropophilic species *Epidermophyton floccosum* or *T. rubrum*, but occasionally by the zoophilic species *T. mentagrophytes.*

The initial clinical lesion is a small, raised, scaly, erythematous patch on the inner aspect of the thigh. This spreads peripherally, often developing numerous tiny vesicles at the advancing margin. It eventually forms bilateral, irregular, sharply bordered patches with hyperpigmented scaly centers. In some cases, particularly in infections with *T. mentagrophytes,* the inflammatory reaction is more intense and the infection may spread beyond the crural region. The scrotum and labia are usually not involved in the infection, an important distinction from candidosis. Pruritus may be severe initially but abates as the inflammatory reaction subsides. Bacterial superinfection may alter the clinical appearance, and erythrasma or candidosis may coexist. Tinea cruris is more prevalent in obese persons and in persons who perspire excessively and wear tight-fitting clothing.

Differential Diagnosis

The diagnosis of tinea cruris is confirmed by culture and by demonstration of septate hyphae on a KOH preparation of epidermal scrapings. The disorder must be differentiated from intertrigo, allergic contact dermatitis, candidosis, and erythrasma. Bacterial superinfection must be precluded when there is a severe inflammatory reaction.

Treatment

Patients should be advised to wear loose cotton underwear. **Topical treatment** with an imidazole twice a day for 3-4 wk is recommended for severe infection, especially because these agents are effective in mixed candidal-dermatophytic infections.

Tinea Pedis
Clinical Manifestations

Tinea pedis (athlete's foot), infection of the toe webs and soles of the feet, is uncommon in young children but occurs with some frequency in preadolescent and adolescent males. The usual etiologic agents are *T. rubrum, T. mentagrophytes,* and *E. floccosum.*

Most commonly, the lateral toe webs (3rd to 4th and 4th to 5th interdigital spaces) and the subdigital crevice are fissured, with maceration and peeling of the surrounding skin (Fig. 666-10). Severe tenderness, itching, and a persistent foul odor are characteristic. These lesions may become chronic. This type of infection may involve overgrowth by bacterial flora, including *Kytococcus sedentarius, Brevibacterium epidermidis,* and Gram-negative organisms. Less commonly, a chronic diffuse hyperkeratosis of the sole of the foot occurs with only mild erythema (Fig. 666-11). In many cases, 2 feet and 1 hand are involved. This type of infection is more refractory to treatment and tends to recur. An inflammatory vesicular type of reaction may occur with *T. mentagrophytes* infection. This type is most common in young children. The lesions involve any area of the foot, including the dorsal surface, and are usually circumscribed. The initial papules progress to

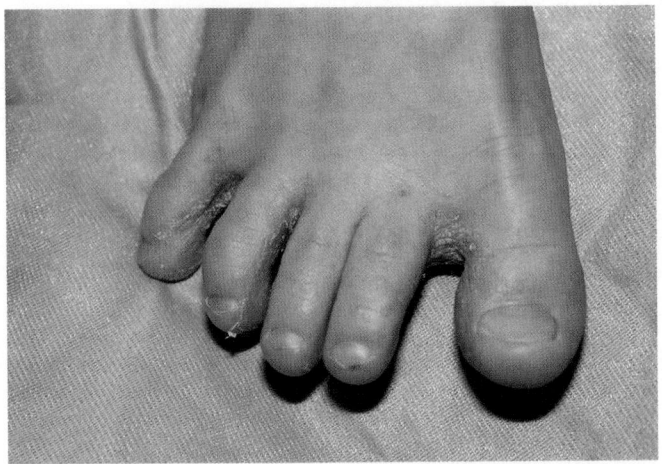

Figure 666-10 Interdigital tinea pedis.

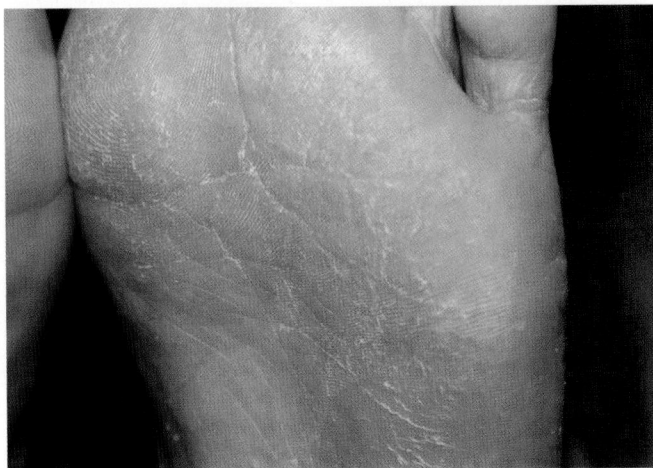

Figure 666-11 Diffuse, minimally erythematous tinea pedis.

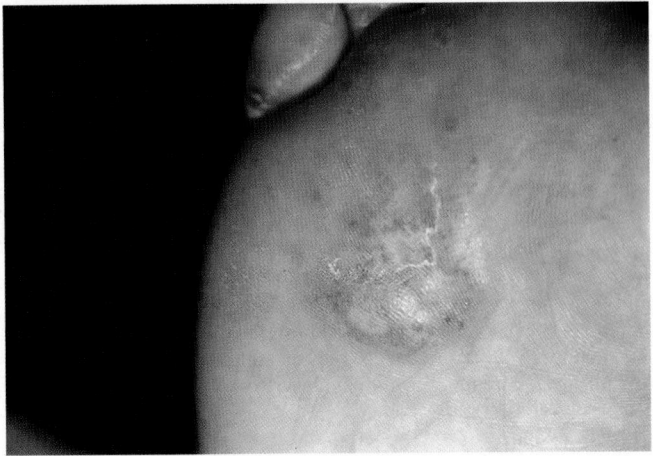

Figure 666-12 Vesicobullous tinea pedis.

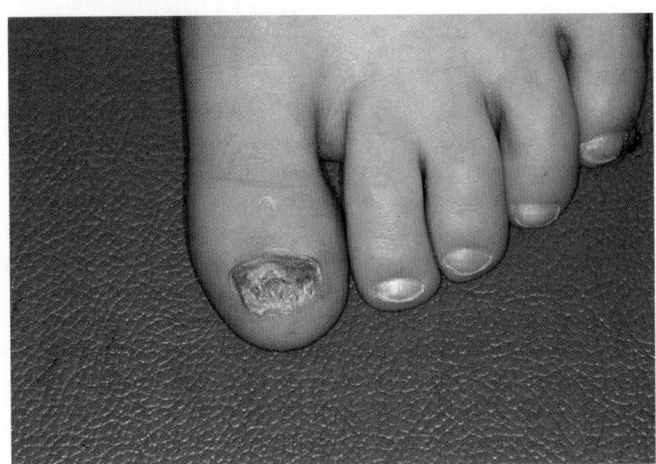

Figure 666-13 Hyperkeratotic nail in onychomycosis.

vesicles and bullae that may become pustular (Fig. 666-12). A number of factors, such as occlusive footwear and warm, humid weather, predispose to infection. Tinea pedis may be transmitted in shower facilities and swimming pool areas.

Differential Diagnosis
Tinea pedis must be differentiated from simple maceration and peeling of the interdigital spaces, which is common in children. Infection with *Candida albicans* and various bacterial organisms (erythrasma) may cause confusion or may coexist with primary tinea pedis. Contact dermatitis, vesicular foot dermatitis, atopic dermatitis, and juvenile plantar dermatitis also simulate tinea pedis. Fungal mycelia can be seen on microscopic examination of a KOH preparation or by culture.

Treatment
Treatment for mild infections includes simple measures such as avoidance of occlusive footwear, careful drying between the toes after bathing, and the use of an absorbent antifungal powder such as zinc undecylenate. Topical therapy with an imidazole is curative in most cases. Each of these agents is also effective against candidal infection. Several weeks of therapy may be necessary, and low-grade, chronic infections, particularly those caused by *T. rubrum*, may be refractory. In refractory cases, oral griseofulvin therapy may effect a cure, but recurrences are common.

Tinea Unguium
Clinical Manifestations
Tinea unguium (onychomycosis) is a dermatophyte infection of the nail plate. It occurs most often in patients with tinea pedis, but it may occur as a primary infection. It can be caused by a number of dermatophytes, of which *T. rubrum* and *T. mentagrophytes* are the most common.

The most superficial form of tinea unguium (i.e., white superficial onychomycosis) is caused by *T. mentagrophytes*. It manifests as irregular single or numerous white patches on the surface of the nail unassociated with paronychial inflammation or deep infection. *T. rubrum* generally causes a more invasive, subungual infection that is initiated at the lateral distal margins of the nail and is often preceded by mild paronychia. The middle and ventral layers of the nail plate, and perhaps the nail bed, are the sites of infection. The nail initially develops a yellowish discoloration and slowly becomes thickened, brittle, and loosened from the nail bed (Fig. 666-13). In advanced infection, the nail may turn dark brown to black and may crack or break off.

Differential Diagnosis
Tinea unguium must be differentiated from various dystrophic nail disorders. Changes as a result of trauma, psoriasis, lichen planus, eczema, and trachyonychia can all be confused with tinea unguium. Nails infected with *C. albicans* have several distinguishing features; most prominently, a pronounced paronychial swelling. Thin shavings taken from the infected nail, preferably from the deeper areas, should be examined microscopically with KOH and cultured. Repeated attempts may be required to demonstrate the fungus. Histologic evaluation of nail clippings with special stains for dermatophytes can be diagnostic.

The long half-life of itraconazole in the nail has led to promising trials of intermittent short courses of therapy (double the normal dose for 1 wk of each mo for 3-4 mo). Oral terbinafine is also used for the treatment of onychomycosis. Terbinafine once daily for 12 wk is more effective than itraconazole pulse therapy. Griseofulvin and application of topical fungistatic agents to the nail bed are often ineffective and are not recommended.

Tinea Nigra Palmaris

Tinea nigra palmaris is a rare but distinctive superficial fungal infection that occurs principally in children and adolescents. It is caused by the dimorphic fungus *Phaeoannellomyces werneckii*, which imparts a gray-black color to the affected palm. The characteristic lesion is a well-defined hyperpigmented macule. Scaling and erythema are rare, and the lesions are asymptomatic. Tinea nigra is often mistaken for a junctional nevus, melanoma, or staining of the skin by contactants. Treatment is with an imidazole antifungal. *Keratolytic agents, such as salicylic acid, once to twice daily* can also be used.

CANDIDAL INFECTIONS (CANDIDOSIS, CANDIDIASIS, AND MONILIASIS)

See Chapter 234.

The dimorphic yeasts of the genus *Candida* are ubiquitous in the environment, but *C. albicans* usually causes candidosis in children. This yeast is not part of the indigenous skin flora, but it is a frequent transient on skin and may colonize the human alimentary tract and the vagina as a saprophytic organism. Certain environmental conditions, notably elevated temperature and humidity, are associated with an increased frequency of isolation of *C. albicans* from the skin. Many bacterial species inhibit the growth of *C. albicans*, and alteration of normal flora by the use of antibiotics may promote overgrowth of the yeast.

Chronic mucocutaneous candidiasis is associated with a diverse group of primary immunodeficiency diseases (Table 666-1). Chronic

Table 666-1	Primary Immunodeficiencies Underlying Fungal Infections			

DISEASE	ASSOCIATED INFECTIONS	IMMUNOLOGIC PHENOTYPE	GENE, TRANSMISSION
CMC			
SCID	Bacteria, viruses, fungi, mycobacteria	No T cells, with or without B and/ or NK cell lymphopenia	>30 genes: *IL2RG*, X-linked; *JAK3*, autosomal recessive; *RAG1*, autosomal recessive; *RAG2*, autosomal recessive; *ARTEMIS*, autosomal recessive; *ADA*, autosomal recessive; *CD3*, autosomal recessive, etc.
CID		T-cell defect	
CD25 deficiency	Viruses and bacteria		*IL2RA*, autosomal recessive
NEMO or iκBγ deficiency	Pyogenic bacteria, mycobacteria, viruses		*NEMO* or *IKBG* X-linked
IκBα GOF mutation			*IKBA*, autosomal dominant
DOCK8 deficiency	Viruses, bacteria and fungi		*DOCK8*, autosomal recessive
TCR-α deficiency	Viruses and bacteria		*TCRA*, autosomal recessive
CRACM1 deficiency	Viruses, mycobacteria, bacteria and fungi		*CRACM1*, autosomal recessive
MST1/STK4 deficiency	Viruses and bacteria		*MST1/STK4*, autosomal recessive
MHC class II deficiency	Viruses, bacteria and fungi		*CIITA, RFXANK, RFXC, RFXAP*, all autosomal recessive
Idiopathic CD4 lymphopenia	*Pneumocystis, Cryptococcus*, virus	CD4 T cells <300 cells/mm^3	*UNC119*, autosomal dominant, *MAGT1* X-linked, *RAG1*, autosomal recessive
SYNDROMIC CMC			
Interleukin-12Rβ1 and interleukin-12p40 deficiencies	*Mycobacteria, Salmonella*	Deficit of interleukin-17–producing T cells	*IL12RB1*, autosomal recessive, *IL12B*, autosomal recessive
STAT3 deficiency (autosomal dominant-HIES)	*Staphylococcus aureus, Aspergillus*	Hyperimmunoglobulin E, deficit of interleukin-17–producing T cells	*STAT3*, autosomal dominant
APECED/APS-1	No	Neutralizing anti–interleukin-17A, anti–interleukin-17F, and/or anti–interleukin-22 autoantibodies	*AIRE*, autosomal recessive
CARD9 deficiency	Dermatophytes, *Candida*, brain abscess	Deficit of interleukin-17–producing T cells	*CARD9*, autosomal recessive
CMCD			
Complete interleukin-17RA deficiency	*S. aureus*	No interleukin-17 response	*IL17RA*, autosomal recessive
Partial interleukin-17F deficiency	*S. aureus*	Impaired interleukin-17F, interleukin-17A/F function	*IL17F*, autosomal dominant
STAT1 GOF mutations	Bacteria, viruses, fungi, mycobacteria	Low interleukin-17–producing T cells	*STAT1*, autosomal dominant

AIRE, autoimmune regulator; APECED, autoimmune polyendocrinopathy-candidiasis-ectodermal dystrophy; APS-1, autoimmune polyendocrinopathy syndrome type 1; CARD9, caspase recruitment domain-containing protein 9; CID, combined immunodeficiency; CMC, chronic mucocutaneous candidiasis; CMCD, chronic mucocutaneous candidiasis disease; CRACM1, calcium release-activated calcium modulator 1; GOF, gain-of-function; HIES, hyperimmunoglobulin E syndrome; IκBα, inhibitor of nuclear factor of kappa light polypeptide gene enhancer in B-cells, alpha; iκBγ, inhibitor of nuclear factor of kappa light polypeptide gene enhancer in B-cells, gamma; MHC, major histocompatibility complex; MST1, macrophage stimulating 1; NEMO, nuclear factor κB essential modulator; NK, natural killer; SCID, severe combined immunodeficiency; STAT, signal transducer and activator of transcription; STK4, serine/threonine protein kinase 4; TCR, T-cell receptor.

From Lanternier F, Cypowyj S, Picard, C, et al: Primary immunodeficiencies underlying fungal infections. Curr Opin Pediatr 25:736–747, 2013.

mucocutaneous candidiasis is characterized by chronic or recurrent *Candida* infections of the oral cavity, esophagus, genitals, nails, and skin. Chronic mucocutaneous candidiasis may also be seen as an acquired infection in patients with HIV infection, and during immunosuppressive treatments.

Oral Candidosis (Thrush)
See Chapter 234.

Vaginal Candidosis
See Chapters 120 and 234.

C. albicans is an inhabitant of the vagina in 5-10% of women, and vaginal candidosis is not uncommon in adolescent girls. A number of factors can predispose to this infection, including antibiotic therapy, corticosteroid therapy, diabetes mellitus, pregnancy, and the use of oral contraceptives. The infection manifests as cheesy white plaques on an erythematous vaginal mucosa and a thick white-yellow discharge. The disease may be relatively mild or may produce pronounced inflammation and scaling of the external genitals and surrounding skin with progression to vesiculation and ulceration. Patients often complain of severe itching and burning in the vaginal area. Before treatment is initiated, the diagnosis should be confirmed by microscopic examination and/or culture. The infection may be eradicated by insertion of nystatin or imidazole vaginal tablets, suppositories, creams, or foam. If these products are ineffective, the addition of one dose of fluconazole (150 mg) is effective.

Congenital Cutaneous Candidosis
See Chapter 234.

Candidal Diaper Dermatitis
Candidal diaper dermatitis is a ubiquitous problem in infants and, although relatively benign, is often frustrating because of its tendency to recur. Predisposed infants usually carry *C. albicans* in their intestinal tracts, and the warm, moist, occluded skin of the diaper area provides an optimal environment for its growth. A seborrheic, atopic, or primary irritant contact dermatitis usually provides a portal of entry for the yeast.

The primary clinical manifestation consists of an intensely erythematous, confluent plaque with a scalloped border and a sharply demarcated edge. It is formed by the confluence of numerous papules and vesicular pustules. Satellite pustules, those that stud the contiguous skin, are a hallmark of localized candidal infections. The perianal skin, inguinal folds, perineum, and lower abdomen are usually involved (Fig. 666-14). In males, the entire scrotum and penis may be involved, with an erosive balanitis of the perimeatal skin. In females, the lesions may be found on the vaginal mucosa and labia. In some infants, the process is generalized, with erythematous lesions distant from the diaper area. In some cases, the generalized process may represent a fungal id (hypersensitivity) reaction.

The **differential diagnosis** of candidal diaper dermatitis includes other eruptions of the diaper area that may coexist with candidal infection. For this reason, it is important to establish a diagnosis by means of KOH preparation or culture.

Treatment consists of applications of an imidazole cream 2 times daily. The combination of a corticosteroid and an antifungal agent may be justified if inflammation is severe but may confuse the situation if the diagnosis is not firmly established. Corticosteroid should not be continued for more than a few days. Protection of the diaper area by an application of thick zinc oxide paste overlying the anticandidal preparation may be helpful. The paste is more easily removed with mineral oil than with soap and water. Fungal id reactions gradually abate with successful treatment of the diaper dermatitis or may be treated with a mild corticosteroid preparation. When recurrences of diaper candidosis are frequent, it may be helpful to prescribe a course of oral anticandidal therapy to decrease the yeast population in the gastrointestinal tract. Some infants seem to be receptive hosts for *C. albicans* and may reacquire the organism from a colonized adult.

Intertriginous Candidosis
Intertriginous candidosis occurs most often in the axillae and groin, on the neck (Fig. 666-15) under the breasts, under pendulous abdominal fat folds, in the umbilicus, and in the gluteal cleft. Typical lesions are large, confluent areas of moist, denuded, erythematous skin with an irregular, macerated, scaly border. Satellite lesions are characteristic and consist of small vesicles or pustules on an erythematous base. With time, intertriginous candidal lesions may become lichenified, dry, scaly plaques. The lesions develop on skin subjected to irritation and maceration. Candidal superinfection is more likely to occur under conditions that lead to excessive perspiration, especially in obese children and in children with underlying disorders, such as diabetes mellitus. A similar condition, interdigital candidosis, commonly occurs in individuals whose hands are constantly immersed in water. Fissures occur between the fingers and have red denuded centers, with an overhanging white epithelial fringe. Similar lesions between the toes may be secondary to occlusive footwear. Treatment is the same as for other candidal infections.

Perianal Candidosis
Perianal dermatitis develops at sites of skin irritation as a result of occlusion, constant moisture, poor hygiene, anal fissures, and pruritus from pinworm infestation. It may become superinfected with *C. albicans,* especially in children who are receiving oral antibiotic or corticosteroid medication. The involved skin becomes erythematous, macerated, and excoriated, and the lesions are identical to those of candidal intertrigo or candidal diaper rash. Application of a topical

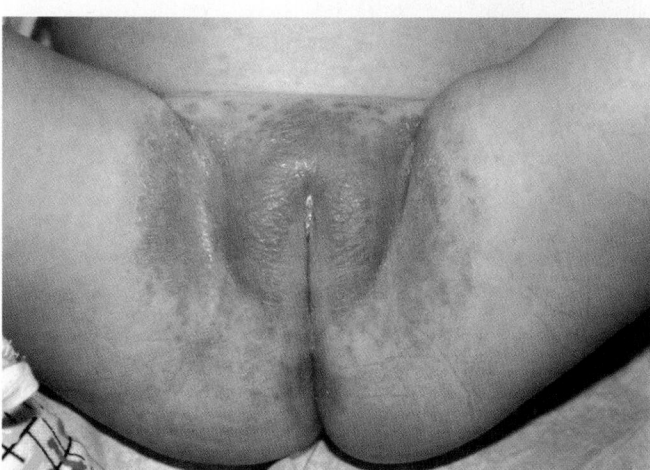

Figure 666-14 Erythematous confluent plaque caused by candidal infection.

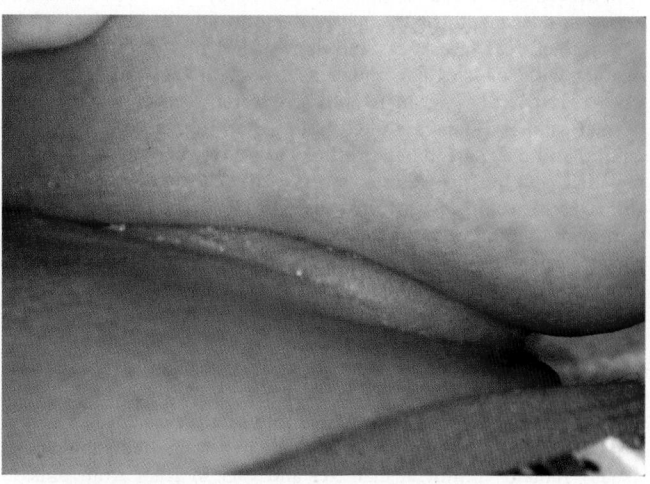

Figure 666-15 Intertriginous candidosis of the neck.

antifungal agent in conjunction with improved hygiene is usually effective. Underlying disorders such as pinworm infection must also be treated (see Chapter 293).

Candidal Paronychia and Onychia
See Chapter 663.

Candidal Granuloma
Candidal granuloma is a rare response to an invasive candidal infection of skin. The lesions appear as crusted, verrucous plaques and hornlike projections on the scalp, face, and distal limbs. Affected patients may have single or numerous defects in immune mechanisms, and the granulomas are often refractory to topical therapy. A systemic anticandidal agent may be required for palliation or eradication of the infection.

Bibliography is available at Expert Consult.

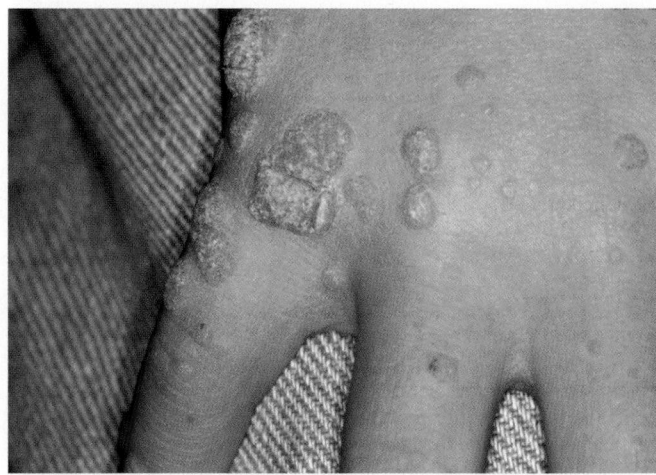

Figure 667-1 Verrucous papules on the back of the hand.

Chapter **667**
Cutaneous Viral Infections
Anna M. Juern and Beth A. Drolet

WART (VERRUCA)
Etiology
Human papillomaviruses (HPVs) cause a spectrum of disease from warts (verrucae vulgaris) to squamous cell carcinoma of the skin and mucous membranes, including the larynx (see Chapter 390.2). The HPVs are classified by genus, species, and type. More than 200 types are known, and the entire genomes of approximately 100 are completely sequenced. The incidence of all types of warts is highest in children and adolescents. HPV is spread by direct contact and autoinoculation; transmission within families and by fomites occurs. The clinical manifestations of infection develop 1 mo or longer after inoculation and depend on the HPV type, the size of the inoculum, the immune status of the host, and the anatomic site.

Clinical Manifestations
Cutaneous warts develop in 5-10% of children. **Common warts** (verruca vulgaris), caused most commonly by HPV types 2 and 4, occur most frequently on the fingers, dorsum of the hands (Fig. 667-1), paronychial areas, face, knees, and elbows. They are well-circumscribed papules with an irregular, roughened, keratotic surface. When the surface is pared away, many black dots representing thrombosed dermal capillary loops are often visible. **Periungual warts** are often painful and may spread beneath the nail plate, separating it from the nail bed (Fig. 667-2). **Plantar warts (verruca plantaris),** although similar to the common wart, are caused by HPV type 1 and are usually flush with the surface of the sole because of the constant pressure from weight bearing. When plantar warts become hyperkeratotic (Fig. 667-3), they may be painful. Similar lesions (palmar–verruca palmaris) can also occur on the palms. They are sharply demarcated, often with a ring of thick callus. The surface keratotic material must sometimes be removed before the boundaries of the wart can be appreciated. Several contiguous warts (HPV type 4) may fuse to form a large plaque, the so-called mosaic wart. Flat warts (verruca plana), caused by HPV types 3 and 10, are slightly elevated, minimally hyperkeratotic papules that usually remain <3 mm in diameter and vary in color from pink to brown. They may occur in profusion on the face, arms, dorsum of the

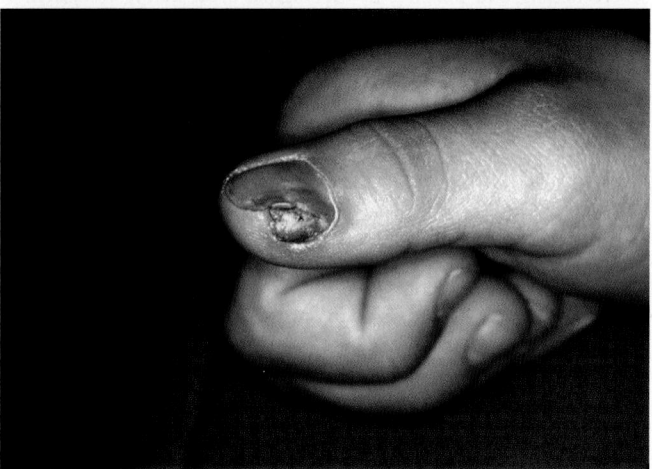

Figure 667-2 Periungual wart with disruption of nail growth.

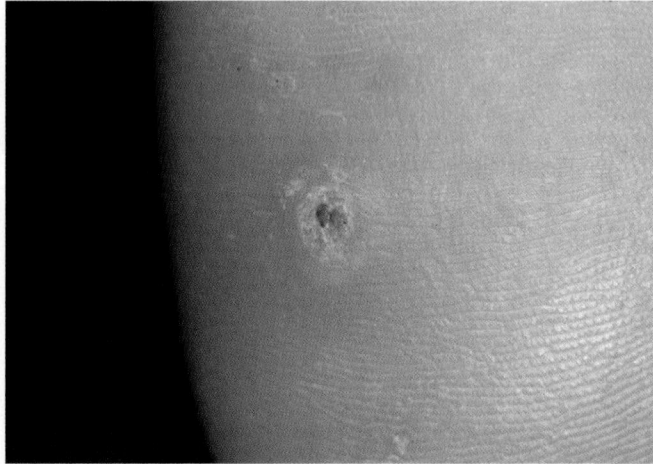

Figure 667-3 Hyperkeratotic plantar wart.

hands, and knees. The distribution of several lesions along a line of cutaneous trauma is a helpful diagnostic feature (Fig. 667-4). Lesions may be disseminated in the beard area and on the legs by shaving and from the hairline onto the scalp by combing the hair. **Epidermodysplasia verruciformis** (*EVER1, EVER2* genes), caused primarily by HPV types 5 and 8 (β-papillomaviruses, species 1), manifests as many diffuse verrucous papules. Wart types 9, 12, 14, 15, 17, 25, 36, 38, 47,

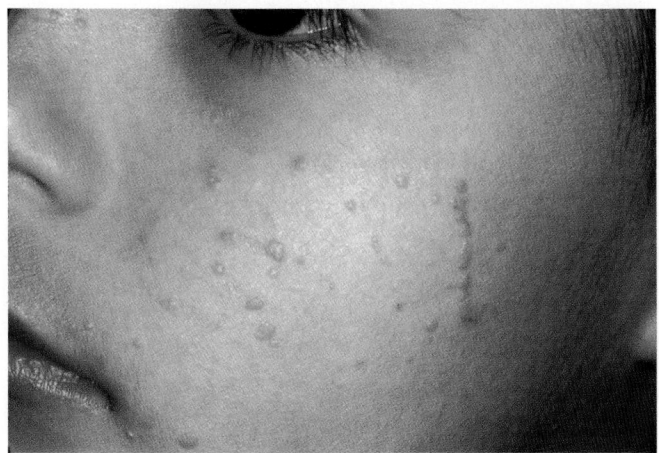

Figure 667-4 Multiple flat warts on the face with lesions in line of trauma.

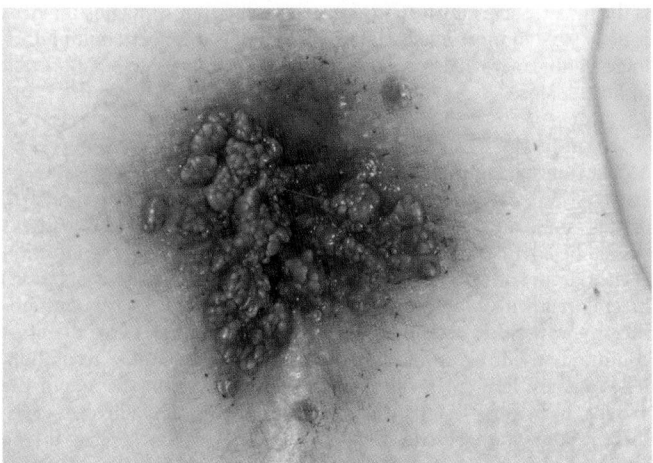

Figure 667-5 Condylomata acuminata in the perianal area of a toddler.

and 50 may also be involved. Inheritance is thought to be primarily autosomal recessive, but an X-linked recessive form also has been postulated. Warts progress to **squamous cell carcinoma** in 10% of patients with epidermodysplasia verruciformis.

Genital HPV infection occurs in sexually active adolescents, most commonly as a result of infection with HPV types 6 and 11. **Condylomata acuminata** (mucous membrane warts) are moist, fleshy, papillomatous lesions that occur on the perianal mucosa (Fig. 667-5), labia, vaginal introitus, and perineal raphe, and on the shaft, corona, and glans penis. Occasionally, they obstruct the urethral meatus or the vaginal introitus. Because they are located in intertriginous areas, they may become moist and friable. When untreated, condylomata proliferate and become confluent, at times forming large cauliflower-like masses. Lesions can also occur on the lips, gingivae, tongue, and conjunctivae. Genital warts in children may occur after inoculation during birth through an infected birth canal, as a consequence of sexual abuse, or from incidental spread from cutaneous warts. A significant proportion of genital warts in children contain HPV types that are usually isolated from cutaneous warts. HPV infection of the cervix is a major risk factor for development of carcinoma, particularly if the infection is caused by HPV type 16, 18, 31, 33, 35, 39, 45, 52, 59, 67, 68, or 70. Immunization against types 6, 11, 16, and 18 is now available. Laryngeal (respiratory) papillomas contain the same HPV types as in anogenital papillomas. Transmission is believed to occur from mothers with genital HPV infection to neonates who aspirate infectious virus during birth and may develop laryngeal papillomatosis.

Histology
The various types of warts share the basic changes of hyperplasia of the epidermal cells and vacuolation of the spinous keratinocytes, which may contain basophilic intranuclear inclusions (viral particles). Warts are confined to the epidermis and do not have "roots." Individuals with impaired cell-mediated immunity are particularly susceptible to HPV infection. Antibodies occur in response to infection but appear to have little protective effect.

Differential Diagnosis
Common warts are most often confused with molluscum contagiosum. Plantar and palmar warts may be difficult to distinguish from punctate keratoses, corns, and calluses. In contrast to calluses, warts obliterate normal skin markings. Juvenile flat warts mimic lichen planus, lichen nitidus, angiofibromas, syringomas, milia, and acne. Condylomata acuminata may resemble condylomata lata of secondary syphilis.

Treatment
Various therapeutic measures are effective in the treatment of warts. More than 65% of warts disappear spontaneously within 2 yr. Warts are epidermal lesions and do not produce scarring unless they are managed surgically or treated in an overly aggressive fashion. Hyperkeratotic lesions (common, plantar, and palmar warts) are more responsive to therapy if the excess keratotic debris is gently pared with a scalpel until thrombosed capillaries are apparent; further paring induces bleeding. Treatment is most successful when performed regularly and frequently (every 2-4 wk).

Common warts can be destroyed by applications of liquid nitrogen or by pulsed dye laser. Daily application of salicylic acid in flexible collodion or as a stick is a slow but painless method of removal that is effective in some patients. Plantar and palmar warts may be treated with 40% salicylic acid plasters. These should be applied for 5 days at a time with a 2-day rest period between applications. Following removal of the plaster and prolonged soaking in hot water, keratotic debris can be removed with an emery board or pumice stone. Condylomata respond best to weekly applications of 25% podophyllin in tincture of benzoin. The medication should be left on the warts for 4-6 hr and then removed by bathing. Keratinized warts near the genitalia (buttocks) do not respond to podophyllin. Imiquimod (5% cream) applied 3 times weekly is also beneficial. Imiquimod is indicated for genital warts but has also been used successfully to treat warts in other locations. For nongenital warts, imiquimod should be applied daily. Cimetidine 30-40 mg/kg/ day has been used in children with multiple warts unresponsive to other treatments. Immunotherapy with intralesional candida or trichophyton antigen may also be employed especially when lesions are numerous or resistant to other tried therapies. Immunotherapy is performed in clinic and multiple treatments every month (at least 3-4) are usually required. With all types of therapy, care should be taken to protect the surrounding normal skin from irritation.

MOLLUSCUM CONTAGIOSUM
Etiology
The poxvirus that causes molluscum contagiosum is a large double-stranded DNA virus that replicates in the cytoplasm of host epithelial cells. The 3 types cannot be differentiated on the basis of clinical appearance, location of lesions, or a patient's age or sex. Type 1 virus causes most infections. The disease is acquired by direct contact with an infected person or from fomites and is spread by autoinoculation. Children age 2-6 yr who are otherwise well and individuals who are immunosuppressed are affected most commonly. The incubation period is estimated to be 2 wk or longer.

Clinical Manifestations
Discrete, pearly, skin-colored, smooth, dome-shaped, papules vary in size from 1-5 mm. They typically have a central umbilication from which a plug of cheesy material can be expressed. The papules may occur anywhere on the body, but the face, eyelids, neck, axillae, and thighs are sites of predilection (Fig. 667-6). They may be found in

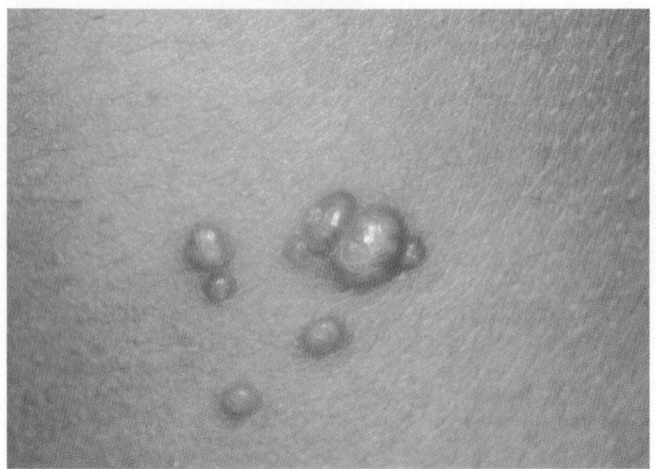

Figure 667-6 Grouped molluscum.

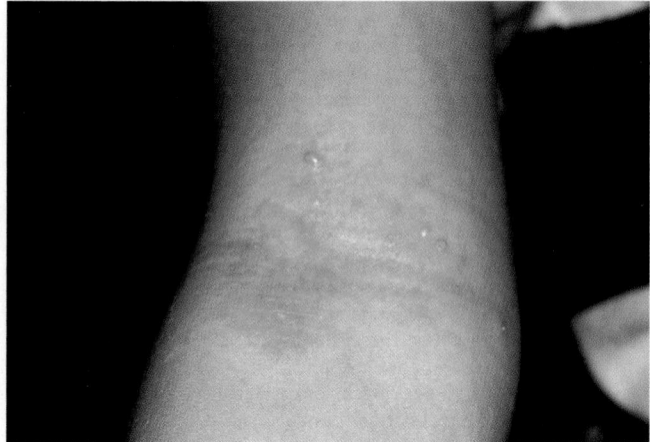

Figure 667-7 Molluscum with surrounding dermatitis.

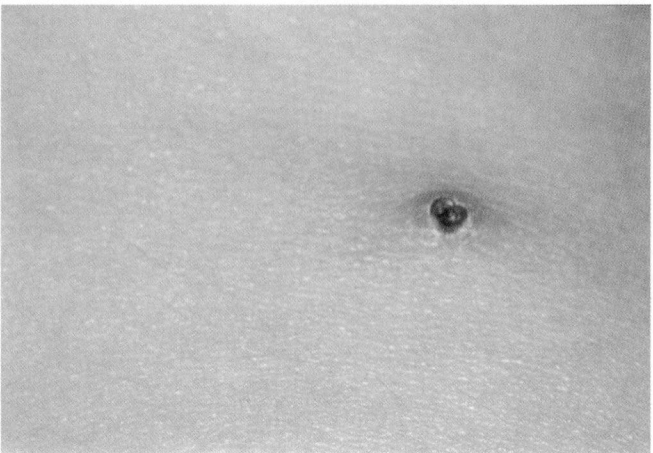

Figure 667-8 Inflamed molluscum. Crusted papule at site of previous molluscum.

is diagnostic. Specific antibody against molluscum contagiosum virus is detectable in most infected individuals but is of uncertain immunologic significance. Cell-mediated immunity is thought to be important in host defense.

Treatment
Molluscum contagiosum is a self-limited disease. The average attack lasts 6-9 mo. However, lesions can persist for years, can spread to distant sites, and may be transmitted to others. Affected patients should be advised to avoid shared baths and towels until the infection is clear. Infection may spread rapidly and produce hundreds of lesions in children with atopic dermatitis or immunodeficiency. Immunotherapy with either candida or trichophyton antigen, is now the most commonly used therapy. This is repeated every 4 wk until resolution. If lesions are limited in number, then depending on the age of the patient, individual lesions can be treated with liquid nitrogen cryotherapy. For younger children, cantharidin may be applied to the lesions and covered with adhesive bandages to prevent unwanted spread of the blistering agent. A blister forms at the site of application, and the molluscum is removed with the blister. Cantharidin should not be used on the face. Cantharidin however, is now very limited or completely unavailable in the United States. Facial molluscum is more cosmetically upsetting to children and parents; imiquimod applied topically is beneficial if not excessively irritating. Molluscum is an epidermal disease and should not be overtreated such that scarring results.

Bibliography is available at Expert Consult.

clusters on the genitals or in the groin of adolescents and may be associated with other venereal diseases in sexually active individuals. Lesions commonly involve the genital area in children but are not acquired by sexual transmission in most cases. Mild surrounding erythema or an eczematous dermatitis may accompany the papules (Fig. 667-7). Lesions on patients with AIDS tend to be large and numerous, particularly on the face. Exuberant lesions may also be found in children with leukemia and other immunodeficiencies. Children with atopic dermatitis are susceptible to widespread involvement in areas of dermatitis. A pustular eruption at the site of individual molluscum lesions is seen (Fig. 667-8). It is not a secondary bacterial infection, but an immunologic reaction to the molluscum virus and it should not be treated with antibiotics. Atrophic scars are often seen after this type of reaction.

Differential Diagnosis
Differential diagnosis of molluscum contagiosum includes trichoepithelioma, basal cell carcinoma, ectopic sebaceous glands, syringoma, hidrocystoma, keratoacanthoma, and warty dyskeratoma. In individuals with AIDS, cryptococcosis may be indistinguishable clinically from molluscum contagiosum. Rarely, coccidioidomycosis, histoplasmosis, or *Penicillium marneffei* infection masquerades as molluscum-like lesions in an immunocompromised host.

Histology
The epidermis is hyperplastic and hypertrophied, extending into the underlying dermis and projecting above the skin surface. The central plug of material, which is composed of virus-laden cells, may be shelled out from a lesion and examined under the microscope. The rounded, cup-shaped mass of homogeneous cells, often with identifiable lobules,

Chapter 668
Arthropod Bites and Infestations

668.1 Arthropod Bites
Anna M. Juern and Beth A. Drolet

Arthropod bites are a common affliction of children and occasionally pose a problem in diagnosis. A patient may be unaware of the source of the lesions or may deny being bitten, making interpretation of the eruption difficult. In these cases, knowledge of the habits, life cycle, and clinical signs of the more common arthropod pests of humans may help lead to a correct diagnosis (Table 668-1).

CLINICAL MANIFESTATIONS

The type of reaction that occurs after an arthropod bite depends on the species of insect and the age group and reactivity of the human host. Arthropods may cause injury to a host by various mechanisms, including mechanical trauma, such as the lacerating bite of a tsetse fly; invasion of host tissues, as in myiasis; contact dermatitis, as seen with repeated exposure to cockroach antigens; granulomatous reaction to retained mouthparts; transmission of systemic disease; injection of irritant cytotoxic or pharmacologically active substances, such as hyaluronidase, proteases, peptidases, and phospholipases in sting venom; and induction of anaphylaxis. Most reactions to arthropod bites depend on antibody formation to antigenic substances in saliva or venom. The type of reaction is determined primarily by the degree of previous exposure to the same or a related species of arthropod. When someone is bitten for the first time, no reaction develops. An immediate petechial reaction is occasionally seen. After repeated bites, sensitivity develops, producing a pruritic papule (Fig. 668-1) approximately 24 hr after the bite. This is the most common reaction seen in young children. With prolonged, repeated exposure, a wheal develops within minutes after a bite, followed 24 hr later by papule, vesicle, or bullae formation. By adolescence or adulthood, only a wheal may form, unaccompanied by the delayed papular reaction. Thus, adults in the same household as affected children may be unaffected. Ultimately, as a person becomes insensitive to the bite, no reaction occurs at all. This stage of nonreactivity is maintained only as long as the individual continues to be bitten regularly. Individuals in whom papular urticaria develops are in the transitional phase between development of primarily a delayed papular reaction and development of an immediate urticarial reaction.

Arthropod bites may occur as solitary, numerous, or profuse lesions, depending on the feeding habits of the perpetrator. Fleas tend to sample their host several times within a small localized area, whereas mosquitoes tend to attack a host as more randomly scattered sites. Delayed hypersensitivity reactions to insect bites, the predominant lesions in the young and uninitiated, are characterized by firm, persistent papules that may become hyperpigmented and are often excoriated and crusted. Pruritus may be mild or severe, transient or persistent. A central punctum is usually visible but may disappear as the lesion ages or is scratched. The immediate hypersensitivity reaction is characterized by an evanescent, erythematous wheal. If edema is marked, a tiny vesicle may surmount the wheal. Certain beetles produce bullous lesions through the action of cantharidin, and various insects, including beetles and spiders, may cause hemorrhagic nodules and ulcers. Bites on the lower extremities are more likely to be severe or persistent or to become bullous than those located elsewhere. Complications of arthropod bites include development of impetigo, folliculitis, cellulitis, lymphangitis, and severe anaphylactic hypersensitivity reactions, particularly after the bite of certain hymenopterans. The histopathologic changes are variable, depending on the arthropod, the age of the lesion, and the reactivity of the host. Acute urticarial lesions tend to show central vesiculation in which eosinophils are numerous. Papules most commonly show dermal edema and a mixed superficial and deep

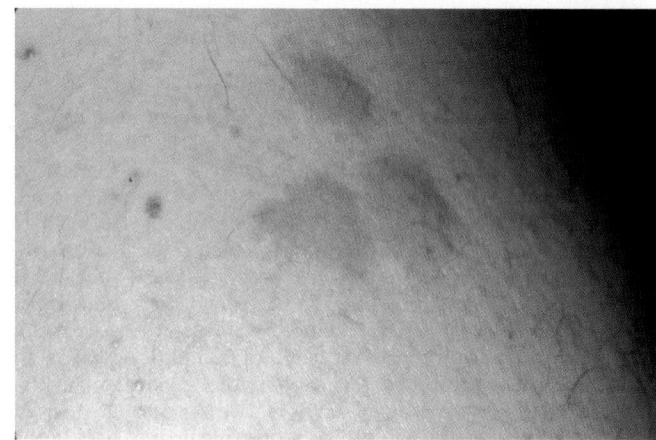

Figure 668-1 Pruritic papules after bedbug bites.

Table 668-1	Bed Bugs vs Other Arthropod Bites: Main Clinical and Epidemiologic Features*			
ARTHROPOD	**CLINICAL FEATURES ON EXAMINATION**	**LOCATION**	**TIMING OF PRURITUS**	**CONTEXT**
Bed bugs	3-4 Bites in a line or curve	Uncovered areas	Morning	Travelling
Fleas	3-4 Bites in a line or curve	Legs and buttocks	Daytime	Pet owners or rural living
Mosquitoes	Nonspecific urticarial papules	Potentially anywhere	*Anopheles* spp. night; *Culex* spp. night; *Aedes* spp. day	Worldwide distribution
Head lice	Live lice on the head associated with itchy, scratched lesions	Scalp, ears, and neck	Any	Children, parents, or contact with children
Body lice	Excoriated papules and hyperpigmentation; live lice inside clothes	Back	Any	Homeless people, developing countries
Sarcoptes scabiei mites (scabies)	Vesicles, burrows, nodules, and nonspecific secondary lesions	Interdigital spaces, forearms, breasts, genitalia	Night	Sexually transmitted, households or institutions
Ticks	Erythema migrans or ulcer	Potentially anywhere	Asymptomatic	Pet owners or hikers
Pyemotes X ventricosus	Comet sign, a linear erythematous macular tract	Under clothes	Any time when inside habitat	People exposed to woodworm contaminated furniture (*Pediculoides ventricosus* is a woodworm parasite)
Spiders	Necrosis (uncommon)	Face and arms	Immediate pain, no itching	Rural living

*It is difficult to diagnose a bite. Diagnosis relies on an array of arguments, none of which is specific by itself; it is the association of elements that is suggestive. Any arthropod bite can be totally asymptomatic.
From Bernardeschi C, Le Cleach L, Delaunay P, Chosidow O: Bed bug infestation. BMJ 346:f138, 2013.

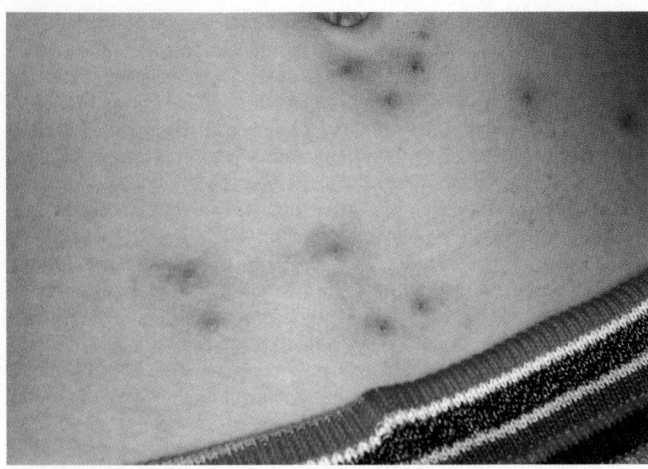

Figure 668-2 Red-brown papules in papular urticaria.

perivascular inflammatory infiltrate, often including a number of eosinophils. At times, however, the dermal cellular infiltrate is so dense that a lymphoma is suspected. Many young children demonstrate extensive dermal but nonerythematous, nontender edema and which responds to oral antihistamines in response to mosquito bites ("skeeter" syndrome), and must be distinguished from cellulitis, which tends to be painful, tender, and red. Retained mouthparts may stimulate a foreign body type of granulomatous reaction.

Papular urticaria occurs principally in the 1st decade of life. It may occur at any time of the year. The most common culprits are species of fleas, mites, bedbugs, gnats, mosquitoes, chiggers, and animal lice. Individuals with papular urticaria have predominantly transitional lesions in various stages of evolution between delayed-onset papules and immediate-onset wheals. The most characteristic lesion is an edematous, red-brown papule (Fig. 668-2). An individual lesion frequently starts as a wheal that, in turn, is replaced by a papule. A given bite may incite an id reaction at distant sites of quiescent bites in the form of erythematous macules, papules, or urticarial plaques. After a season or two, the reaction progresses from a transitional to a primarily immediate hypersensitivity urticarial reaction.

One of the most commonly encountered arthropod bites is that resulting from human, cat, or dog fleas (family *Pulicidae*). Eggs, which are generally laid in dusty areas and cracks between floorboards, give rise to larvae that then form cocoons. The cocoon stage can persist for up to 1 yr, and the flea emerges in response to vibrations from footsteps, accounting for the assaults that frequently befall the new owners of a recently reopened dwelling. Adult dog fleas can live without a blood meal for approximately 60 days. Attacks from fleas are more likely to occur when the fleas do not have access to their usual host; cat or dog fleas are more voracious and problematic when one visits an area frequented by the pet than when the pet is encountered directly. Flea bites tend to be grouped in lines or irregular clusters on the lower extremities. Fleas are often not seen on the body of a pet. Diagnosis of flea bites is aided by examination of debris from the animal's bedding material. The debris is collected by shaking the bedding into a plastic bag and examining the contents for fleas or their eggs, larvae, or feces.

TREATMENT

Treatment is directed at alleviation of pruritus by oral antihistamines and cool compresses. Potent topical corticosteroids are helpful. Topical antihistamines are potent immunologic sensitizers and have no role in the treatment of insect bite reactions. A short course of systemic steroids may be helpful if many severe reactions occur, particularly around the eyes. Insect repellents containing *N,N*-diethyl-3-methylbenzamide (DEET) may afford moderate protection against mosquitoes, fleas, flies, chiggers, and ticks, but are relatively ineffective against wasps, bees, and hornets. DEET must be applied to exposed skin and clothing to be effective. The most effective protection against mosquitoes, the human body louse, and other blood-feeding

Table 668-2	Patient Education to Eliminate Bed Bugs

Detection
- Look for brown insects no bigger than apple seeds on the mattress, sofa, and curtains and in darker places in the room (especially cracks in the walls, crevices in box springs, and furniture)
- Look for black spots on the mattress or blood traces on the sheets

Elimination
- Contact a pest management company
- Wash clothes at 60°C (140°F) or freeze delicate clothing, vacuum, and clean your home before the pest manager visits
- Collaborate with professionals who are used to dealing with bed bug infestation to increase eradication efficacy

Prevention
- Carefully examine secondhand furniture to assure the absence of bed bugs before purchase so as not to contaminate your home
- When sleeping in a hotel, even an upmarket establishment, lift mattresses to look for bed bugs or black spots
- Do not leave luggage in dark places, near furniture, or close to your bed. Before going to bed, close suitcases and put them in the bathroom—in the bathtub or shower stall

From Bernardeschi C, Le Cleach L, Delaunay P, Chosidow O: Bed bug infestation. BMJ 346:f138, 2013.

arthropods is use of DEET and permethrin-impregnated clothing. These measures are not effective, however, against the phlebotomine sand fly, which transmits leishmaniasis. Because of the potential for toxicity, the lowest effective DEET dose should be selected. Additional insect repellents include picaridin (flies, mosquitoes, chiggers, ticks), IR3535 (mosquitoes), oil of lemon, eucalyptus (mosquitoes), and citronella (mosquitoes). Table 668-2 lists methods to eliminate bed bugs.

An effort should be made to identify and eradicate the etiologic agent. Pets should be carefully inspected. Crawl spaces, eaves, and other sites of the house or outbuildings frequented by animals and birds should be decontaminated, and baseboard crevices, mattresses, rugs, furniture, and animal sleeping quarters should be decontaminated. Agents that are effective for ridding the home of fleas include lindane, pyrethroids, and organic thiocyanates. Flea-infested pets may be treated with powders containing rotenone, pyrethroids, Malathion, or methoxychlor. Lufenuron, an agent that prevents fleas from reproducing, is effective for animals in oral and injectable formulations. Fipronil is effective as a topical agent for the prevention of flea infestation.

Bibliography is available at Expert Consult.

668.2 Scabies

Anna M. Juern and Beth A. Drolet

Scabies is caused by burrowing and release of toxic or antigenic substances by the female mite *Sarcoptes scabiei* var. *hominis*. The most important factor that determines spread of scabies is the extent and duration of physical contact with an affected individual. The children and sexual partner of an affected individual are most at risk. Scabies is transmitted only rarely by fomites because the isolated mite dies within 2-3 days.

ETIOLOGY AND PATHOGENESIS

An adult female mite measures approximately 0.4 mm in length, has 4 sets of legs, and has a hemispheric body marked by transverse corrugations, brown spines, and bristles on the dorsal surface. A male mite is approximately half her size and is similar in configuration. After impregnation on the skin surface, a gravid female exudes a keratolytic substance and burrows into the stratum corneum, often forming a shallow well within 30 min. She gradually extends this tract by

0.5-5.0 mm/24 hr along the boundary with the stratum granulosum. She deposits 10-25 oval eggs and numerous brown fecal pellets (scybala) daily. When egg laying is completed, in 4-5 wk, she dies within the burrow. The eggs hatch in 3-5 days, releasing larvae that move to the skin surface to molt into nymphs. Maturity is achieved in approximately 2-3 wk. Mating occurs, and the gravid female invades the skin to complete the life cycle.

CLINICAL MANIFESTATIONS

In an immunocompetent host, scabies is frequently heralded by intense pruritus, particularly at night. The first sign of the infestation often consists of 1-2 mm red papules, some of which are excoriated, crusted, or scaling. Threadlike burrows are the classic lesion of scabies (Fig. 668-3) but may not be seen in infants. In infants, bullae and pustules are relatively common. The eruption may also include wheals, papules, vesicles, and a superimposed eczematous dermatitis (Fig. 668-4). The palms, soles, and scalp are often affected. In older children and adolescents, the clinical pattern is similar to that in adults, in whom preferred sites are the interdigital spaces, wrist flexors, anterior axillary folds, ankles, buttocks, umbilicus and belt line, groin, genitals in men, and areolas in women. The head, neck, palms, and soles are generally spared. Infants will often have a diffuse eczematous eruption that will involve the scalp, neck, and face. Red-brown nodules, most often located in covered areas such as the axillae, groin, and genitals, predominate in the less common variant called nodular scabies. Additional clues include facial sparing, affected family members, poor response to topical antibiotics, and transient response to topical steroids. Untreated, scabies may lead to eczematous dermatitis, impetigo, ecthyma, folliculitis, furunculosis, cellulitis, lymphangitis, and id reaction. Glomerulonephritis has developed in children from streptococcal impetiginization of scabies lesions. In some tropical areas, scabies is the predominant underlying cause of pyoderma. A latent period of approximately 1 mo follows an initial infestation. Thus, itching may be absent and lesions may be relatively inapparent in contacts who are asymptomatic carriers. On reinfestation, however, reactions to mite antigens are noted within hours.

DIFFERENTIAL DIAGNOSIS

Differential diagnosis of scabies can often be made clinically but is confirmed by microscopic identification of mites (Fig. 668-5A), ova, and scybala (Fig. 668-5B) in epithelial debris. Scrapings most often test positive when obtained from burrows or fresh papules. A reliable method is application of a drop of mineral oil on the selected lesion, scraping of it with a No. 15 blade, and transferring the oil and scrapings to a glass slide.

The differential diagnosis depends on the types of lesions present. Burrows are virtually pathognomonic for human scabies. Papulovesicular lesions are confused with papular urticaria, canine scabies, chickenpox, viral exanthems, drug eruptions, dermatitis herpetiformis, and folliculitis. Eczematous lesions may mimic atopic dermatitis and seborrheic dermatitis, and the less common bullous disorders of childhood may be suspected in infants with predominantly bullous lesions. Nodular scabies is frequently misdiagnosed as urticaria pigmentosa and Langerhans cell histiocytosis. The histopathologic appearance of nodular scabies, consisting of a deep, dense, perivascular infiltrate of lymphocytes, histiocytes, plasma cells, and atypical mononuclear cells, may mimic malignant lymphoid neoplasms.

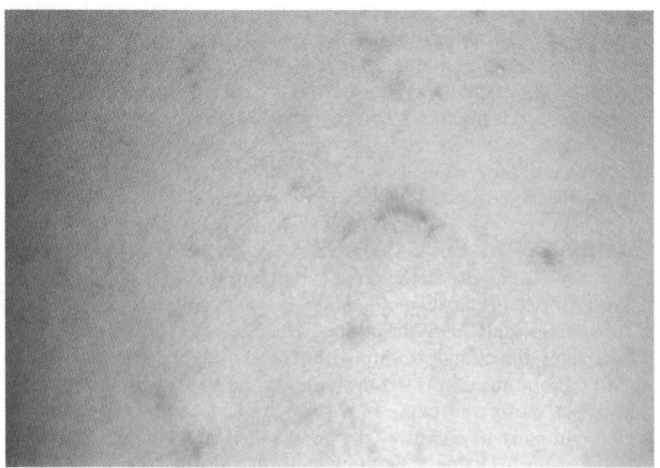

Figure 668-3 Classic scabies burrow.

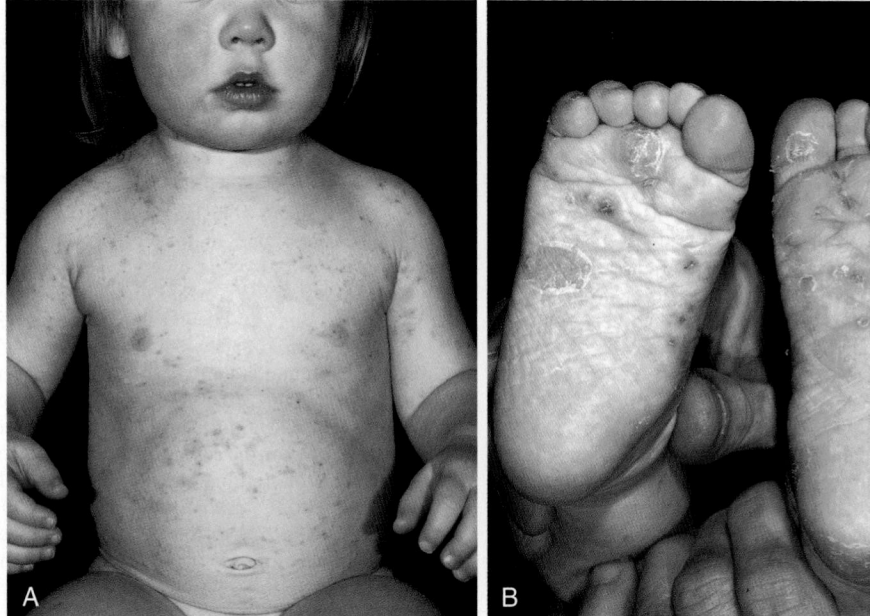

Figure 668-4 A, Diffuse scabies on an infant. The face is clear. The lesions are most numerous around the axillae, chest, and abdomen. **B,** Scabies. Infestation of the palms and soles is common in infants. The vesicular lesions have all ruptured. *(From Habif TP, editor: Clinical dermatology, ed 4, Philadelphia, 2004, Mosby, Figs. 15-8 and 15-9.)*

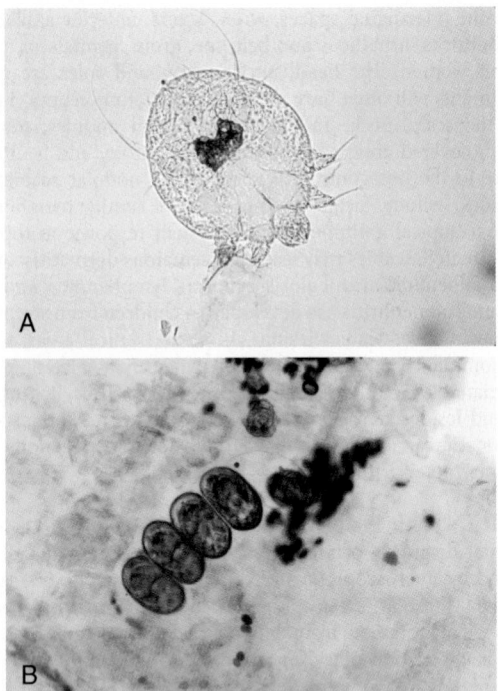

Figure 668-5 A, Human scabies mite obtained from scraping. **B,** Scabies ova and scybala.

TREATMENT

The treatment of choice for scabies is permethrin 5% cream (Elimite) applied to the entire body from the neck down, with particular attention to intensely involved areas, which is also standard therapy. Scabies is frequently found above the neck in infants (younger than 2 yr old), necessitating treatment of the scalp. The medication is left on the skin for 8-12 hr and should be reapplied in 1 wk for another 8-12 hr period. Additional therapies may include lindane 1% lotion or cream, sulfur ointment 5-10%, and crotamiton 10% lotion or cream. For severe infestations and in immunocompromised patients oral ivermectin 200 μg/kg per dose given orally for 2 doses, 2 wk apart can be used (off-label use). Single dose ivermectin (200 μg/kg) has also been effective in immunocompetent patients with improvement (cure) noted in 60% at 2 wk and 89% at 4 wk after treatment.

Transmission of mites is unlikely more than 24 hr after treatment. Pruritus, which is a result of hypersensitivity to mite antigens, may persist for a number of days to weeks, and may be alleviated by a topical corticosteroid preparation. If pruritus persists for >2 wk after treatment and new lesions are occurring, the patient should be reexamined for mites. Nodules are extremely resistant to treatment and may take several months to resolve. The entire family should be treated, as should caretakers of the infested child. Clothing, bed linens, and towels should be washed in hot water and dried using high heat. Clothing or other items (e.g., stuffed animals) that cannot be washed may be dry cleaned or stored in bags for 3 days to 1 wk, as the mite will die when separated from the human host.

NORWEGIAN SCABIES

The Norwegian variant of human scabies is highly contagious and occurs mainly in individuals who are cognitively and physically debilitated, particularly those who are institutionalized and those with Down syndrome; in patients with poor cutaneous sensation (leprosy, spina bifida); in patients who have severe systemic illness (leukemia, diabetes); and in immunosuppressed patients (HIV infection). Affected individuals are infested by myriad mites that inhabit the crusts and exfoliating scales of the skin and scalp. The nails may become thickened and dystrophic. The subungual debris is densely populated by mites. The infestation is often accompanied by generalized lymphadenopathy and eosinophilia. There is massive orthokeratosis and parakeratosis with numerous interspersed mites, psoriasiform epidermal hyperplasia, foci of spongiosis, and neutrophilic abscesses. Norwegian scabies is thought to represent a deficient host immune response to the organism. Management is difficult, requiring scrupulous isolation measures, removal of the thick scales, and repeated but careful applications of permethrin 5% cream. Ivermectin (200-250 μg/kg) has been used successfully as single-dose therapy in refractory cases, particularly in HIV-infected patients. A second dose may be needed a week later. The FDA has not approved this agent for treatment of scabies.

CANINE SCABIES

Canine scabies is caused by *S. scabiei* var. *canis,* the dog mite that is associated with mange. The eruption in humans, which is most frequently acquired by cuddling an infested puppy, consists of tiny papules, vesicles, wheals, and excoriated eczematous plaques. Burrows are not present because the mite infrequently inhabits human stratum corneum. The rash is pruritic and has a predilection for the arms, chest, and abdomen, the usual sites of contact with dogs. Onset is sudden and usually follows exposure by 1-10 days, possibly resulting from development of a hypersensitivity reaction to mite antigens. Recovery of mites or ova from scrapings of human skin is rare. The disease is self-limited because humans are not a suitable host. Bathing and changing clothes are generally sufficient. Removal or treatment of the infested animal is necessary. Symptomatic therapy for itching is helpful. In rare cases in which mites are demonstrated in scrapings from an affected child, they can be eradicated by the same measures applicable to human scabies.

OTHER TYPES OF SCABIES

Other mites that occasionally bite humans include the chigger or harvest mite *(Eutrombicula alfreddugesi),* which prefers to live on grass, shrubs, vines, and stems of grain. Larvae have hooked mouthparts, which allow the chigger to attach to the skin, but not to burrow, to obtain a blood meal, most commonly on the lower legs. Avian mites may affect those who come into close contact with chickens or pet gerbils. Humans may occasionally be assaulted by avian mites that have infested a nest outside a window, an attic, heating vents, or an air conditioner. The dermatitis is variable, including grouped papules, wheals, and vesicular lesions on the wrists, neck, breasts, umbilicus, and anterior axillary folds. A prolonged investigation is often undertaken before the cause and source of the dermatitis are discovered.

Bibliography is available at Expert Consult.

668.3 Pediculosis
Anna M. Juern and Beth A. Drolet

Three types of lice are obligate parasites of the human host: body or clothing lice *(Pediculus humanus corporis),* head lice *(Pediculus humanus capitis),* and pubic or crab lice *(Phthirus pubis).* Only the body louse serves as a vector of human disease (typhus, trench fever, relapsing fever). Body and head lice have similar physical characteristics. They are approximately 2-4 mm in length. Pubic lice are only 1-2 mm in length and are greater in width than length, giving them a crab-like appearance. Female lice live for approximately 1 mo and deposit 3-10 eggs daily on the human host. Body lice, however, generally lay eggs in or near the seams of clothing. The ova or nits are glued to hairs or fibers of clothing but not directly on the body. Ova hatch in 1-2 wk and require another week to mature. Once the eggs hatch, the nits remain attached to the hair as empty sacs of chitin. Freshly hatched larvae die unless a meal is obtained within 24 hr and every few days thereafter. Both nymphs and adult lice feed on human blood, injecting their salivary juices into the host and depositing their fecal matter on the skin. Symptoms of infestation do not appear immediately but develop as an individual becomes sensitized. The hallmark of all types of pediculosis is pruritus.

Pediculosis corporis is rare in children except under conditions of poor hygiene, especially in colder climates when the opportunity to change clothes on a regular basis is lacking. The parasite is transmitted mainly on contaminated clothing or bedding. The primary lesion is a small, intensely pruritic, red macule or papule with a central hemorrhagic punctum, located on the shoulders, trunk, or buttocks. Additional lesions include excoriations, wheals, and eczematous, secondarily infected plaques. Massive infestation may be associated with constitutional symptoms of fever, malaise, and headache. Chronic infestation may lead to "vagabond's skin," which manifests as lichenified, scaling, hyperpigmented plaques, most commonly on the trunk. Lice are found on the skin only transiently when they are feeding. At other times, they inhabit the seams of clothing. Nits are attached firmly to fibers in the cloth and may remain viable for up to 1 mo. Nits hatch when they encounter warmth from the host's body when the clothes are worn again. Therapy consists of improved hygiene and hot water laundering of all infested clothing and bedding. A uniform temperature of 65°C (149°F), wet or dry, for 15-30 min kills all eggs and lice. Alternatively, eggs hatch and nymphs starve if clothing is stored for 2 wk at 23.9-29.4°C (75-85°F).

Pediculosis capitis is an intensely pruritic infestation of lice in the scalp hair. It is the most common form of lice to affect children, in particular those between the ages of 3 and 12 yr. Fomites and head-to-head contact are important modes of transmission. In summer months in many areas of the United States and in the tropics at all times of the year, shared combs, brushes, or towels have a more important role in louse transmission. Translucent 0.5 mm eggs are laid near the proximal portion of the hair shaft and become adherent to 1 side of the shaft (Fig. 668-6). A nit cannot be moved along or knocked off the hair shaft with the fingers. Secondary pyoderma, after trauma from scratching, may result in matting together of the hair and cervical and occipital lymphadenopathy. Hair loss does not result from pediculosis but may accompany the secondary pyoderma. Head lice are a major cause of numerous pyodermas of the scalp, particularly in tropical environments. Lice are not always visible, but nits are detectable on the hairs, most commonly in the occipital region and above the ears, rarely on beard or pubic hair. Dermatitis may also be noted on the neck and pinnae. An id reaction, consisting of erythematous patches and plaques, may develop, particularly on the trunk. Head lice rarely infest African-Americans and this is possibly related to the diameter, shape or twisted nature of their hair shafts (which makes grasping of the shaft more difficult for the louse).

Because of resistance of head lice to pyrethroids, malathion 0.5% in isopropanol is the treatment of choice for head lice and should be applied to dry hair until hair and scalp are wet, and left on for 12 hr. A second application 7-9 days after initial treatment may be necessary. This product is flammable, so care should be taken to avoid open flames. Malathion, like lindane shampoo, is not indicated for use in neonates and infants. Additional approved therapies include spinosad (if >4 yr old), benzyl alcohol lotion (if >6 mo), and ivermectin for difficult-to-treat head lice (Table 668-3). All household members should be treated at the same time. Nits can be removed with a fine-toothed comb after application of a damp towel to the scalp for 30 min. Clothing and bed linens should be laundered in very hot water or dry-cleaned; brushes and combs should be discarded or coated with a pediculicide for 15 min and then thoroughly cleaned in boiling water. Children may return to school after the initial treatment.

Pediculosis pubis is transmitted by skin-to-skin or sexual contact with an infested individual; the chance of acquiring the lice with 1 sexual exposure is 95%. The infestation is usually encountered in adolescents, although small children may occasionally acquire pubic lice on the eyelashes. Patients experience moderate to severe pruritus and may develop a secondary pyoderma from scratching. Excoriations tend to be shallower, and the incidence of secondary infection is lower than in pediculosis corporis. Maculae ceruleae are steel-gray spots, usually <1 cm in diameter, which may appear in the pubic area and on the chest, abdomen, and thighs. Oval translucent nits, which are firmly attached to the hair shafts, may be visible to the naked eye or may be readily identified by a hand lens or by microscopic examination (see Fig. 668-6). Grittiness, as a result of adherent nits, may sometimes be detected when the fingers are run through infested hair. Adult lice are difficult to detect than head or body lice because of their lower level of activity and smaller, translucent bodies. Because pubic lice occasionally may wander or may be transferred to other sites on fomites, terminal hair on the trunk, thighs, axillary region, beard area, and eyelashes should be examined for nits. The coexistence of other venereal diseases should be considered. Treatment with a 10-min application of a pyrethrin preparation is usually effective. Retreatment may be required in 7-10 days. The shampoo form of lindane, which requires a 10 min application time, is an alternative choice, but lindane cream and lotion are no longer recommended for treatment of pubic lice. Infestation of eyelashes is eradicated by petrolatum applied 3-5 times per 24 hr for 8-10 days. Clothing, towels, and bed linens may be contaminated with nit-bearing hairs and should be thoroughly laundered or dry-cleaned.

Bibliography is available at Expert Consult.

668.4 Seabather's Eruption
Anna M. Juern and Beth A. Drolet

Seabather's eruption is a severely pruritic dermatosis of inflammatory papules that develops within ≈12 hr of bathing in saltwater, primarily on body sites that were covered by a bathing suit. The eruption has been described primarily in connection with bathing in the waters of Florida and the Caribbean. Lesions, which may include pustules, vesicles, and urticarial plaques, are more numerous in individuals who keep their bathing suits on for an extended period after leaving the water. The eruption may be accompanied by systemic symptoms of fatigue, malaise, fever, chills, nausea, and headache; in 1 large series, ≈40% of children younger than 16 yr of age had fever. Duration of the pruritus and skin eruption is 1-2 wk. Lesions consist of a superficial and deep perivascular and interstitial infiltrate of lymphocytes, eosinophils, and neutrophils. The eruption appears to be due to an allergic hypersensitivity reaction to venom from larvae of the thimble jellyfish (*Linuche unguiculata*). Treatment is largely symptomatic. Potent topical corticosteroids have been shown to provide relief to some patients.

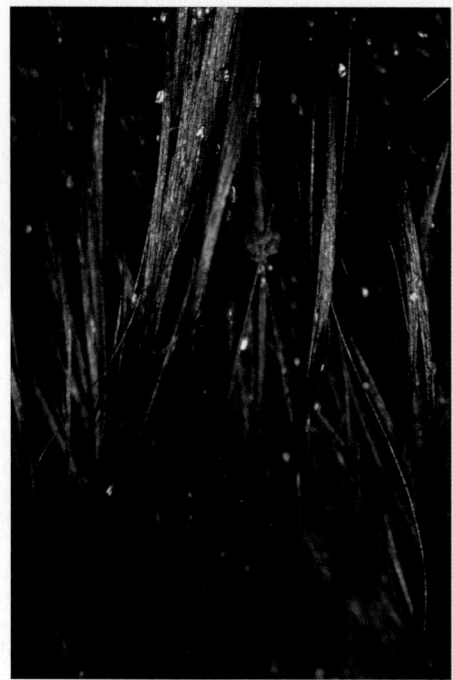

Figure 668-6 Intact nits on human hairs.

Table 668-3	Drugs for Head Lice				
DRUG	**RESISTANCE**	**FDA-APPROVED LOWER AGE OR WEIGHT LIMIT**	**DOSAGE AND ADMINISTRATION**		**COST[a]/SIZE**
Ivermectin 0.5% lotion–Sklice (Sanofi Pasteur)	No[b]	6 months	Apply to dry hair and scalp for 10 min, then rinse		$257.88/4 oz
Ivermectin tablets[c]–Stromectol (Merck)	No	15 kg	200-400 µg/kg PO once; repeat 7-10 days later		9.97[d]
Spinosad 0.9% suspension–Natroba (ParaPro)	No[b]	4 yr	Apply to dry hair for 10 min, then rinse; repeat 7 days later if necessary		219.00/4 oz
Benzyl alcohol 5% lotion–Ulesfia (Shionogi)	No	6 months	Apply to dry hair for 10 min, then rinse; repeat 7 days later		52.62/8 oz
Pyrethrins with piperonyl butoxide shampoo[e,f]–Generic Rid (Bayer)	Yes	2 yr	Apply to dry hair for 10 min, then shampoo; repeat 7-10 days later		12.49/8 oz 19.99/8 oz[g]
Permethrin 1% creme rinse[e]– Generic Nix (Insight)	Yes	2 months	Apply to shampooed, towel-dried hair for 10 min, then rinse; repeat 7 days later		18.49/4 oz 19.99/4 oz[g]
Malathion 0.5% lotion– Generic Ovide (Taro)	Not in U.S.	6 yr	Apply to dry hair for 8-12 hr,[h] then shampoo; repeat 7-9 days later if necessary		152.67/2 oz 160.46/2 oz

[a]Wholesale acquisition cost (WAC). Source: PricePointRx. Reprinted with permission by FDB, Inc. All rights reserved. Copyright 2012. www.firstdatabank.com/support/drug-pricing-policy.aspx. Actual retail prices may be higher. Amount needed may vary.
[b]Product new to market: currently no reports of resistance.
[c]Not FDA-approved for treatment of head lice. Stromectol is available in 3 mg tablets.
[d]Cost of 1 dose for a 30 kg child at the lowest dosage.
[e]Available without a prescription.
[f]Products that contain benzyl alcohol as their vehicle may be more effective.
[g]Cost according to drugstore.com.
[h]One or two 20 min applications have also been effective (Meinking TL, Vicaria M, Eyerdam DH,, et al: Efficacy of a reduced application time of Ovide lotion (0.5% malathion) compared to Nix creme rinse (1% permethrin) for the treatment of head lice, Pediatr Dermatol 21:670–674, 2004.)
 From The Medical Letter: Ivermectin (Sklice) topical lotion for head lice. Med Lett Drugs Ther 54:61–62, 2012.

Chapter 669
Acne
Sheila S. Galbraith

ACNE VULGARIS

Acne, particularly the comedonal form, occurs in 80% of adolescents.

Pathogenesis

Lesions of acne vulgaris develop in sebaceous follicles, which consist of large, multilobular sebaceous glands that drain their products into the follicular canals. The initial lesion of acne is a microcomedone, which progresses to a comedone. A comedone is a dilated epithelium-lined follicular sac filled with lamellated keratinous material, lipid, and bacteria. An open comedone, known as a **blackhead,** has a patulous pilosebaceous orifice that permits visualization of the plug. An open comedone becomes inflammatory less commonly than does a closed comedone or whitehead, which has only a pinpoint opening. An inflammatory papule or nodule develops from a comedone that has ruptured and extruded its follicular contents into the subadjacent dermis, inducing a neutrophilic inflammatory response. If the inflammatory reaction is close to the surface, a papule or pustule develops. If the inflammatory infiltrate develops deeper in the dermis, a nodule forms. Suppuration and an occasional giant cell reaction to the keratin and hair are the cause of nodulocystic lesions. These are not true cysts but liquefied masses of inflammatory debris.

The primary pathogenetic alterations in acne are (1) abnormal keratinization of the follicular epithelium, resulting in impaction of

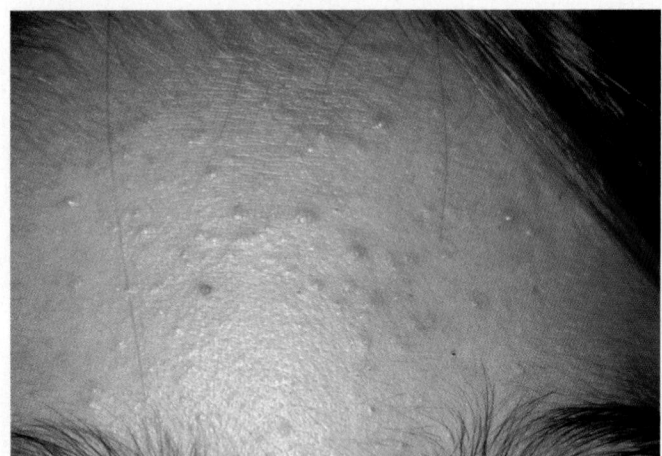

Figure 669-1 Primarily comedonal acne in a 7 yr old girl.

keratinized cells within the follicular lumen; (2) increased sebaceous gland production of sebum; (3) proliferation of *Propionibacterium acnes* within the follicle; and (4) inflammation. Comedonal acne (Fig. 669-1), particularly of the central face, is frequently the first sign of pubertal maturation. At puberty, the sebaceus gland enlarges and sebum production increases in response to the increased activities of androgens of primarily adrenal origin. Most patients with acne do not have endocrine abnormalities. Hyperresponsiveness of the sebocyte to androgens is likely involved in determining the severity of acne in a given individual. Sebocytes and follicular keratinocytes contain 5α-reductase and 3β- and 17β-hydroxyl-steroid dehydrogenase, which are capable of metabolizing androgens. A significant number of women with acne (25-50%), particularly those with relatively mild papulopustular acne, note that their acne flares about 1 wk before menstruation.

Freshly formed sebum consists of a mixture of triglycerides, wax esters, squalene, and sterol esters. Normal follicular bacteria produce lipases that hydrolyze sebum triglycerides to free fatty acids. Those of medium-chain length (C8-C14) may be provocative factors in initiating an inflammatory reaction. Sebum also provides a favorable substrate for proliferation of bacteria. *P. acnes* appears to be largely responsible for the formation of free fatty acids. Skin surface *P. acnes* counts do not correlate with the severity of acne. There is a correlation between reduction of *P. acnes* count and improvement in acne vulgaris. It is probable that bacterial proteases, hyaluronidases, and hydrolytic enzymes produce biologically active extracellular materials that increase the permeability of the follicular epithelium. Chemotactic factors released by the intrafollicular bacteria attract neutrophils and monocytes. Lysosomal enzymes from the neutrophils, released in the process of phagocytizing the bacteria, further disrupt the integrity of the follicular wall and intensify the inflammatory reaction.

Clinical Manifestations

Acne vulgaris is characterized by 4 basic types of lesions: open and closed comedones, papules, pustules (Fig. 669-2), and nodulocystic lesions (Fig. 669-3 and Table 669-1). One or more types of lesions may predominate. In its mildest form, which is often seen early in adolescence, lesions are limited to comedones on the central area of the face.

Lesions may also involve the chest, upper back, and deltoid areas. A predominance of lesions on the forehead, particularly closed comedones, is often attributable to prolonged use of greasy hair preparations (pomade acne) (Fig. 669-4). Marked involvement on the trunk is most often seen in males. Lesions often heal with temporary postinflammatory erythema and hyperpigmentation. Pitted, atrophic, or hypertrophic scars may be interspersed, depending on the severity, depth, and chronicity of the process. Diagnosis of acne is rarely difficult, although flat warts, folliculitis, and other types of acne (drug induced: glucocorticoid agents, anabolic steroids, gold, dactinomycin, isoniazid, lithium, phenytoin, progestins) may be confused with acne vulgaris. The differential diagnosis includes sarcoidosis, angiofibromas, keratosis pilaris, chloracne, rosacea, and fibrofolliculomas.

Treatment

No evidence shows that early treatment, with the exception of isotretinoin, alters the course of acne. Acne can be controlled and severe scarring prevented by judicious maintenance therapy that is continued until the disease process has abated spontaneously. Therapy must be individualized and aimed at preventing microcomedone formation through reduction of follicular hyperkeratosis, sebum production, the *P. acnes* population in follicular orifices, and free fatty acid production. Initial control takes at least 6-8 wk, depending on the severity of the acne (Table 669-2 and Fig. 669-5). It is also important to address the potentially severe emotional impact of acne on adolescents.

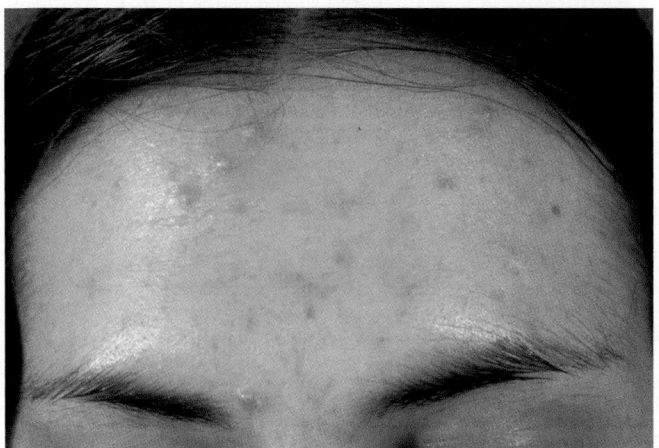

Figure 669-2 Inflammatory papules and pustules.

Table 669-1	Classification of Acne
SEVERITY	**DESCRIPTION**
Mild	Comedones (noninflammatory lesions) are the main lesions. Papules and pustules may be present but are small and few in number (generally <10).
Moderate	Moderate numbers of papules and pustules (10-40) and comedones (10-40) are present. Mild disease of the trunk may also be present.
Moderately severe	Numerous papules and pustules are present (40-100), usually with many comedones (40-100) and occasional larger, deeper nodular inflamed lesions (up to 5). Widespread affected areas usually involve the face, chest, and back.
Severe	Nodulocystic acne and acne conglobata, with many large, painful nodular or pustular lesions, are present, along with many smaller papules, pustules, and comedones.

From James WD: Clinical practice: acne, N Engl J Med 352:1463–1472, 2005.

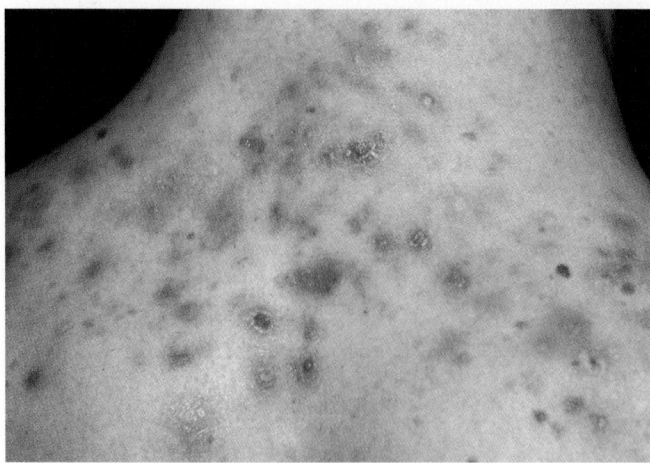

Figure 669-3 Severe nodulocystic acne.

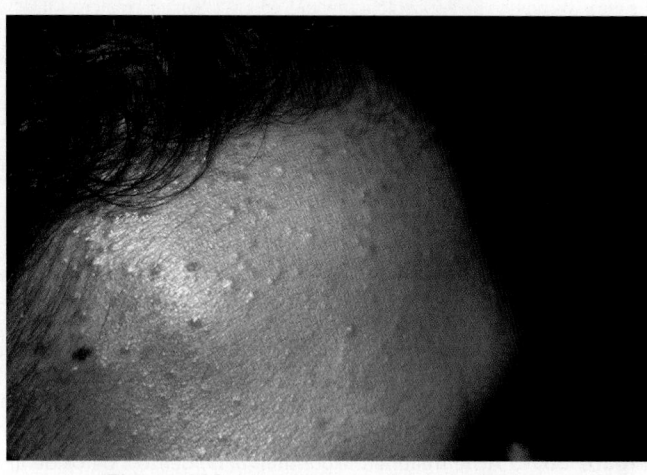

Figure 669-4 Pomade acne along the hairline.

The pediatrician must be aware of the frequently poor correlation between acne severity and psychosocial impact, particularly in adolescents. As adolescents become preoccupied with their appearance, offering treatment even to the youngster whose acne is mild may enhance self-image.

Diet

Little evidence shows that ingestion of particular foods can trigger acne flares. When a patient is convinced that certain dietary items exacerbate acne, it is prudent for the patient to omit those foods.

Climate

Climate appears to influence acne, in that improvement frequently occurs in summer and flares are more common in winter. Remission in summer may relate, in part, to the relative absence of stress. Emotional tension and fatigue seem to exacerbate acne in many individuals;

Table 669-2	Typical Treatment Regimens for Acne

COMEDONAL ACNE
Topical retinoid *or*
Azelaic acid *or*
Salicylic acid

MILD PAPULOPUSTULAR ACNE
Topical retinoid *plus*
Benzoyl peroxide *or*
Benzoyl peroxide/topical antibiotic *or*
Benzoyl peroxide/oral antibiotic

SEVERE PAPULOPUSTULAR OR NODULAR ACNE
Topical retinoid *plus*
Benzoyl peroxide and oral antibiotic *or*
Isotretinoin 1 mg/kg/day

the mechanism is unclear but has been proposed to relate to an increased adrenocortical response.

Cleansing

Cleansing with soap and water removes surface lipid and renders the skin less oily in appearance, but no evidence shows that surface lipid has a role in generating acne lesions. Only superficial drying and peeling are achieved by cleansing, and almost any mild soap or astringent is adequate. Repetitive cleansing can be harmful because it irritates and chaps the skin. Cleansing agents that contain abrasives and keratolytic agents, such as sulfur, resorcinol, and salicylic acid, may temporarily remove sebum from the skin surface. They exert a mild drying and peeling effect and suppress lesions to a limited degree. They do not prevent microcomedones from forming. No evidence shows that preparations containing alcohol or hexachlorophene decrease acne because surface bacteria are not involved in the pathogenesis. Greasy cosmetic and hair preparations must be discontinued because they exacerbate preexisting acne and cause further plugging of follicular pores. Manipulation and squeezing of facial lesions only ruptures intact lesions and provokes a localized inflammatory reaction.

Topical Therapy

All topical preparations must be used for 6-8 wk before their effectiveness can be assessed. Retinoids may be used alone for mild acne, but combination therapy is frequently more effective. A popular and effective combination is use of benzoyl peroxide gel in the morning and a retinoid at night.

Retinoids. A topical retinoid should be the **primary treatment** for acne vulgaris. Topical retinoids have multiple actions, including inhibition of the formation and number of microcomedones, reduction of mature comedones, reduction of inflammatory lesions, and production of normal desquamation of the follicular epithelium. Retinoids should be applied daily to all the affected areas. The main side effects of retinoids are irritation and dryness. Not all patients initially

Global Alliance Acne Treatment Algorithm

Acne severity	Mild		Moderate		Severe
	Comedonal	Mixed and papular/pustular	Mixed and papular/pustular	Nodular(2)	Nodular/conglobate
First choice	Topical retinoid	Topical retinoid + topical antimicrobial	Oral antibiotic + topical retinoid ± BPO	Oral antibiotic + topical retinoid + BPO	Oral isotretinoin[2]
Alternatives(1)	Alt. topical retinoid *or* azelaic acid* *or* salicylic acid	Alt. topical retinoid antimicrobial agent + Alt. topical retinoid *or* azelaic acid*	Alt. oral antibiotic + alt. topical retinoid ± BPO	Oral isotretinoin *or* Alt. oral antibiotic + alt. topical retinoid ± BPO/azelaic acid*	High dose oral antibiotic + topical retinoid + BPO
Alternatives for females(1, 4)	See first choice	See first choice	Oral antiandrogen[5] + topical retinoid/ azelaic acid* ± topical antimicrobial	Oral antiandrogen[5] + topical retinoid/ ± oral antibiotic ± alt. antimicrobial	High dose oral antiandrogen[5] + topical retinoid ± alt. topical antimicrobial
Maintenance therapy	Topical retinoid		Topical retinoid ± BPO		

1. Consider physical removal of comedones. 2. With small nodules (<0.5 cm). 3. Second course in case of relapse. 4. For pregnancy, options are limited. 5. For full discussion, see Gollnick H. et al. JAAD. 2003.49 (Suppl):1-37.

Figure 669-5 Acne treatment algorithm. BPO, benzoyl peroxide. (*From Thiboutot D, Gollnick H; Global Alliance to Improve Acne, et al: New insights into the management of acne: an update from the global alliance to improve outcomes in acne, J Am Acad Dermatol 60:S1–S50, 2009.*)

tolerate daily use of a retinoid. It is prudent to begin therapy every other or every 3rd day and slowly increase the frequency of application as tolerated. Tretinoin, adapalene, and tazarotene (Table 669-3) are the available retinoids. They vary in strength and efficacy, although adapalene tends to be less irritating and tazarotene is more irritating but may be more effective.

Benzoyl Peroxide. Benzoyl peroxide is primarily an antimicrobial agent. It has an advantage over topical antibiotics in that it does not enhance antimicrobial resistance. It is available in multiple formulations and concentrations. The gel formulations are preferred, owing to better stability and more consistent release of the active ingredient. Washes and cleansers are useful for covering large surface areas such as the chest and back. As with retinoids, the main side effects are irritation and drying. Benzoyl peroxide can also bleach clothing.

Topical Antibiotics. Topical antibiotics are indicated for the treatment of inflammatory acne. Clindamycin is the most commonly used. It is not as effective as oral antibiotics. It should not be used as monotherapy because it does not inhibit microcomedone formation and it has the potential to induce antimicrobial resistance. Irritation and dryness are generally less than with retinoids or benzoyl peroxide. Topical antibiotics are best used as combination products. The most common is benzoyl peroxide/clindamycin. A combination tretinoin/clindamycin product may also be used.

Table 669-3	Medications for the Treatment of Acne		
DRUG	**DOSE**	**SIDE EFFECT(S)**	**OTHER CONSIDERATIONS**
TOPICAL AGENTS			
Retinoids			
Tretinoin	Applied once nightly; strengths of 0.025-0.1% available**	Irritation (redness and scaling)	Generics available
Adapalene	Applied once daily, at night or in the morning; 0.01% and 0.3%**	Minimal irritation	0.1% generic available
Tazarotene*	Applied once nightly; 0.05% and 0.1%**	Irritation	Limited data suggest tazarotene more effective than alternatives
Antimicrobials			
Benzoyl peroxide, alone or with zinc, 2.5-10%	Applied once or twice daily	Benzoyl peroxide can bleach clothing and bedding	Available over the counter; 2.5-5% concentrations as effective as and less drying than 10% concentration
Clindamycin, erythromycin[†]	Applied once or twice daily	Propensity to resistance	Most effective for inflammatory lesions (rather than comedones); resistance a concern when used alone
Combination benzoyl peroxide and clindamycin or erythromycin Combination tretinoin and clindamycin	Applied once or twice daily		Combination more effective than topical antibiotics alone; limits development of resistance; use of individual products in combination less expensive and appears similarly effective
Other Topical Agents			
Azelaic acid, sodium sulfacetamide-sulfur, salicylic acid[†]	Applied once or twice daily	Well tolerated	Good adjunctive or alternative treatments
ORAL ANTIBIOTICS[‡]			
Tetracycline[§]	250-500 mg once or twice daily	Gastrointestinal upset, pseudomotor cerebri	Inexpensive; dosing limited by need to take on empty stomach
Doxycycline[§]	50-100 mg once or twice daily	Phototoxicity, pseudomotor cerebri, pill esophagitis, gastrointestinal upset	20 mg dose antiinflammatory only; limited data on efficacy
Minocycline[§]	50-100 mg once or twice daily	Hyperpigmentation of teeth, oral mucosa, and skin; lupus-like reactions with long-term treatment, pseudomotor cerebri, DRESS	
Trimethoprim-sulfamethoxazole	One dose (160 mg trimethoprim, 800 mg sulfamethoxazole) twice daily	Toxic epidermal necrolysis and allergic eruptions	Trimethoprim may be used alone in 300 mg dose twice daily; limited data available
Erythromycin[†]	250-500 mg twice daily	Gastrointestinal upset	Resistance problematic; consensus is that efficacy is limited
HORMONAL AGENTS[¶]			
Spironolactone[§]	50-200 mg in divided doses	Menstrual irregularities, breast tenderness	Higher doses more effective but cause more side effects; best given in combination with oral contraceptives
Estrogen-containing oral contraceptives	Daily	Potential side effects include thromboembolism	

Continued

Table 669-3	Medications for the Treatment of Acne—cont'd			
DRUG	**DOSE**	**SIDE EFFECT(S)**	**OTHER CONSIDERATIONS**

ORAL RETINOID

| Isotretinoin‖ (Accutane) | 0.5-1.0 mg/kg/day in divided doses | Birth defects; adherence to pregnancy prevention program outlined by drug manufacturer, including 2 initial negative pregnancy tests, is essential; hypertriglyceridemia, elevated results on liver function tests, abnormal night vision, benign intracranial hypertension, dryness of the lips, ocular, nasal, and oral mucosa and skin, secondary staphylococcal infections, arthralgias, and mood disturbances are possible common or important side effects; laboratory testing of lipid profiles and liver function tests monthly should be performed monthly until dose is stabilized | Relapse rate higher if patient is younger than age 16 yr at initial treatment, if acne is of high severity and involves the trunk, or if drug is used in adult women |
| Absorica (isotretinoin agent) | 0.5-1 mg/kg/day bid | Same as Accutane | Same as Accutane |

*Tazarotene is in pregnancy category X: contraindicated in pregnancy.
†Clindamycin, erythromycin, and azelaic acid are in pregnancy category B: no evidence of risk in humans.
‡Oral antibiotics are indicated for moderate to severe disease; for the treatment of acne on the chest, back, or shoulders; and in patients with inflammatory disease in whom topical combinations have failed or are not tolerated.
§This drug is in pregnancy category D: positive evidence of risk in humans.
¶Hormonal agents are for use in women only.
‖Isotretinoin is in pregnancy category X: contraindicated in pregnancy. It should be used only in patients with severe acne that does not clear with combined oral and topical therapy.
**As cream or gel.
DRESS, drug rash with eosinophilia and systemic symptoms.
    Modified from James WD: Clinical practice: acne, N Engl J Med 352:1463–1472, 2005.

Azelaic Acid. Azelaic acid (20% cream) has mild antimicrobial and keratolytic properties. It can also help expedite resolution of postinflammatory hyperpigmentation.

Systemic Therapy

Antibiotics, especially tetracycline and its derivatives (see Table 669-3), are indicated for treatment of patients whose acne has not responded to topical medications, who have moderate to severe inflammatory papulopustular and nodulocystic acne, and who have a propensity for scarring. Tetracycline and its derivatives act by reducing the growth and metabolism of *P. acnes.* They also have antiinflammatory properties. For most adolescent patients, therapy may be initiated twice daily, for at least 6-8 wk, followed by a gradual decrease to the minimal effective dose. The drugs should always be administered in combination with a topical retinoid and topical benzoyl peroxide, but not topical antibiotics. Tetracycline absorption is inhibited by food, milk, iron supplements,, and calcium-magnesium salts. It should be taken on an empty stomach 1 hr before or 2 hr after meals. Minocycline and doxycycline may be taken with food. Side effects of tetracycline and derivatives are rare. Side effects of tetracycline include vaginal candidosis, particularly in those who take tetracycline concurrently with oral contraceptives; gastrointestinal irritation; phototoxic reactions, including onycholysis and brown discoloration of nails; esophageal ulceration; inhibition of fetal skeletal growth; and staining of growing teeth, precluding its use during pregnancy and in those younger than age 8 yr. Doxycycline is the most photosensitizing of the tetracycline derivatives and is also more likely to cause pill esophagitis. Rarely, minocycline causes dizziness, intracranial hypertension, bluish discoloration of the skin and mucous membranes, hepatitis, a lupus-like syndrome, and drug reaction with eosinophilia and systemic symptoms. A possible complication of prolonged systemic antibiotic use is proliferation of Gram-negative organisms, particularly *Enterobacter, Klebsiella,*

Escherichia coli, and *Pseudomonas aeruginosa,* producing severe, refractory folliculitis.

Women who have acne and hormonal abnormalities, whose acne is unresponsive to antibiotic therapy, or who are not candidates for isotretinoin therapy should be considered for a trial of hormonal therapy. Combined oral contraceptive pills are the primary form of hormonal therapy. Spironolactone has also shown effectiveness.

Isotretinoin (13-*cis*-retinoic acid; Accutane) is indicated for severe nodulocystic acne and moderate to severe acne that has not responded to conventional therapy. The recommended dosage is 0.5-1.0 mg/kg/day. A standard course in the United States lasts 16-20 wk. At the end of 1 course of isotretinoin, 70-80% of patients are cured, 10-20% need conventional topical and/or oral medications to maintain adequate control, and 10-20% have relapses and need an additional course of isotretinoin. Dosages <0.5 mg/kg/day, or a cumulative dose of <120 mg/kg, are associated with a significantly higher rate of treatment failure and relapse. If the disease process is not in remission 2 mo after the first course of isotretinoin, a second course should be considered. Isotretinoin reduces size and secretion of sebaceous glands, normalizes follicular keratinization, prevents new microcomedone formation, decreases the population of *P. acnes,* and exerts an antiinflammatory effect.

Isotretinoin use has many side effects. It is highly **teratogenic** and is **absolutely contraindicated** in pregnancy. Pregnancy should be avoided for 6 wk after discontinuation of therapy. Two forms of birth control are required, as are monthly pregnancy tests. *Concerns over cases of pregnancy despite warnings have prompted a manufacturer registration program, iPLEDGE (www.ipledgeprogram.com), which requires physician enrollment and careful patient pregnancy screening to prescribe isotretinoin.* Many patients also experience cheilitis, xerosis, periodic epistaxis, and blepharoconjunctivitis. Increased serum triglyceride and cholesterol levels are also common. It is important to rule out

Icepick (V)	Rolling (U)	Boxcar (M)	Keloids	Hypertrophic
Punch excision (deep bases)

Elevation and grafting

Laser resurfacing/ dermabrasion (many scars close together)

Spot TCA peel | **Combined therapy**

Micrograft and subcision

+

± filler

Resurfacing microdermabrasion

Deep-spot TCA peel | **Shallow**
≤3 mm diameter-laser skin resurfacing

>3 mm diameter-laser skin resurfacing ± punch elevation

Deep
≤3 mm diameter-punch excision

>3 mm diameter-punch excision or punch elevation

Fractional thermolysis (deep or shallow)

Dermabrasion CO_2 laser resurfacing | Intralesional corticosteroids

Intralesional 5-FU

Intralesional bleomycin

Compression

Imiquimod after intralesional excision

Cryotherapy

Pulsed-dye laser

Excision + electrotherapy | Intralesional steroids

Intralesional 5-FU

Vascular laser

Intralesional bleomycin

Compression

Imiquimod after intralesional excision |
| Adjunctive treatment: Topical retinoids 2 weeks prior to and following treatment, sunscreens, moisturizers | | | | |

Non-ablative lasers for mild disease; ablative and fractional lasers for moderate scarring

Figure 669-6 Treatment options for acne scars. CO_2, carbon dioxide; FU, fluorouracil; TCA, trichloroacetic acid. *(From Thiboutot D, Gollnick H; Global Alliance to Improve Acne, et al: New insights into the management of acne: an update from the global alliance to improve outcomes in acne, J Am Acad Dermatol 60:S1–S50, 2009.)*

preexisting liver disease and hyperlipidemia before initiating therapy and to recheck laboratory values 4 wk after commencement of therapy. Less common but significant side effects include arthralgias, myalgias, temporary thinning of the hair, paronychia, increased susceptibility to sunburn, formation of pyogenic granulomas, and colonization of the skin with *Staphylococcus aureus,* leading to impetigo, secondarily infected dermatitis, and scalp folliculitis. Rarely, hyperostotic lesions of the spine develop after more than 1 course of isotretinoin. Concomitant use of tetracycline and isotretinoin is contraindicated because either drug, but particularly when they are used together, can cause benign intracranial hypertension. Although no cause-and-effect relationship has been established, drug-induced mood changes and depression and/or suicide have mandated close attention to psychiatric well-being before and during isotretinoin prescription.

Surgical Therapy
Intralesional injection of low-dose (3-5 mg/mL) mid-potency glucocorticoids (e.g., triamcinolone) with a 30-gauge needle on a tuberculin syringe may hasten the healing of individual, painful nodulocystic lesions. Dermabrasion or laser peel to minimize scarring should be considered only after the active process is quiescent. Figure 669-6 describes the management of scarring.

The role of pulsed-dye laser in the treatment of inflammatory acne is controversial and inconclusive.

DRUG-INDUCED ACNE
Pubertal and postpubertal patients who are receiving systemic corticosteroid therapy are predisposed to steroid-induced acne. This monomorphous folliculitis occurs primarily on the face, neck, chest (Fig. 669-7), shoulders, upper back, arms, and, rarely, on the scalp. Onset

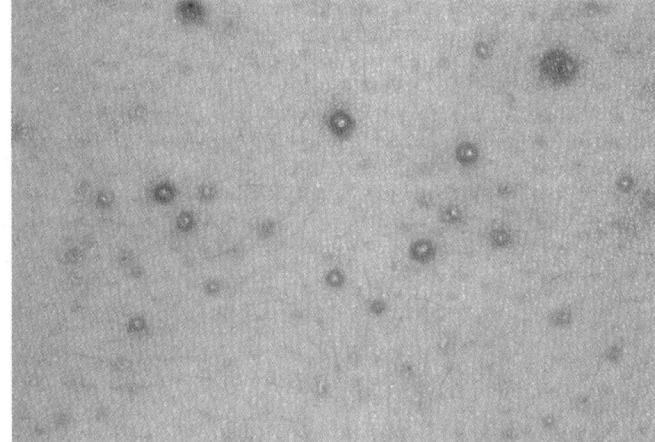

Figure 669-7 Monomorphous papular eruption of steroid acne.

follows the initiation of steroid therapy by approximately 2 wk. The lesions are small, erythematous papules or pustules that may erupt in profusion and are all in the same stage of development. Comedones may occur subsequently, but nodulocystic lesions and scarring are rare. Pruritus is occasional. Although steroid acne is relatively refractory if the medication is continued, the eruption may respond to use of tretinoin and a benzoyl peroxide gel.

Other **drugs** that can induce **acneiform lesions** in susceptible individuals include isoniazid, phenytoin, phenobarbital, trimethadione, lithium carbonate, androgens (anabolic steroids), and vitamin B_{12}.

HALOGEN ACNE

Administration of medications containing iodides or bromides or, rarely, ingestion of massive amounts of vitamin–mineral preparations or iodine-containing "health foods" such as kelp may induce halogen acne. The lesions are often very inflammatory. Discontinuation of the provocative agent and appropriate topical preparations usually achieve reasonable therapeutic results.

CHLORACNE

Chloracne is a result of external contact with, inhalation of, or ingestion of halogenated aromatic hydrocarbons, including polyhalogenated biphenyls, polyhalogenated naphthalenes, and dioxins. Lesions are primarily comedonal. Inflammatory lesions are infrequent but may include papules, pustules, nodules, and cysts. Healing occurs with atrophic or hypertrophic scarring. The face, postauricular regions, neck, axillae, genitals, and chest are most commonly involved. The nose is often spared. In cases of severe exposure, associated findings may include hepatitis, production of porphyrins, bulla formation on sun-exposed skin, hyperpigmentation, hypertrichosis, and palmar and plantar hyperhidrosis. Topical or oral retinoids may be effective; benzoyl peroxide and antibiotics are generally ineffective.

NEONATAL ACNE

Approximately 20% of normal neonates demonstrate acne in the 1st mo of life. Small inflammatory papules and pustules predominate on the cheeks and forehead (Fig. 669-8); comedones are absent. The cause of neonatal acne is unknown but it has been theorized that it may be an inflammatory reaction to *Pityrosporum* species rather than true acne; therefore, the term neonatal cephalic pustulosis has been proposed. Other theories include placental transfer of maternal androgens, hyperactive neonatal adrenal glands, and a hypersensitive neonatal end-organ response to androgenic hormones. The eruption involutes spontaneously over a few months. **Treatment** is usually unnecessary. If desired, the lesions can be treated effectively with topical antifungals, and/or benzoyl peroxide.

INFANTILE ACNE

Infantile acne usually manifests between 3 mo and 2 yr of age, more commonly in boys than in girls. Acne lesions are more numerous, pleomorphic, severe, and persistent than in neonatal acne (Fig. 669-9). Open and closed comedones predominate on the face. Papules and pustules occur frequently, but only occasionally do nodulocystic lesions develop. Pitted scarring is seen in 10-15%. The course may be relatively brief, or the lesions may persist for many months or years, although the eruption generally resolves by age 4 yr. Use of topical benzoyl peroxide gel and tretinoin usually clears the eruption within a few weeks. Oral erythromycin is occasionally necessary. A child with refractory acne warrants a search for an abnormal source of androgens, such as a virilizing tumor or congenital adrenal hyperplasia.

TROPICAL ACNE

A severe form of acne occurs in tropical climates and is believed to be caused by the intense heat and humidity. Hydration of the pilosebaceous duct pore may accentuate blockage of the duct. Affected individuals tend to have an antecedent history of adolescent acne that is quiescent at the time of the eruption. Lesions occur mainly on the entire back, chest, buttocks, and thighs, with a predominance of suppurating papules and nodules. Secondary infection with *S. aureus* may be a complication. The eruption is refractory to acne therapy if the environmental factors are not eliminated.

ACNE CONGLOBATA

Acne conglobata is a chronic progressive inflammatory disease that occurs mainly in men, and more commonly in white than in black individuals, but it may begin during adolescence. Patients usually have a history of preexisting acne vulgaris. The principal lesion is the nodule, although there is often a mixture of comedones with multiple pores, papules, pustules, nodules, cysts, abscesses, and subcutaneous dissection with formation of multichanneled sinus tracts. Severe scarring is characteristic. The face is relatively spared, but in addition to the back and chest, the buttocks, abdomen, arms, and thighs may be involved. Constitutional symptoms and anemia may accompany the inflammatory process. Coagulase-positive staphylococci and β-hemolytic streptococci are frequently cultured from lesions but do not appear to be primarily involved in the pathogenesis. Acne conglobata occasionally occurs in association with hidradenitis suppurativa and dissecting cellulitis of the scalp (as the follicular occlusion triad) and may be complicated by erosive arthritis and ankylosing spondyloarthritis. Endocrinologic studies are not revealing. Routine acne therapy is generally ineffective. Systemic therapy with a corticosteroid may be required to suppress the intense inflammatory activity. Isotretinoin is the most effective form of therapy for some patients but may produce a flare after its initiation.

ACNE FULMINANS (ACUTE FEBRILE ULCERATIVE ACNE)

Acne fulminans is characterized by abrupt onset of extensive inflammatory, tender ulcerative acneiform lesions on the back and chest of male teenagers. The distinctive feature is the tendency for large nodules to form exudative, necrotic, ulcerated, crusted plaques. Lesions often spare the face and heal with scarring. A preceding history of mild papulopustular or nodular acne is noted in most patients. Constitutional symptoms and signs are common, including fever, debilitation, arthralgias, myalgias, weight loss, and leukocytosis. Blood cultures are sterile. Lesions of **erythema nodosum** sometimes develop on the shins. **Osteolytic bone** lesions may develop in the clavicle, sternum, and epiphyseal growth plates; affected bones appear normal or have slight sclerosis or thickening on healing. Salicylates may be helpful for the myalgias, arthralgias, and fever. Corticosteroids (1 mg/kg of

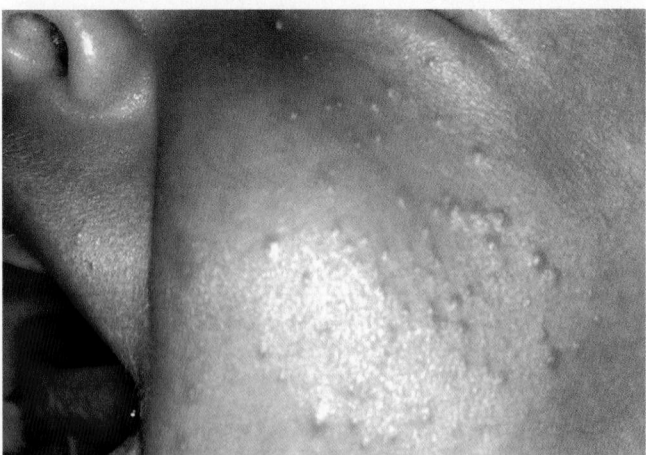

Figure 669-8 Comedonal acne in a neonate.

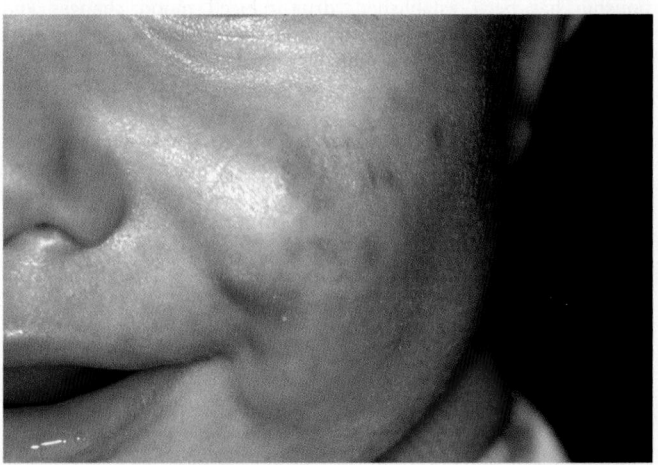

Figure 669-9 Inflammatory infantile acne.

prednisone) are started first. Then 1 wk later, isotretinoin (0.5-1.0 mg/kg) is added. Dapsone may be effective if isotretinoin cannot be used. The corticosteroid dosage is tapered over approximately 6 wk. Antibiotics are not indicated unless there is evidence of secondary infection. Compared with acne conglobata, acne fulminans occurs in younger patients, is more explosive in onset, more commonly has associated constitutional symptoms and ulcerated crusted lesions, and less commonly has multiheaded comedones or involves the face.

Bibliography is available at Expert Consult.

Chapter 670
Tumors of the Skin
Kari L. Martin

See also Chapters 506.2 and 596.

EPIDERMAL INCLUSION CYST (EPIDERMOID CYST)

Epidermoid cysts are the nodules most commonly seen in children. Such a cyst is a sharply circumscribed, dome-shaped, firm, freely movable, skin-colored nodule (Fig. 670-1) often with a central dimple or punctum that is a plugged, dilated pore of a pilosebaceous follicle. Epidermoid cysts form most frequently on the face, neck, chest, or upper back and may periodically become inflamed and infected secondarily, particularly in association with acne vulgaris. The cyst wall may also rupture and induce an inflammatory reaction in the dermis. The wall of the cyst is derived from the follicular infundibulum. A mass of layered keratinized material that may have a cheesy consistency fills the cavity. Epidermoid cysts may arise from occlusion of pilosebaceous follicles, from implantation of epidermal cells into the dermis as a result of an injury that penetrates the epidermis, and from rests of epidermal cells. Multiple epidermoid cysts may be present in Gardner syndrome and the nevoid basal cell carcinoma syndrome. Excision of the cysts with removal of the entire sac and its contents is indicated, particularly if the cyst becomes recurrently infected. A fluctuant, infected cyst should be treated with antibiotics or intralesional corticosteroids. After the inflammation subsides, the cyst should be removed.

MILIUM

Milium is a 1-2 mm, firm, pearly white or yellowish, subepidermal keratin cyst. Milia in newborns is discussed in Chapter 647. Secondary milia occur in association with subepidermal blistering diseases, after dermabrasion or other injury to the skin. They are retention cysts caused by hyperproliferation of injured epithelium and are indistinguishable histopathologically from primary milia. Those that develop after blistering usually arise from the eccrine sweat duct, but they may develop from the hair follicle, sebaceous duct, or epidermis. A milium body differs from an epidermoid cyst only in its small size and superficial location.

FIBROFOLLICULOMAS

These lesions usually appear in late adolescents or in young adults and are characterized by multiple dome-shaped clear-white papules appearing on the nose, cheeks, and neck, and at times the trunk or ears (Fig. 670-2). They are associated with the familial cancer syndrome of Birt-Hogg-Dubé, an autosomal dominant disorder that results from a mutation in the folliculin *(FLCN)* gene. Associated features include pulmonary cysts, pneumothorax, renal cell carcinoma, and other benign or malignant tumors.

PILAR CYST (TRICHILEMMAL CYST)

Pilar cyst may be clinically indistinguishable from an epidermoid cyst. It manifests as a smooth, firm, mobile nodule, predominantly on the scalp (Fig. 670-3). Pilar cysts occasionally develop on the face, neck, or trunk. A cyst may become inflamed and may occasionally suppurate and ulcerate. The cyst wall is composed of epithelial cells with indistinct intercellular bridges. The peripheral cell layer of the wall shows a palisade arrangement, which is not seen in an epidermoid cyst. No granular layer is present. The cyst cavity contains homogeneous eosinophilic keratinous material, and foci of calcification are seen in 25% of cases. The propensity for development of pilar cysts may be inherited in an autosomal dominant manner. More than one cyst generally develops in a patient. Numerous pilar and epidermoid cysts, desmoid tumors, fibromas, lipomas, or osteomas may be associated with colonic polyposis or adenocarcinoma in Gardner syndrome. Pilar cysts shell out easily from the dermis.

PILOMATRICOMA

The second most common nodule seen in children, pilomatricoma is a benign tumor that manifests as a 3-30 mm, firm, solitary, deep dermal or subcutaneous tumor on the head, neck, or upper extremities. The overlying epidermis is usually normal. The tumor may occasionally be located more superficially, however, tinting the overlying skin

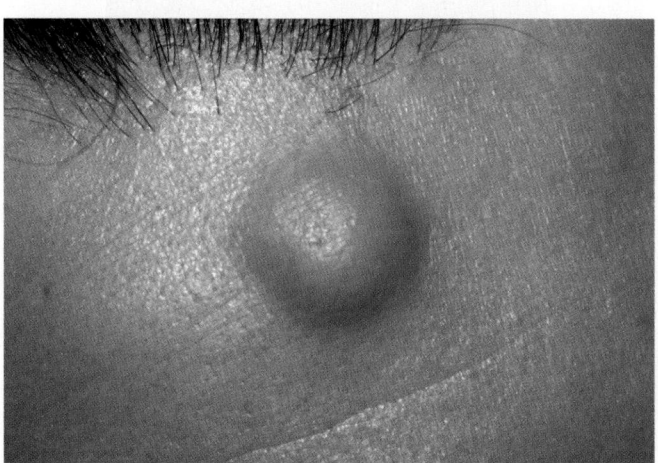

Figure 670-1 Flesh-colored cyst on the forehead.

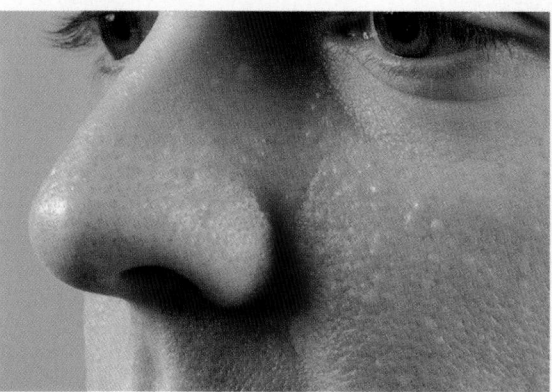

Figure 670-2 Multiple, dome-shaped, whitish papules on the nose and cheeks in a 31 yr old carrier of an *FLCN* mutation. *(From Menko FH, van Steensel MAM, Giraud S, et al: Birt-Hogg-Dubé syndrome: diagnosis and management. Lancet 10:1199–1206, 2009, Fig. 1.)*

blue-red (Fig. 670-4). Multiple pilomatricomas are seen in myotonic dystrophy, Gardner syndrome, Rubinstein-Taybi syndrome, and Turner syndrome. In general, however, pilomatricomas are not hereditary. Histopathologically, irregularly shaped islands of epithelial cells are embedded in a cellular stroma. Calcium deposits are found in 75% of tumors. Pilomatricomas are caused by mutations in β-catenin.

TRICHOEPITHELIOMA

A 2-8 mm, smooth, round, firm, skin-colored papule, trichoepithelioma is derived from an immature hair follicle. Trichoepitheliomas generally occur singly on the face in childhood or early adulthood. Multiple trichoepitheliomas are inherited autosomal dominantly (type 1: *CYLD* gene; type 2: 9p21 gene currently unidentified), appear in childhood or at puberty, and gradually increase in number on the nasofacial folds, nose, forehead, and upper lip and, occasionally, on the scalp, neck, and upper trunk. Microscopically, these benign tumors are characterized by horn cysts composed of a fully keratinized center surrounded by basophilic cells in an adenoid network. Topical imiquimod therapy may be beneficial. Surgical excision is the only other therapy.

ERUPTIVE VELLUS HAIR CYSTS

Eruptive vellus hair cysts are 1-3 mm, asymptomatic, soft, skin-colored follicular papules on the central chest (Fig. 670-5). They may become crusted or umbilicated. Abnormal vellus hair follicles become occluded at the level of the infundibulum, resulting in retention of hairs within an epithelium-lined cystic dilation of the proximal part of the follicle. Most cases are chronic, but spontaneous regression has been reported.

STEATOCYSTOMA MULTIPLEX

An autosomal dominant (*KRT17* gene) condition, steatocystoma multiplex usually manifests in adolescence or early adulthood as numerous soft to firm cystic nodules that are adherent to the underlying skin and are 3 mm to 3 cm in diameter. When punctured, the cysts may drain oily or cheesy material. Sites of predilection include the sternal region, axillae, arms, and scrotal skin. The multiply folded cyst wall is lined on the luminal side with a thick, homogeneous, eosinophilic horny layer and lacks a granular layer. Flattened sebaceous gland lobules are often visible in the cyst wall, and lanugo hairs may be present in the cystic cavity.

SYRINGOMA

The benign tumors known as syringomas are soft, small, skin-colored or yellowish brown papules that develop on the face, particularly in the periorbital regions (Fig. 670-6). Other sites of predilection include the axillae and umbilical and pubic areas. They often develop during puberty and are more frequent in females. Eruptive syringomas develop in crops over the anterior trunk during childhood or adolescence. A

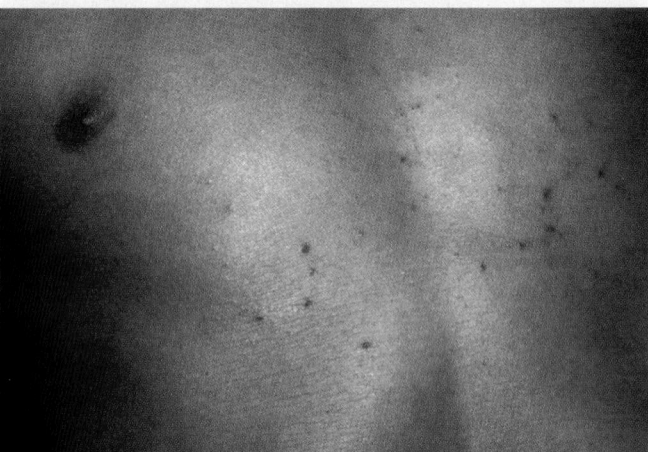

Figure 670-5 Eruptive vellus hair cysts. Multiple papules on the chest.

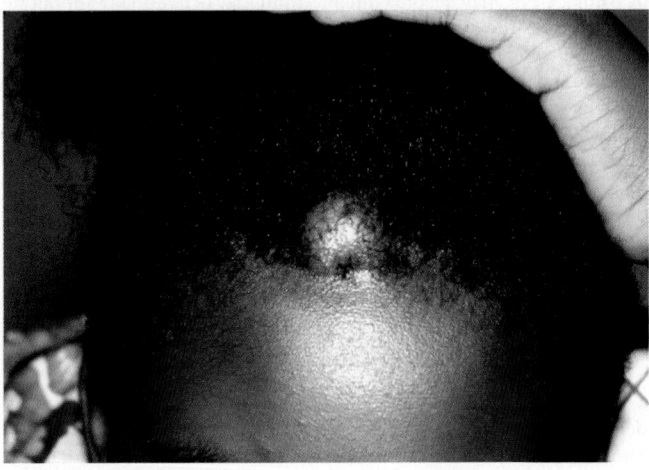

Figure 670-3 Pilar cyst of the anterior scalp.

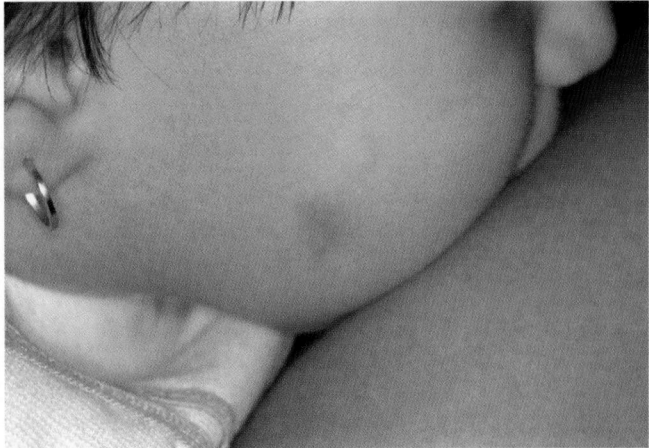

Figure 670-4 Pilomatricoma. Firm tumor with overlying bluish discoloration of the skin.

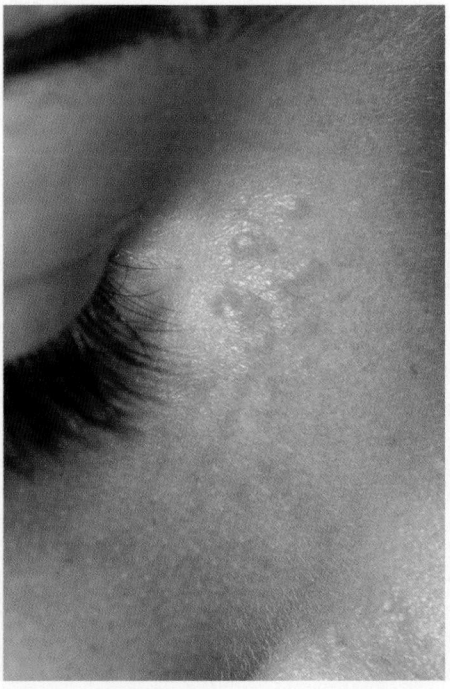

Figure 670-6 Syringomas. Multiple yellow papules near the eye.

syringoma is derived from an intraepidermal sweat gland duct. Syringomas are of cosmetic significance only. Sparse lesions may be excised, but they are often too numerous to remove.

INFANTILE DIGITAL FIBROMA

Infantile digital fibroma is a smooth, firm, erythematous or skin-colored nodule on the dorsal or lateral surface of a distal phalanx of a finger or toe. More than 80% of tumors occur in infancy. They may be present at birth. Lesions may be solitary or multiple and may manifest as "kissing" tumors on opposing digits. They are usually asymptomatic, but flexion deformity of the digits may occur. Clinically, the lesion resembles a fibroma, leiomyoma, angiofibroma, acquired digital fibrokeratoma, accessory digit, or mucous cyst. The diagnosis is confirmed by the finding of numerous spindle-shaped fibroblasts that contain small, round, dense, eosinophilic cytoplasmic inclusion bodies composed of collections of actin microfilaments. Local recurrence after simple excision of this tumor has been reported in 75% of patients. Because the tumor does not metastasize and may regress spontaneously in 2-3 yr, a course of expectant observation is advised. If functional impairment or flexion deformity of the digit becomes apparent, prompt full excision of the tumor is indicated.

DERMATOFIBROMA (HISTIOCYTOMA)

A benign dermal tumor, dermatofibroma may be pedunculated, nodular (Fig. 670-7), or flat and is usually well circumscribed and firm but occasionally feels soft on palpation. The overlying skin is usually hyperpigmented, may be shiny or keratotic, and dimples when the tumor is pinched. Dermatofibromas range in size from 0.5-10.0 mm, arise most frequently on the limbs, and are usually asymptomatic but may occasionally be pruritic. They are composed of fibroblasts, young and mature collagen, capillaries, and histiocytes in varying proportions, forming a nodule in the dermis that has poorly defined edges. The cause of these tumors is unknown, but trauma such as an insect bite or folliculitis appears to induce reactive fibroplasia. The differential diagnosis includes epidermal inclusion cyst, juvenile xanthogranuloma, hypertrophic scar, and neurofibroma. Dermatofibromas may be excised or left intact, according to the patient's preference. They usually persist indefinitely.

JUVENILE XANTHOGRANULOMA

A firm, dome-shaped, yellow, pink, or orange papule or nodule (Fig. 670-8), juvenile xanthogranuloma varies from 5 mm to approximately 4 cm in diameter. The average age at onset is 2 yr. These nodules are 10 times more common in white than in African-American individuals. Sites of predilection are the scalp, face, and upper trunk, where they may erupt in profusion or remain as solitary lesions. Nodular lesions may appear on the oral mucosa. Mature lesions are characterized histopathologically by a dermal infiltrate of lipid-laden histiocytes, admixed inflammatory cells, and Touton giant cells. The lesions may clinically resemble papulonodular urticaria pigmentosa, dermatofibromas, or xanthomas of hyperlipoproteinemia, but can be distinguished from these entities histopathologically.

Affected infants are nearly always otherwise normal, and blood lipid values are not elevated. Café-au-lait macules are found on 20% of patients with juvenile xanthogranuloma. Xanthogranulomatous infiltrates occur occasionally in ocular tissues. This process may result in glaucoma, hyphema, uveitis, heterochromia iridis, iritis, or sudden proptosis. Age less than 2 yr, multiple lesions, and periocular location may heighten concerns for intraocular involvement. There appears to be an association among juvenile xanthogranuloma, neurofibromatosis, and childhood leukemia, most frequently juvenile chronic myelogenous leukemia. There is no need to remove the benign lesions of juvenile xanthogranuloma because most of them regress spontaneously in the 1st few yr. Residual pigmentation and atrophy may result.

LIPOMA

A benign collection of fatty tissue, lipoma appears on the trunk, neck, or proximal portions of the limbs. Lipomas are soft, compressible, lobulated, subcutaneous masses. Multiple lesions may occur occasionally, as in Gardner syndrome. Atrophy, calcification, liquefaction, or xanthomatous change may sometimes complicate their course. A lipoma is composed of normal fat cells surrounded by a thin connective tissue capsule. Lipomas represent a cosmetic defect and may be surgically excised. Multiple lipomas, identical to those that occur singly, are inherited in an autosomal dominant fashion and often appear by the 3rd decade in patients with familial multiple lipomatosis. Lipomas may appear intraabdominally, intramuscularly, and subcutaneously. Congenital lipomatosis manifests in the 1st few mo of life as large subcutaneous fatty masses on the chest, with extension into skeletal muscle. Congenital lipomatosis can also be a manifestation of Proteus syndrome (overgrowth/hyperplasia skin, connective tissue, mutation in *AKT1*). Angiolipomas usually manifest as numerous painful subcutaneous nodules on the arms and trunk.

CLOVES syndrome (congenital lipomatous overgrowth, vascular malformations, epidermal nevi, and scoliosis/skeletal-spinal anomalies) is usually a sporadic disorder with an asymmetric truncal lipomatous mass present at birth. Additional features include macrodactyly, vascular malformations (low flow), linear epidermal nevus and renal anomalies. The differential diagnosis includes Proteus, Klippel-Trenaunay, and Bannayan-Riley-Ruvalcaba syndrome.

BASAL CELL CARCINOMA

Basal cell carcinoma is very rare in children in the absence of a predisposing condition, such as nevoid basal cell carcinoma syndrome, xeroderma pigmentosum, nevus sebaceus of Jadassohn, arsenic intake, or exposure to irradiation. The lesions are smooth, pearly, pink, telangiectatic papules that enlarge slowly and may bleed or ulcerate. Sites of predilection are the face, scalp, and upper back. The differential

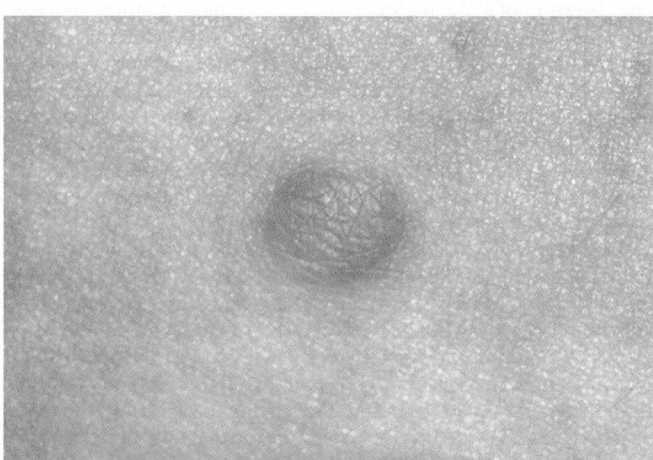

Figure 670-7 Dermatofibroma. Red-brown nodular variant.

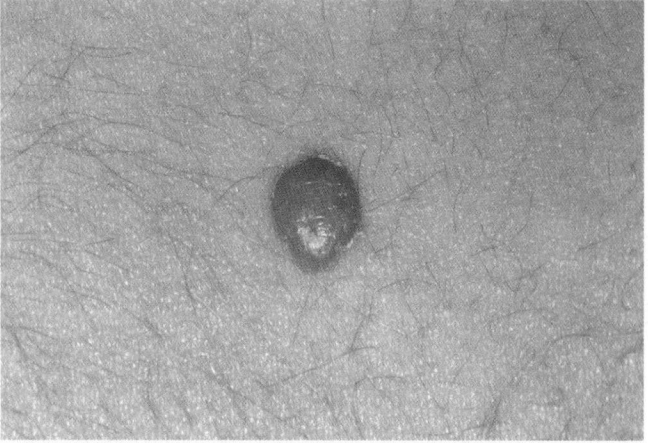

Figure 670-8 Juvenile xanthogranuloma. Solitary orange papule.

diagnosis includes pyogenic granuloma, nevocellular nevus, epidermal inclusion cyst, closed comedo, dermatofibroma, and adnexal tumor. Depending on the site of occurrence and associated disease of the host, electrodesiccation and curettage or simple excision of basal cell epithelioma is usually curative. When the tumor is recurrent, >2 cm in diameter, located on problematic anatomic areas such as the midface or ears, or is an aggressive histopathologic type, Mohs microscopically controlled surgery may be the most appropriate treatment.

NEVOID BASAL CELL CARCINOMA SYNDROME (BASAL CELL NEVUS SYNDROME, GORLIN SYNDROME)

The autosomal dominant entity known as nevoid basal cell carcinoma syndrome is caused by mutations in the *PTCH1* and *PTCH2* ("patched") genes. These tumor-suppressor genes, part of the hedgehog signaling pathway, are important in determining embryonic patterning and cell fate in a number of structures in the developing embryo. Mutations in human patched genes produce dysregulation of several genes involved in organogenesis and carcinogenesis. Consequently, the syndrome includes a wide spectrum of defects involving the skin, eyes, central nervous and endocrine systems, and bones. The predominant features are early-onset basal cell carcinomas and mandibular cysts. Approximately 20% of those in whom a basal cell carcinoma develops before age 19 yr have this syndrome. Basal cell carcinomas appear between puberty and age 35 yr, erupting in crops of tumors that vary in size, color, and number, and may be difficult to distinguish from other types of skin lesions. Sites of predilection are the periorbital skin, nose, malar areas, and upper lip, but the lesions can develop on the trunk and limbs and are not restricted to sun-exposed areas. Ulceration, bleeding, crusting, and local invasion can occur. Small milia, epidermal cysts, pigmented lesions, hirsutism, and palmar and plantar pits are additional cutaneous findings.

The facies of patients with this syndrome are characterized by temporoparietal bossing, prominent supraorbital ridges, a broad nasal root, ocular hypertelorism or dystopia canthorum, and prognathism. Keratinized cysts (odontogenic keratocysts) in the maxilla and mandible occur in most patients. They range in size from a few millimeters to several centimeters, may result in maldevelopment of the teeth, and cause pain, swelling of the jaw, facial deformity, bone erosion, pathologic fractures, and suppurating sinus tracts. Osseous defects such as anomalous rib development, spina bifida, kyphoscoliosis, and brachymetacarpalism occur in 60% of patients, and ocular abnormalities including cataracts, glaucoma, coloboma, strabismus, and blindness occur in approximately 25%. Some males have hypogonadism, and the testes are absent or undescended. Kidney malformations have also been reported. Neurologic manifestations include calcification of the falx, seizures, mental retardation, partial agenesis of the corpus callosum, hydrocephalus, and nerve deafness. The incidence of medulloblastoma, ameloblastoma of the oral cavity, fibrosarcoma of the jaw, teratoma, cystadenoma, cardiac fibroma, ovarian fibroma, and fetal onset rhabdomyoma is higher in patients with nevoid basal cell carcinoma syndrome.

Treatment of these patients requires the participation of various specialists according to individual clinical problems. Basal cell carcinomas should not be treated with irradiation. Most of the basal cell carcinomas have a clinically benign course, and it is often impossible to remove them all. Those with an aggressive growth pattern and those on the central areas of the face, however, should be removed promptly. Treatment options include surgery, Mohs micrographic surgery, laser ablation, cryotherapy, photodynamic therapy, topical 5% imiquimod and oral retinoids (0.5-1.0 mg/kg/day). Vismodegib, which inhibits smoothened protein in the hedgehog pathway, is a targeted therapy available for unresectable basal cell carcinomas. Genetic counseling is also indicated.

MUCOSAL NEUROMA SYNDROME (MULTIPLE ENDOCRINE NEOPLASIA TYPE IIB)

Mucosal neuroma syndrome, an autosomal dominant trait, is characterized by an asthenic or marfanoid habitus with scoliosis, pectus excavatum, pes cavus, and muscular hypotonia. The syndrome is caused by mutations in the tyrosine kinase domain of the *RET* gene. Patients have thick, patulous lips and soft-tissue prognathism simulating acromegaly. Multiple mucosal neuromas or neurofibromas appear as pink, pedunculated or sessile nodules on the anterior third of the tongue, at the commissures of the lips, and on the buccal mucosa and palpebral conjunctiva. Various ophthalmologic defects and intestinal ganglioneuromatosis with recurrent diarrhea are additional common findings. There is a high incidence of medullary thyroid carcinoma in association with high calcitonin levels, pheochromocytoma, and hyperparathyroidism in patients with this syndrome. Periodic screening tests for the associated malignant tumors are mandatory.

Bibliography is available at Expert Consult.

Chapter **671**
Nutritional Dermatoses
Joel C. Joyce

ACRODERMATITIS ENTEROPATHICA

Acrodermatitis enteropathica is a rare autosomal recessive disorder caused by an inability to absorb sufficient zinc from the diet. The genetic defect is in the intestinal zinc-specific transporter gene *SLC39A4*. Initial signs and symptoms usually occur in the 1st few mo of life, often after weaning from breast milk to cow's milk. The cutaneous eruption consists of vesiculobullous, eczematous, dry, scaly, or psoriasiform skin lesions symmetrically distributed in the perioral, acral, and perineal areas (Fig. 671-1) and on the cheeks, knees, and elbows (Fig. 671-2). The hair often has a peculiar, reddish tint, and alopecia of some degree is characteristic. Ocular manifestations include photophobia, conjunctivitis, blepharitis, and corneal dystrophy detectable by slit-lamp examination. Associated manifestations include chronic diarrhea, stomatitis, glossitis, paronychia, nail dystrophy, growth retardation, irritability, delayed wound healing, intercurrent bacterial infections, and superinfection with *Candida albicans*. Lymphocyte function and free radical scavenging are impaired. Without treatment, the course is chronic and intermittent but often relentlessly progressive. When the disease is less severe, only growth retardation and delayed development may be apparent.

The **diagnosis** is established by the constellation of clinical findings and detection of a low plasma zinc concentration. A serum zinc level less than 50 µg/dL is suggestive, but not diagnostic, of acrodermatitis enteropathica. Levels of alkaline phosphatase, a zinc-dependent enzyme, may also be decreased. Histopathologic changes in the skin are nonspecific and include parakeratosis and pallor of the upper epidermis. The variety of manifestations of the syndrome may be because zinc has a role in numerous metabolic pathways, including those of copper, protein, essential fatty acids, and prostaglandins, and that zinc is incorporated into many zinc metalloenzymes.

Oral **therapy** with zinc compounds is the treatment of choice. Replacement for individuals with inherited acrodermatitis enteropathica is with 3 mg/kg/24 hr of elemental zinc found in zinc sulfate, gluconate, or acetate (i.e., 220 mg of zinc sulfate contains 50 mg of elemental zinc). Zinc gluconate carries less risk of gastrointestinal distress. Plasma zinc levels should be monitored every 3-6 mo, however, to individualize the dosage. Zinc therapy rapidly abolishes the manifestations of the disease. A syndrome resembling acrodermatitis enteropathica has been observed in patients with secondary zinc deficiency resulting from long-term total parenteral nutrition without

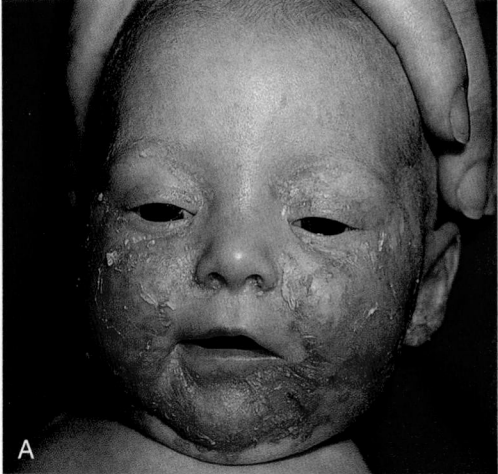

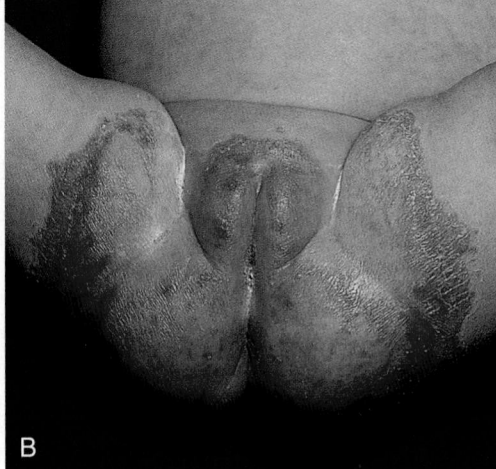

Figure 671-1 A, Periorificial eruption. **B,** Diaper rash. The skin findings are typical of zinc deficiency, in this case caused by low levels of zinc in breast milk. *(From Eichenfield LF, Frieden IJ, Esterly NB: Textbook of neonatal dermatology, Philadelphia, 2001, WB Saunders, Fig. 14-14.)*

supplemental zinc or to chronic malabsorption syndromes. A rash similar to that of acrodermatitis enteropathica has also been reported in infants fed breast milk that is low in zinc and in those with maple syrup urine disease, organic aciduria, methylmalonic acidemia, biotinidase deficiency, essential fatty acid deficiency, severe protein malnutrition (kwashiorkor), and cystic fibrosis. For those individuals with acquired zinc deficiency, oral replacement with 0.5-1.0 mg/kg/24 hr of elemental zinc should be undertaken and the cause of underlying malnutrition should be addressed.

ESSENTIAL FATTY ACID DEFICIENCY

Essential fatty acid deficiency causes a generalized, scaly dermatitis composed of thickened, erythematous, desquamating plaques. Individuals may also show failure-to-thrive, growth retardation, alopecia, thrombocytopenia, and poor wound healing. The eruption has been induced experimentally in animals fed a fat-free diet and has been observed in patients with chronic severe malabsorption, such as in short-gut syndrome, and in those sustained on a fat-free diet or fat-free parenteral alimentation. Linoleic acid (18:2 n-6) and arachidonic acid (20:4 n-6) are deficient, and an abnormal metabolite, 5,8,11-eicosatrienoic acid (20:3 n-9), is present in the plasma. Alterations in the triene:tetraene ratio are diagnostic (arachidonic acid:eicosatrienoic acid ratio greater than 0.4 or linoleic acid:arachidonic acid ratio greater than 2.3). The horny layer of the skin contains microscopic cracks, the barrier function of the skin is disturbed, and transepidermal water loss is increased. Topical application of linoleic acid, which is present in sunflower seed and safflower oils, may ameliorate the clinical and biochemical skin manifestations. Oral and/or parenteral therapy can also be considered. Appropriate nutrition should be provided.

KWASHIORKOR

Severe protein and essential amino acid deprivation in association with adequate caloric intake can lead to kwashiorkor, particularly at the time of weaning to a diet that consists primarily of corn, rice (or rice milk), or beans (see Chapter 46). Children can be fed such a restricted diet for cultural reasons or because of misdiagnosis on the part of the child's parents or healthcare providers of perceived food allergies. Diffuse fine reddish brown scaling (enamel/flaky paint sign) is the classic cutaneous finding. In severe cases, erosions and linear fissures

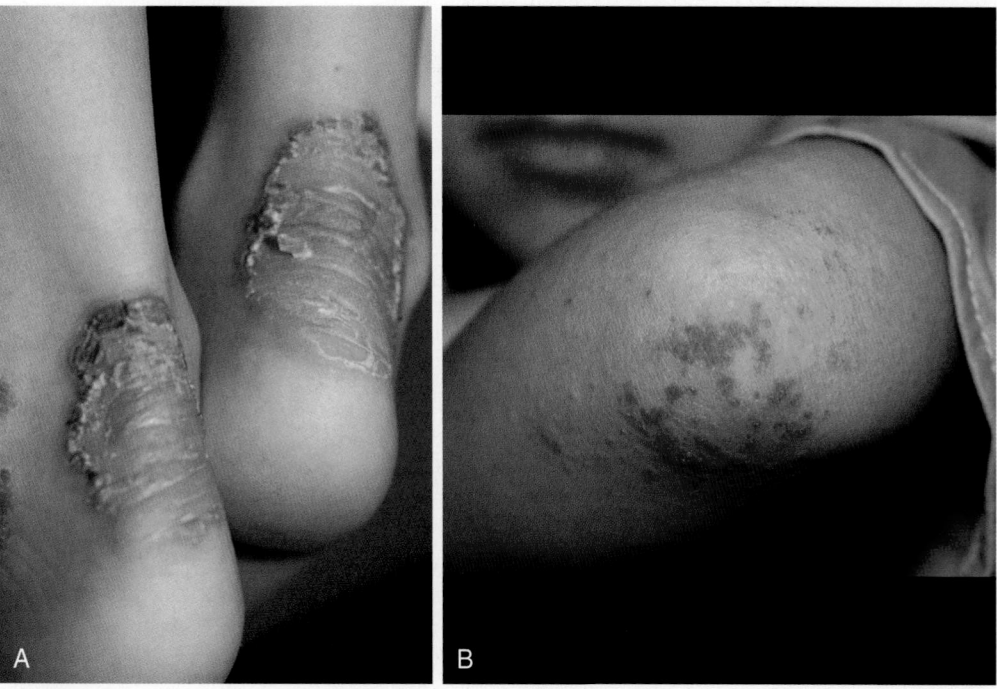

Figure 671-2 A, Psoriasiform lesion of zinc deficiency dermatitis on the ankles. **B,** Similar lesions on the elbows.

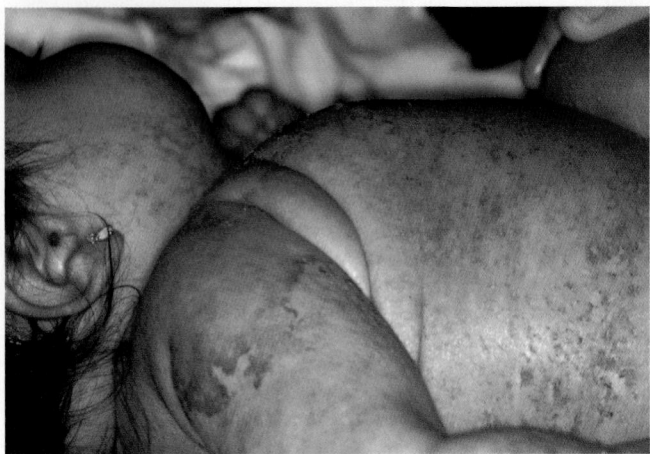

Figure 671-3 Erosions and scaling in kwashiorkor.

develop (Fig. 671-3). Nails are thin and soft, and hair is sparse, thin, and depigmented, sometimes displaying a "flag sign" consisting of alternating light and dark bands that reflect alternating periods of adequate and inadequate nutrition. The cutaneous manifestations may closely resemble those of acrodermatitis enteropathica, however; edema of the extremities and face ("moon facies") and a protuberant abdomen ("pot belly") are key features uniformly observed in kwashiorkor. The serum zinc level is often deficient, and in some cases, skin lesions of kwashiorkor heal more rapidly when zinc is applied topically.

CYSTIC FIBROSIS
See Chapter 403.

Protein-calorie malnutrition develops in 5-10% of patients with cystic fibrosis. Rash in infants with cystic fibrosis and malnutrition is rare but may appear by age 6 mo. The initial eruption consists of scaling, erythematous papules and progresses in 1-3 mo to extensive desquamating plaques. The rash is accentuated around the mouth and perineum and on the extremities (lower > upper). Alopecia may be present, but mucous membranes and nails are uninvolved.

PELLAGRA
See Chapter 49.

Pellagra manifests as edema, erythema, and burning of sun-exposed skin on the face, neck, and dorsal aspects of the hands, forearms, and feet. Lesions of pellagra may also be provoked by burns, pressure, friction, and inflammation. The eruption on the face frequently follows a butterfly distribution, and the dermatitis encircling the neck has been termed "Casal's necklace." Blisters and scales develop, and the skin increasingly becomes dry, rough, thickened, cracked, and hyperpigmented. Skin infections may be unusually severe. Pellagra develops in patients with insufficient dietary intake or malabsorption of niacin and/or tryptophan. Administration of isoniazid, 6-mercaptopurine, or 5-fluorouracil may also produce pellagra. Hartnup disease (see Chapter 85), caused by a mutation in *SLC6A19* that encodes a neutral amino acid transporter, is a rare autosomal recessive disorder that presents in infancy with a "pellagra-like syndrome" as a result of decreased absorption of tryptophan. Nicotinamide supplementation and sun avoidance are the mainstays of therapy in pellagra.

SCURVY (VITAMIN C OR ASCORBIC ACID DEFICIENCY)
See Chapter 50.

Scurvy manifests initially as follicular hyperkeratosis, coiling of the hair on the upper arms, back, buttocks, and lower extremities. Other features are perifollicular erythema and hemorrhage, particularly on the legs and advancing to involve large areas of hemorrhage; swollen, erythematous gums; stomatitis; and subperiosteal hematomas. In children, the most common risk factors are behavioral or psychiatric disease that results in poor nutrition. The best method of confirmation of a clinical diagnosis of scurvy is a trial of vitamin C supplementation.

VITAMIN A DEFICIENCY
See Chapter 48.1.

Vitamin A deficiency manifests initially as impairment of visual adaptation to the dark. Cutaneous changes include xerosis and hyperkeratosis and hyperplasia of the epidermis, particularly the lining of hair follicles and sebaceous glands. In severe cases, desquamation may be prominent.

Bibliography is available at Expert Consult.

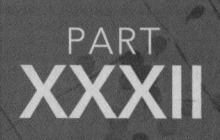

Section 1

Orthopedic Problems

Chapter 672

Growth and Development

Keith D. Baldwin, Lawrence Wells, and John P. Dormans

Statistically, normal is defined as 95% of a population that falls within 2 SD of the mean from any given measurement. Statistically normal should not be confused with ideal in any given person or parent's mind. Table 672-1 lists terms used to describe some common deviations from normal. Congenital anomalies can be categorized into production problems and packaging problems. Production problems include abnormalities caused by malformation, dysplasia, or disruption that will not spontaneously resolve (see Chapter 108). Packaging problems include deformations caused by mechanical causes including in utero positioning and molding, and they usually resolve with time.

IN UTERO POSITIONING

In utero positioning produces temporary joint and muscle contractures and affects the torsional alignment of the long bones, particularly those of the lower extremities. Normal full-term newborns can have up to 20-30 degree hip and knee flexion contractures. These contractures tend to resolve by 4-6 mo of age. The newborn hip externally rotates in extension up to 80-90 degrees and has limited internal rotation to approximately 0-10 degrees. The lower leg often has inward rotation (internal tibial torsion). The face may also be distorted; the spine and upper extremities are less affected by the in utero position. The effects of in utero positioning, therefore, are physiologic in origin and resolve by 3-4 mo of age.

GROWTH AND DEVELOPMENT

Consideration of growth and development helps to formulate treatment strategies designed to preserve or restore normal growth potential. Growth is subject to many variables including genetics, nutrition, general health, endocrine status, mechanical forces, and physiologic age. Growth also varies between 2 anatomic regions and even between 2 bones of the same region.

Bone formation or ossification occurs in 2 different ways. In **endochondral ossification**, mesenchymal cells undergo chondrogenesis to form cartilage that matures to become bone. Most bones in the axial and appendicular skeleton are formed in this manner. In **intramembranous ossification**, osteoblasts are formed by direct differentiation of mesenchymal cells into bone. Flat bones of the skull and clavicle are examples of this pattern of bone formation.

CENTERS OF OSSIFICATION

At the beginning of the fetal period the chondrocytes in the midshaft of the long bones form the **primary** centers of growth from which the bone eventually lengthens. **Secondary** centers of ossification appear in the chondroepiphysis and mostly appear postnatally. They direct the formation of bone throughout growth, particularly joint development. The ossification centers that are typically present at birth are the distal femur, proximal tibia, calcaneus, and talus.

Anatomic Locations: Descriptive Terms

Typical **long bones are divided into** the physis, epiphysis, metaphysis, diaphysis, and perichondrial ring (Fig. 672-1). The physis is the growth plate located at the end of bone. The epiphysis is typically a secondary ossification center that contributes to joint development. The metaphysis is the bone adjacent to the physis on the side away from the joint. The diaphysis is the central part or shaft of long bones. The perichondrial ring contributes to appositional growth.

The articular cartilage also contributes to the growth of the epiphysis. The perichondrial ring, which surrounds the physes, and the perichondrium around the epiphyses and periosteum, which surrounds the metaphysis and diaphyseal regions of the bone, contribute to appositional or circumferential growth. Bones without physes (pelvis, scapulae, carpals, tarsals) grow by appositional bone growth from their surrounding perichondrium and periosteum. Other bones (metacarpals, metatarsals, phalanges, spine) grow by a combination of appositional and endochondral ossification.

Table 672-1	Terminologies for Deviations
TERMINOLOGY	**DESCRIPTION**
Congenital	Anomaly that is apparent at birth
Deformation	A normally formed structure that is pushed out of shape by mechanical forces
Deformity	A body part altered in shape from normal, outside the normal range
Developmental	A deviation that occurs over time; one that might not be present or apparent at birth
Disruption	A structure undergoing normal development that stops developing or is destroyed or removed
Dysplasia	A tissue that is abnormal or wrongly constructed
Malformation	A structure that is wrongly built; failure of embryologic development or differentiation resulting in abnormal or missing structures

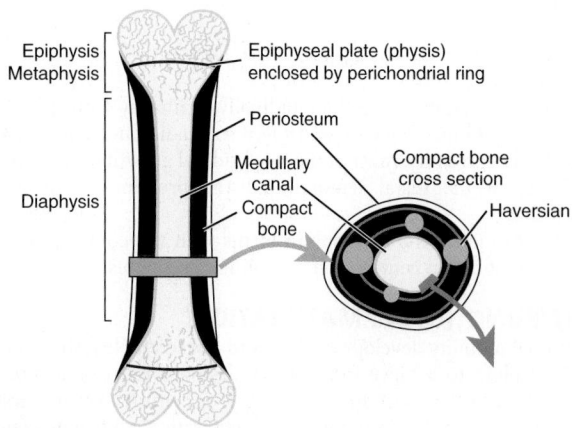

Figure 672-1 Diagram showing typical long bone divisions.

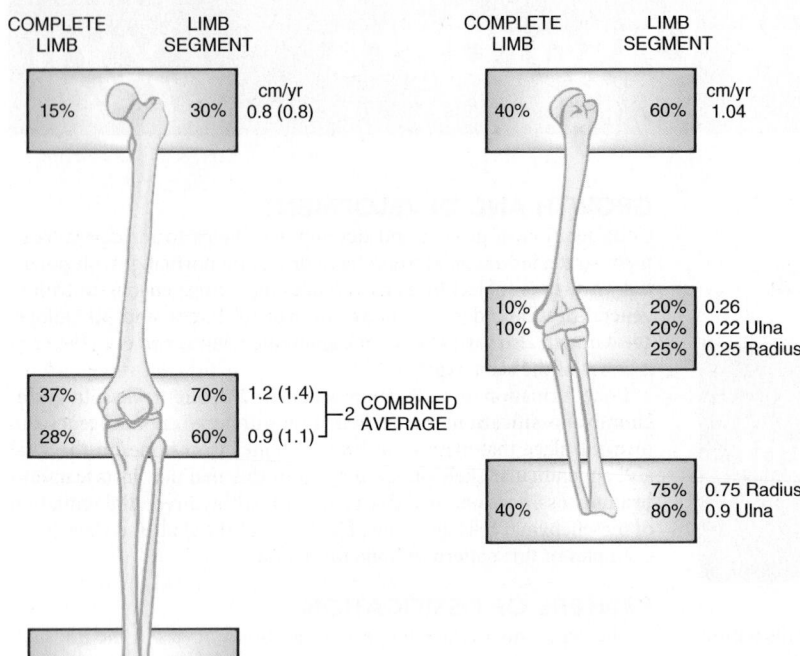

Figure 672-2 The contribution (%) of each physis to the overall length of the extremities. (*From Morrissy R, Weinstein S, editors:* Lovell and Winter's pediatric orthopedics, *ed 5, Philadelphia, 2001, Lippincott Williams & Wilkins.*)

Table 672-2	Skeletal Growth Considerations

- Abnormal stature can be assessed as "proportionate" or "disproportionate" based on comparing the ratio of sitting height with subischial height (lower limbs).
- Normally the arm span is almost equal to standing height.
- The head is disproportionately large at birth and ratio of head height to total height is approximately 1 : 4 at birth, which changes to 1 : 7.5 at skeletal maturity.
- Lower extremities account for approximately 15% of height at birth and 30% at skeletal maturity.
- The rate of height and growth increase is not constant and varies with growth spurts.
- By age 5 yr, birth height usually doubles and the child is approximately 60% of adult height. The child is approximately 80% of final height at 9 yr. During puberty, the standing height increases by approximately 1 cm/mo.
- Bone age is more important than chronologic age in determining future growth potential.

Important Growth and Developmental Milestones

Table 672-2 summarizes some important musculoskeletal growth considerations.

Growth Patterns in Upper and Lower Extremities

The upper extremity grows longitudinally, primarily from physes of the proximal humeral physis and the distal radial and ulnar physes. In the lower extremity, most of the longitudinal growth occurs around the knee, in the distal femoral and the proximal tibial physes (Fig. 672-2).

In the hip joint, the acetabulum forms with the convergence of 3 primary ossification centers: ischium, ilium, and pubis.

GAIT/FUNCTIONAL MATURATION

Functional mobility develops in infants in a predictable fashion (Table 672-3). Failure to achieve functional milestones is an indication for referral to a neurologist to determine if a central nervous system problem exists. Central nervous system maturation contributes significantly to the development of gait. In early ambulation (at 8-15 mo),

Table 672-3	Functional Milestones
MILESTONE	**ACHIEVED BY**
Head control	3-6 months
Sitting	6-9 months
Crawling	8 months
Pulling to stand	8-12 months
Ambulating	12-18 months

the child usually has a wide-based gait with hyperflexion of hips and knees, and initial contact with the heel. By the age of 2 yr, the wide gait diminishes, reciprocal arm swing begins, and there is increased stride length and velocity. Adult fluid gait patterns usually start developing by 3 yr and mature to an adult-like pattern by age 7 yr.

Bibliography is available at Expert Consult.

Chapter **673**
Evaluation of the Child
Keith D. Baldwin, Lawrence Wells, and John P. Dormans

A detailed history and thorough physical examination are critical to the evaluation of a child with an orthopedic problem. The child's family and acquaintances are important sources of information, especially in younger children and infants. Appropriate radiographic imaging and, occasionally, laboratory testing may be necessary to support the clinical diagnosis.

HISTORY

A comprehensive history should include details about the prenatal, perinatal, and postnatal periods. Prenatal history should include maternal health issues: smoking, prenatal vitamins, illicit use of drugs or narcotics, alcohol consumption, diabetes, rubella, and sexually transmitted infections. The child's prenatal and perinatal history should include information about the length of pregnancy, length of labor, type of labor (induced or spontaneous), presentation of fetus, evidence of any fetal distress at delivery, requirements of oxygen following the delivery, birth length and weight, Apgar score, muscle tone at birth, feeding history, and period of hospitalization. In older infants and young children, evaluation of developmental milestones for posture, locomotion, dexterity, social activities, and speech are important. Specific orthopedic questions should focus on joint, muscular, appendicular, or axial skeleton complaints. Information regarding pain or other symptoms in any of these areas should be appropriately elicited (Table 673-1). The family history can give clues to heritable disorders. It also can forecast expectations of the child's future development and allow appropriate interventions as necessary.

PHYSICAL EXAMINATION

The orthopedic physical examination includes a thorough examination of the musculoskeletal system along with a comprehensive neurologic examination. The musculoskeletal examination includes inspection, palpation, and evaluation of motion, stability, and gait. A basic neurologic examination includes sensory examination, motor function, and reflexes. The orthopedic physical examination requires basic knowledge of anatomy of joint range of motion, alignment, and stability. Many common musculoskeletal disorders can be diagnosed by the history and physical examination alone. One screening tool that has been useful in adults has now been adapted and evaluated for use in children, the pediatric gait, arms, legs, spine (pGALS) test, the components of which are listed in Figure 673-1.

Inspection

Initial examination of the child begins with inspection. The clinician should use the guidelines listed in Table 673-2 during inspection.

Palpation

Palpation of the involved region should include assessment of local temperature and tenderness; assessment for a swelling or mass, spasticity or contracture, and bone or joint deformity; and evaluation of anatomic axis of limb and of limb lengths.

Contractures are a loss of mobility of a joint from congenital or acquired causes and are caused by periarticular soft-tissue fibrosis or involvement of muscles crossing the joint. Congenital contractures are common in **arthrogryposis** (see Chapter 682). Spasticity is an abnormal increase in tone associated with hyperreflexia and is common in cerebral palsy.

Deformity of the bone or joint is an abnormal fixed shape or position from congenital or acquired causes. It is important to assess the type of deformity, its location, and degree of deformity upon clinical examination. It is also important to assess whether the deformity is fixed or can be passively or actively corrected and whether there is any associated muscle spasm, local tenderness, or pain on motion. Classification of the deformity depends on the plane of deformity: **varus** (away from midline) or **valgus** (apex toward midline), or **recurvatum** (backward curvature) or **flexion** deformity (sagittal plane). In the axial skeleton, especially the spine, deformity can be defined as scoliosis, kyphosis, hyperlordosis, and kyphoscoliosis.

Range of Motion

Active and passive joint motion should be assessed, recorded, and compared to the opposite side. Objective evaluation should be done with a goniometer and recorded.

Vocabulary for direction of joint motion is as follows:

Abduction: Away from the midline
Adduction: Toward the midline
Flexion: Movement of bending from the starting position
Extension: Movement from bending to the starting position
Supination: Rotating the forearm to face the palm upward
Pronation: Rotating the forearm to face the palm downward
Inversion: Turning the hindfoot inward
Eversion: Turning the hindfoot outward
Plantarflexion: Pointing the toes away from the body (toward the floor)
Dorsiflexion: Pointing the toes toward the body (toward the ceiling)
Internal rotation: Turning inward toward the axis of the body
External rotation: Turning outward away from the axis of the body

Table 673-1	Characterization of Pain and Presenting Symptom

Location: Whether pain is localized to a particular segment or involves a larger area
Intensity: Usually on a pain scale of 1-10
Quality: Tumor pain is often unrelenting, progressive, and often present during the night. Pain at night particularly suggests osteoid osteoma. Pain in inflammation and infection is usually continuous
Onset: Was it acute and related to specific trauma or was it insidious? Acute pain and history of trauma are more commonly associated with fractures.
Duration: Whether transient, only lasting for minutes, or lasting for hours or days. Pain lasting for longer than 3-4 wk suggests a serious underlying problem.
Progress: Whether static, increasing, or decreasing
Radiation: Pain radiating to upper or lower extremities or complaints of numbness, tingling, or weakness require appropriate work-up.
Aggravating factors: Relationship to any activities such as swimming or diving or any particular position
Alleviating factors: Is the pain relieved by rest, heat, and/or medication? Conditions such as spondylolysis, Scheuermann disease, inflammatory spondyloarthropathy, muscle pulls, or overuse are improved by bed rest.
Gait and posture: Disturbances associated with pain

Table 673-2	Guidelines During Inspection of a Child with Musculoskeletal Problem

- The patient should be *comfortable with adequate exposure and well-lit surroundings* (lest some important physical finding be missed). Infants or young children may be examined on their parent's lap so that they feel more secure and are more likely to be cooperative.
- It is important to inspect how the patient moves about in the room before and during the examination, as well as during various maneuvers. *Balance, posture, and gait pattern* should also be checked.
- *General examination* findings should include inspection for skin rashes, café-au-lait spots, hairy patches, dimples, cysts, tuft of hair, or evidence of spinal midline defects that can indicate serious underlying problems that need review.
- *General body habitus*, including signs of cachexia, pallor, and nutritional deficiencies, should be noted.
- Note any obvious spinal asymmetry, axial or appendicular deformities, trunk decompensation, and evidence of muscle spasm or contractures. The *forward bending test* is valuable in assessing asymmetry and movement of the spine.
- It is essential to perform and document a *thorough neurologic examination*. Motor, sensory, and reflex testing should be performed and recorded.
- Any *discrepancies in limb lengths*, as well as *muscle atrophy*, should be recorded.
- The range of motion of all joints, their stability, and any evidence of hyperlaxity, peripheral pulsations, and lymphadenopathy should also be noted in all cases.

Gait

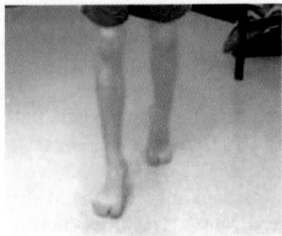 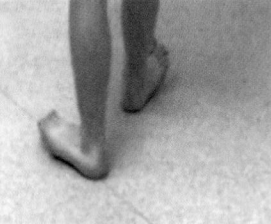

A "Walk on your tip-toes."* Observe the child walking

B "Walk on your heels."* Observe the child walking

Arms

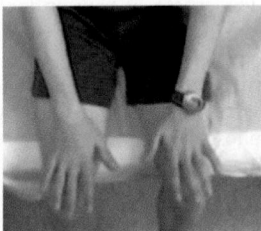 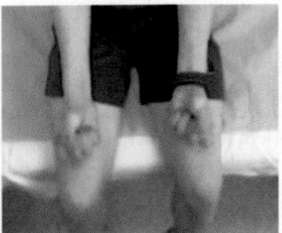 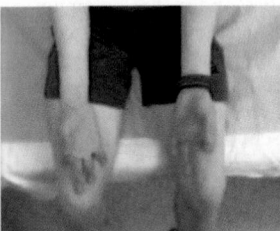 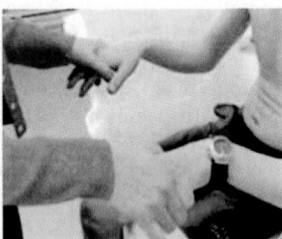

C "Put your hands out in front of you."

D "Turn your hands over and make a fist. Pinch your index finger and thumb together."

E "Touch the tips of your fingers with your thumb."

F Squeeze metacarpophalangeal joints

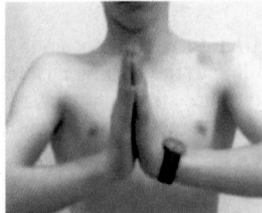 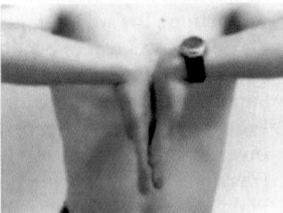 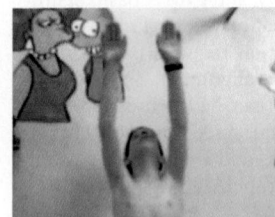 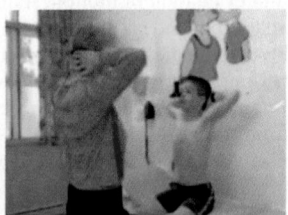

G "Put your hands together."*

H "Put your hands back to back."*

I "Reach up and touch the sky.* Look at the ceiling."

J "Put your hands behind your neck."

Legs

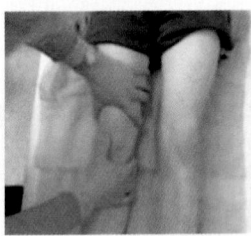 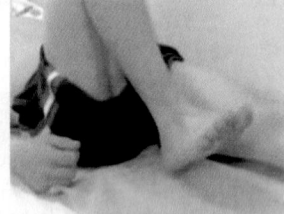 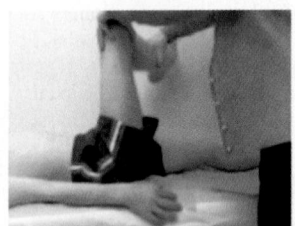

K Feel for effusion at the knee

L "Bend and the straighten your knee." (active movement of knees and examiner feels for crepitus)

M Passive flexion (90 degrees) with internal rotation of hip

Spine

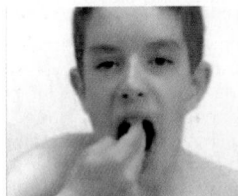 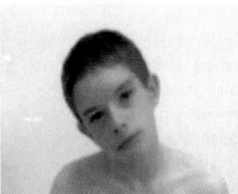 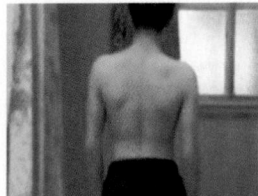 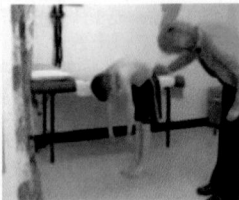

N "Open your mouth and put 3 of your (child's own) fingers in your mouth."*

O Lateral flexion of cervical spine: "Try and touch your shoulder with your ear."

P Observe spine from behind

Q "Can you bend and touch your toes?" Observe curve of spine from side and behind

Figure 673-1 The components of pediatric gait, arms, legs, spine (pGALS) screen, with illustration of movement. Screening questions: (1) Do you have any pain or stiffness in your joints, muscles, or back? (2) Do you have any difficulty getting yourself dressed without any help? (3) Do you have any difficulty going up and down stairs? *Additions and amendments to the original adult gait, arms, legs, spine screen. (*From Foster HE, Kay LJ, Friswell M, et al: Musculoskeletal screening examination [pGALS] for school-age children based on the adult GALS screen,* Arthritis Rheum 55:709–716, 2006.)

Gait Assessment

Children typically begin walking between 8 and 16 mo of age. Early ambulation is characterized by short stride length, a fast cadence, and slow velocity with a wide-based stance. Gait cycle is a single sequence of functions that starts with heel strike, toe off, swing, and heel strike. The 4 events describe 1 gait cycle and include 2 phases: stance and swing. The stance phase is the period during which the foot is in contact with the ground. The swing phase is the portion of the gait cycle during which a limb is being advanced forward without ground contact (see Chapter 672). Normal gait is a symmetric and smooth process. Deviation from the norm indicates potential abnormality and should trigger investigation.

Neurologic maturation is necessary for the development of gait and the normal progression of developmental milestones. A child's gait changes with neurologic maturation. Infants normally walk with greater hip and knee flexion, flexed arms, and a wider base of gait than older children. As the neurologic system continues to develop in the cephalocaudal direction, the efficiency and smoothness of gait increase. The gait characteristics of a 7 yr old child are similar to those of an adult. When the neurologic system is abnormal (cerebral palsy), gait can be disturbed, exhibiting pathologic reflexes and abnormal movements.

Deviations from normal gait occur in a variety of orthopedic conditions. Disorders that result in muscle weakness (e.g., spina bifida, muscular dystrophy), spasticity (e.g., cerebral palsy), or contractures (e.g., arthrogryposis) lead to abnormalities in gait. Other causes of gait disturbances include limp, pain, torsional variations (in-toeing and out-toeing), toe walking, joint abnormalities, and leg-length discrepancy (Table 673-3).

LIMPING

A thorough history and clinical examination are the first steps toward early identification of the underlying problem causing a limp. Limping can be considered as either **painful (antalgic)** or painless, with the differential diagnosis ranging from benign to serious causes (septic hip, tumor). In a painful gait, the stance phase is shortened as the child decreases the time spent on the painful extremity. In a painless gait, which indicates underlying proximal muscle weakness or hip instability, the stance phase is equal between the involved and uninvolved sides, but the child leans or shifts the center of gravity over the involved extremity for balance. A bilateral disorder produces a waddling gait. Trendelenburg gait is produced by weak abnormal hip abductors. In single leg stance, a Trendelenburg sign can often be elicited when abductors are weak.

Disorders most commonly responsible for an abnormal gait generally vary based on the age of the patient. The differential diagnosis of limping varies based on age group (Table 673-4) or mechanism (Table 673-5). Neurologic disorders, especially spinal cord or peripheral nerve disorders, can also produce limping and difficult walking. Antalgic gait is predominantly a result of trauma, infection, or pathologic fracture. Trendelenburg gait is generally caused by congenital, developmental, or muscular disorders. In some cases, limping also may be caused by nonskeletal causes such as testicular torsion, inguinal hernia, and appendicitis.

BACK PAIN

Children frequently have a specific skeletal pathology as the cause of back pain. The most common causes of back pain in children are trauma, spondylolysis, spondylolisthesis, and infection (see Table 679-2). Tumor and tumor-like lesions that cause back pain in children are likely to be missed unless a thorough clinical assessment and adequate work-up are performed when required. Nonorthopedic causes of back pain include urinary tract infections, nephrolithiasis, and pneumonia.

NEUROLOGIC EVALUATION

A careful neurologic evaluation is a part of every pediatric musculoskeletal examination (see Chapter 590). The assessment should include evaluation of developmental milestones, muscle strength, sensory assessment, muscle tone, and deep tendon reflexes. The neurologic evaluation should also assess the spine and identify any deformity, such as scoliosis and kyphosis, or abnormal spinal mobility. The hips and feet should also be examined specifically, along with torsional abnormalities of the lower extremity, which are vastly more common in the neurologically involved population. Specific peripheral nerve examinations may be necessary.

As the nervous system matures, the developing cerebral cortex normally inhibits rudimentary reflexes that are often present at birth (see Chapter 590). Therefore, persistence of these reflexes can indicate neurologic abnormality. The most commonly performed deep tendon reflex tests include biceps, triceps, quadriceps, and gastrocnemius and soleus tendons. Upper motor neuron signs should also be noted. The

Table 673-3	Causes of Abnormal Gait

Limp
Pain
Torsional variations
Toe walking
Joint abnormalities
Leg-length discrepancy
Neuromuscular disorders

Table 673-4	Common Causes of Limping According to Age		
ANTALGIC	**TRENDELENBURG**	**LEG-LENGTH DISCREPANCY**	
TODDLER (1-3 YR)			
Infection	Hip dislocation (DDH)	–	
Septic arthritis	Neuromuscular disease		
Hip	Cerebral palsy		
Knee	Poliomyelitis		
Osteomyelitis			
Diskitis			
Occult trauma			
Toddler's fracture			
Neoplasia			
CHILD (4-10 YR)			
Infection	Hip dislocation (DDH)	+	
Septic arthritis	Neuromuscular disease		
Hip	Cerebral palsy		
Knee	Poliomyelitis		
Osteomyelitis			
Diskitis			
Transient synovitis, hip			
LCPD			
Tarsal coalition			
Rheumatologic disorder			
JRA			
Trauma			
Neoplasia			
ADOLESCENT (11+ YR)			
SCFE		+	
Rheumatologic disorder			
JRA			
Trauma: fracture, overuse			
Tarsal coalition			
Neoplasia			

–, Absent; +, present; DDH, developmental dysplasia of the hip; JRA, juvenile rheumatoid arthritis; LCPD, Legg-Calvé-Perthes disease; SCFE, slipped capital femoral epiphysis.

From Thompson GH: Gait disturbances. In Kliegman RM, editor: Practical strategies of pediatric diagnosis and therapy, Philadelphia, 1996, WB Saunders, pp. 757–778.

Table 673-5	Differential Diagnosis of Limping

ANTALGIC GAIT
Congenital
Tarsal coalition
Acquired
Legg-Calvé-Perthes disease
Slipped capital femoral epiphysis
Trauma
Sprains, strains, contusions
Fractures
Occult
Toddler's fracture
Abuse
Neoplasia
Benign
• Unicameral bone cyst
• Osteoid osteoma
Malignant
• Osteogenic sarcoma
• Ewing sarcoma
• Leukemia
• Neuroblastoma
• Spinal cord tumors
Infectious
Septic arthritis
Reactive arthritis
Osteomyelitis
• Acute
• Subacute
Diskitis
Rheumatologic
Juvenile rheumatoid arthritis
Hip monoarticular synovitis (toxic transient synovitis)

TRENDELENBURG
Developmental
Developmental dysplasia of the hip
Leg-length discrepancy
Neuromuscular
Cerebral palsy
Poliomyelitis

From Thompson GH: Gait disturbances. In Kliegman RM, editor: Practical strategies of pediatric diagnosis and therapy, *Philadelphia, 1996, WB Saunders, pp. 757–778.*

Table 673-6	Ashworth Scale of Spasticity
0	No increase in muscle tone
1	Slight increase in muscle tone, usually a catch or minimal resistance at end range of motion
2	Moderate tone throughout range of motion
3	Considerable increase in tone; passive range of motion difficult
4	Rigid in flexion or extension

Table 673-7	Clinical Scale of Upper-Extremity Motor Control

GRADE	DEFINITION
Grade 1	Hypotonic, no volitional motion
Grade 2	Hypertonic, no volitional motion
Grade 3	Mass flexion or extension in response to a stimulus
Grade 4	Patient can initiate movement but results in mass flexion or extension
Grade 5	Slow volitional movement; stress or rapid movement results in mass action
Grade 6	Volitional control of specific joints/muscles

Ashworth scale is often used to grade spasticity (Table 673-6). Upper-extremity motor control is often graded, and these grades are useful both diagnostically and prognostically. Passive range of motion should be assessed to determine contractures (Table 673-7). Localized or diffuse weakness must be determined and documented. A thorough assessment and grading of muscle strength is mandatory in all cases of neuromuscular disorders.

RADIOGRAPHIC ASSESSMENT
Plain radiographs are the first step in evaluation of most musculoskeletal disorders. Advanced imaging includes special procedures such as nuclear bone scans, ultrasonography, MRI, CT, and positron emission tomography.

Plain Radiographs
Routine radiographs are the first step and consist of anteroposterior and lateral views of the involved area with 1 joint above and below. Comparison views of the opposite side, if uninvolved, may be helpful in difficult situations but are not always necessary. It is important for the clinician to be aware of normal radiographic variants of the immature skeleton. Several synchondroses may be mistaken for fractures. A patient with "normal" plain radiographic appearance but having persistent pain or symptoms might need to be evaluated further with additional imaging studies.

Nuclear Medicine Imaging
A bone scan displays physiologic information rather than pure anatomy and relies on the emission of energy from the nucleotide injected into the patient. Indications include early septic arthritis, osteomyelitis, avascular necrosis, tumors (osteoid osteoma), metastatic lesions, occult and stress fractures, and cases of child abuse.

Total-body radionuclide scan (technetium-99) is useful to identify bony lesions, inflammatory tumors, and stress fractures. Tumor vascularity can also be inferred from the flow phase and the blood pool images. Gallium or indium scans have high sensitivity for local infections. Thallium-201 chloride scintiscans have >90% sensitivity and between 80% and 90% accuracy in detecting malignant bone or soft-tissue tumors.

Ultrasonography
Ultrasonography is useful to evaluate suspected fluid-filled lesions such as popliteal cyst and hip joint effusions. Major indications for ultrasonography are fetal studies of the extremities and spine, including detection of congenital anomalies like spondylocostal dysostosis, fractures suggesting osteogenesis imperfecta, developmental dysplasia of the hip, joint effusions, occult *neonatal* spinal dysraphism, foreign bodies in soft tissues, and popliteal cysts of the knee.

Magnetic Resonance Imaging
MRI is the **imaging modality of choice** for defining the exact anatomic extent of most musculoskeletal lesions (particularly if the structure is soft tissue). MRI avoids ionizing radiation and doing does not produce any known harmful effects. It produces excellent anatomic images of the musculoskeletal system, including the soft tissue, bone marrow cavity, spinal cord, and brain. It is especially useful for defining the extent of soft-tissue lesions, infections, and injuries. Tissue planes are well delineated, allowing more accurate assessment tumor invasion into adjacent structures. Cartilage structures can be visualized (articular cartilage of the knee can be distinguished from the fibrocartilage of the meniscus). MRI is also helpful in visualizing unossified joints in the pediatric population including the shoulders, elbows, and hips of young infants.

Magnetic Resonance Angiography

Magnetic resonance angiography has largely replaced routine angiography in the preoperative assessment of vascular lesions and bone tumors. Magnetic resonance angiography provides good visualization of peripheral vascular branches and tumor neovascularity in patients with primary bone tumors.

Computed Tomography

CT has enhanced the evaluation of multiple musculoskeletal disorders. Coronal, sagittal, and axial imaging is possible with CT including 3-dimensional reconstructions that can be beneficial in evaluating complex lesions of the axial and appendicular skeleton. It allows visualization of the detailed bone anatomy and the relationship of bones to contiguous structures. CT is useful to readily evaluate tarsal coalition, accessory navicular bone, infection, growth plate arrest, osteoid osteoma, pseudoarthrosis, bone and soft tissue tumors, spondylolysis, and spondylolisthesis. CT is superior to MRI for assessing bone involvement and cortical destruction (even subtle changes), including calcification or ossification and fracture (particularly if displacement of an articular fracture is suspected).

LABORATORY STUDIES

Laboratory tests are occasionally necessary in the evaluation of a child with musculoskeletal disorder. These may include a complete blood cell count; erythrocyte sedimentation rate; C-reactive protein assay; Lyme titers; and blood, wound, joint, periosteum, or bone cultures for infectious conditions such as septic arthritis or osteomyelitis. Rheumatoid factor, antinuclear antibodies, and human leukocyte antigen B27 may be necessary for children with suspected rheumatologic disorders. Creatine kinase, aldolase, aspartate aminotransferase, and dystrophin testing are indicated in children with suspected disorders of striated muscle such as Duchenne muscular dystrophy.

Bibliography is available at Expert Consult.

Chapter **674**

The Foot and Toes

Jennifer J. Winell and Richard S. Davidson

Abnormalities affecting the osseous and articular structures of the foot may be congenital, developmental, neuromuscular, inflammatory, or acquired. Problems with the foot and/or toes may be associated with a host of connective tissue diseases and syndromes; overuse syndromes are commonly observed in young athletes. Symptoms may include pain and abnormal shoe wear; cosmetic concerns are common. The foot may be divided into the **forefoot** (toes and metatarsals), the **midfoot** (cuneiforms, navicular, cuboid), and the **hindfoot** (talus and calcaneus). While the tibiotalar joint (ankle) provides plantarflexion and dorsiflexion, the subtalar joint (between the talus and calcaneus) is oriented obliquely, providing inversion and eversion. Inversion represents a combination of plantarflexion and varus, while eversion involves dorsiflexion and valgus. The subtalar joint is especially important for walking on uneven surfaces. Inversion of the transverse tarsal (Chopart) joint locks the midfoot to provide a stable base on which to perform toe off during the gait cycle. Eversion of the transverse tarsal joint unlocks the **hindfoot** to provide accommodation during heel strike of the of the gait cycle. The talonavicular and calcaneocuboid joints connect the midfoot with the hindfoot.

674.1 Metatarsus Adductus

Jennifer J. Winell and Richard S. Davidson

Metatarsus adductus involves adduction of the forefoot relative to the hindfoot. When the forefoot is supinated and adducted, the deformity is termed *metatarsus varus* (Fig. 674-1). The disorder is common in newborns, most frequently caused by intrauterine molding; the deformity is bilateral in 50% of cases. As with other intrauterine positional foot deformities, a careful hip and neck examination should always be performed to look for other abnormalities associated with intrauterine positioning.

CLINICAL MANIFESTATIONS

The forefoot is adducted (occasionally supinated), whereas the midfoot and hindfoot are normal. The lateral border of the foot is convex, and the base of the 5th metatarsal appears prominent. Range of motion at the ankle and subtalar joints is normal. Both the magnitude and the degree of flexibility should be documented. When the foot is viewed from the plantar surface, a line through the midpoint of (and parallel to) the heel should normally extend through the 2nd toe. Flexibility is assessed by stabilizing the hindfoot and midfoot in a neutral position with 1 hand and applying pressure over the 1st metatarsal head with the other. Correction with little pressure is indicative of a more flexible deformity. In the walking child with an uncorrected metatarsus adductus deformity, an in-toe gait and abnormal shoe wear may occur. A subset of patients will also have a dynamic adduction deformity of the great toe (hallux varus), which is often most noticeable during ambulation. This usually improves spontaneously and does not require treatment.

RADIOGRAPHIC EVALUATION

Radiographs are not performed routinely in infants. Older children with residual deformity should have anteroposterior (AP) and lateral weight-bearing or simulated weight-bearing radiographs. The AP radiographs demonstrate adduction of the metatarsals at the tarsometatarsal articulation and an increased intermetatarsal angle between the 1st and 2nd metatarsals.

TREATMENT

The treatment of metatarsus adductus is based on the rigidity of the deformity; most children respond to nonoperative treatment. Deformities that are flexible and overcorrect into abduction with passive manipulation may be observed. Those feet that correct just to a neutral position may benefit from stretching exercises which can be demonstrated to the parents in the office. In a walking child, the parents can try reversing the shoes as well. If this is not effective, reverse-last shoes to maintain the abducted position of foot can be prescribed. These are worn full time (22 hr/day), and the condition is reevaluated in 4-6 wk.

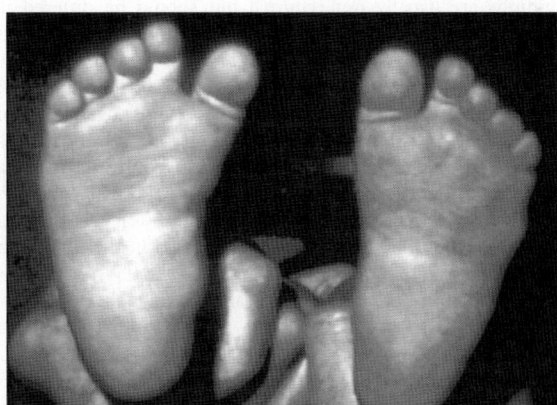

Figure 674-1 Clinical picture of metatarsus adductus with a normal foot on opposite side.

If improvement occurs, treatment can be continued. If there is no improvement, serial plaster casts should be considered. When stretching a foot with metatarsus adductus, care should be taken to maintain the hindfoot in neutral to slight varus alignment to avoid creating hindfoot valgus. Feet that cannot be corrected to a neutral position may benefit from serial casting; the best results are obtained when treatment is started before 8 mo of age. In addition to stretching the soft tissues, the goal is to alter physeal growth and stimulate remodeling, resulting in permanent correction. Once flexibility and alignment are restored, orthoses or corrective shoes are generally recommended for an additional period. A dynamic hallux varus usually improves spontaneously, and no active treatment is required.

Surgical treatment may be considered in the small subset of patients with symptomatic residual deformities that have not responded to previous treatment. Surgery is generally delayed until children are 4-6 yr of age. Cosmesis is often a concern, and pain and/or the inability to wear certain types of shoes may occasionally lead patients to consider surgery. Options for surgical treatment include either soft-tissue releases or osteotomies. An osteotomy (midfoot or multiple metatarsals) is most likely to result in permanent restoration of alignment.

Bibliography is available at Expert Consult.

674.2 Calcaneovalgus Feet

Jennifer J. Winell and Richard S. Davidson

A common finding in the newborn, the calcaneovalgus foot is secondary to in utero positioning. Excessive dorsiflexion and eversion are observed in the hindfoot, and the forefoot may be abducted. There may be an associated external tibial torsion (see Chapter 675).

CLINICAL MANIFESTATIONS
The infant typically presents with the foot dorsiflexed and everted, and occasionally the dorsum of the foot or toes, will be in contact with the anterolateral surface of the lower leg (Fig. 674-2). Dimpling may be indicative of reduced subcutaneous fat at the dorsolateral ankle. Plantarflexion and inversion are often restricted. As with other intrauterine positional deformities, a careful hip examination should be performed; if there is any concern, hip ultrasonography should be considered. When comparing risk for developmental hip dysplasia (DDH) with other congenital foot deformities, congenital calcaneovalgus has the highest association with 19.4% of patients having coexisting DDH. The calcaneovalgus foot may be confused with a congenital vertical talus and may rarely be associated with a posteromedial bow of the tibia. A calcaneovalgus deformity may also be seen in older patients, typically those with a neuromuscular imbalance involving weakness or paralysis of the gastrocsoleus muscle (polio, myelomeningocele).

RADIOGRAPHIC EVALUATION
Radiographs are usually not required but should be ordered if the deformity fails to correct spontaneously or with early treatment. AP and lateral radiographs along with a lateral radiograph of the foot in maximal plantarflexion may help distinguish calcaneovalgus from a congenital vertical talus or congenital oblique talus. Evaluation of the position of the talus in relation to the navicular in both the lateral and maximally plantarflexed lateral view confirm congenital vertical or oblique talus. If a posteromedial bow of the tibia is suspected, AP and lateral radiographs of the tibia and fibula are necessary. In posteromedial bowing of the tibia, the deformity is located in the tibia with the apex of deformity positioned posterior and medial. All three conditions may be confused clinically with calcaneovalgus feet.

TREATMENT
Mild cases of calcaneovalgus foot, in which full passive range of motion is present at birth, require no active treatment. These usually resolve within the 1st few wk of life. A gentle stretching program, focusing on plantarflexion and inversion, is recommended for cases with some

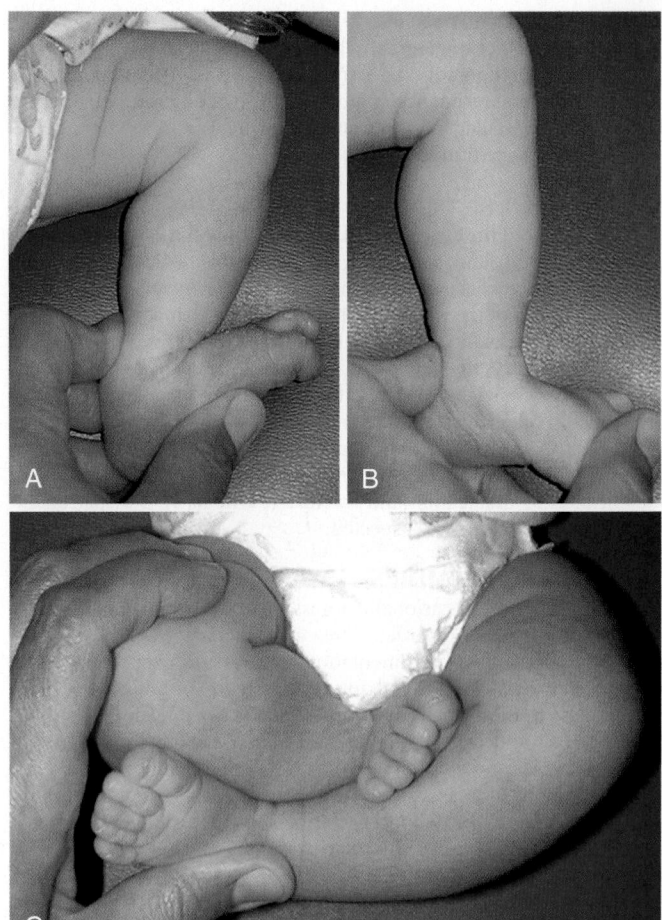

Figure 674-2 Clinical picture of calcaneovalgus foot **(A)** that is passively correctable **(B)** because of intrauterine positioning **(C)**.

restriction in motion. For cases with a greater restriction in mobility, serial casts may be considered to restore motion and alignment. Casting is rarely required in the treatment of calcaneovalgus feet. The management for those cases associated with a posteromedial bow of the tibia is similar.

Bibliography is available at Expert Consult.

674.3 Talipes Equinovarus (Clubfoot)

Jennifer J. Winell and Richard S. Davidson

Clubfoot or congenital talipes equinovarus (CTEV) is the term used to describe a deformity involving malalignment of the calcaneotalar-navicular complex. Components of this deformity may be best understood using the mnemonic **CAVE** (cavus, adductus, varus, equinus). Although this is predominantly a hindfoot deformity, there are plantarflexion (cavus) of the first ray and adduction of the forefoot/midfoot on the hindfoot. The hindfoot is in varus and equinus. The clubfoot deformity may be positional, congenital, associated with a variety of underlying diagnoses (neuromuscular or syndromic) or a focal dysplasia of musculoskeletal tissue distal to the knee.

The **positional (or postural) clubfoot** is a normal foot that has been held in a deformed position in utero and is found to be flexible on examination in the newborn nursery. The **congenital clubfoot** can either be idiopathic or syndromic. There is a spectrum of severity, but clubfoot associated with neuromuscular diagnoses or syndromes is typically rigid and more difficult to treat. Clubfoot is also extremely common in patients with myelodysplasia, arthrogryposis, and other chromosomal syndromes such as trisomy 18 and chromosome 22q11 deletion syndrome (see Chapter 81).

Congenital clubfoot is seen in approximately 1 in 1,000 births and most likely results from a complex multifactorial polygenic inheritance. The risk is approximately 1 in 4 when both a parent and 1 sibling have clubfeet. It occurs more commonly in males (2:1) and is bilateral in 50% of cases. The pathoanatomy involves both abnormal tarsal morphology (plantar and medial deviation of the head and neck of the talus) and abnormal relationships between the tarsal bones in all 3 planes, as well as associated contracture of the soft tissues on the plantar and medial aspects of the foot.

CLINICAL MANIFESTATIONS

A complete physical examination should be performed to rule out coexisting musculoskeletal and neuromuscular problems. The spine should be inspected for signs of occult dysraphism. Examination of the infant clubfoot demonstrates forefoot cavus and adductus and hindfoot varus and equinus (Fig. 674-3). The degree of flexibility varies, and all patients will exhibit calf atrophy. Internal tibial torsion, foot length shortening and leg-length discrepancy (shortening of the ipsilateral extremity) will be observed in a subset of cases. Although classically not associated with DDH (see Chapter 678), there is a higher association of CTEV and DDH than in the general population.

RADIOGRAPHIC EVALUATION

Anteroposterior and lateral radiographs are not recommended for idiopathic clubfoot. For arthrogrypotic or syndromic feet, x-rays may be helpful but must be performed, with the foot held in the maximally corrected position. Multiple radiographic measurements can be made to describe malalignment between the tarsal bones. The navicular bone does not ossify until 3-6 yr of age, so the focus of radiographic interpretation is the relationships between segments of the foot, forefoot to hindfoot. A common radiographic finding is "parallelism" between lines drawn through the axis of the talus and the calcaneus on the lateral radiograph, indicating hindfoot varus. X-ray may be particularly useful for older children with persistent or recurrent deformities that are difficult to assess.

TREATMENT

Nonoperative treatment is initiated in all infants and should be started as soon as possible following birth. Techniques have included taping and strapping, manipulation and serial casting, and functional treatment. Historically, a significant percentage of patients treated by manipulation and casting required a surgical release, which was usually performed between 3 and 12 mo of age. Although many feet remain well aligned after surgical releases, a significant percentage of patients have required additional surgery for recurrent or residual deformities. Stiffness remains a concern at long-term follow-up. While pain is uncommon in childhood and adolescence, symptoms may appear during adulthood. These concerns have led to considerable interest in less-invasive methods for treating the deformity. The Ponseti method of clubfoot treatment, which has now become the standard of initial treatment, involves a specific technique for manipulation and serial casting and may be best described as minimally invasive rather than nonoperative. The order of correction follows the mnemonic **CAVE**. Weekly cast changes are performed; 5-10 casts are typically required. The most difficult deformity to correct is the hindfoot equinus, and approximately 90% of patients will require a percutaneous tenotomy of the heel cord as an outpatient. Following the tenotomy, a long leg cast with the foot in maximal abduction (up to 70 degrees) and dorsiflexion is worn for 3-4 wk; the patient then begins a bracing program. An abduction brace is worn full time for 3 mo and then at nighttime for 3-5 yr. A small subset of patients (up to 20%) with recurrent, dynamic supination deformity will require transfer of the tibialis anterior tendon to the middle cuneiform for recurrence. Although most patients require some form of surgery, the procedures are minimal in comparison with extensive surgical release, which requires lengthening and/or release of muscles and tendons about the ankle and capsulotomy of the major joints to reposition the foot. The results of the Ponseti method are excellent at up to 40 yr of follow-up. Despite casting, children do not have much dysfunction or delay in achieving normal motor milestones. Compliance with the splinting program is essential; recurrence is common if the brace is not worn as recommended. Functional treatment, or the "French method," involves daily manipulations (supervised by a physical therapist) and splinting with elastic tape, as well as continuous passive motion (machine required) while the baby sleeps. While results are promising, it is usually performed in the

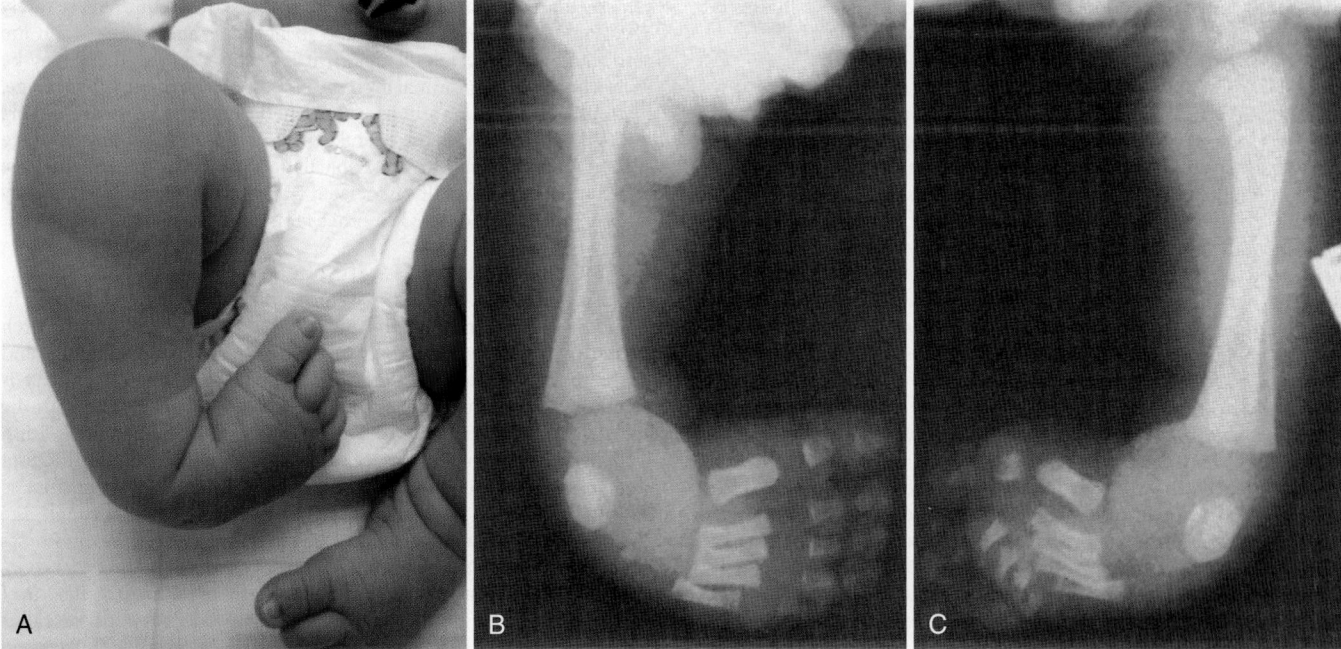

Figure 674-3 Talipes equinovarus in a newborn. **A,** Clinical appearance of an untreated clubfoot. **B** and **C,** Initial radiographic appearance of bilateral untreated clubfeet. *(From Herring JA: Tachdjian's pediatric orthopaedics, ed 5, Philadelphia, 2014, WB Saunders, Fig. 23-42, p. 791.)*

inpatient setting as the method is labor intensive. Implementation on an outpatient basis may be challenging, although just as successful. It remains unclear whether the technique will gain popularity in the United States. These minimally invasive methods are most successful when treatment is begun at birth or during the 1st few mo of life and with good compliance with postmanipulation bracing. As there are varying degrees of severity for idiopathic CTEV, grading systems have been proposed based on rigidity and magnitude of deformity.

Aggressive surgical realignment has a definite role in the management of clubfeet, especially in the minority of congenital clubfeet that have failed nonoperative or minimally invasive methods, and for the rigid neuromuscular and syndromic clubfeet. In such cases, nonoperative methods such as the Ponseti technique may potentially be of value in decreasing the magnitude of surgery required. Common surgical approaches include a release of the involved joints (realignment of the tarsal bones), a lengthening of the shortened posteromedial musculotendinous units, and usually pinning of the foot in the corrected position. The "a la carte" method allows the surgeon to apply the principles to be tailored to the unique characteristics of each deformity. For older children with untreated clubfeet or those in whom a recurrence or residual deformity is observed, bony procedures (osteotomies) may be required in addition to soft-tissue surgery. Triple arthrodesis is reserved as salvage for painful, deformed feet in adolescents and adults.

Bibliography is available at Expert Consult.

674.4 Congenital Vertical Talus
Jennifer J. Winell and Richard S. Davidson

Congenital vertical talus is an uncommon foot deformity in which the midfoot is dorsally dislocated on the hindfoot and the ankle is in fixed equinus. There is nearly an even split between idiopathic cases and cases with an underlying neuromuscular condition or a syndrome. Neurologic causes include myelodysplasia, tethered cord, and sacral agenesis. Other associated conditions include arthrogryposis, Larsen syndrome, multiple pterygium syndrome, and chromosomal abnormalities (trisomy 13-15, 19: see Chapter 81). Depending on the age at diagnosis, the differential diagnosis may include a calcaneovalgus foot, oblique talus (talonavicular joint reduces passively), flexible flatfoot with a tight Achilles tendon, and tarsal coalition. Genetic studies are ongoing regarding abnormal muscle morphology on biopsy.

CLINICAL MANIFESTATIONS
Congenital vertical talus has also been described as a **rocker-bottom foot** (Fig. 674-4) or a Persian slipper foot. The plantar surface of the foot is convex, and the talar head is prominent along the medial border of the midfoot. The fore part of the foot is dorsiflexed (dorsally dislocated on the hindfoot) and abducted relative to the hindfoot, and the hindfoot is in equinus and valgus. There is an associated contracture of the anterolateral (tibialis anterior, toe extensors) and the posterior (Achilles tendon, peroneals) soft tissues. The deformity is typically rigid. A thorough physical examination is required to identify any coexisting neurologic and/or musculoskeletal abnormalities.

RADIOGRAPHIC EVALUATION
AP, lateral, and maximal plantarflexion and dorsiflexion lateral radiographs should be obtained when the diagnosis is suspected. The plantarflexion view helps to determine whether the dorsal subluxation or dislocation of the midfoot on the hindfoot can be reduced passively. The dorsiflexion lateral view confirms the equinus contracture of the ankle. Although the navicular does not ossify until 3-6 yr of age, the relationship between the talus and the 1st metatarsal may be evaluated.

TREATMENT
The initial management consists of serial manipulation and casting, which is started shortly after birth. A "reverse" Ponseti method of casting is particularly useful in stretching out the dorsiflexion and valgus deformities. Open reduction and pin fixation can then stabilize the midfoot allowing simultaneous heel cord tenotomy and dorsiflexion with casting to correct the ankle equinus.

In recalcitrant cases the competing deformities of the midfoot and the hindfoot make conservative treatment difficult. Initially, an attempt is made to reduce the dorsal dislocation of the forefoot/midfoot on the hindfoot. Once this has been achieved, attention can be directed toward stretching the hindfoot contracture. These deformities are typically rigid, and surgical intervention is required in the majority of cases. In such cases, casting helps to stretch out the contracted soft tissues. Surgery is generally performed between 6 and 12 mo of age; a soft-tissue release is performed as a 1 or 2 stage procedure. One component involves release/lengthening of the contracted anterior soft tissues in concert with an open reduction of the talonavicular joint, while the other involves a posterior release with lengthening of the contracted musculotendinous units. Fixation with Kirschner wires is commonly performed to maintain alignment. Postoperatively, casting is employed for a variable period of time; patients often require the use of an orthosis for extended periods, depending on the underlying diagnosis. Salvage options for recurrent or residual deformities in older children include a subtalar or triple arthrodesis.

Bibliography is available at Expert Consult.

674.5 Hypermobile Pes Planus (Flexible Flatfeet)
Jennifer J. Winell and Richard S. Davidson

Flatfoot is a common diagnosis; it has been estimated that up to 23% of the public may be affected, depending on the diagnostic criteria. Three types of flatfeet may be identified: a flexible flatfoot, a flexible flatfoot with a tendo-Achilles contracture, and a rigid flatfoot. Flatfoot describes a change in foot shape, and there are several abnormalities in alignment between the tarsal bones. There is eversion of the subtalar complex. The hindfoot is aligned in valgus. There is midfoot sag at the naviculocuneiform and/or the talonavicular joints. The forefoot is abducted relative to the hindfoot, and the head of the talus is uncovered and prominent along the plantar and medial border of the midfoot/hindfoot. Although hypermobile or flexible pes planus represents a common source of concern for parents, these children are rarely symptomatic. Flatfeet are common in neonates and toddlers and are associated with physiologic ligamentous laxity. Improvement may be seen when the longitudinal arch develops between 5 and 10 yr of age. Flatfoot is less common in societies where shoes are not worn during infancy and childhood. In general, comfortable flexible-soled shoes are recommended for children. Flexible flatfeet persisting into adolescence and adulthood are usually associated with **familial ligamentous laxity** and can often be identified in other family members.

CLINICAL MANIFESTATIONS
Patients typically have a normal longitudinal arch when examined in a non–weightbearing position or standing on the toes, but the arch disappears when standing flat. The hindfoot collapses into valgus, and the midfoot sag becomes evident. Generalized ligamentous laxity is commonly observed. Range of motion should be assessed at both the subtalar and the ankle joints and will be normal in patients with a flexible flatfoot. When assessing range of motion at the ankle, the foot should always be inverted while testing dorsiflexion. If the foot is neutral or everted, spurious dorsiflexion may occur through the midfoot, masking a tendo-Achilles contracture. If subtalar motion is restricted, then the flatfoot is not hypermobile/flexible, and other diagnoses, such as tarsal coalition and juvenile rheumatoid arthritis, must be considered. On occasion, there may be tenderness and/or callus formation under the talar head medially. The shoes should be assessed as well and may have evidence of excessive wear along the medial border.

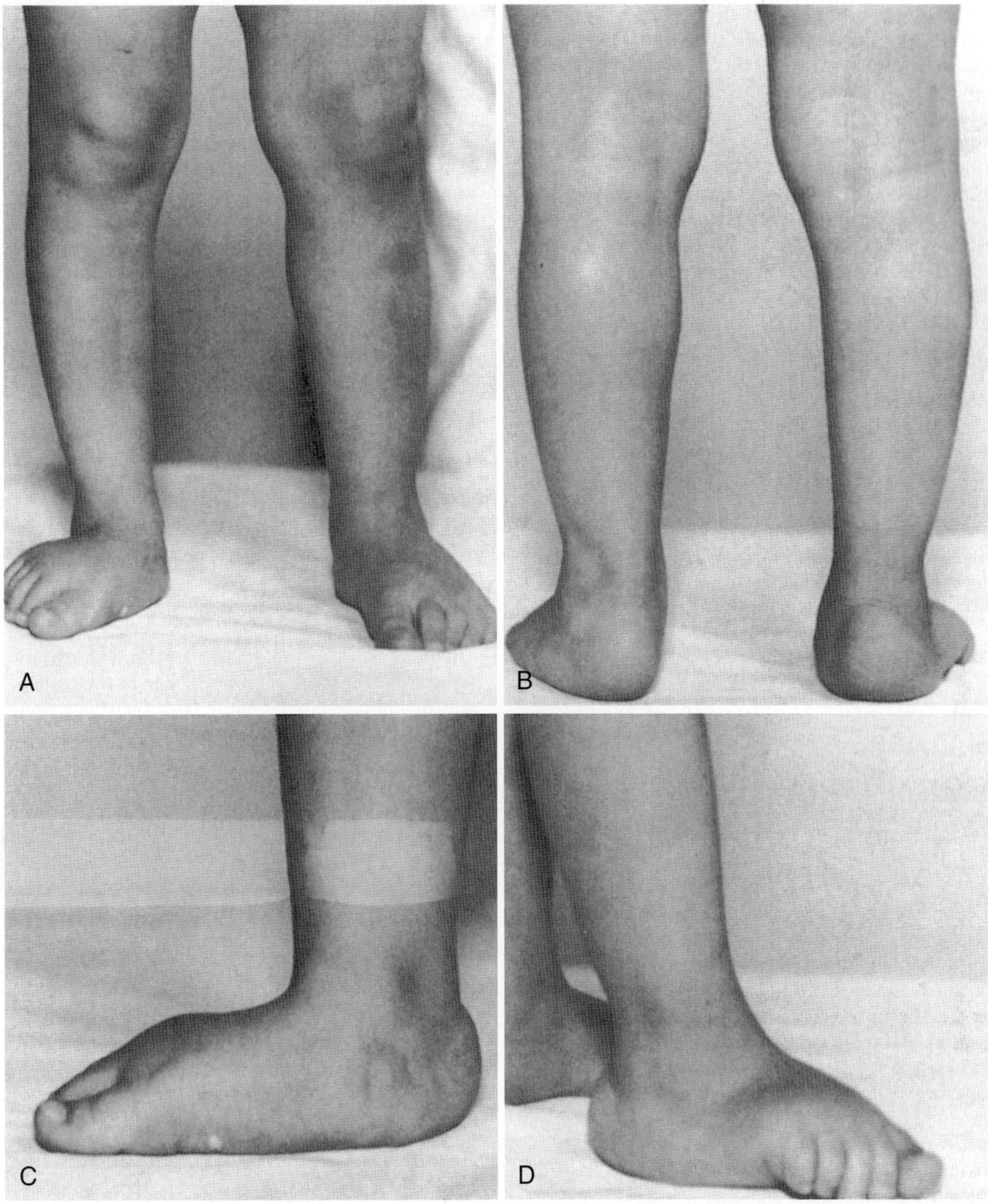

Figure 674-4 Congenital vertical talus. **A,** Pronation of the forefoot. **B,** Valgus of the heel. **C,** Absence of an arch, the rocker bottom deformity. **D,** Elevation of the lateral toes and tight peroneal tendons. *(From Herring JA: Tachdjian's pediatric orthopaedics, ed 5, Philadelphia, 2014, WB Saunders, Fig. 23-67, p. 821)*

RADIOGRAPHIC EVALUATION

Routine radiographs of asymptomatic flexible flatfeet are usually not indicated. If obtained for diagnostic reasons, weightbearing radiographs (AP and lateral) are required to assess the deformity. On the AP radiograph, there is widening of the angle between the longitudinal axis of the talus and the calcaneus, indicating excessive heel valgus. The lateral view shows distortion of the normal straight-line relationship between the long axis of the talus and the 1st metatarsal with sag either of the talonavicular or naviculocuneiform joint, resulting in flattening of the normal medial longitudinal arch (Fig. 674-5).

TREATMENT

Although the natural history of the flexible flatfoot remains unknown, there is little evidence to suggest that this condition results in long-term problems or disability. As such, treatment is reserved for the small

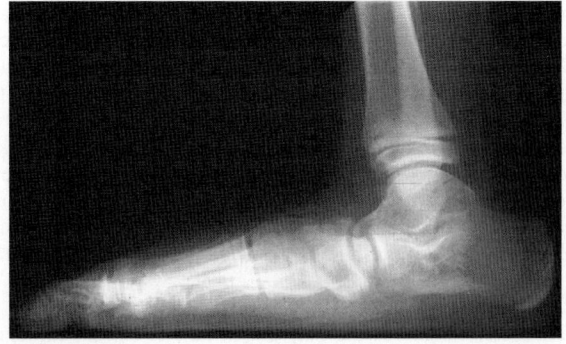

Figure 674-5 Lateral weightbearing radiograph demonstrating features of flatfoot.

subset of patients who develop symptoms. Patients may complain of hindfoot pain, abnormal shoe wear or fatigue after long walking. These patients may benefit from an nonprescription orthosis, such as a medial arch support. Severe cases, often associated with an underlying connective tissue disorder such as Ehlers-Danlos syndrome (see Chapter 659) or Down syndrome (see Chapter 81), may benefit from a custom orthosis such as the UCBL (University of California Biomechanics Laboratory) orthosis to better control the hindfoot and prevent collapse of the arch. Although an orthosis may relieve symptoms, there is no evidence to suggest any permanent change in the shape of the foot or alignment of the tarsal bones. Patients with a flexible flatfoot and a tight tendo-Achilles should be treated with stretching exercises. Many times patients are referred to physical therapy to ensure that the patients are stretching appropriately. On occasion, the muscle will need to be lengthened surgically. For the few patients with persistent pain, surgical treatment can be considered. There has been considerable interest in a lateral column lengthening, which addresses all components of the deformity. The procedure involves an osteotomy of the calcaneus, with placement of a trapezoidal bone graft. A lengthening of the tendo-Achilles is required, often with a plantarflexion osteotomy of the medial cuneiform. This procedure preserves the mobility of the hindfoot joints, in contrast to a subtalar or triple arthrodesis. While a hindfoot arthrodesis may correct the deformity adequately, the stress transfer to neighboring joints may result in late-onset, painful degenerative changes.

Bibliography is available at Expert Consult.

674.6 Tarsal Coalition

Jennifer J. Winell and Richard S. Davidson

Tarsal coalition, also known as **peroneal spastic flatfoot**, is characterized by a painful, rigid flatfoot deformity and peroneal (lateral calf) muscle spasm but without true spasticity. It represents a congenital fusion or failure of segmentation between 2 or more tarsal bones. Any condition that alters the normal gliding and rotatory motion of the subtalar joint may produce the clinical appearance of a tarsal coalition. Thus, congenital malformations, arthritis or inflammatory disorders, infection, neoplasms, and trauma can be possible causes.

The most common tarsal coalitions occur at the medial talocalcaneal (subtalar) facet and between the calcaneus and navicular (calcaneonavicular). Coalitions can be fibrous, cartilaginous, or osseous. Tarsal coalition occurs in approximately 1% of the general population and appears to be inherited as an autosomal dominant trait with nearly full penetrance. Approximately 60% of calcaneonavicular and 50% of the medial facet talocalcaneal coalitions are bilateral.

CLINICAL MANIFESTATIONS

Approximately 25% of patients will become symptomatic, typically during the 2nd decade of life. Although the flatfoot and a decrease in subtalar motion may have been present since early childhood, the onset of symptoms may correlate with the additional restriction in motion that occurs as a cartilaginous bar ossifies. Recurrent "ankle sprains" often accompany the presenting symptoms. The timing of ossification varies between the talonavicular (3-5 yr of age), the calcaneonavicular (8-12 yr of age), and the talocalcaneal (12-16 yr of age) coalitions. Hindfoot pain is commonly observed, especially in the region of the sinus tarsi and also under the head of the talus. Symptoms are activity related and are often increased with running or prolonged walking, especially on uneven surfaces. There may be tenderness over the site of the coalition and/or pain with testing of subtalar motion. The clinical appearance of a flatfoot is seen in both the weightbearing and non–weightbearing positions. There is a restriction in subtalar motion.

RADIOGRAPHIC EVALUATION

AP and lateral weightbearing radiographs and an oblique radiograph of the foot should be obtained (Table 674-1). A calcaneonavicular coalition is seen best on the oblique radiograph (Fig. 674-6). On the

lateral radiograph, there may be elongation of the anterior process of the calcaneus, known as the "anteater sign." A talocalcaneal coalition may be seen on a Harris (axial) view of the heel. On the lateral radiograph, there may be narrowing of the posterior facet of the subtalar joint, or a C-shaped line along the medial outline of the talar dome and the inferior outline of the sustentaculum tali ("C sign"). This "C sign" is made up of the sustentaculum talus of the calcaneus in continuity with the coalition. Beaking of the anterior aspect of the talus on the lateral view is seen with some frequency, and results from an alteration in the distribution of stress. This finding does not imply the presence of degenerative arthritis. Irregularity in the subchondral bony surfaces may be seen in patients with a cartilaginous coalition, in contrast to a well-formed bony bridge in those with an osseous coalition. A fibrous coalition may require additional imaging studies to diagnose. While plain films may be diagnostic, a CT scan is the *imaging modality of choice* when a coalition is suspected (Fig. 674-7). In addition to securing the diagnosis, this study helps to define the degree of joint involvement in patients with a talocalcaneal coalition. Although uncommon, more than one tarsal coalition may be observed in the same patient. Only in young children, MRI may be more effective in identifying either the coalition or a differential diagnosis for the foot pain. MRI offers less radiation exposure but requires more time and may necessitate sedation.

TREATMENT

The treatment of symptomatic tarsal coalitions varies according to the type and extent of coalition, the age of the patient, and the presence and magnitude of symptoms. Treatment is required only for symptomatic coalitions, and the initial management consists of activity

Table 674-1	Radiographic Secondary Signs Associated with Tarsal Conditions

Talar breaking
Posterior subtalar facet narrowing
Rounding and flattening of the lateral talar process
Hypoplasia of the talus, shortening of the talar neck
Anterior nose sign
Ball-and-socket ankle joint
Continuous C-sign
Flatfoot deformity
Altered navicular morphology (wide or laterally tapering)
Dysmorphic sustentaculum tali (enlarged and ovoid on lateral radiograph)

From Slovis TL, editor: Caffey's pediatric diagnostic imaging, ed 11, vol 2, Philadelphia, 2008, Mosby, p. 2604.

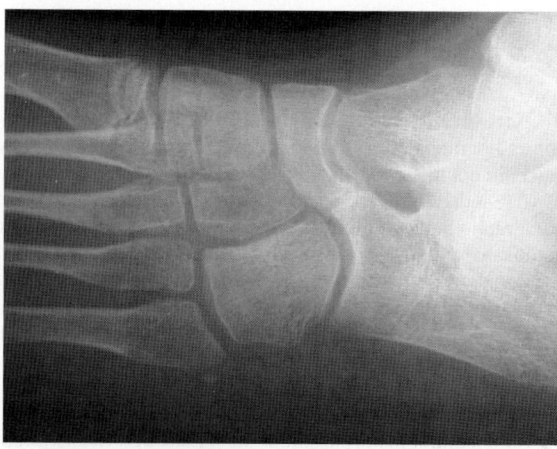

Figure 674-6 Oblique radiograph of the foot demonstrating a calcaneonavicular tarsal coalition.

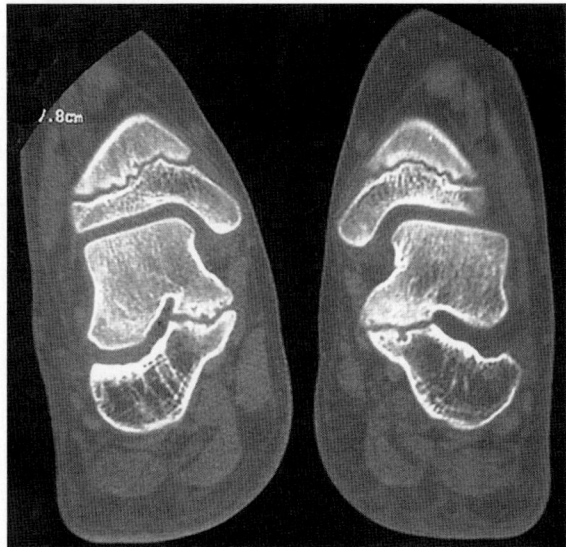

Figure 674-7 CT scan of the talocalcaneal complex demonstrating a talocalcaneal (subtalar).

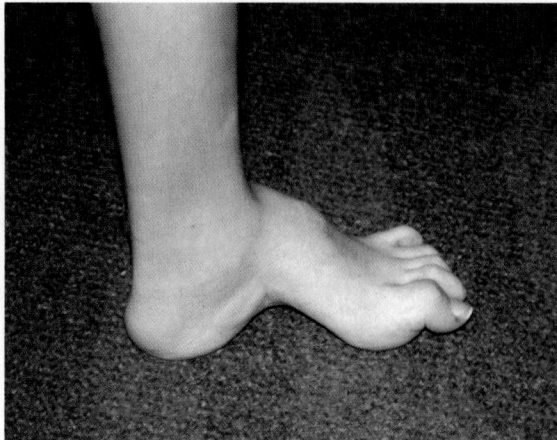

Figure 674-8 Clinical picture demonstrating pes cavus.

restriction and nonsteroidal antiinflammatory medications, with or without a shoe insert. Immobilization in a short leg walking cast for 4-6 wk may be required in patients with more pronounced symptoms. For patients with chronic pain despite an adequate trial of nonoperative therapy, surgical treatment should be considered, and options include resection of the coalition, osteotomy, or arthrodesis. For the calcaneonavicular coalition, resection and interposition of the extensor digitorum brevis muscle have been successful. Often, concomitant hindfoot valgus and contracture of the gastrocnemius-soleus is present. In these patients, more reliable pain relief can be obtained with resection of the coalition, correction of the hindfoot valgus by calcaneal lengthening osteotomy with bank bone graft and lengthening of the gastrocnemius-soleus. For those with extensive involvement of the joint and/or degenerative changes, a triple arthrodesis may be the best option; however, this is rarely needed in adolescents.

Bibliography is available at Expert Consult.

674.7 Cavus Feet
Jennifer J. Winell and Richard S. Davidson

Cavus is a deformity involving plantarflexion of the forefoot or midfoot on the hindfoot and may involve the entire forepart of the foot or just the medial column. The result is an elevation of the medial longitudinal arch (Fig. 674-8). A deformity of the hindfoot will often develop to compensate for the primary forefoot abnormality. While familial cavus may occur, the majority of patients with this deformity will have an underlying neuromuscular etiology. The initial goal is to rule out (and treat) any underlying causes. These diagnoses may relate to abnormalities of the spinal cord (occult dysraphism, tethered cord, polio, myelodysplasia, etc.) and peripheral nerves (hereditary motor and sensory neuropathies [see Chapter 613] such as Charcot-Marie-Tooth [CMT] disease, Dejerine-Sottas disease, or Refsum disease). Although a unilateral cavus foot is most likely to result from an occult intraspinal anomaly, bilateral involvement usually suggests an underlying nerve or muscle disease. Cavus is commonly observed in association with a hindfoot deformity. Two-thirds of CMT patients have pes cavovarus, while 80% of pes cavovarus is most commonly seen in patients with the hereditary motor and sensory neuropathies (CMT), with 80% of CMT patients having pes cavovarus and 65% of patients with cavovarus having CMT. In patients with hereditary motor and sensory

neuropathies, progressive weakness and muscle imbalance result in plantarflexion of the 1st ray/medial column. To obtain a plantigrade foot, the hindfoot must roll into varus. With equinocavus, the hindfoot is in equinus, whereas in calcaneocavus (usually seen in polio or myelodysplasia), the hindfoot is in calcaneus (excessive dorsiflexion).

TREATMENT
Any underlying diagnosis must be identified as this knowledge also helps to address the specific disorder and formulate the proper management strategy. With mild deformities, stretching through physical therapy or serial casting of the plantar fascia and contracted muscles with exercises to strengthen weakened muscles may help to delay progression. An ankle–foot orthosis may be necessary to stabilize the foot and improve ambulation. Surgical treatment is indicated for progressive or symptomatic deformities that have failed to respond to nonoperative measures or in the foot that is no longer braceable. The specific procedures recommended depend on the degree of deformity and the underlying diagnosis. In the case of a progressive neuromuscular condition, recurrence of deformity is commonly observed, and additional procedures may be required to maintain a plantigrade foot. Families should be counseled in detail regarding the disease process and the expected gains from the surgery. The goal of surgery is to restore motion and alignment and to improve muscle balance. For milder deformities, a soft-tissue release of the plantar fascia, often combined with a tendon transfer, may suffice. For patients with a fixed bony deformity of the forefoot, midfoot and/or the hindfoot, 1 or more osteotomies may be required for realignment. A triple arthrodesis (calcaneocuboid, talonavicular, and subtalar) may be required for severe feet (or recurrent deformities) in older patients. Long-term bracing is usually helpful in preventing recurrence.

Bibliography is available at Expert Consult.

674.8 Osteochondroses/Apophysitis
Jennifer J. Winell and Richard S. Davidson

Osteochondroses are idiopathic avascular necrosis of bones which may involve tarsal bones as well. Although rare, they may be observed in the tarsal navicular **(Köhler disease)** or the 2nd or 3rd metatarsal head **(Freiberg infraction)** (Fig. 674-9). These are generally self-limited conditions that commonly result in activity-related pain, which can at times be disabling. The treatment is based on the degree of symptoms and commonly includes restriction of activity. The diagnosis is often made by history and physical exam in conjunction with concordant radiographic findings. The navicular is particularly sensitive

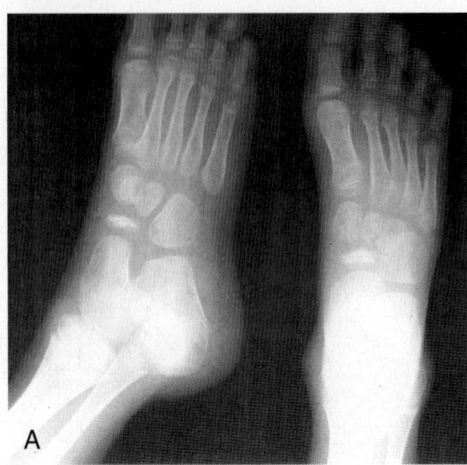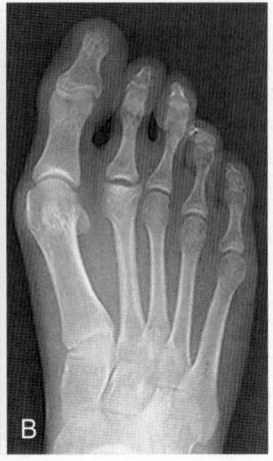

Figure 674-9 Radiographs of Köhler disease **(A)** and Freiberg infraction **(B)**.

as it is the last tarsal bone to ossify which may lead to compression from adjacent ossified bones. For patients with Köhler disease, nonsurgical treatment with a short leg cast for 6-8 wk may provide significant relief. Patients with Freiberg infraction may benefit from a period of casting and/or shoe modifications such as a rocker-bottom sole, a stiff-soled shoe, or a metatarsal bar. Degenerative changes and collapse of the metatarsal head will occasionally occur following the gradual healing process, and surgical intervention is required in a small subset of cases. Procedures have included joint debridement, bone grafting, redirectional osteotomy, subtotal or complete excision of the metatarsal head, and joint replacement.

Apophysitis represents inflammation at the tendinous insertion of a muscle from repetitive tensile loading and is most commonly observed during periods of rapid growth. These stresses result in microfractures at the fibrocartilaginous insertion site, associated with inflammation. Calcaneal apophysitis **(Sever disease)** is the most common cause of heel pain in children; treatment includes activity modification, nonsteroidal antiinflammatory medications, heel cord stretching exercises, and heel cushions or arch supports. **Iselin disease** represents an apophysitis at the 5th metatarsal base where the peroneus brevis attaches and is less common. Even though the mandate for imaging heel pain in all children remains controversial, radiographs should be considered when the symptoms are unilateral or with a failure to respond to treatment. A period of rest (6-8 wk) and avoidance of sports will often resolve symptoms, although recurrence is common until maturity when the apophyses close.

Bibliography is available at Expert Consult.

674.9 Puncture Wounds of the Foot
Jennifer J. Winell and Richard S. Davidson

Most puncture wound injuries to the foot may be adequately managed in the emergency department. **Treatment** involves a thorough irrigation and a tetanus booster, if appropriate; many clinicians will recommend antibiotics. Using this approach, the majority will heal without a complication. A subset of cases may develop cellulitis, most often caused by *Staphylococcus aureus*, and require intravenous antibiotics with or without surgical drainage. Persistent signs of infection should be investigated more thoroughly. Deep infection is uncommon and may be associated with septic arthritis or osteomyelitis. The most common organisms are *S. aureus* and *Pseudomonas aeruginosa*; the treatment involves a thorough surgical debridement followed by a short course (10-14 days) of systemic antibiotics. Although plain radiographs will demonstrate any metallic fragments or other radiopaque foreign bodies, ultrasonography (or advanced imaging such as CT or

MRI) may be necessary to identify radiolucent objects such as glass, plastic, or wood. Routine exploration and removal of foreign bodies is not required, but may be necessary when symptoms are present, with recurrences, or when an infection is suspected. Pain and/or gait disturbance is more likely with superficial objects under the plantar surface of the foot.

A special situation occurs when a puncture wound from a nail comes through a rubber sneaker or running shoe. This situation presents a high risk of a *Pseudomonas* infection, and consideration should be given to a thorough irrigation and debridement under general anesthesia followed by systemic antibiotics for 10-14 days. Foreign-body entrapment of rubber may also occur.

Bibliography is available at Expert Consult.

674.10 Toe Deformities
Jennifer J. Winell and Richard S. Davidson

JUVENILE HALLUX VALGUS (BUNION)
Juvenile hallux valgus is most common in females (~10-fold), and while a family history is uncommon, it is typically associated with familial ligamentous laxity. The etiology is multifactorial, and important factors include genetic factors, ligamentous laxity, pes planus, wearing shoes with a narrow toe box, and occasionally spasticity (cerebral palsy).

Clinical Manifestations
There is prominence of the 1st metatarsophalangeal (MTP) joint and often erythema and callus from chronic irritation. The great toe is in valgus and is usually pronated, and there is splaying of the forefoot. Pes planus, with or without an associated heel cord contracture, is also observed commonly. Although cosmesis is perhaps the most common concern, patients may have pain in the region of the 1st MTP joint and/or difficulty with shoe wear.

Radiographic Evaluation
Weightbearing AP and lateral radiographs of the feet are obtained. On the AP view, common measurements include the angular relationships between the 1st and 2nd metatarsals (intermetatarsal angle, <10 degrees is normal) and between the 1st metatarsal and the proximal phalanx (hallux valgus angle, <25 degrees is normal). The orientation of the 1st metatarsal–medial cuneiform joint is also documented. On the lateral radiograph, the angular relationship between the talus and the 1st metatarsal helps to identify a midfoot break associated with pes planus. Radiographs are more helpful in surgical planning than in establishing the diagnosis.

Treatment

Conservative management of adolescent bunions consists primarily of shoe modifications. It is important that footwear accommodate the width of the forefoot. Patients should avoid wearing shoes with a narrow toe box and/or a high heel. Shoe modifications, such as a soft upper, bunion last, or heel cup, may also be recommended. In the presence of a pes planus, an orthotic to restore the medial longitudinal arch may be beneficial. If a tendo-Achilles contracture is present, stretching exercises are recommended. The value of night splinting remains to be determined. Surgical treatment is reserved for those patients with persistent and disabling pain who have failed a course of nonoperative therapy. Surgery is not advised purely for cosmesis. Surgery is usually delayed until skeletal maturity to decrease the risk of recurrence or overcorrection. Radiographs are essential in preoperative planning to assess both the magnitude of deformity (hallux valgus angle, intermetatarsal angle, distal metatarsal articular angle) and associated features such as obliquity of the 1st metatarsal–medial cuneiform joint. Surgical treatment often involves a soft-tissue release and or rebalancing procedure at the 1st MTP joint, and a single or double osteotomy of the 1st metatarsal to decrease foot width and realign the joints along the medial column of the forefoot. An arthrodesis of the 1st MTP joint may be indicated in patients with spasticity to prevent recurrence.

CURLY TOES

A curly toe is caused by contracture of the flexor digitorum longus, and there is flexion at the MTP and the interphalangeal (IP) joints associated with medial deviation of the toe. The toe usually lies underneath its neighbor, and the 4th and 5th toes are most commonly involved. The deformity rarely causes symptoms, and active treatment (stretching, splinting, or taping) is not required. Most cases improve over time, and a subset will resolve completely. For the rare case in which there is chronic pain or skin irritation, release of the flexor digitorum longus muscle at the distal IP joint may be considered when the child is older.

OVERLAPPING FIFTH TOE

Congenital digitus minimus varus, or varus 5th toe, involves dorsiflexion and adduction of the 5th toe. The 5th toe typically overlaps the 4th. There is also a rotatory deformity of the toe, and the nail tends to point outward. The deformity is usually bilateral and may have a genetic basis. Symptoms are frequent and involve pain over the dorsum of the toe from shoe wear. Nonoperative treatment has not been successful. For symptomatic patients, several different options for reconstruction have been described. Common features include releasing the contracted extensor tendon and the MTP joint capsule (dorsal, dorsomedial, or complete). A partial removal of the proximal phalanx and creation of a syndactyly between the 4th and 5th toes has been performed in conjunction with the release as well.

POLYDACTYLY

Polydactyly is the most common congenital toe deformity and is seen in approximately 2 in 1,000 births and is bilateral in 50% of cases. Polydactyly may be preaxial (great toe) or postaxial (5th toe), and occasionally one of the central toes is duplicated. Associated anomalies are found in approximately 10% of the preaxial and 20% of postaxial polydactyly. One-third of patients will also have polydactyly of the hand. Conditions that may be associated with polydactyly include Ellis-Van Creveld (chondroectodermal dysplasia), longitudinal deficiency of the tibia, and Down syndrome. The extra digit may be either rudimentary or well formed, and plain radiographs of the foot help to define the anatomy and evaluate any coexisting bony anomalies. Treatment is indicated for cosmesis and to allow for fitting with standard shoes. This involves surgical removal of the extra digit, and the procedure is generally performed between 9 and 12 mo of age. Rudimentary digits may be surgically excised earlier, but should not be "tied off."

SYNDACTYLY

Syndactyly involves webbing of the toes, which may be incomplete or complete (extends to the tip of the toes), and the toenails may be

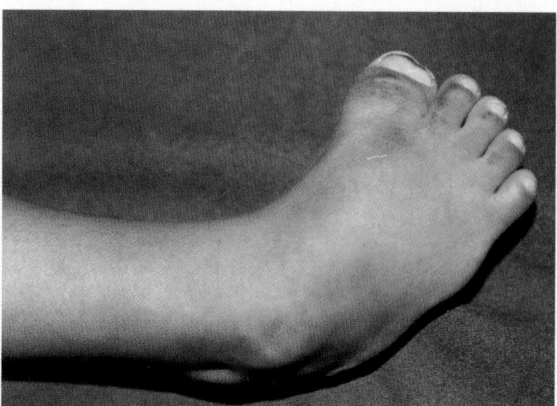

Figure 674-10 Clinical picture of polysyndactyly involving the great toe.

confluent. There is often a positive family history, and the 3rd and 4th toes are involved most commonly. Symptoms are extremely rare, and cosmetic concerns are infrequent. Treatment is only required for a subset of cases in which there is an associated polydactyly (Fig. 674-10). In such cases, the border digit is excised, and the extra skin facilitates coverage of the wound. If the syndactyly does not involve the extra toe, then it can be observed. A complex syndactyly may be seen in patients with Apert syndrome.

HAMMER TOE

A hammer toe involves flexion at the proximal IP (PIP) joint with or without the distal IP (DIP) joint, and the MTP joint may be hyperextended. This deformity may be distinguished from a curly toe by the absence of rotation. The 2nd toe is most commonly involved, and a painful callus may develop over the dorsum of the toe where it rubs on the shoe. Nonoperative therapy is rarely successful, and surgery is recommended for symptomatic cases. A release of the flexor tendons will suffice in the majority of cases. Some authors recommend a transfer of the flexor tendon to the extensor tendon. For severe cases with significant rigidity, especially in older patients, a partial or complete resection of the proximal phalanx and a PIP fusion may be required.

MALLET TOE

Mallet toe involves a flexion contracture at the DIP joint and results from congenital shortening of the flexor digitorum longus tendon. Patients may develop a painful callus on the plantar surface of the tuft. As nonoperative therapy is usually unsuccessful, surgery is required for patients with chronic symptoms. For flexible deformities in younger children, release of the flexor digitorum longus tendon is recommended. For stiffer deformities in older patients, resection of the head of the middle phalanx, or arthrodesis of the DIP joint, may be considered.

CLAW TOE

A claw toe deformity involves hyperextension at the MTP joint and flexion at both the PIP and DIP joints, often associated with dorsal subluxation of the MTP joint. The majority are associated with an underlying neurologic disorder such as CMT disease. The etiology is usually muscle imbalance, and the extensor tendons are recruited to substitute for weakening of the tibialis anterior muscle. If treatment is elected, then surgery is required. Transfer of the extensor digitorum (or hallucis) tendon to the metatarsal neck is commonly performed along with a dorsal capsulotomy of the MTP joint and fusion of the fusion of the PIP joint (IP joint of the great toe).

ANNULAR BANDS

Bands of amniotic tissue associated with amniotic disruption syndrome (early amniotic rupture sequence, congenital constriction band syndrome, annular band syndrome) may become entwined along the

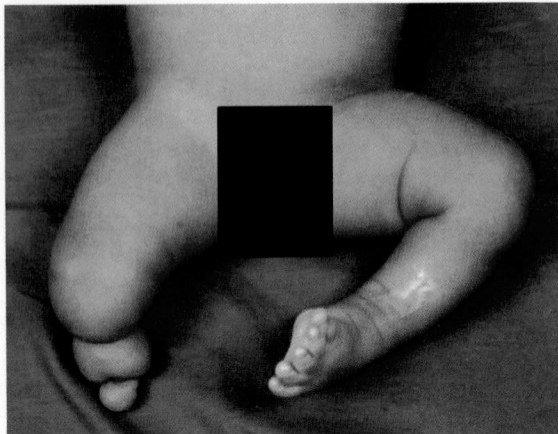

Figure 674-11 Constriction band syndrome with congenital amputation.

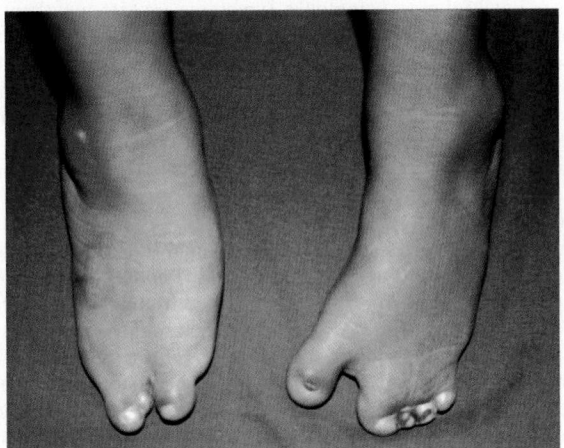

Figure 674-12 Constriction band syndrome with foot involvement.

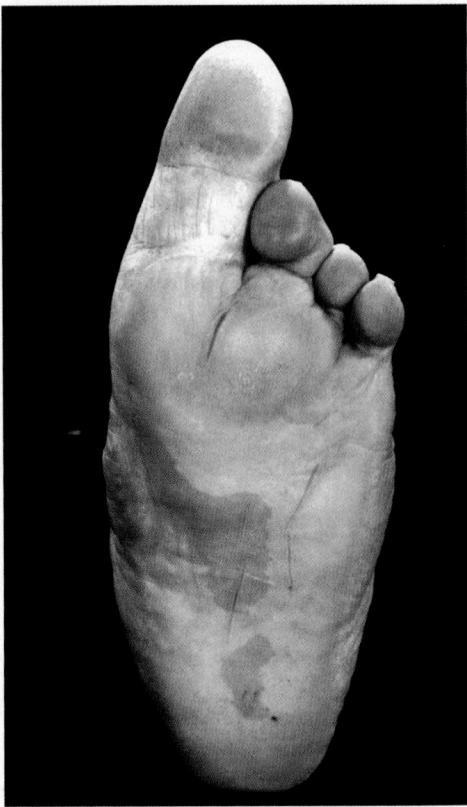

Figure 674-13 Macrodactyly of the great toe in a case of Proteus syndrome.

extremities, resulting in a spectrum of problems from in utero amputation (Fig. 674-11) to a constriction ring along a digit (Fig. 674-12) (see Chapter 108). These rings, if deep enough, may result in impairment of arterial or venous blood flow. Even though concerns regarding tissue viability are less common, swelling from impairment in venous return is often a great problem. The treatment of annular bands usually involves observation; however, circumferential release of the band may be required emergently if arterial inflow is obstructed or electively to relieve venous congestion.

MACRODACTYLY

Macrodactyly represents an enlargement of the toes and may occur as an isolated problem or in association with a variety of other conditions such as Proteus syndrome (Fig. 674-13), neurofibromatosis, tuberous sclerosis, and Klippel-Trenaunay-Weber syndrome. This condition results from a deregulation of growth, and there is hyperplasia of one or more of the underlying tissues (osseous, nervous, lymphatic, vascular, fibrofatty). Macrodactyly of the toes may be seen in isolation (localized gigantism) or with enlargement of the entire foot. In addition to cosmetic concerns, patients may have difficulty wearing standard shoes. The treatment is observation, if possible. This is a difficult condition to treat surgically, and complications are frequent. For involvement of a single toe, the best option may be a resection of the ray (including the metatarsal). For greater degrees of involvement, debulking of the various tissues is required. Often, a growth arrest of the underlying osseous structures is performed. Stiffness and wound problems are common. The rate of recurrence is high, and more than one

debulking may be required. Patients may elect to have an amputation if the process cannot be controlled by less extensive procedures.

SUBUNGUAL EXOSTOSIS

A subungual exostosis is a mass of normal bone tissue that projects out from the dorsal and medial surface of a toe, under the nail. The etiology is unknown but may relate to minor, repetitive trauma. The great toe is involved most often. Patients present with discomfort, and the toenail may be elevated. The lesion may be demonstrated on plain radiographs, and histologically involves normal bone with a fibrocartilaginous cap. The treatment for symptomatic lesions is excision, and the recurrence rate is in the range of 10%.

INGROWN TOENAIL

Ingrown toenails are relatively common in infants and young children and usually involve the medial or lateral border of the great toe. Symptoms include chronic irritation and discomfort, and recurrent infection is seen in some cases. Parents should be instructed when cutting toe nails to cut straight across the distal aspect of the nail, rather than curve inwards at the nail edges. If conservative measures including shoe modifications, warm soaks, and appropriate nail trimming fail to control the symptoms, then surgical removal of a portion of the nail should be considered.

Bibliography is available at Expert Consult.

674.11 Painful Foot
Jennifer J. Winell and Richard S. Davidson

Table 674-2 shows a differential diagnosis for foot pain in different age ranges. In addition to the history and physical examination, plain

Table 674-2	Differential Diagnosis of Foot Pain By Age	
0-6 YR	**6-12 YR**	**12-20 YR**
Poorly fitting shoes	Poorly fitting shoes	Poorly fitting shoes
Foreign body	Sever disease	Stress fracture
Fracture	Enthesopathy (JIA)	Foreign body
Osteomyelitis	Foreign body	Ingrown toenail
Leukemia	Accessory navicular	Metatarsalgia
Puncture wound	Tarsal coalition	Plantar fasciitis
Drawing of blood	Ewing sarcoma	Osteochondroses (avascular necrosis)
Dactylitis	Hypermobile flatfoot	Freiberg
JIA	Trauma (sprains, fractures) Puncture wound	Köhler Achilles tendinitis Trauma (sprains) Plantar warts Tarsal coalition

JIA, juvenile idiopathic arthritis.

radiographs are most helpful in establishing the diagnosis. Occasionally, more sophisticated imaging modalities such as CT or MRI will be required.

674.12 Shoes
Jennifer J. Winell and Richard S. Davidson

In toddlers and children, a well-fitting shoe with a **flexible** sole is recommended. This recommendation is in part based on studies suggesting that the development of the longitudinal arch seems to be best in societies where shoes are not worn and flatfeet are more common in shod children. Well-cushioned, shock-absorbing shoes are helpful in the child and adolescent athlete to decrease the chances of developing an overuse injury. Otherwise, shoe modifications are generally reserved for abnormalities in either alignment between segments of the foot or symptoms from an underlying condition (such as a limb-length discrepancy). Numerous modifications are available.

As a rule, shoes protect the foot from abnormal temperature as well as rough surfaces and sharp objects but have not been shown to help the normal foot develop. Poorly fitting shoes may create problems.

Bibliography is available at Expert Consult.

Chapter 675
Torsional and Angular Deformities

675.1 Normal Limb Development
Keith D. Baldwin and Lawrence Wells

Pediatricians must understand normal limb development so as to recognize pathologic conditions during routine and targeted exams.

During the 7th wk of intrauterine life, the lower limb rotates medially to bring the great toe toward the midline. The hip joint forms by the 11th wk; the proximal femur and acetabulum continue to develop until physeal closure in adolescence. At birth, the femoral neck is rotated forward approximately 40 degrees. This forward rotation is referred to as anteversion (the angle between the axis of the femoral neck and the transcondylar axis). The increased anteversion increases the internal rotation of the hip. Femoral anteversion decreases to 15-20 degrees by 8-10 yr of age. Conditions such as cerebral palsy that involve spasticity of the lower extremities can result in the persistence of fetal anteversion, which results in torsional abnormalities of the lower limb and gait disturbances. The second source of limb rotation is found in the tibia. Infants can have 30 degrees of medial rotation of the tibia, and by maturity the rotation is between 5 degrees of medial rotation and 15 degrees of lateral rotation (Fig. 675-1). Excessive medial rotation of tibia is referred to as **medial tibial torsion**. This is very common, and although very concerning to parents, very rarely requires treatment. Observation is indicated for most cases of medial tibial torsion. The tibial torsion is the angular difference between the axis of the knee and the transmalleolar axis. The medial or lateral rotation beyond ±2 SDs from the mean is considered abnormal rotation. The third source of rotational (axial) abnormalities of the lower extremity comes from the foot. Metatarsus adductus can cause the toes to point inward, and can be assessed by assessing if the medial border of the foot is straight.

Torsional deformity may be simple, involving a single segment, or complex, involving multiple segments. Complex deformities may be additive (internal tibial torsion and internal femoral torsion are additive) or compensatory (external tibial torsion and internal femoral torsion are compensatory).

The normal tibiofemoral angle at birth is 10-15 degrees of physiologic varus. The alignment changes to 0 degrees by 18 mo, and physiologic valgus up to 12 degrees is reached in between 3 and 4 yr of age. The normal valgus of 7 degrees is achieved by 5-8 yr of age (Fig. 675-2). Persistence of varus beyond 2 yr of age may be pathologic and is seen in conditions such as Blount disease. Overall, 95% of developmental physiologic genu varum and genu valgum cases resolve with growth. Persistent genu valgum or valgus into adolescence is considered pathologic and deserves further evaluation.

Bibliography is available at Expert Consult.

675.2 Evaluation
Keith D. Baldwin and Lawrence Wells

In evaluation of concerns relating to the limb, the pediatrician should obtain a history of the onset, progression, functional limitations, previous treatment, evidence of neuromuscular disorder, and any significant family history.

The examination should assess the exact torsional profile and include (1) foot progression angle, (2) femoral anteversion, (3) tibial version with thigh–foot angle, and (4) assessment of foot adduction and abduction.

FOOT PROGRESSION ANGLE
Limb position during gait is expressed as the foot progression angle and represents the angular difference between the axis of the foot with the direction in which the child is walking. Its value is usually estimated by asking the child to walk in the clinic hallway (Fig. 675-3). Inward rotation of the foot is assigned a negative value, and outward rotation is designated with positive value. The normal foot progression angle in children and adolescents is 10 degrees (range: −3 to 20 degrees). The foot progression angle serves only to define whether there is an in-toeing or out-toeing gait.

FEMORAL ANTEVERSION
Measuring the hip rotation with the child in prone position, the hip in neutral flexion or extension, thighs together, and the knees flexed 90

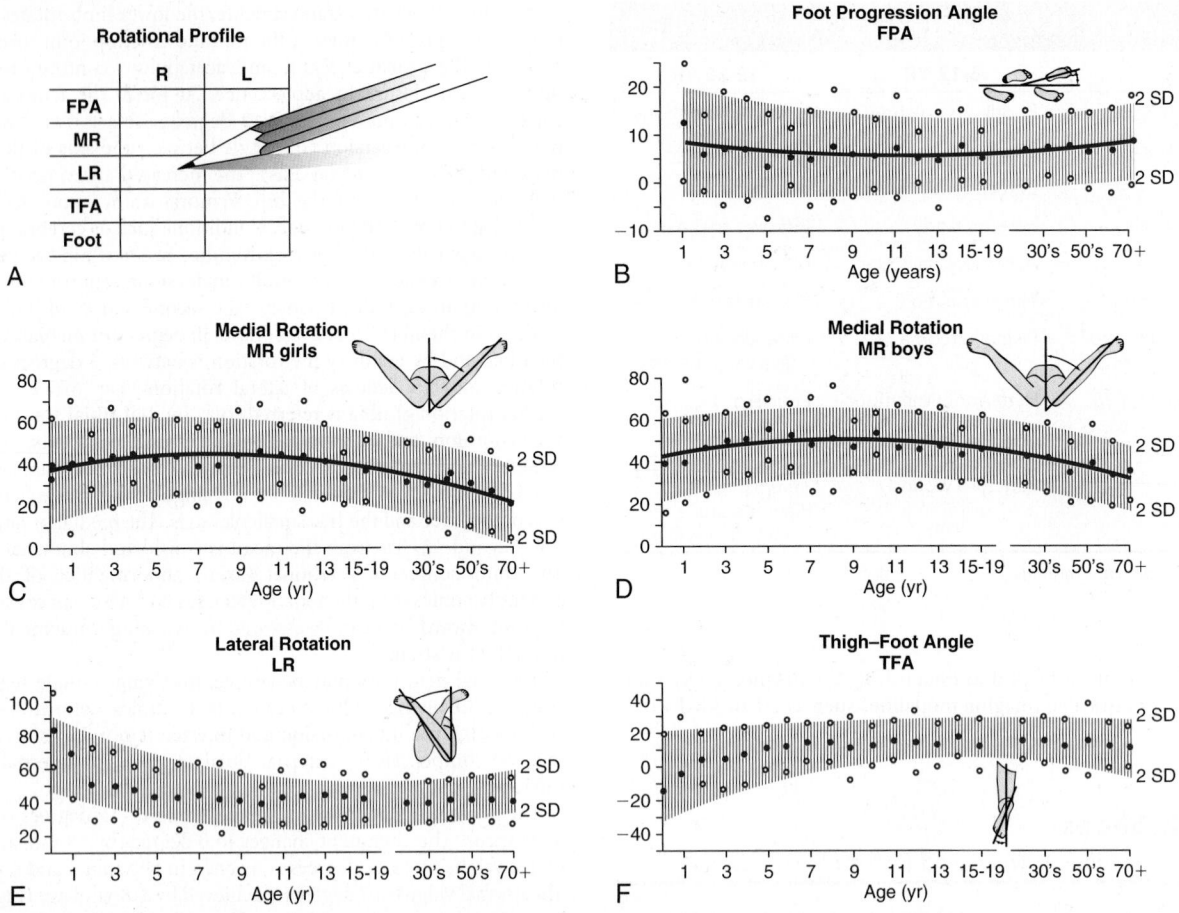

Figure 675-1 A-F, The rotational profile from birth to maturity is depicted graphically. All graphs include 2 SD from the mean for the foot progression angle *(FPA)* for femoral medial rotation *(MR)* and lateral rotation *(LR)* (for boys and girls), and the thigh–foot angle *(TFA). (From Morrissey RT, Weinstein SL, editors:* Lovell and Winter's pediatric orthopaedics, *ed 3, Philadelphia, 1990, Lippincott Williams & Wilkins.)*

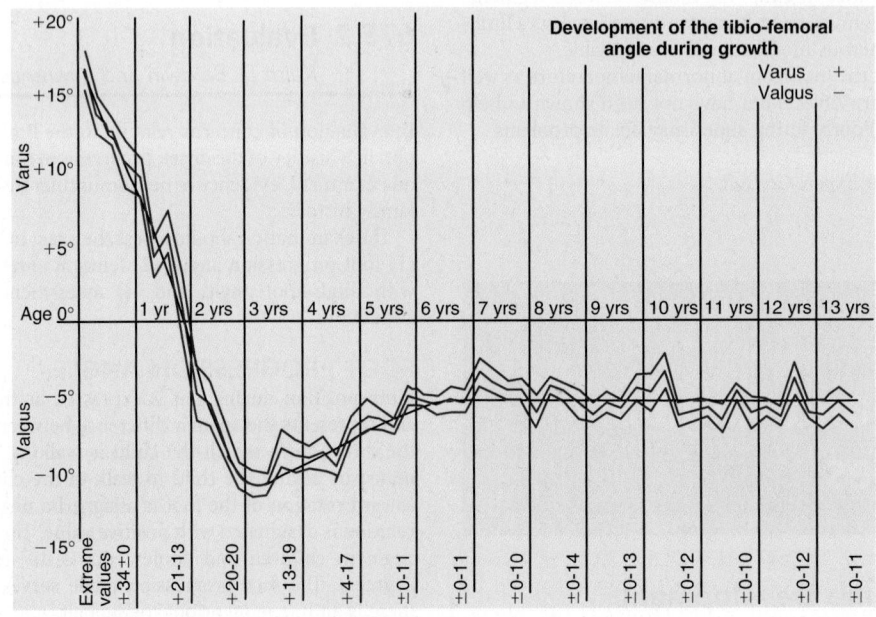

Figure 675-2 The normal coronal alignment of the knee plotted for age. *(From Salenius P, Vanka E: The development of the tibiofemoral angle in children.* J Bone Joint Surg Am *57:259–261, 1975.)*

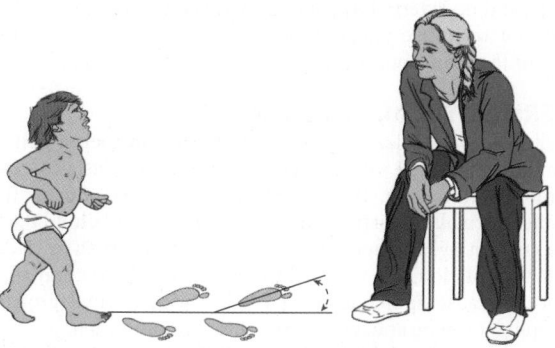

Figure 675-3 Foot progression angle. The long axis of the foot is compared with the direction in which the child is walking. If the long axis of the foot is directed outward, the angle is positive. If the foot is directed inward, the angle is negative and indicates in-toeing. *(From Thompson GH: Gait disturbances. In Kliegman RM, editor:* Practical strategies in pediatric diagnosis and therapy. *Philadelphia, 2004, WB Saunders.)*

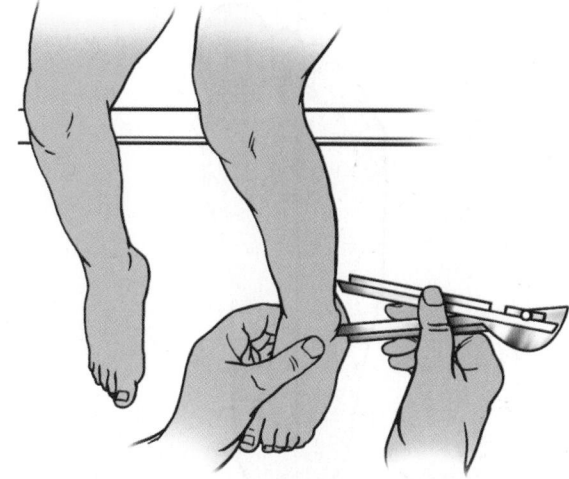

Figure 675-5 The transmalleolar angle is measured with the patient sitting at the edge of the table and the distal femoral condyles aligned with the side of the table. The angle between a line through the medial and lateral malleoli and edge of the table should be approximately 30 degrees external. *(From Bleck EE:* Orthopaedic management in cerebral palsy, *London, 1987, MacKeith Press, p. 55.)*

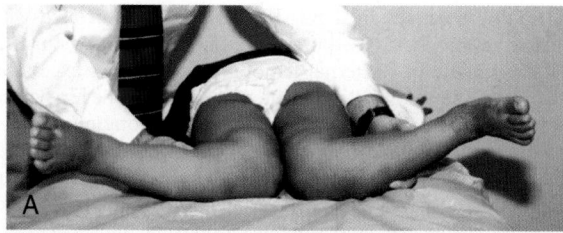

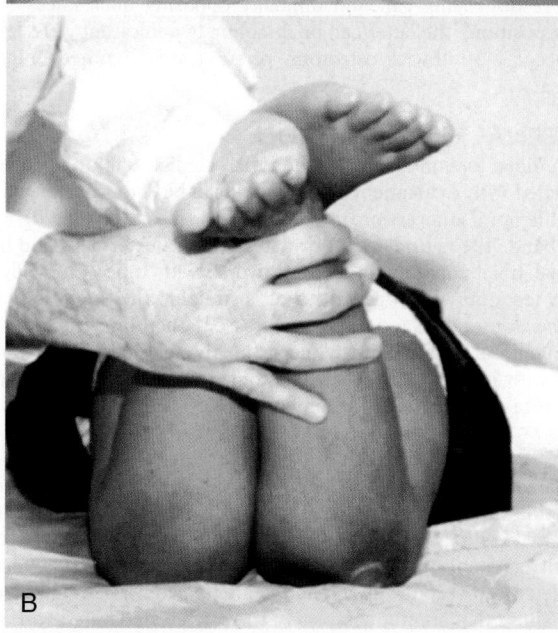

Figure 675-4 Anteversion measured by medial rotation of hip **(A)** and lateral rotation of hip **(B).**

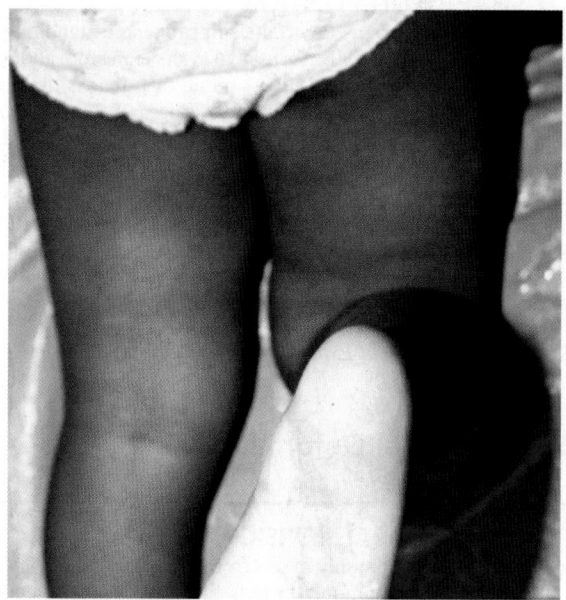

Figure 675-6 Thigh–foot angle.

TIBIAL ROTATION

Tibial rotation is measured using the transmalleolar angle. The transmalleolar angle is the angle between the longitudinal axis of the thigh with a line perpendicular to the axis of the medial and lateral malleolus (Fig. 675-5). In the absence of foot deformity, the thigh–foot angle is preferred (Fig. 675-6). It is measured with the child lying prone. The angle is formed between the longitudinal axis of the thigh and the longitudinal axis of the foot. It measures the tibial and hindfoot rotational status. Inward rotation is assigned a negative value, and outward rotation is designated a positive value. Inward rotation indicates internal tibial torsion, whereas outward rotation represents external tibial torsion. Infants have a mean angle of −5 degrees (range: −35 to 40 degrees) as a consequence of normal in utero position. In mid-childhood through adult life, the mean thigh–foot angle is 10 degrees (range: −5 to 30 degrees).

degrees indirectly assesses the anteversion (Fig. 675-4). Both hips are assessed at the same time. As the lower leg is rotated ipsilaterally, this produces internal rotation of the hip, whereas contralateral rotation produces external rotation. Excessive anteversion increases internal rotation, and, retroversion increases the external rotation. The amount of anteversion can be roughly estimated by palpating the greater trochanter of the hip while internally rotating the limb. The point of maximal prominence of the greater trochanter corresponds to femoral anteversion.

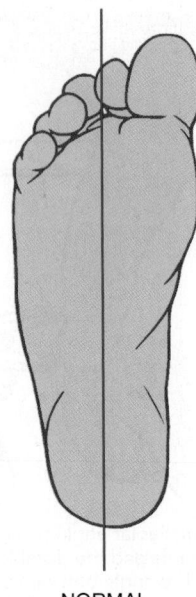

NORMAL

Figure 675-7 Schematic demonstration of heel bisector line.

FOOT SHAPE AND POSITION

The foot is observed for any deformities in prone and standing position. The heel bisector line (HBL) is used to evaluate the foot adduction and abduction deformities. The HBL is a line that divides the heel in 2 equal halves along the longitudinal axis (Fig. 675-7). It normally extends to the 2nd toe. When the HBL points medial to the 2nd toe, the forefoot is abducted, and when the HBL is lateral to the 2nd toe, the forefoot is adducted. Other lower-extremity problems, such as heel varus or valgus, can also make assessment of axial plane issues more difficult.

It is also important to screen every affected child for associated hip dysplasia and neuromuscular problems (cerebral palsy).

Bibliography is available at Expert Consult.

675.3 Torsional Deformities
Keith D. Baldwin and Lawrence Wells

INTERNAL FEMORAL TORSION

In-toeing gait most commonly results from excessive femoral anteversion. It occurs more commonly in girls than boys (2:1) in children 3-6 yr of age. The etiology of femoral torsion is controversial. Some believe that it is congenital and a result of persistent infantile femoral anteversion, whereas others believe it is acquired secondary to abnormal sitting habits. Some children are in habit of sitting in a W position or sleeping prone. On examination, most children with this condition have **generalized ligamentous laxity**. Gait examination reveals that entire leg is inwardly rotated. Internal hip rotation is increased beyond 70 degrees, and consequently the external rotation is restricted to 10-20 degrees. The patellas are pointing inward when the foot is straight, and compensatory external rotation of the tibia is demonstrated. The amount of anteversion can be roughly estimated by palpating the greater trochanter of the hip while internally rotating the limb. The point of maximal prominence of the greater trochanter corresponds to femoral anteversion.

Diagnosis is made clinically on examination; CT can provide objective measurements but is rarely indicated. The treatment is predominantly observation and correction of abnormal sitting habits. The torsion usually corrects with growth by 8-10 yr of age. Persistent deformity, unacceptable cosmesis, functional impairment, anteversion >45

degrees, and no external rotation beyond neutral are some of the indications for operative intervention. Surgery involves derotation osteotomy of the femur but is rarely performed or necessary.

INTERNAL TIBIAL TORSION

Medial (internal) tibial torsion manifests with **in-toeing gait** and is commonly associated with congenital metatarsus varus, genu valgum, or femoral anteversion. This condition is usually seen during the 2nd yr of life. Normally at birth, the medial malleolus lies behind the lateral malleolus, but by adulthood, it is reversed, with the tibia in 15 degrees of external rotation. The treatment is essentially observation and reassurance, because spontaneous resolution with normal growth and development can be anticipated. Significant improvement usually does not occur until the child begins to pull to stand and walk independently. Thereafter, correction can be seen as early as 4 yr of age and in some children by 8-10 yr of age. Persistent deformity with functional impairment is treated with supramalleolar osteotomy, which is rarely necessary.

EXTERNAL FEMORAL TORSION

External femoral torsion can follow a **slipped capital femoral epiphysis**; there is a low threshold to perform radiographs of the hips in children older than 10 yr of age. Femoral retrotorsion, when of idiopathic origin, is usually bilateral. The disorder is associated with an **out-toeing gait** and increased incidence of degenerative arthritis. The clinical examination of external femoral torsion shows excessive hip external rotation and limitation of internal rotation. The hip will externally rotate up to 70-90 degrees, whereas internal rotation is only 0-20 degrees. If slipped capital femoral epiphysis is detected, it is treated surgically. Occasionally, persistent femoral retroversion after slipped capital femoral epiphysis can produce functional impairment such as a severe out-toeing gait and difficulty opposing one's knees in the sitting position. The latter can be disabling to adolescent girls. Should this occur, a Southwick osteotomy or surgical realignment might be necessary.

EXTERNAL TIBIAL TORSION

Lateral tibial torsion is less common than medial rotation and is often associated with a **calcaneovalgus foot**. It can be compensatory to persistent femoral anteversion and idiopathic or secondary to a tight iliotibial band. The natural growth rotates the tibia externally, and hence external tibial torsion can become worse with time. Clinically, the patella faces outward when the foot is straight. The thigh–foot angle and the transmalleolar angle are increased. There may be associated patellofemoral instability with knee pain. Though some correction can occur with growth, extremely symptomatic children need supramalleolar osteotomy, which is usually done by 10-12 yr of age.

METATARSUS ADDUCTUS

Metatarsus adductus (see Chapter 674.1) manifests with forefoot adduction and inversion of all metatarsals. Ten percent to 15% are associated with hip dysplasia. The prognosis is good, because the majority get better with nonoperative intervention. The feet, which are flexible and correctable up to neutral, are treated with stretching exercises. Those that are not completely correctable are treated with serial casting. Rigid deformities, which are not correctable by stretching, are treated with medial capsulotomy of the 1st metatarsal cuneiform joint and soft-tissue release by 2 yr of age. Osteotomies of the base of the metatarsal may be performed after 6 yr of age.

Bibliography is available at Expert Consult.

675.4 Coronal Plane Deformities
Keith D. Baldwin and Lawrence Wells

Genu varum and genu valgum are common pediatric deformities of the knee. Figure 675-2 presents the age-appropriate normal values for

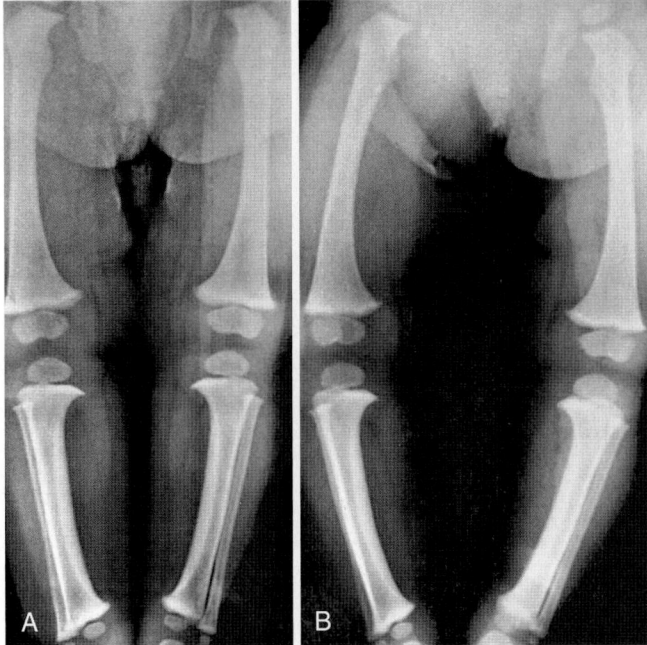

Figure 675-8 A, In recumbent position, tibia and femora are bowed but the legs do not appear bowed. **B,** In erect position during weight bearing and with ankles in apposition, the legs are bowed. *(From Slovis TL, editor:* Caffey's pediatric diagnostic imaging, *ed 11, Philadelphia, 2008, Mosby.)*

knee angle. Tibial bowing is common during the 1st yr, bowlegs are common during the 2nd yr, and knock-knees are most prominent between 3 and 4 yr of age.

GENU VARUM
Physiologic bowleg is a common torsional combination that is secondary to normal in utero positioning (Fig. 675-8). Spontaneous resolution with normal growth and development can be anticipated. Persistence of varus beyond 2 yr of age may be pathologic. The different causes are metabolic bone disease (vitamin D deficiency, rickets, hypophosphatasia), asymmetric growth arrest (trauma, infection, tumor, Blount), bone dysplasia (dwarfism, metaphyseal dysplasia), and congenital and neuromuscular disorders (Table 675-1). It is prudent to differentiate physiologic bowing from Blount disease (Table 675-2). Physiologic bowing should also be differentiated from rickets and skeletal dysplasia. Rickets has classic bone changes with trumpeting widening and fraying of the metaphysis and widening of the physis (see Chapter 51).

TIBIA VARA
Idiopathic tibia vara, or **Blount disease**, is a developmental deformity resulting from abnormal endochondral ossification of the medial aspect of the proximal tibial physis leading to varus angulation and medial rotation of the tibia (Fig. 675-9). The incidence is greater in African-Americans and in toddlers who are overweight, have an affected family member, or started walking early in life. It has been classified into 3 types, depending on the age at onset: infantile (1-3 yr of age), juvenile (4-10 yr of age), and adolescent (11 yr or older). The juvenile and adolescent forms are commonly combined as late-onset tibia vara. The exact cause of tibia vara remains unknown, although it is thought to involve abnormal growth resultant from excessive weight.

The infantile form of tibia vara is the most common; its characteristics include predominance in black females, approximately 80% bilateral involvement, a prominent medial metaphyseal beak, internal tibial torsion, and leg-length discrepancy (LLD). The characteristics of the juvenile and adolescent forms (late onset) include predominance in black males, normal or greater than normal height, approximately

Table 675-1	Classification of Genu Varum (Bowlegs)

PHYSIOLOGIC

ASYMMETRIC GROWTH
Tibia vara (Blount disease)
• Infantile
• Juvenile
• Adolescent
Focal fibrocartilaginous dysplasia
Physeal injury
Trauma
Infection
Tumor

METABOLIC DISORDERS
Vitamin D deficiency (nutritional rickets)
Vitamin D–resistant rickets
Hypophosphatasia

SKELETAL DYSPLASIA
Metaphyseal dysplasia
Achondroplasia
Enchondromatosis

Modified from Thompson GH: Angular deformities of the lower extremities. In Chapman MW (ed): Operative orthopedics, *ed 2, Philadelphia, 1993, JB Lippincott, Tab 222-1, p. 3132.*

Table 675-2	Differentiation of Leg Bowing

PHYSIOLOGIC BOWING	BLOUNT DISEASE
Gentle and symmetric deformity	Asymmetric, abrupt, and sharp angulation
Metaphyseal–diaphyseal angle <11 degrees	Metaphyseal–diaphyseal angle >11 degrees
Normal appearance of the proximal tibial growth plate	Medial sloping of the epiphysis Widening of the physis Fragmentation of the metaphysis
No significant lateral thrust	Significant lateral thrust

50% bilateral involvement, slowly progressive genu varum deformity, pain rather than deformity as the primary initial complaint, no palpable proximal medial metaphyseal beak, minimal internal tibial torsion, mild medial collateral ligament laxity, and mild lower extremity length discrepancy. The infantile group has the greatest potential for progression.

An anteroposterior standing radiograph of both lower extremities with patellas facing forward and a lateral radiograph of the involved extremity should be obtained (Fig. 675-10). Weightbearing radiographs are preferred and allow maximal presentation of the clinical deformity. The metaphyseal–diaphyseal angle can be measured and is useful in distinguishing between physiologic genu varum and early tibia vara (Fig. 675-11). Langenskiöld has 6 stages on radiographs (Fig. 675-12). The differentiation is based on fragmentation of the epiphysis, beaking of the medial tibial epiphysis, depression of the medial tibial plateau, and formation of a bony bar. Occasionally, CT with 3-dimensional reconstructions, or MRI, may be necessary to assess the meniscus, the articular surface of the proximal tibia including the posteromedial slope, or the integrity of the proximal tibial physis.

Management is based on the stage of the disease, the age of the child, and nature of presentation (primary or recurrent deformity). In children younger than 3 yr and Langenskiöld stage <3, bracing is effective and can prevent progression in 50% of these children. A maximal trial of 1 yr of orthotic management is recommended. If complete correction is not obtained after 1 yr or if progression occurs during this

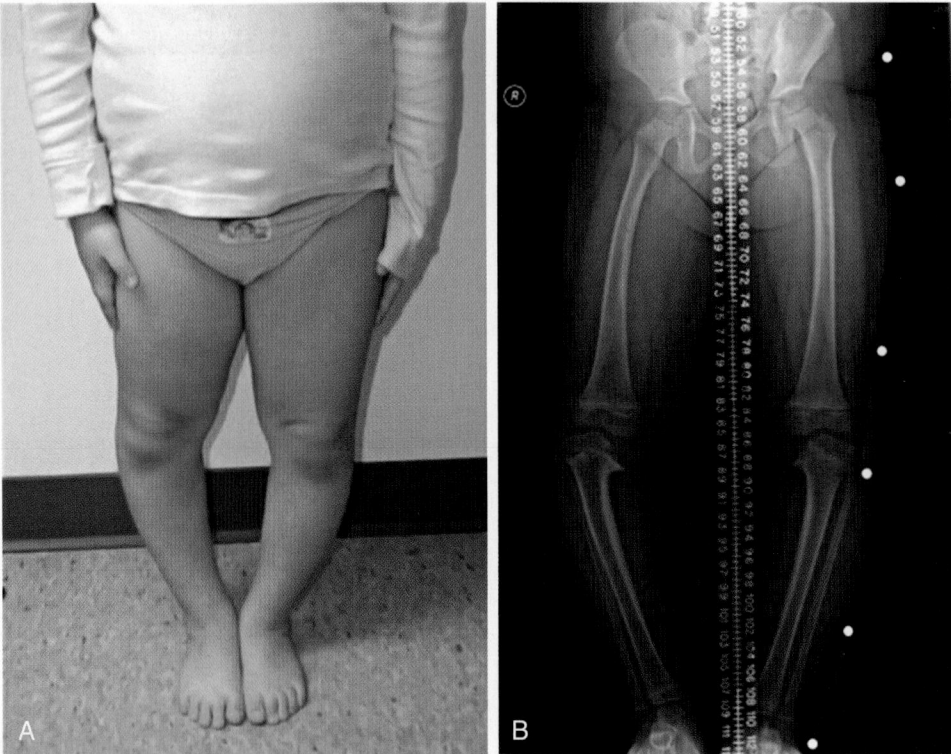

Figure 675-9 Clinical photograph **(A)** and standing anteroposterior radiograph **(B)** of a 5 yr old girl with bilateral early-onset Blount disease. *(From Sabharwal S: Blount disease, J Bone Joint Surg Am 91:1758–1776, 2009.)*

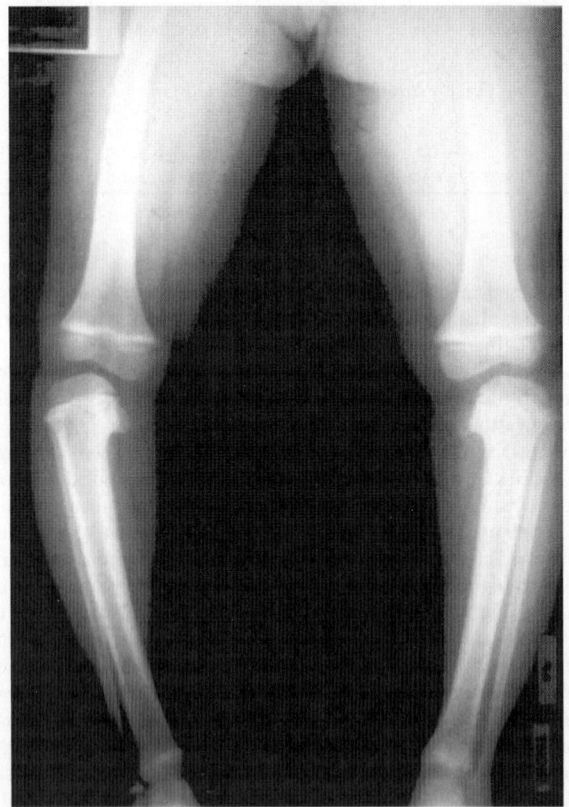

Figure 675-10 Anteroposterior radiograph of both knees in Blount disease.

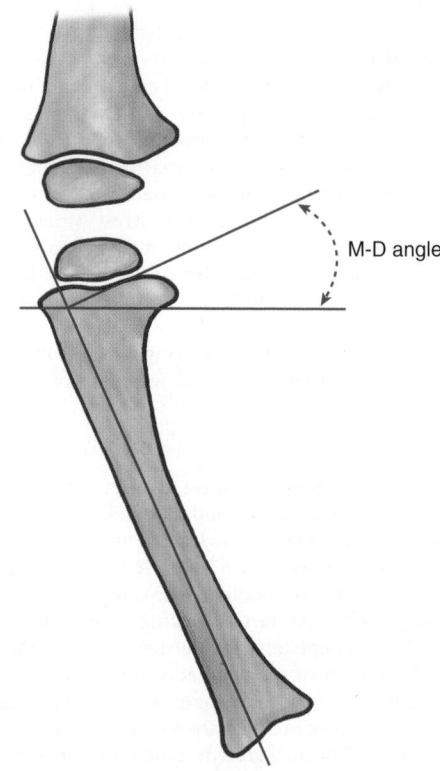

Figure 675-11 Metaphyseal–diaphyseal (M-D) angle. Draw a line on the radiograph through the proximal tibial physis. Draw another line along the lateral tibial cortex. Last, draw a line perpendicular to the shaft line as demonstrated in the diagram. *(From Morrissey RT, Weinstein SL, editors: Lovell and Winter's pediatric orthopaedics, ed 3, Philadelphia, 1990, Lippincott Williams & Wilkins.)*

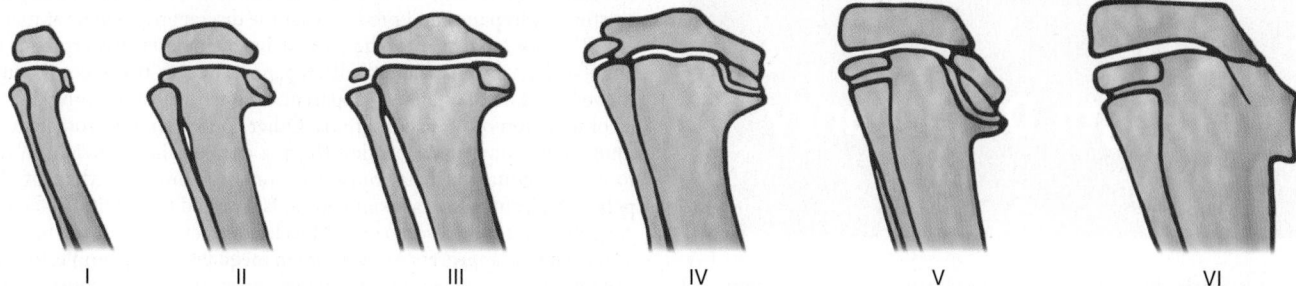

Figure 675-12 Depiction of the stages of infantile Blount disease. *(From Langeskiöld A: Tibia vara (osteochondrosis deformans tibiae): a survey of 23 cases, Acta Chir Scand 103:1, 1952.)*

time, a corrective osteotomy may be indicated. Surgical treatment is also indicated in children >4 yr of age, those at Langenskiöld stage >3, and those with severe deformities. A proximal tibial valgus osteotomy and associated fibular diaphyseal osteotomy are usually the procedures of choice. In late-onset tibia vara, correction is also necessary to restore the mechanical axis of the knee. Hemiplateau elevation with correction of posteromedial slope has also been established as a treatment modality in relapsed cases.

GENU VALGUM (KNOCK-KNEES)
The normal valgus is achieved by 4 yr of age. Variation up to 15 degrees of valgus is possible until 6 yr of age, and thus physiologic valgus has a good chance of correction until this age. The intermalleolar distance with the knees approximated is normally <2 cm, and in a severe valgus deformity it could measure >10 cm. Pathologic conditions leading to valgus are metabolic bone disease (rickets, renal osteodystrophy), skeletal dysplasia, posttraumatic physeal arrest, tumors, and infection. The increased valgus at the knee causes lateral deviation of the mechanical axis with stretching of the medial aspect of the knee leading to knee pain. Deformities >15 degrees and occurring after 6 yr of age are unlikely to correct with growth and require surgical management. In the skeletally immature, medial tibial epiphyseal hemiepiphysiodesis or stapling (guided growth) is attempted for correction. In the skeletally mature, osteotomy is necessary at the center of rotation of angulation and is usually situated in the distal femur. Long-length anteroposterior radiographs of the leg in a weight-bearing stance are necessary for preoperative planning.

Bibliography is available at Expert Consult.

675.5 Congenital Angular Deformities of the Tibia and Fibula
Keith D. Baldwin and Lawrence Wells

POSTEROMEDIAL TIBIAL BOWING
Congenital posteromedial bowing is typically associated with a calcaneovalgus foot and rarely with secondary valgus of the tibia. The exact cause is unknown. Early operative intervention is not indicated because this bowing generally corrects with growth. However, despite the correction of angulation, there is residual shortening in the tibia and fibula. The mean growth inhibition is 12-13% (range: 5-27%). The mean LLD at maturity is 4 cm (range: 3-7 cm). The diagnosis of bowing is confirmed on radiographs, which show the posteromedial angulation without any other osseous abnormalities. The calcaneovalgus deformity of the foot improves with stretching or modified shoe wear and occasionally ankle-foot orthosis. Predicted LLD <4 cm is managed with age-appropriate epiphysiodesis of the normal leg. LLD >4 cm is managed with combination of contralateral epiphysiodesis and ipsilateral lengthening. A corrective osteotomy for distal valgus may be required and can be done in the same setting while correcting LLD.

ANTEROMEDIAL TIBIAL BOWING (POSTAXIAL HEMIMELIA)
Fibular hemimelia is the most common cause of anteromedial bowing of the tibia. The fibular deficiency can occur with complete absence of fibula or a partial development both proximally and distally. It is associated with deformities of femur, knee, tibia, ankle, and foot. The femur is short and has lateral condylar hypoplasia, causing patellar instability and genu valgum deformity. The tibia has anteromedial bowing with reduced growth potential. The keys for management are the ankle stability and foot deformities. The ankle resembles a ball-and-socket joint with lateral instability. The foot deformities are characterized by the absence of lateral digits, equinocavovarus foot, and tarsal coalition.

Various surgical options have been described, and the treatment is tailored to the patient's needs and parents' acceptance. A severely deformed foot could be best managed with Syme or Boyd amputation, with prosthesis as early as 1 yr of age. In the salvageable foot, LLD can be treated with contralateral leg epiphysiodesis or ipsilateral limb lengthening.

ANTEROLATERAL TIBIAL BOWING
Anterolateral tibial bowing is associated with congenital pseudarthrosis of tibia. Fifty percent of the patients have neurofibromatosis, but only 10% of the neurofibromatosis patients have this lesion. The pseudarthrosis or site of nonunion is typically situated at the middle third and distal third of the tibia. Boyd has classified it in increasing severity depending on the presence of cystic and dysplastic changes. The treatment for this condition has been very frustrating, with poor results. Bracing has been recommended to prevent fracture early in the course; however, it has not been successful. Numerous surgical interventions have been attempted to achieve union, such as single- and dual-onlay grafting with rigid internal fixation, intramedullary pinning with or without bone grafting, and an Ilizarov device. With the advent of microsurgery, live fibular grafts have been used with varying results. Because of the poor chances of successful union and considerable LLD, a below-knee amputation with early rehabilitation may be preferred. It is important not to attempt any osteotomy for correction of the tibial bowing.

TIBIAL LONGITUDINAL DEFICIENCY
Tibial longitudinal deficiency follows an autosomal dominant inheritance pattern and has been divided into four types depending on the deficient part of the tibia. The other associated anomalies are foot deformities, hip dysplasia, and symphalangism of the hand. The treatment revolves around presence of proximal tibial anlage and a functional quadriceps mechanism. In type Ia deformity, the proximal tibial anlage is absent and knee disarticulation with prosthesis is recommended. In types Ib and II, the tibial anlage is present and the management consists of an early Syme amputation, followed later by synostosis of the fibula with the tibia, and a below-knee prosthesis. Type III is rare and the principal management is with Syme amputation and a prosthesis. Type IV deformity is associated with ankle diastasis, which requires stabilization of the ankle and correction of LLD at a later stage.

Bibliography is available at Expert Consult.

Chapter **676**
Leg-Length Discrepancy
Richard S. Davidson

A discrepancy in the leg lengths may result from a variety of congenital or acquired conditions (Table 676-1). Although up to 25% of the American public may have a difference of more than 1 cm, only a small percentage have more than a 2 cm difference. The main consequence is gait asymmetry. An increase in vertical pelvic motion is observed, and more energy must be expended during ambulation. Although a small compensatory lumbar curvature may develop, there is little evidence to suggest that leg-length discrepancy results in back pain, structural scoliosis, or degenerative arthritis. The goal of treatment is to have a discrepancy of <2-2.5 cm at skeletal maturity, and a variety of treatment methods are available to achieve this objective. Knowledge of the underlying etiology, coupled with regular follow-up to assess limb growth and skeletal maturity, allows the treating physician to project the discrepancy at skeletal maturity and to plan treatment. A subset of patients will have coexisting abnormalities in the viscera or musculoskeletal system, which must be identified and treated as well.

DIAGNOSIS AND CLINICAL FINDINGS
Gait asymmetry is the most frequent complaint. The long leg is often kept flexed in stance to level the pelvis. The diagnosis is made on

Table 676-1	Causes of Leg-Length Discrepancy

CONGENITAL CAUSES
Defects in Growth
Proximal femoral focal deficiency
Congenital pseudarthrosis of the tibia
Fibular hemimelia (see Fig. 676-8)
Bone Tumors/Disease
Skeletal dysplasia
Multiple hereditary exostoses
Neurofibromatosis
Enchondromatosis (Ollier disease)
Osteogenesis imperfecta
Vascular
Klippel-Trenaunay-Weber syndrome
Russell-Silver syndrome
Miscellaneous
Congenital coxa vara
Proteus syndrome

ACQUIRED CAUSES
Trauma
Overriding fractures
Epiphyseal fractures with growth plate damage
Developmental
Developmental dysplasia of the hip
Neoplastic
Malignant tumors
Tumors across epiphysis
Neurologic
Myelodysplasia
Cerebral palsy
Infections/Inflammatory
Septic arthritis of hip
Osteomyelitis
Rheumatoid arthritis
Miscellaneous
Acquired coxa vara
Fixed pelvic obliquity in scoliosis

physical examination, and specialized radiographs help to quantify the existing discrepancy and predict what the discrepancy will be at maturity The discrepancy may be caused by hypoplasia, hyperplasia, or angular deformity (structural discrepancy), by soft-tissue contracture at the hips, knees, or ankles (apparent or functional shortening), or by a combination of these conditions. Other contributing factors include joint subluxation or dislocation (hip), a decrease in the height of the foot (congenital or neuromuscular) or structural disorders of the pelvis. A careful physical examination is required to identify all factors contributing to the discrepancy. Muscle contracture about the hip will also create the appearance of leg-length inequality. For example, to bear weight on an abducted hip, the patient must hike up the contralateral hip and pelvis, making the contralateral leg appear short.

There are several clinical methods for measuring limb length. Our preference is to perform a standing examination, in which blocks of various sizes are placed under the short leg until the pelvis is leveled (Fig. 676-1). An alternate method is to measure the length of each leg with the patient supine by the Galiazzi and Alis tests. The traditional method of using a tape measure is very inaccurate because of, for example, the line of measurement used, muscle atrophy, and moving patients. The range of motion at the hip, knee, and ankle must be also assessed to identify any causes of apparent discrepancy. A 10 degree fixed abduction (or adduction) contracture of the hip will create an apparent leg-length discrepancy of 2-3 cm. Similarly, a flexion contracture of the hip and/or knee will create apparent shortening of the extremity, while an equinus contracture at the ankle will create apparent lengthening of the extremity. A rigid lumbar scoliosis (suprapelvic contracture) will create pelvic obliquity and an associated limb length inequality. Once a discrepancy is quantified, it must be followed at regular intervals until maturity. Assessments at 6-12 mo intervals are most common.

RADIOGRAPHIC EVALUATION
The radiologic evaluation complements the clinical examination; both are typically employed when making treatment decisions. Five

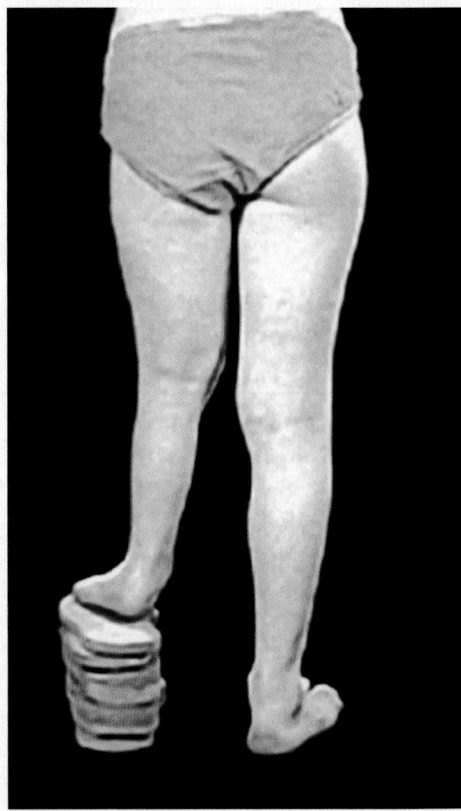

Figure 676-1 Examination with blocks under short leg until the pelvis is squared.

different techniques are available. The *teleoroentgenogram* is a single radiographic exposure of both lower extremities (standing) and requires a long cassette. A ruler is placed on the film, and direct measurements are made, factoring in a 6% magnification error. One advantage is that angular deformities may be assessed. Its primary indication is for young children. Unfortunately, as only one exposure is used for the leg and as the ankle is less dense than the hip, it may be difficult to "see" the whole leg. Additionally, because the x-ray source is at the knee projecting up to the hip and down to the ankle, this method projects the hip and ankle along the ruler making the leg appear longer than it really is, particularly in obese patients. The *orthoroentgenogram* consists of 3 separate exposures of the hips, knees, and ankles on a long cassette. The patient is supine, and a ruler is placed on the cassette for measurement of bone length. However, the patient must lie still for the 3 exposures, which is often difficult to achieve in younger children. Because the x-ray beam is pointed at the hip, knee, and ankle in each of the 3 exposures, the length measurement is accurate and each of the 3 joints can be exposed properly. The x-rays expose from the top of the pelvis to the mid femur, from the mid femur to the mid tibia, and from the mid tibia to below the foot for each of the 3 exposures, respectively, permitting angular deformity assessment in the frontal plane only. The *scanogram* also consists of separate exposures of the hips, knees, and ankles on a cassette with a radiographic ruler; a chest sized film cassette is used (Fig. 676-2). There is no magnification error; patients must remain still for the 3 exposures, and angular deformities cannot be assessed. While *CT* is an accurate technique, the assessment is time-consuming, and the technique is not available in most centers. Additionally a radiologist must normalize the axis of the leg to the screen to accurately measure the limbs. Another technique, called *EOS*, employs a 3D, low-dose ($\frac{1}{7}$ to $\frac{1}{10}$ the radiation) scanner but requires a sophisticated radiologist to correctly align the limbs for computer measurement. Regardless of the technique it is critical that the patellae be pointed forward, that measurements be made in the plane of the limb,

and that the same method be used in sequential measurements to be compared.

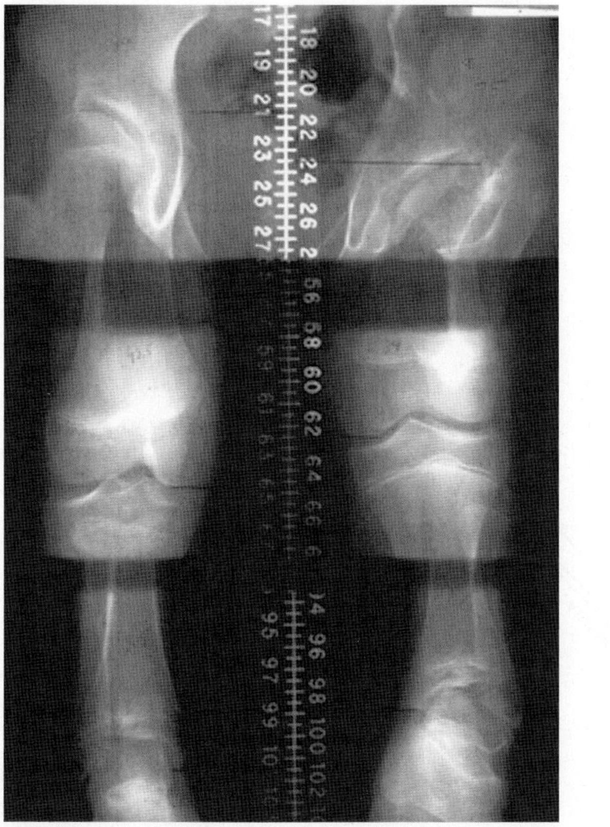

In the presence of flexion or extension deformities, each bone should be x-rayed individually with a ruler where the x-ray beam is perpendicular to the bone and the ruler parallel to the bone.

In addition to quantifying the discrepancy, it is essential to determine skeletal age (bone age). An anteroposterior radiograph of the hand and wrist is usually obtained at each visit and compared with the standards in the Greulich and Pyle Atlas to estimate skeletal age. While more accurate techniques are available, most are time-consuming and impractical for routine clinical application. The range of variability using the atlas is approximately 9 mo, so the method is most accurate when multiple data points have been collected.

TREATMENT

Options for treatment include observation, a shoe lift or custom orthosis, a limb-shortening procedure (acute shortening and internal fixation vs gradual shortening by growth arrest or guided growth), a limb-lengthening procedure (with internal or external fixation), or a combination of these. Deformity correction is often accomplished simultaneously. In the congenital deficiencies (femur, tibia, fibula) in which the predicted limb-length inequality will require more than 3 lengthening operations (more than 20 cm), an early foot amputation may be the best option to achieve an optimal functional outcome. In addition to the magnitude of discrepancy predicted at skeletal maturity, both the anticipated adult height of the patient (estimated from family members) and the desires of the patient and the patient's family are important considerations.

Discrepancies of up to 2.5 cm may be treated by observation or a shoe lift. Up to 1 cm may be placed within the shoe, and up to 5 cm may be placed on the outside of the shoe. Complete correction of inequality is not required, and the height of the lift should be adjusted based on the patient's gait and comfort. An orthotic may be used as a temporizing measure prior to definitive treatment. For extended discrepancies, "foot in foot" prostheses are a reasonable alternative until limb length can be accomplished or for patients who cannot or do not wish to undergo surgical correction.

For patients with a discrepancy between 2 and 5 cm, an **epiphysiodesis** is offered in skeletally immature patients, and an acute shortening may be performed in a skeletally mature patient. Epiphysiodesis refers to a temporary or permanent cessation of growth at 1 or more physes. A permanent growth arrest is most commonly performed as long as sufficient data are available with which to accurately predict when to perform the procedure. Approximately 65% of the growth of the lower extremity comes from the distal femur (37%, 9 mm/yr) and proximal tibia (28%, 6 mm/yr). Males typically grow until 16 yr of age, whereas females grow until 14 yr of age. As such, performing an epiphysiodesis of both the distal femur and the proximal tibia in a patient with 3 yr of growth remaining should achieve approximately 4.5 cm of correction. Techniques used to determine the timing of epiphysiodesis are the Menelaus method ("rule of thumb"), the Green and Anderson method, the Moseley straight-line graph, and the multiplier method (Figs. 676-3, 676-4, and 676-5). The most common surgical technique is the percutaneous epiphysiodesis, in which the physis is ablated with a drill and curette under image intensification. This is an outpatient procedure with few complications. Insertion of plates and screws or just screws across the physis is an alternative but usually requires a second operation to remove the hardware. For patients for whom sufficient data are unavailable or those for whom the underlying diagnosis is associated with an unpredictable pattern of growth, then a reversible technique, such as staples, plates, and/or screws, may be considered. Once equalization has been achieved, the hardware can be removed, allowing growth to resume. When the patient is skeletally mature or if it is deemed appropriate to wait until maturity before treatment, acute shortening may be the best option. Acute shortening is typically performed at the femur (several techniques have been described), given the increased risk of complications (compartment syndrome, neurovascular problems) associated with shortening of the tibia and fibula.

Figure 676-2 Scanogram to demonstrate exact leg-length discrepancy.

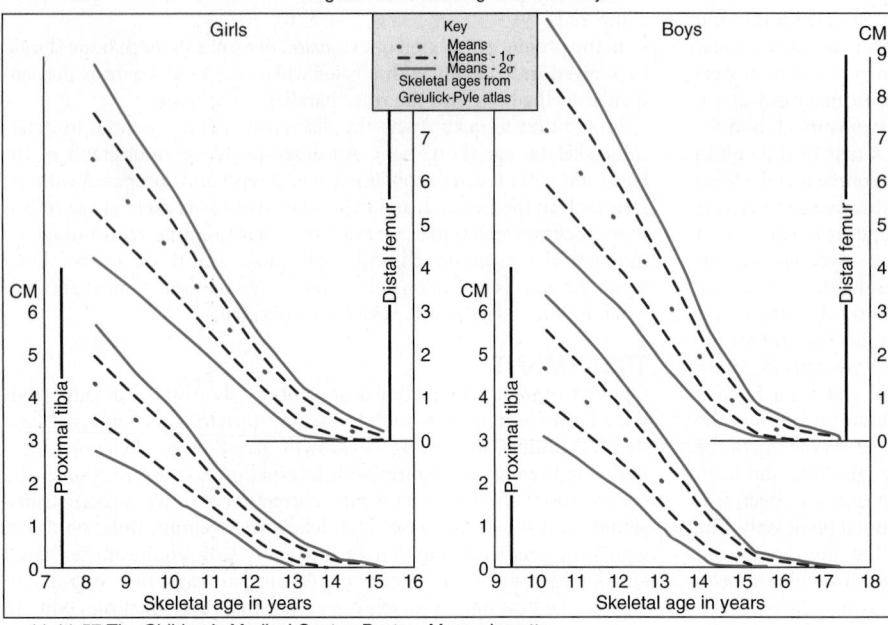

Growth Remaining in Normal Distal Femur and Proximal Tibia Following Consecutive Skeletal Age Levels

Means and standard deviations derived from
longitudinal series 50 girls and 50 boys

11-11-57 The Children's Medical Center, Boston, Massachusetts

Figure 676-3 Growth remaining charts for girls and boys. The growth remaining charts for girls and boys are different. Actual correction is based on growth of the short limb. To use the chart correctly, the discrepancy at maturity and the percentage of growth retardation of the short limb should be calculated. *(Redrawn from Anderson M, Green WT, Messner MB: Growth and predictions of growth in lower extremities. J Bone Joint Surg Am 45:1–4, 1963.)*

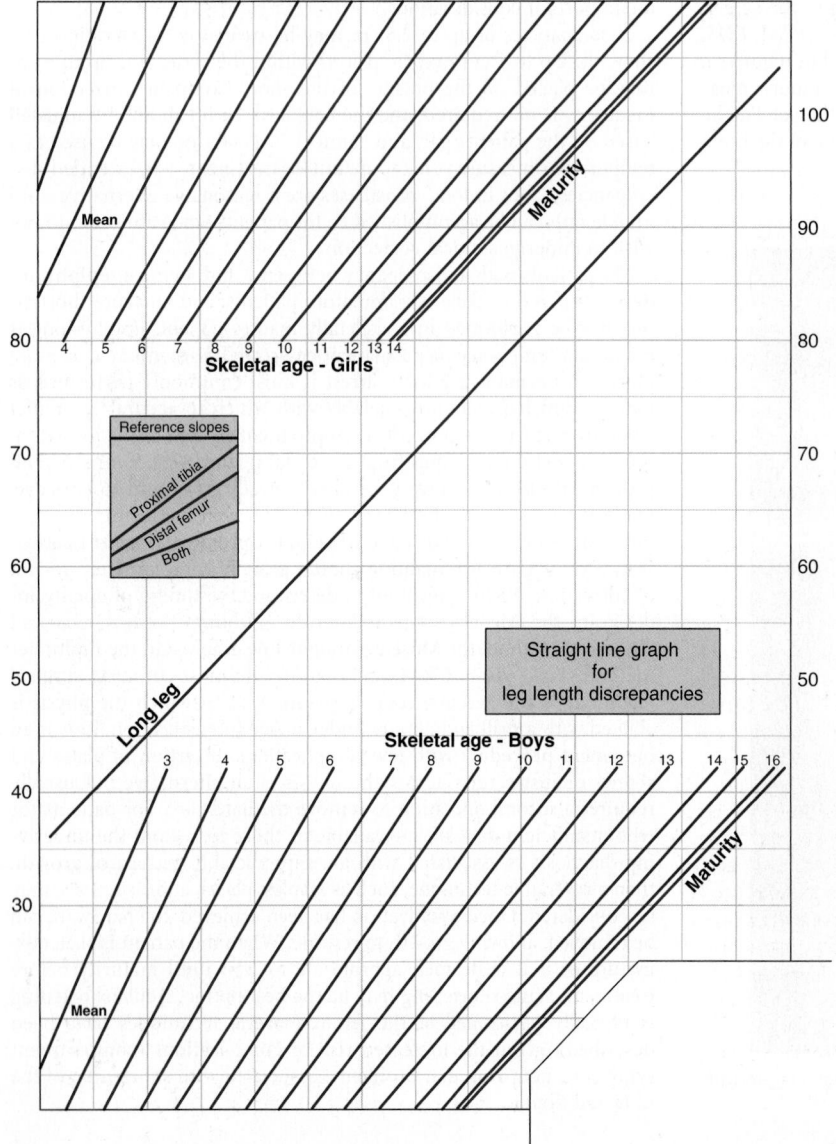

Figure 676-4 The Moseley straight-line graph for the assessment of leg-length inequalities. This allows simultaneous correlation of the normal leg, short leg, and bone age of the child. It will accurately predict lengths of each extremity at skeletal maturity. The reference slopes are used as a guide in determining when appropriate treatment should be performed. *(From Moseley CF: A straight-line graph for leg-length discrepancies. J Bone Joint Surg Am 59:174–179, 1977.)*

Multiplier for Boys and Girls (Paley et al, 1999)				LLD Prediction Formulas
Boys		**Girls**		
Age	Multiplier	Age	Multiplier	
0	5.08	0	4.63	
0.4	4.01	0.3	4.01	
1	3.24	1	2.97	
1.3	2.99	2	2.39	
2	2.59	3	2.05	
3	2.23	3.3	2.00	
4	2.00	4	1.83	
5	1.83	5	1.66	
6	1.68	6	1.53	
7	1.57	7	1.43	
8	1.47	8	1.33	
9	1.38	9	1.26	
10	1.31	10	1.19	
11	1.24	11	1.13	
12	1.18	12	1.07	
13	1.12	13	1.03	
14	1.07	14	1.00	
15	1.03	15	1.00	
16	1.01	16	1.00	
17	1.00			
18	1.00			

LLD Prediction Formulas

Prenatal LLD (congenital)
$$\Delta_m = \Delta \times M$$

Postnatal LLD (developmental)
$$\Delta_m = \Delta + I \times G$$

$$\text{Inhibition} \approx I = 1 - \frac{S - S^\bullet}{L - L^\bullet}$$

$$\text{Growth remaining} = G = L(M - 1)$$

Δ_m = LLD at maturity

Δ = Current LLD

L & S = Current length of long and short leg

$L^\bullet$ & $S^\bullet$ = Length of long and short leg at any other date since LLD began

Figure 676-5 Paley multiplier. This is a simple method of determining the leg-length discrepancy (LLD) at maturation. This is applicable for shortening conditions in which growth retardation is consistent. *(From Paley D, Bhave A, Herzenberg JE, Bowen JR: Multiplier methods for predicting limb-length discrepancy. J Bone Joint Surg Am 82;1432–1446, 2000.)*

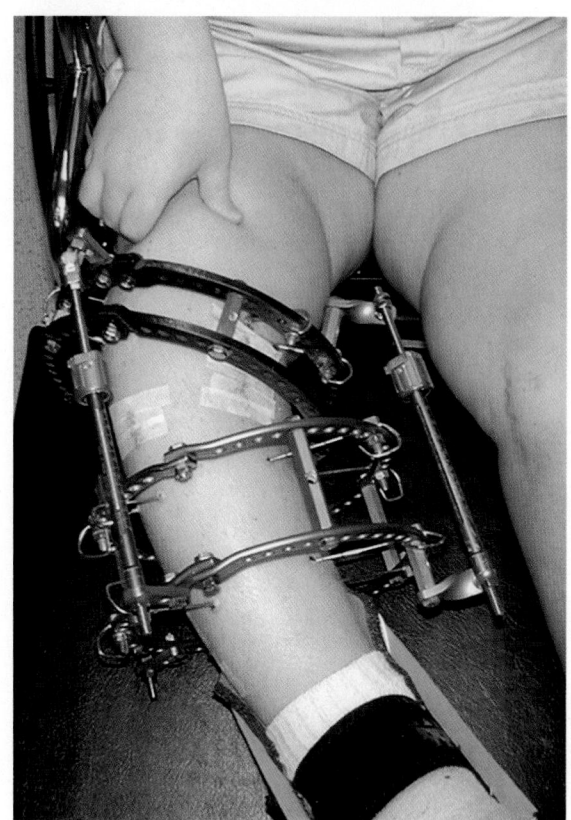

Figure 676-6 Ilizarov device demonstrating bone lengthening by distraction osteogenesis.

For discrepancies >5 cm, lengthening of the short limb is the procedure of choice. An exception would be a discrepancy secondary to overgrowth of 1 limb, in which limb shortening would be preferred so as to preserve body proportions, for which acute or gradual shortening of the abnormal limb is preferred. Patients with anticipated discrepancies greater than 8-10 cm often require 1 or more limb-lengthening procedures (several years apart) with or without an epiphysiodesis. The most common technique used for limb lengthening involves placement of an external fixator, either a ring fixator such as the Ilizarov device or a monolateral device (Fig. 676-6). The bone is cut at the metaphyseal–diaphyseal junction, and lengthening is achieved gradually through distraction at the corticotomy. The usual rate of lengthening is 1 mm/day, and it takes approximately 1 mo wearing the fixator for each centimeter of length gained with a minimum of 3 mo in the fixator. Additional time in the fixation may be required for pathologic bone or for metabolic diseases affecting bone formation. A maximum of 15-25% of the original length of the bone may be gained at each session. An advantage of the circular fixator or multiaxial external fixators is the ability to correct coexisting angular deformities at the same time. Technologic advances have allowed the development of intramedullary lengthening and compression rods driven by external magnets. These may provide improvements in patient satisfaction and reduced complications.

Complications include pin tract infection (most common), wound infection, hypertension, joint subluxation, muscle contracture, premature consolidation, delayed union, implant-related problems, and fractures after implant removal. Finally, early amputation and prosthetic fitting may provide the best long-term function in patients with projected discrepancies in excess of 18-20 cm, especially when there are coexisting deformities or deficiencies of the ipsilateral foot (Figs. 676-7 and 676-8). The alternative would be multiple reconstructive procedures throughout childhood and adolescence. The impact of multiple procedures on the child's psychosocial development must also be kept in mind when formulating the treatment plan in these complex cases.

Bibliography is available at Expert Consult.

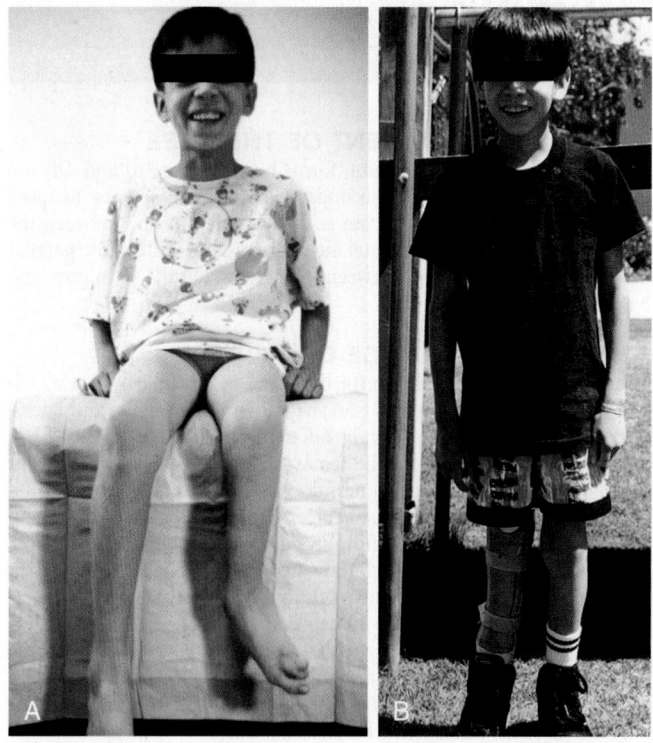

Figure 676-7 Extension prosthesis leg-length discrepancy **(A)** and compensated with extension prosthesis **(B)**.

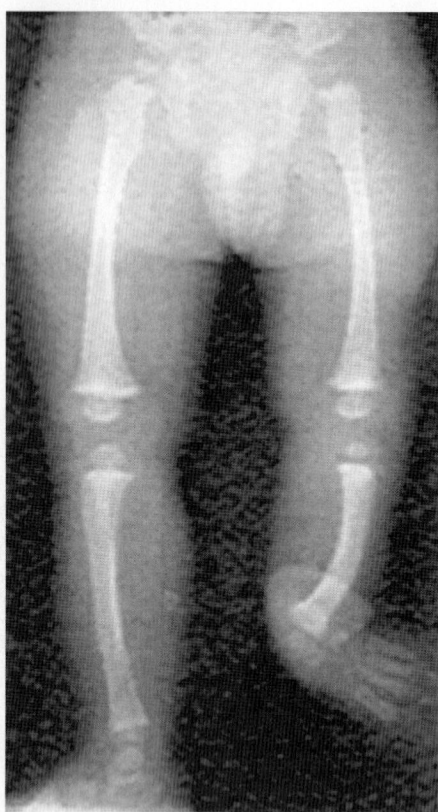

Figure 676-8 Anteroposterior radiograph of fibular hemimelia with leg-length discrepancy.

Chapter 677
The Knee
Eric J. Sarkissian and J. Todd R. Lawrence

NORMAL DEVELOPMENT OF THE KNEE

The knee, a major synovial joint, forms between the 3rd and 4th mo of fetal development, with secondary ossification centers forming between the 6th and 9th fetal mo at the distal femur and between the 8th fetal mo and the 1st postnatal mo at the proximal tibia. The patellar ossification center appears between the ages of 2 and 4 yr in girls and 3 and 5 yr in boys.

ANATOMY AND RANGE OF MOTION

The knee is the largest joint in the body and acts primarily as a modified hinge. The distal femur is cam shaped with the medial and lateral femoral condyles having slightly different shapes. This allows for a posterior gliding motion of the femur on the tibial plateau to occur during knee flexion. This also permits about 8-12 degrees of rotation through the flexion and extension arc. The normal range of motion of the knee is from neutral (or fully straight) to 140 degrees of flexion. Increased ligament laxity including hyperextension of up to 10-15 degrees can be normal in many children. Most activities can be performed in the flexion arc of 0-70 degrees.

The knee consists of three articulations: *patellofemoral, tibiofemoral,* and *tibiofibular.* The anterior and posterior cruciate ligaments as well as medial and lateral collateral ligaments stabilize the knee during movement. The medial and lateral menisci provide support under compressive forces, helping to redistribute the forces from the more rounded distal femur to the more flat proximal tibia. The medial patellofemoral ligament is the primary static soft-tissue restraint against lateral patellar displacement. There are also several bursae located about the knee to cushion and reduce friction on tendons acting across the knee joint.

677.1 Discoid Lateral Meniscus
Eric J. Sarkissian and J. Todd R. Lawrence

Discoid lateral meniscus (DLM) is a congenital anatomic variation of the lateral meniscus that may be asymptomatic or cause the classic *snapping knee syndrome*. Because of asymptomatic cases, the true incidence is difficult to determine, but it is estimated to occur in 3-5% of children and adolescents. Up to 25% of DLM cases may be bilateral. Previously thought to result from a failure of an embryologic sequence of degeneration at the center of the meniscus, discoid menisci have been subsequently shown to not be the developmental precursors for normal menisci.

Anatomically, the normal meniscus (Fig. 677-1A) is attached around its periphery and at the tips of the C anteriorly and posteriorly onto the tibia. During knee motion, the meniscus translates anteriorly and posteriorly to match the slight rollback of the lateral femoral condyle on the tibia with knee flexion. However, with a DLM, the meniscal tissue trapped between the articular surfaces is pushed anteriorly as the knee flexes. These abnormal forces, over time, result in tears in the meniscal tissue or in the posterior attachments, creating excessive meniscal displacement anteriorly during knee flexion. This produces a pop when flexing, usually at about 90-120 degrees of knee flexion as the meniscus is extruded anteriorly, and a loud click or clunk when extending the knee, usually in the last 30 degrees of extension, as the meniscus reduces back between the joint surfaces.

There are 3 types of DLM, according to the widely used **Watanabe classification**. Type I, or **complete, most commonly produces symptoms and** is characterized by a thickened lateral meniscus with complete coverage of the tibial surface (see Fig. 677-1B). Meniscus tissue is always between the joint surfaces. **Type II,** or incomplete, is of variable size and covers a lower percentage of the tibial surface (see Fig. 677-1C) compared to the complete type. Although they can become stretched or torn over time, both the complete and the incomplete types are thought to develop with normal peripheral attachments. Type III, or the Wrisberg ligament type, is a lateral meniscus with no peripheral attachments posteriorly. Instead it is stabilized posteriorly by a prominent meniscofemoral ligament, or ligament of Wrisberg, that secures the posterior horn of the lateral meniscus to the lateral surface of the medial femoral condyle (see Fig. 677-1D). As a result, the Wrisberg ligament type DLM is extremely mobile. Although its shape is not necessarily discoid, the hypermobility of the posterior portion of the meniscus allows it to be extruded anteriorly with flexion and for it to pop back in place with extension, as is characteristic of the other DLM variants.

CLINICAL MANIFESTATIONS AND DIAGNOSIS

The complete and incomplete types of DLM can be asymptomatic, especially if they have stable peripheral attachments. A symptomatic DLM in early childhood is usually caused by a meniscal tear or absent peripheral attachments allowing for the anterior extrusion during flexion and reduction with extension, producing the classical **snapping knee**. These patients can present as early as 2 yr of age, but more commonly present after approximately 6 yr of age; most patients present with symptoms during their teenage years. As these patients gain weight with their adolescent growth spurt, they place increasing static and dynamic loads on the tissue, often with high-level sports. Degeneration in the central portion of the DLM with direct weight bearing makes the meniscus highly susceptible to injury and tears, producing lateral pain and swelling in the knee. Often, the classic popping is not appreciated in these patients.

Younger children usually present with no history of trauma or acute inciting event and with a complaint of popping in the knee with

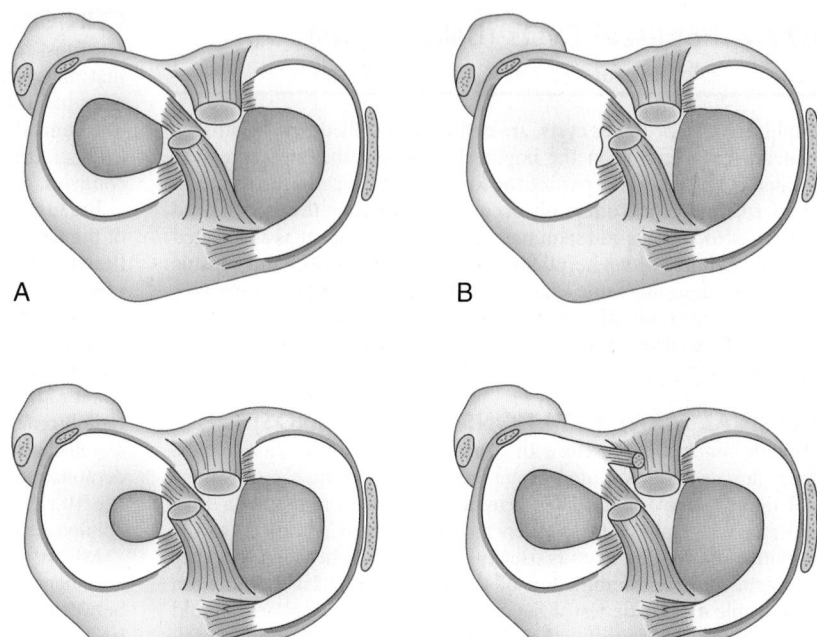

Figure 677-1 The anatomy of the normal meniscus and discoid variants. **A,** The lateral meniscus normally has a C shape with circumferential and root attachments. **B,** A type I, or complete, discoid lateral meniscus covers the entire tibial plateau and has normal attachments. **C,** A type II, or incomplete, discoid lateral meniscus partially covers the tibial plateau and also has normal attachments. **D,** A type III, or Wrisberg ligament type, appears similar in shape to a normal lateral meniscus but lacks sufficient attachments posteriorly resulting in a hypermobile meniscus. The ligament of Wrisberg secures the posterior horn of the meniscus to the lateral aspect of the medial femoral condyle.

occasional swelling. Older children and adolescents often can recall an inciting event and will sometimes report the mechanical popping, but more often note the lateral joint line pain and knee swelling. Physical examination might show a mild effusion and tenderness over the lateral joint line. With knee flexion, a pop with a slight protuberance along the lateral joint line anteriorly can sometimes be appreciated as the meniscus is extruded anteriorly. As the knee is brought back into extension at approximately 20-30 degrees short of full extension, the meniscus can be felt to snap back into the joint and the protuberance at the lateral joint line disappears.

A high index of suspicion is necessary based on history and clinical exam findings. Standard anteroposterior, lateral, merchant (patellar), and 45 degrees flexed posteroanterior (tunnel) views should be obtained if this diagnosis is considered. Radiography of the knee may show widening of the lateral aspect of the knee joint, flattening of the lateral femoral condyle resulting in a squared-off appearance, and cupping of the lateral aspect of the tibial plateau. Because these findings are very nonspecific, with any history or physical examination findings suggestive of a DLM, evaluation with MRI provides a definitive diagnosis.

TREATMENT

Patients with asymptomatic or incidentally found DLM without evidence of a tear or meniscal instability are treated nonoperatively with observation. They should be educated on symptoms to watch out for, but no activity restrictions are often necessary. If knee pain or mechanical symptoms limit activity or a meniscal tear develops, consideration is given for surgical intervention. **Partial meniscectomy**, referred to as **saucerization,** is often performed to reshape the meniscus arthroscopically with the goal of obtaining an anatomically normal-appearing meniscus (Fig. 677-2). Tears remaining in what would be the normal rim of meniscal tissue are either repaired or excised. Meniscal instability is also addressed with repairs as appropriate. If tears extend all the way to the periphery of the meniscus, sometimes a **total meniscectomy**, or complete excision of the meniscus, may be necessary. Because this leaves the joint surfaces unprotected and can lead to early osteoarthritis, addressing DLM tears as soon as they develop and before they extend to the periphery is preferred.

Bibliography is available at Expert Consult.

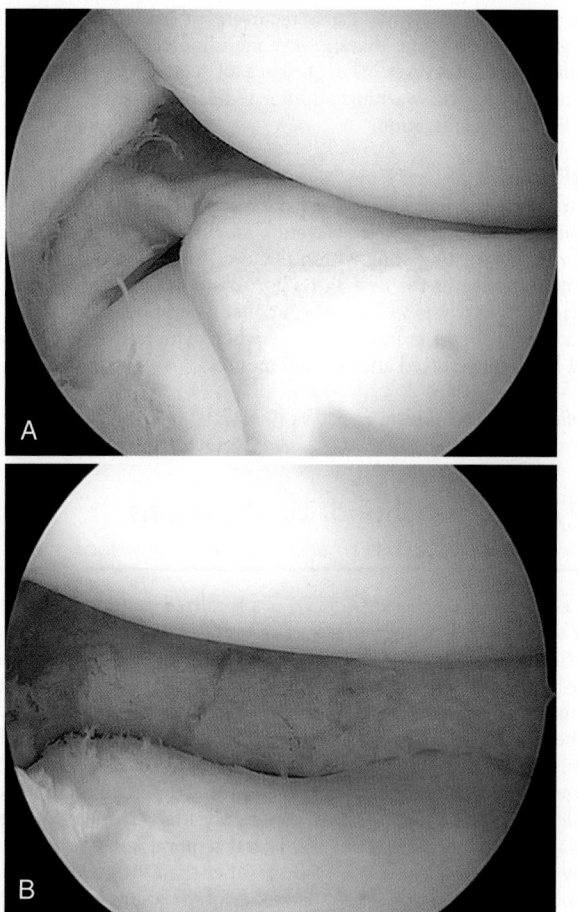

Figure 677-2 Surgical treatment of discoid lateral meniscus. Arthroscopic images of a complete discoid lateral meniscus before **(A)** and after **(B)** partial meniscectomy.

677.2 Popliteal Cysts (Baker Cysts)

Eric J. Sarkissian and J. Todd R. Lawrence

Popliteal cysts, or **Baker cysts,** are cystic masses filled with gelatinous material that develop in the popliteal fossa, the shallow depression located at the posterior part of the knee. They are considered rare in children. They most commonly occur in the region of the medial head of the gastrocnemius and semimembranosus. They occur as an isolated fluid-filled bursa or via herniation through the posterior joint capsule of the knee into this same location. Histologically, the cysts are classified as fibrous, synovial, inflammatory, or transitional. Typically, popliteal cysts resolve spontaneously, although the process may take several years.

CLINICAL MANIFESTATIONS AND DIAGNOSIS

Patients commonly present with a mass behind the knee that may be fairly large when first noted. There are usually no symptoms of internal derangement of the knee. Physical examination reveals a firm mass in the popliteal fossa, often medially located and distal to the popliteal crease. The mass is usually most prominent when the knee is extended. Transillumination of the cyst on physical examination is a simple diagnostic test. Knee radiographs are normal and should be obtained to identify other lesions, such as osteochondromas, osteochondritis dissecans, and malignancies. The diagnosis may be confirmed by ultrasonography, MRI, or aspiration. Ultrasound differentiates a solid mass from a cystic lesion. In the presence of a knee effusion, consideration should be given to an MRI to evaluate for knee intraarticular pathology that may be causing the swelling, such as a meniscal tear or a DLM. These children should also be assessed for *other pathology* that may cause recurrent or intermittent knee effusions, including Lyme disease, juvenile idiopathic arthritis, or other autoimmune processes. The presence of a solid mass detected on ultrasound or MRI warrants additional diagnostic testing and referral for biopsy consideration.

TREATMENT

In most cases, popliteal cysts are observed because they often resolve spontaneously. Rest and leg elevation are beneficial to promote drainage of fluid accumulating within the cyst. If necessary, aspiration can reduce the size of the cyst and a corticosteroid injection can reduce inflammation. Cysts will often recur after aspiration. Surgical excision of a popliteal cyst is indicated only when symptoms are debilitating and have not resolved after several months.

Bibliography is available at Expert Consult.

677.3 Osteochondritis Dissecans

Eric J. Sarkissian and J. Todd R. Lawrence

Osteochondritis dissecans (OCD) is a localized pathologic process of the subchondral bone that secondarily affects the overlying articular cartilage and can progress to cartilage separation and fragmentation. The precise cause for OCD remains unclear, although repetitive microtrauma appears to be the leading candidate. Roles for genetics and ischemia have also been implicated in the etiology. The disorder is being seen with rising frequency in children and adolescents, likely in large part, as a consequence of increased sports participation in young athletes. In the knee, OCD most commonly affects the lateral aspect of the medial femoral condyle. The lateral femoral condyle and patella may also be affected, as well as joints other than the knee, such as the elbow or ankle. Characteristic pathology of the lesion includes an area of avascular necrosis in the subchondral bone, the segment of bone just below the joint surface, and varying degrees of ischemia and fibrosis of the overlying hyaline cartilage. Failure of both the bone and the cartilage surface to heal completely is associated with an increased risk for developing premature osteoarthritis.

CLINICAL MANIFESTATIONS AND DIAGNOSIS

The most common presenting complaint is a vague or **deep knee pain** that may localize along the medial or lateral joint line. If the osteochondral fragment becomes unstable, the patient may also develop **mechanical symptoms**, such as catching or locking. Physical exam findings include effusion, tenderness to palpation over the femoral condyles, quadriceps atrophy, and diminished range of motion.

Because most OCD lesions are located more on the posterior aspect of the femoral condyle, a posteroanterior radiograph with a 45 degree flexed knee (tunnel view) is often required to evaluate for the presence of an OCD. Many of these patients also have some degree of patellar-related pain, necessitating merchant (patellar) view plain films. Thus, standard radiographic evaluation of nontraumatic adolescent knee pain should routinely include anteroposterior, lateral, tunnel, and merchant radiographs of the knee. An early lesion may appear as a small radiolucency at the articular surface. A more advanced lesion may have a well-demarcated segment of subchondral bone with a lucent line demonstrating separation from the condyle. In children younger than age 10 yr, irregularities in the ossification center of the developing epiphysis may be difficult to distinguish from an OCD lesion.

MRI is useful for determining the size of the OCD, integrity of the articular cartilage, and presence of loose bodies. Fluid observed between the fragment and subchondral bone suggests an unstable lesion and high risk for detachment. Any linear signal through the articular cartilage or displacement of the fragment indicates a potentially unstable lesion as well. For an unstable-appearing OCD, either based on the patients' symptoms and signs, or the imaging, arthroscopy should be performed to evaluate the status of the lesion.

TREATMENT

Treatment for juvenile OCD includes nonoperative and surgical management, with treatment decisions being based on many factors, including the growth status and skeletal maturity of the patient, the presence of symptoms, the lesion size, and whether the lesion appears intact and stable or if there is any suggestion of instability. Skeletal immaturity (i.e., younger age), smaller lesion size, and the absence of mechanical symptoms or pain have been associated with a higher likelihood of OCD healing with nonoperative treatment. Unstable lesions will not usually heal with conservative treatment.

Thus, young patients with stable lesions, as evidenced by an intact articular surface on imaging (Fig. 677-3*A*), are deemed to have an acceptable probability of healing and are often initially managed conservatively with a period of non–weightbearing and immobilization, followed by a period of strict activity restriction and physical therapy for 3-6 mo. OCD healing is followed with radiographs, usually at approximately 3 mo intervals, until lesion healing has been noted. If healing has not been radiographically confirmed in 3-6 mo, surgical intervention is often considered. Because of the low rate of healing in skeletally mature patients, even intact lesions are not usually managed conservatively in this patient population, but recommended for surgery.

Although nonsurgical treatment can be successful in intact lesions, surgical treatment of intact lesions is often more successful and induces healing at a faster rate. Consequently, patients often choose to pursue early surgical intervention. For stable and intact lesions, surgical management involves arthroscopic evaluation of the joint followed by either a transarticular or retroarticular drilling to stimulate bony healing by creating channels in the subchondral bone that allow revascularization to occur. Both techniques are comparably effective in producing short-term patient-oriented outcomes and radiographic healing.

More advanced lesions with edema beneath the fragment, subchondral cyst formation, and partial (see Fig. 677-3*B*) or complete (see Fig. 677-3*C*) fragment detachment on arthroscopy are potentially salvageable. Treatment involves drilling or fixation with possible bone grafting. OCD lesions may progress to become unstable and dislodge into the joint space (see Fig. 677-3*D*). Removal of the loose body in addition to cartilage repair and restoration are typically performed for such unsalvageable lesions. In the postoperative period, patients undergo

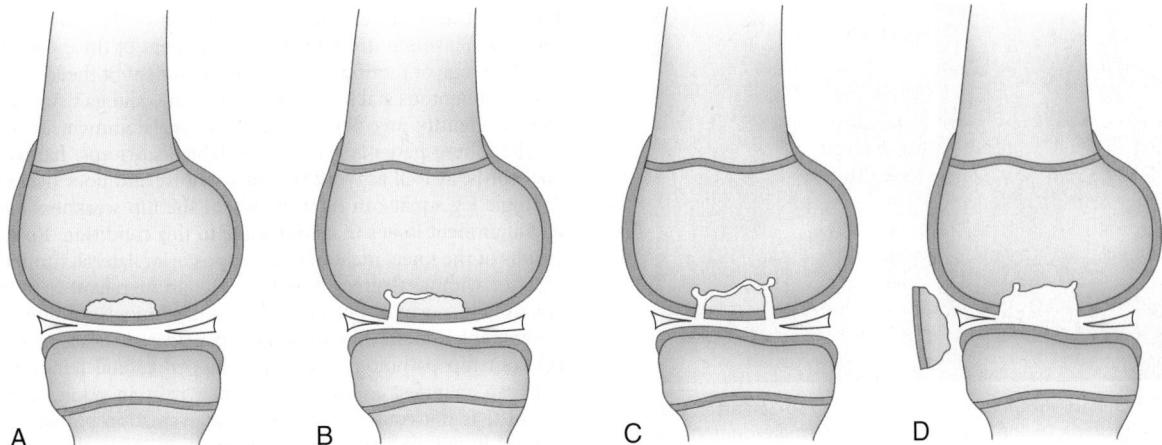

Figure 677-3 The spectrum of osteochondritis dissecans (OCD) pathology of the knee. **A,** A stable and intact lesion without breach of the overlying articular cartilage. **B,** An OCD with fluid beneath the fragment, subchondral cyst formation, and partial fragment detachment. **C,** An unstable but located lesion with fluid beneath the fragment, multiple subchondral cysts, and complete fragment detachment. **D,** A dislodged OCD lesion resulting in a loose body within the knee joint space.

physical therapy to regain strength and range of motion, with a gradual return to baseline activity levels. Treating OCD early and effectively often prevents recurrent symptoms in adulthood and reduces risk for early-onset osteoarthritis.

Bibliography is available at Expert Consult.

677.4 Osgood-Schlatter Disease and Sinding-Larsen-Johansson Syndrome

Eric J. Sarkissian and J. Todd R. Lawrence

In skeletally immature patients, the tibial tubercle is an extension of the proximal tibial epiphysis. As the femur rapidly grows in length, patients often develop tight musculature, particularly of the quadriceps, across the knee joint. These patients also develop movement patterns that preferentially place stress at the knees during activities instead of distributing that stress across other joints in the lower extremity. The repetitive tensile microtrauma sustained during sports or other athletic activities then creates traction injuries at the weak points in the extensor mechanism at the knee, as the stress exceeds the developing skeleton's ability to repair the damage.

Sinding-Larsen-Johansson syndrome is an insertional periostitis at the inferior pole of the patella. **Osgood-Schlatter (OS) disease** is an irritation of the patellar tendon at its insertion into the tibial tubercle or a traction apophysitis of the tibial tubercle growth plate. These conditions typically present during periods of relative accelerated growth. Sinding-Larsen-Johansson syndrome tends to occur in a slightly younger patient population, whereas OS disease presents in slightly older patients with most symptomatic between the ages of 10 and 15 yr. These conditions are most common in very physically active boys. However, as the number and intensity of female athletics has increased, the incidence in females seems to be on the rise.

CLINICAL MANIFESTATIONS AND DIAGNOSIS

Anterior knee pain, very specifically localized to the inferior pole of the patella (Sinding-Larsen-Johansson syndrome) or over the tibial tubercle (OS disease) is the most common patient complaint. Swelling, as well as an eventual firm and fixed increased prominence at the tibial tubercle, may occur with OS disease and may also be part of the initial complaint (Fig. 677-4). There is typically no acute traumatic inciting event. The pain is aggravated by sports activities, but may often persist with daily activities and even at rest. Physical examination reveals point tenderness over the tibial tubercle and the distal portion of the patellar

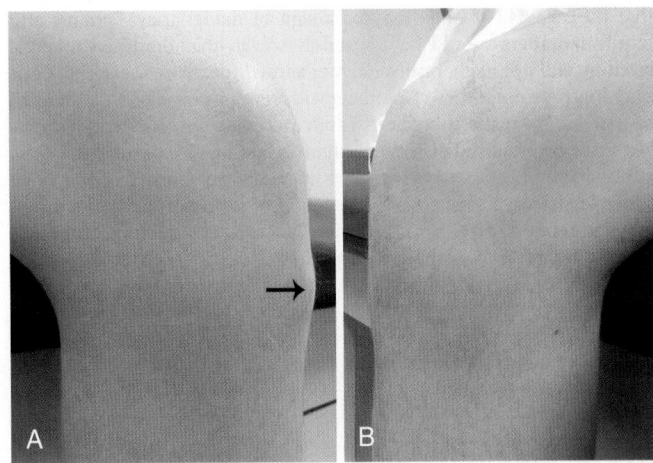

Figure 677-4 Clinical manifestations of Osgood-Schlatter disease. The increased prominence of the tibial tubercle, indicated by the *arrow*, **(A)** from traction apophysitis in a 15 yr old boy's knee is contrasted with the normal appearance of the tibial tubercle **(B)** in his contralateral, unaffected knee.

tendon (OS disease). Diagnosis is usually made clinically, but radiographs may reveal fragmentation of the tibial tubercle and soft tissue swelling (Fig. 677-5).

TREATMENT

In most patients, Sinding-Larsen-Johansson syndrome and OS disease are self-limited processes and resolve with rest. Patients are treated with an escalating treatment regime until they are pain free with activity. If they are pain free with normal daily activities, they may maintain this level of activity for 2 additional wk. In more-severe cases, a knee immobilizer or even crutches with restricted weightbearing are required to get the patient comfortable. Patients are usually advised to maintain a level of activity for 1-2 wk before attempting to advance. Sports and other dynamic activities are restricted until the patient has been pain free to palpation for at least 2 wk. During this rest period, addressing some of the contributing factors, such as muscular tightness, can help prevent recurrence with activity resumption. A self-directed stretching regime concentrating on the quadriceps and hamstrings may be provided. Some patients and resistant cases may benefit from formal instruction in these exercises with a physical therapist.

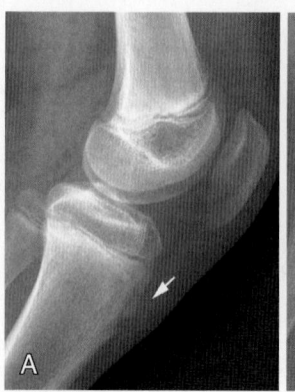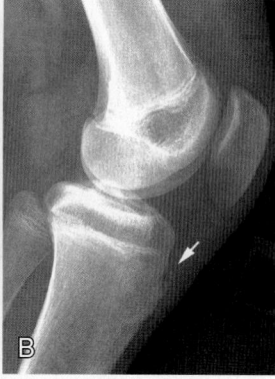

Figure 677-5 Radiographic findings of Osgood-Schlatter disease. **A,** Lateral radiograph of the knee of a 13 yr old male demonstrates a sliver of new bone formation *(arrow)* at the tibial tubercle. **B,** Lateral radiograph of the same child at 15 yr of age demonstrates characteristic fragmentation *(arrow)* of the tibial tubercle.

Reassurance is important, because some patients and parents fear that the swollen tubercle may be a sign of malignancy. Patients and family members should be advised, however, that the tibial tubercle swelling will not likely resolve. Hyperosmolar dextrose local injections may improve outcomes in patients with recalcitrant disease. Removal of ossicles from the tubercle is rarely necessary in pediatric patients but may be required with persistent disabling symptoms in young adults. Complications are rare and include early closure of the tibial tubercle with recurvatum, or hyperextension, deformity, and rarely, patellar tendon rupture or avulsion fracture of the tibial tubercle. Although rare, these complications can have significant long-term consequences and should thus prompt counseling to avoid playing through the pain.

Bibliography is available at Expert Consult.

677.5 Patellofemoral Pain Syndrome

Eric J. Sarkissian and J. Todd R. Lawrence

Also known as anterior knee pain syndrome, patellofemoral pain syndrome (PFPS) is one of the most common causes of knee pain, particularly in adolescent girls. Previously, PFPS was thought to arise from a deranged patellar articular surface, hence, the former term chondromalacia patella. Increasing evidence shows that anterior knee pain is frequently present even with normal articular cartilage of the patella, resulting in more appropriate labeling of the condition. The precise etiology of the knee pain remains unknown and is likely multifactorial.

CLINICAL MANIFESTATIONS AND DIAGNOSIS

Pain beneath or near the patella is the most common symptom. Classically, walking up and down stairs, which puts the patella under high compressive loads, aggravates the pain. Squatting, running, and other vigorous physical activities also exacerbate the anterior knee pain. Sitting in a flexed knee position for an extended period of time, the so-called theater sign, is another common complaint. There is usually no history of antecedent trauma, although falling onto a flexed knee is sometimes noted. Buckling or a sense of the knee *giving way* can occur, but there is rarely any true knee instability. Swelling is not common and if present should prompt further investigation. Pain is often relieved through knee extension.

Physical exam reveals isolated tenderness with palpation about the medial or lateral aspects of the patella. With the knee extended and the quadriceps relaxed, placing pressure on the patella and translating it distally into the top of the trochlear groove, the so-called **grind**

test, often also causes pain. Reproduction of the patient's pain with these maneuvers is an important component of the exam. Active and passive range of motion of the knee, alignment of the lower extremity, knee ligamentous stability, patellar tracking, and gait should be evaluated to identify any obvious causes of malalignment or an unstable patella. These patients often have tight quadriceps, hamstrings, and heel cords, as well as weak hip musculature and poor overall balance. A single leg squat can often highlight the hip weakness and balance and alignment issues that contribute to this condition. Routine radiographs of the knee, including anteroposterior, lateral, tunnel (posteroanterior with 45 degrees flexed knee), and merchant (patellar) views, are usually normal, but are helpful in eliminating other etiologies. Radiographs of the hip should be considered in suspected cases to rule out hip pathology, such as a slipped capital femoral epiphysis, that can manifest as ill-defined knee pain in adolescents as well. An MRI is not routinely required for evaluation but should be considered in any patient with a history of mechanical symptoms or an effusion.

TREATMENT

Several methods of nonoperative treatment are utilized to address PFPS. The mainstay of treatment is continued physiotherapy, involving overall lower-extremity stretching and strengthening, including short-arc quadriceps strengthening, hip and core strengthening, and exercises designed to address balance and overall body positioning during dynamic activities. No one particular regime seems to demonstrate results superior to the others. Home exercise programs can be effective for the properly disciplined and motivated patient, but formal physical therapy should be considered in resistant cases or in patients who may not have the motivation or wherewithal to adhere to a self-directed program. Orthoses, including patellar taping, knee sleeves, customized knee braces, or even shoe inserts are often used in conjunction with physical therapy. However, evidence for long-term benefit from orthotic use is unclear. Treatment with Botulinum toxin injections, nonsteroidal antiinflammatory medications, or therapeutic ultrasound is not substantiated. Most cases of PFPS resolve spontaneously over a period of years. Arthroscopic evaluation of the knee and patellofemoral joint is rarely necessary.

Bibliography is available at Expert Consult.

677.6 Patellofemoral Instability

Eric J. Sarkissian and J. Todd R. Lawrence

Patellofemoral joint stability depends on a balance of the static restraints and the dynamic forces acting on the patella. These include the restraining ligaments and the articular anatomy of the patellofemoral groove that serve to balance the dynamic forces of the quadriceps mechanism and overall limb positioning. During knee flexion, the pull of the quadriceps mechanism tends to place an overall lateral displacing force at the patella. The **Q angle** refers to the deviation between the angle of the patellar tendon and the line of the quadriceps. Wider hips and valgus (knock-kneed) positioning increase the Q angle and thus the lateral force applied at the patella. In extension, the static restraints, including the medial restraining ligaments, primarily the medial patellofemoral ligament, are responsible for guiding the patella into the trochlear grove in the distal femur. The pull of the vastus medialis obliquus is the only dynamic restraint. Once in the trochlea, the bony congruity becomes the primary restraint to the net lateral muscular forces.

Factors that contribute to patellofemoral instability are multifactorial and include vastus medialis insufficiency, ligamentous laxity, shallow sulcus, condylar hypoplasia, patella alta (high riding patella), or malalignment that effectively increases the Q angle, such as genu valgum, internal femoral torsion, or external tibial torsion.

Acute patellofemoral dislocation is the most common acute knee disorder in children and adolescents and often occurs after a sudden valgus strain during a sporting activity but may be the result of direct trauma. **Recurrent patellofemoral subluxation** is more than 1 episode of patellar subluxation without frank dislocation. Lateral malalignment of the quadriceps mechanism is the most common etiologic factor. **Habitual dislocation of the patella** describes patellar dislocation occurring during every knee flexion. A dysplastic knee with contracture of the lateral portion of the quadriceps mechanism is often associated. Several syndromes are associated with patellar instability, including Down syndrome (see Chapter 81), Turner syndrome (see Chapter 81), Kabuki syndrome, and Rubinstein-Taybi syndrome.

CLINICAL MANIFESTATIONS AND DIAGNOSIS

With an acute patellar dislocation, patients will recall the acute event and the sensation that their knee cap was out of place. Straightening the knee is all that is usually required to reduce the patella, but sometimes this requires medical attention. Swelling is usually almost immediate following the injury and appreciable on examination with an effusion. The patella may appear laterally displaced when the knee is fully extended or higher than normal with the knee slightly flexed. Pain along the medial knee from the medial patella to the medial epicondyle of the femur is common. Lateral patellar translocation with the knee slightly flexed should be tested with the **patellar apprehension test**. In the acute setting there will be increased translation and pain as well as a feeling of insecurity. Patellar tracking is also an important component to the exam but may not be possible due to pain in the acute setting. The **J sign** refers to the inverted J-path the patella takes, beginning in a laterally subluxated position and then suddenly shifting medially to engage the femoral groove with early knee flexion. The torsional profile of the patient is also important to assess to rule out possible rotational abnormalities of the femur or tibia.

Radiographs of a patient with patellar instability should include anteroposterior, lateral, and merchant views (obtained with the knee bent 45 degrees, with the beam of the x-ray through the knee from head to toe) of the patella. Radiographs should also be carefully examined for occult fractures. In the presence of a significant knee effusion, mechanical symptoms, acute traumatic patellar dislocation, or uncertainty in the diagnosis, further investigation may warrant an MRI to evaluate for loose bodies or cartilage damage. MRI will illustrate bone bruise patterns typical of patellar dislocation at the medial patellar facet and at the lateral femoral condyle. A tear in the medial patellofemoral ligament may also be seen, especially in cases of an acute patellofemoral dislocation.

TREATMENT

Nonoperative management is initially recommended for acute patellar dislocation and recurrent patellar subluxation, unless an osteochondral fracture or additional intra-articular pathology is seen on imaging studies. Although early physical therapy has also been shown to be successful, a brief 4-6 wk period of immobilization in full extension may help with healing of the medial knee restraints following an initial traumatic dislocation. After this, transition to a patellar stabilizing brace usually improves symptoms. Successful treatment is usually achieved with formal physical therapy aimed at improving extensor muscle tone, particularly the vastus medialis obliquus, activity-related body positioning, and hip and core muscle strengthening. The reported redislocation rate following an initial traumatic patellar dislocation ranges from 15-44%.

Failure to improve after nonoperative treatment and persistent episodes of patellar subluxation or dislocation are indications for surgical intervention to address patellofemoral instability. Patients with loose bodies, osteochondral fractures, or chondral damage are surgical candidates for early intervention. Many different types of surgical procedures exist to prevent lateral excursion of the patella from occurring. These include proximal realignment of the patella, distal realignment of the patellar tendon insertion, lateral release, medial patellofemoral ligament reconstruction, or guided growth techniques. The surgical approach that is selected should be individualized for each patient depending on the pathoanatomy contributing to the recurrent subluxations or dislocations.

Bibliography is available at Expert Consult.

677.7 Anterior Cruciate Ligament Rupture

Eric J. Sarkissian and J. Todd R. Lawrence

Pediatric anterior cruciate ligament (ACL) reconstruction has become more prevalent as ACL tears in skeletally immature patients have greatly increased in recent years. Increased sports participation, increased intensity of training and competition, participation on multiple teams, heightened awareness, and improved methods for diagnosis are all cited as contributing factors to the growing awareness of ACL injuries in children and adolescents.

Females are also known to have a greater risk for ACL injury than males. The gender-specific discrepancy appears to be caused mostly by insufficient neuromuscular activation patterns in females, resulting in increased **genu valgum**, or knock-knee, biased landing and, therefore, a heightened tendency toward landing or stopping in an injury prone position. Various pediatric ACL injury prevention programs show benefit in not only reducing the rate of injuries but also in increasing athletic strength and performance.

CLINICAL MANIFESTATIONS AND DIAGNOSIS

The majority of ACL tears occurs as a result of a noncontact injury. Patients may report a pop associated with the acute onset of knee pain. Later they develop swelling, limited range of motion, and sometimes a sensation of instability. After the initial injury, patients may have surprisingly little pain. On physical exam, the anterior drawer sign or Lachman test may indicate increased anterior tibial translation. The Lachman examination is performed by applying an anteriorly directed force to the proximal tibia with the femur stabilized and the knee flexed 20-30 degrees. The amount of translation and the end point are assessed, with increased translation and an indistinct end point indicating a positive test. A pivot shift test can also be performed to confirm the diagnosis but is rarely successful in the conscious patient. It is conducted by gently bending the knee while just supporting the lower leg. A gentle valgus stress and slight internal rotation can enhance the shift.

Radiographs of the knee are performed, including anteroposterior, lateral, tunnel (posteroanterior with 45 degrees flexed knee), and merchant (patellar) views, to assess for other potential injuries common in pediatric and adolescent patients, such as tibial spine avulsion fractures or OCD. In traumatic injuries, internal and external oblique radiographs can also be helpful. Ultimately, knee MRI can confirm the presence of an intrasubstance ACL tear, as well as meniscal or chondral pathology. Arthroscopic evaluation is the gold standard for diagnosis and treatment.

TREATMENT

The management of ACL injury in this patient population can be challenging and the severity of the ACL tear is important to differentiate. Incomplete ACL tears may be treated nonoperatively and the patient and family's understanding and willingness to adhere to a protocol of bracing and activity restriction are important factors in optimizing outcomes. For complete tears of the ACL, because of the risk of ongoing knee damage if stabilization of the knee is delayed, surgical reconstruction is now recommended for patients who are physically, mentally, and emotionally capable after a thorough discussion with the patient and family about the risks and benefits. All-epiphyseal, partial transphyseal, or traditional transphyseal reconstruction techniques are used based upon the skeletal maturity of the patient to minimize the risk for growth disturbance across the distal femoral and proximal tibial physes.

Depending on the technique used for reconstruction and any associated meniscal pathology addressed, weight bearing is restricted and a brace is used for the 1st 4-6 wk postoperatively. Physical therapy is used postoperatively and continued until strength and functional testing are equal to the contralateral, unaffected limb. Routine follow-up visits and radiographs are conducted to monitor progress and signs of growth disturbance. Patients return to sports typically at a minimum of 9 mo postoperatively and are followed on a yearly basis thereafter until skeletal maturity.

Bibliography is available at Expert Consult.

Chapter **678**
The Hip

Wudbhav N. Sankar, B. David Horn,
Lawrence Wells, and John P. Dormans

Anatomically, the hip joint is a ball-and-socket articulation between the femoral head and acetabulum.

The hip joint is a pivotal joint of the lower extremity, and its functional demands require both stability and flexibility.

GROWTH AND DEVELOPMENT

The hip joint begins to develop at about the 7th wk of gestation, when a cleft appears in the mesenchyme of the primitive limb bud. These precartilaginous cells differentiate into a fully formed cartilaginous **femoral head** and **acetabulum** by the 11th wk of gestation (see Chapter 8). At birth, the neonatal acetabulum is completely composed of cartilage, with a thin rim of fibrocartilage called the **labrum**.

The very cellular hyaline cartilage of the acetabulum is continuous with the triradiate cartilages, which divide and interconnect the 3 osseous components of the pelvis (the **ilium**, **ischium**, and **pubis**). The concave shape of the hip joint is determined by the presence of a spherical femoral head.

Several factors determine acetabular depth, including interstitial growth within the acetabular cartilage, appositional growth under the perichondrium, and growth of adjacent bones (the ilium, ischium, and pubis). In the neonate, the entire proximal femur is a cartilaginous structure, which includes the femoral head and the greater and lesser trochanters. The 3 main growth areas are the physeal plate, the growth plate of the greater trochanter, and the femoral neck isthmus. Between the 4th and 7th mo of life, the proximal femoral ossification center (in the center of the femoral head) appears. This ossification center continues to enlarge, along with its cartilaginous anlage, until adult life, when only a thin layer of articular cartilage remains. During this period of growth, the thickness of the cartilage surrounding this bony nucleus gradually decreases, as does the thickness of the acetabular cartilage. The growth of the proximal femur is affected by muscle pull, the forces transmitted across the hip joint with weight bearing, normal joint nutrition, circulation, and muscle tone. Alterations in these factors can cause profound changes in the development of the proximal femur.

VASCULAR SUPPLY

The blood supply to the capital femoral epiphysis is complex and changes with growth of the proximal femur. The proximal femur receives its arterial supply from intraosseous (primarily the medial femoral circumflex artery) and extraosseous vessels (Fig. 678-1). The **retinacular vessels** (extraosseous) lie on the surface of the femoral neck but are intracapsular because they enter the epiphysis from the periphery. This makes the blood supply vulnerable to damage from septic arthritis, trauma, thrombosis, and other vascular insults. Interruption of this tenuous blood supply can lead to avascular necrosis of the femoral head and permanent deformity of the hip.

678.1 Developmental Dysplasia of the Hip

Wudbhav N. Sankar, B. David Horn, Lawrence Wells,
and John P. Dormans

Developmental dysplasia of the hip (DDH) refers to a spectrum of pathology in the development of the immature hip joint. Formerly called *congenital dislocation of the hip*, DDH more accurately describes the variable presentation of the disorder, encompassing mild dysplasias as well as frank dislocations.

CLASSIFICATION

Acetabular **dysplasia** refers to abnormal morphology and development of the acetabulum. Hip **subluxation** is defined as partial contact between the femoral head and acetabulum. Hip **dislocation** refers to a hip with no contact between the articulating surfaces of the hip. DDH is classified into 2 major groups: **typical** and **teratologic**. Typical DDH occurs in otherwise normal patients or those without defined syndromes or genetic conditions. Teratologic hip dislocations usually have identifiable causes, such as arthrogryposis or a genetic syndrome, and occur before birth.

ETIOLOGY AND RISK FACTORS

Although the etiology remains unknown, the final common pathway in the development of DDH is increased laxity of the joint, which fails to maintain a stable femoroacetabular articulation. This increased laxity is probably the result of a combination of hormonal, mechanical, and genetic factors. A positive family history for DDH is found in 12-33% of affected patients. DDH is more common among female patients (80%), which is thought to be because of the greater susceptibility of female fetuses to maternal hormones such as relaxin, which increases ligamentous laxity. Although only 2-3% of all babies are born

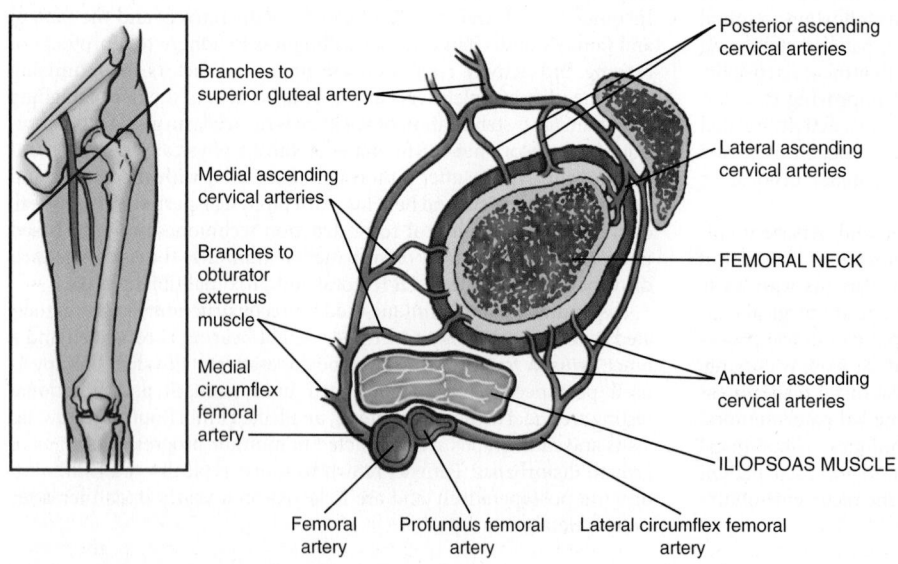

Figure 678-1 Diagram of vascular anatomy of the proximal femur.

in breech presentation, the incidence of DDH in these patients is 16-25%.

Any condition that leads to a tighter intrauterine space and, consequently, less room for normal fetal motion may be associated with DDH. These conditions include oligohydramnios, large birth weight, and 1st pregnancy. The high rate of association of DDH with other *intrauterine molding abnormalities,* such as torticollis and metatarsus adductus, supports the theory that the *crowding phenomenon* has a role in the pathogenesis. The left hip is the most commonly affected hip; in the most common fetal position, this is the hip that is usually forced into adduction by the mother's sacrum.

EPIDEMIOLOGY

Although most newborn screening studies suggest that some degree of hip instability can be detected in 1 in 100 to 1 in 250 babies, actual dislocated or dislocatable hips are much less common, being found in 1-1.5 of 1,000 live births.

There is marked geographic and racial variation in the incidence of DDH. The reported incidence based on geography ranges from 1.7 in 1,000 babies in Sweden to 75 in 1,000 in Yugoslavia to 188.5 in 1,000 in a district in Manitoba, Canada. The incidence of DDH in Chinese and African newborns is almost 0%, whereas it is 1% for hip dysplasia and 0.1% for hip dislocation in white newborns. These differences may be the result of environmental factors, such as child-rearing practices, rather than to genetic predisposition. African and Asian caregivers have traditionally carried babies against their bodies in a shawl so that a child's hips are flexed, abducted, and free to move. This keeps the hips in the optimal position for stability and for dynamic molding of the developing acetabulum by the cartilaginous femoral head. Children in Native American and Eastern European cultures, which have a relatively high incidence of DDH, have historically been swaddled in confining clothes that bring their hips into extension. This position increases the tension of the psoas muscle-tendon unit and might predispose the hips to displace and eventually dislocate laterally and superiorly.

PATHOANATOMY

In DDH, several secondary anatomic changes can develop that can prevent reduction. Both the fatty tissue in the depths of the socket, known as the **pulvinar,** and the ligamentum teres can hypertrophy, blocking reduction of the femoral head. The transverse acetabular ligament usually thickens as well, which effectively narrows the opening of the acetabulum. In addition, the shortened iliopsoas tendon becomes taut across the front of the hip, creating an hourglass shape to the hip capsule, which limits access to the acetabulum. Over time, the dislocated femoral head places pressure on the acetabular rim and labrum, causing the labrum to infold and become thick.

The shape of a normal femoral head and acetabulum depends on a concentric reduction between the two. The more time that a hip spends dislocated, the more likely that the acetabulum will develop abnormally. Without a femoral head to provide a template, the acetabulum will become progressively shallow, with an oblique acetabular roof and a thickened medial wall.

CLINICAL FINDINGS
The Neonate
DDH in the neonate is asymptomatic and must be screened for by specific maneuvers. Physical examination must be carried out with the infant unclothed and placed supine in a warm, comfortable setting on a flat examination table.

The **Barlow** provocative maneuver assesses the potential for dislocation of a nondisplaced hip. The examiner adducts the flexed hip and gently pushes the thigh posteriorly in an effort to dislocate the femoral head (Fig. 678-2). In a positive test, the hip is felt to slide out of the acetabulum. As the examiner relaxes the proximal push, the hip can be felt to slip back into the acetabulum.

The **Ortolani** test is the reverse of Barlow test: The examiner attempts to reduce a dislocated hip (Fig. 678-3). The examiner grasps the child's thigh between the thumb and index finger and, with the 4th and 5th

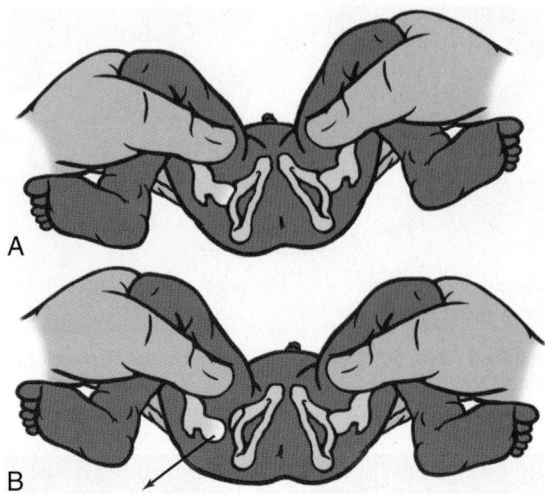

Figure 678-2 The Barlow provocative test is performed with the patient's knees and hips flexed. **A,** Holding the patient's limbs gently, with the thigh in adduction, the examiner applies a posteriorly directed force. **B,** This test is positive in a dislocatable hip.

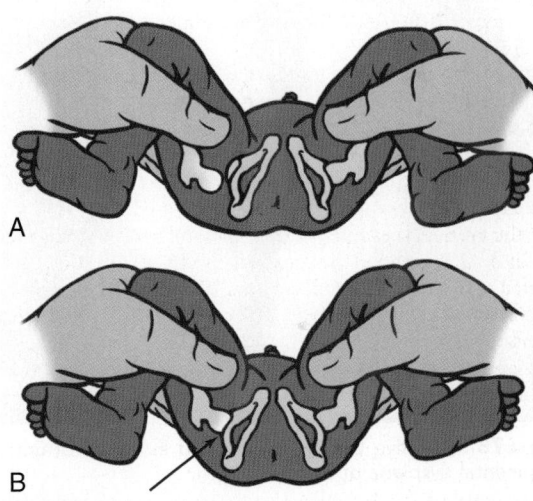

Figure 678-3 The Ortolani maneuver is the sign of the ball of the femoral head moving in and out of the acetabulum. **A,** The examiner holds the patient's thigh and gently abducts the hip while lifting the greater trochanter with 2 fingers. **B,** When the test is positive, the dislocated femoral head falls back into the acetabulum with a palpable clunk as the hip is abducted.

fingers, lifts the greater trochanter while simultaneously abducting the hip. When the test is positive, the femoral head will slip into the socket with a delicate clunk that is palpable but usually not audible. It should be a gentle, nonforced maneuver.

A **hip click** is the high-pitched sensation (or sound) felt at the very end of abduction during testing for DDH with Barlow and Ortolani maneuvers. Classically, a hip click is differentiated from a **hip clunk,** which is felt as the hip goes in and out of joint. Hip clicks usually originate in the ligamentum teres or occasionally in the fascia lata or psoas tendon and do not indicate a significant hip abnormality.

The Infant
As the baby enters the 2nd and 3rd mo of life, the soft tissues begin to tighten and the Ortolani and Barlow tests are no longer reliable. In this age group, the examiner must look for other specific physical findings, including limited hip abduction, apparent shortening of the thigh, proximal location of the greater trochanter, asymmetry of the gluteal

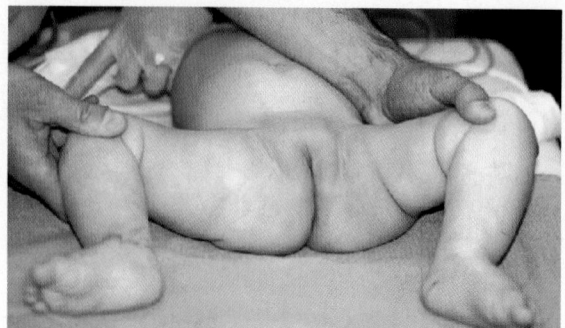

Figure 678-4 Asymmetry of thigh folds in a child with developmental dysplasia of the hip.

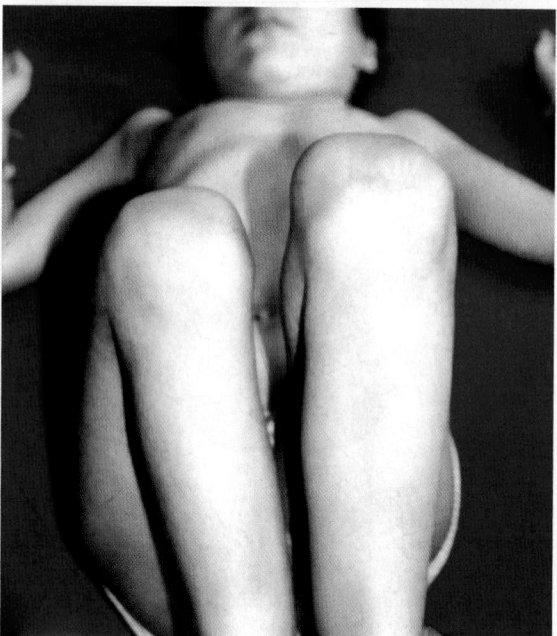

Figure 678-5 Positive Galeazzi sign noted in a case of untreated developmental dysplasia of the hip.

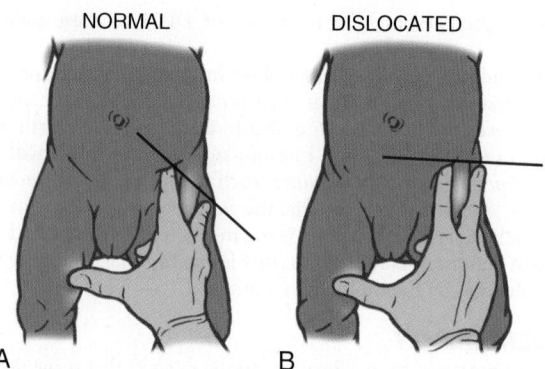

Figure 678-6 Klisic test. **A,** In a normal hip, an imaginary line drawn down through the tip of an index finger placed on the patient's iliac crest and the tip of the long finger placed on the patient's greater trochanter should point to the umbilicus. **B,** In a dislocated hip, this line drawn through the 2 fingertips runs below the umbilicus because the greater trochanter is abnormally high.

or thigh folds (Fig. 678-4), and positioning of the hip. Limitation of abduction is the most reliable sign of a dislocated hip in this age group.

Shortening of the thigh, the **Galeazzi sign,** is best appreciated by placing both hips in 90 degrees of flexion and comparing the height of the knees, looking for asymmetry (Fig. 678-5). Asymmetry of thigh and gluteal skin folds may be present in 10% of normal infants but suggests DDH. Another helpful test is the **Klisic test,** in which the examiner places the 3rd finger over the greater trochanter and the index finger of the same hand on the anterior superior iliac spine. In a normal hip, an imaginary line drawn between the 2 fingers points to the umbilicus. In the dislocated hip, the trochanter is elevated, and the line projects halfway between the umbilicus and the pubis (Fig. 678-6).

The Walking Child
The walking child often presents to the physician after the family has noticed a limp, a waddling gait, or a leg-length discrepancy. The affected side appears shorter than the normal extremity, and the child toe-walks on the affected side. The Trendelenburg sign is positive in these children, and an abductor lurch is usually observed when the child walks. As in the younger child, there is limited hip abduction on the affected side and the knees are at different levels when the hips are flexed (the Galeazzi sign). Excessive lordosis, which develops secondary to altered hip mechanics, is common and is often the presenting complaint.

DIAGNOSTIC TESTING
Ultrasonography
Because it is superior to radiographs for evaluating cartilaginous structures, ultrasonography is the diagnostic modality of choice for DDH before the appearance of the femoral head ossific nucleus (4-6 mo). During the early newborn period (0-4 wk), however, physical examination is preferred over ultrasonography because there is a high incidence of false-positive sonograms in this age group. In addition to elucidating the static relationship of the femur to the acetabulum, ultrasonography provides dynamic information about the stability of the hip joint. The ultrasound examination can be used to monitor acetabular development, particularly of infants in Pavlik harness treatment; this method can minimize the number of radiographs taken and might allow the clinician to detect failure of treatment earlier.

In the Graf technique, the transducer is placed over the greater trochanter, which allows visualization of the ilium, the bony acetabulum, the labrum, and the femoral epiphysis (Fig. 678-7). The angle formed by the line of the ilium and a line tangential to the boney roof of the acetabulum is termed the α **angle** and represents the depth of the acetabulum. Values >60 degrees are considered normal, and those <60 degrees imply acetabular dysplasia. The β **angle** is formed by a line drawn tangential to the labrum and the line of the ilium; this represents the cartilaginous roof of the acetabulum. A normal β angle is <55 degrees; as the femoral head subluxates, the β angle increases. Another useful test is to evaluate the position of the center of the head compared to the vertical line of the ilium. If the line of the ilium falls lateral to the center of the head, the epiphysis is considered reduced. If the line falls medial to the center of the head, the epiphysis is uncovered and is either subluxated or dislocated.

Screening for DDH with ultrasound remains controversial. Although routinely performed in Europe, meta-analyses indicate that data are insufficient to give clear recommendations. In the United States, the current recommendations are that every newborn undergo a clinical examination for hip instability. Children who have findings suspicious for DDH should be followed up with ultrasound. Most authors agree that infants with *risk factors* for DDH (breech position, family history, torticollis) should be screened with ultrasound regardless of the clinical findings.

Radiography
Radiographs are recommended for an infant once the proximal femoral epiphysis ossifies, usually by 4-6 mo. In infants of this age, radiographs have proved to be more effective, less costly, and less operator dependent than an ultrasound examination. An anteroposterior (AP) view of the pelvis can be interpreted with the aid of several classic lines drawn on it (Fig. 678-8).

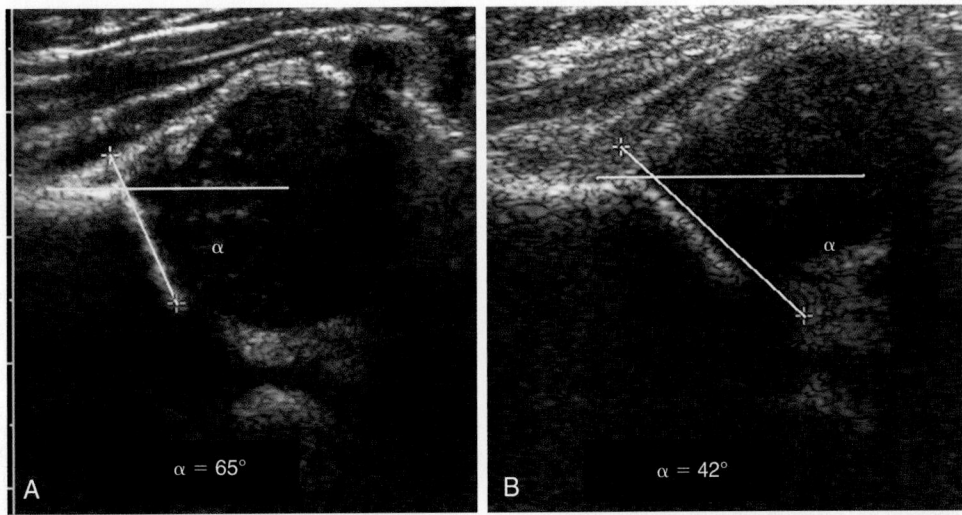

Figure 678-7 A, Normal ultrasonographic image of the hip in an infant. The α angle is >60 degrees. Note that a line drawn tangential to the ilium falls lateral to the center of the femoral head. **B,** In this child with developmental dysplasia of the hip, the left hip demonstrates an α angle of 42 degrees, and a line drawn tangential to the ilium shows that <50% of the femoral head is contained within the acetabulum.

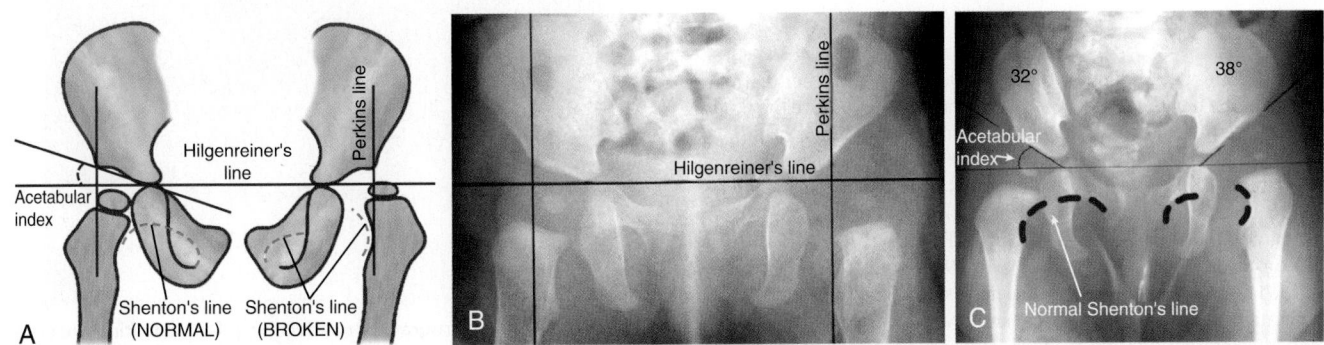

Figure 678-8 A-C, Radiographic measurements are useful in evaluating developmental dysplasia of the hip. Hilgenreiner's line is drawn through the triradiate cartilages. Perkins line is drawn perpendicular to Hilgenreiner's line at the lateral edge of the acetabulum. The ossific nucleus of the femoral head should be located in the medial lower quadrant of the intersection of these 2 lines. Shenton's line curves along the femoral metaphysis and connects smoothly to the inner margin of the pubis. In a child with hip subluxation or dislocation, this line consists of 2 separate arcs and is described as broken. The acetabular index is the angle between a line drawn along the margin of the acetabulum and Hilgenreiner's line; in normal newborns, it averages 27.5 degrees and decreases with age.

Hilgenreiner's **line** is a horizontal line drawn through the top of both triradiate cartilages (the clear area in the depth of the acetabulum). **Perkins line** is a vertical line through the most lateral ossified margin of the roof of the acetabulum, drawn perpendicular to Hilgenreiner's line. The ossific nucleus of the femoral head should be located in the medial lower quadrant of the intersection of these 2 lines. **Shenton's line** is a curved line drawn from the medial aspect of the femoral neck to the lower border of the superior pubic ramus. In a child with normal hips, this line is a continuous contour. In a child with hip subluxation or dislocation, this line consists of 2 separate arcs and is described as "broken."

The **acetabular index** is the angle formed between Hilgenreiner's line and a line drawn from the depth of the acetabular socket to the most lateral ossified margin of the roof of the acetabulum. This angle measures the development of the osseous roof of the acetabulum. In the newborn, the acetabular index can be up to 40 degrees; by 4 mo in the normal infant, it should be no more than 30 degrees. In the older child, the **center-edge angle** is a useful measure of femoral head coverage. This angle is formed at the juncture of the Perkins line and a line connecting the lateral margin of the acetabulum to the center of the femoral head. In children 6-13 yr old, an angle >19 degrees is normal, whereas in children 14 yr and older, an angle >25 degrees is considered normal.

TREATMENT
The goals in the management of DDH are to obtain and maintain a concentric reduction of the femoral head within the acetabulum in order to provide the optimal environment for the normal development of both the femoral head and acetabulum. The later the diagnosis of DDH is made, the more difficult it is to achieve these goals, the less potential there is for acetabular and proximal femoral remodeling, and the more complex the required treatments.

Newborns and Infants Younger Than 6 Months
Newborns hips that are Barlow-positive (reduced but dislocatable) or Ortolani-positive (dislocated but reducible) should generally be treated with a Pavlik harness as soon as the diagnosis is made. The management of newborns with dysplasia who are younger than 4 wk of age is less clear. A significant proportion of these hips normalize within 3-4 wk; consequently, many physicians prefer to reexamine these newborns after a few weeks before making treatment decisions. A study of 128 newborns with mildly dysplastic hips based on the results of an ultrasound (alpha angles between 43 and 50 degrees) who were randomly assigned to receive immediate abduction splinting or active sonographic surveillance from birth with Frejka splinting provided if treatment was subsequently needed revealed no difference in radiologic findings at 6 yr of age.

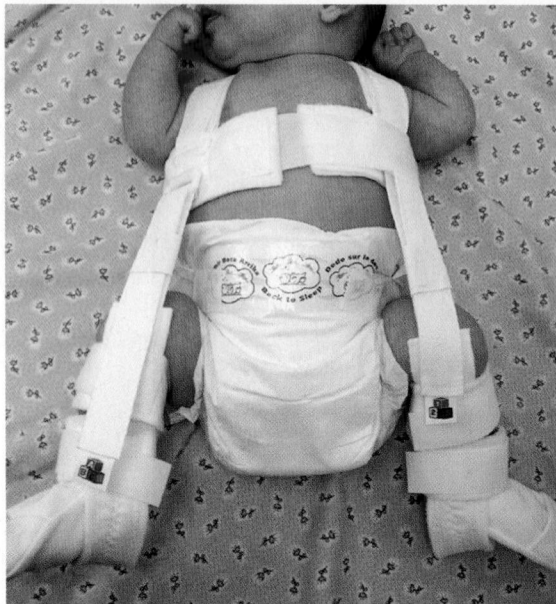

Figure 678-9 Photograph of a Pavlik harness.

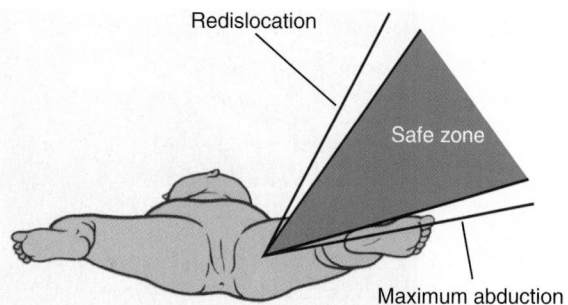

Figure 678-10 Diagram of the safe zone of Ramsey.

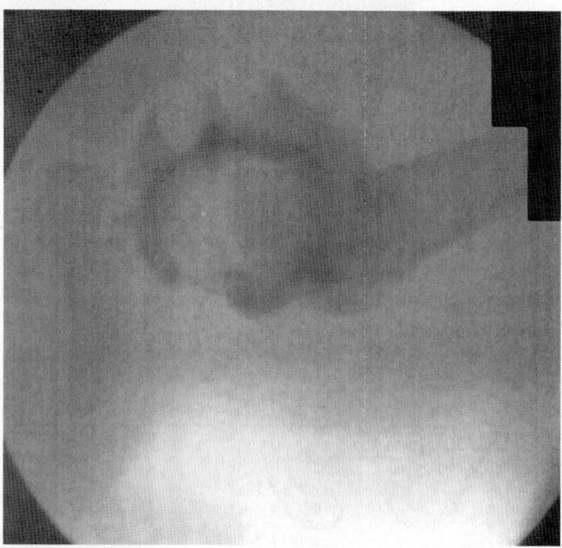

Figure 678-11 Arthrogram of a reduced hip for evaluating the stability of reduction.

Triple diapers or abduction diapers have no place in the treatment of DDH in the newborn; they are usually ineffective and give the family a false sense of security. *Acetabular dysplasia, subluxation, or dislocation can all be readily managed with the Pavlik harness.* Although other braces are available (von Rosen splint, Frejka pillow), the Pavlik harness remains the most commonly used device worldwide (Fig. 678-9). By maintaining the Ortolani-positive hip in a Pavlik harness on a full-time basis for 6 wk, hip instability resolves in 95% of cases. After 6 mo of age, the failure rate for the Pavlik harness is >50% because it is difficult to maintain the increasingly active and crawling child in the harness. Frequent examinations and readjustments are necessary to ensure that the harness is fitting correctly. The anterior straps of the harness should be set to maintain the hips in flexion (usually ~90-100 degrees); excessive flexion is discouraged because of the risk of femoral nerve palsy. The posterior straps are designed to encourage abduction. These are generally set to allow adduction just to neutral, as forced abduction by the harness can lead to avascular necrosis of the femoral epiphysis.

If follow-up examinations and ultrasounds do not demonstrate concentric reduction of the hip after 3-4 wk of Pavlik harness treatment, the harness should be abandoned. Continued use of the harness beyond this period in a persistently dislocated hip can cause *Pavlik harness disease,* or wearing away of the posterior aspect of the acetabulum, which can make the ultimate reduction less stable.

Children 6 Months to 2 Years of Age
The principal goals in the treatment of late-diagnosed dysplasia are to obtain and maintain reduction of the hip without damaging the femoral head. **Closed reductions** are performed in the operating room under general anesthesia. The hip is moved to determine the range of motion in which it remains reduced. This is compared to the maximal range of motion to construct a "safe zone" (Fig. 678-10). An arthrogram obtained at the time of reduction is very helpful for evaluating the depth and stability of the reduction (Fig. 678-11). The reduction is maintained in a well-molded spica cast, with the "human position" of moderate flexion and abduction being the preferred position. After the procedure, single-cut CT or MRI may be used to confirm the reduction. Twelve weeks after closed reduction, the plaster cast is removed; an abduction orthosis is often used at this point to encourage further remodeling of the acetabulum. Failure to obtain a stable hip with a closed reduction indicates the need for an **open reduction**. In patients younger than 2 yr of age, a secondary acetabular or femoral procedure is rarely required. The potential for acetabular development after closed or open reduction is excellent and continues for 4-8 yr after the procedure.

Children Older Than 2 Years
Children 2-6 yr of age with a hip dislocation usually require an open reduction. In this age group, a concomitant femoral shortening osteotomy is often performed to reduce the pressure on the proximal femur and minimize the risk of osteonecrosis. Because the potential for acetabular development is markedly diminished in these older children, a pelvic osteotomy is usually performed in conjunction with the open reduction. Postoperatively, patients are immobilized in a spica cast for 6-12 wk.

COMPLICATIONS
The most important complication of DDH is **avascular necrosis** of the femoral epiphysis. Reduction of the femoral head under pressure or in extreme abduction can result in occlusion of the epiphyseal vessels and produce either partial or total infarction of the epiphysis. Revascularization soon follows, but if the physis is severely damaged, abnormal growth and development can occur. The hip is most vulnerable to this complication before 4-6 mo, when the ossific nucleus appears. Management, as previously outlined, is designed to minimize this complication. With appropriate treatment, the incidence of avascular necrosis for DDH is reduced to 5-15%. Other complications in DDH include redislocation, residual subluxation, acetabular dysplasia, and postoperative complications, including wound infections.

Bibliography is available at Expert Consult.

678.2 Transient Monoarticular Synovitis (Toxic Synovitis)

Wudbhav N. Sankar, B. David Horn, Lawrence Wells, and John P. Dormans

Transient synovitis (toxic synovitis) is a reactive arthritis and is one of the most common causes of hip pain in young children.

ETIOLOGY

The cause of transient synovitis remains unknown. It has been variously described as a nonspecific inflammatory condition or as a postviral immunologic synovitis because it tends to follow recent viral illnesses.

CLINICAL MANIFESTATIONS

Although transient synovitis can occur in all age groups, it is most prevalent in children between 3 and 8 yr of age, with a mean onset at age 6 yr. Approximately 70% of all affected children have had a nonspecific upper respiratory tract infection 7-14 days before the onset of symptoms. Symptoms often develop acutely and usually consist of pain in the groin, anterior thigh, or knee, which may be referred from the hip. These children are usually able to bear weight on the affected limb and typically walk with a painful, limping gait. The hip is not held flexed, abducted, or laterally rotated unless a significant effusion is present. They are often afebrile or have a low-grade fever <38°C (100.4°F).

DIAGNOSIS

Transient synovitis is a clinical diagnosis, but laboratory and radiographic tests can be useful to rule out other more serious conditions. In transient synovitis, infection labs (erythrocyte sedimentation rate, serum C-reactive protein, and white blood cell counts) are relatively normal, but on occasion a mild elevation in the erythrocyte sedimentation rate is observed. AP and Lauenstein (frogleg) lateral radiographs of the pelvis may be acquired and are also usually found to be normal. Ultrasonography of the hip is preferred to x-rays and often demonstrates a joint effusion.

The most important condition to exclude before confirming a diagnosis of toxic synovitis is septic arthritis. Children with septic arthritis usually appear more systemically ill than those with transient synovitis. The pain associated with septic arthritis is more severe, and children often refuse to walk or move their hip at all. High fever, refusal to walk, and elevations of the erythrocyte sedimentation rate, serum C-reactive protein, and white blood cell count all point toward a diagnosis of septic arthritis. If the clinical scenario is suspicious for septic arthritis, an ultrasound-guided aspiration of the hip joint should be performed to make the definitive diagnosis (see Chapter 685). An exception to these criteria is hip septic arthritis due to *Kingella kingae*, which may have minimal inflammation and low grade or no fever (see Chapter 685). MRI may be needed to detect an associated osteomyelitis.

TREATMENT

The treatment of transient monoarticular synovitis of the hip is symptomatic. Recommended therapies include activity limitation and relief of weight bearing until the pain subsides. Antiinflammatory agents and analgesics can shorten the duration of pain. Most children recover completely within 3-6 wk.

Bibliography is available at Expert Consult.

678.3 Legg-Calvé-Perthes Disease

Wudbhav N. Sankar, B. David Horn, Lawrence Wells, and John P. Dormans

Legg-Calvé-Perthes disease (LCPD) is a hip disorder of unknown etiology that results from temporary interruption of the blood supply to the proximal femoral epiphysis, leading to osteonecrosis and femoral head deformity.

ETIOLOGY

Although the underlying etiology remains obscure, most authors agree that the final common pathway in the development of LCPD is disruption of the vascular supply to the femoral epiphysis, which results in ischemia and osteonecrosis. Infection, trauma, and transient synovitis have all been proposed as causative factors but are unsubstantiated. Factors leading to thrombophilia, an increased tendency to develop thrombosis and hypofibrinolysis, and a reduced ability to lyse thrombi have been identified. Factor V Leiden mutation, deficiency of proteins C and S, lupus anticoagulant, anticardiolipin antibodies, antitrypsin, and plasminogen activator might play a role in the abnormal clotting mechanism. These abnormalities in the clotting cascade are thought to increase blood viscosity and the risk for venous thrombosis. Poor venous outflow leads to increased intraosseous pressure, which, in turn, impedes arterial inflow, causing ischemia and cell death.

EPIDEMIOLOGY

The incidence of LCPD in the United States is 1 in 1,200 children with boys 4-5 times more likely to be affected than girls. The peak incidence of the disease is between the ages of 4 and 8 yr. Bilateral involvement is seen in approximately 10% of the patients, but the hips are usually in different stages of collapse. East Asians have the lowest incidence of the disease and whites the highest.

PATHOGENESIS

Early pathologic changes in the femoral head are the result of ischemia and necrosis; subsequent changes result from the repair process. The disease course may have 4 stages, although variations have been described. The **initial** stage of the disease, which often lasts 6 mo, is characterized by synovitis, joint irritability, and early necrosis of the femoral head. Revascularization then leads to osteoclastic-mediated resorption of the necrotic segment. The necrotic bone is replaced by fibrovascular tissue rather than new bone, which compromises the structural integrity of the femoral epiphysis. The second stage is the **fragmentation** stage, which typically lasts 8 mo. During this stage, the femoral epiphysis begins to collapse, usually laterally, and begins to extrude from the acetabulum. The **healing** stage, which lasts approximately 4 yr, begins with new bone formation in the subchondral region. Reossification begins centrally and expands in all directions. The degree of femoral head deformity depends on the severity of collapse and the amount of remodeling that occurs. The final stage is the **residual** stage, which begins after the entire head has reossified. A mild amount of remodeling of the femoral head still occurs until the child reaches skeletal maturity. LCPD often damages the proximal femoral physis leading to a short neck (coxa breva) and trochanteric overgrowth.

CLINICAL MANIFESTATIONS

The most common presenting symptom is a limp of varying duration. Pain, if present, is usually activity related and may be localized in the groin or referred to the anteromedial thigh or knee region. *Failure to recognize that thigh or knee pain in a child may be secondary to hip pathology can cause further delay in the diagnosis.* Less commonly, the onset of the disease may be much more acute and may be associated with a failure to ambulate.

Antalgic gait (a limp characterized by a shortening of gait phase on the injured side to alleviate weight-bearing pain) may be particularly prominent after strenuous activity at the end of the day. Hip motion, primarily internal rotation and abduction, is limited. Early in the course of the disease, the limited abduction is secondary to synovitis and muscle spasm in the adductor group; however, with time and the subsequent deformities that can develop, the limitation of abduction can become permanent. A mild hip flexion contracture of 10-20 degrees may be present. Atrophy of the muscles of the thigh, calf, or buttock from disuse secondary to pain may be evident. An apparent leg-length inequality may be caused by an adduction contracture or true shortening on the involved side from femoral head collapse.

DIAGNOSIS

Routine plain radiographs are the primary diagnostic tool for LCPD. AP and Lauenstein (frogleg) lateral views are used to diagnose, stage, provide prognosis for, and follow the course of the disease (Fig. 678-12). It is important when evaluating disease progression that all radiographs be viewed sequentially and compared with previous radiographs to assess the stage of the disease and to determine the true extent of epiphyseal involvement.

In the initial stage of LCPD, the radiographic changes include a decreased size of the ossification center, lateralization of the femoral head with widening of the medial joint space, a subchondral fracture, and physeal irregularity. In the fragmentation stage, the epiphysis appears fragmented, and there are scattered areas of increased radiolucency and radiodensity. During the reossification stage, the bone density returns to normal by new (woven) bone formation. The residual stage is marked by the reossification of the femoral head, gradual remodeling of head shape until skeletal maturity, and remodeling of the acetabulum.

In addition to these radiographic changes, several classic radiographic signs have been reported that describe a "head at risk" for severe deformity. Lateral extrusion of the epiphysis, a horizontal physis, calcification lateral to the epiphysis, subluxation of the hip, and a radiolucent horizontal V in the lateral aspect of the physis (Gage's sign) are all associated with a poor prognosis.

In the absence of changes on plain radiographs, particularly in the early stages of the disease, MRI is useful to diagnose early infarction and determine the degree of impaired perfusion. During the remodeling or residual stages, MRI is extremely helpful to define the abnormal anatomy and determine the extent of intra-articular injury. Arthrography can be useful to dynamically assess the shape of the femoral head, demonstrate whether a hip can be contained, and diagnose hinge abduction. Table 678-1 outlines the differential diagnosis.

CLASSIFICATION

Catterall proposed a 4-group classification based on the amount of femoral epiphysis involvement and a set of radiographic "head at-risk" signs. Group I hips have anterior femoral head involvement of 25%, no sequestrum (an island of dead bone within the epiphysis), and no metaphyseal abnormalities. Group II hips have up to 50% involvement and a clear demarcation between involved and uninvolved segments. Metaphyseal cysts may be present. Group III hips display up to 75% involvement and a large sequestrum. In group IV, the entire femoral head is involved. Use of the Catterall classification system has been limited because of a high degree of interobserver variability.

The **Herring lateral pillar classification** is the most widely used radiographic classification system for determining treatment and prognosis during the active stage of the disease (Fig. 678-13). Unlike the Catterall system, the Herring classification has a high degree of interobserver reliability. Classification is based on several radiographs taken during the early fragmentation stage. The lateral pillar classification system for LCPD evaluates the shape of the femoral head epiphysis on AP radiograph of the hip. The head is divided into 3 sections or pillars. The lateral pillar occupies the lateral 15-30% of the head width, the central pillar is approximately 50% of the head width, and the medial pillar is 20-35% of the head width. The degree of involvement of the lateral pillar can be subdivided into 3 groups. In group A, the lateral pillar is radiographically normal. In group B, the lateral pillar has some lucency but >50% of the lateral pillar height is maintained. In group C, the lateral pillar is more lucent than in group B and <50% of the pillar height remains. Herring has added a B/C border group to the

Table 678-1	Differential Diagnosis of Legg-Calvé-Perthes Disease

OTHER CAUSES OF AVASCULAR NECROSIS
Sickle cell disease
Other hemoglobinopathies (e.g., thalassemia)
Chronic myelogenous leukemia
Steroid medication
Sequela of traumatic hip dislocation
Treatment of developmental dysplasia of the hip
Septic arthritis

EPIPHYSEAL DYSPLASIAS
Multiple epiphyseal dysplasia
Spondyloepiphyseal dysplasia
Mucopolysaccharidoses
Hypothyroidism

OTHER SYNDROMES
Osteochondromatosis
Metachondromatosis
Schwartz-Jampel syndrome
Trichorhinophalangeal syndrome
Maroteaux-Lamy syndrome
Martsolf syndrome

(From Kim HKW, Herring JA: Legg-Calvé-Perthes Disease. In Herring JA, editor: Tachdjian's pediatric orthopaedics, ed 5. Philadelphia, 2014, WB Saunders, Box 17-6, p. 613.)

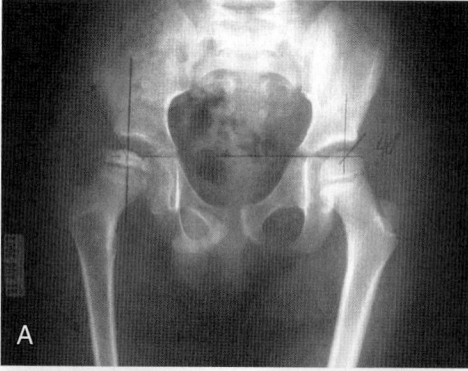
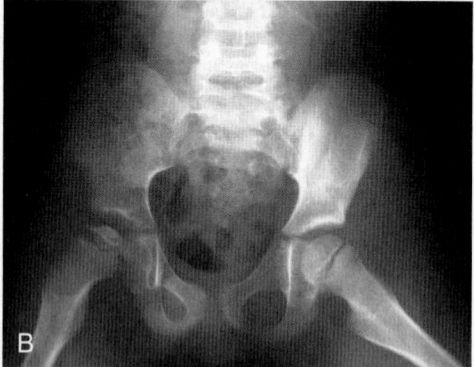

Figure 678-12 A, Anteroposterior radiograph of the pelvis shows epiphyseal fragmentation in the right hip, characteristic of the fragmentation phase of Legg-Calvé-Perthes disease. **B,** The frogleg lateral view demonstrates subchondral fracture, increased density of the femoral head, and some collapse.

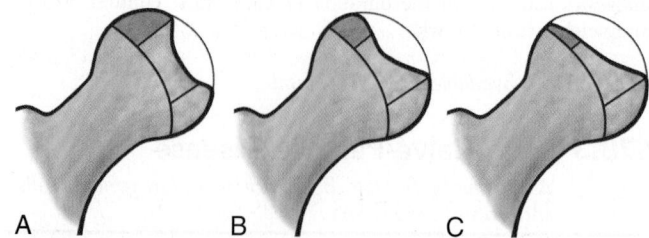

Figure 678-13 Lateral pillar classification for Legg-Calvé-Perthes disease. **A,** There is no involvement of the lateral pillar. **B,** More than 50% of the lateral pillar height is maintained. **C,** Less than 50% of the lateral pillar height is maintained.

classification system to describe patients with approximately 50% collapse of the lateral pillar.

NATURAL HISTORY AND PROGNOSIS

Children who develop signs and symptoms of LCPD before the age of 6 yr tend to recover with fewer residual problems. Patients older than 9 yr of age at presentation usually have a poor prognosis. The reason for this difference is that the remodeling potential of the femoral head is higher in younger children. Greater extent of femoral head involvement and duration of the disease process are additional factors associated with a poor prognosis. Hips classified as Catterall groups III and IV and lateral pillar group C generally have a poor prognosis.

TREATMENT

The goal of treatment in LCPD is preservation of a spherical, well-covered femoral head and maintenance of hip range of motion that is close to normal. Although the treatment of LCPD remains controversial, most authors agree that the general approach to these patients should be guided by the principle of containment. This principle is predicated on the fact that while the femoral head is fragmenting, and therefore in a softened condition, it is best to contain it entirely within the acetabulum; by doing so, the acetabulum acts as a mold for the regenerating femoral head. Conversely, failure to contain the head permits it to deform, with resulting extrusion and impingement on the lateral edge of the acetabulum. To be successful, containment must be instituted early while the femoral head is still moldable; once the head has healed, repositioning the femoral epiphysis will not aid remodeling and can, in fact, worsen symptoms.

Initial options to manage symptoms include activity limitation, protected weightbearing, and nonsteroidal antiinflammatory medications. "Nonoperative" containment can be achieved by using a Petrie cast to restore abduction and to direct the femoral head deeper into the acetabulum. Petrie casts are 2 long-leg casts that are connected by a bar and can be helpful to keep the hips in abduction and internal rotation (the best position for containment). Casting is generally done in conjunction with an arthrogram to confirm containment and a tenotomy of the adductor tendons. After 6 wk, patients can be transitioned into an abduction orthosis with limited weightbearing. Several older studies did not support the efficacy of casting and long-term bracing as a means of containment, but a subsequent large series reported excellent results with this form of treatment.

Surgical containment may be approached from the femoral side, the acetabular side, or both sides of the hip joint. A varus osteotomy of the proximal femur is the most common procedure. Pelvic osteotomies in LCPD are divided into 3 categories: acetabular rotational osteotomies, shelf procedures, and medial displacement or Chiari osteotomies. Any of these procedures can be combined with a proximal femoral varus osteotomy when severe deformity of the femoral head cannot be contained by a pelvic osteotomy alone.

After healing of the epiphysis, surgical treatment shifts from containment to managing the residual deformity. Patients with hinge abduction or joint incongruity might benefit from a valgus-producing proximal femoral osteotomy. Coxa breva and overgrowth of the greater trochanter can be managed by performing an advancement of the trochanter. This helps restore the length–tension relationship of the abductor mechanism and can alleviate abductor fatigue. Patients with femoroacetabular impingement from irregularity of the femoral head can often be helped with an osteoplasty or cheilectomy of the offending prominence.

Bibliography is available at Expert Consult.

678.4 Slipped Capital Femoral Epiphysis
Wudbhav N. Sankar, B. David Horn, Lawrence Wells, and John P. Dormans

Slipped capital femoral epiphysis (SCFE) is a hip disorder that affects adolescents, most often between 10 and 16 yr of age, and involves failure of the physis and displacement of the femoral head relative to the neck.

CLASSIFICATION

SCFEs may be classified temporally, according to onset of symptoms (acute, chronic, acute-on-chronic); functionally, according to patient's ability to bear weight (stable or unstable); or morphologically, as the extent of displacement of the femoral epiphysis relative to the neck (mild, moderate, or severe), as estimated by measurement on radiographic or CT images.

An **acute** SCFE is characterized as one occurring in a patient who has prodromal symptoms for ≤3 wk and should be distinguished from a purely traumatic separation of the epiphysis in a previously normal hip (a true Salter-Harris type I fracture; see Chapter 683). The patient with an acute slip usually has some prodromal pain in the groin, thigh, or knee, and usually reports a relatively minor injury (a twist or fall) that is not sufficiently violent to produce an acute fracture of this severity.

Chronic SCFE is the most common form of presentation. Typically, an adolescent presents with a few-month history of vague groin, thigh, or knee pain and a limp. Radiographs show a variable amount of posterior and inferior migration of the femoral epiphysis and remodeling of the femoral neck in the same direction.

Children with **acute-on-chronic** SCFE can have features of both acute and chronic conditions. Prodromal symptoms have been present for >3 wk with a sudden exacerbation of pain. Radiographs demonstrate femoral neck remodeling and further displacement of the capital epiphysis beyond the remodeled point of the femoral neck.

The stability classification separates patients based on their ability to ambulate and is more useful in predicting prognosis and establishing a treatment plan. The SCFE is considered **stable** when the child is able to walk with or without crutches. A child with an **unstable** SCFE is unable to walk with or without walking aids. Patients with unstable SCFE have a much higher prevalence of osteonecrosis (up to 50%) compared to those with stable SCFE (nearly 0%). This is most likely because of the vascular injury caused at the time of initial displacement.

SCFE may also be categorized by the degree of displacement of the epiphysis on the femoral neck. The head-shaft angle difference is <30 degrees in mild slips, between 30 and 60 degrees in moderate slips, and >60 degrees in severe slips, compared to the normal contralateral side.

ETIOLOGY AND PATHOGENESIS

SCFEs are most likely caused by a combination of mechanical and endocrine factors. The plane of cleavage in most SCFEs occurs through the hypertrophic zone of the physis. During normal puberty, the physis becomes more vertically oriented, which converts mechanical forces from compression to shear. In addition, the hypertrophic zone becomes elongated in pubertal adolescents due to high levels of circulating hormones. This widening of the physis decreases the threshold for mechanical failure. Normal ossification depends on a number of different factors, including thyroid hormone, vitamin D, and calcium. Consequently, it is not surprising that SCFEs occur with increased incidence in children with medical disorders such as hypothyroidism, hypopituitarism, and renal osteodystrophy. Obesity, one of the largest risk factors for SCFE, affects both the mechanical load on the physis and the level of circulating hormones. The combination of mechanical and endocrine factors results in gradual failure of the physis, which allows posterior and inferior displacement of the head in relation to the femoral neck.

EPIDEMIOLOGY

The annual incidence of SCFE is 2 per 100,000 in the general population. Incidence has ranged from 0.2 per 100,000 in eastern Japan to 10.08 per 100,000 in the northeastern United States. The African-American and Polynesian populations are reported to have an increased incidence of SCFE. Obesity is the most closely associated risk factor in the development of SCFE; approximately 65% of the patients are >90th percentile in weight-for-age profiles. There is a predilection for boys to

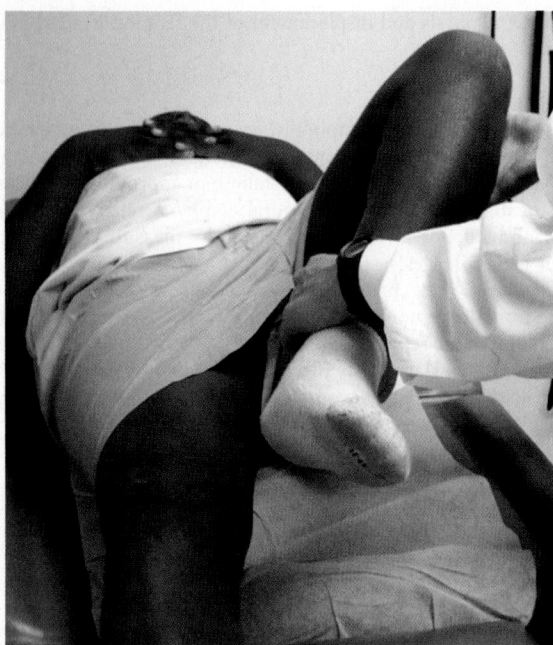

Figure 678-14 Progressive external rotation noted with flexion: the knee-axilla sign.

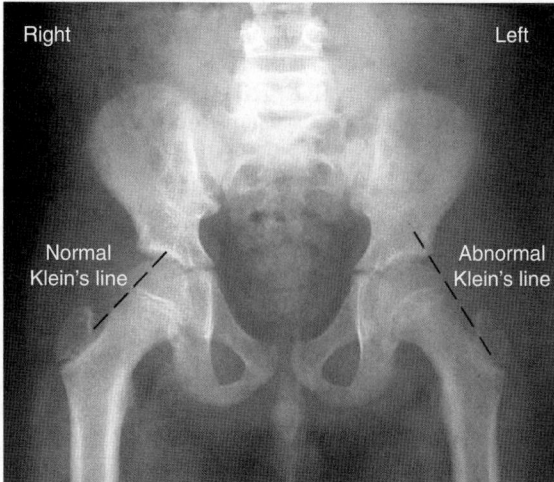

Figure 678-15 Illustration of Klein's line.

be affected more often than girls and for the left hip to be affected more often than the right. Bilateral involvement has been reported in as many as 60% of cases, nearly half of which may be present at the time of initial presentation.

CLINICAL MANIFESTATIONS

The classic patient presenting with a SCFE is an obese, African-American boy between the ages of 11 and 16 yr. Girls present earlier, usually between 10 and 14 yr of age. Patients with chronic and stable SCFEs tend to present after weeks to months of symptoms. Patients usually limp to some degree and have an externally rotated lower extremity. Physical examination of the affected hip reveals a restriction of internal rotation, abduction, and flexion. Commonly, the examiner notes that as the affected hip is flexed, the thigh tends to rotate progressively into more external rotation with increased flexion (Fig. 678-14). Most patients complain of groin symptoms, but isolated thigh pain or knee pain is a common presentation from referred pain along the course of the obturator nerve. Missed or delayed diagnosis often occurs in children who present with knee pain and do not receive appropriate imaging of the hip. Patients with unstable SCFEs usually present in an urgent fashion. Children typically refuse to allow any range of motion of the hip; much like a hip fracture, the extremity is shortened, abducted, and externally rotated.

DIAGNOSTIC STUDIES

AP and frogleg lateral radiographic views of both hips are usually the only imaging studies needed to make the diagnosis. Because approximately 25% of patients have a contralateral slip on initial presentation, it is critical that both hips be carefully evaluated by the treating physician. Radiographic findings include widening and irregularity of the physis, a decrease in epiphyseal height in the center of the acetabulum, a crescent-shaped area of increased density in the proximal portion of the femoral neck, and the "blanch sign of Steel" corresponding to the double density created from the anteriorly displaced femoral neck overlying the femoral head. In an unaffected patient, Klein's line, a straight line drawn along the superior cortex of the femoral neck on the AP radiograph, should intersect some portion of the lateral capital femoral epiphysis. With progressive displacement of the epiphysis, Klein's line no longer intersects the epiphysis (Fig. 678-15). Although

some of these radiographic findings can be subtle, most diagnoses can be readily made on the frogleg lateral view, which reveals the characteristic posterior and inferior displacement of the epiphysis in relation to the femoral neck (Fig. 678-16).

TREATMENT

Once the diagnosis is made, the patient should be admitted to the hospital immediately and placed on bed rest. Allowing the child to go home without definitive treatment increases the risk that a stable SCFE will become an unstable SCFE and that further displacement will occur. Children with atypical presentations (younger than 10 yr of age, thin body habitus) should have screening labs sent to rule out an underlying endocrinopathy.

The goal of treatment is to prevent further progression of the slip and to stabilize (i.e., close) the physis. Although various forms of treatment have been used in the past, including spica casting, the current gold standard for the treatment of SCFE is in situ pinning with a single, large screw (Fig. 678-17). The term *in situ* implies that no attempt is made to reduce the displacement between the epiphysis and femoral neck because doing so increases the risk of osteonecrosis. Screws are typically placed percutaneously under fluoroscopic guidance. Postoperatively, most patients are allowed partial weightbearing with crutches for 4-6 wk, followed by a gradual return to normal activities. Patients should be monitored with serial radiographs to be sure that the physis is closing and that the slip is stable. After healing from the initial stabilization, patients with severe residual deformity may be candidates for proximal femoral osteotomy to correct the deformity, reduce impingement, and improve range of motion.

Because 20-40% of children will develop a contralateral SCFE at some point, many orthopedists advocate prophylactic pin fixation of the contralateral (normal) side in patients with a unilateral SCFE. The benefits of preventing a possible slip must be balanced with the risks of performing a potentially unnecessary surgery. Several recent studies have attempted to analyze decision models for prophylactic pinning, but controversy remains regarding the optimal course of treatment.

COMPLICATIONS

Osteonecrosis and chondrolysis are the 2 most serious complications of SCFE. Osteonecrosis, or avascular necrosis, usually occurs as a result of injury to the retinacular vessels. This can be caused by an initial force of injury, particularly in unstable slips, forced manipulation of an acute or unstable SCFE, compression from intracapsular hematoma, or as a direct injury during surgery. Partial forms of osteonecrosis can also appear following internal fixation; this can be caused by a disruption of the intraepiphyseal blood vessels. Chondrolysis, on the other

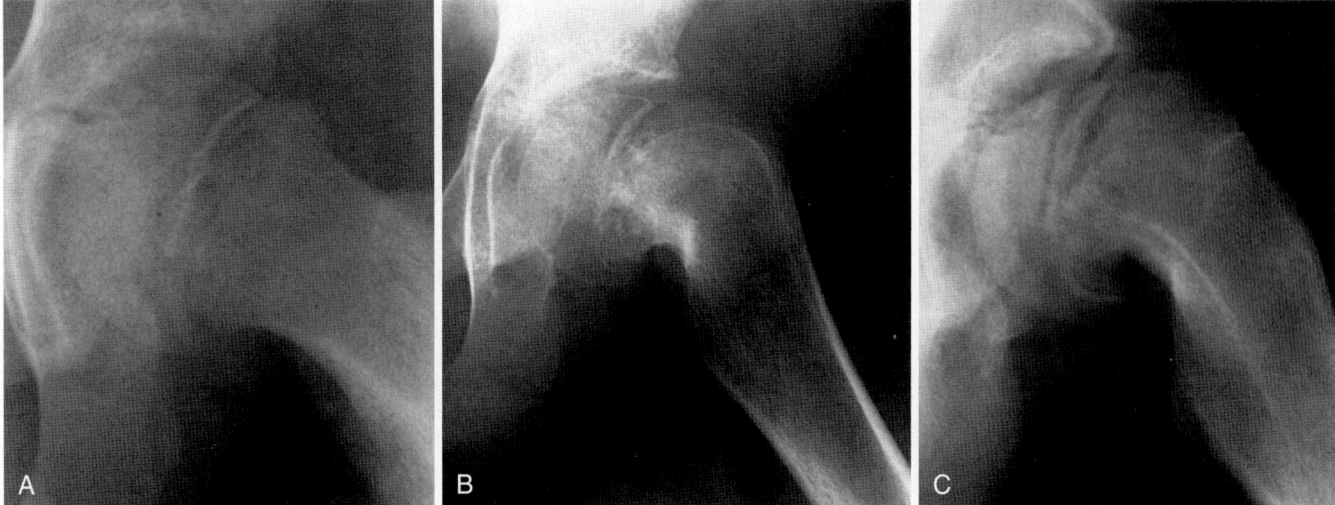

Figure 678-16 Radiographic appearance of slipped capital femoral epiphysis (SCFE) on presentation. **A,** Appearance of acute SCFE on a frogleg lateral view. The displacement of the epiphysis is suggestive of a Salter-Harris type I fracture of the upper femoral physis. There are no secondary adaptive changes noted in the femoral neck. **B,** Frogleg lateral radiographs in a patient with many months of thigh discomfort and a chronic slipped epiphysis. Adaptive changes in the femoral neck predominate, and the epiphysis is centered on the adapted femoral neck. **C,** Frogleg lateral radiographs of a patient with acute-on-chronic SCFE. The patient had several months of vague thigh pain, with sudden, severe exacerbation of that pain. The acute displacement of the epiphysis is evident. Unlike in acute SCFE (see **A**), secondary adaptive remodeling changes are also present in the femoral neck, beyond which the epiphysis has acutely displaced. *(From Herring JA: Slipped capital femoral epiphysis. In Herring JA, editor: Tachdjian's pediatric orthopaedics, ed 5, Philadelphia, 2014, WB Saunders, Fig. 18-1, p. 632.)*

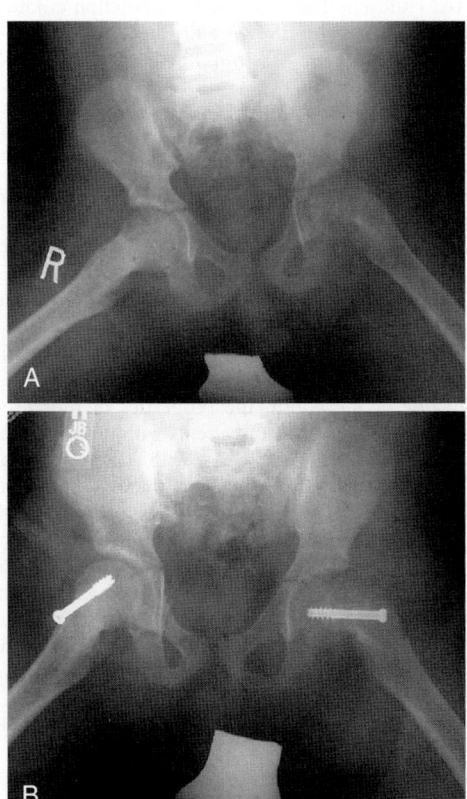

Figure 678-17 Preoperative **(A)** and postoperative **(B)** radiographs demonstrating the in situ pinning in a case of slipped capital femoral epiphysis.

hand, is an acute dissolution of articular cartilage in the hip. There are no clear causes of this complication, but it is believed to be associated with more-severe slips, to occur more commonly among African-Americans and girls, and to be associated with pins or screws protruding out of the femoral head.

Bibliography is available at Expert Consult.

Chapter **679**
The Spine
R. Justin Mistovich and David A. Spiegel

Abnormalities of the spine can result from a variety of causes including congenital, developmental, and traumatic. In addition to spinal deformities, back pain has become increasingly prevalent in childhood and adolescence, and a thoughtful diagnostic evaluation is required to establish the diagnosis while minimizing the overutilization of healthcare resources. The most common deformities are scoliosis and kyphosis. An early diagnosis is important, as a subset of patients may be candidates for "preventive" strategies such as bracing. Early intervention may potentially reduce the number requiring surgery, or at least reduce the magnitude or risks if surgical treatment is required.

Scoliosis may be from congenital bony deformities, may be idiopathic, including infantile, juvenile, or adolescent idiopathic scoliosis, or may be associated with a variety of underlying conditions, including neuromuscular diseases, connective tissue diseases, and genetic

Table 679-1	Classification of Spinal Deformities
SCOLIOSIS	**Myopathies**
Idiopathic	Duchenne muscular dystrophy
Infantile	Arthrogryposis
Juvenile	Other muscular dystrophies
Adolescent	*Syndromes*
Congenital	Neurofibromatosis
Failure of formation	Marfan syndrome
Wedge vertebrae	*Compensatory*
Hemivertebrae	Leg-length discrepancy
Failure of segmentation	
Unilateral bar	**KYPHOSIS**
Block vertebra	Postural kyphosis (flexible)
Mixed	Scheuermann disease
Neuromuscular	Congenital kyphosis
Neuropathic diseases	Failure of formation
Upper motor neuron	Failure of segmentation
Cerebral palsy	Mixed
Spinocerebellar degeneration (Friedreich ataxia, Charcot-Marie-Tooth disease)	
Syringomyelia	
Spinal cord tumor	
Spinal cord trauma	
Lower motor neuron	
Poliomyelitis	
Spinal muscular atrophy	

syndromes (Table 679-1). The pediatrician is often the first to diagnose these conditions. A familiarity with the physical examination, as well as the natural history and treatment options, will help the pediatrician to not only establish an early diagnosis but also to provide basic counseling for the patient and family regarding the diagnosis, general prognosis, and whether any referral and/or further workup might be indicated.

While parents and families are primarily concerned about the resulting cosmetic abnormalities, the physician diagnosing a patient with a spine deformity must carefully consider both the potential for underlying causes requiring treatment and the patient's long-term prognosis. If a certain curve magnitude is crossed in a patient with adolescent idiopathic scoliosis, the curve will be likely to continue to progress in adulthood and may require surgical treatment. Progressive curvatures in the neuromuscular population may result in respiratory insufficiency in addition to a loss of sitting balance. Additionally, while the majority of patients with excessive thoracic kyphosis have benign flexible curves and require no active treatment, a subset will have a progressive or rigid deformity which may require treatment. Parents and the patient must have an understanding of the deformity, how it may progress, and potential complications associated with the diagnosis. Table 679-1 presents a classification of common spinal abnormalities.

NORMAL SPINAL CURVATURES

The spine has curvatures that are anatomically normal in the lateral (sagittal) plane. Cervical lordosis (convex anteriorly), thoracic kyphosis (convex posteriorly), and lumbar lordosis regions are biomechanically advantageous as they maintain relationships of the body relative to the forces of gravity, which is important for balance. These curvatures also help to conserve energy by minimizing the amount of muscular activity required to maintain an upright posture.

Abnormalities affecting these normal curvatures, termed *sagittal plane imbalances*, can be measured on a sagittal spine radiograph. A vertical line, or *plumb line*, drawn from the center of the 7th cervical vertebra should normally fall through the posterosuperior corner of the sacrum. Disorders affecting sagittal alignment include thoracic hyperkyphosis and lumbar hyperlordosis. Although scoliosis is a

3-dimensional deformity, it is most commonly described as a lateral curvature of the spine in the frontal (coronal) plane.

679.1 Idiopathic Scoliosis
R. Justin Mistovich and David A. Spiegel

DEFINITION

The word *scoliosis* takes its origin from the Greek word *skolios*, meaning bent or curved. Medically recognized for centuries, Hippocrates described scoliosis in his treatise *On Articulations*. Scoliosis is a complex 3-dimensional spinal deformity that is defined in the coronal plane as a curve of at least 10 degrees, measured by the Cobb method, on a **posteroanterior (PA)** radiograph of the spine. The deformity also includes rotation of the vertebrae and also malalignment in the sagittal plane, such as a segmental apical lordosis in thoracic curves.

ETIOLOGY

The etiology of idiopathic scoliosis remains unknown; it is likely that the cause is multifactorial with genetic, hormonal, cellular, anatomic, and functional contributions.

A genetic link has been proposed with sex-linked dominant, autosomal dominant and polygenetic inheritance patterns all suggested. Genetic involvement has been substantiated in studies of twins, demonstrating a 73% concordance rate for **adolescent idiopathic scoliosis (AIS)** in monozygotic twins compared to a 36% concordance rate in dizygotic twins.

AIS is 2-10 times more common in females than males. Investigators have attempted to explain this difference as a genetic effect: It has been hypothesized that males are not as susceptible to the involved genes as females. Therefore, affected males must inherit a larger number of susceptibility genes to have a scoliosis phenotype. Males would pass more susceptibility genes onto their children and would therefore have more affected children. This polygenetic prediction is known as the Carter effect; fathers with AIS *transmit* the disease to 80% of their children, but mothers with AIS *transmit* the disease to only 56% of their children.

Certain polymorphisms in the estrogen receptor gene are linked to an increased curve progression and higher risk of requiring operative treatment. Genetic analysis may also be able to determine curve progression, although data concerning the effectiveness and validity of this are limited.

Endocrine factors may have a possible role in the disease pathology. Lower plasma melatonin levels have been noted in patients with progressive curvatures. Abnormal levels of growth hormone and insulin-like growth factor-1 have also been discovered. Leptin, the hormone responsible for satiety, is found at lower levels in patients with AIS.

Cellular structures may be involved in the disease process. Calmodulin, a regulator of the contractile properties of muscle, occurs at increased levels in the platelets of patients with progressive AIS.

MRI studies of the brain in patients with AIS have found that the cerebellum of affected patients is hypertrophied in areas involving the somatosensory tracts, motor control, and response to visual stimulation. These areas of hypertrophy may be a compensation for impaired balance resulting from malalignment of the spine. Other studies have noted a decrease in regional brain volumes and white matter in the corpus callosum and internal capsule between patients affected with AIS and normal adolescents. Girls with AIS have also been noted to have a larger foramen magnum. The importance of these imaging findings remains unclear.

Functional evaluations of patients with AIS have noted abnormalities in proprioception, postural balance, somatosensory function, somatosensory evoked potentials and electromyography. Patients with AIS have differences in vestibular-evoked myogenic potentials, suggesting that otolith system dysfunction may play a role in the disease. Approximately one-third of girls with AIS have osteopenia on dual-energy x-ray absorptiometry studies, and of these, 80% will have life-long osteopenia. Osteopenia is linked to an increased risk of curve progression. It is nonetheless difficult to determine which findings are primary or causative, and which are secondary to the disease.

EPIDEMIOLOGY

The overall prevalence of idiopathic scoliosis in skeletally immature patients ranges from 1-3% of the population. Most curves are mild and do not require treatment, with only 0.5% greater than 20 degrees and 0.3% exceeding 30 degrees. While curves of ≤10 degrees occur equally in males and females, those requiring an intervention occur in a 7:1 female:male ratio.

CLASSIFICATION OF IDIOPATHIC SCOLIOSIS

Idiopathic scoliosis is classified according to the age at onset. **Infantile scoliosis** is rare, comprising 0.5-4% of all cases of idiopathic scoliosis. It describes patients with spinal curves noted from birth to 3 yr of age. Juvenile scoliosis accounts for 8-16% of cases of idiopathic scoliosis and affects children age 3-10 yr. AIS affects patients 11 yr of age and older, and comprises 70-80% of all cases of idiopathic scoliosis.

CLINICAL PRESENTATION OF IDIOPATHIC SCOLIOSIS

When evaluating a patient with a structural spinal curvature, a thorough history and physical examination are required because idiopathic scoliosis is a diagnosis of exclusion. All other potential causes, including congenital bone malformations, neuromuscular and connective tissue diseases, and tumors, must carefully be excluded.

Patients often present after a positive screening by their primary care physician, through a school screening program, or because they (or their family or friends) have noticed a cosmetic deformity. It should be noted that school screening programs have become controversial, as some authors claim that the programs do not change the outcomes of patients requiring intervention, result in unnecessary physician visits and radiographs, and are not cost-effective. The British Orthopaedic Association and the U.S. Preventive Services Task Force have both issued statements recommending against routine screening for the above reasons. However, citing the need for early identification of scoliosis to reduce the risk of operative complications common to correction of large, neglected curves, the Scoliosis Research Society, an international organization of spine surgeons, still advocates for school screening.

Back pain is not commonly a primary presenting complaint of patients with scoliosis, although when questioned, one-third of adolescents with idiopathic scoliosis will endorse some degree of back discomfort at some point in time. To keep this finding in perspective, approximately 35% of healthy adolescents complain of episodes of low back pain and discomfort. However, if a patient presents with the complaint of significant back pain associated with a curvature, the physician must perform a careful physical exam, check spinal radiographs, and evaluate for other causes of pain, including spondylosis, spondylolisthesis, tethered cords or a syrinx, herniated discs, or tumors such as osteoid osteoma or spinal cord tumor (see Chapter 679.5 below).

PHYSICAL EXAMINATION OF IDIOPATHIC SCOLIOSIS

Evaluate the patient in the standing position, from both the front and the side, to identify any asymmetry in the chest wall, trunk, and/or shoulders.

Begin the examination focusing on the back. The earliest abnormality noted on physical exam in patients with scoliosis is asymmetry of the posterior chest wall on forward bending. This test, called the Adams forward-bending test (Fig. 679-1) is performed by placing a scoliometer at the apex of the deformity with the patient bending 45 degrees forward. An inclination measuring 7 degrees or more has been suggested as the cut off for orthopaedic referral. Scoliosis is a 3-dimensional deformity. Patients develop a posterior rib hump on the convex side of the spinal curve as a result of the rotational component of the deformity. The anterior chest wall may be prominent on the concavity of the curve as a result of outward rib rotation. Other

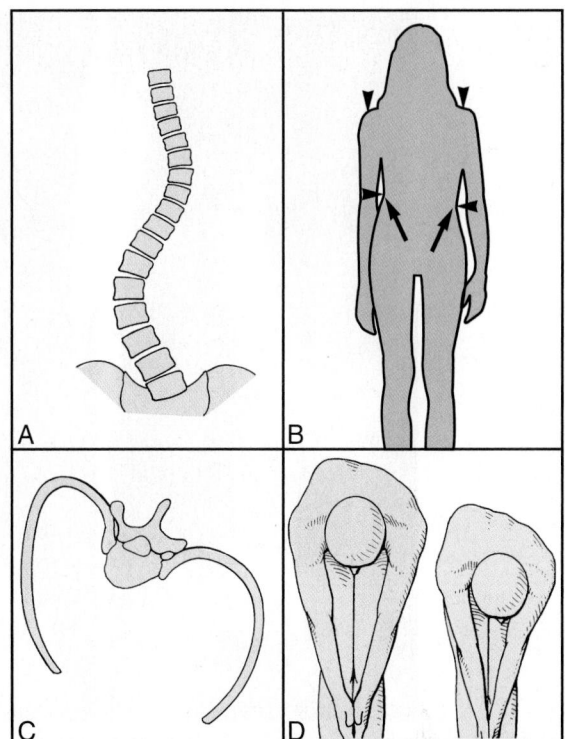

Figure 679-1 Structural changes in idiopathic scoliosis. **A,** As curvature increases, alterations in body configuration develop in both the primary and compensatory curve regions. **B,** Asymmetry of shoulder height, waistline, and elbow-to-flank distance are common findings. **C,** Vertebral rotation and associated posterior displacement of the ribs on the convex side of the curve are responsible for the characteristic deformity of the chest wall in scoliosis patients. **D,** In the school screening examination for scoliosis, the patient bends forward at the waist. Rib asymmetry of even a small degree is obvious. *(From Scoles PV: Spinal deformity in childhood and adolescence. In Behrman RE, Vaughn VC III, editors: Nelson textbook of pediatrics, update 5, Philadelphia, 1989, WB Saunders.)*

associated findings may include elevation of the shoulder, a lateral shift of the trunk, or an apparent leg-length discrepancy. A lumbar curve may also compensate for a primary limb-length discrepancy, with the apex toward the shorter leg.

Next, examine the patient from the side to evaluate the degree of kyphosis and lordosis. The upper thoracic spine normally has a smooth, gently rounded kyphotic curve with an apex in the midthoracic region. The cervical spine and lower lumbar spine have concave, or lordotic curves. The magnitude of these sagittal contours varies both with age and among individuals of the same age. Children have less cervical lordosis and more lumbar lordosis than do adults or adolescents. When examining a patient with idiopathic scoliosis, a common finding is a loss of the normal thoracic kyphosis, resulting in what is called a relative thoracic lordosis. A common benign finding in normal adolescent thoracic spines is a flexible roundback, or postural kyphosis. This can be corrected voluntarily when the patient extends his or her spine. This is different from sharp, abrupt, or accentuated forward angulation in the thoracic or thoracolumbar region, which is indicative of a pathologic kyphotic deformity.

The final exam component is a careful neurologic examination, as scoliosis may be associated with an underlying neurologic diagnosis. Check superficial abdominal reflexes, extremity reflexes, muscle strength, and examine for clonus. A high suspicion is necessary in patients with infantile and juvenile idiopathic scoliosis because 20% have an associated intraspinal abnormality such as a tethered spinal cord or syringomyelia. The index of suspicion for neurologic involvement is further raised in the presence of back pain or neurologic symptoms, café-au-lait spots, a sacral dimple, midline cutaneous

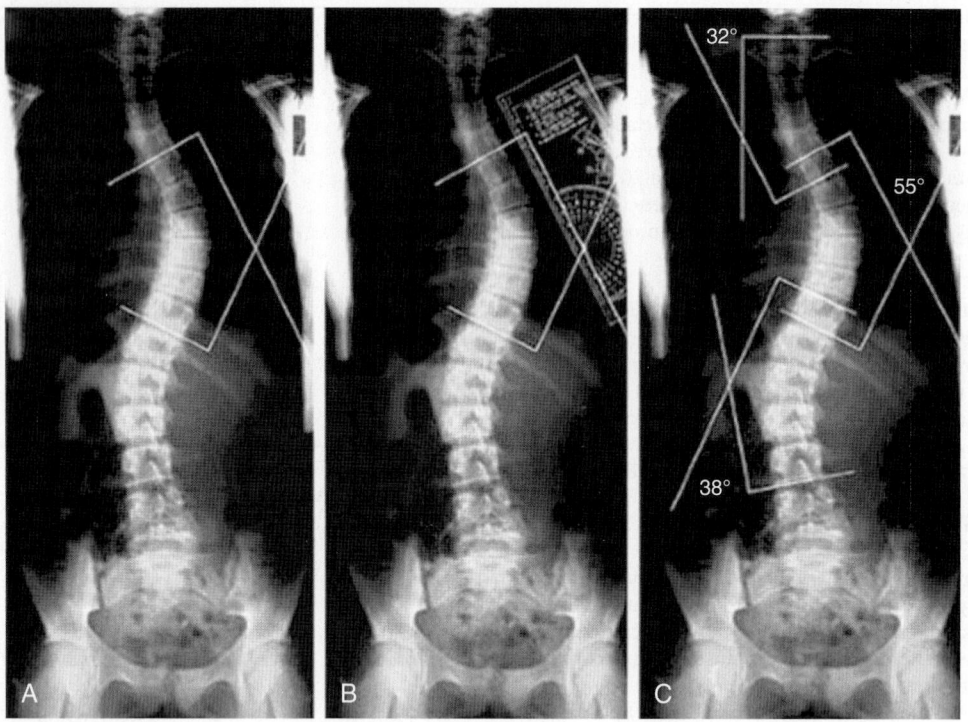

Figure 679-2 A-C, Cobb angles measurements. *(From Morrissy, RT, Weinstein, SL: Lovell & Winter's pediatric orthopaedics, ed 6, Philadelphia, 2006, Lippincott Williams & Wilkins.)*

abnormalities such as a hair patch or skin tag, or a unilateral foot deformity.

RADIOGRAPHIC EVALUATION OF IDIOPATHIC SCOLIOSIS

Standing, high-quality, PA and lateral radiographs of the entire spine are recommended at the initial evaluation for patients with clinical findings suggestive of a spinal deformity. On the PA radiograph, the degree of curvature is determined by the Cobb method, in which the angle between the superior and inferior vertebrae tilted into the curve is measured (Fig. 679-2). A line is drawn across the superior end plate of each end vertebra, and the angle between perpendicular lines drawn from each of these is measured.

Spinal MRI is indicated when there is suspicion of an underlying cause for the scoliosis, such as spinal cord abnormality based on age (infantile or juvenile curves), abnormal findings on the history and physical examination, and atypical radiographic features. Atypical radiographic findings may include certain curve patterns such as a left thoracic curve, double thoracic curves, or high thoracic curves. Other radiographic abnormalities include widening of the spinal canal and erosive or dysplastic changes in the vertebral body or ribs. On the lateral radiograph, an increase in thoracic kyphosis or an absence of segmental lordosis may be suggestive of an underlying neurologic abnormality.

NATURAL HISTORY OF IDIOPATHIC SCOLIOSIS

The decision to treat the patient is based on the natural history of idiopathic scoliosis. Uniquely, infantile idiopathic scoliosis may spontaneously resolve in 20-90% of cases. Patients with infantile scoliosis who have developmental delay, curves presenting after 1 yr of age, and larger magnitude curves are more likely to progress. A radiographic parameter called the *Mehta angle* can also be used to predict curve progression. This measurement examines the vertebra at the apex of the thoracic curve. It measures the angle formed by a line perpendicular from the vertebral end plate and a line down the center of the rib. The measurement is calculated on the convex and concave side, and

the final *rib vertebral angle difference* is calculated by subtracting the convex side from the concave side. A curve with an rib vertebral angle difference <20 degrees will resolve in approximately 80% of cases, whereas a curve with an rib vertebral angle difference >20 degrees will progress in more than 80% of cases. Curves that resolve typically do so before 2 yr of age.

Several factors affect the rate of curve progression in patients with AIS. Curves are more likely to progress in patients with significant growth remaining and skeletal immaturity, meaning that the growth plates, or physes, remain open allowing for continued skeletal growth. Findings associated with significant growth remaining are younger age, premenarchal status, Tanner stage I or II, and Risser sign (a radiographic measurement of ossification of the iliac crest) of 0 or 1. Other factors affecting progression are the curve magnitude, pattern, and patient gender. There is a relationship between curve progression and 3-dimensional spinal measurements of vertebral wedging, axial rotation, and torsion, possibly allowing for better prognostication of curves at risk. In general, female patients are more likely than males to have curves that progress. Younger, premenarchal girls with curves between 20 degrees and 30 degrees have a significantly higher risk of progression than do girls 2 yr after menarche with similar curves, demonstrating the significance of age on progression. The older group is unlikely to have any progression at all while premenarchal girls with the same curve are likely to progress. Thoracic curves <30 degrees rarely progress after skeletal maturity, whereas those >45-50 degrees may progress approximately 1 degree per year through life.

Functionally, there are not many significant, clinically detrimental effects of smaller curves. Idiopathic thoracic curvatures greater than 60-70 degrees may be associated with abnormalities on pulmonary function testing, and curves of higher magnitude may cause clinically significant cardiopulmonary impairment and even cor pulmonale in severe curves. Long-term studies demonstrate that a degree of chronic back pain may be a problem for patients with scoliosis, although there is no definitive connection between pain and the curve magnitude or location. Furthermore, nearly 70% of patients with pain reported low or moderate severity of symptoms, stating that the pain does not interfere with normal activities.

TREATMENT OF IDIOPATHIC SCOLIOSIS

Brace treatment may prevent curve progression in a significant number of patients with AIS and is most successful when an early diagnosis is established. The success rate depends upon the amount of growth remaining; patients with infantile or juvenile scoliosis are much more likely to require a surgical procedure than those with AIS. Adherence with the recommended protocol for wearing the brace will influence the outcome. Although various schedules for brace wear have been reported, from 12-23 hr daily, the brace is generally worn for 16 or more hours per day, maximizing wear when the patient is upright. Adherence can be a challenge in the adolescent population. Braces are offered for treatment of skeletally immature patients with curves >30 degrees at the first visit, or in patients who are being followed and have developed progression of their curvature beyond 25 degrees. Bracing is ineffective in curvatures >45 degrees. The brace is worn until cessation of growth in males, but in females some authors will consider weaning from the brace when the patient is more than 1.5 yr postmenarchal, is a Risser 4 or greater and/or has grown less than 1 cm over the previous 6 mo.

Surgical treatment involves spinal arthrodesis or fusion and is usually recommended for skeletally immature patients with progressive curves >45 degrees and skeletally mature patients with curves >50 degrees. The goals of surgery are to arrest progression of the deformity, to improve cosmesis, and to achieve a balanced spine, all while minimizing the number of vertebral segments that are stabilized.

Implants, including pedicle screws, sublaminar wires, and hooks, are attached to 2 longitudinal rods (Fig. 679-3). These are used to apply mechanical forces to the spine, correcting the deformity in both the frontal and lateral planes. The spine is decorticated and bone graft is placed for the fusion portion of the procedure. Correction also maintains normal frontal and sagittal spinal balance. The strength of the spinal implants maintains correction without requiring a postoperative brace in the majority of cases.

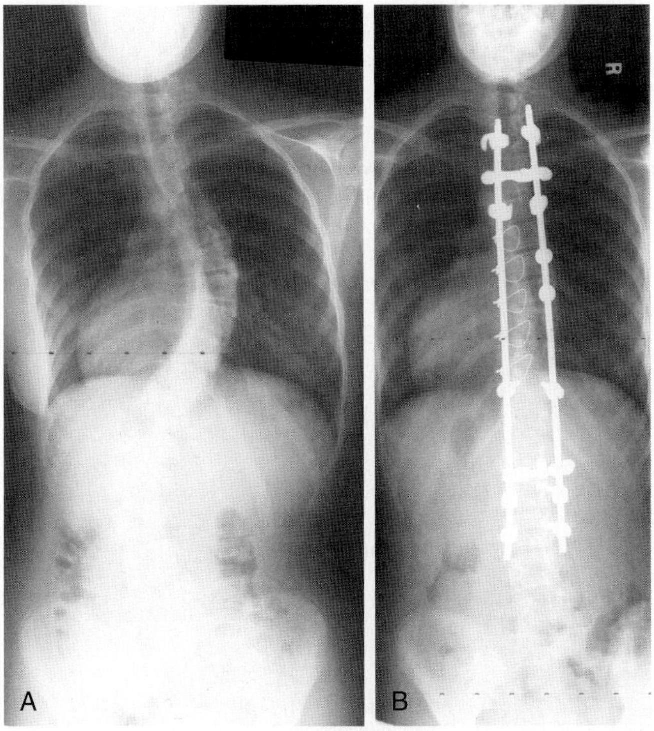

Most procedures are performed posteriorly using pedicle screw fixation, which affords excellent correction, especially of the rotational component of the deformity. Posterior osteotomies are often added to enhance flexibility and improve the degree of correction in stiffer curves. Anterior spinal releases requiring a thoracotomy are performed infrequently. Open anterior thoracic and thoracolumbar procedures violate the chest wall and often the diaphragm, and pulmonary function may take up to 2 yr to return to normal values. Even though thoracoscopic techniques can be utilized to perform anterior spinal release with or without instrumentation and fusion, their use is limited. Patients with conditions such as neurofibromatosis (see Chapter 596.1) and myelomeningocele (see Chapter 591.4) have a higher likelihood of achieving a non-union of their fusion, and an anterior fusion is considered in addition to the posterior fusion in these groups. Younger patients, in whom the triradiate cartilage remain open, are at risk for crankshaft, or progressive deformity/loss of correction as a consequence of continued anterior spinal growth, after a posterior fusion. Traditionally, these patients were treated by simultaneous anterior fusion to remove the growth potential; however, the rigidity of constructs with pedicle screws negates the need for this additional surgery. For idiopathic thoracolumbar and lumbar curves, an anterior fusion with instrumentation can be considered, although the posterior approach with osteotomies and pedicle screw fixation is being used more frequently to avoid the need for anterior surgery. Posterior spinal fusion has been associated with accelerated degeneration of the unfused levels. In many, this remains asymptomatic, but the long-term effects remain unknown.

Several emerging techniques are being evaluated in the management of idiopathic scoliosis. These include new approaches to the spine, attempts to preserve remaining growth in younger patients, and even specialized treatments to save the lives of young patients with curves so significant that they result in mortality secondary to inadequate pulmonary volume. There are techniques to correct curves without limiting future growth and even to modulate spinal growth and prevent future fusion surgeries. The FDA-approved **VEPTR (vertical expandable prosthetic titanium rib)** helps young children with thoracic insufficiency syndrome caused by severe spinal curves with restrictive lung disease, often associated with a high mortality rate (see Chapter 679.2 below). The chest wall device can enlarge the thorax and correct scoliosis without adverse effect to somatic growth, likely triggering lung growth. After implantation, it is lengthened twice a year by minor surgery. Long-term survival rates are favorable for these extremely severe scoliosis patients treated by VEPTR. The device obtains and maintains correction without fusing the spine, which allows for alveolar development and maximizes trunk height prior to definitive spinal fusion.

Growing rods have also been used in young children with scoliosis. These devices have fixation points placed at the proximal and distal ends of the deformity, with expandable rods placed subcutaneously, spanning the length of the deformity. Similar to the VEPTR, growing rods require additional minor operations to lengthen the rods twice a year until skeletal maturity or definitive spinal fusion.

Intervertebral stapling is an experimental technique that attempts to dynamically modify spinal growth in immature individuals with smaller curves. Staples are placed through either an open or thoracoscopic approach across the intervertebral disk space (growth zone) on the convex side of the curve. This technique holds the spine in a corrected position and limits growth on the convex side, preventing further curvature, and achieving correction through concave growth. It remains to be seen whether this technique will play a role in the management of patients with idiopathic scoliosis.

Bibliography is available at Expert Consult.

Figure 679-3 A, Preoperative standing posteroanterior radiograph of a 14 yr old girl who was skeletally immature and developed a 68 degree right thoracic and a 53 degree left lumbar scoliosis. Her trunk was shifted to the right, and the left shoulder was slightly depressed. **B,** Based upon the risk of future progression, she was treated by an instrumented posterior spinal fusion from T3 to L3 with correction of the right thoracic curve to 20 degrees and the left lumbar curve to 10 degrees. Coronal spinal balance was restored, and shoulder height was maintained.

679.2 Congenital Scoliosis

R. Justin Mistovich and David A. Spiegel

DEFINITION

Congenital scoliosis is a spinal deformity that results from abnormal development of the bony spinal column. Asymmetric spinal growth as a result of 1 or more vertebral anomalies leads to spinal curvature. The malformation(s) is (are) present at birth but may not become clinically apparent until a later time as growth progresses.

ETIOLOGY

Although the underlying cause of congenital scoliosis remains unknown, embryologic development of the spine begins at the 5th wk of gestation. An insult to the normal developmental process occurs, resulting in abnormal growth of 1 or more vertebrae.

ASSOCIATED CONDITIONS

The developmental insult is typically not limited to the spine alone: it is extremely common for children with congenital scoliosis to have associated malformations in other organ systems, which must be ruled out. Nearly 60% of patients with congenital scoliosis have other developmental malformations.

Genitourinary abnormalities are identified in 20-40% of children with congenital scoliosis and include unilateral renal agenesis, ureteral duplication, horseshoe kidney, and genital anomalies. Approximately 2% of these patients have a silent obstructive uropathy that may be life-threatening. Renal ultrasonography should be performed early on in all children with congenital scoliosis, and other studies such as CT or MRI may also be required.

Cardiac anomalies are identified in 10-25% of patients. A careful cardiac examination should be performed. Some clinicians recommend routine echocardiography.

Intraspinal anomalies are identified in approximately 15-40% of patients. Spinal dysraphism is the general term applied to such lesions (see Chapters 591 and 606). Examples include diastematomyelia, split-cord malformations, intraspinal lipomas, arachnoid cysts, teratomas, dermoid sinuses, fibrous bands, and tight filum terminale. Cutaneous findings that may be seen in patients with closed spinal dysraphism include hair patches, skin tags or dimples, sinuses, and hemangiomas. Infants with these cutaneous abnormalities overlying the spine may benefit from ultrasonography to rule out an occult spinal dysraphic condition. MRI is indicated in infants, but in the past was delayed in older patients until a clinical indication is present, such as tethering of the spinal cord, which may present as back or leg pain, calf atrophy, progressive unilateral foot deformity (especially cavovarus), and problems with bowel or bladder function.

CLASSIFICATION OF CONGENITAL SCOLIOSIS

Congenital scoliosis is classified by the type of developmental abnormality: either a failure of formation or a failure of segmentation. The deformities are then further described by the anatomic features of the affected vertebra. Failures of formation result in wedge vertebrae or hemivertebrae. Failures of segmentation result in unilateral bars vertebrae, or block vertebrae. Lastly, some instances of congenital scoliosis result from a combination of both failure of formation and failure of segmentation (Fig. 679-4). One or more bony anomalies may occur in isolation or in combination.

NATURAL HISTORY OF CONGENITAL SCOLIOSIS

The risk of progression depends on the growth potential of each anomaly, which may vary considerably. Close radiographic follow-up is required. Progression of these curves is most pronounced during periods of rapid growth associated with the 1st 2-3 yr of life and during the adolescent growth spurt.

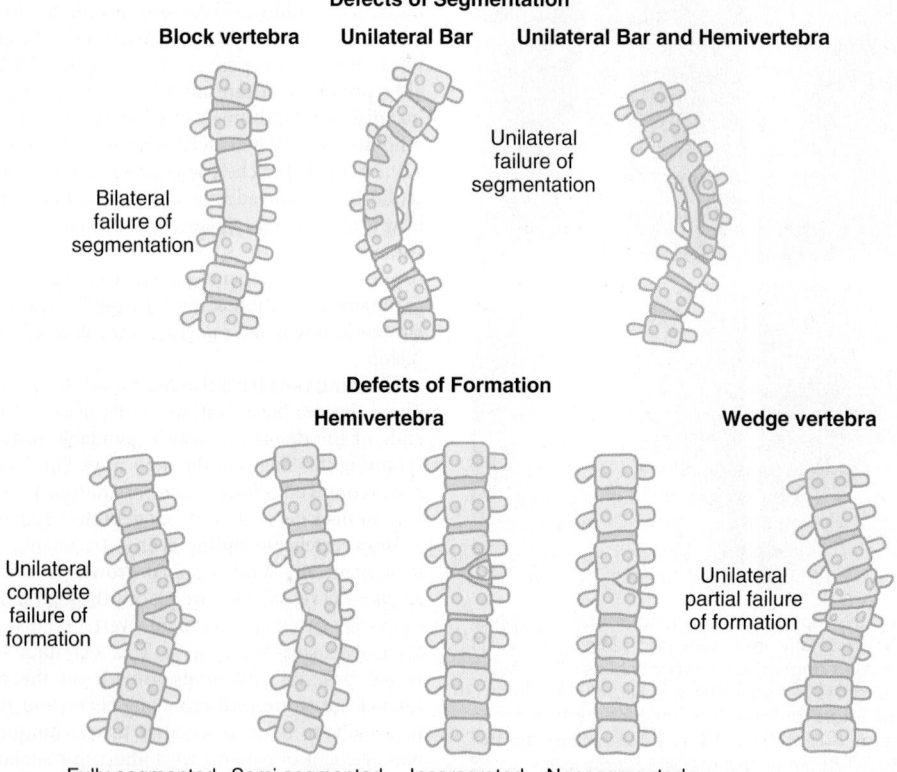

Figure 679-4 The defects of segmentation and formation that can occur during spinal development. *(From McMaster MJ: Congenital scoliosis. In Weinstein SL, editor: The pediatric spine: principles and practice, ed 2, Philadelphia, 2001, Lippincott Williams & Wilkins, p. 163.)*

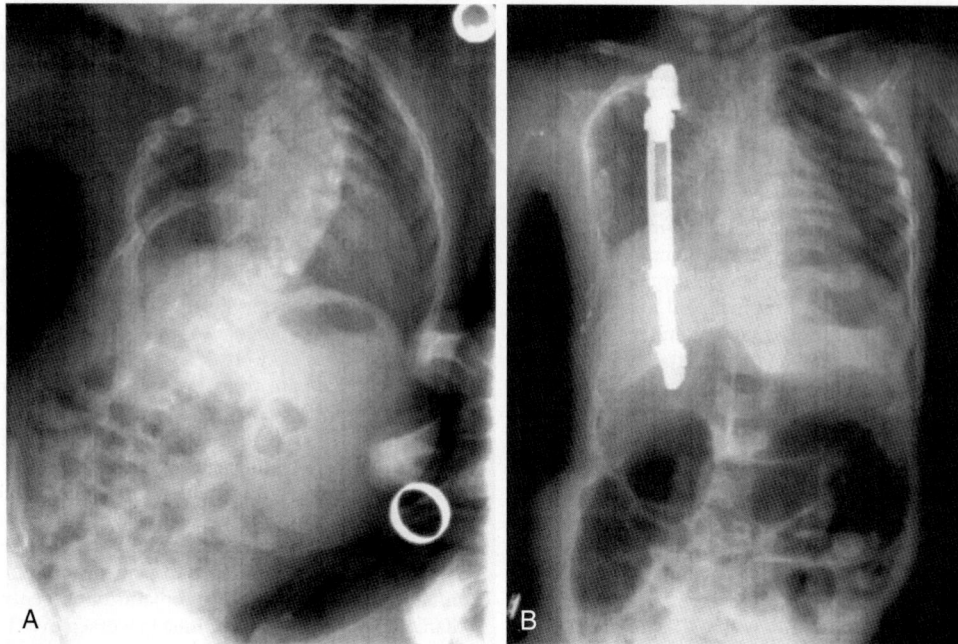

Figure 679-5 A, Anteroposterior preoperative radiograph of a 7 mo old boy with congenital scoliosis and fused ribs. A 3-dimensional reconstruction of a CT scan of the chest of this infant estimated his lung volume to be 173.2 mL³. **B,** Anteroposterior radiograph after implantation of a vertically expandable prosthetic titanium rib and several expansions over 33 mo. The lung volume now measures 330.3 mL³, an increase of 90.7%. *(From Gollogly S, Smith JT, Campbell RM: Determining lung volume with three-dimensional reconstructions of CT scan data: a pilot study to evaluate the effects of expansion thoracoplasty on children with severe spinal deformities. J Pediatr Orthop 23:323–328, 2004.)*

The anatomic characteristics of the malformed vertebra play a significant role in the progression of deformity. The most severe form of congenital scoliosis is a unilateral unsegmented bar with a contralateral hemivertebra. In this anomaly, the spine is fused the side of the unsegmented bar but also has a growth center on the other side at the location of the hemivertebra at the same level. This combination of deformities in the bony spine results in a rapidly progressive curve. As a result, all affected patients usually require surgical stabilization. A unilateral unsegmented bar is also associated with significant progression and in most cases will require surgical intervention. An isolated hemivertebra must be followed closely, and many, but not all, of these will be associated with a progressive deformity that requires surgical intervention. In contrast, an isolated block vertebra has little growth potential and rarely requires treatment.

TREATMENT OF CONGENITAL SCOLIOSIS
Early diagnosis and prompt treatment of progressive curves are essential. Bracing is not indicated for most congenital curves because of their structural nature, except in rare cases to treat additional curves not associated with the congenital abnormality. The treatment of progressive curves is spinal fusion, or *arthrodesis*. Once a bony abnormality is identified that is likely to progress, surgery is performed before progression occurs, preventing development or further inevitable progression of spinal deformity. If the deformity has already developed, surgical correction is difficult to achieve and the risk of neurologic complications is high.

Both anterior and posterior spinal fusion is often required. Other procedures that are employed in selected patients include an isolated posterior spinal fusion. A convex hemiepiphysiodesis can be performed with certain deformities, fusing only 1 side of the spine to allow some correction of the deformity by permitting growth on the noninvolved side of the curve. Complete excision of a hemivertebra, along with fusion of a short segment of the spine, can be performed via a posterior approach and may result in better correction and spinal balance in selected cases.

It should be noted that surgery in these young, syndromic patients is not without risk. One recent study found a complication rate of nearly 85% and a mortality rate of >15% in patients who underwent operative treatment for all types of early onset scoliosis, including those with congenital scoliosis as well as other associated syndromes producing early onset scoliosis.

THORACIC INSUFFICIENCY SYNDROME
When multiple levels of the thoracic spine are involved in the presence of fused ribs, a progressive 3-dimensional deformity of the chest wall may impair lung development and function. This development is termed **thoracic insufficiency syndrome**. As a result of thoracic insufficiency syndrome, the chest wall cannot support normal respiration resulting in decreased life expectancy.

Thoracic insufficiency syndrome may be seen in patients with several recognized conditions such as Jarcho-Levin syndrome (spondylocostal or spondylothoracic dysplasia; see Chapter 108) and Jeune syndrome (asphyxiating thoracic dystrophy; see Chapter 417.3), as well as patients with severe spinal deformities. These difficult cases are being treated with a technique called *expansion thoracoplasty*, in which the thoracic cage is gradually expanded over time by progressive lengthening of the chest wall on the concavity of the spinal deformity (or in some cases on both sides of the spine). The procedure involves an opening wedge thoracostomy, followed by placement of a vertical expandable titanium prosthetic rib. The implant is then lengthened at regular intervals (Fig. 679-5). The primary goal is to gradually correct the chest wall deformity to improve pulmonary function, and a secondary goal is correction of an associated spinal deformity. This technique is currently not approved by the FDA for the treatment of scoliosis in the absence of a thoracic insufficiency, and further study will help to refine and possible expand the indications for this new technique.

Bibliography is available at Expert Consult.

679.3 Neuromuscular Scoliosis, Genetic Syndromes, and Compensatory Scoliosis

R. Justin Mistovich and David A. Spiegel

NEUROMUSCULAR SCOLIOSIS

Scoliosis is frequently identified in children with neuromuscular diseases such as cerebral palsy, muscular dystrophies and other myopathies, spinal muscular atrophy, Friedreich ataxia, myelomeningocele, polio, and arthrogryposis. Children with spinal cord injuries are also at high risk for a progressive curvature. The etiology and natural history of these patients differ from idiopathic and congenital scoliosis. Most cases result from weakness and/or imbalance of the trunk musculature. Spasticity may also contribute to spinal curvatures. In some cases, such as myelomeningocele, coexisting congenital vertebral anomalies may be present, further contributing to curve development.

As might be expected, neuromuscular scoliosis is most common in patients with higher degrees of neurologic impairment, usually those who are nonambulatory and may not have adequate control of their trunk. It is diagnosed in more than 70% of nonambulatory patients with cerebral palsy (see Chapter 598.1), and in more than 90% of patients with Duchenne muscular dystrophy (see Chapter 609.1).

The diagnosis is suspected on physical examination. In nonambulators, the most common curve pattern is a C-shaped thoracolumbar or lumbar curve (Fig. 679-6). This curve is typically associated with pelvic obliquity. In contrast, ambulatory patients with diagnoses such as Friedreich ataxia may have curve patterns more similar to idiopathic scoliosis.

In ambulatory patients, the examination is similar to the previously described physical examination for idiopathic scoliosis. In nonambulators, the back is inspected with the patient sitting upright. Any asymmetry should be noted. These patients often need manual support to maintain an upright position. If any progressive asymmetry is observed, then sitting PA and lateral radiographs are obtained. Because prophylactic treatment cannot alter the natural history of the disease, it is appropriate to establish the diagnosis clinically and obtain radiographs if the curve is noted to progress.

The clinical course of patients with neuromuscular scoliosis depends on the severity of neuromuscular involvement as well as the nature of the underlying disease process. Progressive diseases are often associated with progressive curvatures. The consequences of a progressive

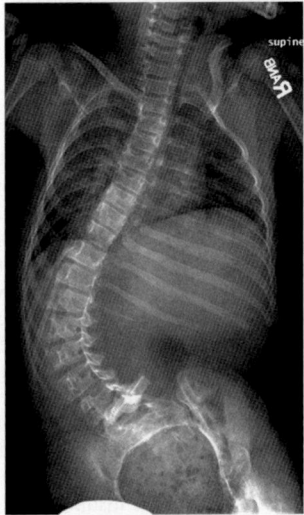

Figure 679-6 Imaging shows a long C-shaped curve with convexity to the left side and significant pelvic obliquity, a curve pattern often seen in patients with neuromuscular scoliosis. *(From Pruthi S: Scoliosis. In Coley BD, editor: Caffey's pediatric diagnostic imaging, ed 12, Philadelphia, 2013, WB Saunders, eFig. 135-10B.)*

scoliosis in the neuromuscular population involve both function, especially sitting and standing balance, as well ease of hygiene and personal care. Pulmonary dysfunction may be expected with the gradual deformation of the rib cage and vertebra–pelvic axis, as well as collapse of the spine with the pelvis impinging on the rib cage. Diaphragmatic function is impaired, and changes in chest volume and chest wall architecture will undoubtedly exacerbate the pulmonary dysfunction owing to underlying muscle weakness. Pulmonary function may be difficult to document in some patient populations, especially those with severe cerebral palsy. Additionally, patients who initially were marginal ambulators may lose the ability to walk altogether as their scoliosis advances. Curves associated with pelvic obliquity result in asymmetric seating pressures, which may limit sitting endurance and may rarely cause skin breakdown and decubitus ulcers. Patients may also experience pain from impingement of the rib cage on the iliac crest.

The treatment of neuromuscular scoliosis depends on the age of the patient, the underlying diagnosis, and the magnitude of the deformity. The goal is to achieve or maintain a straight spine over a level pelvis, especially in patients who are wheelchair bound, and to intervene early before curve magnitude and rigidity become severe. In contrast to idiopathic and congenital scoliosis, neuromuscular curves often continue to progress after skeletal maturity. In general, curves of greater than 40-50 degrees will continue to worsen over time. Brace treatment does not affect the natural history of neuromuscular scoliosis, and standard braces used for idiopathic scoliosis are poorly tolerated in neuromuscular patients. A soft spinal orthosis may improve sitting balance and ease of care, although it does not prevent progression of the curvature.

In general, a spinal arthrodesis is offered to patients with progressive curvatures >40-50 degrees. The indications will differ somewhat based on the underlying diagnosis. For example, patients with Duchenne muscular dystrophy are offered surgery when their curves progress beyond 20-30 degrees, thereby having surgery before the anticipated decline in pulmonary or cardiac function preclude their ability to tolerate it. Ambulatory patients with curvatures similar to those seen in idiopathic scoliosis are managed by similar principles. Patients who are nonambulatory with pelvic obliquity are usually managed by a spinal fusion extending from the upper thoracic spine to the pelvis, similar to that described in the idiopathic scoliosis section. A brace is not required following this procedure. Treatment decisions must be individualized in those nonambulatory patients with spastic quadriplegia, and are based on loss of function, the potential to improve hygiene or personal care, and the desires of the family and/or caregivers.

Although complications are relatively frequent in comparison with patients with nonneuromuscular curves, the available literature suggests that most patients benefit in terms of function and ease of care. To better identify patients at risk of complications, a recent study found that nonambulatory patients and those with curves 60 degrees or greater had a significantly increased risk of postoperative major complications, including ileus, pneumonia, infection, and wound problems. Because of the risks involved and potential for complications, this surgery should ideally be performed at centers with significant experience.

SYNDROMES AND GENETIC DISORDERS

Representative examples of this diverse group of diagnoses include neurofibromatosis, osteogenesis imperfecta, connective tissue diseases including Marfan syndrome (see Chapter 702), Ehlers-Danlos syndrome (see Chapter 659), and Prader-Willi syndrome (see Chapter 81), among many others. Patients with these diagnoses should have their spine examined routinely during visits to their primary care physician. Similar to other types of scoliosis, the follow-up and treatment are based on the age of the patient, the degree of deformity, whether progression has been documented, and the underlying diagnosis.

COMPENSATORY SCOLIOSIS

Leg-length inequality is a common clinical diagnosis and is usually associated with a small compensatory lumbar curvature (see Chapter

676). This is one cause of false-positive screening examinations. Patients with leg-length inequality may have the pelvis become tilted toward the shorter limb and subsequently develop an associated lumbar curve. The apex of the curve points toward the short leg. There is little evidence to suggest that a small compensatory lumbar curve places the patient at risk of progression or back pain. However, children with leg-length inequality may also have idiopathic or congenital scoliosis. A standing radiograph may be obtained with a block under the foot on the short side, which corrects the leg-length discrepancy and levels the pelvis. If the curvature disappears when the limb-length discrepancy is corrected, then a diagnosis of a compensatory curve is made. An alternative is a PA radiograph with the patient seated.

In neuromuscular disorders such as polio or cerebral palsy, an adduction or abduction contracture of the hip, described as a fixed infrapelvic contracture, may have an associated compensatory lumbar scoliosis to maintain standing balance. For patients who ambulate, a 10-degree fixed contracture will result in up to 3 cm apparent leg-length discrepancy.

Bibliography is available at Expert Consult.

679.4 Kyphosis (Round-Back)

R. Justin Mistovich and David A. Spiegel

The normal thoracic spine has 20-50 degrees of kyphosis as measured from T3 to T12. This is measured using the Cobb method on a standing lateral radiograph of the thoracolumbar spine. A thoracic kyphosis in excess of the normal range of values is termed *hyperkyphosis*. These patients may present with cosmetic concerns, back pain, or both. A flexible or postural kyphosis may be overcorrected voluntarily or with postural adjustment, whereas a rigid kyphosis cannot be corrected passively. Causes of rigid kyphosis include Scheuermann disease and congenital kyphosis, among others. Table 679-2 lists conditions associated with hyperkyphosis.

The evaluation and treatment depends on the underlying diagnosis, the degree of deformity and its flexibility, whether the deformity is progressive, and whether any symptoms are present.

FLEXIBLE KYPHOSIS (POSTURAL KYPHOSIS)

Postural kyphosis is a common cosmetic concern and is most often recognized by family and friends. Adolescents with postural kyphosis can correct the curvature voluntarily. A standing lateral radiograph will show an increase in kyphosis but no pathologic changes of the involved vertebrae. There is no evidence to suggest that postural kyphosis progresses to a structural deformity. Although mild aching discomfort is sometimes reported, there is no evidence that the conditions leads to long-term symptoms or alterations in function or quality of life. The mainstay of treatment is reassurance. Physical therapy can be considered for muscular discomfort, although there are no data to suggest that a permanent alteration in alignment can be maintained.

Table 679-2	Conditions Associated with Hyperkyphosis

- Trauma causing spinal fractures
- Spinal infections resulting from bacterial, tuberculosis, and fungal diseases
- Metabolic diseases such as osteogenesis imperfecta or osteoporosis
- Iatrogenic (laminectomy, spinal irradiation)
- Neuromuscular diseases
- Neoplasms
- Congenital/developmental
  - Disorders of collagen such as Marfan syndrome
  - Dysplasias such as neurofibromatosis, achondroplasia, and mucopolysaccharidoses

Neither bracing nor surgery plays a role in the management of this condition.

STRUCTURAL KYPHOSIS
Scheuermann Disease

Scheuermann disease is the most common form of structural hyperkyphosis and is defined by wedging of greater than 5 degrees of 3 or more consecutive vertebral bodies at the apex of the deformity on a lateral radiograph. In addition, the apex of the thoracic kyphosis is lower than expected. Other radiographic findings include irregularities of the vertebral end plates and Schmorl nodes, which are herniations of the vertebral disc into the surface of the vertebral body. The etiology remains unknown but most likely involves the influence of mechanical forces in a genetically susceptible individual. Histologic specimens taken from patients with Scheuermann disease show a disordered pattern of endochondral ossification. However, it remains unclear whether these findings are the primary result of a genetic or metabolic pathologic process, or simply the secondary result of mechanical overload. The reported incidence varies from 0.4-10%, affecting boys 3 times more frequently than girls.

Physical Exam and Clinical Manifestations

Examine the patient from the side. There is a hyperkyphosis of the thoracic spine typically associated with a sharp contour. The apex of the deformity will often be in the lower thoracic spine. Patients are unable to correct the deformity voluntarily. Pain is a relatively common complaint. It is typically mild and near the apex of the kyphosis. The symptoms are intermittent, rarely severe, and occasionally limit certain activities. Neurologic symptoms are uncommon.

Radiographic Evaluation

The standard imaging protocol includes standing PA and lateral radiographs (Fig. 679-7). A specific, standardized technique in which the

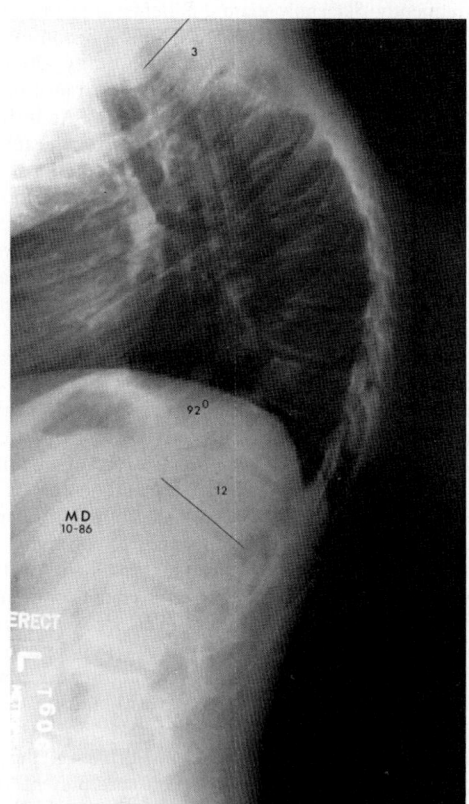

Figure 679-7 Standing lateral radiograph of a 14 yr old boy with severe Scheuermann kyphosis. This measures 92 degrees between T3 and T12. Note the wedging of the vertebrae at T6, T7, T8, and T9. The normal thoracic kyphosis is ≤40 degrees.

arms are folded across the chest is recommended for the lateral view. In addition to the diagnostic findings noted above, a mild scoliosis is commonly seen. Less frequently, a spondylolisthesis may be identified on the lateral radiograph.

Natural History

Treatment depends on the age of the patient, the degree of deformity, and whether any symptoms are present. As adolescents, patients with Scheuermann kyphosis may have more complaints of back pain compared to other adolescents, but this often improves after skeletal maturity. With regard to back pain, several studies have found no difference between Scheuermann patients and controls, whereas others have noted an increased incidence of constant back pain. Patients' self-esteem, participation in activities of daily living and recreational activities, and level of education are not different than in the general population. Kyphotic deformities greater than 90 degrees are more likely to be aesthetically unacceptable, symptomatic, and progressive. Deformities in excess of 100 degrees may be associated with restrictive pulmonary dysfunction.

Treatment

Because there are few absolute guidelines for treatment, treatment decisions must be individualized. Skeletally immature patients with mild deformity may benefit from a hyperextension exercise program, but the effects of this strategy on pain relief and spinal alignment, or the natural history, remain unknown. Patients with more than 1 yr of growth remaining and a kyphosis of greater than 55-60 degrees may benefit from a bracing program. A Milwaukee brace, which extends up to the neck, is recommended for curves with an apex above T7, while curves with a lower apex often may be treated by a thoracolumbar orthosis. The brace should be worn for up to 23 hr daily. Consideration also may be given to a serial casting or stretching program to gain flexibility prior to instituting the brace program. The goal of the brace is to prevent progression. A permanent improvement in alignment is seen less frequently. Skeletally mature patients with little or no pain and acceptable cosmesis are not treated. A spinal fusion may be considered in the rare patient with progressive deformity >70-80 degrees who is dissatisfied with his or her cosmetic appearance or who has persistent back pain despite nonoperative measures. An instrumented posterior spinal fusion from the upper thoracic to the mid lumbar spine is commonly performed, with spinal osteotomies to promote shortening of the spine when correcting with compressive forces. Some surgeons have recommended an anterior spinal release (discectomies and fusion) in addition to the posterior spinal fusion; however, this procedure is performed less frequently because of the increased neurologic risks of this combined procedure as the spine is lengthened during the correction.

CONGENITAL KYPHOSIS

Congenital kyphosis results from congenital anomalies of the vertebrae. In an anterior failure of formation (type I), a portion of the vertebral body fails to form. A kyphosis is typically identified after birth, and there is a high risk of progression and neurologic dysfunction. Spinal cord dysfunction commonly results from compression at the apex of the deformity. The second type of congenital kyphosis involves an anterior failure of segmentation, in which 2 vertebrae are fused (type II). The posterior elements of the spine continue to grow but the anterior spine does not, resulting in a variably progressive kyphosis and a much lower risk of neurologic dysfunction. Patients must be followed closely, and treatment is required in a significant number of cases. Similar to congenital scoliosis, abnormalities of other organ systems should be ruled out.

The treatment depends on the type of malformation, the degree of deformity, and whether neurologic symptoms are present. Bracing is ineffective, and surgical treatment is the only option for progressive curves. Because the natural history is so poor for type I deformities, spinal fusion is usually performed shortly after the diagnosis is made. The surgical goals are to prevent or treat kyphotic deformities, avoid neurologic deterioration, while maximizing spinal growth to the extent possible. This usually involves some form of spinal fusion, which may include anterior and/or posterior components, with or without resection of the vertebral remnant, and spinal instrumentation. Ideally, only a short segment of the spine will be fused to try and maximize trunk height. Deformities caused by anterior failure of segmentation also require spinal stabilization in some cases, but progression is typically slower, and patients are often followed over years to determine whether surgical stabilization will be required.

Bibliography is available at Expert Consult.

679.5 Back Pain in Children
R. Justin Mistovich and David A. Spiegel

With a lifetime prevalence of >70%, only the common cold affects individuals more frequently than back pain. Back pain is a frequent complaint in the pediatric and adolescent patient, affecting approximately 35% of adolescents. Back pain may be a physical manifestation of psychosocial factors in adolescents, similar to adults. Traditionally, the pediatric patient presenting with back pain warranted an aggressive clinical evaluation as the probability of establishing a specific diagnosis was high. Recent literature suggests that the incidence of both pediatric and adolescent back pain is increasing, while the proportion of patients having a diagnosable pathology is decreasing. In fact, a recent large cohort found no diagnosable pathology in 76% of patients. These trends add further complexity to determining the proper approach to diagnosis and treatment. The differential diagnosis is extensive (Table 679-3). Given the potential for serious pathology, a complete history and careful physical exam must be performed on all patients presenting with back pain, with appropriate diagnostic follow-up of concerning findings.

CLINICAL EVALUATION

A full, careful history is very important. Identify the location, character, and duration of symptoms. Any history of acute trauma or repetitive physical activities should be sought. Identify patients with at-risk athletic pursuits, including football lineman and gymnasts, who have a high incidence of spondylolysis (see Chapter 679.6). Symptoms consistent with a neoplastic or infectious etiology include pain that is constant or unrelenting, not relieved by rest, and wakes the patient from sleep. Fevers, chills, or constitutional symptoms of weight loss or malaise are additional red flags for infectious or neoplastic processes.

Symptoms of neurologic dysfunction must also be uncovered. Patients should be questioned about the presence of any radicular symptoms, gait disturbance, muscle weakness, alterations in sensation, and changes in bowel or bladder function.

The physical examination includes a complete musculoskeletal and neurologic assessment. The patient should be adequately undressed for the clinical exam. Inspect the patient from the back and the side, identifying any changes in alignment in the frontal or sagittal plane. Assess range of motion in flexion, extension, and lateral bending. Pain with extension suggests pathology within the posterior elements of the spine such as spondylolysis. Forward flexion will exacerbate pain linked to abnormalities of the anterior column of the spine (vertebral body or disc), such as a herniated disc or discitis. Younger children may be asked to pick up an object off the floor to assess spinal flexion.

Palpation will reveal any areas of point tenderness over the posterior elements or the muscles and identify muscle spasm.

As spinal pain may be referred, an abdominal examination should be performed, and a gynecologic evaluation should also be considered. Pathology at the sacroiliac joint may also mimic low back pain. This joint should be stressed by compression of the iliac wings or by external rotation at the hip (Faber test).

A careful neurologic examination should be performed, including manual muscle testing, sensation, proprioception, and reflexes. Examine for myelopathy by performing the Babinski test, assessing for hyperreflexia, and checking for sustained, or greater than 3 beats, of

Table 679-3	Differential Diagnosis of Back Pain

INFLAMMATORY/INFECTIOUS
Diskitis
Vertebral osteomyelitis (pyogenic, tuberculous)
Spinal epidural abscess
Pyelonephritis
Pancreatitis
Psoas abscess

RHEUMATOLOGIC
Pauciarticular juvenile idiopathic arthritis
Reiter syndrome
Ankylosing spondylitis
Psoriatic arthritis

DEVELOPMENTAL
Spondylolysis
Spondylolisthesis
Scheuermann disease
Scoliosis

TRAUMATIC (ACUTE VERSUS REPETITIVE)
Hip–pelvic anomalies
Herniated disk
Overuse syndromes
Vertebral stress fractures
Upper cervical spine instability

NEOPLASTIC
Vertebral tumors
  Benign
    Eosinophilic granuloma
    Aneurysmal bone cyst
    Osteoid osteoma
    Osteoblastoma
  Malignant
    Osteogenic sarcoma
    Leukemia
    Lymphoma
    Metastatic tumor
Spinal cord, ganglia, and nerve roots
  Intramedullary spinal cord tumor
  Sympathetic chain
  Ganglioneuroma
  Ganglioneuroblastoma
  Neuroblastoma

OTHER
Intraabdominal or pelvic pathology
Following lumbar puncture
Conversion reaction
Juvenile osteoporosis

Table 679-4	Findings Consistent with a Nonmechanical Etiology Warranting Further Evaluation

- History of trauma
- Pain that wakes the patient from sleep
- Constant pain unrelieved by rest
- Constitutional or systemic symptoms of fevers, chills, malaise, weight loss
- Any neurologic dysfunction including weakness, numbness, radicular pain, gait changes, or bowel and bladder changes
- Abnormalities in spinal alignment
- Bony tenderness to palpation or vertebral step-offs
- Significant pain with provocative tests (spinal flexion or extension)
- Positive straight-leg raise test for neurologic symptoms below the knee
- Abnormal neurologic exam

restrictions and nonnarcotic analgesics. Physical therapy for core strengthening can be considered. The patient is asked to return for a follow-up appointment after 4-6 wks. Plain radiographs are commonly obtained at the discretion of individual practitioners, although, if no red flags are present, consider delaying radiographs until the follow-up appointment because of the cumulative adverse effects of radiation exposure. Patients presenting with concerning findings or those who have not improved after 6 wk of conservative care are subject to further investigation.

RADIOGRAPHIC AND LABORATORY EVALUATION

When further workup is indicated, posteroanterior and lateral radiographs of the involved region of the spine are the initial images of choice. Some clinicians will also utilize oblique radiographs of the lumbar spine when spondylolysis is in the differential diagnosis. If plain radiographs are normal, advanced imaging modalities are considered including a 3-phase technetium bone scan, a bone scan with single-photon emission CT if spondylolysis is suspected, CT for viewing osseous detail, and MRI for viewing soft tissue and intraspinal detail. There are advantages and disadvantages with each, and no evidenced-based guidelines are available for the work-up or back pain in the pediatric population.

When systemic signs or constitutional symptoms are present, a complete blood cell count with differential, erythrocyte sedimentation rate, and C-reactive protein should be ordered. In certain cases, laboratory tests to evaluate for inflammatory diseases, such as juvenile idiopathic arthritis, seronegative spondyloarthropathies, and ankylosing spondylitis, are indicated.

Bibliography is available at Expert Consult.

679.6 Spondylolysis and Spondylolisthesis
R. Justin Mistovich and David A. Spiegel

Spondylolysis represents a defect in the pars interarticularis, the segment of bone connecting the superior and inferior articular facets in the vertebra. It is thought to result from repetitive hyperextension stresses, in which compressive forces are transmitted from the inferior articular facet of the superior vertebra to the pars interarticularis of the inferior vertebra. A stress fracture, unilateral or bilateral, may progress to a spondylolysis. In many cases, this stress fracture does not heal, resulting in a pseudarthrosis or false joint, and thereby allowing motion through this bony area where motion should not normally exist.

Spondylolysis is common in athletes who engage in repetitive spinal hyperextension, especially gymnasts, football interior lineman, weight lifters, and wrestlers. Approximately 4-8% of the entire pediatric population is affected, making it the most common cause of back pain in

clonus. The superficial abdominal reflex should be tested by gently stroking the skin on each of the four quadrants surrounding the umbilicus. Normally, the umbilicus will move toward the area stimulated. A normal examination includes symmetry in the response on both sides of the midline, even if the reflex cannot be elicited on either side. An abnormal test suggests the presence of a subtle abnormality of spinal cord function, most commonly syringomyelia. Perform a straight-leg raise test to check for nerve root tension caused by a herniated disk, slipped vertebral apophysis, or other pathology. This examination should reproduce any neurologic symptoms distal to the knee.

MEDICAL DECISION MAKING

A detailed history and physical exam are the most important components of the initial evaluation, and should focus on identifying *red flags* and differentiating between mechanical and nonmechanical back pain. Findings consistent with a nonmechanical etiology, warrant a more aggressive evaluation and/or prompt referral (Table 679-4).

Patients with mechanical back pain and symptoms that are activity-related and improve with rest are typically treated by rest or activity adolescents when a diagnosis can be established. Patients with excessive lordosis in the lumbar spine may be predisposed to developing a spondylolysis, and a genetic component has also been suggested. The lesion is most common at L5, but it may be identified at upper lumbar levels as well.

Spondylolisthesis represents a forward slippage of 1 vertebra on another and is also identified in approximately 4-5% of the population. There are multiple causes of spondylolisthesis, including dysplastic/congenital, isthmic (from a pars stress fracture), traumatic, and neoplastic. In children and adolescents, the most common types are dysplastic and isthmic. Between 5% and 15% of patients with spondylolysis will develop *spondylolisthesis*.

Spondylolisthesis is assessed on a standing lateral radiograph of the lumbosacral junction according to (1) percentage of forward translation of 1 vertebra on the other, (2) rotation of the involved vertebrae in the sagittal plane (slip angle), and (3) relative position of the sacrum during upright posture. For example, a grade 1 slip of L5 on S1 has less than 25% of the width of the vertebral body of L5 translated anteriorly on S1. Similarly, grade 2 is 25-50%, grade 3 is 50-75%, grade 4 is 75-100%. *Spondyloptosis*, or grade 5, describes a complete displacement of 1 vertebral body on the level below. The slip angle, which demonstrates the degree to which the superior vertebra is flexed forward relative to the underlying vertebra, and the verticality of the sacrum, both have a significant effect on sagittal balance or relationship of the sagittal weightbearing axis to the body segments. Abnormalities in sagittal spinal balance may be associated with compensatory flexion of the knees during ambulation, hamstring spasm and/or contracture, and back pain.

CLINICAL MANIFESTATIONS

Spondylolysis may occasionally be asymptomatic and diagnosed incidentally on imaging obtained for other reasons. Usually though, it presents with mechanical low back pain that may radiate to the buttocks, with or without spasm of the hamstring muscles. Neurologic symptoms are rare in patients with spondylolysis. However, patients with spondylolisthesis may experience neurologic symptoms from compression of the nerve roots causing radiculopathy or even the surgical emergency of cauda equina in which bowel and bladder function is affected.

PHYSICAL EXAM

Patients with spondylolysis often have discomfort with spinal extension or hyperextension. Provocative testing may include keeping the spine extended for 10-20 seconds to see if back pain can be reproduced. There may be discomfort with palpation of the spinous process of the involved vertebra. Patients with higher grades of spondylolisthesis demonstrate loss of lumbar lordosis, flattening of the buttocks on visual inspection, and a vertical sacrum caused by posterior rotation of the pelvis. A step off may be palpated between the spinous processes of the involved vertebrae. Hamstring contracture is testing by measuring the popliteal angle. The hip is flexed to 90 degrees while fully extending the contralateral hip to level the pelvis. The knee is then passively extended, and the popliteal angle represents the angle between the thigh (vertical) and the lower leg axis. The involved spinous processes may be tender to palpation. A careful, complete neurologic examination is essential.

RADIOGRAPHIC EVALUATION

The initial evaluation of the lumbar region should include high-quality anteroposterior and lateral radiographs. Some authors also prefer to obtain oblique radiographs, which demonstrate the classic "Scotty dog" finding. One study suggests that a series of 4 views may not offer greater diagnostic accuracy than 2 views. Standing PA and lateral radiographs are obtained if findings suggestive of scoliosis or hyperkyphosis are also present (Figs. 679-8 and 679-9). In patients with normal plain films, a bone scan with single-photon emission CT may help to diagnose a spondylolysis during the earliest stage of a stress reaction, prior to the formation of a stress fracture or an established pseudarthrosis. A CT scan with thin cuts may provide additional information to establish the presence of a pars defect. MRI is indicated in the presence of signs or symptoms of cauda equina or nerve root involvement.

TREATMENT

The asymptomatic patient with spondylolysis requires no treatment. Patients with pain are treated initially by activity modification, physical therapy for core strengthening, and nonnarcotic analgesics. The use of a lumbosacral orthosis, which immobilizes the spine in slight flexion to decompress the posterior elements, may lead to a faster resolution of symptoms. This orthosis is typically worn for 3-4 mo. Participation

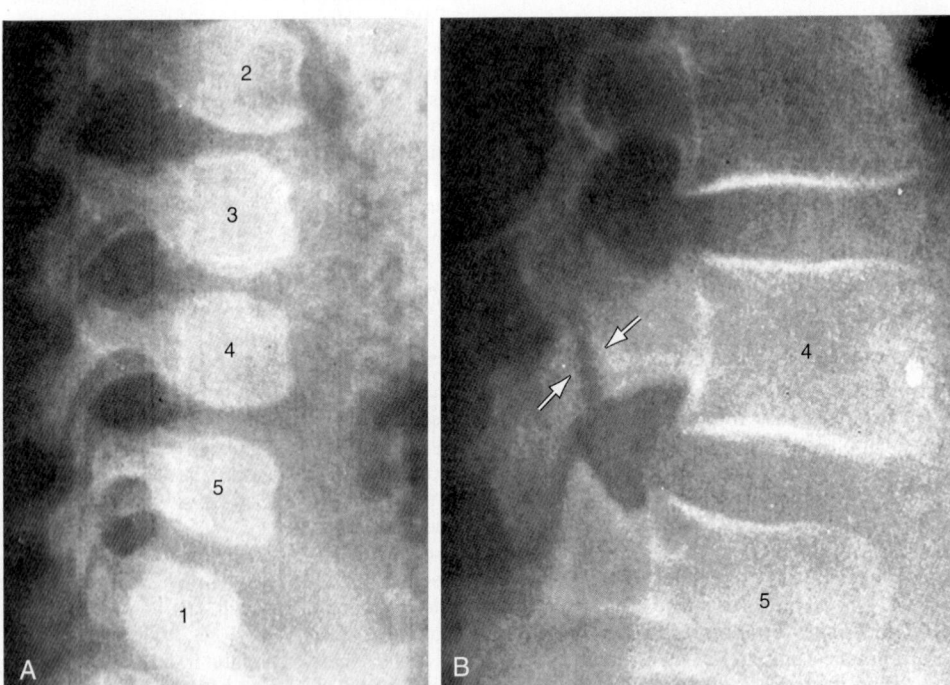

Figure 679-8 A, Normal spine at 9 mo of age. **B,** Spondylolysis in the L4 vertebra at 10 yr of age. *(From Silverman FN, Kuhn JP: Essentials of Caffey's pediatric x-ray diagnosis, Chicago, 1990, Year Book Medical Publishers, p. 94.)*

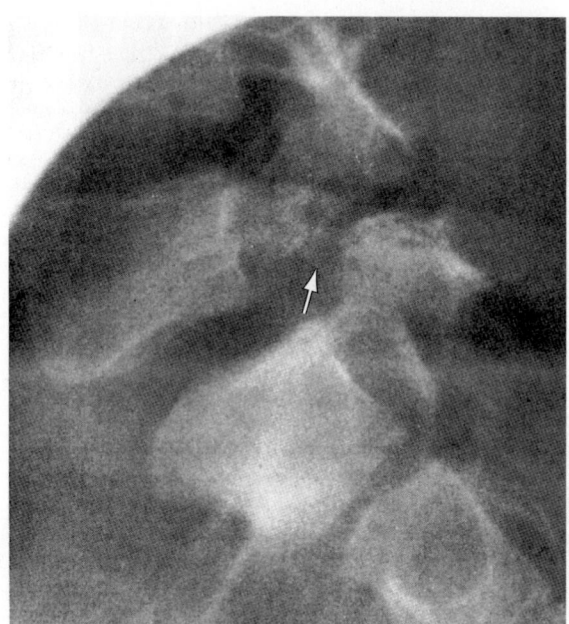

Figure 679-9 Defect in the pars interarticularis *(arrow)* of the neural arch of L5 (spondylolysis) that has permitted the body of L5 to slip forward (spondylolisthesis) on the body of S1. *(From Silverman FN, Kuhn JP: Essentials of Caffey's pediatric x-ray diagnosis, Chicago, 1990, Year Book Medical Publishers, p. 95.)*

in sports or other activities that exacerbate pain should be restricted until the symptoms have resolved.

Most patients experience resolution of their symptoms even though the spondylolysis heals in only a small number of patients. Surgery is offered for chronic, refractory back pain when conservative measures have failed. For those with spondylolysis at L5, a posterior spinal fusion from L5 to S1 is indicated as the mobility at this joint is limited relative to that observed at higher levels in the spine. For the infrequent cases in which the defect is at higher levels in the lumbar spine, techniques for repairing the pseudarthrosis without fusion are considered.

Recommendations for the management of spondylolisthesis depend on the age of the patient, the presence of pain or neurologic symptoms, and the degree of deformity. For low-grade lesions with a slip <50%, the management is similar to that for spondylolysis. As progressive slippage may occur in a subset of skeletally immature patients, patients must be followed through skeletal maturity. Guidelines for the timing of follow-up, and whether or not to obtain routine radiographs at each follow-up, differ between individuals and institutions. The authors typically follow asymptomatic patients yearly with a standing lateral of the lumbosacral junction.

For low-grade slips (<50% translation) with persistent symptoms despite nonoperative measures, an in situ posterior spinal arthrodesis is suggested. Surgery is also offered to skeletally immature patients with a high-grade slip (>50% translation) based on the likelihood of slip progression. The surgical approach for these high-grade slips varies between surgeons and institutions. The main principle is to stabilize the unstable segment of the spine and avoid neurologic complications. The typical components of these complex procedures include (1) posterior decompression of the L5 and S1 nerve roots (laminectomy and takedown of pseudarthrosis), (2) instrumented posterior spinal fusion from L5-S1, (3) discectomy at L5-S1 with placement of anterior column support (transforaminal cage or fibular allograft from sacrum to L5), and (4) reduction of the slippage by positioning the hips in extension or by an "instrumented reduction" utilizing the spinal implants. The risk of neurologic complications is higher when an instrumented reduction is attempted.

Bibliography is available at Expert Consult.

679.7 Spine Infection
R. Justin Mistovich and David A. Spiegel

Spondylitis, meaning inflammation of the vertebrae, is most commonly caused by infectious or autoimmune processes. Both *diskitis* and *vertebral osteomyelitis* are causes within the spectrum of **infectious spondylitis**. Most causes of infectious spondylitis result from hematogenous seeding of osteoarticular structures. Diskitis involves bacterial infection of the disc space and is generally seen in children younger than 5 yr of age. In contrast, vertebral osteomyelitis most often occurs in older children and adolescents and involves the vertebral body. Differences in anatomic location of the infectious focus relate to the vascular development of the spine. Patients in the younger age range have vascular channels between the vertebral end plate and the disc space, explaining the prevalence of discitis. In older children these channels have closed, and the infection remains in the vertebra causing osteomyelitis.

Staphylococcus aureus (see Chapter 181) is the most common organism causing spine infections. Other, less-common organisms include *Kingella kingae,* group A streptococcus, *Bartonella henselae, Salmonella,* and *Escherichia coli.* Blood cultures have a sensitivity of only 30%. Percutaneous or open biopsy of the disc space is positive only 50-85% of the time. The differential diagnosis must include tuberculosis of the spine.

CLINICAL MANIFESTATIONS
A high index of suspicion is required to establish the diagnosis of infectious spondylitis. Patients may experience back pain, abdominal pain, fever, or malaise. Fever is less common and may be present in only 30% of patients. Toddlers may develop a limp, or refuse to walk or sit. In an effort to reduce the pain associated with spinal motion, the child will hold the spine in a rigid position. There may also be paraspinal muscle spasm. Local point tenderness over the affected spinous process is common. There may be a list or leaning of the trunk when the patient is viewed from the front or back, and from the side there may be a loss of lumbar lordosis. Neurologic manifestations are rare and if present suggest that an epidural abscess may be present. The L3-4 or L4-5 spaces are most commonly affected in diskitis.

Spine flexion compresses the anterior elements of the spine and will elicit an increase in pain. Asking a child to pick up an object from the ground is a simple way to elicit this provocative test.

Although the white blood count may remain normal, the erythrocyte sedimentation rate is elevated in 80% of cases, and the C-reactive protein is also elevated.

RADIOGRAPHIC EVALUATION
The earliest radiographic finding is loss of lumbar lordosis. The characteristic features on plain radiographs are disc space narrowing, or loss of disc height, and irregularity of the adjacent vertebral end plates. However, these findings do not develop until 2-3 wk after the onset of symptoms. The diagnosis may be established earlier using either a technetium bone scan or MRI, although MRI is the most sensitive and specific imaging to diagnose osteomyelitis and to identify abscesses and/or neural compression (Fig. 679-10).

TREATMENT
Once the diagnosis is suspected clinically, the treatment involves symptomatic care and empiric antistaphylococcal antibiotics. Blood cultures should be obtained **prior** to the administration of antibiotics. The antibiotic agent may be modified if blood cultures are positive. Symptomatic care includes rest and analgesics, and a spinal orthosis may also be considered. The typical antibiotic course is from 4-6 wk; conversion from intravenous to oral agents may be acceptable after several days of improvement of the clinical course. A CT-guided needle biopsy of the disk space is usually reserved for patients who do not respond to empiric antibiotics. Surgical treatment is rarely required, and indications include establishing the diagnosis in patients who fail to respond

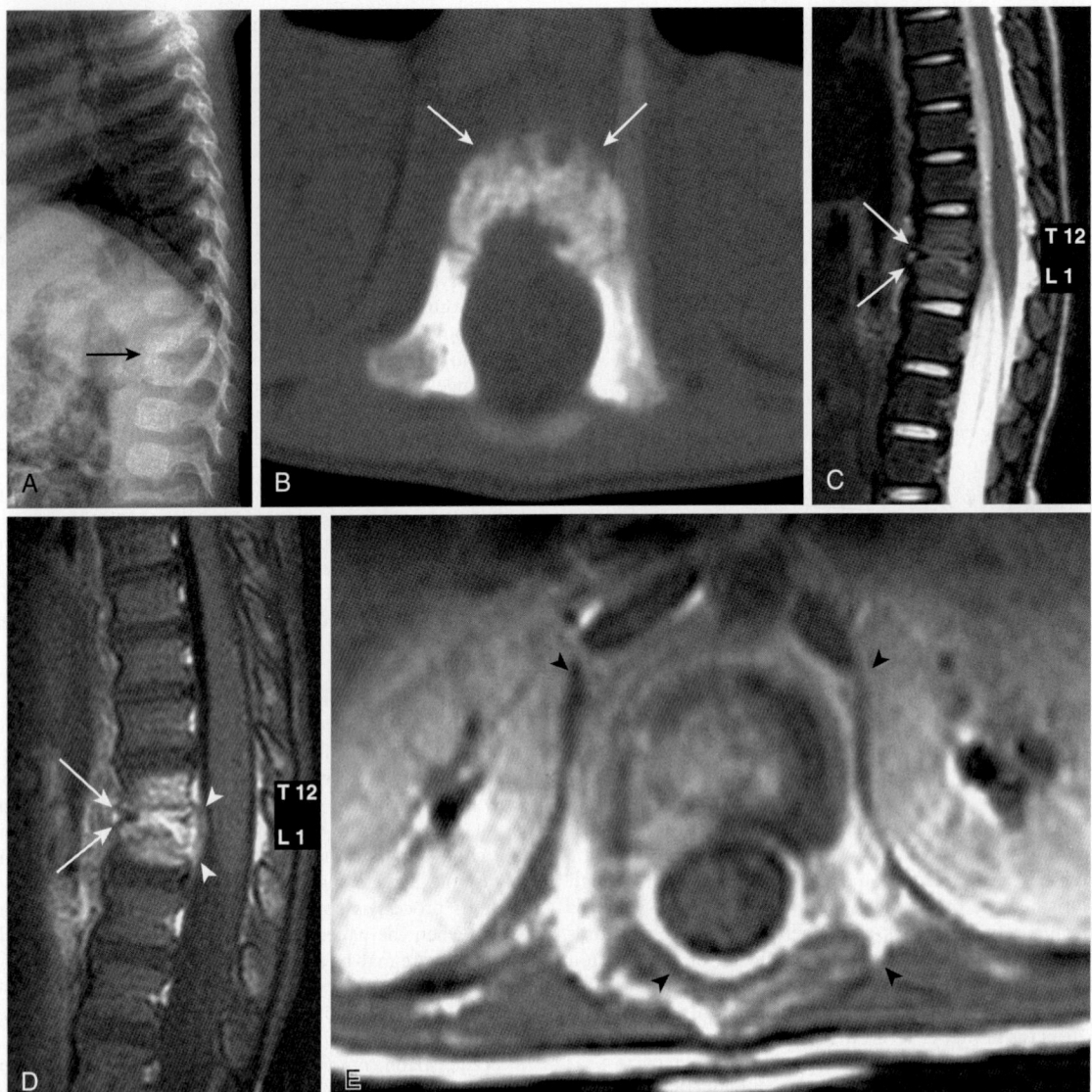

Figure 679-10 A 15 mo old girl with abnormal gait and concern for an intraspinal mass had discitis/osteomyelitis. Lateral spine radiographs demonstrate narrowing of the T12-L1 intervertebral disc space (*arrow* in **A**). An axial bone window from a noncontrast CT scan of the spine demonstrates irregularity to the vertebral end plates (*arrows* in **B**). A sagittal T2-weighted image **(C)**, a sagittal fat-saturated T1-weighted postcontrast image **(D)**, and an axial T1-weighted postcontrast image **(E)** of the thoracolumbar junction demonstrate loss of height of the T12-L1 intervertebral disc space with adjacent T2 prolongation of the adjacent endplates (*arrows* in **C**), with corresponding abnormal enhancement in the same regions (*arrows* in **D**), and surrounding mass-like soft-tissue enhancement (*arrowheads* in **E**). Note the thickening/elevation and enhancement of the posterior longitudinal ligament (*arrowheads* in **D**). (*From Pollock AN, Henesch SM: Infections of the spine and spinal cord. In Cooley BD, editor: Caffey's pediatric diagnostic imaging, ed 12, Philadelphia, 2013, WB Saunders, Fig. 44-6, p. 465.*)

to empiric antibiotics, and in those in whom an abscess and/or neurologic involvement are identified.

Bibliography is available at Expert Consult.

679.8 Intervertebral Disc Herniation/ Slipped Vertebral Apophysis

R. Justin Mistovich and David A. Spiegel

Intervertebral disc herniation is the result of a tear in the outer layer of the vertebral disc, called the *annulus fibrosus*, which then allows for protrusion of the inner *nucleus pulposus*. At times, a free fragment of disc can rupture and compress the nerve roots or spinal cord. Bulging of the annulus without rupture may also be observed, resulting in back pain and occasionally radicular symptoms. Symptoms are from

either direct mechanical compression and/or a local inflammatory response.

Slipped vertebral apophysis, also called a posterior ring apophysis separation, is caused by an injury and is only found in the skeletally immature. A small fragment of osseous or osteocartilagenous material from the posterior corner of the vertebral body apophysis avulses and may cause direct mechanical compression to the spinal cords and/or nerve roots, similar to a disc herniation. Both disc herniations and ring apophysis separations can cause back pain, radicular symptoms (nerve root compression or irritation), and/or spinal cord compression.

ETIOLOGY

The etiology remains unknown, but predisposing activities for both of these conditions include heavy lifting, repetitive axial loading activities, and occasionally traumatic injury such as a fall. Approximately 30-60% of patients with symptomatic herniated discs have a history of a trauma or sports-related injury. Other associations include preexisting disc degeneration, congenital malformation, and genetic or environmental factors. There is also a potential association between disc degeneration and the herpes virus, adding the possibility of an infectious etiology.

CLINICAL MANIFESTATIONS

Symptoms of intervertebral disc herniation or slipped vertebral apophysis in adolescents are similar to adult herniated disc symptoms. The major complaint is back pain, present in nearly 90% of patients. More than 30% of patients complain of radicular symptoms, or radiating sciatic-type pain into the legs. The back pain is often made worse by coughing, a Valsalva maneuver, or sitting. Pain may be relieved by standing or back extension. Inquire about weight loss, fever, or other constitutional symptoms to rule out an infectious or neoplastic etiology.

On physical examination, both paraspinal muscle spasm and a generalized spinal stiffness are common. Patients may lean toward the unaffected side to increase the size of the affected neural foramen thereby partially relieving symptoms. This results in a *reactive scoliosis*, not a true spinal curve, which improves with symptom resolution. Although overt signs of neurologic involvement are absent in most patients, a positive straight-leg raise test, causing radicular pain to shoot down the affected leg, is usually present. Pain is also worsened by spinal flexion.

It is critical perform a full neurologic evaluation. Evaluate sensation to light touch, pinprick, and proprioception. Check muscle strength and reflexes. It is critical to evaluate for perineal numbness, or *saddle anesthesia*. This finding, combined with changes in bowel or bladder function, which is also critical to specifically discern in the history, is indicative of cauda equina syndrome, a surgical emergency in which the nerve roots at the caudal end of the spinal cord are compressed or damaged.

RADIOGRAPHIC EVALUATION

Radiographs often show loss of lumbar lordosis, which is a result of muscle spasm, and sometimes a mild lumbar scoliosis. Other radiographic findings include degenerative changes and a loss of intervertebral disc height. MRI is the best study to establish the diagnosis of a disc herniation. CT is especially helpful to visualize a partially ossified fragment associated with a slipped apophysis.

TREATMENT

The initial treatment is nonoperative in the vast majority of patients—even if symptoms or findings of radiculopathy are observed. Treatment focuses on rest, activity modification, nonsteroidal antiinflammatory drugs, and physical therapy. An orthosis may provide additional symptomatic relief. Complete bed rest is not recommended. **Epidural steroid injection** may be discussed with patients after approximately 6 wk of treatment if symptoms persist; evidence suggests faster short-term pain relief but no difference in long-term outcome. However, if patients elect to undergo an epidural steroid injection, they should only have a single injection, even if the first did not provide any relief. Multiple injections are no more likely to provide relief than a single injection, and multiple injections expose patients to additional risks of infection, scarring, and neural injury. If a patient experiences substantial relief from an epidural steroid injection and has a later recurrence of symptoms, consideration may be given for a repeat injection after performing a complete physical exam and ruling out any new pathology.

Surgical treatment should be considered when nonoperative measures have failed or when a profound neurologic deficit such as cauda equina syndrome is present or evolving. Unfortunately, children and adolescents respond less favorably to nonoperative therapy compared with adults, and a significant percentage will require surgical intervention. Although patients with disc herniation may improve with reduction in the local inflammatory response around the nerve root, and also as the disc material loses water volume and shrinks, which eliminates mechanical compression, patients with symptomatic ring

apophyseal separations have a bony fragment causing their symptoms and are much less likely to improve spontaneously.

The surgical technique involves removing a small area of the lamina via a posterior approach, called a **laminotomy**, which allows exposure of the neural elements and underlying disc. Any loose fragments are removed. A bulging disc may also be opened surgically to decompress the area compressing the neural elements, although a complete discectomy is inadvisable. The surgical approach is similar in the case of a slipped vertebral apophysis, in which fragments of bone and cartilage must also be removed. This often requires a bilateral laminotomy to completely address the pathology.

The initial results are excellent in the majority of patients. Up to one-third of patients may have recurrent herniations and resultant symptoms of back or leg pain with longer-term follow-up. These recurrences are initially treated nonoperatively. A spinal fusion may be required when there is instability, for example, a spondylolisthesis.

Bibliography is available at Expert Consult.

679.9 Tumors
R. Justin Mistovich and David A. Spiegel

Back pain may be the most common presenting complaint in children who have a tumor involving the vertebral column or the spinal cord. Other associated symptoms may include weakness of the lower extremities, scoliosis, and loss of sphincter control. The majority of tumors are benign (see Chapter 501), including osteoid osteoma, osteoblastoma, aneurysmal bone cyst, and eosinophilic granuloma. Malignant tumors involving the vertebral column may be osseous, such as osteosarcoma or Ewing sarcoma. The may involve the spinal cord and sympathetic or parasympathetic nerves, in cases of ganglioneuroma, ganglioneuroblastoma, neuroblastoma. Tumors from other primary sites can also metastasize to the spine.

In addition to high-quality plain radiographs, useful imaging modalities include bone scans, which help with localization and identification of other lesions; MRI, which is helpful to identify soft-tissue extension and neurologic compression; and CT, which provides excellent bony detail.

A biopsy is usually required to establish the diagnosis. Treatment of tumors of the spinal column may require a multidisciplinary approach. These cases should ideally be managed in centers with experience in the care patients with these lesions.

Chapter **680**
The Neck

680.1 Torticollis
Patrick O'Toole and David A. Spiegel

Torticollis, literally meaning *twisted neck*, is not a diagnosis but rather a manifestation of a variety of underlying conditions (Table 680-1). Alternative names associated with this condition include *wry-neck* and *cock-robin* deformity.

CONGENITAL MUSCULAR TORTICOLLIS

Typically diagnosed during infancy, **congenital muscular torticollis (CMT)** is contracture of the sternocleidomastoid muscle, which results in tilting of the head and neck toward the side of the contracted muscle with rotation to the contralateral side. In the majority of cases (75%)

Table 680-1	Differential Diagnosis of Torticollis

CONGENITAL
Muscular torticollis
Positional deformation
Vertebral anomalies (failure segmentation, formation or both)
Unilateral atlantooccipital fusion
Klippel-Feil syndrome
Unilateral absence of sternocleidomastoid
Pterygium colli

TRAUMA
Muscular injury (cervical muscles)
Atlantooccipital subluxation
Atlantoaxial subluxation
C2-3 subluxation
Rotary subluxation
Fractures (C1, others)

INFLAMMATION
Cervical lymphadenitis
Retropharyngeal abscess
Cervical vertebral osteomyelitis or diskitis
Juvenile idiopathic arthritis
Grisel syndrome (nontraumatic rotary subluxation of the atlantoaxial joint caused by inflammation)
Upper lobe pneumonia

NEUROLOGIC
Visual disturbances (nystagmus, superior oblique or lateral rectus paresis)
Dystonic oculogyric drug reactions (phenothiazines, haloperidol, metoclopramide)
Cervical cord tumor
Posterior fossa brain tumor
Acoustic neuroma
Syringomyelia
Wilson disease
Dystonia musculorum deformans

OTHER
Acute cervical disk calcification
Sandifer syndrome (gastroesophageal reflux, hiatal hernia)
Benign paroxysmal torticollis
Bone tumors (eosinophilic granuloma, osteoid osteoma)
Soft-tissue tumor
Psychogenic

the right-hand sided sternocleidomastoid muscle is involved, causing the patient's face and chin to point to the left side.

CMT is thought to be the result of an intrauterine deformation and is more common in first pregnancies and in those with uterine compression syndrome or decreased amniotic fluid volume. CMT may be associated with the presence of a palpable mass (fibrous tissue) within the substance of the sternocleidomastoid muscle in approximately 50% of cases. The mass disappears during infancy and is replaced by a fibrous band. Information from muscle biopsies and magnetic resonance imaging has led to the suggestion that muscle injury from compression and/or stretch may create localized ischemia resulting in fibrosis and subsequent contracture: an intramuscular compartment syndrome. The condition may rarely be caused by hereditary muscle aplasia. Associated findings in CMT include plagiocephaly, facial asymmetry, and positional musculoskeletal deformities such as metatarsus adductus (15%) and calcaneovalgus feet. Hip dysplasia may be identified in 8-20% of CMT cases.

Although standards for screening in patients with a normal hip examination have not been established, as many as 15% of patients with CMT have developmental dysplasia of the hip based on screening ultrasound, some of whom required treatment. Consideration should be given to obtaining either an ultrasound scan (4 wks of age) or a plain radiograph of the hips (4-6 mo of age).

A muscle-stretching program should be successful in more than 90% of patients with CMT, especially when treatment is started within the 1st 3 mo of life. Although firm guidelines for imaging the cervical spine have not been established, consideration may be given to obtaining anteroposterior and lateral radiographs of the cervical spine when the typical clinical features associated with CMT are absent or if the deformity does not respond to treatment, as torticollis in infants may be a result of congenital vertebral anomalies. Surgical release of the sternocleidomastoid is considered in patients with persistent deformity despite nonoperative treatment. The muscle may be released at its insertion on the clavicle (unipolar release) or off both its origin and insertion (bipolar release). There is no agreement as to the most appropriate time for the surgical release, but surgical treatment is typically delayed until after 18 mo of age, and some even suggest waiting until the child is approaching school age. Although range of motion can be improved following surgical release even during the teenage years, remodeling of facial asymmetry and plagiocephaly may be less predictable in patients older than infancy. Surgical management results in adequate function and acceptable cosmesis in more than 90% of patients. However with early diagnosis and medical treatment, surgery should only be required in a minority of cases.

OTHER CAUSES OF TORTICOLLIS
The evaluation of torticollis becomes more complex when the typical findings associated with CMT are absent, the usual clinical response is not observed, or when the torticollis presents at a later age. In addition to a careful history and physical examination, consultation with an ophthalmologist and/or neurologist may be helpful. Plain radiographs should be obtained, and an MRI scan of the brain and cervical spine will be required in a subset of cases.

The differential diagnosis is extensive (see Table 680-1). **Neurogenic torticollis** is uncommon and results from tumors of the posterior fossa or brainstem, syringomyelia (see Chapter 606.3), and Arnold-Chiari malformation (see Chapter 591.11). In addition to the neurologic examination, MRI of the brain and cervical spine is required to establish the diagnosis. **Paroxysmal torticollis of infancy** is also uncommon and may be a result of vestibular dysfunction. Episodes may last from minutes to days, and the side of the deformity may alternate. The condition is self-limiting, and no specific treatment is required other than ruling out other treatable causes.

Torticollis may also be seen in association with discitis or vertebral osteomyelitis, juvenile idiopathic arthritis, cervical disc calcification, visual problems such as congenital nystagmus or paresis of the superior oblique or lateral rectus muscles, benign or malignant bone tumors, and in patients with cerebral palsy and chronic gastroesophageal reflux (Sandifer syndrome).

Atlantoaxial rotatory displacement represents a spectrum of rotational malalignment from subluxation to frank dislocation between the atlas (C1) and the axis (C2), and may best be described as a pathologic stickiness in the arc of joint motion. In some cases there is fixed malalignment between C1 and C2 (atlantoaxial rotary fixation) that results in a 50% loss of cervical rotation. The malalignment is often reducible initially but may become irreducible and fixed after weeks to months. As such, prompt diagnosis and treatment are essential. Atlantoaxial rotatory displacement may be diagnosed after infection or inflammation of the tissues of the upper airway, neck, and/or pharynx (**Grisel syndrome**), following traumatic injuries (usually minor), and as a complication of surgical procedures in the oropharynx, ear, or nose. The diagnosis is established using a dynamic rotational computerized tomography scan, in which axial images are obtained through the upper cervical spine with the head rotated maximally toward both the right and the left. If the patient is seen within a few days of the onset of symptoms, then a trial of analgesics and a soft collar may be attempted. Patients with symptoms for more than a week are often admitted to the hospital for analgesia, muscle relaxants, and a period of cervical traction. If this fails to reduce the displacement, then halo traction may be attempted. If the joint can be reduced, patients are typically immobilized for at least 6 wk in a halo vest. Patients with a fixed deformity may require a posterior atlantoaxial fusion to stabilize the articulation. Most children with Grisel syndrome improve with supportive care (nonsteroidal antiinflammatory drugs, muscle relaxants) and treatment of their head and neck infections.

Bibliography is available at Expert Consult.

680.2 Klippel-Feil Syndrome
Patrick O'Toole and David A. Spiegel

Klippel-Feil syndrome (KFS) includes the classic triad of a low posterior hairline, short neck, and decreased cervical range of motion. These clinical findings are present in <50% of patients with KFS. Patients have a congenital fusion (failure of segmentation) of 1 or more cervical motion segments at the craniocervical junction or in the subaxial spine and often have associated congenital anomalies of the cervical spine and other organ systems (Fig. 680-1). Clinical problems are more common in adults and include pain and/or neurologic symptoms, from spinal instability and/or stenosis. The incidence has been estimated at 1 : 40,000-42,000 births; not every patient with the condition is diagnosed.

ETIOLOGY AND CLASSIFICATION
The etiology is felt to be sporadic when KFS is seen in isolation, but several candidate genes have been proposed in patients with associated anomalies. Additional findings in the cervical spine include occipitocervical synostosis, odontoid abnormalities, and basilar impression (proximal migration of the C2 vertebra). Other associations include **Sprengel's deformity** (congenital elevation of the scapula), congenital scoliosis, genitourinary anomalies (25-35%), sensorineural hearing loss (5%), and congenital heart disease (5-10%). Renal abnormalities include double collecting systems, renal aplasia, and horseshoe kidney. The cervical spine anomalies seen in patients with KFS may also be seen with Goldenhar syndrome, Mohr syndrome, VACTERL (vertebral defects, imperforate anus, congenital heart disease, tracheoesophageal fistula, renal and limb defects) syndrome, and fetal alcohol syndrome.

Traditionally, the classification of KFS has been based on the anatomic distribution of the cervical fusions and the kinematics of the cervical spine in flexion and extension. As more information regarding the genetics of this condition has become available, the classification system has incorporated these changes. KF 1 involves a fusion at C1 with or without a more caudal fusion level (autosomal recessive) and is associated with severe anomalies. KF 2 has a fusion of C2 and C3 with or without a more caudal fusion (autosomal dominant with 100% penetrance). KF 3 is an isolated fusion caudal to C1 and C2/3 (autosomal dominant or recessive). KF 4 (X-linked dominant) is synonymous with **Wildervanck syndrome**, which involves congenital cervical synostosis associated with hearing loss and the **Duane anomaly** (congenital rare type of strabismus).

CLINICAL PRESENTATION
KFS is present at birth but does not usually become clinically apparent until the 2nd or 3rd decades, when patients present with pain, loss of motion, and/or neurologic symptoms. Given that the same physiologic stresses are applied to a smaller number of mobile spinal segments, patients are at risk for the development of hypermobility and often instability, especially at motion segments adjacent to the fused vertebrae. Weakness or clumsiness may be the presenting symptoms. A complete history is essential, including a detailed family and birth history and review of systems.

PHYSICAL EXAMINATION
A comprehensive musculoskeletal and neurologic examination is required, given associated anomalies in the musculoskeletal and visceral systems. Scoliosis is present in more than 50% of patients with KFS, and congenital anomalies may be identified in other regions of the spine as well. The neurologic exam focuses on identifying any signs of radiculopathy or myelopathy. Spinal cord compression (myelopathy) may result from stenosis or instability, and may result in upper motor neuron signs such as hyperreflexia, Babinski's sign, and sustained clonus, with more than 3 beats considered pathologic. Nerve root compression (radiculopathy) may be from stenosis and is identified by weakness or decreased sensation in the muscles or dermatomes served by a particular nerve root, respectively.

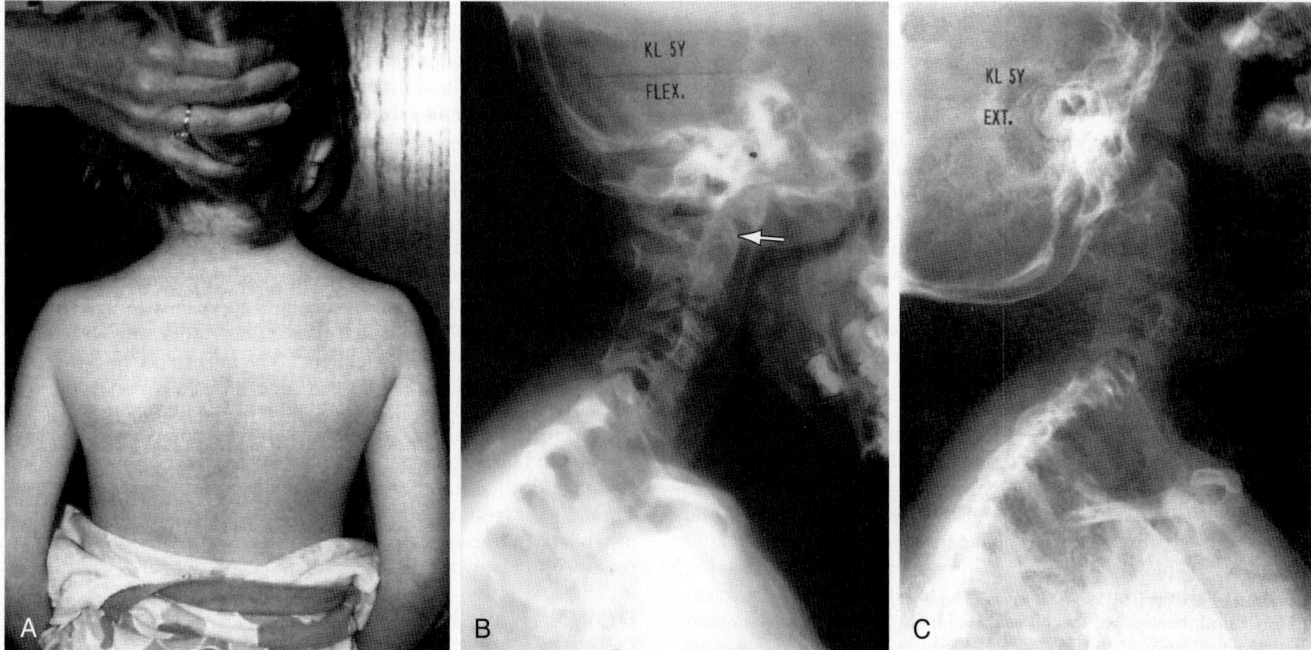

Figure 680-1 Clinical picture of a 5 yr old with Klippel-Feil syndrome. **A,** Note short neck and low hairline. **B** and **C,** Radiographs of the cervical spine (**B,** flexion; **C,** extension) demonstrate congenital fusion and evidence of spinal instability *(arrow). (From Drummond DS: Pediatric cervical instability. In Weisel SE, Boden SD, Wisnecki RI, editors: Seminars in spine surgery, Philadelphia, 1996, WB Saunders, pp. 292–309.)*

RADIOGRAPHIC INVESTIGATION

Initial radiologic evaluation should include an anteroposterior, lateral, and oblique view of the cervical spine. The characteristic finding is a congenital fusion of 2 or more vertebrae (failure of segmentation); however, multiple vertebrae may be involved. Because congenital anomalies may exist in more than 1 region of the spine, radiographs of the thoracic and lumbosacral spine should be routinely obtained. Flexion–extension lateral views of the cervical spine may help to identify segments with excessive motion. Referral to an orthopedist is appropriate if the diagnosis is established. Patients with this condition usually undergo CT and MRI of the spine to accurately characterize the bony anomalies and also identify any coexisting neural pathology. A renal ultrasound is routinely obtained, and additional tests may be indicated.

TREATMENT

The 3 patterns commonly associated with instability include (1) C2/C3 fusion with occipitocervical synostosis, (2) extensive fusion over multiple levels with an abnormal occipitocervical junction, and (3) 2 fused segments separated by an open joint space. Pain may often be controlled by activity restriction, intermittent immobilization, or other nonoperative modalities. Patients who are chronically symptomatic and/or have instability with positive neurologic symptoms and/or findings, or are felt to be at increased risk for neurologic deterioration, are candidates for surgical treatment. Operative interventions include decompression of a nerve root(s) or the spinal cord, and/or spinal fusion to address spinal instability.

Bibliography is available at Expert Consult.

680.3 Cervical Anomalies and Instabilities
Patrick O'Toole and David A. Spiegel

One or more anomalies of the craniovertebral junction and/or lower cervical spine may be seen in isolation or in association with other conditions, including genetic syndromes, skeletal dysplasias, connective tissue disorders, and metabolic disorders. These anomalies may be congenital, resulting from a mutation in the homeobox genes, or developmental. Even though most anomalies remain asymptomatic and undiagnosed, a subset will place the patient at risk of neurologic injury as a result of instability or spinal canal stenosis. The most frequently encountered causes of cervical spine instability in children can be categorized etiologically (Table 680-2). Patients with conditions that have known associations involving the cervical spine should have a complete evaluation, including history, physical examination, and initial radiographic examination.

Patients may complain of neck pain and/or neurologic symptoms. Radicular symptoms include pain, weakness, and numbness within the distribution of a nerve root; myelopathic symptoms may include generalized weakness, gait disturbance, increased fatigue with ambulation, upper-extremity clumsiness, and abnormalities in bowel or bladder function. Physical findings may include a restriction in cervical mobility, cervical tenderness and/or spasm, and neurologic abnormalities.

The upper cervical spine has limited flexion and extension, with roughly 50% of cervical rotation occurring at the atlantoaxial (C1-2) joint. The main constraints to motion in the upper cervical spine are soft tissue (ligaments and joint capsules) rather than osseous, and excessive motion or instability may put neural tissues at risk, and result in compressive injury to the brainstem or spinal cord. Anomalies at the craniovertebral junction include congenital fusion of the occiput to C1 (occipitalization of the atlas), basilar impression and invagination (proximal migration of the C2 vertebra as the result of softening of the bones and with normal bones respectively), and accessory vertebrae. Aplasia or hypoplasia of the atlas or the axis may result in atlantoaxial instability.

Table 680-2	Causes of Pediatric Cervical Instability	
CAUSES	**SUBTYPES**	
Congenital	Cranio-occipital defects (occipital vertebrae, basilar impression, occipital dysplasias, condylar hypoplasia, occipitalized atlas)	
	Atlantoaxial defects (aplasia of atlas arch, aplasia of odontoid process)	
	Subaxial anomalies (failure of segmentation and/or fusion, spina bifida, spondylolisthesis)	
	Syndromic disorders (i.e., Down syndrome, Klippel-Feil syndrome, 22q11.2 deletion syndrome, Larsen syndrome, Marfan syndrome, Ehlers-Danlos syndrome)	
Acquired	Trauma	
	Infection (pyogenic/granulomatous)	
	Tumor (including neurofibromatosis)	
	Inflammatory conditions (i.e., juvenile idiopathic arthritis)	
	Osteochondrodysplasias (i.e., achondroplasia, diastrophic dysplasia, metatropic dysplasia, spondyloepiphyseal dysplasia)	
	Storage disorders (i.e., mucopolysaccharidoses)	
	Metabolic disorders (rickets)	
	Miscellaneous (including osteogenesis imperfecta, postsurgery)	

OS ODONTOIDEUM

Os odontoideum is the most common anomaly of the odontoid peg (dens) and radiographically appears as an oval-shaped, well-corticated, bony ossicle that is positioned cephalad to the body of the axis. There is a discontinuity in the midportion of the dens, and the upper portion of the dens moves with the ring of C1, narrowing the space available for the spinal cord and placing the spinal cord at risk for injury. The body of the dens is mesenchymal in origin and originates from the 1st cervical vertebra, subsequent separation allows it to then fuse with the C2 vertebra. It is formed by 2 separate ossification centers, 1 on either side of the midline, which fuse and are visible at birth. Three etiologies have been proposed: (1) that the os odontoideum represents a fracture nonunion of the odontoid peg; (2) that the os odontoideum represents damage to the epiphyseal plate that has occurred in the 1st yr of life; and (3) that the os odontoideum represents a congenital malformation of the dens itself. The most widely accepted etiology is that a fracture of the dens occurs and subsequently develops a nonunion.

The symptoms and physical findings vary with the location of compression or impingement. In a large series, the average age at presentation was 18.9 yr. The most common presenting symptom was neck pain followed by upper- and lower-limb paresthesia, while torticollis, neck stiffness, gait disturbance, and headaches were uncommon symptoms at presentation. Neurologic examination may reveal a combination of both upper and lower motor neuron signs. Some patients are completely asymptomatic with the anomaly noted incidentally on a lateral cervical spine radiograph.

The radiographic evaluation begins with anteroposterior, lateral, and open mouth (odontoid) views, which may be supplemented by flexion and extension lateral radiographs. CT provides the best bony detail and is useful in defining each anomaly. MRI, including dynamic images in flexion and extension, is best for evaluating neurologic impingement. Symptomatic treatment may be helpful; however, patients with cervical instability and/or neurologic impingement require surgical decompression with or without stabilization.

DOWN SYNDROME

Ligamentous hyperlaxity is a characteristic feature of Down syndrome and may result in hypermobility or instability at the occipitoatlantal or the atlantoaxial joints in 10-30% of patients (see Chapter 81). These patients may also have coexisting congenital or developmental

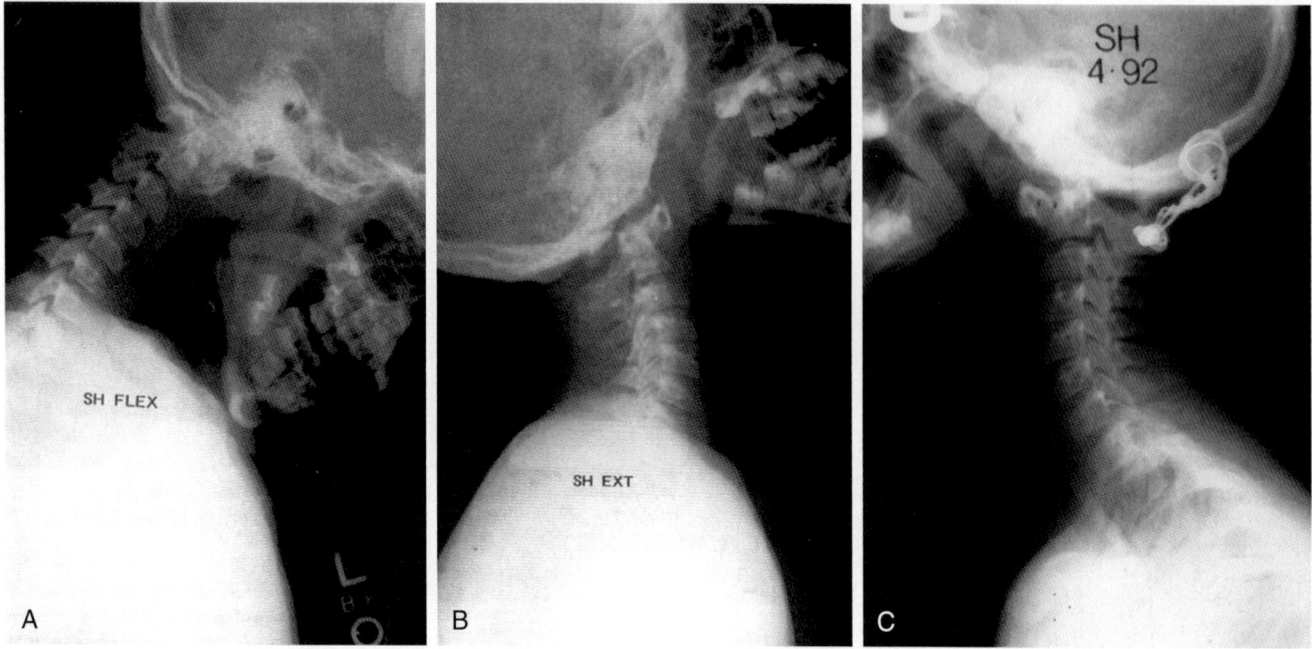

Figure 680-2 Flexion (**A**) and extension (**B**) radiographs of a case of Down syndrome demonstrating atlantooccipital hypermobility and subluxation. **C,** Instability and symptoms were relieved by an occipitoaxial arthrodesis.

anomalies of the cervical spine such as occipitalization of the atlas, atlantal arch hypoplasia, basilar invagination, and os odontoideum.

Even though the natural history of this spectrum of pathology remains unknown, a subset of patients may develop or be at significant risk of developing neurologic dysfunction. The clinical diagnosis of neurologic dysfunction may be challenging, and subtle findings, such as decreased exercise tolerance and gait abnormalities, including increased tripping or falling, may be the earliest signs of myelopathy. In addition to a neurologic examination, focusing on the presence of long tract signs, imaging studies (plain films, MRI) are required to evaluate patients suspected of having neurologic involvement.

All patients require screening by history and physical examination (at regular intervals) and at least a single series of cervical spinal radiographs, including a lateral view in flexion and extension. Plain radiographs are the preliminary imaging modality used to evaluate for hypermobility or instability. The atlantodens interval (ADI) is used to evaluate the relationship between C1 and C2 (atlantoaxial joint) and is measured as the space between the dens and the anterior ring of C1 (ADI) on lateral radiographs in neutral, flexion, and extension (Fig. 680-2). Although the ADI should be 3 mm or less in the population without Down syndrome, a normal ADI in children with Down syndrome is <4.5 mm. Hypermobility is diagnosed as an ADI between 4.5 and 10 mm, while an ADI >10 mm represents instability and carries a significant risk of neurologic injury. MRI is indicated to detect neurologic involvement in patients with radiographic instability. Recommendations for surveillance of the cervical spine in children with Down syndrome remain varied. Routine clinical evaluations, including a neurologic examination, should be performed; the indications for repeating imaging studies in the absence of clinical symptoms or findings have not been defined. Surveillance helps to define the most appropriate level of physical activity and to identify the small subset of those with either progressive hyperlaxity or instability. Although the specific recommendations vary between states, both clinical and radiographic screenings are also required prior to participation in the Special Olympics. Patients with normal radiographs who are also neurologically normal may be allowed to participate in full activity. Those who are diagnosed with hypermobility may be restricted from contact sports and other high-risk activities that increase the risk of trauma to

the cervical spine. Patients with C1-C2 instability with or without neurologic findings are candidates for an atlantoaxial fusion. The risks of a major complication are extremely high for a posterior cervical fusion in this population and include death, neurologic deterioration, and pseudarthrosis with or without graft resorption.

Although hypermobility at the occipitoatlantal joint is present in >50% of children with Down syndrome, most patients do not develop instability or neurologic symptoms. The relationships at this articulation are difficult to measure reliably on plain radiographs and an MRI in flexion and extension is required to evaluate any questionable radiographic findings, especially in the presence of symptoms. Involvement of the subaxial spine is less common and is typically encountered in the adult population of patients with Down syndrome, where degenerative changes and/or instability may result in pain, radiculopathy, and/or myelopathy.

22q11.2 DELETION SYNDROME

The chromosome abnormality deletion of 22q11.2 is a common genetic syndrome, with an overall prevalence of 1 in 5,950 births, and encompasses a wide spectrum of abnormalities. There are characteristic facial features, cleft palate, and cardiac anomalies. Cervical spine anomalies are also common phenotypic features of this syndrome.

At least 1 developmental variation of the occiput or cervical spine is noted in all patients. The occipital variations observed include platybasia (abnormal flattening of the base of the skull) and basilar impression. Variations in anatomy of C1 include dysmorphic shape, an open posterior arch, and occipitalization; axis variations include a dysmorphic dens and "C2 swoosh" (upswept lamina and posterior elements). A range of cervical vertebral fusions is noted in these patients, the most common being at the C2-3 level. Increased segmental motion in the cervical spine is noted in more than half of these patients, and more than a third of patients have increased segmental motion at more than 1 level. With frequent occurrence of upper cervical spine variations in the 22q11.2 deletion syndrome (Fig. 680-3), advanced imaging of the upper cervical spine and regular follow-up of patients to clarify their clinical course is recommended.

Bibliography is available at Expert Consult.

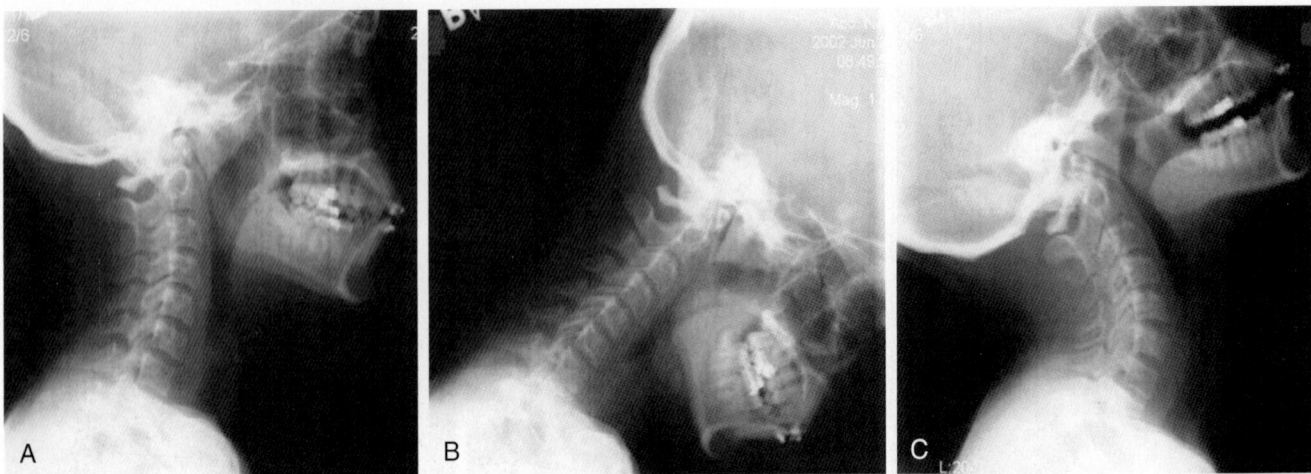

Figure 680-3 Radiographs of the cervical spine in a child with 22q11.2 deletion syndrome showing evidence of platybasia, occipitocervical, and atlantoaxial instability. **A,** Neutral radiograph. **B,** Flexion. **C,** Extension. *(From Drummond DS: Pediatric cervical instability. In Weisel SE, Boden SD, Wisnecki RI, editors: Seminars in spine surgery, Philadelphia, 1996, WB Saunders, pp. 292–309.)*

Chapter **681**
The Upper Limb
Robert B. Carrigan

SHOULDER

The shoulder is a ball-and-socket joint. Although similar to the hip, the shoulder has a greater range of motion because of the size of the humeral head relative to the glenoid, as well as to the presence of scapulothoracic motion. The shoulder positions the hand along the surface of a theoretical sphere in space, with its center at the glenohumeral joint.

Brachial Plexus Birth Palsy
(See also Chapter 99.7.)

Injuries to the brachial plexus can occur in the peripartum time, usually as a result of a stretching mechanism. This palsy is often associated with large fetal size and shoulder dystocia. The incidence is 1-3 per 1,000 live births. The injury can range in severity from neurapraxia, to complete rupture of the nerve roots or avulsion of the nerve root from the spinal cord. More often, the upper roots (C5 and C6) of the brachial plexus are affected, rather than a complete brachial plexus palsy itself (C5-T1). Rarely, in isolation, is a lower plexus injury (C8 and T1) observed. The clinical appearance of a C5-C6 brachial plexus birth palsy (Erb-Duchenne palsy) is the waiter's tip position. The arm is held in a position of shoulder adduction and internal rotation, elbow extension, and wrist flexion.

Treatment
Occupational therapy should be instituted quickly after brachial plexus injury to maintain passive range of motion of the limb and encourage use of the arm. If the biceps muscle does not demonstrate evidence of recovery by 3 mo of age, or shows persistent weakness at 5 mo of age, a more severe nerve injury may be suspected. MRI and electrodiagnostic testing are not consistently reliable for delineation of nerve injury in this setting. Surgical exploration and nerve grafting of the brachial plexus are then indicated.

After complete or incomplete neurologic recovery shoulder dysplasia and dislocation (analogous to developmental dysplasia of the hip) can occur. This occurs as a result of muscle imbalances in the shoulder.

In the typical Erb palsy a child may have a persistent internal rotation contracture of the shoulder as a result of the imbalance of the weak abductors and external rotators and stronger adductors and internal rotators. Infants and older children may require arthroscopic or open reduction of shoulder contractures. Older children with residual weakness in shoulder abduction and external rotation can benefit from muscle transfers. Osteotomies are reserved for children with severely deformed glenohumeral joints and functional impairment from persistent shoulder internal rotation contracture (Fig. 681-1).

Sprengel's Deformity
Sprengel's deformity, or congenital elevation of the scapula, is a disorder of development that involves a high scapula and limited scapulothoracic motion. The scapula originates in early embryogenesis at a level posterior to the 4th cervical vertebra, but it descends during development to below the 7th cervical vertebra. Failure of this descent, either unilateral or bilateral, is Sprengel's deformity. The severity of the deformity depends on the location of the scapula and associated anomalies. The scapula in mild cases is simply rotated, with a palpable or visible bump corresponding to the superomedial corner of the scapula in the region of the trapezius muscle. Function is generally good. In moderate cases, the scapula is higher on the neck and connected to the spine with an abnormal omovertebral ligament or even bone. Shoulder motion, particularly abduction, is limited. In severe cases, the scapula is small and positioned on the posterior neck, and the neck may be webbed. The majority of patients have associated anomalies of the musculoskeletal system, especially in the spine, making spinal evaluation important.

Treatment
In mild cases, treatment is generally unnecessary, although a prominent and unsightly superomedial corner of the scapula can be excised. In more severe cases, surgical repositioning of the scapula with rebalancing of parascapular muscles can significantly improve both function and appearance.

ELBOW
The elbow is the most congruent joint in the body. The stability of the elbow is imparted via this bony congruity as well as through the medial and radial collateral ligaments. Where the shoulder positions the hand along the surface of a theoretical sphere, the elbow positions the hand within that sphere. The elbow allows extension and flexion through the ulnohumeral articulation and pronation and supination through the radiocapitellar articulation.

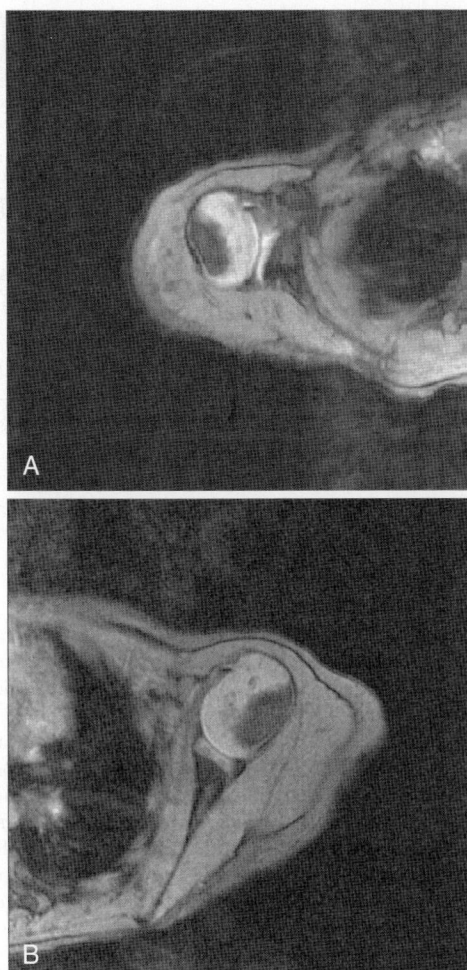

Figure 681-1 A, Shoulder MRI demonstrating glenohumeral dysplasia following brachial plexus birth palsy. **B,** Comparison MRI of uninvolved contralateral shoulder.

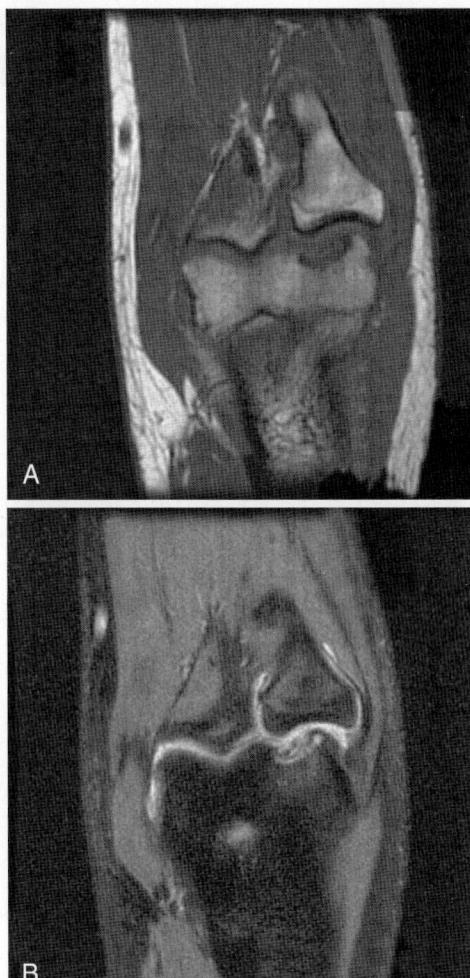

Figure 681-2 T1 **(A)** and T2 **(B)** coronal MRI images of the elbow depicting Panner disease of the elbow.

Panner Disease

Panner disease is a disruption of the blood flow to the articular cartilage and subchondral bone to the capitellum (Fig. 681-2). It typically occurs in boys between the ages of 5 and 13 yr. Presenting symptoms include lateral elbow pain, loss of motion, and, in advanced cases, mechanical symptoms of the elbow (loose bodies).

The mechanism of injury can be impaction or overloading of the joint, as seen with sports such as gymnastics and baseball. It can also be idiopathic. Radiographs of the elbow may be normal, but they may also show a small lucency within the subchondral bone of the capitellum. MRI is the study of choice to evaluate a suspected capitellar lesion. MRI can demonstrate the extent of the involvement in the subchondral bone as well as the integrity of the cartilage of the articular surface.

Treatment

Treatment is typically conservative. Rest, activity modification, and patient education are initial treatment options. In cases where the articular cartilage fragments and loose bodies form, arthroscopy of the elbow is warranted to remove the loose bodies. When the cartilage defect in the capitellum is large and symptomatic, procedures for restoration of the articular cartilage may be considered. These procedures include drilling of the subchondral bone (microfracture) to promote scar cartilage and osteochondral autograft transplantation.

Radial Longitudinal Deficiency

Radial longitudinal deficiency of the forearm comprises a spectrum of conditions and diseases that have resulted in hypoplasia or absence of the radius (Table 681-1). This process was formerly referred to as *radial club hand,* but the name has been changed to *radial longitudinal deficiency,* which better characterizes the condition. Clinical characteristics consist of a small, shortened limb with the hand and wrist in excessive radial deviation. Partial or complete absence of the radial structures of the forearm and hand are observed (Fig. 681-3).

Radial longitudinal deficiency can range in severity from mild to severe and has been classified into 4 types (Table 681-2). Radial longitudinal deficiency can be associated with other syndromes such as Holt-Oram and Fanconi anemia (see Table 681-1).

Treatment

The goals for the treatment of radial longitudinal deficiency include centralizing the hand and wrist on the forearm, balancing the wrist, and maintaining appropriate thumb and digital motion. Shortly after birth, parents are encouraged to passively stretch the wrist and hand to elongate the contracted radial soft tissues. Serial casting and splinting are ineffective at this time, because of the small size of the arm.

Surgery for correction of the wrist deformity remains controversial. Historically, for children with good elbow motion, centralization of the wrist on the forearm was performed. However recurrence of the deformity was often observed. For this reason some surgeons have elected to abandon this procedure.

When considering a centralization procedure, the preoperative plan begins with careful examination of the patient; considerations in regard to thumb and elbow function must be made before surgery. The surgery typically occurs when the child is 1 yr of age. Correction of the

Table 681-1	Syndromic Association with Radial Day Deficiency
SYSTEM	**CONDITION**
Cardiac	Holt-Oram syndrome VACTERL association Ventriculoradial dysplasia
Chromosomal	Trisomies 13, 17, and 18 Deletions 4q and 14q
Craniofacial	Acrorenal–ocular syndrome Craniosynostosis–radial aplasia (Baller-Gerold syndrome) Cleft lip/palate Oculoauriculovertebral dysplasia (Goldenhar syndrome) Orofacial–digital syndrome (Juberg-Hayward syndrome) Roberts SC phocomelia syndrome Treacher Collins syndrome Eye–radial dysplasia (Duane syndrome) Möbius syndrome Hemifacial microsomia
Cutaneous	Rothmund-Thompson syndrome (cutaneous poikiloderma)
Developmental delay	de Lange syndrome
Hematologic	Thrombocytopenia–absent radius syndrome Fanconi anemia Anemia–triphalangeal thumb (Aase-Smith syndrome)
Renal	Renal–radial ray aplasia (Sofer syndrome)
Skeletal	Cervical rib–radial ray defect (Funston syndrome) Costovertebral dysplasia–humeroradial synostosis (Keutel syndrome) Klippel-Feil syndrome VACTERL association
Teratogenic	
Other	IVIC (Instituto Venezolano de Investigaciones Científicas) syndrome

VACTERL, Vertebral abnormalities, anal atresia, cardiac abnormalities, tracheoesophageal fistula and/or esophageal atresia, renal agenesis and dysplasia, and limb defects.
Adapted from Gupta A, Kay SPJ, Scheker LR, editors: The growing hand: diagnosis and management of the upper extremity in children, St Louis, 2000, Mosby, p 147.

Table 681-2	Classification of Radial Longitudinal Deficiency
TYPE	**CHARACTERISTICS**
I	Short radius Minor radial deviation of the hand
II	Hypoplastic radius with abnormal growth at proximal and distal ends Moderate radial deviation of the hand
III	Partial absence of the radius Severe radial deviation of the hand
IV	Complete absence of the radius The most common type

Adapted from Bayne LG, Klug MS: Long-term review of the surgical treatment of radial deficiencies, J Hand Surg Am 12(2):169–179, 1987.

The diagnosis is made by history and physical examination, as radiographs are typically normal.

Treatment

The annular ligament is reduced by rotating the forearm into supination while holding pressure over the radial head. A palpable click or clunk can be felt. The child recovers active supination immediately and usually has immediate relief of discomfort. Immobilization is not required, but recurrent annular ligament subluxations can occur, and the parents should avoid activities that apply traction to the elbows. Parents can learn reduction maneuvers for recurrent episodes to avoid trips to the emergency department or pediatrician's office. Recurrent subluxation beyond 5 yr of age is rare. Irreducible subluxations tend to resolve spontaneously, with gradual resolution of symptoms over days to weeks; surgery is rarely indicated.

WRIST

The wrist is composed of the 2 forearm bones as well as the 8 carpal bones. The wrist allows flexion, extension, and radial and ulnar deviation through the radiocarpal and midcarpal articulations. Pronation and supination occur, at the wrist, through the distal radial ulnar joint. The wrist is a complex joint with numerous ligamentous and soft-tissue attachments. It has complex kinematics that allows for its generous range of motion, but when these kinematics are altered, significant dysfunction can occur.

Madelung Deformity

Madelung deformity is a deformity of the wrist that is characterized as radial and palmar angulations of the distal aspect of the radius (Fig. 681-5). Growth arrest of the palmar and ulnar aspect of the distal radial physis is the underlying cause of this deformity. Bony physeal lesions and an abnormal radiolunate ligament (Vicker's ligament) have been implicated. The deformity can be bilateral and affects girls more than boys.

Treatment

Treatment of Madelung's deformity is typically observation. Mild deformities can be observed until skeletal maturity. Moderate to severe deformities that either are painful or limit function may be candidates for surgical intervention. Surgical treatment for Madelung's deformity is often motivated by appearance. Patients and their families may be concerned about the palmar angulation of the wrist as well as the resulting prominent distal ulna.

There are a multitude of surgical options for treating Madelung's deformity. For the skeletally immature patient, resection of the tethering soft tissue (Vicker's ligament) and physiolysis (fat grafting of any bony lesion seen within the physis) is often the first option. When Madelung's deformity is encountered in skeletally mature patients, an osteotomy may be considered. Dorsal closing wedge, dome, and ulnar

radial deviation as well as centralization of the wrist can be accomplished with a variety of different surgical techniques. These techniques include open release, capsular reefing, and tendon rebalancing. External fixation techniques have also been described.

Nursemaid Elbow

Nursemaid elbow is a subluxation of a ligament rather than a subluxation or dislocation of the radial head. The proximal end of the radius, or radial head, is anchored to the proximal ulna by the annular ligament, which wraps like a leash from the ulna, around the radial head, and back to the ulna. If the radius is pulled distally, the annular ligament can slip proximally off the radial head and into the joint between the radial head and the humerus (Fig. 681-4). The injury is typically produced when a longitudinal traction force is applied to the arm, such as when a falling child is caught by the hand, or when a child is pulled by the hand. The injury usually occurs in toddlers and rarely occurs in children older than 5 yr of age. Subluxation of the annular ligament produces immediate pain and limitation of supination. Flexion and extension of the elbow are not limited, and swelling is generally absent.

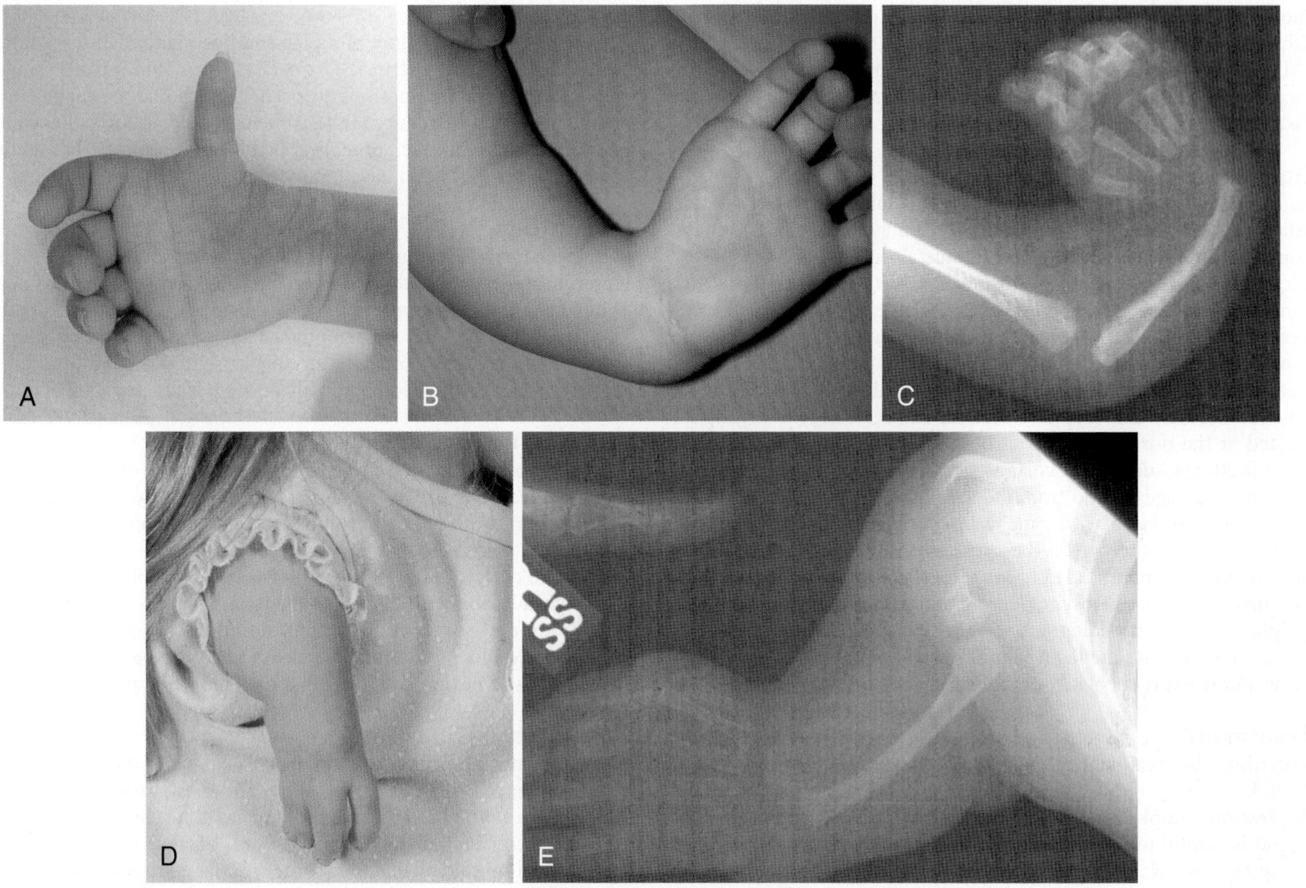

Figure 681-3 Spectrum of phenotypes of radial dysplasia. **A,** Type 1 radius with a hypoplastic thumb. **B,** Type IV radius with an absent thumb. **C,** Radiograph of a type IV radius. **D** and **E,** Phocomelic radial deficiency. *(From Ho C: Disorders of the upper extremity. In Herring JA, editor: Tachdjian's pediatric orthopaedics, ed 5, Philadelphia, 2014, WB Saunders, Fig. 15-72, p. 391.)*

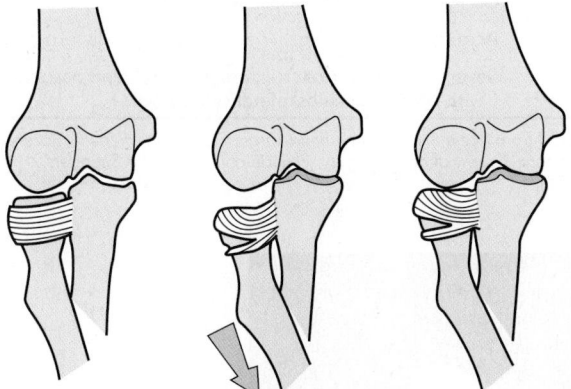

Figure 681-4 The pathology of nursemaid, or pulled, elbow. The annular ligament is partially torn when the arm is pulled. The radial head moves distally, and when traction is discontinued, the ligament is carried into the joint. *(From Rang M: Children's fractures, ed 2, Philadelphia, 1983, JB Lippincott, p. 193.)*

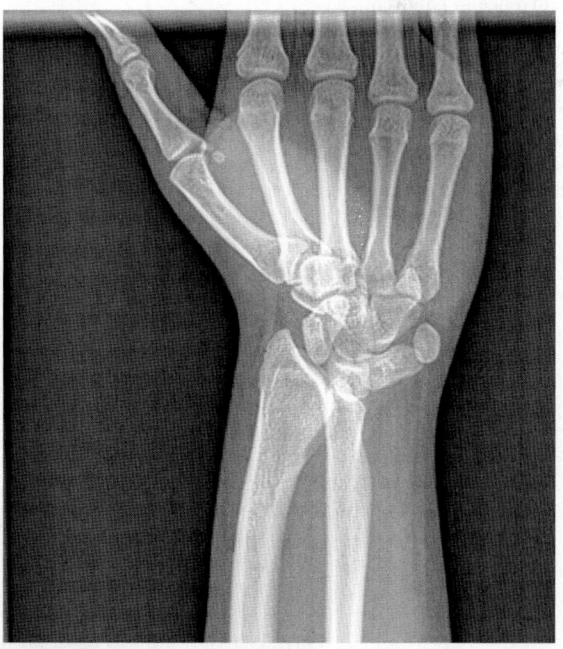

Figure 681-5 Radiograph of an adolescent with Madelung's deformity.

shortening osteotomies may be used alone or in combination to achieve the desired result.

Long-term considerations of Madelung's deformity concern the incongruity of the distal radial ulnar joint and resulting premature distal radial ulnar joint arthritis.

Ganglion

As a synovial joint, the wrist articulation is lubricated with synovial fluid, which is produced by the synovial lining of the joint and maintained within the joint by the joint capsule. A defect in the capsule can allow fluid to leak from the joint into the soft tissues, resulting in a ganglion. The term *cyst* is a misnomer, because this extraarticular collection of fluid does not have its own true lining. The defect in the capsule can occur as a traumatic event, although trauma is rarely a feature of the presenting history. The fluid usually exits the joint in the interval between the scaphoid and lunate, resulting in a ganglion located at the dorsoradial aspect of the wrist. Ganglia can occur at other locations, such as the volar aspect of the wrist, or in the palm as a result of leakage of fluid from the flexor tendon sheaths. Pain is not commonly associated with ganglia in children, and when it is, it is unclear whether the cyst is the cause of the pain. The diagnosis is usually evident on physical examination, especially if the lesion transilluminates. Extensor tenosynovitis and anomalous muscles can mimic ganglion cysts, but radiography or MRI is not routinely required. Ultrasonography is an effective, noninvasive tool to support the diagnosis and reassure the patient and family.

Treatment

Regarding the treatment of ganglia in children, consider the vowels AEIOU.

Aspiration: Simple aspiration of the fluid has a high recurrence rate and is painful for children given the large-bore needle required to aspirate the gelatinous fluid. However, in older children who would like to try and decompress the cyst before considering surgery, this may be reasonable.

Excision: Surgical excision, including excision of the stalk connecting the ganglion to its joint of origin, has a high success rate, although the ganglion can recur.

Injection: Aspiration of the cyst and a simultaneous injection of a corticosteroid have been shown to be effective in treating recurrence in children.

Observation: Up to 80% of ganglia in children younger than 10 yr of age resolve spontaneously within 1 yr of being noticed. If the ganglion is painful or bothersome and the child is older than 10 yr of age, treatment may be warranted.

Ultrasound: For children's parents who are concerned about the mass and want a radiographic study to confirm the diagnosis, ultrasound is a noninvasive test to confirm the diagnosis.

HAND

The hand and fingers allow complex and fine manipulations. An intricate balance among extrinsic flexors, extensors, and intrinsic muscles allow these complex motions to occur. Congenital anomalies of the hand and upper extremity rank just behind cardiac anomalies in incidence, and like cardiac anomalies, if they are not properly identified and remedied, they can have long-term consequences.

Camptodactyly

Camptodactyly is a nontraumatic flexion contracture of the proximal interphalangeal joint that is often progressive. The small and ring fingers are most often affected. Bilateralism is observed two-thirds of the time. The etiology of camptodactyly is varied. Several different hypotheses have been offered as to the cause of this condition. Camptodactyly can be divided into 3 different types (Table 681-3).

Treatment

Nonsurgical treatment is the primary treatment of camptodactyly. Mild contractures of <30 degrees are usually well tolerated and do not need treatment. Serial casting and static and dynamic splinting are the treatments of choice for preventing progression of contractures. This should be performed until the child is skeletally mature.

Surgical treatment is limited to the treatment of severe contractures. At the time of surgery, all contracted and anomalous structures are released. Results of contracture release for camptodactyly are mixed; often a loss of flexion results from an attempt to improve extension.

Clinodactyly

Angular deformity of the digit in the coronal plane, distal to the metacarpophalangeal joint is clinodactyly. The most commonly observed finding is a mild radial deviation of the small finger at the level of the distal interphalangeal joint. This is often because of a triangular or trapezoidal middle phalanx. In some cases, a disruption of the physis at the middle phalanx produces a longitudinal epiphysial bracket. This

Table 681-3	Classification of Camptodactyly
TYPE	**CHARACTERISTICS**
I	Congenital, no sex bias, small finger only
II	Acquired between ages 7 and 11 yr, typically progressive
III	Severe, significant contracture, bilateral, and associated with other musculoskeletal syndromes

Adapted from Kozin SH: Pediatric hand surgery. In Beredjiklian PK, Bozentka DJ, editors: Review of hand surgery, Philadelphia, 2004, WB Saunders, pp. 223–245.

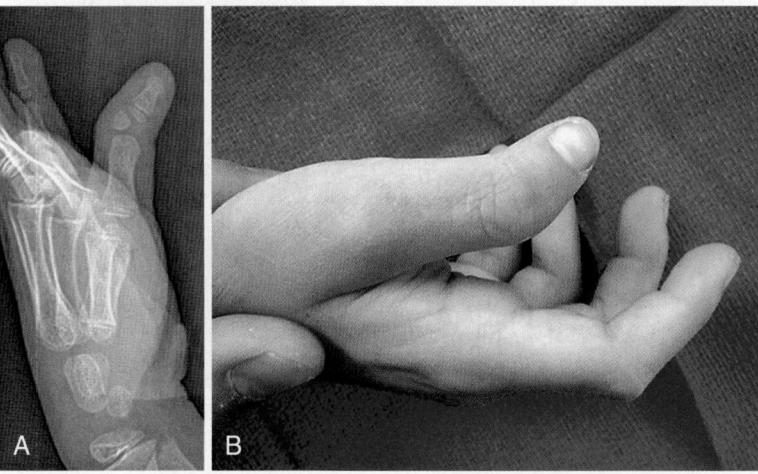

Figure 681-6 Clinodactyly of the thumb.

bracket is thought to be the underlying cause for the formation the "delta phalanx" that is often observed in clinodactyly. Clinodactyly has been observed in other fingers, including the thumb (Fig. 681-6) and ring finger.

Treatment

Often the treatment for clinodactyly is observation and not surgery. For severe deformities and for those affecting the thumb, surgery may be indicated. Surgery is technically demanding. Bracket resections, corrective osteotomies, and growth plate ablations are the most common procedures performed to correct the observed angular deformities. Results are good and recurrences are few when an appropriate procedure is performed.

Polydactyly

Polydactyly or duplication of a digit can occur either as a preaxial deformity (involving the thumb) or as a postaxial deformity (involving the small finger) (Table 681-4; Fig. 681-7). Each has an inherited and genetic component. Duplication of the thumb occurs more often in whites and Asians and is often unilateral, whereas duplication of the small finger occurs more frequently in African-Americans and may be bilateral. Transmission is typically in an autosomal dominant pattern and has been linked to defects in genes localized to chromosome 2.

Duplication of the thumb is subdivided on the basis of the degree of duplication. Table 681-5 lists the 7 types. Small finger duplication has been further subdivided into 2 types. Type A is a well-formed digit. Type B is a small, often underdeveloped supernumerary digit.

Treatment

Thumb and small finger duplication is typically treated with ablation of the supernumerary digit. Treatment options vary based on the

Table 681-4	Syndromes Associated with Polydactyly
Carpenter syndrome	
Ellis-van Creveld syndrome	
Meckel-Gruber syndrome	
Polysyndactyly	
Trisomy 13	
Orofaciodigital syndrome	
Rubinstein-Taybi syndrome	

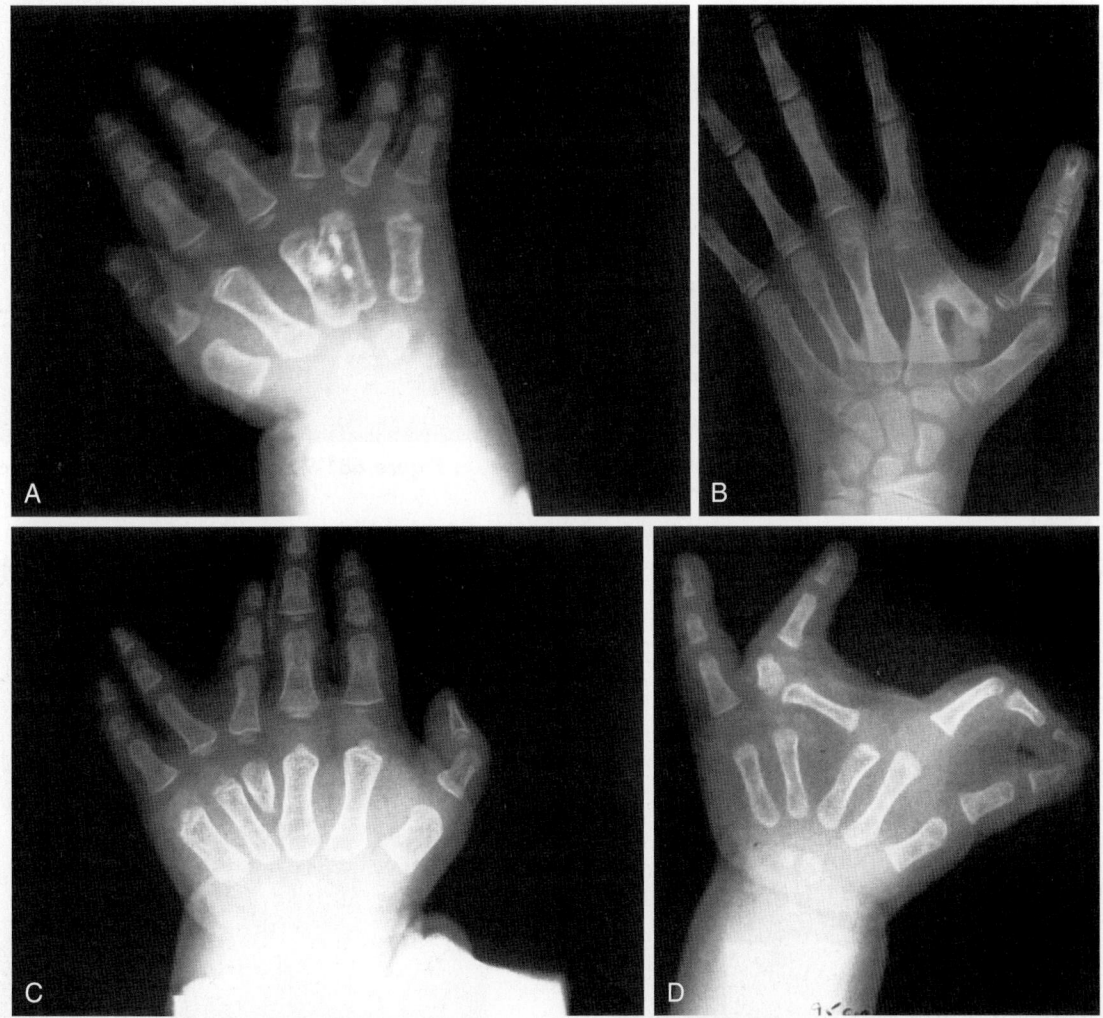

Figure 681-7 Several types of central polydactyly are recognized. Type I central polydactyly is characterized by no skeletal attachment of a soft-tissue mass. (No illustration of this unusual type is provided.) **A,** Type IIA central polydactyly: duplication on a common metacarpal or phalanx without syndactyly. **B,** Type IIB central polydactyly: duplication on a common metacarpal or phalanx with syndactyly to adjacent digits, which is often manifested as an extra digit hidden within a syndactyly. **C,** Type III central polydactyly. A complete duplication, including the metacarpal, is a rare anomaly. **D,** Relationship of central polydactyly and cleft hand. *(From From Ho C: Disorders of the upper extremity. In Herring JA, editor: Tachdjian's pediatric orthopaedics, ed 5, Philadelphia, 2014, WB Saunders, Fig. 15-99, p. 416.)*

degree of involvement. Less-well-formed digits can be treated with suture ligation. Well-formed digits require reconstructive procedures that preserve important structures such as the collateral ligaments and nail folds (Fig. 681-8).

Thumb Hypoplasia

Hypoplasia of the thumb is a challenging condition for both the patient and the doctor. The thumb represents approximately 40% of hand function. A less-than-optimal thumb can severely limit a patient's function as the patient grows and develops. Hypoplasia of the thumb can range from being mild with slight shortening and underdeveloped musculature to complete absence of the thumb (Fig. 681-9). Radiographs are useful to help determine osseous abnormalities. The most important finding on physical exam is the presence or absence of a stable carpometacarpal joint. This finding helps guide surgical treatment.

Treatment

If the thumb has a stable carpometacarpal joint, reconstruction is advised. Key elements of thumb reconstruction include rebuilding the ulnar collateral ligament of the metacarpophalangeal joint, tendon transfers to aid thumb abduction, and procedures to deepen the web space.

If a stable carpometacarpal joint is not present or the thumb is completely absent, **pollicization** (surgical construction of a thumb from a finger) is the definitive treatment. Pollicization is a complex procedure rotating the index finger along its neurovascular pedicle to form a thumb. This procedure is typically performed at around 1 yr of age and may be followed by subsequent procedures to deepen the web space or augment abduction (Fig. 681-10).

Syndactyly

Failure of the individual digits to separate during development produces syndactyly. Syndactyly is one of the more common anomalies

Table 681-5	Wassel Classification of Thumb Duplication
TYPE	**CHARACTERISTICS**
I	Bifid distal phalanx
II	Duplicate distal phalanx
III	Bifid proximal phalanx
IV	Duplicate proximal phalanx
V	Bifid metacarpal
VI	Duplicate metacarpal
VII	Triphalangeal component

Adapted from Wassel, HD: The results of surgery for polydactyly of the thumb. A review, Clin Orthop 125:175–193, 1969.

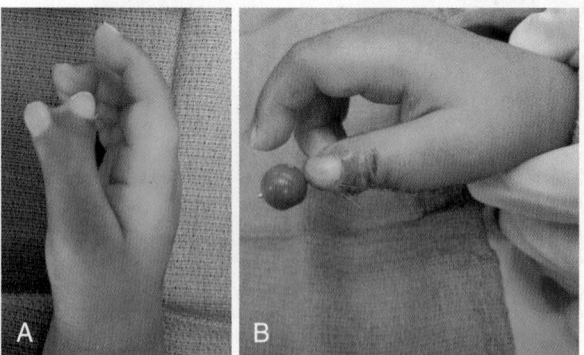

Figure 681-8 Pre- **(A)** and postoperative **(B)** pictures of a Wassel II thumb duplication.

observed in the upper limb (Table 681-6). It is seen in 0.5 of 1,000 live births. Syndactyly can be classified as simple (skin attachments only), complicated (bone and tendon attachments), complete (fusion to the tips, including the nail), or incomplete (simple webbing).

Treatment

Division of the conjoined digits should be considered before the 2nd yr of life. Border digits should be divided earlier (3-6 mo) because of concern for tethered growth of digits of unequal length. Digits of similar size, such as the ring and middle, may wait until the child is older to consider separation. Reconstruction of the web space and nail folds as well as appropriate skin-grafting techniques must be used to ensure the best possible functional and cosmetic result (Fig. 681-11).

Fingertip Injuries

Young children are fascinated with doorjambs or car doors and other tight spaces, making crush injuries to the fingertips quite common.

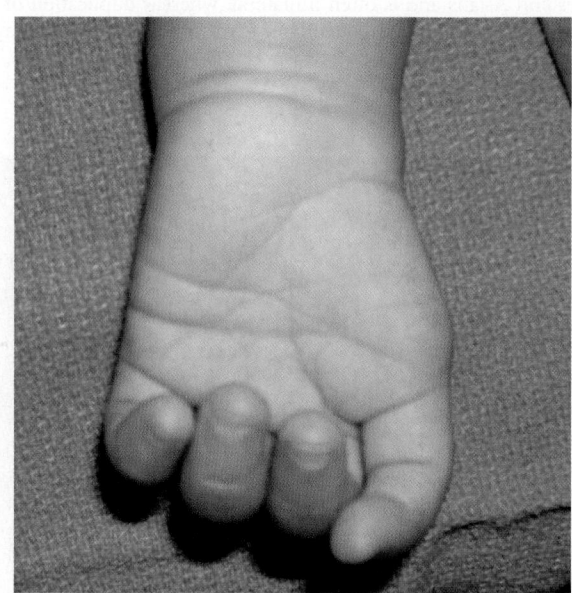

Figure 681-9 Congenital absence of the thumb.

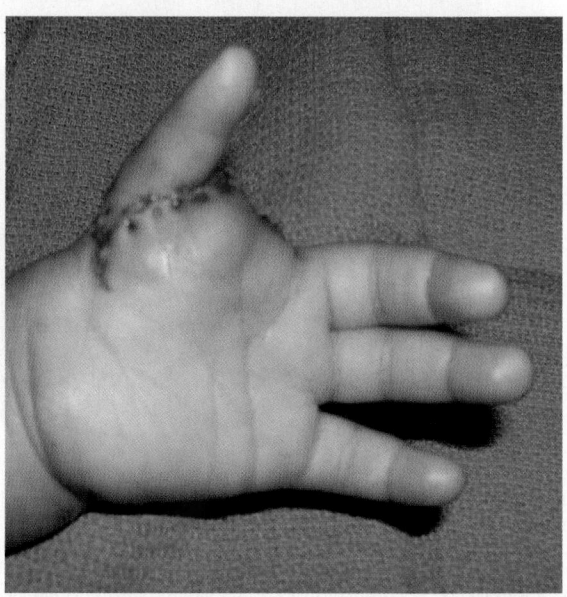

Figure 681-10 Postsurgical image after pollicization.

Injury can range from a simple subungual hematoma to complete amputation of part or the entire fingertip. Radiographs are important to rule out fractures. Physeal fractures associated with nail bed injuries are **open fractures** with a high risk of osteomyelitis, growth arrest, and deformity if not treated promptly with formal surgical debridement and reduction. Tuft fractures involving the very distal portion of the distal phalanx are common and require little specific treatment other than that for the soft-tissue injury.

The treatment of the soft-tissue injury depends on the type of injury. For suture repairs, only absorbable sutures should be used, because suture removal from a young child's fingertip can require sedation or general anesthesia. If a subungual hematoma exists but the nail is normal and no displaced fracture exists, the nail need not be removed for nail bed repair. If the nail is torn or avulsed, the nail should be removed, the nail bed and skin should be repaired with absorbable sutures, and the nail (or a piece of foil if the nail is absent) should be replaced under the eponychial fold to prevent scar adhesion of the eponychial fold to the nail bed that can prevent nail regrowth.

Table 681-6	Syndromes Associated with Syndactyly
Apert syndrome	Trisomy 21
Carpenter syndrome	Fetal hydantoin syndrome
de Lange syndrome	Laurence-Moon-Biedl syndrome
Holt-Oram syndrome	Fanconi pancytopenia
Orofaciodigital syndrome	Trisomy 13
Polysyndactyly	Trisomy 18

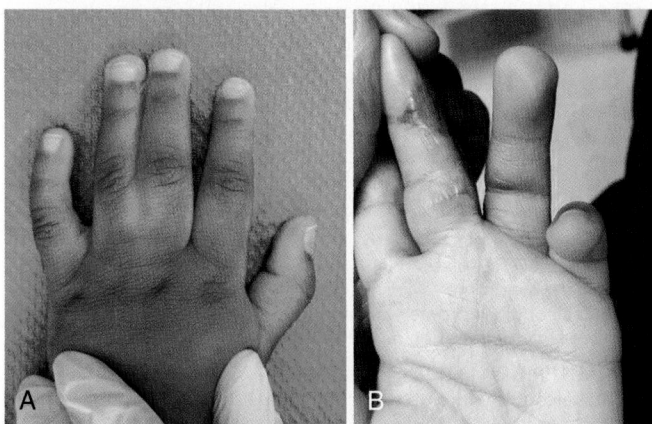

Figure 681-11 Pre- and postoperative pictures of a simple incomplete syndactyly.

If the fingertip is completely amputated, treatment depends on the level of amputation and the age of the child. Distal amputations of skin and fat in children younger than 2 yr of age can be replaced as a composite graft with a reasonable chance of surviving. Similar amputations in older children can heal without replacing the skin as long as no bone is exposed and the amputated area is small. A variety of coverage procedures exist for amputations through the mid-portion of the nail. Amputations at or proximal to the proximal edge of the fingernail should be referred emergently to a replant center for consideration for microvascular replantation. When referring, all amputated parts should be saved, wrapped in saline-soaked gauze, placed in a water-tight bag, and then placed in ice water. Ice should never directly contact the part, because it can cause severe osmotic and thermal injury.

Trigger Thumb and Fingers
The flexor tendons for the thumb and fingers pass through fibrous tunnels made up of a series of pulleys on the volar surface of the digits. These tunnels, for reasons that are not well understood, can become tight at the most proximal or first annular pulley. Swelling of the underlying tendon occurs, and the tendon no longer glides under the pulley. In children, the most common digit involved is the thumb. It has classically been thought to be a congenital problem, but prospective screening studies of large numbers of neonates have failed to find a single case in a newborn child. The incidence of trigger thumb is approximately 3 per 1,000 children at 1 yr of age. Trauma is rarely a feature of the history, and the condition is often painless. Overall function is rarely impaired. A trigger thumb typically manifests with the inability to fully extend the thumb interphalangeal joint. A palpable nodule can be felt in the flexor pollicis longus tendon at the base of the thumb metacarpal phalangeal joint volarly. Other conditions can mimic trigger thumb, including the thumb-in-palm deformity of cerebral palsy. Similar findings in the fingers (index through small) are much less common and may be associated with inflammatory conditions such as juvenile rheumatoid arthritis (Fig. 681-12).

Treatment
Trigger thumbs spontaneously resolve in up to 30% of children in whom they are diagnosed before 1 yr of age. Spontaneous resolution beyond that age is not common. Corticosteroid injections are effective in adults but are not effective in children and risk injury to the nearby digital nerves. Surgical release of the first annular pulley is curative and is generally performed between 1 and 3 yr of age. Treatment of trigger fingers other than the thumb in children involves evaluation and treatment of any underlying inflammatory process and in some cases surgical decompression of the flexor sheath and possible flexor tendon partial excision.

Bibliography is available at Expert Consult.

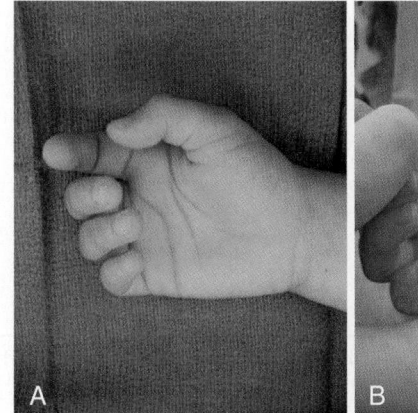
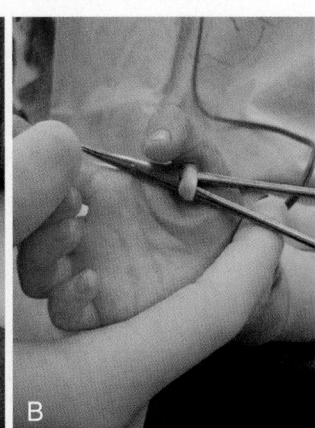
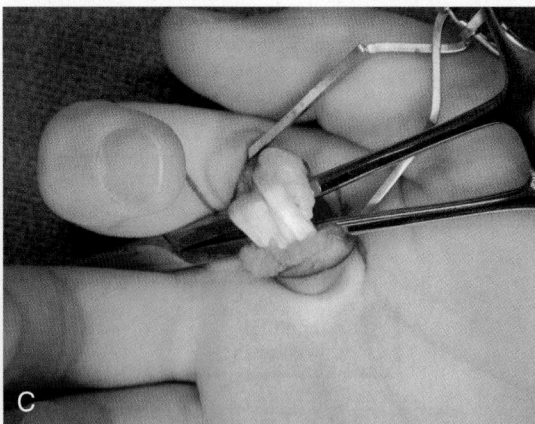

Figure 681-12 A, Clinical picture of trigger thumb in a 2 yr old. Note flexed posture of the interphalangeal joint. **B,** Intraoperative picture of flexor tendon following release of A1 pulley. **C,** Intraoperative picture of benign growth along flexor tendon causing triggering in an index finger.

Chapter 682
Arthrogryposis
Helen M. Horstmann, Christine M. Conroy, and Richard S. Davidson

Arthrogryposis multiplex congenita refers to a heterogeneous group of muscular, neurologic, and connective tissue anomalies that present with 2 or more joint contractures at birth as well as muscle weakness. It is associated with abnormal contraction of muscle fibers, causing reduced mobility with a decreased active and passive arc of motion. Arthrogryposis is not a specific diagnosis but a descriptive term with various etiologies and complex clinical features, including multiple congenital contractures of various limb joints. It is associated with 200-300 different disorders encompassing malformations, malfunction, and neurologic deficiencies.

Approximately 1% of all births show some form of contractures of the joints ranging from unilateral clubfoot to pervasive, crippling contractures due to amyoplasia. Overall incidents of arthrogryposis have been reported to be 1 in 5,000-10,000 live births with equal gender ratios.

Although children with arthrogryposis have many other problems, such as micrognathia, nutrition issues, and sucking issues, here we focus on the orthopedic problems frequently seen in this group of children. In the absence of central nervous system lesions, many children have normal intelligence.

ETIOLOGY
In humans, both the intrinsic and extrinsic causes of arthrogryposis are categorized into 6 groups (Fig. 682-1), including a multitude of disorders (Table 682-1).

Neurologic Abnormalities
As one of the most common causes of arthrogryposis, neurologic abnormalities are present in 70-80% of cases. Patchy damage to the anterior horn cells of the spinal cord can lead to characteristic limb posturing of arthrogryposis. Neurologic disorders, such as spinal muscular atrophy and anterior horn disease, including Werdnig-Hoffmann disease, are associated with arthrogryposis; however, the type of anterior horn cell involvement is usually not from spinal muscular atrophy syndrome (Werdnig-Hoffman disease). Other, less-common neurologic disorders include neonatal myasthenia and myotonic dystrophy.

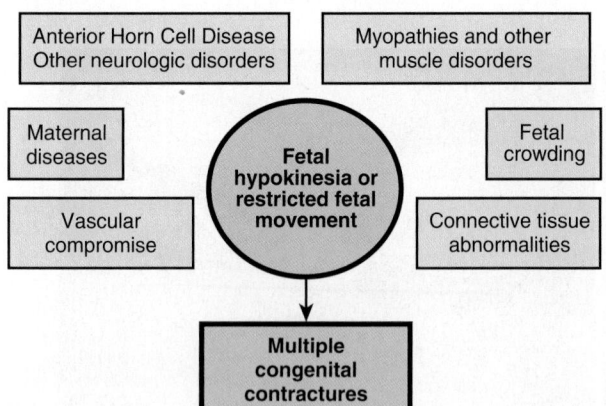

Figure 682-1 Etiology of arthrogryposis. *(Modified from Hall JG: Arthrogryposis multiplex congenital: Etiology, genetics, classification, diagnostic approach, and general aspects. J Pediatr Orthop B 6:159–166, 1996.)*

Table 682-1	Associated Etiologies of Arthrogryposis

ARTHROGRYPOSIS CAUSED BY NERVOUS SYSTEM DISORDERS
- Focal anterior horn cell deficiency
- Generalized anterior horn cell deficiency
- Structural brain disorder/damage
- Uncertain location
(Spastic conditions are excluded)

DISTAL ARTHROGRYPOSIS SYNDROMES
- Type I dominant distal
- Type IIa dominant distal (Gordon syndrome)
- Type IIe distal
- Digitotalar dysmorphism
- Trismus pseudocamptodactyly
- Distal distribution, type not specified

PTERYGIUM SYNDROMES
- Multiple pterygium syndrome
- Lethal multiple pterygium syndrome
- Popliteal pterygium syndrome
- Ptosis, scoliosis, pterygia
- Antecubital webbing syndrome (Liebenberg)

MYOPATHIES
- Emery-Dreifuss muscular dystrophy
- Hypotonia, myopathy, mild contractures

ABNORMALITIES OF JOINTS AND CONTIGUOUS TISSUE
- Congenital contractural arachnodactyly
- Freeman-Sheldon syndrome
- Laxity or hypertonicity with intrauterine dislocation and contractures
- Larsen syndrome
- Spondyloepimetaphyseal dysplasia with joint laxity
- Trisomy 18, extended breech position with bilateral hip dislocation
- Siblings with bifid humeri, hypertelorism, and hip and knee joint dislocations

SKELETAL DISORDERS
- Diastrophic dysplasia
- Parastremmatic dysplasia
- Kniest dysplasia
- Metatropic dysplasia
- Campomelic dysplasia
- Schwartz syndrome
- Fetal alcohol syndrome with synostoses
- Osteogenesis imperfecta with bowing/contractures

INTRAUTERINE/MATERNAL FACTORS
- Fetal alcohol syndrome with contractures
- Infections
- Untreated maternal systemic lupus erythematosus
- Intrauterine fetal constraint
- Deformity (pressure)
- Amniotic fluid leakage
- Multiple pregnancies
- Intrauterine tumors
- Disruption (bands)

MISCELLANEOUS
- Pseudotrisomy 18 with contractures
- Roberts pseudothalidomide syndrome
- Deafness with distal contractures
- VACTERL association
- Multiple abnormalities and contractures not otherwise specified
- ARC

SINGLE JOINT
- Campomelia
- Symphalangism
- "Trigger" finger

ARC, arthrogryposis, renal tubular acidosis, cholestasis; VACTERL, vertebral defects, imperforate anus, congenital heart disease, tracheoesophageal fistula, renal and limb defects.
Modified from Mennen U, Van Heest A, Ezaki MB, et al: Arthrogryposis multiplex congenita. J Hand Surg Br 30:5:468–474, 2005. Copyright 2005 The British Society for Surgery of the Hand.

Muscular Abnormalities

These rare abnormalities affect the function and structure of the muscles. Some muscular diseases associated with arthrogryposis are muscular dystrophies, congenital muscular dystrophies (central core, nemaline, centronuclear), intrauterine myositis and mitochondrial diseases.

Limited Intrauterine Spacing

With a less than 0.1% occurrence rate, uterine constraint is rarely the primary cause of arthrogryposis. Maternal uterine anomalies will occasionally increase contractures of fetal limbs with arthrogryposis already existing. Other known causes are lack of amniotic fluid within the uterus and tumors, such as fibroids that can impinge on uterine space, preventing movement.

Connective Tissue Abnormalities

When the tendons, bones, joints, and joint lining develop atypically, decrease in fetal movement causes congenital contractures. Diseases such as diastrophic dysplasia and metatropic dwarfism result from connective tissue not developing properly. These are specific diagnoses resulting in limited joint motion and not true distal arthrogryposis. Other cases show that individuals who lack normal joint movement have distal joint involvement because the connective tissue develops normally but does not attach to the proper location around a joint bone or joint.

Maternal Diseases

Maternal diseases, such as multiple sclerosis, diabetes mellitus, myasthenia gravis, maternal hyperthermia, infection, drugs, and trauma, are associated with an increased incidence of arthrogryposis. In approximately 10% of neonates born to mothers with myasthenia gravis, maternal antibodies enter the fetal circulation through the placenta, causing transient myasthenia gravis; this inhibits fetal acetylcholine receptors, which leads to damaged fetal muscles.

Intrauterine Vascular Compromise

Inadequate vascular supply to the fetus causes fetal hypoxia resulting in anterior horn cell death, which decreases neurologic and myopathic function, resulting in fetal akinesia and secondary joint contractures. Multiple congenital contractures have been reported in individuals after bleeding throughout pregnancy or after a failed attempt at terminating the pregnancy.

CLASSIFICATION

Arthrogryposis multiplex congenita is divided into subgroups with different signs, symptoms, and causes as a practical way to make a differential diagnosis. Disorders involving primarily limbs such as **amyoplasia** and **distal arthrogryposis** are the most common subgroups (Table 682-2). Disorders involving limbs *and* other body parts typically represent a form of *multiple pterygium,* which is characterized by a web-like membrane that forms across joints affecting a child's ability to extend and causing fixed flexion. Disorders with limb involvement and abnormal neurologic function are caused by atypical central nervous system, peripheral nervous system, and damaged or absent anterior horn cells.

Amyoplasia, also known as *classic arthrogryposis,* is a sporadic symmetric disorder that causes fibrotic replacement of the muscles. Symptoms include internally rotated and adducted shoulders, extended elbows, pronated forearms, flexed fingers and wrists, dislocated hips, feet with severe equinovarus contractures, and extended knees. Involved muscles are hypoplastic and fibrotic. Often patients have midfacial hemangioma. Intelligence is usually normal (Figs. 682-2 and 682-3).

Distal arthrogryposis is an autosomal dominant disorder that primarily affects the distal joints of the limbs. Characteristics of the upper limbs are medially overlapping fingers, clenched fists, ulnar deviation of fingers, camptodactyly, and hypoplasia. Lower limbs show talipes equinovarus, calcaneovalgus, vertical talus, or metatarsus varus (Fig. 682-4).

Ten different types of distal arthrogryposis have been categorized based on specific traits they share with each other.

MANAGEMENT OF ORTHOPEDIC PROBLEMS OF ARTHROGRYPOSIS

When a child is born with arthrogryposis, the many stiff or dislocated joints pose issues of timing and best practices of management.

Table 682-2	Current Labels and OMIM Numbers for the Distal Arthrogryposis Syndromes
SYNDROME	**OMIM NUMBER**
Distal arthrogryposis type 1	108120
Distal arthrogryposis type 2A (Freeman-Sheldon syndrome)	193700
Distal arthrogryposis type 2B (Sheldon-Hall syndrome)	601680
Distal arthrogryposis type 3 (Gordon syndrome)	114300
Distal arthrogryposis type 4 (scoliosis)	609128
Distal arthrogryposis type 5 (ophthalmoplegia, ptosis)	108145
Distal arthrogryposis type 6 (sensorineural hearing loss)	108200
Distal arthrogryposis type 7 (trismus-pseudocamptodactyly)	158300
Distal arthrogryposis type 8 (autosomal dominant multiple pterygium syndrome)	178110
Distal arthrogryposis type 9 (congenital contractural arachnodactyly)	121050
Distal arthrogryposis type 10 (congenital plantar contractures)	187370

From Bamshad M, Van Heest AE, Pleasure D: Arthrogryposis: a review and update. J Bone Joint Surg Am 91 Suppl 4:40–46, 2009, Table 1, p. 43.

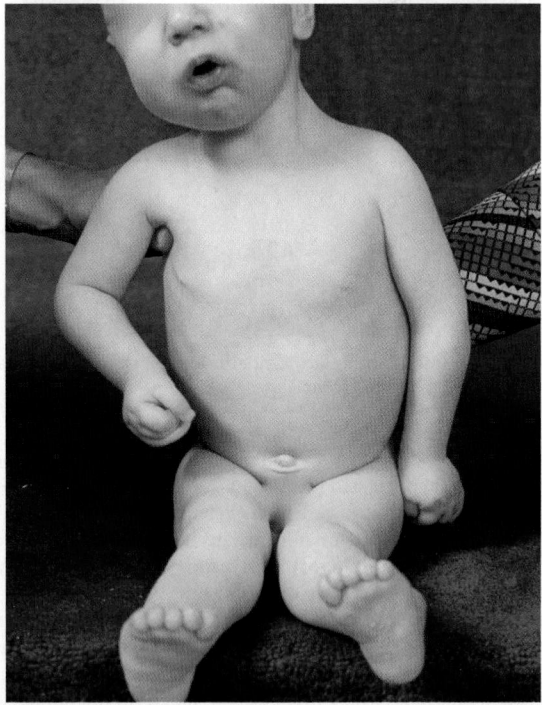

Figure 682-2 Infant with stiff elbows, wrists, fingers, dislocated left hip, valgus stiff knees, and clubfeet.

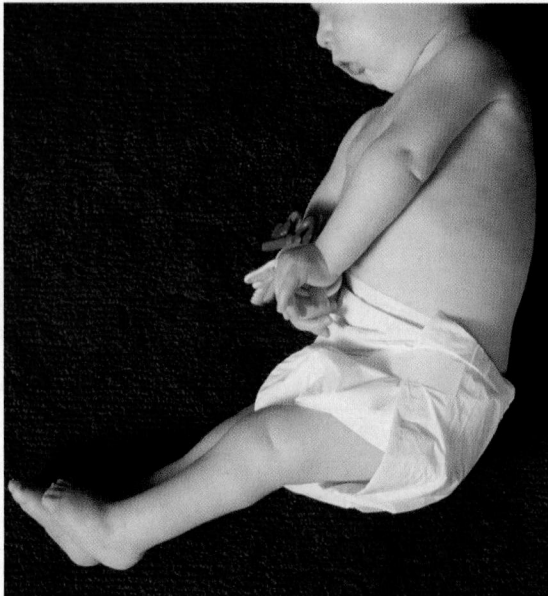

Figure 682-3 Infant with stiff elbows, wrists, fingers, dislocated left hip, clubfeet, and micrognathia.

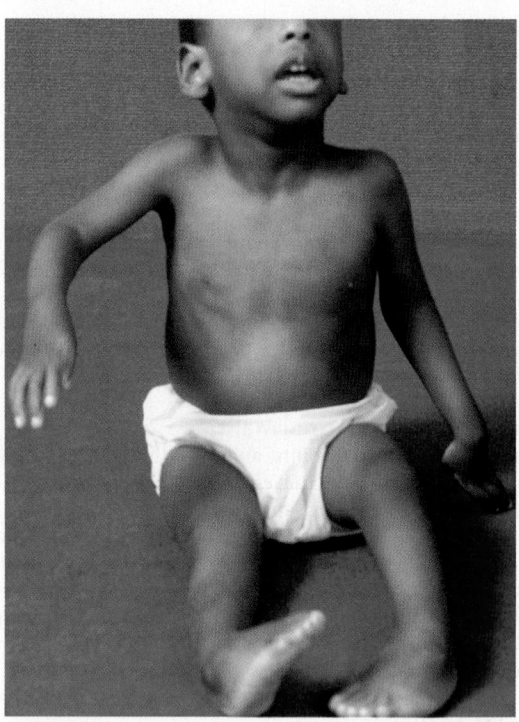

Figure 682-5 Child with stiff elbows, wrists, knees, and clubfeet.

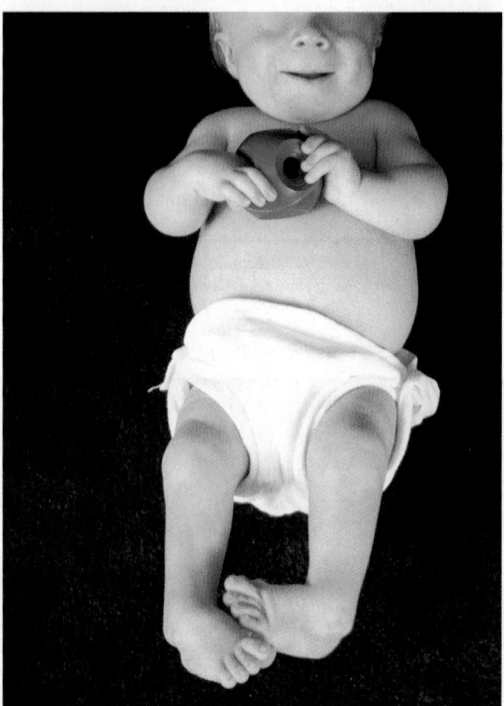

Figure 682-4 Infant with club feet, stiff knees, dislocated hips, stiff fingers, and facial hemangioma.

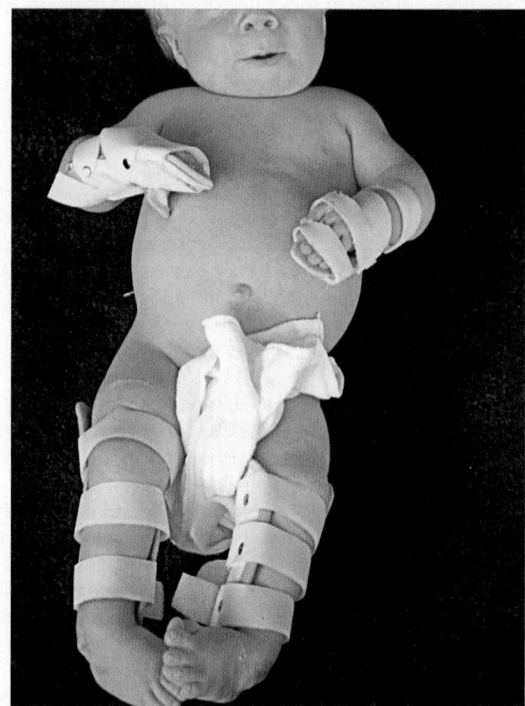

Figure 682-6 Infant with splints to extend metatarsophalangeal joints, wrists, and knees.

Typically a child can have stiff elbows, dislocated hips, dislocated, hyperextended or contracted knees, and clubfeet (Fig. 682-5). The stiffness and deformity need to be aggressively addressed through a combination of modalities. A team of clinicians including therapists for the upper and lower extremities, orthotists, and orthopedic surgeons will be involved.

Initially, passive range-of-motion exercises and judicious splinting directed and assisted by physical and occupational therapy will help to address the various deformities. Splinting and casting can be augmented by a taping program which can be taught to the family so that the taping can be redone frequently to take advantage of improved range of motion. The ingenuity of the therapists and/or orthotist to create the right splints and braces using appropriate thermoplastics, neoprene, Velcro, and other materials can be simple yet effective (Fig. 682-6).

The therapeutic and orthopedic goal for the child with arthrogrypotic limb deformities is to achieve maximal joint motion and to optimize joint position for function. In the lower extremities, the foot needs to be plantigrade. The knees need to have optimal motion for sitting and standing. Hips need to be stabilized especially if the child has walking potential. In the upper extremities, the goals should

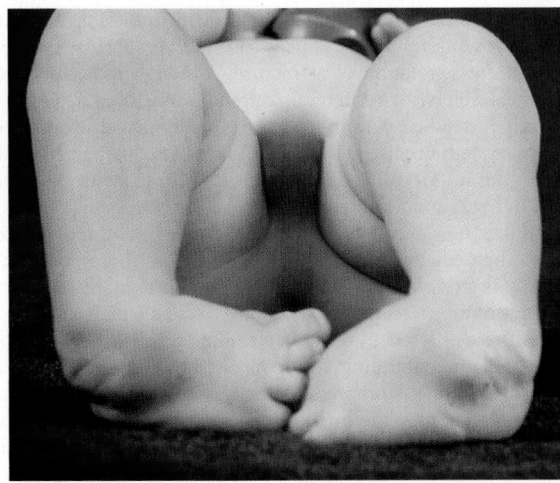

Figure 682-7 Clubfeet in infant with arthrogryposis.

include positioning of 1 arm for feeding and the other for toileting in cases where there is extreme stiffness. Two-handed activities require some symmetry, which can be a challenging goal with extreme contractures and limited muscle strength.

Although scoliosis is common, it usually does not become a problem until adolescence.

FOOT PROBLEMS

Clubfoot deformities are the most commonly seen deformities with arthrogryposis (Fig. 682-7). A clubfoot has components of hindfoot equinus, midfoot varus, and forefoot adduction. Feet in arthrogryposis tend to be resistant to improvement but the traditional methods of treatment are nevertheless employed. Casting is begun shortly after birth in a method known as the Ponseti method. Casts are changed weekly until a plateau is reached and heel cord lengthening is needed. Other deformities such as vertical talus are also seen and are addressed in a similar approach although with appropriately differing techniques.

Persistent stiffness often leads to more comprehensive soft tissue releases. This is typically done around age 6-12 mo and is followed by 3 mo of further casting and additional bracing as needed, especially as the foot is growing. When deformities are not corrected in early childhood, additional bony surgery may be needed later. Some of the approaches to this involve bony wedge osteotomies, lateral column lengthening, bone decancellation or talectomy. Ilizarov ring or multiaxial monolateral external fixation with or without osteotomies are used in late correction of residual deformities.

Children with significant deformities are often in ankle foot orthoses through much of their lives to avoid deformity recurrence and to augment the standing base due to weak leg muscles. A plantigrade, pain free, stable foot is the goal of foot management. Foot stiffness is anticipated and unavoidable in arthrogryposis involving the foot.

KNEE PROBLEMS

Knee issues, including knee extension or flexion, subluxation, and stiffness, respond well to therapy and splinting. Knee flexion is more common in arthrogryposis. Infrequently it can structurally be complex and associated with skin webbing known as pterygiums. Pterygiums are resistant to nonsurgical intervention and require plastic Z lengthenings. In the case of a flexion contracture, the quadriceps musculature is often deficient and weak. Sometimes the casting and splinting of the knee contractures is insufficient. Hamstring lengthenings with additional posterior knee capsular releases are often needed.

In the case of knee hyperextension, the quadriceps are sometimes fibrotic and weak in spite of seeming to overpower the hamstrings. Casting and splinting should begin shortly after birth, which can be done in conjunction with clubfoot casting following the principles of Ponseti. If splinting and therapy fail, lengthening of the quadriceps can

be achieved through release of the lateral medial quadriceps, with proximal detachment of the rectus femoris, lengthening of the quadriceps either percutaneously or through a mini open procedure which may minimize scarring.

Long-standing stiffness may lead to joint surface flattening permanently reducing the arc of motion. Repositioning the arc of motion may improve sitting or standing, a choice to be made by the patient, family and physician. Follow up bracing can help to compensate for weak, fibrotic muscles of the legs.

HIP PROBLEMS

Teratologic hip dislocations are common within the spectrum of arthrogryposis and usually require open reduction of the hip. Hips in a child with less upper-extremity involvement and more supple hips that are not pathologically stiff *may* respond to early treatment with a Pavlik harness. Knee hyperextension can often be treated with physical therapy and serial casting. Careful observation of the hip during knee flexion as tightening of the quadriceps and hip flexors can push the hip into posterior dislocation. Once some knee flexion has been achieved, the Pavlik harness can be useful in further flexing the knee and maintaining hip stability in the infant. Most often the hips are stiff and not reducible closed. For these, open reduction with pelvic reconstruction and femoral osteotomy are commonly required, typically at 1 yr of age. There is some controversy about reducing bilateral hip dislocations as a high failure rate can result in asymmetry of the pelvis, pain, leg length inequality, and stiffness. If a child has little ambulation potential, he may do as well retaining the bilateral hip dislocations and positioning the hips for sitting. Management judgment should be made in conjunction with the family guided by a pediatric hip surgeon.

Ambulation

As would be expected walking is more difficult for children with arthrogryposis due to the muscle weakness and limited joint motion. Children with arthrogryposis who walk have lower activity levels and take fewer steps than their peers. Not surprisingly muscle fatigue and pain on exertion was noted in a study that included adults with distal arthrogryposis.

UPPER-EXTREMITY PROBLEMS

If splinting and a movement exercise program do not result in optimally functional upper extremities, surgical management may improve use of the arms of the child with arthrogryposis. A typical child with arthrogrypotic involvement of the upper extremities has internally rotated arms, extended elbows, flexed wrists, and thumb in palm or clasp thumb deformities (see Figs. 682-2 and 682-3).

Treatment is geared toward optimizing use of the arms and hands particularly for critical activities of daily living, such as feeding and toileting. Therapy to improve motion of the joints is started immediately after birth. Pediatric hand therapists are the optimal leaders of the mobility treatment program. Therapy is augmented by use of splints so that less-extensive surgery will be required. The elbow is the critical length adjuster of the arm, allowing the arm to reach out as is necessary for toileting or to approach the mouth for feeding. If necessary, lack of these motions can be compensated by modified silverware and other adaptive equipment, including arm extenders for grabbing.

Surgery of the Upper Extremity

Surgical correction of arthrogrypotic upper extremity contractures should be started after 1-3 mo and completed by age 12 mo so that the child can optimize his or her motor development. This allows for improved results optimizing the joint growth remodeling plasticity. One-stage procedures yield the best results. Delays in surgery result in more problems of intraarticular adhesions as well as fixed joint incongruity.

Shoulder

Because of the rotational capacity of the shoulder derotation osteotomy of the humerus is only occasionally needed. This is usually done in later childhood.

Elbow

A stiff elbow that does not respond to therapy requires surgical intervention starting with soft tissue and capsular release. Capsulotomy of the posterior elbow combined with a V-Y or Z reconstructive lengthening of the triceps allows improved elbow flexion. The triceps may need to be lengthened. Muscle transfer to the forearm can permit active elbow flexion. Each child needs individual assessment as to available flexor source. Most commonly available is the triceps. An elbow with some flexion is extremely important for arm function. Use of the triceps can create elbow flexion overpowering and contracture.

Wrist

Wrist flexion deformity is improved with soft-tissue balancing as well as partial carpectomies. The carpectomies need to be trapezoidal with more removed from the dorsum and the radial side to balance the wrist flexion contracture as well as the tendency for ulnar deviation. Thumb adduction may require an adductor release with an opponensplasty. Tendon transfers such as transfer of the extensor indicis pollicis to the extensor pollicis longus is helpful for improved function of the thumb in clasp thumb deformity.

Finger stiffness and wrist contractures often respond to therapy and bracing without need for surgery.

Scoliosis

Scoliosis is frequent in arthrogrypotic children, although the reported incidence of between 28% and 66% is probably skewed upward in reports as they reflect the experience of scoliosis surgeons. Scoliosis can be congenital or paralytic. The scoliosis is often accompanied by hip contractures associated with hip dislocation and compensatory lumbar lordosis. Curves <30 degrees can be treated initially with bracing in a thoracolumbar spinal orthosis (TLSO brace). After 40 degrees, spinal fusion is warranted.

Surgical Staging

At Children's Hospital of Philadelphia, surgical treatment of the lower limbs usually begins distally and works proximally. The feet are corrected around 6 mo of age, the knees around 8 mo of age, and the hips around 12 mo of age as pelvic osteotomy is often needed to stabilize the hips properly.

The upper extremities are corrected during infancy when the child is seen early. Hand, physical, and occupational therapy are a critical part of the team to optimize function and function prior to and after surgery. Further surgery as a child may be needed to tweak and optimize functional use of the upper and lower extremities.

Bibliography is available at Expert Consult.

Chapter **683**

Common Fractures

Keith D. Baldwin, Lawrence Wells,
and John P. Dormans

Trauma is a leading cause of death and disability in children older than 1 yr of age (see Chapter 5.1). Several factors make fractures of the immature skeleton different from those involving the mature skeleton. The anatomy, biomechanics, and physiology of the pediatric skeletal system are different from those of adults. This results in different fracture patterns (Fig. 683-1), diagnostic challenges, and management techniques specific to children to preserve growth and function.

Epiphyseal lines, rarefaction, dense growth lines, congenital fractures, and pseudofractures appear on radiographs, which could confuse the interpretation of a fracture. Although most fractures in children heal well with indifferent treatment, some fractures terminate disastrously if handled with inexpertise. The differences in the pediatric skeletal system predispose children to injuries different from those of adults. The important differences are the presence of periosseous cartilage, physes, and a thicker, stronger, more osteogenic periosteum that produces new bone, called *callus*, more rapidly and in greater amounts. The pediatric bone has low density and more porosity. The low density is from lower mineral content and the increased porosity is the result of an increased number of haversian canals and vascular channels. These differences result in a comparatively lower modulus of elasticity and lower bending strength. The bone in children can fail either in tension or in compression; because the fracture lines do not propagate as in adults, there is less chance of comminuted fractures. Hence, pediatric bone can crush, splinter, and break incompletely, as opposed to adult bone which generally breaks like glass and may comminute.

A common teaching is that joint injuries, dislocation, and ligament disruptions are infrequent in children. Although this is generally true, MRI studies show that ligament damage in ankle injuries may not be as unusual as once thought. Damage to a contiguous physis is more likely. Interdigitating mammillary bodies and the perichondrial ring enhance the strength of the physes. Biomechanically, the physes are not as strong as the ligaments or metaphyseal bone. The physis is most resistant to traction and least resistant to torsional forces. The periosteum is loosely attached to the shaft of bone and adheres densely to the physeal periphery. The periosteum is usually injured in all fractures, but it is less likely to have complete circumferential rupture, because of its loose attachment to the shaft. This intact hinge or sleeve of periosteum lessens the extent of fracture displacement and assists in reduction and maintenance of reduction. The thick periosteum can also act as an impediment to closed reduction, particularly if the fracture has penetrated the periosteum, or in reduction of displaced growth plate.

683.1 Unique Characteristics of Pediatric Fractures

Keith D. Baldwin, Lawrence Wells,
and John P. Dormans

FRACTURE REMODELING

Remodeling is the third and final phase in biology of fracture healing, preceded by the inflammatory and reparative phases. This occurs from a combination of appositional bone deposition on the concavity of deformity, resorption on the convexity, and asymmetric physeal growth. Thus, reduction accuracy is somewhat less important than it is in adults (Fig. 683-2). The 3 major factors that have a bearing on the potential for angular correction are skeletal age, distance to the joint, and orientation to the joint axis. The rotational deformity and angular deformity not in the axis of the joint motion are less likely to remodel. Remodeling is best when the fracture occurs close to the physis, the child has more growth remaining, has less deformity to remodel, and is adjacent to a rapidly growing physis (i.e., the proximal humerus). Remodeling typically occurs over the next several months following injury throughout skeletal maturity. Skeletal maturity is reached in girls between 13 and 15 yr of age, and in boys between 14 and 17 yr of age.

OVERGROWTH

Physeal stimulation from the hyperemia associated with fracture healing causes overgrowth. It is usually prominent in long bones such as the femur. The growth acceleration is usually present for 6 mo to 1 yr following the injury. Femoral fractures in children younger than 10 yr of age often overgrow by 1-3 cm. If external fixation or casting is employed, bayonet apposition of bone may be preferred to

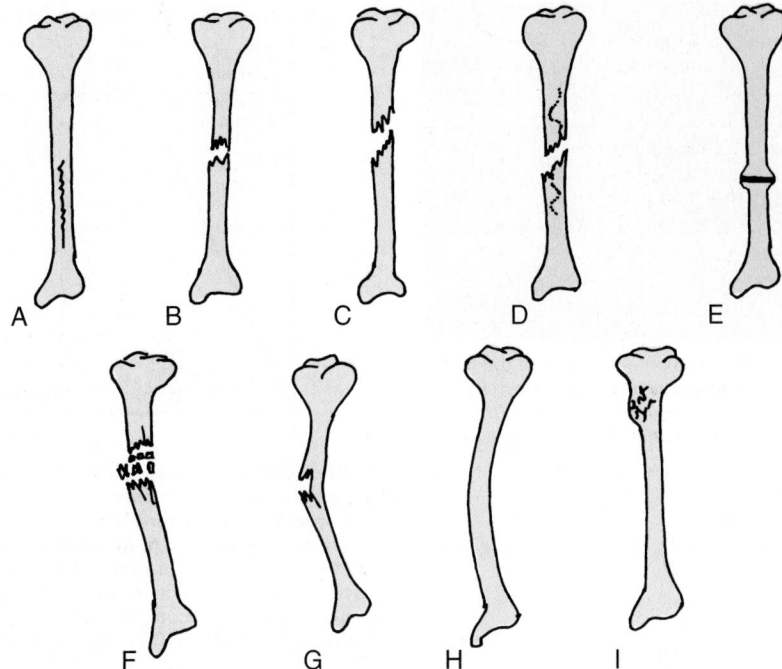

Figure 683-1 Illustration of fracture patterns. **A,** Longitudinal fracture line parallel to bony axis. **B,** Transverse fracture line perpendicular to bony axis. **C,** Oblique fracture line at angle to bony axis. **D,** Spiral fracture line runs a curvilinear course to the bony axis. **E,** Impacted fractured bone ends compressed together. **F,** Comminuted fragmentation of bone into 3 or more parts. **G,** Greenstick bending of bone with incomplete fracture of convex side. **H,** Bowing bone plastic deformation. **I,** Torus buckling fracture. *(From White N, Sty R: Radiological evaluation and classification of pediatric fractures, Clin Pediatr Emerg Med 3:94–105, 2002.)*

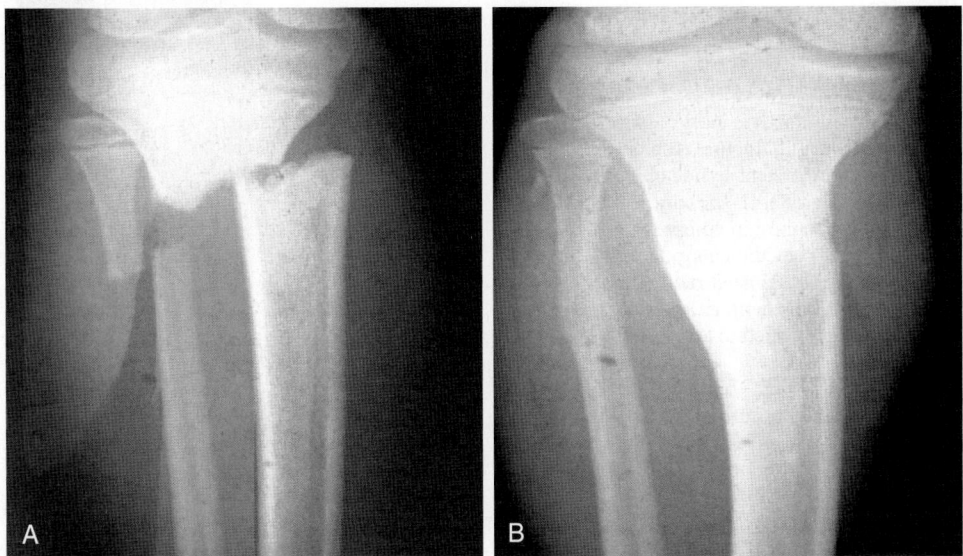

Figure 683-2 Remodeling in children is often extensive, as in this proximal tibial fracture **(A)** and as seen 1 yr later **(B)**. *(From Dormans JP: Pediatric orthopedics: introduction to trauma, Philadelphia, 2005, Mosby, p. 38.)*

compensate for the expected overgrowth. This overgrowth phenomenon will result in equal or near equal limb lengths at the conclusion of fracture remodeling if the fracture shortens less than 2 cm. After 10 yr of age, overgrowth is less of a problem and anatomic alignment is recommended. In physeal injuries, growth stimulation is associated with use of implants or fixation hardware that can cause chronic stimulus for longitudinal growth.

PROGRESSIVE DEFORMITY

Injuries to the physes can be complicated by progressive deformities with growth. The most common cause is complete or partial closure of the growth plate. This can be common in fractures of the distal

ulna, distal femur, and proximal tibia. An MRI can be helpful to diagnose percent of physeal closure after such an injury. Harris growth arrest lines may be observed in the setting of asymmetric growth and will point toward the area of growth arrest (Fig. 683-3). As a consequence, angular deformity, shortening, or both, can occur. The partial arrest may be peripheral, central, or combined. The magnitude of deformity depends on the physis involved and the amount of growth remaining.

RAPID HEALING

Children's fractures heal more quickly than adults as a result of children's growth potential and thicker, more active periosteum. As

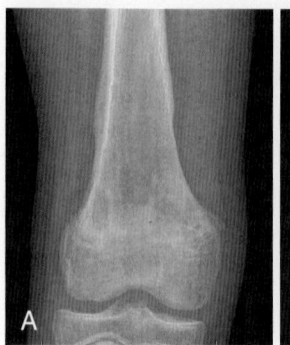
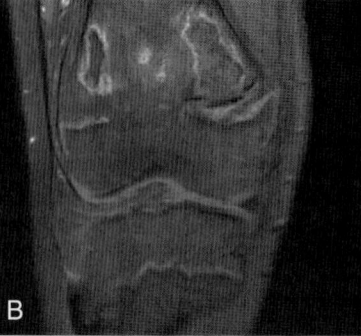

Figure 683-3 A, Harris growth arrest lines on either side of the femur pointing centrally in the femur indicating a central growth arrest. **B,** Corresponding MRI image showing central growth arrest. (*A courtesy of Keith D. Baldwin, MD, MPH, Children's Hospital of Philadelphia.*)

children approach adolescence and maturity, the rate of healing slows and becomes similar to that of an adult.

Bibliography is available at Expert Consult.

683.2 Pediatric Fracture Patterns

Keith D. Baldwin, Lawrence Wells, and John P. Dormans

The different pediatric fracture patterns are the reflection of a child's characteristic skeletal system. The majority of pediatric fractures can be managed by closed methods and heal well.

PLASTIC DEFORMATION
Plastic deformation is unique to children. It is most commonly seen in the ulna and occasionally the fibula. The fracture results from a force that produces microscopic failure on the tensile side of bone and does not propagate to the concave side (Fig. 683-4). The concave side of bone also shows evidence of microscopic failure in compression. The bone is angulated beyond its elastic limit, but the energy is insufficient to produce a fracture. Thus, no fracture line is visible radiographically (Fig. 683-5). The plastic deformation is permanent, and a bend in the ulna of <20 degrees in a 4 yr old child is expected to correct with growth.

BUCKLE OR TORUS FRACTURE
A compression failure of bone usually occurs at the junction of the metaphysis and diaphysis, especially in the distal radius (Fig. 683-6). This injury is referred to as a *torus fracture* because of its similarity to the raised band around the base of a classic Greek column. They are inherently stable and heal in 3-4 wk with simple immobilization.

GREENSTICK FRACTURE
These fractures occur when the bone is bent, and there is failure on the tensile (convex) side of the bone. The fracture line does not propagate to the concave side of the bone (Fig. 683-7). The concave side shows evidence of microscopic failure with plastic deformation. It is necessary to break the bone on the concave side because the plastic deformation recoils it back to the deformed position.

COMPLETE FRACTURES
Fractures that propagate completely through the bone are called *complete fractures*. These fractures may be classified as spiral, transverse, or oblique, depending on the direction of the fracture lines. A rotational force usually creates the spiral fractures, and reduction is easy because of the presence of an intact periosteal hinge. Oblique fractures are in the diaphysis at 30 degrees to the axis of the bone and are inherently unstable. The transverse fractures occur following a 3-point

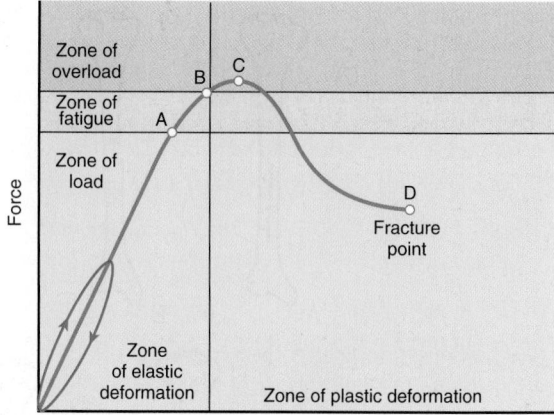

Figure 683-4 Graphic relation of bony deformation (bowing) and force (longitudinal compression) showing that the limit of an elastic response is not a fracture but plastic deformation. If the force continues, a fracture results. **A,** Reversible bowing with stress; **B,** microfractures occur; **C,** point of maximal strength; between **C** and **D,** bowing fractures; **D,** linear fracture occurs. (*Modified from Borden S IV: Roentgen recognition of acute plastic bowing of the forearm in children, Am J Roentgenol Radium Ther Nucl Med 125:524–530, 1975.*)

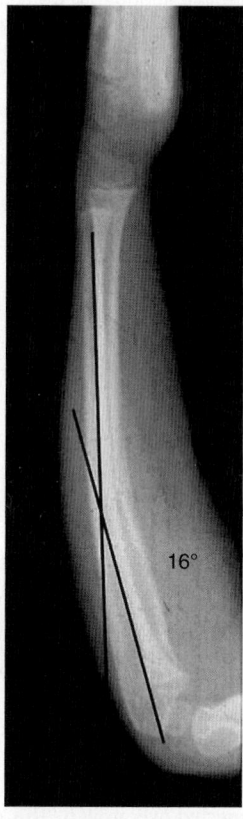

Figure 683-5 Plastic deformation is a microfailure in tension without a visible fracture line. (*Courtesy of Dr. John Flynn, Children's Hospital, Philadelphia.*)

bending force and are easily reduced by using the intact periosteum from the concave side.

EPIPHYSEAL FRACTURES
The injuries to the epiphysis involve the growth plate. There is always a potential for deformity to occur, and hence long-term observation is

necessary. The distal radial physis is the most commonly injured physis. Salter and Harris (SH) classified epiphyseal injuries into 5 groups (Table 683-1 and Fig. 683-8). This classification helps to predict the outcome of the injury and offers guidelines in formulating treatment. SH types I and II fractures usually can be managed by closed reduction techniques and do not require perfect alignment, because they tend to remodel with growth. SH type II fractures of the distal femoral epiphysis need anatomic reduction. The SH type III and IV epiphyseal fractures involve the articular surface and require anatomic alignment (<2 mm displacement) to prevent any step off and realign the growth cells of the physis. SH type V fractures are usually not diagnosed initially. They manifest in the future with growth disturbance. Other injuries to the epiphysis are avulsion injuries of the tibial spine and muscle attachments to the pelvis. Osteochondral fractures are also defined as physeal injuries that do not involve the growth plate.

CHILD ABUSE
(See also Chapter 40.)

Fractures are the second most common manifestation of child abuse after skin injury (bruises, burns/abrasions). The orthopedic surgeon sees 30-50% of physically abused children. Child abuse should be expected in nonambulatory children with lower-extremity long-bone fractures. No fracture pattern or types are pathognomonic for child abuse; any type of fracture can result from nonaccidental trauma. The fractures that suggest nonaccidental injury include femur fractures in nonambulatory children (younger than age18 months), distal femoral metaphyseal corner fractures, posterior rib fractures, scapular spinous process fractures, and proximal humeral fractures. Fractures that were unwitnessed or carry a suspicious or changing story also warrant investigation. A full skeletal survey (as opposed to a "babygram") is essential in every suspected case of child abuse, because it can demonstrate other fractures in different stages of healing. Radiographically, some systemic diseases mimic signs of child abuse, such as osteogenesis imperfecta, osteomyelitis, Caffey disease, and fatigue fractures. Many hospitals have a multidisciplinary team to evaluate and treat patients who are victims of child abuse, these teams are critical to engage early and preferably in the emergency room setting, as difficulty arises managing these emotionally charged issues in a clinic setting. Dedicated teams are most well equipped to identify and manage these issues. It is mandatory to report these cases to social welfare agencies.

Bibliography is available at Expert Consult.

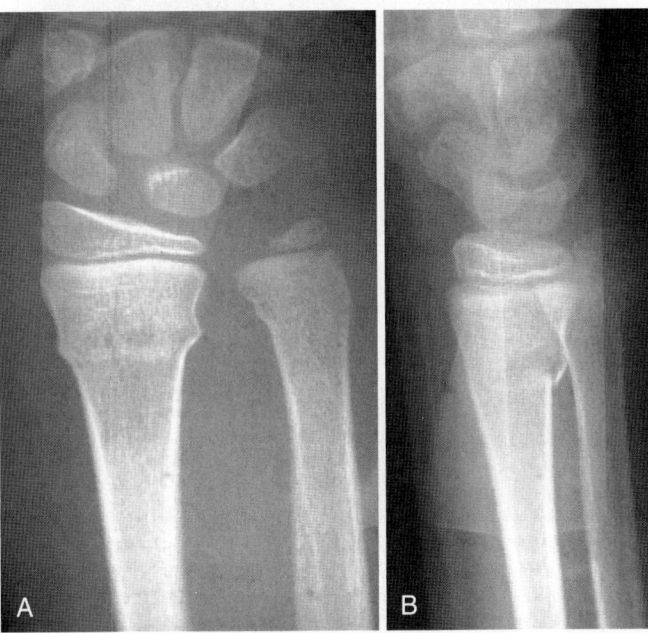

Figure 683-6 Buckle fracture is a partial failure in compression: anteroposterior **(A)** and lateral **(B)** radiographs of the distal radius. *(From Dormans JP: Pediatric orthopedics: introduction to trauma, Philadelphia, 2005, Mosby, p. 37.)*

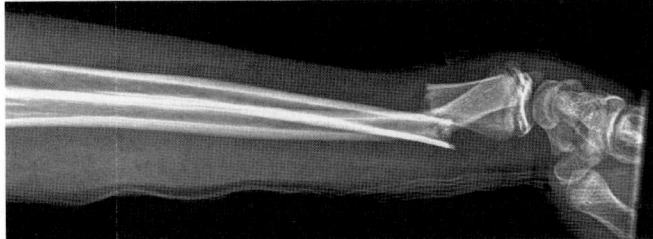

Figure 683-7 This displaced distal radius fracture has an ulna fracture that is a greenstick (complete failure on the tensile side with microscopic failure on the compression side).

Table 683-1	Salter-Harris Classification
SALTER-HARRIS TYPE	**CHARACTERISTICS**
I	Separation through the physis, usually through the zones of hypertrophic and degenerating cartilage cell columns
II	Fracture through a portion of the physis but extending through the metaphyses
III	Fracture through a portion of the physis extending through the epiphysis and into the joint
IV	Fracture across the metaphysis, physis, and epiphysis
V	Crush injury to the physis

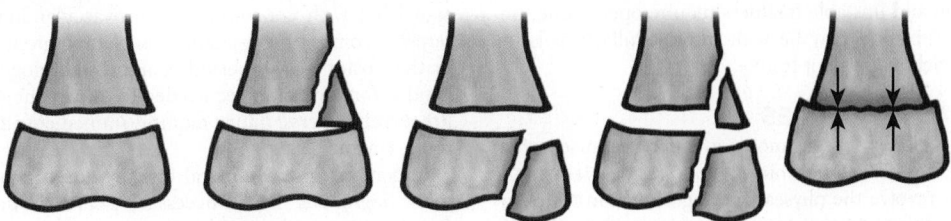

Figure 683-8 Salter-Harris classification of physeal fractures, types I-V.

683.3 Upper Extremity Fractures

Keith D. Baldwin, Lawrence Wells,
and John P. Dormans

PHALANGEAL FRACTURES

The different phalangeal fracture patterns in children include physeal, diaphyseal, and tuft fractures. The mechanism of injury is a direct blow to the finger or a finger trapped in a door (see Chapter 681). Crush injuries of the distal phalanx manifest with severe comminution of the underlying bone (tuft fracture), disruption of the nail bed, and significant soft-tissue injury. These injuries are best managed with antibiotics, tetanus prophylaxis, and irrigation. A mallet finger deformity is the inability to extend the distal portion of the digit and is caused by a hyperextension injury. It represents an avulsion fracture of the physis of the distal phalanx. The treatment is splinting the digit in extension for 3-4 wk. The physeal injuries of the proximal and middle phalanx are similarly treated with splint immobilization. Diaphyseal fractures may be oblique, spiral, or transverse in fracture geometry. They are assessed for angular and rotational deformity with the finger in flexion. The patient should be asked to make a fist. All fingers should point toward the scaphoid. If they do not, a malrotation is suspected, even in the presence of x-rays which appear minimally displaced. Any malrotation or angular deformity requires correction for optimal functioning of the hand. These deformities are corrected with closed reduction, and if unstable, they need stabilization.

FOREARM FRACTURES

Fractures of the wrist and forearm are very common fractures in children, accounting for nearly half of all fractures seen in the skeletally immature. The most common mechanism of injury is a fall on the outstretched hand. Eighty percent of forearm fractures involve the distal radius and ulna, 15% involve the middle third, and the rest are rare fractures of the proximal third of the radius or ulnar shaft. The majority of forearm fractures are torus or greenstick fractures. The torus fracture is an impacted fracture, and there is minimal soft-tissue swelling or hemorrhage. They are best treated in a short arm (below the elbow) cast and usually heal within 3-4 wk. Wrist buckle fractures have also been successfully treated with a removable splint. Impacted greenstick fractures of the forearm tend to be intrinsically stable (no cortical disruption) and may be managed with a soft bandage rather than casting.

Diaphyseal fractures can be more difficult to treat because the limits of acceptable reduction are much more stringent than for distal radial fractures. A significant malunion of a forearm diaphyseal fracture can lead to a permanent loss of pronation and supination, leading to functional difficulties. This is particularly true with malrotation of the fragments. Diaphyseal fractures are vulnerable to rotational malalignment due to insertion of the pronator muscle groups and the supinator groups. This malalignment is particularly hard to assess because the deformity is in the axial plane and is evaluated with anteroposterior (AP) and lateral radiographs (Fig. 683-9). The physical examination focuses on soft-tissue injuries and ruling out any neurovascular involvement. The AP and lateral radiographs of the forearm and wrist confirm the diagnosis. Displaced and angulated fractures require manipulative closed reduction under general anesthesia or conscious sedation. They are immobilized in an above-elbow cast for at least 6 wk. Both bone fractures in older children and adolescents (<10 yr of age) must be followed carefully as they are vulnerable to loss of reduction. Loss of reduction and unstable fractures require open reduction and internal fixation. Fixation may be with intramedullary nails or plate fixation, which yield equivalent results.

DISTAL HUMERAL FRACTURES

Fractures around the elbow receive more attention because more aggressive management is needed to achieve a good result. Many injuries are intraarticular, involve the physeal cartilage, and can result in rare malunion or nonunion. As the distal humerus develops from a

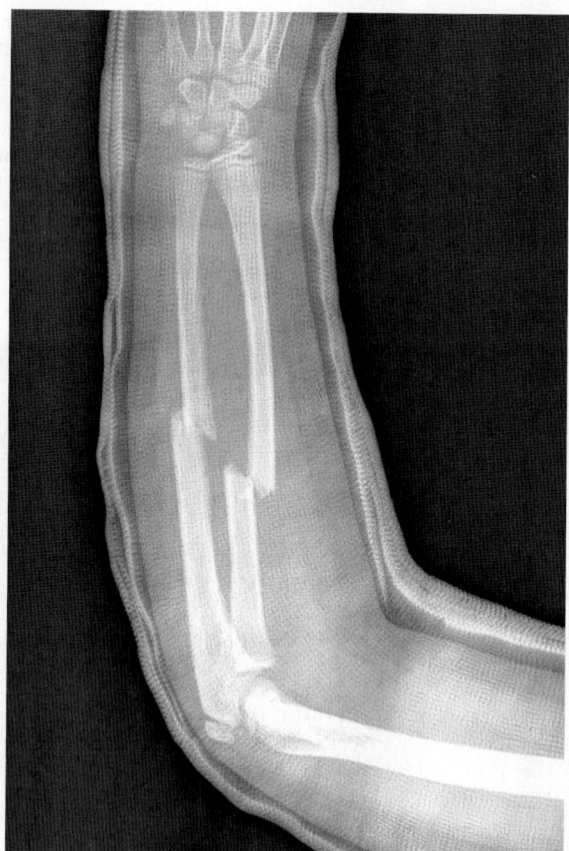

Figure 683-9 A rotationally malaligned forearm fracture that initially had good alignment but lost reduction in the cast. Note that the radial styloid is visible, but the biceps tuberosity is not. The 2 should normally be 180 degrees from one another. These landmarks are sometimes hard to appreciate in children but were visible on other views in this child.

series of ossification centers, these ossification centers can be mistaken for fractures by inexperienced eyes. Careful radiographic evaluation is an essential part of diagnosing and managing distal humeral injuries. Observation of soft-tissue swelling and tenderness is critical to pick up subtle injuries. Common fractures include separation of the distal humeral epiphysis (transcondylar fracture), supracondylar fractures of the distal humerus, and epiphyseal fractures of the lateral condyle or medial epicondyle. The mechanism of injury is a fall on an outstretched arm. The physical examination includes noting the location and extent of soft-tissue swelling, ruling out any neurovascular injury, specifically anterior interosseous nerve involvement or evidence of compartment syndrome. A transcondylar fracture in neonates should raise suspicion of child abuse. AP and lateral radiographs of the involved extremity are necessary for the diagnosis. If the fracture is not visible, but there is an altered relationship between the humerus and the radius and ulna or the presence of a posterior fat pad sign, a transcondylar fracture or an occult fracture should be suspected. Imaging studies such as oblique radiographs, CT, MRI, and ultrasonography may be required for further confirmation. Displaced supracondylar fractures may be associated with concomitant neurovascular injury (Fig. 683-10) or, rarely, a compartment syndrome. Neurologic injury may also appear in the postoperative period. Careful neurologic examination of the hand before and after are needed to document and treat nerve injury. Preoperative nerve injury requires immediate attention and treatment of the fracture.

In general, distal humeral fractures need good restoration of anatomic alignment. This is necessary to prevent deformity and to allow for normal growth and development. Closed reduction alone, or in

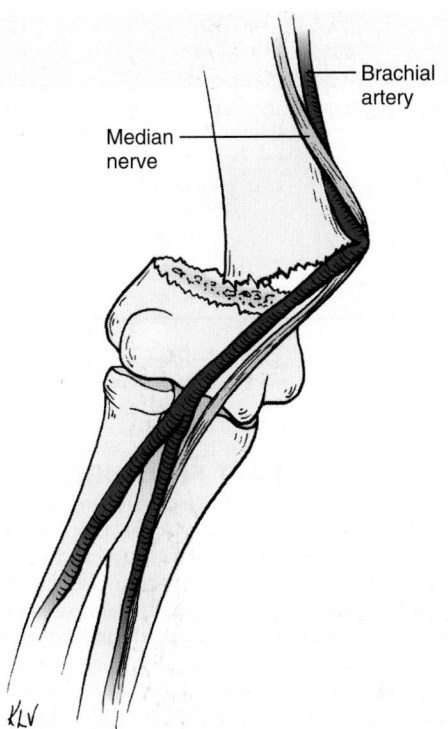

Figure 683-10 Posterolaterally displaced type III (extension-type) supracondylar humeral fracture. The proximal fragment displaces anteromedially. Thus placing the brachial artery and median nerve at risk. *(From Herring JA, Ho C: Upper extremity injuries. In Herring JA, editor: Tachdjian's pediatric orthopaedics, ed 5, Philadelphia, 2014, WB Saunders, Fig. 33-36, p. 1268.)*

association with percutaneous fixation, is the preferred method. Open reduction is indicated for fractures that cannot be reduced by closed methods, fractures with vascular compromise following closed reduction, open fractures, or interarticular fractures, particularly in older children. Inadequate reductions can lead to loss of motion, cubitus varus, cubitus valgus, and rare nonunion or elbow instability. Elbow stiffness is not as common as in adult fractures, but may occur with fractures which are severe or intra-articular.

PROXIMAL HUMERUS FRACTURES

Fractures of the proximal humerus account for <5% of fractures in children. They usually result from a fall onto an outstretched arm. The fracture pattern tends to vary with the age group. Children younger than 5 yr of age have an SH I injury, those 5-10 yr of age have metaphyseal fractures, and children older than 11 yr of age have SH II injury. Examination includes a thorough neurologic evaluation, especially of the axillary nerve. The diagnosis is made on AP radiographs of the shoulder. An axillary view is obtained to rule out any dislocation. Many children are too uncomfortable to tolerate this view. In this case, a Velpeau axillary can be obtained while the arm remains in a sling. SH I injuries do not require reduction because they have excellent remodeling capacity, and simple immobilization in a sling for 2-3 wk is sufficient. The proximal humerus contributes 80% of the growth to the humerus. The metaphyseal fractures usually do not need reduction unless the angulation is >50 degrees. A closed reduction with sling immobilization adequately treats this fracture. SH II fractures with <30 degrees of angulation and <50% displacement are managed in a sling. Displaced fractures are treated with closed reduction and further stabilization if unstable. Occasionally, open reduction is required because of button-holing of the fracture spike through the deltoid or interposition of the tendon of biceps. The majority of longitudinal growth of the limb comes from the proximal humeral physis. Additionally, the glenohumeral joint is capable of a large amount of motion. As such this area is extremely tolerant to deformity. Indications for open reduction are rare. However, as adolescents approach adulthood, these fractures will remodel less.

CLAVICULAR FRACTURES

Neonatal fractures occur as a result of direct trauma during birth, most often through a narrow pelvis or following shoulder dystocia. They can be missed initially and can appear with pseudoparalysis. Childhood fractures are usually the result of a fall on the affected shoulder or direct trauma to the clavicle. The most common site for fracture is the junction of the middle and lateral 3rd clavicle. Tenderness over the clavicle will make the diagnosis. A thorough neurovascular examination is important to diagnose any associated **brachial plexus injury.** Biceps function is important to assess as it is a prognostic indicator for future function.

An AP radiograph of the clavicle demonstrates the fracture and can show overlap of the fragments. Physeal injuries occur through the medial or lateral growth plate and are sometimes difficult to differentiate from dislocations of the acromioclavicular or sternoclavicular joint. Further imaging such as a CT scan may be necessary to further define the injury. Posterior medial clavicular physeal injuries are particularly problematic due to their proximity to the great vessels and the trachea. Closed vs open reduction with a cardiac/thoracic team on standby is necessary. This can be delayed if there is no sign of vascular or respiratory compromise.

The treatment of most clavicle fractures consists of an application of a figure-of-eight clavicle strap or a simple sling. A figure-of-eight strap will extend the shoulders and minimize the amount of overlap of the fracture fragments. Evidence exists for adults — that fractures that are shortened or displaced result in strength loss of the shoulder without anatomic reduction and fixation. Many centers are extending that indication to older adolescents, though the data are currently not as strong as for adults. If a fracture is tenting the skin, or open or resulting in neurovascular compromise, surgery is indicated. The physeal fractures are treated with simple sling immobilization without any reduction attempt. Often, anatomic alignment is not achieved, nor is it necessary. The fractures heal rapidly usually in 3-6 wk. A palpable mass of callus is usually visible in thin children. This remodels satisfactorily in 6-12 mo. Complete restoration of shoulder motion and function is uniformly achieved.

Bibliography is available at Expert Consult.

683.4 Fractures of Lower Extremity

Keith D. Baldwin, Lawrence Wells, and John P. Dormans

HIP FRACTURE

Hip fractures in children account for <1% of all children's fractures. These injuries result from high-energy trauma and are often associated with injury to the chest, head, or abdomen. Treatment of hip fractures in children entails a complication rate of up to 60%, an overall avascular necrosis rate of 50%, and a malunion rate of up to 30%. The unique blood supply to the femoral head accounts for the high rate of avascular necrosis. Fractures are classified by the Delbet classification as transphyseal separations, transcervical fractures, cervicotrochanteric fractures, and intertrochanteric fractures. The management principle includes urgent anatomic reduction (either open or closed), stable internal fixation (avoiding the physis if possible), and spica casting. Urgent management has been associated with a lower rate of avascular necrosis and superior overall outcomes. Capsular decompression also has been advocated as decreasing overall pressure on the epiphyseal vessels, and has been demonstrated experimentally. The clinical results have been mixed.

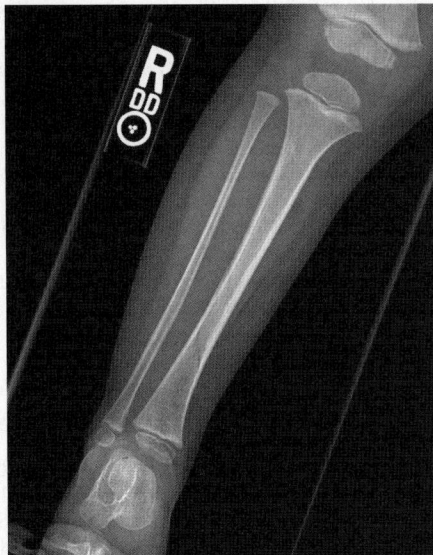

Figure 683-11 A spiral fracture of the tibia in a 3 yr old (toddler fracture). The mechanism was a twisting fall.

TODDLER FRACTURE

Toddler fractures occur in young ambulatory children. The age range for this fracture is typically from around 1-4 yr (Fig. 683-11). The injury often occurs after a seemingly harmless twist or fall and is often unwitnessed. The children in this age group are usually unable to articulate the mechanism of injury clearly or to describe the area of injury well. The radiographs may show no fracture; the diagnosis is made by physical examination. The classic symptom is refusal to bear weight, which can manifest as pulling up the affected extremity or florid display of protest. The AP and lateral views of the tibia–fibula might show a nondisplaced spiral fracture of the distal tibial metaphysis. An oblique view is often helpful because the fracture line may be visible in only 1 of the 3 views. Inflammatory markers may be ordered to rule out infectious processes if the diagnosis is in doubt. Bone scans were employed in the past but impart a large amount of radiation to the child. The fracture is treated with an above-knee cast for approximately 3 wk.

PROXIMAL TIBIA FRACTURES

Proximal tibia fractures can be physeal injuries, metaphyseal injuries, or avulsion injuries of the tibial spine or tubercle. Physeal injuries can be either isolated or as part of tibial tubercle fracture. If the distal segment is displaced posteriorly the trifurcation of the popliteal vessels may be involved. Careful neurovascular examination is warranted both pre- and postreduction. Anatomic reduction and pin fixation is preferred with unstable fractures or displaced Salter-Harris III or IV fractures.

Proximal tibial metaphyseal fractures, or the so-called cozen fracture, are most common in the 3-6 yr old age group. They result in a late valgus deformity even if anatomically reduced. This deformity remodels within 1-2 yr but can cause great distress to parents and treating clinicians.

Tibial eminence fractures are fractures of the bony prominence that is the attachment of the anterior cruciate ligament. The mechanism of injury is similar to that of an anterior cruciate ligament tear in an adult. Displaced fractures require surgical reduction and fixation. This may be done either open or arthroscopically.

Tibial tubercle fractures are common in patients with Osgood-Schlatter syndrome. Care must be taken to observe for compartment syndrome as the injury is associated with injury of the recurrent anterior tibial artery. The injury may be treated non operatively if the fracture is displaced <2 mm and the patient has no extensor lag (rare). Open reduction and internal fixation is preferred otherwise.

Table 683-2	Femoral Shaft Fracture: Treatment Options by Age			
TREATMENT OPTIONS	**0-2 YR**	**3-5 YR**	**6-10 YR**	**>11 YR**
Spica cast	x	x		
Traction and spica cast		x	x	x
Intramedullary rod		x	x	x
External fixator		x*	x*	x*
Screw or plate		x	x	x

*Open fracture.

Modified from Wells L: Trauma related to the lower extremity. In Dormans JP, editor: Pediatric orthopaedics: core knowledge in orthopaedics, Philadelphia, 2005, Mosby, p. 93.

TIBIA AND FIBULA SHAFT FRACTURES

The tibia is the most commonly fractured bone of the lower limb in children. This fracture generally results from a direct injury. Most tibial fractures are associated with a fibular fracture, and the mean age of presentation is 8 yr. The child has pain, swelling, and deformity of the affected leg and is unable to bear weight. Distal neurovascular examination is important in assessment. The AP and lateral radiographs should include the knee and ankle. Closed reduction and immobilization are the standard method of treatment. Most fractures heal well, and children usually have excellent results. Open fractures need to undergo irrigation and debridement, and antibiotic treatment. The tibia is a subcutaneous bone. Severe soft-tissue loss may necessitate plastic surgery consultation. Definitive external fixation vs internal fixation and simultaneous soft-tissue coverage are alternate treatment strategies to minimize infection. Tibia fractures are associated with compartment syndrome. Vigilance is necessary to avoid disastrous outcomes in the setting of missed compartment syndrome. Emergent fasciotomy is indicated as soon as compartment syndrome is diagnosed. Several return trips to the operating room are often necessary to close, vs cover, the fasciotomy wounds.

FEMORAL SHAFT FRACTURES

Fractures of the femur in children are common. All age groups, from early childhood to adolescence, can be affected. The mechanism of injury varies from low-energy twisting type injuries to high-velocity injuries in vehicular accidents. Femur fractures in children younger than age 2 yr should raise the concern for child abuse. A thorough physical examination is necessary to rule out other injuries and assess the neurovascular status. In the case of high-energy trauma, any signs of hemodynamic instability should prompt the examiner to look for other sources of bleeding. AP and lateral radiographs of the femur demonstrate the fracture. An AP radiograph of the pelvis is obtained to rule out any associated pelvic fracture. Treatment of shaft fractures varies with the age group, as described in Table 683-2.

TRIPLANE AND TILLAUX FRACTURES

Triplane and Tillaux fracture patterns occur at the end of the growth period and are based on relative strength of the bone–physis junction and asymmetric closure of the tibial physis. The triplane fractures are so named because the injury has coronal, sagittal, and transverse components (Fig. 683-12). The Tillaux fracture is an avulsion fracture of the anterolateral aspect of the distal tibial epiphysis. Radiographs and further imaging with CT and 3-dimensional reconstructions are necessary to analyze the fracture geometry. The triplane fracture involves the articular surface and hence anatomic reduction is necessary. The reduction is further stabilized with internal fixation. The Tillaux fracture is treated by closed reduction. Open reduction is recommended if a residual intraarticular step-off persists.

METATARSAL FRACTURES

Metatarsal fractures are common in children. They usually result from direct trauma to the dorsum of the foot. High-energy trauma or

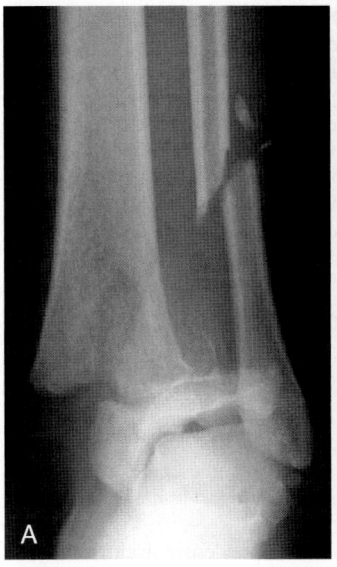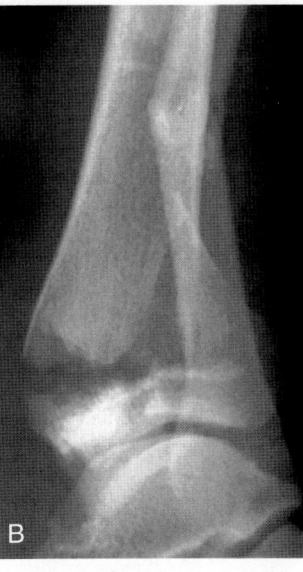

Figure 683-12 The triplane fracture is a transitional fracture: antero-posterior **(A)** and lateral **(B)** radiographs. *(From Dormans JP: Pediatric orthopedics: introduction to trauma, Philadelphia, 2005, Mosby, p. 38.)*

multiple fractures of the metatarsal base are associated with significant swelling. A high index for compartment syndrome of the foot must be maintained and compartment pressures must be measured if indicated. Diagnosis is obtained by AP, lateral, and oblique radiographs of the foot. Most metatarsal fractures can be treated by closed methods in a below-knee cast. Weight bearing is allowed as tolerated. Displaced fractures can require closed or open reduction with internal fixation. Percutaneous, smooth Kirschner wires generally provide sufficient internal fixation for these injuries. If the compartment pressure is increased, complete release of all compartments in the foot is necessary.

TOE PHALANGEAL FRACTURES
Fractures of the lesser toes are common and are usually secondary to direct blows. They commonly occur when the child is barefoot. The toes are swollen, ecchymotic, and tender. There may be a mild deformity. Diagnosis is made radiographically. Bleeding suggests the possibility of an open fracture. The lesser toes usually do not require closed reduction unless significantly displaced. If necessary, reduction can usually be accomplished with longitudinal traction on the toe. Casting is not usually necessary. Buddy taping of the fractured toe to an adjacent stable toe usually provides satisfactory alignment and relief of symptoms. Crutches and heel walking may be beneficial for several days until the soft-tissue swelling and the discomfort decrease.

Bibliography is available at Expert Consult.

683.5 Operative Treatment
Keith D. Baldwin, Lawrence Wells, and John P. Dormans

Surgery is required for 4-5% of pediatric fractures. The common indications for operative treatment in children and adolescents include displaced physeal fractures, displaced intraarticular fractures, unstable fractures, multiple injuries, open fractures, failure to achieve adequate reduction in older children, failure to maintain an adequate reduction, and certain pathologic fractures.

The aim of operative intervention is to obtain anatomic alignment and relative stability. Rigid fixation is not necessary as it is in adults for early mobilization. The relatively stable construct can be supplemented

Table 683-3	Common Indications for External Fixation in Pediatric Fractures

Grades II and III open fractures
Fractures associated with severe burns
Fractures with soft-tissue loss requiring free flaps or skin grafts
Fractures requiring distractions such as those with significant bone loss
Unstable pelvic fractures
Fractures in children with associated head injuries and spasticity
Fractures associated with vascular or nerve repairs or reconstruction

with external immobilization. SH types III and IV injuries require anatomic alignment, and if they are unstable, internal fixation is used (smooth Kirschner wires, preferably avoiding the course across the growth plate). Multiple closed reductions of an epiphyseal fracture are contraindicated because they can cause permanent damage to the germinal cells of the physis.

SURGICAL TECHNIQUES
It is important to take great care with soft tissues and skin. The other indications for open reduction and internal fixation are unstable fractures of the spine, ipsilateral fractures of the femur, neurovascular injuries requiring repair, and, occasionally, open fractures of the femur and tibia. Closed reduction and minimally invasive fixation are specifically used for supracondylar fractures of the distal humerus, phalangeal fractures. Failure to obtain anatomic alignment by closed means is an indication for an open reduction. Percutaneous techniques such as intramedullary fixation and minimally invasive plate osteosynthesis are increasingly popular as well.

As children become older and more similar to adults, techniques become more similar to adult techniques. The classic example of this is the femoral shaft fracture. Newborns may be treated with a soft dressing or Pavlik harness; young children may have a spica cast; older children will often be treated with flexible nails. Adolescents will frequently be treated with rigid intramedullary fixation similar to their adult counterparts.

Table 683-3 summarizes the main indications for external fixation. The advantages of external fixation include rigid immobilization of the fractures, access to open wounds for continued management, and easier patient mobilization for treatment of other injuries and transportation for diagnostic and therapeutic procedures. The majority of complications with external fixation are pin tract infections, chronic osteomyelitis, and refractures after pin removal.

Bibliography is available at Expert Consult.

683.6 Complications of Fractures in Children
Keith D. Baldwin, Lawrence Wells, and John P. Dormans

Complications of fractures in children can be as the result of the injury itself, of treatment, or of late effects of the injury on growth and development of the limb.

The fracture itself may cause growth arrest; this is most common in the proximal tibia, distal femur, and distal ulna. Fractures about the hip may cause avascular necrosis or premature physeal closure. Unacceptable alignment may cause loss of motion or limb malalignment. Fracture healing may cause cosmetically unappealing bumps or curves in the limb. Injuries to the limbs may cause neurovascular compromise or compartment syndrome. Nonunions are rare in children.

Treatment may complicate fractures. Cast immobilization can result in cast ulcers, either from inadequate padding of bony prominences or from patients placing objects in the cast. Casts that are too tight can cause neurovascular compromise. Patients can get cast saw burns from using cast saws that are too dull to remove the cast. Improperly placed casts can promote fracture displacement. Improper follow-up of fractures can result in malunited fractures. Surgical treatment can be complicated by blood loss, neurovascular compromise, iatrogenic physeal damage and hardware complications such as infection or hardware failure.

Late effects of trauma can be from partial or complete closure of the physis. This can lead to limb angular deformity or shortening. Angular deformities can be treated by hemiepiphysiodesis or osteotomy. Reflex sympathetic dystrophy is another poorly understood late effect of trauma but can be debilitating. Physical and occupational therapists are very helpful in managing this condition. Some evidence exists that vitamin C may be useful in the acute setting of high-risk injuries to prevent this complication.

Chapter **684**
Osteomyelitis
Sheldon L. Kaplan

Bone infections in children are relatively common. Early recognition of osteomyelitis in young patients is of critical importance; prompt institution of appropriate medical and surgical therapy before extensive infection develops will minimize permanent damage. The risk is greatest if the physis (the growth plate of bone) is damaged.

ETIOLOGY
Bacteria are the most common pathogens in acute skeletal infections. *Staphylococcus aureus* (see Chapter 181.1) is the most common infecting organism in osteomyelitis among all age groups, including newborns. Community-acquired methicillin-resistant *S. aureus* (CA-MRSA) isolates account for more than 50% of *S. aureus* isolates recovered from children with osteomyelitis in some reports. The USA300 clone of *S. aureus* is the most common among CA-MRSA isolates in the United States and is more likely to cause venous thrombosis in children with acute osteomyelitis than other *S. aureus* clones or other bacteria for reasons that are not known.

Group B streptococcus (see Chapter 184) and Gram-negative enteric bacilli (*Escherichia coli*, see Chapter 200) are also prominent pathogens in neonates; group A streptococcus (see Chapter 183) constitutes <10% of all cases. After 6 yr of age, most cases of osteomyelitis are caused by *S. aureus*, streptococcus, or *Pseudomonas aeruginosa* (see Chapter 205). Cases of *Pseudomonas* infection are related almost exclusively to puncture wounds of the foot, with direct inoculation of *P. aeruginosa* from the foam padding of the shoe into bone or cartilage, which develops as osteochondritis. *Salmonella* species (see Chapter 198) and *S. aureus* are the 2 most common causes of osteomyelitis in children with sickle cell anemia (see Chapter 462.1). *Streptococcus pneumoniae* (see Chapter 182) most commonly causes osteomyelitis in children younger than 24 mo of age and in children with sickle cell anemia, but its frequency has declined because of pneumococcal conjugate vaccines. *Bartonella henselae* (see Chapter 209.2) can cause osteomyelitis of any bone, but especially in pelvic and vertebral bones.

Kingella kingae (see Chapter 193) may be the second most common cause of osteomyelitis in children younger than 5 yr of age in some parts of the world. The organism is increasingly recognized as a cause of osteomyelitis, spondylodiskitis, and septic arthritis, especially when polymerase chain reaction testing is employed. Nearly 90% of identified *K. kingae* infections have been in young children.

Infection with atypical mycobacteria (see Chapter 217), *S. aureus*, or *Pseudomonas* can occur after penetrating injuries. These organisms as well as coagulase-negative staphylococci or Gram-negative enteric bacteria may cause bone infection related to implanted materials such as spinal instrumentation or any orthopedic hardware. Fungal infections usually occur as part of multisystem disseminated disease; *Candida* (see Chapter 234) osteomyelitis sometimes complicates fungemia in neonates with or without indwelling vascular catheters.

A microbial etiology is confirmed in approximately 60% of cases of osteomyelitis. Blood cultures are positive in approximately 50% of patients. Prior antibiotic therapy and the inhibitory effect of pus on microbial growth might explain the low bacterial yield.

EPIDEMIOLOGY
The median age of children with musculoskeletal infections is approximately 6 yr. Bone infections are more common in boys than girls; the behavior of boys might predispose them to traumatic events. Except for the increased incidence of skeletal infection in patients with sickle cell disease, there is no predilection for osteomyelitis based on race.

The majority of osteomyelitis cases in previously healthy children are hematogenous. Minor closed trauma is a common preceding event in cases of osteomyelitis, occurring in approximately 30% of patients. Infection of bones can also follow penetrating injuries or open fractures. Bone infection following orthopedic surgery is unusually associated with an implanted surgical device. Impaired host defenses also increase the risk of skeletal infection. Table 684-1 lists other risk factors.

PATHOGENESIS
The unique anatomy and circulation of the ends of long bones result in the predilection for localization of bloodborne bacteria. In the metaphysis, nutrient arteries branch into nonanastomosing capillaries

Table 684-1	Microorganisms Isolated from Patients with Osteomyelitis and Their Clinical Associations
MOST COMMON CLINICAL ASSOCIATION	**MICROORGANISM**
Frequent microorganism in any type of osteomyelitis	*Staphylococcus aureus* (susceptible or resistant to methicillin)
Foreign body–associated infection	Coagulase-negative staphylococci, other skin flora, atypical mycobacteria, fungi
Common in nosocomial infections	*Enterobacteriaceae, Pseudomonas aeruginosa, Candida* spp.
Decubitus ulcer	*S. aureus*, streptococci, Gram-negative enterics, and/or anaerobic bacteria; polymicrobial infections are common
Sickle cell disease	*Salmonella* spp., *S. aureus*, or *Streptococcus pneumoniae*
Exposure to kittens	*Bartonella henselae*
Human or animal bites	*Pasteurella multocida* or *Eikenella corrodens*
Immunocompromised patients	*Aspergillus* spp., *Candida albicans*, or *Mycobacteria* spp.
Populations in which tuberculosis is prevalent	*Mycobacterium tuberculosis*
Populations in which these pathogens are endemic	*Brucella* spp., *Coxiella burnetii*, fungi found in specific geographic areas (coccidioidomycosis, blastomycosis, histoplasmosis)

Modified From Lew DP, Waldvogel FA: Osteomyelitis, Lancet 364:369–379, 2004.

under the physis, which make a sharp loop before entering venous sinusoids draining into the marrow. Blood flow in this area is thought to be "sluggish," predisposing to bacterial invasion. Once a bacterial focus is established, phagocytes migrate to the site and produce an inflammatory exudate (metaphyseal abscess). The generation of proteolytic enzymes, toxic oxygen radicals, and cytokines results in decreased oxygen tension, decreased pH, osteolysis, and tissue destruction. As the inflammatory exudate progresses, pressure increases spread through the porous metaphyseal space via the haversian system and Volkmann canals into the subperiosteal space. Purulence beneath the periosteum may lift the periosteal membrane of the bony surface, further impairing blood supply to the cortex and metaphysis.

In newborns and young infants, transphyseal blood vessels connect the metaphysis and epiphysis, so it is common for pus from the metaphysis to enter the joint space. This extension through the physis has the potential to result in abnormal growth and bone or joint deformity. During the latter part of the 1st yr of life, the physis forms, obliterating the transphyseal blood vessels. Joint involvement, once the physis forms, can occur in joints where the metaphysis is intra-articular (hip, ankle, shoulder, and elbow), and subperiosteal pus ruptures into the joint space.

In later childhood, the periosteum becomes more adherent, favoring pus to decompress through the periosteum. Once the growth plate closes in late adolescence, hematogenous osteomyelitis more often begins in the diaphysis and can spread to the entire intramedullary canal. Septic arthritis contiguous with a site of osteomyelitis is also seen in older children with *S. aureus* osteomyelitis, which may be related to simultaneous hematogenous inoculation of bone and joint space.

CLINICAL MANIFESTATIONS

The earliest signs and symptoms of osteomyelitis, often subtle and nonspecific, are generally highly dependent on the age of the patient. Neonates might exhibit **pseudoparalysis** or pain with movement of the affected extremity (e.g., diaper changes). Half of neonates do not have fever and might not appear ill. Older infants and children are more likely to have pain, fever, and localizing signs such as edema, erythema, and warmth. With involvement of the lower extremities, limp or refusal to walk is seen in approximately half of patients.

Focal tenderness over a long bone can be an important finding. Local swelling and redness with osteomyelitis can mean that the infection has spread out of the metaphysis into the subperiosteal space, representing a secondary soft-tissue inflammatory response. Pelvic

osteomyelitis can manifest with subtle findings such as hip, thigh, or abdominal pain. Back pain with or without tenderness to palpation overlying the vertebral processes is noted in vertebral osteomyelitis.

Long bones are principally involved in osteomyelitis (Table 684-2); the femur and tibia are equally affected and together constitute almost half of all cases. The bones of the upper extremities account for 25% of all cases. Flat bones are less commonly affected.

Usually only a single site of bone or joint is involved, although multiple sites of osteomyelitis may be noted in up to 20% of children with *S. aureus* infections. In neonates, 2 or more bones are involved in almost half of the cases. Children with subacute symptoms and focal findings in the metaphyseal area (usually of tibia) might have a **Brodie abscess**, with radiographic lucency and surrounding reactive bone. Typically the contents of Brodie abscesses are sterile (Fig. 684-1).

Table 684-2	Sites of Osteomyelitis in Children		
BONE	**PERCENT (%)**	**BONE**	**PERCENT (%)**
Femur	23-28	Carpal bone	<1
Tibia	20-26	Rib	<1
Humerus	8-13	Metacarpal	<1
Radius	5-6	Cuboid	<1
Phalanx	2-4	Cuneiform	<1
Pelvis	5-9	Pyriform aperture	<1
Calcaneus	4-6	Olecranon	<1
Ulna	5-6	Maxilla	<1
Metatarsal	~2	Mandible	<1
Vertebrae	2-4	Scapula	<1
Sacrum	~2	Sternum	<1
Clavicle	1-2	Foot	1
Skull	~1		

Modified from Gafur OA, Copley LA, Hollmig ST, et al: The impact of the current epidemiology of pediatric musculoskeletal infection on evaluation and treatment guidelines, *J Pediatr Orthop* 28(7):777–785, 2008.

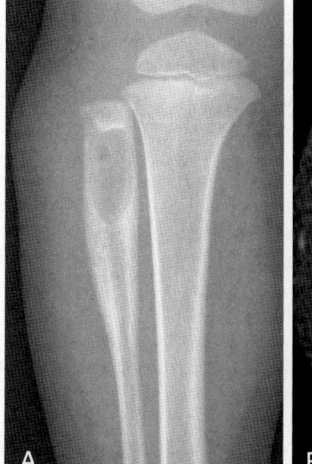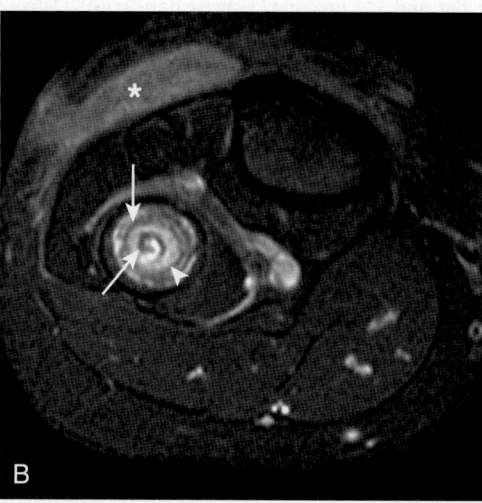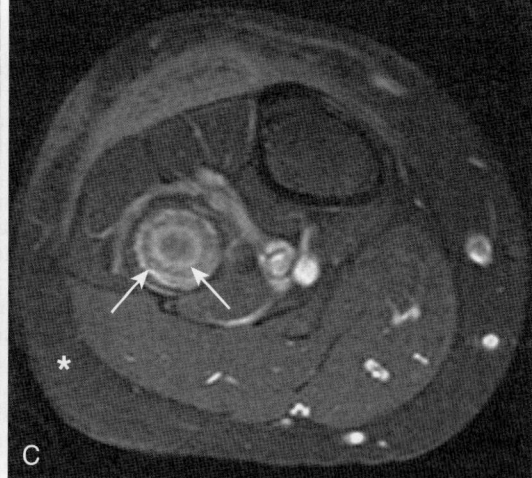

Figure 684-1 A, Radiograph demonstrates a lytic lesion in the proximal fibula with laminated thick periostitis. T2-weighted fat-saturated axial **(B)** and T1-weighted fat-saturated postgadolinium axial **(C)** magnetic resonance images demonstrate a Brodie abscess with sclerotic outer rim (*asterisk*) and inner granulation tissue with enhancement (*arrowhead*). Note the nonenhancing central abscess, which contains a small sequestrum (*arrows*) that is only seen on the T2-weighted fat-saturated sequence. (*From Kan JH, Azouz EM: Musculoskeletal infections. In Coley BD, editor: Caffey's pediatric diagnostic imaging, ed 12, Philadelphia, 2013, WB Saunders, Fig. 138-15, p. 1477.*)

Some patients with an adjacent deep venous thrombosis develop septic pulmonary emboli and are more acutely ill than those with a more insidious onset.

DIAGNOSIS

The diagnosis of osteomyelitis is clinical; **blood cultures should be performed in all suspected cases.** Depending on the results of imaging studies (see later) aspiration or biopsy of bone or subperiosteal abscess for Gram stain, culture, and possibly bone histology provides the optimal specimen for culture to confirm the diagnosis. These specimens are often obtained by the interventional radiologist or at the time of surgical drainage by the orthopedic surgeon. Direct inoculation of clinical specimens into aerobic blood culture bottles can improve the recovery of *K. kingae*, particularly if held for 1 wk. Polymerase chain reaction appears to be the most sensitive technique to detect *K. kingae*, even up to 6 days after antibiotics are initiated.

There are no specific laboratory tests for osteomyelitis. The white blood cell count and differential, erythrocyte sedimentation rate (ESR), or C-reactive protein (CRP) are generally elevated in children with bone infections but are nonspecific and not helpful in distinguishing between skeletal infection and other inflammatory processes. The leukocyte count and ESR may be normal during the 1st few days of infection, and normal test results do not preclude the diagnosis of skeletal infection. However, most children with acute hematogenous osteomyelitis have elevations in the ESR and/or CRP. Monitoring elevated ESR and CRP may be of value in assessing response to therapy or identifying complications.

RADIOGRAPHIC EVALUATION

Radiographic studies play a crucial role in the evaluation of osteomyelitis. Conventional radiographs, MRI, ultrasonography, CT, and radionuclide studies can all contribute to establishing the diagnosis. Plain radiographs are often used for initial evaluation to exclude other causes such as trauma and foreign bodies. The sequence of radionuclide studies or MRI is often determined by age, site, and clinical presentation.

Plain Radiographs

Within 72 hr of onset of symptoms of osteomyelitis, plain radiographs of the involved site using soft-tissue technique and compared to the opposite extremity, if necessary, can show displacement of the deep muscle planes from the adjacent metaphysis caused by deep-tissue edema. Lytic bone changes are not visible on radiographs until 30-50% of the bony matrix is destroyed. Tubular long bones do not show lytic changes for 7-14 days after onset of infection. Infection in flat and irregular bones can take longer to appear.

Computed Tomography and Magnetic Resonance Imaging

CT can demonstrate osseous and soft-tissue abnormalities and is ideal for detecting gas in soft tissues. In selected children who cannot remain still or tolerate sedation, CT is a valuable imaging modality. **MRI is more sensitive than CT or radionuclide imaging in acute osteomyelitis and is the best radiographic imaging technique for identifying abscesses and for differentiating between bone and soft-tissue infection.** MRI provides precise anatomic detail of subperiosteal pus and accumulation of purulent debris in the bone marrow and metaphyses for possible surgical intervention. In acute osteomyelitis, purulent debris and edema appear dark, with decreased signal intensity on T1-weighted images, with fat appearing bright (Figs. 684-2 and 684-3). The opposite is seen in T2-weighted images. The signal from fat can be diminished with fat-suppression techniques to enhance visualization. Gadolinium administration can also enhance MRI. Cellulitis and sinus tracts appear as areas of high signal intensity on T2-weighted images. Short tau inversion recovery MRI is a rapid imaging modality for osteomyelitis (Fig. 684-4). MRI can also demonstrate a contiguous or isolated septic arthritis, pyomyositis, or venous thrombosis.

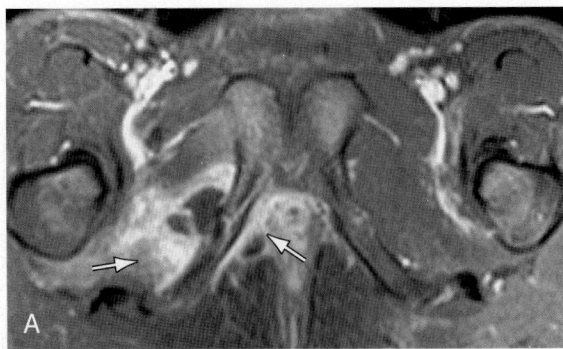

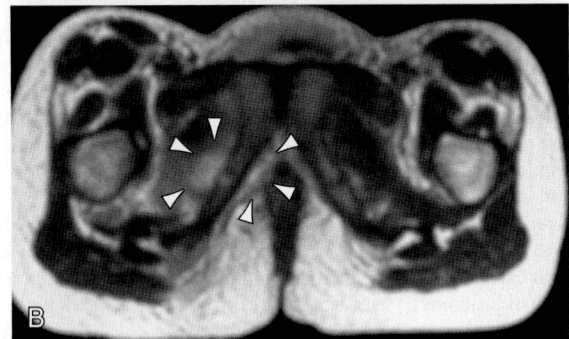

Figure 684-2 MRI of an 8 yr old girl with acute pelvic hematogenous osteomyelitis. **A,** Axial T1-weighted contrast-enhanced MRI with fat saturation reveals a nonenhancing fluid collection adjacent to the inflamed pubic synchondrosis. **B,** The fluid collection appears hyperintense on the corresponding T2-weighted image *(arrowheads)*. In addition, a contrast enhancement within the adjacent internal obturator muscle is seen *(arrow)*, indicating pelvic acute pelvic hematogenous osteomyelitis with complicating adjacent abscess formation and soft-tissue inflammation. *(From Weber-Chrysochoou C, Corti N, Goetschel P, et al: Pelvic osteomyelitis: a diagnostic challenge in children, J Pediatr Surg 42:553–557, 2007.)*

Radionuclide Studies

Radionuclide imaging can be valuable in suspected bone infections, especially early in the course of infection and/or if multiple foci are suspected or an unusual site is suspected, as in the pelvis. Technetium-99 methylene diphosphonate (^{99m}Tc), which accumulates in areas of increased bone turnover, is the preferred agent for radionuclide bone imaging (3-phase bone scan). Osteomyelitis causes increased vascularity, inflammation, and increased osteoblastic activity, resulting in an increased concentration of ^{99m}Tc. Any areas of increased blood flow or inflammation can cause increased uptake of ^{99m}Tc in the 1st and 2nd phases, but osteomyelitis causes increased uptake of ^{99m}Tc in the 3rd phase (4-6 hr). Three-phase imaging with ^{99m}Tc has excellent sensitivity (84-100%) and specificity (70-96%) in hematogenous osteomyelitis and can detect osteomyelitis within 24-48 hr after onset of symptoms. The sensitivity in neonates is much lower, because of poor bone mineralization. Advantages include infrequent need for sedation, lower cost, and the ability to image the entire skeleton for detection of multiple foci.

DIFFERENTIAL DIAGNOSIS

Distinguishing osteomyelitis from cellulitis or trauma (accidental or abuse) is the most common clinical circumstance. Myositis or pyomyositis can also appear similar to osteomyelitis with fever, warm and swollen extremities, and limping; tenderness to palpation of the affected soft-tissue area is generally more diffuse than noted in acute osteomyelitis. Nevertheless, distinguishing myositis and pyomyositis from osteomyelitis clinically may be difficult. Myositis and pyomyositis may be isolated but are often found adjacent to an osteomyelitis on MRI. Pyomyositis is most often caused by *S. aureus* followed by group A streptococcus. The pelvic muscles are a common site of pyomyositis

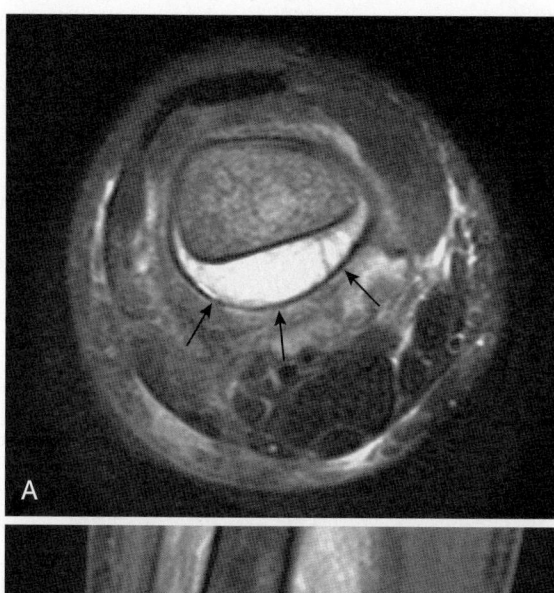

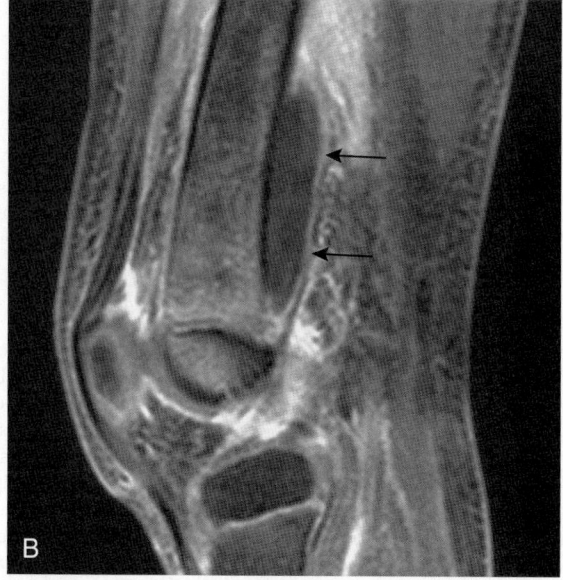

Figure 684-3 Acute osteomyelitis of the distal femur in a 5 yr old boy. **A,** T2-weighted fat-saturated axial MRI shows a large subperiosteal abscess *(arrows)* at the posterior aspect of the femur. Increased signal is seen within the bone, and there is adjacent soft-tissue edema. **B,** T1-weighted fat-saturated postgadolinium sagittal MRI shows the longitudinal extent of the subperiosteal abscess with enhancing wall *(arrows)*. *(From Kan JH, Azouz EM: Musculoskeletal infections. In Coley BD, editor: Caffey's pediatric diagnostic imaging, ed 12, Philadelphia, 2013, WB Saunders, Fig. 138-13, p. 1476.)*

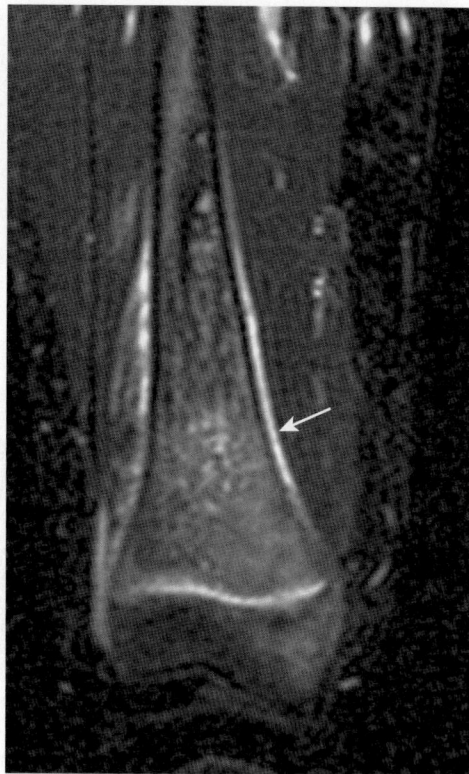

Figure 684-4 Short tau inversion (STIR) recovery coronal magnetic resonance image demonstrates a salt-and-pepper appearance to marrow edema and periosteal reaction *(arrow)*. *(From Kan JH, Azouz EM: Musculoskeletal infections. In Coley BD, editor: Caffey's pediatric diagnostic imaging, ed 12, Philadelphia, 2013, WB Saunders, Fig. 138-14, p. 1477.)*

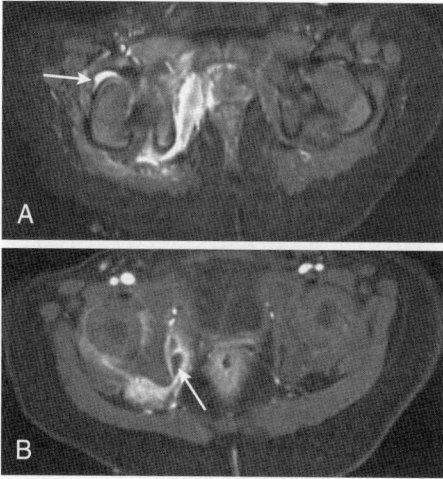

Figure 684-5 A, Axial short tau inversion recovery (STIR) MR demonstrates high signal in the left internal obturator muscle. **B,** Postcontrast fast multiplanar spoiled gradient recalled MR demonstrates a small abscess *(arrow)*. This child had *Staphylococcus aureus* pyomyositis and responded to intravenous antibiotic treatment. *(From Karmazyn B, Loder RT, Kleiman MB, et al: The role of pelvic magnetic resonance in evaluating nonhip sources of infection in children with acute nontraumatic hip pain. J Pediatr Orthop 27:158–164, 2007, Fig. 1, p. 160.)*

and can mimic a pelvic osteomyelitis. MRI is the definitive study to identify and localize pelvic pyomyositis (Fig. 684-5). An iliopsoas abscess can manifest with thigh pain, limp, and fever and must be considered in the differential diagnosis of osteomyelitis. The iliopsoas abscess may be primary (hematogenous: *S. aureus*) or secondary to infection in adjacent bone (*S. aureus*), kidney (*E. coli*) or intestine (*E. coli, Bacteroides* spp.). *Mycobacterium tuberculosis* has been reported in patients with HIV infection. Any child with negative bone imaging and a negative hip aspiration, who presents with fever, limp, and elevated inflammatory marks should be evaluated for pyomyositis.

Appendicitis, urinary tract infection, and gynecologic disease are among the conditions in the differential diagnosis of pelvic osteomyelitis. Children with leukemia commonly have bone pain or joint pain as an early symptom. Neuroblastoma with bone involvement may be mistaken for osteomyelitis. Primary bone tumors need to be considered, but fever and other signs of illness are generally absent except in

Ewing sarcoma. In patients with sickle cell disease, distinguishing bone infection from infarction may be challenging.

Chronic recurrent multifocal osteomyelitis (CRMO) is a nonpyrogenic, sterile inflammatory bone disease that is considered an autoinflammatory disorder (see Chapter 163). It is also associated with a family history of autoimmune disease; the affected patient may also

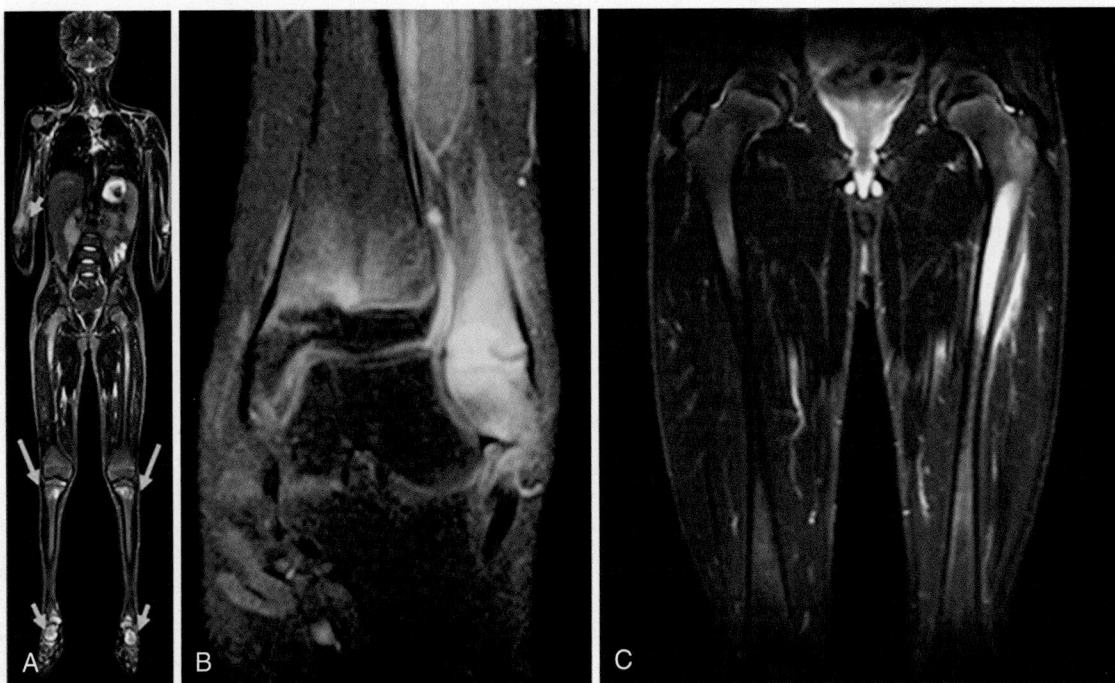

Figure 684-6 MRI in a patient with chronic recurrent multifocal osteomyelitis. **A,** Whole-body image showing multiple foci of osteomyelitis, some of which are distributed symmetrically. **B,** Image of the ankle showing inflammatory metaphyseal and epiphyseal lesions. **C,** Image of the left femur showing involvement of the diaphysis with a soft-tissue reaction. *(From Wipff J, Adamsbaum C, Kahan A, Job-Deslandre C: Chronic recurrent multifocal osteomyelitis. Joint Bone Spine 78:555–560, 2011, Fig. 3, p. 557.)*

have other inflammatory diseases such as Crohn disease, Sweet syndrome, psoriasis, and palmer plantar pustulosis. CRMO in children has many similarities with synovitis, acne, pustulosis, hyperostosis, and osteitis seen in adults. In addition, CRMO has similarities to Majeed syndrome, an autosomal recessive disorder with a microcytic dyserythropoietic anemia and with a deficiency of interleukin-1 receptor antagonist, an autosomal recessive autoinflammatory disease.

In contrast to infectious osteomyelitis, CRMO is multifocal, recurrent, and may involve bones not typical of osteomyelitis (spine, pelvis, clavicle, mandible, calcaneus). Plain radiographs reveal osteolytic lesions or sclerosis; whole-body short tau inversion recovery MRI imaging is the diagnostic study of choice (Fig. 684-6), followed by bone scan.

Pain in CRMO is usually insidious, noted at night; fever is not always present. The mean age of onset is 10 yr. The ESR and CRP may be elevated but are not as high as in bacterial osteomyelitis. Pain usually responds to nonsteroidal antiinflammatory drug agents or, in more severe cases, a short course of prednisone.

TREATMENT
Optimal treatment of skeletal infections requires collaborative efforts of pediatricians, orthopedic surgeons, and radiologists. Obtaining material for culture (blood, periosteal abscess, bone) **before** antibiotics are given is essential. Because most patients with osteomyelitis have an indolent, non–life-threatening condition, optimally cultures should be obtained, even if there is a delay of a few hours in initiating antibiotics.

Antibiotic Therapy
The initial empirical antibiotic therapy is based on knowledge of likely bacterial pathogens at various ages, the results of the Gram stain of aspirated material, and additional considerations. In neonates, an antistaphylococcal penicillin, such as nafcillin or oxacillin (150-200 mg/kg/24 hr divided q6h IV), and a broad-spectrum cephalosporin, such as cefotaxime (150-225 mg/kg/24 hr divided q8h IV), provide coverage for the methicillin-susceptible S. aureus, group B streptococcus, and Gram-negative bacilli. If methicillin-resistant Staphylococcus is

suspected, vancomycin is substituted for nafcillin. If the neonate is a small premature infant or has a central vascular catheter, the possibility of nosocomial bacteria (Gram-negative enteric, Pseudomonas, or S. aureus) or fungi (Candida) should be considered. In older infants and children, the principal pathogens are S. aureus and streptococcus.

A major factor influencing the selection of empirical therapy is the rate of methicillin resistance among community S. aureus isolates. **If methicillin-resistant S. aureus (MRSA) accounts for ≥10% of community S. aureus isolates, including an antibiotic effective against CA-MRSA in the initial empirical antibiotic regimen is suggested.** Vancomycin (60 mg/kg/24 hr divided q6h IV) is the gold standard agent for treating invasive MRSA infections, especially when the child is critically ill. Clindamycin (40 mg/kg/24 hr q8hr) is also recommended when the rate of clindamycin resistance is ≤10% among community S. aureus isolates, the child is not severely ill and bacteremia is not a concern or blood cultures are known to be negative. Cefazolin (100 mg/kg/24 hr divided q8h IV) or nafcillin (150-200 mg/kg/24 hr divided q6h) is the agent of choice for parenteral treatment of osteomyelitis caused by methicillin-susceptible S. aureus. Penicillin is first-line therapy for treating osteomyelitis caused by susceptible strains of S. pneumoniae as well as all group A streptococci. Cefotaxime or ceftriaxone is recommended for pneumococcal isolates with resistance to penicillin and for most Salmonella spp.

Special situations dictate deviations from the usual empirical antibiotic selection. In patients with sickle cell disease with osteomyelitis, Gram-negative enteric bacteria (Salmonella) are common pathogens as well as S. aureus, so a broad-spectrum cephalosporin such as cefotaxime (150-225 mg/kg/24 hr divided q8h) is used in addition to vancomycin or clindamycin. Clindamycin (40 mg/kg/24 hr divided q6h IV) is a useful alternative drug for patients allergic to β-lactam drugs. In addition to good antistaphylococcal activity, clindamycin has broad activity against anaerobes and is useful for treating infections secondary to penetrating injuries or compound fractures. For immunocompromised patients, combination therapy is usually initiated, such as with vancomycin and ceftazidime, or with piperacillin-tazobactam and an aminoglycoside. K. kingae usually responds to β-lactam antibiotics, including cefotaxime. Although the efficacy of treating osteomyelitis caused by *B. henselae* is uncertain, azithromycin plus rifampin may be considered.

When the pathogen is identified and antibiotic susceptibilities are determined, appropriate adjustments in antibiotics are made as necessary. If a pathogen is not identified and a patient's condition is improving, therapy is continued with the initially selected antibiotic. This selection is more complicated currently owing to the presence of MRSA isolates in the community. If a pathogen is not identified and a patient's condition is not improving, reaspiration or biopsy and the possibility of a noninfectious condition should be considered.

Duration of antibiotic therapy is individualized depending on the organism isolated and clinical course. For most infections including those caused by *S. aureus*, the minimal duration of antibiotics is 21-28 days, provided that the patient shows prompt resolution of signs and symptoms (within 5-7 days) and the CRP and ESR have normalized; a total of 4-6 wk of therapy may be required. For group A streptococcus, *S. pneumoniae*, or *Haemophilus influenzae* type b, treatment duration maybe shorter. A total of 7-10 postoperative days of treatment is adequate for *Pseudomonas* osteochondritis when thorough curettage of infected tissue has been performed. Immunocompromised patients generally require prolonged courses of therapy, as do patients with mycobacterial or fungal infection.

Changing antibiotics from the intravenous route to oral administration when a patient's condition clearly has improved and the child is afebrile for ≥48-72 hr may be considered. For the oral antibiotic regimen with β-lactam drugs for susceptible staphylococcal or streptococcal infection, cephalexin (80-100 mg/kg/24 hr q8h) or oral clindamycin (30-40 mg/kg/24 hr q8h) can be used to complete therapy for children with clindamycin-susceptible CA-MRSA or for patients who are seriously allergic or cannot tolerate β-lactam antibiotics. The oral regimen decreases the risk of complications related to prolonged intravenous therapy, is more comfortable for patients, and permits treatment outside the hospital if adherence to treatment can be ensured. Outpatient intravenous antibiotic therapy via a central venous catheter can be used for completing therapy at home, as an alternative; however, catheter-related complications, including infection or mechanical problems, can lead to readmission or emergency department visits.

In children with venous thrombosis complicating osteomyelitis, anticoagulants generally are administered under the supervision of a hematologist until the thrombus has resolved.

Surgical Therapy
When frank pus is obtained from subperiosteal or metaphyseal aspiration or is suspected based on MRI findings, a surgical drainage procedure is usually indicated. Surgical intervention is also often indicated after a penetrating injury and when a retained foreign body is possible. In selected cases, catheter drainage performed by an interventional radiologist is adequate.

Treatment of chronic osteomyelitis consists of surgical removal of sinus tracts and sequestrum, if present. Antibiotic therapy is continued for several months or longer until clinical and radiographic findings suggest that healing has occurred. Monitoring the CRP or ESR is not helpful in most cases of chronic osteomyelitis.

Physical Therapy
The major role of physical medicine is a preventive one. If a child is allowed to lie in bed with an extremity in flexion, limitation of extension can develop within a few days. The affected extremity should be kept in extension with sandbags, splints, or, if necessary, a temporary cast. Casts are also indicated when there is a potential for pathologic fracture. After 2-3 days, when pain is easing, passive range of motion exercises are started and continued until the child resumes normal activity. In neglected cases with flexion contractures, prolonged physical therapy is required.

PROGNOSIS
When pus is drained and appropriate antibiotic therapy is given, the improvement in signs and symptoms is rapid. Failure to improve or worsening by 72 hr requires review of the appropriateness of the antibiotic therapy, the need for surgical intervention, or the correctness of the diagnosis. Acute-phase reactants may be useful as monitors. The serum CRP typically normalizes within 7 days after start of treatment, whereas the ESR typically rises for 5-7 days, and then falls slowly, dropping sharply after 10-14 days. Failure of either of these acute-phase reactants to follow the usual course should raise concerns about the adequacy of therapy. Recurrence of disease and development of chronic infection after treatment occur in <10% of patients.

Because children are in a dynamic state of growth, sequelae of skeletal infections might not become apparent for months or years; therefore, long-term follow-up is necessary with close attention to range of motion of joints and bone length. Although firm data about the impact of delayed treatment on outcome are not available, it appears that initiation of medical and surgical therapy within 1 wk of onset of symptoms provides a better prognosis than delayed treatment.

Bibliography is available at Expert Consult.

Chapter **685**
Septic Arthritis
Sheldon L. Kaplan

Without early recognition and prompt institution of appropriate medical and surgical therapy, septic arthritis in infants and children has the potential to damage to the synovium, adjacent cartilage, and bone, and cause permanent disability.

ETIOLOGY
Historically, *Haemophilus influenzae* type b (see Chapter 194) accounted for more than half of all cases of bacterial arthritis in infants and young children. Since the development of the conjugate vaccine, it is now a rare cause; *Staphylococcus aureus* (see Chapter 181.1) is now the most common infection in all age groups. Methicillin-resistant *S. aureus* accounts for a high proportion (>25%) of community *S. aureus* isolates in many areas of the United States and throughout the world. Group A streptococcus (see Chapter 183) and *Streptococcus pneumoniae* (pneumococcus; see Chapter 182) historically cause 10-20%; *S. pneumoniae* is most likely in the 1st 2 yr of life, but its frequency has declined since the introduction of the pneumococcal conjugate vaccines. *Kingella kingae* is recognized as a relatively common etiology with improved culture and polymerase chain reaction methods in children younger than 5 yr old (see Chapters 193 and 684). In sexually active adolescents, gonococcus (see Chapter 192) is a common cause of septic arthritis and tenosynovitis, usually of small joints or as a monoarticular infection of a large joint (knee). *Neisseria meningitidis* (see Chapter 191) can cause either a septic arthritis that occurs in the 1st few days of illness or a reactive arthritis that is typically seen several days after antibiotics have been initiated. Group B streptococcus (see Chapter 184) is an important cause of septic arthritis in neonates.

Fungal infections usually occur as part of multisystem disseminated disease; *Candida* arthritis can complicate systemic infection in neonates with or without indwelling vascular catheters. Primary viral infections of joints are rare, but arthritis accompanies many viral (parvovirus, mumps, rubella live vaccines) syndromes, suggesting an immune-mediated pathogenesis.

A microbial etiology is confirmed in approximately 65% of cases of septic arthritis. Prior antibiotic therapy and the inhibitory effect of synovial fluid on microbial growth might explain the low bacterial yield. Additionally, some cases treated as bacterial arthritis are actually postinfectious (gastrointestinal or genitourinary) reactive arthritis (see Chapter 157) rather than primary infection. Lyme disease produces an arthritis more like a rheumatologic disorder and not typically suppurative.

EPIDEMIOLOGY

Septic arthritis is more common in young children. Half of all cases occur by 2 yr of age and three-fourths of all cases occur by 5 yr of age. Adolescents and neonates are at risk of gonococcal septic arthritis.

The majority of infections in otherwise healthy children are of hematogenous origin. Infection of joints can follow penetrating injuries or procedures such as trauma, arthroscopy, prosthetic joint surgery, intraarticular steroid injection, and orthopedic surgery, although this is uncommon. Immunocompromised patients and those with rheumatologic joint disease are also at increased risk of joint infection.

PATHOGENESIS

Septic arthritis primarily occurs as a result of hematogenous seeding of the synovial space. Less often, organisms enter the joint space by direct inoculation or extension from a contiguous focus. The synovial membrane has a rich vascular supply and lacks a basement membrane, providing an ideal environment for hematogenous seeding. The presence of bacterial products (endotoxin or other toxins) within the joint space stimulates cytokine production (tumor necrosis factor-α, interleukin-1) within the joint, triggering an inflammatory cascade. The cytokines stimulate chemotaxis of neutrophils into the joint space, where proteolytic enzymes and elastases are released by neutrophils, damaging the cartilage. Proteolytic enzymes released from the synovial cells and chondrocytes also contribute to destruction of cartilage and synovium. Bacterial hyaluronidase breaks down the hyaluronic acid in the synovial fluid, making the fluid less viscous and diminishing its ability to lubricate and protect the joint cartilage. Damage to the cartilage can occur through increased friction, especially for weight-bearing joints. The increased pressure within the joint space from accumulation of purulent material can compromise the vascular supply and induce pressure necrosis of the cartilage. Synovial and cartilage destruction results from a combination of proteolytic enzymes and mechanical factors.

CLINICAL MANIFESTATIONS

Most septic arthritides are monoarticular. The signs and symptoms of septic arthritis depend on the age of the patient. Early signs and symptoms may be subtle, particularly in neonates. Septic arthritis in neonates and young infants is often associated with adjacent osteomyelitis caused by transphyseal spread of infection, although osteomyelitis contiguous with an infected joint can be seen at any age (see Chapter 684).

Older infants and children might have fever and pain, with localizing signs such as swelling, erythema, and warmth of the affected joint. With involvement of joints of the pelvis and lower extremities, limp or refusal to walk is often seen.

Erythema and edema of the skin and soft tissue overlying the site of infection are seen earlier in septic arthritis than in osteomyelitis, because the bulging infected synovium is usually more superficial, whereas the metaphysis is located more deeply. Septic arthritis of the hip is an exception because of the deep location of the hip joint.

Joints of the lower extremity constitute 75% of all cases of septic arthritis (Table 685-1). The elbow, wrist, and shoulder joints are involved in approximately 25% of cases, and small joints are uncommonly infected. Suppurative infections of the hip, shoulder, elbow, and ankle in older infants and children may be associated with an adjacent osteomyelitis of the proximal femur, proximal humerus, proximal radius, and distal tibia because the metaphysis extends intraarticularly.

DIAGNOSIS

Blood cultures should be performed in all cases of suspected septic arthritis. Aspiration of the joint fluid for Gram stain and culture when the history and physical findings indicate septic arthritis remains the definitive diagnostic technique and provides the optimal specimen for culture to confirm the diagnosis. Most large joint spaces are easy to aspirate, but the hip can pose technical problems; ultrasound guidance facilitates aspiration. Aspiration of joint pus provides the best specimen

Table 685-1	Anatomic Distribution of Septic Arthritis		
BONE	**PERCENT (%)**	**BONE**	**PERCENT (%)**
Knee	~40	Interphalangeal	<1
Hip	22-40	Metatarsal	<1
Ankle	4-13	Sacroiliac	<1
Elbow	8-12	Acromioclavicular	<1
Wrist	1-4	Metacarpal	<1
Shoulder	~3	Toe	~1

Modified from Gafur OA, Copley LA, Hollmig ST, et al: The impact of the current epidemiology of pediatric musculoskeletal infection on evaluation and treatment guidelines, J Pediatr Orthop 28:777–785, 2008.

for bacteriologic culture of infection. If gonococcus is suspected, cervical, anal, and throat cultures should also be obtained. In addition to prompt inoculation onto solid media, inoculation of the specimen in blood culture bottles can increase recovery of *K. kingae*. Polymerase chain reaction appears to be the most sensitive method for detecting *K. kingae* in joint fluid.

Synovial fluid analysis for cell count, differential, protein, and glucose has limited usefulness because noninfectious inflammatory diseases, such as rheumatic fever (see Chapter 183.1) and rheumatoid arthritis (see Chapter 155), can also cause exuberant reaction with increased cells and protein and decreased glucose. Nevertheless, cell counts >50,000-100,000 cells/mm^3 generally indicate an infectious process. Synovial fluid characteristics of septic arthritis can suggest infection but are not sufficiently specific to exclude infection. When the joint aspiration is negative, pyomyositis, especially of pelvic muscles, must be excluded by MRI (see Chapter 684).

The white blood cell count and differential, erythrocyte sedimentation rate (ESR), and C-reactive protein (CRP) are generally elevated in children with joint infections but are nonspecific and might not be helpful in distinguishing between infection and other inflammatory processes. The leukocyte count and ESR may be normal during the 1st few days of infection, and normal test results do not preclude the diagnosis of septic arthritis. Monitoring elevated ESR and CRP may be of value in assessing response to therapy or identifying complications. In one study of *S. aureus* septic arthritis, risk features for a site of osteomyelitis contiguous with septic arthritis included a CRP >10 mg/dL at the time of admission, positive blood cultures or more than 2 days of fever following admission.

Radiographic Evaluation

Radiographic studies play a crucial role in evaluating septic arthritis. Conventional radiographs, ultrasonography, CT, MRI, and radionuclide studies can all contribute to establishing the diagnosis (Fig. 685-1).

Plain Radiographs

Plain films of septic arthritis can show widening of the joint capsule, soft-tissue edema, and obliteration of normal fat lines. Plain films of the hip can show medial displacement of the obturator muscle into the pelvis (the obturator sign), lateral displacement or obliteration of the gluteal fat lines, and elevation of Shenton's line with a widened arc.

Ultrasonography

Ultrasonography is particularly helpful in detecting joint effusion and fluid collection in the soft-tissue and subperiosteal regions. Ultrasonography is highly sensitive in detecting joint effusion, particularly for the hip joint, where plain radiographs are normal in more than 50% of cases of septic arthritis of the hip. Ultrasonography can serve as an aid in performing hip aspiration.

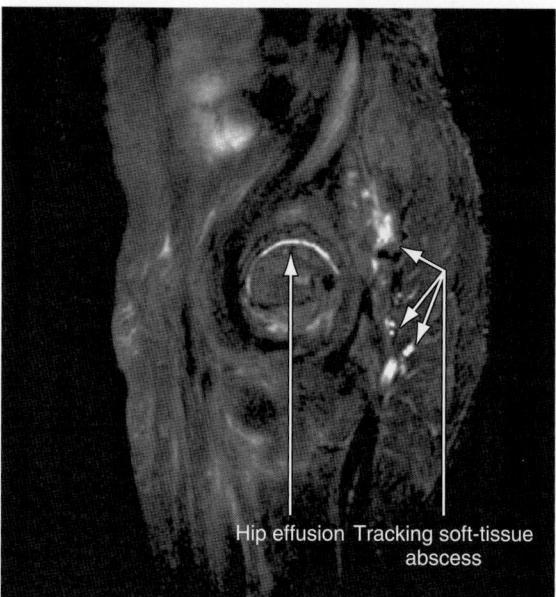

Figure 685-1 MRI of staphylococcal septic arthritis of left hip, with fluid collections between planes of gluteal muscles. *Arrows* indicate fluid collection. *(From Matthews CJ, Weston VC, Jones A, et al: Bacterial septic arthritis in adults,* Lancet *375:846–854, 2010.)*

Hip effusion Tracking soft-tissue abscess

Magnetic Resonance Imaging and Computed Tomography

MRI and CT may be useful in confirming the presence of joint fluid in patients with suspected osteoarthritis infections. MRI may be useful in excluding adjacent osteomyelitis.

Radionuclide Imaging

Radionuclide imaging compared to radiographs is more sensitive in providing supportive evidence of the diagnosis of septic arthritis; a scan may be positive within 2 days of the onset of symptoms. Three-phase imaging with technetium-99 methylene diphosphonate shows symmetric uptake on both sides of the joint, limited to the bony structures adjacent to the joint. Radionuclide imaging is also useful for evaluating the sacroiliac joint.

DIFFERENTIAL DIAGNOSIS

The differential diagnosis of septic arthritis depends on the joint or joints involved and the age of the patient. For the hip, toxic synovitis, pyomyositis, Legg-Calvé-Perthes disease, slipped capital femoral epiphysis, psoas abscess, and proximal femoral, pelvic, or vertebral osteomyelitis as well as diskitis should be considered. For the knee, distal femoral or proximal tibial osteomyelitis, pauciarticular rheumatoid arthritis, and referred pain from the hip should be considered. Knee or thigh pain may be referred from the hip. Other conditions such as trauma, cellulitis, pyomyositis, sickle cell disease, hemophilia, and Henoch-Schönlein purpura can mimic purulent arthritis. When several joints are involved, serum sickness, collagen vascular disease, rheumatic fever, and Henoch-Schönlein purpura should be considered. Arthritis is one of the extraintestinal manifestations of inflammatory bowel disease. Reactive arthritis following a variety of bacterial (gastrointestinal or genital) and parasitic infections, streptococcal pharyngitis, or viral hepatitis can resemble acute septic arthritis (see Chapter 157).

TREATMENT

Optimal treatment of septic arthritis requires cooperation of pediatricians, orthopedic surgeons, and radiologists to benefit the patient.

Antibiotic Therapy

The initial empirical antibiotic therapy is based on knowledge of likely bacterial pathogens at various ages, the results of the Gram stain of aspirated material, and additional considerations. In neonates, an antistaphylococcal penicillin, such as nafcillin or oxacillin (150-200 mg/kg/24 hr divided q6h IV), and a broad-spectrum cephalosporin, such as cefotaxime (150-225 mg/kg/24 hr divided q8h IV), provide coverage for the *S. aureus,* group B streptococcus, and Gram-negative bacilli. If methicillin-resistant *S. aureus* (MRSA) is a concern, vancomycin is selected in stead of nafcillin or oxacillin. If the neonate is a small premature infant or has a central vascular catheter, the possibility of nosocomial bacteria (*S. aureus,* Gram-negative enterics, or *Pseudomonas aeruginosa*) or fungi (*Candida*) should be considered.

In older infants and children with septic arthritis, empirical therapy to cover for *S. aureus,* streptococci, and *K. kingae* includes cefazolin (100-150 mg/kg/24 hr divided q8h) or nafcillin (150-200 mg/kg/24 hr divided q6h).

In areas where methicillin resistance is noted in ≥10% of community-acquired methicillin-resistant *S. aureus* strains (CA-MRSA), including an antibiotic that is effective against CA-MRSA isolates is suggested. Clindamycin (40 mg/kg divided q8h) and vancomycin (15 mg/kg q6 IV) are alternatives when treating CA-MRSA infections. For immunocompromised patients, combination therapy is usually initiated, such as with vancomycin and ceftazidime or with extended-spectrum penicillins and β-lactamase inhibitors with an aminoglycoside. Adjunct therapy with dexamethasone for 4 days with antibiotic therapy appeared to benefit children with septic arthritis in one study but has not been studied in children with CA-MRSA septic arthritis.

When the pathogen is identified, appropriate changes in antibiotics are made, if necessary. If a pathogen is not identified and a patient's condition is improving, therapy is continued with the antibiotic selected initially. If a pathogen is not identified and a patient's condition is not improving, reaspiration or the possibility of a noninfectious condition should be considered.

Duration of antibiotic therapy is individualized depending on the organism isolated and the clinical course. Ten to 14 days is usually adequate for streptococci, *S. pneumoniae,* and *K. kingae;* longer therapy may be needed for *S. aureus* and Gram-negative infections. Normalization of ESR and CRP in addition to a normal examination supports discontinuing antibiotic therapy. In selected patients, obtaining a plain radiograph of the joint before completing therapy can provide evidence (typically periosteal new bone) of a previously unappreciated contiguous site of osteomyelitis that would likely prolong antibiotic treatment. Oral antibiotics can be used to complete therapy once the patient is afebrile for 48-72 hr and is clearly improving.

Surgical Therapy

Infection of the hip is generally considered a surgical emergency because of the vulnerability of the blood supply to the head of the femur. For joints other than the hip, daily aspirations of synovial fluid may be required. Generally, 1 or 2 subsequent aspirations suffice. If fluid continues to accumulate after 4-5 days, arthrotomy or video-assisted arthroscopy is needed. At the time of surgery, the joint is flushed with sterile saline solution. Antibiotics are not instilled because they are irritating to synovial tissue, and adequate amounts of antibiotic are achieved in joint fluid with systemic administration.

PROGNOSIS

When pus is drained and appropriate antibiotic therapy is given, the improvement in signs and symptoms is rapid. Failure to improve or worsening by 72 hr requires review of the appropriateness of the antibiotic therapy, the need for surgical intervention, and the correctness of the diagnosis. Acute-phase reactants may be useful as monitors. Failure of either of these acute-phase reactants to follow the usual course should raise concerns about the adequacy of therapy. Recurrence of disease and development of chronic infection after treatment occur in <10% of patients.

Because children are in a dynamic state of growth, sequelae of skeletal infections might not become apparent for months or years; therefore, long-term follow-up is necessary, with close attention to range of motion of joints and bone length. Although firm data about the impact of delayed treatment on outcome are not available, it appears that initiation of medical and surgical therapy within 1 wk of onset of symptoms provides a better prognosis than delayed treatment.

Bibliography is available at Expert Consult.

Section 2
Sports Medicine

Chapter 686
Epidemiology and Prevention of Injuries
Gregory L. Landry

The Centers for Disease Control and Prevention recommend moderate to vigorous physical activity on a regular basis for all adolescents. Physical activity has favorable effects on hypertension, obesity, and serum lipid levels in youths and is associated with lower rates of cardiovascular disease, type 2 diabetes mellitus, osteoporosis, and colon and breast cancer among adults.

Pediatricians should promote physical activity to their patients, especially those with lower rates of physical activity and sports participation, including children with special healthcare needs (see Chapter 717) and those from lower socioeconomic groups. Physicians also have the responsibility of providing medical clearance for participation in physical activity and sports and for diagnosis and rehabilitation of injuries.

Approximately 30 million children and adolescents participate in organized sports in the United States. Approximately 3 million injuries occur annually if injury is defined as time lost from the sport. Deaths in sports are rare, with the majority of nontraumatic deaths caused by cardiac diseases (see Chapter 436). Nonetheless, approximately 30% of life-threatening injuries in children presenting to an emergency room are sports related. Overall, injury rates and injury severity in sports increase with age and pubertal development, related to the greater speed, strength, and intensity of competition.

Identifying mechanisms of injury and establishing and enforcing rules that reduce the likelihood of that mechanism of injury, including penalizing dangerous play, have reduced catastrophic injury rates. Injury rates also have been reduced by removing environmental hazards, such as trampolines in gymnastics and stationary (vs break-away) bases in softball, and by modifying heat injury rates in soccer tournaments by adding water breaks and reducing the playing time. Wearing equipment such as mouth guards can reduce dental injuries. A common reason for reinjury is lack of rehabilitation of old injuries; appropriate rehabilitation reduces injury rates. Preseason training for high school athletes, with an emphasis on speed, agility, jump training, and flexibility, is associated with lower injury rates in soccer and fewer serious knee injuries in female athletes. Traditional stretching maneuvers or massage have not been demonstrated to reduce the risk of injury or muscle soreness, but ankle taping is helpful particularly to

Table 686-1	Objectives of the Preparticipation Sports Examination

- Determination of the general health of the athlete
- Disclosure of defects that may limit participation
- Detection of conditions that may predispose the athlete to injury
- Determination of optimal level of performance
- Classification of the athlete according to individual qualifications
- Fulfillment of legal and insurance requirements for organized athletic programs
- Evaluation of size and level of maturation of younger athletes
- Improvement of fitness and performance
- Provision of opportunities for students to compete who have either physiologic or pathologic health conditions that may preclude blanket approval
- Provision of the opportunity to counsel youths and answer health and personal questions
- Entry of the athlete into the local sports medicine system establishing a doctor-patient relationship that continues

From Sanders B, Blackburn TA, Boucher B: Preparticipation screening-the sports physical therapy perspective. Int J Sports Phys Ther 8(2):180–193, 2013, Table 1.

prevent reinjury of the ankle. One setting for implementing some of these prevention strategies and for detecting unrehabilitated injuries and medical problems that could affect participation in sports is the preparticipation sports examination.

PREPARTICIPATION SPORTS EXAMINATION
The preparticipation sports examination (PSE) is performed with a directed history and a directed physical examination, including a screening musculoskeletal examination. It identifies possible problems in 1-8% of athletes and excludes fewer than 1% from participation. The PSE is not a substitute for the recommended comprehensive annual evaluation, which looks at behaviors that are potentially harmful to teens, such as sexual activity, drug use, and violence, and assesses for depression and suicidal ideation and addresses broader issues of prevention. Table 686-1 identifies the purposes of the PSE. If possible, the PSE should be combined with the comprehensive annual health visit with emphasis on preventive healthcare (see Chapters 5 and 16).

State requirements for how often a youth needs a PSE differ, ranging from annually to entry to a new school level (middle school, high school, college). At a minimum, a focused, annual interim evaluation should be done on an otherwise healthy young athlete. The PSE is optimally performed 3-6 wk before the start of practice.

History and Physical Examination
The essential components of the PSE are the history and focused medical and musculoskeletal screening examinations. Identified problems require more investigation (Tables 686-2 and 686-3). In the absence of symptoms, no screening laboratory tests are required.

Seventy-five percent of significant findings are identified by the history; a standardized questionnaire given to the parent and athlete is important because the young athlete might not know or might forget important aspects of his or her history. The questionnaire should include questions about previous medical, surgical, cardiac, pulmonary, neurologic, dermatologic, visual, psychologic, musculoskeletal, and menstrual problems, as well as about heat illness, medications, allergies, immunizations, and diet. The most commonly identified problems are **unrehabilitated injuries.** An investigation of previous injuries, including diagnostic tests, treatment, and present functional status, is indicated.

Sudden death during sports can result from undetected cardiac disease such as hypertrophic or other cardiomyopathies (see Chapter 439), anomalous coronary vessels (see Chapter 432.2), or a ruptured aorta in Marfan syndrome (see Chapter 702). In many cases, the underlying heart disease is not suspected, and death is the first sign of heart disease (see Chapter 436). However, in approximately 25-50% of cases,

Text continued on p. 3335

Table 686-2	Preparticipation Sports Examination
COMPONENT OF THE PHYSICAL EXAMINATION	**CONDITION TO BE DETECTED**
Vital signs	Hypertension, cardiac disease, brady- or tachycardia
Height and weight	Obesity, eating disorders, malabsorption
Vision and pupil size	Legal blindness, absent eye, anisocoria, amblyopia
Lymph node	Infectious diseases, malignancy
Cardiac (performed standing and supine)	Heart murmur, prior surgery, dysrhythmia
Pulmonary	Recurrent and exercise-induced bronchospasm, chronic lung disease
Abdomen	Organomegaly, abdominal mass
Skin	Contagious diseases (impetigo, herpes, staphylococcal, streptococcal)
Genitourinary	Varicocele, undescended testes, tumor, hernia
Musculoskeletal	Acute and chronic injuries, physical anomalies (scoliosis)

Table 686-3	Medical Conditions and Sports Participation	
CONDITION	**MAY PARTICIPATE**	**EXPLANATION**
Atlantoaxial instability (instability of the joint between cervical vertebrae 1 and 2)	Qualified yes	Athlete (particularly if the athlete has Down syndrome or juvenile rheumatoid arthritis with cervical involvement) needs evaluation to assess the risk of spinal cord injury during sports participation, especially when using a trampoline
Bleeding disorder	Qualified yes	Athlete needs evaluation
Diabetes mellitus	Yes	All sports can be played with proper attention and appropriate adjustments to diet (particularly carbohydrate intake), blood glucose concentrations, hydration, and insulin therapy Blood glucose concentrations should be monitored before exercise, every 30 min during continuous exercise, 15 min after completion of exercise, and at bedtime
Eating disorders	Qualified yes	Athlete with an eating disorder needs medical and psychiatric assessment before participation
Fever	No	Elevated core temperature can indicate a pathologic medical condition (infection or disease) that is often manifest by increased resting metabolism and heart rate. Accordingly, during the athlete's usual exercise regimen, fever can result in greater heat storage, decreased heat tolerance, increased risk of heat illness, increased cardiopulmonary effort, reduced maximal exercise capacity, and increased risk of hypotension because of altered vascular tone and dehydration. On rare occasions, fever accompanies myocarditis or other conditions that can make usual exercise dangerous
Heat illness, history of	Qualified yes	Because of the likelihood of recurrence, the athlete needs individual assessment to determine the presence of predisposing conditions and behavior and to develop a prevention strategy that includes sufficient acclimatization (to the environment and to exercise intensity and duration), conditioning, hydration, and salt intake, as well as other effective measures to improve heat tolerance and to reduce heat injury risk (e.g., protective equipment and uniform configurations)
HIV infection	Yes	Because of the apparent minimal risk to others, all sports may be played as athlete's state of health allows (especially if viral load is undetectable or very low) For all athletes, skin lesions should be covered properly, and athletic personnel should use universal precautions when handling blood or body fluids with visible blood Certain sports (such as wrestling and boxing) can create a situation that favors viral transmission (likely bleeding plus skin breaks); if viral load is detectable, then athletes should be advised to avoid such high-contact sports
Malignant neoplasm	Qualified yes	Athlete needs individual assessment
Musculoskeletal disorders	Qualified yes	Athlete needs individual assessment

Continued

Table 686-3	Medical Conditions and Sports Participation—cont'd	
CONDITION	**MAY PARTICIPATE**	**EXPLANATION**
Myopathies	Qualified yes	Athlete needs individual assessment
Obesity	Yes	Because of the increased risk of heat illness and cardiovascular strain, obese athletes particularly need careful acclimatization (to the environment and to exercise intensity and duration), sufficient hydration, and potential activity and recovery modifications during competition and training.
Organ transplant recipient (and those taking immunosuppressive medications)	Qualified yes	Athlete needs individual assessment for contact, collision, and limited-contact sports In addition to potential risk of infections, some medications (e.g., prednisone) increase tendency for bruising
Skin infections, including herpes simplex, molluscum contagiosum, verrucae (warts), staphylococcal and streptococcal infections (furuncles [boils], carbuncles, impetigo, methicillin-resistant *Staphylococcus aureus* [cellulitis and/or abscesses]), scabies, and tinea	Qualified yes	During contagious periods, participation in gymnastics or cheerleading with mats, martial arts, wrestling, or other collision, contact, or limited-contact sports is not allowed
Spleen, enlarged	Qualified yes	If the spleen is acutely enlarged, then participation should be avoided because of risk of rupture If the spleen is chronically enlarged, then individual assessment is needed before collision, contact, or limited-contact sports are played
CARDIOVASCULAR		
Carditis (inflammation of the heart)	No	Carditis can result in sudden death with exertion
Hypertension (high blood pressure)	Qualified yes	Those with hypertension >5 mm Hg above the 99th percentile for age, sex, and height should avoid heavy weightlifting and power lifting, bodybuilding, and high-static component sports Those with sustained hypertension (>95th percentile for age, sex, and height) need evaluation The National High Blood Pressure Education Program Working Group report defined prehypertension and stage 1 and stage 2 hypertension in children and adolescents younger than 18 yr of age
Congenital heart disease (structural heart defects present at birth)	Qualified yes	Consultation with a cardiologist is recommended Those who have mild forms may participate fully in most cases; those who have moderate or severe forms or who have undergone surgery need evaluation The 36th Bethesda Conference defined mild, moderate, and severe disease for common cardiac lesions
Heart murmur	Qualified yes	If the murmur is innocent (does not indicate heart disease), full participation is permitted; otherwise, athlete needs evaluation (see structural heart disease, especially hypertrophic cardiomyopathy and mitral valve prolapse)
Dysrhythmia (Irregular Heart Rhythm)		
Long-QT syndrome	Qualified yes	Consultation with a cardiologist is advised. Those with symptoms (chest pain, syncope, near-syncope, dizziness, shortness of breath, or other symptoms of possible dysrhythmia) or evidence of mitral regurgitation on physical examination need evaluation; all others may participate fully
Malignant ventricular arrhythmias	Qualified yes	
Symptomatic Wolff-Parkinson-White syndrome	Qualified yes	
Advanced heart block	Qualified yes	
Family history of sudden death or previous sudden cardiac event	Qualified yes	
Implantation of a cardioverter-defibrillator	Qualified yes	
Structural or Acquired Heart Disease		
Hypertrophic cardiomyopathy	Qualified no	Consultation with a cardiologist is recommended. The 36th Bethesda Conference provided detailed recommendations. Most of these conditions carry a significant risk of sudden cardiac death associated with intense physical exercise. Hypertrophic cardiomyopathy requires thorough and repeated evaluations, because disease can change manifestations during later adolescence. Marfan syndrome with an aortic aneurysm also can cause sudden death during intense physical exercise. An athlete who has ever received chemotherapy with anthracyclines may be at increased risk for cardiac problems owing to the cardiotoxic effects of the medications, and resistance training in this population should be approached with caution; strength training that avoids isometric contractions may be permitted. Athlete needs evaluation
Coronary artery anomalies	Qualified no	
Arrhythmogenic right ventricular cardiomyopathy	Qualified no	
Acute rheumatic fever with carditis	Qualified no	
Ehlers-Danlos syndrome, vascular form	Qualified no	
Marfan syndrome	Qualified yes	
Mitral valve prolapse	Qualified yes	
Anthracycline use	Qualified yes	
Vasculitis, vascular disease	Qualified yes	
Kawasaki disease (coronary artery vasculitis)	Qualified yes	Consultation with a cardiologist is recommended. Athlete needs individual evaluation to assess risk on the basis of disease activity, pathologic changes, and medical regimen
Pulmonary hypertension	Qualified yes	

Table 686-3	Medical Conditions and Sports Participation—cont'd	
CONDITION	**MAY PARTICIPATE**	**EXPLANATION**
EYES		
Functionally 1-eyed athlete	Qualified yes	A functionally 1-eyed athlete is defined as having best-corrected visual acuity worse than 20/40 in the poorer-seeing eye. Such an athlete would suffer significant disability if the better eye were seriously injured, as would an athlete with loss of an eye. Specifically, boxing and full-contact martial arts are not recommended for functionally 1-eyed athletes, because eye protection is impractical and/or not permitted. Some athletes who previously underwent intraocular eye surgery or had a serious eye injury may have increased risk of injury because of weakened eye tissue. Availability of eye guards approved by the American Society for Testing and Materials and other protective equipment might allow participation in most sports, but this must be judged on an individual basis
Loss of an eye	Qualified yes	
Detached retina or family history of retinal detachment at young age	Qualified yes	
High myopia	Qualified yes	
Connective tissue disorder, such as Marfan or Stickler syndrome	Qualified yes	
Previous intraocular eye surgery or serious eye injury	Qualified yes	
Conjunctivitis, infectious	Qualified no	Athlete with active infectious conjunctivitis should be excluded from swimming
GASTROINTESTINAL		
Malabsorption syndromes (celiac disease or cystic fibrosis)	Qualified yes	Athlete needs individual assessment for general malnutrition or specific deficits resulting in coagulation or other defects; with appropriate treatment, these deficits can be treated adequately to permit normal activities
Short-bowel syndrome or other disorders requiring specialized nutritional support, including parenteral or enteral nutrition	Qualified yes	Athlete needs individual assessment for collision, contact, or limited-contact sports Central or peripheral indwelling venous catheter might require special considerations for activities and emergency preparedness for unexpected trauma to the device(s)
Hepatitis, infectious (primarily hepatitis C)	Yes	All athletes should receive hepatitis B vaccination before participation. Because of the apparent minimal risk to others, all sports may be played as the athlete's state of health allows For all athletes, skin lesions should be covered properly, and athletic personnel should use universal precautions when handling blood or body fluids with visible blood
Liver, enlarged	Qualified yes	If the liver is acutely enlarged, participation should be avoided because of risk of rupture If the liver is chronically enlarged, individual assessment is needed before collision, contact, or limited-contact sports are played Patients with chronic liver disease can have changes in liver function that affect stamina, mental status, coagulation, or nutritional status
Diarrhea, infectious	Qualified no	Unless symptoms are mild and athlete is fully hydrated, no participation is permitted, because diarrhea can increase risk of dehydration and heat illness (see fever)
GENITOURINARY		
Kidney, absence of one	Qualified yes	Athlete needs individual assessment for contact, collision, and limited-contact sports Protective equipment can reduce risk of injury to the remaining kidney sufficiently to allow participation in most sports, providing such equipment remains in place during the activity
Ovary, absence of one	Yes	Risk of severe injury to remaining ovary is minimal
Pregnancy and postpartum period	Qualified yes	Athlete needs individual assessment As pregnancy progresses, modifications to usual exercise routines become necessary; activities with high risk of falling or abdominal trauma should be avoided Scuba diving and activities posing risk of altitude sickness should also be avoided during pregnancy After the birth, physiologic and morphologic changes of pregnancy take 4-6 wk to return to baseline
Testicle, undescended or absence of 1	Yes	Certain sports require a protective cup
NEUROLOGIC		
Cerebral palsy	Qualified yes	Athlete needs evaluation to assess functional capacity to perform sports-specific activity
History of serious head or spine trauma or abnormality, including craniotomy, epidural bleeding, subdural hematoma, intracerebral hemorrhage, second-impact syndrome, vascular malformation, and neck fracture	Qualified yes	Athlete needs individual assessment for collision, contact, or limited-contact sports
History of simple concussion (mild traumatic brain injury), multiple simple concussions, and/or complex concussion	Qualified yes	Athlete needs individual assessment Research supports a conservative approach to concussion management, including no athletic participation while symptomatic or when deficits in judgment or cognition are detected, followed by graduated return to full activity
Recurrent headaches	Yes	Athlete needs individual assessment
Seizure disorder, well controlled	Yes	Risk of seizure during participation is minimal

Continued

Table 686-3	Medical Conditions and Sports Participation—cont'd	
CONDITION	**MAY PARTICIPATE**	**EXPLANATION**
Seizure disorder, poorly controlled	Qualified yes	Athlete needs individual assessment for collision, contact, or limited-contact sports The following noncontact sports should be avoided: archery, riflery, swimming, weightlifting, power lifting, strength training, and sports involving heights; in these sports, a seizure during activity can pose a risk to self or others
Recurrent plexopathy (burner or stinger) and cervical cord neuropraxia with persistent defects	Qualified yes	Athlete needs individual assessment for collision, contact, or limited-contact sports; regaining normal strength is an important benchmark for return to play
RESPIRATORY Pulmonary compromise, including cystic fibrosis	Qualified yes	Athlete needs individual assessment but, generally, all sports may be played if oxygenation remains satisfactory during graded exercise test Athletes with cystic fibrosis need acclimatization and good hydration to reduce risk of heat illness
Asthma	Yes	With proper medication and education, only athletes with severe asthma need to modify their participation For those using inhalers, recommend having a written action plan and using a peak flowmeter daily Athletes with asthma might encounter risks when scuba diving
Acute upper respiratory infection	Qualified yes	Upper respiratory obstruction can affect pulmonary function Athlete needs individual assessment for all except mild disease (see fever)
RHEUMATOLOGIC Juvenile rheumatoid arthritis	Qualified yes	Athletes with systemic or polyarticular juvenile rheumatoid arthritis and history of cervical spine involvement need radiographs of C1 and C2 to assess risk of spinal cord injury Athletes with systemic or HLA-B27–associated arthritis require cardiovascular assessment for possible cardiac complications during exercise For those with micrognathia (open bite and exposed teeth), mouth guards are helpful If uveitis is present, risk of eye damage from trauma is increased; ophthalmologic assessment is recommended In visually impaired athletes, guidelines for functionally 1-eyed athletes should be followed
Juvenile dermatomyositis, idiopathic myositis	Qualified yes	Athlete with juvenile dermatomyositis or systemic lupus erythematosus with cardiac involvement requires cardiology assessment before participation. Athletes receiving systemic corticosteroid therapy are at higher risk for osteoporotic fractures and avascular necrosis, which should be assessed before clearance; those receiving immunosuppressive medications are at higher risk for serious infection. Sports activities should be avoided when myositis is active. Rhabdomyolysis during intensive exercise can cause renal injury in athletes with idiopathic myositis and other myopathies. Because of photosensitivity with juvenile dermatomyositis and systemic lupus erythematosus, sun protection is necessary during outdoor activities. With Raynaud phenomenon, exposure to the cold presents risk to hands and feet
Systemic lupus erythematosus	Qualified yes	
Raynaud phenomenon	Qualified yes	
SICKLE CELL Sickle cell disease	Qualified yes	Athlete needs individual assessment In general, if illness status permits, all sports may be played; however, any sport or activity that entails overexertion, overheating, dehydration, or chilling should be avoided Participation at high altitude, especially when not acclimatized, also poses risk of sickle cell crisis
Sickle cell trait	Yes	Athletes with sickle cell trait generally do not have increased risk of sudden death or other medical problems during athletic participation under normal environmental conditions; however, when high exertional activity is performed under extreme conditions of heat and humidity or increased altitude, such catastrophic complications have occurred rarely Athletes with sickle cell trait, like all athletes, should be progressively acclimatized to the environment and to the intensity and duration of activities and should be sufficiently hydrated to reduce the risk of exertional heat illness and/or rhabdomyolysis According to National Institutes of Health management guidelines, sickle cell trait is not a contraindication to participation in competitive athletics, and there is no requirement for screening before participation More research is needed to fully assess potential risks and benefits of screening athletes for sickle cell trait

This table is intended for use by medical and nonmedical personnel. "Needs evaluation" means that a physician with appropriate knowledge and experience should assess the safety of a given sport for an athlete with the listed medical condition. Unless otherwise noted, this need for special consideration is because of variability in the severity of the disease, the risk of injury for the specific sports, or both.

From Rice SG; the Council on Sports Medicine and Fitness, American Academy of Pediatrics: Medical conditions affecting sports participation, Pediatrics 121:841–848, 2008.

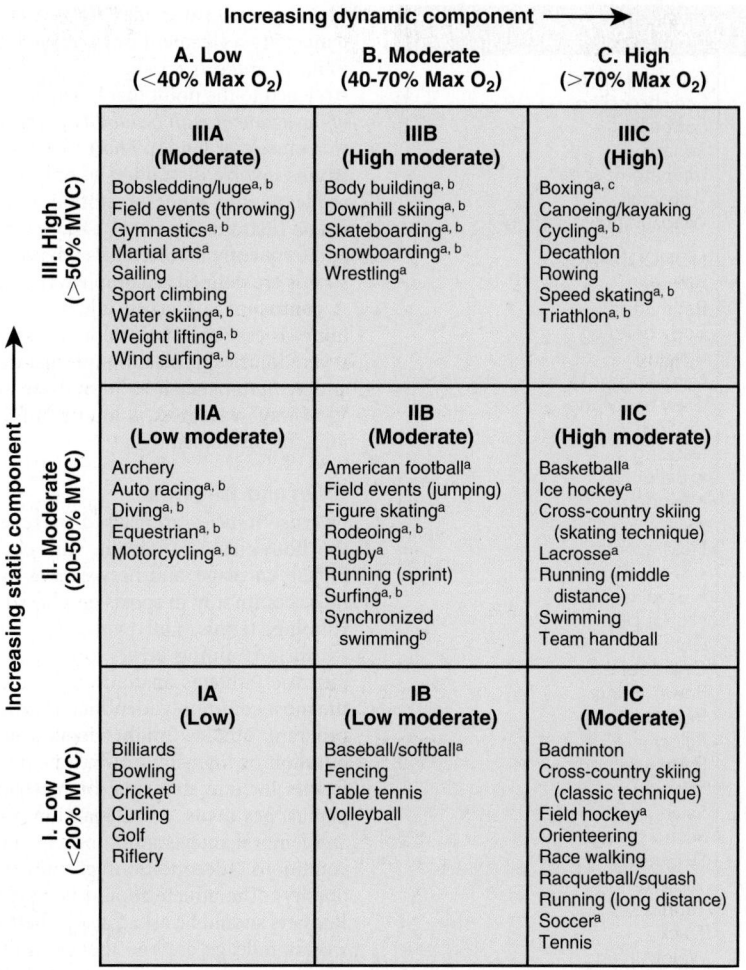

Figure 686-1 Classification of sports according to cardiovascular demands (based on combined static and dynamic components). This classification is based on peak static and dynamic components achieved during competition. The higher values may be reached during training. The increasing dynamic component is defined in terms of the estimated percentage of maximal oxygen uptake (Max O_2) achieved and results in increasing cardiac output. The increasing static component is related to the estimated percentage of maximal voluntary contraction (MVC) reached and results in increasing blood pressure load. Activities with the lowest total cardiovascular demands (cardiac output and blood pressure) are shown in box IA, and those with the highest demands are shown in box IIIC. Boxes IIA and IB depict activities with low to moderate total cardiovascular demands; boxes IIIA, IIB, and IC depict activities with moderate total cardiovascular demands; and boxes IIIB and IIC depict high-moderate total cardiovascular demands. These categories progress diagonally across the graph from lower left to upper right. [a]Danger of bodily collision. [b]Increased risk if syncope occurs. [c]Participation is not recommended by the American Academy of Pediatrics. [d]The American Academy of Pediatrics classifies cricket in the IB box (low static component and moderate dynamic component). *(From Mitchell JH, Haskell W, Snell P, et al: 36th Bethesda conference. Task force 8: classification of sports. J Am Coll Cardiol 45:1364–1367, 2005.)*

in retrospect there were preceding symptoms of dizziness, chest pain, syncope, palpitations, shortness of breath, and/or a family history of early, unexpected death. Chest radiographs, electrocardiograms, and echocardiograms are not recommended as routine screening tests. If there is a **suspicion** of heart disease, such as a history of syncope, presyncope, palpitations, or excessive dyspnea with exercise, or a family history of a condition such as hypertrophic cardiomyopathy or prolonged QT or Marfan syndrome, the evaluation should be complete and include a 12-lead electrocardiogram, an echocardiogram, Holter or event-capture monitoring, and a stress test with electrocardiographic monitoring. Recommendations for participation with identified cardiac disease should be made in consultation with a cardiologist.

Disqualification and limitations for sports participation among various medical conditions are available from the American Academy of Pediatrics (see Table 686-3). Sports may also be classified by intensity (Fig. 686-1) and contact (Table 686-4). Athletes may seek to par-

ticipate in sports against medical advice and have done so successfully for professional sports. Section 504(a) of the Rehabilitation Act of 1973 prohibits discrimination against disabled athletes if they have the capabilities or skills required to play a competitive sport. This was reinforced through the Americans with Disabilities Act of 1990. An amateur athlete has no absolute right to decide whether to participate in competitive sports. Participation in competitive sports is considered a privilege, not a right. *Knapp v Northwestern University* established that "difficult medical decisions involving complex medical problems can be made by responsible physicians exercising prudent judgment (which will be necessarily conservative when definitive scientific evidence is lacking or conflicting) and relying on the recommendations of specialist consultants or guidelines established by a panel of experts."

Bibliography is available at Expert Consult.

Table 686-4	Classification of Sports by Contact

CONTACT OR COLLISION

Basketball	Skateboarding
Boxing*	Snowboarding
Diving	Softball
Field hockey	Squash
Football, tackle	Ultimate Frisbee
Ice hockey†	Volleyball
Lacrosse	Windsurfing or surfing
Martial arts	
Rodeo	**NONCONTACT**
Rugby	Archery
Ski jumping	Badminton
Soccer	Body building
Team handball	Bowling
Water polo	Canoeing or kayaking (flat water)
Wrestling	Crew or rowing
	Curling
LIMITED CONTACT	Dancing
Baseball	• Ballet
Bicycling	• Modern
Cheerleading	• Jazz
Canoeing or kayaking (white	Field events
water)	• Discus
Fencing	• Javelin
Field events	• Shot put
• High jump	Golf
• Pole vault	Orienteering‡
Floor hockey	Power lifting
Football, flag	Race walking
Gymnastics	Riflery
Handball	Rope jumping
Horseback riding	Running
Racquetball	Sailing
Skating	Scuba diving
• Ice	Swimming
• Inline	Table tennis
• Roller	Tennis
Skiing	Track
• Cross-country	Weight lifting
• Downhill	
• Water	

*Participation not recommended by the American Academy of Pediatrics.
†The American Academy of Pediatrics recommends limiting the amount of body checking allowed for hockey players ≤15 yr to reduce injuries.
‡A race (contest) in which competitors use a map and compass to find their way through unfamiliar territory.
From the American Academy of Pediatrics, Committee on Sports Medicine and Fitness: Medical conditions affecting sports participation, Pediatrics 107:1205, 2001.

Chapter **687**

Management of Musculoskeletal Injury

Kevin P. Murphy and Aaron M. Karlin

MECHANISM OF INJURY
Acute Injuries

Sprains, strains, and contusions account for the majority of musculoskeletal injuries. A **sprain** is an injury to a ligament or joint capsule.

Most sprains are grades I-III. A *grade I* sprain is defined as mild damage to a ligament or ligaments without instability of the affected joint. A *grade II* sprain is considered a partial tear to the ligament, stretched to the point that it becomes loose. *Grade III is a complete tear of the ligament with instability to the affected joint.* A **strain** is an injury to a muscle or tendon and these, too, are graded I-III. *Grade I* muscle strains involve disruption of only a few muscle fibers, pain is mild to moderate and range of motion and strength are at or near normal. *Grade II* strains represent a more significant partial tear of the muscle and frequently involve loss of range of motion and strength. *Grade III* strains are defined as complete rupture of the musculotendinous unit. A **contusion** is a crush injury to any soft tissue. The history of the injury is especially helpful in assessing musculoskeletal trauma. More severe injuries, indicating internal derangement, can have acute signs and symptoms such as immediate swelling, deformity, numbness or "give-way" weakness, a loud painful pop, mechanical locking of the joint, or instability.

Overuse Injuries

Overuse injuries are caused by repetitive microtrauma that exceeds the body's rate of repair. This occurs in muscles, tendons, bone, bursae, cartilage, and nerves. Overuse injuries occur in all sports but more commonly in sports emphasizing repetitive motion (swimming, running, tennis, and gymnastics). Factors can be categorized into extrinsic (training errors, poor equipment or workout surface) and intrinsic (athlete's anatomy or medical conditions). Training error is the most commonly identified factor. At the beginning of the workout program, athletes might violate the 10% rule: Do not increase the duration or intensity of workouts more than 10% per week. Intrinsic factors include abnormal biomechanics (leg-length discrepancy, pes planus, pes cavus, tarsal coalition, valgus heel, external tibial torsion, and femoral anteversion), muscle imbalance, inflexibility, and medical conditions (deconditioning, nutritional deficits, amenorrhea, and obesity). The athlete should be asked about the specifics of training. Runners should be asked about their shoes, orthotics, running surface, weekly mileage or time spent running per week, speed or hill workouts, and previous injuries and rehabilitation. When causative factors are identified, they can be eliminated or modified so that after rehabilitation the athlete does not return to the same regimen and suffer reinjury.

For athletes engaged in excessive training that causes an overuse injury (e.g., multiple-sport school athletes), curtailing all exercise may not be necessary. Treatment is a reduction of training load (relative rest) combined with a rehabilitation program designed to return athletes to their sport as soon as possible while minimizing exposure to reinjury. Early identification of an overuse injury requires less alteration of the workout regimen.

The goals of treatment are to control pain and spasm to rehabilitate flexibility, strength, endurance, and proprioceptive deficits (Table 687-1). In many overuse injuries, the role of inflammation in the process is minimal. For most injuries to tendons, the term *tendinitis* is obsolete because there is little or no inflammation on histopathology of tendons. Instead, there is evidence of microscopic trauma to the tissue. Most of these entities are now more appropriately called **tendinosis** and, when the tendon tissue is scarred and very abnormal, **tendinopathy**. With tendinosis, there is less of a role for antiinflammatory medication in the treatment, except as an analgesic.

INITIAL EVALUATION OF THE INJURED EXTREMITY

Initially, the examiner should determine the quality of the peripheral pulses and capillary refill rate as well as the gross motor and sensory function to assess for neurovascular injury. The first priorities are to maintain vascular and skeletal stability.

Criteria for immediate attention and rapid orthopedic consultation include vascular compromise, nerve compromise, and open fracture. The exposed wound should be covered with sterile saline-soaked gauze, and the injured limb should be padded and splinted. Pressure should

Table 687-1	Staging of Overuse Injuries	
GRADE	**GRADING SYMPTOMS**	**TREATMENT**
I	Pain only after activity Does not interfere with performance or intensity Generalized tenderness Disappears before next session	Modification of activity, consider cross-training, home rehabilitation program
II	Minimal pain with activity Does not interfere with performance More localized tenderness	Modification of activity, cross-training, home rehabilitation program
III	Pain interferes with activity and performance Definite area of tenderness Usually disappears between sessions	Significant modification of activity, strongly encourage cross-training, home rehabilitation program, and outpatient physical therapy
IV	Pain with activities of daily living Pain does not disappear between sessions Marked interference with performance and training intensity	Discontinue activity temporarily, cross-training only, oral analgesic, home rehabilitation program, and intensive outpatient physical therapy
V	Pain interferes with activities of daily living Signs of tissue injury (e.g., edema) Chronic or recurrent symptoms	Prolonged discontinuation of activity, cross-training only, oral analgesic, home rehabilitation program, and intensive outpatient physical therapy

be applied to any site of bleeding. Additional criteria include deep laceration over a joint, unreducible dislocation, grade III (complete) tear of a muscle–tendon unit, and displaced, significantly angulated fractures (depends on the bone involved, the degree of displacement and angulation, and neurovascular status of the extremity).

TRANSITION FROM IMMEDIATE MANAGEMENT TO RETURN TO PLAY
Rehabilitation of a musculoskeletal injury should begin on the day of the injury.

Phase 1
Limit further injury, control swelling and pain, and minimize strength and flexibility losses. **PRICE** principles (**P**rotection, **R**est, **I**ce, **C**ompression, and **E**levation) need to be applied. Crutches, air stirrups for ankle sprains, slings for arm injuries and elastic wraps (4-8 inches) for compression are a helpful inventory of office supplies. Ice can be placed directly over the injury as tolerated for 20 min continuously 3-4 times per day until the swelling resolves. Compression limits further bleeding and swelling but should not be so tight that it limits perfusion. Elevation of the extremity promotes venous return and limits swelling. A nonsteroidal antiinflammatory drug or acetaminophen is indicated for analgesia.

Pain-free isometric strengthening and range of motion should be initiated as soon as possible. Pain inhibits full muscle contraction; deconditioning results if the pain and resultant nonuse persist for days to weeks, thus delaying recovery. Education about the nature of the injury and the specifics of rehabilitation exercises, including handouts with written instructions and drawings demonstrating the exercises, are helpful.

Phase 2
Improve strength and range of motion (i.e., flexibility) while allowing the injured structures to heal. Protective devices are removed when the patient's strength and flexibility improve and activities of daily living are pain free. Flexibility can then be improved by a program of specific stretches, held for 15-30 sec for 3-5 repetitions, once or twice daily. A physical therapist or athletic trainer is invaluable in guiding the athlete through this process. Protective devices might need to be used for months during sports participation. Swimming, water jogging, and stationary cycling are good aerobic exercises that can allow the injured extremity to get relative rest or be used pain free while maintaining cardiovascular fitness.

Phase 3
Achieve near-normal strength and flexibility of the injured structures and further improve or maintain cardiovascular fitness. Strength and endurance are improved under controlled conditions using elastic bands and eventually exercise equipment followed by free weights. Sensory proprioceptive training allows the athlete to redevelop the kinesthetic sense critical to joint function and stability.

Phase 4
Return to exercise or competition without restriction. When the athlete has reached nearly normal flexibility, strength, proprioception, and endurance, the athlete can start sports-specific exercises. The athlete will make the transition from the rehabilitation program to functional rehabilitation appropriate for the sport. Substituting sports participation for rehabilitation is inappropriate; rather, there should be progressive stepwise functional return to a full activity or play program. For instance, a basketball player recovering from an ankle injury might begin a walk-run-sprint-cut program before returning to competition. At any point in this progression, if pain is experienced, the athlete needs to stop, apply ice, avoid running for 1-2 days, continue to do ankle exercises, and then resume running at a lower intensity and progress accordingly.

Relative Rest and Return-to-Play Guidelines
Relative rest means that the athlete can do whatever the athlete wants as long as the injured structures do not hurt during or within 24 hr of the activity. Exercising beyond the pain threshold delays recovery.

DIFFERENTIAL DIAGNOSES OF MUSCULOSKELETAL PAIN
Traumatic, rheumatologic, infectious, hematologic, psychologic, congenital, and oncologic processes can cause the presenting complaint of musculoskeletal pain. Symptoms such as fatigue, weight loss, rash, multiple joint complaints, fever, chronic or recent illness, and persistent pain despite conservative care suggests a diagnosis other than sports-related trauma. The possibility of child abuse as an etiology is not to be overlooked permeating all socioeconomic strata. Incongruity between the patient's history and physical examination findings should lead to further evaluation. A negative review of systems with an injury history consistent with the physical findings suggests a sports-related etiology.

Bibliography is available at Expert Consult.

687.1 Growth Plate Injuries

Kevin P. Murphy and Aaron M. Karlin

Approximately 20% of pediatric sports injuries seen in the emergency department are fractures, and 25% of those fractures involve an epiphyseal growth plate or physis (see Chapter 683). Growth in long bones occurs in 3 areas and is susceptible to injury. Immature bone can be acutely injured at the **physis** (Salter-Harris fractures, see Chapter 683.2), the **articular surface** (osteochondritis dissecans), or the **apophysis** (avulsion fractures). Boys suffer about twice as many physeal fractures as girls; the peak incidence of fracture is during peak height velocity (girls: age 12 ± 2.5 yr; boys: age 14 ± 2 yr). The physis is a pressure growth plate and is responsible for longitudinal growth in bone. The apophysis is a bony outgrowth at the attachment of a tendon and is a traction physis. The epiphysis is the end of a long bone, distal or proximal to the long bone, and contains articular cartilage at the joint.

Physeal injuries of the distal radius occur most often in the growing child or adolescent resulting from excessive force applied to the upper extremity. Injuries of this nature can be seen in athletes including those participating in gymnastics, cheerleading, ice skating, hockey and weight lifting. Mechanisms of injury include falls onto an outstretched hand or repetitive dorsiflexion and axial loading through the distal radius (see Chapter 693). Chronic wrist pain can be seen in up to 79% of young gymnasts, particularly female gymnasts between the ages of 12 and 14 yr. With repetitive axial loading temporary metaphyseal ischemia may be induced preventing cartilage calcification and causing the physis to widen. With widening of the distal radial physis, microfractures can develop. Clinical features involve radial wrist pain particularly dorsal with passive and active hyperextension activities relieved with suspension of the offending activity. Tenderness or focal pain around the circumference of the distal radius is often noted. Differential diagnosis includes metacarpal fractures, scaphoid fracture and in the older child, De Quervain tenosynovitis. Juvenile idiopathic arthritis always needs to be considered in a child with a painful swollen wrist not to exclude malignancy or an infectious process. X-rays of the wrist can be helpful particularly when compared to the contralateral extremity. Radiographs can show physeal widening with cystic changes involving the metaphyseal segment, beaking of the distal epiphysis and in later stages, positive ulnar variance. Bone scan may be helpful for stress fractures followed by MRI if subsequently needed. PRICE principles are followed with nonnarcotic pain management. Salter-Harris fractures types I and II can be treated with closed reduction and immobilization. Ulnar shortening osteotomy may be necessary in the athlete with significant ulnar positive variance. Physeal injuries at the knee (distal femur, proximal tibia) are rare. Growth disturbance following a growth plate injury is a function of location and the part of the physis fractured. These factors influence the probability a physeal bar will form, resulting in growth arrest. The areas making the largest contribution to longitudinal growth in the upper extremities are the proximal humerus and distal radius and ulna; in the lower extremities, they are the distal femur and the proximal tibia and fibula. Injuries to these areas are more likely to cause growth disturbance compared with physeal injuries at the other end of these long bones. The type of the physis fracture relative to risk of growth disturbance is described by the Salter-Harris classification system (see Table 683-1). A grade I injury is least likely to result in growth disturbance, and grade V is the most likely fracture to result in growth disturbance.

Osteochondritis dissecans (OCD) affects the subchondral bone and overlying articular surface (see Chapter 683). With avascular necrosis of subchondral bone, the articular surface can flatten, soften, or break off in fragments. The etiology is unknown but may be related to repetitive stress injury in some patients. The condition most commonly affects the knee (lateral aspect of the medial femoral condyle in 70% of patients and lateral femoral condyle in 20%) with the patella in 10%. Other joints where OCD lesions are also seen are the ankle (talus), elbow (usually involving the capitellum), and radial

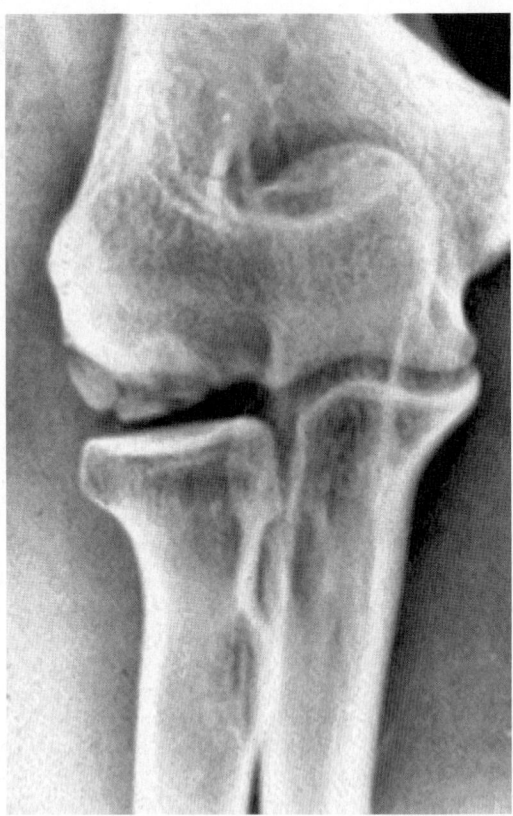

Figure 687-1 Osteochondritis dissecans in the elbow. *(From Anderson SJ: Sports injuries. Curr Probl Pediatr Adolesc Health 35:105–176, 2005.)*

head. OCD classically affects athletes in their 2nd decade. The most common presentation is poorly localized vague knee pain. There is rarely a history of recent acute trauma. Some OCD lesions are asymptomatic (diagnosed on "routine" radiographs), whereas others are manifested as joint effusion, pain, decreased range of motion, and mechanical symptoms (locking, popping, catching). Activity usually worsens the pain.

Physical examination might show no specific findings. Sometimes tenderness over the involved condyle can be elicited by deep palpation with the knee flexed. Diagnosis is usually made with plain radiographs (Fig. 687-1). A tunnel view radiograph can be obtained to better view the posterior two-thirds of the femoral condyle. Treatment of OCD remains controversial. Intact lesions can often be treated symptomatically with or without activity modification or immobilization. Free fragments often require surgical removal. Drilling techniques can be utilized and are helpful in stimulating new bone formation, healing, and return of mobile bodies to their original donor sites. Long-term sequelae can be seen in up to 25% with atypical lesions, older age, effusion, and lesions of large size.

Avulsion fractures occur when a forceful muscle contraction dislodges the apophysis from the bone. They occur most commonly around the hip (Fig. 687-2) and are treated nonsurgically. Acute fractures to other apophyses (knee and elbow) require urgent orthopedic consultation. Chronically increased traction at the muscle–apophysis attachment can lead to repetitive microtrauma and pain at the apophysis. The most common areas affected are the knee (Osgood-Schlatter and Sinding-Larsen-Johansson disease), the ankle (Sever disease) (Fig. 687-3), and the medial epicondyle (Little League elbow). Traction apophysitis of the knee and ankle can potentially be treated in a primary care setting. The main goal of treatment is to minimize the intensity and incidence of pain and disability. Exercises that increase the strength, flexibility, and endurance of the muscles attached at the

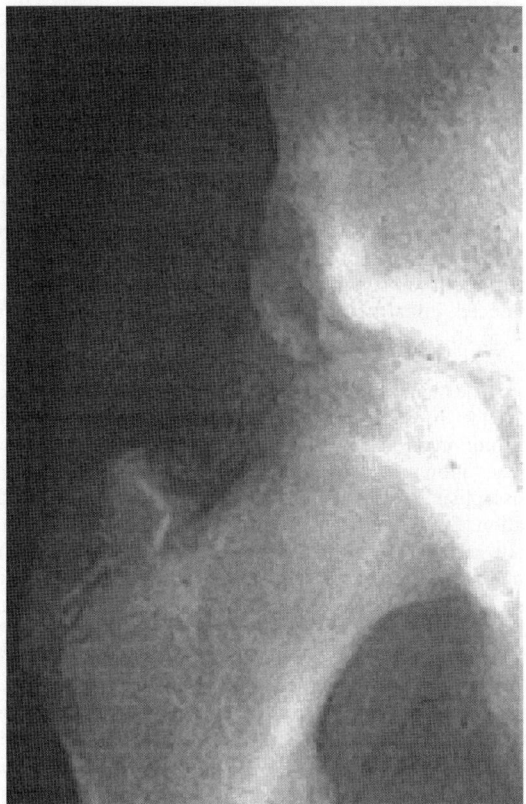

Figure 687-2 Anterior inferior iliac spine avulsion. *(From Anderson SJ: Lower extremity injuries in youth sports. Pediatr Clin North Am 49:62–641, 2003.)*

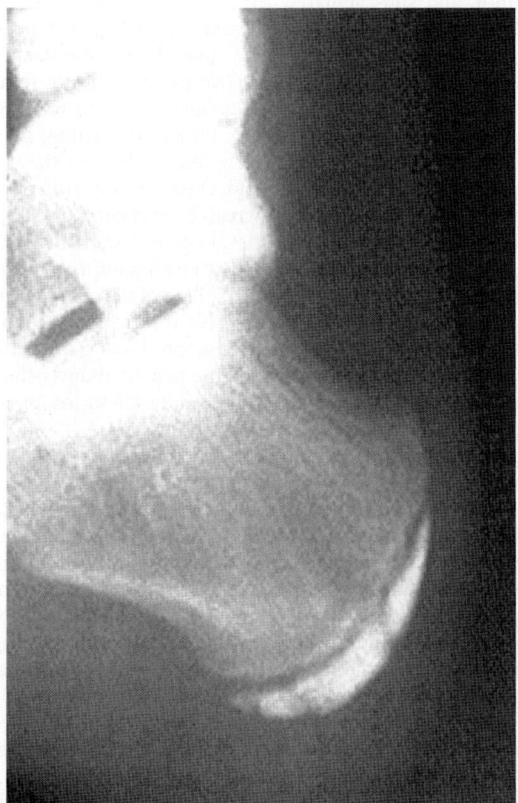

Figure 687-3 Calcaneal apophysitis (Sever disease). *(From Anderson SJ: Sports injuries. Curr Probl Pediatr Adolesc Health 35:105–176, 2005.)*

apophysis, using the relative rest principle, are appropriate. Symptoms can last for 12-24 mo if untreated. As growth slows, symptoms abate.

Bibliography is available at Expert Consult.

687.2 Shoulder Injuries
Kevin P. Murphy and Aaron M. Karlin

Shoulder pain associated with radiating symptoms down the arm should raise the possibility of a neck injury. *Neck pain and tenderness or limitation of cervical range of motion requires that the cervical spine be immobilized and that the athlete be transferred for further evaluation.* If there is no neck pain or tenderness or limitation of motion of the cervical spine, then the shoulder is likely the site of the primary injury.

CLAVICLE FRACTURES
Clavicle fracture is one of the most common shoulder injuries. Injury is usually sustained by a fall on the lateral shoulder, on an outstretched hand, or by direct blow. Approximately 80% of fractures occur in the middle third of the clavicle. With younger children, plastic bowing of the clavicle may be present instead of an overt fracture and should be treated in the same fashion. Treatment is conservative and includes the use of an arm sling for comfort and protection. Healing time is shorter in comparison to adults, generally 4-6 wk. And additional 2-3 wk period of protection from contact/collision activities is recommended after clinical and radiographic healing is achieved to prevent reinjury. If nondisplaced, most medial and lateral clavicular fractures can be managed similar to middle 3rd clavicular fractures. Displaced lateral and medial third fractures require orthopedic consultation because of a higher incidence of acromioclavicular osteoarthritis (lateral) and physeal involvement (medial). Distal clavicular osteolysis is likely an overuse injury associated with slow dissolution and resorption of bone. The cause of injury is unclear, appearing most consistent with a stress reaction or fracture at the site of considerable force. This lesion is commonly seen in weightlifting athletes and can be seen in the older children. Nonoperative treatment including activity limitations, ice, nonsteroidal antiinflammatory agents and cortisone injections can be helpful. Gripping the bar at a greater distance for the weightlifter may be helpful. For those not willing to modify weightlifting activity or with persistent symptoms despite conservative care, surgery can be very successful and involves removal of the distal clavicle (approximately 1 cm) with no loss of strength and full return to activity anticipated.

ACROMIOCLAVICULAR SEPARATION
An acromioclavicular (AC) separation most commonly occurs when an athlete sustains a direct blow to the acromion with the humerus in an adducted position, forcing the acromion inferiorly and medially. Force is directed toward the AC and coracoclavicular ligaments because of the inherent stability of the sternoclavicular joint. Patients have point tenderness at the AC joint, pain with lifting their arms above the level of their shoulder, and may have an apparent step-off between the distal clavicle and the acromion (Fig. 687-4).

Type I AC injuries involve isolated sprain of the AC ligament with the periosteal sleeve intact. There is no visible deformity and radiographs are normal. Pain is elicited with adduction of the humerus across the chest. **Type II** injuries involve the AC ligament and coracoclavicular ligament, as well as partial disruption of the periosteal sleeve. Radiographs may show slight widening of the AC joint though the distance between the clavicle and the coracoid process is unchanged in comparison to the uninjured shoulder. Treatment of type I and type II AC injuries is conservative and nonoperative and consists of ice, nonsteroidal antiinflammatories and a sling for immobilization and pain control acutely. Shoulder range of motion exercises and strengthening of the rotator cuff, deltoid and trapezius musculature are incorporated early in the course once pain free range improves to prevent residual joint stiffness. A short course of physical therapy may be helpful if range of motion limitations are present 2-4 wk out from

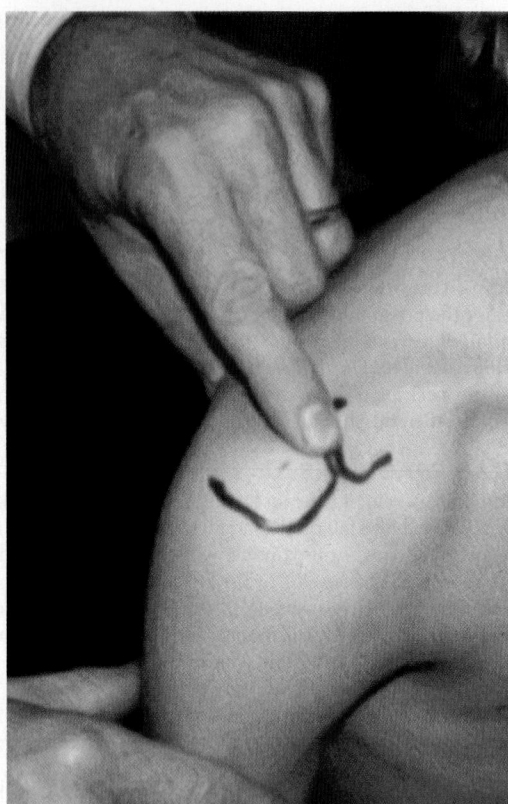

Figure 687-4 Palpitation of acromioclavicular joint. *(From Anderson SJ: Sports injuries,* Curr Probl Pediatr Adolesc Health *35:105–176, 2005.)*

injury. Consideration for return to play is made when the patient no longer has focal AC joint tenderness, exhibits full painless range of motion, has strength sufficient to be functionally protected from a collision or fall, and can perform maneuvers required within their sport. Typically, return to play from a type I AC injury is 1-2 wk, and 2-4 wk for type II.

Type III injury is more severe involving further tearing of the AC and coracoclavicular ligaments and disruption of the periosteal tube with instability of the distal clavicle because of deltotrapezial fascial detachment. Radiographs will commonly show superior displacement of the distal clavicle from the coracoid of 25-100%. Treatment of type III AC injuries is controversial, although many can be treated nonoperatively similar to that described for types I and II AC injuries if there is no damage to the overlying skin or neurovascular compromise to the injured limb. The patient should be counseled regarding this injury, likely resulting in a noticeable defect, to ascertain whether this is acceptable. Surgery for type III AC injuries are uncommon and primarily for cosmetic reasons. **Types IV, V, and VI** AC injuries have progressive worsening of ligamentous and fascial disruption with varied locations of the clavicular displacement. These injuries should be referred to an orthopedist for consultation and operative repair.

ANTERIOR DISLOCATION

The most common mechanism of injury is making contact with another player with the shoulder abducted to 90 degrees and forcefully rotated externally. A common example of the latter is a football player tackling another player only with the arm. Patients complain of severe pain and that their shoulder "popped out of place" or "shifted." Patients with an unreduced anterior dislocation have a hollow region inferior to the acromion and a bulge in the anterior portion of the shoulder caused by anterior displacement of the humeral head. Abnormal sensation of the lateral deltoid region (axillary nerve) and the extensor

surface of the proximal forearm (musculocutaneous nerve) should be noted.

Reduction of a dislocated shoulder should be made expediently assuming no presence of crepitans (concerning for fracture). Numerous safe methods for closed reduction have been described, including the traction–counter traction technique, the Stimson maneuver, and the abduction maneuver. Postreduction radiographs are helpful and may show evidence of a posterior lateral humeral head impaction fracture (Hill-Sachs lesion). Injuries to the surrounding soft tissues, including the anterior capsule and labrum, are best evaluated by MRI, often with an accompanying arthrogram of the glenohumeral joint. Once reduced, initial treatment of a dislocation includes placing the patient into an arm sling for comfort and protection. The duration of immobilization is controversial and may last anywhere from a few days to 4-6 wk. The most significant risk after an acute traumatic dislocation is recurrence. Most sports medicine practitioners encourage early range of motion and strengthening exercises as tolerated. Rehabilitation focuses upon progressive strengthening of the rotator cuff, deltoid, and periscapular muscles at increasing degrees of abduction and external rotation. Strengthening of the rotator cuff muscles is extremely important as they are the dynamic stabilizers of the glenohumeral joint, integral in preventing future dislocation. Plyometric exercises may also be incorporated near the end of rehabilitation to improve proprioceptive function in preparation for return to athletics. Patients can return to play when strength, flexibility, and proprioception are equal to the uninjured shoulder to the extent that they are able to protect the shoulder and perform sports specific activities without pain. Surgery is to be considered in cases of multiple recurrent dislocations or in those individuals that fail to heal adequately after prolonged rehabilitation. Additionally, early operative repair should be considered for athletes participating in contact or collision spots that inherently have higher recurrence rates.

ROTATOR CUFF INJURY

The rotator cuff muscles comprise the supraspinatus, infraspinatus, teres minor, and subscapularis. The function of these muscles is to rotate the humerus and stabilize the humeral head against the glenoid. The supraspinatus is most commonly injured, an acute strain caused by trauma or chronic tendinosis from overuse. Specifically, rotator cuff tendinosis commonly presents with complaint of pain with overhead arc of motion, such as with throwing, lifting, or reaching for objects above one's head. Pain is often poorly localized about the shoulder, although may be referred to the deltoid. Onset of pain is often insidious and commonly associated with increased frequency or duration of overhead throwing or lifting activities. Pain is exacerbated with these or other activities but is often present at rest; nighttime pain in more severe cases. On exam, manual muscle testing of the cuff muscles often produces pain and in some cases weakness in comparison to the uninjured shoulder. Supraspinatus tendinosis produces pain with active abduction against resistance in which the patient abducts the arm to 90 degrees, forward flexes to 30 degrees anterior to the parasagittal plane, and internally rotates the humerus.

Treatment of rotator cuff tendinosis includes relative rest from athletics or activities causing pain, ice, analgesia or nonsteroidal antiinflammatory use. Strengthening of the rotator cuff and scapular stabilizer musculature, modifications of technique, and core strengthening are important components of rehabilitation often supervised by a physical therapist. In the young athlete, rotator cuff pain is most commonly a result of glenohumeral instability and not rotator cuff impingement syndrome, more commonly seen in adults and caused by impingement of the rotator cuff by the bony structures superior to it. As a result, treatment focusing on stretching alone can make symptoms worse. Return to play often includes gradual increases in load placed upon the rotator cuff as the patient resumes their prior activities such as an interval throwing program in baseball.

Glenoid labrum tears may present in similar insidious fashion to rotator cuff tendinosis or be associated with an acute traumatic dislocation. This is frequently manifested with pain in the glenohumeral joint and may be associated with a sensation of clicking or catching in the shoulder. This can frequently be reproduced on exam. One of the most common lesions is a superior labrum anterior and posterior lesion. Throwing athletes are at particular risk. Mechanism of injury is thought to be related to a traction injury along the long head of the biceps at its attachment at the superior glenoid labrum occurring during a throwing cycle. Radiographs are usually normal. MRI with arthrogram is the best study to identify glenoid labrum pathology.

Proximal humeral stress fracture (epiphysiolysis) is an uncommon cause of proximal shoulder pain and is suspected when shoulder pain does not respond to routine measures. Gradual onset of deep shoulder pain occurs in a young (open epiphyseal plates) athlete involved in repetitive overhead motion, such as in baseball, tennis, or swimming, but with no history of trauma. Tenderness is noted over the proximal humerus; the diagnosis is confirmed by detecting a widened epiphyseal plate on plain radiographs, increased uptake on nuclear scan, or edema of the physis on MRI. Treatment is total rest from throwing for 6-8 wk.

Non–sports-related conditions that need to be considered in the child with a painful shoulder include the Sprengel deformity. This deformity involves the scapula, which fails to descend from its cervical region overlying the 1st through 5th ribs. Children often present with a shortened neckline and lack of normal scapular thoracic motion. Malpositioning of a glenoid can cause limited forward flexion and abduction of the shoulder. An omovertebral bar is present in up to 50% of cases. This bar connects the superior medial angle of the scapula and the cervical spine and consists of fibrous cartilaginous tissue or bone. Other regional abnormalities can include scoliosis with a prominent scapula on the convex side, rib anomalies, and Klippel-Feil syndrome. Winging of the scapula always raises the question of muscular dystrophy, particularly scapular thoracic. Family histories can be most helpful. Primary bone tumors (see Chapter 501) common to the upper extremities include Ewing sarcoma of the scapula and osteogenic sarcoma of the proximal humerus, in addition to osteoblastomas and chondroblastomas common to the diaphysis and epiphysis of long bones. The most common presenting manifestations of osteosarcoma are pain, upper limb dysfunction, and swelling. Similar presentations can be seen in Ewing sarcoma, along with weight loss and fever. Symptoms not responding to conservative treatment require further investigation and specialty consultation.

Bibliography is available at Expert Consult.

687.3 Elbow Injuries
Kevin P. Murphy and Aaron M. Karlin

ACUTE INJURIES

The most commonly dislocated joint in childhood is the elbow. Radial head subluxation, or "nurse maid's elbow," comprises the majority of these and is discussed in more depth in Chapter 681. Posterior dislocation is the next most common type of elbow dislocation, with its mechanism being that of falling backward onto an outstretched arm with the elbow in extension. The dislocation may be complete or incomplete, termed "perched," with the trochlea subluxed upon the top of the coronoid process. The ulnar collateral ligament is commonly disrupted along with other components of the soft-tissue capsule about the elbow. Fractures of the olecranon (greater than 80%) or medial epicondyle may be present as well. An obvious deformity is visualized with the olecranon process displaced prominently behind the distal humerus. Careful examination of the distal radius and ulnar pulses to assess vascular integrity of the distal upper arm is important because of the potential for injury to the brachial artery. Sensation to the distal extremity should also be assessed because of possible injury to the radial, median, and ulnar nerves. Reduction should be performed as soon as possible before significant swelling and muscle spasm potentially complicate the procedure. Longitudinal traction is applied to the

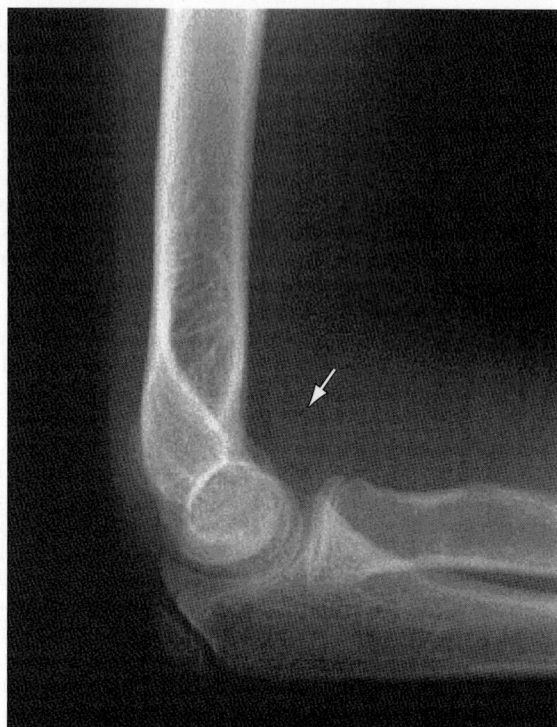

Figure 687-5 Deflection of the coronoid fat pad with a joint effusion (fat pad sign) showing evidence of a fracture. *(From Gomez JE: Upper extremity injuries in youth sports. Pediatr Clin North Am 49:593–626, 2002.)*

forearm with gentle upward pressure on the distal humerus so that the coronoid process clears the trochlea. If reduction is unable to be performed, the arm should be placed in a padded splint and sling and the patient transported to an emergency facility.

Supracondylar humeral fractures can result from the same mechanism of injury as elbow dislocations and can be difficult to distinguish from a posterior dislocation because of significant swelling about the elbow joint. These, too, can be complicated by concomitant injury to the brachial artery and to a lesser extent the median, radial, and ulnar nerves. The injury typically occurs in the 1st decade of life, which is associated with peak hyperlaxity of the elbow joint in children between the ages of 5 and 8 yr. An acute compartment syndrome can develop after these fractures, which is associated with a fat pad sign (Fig. 687-5). These fractures should be referred for orthopedic consultation and are discussed in more depth in Chapter 683.

Direct trauma to the elbow can cause bleeding and inflammation in the olecranon bursa resulting in *olecranon bursitis.* Aspiration is rarely required and this injury can be managed with ice, compressive dressing and analgesia (RICE principles). An overlying elbow pad provides comfort during activity and prevention of reinjury.

Chronic Injuries

Overuse injuries occur primarily in throwing sports and sports that require repetitive wrist flexion or extension or demand weightbearing on hands (gymnastics). "Little League elbow" is a broad term for several different elbow problems.

Throwing overhand creates valgus stress to the elbow with medial opening of the joint and lateral compressive forces.

Medial elbow pain is a common complaint of young throwers, resulting from repetitive valgus overload of the wrist flexor-pronator muscle groups and their attachment on the medial apophysis. In preadolescents who still have maturing secondary ossification centers, *traction apophysitis of the medial epicondyle* is likely. Patients have tenderness along the medial epicondyle; pain is exacerbated by valgus stress or resisted wrist flexion and pronation. Wrist pain may be present in more severe cases. Radiographs may show widening of the growth plate at the medial apophysis in comparison to the uninjured elbow. Treatment includes no throwing for 4-6 wk, pain-free strengthening, and stretching of the flexor–pronator group followed by a 1-2 wk progressive functional throwing program with careful rehabilitation. Incorporation of core strengthening and scapular stabilizing exercise, as well as addressing proper throwing mechanics (to reduce the load upon the medial elbow), are important components of rehabilitation. This problem has to be treated with rest because of the risk of nonunion of the apophysis and chronic pain. If pain occurs acutely, *avulsion fracture of the medial epicondyle* must be considered. Radiographs should be taken in any thrower with acute elbow pain (Fig. 687-6). If the medial epicondyle is avulsed, orthopedic consultation is indicated.

In older adolescents and young adults with a fused apophysis, the vulnerable structure is the *ulnar collateral ligament* (UCL). UCL sprains/tears are common in sports requiring high-velocity throwing or overhead activities. Medial elbow pain primarily worse during the acceleration phase of throwing is common. A sensation of elbow "opening" during throwing is also frequently described. On exam focal tenderness to palpation over the UCL is present. Additionally laxity may be appreciated with valgus stress of the elbow when flexed to 30 and/or 90 degrees. Radiographs are generally unremarkable. MRI with arthrography or ultrasonography is often necessary to assess the integrity of the UCL. Partial tears can be treated with a period of time off from throwing (2-4 wk) followed by careful progressive rehabilitation as discussed above for medial elbow pain. If there is a complete tear, surgical repair is indicated if the athlete desires to continue a pitching career.

Medial epicondylitis (golfer's elbow) is another common cause of medial elbow pain in the individual with fused apophysis. It is commonly caused by overuse of the flexor pronator muscle groups at their origin at the medial humeral epicondyle. This occurs frequently in athletics or activities with repetitive wrist flexion. Tenderness is noted over the medical epicondyle and exacerbated by passive wrist extension or resisted wrist flexion. Treatment includes rest from the inciting activity, ice, stretching and strengthening of the wrist flexors, forearm straps, counterforce bracing, and analgesia. Ulnar nerve dysfunction can be a complication of valgus overload and can occur with any of the diagnoses previously discussed. Persisting paresthesia or motor weakness in the ulnar nerve distribution should be evaluated with electromyography and nerve conduction studies.

Lateral elbow pain can be caused by compression during the throwing motion at the radiocapitellar joint. *Panner disease* is osteochondrosis of the capitellum that occurs between ages 7 and 12 yr (Fig. 687-7). *OCD* of the capitellum occurs at age 13-16 yr (see Fig. 687-1). These 2 entities might represent a continuum of the same disease. Although patients with both conditions present with insidious onset of lateral elbow pain exacerbated by throwing, patients with OCD have mechanical symptoms (popping, locking) and, more commonly, decreased range of motion. Patients with Panner disease have no mechanical symptoms and often have normal range of motion. The prognosis of Panner disease is excellent, and treatments consist of relative rest (no throwing), brief immobilization, and repeat radiographs in 6-12 wk to assess bone remodeling. In OCD, radiographs show a more focal lesion in the capitellum with eventual flattening and potentially fragmentation. MRI scan can be very helpful in the diagnosis early on and with subsequent staging. A diagnosis of OCD requires orthopedic consultation with treatment dependent upon the severity of the lesion and fragmentation.

Lateral epicondylitis (tennis elbow), the most common overuse elbow injury in adults, is relatively uncommon in children and

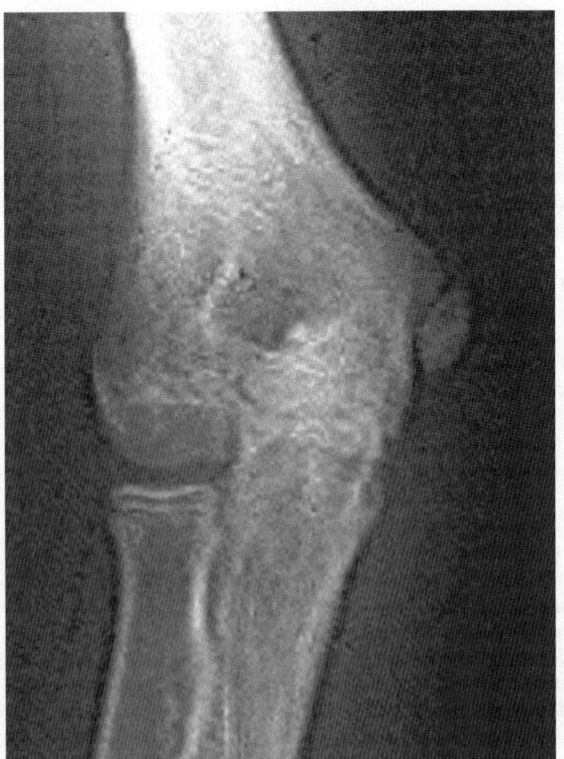

Figure 687-6 Medial epicondylitis. *(From Anderson SJ: Sports injuries. Curr Probl Pediatr Adolesc Health 35:105–176, 2005.)*

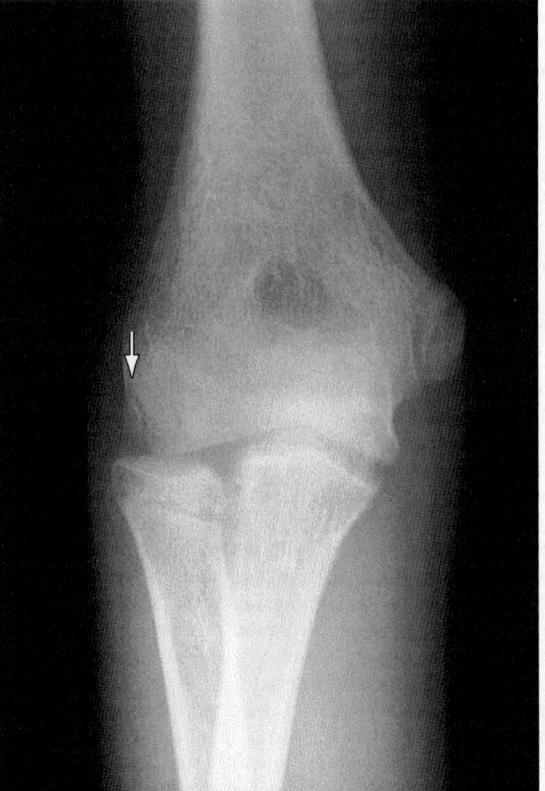

Figure 687-7 Panner disease. Note fragmentation of the humeral capitellum and flattening of the articular surface *(arrow)*. *(Courtesy of Dr. Ralph J. Curtis. From Gomez JE: Upper extremity injuries in youth sports. Pediatr Clin North Am 49:593–626, 2002.)*

adolescents. It is a tendinosis of the extensor muscle origin at the lateral humeral epicondyle commonly found in individuals performing activities requiring repetitive or prolonged grip. Tenderness is localized over the upper lateral epicondyle and is worsened with passive wrist flexion or resisted wrist extension. Treatment includes relative rest, analgesia, and specific stretching and strengthening exercises for the elbow and forearm. Improper equipment (i.e., wrong grip size or overstrung racket) and poor technique can contribute to onset of symptoms. Return to play should be gradual and progressive to prevent reinjury.

Elbow injuries can be minimized but not necessarily prevented by preseason stretching and strengthening exercises. The importance of core strengthening and scapular stabilization with respect to preventing elbow and shoulder injuries in the throwing athlete cannot be overstated. The most important consideration for preventing elbow injuries in throwers is limitation of the number of pitches and advising players, coaches, and athletes that they should stop immediately when they experience elbow pain. If it persists, they need medical evaluation. It has been recommended that a young pitcher have age specific limits on pitch counts including number of pitches thrown per game and per week, as well as maintaining appropriate days off between games pitched. A good rule of thumb is the maximal number of pitches per game should be approximately 6 times the pitcher's age in years.

Other less-common problems that cause elbow pain are ulnar neuropathy/subluxation, tricipital or bicipital tendonitis (distal), olecranon apophysitis, and loose bodies. Non–sports-related injuries that need to be considered in the child with a painful elbow include congenital conditions, such as radial dysplasia, including radial ulnar synostosis and mild persistent brachial plexus palsy. The elbow is not an uncommon site for inflammatory arthritides, including juvenile idiopathic arthritis, sepsis, hemophilia, and sickle cell disease. Neoplasia to consider includes osteoblastomas and chondroblastomas, common in the diaphysis and epiphysis of longer bones, in addition to osteosarcoma. As always, in the child with persistent symptoms who is not responding to conservative care, further diagnostic work up is always indicated.

Bibliography is available at Expert Consult.

687.4 Low Back Injuries
Kevin P. Murphy and Aaron M. Karlin

SPONDYLOLYSIS, SPONDYLOLISTHESIS, AND FACET SYNDROME
Spondylolysis
Spondylolysis, a common cause of back pain in athletes, is a stress fracture of the pars interarticularis (see Chapter 679.6). It can occur at any vertebral level but is most likely at L4 or L5. Complete spondylolysis has never been found in the newborn. Its occurrence increases between the ages of 5.5 and 6.5 yr to a rate of 5%, close to the frequency of 5.8% in the white population. Prevalence in adolescent athletes evaluated for low back pain is 13-47%. Besides acute hyperextension that causes an acute fracture, the mechanism of injury is either a congenital defect or hypoplastic pars, which is exacerbated by lumbar extension loading, or a stress fracture caused by repetitive extension loading. Ballet, weightlifting, gymnastics, and football are examples of sports in which repetitive extension loading of the lumbar spine occurs; it occurs in any activity in which there is repetitive extension loading, including swimming.

Patients often present with pain of insidious onset. However, there may be a precipitating injury such as a fall or single episode of hyperextension. The pain is worse with extension, can radiate to the buttocks, and can eventually affect activities of daily living. Rest or supine positioning usually alleviates the pain.

On examination, the pain is reproduced with lumbar extension while standing, especially when standing on 1 leg (single-leg hyperextension test). Limited forward spinal flexion and tight hamstrings may

be seen. Neurologic examination should be normal. There is well-localized tenderness to deep palpation just lateral to the spinous process on the affected side and is usually at L4 or L5.

The diagnosis is confirmed by finding a pars defect on an oblique lumbar spine radiograph. The defect is rarely seen on anteroposterior (AP) and lateral views. Bone single-photon emission CT is needed to confirm diagnosis if radiographs are normal. A plain CT scan can help to identify the degree of bony involvement and is sometimes used to assess healing.

Treatment includes pain relief and activity restriction. Rehabilitation consisting of trunk strengthening, hip flexor stretching, and hamstring stretching is important in most cases. A thoracic lumbar sacral orthotic on a temporary basis may be helpful for the spondylolytic stress fracture resistant to healing by alternative conservative means.

Spondylolisthesis and Facet Syndrome
Spondylolysis, spondylolisthesis, and facet syndrome are injuries posterior to vertebral elements. *Spondylolisthesis* occurs when bilateral pars defects exist and forward displacement or slippage of a vertebra occurs on the vertebra inferior to it (see Chapter 679.6). *Facet syndrome* has a similar history and physical examination findings as spondylolysis. It is caused by instability or injury to the facet joint, posterior to the pars interarticularis and at the interface of the inferior and superior articulating processes. Facet syndrome can be established by identifying facet abnormalities on CT or by exclusion, requiring a nondiagnostic radiograph and nuclear scan to rule out spondylolysis.

Treatment of posterior element injuries is conservative, directed at reducing the extension-loading activity, often for 2-3 mo. Body mechanics, posture principals, core strengthening, and lumbar pelvic stabilization routines can be very helpful in the functional recovery of the motivated athlete. Walking, swimming and cycling can be appropriate exercises also during the rehabilitation phase. Rarely spinal segmental fusion can be indicated in the athlete with spondylolisthesis and persistent symptomatic segmental instability despite further conservative care.

LUMBAR DISK HERNIATION, STRAIN, AND CONTUSION
Intervertebral disc injury in children and the young athlete is uncommon. In contrast to the selective motor and sensory deficits often observed in adults with disc herniation, athletes younger than 20 yr of age have pain or tenderness less commonly identified over the course of the sciatic nerve. Physical examination findings may be minimal but usually include pain with forward flexion and lateral bending. It is unusual to have a positive straight leg test or any neurologic deficit in the young athlete with an injured disc. There may be tenderness of the vertebral spinous process at the level of the disc. A general aching sensation in the lower back or upper buttocks may be present. MRI usually confirms a clinical diagnosis. Assuming the herniation is not large and the pain is not intractable, the treatment of choice is conservative with analgesia and physical therapy. Surgery is rarely necessary.

Acute lumbar strain or contusion can be seen in the younger athlete and is usually associated with precipitating activity often outside of the normal routine. Physical examination reveals tenderness in the paraspinal and lateral soft tissues often associated with recreating the mechanisms of injury. Thoracic and lumbar strain in the school-age child is associated with obesity, deconditioning, positive family history, and poorly supervised and equipped recreational activity. Up to 20% of youth have experienced back pain at some point in their life (younger than age 15 yr). The school-age backpack is rapidly becoming the most common cause of back pain of a benign nature in children. Up to 74% of school backpackers experience pain. Back pain is more common with the heavy backpack (greater than 10-20% of body weight), female gender, large body mass index, and single shoulder strap.

Treatment is conservative including analgesia, myofascial release, massage, and physical therapy, as tolerated. The natural history of acute back strain in adults is that 50% are better in 1 wk, 80% in 1 mo, and 90% in 2 mo, regardless of therapy. The course of back pain in young athletes is likely similar given the elimination of obvious precipitating influence and/or activities, as discussed above.

SACROILIITIS

Sacroiliitis manifests as pain over the sacroiliac joints; it is usually chronic but occasionally associated with a history of trauma. Patients have a positive result with the **Patrick test,** which includes resting the foot of the affected side on the opposite knee (hip flexed 90 degrees), stabilizing the opposite iliac crest, and externally rotating the hip on the affected side (pushing the knee down and lateral). Symptomatic improvement with knee-to-chest maneuvers and subsequent posterior pelvic tilt may be present. A radiograph of the sacroiliac joints is indicated, and if results are positive, exploration for a rheumatologic disease (ankylosing spondylitis [see Chapter 156], juvenile rheumatoid arthritis [see Chapter 155], ulcerative colitis [see Chapter 336]) is warranted.

Treatment is with relative rest, nonsteroidal antiinflammatory drugs, and physical therapy. Ankylosing spondylitis is more likely if the onset of lower back pain is before age 40 yr, if there is morning stiffness that is associated with improvement with activity, and if the pain has a gradual onset and has lasted longer than 3 mo.

OTHER CAUSES

Non–sports-related causes of low back pain are numerous and include infection (osteomyelitis, diskitis) and neoplasia. These should be considered in patients with fever, weight loss, other constitutional signs, or lack of response to initial therapy. Osteomyelitis of the lower back or pelvis is often, but not always, associated with fever. Scheuermann disease needs to be considered more common in males and younger adolescents, and needs to be distinguished from symptomatic postural roundback and congenital decompensating kyphosis. Atypical Scheuermann disease or thoracolumbar apophysitis can progress and become the pediatric equivalent of an adult compression fracture. Benign tumors of the spine include osteoid osteoma with intense focal nighttime pain, not activity related and almost always relieved by aspirin or nonsteroidal antiinflammatory agents. Osteoblastoma, eosinophilic granuloma, aneurismal bone cyst, and fibrous dysplasia are additional benign tumors not to be excluded. Malignant spinal tumors include the Ewing sarcoma (onion skin appearance) and osteogenic sarcoma (sunburst pattern) both associated with the Codman triangle. Metastatic tumors of the spine include neuroblastoma, spinal cord tumors, leukemia, and lymphoma. Wilms tumor can also metastasize to the spine and be associated with hemihypertrophy. Referred pain to the spine always needs to be considered. Conditions that can refer pain include pyelonephritis, renal osteodystrophy, pneumonia, endocarditis, cholecystitis, nephrolithiasis, pancreatitis, megacolon, constipation/ileus, hiatal hernia/reflux, pelvic inflammatory disease, and sickle cell

crisis. Pregnancy is always a consideration in the age-appropriate female. Psychogenic pain and fibromyalgia can be seen in children. Child abuse can present in the spine with soft-tissue injuries more common than fractures. Posterior rib and spinous process fractures can be seen in up to 30% of abused children. Skeletal survey can be helpful with multiple injuries in multiple stages of healing.

Bibliography is available at Expert Consult.

687.5 Hip and Pelvis Injuries
Kevin P. Murphy and Aaron M. Karlin

Hip and pelvis injuries represent a small percentage of sports injuries, but they are potentially severe and require prompt diagnosis. Hip pathology can manifest as knee pain and normal findings on knee examination.

In children, *transient synovitis* is the most common cause. It usually manifests with acute onset of a limp, with the child refusing to use the affected leg and having painful range of motion on examination. There may be a history of minor trauma. This is a self-limiting condition that usually resolves in 48-72 hr.

Legg-Calvé-Perthes disease (avascular necrosis of the femoral head) also manifests in childhood with insidious onset of limp and hip pain (see Chapter 678.3).

Until the skeleton matures (Table 687-2), younger athletes are susceptible to apophyseal injuries (e.g., the anterior superior iliac spine). *Apophysitis* develops from overuse or from direct trauma. *Avulsion fractures* occur in adolescents playing sports requiring sudden, explosive bursts of speed (see Fig. 687-2). Large muscles contract and create force greater than the strength of the attachment of the muscle to the apophysis. Biomechanical susceptibility of the pelvis allows separation to occur in the cartilaginous region between the apophysis and the adjoining bone. The most common sites of avulsion fractures are the anterior superior iliac spine (sartorius and tensor fasciae lata), anterior inferior iliac spine (rectus femoris), lesser femoral trochanter (iliopsoas), ischial tuberosity (hamstrings), and the iliac crest (abdominal muscles). Symptoms include localized pain and swelling, with decreased strength and range of motion. Bilateral radiographs are important in order to allow for comparison to assess for displacement, if any, of the fracture fragment. Significant displacement or presence of a large fragment may require orthopedic consultation. Initial **treatment** includes ice, analgesics, rest, and pain-free range-of-motion exercises. Crutches are usually needed for ambulation. Surgery is usually not indicated because most of these fractures—even large or displaced ones—heal well. Direct contact to the bone around the hip and pelvis causes exquisitely tender subperiosteal hematomas called

Table 687-2	Age of Appearance and Fusion of Apophyses in Hip and Pelvis		
APOPHYSIS	**APPEARANCE (YR)**	**FUSION (YR)**	**RELATED MUSCLE GROUP(S)**
AIIS	13-15	16-18	Quadriceps
ASIS	13-15	21-25	Sartorius
Lesser trochanter	11-12	16-17	Iliopsoas
Greater trochanter	2-3	16-17	Gluteal
Ischial tuberosity	13-15	20-25	Hamstrings
Iliac crest	13-15	21-25	Abdominal obliques Latissimus dorsi

AIIS, anterior inferior iliac spine; ASIS, anterior superior iliac spine.
From Waite BL, Krabak BJ: Examination and treatment of pediatric injuries of the hip and pelvis, Phys Med Rehabil Clin N Am 19:305–318, ix, 2008.

hip pointers. These injuries are more commonly seen around the anterior superior iliac spine and the iliac crest. Limited active range of motion can be identified about the hip brought on by contracture of locally attached musculature such as hip flexors and hip abductors. Symptomatic care includes rest, ice, analgesia, and protection from reinjury.

Slipped capital femoral epiphysis usually occurs in the 11-15 yr age range during the time of rapid linear bone growth (see Chapter 678.4).

A *femoral neck stress fracture* can manifest as vague progressive hip pain in an endurance athlete. Girls with the female athlete triad are especially at risk. This diagnosis should always be kept in mind in the running athlete with vague anterior thigh pain. On examination, there may be pain with passive stretch of the hip flexors and pain with hip rotation. If radiographs do not demonstrate a periosteal reaction consistent with a stress fracture, a bone scan or MRI may be required. Orthopedic consultation is necessary in femoral neck stress fractures because of their predisposition to nonunion and displacement with minor trauma or continued weight bearing. These fractures carry increased risk of avascular necrosis of the femoral head.

Osteitis pubis is an inflammation at the pubic symphysis that may be caused by excessive side-to-side rocking of the pelvis. It can be seen in an athlete in any running sport and is more common in sports requiring more use of the adductor muscles such as ice hockey, soccer, and inline skating. Athletes typically present with vague groin pain that may be unilateral or bilateral. On physical examination, there is tenderness over the symphysis and sometimes over the proximal adductors. Adduction strength testing causes discomfort. Radiographic evidence (irregularity, sclerosis, widening of the pubic symphysis with osteolysis) might not be present until symptoms are present for 6-8 wk; a bone scan and MRI are more sensitive to early changes. Relative rest for 6-12 wk may be required. Some patients require corticosteroid injection as adjunctive therapy.

Acetabular labrum tears can occur in the hip, similar to glenoid labrum tears in the shoulder. Athletes might have a history of trauma and complain of sharp anterior hip pain associated with a clicking or catching sensation. Clinical diagnosis is difficult; magnetic resonance arthrography is useful for diagnosis.

Snapping hip syndrome is caused by the iliopsoas musculotendinous unit riding over the pectineal eminence of the pelvis, anterior hip capsule or the iliotibial band over the greater trochanter. Lack of flexibility in these muscles results in snapping, as the musculotendinous unit slides over the associated bony prominences. It is commonly seen in ballet dancers and runners; it can occur as an acute or overuse injury (more common). Athletes present with either a painful or painless click or snap in the hip, usually located lateral or anterior and deep in the joint. Examination often reproduces the symptoms. Radiographs are not usually needed in the work-up. Core weakness may be present leading to excessive movement about the hip girdle contributing to increased sliding of the tight muscle over the boney prominence. **Treatment** involves an analgesia, relative rest, biomechanical assessment, core flexibility, with stretching and strengthening of the involved soft tissue. The athlete may return to activity as tolerated. Common soft-tissue injuries around the hip and pelvis include strain and tendinosis of the hip flexors (groin) and hamstrings in addition to quadriceps contusions and greater trochanteric bursitis. Sportsman hernia also needs to be considered in the athlete with insidious onset exertional groin pain, worsening with Valsalva. Pain may radiate into the anterior thigh, inguinal region, rectum, perineum and/or scrotum. Tenderness to deep palpation may or may not be present. Resisted hip flexion and/or half sit ups may be provocative. MRI, CT scan, and bone scan can be helpful in ruling out other diagnoses, but usually are negative with respect to sports hernia pathology. Patients who continue with symptoms despite conservative care may be surgical candidates. Surgical repair can be 95% successful if anatomical lesions are identified. As with any child or adolescent presenting with a painful hip or pelvis, non–sports-related conditions need to be considered. Differential diagnoses may also include the epiphyseal dysplasias, recurrent or undiagnosed congenital or developmental hip dysplasia, additional causes of avascular necrosis including sickle cell anemia, Gaucher

disease, rheumatoid arthritis, and other collagen disorders including steroid therapy. Traumatic hip dislocations are relatively rare in children but not to be overlooked. Leg-length discrepancies can be symptomatic at the hip in an otherwise able bodied child. Common tumors in lower extremities include osteosarcoma along with osteoblastoma, aneurismal bone cysts, and fibrous dysplasia (more common in the pelvis). Metastatic tumors to the lower extremities include neuroblastoma and lymphomas of various types, not to exclude leukemic infiltration with joint arthralgia. Child abuse always needs to be considered in a young patient with musculoskeletal pain no matter what the socioeconomic status.

Bibliography is available at Expert Consult.

687.6 Knee Injuries
Kevin P. Murphy and Aaron M. Karlin

Knee pain is common among adolescents. Acute knee injuries that cause immediate disability are likely to be due to fracture, patellar dislocation, anterior cruciate ligament (ACL) injury, or meniscal tear. The mechanism of injury is usually a weightbearing event. If the knee swells more immediately (within several hours of injury), the swelling is likely caused by a hemarthrosis and more severe injury. The injury most likely to occur with a hemarthrosis is an **ACL** injury. This injury (rare in children younger than 12 yr) is usually caused from being hit directly, landing off-balance from a jump, quickly changing direction while running, or hyperextension. Instability is often present but may be hard to detect in the presence of significant swelling. Girls are more than twice as likely as boys to disrupt their ACL, with a soccer injury a common scenario. Often, these injuries are associated with an avulsion injury of the anterior tibial spine. The majority of athletes with significant ACL injury need orthopedic consultation with consideration of ACL reconstruction. Chronic ACL insufficiency may increase the risk of meniscal injury and further joint dysfunction. Additional physeal-sparing reconstructions with minimal risk of growth arrest or angular deformity have been reported with success in children younger than 12 yr and adolescents.

Posterior cruciate ligament injury occurs from a direct blow to the region of the proximal tibia, such as might occur with a dashboard injury or a fall to the knees in volleyball. Posterior cruciate ligament injuries are rare and are usually treated nonsurgically.

Medial collateral ligament injuries result from a valgus blow to the outside of the knee. Isolated *lateral collateral ligament* injuries are uncommon and result from significant varus knee stress. Because they are extraarticular, lateral collateral ligament injuries should not produce much of a knee effusion and are generally less disabling. Isolated medial and lateral collateral injuries are generally managed nonsurgically with conservative care and appropriate rehabilitation.

Meniscal tears generally occur by the same mechanisms as ACL injuries. They are often associated with less hemarthrosis, significant joint line pain, and increased pain with full knee flexion. MRI scan will often yield the diagnosis; conservative care, including **PRICE** principles, is therapeutic for smaller injuries. Orthopedic consultation is indicated for larger tears not healing with conservative care and causing significant dysfunction inhibiting quality of life. An isolated meniscal tear in a child younger than age 10 yr is unusual, with surgery, again, only if conservative measures fail. The choice is often repair of the meniscus rather than surgical resection because of the increased potential in children for cartilaginous healing. Physeal injuries tend to predominate in younger patients, whereas the more skeletally mature adolescents tend to sustain medial collateral ligament injuries. Discoid meniscus (anatomical variant covering lateral tibial plateau) always needs to be considered, particularly in children younger than age 12 yr.

Patellar dislocation occurs most often as a noncontact injury when the quadriceps muscles forcefully contract to extend the knee while the lower leg is externally rotated. Patellar dislocation is the second most

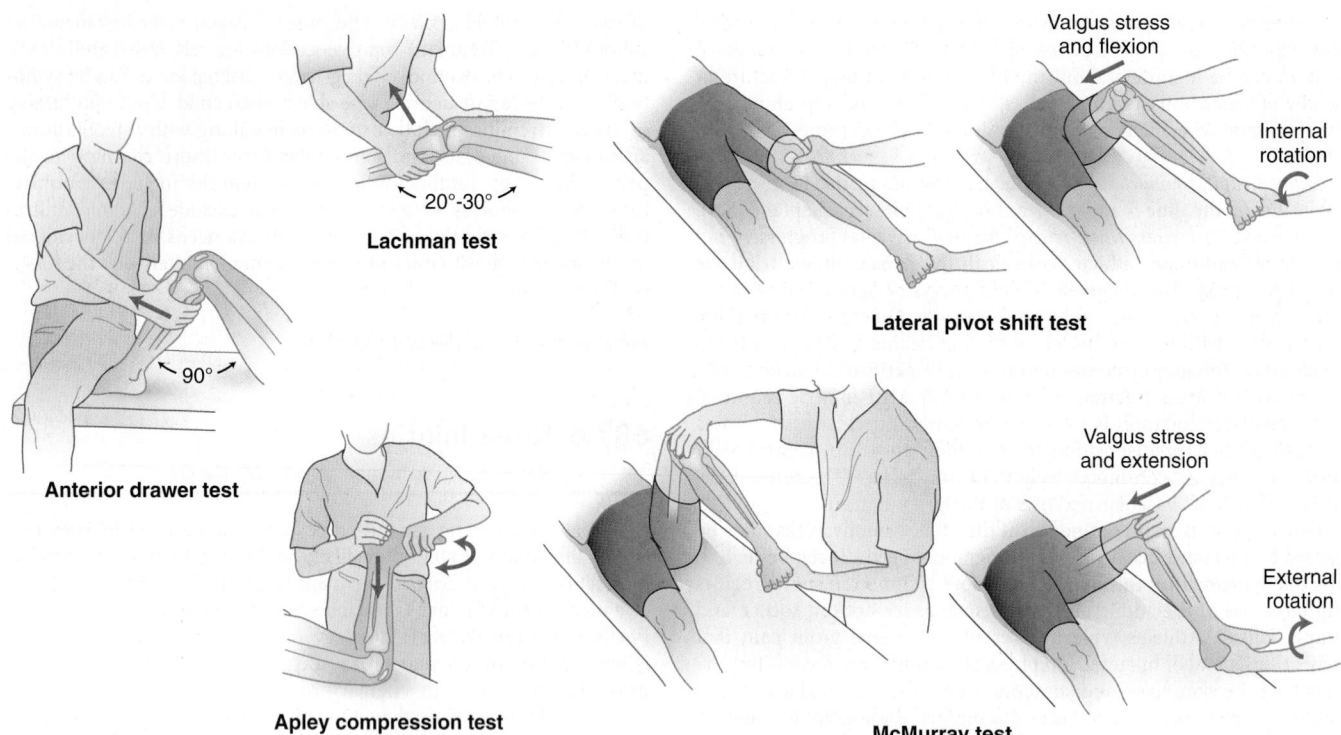

Figure 687-8 Examination maneuvers include the Lachman, anterior drawer, lateral pivot shift, Apley compression, and McMurray tests (the right knee is shown). The Lachman test, performed to detect anterior cruciate ligament (ACL) injuries, is conducted with the patient supine and the knee flexed 20-30 degrees. The anterior drawer test detects ACL injuries and is performed with the patient supine and the knee in 90 degrees of flexion. The lateral pivot shift test is performed with the patient supine, the hip flexed 45 degrees, and the knee in full extension. Internal rotation is applied to the tibia while the knee is flexed to 40 degrees under a valgus stress (pushing the outside of the knee medially). The Apley compression test, used to assess meniscal integrity, is performed with the patient prone and the examiner's knee over the patient's posterior thigh. The tibia is externally rotated while a downward compressive force is applied over the tibia. The McMurray test, used to assess meniscal integrity, is performed with the patient supine and the examiner standing on the side of the affected knee.

common cause of hemarthrosis. The patella is almost always dislocated laterally, and this motion tears the medial patellar retinaculum, causing bleeding in the joint. Recurrent episodes of patellar instability are associated with less swelling. Patellar dislocations are often associated with genu valgum, external tibial torsion, and general ligamentum hyperlaxity. Exercises to strengthen the quadriceps, particularly the vastus medialis, and the use of patella-tracking braces may be helpful. Recurrent instability can require surgical intervention. Surgical stabilization of the medial patellar tissues and lateral retinacular release can be helpful in more difficult cases.

INITIAL TREATMENT OF ACUTE KNEE INJURIES

The physician should inspect for an effusion and obvious deformities; if any deformity is present, the physician should assess neurovascular status and transfer the patient for emergency care as indicated. If no gross deformities are present and neurovascular integrity is intact, initial maneuvers include full passive extension and gentle valgus and varus stress to the knee while in extension. Comparison to the non-injured knee is always helpful for assessing degrees of laxity and range of motion. The patient's ability to contract the quadriceps should be noted. Pain occurring with quadriceps contraction or inability to contract the quadriceps muscle implies an injury to the extensor mechanism. Tenderness over the medial patella, medial retinaculum, or above the adductor tubercle is associated with a patellar dislocation (usually lateral). Point tenderness is consistent with fracture or injury to the underlying structure. Meniscal tears usually manifest as tenderness along the joint line, accentuated with flexion of the knee often beyond 90 degrees. Pain or limitation in either

flexion or extension while rotating the tibia implies a meniscal injury. Ligament injury is manifested as pain or laxity with the appropriate maneuver (Fig. 687-8).

If a patient cannot weight-bear pain free or has clinical signs of instability, significant swelling or other major concern, the knee should be immobilized, crutches provided, and plain radiographs obtained. If the patella is dislocated, reduction may be achieved with gentle active assistive knee extension Straight-leg immobilizers offer no structural support and are only used for comfort and reminding the patient to be careful with any weight-bearing. A derotational hinge brace may be indicated for stabilization such as an injury when both ACL and medial collateral ligament have been traumatized. The leg should be elevated and an elastic wrap can be applied for compression (PRICE principles).

CHRONIC INJURIES
Patellofemoral Stress Syndrome

Patellofemoral stress syndrome (PFSS) is the most common cause of anterior knee pain. PFSS is also known as *patellofemoral pain syndrome* or *patellofemoral dysfunction* (see Chapter 677.5). It is a diagnosis of exclusion used to describe anterior knee pain that has no other identifiable pathology. Chondromalacia may be seen in association with softening of the articular cartilage underneath the patellar surface. Pain is usually difficult to localize. Patients indicate a diffuse area over the anterior knee as the source, or they might feel as if the pain is coming from behind the patella. Bilateral pain is common, and pain is often worse going up stairs, after sitting for prolonged periods, or after squatting or running. There should be a negative history for significant swelling, which would indicate a more serious injury. History of change in activity is common, such as altered training surface or terrain, increased training regimen, or performance of new tasks.

Examination should include evaluation of stance and gait for lower limb alignment, musculature, and midfoot hyperpronation. Flexibility of the hamstrings, iliotibial band (ITB), and gastrocnemius should be assessed, because stress is increased across the patellofemoral joint when these structures are tight. Hip range of motion should be assessed to rule out hip pathology. Medial patellar tenderness or pain with compression of the patellofemoral joint confirms the diagnosis in the absence of a significant effusion and other positive findings. PFSS is a clinical diagnosis usually managed without imaging.

Treatment focuses on assessing and improving flexibility, strength, and gait abnormalities. In the presence of midfoot hyperpronation (ankle valgus), new shoes or use of arch supports can improve patellofemoral mechanics and improve pain. Ice and an analgesic can be used to help control pain. Reduced overall activity or training is important initially in rehabilitation along with limiting knee flexion no greater than 60 degrees as possible. Short arc quadriceps strengthening exercises can be helpful (active knee extension with or without resistance between 0 and 30 degrees of knee flexion). Therapeutic taping techniques to help improve patella tracking within the trochlear groove can be helpful with the assistance of a sports physical therapist.

Osgood-Schlatter Disease

Osgood-Schlatter disease is a traction apophysitis occurring at the insertion of the patellar tendon on the tibial tuberosity (see Chapter 677.4). Because it is also related to overuse of the extensor mechanism, Osgood-Schlatter disease is **treated** like PFSS. A protective pad to protect the tibial tubercle from direct trauma can be used. Therapeutic taping of the tibial tubercle may provide comfort, along with well-fitted knee sleeves and/or straps. Nonsteroidal antiinflammatory drugs are often prescribed as well. Pain-free strengthening of weightbearing soft tissues using more closed-kinetic chain techniques may be best. PRICE principles apply. Make certain that patients and parents are aware that resolution is usually slow, often requiring 12-18 mo. Complications are rare and can include growth arrest with recurvatum deformity and rupture or avulsion of the patellar tendon/tibial tubercle.

Other Chronic Injuries

Sinding-Larsen-Johansson disease is a traction apophysitis occurring at the inferior pole of the patella. It occurs most often in volleyball and basketball athletes. **Treatment** is similar to that of PFSS and Osgood-Schlatter disease.

Patellar tendinosis (jumper's knee) is caused by repetitive microtrauma of the patellar tendon, usually at the inferior pole of the patella. In approximately 10% of the cases, the quadriceps tendon above the patella is affected. It is associated with jumping sports but occurs in runners as well. **Treatment** is similar to that for PFSS. Relative rest is more important in patellar tendinosis because chronic pain can be associated with irreversible changes in the tendon.

ITB friction syndrome is the most common cause of chronic lateral knee pain. Generally it is not associated with swelling or instability. It is from friction of the ITB along the lateral knee, resulting in bursitis. Tenderness is elicited along the ITB as it courses over the lateral femoral condyle or at its insertion at the Gerdy tubercle, along the lateral tibial plateau. Tightness of the ITB is also noted using the Ober test. To perform an Ober test, the athlete lies on one side and the superior hip is extended with the knee flexed. The examiner holds the ankle in midair, and if the knee moves inferiorly, it implies a flexible ITB and a negative Ober test. If the knee and leg stay in midair, the ITB is tight and the Ober test is positive. **Treatment** principles follow those for PFSS, except emphasis is on improving flexibility of the ITB.

Other soft-tissue injuries not to be excluded include prepatellar and pes anserine bursitis, plical syndromes, and Hoffa syndrome. The pes anserine bursa lies just under the conjoined tendon of the sartorius, gracilis, and semitendinosus muscles as it attaches medially to the proximal tibia. In Hoffa syndrome, the fat pad beneath the patella and

posterior to the patella ligament becomes pinched with anterior pain on knee extension. These conditions are generally more common in adolescents, those with genu recurvatum, and long distance runners. Non–sports-related conditions, again, always need to be considered in the context of any child with a painful knee, particularly in a child younger than age 12 yr. These include conditions such as OCD (see Chapter 677.3), which is most common on the lateral aspect of the medial femoral condyle. Inflammatory and infectious arthritis, Baker's cyst (see Chapter 677.2), and hip pain referred to the knee are additional considerations. Tumors more common to the knee joint include osteogenic sarcoma (distal femoral and proximal tibial), histiocytosis X in the diaphysis, and eosinophilic granuloma in the epiphysis of long bones. Metastatic tumors to the lower extremities include neuroblastoma and lymphomas of various types. As with any apparent musculoskeletal injury in a child not responding to conservative care, more in-depth diagnostic pursuit for alternative pathology is mandatory.

Bibliography is available at Expert Consult.

687.7 Lower Leg Pain: Shin Splints, Stress Fractures, and Chronic Compartment Syndrome

Kevin P. Murphy and Aaron M. Karlin

Stress injury to the bones of the lower leg occurs on a continuum from mild injury (shin splints) to stress fracture. All occur by an overuse mechanism.

Shin splints, also known as medial tibial stress syndrome, manifests with pain along the medial tibia or both tibiae and is the most common overuse injury of the lower leg. The pain initially appears toward the end of exercise, and if exercise continues without rehabilitation, the pain worsens and occurs earlier in the exercise period. There is diffuse tenderness over the lower third to half of the distal medial tibia. Any focal tenderness or tenderness of the proximal tibia is suspicious for a stress fracture. A stress fracture tends to be painful during the entire workout. Shin splints can usually be distinguished from a **tibial stress fracture** in which the tenderness is more focal (2-5 cm) and more severe. Shin splints and stress fracture represent a continuum of stress injury to the tibia and are thought to be related to traction of the soleus on the tibia. Eccentric contraction of the medial aspect of the soleus is required to control pronation from initial contact to mid-stance with running. This contraction increases the stress of the fascial origin of the soleus possibly through Sharpey's fibers causing disruption to the tibial periosteum and fibrocartilaginous attachments.

The diagnosis can be made by history and physical examination. Findings on plain radiographs of the tibia are normal with shin splints and in tibial stress fractures within the 1st 2 wk of the injury. Afterward, the radiographs can demonstrate periosteal reaction if a stress fracture is present. Sensitivity of plain radiographs may be increased by obtaining 4 views of the tibia: AP, lateral, and both oblique views. A bone scan is the most sensitive test to diagnose stress fractures; it demonstrates discrete tracer uptake at the site(s) of the stress fracture. Increased uptake may be noted in the presence of shin splints, but in a fusiform pattern along the periosteal surface. If results of the bone scan are normal, the diagnosis is likely to be shin splints or chronic compartment syndrome. MRI has replaced bone scan as the most sensitive tool for diagnosing stress fractures in long bones in many medical centers.

The treatment of shin splints and tibial stress fractures is similar, involving relative rest, correcting training errors and addressing quartile muscle imbalances and abnormal mechanical alignment. Orthotics and/or new shoes may be useful in patients who hyperpronate. Fitness can be maintained with non-weightbearing activities, such as swimming, cycling, and water jogging. With shin splints, after

7-10 days, patients can usually start on the walk–jog program. If pain worsens, 2-3 pain-free days are required before resuming the walk–jog program. Ice should be used daily and an analgesic should be used for pain control. Stretching the plantar flexors, hamstrings and strengthening the ankle dorsiflexors may be useful. Therapeutic taping and wrapping techniques to support the soft-tissue attachments have been useful in some when directed by a skilled sports therapist. Being pain free for 7-10 days is recommended before exercises are commenced. Individuals with pain at rest and not responsive to treatment require continued suspicion for stress fracture.

Chronic compartment syndrome occurs in an athlete in a running sport, usually during a period of heavy training. It is caused by muscle hypertrophy and increased intracompartmental pressure with exercise. There is typically a pain-free period of about 10 min at the beginning of a workout before onset of constant throbbing pain that is difficult to localize. It lasts for minutes to hours after exercise and is relieved by ice and elevation. In a classic case, there is numbness of the foot associated with high pressure within the corresponding muscle compartment. The most common compartment affected is the anterolateral compartment with compression of the fibular nerve followed by the deep posterior compartment. The physical examination in the office is often normal but weakness of the extensor hallucis longus (anterolateral compartment) and decreased sensation between the 1st and 2nd toe may be present. X-rays, bone scan, and MRI are negative and are used to rule out other conditions. Compartment pressure measurements are the test of choice. Treatment involves reduction of activity, antiinflammatory medication, orthotics (hyperpronation), heel cord stretching, light strengthening of distal musculature, optimal footwear, and crosstraining (swimming, cycling and water jogging). Cryotherapy and superficial heat can be of help in addition. Persistent systems, despite conservative care, require fasciotomy (successful in up to 90% of cases).

Bibliography is available at Expert Consult.

687.8 Ankle Injuries
Kevin P. Murphy and Aaron M. Karlin

Ankle injuries are the most common acute athletic injury. Approximately 85% of ankle injuries are sprains, and 85% of those are inversion injuries (foot planted with the lateral fibula moving toward the ground), 5% are eversion injuries (foot planted with the medial malleolus moving toward the ground), and 10% are combined.

EXAMINATION AND INJURY GRADING SCALE
In obvious cases of fracture or dislocation, evaluating neurovascular status with as little movement as possible is the priority. If no deformity is obvious, the next step is inspection for edema, ecchymosis, and anatomic variants. Key sites to palpate for tenderness are the entire length of the fibula; the medial and lateral malleoli; the base of the 5th metatarsal; the anterior, medial, and lateral joint lines; and the navicular and the Achilles tendon complex. Assessment of active range of motion (patient alone) in dorsiflexion, plantar flexion, inversion, and eversion along with gentle resisted range of motion can be helpful.

Provocative testing attempts to evaluate the integrity of the ligaments. In a patient with a markedly swollen, painful ankle, provocative testing is difficult because of muscle spasm and involuntary guarding. It is more useful on the field before much bleeding and edema have occurred. The anterior drawer test assesses for anterior translation of the talus and competence of the anterior talofibular ligament. The inversion stress test examines the competence of the anterior talofibular and calcaneofibular ligaments (Fig. 687-9). In the acute setting, the integrity of the tibiofibular ligaments and syndesmosis is examined by the syndesmosis squeeze test. Pain with squeezing the lower leg implies injury to the interosseous membrane and syndesmosis between the tibia and fibula, making a high ankle sprain or more severe injury suspicious. Athletes with this injury cannot bear any weight and also

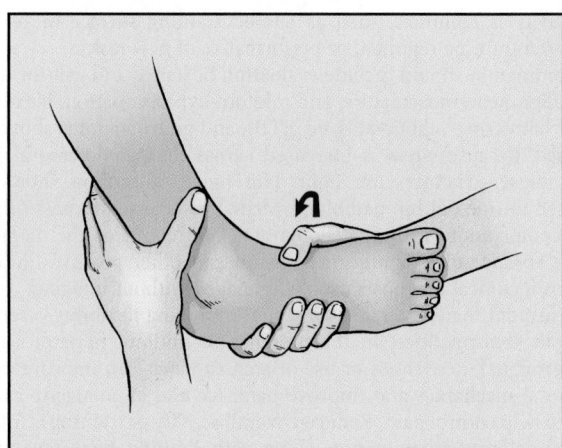

Figure 687-9 Inversion stress tilt test for ankle instability. *(From Hergenroeder AC: Diagnosis and treatment of ankle sprains. A review, Am J Dis Child 144:809–814, 1990.)*

have severe pain with external rotation of the foot. Occasionally, the peroneal tendon dislocates from the fibular groove simultaneously with an ankle sprain. To assess for peroneal tendon instability, the examiner applies pressure from behind the peroneal tendon with resisting eversion and plantar flexion, and the tendon pops anteriorly. If either a significant syndesmotic injury or an acute peroneal dislocation is suspected, orthopedic consultation should be sought.

RADIOGRAPHS
AP, lateral, and mortise views of the ankle are obtained when patients have pain in the area of the malleoli, are unable to bear weight, or have focal bone tenderness over the distal tibia or fibula. The Ottawa ankle rules help define who requires radiographs (Fig. 687-10). A foot series (AP, lateral, and oblique views) should be obtained when patients have pain in the area of the midfoot or bone tenderness over the navicular or 5th metatarsal. It is important to differentiate an avulsion fracture of the proximal 5th metatarsal (Dancer's fracture) from the Jones fracture of the proximal 5th metatarsal (a lucency about 2 cm from the proximal end). The former is treated more like an ankle sprain; the latter fracture has an increased risk of nonunion and requires orthopedic consultation. Injury to the deltoid ligament in the medial ankle (more rare) should raise the question of proximal fibular fracture. In this circumstance more proximal tibial imaging may be necessary. The *talar dome fracture* is manifested as an ankle sprain that does not improve. Radiographs on initial presentation can have subtle abnormalities. Any suspicion on the initial radiographs of a talar dome fracture warrants orthopedic consultation and further imaging. In the early adolescent, always look carefully at the tibial epiphysis. Nondisplaced Salter III fractures can be subtle and need to be recognized early and referred to an orthopedic surgeon promptly.

INITIAL TREATMENT OF ANKLE SPRAINS
Ankle sprains need to be **treated** with **PRICE**. This should be followed for the 1st 48-72 hr after the injury to minimize bleeding and edema. For an ankle injury, this might consist of crutches and an elastic wrap, although other compression devices such as an air stirrup splint work quite well. This allows early weightbearing with protection and can be removed for rehabilitation. It is important to start a rehabilitation program as soon as possible.

Rehabilitation
Rehabilitation should begin the day of injury; for patients who have pain with movement, isometric strengthening can be started. Early phase intervention includes restoration of functional range of motion, strengthening with emphasis on peroneal musculature and early sensory proprioceptive training. Later intervention includes

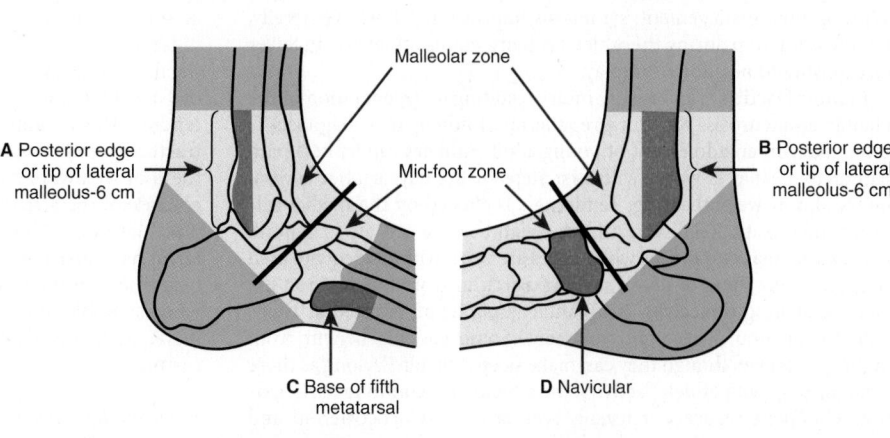

Figure 687-10 Ottawa ankle rules. *(From Bachmann LM, Kolb E, Koller MT, et al: Accuracy of Ottawa ankle rules to exclude fractures of the ankle and mid-foot; systematic review, BMJ 326:417–419, 2003.)*

higher-level balance activities, advanced proprioception exercises, and endurance training. When determining when an athlete is ready for running, there must be full range of motion and nearly full strength compared to the uninjured side. While standing on the uninjured side only, the athlete is instructed to hop 8-10 times, if possible. When this can be achieved without pain on the injured side, the athlete can begin to run, starting out with jogging and gradually progressing in speed, and finally to sprints. The athlete must stop if there is significant pain or limp. Finally, before returning to sport, the athlete must be able to sprint and change directions off the injured ankle comfortably. Performing some sport-related tasks is also helpful in determining readiness for return to play.

Recurrent ankle injuries are more likely in patients who have not undergone complete rehabilitation. Ankle sprains are less likely in players wearing high-top shoes. Proper taping of the ankle with adhesive tape can provide functional support but loosens with use and is often unavailable. Lace-up ankle supports are felt to be more useful for preventing recurrences by many. They are more supportive than tape and can be tightened repeatedly during the course of a practice or a game. Most sports physicians recommend their use indefinitely to help prevent further sprains. Surgery is a consideration for chronic mechanical instability with lateral complex ligamentous laxity in the failure of more conservative care. Salter-Harris grade I distal fibular fractures need careful consideration, particularly in the child younger than 12 yr old. The physeal plates are generally the weakest link in the musculoskeletal chain and tend to slide or pull apart before the surrounding soft tissue and/or ligaments tear in this younger population. Toddler's fracture also needs to be considered especially in those younger than age 8 yr. The proposed mechanism involves sheer stress with lack of displacement because of the periosteum that is relatively strong compared to the elastic bone in younger children. Additional radiographs may be inconspicuous (a faint spiral oblique line) or even normal. After 1 or 2 wk callous develops. The condition can be mistaken for osteomyelitis, transient synovitis, and/or even child abuse. Toddler's fracture usually occurs in the lower third of the tibia, whereas nonaccidental injury typically affects the upper two-thirds or midshaft of the tibia. Other, more rare conditions that cannot be excluded include os fibulare, a congenital unfused secondary ossification center of the distal fibula. This can be seen in younger patients with recurrent ankle sprains, particularly as their body weight and activity increase during the early academic years. Tarsal coalitions can be seen also in the presence of ankle sprains in younger children the most common being

talocalcaneal and calcaneal navicular. More common muscular strains and/or tendinosis remains more prevalent in the older child and adolescent including peroneal, posterior tibialis, and gastrocnemius/Achilles types. Tarsal tunnel syndrome is also more prevalent in the adolescent/younger adult and can be associated with medial ankle pain with burning or tingling into the sole of the foot.

Bibliography is available at Expert Consult.

687.9 Foot Injuries
Kevin P. Murphy and Aaron M. Karlin

Metatarsal stress fractures can occur in any running athlete. The history is insidious pain with activity that is getting worse. Examination reveals point tenderness over the midshaft of the metatarsal, most commonly the 2nd or 3rd metatarsal. Radiographs might not show the periosteal reaction before pain has been present for 2 wk or more. **Treatment** is relative rest for 6-8 wk. Shoes with good arch supports reduce stress to the metatarsals.

Vague dorsal foot pain in an athlete in a running sport can represent a **navicular stress fracture.** Unlike other stress fractures, it might not localize well on examination. If there is any tenderness around the navicular, a stress fracture should be suspected. This stress fracture can take many weeks to show up on plain radiographs, so a bone scan or MRI should be obtained to make the diagnosis. Because this fracture is at high risk of nonunion, immobilization and non-weightbearing for 8 wk is the usual **treatment.** A CT scan should be obtained to document full healing after the period of immobilization.

Sever disease (calcaneal apophysitis) occurs at the insertion of the Achilles tendon on the calcaneus and manifests as activity-related pain (see Fig. 687-3). It is more common in boys (2:1), is often bilateral, and usually occurs between ages 8 and 13 yr. Tenderness is elicited at the insertion of the Achilles tendon into the calcaneus, especially with squeezing the heel (positive squeeze test). Sever disease is associated with tight Achilles tendons and midfoot hyperpronation that puts more stress on the plantar flexors of the foot. **Treatment** includes relative rest, ice, massage, stretching, and strengthening the Achilles tendon. Correcting the midfoot hyperpronation with orthotics, arch supports, or better shoes is important in most athletes with Sever disease. If the foot is neutral or there is mild hyperpronation, in-heel lifts can be helpful to unload the Achilles tendon and its insertion. With optimal management, symptoms improve in 4-8 wk. Generally, if there is no limp during the athletic activity, young athletes with Sever disease should be allowed to play.

Plantar fasciitis is an overuse injury resulting in degeneration of the plantar aponeurosis. Rare in prepubertal children, this diagnosis is more likely in an adolescent or young adult. Athletes report heel pain with activity that is worse with first steps of the day or after several hours of non-weightbearing. Tenderness is elicited on the medial calcaneal tuberosity. Relative rest from weightbearing activity is helpful. Athletes get plantar fasciitis when shoes are worn with inadequate arch supports. New shoes or use of semirigid arch supports often lessen the pain. Stretching the calves and plantar fascia helps, assisted at times with therapeutic ultrasound treatment. Some patients benefit from night splints even though they can make sleep difficult. As long as there is no limping with athletic activity, the athlete may continue participation. Complete recovery is usually seen at 6 mo. Corticosteroid and extracorporeal shock-wave therapy are reserved for severe, chronic cases.

Calcaneal stress fracture is seen in the older adolescent or young adult involved in a running sport. There is heel pain with any weightbearing activity. The physical examination reveals pain with squeezing the calcaneus. Sclerosis can show up on the AP and lateral radiographs after 2-3 wk of pain. A bone scan or MRI needs to be performed to clinch the diagnosis in some cases. The calcaneus is an uncommon location for a stress fracture; it is associated with osteopenia (amenorrheic girls). **Treatment** is rest from running and other weight-bearing activity for at least 8 wk. Immobilization is rarely necessary.

Flatfeet or pes planus may be flexible or rigid. Flexible pes planus is usually asymptomatic, at least in the early years and is the most common type found in children. Scaphoid pads or medial inserts may be helpful to create plantigrade weightbearing posture. Untreated sports progression may occur with compensatory hallux valgus, planovalgus, and secondary bunion and toe deformities. With progression pain may develop, along with shortening in the peroneal musculature. Rigid pes planus is a congenital deformity associated with other anomalies in 50% of cases. It is caused by failure of the tarsal bones to separate leaving a bony cartilaginous or fibrous bridge or coalition between 2 or more tarsal bones. Talocalcaneal coalitions are more symptomatic between 8 and 12 yr of age, whereas calcaneal navicular coalitions are more symptomatic between 12 and 16 yr of age. Symptoms are insidious with occasional acute arch, ankle, and midfoot pain, at times brought on with sports-related activities. The hindfoot often does not align in its normal varus position on tiptoe maneuvers. Patients are predisposed to ankle sprains secondary to limited subtalar motion and stress to the subtalar and transverse tarsal joints frequently causes pain. CT scans are diagnostic and initial treatment is conservative with short leg casting and/or molded orthoses and rest. In the case of failure of conservative care, surgical intervention is usually necessary. Rigid cavus feet can also be associated with metatarsalgia, clawing, and intrinsic muscle atrophy, all possible in the young athlete. With a cavus foot, underlying neurologic conditions, such a Charcot-Marie-Tooth disease, spinal dysraphism, Friedrich ataxia, or other spinal tumor, need be considered. Custom-molded orthotics may be helpful. Family history can be critical. Coleman block test can help determine hindfoot flexibility and more rigid vs flexible pes planus. Plantar fascial surgical release is standard for all cavus foot procedures. Accessory navicular bones and sesamoiditis need to be considered in all symptomatic feet, especially those with rigid components. These conditions are more common in the adolescent or younger adult and can be exacerbated with sporting activities.

Other conditions not to be excluded include Lisfranc sprain and/or dislocation, more common in football linemen or other athletes requiring heavy loading on the mid and forefoot joints and gymnasts using the balance beam. Lisfranc joint is the tarsal metatarsal articulation of the 3 cuneiform bones and the cuboid with the 5 proximal metatarsals. Turf toe can be seen, particularly in the older child and/or adolescent running on artificial or synthetic surfaces. It usually involves hyperextension through the 1st metatarsal phalangeal joint,

spraining the ligaments surrounding the joint often in a football and/or soccer activity.

Iselin apophysitis is an apophysitis that occurs at the tuberosity of the fifth metatarsal. The apophysis at this site appears between the ages of 9 and 14 yr and is located within the insertion of the peroneus brevis tendon. This condition can be a predisposing factor to the Dancer's fracture (see Chapter 687.8). Osteochondroses (see Chapter 674.08) of the foot to always consider include Freiberg disease, which involves collapse of the articular service and subchondral bone, usually of the 2nd metatarsal. Kohler disease involves irregular ossification of the tarsal navicular joint with localized pain and increased density. Freiberg disease is more common in girls between the ages of 12 and 15 yr, whereas Kohler disease occurs in younger individuals, age 2-9 yr, and is frequently reversible with conservative care including orthoses and casting.

Bibliography is available at Expert Consult.

Chapter **688**

Sports-Related Traumatic Brain Injury (Concussion)

Christopher W. Liebig and Joseph A. Congeni

Concussion is defined as a traumatically induced transient disturbance of brain function that involves a complex pathophysiologic process. Concussion may be caused either by a direct blow to the head, face, neck, or elsewhere on the body with an "impulsive" force transmitted to the head, whether these are linear or rotational forces. Concussion is a subset of mild traumatic brain injury; it is important to communicate this fact to families and patients as the word "concussion" unintentionally and incorrectly has been found to communicate to some families that a brain injury has not occurred, resulting in less-than-adequate follow-up.

EPIDEMIOLOGY

At least 1.6-3.8 million concussions occur in the United States each year during competitive sports and other recreational activities. This number is likely to represent only a fraction of the true incidence as there is underreporting of symptoms by athletes from direct withholding of information to continue participation and poor understanding of their symptoms. From 1997 to 2007, visits to emergency departments for sports concussion doubled in the 8-13 yr old group; in 14-19 yr olds, the incidence has increased by more than 200%. Activities include football, bicycling, hockey, lacrosse, soccer, field hockey, basketball, and playground injuries.

PATHOPHYSIOLOGY

The pathophysiologic process following a concussion is best described as an "energy crisis" following a neurometabolic cascade. In animal models, these ionic and metabolic events, along with microscopic axonal injury, results in a desperation use of glucose to begin the healing process. The increased energy demand is met with a decreased cerebral blood flow, resulting in less available energy for other brain processes and a true mismatch of energy supply and demand.

ASSESSMENT OF THE INJURED PLAYER

The most current assessment tools are the Sport Concussion Assessment Tool (SCAT3) and the Child-SCAT3 for children ages 5-12, available at: http://bjsm.bmj.com/content/47/5/259.citation; http://bjsm.bmj.com/content/47/5/263.citation

These tests include the Glasgow coma scale, presence and duration of loss of consciousness, memory of the activity ("Who scored last?" "What team did you play last week?"), general memory/orientation (date, day of week, season), short-term memory (list 3 words and have patient repeat), concentration (give digits: 5-8-3, and have patient repeat backwards or do serial 7s), balance testing (double, single, tandem leg stances), finger to nose coordination, and cognitive testing (repeat list of words).

The signs and symptoms of concussion fall into 4 categories: physical, cognitive, emotional, and sleep (Table 688-1), with the most common symptom reported being headache. Transient loss of consciousness occurs in less than 10% of concussions and does not correlated with severity of injury. Assessment can be challenging as several or only 1 of the symptoms listed are identified. Furthermore, patients with preexisting mental health disorders such as depression or attention-deficit/hyperactivity disorder may experience exacerbations in their symptoms, making them more difficult to control.

A gold-standard assessment of suspected concussion has been difficult to ascertain throughout the years. Particularly difficult is the sideline evaluation where simply recognizing the injury can be most challenging for medical personnel. Initial sideline evaluation should include cervical spine stabilization, 4-limb neurologic testing, and evaluation of ABCs (airway, breathing, circulation). Secondly, discussion of the athlete's symptoms with an accepted sideline assessment tool (SCAT3 or Child-SCAT3) with balance testing should be completed because sensory coordination and vestibular systems are also affected by concussion. When available, preinjury baseline performance can be compared to the individual's postinjury test. Given the variability in concussion presentation, medical personnel are encouraged to err on the side of safety by adapting the phrase *when in doubt, sit them out*. If concussion is suspected, an athlete must be removed from participation and forbidden to return on the day of injury.

Evaluation with neuropsychologic testing provides another objective measurement of brain function. Computerized neurocognitive tests can be most useful to those familiar with the test and when athletes were able to perform baseline testing.

Concussion lacks structural changes with conventional imaging studies (MRI and CT) limiting their usefulness in evaluation. Neuroimaging should be used if suspicion of intracerebral lesion exists. Advances in functional neuroimaging have shown positive findings but require further research before clinical utilization and recommendation. Imaging may be indicated for possible related neck injury (see Chapter 689). CT imaging may be indicated for prolonged loss of consciousness, persistent altered mental status, focal neurologic deficits, suspicion of a skull fracture, or signs of clinical deterioration.

MANAGEMENT AND TREATMENT
Initial Phase

Management of a concussion also continues to evolve and is primarily based on symptom control while protecting the athlete from activities that may slow recovery. Initiating a management plan consisting of complete physical and cognitive rest is paramount. Symptoms may be followed with a postconcussion symptom scale (see Table 688-1), where symptoms are more likely to be reported. Concussed patients will often complain of increased symptoms with cognitive activities such as reading, video games, music, and even texting. They often have difficulty attending school, focusing on schoolwork, and trying to keep up with assignments. Taking standardized tests while recovering from a concussion is discouraged as lower-than-expected scores may occur. Cognitive rest may include shortened school days, reduced workload, or even temporary leave of absence with gradual return to school. Controlling symptoms can be difficult as there is no evidence-based pharmacologic treatment to offer a concussed athlete. However, medication is considered in those with prolonged recovery and specific symptoms. Vestibular therapy consisting of balance and oculomotor exercises has shown results in combating dizziness and vertigo. The duration of rest has been controversial, but one randomized controlled trial suggested that rest for 1-2 days when compared to 5 days resulted in **fewer** daily postconcussive symptoms and **faster** recovery.

Returning to Sport

No athlete should return to sport until clinically and completely asymptomatic at rest and without medication use. Each athlete's return should be individually based as recovery occurs at different rates with the majority of youth fully recovered by 1-3 wk; some may require 1-2 mo, particularly those who have had repeated concussions. Younger athletes may take longer to recover to neurocognitive and symptom baseline than older athletes. A return to play protocol provides a structured guideline that athletes progress through gradually, provided that the athlete remains asymptomatic for 24 hr at each step (Table 688-2). If no symptoms return, the athlete should wait 5 full days to complete and return to play. If symptoms have occurred, the athlete is required to rest until asymptomatic for 24 hr and resume at the previous asymptomatic step. It is important to consider individual factors at this juncture that are suspected to prolong recovery or increase patient

Table 688-1	Postconcussion Symptom Scale						
Headache	0	1	2	3	4	5	6
Nausea	0	1	2	3	4	5	6
Vomiting	0	1	2	3	4	5	6
Balance problems	0	1	2	3	4	5	6
Dizziness	0	1	2	3	4	5	6
Fatigue	0	1	2	3	4	5	6
Trouble falling to sleep	0	1	2	3	4	5	6
Excessive sleep	0	1	2	3	4	5	6
Loss of sleep	0	1	2	3	4	5	6
Drowsiness	0	1	2	3	4	5	6
Light sensitivity	0	1	2	3	4	5	6
Noise sensitivity	0	1	2	3	4	5	6
Irritability	0	1	2	3	4	5	6
Sadness	0	1	2	3	4	5	6
Nervousness	0	1	2	3	4	5	6
More emotional	0	1	2	3	4	5	6
Numbness	0	1	2	3	4	5	6
Feeling "slow"	0	1	2	3	4	5	6
Feeling "foggy"	0	1	2	3	4	5	6
Difficulty concentrating	0	1	2	3	4	5	6
Difficulty remembering	0	1	2	3	4	5	6
Visual problems	0	1	2	3	4	5	6

Scale: 0, no symptoms; 3, moderate; 6, severe.

Use of the postconcussion symptom scale: The athlete should complete the form, on the athlete's own, by circling a subjective value for each symptom. This form can be used with each encounter to track progress toward symptom resolution. Many athletes may have some of these reported symptoms at a baseline, such as concentration difficulties in the patient with attention-deficit disorder or sadness in an athlete with underlying depression. This must be taken into consideration when interpreting the score. Athletes do not need a total score of 0 to return to play if they had symptoms before their concussion. This scale has not been validated to determine concussion severity.

From Halstead ME, Walter KD, Council on Sports Medicine and Fitness. Sport-related concussion in children and adolescents. Pediatrics 126(3):597–615, 2010.

Table 688-2	Graduated Return to Play Protocol	
REHABILITATION STAGE	**FUNCTIONAL EXERCISE AT EACH STAGE OF REHABILITATION**	**OBJECTIVE OF EACH STAGE**
1. No activity	Symptom limited physical and cognitive rest	Recovery
2. Light aerobic exercise	Walking, swimming or stationary cycling keeping intensity <70% maximum permitted heart rate No resistance training	Increase heart rate
3. Sport-specific exercise	Skating drills in ice hockey, running drills in soccer. No head impact activities	Add movement
4. Noncontact training drills	Progression to more complex training drills, e.g., passing drills in football and ice hockey May start progressive resistance training	Exercise, coordination and cognitive load
5. Full-contact practice	Following medical clearance participate in normal training activities	Restore confidence and assess functional skills by coaching staff
6. Return to play	Normal game play	

From McCrory P, Meeuwise WH, Aubry M, et al. Consensus statement on concussion in sport: the 4th International Conference on Concussion in Sport held in Zurich, November 2012. Br J Sports Med 47:250–258, 2013.

susceptibility. Females may be at greater risk for concussion, increased severity, and longer duration of recovery.

After sustaining a concussion, a child is 2-6–fold more likely to sustain another concussion. This risk is heightened while recovering from an initial injury with a rare, yet catastrophic injury known as **second-impact syndrome**. In this injury, seen more frequently in child athletes, a mild impact may result in brain swelling and death. Previous and repeat concussions may be associated with slower recovery with more cognitive, emotional, physical, and sleep symptoms than those who have experienced 1 or no concussions.

Those with multiple concussions may experience a cumulative effect resulting in difficulty in attention and concentration. Prolonged concussive symptoms or postconcussion syndrome is another complication that is most simply noted as symptoms of concussion that persist beyond an expected time frame. Causes and correlations have yet to be determined, making this diagnosis difficult to establish.

PREVENTION
Despite ongoing research and technologic advances, personal protective equipment has not decreased the severity or reduced the incidence of concussion in team sports. Therefore, educating athletes, coaches, officials, and parents to adhere to rule changes should be emphasized. Concussion-related legislations may prove to be the most effective methods in managing and preventing concussion.

Bibliography is available at Expert Consult.

Chapter 689
Cervical Spinal Injuries
Joseph A. Congeni and John H. Lockhart

Sports participation has surpassed motor vehicle crashes as the number 1 cause of cervical spine injuries in youth older than 9 yr of age. American football, hockey, and wrestling have the highest incidence in the United States; internationally, rugby is nearly as high.

The normal cervical spine has a lordotic curve, allowing it to absorb shock and dissipate force. When the neck is flexed forward, the spine straightens, losing this shock-absorbing property. Axial loading is when a force is applied to the top of the head in this flexed position transmitting force through the spine.

SOFT-TISSUE INJURY
The most frequent injury resulting from trauma to the head and neck involves the muscles, tendons, and ligamentous structures. Even though strains, sprains, and contusions are common, proper examination and evaluation is required to rule out more serious injuries. Even without bony abnormalities, the cervical spine may become unstable secondary to soft-tissue injury.

Spinal laxity results when most restraining ligaments are injured. When compared to adjacent vertebra, laxity should horizontally be less than 3.5 mm, and angular displacement less than 11 degrees on plain flexion/extension films. However, younger athletes have more baseline laxity making the criteria less applicable and muscle spasm can acutely mask instability. If subluxation is remotely suspected, a hard cervical collar should be placed and imaging obtained again at 2-4 wk when inflammation and spasm have subsided.

Disk injuries are rare in pediatric patients. Rupture or herniation must be considered in any cervical pain differential (see Chapter 679.8).

SPEAR TACKLER'S SPINE
This clinical entity is characterized by progressive spinal changes secondary to incorrect tackling form. Findings on plain x-ray consist of (1) narrowing of cervical spinal canal, (2) loss or reversal of normal cervical lordosis, and (3) preexisting minor posttraumatic x-ray evidence of bony or ligamentous injury. Although rule changes in collision and contact sports have limited the practice of making contact with a "head-down" neck position, this condition still persists.

Many experts argue that this condition disqualifies athletes from return to play. Others argue that if physical therapy and rehabilitation are able to correct the curvature and improper technique is corrected, then athletes are not at a high risk of reinjury and could return. Data are lacking and more research required for a definitive answer.

CERVICAL FRACTURES
All significant neck injuries should be treated seriously until cleared with appropriate examination and imaging. Although many cervical fractures are stable, improper management or inadequate evaluation could end with catastrophic results. **Until properly evaluated, the patient should be immobilized and treated as if the patient has an unstable cervical fracture.**

STINGERS (BURNERS)
Stingers are unilateral peripheral nerve injuries occurring somewhere between the cervical nerve root and the brachial plexus. Three

proposed mechanisms are traction or tensile stretch injury, compressive injury, and direct trauma. Typical presentation is a transient episode of unilateral pain, with or without paresthesia, in an upper extremity. Symptoms of C5 and C6 roots and upper trunk are most common. Careful examination for weakness should be performed, especially shoulder abduction, external rotation, and elbow flexion. Cervical spine should have pain-free full range of motion and have no tenderness to palpation. Spurling's Compression test, a head-tilting maneuver that when positive differentiates cervical radiculopathy from other causes of upper-extremity pain, may or may not be positive. The test is only 30% sensitive, but specificity is 93%.

Return to play may be considered the same day if the exam is reassuring. This requires complete resolution of symptoms, full range of motion, and normal strength. Multiple stingers, bilateral symptoms, or symptoms persisting for longer than 1 hr should prompt further evaluation before resumption of any physical activities.

TRANSIENT QUADRIPARESIS

Transient quadriparesis (TQ) is a temporary neurologic episode encompassing sensory symptoms with or without motor changes. TQ is also known as *cervical cord neurapraxia, burning hands syndrome, commotio spinalis,* and *spinal cord concussion.* TQ can be divided into 3 types: plegia (complete loss of motor function), paresis (motor weakness), and paresthesia (sensory symptoms only). There is also a 3-part grading system: grade 1 symptoms last <15 min, grade 2 symptoms last 15 min to 24 hr, and grade 3 symptoms persist beyond 24 hr. TQ must be differentiated from just a stinger and the player should be removed from activity and spinal cord injury considered.

Mechanisms of injury include hyperextension, hyperflexion, and axial loading. Anatomically, when the neck is hyperflexed or hyperextended, the spinal canal is narrowed by up to 30%, increasing the likelihood of cord injury.

Burning hands syndrome is the most common presentation. The athlete has intense paresthesias in both upper extremities. This is suggestive of a central cord syndrome and includes burning, tingling, and loss of sensation. Treat athletes with full cervical precautions to prevent injury progression.

Evaluation should start with plain flexion and extension films if stable. CT can be utilized if cervical fracture is suspected. MRI should then be used to evaluate for intrinsic spinal cord abnormalities or ongoing cord or root compression. Spinal stenosis is discussed below.

Return to play for TQ is heavily debated and lacks data to support it. Conservatively, some argue that 1 episode is a contraindication to return to contact sports, whereas others agree with utilizing the Return to Play Table (Table 689-1) for absolute and relative contraindications for return. If allowed to return to play and second episode of TQ occurs, the complete work-up needs repeating.

CONGENITAL SPINAL STENOSIS

Developmental narrowing of the cervical spinal canal predisposes an athlete to higher risk of spinal cord injury. This condition can be found incidentally while working up other conditions. The Torg Ratio, the ratio of vertebral body width to canal width on plain lateral film (cutoff for normal is 0.7 or 0.8, depending on clinical setting), is being evaluated for utility as a diagnostic test. Alternatively, a canal width measuring <13 mm between C3 and C7 can be used to define stenosis, with "normal" being >15 mm.

Functional stenosis can be seen with dynamic MRI in flexion and extension to see if the canal space decreases with movement. The positioning of the canal in flexion or extension causes narrowing from positioning of the vertebra and ligament, respectively. The measured diameter may be irrelevant if disc protrusion or ligament hypertrophy causes compression. This narrow "reserve space" around the spinal cord puts the athlete at greater risk for injury as compared to the same force on a normal spine.

SPINAL CORD INJURY

Spinal cord injury is the most dreaded complication of cervical trauma and is categorized into 4 entities. Hemorrhage and transection are

Table 689-1	Return to Play (RTP) Table
NO CONTRAINDICATION TO RTP	
Healed fractures including:	Healed C1 or C2 fracture with normal cervical spine range of motion (ROM)
	Healed subaxial fracture without sagittal plane deformity
	Asymptomatic clay-shoveler's (C7) spinous process avulsion fracture
Congenital conditions	Klippel-Feil (single-level anomaly not C0/C1 articulation)
	Spina bifida occulta
Degenerative/ postsurgical conditions	Cervical disc disease (no change in baseline neurologic status)
	Single-level anterior cervical fusion (ACF) with/without instrumentation
	Single- or multiple-level posterior cervical laminotomy
Recurrent stingers	Less than 3 episodes lasting <24 hr
	Must have full cervical range of motion
	No persisting neurologic deficit
Transient quadriparesis	Single episode
	Full cervical range of motion
	Normal neurologic exam
	No radiologic instability
	Normal spinal reserve (as evidenced on MRI)
RELATIVE CONTRAINDICATION TO RTP	
Stingers/Burners	Prolonged symptomatic burner/stinger
	Three or more stingers
Transient quadriparesis	Transient quadriparesis lasting >24 hr
	More than 1 episode with symptoms of any duration
Postsurgical	Healed 2-level ACF
	Posterior cervical fusion (PCF) with/without instrumentation
ABSOLUTE CONTRAINDICATION TO RTP	
Transient quadriparesis and any 1 or more of:	Cervical myelopathy
	Continued neck discomfort
	Reduced ROM
	Neurologic deficit from baseline after injury
Surgical procedures	C1 + C2 fusion
	Cervical laminectomy
	Three-level ACF or PCF
Soft-tissue injuries	Asymptomatic ligamentous laxity (>11 degrees of kyphotic deformity)
	C1 + C2 hypermobility with anterior dens >3.5 mm (adult), >4 mm (child), i.e., Down syndrome (see Chapter 680)
	Symptomatic cervical disc herniation
Other conditions including:	Spear tackler's spine
	Multilevel Klippel-Feil anomaly (see Chapter 680)
	Healed subaxial fracture with sagittal kyphosis coronal plane abnormality, or cord encroachment
	Ankylosing spondylitis
	Rheumatoid arthritis with spinal abnormalities
	Spinal cord abnormality (cord edema, compression, etc.)
	Arnold-Chiari syndrome
	Basilar invagination
	Occipital-C1 assimilation (occipitalization or connection)
	Spinal stenosis (canal width <13 mm between C3 and C7)

Adapted from Cantu R, Li YM, Abdulhamid M, Chin LS: Return to play after cervical spine injury in sports. Curr Sports Med Rep 12:14–17, 2013.

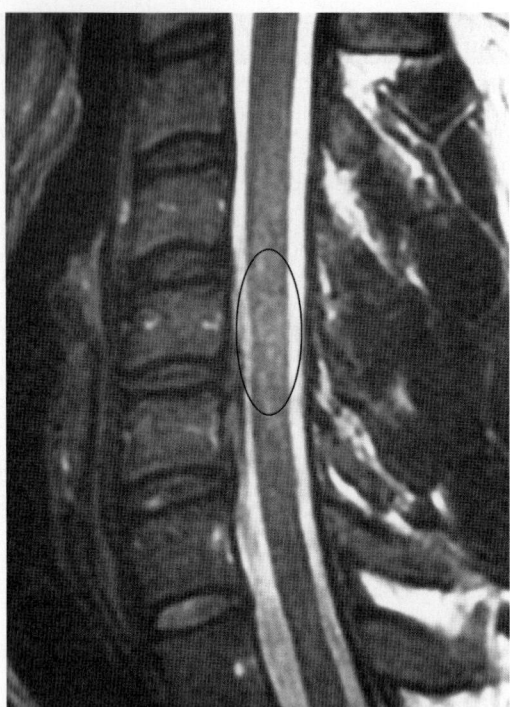

Figure 689-1 A magnetic resonance image (sagittal) demonstrating spinal cord contusion (edema in central portion of spinal cord). *(From Krabak BJ, Kanarek SL: Cervical spine pain in the competitive athlete. Phys Med Rehabil Clin N Am 22:459–471, 2011, Fig. 2.)*

Table 690-1	Spectrum of Heat Illness

Heat cramps and dehydration: Cautious return to play
Muscle cramps
Thirst
Fatigue
Light-headedness
Sweating
Flushed face
Heat Exhaustion: Remove from play
Dizziness
Rapid pulse
Headaches
Nausea
Vomiting
Loss of coordination
Profuse sweating
Core temperature less than 40°C (104°F)
Heat Stroke: Medical emergency, call 911
Core temperature of 40°C (104°F) or higher
Hot dry skin
Multiple system failure
Delirium
Convulsions
Abnormal vital signs

(From Merkel DL, Molony JT Jr. Medical sports injuries in the youth athlete: emergency management. Int J Sports Phys Ther 7:242–251, 2012, Table 4.)

considered irreversible and associated with complete cord injury, whereas contusion and edema (Fig. 689-1) are considered to have more potential for recovery. Steroids and hypothermia are 2 proposed treatments to prevent secondary injury. These severe injuries should be managed by providers with expertise in this area.

Bibliography is available at Expert Consult.

Chapter 690
Heat Injuries
Gregory L. Landry

Heat illness is the third leading cause of death in U.S. high school athletes. It is a continuum of clinical signs and symptoms that can be mild (heat stress) to fatal (heatstroke) (see Chapter 70). Children are more vulnerable to heat illness than adults because they have greater ratio of surface area to body mass and produce greater heat per kilogram of body weight during activity. The sweat rate is lower in children and the temperature at which sweating occurs is higher. Children can take longer to acclimatize to warmer, more humid environments (typically 8-12 near-consecutive days of 30-45 min exposures). Children also have a blunted thirst response compared to adults and might not consume enough fluid during exercise to prevent dehydration.

Three categories for heat illness are generally used: **heat cramps, heat exhaustion,** and **heat stroke** (Table 690-1). However, symptoms of heat illness overlap and advance as the core temperature rises. **Heat cramps** are the most common heat injury and usually occur in mild dehydration and/or salt depletion, usually affecting the calf and hamstring muscles. They tend to occur later in activity, as muscle fatigue is reached and water loss and sodium loss worsen. They respond to oral

rehydration with electrolyte solution and with gentle stretching. The athlete can return to play when ability to perform is not impaired. **Heat syncope** is fainting after prolonged exercise attributed to poor vasomotor tone and depleted intravascular volume, and it responds to fluids, cooling, and supine positioning. **Heat edema** is mild edema of the hands and feet during initial exposure to heat; it resolves with acclimatization. **Heat tetany** is carpopedal tingling or spasms caused by heat-related hyperventilation. It responds to moving to a cooler environment and decreasing respiratory rate (or rebreathing by breathing into a bag).

Heat exhaustion is a moderate illness with core temperature 37.7-39.4°C (100-103°F). Performance is obviously affected, but central nervous system dysfunction is mild, if present. It is manifested as headache, nausea, vomiting, dizziness, orthostasis, weakness, piloerection, and possibly syncope. **Treatment** includes moving to a cool environment, cooling the body with fans, removing excess clothing, and placing ice over the groin and axillae. If a patient is not able to tolerate oral rehydration, IV fluids are indicated. Patients should be monitored, including rectal temperature, for signs of heat stroke. If rapid improvement is not achieved, transport to an emergency facility is recommended.

Heat stroke is a severe illness manifested by central nervous system disturbances and potential tissue damage. It is a medical emergency; *the mortality rate is 50%.* Sports-related heat stroke is characterized by profuse sweating and is related to intense exertion, whereas "classic" heatstroke with dry, hot skin is of slower onset (days) in elderly or chronically ill persons. Rectal temperature is usually >40°C (104°F). Significant damage to the heart, brain, liver, kidneys, and muscle occurs, with possible fatal consequences if untreated. **Treatment** is immediate whole-body cooling via cold water immersion. Airway, breathing, circulation, core temperature, and central nervous system status should be monitored constantly. Rapid cooling should be ceased when core temperature is approximately 38.3-38.9°C (101-102°F). IV fluid at a rate of 800 mL/m^2 in the 1st hr with normal saline or lactated Ringer solution improves intravascular volume and the body's ability to dissipate heat. Immediate transport to an emergency facility is necessary. Physician clearance is required before return to exercise.

Dehydration is common to all heat illness; consequently, measures to prevent dehydration can also prevent heat illness. Thirst is not an adequate indicator of hydration status because it is initiated at 2-3% dehydration. Athletes are advised to be well hydrated before exercise and should drink every 20 min during exercise (5 oz for those

Heat index °F (°C)													
	Relative humidity (%)												
Temperature °F (°C)	40	45	50	55	60	65	70	75	80	85	90	95	100
110 (47)	136 (58)												
108 (43)	130 (54)	137 (58)											
106 (41)	124 (51)	130 (54)	137 (58)										
104 (40)	119 (48)	124 (51)	131 (55)	137 (58)									
102 (39)	114 (46)	119 (48)	124 (51)	130 (54)	137 (58)								
100 (38)	109 (43)	114 (46)	118 (48)	124 (51)	129 (54)	136 (58)							
98 (37)	105 (41)	109 (43)	113 (45)	117 (47)	123 (51)	128 (53)	134 (57)						
96 (36)	101 (38)	104 (40)	108 (42)	112 (44)	116 (47)	121 (49)	126 (52)	132 (56)					
94 (34)	97 (36)	100 (38)	103 (39)	106 (41)	110 (43)	114 (46)	119 (48)	124 (51)	129 (54)	135 (57)			
92 (33)	94 (34)	96 (36)	99 (37)	101 (38)	105 (41)	108 (42)	112 (44)	116 (47)	121 (49)	126 (52)	131 (55)		
90 (32)	91 (33)	93 (34)	95 (35)	97 (36)	100 (38)	103 (39)	106 (41)	109 (43)	113 (45)	117 (47)	122 (50)	127 (53)	132 (56)
88 (31)	88 (31)	89 (32)	91 (33)	93 (34)	95 (35)	98 (37)	100 (38)	103 (39)	106 (41)	110 (43)	113 (45)	117 (47)	121 (49)
86 (30)	85 (29)	87 (31)	88 (31)	89 (32)	91 (33)	93 (34)	95 (35)	97 (36)	100 (38)	102 (39)	105 (41)	108 (42)	112 (44)
84 (29)	83 (28)	84 (29)	85 (29)	86 (30)	88 (31)	89 (32)	90 (32)	92 (33)	94 (34)	96 (36)	98 (37)	100 (38)	103 (39)
82 (28)	81 (27)	82 (28)	83 (28)	84 (29)	84 (29)	85 (29)	86 (30)	88 (31)	89 (32)	90 (32)	91 (33)	93 (34)	95 (35)
80 (27)	80 (27)	80 (27)	81 (27)	81 (27)	82 (28)	82 (28)	83 (28)	84 (29)	84 (29)	85 (29)	86 (30)	86 (30)	87 (31)

Category	Heat index	Possible heat disorders for people in high risk groups
Extreme danger	130°F or higher (54°C or higher)	Heat stroke or sunstroke likely.
Danger	105 - 129°F (41 - 54°C)	Sunstroke, muscle cramps, and/or heat exhaustion likely. Heatstroke possible with prolonged exposure and/ or physical activity.
Extreme caution	90 - 105°F (32 - 41°C)	Sunstroke, muscle cramps, and/or heat exhaustion possible with prolonged exposure and/ or physical activity.
Caution	80 - 90°F (27 - 32°C)	Fatigue possible with prolonged exposure and/or physical activity.

Heat index reference chart provided by the National Weather Service, Tulsa, Oklahoma.
Note: Exposure to full sunshine can increase Heat Index values by up to 15°F

Figure 690-1 Heat stroke index. (*From Jardine DS: Heat illness and heat stroke, Pediatr Rev 28:249–258, 2007.*)

weighing 40 kg, 9 oz for 60 kg, and 10-12 oz for those >60 kg). Free access to cold water should be advocated to coaches. During a football practice, scheduled breaks every 20-30 min with helmets off to get out of the heat can decrease the cumulative amount of heat exposure. Practices and competition should be scheduled in the early morning or late afternoon to avoid the hottest part of the day. Guidelines have been published about modifying activity related to temperature and humidity (Fig. 690-1). Proper clothing such as shorts and T-shirts without helmets can improve heat dissipation. Prepractice and post-practice weight can be helpful in determining the amount of fluid necessary to replace (8 oz for each pound of weight loss).

Water is adequate for most persons who exercise <1 hr, although there is evidence that children drink more water when it is flavored. Fluids with electrolyte and carbohydrate are more important for persons who exercise for longer than 1 hr. Salt pills should not be used by most people because of the risk of their causing hypernatremia and delayed gastric emptying. They may be useful in a person with a high sweat rate or recurrent heat cramps. Prolonged exercise (marathon running) with only water replacement places the athlete at risk of hyponatremia.

Bibliography is available at Expert Consult.

Chapter **691**
Female Athletes: Menstrual Problems and the Risk of Osteopenia

Gregory L. Landry

Physical training in young women can adversely affect reproductive function and bone mineral status especially when combined with calorie restriction (see Chapters 28 and 116).

The majority of bone mass is acquired by the end of the 2nd decade (see Chapter 707). Approximately 60-70% of adult bone mass is genetically determined, and the remaining is influenced by 3 controllable factors: exercise, calcium intake, and sex steroids, primarily estrogen. Exercise promotes bone mineralization in the majority of young women and is to be encouraged. In girls with eating disorders and those who exercise to the point of excessive weight loss with amenorrhea or oligomenorrhea, exercise can be detrimental to bone mineral acquisition, resulting in reduced bone mineral content, or **osteopenia**.

Specifically, bone mineralization is negatively affected by amenorrhea (absence of menstruation for ≥3 consecutive months). This may be influenced by abnormal eating patterns, or "disordered eating." When occurring together, disordered eating, amenorrhea, and osteoporosis form the **female athlete triad**. At health supervision visits and the preparticipation physical examination, special attention should be given to screening for any features of the triad.

Menstrual abnormalities (including **amenorrhea**) results from suppression of the spontaneous hypothalamic pulsatile secretion of gonadotropin-releasing hormone (see Chapter 116.1). It is believed that the amenorrhea results from reduced energy availability, defined as energy intake minus expenditure. Energy availability below a threshold of 30 kcal/kg/day lean body mass is thought to result in menstrual disturbances. Negative energy balance also appears to lower levels of leptin, which affects both nutritional state and the reproductive system. Other causes to be ruled out are pregnancy (see Chapter 118), pituitary tumors, thyroid abnormalities, polycystic ovary syndrome (see Chapter 552), anabolic–androgenic steroid use (see Chapters 114 and 692), and other medication side effects.

The low estrogen state of amenorrhea predisposes the female athlete to osteopenia and puts her at risk for stress fractures, especially of the spine and lower extremity. If left unchecked, bone loss is partially irreversible despite resumed menses, estrogen replacement, or calcium supplements. Routine bone mineral density screening is not recommended but can help guide treatment and return to activity in severe cases.

Normal ovulation and menses can be recovered in athletes with amenorrhea. This usually involves decreasing exercise amount and/or increasing caloric intake. However, many athletes are resistant to a decrease their training, and other methods, such as hormone supplementation, should be discussed. Nutritional counseling is important to help the athlete develop a plan for increasing calories. Calcium intake should be addressed, with the goal being at least 1,500 mg daily. If amenorrhea is present for ≥6 mo, hormone supplementation is recommended.

Three eating disorders can occur in the context of amenorrhea. Anorexia nervosa manifests as weight <85% of estimated ideal body weight with evidence of starvation manifesting as bradycardia, hypothermia, and orthostatic hypotension or orthostatic tachycardia. Bulimia nervosa manifests as recurrent episodes (at least once weekly) of binge eating with a sense of lack of control over eating during an episode with recurrent episodes of compensatory behaviors. A third category, "Unspecified Feeding and Eating Disorder," is a general description for disorders failing to meet the criteria for the 2 previous disorders. With the revised diagnostic criteria for bulimia and anorexia nervosa in the *Diagnostic and Statistical Manual of Mental Disorders, Fifth Edition,* it is anticipated that many young women who previously were diagnosed as "Unspecified Feeding and Eating Disorder" will receive a specific diagnosis of anorexia or bulimia. Signs of an eating disorder are weight loss, food restriction, depression, fatigue, and worsened athletic performance, and preoccupation with calories and weight. The athlete might avoid events surrounding food consumption or might hide and discard food. Signs and symptoms include fat depletion, muscle wasting, bradycardia worsened from baseline, orthostatic hypotension, constipation, cold intolerance, hypothermia, gastric motility problems, and, in some cases, lanugo (see Chapter 28). Electrolyte abnormalities can lead to cardiac dysrhythmias. Psychiatric problems (depression [see Chapter 26], anxiety [see Chapter 25], suicide risk [see Chapter 27]) are of higher incidence in this population.

For **treatment** of eating disorders, control of the symptoms is a central theme. The first step is confronting the athlete about the abnormal behavior and unhealthy weight. Generally, exercise is not recommended if the body weight is <85% of estimated ideal body weight, although there are exceptions, especially if the athlete is eumenorrheic. If the athlete is unable to gain weight with nutrition and medical counseling alone, then psychologic consultation is sought.

Most athletes will not initially admit a problem, and many are unaware of the serious physical consequences. A helpful technique in talking to these athletes is to sensitively point out performance issues. Education about decreased strength, endurance, and concentration can be a motivating factor for treatment. Often, the athlete's family needs to be involved, and the athlete should be encouraged to reveal necessary information to them. Psychology or psychiatry referral is important in the multidisciplinary approach to treatment of disordered eating. It is important for the physician to monitor the athlete's physical health while the mental health professional is caring for the mental aspects of the eating disorder.

Bibliography is available at Expert Consult.

Chapter **692**
Performance-Enhancing Aids

Gregory L. Landry

See also Chapter 114.

Ergogenic aids are substances used for performance enhancement, most of which are unregulated supplements (Table 692-1). The 1994 Dietary Supplement and Health Education Act limited the ability of the U.S. Food and Drug Administration to regulate any product labeled as a supplement. Many agents have significant side effects without proven ergogenic properties. In 2005, the American Academy of Pediatrics published a policy statement strongly condemning their use in children and adolescents. The 2004 Controlled Substance Act outlawed the purchase of steroidal supplements such as androstenediol, and androstenedione, with the exception of dehydroepiandrosterone (DHEA).

The prevalence of lifetime steroid use is highest among boys in the United States; among a large representative sample in 2010, 5.5% of

Table 692-1	Ergogenic Drugs			
ERGOGENIC DRUG	**CATEGORY**	**GOALS OF USE**	**ATHLETIC EFFECT**	**ADVERSE EFFECTS**
Anabolic–androgenic steroids	Controlled substance	Gain muscle mass, strength	Increase muscle mass, strength	Multiple organ systems: infertility, gynecomastia, female virilization, hypertension, atherosclerosis, physeal closure, aggression, depression
Androstenedione	Controlled substance	Increase testosterone to gain muscle mass, strength	No measurable effect	Increase estrogens in men; overlaps systemic risks with steroids
Dehydroepiandrosterone (DHEA)	Nutritional supplement	Increase testosterone to gain muscle mass, strength	No measurable effect	Increase estrogens in men; impurities in preparation
Growth hormone	Controlled substance	Increase muscle mass, strength, and definition	Decreases subcutaneous fat; no performance effect	Acromegaly effects: increased lipids, myopathy, glucose intolerance, physeal closure
Creatine	Nutritional supplement	Gain muscle mass, strength	Increase muscle strength gains; performance benefit in short, anaerobic tasks	Dehydration, muscle cramps, gastrointestinal distress, compromised renal function
Ephedra alkaloids	Possibly returning as nutritional supplement	Increase weight loss, delay fatigue	Increases metabolism; no clear performance benefit	Cerebral vascular accident, arrhythmia, myocardial infarction, seizure, psychosis, hypertension, death

From Calfee R, Fadale P: Popular ergogenic drugs and supplements in young athletes, Pediatrics 117:e577–e589, 2006.

boys in middle school and 6.6% of those in high school report having used steroids for muscle-enhancement. The European School Survey Project on Alcohol and Other Drugs found that 1% of European youth reported any use of steroids. Steroids in oral, injectable, and skin cream form are taken in various patterns. *Cycling* is a term used to describe taking multiple doses of steroids for a period, ceasing, and then starting again. *Stacking* refers to the use of different types of steroids in both oral and injectable forms. *Pyramiding* involves slowly increasing the steroid dose to a peak amount and then gradually tapering down.

Anabolic–androgenic steroids have been used in supraphysiologic doses for their ability to increase muscle size and strength and decrease body fat. An evidence-base does support the increase in muscle mass and strength; the effects appear to be related to the myotrophic action at androgen receptors as well as competitive antagonism at catabolism-mediating corticosteroid receptors. However, they have significant endocrinologic side effects, such as decreased sperm count and testicular atrophy in men and menstrual irregularities and virilization in women. Hepatic problems include elevated aminotransaminases and γ-glutamyl transferase, cholestatic jaundice, peliosis hepatitis, and a variety of tumors, including hepatocellular carcinoma. There is evidence that anabolic–androgenic steroids might cause cardiovascular problems as well, including higher blood pressure, lower high-density lipoprotein, higher low-density lipoprotein, higher homocysteine, and decreased glucose tolerance. The psychologic effects include aggression, several personality disorders, and a variety of other psychologic problems (anxiety, paranoia, mania, depression, psychosis). Physical findings in males include gynecomastia, testicular shrinkage, jaundice, male pattern baldness, acne, and marked striae. Women can develop hirsutism, voice deepening, cliterol hypertrophy, male-pattern baldness, acne, and marked striae.

Testosterone precursors (also known as *prohormones*) include androstenedione and DHEA. Their use in the adolescent population has increased markedly in conjunction with reports of high-profile athletes' use. They are androgenic but have not been proved to be anabolic. If they are anabolic at all, they work by increasing the production of testosterone. They also increase production of estrogenic metabolites. The side effects are similar to those of anabolic–androgenic steroids and far outweigh any ergogenic benefit. Since January 2005, these substances cannot be sold without prescription.

Creatine is an amino acid mostly stored in skeletal muscle. Its key feature is ability to rephosphorylate adenosine diphosphate to adenosine triphosphate, therefore increasing muscle performance. Its use has increased, especially since other supplements have been withdrawn from the market. Thirty percent of high school football players have used creatine. There is evidence that creatine, as a source of increased energy, enhances strength and maximal exercise performance when used during training. There is no evidence that creatine affects hydration or temperature regulation. Concerns about nephritis in case reports have not been supported by controlled studies. However, there are few long-term studies evaluating creatine use.

Caffeine is an active ingredient in energy drinks and some endurance sport supplements. More of a problem as an energy drink when combined with alcohol, excessive caffeine ingestion may result in tachycardia, gastritis, nausea, vomiting, and central nervous system excitation. Overdoses may result in seizures, arrhythmias, and hypotension.

Bibliography is available at Expert Consult.

Chapter 693
Specific Sports and Associated Injuries
Kevin P. Murphy and Aaron M. Karlin

GYMNASTICS

Typically, males and females begin gymnastics participation at 4-5 yr of age. The highest level of competition is in the mid-teens followed by retirement, often by 20 yr for females and mid-twenties for males. Lower-extremity injuries are more common in female gymnasts, whereas upper body injuries occur with higher frequency in male gymnasts. Apparatus competed upon accounts for this discrepancy, such as the horizontal bar and ring exercises for male gymnasts, which place a great deal of stress upon the shoulders. In addition to mechanical or traumatic injuries, female gymnastics commonly have delayed menarche and are at risk for hypothalamic amenorrhea or oligomenorrhea, as well as low body weight for height related to disordered eating. Despite the presence of these 2 components of the *female athlete triad* (see Chapter 691), the third component, reduced bone density or osteoporosis, is not commonly seen. In fact, bone density tends to be high in most gymnasts, which is thought to be secondary to their performance involving repetitive high-impact activities. Nevertheless, stress fractures, in both the upper and lower extremities, are a significant problem. The short stature associated with male and female gymnasts is probably caused by selection bias and not the result of gymnastics training.

Both acute and chronic injuries are seen in gymnasts and commonly involve the ankles, wrists, and spine. The incidence of injury increases with the skill level and is greatest with the floor exercise. The amount of weightbearing through the upper extremities in gymnastics lends itself to the development of both traumatic and overuse injuries. At the wrist, this can manifest as Salter I stress fractures of the distal radial physis (*gymnast's wrist*), triangular fibrocartilage tears, scaphoid fractures, dorsal ganglions, and, most commonly, wrist sprains (see Chapter 683.2). Spine injuries are notable for a high incidence of spondylolysis (stress fracture of the pars interarticularis) and, in less frequent cases, spondylolisthesis, both related to repetitive extension loading of spine (see Chapter 679.6). Ligamentous laxity can predispose to elbow or shoulder dislocation and ankle sprains.

Treatment of many of these injuries includes relative rest from the inciting activity, immobilization, ice, and nonsteroidal antiinflammatory drugs. Imaging begins with radiographs but may include bone scan with single-photon emission computed tomography to evaluate spondylolysis, or MRI to rule out intraarticular tears, loose bodies, ligamentous instability, or physeal injury. A pediatrician should have a low threshold for referral to a sports medicine or orthopedic specialist in a child with a wrist injury not improving with rest.

SWIMMING

Injuries of the shoulder in competitive swimming are most common and generally a result of chronic, overuse. *Swimmer's shoulder* is a combination of subacromial bursitis and tendinosis of the rotator cuff and long-head of the biceps. Commonly, increased laxity of the shoulder capsule and weakness of the scapular stabilizers contribute over time leading to the insidious onset of shoulder pain (see Chapter 687.2). Freestyle, back, and butterfly strokes tend to exacerbate the pain. Pain may be provoked on exam by passively abducting the arm to 90 degrees, forward flexing to 30 degrees, and internally rotating the humerus with the elbow extended while having the patient actively abduct against resistance (*Empty Can* Test). The Hawkins impingement test involves the same position of the shoulder with the elbow flexed to 90 degrees and the examiner internally rotating the humerus. Pain and/or weakness indicates supraspinatus injury. Treatment includes relative rest, ice, and modification of stroke technique. The multi-axial instability of the glenohumeral joint common to swimmers is addressed with rehabilitation focusing upon strengthening of the rotator cuff and scapular stabilizer musculature. Prevention includes monitoring training load, proper technique and strengthening exercises.

Swimmer's ear, or otitis externa, presents with pain and often drainage from the external auditory canal. It is caused by bacterial, or less commonly, fungal infection of the external auditory canal due to chronic, excessive wetness (see Chapter 639).

BASEBALL

Throwing injuries of the elbow and shoulder (particularly among pitchers) are the most common baseball injuries (see Chapters 687.2 and 687.3). Monitoring the number of pitches thrown per game, no more than 6 times the young athlete's age in years and per week based upon the athlete's age, is important. Counseling athletes (and coaches)

to stop all throwing activities if the player experiences elbow pain, with medical evaluation to be sought if there is no resolution with rest, is essential. Death or serious injury in baseball is rare and generally from direct contact by the ball, causing serious head injury or, in the case of chest wall impact, *commotio cordis*. Batting helmets need to be worn properly to try to prevent face and head injuries; modifications to the hardness of baseballs used with younger athletes is also helpful. Injures to catchers can involve traumatic brain injury with various levels of concussion from contact of the ball to the face mask. Catchers are more vulnerable to traumatic sprains of the interphalangeal and metacarpal phalangeal joints along with internal derangement and ligamentous sprain of the knees associated with the deep squatting posture.

DANCE

Dance is a highly demanding activity that may be associated with delayed menarche and disordered eating in females (see Chapter 691). Acute injuries commonly involve the lower extremities. Overuse injuries are likely, due to the repetitive nature of maneuvers incorporated into training and performance. Frequently, kinetic chain dysfunction contributes to injury and this should be considered when evaluating the dancer. Common mistakes in technique can cause injury, such as forcing excessive "turnout" (external rotation at the hip) in ballet can result in undue stress being placed upon the knees (see Chapter 687.6). An unrehabilitated ankle sprain may cause favoring of the affected leg leading to development of a stress fracture of the contralateral tibia. In contrast to injuries in most types of dance, injuries associated with breakdancing more frequently involve the spine and upper extremities than lower extremities. This likely relates to the significant amount of twisting of the torso and weight bearing through the hands inherent in this genre of dance.

Foot problems are not uncommon and include metatarsal stress fractures, subungual hematomas, sesamoiditis, plantar fasciitis, calluses, and bunions (see Chapter 687.9). A *Dancer's fracture* is an avulsion fracture of the distal shaft of the 5th metatarsal. This is treated with immobilization for 4-6 wk, although poor healing, a result of the tenuous blood supply in the area, may necessitate surgical fixation. Common ankle injuries include acute sprains, anterior and posterior impingement syndromes, and osteochondritis dissecans of the talus. Medial tibial stress syndrome ("shin splints") and tibial stress fractures are noted in the lower leg. Patellar malalignment/hypermobility can result in patellofemoral pain syndrome or, less frequently, patellar subluxation/dislocation. Medial snapping hip syndrome, caused by the iliopsoas tendon riding over the anterior hip capsule, and hip flexor (rectus femoris, iliopsoas) tendinosis are commonly noted in addition. Gluteal region pain with sciatica may be a result of *piriformis syndrome*, which occurs because of the repetitive external hip rotation required in ballet (see Chapter 687.5).

The proper timing of allowing a ballet dancer to go *en pointe* is a common question asked by dancers and parent alike. An average age to go en pointe is 12 yr. A functional test should be part of that decision: If the young dancer is able to perform a passé steadily away from the barre as well as being able to maintain an en pointe position without pain or instability the dancer is likely ready to begin dancing en pointe.

WRESTLING

Wrestlers have great fluctuations in weight to meet weight-matched competition standards. Such fluctuations are associated with fasting, dehydration, and then binging. Counseling to wrestlers and their parents regarding impaired performance resulting from these components of disordered eating, especially with respect to decreased speed and strength, is important in order to deter athletes from incorporating them into routine practice.

Wrestling holds apply a variety of torques or forces to the extremities and spine producing a number of common injuries. Takedown maneuvers and subsequent impact with the mat can produce concussions, neck strain/sprain, or spinal cord injury (see Chapter 689). *Stingers* and *burners*, also seen among football players, are caused by stretching or pinching of the brachial plexus (see Chapter 689). Pain at the shoulder often radiates down the arm and is frequently associated with paresthesias and weakness; the latter most commonly involving the deltoid and other C5/C6 innervated muscles. Overall, the 2 most common sites of injury in wrestling are the shoulder and knee.

At the shoulder, subluxation is common. This generally occurs anteriorly with the shoulder forcibly abducted and extended. Patients are commonly aware of their shoulder slipping in and out (see Chapter 687.2).

Injuries to the hand are less common and typically include metacarpophalangeal and proximal interphalangeal joint sprains. Treatment consists of buddy taping and/or splinting.

Knee injuries (see Chapter 687.6) are also common and include prepatellar bursitis, medial and lateral collateral ligament sprains, and medial and lateral meniscus tears. Acute or recurrent traumatic impact to the mat can result in prepatellar bursitis. Swelling is noted over the patella with the patient experiencing limitations to range of motion primarily with knee flexion as a result. If the overlying skin is broken, septic bursitis must be considered. Distinguishing between a traumatic and infected bursitis may require aspiration of the bursa. Treatment of traumatic bursitis includes protective padding upon return to wrestling, ice, nonsteroidal antiinflammatory drugs (NSAIDs), and, on occasion, aspiration if flexion is markedly impaired. Recurrence after aspiration is not uncommon. Rarely, bursectomy is needed if there are several reoccurrences.

Dermatologic problems associated with wrestling include herpes simplex (see Chapter 252: *herpes gladiatorum*), impetigo (see Chapter 665.1), staphylococcal furunculosis or folliculitis, superficial fungal infections, and contact dermatitis. Herpes gladiatorum and impetigo are contraindications to wrestling until the lesions have resolved. Treatment of herpes gladiatorum with oral antiviral medications, such as Acyclovir, for both acute outbreaks and long-term suppression is recommended. Washing of the wrestling mats with appropriate antibacterial and antifungal solution is required after daily wrestling sessions to keep the mats disinfected and protect the spread of dermatologic contagion.

Auricular hematoma is caused by friction or direct trauma to the auricle (see Chapter 642). If allowed to remain without evacuation, irreversible deformity of the auricle often results, termed *cauliflower ear*. Properly fitted headgear is the best means of prevention.

FOOTBALL

Football is the sport with the highest number of injuries, with the greatest number of participants (especially at the high school level) and with a higher rate of injury. The majority of these injuries is relatively minor and compared to many other sports, the injuries are less severe, as evidenced by less number of days lost from injury. The most common football injuries include joint sprains, muscle strains, and contusions, with the lower extremities injured most frequently. Treated appropriately, these injuries generally result in minimal time away from football. An important exception to this, contusions to the arm or thigh muscles can result in the development of a large hematoma if not treated aggressively in the acute stage, resulting in prolonged time away from football. Without the presence of fracture, treatment includes ice and compression for the 1st few days to reduce the expansion of the hematoma. Pain-free stretching and strengthening exercises are then incorporated. Therapeutic ultrasound per physical therapy staff can be helpful in stretching deeper tissue and resolving persistent hematoma limiting further flexibility. Return to contact play is initiated when baseline range of motion and strength are achieved. Large hematomas and those allowed to persist are at risk for development of myositis ossificans.

Although the majority of catastrophic sports injuries in the United States have occurred in football, these injuries are rare. Catastrophic injury is defined as a fatal injury or a severe injury with or without permanent severe functional disability. Disabling injuries include cervical spine and cerebral injuries.

Head and neck injuries in football include concussion, neck sprain, and brachial plexopathy. The latter, also seen among wrestlers, is referred to as a *stinger* or *burner* and represents a brachial plexus

neurapraxia (see Chapter 689). This is the most common nerve injury in football and is often the result of a traction or compression injury to the upper nerve roots of the brachial plexus caused by forceful lateral neck bending. This results in painful arm dysesthesias and deltoid muscle weakness. This is usually transient, resolving in minutes to days, with return to play upon return of full range of motion, comfort and strength.

Compared to other sports, brain injury (**concussions**) occurs with the highest rate in football, a result of the frequent exposure to contact during practices and games. The prevention, diagnosis, and management of this significant injury with potentially lifelong implications are discussed in full in Chapter 688.

Lumbar spine injury manifested as low back pain can indicate spondylolysis (see Chapter 679.6). Shoulder trauma can cause glenohumeral dislocation, the majority of which are anterior dislocations, acromioclavicular joint sprain, and fractures to the clavicle or humerus (see Chapter 687.8). Knee injuries (see Chapter 687.6) are common and include anterior cruciate ligament and, less frequently, posterior cruciate ligament tears along with medial collateral ligament sprains.

Ankle sprains occur frequently, and the risk of reinjury may be reduced by rehabilitation and the use of a lace-up ankle brace (see Chapter 687.6). Turf toe, a sprain to the 1st metatarsophalangeal joint, is caused by forceful dorsiflexion of the toe while wearing soft, lightweight, flexible shoes. Treatment of turf toe includes ice, NSAIDs, and orthotic to limit extension of the great toe, along with rest.

ICE HOCKEY

Ice hockey is classified as a collision sport and is associated with injuries caused by contact from the puck or stick as well as from other players, the ice, or the boards. These injuries commonly include contusions, lacerations, fractures, sprains, or concussions. The risk of injury is reduced by the use of proper equipment (helmets with facemasks) and enforcement of the rules regarding dangerous body contact (checking from behind, high sticking, and fighting).

Specific hockey injuries include ankle sprains (dorsiflexion, eversion, and external rotation in contrast to the usual inversion sprain in other sports), hip adductor strain, osteitis pubis, and various shoulder injuries from body contact. The latter include acromioclavicular joint sprain, glenohumeral dislocation, and clavicle fractures (see Chapter 687.2). The most serious injuries are to the head and neck (see Chapters 688 and 689).

BASKETBALL AND VOLLEYBALL

Common maneuvers of these 2 sports include jumping, pivoting, running and sudden stopping which increase the risk for knee and ankle injuries. Similarly, injury to the fingers may result from the passing, catching, and striking of the ball inherent in these sports.

Knee injuries include those caused by overuse, such as **traction apophysitis** (Osgood-Schlatter disease) and **patellar tendinosis** (*jumper's knee*) (see Chapter 687.6). As with other jumping sports, acute ligament sprains (medial collateral with or without anterior cruciate ligaments) can occur. Shoulder injuries in volleyball players are similar to other overhead athletes and include rotator cuff tendinosis and glenohumeral instability.

Ankle sprain is the most common injury and is usually caused by inversion with plantar flexion, placing the lateral ligaments at high tension. An avulsion fracture of the base of the 5th metatarsal at the insertion of the peroneus brevis tendon is another sequelae of inversion ankle injuries. In terms of overuse injuries at the ankle, Achilles tendinosis is common. Foot pain may be from calcaneal apophysitis (Sever disease), retrocalcaneal bursitis, posterior tibialis tendinosis, accessory tarsal navicular, plantar fasciitis, stress fracture of the tarsal navicular, Jones's stress fracture of the 5th metatarsal, sesamoiditis, blisters, subungual hematoma, and paronychia (see Chapters 687.8 and 687.9).

RUNNING

Running problems are typically caused by an overuse injury related to muscle imbalance; a minor skeletal deformity; repetitive overload trauma; or poor flexibility, strength, endurance, or proprioception. With each step while running, the foot impact ranges from 3-8 times the athlete's body weight. Errors in training, including increasing the distance or intensity of workouts too rapidly, often result in injury to the runner. Minor variations (e.g., malalignment) in anatomy that do not cause problems at rest can predispose to injury at specific sites, such as overpronation, contributing to increased patellofemoral stress. Muscle fatigue, environmental temperature (see Chapter 690), and running surface (grass vs unyielding concrete) also contribute to injury. Prevention of injuries is possible by muscle-strengthening exercises, incorporating periods of rest into training plans, and the use of good-quality running shoes that match an athlete's foot type. Those who overpronate may benefit from a motion control shoe for maximal rearfoot and arch support. Those who mildly overpronate should utilize a stability shoe that combines extra support in the medial midsole with midsole cushion. Those who supinate should wear a neutral, cushioned shoe with increased shock absorption in the midsole and less arch support.

Stress fractures of all bones of the lower extremities can occur in runners (see Chapter 683.4). They have been documented at the femoral neck, inferior pubic rami, subtrochanteric area, proximal femoral shaft, proximal tibia, fibula, navicular, metatarsals, desmoids, and calcaneal apophysis. The most common are in the metatarsals, tibia, and fibula. The anterior proximal tibia, femoral neck, and tarsal navicular are most at risk for nonunion. Muscle strains most frequently affect the hamstrings, followed by the quadriceps, hip adductors, soleus, and gastronomies muscles. Tendinosis is most common in the Achilles tendon, followed by the posterior tibial, peroneal, iliopsoas, and proximal hamstrings. Achilles tendinosis characterized by tenderness and crepitance if acute and nodularity if chronic, initially might get better when running, and must be distinguished from retrocalcaneal bursitis. Treatment includes a period of rest from running (substitute cross-training), a heel lift, Achilles tendon stretching, and NSAIDs.

Knee pain in the runner is frequently anterior in location and commonly caused by patellofemoral stress syndrome (**runner's knee**), which results from excessive dynamic, usually lateral, motion of the patella in relationship to the femoral intracondylar groove (see Chapter 687.6). The athlete's body habitus (i.e., increased Q-angle, overpronation) and presence of core weakness may contribute to this overuse injury. Posterior knee pain can be caused by gastrocnemius strain, while posteromedial pain may be caused by proximal tibial stress fracture or semimembranosus/semitendinosus tendinosis. Lateral knee pain is commonly caused by **iliotibial band syndrome** and less so by popliteal tendinosis. Iliotibial band syndrome may combine both a component of bursitis and tendinosis owing to mechanical friction of the iliotibial band (an extension of the tensor fasciae latae) over the lateral femoral epicondyle. Treatment for knee pain in the runner includes relative rest from running, ice, and stretching of the quadriceps, hamstrings, and, in some cases, the iliotibial band. Strengthening exercises should include the quadriceps, hips, and core muscles. Foot orthotics may be indicated if there is no improvement with this treatment plan.

Shin splints, or medial tibial stress syndrome, is a descriptive term for pain located diffusely over the distal medial tibia and should be distinguished from tibia stress fracture and chronic compartment syndrome. Medial tibial stress syndrome often occurs in new runners with overpronation, or runners that have markedly increased their training duration in a short period of time. See Chapter 687.7 for prevention, diagnosis, and treatment.

Chronic compartment syndromes involve any of the muscle compartments with the most common being anterior. There is typically poorly localized throbbing pain that onsets 10-15 min into a run. Pain typically prevents further training limiting the risk of nerve injury. Physical exam is usually normal. Diagnosis is made by measurement of intracompartmental pressures at rest or during exercise.

Plantar fasciitis is an inflammation of the supporting structures of the longitudinal arch, due to repetitive cyclic loading with foot strike. Pain is typically worst with the first step out of bed in the morning and with running and is located on the medial aspect of the heel. Pes planus and overpronation are common in these patients. Treatment includes relative rest, ice, heel cord stretching, transverse friction massage, proper shoes, use of a posterior night splint, and corticosteroid injection. Therapeutic ultrasound by a trained physical therapist can be helpful in stretching the deep plantar fascia pre-friction massage in certain individuals. Calcaneal stress fracture should be considered, especially in the amenorrheic distance runner (see Chapter 691).

SOCCER

Injuries in soccer include any of the running injuries previously noted as well as abrasions, contusions, muscle strains, and ligament sprains (ankle, knee predominantly), partly from body-to-body contact, falls, running, and kicking. Hip problems include the *hip pointer* (iliac crest contusion), iliac crest apophysitis, and chronic groin pain (muscle strain, hernia, osteitis pubis). Femoral neck stress fractures, slipped femoral capital epiphysis, and avulsion fractures of the pelvis or femur should also be considered in the differential despite being uncommon (see Chapter 687.5). In general, most other upper- and lower-extremity injuries can occur in soccer.

Traumatic brain injury (see the discussion of concussions in Chapter 688) is common in soccer because of contact between players, player and goal post, and player and ground. The American Academy of Pediatrics recommends that youth soccer participants minimize heading the ball until more is known about the risks in young children. Proper heading technique is vital and should be taught in youth soccer. Additional points of play to consider include: On long kicks, the receiving player should trap the ball with the chest or leg, not strike it with the head; players should kick the ball about 5 ft in front of their teammates so that the latter have to come to the ball and trap with their legs; players avoid heading the ball backward toward the goal (with cervical extension); referees, as with all sports, have to keep the game under control and penalize dangerous play; and guidelines for returning to play after a concussion should be followed.

TENNIS

Tennis injuries occur twice as often in the lower extremity compared to the upper extremity with overall injury rates similar for boys and girls. Common areas of injury include the muscles, tendons, and ligaments of the ankle, thigh, elbow, shoulder, back, wrist, and abdomen. The risk of injury is increased by increased training duration and intensity; anatomic considerations (muscle imbalance, malalignment); poorly rehabilitated injuries with resultant deficits in flexibility and strength; and poor technique. Injuries can also be related to improper equipment, such as a racquet that is too big, or trying to learn techniques, such as hitting with top spin or with power before proper coordination and technique have been established.

Acute injuries include ankle sprains, abdominal or extremity muscle strains, and knee sprains. Overuse injuries involve both the upper and lower extremities as well as the back. Lower-extremity injuries are related to the frequent directional changes inherent in the sport, creating significant concentric and eccentric loads on the lower extremities. These include patellofemoral stress syndrome, proximal tibial stress fractures, traction apophysis of the calcaneus (Sever disease), and tibial tubercle (Osgood-Schlatter disease) (see Chapters 687.6 and 687.7)

In the upper extremities, overuse injuries include stress fractures of the humerus, ulna, and metacarpals, as well as traction apophysis at the medial humeral epicondyle. The marked and rapid load and directional change associated with serving in tennis contributes to injuries of the back.

Tennis elbow, or lateral epicondylitis, is from repetitive overload of the wrist extensor-supinator mechanism, especially the extensor carpi radialis brevis (see Chapter 687.3). Medial epicondylitis is caused by repetitive overload of the wrist flexor–pronator muscle groups. This can secondarily involve the ulnar collateral ligament at the elbow. In young athletes, medial epicondylar apophysitis may also be associated with ulnar nerve dysfunction in the presence of an avulsion injury.

Olecranon apophysitis is similar to Osgood-Schlatter disease and is marked by pain at the olecranon with elbow extension.

At the shoulder (see Chapter 687.2), rotator cuff tendinosis is caused by repetitive overuse and may be related to anteroposterior glenohumeral instability. Subluxation of the glenohumeral joint may also be present. Biceps tendinosis can present as anterior shoulder pain. Wrist problems include an enlarged dorsal ganglion cyst, radiocarpal joint capsular (impingement) synovitis, chronic degenerative tears of the triangular fibrocartilage complex, and acute fracture of the hook of the hamate.

Basic treatment includes relative rest, ice, NSAIDs, rehabilitation, learning proper mechanics, use of properly sized racquets, counterforce bracing (elbow, wrist), forearm straps, strengthening exercises, and gradual return to tennis. Corticosteroid injections in the wrist extensor–supinator muscle group for tennis elbow are not recommended as outcomes at 1 yr are poorer than those treated with rehabilitation.

SKIING AND SNOWBOARDING

Injuries are related to falls (concussions, contusions, lacerations), and ski-specific mechanisms. Overall injuries have declined, partly because of better equipment (boots, bindings, poles) and slope conditions. It is strongly advised that children, adolescents, and adults wear helmets for skiing and snowboarding. Wrist protectors are also recommended for snowboarders. Injury patterns differ between these two sports with lower extremity injuries more commonly associated with skiing. Upper-extremity injuries (often from falls onto an outstretched arm) are more common in snowboarding related to the fact that both of the snowboarder's feet are strapped onto the same board reducing torque at the knees. The upper extremities, not poles, are used for balance in snowboarding putting them at increased risk.

Skier's thumb, a sprain of the ulnar collateral ligament of the thumb, often results from a fall with the thumb in abduction and hyperextension. Complete tears with a 45 degree joint opening require surgical intervention. Smaller degrees of joint opening can be treated with immobilization in a thumb spica cast × 4 wk. Care should be taken to rule out a concomitant Salter-Harris III fracture, which would require open reduction and internal fixation if the epiphyseal fracture is displaced. In snowboarding, shoulder dislocation, acromioclavicular joint sprain, and fractures of the wrist or collarbone are common injuries.

Lower-extremity injuries include fractures (often spiral) of the tibia ("boot top") and sprains of the high ankle and anterior cruciate ligament, the latter may include tibial eminence fracture. Hemarthrosis is present in fractures and anterior cruciate ligament injuries. Treatment is described in Chapter 683.4.

CHEERLEADING

Cheerleading injuries are mostly related to the gymnastic component of the sport, primarily stunting, tumbling, and pyramids. Sprains and strains comprise the majority of these injuries followed by fractures and contusions. These injuries involve the upper and lower extremities nearly equally, with the ankle being the most commonly injured joint followed by the head, neck, knee, and lower back. The use of impact-absorbing surfaces for practices reduces the risk of serious injury from falls. Ankle sprains in cheerleading predominantly involve the lateral ligaments with the ankle injured when forced into excessive plantarflexion and inversion during landings.

Similar to gymnasts, the excessive amount of repetitive hyperextension, flexion, rotation, and axial loading of the spine associated with stunting and tumbling maneuvers results in significant stress being placed upon the lower back. Another common mechanism of injury involves the act of spotting or basing another cheerleader during partner or group stunts. This involves the lifting or throwing of a teammate above the level of one's head, followed by catching them upon their descent. Injuries with this activity include sprains and strains to the upper and lower back, contributed to by poor technique, requiring coaching to avoid excessive lordosis and encourage lifting with one's legs. Concussions (brain injury) are not uncommon in cheerleading, primarily due to falls while stunting or from a pyramid. This

sometimes places the cheerleaders on the bottom of these formations at greater risk of injury than those held aloft or thrown. Prevention, diagnosis, and treatment of concussion are described in Chapter 688.

SKATEBOARDING

Injuries associated with skateboarding are predominantly acute including contusions, lacerations, sprains, and fractures, affecting the wrists, forearms, and to a lesser extent, ankles and head. Fractures involving the upper extremities are more common in younger skateboarders, often from a fall onto an outstretched arm (see Chapter 683.3). Lower-extremity fractures and head injuries predominate in the adolescent population, likely because of higher complexity of the often airborne maneuvers attempted. Loss of balance leading to a fall when failing to perform a particular maneuver is generally the primary cause of injury. These falls can occur at high velocities, with speeds up to 40 mph documented in the literature, placing the skateboarder at risk for serious injuries.

Traumatic brain injuries are not uncommon within this sport, the incidence increasing with age as well as more common in males than females. In older children and adolescents, the neglected use of helmets and increased speed of their skating contribute to this fact. The prevention, diagnosis, and treatment of traumatic brain injuries are discussed in Chapter 688.

In addition to helmet use, other safety measures recommended include wrist guards with elbow and knee pads. The building of skateboard parks has been a recent strategy to remove skateboarders from pedestrians, bicyclists, and traffic while also encouraging adult supervision.

Bibliography is available at Expert Consult.

Section 3
The Skeletal Dysplasias

Chapter 694
General Considerations
William A. Horton and Jacqueline T. Hecht

The **skeletal dysplasias**, **bone dysplasias**, and **osteochondrodysplasias** are a genetically and clinically heterogeneous group of disorders of skeletal development and growth with an estimated prevalence of 1 in 4,000 births. They can be divided into the osteodysplasias typified by osteogenesis imperfecta (see Chapter 701) and the chondrodysplasias. The latter result from mutations of genes that are essential for skeletal development and growth. The clinical picture is dominated by skeletal abnormalities. The manifestations may be restricted to the skeleton, but in most cases nonskeletal tissues are also involved. The disorders range in severity from lethal in utero to such mild features as to go undetected.

The chondrodysplasias are distinguished from other forms of short stature by a disproportionality of skeletal manifestations. **Figure 694-1** notes the importance of cartilage in bone formation. There are 2 basic categories: predominantly with short limbs and predominantly with short trunks. Efforts to define the extent of clinical heterogeneity resulted in the delineation of well over 100 distinct entities. Many of these disorders result from mutations of a relatively small group of genes, the *chondrodysplasia genes*. An International Working Group on

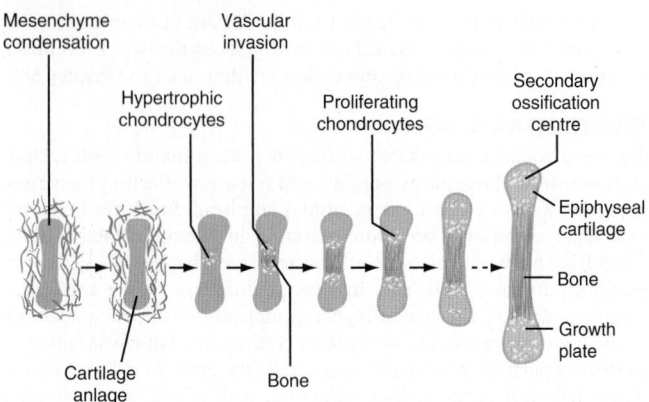

Figure 694-1 The importance of cartilage in bone formation. *(From Horton WA: Skeletal development: Insights from targeting the mouse genome, Lancet 362:560, 2005.)*

Bone Dysplasias has named and classified these disorders into groups based on genetic cause if known or on similarities of clinical and radiographic manifestations, which often imply a common pathogenesis and a common genetic basis, if the cause is unknown (Table 694-1). The better-defined chondrodysplasia groups, such as the achondroplasia and type II collagenopathy groups, contain graded series of disorders that range from very severe to very mild. This may be true for other groups as more mutations are found and the full spectrum of clinical phenotypes associated with mutations of a given gene is defined. These disorders are clinical phenotypes distributed along spectra of phenotypic abnormality associated with mutations of particular genes. For mutations of some genes, such as *COL2A1*, the distribution is fairly continuous, with clinical phenotypes merging into one another across a broad range. There is much less clinical overlap for mutations of some other genes, such as *FGFR3*, in which the distribution is discontinuous. Because most clinicians and most reference materials refer to the disorders as distinct entities, this vernacular continues to be used.

Most chondrodysplasias require the analysis of information from the history, physical examination, skeletal radiographs, family history, and laboratory testing to make a diagnosis. The process involves recognizing complex patterns that are characteristic of the different disorders (Tables 694-2, 694-3, 694-4, and 694-5). Comprehensive descriptions of disorders and references are at the Online Mendelian Inheritance in Man (OMIM) Internet site (http://omim.org/about).

CLINICAL MANIFESTATIONS
Growth
The hallmark of the chondrodysplasias is disproportionate short stature. Although this refers to a disproportion between the limbs and the trunk, most disorders exhibit some shortening of both, and subtle degrees of disproportion may be difficult to appreciate, especially in premature, obese, or edematous infants. Disproportionate shortening of the limbs should be suspected if the upper limbs do not reach the mid pelvis in infancy or the upper thigh after infancy. Disproportionate shortening of the trunk is indicated by a short neck, small chest, and protuberant abdomen. Skeletal disproportion is usually accompanied by short stature (length and height below the 3rd percentile); these measurements are occasionally within the low-normal range early in the course of certain conditions.

There may also be disproportionate shortening of different segments of the limbs; the particular pattern can provide clues for specific diagnoses. Shortening is greatest in the proximal segments (upper arms and legs) in achondroplasia; this is termed **rhizomelic shortening.** Disproportionate shortening of the middle segments (forearms and lower legs) is called **mesomelic shortening; acromelic** shortening involves the hands and feet.

With some exceptions, there is a strong correlation between the age at onset and the clinical severity. Many of the lethal neonatal chondro-

dysplasias are evident during routine fetal ultrasound examinations performed at the end of the 1st trimester of gestation (see Table 694-4). Gestational standards exist for long-bone lengths; discrepancies are often detected between biparietal diameter of the skull and long-bone lengths. Many disorders become apparent around the time of birth; others manifest during the 1st yr of life. A number of disorders manifest in early childhood and a few in late childhood or later.

Non–Growth-Related Manifestations
Most patients also have problems unrelated to growth. Skeletal deformities, such as abnormal joint mobility, protuberances at and around joints, and angular deformities, are common and usually symmetric. Skeletal abnormalities can adversely affect nonskeletal tissues. Impaired growth at the base of the skull and of vertebral pedicles reduces the size of the spinal canal in achondroplasia and can contribute to spinal cord compression. Short ribs reduce thoracic volume, which can compromise breathing in patients with short trunk chondrodysplasias. Cleft palate (see Chapter 310) is common to many disorders, presumably reflecting defective palatal growth.

Manifestations may be unrelated to the skeleton; they reflect expression of mutant genes in nonskeletal tissues. Examples include retinal detachment in spondyloepiphyseal dysplasia congenita, sex reversal in camptomelic dysplasia, congenital heart malformations in Ellis-van Creveld syndrome, immunodeficiency in cartilage-hair hypoplasia, and renal dysfunction in asphyxiating thoracic dystrophy. These nonskeletal problems provide valuable clues to specific diagnoses and must be managed clinically (see Table 694-3).

Family and Reproductive History
A family history might identify relatives with the condition; a mendelian inheritance pattern may be elicited. Because the presentation can vary in some disorders, features that might be related to the disorder should be identified. Special attention should be given to mild degrees of short stature, disproportion, deformities, and other manifestations such as precocious osteoarthritis because they may be overlooked. Physical examination of relatives may be useful, as may the review of their photographs, radiographs, and medical and laboratory records.

A reproductive history might reveal previous stillbirths, fetal losses, and other abnormal pregnancy outcomes resulting from a skeletal dysplasia. Pregnancy complications, such as polyhydramnios or reduced fetal movement, are common in bone dysplasias, especially neonatal lethal variants.

Even though most of the skeletal dysplasias are genetic, it is common to have no family history of the disorder. New mutations are common for autosomal dominant disorders, especially lethal disorders in the perinatal period (thanatophoric dysplasia, osteogenesis imperfecta). Most cases of achondroplasia result from new mutations. Germ cell mosaicism, in which a parent has clones of mutant germ cells, has been observed in osteogenesis imperfecta and in other dominant disorders. A negative family history is usually seen in recessive disorders. Few of these conditions are caused by X-linked mutations. Prenatal diagnosis is available for disorders that have a genetic locus identified. Appropriateness of the testing depends on many factors, and genetic counseling is warranted for these families.

Radiographic Features
Radiographic evaluation for a chondrodysplasia should include plain films of the entire skeleton. Efforts should be made to identify which bones and which parts of bones (epiphyses, metaphyses, diaphyses) are most affected. If possible, films taken at different ages should be examined because the radiographic changes evolve with time. Films taken before puberty are generally more informative because pubertal closure of the epiphyses obliterates many of the signs needed for a radiographic diagnosis. Prenatal diagnosis may also be possible with fetal ultrasound.

DIAGNOSIS
If an infant or child is short with disproportionate features, a diagnosis is established by matching the observed clinical picture (defined

Table 694-1 Genetics of Skeletal Dysplasias

GENE LOCUS	CHROMOSOME LOCATION	PROTEIN	PROTEIN FUNCTION	CLINICAL PHENOTYPE	MIM	DISEASE MECHANISM	INHERIT
COL2A1	12q13.1-q13.3	Type II collagen α_1 chain	Cartilage matrix protein	Achondrogenesis II	200610	Dominant negative	AD*
				Hypochondrogenesis	200610	Dominant negative	AD*
				SED congenital	183900	Dominant negative	AD
				Kniest dysplasia	156550	Dominant negative	AD
				Late-onset SED		Dominant negative	AD
				Stickler dysplasia	108300	Haploinsufficiency	AD
ACG1	15q26.1	Aggrecan	Cartilage matrix protein	SED Kimberley	608361	Haploinsufficiency	AD
				SEMD Aggrecan type	155760	Dominant negative	AR
SEDL	Xp22.2-p22.1	Sedlin	Intracellular transporter	X-linked SED tarda	313400	Loss of function	XLR
COL11A1	1p21	Type XI collagen α_1 chain	Cartilage matrix protein	Stickler-like dysplasia	184840	Dominant negative	AD
COL11A2	6p21.3	Type XI collagen α_2 chain	Cartilage matrix protein	Stickler-like dysplasia	215150	Loss of function	AR
COMP	19p12-p13.1	Cartilage oligomeric matrix protein	Cartilage matrix protein	Pseudoachondroplasia	177170	Dominant negative	AD
				MED	600969	Dominant negative	AD
COL9A2	1p32.2-p33	Type IX collagen α_2 chain	Cartilage matrix protein	MED	600969	Dominant negative	AD
COL9A3	20q13.3	Type IX collagen α_3 chain	Cartilage matrix protein	MED	600969	Dominant negative	AD
MATN3	2p24-p23	Matrilin 3	Cartilage matrix protein	MED	600969	Dominant negative	AD
COL10A1	6q21-q22.3	Type X collagen α_1 chain	Hypertrophic cartilage matrix protein	Schmid metaphyseal chondrodysplasia	156500	Haploinsufficiency	AD
FGFR3	4p16.3	FGF receptor 3	Tyrosine kinase receptor for FGFs	Thanatophoric dysplasia I	187600	Gain of function	AD*
				Thanatophoric dysplasia II	187610	Gain of function	AD*
				Achondroplasia	100800	Gain of function	AD
				Hypochondroplasia	146000	Gain of function	AD
PTHR1	3p21-p22	PTHrP receptor	G protein-coupled receptor for PTH and PTHrP	Jansen metaphyseal chondrodysplasia	156400	Gain of function	AD
DTDST	5q32-q33	DTD sulfate transporter	Transmembrane sulfate transporter	Achondrogenesis 1B	600972	Loss of function	AR*
				Atelosteogenesis II	256050	Loss of function	AR*
				Diastrophic dysplasia	222600	Loss of function	AR
SOX9	17q24.3-q25.1	SRY box 9	Transcription factor	Campomelic dysplasia	114290	Haploinsufficiency	AD
RUNX2†	6p21	Runt-related transcription factor 2	Transcription factor	Cleidocranial dysplasia	119600	Haploinsufficiency	AD
LMX1B	9q34.1		Transcription factor	Nail-patella dysplasia	161200	Haploinsufficiency	AD
CTSK	1q21	Cathepsin K	Enzyme	Pyknodysostosis	265800	Loss of function	AR
RMRP	9p21-p12	Mitochondrial RNA-processing endoribonuclease	RNA-processing enzyme	CHH	250250	Loss of function	AR
DYNC2H1	11q13.5	Dynein, cytoplasmic 2, heavy chain 1	Cytoplasmic cilia-related protein	ATD	208500	Loss of function?	AR
				SRPIII	263510	Loss of function?	AR
TRPV4	12q24.1-12q24.2	Calcium-permeable TRP ion channel	Transmembrane channel protein	Brachyolmia	113500	Gain of function	AD
				SMDK	1842522	Gain of function	AD
				Metatropic dysplasia	156530	Gain of function	AD

*Usually lethal.
†Also called CBFA1.
AD, autosomal dominant; AR, autosomal recessive; ATD, Jeune asphyxiating thoracic dystrophy; CHH, cartilage-hair hypoplasia; DTD, diastrophic dysplasia; FGF, fibroblast growth factor; MED, multiple epiphyseal dysplasia; PTH, parathyroid hormone; PTHrP, parathyroid hormone–related protein; SED, spondyloepiphyseal dysplasia; SEMD, spondyloepimetaphyseal dysplasia; SMDK, spondylometaphyseal dysplasia Kozlowski type; SRPIII, short rib polydactyly syndrome type III; SRY, sex-determining region of the Y chromosome; TRPV4, transient receptor potential vanilloid family 4.

Table 694-2	Major Problems Associated with Skeletal Dysplasias

PROBLEM	EXAMPLE
Lethality*	Thanatophoric dysplasia
Associated anomalies†	Ellis-van Creveld syndrome
Short stature	Common to almost all
Cervical spine dislocations	Larsen syndrome
Severe limb bowing	Metaphyseal dysplasia, Schmid type
Spine curvatures	Metatropic dysplasia
Clubfeet	Diastrophic dysplasia
Fractures	Osteogenesis imperfecta
Pneumonias, aspirations	Camptomelic dysplasia
Spinal cord compression	Achondroplasia
Joint problems (hips, knees)	Most skeletal dysplasias
Hearing loss	Common (greatest with cleft palate)
Myopia/cataracts	Stickler syndrome
Immunodeficiency‡	Cartilage-hair hypoplasia, Schimke immunoosseous dysplasia
Poor body image	Variable, but common to all
Sex reversal	Camptomelic dysplasia

*Mostly a result of severely reduced size of thorax.
†See Table 694-3.
‡At least 4 additional disorders, all involving the metaphyses, can have immunodeficiency.

primarily from clinical, family, and gestational histories; physical examination; and radiographic evaluation) with clinical phenotypes of well-documented disorders. Pediatricians should be able to gather most of this information and, in consultation with a radiologist, diagnose the common chondrodysplasias. A number of reference texts and online databases provide information about the disorders and comprehensive lists of current references (http://www.ncbi.nlm.nih.gov/books/NBK1116/). For less-common disorders and for infants and children whose phenotypes do not closely match well-established clinical phenotypes, consultation with experts in the bone dysplasia field is warranted.

Molecular genetic testing for chondrodysplasias is very useful, especially for disorders in which recurrent mutations occur (typical achondroplasia has the same *FGFR3* mutation). Mutation testing for achondroplasia is available, although the diagnosis is usually made clinically. The greatest utility for testing may be for prenatal diagnosis for couples where both parents have typical (heterozygous) achondroplasia. Their children are at a 25% risk of the much more severe homozygous achondroplasia, which can be detected by mutation analysis. Preimplantation genetic testing can be used to identify double dominant mutations. Another example of testing is in disorders resulting from mutations of *DTDST*. These disorders are inherited in an autosomal recessive manner, and a limited number of mutant alleles have been found. If the mutations are identified in the patient, they should be detectable in the parents and potentially used for prenatal diagnosis. Mutational analysis is now commercially available for many of the skeletal dysplasias and is increasingly used to confirm clinical diagnosis and for future pregnancy planning.

Many of the chondrodysplasias have distinct histologic changes of the skeletal growth plate. Sometimes such tissues obtained at biopsy or discarded from a surgical procedure are helpful diagnostically. It is uncommon to make a diagnosis histologically if it was not already suspected on clinical or radiographic grounds.

Table 694-3	Associated Anomalies in Skeletal Dysplasias

ANOMALY	EXAMPLE
Heart defects	Ellis-van Creveld syndrome, Jeune syndrome
Polydactyly	Short rib polydactyly, Majewski type
Cleft palate	Diastrophic dysplasia
Ear cysts	Diastrophic dysplasia
Spinal cord compression	Achondroplasia
Encephalocele	Dyssegmental dysplasia
Hemivertebrae	Dyssegmental dysplasia
Micrognathia	Camptomelic dysplasia
Nail dysplasia	Ellis-van Creveld syndrome
Conical teeth, oligodontia	Ellis-van Creveld syndrome
Multiple oral frenula	Ellis-van Creveld syndrome
Dentinogenesis imperfecta	Osteogenesis imperfecta
Pretibial skin dimples	Camptomelic dysplasia
Cataracts, retinal detachment	Stickler syndrome
Intestinal atresia	Saldino-Noonan
Renal cysts	Saldino-Noonan
Camptodactyly	Diastrophic dysplasia
Craniosynostosis	Thanatophoric dysplasia
Ichthyosis	Chondrodystrophia punctata
Hitchhiker thumb	Diastrophic dysplasia
Sparse scalp hair	Cartilage-hair hypoplasia
Hypertelorism	Robinow syndrome
Hypoplastic nasal bridge	Acrodysostosis
Clavicular agenesis	Cleidocranial dysplasia
Genital hypoplasia	Robinow syndrome
Tail	Metatropic dysplasia
Omphalocele	Beemer-Langer syndrome
Blue sclera	Osteogenesis imperfecta

Table 694-4	Lethal Neonatal Dwarfism

USUALLY FATAL*
Achondrogenesis (different types)
Thanatophoric dysplasia
Short rib polydactyly (different types)
Homozygous achondroplasia
Camptomelic dysplasia
Dyssegmental dysplasia, Silverman-Handmaker type
Osteogenesis imperfecta, type II
Hypophosphatasia (congenital form)
Chondrodysplasia punctata (rhizomelic form)

OFTEN FATAL
Asphyxiating thoracic dystrophy (Jeune syndrome)

OCCASIONALLY FATAL
Ellis-van Creveld syndrome
Diastrophic dysplasia
Metatropic dwarfism
Kniest dysplasia

*A few prolonged survivors have been reported in most of these disorders.

Table 694-5	Usually Nonlethal Dwarfing Conditions Recognizable at Birth or Within 1st Few Mo of Life

MOST COMMON
Achondroplasia
Osteogenesis imperfecta (types I, III, IV)
Spondyloepiphyseal dysplasia congenita
Diastrophic dysplasia
Ellis-van Creveld syndrome

LESS COMMON
Chondrodysplasia punctata (some forms)
Kniest dysplasia
Metatropic dysplasia
Langer mesomelic dysplasia

MOLECULAR GENETICS

A number of chondrodysplasia genes have been identified (see **Table 694-1**). They encode several categories of proteins, including cartilage matrix proteins, transmembrane receptors, ion transporters, and transcription factors. The number of identified gene loci is smaller than anticipated from the number of recognized clinical phenotypes. The majority of patients have disorders that map to fewer than 10 loci; mutations at 2 loci (*COL2A1* and *FGFR3*) account for more than half of all cases. There may be a limited number of genes whose function is critical to skeletal development, especially linear bone growth; mutations in these genes give rise to a wide range of chondrodysplasia clinical phenotypes. New genes harboring mutations that cause chondrodysplasias continue to be identified with advances in detection technology.

Mutations at the *COL2A1* and *FGFR3* loci illustrate different genetic characteristics. *COL2A1* mutations are distributed throughout the gene, with few instances of recurrence in unrelated persons. In contrast, *FGFR3* mutations are restricted to a few locations within the gene, and occurrence of new mutations at these sites in unrelated persons is the rule. There is a strong correlation between clinical phenotype and mutation site for *FGFR3*, but not *COL2A1*, mutations.

PATHOPHYSIOLOGY

Chondrodysplasia mutations act through different mechanisms. Most mutations involving cartilage matrix proteins cause disease when only 1 of the 2 copies (alleles) of the relevant gene is mutated. These mutations usually act through a dominant negative mechanism in which the protein products of the mutant allele interfere with the assembly and function of multimeric molecules that contain the protein products of both the normal and mutant alleles. The type II collagen molecule is a triple helix composed of 3 collagen chains, which are the products of the type II collagen gene *COL2A1*. When chains from both normal and mutant alleles are combined to form triple helices, most molecules contain at least 1 mutant chain. It is not known how many mutant chains are required to produce a dysfunctional molecule but, depending on the mutation, it theoretically could be as few as 1.

Mutations involving type X collagen differ from the model just described. They map to the region of the chain that is responsible for chain recognition; the chains must recognize each other before they can assemble into collagen molecules. Mutations are thought to disrupt this process. As a result, none of the mutant chains are incorporated into molecules. This mechanism is haploinsufficiency because the products of the mutant allele are functionally absent and the normal allele is insufficient for normal function. Mutations involving ion transport genes also act through a loss of function of the transporters. Mutations of transmembrane receptors studied to date appear to act through a gain of function; the mutant receptors initiate signals in a constitutive manner independent of their normal ligands.

Regardless of genetic mechanism, the mutations ultimately disrupt endochondral ossification, the biologic process responsible for the development and linear growth of the skeleton (see **Fig. 694-1**). Indeed, a wide range of morphologic abnormalities of the skeletal growth plate, the anatomic structure in which endochondral ossification occurs, have been described in the chondrodysplasias.

TREATMENT

The first step is to establish the correct diagnosis. This allows one to predict a prognosis and to anticipate the medical and surgical problems associated with a particular disorder. Establishing a diagnosis helps to distinguish between lethal disorders and nonlethal disorders in a premature or newborn infant (see **Tables 694-4 and 694-5**). A poor prognosis for long-term survival might argue against initiating extreme lifesaving measures for thanatophoric dysplasia or achondrogenesis types Ib or II, whereas such measures may be indicated for infants with spondyloepiphyseal dysplasia congenita or diastrophic dysplasia, which have a good prognosis if the infant survives the newborn period.

Because there is no definitive therapy to normalize bone growth in any of the disorders, management is directed at preventing and correcting skeletal deformities, treating nonskeletal complications, providing genetic counseling, and helping patients and families learn to cope. Each disorder has its own unique set of problems, and consequently management must be tailored to each disorder.

There are a number of problems common to many chondrodysplasias for which general recommendations can be made. Children with most chondrodysplasias should avoid contact sports and other activities that cause injury or stress to joints. Good dietary habits should be established in childhood to prevent or minimize obesity in adulthood. Dental care should be started early to minimize crowding and malalignment of teeth. Children and relatives should be given the opportunity to participate in support groups, such as the Little People of America (http://www.lpoaonline.org) and Human Growth Foundation (http://www.hgfound.org).

Two controversial approaches have been used to increase bone length. Surgical limb lengthening has been employed for a few disorders. Its greatest success has been in achondroplasia in which nonskeletal tissues tend to be redundant and easily stretched. The procedure is usually performed during adolescence. Pharmacologic doses of human growth hormone comparable to those used to treat Turner syndrome have also been tried in several disorders; the results have been equivocal. Animal studies suggest that C-type natriuretic peptide may promote linear bone growth in achondroplasia. Clinical trials are beginning to test the efficacy of this approach.

Bibliography is available at Expert Consult.

Chapter **695**
Disorders Involving Cartilage Matrix Proteins
William A. Horton and Jacqueline T. Hecht

Disorders of cartilage matrix proteins resulting in bone and joint disorders can be classified in 5 categories corresponding to the defective proteins: 3 collagens and the noncollagenous proteins COMP (cartilage oligomeric matrix protein), matrilin 3, and aggrecan. The clinical phenotypes and clinical severity differ between and within the groups, especially the **spondyloepiphyseal dysplasia (SED)** group.

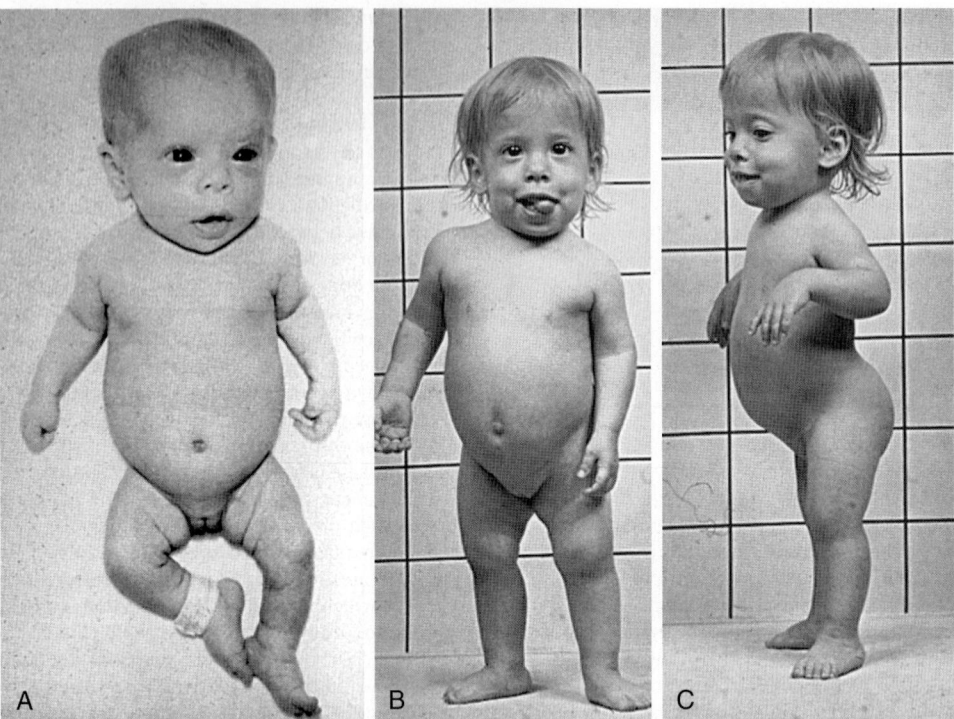

Figure 695-1 Spondyloepiphyseal dysplasia congenita is shown in infancy **(A)** and early childhood **(B, C).** Note the short extremities, relatively normal hands, flat facies, and exaggerated lordosis.

SPONDYLOEPIPHYSEAL DYSPLASIAS

The term *spondyloepiphyseal dysplasia* refers to a heterogeneous group of disorders characterized by shortening of the trunk and, to a lesser extent, the limbs. Severity ranges from achondrogenesis type II to the slightly less-severe hypochondrogenesis (although both types are lethal in the perinatal period) to SED congenita and its variants, including Kniest dysplasia (which is apparent at birth and is usually nonlethal), to late-onset SED (which might not be detected until adolescence or later). The radiographic hallmarks are abnormal development of the vertebral bodies and of epiphyses, the extent of which corresponds to the clinical severity. Most of the SEDs result from heterozygous mutations of *COL2A1*; they are autosomal dominant disorders. The mutations are dispersed throughout the gene; there is a poor correlation between the mutation's location and the resultant clinical phenotype. For familial cases, prenatal diagnosis is possible if the mutation is identified. Schimke immuno-osseous dysplasia may be an exception because it is an autosomal recessive disorder characterized by short stature, hyperpigmented macules, unusual facies, proteinuria and progressive renal failure, cerebral ischemia, and a T-cell defect with lymphopenia and recurrent infections.

Lethal Spondyloepiphyseal Dysplasias

Achondrogenesis type II (MIM 200610) is characterized by severe shortening of the neck and trunk and especially the limbs and by a large, soft head. Fetal hydrops and prematurity are common; infants are stillborn or die shortly after birth. Hypochondrogenesis (MIM 200610) refers to a clinical phenotype intermediate between achondrogenesis type II and SED congenita. It is typically lethal in the newborn period.

The severity of radiographic changes correlates with the clinical severity. Both conditions produce short, broad tubular bones with cupped metaphyses. The pelvic bones are hypoplastic, and the cranial bones are not well mineralized. The vertebral bodies are poorly ossified in the entire spine in achondrogenesis type II and in the cervical and sacral spine in hypochondrogenesis. The pedicles are ossified in both.

Spondyloepiphyseal Dysplasia Congenita

The phenotype of this group, SED congenita (MIM 183900), is apparent at birth. The head and face are usually normal, but a cleft palate is common. The neck is short and the chest is barrel shaped (Fig. 695-1). Kyphosis and exaggeration of the normal lumbar lordosis are common. The proximal segments of the limbs are shorter than the hands and feet, which often appear normal. Some infants have clubfoot or exhibit hypotonia.

Skeletal radiographs of the newborn reveal short tubular bones, delayed ossification of vertebral bodies, and proximal limb bone epiphyses (Fig. 695-2). Hypoplasia of the odontoid process, a short, square pelvis with a poorly ossified symphysis pubis, and mild irregularity of metaphyses are apparent.

Infants usually have normal developmental milestones; a waddling gait typically appears in early childhood. Childhood complications include respiratory compromise from spinal deformities and spinal cord compression because of cervicomedullary instability. The disproportion and shortening become progressively worse with age, and adult heights range from 95-128 cm. Myopia is typical; adults are predisposed to retinal detachment. Precocious osteoarthritis occurs in adulthood and requires surgical joint replacement.

KNIEST DYSPLASIA

The Kniest dysplasia variant of SED (MIM 156550) manifests at birth with a short trunk and limbs associated with a flat face, prominent eyes, enlarged joints, cleft palate, and clubfoot (Fig. 695-3). Radiographs show vertebral defects and short tubular bones with epiphyseal irregularities and metaphyseal enlargement that gives rise to a dumbbell appearance.

Motor development is often delayed because of the joint deformities, although intelligence is normal. Hearing loss and myopia commonly develop during childhood, and retinal detachment can occur as a late complication. Joint enlargement progresses during childhood and becomes painful; it is accompanied by flexion contractures and muscle atrophy, which may be incapacitating by adolescence.

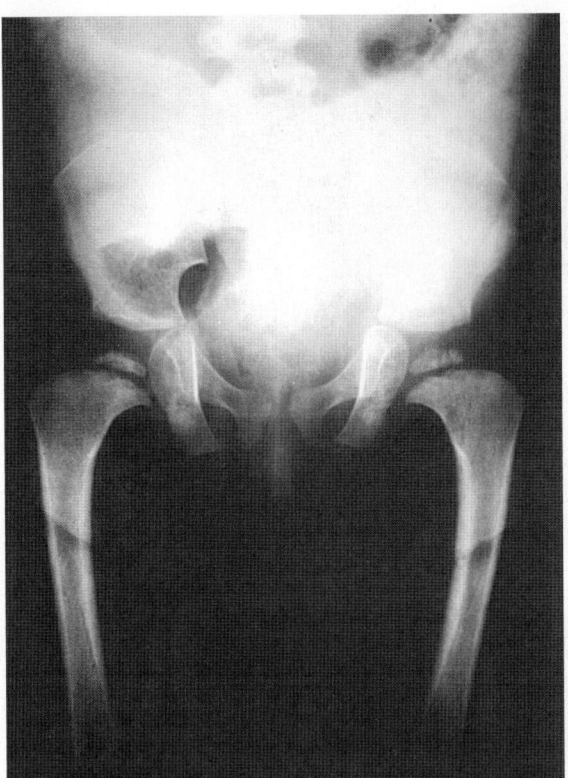

Figure 695-2 Radiograph of spondyloepiphyseal dysplasia congenita pelvis demonstrating squared pelvis, hypoplastic capital femoral epiphyses, and femoral necks that are wide and short.

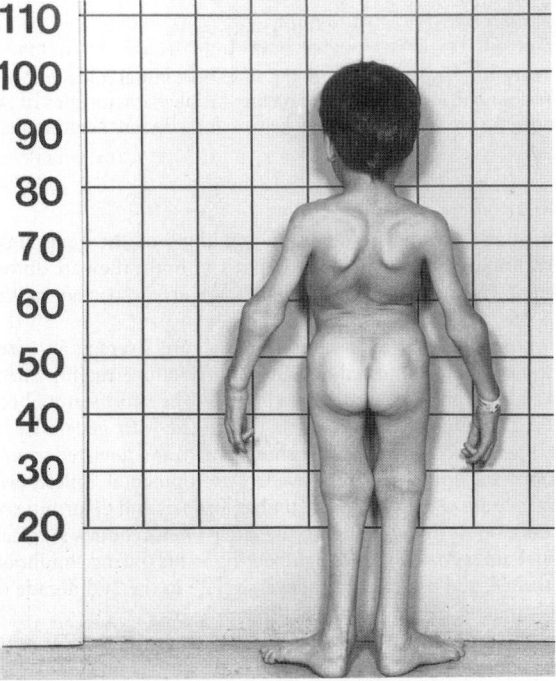

110
100
90
80
70
60
50
40
30
20

Figure 695-3 Patient with Kniest dysplasia. The trunk is short, and the epiphyses are broad. There is contracture of the fingers. *(From Traboulsi EI: Skeletal and connective tissue disorders with anterior segment manifestations. In Krachmer JH, Mannis MJ, Holland EJ, editors: Cornea, ed 3, Philadelphia, 2011, Elsevier, Fig. 60-9.)*

LATE-ONSET SPONDYLOEPIPHYSEAL DYSPLASIA

Late-onset SED is a mild to very mild clinical phenotype characterized by slightly short stature associated with mild epiphyseal and vertebral abnormalities on radiographs. It is typically detected during childhood or adolescence but can go unrecognized until adulthood when precocious osteoarthritis appears. This designation is nosologically distinct from SED tarda, which is clinically similar but results from mutation of the X-linked gene *SEDL*.

AGGRECAN-RELATED SPONDYLOEPIPHYSEAL DYSPLASIAS

Mutations of aggrecan have been detected in 2 SED-like conditions. SED-Kimberley (*MIM 608361*) is relatively mild, with short stature, stocky build, and early onset osteoarthritis of weightbearing joints. A more severe and generalized clinical phenotype with characteristic radiographic changes including widened metaphyses is observed in spondyloepimetaphyseal dysplasia–Aggrecan type (*MIM 612813*).

STICKLER SYNDROME/DYSPLASIA (HEREDITARY OSTEOARTHROOPHTHALMOPATHY)

Short stature is not a feature of Stickler dysplasia (MIM 184840). It resembles SED because of its joint and eye manifestations. Mutations of genes encoding type II (*COL2A1*), type XI (*COL11A1, COL11A2*), and type IX (*COL9A1*) collagens have been identified in Stickler-like disorders (MIM 184840, MIM 215150). Stickler dysplasia is often identified in the newborn because of cleft palate and micrognathia (Pierre Robin anomaly; see Chapter 311). Twenty-five percent of patients with Stickler syndrome have Pierre Robin anomaly; 30% of patients with Pierre Robin anomaly have Stickler syndrome. Infants typically have severe myopia and additional ophthalmologic complications, including choroidoretinal and vitreous degeneration; retinal detachment is common during childhood (Fig. 695-4). Sensorineural hearing loss can arise during adolescence, which is when symptoms of significant osteoarthritis can also begin. Special attention must be given to the eye complications even in childhood. Osteoarticular manifestations include joint hypermobility (especially hip), muscle hypotonia, metaphyseal–epiphyseal dysplasia; progressive osteoarthritis of spine and peripheral joints, which may require hip replacement surgery before age 30 yr and decreased bone density. Similar manifestations may be seen in other diseases with mutations in type II and XI collagen genes (Table 695-1).

Table 695-1	Other Genetic Diseases Associated with Mutations in Type II and Type XI Collagen Genes, with Clinical Presentations Similar to That of Stickler Syndrome

Phenotypes associated with COL2A1 mutations
Achondrogenesis type 2
Hypochondrogenesis
Spondyloepiphyseal dysplasia congenita
Spondyloepimetaphyseal dysplasia, Strudwick type
Kniest dysplasia
Dysplasia with altered vertebral contours
Some of the juvenile joint diseases
Phenotypes associated with COL11A1 mutations
Marshall syndrome
Phenotypes associated with COL11A2 mutations
Otospondylometaphyseal dysplasia
Weissenbach-Zweymuller syndrome
Some cases of isolated sensorineural deafness

From Couchouron T, Masson C: Early-onset progressive osteoarthritis with hereditary progressive ophthalmology or Stickler syndrome. Joint Bone Spine 78:45–49, 2011, Table 1, p. 48.

Daughter

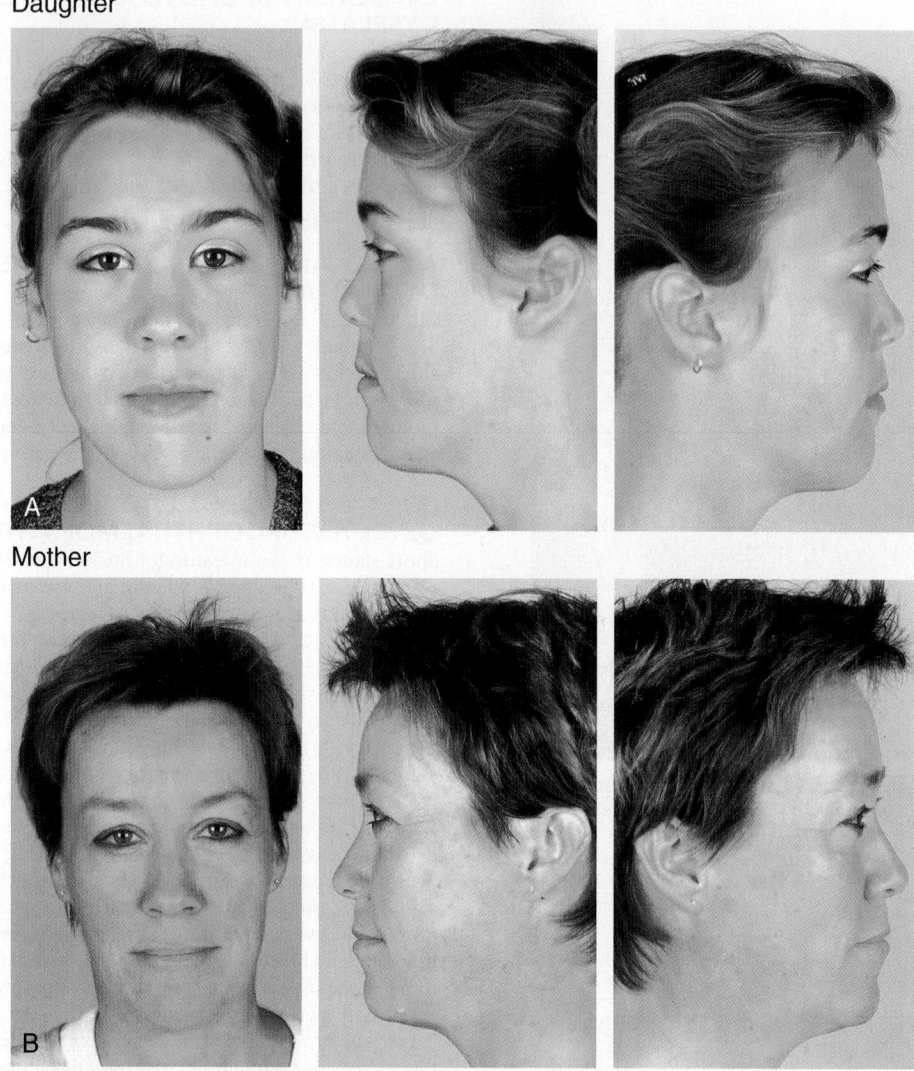

Mother

Figure 695-4 Face and profile of the daughter with Stickler syndrome type I. Note the flat nasal bridge, the mild epicanthal folds and discrete micrognathia. Face and profile of the mother with Stickler syndrome type I. The mother shows at first sight no clear facial characteristics of Stickler syndrome. *(From Baijens LWJ, De Leenheer EMR, Weekamp HH, et al: Stickler syndrome type I and Stapes ankylosis. Int J Pediatr Otorhinolaryngol 68:1573–1580, 2004, Fig. 2.)*

SCHMID METAPHYSEAL DYSPLASIA

Schmid metaphyseal dysplasia (MIM 156500) is one of several chondrodysplasias in which metaphyseal abnormalities dominate the radiographic features. It typically manifests in early childhood with mild short stature, bowing of the legs, and a waddling gait (Fig. 695-5). Joints, such as the wrist, may be enlarged. Radiographs show flaring and irregular mineralization of the metaphyses of tubular bones of the proximal limbs (Fig. 695-6). Coxa vara is usually present and can require surgical correction. Short stature becomes more evident with age and affects the lower extremities more than the upper extremities; the manifestations are limited to the skeleton.

Schmid metaphyseal chondrodysplasia is caused by heterozygous mutations of the gene encoding type X collagen; it is an autosomal dominant trait. The distribution of type X collagen is restricted to the region of growing bone in which cartilage is converted into bone. This might explain why radiographic changes are confined to the metaphyses.

PSEUDOACHONDROPLASIA AND MULTIPLE EPIPHYSEAL DYSPLASIA

Pseudoachondroplasia (MIM 177170) and multiple epiphyseal dysplasia (MED) (MIM 600969) are 2 distinct phenotypes that are grouped together because they result from mutations of the gene encoding COMP. The mutations are heterozygous in both; they are autosomal dominant traits. The clinical phenotypes are restricted to skeletal tissues.

Newborns with pseudoachondroplasia are average in size and appearance. Gait abnormalities and short stature mainly affect the limbs and become apparent in late infancy. The short stature becomes marked as the child grows and is associated with generalized joint laxity (Fig. 695-7). The hands are short, broad, and deviated in an ulnar direction; the forearms are bowed. Developmental milestones and intelligence are usually normal. Lumbar lordosis and deformities of the knee develop during childhood; the latter often requires surgical correction. Pain is common in weightbearing joints during childhood and adolescence, and osteoarthritis develops late in the 2nd decade of life. Adults range in height from 105-128 cm.

Skeletal radiographs show distinctive abnormalities of vertebral bodies and of both epiphyses and metaphyses of tubular bones (Fig. 695-8).

The MED phenotype has skeletal abnormalities that predominantly affect the epiphyses as noted on radiographs. Two classic forms are a severe Fairbank type and a mild Ribbing type. Because of overlap in clinical features and because COMP mutations are found in both types, they may be considered clinical variants. This nomenclature is not generally used now.

The more severe clinical phenotype has its onset during childhood, with mild short-limbed short stature, pain in weightbearing joints, and a waddling gait. Radiographs show delayed and irregular ossification of epiphyses. In more mildly affected patients the disorder might not be recognized until adolescence or adulthood. Radiographic changes may be limited to the capital femoral epiphyses. In the latter case, mild MED must be distinguished from bilateral Legg-Calvé-Perthes disease

(see Chapter 678.3). Precocious osteoarthritis of hips and knees is the major complication in adults with MED. Adult heights range from 136-151 cm.

There are families with clinical and radiographic manifestations of MED that are not caused by mutations of COMP. Some are linked to the gene encoding 1 of the type IX collagen chains. It has been suggested that COMP and type IX collagen interact functionally in cartilage matrix, thus explaining why mutations of different genes produce similar pictures. Mutations of the genes coding for another cartilage

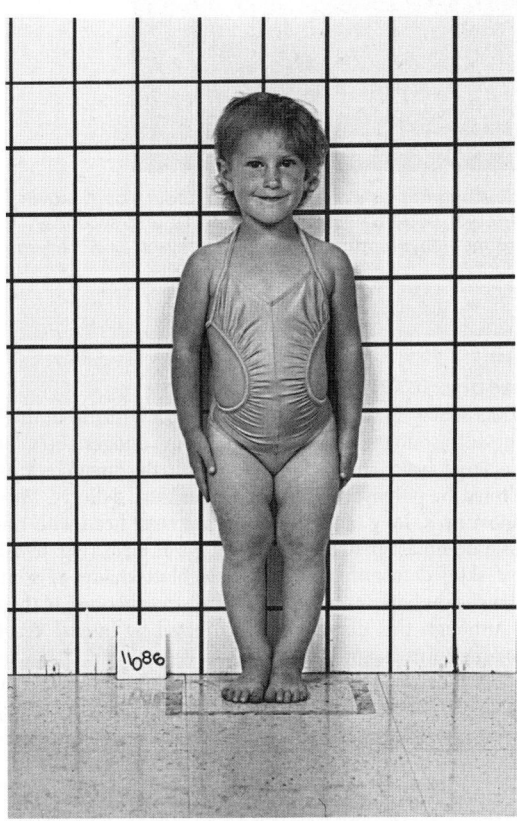

Figure 695-5 Female patient with metaphyseal dysplasia, type Schmid. The facies are normal and stature is mildly reduced. Mild tibia vara is present.

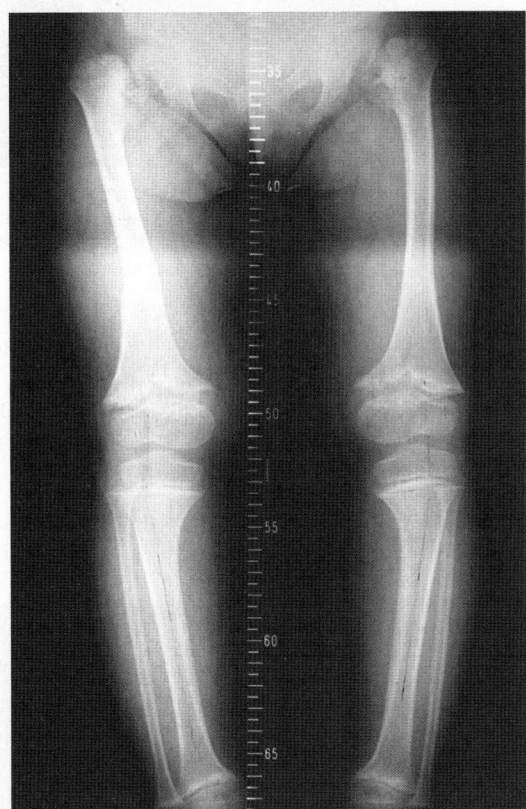

Figure 695-6 Radiograph of lower extremities in Schmid metaphyseal dysplasia showing short tubular bones and metaphyseal flaring and irregularities, abnormal capital femoral epiphyses, and femoral necks. The epiphyses are normal. Coxa vara is present.

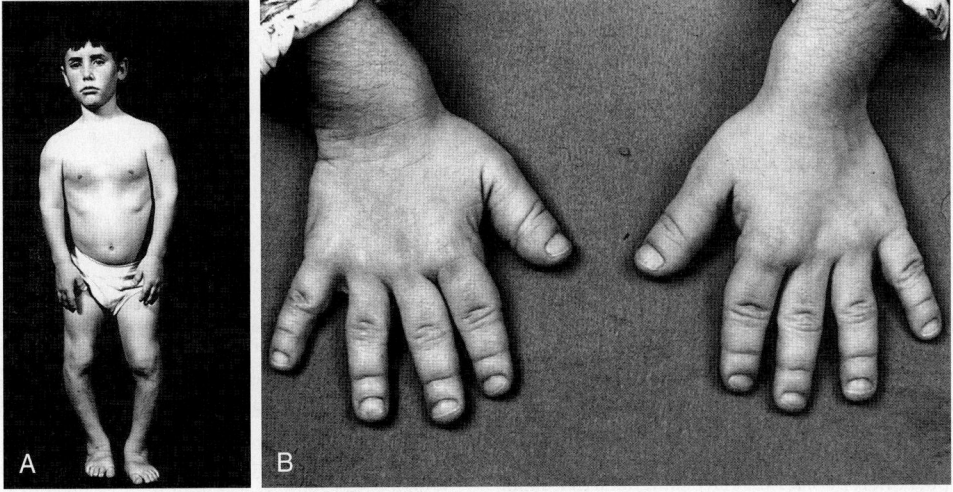

Figure 695-7 A, Pseudoachondroplasia in an adolescent boy. The facies and head circumference are normal. There is shortening of all extremities and bowing of the lower extremities. **B,** Photograph of hands, demonstrating short stubby fingers.

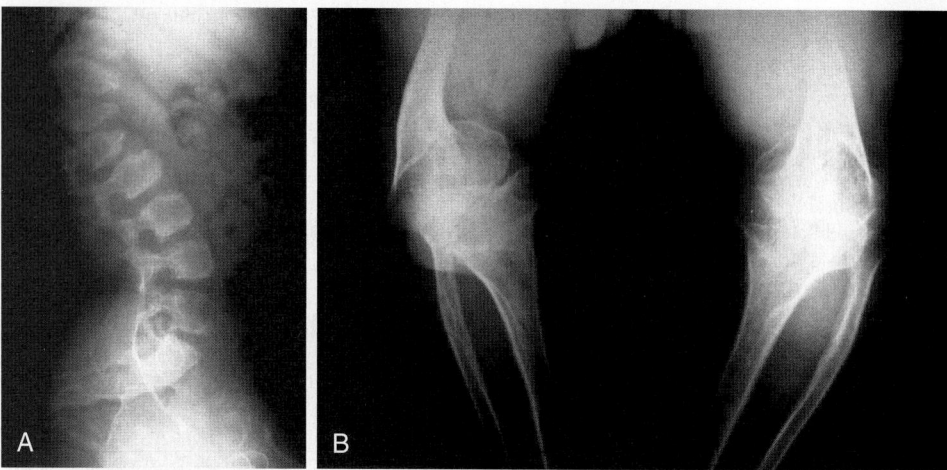

Figure 695-8 A, Lateral thoracolumbar spine radiograph of a patient with pseudoachondroplasia showing central protrusion (tonguing) of the anterior aspect of upper lumbar and lower thoracic vertebrae. Note reduced vertebral body heights (platyspondyly) and secondary lordosis. **B,** Lower-extremity radiograph of patient with pseudoachondroplasia showing large metaphyses, poorly formed epiphyses, and marked bowing of the long bones.

matrix protein, matrilin 3, and the diastrophic dysplasia transporter have also been found in patients with MED. For familial cases of pseudoachondroplasia and MED resulting from mutation in COMP, prenatal diagnosis is available.

Bibliography is available at Expert Consult.

Chapter **696**

Disorders Involving Transmembrane Receptors

William A. Horton and Jacqueline T. Hecht

Heterozygous mutations of genes encoding *FGFR3* (fibroblast growth factor receptor 3) and *PTHR* (parathyroid hormone receptor) result in disorders involving transmembrane receptors. The mutations cause the receptors to become activated in the absence of physiologic ligands, which accentuates normal receptor function of negatively regulating bone growth. The mutations act by gain of negative function. In the *FGFR3* mutation group, in which the clinical phenotypes range from severe to mild, the severity appears to correlate with the extent to which the receptor is activated. *PTHR* and especially *FGFR3* mutations tend to recur in unrelated individuals.

ACHONDROPLASIA GROUP
The achondroplasia group represents a substantial percentage of patients with chondrodysplasias and contains thanatophoric dysplasia (TD), the most common lethal chondrodysplasia, with a birth prevalence of 1 in 35,000 births; achondroplasia, the most common nonlethal chondrodysplasia, with a birth prevalence of 1 in 15,000 to 1 in 40,000 births; and hypochondroplasia. All 3 have mutations in a small number of locations in the *FGFR3* gene. There is a strong correlation between the mutation site and the clinical phenotype.

Thanatophoric Dysplasia
TD (MIM 187600, 187610) manifests before or at birth. In the former situation, ultrasonographic examination in midgestation or later reveals a large head and very short limbs; the pregnancy is often accompanied by polyhydramnios and premature delivery. Very short limbs, short neck, long narrow thorax, and large head with midfacial hypoplasia dominate the clinical phenotype at birth (Fig. 696-1). The cloverleaf skull deformity known as **kleeblattschädel** is sometimes found. Newborns have severe respiratory distress because of their small thorax. Although this distress can be treated by intense respiratory care, the long-term prognosis is poor.

Skeletal radiographs distinguish 2 slightly different forms called TD I and TD II. In the more common TD I, radiographs show large calvariae with a small cranial base, marked thinning and flattening of vertebral bodies visualized best on lateral view, very short ribs, severe hypoplasia of pelvic bones, and very short and bowed tubular bones

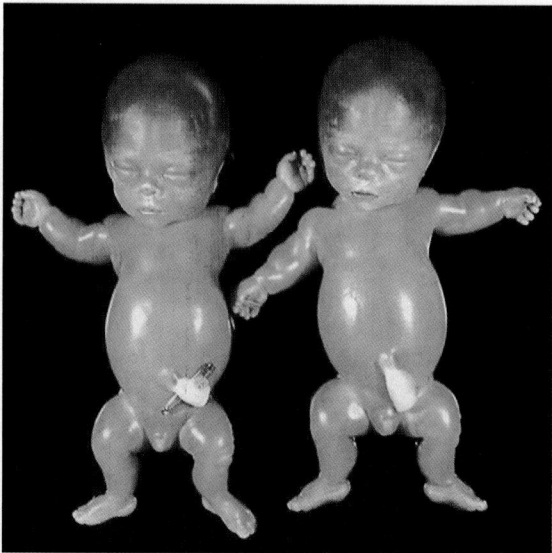

Figure 696-1 Identical twins with type I thanatophoric dysplasia. Disproportionately large head, bell-shaped chest, and micromelia. *(From Gilbert-Barness E, Kapur RP, Oligny LL, Siebert JR, editors: Potter's pathology of the fetus, infant and child, ed 2, Philadelphia, 2007, Elsevier, Fig. 20-47.)*

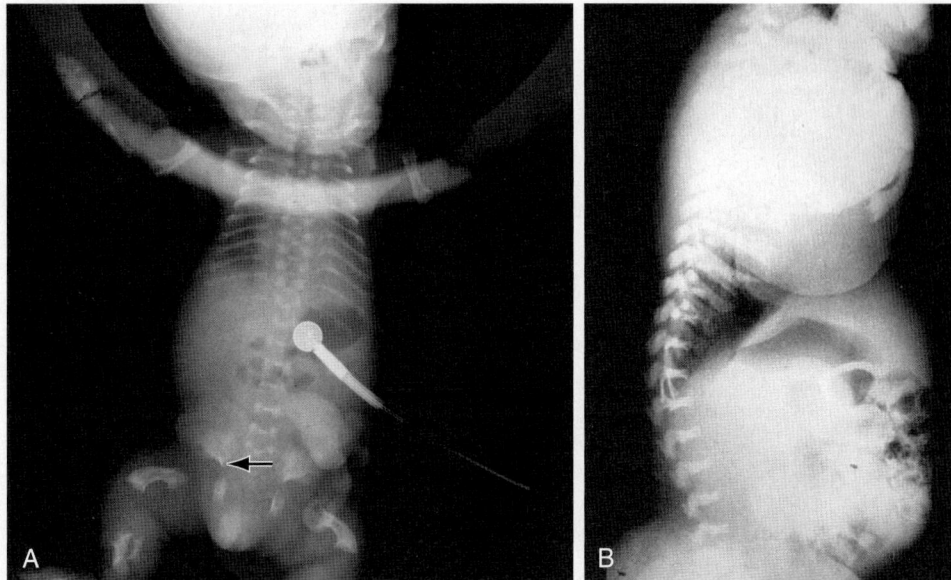

Figure 696-2 A, Neonatal radiograph of a child with thanatophoric dysplasia. Note medial acetabular spurs *(arrow)*, hypoplastic iliac bones, bowed femora with rounded protrusion of proximal femurs, hypoplastic thorax, and wafer-thin vertebral bodies. **B**, Lateral radiograph of the thoracolumbar spine in thanatophoric dysplasia, showing marked vertebral flattening and short ribs. Ossification defect of the central portion of the vertebral bodies is present.

with flared metaphyses (Fig. 696-2). The femurs are curved and shaped like a telephone receiver. TD II differs mainly in that there are longer and straighter femurs.

The TD II clinical phenotype is associated with mutations that map to codon 650 of *FGFR3*, causing the substitution of a glutamic acid for the lysine. This activates the tyrosine kinase activity of a receptor that transmits signals to intracellular pathways. Mutation of lysine 650 to methionine is associated with a clinical phenotype intermediate between TD and achondroplasia, referred to as **severe achondroplasia with developmental delay and acanthosis nigricans**. Mutations of the TD I phenotype mainly map to 2 regions in the extracellular domain of the receptor, where they substitute cysteine residues for other amino acids. Free cysteine residues are thought to form disulfide bonds promoting dimerization of receptor molecules, leading to activation and signal transmission.

TD I and TD II represent new mutations to normal parents. The recurrence risk is low. Because the mutated codons in TD are mutable for unknown reasons and because of the theoretical risk of germ cell mosaicism, parents are offered prenatal diagnosis for subsequent pregnancies.

Achondroplasia

Achondroplasia (MIM 100800) is the prototype chondrodysplasia. It typically manifests at birth with short limbs, a long narrow trunk, and a large head with midfacial hypoplasia and prominent forehead (Fig. 696-3). The limb shortening is greatest in the proximal segments, and the fingers often display a trident configuration. Most joints are hyperextensible, but extension is restricted at the elbow. A thoracolumbar gibbus is often found. Usually, birth length is slightly less than normal but occasionally plots within the low-normal range.

Diagnosis

Skeletal radiographs confirm the diagnosis (see Figs. 696-3 and 696-4). The calvarial bones are large, whereas the cranial base and facial bones are small. The vertebral pedicles are short throughout the spine as noted on a lateral radiograph. The interpedicular distance, which normally increases from the 1st to the 5th lumbar vertebra, decreases in achondroplasia. The iliac bones are short and round, and the acetabular roofs are flat. The tubular bones are short with mildly irregular and flared metaphyses. The fibula is disproportionately long compared with the tibia.

Clinical Manifestations

Infants usually exhibit delayed motor milestones, often not walking alone until 18-24 mo. This is because of hypotonia and mechanical difficulty balancing the large head on a normal-sized trunk and short extremities. Intelligence is normal unless central nervous system complications develop. As the child begins to walk, the gibbus usually gives way to an exaggerated lumbar lordosis.

Infants and children with achondroplasia progressively fall below normal standards for length and height. They can be plotted against standards established for achondroplasia. Adult heights typically are 118-145 cm for men and 112-136 cm for women. Surgical limb lengthening and human growth hormone treatment have been used to increase height; both are controversial. C-type natriuretic peptide may stimulate bone growth in achondroplasia based on studies in animal models. Clinical studies are in the initial phases of testing.

Virtually all infants and children with achondroplasia have large heads, although only a fraction have true hydrocephalus. Head circumference should be carefully monitored using standards developed for achondroplasia, as should neurologic function in general. The spinal canal is stenotic, and spinal cord compression can occur at the foramen magnum and in the lumbar spine. The former usually occurs in infants and small children; it may be associated with hypotonia, failure to thrive, quadriparesis, central and obstructive apnea, and sudden death. Surgical correction may be required for severe stenosis. Lumbar spinal stenosis usually does not occur until early adulthood. Symptoms include paresthesias, numbness, and claudication in the legs. Loss of bladder and bowel control may be late complications.

Bowing of the legs is common and might need to be corrected surgically. Other common problems include dental crowding, articulation difficulties, obesity, and frequent episodes of otitis media, which can contribute to hearing loss.

Genetics

All patients with typical achondroplasia have mutations at *FGFR3* codon 380. The mutation maps to the transmembrane domain of the receptor and is thought to stabilize receptor dimers that enhance receptor signals, the consequences of which inhibit linear bone growth. Achondroplasia behaves as an autosomal dominant trait; most cases arise from a new mutation to normal parents.

Because of the high frequency of achondroplasia among dwarfing conditions, it is relatively common for adults with achondroplasia to

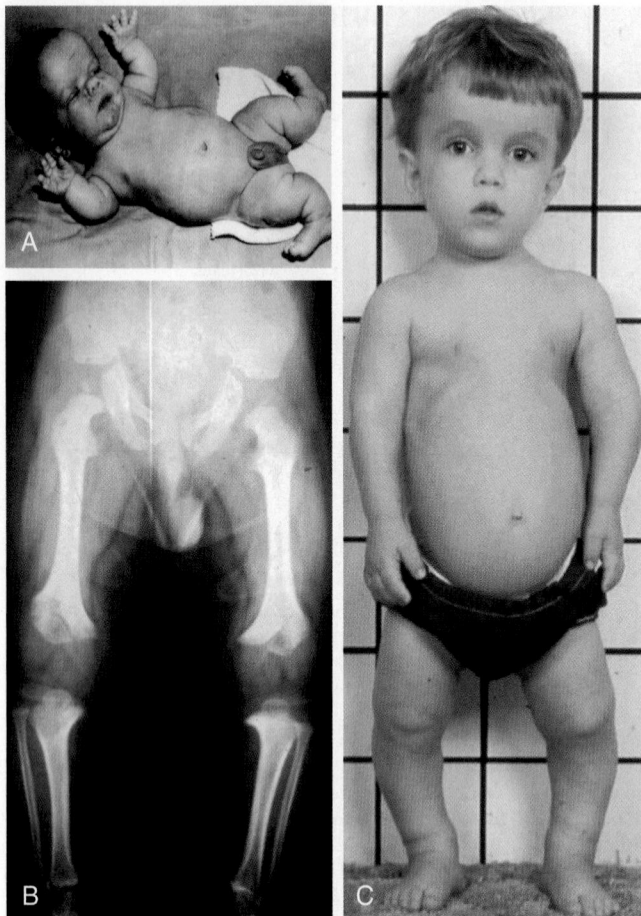

Figure 696-3 Achondroplasia phenotype at different ages. **A,** Infant with achondroplasia with macrocephaly, frontal bossing, midface hypoplasia, small chest, rhizomelic shortening of all the limbs, redundant skin folds, and extreme joint laxity. Note the trident hand with short fingers and abducted hips. **B,** Typical radiographic findings from a child with achondroplasia. All of the tubular bones are short, but the fibula is relatively long compared to the tibia. There is protrusion of the epiphysis into the metaphysis of the distal femur, creating the chevron deformity, and to a lesser extent of the proximal tibia. The iliac bones are rounded, the acetabular roof is horizontal, and the sacrosciatic notches are small. **C,** A 3 yr old with achondroplasia with the typical features shown in **A.** Note that the redundant skin folds are no longer present and that joint laxity has improved. Rhizomelic shortening of the extremities is more pronounced and accompanied by tibial bowing. *(From Horton WA, Hall JG, Hecht JT: Achondroplasia, Lancet 370:162–172, 2007.)*

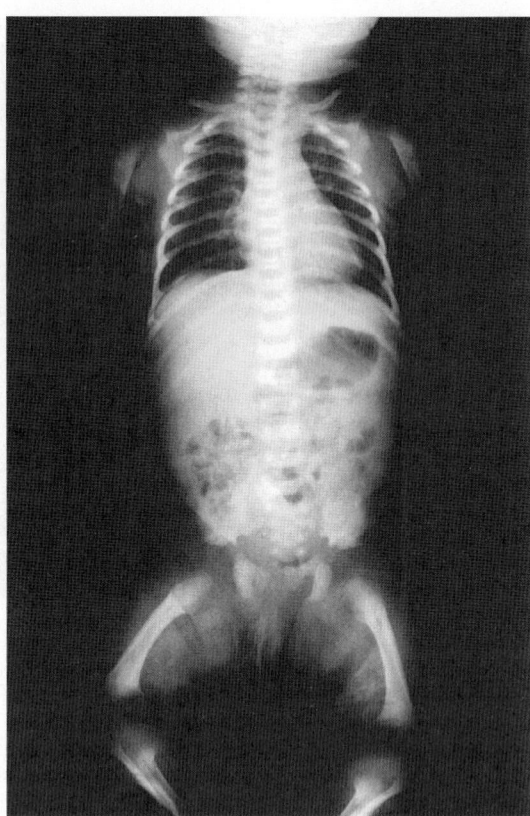

Figure 696-4 Radiograph of infant with achondroplasia, demonstrating interpedicular narrowing of the 1st through 5th lumbar vertebrae, short round iliac bones, and flat acetabular roofs. The tubular bones are short and show mild irregularities of the metaphyses.

marry. Such couples have a 50% risk of transmitting their condition, heterozygous achondroplasia, to each offspring, as well as a 25% risk of **homozygous achondroplasia**. The latter condition exhibits intermediate severity between TD and heterozygous achondroplasia and is usually lethal in the newborn period. Prenatal diagnosis is available and has been used to diagnose homozygous achondroplasia. Preimplantation genetic testing can be used to identify double dominant mutations.

Hypochondroplasia

Hypochondroplasia (MIM 146000) resembles achondroplasia but is milder. Usually, it is not apparent until childhood, when mild short stature affecting the limbs becomes evident. Children have a stocky build and slight frontal bossing of the head. Learning disabilities may be more common in this condition. Radiographic changes are mild and consistent with the mild achondroplastic phenotype. Complica-

tions are rare; in some patients the condition is never diagnosed. Adult heights range from 116-146 cm. An *FGFR3* mutation at codon 540 has been found in many patients with hypochondroplasia. Genetic heterogeneity exists in hypochondroplasia; that is, *SHOX* mutations are associated with a very similar clinical phenotype. Recombinant growth hormone therapy may enhance growth and improve body disproportion.

JANSEN METAPHYSEAL DYSPLASIA

Jansen metaphyseal chondrodysplasia (MIM 156400) is a rare, dominantly inherited chondrodysplasia characterized by severe shortening of limbs associated with an unusual facial appearance. Sometimes it is accompanied by clubfoot and hypercalcemia. At birth, a diagnosis can be made from these clinical findings and radiographs that show short tubular bones with characteristic metaphyseal abnormalities that include flaring, irregular mineralization, fragmentation, and widening of the physeal space. The epiphyses are normal.

The joints become enlarged and limited in mobility with age. Flexion contractures develop at the knees and hips, producing a bent-over posture. Intelligence is normal, although there may be hearing loss.

Jansen metaphyseal chondrodysplasia is caused by activating mutations of *PTHR1*. This G-protein–coupled transmembrane receptor serves as a receptor for both parathyroid hormone and parathyroid hormone-related peptide. Signaling through this receptor serves as a brake on the terminal differentiation of cartilage cells at a critical step in bone growth. Because the mutations activate the receptor, they enhance the braking effect and thereby slow bone growth. Loss-of-function mutations of *PTHR1* are observed in Blomstrand chondrodysplasia, whose clinical features are the mirror image of Jansen metaphyseal chondrodysplasia.

Bibliography is available at Expert Consult.

Chapter **697**
Disorders Involving Ion Transporters
William A. Horton and Jacqueline T. Hecht

The disorders involving ion transporters result from the functional loss of the sulfate ion transporter called *diastrophic dysplasia sulfate transporter* (DTDST), which is also referred to as *SLC26A2* (solute carrier family 26, member 2). This protein transports sulfate ions into cells and is important for cartilage cells that add sulfate moieties to newly synthesized proteoglycans destined for cartilage extracellular matrix. Matrix proteoglycans are responsible for many of the properties of cartilage that allow it to serve as a template for skeletal development. The clinical manifestations result from defective sulfation of cartilage proteoglycans. In order of decreasing severity, the disorders include: achondrogenesis type 1B, atelosteogenesis type II, diastrophic dysplasia, and a rare recessive form of multiple epiphyseal dysplasia (MIM 226900).

A number of mutant alleles have been found for the *DTDST* gene; they variably disturb transporter function. The disorders are recessive traits requiring the presence of 2 mutant alleles. The phenotype is determined by the combination of mutant alleles; some alleles are present in more than one disorder.

DIASTROPHIC DYSPLASIA

Diastrophic dysplasia (MIM 22600) is a well-characterized disorder recognized at birth by the presence of very short extremities, clubfoot, and short hands, with proximal displacement of the thumb producing a hitchhiker appearance (Fig. 697-1). The hands are usually deviated in an ulnar direction. Bony fusion of the metacarpophalangeal joints (symphalangism) is common, as is restricted movement of many joints, including hips, knees, and elbows. The external ears often become inflamed soon after birth. The inflammation resolves spontaneously but leaves the ears fibrotic and contracted (cauliflower ear deformity). Many newborns have a cleft palate.

Radiographs reveal short and broad tubular bones with flared metaphyses and flat, irregular epiphyses (Fig. 697-2). The capital femoral epiphyses are hypoplastic, and the femoral heads are broad. The ulnas and fibulas are disproportionately short. Carpal centers may be developmentally advanced; the 1st metacarpal is typically ovoid, and the metatarsals are twisted medially. There may be vertebral abnormalities, including clefts of cervical vertebral lamina and narrowing of the interpedicular distances in the lumbar spine.

Complications are primarily orthopedic and tend to be severe and progressive. The clubfoot deformity in the newborn resists usual treatments, and multiple corrective surgeries are common. Scoliosis typically develops during early childhood. It often requires multiple surgical procedures to control, and it sometimes compromises respiratory function in older children. Despite the orthopedic problems, patients typically have a normal life span and reach adult heights in the 105-130 cm range, depending on the severity of scoliosis. Growth curves are available for diastrophic dysplasia.

Some patients are mildly affected and exhibit slight short stature and joint contractures, no clubfoot or cleft palate, and correspondingly mild radiographic changes. The mild phenotype tends to recur within families. The recurrence risk of this autosomal recessive condition is 25%. Ultrasonographic examination can be employed for prenatal diagnosis, but if *DTDST* mutations can be identified in the patients or parents, molecular genetic diagnosis is possible.

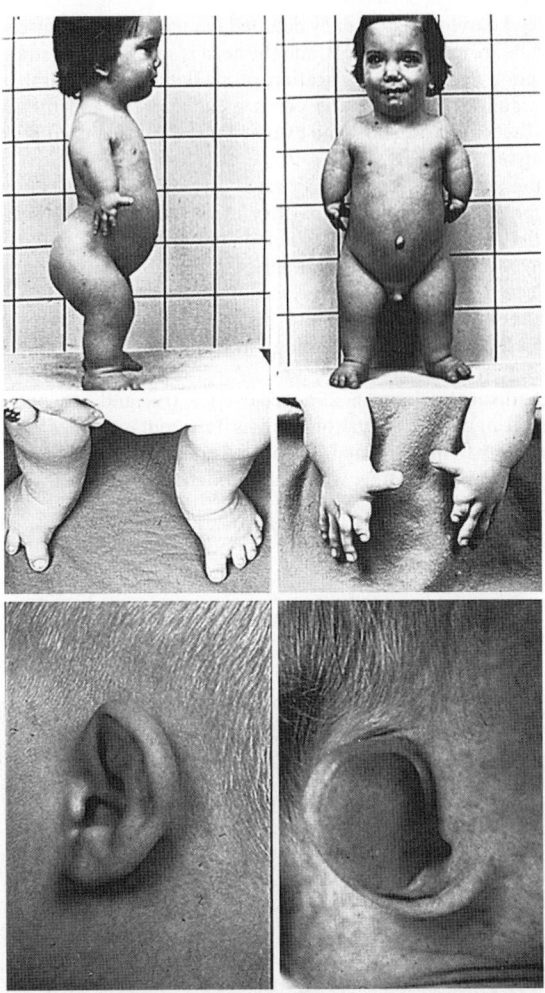

Figure 697-1 Child with diastrophic dysplasia. The extremities are dramatically shortened *(top)*. Clubfoot is commonly observed *(middle left)*. The fingers are short, especially the index finger; the thumb characteristically is proximally placed and has a hitchhiker appearance *(middle right)*. The upper helix of the ears becomes swollen 3-4 wk postnatally *(lower left)*, and this inflammation spontaneously resolves, leaving a cauliflower deformity of the pinnae *(lower right)*.

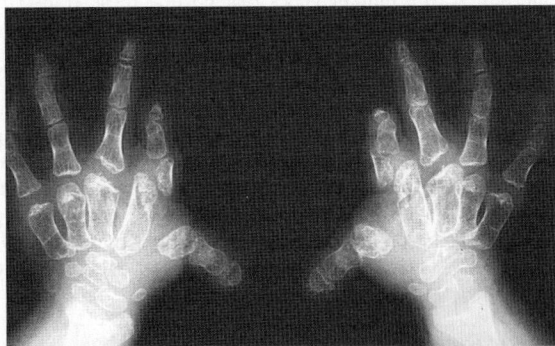

Figure 697-2 Radiograph of hands in diastrophic dysplasia. The metacarpals and phalanges are irregular and short. The 1st metacarpal is ovoid.

ACHONDROGENESIS TYPE 1B AND ATELOSTEOGENESIS TYPE II

Achondrogenesis type 1B (MIM 600972) and atelosteogenesis type II (MIM 256050) are rare recessive lethal chondrodysplasias. The most serious is achondrogenesis type 1B, which demonstrates a severe lack of skeletal development usually detected in utero or after a miscarriage. The limbs are extremely short, and the head is soft. Skeletal radiographs show poor to missing ossification of skull bones, vertebral bodies, fibulas, and ankle bones. The pelvis is hypoplastic, and the ribs are short. The femurs are short and exhibit a trapezoid shape with irregular metaphyses.

Infants with atelosteogenesis type II are stillborn or die soon after birth; prematurity is common. They exhibit very short limbs, especially the proximal segments. Clubfoot and dislocations of the elbows and knees may be detected. Hypoplasia of vertebral bodies, especially in the cervical and lumbar spine, is found on radiographs. The femora and humeri are hypoplastic and display a club-shaped appearance. The distal limb bones, including the ulna and fibula, are poorly ossified.

Both disorders carry a 25% recurrence risk and are potentially detectable in utero by mutation analysis if the mutant alleles are identified in the parents. Prenatal diagnosis is possible with fetal imaging and/or mutational testing, which is commercially available.

Bibliography is available at Expert Consult.

Chapter **698**
Disorders Involving Transcription Factors

William A. Horton and Jacqueline T. Hecht

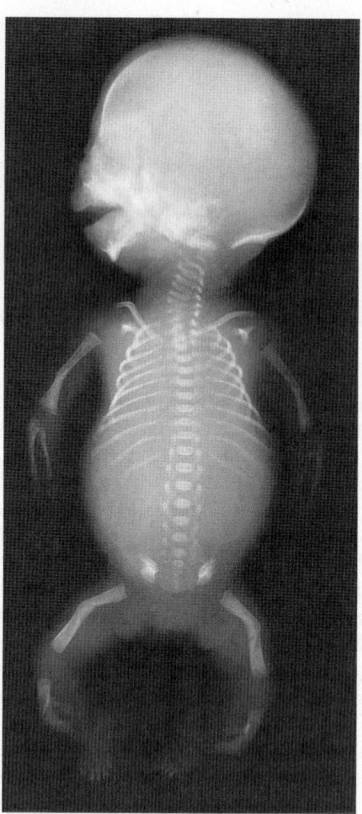

Figure 698-1 A fetus of 21 weeks' gestation with campomelic dysplasia. Radiographic findings include a large skull with a small face; hypoplastic/absent scapular bodies; 11 ribs; poorly ossified thoracic pedicles; tall, narrow iliac wings; and short extremities with proportionately long, bowed femurs. *(From Dwek J, Lachman R: Skeletal dysplasias and selected chromosomal disorders. In Coley BD, editor: Caffey's pediatric diagnostic imaging, ed 12, Philadelphia, 2013, WB Saunders, Fig. 133-34.)*

There are 3 well-delineated disorders involving transcription factors that result in bone dysplasias. **Campomelic dysplasia** is historically considered a chondrodysplasia while **cleidocranial dysplasia** and **nail-patella syndrome**, have been regarded as dysostoses, or abnormalities of single bones. The mutant genes that encode these transcription factors, *SOX9*, *RUNX2 (CBFA1)*, and *LMX1B*, respectively, are members of much larger gene families. *SOX9* is a member of the *SOX* family of genes related to the *SRY* (sex-determining region of the Y chromosome) gene; *RUNX2 (CBFA1)* belongs to the runt family of transcription factor genes, and *LMX1B* is one of the LIM homeodomain gene family. All 3 disorders are a result of haploinsufficiency of the respective gene products; the disorders are dominant traits. For familial cases of cleidocranial dysplasia and nail-patella syndrome, prenatal diagnosis is possible if the mutations are identified. Campomelic dysplasia results from new mutational events and has a low risk of recurrence in subsequent pregnancies.

CAMPOMELIC DYSPLASIA
Campomelic dysplasia (MIM 114290) is apparent at birth owing to bowing of long bones (especially in the lower legs), short bones, respiratory distress, and other anomalies that include defects of the cervical spine, central nervous system, heart, and kidneys. In some cases, femoral bowing is minimal (acampomelic campomelic dysplasia). Cases of sex reversal of XY males have been reported; 75% of those with a male karyotype have partial or complete sex reversal. Radiographs confirm the bowing and often show hypoplasia of the scapulae and pelvic bones (Fig. 698-1). Affected infants usually die of respira-

tory distress in the neonatal period. Complications in children and adolescents who survive include short stature with progressive kyphoscoliosis, hip dislocation, recurrent apnea and respiratory infections, and mild to moderate learning difficulties. Mutational testing is commercially available.

CLEIDOCRANIAL DYSPLASIA
Cleidocranial dysplasia (MIM 114290) is recognized in infants because of drooping shoulders, open fontanelles, prominent forehead, mild short stature, and dental abnormalities (Fig. 698-2). Radiographs reveal hypoplastic or absent clavicles, delayed ossification of the cranial bones with multiple ossification centers (wormian bones), and delayed ossification of pelvic bones. The course is usually uncomplicated except for dislocations, especially of the shoulders, and dental anomalies (numerous teeth) that require therapy.

NAIL-PATELLA SYNDROME
Dysplasia of the nails, absence or hypoplasia of the patella, abnormalities of the elbow, and spurs or "horns" extending from the iliac bones characterize the nail-patella syndrome (MIM 119600), which is also called *osteo-onychodysostosis*. Some patients have nephritis that resembles chronic glomerulonephritis. There is a wide spectrum of severity; some patients present in early childhood, whereas others are asymptomatic as adults.

Bibliography is available at Expert Consult.

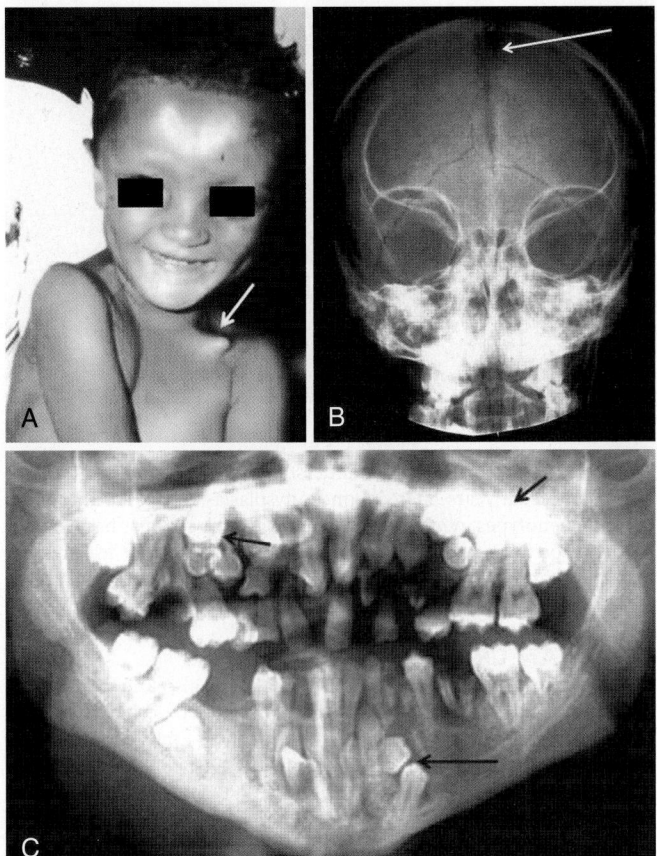

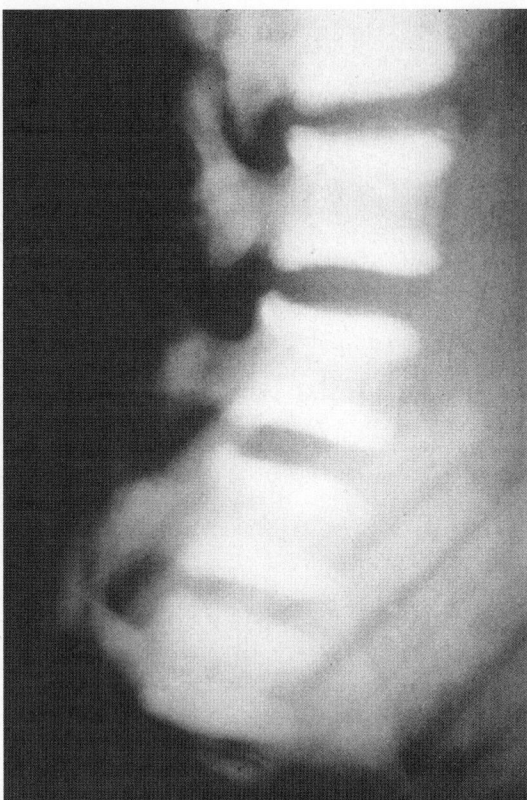

Figure 699-1 Lateral radiograph showing bone-in-bone appearance that is characteristic of osteopetrosis.

Figure 698-2 Features of cleidocranial dysplasia displayed. **A,** The forehead is bulky with a central depression, the eyes are widely spaced and the jaw is pointed. The clavicle is misshapen *(arrow).* **B,** Note patency of the anterior fontanelle. **C,** Hyperdontia pantomogram of an affected male showing supernumerary teeth. *(From Roberts T, Stephen L, Beighton P. Cleidocranial dysplasia: a review of the dental, historical, and practical implications with an overview of the South African experience. Oral Surg Oral Med Oral Pathol Oral Radiol 115(1):46–55, 2013, Figs. 1, 4, and 6.)*

Chapter **699**
Disorders Involving Defective Bone Resorption

William A. Horton and Jacqueline T. Hecht

Osteopetrosis, which has many subtypes, and pyknodysostosis result from defective bone resorption. Overall, bone dysplasias displaying increased bone density are rare.

OSTEOPETROSIS

Two main forms of osteopetrosis have been delineated: a severe autosomal recessive form (MIM 259700) with an incidence of approximately 1 in 250,000 births and a mild autosomal dominant form (MIM 166600) with an incidence of approximately 1 in 20,000 births. Intrinsic disturbances of osteoclast function due to mutations in genes encoding osteoclast-specific subunits of the vacuolar proton pump (*TCIRG1, CLCN7*) are found in most patients with the recessive form. Mutations of *CLCN7* are observed in the dominant form of osteopetrosis. Both types of mutations lead to disturbances of acidification needed for normal osteoclast function. Rarely, patients lack bioactive RANKL (receptor activator of nuclear factor kappa B ligand), the master osteoclastogenic cytokine produced mainly by osteoblasts.

The severe form is usually detected in infancy or earlier because of macrocephaly, hepatosplenomegaly, deafness, blindness, and severe anemia. Radiographs reveal diffuse bone sclerosis and low serum calcium and phosphorus levels with elevated parathyroid hormone levels and normal vitamin D levels. may be detected. Later films show the characteristic bone-within-bone appearance (Fig. 699-1). With time, infants typically fail to thrive and show psychomotor delay and worsening of cranial neuropathies and anemia. Dental problems, osteomyelitis of the mandible, and pathologic fractures are common. Untreated, the most severely affected patients die during infancy; less severely affected patients rarely survive beyond the 2nd decade. Those who survive beyond infancy usually have learning disorders but might have normal intelligence despite hearing and vision loss.

Clinical Manifestations

Most of the manifestations are from failure to remodel growing bones. This leads to narrowing of cranial nerve foramina and encroachment on marrow spaces, which results in secondary complications, such as optic and facial nerve dysfunction, and anemia accompanied by compensatory extramedullary hematopoiesis in the liver and spleen. The unusually dense bones are weak, leading to increased risk of fractures.

The autosomal dominant form of osteopetrosis (Albers-Schönberg disease, osteopetrosis tarda, or marble bone disease) usually manifests during childhood or adolescence with fractures and mild anemia and, less often, as cranial nerve dysfunction, dental abnormalities, or osteomyelitis of the mandible. Skeletal radiographs reveal a generalized

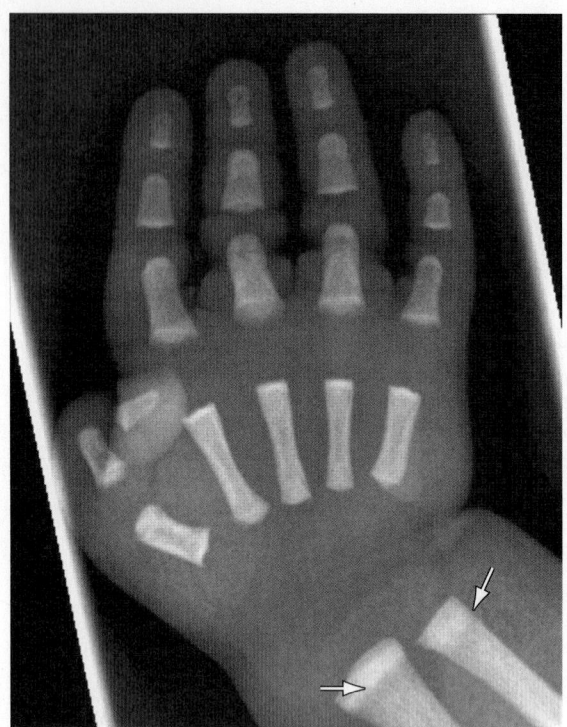

Figure 699-2 Right-hand radiograph of infant age 2 wk. Note metaphyseal lucent bands in the distal ulna and radius *(arrows)* and short tubular bones. *(From Stark Z, Savarirayan R: Osteopetrosis, Orphanet J Rare Dis 4:5, 2009.)*

increase in bone density and clubbing of metaphyses. Alternating bands of lucent and dense bands produce a sandwich appearance to vertebral bodies. The radiographic changes are sometimes incidental findings in otherwise asymptomatic adolescents and adults.

Treatment
Most of the bone manifestations in severe osteopetrosis caused by intrinsic osteoclast defects can be prevented or reversed by hematopoietic stem cell transplantation, if carried out before development of irreversible secondary complications, such as visual impairment. RANKL replacement therapy may be useful in patients with RANKL deficiency. Calcitriol and interferon-γ have also been used with equivocal results. Symptomatic care, such as dental care, transfusions for anemia, and antibiotic treatment of infections, is important for patients who survive infancy.

PYKNODYSOSTOSIS
An autosomal recessive bone dysplasia, pyknodysostosis (MIM 265800) manifests in early childhood with short limbs, characteristic facies, an open anterior fontanel, a large skull with frontal and occipital bossing, and dental abnormalities. The hands and feet are short and broad, and the nails may be dysplastic. The sclerae may be blue. Minimal trauma often leads to fractures. Treatment is symptomatic and focused mainly on the management of dental problems and fractures. The prognosis is generally good, and patients typically reach heights of 130-150 cm.

Skeletal radiographs show a generalized increase in bone density. In contrast to many disorders in this group, the metaphyses are normal. Other changes include wide sutures and wormian bones in the skull, a small mandible, and hypoplasia of the distal phalanges (Fig. 699-2).

Several mutations have been found in the gene encoding cathepsin K, a cysteine protease that is highly expressed in osteoclasts. The mutations predict loss of enzyme function, suggesting that there is an inability of osteoclasts to degrade bone matrix and remodel bones.

Bibliography is available at Expert Consult.

Chapter **700**
Disorders for Which Defects Are Poorly Understood or Unknown
William A. Horton and Jacqueline T. Hecht

Despite great advances in our understanding of the genetic basis of disease in recent years, many chondrodysplasias, or chondrodysplasia clinical phenotypes, remain for which the genetic cause or basic mechanism is poorly understood or not known. Many illustrate features not found in other disorders and have historical significance in the evolution of chondrodysplasia nomenclature and classification.

ELLIS–VAN CREVELD SYNDROME
The Ellis-van Creveld syndrome (MIM 225500), also known as **chondroectodermal dysplasia**, is a skeletal and an ectodermal dysplasia. The skeletal dysplasia presents at birth with short limbs, especially the middle and distal segments, accompanied by postaxial polydactyly of the hands and sometimes of the feet (Fig. 700-1). Nail dysplasia and dental anomalies (including neonatal, absent, and premature loss of teeth and upper lip defects) constitute the ectodermal dysplasia. Common manifestations also include atrial septal defects and other congenital heart defects.

Skeletal radiographs reveal short tubular bones with clubbed ends, especially the proximal tibia and ulna (Fig. 700-2). Carpal bones display extra ossification centers and fusion; cone-shaped epiphyses are evident in the hands. A bony spur is often noted above the medial aspect of the acetabulum.

Ellis-van Creveld syndrome is an autosomal recessive trait that occurs most often in the Amish. Mutations have been identified in 1 of 2 genes, *EVC (EVC1)* or *EVC2*, which map in a head-to-head configuration to chromosome 4p. Mutations of *EVC2* are detected in the allelic condition Weyers acrofacial dysostosis. EVC and EVC2 proteins are thought to influence hedgehog signaling in cilia.

Approximately 30% of patients die of cardiac or respiratory problems during infancy. Life span is otherwise normal; adult heights range from 119-161 cm.

ASPHYXIATING THORACIC DYSTROPHY
(see also Chapter 417.3)
Asphyxiating thoracic dystrophy (MIM 208500), or **Jeune syndrome**, is an autosomal recessive chondrodysplasia that resembles Ellis-van Creveld syndrome. Newborn infants present with a long, narrow thorax and respiratory insufficiency associated with pulmonary hypoplasia. Neonates often die. Other neonatal manifestations include slightly short limbs and postaxial polydactyly. This condition results from a disturbance of primary cilia, most often from mutations of the gene encoding cytoplasmic dynein 2 heavy chain 1 (*DYNC2H1*).

Skeletal radiographs show very short ribs with anterior expansion. Tubular limb bones are short with bulbous ends; cone-shaped epiphyses occur in hand bones. The iliac bones are short and square with a spur above the medial aspect of the acetabulum.

If infants survive the neonatal period, respiratory function usually improves as the rib cage grows. Surgery that produces lateral thoracic expansion improves rib growth and enhances chest wall dimensions. Progressive renal dysfunction often develops during childhood. Intestinal malabsorption and hepatic dysfunction have also been reported.

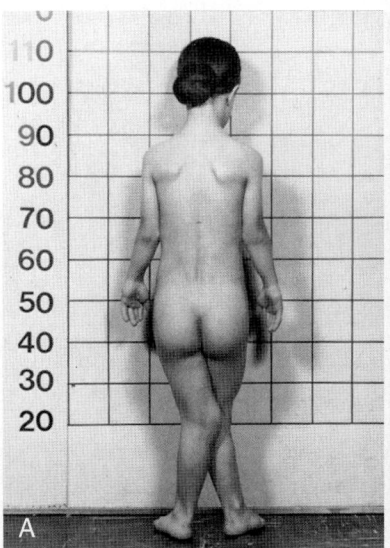
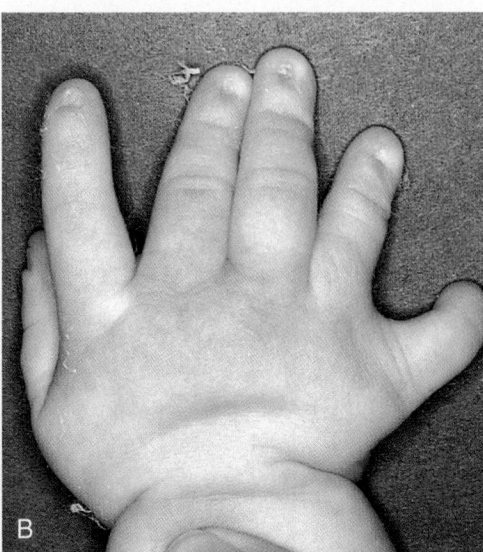

Figure 700-1 A, Ellis-van Creveld syndrome in a young woman. Note short stature, joint contractures at the elbows, and marked genu valgum. **B,** Multiple digits (polydactyly) in a different patient with Ellis-van Creveld syndrome. (**A** *from Zipes DP, Libby P, Bonow R, Braunwald E, editors: Braunwald's heart disease: a textbook of cardiovascular medicine, ed 7, Philadelphia, 2004, WB Saunders, Fig 70-6;* **B** *from Beerman LB, Kreutzer J, Allada V: Cardiology. In Zitelli BJ, McIntire SC, Nowalk AJ, editors: Zitelli and Davis' atlas of pediatric physical diagnosis, ed 6, Philadelphia, 2012, Elsevier, Fig 5-6.)*

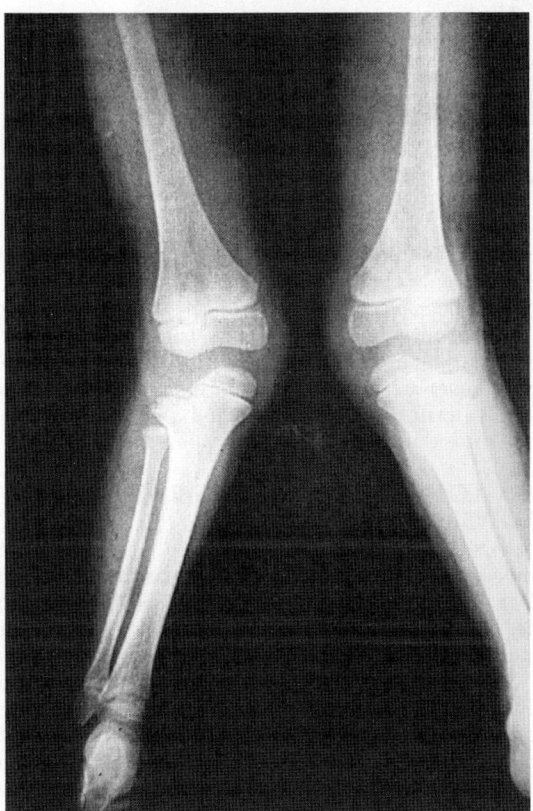
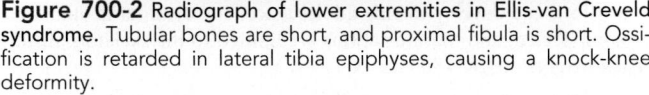

Figure 700-2 Radiograph of lower extremities in Ellis-van Creveld syndrome. Tubular bones are short, and proximal fibula is short. Ossification is retarded in lateral tibia epiphyses, causing a knock-knee deformity.

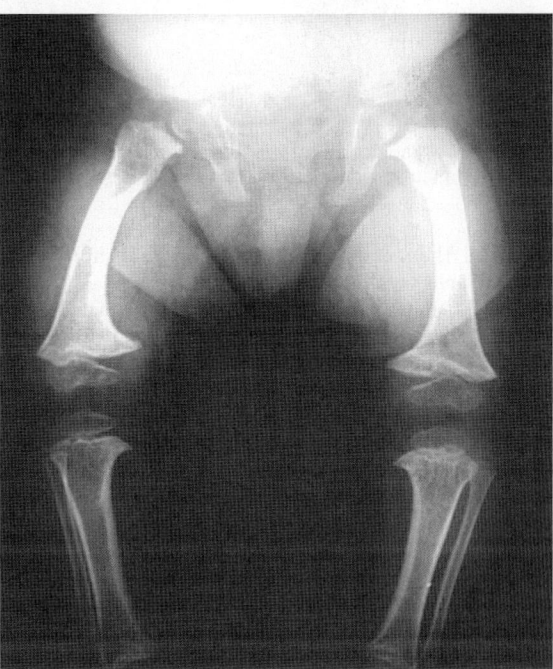

Figure 700-3 Radiograph of lower extremities in cartilage-hair hypoplasia. The tubular bones are short and the metaphyses are flared and irregular. The fibula is disproportionately long compared with the tibia. The femoral necks are short.

SHORT-RIB POLYDACTYLY SYNDROMES

These conditions, which share the clinical features of constricted thoracic cage, short ribs, polydactyly, very short extremities, lethality during the newborn period and autosomal recessive inheritance, were originally grouped into 4 syndromes (SRP-I-IV). However, this classification is in flux as mutations that map to cilia-related genes *IFT80* and *DYNCH2H1* similar to those observed in Jeune syndrome have been detected in infants with SRP II and III. Mutations of two other cilia-related genes *NEK1* and *WDR34* have also been found in this group of disorders.

CARTILAGE-HAIR HYPOPLASIA

Cartilage-hair hypoplasia (CHH; MIM 250250) is also known as **metaphyseal chondrodysplasia–McKusick type**. It is recognized during the 2nd yr because of growth deficiency affecting the limbs, accompanied by flaring of the lower rib cage, a prominent sternum, and bowing of the legs. The hands and feet are short, and the fingers are very short with extreme ligamentous laxity. The hair is thin, sparse, and light colored, and nails are hypoplastic. The skin is hypopigmented.

Radiographs show short tubular bones with flared, irregularly mineralized, and cupped metaphyses (Fig. 700-3). The knees are more affected than are the hips, and the fibula is disproportionately longer

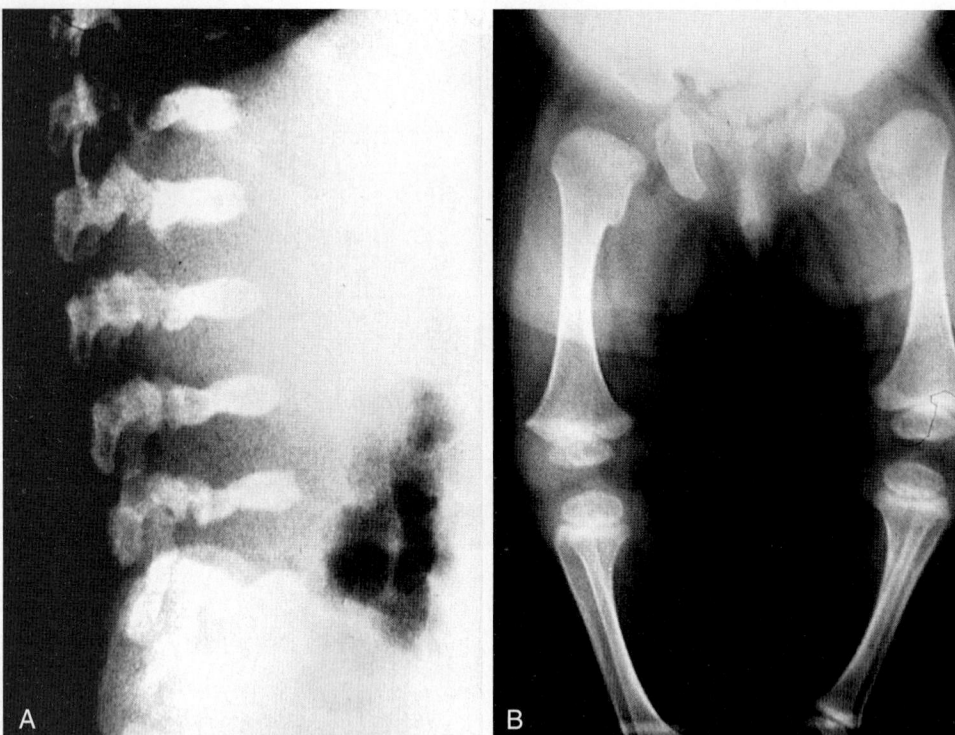

Figure 700-4 A, Radiograph of the lateral thoracolumbar spine in metatropic dysplasia showing severe platyspondyly. **B,** Radiograph of lower extremities in metatropic dysplasia showing short tubular bones with widened metaphyses. The femurs have a dumbbell appearance.

than the tibia. The metacarpals and phalanges are short and broad. Spinal radiographs reveal mild platyspondyly.

Nonskeletal manifestations associated with CHH include immunodeficiency (T-cell abnormalities, neutropenia, leukopenia, and susceptibility to chickenpox; children also may have complications from smallpox and polio vaccinations), malabsorption, celiac disease, and Hirschsprung disease. Adults are at risk for malignancy, especially non-Hodgkin lymphoma and skin tumors. Adults reach heights of 107-157 cm.

CHH shows autosomal recessive inheritance. Its highest prevalence is in the Amish and Finnish populations. It results from mutations of a gene coding for a large untranslated RNA component of an enzyme complex involved in processing mitochondrial RNA. Loss of this gene product interferes with processing of both messenger RNA and ribosomal RNA. Loss of ribosomal RNA processing correlates with the extent of bone dysplasia, whereas loss of messenger RNA processing correlates with degree of hair hypoplasia, immunodeficiency, and hematologic abnormality. Mutations of the RNA component of mitochondrial RNA processing are occasionally detected in patients with mild metaphyseal dysplasia lacking the extraskeletal features characteristic of CHH. Prenatal diagnosis is available if the mutation is identified either in the patient or parents.

METATROPIC DYSPLASIA

Metatropic dysplasia (MIM 156530) is an autosomal dominant disorder resulting from heterozygous mutations of *TRPV4* (transient receptor potential vanilloid family 4), which encodes a calcium-permeable cation channel. Newborn infants present with a long narrow trunk and short extremities. A tail-like appendage sometimes extends from the base of the spine. Odontoid hypoplasia is common and may be associated with cervical instability. Kyphoscoliosis appears in late infancy and progresses through childhood, often becoming severe enough to compromise cardiopulmonary function. The joints are large and become progressively restricted in mobility, except in the hands. Contractures often develop in the hips and knees during childhood. Although severely affected infants can die at a young age from respiratory failure, patients usually survive, although they can become

disabled as adults from the progressive musculoskeletal deformities. Adult heights range from 110-120 cm.

Skeletal radiographs show characteristic changes dominated by severe platyspondyly and short tubular bones with expanded and deformed metaphyses that exhibit a dumbbell appearance (Fig. 700-4). The pelvic bones are hypoplastic and exhibit a halberd appearance because of a small sacrosciatic notch and a notch above the lateral margin of the acetabulum.

SPONDYLOMETAPHYSEAL DYSPLASIA, KOZLOWSKI TYPE

The Kozlowski type of spondylometaphyseal dysplasia (MIM 184252) is an autosomal dominant allelic disorder to metatropic dysplasia caused by *TRPV4* mutations. Mutations of *TRPV4* have also been identified in autosomal dominant brachyolmia, whose phenotype is dominated by progressive scoliosis and platyspondyly on x-rays.

The Kozlowski type of spondylometaphyseal dysplasia manifests in early childhood with mild short stature involving mostly the trunk and a waddling gait. The hands and feet may be short and stubby. Radiographs show flattening of vertebral bodies. The metaphyses of tubular bones are widened and irregularly mineralized, especially at the proximal femur. The pelvic bones manifest mild hypoplasia.

Scoliosis can develop during adolescence. The disorder is otherwise uncomplicated, and manifestations are limited to the skeleton. Adults reach heights of 130-150 cm.

DISORDERS INVOLVING FILAMINS

Mutations of genes encoding filamin A and filamin B proteins have been detected in diverse disorders of skeletal development: filamin A mutations in otopalatodigital syndromes type 1 and 2 frontometaphyseal dysplasia and Melnick-Needles syndrome (MIM 311300, 304120, 305620, 309350) and filamin B mutations in Larsen syndrome and perinatal lethal atelosteogenesis types I and III and Boomerang dysplasia (MIM 150250, 108720, 108721, 112310). Filamins functionally connect extracellular to intracellular structural proteins, thereby linking cells to their local microenvironment, which is essential for skeletal development and growth.

Table 700-1	Juvenile Osteochondroses	
EPONYM	**AFFECTED REGION**	**AGE AT PRESENTATION**
Legg-Calvé-Perthes disease	Capital femoral epiphysis	3-12 yr
Osgood-Schlatter disease	Tibial tubercle	10-16 yr
Sever disease	Os calcaneus	6-10 yr
Freiberg disease	Head of second metatarsal	10-14 yr
Scheuermann disease	Vertebral bodies	Adolescence
Blount disease	Medial aspect of proximal tibial epiphysis	Infancy or adolescence
Osteochondritis dissecans	Subchondral regions of knee, hip, elbow, and ankle	Adolescence

JUVENILE OSTEOCHONDROSES

The juvenile osteochondroses are a heterogeneous group of disorders in which regional disturbances in bone growth cause noninflammatory arthropathies. Table 700-1 summarizes the juvenile osteochondroses. Some have localized pain and tenderness (Freiberg disease, Osgood-Schlatter disease [see Chapter 677.4], osteochondritis dissecans [see Chapter 677.3]), whereas others present with painless limitation of joint movement (Legg-Calvé-Perthes disease [see Chapter 678.3], Scheuermann disease [see Chapter 679.4]). Bone growth may be disrupted, leading to deformities. The diagnosis is usually confirmed radiographically, and treatment is symptomatic. The pathogenesis of these disorders is believed to involve ischemic necrosis of primary and secondary ossification centers. Although familial forms have been reported, these disorders usually occur sporadically.

CAFFEY DISEASE (INFANTILE CORTICAL HYPEROSTOSIS)

This is a rare disorder of unknown etiology characterized by cortical hyperostosis with inflammation of the contiguous fascia and muscle. It is often sporadic, but both autosomal dominant and autosomal recessive inheritance have been reported. In 3 unrelated families with autosomal dominant inheritance, a linkage to mutations of the *COL1A1* gene (codes for the α_1 chain of type I collagen) has been reported.

Prenatal and more often postnatal onset have been described. Prenatal onset may be mild (autosomal dominant) or severe (autosomal recessive). Severe prenatal disease is characterized by typical bone lesions, polyhydramnios, hydrops fetalis, severe respiratory distress, prematurity, and high mortality. Onset in infancy (younger than 6 mo; average: 10 wk) is most common; manifestations include the sudden onset of irritability, swelling of contiguous soft tissue that precedes the cortical thickening of the underlying bones, fever, and anorexia. The swelling is painful with a wood-like induration but with minimal warmth or redness; suppuration is absent. There are unpredictable remissions and relapses; an episode can last 2 wk to 3 mo. The most common bones involved include the mandible (75%) (Fig. 700-5), the clavicle, and the ulna. If swelling is not prominent or visible, the diagnosis might not be evident.

Laboratory features include elevated erythrocyte sedimentation rate and serum alkaline phosphatase as well as, in some patients, increased serum prostaglandin E levels. There may be thrombocytosis and anemia. The **radiographic features** include soft-tissue swelling and calcification and cortical hyperostosis (Fig. 700-6). All bones may be affected except the phalanges or vertebral bodies. The **differential diagnosis** includes other causes of hyperostosis such as chronic vitamin A intoxication, prolonged prostaglandin E infusion in children with ductal dependent congenital heart disease, primary bone tumors, and scurvy.

Complications are unusual but include pseudoparalysis with limb or scapula involvement, pleural effusions (rib), torticollis (clavicle), mandibular asymmetry, bone fusion (ribs or ulna and radius), and bone angulation deformities (common with severe prenatal onset).

Treatment includes indomethacin and prednisone (if there is a poor response to indomethacin).

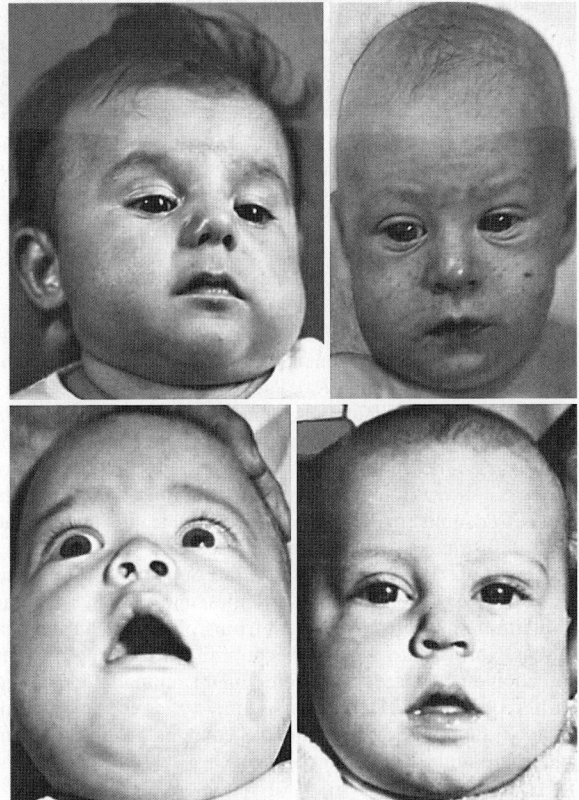

Figure 700-5 Facies in infantile cortical hyperostosis. In almost all cases, the changes have appeared before the 5th mo of life. Unilateral swelling of the left cheek and left side of the jaw in an infant 12 wk of age. *(From Slovis TL:* Caffey's pediatric diagnostic imaging, *ed 11, Philadelphia, 2008, Mosby.)*

FIBRODYSPLASIA OSSIFICANS PROGRESSIVE

Fibrodysplasia ossificans progressive (FOP) (MIM 135100) is a rare and severely disabling disorder characterized by progressive extraskeletal bone formation in soft connective tissues including muscles, tendons, ligaments, fascia, and aponeuroses. With exception of deformity of the large toes, infants are normal at birth. Episodes of painful soft-tissue swelling with inflammation usually begin in early childhood initially involving the upper back and neck and later the entire trunk and extremities. Repeated episodes (flare-ups) slowly transform the soft tissues into bands or plates of bone that span joints and progressively limit movement and mobility. Episodes are often triggered by injury, intramuscular injections and viral infection. Most patients are wheelchair bound by their late teens. The average life span is approximately 40 yr, with death usually resulting from complications of thoracic insufficiency.

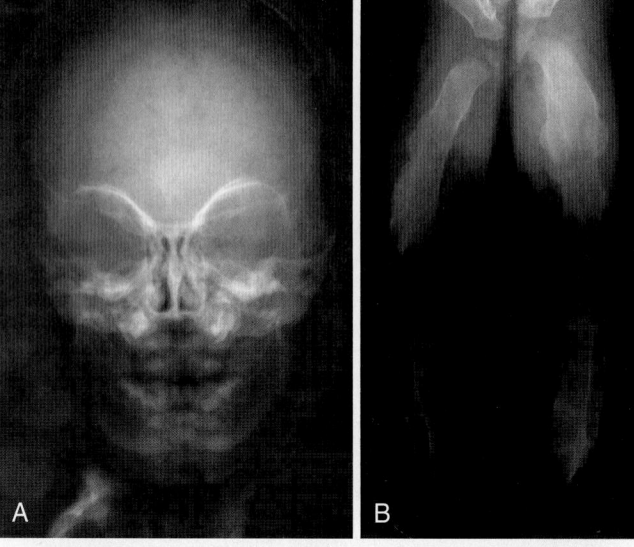

Figure 700-6 A, X-ray of a 5 mo old infant showing hyperostosis of the mandible. **B,** X-ray of a 5 mo old infant shoeing hyperostosis of both legs. *(From Kamoun-Goldrat A, le Merrer M: Infantile cortical hyperostosis (Caffey disease): a review. J Oral Maxillofac Surg 66:2145–2150, 2008, Figs. 1 and 2.)*

FOP results from heterozygous activating mutations of the gene encoding the bone morphogenetic protein (BMP) type I receptor, activin A receptor type I (*ACVR1*). Patients with classic FOP have the same missense *ACVR1* mutation, which enhances BMP signaling, which, in turn, induces inflammation and aberrant endochondral ossification through mechanisms that are poorly understood. Environmental factors such as injury play an important role in triggering these events. *ACVR1* mutations usually occur sporadically, but autosomal dominant transmission has rarely been observed.

There is no definitive treatment for FOP. Supportive care includes avoidance of injury-prone physical activities, intramuscular injections including immunizations and overstretching of the jaw during dental procedures. Corticosteroids and other antiinflammatory agents reduce inflammation during flare-ups. Studies in FOP animal models suggest that BMP type I kinase inhibitors and retinoic acid receptor γ agonists, which block chondrogenesis, the initial step in endochondral ossification, may be useful therapies in the future.

Bibliography is available at Expert Consult.

Chapter **701**
Osteogenesis Imperfecta
Joan C. Marini

Osteoporosis is fragility of the skeletal system and a susceptibility to fractures of the long bones or vertebral compressions from mild or inconsequential trauma. **Osteogenesis imperfecta** (**OI**) (brittle bone disease), the most common genetic cause of osteoporosis, is a generalized disorder of connective tissue. The spectrum of OI is extremely broad, ranging from forms that are lethal in the perinatal period to a mild form in which the diagnosis may be equivocal in an adult.

ETIOLOGY
Structural or quantitative defects in type I collagen cause the full clinical spectrum of OI (types I-IV). Type I collagen is the primary component of the extracellular matrix of bone and skin. Between 10 and 15% of patients clinically indistinguishable from OI do not have a molecular defect in type I collagen (Table 701-1). These cases are caused by defects in genes whose protein products interact with type I collagen. One group of patients has overmodified collagen, with similar biochemical findings to those with collagen structural defects and severe or lethal OI bone dysplasia. These cases are caused by recessive null mutations in any of the 3 components of the collagen prolyl 3-hydroxylation complex, prolyl 3-hydroxylase 1 (coded by the *LEPRE1* gene on chromosome 1p34.1) or its associated protein, CRTAP, or cyclophilin B (CyPB, encoded by *PPIB*). A second set of cases without collagen defects have biochemically normal collagen. Defects in *IFITM5* and *SERPINF1* account for defects in mineralization in types V and VI OI, while mutations in *SERPINH1*, encoding the collagen chaperone HSP47, and *FKBP10*, encoding the peptidyl-prolyl *cis-trans* isomerase FKBP65, cause types X and XI OI, respectively. Rare mutations in *BMP1*, *TMEM38B* and *WNT1* also cause recessive OI; the genetic defect in some individuals is still unknown.

EPIDEMIOLOGY
The autosomal dominant forms of OI occur equally in all racial and ethnic groups, whereas recessive forms occur predominantly in ethnic groups with consanguineous marriages. The West African founder mutation for type VIII OI has a carrier frequency of 1 in 200-300 among African-Americans. The incidence of OI detectable in infancy is approximately 1 in 20,000. There is a similar incidence of the mild form OI type I.

PATHOLOGY
The collagen structural mutations cause OI bone to be globally abnormal. The bone matrix contains abnormal type I collagen fibrils and relatively increased levels of types III and V collagen. Several noncollagenous proteins of bone matrix are also reduced. Bone cells contribute to OI pathology, with abnormal osteoblast differentiation and increased numbers of active bone resorbing osteoclasts. The hydroxyapatite crystals deposited on this matrix are poorly aligned with the long axis of fibrils, and there is paradoxical hypermineralization of bone.

PATHOGENESIS
Type I collagen is a heterotrimer composed of 2 α1(I) chains and 1 α2(I) chain. The chains are synthesized as procollagen molecules with short globular extensions on both ends of the central helical domain. The helical domain is composed of uninterrupted repeats of the sequence Gly-X-Y, where Gly is glycine, X is often proline, and Y is often hydroxyproline. The presence of glycine at every third residue is crucial to helix formation because its small side chain can be accommodated in the interior of the helix. The chains are assembled into trimers at their carboxyl ends; helix formation then proceeds linearly in a carboxyl to amino direction. Concomitant with helix assembly and formation, helical proline and lysine residues are hydroxylated by prolyl 4-hydroxylase and lysyl hydroxylase and some hydroxylysine residues are glycosylated.

Collagen structural defects are predominantly of 2 types: 80% are point mutations causing substitutions of helical glycine residues or crucial residues in the C-propeptide by other amino acids, and 20% are single exon splicing defects. The clinically mild OI type I has a quantitative defect, with null mutations in 1 α1(I) allele leading to a reduced amount of normal collagen.

The glycine substitutions in the 2 α chains have distinct genotype–phenotype relationships. One-third of mutations in the α_1 chain are lethal, and those in α2(I) are predominantly nonlethal. Two lethal regions in α1(I) align with major ligand binding regions of the collagen helix. Lethal mutations in α2(I) occur in 8 regularly spaced clusters along the chain that align with binding regions for matrix proteoglycans in the collagen fibril.

Table 701-1	Osteogenesis Type, Gene Defects, and Phenotypes	
OSTEOGENESIS IMPERFECTA TYPE	**GENE DEFECT**	**PHENOTYPE**
DOMINANT INHERITANCE		
Classical Sillence Types		
I	COL1A1 null allele	Mild, nondeforming
II	COL1A1 or COL1A2	Lethal perinatal
III	COL1A1 or COL1A2	Progressively deforming
IV	COL1A1 or COL1A2	Moderately deforming
COL1-Mutation Negative		
V	IFITM5	Distinct histology
RECESSIVE INHERITANCE		
Mineralization Defect		
VI	SERPINF1	Distinct histology
3-Hydroxylation Defects		
VII	CRTAP	Severe to lethal
VIII	LEPRE1	Severe to lethal
IX	PPIB	Moderate to lethal
Chaperone Defects		
X	SERPINH1	Severe
XI	FKBP10	Progressive deforming, Bruck syndrome 1
C-Propeptide Cleavage Defect		
XII	BMP1	Severe, high bone mass case
UNCLASSIFIED		
Zinc-finger transcription factor defect	SP7	Moderate
Cation channel defect	TMEM38B	Moderate to severe
WNT signaling pathway defect	WNT1	Moderate, progressively deforming

From Marini JC, Blissett AR: New genes in bone development: what's new in osteogenesis imperfecta. J Clin Endocrinol Metab 98:3095–3103, 2013, Table 1, p. 3096.

Classical OI (Sillence types I-IV) is an autosomal dominant disorder, as is type V OI. Some familial recurrences of OI are caused by parental mosaicism for dominant collagen mutations. Recessive OI accounts for 5-7% of new OI in North America. Three recessive types are caused by null mutations in the genes coding for the components of the collagen prolyl 3-hydroxylation complex in the endoplasmic reticulum (*LEPRE1, CRTAP,* or *PPIB*). It is not yet clear whether absence of the complex itself or of the modification is the crucial feature of these types of recessive OI. Other recessive types are caused by null mutations in genes whose products are involved in collagen folding (*SERPINH1, FKBP10*), or mineralization (*SERPINF1*).

CLINICAL MANIFESTATIONS

Classical OI was described with the triad of fragile bones, blue sclerae, and early deafness, although most cases do not have all of these features. The Sillence classification divides OI into 4 types based on clinical and radiographic criteria. Types V and VI were later proposed based on histologic distinctions. Subsequent types VII-XII were based on identification of the molecular defect, followed by clinical description.

Osteogenesis Imperfecta Type I (Mild)
OI type I is sufficiently mild that it is often found in large pedigrees. Many type I families have blue sclerae, recurrent fractures in childhood, and presenile hearing loss (30-60%). Both types I and IV are divided into A and B subtypes, depending on the absence (A) or presence (B) of **dentinogenesis imperfecta**. Other possible connective tissue abnormalities include hyperextensible joints, easy bruising, thin skin, joint laxity, scoliosis, wormian bones, hernia, and mild short stature compared with family members. Fractures result from mild to moderate trauma but decrease after puberty.

Osteogenesis Imperfecta Type II (Perinatal Lethal)
Infants with OI type II may be stillborn or die in the 1st yr of life. Birthweight and length are small for gestational age. There is extreme fragility of the skeleton and other connective tissues. There are multiple intrauterine fractures of long bones, which have a crumpled appearance on radiographs. There are striking micromelia and bowing of extremities; the legs are held abducted at right angles to the body in the frogleg position. Multiple rib fractures create a beaded appearance, and the small thorax contributes to respiratory insufficiency. The skull is large for body size, with enlarged anterior and posterior fontanels. Sclerae are dark blue-gray. The cerebral cortex has multiple neuronal migration and other defects (agyria, gliosis, periventricular leukomalacia).

Osteogenesis Imperfecta Type III (Progressive Deforming)
OI type III is the most severe nonlethal form of OI and results in significant physical disability. Birthweight and length are often low normal. Fractures usually occur in utero. There is relative macrocephaly and triangular facies (Fig. 701-1). Postnatally, fractures occur from inconsequential trauma and heal with deformity. Disorganization of the bone matrix results in a "popcorn" appearance at the metaphyses (Fig. 701-2). The rib cage has flaring at the base, and pectal deformity is frequent. Virtually all type III patients have scoliosis and vertebral compression. Growth falls below the curve by the 1st yr; all type III patients have extreme short stature. Scleral hue ranges from white to blue. Dentinogenesis imperfecta, hearing loss, and kyphoscoliosis may be present or develop over time.

Osteogenesis Imperfecta Type IV (Moderately Severe)
Patients with OI type IV can present at birth with in utero fractures or bowing of lower long bones. They can also present with recurrent fractures after ambulation and have normal to moderate short stature. Most children have moderate bowing even with infrequent fractures. Children with OI type IV require orthopedic and rehabilitation intervention, but they are usually able to attain community ambulation skills. Fracture rates decrease after puberty. Radiographically, they are osteoporotic and have metaphyseal flaring and vertebral compressions. Patients with type IV have moderate short stature. Scleral hue may be blue or white.

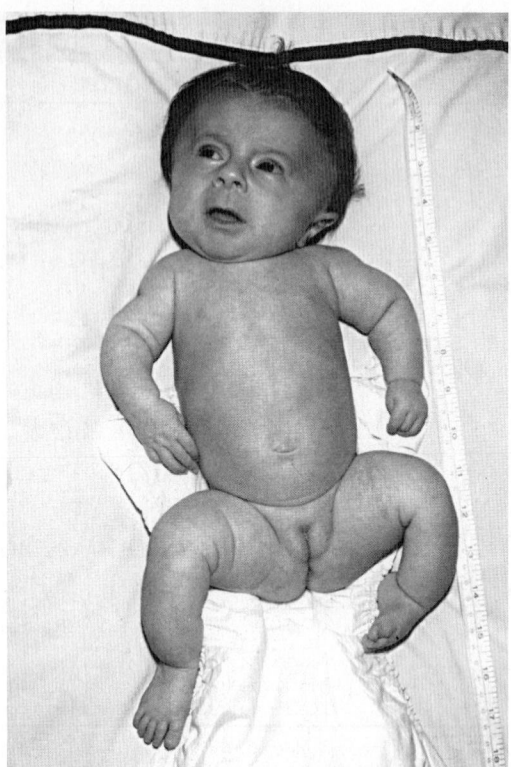

Figure 701-1 Infant with type III osteogenesis imperfecta displays shortened bowed extremities, thoracic deformity, and relative macrocephaly.

Osteogenesis Imperfecta Type V (Hyperplastic Callus) and Type VI Hyperosteoidosis (Mineralization Defect)

Types V and VI OI patients clinically have OI similar in skeletal severity to type IV, but they have distinct findings on bone histology. Type V patients also usually have some combination of hyperplastic callus, calcification of the interosseous membrane of the forearm, and/or a radiodense metaphyseal band. They constitute <5% of OI populations. All type V OI patients are heterozygous for the same mutation in *IFITM5*, which generates a novel start codon for the bone protein Bril. Ligamentous laxity may be present; blue sclera or dentinogenesis imperfect are not present. Patients with type VI OI have progressive deforming OI that does not manifest at birth. They have distinctive bone histology with broad osteoid seams and fish-scale lamellation under polarized light.

Osteogenesis Imperfecta Types VII, VIII, and IX (Autosomal Recessive)

Types VII and VIII patients overlap clinically with types II and III OI but have distinct features including white sclerae, rhizomelia, and small to normal head circumference. Surviving children have severe osteochondrodysplasia with extreme short stature and dual-energy x-ray absorptiometry L1-L2 z-score in the −6 to −7 range. Type IX OI is very rare (only 8 cases reported). The severity is quite broad, ranging from lethal to moderately severe. These children have white sclerae but do not have rhizomelia.

Osteogenesis Imperfecta Types X and XI (Autosomal Recessive)

Only 1 patient with type X OI has been reported; the child had severe OI with white sclerae and died of respiratory causes at age 3 yr. Type XI OI is a more prevalent recessive form with a moderate to severe skeletal phenotype, including white sclerae and normal teeth. Congenital contractures of large joints may occur with the same mutations that cause only skeletal fragility, even in sibships. At the opposite end of the spectrum, a deletion of a single tyrosine residue causes Kuskokwim syndrome, a congenital contracture disorder with very mild vertebral findings and osteopenia.

High Bone Mass Osteogenesis Imperfecta (Cleavage of the Procollagen C-Propeptide)

Autosomal dominant mutations in the C-propeptide cleavage site of procollagen or in the enzyme responsible for its cleavage cause bone fragility with normal or elevated dual-energy x-ray absorptiometry bone density z-scores. Individuals with dominant mutations have normal stature, white sclerae and teeth and mild to moderate OI. Null mutations in *BMP1* lead to a more severe skeletal phenotype with short stature, scoliosis and bone deformity, because *BMP1* has other substrates in addition to type I collagen.

Other Genes for Osteogenesis Imperfecta

A very small percentage of OI patients have bone dysplasia that cannot be accounted for by mutations in the genes described above.

LABORATORY FINDINGS

DNA sequencing is the first diagnostic laboratory test; several diagnostic labs offer panels to test for dominant and recessive OI. Mutation identification is useful to determine the type with certainty and to facilitate family screening and prenatal diagnosis. It is also possible to screen for type VI OI by determination of serum pigment epithelium-derived factor level, which is severely reduced in this type.

If dermal fibroblasts are obtained these can be useful for determining the level of transcripts of the candidate gene and also for collagen biochemical testing, which is positive in most cases of types I-IV and IX OI and all cases of VII/VIII OI. In OI type I, the reduced amount of type I collagen results in an increase in the ratio of type III to type I collagen on gel electrophoresis.

Severe OI can be detected prenatally by level II ultrasonography as early as 16 wk of gestation. OI and thanatophoric dysplasia may be confused. Fetal ultrasonography might not detect OI type IV and rarely detects OI type I. For recurrent cases, chorionic villus biopsy can be used for biochemical or molecular studies. Amniocytes produce false-positive biochemical studies but can be used for molecular studies in appropriate cases.

In the neonatal period, the normal to elevated alkaline phosphatase levels present in OI distinguish it from hypophosphatasia.

COMPLICATIONS

The morbidity and mortality of OI are cardiopulmonary. Recurrent pneumonias and declining pulmonary function occur in childhood, and cor pulmonale is seen in adults.

Neurologic complications include basilar invagination, brainstem compression, hydrocephalus, and syringohydromyelia. Most children with OI types III and IV have basilar invagination, but brainstem compression is uncommon. Basilar invagination is best detected with spiral CT of the craniocervical junction (Fig. 701-3).

TREATMENT

There is no cure for OI. For severe nonlethal OI, active physical rehabilitation in the early years allows children to attain a higher functional level than orthopedic management alone. Children with OI type I and some with type IV are spontaneous ambulators. Children with types III, IV, V, VI, and XI OI benefit from gait aids and a program of swimming and conditioning. Severely affected patients require a wheelchair for community mobility but can acquire transfer and self-care skills. Teens with OI can require psychologic support with body image issues. Growth hormone improves bone histology in growth-responsive children (usually types I and IV).

Orthopedic management of OI is aimed at fracture management and correction of deformity to enable function. Fractures should be promptly splinted or cast; OI fractures heal well, and cast removal should be aimed at minimizing immobilization osteoporosis. Correction of long bone deformity requires an osteotomy procedure and placement of an intramedullary rod.

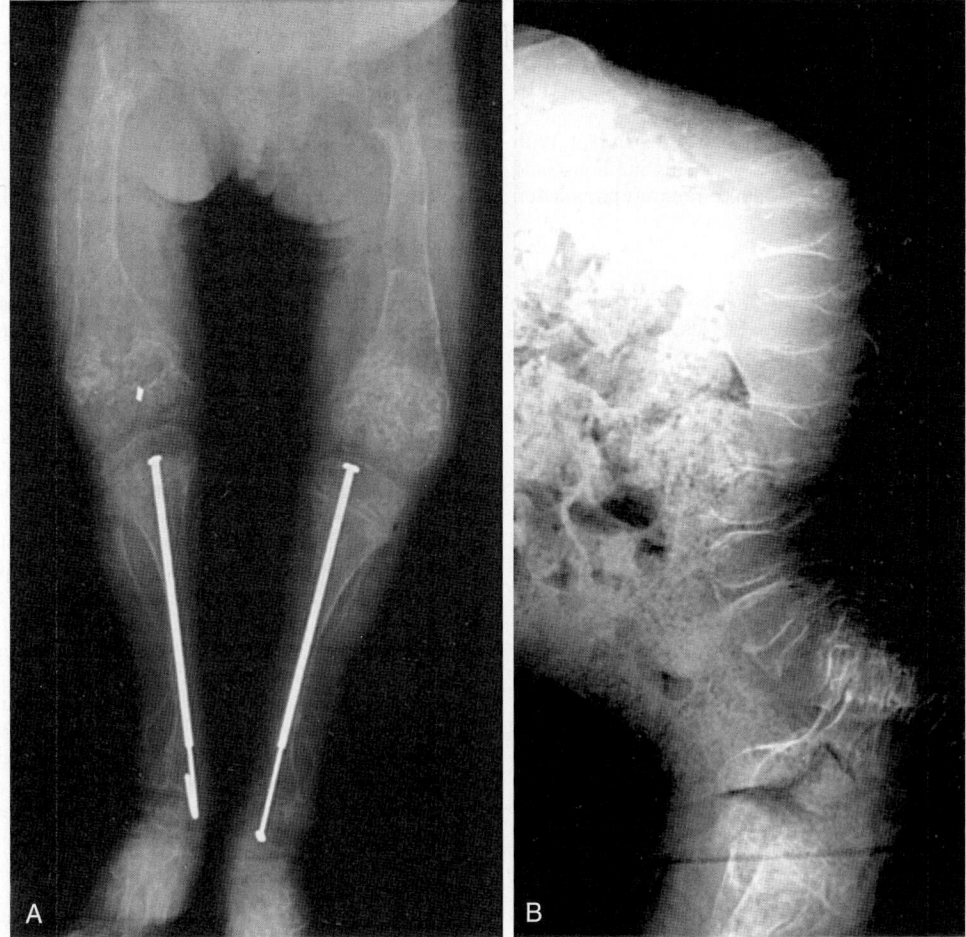

Figure 701-2 Typical features of type III osteogenesis imperfecta radiographs in a 6 yr old child. **A,** Lower long bones are osteoporotic, with metaphyseal flaring, "popcorn" formation at growth plates, and placement of intramedullary rods. **B,** Vertical bodies are compressed and osteoporotic.

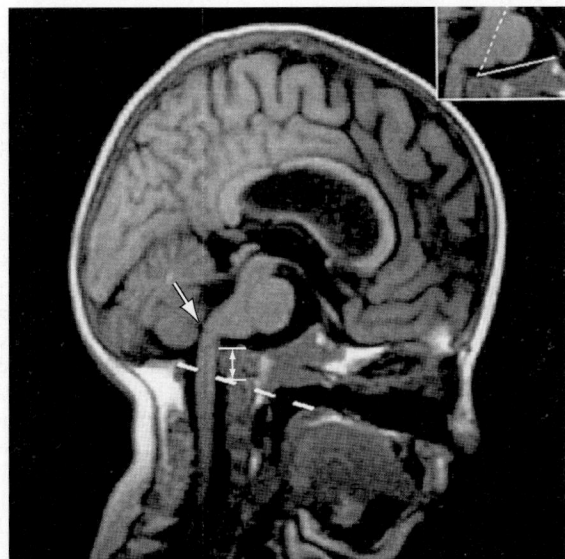

Figure 701-3 Typical feature of basilar invagination shown in the sagittal MRI of an asymptomatic child with type III osteogenesis imperfecta. There is invagination of the odontoid above the Chamberlain line, causing compression and kinking at the pontomedullary junction *(arrow).*

A several-year course of treatment of children with OI with bisphosphonates (IV pamidronate or oral olpadronate or risedronate) confers some benefits. Bisphosphonates decrease bone resorption by osteoclasts; OI patients have increased bone volume that still contains the defective collagen. Bisphosphonates are more beneficial for vertebrae (trabecular bone) than long bones (cortical bone). Treatment for 1-2 yr results in increased L1-4 dual-energy x-ray absorptiometry and, more importantly, improved vertebral compressions and area, which can prevent or delay the scoliosis of OI. Relative risk of long bone fractures is modestly decreased. However, the material properties of long bones are weakened by prolonged treatment and nonunion after osteotomy is increased. There is no effect of bisphosphonates on mobility scores, muscle strength, or bone pain. Limiting treatment duration to 2-3 yr in mid-childhood can maximize benefits and minimize detriment to cortical material properties. Benefits appear to persist several years after the treatment interval. Side effects include abnormal long bone remodeling, increased incidence of fracture nonunion, and osteopetrotic-like brittleness to bone.

PROGNOSIS

OI is a chronic condition that limits both life span and functional level. Infants with OI type II usually die within months to a year of life. An occasional child with radiographic type II and extreme growth deficiency survives to the teen years. Persons with OI type III have a reduced life span with clusters of mortality from pulmonary causes in early childhood, the teen years, and the 40s. OI types I, IV, and V OI are compatible with a full life span. The oldest reported individuals with type VIII are in their 3rd decade, and some with type XI are in their 4th decade. The long-term prognosis for most recessive types is still emerging, and many adults with OI have not had molecular testing.

Individuals with OI type III are usually wheelchair dependent. With aggressive rehabilitation, they can attain transfer skills and household ambulation. OI type IV children usually attain community ambulation skills either independently or with gait aids.

GENETIC COUNSELING

For autosomal dominant OI, the risk of an affected individual passing the gene to the individual's offspring is 50%. An affected child usually has about the same severity of OI as the parent; however, there is variability of expression, and the child's condition can be either more or less severe than that of the parent. The empirical recurrence risk to an apparently unaffected couple of having a second child with OI is 5-7%; this is the statistical chance that 1 parent has germline mosaicism. The collagen mutation in the mosaic parent is present in some germ cells and may be present in somatic tissues. If a parent is a mosaic carrier, the risk of recurrence may be as high as 50%.

For recessive OI, the recurrence risk is 25% per pregnancy. No known individual with severe nonlethal recessive OI has had a child.

Bibliography is available at Expert Consult.

Chapter **702**
Marfan Syndrome

Alexander Doyle, Jefferson J. Doyle, and Harry C. Dietz III

Marfan syndrome (MFS) is an inherited, systemic, connective tissue disorder caused by mutations in the gene encoding the *extracellular matrix* (ECM) protein fibrillin-1. It is primarily associated with skeletal, cardiovascular, and ocular pathology. The diagnosis is based on clinical findings, some of which are age dependent.

EPIDEMIOLOGY

The incidence is reported to be 1 in 10,000 live births and approximately one-fourth of cases are sporadic. The disorder shows autosomal dominant inheritance, with high penetrance, but variable expression; both interfamilial and intrafamilial clinical variation is common. There is no racial or gender preference.

PATHOGENESIS

MFS is associated with abnormal production, matrix deposition and/or stability of fibrillin-1, a 350-kDa ECM protein that is the major constituent of microfibrils, with prominent disruption of microfibrils and elastic fibers in diseased tissues. The *fibrillin-1 (FBN1)* locus resides on the long arm of chromosome 15 (15q21), and the gene is composed of 65 exons. Linkage analysis suggests an absence of locus heterogeneity and the involvement of *FBN1* has been demonstrated in >90% of cases, with more than 1,000 disease-causing mutations identified to date (the majority of which are missense point mutations and unique to a given family). With the exception of an early onset and severe presentations of the disease associated with some mutations in exons 26-27 and 31-32, no clear genotype–phenotype correlation has been identified. Given that there is considerable intrafamilial variability, genetic, epigenetic, environmental or other unidentified factors may influence expression of the disease.

MFS was traditionally considered to result from a structural deficiency of connective tissues. Reduced fibrillin-1 was thought to lead to a primary derangement of elastic fiber deposition, because both skin

and aorta from affected patients show decreased elastin, along with elastic fiber fragmentation. In response to stress (such as hemodynamic forces in the proximal aorta), affected organs were thought to manifest this structural insufficiency with accelerated degeneration. Additional research identified a cytokine-regulatory role for fibrillin-1 that appears to have important implications for MFS. The *transforming growth factor beta (TGF-β)* family of cytokines influences a diverse repertoire of cellular processes, including cell proliferation, migration, differentiation, survival and synthetic activity. The *TGF-β* ligands (TGF-β_1, -β_2, or -β_3) are synthesized as inactive precursor complexes and sequestered by ECM proteins, including fibrillin-1. Mice heterozygous for a mutation in the fibrillin-1 gene, typical of those that cause MFS in humans, display many of the classic features of MFS including aortic root aneurysm, which associates with a tissue signature for increased TGF-β signaling, suggesting that failed ECM sequestration of latent TGF-β by fibrillin-1 leads to increased TGF-β activation and signaling. Furthermore, pharmacologic antagonism of TGF-β signaling ameliorates aortic aneurysm in mouse models of MFS, demonstrating that high TGF-β signaling is a cause rather than a consequence of disease progression.

Aberrant TGF-β signaling might also play a role in the wider spectrum of manifestations of MFS. Increased TGF-β signaling has been observed in other tissues in MFS mice, including the developing lung, mitral valve, and skeletal muscle. Treatment of these mice with agents that antagonize TGF-β attenuates or prevents pulmonary emphysema, myxomatous degeneration of the mitral valve, and skeletal muscle myopathy. The prominent role of TGF-β dysregulation in the pathogenesis of MFS was further validated by the discovery and characterization of another aortic aneurysm syndrome, **Loeys-Dietz syndrome**, in which patients have mutations in the TGF-β receptors and share many overlapping clinical features with MFS (see "Differential Diagnosis" below).

CLINICAL MANIFESTATIONS

MFS is a multisystem disorder, with cardinal manifestations in the skeletal, cardiovascular, and ocular systems.

Skeletal System

Overgrowth of the long bones (dolichostenomelia) is often the most obvious manifestation of MFS and may produce a reduced *upper segment: lower segment ratio* (US:LS) or an arm span to height ratio >1.05 times. Abnormal ratios are US:LS <1 for ages 0-5 yr, US:LS <0.95 for ages 6-7 yr, US:LS <0.9 for ages 8-9 yr, and <0.85 above age 10 yr. Anterior chest deformity is likely the result of excessive rib growth, pushing the sternum either outward (pectus carinatum) or inward (pectus excavatum). Abnormal curvatures of the spine (most commonly thoracolumbar scoliosis) may also partly result from increased vertebral growth. Other skeletal features include an inward bulging of the acetabulum into the pelvic cavity (protrusio acetabuli), flatfeet (pes planus), and joint hypermobility or joint contractures. Long and slender fingers in relation to the palm of the hand (arachnodactyly) is generally a subjective finding. The combination of arachnodactyly and hypermobile joints is examined by the Walker-Murdoch or wrist sign, which is positive if there is full overlap of the distal phalanges of the thumb and fifth finger when wrapped around the contralateral wrist (Fig. 702-1), and the Steinberg or thumb sign, which is present when the distal phalanx of the thumb fully extends beyond the ulnar border of the hand when folded across the palm (Fig. 702-1). Contracture of the fingers (camptodactyly) and elbows is commonly observed. A selection of craniofacial manifestations may be present including a long narrow skull (dolichocephaly), deep-set eyes (enophthalmos), recessed lower mandible (retrognathia) or small chin (micrognathia), flattening of the midface (malar hypoplasia), a high-arching palate, and downward-slanting palpebral fissures (Fig. 702-2).

Cardiovascular System

Within the heart, thickening of the atrioventricular valves is common and often associated with valvular prolapse. Variable degrees of regurgitation may be present. In children with early onset and severe MFS,

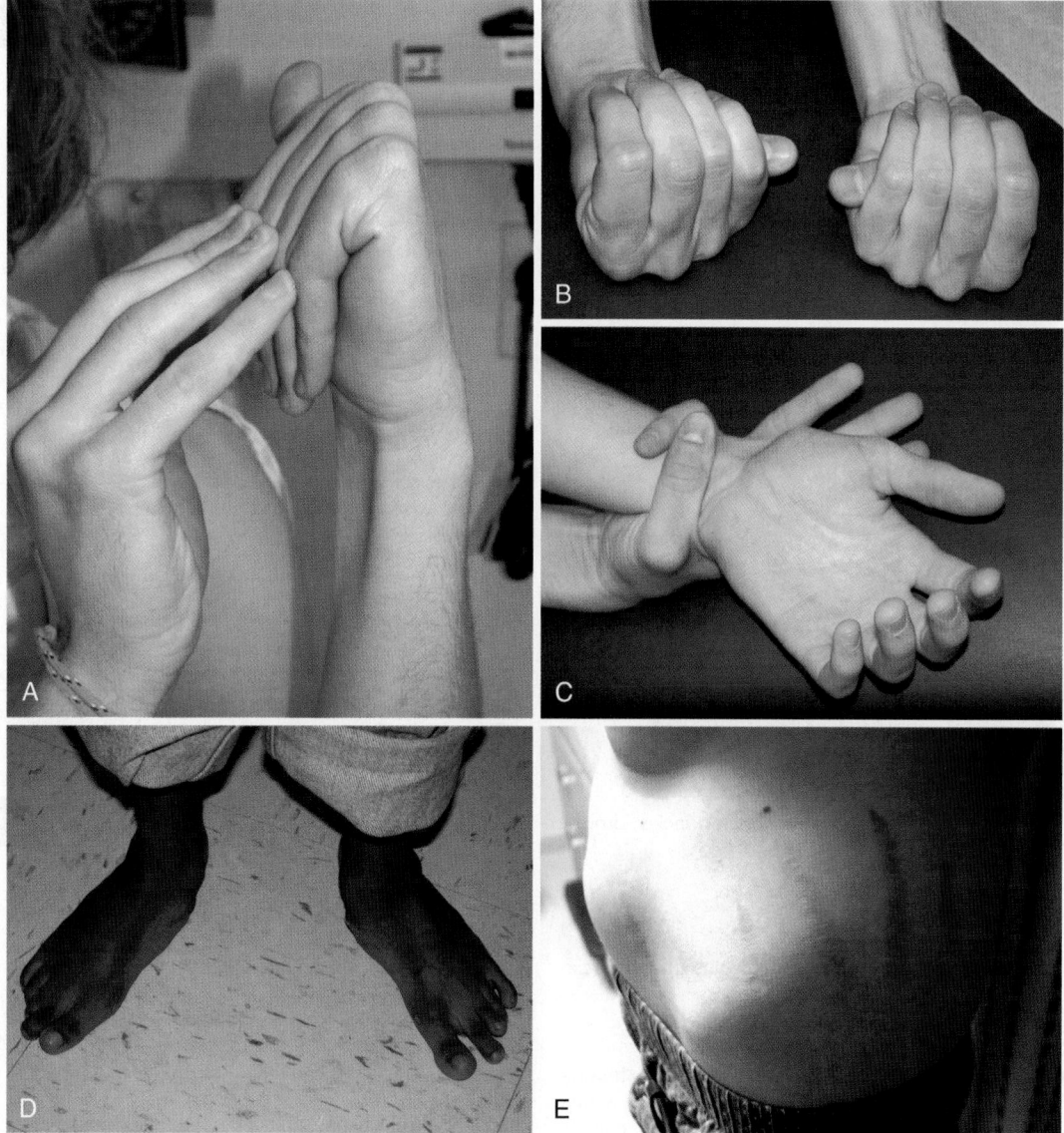

Figure 702-1 Note the joint laxity **(A)**, Steinberg thumb sign **(B)**, ability to join thumb and fifth finger around the wrist (Walker-Murdoch sign) **(C)**, pes planus **(D)**, and striae over hips and back **(E)**. *(From Jones KL, Jones MC, del Campo M: Smith's recognizable patterns of human malformation, ed 7, Philadelphia, 2013, WB Saunders, Fig. 2, p. 616; A-D courtesy Dr. Lynne M. Bird, Rady Children's Hospital, San Diego, CA.)*

insufficiency of the mitral valve can lead to congestive heart failure, pulmonary hypertension and death in infancy; this manifestation is the leading cause of morbidity and mortality in young children with the disorder. Supraventricular arrhythmias and ventricular dysrhythmias may be seen in association with mitral valve dysfunction, and there is an increased prevalence of prolonged QT interval. Dilated cardiomyopathy occurs with increased prevalence in patients with MFS, most often attributed to volume overload imposed by valve regurgitation. Aortic valve dysfunction is generally a late occurrence and attributed to stretching of the aortic annulus by an expanding aortic root aneurysm.

Aortic aneurysm, dissection and rupture, principally at the level of the sinuses of Valsalva (aortic root), remains the most life-threatening manifestations of MFS, prompting lifelong monitoring by echocardiography or other imaging modalities. In severe cases, the aneurysm may be present in utero, but in mild examples, it may be absent or never exceed dimensions that require clinical intervention. Aortic dimensions must be interpreted in comparison to age-dependent nomograms. The most important risk factor for aortic dissection are the maximal aortic root size and a positive family history. The

characteristic histologic findings from aortae of patients with MFS include cystic medial necrosis of the tunica media and disruption of elastic lamellae. Cystic medial necrosis describes the focal apoptosis and disappearance of vascular smooth muscle cells and elastic fibers from the of the tunica media of the aortic wall, and subsequent deposition of mucin-like material in the cystic space. These changes produce a thicker, less distensible and stiffer aorta, which is more prone to aortic dissection. Most patients experiencing acute aortic dissection present with classic symptoms including sudden-onset, severe, tearing chest pain, often radiate into the back. The dissection typically starts at the aortic root and may remain confined to the ascending aorta (type II) or continue into the descending aorta (type I). Acute-onset congestive heart failure may occur if aortic valve function is compromised and patients may suffer cerebrovascular injury depending on the involvement of the carotid arteries. Involvement of the coronary arteries may herald sudden cardiac death, secondary to myocardial infarction or rupture into the pericardial sac with subsequent pericardial tamponade. Chronic aortic dissection usually occurs more insidiously, often without chest pain. Dilation of the main pulmonary artery is common but does not typically cause any clinical sequelae. Enlargement of the

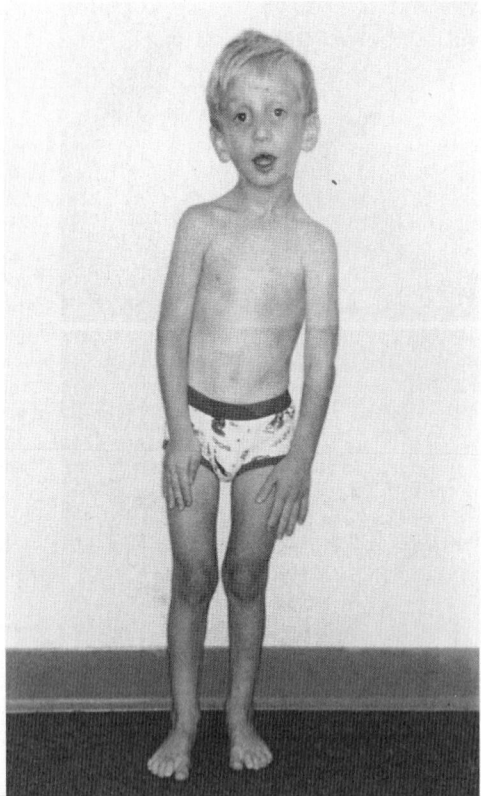

Figure 702-2 Marfan syndrome. Note the elongated facies, droopy lids, apparent dolichostenomelia, and mild scoliosis.

descending thoracic or abdominal aorta can also occur, although relatively rarely.

Ocular System
Dislocation of the ocular lens (ectopia lentis) occurs in approximately 60-70% of patients, although it is not unique to the disorder. Other ocular manifestations include early and severe myopia, flat cornea, increased axial length of the globe, hypoplastic iris, and ciliary muscle hypoplasia, causing decreased miosis. Patients are also predisposed to retinal detachment and early cataracts or glaucoma.

Other Systems
There is an increased incidence of pulmonary disease in MFS: progressive anterior chest deformity or thoracic scoliosis may contribute to a restrictive pattern of lung disease. A widening of the distal airspaces predisposes patients to spontaneous pneumothorax, which occurs in up to 15% of patients. Assessment of pulmonary volumes and function should account for long bone overgrowth affecting the lower extremities, which can lead to a reduction in the normalized forced vital capacity and total lung capacity. If normalized to thoracic size or sitting height, pulmonary function testing is often normal in patients with the disorder.

MFS patients typically have normal skin texture and elasticity. The most common skin finding is stretch marks—pinkish, scar-like lesions that later become white (striae atrophicae), which occur in about one-third of patients (see Fig. 702-1). These may occur in the absence of obesity, rapid gain in muscle mass, or pregnancy, and at sites not associated with increased skin distention (i.e., the anterior shoulder or lower back). Another common manifestation is congenital or acquired inguinal hernia. There is also an increased risk of surgical and recurrent hernias in the Marfan population.

Widening of the dural sac or root sleeves (dural ectasia) is present in 63-92% of MFS patients. Although dural ectasia can result in lumbar

Table 702-1	Diagnostic Criteria for Marfan Syndrome

In the absence of a family history of MFS, a diagnosis can be established in 4 distinct scenarios:
1. Aortic root Z score >2 *and* ectopia Lentis*
2. Aortic root Z score >2 *and* a bona fide *FBN1* mutation
3. Aortic root Z score >2 *and* a systemic score >7*
4. Ectopia lentis *and* a bona fide *FBN1* mutation known to cause aortic disease

In the presence of a family history of MFS, a diagnosis can be established in the presence of:
1. Ectopia lentis
2. A systemic score >7*
3. Aortic root Z score >2 if older than 20 yr or >3 if younger than 20 yr*

In the absence of a family history of MFS, alternative diagnoses include:
1. Ectopia lentis ± systemic score *and* *FBN1* mutation not known to associate with aortic aneurysm or no *FBN1* mutation = ectopia lentis syndrome
2. Aortic root Z score <2 *and* a systemic score >5 (with at least 1 skeletal feature) without ectopia lentis = MASS (mitral valve prolapse, myopia, borderline and nonprogressive aortic enlargement, and nonspecific skin and skeletal findings) phenotype
3. Mitral valve prolapse *and* aortic root Z score <2 *and* a systemic score <5 without ectopia lentis = mitral valve prolapse syndrome

*Denotes caveat that features suggestive of an alternative diagnosis must be excluded and appropriate alternative molecular testing should be performed.

Table 702-2	Scoring of Systemic Features in Points

- Wrist *and* thumb sign = 3 (wrist *or* thumb sign = 1)
- Pectus carinatum deformity = 2 (pectus excavatum or chest asymmetry = 1)
- Hind foot deformity = 2 (plain pes planus = 1)
- Pneumothorax = 2
- Dural ectasia = 2
- Protrusio acetabuli = 2
- Reduced US : LS *and* increased arm : height *and* no severe scoliosis = 1
- Scoliosis or thoracolumbar kyphosis = 1
- Reduced elbow extension = 1
- Facial features (3/5) = 1 (dolichocephaly, enophthalmos, downslanting palpebral fissures, midface hypoplasia, retrognathia)
- Skin striae = 1
- Myopia >3 diopters = 1
- Mitral valve prolapse (all types) = 1

Maximum total: 20 points; score ≥7 indicates systemic involvement.
US:LS, upper segment:lower segment ratio.

back pain, it is often asymptomatic and should be assessed by lumbosacral imaging with CT or MRI.

DIAGNOSIS
Given the complexity of the clinical examination in MFS and the relevant differential diagnoses, evaluation should be coordinated by a professional with extensive experience, such as a geneticist, cardiologist, or ophthalmologist. The diagnosis is based on a defined set of clinical criteria drawn up by an international panel of experts: revised Ghent nosology for the MFS (Table 702-1).

In the absence of a conclusive family history of MFS, the diagnosis can be established in 4 distinct scenarios:
1. The presence of either aortic root dilation when standardized to age and body size (an aortic root Z score ≥2) or aortic dissection combined with ectopia lentis allows for the unequivocal diagnosis of MFS, irrespective of the presence or absence of any systemic features (Table 702-2), except when these are indicative of an alternate diagnosis.

Table 702-3	Criteria for Causal *FBN1* Mutation

- Mutation previously shown to segregate in a Marfan family
- Any 1 of the following de novo mutations (with proven paternity and absence of disease in parents):
  - Nonsense mutation
  - Inframe and out of frame deletion/insertion
  - Splice site mutations affecting canonical splice sequence or shown to alter splicing on mRNA/cDNA level
  - Missense mutation affecting/creating cysteine residues
  - Missense mutation affecting conserved residues of the EGF consensus sequence [(D/N)X(D/N)(E/Q)Xm(D/N)Xn(Y/F) with m and n representing variable number of residues; D representing aspartic acid; N representing asparagine; E representing glutamic acid; Q representing glutamine; Y representing tyrosine; F representing phenylalanine; X representing any amino acid]
  - Other missense mutations: segregation in family if possible *and* absence in 400 ethnically matched control chromosomes; if no family history, absence in 400 ethnically matched control chromosomes
  - Linkage of haplotype for n ≥6 meioses to the *FBN1* locus

cDNA, complementary DNA; mRNA, messenger RNA;
From Loeys BL, Dietz HC, Braverman AC, et al: The revised Ghent nosology for the Marfan syndrome. J Med Genet 47:476–485, 2010.

2. The presence of aortic root dilation (Z score ≥2) or aortic dissection and the identification of a bona fide *FBN1* mutation (Table 702-3) are sufficient to establish the diagnosis even if ectopia lentis is absent.
3. When aortic root dilation (an aortic root Z score ≥2) or aortic dissection is present, but ectopia lentis is absent and the *FBN1* status is either unknown or negative, the diagnosis may be confirmed by the presence of sufficient systemic findings (a systemic score ≥7 points; see Table 702-2). However, features suggestive of an alternate diagnosis must be excluded and the appropriate alternative molecular testing should be performed.
4. In the presence of ectopia lentis, but absence of aortic root dilation or aortic dissection, an *FBN1* mutation, which has previously been associated with aortic disease, is required before the diagnosis can be made. If the *FBN1* mutation is not unequivocally associated with cardiovascular disease in either a related or unrelated proband, the patient should be classified as *isolated ectopia lentis syndrome*.

Despite these diagnostic criteria, on occasion young (<20 yr) sporadic cases may not fit in 1 of the 4 proposed scenarios detailed above. If insufficient systemic features (systemic score <7) and/or borderline aortic root measurements (Z score <3) are present without documented evidence of a bona fide *FBN1* mutation, the term *nonspecific connective tissue disorder* is recommended. In those instances when a *FBN1* mutation is identified, the term *potential MFS* should be used instead.

In an individual with a positive family history of MFS (where a family member has been independently diagnosed using the above criteria), the diagnosis can be established in the presence of:
1. Ectopia lentis
2. A systemic score >7 points (see Table 702-1)
3. Aortic root dilation with Z score ≥2 in adults (≥20 yr old) or Z score ≥3 in individuals younger than 20 yr old

In the case of scenarios 2 and 3, features suggestive of an alternative diagnosis must again be excluded and appropriate alternative molecular testing should be performed.

DIFFERENTIAL DIAGNOSIS

The differential diagnosis of MFS includes disorders with aortic aneurysm (Loeys-Dietz syndrome, familial thoracic aortic aneurysm syndrome, Shprintzen-Goldberg syndrome); ectopia lentis (ectopia lentis syndrome, Weill-Marchesani syndrome, and homocystinuria [see Chapter 85.3]); or systemic manifestations of MFS (congenital contractural arachnodactyly and MASS phenotype) (Table 702-4).

Aortic Aneurysm Syndromes
An important differential diagnosis is **Loeys-Dietz syndrome (LDS)**, a systemic connective tissue disorder characterized by the triad of arterial tortuosity and aggressive aneurysm disease, hypertelorism, and bifid uvula or cleft palate, as well as many of the craniofacial and skeletal features found in MFS. The diagnosis may be classified into LDS type 1 or LDS type 2 depending on whether the mutant locus resides in the *TGFBR1* or the *TGFBR2* gene, which encode the type 1 or the type 2 TGF-β receptors respectively. Two new LDS variants have been described, LDS type 3 and LDS type 4, which are caused by heterozygous mutations in the genes encoding the TGF-β intracellular signaling molecule SMAD3 and the extracellular ligand TGF-β$_2$, respectively. These new subtypes are also characterized by widespread arterial tortuosity and aneurysm disease, aortic dissection, as well as typical craniofacial and skeletal abnormalities. Patients with *SMAD3* mutations also appear predisposed to early onset osteoarthritis and supraventricular arrhythmias. Distinguishing between MFS and the various LDS subtypes is important because aneurysms tend to dissect at younger ages and smaller dimensions in LDS patients, necessitating more aggressive management.

Like MFS, **familial thoracic aortic aneurysm** syndrome segregates as an autosomal dominant trait characterized aortic root aneurysm and dissection. Other systemic manifestations of MFS are typically absent and the disorder has reduced penetrance. Disease-causing heterozygous mutations have been identified in several genes with roles in the vascular smooth muscle contractile apparatus, including *MYH11*, *ACTA2*, and *MYLK*, which encode smooth muscle myosin heavy chain 11, vascular smooth muscle α-actin, and myosin light chain kinase. However, these genes only account for a fraction of cases of nonsyndromic familial thoracic aortic aneurysm. In most cases, the management principles that have been generated for MFS have proved effective for this form of familial aortic aneurysm.

Shprintzen-Goldberg syndrome is a systemic connective tissue disorder that includes virtually all the craniofacial, skeletal, skin and cardiovascular manifestations of MFS and LDS, with the additional findings of craniosynostosis, hydrocephalus, mental retardation and severe skeletal muscle hypotonia. The majority of cases are caused by heterozygous mutations in the *SKI* gene, which encodes an intracellular repressor of TGF-β signaling. Vascular involvement tends to be less prevalent and less severe when compared to MFS or LDS.

Ectopia Lentis Syndromes
Both **ectopia lentis syndrome** and **Weill-Marchesani syndrome** may also be caused by heterozygous mutations in *FBN1*. Compound heterozygous or homozygous mutations at a second locus, *ADAMTSL4*, have been shown to cause ectopia lentis associated with slightly younger age at diagnosis. Interestingly, the same *FBN1* mutation produces classical MFS, ectopia lentis, and ectopia lentis combined with skin, but not cardiovascular, manifestations of MFS, suggesting that these presentations are part of a spectrum of clinical features of the same disease.

Weill-Marchesani syndrome is a systemic connective tissue disorder characterized by skin, skeletal, and ocular abnormalities, including microspherophakia, ectopia lentis, and myopia. Features inconsistent with the diagnosis of MFS include short stature and brachydactyly. As well as *FBN1* mutations (type 2), the syndrome may be caused by homozygous or compound heterozygous mutations in *ADAMTS10* (type 1) or homozygous mutations in *LTBP2* (type 3).

Homocystinuria is a metabolic disorder caused by homozygous or compound heterozygous mutations in the gene encoding cystathionine β-synthase, which leads to increases in both homocysteine and methionine. The clinical features of untreated homocystinuria include ectopia lentis and skeletal abnormalities resembling MFS. However, in contrast to MFS, affected persons often suffer from developmental delay, a predisposition to thromboembolic events, and a high incidence of coronary artery disease.

Table 702-4	Differential Diagnosis of Marfan Syndrome		
DIFFERENTIAL DIAGNOSIS	**CARDIAC FEATURES**	**VASCULAR FEATURES**	**SYSTEMIC FEATURES**
AORTIC ANEURYSM SYNDROMES			
Loeys-Dietz syndrome (MIM 609192)	Patent ductus arteriosus Atrial septal defect Bicuspid aortic valve	Aortic root aneurysm Arterial tortuosity Widespread aneurysms Vascular dissection at relatively young ages and small aortic dimensions	Hypertelorism Cleft palate Broad or bifid uvula Craniosynostosis Midface hypoplasia Blue sclerae Arachnodactyly Pectus deformity Scoliosis Joint hypermobility Pes planus Rarely Easy bruising Dystrophic scars Translucent skin Rarely developmental delay
Familial thoracic aortic aneurysm (MIM 132900)	Generally none Rare forms with patent ductus arteriosus	Aortic root aneurysm Ascending aortic aneurysm	Generally none Rarely livedo reticularis and iris flocculi
Shprintzen-Goldberg syndrome (MIM 182212)	None	Aortic root aneurysm	Hypertelorism Craniosynostosis Arched palate Arachnodactyly Pectus deformity Scoliosis Joint hypermobility Developmental delay
Bicuspid aortic valve with aortic aneurysm (MIM: 109730)	Bicuspid aortic valve	Aortic root aneurysm Ascending aortic aneurysm	
Ehlers-Danlos syndrome, type IV (MIM: 130050)	Mitral valve prolapse	Aneurysm and rupture of any medium to large muscular artery No predisposition for aortic root enlargement	Joint hypermobility Atrophic scars Translucent skin Easy bruising Hernias Rupture of hollow organs
ECTOPIA LENTIS SYNDROMES			
Familial ectopia lentis (MIM 129600)	None	None	Nonspecific skeletal features
Homocystinuria (MIM 236200)	Mitral valve prolapse	Intravascular thrombosis	Tall stature Ectopia lentis Long-bone overgrowth Developmental delay
SYNDROMES WITH SYSTEMIC MANIFESTATIONS OF MFS			
MASS phenotype (MIM 604308)	Mitral valve prolapse	Borderline or nonprogressive	Nonspecific skin and skeletal findings Myopia

Syndromes with Systemic Manifestations of Marfan Syndrome

Congenital contractural arachnodactyly is a connective tissue disorder caused by heterozygous mutations in the gene encoding fibrillin-2 (*FBN2*). There are a number of clinical features overlapping with MFS including dolichostenomelia, anterior chest deformity, scoliosis, joint contractures, and arachnodactyly, as well as some craniofacial malformations, including highly arched palate and retrognathia. In addition, both may suffer from severe cardiovascular abnormalities leading to premature death, but the specific cardiac anomalies are quite different; valvular insufficiency and aortic root dilation in MFS whereas congenital heart defects are more common in congenital contractural arachnodactyly. Patients with congenital contractural arachnodactyly also suffer from crumpled auricular helices (a hallmark of this condition).

Many patients referred for possible MFS are found to have evidence of a systemic connective tissue disorder, including long limbs, deformity of the thoracic cage, striae atrophicae, mitral valve prolapse, and borderline but nonprogressive dilation of the aortic root, but do not

meet diagnostic criteria for MFS. This constellation of features is referred to by the acronym **MASS** phenotype (mitral valve prolapse, myopia, borderline and nonprogressive aortic enlargement, and nonspecific skin and skeletal findings). The MASS phenotype can segregate in large pedigrees and remain stable over time. The diagnosis is particularly challenging in the context of a young, sporadic patient in whom careful follow-up is needed to distinguish MASS phenotype from emerging MFS. Familial mitral valve prolapse syndrome can also be caused by mutations in the gene encoding fibrillin-1 and include subdiagnostic systemic manifestations.

LABORATORY FINDINGS

Laboratory studies should document a negative urinary cyanide nitroprusside test or specific amino acid studies to exclude cystathionine β-synthase deficiency (homocystinuria). Although it is estimated that most, if not all, people with classic MFS have an *FBN1* mutation, the large size of this gene and the extreme allelic heterogeneity in MFS have frustrated efficient molecular diagnosis. The yield of mutation screening varies based on technique and clinical presentation. It remains unclear whether the "missing" mutations are simply atypical in character or location within *FBN1* or located in another gene. Other differential diagnoses, such as MASS phenotype, ectopia lentis, Weill-Marchesani syndrome, and Shprintzen-Goldberg syndrome, are associated with mutations in the *FBN1* gene. It is often difficult or impossible to predict the phenotype from the nature or location of a *FBN1* mutation in MFS. Hence, molecular genetic techniques can contribute to the diagnosis, but they do not substitute for comprehensive clinical evaluation and follow-up. The absence or presence of an *FBN1* mutation is not sufficient to exclude or establish the diagnosis, respectively.

MANAGEMENT
Management focuses on preventing complications and genetic counseling. Referral to a multidisciplinary center where a geneticist with experience in MFS works in concert with subspecialists to coordinate a rational approach to monitoring and treatment is advisable given the complex nature of some patient's disease. Yearly evaluations for cardiovascular disease, scoliosis, or ophthalmologic problems are imperative.

CURRENT THERAPIES
Most therapies currently available or under investigation aim to diminish cardiovascular complications, which can be categorized into activity restrictions, aortic surgery, endocarditis prophylaxis, and current pharmacologic approaches.

Activity Restrictions
Physical therapy can improve cardiovascular performance, neuromuscular tone, and psychosocial health, and so aerobic exertion in moderation is recommended. However, strenuous physical exertion, competitive or contact sports and particularly isometric activities, which invoke a Valsalva maneuver, such as weight lifting, should be avoided.

Aortic Surgery
Surgical outcome is more favorable if undertaken on an elective rather than an urgent or emergent basis (mortality of 1.5% vs 2.6% and 11.7%, respectively). Therefore, aortic surgery should be recommended for adult patients when their aortic root diameter approaches 50 mm, and early intervention considered for those with a rapid rate of enlargement (>5-10 mm per year) or a family history of early aortic dissection. There are no definitive criteria guiding the timing of surgery in children in whom dissection is extremely rare, irrespective of aortic size. This has prompted many centers to adopt the adult criterion of 50 mm, although early surgery may be undertaken in the presence of a rapid rate of growth (>10 mm per year) or the emergence of significant aortic regurgitation. Preserving the native aortic valve at the time of repair is desirable to avoid the need for lifelong anticoagulation. Replacement of the aortic root with a pulmonary root autograft (a Ross procedure) is not recommended as the neoaorta can undergo progressive enlargement and autograft failure once exposed to the systemic blood pressure. Mitral valve repair or replacement is advised for severe mitral valve regurgitation with associated symptoms or progressive left ventricular dilation or dysfunction.

Pregnancy
There is higher risk of aortic dissection during pregnancy in women with MFS. However, improved awareness and more recent analyses have indicated the risk is low in patients with an aortic root diameter <40 mm. Prophylactic aortic root replacement can minimize the risk of aortic dissection and death in women with MFS who wish to become pregnant.

Endocarditis Prophylaxis
The American Heart Association no longer recommends the use of antibiotic prophylaxis for persons with structural or valvular heart disease, but exceptions are made for select groups at the greatest risk for bad outcomes from infectious endocarditis. The Professional Advisory Board of the National Marfan Foundation believes that patients with MFS should continue to receive prophylaxis for bacterial endocarditis, in part because it remains unknown, but possible, that the myxomatous valves typical of MFS are a preferred substrate for bacterial infection.

Current Pharmacologic Approaches
β-Blockers have traditionally been considered the standard of care in MFS and multiple small observational studies suggest there is a protective effect on aortic root growth, with the dose typically titrated to achieve a resting heart rate <100 beats/min during submaximal exercise. Given the putative role of hemodynamic stress in aortic dilation and aortic dissection in MFS, these effects are attributed to the negative inotropic and chronotropic effects of β-blockade.

EMERGING THERAPEUTIC STRATEGIES
Angiotensin II Receptor Type 1 Blockers
There is extensive evidence linking angiotensin II signaling to TGF-β activation and signaling. In a mouse model of MFS, the **angiotensin II receptor type 1 blocker losartan** completely prevents pathologic aortic root growth and normalizes both aortic wall thickness and architecture. In support of its relevance to humans, a retrospective study assessing the effect of angiotensin II receptor type 1 blockers in a small cohort of pediatric patients with MFS who had severe aortic root enlargement despite previous alternate medical therapy, showed that angiotensin II receptor type 1 blockers significantly slowed the rate of aortic root and sinotubular junction dilation (both of which occur in MFS), whereas the distal ascending aorta (which does not normally become dilated in MFS) remained unaffected. Further evidence of a beneficial effect from losartan therapy is provided by 3 prospective clinical trials that demonstrated that losartan treatment alone or in combination with β-blockade slows the progression of aortic root dilation in patients with MFS. Nonetheless when compared to atenolol, losartan therapy in children and young adults with Marfan syndrome and aortic root dilation demonstrated equivalent rates of aortic root dilation during a 3-yr study.

PROGNOSIS
The major cause of mortality is aortic root dilation, dissection, and rupture, with the majority of fatal events occurring in the 3rd and 4th decade of life. A reevaluation of life expectancy in MFS suggests that early diagnosis and refined medical and surgical management has greatly improved the prognosis for patients with the condition. Nevertheless, MFS continues to be associated with significant morbidity and selected subgroups are refractory to therapy and continue to show early mortality. In a review of 54 patients diagnosed during infancy, 89% had serious cardiac pathology; cardiac disease was progressive despite standard care (22% died during childhood, 16% before age 1 yr). In the more classic form of MFS, it is estimated that more than 90% of individuals will have a cardiovascular event during their lifetime, placing both physical and mental stresses on patients and their families. Awareness of these issues and referral for support services can facilitate a positive perspective toward the condition.

GENETIC COUNSELING
The heritable nature of MFS makes recurrence risk (genetic) counseling mandatory. Fathers of these sporadic cases are, on average, 7-10 yr older than fathers in the general population. This paternal age effect suggests that these cases represent new dominant mutations with minimal recurrence risk to the future offspring of the normal parents. Owing to rare reports of gonadal mosaicism in a phenotypically normal parent, the recurrence risk for parents of a sporadic case can be reported as low, but not zero. Each child of an affected parent, however, has a 50% risk of inheriting the MFS mutation and thus being affected. Recurrence risk counseling is best accomplished by professionals with expertise in the issues surrounding the disorder.

Bibliography is available at Expert Consult.

Section **4**

Metabolic Bone Disease

Chapter **703**

Bone Structure, Growth, and Hormonal Regulation

Russell W. Chesney

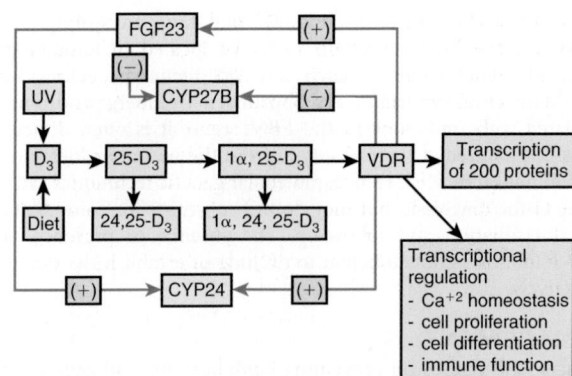

Figure 703-1 Vitamin D metabolism. Vitamin D can be synthesized in the skin under the influence of UV irradiation, or it can be absorbed from the diet. It is converted to $25(OH)D_3$ (vitamin D_3) in the liver and then further converted by the kidney. The enzyme cytochrome P450 (CYP) 27B converts $25(OH)D_3$ to $1\alpha,25\text{-}(OH)_2D_3$. $1,25(OH)_2D_3$ binds to vitamin D receptor (VDR), which, after transport to the nucleus, acts to induce the transcription of more than 200 proteins. The functions of some of the proteins are indicated. VDR activation leads to productions of fibroblast growth factor 23 (FGF23). FGF23 induces phosphaturia (not shown), upregulates CYP 24, and downregulates CYP 27B.

See also Chapters 51 and 570.

Bone is a rigid organ but metabolically active in that it is constantly being formed (**modeling**) and reformed (**remodeling**). It is capable of rapid turnover, bearing weight, and withstanding the stresses of various physical activities. Bone is the major body reservoir for calcium, phosphorus, and magnesium. Other functions of bone include organ protection, structure, movement, and sound transmission. It is also an endocrine organ that produces fibroblast growth factor 23 (FGF23), which regulates renal phosphate handling. Disorders that affect this organ and the process of mineralization are designated **metabolic bone diseases**.

The human skeleton consists of a protein matrix, largely composed of a collagen-containing protein, osteoid, on which is deposited a crystalline mineral phase. Collagen-containing osteoid accounts for 90% of bone protein; other proteins, including osteocalcin, which contains γ-carboxyglutamic acid, are also present. Synthesis of osteocalcin depends on vitamin K and vitamin D; in states with high bone turnover, serum osteocalcin values are often elevated. Osteocalcin itself acts on insulin secretion and reduction of fat stores.

The microfibrillar matrix of osteoid permits deposition of highly organized calcium phosphate crystals, including hydroxyapatite $[C_{10}(PO_4)_6\cdot6H_2O]$ and octacalcium phosphate $[Ca_8(H_2PO_4)_6\cdot5H_2O]$, plus less-organized amorphous calcium phosphate, calcium carbonate, sodium, magnesium, and citrate. Hydroxyapatite is deep within bone matrix, whereas amorphous calcium phosphate coats the surface of newly formed or remodeled bone.

Because bone growth and turnover rates are high during childhood, many clinical and osseous features of metabolic bone diseases are more prominent in children than in adults.

The growth pattern of bones is an acceleration of bone growth (length) of the limbs during prepubescence, increased growth (length) of the trunk (spine) during early adolescence, and increased bone mineral deposition in late adolescence. The use of dual-energy x-ray absorptiometry or quantitative CT permits measurement of both mineral content and bone density in healthy subjects and in children with metabolic bone disease. Dual-energy x-ray absorptiometry scanning exposes the patient to less radiation than a chest radiograph.

Bone growth occurs in children by the process of calcification of the cartilage cells present at the ends of bone. In accord with the prevailing extracellular fluid calcium and phosphate concentrations, mineral is deposited in chondrocytes or cartilage cells set to undergo mineralization. The main function of the vitamin D–parathyroid hormone (PTH)–FGF23–endocrine axis is to maintain the extracellular fluid calcium and phosphate concentrations at appropriate levels to permit mineralization.

Other hormones also appear to regulate the growth and mineralization of cartilage, including growth hormone acting through insulin-like growth factors, thyroid hormones, insulin, leptin, ghrelin, and androgens and estrogens during the pubertal growth spurt. Supraphysiologic concentrations of glucocorticoids impair cartilage function and bone growth and augment bone resorption.

Rates of bone formation are coordinated with alterations in mineral metabolism in both the intestine and kidneys, where a number of hormones regulate the processes. Inadequate dietary intake or intestinal absorption of calcium causes a fall in serum levels of calcium and its ionized fraction. This serves as the signal for PTH synthesis and secretion, resulting in greater bone resorption (which raises the serum calcium level), enhanced distal tubular reabsorption of calcium, and promotes higher rates of renal synthesis of $1,25(OH)_2D$ or calcitriol, the most active metabolite of vitamin D (Fig. 703-1). Calcium homeostasis thus is controlled by the intestine because the availability of $1,25(OH)_2D$ ultimately determines the fraction of ingested calcium that is absorbed.

Phosphate homeostasis is regulated by the kidneys because intestinal phosphate absorption is nearly complete and renal excretion determines the serum level of phosphate. Excessive intestinal phosphate absorption causes a fall in serum levels of ionized calcium and a rise in PTH secretion, resulting in phosphaturia, thus lowering the serum phosphate level and permitting the calcium level to rise. Hypophosphatemia blocks PTH secretion and promotes renal $1,25$-dihydroxyvitamin D $[1,25(OH)_2D]$ synthesis. This latter compound also promotes greater intestinal phosphate absorption. The important role of FGF23 in phosphate homeostasis is described below.

Vitamin D can be synthesized in the skin under the influence of UV irradiation, or it can be absorbed from the diet. It is converted to $25(OH)D_3$ (vitamin D_3) in the liver and then further converted by the kidney. An understanding of the metabolism of vitamin D is necessary to appreciate mineral homeostasis and metabolic bone disease and rickets. The skin contains 7-dehydrocholesterol, which is converted to vitamin D_3 $[25(OH)D_3]$ by UV radiation; other inactive vitamin D sterols are also produced (see Chapter 51). Vitamin D_3 is then transported in the bloodstream to the liver by a vitamin D–binding protein (DBP); DBP binds all forms of vitamin D. The plasma concentration of free or nonbound vitamin D is much lower than the level of DBP-bound vitamin D metabolites.

Vitamin D also can enter the metabolic pathway by ingestion of dietary vitamin D_2 (ergocalciferol) or vitamin D_3 (cholecalciferol), both of which are absorbed from the intestine because of the action of bile salts. After absorption, ingested vitamin D is transported by chylomicrons to the liver, where, along with skin-derived vitamin D_3, it is converted to 25-hydroxyvitamin D [25(OH)D] by the action of a hepatic microsomal enzyme requiring oxygen, nicotinamide adenine dinucleotide phosphate, and magnesium to hydroxylate vitamin D at the 25th carbon atom. The 25(OH)D is next transported by DBP to the kidneys, where it undergoes further metabolism. 25(OH)D is the main circulating vitamin D metabolite in humans (Table 703-1). Because the synthesis of 25(OH)D is weakly regulated by feedback, its plasma level rises in summer and falls in winter. High vitamin D intake raises the plasma level of 25(OH)D to many times above normal, but the parent vitamin D compound itself is absorbed by adipose tissue.

In the kidneys, 25(OH)D undergoes further hydroxylation, depending on the prevailing serum concentration of calcium, phosphate, PTH and FGF23. If the calcium or phosphate level is reduced or the PTH level is elevated, the enzyme 25(OH)D-1-hydroxylase is activated and $1,25(OH)_2D$ is formed. The enzyme cytochrome P450 (CYP) 27B1 converts $25(OH)D_3$ to $1\alpha,25-(OH)_2D_3$. $1,25(OH)_2D_3$ binds to vitamin D receptor, which, after transport to the nucleus, acts to induce the transcription of 200-400 proteins and peptides. The functions of some of the proteins are known.

Another class of proteins important in the regulation of mineral balance and vitamin D synthesis are the phosphatonins. Among these are FGF23, sFRP-4 (secreted Frizzled-related protein 4), and MEPE (matrix extracellular phosphoglycoprotein). Overexpression of FGF23 results in hypophosphatemia, phosphaturia, reduced serum $1,25(OH)_2D$ values, and some forms of rickets. Disorders of phosphate balance, including hyper- and hypophosphatemia, can relate to loss or gain of function of these phosphatonins (see Fig. 703-1).

Vitamin D receptor activation by $1,25(OH)_2D$ leads to production of FGF23. FGF23 is produced by osteocytes and targets another organ,

the kidney, to promote phosphaturia. FGF23 reduces expression/insertion of 2 sodium phosphate transporters into the renal proximal tubule, resulting in higher levels of urinary phosphate excretion. This bone-derived hormone also inhibits renal hydroxylase activity (CYP 27B1) and promotes 24-hydroxylase activity. Consequently, circulating $1,25(OH)_2D$ levels fall.

A gene termed *Klotho* codes for a single-pass transmembrane protein that is an aging suppressor in mice. Klotho protein also influences interaction of FGF23 with its receptor FGF23R. FGF23 is then able to inhibit the action of CYP27B1 and the sodium-dependent phosphate transporter in the kidney. The net result of Klotho FGF23 interaction is reduced $1,25(OH)_2D$ values and phosphaturia.

The active metabolite, $1,25(OH)_2D$, circulates at a level that is only 0.1% of the level of 25(OH)D (see Table 703-1) and acts on the intestine to increase the active transport of calcium and stimulate phosphate absorption. Because 1α-hydroxylase is a mitochondrial enzyme that is tightly feedback regulated, the synthesis of $1,25(OH)_2D$ declines after serum calcium or phosphate values return to normal. Excessive $1,25(OH)_2D$ is converted to an inactive metabolite. In the presence of normal or elevated serum calcium or phosphate concentrations, the renal 25(OH)D-24-hydroxylase is activated, producing 24,25-dihydroxyvitamin D [$24,25(OH)_2D$], which is a pathway for the removal of excess vitamin D; serum levels of $24,25(OH)_2D$ (1-5 ng/mL) increase after ingestion of large amounts of vitamin D (see Fig. 703-1), or in the presence of increased concentrations of FGF23. Although hypervitaminosis D and production of inactive metabolites can occur after oral dosing, extensive skin exposure to sunlight does not usually produce toxic levels of $25(OH)D_3$, suggesting natural regulation of the production of this metabolite in cutaneous tissue.

Serum $1,25(OH)_2D$ levels are higher in children than in adults, are not as subject to seasonal variability, and peak in the 1st yr of life and again during the adolescent growth spurt. These values must be interpreted in light of the prevailing serum calcium, phosphate, and PTH values, and with regard to the entire vitamin D metabolite profile.

Mineral deficiency prevents the normal process of bone mineral deposition. If mineral deficiency occurs at the growth plate, growth slows and bone age is retarded, a condition called *rickets*. Poor mineralization of trabecular bone resulting in a greater proportion of unmineralized osteoid is the condition of osteomalacia. Rickets is found only in growing children before fusion of the epiphyses, whereas osteomalacia is present at all ages. All patients with rickets have osteomalacia, but not all patients with osteomalacia have rickets. These conditions should not be confused with osteoporosis, a condition of equal loss of bone volume and mineral (see Chapter 707).

Rickets may be classified as calcium-deficient or phosphate-deficient rickets. Because both calcium and phosphate ions constitute bone mineral, the insufficiency of either type in the extracellular fluid that bathes the mineralizing surface of bone results in rickets and osteomalacia. The 2 types of rickets are distinguishable by their clinical manifestations (Table 703-2). Rickets can also occur in the face of mineral deficiency, despite adequate vitamin D stores. True dietary calcium deficiency rickets is found in some parts of Africa but rarely in North America or Europe. A form of phosphate-deficiency rickets can occur in infants given prolonged administration of phosphate-sequestering aluminum salts as a treatment for colic or gastroesophageal reflux. This results in the phosphate depletion syndrome.

Bibliography is available at Expert Consult.

METABOLITE	PLASMA VALUE
Vitamin D_2	1-2 ng/mL
Vitamin D_3	1-2 ng/mL
$25(OH)D_2$	4-10 ng/mL
$25(OH)D_3$	26-70 ng/mL
TOTAL 25(OH)D	30-80 ng/mL [The 2010 Institute of Medicine report states that a value of 25(OH)D above 20 ng/mL is the lower limit of normal.]
$24,25(OH)_2D$	1-4 ng/mL
$1,25(OH)_2D$	
Infancy	70-100 pg/mL
Childhood	30-50 pg/mL
Adolescence	40-80 pg/mL
Adulthood	20-35 pg/mL

Table 703-1 Vitamin D Metabolic Values in Plasma of Normal Healthy Subjects

Table 703-2 | Clinical Variants of Rickets and Related Conditions

TYPE	SERUM CALCIUM LEVEL	SERUM PHOSPHORUS LEVEL	ALKALINE PHOSPHATASE ACTIVITY	URINE CONCENTRATION OF AMINO ACIDS	GENETICS	GENE DEFECT KNOWN
CALCIUM DEFICIENCY WITH SECONDARY HYPERPARATHYROIDISM [DEFICIENCY OF VITAMIN D; LOW 25(OH)D AND NO STIMULATION OF HIGHER 1,25(OH)₂D VALUES]						
Lack of Vitamin D						
Lack of exposure to sunlight	N or L	L	E	E		
Dietary deficiency of vitamin D	N or L	L	E	E		
Congenital	N or L	L	E	E		
Other Deficiencies						
Malabsorption of vitamin D	N or L	L	E	E		
Liver diseases	N or L	L	E	E		
Anticonvulsant drug	N or L	L	E	E		
Renal osteodystrophy	N or L	E	E	V		
Vitamin D–dependent type I	L	N or L	E	E	AR	Y
PRIMARY PHOSPHATE DEFICIENCY (NO SECONDARY HYPERPARATHYROIDISM)						
Genetic Primary Hypophosphatemia	N	L	E	N	XI, AD, AR	Y
X-linked hypophosphatemic rickets					XL	Y
Autosomal dominant hypophosphatemic rickets					AD	Y
Autosomal recessive hypophosphatemic rickets					AR	Y
Fanconi Syndrome						
Cystinosis	N	L	E	E	AR	Y
Tyrosinosis	N	L	E	E	AR	Y
Lowe syndrome	N	L	E	E	XR	Y
Acquired	N	L	E	E		
Phosphate Deficiency or Malabsorption						
Parenteral hyperalimentation	N	L	E	N		
Low phosphate intake	N	L	E	N		
Other						
Renal tubular acidosis, type II proximal	N	L	E	N		Y
Tumor-induced osteomalacia	N	L	E	N		Y
END-ORGAN RESISTANCE TO 1,25(OH)₂D₃						
Vitamin D-dependent type II (several variants)	L	L or N	E	E	AR	Y
RELATED CONDITIONS RESEMBLING RICKETS						
Hypophosphatasia	N	N	L	Phosphoethanolamine elevated	AR	Y
Metaphyseal Dysostosis						
Jansen type		N	E	N	AD	Y
Schmid type		N	E	N	AD	Y

AD, autosomal dominant; AR, autosomal recessive; E, elevated; L, low; N, normal; V, variable; XL, X-linked; Y, yes.

Chapter 704
Primary Chondrodystrophy (Metaphyseal Dysplasia)

Russell W. Chesney

Skeletal dysplasias are classified under 3 major categories: **osteodysplasias, chondrodysplasias,** and **dysostoses.** The osteodysplasias affect bone density and often lead to osteopenia. The chondrodysplasias are genetic disorders of cartilage and result in deficient linear growth. The dysostoses affect a single bone.

In primary chondrodystrophy, which is an autosomal dominant condition, bowing of the legs, short stature, and a waddling gait appear in the absence of abnormalities of serum levels of calcium and phosphate, alkaline phosphatase activity, or vitamin D metabolites. Metaphyseal chondrodysplasia (**Jansen type**) is very rare and is typified by cupped and ragged metaphyses, which develop mottled calcification at the distal ends of bone over time (Fig. 704-1). Hypercalcemia, with serum values of 13-15 mg/dL, can occur. The spine can also be deformed by the irregular growth of vertebrae. Three different mutations, resulting in ligand independent activation, have been identified in parathyroid hormone receptor type I as the molecular cause of this syndrome, as have some of the downstream target genes that can contribute to the pathogenesis of the disease. The **Schmid type** of metaphyseal chondrodysplasia is less severe, although the radiographic appearance of the knees and extreme bowing of the lower limbs resemble signs seen in patients with familial hypophosphatemia. It is associated with defects in collagen type X, alpha 1, and the hip abnormalities are more debilitating than in Jansen metaphyseal chondrodysplasia. Patients with both types of metaphyseal chondrodysplasia have lifelong short stature.

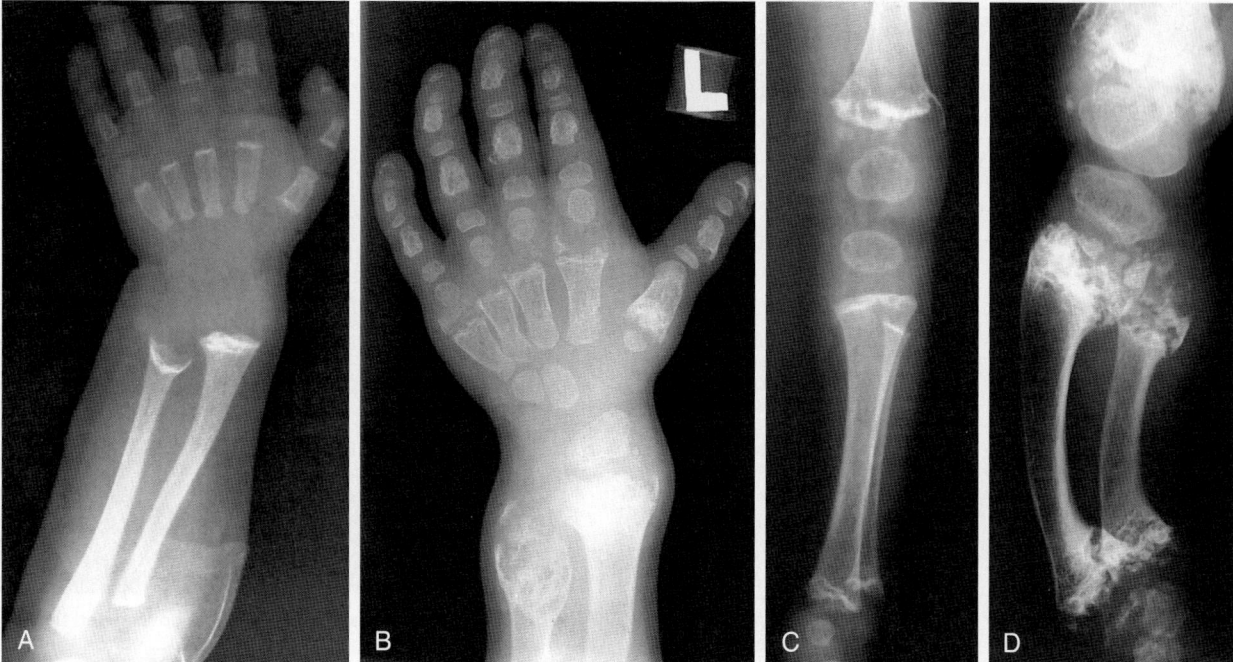

Figure 704-1 Radiographic findings in Jansen-type metaphyseal chondrodysplasia. **A,** At age 1 yr there is severe metaphyseal cupping and splaying at the wrists and also in the hand bones. **B,** At age 7 yr there is increasing metaphyseal change at the wrists with enlarged epiphysis; enlarged epiphyses with wide epiphyseal plates are also present in the hands. **C,** At age 1 yr there are severe metaphyseal irregularities at knees and ankles (femur, tibia, and fibula) and enlarged, rounded epiphyses. **D,** At age 7 yr there are severely fragmented, sclerotic metaphyses, wide epiphyseal plates, and enlarged epiphyses. Radiographic findings in Jansen-type metaphyseal chondrodysplasia. *(From Slovis TL, editor: Caffey's pediatric diagnostic imaging, ed 11, Philadelphia, 2008, Mosby.)*

Metaphyseal dysostosis, or **Pyle disease,** results from defects in endochondral bone formation and metaphyseal modeling. The long ends of bones are splayed, resulting in an "Erlenmeyer flask" defect. Short stature is not necessarily characteristic, and serum chemical levels are normal. Leonine features often develop if the facial bones are involved. Metaphyseal dysostosis may also be a clinical feature of Shwachman-Diamond syndrome, a rare autosomal recessive disorder characterized by neutropenia, pancreatic exocrine insufficiency, bone marrow dysfunction, and sometimes severe hematologic complications (see Chapter 448). Allogeneic bone marrow transplantation has been used as a therapeutic approach, with mixed results.

There are no other currently available forms of treatment known to be effective for the chondrodystrophies or dysostosis.

Bibliography is available at Expert Consult.

Chapter **705**
Hypophosphatasia
Russell W. Chesney

Hypophosphatasia, which radiographically resembles rickets, is defined by low serum alkaline phosphatase activity and mainly affects the skeleton and teeth. This inherited disorder (with both autosomal recessive and dominant forms) is an inborn error of metabolism in which activity of the tissue-nonspecific (liver, bone, kidney) alkaline phosphatase isoenzyme (TNSALP) is deficient, although activity of the intestinal and placental isoenzymes is normal. Single-point mutations of the gene prevent expression of the activity of this enzyme in vitro and indicate its necessity for normal skeletal mineralization. A large proportion of the more than 100 mutations of the gene identified to date are missense

mutations, although splice-site mutations, small deletions, and frameshift mutations also have been found. The only phenotype associated with these mutations is hypophosphatasia. Some patients have a regulatory defect involving this enzyme rather than a mutation.

There is considerable heterogeneity in the severity of the disease and 6 forms of the condition are described. Some cases appear at birth, and diagnosis has even been made in utero by radiographic examination of a fetus. The disease can appear in a lethal neonatal or perinatal form **(congenital lethal hypophosphatasia),** a severe infantile form, or a milder form occurring in childhood or late adolescence **(hypophosphatasia tarda)** (Fig. 705-1). The lethal form is characterized by a moth-eaten appearance at the ends of the long bones, severe deficiency of ossification throughout the skeleton, and marked shortening of the long bones. Patients with mild disease can present with bowing of the legs and variable statural shortening. Hypercalcemia is common in the neonatal and infantile forms, and because calcium accumulation by mature chondrocytes does not occur, patients might appear to have rickets.

Unusual clinical manifestations include wormian bones in the calvariae; poor calcification of the frontal, parietal, and occipital bones; and premature loss of deciduous or permanent teeth, due to hypoplasia of dental cementum. Because of the hypercalcemia in the infantile form, nephrocalcinosis is also found.

In the childhood form, bone pain, frequent fractures, and milder skeletal deformities are evident, as well as premature tooth loss. The metaphyseal defect consists of irregular ossification, punched-out areas, and metaphyseal cupping.

There is an adult form, manifesting in middle age, which is characterized by recurrent metaphyseal stress fractures and femoral pseudofractures. The lethal and infantile forms are autosomal recessive. The milder forms can be either autosomal recessive or dominant.

In hypophosphatasia, large quantities of phosphoethanolamine are found in the urine because this compound cannot be degraded in the absence of TNSALP activity. Plasma inorganic pyrophosphate and pyridoxal-5-phosphate levels are also elevated for the same reason. Pyridoxal-5-phosphate levels tend to be lower than normal in most

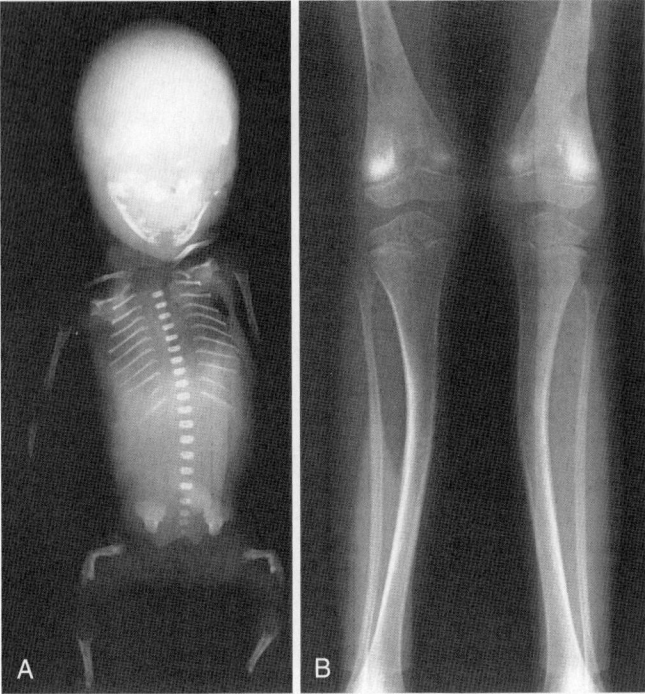

Figure 705-1 A, Fetus with congenital lethal hypophosphatasia showing thin wavy ribs, platyspondyly, missing cervical vertebrae, ossification, and bent femurs. **B,** A 7 yr old with hypophosphatasia tarda showing osteopenia, bent tibias, and punched-out metaphyseal lesions.

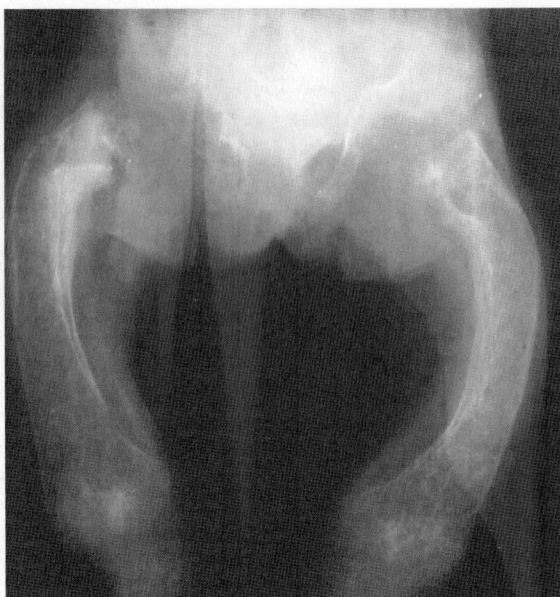

Figure 706-1 Hyperphosphatasia showing bowing and thickening of the diaphyses and osteopenia. *(From Slovis TL, editor: Caffey's pediatric diagnostic imaging, ed 11, Philadelphia, 2008, Mosby, Fig. 167-26, p. 2744.)*

other bone diseases and hence can aid in the differential diagnosis of hypophosphatasia. Seizures in patients with the lethal and infantile forms of the disease may be related to impaired pyridoxine metabolism. Although no satisfactory therapy has been found, infusion of plasma rich in alkaline phosphatase activity has been helpful in healing bone in short-term studies. Enzyme replacement therapy with recombinant human TNSALP improves skeletal healing and mineral content, pulmonary status, and overall physical activity. Bone marrow transplantation has been successful using donors with normal TNSALP values. The clinical course of this condition often improves spontaneously as an affected child matures, although early death from renal failure or flail chest leading to pneumonia can occur in the severe infantile form of the disorder.

Rare patients presenting with identical clinical and radiographic patterns have normal serum alkaline phosphatase activity. Their disease has been labeled **pseudohypophosphatasia** and might represent the presence of a mutant alkaline phosphatase isoenzyme that reacts to artificial substrates in an alkaline environment (in a test tube) but not in vivo with natural substrates.

Bibliography is available at Expert Consult.

Chapter 706
Hyperphosphatasia
Russell W. Chesney

Hyperphosphatasia is defined by excessive elevation of the bone isoenzyme of alkaline phosphatase in serum and significant growth failure. Osteoid proliferation in the subperiosteal portion of bone results in separation of the periosteum from the bone cortex. Bowing and thickening of the diaphyses are common, along with osteopenia

(Fig. 706-1). The disease usually has its onset by 2-3 yr of age, when painful deformity developing in the extremities leads to abnormal gait and sometimes fractures. Other common findings include pectus carinatum, kyphoscoliosis, and rib fraying. The skull is large, and the cranium is thickened (widened diploë) and may be deformed. Skull involvement can lead to progressive and profound hearing loss. Radiographically, the bony texture is variable; dense areas (showing a teased cotton-wool appearance) are interspersed with radiolucent areas and general demineralization. Long bones appear cylindrical, lose metaphyseal modeling, and contain pseudocysts that show a dense, bony halo. There exist several clinical phenotypes.

In this autosomal recessive disorder, serum levels of both calcium and phosphate are normal, whereas urinary leucine amino acid peptidase activity and serum acid phosphatase levels are increased. This disorder is often called **juvenile Paget disease** because, as in adult-onset Paget disease, calcitonin can reduce the rapid bone turnover found in this disorder; in children, the disorder is more generalized and symmetric. This disorder is distinct from Paget disease because histology of bone reveals a lack of normal cortical bone remodeling and an absence of the classic mosaic pattern of lamellar bone found in the adult condition. Hence, the term *juvenile Paget disease* is inappropriate. A case has been reported in which intense intravenous bisphosphonate (ibandronate) therapy administered over a 3 yr period arrested progression of idiopathic hyperphosphatasia, preventing deformity and disability and improving hearing.

Transient hyperphosphatasia occurs between 2 mo and 2 yr of age, has no associated manifestations other than some mild gastrointestinal symptoms; it is usually detected during routine (screening) laboratory evaluation for some unrelated complaint. Liver and bone isoenzyme fractions are elevated; there are no other manifestations of hepatic or bone dysfunction. Serum alkaline phosphatase values as high as 3,000-6,000 IU/L may be encountered. The cause is unknown. Resolution usually occurs within 4-6 mo.

Familial hyperphosphatemia, an autosomal dominant trait, is another benign condition that is distinguished from the transient infantile form by persistent and asymptomatic elevations of serum alkaline phosphatase levels.

A more serious autosomal dominant variant, expansile skeletal hyperplasia, is characterized by early-onset deafness, premature loss of teeth, progressive hyperostotic widening of long bones causing painful phalanges in the hands, episodic hypercalcemia, and enhanced bone remodeling. A defect in the gene that encodes receptor activation of nuclear factor γB is relevant. This gene appears to be necessary for osteogenesis, and the defect leads to increased activity of nuclear factor γB in the skeleton.

Bibliography is available at Expert Consult.

Chapter **707**
Osteoporosis
Russell W. Chesney

Osteoporosis, the most common bone disorder in adults, is relatively uncommon in children. This disorder is characterized by diminished bone volume and a marked increase in the prevalence of fractures. In contrast to osteomalacia, which shows undermineralization and normal bone volume, histologic sections of bone in all forms of osteoporosis reveal a normal degree of mineralization but a reduction in the volume of bone, especially trabecular bone (vertebral bone). There is a reduction in trabecular bone turnover as well. In osteoporosis, by definition, there is a reduced amount of bone tissue (termed *osteopenia*), which is associated with atraumatic (pathologic) fractures. Osteoporosis in children may be primary or secondary (Table 707-1). The primary osteoporoses can be divided into heritable disorders of connective tissue, including osteogenesis imperfect (see Chapter 701), Bruck syndrome, osteoporosis-pseudoglioma syndrome, Ehlers-Danlos syndrome (see Chapter 659), Marfan syndrome (see Chapter 702), homocystinuria, and idiopathic juvenile osteoporosis. Secondary forms of osteoporosis include various neuromuscular disorders, chronic illness, endocrine disorders, and drug-induced and inborn errors of metabolism, including lysinuric protein intolerance and Gaucher disease.

When no obvious primary or secondary cause can be detected, **idiopathic juvenile osteoporosis** should be considered, especially if the following clinical features are evident: onset before puberty, long-bone and lower back pain, vertebral fractures, long-bone and metatarsal fractures, a washed-out appearance of the spine and appendicular skeleton, and improvement after puberty. Trabecular bones such as the spine and metatarsals are particularly affected by atraumatic fractures.

In general, blood values of minerals, vitamin D metabolites, alkaline phosphatase, and parathyroid hormone are normal. Evaluation of bone mineral content and bone density by dual-energy x-ray absorptiometry or, less often, quantitative CT shows markedly reduced values. Several modes of therapy (including oral calcium supplements, calcitriol, bisphosphonates, and calcitonin) have been used with some success in individual conditions, but the effect of these treatments is difficult to gauge because spontaneous recovery occurs after the onset of puberty in more than 75% of cases.

Osteoporosis-pseudoglioma is an autosomal recessive disorder manifested by variable age at onset, low bone mass, fractures in childhood, and abnormal eye development; the defective gene has been

Table 707-1	Risks for Osteoporosis

ENDOCRINE DISORDERS	**CONNECTIVE TISSUE/BONE DISORDERS**
Female Hypogonadism	Juvenile osteoporosis
Turner syndrome	Osteogenesis imperfecta
Hypothalamic amenorrhea (athletic triad)	Ehlers-Danlos syndrome
Anorexia nervosa	Marfan syndrome
Premature and primary ovarian failure	Homocystinuria
Depot medroxyprogesterone acetate therapy	Fibrous dysplasia
Estrogen receptor α (*ESR1*) mutations	Previous or recurrent low impact fractures
Hyperprolactinemia	Early onset osteoporosis with *WNT1* mutations
Male Hypogonadism	X-linked osteoporosis with fractures with *PLS3* mutations
Primary gonadal failure (Klinefelter syndrome)	
Secondary gonadal failure (idiopathic hypogonadotropic hypogonadism)	**DRUGS**
Delayed puberty	Alcohol
Hyperthyroidism	Heparin
Hyperparathyroidism	Glucocorticosteroids
Hypercortisolism (therapeutic or Cushing disease)	Thyroxine
Growth hormone deficiency	Anticonvulsants
Thyrotoxicosis	Gonadotropin-releasing hormone agonists
	Cyclosporine
INFLAMMATORY DISORDERS	Chemotherapy
Dermatomyositis	Cigarettes
Chronic hepatitis	
Systemic lupus erythematosus	**MISCELLANEOUS DISORDERS**
	Immobilization (cerebral palsy, spinal muscular atrophy, Duchenne dystrophy)
GASTROINTESTINAL DISORDERS	Rheumatoid arthritis
Malabsorption syndromes (cystic fibrosis, celiac disease, biliary atresia)	Renal disease
True or perceived milk intolerance	Glycogen storage disease type 1
Inflammatory bowel disease	Chronic hepatitis
Chronic obstructive jaundice	Low calcium dietary intake
Primary biliary cirrhosis and other cirrhoses	Gaucher disease
Alactasia	Severe congenital neutropenia
Subtotal gastrectomy	
BONE MARROW DISORDERS	
Bone marrow transplant	
Lymphoma	
Leukemia	
Hemolytic anemias (sickle cell anemia, thalassemia)	
Systemic mastocytosis	

mapped to chromosome 11q12-13. The mutation is a loss of function in the gene for low-density lipoprotein receptor-related protein 5. Interestingly, gain-of-function mutations result in a gene product that increases bone density.

The life-cycle implications of either significant demineralization or osteoporosis in childhood need to be stressed. Events in childhood influence peak bone mass, and late adolescence is a period of rapid bone mineral accretion. Peak bone mass is achieved by 20-35 yr of age (depending on the bone measured), and the contribution during childhood is considerable. A number of measures influence bone mass: vitamin D (400-800 IU daily), calcium intake (≥1,200 mg/day in adolescents), and weightbearing exercise throughout childhood. Weightbearing exercise enhances bone formation and reduces bone resorption. Other factors that can prevent acquisition of peak bone mass include use of alcohol and tobacco. Excellent sources of dietary calcium include mainly dairy products but also bony fish, green vegetables, and calcium-supplemented drinks (e.g., orange juice). Yogurt and cheeses can be used in lactase-deficient children. Because it appears that adult-onset osteoporosis is the result of a number of genetic factors, thus forming a complex trait interaction, specific interventions during childhood to influence bone mass are not available.

The treatment of secondary osteoporosis is best achieved by treating the underlying disorder when feasible. Hypogonadism should be treated with hormone replacement therapy, especially in thin athletic women (see Chapter 691). Calcium intake should be increased to 1,500-2,000 mg/day. In glucocorticoid-induced osteoporosis, an emphasis on the lowest possible dose to prevent disease activity (inflammatory bowel disease) with alternate-day or topical therapy and the use of inhaled glucocorticoids in asthma is essential. Special diets for inborn errors of metabolism are also appropriate. Celiac disease may be overrepresented in adults with osteoporosis and should be screened for and treated appropriately (see Chapter 338.2). Treatment with bisphosphonates that inhibit bone resorption in certain secondary (glucocorticoid-induced) and adult-onset osteoporosis has been successful. Bisphosphonate therapy is also beneficial in osteogenesis imperfecta and cerebral palsy.

Bibliography is available at Expert Consult.

Rehabilitation Medicine

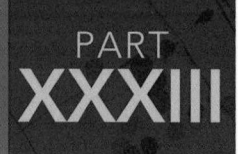

PART XXXIII

Chapter **708**

Principles of Rehabilitation Medicine

Dennis J. Matthews

Pediatric rehabilitative medicine is dedicated to improving the lives and daily function of children with acute and chronic disabilities and to maximizing their potential. It is based on an understanding of the importance of early intervention among those children identified as needing or potentially needing additional support; the development of simpler, culturally relevant surveillance systems that function well in all nations and within all populations within nations; and expanding intervention programs in the scope of services offered and reach of programs.

EPIDEMIOLOGY

The Centers for Disease Control estimates that the prevalence of developmental disabilities in the United States increased by 17% between 1997-1999 and 2006-2008 (Table 708-1). Over the past 3 decades, mortality rates have plummeted among children in lower- and middle-income nations (see Chapter 1). A least a portion of those who formerly would not have survived early childhood have disabilities; it is estimated that more than 200 million children from lower- and middle-income nations have developmental delays or disabilities.

APPROACH

Rehabilitation requires knowledge of the enabling/disabling process and the interrelationships of pathology, impairment, functional ability, and social participation, superimposed on normal development. Rehabilitation management of children with impairments requires the integration and identification of their functional capabilities and selection of the best rehabilitation intervention strategies. A well-designed rehabilitation program can reverse many disabling conditions and can help patients cope with deficits that cannot be reversed by medical care. *The goal of rehabilitation is to maximize an individual's function and participation in society.*

Pediatric rehabilitation medicine uses an interdisciplinary approach to address the prevention, diagnosis, treatment, and management of congenital and childhood-onset impairments, including related or secondary medical, physical, functional, cognitive, psychosocial, and vocational limitations or conditions, with an understanding of the life course of the disability. It requires identifying and managing common pediatric rehabilitation medical conditions and complications, including nutrition, bowel management, bladder management, gastroesophageal reflux, skin protection, pulmonary hygiene and protection, sensory impairments, sleep disorders, spasticity, swallowing dysfunction, and behavioral problems.

Therapeutic treatment includes (1) early intervention, (2) age-appropriate functional training, (3) programs of therapy, (4) play, (5) therapeutic exercise, (6) electrical stimulation and other modalities, (7) communication strategies, (8) oral motor interventions, (9) educational and vocational planning, (10) transitional planning, (11) adjustment to disability support, and (12) prevention strategies.

SCOPE OF PRACTICE

Rehabilitation management of common pediatric problems includes musculoskeletal disorders and trauma, cerebral palsy, spinal dysraphism and other congenital anomalies, spinal cord injury, traumatic and other acquired brain injuries (see Chapter 710), limb deficiency/amputation, neuromuscular disorders, peripheral nerve injuries, and spasticity management.

A significant deleterious effect of childhood disability is inactivity. This is defined as a reduced functional capacity of musculoskeletal and other body systems. It should be considered a distinct diagnosis from the original condition that has led to a curtailment of normal physical function. The main adverse effects are muscle atrophy and weakness, joint contracture, and immobilization osteoporosis.

PREVENTION OF MUSCLE WEAKNESS

Muscle weakness can be reduced by prescribing progressive resistance, stretching, and aerobic exercises. A minimum of once-a-day muscle contraction at 30-50% of maximal strength for 3-5 min, 3 times per wk for a single muscle group, may suffice to prevent muscle loss and weakness. For chronic disuse atrophy with weakness and stiffness, strengthening and stretching exercises may be required for many months, and even then, the child is unlikely to gain normal strength and range of motion.

Stretching to maintain optimal muscle resting length as well as viscoelastic properties is important for maintaining muscle function. Muscles that cross 2 joints, such as the hamstring, gastrocnemius, biceps, and long back extensor muscles, are particularly prone to stiffness. Once a contracture has developed, the treatment is active and passive range-of-motion exercises combined with a sustained terminal stretch on a daily basis. The daily stretching can prevent the loss of sarcomeres in series of immobilized muscles and maintain elongation properties of muscle fibers and surrounding connective tissue, maintaining range of motion.

Stretching techniques include ballistic, static, or passive and neuromuscular facilitation. Prevention of injury and treatment of specific joint injury, as well as the presence and effects of pain or muscle spasms, require modification. The intensity should be a mild degree of tightness without discomfort. Static stretches are held 15-60 sec. Passive and neuromuscular facilitation is a 6 sec contraction followed by 10-30 sec of assisted stretch. Stretching is generally more successful when used in combination with the application of deep heat (i.e., ultrasound). Sustained stretching lasting 2 hr can be obtained by splinting (orthotics, serial casting). In patients with spasticity, chemical denervation (botulinum toxin, phenol blocks) may improve positioning inside the cast or orthotic to improve the tolerance for wearing.

Dynamic splinting provides tension in the desired direction with the use of springs or elastic bands. This type of splinting is often used in the hand and arm because it allows a measure of function while providing stretching. To achieve optimal joint position, it is sometimes necessary to surgically lengthen the contracted tendon.

Maintenance of skeletal mass depends largely on mechanical loading applied to the bone by muscle pull and the force of gravity. Bone mass only increases with repeated loading and increase in muscle strength. Disuse osteoporosis can be prevented by regular use of isotonic exercises, weight bearing, and functional training. Passive loading and standing are of little benefit.

A variety of therapeutic exercise techniques have been developed to address central nervous system dysfunction. Most commonly used are neurodevelopmental techniques using reflex inhibitory patterns to inhibit increased tone along with advanced postural reactions to stimulate recovery. Other therapeutic programs include proprioceptive neuromuscular facilitation. There is no convincing evidence that any

Table 708-1	Specific Developmental Disabilities in U.S. Children Ages 3-17 Yr
DISABILITY	**PERCENT CHANGE BETWEEN 1997-1999 AND 2006-2008**
Any developmental disability	17.1%*
Attention-deficit/ hyperactivity disorder	33.0%*
Autism	289.5%*
Blind/unable to see at all	18.2%
Cerebral palsy	—
Moderate to profound hearing loss	−30.9%
Learning disability	5.5%
Intellectual disability	−1.5%
Seizures, past 12 mo	9.1%
Stuttered or stammered, past 12 mo	3.1%
Other developmental delay	24.7%*

*Statistically significant trend over 4 time periods: 1997-1999, 2000-2002, 2003-2005, and 2006-2008.
   From Centers for Disease Control and Prevention, National Center for Health Statistics, NHIS, 1997-2008, https://iacc.hhs.gov/events/2011/slides_coleen _boyle_071911.pdf.

of these methods actually alter the natural history of recovery. These approaches to therapy seem to be most useful in enabling the child to develop compensatory techniques. Using these methods, patients improve performance in and gain independence with such tasks as making transfers, stretching, bed mobility, and safe ambulation.

OTHER ASSIST DEVICES

Rehabilitation often includes prescribing age-appropriate assistive devices and technology to assist environmental accessibility, including orthotics, prosthetics, wheelchairs, positioning, activities of daily living aids, interfaces and environmental controls, and augmentative communication devices. The goal of all assistive devices is to overcome the limitations and improve function and community participation.

Rehabilitation management of children with developmental or acquired disabilities is best accomplished through a medical home and team approach seeking to maximize the child's level of motor, intellectual, emotional, and social functioning.

Bibliography is available at Expert Consult.

Chapter 709

Evaluation of the Child for Rehabilitative Services

Michael A. Alexander

CHILD CHARACTERISTICS

A rehabilitation evaluation starts with *determining physiologic impairments and strengths.* The strengths may turn out to be pivotal in how well the individual compensates for his or her actual impairments. Physiologic impairments are the biologic shortfalls, which limit the

child. Many assessment tools are available and professional organizations have developed compendiums of such tools.

The assessment begins with **cognitive issues**. Where is the child in the developmental spectrum in language, social, and emotional abilities? How does the child function in the family, school, and community? Does the presence of an impairment act as an impediment to social acceptance? Poor impulse control, stuttering, or speaking loudly, perhaps because of hearing loss, will all distance a child from other children of the same age group.

Sensory issues need to be evaluated. Are vision, hearing, and other senses present and meeting the needs of the child? Impairment of the sense of touch and position sense may affect the child's extremity function, particularly in the area of fine motor activities. Deficiencies in these skills can also affect how others perceive the child.

For a child who has significant disabilities, the evaluation team needs to include educators, neuropsychologists, social workers, physical therapists, occupational therapists, speech therapists, augmentative communication and device technicians, and seating and adaptive equipment specialists, as well as the physician. The pediatric rehabilitation evaluation is a process that not only looks at the actual impairments but looks to see how they affect the functioning of the individual. Functional substitutions and adaptive equipment and strategies need to be applied by the team to minimize the overall impact of the child's impairments on the child's function, maturation, and separation from family and, ultimately, on the child's function as an adult.

Upper-extremity function is assessed to determine strength, range of motion, and agility. Obviously, weakness of both the arms and legs will result in a greater degree of dysfunction than weakness of only the arms or only the legs. Lower-extremity function affects movement in other environments as well.

For one child, a manual wheelchair may enhance mobility. But children with arm weakness may need electric wheelchairs, with their associated complications. Problems of accessibility, transport, and cost can become significant issues for the family. Fine motor and prehension (the highly complex motor and sensory tasks performed by the hand) tasks are closely assessed because some of these children may need to rely on their ability to interface with access joysticks and computers and strength in these areas may compensate for physical weaknesses.

Skeletal deformities, range-of-motion limitations, and contractures may affect gross motor function, balance, sitting, walking, and climbing. Scoliosis, kyphosis, and pelvic obliquity may limit sitting balance and tolerance, which can secondarily affect upper-extremity function and the amount of time a child is able to socialize.

FAMILY CHARACTERISTICS

The education, vocation, and mental well-being of the parents or caregivers have a dramatic impact on the child. We know that if a child with impairment is to reach maximum potential, a stable and loving family structure facilitates the child's outcome. Does the family have other stressors, such as illness, death, divorce, and legal problems? What are their health care resources?

THE PHYSICAL ENVIRONMENT

Environment assessment begins with the child's room and home. Access to and inside the home should be discussed. How is this child transported? If the child uses power mobility, does the chair travel with the child or does it need to reside at the school or home or elsewhere? How is the child mobile in environments in which the power chair is not available? Is the transport of the child the problem? What is the adequacy, cost, and reliability of the van that is being used by the family? How the child gets in and out of the wheelchair is a significant part of the evaluation. Does the child assist with this, or is the child totally and passively dependent on an adult to move the child from, for example, a toilet seat back to the wheelchair?

In the school, does the child have access to all of the building and can the child participate in all activities in the building, such as those in the art and music rooms, cafeteria, science lab, and stage? Does the child participate in clubs, teams, and other activities outside of the home?

THE PREVIOUSLY HEALTHY CHILD

For children who have established themselves in the general community and functioned in their environment in a normal capacity but then acquire a significant impairment, it becomes incredibly important to understand what their world looked like before they were affected by this new set of problems. If the child is old enough to remember what life had been like, the loss of function can be devastating. Coping with "what could have been" coupled with what was lost will require the help of skilled psychosocial clinicians.

Chapter **710**
Severe Traumatic Brain Injury

Linda E. Krach

Medical rehabilitation is an integral part of the process of assisting families and their children in transitioning from acute medical care after a severe traumatic brain injury (TBI) to reintegration into the community. Table 710-1 lists the quality of care indicators for inpatient pediatric TBI rehabilitation based on a review of evidence and the application of the RAND/UCLA modified Delphi Method.

ETIOLOGY

The cause of TBI varies by age. For young children, ages 0-4 yr, falls and nonaccidental trauma are the most common causes. The major cause of TBI among adolescents >14 yr is motor vehicle traffic. TBI is more common in males than females at all ages.

PATHOPHYSIOLOGY

Brain injury from trauma results from a combination of primary and secondary injury. The mechanism of injury can be different in children because of factors that differentiate them from adults; very young children have open sutures, so they can accommodate some increase in intracranial pressure by an increase in their head circumference or widening of the sutures. Compared with adults, children also have a larger head size compared to their neck musculature, higher brain water content, and less myelination, all of which are thought to contribute to greater brain distortion with resultant injury.

Table 710-1	Quality of Care Indicators for Pediatric Rehabilitation Care After Traumatic Brain Injury

- Dedicated pediatric specialty unit that has at least 1 inpatient with a TBI 90% of the time
- Physical accommodations for family to remain on-site 24 hr/day
- Age-appropriate therapeutic and adaptive equipment
- On-site classroom
- Medical director experienced in pediatric rehabilitation medicine
- Therapists with pediatric training/certification
- Pediatric clinical psychologist, at least 1 certified rehabilitation registered nurse
- 24 hr access to:
  - pharmacy
  - respiratory therapy
  - neurosurgery
  - neurology
  - radiology

ACUTE REHABILITATION

The acute rehabilitation course for children with severe TBI includes addressing multiple medical issues related to the injury in addition to the provision of rehabilitation services. One of these issues is the possibility of seizure activity. Although it is common practice to initiate prophylactic anticonvulsant therapy early after injury, it is appropriate to consider discontinuing this treatment if late seizures have not occurred. Among children, early seizures do not correlate with the later development of epilepsy. The severity of injury, the presence of severe edema, and a very young age at injury increase the likelihood of the later development of **posttraumatic seizures**.

Sleep disturbance is common after TBI and can have an effect on the individual's ability to function (Fig. 710-1). Various approaches, including sleep hygiene, sleep aids, strategic stimulants, cognitive behavioral therapy, strategic caffeine, and naps, can be tried for both the initiation and maintenance of sleep. Other chronotherapy techniques (coordinating the biologic rhythms of a child's body with his/her medical therapy) may be necessary to address sleep–wake cycle abnormalities.

Children with severe TBI may also experience **autonomic dysfunction** characterized by elevated temperature, heart rate, respiratory rate, and blood pressure, accompanied by diaphoresis and posturing. Autonomic dysfunction is a diagnosis of exclusion and is associated with poor outcome after acquired brain injury in children. Autonomic dysfunction develops in approximately 13% of children with acquired brain injury, 10% of those with TBI, and 31% of those with injury as a result of cardiac arrest. Autonomic dysfunction is associated with longer hospital lengths of stay and poorer outcomes.

Acute inpatient rehabilitation emphasizes functional goals and community reintegration. The child and family are integral members of the rehabilitation team. Community reintegration involves careful consultation and planning with the school system to facilitate the transition from hospital to school. In the United States, federal law requires that a physician document that a child had a TBI to qualify for special education services under this disability category. Rehabilitation team consultation with the school team is essential for optimal and expeditious transition back to the school setting. Participation in school is essential for peer interaction and a step toward normalization of the child's life. Schools can adapt to the child's needs rather than providing services in an isolating homebound manner.

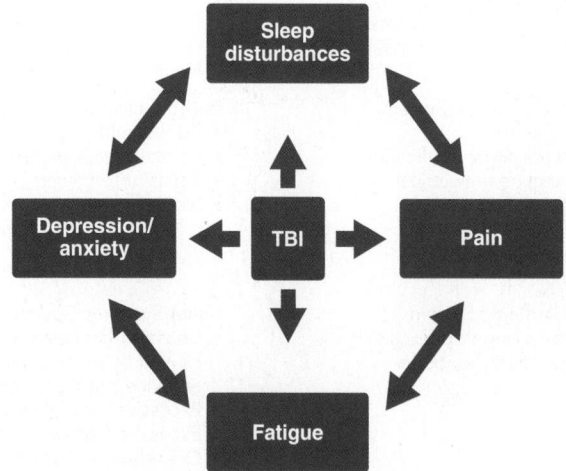

Figure 710-1 Relationship of sleep-related issues among patients recovering from traumatic brain injury. *(From Viola-Saltzman M, Watson NFL: Traumatic brain injury and sleep disorders. Neurol Clin 30(4):1299–1312, 2012, Flowchart 2.)*

OUTCOMES ASSOCIATED WITH SEVERE TRAUMATIC BRAIN INJURY

The most disabling consequences of TBI are cognitive, particularly those associated with executive function.

In severe TBI, cognition is often the most affected area of functioning and outcomes are associated with preinjury adaptive functioning and family function. Attentional skills may remain impaired in children 10 yr after sustaining a TBI. Subsets of attention appear to be more impaired after TBI, particularly divided and sustained attention.

Other areas of long-term impairment of cognitive performance after pediatric TBI include overall intellectual performance, learning, metamemory, working memory, social competence, and a variety of behavioral concerns. Impairments have been noted in ability to perform self-care activities, communicate, and participate in community and social activities.

PEDIATRIC TRAUMATIC BRAIN INJURY AND PLASTICITY

In the past there has been an assumption that sustaining a TBI at a young age compared to more advanced age would allow for better outcomes because of plasticity. In fact, plasticity may actually be related to poorer outcomes in those injured at a very young age. The major task of childhood is development and learning; a significant TBI can impact the child's ability to learn. Likewise, children do not have over-learned material to fall back on as do adults. There is some evidence that the anticipated changes associated with brain maturation, including cortical thinning of specific regions, do not occur in children who have had TBI at a young age. There are potentially critical periods in development during which a child is more at risk for the effects of a brain injury. Because children are expected to develop cognitive skills over time, the full extent of the impairment from injury might not be recognized until a significant amount of time has elapsed following the injury. For example, if executive function were impaired, one wouldn't expect to see the manifestations of that until adolescence.

Bibliography is available at Expert Consult.

Chapter **711**

Spinal Cord Injury and Autonomic Crisis Management

David W. Pruitt and Mary A. McMahon

EVALUATION

The most accurate way to assess a patient who has sustained a **spinal cord injury (SCI)** is by performing a standardized physical examination as endorsed by the International Standards for Neurological and Functional Classification of Spinal Cord Injury (Fig. 711-1). These standards provide the basic definitions of the terms utilized by clinicians caring for patients with SCI. Caution is recommended in utilizing and trusting the anorectal examination portion of this examination in children and youth because of poor interrater reliability.

CLINICAL MANIFESTATIONS

Children with neurologic levels of injury at T6 or above are particularly at risk for interruption and decentralization of the autonomic nervous system. The most common manifestations include bradycardia, hypotension, temperature dysregulation, and, once spinal shock has resolved, **autonomic dysreflexia (AD).** Children and adolescents with cervical and upper level SCI have lower baseline blood pressure compared with the general population. Blood pressure elevations of 20-40 mm Hg above baseline may be considered a sign of AD. AD is a sustained sympathetic response in relation to a noxious stimulus *below* the level of injury. Symptoms resulting from AD typically include hypertension, bradycardia, headache, and flushing of skin above the level of injury. Noxious stimuli are most often localized to bladder or rectal distention, but may include a number of other causes (Table 711-1). Identification and treatment of the noxious stimulus is

Table 711-1	Potential Etiologies of Noxious Stimuli Causing Autonomic Dysreflexia

Urinary System	Gastrointestinal System	Integumentary System
• Bladder distention	• Bowel distention	• Constrictive clothing, shoes, or orthotics
• Bladder or kidney stones	• Bowel impaction	• Blisters
• Blocked/kinked catheter	• Gallstones	• Burns, sunburn, or frostbite
• Detrusor sphincter dyssynergia	• Appendicitis	• Ingrown toenail
• Urinary tract infection	• Gastric ulcers	• Insect bites
• Urologic instrumentation	• Gastritis	• Pressure ulcers
• Shock wave lithotripsy	• Gastrointestinal instrumentation	
	• Hemorrhoids	
Musculoskeletal System	**Reproductive System–Male**	**Reproductive System–Female**
• Fractures	• Epididymitis	• Menstruation
• Heterotopic ossification	• Scrotal compression (sitting on scrotum)	• Pregnancy, especially labor and delivery
• Functional electrical stimulation	• Sexual intercourse	• Vaginitis
	• Sexually transmitted infections	• Sexual intercourse
		• Sexually transmitted infections
Hematologic System	**Other Systemic Causes**	
• Deep vein thrombosis	• Boosting (an episode of autonomic dysreflexia intentionally caused by an athlete with spinal cord injury in an attempt to enhance physical performance).	
• Pulmonary embolus	• Excessive alcohol intake	
	• Excessive caffeine or diuretic intake	
	• Over-the-counter or prescribed stimulants	
	• Substance abuse	

From Consortium for Spinal Cord Medicine: Acute management of autonomic dysreflexia: individuals with spinal cord injury presenting to health-care facilities, Washington, DC, 2001, Paralyzed Veterans of America, pp 10-11.

Patient Name _____ Date/Time of Exam _____

Examiner Name _____ Signature _____

RIGHT

MOTOR KEY MUSCLES

SENSORY KEY SENSORY POINTS
Light Touch (LTR)   Pin Prick (PPR)

C2
C3
C4

UER (Upper Extremity Right)

Elbow flexors **C5**
Wrist extensors **C6**
Elbow extensors **C7**
Finger flexors **C8**
Finger abductors (little finger) **T1**

Comments (Non-key Muscle? Reason for NT? Pain?):

T2
T3
T4
T5
T6
T7
T8
T9
T10
T11
T12
L1

LER (Lower Extremity Right)

Hip flexors **L2**
Knee extensors **L3**
Ankle dorsiflexors **L4**
Long toe extensors **L5**
Ankle plantar flexors **S1**

S2
S3
S4-5

(VAC) Voluntary anal contraction (Yes/No)

RIGHT TOTALS (MAXIMUM)   (50)   (56)   (56)

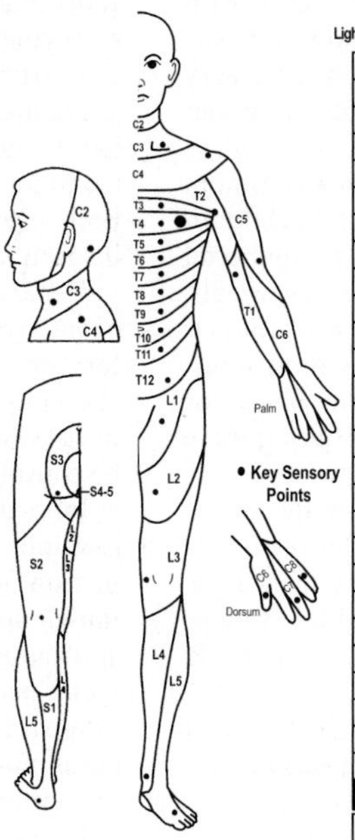

LEFT

SENSORY KEY SENSORY POINTS
Light Touch (LTL)   Pin Prick (PPL)

MOTOR KEY MUSCLES

C2
C3
C4

C5 Elbow flexors
C6 Wrist extensors
C7 Elbow extensors
C8 Finger flexors
T1 Finger abductors (little finger)

UEL (Upper Extremity Left)

T2
T3
T4
T5
T6
T7
T8
T9
T10
T11
T12
L1

MOTOR
(SCORING ON REVERSE SIDE)
0 = total paralysis
1 = palpable or visible contraction
2 = active movement, gravity eliminated
3 = active movement, against gravity
4 = active movement, against some resistance
5 = active movement, against full resistance
5* = normal corrected for pain/disuse
NT = not testable

SENSORY
(SCORING ON REVERSE SIDE)
0 = absent   2 = normal
1 = altered   NT = not testable

L2 Hip flexors
L3 Knee extensors
L4 Ankle dorsiflexors
L5 Long toe extensors
S1 Ankle plantar flexors

LEL (Lower Extremity Left)

S2
S3
S4-5

(DAP) Deep anal pressure (Yes/No)

LEFT TOTALS (MAXIMUM)   (56)   (56)   (50)

• Key Sensory Points

Palm

Dorsum

MOTOR SUBSCORES

UER ___ + UEL ___ = UEMS TOTAL ___   LER ___ + LEL ___ = LEMS TOTAL ___
MAX (25)   (25)   (50)   MAX (25)   (25)   (50)

SENSORY SUBSCORES

LTR ___ + LTL ___ = LT TOTAL ___   PPR ___ + PPL ___ = PP TOTAL ___
MAX (56)   (56)   (112)   MAX (56)   (56)   (112)

NEUROLOGICAL LEVELS	R	L	3. NEUROLOGICAL LEVEL OF INJURY (NLI)	4. COMPLETE OR INCOMPLETE? Incomplete = Any sensory or motor function in S4-5	ZONE OF PARTIAL PRESERVATION Most caudal level with any innervation	R	L
Steps 1-5 for classification as on reverse					SENSORY		
1. SENSORY				5. ASIA IMPAIRMENT SCALE (AIS)	MOTOR		
2. MOTOR							

This form may be copied freely but should not be altered without permission from the American Spinal Injury Association.   REV 02/13

Muscle Function Grading

0 = total paralysis

1 = palpable or visible contraction

2 = active movement, full range of motion (ROM) with gravity eliminated

3 = active movement, full ROM against gravity

4 = active movement, full ROM against gravity and moderate resistance in a muscle specific position

5 = (normal) active movement, full ROM against gravity and full resistance in a functional muscle position expected from an otherwise unimpaired person

5* = (normal) active movement, full ROM against gravity and sufficient resistance to be considered normal if identified inhibiting factors (i.e. pain, disuse) were not present

NT = not testable (i.e. due to immobilization, severe pain such that the patient cannot be graded, amputation of limb, or contracture of > 50% of the normal range of motion)

Sensory Grading

0 = Absent

1 = Altered, either decreased/impaired sensation or hypersensitivity

2 = Normal

NT = Not testable

Non Key Muscle Functions (optional)

May be used to assign a motor level to differentiate AIS B vs. C

Movement	Root level
Shoulder: Flexion, extension, abduction, adduction, internal and external rotation **Elbow:** Supination	C5
Elbow: Pronation **Wrist:** Flexion	C6
Finger: Flexion at proximal joint, extension. **Thumb:** Flexion, extension and abduction in plane of thumb	C7
Finger: Flexion at MCP joint **Thumb:** Opposition, adduction and abduction perpendicular to palm	C8
Finger: Abduction of the index finger	T1
Hip: Adduction	L2
Hip: External rotation	L3
Hip: Extension, abduction, internal rotation **Knee:** Flexion **Ankle:** Inversion and eversion **Toe:** MP and IP extension	L4
Hallux and Toe: DIP and PIP flexion and abduction	L5
Hallux: Adduction	S1

ASIA Impairment Scale (AIS)

A = Complete. No sensory or motor function is preserved in the sacral segments S4-5.

B = Sensory Incomplete. Sensory but not motor function is preserved below the neurological level and includes the sacral segments S4-5 (light touch or pin prick at S4-5 or deep anal pressure) AND no motor function is preserved more than three levels below the motor level on either side of the body.

C = Motor Incomplete. Motor function is preserved below the neurological level**, and more than half of key muscle functions below the neurological level of injury (NLI) have a muscle grade less than 3 (Grades 0-2).

D = Motor Incomplete. Motor function is preserved below the neurological level**, and at least half (half or more) of key muscle functions below the NLI have a muscle grade ≥ 3.

E = Normal. If sensation and motor function as tested with the ISNCSCI are graded as normal in all segments, and the patient had prior deficits, then the AIS grade is E. Someone without an initial SCI does not receive an AIS grade.

** For an individual to receive a grade of C or D, i.e. motor incomplete status, they must have either (1) voluntary anal sphincter contraction or (2) sacral sensory sparing with sparing of motor function more than three levels below the motor level for that side of the body. The International Standards at this time allows even non-key muscle function more than 3 levels below the motor level to be used in determining motor incomplete status (AIS B versus C).

NOTE: When assessing the extent of motor sparing below the level for distinguishing between AIS B and C, the **motor level** on each side is used; whereas to differentiate between AIS C and D (based on proportion of key muscle functions with strength grade 3 or greater) the **neurological level of injury** is used.

Steps in Classification

The following order is recommended for determining the classification of individuals with SCI.

1. Determine sensory levels for right and left sides.
The sensory level is the most caudal, intact dermatome for both pin prick and light touch sensation.

2. Determine motor levels for right and left sides.
Defined by the lowest key muscle function that has a grade of at least 3 (on supine testing), providing the key muscle functions represented by segments above that level are judged to be intact (graded as a 5).
Note: in regions where there is no myotome to test, the motor level is presumed to be the same as the sensory level, if testable motor function above that level is also normal.

3. Determine the neurological level of injury (NLI)
This refers to the most caudal segment of the cord with intact sensation and antigravity (3 or more) muscle function strength, provided that there is normal (intact) sensory and motor function rostrally respectively.
The NLI is the most cephalad of the sensory and motor levels determined in steps 1 and 2.

4. Determine whether the injury is Complete or Incomplete.
(i.e. absence or presence of sacral sparing)
If voluntary anal contraction = No AND all S4-5 sensory scores = 0 AND deep anal pressure = No, then injury is Complete.
Otherwise, injury is Incomplete.

5. Determine ASIA Impairment Scale (AIS) Grade:

Is injury Complete?   If YES, AIS=A and can record ZPP (lowest dermatome or myotome on each side with some preservation)

NO ↓

Is injury Motor Complete?   If YES, AIS=B
NO ↓ (No=voluntary anal contraction OR motor function more than three levels below the motor level on a given side, if the patient has sensory incomplete classification)

Are at least half (half or more) of the key muscles below the neurological level of injury graded 3 or better?

NO ↓   YES ↓
AIS=C   AIS=D

If sensation and motor function is normal in all segments, AIS=E
Note: AIS E is used in follow-up testing when an individual with a documented SCI has recovered normal function. If at initial testing no deficits are found, the individual is neurologically intact; the ASIA Impairment Scale does not apply.

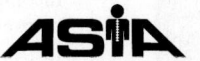

ASIA
INTERNATIONAL STANDARDS FOR NEUROLOGICAL
CLASSIFICATION OF SPINAL CORD INJURY

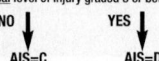

ISCOS INTERNATIONAL SPINAL CORD SOCIETY

Figure 711-1 American Spinal Injury Association flow sheet. *(From American Spinal Injury Association/International Medical Society of Paraplegia. International standards for neurological and functional classification of spinal cord injury patients. Chicago, 2013, http://www.asia-spinalinjury.org/elearning/ISNCSCI.php.)*

typically associated with resolution of symptoms without the use of antihypertensive medication. If necessary, antihypertensive agents with a rapid onset and short duration, including nifedipine and nitropaste, are advocated (Fig. 711-2). Emergent management of AD is necessary owing to the risk of cerebrovascular accident and additional organ damage as a result of sustained hypertension.

Deep venous thrombosis and **pulmonary embolism** are common, potentially life-threatening conditions in patients with SCI. In children and youth, deep venous thromboses are more common in postpubertal children. Prophylactic treatment, including low-molecular-weight heparin and calf compression pumps, during acute rehabilitation is recommended. Late-occurring deep venous thrombosis most commonly occurs with increased immobilization related to illness or surgery and prophylactic measures should be considered during these situations as well.

Following SCI, the **bladder** can be **areflexic** or **hyperreflexic** and detrusor sphincter dyssynergia is possible. Clean intermittent catheterization is typically used 4-6 times/day to keep bladder volumes below capacity. Anticholinergic medications can improve bladder storage. Asymptomatic bacteriuria, without vesicoureteral reflux, is generally not treated.

Bowel continence requires optimal consistency through the use of diet and medications and planned evacuation, employing aids includ-

ing gastrocolic reflex, digital stimulation, suppositories, and enemas. Individuals with SCI have increased risk for dysphagia, delayed gastric emptying, ileus, gastric ulceration, pancreatitis, and superior mesenteric artery syndrome.

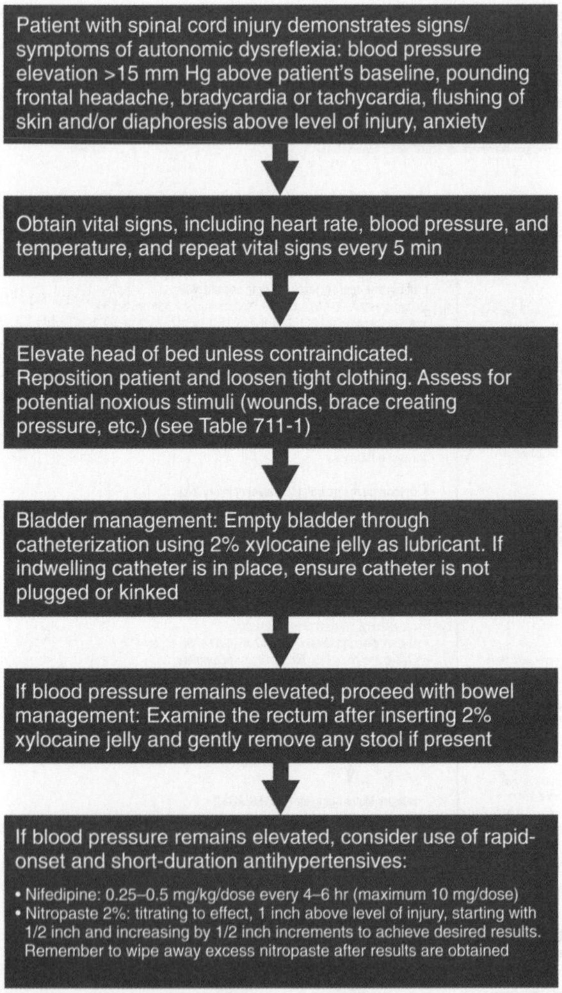

Frequent monitoring for **skin breakdown** and **pressure ulcers** is necessary both acutely as well as lifelong in individuals with SCI. Common locations include the occiput, elbows, sacrum, ischium, and heels. Devices such as halo vests and splints increase risk. Frequent inspection and repositioning are important means of minimizing risk.

Depending upon the level of the lesion, paralysis of the diaphragm or intercostal and abdominal muscles can result in restrictive ventilatory impairment and ineffective cough. Respiratory muscle training, abdominal binders, and noninvasive ventilation and airway clearance devices, such as the insufflator–exsufflator cough assist device, should be considered in select patients.

Immediately following SCI there is a period of **spinal shock** with low tone and absent reflexes. Eventually, signs of an upper motor neuron lesion will increase, including spasticity and involuntary muscle spasms. Symptoms typically increase with noxious stimulation and can interfere with sleep, comfort, positioning, and care. Management includes pharmacologic therapy, stretching, splinting, and positioning. Focal spasticity can be treated with chemodenervation using botulinum toxin or phenol. Intrathecal baclofen should be considered for severe generalized spasticity.

Increased bone resorption occurs as a result of immobilization. If excessive calcium is not adequately excreted by the kidneys, insidious onset of abdominal pain, nausea, vomiting, lethargy, polydipsia, and polyuria may occur. This **immobilization hypercalcemia** is managed with intravenous fluid hydration at 1.5-2 times the maintenance rate, as well as use of furosemide to hasten the renal excretion of calcium. Complications include nephrocalcinosis, urolithiasis, and renal failure.

Osteopenia begins immediately after an SCI occurs and plateaus 6-12 mo later. **Pathologic fractures** occur as a consequence of loss of bone mineral density. The most common sites of fracture include the supracondylar region of the femur and the proximal tibia; fracture is often associated with gait training, minor trauma, and range of motion. Treatment should include use of removable splints or casts that are well padded over bony prominences to prevent skin breakdown. Prevention through weight bearing and calcium and vitamin D supplementation is encouraged.

Development of spine deformity and scoliosis is prevalent in patients sustaining SCI prior to puberty and many of these individuals will require surgical correction. Because of the high incidence of scoliosis, radiographs of the thoracolumbar-sacral spine should be obtained every 6 mo prior to skeletal maturity and every 12 mo thereafter.

An SCI will impact the child's social-emotional development, so adjustment should be monitored closely. Positive coping strategies and strong social supports are associated with greater social participation. Education regarding sexual development and function with SCI injury should be provided.

PROGNOSIS

Prognosis for recovery of neurologic deficits resulting from SCI depends on the neurologic level of injury and level of completeness. Examination at least 72 hr after injury has been determined a better indicator of the prognosis than examinations done earlier. It is prudent for those determining and communicating the diagnosis to understand the particularities and limitations of the anorectal examinations, and thus completeness of injury, unique to children. Those individuals with incomplete injury tend to have increased likelihood of neurologic recovery. The neurologic level of injury can be assistive in determining the level of independence with functional activities (Table 711-2).

Bibliography is available at Expert Consult.

Figure 711-2 Algorithm for management of autonomic dysreflexia.

The flowchart contains the following boxes:

Patient with spinal cord injury demonstrates signs/symptoms of autonomic dysreflexia: blood pressure elevation >15 mm Hg above patient's baseline, pounding frontal headache, bradycardia or tachycardia, flushing of skin and/or diaphoresis above level of injury, anxiety

Obtain vital signs, including heart rate, blood pressure, and temperature, and repeat vital signs every 5 min

Elevate head of bed unless contraindicated. Reposition patient and loosen tight clothing. Assess for potential noxious stimuli (wounds, brace creating pressure, etc.) (see Table 711-1)

Bladder management: Empty bladder through catheterization using 2% xylocaine jelly as lubricant. If indwelling catheter is in place, ensure catheter is not plugged or kinked

If blood pressure remains elevated, proceed with bowel management: Examine the rectum after inserting 2% xylocaine jelly and gently remove any stool if present

If blood pressure remains elevated, consider use of rapid-onset and short-duration antihypertensives:
• Nifedipine: 0.25–0.5 mg/kg/dose every 4–6 hr (maximum 10 mg/dose)
• Nitropaste 2%: titrating to effect, 1 inch above level of injury, starting with 1/2 inch and increasing by 1/2 inch increments to achieve desired results. Remember to wipe away excess nitropaste after results are obtained

Table 711-2	Projected Functional Outcomes at 1 Yr after Injury and/or Diagnosis According to Neurologic Level of Injury				
	C1-C4	**C5**	**C6**	**C7**	**C8-T1**
Feeding	Dependent	Independent with adaptive equipment after set-up	Independent with or without adaptive equipment	Independent	Independent
Grooming	Dependent	Minimal assistance with equipment after set-up	Some assistance to independent with adaptive equipment	Independent with adaptive equipment	Independent
Upper-extremity dressing	Dependent	Requires assistance	Independent	Independent	Independent
Lower-extremity dressing	Dependent	Dependent	Requires assistance	Some assistance to independent with adaptive equipment	Usually independent
Bathing	Dependent	Dependent	Some assistance to independent with equipment	Some assistance to independent with equipment	Independent with equipment
Bed mobility	Dependent	Assistance	Assistance	Independent to some assistance	Independent
Weight shifts	Independent in power; dependent in manual wheelchair	Assistance unless in power wheelchair	Independent	Independent	Independent
Transfers	Dependent	Maximum assistance	Some assistance to independence on level surfaces	Independence with or without board for level surfaces	Independent
Wheelchair propulsion	Independent with power Dependent with manual	Independent in power; independent to some assistance in manual with adaptations on level surfaces	Independent–manual with coated rims on level surfaces	Independent–except curbs and uneven terrain	Independent
Driving	Unable	Independent with adaptations	Independent with adaptations	Car with hand controls or adapted van	Car with hand controls or adapted van
	T2-T9		**T10-L2**		**L3–L5**
Activities of daily living (grooming, feeding, dressing, bathing)	Independent		Independent		Independent
Bowel/bladder	Independent		Independent		Independent
Transfers	Independent		Independent		Independent
Ambulation	Standing in frame, tilt table, or standing wheelchair Exercise only		Household ambulation with orthosis		Community ambulation is possible

From Kirshblum SC, Ho C, Druin E, et al: Rehabilitation after spinal cord injury. In Kirshblum SC, Campagnolo D, DeLisa JE, editors: Spinal cord medicine, Philadelphia, 2002, Lippincott Williams & Wilkins, pp 275–298.

Chapter 712
Spasticity
Joyce L. Oleszek and Loren T. Davidson

Spasticity is a component of the upper motor neuron syndrome characterized by velocity-dependent resistance to passive range of motion resulting in tonic stretch reflexes and accompanied by exaggerated tendon jerks. Spasticity management is determining what degree of spasticity may be tolerable and of functional benefit vs counterproductive and potentially injurious. When devising a treatment plan, both the positive and negative effects of spasticity on function must be considered; treatment should maximize function while minimizing sedation and adverse effects.

ORAL MEDICATIONS

Oral medications are often used as an early treatment for generalized spasticity (Table 712-1). Although efficacy of certain antispasmodics has been demonstrated, their use should be contingent upon functional benefit as adverse effects are quite common. Frequently used medications include baclofen, benzodiazepines (diazepam, clonazepam), dantrolene sodium, tizanidine, and clonidine.

GABAergic Medications

γ-Aminobutyric acid (GABA) is an inhibitory neurotransmitter of the central nervous system. The 2 most relevant GABA receptors for the purposes of pharmacologic management of spasticity are $GABA_A$ and $GABA_B$. **Benzodiazepine medications** exert their effect through

Table 712-1	Dosing Guidelines, Pharmacologic Actions, and Adverse Event Profile of Commonly Prescribed Oral Antispasmodic Medications for Children	
ORAL MEDICATION (DOSE/FREQ., AGE/ WEIGHT RANGE)	**MODE OF ACTION**	**ADVERSE EVENTS/PRECAUTIONS**
Baclofen (0.125-1 mg/kg/day) *Dosing guideline* *2-7 yr* 2.5-10 mg tid-qid (10-40 mg/day) *8-12 yr* 5-15 mg tid-qid (15-60 mg/day) *12-16 yr* 5-20 mg tid-qid (20-80 mg/day) *Note:* Caution advised with renal impairment, consider reducing dose.	Centrally acting, structural analog of γ-aminobutyric acid (GABA), binds to $GABA_B$ receptors of presynaptic excitatory interneurons (and postsynaptic primary afferents) causing presynaptic inhibition of monosynaptic/polysynaptic spinal reflexes. Rapid absorption, blood level peaks in 1 hr, half-life 5.5 hr. Renal (70-80% unchanged) and hepatic (15%) excretion.	Central nervous system (CNS) depression (sedation, drowsiness, fatigue), nausea, headache, dizziness, confusion, euphoria, hallucinations, hypotonia, ataxia, paresthesias. **Note: Abrupt withdrawal** may cause seizures, hallucinations, rebound muscle spasms, and hyperpyrexia.
Diazepam (0.12-0.8 mg/kg/day) *Dosing guideline* *6 mo-12 yr* 0.12-0.8 mg/kg/day PO divided q6-8h *>12 yr* 2-10 mg PO bid-qid *Note:* Prescription of a *qhs* dose only or proportionately larger dose at bedtime may limit excessive daytime sedation.	Centrally acting; binds to $GABA_A$ receptors mediating presynaptic inhibition in brainstem reticular formation and spinal polysynaptic pathways. Rapid absorption; blood level peaks in 1 hr, with half-life of 30-60 hr. Metabolized in liver, producing pharmacologically active metabolites with long duration of action. Increased potential for adverse effects with low albumin levels as a result of being 98% protein bound.	CNS depression (sedation, impaired memory and attention), ataxia. Dependence/potential for substance abuse/ overdose. Withdrawal syndrome (including anxiety, agitation, irritability, tremor, muscle twitching, nausea, insomnia, seizures, hyperpyrexia).
Dantrolene Sodium (3-12 mg/kg/day) *Dosing guideline (for children >5 yr old):* *6-8 mg/kg/day PO divided bid-qid* In children >5 yr old Start 0.5 mg/kg qd-bid for 7 days, then 0.5 mg/kg tid for 7 days, then 1 mg/kg tid for 7 days, then 2 mg/kg tid to a maximum of 12 mg/kg/day or 400 mg/day.	Peripheral action, blocking release of calcium from sarcoplasmic reticulum with uncoupling of nerve excitation and skeletal muscle contraction. Blood level peaks in 3-6 hr (active metabolite 4-8 hr), with half-life of approximately 15 hr. Metabolized largely in liver, with 15-25% of nonmetabolized drug excreted in urine.	Malaise, fatigue, nausea, vomiting, diarrhea, muscle weakness with high dose. *Note:* Hepatotoxicity (baseline liver function tests **must** be checked prior to starting dantrolene, tested weekly during dose titration, and regularly every 1-2 mo thereafter). Drug *should be discontinued* promptly if liver enzymes become elevated.
Tizanidine *Dosing guideline* In children <10 yr: Commence 1 mg orally at bedtime initially, increasing to 0.3-0.5 mg/ kg in 4 divided doses. In children >10 yr: Commence 2 mg orally at bedtime initially, increased according to response, maximum 24 mg/day in 3-4 divided doses.	Centrally acting, α_2-adrenoceptor agonist activity at both spinal and supraspinal sites. Prevents release of excitatory amino acids, facilitating presynaptic inhibition. Good oral absorption, blood level peaks in 1-2 hr, with a half-life of 2.5 hr. Extensive first-pass hepatic metabolism with urinary excretion of inactive metabolites.	Dry mouth, drowsiness, tiredness, headache, dizziness, insomnia, anxiety, aggression, mood swings, visual hallucinations, risk of hypotension (although 10 times less antihypertensive potency than clonidine), nausea, vomiting, and constipation. Liver function tests should be monitored at baseline, 1, 3, and 6 mo. Then periodically.
Clonidine *Dosing guideline* 0.025-0.1 mg in 2-3 divided doses. *Note:* A retrospective chart review of literature about clonidine in children reported an average dosage based on weight was 0.02-0.03 mg/kg/day (0.4- 0.5 mg/day), with a range of 0.0014- 0.15 mg/kg/day.	Centrally acting, mixed α-adrenoceptor agonist with predominant α_2 activity causing membrane hyperpolarization at multiple sites in brain, brainstem, and dorsal horns of spinal cord. Inhibition of substance P may also contribute to tone reduction via an antinociceptive effect. Rapidly absorbed orally, blood level peaks in 1-1.5 hr, with a half-life of 6-20 hr.	Drowsiness, dry mouth, bradycardia, orthostatic hypotension. Abrupt cessation may result in rebound hypertension.

GABA$_A$ receptors by increasing the affinity of GABA for the GABA$_A$ receptor. This results in presynaptic inhibition and a net inhibitory effect at both spinal and supraspinal levels. Of the benzodiazepines, **diazepam** is the oldest and most commonly used medication to treat spasticity because of its long half-life and need for less-frequent administration. In children <2 yr of age, **clonazepam** is a good option because of the availability of a liquid formulation and dosing guidelines. The cognitive effects of benzodiazepines limit its use in persons with severe spasticity as dose escalation results in increased sedation. Furthermore, sedation and cognitive slowing limit the usefulness of benzodiazepines in persons with spasticity of cerebral origin as it may impede recovery in acquired brain injury and cognitive development in congenital developmental delay. The use of benzodiazepines may lead to physiologic dependence, and, thus, abrupt discontinuation should be avoided to prevent withdrawal.

Baclofen is a GABA$_B$ agonist and is a preferred agent in the treatment of spasticity of spinal origin. Baclofen exerts an inhibitory effect on both monosynaptic and polysynaptic spinal reflexes. Unfortunately, supraspinal receptor sites also exist, resulting in sedation, which is common to all GABAergic medications. In most instances, daytime dosing of oral baclofen is better tolerated than benzodiazepines with regard to sedation. Intrathecal administration of baclofen via a baclofen pump (see below) allows greater selectivity of spasticity reduction while minimizing adverse cognitive effects. Abrupt cessation of both oral and intrathecal baclofen therapy *must be avoided* as it may result in a life-threatening withdrawal response.

α$_2$-Adrenergic Agents

Clonidine and **tizanidine** are examples of centrally acting α$_2$-adrenergic agents that decrease spasticity and have an antinociceptive effect. Clonidine is the older of the 2 agents and is used more frequently as an antihypertensive agent. Clonidine exerts its effect on spasticity via both presynaptic inhibition of sensory afferents, as well as release of glutamate at the level of the spinal cord. Adverse effects of clonidine that limit its use as an antispasmodic include hypotension, bradycardia, sedation, cognitive impairment, and xerostomia.

Tizanidine is an α$_2$-noradrenergic agonist that is as effective as diazepam and baclofen in tone reduction. In comparison to clonidine, tizanidine has less-potent hemodynamic effects, which is desirable when it is used primarily for spasticity reduction. The half-life of tizanidine is approximately 2.5 hr, requiring frequent dosing to maintain a steady state. Adverse effects of tizanidine include hypotension, sedation, xerostomia, dizziness, hallucination, and hepatotoxicity.

Peripherally Acting Calcium Blockers

Dantrolene sodium works at the level of skeletal muscle to block calcium release from the sarcoplasmic reticulum. Despite its peripheral site of action, dantrolene may induce sedation, although to a lesser degree than other centrally acting agents. Dantrolene is effective at decreasing both clonus and spasticity but achieves this by weakening skeletal muscle in a nonselective fashion. The resultant generalized weakness seen with dantrolene use limits its utility in ambulatory patients. Dantrolene has a rare but significant adverse event of fatal hepatotoxicity in less than 1% of patients. Hepatotoxicity risk increases with increasing age, increasing dose, and female sex.

Pediatric dosing of spasticity medications is quite variable and needs to be tailored to the response of the child. The choice of medication is often based on personal experience and the impact of benefit vs potential adverse effects. See Table 712-1 for dosing guidelines.

SURGICAL MANAGEMENT

Surgical management of spasticity should be considered when spasticity causes significant functional impairments that are refractory to more conservative management. Combining treatment options such as injections and systemic medications can be very effective.

Botulinum toxin (BTX) intramuscular injections and **phenol/alcohol neurolysis** are used to treat focal areas of spasticity. These injections are most effective in children with hypertonia localized to specific muscles and those without significant contracture. BTX blocks signal transmission at the neuromuscular junction by preventing the release of acetylcholine from the presynaptic axon of the motor end plate. Treatment with BTX type A is most common but BTX type B is also used. The period of clinically useful relaxation is usually 12-16 wk and it is recommended that injections be spaced a minimum of 3 mo apart because of concern for neutralizing antibody formation. Adverse events related to BTX are rare and include injection-site pain and focal muscle weakness. The FDA requires black box labeling on BTX products cautioning that the effects of the BTX may spread from the area of injection to other areas of the body, causing symptoms similar to botulism. Coadministration of BTX and aminoglycosides or other agents interfering with neuromuscular transmission (curare-like nondepolarizing blockers, lincosamides, polymyxins, quinidine, magnesium sulfate, anticholinesterases, succinylcholine chloride) should be performed with caution as the effect of the toxin may be potentiated. BTX-A is an effective and generally safe treatment for spasticity of the upper and lower extremities; evidence regarding functional improvement is conflicting. Long-term use of BTX-A with repeated rounds of injections in children with cerebral palsy is safe and efficacious. BTX-A injections into the gastrocnemius can be combined with serial casting to help improve ankle range and gait.

Phenol perineural injections are typically performed in the large proximal muscles (biceps brachii, hip adductors, hamstrings) and duration of clinical effect may be longer than BTX, varying between 3 and 18 mo. Phenol injection of the anterior branch of the obturator nerve in children with cerebral palsy is safe and effective. The low cost of phenol is a significant advantage over BTX, but the need for electrical stimulation guidance and general anesthesia may offset any cost savings. Combining phenol injections with BTXs allows an increased number of affected muscles to be injected at the maximal recommended dose during one procedure. Phenol is safe in children, but transient sensory dysesthesias occur rarely.

Intrathecal baclofen (ITB) is highly effective in treating severe spasticity. ITB is delivered to the intrathecal space via a surgically implanted infusion pump and catheter. This method of delivery confers an advantage over enteral baclofen in that central nervous system depressive effects are minimized and dosages can be titrated to functional effect. A preoperative screening bolus dose of baclofen can be delivered via lumbar puncture and is used to evaluate responsiveness and impact on functional abilities. Goals of treatment, whether they are to improve function, comfort, and/or care, need to be firmly established. Cost and maintenance can be prohibitive for some families. Catheter tips are typically positioned at C5-T2 but can be placed intraventricularly for severe dystonia. ITB is effective in children with cerebral palsy; there may be a significant reduction in upper- and lower-extremity spasticity for up to 10 yr. Speech, communication, and saliva control can improve after ITB. The most frequent and serious adverse events related to device and implant procedures are catheter dislodgement from the intrathecal space, catheter break/cut, and implant site infection, including meningitis. Electromagnetic interference and MRI may cause transient operational changes to the pump and changes in flow rate. Although baclofen pumps do not prohibit MRI imaging, it is recommended that the pump be "interrogated" by a programmer after MRI as a precaution. ITB pumps need to be replaced every 5-7 yr for end of battery life. The pump comes in a 20 mL and 40 mL size, both of which measure 8.75 cm in diameter. The baclofen pump requires regular refills at 2-6 mo intervals depending on dose rate and pump size, and refills are readily performed in an outpatient clinic setting. **ITB withdrawal** is a medical emergency and needs to be identified early and managed aggressively. Sequelae can include high fever, altered mental status, exaggerated rebound spasticity, and muscle rigidity that, in rare cases, can advance to rhabdomyolysis, multiple organ–system failure, and death. Prevention of abrupt discontinuation of ITB requires careful attention to programming and monitoring of the infusion system, refill scheduling, and pump alarms. Caregivers need to be educated about the early symptoms of baclofen withdrawal.

Selective dorsal rhizotomy (SDR) is a surgical procedure that has been widely used as a treatment for spasticity. The surgical technique involves single-level or multilevel osteoplastic laminectomies exposing the L2-S1 nerve roots. Typically, 25-70% of dorsal rootlets are selectively cut with the aid of electrophysiologic monitoring. Children 3-8 yr of age with spastic diplegia, minimal upper-limb involvement, good selective motor skills and strength, and minimal contractures are the best candidates for SDR. The preoperative ability to rise from a squatted position with minimal support or a younger child's ability to crawl on hands and knees are positive predictors for a good outcome with SDR. Children must have the cognitive and social capacity for the requisite intensive postoperative therapy program. Long-term outcomes 5 and 20 yr after SDR in children show an improvement in spasticity, motor function, and gait pattern. SDR can reduce the need for orthopedic surgeries, with 35% of children avoiding surgery; this might be more likely if SDR is performed before the age of 5 yr. Long-term complications such as sensory dysfunction, bladder or bowel dysfunction, or back pain are infrequent. A concern with multilevel laminectomies is the potential increased risk of spinal deformities, but there is no clear evidence to support this.

Bibliography is available at Expert Consult.

Chapter 713
Birth Brachial Plexus Palsy
Maureen R. Nelson

Birth brachial plexus palsy (BBPP) may cause significant arm weakness and subsequent functional deficits in children. The nerves to the arm are affected with variable degrees of weakness and sensory loss. Most children will have good recovery spontaneously, but functional deficits will remain in 20-30% of children with BBPP (see Chapter 99.7).

The mechanism for birth brachial plexus injury appears to be a lateral stretch of the plexus for the vast majority of cases. Anatomic variations in bones, blood vessels, and tendons lead to a very small number of cases. The incidence of BBPP is reported as 0.5-4.6 per 1,000 live births, with variability thought to be attributable to the type of obstetric care and the size of infants around the world.

Risk factors for birth brachial plexus injury include prior infants with BBPP, shoulder dystocia, birthweight greater than 4 kg, multiparous mothers, mothers with excessive weight gain, and diabetic mothers. Delivering twins or triplets, as well as cesarean sections, have been described as protective from BBPP.

Nerve injuries include neurapraxia, neurotmesis, and axonotmesis. *Neurapraxia* is the least severe of these types and is a reversible loss of nerve conduction. This type will recover. *Neurotmesis* is the most severe and is a total and complete disruption of the nerve; an *avulsion* describes a rupture of a preganglionic lesion, and a *rupture* describes the same event in a postganglionic lesion. *Axonotmesis* is the intermediate form and the most difficult to delineate. There is disruption of the epineurium with variable injury to the axons (Fig. 713-1). Nerves are made of groups of fascicles, which, in turn, are made of groups of axons. This type of lesion contributes greatly to the diagnostic dilemma and difficulty in prediction of recovery.

The brachial plexus consists of the anterior primary rami, or roots, from C5, C6, C7, C8, and T1 (Fig. 713-2). The trunks of the brachial plexus consist of C5-C6 forming the upper trunk, C7 forming the middle trunk, and C8-T1 forming the lower trunk; each trunk has anterior and posterior divisions. The posterior cord is formed from the posterior division of each trunk. The medial cord comes from the anterior division of the lower trunk. The lateral cord is formed from the anterior divisions of the upper and middle trunks. Evaluation of

the roots, trunks, and cords from which the nerves arise helps determine the site of injury.

Erb palsy is generally described as the upper trunk or C 5-6 palsy. It is by far the most common injury seen in birth brachial plexus injury, present in three fourths of infants. It also demonstrates the greatest recovery rate at >80% with a functional arm. *Klumpke palsy,* C8-T1, is extremely rare in BBPP, likely not occurring except in the case of anatomic variation. If a baby presents with a C8-T1 deficit, the baby most likely originally had a complete C5-T1 BBPP and then had recovery of the upper portion of the plexus. This can happen because C4, C5, C6, and sometimes C7 are protected coming out from the spinal cord, held in a gutter along the transverse processes by connective tissue, whereas C8 and T1 are not. The sensory fibers are also relatively protected compared to the motor fibers because the sensory fibers run together until outside of the spinal cord into the dorsal root ganglion where their cell bodies lie. The motor fibers have the cell bodies within the spinal cord and so are not as cohesive in their path. Therefore the sensory fibers may be spared while motor fibers show clinical deficits. A C8-T1 deficit may also result from a spinal cord injury. Consequently, it is important to check for any other indications of spinal cord injury throughout the body. Consideration also must be given to the potential of an anatomic variation, such as an anomalous rib, that may actually cause a C8-T1 deficit alone.

Because various parts of the brachial plexus have different risks of injury, the clinical presentation can be quite variable, causing the diagnosis to be challenging. The phrenic nerve may also be involved with its innervation from C3, C4, and C5, with potential respiratory concerns.

Included in the differential diagnosis of an infant with an arm deficit is the possibility of a fracture of the humerus or clavicle, osteomyelitis, a tumor, or congenital varicella infection, all of which may lead to the limited ability to move the arm.

PHYSICAL EXAMINATION
The physical examination of the child begins with observation. Examination for sensation, particularly examining for sharp sensation, useful in its own right, will also frequently help with active motor evaluation in infants. Assessment of muscle stretch reflexes is important in that infants with a brachial plexus palsy will be areflexive or hyporeflexive in the involved arm. Evaluation of primitive reflexes, particularly the Moro reflex, is helpful as most of these infants will have C5-6 involvement and therefore the Moro may show shoulder abduction and elbow flexion on 1 side but not the involved side. Range-of-motion examination is critical. Deficits are commonly seen because of the imbalance of muscles that are active and those that are not. Shoulder adduction and internal rotation is a common position, as is elbow flexion, forearm pronation, and wrist and finger flexion. The size of the involved arm may also be smaller because of muscle atrophy and sometimes shorter length and smaller diameter of the bone. In children with very severe deficits, the arm may be cooler because of the sympathetic nervous system outflow at T1. **Torticollis** is commonly present and almost always with the face turned away from the involved arm.

Among older infants and children, compensatory movements of the arm may be noted. Common examples are use of trunk momentum to move (particularly to rotate) the proximal arm, hyperlordosis of the lumbar spine to position the arm more advantageously, use of the pectoralis muscle to flex the shoulder, and use of the knee to physically flex the elbow. Examination of the back for symmetry, along with the scapulae for winging, is also relevant. Having the older child manipulate buttons, snaps, or zippers, throw and catch a ball, and write, print, or color may be revealing.

LABORATORY EXAMINATION
Radiographic evaluation may be needed. Plain films can be viewed immediately if there is reason to consider clavicle or humerus fracture, infection, osteomyelitis, or tumor. Ultrasound shows the nerves and this is improving as technology advances. MRI and CT myelogram are used for evaluation of nerve roots and nerves.

Electrodiagnostic evaluation may also contribute to the diagnosis. Sensory nerve conduction studies are very useful in a child with severe

Anatomy of Peripheral Nerve

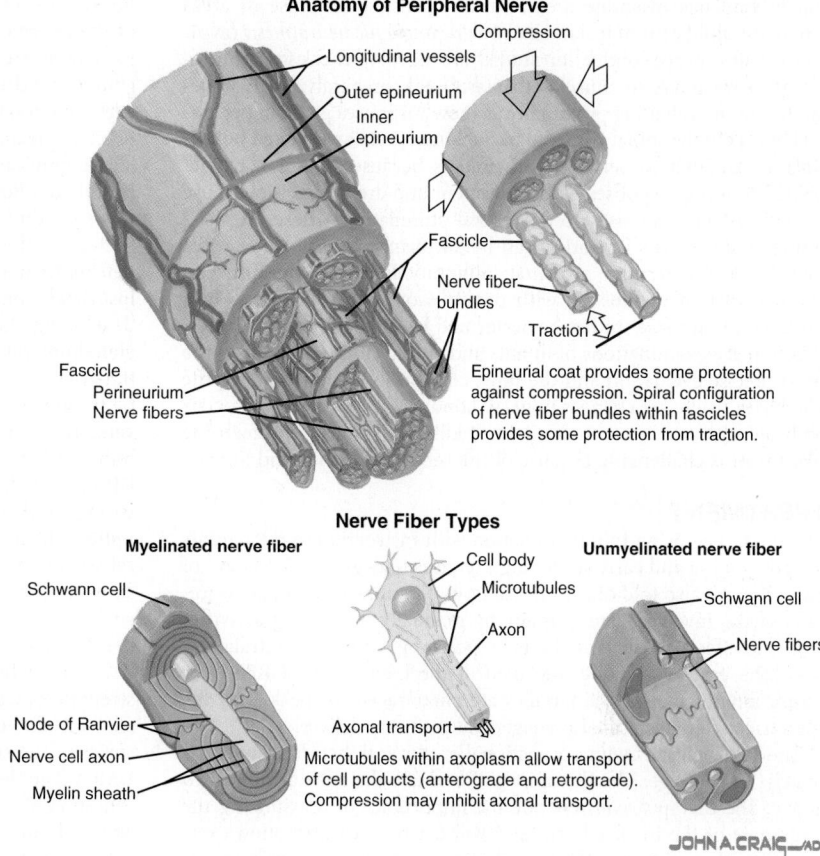

Nerve Fiber Types

Figure 713-1 Anatomy of peripheral nerve. *(Netter illustration from www.netterimages.com. Elsevier, Inc. All rights reserved.)*

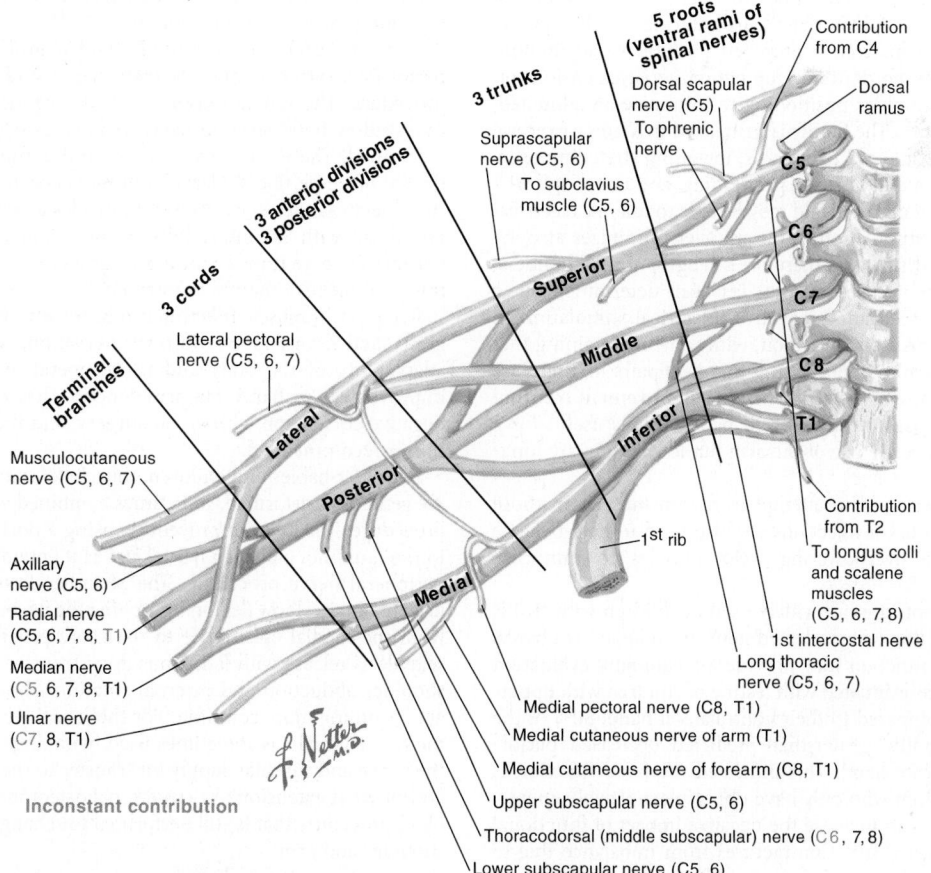

Figure 713-2 Schematic of the brachial plexus. *(Netter illustration from www.netterimages.com. Elsevier, Inc. All rights reserved.)*

injury who has insensate areas. Normal sensory response in areas where the child cannot feel indicates a *preganglionic neurotmesis* (avulsion). Motor nerve conduction studies are useful to check for continuity of nerve fibers to muscles that are weak or paralyzed. F waves are useful in evaluating proximally as these responses go from peripheral nerves to the spinal cord and back. **Somatosensory evoked potentials** are difficult to perform with infants because of motor artifact obliterating the responses with movement and are imprecise because of overlapping responses to peripheral stimulation. These are used intraoperatively as stimulation can be performed on the nerve roots themselves to determine proximal continuity. **Electromyography** can show activation in muscles with paralysis or severe weakness. It is important that these studies be performed by someone who is experienced in the examinations of infants and young children, both for the most precise evaluation and the most comfortable experience for the youngster. There are changes in nerve conduction velocities that occur with age, distances are nonclassic for traditional studies, and electrode placement is challenging because of the very small hands and limbs.

TREATMENT

Treatment begins on initial evaluation with instruction to the parents for positioning and early stretching exercises to begin at 10-14 days of age. They are also told of the critical task of maintaining infant awareness of the involved arm, initially by manually mimicking activities with the affected arm that the baby performs with the contralateral arm. The parents also are informed of the higher risk of BBPP for future infants, and so the families are encouraged to speak with the obstetrician about optimal management in future deliveries.

The baby will start with occupational or physical therapy at approximately 2 wk of age. The therapist will evaluate the baby as described above. The therapist will reiterate the importance of maximizing the awareness of the involved arm and will teach range-of-motion exercises. The therapist will often do splinting, commonly for wrist extension in a baby with wrist-drop, and possibly extending the fingers and abducting the thumb as well. Over time other splinting needs may be evident. There may be a supinator strap used during the therapeutic activities to turn the arm from a pronated position to supination. Therapeutic taping may be done for supination, wrist extension, or, most commonly, for shoulder positioning to minimize an adducted, internally rotated posture. The family is instructed in a home exercise program to be carried out on a daily basis, including stretching exercises, strengthening as a child is able, positioning, and use of splints.

After a few months of age the child may be able to tolerate electrical stimulation. Electrical stimulation to the muscles minimizes atrophy and promotes increased size, and therefore strength, of muscle fibers. Specific parameters for its use have not yet been determined but a 20-30 min twice-daily program is effective. Electrical stimulation to the nerves remains an area of contention, with some maintaining that it improves recovery while others stating that it impairs it. There are also proponents of the use of **constraint-induced movement training** to increase the active use of the involved hand. This is useful for a short-term increase in active use of the arm but less certain are long-term improvements.

Biofeedback has been used to attempt to retrain muscles in those with BBPP. Botulinum toxin injections are also used to help balance out muscles that are overpowering weak muscles to minimize contractures.

Functional assessments are not widely used in children with BBPP. Computer adaptive testing using selected items from large item banks relevant to the child's function may provide a meaningful evaluation tool. Hand function was evaluated with testing of children with upper-plexus involvement compared to their contralateral hand; 80% of the children had significantly greater-than-predicted decreased performance from the opposite hand. This indicated the hand function is impaired even in children who only have upper-plexus involvement.

Secondary problems can increase the negative impact of functional deficits in children with BBPP. Contractures from imbalance due to muscle weakness or paralysis, including shoulder adduction and internal rotation, elbow flexion, forearm pronation, and wrist and finger

flexion, are all seen and interfere with function. A decrease in growth of the affected arm in length and atrophy of muscles are often seen. Lack of awareness of the arm, sometimes called *developmental disregard*, in children can have a significant impact on active use of the arm, with functional loss as a consequence. Pain is not usually seen in birth brachial plexus as opposed to injuries, which occur later in life. Scapular winging can be problematic both socially and clinically. The change in child development overall can be problematic. Toddlers with sensory loss sometimes chew on their fingers, causing injury.

Because the shoulder joint develops as the infant and toddler grows, deficits frequently develop. Shoulder deformity is a common musculoskeletal complication of BBPP. Muscular imbalance across the developing shoulder results in deformity of the skeletally immature glenohumeral joint. The weakness of shoulder external rotation, combined with strong internal rotation, leads to this difficulty. There can be progressive glenohumeral dysplasia, with increased glenoid retroversion, humeral head flattening, and posterior subluxation of the humeral head. The natural history of this deformity is progression if left untreated. This leads to further functional limitations even with a strong hand. Treatment aims to minimize this progression. Treatment options include botulinum toxin injections, arthroscopic surgeries, release of contracture, muscular tendinous lengthening (frequently a subscapularis slide), tendon transfers (commonly transfer of the latissimus dorsi to increase external rotation and abduction strength), and derotational humeral osteotomy.

Infants who do not show satisfactory improvement in muscle strength are candidates for surgical intervention. Classically the lack of elbow flexion to three fifths or greater strength merits referral for nerve surgery. The specific criteria and timing remain under debate. Those with a complete brachial plexus palsy with a flaccid arm and lack of sensation are under consideration for surgery between 2 and 4 mo of age, and those with upper-plexus involvement are considered between 3 and 6 mo of age. The surgical strategy for complete palsy is early microsurgery with the focus first on hand reinnervation. If the shoulder and elbow have continued deficits later, they will undergo secondary musculotendinous procedures.

Nerve transfers, nerve grafting, and neurolysis all are commonly performed. Intraoperative electrical nerve studies can help guide the procedure. The somatosensory evoked potentials and nerve conduction studies, both nerve-to-nerve and nerve-to-muscle, are commonly performed. These can assist in determining functional electrical continuity of nerve fibers. Nerve grafting is commonly performed using sural nerve fascicles, with several fascicles attached at each root level. For those with no intact nerve roots, intercostal nerve and other peripheral nerve transfers or grafts, or a cross C7 graft (from the contralateral plexus), may be performed.

Recovery of muscle function can occur with extremely varied nerve grafts and transfers providing innervation, showing the amazing adaptability of the body and its recuperative power. Postoperative improvement in hand and arm function has been shown to have a negative correlation with age at surgery, and therefore early intervention is recommended.

For older babies and children, muscle tendon and bony procedures are generally performed, sometimes combined with a peripheral nerve procedure. The Oberlin procedure, using a portion of the ulnar nerve to the musculocutaneous nerve, just as it enters the biceps, is a classic peripheral nerve procedure. The Steindler flexorplasty is sometimes used to obtain elbow flexion by moving the flexor and pronator muscles from the medial epicondyle to the more proximal humerus. A subscapularis release with latissimus dorsi transfer is commonly used for shoulder abduction and external rotation. Shoulder joint procedures are becoming more common. For those with very severe arm involvement, the gracilis is sometimes used by taking this muscle along with the nerve and vascular supply for transfer to the arm for elbow flexion and/or wrist extension. A derotational osteotomy of the humerus is an older procedure that is still performed for changing the position of the shoulder and arm.

Bibliography is available at Expert Consult.

Chapter 714

Traumatic and Sports-Related Injuries of the Lower Extremity

See Chapters 687 and 693.

Chapter 715

Meningomyelocele (Spina Bifida)

Pamela Wilson and Janet Stewart

See also Chapter 591.

Meningomyelocele, or spina bifida, is a congenital neural tube defect that results in the malformation of the spine and spinal cord. It is the second most common disability in children and can range from spina bifida occulta (see Chapter 591.2) to anencephaly (see Chapter 591.6).

ETIOLOGY
See Chapter 591.1.

PREVENTION
See Chapter 591.1.

PRENATAL SCREENING
Prenatal screening is recommended for all pregnant women to detect neural tube defect. A simple blood test is done in the 2nd trimester to evaluate α-fetoprotein, human chorionic gonadotropin, estriol, and inhibin. If a neural tube defect is present, the α-fetoprotein is often elevated and further screening using high-resolution ultrasound is indicated. Ultrasound may reveal not only a spinal defect but also abnormal brain development, including the *lemon* and *banana signs*. The lemon sign is related to the shape of the head, whereas the banana sign is associated with hindbrain herniation of the cerebellum into the foramen magnum. The importance in early identification allows families to plan for delivery and consider fetal interventions, mainly prenatal closure of the defect. The Management of Meningomyelocele trial studied the safety and efficacy of prenatal spinal defect closure and the results suggest that prenatal closure may decrease the need for a shunt and lower the incidence of severe Arnold-Chiari malformations along with improved motor outcomes. However, study data show an increased incidence of preterm delivery and a risk for uterine dehiscence.

CLINICAL IMPLICATIONS
Spina bifida is often a multisystem problem that is most frequently associated with central nervous system abnormalities. The neurologic lesion is assessed by the actual anatomic level and then neurologic or functional level. Lesions associated with spina bifida are often grouped together as thoracic, upper lumbar (L1-2), midlumbar (L3), lower lumbar (L4-5), and sacral. Based on this information 1 can make inferences on the functional capabilities of the child and answer pertinent questions during the initial encounters (Table 715-1). The most basic question all families ask is: "Will my child walk?"

The first issue that must be dealt with after delivery is closure of the back defect. This is generally done the 1st day of life. Once the back is closed the child will be monitored to see if hydrocephalus develops. Hydrocephalus is very common in spina bifida and is related to hindbrain herniation. Hydrocephalus may develop most rapidly in the 1st postnatal mo; ventricular dilation may precede a change in head circumference or signs of increased intracranial pressure. The occurrence of hydrocephalus has been noted to be anywhere from 77-95% and does appear to have an association with level of lesion. Treatment is placement of a ventricular shunt or endoscopic third ventriculostomy. The risk for shunt revision in the 1st 2 yr is 30-50%, which decreases to 10% after 2 yr.

Hindbrain herniation or the **Chiari type II malformation** is seen in 80-90% of individuals with myelomeningocele. The classic manifestations include caudal displacement of the cerebellum, pons, and medulla and elongation of the fourth ventricle. This can impede cerebrospinal fluid flow and is involved in the development of hydrocephalus. The Chiari II malformation is symptomatic (from brainstem herniation/compression) in approximately 20% of children. Respiratory symptoms may be seen at birth or develop in the 1st few mo. These include stridor, vocal cord dysfunction, and central or obstructive apnea. Swallowing and feeding problems may require gastrostomy tube placement. If the child has a symptomatic Chiari II malformation, surgical

Table 715-1	Prognosticating in Myelomeningocele			
MOTOR LEVEL SPINAL CORD SEGMENT	CRITICAL MOTOR FUNCTION PRESENT	MOBILITY: SCHOOL AGE	RANGE: ADULT	ACTIVITY: ADOLESCENT
T12	Totally paralyzed lower limbs	Standing brace, wheelchair	Wheelchair	Wheelchair, no ambulation
L1-2	Hip flexor muscles	Crutches, braces, wheelchair	Wheelchair, household ambulation	Wheelchair, nonfunctional ambulation
L3-4	Quadriceps muscles	Crutches, braces, household ambulation, wheelchair	Crutches, household ambulation, wheelchair	50% Wheelchair, household ambulation with crutches
L5	Medical hamstrings, anterior tibial muscles	Crutches, braces, community ambulation	Crutches, community ambulation	Community ambulation with crutches
S1	Lateral hamstring and peroneal muscles	Community ambulation	Community ambulation	Community ambulation 50% crutch or cane
S2-3	Mild loss of intrinsic foot muscles possible	Normal	Normal	Limited endurance because of late foot deformities

From Braddon RL, editor: Physical medicine & rehabilitation, ed 4, Philadelphia, 2011, WB Saunders, Table 54-1, p. 1284.

decompression is indicated. All children with spina bifida are at risk for **tethered cord syndrome**. After shunt malfunction, this is the second most common cause for neurologic decline. Clinical manifestations of tethered cord syndrome include any change in gait or bowel or bladder function, increasing scoliosis, back pain, or orthopedic changes. Surgical detethering procedures are indicated in those with neurologic decline but the success rate is variable.

The **orthopedic complications** of myelomeningocele are common and have predictable patterns. The spine deformities include scoliosis, lordosis, and kyphosis (see Chapter 679). The development of scoliosis has an association with the neurologic level. Children with thoracic level defects have an 80-100% risk, whereas those with a sacral level are at very low risk. Spine deformities tend to increase more rapidly during growth and puberty. Treatment of scoliosis includes both non-surgical and surgical options. Braces, such as **thoracic-lumbar-sacral orthotics**, therapy, and proper seating options may be beneficial. Surgically implanted growing rods to support the developing spine have been used in younger children. Spine surgery should definitely be considered if the scoliotic spine curvature reaches 45 degrees; the child who is nearing skeletal maturity is a better candidate for spine surgery. Realistic expectations need to be discussed with the child and family. Correction of the spine may improve sitting, posture, and pelvic obliquity, but may have a negative impact on function and ambulation.

The **development of the hip** is also influenced by neurologic level (see Chapter 678). The risk for dislocation is highest in the L3 level followed by the L1-L2. Unilateral hip dislocations should be fixed surgically as they may result in pelvic obliquity and problems with sitting, whereas bilateral dislocations generally do not require interventions. Contractures of soft tissues are commonly seen in children with higher lesion levels. Hip flexors and knee flexors are commonly involved.

Abnormalities in the foot occur in approximately 90% of children and adolescents. The goal of treatment is to achieve a plantar grade foot for weight bearing and allow shoe wear. Clubfoot deformities are common in babies and treatment commonly includes serial casting and orthotics (see Chapter 674.3). The results are often suboptimal and surgery may be needed. In addition congenital vertical talus (rocker-bottom feet) are often encountered and need to be addressed (see Chapter 674.4).

Osteoporosis (see Chapter 707) begins to develop in childhood and is more severe in the higher-level injuries. Fractures of the lower extremities are most common in the femur followed by the tibia. Preventive treatment includes use of supplemental calcium and vitamin D. Those with documented fractures should undergo a diagnostic evaluation (see Table 707-1), including dual-energy x-ray absorptiometry. The use of bisphosphonates may be considered if the diagnostic evaluation does not reveal other underlying causes. The utility of early weight bearing has been advocated, but passive standing may have little impact on bone density.

Neurogenic bladder and bowel can be anticipated (see Chapters 543 and 606.1). The goals of treatment interventions are to protect kidney function and achieve social continence. The introduction of clean intermittent catheterization is the mainstay of management. It is not atypical for newborn babies to be started on a clean intermittent catheterization program. Urodynamics and renal ultrasounds are routinely used to monitor for hydronephrosis and track intravesicular pressures. Medications may be used to reduce bladder contractions and improve volume capacity. Surgical techniques are being used to improve continence, including bladder augmentation and the Mitrofanoff procedure (appendicovesicostomy). Symptomatic urinary tract infections should be treated with appropriate antibiotics. These children tend to have colonized bladders and should only be treated for symptoms and not the urinalysis or culture. A good bowel program is generally needed to achieve bowel continence. Nonsurgical interventions include adequate hydration, dietary manipulation, fiber regulation, and use of laxatives. Surgical interventions, such as the antegrade continence enema, have improved continence in many of these children and adolescents.

Latex allergies are fairly common in this population. The etiology may be multifactorial but increased exposure may play a role in development of severe reactions (see Chapter 149). Care providers need to be keenly aware of products that contain latex or that have a cross reactivity such as foods mixed with avocado, bananas or Kiwi fruit. **Radioallergosorbent testing** is used for identification of potential severe allergens.

Spina bifida is known to be associated with specific **neuropsychologic problems**. Various cerebral neuronal dysplasias may be present. The hallmark is a nonverbal learning disorder characterized by difficulties in math reasoning, visual spatial perception, and time concepts. In addition there are weaknesses in executive function, processing speed, and organizational skills. Children with spina bifida typically fall within the average IQ range although those with a higher lesion tend to cluster on the lower range. Hydrocephalus itself has an impact on cognition as noted by deficits in learning, memory, and executive function. Young children with spina bifida tend to do well early on as they have good verbal skills but as the academic demands increase school problems become more obvious. It is important to have appropriate neuropsychologic/educational testing done to identify difficulties each child or adolescent may encounter. Appropriate early intervention and support programs should be put in place and **individual education plans** or 504 plans developed (see Chapter 36). Structure in the home environment plays a key role in teaching self-care, dressing, and mobility skills. The importance of these early interventions cannot be underestimated as they will impact the quality of life and independence in adolescence and transition to an independent adulthood.

ADOLESCENCE AND TRANSITION INTO ADULTHOOD

Clinical care has increased the life span of individuals with spina bifida and the majority are living into adulthood. The physical problems in association with the learning disorders make the transition into independent living and competitive employment very difficult. The pediatrician in conjunction with specialty services plays a pivotal role in developing future planning. It is important to discuss early on strategies to encourage developmentally appropriate independence and self-help skills. Long-term financial arrangements, such as Special Needs Trusts, should be discussed. Transitioning primary and specialty care will need to be researched and introduced to the individual and family. Young adults may have depression and suicidal ideation.

Bibliography is available at Expert Consult.

Chapter **716**
Ambulation Assistance
Marisa Osorio and Susan Apkon

Assistive devices, such as orthoses, prostheses, walkers, crutches, and wheelchairs, are key components of the therapeutic prescription for children with physical disabilities. The type of device chosen depends on the underlying diagnosis, functional level of the child, prognosis for improvement, tone abnormalities, range of motion, strength, and the overall gait pattern. Physicians, licensed independent practitioners, and physical therapists perform the evaluation of a child requiring mobility assistance. The physician or licensed independent practitioner is ultimately responsible for writing the prescription for the assistive device.

ORTHOSES

An orthosis is a device that is applied to the surface of the body to maintain alignment or position, to prevent or assist movement of the body part, or to provide support. Orthoses can be static, indicating the brace is rigid and does not allow movement, or they can be dynamic, allowing movement of the limb to occur. Orthoses are named for the body parts covered. For example, "AFO" stands for *ankle–foot orthosis*, a brace worn on the foot that extends from the toes to the midcalf position (Fig. 716-1). Orthoses are custom made by an orthotist and can be obtained either directly through the orthotist or through the child's physical therapist. The orthosis is replaced during periods of growth or changes in function. All braces must be prescribed by a physician or licensed independent practitioner.

The type of lower-extremity orthosis prescribed is based on evaluation of the child's gait, strength, tone, and range of motion. There are many types of braces that have specific functions to improve gait. Table 716-1 lists examples of these orthoses and their potential uses.

Solid and articulated AFOs are the most commonly prescribed braces. Solid AFOs are used for children with hypertonicity, as they help to biomechanically reduce tone and provide stability with standing. Solid-ankle AFOs are also used in children who are nonambulatory to maintain range of motion of the ankle.

Articulated (hinged) AFOs allow the child with active ankle dorsiflexion to achieve heel strike and a more typical-appearing gait pattern by allowing forward movement of the tibia. This design makes ambulating on uneven surfaces and using stairs easier because of the movement allowed at the ankle, while still supporting the foot position and medial-lateral stability of the ankle. Articulated AFOs should not be used in children with cerebral palsy, spina bifida, or other disorders if

they have a crouched gait pattern because the braces do not prevent crouching and may, in fact, allow further crouching. With crouched gait the hips and knees are held in flexion and ankles in dorsiflexion throughout the gait cycle.

PROSTHESES

A prosthesis is a device that replaces a missing body part, such as an arm or a leg. Lower-extremity prostheses are used to improve mobility, while upper-limb prostheses are not always needed to improve function as children can be quite independent with a single upper limb. Lower-limb prostheses are used in children with congenital amputations, limb deficiencies such as fibular longitudinal deficiency, and acquired amputations as a result of trauma or cancer.

There are multiple components to lower-limb prostheses, which include the socket and foot, but may also include a hip and knee joint depending on the level of amputation. A prosthetist works with the child and family to fabricate the prosthesis. A physician or licensed independent practitioner with experience in prostheses provides the prescription for this device.

The type of prosthesis and the age at which a child is fit for the device depends on the etiology of the amputation, healing after surgery, and weight-bearing restrictions. In very young children, use of a lower-extremity prosthesis follows developmental milestones, with the first prosthesis prescribed at the time the child is pulling to stand. Addition of joints to the prosthesis also occurs when developmentally appropriate, such as use of a knee joint around the age of 3 when the child is learning to use stairs.

Advances in technology are helping children who use prostheses achieve a fluid gait pattern that makes their prosthetic use virtually undetectable to the untrained eye. New components and designs allow amputees to lead active lifestyles, including running, swimming, biking, and mountain climbing.

ASSISTIVE DEVICES

The purpose of assistive devices is to provide a wider base of support to improve stability during ambulation. The least supportive device is a traditional single-point cane commonly used following an orthopedic injury. For most children with gait abnormalities secondary to neurologic disorders, this is not a functional option. More supportive gait aids, such as forearm or Lofstrand crutches, are appropriate in these children; however, use of these devices requires good coordination and strength. Children with cerebral palsy and spina bifida may benefit from these devices.

Walkers provide more support than crutches and canes; they do not require as much strength and coordination to operate. Children with cerebral palsy, for example, may use a reverse walker, which they pull behind them. This reverse configuration provides a wide base of support and stability, helps to maintain an erect posture, and allows the child to engage with the environment without the barrier of the walker in front of them. Having the walker behind them also reduces the risk for more serious injury after a forward fall.

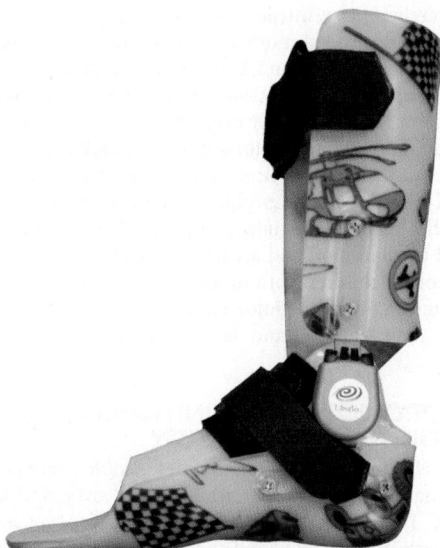

Figure 716-1 Hinged ankle-foot orthosis. *(Courtesy of Ultraflex Systems, Inc., Pottstown, PA.)*

Table 716-1	Orthotic Options	
ORTHOSIS	**FUNCTION**	**COMMENTS**
Foot orthosis	Provides support of foot only	Not typically customized
Supramalleolar orthosis	Provides medial-lateral support	Appropriate for children with low tone such as in Down syndrome
Ankle–foot orthosis	Provides support at the ankle and reduces footdrop or plantarflexion tone	Commonly used for ambulatory and nonambulatory children
Ground reaction ankle–foot orthosis	Provides knee extension moment to reduce crouching	Appropriate for children with spina bifida who crouch when walking
Knee–ankle–foot orthosis	Provides support at the knee when there is quadriceps weakness	Less commonly used because of large size of brace

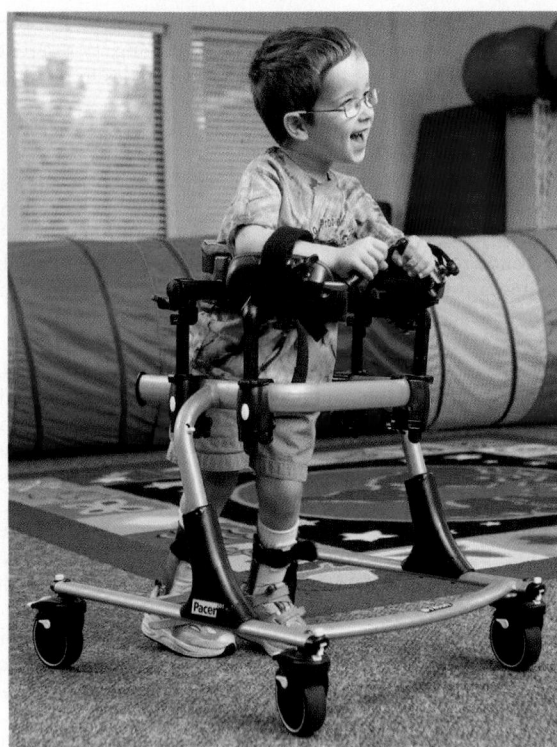

Figure 716-2 Gait trainer. *(Photo copyright 2013 by Rifton Equipment, http://www.rifton.com.)*

For children who require a significant amount of support, gait trainers are often used. These devices allow the child to work on leg movements while the trunk and pelvis are stabilized (Fig. 716-2).

WHEELCHAIRS
Wheelchairs should be considered as a means of mobility when ambulation is not possible or is difficult outside of the home setting. Children with spinal cord injuries, spina bifida, neuromuscular diseases, or cerebral palsy may benefit from the use of a wheelchair. The goal is to provide a wheelchair that will allow the child to move independently about the environment, including home, school, and the community. Children as young as age 2 yr can self-propel a manual wheelchair and drive a power wheelchair. The type of wheelchair will depend on the child's underlying diagnosis, cognitive abilities, vision, motor skills such as head and trunk control, ability to manually propel a wheelchair, strength and endurance, musculoskeletal deformities if present, and medical comorbidities. One must also consider future growth or anticipated changes in function over time as well as the family's ability to transport the chair. Unique to pediatric wheelchairs is the adjustability to accommodate growth. A typical wheelchair may last 3-5 yr with periodic adjustments to growth by a seating specialist. There are many components that can be added in order to provide more support in the wheelchair, including head rests, lateral trunk support, hip guides, antitippers that prevent the wheelchair from tipping backwards, and specialized tires. The seating system is considered a separate item from the wheelchair itself and should be properly fit for the child's current size and seating needs. Seats that are too large for the child can cause pressure ulcers, worsen scoliosis, and make it more difficult for the child to maneuver or propel.

Bibliography is available at Expert Consult.

Chapter 717
Health and Wellness for Children with Disabilities
Margaret A. Turk

See also Chapter 42.

The number of children with developmental disabilities in the United States has increased by 17% in the past 20 yr, with nearly 3 million being of school age. Despite available medical support, many of these children and their families do not receive recommended childhood preventive care and anticipatory guidance, health education, discussions about appropriate activity and exercise, or an opportunity to engage in or learn about health promotion.

The expansion of the disability definition to include children with special healthcare needs, chronic conditions, and activity limitations from any cause (e.g., limitations in usual daily activities such as age-appropriate self-care, mobility, communication, and cognition) has made the health issues of the more traditional childhood disability types (e.g., cerebral palsy, intellectual disability, spina bifida, congenital musculoskeletal disorders) more difficult to identify. U.S. data identify developmental, emotional, and behavioral conditions as the leading conditions with activity or functional limitations, with physical health conditions comprising a smaller proportion of self-identified disabilities (although mobility and motor control issues may be noted among the aforementioned nonphysical conditions). Childhood cognitive, mental, and physical health problems contribute to continued economic and health problems into adulthood. Because these problems can respond to childhood and adolescent health promotion interventions, monitoring children with disabilities throughout their development is helpful in providing information and support to children and adolescents, their parents, and families to promote health over a lifetime.

HEALTH PROMOTION DEFINITIONS AND BACKGROUND FOR DISABILITY
The World Health Organization defines *health promotion* as "the process of enabling people to increase control over, and to improve, their health." For people with disabilities, this concept is important because they are both underserved and have comparatively large health disparities. The World Health Organization further defines health promotion approaches as including more than health education, and consisting of community action, supportive and accessible environments, policy changes, health service modifications, and development of personal skills. Health and wellness programs also include traditional preventive management strategies, such as anticipatory guidance. There is ample evidence that engaging in specific areas of health promotion results in improvement, although the evidence for its influence on adult health is less robust.

Children with disabilities encounter many barriers to healthy behaviors (Table 717-1). Both broad and focused health promotion programs consider severity of condition, barriers and resources, and self-efficacy and resiliency, to achieve health-promoting behaviors. Children with disabilities may also require modeling or assistance to apply healthy behaviors to their particular disability or economic, social, and environmental circumstances.

Children and adults (and their families) often view health differently than those without disabilities. Disability may influence health and vice versa, but their perception of their own health and wellness does not equate with their level of disability. Children with congenital or

Table 717-1	Barriers and Facilitators for Children to Engage in Healthy Behaviors

BARRIERS	FACILITATORS
• Lack of knowledge and skills • Fear of injury or failure • Negative attitudes by parents, peers, healthcare providers • Poor parental healthy behaviors • Stress in the close family network • Personal choices • Fatigue • Lack of initiative • Limited function or capability • Inability to control behaviors • Inaccessible facilities or resources • Needing adult or aid assistance • Economic restrictions • Policies and procedures of facilities or programs	• Education or knowledge about healthy behaviors • Engaging child in discussions and decisions • Promotion of activities by rehabilitation and other healthcare professionals • Family support and participation • Involvement of friends and peers in activities • Desire to be active • Models or directions for participation with adaptations • Creative and knowledgeable professionals • Making activities a part of the routine—repetition and consistency promote ongoing activities • Accessible facilities and opportunities, with knowledgeable staff • Policies and resources promoting participation

acquired disabilities have a narrow view of healthy living, concentrating on nutrition and secondarily on physical activity, with little understanding of how they apply to their own condition. Experiences as a child with a disability often foreshadow adult behaviors, especially negative attitudes toward therapy, exercise, and activity. Beliefs of parents, families, and healthcare providers also influence the views of health by children with disabilities. Health promotion programs for these children must (1) understand and support the role and well-being of parents, (2) recognize that parents of children with more functional limitations may require more resources and support, (3) involve children with disabilities in design of programs and decisions about participation, and (4) address barriers to participation, perceived and real (see Table 717-1). Because many healthcare providers have a poor understanding of the needs of people with disabilities, engaging experienced rehabilitation health professionals in designing and promoting a health and wellness agenda is an important strategy.

An effective health and wellness program should involve multiple approaches and opportunities for success, including partnerships with families, school staff, and rehabilitation providers. Competency requires addressing any mismatch between the child's positive sense of health and well-being and that expected by the healthcare providers; limitations of an education-only model; engaging the child in discussions about the importance of healthy behaviors, ways to engage in healthy behaviors related to the child's disability and circumstances, and decisions about participation; and parent and family involvement coupled with sensitivity for the already overwhelming support a family provides for the child with a disability.

ANTICIPATORY GUIDANCE, COUNSELING, AND PREVENTIVE CARE
Preventive healthcare through health education, anticipatory guidance, and participation in screening and immunization schedules is the mainstay of pediatric public health programs (see Chapter 16). *Bright Futures,* developed by the American Academy of Pediatrics and their collaborators and supported by the Maternal and Child Health Bureau, Health Resources and Services Administration, provides a knowledge base for pediatric healthcare providers and the public about anticipatory guidance, health promotion, and prevention for children and adolescents; but it has few references to disability. Anticipatory guidance refers to general information related to growth/development and healthy practices. Counseling refers to advice given regarding specific conditions, which could include discussions of applications of general guidance to children with disabilities. For the general population, 25% of parents receive no information and <50% receive all recommended guidance. Although parents of children with special healthcare needs (the broad inclusive definition of disabilities) report similar or better receipt of general preventive information, it is not clear whether those with higher severity of functional limitations receive this guidance or counseling, and whether it is provided in the context of disability and other circumstances.

Children with special healthcare needs require typical prevention, as well as more specific counseling related to their disability. Some of this more specific counseling can be managed by specialty care providers, although children with special healthcare needs have difficulty obtaining appropriate specialty outpatient services. Additional barriers to care, especially with increasing age of the child, are the lack of accessible medical equipment and facilities. Although discussions of health risks with adolescents about smoking, drinking, and protected sexual activity should be undertaken, the discussions may require a different focus for adolescents with disabilities. Higher violence and abuse rates toward children with disabilities are reported for which providers must be vigilant.

The recommendation is to recognize the need for modifications to typical guidance, to be alert for any signs of violence, and to broaden counseling to include questions and discussions about conditions associated with the specific disabilities (e.g., epilepsy or cognitive impairments often seen with cerebral palsy, or neurogenic bladder and bowel in spinal cord dysfunction) or secondary conditions, such as pain, osteoporosis/fractures, or fatigue seen in many children and adolescents with disabilities. Although the patient-centered medical home may provide this inclusive support, it risks decreased access to the specialty physicians and healthcare providers who will provide much of this information.

PHYSICAL ACTIVITY AND EXERCISE
National health guidelines recommend at least 60 min of physical activity daily for children, and they suggest that specific advice from health professionals is needed for children with disabilities. Exercise and activity have shown to increase aerobic capacity, functional ability, and quality of life for children with many kinds of disabilities and chronic diseases (e.g., cerebral palsy, spinal cord dysfunction, cystic fibrosis, asthma, intellectual disabilities, diabetes). The vast majority of study participants noted benefits. And yet, most healthcare providers expect sedentary lifestyles for children and adolescents with disabilities, whatever their functional abilities. For children with disabilities, school physical education and recess programs can support activities at or greater than the recommendation, and school requirements can reinforce activity expectations. Despite this potential, most children with disabilities engage in very limited physical activity even in supported school environments. School and public playgrounds are not sufficiently accessible to support community physical activity.

Physical activity for children and adolescents improves fitness and quality of life for youth with developmental disabilities (Table 717-2). The described exercise and fitness programs require 2-3 mo of participation at least twice a week to achieve any changes, and many of the changes achieved are longer lasting than expected. These programs are not traditional therapy, and participation in therapy is not a substitute. The focused fitness and exercise programs cited here generally required the support and direction of rehabilitation professionals, although programs can be community based in nonmedical surroundings.

Table 717-2	Examples of Effective Exercise Programs for Children with Disabilities	
PROGRAM	**DESCRIPTION**	**OUTCOMES/COMMENTS**
Center-based fitness program and home program*	Children with a variety of disabilities Group exercise: 2×/wk for 14 wk; warm-up, aerobics, strengthening, cool down Home program: 2×/wk for 12 wk using video exercises	Improved walking efficiency, strength, general function Group treatment more effective by measures and by satisfaction
Group aquatics aerobic exercise program†	Children with a variety of disabilities, >50% able to walk 2×/wk for 14 wk Recreation to achieve target heart rate; aquatic strengthening program	Improved walk/run, not strength to isometric testing Required adults monitoring to maintain target heart rates
Group training class‡	Children with cerebral palsy able to walk 2×/wk for 4 wk Warm-up, circuit training stations (treadmill, balance, stairs, closed-chain exercises)	Improved muscle strength, mobility, function except fine-motor test–maintained 8 wk later Therapists conducted and monitored
Strength training§	Children with cerebral palsy, including a majority able to walk with assistive devices 3×/wk for 6 wk Progressive strength training program, conducted in the home	Improved perceptions of strength, walking, stair management and improved psychologic benefits Clinicians to monitor, problem solve; some need for direct parental involvement
Walking–jogging program‖	Children with Down syndrome 3×/wk for 10 wk 30 min sessions, achieving 65-70% peak heart rate	Difficulty promoting increasing activity intensity Improved peak exercise time and grade, but not in aerobic capacity; improved walking capacity
Treadmill training program¶	Children with intellectual disabilities Daily for 2 mo Progressive treadmill use with goal of 20-30 min	Improved heart rate with and without activities Therapist developed and monitored, community staff implemented
Peer-guided exercise**	Adolescents with intellectual disabilities 2×/wk for 15 wk Typical adolescents and those with disabilities paired to support each other in 1 hr aerobic, weight-training, flexibility activities	Improved curl-ups, 6 min walk, and body mass index High attendance, less compliance with weight training

*Fragala-Pinkham MA, Haley SM, Rabin J, Kharasch VS. A fitness program for children with disabilities. Phys Ther 85(11):1182–1200, 2005.
†Fragala-Pinkham M, Haley SM, O'Neil ME. Group aquatic aerobic exercise for children with disabilities. Dev Med Child Neurol 50(11):822–827, 2008.
‡Blundell SW, Shepherd RB, Dean CM, Adams RD, Cahill BM. Functional strength training in cerebral palsy: a pilot study of a group circuit training class for children aged 4-8 years. Clin Rehabil 17(1):48–57, 2003.
§McBurney H, Taylor NF, Dodd KJ, Graham HK. A qualitative analysis of the benefits of strength training for young people with cerebral palsy. Dev Med Child Neurol 45(10):658–663, 2003.
‖Millar AL, Fernhall B, Burkett LN. Effects of aerobic training in adolescents with down syndrome. Med Sci Sports Exerc 25(2):270–274, 1993.
¶Lotan M, Isakov E, Kessel S, Merrick J. Physical fitness and functional ability of children with intellectual disability: effects of a short-term daily treadmill intervention. ScientificWorldJournal 4:449–457, 2004.
**Stanish HI, Temple VA. Efficacy of a peer-guided exercise programme for adolescents with intellectual disability. J Appl Res Intellect Disabil 25(4):319–328, 2012.

Recreation and organized sports are other areas where children and adolescents with disabilities can engage successfully, at times with modifications. Participation improves cardiopulmonary parameters, motor function, social competence, and general sense of well-being. Programs through Special Olympics International are an opportunity for children and adolescents to engage in supportive and monitored environments for sport and recreation.

NUTRITION AND OBESITY

Managing the combination of nutrition and physical activity is the key ingredient of weight control. Obesity is a significant problem affecting a large portion of the general population, including children with special needs. Estimates suggest that children with physical activity limitations were twice as likely as the general population to be overweight and youth with cognitive impairments are at increased risk. It is unclear if obesity is a cause for the activity limitations or is a result of the limited activity, which may be an important distinction in developing interventions. The concern with obesity contrasts with early life weight gain needs of many children with disabilities, and may pose important management confusion for parents and families with the change of focus to weight decrease. Confounding factors include (1) the propensity of some disabilities, usually those that are genetically mediated, to be associated with obesity; (2) standards of measurement may not be appropriate for certain diagnoses or disability types (e.g., expected body composition differences, short statures, contractures, or

limb deficiencies or amputations); (3) obesity may be a side effect of medication and must be weighed against benefits (e.g., antidepressants, mood stabilizers, steroids); and (4) the social network of family, friends, schools, and healthcare providers may unwittingly influence healthy habits in a negative way, including use of food as reward for behavior management.

EMOTIONAL HEALTH AND LEISURE ACTIVITIES

Emotional health is often overlooked in children with disabilities, unless mental health or challenging behaviors are the cause for the disability. Youth and adolescents with disabilities appear to be at higher risk for feeling low, stressed, or anxious (especially those with higher levels of limitations), and those with mental health needs may have lower adaptive functioning, a family history of mental illness, or a diagnosis of autism spectrum disorder. Adolescents with physical disabilities participate in fewer social activities, have fewer close or intimate friends, and have few plans for ongoing education. There is a risk for continued isolation into adulthood. Medications may be considered, but effectiveness is not guaranteed and unwanted side effects may produce more health conditions. Counseling requires insurance support or discretionary funding.

Leisure and recreational activities provide social supports, additional stress-coping mechanisms, and ability to develop social skills and a stronger personal identity. Girls with disabilities tend to engage

Table 717-3	Targeting Healthy Behaviors for Children with Disabilities
HEALTH ACTIVITY TARGET	**RELEVANCE TO CHILDREN WITH DISABILITIES**
General prevention	• Recognize risks for less healthy behaviors and barriers and facilitators about behavior changes and participation • Cover typical topics for all children; counsel regarding disability or situation context • Specifically monitor for abuse and violence • Provide typical age-appropriate adolescent information about smoking, drinking, substance abuse, sexual contacts; refer if unable to provide • Monitor for disability-specific health conditions; may require referral
Physical activity	• Promote exercise and activity—should be an expectation for activity • Ensure that family and child/adolescent are knowledgeable about benefits and possible adaptation • Review need for possible dietary changes • Consider engaging rehabilitation professionals
Nutrition and obesity	• Recognize obesity can cause limitations, and can be the result of poor dietary habits and limited activity • Ensure that family and child/adolescent are knowledgeable about healthy nutrition • Consider referral to nutritionist or other professional to engage patient and family in modeling/direction or behavior suggestions • Review need for increased activity level with dietary changes
Emotional health	• Question for sense of anxiety/feeling low, stress management and ability to adapt, social activities • Consider medications and counseling based on expected effect, monitor effects/side effects; consider referral, making sure that insurance/payment coverage is available • Consider recreation and leisure activities to promote social support and ability to develop social skills
Recreation and leisure	• Question about social activities outside the home; promote importance for development of social skills, sense of self, support • Consider referral to community programs or rehabilitation professionals
Dental	• Discuss more than preventive dental care • Suggest behavior strategies if there are problems engaging in dental appointments and refer for this service as needed

in social or skill-based activities, and boys in physical activities, with decreasing participation with increasing age. Rehabilitation professionals can assist with problem-solving activities, such as using computerized technologies (e.g., Wii, Xbox), adaptation of equipment (e.g., modified upper-limb prosthesis to allow baseball glove use), and knowledge of adapted recreation programs in the area (e.g., horseback riding, winter/water sports) to increase participation.

DENTAL CARE
Dental care is a frequently unmet health care need for children with disabilities. The principal deficits are in receipt of further or specific dental care (not preventive services) and that condition severity and low income may be associated with unmet dental needs. Challenging behaviors often limit dental care, and the use of behavior management techniques and education programs have been effective in allowing both preventive and additional dental care.

ROLE OF HEALTHCARE PROVIDERS
Healthcare providers should have higher expectations for health and healthy behaviors for children with disabilities. Healthy behaviors do not come naturally to most people, including children with disabilities and their families, and there is a role for healthcare providers in providing a better understanding of health and behavior change concepts. Primary care and other healthcare providers should be mindful of discussing and promoting health and healthy behaviors with children and adolescents with disabilities and their families (Table 717-3).

Bibliography is available at Expert Consult.

Environmental Health Hazards

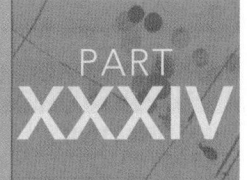

Chapter **718**

Biologic Effects of Radiation on Children

Thomas L. Slovis and Donald P. Frush

BASIC PRINCIPLES

Radiation exposure occurs from both natural (50%) and manmade (50%) sources. Radon gas accounts for the majority (37%) of natural radiation. The contribution of medical radiation has dramatically increased to 50% in 2006 from 15% in the mid-1980s. CT is responsible for 24% of all radiation exposure and almost half of manmade radiation (Fig. 718-1). Medical radiation is concerning. Estimates of dose risks ranging from no risk to as much as 2% of all cancers in the United States may be attributable to radiation from CT studies. Studies implicate CT examinations in childhood with subsequent development of cancer. In addition, radiation doses from medical imaging can be poorly understood. Seventy-five percent of radiologists and emergency department physicians are reported to underestimate the radiation dose from CT. Some imaging procedures do not produce radiation (Table 718-1), and not all radiation-producing modalities expose a child to the same amount of radiation (Table 718-2).

Nuclear medicine and positron emission tomography examinations are described by the amount of radioactivity injected (millicuries or becquerels) or are converted to effective dose (milliSieverts). The units of absorbed dose, as defined by the International Commission of Radiation Units, are the **rad,** introduced in the 1960s, and the **Gray** (Gy), introduced in 1985. The metric used in denoting biologic response is the rem (older unit) and the Sievert (Sv) (Table 718-3). Equivalent dose and effective dose are measured in Sv and mSv. Not all radiation has the same effect on biologic tissue for a given dose. Beta rays are quite superficial; alpha particles and protons cause significantly more damage than gamma radiation (x-rays) for a given absorbed dose. Diagnostic imaging uses x-rays (gamma rays). Each dose has a modifier, for example, skin dose, whole-body dose, organ dose, or effective dose. **Effective dose** considers specific tissues and their radiosensitivity.

BIOLOGIC EFFECTS OF RADIATION

Biologic effects of radiation are divided into 2 types. **Tissue reactions** (previously **deterministic effects**) (determined by the dose) are characterized by a threshold dose and severity is directly related to the magnitude once the threshold is exceeded. For example, cataracts have traditionally been reported to occur with an acute exposure to >2.0 Gy or with long-term exposure to >5.0 Gy (Table 718-4), although publications indicate lower thresholds as well as debate about these thresholds. Tissue reactions never occur from the radiation organ doses generally used in single diagnostic examinations (<100 mGy), but invasive procedures (therapeutic and interventional) have on rare occasions led to these effects. **Stochastic** (random) **effects** are of concern because they can occur at any dose; that is, there is no threshold, with the probability of an effect increasing with rising dose. These effects can be caused by any radiation striking vulnerable tissue (most importantly DNA, but cytoplasm also may be at risk) and causing irreversible damage. These effects lead to the **linear no (dose)**

threshold model, which states that radiation damage increases with rising dose in a linear fashion. This concept stresses that no level of radiation exposure can be considered to be absolutely safe.

Radiation can cause permanent cell injury, carcinogenesis, genetic mutations, or cell death. The biologic effects of radiation result primarily from damage to DNA directly (**direct effect**) through interaction of fast recoil electrons caused by the absorption of x-rays (one third of the damage) or secondarily by the formation of free radicals (**indirect effect**). Approximately 80% of the cell is water, so most of the energy deposited in a cell results in production of aqueous free radicals. The reactions are rapid (10^{-18} to 10^{-3} sec). A dose of 10 mGy results in approximately 10^3 ionizations per cell type. The biochemical and physiologic changes that follow take hours or days, whereas the induction of cancer may take a few years to decades.

The manifestations of DNA injury are variable. The cell containing the damaged DNA might die; cell death (apoptosis) is a mechanism for eliminating heavily damaged and potentially mutable cells. Damage to a base pair is the most prevalent and least significant effect. Breaks of a single strand of DNA usually have little biologic significance because each strand is repaired with use of the opposite strand as a template, but a mutation can result if misrepair occurs.

Breakage of both strands of DNA (the least-common event) is more problematic. The end result seems to depend on the proximity of the break in each strand. If widely separated, repairs occur as with a single-strand break. If the breaks in the 2 strands are opposite each other (or separated by only a few base pairs) repair is more difficult without a template. This type of break is the mechanism of radiation-induced cell death, chromosomal damage leading to mutations, and carcinogenesis.

When DNA damage occurs, aberrations are produced in chromosomes, resulting in an *unstable aberration* (usually lethal to dividing cells) or *stable aberration*. Stable aberrations can result in failure of chromosomes to reunite (leading to deletions) or in abnormal rearrangement of chromosomes, such as reciprocal translocation or aneuploidy. Although it is logical to think that these abnormalities in chromosomes lead to mutations that can activate oncogenes or proto-oncogenes or cause mutations in tumor-suppressor genes (see Chapter 492), few radiation-induced cancers show specific translocations such as would be associated with activation of specific oncogenes or known tumor-suppressor genes. An exception is the radiation induction of papillary thyroid carcinoma in children, which probably results from activation of the RET oncogene (see Chapter 506).

Radiation carcinogenesis seems to be a progressive multistep process composed of 3 independent stages: morphologic changes, cellular immortality, and tumorigenicity. Radiation exposure induces cellular genomic instability. This instability is transmitted to a cell's progeny, resulting in a continued elevation in the rate at which genetic changes arise in the subsequent generations of the irradiated cell (Fig. 718-2).

A longitudinal study of the lifetime risks of excess cancer mortality secondary to irradiation has been evaluated in *atomic bomb survivors*. More than 86,000 survivors have been followed for more than 65 yr since exposure. Individual radiation doses were estimated by considering the person's location in relation to distance from the epicenter and individual shielding situations. Most of the exposure was direct gamma irradiation, with some neutron exposure. Age at exposure and ethnic differences in cancer occurrence influence the sensitivity to radiation-induced cancers (Fig. 718-3). Compared with the middle-aged adult, children are 2-10 times more sensitive to radiation-induced carcinogenesis, and the youngest neonate is more sensitive than the older child. Because of the higher risks associated with breast and thyroid cancer, girls are more sensitive than boys. It must be understood that cancer rates in this study are mortality figures. The incidence of cancer in this population is approximately 2 times greater than mortality incidence.

The doses used in *diagnostic radiology for multidetector CT* scans overlap with low-dose induced cancer in atomic bomb survivors (Fig. 718-4). Estimates for lifetime risk of cancer following head and abdominal CT scans in children vary widely, from as low as 1:500 to more than 1:10,000 (including the possibility that these doses do not incur a risk). Therefore, since stochastic effects are random but increase with rising dose, it is mandatory that we use the lowest dose necessary to get sufficiently diagnostic images. The advent of digital picture archiving communication systems utilizes postprocessing algorithms and can make all images diagnostic, even those with higher-than-necessary exposures. Since the elimination of film-based systems, where overexposures were evident as "dark" films, digital technology eliminates the imager's ability to know whether enough or too much radiation was given. It does not allow the imager to determine whether the patient received "as low as reasonably achievable" radiation dosing. It is for this reason that some radiation metric (and familiarity with this metric) should appear on each image.

Increased biologic vulnerability to radiation can be seen in the fetus exposed in utero through maternal radiation. In utero radiation exposure is associated with a 92% excess risk of dying from leukemia

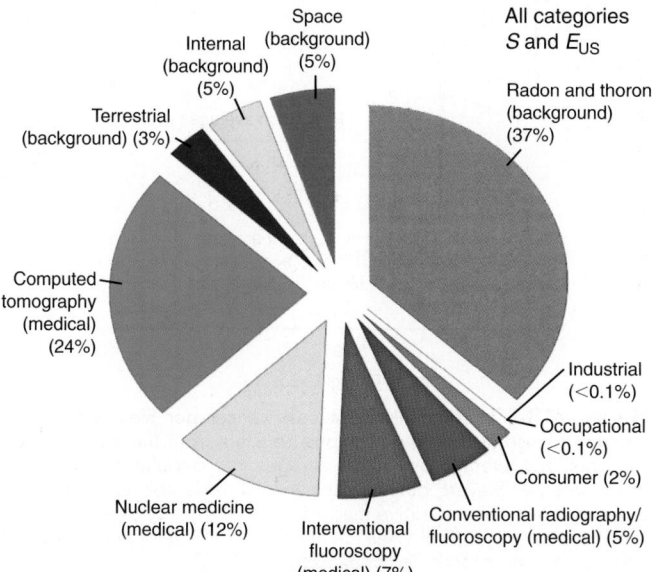

Figure 718-1 All exposure categories collective effective dose (percentage) 2006. *(From the National Council on Radiation Protection and Measurements. Ionizing Radiation Exposure of the Population of the United States (NCRP report 160), Bethesda, MD, National Council on Radiation Protection and Measurements http://pubs.rsna.org/doi/full/10.1148/radiol.2532090494.)*

Table 718-1	Imaging Modalities	
MODALITY	**SOURCE**
Plain film	Radiation (x-ray)
Angiography/fluoroscopy	Radiation (x-ray)
Ultrasound	Sound beams
Computed tomography	Radiation (x-ray)
Magnetic resonance imaging	Magnetic field; radiofrequency
Nuclear medicine (including positron emission tomography)	Radiation (injected isotope)

Table 718-2	Radiation Dose by Imaging Test*	
EXAMINATION	**DOSE**	**SITE MEASURED**
Chest—2 views	0.1-0.2 mGy	Entrance (skin)
Abdominal—2 views	0.5-1.0 mGy	Entrance (skin)
Fluoroscopy		Entrance (skin)
Nonpulsed	3-5 mGy/min	
Pulsed	1-3 mGy/min	
Computed tomography[†]		
Head (2 yr old)	20-30 mGY	Middiameter of phantom of 16 cm
Abdomen (2 yr old)	2-3 mGY	Middiameter of phantom of 32 cm
Nuclear medicine[‡] (technetium ^{99m}Tc mercaptoacetyltriglycine–renal)	120 mSv	Effective dose
Positron emission tomography[‡] (brain fludeoxyglucose ^{18}F)	185 mSv	Effective dose, whole body

*Background radiation = 0.01 mSv/day or 3 mSv/yr.
[†]Scan explained as CT dose index (CTDI). First dose is with adult factors; second dose, shown in parentheses, is examination adjusted for children.
[‡]Expressed as effective dose. These are rough guidelines for dose given to a 5 yr old with normal renal function.
From Valentin J: Radiation dose to patients from radiopharmaceuticals. (Addendum 2 to ICRP Publication 53.) ICRP Publication 80. Approved by the Commission in September 1997. Ann ICRP 28:1, 1998.

Table 718-3	Radiation Measurements			
UNITS	**RADIOACTIVITY**	**ABSORBED DOSE**	**DOSE EQUIVALENT**	**EXPOSURE**
Common units	curie (Ci)	rad	rem	roentgen (R)
New units	Becquerel (Bq)	Gray (Gy)	Sievert (Sv)	coulombs/kg

CONVERSION EQUIVALENTS
1 millicurie (mCi) = 37 megabecquerels (MBq)*
100 rad = 1 Gy
1 rad = 1 cGy
100 rem = 1 Sv
1 rem = 10 mSv
Background radiation dose is approximately 1 millirad/day

*To convert mBq to mSv, use conversion table:
  1 mrad = millirad = 1/1,000 of a rad.
  rem = rad × radiation factor; weighting for gamma and x-ray, this factor is 1.
  rem = rad × 1.

Table 718-4	Deterministic Dose Rates
INJURY	**APPROXIMATE THRESHOLD**
SKIN	
Transient erythema	200 rad (2 Gy)
Dry desquamation	1,000 rad (10 Gy)
Moist desquamation	1,500 rad (15 Gy)
Temporary epilation	200 rad (2 Gy)
Permanent epilation	700 rad (7 Gy)
EYES	
Cataracts (acute)	>200 rad (2.0 Gy)*

*Has been reported as occurring between 0.5 and 1.0 Gy.
Modified from Hall EJ: Radiobiology for the radiologist, ed 5, Philadelphia, 2000, Lippincott Williams & Wilkins.

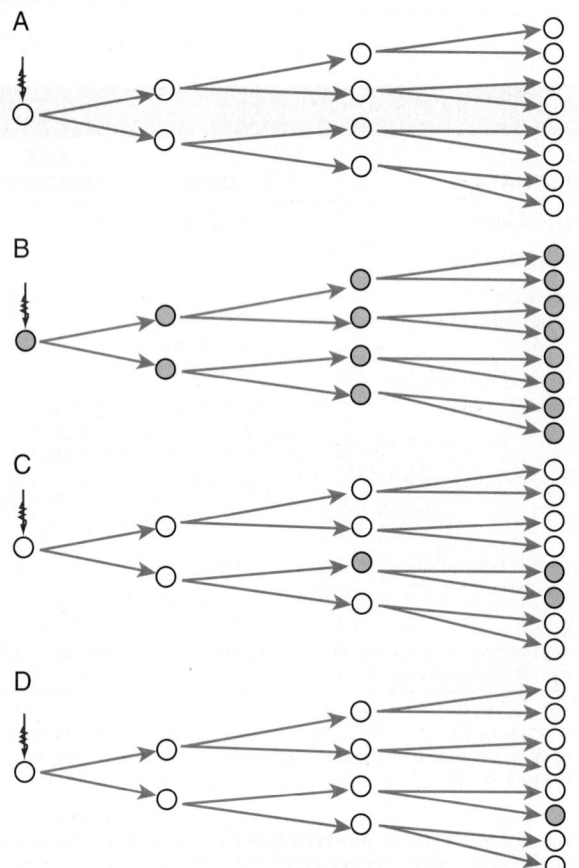

Figure 718-2 Schematic of radiation-induced mutagenesis. *Open circles* represent normal wild-type cells, whereas *solid blue circles* represent mutated cells. **A,** Most of the cells in an irradiated population retain the wild-type phenotype. **B,** Example of a cell directly mutated by radiation exposure; the mutation is transmitted to all of its progeny. **C** and **D** are examples of mutations arising as a result of radiation-induced genomic instability. The irradiated cell and its immediate progeny are wild type, but the frequency with which mutations arise among the more distant descendants of the irradiated cell is elevated. *(From Little JB: Ionizing radiation. In Kufe DW, Pollock RE, Weichselbaum RR, et al, editors: Holland-Frei cancer medicine, ed 3, Ontario, Canada, 2003, BC Decker.)*

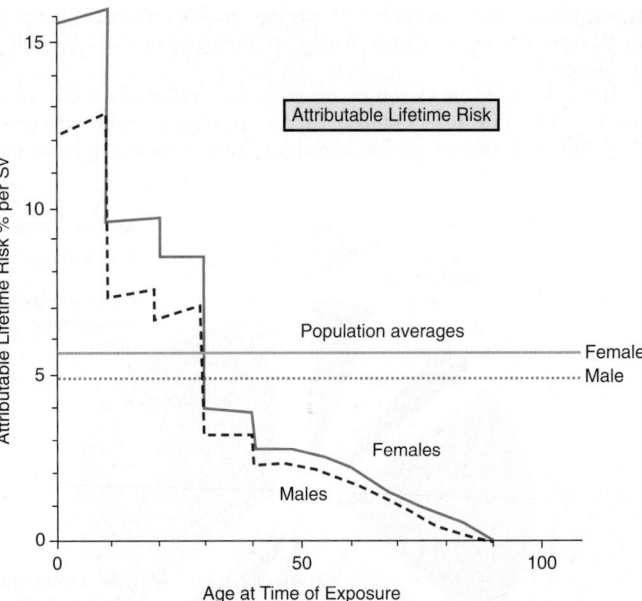

Figure 718-3 Lifetime risk of excess cancer per Sievert (Sv) as a function of age at the time of exposure. Data from the atomic bomb survivors. The average risk across all ages in a population is approximately 5% per Sievert, but the risk varies considerably with age: children are much more sensitive than adults. At early ages, girls are more sensitive than boys. *(From Hall EJ: Introduction to session I: Helical CT and cancer risk, Pediatr Radiol 32:225–227, 2002.)*

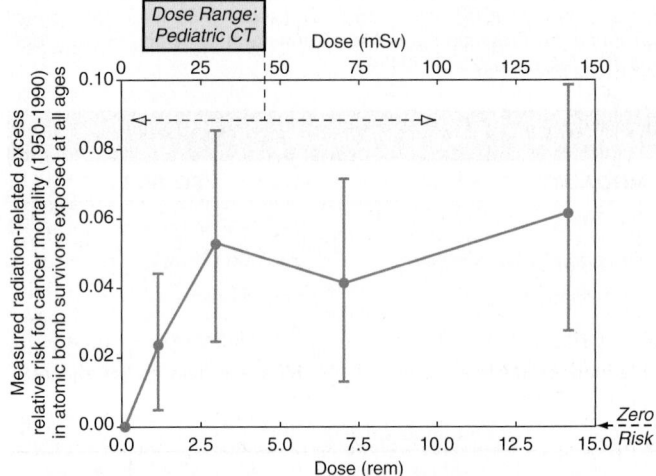

Figure 718-4 Relevant dose range for pediatric CT: 6-100 mSv (0.006-0.1 Sv). There is direct, statistically significant evidence for risk in the dose range from 0-0.1 Sv. *(From Brenner DJ: Estimating cancer risks from pediatric CT: going from the qualitative to the quantitative, Pediatr Radiol 32:228–231, 2002.)*

before age 10 yr and a 180% excess risk of dying from other malignant diseases. Even 40 yr later there is a 228% increased relative risk of cancer associated with radiation in utero.

The fetus and infant are most vulnerable to radiation-induced cancer because (1) they are growing rapidly, with many cells undergoing mitotic activity; (2) radiation-induced tumors (except leukemia) take a long time to develop and children have a longer lifetime; and (3) there is a greater time to have imaging studies, with accumulation of the risks related to doses.

Most childhood tumors occur sporadically, but 10-15% of cases have a strong familial association. Familial tumors have specific chromosomal deletions in common. In some of these tumors (retinoblastoma), the 2-hit hypothesis by Knudson is apparent (see Chapter 491). It is not coincidental that individuals with many of the congenital diseases are at risk for the development of tumors after irradiation.

Table 718-5	Inherited Human Syndromes Associated with Sensitivities to X-Rays
Ataxia-telangiectasia Basal cell nevoid syndrome Cockayne syndrome Down syndrome	Fanconi anemia Gardner syndrome Nijmegen breakage syndrome Usher syndrome

Modified from Slovis TL, Frush DP, Berdon WE, et al: Biologic effects of diagnostic radiation on children. In Slovis TL, editor: Caffey's pediatric diagnostic imaging, ed 11, Philadelphia, 2008, Mosby, p. 5; and Hall EJ: Radiobiology for the radiologist, ed 6, Philadelphia, 2006, Lippincott Williams & Wilkins, p. 41.

Table 718-5 lists diseases that are associated with sensitivity to radiation.

DECREASING UNNECESSARY DIAGNOSTIC RADIATION IN CHILDREN WHILE STILL OBTAINING DIAGNOSTIC IMAGES

Selecting the correct examination is the responsibility of the ordering physician and may involve consultation with the radiologist, preferably with pediatric expertise. Evidence-based medicine has shown little yield from an imaging work-up (including CT) of a child with a single nonfebrile seizure without other neurologic abnormalities. This is especially true if there is no antecedent history of abnormal behavior or of personality or developmental change. CT does not detect as many abnormalities as MRI, and CT involves ionizing radiation. MRI detects the subtle changes of congenital or acquired anomalies that may be responsible for seizures much more easily. Therefore, it is appropriate, **except** in an emergency situation, to obtain MRI within a reasonable time frame instead of performing 2 tests (CT followed by an MRI).

It has been estimated that perhaps up to 30% of imaging examinations, including CT examinations, are questionably indicated, and may be replaced by another, non–radiation-producing modality, or are performed without evidence-based indications.

Reducing Radiation from the CT Examination

The most common source of medical radiation is CT. We have progressed from a single-slice scanner to scanners that can obtain up to 320 slices in subsecond time. The images have excellent detail, including multiplanar and 3-dimensional reconstruction of the acquired data. It once took more than 30 min to obtain 10-12 images, but now hundreds to thousands of images are generated in seconds. When adult parameters for CT settings are used for children, the dosage for children is actually higher than the dosage for adults. This occurs because lower-energy x-rays that would have been absorbed in the near field in an adult pass into the entire child, irradiating all organs. When comparing dosages given to newborns and adults during CT scanning of the head, with the same parameters in both groups, the dosage given to newborns is 4 times that of the dosage given to adults. With abdominal imaging, the dosage is increased by 60%.

It is the role of the radiologist to tailor the examination to the pediatric patient. One can determine whether the examination is tailored to the pediatric patient by looking at the dose report or the parameters of tube current (milliamperage/second [mAs]) and peak kilovoltage (kVp). Scanning range should be limited to only the necessary area. Multiphase scanning should only be obtained when necessary. The radiologist has many ways to decrease parameters so that children receive diagnostic imaging without excessive radiation. In some instances, reducing the radiation dose by half, even in adults receiving CT, does not change the diagnostic efficacy of the study and the radiologist's ability to make the proper diagnosis.

RADIATION THERAPY—ACUTE AND LATE EFFECTS

Radiation therapy uses high doses to kill malignant cells. The sensitivity of normal cells is quite close to that of malignant cells, and to achieve significant cure rates, radiation oncologists must accept a given

Table 718-6	Late Effects of Radiation Therapy in Children Treated for Cancer	
SYSTEM	**LATE EFFECT**	**DOSE (Gy)**
Musculoskeletal	Muscular hypoplasia	>20
	Scoliosis, kyphosis, lordosis	10-20
	Osteocartilaginous exostosis	?
Neuroendocrine (cranial or cranial spinal)	Impaired growth hormone	>18
	Adrenocorticotropic hormone deficiency	>40
	Thyrotropin-releasing deficiency	>40
	Precocious puberty (females mostly)	>20
	Gonadotropin deficiency	<40
Gonad failure	Ovarian failure	4-12
	Testicular failure	>3
Central nervous system dysfunction*	Structured changes	>18
	Cognitive changes	?
Other	Pulmonary fibrosis	
	Nephropathy	
	Liver failure	
	Arteritis	
	Eye impairment	
	Ear impairment	
	Bone marrow dysfunction	
	Cardiac impairment	

*With intrathecal chemotherapy (methotrexate).
Derived from Halperin EC, Constine LS, Tarbell NJ, et al, editors: Pediatric radiation oncology, ed 3, Philadelphia, 1999, Lippincott Williams & Wilkins.

percentage of serious complications (5-10%). Radiation causes tissue loss plus injury to the underlying vasculature. The vascular change may be progressive, leading to arteriocapillary fibrosis and irreparable injury, in turn leading to further tissue loss.

The acute effects of therapy (occurring less than 3 mo after therapy begins) are usually related to the area of the body being irradiated (except fatigue, which can begin during this time period). These acute effects include radiation-caused pneumonitis, dermatitis, mucositis and esophagitis, cerebral edema, and swelling of the organ irradiated. There may be changes in bowel movement patterns. Of these, one of the most severe acute reactions is pneumonitis. It can be manifest within 24 hr of irradiation when there is an exudation of proteinaceous material into the alveoli and intraalveolar edema. Most often, however, radiation pneumonitis begins 2-6 mo after the beginning of radiation with a clinical presentation of fever, cough, congestion, and pruritic pain. The late effects of therapy (beginning more than 3 mo after therapy) are numerous (Table 718-6). The most common are abnormalities of pulmonary function, hearing loss, endocrine/reproductive function, cardiac function, and neurocognitive loss.

Annually, childhood cancer affects 70-160 per million children between the ages of 0 and 14 yr. Because of earlier diagnosis and improved therapy, more than 79% of children who were diagnosed from 1995-2001 with cancer are long-term survivors. Approximately 1 in 570 young adults is a long-term survivor of cancer, and up to 25% have a complication related to their therapy. Second cancers account for 6-10% of all cancers in children or adults. Among children in the Childhood Cancer Survivor Study, there is a cumulative incidence of second neoplasms of 3.2% at 20 yr from original diagnosis. Primary malignancies with the highest cumulative incidence of a second neoplasm in the order of frequency are Hodgkin disease (7.6), soft tissue

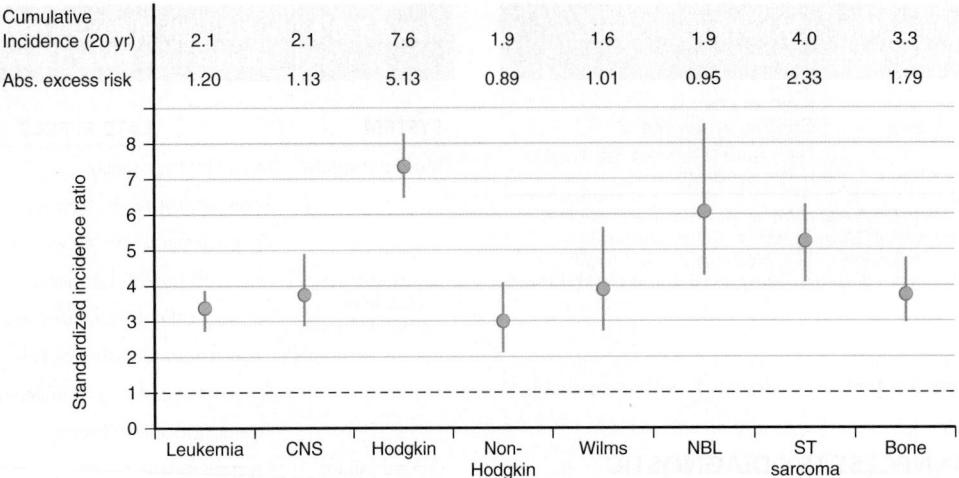

Figure 718-5 Second malignancies among the Childhood Cancer Survivor Study cohort. CNS, central nervous system; NBL, neuroblastoma; ST, soft tissue. *(From Robison LL: Treatment-associated subsequent neoplasms among long-term survivors of childhood cancer: the experience of the Childhood Cancer Survivor Study, Pediatr Radiol 39[Suppl 1]:S32–S37, 2009, Fig. 1.)*

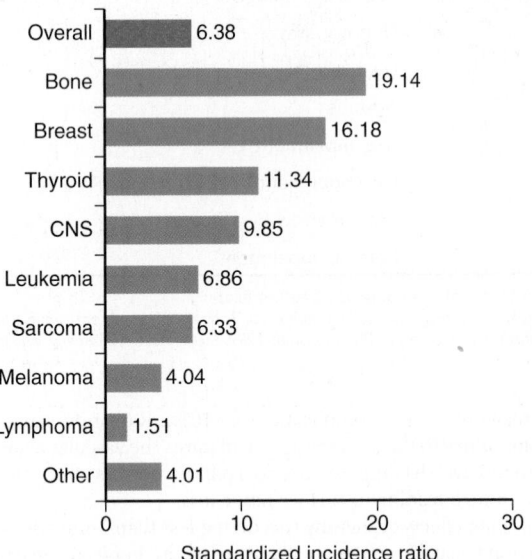

Figure 718-6 Standardized incidence ratio by type of second malignancy. CNS, central nervous system. *(Robison LL: Treatment-associated subsequent neoplasms among long-term survivors of childhood cancer: the experience of the Childhood Cancer Survivor Study, Pediatr Radiol 39[Suppl 1]:S32–S37, 2009, Fig. 2.)*

sarcoma (4.0), cancers of bone (3.3), leukemia (2.1), central nervous system (CNS) cancers (2.1), and non-Hodgkin disease lymphoma (1.9). This reflects an overall standard incidence rate of 6.38% (Fig. 718-5). The most prevalent second tumors are bone, breast, thyroid, and CNS lesions (Fig. 718-6). Table 718-7 relates second cancers to primary cancer and latency period. Almost 70% of the second neoplasms are in the field of the original irradiation. Radiation therapy increases the risk of second cancers in a dose-dependent manner for nongenetic neoplasms.

The exact complications depend on the location of the treatment field. In children, because of the location of many childhood tumors, the normal brain is commonly in the treatment field. Standard irradiation of the brain in children results in cortical atrophy in more than half of patients who receive 2,000-6,000 rads; 26% are left with white matter changes (leukoencephalopathy) and 8% with calcifications. The younger the child is at the time of irradiation, the greater is the

atrophy. Some patients also demonstrate mineralizing microangiopathy. Radiation-induced changes of the brain are potentiated by methotrexate administered before, during, or after radiation therapy.

Cerebral necrosis is a serious complication of radiation-induced vascular disease. It usually is diagnosed 1-5 yr after irradiation but can occur up to a decade later. Brain necrosis may manifest as headache, increased intracranial pressure, seizures, sensory deficits, and psychotic changes.

Spinal cord irradiation may result in **radiation myelitis,** which may be either transient or permanent. Acute transient myelitis often appears 2-4 mo after irradiation. Patients with myelitis usually present with **Lhermitte sign,** a sensation of little electrical shocks in the arms and legs occurring with neck flexion or other movements that stretch the spinal cord. Reversal of transient myelopathy usually occurs between 8 and 40 wk and does not necessarily progress to delayed necrosis.

Delayed myelopathy occurs after a mean latent period of 20 mo but can occur earlier if the total dose or the dose per fraction is high. It usually manifests as discontinuous deterioration and is irreversible. In the cervical and thoracic regions, sensory dissociation develops, followed by spastic and then flaccid paresis. In the lumbar cord, flaccid paresis is dominant. The mortality for high thoracic and cervical lesions reaches 70%, death being due to pneumonia and urinary tract infections.

Central nervous system irradiation may also affect growth by compromising function of the pituitary-hypothalamic axis and leading to diminishing growth hormone production and release. Non–growth hormone trophins may also be affected by CNS irradiation, leading to gonadotrophin deficiency or precocious puberty. Central hypothyroidism can also develop. CNS irradiation also compromises bone mineral deposition both locally (in the radiation field) and systemically.

Irradiation also has other effects specific to children (see Table 718-6). Scoliosis and hypoplasia of bones may occur if fractionated treatment schemes exceed 4,000 rad. Fractionated doses higher than 2,500 rad can result in slipped capital femoral epiphyses. An increase in the incidence of benign osteochondromas also has been reported after childhood irradiation. Chest wall irradiation of girls (besides causing breast cancer) may impair breast development and/or cause fibrosis and atrophy of breast tissue.

WHOLE-BODY IRRADIATION
Uncontrolled Large- or Small-Scale Exposure to Radiation

Large-scale exposure to radiation can occur in an event of nuclear accidents, war, or terrorist attacks (see Chapters 39.2 and 723). Radiation as well as explosive and thermal injury need to be considered.

Table 718-7	Second Cancers and Their Relationship with Primary Cancers		
SECOND CANCERS	**PRIMARY CANCERS**	**LATENCY (MEDIAN IN Yr)**	**RISK FACTORS**
Brain tumors	ALL; brain tumors; HD	9-10	Radiation; younger age
Myelodysplastic syndromes/acute myelogenous leukemia	ALL; HD; bone tumors	3-5	Topoisomerase II inhibitors; alkylating agents
Breast cancer	HD; bone tumors; soft-tissue sarcomas; ALL; brain tumors; Wilms tumors; NHL	15-20	Radiation; female gender
Thyroid cancer	ALL: HD; neuroblastoma; soft-tissue sarcomas; bone tumors; NH: L	13-15	Radiation; younger age; female gender
Bone tumors	Retinoblastoma (heritable); other bone tumors; Ewing sarcoma; soft-tissue sarcomas; ALL	9-10	Radiation; alkylating agents; removal of the spleen
Soft-tissue sarcomas	Retinoblastoma (heritable); soft-tissue sarcomas; HD; Wilms tumors; bone tumors; ALL	10-11	Radiation; younger age; anthracyclines

ALL, acute lymphocytic leukemia; HD, Hodgkin disease; NHL, non-Hodgkin lymphoma.
From Bhatia S, Sklar S: Second cancers in survivors of childhood cancer. Nat Rev Cancer 2:124–132, 2002.

Table 718-8	Dose–Effect Relationships After Acute Whole-Body Irradiation from Gamma Rays or X-Rays
WHOLE-BODY ABSORBED DOSE, RAD (Gy)	**FINDINGS**
5 (0.05)	Asymptomatic
15 (0.15)	Asymptomatic (but chromosome aberrations may be present in cultured peripheral lymphocytes)
50 (0.5)	Asymptomatic (minor depression of white blood cell and platelet counts in a few persons)
100 (1.0)	Nausea and vomiting in approximately 10% of patients within 2 days of exposure
200 (2.0)	Nausea and vomiting in most persons exposed, with clear hematologic depression
400 (4.0)	Nausea, vomiting, and diarrhea within 48 hr; 50% mortality without medical treatment
600 (6.0)	100% mortality within 30 days from bone marrow failure without medical treatment
5,000 (50.0)	Cardiovascular collapse and central nervous system damage, with death in 24-72 hr

Table 718-9	Expected Outcome Based on Absolute Lymphocyte Count After Acute Penetrating Whole-Body Irradiation
MINIMAL LYMPHOCYTE COUNT WITHIN FIRST 48 HR AFTER EXPOSURE	**PROGNOSIS**
1,000-3,000 (normal range)	No significant injury
1,000-1,500	Significant but probably nonlethal injury, good prognosis
500-1,000	Severe injury, fair prognosis
100-500	Very severe injury, poor prognosis
<100	Lethal without compatible bone marrow donor

Clinical Manifestations

Table 718-8 presents dose–effect relationships for acute whole-body penetrating radiation. A large single exposure of penetrating radiation can result in **acute radiation syndrome.** The signs and symptoms of this syndrome result from damage to major organ systems that have different levels of radiation sensitivity, modulated by the rate at which the radiation exposure occurred. Delivery of 100 rads in 1 min would be symptomatic, but delivery of 1 rad/day for 100 days would not be symptomatic.

The **hematopoietic syndrome** results from acute whole-body doses above 200 rad. A prodromal phase consists of nausea and vomiting within the 1st 12 hr, with symptoms usually lasting up to 48 hr. A latent period of 2-3 wk, during which patients may feel quite well, follows. Although patients are asymptomatic, bone marrow impairment has occurred. The most obvious laboratory finding is lymphocyte depression (Table 718-9). Maximal bone marrow depression occurs approxi-

mately 30 days after exposure, when hemorrhage and infection can be major problems. If the bone marrow was not completely eradicated, a recovery phase then ensues. This radiation effect is similar to what occurs when whole-body irradiation (given as 1,200 rads in 2 treatments) is used to obliterate the bone marrow in children with leukemia before bone marrow transplantation.

The **gastrointestinal syndrome** occurs from acute whole-body doses above 800 rads. Prompt onset of nausea, vomiting, and diarrhea follows. There is a latent period of approximately 1 wk followed by recurrence of gastrointestinal symptoms, sepsis, and electrolyte imbalance, which may result in death.

At dose levels exceeding 3,000 rad, the **cardiovascular/CNS syndrome** predominates. Nausea, vomiting, prostration, hypotension, ataxia, and convulsions are almost immediate. Death usually occurs promptly.

Treatment

For the hematopoietic and gastrointestinal syndromes, treatment is supportive, involving transfusions, fluids, antibiotics, and antiviral agents.

Localized Irradiation
Clinical Manifestations

Because localized exposure involves a small amount of tissue, systemic manifestations may be less severe and patients may survive even if locally absorbed doses are very high. The hand is the most common

Table 718-10	Skin Changes After a Single, Acute, Localized Radiation Exposure

ABSORBED DOSE (Gy)	CHANGE
3-4	Epilation in 2-3 wk
10-15	Threshold for erythema; appears 18-20 days after exposure at lower doses; may appear within a few hours at higher doses
20	Moist desquamation, possible ulceration
25	Ulceration with slow healing
30-50	Blistering, necrosis at 3 wk
100	Blistering, necrosis at 1-2 wk

Data from Gusev I, Guskova AK, Mettler FA Jr, editors: Medical management of radiation accidents, ed 2, Boca Raton, FL, 2001, CRC Press.

site for accidental localized irradiation injuries, usually as a result of picking up or playing with lost radiation sources. The second most common accidental site is the thigh and buttocks, predominantly from placing unsuspected highly radioactive sources in the pockets.

Table 718-10 lists the skin changes that occur after a single acute, localized irradiation. As opposed to other forms of thermal burns, signs of irradiation appear a period of days *after* the exposure. Vascular insufficiency may appear months to years later and cause ulcerations or necrosis in formerly healed areas. The penetrability of the radiation is an important factor in the outcome of local radiation injury. Beta rays from heavy radiation fallout can cause superficial skin burns because they have low penetrability.

Some tissues that may receive localized radiation exposure are relatively radiosensitive. **Cataract formation** (see Chapter 628) may occur with single gamma ray exposures in the range of less than 1 Gy to several Gy. Such cataracts usually take from 2 mo to several years to develop. **Oligospermia** may take up to 2 mo to develop. Transient infertility in men may result from doses as low as 15 rad, and permanent sterility may occur in men at dose levels between 300 and 600 rad.

Treatment
Skin therapy is directed at prevention of infections. Treatment of localized injuries usually involves plastic surgery and grafting, if the radiation exposure was not very penetrating (see Chapter 75). The nature of the surgery depends on the dose at various depths in tissue and the location of the lesion. The full expression of radiation injury often is not apparent for 1-2 yr, owing to slow arteriolar narrowing that can cause delayed necrosis. After relatively penetrating radiation, amputation may be necessary because of obliterative changes in small vessels.

INTERNAL CONTAMINATION
Epidemiology
Accidents involving internal contamination are rare and are usually the result of misadministration in hospital settings or voluntary ingestion of unsuspected contaminated radioactive materials. Other possible causes of internal contamination of children include ingestion of breast milk from mothers who have had diagnostic nuclear medicine scans and radiation exposure when a parent or sibling receives a therapeutic dose of iodine-131.

Clinical Manifestations
The hazards from internal contamination depend on the nature of both the radionuclide (particularly in terms of its solubility in water, half-life, and radioactive emission) and the chemical compound.

Treatment
The most effective treatment requires knowledge of both the radionuclide and the chemical form. Treatment must be instituted quickly to

Table 718-11	Specific Therapy for Internal Radiation Contamination

RADIONUCLIDE	THERAPEUTIC APPROACH
Tritium	Dilution (force fluids)
Iodine-125 or iodine-131	Blockage (saturated solution of potassium iodide or potassium iodide), mobilization (antithyroid drugs)
Cesium-134 or cesium-137	Reduction of gastrointestinal absorption (Prussian blue)
Strontium-89 or strontium-90	Reduction of absorption (aluminum phosphate gel antacids), blockage (strontium lactate), displacement (oral phosphate), mobilization (ammonium chloride or parathyroid extract)
Plutonium and other transuranic elements	Chelation with zinc or calcium diethylenetriamine pentaacetic acid (investigational agents)
Unknown	Reduction of absorption (emetics, lavage, charcoal, or laxatives) in cases of ingestion

From Mettler FA, Voelz GL: Major radiation exposure—what to expect and how to respond. N Engl J Med 346:1554, 2002.

be effective (Table 718-11). **Removal treatment** involves cleaning a contaminated wound and performing stomach lavage or administration of cathartics in the case of ingestion. Administration of alginate-containing antacids (e.g., Gaviscon) also usually helps in removal by decreasing absorption in the gastrointestinal tract. An example of **blocking therapy** is the administration of potassium iodine or other stable iodine-containing compounds to patients with known internal contamination with radioactive iodine. The stable iodine effectively blocks the thyroid, although its effectiveness decreases rapidly as time elapses after the contamination. The recommended dose of potassium iodine is 16 mg for neonates; 32 mg for children ages 3 yr or younger; and 65 mg for children ages 3-18 yr. Each dose protects for only 1 day. **Dilution therapy** is used in cases of tritium (radioactive hydrogen as water) contamination. Forcing fluids promotes excretion. Cases of internal contamination with transuranic elements (americium and plutonium) may require **chelation therapy** with calcium diethylene triamine pentaacetic acid.

Prussian blue is a drug approved by the FDA for patients with internal contamination with cesium or thallium. It can speed fecal elimination of radioactive cesium from the body. It acts by intercepting the cesium coming into the gut from the bile. Prussian blue prevents the cesium from being absorbed again from the gut. Prussian blue can be given days after ingestion, unlike potassium iodine, which must be given initially in the 1st 12-24 hr after exposure.

EXTERNAL CONTAMINATION
The presence of external radioactive contamination on a patient's skin is not an immediate medical emergency. Management involves removing and controlling the spread of radioactive materials. If a patient has suspected surface contamination and no physical injuries, decontamination can be performed relatively easily. If substantial physical trauma or other life-threatening injuries are combined with external contamination, surface decontamination should proceed only after the patient has been stabilized physiologically. In many accident situations, essential medical care is delayed inappropriately by hospital emergency staff because of fear of radiation or spread of contamination in the hospital. After a radiation accident, triaging of patients is critical and is based on exposure and symptoms (Fig. 718-7).

Bibliography is available at Expert Consult.

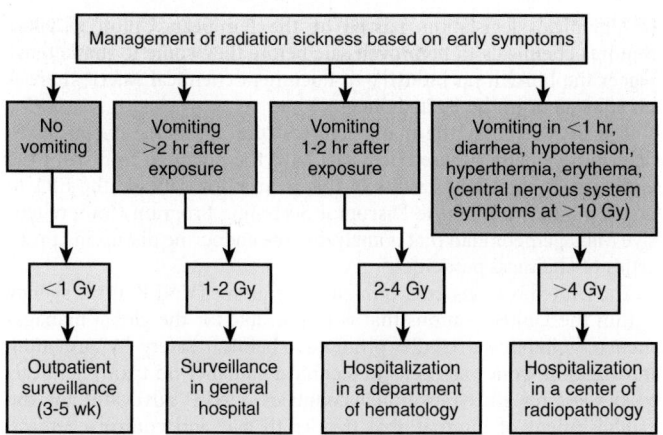

Figure 718-7 Management of radiation sickness at different levels of medical care, depending on the appearance of early symptoms and the estimated radiation dose to the whole body. *(From Turai I, Veress K, Günalp B, et al: Medical response to radiation incidents and radio-nuclear threats, BMJ 328:568–572, 2004.)*

Chapter **719**
Chemical Pollutants
Philip J. Landrigan and Joel A. Forman

More than 85,000 new synthetic chemicals have been developed in the past 75 yr. Most did not previously exist in nature. These chemicals are used today in millions of products ranging from food packaging to clothing, building materials, motor fuels, cleaning products, cosmetics, medical products, toys, and baby bottles.

Synthetic chemicals are widely disseminated in the environment. The Toxic Release Inventory of the U.S. Environmental Protection Agency (EPA) reports that in 2011 more than 4 billion pounds of toxic chemicals were discharged to air, water, and land in the United States.

Human exposure to toxic synthetic chemicals is widespread. Children are especially likely to be exposed to the nearly 3,000 chemicals that are produced in amounts of 1 million pounds or more per yr. These are designated by the EPA as high-production-volume chemicals. Biomonitoring data on blood and urine levels of more than 200 high-production-volume chemicals are obtained annually by the Centers for Disease Control and Prevention in a sample of the U.S. population through the National Health and Nutrition Examination Survey. These data document that American children are exposed to a broad array of synthetic chemicals.

Toxic chemicals are being exported in ever-increasing quantities to the world's poorer countries as these countries pass through industrial development. Environmental safeguards in those countries are typically not as stringent as in the industrially developed nations, and the potential for serious exposure to children there is therefore high.

SYNTHETIC CHEMICALS AND HUMAN HEALTH

Some synthetic chemicals have greatly benefitted human health. Antibiotics have helped control the major communicable diseases. Chemical disinfectants have reduced deaths from dysentery. Chemotherapeutic agents have made possible the cure of many childhood cancers.

But new chemicals have also been responsible for tragic episodes of disease, death, and environmental degradation. Many of these episodes have resulted in severe injury to children. A recurrent pattern has been that new chemicals were brought to market with great enthusiasm,

were presumed harmless, and underwent little or no premarket safety testing. Then yr or decades later, after they had come into wide use, established markets, and become widely disseminated in the environment, the chemicals were found to have harmful effects.

Historical examples of synthetic chemicals that were initially hailed as beneficial but later found to cause great harm include *thalidomide*, a mild sedative that proved very effective at suppressing "morning sickness" in the 1st trimester of pregnancy, but later was found to have caused an epidemic of phocomelia in infants exposed in utero; *tetraethyl lead*, which was added to gasoline in the United States from the early 1930s until 1980 and was responsible for widespread lead poisoning with subclinical neurotoxicity and reduction in IQ across 2 generations of U.S. children (see Chapter 721); the pesticide *dichloro-diphenyltrichloroethane (DDT)*, the environmental toxicity of which very nearly led to extinction of the osprey and the American bald eagle and that more recently was linked to increased risk for human breast cancer; the *polychlorinated biphenyls (PCBs)*, highly persistent pollutants of which production was banned in 1977 but which continue today to contaminate major lakes and rivers and which have been found also to be responsible for loss of IQ and disruption of behavior in U.S. children; *diethylstilbestrol (DES)*, which was administered to pregnant women to prevent miscarriage and later found to cause adenocarcinoma of the vagina in girls and young women who had been exposed in utero; and the ozone-destroying *chlorofluorocarbons*.

Other examples of synthetic chemicals that came into wide use with little assessment of their potential hazards include the *phthalates*, plasticizers widely used in plastics, cosmetics, and common household products, which are linked to increased risk for reproductive abnormalities in baby boys and to heightened risk of behavioral abnormalities that resemble attention-deficit/hyperactivity disorder (see Chapter 33); *polybrominated diphenyl ethers*, a class of chemicals widely used as flame retardants in carpets, furniture, and electronic equipment that are linked to persistent loss of intelligence and disruption of behavior; and *bisphenol A*, a plastics chemical that has been linked to neurodevelopmental disorders. These chemicals are all produced in volumes of millions of tons per yr, are widely disseminated in the environment, and are detectable in the bodies of nearly all Americans. Only now, decades after their introduction, are their possible hazards to children's health beginning to be assessed.

CHILDREN'S UNIQUE SUSCEPTIBILITY TO SYNTHETIC CHEMICALS

The health effects of synthetic chemicals are especially serious when exposure occurs in early life—during pregnancy, in infancy, or in early childhood. Children are uniquely vulnerable to chemical pollutants for several reasons:

1. Children have proportionally greater exposures to many environmental pollutants than adults. Because they drink more water, eat more food, and breathe more air per kilogram of body weight, children are more heavily exposed to pollutants in water, food, and air. Children's hand-to-mouth behavior and their play close to the ground further magnify their exposures.
2. Children's metabolic pathways, especially in the 1st few mo after birth, are immature. Although in some instances children are better able than adults to cope with environmental toxicants because they are unable to metabolize them to their active form, children are frequently less able to detoxify and excrete chemical pollutants.
3. Infants and children are growing and developing, and their complex, fast-moving, and highly choreographed developmental processes are uniquely sensitive to disruption by chemical pollutants. Exposures to even minute doses of toxic chemicals during windows of exquisite vulnerability in early development have been shown to cause a wide array of diseases in childhood and also to increase risk for chronic disease and disability lifelong (Table 719-1).
4. Because children have many future years of life, they have time for the development of multistage chronic diseases that may be triggered by early exposures.

Table 719-1	Effects of Selected Chemical Pollutants on Infants and Children
CHEMICAL POLLUTANT	**EFFECT(S)**
Air pollution	Asthma, other respiratory diseases, sudden infant death syndrome
Asbestos	Mesothelioma and lung cancer
Benzene, nitrosamine, vinyl chloride, ionizing radiation	Cancer
Diethylstilbestrol	Adenocarcinoma of the vagina after intrauterine exposure
Environmental tobacco smoke	Increased risk of sudden infant death syndrome and asthma
Ethyl alcohol	Fetal alcohol syndrome after intrauterine exposure
Lead	Neurobehavioral toxicity from low-dose exposure
Methyl mercury	Developmental neurotoxicity
Organophosphate insecticides	Developmental neurotoxicity
Polychlorinated biphenyls	Developmental neurotoxicity
Polybrominated diphenyl ethers	Developmental neurotoxicity
Phthalates	Developmental neurotoxicity and reproductive impairment
Thalidomide	Phocomelia after intrauterine exposure
Trichloroethylene	Elevated risk of leukemia after intrauterine exposure

The unique susceptibility of infants and children to toxic chemicals—susceptibility that is both quantitatively and qualitatively different from that of adults—is summarized in the phrase "children are not little adults."

SAFETY TESTING OF SYNTHETIC CHEMICALS

A fundamental problem in environmental pediatrics is that only approximately 65% of high-production-volume chemicals have been tested for their potential hazards to human health, and fewer than 30% have been assessed for their pediatric or developmental toxicity. In the United States, chemicals are regulated under the 1976 Toxic Substances Control Act. Unfortunately, this law is obsolete, broken, and fails to protect children's health against toxic synthetic chemicals.

At the time of its passage, the Toxic Substances Control Act was intended to be pioneering legislation that would require chemicals already in commerce to be tested for potential toxicity and that would also require premarket safety testing of all new chemicals. The Toxic Substances Control Act never fulfilled these noble intentions. A particularly egregious lapse was a decision by the Congress to "grandfather in" 62,000 chemicals already on the market without any toxicity testing. These chemicals were simply presumed to be safe and allowed to remain in commerce unless the EPA made a finding that they posed an "unreasonable risk." Under the Toxic Substances Control Act, only 5 chemicals have been banned in the United States in the past 35 yr: PCBs, the ozone-destroying chlorofluorocarbons, dioxin, asbestos, and hexavalent chromium.

In consequence of the failure of current chemical safety legislation in the United States, chemicals are de facto presumed to be safe until they are proven beyond any shadow of doubt to cause harm. New chemicals are brought to the market with little or no safety testing. By contrast, the Registration, Evaluation, Authorization, and Restriction

of Chemicals legislation, passed by the European Union in 2006, requires chemicals to be proven safe before they come to market and places the burden on industry to document chemical safety; there is no equivalent in the United States.

The EPA requires the manufacturers of 67 pesticide chemicals to determine whether these chemicals have the potential to disrupt the endocrine system. The results of this request for data led the EPA to develop a new Endocrine Disruptor Screening Program Comprehensive Management Plan that is analyzing the endocrine disrupting properties of chemical pesticides.

The United Nations Environment Programme (UNEP) is the agency within the United Nations that is responsible for the global management of chemicals. UNEP promotes chemical safety by providing information, policy advice, and technical guidance on toxic chemicals to developing and transitional countries. UNEP advocates for the establishment of international treaties to ban and control chemical substances. UNEP coordinates with other international organizations such as the Food and Agriculture Organization of the United Nations. UNEP has been centrally involved in partnership with the World Health Organization in coordinating the global effort to remove lead from gasoline in countries around the world.

SYNTHETIC CHEMICALS AND DISEASE IN CHILDREN

A large and growing body of evidence accumulated over the past 5 decades documents that chemical pollutants in the environment can cause disease and dysfunction in children. High-dose exposures can cause acute, clinically evident disease. Lower-dose exposures can cause subclinical injury—injury that is very real but detectable only through special testing—such as decreases in intelligence, shortening of attention span, and disruption of behavior. When exposure to a chemical pollutant is widespread, subclinical toxicity can reduce intelligence and cause other adverse effects across entire societies (Fig. 719-1).

CHEMICAL POLLUTANTS OF MAJOR CONCERN
Air Pollutants

The outdoor air pollutants of greatest concern are photochemical oxidants (especially ozone), oxides of nitrogen, fine particulates, sulfur oxides, and carbon monoxide. These pollutants result principally from the combustion of fossil fuels. Automotive emissions are the major source of air pollution worldwide, followed by stationary sources such as coal-fired power plants and other industrial sources.

Elevated values of air pollutants, especially fine particulates, ozone, and oxides of nitrogen, are associated with respiratory problems in children, including decreased pulmonary expiratory flow, wheezing, and exacerbations of asthma. Fine particulate air pollution, even at low levels, is associated with slight increases in cardiopulmonary mortality and with an increased death rate from sudden infant death syndrome (see Chapter 375). A prospective cohort study of air pollution and lung development in California found an association between pollution and reduced lung growth from ages 10-18 yr, which leads to clinically significant decreases in lung function that persist into adulthood. It is notable that these effects were seen at air toxic levels below the National Ambient Air Quality Standards set by the EPA under the Clean Air Act.

Indoor air also can be an important source of respiratory irritation, because many children spend 80-90% of their time indoors. Globally, indoor air pollution is largely caused by household use of solid fuel, such as wood, charcoal, or dung. According to the World Health Organization, globally more than 2 million children < age 5 yr die each year from acute respiratory infections of which 50% are attributable to the indoor burning of biomass fuels. Indoor air pollution has become especially important in the United States since the energy crises of the 1970s, which led to the construction of tighter, more energy-efficient homes. Second-hand cigarette smoke is an especially hazardous constituent of indoor air and a powerful asthma trigger. Allergens in indoor air can contribute to respiratory problems and include cockroach, mite, mold, and cat and dog allergens.

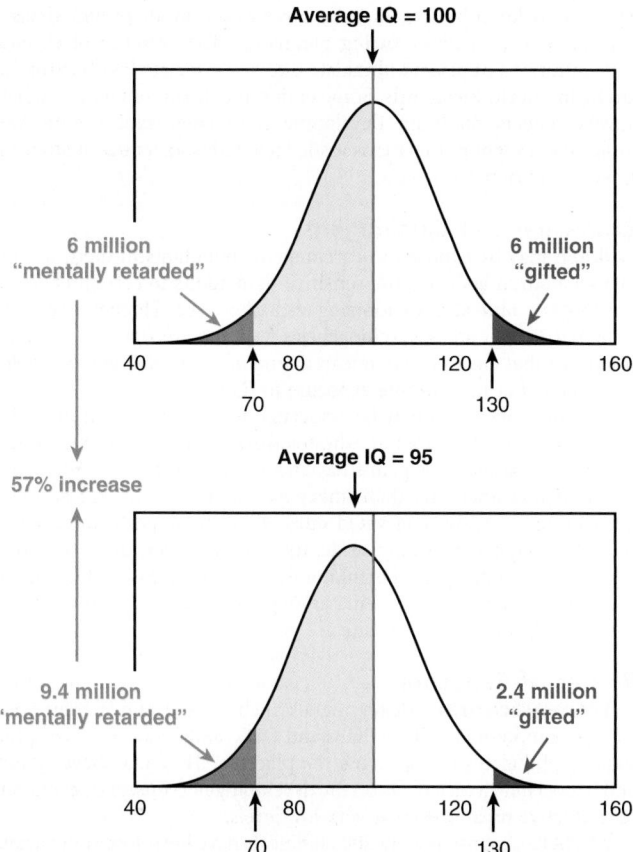

Figure 719-1 Societal impact of subclinical neurotoxicity. Widespread exposure to a neurotoxic chemical pollutant that reduces average IQ by 5 points can reduce the number of children in a society with truly superior intelligence (IQ scores above 130 points) by more than 50% and likewise cause a more than 50% increase in the number with IQ scores below 70, thus increasing the number of children who do poorly in school, require special education and other remedial programs, and cannot contribute fully to society when they become adults. Although subclinical effects may be small at the individual level, the aggregate effects at a population level can have far-reaching consequences. And until the toxicity is recognized, the damage can proceed unchecked for many years. *(From Schettler, T Stein J, Reich F, Valenti M. In harm's way: toxic threats to child development. A report by Greater Boston Physicians for Social Responsibility, 2000, p 25. Available at: http://www.psr.org/chapters/boston/resources/in-harms -way.html.)*

Oil Spill Hazards

Through 2014, there have been at least 36 crude oil spills worldwide. Ten of these spills have occurred since 1980, the largest in 2010. Although specific composition and concentrations vary, crude oil contains many toxic chemicals that are of concern to human health, including metals (e.g., zinc, cadmium, and lead) (see Chapters 720 and 721), volatile organic compounds (including benzene, toluene, ethyl benzene, and styrene), and semivolatile organics (such as polycyclic aromatic compounds). Several of these compounds are classified as possible or potential carcinogens, endocrine disruptors, and neurotoxins. Chemical dispersants—mixtures of detergents and organic solvents—are often used to break up spilled oil and may also have potential adverse effects on health. Toxic effects may occur from exposure during contact with the skin, eyes, or respiratory tract or in a person's diet (e.g., drinking of contaminated water or eating of contaminated seafood).

Commonly reported symptoms from direct exposure to crude oil include eye redness and burning, rashes, sore throat, respiratory difficulty, and acute neurologic symptoms such as headache and nausea. Children with asthma may be particularly vulnerable to respiratory

toxicity. The amount and duration of exposure along with individual genetic variability influence the degree of symptoms.

Most information on health effects of oil spills comes from studies of exposed adult workers; there are few studies of health effects, acute or long term, in children. Studies of workers exposed to spilled oil have noted elevated blood concentrations of heavy metals such as lead and cadmium, evidence of genotoxic effects, and endocrine disruption (as manifested by changes in prolactin and cortisol levels). Children and teens are at risk for exposure in a variety of settings, including recreational activities like swimming and boating as well as clean-up efforts. Children should not be allowed to play in or around areas where the water or beach contains oil or sludge. In light of teenagers' propensity to not adhere as well as adults to workplace safety regulations, teens should not be directly involved in spill clean-up efforts.

Lead
See Chapter 721.

Mercury
See Chapter 720.

Asbestos
Between 1947 and 1973, asbestos was sprayed as insulation on classroom walls and ceilings in approximately 10,000 schools in the United States. Subsequent deterioration of this asbestos has released asbestos fibers into the air. Asbestos is not a health hazard so long as it is intact, but once it becomes airborne, it can be inhaled by children to produce adverse health effects. Asbestos is a human carcinogen, and the 2 principal cancers caused by asbestos are lung cancer and mesothelioma. U.S. federal law requires that all schools be inspected periodically for asbestos and that the results be made public. Removal is required only when asbestos is visibly deteriorating or is within the reach of children. In most cases, placement of barriers (drywall walls or drop ceilings) provides appropriate protection.

Second-Hand Tobacco Smoke
Smoking during pregnancy poses a hazard to the fetus (see Chapter 96). Infants born to women who smoke are, on average, 10% smaller than infants born to nonsmoking women. Infants of parents who smoke have a higher risk of sudden infant death syndrome. Nicotine from tobacco smoke appears to be a developmental neurotoxin.

Second-hand smoke exposure is also a hazard to children. The United States has made substantial progress in reducing exposure to second-hand smoke over the last 15 yr and serum cotinine levels have declined by 70% in U.S. nonsmokers of all ages. Children <12 yr old continue to have mean cotinine levels twice those of adults, highlighting their unique vulnerability. Children exposed to second-hand tobacco smoke have increased frequency of lower respiratory illness, more middle-ear effusions, and more viral respiratory illnesses than unexposed children.

Pesticides
Pesticides are a diverse group of chemicals used to control insects, weeds, fungi, and rodents. Approximately 600 pesticides are registered with the EPA for use in the United States.

Diet is a major route of children's exposure to pesticides, because children are exposed to residues of multiple pesticides on fruit and vegetables, especially fruits and vegetables imported from countries where pesticide use is heavier than in the United States. Children also may be exposed in homes or schools, on lawns, and in gardens. They may be exposed to pesticide drift from agricultural areas that have been sprayed. Children employed in agriculture or living in migrant farm camps are at risk of direct exposure to many pesticides.

Children can be acutely overexposed to pesticides. High-dose exposure to both organophosphates and carbamate pesticides can cause acute neurotoxicity. Both of these classes of pesticides act through inhibition of acetylcholinesterase and are responsible for the largest number of acute poisoning cases. Symptoms include meiosis (although not in all cases), excess salivation, abdominal cramping, vomiting, diarrhea, and muscle fasciculation. In severe cases, the child may experience loss of consciousness, cardiac arrhythmias, and death by respiratory arrest. The war gas sarin is an organophosphate. See Chapter 63 for treatment of poisoning from drugs, chemicals, and plants.

Pesticides can also cause a range of chronic toxic effects: polyneuropathy and central nervous system dysfunction (organophosphates); hormonal disruption and reproductive impairment (DDT, kepone, dibromochloropropane); cancer (aldrin, dieldrin, chlorophenoxy herbicides [2,4,5-T]); and pulmonary fibrosis (paraquat). Prenatal exposure to organophosphate pesticides at levels that produce no evident toxicity in pregnant women has been associated with neurodevelopmental disability in children, with reduction in IQ and disordered executive function.

Children's exposures to pesticides can be reduced by minimizing applications to lawns, gardens, schools, and playgrounds; adapting techniques of integrated pest management; and reducing pesticide applications to food crops. Consumption of organic produce dramatically reduces organophosphate pesticide exposure in school-age children. Exposure to herbicides may increase due to an EPA decision to expand their use in agriculture.

Polychlorinated Biphenyls, DDT, Dioxins, Brominated Flame Retardants, and Other Halogenated Hydrocarbons

Chlorinated hydrocarbons are used as insecticides (DDT), plastics (polyvinyl chloride), electrical insulators (PCBs), and solvents (trichloroethylene). Highly toxic dioxins and furans are formed during synthesis of chlorinated herbicides or as by-products of plastic combustion. All of these materials are widely dispersed in the environment. Brominated flame retardants are used in carpets, furniture, and computers. DDT, PCBs, and dioxins are highly persistent.

The embryo, fetus, and young child are at particularly high risk of injury from halogenated hydrocarbons. All of these compounds are lipid-soluble. They readily cross the placenta, and they accumulate in breast milk. Intrauterine exposure to PCBs and brominated flame retardants has been linked to persistent neurobehavioral dysfunction in children.

Fish from contaminated waters are a major source of children's exposure to PCBs. Children can be exposed in utero or through breast milk. To protect children and pregnant women in the United States against PCBs in fish, government agencies have issued advisories concerning fish consumption for certain lakes and rivers. Combustion of medical wastes containing polyvinyl chloride and the use of chlorine to bleach paper products are major preventable sources of environmental dioxin and should be discouraged. Older fluorescent light ballasts that were installed decades ago in schools in the United States are another source of PCB exposure. PCB-containing ballasts should be removed from schools as soon as possible to prevent environmental contamination. Removal must be performed by trained workers.

Endocrine Disruptors

A number of chemicals have been shown to adversely affect the endocrine systems of animals and humans, including DES, DDT, PCBs, and dioxins. Other chemicals, such as other pesticides and phthalates (plasticizers), are also suspected of possessing endocrine disruptor effects. Phthalates have been associated with obesity in animal experiments. Higher urinary levels of bisphenol A are associated with obesity-related outcomes, such as cardiovascular disease, in a cross-sectional analysis of National Health and Nutrition Examination Survey 2003-2004 data in adults. The many effects of endocrine disruptors on wildlife include eggshell thinning in birds, sterility in seals, feminization and cryptorchidism in panthers, and low hatching rates in alligators. In humans, endocrine disruption is implicated in the epidemiologic observations of a trend toward earlier thelarche and menarche in girls (see Chapter 14), the rising rates of testicular cancer and hypospadias, and diminishing sperm counts. The most clearly observed effects include adenocarcinoma of the vagina in women and cryptorchidism in men whose mothers took DES and shortening of the anogenital distance, a measure

of in utero feminization, in baby boys whose mothers had elevated exposures to phthalates during pregnancy. The presence of elevated concentrations of plasma phthalate esters is associated with early thelarche in Puerto Rican girls. Some endocrine disruptors may also have adverse effects on brain development. Prenatal exposure to low-molecular-weight phthalates is associated with shortening of attention span in children 4-9 yr old.

Environmental Carcinogens

Children may be exposed to carcinogenic pollutants in utero or after birth. Children appear more sensitive than adults to certain chemical carcinogens and also to ionizing radiation (see Chapter 718). The potential for in utero carcinogenesis was first recognized with the discovery that clear cell adenocarcinoma of the vagina could develop in women after intrauterine exposure to DES.

Carcinogenesis also may be associated with exposures in the home and community. Children of asbestos workers and children who have grown up near asbestos plants have been found to have a higher incidence of mesothelioma than unexposed populations. Children who grow up on farms have elevated rates of leukemia; pesticides are suspected of playing an etiologic role. Intrauterine exposure to trichloroethylene via contaminated drinking water has been associated with an increased incidence of leukemia among girls living near an industrial facility and industrial waste site.

Routes of Exposure

Transplacental. Heavy metals such as lead and mercury, fat-soluble compounds such as PCBs and DDT, and endocrine disruptors such as phthalates readily cross the placenta. They may have serious and irreversible toxic effects on the developing nervous, endocrine, and reproductive organs, even at very low levels.

Water. Approximately 200 chemicals have been found in various amounts in water supplies. Lead is especially common. In some older neighborhoods, lead in water derives from lead pipes. More commonly, it is dissolved (leached) by soft, acidic water from lead-containing solder. The highest levels of lead occur in water that has been standing in pipes overnight. It is wise therefore to run water for 2-3 min each morning before making up infant formula. Solvents and components of gasoline such as methyl tertiary-butyl ether and benzene are commonly encountered in groundwater. Herbicides, like atrazine, are commonly found contaminants in drinking water in agricultural areas.

Air. Vehicular emissions are the major source of urban air pollution. Diesel exhaust is a human carcinogen. In rural areas, wood smoke can contribute to air pollution. Children living in the vicinity of smelters and chemical production plants can be exposed to toxic industrial emissions such as lead, benzene, and 1,3-butadiene.

Food. Many chemicals are intentionally added to food to improve appearance, taste, texture, or preservation, but many such chemicals have been poorly tested for potential toxicity. Residues of many pesticides are found in both raw and processed foods. Levels of pesticides are lower in organic produce than in conventionally grown fruits and vegetables. Children who consume organic produce have substantially lower urinary pesticide levels than children who eat conventional produce.

Work Clothes. Illnesses in children sometimes may be traced to contaminated dust from parents' work clothes; toxicity from lead, beryllium, dioxin, organophosphate pesticides, and asbestos has occurred. Such exposure (termed "fouling the nest") can be prevented by providing facilities at work for changing and showering.

Schools. Children may be exposed in schools, kindergartens, and nurseries to lead paint, molds, asbestos, environmental tobacco smoke, pesticides, and hazardous arts and crafts materials. Substantial opportunities for prevention exist in the school environment, and pediatricians are often consulted for advice.

Child Labor. Four to 5 million children and adolescents in the United States work for pay, and child labor is widespread around the world. Working children are at high risk of physical trauma and injury. They also may be exposed to a wide range of toxic chemicals, including pesticides in agriculture and lawn work, asbestos in construction and building demolition, and benzene in pumping gasoline.

THE PHYSICIAN'S ROLE

Pediatricians have time and again played key roles in the initial recognition of diseases caused by toxic chemicals. Every pediatrician needs to be an "alert clinician" ever open to the possibility of discovering new diseases in children caused by exposures in the environment. In considering the origins of noninfectious disease, pediatricians should ask about the home environment, parental occupation, unusual exposures, and neighborhood factories. An environmental cause is particularly likely when several unusual cases of disease or constellations of findings occur together. Any adolescent with a traumatic injury may have been injured at work.

The history is the single most important instrument for obtaining information on environmental exposures. Information about current and past exposures (including questions about work and travel to or residence in developing countries) should be sought routinely on every new patient and on every patient with illness of unclear causation through a few brief screening questions. Changes in patterns of exposure or new exposures may be especially important. If suspicious information is elicited, more detailed follow-up should be pursued. Referral to a pediatric environmental health specialty unit may be indicated (http://aoec.org/PEHSU/index.html). Accurate diagnosis of an environmental cause of disease can lead to better care of sick children and prevention of disease in other children.

Bibliography is available at Expert Consult.

Chapter **720**
Heavy Metal Intoxication
Prashant V. Mahajan

Lead, mercury, arsenic, and cadmium, 4 of the World Health Organization's (WHO) "10 chemicals of greatest public health concern," are the heavy metals posing the greatest threats to humans. The most prevalent of these exposures is lead (see Chapter 721). This chapter discusses mercury and arsenic.

Heavy metal intoxication results in diverse multiorgan toxicity through widespread disruption of vital cellular functions. A meticulous history of environmental exposure may be necessary to correctly identify heavy metals as the source of the protean manifestations associated with such exposure. Arsenic exposure can occur from contaminated food or water; globally, more than 100 million people are estimated to be chronically exposed to drinking water containing high arsenic levels. Mercury exposure occurs primarily through food; fish is a major source of methyl mercury exposure.

ARSENIC
Epidemiology

Arsenic is a metalloid that exists in 4 forms: elemental arsenic, arsine gas, inorganic arsenic salts (pentavalent arsenate form or trivalent arsenite form), and organic arsenic compounds. Toxic manifestations are higher in the more soluble and higher-valence compounds. **Arsine gas** is the most toxic form of arsenic. Mass poisonings from exposure to arsenic have occurred throughout history, including one in 1998 in Wakayama, Japan, in which 70 people were poisoned. Children may be poisoned after exposure to inorganic arsenic found in pesticides, herbicides, dyes, homeopathic medicines, and certain contaminated folk remedies from China, India, and Southeast Asia (see Chapter 64). Soil deposits contaminate artesian well water. Groundwater contamination with arsenic is a common problem in developing countries and has been reported to be a common well contaminant in Alaska, Maine,

North Carolina, and areas in western United States. Food products (e.g., rice, organic brown rice syrup, fruit juices) cooked in contaminated water may actually absorb arsenic, thus concentrating it in the food. The WHO has set 10 μg/L as the upper limit of safety. In many parts of Asia and South America, this limit is frequently exceeded. Arsenic concentrations in one quarter of the wells in Bangladesh exceed 50 μg/L and 35-77 million of the 125 million inhabitants of Bangladesh regularly consume arsenic-contaminated water. Occupational exposure may occur in industries involved in the manufacturing, mining, smelting, or refining of glass, pottery, electronic and semiconductor components, and lasers. Although arsenic is no longer produced in the United States, it is produced in many countries and is imported into the United States for industrial use. Organic arsenic compounds may be found in seafood, pesticides, and some veterinary pharmaceuticals. In contrast to mercury, the organic forms of arsenic found in seafood are nontoxic.

Pharmacokinetics

Elemental arsenic is insoluble in water and bodily fluids and, therefore, is insignificantly absorbed and nontoxic. Inhaled arsine gas is rapidly absorbed through the lungs. The inorganic arsenic salts are well absorbed through the gastrointestinal tract, lungs, and skin. The organic arsenic compounds are well absorbed through the gastrointestinal tract. After acute exposure, arsenic initially is bound to the protein portion of hemoglobin in the red blood cells (RBCs) and rapidly distributed to all tissues. Inorganic arsenic is methylated and is eliminated predominantly by the kidneys, with approximately 95% excreted in the urine and 5% excreted in the bile. Most of the arsenic is eliminated in the 1st few days, with the remainder slowly excreted over a period of several weeks. Arsenic concentrates in hair, nails, and skin. Measurement of the distance of **Mees lines** (transverse white striae on the nail) from the nail bed can provide an estimate of time of exposure (nails grow at the rate of 0.4 mm/day).

Pathophysiology

After exposure to arsine gas, absorbed arsine enters RBCs and is oxidized to arsenic dihydride and elemental arsenic. Complexing of these derivatives with red cell sulfhydryl groups results in cell membrane instability and massive hemolysis. The inorganic arsenic salts poison enzymatic processes vital to cellular metabolism. Trivalent arsenic binds to sulfhydryl groups, resulting in decreased production of adenosine triphosphate through the inhibition of enzyme systems such as the pyruvate dehydrogenase and α-ketoglutarate complexes. Pentavalent arsenic may be biotransformed to trivalent arsenic or substituted for phosphate in the glycolytic pathway, resulting in uncoupling of oxidative phosphorylation.

Clinical Manifestations

Arsine gas is colorless, odorless, nonirritating, and highly toxic. Inhalation causes no immediate symptoms. After a latent period of 2-24 hr, exposed individuals experience massive hemolysis, malaise, headache, weakness, dyspnea, nausea, vomiting, abdominal pain, hepatomegaly, pallor, jaundice, hemoglobinuria, and renal failure (Table 720-1). Acute ingestion of arsenic produces gastrointestinal toxicity within minutes to hours and is manifested as nausea, vomiting, abdominal pain, and diarrhea. Hemorrhagic gastroenteritis with extensive fluid loss and third spacing may result in hypovolemic shock. Cardiovascular toxicity includes QT interval prolongation, polymorphous ventricular tachycardia, congestive cardiomyopathy, pulmonary edema, and cardiogenic shock. Acute neurologic toxicity includes delirium, seizures, cerebral edema, encephalopathy, and coma. Lethal doses of arsenates are 5-50 mg/kg; lethal doses of arsenites are <5 mg/kg.

Late sequelae include hematuria, proteinuria, and acute tubular necrosis. A delayed sensorimotor peripheral neuropathy may appear days to weeks after acute exposure, secondary to axonal degeneration. Neuropathy manifests as painful dysesthesias followed by diminished vibratory, pain, touch, and temperature sensation; decreased deep tendon reflexes; and, in the most severe cases, an ascending paralysis with respiratory failure mimicking Guillain-Barré syndrome (see

Chapter 616). Adult survivors of infant arsenic poisoning experience higher mortality from disorders of the nervous system compared to adults without such exposure.

Subacute toxicity is characterized by prolonged fatigue, malaise, weight loss, headache, chronic encephalopathy, peripheral sensorimotor neuropathy, leukopenia, anemia, thrombocytopenia, chronic cough, and gastroenteritis. Mees lines in the nails become apparent 1-2 mo after exposure in approximately 5% of patients. Dermatologic findings include alopecia, oral ulceration, peripheral edema, a pruritic macular rash, and desquamation.

Chronic arsenic toxicity causes significant morbidity in children resulting in skin lesions, lung disease, and defect in intellectual function. **Chronic exposure** to low levels of arsenic is usually from environmental or occupational sources. Over the course of years, dermatologic lesions develop, including hyperpigmentation, hypopigmentation, hyperkeratoses (especially on the palms and soles), squamous and basal cell carcinomas, and **Bowen disease** (cutaneous squamous cell carcinoma in situ). Encephalopathy and peripheral neuropathy may be present. Hepatomegaly, hypersplenism, noncirrhotic portal fibrosis, and portal hypertension occur. **Blackfoot disease** is an obliterative arterial disease of the lower extremities associated with chronic arsenic exposure that has been described in Taiwan. Carcinogenicity of chronic arsenic exposure is reflected in increased rates of cancers of the skin, lung, liver, bladder, and kidney as well as of angiosarcomas. The effects of prenatal exposure to arsenic are uncertain but may include low birthweight.

Laboratory Findings

The diagnosis of arsenic intoxication is based on characteristic clinical findings, a history of exposure, and elevated urinary arsenic values, the last of which confirm the exposure. A spot urine arsenic level should be determined for symptomatic patients before chelation, although initially the result may be negative. Because urinary excretion of arsenic is intermittent, definitive diagnosis depends on a 24 hr urine collection. Concentrations greater than 50 μg/L in a 24 hr urine specimen are consistent with arsenic intoxication (Table 720-2). Urine specimens must be collected in metal-free containers. Ingestion of seafood containing nontoxic arsenobetaine and arsenocholine can cause elevations of urinary arsenic. Blood arsenic levels rarely are helpful because of their high variability and the rapid clearance of arsenic from the blood in acute poisonings. Elevated arsenic values in the hair or nails must be interpreted cautiously because of the possibility of external contamination. Abdominal radiographs may demonstrate ingested radiopaque arsenic.

Later in the course of illness, a complete blood cell count may show anemia, thrombocytopenia, and leukocytosis, followed by leukopenia, karyorrhexis, and basophilic stippling of RBCs. The serum concentrations of creatinine, bilirubin, and transaminases may be elevated; urinalysis may show proteinuria, pyuria, and hematuria; and examination of the cerebrospinal fluid may show protein elevations.

MERCURY
Epidemiology

Mercury exists in 3 forms: elemental mercury, inorganic mercury salts, and organic mercury (Table 720-3). **Elemental mercury** is present in thermometers, sphygmomanometers, barometers, batteries, and some latex paints produced before 1991. Workers in industries producing these products may expose their children to the toxin when mercury is brought home on contaminated clothing. Vacuuming of carpets contaminated with mercury and breaking of mercury fluorescent light bulbs may result in elemental mercury vapor exposure. Severe inhalation poisonings have resulted from attempts to separate gold from gold ore by heating mercury and forming a gold-mercury amalgam. Elemental mercury has been used in folk remedies by Asian and Mexican populations for chronic stomach pain, by Latin Americans and Caribbean natives in occult practices, and as a skin-lightening agent. Dental amalgams containing elemental mercury release trace amounts of mercury. An expert panel for the National Institutes of Health concluded that existing scientific evidence does not indicate that dental amalgams pose a health risk and should not be replaced merely to decrease mercury exposure. A 2009 WHO expert panel concluded that a global near-term ban on amalgam would be problematic for public and dental health. However, this committee recommended that alternatives to amalgam should be sought as part of a phase-out of the use of mercury-containing amalgams.

Inorganic mercury salts are found in pesticides, disinfectants, antiseptics, pigments, dry batteries, and explosives and as preservatives in some medicinal preparations. **Organic mercury** in the diet, especially fish containing methyl mercury, is a major source of mercury exposure among the general population. Industries that may produce mercury-containing effluents include chlorine and caustic soda production, mining and metallurgy, electroplating, chemical and textile manufacturing, paper and pharmaceutical manufacturing, and leather tanning. Mercury compounds in the environment are methylated to methyl

Table 720-1	Effects of Arsenic on Organ Systems
ORGAN SYSTEM	**EFFECTS OF ARSENIC**
Gastrointestinal system	Submucosal vesicles, watery or bloody diarrhea, severe hematemesis
Cardiovascular system	Reduced myocardial contractility, prolonged QT intervals, tachyarrhythmias
	Vasodilation, hypotension
Kidneys	Hematuria, proteinuria, acute tubular necrosis
Nervous system	Toxic encephalopathy with seizures, cerebral edema, and coma
	Chronic exposure: peripheral painful sensorimotor neuropathy
Hematologic and lymphatic system	Anemia and thrombocytopenia; acute hemolysis with arsine gas
Liver	Fatty degeneration with central necrosis
Skin	Desquamation, alopecia, hyperkeratosis, nail changes
	Chronic exposure: hyperkeratosis, hyperpigmentation
Teratogenic	Neural tube defects in the fetus
Oncologic	Urologic cancer, other malignancies

Table 720-2	Acceptable and Toxic Levels of Arsenic and Mercury		
		ARSENIC	**MERCURY**
Molecular weight		74.9 Da	200.59 Da
Acceptable blood level		<5 μg/L (<0.665 nmol/L)	<10 μg/L (<50 nmol/L)
Acceptable urine level		<50 μg/L (<6.65 nmol/L) 24 hr urine sample	<20 μg/L (<100 nmol/L)
Intervene at blood level			>35 μg/L (>175 nmol/L)
Intervene at urine level		>100 μg/L (>13.3 nmol/L) 24 hr urine sample	>150 μg/L (>750 nmol/L)

Table 720-3 | Differential Characteristics of Mercury Exposure

	ELEMENTAL	INORGANIC (SALT)	ORGANIC (ALKYL)
Primary route of exposure	Inhalation	Oral	Oral
Primary tissue distribution	CNS, kidney	Kidney	CNS, kidney, liver
Clearance	Renal, GI	Renal, GI	Methyl: GI Aryl: renal, GI
Clinical effects:			
CNS	Tremor	Tremor, erethism (irritability)	Paresthesias, ataxia, tremor, tunnel vision, dysarthria
Pulmonary	+++	—	—
Gastrointestinal	+	+++ (caustic)	+
Renal	+	+++ (acute tubular necrosis)	+
Acrodynia	+	++	—
Therapy	BAL, DMSA	BAL, DMSA	DMSA (early)

BAL, British antilewisite; CNS, central nervous system; DMSA, 2,3-dimercaptosuccinic acid; GI, gastrointestinal; +, mild; ++, moderate; +++, severe.
From Sue YJ: Mercury (heavy metals). In Nelson LS, Lewin NA, Howland MA, et al, editors: Goldfrank's toxicologic emergencies, *ed 9, New York, 2011, McGraw-Hill, Tab 96-4, p. 1330.*

mercury by soil and water microorganisms. Methyl mercury in the water rapidly accumulates in fish (swordfish, king mackerel, fresh tuna, tile fish, shark) and other aquatic organisms, which are in turn consumed by humans. To address concerns that maternal consumption of large quantities of fish during pregnancy may expose the fetus to concentrations of mercury with adverse consequences, the longitudinal Seychelles Child Development Study has been ongoing since the late 1980s. The first cohort of the study involved nearly 800 mother–child pairs, with subsequent cohorts enrolled. Despite a high maternal fish intake (mean of 12 fish meals per wk), follow-up of children at least through 9 yr of age has revealed no consistent adverse developmental effects. Well-known large outbreaks of methyl mercury intoxication include the incidents in Japan in the 1950s (**Minamata disease,** from consumption of contaminated seafood) and in Iraq in 1971 (from consumption of grain treated with a methyl mercury fungicide).

Thimerosal is a mercury-containing preservative used in some vaccines. Thimerosal contains 49.6% mercury by weight and is metabolized to ethyl mercury and thiosalicylate. During an ongoing review of biologic products in response to the U.S. Food and Drug Administration (FDA) Modernization Act of 1997, the FDA determined that infants who received thimerosal-containing vaccines at multiple visits might have been exposed to more mercury than recommended by federal guidelines. As a precautionary measure, the American Academy of Pediatrics, American Academy of Family Physicians, Advisory Committee on Immunization Practices, and U.S. Public Health Service issued a joint recommendation in 1999 that thimerosal be removed from vaccines as quickly as possible. *In the United States, thimerosal has been removed from all vaccines in the recommended childhood immunization schedule.* Infants and children who have received thimerosal-containing vaccines do not need to undergo blood, urine, or hair testing for mercury because the concentrations of mercury would be quite low and would not require treatment. The benefits and risks of vaccines containing thimerosal should be discussed with parents (as with all vaccines). The larger risks of not vaccinating children far outweigh any known risk of exposure to thimerosal-containing vaccines. Studies do *not* demonstrate a link between thimerosal-containing vaccines and autistic spectrum disorders (see Chapter 30.1), and no evidence supports a change in the standard of practice with regard to administration of thimerosal-containing vaccines in areas of the world where they are used. A rise in blood mercury levels following a single dose of hepatitis vaccine was seen in preterm infants, but the clinical significance is unknown.

Pharmacokinetics

Inhaled elemental mercury vapor is 80% absorbed by the lungs and is distributed rapidly to the central nervous system because of its high lipid solubility. The elemental mercury is oxidized by catalase to the mercuric ion, which is the reactive form that causes cellular toxicity. Elemental mercury liquid is poorly absorbed from the gastrointestinal tract, with less than 0.1% being absorbed. The half-life of elemental mercury in the tissues is approximately 60 days, most of the excretion occurring in the urine.

Inorganic mercury salts are approximately 10% absorbed from the gastrointestinal tract and cross the blood–brain barrier to a lesser extent than elemental mercury. Mercuric salts are more soluble than mercurous salts and, therefore, produce greater toxicity. Elimination occurs primarily in the urine, with a half-life of approximately 40 days.

Methyl mercury is the most avidly absorbed of the organic mercury compounds, with approximately 90% absorbed from the gastrointestinal tract. The lipophilic, short-chain alkyl structure of methyl mercury allows it to distribute rapidly across the blood–brain barrier and placenta. Methyl mercury is approximately 90% excreted in the bile, with the remainder being excreted in the urine. The half-life is 70 days.

Pathophysiology

After absorption, mercury is distributed to all tissues, particularly the central nervous system and kidneys. Mercury reacts with sulfhydryl, phosphoryl, carboxyl, and amide groups, resulting in disruption of enzymes, transport mechanisms, membranes, and structural proteins. Widespread cellular dysfunction or necrosis results in the multiorgan toxicity characteristic of mercury poisoning.

Clinical Manifestations

Five syndromes describe the clinical presentation of mercury poisoning. **Acute inhalation of elemental mercury vapor** results in rapid onset of cough, dyspnea, chest pain, fever, chills, headaches, and visual disturbances. Gastrointestinal findings include metallic taste, salivation, nausea, vomiting, and diarrhea. Depending on the severity of the exposure, the illness may be self-limited or may progress to necrotizing bronchiolitis, interstitial pneumonitis, pulmonary edema, and death from respiratory failure. Younger children are more susceptible to pulmonary toxicity. Survivors may demonstrate restrictive lung disease. Renal dysfunction and neurologic disturbances (ataxia, persistent weakness, emotional lability) may develop subacutely. Chronic exposure to volatilized elemental mercury in dental amalgams has not been found to be of any clinical significance.

Acute ingestion of inorganic mercury salts (typically secondary to ingestion of a button battery) can manifest in a few hours as corrosive gastroenteritis, signified by metallic taste, oropharyngeal burns, nausea, hematemesis, severe abdominal pain, hematochezia, acute tubular necrosis, cardiovascular collapse, and death.

Chronic inorganic mercury intoxication produces the **classic triad** consisting of tremor, neuropsychiatric disturbances, and gingivostomatitis. The syndrome may result from long-term exposure to elemental mercury, inorganic mercury salts, or certain organic mercury compounds, all of which may be metabolized to mercuric ions. The tremor starts as a fine intention tremor of the fingers that is abolished during sleep but that may later involve the face and progress to choreoathetosis and spasmodic ballismus. Mixed sensorimotor neuropathy and visual disturbances may also be present. The neuropsychiatric disturbances include emotional lability, delirium, headaches, memory loss, insomnia, anorexia, and fatigue. Renal dysfunction ranges from asymptomatic proteinuria to nephrotic syndrome.

Acrodynia, or **pink disease,** is a rare idiosyncratic hypersensitivity reaction to mercury that occurs predominantly in children exposed to mercurous powders. The symptom complex includes generalized pain, paresthesias, and an acral (hands, feet) rash that may spread to involve the face. The rash typically is red-pink, papular, pruritic, and painful; it may progress to desquamation and ulceration. Morbilliform, vesicular, and hemorrhagic variants have been described. Other important features include anorexia, apathy, photophobia, and hypotonia, especially of the pectoral and pelvic girdles. Irritability, tremors, diaphoresis, insomnia, hypertension, and tachycardia may be present. Some cases initially were diagnosed as pheochromocytoma. The outcome is good after removal of the source of mercury exposure.

Methyl mercury intoxication (also known as **Minamata disease** after the widespread mercury poisoning that occurred at Minamata Bay in Japan in people who had ingested contaminated fish) manifests as delayed neurotoxicity that appears after a latent period of weeks to mo. It is characterized by ataxia; dysarthria; paresthesias; tremors; movement disorders; impairment of vision, hearing, smell, and taste; memory loss; progressive dementia; and death. Infants exposed in utero are the most severely affected, with low birthweight, microcephaly, profound developmental delay, cerebral palsy, deafness, blindness, and seizures. Although there is significant residual morbidity from methyl mercury neurotoxicity, observations on long-term follow-up of children exposed in Iraq reveal complete or partial resolution in most cases.

Laboratory Findings

The diagnosis of mercury intoxication is based on characteristic clinical findings, a history of exposure, and elevation of whole blood or urine mercury values, the last of which confirms the exposure. Thin-layer and gas chromatographic techniques can be used to distinguish organic from inorganic mercury. Blood should be collected in special tubes for trace elements from laboratories that are capable of performing those tests. Levels <10 µg/L in whole blood and <20 µg/L in a 24 hr urine specimen are considered normal (see Table 720-2). Although blood mercury levels may reflect acute exposure, they decrease as mercury redistributes into the tissues. Urine mercury levels are most useful for identifying long-term exposures, except in the case of methyl mercury, which undergoes minimal urinary excretion. Urinary mercury levels are used in monitoring efficacy of chelation therapy, whereas blood levels are used primarily in monitoring organic mercury poisonings. Hair analysis for mercury is not reliable because hair reflects both endogenous and exogenous mercury exposure (hair avidly binds mercury from the environment). Abdominal radiographs may demonstrate ingested radiopaque mercury.

Urinary markers of early nephrotoxicity include microalbuminuria, retinol-binding protein, β_2-microglobulin, and N-acetyl-β-D-glucosaminidase. Early neurotoxicity may be detected with neuropsychiatric testing and nerve conduction studies, whereas severe central nervous system toxicity is apparent on CT or MRI.

TREATMENT OF ARSENIC AND MERCURY INTOXICATION

The principles of management for arsenic and mercury intoxication include prompt removal from the source of poisoning, aggressive stabilization and supportive care, decontamination, and chelation therapy when appropriate. Once the diagnosis is suspected, the local poison control facility should be contacted, and care coordinated with physicians who are familiar with the management of heavy metal poisoning.

Supportive care for patients exposed to arsine gas requires close monitoring for signs of hemolysis, including evaluation of the peripheral blood smear and urinalysis. Transfusion of packed RBCs may be necessary, as may administration of intravenous fluids, sodium bicarbonate, and mannitol to prevent renal failure secondary to the deposition of hemoglobin in the kidneys. After inhalation of elemental mercury vapor, patients require careful monitoring of respiratory status, which may include pulse oximetry, arterial blood gas analysis, and chest radiography. Supportive care involves administration of supplemental oxygen and, in severe cases, intubation and mechanical ventilation.

Acute ingestion of inorganic arsenic and mercury salts results in hemorrhagic gastroenteritis, cardiovascular collapse, and multiorgan dysfunction. Fluid resuscitation, pressor agents, and transfusion of blood products may be required for management of cardiovascular instability. Severe respiratory distress, coma with loss of airway reflexes, intractable seizures, and respiratory paralysis are indications for intubation and mechanical ventilation. Renal function must be monitored carefully for signs of renal failure and the need for hemodialysis.

Gastrointestinal decontamination after ingestion of the inorganic arsenic and mercury salts has not been well studied. Because of the corrosive effects of these compounds, induced emesis is not recommended, and endoscopy may be considered before gastric lavage. Arsenic and mercury are not well adsorbed to activated charcoal, but its use may be helpful if coingestants are suspected. Whole-bowel irrigation is used to remove any radiopaque material remaining in the gastrointestinal tract.

Chelation for acute arsenic and mercury poisoning is most effective when administered as soon as possible after the exposure. Chelation should be continued until 24 hr urinary arsenic or mercury levels return to normal (<50 µg/L for arsenic and <20 µg/L for mercury), the patient is symptom-free, or the remaining toxic effects are believed to be irreversible. The efficacy of chelation in long-term exposures is reduced because heavy metal in the tissue compartment is relatively unexchangeable and some degree of irreversible toxicity has already occurred.

Dimercaprol, also known as *2,3-dimercaptopropanol* or *British antilewisite (BAL),* is the chelator of choice for a patient who cannot tolerate oral therapy, as often is true for critically ill patients and after ingestion of the corrosive inorganic arsenic and mercury salts. BAL is available suspended in peanut oil and benzyl benzoate in 3 mL ampules at a concentration of 100 mg/mL for deep intramuscular (IM) injection. For **arsenic poisoning,** the recommended regimen of BAL is 2.5 mg/kg IM q6h for the 1st 2 days, 2.5 mg/kg IM q12h on the 3rd day, and then 2.5 mg/kg/day IM for 10 days. For severe arsenic poisoning, the dose of BAL is increased to 3 mg/kg IM q4h for 2 days, 3 mg/kg IM q6h on day 3, and then 3 mg/kg IM q12h for 10 days. The dose of BAL for **inorganic mercury poisoning** is 5 mg/kg IM on the 1st day, and then 2.5 mg/kg IM q12-24h for 10 days. The BAL–heavy metal complex is excreted in the urine and bile. A period of 5 days between courses of chelation is recommended. Adverse effects of BAL include pain at the injection site, hypertension, tachycardia, diaphoresis, nausea, vomiting, abdominal pain, a burning sensation in the oropharynx, and a feeling of constriction in the chest. BAL may cause hemolysis in glucose-6-phosphate dehydrogenase–deficient individuals. It is important to note that BAL is contraindicated for chelation of methyl mercury because BAL redistributes methyl mercury to the brain from other tissue sites, resulting in increased neurotoxicity.

D-Penicillamine is an orally administered chelator that can be considered for less-severe mercury poisoning or as an adjunct to BAL therapy in arsenic poisoning, but its use is largely restricted because of the potential for significant leukopenia, thrombocytopenia, and proteinuria. A newer investigational analog, N-acetyl-D,L-penicillamine, is used with variable success in mercury poisoning.

Oral chelating agents are used to replace the painful BAL injections when the patient is stable enough to tolerate oral therapy and prolonged chelation is necessary. **Succimer,** also known as *2,3-dimercaptosuccinic acid* (DMSA), is an orally administered water-soluble derivative of BAL. DMSA is available in 100 mg capsules. The recommended regimen of DMSA is 10 mg/kg orally every 8 hr for 5 days. The DMSA–heavy metal complex is excreted in the urine and bile. A period of 2 wk between courses of chelation is recommended. Mild adverse effects include nausea, vomiting, diarrhea, loss of appetite, and transient elevations in liver enzyme levels. DMSA also may cause hemolysis in glucose-6-phosphate dehydrogenase–deficient patients. Patients with ingestion of elemental mercury require no follow-up unless there is an underlying disease that decreases the gastrointestinal transit time. Serial abdominal radiographs to document the progression of the metal are recommended. Acute inhalation of mercury fumes and ingestion of inorganic mercury require hospitalization to monitor the respiratory and gastrointestinal status, respectively. Therapeutic abortion may be considered in pregnant patients, because of the teratogenic effect of mercury.

Bibliography is available at Expert Consult.

Chapter 721
Lead Poisoning
Morri Markowitz

Lead is a metal that exists in 4 isotopic forms. Clinically, it is purely a toxicant; no organism has an essential function that is lead dependent. Chemically, its low melting point and ability to form stable compounds have made it useful in the manufacture of hundreds of products; this commercial attractiveness has resulted in the processing of millions of tons of lead ore, leading to widespread dissemination of lead in the human environment.

The blood lead level (BLL) is the gold standard for determining health effects. However, the threshold level at which lead begins to cause biochemical, subclinical, or clinical disturbance remains to be determined. The Centers for Disease Control and Prevention (CDC), recognizing that a BLL of 10 μg/dL qualifies neither as a threshold of toxicity nor as a protective parameter of children with lead exposure, changed its standard. It no longer refers to a level of concern or toxicity but has designated 5 μg/dL as the *"reference value based on the 97.5th percentile of the population BLL in children aged 1-5 years to identify children living or staying for long periods in environments that expose them to lead hazards."* As a measure of the distribution of BLLs in young children, this number will change in a manner dependent on the epidemiology of BLLs rather than on identification of the starting point for toxicity.

Although stated as a reference value, it is likely that clinicians and departments of health will consider this a threshold for action. It is important to recognize that lead toxicity occurs at levels below 5 μg/dL; no safe level has been identified. In part, this reflects the accuracy limitations of available clinical laboratory methodologies.

PUBLIC HEALTH HISTORY
In the late 1970s, nearly all preschool-age children in the United States had BLLs above the current reference value of 5 μg/dL. Around that time government regulations were issued that resulted in the significant reduction of 3 main contributors to lead exposure by means of (1) the elimination of the use of tetraethyl lead as a gasoline additive, (2) the banning of lead-containing solder to seal cans of food and beverages, and (3) the application of a federal rule that limited the amount of lead allowed in paint intended for household use to less than 0.06% by weight (further reduced by the Consumer Product Safety Commission to 0.009% in 2008). Surveillance by many of the states in the United States and by national health surveys conducted by the CDC has shown that the prevalence of elevated BLLs has declined markedly. Approximately 535,000 young children currently have BLLs ≥5 μg/dL. Including all children <18 yr of age yields an estimated 705,000 with levels above the reference value (National Health and Nutritional

Examination Surveys show that for 2007-2010, 0.95% of children < age 18 yr have BLL ≥5 μg/dL). Several subgroups remain at higher risk for lead poisoning. The mean BLL of non-Hispanic black children (1.8 μg/dL) is greater than that of either non-Hispanic white children (1.3 μg/dL) or Mexican American children (1.3 μg/dL); the mean BLL among poor children (1.6 μg/dL) is higher than among more well-to-do children (1.2 μg/dL). Another high-risk group that has been identified consists of recent immigrants from less-wealthy countries, including adoptees. Fortunately, children with levels high enough to be life-threatening (>100 μg/dL) are rarely seen in the United States.

As of 2014 only 6 countries continue to use leaded gasoline (Afghanistan, Algeria, Iraq, North Korea, Myanmar, and Yemen) and these are expected to phase out its use. In all countries examined, the end of this source of exposure was associated with a marked decrease in average BLLs at all ages. In Malta, after the import of red lead paint was banned and the use of lead-treated wood for fuel in bakeries was prohibited, mean BLLs of pregnant women and newborns decreased by 45%. After it was documented that children living in the neighborhood of a battery factory in Nicaragua had a mean BLL of 17.2 μg/dL whereas children in the control community had a mean BLL of 7.4 μg/dL, the factory was closed. Despite these advances, the World Health Organization estimates that nearly a quarter billion people have BLLs above 5 μg/dL; of those who are children, 90% live in developing countries, where, in some regions, BLLs may be 10-20–fold higher than in developed countries.

In 2010, the CDC and World Health Organization, after being alerted by Doctors Without Borders, identified numerous lead-contaminated villages in northern Nigeria. The grinding of ore to extract gold caused widespread leaded dust dissemination. It is likely that hundreds of children died as a consequence of this activity, and all remaining children in the villages assessed to date were lead poisoned, with 97% having a BLL ≥45 μg/dL.

SOURCES OF EXPOSURE
Lead poisoning may occur in utero, because lead readily crosses the placenta from maternal blood. The spectrum of toxicity is similar to that experienced by children after birth. The source of maternal blood lead content is either redistribution from endogenous stores (i.e., the mother's skeleton) or lead newly acquired from ongoing environmental exposure.

Several hundred products contain lead, including batteries, cable sheathing, cosmetics, mineral supplements, plastics, toys (Table 721-1),

Table 721-1	Sources of Lead

Paint chips
Dust
Soil
Parent's or older child's occupational exposure (auto repair, battery manufacturing or recycling, smelting, construction, mining, remodeling, plumbing, gun/bullet exposure, indoor firing ranges, painting)
Glazed ceramics
Herbal remedies (e.g., Ayurvedic medications)
Home remedies, including antiperspirants, deodorants (e.g., litargirio)
Jewelry (as toys or belonging to parents)
Stored battery casings (or living near a battery smelter)
Lead-based gasoline
Moonshine alcohol
Contaminated foods (e.g., Mexican candies; Ecuadorian chocolates, imported rice)
Indoor firing ranges
Imported spices (svanuri marili, saffron, kuzhambu)
Cosmetics (kohl, surma, kajal, tiro, lipstick)
Lead plumbing (water)
Imported foods in lead-containing cans
Imported toys
Home renovations
Antique toys or furniture

| Table 721-2 | Cases of Lead Encephalopathy Associated with Traditional Medicines by Type of Medication |

TRADITIONAL MEDICAL SYSTEM	CASES OF LEAD ENCEPHALOPATHY N (%)	N (%) PEDIATRIC CASES WITHIN CAM SYSTEM OR MEDICATION
Ayurveda	5 (7)	1 (20)
Ghasard	1 (1)	1 (100)
Traditional Middle Eastern practices	66 (87)	66 (100)
Azarcón and greta	2 (3)	2 (100)
Traditional Chinese medicine	2 (3)	2 (100)
Total	76 (100)	72 (95)

CAM, complementary and alternative medicines.
From Karri SK, Saper RB, Kales SN: Lead encephalopathy due to traditional medicines, Curr Drug Saf 3:54–59, 2008.

and traditional medicines (Table 721-2). Major sources of exposure vary among and within countries; the major source of exposure in the United States remains old lead-based paint. Approximately 38 million homes, mainly built before 1950, have lead-based paint (2000 estimate). As paint deteriorates, it chalks, flakes, and turns to dust. Improper rehabilitation work of painted surfaces (e.g., sanding) can result in dissemination of lead-containing dust throughout a home. The dust can coat all surfaces, including children's hands. All of these forms of lead can be ingested. If heat is used to strip paint, then lead vapor concentrations in the room can reach levels sufficient to cause lead poisoning via inhalation.

METABOLISM

The nonnutritive hand-to-mouth activity of young children is the most common pathway for lead to enter the body. In nearly all cases, lead is ingested as a component of solids or dissolved in liquids. Cutaneous contamination with inorganic lead compounds, such as those found in pigments, does not result in a substantial amount of absorption. Organic lead compounds, such as tetraethyl lead, may penetrate through skin, however. This is rarely encountered in the United States.

The percentage of lead absorbed from the gut depends on several factors: particle size, pH, other material in the gut, and nutritional status of essential elements. Large paint chips are difficult to digest and are mainly excreted; this is fortunate as a single chip may contain a lethal dose of lead. Fine dust can be dissolved more readily, especially in an acid medium. Lead eaten on an empty stomach is better absorbed than that taken with a meal. The presence of calcium and iron may decrease lead absorption by direct competition for binding sites; iron (and probably calcium) deficiency results in enhanced lead absorption, retention, and toxicity.

After absorption, lead is disseminated throughout the body. Most retained lead accumulates in bone, where it may reside for years. It circulates bound to erythrocytes; approximately 97% in blood is bound on or in the red blood cells. The plasma fraction is too small to be measured by conventional techniques employing atomic absorption spectroscopy or anodic stripping voltammetry; it is presumably the plasma portion that may enter cells and induce toxicity. Thus, clinical laboratories report the BLL, not the serum or plasma lead level. It is possible, but not yet sufficiently shown by testing, that some of the variance in the relationship between BLLs and outcome measures of toxicity is a result of the limitations of using BLLs to assess risk. Studies that examine plasma lead concentrations in relation to its toxicity are needed.

Lead has multiple effects in cells. It binds to enzymes, particularly those with available sulfhydryl groups, changing the contour and diminishing function. For example, the heme pathway, present in all cells, consists of 8 enzymes, 3 of which are susceptible to lead inhibitory effects. The accumulation of excess amounts of heme precursors also is toxic (see Chapter 91). The last enzyme in this pathway, ferrochelatase, enables protoporphyrin to chelate iron, thus forming heme. Heme is essential for multiple metabolic pathways and not merely as a component of hemoglobin. Erythrocyte protoporphyrin levels higher

than 35 µg/dL are abnormal and are consistent with lead poisoning, iron deficiency, or recent inflammatory disease.

Erythrocyte protoporphyrin levels begin to rise several weeks after BLLs have reached 20 µg/dL in a susceptible portion of the population, and are elevated in nearly all children with BLLs higher than 50 µg/dL. A drop in erythrocyte protoporphyrin levels also lags behind a decline in BLLs by several weeks, because it depends on both cell turnover and cessation of further overproduction by marrow red blood cell precursors. Measurement of the erythrocyte protoporphyrin level is, therefore, a useful tool for monitoring more severe biochemical lead toxicity.

A second mechanism of lead toxicity works via its competition with calcium. Many calcium-binding proteins have a higher affinity for lead than for calcium. Lead bound to these proteins may alter function, resulting in abnormal intracellular and intercellular signaling. Neurotransmitter release is, in part, a calcium-dependent process that is adversely affected by lead.

Although these 2 mechanisms of toxicity may be reversible, a third mechanism prevents the development of the normal tertiary brain structure. In immature mammals the normal neuronal pruning process that results in elimination of multiple intercellular brain connections is inhibited by lead. Failure to construct the appropriate tertiary brain structure during infancy and childhood may result in a permanent abnormality. A longitudinal study of childhood lead poisoning that followed a cohort from birth and into their 20s performed MRI and functional MRI–phosphorus magnetic resonance spectroscopy assessments confirmed the association of early childhood lead exposure and subsequent decreased gray and white matter volume and neuronal function. The investigators concluded that early lead exposure in life causes a persistent reorganization of brain architecture and diminished function.

CLINICAL EFFECTS

The BLL is the best-studied measure of the lead burden in children. Although subclinical and clinical findings correlate with BLLs in populations, there is considerable interindividual variability in this relationship. Lead encephalopathy is more likely to be observed in children with BLLs higher than 100 µg/dL; however, 1 child with a BLL of 300 µg/dL may have no symptoms, whereas another with the same level may be comatose. Susceptibility may be associated with polymorphisms in genes coding for lead-binding proteins, such as Δ-aminolevulinic acid dehydratase, an enzyme in the heme pathway.

Several subclinical effects of lead have been demonstrated in cross-sectional epidemiologic studies. Hearing and height are inversely related to BLLs in children. As BLLs increased in the study population, more sound (at all frequencies) was needed to reach the hearing threshold. Children with higher BLLs are shorter than those with lower levels; for every 10 µg increase in the BLL, the children are 1 cm shorter. Chronic lead exposure also may delay puberty. However, these associations with rising BLLs do not reach a point that would bring an individual child to medical attention.

Several longitudinal studies have followed cohorts of children from birth for as long as 20 yr and examined the relationship between BLLs and cognitive test scores over time. In general, there is agreement that BLLs, expressed either as levels obtained at around 2 yr of age or as a measure that integrates multiple BLLs drawn from subjects over time, are inversely related to cognitive test scores. On average, for each 1 µg/dL elevation in BLL the cognitive score is approximately 0.25-0.50 points lower. Because the BLLs from early childhood are predictors of the cognitive test results performed years later, this finding implies that the effects of lead can be permanent. Concurrent testing of lead levels and cognition sometimes also shows an inverse association.

The effect of in utero lead exposure is less clear. Scores on the Bayley Scale of Mental Development were obtained repeatedly every 6 mo for the 1st 2 yr of life in a cohort of infants born to middle-class families. Results correlated inversely with cord BLLs, a measure of in utero exposure, but not with BLLs obtained concurrently at the time of developmental testing. After 2 yr of age, all other cognitive tests performed on the cohort over the next 10 yr correlated with the BLLs at age 2 yr but not with cord BLLs, indicating that the effects of prenatal lead exposure on brain function were superseded by early childhood events and later BLLs. Later studies, performed in cohorts of Mexican children monitored from the prenatal period, confirm the association between in utero lead exposure and later cognitive outcomes. No threshold for BLL was identified in these studies; maternal BLLs between 0 and 10 µg/dL, even as early as the 1st trimester, were associated with about a 6-point drop in cognitive test score results when the children were tested up to age 10 yr.

Behavior also is adversely affected by lead exposure. Hyperactivity is noted in young school-age children with histories of lead poisoning or with concurrent elevations in BLL. Older children with higher bone lead content are more likely to be aggressive and to have behaviors that are predictive of later juvenile delinquency. Multiple reports support the concept of long-term effects of early lead exposure. In 1 longitudinal study, the mothers of a cohort were enrolled during their pregnancies. BLLs were obtained early in pregnancy, at birth, and then multiple times in the offspring during the 1st 6 yr. The investigators report that the relative rate of arrests, especially for violent crimes, increased significantly in relationship to the presence of these BLLs early in life. For every 5 µg/dL increase in BLL the adjusted arrest rate was 1.40 for prenatal BLLs and 1.27 for 6 yr BLLs. Epidemiologic data support the findings in this observational study. In an analysis that combined 2 national data sets, total annual leaded gasoline use (U.S. Geological Survey) and total reported violent criminal acts (U.S. Department of Justice), the amount of leaded gasoline used yearly was found to be strongly associated with violent criminal behavior with a lag time of 23 yr; that is, early exposure was followed 2 decades later by violent behavior rising and falling in close tandem. A similar association was found, this time between urban air lead levels and later violent crime, with a similar best-fit model employing a lag of approximately 22 yr.

An intervention study, in which children with moderate lead poisoning and initial BLLs of 20-55 µg/dL were aggressively managed over 6 mo, addressed the issue of the effects of treatment on cognitive development. Components of treatment included education regarding sources of lead and its abatement, nutritional guidance, multiple home and clinic visits, and, for a subset, chelation therapy. Average BLLs declined and cognitive scores were inversely related to the change in BLLs. For every 1 µg/dL fall in BLLs, cognitive scores were 0.25 point higher. A randomized placebo-controlled treatment study of 2 yr old children with initial BLLs of 20-44 µg/dL that employed the chelating agent succimer administered over 6 mo found no difference in *mean* cognitive scores at age 4 yr. However, as in the earlier treatment study, regression analysis did find an inverse relation between *change* scores; that is, a change in BLLs was associated with a change in cognitive scores.

Whether the behavioral effects of lead are reversible is unclear. In one small, short-term study, 7 yr old hyperactive children with BLLs in the 20s were randomly allocated to receive a chelating agent (penicillamine), methylphenidate, or placebo. Teacher and parent ratings of behavior improved for the first 2 groups but not the placebo group.

BLLs declined only in the chelated group. Lead-poisoned children age 2 yr old who were enrolled in a placebo-controlled trial of the chelating agent succimer showed no mean difference in behavior at 4 or 7 yr of age. However, mean BLLs were also not different in the 2 groups at those ages.

CLINICAL SYMPTOMS
Gastrointestinal Tract and Central Nervous System

Gastrointestinal symptoms of lead poisoning include anorexia, abdominal pain, vomiting, and constipation, often occurring and recurring over a period of weeks. Children with BLLs higher than 20 µg/dL are twice as likely to have gastrointestinal complaints as those with lower BLLs. **Central nervous system symptoms** are related to worsening cerebral edema and increased intracranial pressure. Headaches, change in mentation, lethargy, papilledema, seizures, and coma leading to death are rarely seen at levels lower than 100 µg/dL but have been reported in children with a BLL as low as 70 µg/dL. The last-reported death directly attributable to lead toxicity in the United States was in 2006 in a child with a BLL of 180 µg/dL. There is no clear cutoff BLL value for the appearance of hyperactivity, but it is more likely to be observed in children who have levels higher than 20 µg/dL.

Other organs also may be affected by lead toxicity, but symptoms usually are not apparent in children. At high levels (>100 µg/dL), **renal tubular dysfunction** is observed. Lead may induce a reversible Fanconi syndrome (see Chapter 529). In addition, at high BLLs, **red blood cell survival** is shortened, possibly contributing to a hemolytic anemia, although most cases of anemia in lead-poisoned children are a result of other factors, such as iron deficiency and hemoglobinopathies. Older patients may develop a peripheral neuropathy leading to wrist drop and footdrop.

DIAGNOSIS
Screening

It is estimated that 99% of lead-poisoned children are identified by screening procedures rather than through clinical recognition of lead-related symptoms. Until 1997 universal screening by blood lead testing of all children at ages 12 mo and 24 mo was the standard in the United States. Given the national decline in the prevalence of lead poisoning, the recommendations have been revised to target blood lead testing of high-risk populations. High risk is based on an evaluation of the likelihood of lead exposure. Departments of health are responsible for determining the local prevalence of lead poisoning, as well as the percentage of housing built before 1950, the period of peak leaded paint use. When this information is available, informed screening guidelines for practitioners can be issued. For instance, in the state of New York, where a large percentage of housing was built before 1950, the Department of Health mandates that all children be tested for lead poisoning via blood analyses. *In the absence of such data the practitioner should continue to test all children at both 12 mo and 24 mo.* In areas where the prevalence of lead poisoning and old housing is low, targeted screening may be performed on the basis of a risk assessment. Three questions form the basis of most published questionnaires (Table 721-3), and items that are pertinent to the locale or individual may be added. If there is a lead-based industry in the child's neighborhood, the child is a recent immigrant from a country that still permits use of leaded

Table 721-3	Minimum Personal Risk Questionnaire

1. Does the child live in or visit regularly a house that was built before 1950? (Include settings such as daycare, babysitter's or relative's home.)
2. Does the child live in or regularly visit a house built before 1978 with recent (past 6 mo) or ongoing renovations or remodeling?
3. Does the child have a sibling or playmate that has or did have lead poisoning?

From Screening young children for lead poisoning: guidance for state and local public health officials, Atlanta, 1997, Centers for Disease Control and Prevention.

gasoline, or the child has pica or developmental delay, blood lead testing would be appropriate. All Medicaid-eligible children should be screened by blood lead testing. Unfortunately, answers on questionnaires are not more successful at identifying children with lead poisoning than is chance. Venous sampling is preferred to capillary sampling because the chances of false-positive and false-negative results are less with the former.

TREATMENT

Once lead is in bone, it is released slowly and is difficult to remove even with chelating agents. Because the cognitive/behavioral effects of lead may be irreversible, the main effort in treating lead poisoning is to **prevent** it from occurring and to **prevent** further ingestion by already-poisoned children. The main components in the effort to eliminate lead poisoning are universally applicable to all children (and adults) and are as follows: (1) identification and elimination of environmental sources of lead exposure, (2) behavioral modification to reduce nonnutritive hand-to-mouth activity, and (3) dietary counseling to ensure sufficient intake of the essential elements calcium and iron. For the small minority of children with more-severe lead poisoning, drug treatment is available that enhances lead excretion.

During health maintenance visits a limited risk assessment is warranted, which includes questions pertaining to the most common sources of lead exposure: the condition of old paint, secondary occupational exposure via an adult living in the home, and/or proximity to an industrial source of pollution. If such a source is identified, its elimination usually requires the assistance of public health and housing agencies as well as education for the parents. The family should move out of a lead-contaminated apartment until repairs are completed. During repairs, repeated washes of surfaces and the use of high-efficiency particle accumulator vacuum cleaners help reduce exposure to lead-containing dust. Careful selection of a contractor who is certified to perform lead abatement work is necessary. Sloppy work can cause dissemination of lead-containing dust and chips throughout a home or building and result in further elevation of a child's BLL. After the work is completed, dust wipe samples should be collected from floors and windowsills or wells to verify that the risk from lead has abated.

A single case of lead poisoning is often discovered in a household with multiple affected family members, including other young children, even in a household with a common source of exposure such as peeling lead-based paint. The mere presence of lead in an environment does not produce lead poisoning. Parental efforts at **reducing the hand-to-mouth activity** of the affected child are necessary to reduce the risk of lead ingestion. Handwashing effectively removes lead, but in a home with lead-containing dust, lead rapidly begins to reaccumulate on the child's hands after washing. Therefore, handwashing is best limited to the period immediately before nutritive hand-to-mouth activity occurs.

Because there is competition between lead and essential minerals, it is reasonable to promote a healthy diet that is sufficient in calcium and iron. The recommended daily intakes of these metals vary somewhat with age. In general, for children 1 yr of age and up a calcium intake of about 1 g/day is sufficient and convenient to remember (roughly the calcium content of a quart of milk [≈1,200 mg/qt] or calcium-fortified orange juice). Calcium absorption is vitamin D dependent; milk is fortified with vitamin D, but other nutritional sources of calcium often are not. A multivitamin containing vitamin D may be prescribed for children who do not drink sufficient milk or who have inadequate sunlight exposure. Iron requirements also vary with age, ranging from 6 mg/day for infants to 12 mg/day for adolescents. For children identified biochemically as being iron deficient, therapeutic iron at a daily dose of 5-6 mg/kg for 3 mo is appropriate. Iron absorption is enhanced when iron is ingested with ascorbic acid (citrus juices). Giving additional calcium or iron above the recommended daily intakes to mineral-sufficient children has not been shown to be of therapeutic benefit in the treatment of lead poisoning.

Drug treatment to remove lead is lifesaving for children with lead encephalopathy. In nonencephalopathic children, it prevents symptom progression and further toxicity. Guidelines for chelation are based on the BLL. *A child with a venous BLL of 45 µg/dL or higher should be treated.* Four drugs are available in the United States: 2,3-dimercaptosuccinic acid (DMSA [succimer]), CaNa$_2$EDTA (versenate), British antilewisite (BAL [dimercaprol]), and penicillamine. DMSA and penicillamine can be given orally, whereas CaNa$_2$EDTA and BAL can be administered only parenterally. The choice of agent is guided by the severity of the lead poisoning, the effectiveness of the drug, and the ease of administration (Table 721-4). Children with BLLs of 44-70 µg/dL may be treated with a single drug, preferably DMSA. Those with BLLs of 70 µg/dL or greater require 2-drug treatment: CaNa$_2$EDTA in combination with either DMSA or BAL for those without evidence of encephalopathy, or CaNa$_2$EDTA and BAL for those with encephalopathy. Published data on the combined treatment with CaNa$_2$EDTA and DMSA for children with BLLs higher than 100 µg/dL are very limited. However, anecdotal information derived from the treatment of hundreds of severely lead poisoned children in northern Nigeria indicates that single-drug treatment with DMSA is lifesaving, although the degree of residual damage in survivors has not been reported.

Acute drug-related toxicities are minor and reversible. These include gastrointestinal distress, transient elevations in transaminases, active urinary sediment, and neutropenia. These types of events are least common for CaNa$_2$EDTA and DMSA and more common for BAL and

Table 721-4	Chelation Therapy		
NAME	**SYNONYM**	**DOSE**	**TOXICITY**
Succimer	Chemet, 2,3-dimercaptosuccinic acid (DMSA)	350 mg/m² body surface area/dose *(not 10 mg/kg)* q8h, PO for 5 days, then q12h for 14 days	Gastrointestinal distress, rashes; elevated LFTs, depressed white blood cell count
Edetate*	CaNa$_2$EDTA (calcium disodium edetate), versenate	1,000-1,500 mg/m² body surface area/day; IV infusion—continuous or intermittent; IM divided q6h or q12h for 5 days	Proteinuria, pyuria, rising blood urea nitrogen/creatinine—all rare. Hypercalcemia if too rapid an infusion. Tissue inflammation if infusion infiltrates
British antilewisite (BAL)	Dimercaprol	300-500 mg/m² body surface area/day; **IM only** divided q4h for 3-5 days. Only for BLL ≥70 µg/dL	Gastrointestinal distress, altered mentation; elevated LFTs, hemolysis if glucose-6-phosphate dehydrogenase deficiency; no concomitant iron treatment
D-Pen	Penicillamine	10 mg/kg/day for 2 wk increasing to 25-40 mg/kg/day; oral, divided q12h. For 12-20 wk	Rashes, fever; blood dyscrasias, elevated LFTs, proteinuria. Allergic cross reactivity with penicillin

*Always given as the calcium salt; never as the sodium salt without calcium.
BLL, blood lead level; IM, intramuscularly; IV, intravenously; LFT, liver function test; PO, by mouth.
From Markowitz ME: Lead poisoning, Pediatr Rev 21:327–335, 2000.

penicillamine. All of the drugs are effective in reducing BLLs when given in sufficient doses and for the prescribed time. These drugs also may increase lead absorption from the gut and should be administered to children in lead-free environments. *Some authorities also recommend the administration of a cathartic immediately prior to or concomitant with the initiation of chelation to eliminate any lead already in the gut.*

None of these agents removes all lead from the body. Within days to weeks after completion of a course of therapy the BLL rises, even in the absence of new lead ingestion. The source of this rebound in the BLL is believed to be bone. Serial examinations of bone lead content have shown that chelation with CaNa₂EDTA is associated with a decline in bone lead levels but that residual bone lead remains detectable even after multiple courses of treatment.

Repeat chelation is indicated if the BLL rebounds to 45 µg/dL or higher. Children with initial BLLs higher than 70 µg/dL are likely to require more than 1 course. A minimum of 3 days between courses is recommended to prevent treatment-related toxicities, especially in the kidney.

The indication for chelation therapy for children with BLLs <45 µg/dL is less clear. Although use of these drugs in children with BLLs from 20-44 µg/dL will result in transiently lowered BLLs, and in some cases reversal of lead-induced enzyme inhibition, few such children increase their excretion of lead significantly during chelation, raising the question of whether any long-term benefit is achieved. A study of 2 yr old children with BLLs of 20-44 µg/dL who were randomized to receive either DMSA or placebo found that the drop in BLLs was greater in the 1st 6 mo after enrollment in the DMSA-treated group, but the levels converged by 1 yr of follow-up. Mean cognitive test scores obtained at 4 and 7 yr of age were not statistically different between the groups. Chelation with DMSA (and CaNa₂EDTA) is not recommended for all children with BLLs <45 µg/dL. It remains to be demonstrated whether other chelating agents available in the United States or elsewhere are effective at either substantially reducing body stores (bone) of lead or at reversing the cognitive deficits attributable to lead at these BLLs.

With successful intervention (with or without chelation), BLLs decline, with the greatest fall in BLL occurring in the 1st 2 mo after therapy is initiated. Subsequently, the rate of change in BLL declines slowly so that by 6-12 mo after identification, the BLL of the average child with moderate lead poisoning (BLL >20 µg/dL) will be 50% lower. Children with more markedly elevated BLLs may take years to reach the CDC reference level, 5 µg/dL, even if all sources of lead exposure have been eliminated, behavior has been modified, and nutrition has been maximized. Early screening remains the best way of avoiding and therefore obviating the need for the treatment of lead poisoning.

Bibliography is available at Expert Consult.

Chapter **722**
Nonbacterial Food Poisoning

722.1 Mushroom Poisoning

Denise A. Salerno and Stephen C. Aronoff

Mushrooms are an ideal food. They are low in calories, fat free, and high in protein, making them a great source of nutrition. Unfortunately, some are highly toxic if ingested. Picking and consumption of wild mushrooms are increasingly popular in the United States. This rise in popularity has led to increased reports of severe and fatal mushroom poisonings.

The clinical syndromes produced by mushroom poisoning are divided according to the rapidity of onset of symptoms and the predominant system involved (Table 722-1). The symptoms are caused by the principal toxin present in the ingested mushrooms. The 8 major toxins produced by mushrooms are categorized as cyclopeptides, monomethylhydrazine, muscarine, hallucinogenic indoles, isoxazole, coprine (disulfiram-like reaction), orellanine, and gastrointestinal tract–specific irritants. The edible wild mushroom *Tricholoma equestre* is associated with delayed rhabdomyolysis, and *Clitocybe amoenolens* and *Clitocybe acromelalga* have been reported to cause erythromelalgia. The toxins responsible for these effects are unknown. An enzyme-linked immunosorbent assay immunoassay is available to detect amanitatoxin; additional rapid tests are becoming available to identify other specific toxins.

Symptoms after eating mushrooms may not be the direct effect of a toxin but may be an allergic reaction or a toxic effect of pesticides or other contaminants. In addition, all who ate the same mushroom may not become sick or if they do they may become sick at different intervals. Table 722-2 lists general principles of management.

GASTROINTESTINAL: DELAYED ONSET
Amanita Poisoning

Poisonings by species of *Amanita* and *Galerina* account for 95% of the fatalities from mushroom intoxication; the mortality rate for this group is 5-10%. Most species produce 2 classes of cyclopeptide toxins: (1) phallotoxins, which are heptapeptides believed to be responsible for the early symptoms of *Amanita* poisoning, and (2) amanitatoxin, an octapeptide that inhibits nuclear RNA polymerase II and subsequent production of messenger RNA leading to impaired protein synthesis and cell death. Cells with high turnover rates, such as those in the gastrointestinal mucosa, kidneys, and liver, are the most severely affected. Other suggested toxin effects are induction of apoptosis, glutathione depletion in the liver, and oxygen free radical formation. Acute yellow atrophy of the liver and necrosis of the proximal renal tubules are found in lethal cases.

The **clinical course** of poisoning with *Amanita* or *Galerina* species is biphasic. Nausea, vomiting, and severe abdominal pain ensue 6-24 hr after ingestion. Profuse watery diarrhea follows shortly thereafter and may last for 12-24 hr or longer. During this time, patients become severely dehydrated. From 24-48 hr after poisoning, jaundice, hypertransaminasemia (peaking at 72-96 hr), renal failure, and coma occur. Death occurs 4-7 days after the ingestion. A prothrombin time less than 10% of control is a poor prognostic factor.

Treatment

Treatment for *Amanita* poisoning is both supportive and specific. Fluid loss from severe diarrhea during the early course of the illness is profound, requiring aggressive correction of fluid loss, electrolytes, and acid–base disturbances. In the late phase of the disease, management of renal and hepatic failure is also necessary.

Specific therapy for *Amanita* poisoning is designed to remove the toxin rapidly and to block binding at its target site. Oral activated charcoal is recommended as part of the initial treatment for children with *Amanita* poisoning. Forced diuresis should be avoided, as this increases renal exposure. For significant ingestions, consider silibinin (5 mg/kg IV over 1 hr followed by a continuous intravenous infusion of 20 mg/kg/24 hr) for 3 days postingestion. If silibinin is not available, intravenous penicillin G (400,000 units/kg/24 hr) may be used. Silibinin and penicillin G inhibit binding of both toxins, interrupt enterohepatic recirculation of amanitatoxin, and protect the liver from further injury. Acetylcysteine has shown promise in some studies. Hemodialysis and hemoperfusion are also recommended as part of the initial treatment for intoxicated children. Orthotopic liver transplantation is recommended for children with severe hepatic failure.

Monomethylhydrazine Intoxication

Species of *Gyromitra* contain gyromitrin which decomposes in the stomach to form monomethylhydrazine (CH₃NHNH₂) and inhibits

Table 722-1	Summary of Common Mushroom-Associated Syndromes		
SYNDROME	**CLINICAL COURSE**	**TOXIN(S)**	**TYPICAL CAUSATIVE MUSHROOM(S)**
Delayed gastroenteritis followed by hepatorenal syndrome	Stage 1: 24 hr after ingestion: onset of nausea, vomiting, profuse cholera-like diarrhea, abdominal pain, hematuria Stage 2: 12-48 hr after ingestion: apparent recovery; levels of hepatic enzymes are rising during this stage Stage 3: 24-72 hr after ingestion: progressive hepatic and renal failure, coagulopathy, cardiomyopathy, encephalopathy, convulsions, coma, death	Cyclopeptides, principally amatoxins	"Deadly *Amanitas*," *Galerina* species
Hyperactivity, delirium, coma	30 min to 2 hr after ingestion: delirium, hallucinations, and coma	Muscimol, ibotenic acid	*Amanita muscaria, Amanita pantherina*
Delayed gastroenteritis with central nervous system abnormalities	6-24 hr after ingestion: nausea, vomiting, diarrhea, abdominal pain, muscle cramps, delirium, convulsions, coma; hemolysis and methemoglobinemia may occur	Gyromitrin	*Gyromitra esculenta* ("false morel")
Cholinergic syndrome	30 min to 2 hr after ingestion: bradycardia, bronchorrhea, bronchospasm, salivation, perspiration, lacrimation, convulsions, coma	Muscarine	*Boletus* species, *Clitocybe* species, *Inocybe* species, *Amanita* species
Disulfiram-like reaction with ethanol	30 min after drinking ethanol (may occur up to 1 wk after eating coprine-containing mushrooms): flushing of skin of face and trunk, hypotension, tachycardia, chest pain, dyspnea, nausea, vomiting, extreme apprehension	Coprine	*Coprinus atramentarius*
Hallucinations	30 min to 3 hr after ingestion: hallucinations, euphoria, drowsiness, compulsive behavior, agitation	Psilocybin and psilocin	*Psilocybe* species
Delayed gastritis and renal failure	Abdominal pain, anorexia, vomiting starting over 30 hr after ingestion, followed by progressive renal failure 3-14 days later	Orelline, orellanine	*Cortinarius* species
Immune-mediated hemolytic anemia	Syncope, gastroenteritis, oliguria, hemoglobinuria, back pain, hemolysis	Immunoglobulin mediated	*Paxillus involutus*
General gastrointestinal irritants	30 min to 2 hr after ingestion: nausea, vomiting, abdominal cramping, diarrhea; may recover without treatment	Unidentified, probably multiple	*Chlorophyllum molybdites*, backyard mushrooms ("little brown mushrooms"), many others

From Brent J, Palmer RB: Mushrooms. In Shannon MW, Borron SW, Burns MJ, editors: Haddad and Winchester's clinical management of poisoning and drug overdose, ed 4, Philadelphia, 2007, WB Saunders, Table 23-1.

Table 722-2	General Management of Mushroom Ingestion

1. Determine history of ingestion: how many types of mushrooms ingested, what time, if anyone else ate them, and what symptoms are present.
2. Attempt to determine which of the possible syndromes (see Table 722-1) the patient may have. For example, gastrointestinal symptoms occurring more than 6 hr after ingestion strongly suggest cyclopeptide, gyromitrin, or *Cortinarius* poisoning.
3. Administer activated charcoal. If the patient has diarrhea, do not give a cathartic. If a cathartic is used, give it only with the first dose of activated charcoal. Use repeated doses of activated charcoal for suspected amatoxin poisonings.
4. If feasible and when indicated, send gastric aspirate or emesis, along with any remaining mushrooms, to a mycologist for identification.
5. Try to perform a preliminary identification of mushroom and spores. Start to develop a spore print as soon as possible.
6. Maintain supportive measures, including airway support, intravenous fluids, and vasopressors (if needed). Monitor volume status.
7. Avoid antispasmodics for gastrointestinal symptoms.
8. Anticipate the clinical course.

From Brent J, Palmer RB: Mushrooms. In Shannon MW, Borron SW, Burns MJ, editors: Haddad and Winchester's clinical management of poisoning and drug overdose, ed 4, Philadelphia, 2007, WB Saunders, Box 23-1.

central nervous system (CNS) enzymatic production of γ-aminobutyric acid. Monomethylhydrazine also oxidizes iron in hemoglobin, resulting in methemoglobinemia. Children with *Gyromitra* poisoning experience vomiting, diarrhea, hematochezia, and abdominal pain within 6-24 hr of ingestion of the toxin. CNS symptoms such as vertigo, diplopia, headache, ataxia, and seizures develop later in the clinical course. Hemolysis and methemoglobinemia (see Chapter 462.6) are rare but potential life-threatening complications of gyromitrin poisoning.

Treatment
Hypovolemia from gastrointestinal fluid losses and seizures require supportive intervention. Pyridoxal phosphate, the coenzyme that catalyzes the production of γ-aminobutyric acid, can reverse the effects of monomethylhydrazine when administered in high doses. **Pyridoxine hydrochloride (25 mg/kg infused over 30 min)** is given at a frequency that is dependent on clinical improvement. Diazepam is given for persistent seizures. Parenteral administration of methylene blue is indicated if the methemoglobin concentration exceeds 30%; severe methemoglobinemia may require dialysis. Blood transfusions may be required for significant hemolysis.

RENAL: DELAYED ONSET
Orellanine Poisoning
Species of *Cortinarius* contain the heat-stable toxin bipyridyl orellanine, which causes severe nonglomerular renal injury characterized by

interstitial fibrosis and acute tubular necrosis. Although the exact mechanism of injury is not fully understood, a metabolite of orellanine is thought to inhibit renal protein synthesis. *Cortinarius* poisoning is characterized by nausea, vomiting, and diarrhea that manifest 36-48 hr after ingestion. Although the initial symptoms may be trivial, more serious renal toxicity occurs in several days. Acute renal failure occurs in 30-50% of those affected, beginning with polyuria and progressing to renal failure (see Chapter 535).

Treatment
Treatment for orellanine poisoning is supportive. Early presentation, within 4-6 hr after ingestion, can be treated with activated charcoal and gastric lavage. Hemodialysis may be needed in patients suffering from renal failure. Most patients recover within 1 mo but chronic renal insufficiency develops in one third to one half of patients who subsequently require renal transplantation.

AUTONOMIC NERVOUS SYSTEM: RAPID ONSET
Muscarine Poisoning
Mushrooms of the genera *Inocybe* and, to a lesser degree, *Clitocybe* contain muscarine or muscarine-related compounds. These quaternary ammonium derivatives bind to postsynaptic receptors, producing an exaggerated cholinergic response.

The onset of symptoms is rapid (30 min to 2 hr after consumption) and intoxication is characterized by a hypercholinergic response: diaphoresis, excessive lacrimation, salivation, miosis, bradycardia, hypotension, urinary and fecal incontinence, and vomiting. Respiratory distress caused by bronchospasm and increased bronchopulmonary secretions is the most serious complication. The symptoms subside spontaneously within 6-24 hr.

Treatment
Atropine sulfate, the specific antidote, is administered intravenously (0.01 mg/kg; maximum: 2 mg). This is repeated until the pulmonary symptoms resolve or the patient becomes overtly tachycardic.

Coprine Ingestion
Coprinus atramentarius and *Clitocybe clavipes* contain coprine. Like disulfiram (Antabuse; Odyssey Pharmaceuticals, Inc.), coprine inhibits the metabolism of acetaldehyde after ethanol ingestion. The clinical manifestations result from accumulation of acetaldehyde.

Coprine intoxication becomes apparent after ethanol ingestion and may occur up to 5 days after consumption of the mushroom. Hyperemia of the face and trunk, tingling of the hands, metallic taste, tachycardia, and vomiting occur acutely. Hypotension may result from intense peripheral vasodilation.

The syndrome typically is self-limited and lasts only several hours. No specific antidote is available. If hypotension is severe, vascular reexpansion with isotonic parenteral solutions may be required. Small oral doses of propranolol have also been suggested.

CENTRAL NERVOUS SYSTEM: RAPID ONSET
Isoxazole Intoxication
Although *Amanita muscaria* and *Amanita pantherina* may contain muscarine, the toxins responsible for the CNS symptoms after ingestion of these mushrooms are muscimol and ibotenic acid, the heat-stable derivatives of the isoxazoles. Muscimol, a hallucinogen, and ibotenic acid, an insecticide, act as γ-aminobutyric acid agonists. From 30 min to 3 hr after ingestion, CNS symptoms appear: obtundation, alternating lethargy and agitation, and, occasionally, seizures. Nausea and vomiting are uncommon. If large amounts of muscarine are contained in the mushroom, symptoms of cholinergic crisis also may occur.

Specific therapy must be carefully selected. If an exaggerated cholinergic response is observed, atropine should be administered. Because ingestions of *A. muscaria* often are associated with anticholinergic findings, the acetylcholinesterase inhibitor physostigmine is often used to reverse the delirium and coma. Benzodiazepines also are used for the agitation and delirium. Seizures can be controlled with diazepam. In most cases, however, early treatment with ipecac (if the patient is conscious) and close observation are all that is required.

Indole Intoxication
Mushrooms belonging to the genus *Psilocybe* ("magic mushrooms") contain psilocybin and psilocin, 2 psychotropic compounds. Within 30 min after ingestion, patients experience euphoria and hallucinations, often accompanied by tachycardia and mydriasis. Fever and seizures have also been observed in children with psilocybin poisoning. These symptoms are short lived, usually lasting for 6 hr after consumption of the mushroom. Treatment consists of rest and observation in a quiet environment. Severely agitated patients may show response to diazepam.

GASTROINTESTINAL: RAPID ONSET
Many mushrooms from various genera produce local gastrointestinal manifestations. The causative toxins are diverse and largely unknown. Within 1 hr of ingestion, patients experience acute abdominal pain, nausea, vomiting, and diarrhea. Symptoms may last from hours to days, depending on the species of mushroom.

Treatment is mainly supportive. Children with large fluid losses may require parenteral fluid therapy. It is imperative to differentiate ingestion of mushrooms of this class from ingestion of *Amanita* and *Galerina* species containing cyclopeptide toxins.

Bibliography is available at Expert Consult.

722.2 Solanine Poisoning
Denise A. Salerno and Stephen C. Aronoff

Potatoes exposed to light and allowed to turn green and/or sprout produce a number of alkaloid glycosides containing the cholesterol derivative solanidine. Two of these glycosides, α-solanine and α-chaconine, are found in highest concentration in the peels of greened potatoes and in the sprouts. Some solanine can be removed by boiling but not by baking. The major effect of α-solanine and α-chaconine is the reversible inhibition of cholinesterase. Cardiotoxic and teratogenic effects have also been reported.

Clinical manifestations of solanine and chaconine poisoning intoxication occur within 7-19 hr after ingestion. The most common symptoms are vomiting, abdominal pain, and diarrhea; in more severe instances of poisoning, neurologic symptoms, including drowsiness, apathy, confusion, weakness, and vision disturbances, are rarely followed by coma or death.

Treatment of solanine poisoning is largely supportive. In the most severe cases, symptoms resolve within 11 days.

Bibliography is available at Expert Consult.

722.3 Seafood Poisoning
Denise A. Salerno and Stephen C. Aronoff

CIGUATERA FISH POISONING
The most frequently reported seafood-toxin illness in the world, ciguatera fish poisoning, has been reported in Florida, Hawaii, French Polynesia, the Marshall Islands, Caribbean and South Pacific islands, and the Virgin Islands. With modern methods of transportation, the illness now occurs worldwide. Grouper is the most commonly identified source of the toxin, followed by snapper, kingfish, amberjack, dolphin, eel, and barracuda. Poisoning has also been associated with farm-raised salmon.

The dinoflagellate *Gambierdiscus toxicus,* a microscopic unicellular organism found along coral reefs, produces high concentrations of ciguatoxin and maitotoxin. The toxins are passed along the food chain

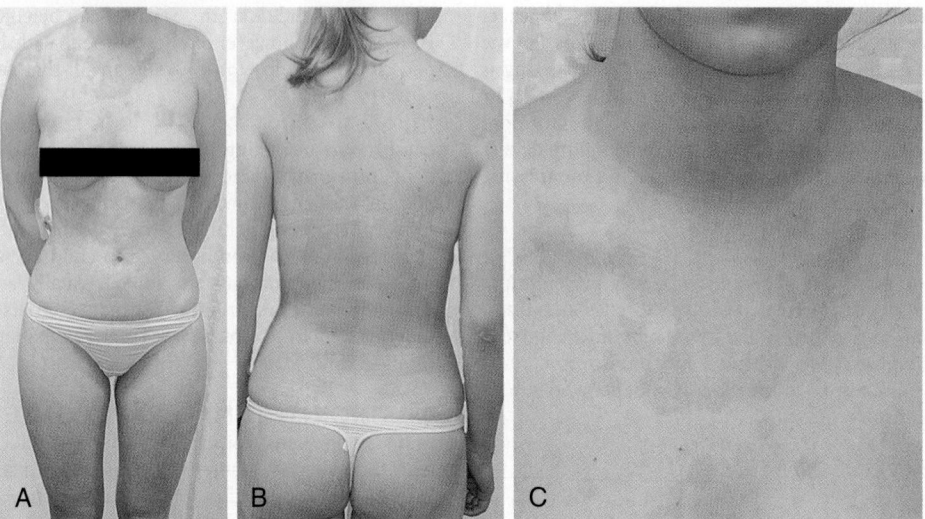

Figure 722-1 A and **B,** Widespread erythematous rash predominantly on the face (not shown) and trunk of patient 1. **C,** Close-up view of the upper chest area. Note the absence of wheals. *(From Jantschitsch C, Kinaciyan T, Manafi M, Safer M, Tanew A. Severe scombroid fish poisoning: an underrecognized dermatologic emergency. J Am Acad Dermatol 65(1):246–247, 2011, Fig. 1.)*

from small herbivorous fish that consume the dinoflagellate to larger predatory fish and then to humans. These toxins are harmless in fish but produce distinct clinical symptoms in humans.

The lipid ciguatoxin-1 is odorless, colorless, and tasteless and is not destroyed by cooking or freezing. Ciguatoxin-1 increases the sodium ion permeability of excitable membranes and depolarizes nerve cells, actions that are inhibited by calcium and tetrodotoxin.

Between 2 and 30 hr after ingestion, ciguatoxin poisoning typically produces a biphasic illness. The initial symptoms are not specific and are of gastrointestinal origin (diarrhea, vomiting, nausea, and abdominal pain). The second phase occurs within a few days of ingestion and consists of intense itching, anxiety, myalgias, painful intercourse, and rash on palms and soles; the neurologic symptoms of circumoral or extremity dysesthesias (characterized by reversal of hot and cold sensation) are characteristic of this disease and may last for months. Tachycardia, bradycardia, hypotension, and death occur infrequently. Eating fish organs, roe, or viscera is associated with greater symptom severity. The diagnosis of ciguatera fish poisoning is based on clinical presentation and a compatible epidemiologic history; the diagnosis is confirmed by testing the ingested fish for toxin. There is no human biomarker to confirm ciguatera fish poisoning.

Treatment
Treatment of ciguatera fish poisoning is supportive. Gastric lavage is recommended to remove any remaining toxin. Intravenous fluids may be required for severe diarrhea, and parenteral administration of calcium can be used to treat hypotension. Once adequate hydration is established, mannitol (0.5-1.0 g/kg, IV over 30-45 min) given within 48-72 hr of the toxic fish ingestion is recommended for reduction of acute symptoms (especially neurologic symptoms) and possible prevention of chronic neurologic symptoms. Various other medications and herbal remedies have been tried, with variable results. Most cases are self-limited, and death occurs in less than 0.1% of cases.

SCOMBROID (PSEUDOALLERGIC) FISH POISONING
Ingestion of members of the Scomberesocidae and Scombridae families, including albacore, mackerel, tuna, bonita, and kingfish, have been linked to major outbreaks of pseudoallergy fish poisoning. Nonscombroid fish and marine mammals, such as mahi-mahi (dolphin fish), swordfish, and bluefish, also are associated with poisoning.

Scombrotoxin, either histamine or the product of the action of the toxin on fish flesh, is responsible for the clinical syndrome. Histidine

is found in high concentrations in the flesh of scombroid fish; the action of bacterial decarboxylases during putrification converts the histidine to histamine. Fish containing more than 20 mg of histamine per 100 g of flesh are toxic. In patients receiving isoniazid, a potent histaminase blocker, ingestion of fish flesh containing a lower concentration of histamine may be toxic.

The onset of **clinical manifestations** is acute and occurs within 10 min to 2 hr of ingestion. The most common symptoms and signs are diarrhea, erythema, sweating, flushing, diaphoresis, urticaria, nausea, and headache (Fig. 722-1). Abdominal pain, tachycardia, oral burning or numbness, dizziness, respiratory distress, hives, and facial swelling also occur. The illness is usually self-limited, terminating within 8-24 hr.

Treatment
Treatment is mainly supportive. Gastric lavage decreases continued absorption of histamine. With severe diarrhea, fluid replacement may be necessary. Antihistamines have been variably successful. Four patients with severe toxicity treated with cimetidine (a histamine blocker) showed rapid response. Because data on these possible treatments are limited, cimetidine or ranitidine should be reserved for severe cases.

PARALYTIC SHELLFISH POISONING
Mussels, clams, oysters, scallops, and other filter-feeding mollusks may become contaminated during dinoflagellate blooms or "red tides." During periods of contamination, water in coastal areas can be colored red by the algae; this sign is the origin of the term *red tide*. (Such discoloration does not necessarily indicate the presence of toxin, and toxin may be present in high quantities without discoloration.) Nonetheless, discolored water should be regarded with suspicion.) The dinoflagellates *Alexandrium* spp. and *Gymnodinium catenatum* often are responsible for these red tides and contain several potent neurotoxins. Paralytic shellfish poisoning is a distinctive neurologic illness caused by 20 closely related heat-stable paralytic shellfish toxins. Saxitoxin is the most potent of the neurotoxins responsible for paralytic shellfish poisoning. This toxin prevents nerve conduction by inhibiting the sodium–potassium pump. Other toxins may be bioconverted to less toxic compounds. Consumption of bivalves, such as mussels, scallops, and clams, is the usual pathway of intoxication, although crustaceans and fish have been implicated as well.

The onset of **clinical manifestations** of paralytic shellfish poisoning occurs rapidly, 30 min to 2 hr after ingestion. Abdominal pain and nausea are common. Paresthesias are common and occur circumorally or in a stocking–glove distribution, or both. Perioral numbness or tingling, diplopia, ataxia, dysarthria, and the sensation of floating are seen less commonly. Hot-cold reversal in temperature sensation is not unusual. In severe cases, respiratory failure from diaphragmatic paralysis may result. Swimming in the water during a red tide episode does not appear to have neurologic sequalae, although skin or mucosal irritation may result.

Treatment
No antidote for paralytic shellfish poisoning is known. Supportive care, including mechanical ventilation, may be needed. Although the symptoms are usually self-limited and short-lived, weakness and malaise may persist for weeks after ingestion.

NEUROTOXIC SHELLFISH POISONING
Neurotoxic shellfish poisoning is a rare disease caused by molluscan shellfish contaminated with brevetoxins. Shellfish harvested along the Gulf of Mexico during or right after a red tide are at risk of contamination with brevetoxins produced by the dinoflagellate *Karenia brevis*. There has also been recent evidence of brevetoxin production by raphidophytes (*Chattonella* spp.). Brevetoxins are a group of more than 10 lipid-soluble neurotoxins that activate sodium ion channels, causing nerve membrane depolarization. Shellfish are not affected by the brevetoxins. Rinsing, cleaning, cooking, and freezing do not destroy the toxins. Consumption of contaminated shellfish goes unnoticed because the brevetoxins cannot be detected by taste or smell.

The onset of **clinical manifestations** of neurotoxic shellfish poisoning occurs from within a few min up to 18 hr after consumption. The majority of symptoms are gastrointestinal (nausea, vomiting, and diarrhea) or neurologic (numbness and tingling of the lips, mouth, face, and extremities, ataxia, partial limb paralysis, reversal of hot and cold sensation, slurred speech, headache, and fatigue). Neurotoxic shellfish poisoning is similar to a mild case of paralytic shellfish poisoning.

Treatment
There are no specific antidotes for brevetoxins. Treatment involves mostly supportive care. Brevenal, a natural antagonist of brevetoxin produced by *K. brevis*, may be used as a form of treatment in the future.

DIARRHETIC SHELLFISH POISONING
Several outbreaks of diarrhetic shellfish poisoning have been reported in Europe after consumption of mussels, cockles, and other shellfish. The dinoflagellates *Dinophysis* and *Prorocentrum* produce okadaic acid and its derivatives, the dinophysistoxins. These compounds inhibit protein phosphatases. The intracellular accumulation of phosphorylated proteins causes increased fluid secretion by gut cells via calcium influx, which is mediated by cyclic adenosine monophosphate and prostaglandins.

Patients have severe diarrhea. Care is supportive and directed at rehydration. The illness is self-limited, and recovery occurs in 3-4 days; few patients require hospitalization.

AMNESIC SHELLFISH POISONING
Amnesic shellfish poisoning was first reported in 1987 in Canada when a group of people demonstrated severe gastroenteritis as well as neurologic symptoms, including memory loss, after eating mussels from Prince Edward Island. Subsequent cases have been identified after consumption of shellfish from the United States, Spain, and the United Kingdom. The responsible toxin, domoic acid, comes from a diatom, *Pseudonitzschia multiseries,* and is a potent glutamate agonist, disrupting neurochemical transmission in the brain. It also binds to glutamate receptors, which increase calcium influx, producing neuronal swelling in the hippocampal area of the brain and death.

The initial **clinical manifestations** are gastrointestinal. Memory loss is closely related to advanced age. Those patients <40 yr are more likely to suffer only from diarrhea, whereas those >50 yr suffer from short-term memory loss lasting months to years.

AZASPIRACID POISONING
The azaspiracids are a class of algal toxins. Azaspiracid poisoning results from ingestion of contaminated bivalve shellfish, especially mussels. Azaspiracid toxins are distributed throughout the muscle tissue in the shellfish. Azaspiracid is cytotoxic to cells and an inhibitor of Ca^{++} channels in plasma membranes. Symptoms start 6-18 hr after ingestion and include nausea, vomiting, severe stomach cramps, and diarrhea, which often persist up to 5 days.

Bibliography is available at Expert Consult.

722.4 Melamine Poisoning
Denise A. Salerno and Stephen C. Aronoff

Melamine (1,3,5-triazine-2,4,6-triamine, or $C_3H_6N_6$), a compound developed in the 1830s, is found in many plastics, adhesives, laminated products, cement, cleansers, fire retardant paint, and more. Melamine poisoning from food products was unheard of until 2007, when melamine-tainted pet food caused the death of many dogs and cats in the United States. In 2008, feeding of melamine-tainted infant formula to more than 300,000 children resulted in kidney injuries, 50,000 hospitalizations, and 6 deaths in China. This was the first reported epidemic of melamine-tainted milk products.

Melamine contains 66% nitrogen by mass. The illegal addition of melamine to infant formula can give the formula a milky appearance and falsely raise the protein content as measured by nitrogen testing.

Melamine, combined with cyanuric acid, forms cyanurate crystals in the kidneys. Along with protein, uric acid, and phosphate, melamine forms renal calculi.

Clinical manifestations are initially subtle and nonspecific. The severity is dose related. The first symptoms in affected infants are unexplained crying (especially when urinating), vomiting, and discolored urine caused by the formation of stones and gravel in the urinary tract. Urinary obstruction and acute renal failure follow. In the absence of a specific diagnosis, death from renal failure occurs. Whether children with melamine-induced renal failure will have chronic sequelae is currently unknown. Animal studies have shown that melamine may cause cognitive impairment but further investigation is needed.

The melamine stones and gravel can be treated with hydration, alkalinization, or lithotripsy. Acute renal failure requires supportive care and dialysis if needed.

Bibliography is available at Expert Consult.

Chapter 723
Biologic and Chemical Terrorism
Theodore J. Cieslak and Frederick M. Henretig

Tragically, increasing numbers of children are being victimized by terrorist actions. Brought to the forefront of American consciousness by Timothy McVeigh's references to child fatalities as "collateral damage" during the Oklahoma City bombing in April 1995, the intentional targeting of children became firmly ensconced as a global reality with the attack upon a school in Beslan, Russia, in September 2004. The attack, which left 334 (Including 186 children) dead, presaged additional attacks specifically directed against children at an Amish School in Pennsylvania in 2006, at a camp for teenagers in Utoya, Norway, in

2011, and at Sandy Hook Elementary School in Connecticut in 2012, among others.

Paralleling the targeting of children is an apparent trend toward the use of "unconventional" weapons of terror. In 1984, members of the Rajneeshee cult employed *Salmonella typhi* in a wave of intentional poisonings that affected 751 persons, including 142 teenage patrons of a popular pizza parlor. In 1995, the Aum Shinrikyo cult killed 12 and sickened thousands by intentionally releasing sarin nerve agent in the Tokyo subway system. A disgruntled scientist deployed anthrax spores via the U.S. mail in October 2001, killing 5 and injuring 17 in an attack upon a nation already reeling in the wake of the 9/11 attacks.

These developments remind us that terrorists can strike at any time utilizing any number of unconventional weapons, including biologic and chemical agents. Children will not be spared in these attacks on civilians, and, indeed, schools and daycare sites may be the targets of these actions.

ETIOLOGY

Terrorists may choose to use **weapons of opportunity,** agents that for some reason are readily available to some member of the terrorist group. The motives of terrorists often are obscure and difficult to predict. Prevention and response strategies should thus concentrate not on those agents most likely to be used but, rather, on those agents that, if used, would constitute the gravest potential threats to public health and security.

Biologic threat agents, including pathogens and toxins, have been divided by the Centers for Disease Control and Prevention into 3 categories, with **category A** including diseases caused by those 6 agents posing the greatest threat: anthrax, plague (see Chapter 203.3), tularemia (see Chapter 206), smallpox, botulism (see Chapter 210), and the viral hemorrhagic fevers (see Chapter 271).

Terrorists could also procure and release a vast array of potentially harmful chemicals. Tank cars full of flammable industrial gases and liquids, corrosive industrial acids and bases, poisonous compounds such as cyanides and nitrites, pesticides, dioxins, and explosives traverse our railways and roads daily. Four classes of "military-grade" chemicals with a history of use in warfare or manufactured specifically for use as weapons include the organophosphate-based nerve agents, vesicants, "blood agents" (cyanides), and certain pulmonary irritants or "choking agents."

EPIDEMIOLOGY AND PEDIATRIC-SPECIFIC CONCERNS

Large-scale attacks on civilian targets will likely involve pediatric victims, and children may be more susceptible than adults to the effects of certain biologic and chemical agents (see Chapter 719). A thinner and less-keratinized epidermis makes dermally active chemical agents, such as mustard, a greater risk to children than adults. A larger surface area per unit volume further increases the problem. A small relative blood volume makes children more susceptible to the volume losses associated with enteric infections such as cholera and to gastrointestinal intoxications such as might be seen with exposure to the staphylococcal enterotoxins. Children's high minute ventilation, compared with that of adults, increases the threat of agents delivered via the inhalational route. The fact that children live "closer to the ground" compounds this effect when heavier-than-air chemicals are involved. An immature blood–brain barrier may heighten the risk of central nervous system toxicity from nerve agents. Developmental considerations make it less likely that a child would readily flee an area of danger, thereby increasing exposure to these various adverse effects.

Children appear to have a unique susceptibility to certain potential agents that might be used by terrorists. Although adults generally suffer only a brief, self-limited incapacitating illness after infection with Venezuelan equine encephalitis virus, young children are more likely to experience seizures, permanent neurologic sequelae, and death. In the case of smallpox, waning herd immunity may disproportionately affect children. Vaccine-induced immunity to smallpox probably diminishes significantly after ages 3-10 yr. Although most adults are considered susceptible to smallpox, given that routine civilian immunization

ceased in the early 1970s, older adults may have some residual protection from death, if not from the development of disease. Today's children are among the first to grow up in a world without any individual or herd immunity to smallpox.

Children also may experience unique disease manifestations not seen in adults; suppurative parotitis is a common characteristic ring among children with melioidosis but is not generally seen in adults with *Burkholderia pseudomallei* infection (see Chapter 205.2).

Pediatricians are likely to experience unique problems in managing childhood victims of biologic or chemical attack. Many of the drugs useful in treating such casualties are unfamiliar to pediatricians or have relative contraindications in childhood. The fluoroquinolones and tetracyclines are commonly cited as agents of choice in the treatment and prophylaxis of anthrax, plague, tularemia, brucellosis, and Q fever. Both drug classes are often avoided in children, although the risk of morbidity and mortality from diseases induced by agents of bioterrorism far outweighs the minor risks associated with short-term use of these agents. Ciprofloxacin received, as its first licensed pediatric indication, FDA approval for use in the prophylaxis of anthrax after inhalational exposure during a terrorist attack. Doxycycline and levofloxacin are licensed specifically in children for the same indication and levofloxacin is also licensed for postexposure prophylaxis of children against plague. Immunizations potentially useful in preventing biologic agent–induced diseases are often not approved for use in pediatric patients. The available anthrax vaccine is licensed only for those between 18 and 65 yr of age. The plague vaccine, currently out of production and probably ineffective against inhalational exposures, was approved only for individuals ages 18-61 yr. The smallpox vaccine, a live vaccine employing vaccinia virus, can cause fetal vaccinia and demise when given to pregnant women.

Many otherwise useful pharmaceutical agents are not available in pediatric dosing regimens. The military distributes nerve agent antidote kits consisting of prefilled autoinjectors designed for the rapid administration of atropine and pralidoxime. Many emergency departments and some ambulances stock these kits. The doses of agents contained in the nerve agent antidote kit are calculated for soldiers and thus are far in excess of those appropriate for young children, and pediatric pralidoxime autoinjectors are not yet available. Atropine autoinjectors specifically formulated for children are approved by the FDA and are available.

Although physical protective measures and devices (e.g., "gas masks") are likely to be of little utility in a civilian terrorism setting, such commercially available devices are not often available in pediatric sizes. The Israeli experience during the first Gulf War suggests that frightened parents may improperly use such masks on their children, resulting in inadvertent suffocation.

In the event of a large-scale terrorist attack, there may be an insufficient number of pediatric hospital beds. In any large disaster, excess bed capacity might potentially be provided at civilian and veterans hospitals under the auspices of the National Disaster Medical System, but that system makes no specific provision for pediatric beds.

CLINICAL MANIFESTATIONS

Should a terrorist attack occur, clinicians may be called on to make prompt diagnoses and render rapid lifesaving treatments before the results of confirmatory diagnostic tests are available. Although each potential agent of terrorism produces its own unique clinical manifestations, it is useful to consider their effects in terms of a limited number of distinct clinical syndromes. This approach helps clinicians make prompt, rational decisions regarding empirical therapy. Casualties resulting from a terrorist attack would either experience symptoms immediately upon exposure to an agent (or within the 1st several hr after exposure) or, alternatively, would see their symptoms develop slowly over a period of days to weeks. In the former case, the sinister nature of the event is often obvious and the etiology more likely to be conventional or chemical in nature. Biologic agents differ from conventional, chemical (see Chapter 719), and nuclear (see Chapter 718) weapons in that they have inherent incubation periods. Consequently, patients are likely to present removed in time and place from the point

Table 723-1	Diseases Caused By Agents of Chemical and Biologic Terrorism, Classified By Syndrome		
	NEUROMUSCULAR SYMPTOMS PROMINENT	**RESPIRATORY SYMPTOMS PROMINENT**	**DERMATOLOGIC FINDINGS PROMINENT**
Sudden-onset	Nerve agents	Chlorine Phosgene Cyanide	Mustard Lewisite
Delayed-onset	Botulism	Anthrax Plague Tularemia Ricin	Smallpox

of an unannounced and unnoticed exposure to a biologic agent. Whereas traditional first responders, such as firefighters and paramedics, may be at the forefront of a conventional or chemical terrorism response, the primary care physician is likely to constitute the first line of defense against the effects of a biologic agent.

Casualties can thus be categorized as either immediate or delayed in presentation. Within each of these categories, patients can be further classified as having primarily respiratory, neuromuscular, or dermatologic manifestations (Table 723-1). A limited number of agents may cause each particular syndrome, permitting institution of empiric therapy targeted at a short list of potential etiologies. The viral hemorrhagic fevers might manifest as fever and a bleeding diathesis; these agents are considered separately in Chapter 271. In most cases, supportive care is the mainstay of hemorrhagic fever treatment.

Sudden-Onset Neuromuscular Syndrome: Nerve Agents

The very rapid onset of neuromuscular symptoms after an exposure should lead the clinician to consider nerve agent intoxication. The nerve agents (*tabun, sarin, soman,* and *VX*) are **organophosphate** analogs of common pesticides that act as potent inhibitors of the enzyme acetylcholinesterase. They are hazardous via ingestion, inhalation, or cutaneous absorption (see Chapter 63).

The inhibition of cholinesterase by these compounds results in the accumulation of acetylcholine at neural and neuromuscular junctions, causing excess stimulation. The resultant **cholinergic syndrome** involves central, nicotinic, and muscarinic effects. Central effects include altered mental status progressing rapidly to lethargy and coma, as well as ataxia, convulsions, and respiratory depression. Studies on pesticide exposure suggest that children may be more prone to central neurologic dysfunction with organophosphate toxicity than adults. Nicotinic effects include muscle fasciculations and twitching, followed by weakness, which can progress to flaccid paralysis as muscles fatigue. Muscarinic effects include miosis, visual blurring, profuse lacrimation, and watery rhinorrhea. Bronchospasm and increased bronchial secretions lead to cough, wheezing, dyspnea, and cyanosis. Cardiovascular manifestations include bradycardia, hypotension, and atrioventricular block. Flushing, sweating, salivation, nausea, vomiting, diarrhea, abdominal cramps, and urinary incontinence are also seen. In the absence of prompt intervention, death can quickly result from a combination of central effects and respiratory muscle paralysis.

Delayed-Onset Neuromuscular Syndrome: Botulism

The delayed onset (hours to days after exposure) of neuromuscular symptoms is characteristic of botulism. Botulism occurs after exposure to 1 of 7 related neurotoxins produced by certain strains of *Clostridium botulinum,* a strictly anaerobic, spore-forming, Gram-positive bacillus commonly found in soil. Naturally occurring botulism (see Chapter 210) usually follows ingestion of preformed toxin (food poisoning) or results from intestinal toxin production (infantile botulism). An aerosol exposure would likely result in a case of clinical botulism indistinguishable from that caused by natural exposures.

Following exposure to botulinum toxin, clinical manifestations typically begin with bulbar palsies, causing patients to complain of

ptosis, photophobia, and blurred vision resulting from difficulty in accommodation. Symptoms can progress to include dysarthria, dysphonia, and dysphagia and, finally, a descending symmetric paralysis. Sensation and sensorium are typically not affected. In the absence of intervention, death often results from respiratory muscle failure.

Sudden-Onset Respiratory Syndrome: Chlorine, Phosgene, and Cyanide

The acute onset of respiratory symptoms shortly after exposure should prompt the clinician to consider a range of potential chemical agents. Of note, nerve agents, discussed previously, may affect respiration via massive bronchial hypersecretion, bronchospasm, and respiratory muscle paresis. However, the nerve agent casualty will likely have generalized muscle involvement and central nervous system manifestations. In contrast, the toxic inhalants chlorine and phosgene produce respiratory distress without neuromuscular involvement.

Chlorine is a dense, acrid, yellow-green gas that is heavier than air. After mild to moderate exposure, ocular and nasal irritation occurs, followed by cough, a choking sensation, bronchospasm, and substernal chest tightness. Pulmonary edema, mediated by hydrochloric acid and free oxygen radical generation, follows moderate to severe exposures within 30 min to several hours. Hypoxemia and hypovolemia secondary to pulmonary edema are the factors responsible for death when it occurs.

Phosgene, like chlorine, is a common industrial compound that was used as a weapon on the battlefields of World War I. Its odor has been described as similar to "new-mown hay." Like chlorine, phosgene also is thought to result in the generation of hydrochloric acid, contributing particularly to upper airway, nasal, and conjunctival irritation. Acylation reactions caused by the effects of phosgene on the pulmonary alveolar-capillary membrane lead to pulmonary edema. Phosgene lung injury also may be mediated, in part, by an inflammatory reaction associated with leukotriene production. Patients with mild to moderate exposures to phosgene may be asymptomatic, a fact that may cause victims to remain in a contaminated area. Pulmonary edema occurs 4-24 hr after exposure and is dose dependent, with heavier exposures causing earlier symptoms. Dyspnea may precede radiologic findings. In severe exposures, pulmonary edema may be so marked as to result in hypovolemia and hypotension. As in the case of chlorine, death results from hypoxemia and asphyxia.

Cyanide is a cellular poison, with protean clinical manifestations. Initially, cyanide toxicity is most likely to manifest as tachypnea and hyperpnea, progressing rapidly to apnea in cases with significant exposure (see Chapter 63). The efficacy of cyanide as a chemical terrorism agent is limited by its volatility in open air and relatively low lethality in comparison with nerve agents. Released in a closed room, however, cyanide could have devastating effects, as evidenced by its use in the Nazi gas chambers during World War II. Cyanide inhibits cytochrome a_3, interfering with normal mitochondrial oxidative metabolism and leading to cellular anoxia and lactic acidosis. In addition to respiratory distress, early findings among cyanide victims include tachycardia, flushing, dizziness, headache, diaphoresis, nausea, and vomiting. With greater exposure, seizures, coma, apnea, and cardiac arrest may follow within min. An elevated anion gap metabolic acidosis is typically present, and decreased peripheral oxygen utilization leads to an elevated mixed venous oxygen saturation value.

Delayed-Onset Respiratory Syndrome: Anthrax, Plague, Tularemia, and Ricin

A delayed onset of respiratory symptoms (days after exposure) is characteristic of several infectious diseases and 1 toxin that might be adapted for sinister purposes by terrorists. Among the most threatening and problematic of these are anthrax, plague, tularemia, and ricin, the latter having garnered considerable media attention in recent years.

Anthrax is caused by infection with the Gram-positive spore-forming rod *Bacillus anthracis*. Its ability to form a spore enables the anthrax bacillus to survive for long periods in the environment and enhances its potential as a weapon.

The vast majority of naturally occurring anthrax cases are cutaneous, acquired by close contact with the hides, wool, bone, and other by-products of infected ruminants (principally cattle, sheep, and goats). Cutaneous anthrax is amenable to therapy with a variety of antibiotics and is readily recognizable to experienced clinicians in endemic areas; consequently, it is rarely fatal. Although it is common in parts of Asia and sub-Saharan Africa, only 2 cases of cutaneous anthrax had occurred in the United States in the 9 yr that preceded the attacks of 2001 (when 11 cutaneous cases were seen). Gastrointestinal anthrax, which has never been described in the United States, can occur after the ingestion of contaminated meat. In the past, inhalational anthrax, or **woolsorters' disease**, was an occupational hazard of abattoir and textile workers. Now eliminated as a naturally occurring disease in the United States, it is this inhalational form of anthrax that poses the greatest terror threat. Following an inadvertent release in 1979 from a bioweapons facility at Sverdlovsk in the former Soviet Union, 66 of 77 (86%) known adult victims of inhalational anthrax died. In the 2001 attacks involving contaminated mail in the United States, 5 of 11 (46%) patients with inhalational anthrax died. Whether better intensive care modalities, changes in antibiotic therapy, or earlier recognition accounted for this improved mortality rate remains unknown.

Symptomatic inhalational anthrax typically begins 1-6 days after exposure, although incubation periods of up to several weeks have been reported. The disease begins as a flu-like illness, characterized by fever, myalgia, headache, and cough. A brief intervening period of improvement sometimes follows, but rapid deterioration then ensues; high fever, dyspnea, cyanosis, and shock mark this second phase. Hemorrhagic meningitis occurs in up to 50% of cases. Chest radiographs obtained late in the course of illness may reveal a widened mediastinum or prominent mediastinal lymphadenopathy; pleural effusions also may be seen. Bacteremia is often so profound that Gram stains of peripheral blood may demonstrate the organism at this stage. Prompt treatment is imperative; death occurs in as many as 95% of inhalational anthrax cases if such treatment is begun more than 48 hr after the onset of symptoms.

Whereas inhalational anthrax is a disease primarily of mediastinal lymphatic tissue, exposure to aerosolized plague bacilli typically leads to a primary pneumonia. Endemic **plague** is usually transmitted via the bites of fleas and is discussed in Chapter 203.3. The causative organism of all forms of human plague, *Yersinia pestis,* is a bipolar-staining, Gram-negative facultative intracellular bacillus. An ability to survive within the macrophage aids its dissemination to distant sites following inoculation or inhalation. "Buboes," markedly swollen, tender regional lymph nodes in the distribution of a bite, are the hallmark feature of bubonic plague. Fever and malaise are typically present, and septicemia often develops as bacteria gain access to the circulation. Petechiae, purpura, and overwhelming disseminated intravascular coagulopathy commonly occur, and 80% of bubonic plague victims ultimately have positive blood culture results. Plague is extremely infective and lethal, as illustrated by the fact that the "Black Death" eliminated one third of the population of Europe during the Middle Ages.

Intentional aerosol dissemination of *Y. pestis* would likely result in a preponderance of pneumonic plague cases. Pneumonic plague may also arise secondarily after seeding of the lungs of septicemic patients.

Symptoms include fever, chills, malaise, headache, and cough. Chest radiographs may reveal a patchy consolidation, and the classic clinical finding is blood-streaked sputum. Disseminated intravascular coagulation and overwhelming sepsis typically develop as the disease progresses. Untreated pneumonic plague has a fatality rate approaching 100%.

Tularemia is a highly infectious disease caused by the Gram-negative coccobacillus *Francisella tularensis*. Naturally occurring tularemia is discussed in Chapter 206. The high degree of infectivity of *F. tularensis* (<10 organisms are thought to be necessary to produce infection via inhalation), as well as its survivability in the environment, contributes to its inclusion on the list of agents of concern. Several clinical forms of endemic tularemia are known, but inhalational exposure resulting from a terrorist attack would likely lead to a plague-like primary pneumonia or to typhoidal tularemia, manifesting as a variety of nonspecific symptoms including fever, malaise, and abdominal pain.

Ricin is a protein toxin derived from the castor bean plant (*Ricinus communis*) that inhibits ribosomal protein synthesis. It is highly toxic in animal studies when inhaled and may result in the delayed onset of respiratory distress, pulmonary edema, and acute respiratory failure. One case series of 8 persons from the 1940s described a febrile respiratory illness after inhalational exposure. If injected it may cause a sepsis-like syndrome that may progress to multiorgan system failure; ingestion can lead to severe gastroenteritis. Ricin-containing letters were mailed to a U.S. Senate office building in 2004, and again to President Obama and New York City Mayor Bloomberg in 2013, although no persons were sickened in either attack.

Sudden-Onset Dermatologic Syndrome: Mustard and Lewisite

The development of skin lesions shortly after exposure is characteristic of the chemical vesicants. These compounds, often referred to as *blistering agents*, are cellular poisons and include the alkylating agent mustard and the organic arsenical agent lewisite. Tissue injury to rapidly reproducing cells begins within minutes of contact with these agents. Clinical effects typically become evident several hours after exposure to mustard, whereas patients exposed to lewisite feel immediate pain. Both mustard and lewisite affect the eyes and respiratory tract and their inadvertent ingestion may produce significant gastrointestinal symptoms. Mustard exposure may lead to bone marrow suppression.

Delayed-Onset Dermatologic Syndrome: Smallpox

The appearance of an exanthem days to weeks after exposure is likely to be a presenting feature of smallpox. Caused by infection with variola virus, a member of the orthopoxvirus family, smallpox has an incubation period of 7-17 days. This would likely permit the wide dispersal of asymptomatic exposed persons, thus contributing to the spread of an outbreak. During the incubation period, virus replicates in the upper respiratory tract. A primary viremia ensues, during which time seeding of the liver and spleen occurs. A secondary viremia then develops, the skin is seeded, and the classic exanthem of smallpox appears.

Symptoms of smallpox begin abruptly during the phase of secondary viremia and include fever, rigors, vomiting, headache, backache, and extreme malaise. Within 2-4 days, macules appear on the face and extremities and then progress in synchronous fashion to papules, pustules, and finally scabs. As the scabs separate, survivors often are left with disfiguring, depigmented scars. The synchronous nature of the rash and its centrifugal distribution distinguish smallpox from chickenpox, which has a centripetal distribution. Historically, smallpox had a 30% mortality rate, with death typically resulting from visceral organ involvement.

DIAGNOSIS

In some cases, the terrorist nature of a chemical or biologic attack may be obvious, for example, a chemical attack in which victims succumb in close temporal and geographic proximity to a dispersal device or terrorists announce their attack. In other instances, the clinician may need to rely on epidemiologic clues to suspect an intentional release of chemical or biologic agents. The presence of large numbers of victims clustered in time and space should raise the index of suspicion, as should cases of unexpected death or unexpectedly severe disease. Diseases unusual in a given locale, in a given age group, or during a certain season likewise may warrant further investigation. Simultaneous outbreaks of a disease in noncontiguous areas should cause one to consider an intentional release, as should outbreaks of multiple diseases in the same area. Even a single case of a rare disorder such as anthrax or certain viral hemorrhagic fevers would be suspicious, and a single case of smallpox would almost certainly be the result of an intentional dissemination. Large numbers of dying animals might provide evidence of an unnatural aerosol release, as would evidence of disparate attack rates between those known to be indoors and outdoors at a given time.

In a mass casualty setting, diagnoses may be made largely on clinical grounds. The diagnosis of nerve agent intoxication is based primarily on clinical recognition and patient response to antidotal therapy. Several simple rapid detection devices developed for military use can detect the presence of nerve agents. Some of these are now commercially available and are stocked in certain emergency departments and public safety vehicles. Measurements of acetylcholinesterase in plasma or erythrocytes of nerve agent victims may be helpful in long-term prognostication, but correlation between cholinesterase levels and clinical effects is often poor, and the test rarely is available on an emergency basis.

Botulism should be suspected clinically among patients presenting with a symmetric, descending, flaccid paralysis. Although the differential diagnosis of botulism includes other uncommon neurologic disorders, such as myasthenia gravis and the Guillain-Barré syndrome, the presence of multiple casualties with similar symptoms should aid in the determination of a botulism outbreak.

Initially, the diagnosis of **cyanide poisoning** also will likely be made on clinical grounds in the presence of the appropriate toxidrome. An unusually high anion gap metabolic acidosis with elevated serum lactate and an oxygen concentration greater than expected in mixed venous blood lend support to the clinical diagnosis. Elevated blood cyanide concentrations can confirm the clinical suspicion.

Anthrax should be suspected upon finding Gram-positive bacilli in skin biopsy material (in the case of cutaneous disease), blood smears, pleural fluid, or spinal fluid. Chest radiographs demonstrating a widened mediastinum in the context of fever and constitutional signs, and in the absence of another obvious explanation (e.g., blunt trauma or postsurgical infection), should also lead one to consider the diagnosis. Confirmation can be obtained by blood culture. State health laboratories and federal facilities at the U.S. Centers for Disease Control and Prevention and at the U.S. Army Medical Research Institute of Infectious Diseases can confirm a diagnosis of anthrax by polymerase chain reaction and immunohistochemical assay.

A diagnosis of **plague** can be suspected on finding bipolar "safety-pin"–staining bacilli in Gram or Wayson stains of sputum or aspirated lymph node material; confirmation is obtained by culturing Y. pestis from blood, sputum, or lymph node aspirate. The organism grows on standard blood or MacConkey TRA agars but it is often misidentified by automated systems. F. tularensis grows poorly on standard media; its growth is enhanced on media containing cysteine. Because of its extreme infectivity, however, many laboratories prefer to make a diagnosis via polymerase chain reaction or serologically using an enzyme-linked immunosorbent assay or serum agglutination assay.

Smallpox should be suspected on clinical grounds and can be confirmed by culture or electron microscopy of scabs or vesicular fluid, although the manipulation of clinical material from suspected smallpox victims should be attempted only at public health laboratories able to employ maximum biocontainment (Biosafety Level 4) precautions. Similar caution should be exercised with specimens from patients with various viral hemorrhagic fevers.

PREVENTION

Preventive measures can be considered in both a preexposure and a postexposure context. **Preexposure protection** against a chemical or biologic attack may consist of physical, chemical, or immunologic measures. **Physical protection** against primary attack often involves gas masks and protective suits; such equipment is used by the military and by certain hazardous materials response teams but it is unlikely to be available to civilians at the precise moment that a release occurs. Medical personnel need to understand the principles of physical protection as they apply to infection control and the spread of contamination.

Pneumonic plague is spread through respiratory droplets. Droplet precautions, including the use of simple surgical masks, are thus warranted for providers caring for patients with plague. Smallpox is transmitted by droplet nuclei. Airborne precautions, including (ideally) a high-efficiency particulate air filter mask, are thus warranted with smallpox victims. Similarly, patients with viral hemorrhagic fever should, in general, be managed with use of contact precautions. Most other biologic agent victims can be safely cared for with use of standard precautions. In the case of chemical agents, residual mustard or nerve agent on the skin or clothing of victims might potentially pose a hazard to medical personnel. For such victims, whenever possible, clothing should be removed and the patients decontaminated using copious amounts of water before extensive medical care is rendered. Most other chemical agents are volatile enough that spread of an agent among patients or from patient to caregiver is unlikely.

Preexposure chemical prophylaxis might be used on the basis of credible intelligence reports. Should officials deem that the threatened release of a specific biologic agent appears imminent, antibiotics might be distributed to a population preemptively. Opportunities to employ such a strategy are likely to be limited, although federal and state officials are examining various mechanisms for such employment.

Although licensed vaccines (**preexposure immunologic measures**) against anthrax and smallpox have been developed, widespread use of either vaccine is likely to be problematic, especially in children. The anthrax vaccine is licensed only for those persons age 18 yr and older, is given as a 5 dose series over 18 mo, and requires annual booster doses. These considerations make civilian employment of the current anthrax vaccine on a large scale unlikely, although a new recombinant anthrax vaccine is in development and being studied as a 3 dose series.

Significant obstacles to the widespread employment of smallpox vaccine also exist, although public health officials have contemplated the resumption of a smallpox vaccination campaign. Whereas in the past smallpox vaccine (prepared from vaccinia virus, an orthopoxvirus related to variola) was used safely and successfully in young infants, it has a relatively high rate of serious complications in certain patients. Fetal vaccinia and demise can occur when pregnant women are vaccinated. Vaccinia gangrenosa, an often fatal complication, can occur when immunocompromised persons are vaccinated. Eczema vaccinatum occurs in those with preexisting dermatoses (atopic dermatitis). Severe vaccine-related encephalitis was well known during the era of widespread vaccination; because it occurs only in primary vaccinees, it would disproportionately affect pediatric patients. Auto-inoculation can occur when virus present at the site of vaccination is manually transferred to other areas of skin or to the eye. Young children would presumably be at greater risk for such inadvertent transmission. Myocarditis has been reported following vaccinations of military recruits.

To manage these complications, vaccinia immune globulin should be available when one is undertaking a vaccination campaign. Vaccinia immune globulin (0.6 mg/kg IM) may be given to vaccine recipients who experience severe complications or to significantly immunocompromised individuals exposed to smallpox and in whom vaccination would be unsafe. A compound, ST-246, has been used successfully under an Investigational New Drug permit to treat persons (including children) experiencing severe complications from vaccine. The current cell-culture–derived vaccine (ACAM2000), as well as vaccinia immune globulin and ST-246, can be obtained as needed upon consultation with officials at the Centers for Disease Control and Prevention. In addition to a potential role in preexposure prophylaxis, vaccination may be effective in postexposure prophylaxis if given within the 1st 4 days or so after exposure.

| Table 723-2 | Critical Biologic Agents of Terrorism |

DISEASE	CLINICAL FINDINGS	INCUBATION PERIOD (DAYS)	ISOLATION PRECAUTIONS	INITIAL TREATMENT	PROPHYLAXIS
Anthrax (inhalational)* Patients who are clinically stable after 14 days can be switched to a single oral agent (ciprofloxacin or doxycycline) to complete a 60-days course[†]	Febrile prodrome with rapid progression to mediastinal lymphadenitis and mediastinitis, sepsis, shock, and meningitis	1-5	Standard	Ciprofloxacin[‡] 10-15 mg/kg IV q12h *or* doxycycline 2.2 mg/kg IV q12h *and* clindamycin[§] 10-15 mg/kg IV q8h *and* penicillin G[‖] 400-600 kU/kg/day IV q4h plus raxibacumab	Ciprofloxacin 10-15 mg/kg PO q12h or doxycycline 2.2 mg/kg PO q12h
Plague (pneumonic)	Febrile prodrome with rapid progression to fulminant pneumonia, hemoptysis, sepsis, disseminated intravascular coagulation	2-3	Droplet (for 1st 3 days of therapy)	Gentamicin 2.5 mg/kg IV q8h *or* doxycycline 2.2 mg/kg IV q12h *or* ciprofloxacin 15 mg/kg IV q12h	Doxycycline 2.2 mg/kg PO q12h *or* ciprofloxacin 20 mg/kg PO q12h
Tularemia	Pneumonic: abrupt onset of fever with fulminant pneumonia Typhoidal: fever, malaise, abdominal pain	2-10	Standard	Same as for plague	Same as for plague
Smallpox	Febrile prodrome with synchronous, centrifugal, vesiculopustular exanthema	7-17	Airborne (+ contact)	Supportive care	Vaccination may be effective if given within the 1st several days after exposure
Botulism	Afebrile descending symmetric flaccid paralysis with cranial nerve palsies	1-5	Standard	Supportive care; antitoxin (see text) may halt the progression of symptoms but is unlikely to reverse them	None
Viral hemorrhagic fevers	Febrile prodrome with rapid progression to shock, purpura, and bleeding diatheses	4-21	Contact (consider airborne in cases of massive hemorrhage)	Supportive care; ribavirin may be beneficial in select cases	None

*In a mass casualty setting, in which resources are severely constrained, it may be necessary to substitute oral therapy for the preferred parenteral option.

[†]Assuming the organism is sensitive, children may be switched to oral amoxicillin (80 mg/kg/day ÷ q8h) to complete a 60-day course. We recommend that the 1st 14 days of therapy or postexposure prophylaxis, however, include ciprofloxacin and/or doxycycline regardless of age.

[‡]Levofloxacin or ofloxacin may be an acceptable alternative to ciprofloxacin.

[§]Rifampin or clarithromycin may be an acceptable alternative to clindamycin as a drug that targets bacterial protein synthesis. If ciprofloxacin or another quinolone is employed, doxycycline may be used as a second agent because it also targets protein synthesis.

[‖]Ampicillin, imipenem, meropenem, or chloramphenicol may be an acceptable alternative to penicillin as a drug with good central nervous system penetration.

Anthrax vaccine might similarly be employed in a postexposure setting. Some authorities recommend 3 doses of this vaccine as an adjunct to postexposure chemoprophylaxis after documented exposure to aerosolized anthrax spores. Nonetheless, postexposure administration of oral antibiotics constitutes the mainstay of management for asymptomatic victims believed to have been exposed to anthrax as well as to other bacterial agents such as plague and tularemia. Table 723-2 lists appropriate prophylactic regimens for various biologic exposures.

TREATMENT

Tables 723-2 and 723-3 provide recommended therapies for overt diseases caused by various chemical and biologic agents. It is likely that the clinician attending to victims will need to make therapeutic decisions before the results of confirmatory diagnostic tests are available and in situations in which the diagnosis is not known with certainty. In particular, decontamination by hospital personnel in appropriate personal protective equipment is required for patients exposed to chemical agents who have not been adequately decontaminated in the prehospital setting (see Table 723-3). In such cases, it is useful to note that many diseases and symptoms caused by chemical and biologic agents will resolve spontaneously, with only supportive care required. Most cases of chlorine or phosgene exposure can be successfully

managed by providing meticulous attention to oxygenation and fluid balance. Mustard victims may require intensive multisystem support, but no specific antidote or therapy is available. Many viral diseases, such as smallpox, most viral hemorrhagic fevers, and the equine encephalitides, are also managed supportively.

In addition to ensuring adequate oxygenation, ventilation, and hydration, the clinician may need to provide specific empiric therapies on an urgent basis. Patients suffering from the sudden onset of severe neuromuscular symptoms may have nerve agent intoxication and should be given atropine (0.05 mg/kg) promptly for its antimuscarinic effects. Although atropine relieves bronchospasm and bradycardia, reduces bronchial secretions, and ameliorates the gastrointestinal effects of nausea, vomiting, and diarrhea, it does not improve skeletal muscle paralysis. Pralidoxime (also known as *2-PAM*) cleaves the organophosphate moiety from cholinesterase and regenerates intact enzyme if "aging" has not occurred. The effect is most prominent at the neuromuscular junction and leads to improved muscle strength. Its prompt use (at a dose of 25 mg/kg) as an adjunct to atropine is recommended in all serious cases.

Ideally, both atropine and pralidoxime should be administered intravenously in severe cases, although the intraosseous route may be acceptable. Some experts recommend that atropine be given intramuscularly in the presence of hypoxia to avoid arrhythmias associated with

| Table 723-3 | Critical Chemical Agents of Terrorism |

AGENT	TOXICITY	CLINICAL FINDINGS	ONSET	DECONTAMINATION*	MANAGEMENT
NERVE AGENTS					
Tabun, sarin, soman, VX	Anticholinesterase: muscarinic, nicotinic, central nervous system effects	Vapor: miosis, rhinorrhea, dyspnea Liquid: diaphoresis, vomiting Both: coma, paralysis, seizures, apnea	Seconds: vapor Minutes to hours: liquid	Vapor: fresh air, remove clothes, wash hair Liquid: remove clothes, wash skin, hair with copious soap and water, ocular irrigation	ABCs. Atropine: 0.05 mg/kg IV†, IM‡ (min: 0.1 mg, max: 5 mg), repeat q2-5 min prn for marked secretions, bronchospasm Pralidoxime: 25 mg/kg IV, IM§ (max: 1 g IV; 2 g IM), may repeat within 30-60 min prn, then again q1h for 1 or 2 doses prn for persistent weakness, high atropine requirement Diazepam: 0.3 mg/kg (max: 10 mg) IV; lorazepam: 0.1 mg/kg IV, IM (max: 4 mg); midazolam: 0.2 mg/kg (max: 10 mg) IM prn for seizures or severe exposure
VESICANTS					
Mustard	Alkylation	Skin: erythema, vesicles Eye: inflammation Respiratory tract: inflammation	Hours	Skin: soap and water Eyes: water (effective only if done within minutes of exposure)	Symptomatic care
Lewisite	Arsenical		Immediate pain		Possibly British antilewisite (BAL) 3 mg/kg IM q4-6h for systemic effects of lewisite in severe cases
PULMONARY AGENTS					
Chlorine, phosgene	Liberate hydrochloric acid, alkylation	Eye, nose, and throat irritation (especially chlorine) Respiratory: bronchospasm, pulmonary edema (especially phosgene)	Minutes: eye, nose, and throat irritation, bronchospasm Hours: pulmonary edema	Fresh air Skin: water	Symptomatic care (see text)
CYANIDE					
	Cytochrome oxidase Inhibition: cellular anoxia, lactic acidosis	Tachypnea, coma, seizures, apnea	Seconds	Fresh air Skin: soap and water	ABCs, 100% oxygen Na bicarbonate prn metabolic acidosis; hydroxycobalamin 70 mg/kg IV (max: 5 g) or nitrite/thiosulfate, given as follows (see text): *Na nitrite (3%): dose (mL/kg) (max: 10 mL)* / *Estimated hemoglobin concentration (g/dL)* 0.27 / 10 0.33 / 12 (estimated for average child) 0.39 / 14 followed by Na thiosulfate (25%): 1.65 mL/kg (max: 50 mL)

*Decontamination, especially for patients with significant nerve agent or vesicant exposure, should be performed by healthcare providers garbed in adequate personal protective equipment. For emergency department staff, this equipment consists of a nonencapsulated, chemically resistant body suit, boots, and gloves with a full-face air-purifier mask/hood.
†Intraosseous route is likely equivalent to intravenous.
‡Atropine might have some benefit via endotracheal tube or inhalation, as might aerosolized ipratropium. See also Table 723-4.
§Pralidoxime is reconstituted to 50 mg/mL (1 g in 20 mL water) for IV administration, and the total dose infused over 30 min, or may be given by continuous infusion (loading dose 25 mg/kg over 30 min, and then 10 mg/kg/hr). For IM use, it might be diluted to a concentration of 300 mg/mL (1 g added to 3 mL water—by analogy to the U.S. Army's Mark 1 autoinjector concentration), to effect a reasonable volume for injection. See also Table 723-4.
ABCs, airway, breathing, and circulatory support; max, maximum; min, minimum; prn, as needed.
Adapted from Henretig FH, Cieslak TJ, Eitzen EM: Biological and chemical terrorism, J Pediatr 141:311–326, 2002.

intravenous administration. Many emergency management services stock military-style autoinjector kits consisting of atropine and 2-PAM for intramuscular injection. Pediatric atropine autoinjectors are licensed, although kits intended for adults (with 2 mg of atropine and 600 mg of pralidoxime) might be used in children >2-3 yr (Table

723-4). Animal studies support the routine prophylactic administration of anticonvulsant doses of benzodiazepines, even in the absence of observable convulsive activity.

Delayed neuromuscular symptoms in the setting of terrorism might be due to botulism. Supportive care, with meticulous attention

Table 723-4	Pediatric Autoinjector Recommendations for Mass Casualties or Prehospital Care*

ATROPINE AUTOINJECTOR THERAPY

APPROXIMATE AGE	APPROXIMATE WEIGHT (kg)	AUTOINJECTOR SIZE (mg)
<6 mo	<7.5	0.25
6 mo-4 yr	7.5-18	0.5
5-10 yr	18-30	1.0
>10 yr	>30	2.0

PRALIDOXIME AUTOINJECTOR THERAPY

APPROXIMATE AGE (yr)	APPROXIMATE WEIGHT (kg)	NUMBER OF AUTOINJECTORS	PRALIDOXIME DOSE (mg/kg)
3-7	13-25	1	24-46
8-14	26-50	2	24-46
>14	>50	3	<35

*Consider adult pralidoxime autoinjector use for severely affected mass casualties when IV access or more precise mg/kg IM dosing is logistically impractical. The initial dose using atropine autoinjectors is 1 autoinjector of each recommended size. The initial dose using pralidoxime autoinjectors is the recommended number of (adult-intended, 600 mg) autoinjectors. These latter may also be injected into an empty sterile vile; the contents redrawn through a filter needle into a small syringe may then provide a ready source of concentrated (300 mg/mL) pralidoxime solution for IM injection to infants. Autoinjectors may become available that provide adult doses of both atropine and pralidoxime in one injector; these could be used in children ≥3 yr in lieu of two individual injectors and dosed as noted above for pralidoxime alone.

to ventilatory support, is the mainstay of botulism treatment. Such support may be necessary for several mo, making the management of a large-scale botulism outbreak especially problematic in terms of medical resources. A licensed heptavalent antitoxin (types A-G) is available through the Centers for Disease Control (1-800-232-4636). Administration of this antitoxin is unlikely to reverse disease in symptomatic patients but may prevent further progression. In addition, a pentavalent (containing antibody against toxin types A to E; but licensed only for treatment of type A or B intoxication) product, Botulism Immune Globulin Intravenous (Human), BabyBIG, is available through the California Department of Health Services (1-916-327-1400) specifically for the treatment of infant botulism.

The **rapid onset of respiratory symptoms** may signal an exposure to chlorine, phosgene, cyanide, or a number of other toxic industrial chemicals. Although the mainstay of therapy in virtually all of these exposures consists of removal to fresh air and intensive supportive care, cyanide intoxication often requires the administration of specific antidotes.

The classic cyanide antidote utilizes a nitrite along with sodium thiosulfate and is given in 2 stages. The methemoglobin-forming agent (e.g., sodium nitrite) is administered first, because methemoglobin has a high affinity for cyanide and causes it to dissociate from cytochrome oxidase. Nitrite dosing in children should be based on body weight to avoid excessive methemoglobin formation and nitrite-induced hypotension. For the same reasons, nitrites should be infused slowly over 5-10 min. A sulfur donor, such as sodium thiosulfate, is given next. This compound is used as a substrate by the hepatic enzyme rhodanese, which converts cyanide to thiocyanate, a less toxic compound excreted in the urine. Thiosulfate treatment itself is efficacious and relatively benign and may be used alone for mild to moderate cases. Sodium nitrite and sodium thiosulfate are packaged together in standard antidote kits, along with amyl nitrite, a sodium nitrite substitute that can be inhaled in prehospital settings in which intravenous access is not available.

Another antidote available in the United States is hydroxocobalamin, which exchanges its hydroxy group for cyanide, forming harmless cyanocobalamin (vitamin B_{12}), which is subsequently excreted by the kidneys. Hydroxycobalamin use is not complicated by the potential for nitrite-induced hypotension or methemoglobinemia, and it has low toxicity. The recommended dose is 5 g in adults or 70 mg/kg in children, administered IV over 15 min. A second dose (2.5-5 g in adults; 35-70 mg/kg in children) may be repeated in severely affected patients. Side effects include modest hypertension and reddening of skin, mucous membranes, and urine that may last several days. Although no human controlled trials are currently available to compare

hydroxocobalamin with nitrite/thiosulfate-based therapies, many authorities believe that hydroxocobalamin's efficacy and safety profile favor it as the cyanide antidote of choice, especially for children in the mass casualty context.

Animal research suggests a modest benefit of steroid therapy in mitigating lung injury after chlorine inhalation, and thus steroids may be considered for patients with chlorine exposure, especially as an adjunct to bronchodilators in those manifesting bronchospasm and/or a history of asthma. Further, symptomatic relief has also been reported following chlorine exposure with nebulized 3.75% sodium bicarbonate therapy, though the impact of this regimen on pulmonary damage is unknown. Animal models have also suggested a benefit from antiinflammatory agents, including ibuprofen and N-acetylcysteine, which appear to ameliorate phosgene-induced pulmonary edema, as well as the utilization of low tidal volume ventilation (protective ventilation), although the results of such interventions have not yet been reported in clinical trials.

In cases in which the **delayed onset of respiratory symptoms** may be the result of a terrorist attack, consideration should be given to the empirical administration of an antibiotic effective against anthrax, plague, and tularemia. Ciprofloxacin (10-15 mg/kg IV q12h), levofloxacin (8 mg/kg IV q12h), or doxycycline (2.2 mg/kg IV q12h) is a reasonable choice. Although naturally occurring strains of B. anthracis usually are quite sensitive to penicillin G, these agents are chosen because penicillin-resistant strains of B. anthracis exist. Moreover, ciprofloxacin and doxycycline are effective against almost all known strains of Y. pestis and F. tularensis. Concerns about inducible β-lactamases in B. anthracis have led some experts to recommend 1 or 2 additional antibiotics in patients with inhalational anthrax. Rifampin, vancomycin, penicillin or ampicillin, clindamycin, imipenem, and clarithromycin are reasonable choices based on in vitro sensitivity data. Because B. anthracis relies on the production of 2 protein toxins, edema toxin, and lethal toxin, for its virulence, drugs that act at the ribosome to disrupt protein synthesis (e.g., clindamycin, the macrolides) provide a theoretical advantage. Frequent meningeal involvement among inhalational anthrax victims makes agents with superior central nervous system penetration desirable. A combination of ciprofloxacin plus clindamycin plus penicillin G is a good initial empiric therapy for presumed inhalational anthrax. Ciprofloxacin, levofloxacin, or doxycycline monotherapy is probably adequate in cases of cutaneous anthrax, although patients with cutaneous disease resulting from a terrorist attack initially should receive multidrug therapy, because of the possibility of concomitant inhalational exposure.

Raxibacumab, a monoclonal antibody that inhibits anthrax antigen binding to cell receptors, thus preventing toxins from entering cells, is approved for the treatment of inhalation anthrax in combination with antibodies. The adult dose is 40 mg/kg given IV over 2 hr and 15 min. The dose for children is weight based; ≤15 kg: 80 mg/kg; >15-50 kg: 60 mg/kg; >50 kg: 40 mg/kg. Premedication with diphenhydramine IV or PO is recommended 1 hr before the infusion.

In patients in whom a diagnosis of plague or tularemia is established, streptomycin (15 mg/kg IM q12h) has historically been considered the drug of choice. Because this drug is generally unavailable, many experts consider gentamicin (2.5 mg/kg IV/IM q8h) the preferred choice for therapy. In addition to ciprofloxacin, levofloxacin, or doxycycline, chloramphenicol (25 mg/kg IV q6h) should be employed in the 6% of pneumonic plague cases with concomitant meningitis. To be effective, therapy for pneumonic plague must be initiated within 24 hr of the onset of symptoms. There is little clinical experience with ricin-induced pulmonary injury. The mainstay of therapy is expected to be supportive care.

The management of **vesicant-induced injury** is similar to that for burn victims and is largely symptomatic (see Chapter 75). Mustard victims will benefit from the application of soothing skin lotions such as calamine and the administration of analgesics. Early intubation of severely exposed patients is warranted to guard against edematous airway compromise. Oxygen and mechanical ventilation may be needed, and meticulous attention to hydration is of paramount importance. Ongoing research suggests a role for oral *N*-acetylcysteine in mitigating chronic pulmonary effects due to mustard injury. Lewisite victims can be managed in much the same manner as mustard victims. In addition, dimercaprol (British antilewisite) in oil, given intramuscularly, may help ameliorate the systemic effects of lewisite.

The management of symptomatic smallpox victims also is largely supportive, with attention to pain control, hydration status, and respiratory sufficiency again of primary importance. The parenteral antiviral compound cidofovir, licensed for the treatment of cytomegalovirus retinitis in HIV-infected patients, has in vitro efficacy against variola and other orthopoxviruses. Its utility in treating smallpox victims is untested. Moreover, in the face of a large outbreak of disease, wide parenteral use of this drug would be problematic. ST-246, mentioned previously, demonstrates excellent in vitro activity against orthopoxviruses, but its utility in treating patients with smallpox is likewise untested.

Bibliography is available at Expert Consult.

Chapter 724
Animal and Human Bites
Charles M. Ginsburg and David A. Hunstad

Many animals besides domestic and stray dogs and cats inflict bites on humans. The profile of such bites varies by country and region, based on living conditions, indigenous species, and opportunity for encounter.

EPIDEMIOLOGY
Worldwide there are tens of millions of **dog bites**, resulting in approximately 55,000 deaths from rabies (see Chapter 274). Dog bites represent approximately 80-90% of all bites in the United States; 5-15% are from cats, 2-5% from rodents, and the remainder from rabbits, ferrets, farm animals, monkeys, and reptiles. An estimated 4.5 million persons in the United States are bitten by dogs annually; approximately 885,000 of those bitten seek medical care. Bites from dogs are also most common in Bangladesh, India, Pakistan, and Myanmar, whereas in Nepal, cattle and buffalo account for more than half of bites, followed

by dogs, pigs, and horses. Approximately 1% of dog bite wounds and 6% of cat bite wounds in the United States require hospitalization. During the past 3 decades, there have been approximately 20 deaths per year in the United States from dog-inflicted injuries; 65% of these occurred in children < age 11 yr. The breed of dog involved in attacks on children varies; Table 724-1 depicts the risk index of fatal dog bites by breed. Compared with other breeds, bites by pit bulls account for higher rates of hospital admission, higher Glasgow scores at admission, and an increased risk of death. Unaltered male dogs account for approximately 75% of attacks; nursing dams often inflict injury to humans when children attempt to handle their puppies.

The majority of dog attacks on children in the United States occur between the ages of 6 and 11 yr, with a slight predominance of males. Approximately 65% of the attacks occur around the home, 75% of the biting animals are known by the children, and almost 50% of the attacks are said to be unprovoked. Similar statistics apply in Canada, where 70% of all bites reported in 1 study were sustained by children between ages 2 and 14 yr; 65% of the dogs involved in the biting were part of the family or extended family, and the bite occurred in someone's home.

Of the approximately 450,000 reported **cat bites** per year occurring in the United States, nearly all are inflicted by known household animals. Because rodent bites (rat, mouse, gerbil) do not represent reportable conditions, little is known about the epidemiology of these injuries or the incidence of infection after rodent-inflicted bites or scratches.

Few data exist on the incidence and demographics of **human bite** injuries in pediatric patients; however, preschool and early school-age children appear to be at greatest risk of sustaining an injury from human bites, often in daycare or preschool settings. In some series, the proportion of human bites is highest among adolescents, an age group in which fist-to-tooth injuries (so-called fight bites) become more common.

CLINICAL MANIFESTATIONS
Dog bite–related injuries can be divided into 3 categories of almost equal incidence: abrasions, puncture wounds, and lacerations with or without an associated avulsion of tissue. Dog bites may also involve crush injury to tissues. In contrast, the most common type of injury from cat and rat bites is a puncture wound. Cat bites often penetrate to deep tissue. Human bite injuries are of 2 types: an occlusion injury that is incurred when the upper and lower teeth come together on a body part, or a clenched-fist injury that occurs when the injured fist, usually on the dominant hand, strikes the teeth of another individual.

DIAGNOSIS
Management of the bite victim should begin with a thorough history and physical examination. Careful attention should be paid to the circumstances surrounding the bite event (e.g., species and number of animals, type of animal [domestic or wild], whether the attack was provoked or unprovoked, location of the attack); a history of drug allergies; and the immunization status of the child (tetanus) and animal (rabies). During physical examination, meticulous attention should be paid to the type, size, and depth of the injury; the presence of any foreign material in the wound; the status of underlying structures; and, when the bite is on an extremity, the exact location of the injury, an assessment of possibly involved structures, and the range of motion of the affected area. A diagram of the injury should be recorded in the patient's medical record. Radiographs of the affected part should be considered if there is likelihood that a bone or joint was penetrated or fractured, or if foreign material is present. The possibility of a fracture or penetrating injury of the skull should particularly be considered in infants who have sustained dog bite injuries to the face or head.

COMPLICATIONS
Infection is the most common complication of bite injuries, regardless of the species of biting animal. The decision to obtain material for culture from a wound depends on the species of the biting animal, the

Table 724-1	Breed of Dog Associated with Involvement in Fatal Attacks, 2007 National Registration Data from the American Kennel Club, and Relative Risk of Fatal Attack		
BREED*	**NUMBER OF DOGS INVOLVED IN FATAL ATTACKS**	**NUMBER OF DOGS REGISTERED AKC**	**RELATIVE RISK OF FATAL ATTACK PER DOG‡**
Pit Bull†	113	2239	2520†
Neapolitan Mastiff	2	357	280
Chow Chow	2	1567	65
Rottweiler	18	14,211	65
Great Pyrenees	2	1916	50
Parson Russell Terrier	1	1096	45
Old English Sheepdog	1	1206	40
Siberian Husky	6	9048	35
Bullmastiff	1	3735	15
Doberman Pinscher	2	11,381	10
Australian Shepherd or Mix	1	6471	10
Mastiff Mix	1	7160	5
German Shepherd Dog	4	43,376	5
Boxer	1	33,548	1.5
Golden Retriever or Mix	1	39,659	1.5
Labrador Retriever or Mix	2	114,110	1
Total	158		

*Data presented only for dog breeds for which registration information is available from the American Kennel Club (AKC). The AKC does not register the Perro de Presa Canario, Wolf Hybrids, or dogs of unknown mixed breed.
†The term pit bull refers to dogs from the following breeds: American Pit Bull Terrier, American Staffordshire Terrier, and Staffordshire Bull Terrier.
‡Data for Labrador Retrievers and Labrador Mix are combined. Relative Risk is normalized to Labrador Retriever and Labrador Mix.
AKC, American Kennel Club.
From Bini JK, Cohn SM, Acosta SM, McFarland MJ, Muir MT, Michalek JE; TRISAT Clinical Trials Group. Mortality, mauling, and maiming by vicious dogs. Ann Surg 253(4):791–797, 2011, Table 2.

length of time that has elapsed since the injury, the depth of the wound, the presence of foreign material contaminating the wound, and whether there is clinical evidence of infection. Although potentially pathogenic bacteria have been isolated from up to 80% of dog bite wounds that are brought to medical attention within 8 hr after the bite, the infection rate for wounds receiving medical attention in <8 hr is relatively low (2.5-20%). If the dog bite(s) is(are) not deep and/or extensive, wounds that are <8 hr old do not require cultures unless there are early signs of infection or the patient is immunocompromised. *Capnocytophaga canimorsus* is isolated from approximately 5% of infected wounds in immunocompromised patients and can cause serious systemic infection in these individuals. The infection rate in **cat bite** wounds, even those that receive prompt medical attention, is >50%; therefore, it is prudent to obtain material for culture from all but the most trivial cat-bite wounds. Cultures should be taken from **all** other animal bite wounds that are not brought to medical attention within 8 hr, regardless of species.

The rate of infection after **rodent bite** injuries is not known. Most of the oral flora of rats is similar to that of other mammals; however, approximately 50% and 25% of rats harbor strains of *Streptobacillus moniliformis* and *Spirillum minus,* respectively, both of which cause **rat bite fever** (see Chapter 724.1).

All human bite wounds, regardless of the mechanism of injury, should be regarded as carrying a high risk for infection and should be cultured. Because of the high incidence of anaerobic infection after bite wounds, it is important to obtain material for anaerobic as well as aerobic cultures.

Table 724-2 lists common causes of soft tissue bacterial infections after dog, cat, or human bites. Bites of humans or cats, those in which treatment is delayed, those in immunocompromised patients, and those associated with deep puncture wounds or significant crush injury carry higher risk for infection. An elevated risk for infection is also present if the bite is to certain anatomic regions (e.g., hand, foot, or genitals) or there is penetration of bone or tendons.

TREATMENT

Table 724-3 describes the prophylactic management of human or animal bite wounds to prevent infection.

After appropriate material has been obtained for culture, the wound should be anesthetized, cleaned, and vigorously irrigated with copious amounts of sterile saline. Irrigation with antibiotic-containing solutions provides no advantage over irrigation with saline alone and may cause local irritation of the tissues. Puncture wounds should be thoroughly cleansed and gently irrigated with a catheter or blunt-tipped needle; high-pressure irrigation should not be employed. Avulsed or devitalized tissue should be debrided and any fluctuant areas incised and drained.

Insufficient data exist to settle questions of whether bite wounds should undergo primary closure, delayed primary closure (3-5 days), or healing by secondary intention. Factors to be considered are the type, size, and depth of the wound; the anatomic location; the presence of infection; the time since the injury; and the potential for cosmetic disfigurement. Appropriate surgical consultation (e.g., general pediatric surgery; plastic, hand, or orthopedic surgery) should be obtained for all patients with deep or extensive wounds; wounds involving the hands, face, or bones and joints; and infected wounds that require open drainage. Although there is general agreement that **visibly infected wounds and those that are more than 24 hr old should not be sutured**, there is variation in practice regarding the efficacy and safety of closing wounds <8 hr old with no evidence of infection. Because all **hand wounds** are at high risk for infection, particularly if there has been disruption of the tendons or penetration of the bones, surgical

Table 724-2	Microorganisms Associated with Bites

DOG BITES
Staphylococcus species
Streptococcus species
Eikenella species
Pasteurella species
Proteus species
Klebsiella species
Haemophilus species
Enterobacter species
Capnocytophaga canimorsus
Bacteroides species
Moraxella species
Corynebacterium species
Neisseria species
Fusobacterium species
Prevotella species
Porphyromonas species

CAT BITES
Pasteurella species
Actinomyces species
Propionibacterium species
Bacteroides species
Fusobacterium species
Clostridium species
Wolinella species
Peptostreptococcus species
Staphylococcus species
Streptococcus species

HERBIVORE BITES
Actinobacillus lignieresii
Actinobacillus suis
Pasteurella multocida
Pasteurella caballi
Staphylococcus hyicus subsp. hyicus

SWINE BITES
Pasteurella aerogenes
Pasteurella multocida
Bacteroides species
Proteus species
Actinobacillus suis
Streptococcus species
Flavobacterium species
Mycoplasma species

RODENT BITES—RAT BITE FEVER
Streptobacillus moniliformis
Spirillum minus

PRIMATE BITES
Bacteroides species
Fusobacterium species
Eikenella corrodens
Streptococcus species
Enterococcus species
Staphylococcus species
Enterobacteriaceae
Simian herpesvirus

LARGE REPTILE (CROCODILE, ALLIGATOR) BITES
Aeromonas hydrophila
Pseudomonas pseudomallei
Pseudomonas aeruginosa
Proteus species
Enterococcus species
Clostridium species

Adapted from Perkins Garth A, Harris NS: Animal bites. Available at: http://emedicine.medscape.com/article/768875-overview. Reprinted with permission from eMedicine.com, 2009.

consultation is almost always indicated, and delayed primary closure is recommended for many bite wounds of the hands. **Facial lacerations** are at smaller risk for secondary infection because of the more luxuriant blood supply to this region. Given this fact and cosmetic considerations, many plastic surgeons advocate primary closure of facial bite wounds that have been brought to medical attention within 6 hr and after thorough irrigation and debridement.

Similarly, there are few studies addressing the efficacy and selection of antimicrobial agents for **prophylaxis** of bite injuries. The bacteriology of bite wound infections is primarily a reflection of the oral flora of the biting animal more than the skin flora of the victim (see Table 724-2). Because many of the aerobic and anaerobic bacterial species colonizing the oral cavity of the biting animal have the potential to invade local tissue, multiply, and cause tissue destruction, most bite wound infections are polymicrobial.

Despite the large degree of homology in the bacterial flora of the oral cavity among humans, dogs, and cats, important differences exist between the biting species, and they are reflected in the type of wound infections that occur. The predominant bacterial species isolated from infected dog bite wounds are *Staphylococcus aureus* (20-30%), *Pasteurella multocida* (20-30%), *Staphylococcus intermedius* (25%), and *C. canimorsus*; approximately one half of dog bite wound infections also contain mixed anaerobes. Similar species are isolated from infected cat bite wounds; however, *P. multocida* is the predominant species in at least 50% of cat bite wound infections. At least 50% of rats harbor strains of *S. moniliformis* in the oropharynx, and approximately 25% harbor *Spirillum minor*, an aerobic Gram-negative organism. In human bite wounds, nontypable strains of *Haemophilus influenzae*, *Eikenella corrodens*, *S. aureus*, α-hemolytic streptococci, and β-lactamase–

Table 724-3	Prophylactic Management of Human or Animal Bite Wounds to Prevent Infection

CATEGORY OF MANAGEMENT	MANAGEMENT
Cleansing	Remove visible dirt. Cleanse the wound surface with soap and water, saline, 1% povidone–iodine, or 1% benzalkonium chloride. Irrigate with a copious volume of sterile saline solution by high-pressure syringe irrigation.* Do not irrigate puncture wounds; Standard Precautions should be used.
Wound culture	No, for fresh wounds, unless signs of infection exist. Yes for wounds that appear infected.†
Diagnostic Imaging	Indicated for penetrating injuries overlying bones or joints, for suspected fracture, or to assess foreign body inoculation.
Debridement	Remove superficial devitalized tissue.
Operative debridement and exploration	Yes if any of the following: • Extensive wounds (devitalized tissue) • Involvement of the metacarpophalangeal joint (clenched-fist injury) • Cranial bites by large animal
Wound closure	Yes for selected fresh, nonpuncture bite wounds.
Assess tetanus immunization status	Yes.
Assess risk of rabies from animal bites	Yes.
Assess risk of hepatitis B virus infection from human bites	Yes.
Assess risk of human immunodeficiency virus from human bites	Yes.
Initiate antimicrobial therapy	Yes for: • Moderate or severe bite wounds, especially if edema or crush injury is present • Puncture wounds, especially if penetration of bone, tendon sheath, or joint has occurred • Face, hand, foot, and genital bites • Wounds in immunocompromised and asplenic persons • Wounds with signs of infection
Follow-up	Inspect wound for signs of infection within 48 hr

*Use of an 18-gauge needle with a large-volume syringe is effective. Antimicrobial or antiinfective solutions offer no advantage and may increase tissue irritation.
†Both aerobic and anaerobic bacterial culture should be performed.
From American Academy of Pediatrics: Red Book: 2012 report of the Committee on Infectious Diseases, ed 29, Elk Grove Village, IL, 2012, American Academy of Pediatrics, Table 2-18.

producing aerobes (~50%) are the predominant species. Clenched-fist injuries are particularly prone to infection by *Eikenella* spp. (25%) and anaerobic bacteria (50%).

The choice between oral and parenteral antimicrobial agents should be based on the severity of the wound, the presence and degree of overt infection, signs of systemic toxicity, and the patient's immune status. Amoxicillin–clavulanate is an excellent choice for empirical oral therapy for human and animal bite wounds, because of its activity against most bacteria that have been isolated from infected bites. Similarly, ticarcillin–clavulanate or ampicillin–sulbactam is preferred for patients who require empirical parenteral therapy. Penicillin G remains the drug of choice for prophylaxis and treatment of rat-inflicted injuries, as this agent has excellent activity against *S. moniliformis* and *S. minor*. Because 1st-generation cephalosporins have limited activity against *P. multocida* and *E. corrodens*, they should not be used for prophylaxis or empirical initial therapy of bite wound infections. Therapeutic alternatives for penicillin-allergic patients are limited, because the traditional alternative agents are generally inactive against 1 or more of the multiple pathogens that cause bite wound infections. Clindamycin plus trimethoprim–sulfamethoxazole is the most commonly suggested regimen for these patients. Tetracycline is the drug of choice for penicillin-allergic patients who have sustained rat bite injuries.

Although **tetanus** occurs only rarely after human or animal bite injuries, it is important to obtain a careful immunization history and to provide tetanus toxoid to all patients who are incompletely immunized or in whom it has been longer than 5 yr since the last tetanus immunization. The need for postexposure **rabies** vaccination in victims of dog and cat bites depends on whether the biting animal is known to have been vaccinated and, most importantly, on local experience with rabid animals in the community. Bites from bats, foxes, skunks, and raccoons should be considered to carry a high risk of rabies, and postexposure prophylaxis is indicated. For dogs, cats, and other animals that are known or can be captured, observation for 7-10 days by the local animal control department is indicated. If a biting dog or cat has escaped, a decision about rabies prophylaxis can be based on the circumstances surrounding the bite and advice from local infectious diseases specialists and/or health department officials. Annually

Table 724-4	Measures for Preventing Dog Bites

- Realistically evaluate environment and lifestyle and consult with a professional (e.g., veterinarian, animal behaviorist, or responsible breeder) to determine suitable breeds of dogs for consideration.
- Dogs with histories of aggression are inappropriate in households with children.
- Be sensitive to cues that a child is fearful or apprehensive about a dog and, if so, delay acquiring a dog.
- Spend time with a dog before buying or adopting it. Use caution when bringing a dog or puppy into the home of an infant or toddler.
- Spay/neuter virtually all dogs (this frequently reduces aggressive tendencies).
- Never leave infants or young children alone with any dog.
- Properly socialize and train any dog entering the household. Teach the dog submissive behaviors (e.g., rolling over to expose abdomen and relinquishing food without growling).
- Immediately seek professional advice (e.g., from veterinarians, animal behaviorists, or responsible breeders) if the dog develops aggressive or undesirable behaviors.
- Do not play aggressive games with your dog (e.g., wrestling).
- Teach children basic safety around dogs and review regularly:
  - Never approach an unfamiliar dog.
  - Never run from a dog and scream.
  - Remain motionless when approached by an unfamiliar dog (e.g., "be still like a tree").
  - If knocked over by a dog, roll into a ball and lie still (e.g., "be still like a log").
  - Never play with a dog unless supervised by an adult.
  - Immediately report stray dogs or dogs displaying unusual behavior to an adult.
  - Avoid direct eye contact with a dog.
  - Do not disturb a dog who is sleeping, eating, or caring for puppies.
  - Do not pet a dog without allowing it to see and sniff you first.
  - If bitten, immediately report the bite to an adult.

From Centers for Disease Control and Prevention: Dog bite-related fatalities—United States, 1995-1996, MMWR Morb Mortal Wkly Rep 46:463–467, 1997.

worldwide, animal bites and contacts result in more than 10 million postexposure courses. Postexposure prophylaxis for hepatitis B should be considered in the rare instance in which a susceptible individual has sustained a human bite from an individual who is at high risk for hepatitis B.

PREVENTION
It is possible to reduce the risk of animal bite injury with anticipatory guidance (Table 724-4). Parents should be routinely counseled during prenatal visits and routine health maintenance examinations about the risks of having potentially biting pets in the household. All patients should be cautioned against harboring exotic animals for pets. Additionally, parents should be made aware of the proclivity of certain breeds of dogs to inflict serious injuries and the protective instincts of nursing dams. All young children should be closely supervised, particularly when in the presence of animals, and from a very early age should be taught to respect animals and to be aware of their potential to inflict injury. Reduction of the rate of human bite injuries, particularly in daycare centers and schools, can be achieved by good surveillance of the children and adequate teacher : child ratios.

Bibliography is available at Expert Consult.

724.1 Rat Bite Fever
Charles M. Ginsburg and David A. Hunstad

ETIOLOGY
Rat bite fever is a generic term that has been applied to at least 2 distinct clinical syndromes, each caused by a different microbial agent. Rat bite fever caused by *S. moniliformis* is most commonly reported in the United States, as well as in Brazil, Canada, Mexico, Paraguay, Great Britain, and France; it has been identified elsewhere in Europe and in Australia. *S. moniliformis* is a Gram-negative bacillus that is present in the nasopharyngeal flora of many laboratory and wild rats. Infection with *S. moniliformis* most commonly occurs following the bite of a rat; however, infection has also been reported in individuals who have been scratched by rats, in those who have handled dead rats, and in those who have ingested milk contaminated with the bacterium (termed **Haverhill fever**). Rat bite fever may also be transmitted by bites from wild mice. Rat bite fever caused by *S. minus*, called **sodoku**, is most commonly reported in Asia. *S. minus* is a small, spiral, aerobic Gram-negative organism. Reports of rat bite fever from Africa are rare, suggesting underrecognition rather than absence of the disease.

CLINICAL COURSE
The incubation period for the streptobacillary form of rat bite fever is variable, ranging from 3-10 days. The illness is characterized by an abrupt onset of fever up to 41°C (105.8°F) (fever occurring in more than 90% of reported cases), severe throbbing headache, intense myalgia, chills, and vomiting. In virtually all instances, the lesion at the cutaneous inoculation site has healed by the time the systemic systems first appear. Shortly after the onset of the fever, a polymorphous rash occurs in up to 75% of patients. In most patients, the rash consists of blotchy, red maculopapular lesions that often have a petechial component; the distribution of the rash is variable but is typically most dense on the extremities. Hemorrhagic vesicles may develop on the hands and feet and are very tender to palpation (Fig. 724-1).

Approximately 50% of patients have arthritis, which first manifests toward the end of the 1st wk of disease; early on, the arthritis may be migratory. If untreated, fever, rash, and arthritis last from 14-21 days, often with a biphasic pattern to the fever and arthritis. A wide range of complications are reported in patients with rat bite fever, the most common being pneumonia, persistent arthritis, brain and soft tissue abscesses, and, less commonly, myocarditis or endocarditis. The mortality rate of untreated rat bite fever is estimated to be approximately 13%.

The incubation period of sodoku is longer (14-21 days) than that of the streptobacillary form of disease. The hallmark of *Spirillum*-induced

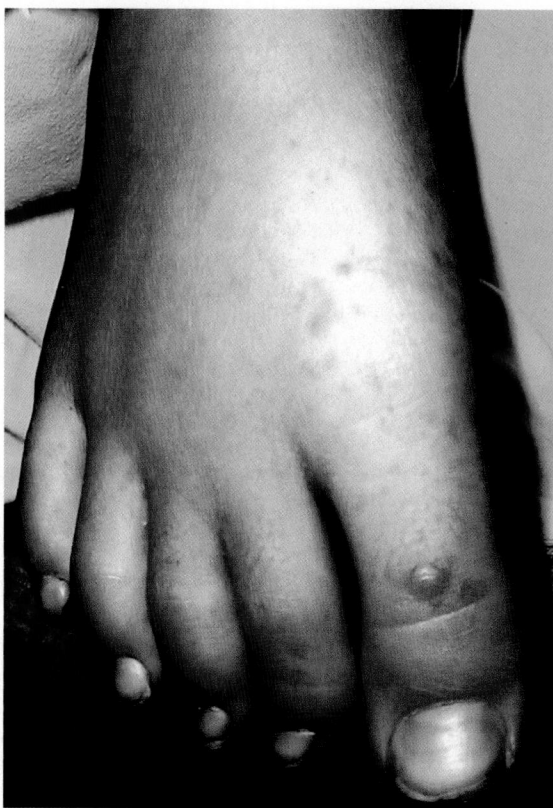

Figure 724-1 Hemorrhagic vesicles on the 1st and 3rd toes of a patient with advanced rat bite fever. *(From Elliott SP: Rat bite fever and Streptobacillus moniliformis. Clin Microbiol Rev 20:13–22, 2007, Fig. 3.)*

disease is fever associated with an indurated, often suppurative, non-healing lesion at the bite site. Lymphadenitis and lymphadenopathy invariably are present in the regional nodes that drain the inoculation site, and many patients have a generalized macular rash most prominent when fever is present. In untreated patients, sodoku has a relapsing and remitting course; symptoms abate after 5-7 days of chills and fever but recur 7-10 days later. There may be multiple cycles if the disease is not recognized and treated.

DIAGNOSIS
Diagnosis of the streptobacillary form of rat bite fever is difficult, because the disease is uncommon and can be confused with Rocky Mountain spotted fever or (less commonly) meningococcemia. Furthermore, *S. moniliformis* is difficult both to isolate and to identify with classic bacteriologic techniques. The organism is fastidious, requires enriched media for growth, and is inhibited by sodium polyanethol sulfonate, an additive present in many commercial blood culture bottles. A definitive diagnosis is made when the organism is recovered from blood or joint fluid or is identified in human samples with molecular technology such as polymerase chain reaction analysis, which has been used successfully in humans and laboratory animals.

Diagnosis of sodoku is made on clinical grounds, because there are no diagnostic serologic tests and *S. minus* has not been cultured on artificial media. Rarely, the organism may be identified in Gram-stained smears of pus from the inoculation site.

TREATMENT
Penicillin is the drug of choice for both forms of rat bite fever. Intravenous penicillin G or intramuscular penicillin G procaine is recommended for 7-10 days; a regimen of IV penicillin G for 5-7 days followed by oral penicillin V for an additional 7 days has also been used. Doxycycline, gentamicin, or streptomycin represent effective alternatives for penicillin-allergic patients. Patients with endocarditis

caused by *S. moniliformis* require high-dose penicillin G for 4 wk; the addition of streptomycin or gentamicin might be helpful.

Bibliography is available at Expert Consult.

724.2 Monkeypox
Charles M. Ginsburg and David A. Hunstad

ETIOLOGY
Monkeypox virus, causing the disease monkeypox, is the most important member for humans of the genus *Orthopoxvirus* since the eradication of smallpox (variola). Monkeys are the predominant host for the virus; however, it may be endemic in African rainforest squirrels and is present in African rats, mice, domestic pigs, hedgehogs, and opossums. It also has been identified in and transmitted by prairie dogs in the United States, and has affected elephants in zoos. Severity of infection varies by viral strain and by host; for example, disease is relatively mild in cynomolgus monkeys but severe in orangutans.

Monkeypox virus was first observed in humans from West and Central Africa in the 1970s at the time that smallpox had been eradicated from the area. In the 1970s, the secondary attack rate was around 3% (a stark comparison to the 80% seen in unvaccinated smallpox contacts). Few cases were observed over the next 2 decades; however, during a subsequent outbreak in the 1990s when immunity to smallpox was no longer prevalent in the population, the secondary attack rate exceeded 75%. Monkeypox outbreaks have also been reported in the Sudan. Monkeypox was inadvertently introduced into the United States in 2003, presumably through rodents from Ghana that infected prairie dogs who were distributed as pets; this outbreak affected more than 70 persons. Primary transmission of the disease from infected animal to human is by bite or by human contact with an infected animal's blood, wound discharge, or other body fluids. Human-to-human transmission of infection is uncommon but is believed to have been an important source for transmission of new cases during the United States outbreak.

CLINICAL COURSE
The clinical signs, symptoms, and course of monkeypox are similar to those of smallpox, although typically milder. After a 10-14 day incubation period during which the virus replicates in lymphoid tissues, humans experience an abrupt onset of malaise, fever, myalgia, headache, and severe backache. Nonproductive cough, nausea, vomiting, and abdominal pain may be present. Generalized lymphadenopathy, a finding unusual in smallpox, is invariably present during the acute stages of monkeypox illness. After a 2-4 day prodrome, an exanthem appears in cephalad-to-caudal progression. As the rash progresses, fevers begin to abate. The rash is initially macular, but transforms within hours to firm papules that rapidly vesiculate and become pustular over 2-3 days. Unlike smallpox lesions, but similar to chickenpox lesions, the lesions of monkeypox tend to occur in crops (Fig. 724-2). Late into the 2nd wk of illness, the lesions begin to desiccate, crust, scab, and fall off.

Monkeypox should be suspected in any child who has the characteristic prodrome associated with an atypical form of chickenpox and a history of contact with prairie dogs or exotic mammals such as Gambian rats and rope squirrels. Diagnosis is by isolation of monkeypox virus in culture, demonstration by polymerase chain reaction of viral DNA in a clinical specimen, or microscopic demonstration of an orthopoxvirus in a clinical specimen in the absence of other orthopoxvirus exposure.

TREATMENT
There is no proven effective therapy for monkeypox. Despite evidence that preexposure administration of smallpox vaccine is 85% effective in preventing or attenuating monkeypox disease, the rarity of monkeypox infection does not warrant universal vaccination. In instances of known exposure or in outbreak situations, there may be an indication

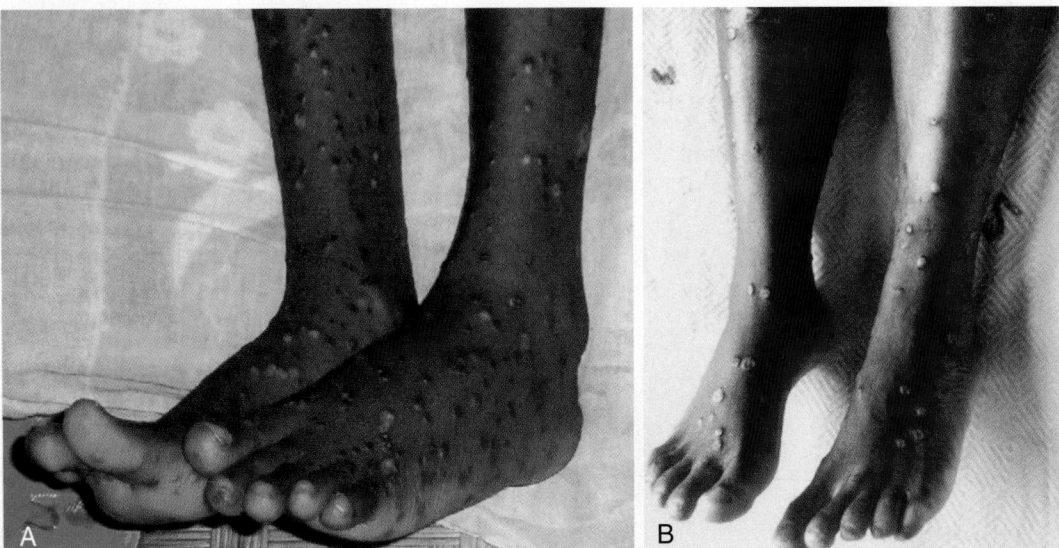

Figure 724-2 A, Legs and feet of monkeypox patient. **B,** Legs and feet of smallpox patient at similar stage of rash (pustular). (**A** *courtesy of Joseph M. Harvey, MD; **B** courtesy of J. Nobel, Jr, MD, Centers for Disease Control and Prevention.*)

for administering smallpox vaccine. Consideration should be given to vaccinating close family contacts and health care workers who provide care to infected individuals. Vaccine is said to be preventive if given within 2 wk of exposure. Individuals with a compromised immune system and those with life-threatening allergies to latex or to smallpox vaccine or any of its components (polymyxin B, streptomycin, tetracycline, neomycin) also should not receive smallpox vaccine.

Although there are data indicating that cidofovir has in vitro activity against monkeypox virus and has been effective in preventing monkeypox infection in animals, there are no data to support its effectiveness in humans. Careful attention should be paid to skin hygiene, maintenance of adequate nutrition and hydration, and prompt implementation of local or systemic therapy of secondary bacterial infection that may occur. For prevention of human-to-human spread of disease, a combination of contact, droplet, and airborne infection control procedures should be implemented.

Bibliography is available at Expert Consult.

Chapter **725**

Envenomations

Bill J. Schroeder and Robert L. Norris

Being bitten or stung by a venomous animal or insect is frightening for an adult, a child, or a child's parent or care provider. Although most bites and stings by spiders, snakes, scorpions, and other venomous animals cause little more than local pain and do not require medical attention, there are thousands of species of potentially harmful or deadly venomous creatures worldwide. Each country/region has its own array of medically important organisms.

The terms *venomous* and *poisonous* are not synonymous. *Venom* is produced in specialized glands of the host and is usually injected by means of a bite or sting. *Poisonous* refers to detrimental effects from consuming or touching a plant, animal, or insect. Poison is generally found throughout the animal and venom is isolated to the specialized glands.

Not every bite from a venomous creature is harmful. In many cases no venom is injected, so-called dry bites. A dry bite may occur for many reasons, including failure of the venom delivery mechanism and depletion of venom. Up to 20% of pit viper, 80% of coral snake, and approximately 50% of all venomous snake bites are dry.

In the 2011 report of the American Association of Poison Control Centers, more than 60,000 consultations were related to bites and stings of various creatures, with approximately one third involving victims < age 19 yr. There were 2 deaths, both from snake bites in adult males, 1 from the genera *Crotalus* (rattlesnake) and 1 from the genera *Agkistrodon* (copperhead or cottonmouth).

GENERAL APPROACH TO THE ENVENOMATED CHILD

Children may be bitten or stung as they play and explore their environment. The evaluation may be hampered by an unclear history of the circumstances and the possible offending organism, particularly with preverbal children. The overall effects of some venomous bites and stings may be relatively more severe in children than in adults, because children generally receive a similar venom load from the offending animal yet have less circulating blood volume to dilute its effects.

General Management

When faced with an envenomated child, the treating physician should anticipate a dynamic clinical syndrome that may progress with time, with important, potentially subtle, findings. Treatment of an envenomated child should start with assessing and managing as necessary the airway, breathing, and circulation (ABCs). Most envenomations require little more than local wound care, pain control, reassurance, and possibly observation. The severely envenomated child may need airway and respiratory protection and support (e.g., high-concentration oxygen administration and endotracheal intubation) and adequate IV access in an unaffected extremity if possible (see Chapters 70 and 71). Early hypotension tends to be related to vasodilation and should be treated with volume expansion using appropriate infusion of physiologic saline solutions (normal saline boluses of 20 mL/kg body weight; repeated as needed up to 3 times). Shock unresponsive to volume repletion may require addition of a vasoactive pharmacologic agent such as epinephrine or dopamine (in addition to antivenom administration as appropriate). If the presentation is suspicious for an anaphylactic reaction to venom, appropriate treatment (including epinephrine) should be initiated as soon as possible (see Chapter 149). Occasionally, it is difficult to determine the precise etiology for sudden collapse after a venomous bite or sting–venom toxicity vs anaphylaxis. In such cases, treatment for both should be started.

The affected body part should be immobilized in a position of function and any areas of edema should be marked, measured, and monitored. If antivenom (AV) is available for the envenomation, efforts should be initiated to locate and secure an adequate amount to treat the patient (at least a starting dose). In the United States, regional poison control centers can facilitate this effort and are especially helpful if the offending species is exotic. Guidance in dosing the appropriate AV can generally be found in the package insert that accompanies the agent, although the advice in inserts for some products from developing countries may contain inaccurate and incorrect recommendations. Physicians who do not regularly treat venomous bites and stings should consult local or regional experts for assistance.

Antivenom Administration

Specific AVs are available for many venomous creatures of the world, particularly snakes, spiders, and scorpions. These products essentially impart passive immunity to the victim and should be given in cases of significant envenomation as early in the process as possible, because AV is capable of neutralizing only circulating, unbound venom components in the blood.

AVs may be either in liquid form or lyophilized (requiring reconstitution prior to administration). Most AVs are given intravenously. *There is no benefit to giving any AV locally at the bite site.* As soon as the need for AV is established, it should be placed into solution (generally diluted in a quantity of normal saline equivalent to 20 mL/kg body weight, up to 250-1,000 mL total).

As heterologous serum products, AVs carry some variable risk of inducing nonallergic or allergic anaphylactic reactions. Therefore, the patient should be closely monitored, and a physician should be present during the infusion, with access to all the appropriate equipment and medications needed to reverse such a reaction. Skin tests, often recommended by AV manufacturers, are unreliable and should be omitted.

Intravenous AV should be started slowly, and the rate gradually increased as tolerated by the patient, with a goal to administer the entire dose in approximately 1 hr.

If the victim experiences a reaction to the product, it should be temporarily stopped. Intramuscular epinephrine and intravenous antihistamines and steroids should be given. Then the AV should be restarted, possibly at a slower rate and in a more dilute solution. If the reaction is severe, the decision must be made as to whether the benefits of AV outweigh the risks of anaphylaxis on the basis of the patient's clinical condition. If AV is deemed critical for the patient's survival despite the occurrence of anaphylaxis, the patient should be placed in an intensive care setting with close, possibly invasive, monitoring, and should receive simultaneous administration of AV and an epinephrine infusion.

AV can also cause delayed immunoglobulin G and M–mediated serum sickness in some patients (see Chapter 150). Serum sickness occurs 1-2 wk after AV administration, manifesting as fever, myalgias, arthralgias, urticaria, and potential renal and neurologic involvement. It is easily treated with oral steroids, antihistamines, and acetaminophen.

General Wound Care

Bites and stings require basic wound care, including copious tap water or normal saline irrigation under pressure when possible. For small puncture wounds this is impractical, but the skin should still be cleaned with soap and water. Tetanus immunization should be updated as needed. Intact blisters should be left to act as natural bandages and help prevent infection, whereas broken blisters should be debrided. Exposed tissue should be covered with wet to dry dressings. Necrotic wounds, such as those that might follow some snake and spider bites, should be judiciously debrided, with removal of only clearly necrotic tissue. Reconstructive surgery with skin grafts or muscle/tendon grafts may be necessary. Prophylactic antibiotics are not necessary except, perhaps, in cases in which an ill-informed "rescuer" cut into the bite and applied mouth suction. Antibiotics should generally be reserved for signs of established secondary infection.

SNAKE BITES

Most snake bites are inflicted by nonvenomous species and are of no more consequence than a potentially contaminated puncture wound (Fig. 725-1). Venomous snakes, however, kill many tens of thousands of people in the world each year. The precise number is difficult to ascertain, because the toll in human suffering is far greatest in developing nations. Developed nations, with established medical care systems, have relatively few fatalities each year.

Most of the world's medically significant venomous snakes belong to 1 of 2 families—Viperidae and Elapidae (Table 725-1). In developing nations, most snake envenomations occur in agricultural workers who inadvertently contact snakes while in the fields. Many victims of snake envenomation in developed nations are adolescent or young adult males, frequently intoxicated, who are attempting to handle or catch the snake. Bites are located on an extremity in more than 95% of cases. In the United States, approximately 98% of venomous snake bites are inflicted by pit vipers (family Viperidae; subfamily *Crotalinae*). A small fraction of bites are caused by coral snakes (family Elapidae) in the South and Southwest, and by exotic snakes that have been imported.

Venoms and Effects

Snake venoms are complex mixtures of proteins including large enzymes that cause local tissue destruction and low-molecular-weight polypeptides that have the more lethal systemic effects. The symptoms and severity of an envenomation vary according to the type of snake, the amount of venom injected, and the location of the bite. The fear caused by a snake bite can result in nausea, vomiting, diarrhea, cold/clammy skin, and even syncope regardless of whether or not venom was injected. In general, viper venoms can have deleterious effects on almost any organ system. Most viper bites cause significant local pain, swelling, and ecchymosis and may result in variable necrosis of the bitten extremity (Fig. 725-2). The pain and swelling typically begin quickly after the bite and progress over hours to days. Serious envenomations may result in a consumptive coagulopathy, hypotension, and respiratory distress. In contrast, venoms from the **Elapidae** tend to be more neurotoxic with little or no local tissue damage. These bites cause variable local pain and the onset of systemic effects can be delayed for hours. Manifestations of neurotoxicity generally are caused by curare-like blockade at the neuromuscular junction. Symptoms usually begin with cranial nerve palsies such as ptosis, dysarthria, and dysphagia and may progress to respiratory failure and complete paralysis. There are exceptions; some members of the Elapidae family cause little or no neurotoxicity but rather severe tissue necrosis (e.g., African spitting cobras). Some vipers, including the southern Pacific rattlesnake (*Crotalus oreganus helleri*), western diamondback rattlesnake (*Crotalus atrox*), timber rattlesnake (*Crotalus horridus horridus*), and some populations of the Mohave rattlesnake (*Crotalus scutulatus*), cause significant neurotoxicity. Physicians should proactively learn the important species in their regions, including how the species can be identified, the expected effects of their venoms, and proper approaches to management.

Management

Prehospital care should focus on rapid transport to the emergency department while supporting the victim's vital signs as needed. Constrictive clothing, jewelry, and watches should be removed, and the injured body part should be immobilized in a position of function at the level of the heart. *All proposed field treatments for snake bites, such as tourniquets, ice, electric shock, incision, and suction, have proven problematic, with most being ineffective and deleterious.*

At the hospital, attention is directed to the ABCs and supportive care as needed. An effort should be made to identify the offending snake and then to secure the appropriate AV. Intravenous access should be established in an unaffected extremity, and standard laboratory specimens should be obtained, including those for a complete blood count, coagulation studies, fibrinogen concentration, and serum chemistry

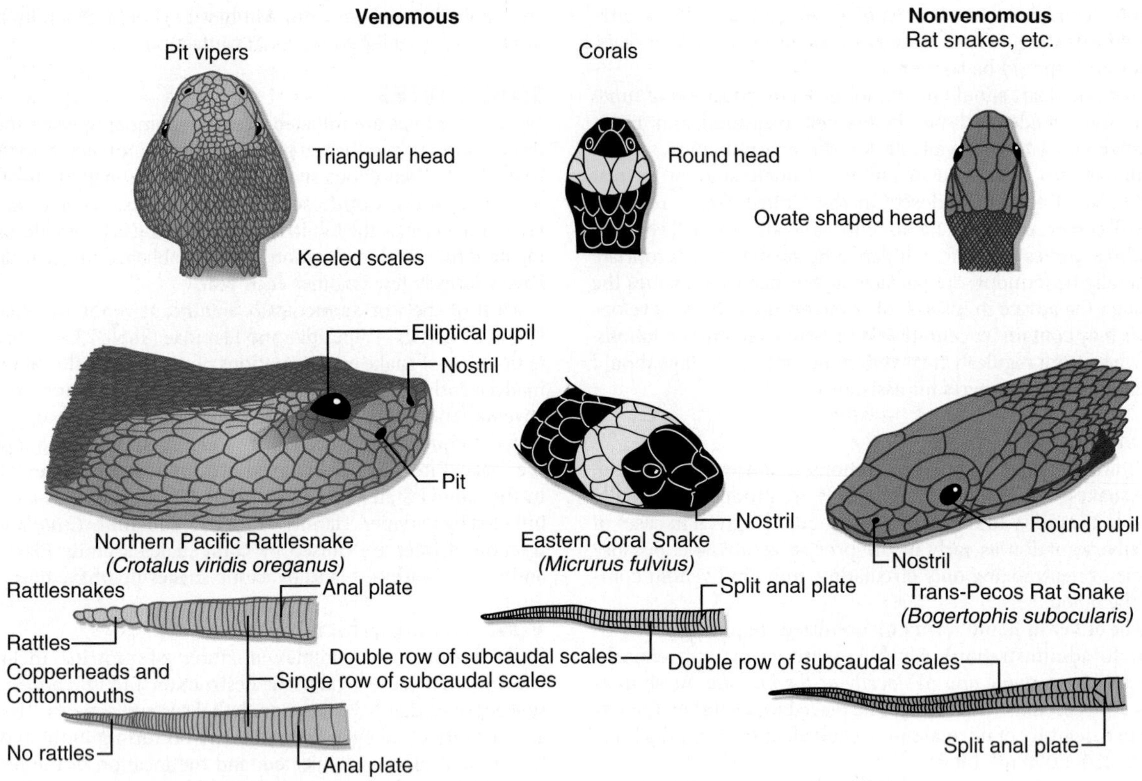

Figure 725-1 Anatomic comparison of pit vipers, coral snakes, and nonvenomous snakes of the United States. (Note: the northern Pacific rattlesnake is now classified as *Crotalus oreganus oreganus*.) (*Modified from Adams JG, et al, editors:* Emergency medicine, *Philadelphia, 2008, WB Saunders. Drawing by Marlin Sawyer.*)

Table 725-1	Medically Important Snake Families			
FAMILY	**VENOMOUS?**	**LOCATION**	**EXAMPLES**	**TOXIN EFFECTS/OTHER COMMENTS**
Colubridae	Some species	Most parts of the world	Garter snakes (*Thamnophis* spp.), king snakes and milk snakes (*Lampropeltis* spp.)	Largest family of snakes; most are considered harmless to humans; a few species are dangerously toxic (e.g., African boomslang [*Dispholidus typus*])
Boidae	None	Most parts of the world	*Boa* species, *Python* species	Constrictors; unsupervised children should not be allowed access to large constrictors
Viperidae Subfamily *Crotalinae* (pit vipers)	All	Americas, Asia	Rattlesnakes (*Crotalus* and *Sistrurus* spp.), cottonmouths and copperheads (*Agkistrodon* spp.), Lancehead pit vipers (*Bothrops* spp.)	Heat-sensing "pit" between each eye and nostril
Subfamily *Viperinae* (true vipers)	All	Europe, Africa, Middle East, Asia	Puff adder (*Bitis arietans*), Gaboon viper (*Bitis gabonica*)	No heat-sensing pits
Elapidae	All	Americas, Africa, Middle East, Asia	Cobras (*Naja* spp.), mambas (*Dendroaspis* spp.), kraits (*Bungarus* spp.), coral snakes (*Micrurus* spp.), and the venomous snakes of Australia	Highly variable venom effects—some largely neurotoxic, others causing severe local tissue damage
Hydrophiidae	All	Warm waters of the Pacific Ocean, Indian Ocean, and Oceana (none in the Atlantic Ocean)	Sea snakes including the pelagic sea snake (*Pelamis platurus*)	Neurotoxins and myotoxins; rarely bite humans unless provoked

analysis including total creatine kinase. A blood sample should be sent for typing and screening, although blood products are rarely actually required in management of snake bite. Samples collected later in the clinical course may be hard to cross match because venom and AV can interfere with the testing. Tourniquets placed in the field by laypeople should be cautiously removed after venous access is obtained, to watch for and treat adverse effects that may follow a sudden bolus of acidotic, hyperkalemic blood mixed with venom into the systemic circulation. The bitten extremity should be marked at 2 or more sites proximal to the bite, and the circumferences at these locations should be assessed every 15 min to monitor for progressive edema—indicative of ongoing venom effects. Occasionally, the sharp, recurved teeth of snakes, including nonvenomous snakes, are left behind in wounds; they should be identified (using soft tissue radiographs or ultrasound as needed) and removed.

Assessing the severity of the envenomation in the field and at the hospital is essential (Table 725-2).

AVs are relatively specific for the snake species against which they are designed to protect. *There is no benefit to administering an AV for an unrelated species,* and doing so certainly involves unacceptable risk (e.g., anaphylaxis) and expense. If it is determined that the child

requires AV, a search for the appropriate product should begin as soon as possible—checking the hospital pharmacy, regional poison control center, and perhaps local zoos and museums that keep captive snakes. Table 725-3 lists the indications for administering AV.

In October 2000, Crotalidae polyvalent immune Fab known as CroFab was approved by the FDA for use in crotaline envenomations. CroFab is derived from sheep (ovine) antibodies and replaces the previously used AV derived from horses (equine-derived AV). The most important advantage of this AV is fewer hypersensitivity reactions, including both immediate and delayed reactions. A metaanalysis showed only 8% immediate hypersensitivity reactions and 13% delayed or serum sickness reactions after administration of CroFab, compared to an estimated 23-56% from the previous equine-derived AV.

CroFab is derived from 4 snakes, 3 from the genera *Crotalus* (the eastern diamondback rattlesnake, the western diamondback rattlesnake, and the Mohave rattlesnake) and 1 from the genera *Agkistrodon* (the cottonmouth water moccasin). It is effective against the venoms of all pit vipers in the United States. There is controversy regarding the use of CroFab in bites from copperheads (*Agkistrodon contortrix*) because they tend to cause fewer systemic effects. Most copperhead envenomations cause only local tissue swelling, ecchymosis, and pain, and generally do well even without AV. Serious envenomations, including fatalities, have followed copperhead bites, and any child with evidence of systemic toxicity should receive CroFab.

The half-life of CroFab is considerably shorter than that of crotaline venom constituents, and redosing is frequently needed to prevent or treat recurrence of venom effects. Patients with significant envenomation should be followed for late hematologic abnormalities (coagulopathy) that can occur up to 2 weeks after the bite. Although these

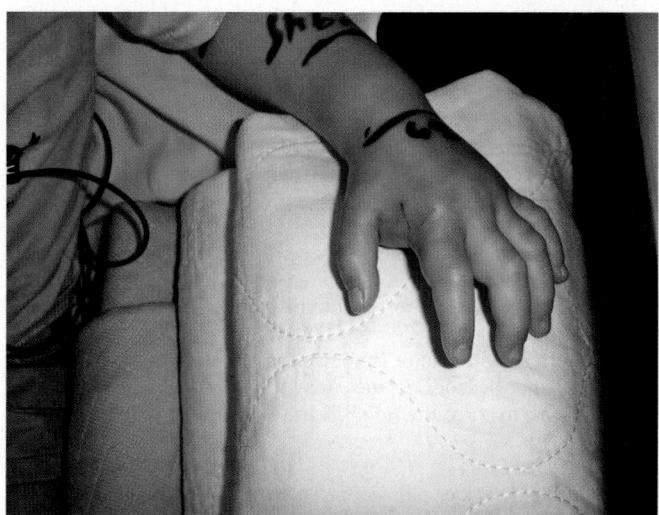

Figure 725-2 Southern Pacific rattlesnake bite *(Crotalus oreganus helleri)* in a 2 yr old boy. Note the fang marks, swelling, and bruising of the tissues (photograph taken 2 hr following the bite). *(Courtesy of Sean Bush, MD.)*

Table 725-3	Indications for Snake Antivenom Administration
Evidence of systemic toxicity:	
Hemodynamic or respiratory instability	Hypotension, respiratory distress
Hemotoxicity	Clinically significant bleeding or abnormal coagulation studies
Neurotoxicity	Any evidence of toxicity: usually beginning with cranial nerve abnormalities and progressing to descending paralysis including the diaphragm
Evidence of worsening local toxicity	*Progressive* soft tissue swelling

Table 725-2	Crotaline Envenomation: Determining the Degree of Envenomation		
DEGREE OF ENVENOMATION	**CONTIGUOUS MANIFESTATIONS**	**SYSTEMIC MANIFESTATIONS**	**LABORATORY ABNORMALITIES**
None or trivial ("dry bite")	Punctures or abrasions; pain and tenderness at bite	None	None
Mild or minimal	Punctures or abrasions; pain, tenderness, edema, and erythema at and adjacent to bite	None	None
Moderate	Punctures or abrasions; pain, tenderness, edema, and erythema beyond area adjacent to bite	Perioral paresthesias; peripheral paresthesias; gustatory changes; nausea; emesis; diarrhea; weakness; light-headedness; diaphoresis; chills	↑PT; ↑PTT; ↓platelets; ↓fibrinogen; ↑hemoglobin
Severe	Punctures or abrasions; pain, tenderness, edema, and erythema of entire extremity	Ventilatory insufficiency; hypotension; shock; bleeding; altered mental status; fasciculations; seizures	↑↑PT; ↑↑PTT; ↓↓platelets; ↓↓fibrinogen; ↑↓hemoglobin

↑, increased; ↑↑, very increased; ↑↓, increased or decreased; ↓, decreased; ↓↓, very decreased; PT, prothrombin time; PTT, partial thromboplastin time.
From Walter FG, Chase PB, Fernández MC, McNally J: Venomous snakes: North American Crotalinae envenomation. In Shannon MW, Borron SW, Burns MJ, editors: Haddad and Winchester's clinical management of poisoning and drug overdose, ed 4, Philadelphia, 2007, WB Saunders, Table 21A-9.

Table 725-4	Indications for Administration of Additional Antivenom in Patients with Recurrent Coagulopathy or Thrombocytopenia After Initial Control

- Evidence of clinically significant bleeding
- Platelet count below 25,000/cu mm
- International normalized ratio (INR) greater than 3
- Activated partial thromboplastin time (aPTT) greater than 50 sec
- Fibrinogen less than 50 mg/dL
- Presence of multicomponent coagulopathy
- Worsening trend in a patient with prior severe coagulopathy
- High-risk behavior for trauma
- Certain comorbid conditions (e.g., systemic vasculitis, seizure disorders, prior stroke)

From Norris RL, Bush SP, Smith J: Bites by venomous reptiles in Canada, the U.S. and Mexico. In Auerbach PS, editor: Wilderness medicine, ed 6, Philadelphia, 2012, Elsevier.

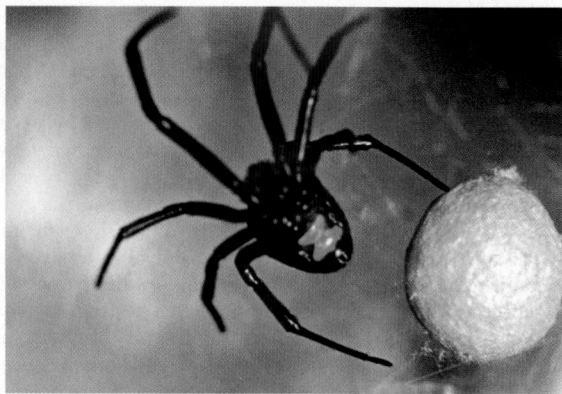

Figure 725-3 Female black widow spider (*Latrodectus mactans*). Note the red hourglass-shaped marking on the underside of her abdomen. (*From The Centers for Disease Control and Prevention Public Health Image Library, Image #5449.*)

tend to be mild laboratory coagulopathies without clinical bleeding, rare cases of intracranial bleeding have been reported. Further AV therapy should be considered for such delayed onset or recurrent coagulopathy as outlined in Table 725-4.

Disposition

Any child with a potential venomous snake bite should be admitted to a closely observed setting for at least 24 hr, regardless of whether evidence of envenomation exists or AV has been given. Children with evidence of systemic toxicity should initially be admitted to an intensive care setting until stabilized.

SPIDER BITES

More than 20,000 venomous spiders have been identified, but most lack either potent venom or fangs long enough to penetrate human skin, and are therefore of no medical significance. No spiders can be considered truly deadly, meaning that an untreated bite in a human would be expected to cause death. The spiders of medical significance can be broadly divided into 2 major groups: those that cause a neurotoxic syndrome and those that cause tissue necrosis. In the United States, the only significant morbidities are caused by 1 genus of spider from each group: *Latrodectus* (the widow spiders) and *Loxosceles* (the fiddleback or recluse spiders).

Neurotoxic Spiders

The major neurotoxic spiders are the widow spiders (*Latrodectus* spp.), the funnel web spiders (*Atrax* and *Hydronyche* spp.—found in Australia), and the banana spiders (*Phoneutria* spp.—indigenous to Latin America).

Venoms and Effects

Neurotoxic spiders all possess venoms that act at neural synapses, both at neuromuscular junctions and at autonomic nervous system junctions. All of the widow spiders (*Latrodectus* spp., including the well-studied black widow [*Latrodectus mactans*; Fig. 725-3]) and the Australian red-back spider [*Latrodectus hasselti*]) possess very similar venoms, with the most important neurotoxin being α-latrotoxin. The neurotoxin of the Sydney funnel web spider (*Atrax robustus*) is robustoxin.

Bites by the neurotoxic spiders tend to be very painful, and the offending spider is often seen. Systemic effects may include hypertension, tachycardia, bradycardia, hypersalivation, diaphoresis, and diffuse muscle spasms.

Management

Management of neurotoxic spider envenomation centers on sound supportive care. Several *Latrodectus* AVs are available, and each appears to be effective regardless of which species of widow spider was responsible for the bite. There is also an AV for the Sydney funnel web spider, the only species of funnel web that has caused human fatalities (none since the introduction of the AV), and a polyspecific AV for the banana spider in South America. These AVs should be used in significant bites with potentially serious systemic effects. The package insert for the appropriate product is used to guide therapy.

In the United States, *Latrodectus* AV is administered to reverse serious systemic effects of widow spider envenomation. One vial is given either intramuscularly (IM) or IV. Efficacy is usually noted within 1 hr of administration, reversal of systemic toxicity and relief of pain being noted. Occasionally, a second vial is necessary. There have been deaths related to acute nonallergic anaphylactic reactions to the U.S. AV, so its administration should be undertaken with due caution and close monitoring.

If AV is to be withheld or is not available, generous doses of opioid analgesics and benzodiazepines may be used to ease symptoms (although this may require up to 72 hr of therapy).

Disposition

Most neurotoxic spider bite victims, even those requiring AV, can be discharged from the emergency department if they have a satisfactory response to therapy. Parents should be warned to bring their child back for any reoccurrence of venom effects. Children with more-severe cases should be admitted for 24 hr of monitoring.

Necrotizing Spiders
Venoms and Effects

Although many spiders may cause a small amount of local tissue damage after their bites, the spiders most notorious for their dermonecrotic potential are the violin or recluse spiders of the genus *Loxosceles*. The best known member of this genus is the brown recluse (*Loxosceles reclusa*; Fig. 725-4), found in the midwestern and southern portions of the United States. The venom of *Loxosceles* spiders contains a phospholipase enzyme, sphingomyelinase D, which attacks cell membranes and can cause local tissue damage that can occasionally be severe. The bite of this spider, most common between April and October, is generally painless and initially goes unnoticed. A few hours after the bite, pain related to focal ischemia begins at the site. Within a day, the site may have a central clear or blood-filled vesicle with surrounding ecchymosis and a rim of pale ischemia. The lesion may gradually expand over a period of days to weeks until necrotic tissue sloughs and healing begins (Fig. 725-5).

Rare cases of systemic loxoscelism appear to be more common in young children than adults. Patients present with systemic toxicity, including fever, chills, nausea, malaise, diffuse macular rash, and petechiae, and may experience hemolysis, coagulopathy, and/or renal failure.

In cases of suspected necrotic arachnidism, when no spider was actually seen by the patient, a broad differential diagnosis must be considered to ensure appropriate management of the true etiology. The differential diagnosis includes skin infections (particularly methicillin-resistant *Staphylococcus aureus;* see Chapter 181), bites by other arthropods (e.g., fleas, ticks), pyoderma gangrenosum, or ecthyma gangrenosum.

Management

For necrotizing spider bites, management of the wound involves sound supportive care, including intermittent local ice therapy for the 1st 72 hr and administration of antibiotics if there is any question of secondary bacterial infection. Daily wound cleansings, combined with

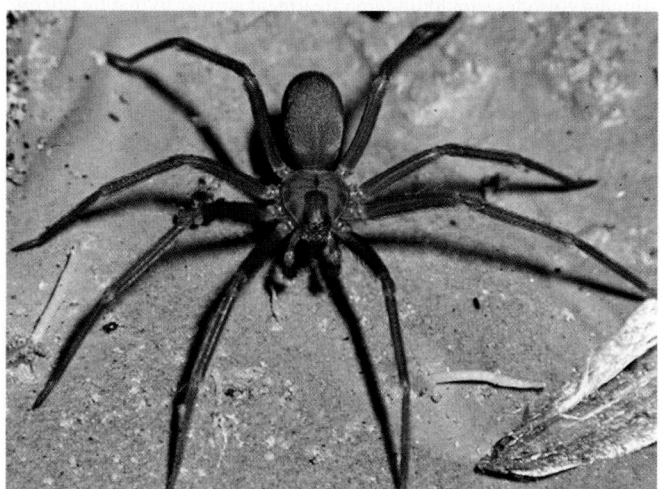

Figure 725-4 Male recluse spider (*Loxosceles* spp.). Note the distinct violin-shaped marking on the dorsum of the cephalothorax. *(Courtesy of Michael Cardwell/Extreme Wildlife Photography.)*

splinting of the bitten area, should be performed until the wound is healed.

Nothing has been definitively proven effective in limiting the extent of necrosis following a spider bite. There is no role for steroids in managing necrotic arachnidism. Dapsone, although used anecdotally in managing *Loxosceles* bites in adults, is not approved for use in children and should not be prescribed.

Children appearing systemically unwell should be admitted and undergo laboratory evaluation (complete blood count, coagulation studies, and urinalysis). Systemic loxoscelism is managed with intravenous hydration, management of renal failure as needed, and a brief course of systemic steroids to stabilize red blood cell membranes. Although there are documented fatalities following bites by the South American violin spider (*Loxosceles laeta*), there has never been a definitively proven fatality following a brown recluse bite in the United States. No AV is commercially available in the United States for management of necrotizing spider bites such as those from *Loxosceles* species.

Disposition

Victims with potentially necrotic bites should be monitored for a few days with daily wound checks. Local, intermittent cooling therapy should be continued for approximately 72 hr. Any child with a probable necrotizing spider bite and evidence of systemic involvement should be admitted to be watched for hemolysis and coagulopathy.

SCORPION STINGS

Of the more than 1,200 species of scorpions worldwide, only a few cause more than a painful sting. In the United States, there is 1 medically significant scorpion, the bark scorpion (*Centruroides sculpturatus* [formerly *Centruroides exilicauda*]). Although this scorpion has caused death in children in the past, such an outcome is exceedingly rare. It is found only in Arizona and small areas of immediately surrounding states. In other regions of the world, especially Latin America, Africa, the Middle East, and Asia, a number of scorpions regularly cause fatalities, particularly in small children.

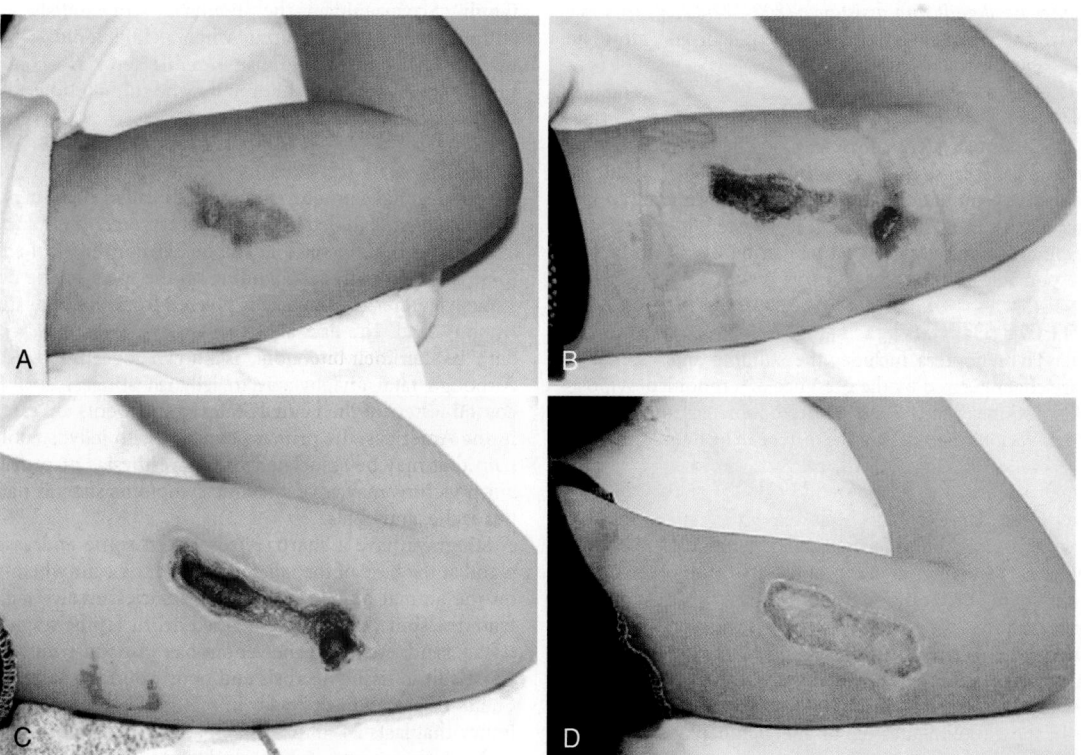

Figure 725-5 Progression of cutaneous loxoscelism in a Brazilian patient who was bitten inside a house while putting on a shirt. Ulceration and necrosis at day 1 **(A)**, day 9 **(B)**, day 16 **(C)**, and day 25 **(D)**. *(From Isbister G, Fan HW: Spider bite. Lancet 378:2039–2046, 2011, Fig. 3. Photographs by Ceila MS Malaque.)*

Venoms and Effects

The major components of important scorpion venoms are neurotoxins that alter neural membrane ionic channels, causing autonomic and cardiovascular dysfunction through the release of acetylcholine and catecholamines. Manifestations of scorpion stings in children vary from mild to severe and may include pain, paresthesias, roving eye movements, cranial nerve dysfunction, opisthotonos/emprosthotonos, seizures, hypertensive crisis, cardiovascular collapse, and respiratory failure. Two important ingestions that can be confused with a bark scorpion envenomation are organophosphate poisoning (see Chapter 63) and methamphetamine intoxication (see Chapter 114). The opsoclonus-like roving eye movements seen in bark scorpion envenomations are not seen in the above ingestions and may help differentiate these conditions.

Management

Most stings require only pain control and respond well to ice, immobilization, and analgesics. Management of severe stings should begin with the ABCs. Opioid analgesics may have some synergy with scorpion neurotoxins and should be used with caution. Benzodiazepines may be more useful, especially for severe muscle spasms or sedation of the agitated child. Approximately 20 different scorpion AVs are available worldwide, but their use is controversial because of variable efficacy and the risk of potential nonallergic anaphylaxis. Practitioners should be familiar with the local standard of care for treating the stings of their indigenous scorpions and should consult a local or regional expert for assistance as necessary. In August 2011, the FDA approved a bark scorpion–specific AV, Anascorp, for use in the United States. It is manufactured in Mexico and marketed there under the name Alacramyn. The AV is generally given to any patient with cranial nerve or somatic skeletal neuromuscular dysfunction. The starting dose is 3 vials given IV, followed by another vial if symptoms still persist 30-60 min later and up to 5 vials were used in the initial study. Anascorp is currently only approved for IV administration; however, there are case reports of it being given IM and IO in children without IV access. *For more specific information about the administration of Anascorp, the practitioner should contact the Arizona Poison and Drug Information Center for details and assistance (800-222-1222).* In some regions of the world, prazosin is used in severe scorpion stings to ameliorate acute cardiovascular effects.

Disposition

The child with evidence of systemic toxicity following a scorpion sting should be admitted for at least 24 hr of monitoring (including cardiac monitoring) and, if envenomation is severe, should be monitored in a pediatric intensive care unit. In the absence of systemic toxicity and with adequate pain control, children >1 yr can be discharged to go home with a responsible adult.

HYMENOPTERA STINGS

The insect order Hymenoptera includes the stinging ants, bees, and wasps, which are characterized by the presence of a modified ovipositor (the "sting" or "stinger") at the end of the abdomen through which venom is injected. Various members of the order can be found throughout the world.

Venoms and Effects

Hymenoptera venoms, mixtures of proteins and vasoactive substances, are not very potent. Most stings result in only local pain, redness, and swelling, followed by itching and resolution. Some patients experience a large local reaction in which swelling progresses beyond the sting site, possibly involving the entire extremity. Approximately 0.4-0.8% of children are at risk for acute, life-threatening allergic reactions as a result of hymenoptera venom sensitivity. Each year, an estimated 50-150 people in the United States die of allergic anaphylaxis caused by hymenoptera stings (see Chapter 70). Rare cases of delayed serum sickness can follow hymenoptera stings (see Chapter 150). Finally, with the spread of Africanized honey bees (*Apis mellifera scutellata),* massive stinging episodes resulting in systemic venom toxicity (hypotension,

respiratory failure, shock, hemolysis, and renal failure) appear to be increasing in Latin America and the southwestern U.S. states.

Management

Children with typical local reactions can be treated with application of cold compresses and with analgesics and antihistamines as needed. Children with large local reactions should also receive a 5 day course of oral corticosteroids and a prescription for an epinephrine autoinjection kit (and instructions in its use) prior to discharge. Patients presenting with urticaria, angioedema, wheezing, or hypotension should be treated aggressively for an immediate hypersensitivity reaction with intramuscular epinephrine (0.01 mg/kg, up to 0.3-0.5 mg of 1 : 1,000 formulation), airway management as needed, oxygen, intravenous fluids, antihistamines, and corticosteroids. Children suffering massive stinging episodes should undergo treatment similar to that for allergic anaphylaxis.

Disposition

Children with local reactions (limited or large local) can be discharged with continued care as outlined previously and instructions for wound precautions. More difficult disposition decisions are involved for children with systemic manifestations. Children with only diffuse urticaria, who are stable after a period of observation, can be discharged in the care of a responsible adult to continue antihistamines and steroids and to carry an epinephrine self-administration kit. These children seem to be at little risk for progressing to systemic anaphylaxis with future stings. Children suffering more than simple hives (e.g., wheezing, evidence of laryngeal edema or cardiovascular instability) should be admitted for 24 hr of observation and should receive a referral to an allergist for testing for hymenoptera venom sensitivity and possible immunotherapy. Immunotherapy reduces the risk of systemic anaphylaxis from future stings in high-risk patients from somewhere between 30% and 60% to less than 5%.

MARINE ENVENOMATION

The most commonly encountered venomous marine creatures are the jellyfish (Cnidaria), stingrays (Chondrichthyes), and members of the family Scorpaenidae—the lionfish, scorpionfish, and stonefish. Although most injuries occur when a child ventures into the animal's natural environment, lionfish (*Pterois* spp.) are commonly kept in private aquariums and children may be stung if they attempt to handle these beautiful fish.

Venoms and Effects

All jellyfish have unique stinging cells called **nematocysts**. These cells contain a highly folded tubule that everts on contact and injects venom. The venom is antigenic and can be dermonecrotic, hemolytic, cardiotoxic, or neuropathic, depending on the species. The nematocysts can sting even after the tentacle is severed from the body and after the jellyfish is dead. The Pacific box jellyfish (*Chironex fleckeri*) of Australia, with its cardiotoxic venom, is known to cause rapidly fatal stings. Although fatal anaphylaxis to jellyfish stings has been reported in coastal waters of the United States, these events are rare. For clinicians in the Americas, the primary concern with jellyfish stings is localized pain that may be associated with paresthesias or pruritus. Rarely, jellyfish victims may have systemic symptoms such as nausea, vomiting, headache, and chills.

Stingrays have a sharp, retroserrated spine and associated venom gland at the base of the tail. Stings tend to occur when the victim steps on the animal hidden in the surf. Injuries involve jagged lacerations from the spine, often with retained debris (spine fragments, glandular tissue, sand, etc.), and the venom has vasoconstrictive properties that can result in tissue necrosis and poor wound healing. Stingray envenomations are noteworthy for immediate and intense pain at the site of injury that lasts 24-48 hr. Some patients experience nausea, vomiting, and muscle cramps, and, rarely, hypotension or seizures.

The Scorpaenidae have venomous dorsal, pelvic, and anal spines that become erect when threatened. The glands associated with these spines contain venoms that result in direct myotoxicity leading to paralysis of cardiac, involuntary, and skeletal muscles. Envenomation causes immediate pain that may persist for hours or days. Victims may experience intense local tissue destruction in which superinfections are common. Systemic symptoms include vomiting, abdominal pain, headache, delirium, seizures, and respiratory failure.

Management

Treatment of jellyfish stings begins in the ocean. The involved skin should be quickly rinsed *in seawater (fresh water may stimulate further nematocyst firing)*. Dousing the sting site with vinegar or rubbing alcohol can inhibit nematocyst discharge. Visible tentacle fragments should be removed with a gloved hand or forceps, and microscopic fragments may be removed by gently shaving the affected area. Folk remedies such as rubbing the sting with sand and applying urine are not helpful and cause more irritation. Meat tenderizer is not effective. Antihistamines and corticosteroids are indicated for swelling and urticaria. An apparent, acute allergic reaction should be treated with intramuscular epinephrine. Antibiotics are not needed.

Treatment of stingray and Scorpaenidae stings is similar. These toxins are heat labile, and immersion in hot water (approximately 42°C [107.6°F]) for 30-60 min denatures the protein constituents and decreases pain significantly. The wounds should be thoroughly cleaned and explored with use of local or regional anesthesia to rule out retention of spine or integument fragments. Stingray spines are radiopaque and may be seen on plain films of the wounded area or identified by ultrasonography. Lacerations should be treated with delayed primary closure or allowed to heal by secondary intention. Systemic analgesia should be provided as needed. Because of the risk of secondary bacterial infection, there should be a low threshold for administering prophylactic antibiotics to cover *Staphylococcus, Streptococcus,* and *Vibrio* species, and wounds should be rechecked daily for a few days.

Disposition

After wound care, most victims can be discharged home with responsible adults. If there are significant systemic effects after pain control is achieved, the child should be admitted for monitoring and further care as needed.

Bites and stings by venomous creatures are common occurrences in children, but they uncommonly cause major morbidity or mortality. The majority of such injuries do very well with sound supportive care. In serious cases, aggressive management of the ABCs combined with specific interventions (such as AVs when available) maximize the potential for an optimal outcome. A low threshold should be maintained for consulting specialists in envenomation medicine, available through regional poison control centers.

Bibliography is available at Expert Consult.

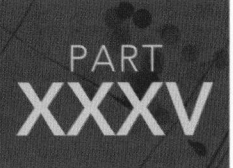

Chapter 726
Laboratory Testing in Infants and Children

Stanley F. Lo

"Normal values" (reference intervals) are difficult to establish within the pediatric population. Differences in genetic composition, physiologic development, environmental influences, and subclinical disease are variables that need to be considered when developing reference intervals. Other considerations for further defining reference intervals include partitioning based on sex and age. The most commonly used reference range is generally given as the mean of the reference population ±2 standard deviations (SD). This is acceptable when the distribution of results for the tested population is essentially gaussian. The serum sodium concentration in children, which is tightly controlled physiologically, has a distribution that is essentially gaussian; the mean value ±2 SD gives a range very close to that actually observed in 95% of children (Table 726-1). However, not all analytes have a gaussian distribution. The serum creatine kinase level, which is subject to diverse influences and is not actively controlled, does not show a gaussian distribution, as evidenced by the lack of agreement between the range actually observed and that predicted by the mean value ±2 SD. In these cases, a reference interval defining the 2.5-97.5 percentiles is typically used.

Reference cutoffs are typically established from large studies with a large reference population. Examples of these cutoffs are illustrated by reference cutoffs established for cholesterol, lipoproteins, and neonatal bilirubin. Patient results exceeding these cutoffs have a future risk of acquiring disease. A final modification needed for reporting reference intervals is referencing the Tanner stage of sexual maturation, which is most useful in assessing pituitary and gonadal function.

The establishment of common reference intervals remains an elusive target. Although some patient results are directly comparable between laboratories and methods, most are not. Careful interpretation of patient results must consider when testing was performed and what method was used. Higher-order methods, methods that are more accurate and precise, continue to be slowly developed. These will be critical to the standardization of tests and the establishment of common reference intervals.

ACCURACY AND PRECISION OF LABORATORY TESTS

Technical accuracy, or trueness, is an important consideration in interpreting the results of a laboratory test. Because of improvements in methods of analysis and elimination of analytic interference, the accuracy of most tests is limited primarily by their precision. **Accuracy** is a measure of the nearness of a test result to the actual value, whereas **precision** is a measure of the reproducibility of a result. No test can be more accurate than it is precise. Analysis of precision by repetitive measurements of a single sample gives rise to a gaussian distribution with a mean and an SD. The estimate of precision is the coefficient of variation (CV):

$$CV = \frac{SD}{Mean} \times 100$$

The CV is not likely to be constant over the full range of values obtained in clinical testing, but it is approximately 5% in the normal range. The CV is generally not reported, but is always known by the laboratory. It is particularly important in assessing the significance of changes in laboratory results. For example, a common situation is the need to assess hepatotoxicity incurred as a result of the administration of a therapeutic drug and reflected in the serum alanine aminotransferase (ALT) value. If serum ALT increases from 25 units/L to 40 units/L, is the change significant? The CV for ALT is 7%. Using the value obtained $\pm 2 \times CV$ to express the extremes of imprecision, it can be seen that a value of 25 units/L is unlikely to reflect an actual concentration of >29 units/L, and a value of 40 units/L is unlikely to reflect an actual concentration of <34 units/L. Therefore, the change in the value as obtained by testing is likely to reflect a real change in circulating ALT levels. Continued monitoring of serum ALT is indicated, even though both values for ALT are within normal limits. *Likely* in this case is only a probability. Inherent biologic variability is such that the results of 2 successive tests may suggest a trend that will disappear on further testing.

The precision of a test may also be indicated by providing confidence limits for a given result. Ordinarily, 95% confidence limits are used, indicating that it is 95% certain that the value obtained lies between the 2 limits reported. Confidence limits are calculated using the mean and SD of replicate determinations:

$$95\% \text{ confidence limits} = \text{Mean} \pm t \times SD$$

where t is a constant derived from the number of replications. In most cases, $t = 2$.

Accuracy is expressed by determining the difference, or bias, between results from a comparative method and a definitive or reference method. A definitive or reference method provides results with increased precision and accuracy compared to the clinical laboratory. When these methods are used, along with highly purified materials (i.e., Standard Reference Materials from the National Institute of Standards and Technology) to establish values for assay calibrators used in the clinical laboratory, the accuracy of patient results is improved. Creatinine, hemoglobin A_{1c}, and neonatal bilirubin are examples in which the accuracy of these tests has been improved.

SENSITIVITY, ACCURACY, AND ANALYTIC TESTING

In some circumstances, the sensitivity and accuracy of an analysis are reduced or increased as functions of clinical purpose. For example, ion exchange chromatography of plasma amino acids for the diagnosis of inborn errors of metabolism is usually performed at an analytic sensitivity that allows measurement of all of the amino acids with a single set of standards. The range of values is approximately 20-800 µmol/L, and accuracy is poor at values ≤20 µmol/L. The detection of homocysteine in this type of analysis suggests an inborn error of methionine metabolism. If the analysis is adjusted to achieve greater analytic sensitivity, it is possible to measure homocysteine accurately in normal plasma (3-12 µmol/L). This more sensitive test is used to assess cobalamin status and analyze risk factors for atherosclerotic cardiovascular disease.

PREDICTIVE VALUE OF LABORATORY TESTS

Predictive value (PV) theory deals with the usefulness of tests as defined by their clinical sensitivity (ability to detect a disease) and specificity (ability to define the absence of a disease).

$$\text{Sensitivity} = \frac{\text{Number positive by test}}{\text{Total number positive}} \times 100$$

Table 726-1	Gaussian and Nongaussian Laboratory Values in 458 Normal School Children 7-14 Yr of Age	
	SERUM SODIUM (mmol/L)	**SERUM CREATINE KINASE (units/L)**
Mean	141	68
SD	1.7	34
Mean ±2 SD	138-144	0-136
Actual 95% range	137-144	24-162

$$\text{Specificity} = \frac{\text{Number negative by test}}{\text{Total number without disease}} \times 100$$

$$\text{PV of a positive test result} = \frac{\text{True-positive results}}{\text{Total positive results}} \times 100$$

$$\text{PV of a negative test result} = \frac{\text{True-negative results}}{\text{Total negative results}} \times 100$$

The problems addressed by PV theory are false-negative and false-positive test results. Both are major considerations in interpreting the results of screening tests in general and neonatal screening tests in particular.

Testing for HIV seroreactivity illustrates some of these considerations. If it is assumed that approximately 1,100,000 of 284,000,000 residents of the United States are infected with HIV (prevalence = 0.39%) and that 90% of those infected demonstrate antibodies to HIV, then we can consider the usefulness of a simple test with 99% sensitivity and 99.5% specificity (see Chapter 276). If the entire population of the United States were screened, it would be possible to identify most of those infected with HIV.

$$1,100,000 \times 0.9 \times 0.99 = 980,100 \, (89.1\%)$$

However, there will be 119,900 false-negative test results. Even with 99.5% specificity, the number of false-positive test results would be larger than the number of true-positive results:

$$284,000,000 \times 0.0005 = 1,420,000$$

In addition, there will be 281,480,000 true-negative results:

$$\text{PV of positive test result} = \frac{980,100}{(980,100 + 1,420,000)} \times 100 = 41\%$$

$$\text{PV of negative test result} = \frac{281,480,000}{(281,480,000 + 119,900)} \times 100$$
$$= 99.96\%$$

Given the high cost associated with follow-up and the anguish produced by a false-positive result, it is easy to see why universal screening for HIV seropositivity received a low priority immediately after the introduction of testing for HIV infection.

By contrast, we can consider the screening of 100,000 individuals from groups at increased risk for HIV in whom the overall prevalence of disease is 10%, with all other considerations being unchanged.

$$\text{True-positive results} = 0.9 \times 0.99 \times 10,000 = 8,910$$

$$\text{False-positive results} = 0.005 \times 90,000 = 450$$

$$\text{False-negative results} = 10,000 - 8,910 = 1,090$$

$$\text{PV of positive test result} = \frac{8,910}{8,910 + 450} \times 100 = 95\%$$

$$\text{PV of negative test result} = \frac{89,500}{89,550 + 1,090} \times 100 = 99\%$$

These 2 hypothetical testing strategies show that the diagnostic efficiency of testing depends heavily on the prevalence of the disease being tested for, even with a superior test, such as the test for HIV antibodies. Because the treatment of pregnant women infected with HIV is effective in preventing vertical transmission of the infection, screening has now been expanded to all pregnant women. The proven effectiveness of current therapy in preventing neonatal infection has intensified screening for HIV early in pregnancy.

However, because of the long time needed to test for HIV antibodies, it was difficult to screen women during labor and provide the necessary therapy. Recently, rapid HIV antibody testing procedures using a fingerstick or venipuncture to obtain whole blood, plasma, or serum, and tests using oral fluid were approved (Table 726-2). The HIV test results are usually obtained in <20 min. The collection of oral fluid samples provides an alternative for individuals who avoid HIV testing because of their dislike of needlesticks. HIV testing using whole blood or oral fluid is classified as a waived test under the **Clinical Laboratory Improvement Amendments of 1988,** and these tests are allowed in a point-of-care setting. Waived tests are simple laboratory procedures that use methodologies that are so simple and accurate as to render the likelihood of an erroneous result by the user negligible. A positive rapid HIV test result is then confirmed by Western blot analysis or immunofluorescence assay.

According to the U.S. Centers for Disease Control and Prevention, 162 infants were born with HIV in 2010 in the United States. Rapid HIV testing during labor allows for implementation of antiretroviral therapy for HIV-infected women who have not been tested or are unaware of their HIV status. The initiation of therapy at the time of labor or within the 1st 12 hr of an infant's birth significantly reduces the risk of mother-to-child transmission. In the mother–infant rapid intervention at delivery study, it was shown that the sensitivity and specificity of a rapid whole blood test for HIV during labor were 100% and 99.9%, respectively, with a positive PV of 90%. The median turnaround time for obtaining results from blood collection to patient notification was only 66 min. The performance of the rapid blood test was better than that of the standard HIV enzyme immunoassay, which had sensitivity and specificity of 100% and 99.8%, respectively, with a positive PV of 76%. In addition, the median turnaround time from blood collection to patient notification was 28 hr. As a result, rapid whole blood HIV testing is now the standard of care for women in labor with undocumented HIV status.

Rapid HIV testing can also be used in developing countries. In resource-poor settings, because of the lack of properly equipped laboratories, skilled technologists, and basic resources, such as electricity and water, these self-contained, point-of-care HIV tests are very attractive. In areas of Asia and Africa in which HIV is epidemic, screening pregnant women with rapid HIV tests and offering antiretroviral therapy can significantly reduce the transmission of HIV to hundreds of thousands of infants.

NEONATAL SCREENING TESTS

Almost all of the diseases detected in neonatal screening programs have a very low prevalence, and for the most part, the tests are quantitative rather than qualitative. In general, the strategy is to use the initial screening test to separate a highly suspect group of patients from normal infants (i.e., to increase the prevalence) and then to follow this suspect group aggressively. There are 2 common strategies used to detect congenital hypothyroidism (see Chapter 568.2): 1 uses thyroid-stimulating hormone for the initial screen and the other uses thyroxine. In the thyroxine strategy for congenital hypothyroidism, which has a prevalence of 25 in 100,000 liveborn infants, the initial test performed is for thyroxine in whole blood. Infants with the lowest 10% of test results are considered suspect. If all infants with hypothyroidism were included in the suspect group, the prevalence of disease in this group would be 250 in 100,000 infants. The original samples obtained from the suspect group are retested for thyroxine and are tested for thyroid-stimulating hormone. This second round of testing results in an even more highly suspect group composed of 0.1% of the infants screened and having a prevalence of hypothyroidism of 25,000

Table 726-2	Rapid HIV Antibody Tests and Status Under the Clinical Laboratory Improvement Amendments of 1988 (CLIA)				
RAPID HIV TEST	**SPECIMEN TYPE**	**CLIA CATEGORY**	**TIME FOR PERFORMING ASSAY**	**WAIT TIME TO READ RESULTS**	**MANUFACTURER**
OraQuick ADVANCE Rapid HIV-1/2 Antibody Test	Oral fluid	Waived	<5 min	20-40 min	OraSure Technologies, Inc. www.orasure.com
	Whole blood (fingerstick or venipuncture)	Waived			
	Plasma	Moderate complexity			
Uni-Gold Recombigen HIV-1	Whole blood (fingerstick or venipuncture)	Waived	<5 min	10-12 min	Trinity Biotech www.unigoldhiv.com
	Serum and plasma	Moderate complexity			
Reveal G-2 Rapid HIV-1 Antibody Test	Serum and plasma	Moderate complexity	<5 min	Read result immediately	MedMira, Inc. www.medmira.com
MultiSpot HIV-1/HIV-2 Rapid Test	Serum and plasma	Moderate complexity	10-15 min	Result can be read immediately or up to 4 hr later	BioRad Laboratories www.bio-rad.com
Clearview HIV 1/2 STAT-PAK	Whole blood (fingerstick or venipuncture)	Waived	5 min	15-20 min	Chembio Diagnostic Systems, Inc; distributed by Alere www.alere.com
	Serum and plasma	Waived	5 min	15-20 min	Chembio Diagnostic Systems, Inc; distributed by Alere www.alere.com
Clearview COMPLETE HIV 1/2	Whole blood (fingerstick or venipuncture)	Waived	5 min	15-20 min	Chembio Diagnostic Systems, Inc; distributed by Alere www.alere.com
	Serum and plasma	Waived	5 min	15-20 min	Chembio Diagnostic Systems, Inc; distributed by Alere www.alere.com

in 100,000 subjects. This final group is aggressively pursued for further testing and treatment. Even with a 1,000-fold increase in prevalence, 75% of the aggressively tested population is euthyroid. The justifications advanced for the program are that treatment is easy and effective and that the alternative, if congenital hypothyroidism is undetected and untreated—long-term custodial care—is both unsatisfactory and expensive.

At its inception, newborn screening was driven by the selection of genetic diseases whose clinical manifestations developed postnatally, such as phenylketonuria, galactosemia, and hypothyroidism. Diseases selected for screening typically had to meet certain criteria. The prevalence of disease had to meet a minimum, typically 1 in 100,000. Disease selection required demonstrated reduction in morbidity and mortality in the neonatal period. Effective therapies needed to be available, and the cost of screening and the feasibility of laboratory testing were also considerations in this selection process.

More common diseases have also become targets for neonatal screening programs. Sickle cell disease (see Chapter 462.1), easily detected using liquid chromatography or isoelectric focusing, can be treated more effectively if it is diagnosed before clinical signs appear. In addition, the results of neonatal screening for cystic fibrosis (CF; see Chapter 403) show that there are clear benefits associated with preclinical diagnosis, but also that there are some inherent difficulties associated with genetic screening for complex autosomal recessive diseases that are common and are caused by a rather large number of mutations (>1,500) of a single gene. The definitive diagnostic test for CF is the measurement of concentrations of chloride in sweat, a test that is not practical during the 1st wk of life. Neonates with CF generally have elevations in whole blood trypsinogen. This test allows the identification of a group of neonates at risk for CF. Unfortunately, trypsinogen as an initial screening test has a high false-positive rate, an unfavorable characteristic that creates unnecessary anxiety among newborn parents and families, and is costly because of the time and expense for medical follow-up. Performing DNA analysis for common mutations that cause CF reduces the size of the suspect group and identifies neonates with a higher likelihood of disease. This 2-tiered strategy identifies a manageable number of infants on whom to perform sweat tests. Problems include the following: (1) Uncommon mutations are not included in the screening panel (thus, cases of CF caused by these mutations can be missed); (2) common mutations that cause clinically innocent elevations of whole blood trypsinogen in heterozygous neonates cause potentially alarming false-positive findings; and (3) CF in patients with normal sweat test results is rare but is likely to be missed.

Tandem mass spectrometry (MS/MS) is a technically advanced method in which many compounds are initially fragmented and separated by molecular weight. Each compound is then fragmented again. Identification of compounds is based upon characteristic fragments. The process requires roughly 2 min per sample and can detect 20 or more inborn errors of metabolism. The effects of prematurity, neonatal illness, and intensive neonatal management on metabolites in blood complicate the interpretation of results. The PV of a positive screening result is likely to be <10%; that is, 90% of positive results are not indicative of a genetic disorder of metabolism. Nonetheless, MS/MS permits a diagnosis to be made before clinical illness develops and has revolutionized the purpose and ability of newborn screening. MS/MS is not directed toward diseases defined as treatable, but it is directed toward all of the diseases, each of which is rare, that the technique can identify.

Electrospray MS/MS permits the detection of rare inborn errors of metabolism and has been introduced as a newborn screening tool all around the world. Since 1998, when mass spectrometry was implemented in Australia, the rate of detection per 100,000 births has been 15.7, significantly higher than the rate of 8.6-9.5 in the 6 preceding 4 yr periods. Disorders of fatty acid oxidation, particularly medium-chain acyl coenzyme A dehydrogenase deficiency (see Chapter 86), accounted for the majority of increased diagnoses.

Table 726-3	American College of Medical Genetics Core Panel

Isovalericacidemia
Glutaric aciduria type 1
3-Hydroxy-3-methylglutaricaciduria
Multiple coenzyme A (CoA) carboxylase deficiency
Methylmalonic acidemia (mutase deficiency)
3-Methylcrotonyl CoA carboxylase deficiency
Methylmalonic acidemia (cobalamin [Cbl] A, B)
Propionicacidemia
β-Ketothiolase deficiency
Medium-chain acyl-CoA dehydrogenase deficiency
Very-long-chain acyl-CoA dehydrogenase deficiency
Long-chain L-3-hydroxy acyl-CoA dehydrogenase deficiency
Trifunctional protein deficiency
Carnitine uptake deficiency
Phenylketonuria
Maple syrup urine disease
Homocystinuria (because of cystathionine β-synthase deficiency)
Citrullinemia
Argininosuccinic acidemia
Tyrosinemia type 1
Sickle cell anemia (Hb SS disease)
Hemoglobin (Hb) S/β-thalassemia
Hb S/C disease
Congenital hypothyroidism
Biotinidase deficiency
Congenital adrenal hyperplasia (21-hydroxylase deficiency)
Classical galactosemia
Hearing loss
Cystic fibrosis

Expanded newborn screening programs using MS/MS increase the detection of inherited metabolic disorders. All states in the United States use MS/MS in their neonatal screening programs. The metabolic conditions screened for by states using MS/MS vary, ranging from 31 to >50.

In an attempt to standardize newborn screening programs, the American College of Medical Genetics recommends that every baby born in the United States be screened for a core panel of 29 disorders (Table 726-3). An additional 25 conditions were recommended as secondary targets because they may be identified while screening for the core panel disorders. The March of Dimes and the American Academy of Pediatrics also endorse the recommendation by the American College of Medical Genetics. However, expansion of the screening test menu raises several issues. The cost of implementation can be significant because many states will need multiple MS/MS systems. Staffing the laboratory with qualified technical personnel to run the MS/MS system and qualified clinical scientists to interpret the profiles can be a challenge. A number of false-positive results will also be obtained with these newborn screening programs. Many of these findings are the result of parenteral nutrition, biologic variation, or treatment, and are not the result of an inborn error of metabolism. Consequently, qualified staff will be needed to ensure that patients with abnormal results are contacted and receive follow-up testing and counseling, if needed. Even with these concerns, the American College of Medical Genetics report is a step in the right direction toward standardizing guidelines for state newborn screening programs.

TESTING IN REFINING A DIFFERENTIAL DIAGNOSIS

The use of laboratory tests in refining a differential diagnosis satisfies PV theory because a correct differential diagnosis should result in a relatively high prevalence of the disease under consideration. An example of testing in refining a differential diagnosis is the measurement of urinary vanillylmandelic acid (VMA) for the diagnosis of neuroblastoma (see Chapter 498). A simple spot test for VMA is not useful in general screening programs because of the low prevalence of neuroblastoma (3 cases/100,000) and the low sensitivity of the test (69%). Even though the specificity of urinary VMA is 99.6%, testing of 100,000 children would produce 2 true-positive test results, 400 false-positive results, and 1 false-negative result. The PV of a positive result in this setting is 0.5%, and the PV of a negative result is 99.99%, not much different from the assumption that neuroblastoma is not present. Testing for urinary VMA in a 3 yr old child with an abdominal mass, however, gives a useful result because the prevalence of neuroblastoma is at least 50% in 3 yr old children with abdominal masses. If 100 such children are tested and the prevalence of neuroblastoma in the group is assumed to be 50%, then a satisfactory PV is obtained.

$$\text{PV of positive test result} = \frac{0.69 \times 50}{0.69 \times 50 + (0.004 \times 50)} \times 100 = 99\%$$

$$\text{PV of negative test result} = \frac{0.996 \times 50}{0.996 \times 50 + (0.31 \times 50)} \times 100 = 76\%$$

Thus, in this situation, a test with low sensitivity is powerful in refining the differential diagnosis because the PV of a positive result is almost 100% in the setting of high prevalence.

Serologic Testing

Using laboratory testing to refine a differential diagnosis poses problems, as exemplified by serologic testing for Lyme disease, which is a tick-borne infection by *Borrelia burgdorferi* that has various manifestations in both early and late stages of infection (see Chapter 222). Direct demonstration of the organism is difficult, and serologic test results for Lyme disease are not reliably positive in young patients presenting early with erythema chronicum migrans. These results become positive after a few weeks of infection and remain positive for a number of years. In an older population being evaluated for late-stage Lyme disease, some individuals will have recovered from either clinical or subclinical Lyme disease and some will have active Lyme disease, with both groups having true-positive serologic test results. Of individuals without Lyme disease, some will have true-negative serologic test results, but a significant percentage will have antibodies to other organisms that cross react with *B. burgdorferi* antigens.

This set of circumstances gives rise to a number of problems. First, the protean nature of Lyme disease makes it difficult to ensure a high prevalence of disease in subjects to be tested. Second, the most appropriate antibodies to be detected are imperfectly defined, leading to a wide variety of tests with varying false-positive and false-negative rates. Third, the natural history of the antibody response to infection and the difficulty of showing the causative organism directly combine to make laboratory diagnosis of early Lyme disease difficult. Fourth, in the diagnosis of late-stage Lyme disease in older subjects, the laboratory diagnosis is plagued by misleading positive (either false-positive or true-positive, but not clinically relevant) results, typically an enzyme-linked immunosorbent assay that uses whole *B. burgdorferi* organisms. In a review of 788 patients referred to a specialty clinic with the diagnosis of Lyme disease, the diagnosis was correct in 180 patients, 156 patients had true seropositivity without active Lyme disease, and 452 had never had Lyme disease, even though 45% of them were found to be seropositive by at least 1 test before referral.

A 2-step approach, similar to that used in HIV testing, is commonly used: a screening test that has high sensitivity (e.g., enzyme-linked immunosorbent assay) and excellent negative PV, followed by a very specific confirmatory test for verification of positive screening test results (e.g., Western blot to detect antibodies to selected bacterial antigens). Negative screening test results and negative verification test results are reported as negative. Positive verification test results are reported as positive. However, standardization of the testing procedures is difficult in North America, where only 1 pathogenic strain of *B. burgdorferi* is found, and is more difficult elsewhere in the Northern hemisphere, where as many as 3 pathogenic strains are present. Identification of microbial DNA in body fluids by polymerase chain reaction is definitive but invasive.

Table 726-4	Laboratory Profile as a Review of Systems
LABORATORY TEST	**ASSESSMENT FACILITATED BY TESTS**
Complete blood cell count and platelets	Nutrition, status of formed elements
Complete urinalysis	Renal function/genitourinary tract inflammation
Albumin and cholesterol	Nutrition
ALT, bilirubin, GGT	Liver function
BUN, creatinine	Renal function, nutrition
Sodium, potassium, chloride, bicarbonate	Electrolyte homeostasis
Calcium and phosphorus	Calcium homeostasis

ALT, alanine aminotransferase; BUN, blood urea nitrogen; GGT, γ-glutamyltransferase.

Table 727-1	Prefixes Denoting Decimal Factors in Table 727-5	
PREFIX	**SYMBOL**	**FACTOR**
Mega-	M	10^6
Kilo-	k	10^3
Hecto-	h	10^2
Deka-	da	10^1
Deci-	d	10^{-1}
Centi-	c	10^{-2}
Milli-	m	10^{-3}
Micro-	μ	10^{-6}
Nano-	n	10^{-9}
Pico-	p	10^{-12}
Femto-	f	10^{-15}

Laboratory Screening

Screening profiles (Table 726-4) are used as part of a complete review of systems, to establish a baseline value, or to facilitate patient care in specific circumstances, such as (1) when a patient clearly has an illness, but a specific diagnosis remains elusive; (2) when a patient requires intensive care; (3) for postmarketing surveillance and evaluation of a new drug; and (4) when a drug is used that is known to have systemic adverse effects. Laboratory screening tests should be used in a targeted manner to supplement, not supplant, a complete history and physical examination.

ACKNOWLEDGMENTS

The author gratefully acknowledges the original contributions by Michael A. Pesce, on which portions of this chapter are based.

Bibliography is available at Expert Consult.

Chapter **727**

Reference Intervals for Laboratory Tests and Procedures

Stanley F. Lo

In Tables 727-1 through 727-5, the reference intervals apply to infants, children, and adolescents when possible. For many analyses, separate reference intervals for children and adolescents are not well delineated. When interpreting a test result, the reference interval supplied by the laboratory performing the test should always be used as these intervals are instrument and/or method dependent. Figures 727-1 and 727-2 provide estimations related to dosages. Figure 727-3 is a nomogram for risk assessment of hyperbilirubinemia.

Bibliography is available at Expert Consult.

Table 727-2	Abbreviations Used in Table 727-5		
Ab	Absorbance	mm Hg	Millimeters of mercury
AU	Arbitrary unit	mmol	Millimole
BB	Brain isoenzyme of creatine kinase	mo	Month, months
		mol	Mole
cap	Capillary	mOsm	Milliosmole
CH_{50}	Dilution required to lyse 50% of indicator red blood cells; indicates complement activity	MW	Relative molecular weight
		ND	Not detected
Cr	Creatinine	nm	Nanometer (wavelength)
CSF	Cerebrospinal fluid	Pa	Pascal
F	Female	pc	Postprandial
g	Gram	RBC	Red blood cell(s), erythrocyte(s)
Hb	Hemoglobin		
HbCO	Carboxyhemoglobin	RT	Room temperature
hpf	High-power field	SD	Standard deviation
hr	Hour, hours	sec	Second, seconds
IU	International unit of hormone activity	Tr	Trace
		U	International unit of enzyme activity
L	Liter		
M	Male	V	Volume
MB	Heart isoenzyme of creatine kinase	WBC	White blood cell(s)
		WHO	World Health Organization
mEq/L	Milliequivalents per liter		
		wk	Week, weeks
min	Minute, minutes	yr	Year, years
mm^3	Cubic millimeter, microliter (μL)		

Table 727-3	Abbreviations for Specimens in Table 727-5		
S	Serum	(C)	Citrate
P	Plasma	(O)	Oxalate
(H)	Heparin	W	Whole blood
(LiH)	Lithium heparin	(NH₄H)	Ammonium heparinate
(E)	Ethylenediaminetetraacetic acid (EDTA)		

Table 727-4	Key to Comments Section of Table 727-5		
30°C, 37°C	Temperature of enzymatic analysis (Celsius)	l	Fluorometric method
a	Values obtained are significantly method dependent	m	Fluorescence-activated cell sorting (FACS)
		n	Fluorescence polarization
b	Values in older males are higher than those in older females	o	Gas chromatography
c	Values in older females are higher than those in older males	p	High-performance liquid chromatography (HPLC)
		q	Indirect fluorescence antibody (IFA) assay
d	Atomic absorption	r	Ion-selective electrode
e	Borate affinity chromatography	s	Nephelometry
f	Cation-exchange chromatography	t	Optical density
g	Vitros, a proprietary analytic system of Ortho Clinical Diagnostics, Inc.	u	Radial immunodiffusion (RID)
		v	Radioimmunoassay (RIA)
i	Electrophoresis	w	Spectrophotometry
j	Enzymatic assay		
k	Enzyme-amplified immunoassay		

Table 727-5	Reference Intervals*				
ANALYTE OR PROCEDURE	**SPECIMEN**	**REFERENCE VALUES (US)†**	**CONVERSION FACTOR**	**REFERENCE VALUES (SI)†**	**COMMENTS**
COMPLETE BLOOD COUNT					
Hematocrit (HCT, Hct)	W(E)	% of packed red cells (V red cells/V whole blood cells × 100)		Volume fraction (V red cells/V whole blood)	
Calculated from mean corpuscular volume (MCV) and RBC count (electronic displacement or laser)	0-30 days 1-23 mo 2-9 yr 10-17 yr M F >18-99 yr M F	44-70% 32-42% 33-43% 36-47% 35-45% 42-52% 37-47%	×0.01	0.44-0.70 0.32-0.42 0.33-0.43 0.36-0.47 0.35-0.45 0.42-0.52 0.37-0.47	
Hemoglobin (Hb)	W(E)	g/dL		mmol/L	
		0-30 days 1-23 mo 2-9 yr 10-17 yr M F >18-99 yr M F	15.0-24.0 10.5-14.0 11.5-14.5 12.5-16.1 12.0-15.0 13.5-18.0 12.5-16.0	×0.155	2.32-3.72 1.63-2.17 1.78-2.25 1.93-2.50 1.86-2.32 2.09-2.79 1.93-2.48	MW Hb = 64,500
	P(H)	See Chemical Elements			

Continued

Table 727-5 | Reference Intervals—cont'd

ANALYTE OR PROCEDURE	SPECIMEN	REFERENCE VALUES (US)[†]		CONVERSION FACTOR	REFERENCE VALUES (SI)[†]	COMMENTS
Erythrocyte indices (RBC indices)						
Mean corpuscular hemoglobin (MCH)	W(E)		pg/cell	×0.0155	fmol/cell	
		0-30 days	33-39		0.51-0.60	
		1-23 mo	24-30		0.37-0.46	
		2-9 yr	25-31		0.39-0.48	
		10-17 yr M	26-32		0.26-0.32	
		F	26-32		0.26-0.32	
		>18-99 yr M	27-31		0.27-0.31	
		F	27-31		0.27-0.31	
Mean corpuscular hemoglobin concentration (MCHC)	W(E)		% Hb/cell or g Hb/dL RBC		mmol Hb/L RBC	
			32-36	×0.155	4.96-5.58	
Mean corpuscular volume (MCV)	W(E)		μm^3		fL	
		0-30 days	99-115	×1	99-115	
		1-23 mo	72-88		72-88	
		2-9 yr	76-90		76-90	
		10-17 yr	78-95		78-95	
		>18-99 yr	78-100		78-100	
Leukocyte count (WBC count)	W(E)	×1,000 cells/mm^3 (μL)			×109 cells/L	
		0-30 days	9.1-34.0	×1	9.1-34.0	
		1-23 mo	6.0-14.0		6.0-14.0	
		2-9 yr	4.0-12.0		45.0-12.0	
		10-17 yr	4.0-10.5		4.0-10.5	
		18-99 yr	4.0-10.5		4.0-10.5	
Leukocyte differential	W(E)	%			Number fraction	
Myelocytes		0%		×0.01	0	
Neutrophils ("bands")		3-5%			0.03-0.05	
Neutrophils ("segs")		54-62%			0.54-0.62	
Lymphocytes		25-33%			0.25-0.33	
Monocytes		3-7%			0.03-0.07	
Eosinophils		1-3%			0.01-0.03	
Basophils		0-0.75%			0-0.0075	
		Cells/mm^3 (μL)			×106 cells/L	
Myelocytes		0		×1	0	
Neutrophils ("bands")		150-400			150-400	
Neutrophils ("segs")		3,000-5,800			3,000-5,800	
Lymphocytes		1,500-3,000			1,500-3,000	
Monocytes		285-500			285-500	
Eosinophils		50-250			50-250	
Basophils		15-50			15-50	
Platelet count (thrombocyte count)	W(E)	×103/mm^3 (μL)			×109/L	
		Newborn 84-478 (after 1 wk, same as adult)		×106	84-478	(Buck, 1996)
		Adult 150-400			150-400	
Reticulocyte count	W(E,H,O)	Adults 0.5-1.5% of erythrocytes or 25,000-75,000/mm^3 (μL)		×0.01 ×106	0.005-0.015 (number fraction) or 25,000-75,000 × 106/L	
	W(cap)	%			Number fraction	
		1 day	0.4-6.0	×0.01	0.004-0.060	
		7 days	<0.1-1.3		<0.001-0.013	
		1-4 wk	<1.0-1.2		<0.001-0.012	
		5-6 wk	<0.1-2.4		<0.001-0.024	
		7-8 wk	0.1-2.9		0.001-0.029	
		9-10 wk	<0.1-2.6		<0.001-0.026	
		11-12 wk	0.1-1.3		0.001-0.013	

Table 727-5	Reference Intervals—cont'd					
ANALYTE OR PROCEDURE	**SPECIMEN**	**REFERENCE VALUES (US)†**		**CONVERSION FACTOR**	**REFERENCE VALUES (SI)†**	**COMMENTS**
Alanine aminotransferase (ALT, SGPT)	S	0-7 days 8-30 days M F 1-12 mo 1-19 yr	6-40 U/L 10-40 8-32 12-45 5-45	×1	6-40 U/L 10-40 8-32 12-45 5-45	37°C, bgw (Soldin, Savwoir, Guo, 1997) (Lockitch, Halstead, Albersheim, 1988)
Albumin (BCG)	P	Premature 1 day Full term <6 days 8 days-1 yr 1-3 yr 4-19 yr	1.8-3.0 g/dL 2.5-3.4 1.9-4.9 3.4-4.2 3.5-5.6	×10	18-30 g/dL 25-34 19-49 34-42 35-56	g (Meites, 1989) (Soldin Morse, 1998) (Lockitch, Halstead, Albersheim, 1988)
Ammonia	P		11-35 µmol/L	×1	11-35 µmol/L	g
Amylase	S,P	1-19 yr	30-100 U/L % pancreatic fraction	×1	30-100 U/L % pancreatic fraction	(Lockitch, Halstead, Albersheim et al, 1988; Gillard, Simbala, Goodglick, 1983)
Amylase isoenzymes	S,P(H)	Cord-8 mo 9 mo-4 yr 5-19 yr	0-34% 5-56% 23-59%	×0.01	0-0.34% 0.05-0.56% 0.23-0.59%	
Anion gap (sodium − [chloride + bicarbonate])	P(H)	7-16 mEq/L		×1	7-16 mEq/L	
Antideoxyribonuclease B titer (anti-DNase B titer)	S	Age 4-6 yr 7-12 yr	Upper limit of normal 240-480 U 480-800 U	×1	Upper limit of normal 240-480 U 480-800 U	(Kaplan, Rothermel, Johnson, 1998)
Antidiuretic hormone (hADH, vasopressin)	P(E)	Plasma osmolarity (mOsm/kg) 270-280 280-285 285-290 290-295 295-300	Plasma ADH (pg/mL) <1.5 <2.5 1-5 2-7 4-12	×1	Plasma ADH ng/L <1.5 <2.5 1-5 2-7 4-12	
Antistreptolysin-O titer (ASO titer)	S	Age 2-5 yr 6-9 yr 10-12 yr	Upper limit of normal 120-160 Todd units 240 Todd units 320 Todd units	×1	Upper limit of normal 120-160 Todd units 240 Todd units 320 Todd units	(Kaplan et al, 1998)
Aspartate aminotransferase (AST, SGOT)	S	0-7 days M F 8-30 days 1-12 mo 1-3 yr 3-9 yr 10-15 yr 16-19 yr M F	U/L 30-100 24-95 22-71 22-63 20-60 15-50 10-40 15-45 5-30	×1	U/L 35-100 24-95 22-71 22-63 20-60 15-50 10-40 15-45 5-30	37°C, g (Soldin, Savwoir, Guo, 1997) (Lockitch, Halstead, Albersheim, 1988)
Base excess	W(H)	 Newborn Infant Child Thereafter	mmol/L (−10)-(−2) (−7)-(−1) (−4)-(+2) (−3)-(+3)	×1	mmol/L (−10)-(−2) (−7)-(−1) (−4)-(+2) (−3)-(−3)	
Bicarbonate	S,P	 Arterial Venous	mmol/L 21-28 22-29	×1	mmol/L 21-28 22-29	

Continued

Table 727-5	Reference Intervals—cont'd

ANALYTE OR PROCEDURE	SPECIMEN	REFERENCE VALUES (US)[†]		CONVERSION FACTOR	REFERENCE VALUES (SI)[†]		COMMENTS
Bilirubin, total	S		mg/dL		µmol/L		
		Newborn	See Bhutani nomogram (Fig. 727-3)	×17.1			(Bhutani, Johnson, Sivieri, 1999)
		1 mo-adult	<1.0		<17		
C-reactive protein (high sensitivity)	S						(Soldin, et al, 2004)
			M (mg/dL)	F (mg/dL)	M (mg/L)	F (mg/L)	
		0-90 days	0.08-1.58	0.09-1.58	×10	0.8-15.8	0.9-15.8	
		91 days-12 mo	0.08-1.12	0.05-0.79		0.8-11.2	0.5-7.9	
		13 mo-3 yr	0.08-1.12	0.08-0.79		0.8-11.2	0.8-7.9	
		4-10 yr	0.06-0.79	0.5-1.0		0.6-7.9	0.5-10.0	
		11-14 yr	0.08-0.76	0.06-0.81		0.8-7.6	0.6-8.1	
		15-18 yr	0.04-0.79	0.06-0.79		0.4-7.9	0.6-7.9	
Calcium, ionized (Ca)	S,P(H),W(H)		mg/dL		mmol/L		
		Cord blood	5.0-6.0	×0.25	1.25-1.50		
		Newborn, 3-24 hr	4.3-5.1		1.07-1.27		
		24-48 hr	4.0-4.7		1.00-1.17		
		Thereafter	4.8-4.92		1.12-1.23		
		or	2.24-2.46 Eq/L	×0.5	1.12-1.23		
Calcium, total	S		mg/dL		mmol/L		
		Cord blood	9.0-11.5	×0.25	2.25-2.88		
		Newborn, 3-24 hr	9.0-10.6		2.3-2.65		
		24-48 hr	7.0-12.0		1.75-3.00		
		4-7 days	9.0-10.9		2.25-2.73		
		Child	8.8-10.8		2.20-2.70		
		Thereafter	8.4-10.2		2.10-2.55		
Carbon dioxide, partial pressure (pCO₂)	W(H)		mm Hg		kPa		
		Newborn	27-40	×0.1333	3.6-5.3		
		Infant	27-41		3.6-5.5		
		Thereafter M	35-48		4.7-6.4		
		F	32-45		4.3-6.0		
Carbon monoxide (carboxyhemoglobin)	W(E)	Nonsmoker	<2% HbCO	×0.01	HbCO fraction <0.02		
		Smoker	<10%		<0.10		
		Lethal	>50%		>0.5		
Chloride	S,P(H)	Cord blood	96-104 mmol/L	×1	96-104 mmol/L		
		Newborn	97-110		97-110		
		Thereafter	98-106		98-106		
Chloride, sweat	Sweat		mmol/L				(Farrell, et al, 2008)
		0-5 mo	≤29	CF unlikely			
			30-59	intermediate			
			≥60	indicative of CF			
		≥6 mo	≤39	CF unlikely			
			40-60	intermediate			
			≥60	indicative of CF			
Cortisol	S,P(H)		µg/dL		nmol/L		
		Newborn	1-24	×27.59	28-662		
		Adults, 8:00 AM	5-23		138-635		
		4:00 PM	3-15		82-413		
		8:00 PM	<50% of 8:00 AM	×0.01	Fraction of 8:00 AM ≤0.50		
Creatine kinase	S	Cord blood	70-380 U/L	×1	70-380 U/L		30°C, b (Jedeikin, et al, 1982)
		5-8 hr	214-1,175		214-1,175		
		24-33 hr	130-1,200		130-1,200		
		72-100 hr	87-725		87-725		
		Adult	5-130		5-130		
Creatine kinase isoenzymes	S		% MB		% BB		
		Cord blood	0.3-3.1		0.3-10.5		
		5-8 hr	1.7-7.9		3.6-13.4		
		24-33 hr	1.8-5.0		2.3-8.6		
		72-100 hr	1.4-5.4		5.1-13.3		
		Adult	0-2		0		

Table 727-5	Reference Intervals—cont'd

ANALYTE OR PROCEDURE	SPECIMEN	REFERENCE VALUES (US)[†]		CONVERSION FACTOR	REFERENCE VALUES (SI)[†]		COMMENTS
Creatinine (IDMS)							
Enzymatic	S,P		mg/dL			μmol/L	g
		0-4 yr	0.03-0.50	×88.4		2.65-44.2	
		4-7 yr	0.03-0.59			2.65-52.2	
		7-10 yr	0.22-0.59			19.4-52.2	
		10-14 yr	0.31-0.88			27.4-77.8	
		>14 yr	0.50-1.06			44.2-93.7	
Creatinine clearance (endogenous)	S,P,U	Newborn 40-65 mL/min/1.73 m^2 <40 yr, M 97-137 F 88-128 Decreases <6.5 mL/min/decade					
Ferritin	S		ng/mL			μg/L	
		0-6 wk	0-400	×1		0-400	
		7 wk-365 days	10-95			10-95	
		1-9 yr	10-60			10-60	
		10-18 yr M	10-300			10-300	
		F	10-70			10-70	
Folate	S	Newborn 7.0-32 ng/mL Thereafter 1.8-9.0		×2.265	15.9-72.4 nmol/L 4.1-20.4		
	W(E)	150-450 ng/mL RBCs			340-1,020 nmol/L cells		
Glucose	S		mg/dL			mmol/L	
		Cord blood	45-96	×0.0555		2.5-5.3	
		Premature	20-60			1.1-3.3	
		Neonate	30-60			1.7-3.3	
		Newborn					
		1 day	40-60			2.2-3.3	
		>1 day	50-90			2.8-5.0	
		Child	60-100			3.3-5.5	
		Adult	70-105			3.9-5.8	
	W(H)	Adult	65-95			3.6-5.3	
Glucose, 2 hr post	S	<120			<6.7		

ANALYTE OR PROCEDURE	SPECIMEN	REFERENCE VALUES (US)[†]			CONVERSION FACTOR	REFERENCE VALUES (SI)[†]			COMMENTS
Glucose tolerance test (GTT) (see Chapter 589) Oral dose Adult: 75 g Child: 1.75 g/kg of ideal weight, up to a maximum of 75 g	S		mg/dL				mmol/L		
			Normal	Diabetic			Normal	Diabetic	
		Fasting	70-105	≥126	×0.0555		3.9-5.8	≥7.0	(Diabetes Care, 2010)
		120 min	70-120	≥200			3.9-6.7	≥11	

ANALYTE OR PROCEDURE	SPECIMEN	REFERENCE VALUES (US)[†]		CONVERSION FACTOR	REFERENCE VALUES (SI)[†]		COMMENTS
Glucose-6-phosphate dehydrogenase (G6PD) in erythrocytes	W(E,H,C)						
Bishop, modified		Adult 3.4-8.0 U/g Hb 98.6-232 U/1012 RBC 1.16-2.72 U/mL RBC Newborn: 50% higher		×0.0645 ×10−3 ×1	Adult 0.22-0.52 mU/mol Hb 0.10-0.23 nU/106 RBC 1.16-2.72 kU/L RBC Newborn: 50% higher		
γ-Glutamyl transpeptidase (GGT, GGTP)	S		U/L			U/L	37°C, b (Knight and Haymond, 1981)
		Cord blood	37-193	×1		37-193	
		0-1 mo	13-147			13-147	
		1-2 mo	12-123			12-123	
		2-4 mo	8-90			8-90	
		4 mo-10 yr	5-32			5-32	
		10-15 yr	5-24			5-24	
Immunoglobulin A (IgA)	S		mg/dL			mg/L	s (Meites, 1989)
		Cord blood	1.4-3.6	×10		14-36	
		1-3 mo	1.3-53			13-530	
		4-6 mo	4.4-84			44-840	
		7 mo-1 yr	11-106			110-1,060	
		2-5 yr	14-159			140-1,590	
		6-10 yr	33-236			330-2,360	
		Adult	70-312			700-3,120	

Continued

Table 727-5 | Reference Intervals—cont'd

ANALYTE OR PROCEDURE	SPECIMEN	REFERENCE VALUES (US)[†]		CONVERSION FACTOR	REFERENCE VALUES (SI)[†]		COMMENTS
Immunoglobulin D (IgD)	S	Newborn: none detected			None detected		
		Thereafter: 0-8 mg/dL		×10	0-80 mg/L		
Immunoglobulin E (IgE)	S	M 0-230 IU/mL		×1	0-230 kIU/L		
		F 0-170			0-170		
Immunoglobulin G (IgG)	S		mg/dL		g/L		
		Cord blood	636-1,606	×0.01	6.36-16.06		s (Meites, 1989)
		1 mo	251-906		2.51-9.06		
		2-4 mo	176-601		1.76-6.01		
		5-12 mo	172-1,069		1.72-10.69		
		1-5 yr	345-1,236		3.45-12.36		
		6-10 yr	608-1,572		6.08-15.72		
		Adult	639-1,349		6.39-13.49		
Immunoglobulin M (IgM)	S		mg/dL		mg/L		
		Cord blood	6.3-25	×10	63-250		s (Meites, 1989)
		1-4 mo	17-105		170-1,050		
		5-9 mo	33-126		330-1,260		
		10 mo-1 yr	41-173		410-1,730		
		2-8 yr	43-207		430-2,070		
		9-10 yr	52-242		520-2,420		
		Adult	56-352		560-3,520		
Iron	P	All ages	22-184 µg/dL	×0.1791	4-33 µmol/L		(Lockitch, Halstead, Wadsworth, et al, 1988)
Iron-binding capacity, total (TIBC)	S	Infant 100-400 µg/dL		×0.179	17.90-71.60 µmol/L		
		Thereafter 250-400			44.75-71.60		
L-lactate (perchloric acid)	W		mg/dL		mmol/L		
		1-12 mo	10-21	×1	1.1-2.3		(Bonnefont, et al, 1990)
		1-7 yr	7-14		0.8-1.5		
		7-15 yr	5-8		0.6-0.9		
D-lactate	P(H)						j (Rosenthal and Pesce, 1985)
		6 mo-3 yr	0.0-0.3	×1	0.0-0.3		
Lactate dehydrogenase	S		U/L		U/L		
		<1 yr	170-580	×1	170-580		37°C, a (Meites, 1989)
		1-9 yr	150-500		150-500		
		10-19 yr	120-330		120-330		
Isoenzymes	S	% of total activity					
			1-6 yr	7-19 yr			
		LD1	20-38	20-35			
		LD2	27-38	31-38			
		LD3	16-26	19-28			
		LD4	5-16	7-13			
		LD5	3-13	5-12			
Lead	W(H)		µg/dL		mmol/L		
		Child	<5	×0.0483	<0.0024		
		Toxic	≥70		≥3.38		
Lipase	P,S	1-18 yr	145-216 U/L	×1	145-216 U/L		(Ghoshal and Soldin, 2003)
Magnesium	P(H)		mg/dL		mmol/L		
		0-6 days	1.2-2.6	×0.411	0.48-1.05		w (Meites, 1989)
		7 days-2 yr	1.6-2.6		0.65-1.05		
		2-14 yr	1.5-2.3		0.60-0.95		
		0.78 ± 0.37% of total Hb		×0.01	0.0078 ± 0.0037 (mass fraction)		
Osmolality	S	Child, adult					
		275-295 mOsm/kg H_2O					
Phosphatase, alkaline	S		U/L		U/L		
		1-9 yr	145-420	×1	145-420		37°C, aw
		10-11 yr	140-560		140-560		
			M	F		M	F
		12-13 yr	200-495	105-420		200-495	105-420
		14-15 yr	130-525	70-230		130-525	70-230
		16-19 yr	65-260	50-130		65-260	50-130

Table 727-5	Reference Intervals—cont'd				
ANALYTE OR PROCEDURE	**SPECIMEN**	**REFERENCE VALUES (US)**[†]		**CONVERSION FACTOR**	**REFERENCE VALUES (SI)**[†]	**COMMENTS**

ANALYTE OR PROCEDURE	SPECIMEN	REFERENCE VALUES (US)[†]		CONVERSION FACTOR	REFERENCE VALUES (SI)[†]	COMMENTS
Phosphorus, inorganic	S,P(H)		mg/dL	×0.3229	mmol/L	w (Meites, 1989)
		0-5 days	4.8-8.2		1.55-2.65	
		1-3 yr	3.8-6.5		1.25-2.10	
		4-11 yr	3.7-5.6		1.20-1.80	
		12-15 yr	2.9-5.4		0.95-1.75	
		16-19 yr	2.7-4.7		0.90-1.50	
Potassium	S		mmol/L		mmol/L	(Greeley, et al, 1993)
		0-1 wk	3.2-5.5	×1	3.3-5.5	Increased by hemolysis; serum values systematically higher than plasma values
		1 wk-1 mo	3.4-6.0		3.4-6.0	
		1-6 mo	3.5-5.6		3.5-5.6	
		6 mo-1 yr	3.5-6.1		3.5-6.1	
		>1 yr	3.3-4.6		3.3-4.6	
	P(H)	3.5-4.5 mmol/L			3.5-4.5 mmol/L	
Prealbumin (transthyretin)	S		mg/dL		mg/L	s (Lockitch, Halstead, Quigley, et al, 1988)
		0-5 days	6.0-21.0	×10	60-210	
		1-5 yr	14.0-30.0		140-300	
		6-9 yr	15.0-30.0		150-300	
		10-13 yr	20.0-36.0		200-360	
		14-19	22.0-45.0		220-450	
Protein, total	S		g/dL		g/L	(Meites, 1989)
		Premature	4.3-7.6	×10	43-76	
		Newborn	4.6-7.4		46-74	
		1-7 yr	6.1-7.9		61-79	
		8-12 yr	6.4-8.1		64-81	
		13-19 yr	6.6-8.2		66-82	
Pyruvate (perchloric acid)	W	7-17 yr	0.076 ± 0.026 mmol/L	×1	0.076 ± 0.026 mmol/L	(Pianosi, Seargeant, Haworth, 1995)
Sodium	S,P (LiH, NH₄H)		mmol/L		mmol/L	g (Greely, Snell, Colaco, 1993)
		Newborn	133-146	×1	133-146	
		Infant	134-144		134-144	
		Child	134-143		134-143	
		Thereafter	135-145		135-145	
Thyroid-stimulating hormone	S		μIU/L		μIU/L	g (Dugaw, Jack, Rutledge, 2001)
		0-3 days	1.00-20.00	×1	1.0-20.00	
		3-30 days	0.5-6.5		0.50-6.50	
		1-5 mo	0.5-6.0		0.5-6.0	
		6 mo-18 yr	0.5-4.5		0.5-4.5	
Thyroid uptake of radioactive iodine	Activity over thyroid gland	2 hr	<6%	×0.01	2 hr <0.06	
		6 hr	3-20%		6 hr 0.03-0.20	
		24 hr	8-30%		24 hr 0.08-0.30	
Thyroid uptake of technetium-99m	Activity over thyroid gland	After 24 hr	0.4-3.0%	×0.01	Fractional uptake 0.004-0.030	
Thyrotropin-releasing hormone (TRH)	P	5-60 pg/mL		×2.759	14-165 pmol/L	
Thyroxine-binding globulin (TBG)	S		mg/dL		mg/L	
		Cord blood	1.4-9.4	×10	14-94	
		1-4 wk	1.0-9.0		10-90	
		1-12 mo	2.0-7.6		20-76	
		1-5 yr	2.9-5.4		29-54	
		5-10 yr	2.5-5.0		25-50	
		10-15 yr	2.1-4.6		21-46	
		Adult	1.5-3.4		15-34	

Continued

Table 727-5 | Reference Intervals—cont'd

ANALYTE OR PROCEDURE	SPECIMEN	REFERENCE VALUES (US)†		CONVERSION FACTOR	REFERENCE VALUES (SI)†	COMMENTS
Thyroxine, total	S		μg/dL		nmol/L	g (Dugaw, Jack, Rutledge, 2001)
		0-3 days	8.0-20.0	×12.9	103-258	
		3-30 days	5.0-15.0		64-193	
		31-365 days	6.0-14.0		77-180	
		1-5 yr	4.5-11.0		58-142	
		6-18 yr	4.5-10.0		58-129	
Thyroxine, free	S		ng/dL		pmol/L	g (Dugaw, Jack, Rutledge, 2001)
		0-3 days	2.00-5.00	×12.9	25.7-64.3	
		3-30 days	0.90-2.20		11.6-28.3	
		31 days-18 yr	0.7-2.00		9.0-25.7	
Thyroxine, total	W	Newborn screen (filter paper) 6.2-22.0 μg/dL		×12.9	80-283 nmol/L	
Triiodothyronine, free	S		pg/dL		pmol/L	
		Cord blood	20-240	×0.01536	0.3-3.7	
		1-3 days	200-610		3.1-9.4	
		6 wk	240-560		3.7-8.6	
		Adult (20-50 yr)	230-660		3.5-10.0	
Triiodothyronine resin uptake test (T3RU)	S		Fractional uptake			
		Newborn 26-36%		×0.01	0.26-0.36	
		Thereafter 26-35%			0.26-0.35	
Triiodothyronine, total	S		ng/dL		nmol/L	g (Dugaw, Jack, Rutledge, 2001)
		0-3 days	60-300	×0.0154	0.9-4.7	
		4-365 days	90-260		1.4-4.0	
		1-6 yr	90-240		1.4-3.7	
		7-11 yr	90-230		1.4-3.6	
		12-18 yr	100-210		1.5-3.3	
Urea nitrogen	S,P		mg/dL		mmol/L	
		Cord blood	21-40	×0.357	7.5-14.3	
		Premature (1 wk)	3-25		1.1-9.0	
		Newborn	3-12		1.1-4.3	
		infant or child	5-18		1.8-6.4	
		Thereafter	7-18		2.5-6.4	
Uric acid	S		mg/dL		μmol/L	(Lockitch, Halstead, Albersheim, et al, 1988)
		1-3 yr	1.8-5.0	×59.48	100-300	
		4-6 yr	2.2-4.7		130-280	
		7-9 yr	2.0-5.0		120-295	
		10-11 yr M	2.3-5.4		135-320	
		10-11 yr F	3.0-4.7		180-280	
		12-13 yr	2.7-6.7		160-400	
		14-15 yr M	2.4-7.8		140-465	
		12-15 yr F	3.0-5.8		180-345	
		16-19 yr M	4.0-8.6		235-510	
		16-19 yr F	3.0-5.9		180-350	

*In preparing the reference range listings, a number of abbreviations, symbols, and codes were used (see Table 727-2).
†Reference values are shown in SI units (International System of Units) and US units (Traditional Units).]

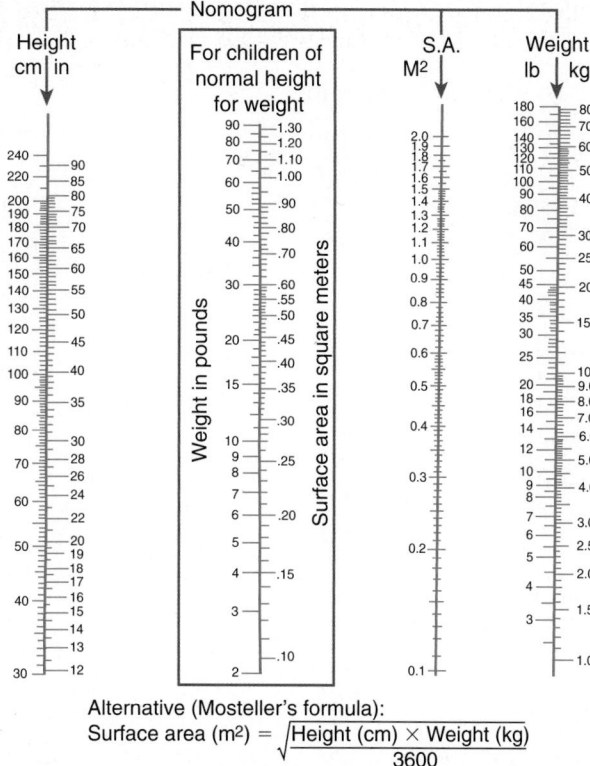

Alternative (Mosteller's formula):
$$\text{Surface area (m}^2) = \sqrt{\frac{\text{Height (cm)} \times \text{Weight (kg)}}{3600}}$$

Figure 727-1 Nomogram for the estimation of surface area. The surface area is indicated where a straight line that connects the height and weight levels intersects the surface area column, or if the patient is roughly of average size, from the weight alone *(enclosed area)*. *(Nomogram modified from the data of E. Boyd by C.D. West. See also Briars GL, Bailey BJ: Surface area estimation: pocket calculator v nomogram, Arch Dis Child 70:246–247, 1994.)*

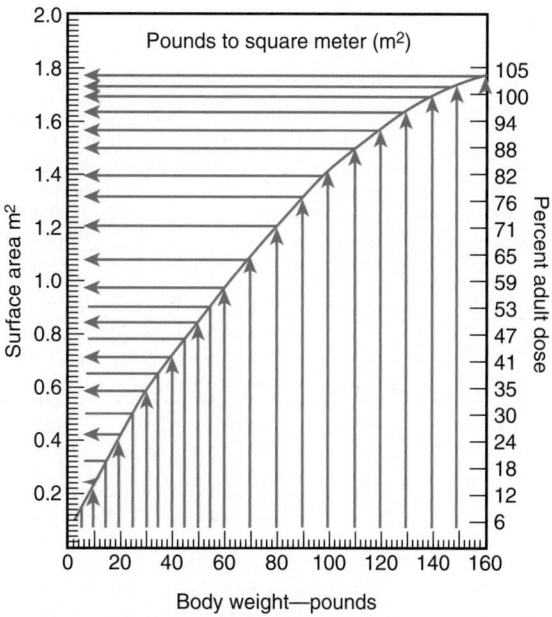

Figure 727-2 Relationships among body weight (lb), body surface area, and adult dosage. The surface area values correspond with those set forth by Crawford JD, Terry ME, Rourke GM: Simplification of drug dosage calculation by application of the surface area principle, *Pediatrics 5:783–790, 1950.* Note that the 100% adult dose is for a patient weighing approximately 140 lb and having a surface area of approximately 1.7 m². *(From Talbot NB, Richie RH, Crawford JH: Metabolic homeostasis: a syllabus for those concerned with the care of patients, Cambridge, MA, 1959, Harvard University Press.)*

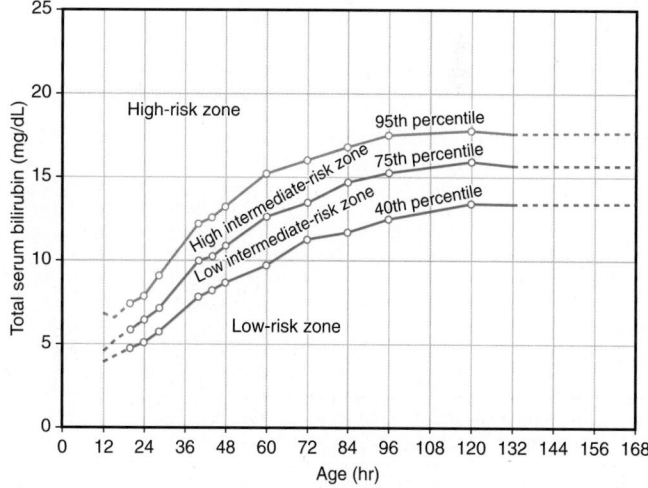

Figure 727-3 Nomogram for risk assessment of hyperbilirubinemia. *(From Bhutani VK, Johnson L, Sivieri EM: Predictive ability of a predischarge hour-specific serum bilirubin for subsequent significant hyperbilirubinemia in healthy term and near-term newborns, Pediatrics 103:6–14, 1999, Fig. 2, p. 9.)*

Index

Page numbers followed by "*f*" indicate figures, "*t*" indicate tables, and "*b*" indicate boxes.

Volume 1 • pp 1–1756 • Volume 2 • pp 1757–3474

I1

Anti-*N*-methyl-D-aspartate receptor encephalitis, 2906*t*, 2907, 2908*t*
Anti-Ro ± anti-La pregnancy, 1181*f*
Antiandrogens, in polycystic ovary syndrome, 2619*f*, 2621-2622
Antiarrhythmic therapy, 2250-2251
Antibiotic-associated diarrhea, microbiome during, 1240-1241
Antibiotic treatment
  for acute bacterial meningitis (postneonatal), 2945*t*
    duration of therapy, 2941-2944
    initial therapy, 2941
  for bacterial conjunctivitis, 3039*t*
  for Crohn disease, 1830
  for cystic fibrosis
    aerosolized therapy, 2108
    intravenous therapy, 2108-2109
    oral therapy, 2108
  for diarrhea, 1873
  for infectious diarrhea, 1874*t*
  for Lyme disease, 1486-1487
  for meningococcal infection, 1360-1361
  for osteomyelitis, 3326-3327
  for persistent diarrhea, 1882*t*
  for pertussis, 1380
  for pharyngitis, 2020*t*
  principles of therapy, 1298-1315
    age- and risk-specific use of antibiotics, 1299-1301
    antibiotics commonly used in pediatric practice, 1301-1315
  prophylactic regimens
    for dental procedure, 2269*t*
    for *Neisseria meningitidis* infection, 1363*t*
  resistance, of *Haemophilus influenzae*, 1372
  for rheumatic fever, 1336
  for septic arthritis, 3329
  topical, for acne, 3231
  for typhoid fever, 1392*t*
  for vulvovaginal infections, 2610*t*
Antibiotics. *See also specific types of antibiotics*
  causing serum sickness, 1136*t*
  intrapartum, 913, 919*t*
  perioperative prophylactic, 1263*t*
  preoperative, in appendicitis, 1893
  reactions to, 1147
  in stabilization of severe acute malnutrition, 304*t*
  topical, 3115
Antibodies
  anti-glomerular basement membrane, 2087
  antiganglioside, 3011*t*
  cold, 2328*t*-2329*t*
  EBV specific, 1589-1590
  IgG, 1000-1001
  in induction therapy
    IL-2, 2550
    T-cell, 2549-2550
  primary defects in production of, 1012-1018
  TSH receptor-blocking, 2667
  warm, 2328*t*-2329*t*
Antibody deficiencies, 1005*t*
  genetic basis of primary disorders of, 1013*t*
  main phenotypes of, 1016*t*
Antibody response, primary and secondary, 1011
Anticholinergic agents
  for allergic diseases, 1084
  for asthma, 1112
  poisoning, 453*t*-454*t*
Anticholinergic syndromes, 953*t*
Anticipation, genetic, 602*f*
Anticipatory guidance
  for children in foster care, 229*t*
  for children with disabilities, 3413
  for establishing healthy eating habits, 316*t*

Anticipatory guidance *(Continued)*
  injury prevention topics, 43*t*
  in palliative care, 258-267
  in well-child care, 38
Anticipatory guidance: sickle cell disease
  echocardiography, 2345
  hydroxyurea, 2345
  immunizations, 2344-2345
  prophylactic penicillin, 2344
  pulmonary and asthma screening, 2345
  regular blood transfusion therapy, 2345
  renal, 2345
  retinopathy, 2345
  spleen palpation, 2344
  transcranial Doppler ultrasound, 2345
Anticoagulant therapy, 2395-2397
  in cerebral sinovenous thrombosis, 2929-2930
Anticoagulants, reference values, 2383*t*
Anticonvulsants, for migraine headaches, 2869*t*-2870*t*
Antidepressants
  for attenuated psychosis syndrome, 187
  atypical
    for depression and anxiety symptoms, 130*t*
    poisoning, 462-463
  in pain management, 439-440
  for psychiatric disorders, 130-131
  tricyclic. *See* Tricyclic antidepressants
Antidiuretic hormone. *See* Arginine vasopressin
Antidopaminergic drugs, for migraines, 2871
Antidotes for poisoning, 453*t*-454*t*
  cyanide antidote kit, 466, 3446
Antiepileptic drugs
  adverse effects, 2846*t*
  choosing
    according to seizure type, 2840-2841
    based on comparative effectiveness, 2841-2844
  discontinuation, 2848
  dosages, 2844*t*-2845*t*
    in status epilepticus, 2855*t*
  hormones and, 2633
  initiating and monitoring therapy, 2844-2847
  mechanisms of action, 2839-2840
  in pain management, 440
  side effects, 2847-2848
  teratogenesis and perinatal outcomes of, 2843*t*
Antifibrinolytics, 2392*t*
Antifungal therapy
  for allergic bronchopulmonary aspergillosis, 2083-2084
  azoles
    fluconazole, 1513
    itraconazole, 1513-1514
    posaconazole, 1514
    voriconazole, 1514
  dosing of antifungal agents for treatment of invasive disease, 1518*t*
  echinocandins
    anidulafungin, 1515
    caspofungin, 1514-1515
    micafungin, 1515
  empirical, for invasive *Aspergillus* infections, 1525
  polyenes, amphotericin B, 1512-1513
  pyrimidine analogs, 5-fluorocytosine, 1513
  topical agents, 3115
Antigen challenge, by inhalation, 2070
Antigen deficiencies
  MHC class I, 1026
  MHC class II, 1026-1027
Antigen detection tests, 1235-1236
  Coccidioides, 1530
Antigen-presenting cells (APCs), 1010
  in allergic disease, 1075-1076
Antigen sources, associated with hypersensitivity pneumonitis, 2068*t*

Antihistamines
  for allergic diseases, 1084-1085
  for allergic rhinitis, 1090-1091
  for atopic dermatitis, 1119
  in management of anaphylaxis, 1135*t*
  second-generation, 1092*t*
Antihypertensives
  management of severe hypertension, 2303*t*
  recommended doses, 2301*t*
Antiimmunoglobulin E, 1086
  for asthma, 1110-1111
Antiinflammatory agents
  for cystic fibrosis, 2109
  for rheumatic fever, 1336
Antiinflammatory cytokines, 1009*t*
Antimetabolites, for atopic dermatitis, 1120
Antimicrobial agents
  for acne, 3231*t*-3232*t*
  for brucellosis, 1421*t*
  for cholera, 1402*t*
  for cystic fibrosis lung infection, 2108*t*
  for *M. pneumoniae*, 1489-1490
  for otitis media
    first-line treatment, 3092-3093
    second-line treatment, 3094
  parenteral, treatment of *S. aureus* infections, 1319*t*
Antimicrobial prophylaxis, in vesicoureteral reflux, 2565-2566
Antimicrobial resistance
  of enterococci, 1343
  of *N. gonorrhoeae*, 1368
  in neonates, 924
  patterns of, 1298-1299
  prevention of, 925
Antimicrobial susceptibility testing, 1234
Antimony, foodborne illness, 1863*t*
Antimotility agents, in diarrhea treatment, 1873
Antimüllerian hormone (AMH), 2730, 2733, 2736, 2750
Antineutrophil cytoplasmic antibody (ANCA)
  in diffuse alveolar hemorrhage, 2121
  in eosinophilic granulomatosis with polyangiitis, 2082
Antineutrophil cytoplasmic antibody (ANCA)-associated vasculitis, 1215*t*, 1221-1224
Antinuclear antibody (ANA)
  in JIA, 1163, 1164*t*
  in rheumatic disease, 1152
  in SLE, 1177, 1179
Antioxidant deficiency, and porphyria cutanea tarda, 767
Antiparasitic therapy, for persistent diarrhea, 1882*t*
Antiphospholipid antibodies, in SLE, 1179
Antiplasmin deficiency, 2389
Antiplatelet therapy, 2397
Antipsychotics
  for aggressive behaviors, 174
  atypical, 131, 132*t*
  for autism spectrum disorder, 183*t*
  in pain management, 441
  poisoning, 463
  for schizophrenia, 188
  typical, 131, 131*t*
Antiquitin deficiency, 675
Antiretroviral therapy
  adherence to, 1661
  changing regimens, 1661
  combination, 1654-1661
  dosing, 1661
  drug summaries, 1655*t*-1660*t*
  highly active, and development of IRIS, 1455
  hypersensitivity to agents used in, 1148
  initiation of therapy, 1661
  monitoring, 1662
  and number of AIDS-related deaths over time, 5*f*

Dysplasias *(Continued)*
  fibrous, 2475
    polyostotic, 2660-2661
  focal cortical, 2809
  focal facial dermal, 3120
  intestinal neuronal, 1811
  osteofibrous, 2475
  radial, 3305*f*
  renal, 2554-2556
  Schimke immunoosseous, 2369
  skeletal. *See* Skeletal dysplasias
Dyspnea, in palliative care
  medications for, 262*t*-264*t*
  nonpharmacologic approach to, 265*t*
Dysthymia, 152
Dystonia, 141*t*
  causes of, 2892*t*
  dopa-responsive
    autosomal dominant form, 667
    autosomal recessive form, 666-667
  drug-induced, 2894
  inherited primary, 2891-2894
  metabolic disorders, 2894
  in symptoms of CRPS, 2894-2895
Dystrophic epidermolysis bullosa, 3146-3147

E
E$_3$ subunit deficiency, 651
Eagle-Barrett syndrome, 2572-2573
Ear disorders. *See also* Hearing loss; Otitis media
  clinical manifestations, 3069
  congenital malformations, 3081-3083
  external otitis, 3083-3085
  facial paralysis due to, 3069
  inner ear and diseases of bony labyrinth,
    3100-3101
  mucopolysaccharidoses, 743*t*
  tumors, 3103
Earlobe, keloid of, 3175*f*
Early childhood
  development of microbiome, 1237-1238
  and infancy, well-child care and, 38-40
  trauma, and poor health outcomes for children in
    foster care, 227-228
Early detection of cancer, 2425
Early disseminated Lyme disease, 1485
Early form of multiple carboxylase deficiency, 652
Early localized Lyme disease, 1484-1485
Early-onset hereditary nonsyndromic sensorineural
  hearing loss, 3072*t*-3073*t*
Early-onset neonatal infection, 912-914
Early-onset sarcoidosis, 1207, 1209
Ears
  assessment in newborn, 796
  minor anomalies, 908*t*
  physical examination, 3069-3071
  and temporal bone, traumatic injuries, 3101-3103
East Asian population
  cultural norms, 34*t*-35*t*
  disease beliefs, 35*t*
EAST syndrome, 361, 364
Eastern equine encephalitis, 1622-1624, 1626
Eating. *See also* Failure to thrive; Feeding; Nutrition
    issues
  healthy habits regarding, 316*t*
  at home and at school, 292
  outside of home, 292
  related concerns in adoptive children, 225
Eating disorder, not otherwise specified, 163
Eating disorders, 162
  among GLB youth, 936
  clinical manifestations, 164
  commonly reported symptoms, 166*t*
  complications, 168
  definitions, 163

Eating disorders *(Continued)*
  differential diagnosis, 164-168
  eating and weight control habits in, 165*t*
  epidemiology, 163-164
  in female athletes in context of amenorrhea, 3356
  laboratory findings, 168
  pathology, 164
  physical signs, 167*t*
  prognosis and prevention, 170
  and sports participation, 3331*t*-3334*t*
  in T1DM, 2779-2780
  treatment, 168-170
Eaton-Lambert syndrome, 2994
Ebola hemorrhagic fever, 1634-1636
Ebola virus disease, 1634-1635
EBS (epidermolysis bullosa simplex), 3144
Ebstein anomaly of tricuspid valve
  clinical manifestations, 2221-2222
  diagnosis and treatment, 2222
  pathophysiology, 2221
EBV. *See* Epstein-Barr virus (EBV)
Ecchymosis, and eyelid edema, 3064
Eccrine sweat glands, 3105
  disorders of, 3190-3192
ECF (extracellular fluid), 346
  osmotic equilibrium with ICF, 347
ECG. *See* Electrocardiography (ECG)
Echinocandins
  anidulafungin, 1515
  caspofungin, 1514-1515
  micafungin, 1515
Echinococcosis
  clinical manifestations, 1754-1755
  diagnosis, 1755
  etiology and epidemiology, 1753-1754
  pathogenesis, 1754
  prognosis and prevention, 1755-1756
  treatment, 1755-1756
Echinococcus, E. granulosus and *E. multilocularis,*
  1753-1756
Echocardiography
  of AV septal defect, 2193*f*
  of coarctation of aorta, 2206*f*
  of d-TGA, 2224*f*
  Doppler, 2176-2177
  of Ebstein anomaly of tricuspid valve, 2222*f*
  fetal, 2178
  of hypoplastic left-heart syndrome, 2231*f*
  in Kawasaki disease, 1212
  M-mode, 2175-2176
  in newborn with PDA, 2198*f*
  of pericardial effusion, 2281*f*
  of perimembranous VSD, 2195*f*
  of rhabdomyomas, 2282*f*
  in secundum ASD, 2190*f*
  in sickle cell anemia, 2345
  of tetralogy of Fallot, 2213*f*
  three-dimensional, 2178
  of total anomalous pulmonary venous return,
    2228*f*
  transesophageal, 2178
  of tricuspid atresia, 2219*f*
  two-dimensional, 2176
  of valvar aortic stenosis with regurgitation, 2204*f*
  of valvar pulmonic stenosis, 2201*f*
Ecobiodevelopmental framework
  biologic influences, 48-49
  developmental domains and theories of emotion
    and cognition, 51-52
  psychologic influences, 49-50
  social factors, 50
  statistics used in describing growth and
    development, 52-54
  unifying concepts, 50-51
Ecologic model of development, 50

Ecstasy. *See* Methylenedioxymethamphetamine
    (MDMA)
Ecthyma, 3207-3208
Ectodermal dysplasia
  anhydrotic, with associated immunodeficiency
    (EDA-ID), 1017
  autoimmune polyendocrinopathy-candidiasis,
    1022
  hidrotic, 3122
  hypohidrotic, 3121
  with oral manifestations, 1772-1773
Ectoparasites, genital lesions and, 988-989
Ectopia, ureteral, 2563*f*
Ectopia cordis, 2239
Ectopia lentis, 3047
  syndromes, 3387
Ectopic kidney, 2556*f*
Ectopic pregnancy, 980
Ectopic thyroid tissue, hyperthyroidism caused by,
    2681*t*
Ectopic ureter, 2571, 2584*f*-2585*f*
Ectropion, 3034
Eczema
  atopic. *See* Atopic dermatitis
  thrombocytopenia and, immunodeficiency with,
    1027
Eczema herpeticum, 1575*f*
Eczematous disorders
  acute palmoplantar eczema, 3154
  contact dermatitis, 3150-3153
  lichen simplex chronicus, 3153-3154
  nummular eczema, 3153
  pityriasis alba, 3153
  seborrheic dermatitis, 3154-3155
Edema
  acute hemorrhagic, 1217, 1218*f*
  bilateral, 300-306
  cerebral
    complication of hepatic encephalopathy, 1968
    due to correction of hypernatremic dehydration,
      391
    HACE, 553-554, 557
    in T1DM, 2775
  in erythromelalgia, 1229*f*
  indurative, in Kawasaki disease, 1211*f*
  in newborn, 794, 892
  pulmonary, 2061-2063
    HAPE, 553-554, 557-560
  resulting from nephrotic syndrome, 2521-2522,
    2525
Edinburgh postnatal depression scale, 64*t*
Edmonton protocol, 2782-2783
Edrophonium chloride, 2994-2995
Education
  on allergen avoidance, 1136
  for child with intellectual disability, 221-222
  continuing
    for healthcare workers, 11
    for office staff, 477-478
  diabetes, 2772-2773
  mother's, and under-5 mortality rate, 4*f*
  outreach, of pediatric transport programs, 483
  parent and family, in pain management, 441-442
  patient, for asthma, 1102
  sexual, for girls with special needs, 2632-2633
  and teen mothers, 981
Edwards syndrome, 611*t*
EEG (electroencephalography)
  amplitude-integrated, 839-840
  associated with partial seizures, 2834*f*
  in diagnosis of neonatal seizures, 2852
  in evaluation of patient with febrile seizures,
    2830
  in neurologic examination, 2800-2802
  showing extreme delta brush, 2907*f*

Retractions
   eardrum, 3070
   eyelid, 3034
   sign of respiratory disease, 1987t
Retrocochlear hearing loss, 3071
Retropharyngeal abscess, 2021-2022
Rett syndrome, 2916-2917
Return to play
   contraindications, after cervical spine injury, 3353t
   graduated, after TBI, 3352t
   transition from immediate management to, 3337
Reverse cholesterol transport, HDLs and, 694
Reverse sequence screening for syphilis, 991, 992f
Reverse transcriptase inhibitors
   nonnucleoside, 1655t-1660t
   nucleoside/nucleotide, 1655t-1660t
Reversible cerebral vasoconstriction syndrome, 2936t
Reversible infantile cytochrome C oxidase deficiency
      myopathy, 2902
Revised pediatric emergency assessment tool, 484
Reye syndrome, 1960t, 2902-2904
Reynolds number, turbulence dependent on, 1984
Rh deficiency syndrome, 2334
Rh incompatibility, hemolytic disease of newborn
      caused by, 883-886
Rh sensitization, prevention of, 886
Rhabdoid tumor of kidney, 2467
Rhabdomyolysis, 2987t
   in toxicologic diagnosis, 452t
Rhabdomyomas, 2281
Rhabdomyosarcomas
   clinical manifestations, 2468-2469
   diagnosis and treatment, 2469-2470
   in ear, 3103
   epidemiology, 2468
   pathogenesis, 2468
   prognosis, 2470
   uterine, 2625-2626
Rheumatic disease
   anesthetic implications, 417t
   in differential diagnosis of Kawasaki disease, 1212t
   eosinophilia caused by, 1039t
   nailfold capillary pattern in, 1183f
Rheumatic disease: suspected
   autoantibody specificity and disease associations,
      1152t
   diagnosis, evaluation based on, 1153t
   imaging studies, 1152-1153
   laboratory testing, 1151-1152
   signs suggestive of, 1150-1151
   symptoms suggestive of, 1150
Rheumatic disease: treatment
   biologic agents
      B cell depletion, 1159
      IL-1 antagonists, 1159
      IL-6 receptor antagonist, 1159
      IVIG, 1159
      modulator of T cell activation, 1159
      TNF-α antagonists, 1158-1159
   cytotoxics
      azathioprine, 1159-1160
      cyclophosphamide, 1159
   multidisciplinary teams and primary care
      physicians, 1153-1154
   nonbiologic drugs
      glucocorticoids, 1158
      hydroxychloroquine, 1157
      leflunomide, 1158
      methotrexate, 1154-1157
      mycophenolate mofetil, 1158
      sulfasalazine, 1158
   NSAIDs, 1154
Rheumatic fever
   clinical manifestations and diagnosis, 1333-1335
   complications, 1336

Rheumatic fever (Continued)
   epidemiology, 1332-1333
   etiology, 1332
   major diagnostic criteria
      carditis, 1334
      chorea, 1334
      erythema marginatum, 1335
      migratory polyarthritis, 1334
      subcutaneous nodules, 1335
   minor diagnostic criteria
      differential diagnosis, 1335
      recent GAS infection, 1335
   pathogenesis, 1333
   prevention, 1336-1337
   prognosis, 1336
   treatment
      antibiotic, 1336
      antiinflammatory, 1336
      for Sydenham chorea, 1336
Rheumatic heart disease
   aortic insufficiency, 2271
   mitral insufficiency, 2269-2270
   mitral stenosis, 2270-2271
   pulmonary valve disease, 2271
   tricuspid valve disease, 2271
Rheumatoid arthritis, and sports participation,
      3331t-3334t
Rhinitis, in asthma, 1105
Rhinoconjunctivitis, food-induced, 1141
Rhinorrhea, in common cold, 2013
Rhinosinusitis
   bacterial, 2016f
   in cystic fibrosis, 2112
Rhinoviruses
   clinical manifestations, 1613
   diagnosis and treatment, 1613
   epidemiology, 1613
   etiology, 1612-1613
   pathogenesis, 1613
Rhizomelic chondrodysplasia punctata, 686-687, 688t
Rhizotomy, selective dorsal, 2899f, 3405-3406
Rhododendron toxicity, 467t
RhoH deficiency, 1021
Rhombencephalosynapsis, 2811
Rhus dermatitis, 3152
Rhythm disorders. See also Arrhythmias
   AV block, 2260-2261
   diagnostic ECG, 2258t
   long QT syndromes, 2258-2259
   postoperative, 2244
   principles of antiarrhythmic therapy, 2250-2251
   sinus node dysfunction, 2259-2260
   supraventricular tachycardia, 2254-2257
   ventricular tachyarrhythmias, 2257-2258
Rhythm strip, ECG, 2172
Rhythmic movements, sleep-related, 120
Ribavirin, 1541-1542
   plus peginterferon, for hepatitis C, 1950
Riboflavin (vitamin B₂)
   deficiency, 322-324
   dietary reference intake, 275t-280t
   dietary sources, 323t-324t
   for migraine headaches, 2869t-2870t
Ribonucleic acid (RNA)
   flow of information from DNA to, 589f
   messenger, 588-589
   site of action of anticancer drugs, 2431f
Ribose-5-phosphate isomerase deficiency, 733-734
Ribs
   congenital anomalies, 2146
   fractures
      abusive, 240f
      and hemothorax, 2140f
   wavy, in hypophosphatasia, 3394f
Richner–Hanhart syndrome, 641, 3175

Ricin, delayed-onset Respiratory syndrome, 3442
Rickets, 331-336
   associated with renal tubular acidosis, 2532
   autosomal dominant hypophosphatemic, 339
   autosomal recessive hypophosphatemic, 339
   calcium- or phosphate-deficient, 3391
   clinical variants and related conditions, 3392t
   hereditary hypophosphatemic, with hypercalciuria,
      339
   hypophosphatemic, with hypercalciuria, 367
   of prematurity, 339-340
   vitamin D-dependent (type 1), 337
   vitamin D-dependent (type 2), 337
   X-linked hypophosphatemic, 338-339
Rickettsia
   R. akari, 1504
   R. conorii, 1503
   R. prowazekii, 1506-1507
   R. rickettsii, 1500-1503
   R. typhi, 1505-1506
Rickettsial infection
   associated with hemophagocytic syndrome,
      2485t
   ehrlichiosis and anaplasmosis, 1507-1509
   pneumonia, 2090t
   Q fever (Coxiella burnetii), 1509-1511
   scrub typhus (Orientia tsutsugamushi), 1504-1505
   spotted fever group rickettsioses, 1497-1504
      boutonneuse fever, 1503
      rickettsialpox (Rickettsia akari), 1504
      Rocky Mountain spotted fever, 1500-1503
   typhus group rickettsioses
      epidemic (louse-borne) typhus, 1506-1507
      murine (endemic or flea-borne) typhus,
         1505-1506
Rickettsialpox, 1498t, 1504
Rickettsioses
   spotted fever group, 1497-1504
   typhus group, 1505-1507
Rifampin, 1299
   against M. tuberculosis, 1441, 1457t
Rifamycins, against M. tuberculosis, 1440-1441
Rifaximin, 1299
RIFLE criteria, pediatric-modified, 2539t
Rift Valley fever, 1634, 1636
Right aortic arch, 2235-2237
Right isomerism, heterotaxy syndromes, 2235t
Right to consent, by minors, 941
Right-to-left shunt, in newborn, 832t
Right ventricle
   arrhythmogenic right ventricular dysplasia, 2261
   double-chamber, 2202
   double-outlet, 2183t, 2220
      with malposition of great arteries, 2226-2227
      without pulmonary stenosis, 2226
   hypertrophy, 2173
Rigid cavus feet, 3350
Riley-Day syndrome, 3044f
Rimantadine, 1542
Ring chromosomes, 620, 3135t-3136t
Ring sideroblast, 2326f
Ringworm, black-dot, 3214f
Risk adjustment, 24
   in EMS for children, 484
Risk assessment
   for corticosteroid adverse effects, 1109t
   of hyperbilirubinemia, nomogram for, 3473f
   for hyperlipidemia, 702-705
Risk factors
   for adolescent health behaviors, 937t
   for allergic rhinitis, 1088-1089
   for AMS, 555-557
   for anaerobic bacterial infections, 1437t
   for anaphylaxis, 1133t
   for arterial ischemic stroke, 2927t